PEREZ AND BRADY'S PRINCIPLES AND PRACTICE OF RADIATION ONCOLOGY

SIXTH EDITION

EDITORS

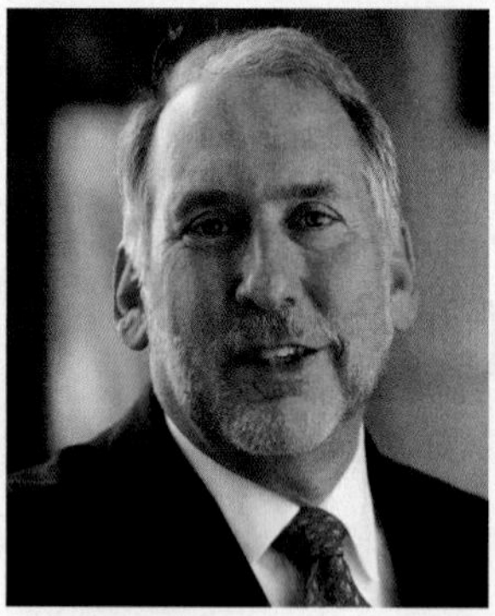

Edward C. Halperin, MD, MA
Chancellor for Health Affairs and Chief Executive Officer
New York Medical College
Professor of Radiation Oncology, Pediatrics, and History
Provost for Biomedical Affairs
Touro College and University
Valhalla, New York

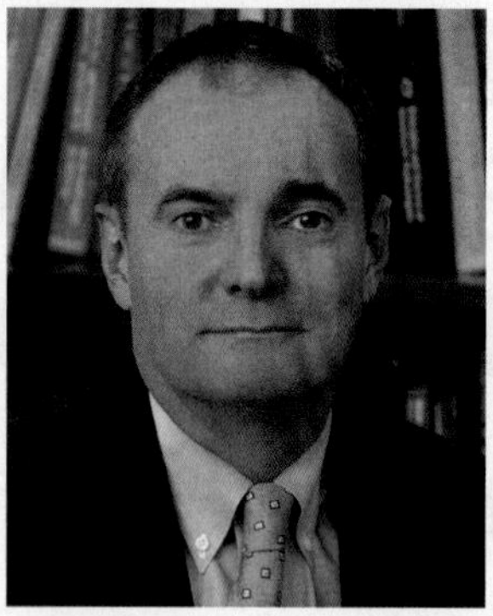

David E. Wazer, MD, FASTRO
Professor and Chairman
Radiation Oncologist-in-Chief
Department of Radiation Oncology
Tufts Medical Center
Tufts University School of Medicine
Boston, Massachusetts
Rhode Island Hospital
Alpert Medical School of Brown University
Providence, Rhode Island

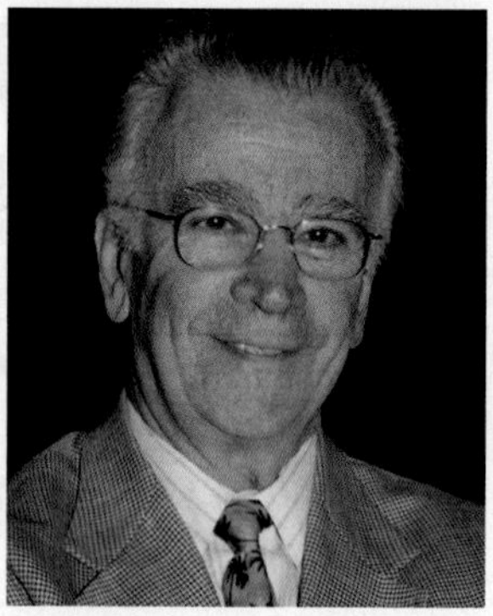

Carlos A. Perez, MD
Professor Emeritus
Mallinckrodt Institute of Radiology
Siteman Cancer Center
Washington University
St. Louis, Missouri

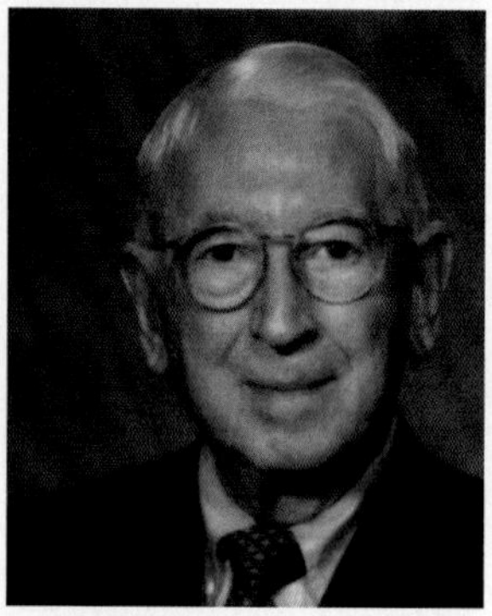

Luther W. Brady, MD
Distinguished University Professor
Hylda Cohn/American Cancer Society Professor of Clinical Oncology
Professor, Department of Radiation Oncology
Drexel University College of Medicine
Philadelphia, Pennsylvania

PEREZ AND BRADY'S

PRINCIPLES AND PRACTICE OF RADIATION ONCOLOGY

SIXTH EDITION

Wolters Kluwer Health | Lippincott Williams & Wilkins

Philadelphia • Baltimore • New York • London
Buenos Aires • Hong Kong • Sydney • Tokyo

Senior Executive Editor: Jonathan W. Pine, Jr.
Senior Product Manager: Emilie Moyer
Production Project Manager: David Orzechowski
Marketing Manager: Alexander Burns
Senior Designer: Stephen Druding
Production Service: Aptara, Inc.

Two Commerce Square
2001 Market Street
Philadelphia, PA 19103 USA
LWW.com

Printed in China

Library of Congress Cataloging-in-Publication Data
Perez and Brady's principles and practice of radiation oncology / editors,
Edward C. Halperin . . . [et al.]. – 6th ed.
p. ; cm.
Principles and practice of radiation oncology
Includes bibliographical references and index.
ISBN 978-1-4511-1648-9 (alk. paper)
I. Halperin, Edward C. II. Perez, Carlos A., 1934- III. Title: Principles and practice of radiation oncology.
[DNLM: 1. Neoplasms–radiotherapy. 2. Radiometry. 3. Radiotherapy–methods. QZ 269]
RC271.R3
616.99'40642–dc23

2012049568

To purchase additional copies of this book, call our customer service department at (800) 638-3030 or fax orders to (301) 223-2320. International customers should call (301) 223-2300.

Visit Lippincott Williams & Wilkins on the Internet: at LWW.com. Lippincott Williams & Wilkins customer service representatives are available from 8:30 am to 6 pm, EST.

10 9 8 7 6 5 4 3 2

CCS0115

To our patients, who have taught us with their courage and suffering,
To our teachers, who inspired us with their knowledge and wisdom,
To our trainees, who will make tomorrow better than today,
To our families, who unselfishly endorsed our endeavors:
This book is gratefully dedicated.

Contributors

David J. Adelstein, MD
Professor of Medicine
Cleveland Clinic Lerner College of Medicine of Case Western Reserve University
Cleveland, Ohio

Anesa Ahamad, MD
Associate Lecturer
Faculty of Medical Sciences
University of the West Indies
St. Augustine, Trinidad Tobago

Kaled M. Alektiar, MD
Department of Radiation Oncology
Memorial Sloan Kettering Cancer Center
New York, New York

Robert J. Amdur, MD
Department of Radiation Oncology
College of Medicine
University of Florida
Gainesville, Florida

K. Kian Ang, MD, PhD
Professor
Department of Radiation Oncology
The University of Texas MD Anderson Cancer Center
Houston, Texas

Douglas W. Arthur, MD
Professor and Vice Chairman
Virginia Commonwealth University
VCU Massey Cancer Center
Richmond, Virginia

Elizabeth H. Baldini, MD, MPH
Associate Professor
Harvard Medical School
Radiation Oncology Director
Bone and Soft Tissue Sarcoma Program
Dana-Farber Cancer Institute and Brigham and Women's Hospital
Boston, Massachusetts

Michael Baumann, MD
Medical Faculty and University Hospital Carl Gustav Carus
Department of Radiation Oncology and OncoRay
National Center for Radiation Research in Oncology Dresden
Technical University of Dresden
Dresden, Germany

Jose G. Bazan, MD, MS
Resident, Department of Radiation Oncology
Stanford Cancer Center
Stanford, California

Stanley Benedict, PhD
Director, Radiological Physics
Department of Radiation Oncology
University of Virginia Health System
Charlottesville, Virginia

Ross Berkowitz, MD
Brigham and Women's Hospital/Dana-Farber Cancer Institute
Harvard Medical School
Boston, Massachusetts

Eric J. Bernhard, PhD
Chief, Radiotherapy Development Branch
Radiation Research Program, Division of Cancer Treatment and Diagnosis (DCTD)
National Cancer Institute
Washington, D.C.

Jeffrey D. Bradley, MD
Washington University School of Medicine
St. Louis, Missouri

Luther W. Brady, MD
Distinguished University Professor
Hylda Cohn/American Cancer Society Professor of Clinical Oncology
Professor, Department of Radiation Oncology
Drexel University College of Medicine
Philadelphia, Pennsylvania

John C. Breneman, MD
Charles M. Barrett Professor of Radiation Oncology and Adjunct Professor of Neurosurgery
University of Cincinnati College of Medicine
Cincinnati Children's Hospital Medical Center
Cincinnati, Ohio

David J. Brenner, PhD, DSc
Center for Radiological Research
Columbia University Medical Center
New York, New York

James D. Brierley, MS, MB, FRCP, FRCR, FRCPC
Professor, Department of Radiation Oncology
University of Toronto
Princess Margaret Hospital
Toronto, Ontario, Canada

David M. Brizel, MD
Leonard R. Prosnitz Professor of Radiation Oncology
Department of Radiation Oncology
Duke University Medical Center
Durham, North Carolina

Richard T. Bryan, MBChB, PhD, MRCS
Senior Research Fellow
School of Cancer Sciences
University of Birmingham
Edgbaston, Birmingham, United Kingdom

Thomas A. Buchholz, MD, FACR
Division Head
Radiation Oncology
The University of Texas MD Anderson Cancer Center
Houston, Texas

Jeffrey Buchsbaum, MD, PhD, AM
Associate Professor
Departments of Radiation Oncology, Pediatrics, and Neurological Surgery
Indiana University School of Medicine
Indiana University Health Proton Therapy Center
Bloomington, Indiana

Theresa M. Busch, PhD
Department of Radiation Oncology
University of Pennsylvania
Philadelphia, Pennsylvania

Jacek Capala, PhD, DSc
Program Director, Clinical Radiation Oncology Branch
Radiation Research Program
Division of Cancer Treatment and Diagnosis
National Cancer Institute/National Institutes of Health
Rockville, Maryland

Christian Carrie, MD
Head, Radiotherapy Department
Medical Director
Centre Leon Berard
Lyon, France

Barrie R. Cassileth, PhD, MS
Integrative Medicine Service
Memorial Sloan-Kettering Cancer Center
New York, New York

Keith A. Cengel, MD, PhD
Department of Radiation Oncology
University of Pennsylvania
Philadelphia, Pennsylvania

K.S. Clifford Chao, MD
Chu H. Chang Distinguished Professor and Chairman
Radiation Oncology
College of Physicians and Surgeons
Columbia University
Professor and Chief
Radiation Oncology
Weill Cornell Medical College
Cornell University
Chairman, Radiation Oncology
New York-Presbyterian Hospital
New York, New York

Zhe Chen, PhD
Associate Professor, Department of Therapeutic Radiology
Hunter Radiation Therapy Center
Yale University School of Medicine
New Haven, Connecticut

Skye H. Cheng, MD
Chief
Department of Radiation Oncology
Koo Foundation Sun Yat-Sen Cancer Center, Taipei, Taiwan
Clinical Professor
Radiation Medicine
National Yang-Ming Medical University, Taipei, Taiwan
Adjunct Associated Professor, Department of Radiation Oncology
Duke University Medical Center
Durham, North Carolina

Sravana Chennupati, MD
Resident
Department of Radiation Medicine
Oregon Health & Science University
Portland, Oregon

Indrin J. Chetty, PhD
Department of Radiation Oncology
Henry Ford Health System
Detroit, Michigan

Junzo P. Chino, MD
Assistant Professor
Department of Radiation Oncology
Duke University Medical Center
Durham, North Carolina

Hak Choy, MD
Professor and Chairman
Department of Radiation Oncology
University of Texas Southwestern Medical Center
Dallas, Texas

Jared D. Christensen, MD
Assistant Professor
Department of Radiology Cardiothoracic Division
Duke University Medical Center
Durham, North Carolina

Hans T. Chung, MD, FRCPC
Assistant Professor
Department of Radiation Oncology
University of Toronto
Odette Cancer Centre
Sunnybrook Health Sciences Centre
Toronto, Ontario, Canada

John J. Coen, MD
Department of Radiation Oncologist
Hartford Radiation Oncology Associates, PC
Hartford, Connecticut

C. Norman Coleman, MD
Associate Director
Radiation Research Program
Division of Cancer Treatment and Diagnosis
National Cancer Institute
Bethesda, Maryland

Stephanie E. Combs, MD
Vice Chairman
Department of Radiation Oncology
University Hospital of Heidelberg
Heidelberg, Germany

Louis S. Constine, MD
Professor and Vice Chair, Department of Radiation Oncology
Professor, Department of Pediatrics
James P. Wilmot Cancer Center
University of Rochester Medical Center
Rochester, New York

Jay S. Cooper, MD
Director
Department of Radiation Oncology
Maimonides Cancer Center
Brooklyn, New York

Nils Cordes, MD, PhD
Head, Molecular Targeting Group
OncoRay Center for Radiation Research in Oncology Medical Faculty Carl Gustav Carus
University of Technology Dresden
Dresden, Germany

Edwin Crandley, MD
Department of Radiation Oncology
University of Virginia
Charlottesville, Virginia

Bernard J. Cummings, MB, ChB, FRCPC
Professor, Department of Radiation Oncology
University of Toronto
Toronto, Ontario, Canada

Brian G. Czito, MD
Associate Professor
Department of Radiation Oncology
Duke University Medical Center
Durham, North Carolina

Roi Dagan, MD
Department of Radiation Oncology,
College of Medicine, University of Florida
Gainesville, Florida

Megan E. Daly, MD
Assistant Professor
Department of Radiation Oncology
UC Davis Medical Center
Sacramento, California

Rupak K. Das, PhD
Professor
Department of Human Oncology
University of Wisconsin
Madison, Wisconsin

Barnali Dasgupta, MD
Research Fellow
Department of Radiation Oncology
Indiana University School of Medicine
Indianapolis, Indiana

Roy H. Decker, MD, PhD
Assistant Professor
Department of Therapeutic Radiology
Yale University School of Medicine
New Haven, Connecticut

Gary Deng, MD, PhD
Integrative Medicine Service
Memorial Sloan-Kettering Cancer Center
New York, New York

Albert S. DeNittis, MD
Chief, Department of Radiation Oncology
Lankenau Hospital
Associate Professor
Lankenau Institute for Medical Research
Wynnewood, Pennsylvania

Phillip M. Devlin, MD, FACR
Chief, Division of Brachytherapy
Dana-Farber/Brigham and Women's Cancer Center
Associate Professor
Harvard Medical School
Boston, Massachusetts

Mark W. Dewhirst, DVM, PhD
Professor of Pathology and Biomedical Engineering
Gustavo S. Montana Professor
Director of Tumor Microcirculation Laboratory
Department of Radiation Oncology
Duke University Medical Center
Durham, North Carolina

James A. Deye, PhD
Radiation Research Program
National Cancer Institute
Rockville, Maryland

James J. Dignam, PhD
Associate Professor, Biostatistics
Department of Health Studies
The University of Chicago
Chicago, Illinois
Group Statistician
Radiation Therapy Oncology Group
American College of Radiology
Philadelphia, Pennsylvania

Bernadine R. Donahue, MD
Department of Radiation Oncology
Maimonides Cancer Center
Brooklyn, New York
Department of Radiation Oncology
New York University School of Medicine
New York, New York

Sarah S. Donaldson, MD
Catharine and Howard Avery Professor
Department of Radiation Oncology
Stanford University School of Medicine
Department of Radiation Oncology
Stanford, California

Lei Dong, PhD
Department of Radiation Physics
The University of Texas MD Anderson Cancer Center
Houston, Texas

James G. Douglas, MD, MS
Professor
Department of Radiation Oncology
Indiana University School of Medicine
Medical Director
Indiana University Health Proton Therapy Center
Bloomington, Indiana

Dan G. Duda, DMD, PhD
Assistant Professor of Radiation Oncology
Edwin L. Steele Laboratory for Tumor Biology
Department of Radiation Oncology
Massachusetts General Hospital and Harvard Medical School
Boston, Massachusetts

Tony Y. Eng, MD
Professor and Vice Chair
Radiation Oncology Department
University of Texas Health Science Center at San Antonio
Cancer Therapy and Research Center
San Antonio, Texas

Joshua Evans, PhD
Assistant Professor of Medical Physics
Department of Radiation Oncology
Virginia Commonwealth University
Richmond, Virginia

Jean-Pierre Farmer, MD
Professor of Neurosurgery and Oncology
McGill University
Montreal, Quebec, Canada

Jarod C. Finlay, PhD
Assistant Professor
Department of Radiation Oncology
University of Pennsylvania
Philadelphia, Pennsylvania

John C. Flickinger, MD
Professor of Radiation Oncology
University of Pittsburgh School of Medicine
Pittsburgh, Pennsylvania

Franklin P. Flowers, MD
Professor Emeritus of Dermatology
University of Florida College of Medicine
Gainesville, Florida

Silvia C. Formenti, MD
Sandra and Edward Meyer Professor and Chair
Department of Radiation Oncology
New York University School of Medicine
New York, New York

Steven J. Frank, MD
Associate Professor
Department of Radiation Oncology
The University of Texas MD Anderson Cancer Center
Houston, Texas

Carolyn R. Freeman, MBBS, FRCPC
Professor of Oncology and Pediatrics
Mike Rosenbloom Chair in Radiation Oncology
McGill University
Montreal, Quebec, Canada

C. David Fuller, MD
Assistant Professor
Department of Radiation Oncology
The University of Texas MD Anderson Cancer Center
Houston, Texas

Hiram Gay, MD
Assistant Professor
Department of Radiation Oncology
Washington University School of Medicine
St. Louis, Missouri

Iris C. Gibbs, MD
Associate Professor
Stanford University
Stanford, California

Maura L. Gillison, MD, PhD
Professor and Jeg Coughlin Chair of Cancer Research
Ohio State University Comprehensive Cancer Center
Columbus, Ohio

Daniel R. Gomez, MD
Assistant Professor
Department of Radiation Oncology
The University of Texas MD Anderson Cancer Center
Houston, Texas

Vanai Gondi, MD
Chief Resident
Department of Human Oncology
University of Wisconsin Comprehensive Cancer Center
Madison, Wisconsin

Sharad Goyal, MD, MS
Assistant Professor
Department of Radiation Oncology
University of Medicine & Dentistry of New Jersey–Robert Wood Johnson Medical School
Cancer Institute of New Jersey
New Brunswick, New Jersey

Sean Grimm, MD
Assistant Professor
Department of Neurology
Northwestern University Feinberg School of Medicine
Chicago, Illinois

Amitabh Gulati, MD
Department of Anesthesia
Memorial Sloan-Kettering Cancer Center
New York, New York

Bruce G. Haffty, MD
Professor and Chairman
Department of Radiation Oncology
University of Medicine & Dentistry of New Jersey–Robert Wood Johnson Medical School
Associate Director
The Cancer Institute of New Jersey
New Brunswick, New Jersey

Caroline L. Halloway, MD, FRCR(C)
Clinical Assistant Professor
University of British Columbia
Radiation Oncologist
BC Cancer Agency
Victoria, British Columbia, Canada

Edward C. Halperin, MD, MA
Chancellor for Health Affairs and Chief Executive Officer
New York Medical College
Professor of Radiation Oncology, Pediatrics, and History
Provost for Biomedical Affairs
Touro College and University
Valhalla, New York

Timothy P. Hanna, MD, MSc, FRCPC
Radiation Oncology Research Fellow
Collaboration for Cancer Outcomes Research and Evaluation (CCORE)
Liverpool Hospital
New South Wales, Australia

James E. Hansen, MD, MS
Chief Resident in Therapeutic Radiology
Yale University School of Medicine
New Haven, Connecticut

Paul M. Harari, MD
Jack Fowler Professor and Chairman of Human Oncology
University of Wisconsin
Madison, Wisconsin

William F. Hartsell, MD
Medical Director
CDH Proton Center, A ProCure Center
Warrenville, Illinois

Laura J. Havrilesky, MD, MHSc
Associate Professor
Department of Obstetrics and Gynecology, Division of Gynecologic Oncology
Duke University Medical Center
Durham, North Carolina

Jaroslaw T. Hepel, MD
Department of Radiation Oncology
Brown University
Rhode Island Hospital
Providence, Rhode Island
Tufts University
Tufts Medical Center
Boston, Massachusetts

Felix Ho, BS
Research Assistant
Department of Radiation Oncology
Memorial Sloan-Kettering Cancer Center
New York, New York

David C. Hodgson, MD, PRCPC
Department of Radiation Oncology
University of Toronto
Princess Margaret Hospital
Toronto, Ontario, Canada

Henry T. Hoffman, MD
Professor of Otolaryngology, Head and Neck Surgery
University of Iowa
Iowa City, Iowa

Richard T. Hoppe, MD
The Henry S. Kaplan-Harry Lebeson Professor in Cancer Biology
Professor and Chairman
Department of Radiation Oncology
Stanford University
Stanford, California

Jiayi Huang, MD
Assistant Professor
Department of Radiation Oncology
Washington University School of Medicine in St. Louis
St. Louis, Missouri

Andrew T. Huang, MD
President and CEO
Koo Foundation Sun Yat-Sen Cancer Center
Taipei City, Taiwan
Professor of Medicine
Duke University
Durham, North Carolina

Syed A. Hussain, MD
Clinical Senior Lecturer and Consultant in Medical Oncology
University of Liverpool and Clatterbridge Centre for Oncology
Liverpool, United Kingdom

Hirota Inaba, MD, PhD
Associate Member
Leukemia/Lymphoma Division
Department of Oncology
St. Jude Children's Research Hospital
Memphis, Tennessee

Siavash Jabbari, MD
Radiation Oncologist
Barnhart Cancer Center
Sharp Chula Vista Medical Center
Chula Vista, California

Rakesh K. Jain, PhD
A.W. Cook Professor of Tumor Biology
Director, Edwin L. Steele Laboratory for Tumor Biology
Department of Radiation Oncology
Massachusetts General Hospital and Harvard Medical School
Boston, Massachusetts

Nicholas James, BSc, MBBS, PhD, FRCP, FRCR
Professor of Clinical Oncology
School of Cancer Sciences
University of Birmingham
Honorary Consultant in Clinical Oncology
Edgbaston, Birmingham, United Kingdom

John A. Kalapurakal, MD
Professor
Radiation Oncology
Northwestern University Feinberg School of Medicine
Chicago, Illinois

Tadashi Kamada, MD, PhD
Director
Research Center for Charged Particle Therapy
National Institute of Radiological Sciences
Chiba, Japan

Josephine Kang, MD, PhD
Attending Physician
Flushing Radiation Oncology Services
Queens, New York

Rojano Kashani, PhD
Instructor
Department of Radiation Oncology
Washington University School of Medicine
St. Louis, Missouri

Brian D. Kavanagh, MD, MPH
Professor of Radiation Oncology
University of Colorado School of Medicine
Aurora, Colorado

Christopher R. Kelsey, MD
Assistant Professor
Department of Radiation Oncology
Duke University Medical Center
Durham, North Carolina

D. Nathan Kim, MD, PhD
Assistant Professor
Department of Radiation Oncology
University of Texas Southwestern Medical Center
Dallas, Texas

Youn H. Kim, MD
Professor of Dermatology
Stanford University School of Medicine
Stanford, California

Thomas J. Kinsella, MS, MD
Research Scholar Professor
Department of Radiation Oncology
Warren Alpert Medical School of Brown University
Rhode Island Hospital
Providence, Rhode Island

John P. Kirkpatrick, MD, PhD
Associate Professor and Clinical Director
Department of Radiation Oncology
Duke University Medical Center
Durham, North Carolina

Jessica M. Kirwan, MA
Research Coordinator
Department of Radiation Oncology
University of Florida
Gainesville, Florida

Eric E. Klein, PhD
Professor
Department of Radiation Oncology
Washington University School of Medicine
St. Louis, Missouri

Mechthild Krause, MD
OncoRay–National Center for Radiation Research in Oncology
Medical Faculty Carl Gustav Carus
Technische Universität
Dresden, Germany

Timothy J. Kruser, MD
Resident Physician
Department of Human Oncology
University of Wisconsin
Madison, Wisconsin

Abraham Kuten, MD
Director, Department of Oncology
RAMBAM Health Care Campus
Haifa, Israel

Young Kwok, MD
Associate Professor
Department of Radiation Oncology
University of Maryland School of Medicine
Baltimore, Maryland

Chelsea D. Landon, MS
Department of Pathology
Duke University Medical Center
Durham, North Carolina

Corey J. Langer, MD
Professor of Internal Medicine
Hospital of the University of Pennsylvania
Director of Thoracic Oncology
Department of Medicine
Perelman Center for Advanced Medicine
Abramson Cancer Center
Philadelphia, Pennsylvania

Brian D. Lawenda, MD
Clinical Director
21st Century Oncology
Las Vegas, Nevada
Adjunct Assistant Professor
Department of Radiation Oncology
Indiana University School of Medicine
Indianapolis, Indiana

Yaacov Richard Lawrence, MA, MBBS, MRCP
Director
Center for Translational Research in Radiation Oncology
Sheba Medical Center, Israel
Assistant Professor (Adjunct)
Department of Radiation Oncology
Jefferson Medical College of Thomas Jefferson University
Philadelphia, Pennsylvania

Nancy Y. Lee, MD
Department of Radiation Oncology
Memorial Sloan-Kettering Cancer Center
New York, New York

Larissa Lee, MD
Brigham and Women's Hospital/Dana-Farber Cancer Institute
Harvard Medical School
Boston, Massachusetts

X. Allen Li, PhD, DABMP, FAAPM
Professor and Chief of Medical Physics
Director, Physics Residency Program
Medical College of Wisconsin
Milwaukee, Wisconsin

Zuofeng Li, PhD
University of Florida Proton Therapy Institute
Jacksonville, Florida

Bruce Libby, PhD
Department of Radiation Oncology
University of Virginia
Charlottesville, Virginia

Yolande Lievens, MD, PhD
Head of Department of Radiotherapy
University Hospital Ghent
Professor in Radiotherapy
Ghent University
Ghent, Belgium

Ray Lin, MD
Medical Director
Department of Radiation Oncology
Scripps Green Hospital
La Jolla, California

Mirrorer M. Liu, MD
Assistant Member of Koo-Foundation Sun Yat-Sen Cancer Center
Taipei City, Taiwan

Benjamin H. Lok, MD
New York University School of Medicine
Memorial Sloan-Kettering Cancer Center
New York, New York

Laurel J. Lyckholm, MD
Sydney Page Professor of Bioethics and Humanities
Division of Hematology/Oncology & Palliative Care Medicine
Virginia Commonwealth University Health System
Richmond, Virginia

Roger M. Macklis, MD
Staff Physician
Department of Radiation Oncology
Taussig Cancer Institute, Cleveland Clinic
Professor of Medicine
Cleveland Clinic Lerner College of Medicine
Cleveland, Ohio

Anthony A. Mancuso, MD
Professor and Chairman
Department of Radiology
Professor of Otolaryngology
University of Florida College of Medicine
Gainesville, Florida

Rafael R. Mañon, MD
Section Leader
Head and Neck and Gynecologic Radiation Oncology
MD Anderson Cancer Center—Orlando
Orlando, Florida

David B. Mansur, MD
Associate Professor and Vice Chair for Education
Department of Radiation Oncology
Case Western Reserve University School of Medicine
Director of Pediatric and Hematologic Radiation Oncology
University Hospitals Seidman Cancer Center
Rainbow Babies and Children's Hospital
Cleveland, Ohio

Robert B. Marcus, Jr., MD
Gulf Region Radiation Oncology Centers
Pensacola, Florida

Timothy D. Marinetti, PhD
Senior Grants Manager and Editor
Department of Radiation Oncology
College of Physicians and Surgeons
Columbia University
New York, New York

Peter W. Marks, MD
Department of Internal Medicine
Yale University School of Medicine
New Haven, Connecticut

Lawrence B. Marks, MD, FASTRO
Professor and Chair
Department of Radiation Oncology
University of North Carolina School of Medicine
North Carolina Cancer Hospital
Chapel Hill, North Carolina

Ursula Matalonis, MD
Brigham and Women's Hospital/Dana-Farber Cancer Institute
Harvard Medical School
Boston, Massachusetts

William H. McBride, PhD, DSc
Department Radiation Oncology
David Geffen School Medicine
University of California
Los Angeles, California

Minesh P. Mehta, MD
Professor, Radiation Oncology
University of Maryland
Director
Maryland Proton Therapy Center
Baltimore, Maryland

Loren K. Mell, PhD
Associate Professor and Director
Division of Clinical and Translational Research
Department of Radiation Medicine and Applied Sciences
UC San Diego Moores Cancer Center
La Jolla, California

Nancy Price Mendenhall, MD
Medical Director
Proton Therapy Institute
Jacksonville, Florida

William M. Mendenhall, MD
Department of Radiation Oncology
University of Florida College of Medicine
Gainesville, Florida

Monika L. Metzger, MD, MSc
Associate Member
Department of Oncology
St. Jude Children's Research Hospital
Memphis, Tennessee

Jeff M. Michalski, MD, MBA, FACR, FASTRO
The Carlos A. Perez Distinguished Professor of Radiation Oncology
Vice Chair and Director of Clinical Programs
Department of Radiation Oncology
Washington University School of Medicine
Siteman Cancer Center and Barnes-Jewish Hospital
St. Louis, Missouri

Joseph Mikhael, MD
Department of Hematology and Medical Oncology
Mayo Clinic Arizona
Scottsdale, Arizona

Michael T. Milano, MD
Associate Professor
Department of Radiation Oncology
James P. Wilmot Cancer Center
University of Rochester Medical Center
Rochester, New York

Radhe Mohan, PhD, FAAPM
Professor
Department of Radiation Physics
Division of Radiation Oncology
The University of Texas MD Anderson Cancer Center
Houston, Texas

Gustavo S. Montana, MD
Professor
Department of Radiation Oncology
Duke University Medical Center
Durham, North Carolina

Gerard C. Morton, MB BCh BAO, MRCPI, FRCPC, FFRRCSI
Associate Professor
Department of Radiation Oncology
University of Toronto
Sunnybrook Odette Cancer Centre
Toronto, Ontario, Canada

Ben Movsas, MD
Chairman, Department of Radiation Oncology
Henry Ford Health System
Detroit, Michigan

Arno J. Mundt, III, MD, FACRO
Professor and Chair
Department of Radiation Medicine and Applied Sciences
University of California San Diego
Rebecca and John Moores Comprehensive Cancer Center
La Jolla, California

Jeffrey N. Myers, MD, PhD, FACS
Professor
Department of Head and Neck Surgery
Division of Surgery
The University of Texas MD Anderson Cancer Center
Houston, Texas

Subir Nag, MD, FACR, FACRO
Director of Brachytherapy Services
Department of Radiation Oncology
Kaiser Permanente
Santa Clara, California
Clinical Professor (Affiliated)
Department of Radiation Oncology
Stanford School of Medicine
Stanford, California

Elizabeth M. Nichols, MD
Chief Resident
Department of Radiation Oncology
University of Maryland School of Medicine
Baltimore, Maryland

Ajay Niranjan, MD, MBA
Associate Professor of Neurological Surgery
Director, UPMC Brain Mapping Center (MEG)
Associate Director, Center for Image-Guided Neurosurgery
Director of Radiosurgery Research
Department of Neurological Surgery
University of Pittsburgh
Pittsburgh, Pennsylvania

William P. O'Meara, MD, MPH
Lahey Clinic Medical Center
Burlington, Massachusetts

Nitin A. Pagedar, MD
Assistant Professor of Otolaryngology, Head and Neck Surgery
University of Iowa
Iowa City, Iowa

Manisha Palta, MD
Assistant Professor
Department of Radiation Oncology
Duke University Medical Center
Durham, North Carolina

Roy A. Patchell, MD
Chairman of Neurology
Barrow Neurological Institute
Phoenix, Arizona

Prashant Patel, MBBS, FRCSEd (Urol), PhD
Consultant Urological Surgeon and Senior Lecturer
Department of Urology
Queen Elizabeth Hospital NHS Trust
School of Cancer Sciences
University of Birmingham
Birmingham, United Kingdom

Todd Pawlicki, PhD
Associate Professor
Director of Medical Physics
Director of Clinical Operations
Department of Radiation Oncology
University of California, San Diego
San Diego, California

Carlos A. Perez, MD
Professor Emeritus
Department of Radiation Oncology
Mallinckrodt Institute of Radiology
Siteman Cancer Center
Washington University
St. Louis, Missouri

Pascal Pommier, MD, PhD
Department of Radiation Oncology
Centre Léon Bérard
Lyon, France

Leonard R. Prosnitz, MD
Professor and Chairman, Emeritus
Department of Radiation Oncology
Duke University Medical Center
Durham, North Carolina

James A. Purdy, PhD
Professor and Vice Chairman
Department of Radiation Oncology
Director, Physics Division
University of California, Davis
Sacramento, California

Harry Quon, MD
Department of Radiation Oncology and Molecular Radiation Sciences
Department of Otolaryngology-Head and Neck Surgery
The Johns Hopkins University
Baltimore, Maryland

Ramji R. Rajendran, MD, PhD
Department of Radiation Oncology
The Cancer Institute at Alexian Brothers Medical Center
Elk Grove Village, Illinois

Shyam S. Rao, MD, PhD
Assistant Attending
Department of Radiation Oncology
Memorial Sloan-Kettering Cancer Center
New York, New York

William F. Regine, MD
Professor and Chairman
Department of Radiation Oncology
University of Maryland Medical Center
Baltimore, Maryland

Ramesh Rengan, MD, PhD
Assistant Professor
Chief, Thoracic Service
Department of Radiation Oncology
Hospital of the University of Pennsylvania
Perelman Center for Advanced Medicine
Philadelphia, Pennsylvania

Nadeem Riaz, MD, MSc
Resident
Department of Radiation Oncology
Memorial Sloan-Kettering Cancer Center
New York, New York

Mack Roach, III, MD
Professor and Chairman
Department of Radiation Oncology
University of California, San Francisco
San Francisco, California

Kenneth B. Roberts, MD
Associate Professor of Therapeutic Radiology
Yale University School of Medicine
New Haven, Connecticut

Cliff Robinson, MD
Assistant Professor
Department of Radiation Oncology
Washington University in St. Louis
St. Louis, Missouri

Joseph K. Salama, MD
Associate Professor
Department of Radiation Oncology
Duke University
Durham, North Carolina

Nicholas J. Sanfilippo, MD
Assistant Professor
Department of Radiation Oncology
New York University School of Medicine
New York, New York

Paul J. Schilling, MD, FACRO
Community Cancer Center of North Florida
Gainesville, Florida

Granger R. Scruggs, MD
Department of Radiation Oncology
Baylor University Medical Center—Dallas
Texas Oncology
Dallas, Texas

Stuart Seropian, MD
Associate Professor of Medicine (Hematology)
Yale Cancer Center
New Haven, Connecticut

Jeremy Setton, MD
Department of Radiation Oncology
Memorial Sloan-Kettering Cancer Center
New York, New York

Hiral K. Shah, MD
Radiation Oncologist
Pinellas Radiation Oncology Associates
Clearwater, Florida

Lawrence J. Sheplan Olsen, MD
Resident
Department of Radiation Oncology
Cleveland Clinic
Cleveland, Ohio

Charles B. Simone, II, MD
Assistant Professor
Department of Radiation Oncology
Perelman School of Medicine at the University of Pennsylvania
Philadelphia, Pennsylvania

Heath D. Skinner, MD, PhD
Assistant Professor
Department of Radiation Oncology
Division of Radiation Oncology
The University of Texas MD Anderson Cancer Center
Houston, Texas

William Y. Song, PhD
Associate Professor
Center for Advanced Radiotherapy Technologies (CART)
Department of Radiation Oncology
University of California, San Diego
La Jolla, California

Tod W. Speer, MD
Department of Human Oncology
Radiation Oncology
University of Wisconsin School of Medicine and Public Health
Madison, Wisconsin

Paul Stauffer, MSEE, CCE
Professor and Director Hyperthermia Physics
Department of Radiation Oncology
Duke University Medical Center
Durham, North Carolina

Alexandra J. Stewart, DM, MRCP, FRCR
Consultant Clinical Oncologist
St Luke's Cancer Centre
Royal Surrey County Hospital
Senior Lecturer
University of Surrey
Guildford, United Kingdom

Michael Story, PhD
Associate Professor
Department of Radiation Oncology
University of Texas Southwestern Medical Center
Dallas, Texas

Jeremy Sugarman, MD, MPH, MA
Harvey M. Meyerhoff Professor of Bioethics and Medicine
The Johns Hopkins Berman Institute of Bioethics
Baltimore, Maryland

Roger E. Taylor, MA, FRCP, FRCR
Professor of Radiation Oncology
University of Wales
Swansea, United Kingdom

Stephanie Terezakis, MD
Johns Hopkins School of Medicine
Baltimore, Maryland

Chris H.J. Terhaard, MD, PhD
Associate Professor
Radiation Oncologist
University Medical Center, Utrecht
Utrecht, The Netherlands

Bruce Thomadsen, PhD
Departments of Medical Physics, Engineering Physics, Biomedical Engineering and Industrial and Systems Engineering
University of Wisconsin
Madison, Wisconsin

Charles R. Thomas, Jr., MD
Professor and Chairman
Department of Radiation Medicine
Knight Cancer Institute
Oregon Health and Science University
Portland, Oregon

Patrick R.M. Thomas, MD, FACR
Former Professor and Chair
Department of Radiation Oncology Temple University School of Medicine
Radiation Oncologist
Bayfront Cancer Care
Bayfront Medical Center
St. Petersburg, Florida

Wade L. Thorstad, MD
Associate Professor
Department of Radiation Oncology
Washington University in St. Louis
St. Louis, Missouri

Robert D. Timmerman, MD
Professor of Radiation Oncology and Neurosurgery
Effie Marie Cain Distinguished Chair in Cancer Therapy Research
University of Texas Southwestern Medical Center
Dallas, Texas

Prabhakar Tripuraneni, MD, FACR, FASTRO
Head, Radiation Oncology
Scripps Clinic
La Jolla, California

Filip T. Troicki, MD
Resident Physician in Radiation Oncologist
Bala Cynwyd, Pennsylvania

Richard W. Tsang, MD, FRCPC
Department of Radiation Oncology
University of Toronto
Princess Margaret Hospital
Toronto, Ontario, Canada

Richard K. Valicenti, MD, MA
Professor and Chairman
Department of Radiation Oncology
UC Davis School of Medicine
Sacramento, California

Gregory M.M. Videtic, MD, CM, FRCPC
Staff Physician
Department of Radiation Oncology
Taussig Cancer Institute
Cleveland Clinic
Associate Professor of Medicine
Cleveland Clinic Lerner College of Medicine
Cleveland, Ohio

Bhadrasain Vikram, MD
Clinical Radiation Oncology Branch
Radiation Research Program
Division of Cancer Treatment and Diagnosis
National Cancer Institute
Rockville, Maryland

Richard Viney, MBChB, MSc, FRCS (Urol)
Senior Lecturer in Urology
Queen Elizabeth Hospital
Birmingham, United Kingdom

Akila N. Viswanathan, MD, MPH
Director, Gynecologic Radiation
Associate Professor of Radiation Oncology
Harvard Medical School
Department of Radiation Oncology
Brigham and Women's Hospital
Boston, Massachusetts

Michael A. Vogelbaum, MD, PhD, FACS
Associate Director
Burkhardt Brain Tumor and Neuro-Oncology Center
Associate Professor of Surgery (Neurosurgery)
Cleveland Clinic Foundation
Cleveland, Ohio

Zelijko Vujaskovic, MD, PhD
Professor of Radiation Oncology
Director of the Division of Translational Radiation Sciences
University of Maryland School of Medicine
Baltimore, Maryland

Tony J. C. Wang, MD
Chief Resident
Department of Radiation Oncology
Columbia University
New York, New York

David E. Wazer, MD, FASTRO
Professor and Chairman
Radiation Oncologist-in-Chief
Department of Radiation Oncology
Tufts Medical Center
Tufts University School of Medicine
Boston, Massachusetts
Rhode Island Hospital
Alpert Medical School of Brown University
Providence, Rhode Island

Maria Werner-Wasik, MD
Department of Radiation Oncology
Thomas Jefferson University Hospital and Kimmel Cancer Center
Philadelphia, Pennsylvania

John W. Werning, MD, DMD, FACS
Associate Professor and Chief, Division of Head and Neck Oncologic Surgery Department of Otolaryngology
University of Florida College of Medicine
Gainesville, Florida

Christopher G. Willett, MD
Professor and Chair
Department of Radiation Oncology
Duke University Medical Center
Durham, North Carolina

Jeffrey F. Williamson, PhD, FAAPM, FACR
Professor of Radiation Oncology
Department of Radiation Oncology
Virginia Commonwealth University
Richmond, Virginia

Lynn D. Wilson, MD, MPH
Professor, Clinical Director, and Vice-Chairman of Therapeutic Radiology
Yale University School of Medicine
Smilow Cancer Hospital
New Haven, Connecticut

Karen M. Winkfield, MD, PhD
Instructor of Radiation Oncology
Harvard Medical School
Massachusetts General Hospital
Boston, Massachusetts

H. Rodney Withers, AO, MD, DSc
Professor and Chair Emeritus
Department of Radiation Oncology
University of California at Los Angeles
Los Angeles, California

Theodore E. Yaeger, MD, FACRO, FRSM
Associate Professor Radiation Oncology
Wake Forest University School of Medicine
Winston-Salem, North Carolina

Santosh Yajnik, MD
Section Chief of Radiation Oncology
Advocate, Illinois Masonic Medical Center
Chicago, Illinois

David S. Yoo, MD, PhD
Medical Instructor
Department of Radiation Oncology
Duke University Medical Center
Durham, North Carolina

Michael J. Zelefsky, MD
Professor of Radiation Oncology
Chief, Brachytherapy Service
Department of Radiation Oncology
Memorial Sloan-Kettering Cancer Center
New York, New York

Timothy C. Zhu, PhD
Department of Radiation Oncology
University of Pennsylvania
Philadelphia, Pennsylvania

Daniel Zips, MD
Department of Radiation Oncology and OncoRay
National Center for Radiation Research in Oncology
Dresden, Germany

Preface

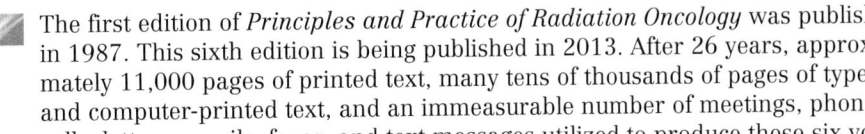

The first edition of *Principles and Practice of Radiation Oncology* was published in 1987. This sixth edition is being published in 2013. After 26 years, approximately 11,000 pages of printed text, many tens of thousands of pages of typed and computer-printed text, and an immeasurable number of meetings, phone calls, letters, emails, faxes, and text messages utilized to produce these six volumes, many things have changed and others have stayed the same.

What has stayed the same? For 26 years radiation therapy has remained a major component of the curative and palliative therapy of cancer and plays a major role in the management of many benign diseases. Patients with cancer are generally best managed by a combined modality approach that requires the participation of a well-informed, well-trained, and well-equipped radiation oncologist directing a radiation oncology team. The radiation oncologist must be capable of taking a detailed medical history; performing a thorough and accurate physical examination of the patient; assessing and integrating the information from diagnostic imaging, gross and microscopic pathology, and clinical chemistry; and formulating and implementing a treatment plan that is cognizant of the wishes of the patient and realistic in its goals. For this book in particular, what has also stayed the same since its inception is the vision and participation of Carlos A. Perez and Luther W. Brady.

What has changed? There has been an explosion of knowledge concerning the molecular biology of cancer and tumor physiology. Concepts that were unknown in the 1980s are now considered fundamental building blocks of knowledge concerning cancer. As it concerns the technology of this specialty, when the first edition of this book was published, cobalt-60 machines remained in widespread use; simulation using diagnostic radiographs still vied with clinical setups of treatment fields using surface anatomy; and many radiation oncologists carried slide rules, protractors, and rulers to calculate and map radiation dose distributions. Now, elaborate linear accelerators with multileaf collimators, particle machines, intensity-modulated and/or image-guided radiation therapy, complex brachytherapy devices, dose painting, image fusion, metabolic imaging, and increasingly powerful computers that support the preceding list of technologies have become the norm in the developed world. (And, unfortunately, the paucity of even the most minimal radiation therapy services in many parts of the world persists.) In some diseases, the diagnostic and staging workup has changed profoundly in the past quarter of a century—for example, the role of staging laparotomy in Hodgkin disease. In other diseases, the role of radiotherapy in treatment has shifted dramatically, as demonstrated by the decline in the role of radiation therapy in the management of retinoblastoma and the change in the use of radiation therapy for breast and prostate cancer. The editors have also changed: Edward C. Halperin joined the editorial team with the fourth edition and David Wazer with the fifth edition.

The editors have striven to be cognizant of change by constantly adding and pruning chapters to document the current state of knowledge of cancer biology; medical radiation physics; clinical radiation oncology; and radiation oncology economics, ethics, and policy. Particular attention in the fifth and sixth editions has been devoted to an attractive and useable design of the printed version of this book and the new electronic versions. We have taken care to have this book evolve with the times, and we have simultaneously striven to be true to the core mission of being "the book of record" for clinical care, providing the data that justifies treatment recommendations as well as comprehensive illustrations and references in radiation oncology.

We have been gratified by the public reception of this book. Sales of the fifth edition rose dramatically compared to the fourth edition—an atypical pattern in the medical book business. It is, we like to believe, evidence that the pact wordlessly exchanged between the editors, the chapter authors, and our readers is being honored by all parties.

The editors sincerely hope that this sixth edition of *Principles and Practice of Radiation Oncology* will continue to advance understanding of the causes, prevention, and treatment of human cancer. We pray that this new edition will contribute to the cure of some malignancies, the amelioration of suffering for many patients and their families, the relief of pain, and the ultimate triumph of human knowledge over cancer.

Edward C. Halperin, MD, MA
David E. Wazer, MD, FASTRO
Carlos A. Perez, MD
Luther W. Brady, MD

Preface to the First Edition

Fifty to sixty percent of all cancer patients in the United States receive radiation therapy each year as definitive therapy, for palliation, or as an adjunct to surgery or chemotherapy. In 1986, according to American Cancer Society estimates, 960,000 new cases of invasive cancer, 45,000 new cases of carcinoma *in situ* of the uterine cervix, 5,000 new cases of carcinoma *in situ* of the female breast, and 400,000 new cases of non-melanomatous skin cancer were diagnosed in the United States. About 71% of patients with invasive cancer presented with disease apparently limited to the local region; 29% had metastases at the time of the initial presentation. Of those who presented with locoregional disease, 56% will be cured and 44% will develop recurrent cancer. Therefore, a substantial portion of the resources in cancer care should be devoted to control of the locoregional tumor, including the use of radiation therapy.

The management of the patient with cancer has evolved into a complex, closely integrated application of sophisticated technology to evaluate and stage the tumor and, using various modalities, to obtain optimal therapeutic results, emphasizing the quality of life of the patient. *Principles and Practice of Radiation Oncology* is designed to contribute to a better understanding of the physical methods of radiation application, of the effects of irradiation on normal tissues, and of the most judicious ways in which radiation therapy can be employed in the case of any particular patient, either as a single modality or as part of a multimodality treatment program.

Chapters are included on basic radiation biology, radiation therapy physics and treatment planning, multimodal integrated programs for patient management, and such technical applications of irradiation as electron beam therapy, brachytherapy, and high LET radiations.

The chapters discussing disease by anatomical site are all organized in a similar fashion to enable complete coverage of pertinent information on each tumor. The format includes sections on epidemiology, pathology, diagnostic workup, treatment techniques, the applications of surgery and chemotherapy, the end results of treatment, and pertinent clinical trials.

We recognize that there is a great deal of individuality in the techniques of irradiation, and we have attempted to include descriptions of various technical approaches, leaving to the individual reader the critical task of selecting the most appropriate one for the particular patient under consideration. We believe that the comprehensive and rigorous approach to the assessment of each tumor site set forth in this text provides the foundation for proper application of radiation therapy techniques and multimodal programs in the treatment of patients with cancer.

It is our intent that *Principles and Practice of Radiation Oncology* should advance the effort to apply clinical and research activities in cancer management in a manner compatible with the current state of knowledge. It is our hope that this contribution will help foster new knowledge that will lead to improved delivery for radiation therapy and ultimately to a reduction in the time lost from other activities, in cost to the health care system, and in the human suffering occasioned by cancer.

Carlos A. Perez, MD
Luther W. Brady, MD

Acknowledgments

We are grateful for the scholarly, meticulous, and thorough work of the contributors to this volume. Through six editions, this book has become the "book of record" for the specialty of radiation oncology. It has achieved that distinction through the hard work of the individual chapter authors.

Jonathan Pine, Emilie Moyer, Grace Caputo, and Indu Jawwad of Lippincott Williams & Wilkins and their associated companies have professionally seen this work through from planning to distribution. We are in their debt.

Our fellow faculty members, residents, and medical students have supported our work, providing consistent intellectual stimulation, valuable suggestions, and materials that have contributed to this book.

Rupert K. Schmidt-Ullrich, MD, of the Medical College of Virginia/Virginia Commonwealth University served as co-editor of the fourth edition. A consummate physician-scientist and a valued colleague, he died in 2005. His positive contributions live on. Ruth Aultman faithfully served as secretary to Dr. Halperin for 21 years and diligently worked on the fourth through sixth editions. She died in 2012 and was working on the manuscript for Chapter 1 until shortly before her death.

Special recognition is due to Vilma Bordonaro, Deborah Habberfield, Susan Pfeifer, and Mary Lou Chin, who diligently worked on the preparation of materials for this volume.

Our families have patiently endured the loss of time and attention to other matters that occurs as a result of the demands of a project of this magnitude. To them, especially, we express our gratitude and love.

Edward C. Halperin, MD, MA
David E. Wazer, MD, FASTRO
Carlos A. Perez, MD
Luther W. Brady, MD

Contents

PART G: GASTROINTESTINAL

PART H: URINARY TRACT

PART I: MALE GENITOURINARY

PART J: GYNECOLOGIC

PART K: RETROPERITONEUM AND ADRENAL GLAND

PART L: LYMPHOMA AND HEMATOLOGIC TUMORS

PART M: BONE AND SOFT TISSUE

PART N: PEDIATRIC

SECTION I OVERVIEW AND BASIC SCIENCE OF RADIATION ONCOLOGY

Chapter 1
The Discipline of Radiation Oncology

Edward C. Halperin, David E. Wazer, and Carlos A. Perez

HISTORICAL FIGURES

Wilhelm Conrad Röntgen

On March 27, 1845, in Lennep, Germany, a son, Wilhelm Conrad, was born to the merchant Friedrich Conrad Röntgen and his wife, Charlotte Constanze (Fig. 1.1). Röntgen's father was a textile merchant, and when Wilhelm was 3, the family moved from Prussia to Apeldoorn in the Netherlands, about 100 miles to the northwest, where Wilhelm's maternal grandparents had made their home. Wilhelm enrolled in the Utrecht Technical School in 1862. A fellow student caricatured a teacher on the fire screen of the schoolroom. The schoolmaster demanded the name of the unflattering artist, but Wilhelm refused to betray his classmate and was expelled. It seemed that his education would come to an end after this episode. Fortunately, however, the Polytechnical School in Zurich, Switzerland, accepted students based on stiff entrance examinations. The black mark of expulsion from Holland served as no impediment. Röntgen began classes in 1865 and received his diploma in mechanical engineering in 1868.[167,175]

Röntgen's considerable skill in designing and constructing precision instruments for measuring physical phenomena attracted the attention of Dr. August Kundt, a theoretical physicist. Röntgen became Kundt's assistant at the University of Zurich. When Kundt moved, in turn, to the University of Würzburg and then to the University of Strasbourg, Röntgen followed. In 1879, Röntgen struck out on his own as a professor at the University of Giessen.

In 1888, Röntgen accepted a professorship of theoretical physics at the University of Würzburg (Fig. 1.2). On November 8, 1895, Röntgen saw the effects of an unusual phenomenon while doing laboratory experiments. He presented his results to the president of the Physical Society at Würzberg on December 28, 1895[174,175,325] (Fig. 1.3).

There are various accounts of Röntgen's discovery. Among the multitude of reporters who rushed to interview Röntgen was H. J. W. Dam, an Englishman who was a correspondent for the Canadian *McClure's Magazine*. Dam had a letter of introduction from the Royal Institution of Great Britain but, like all other reporters, when he arrived in Würzberg he was turned away. Dam, however, was persistent and wrote a letter in French to Röntgen insisting upon an interview. "You are very difficult, much more difficult than Berthlot, Pasteur, Dewar, and other men of science about whose discoveries I have written." Apparently taken by Dam's audacity and, perhaps, willing to have a sensible article written by a knowledgeable reporter, Röntgen granted Dam an exclusive interview.

Dam's lead story in the April 1896 *McClure's* is generally regarded as an accurate depiction.[104] Dam told his readers that "in all the history of scientific discovery there has never been, perhaps, so general, rapid, and dramatic an effect wrought on the scientific centers of Europe as has followed, in the past four weeks, upon an announcement made to the Wurzburg Physio-Medical Society, at their December meeting, by Professor William Konrad Röntgen, professor of physics at the Royal University of Wurzberg.... Röntgen's own report arrived, so cool, so business-like, and so truly scientific in character, that it left no doubt either of the truth or of the great importance of the preceding [newspaper] reports."[325]

Dam, who was able to converse with Röntgen in English, French, and German, conducted an on-site interview in Röntgen's laboratories and had him describe the circumstances related to the discovery. Dam's charming description, excerpted here, gives an excellent insight into Röntgen the man and the nature of his scientific inquiry.

> "Now, Professor," said I, "will you tell me the history of the discovery?"
>
> "There is no history," he said. "I have been for a long time interested in the problems of the cathode rays from a vacuum tube as studied by Hertz and Lenard. I had followed theirs and other researches with great interest, and determined as soon as I had time to make some researches of my own. This time I found at the close of last October. I had been at work for some days when I discovered something new."
>
> "What was the date?"
>
> "The eighth of November."
>
> "And what was the discovery?"
>
> "I was working with a Crookes' tube covered with a shield of black cardboard. A piece of barium platinocyanoide paper lay on the bench there. I had been passing a current through the tube and I noticed a peculiar black line across the paper."
>
> "What of that?"
>
> "The effect was one which could only be produced, in ordinary parlance, by the passage of light. No light could come from the tube, because the shield which covered it was impervious to any light known, even that of the electric arc."
>
> "And what did you think?"
>
> "I did not think; I investigated. I assumed that the effect must have come from the tube, since its character indicated that it could come from nowhere else. I tested it. In a few minutes there was no doubt about it. Rays were coming from the tube which had a luminescent effect on the paper. I tried it successfully at greater and greater distances, even at two metres. It seemed at first a new kind of invisible light. It was clearly something new, something unrecorded."
>
> "Is it light?"
>
> "No."
>
> "Is it electricity?"
>
> "Not in any known form."
>
> "What is it?"
>
> "I don't know. Having discovered the existence of a new kind of rays, I of course began to investigate what they would do. It soon appeared from the tests that the rays had penetrative power to a degree hitherto unknown. They penetrated paper, wood and cloth with ease, and the thickness of the substance made no perceptible difference within reasonable limits. The rays passed through all the metals tested with the facility varying, roughly speaking, with the density of the metal. These phenomena I have discussed carefully in my report to the Würzburg Society and you will find all the technical results therein stated. Since the rays had this great penetrative power, it seemed natural that they should penetrate flesh, and so it proved in photographing the hand I showed you."

A detailed discussion of the characteristics of his rays the professor considered unprofitable and unnecessary. He believes, though, that these mysterious radiations are not light, because their behavior is essentially different from that of light

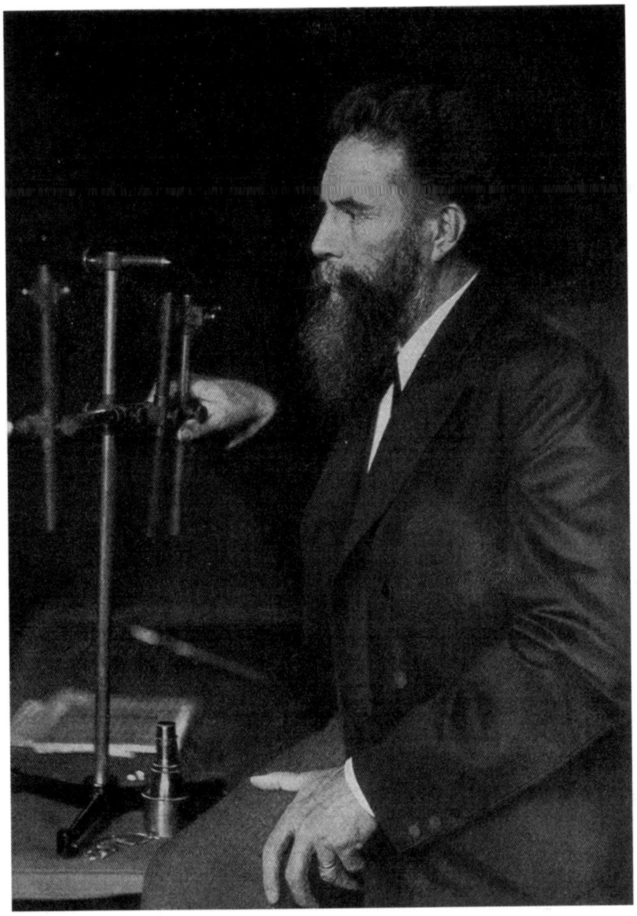

FIGURE 1.1. Wilhelm Conrad von Röntgen was born in Lennep, Germany, in 1845. He studied under Kundt in Zurich and was appointed professor of physics at Giessen in 1879 and at Würzberg in 1888. In 1895, while investigating cathode rays, he noted a new ray of greater penetrating power coming from the cathode tube. Röntgen announced his findings concerning the x-ray before the Würzberg Physical Society in 1895. He received the first Nobel Prize for Physics in 1901. Röntgen died in 1923. He is shown in this photograph with physics instruments. (From Glasser O. *Wilhelm Conrad Röntgen and the early history of the Roentgen rays.* Springfield, IL: Charles C. Thomas, Publisher, Ltd., 1934, with permission.)

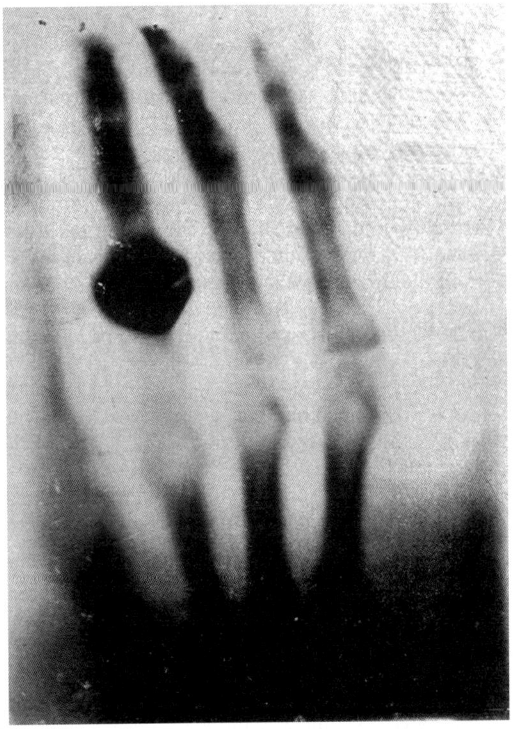

FIGURE 1.3. Röntgen made this image on December 22, 1895, and sent it to Vienna physicist F. Exner. (From Glasser O. *Wilhelm Conrad Röntgen and the early history of the Roentgen rays.* Springfield, IL: Charles C. Thomas, Publisher, Ltd., 1934, with permission.)

ways, even those light rays that are themselves invisible. The Röntgen rays cannot be reflected by reflecting surfaces, concentrated by lenses, or refracted or diffracted. They produce photographic action on a sensitive film, but their action is weak as yet, and herein lies the first important field of their development. The professor's exposures were comparatively long—an average of 15 minutes in easily penetrable media, and half an hour or more in photographing the bones of the hand. Concerning vacuum tubes, he said that he preferred the Hittorf, because it had the most perfect vacuum, the highest degree of air exhaustion being the consummation most desirable. In answer to the question, "What of the future?" he said:

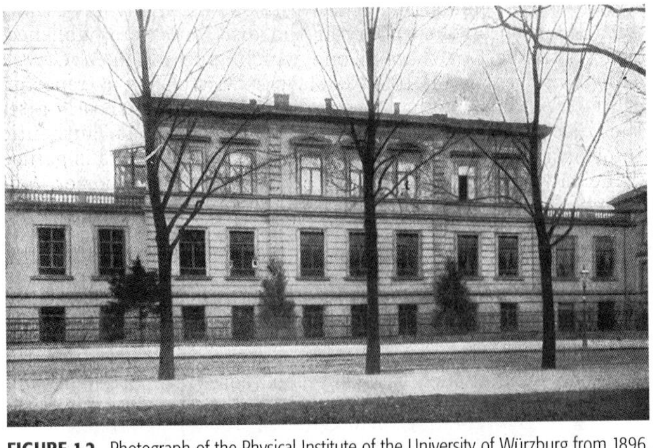

FIGURE 1.2. Photograph of the Physical Institute of the University of Würzburg from 1896. Professor Röntgen and his wife lived on the top floor. On the left side of the upper story can be seen the conservatory, of which Röntgen and his wife were particularly fond. (From Glasser O. *Wilhelm Conrad Röntgen and the early history of the Roentgen rays.* Springfield, IL: Charles C. Thomas, Publisher, Ltd., 1934, with permission.)

> "I am not a prophet, and I am opposed to prophesying. I am pursuing my investigations, and as fast as my results are verified I shall make them public."
>
> "Do you think the rays can be so modified as to photograph the organs of the human body?"
>
> In answer he took up the photograph of the box of weights. "Here are already modifications," he said, indicating the various degrees of shadow produced by the aluminum, platinum, and brass weights, the brass hinges, and even the metallic stamped lettering on the cover of the box, which was faintly perceptible.
>
> "But, Professor Neusser has already announced that the photographing of the various organs is possible."
>
> "We shall see what we shall see," he said; "we have the start now; the developments will follow in time."
>
> "You know the apparatus for introducing the electric light into the stomach?
>
> "Yes."
>
> "Do you think that this electric light will become a vacuum tube for photographing, from the stomach, any part of the abdomen or thorax?"
>
> The idea of swallowing a Crookes tube, and sending a high frequency current down into one's stomach, seemed to him exceedingly funny. "When I have done it, I will tell you," he said, smiling, resolute in abiding by results.
>
> "There is much to do, and I am busy, very busy," he said in conclusion. He extended his hand in farewell, his eye already wandering toward his work in the inside room. And his visitor promptly left him; the words, "I am busy," said in all sincerity, seeming to describe in a single phrase the essence of his character and the watchword of a very unusual man.[104]

Overview and Basic Science of Radiation Oncology

Kaiser Wilhelm II invited Röntgen to the imperial court at Potsdam in January 1896, <2 weeks after the scientist had mailed out reprints to prominent physicists. Röntgen demonstrated his findings and was decorated with the Prussian Order of the Crown, Second Class. On January 23, he gave a lecture to the Würzburg Physical-Medical Society and was startled and overwhelmed by the cheers of the audience. At the end of the talk, Röntgen invited Albert von Killiker, one of Germany's most distinguished anatomists, to come to the podium and have his hand x-rayed. When the audience saw the bones of his hand, it erupted in thunderous applause. This was one of Röntgen's last formal lectures on x-rays. He became flustered before large groups and, when lecturing to small groups of students, was generally regarded as lusterless and dull.

Röntgen received the Nobel Prize in Physics in 1901 from the Swedish king. He thanked him but gave no speech. He willed the prize money to the University of Würzburg.[167] In the presentation speech, the president of the Royal Swedish Academy of Sciences, C. T. Odhner, commented on the enormous potential of Röntgen's discovery for diagnosis and therapy.

> The Academy awarded the Nobel Prize in Physics to Wilhelm Conrad Röntgen, Professor in the University of Wurzburg, for the discovery with which his name is linked for all time: the discovery of the so-called Röntgen rays, or, as he himself called them, x-rays. These are, as we know, a new form of energy and have received the name "rays" on account of their property of propagating themselves in straight lines as light does. The actual constitution of this radiation of energy is still unknown. Several of its characteristic properties, however, have been discovered first by Röntgen himself and then by other physicists who have directed their research into this field. And there is no doubt that much success will be gained in physical science when this strange energy form is sufficiently investigated and its wide field has been thoroughly explored. Let us remind ourselves of one of the properties that has been found in Röntgen rays—the basis of the extensive use of x-rays in medical practice. Many bodies, just as they allow light to pass through them in varying degrees, behave likewise with x-rays but with the difference that some that are totally impenetrable to light can be penetrated easily by x-rays, whereas other bodies stop them. Thus, for example, metals are impenetrable to them; wood, leather, cardboard, and other materials are penetrable as are the muscular tissues of animal organisms. Now, when a foreign body impenetrable to x-rays (e.g., a bullet or a needle) has entered these tissues, its location can be determined by illuminating the appropriate part of the body with x-rays and taking a shadowgraph of it on a photographic plate, whereupon the impenetrable body is detected immediately. The importance of this for practical surgery and how many operations have been made possible and facilitated by it is well known to all. If we add that in many cases severe skin diseases (e.g., lupus) have been treated successfully with Röntgen rays, we can say at once that Röntgen's discovery already has brought so much benefit to mankind that to reward it with the Nobel Prize fulfills the intention of the testator to a very high degree.[325]

Henri Becquerel, Marie Sklodowska Curie, and Pierre Curie

Following Röntgen's discovery, clinical and technologic advances accumulated more rapidly than did basic biologic knowledge (Figs. 1.4 and 1.5). Several scientists began investigating whether or not rays similar to x-rays might be produced by ordinary fluorescent or phosphorescent substances. Henri Becquerel placed fluorescent mineral crusts on photographic plates wrapped in light-tight black paper, exposed them to sunlight, and observed an image on the plates. In February 1896, when poor weather prevented exposing his plates to sunlight, Becquerel put the prepared plates and minerals away in a drawer. On March 1, 1896, he removed them and, for an unknown reason, developed them before any exposure to sunlight. He saw images of the crust shapes on the developed plates and concluded that neither sunlight, fluorescence, nor phosphorescence was necessary to produce the effect. This form of radiation, initially called Becquerel rays, could penetrate thin strips of aluminum and copper.[31] The next day, he presented his findings at the French Academy of Sciences. Becquerel noted the first biologic effect of radium in human tissue; after carrying a small amount of the element in his shirt pocket he observed skin erythema, followed by moist desquamation and ulceration.[32]

Marya Sklodowska was born in Warsaw on November 7, 1867. The youngest of four sisters and a brother, she lived under Russian rule in partitioned Poland. At 17 she left home to work as a governess to the daughters of the supervisor of a large sugar beet factory northeast of Warsaw in order to save enough money to attend university. In 1891 Sklodowska enrolled at the Faculte des Sciences at the Sorbonne in Paris—one of just 23 women in a student body of about 1800. She completed degrees in mathematics and physics and in 1893 was hired by the Society for the Encouragement of National Industry to study the magnetic properties of steel. While in the process of securing additional laboratory space, she was introduced to Pierre Curie.

Curie was the son of a physician who had worked in the laboratory of Louise Pierre Gratiolet (1815–1865), who described the occipital visual pathways. Pierre Curie's doctoral thesis, "Magnetic Properties of Bodies at Diverse Temperatures," evaluated changes in magnetic properties of materials heated to high temperatures. He found that the magnetic properties of a substance change at a very specific temperature. This temperature is called the "Curie point" and is of great importance in studying plate tectonics, understanding extraterrestrial magnetic fields, and measuring the chemical contents of liquids. Curie also found that when crystals were pressed along their axis of symmetry, they produced an electric charge. This phenomenon is called "piezoelectricity," from the Greek word *piezin*, meaning "to squeeze," and is of importance in the operation of quartz watches, inkjet printers, autofocus cameras, and medical ultrasound.

Marya Sklodowska (now using the French form of her first name, "Marie") and Pierre Curie wed on July 26, 1895. For her doctoral thesis, Marie chose to investigate Becquerel's rays. She found that the intensity of the rays was affected neither by

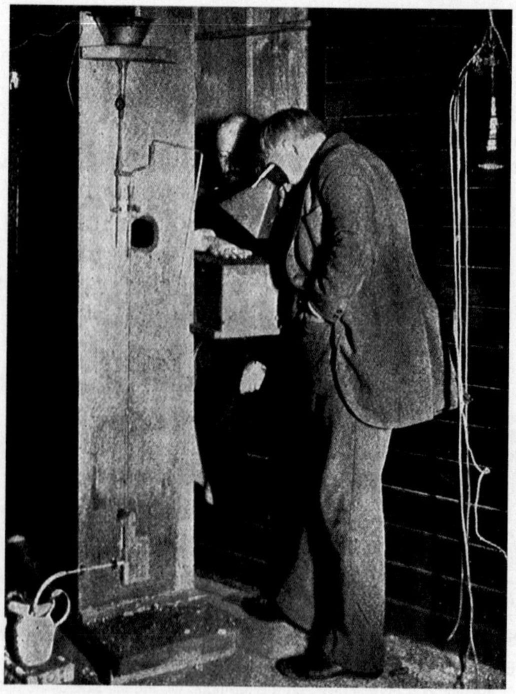

FIGURE 1.4. Thomas A. Edison experimenting with x-rays with, obviously, no radiation protection. (From Glasser O. *Wilhelm Conrad Röntgen and the early history of the Roentgen rays.* Springfield, IL: Charles C. Thomas, Publisher, Ltd., 1934, with permission.)

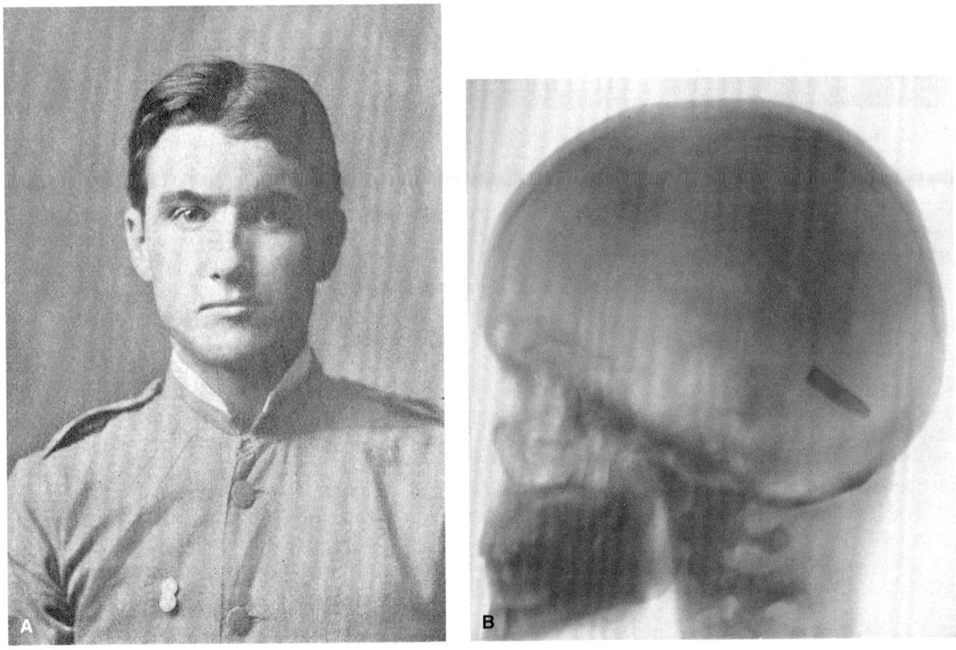

FIGURE 1.5. **A** and **B:** Private John Gretzer, Jr., Company D, First Nebraska volunteer injury, wounded above his left eye at long range in combat at Mariboa, Philippines. Five months after the injury he returned to duty in the military mail service. Diagnostic x-ray units were utilized by the U.S. Army Medical Department in the 1898 war with Spain and the Philippine insurrection–within 4 years of the discovery of the x-ray. (From *The use of the Roentgen ray by the Medical Department of the United States Army in the war with Spain (1898)*. Washington, DC: Government Printing Office, 1900.)

external conditions nor by any chemical process—they were an atomic property of the element. Marie observed that "it was obvious that a new science was in the course of development.... I coined the word *radioactivity*."[372]

After confirming Becquerel's observations, Marie and Pierre Curie in 1898 published a paper entitled "Sur une substance fortement nouvelle radio-active, continue dans la pechblende (on a new, strongly radio-active substance contained in pitchblende)." The new radioactive substance was called polonium (named in honor of Poland). In November and December 1898, while working on polonium, they noticed another substance, chemically akin to barium and more radioactive than polonium. Demarcay found specific spectral characteristics of this new element, which was called radium (from the Latin word for "ray"). The Curies declined to patent their findings. Pierre said "it would be contrary to the scientific spirit." In 1903–1904, radium-226 began to be used in the treatment of patients with skin cancer and uterine cancer.[293] On June 25, 1903, Marie defended her thesis "Researches on Radioactive Substances" and became the first woman in France to receive a doctorate. Later that year the Curies and Becquerel were awarded the Nobel Prize in Physics.

On April 19, 1905, Pierre Curie was killed while crossing the Rue Dauphine near the Seine—run down by a horse-drawn carriage carrying 13,000 pounds of military equipment. Marie returned to work and described the radioactive decay series of polonium. In 1911 she became the first person to win the Nobel Prize twice, this time in chemistry. When France entered World War I, Marie assembled hospital and mobile x-ray units for the care of the wounded. The mobile units were dubbed "petites Curies."[372] In March 1912 a glass tube containing 20 mg of radium was declared the international radium standard after comparison with a similar standard prepared in Vienna. The radioactivity unit was called Curie and defined as the emanation in equilibrium with 1 g of radium. In 1975 the International Commission on Radiation Units and Measurements replaced the Curie with the Becquerel (1 Curie = 3.7×10^{10} Bq).

In 1924 Marie and Pierre's eldest daughter, Irène, married Lieutenant Frederic Joliot. They investigated the transformation of aluminum, bombarded with alpha particles, into a radioactive state. Marie Curie died on July 4, 1934, from radiation poisoning. In 1935 her daughter and son-in-law were awarded the Nobel Prize for the discovery of artificial radioactivity.[103,372,448]

RADIATION THERAPY BEGINS

External-beam radiation therapy quickly showed itself to be a useful form of cancer treatment. Only 8 years after Röntgen's discovery, Dr. Charles L. Leonard, in 1903, observed that

> in spite of the most diligent study, there is nothing known of the etiology and histology of malignant disease that aids its treatment. Its development and fatal termination cannot be retarded, if the diseased tissue be permitted to remain in the body. Total extirpation by surgical intervention has been the only chance of cure. Leonard, however, discerned some promise in a new form of treatment. The results obtained by the use of the Röntgen rays seems to... have demonstrated their power to alter the character of malignant cells, to prevent their spread and development, and to produce retrograde changes that result in fatty and cystic degeneration or absorption, and often terminate in a restoration of the affected part to a nearly normal state.... The Röntgen treatment applied as a palliative in many hopeless, operatively impossible cases, has resulted frequently in cures, that, if not permanent, have at least restored the patient to health and given months and even years of usefulness.... The results so far obtained are, therefore, very encouraging. An agent has been found which has a greater influence in retarding the growth of malignant tumors than any heretofore known. Many remarkable and apparently permanent cures have been obtained.[265]

Although it is controversial, most likely Leopold Freund was the first to report, in 1897, the use of ionizing radiation to "cure" a large nevus pigmentosus on the back of a young girl. Unfortunately, she later developed skin ulceration and scars.[166] Another pioneer in the therapeutic use of x-rays was Victor Despeignes who, in 1896 published on the treatment of a 52-year-old man who had an advanced stomach tumor (likely a lymphoma), with "considerable improvement in the condition of the patient."[112]

At the International Congress of Oncology in Paris in 1922, Coutard[99] and Hautant presented evidence that advanced laryngeal cancer could be cured without disastrous, treatment-induced sequelae. By 1934, Coutard[100] had developed a protracted, fractionated scheme that remains the basis for current radiation therapy and, in 1936, Paterson[347] published results on the treatment of cancer with x-rays.

The use of brachytherapy, starting with radium-226 (^{226}Ra) needles and tubes, has increased steadily in the treatment of

Box 1.1

A Call to Arms

An Institute on Cancer meeting was conducted at the University of Wisconsin in Madison in 1936. Among the prominent scientists in attendance were James Ewing, professor of oncology at Cornell University Medical College, after whom Ewing sarcoma is named; Gioacchino Failla, the famous radiation physicist of the Memorial Hospital for Cancer and Allied Diseases of New York; and Henri Coutard, pioneer radiation therapist of the Curie Institute of Paris. Glenn Frank, president of the University of Wisconsin, addressed the scientists on the first day of the meeting. Seventy-five years later, Frank's opening address remains a moving call to arms for basic science, translational, and clinical researchers, physicists, and clinicians.[353]

"Down the ages, cancer has been the most hideously persistent and the most persistently hideous enemy of mankind, the suffering it lays upon men intolerably horrible, its toll of life progressively devastating, its blows falling so often just when men have reached the years of ripest usefulness to family and state. But not all these tragic consequences together are the worse evil wrought by cancer. For every *body* that is *killed* by the *fact* of cancer, multiplied thousands of *minds* are *unnerved* by the *fear* of cancer. What cancer, as an unsolved mystery, does to the morale of millions who may never know its ravages is incalculable. This is an incidence of cancer that cannot be reached by the physician's medicaments, the surgeon's knife, or any organized advice against panic. Nothing but the actual conquest of cancer itself will remove this sword that today hangs over every head. I can remember, as a boy in rural Missouri, that death from cancer was rarely mentioned and then only with bated breath. I realize now that this reaction was born of a feeling of utter helplessness and awe in the presence of a mysterious enemy. That almost primitive reaction to cancer has happily vanished. We have not penetrated the mystery, but, thanks to you and your colleagues the world over, we have made notable rents in the veil surrounding the mystery. The world is determined to conquer this thing that steals upon men like a thief in the night and without warning strikes down the strong and weak alike. By one thing alone can this conquest come, and that is by the tireless, painstaking, and self-sacrificing genius of scientists who, like yourselves, go to their laboratory tables as to an altar and sink their lives in the great adventure of emancipating mankind from the fact and fear of this plague. Surely, if anywhere in the secular activities of men, there is a spark of divinity in lives so dedicated!"[253]

malignant tumors in many anatomic locations. Isotopes such as cesium, iridium-192 (^{192}Ir), iodine-125 (^{125}I), and palladium-103 (^{103}Pd) were generated from nuclear reactors, and the use of afterloading techniques, including remote afterloading devices and high–dose-rate brachytherapy, brought a revival of this important treatment modality.

With time, ionizing radiation became more precise; high-energy photons, electrons, protons, neutrons, and carbon ions became available; and treatment planning and delivery became more accurate and reproducible. Advances in computer and electronic technology fostered the development of more sophisticated treatment-planning and delivery techniques, leading to the development and eventually broad implementation of three-dimensional conformal radiation therapy (3DCRT) and intensity-modulated radiation therapy (IMRT) (Box 1.1).

A DEFINITION OF RADIATION ONCOLOGY

Radiation oncology is that discipline of human medicine concerned with the generation, conservation, and dissemination of knowledge concerning the causes, prevention, and treatment of cancer and other diseases involving special expertise in the therapeutic applications of ionizing radiation. As a discipline that exists at the juncture of physics and biology, radiation oncology addresses the therapeutic uses of ionizing radiation alone or in combination with other treatment modalities such as biologic therapies, surgery, drugs, oxygen, and heat. Furthermore, radiation oncology is concerned with the investigation of the fundamental principles of cancer biology, the biologic interaction of radiation with normal and malignant tissue, and the physical basis of therapeutic radiation. As a learned profession, radiation oncology is concerned with clinical care, scientific research, and the education of professionals within the discipline.

Box 1.2

The Etymology of *Radiate*

The defining verb of the discipline of radiation oncology, *radiate*, is derived from the Latin verb *radiatus*. *Radiatus* is the participial stem. Some dictionaries cite the origin of the word *radiate* as being from other tenses of the verb such as the present infinitive *radiarae* or the first-person singular present indicative *radio*. Radiate is defined as "to spread from the common center" or "to diverge or spread from the common point" or "to issue and raise." Radiate shares a common root and related meanings with other English words such as *ray*, *radius*, and *radial*. The verb *radiate* is more distantly related to other words. For example, if one proceeds along the ray from the political center to the extreme, then one is called *radical*.

The verb *irradiate* means "to direct rays upon" or "to cause rays to fall upon something." In Latin, the prefix *in* conveys the meaning of in, within, on, upon, or against. When the prefix *in* is used with the word that begins with the letter *r*, the letter *r* is substituted for the letter *n* in the prefix to assimilate the initial sound of the verb. Thus, the verb that indicates the placement of water within or on the ground changed from *inrigate* to *irrigate*. Similarly, *inradiate* was changed to *irradiate*.

An object may be said to radiate something or to emit a ray. For example, "The block of cobalt 60 radiates gamma rays." The verb that indicates directing rays on or into an object is *irradiate*. An example of proper usage would be "I recommend that we irradiate the tumor to a total dose of 45 Gy." Incorrect usage would be "I think the primary tumor should be radiated to a dose of 45 Gy."[200]

Radiation therapy is a clinical modality dealing with the use of ionizing radiations in the treatment of patients with malignant neoplasias (and occasionally benign diseases). The aim of radiation therapy is to deliver a precisely measured dose of irradiation to a defined tumor volume with as minimal damage as possible to surrounding healthy tissue, resulting in eradication of the tumor, a high quality of life, and prolongation of survival at a reasonable cost. In addition to curative efforts, radiation therapy plays a major role in cancer management in the effective palliation or prevention of symptoms of the disease: pain can be alleviated, luminal patency can be restored, skeletal integrity can be preserved, and organ function can be re-established with minimal morbidity[94] (Box 1.2).

In 1962, Buschke[69] defined a radiotherapist as a physician whose practice is limited to radiation therapy. He emphasized the active role of the radiation oncologist:

> While the patient is under our care we take full and exclusive responsibility, exactly as does the surgeon who takes care of a patient with cancer. This means that we examine the patient personally, review the microscopic material, perform examinations and take a biopsy if necessary. On the basis of this thorough clinical investigation we consider the plan of treatment and suggest it to the referring physician and to the patient. We reserve for ourselves the right to an independent opinion regarding diagnosis and advisable therapy and if necessary, the right of disagreement with the referring physician.... During the course of treatment, we ourselves direct any additional medication that may be necessary... and are ready to be called in an emergency at any time.

To integrate the various disciplines and provide better care to patients, the radiation oncologist must cooperate closely with other specialists.[64,395]

THE PLANNING AND CONDUCT OF A COURSE OF RADIATION THERAPY

When a physician proposes administering radiation therapy to a patient, six fundamental questions must be answered. Once these questions have been answered, an appropriate first step has been taken toward the development of a comprehensive justification and plan for the conduct of a course of radiation therapy. The six questions are:

1. What is the *indication* for radiation therapy?
2. What is the *goal* of radiation therapy?

3. What is the planned treatment *volume*?
4. What is the planned treatment *technique*?
5. What is the planned treatment tumor *dose* and fractionation?
6. What is the radiation *tolerance* of surrounding normal tissues (organs at risk)?

The *indication* for radiation therapy is that body of data that can be brought to bear showing that radiation therapy would be efficacious for the patient's condition. Such data might exist in the form of retrospective single-institution reviews of the specific malignancy, which provide evidence favoring the role of radiotherapy. Phase I and II studies demonstrating safety and possible efficacy could be invoked to justify a course of radiation therapy. For many physicians the gold standard, however, is a prospective, randomized, phase III trial that demonstrates the value of radiation therapy. (The quality of clinical evidence is discussed in Chapter 98). There remains a role for sound personal clinical experience. Although there is increasing reliance on published trials, and special deference is given to double-blind, prospective, randomized phase III trials, it is still appropriate for a physician to rely firmly on his or her clinical experience in the context of an intimate knowledge of the patient's problems. A sound scientific basis and an extensive knowledge of clinical research augment the essential nature of the physician–patient relationship, but they do not substitute for it.

Radiation therapy can be justified either because it improves local tumor control, ameliorates a specific symptom, improves the quality of life, or increases the probability of cure. Any data used to justify a course of radiation therapy must have a clearly defined end point, appropriate data analysis, and accepted statistical methodology. It is incumbent on the radiation oncologist to know how to critically evaluate the scientific literature and synthesize it in the best interest of the patient.

There are two possible *goals* of radiation therapy. *Curative* radiation therapy is used for the purpose of curing the patient where one is willing to engender a small risk of significant side effects in return for the possibility of cure. An example is the use of radiation therapy for the treatment of early-stage breast cancer. In return for a high probability of cure, one is willing to engender a very small risk of pneumonitis. *Palliative* radiation therapy is designed to ameliorate a specific symptom such as pain, obstruction, or bleeding. In palliative radiation therapy used in the context of an incurable malignancy, one is not willing to engender a significant risk of side effects to achieve a palliative goal. Thus, if one wishes to relieve pain from lung cancer metastatic to a bone, one would pick a dose and technique of radiation therapy sufficient to relieve pain but not enough to run a risk of radiation osteonecrosis.

The questions of *indication* and *goal* are generic. They should be answered irrespective of the modality of therapy being used for the treatment of malignancy. It is reasonable to ask for indications and goal if one is planning on using chemotherapy, surgery, hyperthermia, biologic therapy, or radiation therapy. Oncologists are often better at formulating indications for curative than for palliative therapy. It is not good palliative medicine to make the patient ill from therapy while making asymptomatic metastatic masses smaller. In palliative cancer treatment, one must treat the patient and his or her symptoms and not treat the mass devoid of its context.

The next three of the six major questions, *volume, dose,* and *technique,* are not generic—they are specific to the discipline of radiation oncology. First, the radiation oncologist must consider *volume* (Fig. 1.6). What is the appropriate volume of tissue that needs to be irradiated for the purpose of achieving the desired curative or palliative goal in the context of the justification? Does one need to treat strictly the visualized or palpable tumor mass? Is it also appropriate to treat the mass and surrounding lymphatic drainage? Does one have to worry about the routes of spread of microscopic disease? All of these are crucial questions in formulating a plan for a course of radiation therapy. If radiation oncologists only needed to treat visible or palpable masses, then radiation oncology would be more of a physics exercise than an exercise in human medicine. Understanding a cancer's routes of spread and the tolerance of organs surrounding the cancer requires honed clinical judgment.

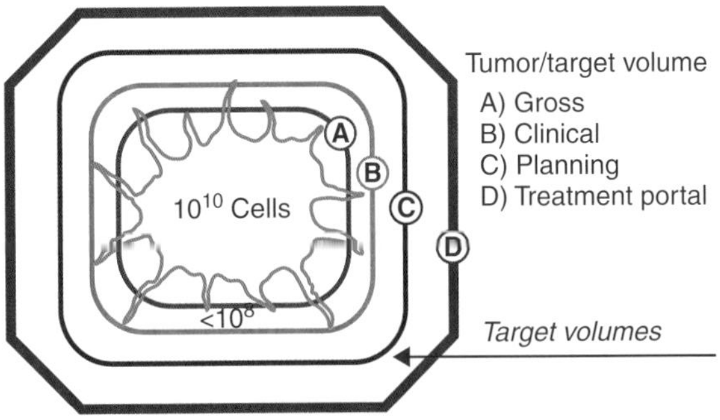

FIGURE 1.6. Schematic representation of "volumes" in radiation therapy. The treatment portal volume includes the tumor volume, potential areas of local and regional microscopic disease around the tumor, and a margin of surrounding normal tissue. (Modified from Perez CA, Purdy JA. Rationale for treatment planning in radiation therapy. In: Levitt SH, Khan FM, Potish RA, eds. *Levitt and Tapley's technological basis of radiation therapy: practical clinical applications,* 2nd ed. Philadelphia: Lea & Febiger, 1992, with permission.)

An example of the problem of volume in the radiation therapy of cancer is medulloblastoma, a tumor that arises in the posterior fossa of the human brain. If, however, one treats with resection alone, patients almost uniformly relapse both locally and by leptomeningeal dissemination via the cerebrospinal fluid. Thus, the treatment volume for radiation therapy of medulloblastoma, in children >3 years old, is the area within the posterior fossa wherein the tumor arises and the entire craniospinal axis. Another example of the problem of treatment volume would be in head and neck cancer. Many of these tumors, by physical examination and by diagnostic imaging, appear to be localized at their site of origin. For many of these squamous cell cancers there is, however, a high incidence of dissemination to the lymph nodes of the neck. Thus, the appropriate radiation therapy treatment volume would include both the primary tumor site and the neck.

The next question that the radiation oncologist must face is what is the appropriate *technique*? Radiation oncologists, in general, have two techniques at their disposal. The first, *teletherapy,* has a similar etymology to telephone, telegraph, and telepathy. It refers to the projection of radiation through space. Teletherapy is administered with external-beam sources such as a cobalt-60 (^{60}Co) machine or a linear accelerator. If one elects to treat a patient with teletherapy, one must derive appropriate external-beam treatment plans. These plans include considerations such as whether the patient should be treated with photons, electrons, neutrons, carbon ions, or protons; with parallel-opposed fields, four fields, or multiple oblique fields; with IMRT; with or without respiratory gating; with or without compensators; and the like. There has been an explosion of interest in new techniques of external-beam radiation therapy (EBRT) related to improvements in diagnostic imaging and the increasing power of computers to allow manipulation of vast amounts of data.

Another technique of radiation therapy is *brachytherapy.* The word brachytherapy shares an etymology with words such as brachycephaly and brachydactyly. It refers to short or slow therapy (i.e., a radioactive implant). There are several broad categories of brachytherapy. These include *interstitial* brachytherapy, *intracavitary* brachytherapy, and *mold* therapy. Interstitial brachytherapy refers to the placement of radioactive sources directly into tissue. An example might be the implantation of the tumor bed for breast cancer or soft-tissue sarcoma. Intracavitary radiotherapy refers to the placement of a radioactive source in a body cavity such as sources placed within the nasopharynx or against and through the os of the uterine cervix. Mold brachytherapy refers to the placement of radioactive sources on the skin surface, such as treatment utilized for a superficial malignancy on the back of the hand. If brachytherapy is used, the radiation oncologist must determine the appropriate isotope and whether that isotope is to be delivered by an afterloading technique or by a direct radioactive application (a hot implant).

Once the radiation oncologist has determined the appropriate treatment volume and the treatment technique(s), he or she must determine the appropriate radiation *dose.* Radiation dose selection is a complex issue. One must determine the correct number of fractions of radiation per day, the correct dose per fraction, and the proposed total dose of irradiation. Furthermore, in certain situations, the dose rate (i.e., the number of cGy per minute) matters, such as in total body irradiation (TBI) for bone marrow transplantation and in brachytherapy. Decisions concerning dose will, in part, be driven by decisions concerning treatment volume and technique. Paramount in the physician's mind will be the goal of treatment. The physician must determine what the correct dose is to achieve the proposed curative or palliative goal. In broad terms, the radiation oncologist must consider what is known about the dose–response relationship for tumor control in a particular clinical situation. This subject, addressed in detail elsewhere in this chapter, concerns the probability of tumor control within a radiation therapy field as a function of the dose administered.

Finally, the radiation oncologist must consider normal tissue *tolerance.* In general terms, the probability of acute and late ill effects of radiation is a function of dose. Ultimately, the prescription of a dose requires the radiation oncologist to engage in a balancing act between a sufficient dose of radiation to achieve the desired treatment goal and not giving so much dose as to engender an unacceptable risk of side effects.

The fundamental questions of radiation therapy are not for the physician alone. A patient has the right to be apprised of the physician's views on these questions, probability of tumor control (cure, if possible), and sequelae. This information should be presented to the patient in an appropriate intellectual, social, and cultural context (i.e., in a manner in which the patient can understand) so that the patient becomes a full partner in his or her care. The signing of an informed consent document by the patient is the norm.

EXTERNAL-BEAM RADIATION TREATMENT PLANNING

Treatment Volume

Tumor cell killing by ionizing radiation is an exponential function of dose. The dose required for a certain level of tumor control probability (TCP, or local control) is proportional to the logarithm of the number of clonogenic cells in the tumor. Subclinical extensions of tumor (also called microscopic disease or disease below the level of ready clinical detection) should be controlled, in general, by a lower dose of external-beam radiation than is required for a palpable tumor mass. Microscopic tumor extensions may be less likely than bulky tumors to contain hypoxic cells. This also means that they may be more readily controlled by radiation.

Insofar as the dose tolerated by normal tissue is inversely related to the volume of normal tissue irradiated, delivering a uniform physical dose of radiation requires that one choose between the risks of marginal recurrence around small volumes of high dose, central recurrences in large volumes of low dose, or excessive normal tissue damage and large volumes of high dose. We may conclude that different doses of radiation are required for a given probability of tumor control, depending on the type and initial number of clonogenic cells present.

A shrinking field technique is a rational approach to the problem of heterogeneous tumor distribution (Fig. 1.7). Withers and Taylor[508] have argued that "in the ideal case, the doses would be graded to provide a homogeneous TCP throughout the treatment volume rather than a homogeneous physical dose distribution." We are entering an era of "dose painting" where a heterogenous dose will be layered on a tumor as determined by sophisticated imaging tools.[40] The radiation oncologist delivers varying radiation doses to certain portions of the tumor (periphery vs. central portion or metabolically active vs. inactive on computed tomography [CT]/positron emission tomography [PET]) or may vary the dose in cases in which gross tumor has been surgically removed.

The International Commission on Radiation Units and Measurements (ICRU) Report 50 has recommended definitions of terms and concepts for radiation therapy treatment volumes and margins:[229]

- The gross tumor volume (GTV) denotes demonstrable tumor. It includes all known gross disease including abnormally enlarged regional lymph nodes. In the determination of GTV, it is important to use the appropriate CT and/or magnetic resonance imaging (MRI) settings and, if appropriate, PET scan to give the maximum dimension of what is considered potential gross disease.

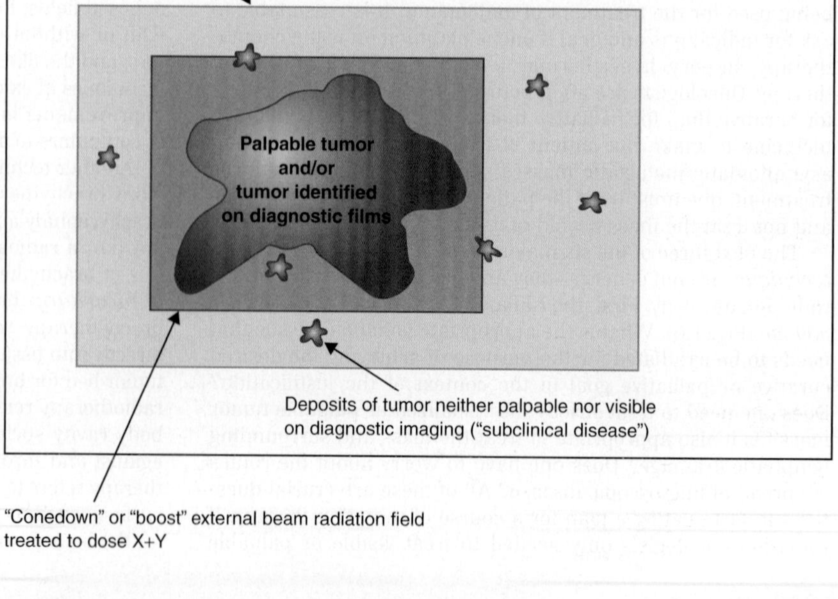

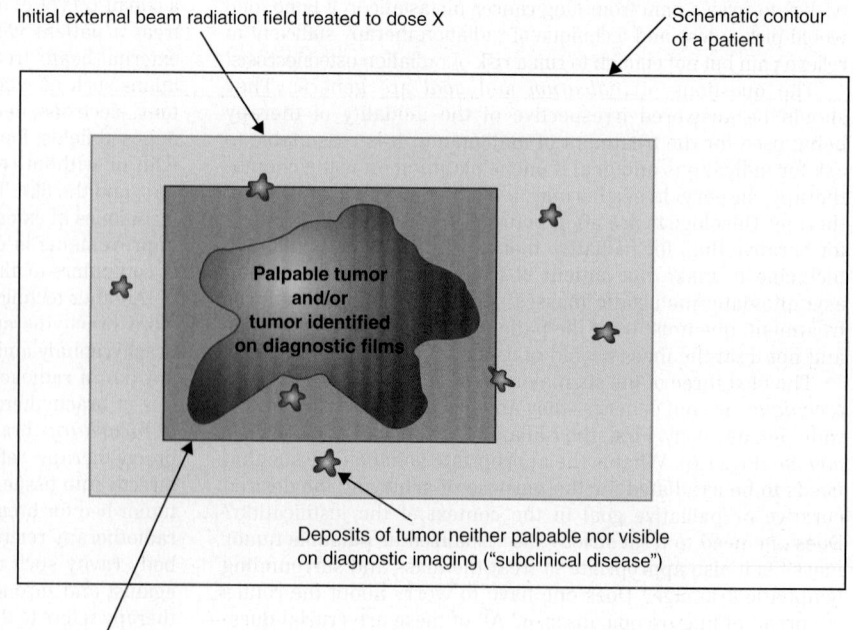

FIGURE 1.7. Cell killing by ionizing radiation is an exponential function of dose. It follows that the dose required for a certain level of tumor control probability (TCP) is directly proportional to the logarithm of the number of clonogenic cells in the tumor deposit. It would be reasonable to expect that subclinical extensions of disease could be controlled by a lower dose of irradiation than what is required for a bulky palpable tumor mass. It has been argued by some researchers that microscopic tumor extensions are less likely to contain hypoxic foci that will minimize the requirement for reoxygenation for their control–but this is controversial. Insofar as the dose tolerated by a tissue is inversely related to the volume of tissue irradiated, delivering a uniform physical dose requires that one choose between the risk of marginal recurrences around small volumes of high dose, central occurrences in large volumes of low dose, or excessive normal tissue damage in large volumes of high dose. A reasonable approach is to use a shrinking-field technique in which one delivers an initial external-beam field that is treated to dose X and then "cones down" to a smaller field to treat to dose X + Y. In the ideal case, doses are graded to provide a homogeneous TCP throughout the treatment volume rather than a homogeneous physical dose distribution. (Based on a concept articulated by Withers HR, Peters LJ. Biologic aspects of radiotherapy. In: Fletcher GH, ed. *Textbook of radiotherapy,* 3rd ed. Philadelphia: Lea & Febiger, 1980:142.)

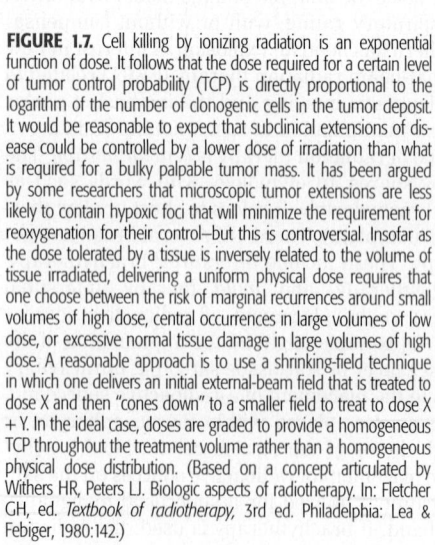

- The clinical target volume (CTV) denotes the GTV and subclinical disease (i.e., volumes of tissue with suspected tumor).
- The planning target volume (PTV) denotes the CTV and includes margins for geometric uncertainties. One also should account for variation in treatment setup and other anatomic motion during treatment such as respiration.

Because the PTV does not account for treatment machine characteristics, the actual treated volume is that volume enclosed by an isodose surface that is selected and specified by the radiation oncologist as being appropriate to achieve the goal of treatment. It is impossible to design a radiation therapy treatment plan that limits the prescribed dose to the PTV only. Some tissues en route to the target or near the target also will be irradiated to the same dose as the target. The treated volume is, therefore, almost always larger than the PTV and usually has a somewhat simpler shape.

- The irradiated volume is that volume of tissue that receives a dose considered significant in relationship to tissue tolerance. This would include tissues in the exit region of unopposed photon beams or in the penumbra region of a beam.
- The planning organ at risk volume refers to the definition of margins around organs at risk for injury by radiation. For example, one might define a 0.5-cm margin around the optic chiasm to avoid the risk of blindness.

Uncertainties

There are, inevitably, uncertainties in the planning and delivery of a course of radiation therapy. These were well characterized by the esteemed dosimetrist Gunilla Bentel[38,39] (1936–2000), to whom we are grateful for the following discussion.

Uncertainties are divided into two general categories. First, there are uncertainties related to the delivery of dose. These include inhomogeneities in the beam, problems related to dose calculations, variables in the output of treatment machines, instability of the beam monitoring technique, and problems related to beam flatness. Spatial uncertainties in the delivery of radiation therapy may be divided into those related to mechanical inaccuracies in the equipment and those related to the patient.

Mechanical Uncertainties

- *Field size settings.* There can be errors related either to mechanical dials or digital settings in which the field size set on the machine is not precisely the same as that delivered.
- *Rotational settings.* Mechanical or digital settings that display the degree of angulation of the gantry or the collimator may be in error.
- *Cross hairs.* Wires in the linear accelerator designed to show the central axis or the field edges may become displaced.
- *Isocenter.* Deviations in the position of the isocenter may occur as a result of sagging of the gantry head.
- *Light-beam congruence.* The light beam within the linear accelerator may be in error. These misalignments may be caused by small shifts in the mirror or the light bulb.
- *Alignment systems.* The laser beam systems used for alignment may be in error. They may not intersect exactly at the isocenter, they may not be perpendicular, and some systems may display relatively thick lines allowing for errors in judgment.
- *Couch top.* There can be differences in sag between radiation treatment couches. In addition, there may be differences in sag between the simulator couch, the CT couch used for 3D or IMRT planning, and the accelerator couch. Sometimes, in the treatment room, a tennis racket–type insert is used. Over time, couch tops can become tilted from side to side or from end to end.
- *Beam-shaping blocks or collimators.* If blocks are used rather than a multileaf collimator, there may be errors in constructing the blocks related to user error or because the cutting wire becomes too hot or is moved too fast around a corner when the Styrofoam mold is cut. If multileaf collimators are used, there may be errors in alignment.

Patient-Related Uncertainties

- *Target delineation.* No matter how sophisticated the computerized treatment-planning system, it will be to no avail if the physician is uncertain about where the tumor is located. The inherent problems related to PET, MRI, CT, and our ability to make correlations between anatomic and functional imaging, and the location of tumor may result in difficulty determining the extent of tumor as well as in transferring anatomic information from imaging studies to the 3D or IMRT treatment-planning system.
- *Organ motion.* Organ motion can occur from respiration or heartbeat. In addition, it can occur from changes in the size or shape of an organ as a function of digestive or excretory function (i.e., changes in the size and position of the stomach, intestines, bladder, and rectum, and, in the last case, its influence on prostate position) (Fig. 1.8).
- *Skin marks.* Skin marks can shift relative to deeper tissues. This can change as a result of alterations in patient weight, patient positioning, or the use of steroids during a course of radiation therapy. A particular problem is related to the width of setup lines drawn by therapists on the patient's skin. Variation in the width of the lines drawn and variation in the position of the light fields in relationship to the lines can cause uncertainty in treatment delivery.

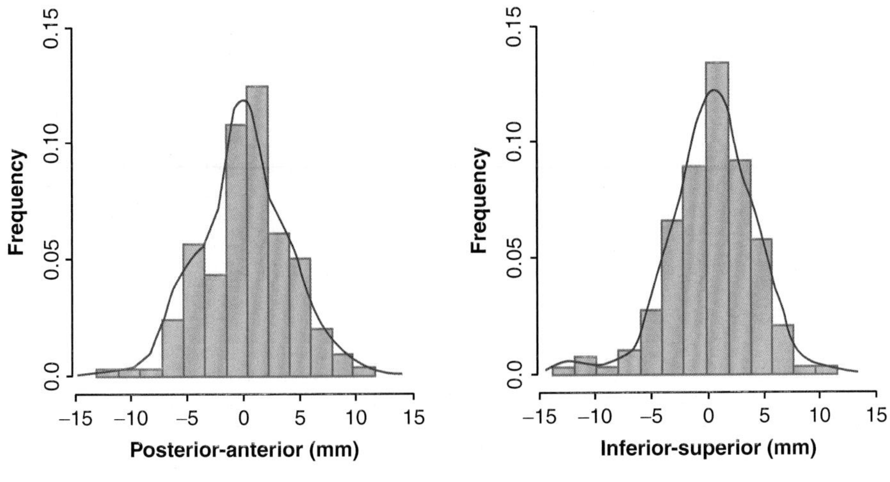

FIGURE 1.8. Precision radiotherapy treatment planning must take physiologic target motion into account. Wu et al. evaluated the treatment errors from setup and interfraction prostatic motion with port films and implanted prostate fiducial markers during conformal radiotherapy for localized prostate cancer. These histograms show the frequency distribution of prostate motion in the anteroposterior and superoinferior planes. Prostate motion can contribute to setup and treatment error in external-beam radiotherapy. (From Wu J, Haycocks T, Alasti H, et al. Position errors and prostate motion during conformal prostate radiotherapy using on-line isocentre set-up verification and implanted prostate markers. *Radiother Oncol* 2001;61:127–133.)

- *Repositioning.* Day-to-day problems in reproducing the position may occur.
- *Patient motion.* Some patients simply will not hold still during radiation therapy. Whether this is related to the patient being anxious, in pain, demented, or subject to a neurologic disorder, it can lead to uncertainties in radiation therapy treatment delivery.

Immobilization

The magnitude of uncertainties in radiation therapy treatment delivery varies. Furthermore, some uncertainties may be additive and some may cancel each other out. The net effect, on any given day, can be quite variable.

To irradiate a tumor while minimizing the radiation dose to uninvolved normal tissue, control of patient movement must be precise and absolute. Sophisticated tumor localization, 3D treatment planning, radiosurgery, and/or IMRT will be of no use if the patient is not holding still. Often, positioning and mobilization can be the weakest link in the chain of treatment planning.[201] Quality radiotherapy demands that a daily setup accuracy of a few millimeters be ensured.

Mechanical immobilization of the awake radiotherapy patient is an adjunct to patient education and psychological preparation of the patient. Although not a substitute for education and psychological preparation, mechanical aids can greatly facilitate accurate treatment. The ideal mechanical aid for patient positioning will achieve the following goals:[201]

1. The patient must be comfortable and secure. There must be no danger of falling. The patient should not become claustrophobic.
2. The device must satisfy the radiotherapy treatment plan regarding patient position for correct geographic irradiation.
3. The setup should be quick and easy for the radiation therapist.
4. The body part treated should be rendered immobile.
5. Position of the body part should be reproducible for daily treatment.
6. Construction of the device should be reasonably quick. It should not be difficult to train therapists, dosimetrists, and physicians in the construction procedure.
7. The stabilization device should not adversely affect beam buildup and backscatter characteristics.
8. This system should be economical.
9. If anesthesia is being used, the device must not interfere with the establishment of a secure airway, intravenous access, or the use of monitoring equipment.

A variety of immobilization devices meet these stated criteria to varying degrees. There is no perfect system. Techniques will vary among institutions. It is reasonable to expect, however, that the radiation oncologist should be knowledgeable in several techniques that can be brought to bear as the situation demands.

There are a variety of stabilization devices. These include commercially available accessories such as plastic headholders and sponges, bite blocks, thermoplastics, plaster of Paris, vacuum-molded thermoplastics, polyurethane foams, vacuum bags, intrarectal balloons to stabilize the prostate and rectal wall during prostate radiotherapy, gated radiotherapy and therapy while breath holding to minimize respiratory excursion, and mechanical devices to compensate for patient movement by compensatory couch movement or collimator leaf movement.

Accuracy of external-beam placement was typically assessed periodically with portal (localization) films. It is now more common to use online imaging verification (electronic portal imaging) devices, or online CT, fluoroscopy, or ultrasound.[302,475] Portal localization errors may be systematic or occur at random. Online electronic portal imaging has been used to document inter- or intratreatment portal displacement.

Patient movement clearly adversely influences the quality of external-beam radiotherapy. In a review of 48 patients on whom multiple digital portal verification images were obtained, Bissett et al.[45] noted that displacements of the field were 2.9 mm in the transverse and 3.4 mm in the craniocaudal dimensions. Mean rotational displacement was 2 degrees. The mean treatment field coverage was 95%. There were some variations in the assessment of the translational errors when observations of several radiation oncologists were analyzed. Rabinowitz et al.,[371] in a comparison of simulator and portal films of 71 patients, noted some discrepancies between the simulator and the localization (treatment) portal films. With an average value of 3-mm standard deviation of the variations, the mean worst case discrepancy averaged 3.5 mm in the head and neck region, 9.2 mm in the thorax, 5.1 mm in the abdomen, 8.4 mm in the pelvis, and 6.9 mm in the extremities. Other investigators have documented similar localization errors on the basis of portal film review analysis.[285,286,414] Hendrickson[216] reported a 3.5% error frequency in multiple parameters (setting of field size, timer, gantry and collimator angles, and patient positioning) with one technologist working. The error rate declined to 0.82% when two technologists worked together.

Doss,[122] in a study of patients with upper airway carcinoma, showed that in 21/28 patients (75%) with treatments in which 30% or more portals exhibited a blocking error, a recurrence developed, whereas tumor failure was noted in only 2/12 patients (17%) without such errors. Perez et al.[384] also reported a higher incidence of failures in patients with carcinoma of the nasopharynx on whom shielding of the ear inadvertently caused some blocking of tumor volume.

A growing body of evidence supports the benefit of stabilization devices in reducing patient motion. Marks et al.[285,286] demonstrated, by systematic use of verification films, a high frequency of localization errors in patients irradiated for head and neck cancer or malignant lymphomas. These errors were corrected with improved patient immobilization; with the use of a bite block in patients with head and neck tumors, localization errors were reduced from 16% to 1%[286] (Table 1.1). The growing popularity of 3DCRT and IMRT, as well as the emphasis on stereotactic body radiosurgery, has led to several excellent contributions to the literature assessing the value of stabilization devices. Such devices are particularly important in the treatment of lung, liver, and paraspinal tumors. Often, these devices include a combination of a thermoplastic body cast, vacuum pillow, arm and leg support, wooden backing and/or sides, or a carbon plate. It has been demonstrated that such devices can

TABLE 1.1 THE IMPACT OF STABILIZATION DEVICES ON EXTERNAL-BEAM SETUP REPRODUCIBILITY

	Number of Position Adjustments Per Number of Times Tested (%)	*P*
Hodgkin's disease (n = 56)[a]		
Short cradle stabilization device	48/237 (20)	0.009
Whole-torso cradle stabilization device	21/213 (10)	–
Head and neck cancer (n = 71)[b]		
Three casting strip stabilization device	55/307 (18)	0.23
Customized mask device	40/291 (14)	–
Lung cancer (n = 60)[c]		
No stabilization device	17/119 (14)	0.139
Cradle	14/171 (8)	–

[a]Bentel GC, Marks LB, Krishnamurthy R, et al. Comparison of two repositioning devices used during radiation therapy for Hodgkin's disease. *Int J Radiat Oncol Biol Phys* 1997;38(4):791–795.

[b]Bentel GC, Marks LB, Hendren K, et al. Comparison of two head and neck immobilization systems. *Int J Radiat Oncol Biol Phys* 1997;38(4):867–873.

[c]Bentel GC, Marks LB, Krishnamurthy R. Impact of cradle immobilization on setup reproducibility during external beam radiation therapy for lung cancer. *Int J Radiat Oncol Biol Phys* 1997;38(4):527–531.

TABLE 1.2 INTRAFRACTIONAL PATIENT MOTION AS A FUNCTION OF THE IMMOBILIZATION DEVICE[a]

Immobilization Device	*Patient Motion*
Alpha cradle	5.0 mm
Bean bag	6.8 mm
Head Aquaplast	3.6 mm
Duncan head rest	7.0 mm
Modified Gill–Thomas-Costman Frame	1.8 mm
Prone craniospinal head support	3.0 mm
Head Aquaplast with bite block	2.9 mm
Wing board	5.9 mm

[a]Based on an analysis of >10,000 fields, there is a 95% chance that the change in patient position between the initial patient setup and the position before the next treatment field is set up will be less than the measurement shown.

Modified from Engelsman M, Rosenthal SJ, Michaud SL, et al. Intra and inter-fractional patient motion for a variety of immobilization devices. *Med Phys* 2005;32:3468–3474.

achieve setup errors and deviations in the 1- to 3-mm range.[279,404] Some institutions rely on vacuum-molded plastic shells. These devices, similarly, will achieve displacements on the order of 1 to 3 mm.[226]

In a randomized trial from the Karolinska University Hospital in Stockholm, Sweden, patients with head and neck cancer were randomly assigned to be stabilized with a thermoplastic head mask or a thermoplastic head and shoulder mask. Reproducibility was assessed by comparing port films in these three-dimensionally planned patients with simulator films. This was done twice during treatment and by comparing the actual treatment table positions weekly. Patient tolerance and skin reactions were also assessed. A total of 241 patients were evaluated. There were no statistically significant differences between the head mask stabilization device or the head and shoulder mask stabilization device in terms of reproducibility. It was of note, however, that patients with the thermoplastic mask extending over the head and shoulders experienced significantly more claustrophobic reactions and greater skin reactions. This study has been criticized for its reliance on thermoplastic devices rather than the vacuum-formed clear polyethylene masks.[383]

Because different stabilization devices are utilized in different clinical situations, there is no simple way to know which is the best stabilization device. An excellent comparative study done at the Northeast Proton Therapy Center analyzed the length for which there is a 95% probability that the total displacement will be smaller as a result of intrafractional patient motion. It is reasonable to expect that customized closely fitting molds should achieve intrafractional stabilization of 2 to 7 mm, with the best stabilization being obtained in precision treatment of the brain utilizing a rigid halo and bite block (Table 1.2).[144]

We may expect further benefits from research on stabilization. For example, air-filled rectal balloons have been shown to decrease prostate motion during prostate radiotherapy. The perturbation of the radiation dose near the air–tissue interface appears to produce some sparing of the rectal mucosa without incremental detriment to the dose to the prostate.[443] Active breathing control, gated radiotherapy, and compensatory motion of the treatment couch to account for patient motion are also all under active investigation.[126]

Respiratory-Dampened, Respiratory-Gated, and Respiration-Synchronized Radiotherapy

The movement associated with respiration affects the position of multiple organs. If the radiation oncologist wishes to administer highly conformal fractionated or single-fraction treatment(s) to tumors of the liver, lung, pancreas, kidney, retroperitoneum, thoracic wall, mediastinal region, and adjacent structures, it will be necessary to either account for respiration-induced movement by putting a larger margin around the tumor or use an intervention to reduce this movement.

TABLE 1.3 AVERAGE DIAPHRAGM MOTION DURING ACTIVE BREATHING CONTROL (ABC) (MEAN, RANGE)[106,131,514]

By Fluoroscopy at Simulation	*By Fluoroscopy During Treatment*	*Beam's Eye View During Treatment*
1.4 mm (0–3.4 mm)	1.2 mm (0.4–2.5 mm)	0.5 mm (0–4.2 mm)

One method for limiting respiratory motion during radiotherapy is the *abdominal compression method.* This involves placing a plate or some other restrictive device above or around the abdomen and chest, sometimes in association with supplemental oxygen, in an effort to minimize the amount of diaphragmatic motion during radiotherapy.[31] This is also referred to as *respiratory-dampened radiotherapy.*[454] Another technique involves general anesthesia and high-frequency jet ventilation to minimize diaphragm motion during liver radiosurgery.[169]

Respiratory-gated radiotherapy involves turning the beam on only during portions of the respiratory cycle. One such method calls for the patient to hold his or her breath during the irradiation. A device called the Active Breathing Coordinator (ABC, Elekta, Norcross, GA) attempts to standardize breath holding. The patient is coached to hold his or her breath at a certain consistent depth of inspiration by watching a monitor. The ABC device uses a mouth piece, nose plug, bacterial filter, tubing, and balloon valve that, when triggered to inflate by the caregiver, will prevent airflow to and from the patient. The patient controls the switch, which must be enabled to allow the operation of the device. Using the ABC system, the caregiver can initiate a patient's breath hold at a predetermined title volume. At the time of simulation, the patient practices inhale-exhale breath hold under guidance of the radiation therapist. At the moment of fixed inspiration, a valve device engages to prevent additional inspiration or expiration. The beam-on time is coordinated with breath holding.[107,131,514]

Investigation of the ABC system has focused on treatment of lung and liver. As seen in Table 1.3, the system can be used to minimize diaphragmatic motion and, therefore, reduce the amount of hepatic excursion during precision radiation therapy.

DNA DAMAGE BY IONIZING RADIATION

The biologic effects of ionizing radiation are largely the result of DNA damage, which is caused directly by ionization within the DNA molecule or indirectly from the action of chemical radicals formed as a result of local ionizations in water. The general forms of DNA damage are base damage, DNA-protein cross-links, single-strand breaks, double-strand breaks, and complex combinations of all of these.

Normal mammalian cells repair a significant proportion of radiation-induced DNA damage. Long-term biologic consequences are the result of those injuries, which are irreparable or misrepaired. The cell will attempt to repair DNA injury induced by radiation via several pathways. Key genes affecting these radiation-repair pathways include ATM (associated with ataxia telangiectasia), Ku (involved in repair of double-strand DNA breaks), and XRCC2.

There is some evidence that clustered local damage to DNA, such as a double-strand break accompanied by additional breaks, base damage, or DNA-protein cross-links, is especially difficult for cells to repair. Even lesions that are potentially repairable may be repaired incorrectly (misrepaired) if lesions are accumulating very rapidly because of high–dose-rate or dose-rate radiation or if the cell enters M phase and attempts DNA synthesis while repair is in progress. Conversely, radiation, which is given at a low dose rate or is highly fractionated,

TABLE 1.4 THE MICROENVIRONMENT AND THE RADIATION RESPONSE

Issues and Problems

Tumor and its interaction with normal tissue and stroma
- Identifying tumor from normal tissue
- Abnormal physiology; stress response and epigenetic changes
- Normal tissue and stromal component–cytokines, growth factors, cell–cell contact
- Immunologic response
- Inflammatory processes
- Interstitial pressure–a barrier to therapy?
- Drug distribution–depends on size, charge, solubility
- Heterogeneity–very complex and hard to replicate in the lab
- Instability–genetic, environmental; inherent cellular genetic instability also is subject to dynamic changes (e.g., ischemia-reperfusion)

New Opportunities

Laser-capture microscopy–analyze heterogeneity
cDNA microarray–molecular phenotype and identification of families of genes and genes that modify the impact of mutated genes
Protein function depends on conformation such that a normal gene product may function abnormally in the tumor microenvironment
Tumor progression may be the result of a combination of tumor and stromal cell factors
Normal tissues within the tumor may become therapeutic target (e.g., endothelial cells)
Immunologic response–adoptive immunotherapy, enhancing immunogenicity with costimulatory molecules and factors and possibly with radiation to increase antigen expression
Heterogeneity of radiation dose intensity within tumor–intensity-modulated radiation therapy, brachytherapy, radiolabeled molecules (antibodies, ligands, peptides)
Inflammatory processes and inflammatory molecules and their role in tumor resistance to therapy
Late effects; these may be a continuous/continual "chronic active" process
Interstitial space analysis–microdialysis, pharmacokinetics
Drug/nutrient distribution–target abnormal tumor physiology with hypoxia activation of drugs and genes
Instability–genetic, environmental
Need to understand selection pressure based on environment; successful treatment or prevention strategies may require abrogating the tumor cell's ability to evolve a more malignant phenotype

From Coleman CN. International Conference on Translational Research and Preclinical Strategies in Radio-Oncology (ICTR): conference summary. *Int J Radiat Oncol Biol Phys* 2001;49:301–309.

provides the best opportunity for repair of radiation-induced lesions and recovery from injury. DNA damage that is not repaired may cause cell death, prevent cell division, or permanently give rise to heritable lesions such as point mutations, small and large deletions and translocations of DNA sequences, and a wide variety of DNA aberrations[276] (Tables 1.4 and 1.5).

RELEVANCE OF RADIOBIOLOGIC CONCEPTS IN CLINICAL RADIATION THERAPY

Radiation and Cancer Biology's Contributions to the Clinical Practice of Radiation Oncology

Generations of radiation oncologists have grappled with the question of radiation and cancer biology's contribution to the clinical practice of radiation oncology. The question was posed and addressed in two classic lectures: first by Stanford's Henry S. Kaplan[244] in his 1970 Failla lecture to the Radiation Research Society and then by Harvard's Herman D. Suit[429] in his 1983 Failla lecture. Treading on the ground prepared for us by Kaplan and Suit, we will reconsider the question in the context of the explosion of knowledge concerning the molecular and cellular basis of cancer at the start of the 21st century.

One can look at the history of cancer biology's contribution to the clinical practice of radiation oncology in terms of two debates: *empiricism versus research-based radiation oncology* and *biology versus physics.*

TABLE 1.5 THE NANO-TO-PICO ENVIRONMENT AND THE RADIATION RESPONSE

Issues and Problems

Where the real action is
- Subcellular dosimetry–heterogeneity at nano-level where dense ionizations occur
- Multiple molecular target beyond DNA
- Molecular pharmacology–cell is highly compartmentalized
- For effective cancer treatment both drug- and radiation therapy–induced radical or other biochemical perturbation–must be at right concentration, right place, at right time

New Opportunities

Subcellular dosimetry–understanding of molecular dosimetry, tracks, and impact of dense ionization on non-DNA processes
Fractionation effects–low-dose hypersensitivity, adaptive response, and bystander effect–what is impact on normal tissue and tumors
Molecular targets beyond DNA
New drug discovery
- Designer molecules synthesized using specific target and structural biology
- Combinatorial molecules can create many molecules and then one sorts out activity

Imaging–functional and molecular of tumor and normal-tissue positron emission tomography, magnetic resonance, electron paramagnetic resonance, etc. (e.g., image oxygen)
Nanotechnology–biomolecular sensors/probes (e.g., imaging biochemical processes)
Targeting radioisotopes–select isotope (α, β, or γ) by desired path length
Ultimate planning of biology plus physics will be *Nano inverse planning*
Radiation oncology more than technology; we need to convey the concept of "focused biology" to colleagues

From Coleman CN. International Conference on Translational Research and Preclinical Strategies in Radio-Oncology (ICTR): conference summary. *Int J Radiat Oncol Biol Phys* 2001;49:301–309.

Empiricism Versus Research-Based Radiation Oncology

Empiricism harkens to the views of David Hume (1711–1776) and other British philosophers of the 17th and 18th centuries and their distrust of the power of unaided reason. In the philosopher's view of empiricism, the best contact between one's understanding of knowledge and the world is not the point at which a mathematical proof crystallizes, but the point at which you see and touch a familiar object. Their paradigm was knowledge by sensory experience rather than by reason alone.[47,315,419]

Empirical radiation oncologists rely on accumulated clinical experience, also known as "what has worked in the past." They are suspicious of therapies based on theories and laboratory research and feel safest when treading the pathway of tested experience. One can find very strong signs of empiricism in the radiation oncology literature: case reports; single-institution retrospective clinical series; and a marked concern with retrospective clinical analyses of radiation therapy that mine clinical experience to aid the selection of radiation treatment volume, dose, and treatment techniques.

There can be no doubt that the development of radiation oncology has been extensively based on empiricism. As Fowler wrote: "If therapists had waited for a fully scientific basis for treating the first patient, radiotherapy would not have started yet."[158,159] We must note, however, that radiation biologists worked closely with the early radiation oncologists. It would be erroneous to suggest that the early history of radiation oncology was completely devoid of reliance on radiation biology.

The theme of hostility to empiricism and support for finding a firm basis for clinical radiation oncology in radiation and cancer biology research is also easily identified in the development of the specialty. "Some people do the same thing wrong for 30 years and then call it accumulated clinical experience," said one critic; or it has been said, "If radiation oncologists were put in charge of the war against polio, they certainly would have perfected the iron lung by now." Knowledge of the genome, proteomics, secondary messengers, solid tumor biology, angiogenesis, oxygenation, and cell-cycle control are changing the present and future of medicine. If clinical radiation oncologists have a future, these individuals say, then they must actively participate in the investigation of the molecular and cellular basis of cancer and in translational research.

Physics Versus Biology

One also may formulate the debate over the role of basic biology in clinical radiation oncology as a pull and tug between physics and biology. Medical radiation physics has dominated the thinking of clinical radiation oncologists. Among the major achievements of this discipline are the following:

- The identification and characterization of physical units of radiation dose.
- Significant changes in photon and electron radiation therapy apparatus (initially, kilovoltage and later ^{60}Co, high-energy linear accelerators, the Gamma Knife [Elekta Corp., Stockholm, Sweden], and the CyberKnife [Accuray, Sunnyvale, CA]).
- The development of 3D treatment planning for identification of tumor volume and characterization of irradiated normal tissue.
- IMRT for improved conformality of treatment beams.
- Particle therapy including neutrons, protons, pions, and stripped nuclei.
- Improved stabilization devices to aid the reproducibility of treatment.
- Advances in brachytherapy technology including new isotopes, the afterloading technique, and remote high–dose-rate machines.
- The apparatus for intraoperative radiation therapy (IORT).
- Equipment for heat deposition in tumors leading to the clinical applications of hyperthermia.

At present, a considerable effort in clinical radiation oncology is focused on the tools and techniques provided to the physician by the physicist. Radiation oncology meetings are dominated by discussions of IMRT, radiosurgery/conformal radiation, and innovations in equipment. Simply put, these techniques all offer better radiation dose distributions, which, one hopes, will lead to an increase in local control of tumors and a decrease in normal tissue toxicity. At present, a better dose distribution is the solution physics offers to the problems of oxygenation, monitoring of tumor blood flow, tumor pH, secondary messengers, tumor-suppressor genes, oncogenes, the biology of metastasis, normal tissue radioprotectors, and tumor radiosensitizers. Could it be that "if all you have is a hammer, then everything looks like a nail"?

What has cancer biology ever done for the clinical radiation oncologist? It is, we think, a generally fair question, although it might be characterized as somewhat narcissistic, along the lines of "What have you done for me lately?"[158,159,429,486] Among the areas one should consider on the list of laboratory contributions to the clinic are the following:

- As early as 1906, Bergonie and Tribondeau[42] enunciated a series of famous laws of radiosensitivity. This was followed by the work of the French investigators Regaud and Ferroux,[373] who demonstrated that whereas a single dose of radiation to the testes always produced maximal damage to the scrotal skin, fractionated exposure spared the skin but destroyed spermatogenesis. They speculated that this same technique of fractionation might be differentially advantageous in the treatment of tumors. This led to Coutard's[98–100] studies that culminated in the fractionated EBRT techniques of today.
- The identification of the relationship between radiation dose and cell kill led to the characterization of the radiation cell survival curve. This contributed to our understanding of radiation therapy dose and fractionation and, consequently, contributed to our understanding of radiation repair. This development placed our understanding of radiation fractionation on sound footing and led to investigations of alternative fractionation schemes. This has contributed to improved tumor control as well as limitation of normal tissue toxicity. Ultimately, the radiation cell survival curve also provided the underpinnings for our understanding of elements of the dose response relationship for tumor control and normal tissue toxicity.
- In 1909, Schwarz[400] demonstrated that compression of the skin to diminish capillary blood flow reduces severity of cutaneous radiation reactions. This may have been the first demonstration of the "oxygen effect."[336] L. H. Gray[185] pointed out the relevance of the "oxygen effect" to radiation oncology by identifying the fact that human neoplasms contain a significant subpopulation of hypoxic cells.[451] A series of important developments has driven home the centrality of hypoxia to our understanding of radiation's effects on tumors. Clearly, histopathologic studies and invasive measurements of intratumoral partial oxygen pressure have shown that many human tumors contain regions with low oxygen tension.[61] We now believe that there are at least two different mechanisms, called *diffusion-limited* and *perfusion-limited* hypoxia, behind this observation. Some have called these *permanent* and *transient* hypoxia.[336] Diffusion-limited hypoxia results from inadequate angiogenesis, whereas perfusion-limited hypoxia is associated with intermittent closure of tumor vessels, leading to acute hypoxic conditions for tumor cells downstream from the obstruction. In addition, we now understand how hypoxia activates genes and may produce tumor differentiation and increase a tumor's metastatic potential. Clinical studies have associated the prognostic value of hemoglobin level with tumor local control.[219,336] The characterization of the hypoxia problem has led to a variety of strategies to overcome it. One has been to have the patient breathe high–oxygen-content gas mixtures or to irradiate patients in hyperbaric oxygen chambers. Another option involves the use of oxygen-mimetic chemicals. Other treatment strategies include blood transfusions or the specific use of hypoxic-specific cytotoxins such as mitomycin-C.
- There has been considerable growth in our understanding of cell proliferation, the cell cycle, and cell repair mechanisms. We now understand that cells are more sensitive to radiation in M phase and more sensitive to hyperthermia in S phase. Our understanding of the differential sensitivity of cells to radiation during the cell cycle helps provide a rational basis for the use of radiation and chemotherapy. Furthermore, our understanding of the influence of the cell cycle on sensitivity has led to work on the halogenated pyrimidine analogs, which appear to sensitize cells to radiation's lethal effects by increasing the yield of nonrepairable double-strand breaks.[262] A large number of clinical trials have resulted. Although this line of research has not, to date, borne major clinical fruit, it has been a rationally based area of investigation that may yet prove itself.
- As an extension of the knowledge associated with the radiation cell survival curve, clinicians obviously need to have a good understanding of the radiation dose and response for both normal and malignant tissue. The development of research involving the lethal dose 50% (LD50), local control rates, and normal tissue toxicity in animal models has led to an improved understanding of the radiation dose–response relationship. Correlates of this understanding have included the use of the progressive shrinking-field technique; IORT; brachytherapy as "boost"; and the use of increasingly conformal beams associated with our improved understanding of how radiation dose should be associated with tumor volume and dose painting. One expects, in the future, to see increasing work in intentional dose heterogeneity as a technique for improving local control.

TABLE 1.6 PRINCIPLES OF RADIATION ONCOLOGY DERIVED FROM THE INITIAL WORK OF SUIT

1956	*1982*	*2013*
1. Aim for uniform dose throughout the treatment volume. Treatment volume is constant for entire treatment (i.e., no shrinking field).	1. Use shrinking-field technique (i.e., a nonuniform dose distribution related to number of tumor cells).	1. Moderate, conform, and "paint" the external-beam or brachytherapy dose distribution in accordance with the viable tumor-cell distribution.
2. Initial large treatment volume is carried to tolerance.	2. Dose to the initial volume is usually less than tolerance. Only the final treatment volume is carried to tolerance dose level.	2. Dose to the initial volume is less than tolerance and may be moderated because of the specific host and treatment factors affecting tolerance.
3. No special emphasis to push dose to higher levels for larger tumors.	3. Dose aim is planned on the basis of tumor size or estimated tumor cell number. a. Maximum doses (with higher risk of morbidity) for large tumors. b. Modest well-tolerated dose levels for subclinical disease. c. For combination of radiation and surgery use less than radical dose level.	3. Dose aim is planned on the basis of tumor size, estimated tumor cell number, extent and completeness of surgical resection, biologic and genetic predictors of tumor aggressiveness, and response to induction chemotherapy. a. Maximum doses (with higher risk of morbidity) for large and more aggressive tumors. b. Modest well-tolerated dose levels for subclinical disease. c. For combinations of radiation and surgery, chemotherapy, and/or biologic therapy one might use less than radical dose level in certain situations. d. For combinations of external-beam radiation therapy and brachytherapy or radiation therapy and hyperthermia, the dose of each modality is modified as a function of the other modalities used.
4. Little priority given to planned combinations of radiation and surgery.	4. Major emphasis on planned combinations of radiation and surgery.	4. Major emphasis on planned combinations of radiation, surgery, chemotherapy, hormonal therapy, and biologic therapy.
5. Treatment fields are square or rectangular.	5. Secondary collimation is utilized on virtually all fields to reduce irradiation of tissues not suspected of involvement by tumor.	5. Multileaf collimators and intensity modulation are used on virtually all fields in an attempt to improve conformality of the radiation and reduce irradiation of tissue not suspected of being involved with tumor. Radiation dose distribution is based on sophisticated imaging technologies.
6. Radiation alone is the general rule.	6. Multidisciplinary approach accepted as most effective for most tumor problems.	6. The radiation oncologist is expected to be trained in and make use of pathology for tumor subtyping and grading; anatomic and molecular staging; diagnostic imaging; and the therapeutic role of chemotherapy, hormonal therapy, biologic therapy, and surgical therapy.
7. Results of treatment described almost exclusively in terms of absolute survival at a fixed period (e.g., 5 years).	7. Results analyzed on basis of detailed assessment of causes of failure (e.g., local persistence or regrowth, local complication, marginal miss, regional spread, distant metastases, intercurrent disease).	7. The phase III randomized prospective trial is the gold standard for clinical decision making. Decisions based on properly planned and conducted cancer trials concerning radiation therapy dose, volume, and technique are most appropriate. It is expected that evidence-based medicine will guide clinical decision making. If such trials are not available or are inadequate, then phase II trials or retrospective reviews involving survival, local control, patterns of failure, and multivariate analysis of outcome are often useful. The future will depend on basic and translational research in cancer biology and medical physics being brought to the clinic.

In his 1983 Failla lecture, Herman Suit[429] considered the evolution of the principles of clinical radiation therapy. He prepared a table in which he attempted to articulate the principles of radiation therapy invoked in the United States in 1956 and 1982. This is reproduced in the first two columns of Table 1.6. The authors of this chapter have added a third column identifying the appropriate principles for 2013. One can see, by scanning across the table, the significant changes that have taken place in our discipline. It is clear that the future holds a role both for empiricism and for research-based radiation oncology as well as a role for improvements in physics and biology. Through cooperation and constructive dialogue, all may contribute to the future of cancer care. Box 1.3 and Table 1.7 explain logarithmic cell kill.

Coleman,[91] in a summary of the International Conference on Translational Research in Radiation Oncology, emphasized the importance of radiation oncologists remaining current with newer scientific findings that will be critical in the development of improved therapeutic strategies. Approaches that alter the content of cyclins or activation of cyclin p34 may overcome cellular resistance. By exploitation of cellular mechanisms related to apoptosis, it may be possible to kill cells with irradiation by inducing changes other than unrepaired DNA damage. With understanding of the tumor microenvironment and new techniques such as complementary DNA (cDNA) microarrays, as well as an understanding of how growth factors may alter cellular processes, innovative bioinformatics and improved combined-modality strategies may emerge. The ability to study many genes simultaneously will provide information beyond the era when biologic effects were attributed to a single gene. Better understanding of hypoxia may improve clinical outcome with antihypoxia strategies, including hypoxic cell radiosensitizers and hypoxic cytotoxic agents. Cyclins and growth factors may be useful as clinical radiation modifiers.

There is a critical need to balance the investment in technical aspects of radiation therapy with concepts and innovative approaches derived from better understanding of cancer biology. Coleman[91,92] has presented a complex model of the biologic factors influencing radiation oncology. These scientific developments will greatly alter the way in which we practice our discipline.

Box 1.3

Logarithmic Cell Kill

Among the simplest exercises a radiation oncologist-in-training can undertake is the creation of a table of logarithmic cell kill. At first, such an exercise seems trivial. The effort expended on this somewhat tedious exercise will, however, be repaid many times over.

Let us assume that we have a tumor that follows a typical cell survival curve. These tumor cells have a 50% probability of cell survival after a radiation dose of 2 Gy. If we assume, for the purpose of this exercise, that there are no changes in the probability of cell kill wrought by changes in tumor oxygenation, pH, or other factors during the course of treatment; that there is no accelerated repopulation; and that only the simplest conditions apply (i.e., that there is 50% kill for each dose), then we can create a table showing the number of cells killed and the number of cells remaining after each dose (Table 1.7).

Let us assume that we begin with a relatively small tumor (i.e., a spherical tumor a bit more than 1 cm in diameter containing, say, 10^9 cells). At each dose of 2 Gy, 50% of the cells are killed. Thus, after the first dose, 500 million cells are killed and 500 million cells remain. At each successive dose 50% of the cells are killed. Therefore, by the end of the course of radiation, very few cells are killed with each individual dose.

One can see, from going through the exercise, that even for a very small tumor the number of initial cells is very large and the marginal killing of the absolute number of cells, with the last few doses, is small. It is not surprising, therefore, that for a tumor of average radiation sensitivity, quite a high dose of radiation is required.

Obviously, the exercise would change if we were to use a different radiation dose per fraction, producing a different probability of survival, or if the intrinsic radiosensitivity of the tumor cell line were different and the probability of survival were different.

Based on Suit HD. Radiation biology: a basis for radiotherapy. In Fletcher GH, ed. *Textbook of radiotherapy.* Philadelphia: Lea & Febiger, 1966.

TABLE 1.7 VARIOUS LEVELS OF IRRADIATION WILL YIELD DIFFERENT PROBABILITIES OF TUMOR CONTROL, DEPENDING ON THE SIZE OF THE LESION

Cumulative Dose (Gy)	*Initial Cell Number*	*Probability of Survival*	*Remaining Cell Number*
2	1,000,000,000	× 0.5 =	500,000,000
4	500,000,000	× 0.5 =	250,000,000
6	250,000,000	× 0.5 =	125,000,000
8	125,000,000	× 0.5 =	62,500,000
10	67,500,000	× 0.5 =	31,250,000
12	33,750,000	× 0.5 =	15,625,000
14	15,625,000	× 0.5 =	7,812,500
16	7,823,500	× 0.5 =	3,906,250
18	3,906,250	× 0.5 =	1,953,125
20	1,953,125	× 0.5 =	976,562
22	976,562	× 0.5 =	488,281
24	488,281	× 0.5 =	244,140
26	244,140	× 0.5 =	122,070
28	122,070	× 0.5 =	61,035
30	61,035	× 0.5 =	30,517
32	30,517	× 0.5 =	15,258
34	15,258	× 0.5 =	7,629
36	7,629	× 0.5 =	3,814
38	3,814	× 0.5 =	1,907
40	1,907	× 0.5 =	953
42	953	× 0.5 =	476
44	476	× 0.5 =	238
46	238	× 0.5 =	119
48	119	× 0.5 =	59
50	59	× 0.5 =	29
52	29	× 0.5 =	15
54	15	× 0.5 =	7
56	7	× 0.5 =	4
58	4	× 0.5 =	2
60	2	× 0.5 =	1
62	1	× 0.5 =	<1

RADIOSENSITIVITY AND RADIOCURABILITY

In 1906, Bergonie and Tribondeau[42] formulated a law relating radiosensitivity to reproductive capacity of cells, based on their experiments on rat testis in which they were able to destroy the germinal cells while the interstitial tissue and Sertoli syncytium remained unimpaired. They wrote that "X-rays are more effective on cells which have a greater reproductive activity; the effectiveness is greater on those cells which have a longer dividing future ahead.... From this law, it is easy to understand that roentgen radiation destroys tumors without destroying healthy tissues." Fletcher[150] felt that this observation, which was interpreted to indicate that radiosensitivity of tumors was linked to that of the mother organ, did much harm to clinical radiation therapy, leading to the erroneous concept that undifferentiated tumors with mitotic activity were radiosensitive and that more differentiated tumors were radioresistant.

In 1914, Schwarz[399] introduced the concept of fractionation by postulating that it was inefficient to deliver the total radiation dose in one treatment because cells were in different states of radiosensitivity and because there was a better chance that multiple exposures could hit the cells in a radiosensitive phase (e.g., mitosis). Fractionation was assumed to create a favorable therapeutic ratio because the tolerance of normal tissues increased relative to that of tumors and because malignant cells had a greater reproductive capacity and were, therefore, more likely to be in a radiosensitive phase.

Based on these and other observations, the term *radiocurability* was coined. It refers to the eradication of tumor at the primary or regional site and reflects a direct effect of the irradiation; this does not necessarily equate with the patient's cure from cancer. In contrast, *radiosensitivity* is a measure of tumor–radiation response, thus describing the degree and speed of regression during and immediately after radiotherapy. However, for most malignant tumors no significant correlation exists between the responsiveness of a tumor to irradiation and its radiocurability.

The response of human tumors to irradiation is a key issue for radiation oncologists and has been addressed by many leading radiobiologists. At least four explanations have been considered that could alone or in combination account for the different radiosensitivities of tumors:[194,457]

1. *Hypoxia.* To explain the spectrum of clinical radioresponsiveness on this basis, it is likely that the less responsive tumors either have a high hypoxic fraction, have failed to reoxygenate during fractionated treatment, or both.[423] Direct oxygen electrode measurements have shown that cervical cancer, breast cancer, and squamous cell cancers are human tumors reported to have mean oxygen pressures below those of the surrounding tissue.[220,239,240,474] Despite a wide range of values, the oxygen pressure in tumors tends to decrease with increasing tumor size.[473] Although it is not possible to prove that hypoxia is unimportant in conventional radiation therapy, some doubts about its importance have been expressed based on the limited success of neutron therapy or hypoxic cell radiosensitizers.[111,127] Recent studies have shown that hypoxia can act as an important determinant of selecting for tumor cells of a more malignant phenotype that is likely to adversely affect treatment outcome.[111,239,240]
2. *Proportion of clonogenic cells.* Proliferating cells are more radiosensitive and have a greater turnover (cell loss) rate. Tumor regression during irradiation may be proportional to the total number of proliferating cells (growth fraction) or the proliferative rate, which may accelerate for certain tumor cells as a result of adaptive processes (accelerated repopulation) during fractionated irradiation.
3. *Inherent radiosensitivity of tumor cells.* Fertil and Malaise[147] and Deacon et al.[108] established a positive correlation

between the steepness of the initial slope of the oxic cell survival curve for human tumor cells and their response to radiation. The magnitude of differences between cell lines at low doses is sufficient to explain the range of curability observed clinically. Steel and Peacock[423] analyzed human tumor radiosensitivity in light of existing concepts of cell killing based on the linear-quadratic (LQ) equation. However, despite encouraging correlations in some studies, these radiobiologic parameters have not been accepted for routine clinical use.

4. *Repair of radiation damage.* Repair of sublethal damage (split-dose effect) is observed in almost all tumor cell lines.[134,135] Potentially lethal damage repair after a single dose varies considerably from one cell line to another and has been reported by Weichselbaum and Little[492] to correlate with clinical radiocurability, with less curable tumors showing the greatest degree of potentially lethal damage recovery. To date, these repair parameters have not been confirmed in larger clinical experiences to justify their use as predictors of radiotherapy outcomes (see later in this chapter).

Some investigators have reported a correlation between the clinical or pathologic response of a tumor after the completion of irradiation with ultimate probability of local tumor control.[432] For this analysis to be valid, it is necessary to compare patients with the same initial stage because, in general, more advanced lesions have a greater probability of tumor persistence at the completion of radiation therapy, and local recurrence may be more frequent. Barkley and Fletcher[27] reported 82% tumor control in 88 patients with tumors of the oropharynx that had regressed completely at the end of therapy, in contrast to 41% in 237 patients with persistent tumor at completion of therapy. Sobel et al.[418] concluded that local tumor control in head and neck carcinomas could be predicted with the greatest accuracy and consistency 1 to 3 months after completion of radiotherapy. They noted that the prediction was 80% accurate in favorable tumors (T1 and T2) but decreased to 50% to 60% in more advanced primary lesions; complete tumor clearance was a more accurate predictor of tumor control. This was confirmed for the radiotherapeutic management of N2 (>3 cm) neck disease, where complete clinical resolution of tumor within 8 weeks of completion of irradiation correlated with a >90% freedom from neck failures.[305]

Tumor Radiosensitivity and Predictive Assays

Since the inception of the use of ionizing radiation, many investigators have categorized the response of tumors according to their sensitivity to irradiation. Wetterer[498] in 1913 characterized tumor radiosensitivity based on histologic types, and Paterson[347] divided tumors into three groups: radiosensitive, intermediate, and radioresistant. The first category included germ cell tumors and reticuloses; the second included squamous cell and adenocarcinomas; and the third group included soft-tissue and bone sarcomas and melanomas. However, depending on variation in proliferative rates and cell loss, end points for response assessment may vary substantially, as has been pointed out for malignant melanoma.[395] Attempts have been made to predict the response of tumors to radiation depending on several parameters, such as the assay proposed by Glucksmann[177] consisting of differential cell counts of mitotic, resting, and degenerating cells in biopsy samples from the growing edge of the tumor before and after initiation of radiotherapy. It is generally accepted that tumors contain mixed-cell populations of stem cells with differing sensitivity to antineoplastic agents and that therapy can be selected for resistant cell populations or, in the case of certain cytotoxic agents, to induce cellular resistance.[73] Peters et al.[356,357] described a predictive assay to assess tumor response *in vitro* and the difficulties in predicting the probability of tumor control by irradiation in a given patient. Unfortunately, despite promising correlations between radiosensitivity *in vitro* and radioresponsiveness of normal tissues and tumors,[41,461] sufficiently powered predictive assays have not been identified. Given the inherent intertumor variability of predictive parameters, such as SF_2[46,283] or T_{POT},[379,380] a single predictive assay is unlikely to carry sufficient predictive power. The incorporation of multiple radiobiologic tumor–cell parameters (e.g., markers for radiosensitivity and proliferation potential) into TCP (see later in this chapter) models appears more promising but awaits broader validation in clinical trials.[66]

Probability of Tumor Control

For many histologic types of cancer, higher radiation doses produce better tumor control. Numerous dose–response curves for a variety of tumors have been published. The first dose–response data were reported for skin cancer by Miescher[303] in 1934; 10 years later Strandqvist[428] published a dose–response curve for skin cancer. The Strandqvist plots were refined by von Essen,[479] who demonstrated from a large skin carcinoma experience that the slopes for 97% tumor control and 3% skin necrosis differed and permitted, through appropriate fractionation schedules also considering the volume of disease, a dissociation of the two end points. As Fletcher[151] pointed out, meaningful dose–response curves can be generated only when a group of homogeneous tumors is given a range of radiation doses, indicating that tumor control is a probabilistic event. For every increment of radiation dose, a certain fraction of cells will be killed; therefore, the total number of surviving clonogenic cells will be proportional to the initial number present and the fraction killed with each dose.[134,135] Thus, various levels of irradiation will yield different probabilities of tumor control, depending on the extent of the lesion (number of clonogenic cells present). For subclinical disease in squamous cell carcinoma of the upper respiratory tract or for adenocarcinoma of the breast, doses of 45 to 50 Gy will result in disease control in more than 90% of patients.[151,301] Subclinical disease has been referred to as deposits of tumor cells that are too small to be detected clinically and even microscopically but, if left untreated, subsequently may evolve to clinically apparent tumor.[344] It must be emphasized that microscopic evidence of tumor, such as at the surgical margin, should not be regarded as subclinical disease; cell aggregates $\geq 10^6/cm^3$ are required for the pathologist to detect them. Therefore, these volumes must receive higher doses of irradiation, in the range of 60 to 65 Gy, in 6 to 7 weeks for epithelial tumors. This distinction of disease extent is re-emphasized by clinical results, demonstrating the need for irradiating patients with likely subclinical carcinoma to postoperative doses near 60 Gy.[506]

For clinically palpable head and neck tumors, doses of 65 (for T1) to 75 to 80 Gy or higher (for T4 tumors) are required at 2 Gy/day using five fractions weekly. This dose range and probability of tumor control have been documented for squamous cell carcinoma and adenocarcinoma.[150,151–152,301,405–407] Even with preoperative irradiation, the dose effect on probability of tumor control can be documented.

Baclesse[24,25] introduced the concept of different doses of irradiation for various portions of the tumor. The higher dose administered through small portals to residual disease is called a *boost,* which is delivered in an effort to achieve the same probability of tumor control as for subclinical aggregates.[151] One consequence of the concepts discussed earlier is use of portals that are progressively reduced in size. This *shrinking field* technique administers higher radiation doses to the entire gross tumor where more clonogenic cells (including hypoxic cells) reside, relative to lower doses to tissues in the immediate proximity of the clinically apparent (gross) tumor. The tissues making up the "tumor margin" contain a lower number of tumor clonogens that are better oxygenated (see Fig. 1.3).

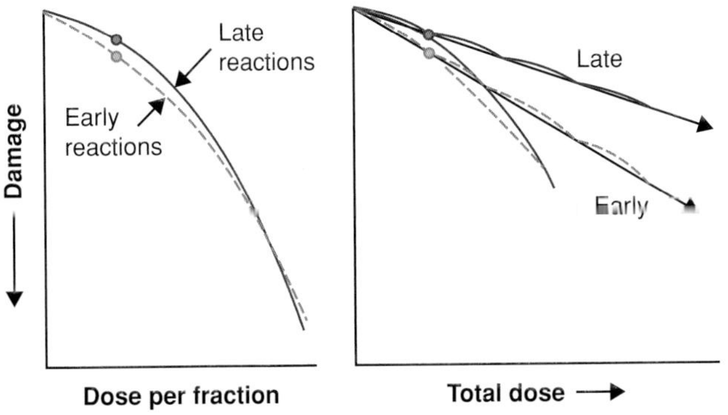

FIGURE 1.9. Difference in cell survival curves for acute and late radiation effects with single or multifractionated doses of irradiation. (From Fowler JF. Fractionation and therapeutic gain. In: Steel GG, Adams GE, Peckham MT, eds. *Biological basis of radiotherapy.* Amsterdam: Elsevier Science, 1983:181–194, with permission.)

Normal Tissue Effects

A variety of normal tissue changes are induced by ionizing radiation, depending on the total dose, fractionation schedule (daily dose and overall treatment time), and volume treated. These factors are closely interrelated (Fig. 1.9).

It has been postulated that for many normal tissues the radiation dose necessary to produce a particular sequela increases as the irradiated fraction of volume of the organ decreases. This concept was demonstrated for skin by Paterson,[345] who plotted doses delivered with orthovoltage x-rays that would produce moist desquamation (Fig. 1.10). The same phenomenon later was reported for supervoltage irradiation of other organs[421] and for brachytherapy.

Several authors have observed higher tolerance doses (TDs) than initially reported for a variety of organs,[305,315,333,382,406,407] which stresses the importance of updating this information in light of more precise treatment planning and delivery of irradiation and more accurate evaluation and recording of sequelae. Excellent examples are radiation dose escalation studies, using conformal radiotherapy delivery techniques, for prostate[204] and lung carcinomas (Radiation Therapy Oncology Group [RTOG] trial 93–11). A compilation from the literature of data on tolerance doses for whole or partial organ irradiation was published by Emami et al.[141] The comprehensive update of this compilation, QUANTEC, is described in Chapter 13.

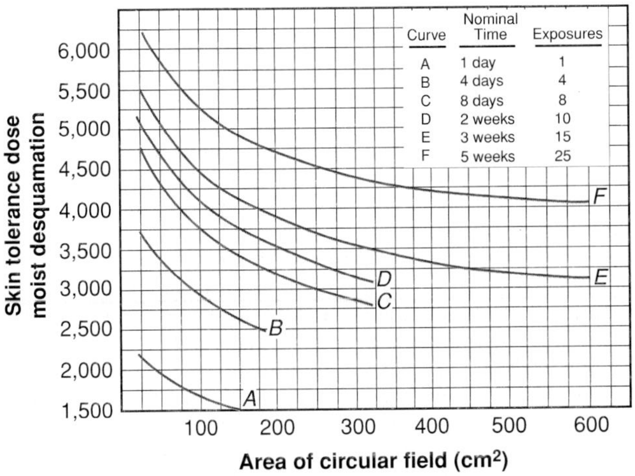

FIGURE 1.10. Graph showing the relationship between dose and size of area irradiated (healthy skin in an "average" site) to produce moist desquamation for various overall treatment times (daily irradiation at about 50 R/min for each exposure with radiation of half-value layer 1.5 mm Cu). (From Paterson R. *The treatment of malignant disease by radium and x-rays.* Baltimore: Williams & Wilkins, 1949:39, with permission.)

In studying late radiation effects, an organ can be considered to be made up of multiple functional subunits (FSUs) that are arranged serially or in parallel.[398,508] For serially structured organs, such as gastrointestinal tract or nervous tissue, damage to one portion of the organ may render the entire organ dysfunctional. In contrast, in organs with parallel structure, FSU damage may not impair the entire organ function because the remaining FSUs operate independently from the damaged group, and clinical injury occurs only when a critical volume of the organ (or proportion of FSUs) is damaged and the surviving FSUs are unable to maintain organ function. Therefore, the sensitivity of an organ depends on the number of FSUs. Marks[287] discussed the importance of organ structure in determining late radiation effects and pointed out that conventional dose–volume histograms (DVHs) and normal tissue complication probability (NTCP) models are frequently inadequate because they ignore functional and structural heterogeneities. Such considerations will be particularly important for partial irradiation of lung, liver, and kidney to doses that approach the tolerance of the organs' functional units. Yorke et al.[526] developed a biologically based model for NTCP as a function of dose and irradiation volume fractions for kidney and lung in which the organ was assumed to be composed of FSUs arranged in a parallel architecture. Jackson et al.[232] presented a thorough discussion of the subject, including its mathematical basis, and addressed the problem of calculating NTCP for inhomogeneously irradiated organs with parallel architecture. They showed that variations in FSUs and functional reserve in a patient population may produce NTCP dose–response curves, the widths of which are comparable with those observed clinically.

Structural alterations without anatomic or functional impairment may be noted, whereas in other instances substantial injuries with tissue destruction, severe dysfunction, or even death may occur.[143] Normal tissues have a substantial capacity to recover from sublethal or potentially lethal damage induced by radiation (at tolerable dose levels). Injury to normal tissues may be caused by the radiation effect on the microvasculature or the support tissues (stromal or parenchymal cells).[457]

Rubin et al.[387,388] indicated the usefulness of assigning a certain percentage of risk of complication, depending on the dose of the radiation. The minimal tolerance dose is defined as $TD_{5/5}$, which represents the dose of radiation that could cause no more than a 5% severe complication rate within 5 years after treatment. (Some authors use the equivalent terms "tissue tolerance dose," or $TTD_{5/5}$. Both the $TD_{5/5}$ and the $TTD_{5/5}$ are based on treatment at 2 Gy per fraction, five fractions per week.) An acceptable complication rate for severe injury is 5% in most curative clinical situations. Moderate sequelae are noted in varying proportions (10% to 25% of patients), depending on the dose of irradiation given and the organs at risk.

Chronologically, the effects of irradiation are subdivided into acute (first 3 months) and late effects (more than 3 months after irradiation), according to the National Cancer Institute Common Toxicity Criteria. The gross manifestations depend on the kinetic properties of the cells (slow or rapid renewal) and the total radiation dose given.

Early applications of time–dose considerations were applied by Baclesse[24,25] based on observations by Coutard[98–100] that various degrees of mucositis and moist desquamation were repaired by re-epithelialization of the mucosa and skin from the periphery of the irradiated field and from cells surviving in the center of the field. Protracted fractionation schedules for carcinoma of the breast with lower daily doses over 10 to 12 weeks were successful in avoiding acute moist desquamation,[24] but the higher radiation doses caused severe tissue damage in a large number of patients.[70]

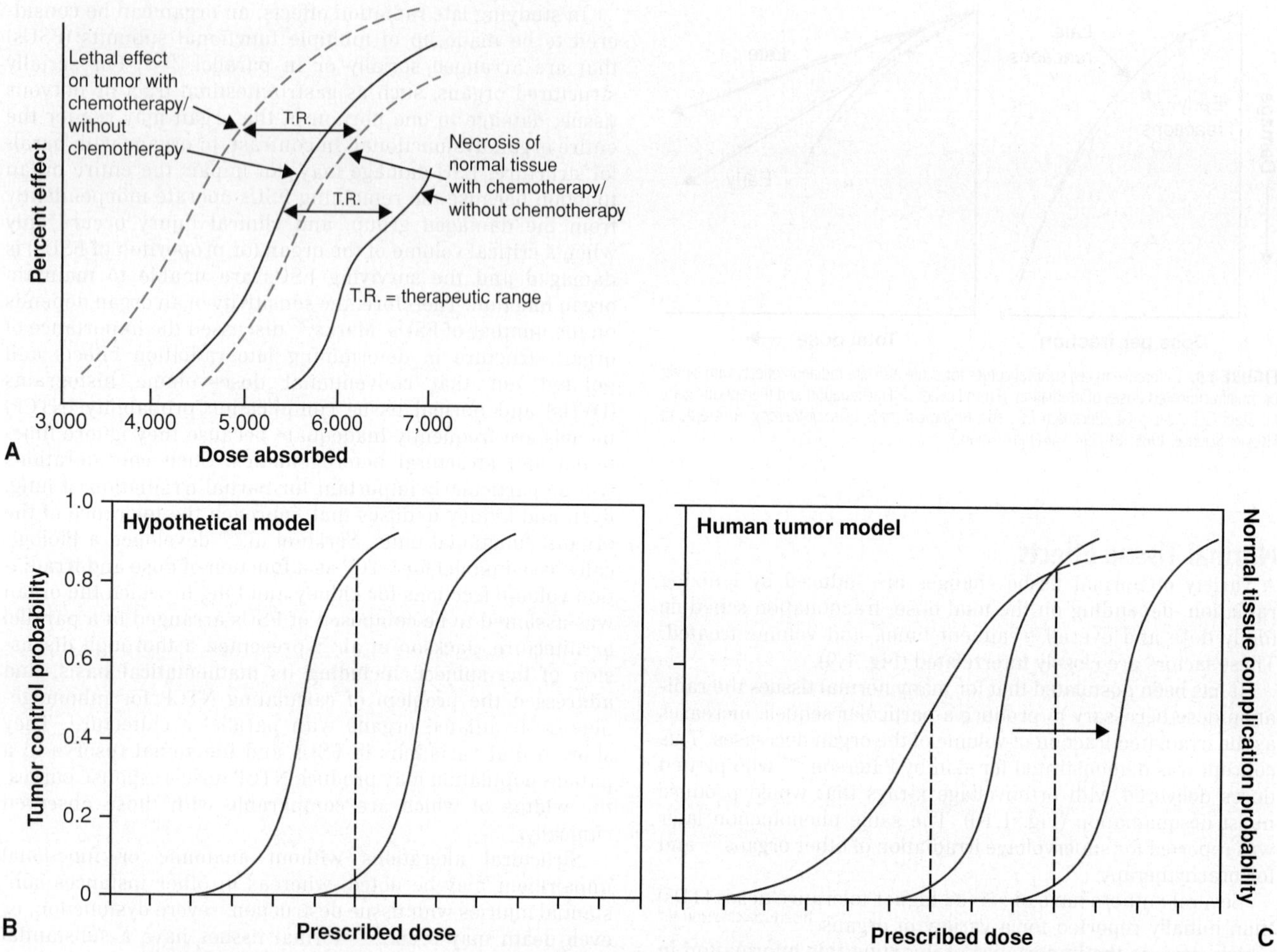

FIGURE 1.11. A: Theoretical curves for tumor control and complications as a function of radiation dose with and without chemotherapy. *TR* is the therapeutic ratio, or the difference between tumor control and complication frequency. (From Perez CA, Thomas PRM. Radiation therapy: basic concepts and clinical implications. In: Sutow WW, Fernbach DJ, Vietti TJ, eds. *Clinical pediatric oncology,* 3rd ed. St. Louis, MO: CV Mosby, 1984:167–209.) **B:** Hypothetical dose–response curves for tumor control and for normal tissue injury. Because the tumor control and the normal tissue complication curves are approximately parallel in shape and are sufficiently separated, the dose levels necessary to cure a high percentage of patients can be administered without producing excessive normal tissue damage (indicated by the *vertical dotted line*). **C:** Human tumor model. The slope of the tumor-control curve is less steep than the normal tissue–complication curve; thus, for an acceptable level of normal tissue injury, the probability of tumor control is decreased compared to the hypothetical model. Because of the volume effect, reducing the volume of normal tissues shifts the curve to the higher dose region, thereby effectively increasing the separation of the dose–response curves. Consequently, a higher dose can be given to the tumor, improving the probability of tumor control without increasing the probability of normal tissue injury. (From Leibel SA, Fuks Z, Zelefsky MJ, et al. Intensity-modulated radiotherapy. *Cancer J* 2002;8[2]:60–166, with permission.)

No correlation has been established between the incidence and severity of acute reactions and the occurrence of late effects. In 286 patients irradiated for head and neck carcinomas, Geara et al.[173] observed no significant difference in local tumor failure rates in patients with maximum grade 1 or 2 versus grade 3 or 4 acute mucositis (28% and 18%, respectively) ($p = .17$). Also, no correlation was found between severity of late reactions and local tumor control. Withers et al.[511] compiled data depicting isoeffect lines for acute or late effects in several organs. The slopes for late reactions were steeper than for acute effects, and there was a lack of correlation between the doses producing similar severities of acute or late effects.[445,446] This may result from the difference in the slopes of cell survival curves for acute or late-reacting tissues[158] (Fig. 1.11).

Combining irradiation with surgery or cytotoxic agents frequently modifies the tolerance of normal tissues to a given dose of irradiation, which may necessitate adjustments in treatment planning and dose prescription. The lack of correlation between acute and late-reacting tissues represents one rationale for combining radiotherapy with chemotherapy. As long as the enhanced acute toxicities of combined treatment can be managed, no significant increased damage in late-reacting tissues is expected.[446]

QUANTITATION OF TREATMENT TOXICITY

There is a critical need to accurately assess and record morbidity of treatment because this, in addition to therapeutic efficacy, is a crucial parameter in the evaluation of new regimens and in the selection of therapy for an individual patient. Multiple schemata have been developed, although a complete consensus has not been reached as to ideal grading scores. Toxicity grading systems for various organs were developed by RTOG and the European Organisation for Research and Treatment of Cancer (EORTC). Overgaard and Bartelink[337] stressed the importance of proper recording of morbidity in clinical radiation oncology, with quantification of the normal tissue effects and description of the treatment-related factors correlating with morbidity.

The evolution of radiation treatment planning and delivery, with innovative techniques (3DCRT, IMRT, image-guided radiation therapy, image-guided brachytherapy) allowing for better definition of target and sensitive structure volumes and more precise quantitation of dose, has introduced more complexity into the evaluation of radiation effects on organs at risk. Recently a supplement of the *International Journal of Radiation Oncology, Biology, and Physics* (Vol. 70 [Supplement 3], 2010) was dedicated to a series of articles on the "Quantitative

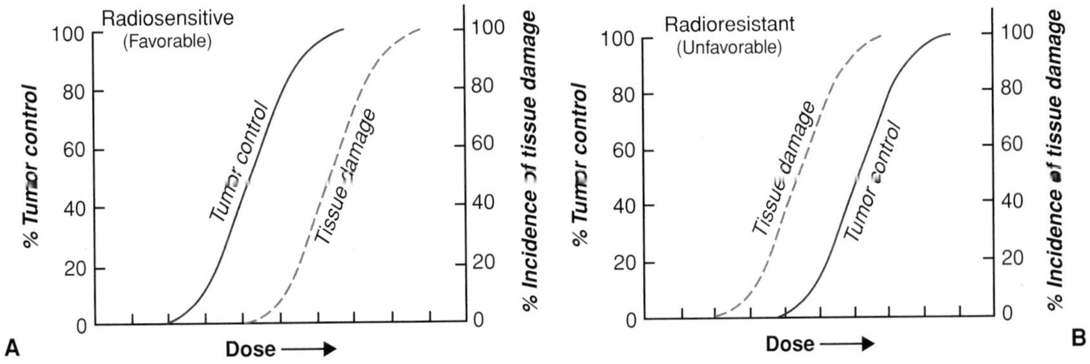

FIGURE 1.12. Different therapeutic ratios exist in different clinical circumstances depending on the radiosensitivity (dose–response curves) for the tumor versus critical normal tissue in the treatment field. **A:** Favorable. **B:** Unfavorable. (From Rubin P. *Clinical oncology: a multidisciplinary approach for physicians and students,* 7th ed. Philadelphia: W.B. Saunders, 1993, with permission.)

Analysis of Normal Tissue Effects in the Clinic (QUANTEC)," which provided an updated review of knowledge in this area and practical guidance on toxicity risks, and attempted to identify future research to elucidate radiation effects in normal tissues and organs. (See Chapter 13.)

Therapeutic Ratio (Gain)

The improved definitions of TCP and NTCP[332] imply that there is an optimal radiation dose that produces a maximum tumor control with a minimum (reasonably acceptable) frequency of complications, also called treatment sequelae. The farther the TCP and NTCP curves diverge, the more favorable is the therapeutic ratio (Fig. 1.12). The therapeutic ratio or therapeutic gain factor (TGF) of a given regimen could be expressed as a ratio:

$$\text{TGF} = \frac{\%\text{ tumor control with therapy A versus therapy B}}{\%\text{ complications with therapy A versus therapy B}}$$

The higher the TGF, the more efficient a particular therapy. Such a quantitative expression could be used to compare different therapeutic strategies. Mendelsohn[300] expressed this concept in terms of "uncomplicated tumor ablation" (Fig. 1.13). The selection of a dose must weigh the probability of major complications for any potential enhancement of tumor control. Models for decision making, using Bayesian theory, incorporate values assigned to positive or negative outcomes.[300] Positive outcome is considered tumor cure without complication, whereas negative outcomes include tumor cure with significant complications or tumor recurrence with or without complications.

Impact of Local Tumor Control on Survival

Over the past two decades, systemic chemotherapy was emphasized as a therapy that could improve survival of cancer through control of systemic metastatic disease. The effect of locoregional tumor control on patient survival has been emphasized repeatedly.[212,488] Clinical experiences and randomized trials[394] demonstrate for cancers with high metastatic potential, such as breast, prostate, and lung, that improved locoregional control by radiotherapy with or without chemotherapy enhances overall survival. This has revived the interest in locoregional radiotherapy as a survival-prolonging treatment modality, also confirming earlier clinical experiences in patients with carcinoma of the lung, prostate, and uterine cervix.

Because of the emphasis on control of systemic disease, assessment of the importance of locoregional tumor control in patients with malignant tumors has been relatively underemphasized. In a large proportion of patients with cancer seen in the United States, locoregional recurrence is just as prevalent (69% of patients dying with locoregional disease)

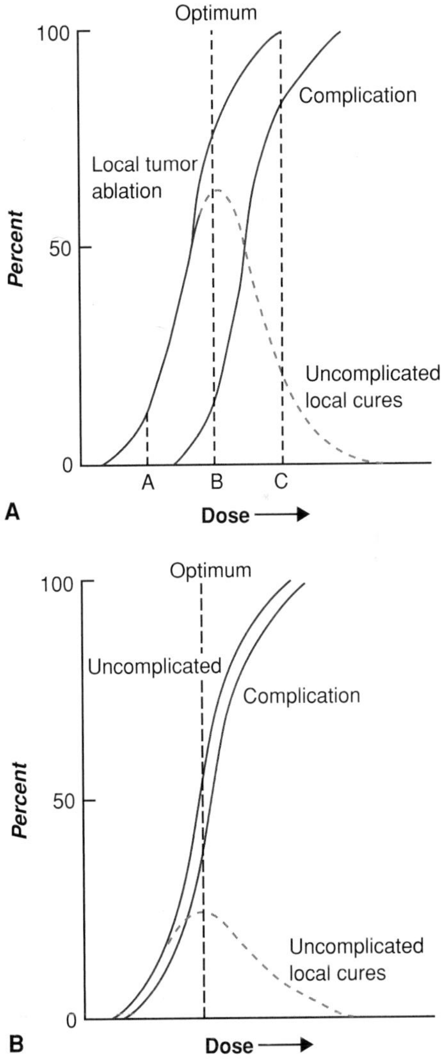

FIGURE 1.13. Treatment outcomes. Uncomplicated curves (*dashed line*) are the desired results of treatment. This is illustrated as a function of the therapeutic ratio; that is, the greater the separation of the tumor-control curve and the normal tissue–complication curve, the greater the number of uncomplicated cures that will result. The letters *A, B,* and *C* represent three different dose levels, which, if chosen, would lead to three different outcomes: *A* would result in few tumor cures but no complications; *C* would lead to complete cure in many cases, but virtually all patients would suffer complications. The optimal choice in this group of dose levels is *B,* which would result in the greatest number of cured patients without complications. (From Mendelsohn ML. The biology of dose-limiting tissues. In: *Time and dose relationships in radiation biology as applied to radiotherapy. Brookhaven National Laboratory (BNL) Report 5023 (C-57).* Upton, NY: Brookhaven National Laboratory, 1969:154–173.)

as distant metastases. A large proportion of patients (50%) have both locoregional recurrence and distant metastases (see Table 1.6).

Clinical data have matured over the past decade, demonstrating that tumor persistence after initial therapy does, because of tumor progression, carry as poor a prognosis as treatment of a more advanced cancer. In addition, radiotherapy has been shown for tumor with high metastatic potential, such as breast, prostate, and lung, to prolong overall survival if higher radiation doses are delivered and achieve improved local control rates.[92,204,395]

DOSE–TIME FACTORS

Dose–time considerations constitute complex relationships that express the interdependence of total dose, time, and number of fractions in the production of a biologic effect within a given tissue volume. This phenomenon, from a radiobiologic viewpoint, is closely related to the four Rs of ionizing radiation:

1. *Repair* of sublethal and potentially lethal damage;
2. *Repopulation* of cells between fractions;
3. *Redistribution* of cells throughout the cell cycle (partially the result of radiation-induced synchrony secondary to transient arrest at cell-cycle checkpoints and cell-cycle–dependent cell killing); and
4. *Reoxygenation* occurring during repeated radiation exposures.

The advantages of dose fractionation include:

1. Reduction in the number of hypoxic cells occurs through cell killing and reoxygenation. There is increased oxygenation in the tumor after irradiation, whereas changes in normal tissue oxygen are slight or nonexistent.[79]
2. Reduction in the absolute number of clonogenic tumor cells by the preceding fractions with the killing of the better-oxygenated cells. Assuming a constant supply of oxygen, fewer cancer cells will have access to an increased amount of oxygen.
3. Blood vessels compressed by a growing cancer are decompressed secondary to tumor regression, thus permitting better oxygenation despite the constant diffusion distance of oxygen in tissue near 200 μm.
4. Fractionation exploits the difference in recovery rate between normal, acute, and late-reacting tissues and tumors. Radiation-induced redistribution of cells within the cell cycle tends to sensitize rapidly proliferating cells as they move into the more sensitive phases of the cell cycle.
5. The acute normal tissue toxicity of single radiation doses can be decreased with fractionation. Thus, patients' tolerance of radiotherapy will improve with fractionated irradiation.

In general, fractionated irradiation will spare acute reactions because of compensatory proliferation in the epithelium of the skin or the mucosa, acceleration of which can be measured experimentally 2 or 3 weeks after initiation of therapy, but most likely starts with initiation of irradiation.[41,110,161,396] However, a prolonged course of therapy with small daily fractions will decrease early acute reactions but not necessarily protect from serious late damage to normal tissues. This approach also promotes accelerated repopulation and permits the growth of rapidly proliferating tumors. A major research effort in clinical radiobiology is and will be devoted to the optimization of dose–time-fractionation schedules for various tumors that are individualized depending on cell kinetic characteristics, molecular biology, and clinical observations.[66,101,459] Fowler[159] published theoretic considerations based on a series of assumptions of the values used in the LQ equation with a time factor in which he attempted to predict the optimal dose-fractionation schedules for tumors with various cell-doubling times. He concluded that optimal overall times depend primarily on the doubling time of the tumor cells and intrinsic radiosensitivity, alpha (assumed to be proportional to α/β). Short overall treatment times are required for tumors with a low α/β ratio or fast proliferation. For median potential doubling times of 5 days and intermediate radiosensitivity, overall times of 2.5 to 4 weeks would be optimal. More slowly proliferating tumors should be treated with longer overall times (Fig. 1.14). *In vitro* techniques to assess tumor radiosensitivity in biopsy specimens ultimately may be helpful as predictive assays.

Altered Fractionation

Without a solid biologic basis and out of empiricism and convenience, the "standard fractionation" for radiation therapy has evolved into five fractions weekly. Other fractionation schedules have been proposed that deliver multiple fractions daily or six fractions weekly or use a hyperfractionation split-course regimen (Fig. 1.15). The characteristics for hyperfractionation, accelerated fractionation, or split-course schedules as well as potential advantages or disadvantages are summarized in

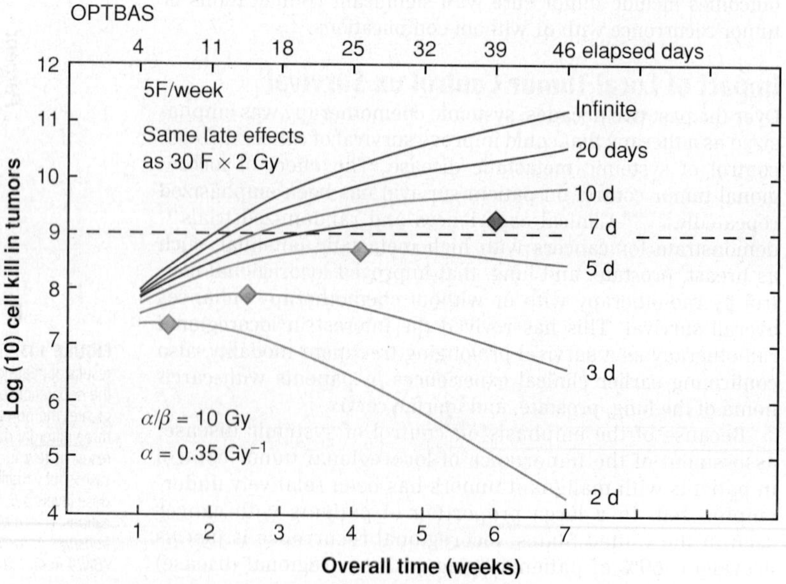

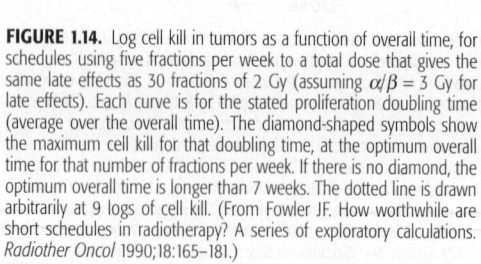

FIGURE 1.14. Log cell kill in tumors as a function of overall time, for schedules using five fractions per week to a total dose that gives the same late effects as 30 fractions of 2 Gy (assuming $\alpha/\beta = 3$ Gy for late effects). Each curve is for the stated proliferation doubling time (average over the overall time). The diamond-shaped symbols show the maximum cell kill for that doubling time, at the optimum overall time for that number of fractions per week. If there is no diamond, the optimum overall time is longer than 7 weeks. The dotted line is drawn arbitrarily at 9 logs of cell kill. (From Fowler JF. How worthwhile are short schedules in radiotherapy? A series of exploratory calculations. *Radiother Oncol* 1990;18:165–181.)

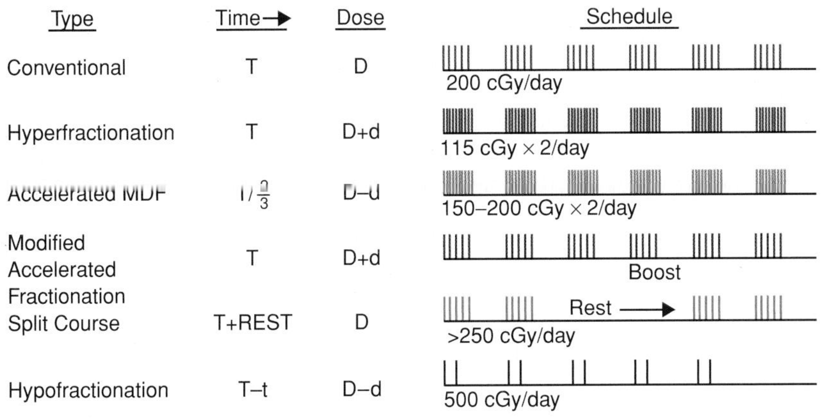

FIGURE 1.15. Various types of fractionation used in radiation therapy.

Table 1.8. Based on the narrow window between improvements in tumor control and enhanced normal tissue toxicities,[355] any altered fractionation schedule is potentially harmful and must be approached with great caution. However, the improved quality of clinical trials by national study groups and by individual institutions has generated a growing body of clinical outcome data that, together with improved biologic modeling, allows relatively accurate predictions of clinical outcomes based on relative biological effectiveness (RBE) calculations.[308]

Multiple daily fractions are likely to be more effective in rapidly growing tumors with a high growth fraction. Normal tissues behave as actively proliferating cells for expression of acute reactions but as slowly proliferating cells in the manifestation of late injury.[509] As suggested by several biologic studies,[163] clinical trial results conducted by EORTC and RTOG demonstrated that a minimum of 6 hours interfraction interval should be allowed when multiple daily fractions are used to allow maximum repair of normal tissues. This is supported by reduced complication rates in patients irradiated for carcinoma of the lung and a highly uniform cohort of patients with tonsillar squamous cell carcinomas.[160,506]

Accelerated fractionation aims at shortening the overall treatment time. Schedules may use larger than standard size fractions five times weekly or more than five fractions per week of 2 Gy. In addition, multiple fractions of radiation may be given daily exclusively or in combination with standard fractions of 2 Gy. Some reduction in the total dose delivered may have to be used for fractions >2 Gy for normal tissue sparing. These schedules may be preferable with hypoxic cell sensitizers or other chemical modifiers of radiation response that require the presence of a high concentration of the compound in the tumor at the time of the radiation exposure.

With hyperfractionation, a larger number of smaller-than-conventional dose fractions are given daily; the total daily dose is usually 10% to 20% greater than with standard fractionation; the total period of time is minimally changed; and the total dose needs to be escalated to achieve tumor toxicity similar to that of standard fractionation. The aim of hyperfractionation is to achieve the same incidence of late effects on normal tissue as observed with a comparable conventional regimen while increasing the probability of tumor control through dose escalation.[507]

Accelerated Repopulation

Withers and Taylor[508] described experimental observations documenting accelerated repopulation of tumor cells during fractionated radiotherapy and provided convincing evidence that this phenomenon occurs in clinical situations (Figs. 1.16–1.18). Although Withers and Taylor's analyses suggested that accelerated repopulation occurs preferentially after the 4th week of radiotherapy, reanalysis of the same data by Bentzen[40] and Thames et al.[445] and independent derivations by Fowler[161] suggested that repopulation starts early during fractionated irradiation. The latter is supported by experimental data of Schmidt-Ullrich et al.,[396] showing that molecular processes of accelerated repopulation, mediated through radiation-induced receptor activation and cellular growth stimulation, occur after a single radiation exposure of 2 Gy. The effectiveness of a course of fractionated irradiation depends in part on the killing by individual fractions as well as on the rate of proliferation of surviving cells between irradiation fractions. Neoadjuvant chemotherapy also may lead to increased proliferation of surviving tumor cells after partial regression of the lesion, which could result in decreased cell killing by subsequent fractionated irradiation.

Isoeffect Graphs

To express an equal biologic effect produced by various fractionation schedules, isoeffect lines have been generated. Kronig and Friedrich[254] first published the observation that a specific physical dose of irradiation is less biologically effective if given in multiple fractions, which embodies the original concept of recovery between fractions. Later, MacComb and

TABLE 1.8 COMPARISON OF VARIOUS FRACTIONATION SCHEDULES

	Conventional	Split-Course	Accelerated Fractionation	Hyperfractionation
Indication, in tumors, of growth rate	Average	Average or slow	Rapid	Slow (with large cell-loss factors)
Normal tissue effects, acute	Standard	Standard or greater	Greater	Standard or greater
Normal tissue effects, late	Standard	Greater	Standard (if complete repair of sublethal damage occurs) or greater	Lower
Advantages	–	Shorter actual treatment time (fewer fractions)	Destroys more tumor cells; prevents tumor cell repopulation; less overall treatment time	Lower OER with small doses; spares late damage; allows reoxygenation; allows stem cell repopulation
Disadvantages	–	May permit tumor repopulation	–	More fractions

OER, oxygen enhancement ratio.

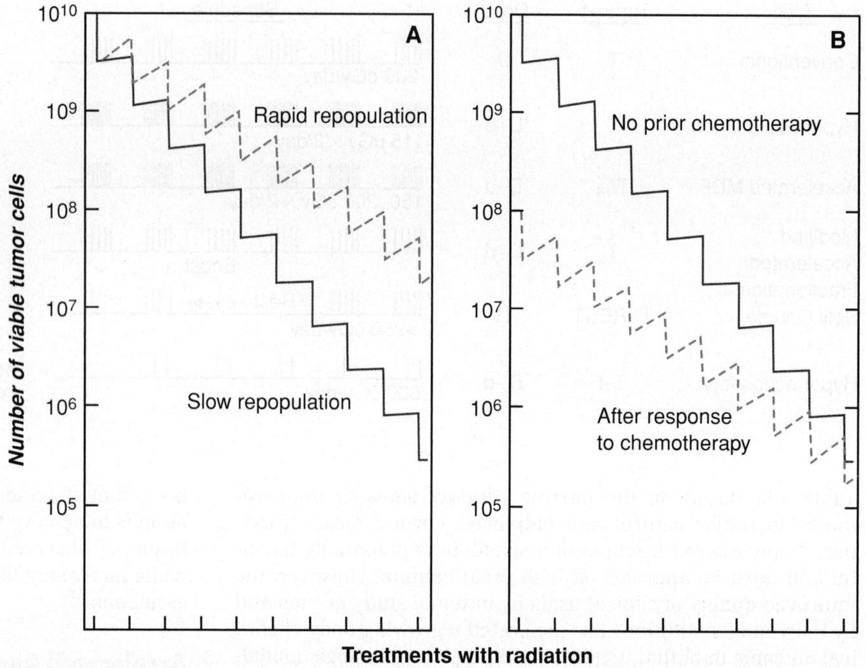

FIGURE 1.16. A: Schematic diagram indicating that cell survival during a course of fractionated irradiation depends not only on the proportion of cells killed with each dose (equal for the two curves shown) but also on the rate of proliferation of surviving cells between dose fractions, which differs for the two curves. **B:** Hypothetical diagram to illustrate the number of surviving cells in a tumor during treatment with irradiation alone (*solid line*) or during radiation therapy delivered to a tumor that has responded to chemotherapy (i.e., cell number reduced to 1% at start of irradiation) but where proliferation has been stimulated (*dashed line*). Note that cell survival is similar after fractionated irradiation, despite the initial response to drugs. (From Tannock IF. Combined modality treatment with radiotherapy and chemotherapy. *Radiother Oncol* 1989;16:83–101.)

Quimby[281] and Reisner[374] established the rate of recovery in experimentally produced skin reactions in patients.

In 1944, Strandqvist[428] published a monograph describing the results of treatment of 280 patients with skin cancer (squamous cell and basal cell carcinoma); most tumors were treated within 14 and 29 days, and only one was treated within 45 days. An isoeffect line was drawn, with a slope of 0.22. He fitted the recovery factors of MacComb and Quimby and Reisner using an extrapolated value of 0.35 per day as the time for a single dose. He also produced a graph for various degrees of radiation reaction on the skin, ranging from erythema to necrosis (Fig. 1.19). It should be emphasized that in these curves, the vertical coordinate represents the total dose given, and the abscissa represents the total duration in days after the first irradiation. However, some authors have plotted similar graphs representing the number of fractions in the horizontal coordinate. It is critical to identify these two parameters because one could deliver 60 Gy in 6 weeks in 30 fractions given five times weekly or the same dose delivered in 18 fractions given three times weekly. The effects on normal tissues certainly would be different. Von Essen,[479] using the Strandqvist data as well as his own, pointed out the importance of the volume irradiated when isoeffect parameters are studied and generated a 3D display of these data.

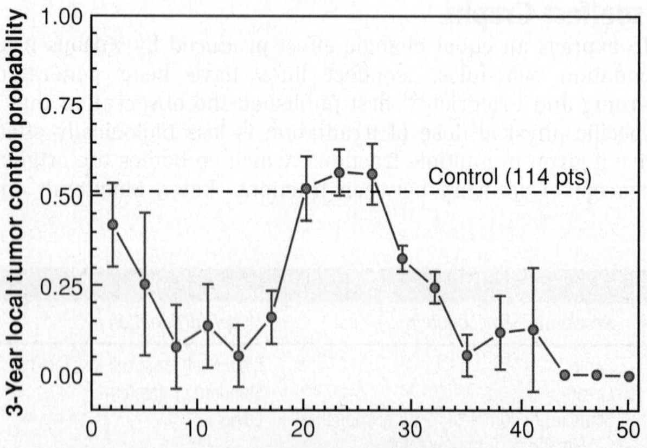

FIGURE 1.17. Dependence of tumor control probability (TCP) on the position of a single treatment gap in 533 patients. Gap duration ranged from 3 to 20 days. Position of a gap is defined by its starting point. Each point shows the TCP averaged over 3 consecutive days (± SD). (From Skladowski K, Law MG, Maciejewski B, et al. Planned and unplanned gaps in radiotherapy: The importance of gap position and gap duration. *Radiother Oncol* 1994;30:109–120.)

Dutreix et al.[130] published observations on the influence of fraction size in patients with cancer of the lung, on whom one of the supraclavicular areas received a single exposure and the other area received two exposures separated by 6 hours. They noticed that two fractions of 1 Gy produced the same skin reaction as one fraction of 2 Gy. As the fraction size increased, however, it took a higher dose in the two-fraction schedule to produce the same reaction as with the single-fraction schedule. With mucositis of the faucial arch used as an end point, researchers at M.D. Anderson Cancer Center observed that 10 Gy per week given in five fractions of 2 Gy is equivalent to 11 Gy given in 10 fractions, twice a day, separated by 3 hours.[150]

The slopes for reactions for various normal tissues differ, as do slopes of tumor curability and normal tissue late effects. In general, the slope for tumor curability is less steep than that for normal tissue reactions. Isoeffect lines for various squamous cell carcinomas of the head and neck, different stages, have slopes varying from 0.33 to 0.38.[152,421] Furthermore, as stated earlier, tolerance of normal tissues is strongly related to the volume irradiated. Whereas 60 Gy could be given safely in 5 weeks for a small glottic tumor with a 5-cm by 4-cm portal, the same dose delivered in the same period for a supraglottic carcinoma, with a larger portal covering the entire larynx, would result in more severe acute and late sequelae[152] (Box 1.4).

Linear-Quadratic Equation (α/β Ratio)

Formulations based on dose survival models have been proposed to evaluate the biologic equivalence of various doses and fractionation schedules. These assumptions are based on an LQ survival curve represented by the equation:

$$\text{Log}_e\, S = \alpha D + \beta D^2,$$

in which α represents the *linear* (i.e., first-order dose-dependent) component of cell killing, and β represents the *quadratic* (i.e.,

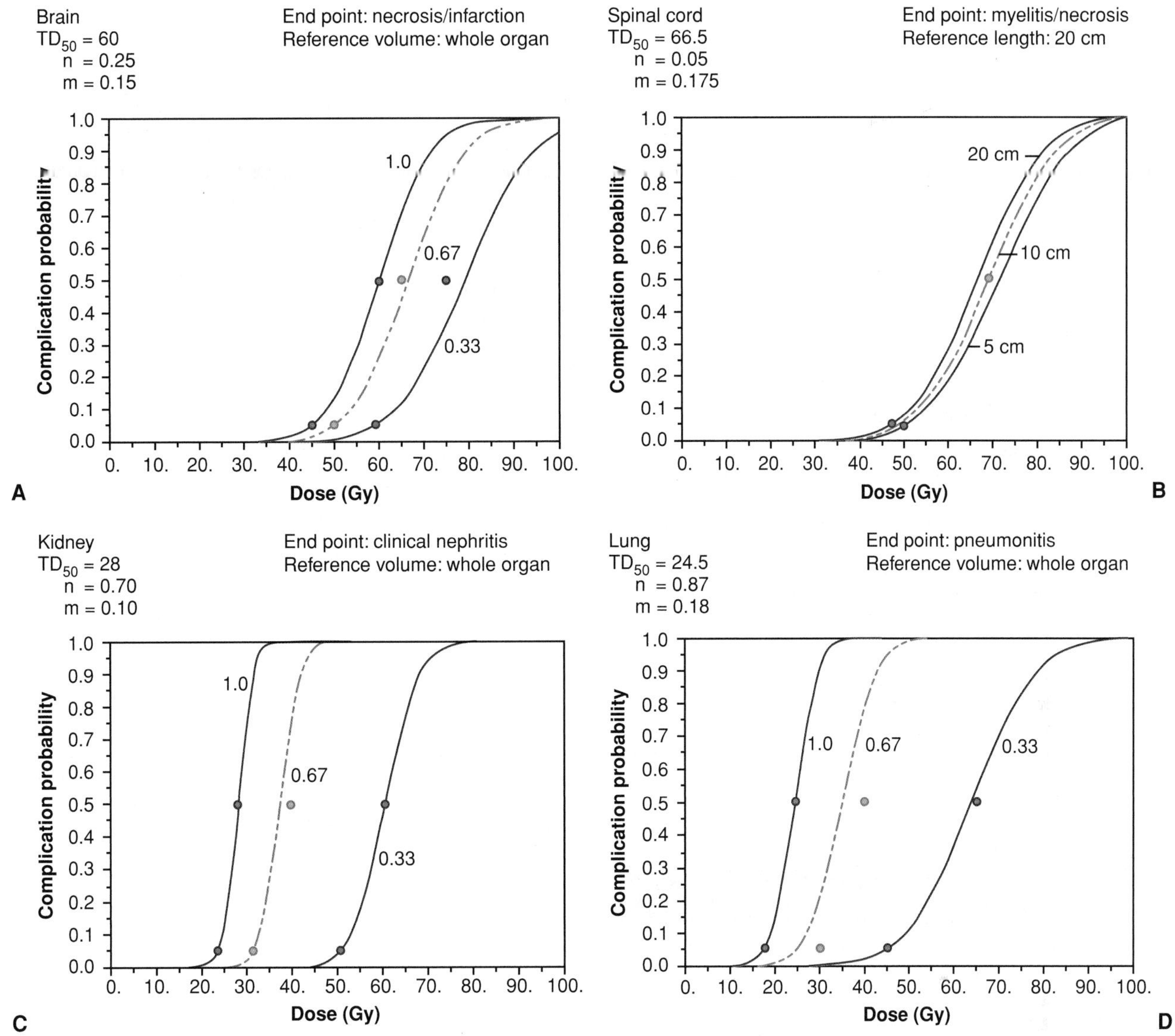

FIGURE 1.18. Complication probability correlated with irradiation dose for **(A)** brain, **(B)** spinal cord, **(C)** kidney, and **(D)** lung. (From Burman C, Kutcher GJ, Emami B, et al. Fitting of normal tissue tolerance data to an analytic function. *Int J Radiat Oncol Biol Phys* 1991;21:123–135.)

second-order dose-dependent) component of cell killing. Thus, β represents the more reparable (over a few hours) component of cell damage (Figs. 1.20–1.22). The dose at which the two components of cell killing are equal constitutes the α/β ratio.

In a study of 17 human tumor cell lines, Steel and Peacock[423] observed that the average surviving fraction at 2 Gy is 0.44 from the α component and 0.88 from the β component. The β effect at that dose level appears to be similar in radiosensitive and radioresistant tumors; thus, among radiosensitive tumors in which the survival from the α component is below 0.3, the β effect makes a very small contribution to overall radiosensitivity in the lower dose region. The overall effect of many small

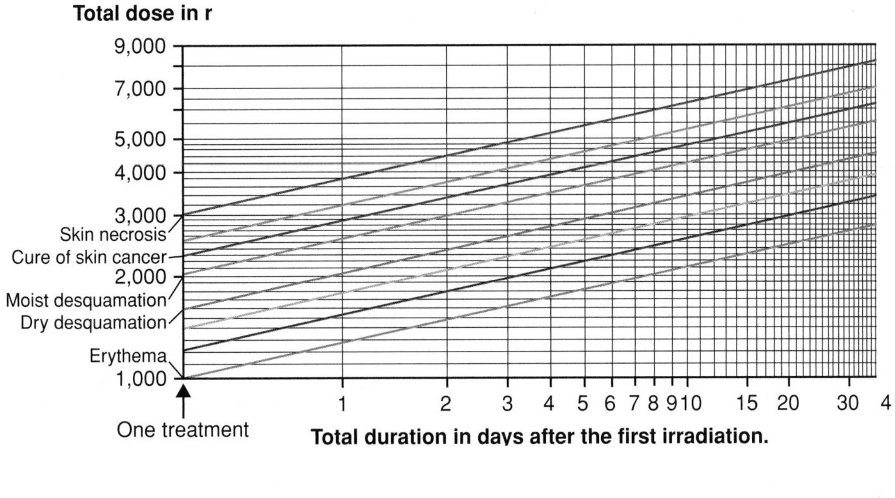

FIGURE 1.19. Strandqvist's curves on log paper. The slope of the curves (0.22) is the same for the tumoricidal dose for squamous cell carcinoma for various degrees of skin reactions. (From Strandqvist M. Sutdien uber die kumulative wirkung der rontgenstrahlen bie frakionierung. *Acta Radiol [Stockh]* 1944;55[Suppl]:1–300.)

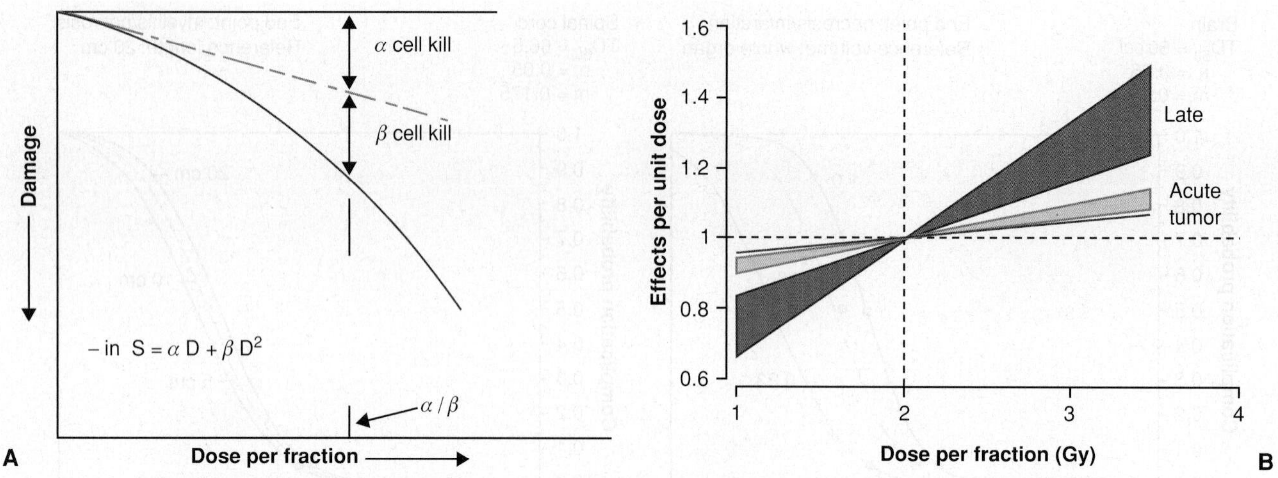

FIGURE 1.20. A: At a dose equal to the α/β ratio, the log cell kill due to the α-process (nonreparable) is equal to that due to the β-process (reparable injury); α/β is thus a measure of how soon the survival curve begins to bend over significantly. The α/β ratio for late effects on normal tissue generates a "curvier curve" than the α/β ratio for radiation's effects on acutely reacting normal tissue and tumor cells. Thus, the relative effect of dose per fraction is higher for late-responding tissue than for acutely responding tissues. In particular, for the central nervous system, high-dose-per-fraction radiation therapy is associated with an increased risk of late effects. An α/β ratio of 2 to 3 commonly is used in calculations of radiation effects on late-reacting tissue, whereas the ratio of 10 is used more commonly for acute-responding tissues or tumor. (From Fowler JR. Fractionation and therapeutic gain. In: Steel GG, Adams GE, Peckham MJ, eds. *The biological basis of radiotherapy.* Amsterdam: Elsevier Science, 1983:181–194.) **B:** A schematic representation of biologic data relating dose per fraction to effect on tumors, early reacting, and late-reacting normal tissues. (From Saunders MI. Programming of radiotherapy in the treatment of non-small-cell lung cancer—a way to advance cure. *Lancet Oncol* 2001;2[7]:401–408.)

fractions is to amplify the dominance of the α component. The β effect is unimportant because repair will be almost complete. In the more radiocurable tumors, cell killing by the α component represents the predominant fraction of tumor cell killing.

Box 1.4

Nominal Standard Dose and Time–Dose Factor

The nominal standard dose (NSD) concept is of historic interest. For 20 years NSD was used frequently to express equivalency of clinical doses of irradiation based on human skin tolerance and curability of squamous cell carcinoma. Cohen[89] pointed out that the regression coefficient for squamous cell carcinoma was different from that of normal skin (0.24). In 1969, Ellis[137] suggested that if one number could be used to represent the dose of irradiation that reached normal tissue tolerance, this would be advantageous in comparing different techniques. This figure should represent the normal connective tissue tolerance because this was, in his thinking, the limiting factor in most tumor therapies.

The unit for NSD expression was the *ret.* It could never be assumed that the NSD value represented a "single equivalent dose" because the isoeffect time calculated by Ellis used data from four to 30 fractions. Another flaw of the NSD calculation was that it did not allow for the effect of variations in volume treated or for interruptions of therapy (split-course therapy). Orton[330] estimated that NSD calculations were misused about 50% of the time by unaware clinicians comparing different radiation therapy regimens. The NSD formula did not predict isoeffect in pig skin irradiation with ^{60}Co using two to five fractions per week. Moreover, early reactions did not predict the magnitude of late damage when dose fractionation was altered from conventional daily schedules.

In 1973, Orton and Ellis[334] published a simplification of the NSD concept more applicable to clinical radiation therapy, stating that when a treatment did not result in normal connective tissue tolerance, treatment effectiveness should be described in terms of partial tolerance. Although there was no definite basis for the application of the time–dose factor (TDF) concept to clinical radiation therapy, equivalency of various dose schedules is sought constantly. For split-course regimens, the TDF values (in units of ret) were used by adding the TDF value for each of the partial tolerance factors corresponding to each component of the treatment and correcting for the decay of the first part of the treatment TDF.

In 1974, Orton[332] defined TDF values for continuous irradiation that could be used with temporary or permanent brachytherapy implants, using various isotopes. A standard radium therapy regimen of 60 Gy in 168 hours was used for comparison with other equivalent techniques. According to Ellis,[139] this was equivalent to 1,800 ret of fractionated external irradiation.

The shape of the dose survival curve with photons differs for acutely and slowly responding normal tissues. This difference in shape is not observed with neutrons. The severity of late effects changes more rapidly with a variation in the size of dose per fraction when a total dose is selected to yield equivalent acute effects. With a decreasing size of dose per fraction, the total dose required to achieve a certain isoeffect increases more

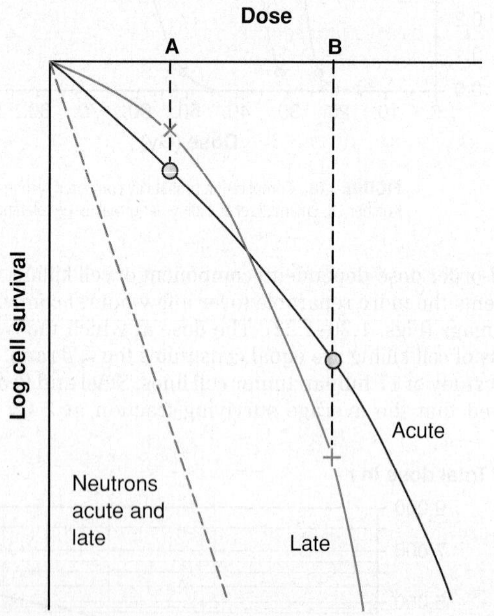

FIGURE 1.21. Hypothetical survival curves for the target cells for acute and late effects in normal tissues exposed to x-rays or neutrons. The α/β ratio in the equation for surviving fractions ($SF = e^{-(\alpha D + \beta D^2)}$) is higher for late effects than for acute effects in x-irradiated tissues, resulting in a greater rate of change in effect in late-responding tissues with change in dose. At dose A, survival of target cells is higher in late-effects than in acute-effects tissues, whereas at dose B, the reverse is true. Therefore, increasing the dose per fraction from A to B results in a relatively greater increase in late rather than acute injury. In the case of neutrons, the α/β ratio is low, with no detectable influence on the quadratic function ($e\beta D \pm D2$) over the first two decades of reduction in cell survival, implying that accumulation of sublethal injury plays a negligible role in cell killing by doses of neutrons of clinical interest. At these doses, the relative biologic effectiveness is higher for late effects than it is for acute effects. (From Fowler JR. Fractionation and therapeutic gain. In: Steel GG, Adams GE, Peckham MJ, eds. *The biological basis of radiotherapy.* Amsterdam: Elsevier Science, 1983:181–194.)

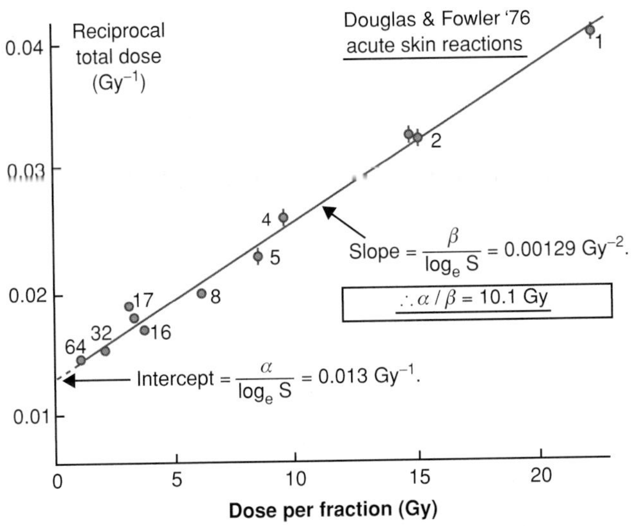

FIGURE 1.22. Values of α and β. If the reciprocal of total dose (for several multifraction schedules) is plotted against dose per fraction, a straight line will be obtained. The intercept of this line with the zero dose-per-fraction axis is proportional to α (α/ln S). The slope is proportional to β (β/ln S). The α/β ratio is readily determined. For absolute values of α and β, clonogenic assay is necessary for the end point. (From Fowler JR. Fractionation and therapeutic gain. In: Steel GG, Adams GE, Peckham MJ, eds. *The biological basis of radiotherapy.* Amsterdam: Elsevier Science, 1983:181–194.)

for late-responding tissues than for acutely responding tissues. Thus, in hyperfractionated regimens, the tolerable dose would be increased more for late effects than for acute effects. Conversely, if large doses per fraction are used, the total dose required to achieve isoeffects in late-responding tissues would be reduced more for late effects than for acute effects. In general, tumors and acutely reacting tissues have a high α/β ratio (8 to 15 Gy), whereas tissues involved in late effects have a low α/β ratio (1 to 5 Gy). Some values obtained in animal experiments and clinical studies are summarized in Table 1.9.

The values for α and β can be obtained from graphs in which the reciprocal of the total dose (Gy^{-1}) and the dose per fraction (Gy) are plotted. A straight line is obtained. The intercept of this line with the zero dose-per-fraction axis is proportional to α and equal to α/ln S, wherein S is the natural logarithm of survival. The slope is proportional to β and equal to β/ln S.

The algebraic functions to derive the straight line from the reciprocal total dose per fraction plot are as follows: Tumor cell survival following n fractions, each of dose d:

$$\begin{aligned}-\ln S &= n(\alpha d + \beta d)^2\\ &= \alpha nd + \beta nd^2\\ &= nd(\alpha + \beta d)\end{aligned}$$

TABLE 1.9 RATIO OF LINEAR (α) TO QUADRATIC (β) TERMS FROM MULTIFRACTION EXPERIMENTS AND CLINICAL DATA

	α/β Ratio (Gy)	
Tissue	*Experimental*	*Clinical*
Early Reactions		
Skin/subcutaneous tissues	9–12	5–10
Jejunum	6–10	2.2–8
Colon	10–11	–
Testis	12–13	–
Callus	9–10	–
Late Reactions		
Spinal cord	1.0–4.9	3.3
Kidney	1.5–2.4	–
Lung	2.4–6.3	4.2–4.7
Bladder	3.1–7.0	3.4–4.5

Modified from Fowler JF. Fractionation and therapeutic gain. In: Steel GE, Adams GE, Peckham MT, eds. *Biological basis of radiotherapy.* Amsterdam: Elsevier Science, 1983:181–194.

Dividing both sides by total dose nd:

$$\frac{-\ln S}{nd} = \alpha + \beta d$$

↑ Intercept ↑ Slope.

Withers et al.[506] proposed a method for using these survival curve parameters for calculating the change in total dose necessary to achieve an equal response in tissue when the dose per fraction is varied, using the α/β ratios. This calculation accounts only for the effect of repair of cellular injury. The isoeffect curves vary for different tissues. A biologically equivalent dose (BED) can be obtained using this formula:

$$\text{BED} = \frac{\ln S}{\alpha}$$

$$\text{BED} = nd[1 + d/(\alpha/\beta)]$$

If one wishes to compare two treatment regimens, the following formula can be used:

$$\frac{Dr}{Dx} = \frac{\alpha/\beta + dx}{\alpha/\beta + dr}$$

in which Dr is the known total dose (reference dose), Dx is the new total dose (with different fractionation schedule), dr is the known fractionation (reference), and dx is the new fractionation schedule.

Let's consider an example of the use of this formula (with some reservations). Suppose 50 Gy in 25 fractions is delivered to yield a given biologic effect. If one assumes that the subcutaneous tissue is the limiting parameter (late reaction), it is desirable to know what the total dose to be administered will be using 4-Gy fractions. Assume α/β for late fibrosis equals 2 Gy.

Using the above formula:

$$Dx = \frac{Dr(\alpha/\beta + dr)}{\alpha/\beta + dx}$$

Thus,

$$Dx = 50\text{ Gy}\left(\frac{5+2}{5+4}\right) = 39\text{ Gy}$$

The basic LQ equation addresses the inactivation of a homogeneous population of cells. One should be wary, however, of accepting the basic equation as being complete. Because it is likely that accelerated repopulation of tumor clonogens occurs during the course of radiotherapy, and that cell-cycle redistribution and reoxygenation also occur, we should consider how these factors can be accounted for in the formula.[58,194,522]

Repopulation may be accounted for, in broad approximation, by describing the number of clonogens (N) at time t as being related to the initial number of clonogens (No).

Then,

$$N = No^{e\lambda t}$$

The parameter λ determines the speed of cell repopulation and is given by

$$\lambda = \frac{\log e^2}{Tpot} = \frac{0.693}{Tpot}$$

where Tpot is the effective doubling time of cells in the tumor. If we ignore spontaneous cell loss, then Tpot is approximately the same as the measurable *in vitro* doubling time of tumor cells. Reported values of Tpot are 2 to 25 days with a median value of approximately 5 days. For late-responding tissues, Tpot is so large that λ is effectively zero.

Incorporating the allowance for tumor proliferation, with t representing time, the LQ equation becomes

$$\text{BED} = nd\left(1 + \frac{d}{\alpha/\beta}\right) - \frac{0.693t}{\alpha\,\text{Tpot}}$$

Let's assume an α/β for an acutely reacting tissue, such as a tumor, of 10, and an α of 0.3 with a Tpot of 5. The BED of 70 Gy of 2 Gy/fraction, five fractions per week, in 46 days, is

$$\text{BED} = 70(1 + 0.2) = 84\ \text{Gy}_{10}.$$

Now let's add the correction for tumor repopulation during the course of treatment:

$$\text{BED} = 70\left(1 + \frac{2}{10}\right) - \frac{0.693}{0.3} \times \frac{46}{5}$$

$$\text{BED} = 84 - 21 = 63\ \text{Gy}_{10}$$

The decrease in clonogens by radiotherapy is attenuated, in part, by the repopulation of the surviving clonogens.

In the LQ equation, redistribution in the cell cycle and reoxygenation may be modeled by a single term called *resensitization.* Immediately after a dose of radiation, the average radiosensitivity of the cell population falls and then gradually returns to greater sensitivity. In contrast to tumor proliferation, resensitization probably increases as overall treatment time increases. Not enough is known about resensitization's clinical importance to make it useful to incorporate a numeric value for it in the LQ formula.

The LQ model can be used to construct a biologically oriented dose distribution algorithm for clinical radiation therapy.[280] A physical dose distribution can be translated to a BED using published biologic parameters. We are certainly not in a position to begin the routine use of this approach in clinical radiation therapy, although it may help clinicians to optimize treatment plans, and the technique may be used for outcome analysis in clinical research when the biologic parameters and the assumptions can be validated.

DOSE RATE

The radiation dose rate may significantly influence the biologic response, particularly for sparsely ionizing radiations such as x-rays and γ-rays. Three main biologic processes are involved in the dose-rate effect (Figs. 1.23 and 1.24).[194,212]

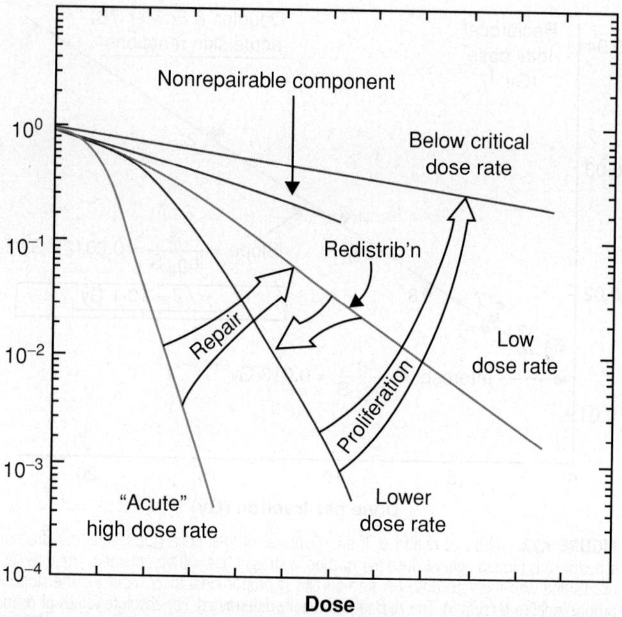

FIGURE 1.23. The dose-rate effect as a result of repair of sublethal damage, redistribution in the cycle, and cell proliferation. The dose–response curve for acute exposures is characterized by a broad initial shoulder. As the dose rate is reduced, the survival curve becomes progressively shallower as more and more sublethal damage is repaired, but cells are "frozen" in their positions in the cycle and do not progress. As the dose rate is lowered further and for a limited range of dose rates, the survival curve steepens again because cells can progress through the cycle to pile up at a block in G2, a radiosensitive phase, but still cannot divide. A further lowering of dose rate allows cells to escape the G2 block and divide; cell proliferation then may occur during the protracted exposure, and survival curves become shallower as cell birth from mitosis offsets cell killing from the irradiation. (Based on the ideas of Dr. Joel Bedford, and from Hall EJ. *Radiobiology for the radiologist,* 4th ed. Philadelphia: J.B. Lippincott, 1994, with permission.)

1. Repair of sublethal damage occurs when radiation is delivered at a low dose rate, and the treatment time is extended to a point where it is comparable to the repair half-time. As the dose rate is reduced, more sublethal damage is repaired because the radiation injury is spread over a longer period. The cell survival curves become progressively less steep, and at the same time the extrapolation number approaches unity.
2. Cell proliferation occurs during protracted radiation exposure if the dose rate is low enough or the cell cycle time is short enough.

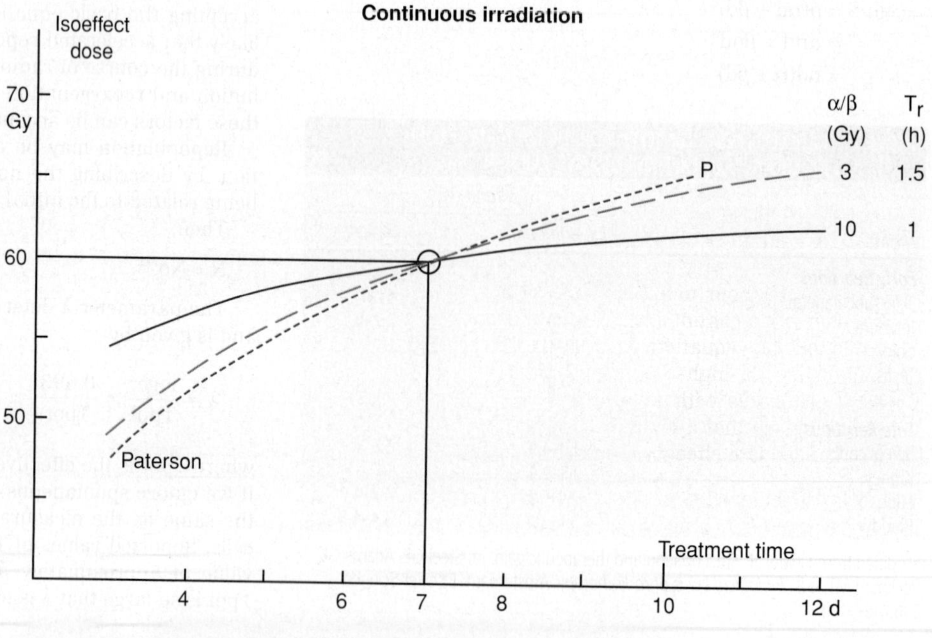

FIGURE 1.24. Low–dose-rate irradiation. Isoeffect dose equivalent to 60 Gy in 7 days. Two sets of parameters have been considered for the computation, which would presumably correspond to skin and mucosa early reactions and to the effect on the epithelioma (α/β = 10 Gy, Tr = 1 hour) and to late reactions (α/β = 3 Gy, Tr = 1.5 hour). (From Dutreix J. Expression of the dose rate effect in clinical curietherapy. *Radiother Oncol* 1989;15:25–37.)

3. Redistribution and accumulation of cells throughout the cell cycle occur with a low dose rate in which proliferation is decreased because cells are arrested and accumulate in G^2. This phase of the cycle is relatively radiosensitive. As a result, cell killing may be greater for a lower dose rate. This effect occurs over a narrow dose-rate range and is known as the inverse dose rate effect.

With the advent of moderate– and high–dose-rate remote control afterloading devices, increased emphasis has been placed on the biologic effects of dose rate. Many *in vitro* and *in vivo* experimental observations indicate variations in cell killing and repair of sublethal or potentially lethal damage with varying dose rates. The so-called dose-rate effect is most dramatic between 1 cGy/minute and 1 Gy/minute.[191] The biologic effect achieved by a given irradiation dose decreases as the dose rate diminishes, chiefly as a result of the increase in cell repair that occurs during continuous prolonged irradiation, because cell proliferation is virtually negligible in the range of treatment times used in low–dose-rate brachytherapy.[129]

In some experiments, a bending of the cell survival curve at very low dose rates has been noted, instead of the expected exponential result, possibly because of cell redistribution[529] or a decline in the repair capacity with large doses.[470] At a very low dose rate, because the cell killing is caused only by direct lethal events that are considered independent of the dose rate, cell repair is also negligible. The induction of sublethal injury is relatively slow compared with the rate of repair, and cell killing, by accumulation of sublethal injury, remains minimal. Variation of the isoeffect dose occurs mainly in the range of medium dose rates (1 to 10 Gy/hour), and it vanishes at very high dose rates because the cell repair is negligible during the short treatment time.[129]

The dose-rate effect in clinical brachytherapy was described initially by Green and Paterson and reiterated by Ellis and Orton.[138,332,346] The historic isoeffect curve showed a significant increase in dose when time was increased from 2 to 7 days. However, the validity of Paterson's curve was questioned by Pierquin et al.,[360] who used the same dose of 70 Gy with treatment times ranging from 3 to 8 days for the treatment of head and neck tumors with ^{192}Ir implants and did not observe any difference in the control rate or incidence of necrosis. The agreement with Paterson's curve is acceptable when the α/β value equals 3 Gy and repair half-time (T_r) equals 1.5 hours, but the curve is shallower when α/β equals 10 Gy and T_r equals 1 hour. One should expect Paterson's curve to correspond to late reactions and to overestimate the variation for early reactions and control of squamous cell carcinoma.

Several important concepts should be considered regarding the clinical relevance of dose rate:[58,191]

1. At ultra-high doses and instantaneous dose rates (i.e., 10 Gy pulsed in nanoseconds), the rapid deposition of energy consumes oxygen too quickly for diffusion to maintain an adequate level of oxygenation, and dose–response curves are characteristic of hypoxia. There is little interest in clinical application of this approach.
2. Based on laboratory data, it may be possible to design schedules with a pulse width of several minutes and a pulse interval of about 1 hour to achieve cell killing equivalent to that obtained with a continuous 30 Gy in 60 hours (0.5 Gy/hour).
3. Using the LQ equation, it is possible to estimate the equivalency of high–dose-rate (HDR) and low–dose-rate (LDR) exposures with a variety of fractionation schedules (remembering that a lower number of fractions may result in enhanced late effects).

Special consideration should be given to the effect of HDR brachytherapy on normal tissues. The tumor dose must be decreased 30% to 50% in comparison with that delivered with conventional low dose rates.[333,335] (For further discussion, see Chapters 22–25.)

In the past, there was some interest in continuous LDR irradiation with external cobalt units.[505] Pierquin et al.[359] used a modified ^{60}Co unit with a small industrial source (activity 45 Ci). Radiation was delivered at 1 to 1.39 Gy/hour to administer daily tumor doses of 8 to 10 Gy in 7 to 8 hours. A minimum of five treatments was given per week, although occasionally weekends and holidays caused schedule modifications. Patients were given short rest periods every 1 or 2 hours. Tumor doses of approximately 63 Gy were delivered in eight to 11 fractions, with the volume reduced to 8 by 10 cm after 45 Gy. Nineteen patients with advanced tumors of the mouth and pharynx were treated; 15 had no evidence of tumor 3 months after treatment. Only three patients developed recurrences. Of 19 patients, two developed moist desquamation and six developed dry desquamation; the others had only erythema. No significant late effects on the skin or the subcutaneous tissues were noted; 16/19 patients developed severe mucositis. Seven patients developed necrosis, six in large areas of the oral cavity and pharynx and, in several instances, at the tumor site.

IMPORTANCE OF TREATMENT PLANNING IN RADIATION THERAPY

The predicted consequences of external-beam radiation therapy are based on the precision with which the dose and the irradiated volume are defined. An imprecise treatment system could lead to a high incidence of necrosis with, paradoxically, a low probability of tumor control (Fig. 1.25).[331] Decreasing irradiation doses to avoid complications will further reduce the probability of achieving tumor control if such action is based on the wrong assumption that the tumor control/complication ratio is related only to radiation dose levels. The ICRU recommends a ± 5% accuracy for dose-delivery computations.[229]

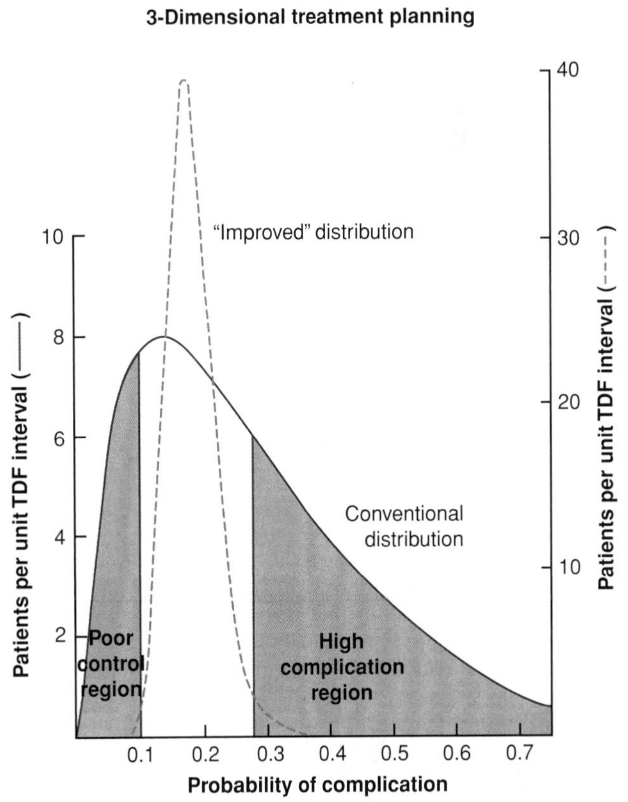

FIGURE 1.25. Frequency distribution of patients treated to different probabilities of complication. (From Orton CG. Other considerations in 3-dimensional treatment planning. In: Bagne F, ed. *Computerized treatment planning systems.* HHS Publication FDA 84-8223. Washington, DC: U.S. Government Printing Office, 1984:136–141.)

However, every effort should be made to develop accurate dose-calculation algorithms, including methods to correct for inhomogeneities in tissue density and the shape of the patient's body, and to develop practical treatment-planning capabilities to obtain the highest possible dose optimization in the irradiated volume (tumor and normal tissues). There are benefits of reducing the treatment volume in an effort to deliver higher doses of irradiation. This may improve the quality of tumor control without excessively irradiating surrounding normal tissues, thereby decreasing treatment-related morbidity.

Various steps can be taken to decrease toxicity in normal tissues, including precise treatment-planning and irradiation techniques, selective decreased volume receiving higher doses dictated by estimated cell burden, and maneuvers to exclude sensitive organs from the irradiated volume. With the emphasis on organ preservation, treatment planning is critical to achieve maximum TCP and satisfactory cosmetic results.

Optimal dose distribution may be achieved by a combination of multiple stationary beams or by moving-beam therapy, such as in arc or full-rotational techniques or IMRT. In addition, the optimal dose distribution in many tumors requires more than one modality or beam energy. A combination of external beams and intracavitary or interstitial therapy also may be required, depending on the location of the tumor.

Three-Dimensional Treatment Planning

Advances in computer technology have augmented accurate and timely computation, display of 3D radiation dose distributions, and DVHs.[182,368] These developments have stimulated sophisticated 3D treatment-planning systems, which yield relevant information in evaluation of tumor extent, definition of target volume, delineation of normal tissues, virtual simulation of therapy, generation of digitally reconstructed radiographs, design of treatment portals and aids (e.g., compensators, blocks), calculation of 3D dose distributions and dose optimization, and critical evaluation of the treatment plan.[180,351,370]

The potential benefits of 3D planning and delivery systems are great. It is, however, not clear which specific disease sites and treatment situations will be benefited by 3D planning.[412] With advanced computerized and display technologies, contiguous CT slices are used to define anatomic structures and target volumes. External radiation beams of any possible orientation are simulated. A significant feature of these systems is the so-called beam's eye view, in which patient contours are viewed as if the observer's eye is placed at the source of radiation looking out along the axis of the radiation beam.[369] These systems allow simulation of the geometric setup; evaluation of the plan for dose optimization still is made on the merits of volumetric dose distributions.

Quantitative treatment-planning evaluation is crucial in selection of the best portals and radiation beams to deliver an optimal dose to the tumor with relative sparing of normal tissues. The ICRU Report 50 and its supplement G2 define 3D volumes for the prescription and reporting of EBRT.[229] The GTV is defined as the gross demonstrable extent and location of malignant growth; the CTV allows a margin around the GTV for subclinical disease; the PTV allows margins on the CTV for variation in position, size, and shape so that the prescribed dose is received by the CTV; and the treated volume is that area receiving a dose considered appropriate to the purpose of treatment such as tumor eradication or palliation (see Fig. 1.2).

The DVH is useful as a means of dose display, particularly in assessing several treatment plan dose distributions.[85] A DVH provides a complete summary of the entire 3D dose matrix, showing the amount of target volume or critical structure receiving more than a specified dose level. Because a DVH does not provide spatial dose information, it cannot replace the other methods of dose display; it can only complement them.

Models for optimization of 3D dose distribution using biologic models of tumor and normal tissue responses correlated with physical radiation doses have been described.[384] Mohan et al.,[308] in a theoretical analysis, concluded that for certain clinical situations it is not sufficient to specify objectives of optimization purely on the basis of pattern of irradiation dose and that dose–volume effects and biologic indices also must be incorporated into the formulation.

Niemierko et al.[324] described a technique for optimization of 3D conformal radiation therapy plans with biologic models of tumor and normal tissue response to irradiation as well as with scores based on physical dose. Optimization programs attempted to minimize dose gradient across the target volume, match specified isodose contours to the target and critical organs, match specified dose–volume constraints, minimize integral dose to the entire volume of patient treated, minimize maximum dose to critical organs, and constrain dose to specified normal tissues below a tolerance-dose level. The solutions were based on TCP, NTCP, various dose levels given to specified volumes of the patient, discrete or continuous values of beam parameters, number of beams, and logical combination of any constraints.

Intensity-Modulated Radiation Therapy

An increasingly popular approach to 3D treatment planning and conformal therapy optimizes the delivery of irradiation to irregularly shaped volumes through a process of complex inverse (or forward) treatment planning and dynamic delivery of irradiation that results in modulated fluence of photon beam profiles and a more conformal dose to the target volume(s), with enhanced sparing of surrounding normal tissues.[56]

Treatment planning begins with the determination of the GTV and the CTV, which contains the GTV, and an estimate of where the tumor may spread. CT, MRI, and fluorodeoxyglucose positron emission tomography (FDG-PET) imaging along with image fusion have enhanced the possibilities for determining the target more accurately. The PTV accounts for inaccuracies in positioning patients and organ motion.

In "forward" planning, software calculates the dose distribution, displays it with a 3D anatomic model, and provides analytical and graphical metrics for assessing the adequacy of tumor treatment and normal tissue avoidance. The physician decides if the plan is acceptable. If not, an alteration is made in the beam arrangement, and the process is repeated.

Computerized optimization techniques have led to "inverse" planning. Goals of an acceptable treatment plan are delineated, and the inverse planning algorithm searches through many thousands of possibilities to find a plan that best satisfies the goals. In IMRT, the beams are broken up into "beamlets" (on the order of 0.5 by 0.5 or 1 by 1 cm) that can each have a different intensity. IMRT may improve the ability to treat with a high radiation dose while minimizing dose to nearby critical structures.

There are a variety of forms in which IMRT can be administered:

1. The North American Scientific (NOMOS) Corporation (Chatsworth, CA) Peacock system: an array of individual beamlets, each consisting of a narrow incident arc photon beam that exposes the target. The radiation fluence is modulated with a small dynamic multileaf collimator (MLC) (MIMiC) activated by a preprogrammed controller.
2. A linear accelerator and multileaf collimation, with a variety of beam configurations at various angles, may be used; the MLC determines the portal shape of each of the portals. Photon-modulated fluency may be obtained (a step-and-shoot method).
3. Dynamic computer-controlled IMRT is delivered when the configuration of the beams outlined with the MLC is changing at the same time that the gantry or the accelerator is changing positions around the patient.

4. In helical tomotherapy, the photon fan beam continually rotates around the patient as the couch transports the patient longitudinally through the ring gantry. The verification processes for helical tomotherapy are enabled by the use of the ring gantry; the geometry of a CT scanner allows tomographic processes to be reliably performed. Dose reconstruction is a key process of tomography; the treatment detector sinogram computes the actual dose deposited in the patient. The length of the beam is 40 cm at the central axis and has a width that can vary between 0.5 and 5 cm. Like the NOMOS MIMiC MLC, the lengths of the MLC in helical tomography are temporarily modulated or binary in the sense that they are rapidly driven either in or out by air system actuators rather than beam slowly pushed by motors driving lead screws as in the conventional MLC.
5. The robotic IMRT system consists of a miniaturized 6-MV photon linear accelerator mounted on a highly mobile arm and a set of ceiling-mounted x-ray cameras to provide near real-time information on patient position and target exposure during treatment.

The majority of the IMRT systems use 6-MV x-rays, but energies of 8 to 10 MV may be more desirable in some anatomic sites (to decrease skin and superficial subcutaneous tissue dose). Higher energies will increase neutron contamination of the therapeutic beam(s). The dose distribution and field-shaping parameters are based on inverse 3D planning using a specially defined minimal dose to target and dose constraints for surrounding normal tissues.[57,77,526] Inverse planning starts with an ideal dose distribution and finds through trial and error or multiple iterations (simulated annealing) the beam characteristics (fluence profiles), then produces the best approximation to the ideal dose defined in a 3D array of dose voxels organized in a stack of two-dimensional (2D) arrays.[337,491]

A back-projection technique through careful choice of filters, beam placement, and shaping of the portals conforms the irradiation dose to the shape of the tumor, minimizing dose to critical adjacent structures. When this technique is used, it is critical to adhere to basic concepts of treatment planning and evaluation of the pathobiology of malignant disease. Well-designed treatment plans based on radiographic imaging (CT or MRI), which in most instances demonstrates gross disease, are necessary to minimize the risk of missing or underirradiating adjacent microscopic or subclinical tumor.

Given the added time and labor involved in IMRT, numerous issues require study:

1. Can the tumor be localized with sufficient accuracy to take advantage of the improved dose localization?
2. Treatment plans that produce a rapid drop in dose between the edge of the tumor and the normal tissue require more exact patient positioning; otherwise, there is a high risk of underdosing the tumor or overdosing normal tissue.
3. Some IMRT plans treat the center of the tumor with a very high dose to achieve an acceptable dose at the edge. This may not be optimal.
4. Many IMRT techniques spread a low dose over a larger volume or normal tissue. This may increase the risk of secondary malignancies years later.

HEAVY PARTICLE BEAMS

The vast majority of radiation therapy is administered with photon or electron external beams or photon-generating brachytherapy sources. Physicians and physicists have explored the possibility that alternative forms of ionizing radiation might be clinically useful.

One can imagine two possible mechanisms by which one could improve on therapeutic x-rays with an alternative particle. First, the alternative particle could have energy deposition characteristics that lead to a superior dose distribution. A beam, conceivably, could have more skin sparing than x-rays, better stopping characteristics, and/or less side scatter. This might allow a more conformal therapy. Second, the alternative particle could have advantageous radiobiologic properties. It might be more toxic than x-rays to hypoxic cells or cells in the late S phase of the mitotic cell cycle. Such a particle would have, perhaps, a lower oxygen enhancement ratio (OER) and a higher RBE than x-rays. These two possible mechanisms of improving on x-rays are not mutually exclusive. A particle could have both superior physical dose distribution and radiobiologic properties.

The effort to identify improved alternatives to x-rays has focused on the group of particles called hadrons. These are particles constituted of strongly interacting particles called quarks and gluons. The hadrons include the mesons and the baryons. The latter include protons, neutrons, negative pions, and the nuclei of heavier atoms such as He^2 (helium), C^6 (carbon), O^8 (oxygen), Ne^{10} (neon), and Ar^{18} (argon). All of these forms of radiation are distinguished from x-rays and electrons by their greater masses. These alternative radiation modalities are relatively difficult to produce, are expensive, and are considerably more difficult to control.

Proton, heavy ion, and hadron beams have attracted radiation oncologists because they offer interesting and potentially beneficial dose distribution characteristics. Radiobiologically, their properties are not significantly different from x-rays. When a heavy particle beam traverses tissue, the dose is deposited in an approximately constant rate. The rate of energy loss (also called the "stopping power") of a heavy charged particle is proportional to the square of the particle charge and inversely proportional to the square of its velocity. As a proton or heavy ion slows down, its rate of energy loss increases and so does the ionization or absorbed dose to the tissue. Near the end of the proton's range, the deposition of energy rises very sharply before dropping to almost zero. This peaking of dose near the end of the particle range is called the Bragg peak. As a result of the Bragg peak effect and minimal scattering, the proton offers the potential advantage and the ability to concentrate dose inside and immediately adjacent to the tumor volume and minimize dose to surrounding normal tissues. There are proton treatment facilities operational and under construction throughout the economically developed world. The technology has been evaluated most extensively in the management of choroidal melanoma, base of skull tumors, soft-tissue sarcomas, and prostate cancer. Box 1.5 provides a helpful glossary of terms related to heavy particle beam radiation therapy.

This section of Chapter 1 offers only the briefest overview of proton and neutron therapy. For a thorough discussion of these two forms of radiation, as well as a consideration of pi meson therapy and charged nuclei therapy such as helium ions and neon ions, the reader is referred Chapters 19 and 20 of this volume.

BORON NEUTRON CAPTURE THERAPY

The fundamental concept of boron neutron capture therapy is the production of high–linear energy transfer (LET) particles ($^{7}Li^{3+}$ and $^{4}He^{2+}$) when one "tags" or "labels" a tumor cell with a compound having a large cross-section capable of capturing a "slow" (thermal) neutron. After the compound captures the neutron, it goes into an excited state. The excited fission of the ^{11}B nucleus will release energy, which drives the heavy ion products over short distances comparable to the dimensions of one cell. A 0.48-MeV photon is also produced in 94% of the fission events. This is useful for monitoring the reaction but is of little consequence for cell killing (Fig. 1.26).

The neutron has a mass of 0.782 MeV, more than that of the proton. Neutrons were identified in 1932 by Chadwick[81] at Cambridge University's Cavendish Laboratory. Subsequently, Fermi[146] discovered that neutrons react most efficiently with a

Box 1.5

A Glossary of Terms Pertinent to Heavy Particle Beam Radiation Therapy

Baryon: A hadron made from three quarks. The proton and the neutron are both baryons. They also may contain additional quark–antiquark pairs.

Bragg, William Henry (1862–1942): He was born in Westward, Cumberland, and educated at King William's College, Isle of Mann; Trinity College, Cambridge; and the Cavendish Laboratory. In collaboration with his son (*vide infra*), he developed techniques of systematically analyzing crystal structures using x-rays. This was recognized by the awarding of the Nobel Prize in Physics jointly to father and son in 1915.

Bragg, William Lawrence (1890–1971): He was born in Adelaide, South Australia, where his father was a professor. He came to England with his father (*vide supra*) and entered Trinity College, Cambridge. He and his father published *X-rays and Crystal Structure* in 1915. Later in his career he used x-ray analysis to investigate the structure of proteins. Having been awarded the Nobel Prize with his father, he was, at 25 years of age, the youngest-ever Nobel laureate.

Bragg peak: The region of high dose at the end of the range of a heavy charged particle.

Charge: A quantum number carried by a particle. Determines whether the particle can participate in an interaction process. A particle with electric charge has electrical interactions, one with strong charge has strong interactions, and so forth.

Electric charge: The quantum number that determines participation in electromagnetic interactions.

Electromagnetic interaction: The interaction resulting from electric charge; this includes magnetic effects that have to do with moving electric charges.

Electron: The least massive electrically charged particle, hence absolutely stable. It is the most common lepton, with electric charge –1.

Fermion: Any particle that has odd-half-integer (1/2, 3/2, ...) intrinsic angular momentum (spin). As a consequence of this peculiar angular momentum, fermions obey the Pauli exclusion principle, which states that no two fermions can exist in the same state at the same place and time. Many of the properties of ordinary matter arise because of this rule. Electrons, protons, and neutrons are all fermions, as are all the fundamental matter particles, both quarks and leptons.

Gluon: The carrier particle of strong interactions.

Hadron: A particle made of strongly interacting constituents (quarks and/or gluons). These include the mesons and baryons. Such particles participate in residual strong interactions.

Lepton: A fundamental fermion that does not participate in strong interactions. The electrically charged leptons are the electron, the muon, the tau, and their antiparticles. Electrically neutral leptons are called neutrinos.

Meson: A hadron made from an even number of quark constituents. The basic structure of most mesons is one quark and one antiquark.

Neutron: A baryon with electric charge zero; it is a fermion with a basic structure of two down quarks and one up quark (held together by gluons). The neutral component of an atomic nucleus is made from neutrons. Different isotopes of the same element are distinguished by having different numbers of neutrons in their nucleus.

Nucleon: A proton or a neutron; that is, one of the particles that makes up a nucleus.

Nucleus: A collection of neutrons and protons that forms the core of an atom.

Particle: A subatomic object with a definite mass and charge.

Photon: The carrier particle of electromagnetic interactions.

Pion: The least massive type of meson, pions can have electric charges +1 or 0.

Proton: The most common hadron, a baryon with electric charge (+1) equal and opposite to that of the electron (–1). Protons have a basic structure of two up quarks and one down quark (bound together by gluons). The nucleus of a hydrogen atom is a proton. A nucleus with electric charge Z contains Z protons; therefore, the number of protons is what distinguishes the different chemical elements.

Quark: A fundamental fermion that has strong interactions. Quarks have electric charge of either +2/3 (*up, charm, top*) or –1/3 (*down, strange, bottom*) in units where the proton charge is +1.

Strong interaction: The interaction responsible for binding quarks, antiquarks, and gluons to make hadrons. Residual strong interactions provide the nuclear binding force.

Subatomic particle: Any particle that is small compared to the size of the atom.

These definitions are derived from Welsh JS. Quarks, leptons, fermions, bosons: the subatomic pharmacology of radiation therapy. *Science Med* 2005;10:124–136; The Nobel Museum (www.nobel.se/physics/laureates); The Atlas Experiment (http://atlasexperiment.org/glossary.html); and Khan FM. *The physics of radiation therapy,* 3rd ed. Philadelphia: Lippincott Williams & Wilkins, 2003.

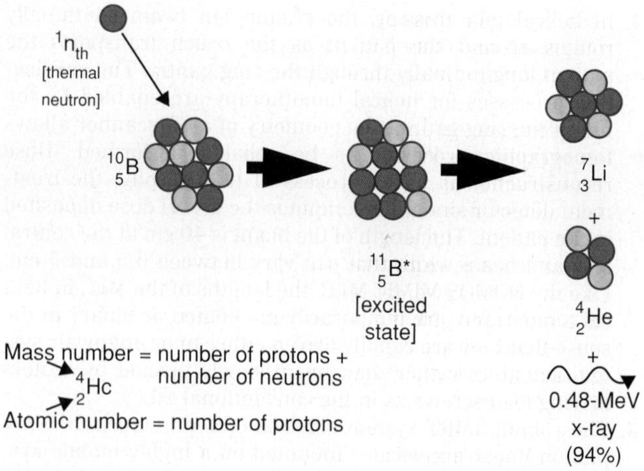

FIGURE 1.26. The bombardment of stable Bo[10] by a thermal neutron results in a nuclear reaction. This reaction yields Li[7] nuclei and α-particles. These fission products have short path links and a high linear energy transfer (LET). This high-LET radiation, over a short path length, offers the possibility of a lethal effect highly localized within a cell.

number of elements after they are slowed by passage through a hydrogen-rich substance such as paraffin. Chadwick and Goldhaber,[82] Taylor and Goldhaber,[441] and Burcham and Goldhaber,[67] showed that slow neutron bombardment of specific stable isotopes of boron, lithium, and nitrogen yield charged particle tracts in photographic plates. The tracts from boron's interaction with neutrons were short and straight and were consistent with the formation of two particles traveling in opposite trajectories. In photographic gelatin, their average travel distance was 7.6 μm. The boron neutron capture process is highly localized. In principle, one could kill a tumor cell containing boron while sparing an adjacent normal cell that does not contain boron. Box 1.6 provides a glossary of terms related to neutron capture therapy.

The complete chemical reaction is as follows:

$$^{10}B + {}^{1}n \rightarrow {}^{7}Li + {}^{4}He + \gamma + 2.4\ MeV.$$

The attraction of boron neutron capture therapy (BNCT), for many clinicians, has been the notion of the "magic bullet." The idea that one could specifically label tumor cells with a compound

Box 1.6

A Glossary of Terms Pertinent to Neutron Capture Therapy

Epithermal neutrons: Energetic neutrons pass through an intermediate energy range on the way to becoming slow or thermal neutrons. This intermediate energy range is called epithermal.

Fast neutrons: Fast neutrons are highly energetic and travel quickly.

Moderation: Neutrons generated from the fission process or from particle bombardment of materials have significant energy. They lose that energy by colliding with atoms in their environment and create energetic recoil atoms. After a sufficient number of collisions, the neutrons lose essentially all of their energy and become thermal. This process of energy loss is called moderation. The material that provides the atoms the fast neutrons collide with is called a moderator. Water is the usual moderator.

Slow neutrons: Slow neutrons have little energy. They also are referred to as thermal neutrons because they have the same average kinetic energy as gas molecules in their environment.

Thermalize: Epithermal neutron beams, as they penetrate tissue, become additionally moderated. This is called becoming thermalized.

From Yanch JC, Shefer RE, Busse PM. Boron neutron capture therapy. *Science Med* 1999; January/February:18–27.

with an enlarged cross-sectional area, not label surrounding normal tissue, and therefore deposit radiation only in the tumor is most attractive. Unfortunately, reality is far different from the ideal.

Fast neutrons differ from x-rays in the mode of their interaction with tissue. Whereas x-ray photons interact with the orbital electrons of atoms via the Compton or photoelectric process and set fast electrons in motion, neutrons interact with the nuclei of the atoms of the absorbing tissue. Neutrons put fast recoil protons, α-particles, and heavier nuclear fragments in motion. At energies above about 6 MeV, inelastic scattering by neutrons takes place. A neutron may interact, for example, with a carbon or an oxygen nucleus to produce α-particles. These lead to nuclear fragments called spallation products. The LET is considerably higher for neutrons than for x-rays. Because the LET of neutron radiation is higher, the slope of the cell survival curve becomes steeper and the size of the initial shoulder gets smaller. This produces a beam with a lower OER than x-rays—neutrons are considerably more toxic to hypoxic cells than x-rays. Also, neutrons are more toxic to cells in phases of the cell cycle that are relatively radioresistant to x-rays. Thus, the RBE of neutrons is higher than x-rays.

In 1936, Locher[278] published a theoretical account of the possible biologic effects and therapeutic possibilities of boron neutron capture. In a prescient comment, he wrote:

> The possibility of destroying or weakening cancerous cells, by the general or selective absorption of neutrons by themselves and particularly there is the possibility of introducing small quantities of neutron absorbers into the regions where it is desired to liberate ionizing energy. A simple illustration would be the injection of a soluble non-toxic compound of boron, lithium, or gold into a superficial cancer followed by bombardment with slow neutrons.

In a 1950 paper by Conger and Giles[95] from Oakridge National Laboratories, they reported that the trace amounts of boron normally present in lily bulbs were responsible for most of the radiation changes in the plants following exposure to slow neutrons. This demonstrated the biologic fact clearly and led William H. Sweet[436] and others to see if the normal brain could exclude enough boron and if tumor tissue could take up enough boron to produce an appropriate therapeutic ratio.

Sweet began work at the Brookhaven National Laboratory in New York with a 20-MW nuclear reactor in 1950. He initially treated 10 glioblastoma multiforme patients who had undergone gross total resection of their tumors at the Massachusetts General Hospital in Boston. Sweet described the initial clinical work:

> A portion of the shielding atop the reactor was removed to permit placing the lateral aspect of the patient's intact scalp and skull at the specially designed portal. To prevent scalp damage, we tied off the external carotid arteries and covered the entire scalp with tight elastic bandages in an attempt to prevent boron-containing blood from entering the scalp. These tactics, however, did not prevent the development of several large radiation erosions of the scalp. Five patients received a single radiation dose and the remaining 5 were given the treatment in 2 to 4 fractions. Although there were no life threatening complications of therapy, all of the patients died from 6 to 21 weeks after the first session of neutron capture therapy, which was usually the case in the 1950s for glioblastoma patients treated by any means. Postmortem studies done in 6 of the patients showed abundant viable tumor. Their painful scalp lesions together with the inadequacy of the radiation dose lead us to attempt to deliver the thermal neutron beam directly to the grossly normal but microscopically tumor-infiltrated brain. The Rockefeller Foundation made this approach possible with a $500,000 gift to the Massachusetts Institute of Technology [MIT] to provide additional features to a nuclear reactor that was then being constructed. Included was a surgical operating room immediately beneath the reactor core. This permitted us to turn down the scalp, bone, and dural flap used in the prior removal of gross tumor. At reopening the cerebrospinal fluid replacing tumor was also drained away to give maximally unimpeded access of the thermal neutrons through sterile air to the tumor-infiltrated brain.[436]

Sweet treated 18 patients at MIT. They died from 10 days to 11.5 months after radiation. In every patient the cause of death was cerebral, and extensive irradiation necrosis of the brain was induced in nine cases. In two cases only recurrent tumor was seen, and in one patient there was extensive radiation necrosis and tumor.

Some of the initial work with BNCT was highly controversial and, decades later, led to investigations concerning the nature of informed consent for these human experiments. President William J. Clinton created, by executive order, a commission to study the ethics of cold war–era medical experimentation using radiation. One of the collateral effects of this commission's report was that Sweet and his colleagues were sued for malpractice 40 years after the BNCT experiments. Although the plaintiffs were awarded substantial damages at trial, the decision was eventually overturned on appeal.[199]

Clinical trials, largely in Japan, have argued that there is benefit to BNCT of glioblastoma multiforme. However, to date, no randomized clinical trials of BNCT have been performed. Although Japanese investigators have reported a survival rate for grade 3 and 4 malignant glioma patients as high as 58% with BNCT, this has been called into question by Laramore et al.[258] They investigated 14 U.S. patients who were treated with BNCT for glioblastoma multiforme in Japan. A comparison of the survival of these patients with a matched set of conventionally treated patients using the prognostic factors of the RTOG showed no statistical difference compared to the BNCT patients. This is almost certainly the result of patients with relatively favorable characteristics being selected for BNCT such as lower histologic grade, young age, good functional status, and superficial location. A 2011 report from Ibaragi, Japan, of 23 glioblastoma multiforme patients treated with 15 to 18 Gy of BNCT described a median survival time of 20 months and a 6% 5-year survival.[242] Because neutron beams have a significant normal tissue toxicity, and because their depth-dose characteristics are not superior to x-rays, their applicability has been limited, and clinical results, to date, have been quite mixed. Clinical studies have been reported concerning the use of neutrons in salivary gland and other head and neck tumors, soft-tissue sarcomas, and prostate cancer.

Lack of progress in BNCT may be attributed to two primary factors: inadequate tumor specificity of the boron compounds used to localize in the tumor and poor penetration into tissue of the thermal neutrons. In addition, the thermal and antithermal neutron beams produced by nuclear reactors have considerable contamination with γ-rays and fast neutrons. These can cause normal tissue damage even in the absence of boron concentration in tissues. In addition, there are a number of compounds in normal tissue that can interact with thermal neutrons and have capture events of their own, producing biologic damage even to non–boron-containing tissue.

The development of suitable boron-carrying agents remains a stumbling block to clinical programs. The ideal agent will be nontoxic, will have a high tumor-to-normal-tissue ratio, and will have a high absolute boron concentration. Three classifications are helpful for defining boron agents:

1. *Global agents* have little selectivity for tumor cells. The clinician is relying on a conformal neutron beam to achieve selectivity rather than selective accretion of boron.
2. *Tumor-selective agents* accumulate selectivity in tumors. L-4-dihydroxyborylphenylanine has been used as a boron-carrying agent (Fig. 1.27). This compound is a dopamine analog in the melanin synthetic pathway and concentrates in pigmented tumors. It was synthesized over 50 years ago and was first used clinically in 1988–1989.[30] It has been thought to be of potential use in the treatment of

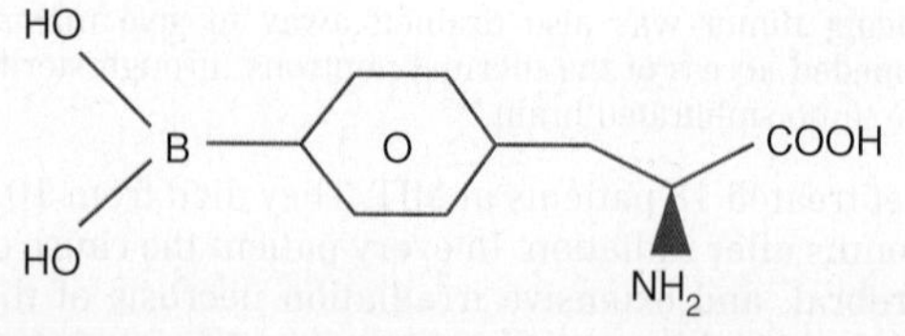

FIGURE 1.27. P-borophenylallanine (BPA) was synthesized in the late 1950s for use in boron neutron capture therapy. It has been shown to accumulate selectively in B16 melanoma cells both *in vivo* and *in vitro*. Clinical trials have been performed of BPA-mediated boron neutron capture therapy for cutaneous melanoma. The compound also has been studied in brain tumor therapy.

melanoma, and initial clinical trials are under way. Tumor-selective agents include, in addition to borylphenylalanine compounds, investigations of boronated porphyrins, amino acids, and nucleic acids that are borinated. Melanin is an intracellular protein synthesized from the amino acid tyrosine. Incorporating boronic acid into the paraposition of phenylalanine, producing p-borophenylallanine, would result in a molecule that behaved like tyrosine and might be able to selectively put boron-10 into melanoma cells. These compounds are capable of achieving a tumor-to-normal-tissue ratio of 3 or 4 to 1. It is not, however, because they are a substrate for tyrosinase, the first enzyme in the pathway to melanin. Nonetheless, they are capable of producing high levels of boron-10 in tumors. For brain tumors, drug uptake may be superior with intracarotid administration.[30]

3. *Tumor-targeted and delivery agents* have a structural feature that either binds to a specific portion of the cancer cell or facilitates drug delivery. Tumor-targeted agents include the use of polycomplex peptides, known as starburst dendrimers, which may allow boron to be attached to an antibody without causing a loss of specificity and carry boron in low-density lipoprotein vesicles. Other techniques for drug delivery include carbon nanotubes and gold nanoparticles.[72]

Investigations of improved ways of delivering thermal neutrons have centered on two areas: the use of nuclear reactors and useful alternatives to reactors. For reasons of safety, reactors generally use a low enriched fuel with uranium. However, one would have considerable doubts about the political and social feasibility of the placement of such units in major medical centers in populated areas. Therefore, some investigators have been pursuing nonreactive sources of thermal and epithermal neutrons with a sufficiently high flux to be used for BNCT.

The most intense way to generate a neutron beam is with a nuclear reactor. Despite the high neutron intensities available from these reactors, it is widely recognized that alternative neutron sources will be necessary for BNCT to be performed. First of all, there are few suitable nuclear reactors in operation. A patient would have to travel a long distance for treatment. Second, nuclear reactors, for political and social reasons, are not likely to be sited near major population centers in the future. A major reactor facility located far from a population center would have to be provided with its own clinical infrastructure, and it is not obvious that the target patient population would be large enough to support the operation of more than a few medical reactors. Therefore, some investigators have been pursuing nonreactive sources of thermal and epithermal neutrons with a sufficiently high flux to be used for boron neutron capture therapy.[88,258,436,489]

An alternative to the reactor would be a neutron source from radioactive decay such as californium-252 (^{252}Cf). However, production of a neutron beam with sufficient intensity for BNCT would require more than the entire present annual supply of ^{252}Cf. Another alternative source is a particle accelerator. Accelerator-based neutron beams are created when light ions such as protons or deuterons are accelerated in an electric field and are made to bombard target materials. Several accelerator techniques now exist that may be capable of producing intense beams for boron neutron capture therapy.

Several current clinical protocols are under way, or have recently been completed, concerning BNCT. These trials attempt to evaluate patients with advanced-stage melanoma of the extremities and are designed to determine the maximally tolerated dose of boron neutron capture therapy to the skin and overlying connective tissue. Other studies are evaluating treatment with BNCT of glioblastoma multiforme or brain metastasis from malignant melanoma. Animal studies and phantom dosimetry calculations have been reported on BNCT synovectomy for treatment of rheumatoid arthritis.[206,489,516]

EFFECTS OF IRRADIATION ON CELLS

The radiation-induced lesion most detrimental to cell survival involves damage to the DNA. This may result in either mitotic cell death or apoptosis. If the cell survives and repairs the damage, it may achieve a normal status. If there is misrepair, it may be associated with permanent mutations and induction of carcinogenesis. The physical interaction of ionizing radiation with the molecular infrastructure of the cell results in chemical reactions that occur within 10^{-18} to 10^{-3} seconds.[485] Absorption of the photon energy destabilizes the target molecule, resulting in molecular breaks or release of energetic electrons and secondary energy-attenuated photons, which may interact with other cellular molecules, leading to a chain reaction that produces a variety of short-lived ions and chemically unstable free radicals. The most common radicals are produced from the radiolysis of cellular water and include hydroxyl radicals ($^{\bullet}$OH), hydrated electrons (e_{aq}), hydrogen atoms (H$^{\bullet}$), and hydrogen peroxide (H_2O_2). Free radicals are extremely unstable and interact nearly instantaneously with neighboring molecules to produce chemically stable lesions. This process can be modified by free radical scavengers or by oxygen, which have opposing effects on the number of stable lesions and on the level of cellular radiosensitivity. However, if all factors remain constant, the permanent damage is linear with dose. Experiments in which the cell nucleus and the cytoplasm were selectively irradiated show that the dose required in the cytoplasm to kill a cell is larger than doses required in the nucleus.[91,312] It is generally accepted that most target molecules for radiation-induced cell killing are located in the nucleus and involve damage to the DNA.[114] However, other targets such as the cell membrane and the membrane of mitochondria have been proposed as the origin of apoptotic cascades that follow irradiation also contributing to cell death.

In many cells, radiation-induced lethality is not instantaneous because cells continue to function and even undergo several divisions before final mitotic death occurs.[410] Noncycling lymphocytes, thymocytes, and hematopoietic cells were shown to undergo an interphase cell death without progressing through the mitotic phase of the cell cycle.[9,513] Two patterns of morphologic changes are associated with cell death in mammalian cells. Cell necrosis, which is degenerative, is the most usual type of cell damage. Necrotic cell death results from collapse of cellular metabolism and depletion of its adenosine triphosphate storage.[508] The final events of necrosis involve membrane rupture, loss of lysosomal enzymes, degradation of nuclear chromatin, and karyolysis. The other process of radiation-induced cell death is apoptosis. Programmed cell death, or apoptosis, is a physiologic process that involves a series of characteristic, genetically controlled steps. These include chromatin condensation and segmentation, fragmentation of the nucleus into apoptotic bodies, cell shrinkage, and loss of cellular contact with neighboring cells.[243,244,518,519] Apoptosis culminates in the engulfment of the cell by neighboring cells, such as macrophages, without a concomitant inflammatory response.[289] Apoptosis occurs spontaneously in various solid tumors and contributes to the balance between tumor cell gain and cell loss.[248]

TABLE 1.10 APPLICATION OF RADIOBIOLOGIC CONCEPTS TO RADIATION THERAPY

Process	*Potential Manipulation*	*Examples of Therapy*[a]
DNA damage	Increase damage in tumor cells	Hypoxic-cell sensitizers, thymidine analogs
DNA repair	Decrease repair in tumor cells	Fluoropyrimidines, hydroxyurea, cisplatin
Signal transduction	Inhibit protective signaling cascades in tumor cells	Protein kinase C inhibitors (?), phosphotyrosine kinase inhibitors (?)
Radiation-induced gene expression	Use gene therapy	Tumor necrosis factor linked to radiation-responsive promoter (?)
Growth factor expression	Administer or increase expression of protective factors	Interleukin-1, granulocyte colony-stimulating factor, granulocyte-macrophage colony-stimulating factor, basic fibroblast growth factor (?)
	Block expression of factors producing long-term toxicity	Antibodies or antisense RNA against epidermal growth factor, transforming growth factor-β (?)
Apoptosis	Force tumor cells to undergo apoptosis	Transfection of wild-type p53 (?)
Cell cycle	Synchronize tumor cells in sensitive phase of cycle (early S or M phase)	Antimetabolites (early S phase), paclitaxel phase (M), cyclin inhibitors (G_1 to S phase) (?)
	Prevent G_2 arrest in tumor cells	Cyclin inhibitors (G_2 to M phase) (?)

[a]A question mark indicates potential therapy.

From Lichter AS, Lawrence TS. Recent advances in radiation oncology. *N Engl J Med* 1995;332:371–379.

Within minutes after irradiation, signal transduction pathways mediated by protein kinase C and tyrosine kinase are stimulated.[83] Genes and enzymes involved in genetic control of radiation damage repair are activated, stress genes are induced, and growth factors and cytokines that modulate response of mammalian cells to ionizing radiation are activated.[177] Radiation-induced stimulation is probably critical to induction of many genes and proteins, including early response genes, which, in turn, activate other genes, including those for tumor necrosis factor, fibroblast growth factor, and transforming growth factor.[91] In addition, new proteins, such as tissue plasminogen activator, are synthesized.[157] This cascade of gene activation and transcription and protein synthesis is related to key cellular functions that the cell invokes in an attempt to survive a dose of radiation[157] (Table 1.10).

Modifiers of Radiation Response

Several approaches have been used to enhance the therapeutic ratio in radiation therapy:

1. *Physical modifiers of low-LET radiations.* IMRT, three-dimensional treatment planning, improvements in anatomic and functional imaging, the increasing power of computer hardware and software, and linear accelerator improvements have led to better photon and electron dose distributions; less side scatter; less differential absorption in bone and normal tissues; and, with charged heavy particles, selective energy deposition at specific depths.
2. *High-LET radiations.* The importance of tumor hypoxia and cells residing in relatively resistant phases of the mitotic cycle are factors that are less likely to cause unsatisfactory results with neutrons, pi mesons, and heavy ions than with standard radiation doses delivered with low-LET beams.[162]
3. *Hyperbaric oxygen or tourniquet techniques.* These techniques involve use of increased oxygen tension to improve the effects of irradiation on the tumor or use of a tourniquet to produce severe hypoxia in the surrounding normal tissues so that higher irradiation doses can be delivered.[435] Theoretically, these approaches yield better tumor control without damaging normal tissues. Interest in the tourniquet technique waned years ago. Some investigators continue to evaluate hyperbaric oxygen. The logistics are formidable, and clinical trials have not been conclusive.[87,116,217,469]
4. *Hypoxic sensitizers.* Compounds with electron affinity, from the nitroimidazole group, theoretically produce free radicals in a manner similar to that of oxygen, selectively sensitizing hypoxic cells to radiation. Misonidazole (RO-07–0582) was evaluated in numerous clinical trials by the RTOG, with no evidence of clinical efficacy;[489] however, in the Danish Head and Neck Cancer trial there was a highly significant survival benefit in the subgroup of patients with pharynx tumors.[339] New compounds, such as SR-2508, have been tested in phase I and II studies without clearly positive results.
5. *Perfluorocarbons.* These agents are administered in emulsion (they are insoluble in water) in sufficient concentrations coupled with inhalation of 95% to 100% oxygen to enhance oxygen transport and release in the presence of low oxygen tension. Their potential application in the treatment of patients with cancer is under evaluation.[249,384]
6. *Cytotoxic agents.* Actinomycin-D, doxorubicin, 5-fluorouracil, cyclophosphamide, cisplatin, methotrexate, bleomycin, and others have been shown to interact with radiation in several forms to maximize tumor cell killing. In some instances, increased normal tissue reactions have been observed.
7. *Epidermal growth factor receptor (EGFR).* EGFR, a member of the ErbB family of receptor tyrosine kinases, is activated in several epithelial cancers. Radiotherapy increases the expression of EGRF in cancer cells and blockade of EGFR signaling can sensitize cells to radiation. Cetuximab is a chimeric monoclonal antibody that targets EGFR. The drug appears to improve locoregional tumor control and survival in locally advanced squamous cell carcinoma of the head and neck.[6]
8. *Radioprotectors.* Sulfhydryl-containing compounds, such as cystine and cysteamine, have been used in animals to protect normal tissues against irradiation. Amifostine (WR-2721), a thiophosphate derivative of cysteamine, has been shown to selectively protect normal tissues, including bone marrow, salivary glands, and intestinal mucosa, in animals, with little effect on tumor response to irradiation.[466] Amifostine undergoes dephosphorylation by cellular-bound alkaline phosphatase to an active metabolite, WR-1065. This alkaline phosphatase–dependent activation is thought to contribute to selective normal tissue protection because of a higher concentration of alkaline phosphatase in normal tissue. Cytoprotection is believed to be the result of the elimination of free radicals.[412] The compound was widely investigated in phase II and III clinical trials.[60] It is now approved by the U.S. Food and Drug Administration (FDA) and the European Medicines Agency for the reduction of xerostomia in patients with head and neck cancer undergoing radiotherapy.[412] A meta-analysis has shown that amifostine does not reduce overall or progression-free survival in patients treated with radiotherapy or chemoradiotherapy—arguing against amifostine protecting tumor tissue.[52]
9. *Hyperthermia.* Heat at temperatures of more than 42.5°C kills cells by itself or enhances the effects of irradiation and numerous cytotoxic agents. Heat selectively kills cells that are chronically hypoxic, acidotic, and nutritionally deficient—characteristics shared by tumor cells in comparison with the better-oxygenated and better-nourished normal cells. Furthermore, heat preferentially kills cells in the

S phase of the proliferative cycle, which are known to be relatively resistant to irradiation.[113,444]

A complete review of these topics will be found in Chapters 29, 31, and 32.

GENES AND THE BIOLOGY OF CANCER

The infectious nature of some cancers was demonstrated by Francis Peyton Rous (1879–1970) in a 1910 experiment showing that defined, submicroscopic, filterable agents (viruses) isolated from a chicken sarcoma could induce new sarcomas in healthy chickens. Rous and his work languished in obscurity before being rediscovered and recognized with the Nobel Prize in Physiology or Medicine in 1966 (Fig. 1.28).[326] In his Nobel Lecture, "The Challenge to Man of the Neoplastic Cell," Rous considered the possible existence of growth-promoting genes—what he called oncogens and what are now called oncogenes.

> Tumors destroy man in a unique and appalling way, as flesh of his own flesh which has somehow been rendered proliferative, rampant, predatory and ungovernable. They are the most concrete and formidable of human maladies, yet despite more than 70 years of experimental study they remain the least understood. This is the more remarkable because they can be evoked at will for scrutiny by any one of a myriad chemical and physical means which are left behind as tumors grow. These had acted merely as initiation. Few situations are more exasperating to the inquirer than to watch a tiny nodule form on a rabbit's skin at a spot from which the chemical agent inducing it has long since been gone, and to follow the nodule as it grows, and only too often becomes a destructive epidermal cancer. What can be the why for these happenings?
>
> Every tumor is made up of cells that have been so singularly changed as to no longer obey the fundamental law whereby the cellular constituents of an organism exist in harmony and act together to maintain it. Instead the changed cells multiply at its expense and inflict damage that can be mortal. We term the lawless cells neoplastic because they form new tissue, and the growth itself is a neoplasm; but on looking into medical dictionaries, hoping for more information, we are told, in effect, that *neoplastic* means "of or pertaining to a neoplasm," and turning to *neoplasm* learn that it is "a growth which consists of neoplastic cells." Ignorance could scarcely be more stark.
>
> The chemical and physical initiators ordinarily are called *carcinogens;* but this is a misleading term because they not only induce the malignant epithelial growths known as carcinomas but also other neoplasms of widely various kinds. In this chapter the less often used term oncogenes will be used, meaning "thereby capable of producing a tumor." It hews precisely to the fact....
>
> What can be the nature of the generality of neoplastic changes, the reason for their persistence; for their irreversibility; and for the discontinuous, steplike alterations that they frequently undergo? A favorite explanation has been that oncogenes cause alterations in the genes of the body—somatic mutations as these are termed. But numerous facts, when taken together, decisively exclude this supposition.[326]

Rous, it turned out, was unequivocally wrong about oncogenes. Theodor Boveri[53] was right. In 1914 he used his studies of normal mitosis in sea urchins and worms as a platform for suggesting that cancer might be caused by the abnormal gain or loss of chromosomes and their function. In a 1929 English translation of his 1926 book, *The Origin of Malignant Tumors,* Boveri wrote:

> The unlimited tendency to rapid proliferation in malignant tumor cells [could result] from a permanent predominance of the chromosomes that promote division.... Another possibility [to explain cancer] is the presence of definite chromosomes which inhibit division.... Cells of tumors with unlimited growth would arise if those "inhibiting chromosomes" were eliminated ... [since] each kind of chromosome is represented twice in the normal cell, the depression of only one of these two might pass unnoticed.[53]

Boveri predicted that the genetic abnormalities leading to the development of cancer are of two sorts: growth-promoting genes and growth-suppressing genes. If the growth-promoting genes are excessive in number or activity, they lead to cell proliferation. If, however, the growth-suppressing genes are defective in amount or activity, they fail to halt cell proliferation and lead to unbridled cell replication (Fig. 1.29). These growth-promoting genes are called *oncogenes.* The growth-suppressing genes are called *tumor-suppressor genes.*

We may think of oncogenes and tumor-suppressor genes as analogous to the accelerator pedal and the brake pedal of an automobile. The car can move forward when it is idling with the transmission in drive either by pushing on the accelerator

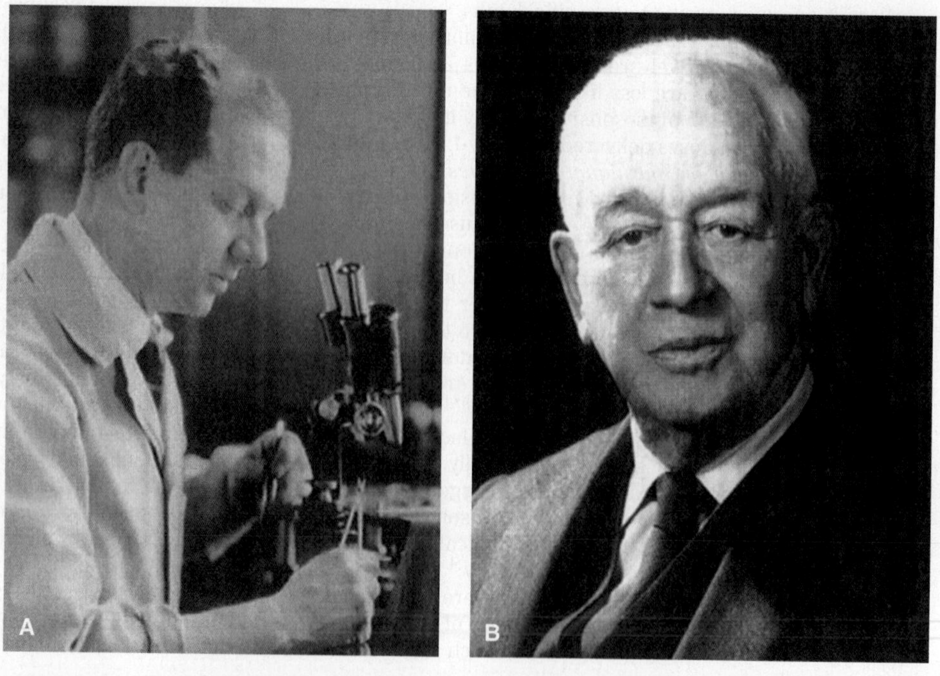

FIGURE 1.28. Peyton Rous won the Nobel Prize in 1966 for experiments he began in 1910. He demonstrated that a sarcoma could be transmitted from one chicken to another via a very small carcinogenic agent–a virus. (**A:** Rous as a young investigator; **B:** At the time of the receipt of the Noble Prize) (From Weinberg RA. *The biology of cancer.* New York: Garland Science, Taylor and Francis Group, 2007.)

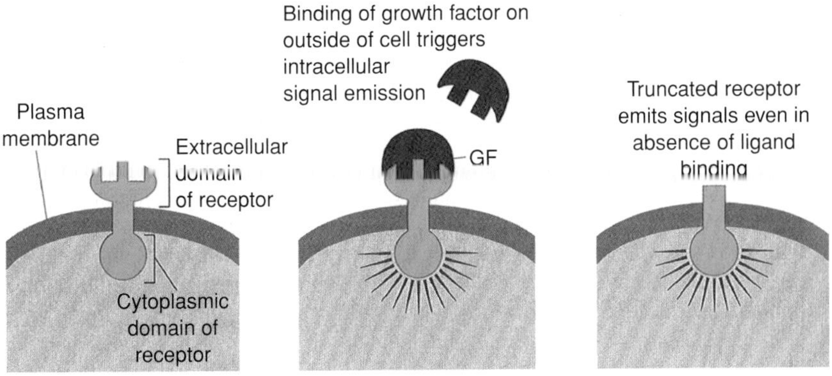
Binding of growth factor on
outside of cell triggers
intracellular
signal emission
Plasma
membrane
Extracellular
domain
of receptor
GF
Truncated receptor
emits signals even in
absence of ligand
binding
Cytoplasmic
domain of
receptor

FIGURE 1.29. Oncogenes can act in multiple ways. One method is for a growth factor receptor, which ordinarily is only active when it binds to a ligand, to become active all the time even in the absence of a growth factor binding to it. This is called "being constitutively active" and is the result of an oncogenic mutation. (From Weinberg RA. *The biology of cancer.* New York: Garland Science, Taylor and Francis Group, 2007.)

pedal, by taking pressure off the brake pedal, or by doing both simultaneously. Similarly, cell growth and proliferation, leading to cancer, can occur either by the activity of the oncogenes or inactivity of the suppressor genes.

There are clearly a wide variety of physiologic conditions that call for the effective use of growth-promoting and growth-suppressing genes. There must be a mechanism to cause the fetus to grow and then, at the appropriate time, to restrain growth. There must be a way of causing fibroblasts to proliferate to heal a wound and then, at the appropriate time, halt the fibroblasts (except in the case of keloid formation). Uncontrolled cell growth, or cancer, may be thought of as a set of physiologic controls of cell growth gone awry.

Oncogenes

The experiments that initially identified oncogenes were based largely on transformed retroviruses in transplantable tumors in chickens, mice, and rats.[257] Oncogenes were described as the genetic material carried by RNA tumor viruses that resulted in rapid malignant transformation of target cells. The name oncogene was given to virus-encoded single genes that alone or in combination with other genes induced a transformed phenotype in affected cells.[38]

The definition of an oncogene (from the Greek *onkos,* a "mass" or "tumor") is still under debate. Many oncogenes are those found in retroviruses. However, not all cellular genes capable of transforming cells have been identified within the genome of known retroviruses. It is accepted that an oncogene is a gene capable of contributing directly to the conversion of a normal cell to a tumorigenic one and that a proto-oncogene is a cellular gene convertible to an oncogene by various molecular mechanisms: sequence mutations, gene amplification, chromosomal translocation, viral transduction, and insertional mutagenesis. In general, these perturbations result in two net effects: altered regulation or augmented expression of an oncogene through mutation or rearrangement of the nucleotide sequences that constitute signals for control of transcription, messenger RNA (mRNA) processing, and stability via insertion of a strong foreign promoter or by increased gene dosage; and altered biochemical function or ectopic expression of a protein product as a result of a mutation or translocation within the protein-coding region of the oncogene. Proto-oncogene products are involved in the regulation of normal cellular growth and differentiation.

A large number of viral oncogenes have been identified. In addition, oncogenes have been identified that are not associated with RNA tumor viruses but are recognized either by their activity in transformation or by their association with chromosome translocations.[326] When DNA-probing techniques were used, it was found that sequences homologous to the oncogene region of the virus were present in the DNA of all tissues of virus-free chickens. The normal cellular sequences are proto-oncogenes.[427] The oncogene carried by a virus is referred to as *v-onc,* whereas the proto-oncogene is referred to as *c-onc.* In the normal cell the expression of proto-oncogene is well controlled and appears to play a role in the growth and development of the organism. The function of some of these genes has been determined, whereas for others a close association between cell proliferation and gene expression has been established.

Stimulation of a nonmalignant cell into a proliferative state often depends on an external signal, which is received by a receptor on the cell membrane and transferred through the membrane into the cytoplasm and ultimately to the nucleus where DNA synthesis is initiated. Proto-oncogenes have been found that function at each step of this pathway. The *erb*-B oncogene is homologous to the gene encoding for cell membrane receptor of epidermal growth factor (EGF). The interaction of EGF with this receptor reduces the proliferation of epidermal cells such as breast epithelium.

Strong evidence suggests that malignancy induction may be associated with genetic changes in the cell. Examples of this are the finding of specific chromosome abnormalities in malignant cells, association of tumor development with DNA-damaging agents such as ionizing irradiation and chemical carcinogens, and increasing incidence of cancer in hereditary diseases such as xeroderma pigmentosum. It is recognized that oncogenes are normal cellular genes that may contribute to the development of the malignant cell if their expression is altered through mutation, translocation, amplification, or some other mechanism. Evidence suggests that several genetic changes are needed to produce a cancer cell, and oncogene studies support this concept.

Chromosome translocations occur at a high frequency in some types of tumors, suggesting that they may play a role in their development. Examples of translocations are the t(9;22) Philadelphia chromosome in chronic myelogenous leukemia (CML), the t(15;17) in promyelocytic leukemia, and several translocations involving chromosome 8 seen in lymphatic malignancies. Common sites of translocations in malignant cells are frequently near an oncogene.[386] Those translocations such as the t(9;22) in CML can result in the formation of a new protein that is intimately involved in the tumorigenic transformation of the cell. In the CML example, the *ber*-gene is translocated next to the *abl*-oncogene, forming the new *bcr-abl* gene. The proteinaceous product of this newly formed gene is a hyperactive protein kinase that provides permanent growth signals to the cell.

Role of Proto-Oncogenes in Normal and Transformed Cells

Proto-oncogenes are genes with apparent oncogenic potential, and because they are apparently present in all animals, it is speculated that some kind of activation of proto-oncogenes could be associated with the initiation and progression of neoplasia. Activated oncogenes are detected in a large percentage of human tumors, suggesting a prominent role of these genes in their development; association between activated oncogenes and neoplastic diseases must have some kind of specificity for both the oncogene and the tumor.

Proto-oncogenes can be activated by genetic changes that affect either protein expression or structure. As succinctly stated by Weinberg:

> The somatic mutations that caused proto-oncogene activation could be divided into two categories—those that caused changes in the structure of encoded proteins and those that led to elevated, deregulated expression of these proteins. Mutations affecting structure included the point mutations affecting ras proto-oncogenes and the chromosomal translocations that yielded hybrid genes such as bcr–abl. Elevated expression could be achieved in human tumors through gene amplification or chromosomal translocations, such as those that place the myc gene under the control of immunoglobulin enhancer sequences....
>
> Gene amplification occurs through preferential replication of a segment (the amplicon) of chromosomal DNA. The result may be repeating end-to-end linear arrays of the segment, which appear as homogeneously staining regions (HSRs) of a chromosome when viewed under the light microscope. Alternatively, the region carrying the amplified segment may break away from the chromosome and can be seen as small, independently replicating, extra-chromosomal particles (double minutes). Gene amplification does not always result in overexpression of the gene....
>
> A variety of structural changes in proteins can also lead to oncogene activation. Examples include alterations in the structure of growth factor receptors (such as the EGF receptor) and translocations that fuse two distinct reading frames to yield a hybrid protein (such as Bcr-Abl). Both types of alterations deregulate the proteins, causing them to emit growth-promoting signals in a strong, unremitting fashion.[494]

Oncogene protein products can be grouped into several classes depending on their location and reactivity: nuclear, cytoplasmic, and membrane protein kinases; cytoplasmic guanosine triphosphate–binding proteins; growth factors; and others. The protein products of the proto-oncogenes *src, abl,* and *ras* are cytoplasmic in location. The proto-oncogene products of *myc, fos, ski,* and *myb* are nuclear in location and are believed to play an important role in the control of cell division. The expression of these genes may be responsible for the entry of the cell into DNA synthesis. Growth factors are proteins that act at the cell surface to stimulate cell growth.

Current evidence suggests that *ras* oncogenes contribute to both initiation and progression of human neoplasia. The incidence of proto-oncogene amplifications in biopsy specimens from tumors, although highly variable, is usually low. However, there may be a tendency toward association of amplification of specific proto-oncogenes and particular types of tumors. Amplifications of the c-*erb*-B-2/*neu* proto-oncogene (also referred to as *her*-2) may be involved in the etiology of human breast, salivary gland, and ovarian cancers and might serve as a useful prognostic marker for these malignancies.[410] Slamon et al.[411] observed that the *erb*-B-2/*neu* locus is amplified in 30% of primary breast carcinomas and that amplification is associated with a worse prognosis.

Amplification of another proto-oncogene, C-*myc,* occurs mainly in adenocarcinomas, squamous cell carcinomas, and sarcomas but not in hematologic malignancies, whereas N-*myc* amplification occurs most frequently in neuroblastomas and occasionally in retinoblastomas and a few small-cell lung carcinomas.

Tumor-Suppressor Genes

The concept that a gene product could inhibit or suppress proliferation of cells in a tumor was derived from experiments using somatic cell genetics.[207] Different chromosomes from normal human cells carry tumor suppression genes that are able to block tumor formation by the cancer cell. The cancer cells must sustain mutation in both alleles of these genes to develop the ability to produce tumors.[267]

These somatic cell genetic experiments relied on cell fusion. In the first type of experiment, a cancerous cell that was able to form a tumor in an animal was fused with a normal cell. The hybrid cell no longer produced tumors in animals. One could conclude that there was an element in the normal cell that was able to suppress the tumorigenic potential of the cancerous cell. It was found that, on occasion, one of the hybrid cell lines produced by fusion of cancerous and normal cells was tumorigenic. Why? These malignant cell lines were missing genetic material supplied by the normal parent cells. Further investigation identified the presence of tumor-suppressing genes from the normal parent. Eventually, several specific tumor-suppressor genes were identified and named.

The next important part of the story of tumor-suppressor genes comes from studies of the ocular tumor of infancy—retinoblastoma. Retinoblastoma can be either unilateral and unifocal or bilateral and multifocal. The disease also can be heritable or nonheritable based on the presence of a positive family history. In a classic study, Alfred Knudson[250] noted that heritable retinoblastoma was more often bilateral and multifocal and occurred in younger children rather than nonheritable unilateral retinoblastoma, which occurred in older children. Knudson postulated that there was a gene that renders children susceptible to retinoblastoma. Patients with early-onset bilateral, multifocal disease inherit one defective copy of this gene and one normal allele. With a very high frequency, mutations develop in the normal allele, and children develop the tumor. However, patients with nonheritable retinoblastoma inherit two normal alleles. Only if two independent mutations develop in the same gene, completely obliterating the function of that gene, will a cancer arise.

Knudson concluded that it requires two genetic injuries in two alleles to produce retinoblastoma. This is called the "Knudson two hit" hypothesis. The hypothesis predicts that if only one of the two gene copies remains active, there is sufficient growth suppression activity to keep the cell normal. Only if both copies are inactivated is there sufficient loss of genetic activity to allow unbridled cell proliferation. The retinoblastoma gene, *Rb,* was isolated on the long arm of chromosome 13. Because the short arm of chromosomes is abbreviated as p and the long arm as q, the deletion of the *Rb* gene is abbreviated as 13q-.

How could one find tumor-suppressor genes when their existence was most apparent by their absence? Robert Weinberg explains:

> The dominantly acting oncogenes, in stark contrast, could be detected far more readily through their presence in a retrovirus genome, through the transfection-focus assay, or through their presence in a chromosomal segment that repeatedly undergoes gene amplification in a number of independently arising tumors....
>
> A more general strategy was required that did not depend on the chance observation of interstitial chromosomal deletions or the presence of a known gene ... that, through good fortune, lay near a tumor suppressor gene on a chromosome. Both of these conditions greatly facilitated the isolation of the Rb gene. In general, however, the searches for most tumor suppressor genes were not favored by such strokes of good luck.
>
> The tendency of tumor suppressor genes to undergo LOH [loss of heterozygosity] during tumor development provided cancer researchers with a novel genetic strategy for tracking them down. Since the chromosomal region flanking a tumor suppressor gene seemed to undergo LOH together with the tumor suppressor gene itself, one might be able to detect the existence of a still-uncloned tumor suppressor gene simply from the fact that an anonymous genetic marker lying nearby on the chromosome repeatedly undergoes LOH during the development of a specific type of human tumor.
>
> The use of more powerful mapping techniques allowed geneticists to plant polymorphic markers more densely along the genetic maps of each chromosomal arm. Within a given

TABLE 1.11 PROPERTIES OF PROTO-ONCOGENES AND TUMOR-SUPPRESSOR GENES

Property	*Proto-Oncogenes*	*Tumor-Suppressor Genes*
Number of mutational events required to contribute to the cancer	One	Two
Function of the mutant allele	Gain of function, acts in a dominant fashion	Loss of function, acts in a recessive fashion
Mutant allele may be inherited through the germ line	No examples at this time	Frequently has an inherited form
Somatic mutation contributes to cancer	Yes	Yes
Tissue specificity of mutational event	Some, but can act in many tissues	Inherited form commonly has a tissue preference

From Levine AJ. Tumor suppressor genes. In: Mendelsohn J, Howley PM, Israel MA, et al., eds. *The molecular basis of cancer.* Philadelphia: W.B. Saunders, 1995:86–104.

chromosomal arm, some markers were found to undergo LOH far more frequently than others. Clearly, the closer these markers were to a sought-after tumor gene (i.e., the tighter the genetic linkage), the higher was the probability that such markers would undergo LOH together with the tumor suppressor gene. Conversely, markers located further away on a chromosomal arm were less likely to LOH together with the tumor suppressor gene. To date, genetic analyses of DNAs prepared from various types of human tumors have revealed a large number of chromosomal regions that frequently suffer LOH. A subset of these regions have yielded to the attacks of the gene cloners, resulting in the isolation of more than 30 tumor suppressor genes.[494]

A number of distinctions separate the oncogenes from the tumor-suppressor genes (Table 1.11). It is almost certain that, in most human cancers, there is a multistep pathway to tumor development, which involves the accumulation of mutations in a series of oncogenes and suppressor genes.[267]

Over 30 tumor-suppressor genes have been cloned (APC, BRCA, DCC, MLM, NF1, NF2, Rb, p53, VHL, and WT1). The suppressor p53 gene resides in 20 kilobase (kb) of DNA located in chromosome 17p13.1. The gene is a nuclear phosphoprotein composed of 393 amino acid residues in humans.[267] p53 mutations have been detected in a wide variety of malignant human tumors. The p53 gene encompasses 16 to 20 kb of DNA on the short arm of human chromosome 17. Loss of normal p53 function is associated with cell transformation *in vitro* and development of neoplasms *in vivo.* Abrogation of the normal p53 pathway is a common feature in human cancers, and it appears to be critical in the pathogenesis and progression of these tumors.[73] In some cases, candidate tumor-suppressor genes have been identified based on an association between loss or inactivation and tumor development, the causal connection being only inferred.

Cell-Cycle Control

The cell cycle, which consists of four phases (G1, S, G2, and M), regulates the duplication of genetic information and distribution of duplicated chromosomes to daughter cells. The phrases "cell-cycle control" or "cell-cycle clock" are used to describe the cell's molecular circuits operating in the nucleus that process and integrate afferent signals and decide if the cell will actively proliferate or remain quiescent. If the "go/no go" decision is to "go" into proliferation, the circuitry is engaged to launch the biochemical changer necessary to allow the cell to double its contents and divide into two daughter cells. Key providers of the afferent information are tyrosine kinase receptors, G-protein-coupled receptors, transforming growth factor-β receptors, integrins, and the cell's nutritional status[494] (Fig. 1.30).

The Nobel Prize in Physiology or Medicine for 2001 was awarded to Leland H. Hartwell, R. Timothy Hunt, and Sir Paul M. Nurse for their discoveries regarding the control of the cell cycle. The Nobel presentation speech by Professor Anders Zetterberg succinctly describes the important controls of cell replication elucidated by these three scientists.

> Cell division is a fundamental process of life. All living organisms on earth are descended from an ancestral cell that appeared about 3 billion years ago, and which has undergone an unbroken series of cell divisions since then. Each human being also began life as one single cell—a cell

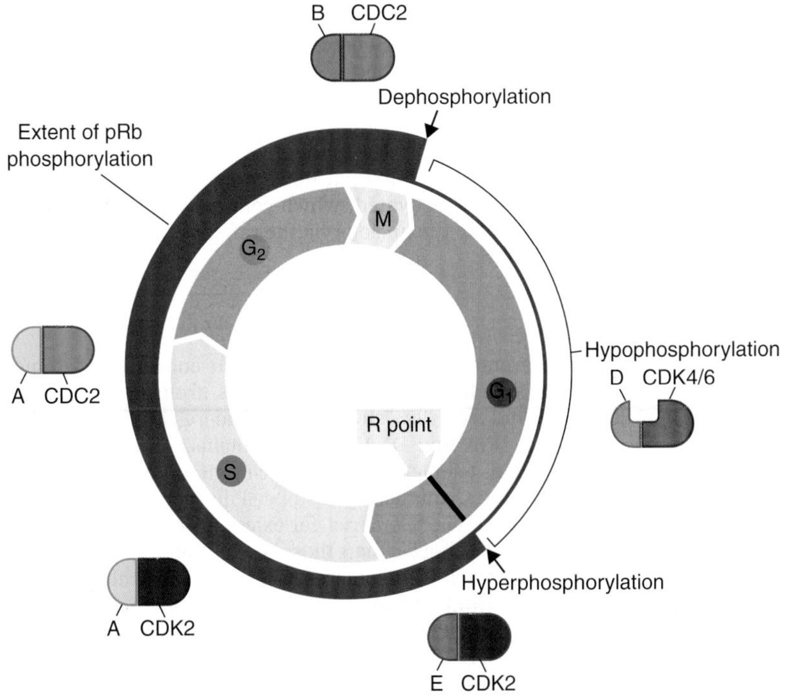

FIGURE 1.30. The phosphorylation of the retinoblastoma gene product protein, depicted as the red circle, helps to control the cell cycle. As the cell moves from M to G1, the protein is unphosphorylated; as the cell progresses through G1, the protein is hypophosphorylated; and after passing the R point (the restriction point), it is hyperphosphorylated. This process of phosphorylation is controlled by cyclins. (From Weinberg RA. *The biology of cancer.* New York: Garland Science, Taylor and Francis Group, 2007.)

that divided repeatedly to give rise to all one hundred thousand billion cells that we consist of.... Every second millions of cells divide in our body.

The cycle of events that a cell completes from one division to the next is called the cell cycle. During the cell cycle the cell grows in size, duplicates its hereditary material—that is, it copies the DNA molecules in the chromosomes—and divides into two daughter cells.

This year's Nobel Laureates have discovered the key regulators of the cell cycle—cyclin dependent kinase (CDK) and cyclin. Together these two components form an enzyme, in which CDK is comparable to a "molecular engine" that drives the cell through the cell cycle by altering the structure and function of other proteins in the cell. Cyclin is the main switch that turns the "CDK engine" on and off. This cell-cycle engine operates in the same way in such widely disparate organisms as yeast cells, plants, animals, and humans.

How were the key regulators CDK and cyclin discovered? Lee Hartwell realized the great potential of genetic methods for cell-cycle studies. He chose baker's yeast as a model organism. In the microscope he could identify genetically altered cells—mutated cells—that stopped in the cell cycle when they were cultured at an elevated temperature. Using this method Hartwell discovered, in the early 1970s, dozens of genes specific to the cell-division cycle, which he named CDC genes. One of these genes, CDC28, controls the initiation of each cell cycle, the "start" function. Hartwell also formulated the concept of "checkpoints," which ensure that cell-cycle events occur in the correct order. Checkpoints are comparable to the program in a washing machine that checks if one step has been properly completed before the next can start. Checkpoint defects are considered to be one of the reasons behind the transformation of normal cells into cancer cells.

Paul Nurse also used the genetic approach in his cell-cycle studies but in a different kind of yeast. In the late 1970s and early 1980s he discovered the gene CDC2, which could be mutated in two different ways. Either the cells did not divide, or they divided too early. From this he correctly concluded that CDC2 controls cell division. He later discovered that CDC2 not only controls cell division, the final event of the cell cycle; it also has a key regulatory function for the whole cell cycle, including that described for CDC28 in baker's yeast. This key function was shown to be that of CDK in the cell-cycle engine. By moving human genes into yeast cells, in 1987 Nurse isolated a human CDC2 gene. This human CDC2 gene functioned perfectly in yeast cells. Thus, the CDK function in the cell-cycle engine had been conserved through more than 1 billion years of evolution—from yeast to man.

Tim Hunt discovered the other key component of the cell-cycle engine, the protein cyclin, which regulates the function of the CDK molecule. Working with sea urchin eggs as a model organism, in 1982 he discovered a specific protein that increased in amount before cell division but disappeared abruptly when the cells divided. Because of these cyclic variations, he named the protein cyclin. These experiments not only led to the discovery of cyclin, but also demonstrated the existence of periodic protein degradation in the cell cycle—a fundamental control mechanism. Hunt also showed the existence of cyclins in other, unrelated species. Thus cyclins, like CDK, had been conserved during evolution.

It is now almost 50 years since the structure of the DNA molecule—the double helix—was discovered, leading to a molecular explanation of how a gene can make a copy of itself. With the discoveries of CDK and cyclin we are now beginning to understand, at the molecular level, how the cell can make a copy of itself.[326]

To ensure that the daughter cells possess a full complement of genetic information, checkpoints exist to ensure fidelity of DNA duplication and accuracy of chromosome segregation.[312] Checkpoint pauses permit editing and repair of genetic information so that each daughter cell receives a full complement of genetic information identical to the parent cell (see Fig. 1.30). In some cells, there are checkpoints for initiation of mitosis. Mutation of the checkpoint genes allows the cell to enter mitosis after x-irradiation.[313] For example, the rad-9 gene is a G2/M checkpoint gene because it responds to two different types of signals.[314] Experimental observations suggest that the p53 gene, shown to be a transcriptional activator,[366] may be critical for G1 checkpoint control. p53 has been shown to induce transcription of p21, which in turn inhibits the association of CDK 4,6 with proliferating cell nuclear antigen and cyclin D. As a consequence, the retinoblastoma protein cannot be phosphorylated and stays in complex with the transcription factor E2 F, effectively blocking the transcription of cell-cycle-promoting proteins and causing a cell-cycle arrest.

Checkpoints are signal-transduction systems that must receive a signal, amplify it, and transmit it to other components that regulate the cell cycle. Double-strand DNA breaks, unexcised ultraviolet light-induced dimers in DNA, and centromeres not engaged by the spindle are potential signals.[36,209] Checkpoints ensure the fidelity of genomic replication and segregation. Biologically significant levels of spontaneous damage require checkpoint control for cells to maintain a high fidelity of chromosome transmission. Therefore, restoration of compromised checkpoints could slow cancer cell evolution even in the absence of exogenous sources of DNA damage.[209] Many signal-transduction systems, including checkpoint controls, exhibit adaptation; that is, in the presence of a constant stimulus, the response diminishes with time. As a consequence, the cell may proceed through the cell cycle, although the original perturbation has not been removed or cannot be repaired.[223] Checkpoint activation may induce a variety of cell responses, including cell death. The checkpoint controlling entry into S phase in mammalian cells includes p53. One function under the control of this pathway is apoptosis. Restoration of defective checkpoints could restore the apoptotic response of cancer cells and increase their sensitivity to DNA-damaging agents. It may be possible to achieve specificity for certain types of cancer cells because not all cells respond to the same apoptotic signals.[504,518,519]

Growth Factors and Signal Transduction

Transmission of biochemical signals to the cellular nucleus leads to altered expression of a wide variety of genes involved in microgenic and differentiation responses.[417] A number of growth factors exert their effects through receptors possessing intrinsic protein tyrosine kinase activity. On activation, these receptors phosphorylate both themselves and other intracellular proteins on the amino acid tyrosine. Among the receptors for growth factors are epidermal growth factor, platelet-derived growth factor, insulin, nerve growth factor, and macrophage colony stimulatory factor. The mitogenic signaling pathway activated by protein tyrosine kinase receptors involves the activation of ras proteins. Ras undergoes conformational change and interacts with additional downstream targets. A protein kinase cascade is activated, which conveys the growth factor–initiated signal to the nucleus via the raf, mek, map kinase, and other proteins.

Telomeres

Human chromosomes are linear. At each end of the chromosome are structures known as telomeres, from the Greek *telo* for "end" and *mere* for "structure." Telomeres are composed of specialized DNA and DNA-binding proteins. As chromosomes are replicated, telomeres shorten each time during the process of cell division. Continued cycles of cell division result in shortened telomeres. The telomeres, for example, in the fibroblasts of older adults are shorter than those in children. Normal human cells senesce when the telomeres shorten to a critical length.

Stem cells and cancer cells must maintain their telomere lengths to prevent senescence. Two mechanisms of telomere maintenance have been identified: expression of the telomerase enzyme, and the recombination of telomeres.

The telomere hypothesis states that critical telomere shortening prevents somatic cells from dividing. In contrast, the maintenance of telomere length allows cancer cells to continue to divide. An increasing body of experimental evidence supports the telomere hypothesis and its association with cancer.

The capacity of cells to respond to ionizing radiation is determined by multiple factors. There are a variety of syndromes associated with molecular defects that are characterized by clinical radiosensitivity. These include ataxia, telangiectasia, Nijmegen breakage syndrome, and ataxia telangiectasia–like disorder. These syndromes all have defective telomere maintenance in common. It has been hypothesized, therefore, that the radiosensitivity phenotype and the telomere dysfunction phenotype may be linked. A variety of experimental models suggest that telomere maintenance and radiosensitivity are associated, and this may offer the opportunity for a therapeutic target.

Apoptosis

Apoptosis or programmed cell death, a phenomenon distinct from necrosis, was described in 1972 by Kerr et al.[248] Apoptosis is programmed by specific signals in the cell that cause an endonuclease to cleave DNA at internucleosomal sites.

Apoptosis is detected by histologic evaluation of membrane blebbing and chromatin condensation, by flow cytometry using fluorescent nucleotides and terminal transferase to detect fragmented DNA, by detecting apoptotic cells that are usually very small with characteristic profiles of right-angle and forward light scattering, or by using DNA fluorochrome to detect a decrease in fluorescence as small DNA fragments diffuse from the cell that is undergoing apoptosis.[86,518,520] An early change in apoptosis, the flip-flop of the phospholipid phosphatidylserine (PS) from the inner to the outer leaflet of the bilayer membrane, also can be detected using a fluorescently labeled annexin V protein that has a high binding affinity to PS. Several oncogenes, cytokines, and growth factors have been reported to play a role in promoting or reducing radiation-induced apoptosis.[114]

Most radiation-induced cell lethality (loss of reproductive integrity) for dividing cells appears to be caused by mitotic-linked death resulting in loss of genetic information as cells with chromosomal aberrations divide. Apoptosis, frequently seen within 4 to 6 hours after irradiation, occurs spontaneously and is enhanced by radiation as observed *in vivo* in the intestinal crypt and salivary and lacrimal glands with nondividing cells and nondividing lymphocytes. Apoptotic cells are eliminated rapidly *in vivo,* making it difficult to quantify. In contrast, this cell death mechanism is easy to quantify *in vitro* because apoptotic cells persist in culture for many hours. However, cell division of nonapoptotic cells complicates quantification.[114] In cell lines susceptible to apoptosis, this process sometimes occurs early before cells enter mitosis or later after the cells divide. Late apoptosis may be associated with mitotically linked death and, in fact, may be triggered by chromosomal aberrations. Apoptosis may be quite important for clinically relevant doses of fractionated irradiation, even if it causes a relatively small reduction in clonogenic survival. However, this requires that cells be recruited into the apoptotic-susceptible fraction after each dose fraction.

It appears that with progression of certain tumors, spontaneous and therapy-related apoptosis occurs less frequently. The apoptotic response to irradiation can be modified by cytokines to protect normal tissues[171] or to induce tumor cell killing.[197,214,215] Tumor necrosis factor increases apoptosis after irradiation in some tumors while protecting the hematopoietic compartment, possibly by blocking apoptosis.[321] Irradiation prevents extensive cellular proliferation by increasing differentiation in both tumors and normal tissues. Also, irradiation appears to increase the aging of normal cells. Another mechanism of reversible loss of proliferative capacity induced by irradiation is necrosis, which occurs with high doses of irradiation and is a major mechanism seen with large dose fractions such as in stereotactic irradiation.

THE BIOLOGY OF METASTASIS

The prefix *meta* is of Greek origin and is defined as "after," "beyond," or "over." It is used to denote change or transformation. The word *stasis* means "stand" or "stationary." Thus, when the two words are combined to form *metastasis,* the new word is used to represent a change in location of a disease or its manifestations. It also means the transfer of a disease from one organ or body part to another organ or body part not directly connected. The oncologist uses the term *metastasis* to refer to the manifestation of malignancy that arises from the primary growth but is now in a secondary site.

It is clear that the pattern of metastatic spread of cancer is not random. The distribution of some secondary tumor deposits can be explained on mechanistic grounds (i.e., that the tumor cells are shed into the bloodstream and lodge in the first narrow capillary network that they encounter downstream). This would explain, for example, why the liver is the most common site for secondary tumors in patients with primary cancer within the catchment area of the hepatic portal vein, such as gastrointestinal malignancies. Similarly, the lung would be a favored site in patients with primary tumor spilling into the systemic veins. There can be no doubt that vascular drainage patterns influence the distribution of secondary tumor deposits from some types of primary cancer.

It is also clear, however, that the distribution of some metastatic tumors cannot be explained solely by patterns of encountering and lodging in the nearest narrow capillary bed. This is called "metastatic tropism": carcinomas form detectable metastases in only a limited subset of possible distant organ sites. The seminal paper addressing this problem was by Stephen Paget (1855–1926). Paget was the fourth and youngest son of the famous British physician Sir James Paget. Stephen Paget worked as an assistant surgeon at the West London and Metropolitan Hospitals in England. Later in life, he devoted himself to public health issues and became a highly regarded biographer and essayist.[341] Writing in the *Lancet* on March 23, 1889, on "The Distribution of Secondary Growth in Cancer of the Breast," Paget wondered:

> The question ought to be asked, and if possible answered: "What is it that decides what organs shall suffer in a case of disseminated cancer?" If the remote organs in such a case are all alike passive and, so to speak, helpless—all equally ready to receive and nourish any particle of the primary growth which may "slip through the lungs," and so be brought to them—then the distribution of cancer throughout the body must be a matter of chance. But if we can trace any sort of rule or sequence in the distribution of cancer, any relation between the character of the primary growth and the situation of the secondary growths derived from it, then the remote organs cannot be altogether passive or indifferent as regards embolism.... Every single cancer cell must be regarded as an organism, alive and capable of development. When a plant goes to seed, its seeds are carried in all directions; but they can only live and grow if they fall on congenial soil.[342]

Paget observed, in a large number of autopsies of women with breast cancer, that the lymph nodes, liver, lung, bone, and brain commonly were involved. However, he found that the kidney and spleen rarely were involved despite receiving a significant amount of blood flow. He was struck by the discrepancy between the relative blood supplies and the relative frequencies of metastatic tumors in various organs. From his data, Paget expounded his "seed and soil hypothesis." He argued that metastasis required both a willing seed (intrinsic cellular factors) and hospitable soil (host organ). There must be intrinsic cellular factors that lead to a satisfactory interaction between the tumor cell and the host organ resulting in successful metastasis. In contemporary terms, we understand this to mean that the tumor cell must have favorable adhesion molecules, and the host organ must be accepting receptors on its endothelial cells, which results in appropriate sites for the circulating tumor cells to bind, migrate into the organ, and subsequently grow, or, perhaps, that tumor cells promote up-regulation of adhesion receptors in specific stromal cells.

Metastasis formation is an inefficient process. Fidler and colleagues[148] injected melanoma cells into the peripheral vein of a mouse whose DNA had been labeled with radioactive iodine. They found that, shortly after the injection, most of the injected cells rested in the lung (i.e., the nearest narrow capillary bed). Most of the tumor cells, however, went on to die in the lung. Only a few live cells continued to circulate. Within a day, only 1% of the injected cells were alive, and after 2 weeks, no known metastasis could be seen in the lungs. Only 0.1% of the cells originally injected were still alive.[148] Bloodborne metastasis must be a highly selective process. Only a very small proportion of malignant cells that enter into the bloodstream are able to survive and grow.

There are three major pathways of metastasis. They are:

- Across body cavities such as the peritoneal cavity or within the cerebrospinal fluid. This is the way, for example, that medulloblastoma disseminates via the leptomeninges or that ovarian tumors form on the peritoneal surface of the intestine.
- Via the lymphatic system. Axillary masses following breast cancer, that are easily palpable, would be a common example.
- Hematogenously, usually via veins rather than arteries. The spread of a limb sarcoma to the lungs would be an example (Fig. 1.31).

The molecular mechanism of tumor metastasis is a multistep process involving many tumor cells—host–cell interactions as well as cell–matrix associations.[427] This process is sometimes called the invasion-metastasis cascade. The crucial processes are as follows:

- Tumor cell adhesion to other tumor cells at the site of the primary malignancy, host cells, or components of the extracellular matrix;
- Proteolysis of the extracellular matrix during invasion;
- Tumor cell motility through the extracellular matrix to reach the vascular or lymphatic endothelium;
- Intravasation into the lumina of blood vessels or lymphatics—this is facilitated by molecular changes that promote the ability of carcinoma cells to cross the pericytes and endothelial cell barriers;
- Embolism into the lymphatic system and/or the blood circulation;
- Tumor cell survival despite both the mechanical trauma endured by the cell in transit in the vascular system as well as the body's immunologic assault directed against the circulating tumor cell (insofar as most tumor cells have a diameter of 20 to 30 μm and capillaries have a diameter of ~ 8 μm, most tumor cells in circulation are probably quickly trapped in capillary beds);
- Adherence to the endothelium when the tumor cell comes to rest at the metastatic site in the secondary organ;
- Dissolution of the cell–cell junction and the basement membrane of the blood vessel or lymphatic into the organ parenchyma;
- Survival in the new host organ microenvironment and interaction with that new microenvironment in the host organ to permit growth of the tumor deposit; and

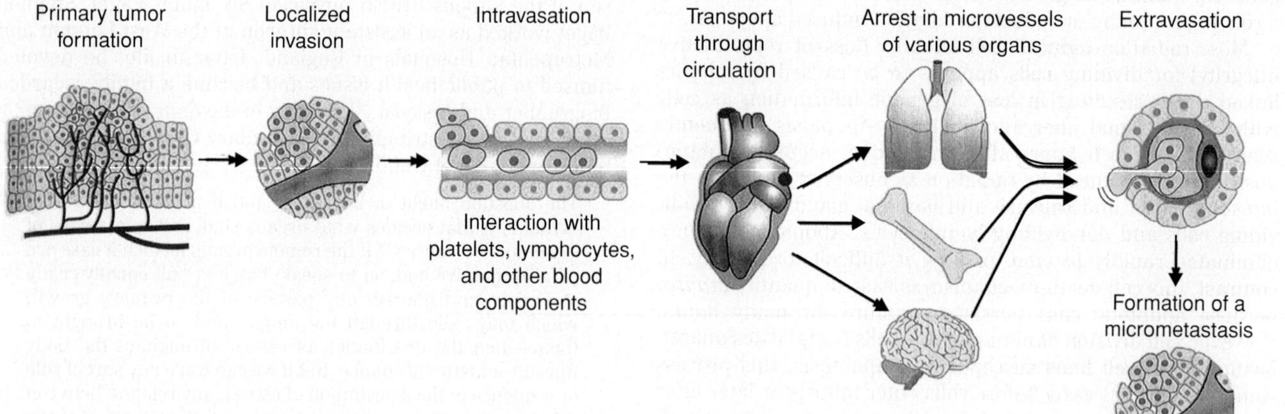

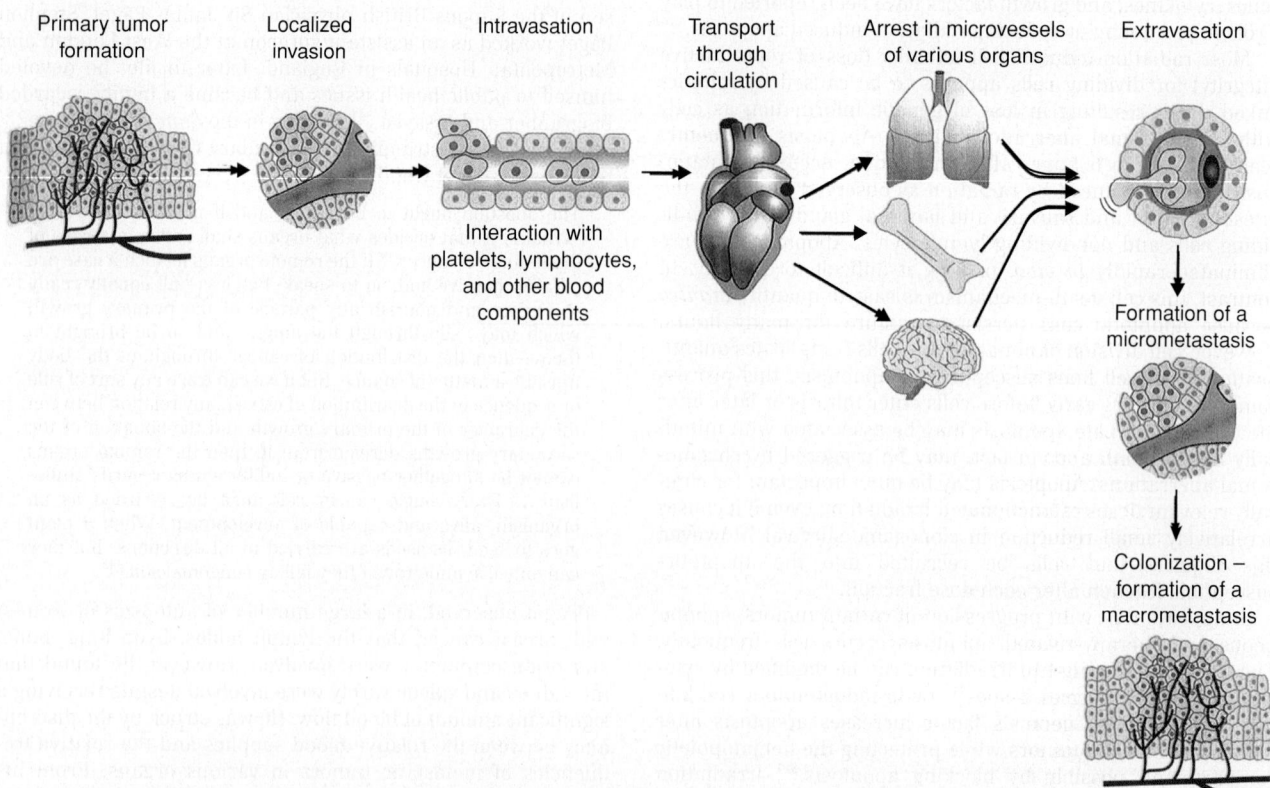

FIGURE 1.31. The development of metastasis is a multistep process that is highly inefficient. In order to form a metastasis, the tumor must breach the basement membrane and enter either a blood vessel or a lymphatic, travel through the bloodstream or the lymphatics and not be destroyed either by attack of the immune system or mechanical trauma, adhere to the endothelium at a distant anatomic site, invade the organ parenchyma, draw a blood supply into the metastatic deposit, and colonize the new organ. (From Weinberg RA. *The biology of cancer.* New York: Garland Science, Taylor and Francis Group, 2007.)

- Tumor cell proliferation in the new organ and angiogenesis to achieve metastatic colonization.

Only if all of these steps can be negotiated successfully can the tumor cell ultimately "set up shop" as a metastatic focus. The fact that only a small fraction of tumor cells survive and successfully establish a metastasis would suggest that the ultimately successful cells must be quite unusual. It would be reasonable to believe that they represent a subpopulation of tumor cells that are endowed with particular characteristics that make for successful metastasis. As the population of tumor cells evolves, it is likely that aggressive subpopulations, having diverse properties, will arise and that their frequency in the population increases under selective pressure of the host immune defenses. This will lead, ultimately, to the emergence of cells with enhanced malignancy.[427] Many people believe that tumor cells evolve via a Darwinian selection. Genetic variation continuously occurs in the tumor population and clones with a survival advantage become overrepresented. These cells have "metastasis virulence genes" enabling their spread. The successful metastatic cells will possess characteristics of neoplastic transformation—the ability to turn on an angiogenic switch, an invasive phenotype, and the capacity to evade the immune response—as well as favorable cell adhesion and motility characteristics.[154–156,467,494]

Metastatic progress involves not only the tumor's cells but also those cells' ability to recruit the aid of stromal cells. As tumors progress the stroma becomes increasingly "reactive"—akin to the tissue of wound healing or chronic inflammation.

THE MOLECULAR BIOLOGY OF THE METASTATIC PHENOTYPE AND ANGIOGENESIS

Tumor progression is the acquisition of permanent, irreversible, qualitative changes in one or more characteristics of neoplasm that ultimately will lead to the tumor becoming more autonomous and malignant.[426] A genetic analysis of the stages of tumor progression has led scientists to formulate the multistep theory of tumorigenesis. The multistep theory involves activation of oncogenes, inactivation of tumor suppression genes, and identification of many tumor-associated molecules. The metastatic phenotype appears to require cells to have the additive effect of positive modulators (oncogenes) as well as the loss of negative effectors (tumor-suppressor genes, invasion- and metastasis-suppressor genes). Thus, the molecular biology of a metastatic cell is clearly a multistep process of diversification and clonal selection for aggressive cells.

The mutated *ras* oncogene sequences, when transfected into mouse embryo-derived fibroblasts (NIH 3T3 cells), cause those transfected cells to produce numerous metastases.[509] This finding has been confirmed in both fibroblasts and epithelial cells of human and rodent origin. A number of other metastasis-associated genes have been described. These include NM23-1 and stomelysm-3 (ST-3). NM23-1 has features similar to a transcription factor and may play a role not only in *c-myc* expression but also in the response of cells to transforming growth factor-β. ST-3 is a member of the matrix proteinase family.[426]

It would be far too simplistic to conclude that the metastatic phenotype arises only from genetic alterations associated with the acquisition of aggressive tumorigenicity. Cells clearly can be transformed by oncogene transfection, but not all cells acquire a metastatic phenotype after this oncogene transfection. Simply stated, we must bear in mind that there is separation between the genetic changes that drive tumorigenicity and the metastatic phenotype. Invasion and metastasis will require the activation of additional effector genes or loss of suppressor local inhibitors above those genetic changes required for uncontrolled growth alone.

The successful development of a metastatic focus requires new blood vessel growth. Recent evidence has identified angiogenesis promoters and inhibitors that may be modified or removed during the tumor-induced angiogenic response. Tumor angiogenesis in the nascent metastasis is a tightly regulated process in a delicate balance between the pro- and antiangiogenic factors.[268]

Angiogenesis

The success of growth of a tumor is, in part, governed by a complex interplay between the tumor cells and the surrounding normal tissue. A dramatic example of this interplay is the process of tumor angiogenesis (also called tumor neovascularization).

The growth of the tumor depends on the tumor's access to nutrients and oxygen as well as its ability to eliminate metabolic waste and carbon dioxide. In very small tumors, these requirements are addressed by diffusion. As the tumor enlarges, however, diffusion is inadequate. The growing tumor requires direct access to the circulatory system.

Tumor access to the circulatory system is secured through angiogenesis, through which the tumor cells encourage the ingrowth of capillaries and larger vessels from the adjacent normal tissue. The tumor cells recruit these vessels through the release of angiogenic factors. These cause the proliferation of endothelial growth factor and, almost certainly, tissue growth factor-β. The generation of tumor vessels is the result of a delicate balance between angiogenesis-promoting factors and angiogenesis-inhibiting factors. These factors have now provided a growing body of therapeutic targets in the treatment of cancer.

Some authorities encourage us to think about the tumor as a structure composed of varied compartments including the actual clonogenic cells, a connective structure, and the blood vessels. Utilizing this way of thinking about tumors, we envision cancer treatment as striking at different components of the tumor (i.e., antiangiogenesis agents directed against the vasculature and anticlonogenic agents directed against proliferating cells). Experimental evidence suggests that, in certain tumor systems, the combination of radiation and antiangiogenic agents is a fruitful way of treating cancer. We may expect to see an increasing body of evidence for the use of combinations of radiation, chemotherapy, hormonal therapy, and antiangiogenesis agents in the coming years.

The hallmark of an invasive cancer is its ability to disrupt the epithelial basement membrane and the presence of cancer cells in the stromal compartment. It makes sense, therefore, that two broad classes of molecules have been implicated repeatedly in contributing to the metastatic ability: cell–cell adhesion molecules and motility molecules play a crucial role in the development of metastatic potential.[55] The ability of tumor cells to adhere to other tumor cells, cells of the host, or components of the extracellular matrix affect multiple components of the metastatic cascade. These interactions depend on several classes of molecules expressed on the cell surface. Cadherins are calcium-dependent molecules that mediate homophilic cell–cell adherence. Integrins are heterodimeric transmemory proteins that are formed by the noncovalent association of α- and β-subunits. The binding of the extracellular matrix ligands to integrins is known to initiate similar transduction pathways. These pathways lead to cell proliferation, differentiation, migration, or cell death. Selectins act through a terminal calcium-dependent lexon domain. They are prominently involved in heterotypic cell–cell adhesion between blood cells and endothelial cells.[65]

Tumor adherence to the extracellular matrix and cell motility is the next crucial component of the metastatic cascade. Tumor cells are able to attach to a specific lipoprotein of the extracellular matrix such as fibronectin, collagen, and laminin. These adherences are formed either through integrin or nonintegrin cell-surface receptors. CD44 is a crucial transmembrane glycoprotein

Box 1.7

Antiangiogenesis Therapy of Cancer

Tumor vessels are fundamentally different from normal blood vessels insofar as they are usually irregular and disorganized. In vessels that are leaky, hemorrhagic, or tortuous or in those containing poorly oxygenated blood that may flow backward and forward in the same vessel, tumor vasculature may provide an interesting therapeutic target. The general public and the scientific community have recently experienced a wave of considerable excitement associated with the possibility that antiangiogenesis agents may be employed clinically to disrupt tumor angiogenesis. This form of therapy may complement existing cancer treatments. Vascular endothelial growth factor (VEGF) is a key element in the stimulation of angiogenesis. VEGF binds to a receptor on endothelial cells (VEGFR), which stimulates tyrosine kinase activity, which in turn stimulates downstream signaling and activation of endothelial cells. The drugs in the therapeutic pipeline may be categorized as follows:

- Anti-VEGF agents: Some drugs prevent the binding of VEGF to its receptors. *Bevacizumab (Avastin)* is a monoclonal antibody that binds to VEGF, prevents it binding to VEGFR, and inhibits VEGFR activation. It is being utilized in the therapy of a variety of human malignancies.[179]
- Anti-VEGFR agents: Several receptors bind to VEGF: VEGFR1, VEGFR2, NRP-1, and NRP-2. VEGR2 is thought to mediate most of the angiogenic properties of VEGF and is expressed at high levels on the endothelial cells of tumor vasculature. Several monoclonal antibodies are under investigation in animal models to target the VEGF receptor.
- Receptor tyrosine kinase inhibitors: An antiangiogenesis strategy is to target the downstream activity of the binding of the VEGFR by inhibition of tyrosine kinase activity. The following drugs, now in human clinical trials, fall into this category: Cediranib or Recentin (AZD2171), Pazopanib, BIBF 1120, Sorafenib, and Sunitib (SU11248).

with a large echo domain and a single cytoplasm domain. CD44 is involved in cell adhesion to hyaluronan[416] (Box 1.7).

The potentially metastatic cell must overcome a series of tissue barriers. These include the basement membrane and connective tissue. These must be traversed by the tumor cells during the metastatic process. Five classes of naturally occurring proteinases have been associated with aggressive tumor cells and implicated in metastases. These include members of the gene family of matrix metalloproteinases. These enzymes, each of which is secreted by a proenzyme that subsequently requires activation, may be divided into three general subclasses: interstitial collagenase, type 4 collagenase (gelatinases), and stromelysins. Once having dissolved barriers, active tumor cell motility is required for the penetration of the basement membrane and the interstitial stoma. Successful migration of metastatic cells requires transition of propulsive force from the extracellular matrix to the cytoskeleton. Tumor cells exhibit amoeboid movement, which is characterized by pseudopod extension. For the protrusion and retraction of pseudopods, the network of intracellular polymerized cross-linked filaments must be disassembled and then reassembled.[427]

MANAGEMENT OF THE PATIENT WITH CANCER

The optimal care of cancer patients is a multidisciplinary effort that may combine two or more disciplines: surgery, radiation therapy, and chemotherapy. Many professionals, including physicians, physicists, laboratory scientists, nurses, rehabilitation staff, sociologists, and social workers, are intimately involved. Pathologists, radiologists, clinical laboratory physicians, and immunologists are integral members of the team that renders the correct diagnosis. Biology, biochemistry, and pharmacology have contributed greatly to the advancement of methods used to evaluate and treat cancer patients (e.g., biomarkers, cell kinetics indicators, oncogenes).

The radiation oncologist, like any other physician, must assess all conditions relative to the patient and the tumor under consideration for treatment and systematically review the need for diagnostic and staging procedures as well as the best therapeutic strategy. This has been well illustrated in a series of "decision trees" designed by the Patterns of Care Study Group for radiation therapy.[224] In several instances, a clear relationship existed between compliance with guidelines for diagnostic or therapeutic procedures (best current management consensus) and therapy outcome, as defined by survival, recurrence patterns, or complications of treatment.

Emphasis on screening and early diagnosis of cancer, as well as improvements in therapeutic strategies, has had a significant positive impact on the survival of patients with cancer. In the United States, results of the Surveillance Epidemiology and End Results program have shown a small but steady improvement in survival for a variety of tumor sites. Relative survival of patients with cancer at various times after diagnosis has improved substantially since 1960.

Combination of Therapeutic Modalities

Irradiation and Surgery

The rationale for *preoperative radiation therapy* relates to its potential ability to eradicate subclinical or microscopic disease beyond the margins of the surgical resection, to diminish tumor implantation by decreasing the number of viable cells within the operative field, to sterilize lymph node metastases outside the operative field, to decrease the potential for dissemination of clonogenic tumor cells that might produce distant metastases, and to increase the possibility of resectability. The disadvantages of preoperative irradiation are that it may interfere with normal healing of the tissues affected by the radiation, it delays surgery, and it may disrupt surgical staging of the tumor and/or the expression of histologic or immunohistochemical prognostic factors.

The rationale for *postoperative irradiation* is based on the fact that it is possible to eliminate subclinical foci of tumor cells in the tumor bed (including lymph node metastases). By delivering higher doses to the volume of high-risk or known residual disease than can be achieved with preoperative irradiation, a greater tumor control may be obtained. For example, improved survival rates have been reported in patients with head and neck tumors treated with combined therapy in comparison with surgery alone.[151]

The potential disadvantages of postoperative irradiation are related to the delay in initiation of radiation therapy until wound healing is completed. Theoretic and experimental evidence suggests that the radiation effect may be impaired by vascular changes produced in the tumor bed by surgery. Experimental data suggest that preoperative irradiation may be more effective than postoperative irradiation[392] (Fig. 1.32).

Irradiation and Chemotherapy

Tumor or *normal tissue enhancement* describes any increase in effect greater than that observed with either chemotherapy or irradiation alone.[358] Agents used in chemoirradiation include those with cytotoxic activity against the tumor, which may show additive, subadditive, or supra-additive effects, such as 5-fluorouracil or mitomycin-C in anal carcinoma; agents with minimal or no significant activity against a specific tumor, which may, however, enhance the irradiation effect; radiation hypoxic cell cytotoxins or bioreductive agents; and radioprotectors.

Chemotherapy alone or combined with irradiation may be used in several settings.[438] *Primary chemotherapy* is used as part of the primary lesion treatment (even if later followed by other local therapy) and when the primary tumor response to the initial treatment is the key identifier of systemic effects. *Adjuvant chemotherapy* is used as an adjunct to other local modalities as part of the initial curative treatment. The term *neoadjuvant chemotherapy* is used when this modality is used in the initial treatment of patients with localized tumors, before surgery or irradiation.

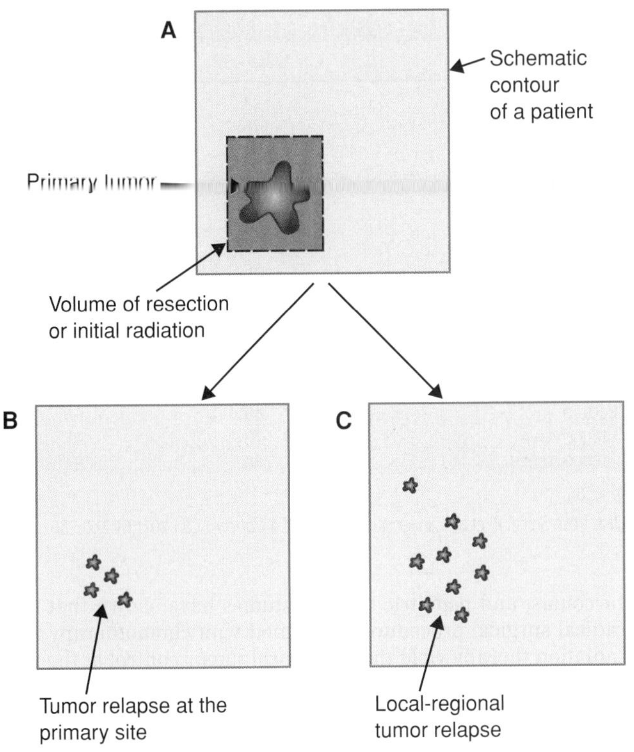

FIGURE 1.32. A: A pattern of failure analysis is useful to improve treatment of malignancies. **B:** If the tumor after surgery and/or radiotherapy tends to relapse at the primary site within the volume treated, it would suggest that the local therapy is insufficiently intense. **C:** If, however, there is a local-regional tumor relapse, it would suggest that the initial surgery or radiotherapy field size is insufficient to cover microscopic extension of disease that has the potential to be controlled. A pattern of failure as shown in panel (C) is not, by itself, sufficient to make the case for extended field radiation. One must have a pattern of failure such as that which is seen in panel (C) and also be able to show that intervention with large field irradiation can alter that pattern in a favorable manner.

The effects of combined radiation therapy–chemotherapy can be independent, additive, or interactive. Chemotherapy and irradiation can be administered sequentially or concomitantly. Sequencing of treatment at the appropriate time is significantly related to the residual tumor cell burden at the point of introduction of each new treatment program.[515]

Administration of chemotherapy before irradiation may produce cell killing and reduce the number of cells to be eliminated by the irradiation. Use of chemotherapy concurrently with radiation therapy has a strong rationale because it could interact with the local treatment (additive and even supra-additive action) and also could affect subclinical disease early in treatment. However, the combination of modalities may enhance normal tissue toxicity. When agents with added toxicity are used, lower tumor control may result because the added morbidity requires lowering the doses of the effective agents or prolonging overall irradiation treatment time. When fatal toxicity from chemotherapy occurs, it prevents some dying patients from demonstrating tumor response that could have been observed had they survived. Overall patient survival may be compromised as well.

Biologic Considerations in Combinations of Chemotherapy and Irradiation

Many experimental animal studies have shown therapeutic benefit from a combination of irradiation and drugs, but most are phenomenologic. Therapeutic benefit requires differential properties on tumor and normal tissues, which may be exploited for therapeutic gain. These include genetic instability of tumors compared with normal tissues, differences in cell proliferation (particularly cell repopulation during fractionated radiation therapy), and environmental factors such as hypoxia and acidity (which usually are confined to tumors). There are variations in sensitivity or resistance to irradiation or drugs. The mechanisms for resistance to these agents may be shared in some tumors and different in other tumors. Resistance to anticancer drugs may have implications for resistance to radiation therapy; many drug mechanisms for resistance are multifactorial, such as in cisplatin, in which this phenomenon may be the result of decreased drug uptake, increased repair of DNA, increased expression of sulfhydryl compounds such as glutathione and metallothionein, and increased expression of glutathione-S-transferase. Combined treatment with radiation and drugs might result in an improved therapeutic index if mechanisms of resistance are independent.[440]

Oxygen, pH, and nutrient supply can play an important role in the combined effects of chemotherapy and irradiation on tumor cells.[128] Hypoxic cells are less radiosensitive and chemosensitive to many drugs, and chronic hypoxia can alter cell-cycle age distribution and proliferation rate—both important modifiers of cellular response to ionizing radiation and drugs. In addition, chronic hypoxia can affect cellular ability to repair radiation- and drug-induced DNA damage. Bioreductive drugs such as mitomycin-C are activated to toxic species and affect solid animal tumors under hypoxic conditions. DNA repair, cell-cycle age distribution, and the activity and stability of some chemotherapeutic drugs may be pH dependent; thus, this factor plays a role in the sensitivity of cells to irradiation and cytotoxic agents.

Hypoxic conditions, which commonly exist in tumors, may lead to amplification of genes. Under hypoxic conditions hypoxia-inducible factor 1 (HIF-1) occur, levels rise and functional HIF-1 transcription factor complexes induce angiogenesis, erythrocytopoiesis, glycolysis, and glucose transport into cells—all techniques to allow the cell to survive hypoxia. HIF-1 induces the genes encoding vascular endothelial growth factor (VEGF), platelet-derived growth factor, and transforming growth factor.[494] Some cytokines such as tumor necrosis factor-α or interleukin[513] and growth factors such as platelet-derived and fibroblast growth factors are seen in malignant and normal human cells after irradiation.[512] These cytokines and growth factors enhance the cytotoxic effects of irradiation and chemotherapy in tumor cells[256] or offer radioprotection in normal cells.[322]

Possible molecular or cellular mechanisms of interaction of chemotherapy and irradiation include:

1. Modification of the slope of the dose–response curves, such as has been shown with actinomycin D, cisplatin, doxorubicin, mitomycin-C, 5-fluorouracil, and other agents.
2. Decreased accumulation or inhibition of repair of sublethal damage, as induced by actinomycin D, cisplatin, bleomycin, hydroxyurea, and nitrosoureas.[76,246,408] Doxorubicin and other DNA intercalators decrease the shoulder widths but do not decrease the slope or suppress the repair of lethal damage in *in vitro* studies.[121]
3. Inhibition of repair of potentially lethal damage, as has been shown with actinomycin D, doxorubicin, and cisplatin.[124,482]
4. Perturbation of cell kinetics, for example, after treatment with hydroxyurea, which kills cells in the S phase, when cells may become partially synchronized and blocked at the G1/S phase of the cell cycle. If irradiation is delivered during this sensitive phase, as the cells subsequently emerge from the block, an enhanced cytotoxic effect may be expected.
5. Selective cytotoxicity and radiosensitization of hypoxic cells, which have been reported with mitomycin-C and cisplatin.[252]
6. Inhibition of cell repopulation.
7. Decrease in tumor bulk leading to improved blood supply, reoxygenation, and cell-cycle recruitment, resulting in increased radiosensitivity and chemosensitivity.

A possible danger in the administration of cytotoxic drugs before radiation therapy is accelerated cell proliferation or repopulation. Because some tumor regression is induced by the cytotoxic agent (drugs or irradiation), the distance between

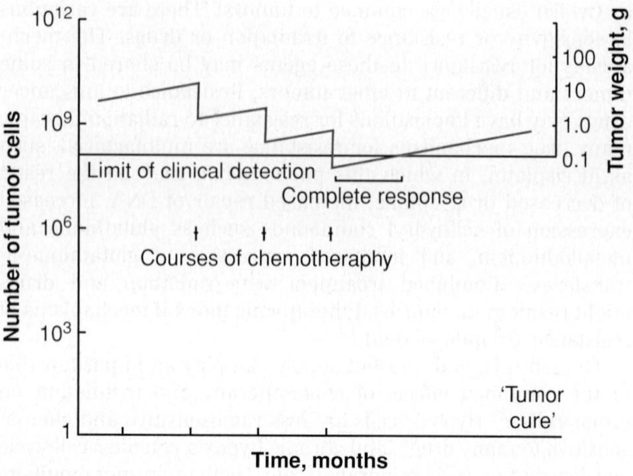

FIGURE 1.33. Relationship between clinical remission and cure. A 10-g tumor containing 10^{10} cells is treated with three courses of chemotherapy, each of which kills 90% of the tumor cells present. After three courses, the number of viable tumor cells is $<10^8$ (<0.1 g) and the patient is judged to be in clinical and radiologic complete remission. Note that this is a small step toward tumor cure. Moreover, additional chemotherapy may not be helpful if drug-resistant cells have been selected after three courses of chemotherapy. (From Tannock IF. Combined modality treatment with radiotherapy and chemotherapy. *Radiother Oncol* 1989;16:83–101, with permission.)

the tumor cells, and decreases in adjacent functional capillaries, this may induce tumor cell proliferation so that higher doses of irradiation would be required to produce a given tumor control. This may occur because, during radiation therapy, tumor cells surviving neoadjuvant chemotherapy may be stimulated to repopulate at a faster rate. Because of this effect, the initial advantage in cell killing by drugs is lost, and the survival curves for fractionated radiation therapy may come together or even cross over. As pointed out by Tannock,[440] although this mechanism is hypothetical, it suggests caution in the use of induction chemotherapy and explains why an initial tumor response may not necessarily translate to a therapeutic advantage with combined-modality treatment given in this fashion. In the example in Figure 1.33, three courses of induction chemotherapy reduced tumor cell numbers from 10^{10} to 10^8 (from 10 g to about 0.1 g), which is considered a complete clinical tumor regression. Even a pathologic complete response has limited long-term implications; a complete pathologic regression is consistent with the presence of about 106 tumor cells per gram, a substantial biologic cell burden.

Integrated Multimodality Cancer Management and Organ Preservation

Combinations of two or all three of the classic modalities frequently are used to improve tumor control and patient survival. Steel and Peckham[424] postulated the biologic basis of cancer therapy as spatial cooperation, in which an agent is active against tumor cells spatially missed by another agent, addition of antitumor effects by two or more agents, and nonoverlapping toxicity and protection of normal tissues. Large primary tumors or metastatic lymph nodes must be removed surgically or treated with definitive radiation therapy. Regional microextensions are eliminated effectively by irradiation without the anatomic and at times physiologic deficit produced by equivalent medical surgery. Chemotherapy is applied mainly to control disseminated subclinical disease, although it also has an effect on some larger tumors.

Organ preservation is being vigorously promoted because it enhances the quality of life and psychoemotional feelings of patients with excellent tumor control and survival. In some types and stages of head and neck tumors, breast cancer, gastrointestinal malignancies, genitourinary tumors, soft-tissue

TABLE 1.12 TRENDS IN 5-YEAR U.S. CANCER SURVIVAL RATES (%)

Site Diagnosed	*1975–1977*	*1999–2006*
Brain	24	36[a]
Breast (female)	75	90[a]
Colon	52	66[a]
Esophagus	5	19[a]
Hodgkin's disease	74	87
Larynx	67	63
Lung and bronchus	13	16[a]
Multiple myeloma	26	39[a]
Non-Hodgkin lymphoma	48	69[a]
Oral cavity	53	63[a]
Ovary	37	45[a]
Pancreas	3	6[a]
Prostate	69	100[a]
Rectum	49	65[a]
Uterine cervix	70	71[a]
Uterine corpus	88	84[a]

[a] $p < .05$.

Data from Siegel R, et al. Cancer statistics 2011. *CA Cancer J Clin* 2011;61:212–236.

sarcomas, and pediatric tumors, studies have shown that less radical surgical procedures combined with chemotherapy and radiation therapy yield the same local tumor control at the primary site and survival as did radical procedures. Advances in reconstructive surgery have greatly improved our ability to repair defects of radical surgery.

CANCER PREVENTION

Cancer is a largely preventable disease. Epidemiologic studies have identified the causative agents for a significant proportion of adult cancers (Tables 1.12 and 1.13). Approximately 30% to 35% of cases of cancer in the United States are associated with tobacco use. Another 30% to 35% of cases are associated with excessive dietary fat and obesity. Approximately 5% of cancer is related to alcohol use. Another 5% is associated with exposure to viral agents.[119] Among the other causative factors of cancer, each responsible for a small percentage of malignancies, are occupational exposures, a family history of cancer, environmental pollution, ionizing and ultraviolet irradiation, prescription drugs, and medical procedures.

There are two general approaches to cancer prevention. They are referred to as *primary prevention strategies* and *secondary prevention strategies*. A primary preventive strategy may be invoked when there is an explicit and indisputable behavior that should be avoided or adopted because of its

TABLE 1.13 ESTIMATED NEW U.S. CANCER CASES AND DEATHS, 2011

	New Cases	*Deaths*
All sites	1,596,670	571,950
Oral cavity and pharynx	39,400	7,900
Digestive system	277,570	139,250
Respiratory system	239,520	161,250
Bones and joint	2,810	1,490
Soft tissue (excluding heart)	10,980	5,920
Skin (excluding basal and squamous)	76,330	11,980
Breast	232,620	39,970
Genital system	338,620	63,980
Urinary system	132,900	28,970
Eye and orbit	2,570	240
Brain and other nervous system	22,340	13,110
Endocrine system	50,400	2,620
Lymphoma	75,190	20,620
Multiple myeloma	20,520	10,610
Leukemia	44,600	21,780
Other and unspecified primary sites	30,500	44,260

Data from Siegel R, et al. Cancer statistics 2011. *CA Cancer J Clin* 2011;61:212–256.

association with a predictable and certain reduction in cancer risk for an individual. A secondary prevention is distinguished from primary prevention in that it is an intervention focused on altering the natural history of a disease and thus avoiding disease-related adverse outcomes.[97] The most commonly used secondary prevention strategy is broad-based or targeted population screening.

The principal primary prevention strategies are directed against cancers that have been associated with certain behaviors. They begin, first and foremost, with avoidance of tobacco. Tobacco use, either in the form of cigarette, pipe, or cigar smoking or the use of snuff or chewing tobacco, is strongly associated with carcinoma of the lung, larynx, pharynx, oral cavity, and esophagus. Tobacco also appears to be an important contributing factor in cancer of the pancreas, bladder, kidney, stomach, colon, and uterine cervix. In addition to its role in the etiology of cancer, tobacco also is associated with coronary heart disease, chronic lung disease, stroke, and other maladies. Tobacco is the single largest preventable cause of death in the Western world today.

In recent years, we have come to understand the role of excessive fat consumption and obesity in the etiology of cancer. Studies suggest a direct correlation between average dietary fat intake in various countries and the incidence of breast cancer. Classic studies have shown that the incidence of stomach cancer among the Japanese decreases when Japanese individuals migrate to Hawaii. Second-generation Japanese residents of Hawaii have an incidence of stomach cancer equivalent to that of the White population.[297] Clearly, a more healthy diet could reduce the incidence of cancer.[292]

Excessive alcohol consumption also is associated with cancer. Alcohol consumption is particularly harmful among cigarette smokers. It appears that smoking acts as an initiator, producing injurious mutations, and alcohol acts as a promoter in cancer of the oral cavity, oropharynx, pharynx, larynx, and esophagus.

A variety of occupational exposures also are associated with specific cancers. These include cancer in asbestos miners and workers, various forms of cancer in workers in the chemical industry, cancers associated with pesticide exposure in agricultural workers, and radiation-associated cancers in uranium miners. An obvious preventive strategy is to minimize or eliminate such harmful exposures in the workplace.

In recent years, scientists have become increasingly aware of various genetic syndromes associated with the etiology of cancer. These include the multiple endocrine neoplasia syndromes and their association with medullary cancer of the thyroid, susceptibility genes that increase the risk of colon cancer, and the association of the BRCA1 and BRCA2 genes with carcinoma of the breast and ovary. For some of these genetic susceptibility traits, the best that the physician can offer is close follow-up. There are certain situations where the avoidance of a potentially lethal cancer may lead an individual to consider prophylactic surgery. For example, consider the problem of a woman who is treated for breast-conserving surgery followed by radiotherapy for breast cancer. She subsequently is found to have a deleterious mutation of BRCA1 or BRCA2. The patient has a risk of relapse in the treated breast, development of a tumor in the contralateral breast, and development of ovarian cancer. Is the patient best handled by close follow-up? Should bilateral mastectomies be offered?[316] At present, the answer is unclear. In a study reported in 2002, investigators found that prophylactic salpingo-oophorectomy in women with BRCA1 and BRCA2 mutations significantly reduced their risk of not only ovarian cancer but also breast cancer.[8,294] This effect, presumably, is the result of decreasing endogenous estrogen exposure in the setting of BRCA genes, rendering the breast susceptible to estrogen-induced DNA damage.[54]

An exciting development in cancer prevention is the successful clinical trial of a vaccine capable of reducing, by about 70%, the incidence of human papillomavirus (HPV)-associated cervical cancer. The U.S. Food and Drug Administration approved this vaccine for clinical use in summer 2006. This vaccine, along with the use of routine Pap testing, has the potential to make invasive cervical cancer an exceedingly rare event.

Cancer screening is the most frequently considered secondary preventive strategy. A cancer screening procedure should lead to the early detection of an asymptomatic or unrecognized disease by the application of simple, inexpensive tests or examinations in a targeted population. For cancer screening to be appropriate and successful, several criteria should be met. These include the following:

1. The cancer for which one is screening should have a substantial morbidity and/or mortality rate that warrants the screening procedure.
2. The cancer for which one is screening should have a sufficiently high prevalence in a detectable, preclinical state to warrant screening.
3. Once the cancer is detected by a screening procedure, there should be an effective treatment related to early detection. This criterion is quite important because there is little value in screening for an untreatable malignancy.
4. The screening test should have a high sensitivity and specificity.
5. The screening test should be of low cost such that the expense of screening a large population would be more than offset by the reduced cost to society of treating early rather than advanced malignancy.
6. Individuals screened should suffer little inconvenience and discomfort.

There is no perfect screening test. Those tests currently used generally meet most, but not all, of the aforementioned criteria.[97,377]

There are several examples of currently used screening tests. For breast cancer, these include self-examination, examination by a trained health practitioner, and mammography, augmented, when appropriate, by ultrasound and MRI. The value of these tests in various populations of women is currently highly disputed. In screening for colorectal cancer, the tools available to the clinician include testing for fecal occult blood, sigmoidoscopy, colonoscopy, and barium enema studies, and the developing field of virtual colonoscopy. There is a general consensus that screening for fecal occult blood and, in the appropriate aged population, screening colonoscopy are worthwhile. Among the most controversial areas for cancer screening is the role of screening in the detection of early prostate cancer. There was rapid general acceptance of the use of physical examination and prostate-specific antigen (PSA) testing to ascertain the presence of early prostate cancer. On further consideration, however, many investigators fear that we have, as a society, successfully identified large numbers of men who would never have been diagnosed with symptomatic prostate cancer in their remaining lifetime or required treatment. The appropriate role of screening for prostate cancer has generated as much controversy as the debate over mammography in breast cancer. A considerable amount of anxiety has been generated in asymptomatic men compulsively watching their PSA levels. By the fall of 2011, the U.S. oncology community was engaged in a very public debate over the recommendation of the U.S. Preventive Services Task Force to rescind a recommendation in favor of the widespread use of PSA for screening. The task force report, released in October 2011, advised that healthy men should no longer receive the PSA blood test to screen for prostate cancer because the test does not save lives overall and often leads to more tests and treatments that needlessly cause pain, impotence, and incontinence in many.

The draft recommendation was based on the results of five clinical trials and could substantially change the care given to men age 50 years and older. There are 44 million such men in the United States, and 33 million of them have already had a PSA test—sometimes without their knowledge—during routine physicals.

It is likely that, in the future, efforts will be expended to identify that subset of men with biologic markers suggesting that they might benefit from PSA screening and, if diagnosed, treatment compared to those who are "best left alone."

Far less controversial, however, has been the use of the Pap test for early detection of carcinoma of the cervix. Where properly used, the test appears to have resulted in a decrease of mortality from this malignancy.

Cancer chemoprevention is defined as a pharmacologic intervention with specific nutrients or other chemicals intended to suppress or reverse carcinogenesis and to prevent the development of invasive cancer. Trials involving chemopreventive therapy require large numbers of individuals who are at high risk for malignancy because of family history, carcinogenic exposure, or the presence of a mutated gene. The ideal chemopreventive agent would have minimal side effects because it would be given to a considerable number of people, none of whom have cancer. Chemoprevention trials differ from other types of cancer prevention studies and from therapeutic studies in important ways. The participants are healthy volunteers, and one seeks to measure a reduction in morbidity and mortality in the long run. Chemoprevention trials are, by definition, large. There are strict enrollment criteria that reflect the group of interest. These studies are often long term and expensive. To date, the best-studied agents in human preventive trials are retinoids (the natural derivatives and synthetic analogs of vitamin A) and one member of the carotenoid class, β-carotene. A number of randomized cancer prevention trials involving carotenoids and retinoids have been completed. Some of these trials have reported chemopreventive effects for various retinoids and for β-carotene, particularly in oral premalignancy. Other trials have been negative or even have suggested cancer promotional effects by β-carotene.[292]

CLINICAL TRIALS

These studies have been classified as phase I (toxicity), phase II (dose/efficacy), and phase III (efficacy and toxicity of a new drug compared with an established standard). Randomized phase III clinical trials and meta-analyses are the two most accepted sources of scientific information in evidence-based medicine. These randomized clinical studies, with sometimes complicated treatment schemas, large numbers of patients, defined end points, and rigorous statistical testing, which are increasingly required by the U.S. Food and Drug Administration to document the efficacy and safety of new drugs (and, we would add, should be required for medical devices), are logistically difficult and expensive to conduct. Suit and others have suggested replacing them with trials in humanized experimental animals. RTOG has been a major contributor, along with any participating institutions, investigators, and associated staff, to clinical investigation centered on the application of ionizing radiations, alone or combined with surgery or cytotoxic agents, hormones, and so forth, to improve the management of patients with cancer.

It is the responsibility of practicing radiation oncologists in academic and community centers to be active contributors, with both scientific input and encouragement of their patients to participate in many of these trials.

RADIATION-INDUCED SECOND PRIMARY MALIGNANT TUMORS

Patients cured of cancer have a significant probability of developing other cancers. Many publications document the frequency of second malignant neoplasms, associated with

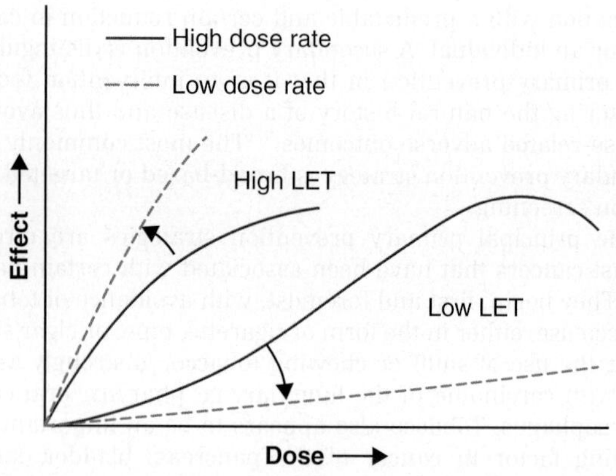

FIGURE 1.34. Dose–response curves for incidence of tumors in relation to dose and dose rate of high–linear energy transfer (LET) and low-LET irradiation. (From Upton AC. Biological aspects of radiation carcinogenesis. In: Boice JD, Fraumeni JF, eds. *Radiation carcinogenesis: epidemiology and biological significance.* New York: Raven, 1984:9.)

radiation therapy, in cancer survivors.[201] Several principles characterize radiation-induced cancers:

1. A wide variety of histologic types of cancers can be induced by radiation therapy. The current state of knowledge does not allow us to distinguish these tumors, morphologically, from "naturally" occurring cancers. In the future, it may be possible to identify specific genetic changes associated with radiation-induced malignancy. This future technology, termed *molecular forensics,* may, ultimately, affect our understanding of attributable risk of radiation-induced malignancies.[20,51]
2. The dose incidence curve for carcinogenesis generally rises more steeply with high-LET radiation doses than with low-LET doses, especially at low dose rates (Fig. 1.34).[465] In a liver cancer model in mice, neutron irradiation produces a greater incidence of hepatomas than gamma irradiation.[502] Low-LET radiation becomes less effective at carcinogenesis per cGy as the dose falls. High-LET radiation, however, does not.[251]
3. When one compares the frequency of second malignant neoplasms over time, it appears that orthovoltage radiation therapy is more likely to be carcinogenic than megavoltage therapy. This may be a dose-related phenomenon insofar as orthovoltage irradiation gives a higher dose to bone. It is also possible that the longer-term follow-up available for survivors of orthovoltage irradiation may, somewhat artifactually, lead to a higher reported incidence of tumors.[210,292,362]
4. The sensitivity of tissues to radiation-induced malignancies is not uniform. Current evidence indicates that the thyroid gland and the breast are sensitive to cancer induction at relatively low doses of radiation; lymphoid tissue, lung, and liver require moderate doses; and bone requires the highest dose. It also seems likely that the relationship between dose and response may vary according to the type of induced tumor. One can estimate the cancer risk from radiation either per unit dose measured in Gy or per unit dose equivalent measured in sievert. When one measures in sieverts, a quality factor (Q) is used to take account of the varying biologic effectiveness of the different forms of radiation. For example, for a conventional γ-ray or x-ray, Q = 1. For neutron irradiation, Q = 20. A review of the available literature indicates that the lifetime cancer mortality risk for a working population of both sexes is 0.008 per Sv for high doses and 0.004 per Sv for low doses.[196] The cancer mortality risk for the general population after whole-body exposure is 0.0001 to 0.0004 per cGy per person.
5. One of the most puzzling aspects of radiation-induced cancer concerns the issue of the relation of low radiation dose

to carcinogenesis. Most of the data we have concerns relatively high doses. Much of the public debate, however, concerns exposure to relatively low doses. Because we have few exact data regarding low doses, extrapolation is, for the most part, used to predict risk at low doses. This can be a particularly vexing problem in litigation where a plaintiff sues for an alleged radiation-induced malignancy following relatively low-dose exposure to radiation.

6. Any assessment of the radiation-dose–response curve for the production of second malignant neoplasms has to take into account the fact that neoplasms also can be induced by agents other than radiation. These include chemotherapy, environmental exposures, and hereditary disposition.
7. Because the risk of radiation-induced carcinogenesis is very small, a large denominator of radiated patients followed for a long period with thorough follow-up would be necessary to calculate risk with any reliability.
8. Latent periods for the production of radiation-induced tumor vary according to the type of induced tumor. One type of latency is exemplified by the risk of leukemia in survivors of the atomic bomb. This consisted of an early pulse of increased risk followed by a gradual decline to baseline levels. The second pattern of occurrence, more typical of solid tumors, is an increase in the relative risk of second malignant neoplasms over many years that remains constant over time thereafter. It is important to remember, therefore, that the duration of follow-up for any study population is very likely to influence the frequency of tumors seen.
9. Age is a critical factor in determining radiation risk. In children, second cancers would be more likely to occur in tissues undergoing rapid proliferation such as bone and thyroid tissue.

There are several classically cited episodes of human radiation carcinogenesis. These include:

1. Individuals who are treated with radiation for ankylosing spondylitis suffered from an increase in leukemia. Mortality from colon cancer, which is associated with spondylitis through a common association with ulcerative colitis, was increased in irradiated patients. Mortality for patients with cancers other than leukemia or colon cancer also rose.[105]
2. Diagnostic x-rays of the abdomen and pelvis taken of a pregnant woman to ascertain the size of the pelvic outlet before delivery are associated with an increased risk of malignancy in the offspring.
3. A large number of immigrants entered the State of Israel following its founding in 1948. X-ray epilation was used to treat tinea capitis. There was an increased incidence of brain and nervous system tumors (1.8 excess risk per 10,000 persons per year) in 10,834 children irradiated for tinea capitis compared with the same number of nonirradiated matched controls and 5,392 siblings. There were 12 malignant brain tumors in the irradiated patients versus five and one suspected in nonirradiated people. The average dose received was 4 Gy in 5 consecutive days. Irradiation doses of 1 to 2 Gy significantly increased the risk of neurologic tumors.[382]
4. The United States dropped atomic bombs on Hiroshima and Nagasaki in Japan in August 1945. Radiation-related risks among bomb survivors show that the incidence of leukemia rose. The increased risk appeared 1 to 3 years after the bombing and peaked at 6 to 7 years. In solid tumors, excess tumor risk was manifest only after exposed individuals reached the age at which the cancer was normally prone to develop.
5. Uranium miners suffered an increase of lung cancer as a result of inhalation of radon gas. Workers who painted luminous radium dials on watch faces developed bone sarcomas because of the habit of shaping the paintbrush in the mouth and ingesting bone-seeking radium.[170]
6. In the past, thorotrast was used as a contrast medium in diagnostic radiology. This material is a colloidal suspension of the α-emitter thorium dioxide. The compound was associated with the late development of angiosarcoma.
7. Canadian studies of women with tuberculosis who were fluoroscoped repeatedly for monitoring of an induced pneumothorax demonstrated an increased incidence of breast cancer.
8. The Chernobyl Nuclear Power Plant accident of April 26, 1986, appears to be associated with an increased risk of thyroid cancer in Belarus and Ukraine.

An important review of radiation-induced sarcomas was published by Cahan et al.[71] in 1948. Cahan's criteria, which were used to define a radiation-induced sarcoma, have wide applicability and are used, by some investigators, as the standard for demonstration of any alleged radiation-induced malignancy. The Cahan Criteria,[71] modified from his original definition, are:

a. A radiation-induced malignancy must have arisen in an irradiated field.
b. A sufficient latent period, preferably longer than 4 years, must have elapsed between the initial irradiation and the alleged induced malignancy.
c. The treated tumor must have been biopsied. The alleged induced tumor must have been biopsied. The two tumors must be of different histologies.
d. The tissue in which the alleged induced tumor arose must have been normal (i.e., metabolically and genetically normal) prior to radiation exposure.

QUALITY AND SAFETY

Quality and safety have always been important topics in the radiotherapy community. The issue of patient safety for radiation therapy and diagnostic imaging has been pulled to the forefront by reports in the lay press and associated congressional hearings. A number of misadministrations described in a series of *New York Times* articles triggered increased interest in improved patient safety in radiation oncology.[49,50] These articles have highlighted some of the risks inherent to advanced radiation therapy treatment-planning and delivery systems and techniques. Many new patient safety initiatives, meetings, and other efforts have been organized to address the need to continue to enhance the safety of patients undergoing radiation therapy.

As part of this effort, the American Society for Radiation Oncology (ASTRO) commissioned a series of "Safety White Papers" to help identify areas where improvements are necessary, so that patient safety is continually enhanced.[14] The white papers have been written by small interdisciplinary teams, reviewed by groups of experts, and subjected to a public comment period. The first paper in this series, "Safety Considerations for Intensity Modulated Radiation Therapy: Executive Summary," by Moran et al.,[310] addressed safety and quality issues for IMRT. Other white papers to follow address stereotactic body radiation therapy, high–dose-rate brachytherapy, IGRT, and peer review in radiation oncology. It is planned that additional reports and updates will continue to follow as radiation therapy techniques and devices evolve. Safety issues for any of these complex technologies cannot be summarized briefly. Thus, the goals of the white papers are as follows: (a) to provide an overview of issues that should be addressed within a broad safety program for these kinds of treatments (e.g., IMRT) and (b) to make recommendations to the radiation oncology community that identify issues that require new approaches, new guidance, or other modifications of current safety and quality assurance methods. The intended audience is radiation oncology professionals, including radiation oncologists, physicists, therapists, dosimetrists, nurses, radiation oncology administrators, and vendors.

Safety and quality are different but related concepts. Safety generally relates to preventing errors that can have major therapeutic implications (e.g., treatment of the wrong patient, treatment with the wrong plan, incorrect placement of a block or wedge, failure to correctly transfer electronic data between the various computer systems). In contrast, quality often relates more to somewhat subjective issues such as ensuring that the defined volumes, doses, beams, and so forth are clinically appropriate, and that the treatment is delivered as prescribed within acceptable clinical tolerance limits. To reconcile these concepts, in May of 2011, ASTRO sponsored the Intersociety Council to review and update previously published guidelines concerning the role of radiation oncology in integrated cancer management. In this updated document, entitled "Safety Is No Accident," every facet of patient evaluation, treatment planning, and treatment delivery were described with the specific goal of maximizing patient safety.[231] The process of care, the roles and responsibilities of staff, staff training and maintenance of competency, requirements for facilities and equipment, and the management of quality assurance were formally recognized as inextricably linked to the provision of safe, efficient, and effective radiation therapy. These ASTRO initiatives have involved cooperation with other organizations, including the American Association of Physicists in Medicine (AAPM), the American Brachytherapy Society, the American College of Radiology (ACR), the American College of Radiation Oncology, the American Board of Radiology, the American Society of Radiation Technologists, and the Society of Radiation Oncology Administrators.

Modern radiation therapy is complex and rapidly evolving. The safe delivery of radiation therapy requires the concerted and coordinated efforts of many individuals with varied responsibilities. Thus, all team members need to work together to create a *safe, high-quality,* and *efficient* clinical environment and workflow.

THE PROCESS OF CARE IN RADIATION ONCOLOGY

The "process of care" in radiation oncology refers to a conceptual framework for ensuring the appropriateness, quality, and safety of all patients treated with radiation for therapy. Each of the aspects of the process of care in radiation oncology requires knowledge and training in the natural history of cancer and certain benign diseases, radiobiology, medical physics, and radiation safety that can only be achieved by board certification in radiation oncology (or equivalent training) to synthesize and integrate the necessary knowledge base to safely and completely deliver care. This high level of training and board certification apply as a recommendation for all of the specialists on the radiation oncology team. The medical therapeutic application of ionizing radiation is irreversible, may cause significant morbidity, and is potentially lethal. Use of ionizing radiation in medical treatment, therefore, requires direct or personal physician management, as the leader of the radiation oncology team, as well as input from various other essential coworkers.

The radiation oncology process of care can be separated into five categories:

- Patient evaluation
- Preparing for treatment
  - Therapeutic simulation
  - Treatment planning
  - Pretreatment quality assurance (QA) and plan verification
- Radiation treatment delivery
- Radiation treatment management
- Follow-up care management

A course of radiation therapy is composed of a series of distinct activities of varying complexity and is a function of the individual patient situation. All components of care involve intense cognitive medical evaluation, interpretation, management, and decision making by the radiation oncologist and other members of the clinical team. Each time a procedure is approved and reported, its level of effort/complexity should be appropriately documented in the patient record.

The clinical team, led by the radiation oncologist, provides the medical services associated with the process of care. Other team members involved in the patient's planning and treatment regimen include the medical physicist, dosimetrist, radiation therapist, and nursing staff. Many of the procedures within each phase of care will be carried to completion before the patient's care is taken to the next phase. Others will occur and recur during the course of treatment, and they are by necessity repeated during treatment due to patient tolerance, changes in tumor size, need for boost fields or port size changes, or protection of normal tissue, or as required by other clinical circumstances (i.e., certain procedures may need to occur multiple times during the treatment course). Each phase of care involves medical evaluation, interpretation, management, and decision making by the radiation oncologist as well as other team members.

Patient Evaluation

Patient evaluation is a service provided by a physician at the request of another physician, the patient, or an appropriate source to either recommend care for a specific condition or problem or to determine whether to accept responsibility for ongoing management of the patient's entire care or for the care of a specific condition or problem. The physician as part of this process will review the pertinent radiologic and pathologic studies, the patient's complaints, and physical findings. This initial visit can also be used for patient counseling, coordinating care, and making recommendations about other aspects of oncologic management or staging.

Preparing for Treatment

The selection of a comfortable and appropriate patient position for treatment is an important part of the simulation processes. The selected position should consider the location of the target and anticipated orientation of the treatment beams. Appropriate immobilization devices provide comfort, support, and reproducibility. Immobilization of the patient in a comfortable position for treatment might involve the construction or selection of certain treatment devices for helping the patient remain in position during treatment. This step must consider the potential treatment-planning considerations so that the treatment aids do not restrict the treatment techniques.

Simulation is the process of determining critical information about the patient's geometry, to permit safe and reproducible treatments on a megavoltage machine. Simulation for external-beam radiation treatment is always image based. Most simulation procedures have now shifted away from the direct use of the treatment beam to using x-rays in the diagnostic range of energies. In general, this part of the overall process of care determines the relationship between the position of the target or targets and the surrounding critical structures. When a simulator of conventional design is used that mimics the geometry of the treatment unit or when direct simulation is performed on the treatment machine, this relationship is often determined indirectly through observation of skeletal anatomy that can act as a surrogate for the target position. Modern conventional simulators, like the CT simulator, can include the ability to produce volumetric data in addition to 2D images.

The preparation for external-beam treatment can also depend on other imaging modalities that are directly or indirectly introduced in the simulation process. MRI, ultrasound, and/or PET are now available, and treatment-planning systems that include image registration capabilities allow combining of information from other imaging modalities with the standard CT dataset obtained during simulation in appropriate situations. It is now possible to produce image datasets that quantify the motion of structures and targets due to respiration, cardiac motion, and physiologic changes in the body.

For most brachytherapy, treatment preparation is similar to the procedure described earlier for EBRT. The simulation process is also image based. Multiple imaging modalities may be important for some brachytherapy procedures, and these studies can be obtained as part of the preplanning imaging process. For clinical situations where therapy is delivered by unencapsulated radionuclides, a separate and distinct treatment-planning process is necessary due to its multidisciplinary execution.[2]

Clinical treatment planning is a comprehensive, cognitive team effort performed under the direction of the radiation oncologist for each patient undergoing radiation treatment. The radiation oncologist is responsible for understanding the natural history of the patient's disease, knowing the extent of the disease relative to the adjacent normal anatomic structure, and integrating the patient's overall medical condition and associated comorbidities. A detailed understanding of the integration of chemotherapeutic and surgical treatment modalities with radiation therapy is also essential.

The skills of the trained and appropriately credentialed dosimetrist relate to the efficient and effective use of the complex treatment-planning system hardware and software. This individual must also understand the clinical aspects of radiation oncology in order to interact with the radiation oncologist during the planning process. The role of the medical physicist is to guarantee proper functioning of the hardware and software used for the planning process, consult with the radiation oncologist and dosimetrist, check the accuracy of the selected treatment plan, and perform measurements and other checks aimed at ensuring accurate delivery of the plan.

For either EBRT or brachytherapy, treatment planning starts with a complete, formally documented, and approved directive. Details including total dose to all targets and organs at risk (OARs), fractionation, treatment modality, energy, time constraints, and all other aspects of the radiation prescription in a written or electronic format must be provided by the radiation oncologist prior to the start of treatment planning. In some cases, this prescription can require modification based on the results of the treatment-planning process.

Clinical treatment planning for either EBRT or brachytherapy is an important step in preparing for radiation oncology treatment. This planning includes the following components: determining the disease-bearing areas based on the imaging studies and pathology information, identifying the type (brachytherapy, photon beam, particle beam, other) and method of radiation treatment delivery, specifying areas to be treated, and specifying the dose and dose fractionation. In developing the clinical treatment plan, the radiation oncologist may use information obtained from the patient's clinical evaluation as well as any additional tests, studies, and procedures that are necessary to complete treatment planning. Studies ordered as part of clinical treatment planning may or may not be associated with studies necessary for staging the cancer and may be needed to obtain specific information to accomplish the clinical treatment plan. Review of imaging studies and lab tests must be performed to determine treatment volume and critical structures in close proximity to the treatment area.

At various steps in the treatment-planning process, the radiation oncologist is presented with one or more treatment plans for review and selection. This process is often iterative and requires additional treatment planning. The radiation oncologist is responsible for selecting and formally approving the plan to be used for treatment.

The quality assurance steps taken after completion of treatment planning and before the start of treatment are critical for guaranteeing patient safety. In the past, treatment verification consisted of field aperture imaging using radiographic film. These images are referred to as portal images or port films. With the introduction of IMRT, imaging of individual apertures is no longer practical. However, the traditional method of verifying the plan isocenter position using orthogonal imaging is often used for both 3DCRT and IMRT. For IMRT, this important QA technique is not considered to be sufficient to guarantee patient safety. In addition to this isocenter check procedure, for IMRT and other complex delivery techniques that use inverse treatment planning, patient-specific QA measurements are also required. In terms of clearly organizing the different steps in the process of care for radiation oncology, a blurring of the separation between the verification and treatment delivery occurs on the first day of treatment and whenever the treatment plan is changed.

Radiation Treatment Delivery

The physician is responsible for verification and documentation of the accuracy of treatment delivery as related to the initial treatment-planning and setup procedure. Image guidance (IGRT) may be performed to ensure accurate targeting of precise radiation beams. IGRT requires a target that is expected to move from day to day and can be reliably identified by the selected imaging modality. The physician is responsible for the supervision and review of these images and prescribing necessary positional shifts to ensure the therapy delivered conforms to the originally planned dosimetric constraints. Similarly, management of organ motion during treatment delivery is the responsibility of the treating physician.

Radiation Treatment Management

Radiation treatment management encompasses the radiation oncologist's overall management of the course of treatment and care for the patient as well as checks and approvals provided by other members of the radiation therapy team that are necessary at various points in the process. For the radiation oncologist, radiation treatment management requires and includes a minimum of one examination of the patient for medical evaluation and management. The professional services furnished during treatment management typically include:

- Review of portal images;
- Review of dosimetry, dose delivery, and treatment parameters;
- Review of patient treatment setup; and
- Patient evaluation visit.

Not all of these elements of treatment management are required for all patients for each week of management (except for the patient evaluation visit) because the clinical course of care may differ due to variation in treatment modality and individual patient requirements. Examinations and evaluations may be required more often than once weekly.

Follow-Up Care

Continued follow-up care of patients who have completed radiation therapy is necessary to manage acute and chronic morbidity resulting from treatment as well as to monitor the patient for tumor recurrence.

THE RADIATION ONCOLOGY TEAM

The radiation oncology team ensures every patient undergoing radiation treatment receives the appropriate level of medical, emotional, and psychological care before, during, and after treatment, through a collaborative multidisciplinary approach.

The radiation oncology team consists of but is not limited to radiation oncologists, physicists, dosimetrists, oncology nurses, and radiation therapists. The process of care in radiation oncology involves close collaboration of a team of qualified professionals. On-site or by consultation services can be provided by nonphysician providers, including nurse practitioners, clinical nurse specialists, advanced practice nurses and physician assistants, dentists, clinical social workers, psychologists/psychiatrists,

TABLE 1.14 STAFFING LEVELS FOR RADIATION ONCOLOGIST, MEDICAL PHYSICIST, DOSIMETRIST, AND RADIATION THERAPY TECHNOLOGIST

Clinical FTE[a]	*Approximate Maximum # of Patients Treated per FTE per Year*
Radiation oncologist	250
Physicist	250
Dosimetrist	250
Therapist	90
Nurse	250
Treatment machine	300[b]
Therapists/treatment machine	3.5[c]

FTE, full-time equivalent.

[a]It is recommended that a minimum of two qualified individuals be present for any external-beam patient treatment.

[b]Each treatment machine is assumed to be operational for 9 hours a day.

[c]The number of therapists per treatment machine is the ratio of the total number of therapists and the number of treatment delivery machines, not including the simulator.

nutritionists, speech/swallowing therapists, physical therapists, occupational therapists, genetic counselors, integrative medicine specialists, and pastoral care providers.

Board certification is the primary consideration for establishing proper qualifications and training for any professional working in radiation oncology. The relevant professional societies will establish the eligibility requirements to sit for a board exam. This may include education and training requirements such as a clinical residency. In addition, in some jurisdictions, professionals must meet requirements for obtaining appropriate licensure.

The applications, technologies, and methods of radiation oncology continue to expand and develop. Lifelong learning is vital to ensure incorporation of new knowledge into clinical practice. Therefore, each member of the interdisciplinary radiation oncology team should participate in available Continuing Education (CE) and Maintenance of Certification (MOC) programs. Each facility should have a policy regarding orientation, competency, credentialing, and periodic competency evaluations of all team members.

Staffing Requirements

Starting in 1986, the Intersociety Council for Radiation Oncology published a set of guidelines in a small pamphlet titled "Radiation Oncology in Integrated Cancer Management," often referred to as the "Blue Book."[230] This subsequently has been updated several times, most recently in May of 2011. The document offers guidelines for staffing requirements and equipment utilization. The staffing needs of each facility are unique based on the patient mix and complexity of the services offered. The patient load, number of machines, and satellite clinics and affiliated treatment centers will influence the demand on management and clinical staff (Figs. 1.35 and 1.36) The minimum personnel requirements for a radiation oncology facility specify the need for one medical director (radiation oncologist), chief medical physicist, and department manager per program.[231] Table 1.14 presents an estimate of the maximum number of patients treated per FTE per year.

MANAGEMENT AND QUALITY ASSURANCE IN RADIATION ONCOLOGY

Quality assurance in radiation oncology is a set of processes and procedures designed to improve the practice of radiation therapy by confirming that radiation therapy will be or was administered appropriately and safely and documented properly. The overall goal of a QA process is the delivery of high-quality radiation oncology treatment to all patients. Note that QA is an all-encompassing term that is often used to describe some or all of the different elements involved in quality management and a culture of safety.

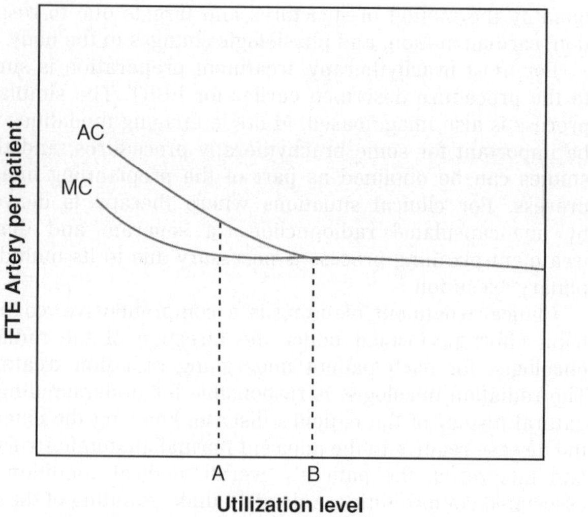

FIGURE 1.35. The theoretical relation between the cost per patient and rate of use of a linear accelerator for cancer therapy. As the rate of use of a linear accelerator increases, the average cost (AC) of treatment per patient declines until all economies of scale have been achieved (*point B*). The average cost of a radiotherapy treatment will fall as long as any additional patients can be treated at a marginal cost (MC) lower than the AC. It is important to remember that point B represents only the minimized cost of operating the linear accelerator. If you add in costs such as the travel time for a patient to go a considerable distance to reach the linear accelerator, the lost time from work for the patient and anyone traveling with him or her, child care costs, and stress, then the total societal expenditure for a linear accelerator will not be minimized at point B. It will, instead, be reached at point A. We are, however, quite poor at accounting for costs such as travel, loss of work time, and stress, so it is difficult to determine point B and, in turn, the need for a new linear accelerator. If you wish to persuade a government regulatory agency to grant a certificate of need for a piece of radiotherapy equipment at a moderate distance from an existing facility, then you will have an economic incentive to inflate the importance of travel and inconvenience. In the United States, this behavior is increasing as institutions try to justify the need for linear accelerators, radiosurgery, and proton therapy units. The corporations that manufacture and market these units have a vested interest in contributing to this exaggeration of need. (Modified from Suit HD, Urie M. Proton beams in radiation therapy. *J Natl Cancer Inst* 1992;84:155–164.)

A radiation oncology facility must satisfy numerous requirements:[231]

- A department must provide adequate clinic space, exam rooms and equipment, patient waiting and changing space, convenient patient parking, treatment rooms, simulation and imaging space, brachytherapy source preparation and storage space, dosimetry/treatment-planning rooms, office space for professional staff, and medical physics laboratory and equipment storage space. The extent of facilities should be appropriate for the volume of patients seen and treated.
- Treatment rooms (for linear accelerators or other treatment machines) must be carefully designed for radiation shielding, environmental conditions, adequate storage space for spare parts, testing and dosimetry equipment, and patient access and safety.
- There must be access to CT imaging for treatment planning.
- Rooms used for brachytherapy procedures require special attention to the specific radiation protection requirements associated with the particular brachytherapy modalities to be used. If the brachytherapy procedure load warrants it, a brachytherapy suite should be available, including patient waiting space, procedure rooms, recovery rooms, and brachytherapy source preparation and storage areas.
- Each department must have electronic access to the hospital or clinic information system and picture archiving and communication system (PACS).

Every radiation oncology program should be accredited by the ASTRO/ACR accreditation process.[231] Accreditation will verify that crucial basic capabilities and procedures are performed that are generally recognized as necessary for high-quality radiotherapy. The following specific capabilities and methods for various aspects of the radiotherapy process are considered essential:[231]

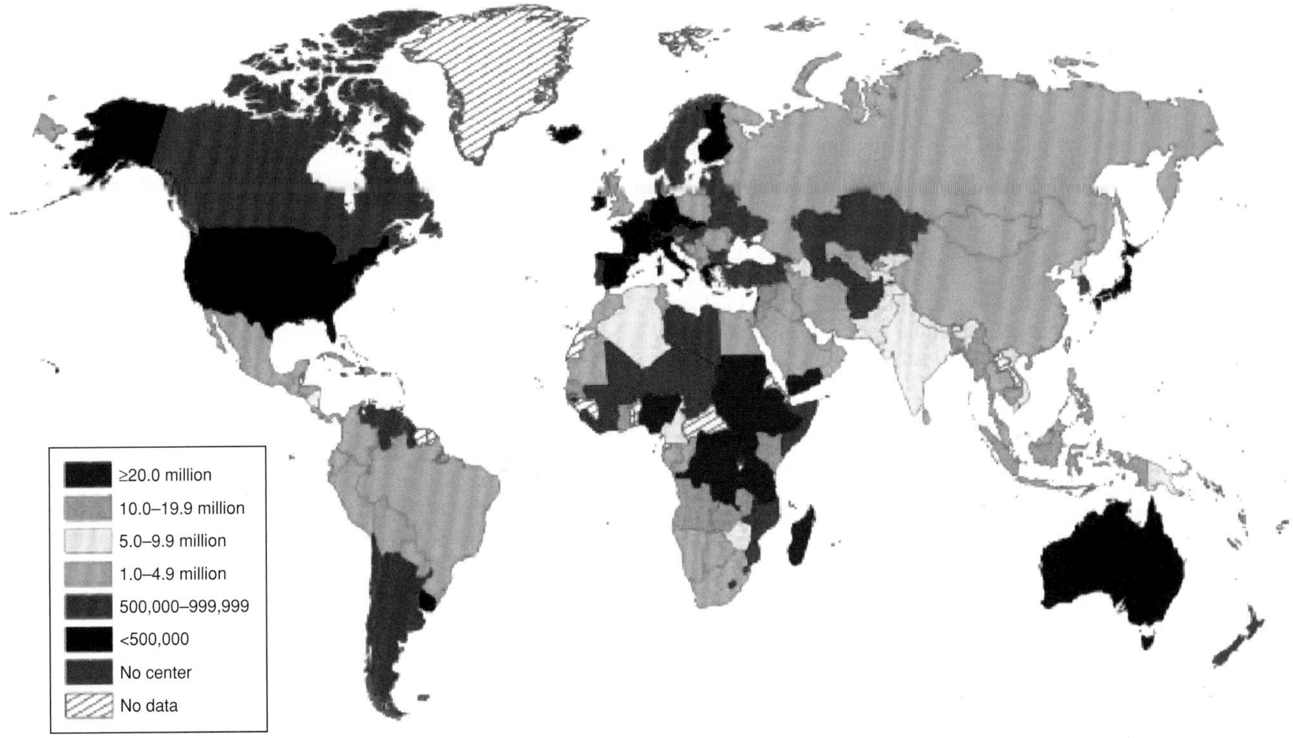

FIGURE 1.36. The number of people served by each radiation therapy center by country. (From Jemal A, Bray F, Center MM, et al. Global cancer statistics. *CA Cancer J Clin* 2011;61:69–90. Based on data from the International Atomic Energy Agency, Directory of Radiotherapy Centers, http://www-nawebiaea.org/nuhu/dirac/; Population Division of the Department of Economic and Social Affairs of the United Nations Secretariat, World Population Prospects: The 2008 Revision, http://esa.un.org/unpp.)

- Calibration of treatment machines, CT and MRI scanners, treatment-planning systems, and brachytherapy sources is to be carefully accomplished according to the appropriate protocols described by scientific/professional organizations.
- A safety program designed to monitor patient safety, avoid radiation incidents, and prevent errors in the treatment process should be in place and subject to periodic review and update.
- A system for documenting radiotherapy treatment and other aspects of the patient's medical care should be rigorous and be subject to periodic review and update.
- High-quality and comprehensive treatment planning, using 3D computerized treatment planning for dose calculations, imaging, and other aspects of the planning process.
- A comprehensive quality management program, including QA, quality control (QC), and other quality improvement tools.
- Radiation monitoring of simulators and treatment machines. A system to carefully control and monitor all radioactive sources in accordance with the requirements of regulatory agencies.
- A program for maintenance and repair of equipment.
- Staff training that is comprehensive, ongoing, and well documented.
- A well-developed process for continuous peer review. This should include a mechanism for peer review of the entire department and its procedures as well as for individual clinical care decisions.
- Access to medical oncology, surgical oncology, and other physician and nonphysician specialists involved in the multidisciplinary care and follow-up of the patient.
- Each department must implement careful and well-described policies and procedures for every aspect of patient care, for QA of the patient care process, for staff behavior, and for any issues that may impact the safety of patients and/or staff. Each specific treatment modality (e.g., IMRT, IGRT, stereotactic body radiation therapy [SBRT], etc.) should have detailed documentation of its treatment planning and delivery process including a description of the roles and responsibilities of each team member in that procedure, QA checklists, and a plan for continuous quality improvement and safety.

One of the most crucial activities in a quality radiation oncology department is the organized review and monitoring of all aspects of safety, errors, and outcome. Creating a "culture of safety" depends on guidance, direction, and financial support from the leadership of the institution and of the radiotherapy department, on individual effort by every member of the department, and on organized support for quality and safety at every level in the institution.

Each department should have a department-wide review committee that monitors specific quality metrics including near misses and errors in treatment, diagnosis, patient care, or other procedural problems that might lead to errors. This committee should organize the collection and analysis of such events, work to identify potential problems in devices or processes, and then try to mitigate these problems by modifying processes or adding new checks or actions to minimize the likelihood of further problems. Radiation oncology departments should hold regularly scheduled rounds to review patient morbidity and mortality, dose discrepancies, and any incident reports that involved an accident or injury to a patient. Morbidity and mortality include unusual or severe complications of treatment, unexpected deaths, or unplanned interruptions of treatment. Staff included should represent all the team members, including radiation oncologists, nurses, physicists, dosimetrists, therapists, and administrators.

Professional Performance Review of Radiation Oncologists and Physicists

Over the past several years, there has been increasing interest on the part of the general public and government agencies in requirements for greater oversight for physicians and other health care providers. In response to these concerns, the American Board of Medical Specialties has mandated that all medical specialties must develop MOC programs to replace current recertification initiatives. The American Board of Medical Specialties has defined four components of MOC: professional standing, lifelong learning and self-assessment, cognitive expertise, and practice quality improvement (PQI).[11]

ASTRO and AAPM offer several opportunities for radiation oncologists and physicists to satisfy the requirements of MOC. ASTRO and other professional organizations have developed online courses with self-assessment modules (SAMs) to satisfy the lifelong learning requirements and a special program called the Performance Assessment for the Advancement of Radiation Oncology Treatment (PAAROT)[14] to satisfy the PQI requirements. AAPM offers similar initiatives for medical physicists.

One important aspect of these programs is the use of peer review to help individuals learn from other practitioners in the field. Peer review is relevant in a number of different aspects of clinical practice including overall review of the behavior of the practice, review of individual skills and methods, and review of physician clinical decisions that occur at weekly chart rounds. Peer review is a quality improvement tool that has application throughout the process of radiotherapy.[245]

Radiation oncology is a highly technical field that is dependent on many well-trained and highly skilled individuals. It is, therefore, advisable that all members of the team maintain the proper credentials as reflected in their skills and training through demonstrated competency on an annual basis. In some cases (e.g., therapists moving between different kinds of treatment machines), additional training or review sessions in the use of specific devices may be necessary more often than annually.[311]

Equipment and Device Quality Management

The delivery of radiation therapy relies on computer-controlled treatment machines, interconnected imaging, delivery and planning systems, and complex ancillary devices. Any new radiotherapy system should go through the following processes as it is prepared for clinical use:[1–4]

- Each system should be carefully specified before acquisition, purchase, or development, including design, expectations, capabilities, tolerances, hazards, necessary training, usability, and technical specifications.
- To prevent data communication errors and clinical efficiency issues, each system must be interoperable and connectable with other systems in the clinic.
- Acceptance testing must be performed to document that the new system satisfies the specifications. Often, the acceptance criteria and/or testing methods should be documented as part of the specification for the system.
- Clinical commissioning includes all the activities that must be performed to understand, document, characterize, and prove that a given system is ready to be used clinically. Standard operating procedures, training, and hazard analysis should be part of the commissioning process.
- Each new system, device, and process must be formally released for clinical use after clinical commissioning has been completed.

Clinical use of a device, system, or process must involve the creation and application of a safety- and quality-oriented program designed to ensure that the machine or device is functioning in accordance with accepted standards:[1–4]

- Quality management (QM) is defined as the overall program to organize the oversight of the use of any system or process in radiation oncology. The QM program should include hazard analysis, quality control, quality assurance, training and documentation, and ongoing quality improvement efforts.
- Hazard analysis is the active evaluation of the potential for failures that will cause incorrect results or harm to the patient and should be performed for any new system.
- QC checks on the data that are input into a decision or process and is designed to prevent the propagation of error.
- QA is the typical shorthand term for the entire QM program and addresses quality checks that confirm that a given process is reasonable and generates appropriate results. QA checks, along with QC, are essential parts of the QM process for most devices and systems, as they can check the output of potentially very complicated decisions or actions performed by the system.
- Training of staff in goals, methods, results, operation, and evaluation of the quality of the output is important for the proper use of any system.

Patient-Related Quality Management

Within the complex and many-step process with which radiotherapy patients are treated, patient-specific issues must be carefully and comprehensively analyzed, documented and verified. Each radiation oncology facility, regardless of its location or size, must appropriately manage and adhere to high-quality standards of practice for general medical issues,[6] including:

- Drug allergies;
- Medication reconciliation;
- Do-not-resuscitate codes;
- Cleanliness and efforts to reduce infection; and
- Patient confidentiality and security of protected health information.

Modern oncology patient care very often involves multiple modalities and requires the review and discussion of experts in various oncology-related disciplines. It is critical that the management of most cancer be addressed by the appropriate mix of disciplines. Regular presentation of these cases to a multidisciplinary tumor board is the standard of care and should be performed for most cancer cases to determine the appropriate combination (and coordination) of therapies for each individual case.

The details of the patient care process in radiation oncology varies from institution to institution. However, maintenance of the safety and quality of the radiotherapy process for most patients requires that a number of procedures be performed.[231] These include:

- A new patient conference that consists of a brief presentation of the details of each patient's history and physical examination, disease status, and plan for therapy to the other physicians and staff involved in patient care is used as an initial peer review for the basic treatment decisions and plan.
- The physician must obtain a clear, accurate, and detailed description of the patient's chief complaint and pertinent history in conjunction with an appropriate physical examination as part of the decision process for radiation therapy.
- Virtually all patients who receive radiation therapy should receive a CT- or MRI-based simulation.
- After the physician defines target volumes and other normal tissues (contouring), this should be peer reviewed and confirmed before treatment planning begins.
- After treatment planning is complete, the physician and members of the planning team should review the plan and verify that it satisfies the clinical requirements and prescription(s) from the physician and that it can be carried out accurately.
- On-treatment visits of the patient by the physician are essential for continuity of care and monitoring of tumor response and normal tissue toxicity. Typically, this occurs every five fractions, but some situations may require more frequent visits.

- Patient chart rounds are an important peer review procedure used involving weekly review of all patients under treatment by the radiotherapy team, including physicians, therapists, nurses, dosimetrists, and physicists.
- Follow-up visits are a critical component of care for the radiotherapy patient. The frequency of follow-up visits will vary in accordance with the type of cancer, stage, degree of tumor response, normal tissue reactions, and other factors.
- Documentation is required of all the relevant details of patient care. Maintenance and continuous improvement of the quality and accessibility of the treatment record are essential.

The overall performance status of the patient prior to treatment should be recorded. Assessment of tumor response and normal tissue toxicity should occur both during and after treatment. Clinical assessment of patient response is a valuable independent check on the success of the overall quality management system as unexpected outcomes may identify issues related to technique or equipment performance.

External-Beam Quality Assurance

Nearly all external-beam treatment requires the following steps, each of which must be carefully confirmed as part of the patient-specific QA process: determination of patient setup position and immobilization; cross-sectional imaging (CT simulation); creation of the anatomic model (contouring); specification of the treatment intent; creation of the planning directive and treatment prescription by the physician; computerized treatment planning and dose calculation; monitor unit calculation and/or IMRT leaf sequencing; plan and (electronic chart) preparation; plan evaluation; download to treatment management system (TMS); patient-specific QA as typically performed for IMRT, stereotactic radiosurgery [SRS], or SBRT; patient setup and delivery; plan verification checks; plan adaptation and modifications; chart checks; and more. The details associated with these processes have been described in a series of guideline reports.[3,4,208,317]

Brachytherapy Quality Assurance

The QA process for brachytherapy is similar to that of external beam and involves several components that must be confirmed as part of the patient-specific QA management: treatment planning; treatment delivery systems; applicator commissioning and periodic checks; cross-sectional imaging (CT simulation); specification of the treatment intent, planning directive, and treatment prescription by the physician; plan preparation; plan evaluation; download to TMS; plan verification checks; plan modifications; and chart checks. The details of these processes have been described in a series of guideline reports.[145,317,318,447,477,478,524]

LEGAL PRINCIPLES CONCERNING MALPRACTICE IN RADIATION ONCOLOGY

A plaintiff initiates a radiation oncology malpractice lawsuit by filing papers with the court claiming that he or she was harmed by the radiation oncologist and is entitled to legal redress. The claim of malpractice must be set out in the plaintiff's *prima facie* case. This will include a statement of the facts and legal theories that establish that the plaintiff believes he or she is legally entitled to enforceable claims against the physician.

There are four essential elements to a *prima facie* case of medical malpractice. They are the establishment of duty, breach, causation, and damages. To demonstrate medical malpractice, a plaintiff–patient must show that the radiation oncologist had a duty to provide nonnegligent care to the patient, that the provider breached that duty by providing negligent care, and that this breech caused the patient injury or damage.[376]

To establish a *duty*, the plaintiff must have facts that demonstrate a legal relationship between the radiation oncologist and the patient. It is a basic rule of Anglo-American law that there is no duty to another person unless there is a legally recognized relationship with that person. The plaintiff–patient must demonstrate the existence of a physician–patient relationship.[376]

To establish a *breach*, the patient–plaintiff must demonstrate facts that illustrate the radiation oncologist breached the legal duties implied in the physician–patient relationship or duties that would be generally imposed on members of society. The plaintiff must establish that the appropriate standard of care was violated. Although, in theory, the establishment of the standard of care and the breach of that standard are legally separate, in reality, unless there is a factual question about what the radiation oncologist actually did, the proof of the standard of care also would demonstrate the defendant's breach. Most commonly, in law, the definition of *standard of care* is how similarly qualified radiation oncologists would have managed the patient's care under the same or similar circumstances. In most medical malpractice cases, both the standard of care and the breach are established through the testimony of expert witnesses.[269]

Negligence is defined as "the omission to do something which a reasonable man guided by those ordinary considerations which ordinarily regulate human affairs would do, or the doing of something which a reasonable and prudent man would not do." The person who brings a malpractice claim is asserting that he or she is owed some duty by the defendant physician and that the violation of that duty by the physician must have caused injury. The court will make a determination concerning the propriety or impropriety of the defendant physician's performance on the basis of "the reasonable man" had he or she been in the same situation as the individual being judged. Negligence may derive from the physician's lack of training or experience. It may also result from the physician's carelessness or inadvertence.[48]

To understand the concept of an expert witness, we must consider the legal doctrines of the *school of practice*, the *locality rule*, and the concept of the *qualifications of an expert*. The legal doctrine of the school of practice is designed to deal with the historic problem of the competing interests of physicians. Physicians generally do not want to testify against their colleagues, but they often are tempted to try to run their competitors out of business. Allopathic physicians were happy to label homeopathic physicians as quacks, and many medical doctors would be happy to dispute the competence of a chiropractor. To deal with the problem, the courts use the legal doctrine of the *school of practice* in which they refuse to allow physician experts to question a different school based on philosophic or psychologic beliefs.[376] The school of practice rule now generally is used to differentiate physicians in the self-designated specialties (we use the term *self-designated* because few state licensing boards recognize specialties or limit physicians' rights to practice the specialties in which they have been trained).

The *locality rule* refers to the concept that a physician's competence should be determined by comparison with other physicians in the community or in similar neighboring communities.[376] However, with the development of national standards for the practice of radiation oncology, there is no justification for rules that shelter substandard medical decision making by using an excuse that it is the norm for a given community. A radiation oncologist, for example, could not be held at fault for failing to treat a patient with an unusual or exotic technology if that technology were not available in his or her local community. However, physicians are required to inform the patients of the limitations of the available facilities and recommend prompt transfer if indicated. Failure to refer patients when a provider lacks the experience to appropriately treat may create malpractice liability. Furthermore, if a radiation oncologist does not give a patient information about the potential result associated with not seeing a subspecialist able to use a specific technology, then the initial radiation oncologist may be held liable. Physicians must recognize when a particular medical problem is beyond their capacity for diagnosis or treatment. They are responsible for obtaining timely and adequate consultations when indicated and for referring the patient to an appropriate specialist or facility whenever the requirements for the appropriate or specialized care cannot be satisfied at the available facilities. The continued expansion of knowledge in radiation oncology and the increasingly specialized training of physicians make it essential that the radiation oncologist be able to recognize any limitations in his or her capabilities or ability to treat a given patient with what is perceived to be standard of care. Failure to obtain an appropriate consultation or make an appropriate referral may denote negligence.[17,18,261]

Qualified experts sometimes disagree as to the standard of care. When alternative schools of thought exist, the physician defendant is entitled to be judged by the tenants of the school he or she follows. In such states, this is called the *minority practice doctrine*. With this doctrine, also called the *respectable minority rule*, the physician may show that although the course of therapy followed was not the same as other practitioners would have followed, it was one that was accepted by a respectable minority group of practitioners.[376]

A problem that is increasingly facing physicians in the United States has been the pressure radiation oncologists face from health maintenance organizations (HMOs) and insurance companies to conform their proposed care to a predetermined regimen. Despite legislative initiatives to hold managed care organizations accountable, the radiation oncologist will, for the most part, carry a significant portion of the risk of liability in cases where the patient asserts that he or she was unable to obtain the most accurate and appropriate diagnostic and therapeutic measures. It is essential that the radiation oncologist come to his or her own conclusions about the standard of care irrespective of any pressures applied by an HMO or an insurance company. In litigation, the radiation oncologist's best defense against a claim of malpractice is if he or she can demonstrate action only in the interest of the patient, regardless of any financial consideration or bureaucratic restraint imposed by an insurance company, an HMO, or any other financial consideration. If a conflict arises between the radiation oncologist's recommendations for the best course of treatment and the level of care authorized by the HMO, the physician must give the best care to the patient even if it means he or she will not ultimately be compensated.[225]

Radiation oncologists will, on occasion, be called on to serve as expert witnesses in malpractice cases. Physicians, trained to give opinions, may find the give and take of the court room offputting. For an expert witness, the foremost qualifications are effective presentation and teaching ability. The radiation oncologist, serving as an expert witness, must educate the attorneys, judge, and jury. Once there is a perception of understanding, the radiation oncologist may be able to convince the judge and jury that they can make an independent decision that his or her testimony is correct.

Both the plaintiff's attorney and the defense attorney will retain expert witnesses who will be persuaded to "take sides." The expert witness will be asked to swear, under oath, what influence the radiation dose, volume, or technique had on the risk of an ill effect of radiation therapy on normal tissue or alleged failure to control the tumor. This expert witness system troubles many physicians who feel that they can bring a dispassionate and scientific view to such cases and come to a reasonable conclusion about whether or not malpractice occurred outside the process of litigation.[225] Whatever the wishes of the physician, a trial is an adversarial process. The physician is best advised, therefore, to state his or her opinion about the case frankly and not attempt to predict or handicap how a trial will turn out. The physician should do his or her best to provide an opinion and then step aside to let a system, in which he or she has little expertise, run its course in the hands of the attorneys and judge. Although often frustrating and distressing, the physicians will find themselves out of their league if they attempt to act as attorney or judge.

Each physician must make a determination as to whether he or she feels comfortable participating in the legal process as an expert witness. Some radiation oncologists accept employment as expert witnesses in both plaintiffs' actions and in defense. Some only choose to participate as expert witnesses for the defendant physicians or simply wash their hands of the matter and will have nothing to do with the process. The lure of money is strong and serving as an expert witness can be quite lucrative. Each physician must, however, determine for him- or herself whether the financial compensation for serving as an expert witness outweighs the considerable effort and troubling aspects of the process.

It is important that radiation oncologists understand that the concept in malpractice law of *res ipsa loquitur*,[376] roughly translated as "the thing speaks for itself," is used to deal with cases in which the actual negligent act may not be proved, but it is clear that the injury was caused by negligence. In law, this doctrine was first recognized in the case of a man who was injured when a barrel rolled out of a second-story window of a warehouse. The defense attorney argued that the plaintiff did not know what events preceded the barrel rolling out of the window and, therefore, it could not be proven that an employee of the warehouse was negligent. The plaintiff, however, countered that barrels do not normally fall out of second-story warehouse windows. The simple fact that the barrel fell from the window and caused an injury "spoke for itself" and demonstrated that someone must have been negligent.

In medical malpractice law, *res ipsa loquitur* is used to shift the burden of proof to the defendant's position regarding causation. *Res ipsa loquitur* can be invoked if the patient suffers an injury that is not an expected complication of medical care, the injury does not normally occur unless someone has been negligent, and the defendant was responsible for the patient's well-being at the time of the injury. Examples in which this concept has been invoked include the dislocation of a patient's shoulder while aligning it for a chest x-ray, knocking out a patient's tooth while the patient was under anesthesia for a tonsillectomy, nerve injury due to a hypodermic injection, leaving a sponge in the abdomen during an operation, or fracturing a patient's jaw while extracting a tooth.[376]

An *intentional tort* is an action that can result in harm to the plaintiff. The classic intentional tort in medical malpractice law is forcing unwanted medical care on a patient. Even if care clearly would benefit a patient, if that care were refused and the radiation oncologist had no state mandate to force care on the patient, but did so anyway, the patient might sue for intentional tort. The most common intentional tort is *battery*. The legal standard for a battery is "an intentional unconsented touching."[269]

Battery is not the same, in law, as *assault*. Assault is the act of putting a person in fear of bodily harm. Most battery claims against physicians are based on real attacks. However, battery claims also can be created by the circumstances of the medical treatment. The legal standard of care is that male health care providers do not examine female patients without a female attendant present. Although the standard frequently is ignored, it should not be. An attorney representing a plaintiff–patient may attempt to demonstrate that allowing an unattended examination of a female patient by a male radiation oncologist is concrete evidence that, at the very least, the physician has very poor judgment.

Of particular concern to radiation oncologists, in the realm of malpractice, is the concept of *loss of chance*. This usually is evoked in circumstances where physicians failed to diagnose a terminal illness. The loss of chance stems from the failure to diagnose in time for the patient to have a chance of cure. Not all states recognize this standard. In those states that do, however, the patient must show that the loss of chance is statistically significant.[376]

It is generally viewed that any patient injured by exposure to a defective x-ray machine will be compensated as a matter of law.[48] If, however, the radiation oncologists did not know or could not have reasonably been expected to know that a machine was defective, they will generally not be held liable if they used the machine properly.[19] Radiation oncologists are bound by the usual standards of skill, knowledge, and appropriate diligence that apply to the specialists within the field.

If a patient is hypersensitive to radiation therapy, and in the absence of any reasonable way to predict this, the radiation oncologist will not be expected to predict or prevent it.[21,390,503] There is, however, the possibility that the plaintiff's attorney will invoke *res ipsa loquitur* in certain circumstances.[96] For example, in a patient who received radiation therapy for a benign condition and suffered a severe radiation cutaneous reaction that required bilateral amputation, the radiation oncologist was found to be negligent.[480] In the employment of diagnostic radiation, minimal exposure is involved, and it is not expected that a skin reaction will be produced. Thus, if a skin reaction does ensue, many courts would infer negligence.[28] If a part of the body is unintentionally irradiated and injured, liability will generally follow. For example, a patient who is undergoing radiation therapy to the head and neck was compensated when he suffered severe injury to the arms.[290] A patient given radiation therapy to the ear suffered reaction of the head, face, and neck. Liability was also imposed.[142] It is reasonable to expect that patients give informed consent for radiation therapy and will accept a certain risk of ill effects. This does not mean that the patient assumes a risk of negligent care.[188,223]

In a case where a patient with carcinoma of the rectum was given radiation therapy at a dose above that recognized as proper and suffered severe ill effects, the radiation oncologist offered a defense that such dosage had been given in accordance with the recommendation of a recently delivered scientific paper. The court rejected this claim. In the court's view, this was not a generally accepted course or program of therapy, and the patient's specific consent to the variance in therapy had not been obtained.[7]

One must be particularly cautious in dealing with a woman of childbearing age concerning the possibility of pregnancy before exposing her to radiation therapy. Because the fetus might be injured, producing birth defects or necessitating an abortion, the patient has a right to refuse or at least should be given the full chance of providing informed consent.[392]

One must also be wary of injury through other forms of negligence involving radiation therapy. Injuries of this type include allowing the patient to fall, unstrapped, off the couch of a linear accelerator as it is being moved into the correct position, being struck by a fluoroscopic screen or other equipment from a treatment machine or a simulator, being shocked or burned, or being permitted to come in contact with high-tension electrical wires.

There are some data concerning the types of malpractice claims brought in radiation oncology. From 1975 through 1994, a total of 18,860 malpractice suits were brought in Cook County, Illinois, naming at least one codefendant physician; 8% named a radiation oncologist as one of the defendants. The number of suits directed against radiation oncologists fell sharply in Cook County after 1982. At that time allegations that thyroid cancer in adults developed from tonsillar irradiation administered in childhood for benign disease halted when such suits proved unsuccessful. The most common complaints initiating radiation oncology suits in recent years relate to:

a. Alleged complications of radiation therapy;
b. Alleged administration of radiation therapy for inappropriate indications, and
c. Alleged inappropriate withholding of radiation therapy.[43]

An interesting survey of 107 radiation oncology lawsuits conducted by the Fletcher Society found that 59% of the plaintiff patients were female. The four most common organ sites involved in the suits were gynecologic (17%), breast (16%), head and neck (14%), and urologic (12%). The actuarial probability of a radiation oncologist remaining free of a lawsuit after 30 years in practice was 35%.[403]

The National Association for Insurance Commissioners conducted an extensive study of medical liability claims and insurance indemnity. It was published yearly between 1977 and 1980. The final report was based on data collected from over 70,000 medical liability claims arising from over 62,000 alleged injuries or incidences that were closed with payments to the plaintiffs by insurers. These data show that 4% of paid claims were related to external-beam radiation therapy.[319]

Brachytherapy as the origin of a malpractice action poses particular problems for the radiation oncologist. Brachytherapy procedures are relatively rare. Therefore, expertise is often limited and the individual experience of the practicing radiation oncologist may be minimal. The existence of postimplant films, which document the location of the radioactive material, can be used to challenge the quality of the implant procedure. Brachytherapy complications can take years to occur and, because brachytherapy is often employed in treatment of carcinoma of the prostate, cervix, and uterus, the development of fistulas in long-term survivors can be the cause of a malpractice action.

Radiation oncologists conduct their practice with the assistance of others: physicists, dosimetrists, nurses, and therapists. It is necessary, therefore, for radiation oncologists to understand *vicarious liability*. In general, employers are responsible for the actions of their employees. This is called *respondent superior*—also called the master–servant relationship.[284] The fundamental issue that determines whether a person is legally treated as an employee is the extent to which the person hiring the worker may control the details of that work. Nurses, physician assistants, radiation therapists, and other physician extenders are professionals, but in most states in which they are licensed, they generally have a limited license. The extent to which they make medical decisions is determined by state law, but they usually must work under the supervision of a practicing physician. The physician's license, however, is unlimited. The physician, for example, may perform nursing tasks without violating nursing practice laws. Injury caused by extenders may, ultimately, lead to a malpractice claim against the physician. Physician liability for the actions of hospital employees is particularly problematic for radiation oncologists. Many radiation oncologists practice in hospital-based clinics. In general, the *doctrine of the borrowed-servant* or the *captain of the ship doctrine* states that all actions of hospital employees are attributable to the patient's attending physician. Under such a doctrine, the radiation oncologist may be found liable for the actions of a nurse, dosimetrist, or radiation therapist who the physician can neither hire, fire, nor otherwise directly control.[269]

When radiation oncologists are directors of clinical services, they also should be aware of the fact that they may be vicariously liable for the behavior of employees if they tolerate inappropriate activity or do not properly screen employees for dangerous tendencies. If, for example, a therapist has assaulted persons in the past and the radiation oncologist was negligent in discovering this, the radiation oncologist could be held liable under the theory of negligent hiring. The radiation oncologist also could be held liable for negligent retention if there were complaints about the behavior of the therapist and the physician failed to act on them.[376]

The captain of the ship doctrine means that physicians may have responsibility for the mistakes of their radiation therapists, dosimetrists, physicists, nurses, and fellow practicing physicians allegedly under their supervision or control. It is, therefore, incumbent upon the responsible radiation oncologist to take care in staff selection, training, and supervision. There is a risk in delegating such matters to an office manager. Ultimately, the physician must maintain an active role in ascertaining that he or she can fully trust the person selected to assist in all aspects of patient care. This means that the radiation oncologist must protect against allegations of sexual misconduct or abuse, alcohol or drug impairment, or mental illness potentially affecting patient care; because the physician is ultimately liable for the care given to a patient, the radiation oncologist must play an active role in ongoing training and professional development of his or her staff.

If an accident or allegation of misconduct occurs, the radiation oncologist must have a thorough, efficient, and adequate means of investigation of the matter and, if necessary, discipline or dismissal. Adequate employment records must be maintained.[225]

One of the most vexing problems now facing the practicing radiation oncologist is the matter of substance and alcohol abuse in the workplace and potential criminal records of employees. Some practices are instituting mandatory preemployment screening for alcohol and drug abuse and criminal background checks. These issues, however, are extremely complicated, and it is not yet clear which drugs should be tested for, when the testing should occur, who should be evaluated for a potential criminal background, which positive criminal background checks merit a decision not to employ an individual or to dismiss the person, under what circumstances a person can be felt to have paid his or her debt to society in a way that allows the individual to practice in a health care environment, and to what extent a radiation oncologist can be held liable for failure to exercise due caution in this process. Obtaining sound advice from an expert in personnel relations and legal counsel is advisable.[43]

It is well recognized that no radiation oncologist can be available at all times and in all circumstances. A physician may arrange, during his or her absence for vacation or ill health, for practice coverage by another physician. When one radiation oncologist "covers" for another, there are risks to patient safety, and possible susceptibility to malpractice claims, if clinical care "falls through the cracks." To minimize the risk of malpractice claims, the following guidelines should be followed:

- When you are away from your practice, you should select a covering radiation oncologist who possesses knowledge and skill at least equal to yours.
- Inform and obtain consent from those patients who will be affected.
- Apprise your covering physician of any important clinical information pertaining to patients he or she will see in your absence.
- The covering physician is expected to do more than just "fill in." He or she must apply the same degree of medical skill and care as the regular radiation oncologist.
- When the regular radiation oncologist returns, he or she should receive a report of any noteworthy patient care events, laboratory tests or diagnostic imaging results that deserve follow-up, and any other "loose-ends."[37]

It cannot be overemphasized that well-maintained medical records are crucial to a satisfactory legal defense in malpractice claims in radiation oncology. In law, the concept of *spoliation* refers to the destruction of evidence of significance or a meaningful alteration of a document. In medical malpractice cases, this would refer to the absence or disappearance of medical records. One radiation oncologist wisely counseled: now and then pick up an old chart, see if you can trace all of your steps in making decisions and executing treatments. Would this chart be sufficient to defend yourself against a malpractice claim?[403]

The Nature of Grievances and Malpractice Claims in Radiation Oncology

Dissatisfied patients might ignore their physician's advice or seek a new physician. Assertive patients may confront their physician. It is also commonplace for patients to discuss their complaints about physicians with friends and relatives.

In Anglo-American law and custom, patients whose dissatisfaction prompts formal action have several options. These include bringing a malpractice claim and seeking redress in courts. Other options include filing a complaint with a government medical board; filing a complaint with the "patient relations office" of a hospital or group practice; directing a complaint to a hospital's chief of medical staff or credentials office; or submitting a grievance to the local, state, district, or national medical society. Why some dissatisfied patients do nothing and others take formal action is not well studied. The general nature of patient grievances against physicians, however, has been evaluated by several authors.[198] Complaints fall into several broad categories:

- Alleged failure of physicians to fulfill the patient's expectations for examination and treatment (i.e., inadequate therapy, failure to obtain informed consent prior to a procedure, inadequate physical examination, or lack of prompt attention following hospitalization);
- Alleged failure to make a prompt diagnosis;
- Alleged rude or discourteous behavior;
- Alleged unacceptable practice behavior, such as producing excessive pain or practicing outside an area of expertise;
- Alleged inappropriate behavior related to billings and collections;
- Alleged physician's use of alcohol or drugs;
- Alleged sexual misconduct;
- Alleged errors in prescribing; and
- Alleged insurance fraud.

Formal complaints, including malpractice suits, represent only the tip of the iceberg of patient dissatisfaction. Patients far more often deal with their dissatisfaction by complaining to family and friends or switching doctors than by submitting a written complaint. A study by the Harvard Medical Practice Study Group, for example, found that <2% of patients who had adverse events because of medical malpractice ever filed malpractice claims.[277] Patients pursued medical malpractice claims for a variety of reasons. The four most common include an attempt to hold the offending caregiver accountable, to seek a more complete or satisfying explanation for the adverse event, to stop similar events from occurring to other patients, and to obtain financial compensation[476] (Boxes 1.8 and 1.9).

A disagreement between a patient and his or her radiation oncologist may cause the patient to have diminished trust in the physician, to be dissatisfied with the clinical results, to

Box 1.8

Systematic Radiation Therapy Overdose and Underdose: Recent Events in the United Kingdom

It was discovered in 1998 at Exeter that 207 patients were given a radiation dose >25% than that generally deemed appropriate for the treatment of breast cancer. Some patients had more marked radiation reactions than appropriate. When this became known, adverse publicity appeared in the press. At Stafford ~1,000 patients received ~25% underdosing over a 20-year period. An investigation concluded that in ~500 patients there was a real possibility that underdosage may have affected the outcome of treatment and, in a small number of patients, produced a cancer recurrence higher rate than that expected.[22,255]

The causes of these two incidents were analyzed in great detail and may have been related to inadequate medical physics staffing. A Royal College of Radiologists survey showed that radiation oncologists in many U.K. radiotherapy departments were seeing ≥600 new patients per year as compared to the usual 250 to 300 patients seen in France, Germany, and the United States.

Box 1.9

The RAGE Campaign

In 1991, a group of women formed an organization in the United Kingdom called RAGE (Radiation in Action Group Exposure). Their campaign began when a patient developed serious brachial plexus damage following surgery and radiotherapy for breast cancer. The patient wrote a letter to several newspapers describing these events and criticizing the medical and legal processes. This produced an outpouring of concern from other patients who claimed to have suffered from the same side effects. RAGE called for significant changes in the use of radiotherapy for the treatment of breast cancer.[373] The group successfully applied to the legal aid board for funds to undertake research toward a group legal action and, in 1995, constituted a group of plaintiffs in a malpractice case. Publicity associated with the litigation prompted the Royal College of Radiology to establish a multidisciplinary working party that made recommendations to ensure that patients with symptoms that might be due to radiation-associated brachial plexus injury had access to a network of health care professionals and cancer centers with the necessary skills for diagnosis, functional assessment, and treatment. The case highlighted the risks of high-dose-per-fraction radiation therapy used in the 1970s and 1980s. When the case eventually came to judgment, Justice Ebsworth concluded that there was no negligence and costs were directed against the plaintiffs. The justice commented that "it was unfortunate that litigation in terms of medical negligence was felt to be the only mechanism available," particularly in view of the fact that the cost of litigation exceeded £4 million. The case is instructive on several grounds:

1. The ill effects of radiation therapy may take a long time to become manifest.
2. Communication with patients concerning the causes and treatment of an injury is crucial.
3. The cost of litigation is quite high, and one would certainly hope that in the future society can derive alternative mechanisms to costly malpractice actions to allow patients to understand how and why injuries occur.[22,117,255]

Box 1.10

***The New York Times* Investigates Radiation Therapy**

Radiation therapy practice was severely shaken when *The New York Times* published an article on June 21, 2009, titled "At V.A. Hospital, a Rogue Cancer Unit" and a second article on January 23, 2010, titled "Radiation Offers New Cures, and Ways to Do Harm." Both articles were authored by Walt Bogdanich.[49,50]

The first article described allegations that the prostate brachytherapy program at the Philadelphia V.A. Medical Center was "a rogue cancer unit at the hospital, one that operated with virtually no outside scrutiny and botched 92 of 116 cancer treatments over a span of more than six years—and then kept quiet about it. . . ." The article described allegations of repetitive misplacement of prostate brachytherapy seeds, the changing of treatment plans to cover up the alleged errors, lack of peer review and quality assurance procedures, and the development of severe complications in patients.

The second article focused on the death of a 43-year-old man who had been irradiated at St. Vincent's Hospital in Manhattan for a tongue carcinoma and a 32-year-old female breast cancer patient treated at the State University of New York Downstate Medical Center. In the former case, the multileaf collimator was left fully open during intensity-modulated radiation therapy. In the latter case, a wedge was left out of the linear accelerator. Both patients were significantly overdosed and the tongue cancer patient died of radiation injuries. Bogdanich explores the causes of the errors: possible software malfunctions, human error, and lack of quality assurance and safety check procedures. Furthermore, the reporter raised the serious question of whether or not governmental oversight was sufficient to ensure the safety of clinical radiation therapy.

The articles made the safety of radiation therapy a national concern and have produced considerable soul searching in the medical physics and clinical radiation therapy communities. Efforts are under way at many levels to understand what can go wrong in radiation therapy, what can be done to prevent these errors, how much can be done to engineer procedures to prevent machine and human error, and what types of oversight are necessary to minimize error. We must never forget the Hippocratic admonishment *primo non nocere:* "First do no harm."

change physicians or health plans, to file a complaint, or to undertake litigation. For physicians, however, disagreements with patients may result in frustration, anger, a feeling of loss of control, and career dissatisfaction.

It is important to document your explanation of the risks and benefits of radiation therapy and to obtain the patient's written authorization to proceed, with a full understanding of those risks. In discussing any procedure or treatment with the patient or his or her guardian, the radiation oncologist should endeavor to explain all of the risks in sufficient detail to permit the patient to make a well-educated decision. Written informed consent should be obtained. But simply having the patient sign a standard form is not the end of the matter. The forms need to be easily understood and written in clear language. It is unwise for a physician to adopt standard printed forms without giving them proper scrutiny. Radiation oncologists must also be sure that the consent form is properly filled out. If, for example, there are blanks for explanations of particular risks involved for the procedure, they should be properly filled in.[225]

It is essential that radiation oncologists use fundamental communication skills to avoid grievances and malpractice claims, understand the patient's worries and concerns, express empathy, actively discuss care options, negotiate differences of opinion, and allow time for adequate conversation. The challenge for radiation oncologists is to recognize patients' unfulfilled expectations and to engage patients in a discussion with the goal of identifying and avoiding dissatisfaction while building a trusting therapeutic relationship (Box 1.10).

Health Insurance Portability and Accountability Act

Since the Health Insurance Portability and Accountability Act of 1996 (HIPAA) has come fully into effect, considerable changes have occurred in the area of health care fraud and abuse. HIPAA created new criminal offenses and brought civil remedies while strengthening existing ones. More important for the practicing radiation oncologist, however, HIPAA is part of a larger political initiative in which health care fraud and abuse became a top law enforcement priority. Large numbers of civil investigations have been brought regarding alleged abuses of Medicare and Medicaid. Many physicians and organizations have been excluded from federally funded health care programs, and there have been criminal convictions and collection of large amounts of money in criminal fines.

RISK MANAGEMENT IN RADIATION ONCOLOGY

In an era of increasing litigation and, unfortunately, a growth in adversarial situations between physicians and patients, it is critical for the radiation oncologist and staff to make every effort to decrease professional liability risks.

The origins of medical malpractice suits include:[242]

- Medical accidents that may not be adequately understood by the patient or explained by the treating physician.
- Less than successful or unexpected adverse results of treatment.
- Poor results from previous treatment elsewhere and ill-advised comments by other physicians or health care personnel.
- Rejection of a plan of therapy without appropriate documentation that the physician has advised the patient of the consequences of declining treatment. Some physicians document this discussion in the chart and send a certified letter advising the patient of the consequences of rejection of treatment.
- Complaint of experimentation when the patient has not been appropriately informed of the nature of the therapy to be administered.
- An angry patient who may find this a way to vent anger or frustration about any events surrounding treatment, including lack of communication, discourteous treatment by the physician or staff, or the amount of the medical bill.

The best prevention against a lawsuit is good rapport with the patient and relatives, effective communication and QA programs in all activities related to patient management, and clear and accurate documentation of all procedures, discussions, and events that take place before, during, and after treatment.

After appropriate clinical assessment, the histologic diagnosis of the patient must be confirmed at the treating institution; this often includes review of outside pathologic slides. Rationale of therapy and any changes in treatment plan should be duly explained and documented in the record. All procedures performed on the patient should be recorded in the chart, including details of daily treatments, such as use of special treatment aids (i.e., bright blocks, testicular shields, eye shields, immobilization devices), and any problems related to equipment operation. All treatment parameters and calculations should be accurately recorded and verified by a physicist or dosimetrist, in addition to the radiation oncologist. We should remember that, as professional liability attorneys say, "If it is not recorded on the chart, we may assume it never happened."

The physician and staff may help in their own professional liability defense in case a lawsuit occurs. It is extremely important for the physician to understand and, at an appropriate time, identify early warning signs of an impending malpractice suit. The physician should promptly contact his or her attorney, risk management office, and insurance carrier.

The physician should prepare an incident report in anticipation of potential litigation, describing the potential liability, including dates when events took place and actors and witnesses to be identified by name, affiliation, and status. Incident reports are confidential information between the physician and the attorney, risk manager, or insurance carrier. The report should be prepared while the facts are still fresh so that documentation will be optimal.

Clear and well-kept records with notes documenting every discussion and procedure that is performed on the patient should help in case of a lawsuit. A full discussion with the patient and relatives regarding planned therapy, particularly side effects of irradiation, and a well-documented informed consent form are valuable in risk management.

Informed Consent

The need to obtain informed consent for treatment is based on the patient's right to self-determination and the fiduciary relationship between the patient and physician.[375] The law requires that the treating physician adequately apprise every patient of the nature of the disease requiring treatment, recommended course of therapy and details regarding it, alternative treatments available, benefits of recommended treatment, and all minor and major risks (acute and late effects) associated with the recommended therapy (Table 1.15). If the plan of therapy is modified, this should be discussed with the patient, and, if warranted, a second informed consent may be required. It is advisable to discuss the informed consent contents in the presence of a witness and have that person sign an informed consent form or the chart verifying that the information was discussed with the patient.

Informed consent is a process, not a form. A consent form documents and codifies the process but does not substitute for clear and appropriate provision of information to the patient with adequate time for questions, answers, and free discussion and exchange. Ultimately, the competent adult patient or a legal representative must agree to the treatment and give approval. For unemancipated minors or legally incompetent adults, informed consent must be signed by the parents, adult brothers or sisters, or a responsible near relative or legal guardian. For incompetent adults, spouses may be allowed by the state to sign. Emancipated minors may provide their own consent. It is extremely important for the radiation oncologist and the staff to spend as much time as is needed to ensure that the patient and, if necessary, relatives understand all aspects of the radiation therapy, particularly the specific description of the various potential deleterious effects of this modality. Many physicians indicate which situations may require surgery to treat a complication and, specifically, when a gastrostomy, colostomy, ileal bladder, or other organ-substituting operation may be necessary to correct sequelae of therapy.

The radiation oncologist is always balancing a full disclosure of risks and options without overwhelming the patient with

TABLE 1.15 POSSIBLE SPECIFIC SEQUELAE OF THERAPY DISCUSSED IN INFORMED CONSENT

Anatomic Site	*Acute Sequelae*	*Late Sequelae*
Brain	Earache, headache, dizziness, hair loss, erythema	Hearing loss Damage to middle or inner ear Pituitary gland dysfunction Cataract formation Brain necrosis
Head and neck	Odynophagia, dysphagia, hoarseness, xerostomia, dysgeusia, weight loss	Subcutaneous fibrosis, skin ulceration, necrosis Thyroid dysfunction Persistent hoarseness, dysphonia, xerostomia, dysgeusia Cartilage necrosis Osteoradionecrosis of mandible Delayed wound healing, fistulae Dental decay Damage to middle and inner ear Apical pulmonary fibrosis Rare: myelopathy
Lung and mediastinum or esophagus	Odynophagia, dysphagia, hoarseness, cough Pneumonitis Carditis	Progressive fibrosis of lung, dyspnea, chronic cough Esophageal stricture Rare: chronic pericarditis, myelopathy
Breast or chest wall	Odynophagia, dysphagia, hoarseness, cough Pneumonitis (asymptomatic) Carditis Cytopenia	Fibrosis, retraction of breast Lung fibrosis Arm edema Chronic endocarditis, myocardial infarction Rare: osteonecrosis of ribs
Abdomen or pelvis	Nausea, vomiting Abdominal pain, diarrhea Urinary frequency, dysuria, nocturia Cytopenia	Proctitis, sigmoiditis Rectal or sigmoid stricture Colonic perforation or obstruction Contracted bladder, urinary incontinence, hematuria (chronic cystitis) Vesicovaginal fistula Rectovaginal fistula Leg edema Scrotal edema, sexual impotency Vaginal retraction or scarring Sterilization Sexual impotence Damage to liver or kidneys
Extremities	Erythema, dry/moist desquamation	Subcutaneous fibrosis Ankylosis, edema Bone/soft-tissue necrosis

data and causing distress. It is reasonable to expect the patient to come away from a meeting with the treating radiation oncologist with a general realistic hope regarding the proposed course of treatment and honest understanding of the side effects, and a sense of trust for the physician and the organization.[225] Good documentation is crucial and, if a malpractice action were to occur, liability may hinge on who said what to whom at what point of the treatment process. Absent or lost records will reflect extremely poorly on the radiation oncologist.[225]

It must be stressed that in dealing with children or mentally incompetent adults, a thorough discussion of the plan of therapy and sequelae should be held with the parents, relatives, or legal guardian of the patient. Also, they must sign the informed consent.

Although, in case of a lawsuit, having a properly executed informed consent form in the record is helpful, more important is the incontrovertible documentation in the chart of the pertinent discussion held with the patient. Table 1.15 describes many of the specific sequelae in several anatomic sites that should be included in the informed consent. Radiation oncologists also should be aware of court decisions that place a greater burden on the physician to disclose statistical life-expectancy information to critically ill patients as part of the informed consent and as an affirmation of patient-centered decision making (regarding treatment) in the context of a physician–patient relationship based on trust.[16]

SMART RADIATION ONCOLOGY IS COMING

Sequencing of the human genome is now complete. There are now vigorous efforts under way to catalog specific genes and to identify the protein makeup of cells—disciplines called genomics and proteomics.

What do genomics and proteomics mean for the future of radiation oncology? Engaging in predictions is a highly risky endeavor. We think it is reasonable, however, to expect the development of a new, more individualized, smarter radiation oncology.

First, we think that there will continue to be a movement away from anatomic staging of cancer toward molecular staging. When cancer staging was first developed, it was based on whether tumors could be labeled "operable" or "inoperable." Our discipline then moved toward anatomic staging, in which an assessment of the status of the tumor was made by inspection and palpation. Typical examples of this were the Jewett system for prostate cancer or the League of Nations system for cervical cancer. Staging now has developed into a system based on physical examination, radiographic studies, and, in some cases, pathologic assessment. The most widely used system includes an assessment of tumor status (T), nodal status (N), and the presence or absence of distant metastasis (M).

There is a trend toward a more molecular-based staging of cancer in which one assesses the genetic component of an individual tumor as a predictor of outcome and as a guide toward treatment. We see evidence of this trend in the use of hormone receptors, DNA ploidy, presence or absence of n-*myc*, presence or absence of H-erb-2B, and study of subtypes of gene rearrangements in the staging of leukemias and solid tumors. With more detailed molecular staging, one will be able to more finely tailor therapy to the specific needs of the patient.[500]

There will be an increasing trend toward the use of genomics and proteomics to prospectively identify high-risk patients for development of cancer. There are many cancers that have an obvious genetic basis. Population screening tests based on the presence or absence of a gene could change significantly the stage distribution of malignancies the clinician faces.[145] It is hoped that screening will allow us to identify earlier cases that would be more amenable to treatment. It certainly will be

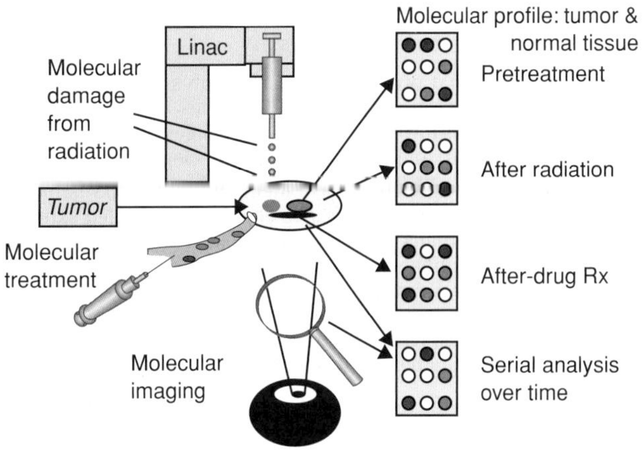

FIGURE 1.37. New developments in biotechnology will permit an analysis of how the genome or proteome of a tumor changes with treatment. This may allow researchers to identify novel therapeutic targets or find predictors of treatment outcome. The interaction between ionizing radiation and a biologic system may be thought of as a molecular event. Before, during, and after radiation, gene expression profiles using microarrays may be generated. (From Coleman CN. Radiation oncology–linking technology and biology in the treatment of cancer. *Acta Oncol* 2002;41:6–13.)

preferable to have a clear-cut genetic test for the early detection of colorectal cancer, for example, rather than the cumbersome, uncomfortable, and relatively expensive use of colonoscopy.

Developments in genetics and proteomics are highly likely to modify the clinician's use of drugs and radiation (Fig. 1.37). In many situations physicians treat individuals as a statistically average person. Medications are prescribed because they are thought, on average, to bring about a certain effect in the average patient and have a known risk of side effects. It would be preferable to understand the genetic profile of the individual patient and to more precisely predict whether he or she will respond to a drug and whether he or she would be more or less likely to have side effects from the medication. Genomics offers the possibility of developing a personalized medicine in which one would match medication-prescribing practices to the specific DNA profile of an individual patient. This evolving discipline is called pharmacogenomics.

Predictive assays for tumor control and the risk of normal tissue complications are under active investigation. Among the hypotheses being explored are the possible correlation of gene activity promoting or inhibiting apoptosis with tumor response to radiation, the correlation of the presence or absence of tumor markers for hypoxia with the chance of local tumor control with radiation, whether skin fibroblast radiosensitivity correlates with normal tissue complication risk from radiotherapy, the possible association of transforming growth factor β-1 polymorphisms with the risk of radiation-induced normal tissue damage, the possible correlation between *in vitro* chromosomal radiosensitivity of lymphocytes and normal tissue damage following external-beam radiotherapy, the pretreatment predictive power of microarray technology for gene expression in tumors, and protein expression profiling (proteomics) of tumors and normal tissue. These latter two technologies, because of their ability to measure many genes or proteins quickly, may allow the clinician of the future to obtain profiles of the tumor before, during, and after treatment; predict outcome; and, perhaps, tailor treatment according to the molecular response of the tumor.[26,102,190,265,266,379]

Finally, we may hope to understand the fine tuning of the individual patient's and his or her tumor's genome to influence or direct (epigenetics) therapy. Overproduction of oncogenes or inadequate production of tumor-suppressor genes might be genetically modified to place tumors in remission. Such activities are, almost certainly, far off in the future and will be enormously complex. One biotechnology executive artfully characterized the problem, as it regards the p53 tumor-suppressor gene, as follows:

> This is a gene that produces a tumor suppressor protein.... If it is under expressed [the cell] becomes cancerous. So when your p53 is lowered, the whole intelligence network of the cell is altered, and that's where cancer begins.
>
> However, researchers now have identified that if p53 is too high, that same gene produces osteoporosis, wrinkled skin, and shriveled organs—results that are linked to premature aging and a number of other diseases. A healthy human being, then, has an exact regulation of the p53 gene. There appears only to be a fine line between premature old age and cancer. It's obviously a very important gene, but we don't know much about how it works yet.[499]

One of the evolving areas in external-beam radiotherapy will, undoubtedly, be the attempt to develop *dose painting* or *biologically based optimization.* These techniques strive to marry diagnostic imaging, which identifies the tumor location, with metabolic imaging to show tumor activity (PET and PET/CT), along with calculations of tumor control probability, normal tissue complication probability, and uncomplicated tumor control probability. The software packages for these techniques strive to conform the radiation dose not only to the anatomic location of the tumor but also to the most metabolically active areas of the tumor while, at the same time, minimizing the dose to those areas of normal tissue most likely to produce complications.[379]

A new, smart form of radiation oncology offers enormous promise to the practicing clinician. An exciting age of medicine is before us. Obviously, developments in biotechnology pose formidable ethical problems that will vex the clinician. How much will be known about each individual patient's genetic makeup? How will that information be shared with the patient's family, insurance company, and employer? What protection will be built into a system in which enormous amounts of very private information will exist in electronic form? We must make sure that ethics and law keep up with scientific progress.

Radiation oncologists must enrich training programs with more exposure to basic science investigation and nurture research that will provide new directions for the personalized applications of radiation therapy to the treatment of malignant neoplasias in specific patients.

SELECTED REFERENCES

A full list of references for this chapter is available online.

24. Baclesse F. Carcinoma of the larynx. *Br J Radiol* 1949;3:1–62.
31. Becquerel H. Sur les radiations invisible emises par les sources d'uranium. *Cr Acad Sci Paris* 1896;122:689–694.
32. Becquerel H, Curie P. L'action physiologique des rayons du radium. *Cr Acad Sci Paris* 1901;132:1289–1291.
38. Bentel GC. *Patient positioning and immobilization in radiation oncology.* New York: McGraw-Hill, 1999.
39. Bentel GC. *Radiation therapy planning,* 2nd ed. New York: McGraw-Hill, 1996.
40. Bentzen SM. Dose-painting by numbers. Theranostic imaging for radiation oncology. *Lancet Oncol* 2005;6:112–117.
42. Bergonie J, Tribondeau L. Interpretation of some results of radiotherapy and an attempt at determining a logical technique of treatment. *Radiat Res* 1959;11:587–588. [Translation of original article in *CR Acad Sci* 1906;143:983.]
53. Boveri T. *The origin of malignant tumors.* Baltimore: Williams & Wilkins, 1929.
80. Catterall M. Neutron therapy at Hammersmith Hospital 1970 to 1985: a re-examination of results. *Strahlenther Onkol* 1989;165:298–301.
81. Chadwick J. The existence of a neutron. *Proc Roy Soc London* 1932;136:692–708.
82. Chadwick J, Goldhaber M. Disintegration by slow neutrons. *Nature* 1935;135:65.
91. Coleman CN. International Conference on Translational Research and Preclinical Strategies in Radio-Oncology (ICTR): conference summary. *Int J Radiat Oncol Biol Phys* 2001;49:301–309.
92. Coleman CN, Stevenson MA. The hallmark of modern radiation oncology. *Int J Radiat Oncol Biol Phys* 1994;30:1247–1249.
98. Coutard H. Cancer of the larynx: results of roentgen therapy after five and ten years of control. *Am J Roentgenol* 1938;40:509.
99. Coutard H. Principles of x-ray therapy of malignant diseases. *Lancet* 1934;2:1–8.
100. Coutard H. Roentgentherapy of epitheliomas of the tonsillar region, hypopharynx and larynx from 1920 to 1926. *Am J Roentgenol* 1932;28:313–331.
103. Curie P, Curie MP, Bemont G. Sur une nouvelle substance fortement radioactive contenue dans la pechblende (note presented by M. Becquerel). *Compt Rend Acad Sci (Paris)* 1898;127:1215–1217.
104. Dam HJW. The new marvel in photography. *McClure's Magazine* 1896;6:403.
119. Doll R, Peto R. *The causes of cancer: quantitative estimates of avoidable risks of cancer in the United States.* Oxford: Oxford University Press, 1981.
120. Donaldson S. Lessons from our children. *Int J Radiat Oncol Biol Phys* 1993;26:739–749.
140. Emami B, Lyman J, Brown A, et al. Tolerance of normal tissue to therapeutic irradiation. *Int J Radiat Oncol Biol Phys* 1991;21:109–122.
146. Fermi E. Artificial radioactivity produced by neutron bombardment. In: Holberg MA, ed. *Les Prix Nobel in 1939.* Stockholm: Norstedt and Söner, 1939.
148. Fidler IJ, Hart IR. Biological diversity in metastatic neoplasms: origins and implications. *Science* 1982;217:998–1003.
149. Fletcher GH. Clinical dose-response curve of human malignant epithelial tumors. *Br J Radiol* 1973;46:1–12.
151. Fletcher GH. Keynote address: the scientific basis of the present and future practice of clinical radiotherapy. *Int J Radiat Oncol Biol Phys* 1983;9:1073–1082.
152. Fletcher GH, Shukovsky LJ. The interplay of radiocurability and tolerance in the irradiation of human cancers. *J Radiol Electrol* 1975;56:383–400.
155. Folkman J. Tumor angiogenesis: therapeutic implications. *N Engl J Med* 1971; 285:1182.
163. Fowler JF. The linear quadratic formula and progress in fractionated radiotherapy: a review. *Br J Radiol* 1989;62:679–694.
168. Friend SH, Dryja TP, Weinberg RA. Oncogenes and tumor-suppressing genes. *N Engl J Med* 1988;318:618–622.
170. Fry SA. Studies of US radium dial workers: an epidemiological classic. *Radiat Res* 1998;150:521–529.
171. Fuks Z, Alfieri A, Haimovitz-Friedman A, et al. Intravenous basic fibroblast growth factor protects the lung but not mediastinal organs against radiation-induced apoptosis. *Cancer J Sci Am* 1995;1:62–72.
175. Glasser O. *Wilhelm Conrad Röntgen and the early history of the Roentgen rays.* Springfield: Charles C. Thomas, 1934.
185. Gray LH. Oxygenation in radiotherapy. I. radiobiological considerations. *Br J Radiol* 1957;30:403–406.
199. Halperin EC. Historical review: particle therapy for cancer. *Lancet Oncol* 2006;7: 676–685.
212. Hellman S. Roentgen Centennial Lecture: discovering the past, inventing the future. *Int J Radiat Oncol Biol Phys* 1996;35:15–20.
213. Hellman S, Vokes EE. Advancing current treatments for cancer. *Sci Am* 1996; 275:118–123.
214. Hellman S, Weichselbaum RR. Radiation oncology. *JAMA* 1996;275:1852–1853.
215. Hellman S, Weichselbaum RR. Radiation oncology and the new biology. *Cancer J Sci Am* 1995;1:174–179.
243. Kaplan HS. Historic milestones in radiobiology and radiation therapy. *Semin Oncol* 1979;6(4).
244. Kaplan HS. Radiobiology's contribution to radiotherapy: promise or mirage? Failla Memorial Lecture. *Radiat Res* 1970;43:460–476.
250. Knudson AG Jr. Mutation and cancer: statistical study of retinoblastoma. *Proc Natl Acad Sci U S A* 1971;68:820–823.
251. Kohn HI, Fry RJM. Radiation carcinogenesis. *N Engl J Med* 1984;310:504–511.
252. Korbelik M, Skov KA. Inactivation of hypoxic cells by cisplatin and radiation at clinically relevant doses. *Radiat Res* 1989;119:145–156.
258. Laramore GE. The use of neutrons in cancer therapy: a historical perspective through the modern era. *Semin Oncol* 1997;24:672–686.
267. Levine AJ. Tumor suppressor genes. In: Mendelsohn J, Howley PM, Israel MA, et al., eds. *The molecular basis of cancer.* Philadelphia: W.B. Saunders, 1995: 86–104.
270. Lichter AS, Lawrence TS. Recent advances in radiation oncology. *N Engl J Med* 1995;332:371–379.
273. Liotta LA. Tumor invasion and metastases: role of the extracellular matrix: Rhoads Memorial Award Lecture. *Cancer Res* 1986;46:1–7.
310. Moran JM, Elshaikh MA, Lawrence TS. Radiotherapy: what can be achieved by technical improvements in dose delivery? *Lancet Oncol* 2005;6:51–58.
334. Orton CG, Ellis F. A simplification in the use of the NSD concept in practical radiotherapy. *Br J Radiol* 1973;46:529–537.
339. Overgaard J, Horsman MR. Modification of hypoxia-induced radio-resistance in tumors by the use of oxygen and sensitizers. *Semin Radiat Oncol* 1996;6: 10–21.
342. Paget S. The distribution of secondary growths in cancer of the breast. *Lancet* 1889;1:571–573.
347. Paterson RP. The radical x-ray treatment of the carcinomata. *Br J Radiol* 1936; 9:671–679.
367. Puck TT, Marcus PI. Actions of x-rays on mammalian cells. *J Exp Med* 1956; 103:653–666.
373. Regaud C, Ferroux R. Discordance des effects de rayons X, d'une part dans le testicule, par le fractionnement de la dose. *CR Soc Biol* 1927;97:431–434.
381. Roentgen WC. On a new kind of rays (preliminary communication). Translation of a paper read before the Physikalische-medicinischen Gesellschaft of Würzburg on December 28, 1985. *Br J Radiol* 1931;4:32.
428. Strandqvist M. Sutdien uber die kumulative wirkung der rontgenstrahlen bie frakionierung. *Acta Radiol (Stockh)* 1944;55(Suppl):1–300.
429. Suit H. Radiation biology: the conceptual and practical impact on radiation therapy. *Radiat Res* 1983;94:10–40.
432. Suit HD, Westgate SJ. Impact of improved local tumor control on survival. *Int J Radiat Oncol Biol Phys* 1986;12:453–458.
434. Suit HD. A personal philosophy of a radiation oncologist. *Radiother Oncol* 2011; 100:10–14.
436. Sweet WH. Early history of development of boron neutron capture therapy of tumors. *J Neuro Oncol* 1997;33:19–26.
437. Tannock IF. Eradication of a disease: how we cured symptomless prostate cancer. *Lancet* 2002;359:1341–1342.
445. Thames HD, Withers HR, Mason KA, et al. Dose-survival characteristics of mouse jejunal crypt cells. *Int J Radiat Oncol Biol Phys* 1981;7:1591–1597.
471. Varmus H, Weinberg RA. *Genes and the biology of cancer.* New York: Scientific American Library, 1993.
479. Von Essen CF. A spatial model of time-dose-area relationships in radiation therapy. *Radiology* 1963;81:881–883.
484. Wang CC, Blitzer PH, Suit HD. Twice-a-day radiation therapy for cancer of the head and neck. *Cancer* 1985;55:2100–2104.
487. Wasserman TH, Brizel DM. The role of amifostine as a radioprotector. *Oncology* 2001;15:1349–1354.
494. Weinberg RA. *The biology of cancer.* New York: Garland Science, Taylor and Francis Group, 2007.
495. Weinberg RA. Tumor suppressor genes. *Science* 1991;254:1138–1146.

Part A Cancer Biology

Chapter 2
Biologic Basis of Radiation Therapy

William H. McBride and H. Rodney Withers

INTRODUCTION

Clinically Relevant Physicochemical Events

Ionizing radiation (IR) interacts with matter in many different ways; however, for high-energy photons, a two-step process dominates. Energetic ionizing electrons are produced that directly ionize atoms and break chemical bonds. Subsequent physicochemical reactions involve production of free radical and other reactive species that are heavily influenced by the intracellular milieu, such as free radical scavengers and the quaternary structure of the biologic target. For low linear energy transfer (LET) x- or γ-rays, 1 Gy represents about 1,000 ionization tracks, and most of the free radicals formed such as hydroxyl radicals, singlet oxygen, superoxide, and hydrogen peroxide are from ionization of water, a cell's major (about 90%) constituent. These oxygen-containing molecules are collectively, although not totally accurately, often referred to as reactive oxygen species (ROS). They generate oxidative damage within a cell by virtue of their unpaired valence shell electrons and are the major cause of low LET radiation damage (perhaps 70%)—the radiation acts largely indirectly, which has numerous implications for the biologic effectiveness of radiation therapy (RT).

The importance of the indirect pathway varies with the type (quality) of radiation as the density at which energy is deposited determines the amount and type of damage caused. For all IRs, the density is especially high at the end of the electron tracks. For high LET radiations, such as α-particles, dense ionizing takes place along and close to tracks, which number about four for each Gy. As a result, more energy is deposited directly in biologic molecules, and more direct rather than indirect damage results.

Because free radicals are involved, the biologic microenvironment where these events take place contributes to the outcome. If oxygen, or other electron-affinic molecules, is present,[1] it can participate in the free radical cascadic reactions, but its major effect is probably to "fix" chemical damage in biologic molecules and limit chemical repair. Oxygen is therefore a potent radiosensitizer, whereas hypoxia will limit radiation damage. Within tumors, hypoxia is a potential cause of failure of RT. Considerable effort has gone into the search for oxygen mimetic drugs that might penetrate into tumor hypoxic regions; some, such as the imidazoles, have been used clinically with effect, although they are not without toxicity.

Conversely, antioxidants such as glutathione, which is present in millimolar amounts in cells, scavenge radiation-induced free radicals to limit damage. The nuclear bomb era prompted searches for radioprotectors of normal tissue. The organic thiophosphates, such as WR2721, which is hydrolyzed in vivo by alkaline phosphatase to the thiol metabolite WR-1065, received much attention. Its commercial version, Amifostine, has been approved by the Food and Drug Administration (FDA) for reduction of xerostomia in patients receiving RT for head and neck cancer, although its use has not gained general acceptance.

Free radicals react with substrates in many different ways and at different rates; however, in general, IR has an oxidizing effect that lowers buffering power of the antioxidants in a cell and changes its redox status. The sensitivity of cells to IR depends on the levels and redox potential of many molecules, and this may be heavily influenced by the cell's metabolic state. For example, quiescent stem cells appear to have high levels of free radical scavengers and antioxidants that may account for their relative radioresistance.[2] Cells contain many molecular sensors for redox changes. These may make conformational changes to initiate rapid molecular responses through activation of transcriptional and translational pathways.

DNA as a Biologic Target of Radiation

Whereas the primary ionization and excitation events associated with IR exposure are over within a second or so, the biologic consequences may last for life. IR will damage all cellular organelles, but its biggest footprint is in DNA. Indeed, the efficiency with which IR causes complex DNA damage, as opposed to other lesions, in both cycling and noncycling cells is why it is such an effective cytotoxic agent. Complex or clustered damage (also referred to as multiply-damaged sites) are multiple lesions located within about one helical turn of the DNA that involve both DNA strands and about 15 to 20 base pairs. These are a direct consequence of the characteristic way that IR spatially deposits energy in dense "packets." For sparse IR about 30% of events are of this form, whereas it is >90% for α-particles. Few complex lesions result from everyday oxidative and chemical damage. Instead, of the 10,000–20,000 DNA lesions produced per cell per day, the preponderance is single-strand breaks (SSBs) and base damage. Many agents produce DNA damage—even breathing; however, IR is exceptional in that it causes a relatively large number of complex lesions in DNA that are frequently lethal and all cell cycle phases are affected, although not equally when it comes to survival.

Safeguarding the integrity of DNA so as to minimize mutation is a biologic imperative. A complex group of highly efficient DNA repair mechanisms have evolved to achieve this, with each focused largely on a type of DNA lesion. SSBs and base damages formed by IR (1,000 per cell per Gray), as with everyday oxidative damage, are rapidly and faithfully repaired using processes such as base excision repair (BER), which uses the complementary undamaged DNA strand as a template.

DNA double-strand breaks (DSBs) at 15 to 20 per cell per Gray are more significant than SSBs for lethality and carcinogenesis following radiation exposure; however, many of these also can be repaired. The two major DSB repair pathways are nonhomologous end joining (NHEJ), which is error-prone but efficient, and homologous recombination (HR), which contributes in the late S/G2 cell cycle phase. HR is error free because it uses the sister chromatid as a template but has slower kinetics. These are canonical mechanisms that exist to deal with DSBs produced physiologically during meiosis (HR), DNA replication (HR), and for the generation of specific immune receptors (NHEJ), as well as by pathologic oxidative damage. The key proteins required for both NHEJ (Ku70, Ku80, DNA-PKcs, XRCC4, XLF, DNA ligase IV) and HR (Rad51, Rad52, Rad54, BRCA2, RPA) have been identified by a combination of genetic experiments and examination of the composition of ionizing radiation–induced foci (IRIF) that form at sites of DSBs. MRE11, Rad50, and NBS1 act as a complex (MRSN) to participate in both HR and NHEJ. Many other molecules play important roles in DSB repair, including the protein mutated in ataxia telangiectasia (ATM), whose loss gives rise to extreme radiosensitivity in humans. Analysis of IRIFs has shown that their composition and number vary depending on whether the DSB is in euchromatin or heterochromatin and on the phase of the cell cycle when irradiation occurs.

On the other hand, complex IR-induced DNA damage is highly diverse and presents an especially difficult challenge for repair mechanisms. Breaks resolve slowly with time, and non-DSB lesions can sometimes convert to DSBs during processing. For example, SSBs may be converted into DSBs at replication forks, making BER relevant to the irradiation outcome. One consequence of this complexity is that the time taken for DNA repair varies with the repair mechanism and site of damage. "Fast" and "slow" components are the minimum consideration, with the latter having estimated half-lives of up to 4 hours and the former 50 minutes to 1 hour. Estimates of "repair" rates within a tissue are therefore very uncertain, and when the times for repair during clinical fractionated treatments are discussed, this usually refers to tissue recovery rather than DNA repair rates.

The complexity of the different DNA DSB repair mechanisms and their involvement at different cell cycle phases has major ramifications for cancer treatments. Chemotherapy agents frequently target cells in the S phase and emphasize the importance of the HR mechanism especially when combined with RT, even though NHEJ is the predominant repair mechanism overall because most cells are in the G0-G1 phase. Tumors that carry BRCA1 or BRCA2 mutations that compromise their ability to perform HR are sensitive to PARP-1 inhibitors that block BER mechanisms through a process known as synthetic lethality, which is where a mutation in either of two genes is not lethal but mutations in both cause cell death. These drugs are in clinical trials in combination with RT. Finally, critical defects in DNA damage and repair are not always easy to detect because they may affect only one cell cycle phase or one mechanism. For example, ATM or BRCA1 mutated cells do not always show radiosensitivity in terms of DNA damage or rate of DNA repair. The detection of such mutations also indicates the lesser role of these genes in DNA repair compared to certain others where the mutations cause fetal lethality.

Our ability to interrogate DNA repair mechanisms has been greatly enhanced by the use of IRIF assays. One early IRIF event is phosphorylation of a histone 2A subtype, H2AX, by one of several phosphoinositol 3-kinase-related protein kinases (PIKKs), including the ATM checkpoint kinase, DNA-PK, and ATR. Gamma-H2AX molecules bind to DSB over several megabases of the flanking chromatin and can easily be detected using specific antibody. This sensitive assay has become a routine way to measure DSB formation and repair.[3] More importantly, this histone provides interaction surfaces for other repair and checkpoint molecules and activates kinase-dependent pathways that lead to a coherent downstream DNA damage responses (DDRs). The classical DDR through ATM drives activation of p53, whose primordial function was transcriptional activation of stress responses. Cell cycle checkpoints are activated to allow time for repair, as are cell death pathways to remove highly damaged cells.

Other Biologic Targets of Radiation

RT targets cellular structures other than DNA to activate signaling pathways. As mentioned earlier, some of these are driven by changes in redox. In fact, although IR is an oxidative stress, most of the ROS and reactive nitrogen species (RNS) that are generated by IR can come from secondary sources such as damaged mitochondria, activation of cation membrane channels and activation of NADPH and other oxidases, alterations in cellular metabolism, induction of nitric oxide synthetase, and proinflammatory cytokines such as members of the tumor necrosis factor (TNF) family (e.g., TNF-α, fasL, Trail) that can be generated by radiation. Low levels of ROS and RNS are an integral part of metabolism and participate in most cellular processes, including cell signaling. Higher levels can precipitate cell death. It is not surprising that through inducing oxidative stress, IR can activate redox-sensitive transcription factor systems, such as NF-κB, AP-1, HIF-1α, Nrf2, PPARγ, p53, Sp1, c-abl, and STAT3, and other molecules including membrane receptors such as epidermal growth factor receptor (EGFR). As a result, primary (also known as immediate early response) genetic programs can be activated rapidly without de novo protein synthesis following IR exposure. These rapid and relatively promiscuous responses become consolidated where appropriate by the generation of more restricted secondary gene programs. Importantly, these pathways couple molecular damage to DNA repair, cell cycle arrest, phenotypic changes, and cell death. They also serve to signal "danger" to the body through tissue damage responses (TDRs).

Cellular Damage Responses After Irradiation

The ways that cells and tissues "perceive" radiation damage influence the final outcome. In other words, they depend on pre-existing internal "sensors" that are influenced by metabolic status and the external molecular signals from hypoxia, cytokines, cell–cell and cell extracellular matrix interactions, the signaling pathways that are activated, and so forth. Because tumorigenesis involves mutations in molecular pathways that govern DNA repair, cell cycle, and cell death, it follows that genetic alterations associated with cancer frequently alter the cellular response to RT. These pathways are activated by stresses other than IR, including chemotherapy, hyperthermia, and inflammation making these interactions complex. Given the complexity of the biologic system, clinical outcomes cannot be predicted from the amount of physical energy deposited, but only from the biologic context. This is why what is known as "biologic dose" differs considerably from "physical dose."

Because IR causes a relatively large number of complex lesions in DNA that are frequently lethal, it is a highly effective cytotoxic agent, and loss of reproductive ability of tumor cells is the desired therapeutic outcome. This can occur in several different ways, depending on the dose and the cell type. In 1956, Puck and Marcus[4] noted: "Cells in which the ability to reproduce has been destroyed by doses below 800r can still multiply several times. At higher doses, even a single cell division is precluded. The mitotic death that they observed is the most common form of cell death caused by IR.[5] It is a slow process that contrasts with rapid interphase death that is over in about 4 to 6 hours in certain cell types, including many lymphocytes, endothelial cells, and some cells in the salivary gland, thyroid, intestinal crypt, and hair follicles. Interphase death is now known to be by rapid apoptosis.[6–7,8–9] Mitotic death, however, can be caused by any of several mechanisms—for example, failure of spindle formation in the M phase, loss of the G2 checkpoint leading to "mitotic catastrophe," or improper chromosome segregation from damage and loss of genetic material—and the molecular machinery that is employed can be apoptotic, necrotic, or involve other mechanisms.

Radiation-induced apoptosis in normal tissues is often, although not always, dependent on activation of the DDR through p53 and its downstream effectors Bax and Bak.[10] These disrupt mitochondrial membranes, releasing factors that activate the caspase cascade of proteolytic enzymes and endonucleases that cleave DNA between nucleosomes to commit cellular "suicide."[10] Apoptosis can therefore be recognized morphologically by cell shrinkage or by labeling the 5'-ends of apoptotic DNA strand breaks using terminal deoxynucleotidyl transferase (TdT) (TUNEL technique). This intrinsic mitochondrial factor activates caspase 9 to lead to apoptosis and often overlaps mechanistically with an extrinsic pathway activated through tumor necrosis factor receptor (TNFR) family members in the plasma membrane that activates caspase 8. Most notably, both utilize the same final executioner caspase 3–dependent pathway.

Because radiation can induce expression of both TNF and TNFR family members, these pathways may form an additional indirect pathway leading to death or survival of some cell types following irradiation.[11,12] For example, mice lacking TNFR2, which does not have a death domain and drives cell survival, are particularly sensitive to late effects of IR to the brain.[13] The cytotoxicity of certain chemotherapeutic agents, such as 5-fluorouracil (5-FU) and cisplatin, can also involve TNF-α.[14]

Apoptosis is a form of programmed cell death that during development shapes organs. In adults, its role is in physiologic homeostatic control—for example, removing excess cells at sites of proliferation and self-reactive lymphocytes. Pathologically stressed cells may use also this form of cell death (e.g., after IR exposure). Interestingly, IR-induced apoptosis signals "danger" in tissues through inflammatory signaling, whereas cells that die by physiologic apoptosis are immunologically silent. Many cells are protected against apoptosis. Only cells that have their internal molecular "rheostat" on a proapoptosis setting undergo this form of death in response to IR. Therefore, IR increases the frequency of apoptosis, although only in cells that have the relevant molecular circuitry—for example, lymphomas die in this way, whereas glioma cells tend not to. Tumors formed of cells that are predisposed to apoptosis often are among the most clinically sensitive.

In contrast to apoptosis, necrosis is a purely pathologic tissue injury process that does not involve activation of cellular pathways. Membrane integrity is lost, cells increase in size, lysosomal enzymes are released, vasculature is damaged, and inflammatory responses are generated. DNA is cleaved in an indiscriminatory fashion.

Autophagy is another possible alternative death style following IR exposure. This is a primordial survival response in which cells internalize their cellular organelles within vacuoles and digest them; it is most often seen in nutrient deprivation. Cells can be rescued from autophagy, although they die if taken to excess. Another important alternative radiation-induced outcome is *senescence,* which involves activation of cell cycle checkpoint molecules such as p21 and p16 and can be promoted by cytokine transforming growth factor beta (TGF-β),[15,16] which drives collagen production. IR-induced senescence is therefore highly relevant to IR-induced fibrosis.[17]

Under normal circumstances, cell death in tissues is balanced by cell production and survival. Signals in the cell's environment, such as growth factors, cell–cell contact, and extracellular matrix, are critical for survival, and their loss may lead cells to exit the cell cycle and cell death by anoikis,[18] or "homelessness," which may occur by any mechanism.

Apoptosis, autophagy, and senescence all have the effect of removing damaged cells from the reproductive pool. This may limit the chances of radiocarcinogenesis, but cells in senescence and autophagy may retain function for some time. The long-term outcome may be IR-induced fibrosis through enhanced collagen production,[17] or re-entry into the cell cycle, or in the case of tumor cells, re-entry into a stem cell phase and subsequent tumor regrowth.

Because cells need positive signals to proliferate and survive, these pathways often promote radioresistance, and blocking them often results in radiosensitization. This is an oversimplification of complex biology, but it may help to explain why blocking EGFR tyrosine kinase signaling with cetuximab or gefitinib (Iressa), or NF-κB activation with bortezomib, may radiosensitize tumor cells. Survival pathway signaling may underlie some of the phenomena ascribed to potentially lethal damage repair (PLDR) following irradiation. In PLDR, the cellular microenvironment determines the likelihood of cell death. Classically, PLDR occurs when cells are irradiated and maintained in a contact-inhibited, plateau-phase culture. If such contact-inhibited cells are trypsinized immediately, or soon after irradiation, survival is compromised. One interpretation is that the cells are rendered homeless by trypsinization and are more likely to die. It must be noted, however, that PLDR, like autophagy, has been invoked as a mechanism that increases survival under diverse sets of experimental conditions and that multiple mechanisms contribute to the final outcome.

TISSUE DAMAGE RESPONSES

Molecular and Cellular Aspects

In tissues, cellular apoptosis can often be observed within hours of IR exposure. This is generally restricted to specific sites within the tissue. Radiation-induced rapid apoptosis in the mouse small intestine is maximal around position 4 from the base of the crypt,[19] which is the site of most proliferation and most spontaneous apoptosis. In contrast, apoptosis is not so marked in the colon and is not seen in the proliferative region. Indeed, the antiapoptotic molecule Bcl-2 is expressed by cells in this region.[20] In the thymus, about 98% of the cells that are generated die (about 5×10^7 cells per day in a young adult mouse), and after irradiation, there is massive rapid, p53-dependent apoptosis of T cells in the cortex but less in the medulla, which contains more mature cells. Concordance with the p53-related DDR is obvious in some tissues but not others. In lymphoid tissues, small intestine, hair follicles, and ependyma, the position of radiation-induced apoptotic cells correlates with up-regulated p53.[19,21,22] In subpopulations of cells in other tissues, p53 can be up-regulated with little evidence of rapid apoptosis, whereas most cells in liver, skeletal muscle, and brain show neither p53 nor much apoptosis.[10,14]

The role of apoptosis in normal tissue responses to IR is still controversial. It may depend on the physiologic role of the proapoptotic cells. If they are superfluous to needs, IR-induced cell death may have little impact; however, if they are critical to tissue function, the opposite will be true. Although little information is available in humans, acute parotitis can develop in the first 24 hours of treatment of patients receiving head and neck irradiation, which reflects apoptotic death of serous cells.[23] There is no such acute death in mucous cells; hence, the mouth is dry and the saliva more viscous.

The role of the vasculature in radiation responses is a longstanding controversy. The arguments have recently been resurrected by the suggestion that radiation-induced endothelial cell apoptosis through ceramide activation is critical for both normal tissue and tumor damage.[24,25–27] There is little doubt that IR causes vascular damage, and in particular microvascular "pruning," and this is an important aspect of tissue responses to IR, as well as to any ensuing hypoxia; however, parenchymal cell responses are also obviously relevant. A balanced view is that what is most critical is the integrated tissue response.

Part of the TDR occurs through the generation of pro-oxidant conditions that signal "danger" in damaged tissues through elaboration of proinflammatory chemokines and cytokines such as TNF-α and IL-1, as well as proteases, cell adhesion molecules, and extracellular matrix materials.[28,29] This regulated acute tissue reaction has its roots in fighting tissue infection by processes of cell death, inflammation, cell proliferation, and wound healing with tissue regeneration and remodeling. IR doses above approximately 6 to 7 Gy are especially proinflammatory.[30,31] Indeed, 2 Gy may have become a popular fraction size in the early days of RT simply because it minimized skin inflammation, the power output of x-ray tubes being low, and radiation dose to the skin being high.

This danger signaling can extend beyond the radiation field and may generate tumor-specific immunity by similar mechanisms to those that generate antipathogen immunity. These may be observed as "abscopal" effects of IR.[32,33] Cytokine-mediated responses can play many roles that could influence the overall outcome of RT. For example, radiation-induced basic fibroblast growth factor (bFGF) may act through autocrine pathways to promote survival of endothelial cells.[34] In vivo, antagonists of radiation-induced IL-1 and TNF-α increase the intrinsic sensitivity of mice to bone marrow death after irradiation,[35,36] suggesting that such responses have an adaptive survival value. On the other hand, radiation-induced TNF-α can cause certain cells to apoptose[11] and may trigger clinical symptoms that are not associated with cell death. Examples are nausea or vomiting that can occur within hours of RT involving the upper abdomen; acute erythema and edema associated with vascular leakage; fatigue in patients receiving RT to a large volume, especially within the abdomen; and somnolence that can develop within a few hours of cranial irradiation. Radiation-induced proliferative responses such as gliosis[37] or certain forms of fibrosis could also cause symptoms unrelated to cell depletion.

In the longer term, danger signaling by IR can set in motion a train of events culminating in continued proinflammatory responses in tissues long after exposure. Dose-related oscillating waves of inflammatory responses have been observed for months after IR tissue exposure. Failure to control these can be very damaging. Just as IR-induced redox imbalances are countered in time by antioxidant responses (e.g., superoxide dismutase, catalase, glutathione peroxidase, thioredoxin reductase, peroxidase), inflammation is controlled by anti-inflammatory mechanisms that critically mediate wound healing and tissue repair, and continuing waves of proinflammatory cytokines presumably reflect continual failing attempts at tissue recovery and remodeling.[38] Again, the inflammatory aspects of the TDR can extend outside the irradiated site to mediate bystander regional and systemic effects of local RT; because of their persistence, late radiation effects can be considered to have a chronic inflammatory component.[28,33]

Cytokines and growth factors are important mediators of late IR effects. For example, signaling through the TNFR2 protects mice from late effects of brain irradiation.[13] Anscher[39] has reported that lung cancer patients with elevated plasma levels of TGF-β prior to RT are more likely to develop radiation pneumonitis, illuminating the systemic influence on local radiation damage. Elevated TGF-β levels could be from the tumor or the stromal cells that invade it, or may be IR induced; the outcome may be the same. Not surprisingly, inhibition of TGF-β activation during RT is being investigated as a strategy to lower the risk of pneumonitis in patients with non–small cell lung cancer.[40] In addition, dose escalation is being attempted in patients whose TGF-β levels normalize during a course of RT.

Kinetics of Normal Tissue Radiation Injury

Although these more pathologic aspects of RT are an important aspect of the TDR, the time for a given tissue to express complications (latency) is determined in large part by the physiologic cell turnover rates—that is, on the kinetics of cell differentiation, loss, and renewal. As a result, the latency time to a complication is quite similar between individuals—for example, mucosal reactions generally occur at similar time intervals after the start of RT.

The terms *acute, subacute,* and *late* are commonly used to describe the time to occurrence of functional inadequacy after RT and reflect the major kinetic differences between tissues. The terms are also often loosely used to describe the tissues in which such effects are seen, as in "acute effects tissue," but are misleading because tissues and organs comprise more than one cell type, each with its own turnover rate characteristics. Any one tissue can therefore express both acute and late symptoms of radiation damage, depending on the cell type that is limiting function at that time. In addition, a severe acute radiation injury can lead to nonspecific late (consequential) changes such as fibrosis, atrophy, or ulceration (e.g., stenosis consequent to mucosal ulceration of the bowel, or fibrosis or necrosis of skin or oropharyngeal tissues consequent to desquamation and acute ulceration).

Acute Responses

Acute responses to RT are defined as occurring during a standard 6- to 8-week course of treatment and are seen in tissues with large populations of cells that turn over rapidly (gastrointestinal mucosa, bone marrow, skin, oropharyngeal and esophageal mucosa). Hierarchical organization exists in such tissues with a small number of relatively quiescent stem cells that proliferate slowly to produce a highly proliferative compartment of progenitor cells that differentiate into mature, nonproliferative, functional cells. IR generally depletes the more radiation-sensitive progenitor cell pool first. Nonproliferating, differentiated cells, however, maintain tissue function until they are lost through continuing physiologic cell turnover. In many circumstances, such as after lethal doses of whole body irradiation, depletion of the progenitor pool may be the critical event leading to death through loss of function, not loss of stem cells per se. The recent discovery of stem cell markers is currently allowing these responses to be evaluated in many different tissues.

After irradiation, there is homeostatic proliferation in most tissues in an attempt to re-equilibrate, in particular with respect to the generation of sufficient functional cells. Depleted stem and progenitor cells may, however, first reconstitute their own numbers before differentiating to restore function, although this seems to vary with the tissue. A useful model to consider is that under normal steady-state circumstances (i.e., not growing or involuting), tissues have, by definition, a cell loss factor (ϕ) of 1. The only requirement for tissue growth is a decrease in (ϕ) to <1, which is characteristic of embryos and fetuses, tissue regeneration, and malignancy. After IR exposure, some tissues (e.g., jejunal crypts) appear to reduce (ϕ) to zero and regenerate quickly; others (e.g., skin) may reduce it to about 0.5 and regenerate less quickly, continuously producing some functional cells; others such as seminiferous epithelium show little change in (ϕ) and mostly continue in steady state, producing sperm in numbers that are reduced for months or years in direct proportion to the extent of stem cell depletion. This, however, is simply a model that requires further confirmation using defined stem cell markers.

Because acute-responding tissues are organized in a hierarchical fashion, the *severity* of radiation injury depends on both the extent of stem/progenitor cell depletion and the length of the delay before new functional cells are generated. Severity of injury increases with dose; however, providing the proliferative pool does not fall below a critical value, symptoms are transient and recovery can be complete. Dose fractionation can lessen the severity of acute effects by allowing regeneration from the stem/progenitor cell compartment during the course of therapy. Unlike the *extent* of injury, the *rate* at which acute injury develops and the latent time to the appearance of symptoms is relatively, although not completely, independent of dose because latency is mainly determined by the rate of loss of differentiated cells. For example, in hematopoiesis, leukocyte and platelet numbers drop quickly after bone marrow irradiation because they have a fast turnover rate, whereas anemia is not an obvious acute effect because red cells turn over slowly. In the testis, each spermatogenic stem cell division ultimately produces more than 1,000 sperm through successive divisions of spermatogonia and spermatocytes—a process that in humans takes more than 60 days. Early differentiating spermatogonia are few in number and are more radiosensitive than mature stages of spermatogenesis. This is why sperm counts remain normal for several weeks after exposure, falling steeply only at the time when the progeny of the irradiated spermatogonia would normally have reached the seminal vesicles. In the mucosa of the small bowel, because crypt cells divide rapidly (an average of more than once daily in humans), they are lost within days if sterilized by radiation. The nonproliferative villus shows no immediate effect of irradiation, with shortening becoming evident only as differentiated cells are shed into the lumen in the absence of renewal from the crypts. This is why symptoms take about 2 weeks to appear in patients undergoing abdominal RT.

Subacute Responses

Certain tissues may display subacute reactions several months after RT. Symptoms are generally reversible, although in some instances they may be associated with severe damage and even death. Examples of transient effects are Lhermitte's syndrome after spinal cord irradiation and subacute pneumonitis 2 to 3 months after the start of lung irradiation. The target population appears to have a longer turnover time, and transient symptoms are considered due to a lag between loss of functional populations and stem/progenitor cell recovery, although production of proinflammatory cytokines driven by continuing cell loss and hypoxia due to microvasculature pruning may play a considerable role, as will the genetically determined mechanisms that control these responses.

Late Responses

Late reactions to RT in normal tissues can be severe, and recovery is often limited. They are generally considered to be the result of the depletion of slowly proliferating "target" cells that are lost from the tissue at a slow rate—for example, from central (oligodendroglia) or peripheral (Schwann cells) nervous tissue, kidney (tubule epithelium), blood vessels (endothelium), dermis (fibroblasts), and bones (osteoblasts and chondroblasts). Some lesions, such as those associated with atherosclerosis and heart disease, may occur decades after RT and are an increasing problem as patients live longer following therapy. Pathologic findings associated with late effects can be quite variable. For instance, late demyelination after brain irradiation has often been ascribed to loss of oligodendrocytes, and subsequently of neurons, but proliferation of astrocytes and microglial cells can be observed,[41] as can vascular lesions with edema, hemorrhage, or inflammatory infiltrates. Infiltrating cells may contribute to the pathogenesis of radiation injury as is illustrated by their involvement in radiation pneumonitis, or recovery from injury as in the slower healing of skin wounds in mice receiving total body irradiation compared with those irradiated only locally.

Unlike acute-responding hierarchical tissues, slowly proliferating tissues, in which late effects occur, contain cells that are usually both functional and able to proliferate on demand. In an operational sense, such tissues can be regarded as "flexible." This does not deny the presence of stem cells with limited function or functional cells that do not proliferate; however, the roles of such cells are probably of lesser importance than in hierarchical tissues. The more chronic and debilitating nature of late reactions may be because of their relative inability to be repopulated from a stem cell pool. Alternatively, regeneration may be compromised by inflammation and fibrosis that is an alternative healing response for slow-responding tissues.

Because the proliferative cells may also be functional, dose has a greater apparent influence on *latency* in late reactions, with injury developing more quickly with increase in dose. This may be because the greater the dose, the fewer the number of division cycles the cells can successfully negotiate before death. Another reason may be that as cells die, residual (mostly lethally injured) target cells are increasingly recruited to the proliferative pool, causing a cascade or "avalanche" of cell death and functional tissue failure. A third possible explanation is that because late effects are complex and involve interactions between many cell types, the nature of the lesion may change with time depending on which cell type is critically limiting. The time course to development of injury can be accelerated and the severity increased by various insults such as surgery, chemotherapy, infection, or physical trauma. Indeed, such factors may play a major role in precipitating the onset of late effects in humans (e.g., necrotic, nonhealing ulcers after trauma). Conversely, slowing the proliferation process and decreasing stress may reduce their incidence and severity.

An issue of growing clinical importance is the extent to which late radiation effects can be reversed. It has been shown recently that certain agents given late after radiation can modify injury in tissues. For example, captopril, an angiotensin-converting enzyme inhibitor, slows the development of radiation-induced nephritis and lung fibrosis in rats. Steroids also can prevent death from radiation pneumonitis in animals, although their withdrawal before the end of the usual period of pneumonitis can result in accelerated mortality. Pentoxifylline, alone or in combination with vitamin E, protects against radiation-induced late effects in some experimental models. In a clinical study, the combination, but neither agent alone, reversed chronic radiation-induced fibrosis. It is not clear how these agents act, but such studies point to ways to improve the future management of late complications of RT.

Whereas a severe early response in a rapidly proliferating tissue permits adjustment of the dose schedule during the standard course of RT, this is not the case for late injuries because they occur after completion of treatment. Furthermore, because cell turnover kinetics determines the time to a normal tissue effect, latency is not an indicator of radiosensitivity.

Tolerance Doses and Functional Subunits

Normal tissue tolerance doses have not been precisely defined, even though generally accepted dose limits exist for various organs.

The tolerance of a tissue to IR is determined not only by its intrinsic radiosensitivity but also by the number of cells with regenerative potential and the way they are organized. Tissues can be thought of as being composed of functional subunits (FSU)—the minimum clonogenic entity required for regeneration of a structure. For example, epilation requires doses lower than those for desquamation, primarily because there is a smaller number of clonogenic cells in the FSU that produces a hair than in the sheet of basal cells that is capable of self-regeneration. Similarly, hair is depigmented by lower doses of radiation than the epidermis because each hair follicle contains a smaller number of melanocytes, sometimes only one.

In the kidney, each nephron is an FSU. If a tubule is completely de-epithelialized, it is lost permanently because it is not repopulated from adjacent nephrons. Therefore, the tolerance dose for the kidney is determined more by the number of tubule stem/progenitor cells per nephron than the number of nephrons. For example, if the kidney contained 10^{11} clonogenic tubule cells distributed as 10^4 cells in each of 10^7 nephrons, then most tubules should regenerate after a dose that reduced survival to 10^{-4}. Because of the random nature of IR events, from Poisson distribution statistics, 37% of FSU nephrons would be eliminated. If on the other hand, 10^{11} clonogenic tubule cells were distributed as 10^7 cells in each of 10^4 nephrons, the dose required to eliminate 37% of the nephrons would have to reduce survival to 10^{-7}. In a multifractionated dose regimen, during which a logarithmic decline in cell number occurs, this is $7/4$ (1.75) times higher. Tolerance doses can therefore vary greatly among tissues and organs, even if the target cells have the same intrinsic radiosensitivity. In mouse skin, the survival of about 10 out of approximately 10^6 basal stem/progenitor cells per cm^2 is required to prevent overt desquamation. Therefore, the FSU would be about $1/10$ cm^2.

Organs with more tubular architecture (e.g., salivary glands, pancreas, sweat glands, testis, mammary epithelium, lung, and perhaps liver) may resemble the kidney in having better-defined FSUs organized "in series," whereas the target cells in dermis, mucosa, gut epithelium, and epidermis may be considered to be organized "in parallel." These lack restricting physical barriers to cell migration, which may assist tissue regeneration. Structurally well-defined organs appear to have small FSUs, whereas those in the spinal cord are intermediate and the dermis large. A tumor behaves as just one FSU, as one surviving stem/progenitor cell can lead to recurrence. The number of such cells will therefore play a big role in determining local tumor control. For metastatic deposits, in general a larger number of small metastatic deposits will be cured with lower radiation doses than a small number of larger metastases even if the total cell number is the same in the two cases.

Volume Effects

Traditionally, radiation oncologists have reduced the total dose when treating large volumes of normal tissue. In fact, the now widespread use of 1.8 rather than 2 Gy had its origin in a volume effect; the longer treatment duration enhanced mucosal tolerance in large head and neck treatment fields. In the orthovoltage era, a reduction in dose with increase in treatment volume was generally recommended but became less important with the advent of skin-sparing megavoltage beams. Modern intensity-modulated radiation therapy (IMRT) treatment planning gives a readout for dose-volume histograms for various normal tissues that are useful for avoiding excessive dose to too high a volume. However, they are limited because there is no spatial information and as a result do not predict toxicity well.

In reality, the concept of decreasing dose with increasing treatment volume has little cellular radiobiologic basis, except in specific circumstances. For example, if FSUs are arranged in series, as in tubular structures such as nerve tracts, the spinal cord, and the peritoneal sheath, the loss of one subunit may results in an overt expression of injury regardless of the state of the other subunits in the series. The probability of injury increases with volume (number of FSUs exposed) (Fig. 2.1). Such a volume effect has been demonstrated clinically for small bowel obstruction and experimentally for myelitis.

Experimental studies on volume effects of radiation in spinal cord of rats have indicated a steep volume effect for rat spinal cord at <10 mm of length and an interesting "bath-and-shower" effect[42] for small fields with high tolerance for IR-induced paralysis. In such models, if an additional modest "bath" dose (about 4 Gy) is administered to 4-mm segments of spinal cord surrounding a targeted "shower" 2 mm in size, the effective dose for 50% paralysis (ED_{50}) dramatically decreases from 88 to 61 Gy. The mechanism underlying this bath effect is not known, although inhibition of angiogenesis and cell migration are possible explanations.

Spinal cord has been a favorite model for volume effects. One recent study showed that IR-induced motor deficit in pigs

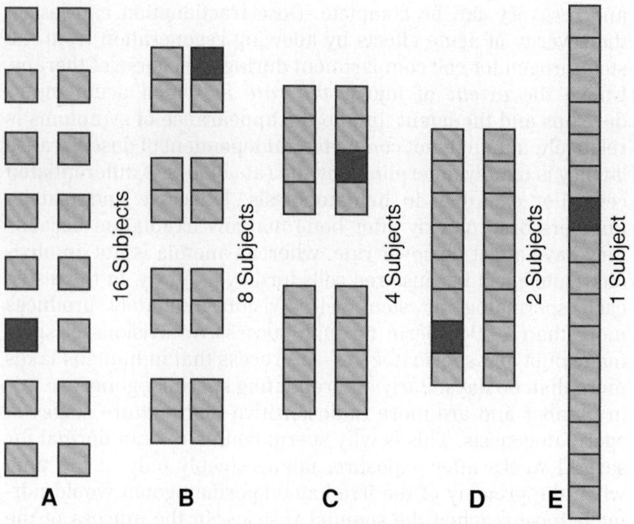

FIGURE 2.1. Diagrammatic representation of the influence on the probability of a complication from increasing the treatment volume in a tissue where FSUs are arranged serially. The average survival of FSUs was 1 in 16, with sterilized FSUs being denoted by the black squares. With the small volumes **(A)**, the probability of myelitis was 6% (1/16), whereas it would approach 100% if 16 FSUs in one patient were exposed **(E)**. The actual probabilities can be calculated using the equation in the text. (From Withers HR, Taylor JMG, Maciejewski B. Treatment volume and tissue tolerance. *Int J Radiat Oncol Biol Phys* 1988;14:751.)

appears to be independent of the irradiated volume in the lateral direction, with around 20 Gy being the effective dose for paralysis. This is of considerable clinical relevance because it suggests that even partial spinal cord irradiation can have deleterious effects. However, in general, preclinical spinal cord dose-volume studies indicate that dose distribution may be more critical than the volume irradiated, suggesting that neither dose-volume histogram analysis nor absolute volume constraints will be fully effective in predicting complications.

The relationship between the number of FSUs irradiated (n) and the probability of a complication (P) can be quantified by:

$$P = 1 - (1 - p)^n,$$

where p is the probability of the loss of one FSU. This relationship is illustrated in Figure 2.2. When the average number of surviving cells per FSU is reduced to almost one, increasing the volume (number of FSUs exposed) reduces the dose necessary

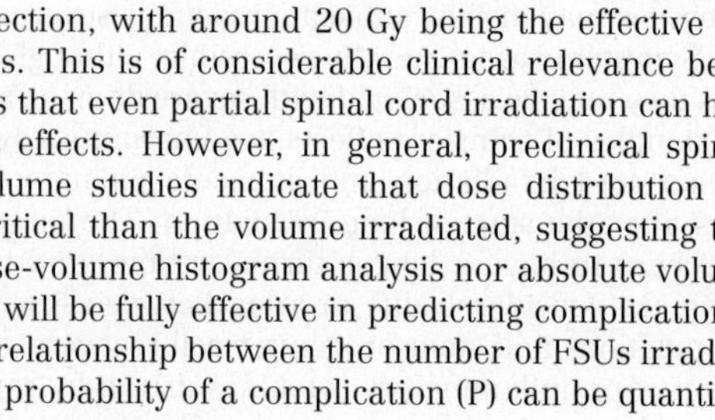

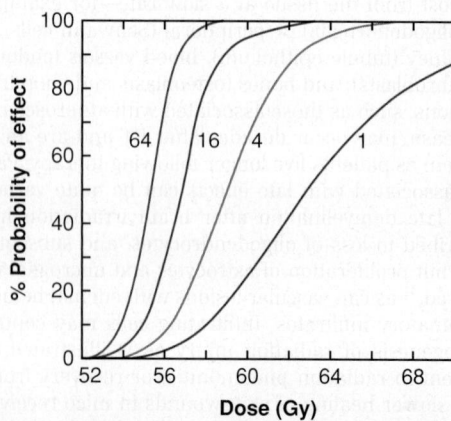

FIGURE 2.2. Curves illustrating how the probability of producing a complication increases with increase in the number of serially arranged FSUs included in the treatment volume. The curves were positioned by assuming that 58 Gy in 2-Gy fractions sterilized 10% of FSUs and that for a series of 2-Gy fractions, the effective D_0 for the target cells was 4 Gy. The curves are shifted to the left and are steeper with increase in number of FSUs exposed; however, this effect becomes less obvious once large numbers of subunits are involved. (From Withers HR, Taylor JMG, Maciejewski B. Treatment volume and tissue tolerance. *Int J Radiat Oncol Biol Phys* 1988;14:751.)

to produce a complication and increases the steepness of the dose-response curves. This may be less true for the small bowel than for spinal cord.

There is no evidence that cellular radiosensitivity is affected by an increase in treatment volume. The radiosensitivity of skin epithelium is constant over a 5,000-fold range of treatment area. In addition, no evidence exists for an increased role for vascular damage as volume increases. On the other hand, nonradiobiologic "volume effects" can be seen when:

1. A small area of injury (such as ulceration) is tolerated better than a large area of the same severity, even though the severity of the radiation response is independent of volume treated. In this case, pain, exudation, and infection may be worse; healing may be slower; and consequential contraction and scarring may be more of a problem.
2. As volume increases, so does dose heterogeneity across the field. A tumor dose prescribed at the 80% level may lead to a 25% higher dose at D_{max}. If the threshold-sigmoid curve of the probability of normal tissue complications against dose is as steep as in experimental studies,[20] a 25% increase in total dose could produce a marked change in the incidence of complications. Any increase is further compounded by the biologic effectiveness of each dose per fraction or the "double trouble" of increased physical and biologic dose that will depend on the size of the dose per fraction and the type of normal tissue, but it will be greatest in late-responding normal tissues for reasons that will be explained later. Because this additional augmentation of biologic doses is not evident from physical isodose contours, an increased biologic effect may be erroneously attributed to the large volume being treated per se. In addition, with large fields, large variations in contour may exist that could cause a high dose region where tissue thickness is less than that measured at the mid-plane; as, for example, in the spinal cord at the thoracic inlet in thoracic irradiation and in tangential fields for treatment of the breast.
3. If organ "reserve" is obliterated as volume is increased (e.g., lung, salivary gland). This is not a true volume effect because sequelae are determined by the volume and functional status of the tissue *excluded* from the treatment volume, not the volume irradiated.

Regeneration (Repopulation)

The time to onset of repopulation after RT and the rate at which it proceeds varies in different normal tissues. Both can be measured experimentally by a split-dose technique in which two doses are given separated in time. The size of the second dose required to produce a certain constant level of effect (isoeffect) increases with time after the first dose because of regeneration/repopulation.

In acute-responding tissues, repopulation starts early because cell loss is rapid. In the irradiated jejunal mucosa, the lag time may be <24 hours. In the colon and stomach, it is slightly longer. In mouse renal tubules, there is no histologic evidence of cell depletion for many months after irradiation; there is a long lag period, and it takes more than 12 months to reconstitute a tubule.[43] The rate of repopulation has not been well quantified in tissues. In mice, some approximate doubling times for clonogenic cells are 8, 12, and 22 hours for jejunum,[44] colon, and skin,[45] respectively.

In humans, tissue turnover kinetics are slower than in mice. They have been approximated for oropharyngeal mucosa from consideration of responses to various dose fractionation regimens. Mucositis begins to appear 14 to 21 days after the start of a regimen of 2 Gy given five times per week, but repopulation begins at about 10 to 12 days.[46] High initial doses may shorten the lag period, although only by 1 or 2 days. Repopulation can increase the tolerance of the mucosa to a conventional dose regimen by an *average* of at least 1 Gy per day, which is equivalent to approximately a doubling of clonogenic cell numbers every 2 days, and it may be significantly faster.[47] If daily irradiation is suspended (e.g., during a 10- to 14-day break in a split-course accelerated regimen), clonogenic cells may repopulate at two or three times this rate.[46–48] Figure 2.3 shows values for lengths of lag time and repopulation rates; however, they are, at best, estimates. The critical point is that there is a lag period

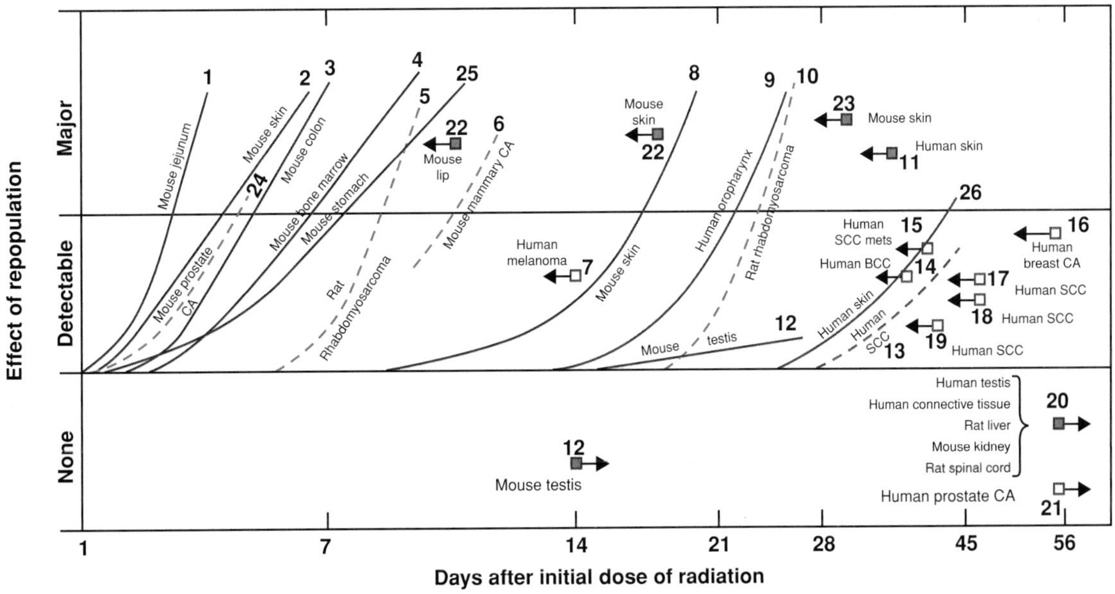

FIGURE 2.3. Representation of the approximate kinetics of regeneration of irradiated normal tissues (*solid lines, solid symbols*) and tumors (*dashed lines, open symbols*). Curves are based on measurements or estimates of regeneration; symbols denote times at which an effect of regeneration has already appeared (*left-pointing arrow*) or has not yet appeared (*right-pointing arrow*). The logarithmic abscissa is for convenience of presentation only and has no biologic rationale. In general, the human data are displaced to the right of experimental animal data, reflecting a slower initiation of repopulation. Because human tissues proliferate more slowly than do their rodent counterparts, they were exposed to protracted dose regimens, and less-sensitive end points were used to detect onset of repopulation in humans. Numbers on the curve and symbols refer to different sources of data. These come from many sources. Further details are in the previous editions of this book.

followed by a phase of rapid exponential growth. In general, the lag period is shorter for chemotherapy, hyperthermia, and surgery because the cell depletion that stimulates regeneration occurs more rapidly than after irradiation.

The importance of repopulation is implicit in the history of RT. The current standard protracted overall treatment times confer a benefit by allowing regeneration of acute-responding tissues, which reduces toxicity. When attempts are made to deliver curative therapy more quickly, acute responses become more severe and dose limiting.

Growth factors may shorten the apparent lag phase and accelerate recovery in irradiated tissues. Hematopoietic growth factors such as G-CSF, GM-CSF, erythropoietin, and IL-11 can accelerate proliferation of hematopoietic cells.[49] In doing so, they minimize the danger of infection. In epithelial tissues, keratinocyte growth factor (KGF), which is specific for epithelial cells, has similar potential. It protects the oral mucosa, small intestine, lung, and hair follicles against chemo- or radiation injury[50–52] in preclinical models and has shown efficacy in clinical bone marrow transplantation trials. There is ongoing interest in the discovery of mitigators of radiation damage that can be given at least 24 hours after exposure of individuals in nuclear accidents or radiologic terrorist attacks.

"Remembered" Dose: Tolerance to Retreatment

Conventional wisdom in radiation oncology has been that a heavily irradiated tissue will not tolerate retreatment. The postulated reason was that the basis of late effects was irreversible vascular damage. Although irradiation may limit the tolerance of a tissue to retreatment, retreatment is often possible and may be better tolerated than previously expected.[42] Factors that determine the extent to which residual injury will limit retreatment tolerance include the amount of cell depletion caused by prior treatment, the time elapsed since that treatment and therefore the extent of regeneration, and the tissue at risk. High prior doses, short intervals between treatment courses, and slow regeneration of target cells will reduce retreatment tolerance.

Some data for experimental radiation myelitis are shown in Figure 2.4. The plot shows the effect of size of the first dose on the dose required to produce myelitis in a second regimen. Recovery is complete after low doses but is progressively compromised as the initial dose approaches tissue tolerance.[54] It should be remembered that clinical "tolerance" doses for the spinal cord of 45 to 50 Gy in 1.8- to 2-Gy fractions are low in terms of the injury evaluated in Figure 2.4 (50% incidence of myelitis). The time to recovery for the spinal cord is not accurately known; however, in rats, at 100 days it is about half of what it reaches by 200 days.[55] In monkeys, there was extensive recovery from 44 Gy in 2.2-Gy fractions by 2 years, but a detailed profile of the time course could not be established.[56]

Not all tissues, or elements within tissues, recover at an equal rate or to an equal extent after irradiation. Acute-responding epithelial and hemopoietic tissues generally recover quickly and demonstrate a high tolerance to retreatment. However, the fibrovascular support in skin and mucosa and the stroma in bone marrow are less tolerant to retreatment because they respond more slowly. The kidney shows poor retreatment tolerance as assessed functionally in mice.[57] Reirradiation tolerance in this organ is inversely related to the initial dose, although tolerance decreases significantly with increasing interval between treatments, suggesting progression rather than recovery from the initial damage.

Because different tissues show different levels of tolerance to retreatment, caution should be exercised in the application of these concepts to the clinic. In addition, the experimental studies deal with well-defined end points within a limited time scale. If different end points in the same tissue are examined or the time is extended, the same guidelines may not apply. It should also be noted that if slowly proliferating cells involved in late responses are extensively depleted, recovery may be permanently incomplete and the organ will be vulnerable to further injury, whether from radiation, trauma, cytotoxic drugs, or any other insult. For example, hyperthermia can precipitate myelitis in a patient who has had high but otherwise tolerable doses of x-irradiation, and trauma from dental intervention frequently precipitates mandibular necrosis.

Reproducible differences in tolerance of acute- and late-responding normal tissues and between different types of tumors to the same physical dose of IR are important because they define the basis of the biologic advantage of dose fractionation in conventional RT. This radiobiologic rationale has been encapsulated in the 4 "Rs" (repair, repopulation, redistribution, and reoxygenation).[58]

TUMOR RADIOBIOLOGY

Kinetics

Tumor Cell Death and Survival

As is obvious from clinical practice, the doses of irradiation required for a certain control rate vary widely among human tumors. Tumor types that are traditionally radiocurable tend to show greater cellular radiosensitivity in vitro.[59] However, within one tumor type, there is a wide spectrum of radiosensitivities.[60] Considerable effort has therefore been expended to develop molecular or cellular assays for molecules involved in cell death/survival, proliferation/arrest, and DNA repair so as to predict clinical responses to RT, as well as to identify potential targets for tumor radiosensitization.

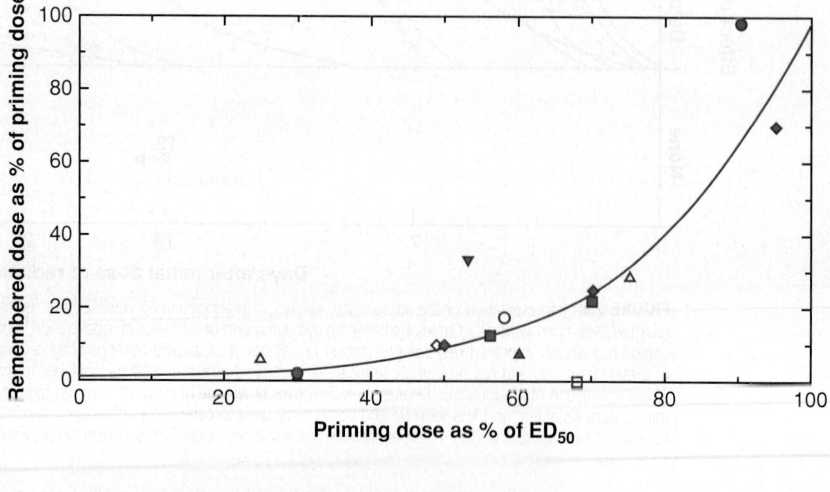

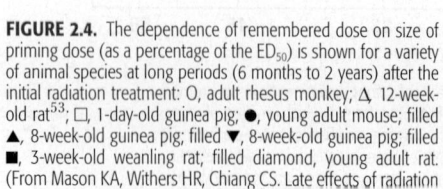

FIGURE 2.4. The dependence of remembered dose on size of priming dose (as a percentage of the ED_{50}) is shown for a variety of animal species at long periods (6 months to 2 years) after the initial radiation treatment: O, adult rhesus monkey; Δ, 12-week-old rat[53]; □, 1-day-old guinea pig; ●, young adult mouse; filled ▲, 8-week-old guinea pig; filled ▼, 8-week-old guinea pig; filled ■, 3-week-old weanling rat; filled diamond, young adult rat. (From Mason KA, Withers HR, Chiang CS. Late effects of radiation on the lumbar spinal cord of guinea pigs: re-treatment tolerance. *Int J Radiat Oncol Biol Phys* 1993;26:643.)

Part of the heterogeneity between tumor radiation responses is because differences in mutations in oncogenes and tumor suppressor genes that affect pathways integral to cell death and proliferation alter intrinsic radiosensitivity. However, in addition, many cancers show an epithelial hierarchy similar to what is found in normal tissues. For example, in breast, undifferentiated estrogen receptor–negative mammary stem cells (MaSCs) maintain themselves through self-renewal and also differentiate into committed progenitors that ultimately give rise to mature ductal and alveolar cells, which belong to the luminal epithelial cell lineage that line the lumen of the mammary gland, and the mature myoepithelial cells, which surround the luminal epithelium.

Breast cancer is a heterogeneous disease with distinct molecular entities or "intrinsic" subtypes that have recently been linked to these developmental pathways by genomically defined tumor profiles and expression patterns of luminal, mesenchymal or claudin-low, and basal-like cells, with distinct blocks imposed by BRCA1 loss and HER2 amplification.[61] These findings generally support the cancer stem cell (CSC) hypothesis that a cancer can arise from transformation of a normal stem or progenitor cell and give rise to a heterogeneous population of tumor cells. Alternatively, a differentiated cancer cell within a heterogeneous tumor may acquire stem cell–like features through self-renewal mechanisms prompted by oncogene expression, RT, chemotherapy, or hypoxia. Either way, the conclusion is that the bulk of hierarchically organized tumors is composed of more differentiated cells with limited proliferative potential, whereas the CSC compartment maintains the tumor and contributes to treatment resistance owing to its unique biologic properties. The importance of this concept is that tumor cure and regrowth is dependent on what may be a small minority of relatively quiescent cells.

No single marker is currently adequate to define CSCs of any histology; however, combinations of markers can be used, and in several tumor types, CSCs have been shown to be very radioresistant and chemoresistant.[62] They are more tumorigenic and responsible for metastatic growths, and in general, the more primitive CSCs are more aggressive and more radioresistant. In vitro clonogenic assays are generally not good surrogates for CSC identification.

In the future, prediction of tumor behavior and response to therapy and the identification of biologic targets will require CSCs to be defined in molecular terms linked to normal developmental pathways and cancer-related mutations. A similar example of the importance of molecular profiling is the demonstration that patients with human papillomavirus (HPV)-positive oropharyngeal squamous cell carcinoma (OPSCC) have improved outcomes over those with HPV-negative tumors when treated with concurrent chemoradiation.[63] Obviously, if CSCs are critical for cancer cure, then they have to be a prime target of any treatment. Therapies that fail to target them will be inadequate to affect cure even if they cause dramatic tumor shrinkage.

The mechanism of cell death may be important for both tumor cure and failure through stem cell reprogramming. Tumors of those histologic types that are traditionally radiocurable have a tendency to apoptose.[8] Lymphocytic tumors generally apoptose more than carcinomas, whereas melanomas, sarcomas, and astrocytomas are relatively resistant.[64] Importantly, apoptotic cells reappear between fractionated exposures.[65] In addition, genetic modification of cells to introduce a proapoptotic phenotype frequently, although not always, radiosensitize.[66] Despite these findings, studies specifically designed to find relationships between molecular markers of apoptosis and radiocurability of human tumors have yielded mixed and sometimes contradictory results.[67] This may be because the CSCs do not express this phenotype. In contrast, cells that senesce or undergo autophagy or go through several divisions after RT may have a greater chance of surviving and undergoing CSC reprogramming.

In Vivo Kinetics of Tumor Responses

Most tumors regress during a course of RT and are considered analogous to acute-responding normal tissues in their radiation dose-fractionation responses. However, it has been known for decades that some tumors, such as melanoma, soft tissue sarcoma, and liposarcoma, behave similar to late-responding tissues and have a low α/β ratio (see later).[68] More recently, prostate[69] and breast[70] cancers have been added to the list. Such tumors have a relatively slow turnover rate.

Regression of a tumor after RT reflects the *rate* of cell loss, which is determined by turnover kinetics, in the same way as for normal tissues. Thus, tumors with a small cell loss factor can respond slowly after RT, even though all CSCs have been sterilized, as evidenced by their failure to recur.

The kinetics of tumor responses to RT will depend on whether the cell of origin is an early or a more differentiated (progenitor) CSC as well as the effects of the cancer-related mutations.

Cell Loss Factors in Tumors

A cell loss factor (ϕ) of <1 is characteristic of tissue growth. In tumors—for example, head and neck carcinomas—ϕ is actually close to 1,[71] which is why their growth rate is much slower (on average, doubling times of about 60 days)[72] than could be predicted by their proliferative activity. Mitotic count, S-phase count, or labeling index (LI) would suggest a potential doubling time (Tpot) of about 3 to 7 days. It follows that a high proliferative index is not necessarily evidence of a tumor that will grow rapidly in size. A classic example is the slow-growing basal cell skin carcinoma, in which numerous mitotic figures are commonly visible. They have a high ϕ owing to extensive apoptosis.[73,74]

Tumor Regression After Irradiation

Tumors with a high rate of cell loss will regress rapidly during and after RT, regardless of pretreatment growth rate; providing the overall treatment duration is not unduly protracted, the prognosis is generally good.[71,75] On the other hand, rapid regression would also be expected in a tumor with a low cell loss rate if a large proportion of its cells are actively cycling and it is growing quickly; however, in this case, the prognosis is poor. Rapid regression is therefore not a universal prognostic indicator,[75] although it is usually a favorable prognostic sign.

Similar arguments can be applied to tumors that regress slowly, such as prostate carcinoma, some cases of nodular sclerosing Hodgkin's disease, teratocarcinomas of testis, some soft tissue sarcomas, choroidal melanomas, meningiomas, pituitary adenomas, chordomas, or glomus tumors. Slow regression may reflect slow proliferation, low cell loss factor, residual stroma, or, sometimes, treatment failure.

Repopulation occurs as a homeostatic response to cell depletion caused by treatment. The rate of cell loss slows (the cell loss factor decreases), as in acute-responding normal tissues, during rapid repopulation. Tumors with a high rate of cell production and a large cell loss factor are likely to regress quickly but recur early and regrow rapidly after unsuccessful irradiation, chemotherapy, or surgery.[76]

A practical implication of the complex reasons for different rates of tumor response to RT is that it is not a good idea to reduce the total dose just because a tumor regresses rapidly.[77] In addition, local control of tumors that grow slowly because of high cell loss factors may initiate an early repopulation response, and local control may be prejudiced by protraction of treatment time beyond normal, just as it is for fast-growing tumors that are initially fast growing.[78,79] Well-differentiated tumors (which have a high cell loss factor) are more prone to an early reduction in cell loss factor and, consequently, an early repopulation response that prejudices local control, especially if overall duration of treatment is protracted.[80]

Tumor Regeneration After Irradiation

Potential Doubling Time

The potential regeneration rate of tumors after cytotoxic injury is better predicted by pre-RT proliferative activity than by pre-RT tumor growth rate. The Tpot,[81–83] which is the time that would be required for the number of clonogenic cells to double if the cell loss factor were zero, is a measure of this and can be estimated from the average duration of the S phase (Ts) and the fraction of cells in S phase, measured by LI:

Tpot = lTs/LI,

where l is a correction factor for the cell cycle distribution of the population.

Tpot is a logical predictor of the kinetics of a regenerative response, and attempts were made to use it to predict which tumors would benefit from acceleration of treatment that aims to minimize such repopulation.[81,83,84] Early results indicated that it might be of some value, although later analyses indicate otherwise.[85] This may be because the cell cycle time measured in an unperturbed tumor before treatment is different from that during or after treatment. More likely, without knowledge of the behavior of the CSC compartment, gross observations on whole tumor populations are likely to mislead.

Growth Fraction

The *growth fraction*[86] is simply the fraction of tumor cells that are cycling. In solid tumors, this is usually a small proportion of the total (e.g., 20%). These are not the CSCs that are generally quiescent but more likely are progenitor cells. The growth fraction may decrease as tumors enlarge and grow more slowly (see control curve, Fig. 2.5). This changing growth rate can be approximated by a Gompertz equation.[71] In contrast, after cytoreductive therapy, the growth fraction probably increases, CSCs can be induced to proliferate, and these contribute to accelerated tumor regrowth. Treatment may therefore accelerate tumor growth. An analogous response is found in some

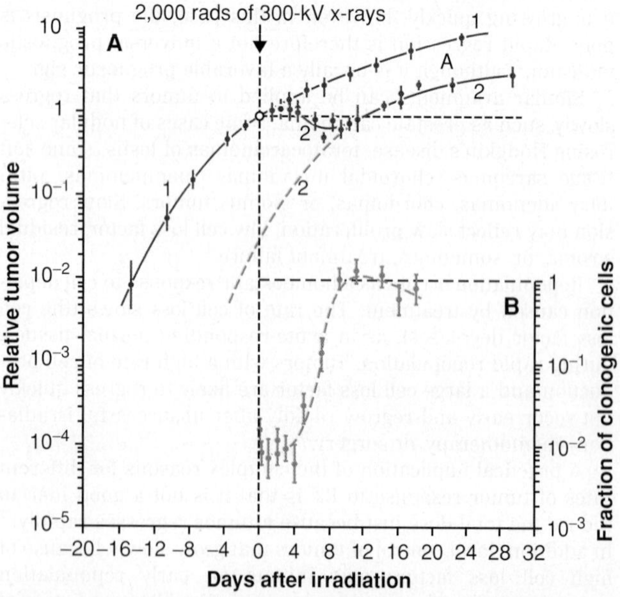

FIGURE 2.5. Growth curves for a rat rhabdomyosarcoma and its constituent clonogenic cells after a dose that reduced survival to 1%. The upper curve (1) shows unperturbed growth of tumors; the middle curve (2) shows regression and regrowth of tumors irradiated on day 0 with a dose that reduced cell survival to 1%; the lower curve (B) traces the repopulation of the tumor by surviving clonogens. Exponential regrowth of the surviving clonogenic cells occurs while the gross tumor is regressing. (From Hermens AF, Barendsen GW. Changes of cell proliferation characteristics in a rat rhabdomyosarcoma before and after x-irradiation. *Eur J Cancer* 1969;5:173. © 1969 Pergamon Press, Ltd.)

normal tissues (liver, dermis), which have only a small fraction of cells in cycle but can regenerate rapidly through recruiting resting, G0-phase cells into cycle.

Regeneration in Experimental Tumors

Hermens and Barendsen[87] showed a rapid exponential increase of surviving clonogenic tumor cells in a rat rhabdomyosarcoma several days after irradiation. Because only 1% of the initial clonogens survived, tumors did not enlarge; rather, the tumor mass was still regressing when repopulation began (Fig. 2.5). This was later confirmed in other experiential tumors,[88,89] and the same probably occurs during regression of clinical tumors. It would be important to revisit these experiments in light of the CSC hypothesis. In vitro fractionated daily irradiation can select for CSCs[2] and also promote reprogramming from more differentiated tumor cells.

Regeneration in Human Tumors

Clonogen regeneration in human tumors can be assessed by an increase in dose required for tumor control as treatment duration is increased.[90] Alternatively, if a constant dose has been used, the decrease in tumor control rate as treatment time is extended. These techniques have been used to derive evidence for accelerated regrowth during a standard RT regimen for head and neck cancer, although it is likely to occur in all tumor sites. The magnitude and timing of regeneration will vary from tumor to tumor of the same type and among different types.

The concept of accelerated repopulation by human tumor clonogens during and after a course of fractionated RT is supported by several observations and is of particular concern when delivery time is prolonged.

1. *Time to Tumor Recurrence*
   If 10^4 tumor cells survived RT, they would have to undergo 15 doublings to present as a recurrence. Because most local recurrences of head and neck cancer are detectable within 12 months after RT, the *average* tumor volume doubling time would have to be about 2 weeks. Because the median volume doubling time for tumors at presentation is about 2 months,[41] the growth rate of residual clonogens must accelerate following unsuccessful treatment. Similar rapid regrowth was seen in pulmonary metastases after subcurative RT.[91]
2. *Split-Course Treatment*
   Split-course regimens for head and neck squamous cell carcinomas (SCCs) give lower local control rates than continuous regimens of the same total dose,[92] suggesting that tumor regrowth occurred rapidly during the time extension. This does not happen for prostate cancer.[92,93]
3. *Protracted Treatment*
   Protraction of treatment time decreased the rate of locoregional control for head and neck cancer in several retrospective analyses,[79,94–97] which is consistent with accelerated tumor regeneration. The analyses were of three types:
   a. *Scattergram analysis.* Protracting treatment time for OPSCC led to worse outcome[95] (Fig. 2.6). For treatment durations of 30 to 55 days, each day's extension required the total dose to be increased by about 0.6 Gy to achieve a constant rate of tumor control. Assuming that between 1.8 Gy and 2.4 Gy reduces cell survival by 50%, an increase of 0.6 Gy per day is consistent with clonogens doubling every 3 to 4 days. Because tumors at presentation have a doubling time of about 2 months,[41] there must be a dramatic change in growth rate during RT. The same pattern (Fig. 2.6) was seen in 11 other subsets of patients with oropharyngeal cancers[95] and carcinomas of the supraglottic larynx,[98] as well as in reanalyses of earlier data,[79] and for SCC of tonsil collected from nine centers in the United States, Canada, and England.[97] The multicenter study of SCC of tonsil is important because differences

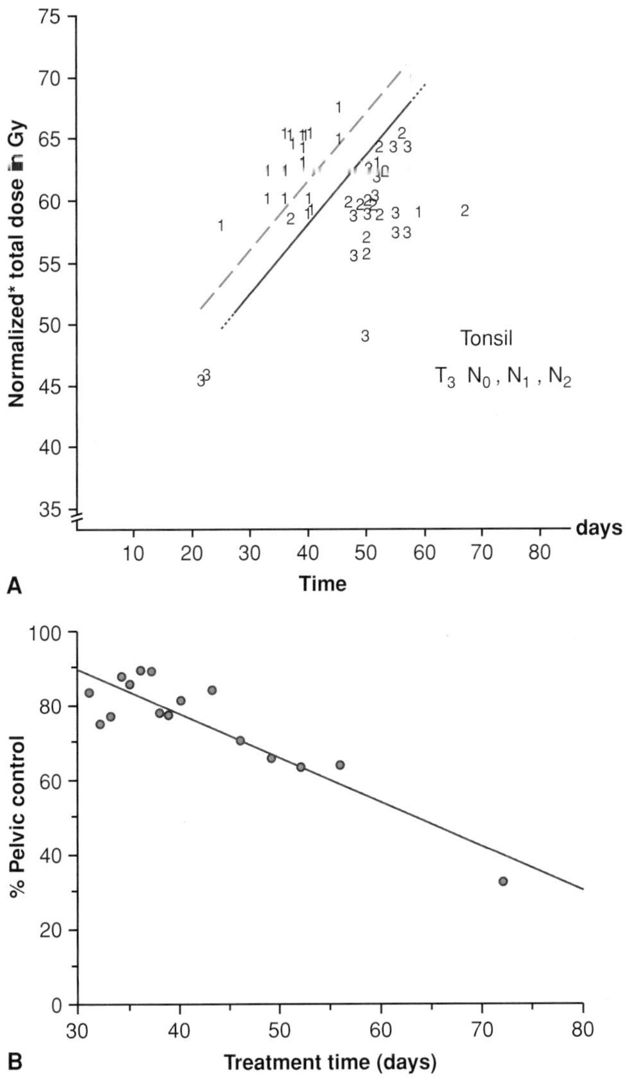

FIGURE 2.6. **A:** Scattergram with TCD_{50} and TCD_{90} (tumor control dose) curves for 3-year local control of SCC of the tonsil (1, local control; 2, recurrence; 3, persistence of detectable disease). For a given total dose, local control decreased with protraction of overall treatment time. For a given overall time, local control improved with increase in dose. The total doses were normalized to be equivalent to the total dose in 2.5-Gy fractions using the LQ isoeffect curve (Fig. 2.22). An α/β value of 2.5 Gy was used, being the best estimate from these and other data. (From Maciejewski B, Withers HR, Taylor JMG. Dose fractionation and regeneration in radiotherapy for cancer of the oral cavity and oropharynx. I. Tumor dose-response and repopulation. *Int J Radiat Oncol Biol Phys* 1989;16:831.) **B:** Pelvic control as a function of treatment time for 621 patients treated with a total dose of 85 Gy. (From Keane TJ, Fyles A, O'Sullivan B, et al. The effect of treatment duration on local control of squamous carcinoma of the tonsil and carcinoma of the cervix. *Semin Radiat Oncol* 1992;2:27.)

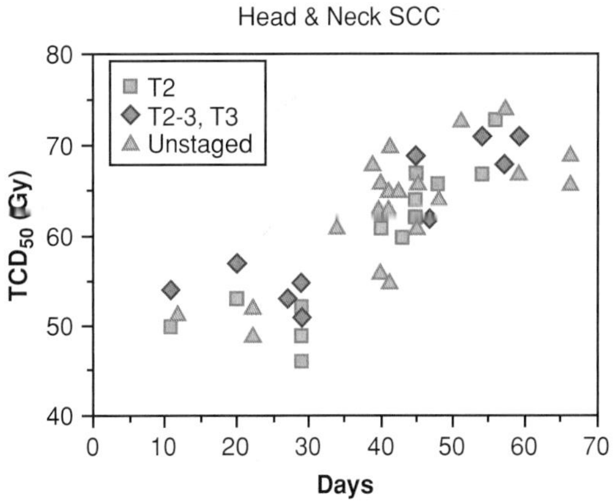

FIGURE 2.7. Estimated TCD_{50} (tumor control dose) values as a function of treatment duration from published results of radiation therapy for squamous carcinomas of the head and neck excluding nasopharynx and true vocal cord. TCD_{50} values are expressed as $LQED_{2Gy}$ (the equivalent dose given in 2-Gy fractions calculated using the LQ model). Total doses for an isoeffect increase steeply with protraction of treatment duration, implying accelerated repopulation by surviving tumor clonogens, consistent with the 3- to 4-day average doubling time calculated from scattergrams (Fig. 2.6A). The relatively constant TCD_{50} value for treatments lasting up to 4 weeks is consistent with an average time of onset of accelerated growth at about 4 weeks. Growth of clonogens at the average preirradiation doubling rate of 2 months would have little detectable effect on TCD_{50} values (about 2.5-Gy increase in 8 weeks). (From Withers HR, Taylor JMG, Maciejewski B. The hazard of accelerated tumor clonogen repopulation during radiotherapy. *Acta Oncol* 1988;27:131.)

in overall treatment duration predominantly reflect institutional policy; selection of longer treatments for worse tumors cannot explain the increase of tumor control dose 50 (TCD_{50}) with extension of overall treatment time.

b. *TCD_{50} analysis.* Figure 2.7 presents TCD_{50} values for SCC of head and neck calculated from the literature.[79] They are independent of treatment duration up to about 28 days, after which they increase rapidly (consistent with 0.6 Gy per day). The suggestion is that *on average,* head and neck SCCs exhibit a lag period of 3 to 4 weeks before beginning to repopulate, with an average doubling time of 3 to 4 days.

c. *Analysis of primary tumor control rate.* When a standard prescription (e.g., 50 Gy in 20 fractions in 4 weeks) is given but overall duration of therapy is extended for whatever reason, the control rate decreases, commonly by 1% to 2% per day for head and neck and cervix cancer (Fig. 2.6b).[99,100]

It should be noted that a lag period of up to 4 weeks and thereafter a 0.6 Gy per day increase in the "isocontrol" dose are *not* evidence that RT for head and neck cancer is best given in 4 weeks. Repopulation of mucosa begins at about 10 to 12 days and is more rapid than tumor, requiring thereafter an average daily dose increment of at least 1 Gy for a mucosal isoresponse.[79] Thus, a therapeutic gain in mucosal tolerance relative to tumor control is still achieved by extending treatment beyond 4 weeks. It is only late-responding tissues, which do not benefit from repopulation, that lose out. The overall therapeutic differential will be greatest if the tolerance dose for the critical late-responding tissue is delivered in the shortest overall time consistent with an acceptable acute response,[75,79] and without compromising the total dose delivered to the tumor.

4. *Accelerated Treatment*
If accelerated tumor growth contributes to treatment failure, it may be neutralized by acceleration of RT. In nonrandomized studies, shortening the overall duration of treatment improved the local control in inflammatory breast cancer,[101] melanoma metastases to brain,[102] and head and neck cancer.[47,103,104] Randomized studies of accelerated treatment of head and neck cancer validated the benefit. Exceptions may be cancer of the prostate, which is slow growing,[92,93] although hypofractionation with stereotactic body radiation therapy (SBRT) for prostate cancer has shown promise.[105]

Dose-intensity studies[106,107,108] suggest that chemotherapy also accelerates tumor regrowth. Furthermore, the lack of benefit from neoadjuvant chemotherapy given for two or three cycles before the start of RT for head and neck cancer, despite shrinkage of the gross tumor mass, is consistent with accelerated regrowth of subclinical residual CSCs.

Cell Cycle Redistribution After Radiation Therapy

Cells change in their radiosensitivity as they traverse the division cycle[109] (Fig. 2.8). The difference in radiosensitivity between late S-phase and G_2-M cells is greater than that between euoxic and hypoxic cells. After exposure of an asynchronous population of cells to 2 Gy, the survivors will be partially synchronized in

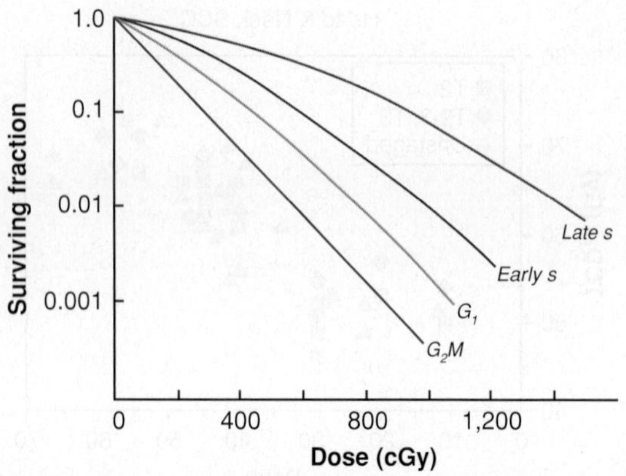

FIGURE 2.8. Radiation dose survival curves for one line of mammalian cells (V-79 Chinese hamster) synchronized in four positions in the division cycle. Significant differences occur in the survival of cells at different ages, with the differences relative to absolute survival being greatest at lower doses. The survival ratio between late S and G_2M cells after 2 Gy is approximately 5. (From Withers HR, Peters LJ. Biological aspects of radiation therapy. In: Fletcher GH, ed. *Textbook of radiotherapy,* 3rd ed. Philadelphia: Lea and Febiger, 1980.)

relatively radioresistant cell cycle phases (because of the preferential killing of cells in sensitive phases). When these survivors resume their progression through the division cycle, they move into more sensitive phases. If they were to do so in a synchronized fashion, this could be exploited.[110] Unfortunately, they do not. However, a greater proportion of the surviving population will be in sensitive phases of the division cycle than immediately after irradiation, which will produce a net "self-sensitization" effect. Dose fractionation will enhance the therapeutic ratio by permitting redistribution among tumor cells but not nonproliferating cells in late-responding normal tissues.[111] The differential is greater the smaller the dose per fraction, and it is amplified as an exponential function of the number of fractions delivered. This amplification of small differentials between cycling tumor cells and the nonredistributing target cells in late-responding normal tissues was the initial rationale for clinical trials of hyperfractionation,[111] before important intrinsic differences in response to low-dose fractionation between late-responding normal tissues and tumors were appreciated.[112]

The effect of cell cycle redistribution on tumor responses to multifraction irradiation is difficult to demonstrate.[113] This may be because of intratumoral heterogeneity and timing. CSCs are believed to exist in the G0-phase of the cell cycle and to cycle slowly because of their intrinsic metabolic state influences from the niche in which they reside. Niches for most CSCs have yet to be convincingly demonstrated; however, glioma CSCs appear to reside in a perivascular location,[114–116] although there is also evidence for hypoxic niches.[117] Most CSCs are negative for the proliferation marker Ki67,[118] but multiple fractions of IR may promote recruitment of CSCs from the niche and increase the proportion of cycling cells,[118] with a possible concomitant increase in radiosensitivity. Therefore, for CSCs, redistribution following irradiation may be tied to their mobilization into the cell cycle and thus regeneration. This raises the interesting possibility that this may be strategy for increasing their radiosensitivity.

The Oxygen Effect

In 1909, Schwarz reported that restricting the blood flow to a tissue decreased its radiation response.[119] It was thought that this was a metabolic effect; however, in 1951, Read[120] showed that oxygen sensitized cells through a radiochemical mechanism. Now, oxygen is recognized as a potent chemical modifier of radiosensitivity.[121,122] The relationship between oxygen tension and radiosensitivity varies, but a radiosensitivity halfway between that of hypoxic and euoxic (aerobic) cells (the k value[5]) is achieved with oxygen concentrations ranging from about 3 to 10 mm Hg[1,121,122] (Fig. 2.9). The curve relating metabolic activity to oxygen concentration is steeper and to the left of this.

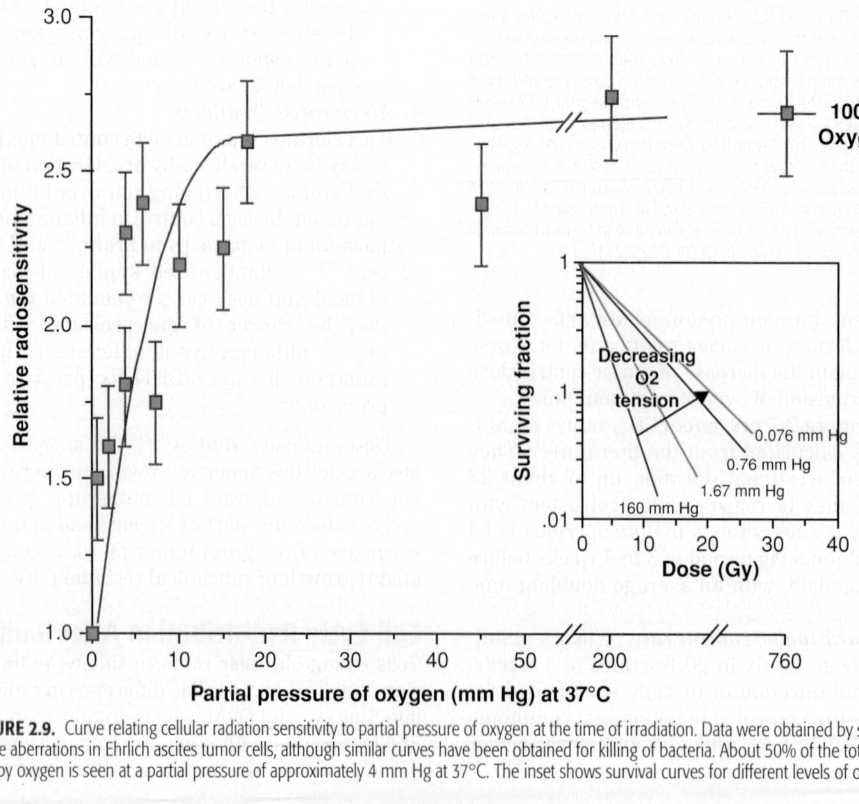

FIGURE 2.9. Curve relating cellular radiation sensitivity to partial pressure of oxygen at the time of irradiation. Data were obtained by scoring anaphase aberrations in Ehrlich ascites tumor cells, although similar curves have been obtained for killing of bacteria. About 50% of the total sensitization by oxygen is seen at a partial pressure of approximately 4 mm Hg at 37°C. The inset shows survival curves for different levels of oxygenation.

Therefore, hypoxic radioresistant cells can be metabolically normal and viable. The inset in Figure 2.9 shows how survival curves are modified by oxygen concentration. The ratio of doses required to produce the same level of effect (e.g., cell survival) in hypoxic, as in euoxia, conditions is called the oxygen enhancement ratio (OER). The OER is between 2.5 and 3 for cells exposed to high doses of x- or γ-rays and does not change much as cells progress through the cell cycle. At low doses or low dose rates,[123] the OER is slightly lower. The reason may be that electrons scattered by photons may be regarded operationally as a mixture of low and high LET particles. At the ends of electron tracks, there is a densely ionizing component that will be relatively more important at low doses or low dose rates, and this may result in a lower OER. The OER for neutrons used in clinical trials is approximately 1.6 and 1 or close to it for α-particles or beams of stripped nuclei.

The property of oxygen critical to radiosensitization is its electron affinity. After this was realized, radiochemists developed oxygen-mimetic, electron-affinic radiosensitizers, such as metronidazole, misonidazole, etanidazole, nimorazole, and other nitroimidazoles. These radiosensitizers are easier to administer than oxygen, are less rapidly metabolized, and can therefore diffuse further from blood vessels into the hypoxic regions of the tumor. Toxicity has somewhat limited their use, but there is evidence of clinical efficacy. Recently, drugs have been developed, such as tirapazamine, that are selectively toxic to hypoxic cells and may both radiosensitize and chemosensitize them.[124]

Relevance of Hypoxia to Clinical Radiation Therapy

Tissue oxygenation is critically dependent on capillary blood flow. If blood is stagnant, as it can be in tumor capillaries, then arterial and venous oxygen tension are of secondary relevance.[125,126,127] It is therefore not surprising that solid tumors contain hypoxic foci.[90,126,128,129] These may be due to the tumor outgrowing the blood supply, necrosis, sluggish blood flow, shunts, or temporary occlusion.[127] Temporary occlusion and blood shunting cause transient hypoxia that may be as, or more, important to the overall response as chronic hypoxia caused by limited diffusion.

Hypoxia has been demonstrated by a variety of methods. When single high doses of radiation of varying magnitude are given to experimental tumors and clonogenic survival assessed in vitro, the dose survival curve has two components: an initial, relatively rapid decline as euoxic cells are killed, and a second slower decline resulting from the less efficient killing of radioresistant hypoxic cells.[129] Polarographic oxygen electrodes have been used to measure oxygen tension (pO_2) within human and experimental tumors,[126] as have DNA strand break (Comet) assays,[130,131] detection of binding of the 2-nitroimidazole by immunohistochemistry (EF5)[132] or PET imaging, and immunohistochemistry for localized expression of hypoxia-inducible factor-1α (HIF-1α) or its downstream effectors. HIF-1 expression is stabilized under hypoxia, and it acts as a transcription factor to up-regulate several genes that promote cell and tissue survival. These include glycolysis enzymes and vascular endothelial growth factor (VEGF), which promotes angiogenesis. It is a metabolic switch mechanism that may also be produced in the presence of oxygen under inflammatory conditions under the direction of the transcription factor NF-κB (nuclear factor κB). HIF-1 may therefore be best regarded as a factor whose expression is dysregulated in cancer and has wider implications than promoting radioresistance.

Hypoxia is being increasingly linked with clinical outcome. Hyperbaric oxygen[133,134] or correction of anemia[133,135] has been reported to improve outcome, although the use of erythropoietin has been reported to have the opposite effect,[136] most likely because it supports CSC proliferation and survival.[137] High hypoxic fraction[126] portends poor local control and survival rates in head and neck and cervix cancer treated with RT.[95,138] However, outcome of patients with uterine cervix cancers treated with surgery only also correlated with hypoxia.[139] In addition, hypoxia provides a growth advantage for cells with mutated p53[140] and can select for, and be a marker for, more aggressive tumors.

Despite the probable existence of hypoxic cells within many, if not all, solid tumors of humans, the importance of hypoxia as a predictor of individual response to RT has yet to be established. CSCs have been shown to have a high level of antioxidants and respond less to IR with ROS production.[2] This may make them resistant to oxygen-enhanced radiosensitization.

RT may also actually induce hypoxia, as may other treatments. Fuks and Kolesnick[24] noted "rapid endothelial cell death in tumor displays an apparent threshold at 8–10 Gy and a maximal response at 20–25 Gy." This apoptosis was observed within hours, and loss of microvasculature after RT has been reported after a few weeks.[141] The failure of normal tissues irradiated with <20 Gy to support angiogenesis has been known for decades as the tumor bed effect.[142] In light of this, tumor regrowth during or after RT may depend on vasculogenesis more than angiogenesis.[143,144] Vasculogenesis is a relatively inefficient process, and an increase in hypoxia is a possible outcome.

How common these radiation-induced alterations in the tumor microenvironment are in clinical reality and their relationship to tumor cure has yet to be fully established. Dose may play a major role, as suggested by Fuks and Kolesnick,[24] although Tsai et al.[144] showed that modest fractionated protocols caused vascular loss similar to that of high single doses. Again, proinflammatory cytokines such as TNF-α may be particularly important after high doses because they target vasculature.[145] In fact, it is not definite that chronic hypoxia leads to radioresistance, because it has been shown to decrease DNA DSB repair, in particular RAD51-mediated HR.[146] The nature of the hypoxia may therefore be critical, and transient acute hypoxia due to intermittent vessel closure that may reoxygenate rapidly could be more clinically relevant than chronic hypoxia, which is owing to the limitation of oxygen diffusion.

An important issue is whether reoxygenation occurs during a course of fractionated RT. If hypoxia is simply a marker of tumor aggression, then reoxygenation may not be important for outcome; however, if hypoxia is radiobiologically relevant, the rate and extent of reoxygenation will be critical.

Tumor Reoxygenation

If 30% of tumor cells were hypoxic and 70% euoxic, and no change were to occur in the distribution of oxygenation during a course of conventional RT, most surviving cells would be hypoxic after the first few fractions and 70 Gy would reduce survival to $<10^{-4}$. This is providing that the CSCs are sensitized by oxygen in vivo in the same way that many other cells are in vitro and are equivalent to clonogenic cells. These are large assumptions and probably incorrect; however, reoxygenation may still be relevant to tumor control in the clinic. The possible magnitude of the effect of reoxygenation on the response to multiple dose fractions can be appreciated from Table 2.1. For example, the dose to a tumor that repeatedly returns to an 80-to-20 euoxic-to-hypoxic cell mixture would need to be 15%

TABLE 2.1 RATIOS OF DOSE FOR ISOSURVIVAL EQUIVALENT TO THAT FROM 2 GY IN OXIC CONDITIONS[a]

Ratio of Euoxic to Hypoxic Cells	Dose Modification Factor
100/0	1.0
90/10	1.07
80/20	1.15
70/30	1.23
60/40	1.35

[a]Assuming a constant OER of 2.5 at all doses.

higher than it would if all tumor cells were oxic. Reoxygenation may require reduction in total tumor cells with less loss of blood vessels, decreased interstitial tumor pressure, and better oxygen diffusion as a result of less temporary occlusions.[125] It should be noted that free radicals generated during reoxygenation may be particularly toxic to cells. This may be why CSCs can exist in a perivascular niche, being more resistant to redox changes.[62]

Most studies on the kinetics of reoxygenation in animal tumors have used relatively large dose fractions and indicate considerable variation between tumors. In most cases, reoxygenation occurs rapidly and is completed within 6 to 24 hours.[147] In human tumors, it is still a matter of controversy.[148] The variation between tumors and tumor sites seems considerable.

It seems unlikely that the beneficial effects of reoxygenation are compromised much by changes in dose fractionation. In pure hyperfractionation, where the dose per fraction is small, responses will be little affected by 10% to 20% of the cells being hypoxic.[149] The overall duration of the course of RT is not shortened; therefore, the time available for reoxygenation will be the same. In accelerated regimens, the theoretical problem of the proportion of surviving hypoxic cells increasing with time is of more concern. However, the rapid reoxygenation kinetics observed in experimental tumors, as well as high control rates achieved experimentally and clinically with brachytherapy and in centers using 3- or 4-week overall treatment durations, suggest that reoxygenation is adequate in most tumors, even with short courses of fractionated or low dose rate irradiation, or it is not a problem.

Where large dose fractions are given as a single exposure, as in intraoperative RT, single-dose stereotactic radiosurgery, and high dose rate brachytherapy, outcome may be more compromised by hypoxia. However, results show that local control is often achieved, suggesting that advantageous physical factors outweigh any lack of reoxygenation. In chemoradiotherapy or bioradiotherapy protocols that target tumor vasculature or angiogenesis, the extent of reoxygenation might also be an issue.

QUANTITATIVE RADIOBIOLOGY AND DOSE FRACTIONATION

Random Nature of Cell Killing

Our earliest understanding of dose-response relationships for irradiated cells came from studies with bacteria.[150] Bacterial cell survival decreases geometrically with dose. In other words, the dose that reduces the survival rate to 50% will, when doubled, reduce it to 25%, and if tripled, to 12.5%, and so forth. When such a relationship is plotted semilogarithmically, a straight line results. Such a dose-survival relationship reflects a random cell kill process, which means that if 100 lethal lesions are distributed randomly throughout 100 equally radiation-sensitive cells (mean lethal dose = 1), by Poisson statistics, 37 cells will be spared; 37 will have one lethal lesion; 18 will have two; 6 will have three, and the like (Fig. 2.10). It is immaterial whether a cell is killed by one or more lethal lesions; however, the survival rate of 37% recurs for each additional mean lethal dose, which ensures the semilogarithmic relationship.

The mathematic bent of early radiation biologists, many of whom were also physicists, caused them to describe the slope of survival curves in terms of the mean lethal dose (D_{37} or D_0), which reduces survival by one natural logarithm (e^{-1}), rather than D_{10}, which reduces it by one common logarithm and is an easier term for biologists to think in. It is useful to remember that D_{10} is about 2.3 times D_0.

Mammalian Cell Survival Curves

Puck and Marcus[4] published the first survival curve for mammalian cells in 1956. Logarithmic decreases in cell survival with dose were found that fitted the model described for bacteria, although with two important differences. D_0 values for cells are generally between 0.75 and 2 Gy, which is less than one-tenth of those for bacteria, largely reflecting the latter's smaller target size (less DNA). In addition, unlike those for bacteria, mammalian cell survival curves most often have a shoulder before the logarithmic decline (Fig. 2.11). The biologic basis for the shoulder is not firmly established; however, it is consistent with mechanistic view of Catcheside et al.[150] that radiation-induced cell kill has a linear, single-hit, α-type killing term plus a quadratic, multihit, β-type killing term relating it to dose. At low clinical doses of around 2 Gy, most killing is single hit. At higher doses, there is additional accumulation of ionization multihit lesions from other electron tracks (intertrack). This "sublethal" injury can be converted into additional lethal injury.

An additional complexity in dose-response curves is that hyperradiosensitivity to very low radiation doses (<10 cGy) has been shown in some systems; however, as dose increases above about 30 cGy, radioresistance increases until about 1 Gy, when cell survival begins to follow the usual downward-bending curve with increasing dose.[151,152] This phenomenon is not universal but has been seen in many human cell lines in vitro and in experimental studies in mouse skin, kidney, and lung. The precise mechanisms are still unclear, although low-dose hypersensitivity may be due to a failure to activate G2-phase cell cycle checkpoints.[17]

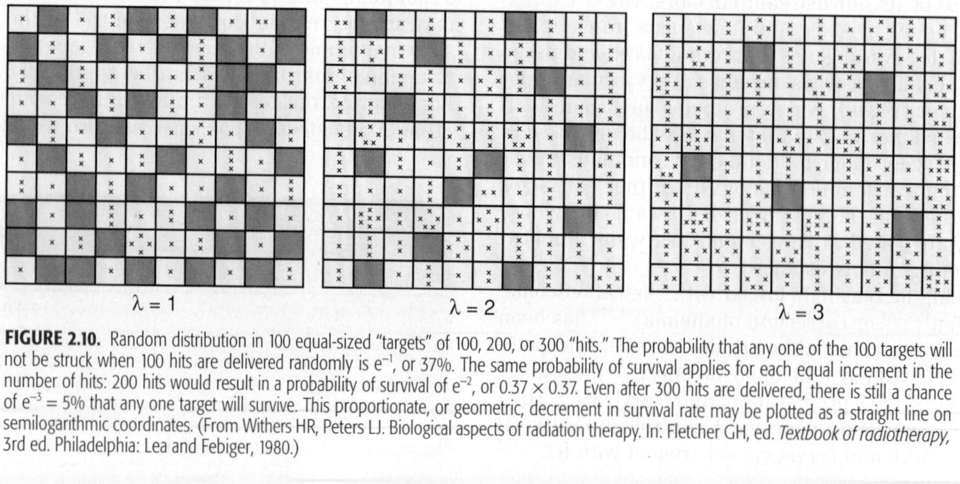

FIGURE 2.10. Random distribution in 100 equal-sized "targets" of 100, 200, or 300 "hits." The probability that any one of the 100 targets will not be struck when 100 hits are delivered randomly is e^{-1}, or 37%. The same probability of survival applies for each equal increment in the number of hits: 200 hits would result in a probability of survival of e^{-2}, or 0.37×0.37. Even after 300 hits are delivered, there is still a chance of e^{-3} = 5% that any one target will survive. This proportionate, or geometric, decrement in survival rate may be plotted as a straight line on semilogarithmic coordinates. (From Withers HR, Peters LJ. Biological aspects of radiation therapy. In: Fletcher GH, ed. *Textbook of radiotherapy*, 3rd ed. Philadelphia: Lea and Febiger, 1980.)

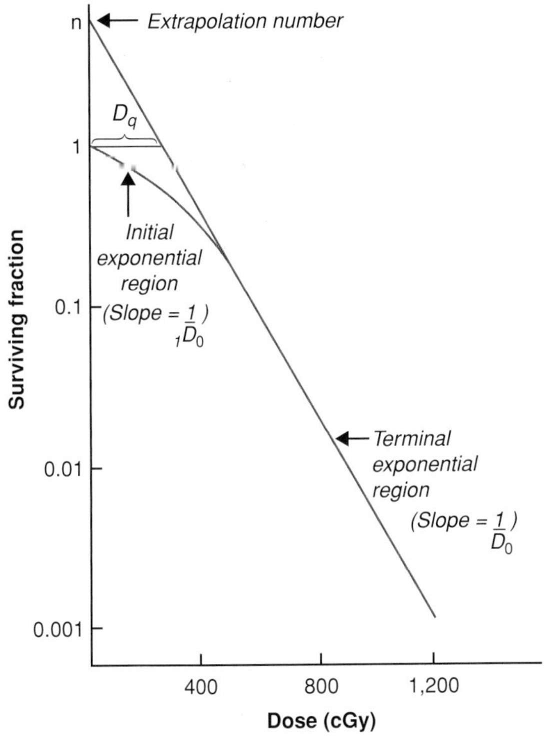

FIGURE 2.11. A two-component survival curve for mammalian cells is characterized by a "shoulder" followed by a terminal exponential region, the slope of which is defined by a D_0 value (slope = $1/D_0$). The position of the curve on the radiation dose axis can be fixed by the intercepts of the terminal exponential region extrapolated back to the zero dose axis (n) or to the 100% survival level (D_q): n is termed the extrapolation number, and D_q the quasi-threshold dose. Although n and D_q are parameters that define the width of the shoulder on the survival curve, they do not indicate its shape, which is of prime importance in RT. The survival curve shoulder can be considered to consist of an initial exponential region (the slope of which is defined by ${}_1D_0$), followed by a downward-bending segment that merges asymptotically into the final exponential region of the survival curve. (From Withers HR, Peters LJ. Biological aspects of radiation therapy. In: Fletcher GH, ed. *Textbook of radiotherapy,* 3rd ed. Philadelphia: Lea and Febiger, 1980.)

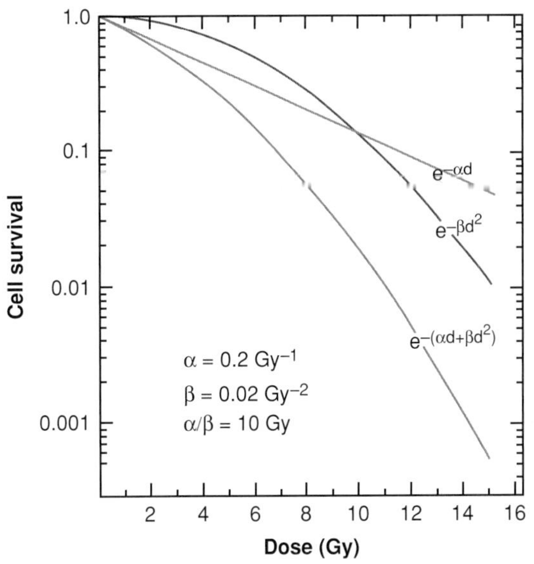

FIGURE 2.12. Model dose survival curves for mammalian cells showing that the experimentally determined curve for acute exposures (lowest curve) is the product of two mechanisms: single-hit injury described by an exponential curve ($e^{-\alpha d}$), and multihit, or cumulative, injury described by a continuously bending curve related by a coefficient, β, to the square of the dose. At doses of clinical relevance, cell death from the single-hit mechanism predominates. The rate at which the survival curve bends from an initial, essentially exponential region depends on the ratio (α/β) of the coefficients for single-hit and multihit killing: the lower the value, the sooner and more steeply the curve bends. The value of α/β is the dose at which single- and multihit mechanisms contribute equally to cell killing. In these curves, $\alpha/\beta = 10$ Gy, which is a value characteristic of acutely responding tissues. Target cells in late-responding normal tissues are characterized by low α/β values; hence, their survival curves are curvier. The flexure dose, D_f, is the dose at which deviation from the initial exponential part of the curve is difficult to detect and, for available biologic assay systems, is about one-tenth of α/β. When doses in a multifraction regimen are less than D_f, further dose fractionation does not produce detectable "sparing" (because cell killing is essentially all the result of single-hit events, the lesions potentially contributing to multievent killing being completely repaired during the fractionation intervals). The lower the α/β value, the lower the dose at which multihit mechanisms cause cell death, the lower the value of D_f, and the lower the dose per fraction below which a sparing effect of dose fractionation is lost. The curve for single-hit killing ($e^{-\alpha d}$) can be measured experimentally using very small dose fractions or a continuous low dose rate exposure; however, the curves for multihit killing ($e^{-\beta d^2}$) can be determined only indirectly from a knowledge of the other two curves.

Other phenomena also challenge any simple relationship between DNA lesions and radiation response. One is radiation-induced genomic instability where the rate of genomic alterations increases with increasing number of divisions of irradiated cells, as manifested by chromosomal rearrangements, formation of micronuclei, gene amplification, or cell killing.[153] Another is the nontargeted radiation effect in which cells that were not irradiated but were "bystanders" at the time of irradiation are affected. In some but not all cases, culture medium from irradiated cells is active.[154,155] Again, chromosome-related alterations, mutations, gene induction, and cell killing are observed end points. The relevance of low-dose hypersensitivity, adaptive responses, induced genetic instability, and bystander effects to clinical radiotherapy has yet to be fully evaluated; however, they challenge classical radiobiologic paradigms. They are probably more relevant to radiation-induced carcinogenesis, where they can explain the higher than expected frequency of postradiation chromosomal aberrations; in the future, they may provide novel opportunities for therapeutic intervention. In any event, they do not significantly impact the mathematical models that have been proposed for RT, which were derived to fit existing data within the clinically relevant dose range.

Linear Quadratic Formula

Lea[150] and Read[120,156] quantified biologic responses to irradiation in terms of a linear dose coefficient (α) and a coefficient (β) for the square of the dose so that effect is proportional to $\alpha D + \beta D^2$. This can be used to fit a continuously bending curve to cell survival data:

$$\text{S.F. (survival fraction)} = e^{-(\alpha D+\beta D^2)}$$

The linear component (αD) is of major significance if RT is delivered in fractions of about 2 Gy (Fig. 2.12). Its importance was largely ignored in the 1960s but was "rediscovered" in the early 1970s when Dutreix et al.[157] demonstrated that reducing doses per fraction below 3 Gy did not result in additional sparing of acute effects in human skin. Now it is accepted that low-dose brachytherapy or standard fractionated RT could not eradicate cancer without single-lethal-hit damage.[158,159]

The survival curve at low doses is essentially linear because α-type lethality predominates and there is little opportunity for accumulated (β-type) injury. Likewise, exposure to low dose rate continuous irradiation results predominantly in α-type lethality because of continuous repair. Under these circumstances, the effective survival curve is linear and defined by α.

The dose range over which the linear component dominates depends on the relative values of α and β. The α/β ratio defines the dose at which cell killing by linear and quadratic components are equal. The higher the α/β ratio, the more linear and steeper is the dose-response curve and the less sensitive it is to dose fractionation. If the α/β coefficient is low, the survival curve will be "curvier," bending down only after an initial linear region; there will also be a marked sparing effect of dose fractionation (Figs. 2.13 and 2.14). The parameters can be estimated from multifraction data if the reciprocal of the total dose 1/nd is plotted against dose per fraction (d) (Fe plot).[160] The intercept on the ordinate is $\alpha/\log_e S$ and the slope is $\beta/\log_e S$. The ratio of the intercept to slope gives the α/β ratio. Late-responding tissues generally have a low α/β ratio and show a large fractionation effect. Acute-responding tissues generally

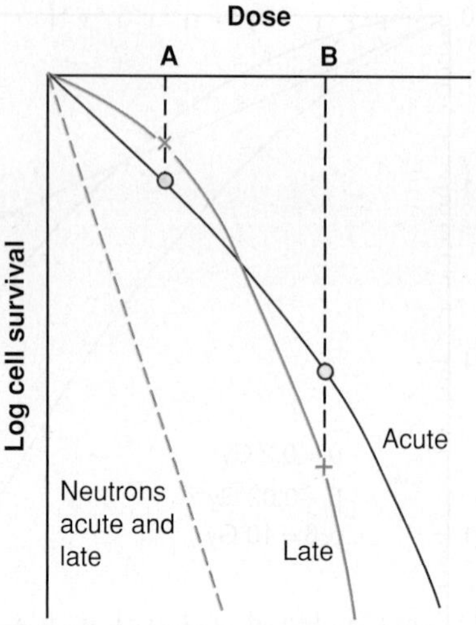

FIGURE 2.13. Hypothetical survival curves for the target cells for acute and late effects in normal tissues exposed to X-rays or neutrons. The α/β ratio is lower for late effects than for acute effects in x-irradiated tissues, resulting in a greater change in effect in late-responding tissues with change in dose. At dose A, survival of target cells is higher in late-effects than in acute-effects tissues; at dose B, the reverse is true. Increasing the dose per fraction from A to B results in a relatively greater increase in late than acute injury. For neutrons, the α/β ratio is high, with no detectable influence of the quadratic function (βd^2) over the first two decades of reduction in cell survival, implying that accumulation of sublethal injury plays a negligible role in cell killing by doses of neutrons of clinical interest. (From Withers HR, Thames HD, Peters LJ. Biological bases for high RBE values for late effects of neutron irradiation. *Int J Radiat Oncol Biol Phys* 1982;8:2071.)

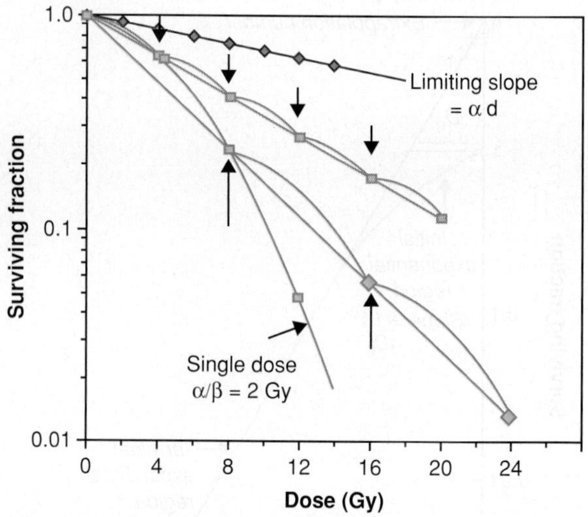

FIGURE 2.14. Multifraction-dose survival curves compared with a single-dose curve. Effective survival curves for multifraction regimens that produce an equal (proportionate) decrement in survival from each dose are linear, with shallower slopes than the single-dose curve at the same dose. Slopes of the multifraction curves become less steep with a decrease in fraction size until the dose per fraction is so low that multihit killing contributes negligibly and the slope is the limiting one determined by single-hit killing (and ${}_eD_0 = 1/\alpha$). The dose per fraction below which the effective survival curve becomes no shallower is a function of the curviness of the single-dose survival curve and is lower than the α/β value.

have a large α/β ratio, as do many tumors, although they show considerable variation (Table 2.2) with melanoma, soft tissue sarcoma, and liposarcoma tending to have low α/β ratios,[68] as do prostate[69] and breast[70] cancers. The considerable variation observed within any one tumor type may be caused by failure to take into account their CSC origin.[61]

Two-Component Model

Dose survival curves can be well fitted by equations other than the linear quadratic (LQ) model. The most common is the two-component (TC) model. This combines a single-hit component $e^{-D/_1D_0}$, where ${}_1D_0$ is the dose necessary to reduce survival to $0.37(e^{-1})$ in the initial region of the curve, with a multiple-event cell killing model $e^{-(1-e^{-D/_nD_0})^n}$, where ${}_nD_0$ is the dose needed to reduce survival to e^{-1} in the final region of the curve and n is the extrapolation number (Fig. 2.11).

$$S.F. = e^{-D/_1D_0} \cdot (1 - [e^{-D_n/D_0}]^n)$$

Comparison of the Linear Quadratic and Two-Component Survival Models

Over a limited dose range (e.g., 2 to 8 Gy), including the region that matters in most clinical radiotherapy, both the TC and LQ models "fit" data indistinguishably (Fig. 2.15). At high doses, the LQ model fits some cell survival curves better because they appear to continue to bend, whereas the TC model better fits those that seem more linear. However, the experimental data suggest that isoeffective curves are not very linear over a wide range of dose per fraction for many normal tissue responses and that extrapolation from 2 Gy to more than 7-Gy fractions or single doses as in SBRT is unlikely to give realistic equivalent doses,[161] although there are other opinions.[162] In addition, the models differ significantly at predicting responses to doses <2 Gy using data from doses >2 Gy. The differences may appear small but would be amplified if a dose of 1.15 Gy, for example, were repeated 70 times or more, as could happen in a hyperfractionated RT regimen (Fig. 2.16).

TABLE 2.2 α/β VALUES

Early-Responding Tissues	α/β *(Gy)*	*Late-Responding Tissues*	α/β *(Gy)*
Skin (desquamation)	9.4–21.0	Spinal cord (paresis)	1.6–5
Skin–pig (desquamation)		–Cervical	2–3.4
–Time ≤16 days	8.7	–Lumbar	4–5
–Time >16 days	0.9	Brain (LD_{50}/10 mo)	2.1
Lip mucosa (desquamation)	7.9	Kidney (multiple end points)	0.4–5
Jejunal mucosa (clones)	7–13	Lung (pneumonitis)	1.6–4.5
Tongue mucosa (ulceration)	11.6	Lung (fibrosis)	2.3
Colonic mucosa (clones)	7–8.5	Heart failure	3.7
Hair follicles (epilation)		Liver (clones)	2.5
–Anagen	7.5	Bladder (frequency)	7.2
–Telogen	5.5	Bladder (contraction)	5.8–11.0
Testis (clones)	13.9	Bowel (stricture/perforation)	3.5–5
Spleen (clones)	8.9	Bowel (fistula/obstruction)	10.7
Bone marrow (clones)	9.0	Bowel (rectal stenosis, <5 d)	6.2
Melanocytes (depigmentation)	6.5	Bowel (rectal stenosis, >5 d)	1.1
Tumors (cure)		Dermal contraction	1.5–3.5
Experimental tumors	10–35	Dermal wound healing	2.5
Most human tumors	6–25	Eye cataracts	1.2
Human prostate cancer	1.5	Bone (human fracture)	2.2
		Cartilage and submucosa	1–4.9
		Total body irradiation (LD_{50}/1 y)	5.1

These values represent a synthesis from many sources. Individual values are means from one study. Where a range is given, it represents mean values from multiple studies. Further details can be obtained from the Chapter by Ang and Thames, and from Table 2.2 of the 4th edition Perez.

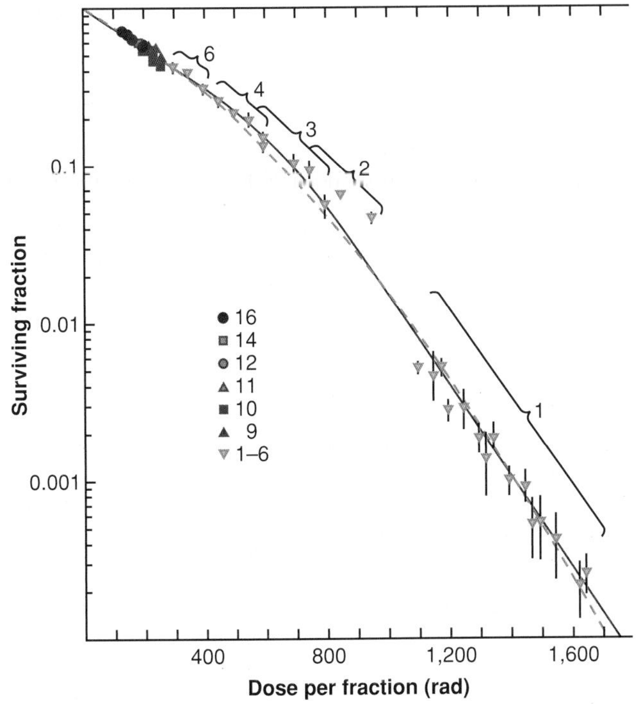

FIGURE 2.15. Effective single-dose survival curves for clonogenic cells of jejunal crypts fitted to multifraction data using LQ (*broken curves*) and TC (*solid lines*) models. Numbered brackets illustrate that the data were from experiments using that number of fractions. Mean survival curve parameters are as follows: for LQ model, □ $\alpha = 0.23$ Gy, $\beta = 0.018$ Gy^{-2}; for TC model, ${}_1D_0 = 3.57$ Gy, $D_0 = 1.43$ Gy, ${}_nD_0 = 2.37$ Gy, and n = 20.4. (From Thames HD, Withers HR, Mason KA, et al. Dose-survival characteristics of mouse jejunal crypt cells. *Int J Radiat Oncol Biol Phys* 1981;7:1591.)

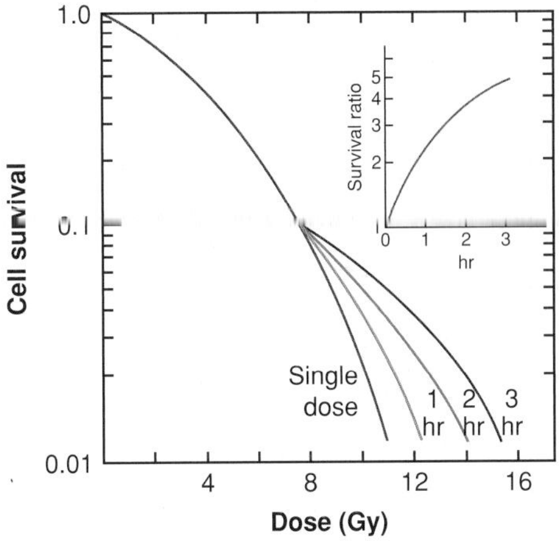

FIGURE 2.17. Recovery curves of the type first described by Elkind and Sutton.[165] The repair of sublethal injury begins immediately and can be measured in terms of survival ratio (*inset*) or the increment in dose to achieve isosurvival.

The LQ model has gained popularity[112,160,163–165] because it is simpler and because α/β ratios can be determined from in vivo multifraction experiments even though the absolute values of each coefficient are unknown. Adding to the utility of the LQ model is that responses of tissues to change in dose fractionation can be predicted from just the α/β ratio.[112]

Multifraction Survival Curves

In 1959, Elkind and Sutton[110] showed that sublethal damage (SLD) can be repaired, given a few hours of normal metabolic activity. The extent and rate of repair of SLD can be estimated by the change in survival fraction with increasing time between two dose fractions or by the increase in total dose necessary to achieve the same level of cell survival (D2-D1) (Fig. 2.17). If two doses are separated by enough time to permit complete repair of SLD, it is as though the survivors of the first dose had not been previously irradiated and harbor no residual injury. Net survival is the product of the survival after each exposure. In other words, if 2 Gy reduces survival to 50% ($S.F._{2Gy} = 0.5$), two doses of 2 Gy would reduce it to $(0.5)^2$ and n doses to $(0.5)^n$—that is, there is an equally proportionate decrease in the survival rate with each equal increment in dose. Although this and the absence of regeneration between doses are not universally accurate assumptions, they are sufficient for modeling purposes. Thus, the dose-survival relationship for a series of equal dose fractions can be considered to

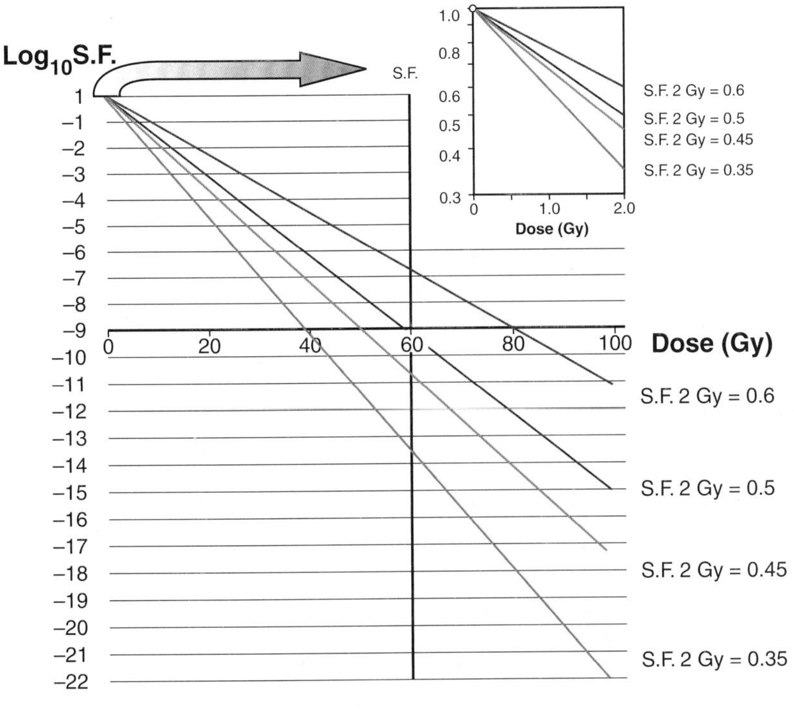

FIGURE 2.16. Effective multifraction-dose survival curves for cell populations, the survival of which from 2 Gy varies from 0.65 to 0.35. When survival from 2 Gy is 0.5, survival from 30 × 2 Gy is $(0.5)^{30}$ = approximately 10^{-9}. When this figure was constructed, this survival value was taken as an arbitrary standard against which the relative survival of other populations exposed to 30 × 2 Gy was plotted. The abscissa at the standard survival shows the total doses in 2-Gy fractions necessary to achieve that standard survival level in different cell populations. In all cases, an equal effect per dose fraction was assumed. The ratios of cell survival after a total dose of 60 Gy illustrate the exponential amplification of survival differences with increasing dose. Thus, dose fractionation can transform small differences in response at low doses (2 Gy) to large ultimate differences; measurements must be made accurately after a dose of 2 Gy to predict accurately the ultimate outcome of high-dose multifraction irradiation. (From Withers HR. Predicting late normal tissue responses. *Int J Radiat Oncol Biol Phys* 1986;12:693.)

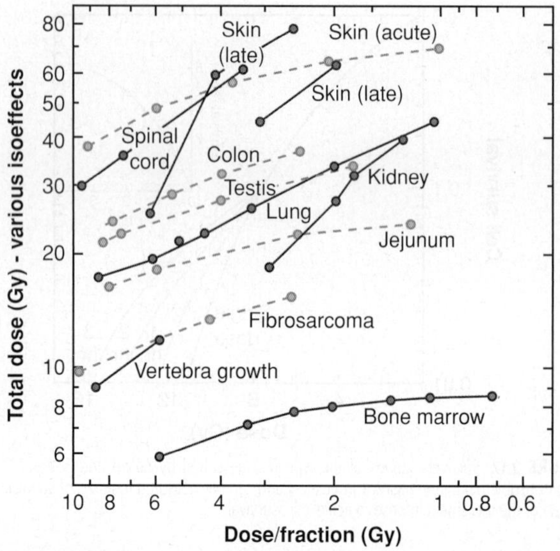

FIGURE 2.18. Isoeffect curves in which the total dose necessary for a certain effect in various tissues is plotted as a function of dose per fraction (late effects, *solid lines*; acute effects, *broken lines*). Data were selected to exclude an influence on the total dose of regeneration during the multifraction experiments. The isodoses for late effects increase more rapidly with decrease in dose per fraction than is the case for acute effects. (From Withers HR. Biologic basis for altered fractionation schemes. *Cancer* 1985;55:2086.)

give a straight line when plotted on semilogarithmic coordinates (Fig. 2.18). The multifraction survival curve extrapolates to 1 (n = 1) from any dose level, unlike most single-dose low LET survival curves. The slope of such a linear multifraction curve is always less than that for the single-dose curve at an equivalent total dose and becomes shallower the smaller the dose per fraction (Fig. 2.14).

The slope of a linear multifraction cell survival curve can be described by an "effective D_0" ($_{eff}D_0$, or $_eD_0$), which is the dose that reduces survival to e^{-1} for a particular fractionation regimen. In clinical RT, where most treatment involves multiple dose fractions, $_{eff}D_0$ values are much more relevant than D_0 values. If $S.F._{2Gy}$ were 0.5, the corresponding $_eD_0$ value for a series of 2-Gy fractions would be 2.9 Gy ($S.F. = e^{-D/_{eff}D_0}$). If the $S.F._{2Gy}$ values ranged from 0.45 to 0.67, the $_{eff}D_0$ values would range from 2.5 to 5.0 Gy. In mice, $S.F._{2Gy}$ values for jejunal crypt and spermatogenic stem cells are about 0.6 and for colonic cells about 0.65, giving $_{eff}D_0$ values for 2-Gy fractions of about 3.9 and 5.0 Gy, respectively. It can be calculated, in two ways, that 30 fractions of 2 Gy would reduce survival of jejunal crypt cells to 2×10^{-7}:

$$S.F.\text{ after } 30 \times 2\text{ Gy} = (S.F._{2\text{ Gy}})^{30} = (0.6)^{30} = 2 \times 10^{-7} \text{ or}$$

$$S.F.\text{ after 60 Gy in 2-Gy fractions} = e^{-60/_{eff}D_0} = e^{-60/3.9} = 2 \times 10^{-7}$$

Small differences between cell types in their intrinsic radiosensitivity to dose fractions of 2 Gy could amplify into large differences after many fractions if there is equal effect per fraction. This could have a major influence on the outcome of therapy. For example, if $S.F._{2Gy}$ in one tissue were 0.6 and in another 0.5, the ratio of cell survival after 30 doses of 2 Gy would be $(\frac{0.6}{0.5})^{30}$, or 237-fold. For 35 doses, the difference would increase to 590-fold. The effect of differences in $S.F._{2Gy}$ ranging from 0.35 to 0.6 on outcome after 30 fractions is shown in Figure 2.16.[166] These very large differences can be judged from the ratios of cell survival rate (on the ordinate), or the range of total doses needed to achieve the same level of cell survival (approximately 10^{-9}) (abscissa).

Common Logarithms and $_eD_{10}$

The effective survival curve for a multifraction regimen is more easily considered in terms of $_eD_{10}$, which reduces survival to 10% (10^{-1}), than in $_eD_0$. An approximate value for $_eD_{10}$ for 2-Gy fractions is 6.5 to 7 Gy, which corresponds with $S.F._{2Gy}$ of about 0.5. Remembering that about 10^9 tumor cells tightly packed would have a volume of about 1 cm^3 and that 10^{10} cells would form a sphere about 2.2 cm diameter, then an average T_3 tumor would contain about 10^{10} clonogenic cells. Assuming an $_eD_{10}$ of 7 Gy, a T_3 tumor treated with 70 Gy would have its surviving clonogen number reduced by 10^{-10} ($10^{-70/7}$), or to an average of 1 clonogen per tumor. Because of the random nature of cell survival, 37% of such tumors would contain 0 clonogens and would be eliminated. If $_eD_{10}$ were 6.5 Gy, then 65 Gy would be sufficient to cure 37% of tumors containing 10^{10} cells, and a dose of (65 + 6.5) = 71.5 Gy would reduce cell survival to 10^{-11}, resulting in a 90% local control rate.

Tumor Response and Dose Fractionation

As has already been mentioned, there is a wide spectrum of radiosensitivities within and between tumor types and variation in their α/β ratios (Table 2.2). There is also uncertainty in the weight that should be attributed to each of the four "Rs" affecting survival of tumor cells during a course of RT[58]: *repair* of SLD, *repopulation, redistribution* through the division cycle, and *reoxygenation* of hypoxic tumor clonogens. If the effects of such phenomena on the response to each dose were constant throughout the course of a multifraction regimen, the resulting survival curve would be linear and the slope would depend on the extent to which each phenomenon affected the response. More likely, their influence, and particularly the effect of reoxygenation and regeneration, varies with time as treatment progresses. In some normal tissues (e.g., oropharyngeal mucosa), regeneration of surviving clonogenic cells late in a course of 1.8- to 2-Gy fractions may outstrip the cytocidal effect of treatment and the net survival curve will have a positive slope. The same phenomenon may occasionally happen within a tumor during treatment. Despite the uncertainties, it is possible to model dose-response relationships for tumors and to use these models to guide treatment.

Tumor Control Probability

Tumor Control Probability for Clinically Detectable Disease

The probability of tumor control increases as radiation dose increases, although not linearly. Success or failure depends on killing the last surviving clonogen. Permanent tumor control (not palliation) is achieved abruptly as the last clonogen is sterilized. A plot of tumor control probability (TCP) versus dose for a single tumor therefore shows no response up to a certain dose and then an immediate increase to 100% at death of the last clonogen. For a series of patients, even if they have identical tumors, the shape of the TCP curve is different because cell killing is a random process. After a certain dose of irradiation, the numbers of surviving clonogens per tumor will begin to follow a Poisson distribution. For example, if cell survival is reduced to an average of one clonogen per tumor, there would be, on average, 37% with no survivors, 37% with one, 18.4% with two, 6.1% with three, and 1.5% with four or more surviving clonogens. Obviously, the local control rate would be 37%, not 0%. Poisson statistics correlate probability of tumor control with cell survival rate by:

$$P_{cure} = e^{-x} = e^{-(SF \cdot M)},$$

where x is the average number of surviving clonogens per tumor, which in turn is the product of S.F. (fraction of cells surviving) and M (initial cell number). For example, if a tumor contains 10^{10} clonogens, doses that reduce survival to 10^{-10} would give an average cell survival of 1 and P_{cure} to $e - (10^{10} \cdot 10^{-10}) = e^{-1} = 0.37$, or 37%.

If the total dose were increased by two $_{eff}D_0$ values, cell survival would be further reduced by two natural logarithms, from 1 to $1 \times e^{-2}$, that is, to an average of 0.135 cells per tumor, and $P_{cure} = e^{-0.135} = 0.87$, or 87%. It can be calculated that an

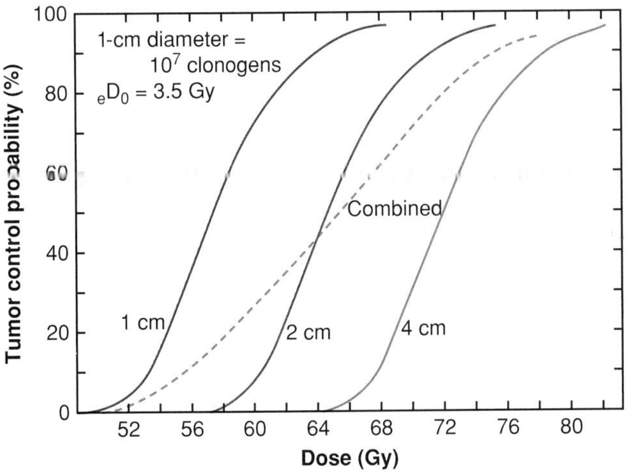

FIGURE 2.19. Theoretic tumor control probability (TCP) curves for three sizes of spherical tumors (*solid lines*) and one that would result from a study incorporating into the dose-response analysis all three tumor sizes in equal proportions (*broken line*). They were calculated on the assumptions that the dose was given in 2-Gy fractions, that the $_eD_0$ value for 2 Gy per fraction was 3.5 Gy, and that a 1-cm diameter spherical tumor contained 10^7 clonogens. As tumor volume increases, so does the dose required for a certain probability of control. The cell number increases by 8 times and 64 times as the spherical tumor increases from 1-cm diameter to 2 and 4 cm, respectively. An exponential increase in clonogen number is related to a linear increase in dose for an isoeffect. Heterogeneity of even one factor, initial clonogen number, causes the TCP curve to be shallower (*broken line*). Retrospective clinical studies incorporate a large number of causes for heterogeneity of response.

increase in dose by three $_{eff}D_0$ values is sufficient to increase the probability of cure from 10% to 90%. If $P_{cure} = 10\% = 0.1 = e^{-x}$ then x = 2.3. In other words, at 10% local control rate, there is an average of 2.3 clonogens per tumor. After an increase in dose by three $_{eff}D_0$ values, $P_{cure} = e^{-(2.3 \cdot e^{-3})} = e^{-(0.115)} = 0.89$, or 89%.

This relationship between probability of cure and dose, above a certain threshold, is described by a sigmoid curve (Fig. 2.19). It is obvious from the previous equations and calculations that the slope of the curve is a function of the $_{eff}D_0$ values for the last few surviving tumor clonogens. It is steeper for neutrons or for single-dose x-ray treatments than for multifraction x-ray exposures and steeper (by the OER) for euoxic than for hypoxic cells.

The dose that yields a 50% control rate is known as the TCD_{50}. A higher rate is usually sought in clinical practice; however, for experimental studies, the TCD_{50} is useful because it is in a steep part of the TCP curve and is sensitive to small changes in the effectiveness of therapy. (Actually, the curve is steepest at TCD_{37}, where an average of one clonogenic cell survives per tumor.)

TCP curves from experimental animal data are steep, although those for human tumor control are shallower than would be predicted.[53,168–176] This reflects heterogeneity in tumor characteristics and treatment prescriptions, which give a wider spread of responses to a given (nominal) dose. However, even in recent analyses where variation in tumor characteristics and treatment parameters has been minimized or adjusted for, and uniformity facilitated by analyzing a body of data large enough to allow relatively homogeneous stages of disease to be studied independently, the TCP curves have been fairly shallow, indicating a need for even better tumor profiling. Heterogeneity may come from molecular cancer-related differences, cancer origin, or numbers of CSCs that would impact their intrinsic radiosensitivity, redistribution and repopulation kinetics, reoxygenation rates, or physical parameters such as dose rate, dose calculation, inhomogeneities of dose distribution, inconsistency of methods of dose prescription, geographic misses, overall time, and more. Of course if RT were perfect, the TCP curve would be flat at a high level of control. As it is, treatment is often individualized (e.g., by prescribing higher doses for larger tumors), which tends to flatten TCP curves.

The effect of constructing TCP curves for a series of tumors nonhomogeneous in only one characteristic—volume (T-stages)—is illustrated in Figure 2.19. If tumors of three sizes varying in diameter by factors of 2 are stratified carefully, three distinct steep TCP curves would be obtained. If an equal number of tumors of all three sizes are analyzed together, the TCP curve obtained would be flat, as shown as a broken line. It would not be appropriate to include tumors with a 64-fold range of volumes in a clinical TCP analysis, although the range in CSC numbers in human cancers of similar T-stage may be of this magnitude. Further variation in the effective number of CSCs would also arise from differences in inherent growth and accelerated repopulation kinetics of surviving cells during RT.

Normal tissue dose-response curves for the incidence of a certain complication are also sigmoid above a certain threshold. Such curves are used for estimating LD_{50} or ED_{50} values, the doses that cause in 50% of cases lethality or any specified effect, respectively. Because normal tissues are more homogeneous than tumors in their composition and radiation responses, complication probability curves are steeper than those for tumor control.[20]

The art of RT can be quantified in a risk-benefit analysis as a balance between the TCP and the probability of complications, NTCP (both represented by sigmoid curves illustrated in Fig. 2.20), with many factors involved. Different points illustrate this:

1. If there is to be therapeutic gain, the biologic effectiveness of RT must be greater in the tumor than in normal tissues—that is, normal tissues must be preferentially spared.
2. In the steep midrange of TCP or complication frequency, a small change in the biologic effectiveness of therapy can give a substantial change in clinical outcome. Conversely, if a change in treatment produces a modest difference in TCP or frequency of complications, it should not be interpreted as being from a large change in biologic effectiveness. Effectiveness is expressed more appropriately as change in dose to achieve a certain isoeffect—that is, by quantifying the lateral shift of the TCP or NTCP curve. The ratio of isoeffect doses is the dose-modification factor.
3. At incidences of less than about 10% and greater than about 85%, changes in biologically effective dose will appear less than in the midrange. For example, if the TCP is 90%, minor therapeutic gain would be achieved from an increase in dose, and perhaps a therapeutic disadvantage if there was an associated incidence of severe complications that already lay on the bottom part of the NTCP curve.

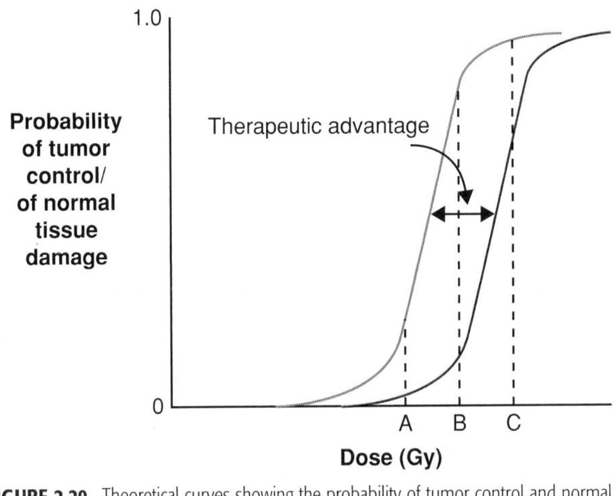

FIGURE 2.20. Theoretical curves showing the probability of tumor control and normal tissue complications. Both curves have a threshold and are log sigmoid in nature. The art of radiotherapy is to increase the distance between these two curves–that is, to derive a therapeutic benefit. If the normal tissue damage curve is to the left of that for TCP, tumor control is unlikely without unacceptable normal tissue complications.

4. Because TCP and NTCP curves are generally close together, it is usually inappropriate to produce no complications. Within the treatment volume, a certain incidence of injury to normal tissues sufficient to be defined as a complication is a prerequisite to good curative RT under most circumstances where the TCP is not close to 100%.
5. If the TCP is to the right of the NTCP curve, tumor control without a high incidence of complications is unlikely and other modalities should be used, either independently or as adjuvants. For example, if the TCP curves for large tumors lie to the right of those for complications, whereas those for smaller tumors are to the left, a therapeutic gain might be derived from excision of the large tumor or some form of chemotherapy that would add to the effect of RT without increasing normal tissue toxicity. However, a 50% or even 90% debulking is of modest value. A 90% reduction in tumor volume represents only a one-decade decrease in cell number, equivalent to about 6.5 to 7 Gy in 2-Gy fractions, other things being equal.
6. It defies biologic rationale to deny the existence of a potential benefit from maximizing the dose in a patient considered to have some finite chance of tumor control merely because retrospective studies show a shallow TCP curve.

Tumor Control Probability for Subclinical Disease

The threshold-sigmoid TCP curve for clinically detectable tumors is not appropriate for subclinical metastases. If 10^n clonogens represent the upper limit of clinical undetectability of metastases, then patients who harbor subclinical metastases must have a tumor burden of between 1 and 10^n cells. Given that micrometastases grow exponentially, it is reasonable (as a working hypothesis) to assume that an even distribution of the logarithm of metastatic clonogens (between 1 and 10^n cells) exist within a series of patients.[177,178]

If a reasonable value for n is 9, then 11% of patients with subclinical metastases would have between 1 and 10 metastatic clonogens, another 11% between 10 and 100, another 11% of patients between 10^2 and 10^3, and so forth. Based on this simple model, the TCP curve would exhibit no threshold and would be shallow. The lack of a detectable threshold would reflect the existence of a very small number of metastatic cells in some patients, and the shallow slope would reflect the wide variation in cell burden within the population harboring subclinical metastases. The model in Figure 2.21A illustrates these concepts. Although this distribution could be modified by many factors (notably gompertzian growth of micrometastases), it is generally consistent with results of RT of subclinical metastases (Fig. 2.21B).

TIME-DOSE ISOEFFECT FORMULAS AND DOSE FRACTIONATION

History

Early isoeffect curves related the total dose required to produce certain skin reactions or to achieve a certain TCP to the treatment time over which the dose regimen was delivered.[179] That work preceded the demonstration by Puck and Marcus[4] in 1956 that mammalian cell survival curves had a shoulder. It also preceded the work of Elkind and Sutton[180] demonstrating that sublethal injury could be repaired and therefore that the number of fractions, not just overall time, was important. Fowler and Stern[181] varied the number of fractions (N) and overall time (T) experimentally and showed that they were independent variables. Ellis[182] developed the nominal standard dose (NSD) formula to incorporate these two variables into an isoeffect curve that was thought to be more clinically relevant than the original Strandqvist curves.[179]

More recently, isoeffect curves that are based on parameters of dose survival curves only[112,160,165,183] or that include other biologic parameters, such as regeneration, have been proposed.[184,185] We now understand that there can be no single universally applicable isoeffect equation or curve because tissues (and tumors) differ in the characteristics that determine their fractionation responses and repopulation kinetics.

Acute- Versus Late-Responding Tissues

The most general biologic phenomenon influencing the fractionation response is repair of sublethal injury.[110] This varies among tissues, with slow-responding tissues consistently showing a greater capacity than rapidly responding tissues.[112,165,186–188] This may be because surviving cells in early-responding tissues redistribute through the division cycle during the interfraction interval and express unrepaired damage as they do so, or they may move into cell cycle phases that are more radiation sensitive. Alternatively, repair of sublethal injury may be more complete in late-responding than in

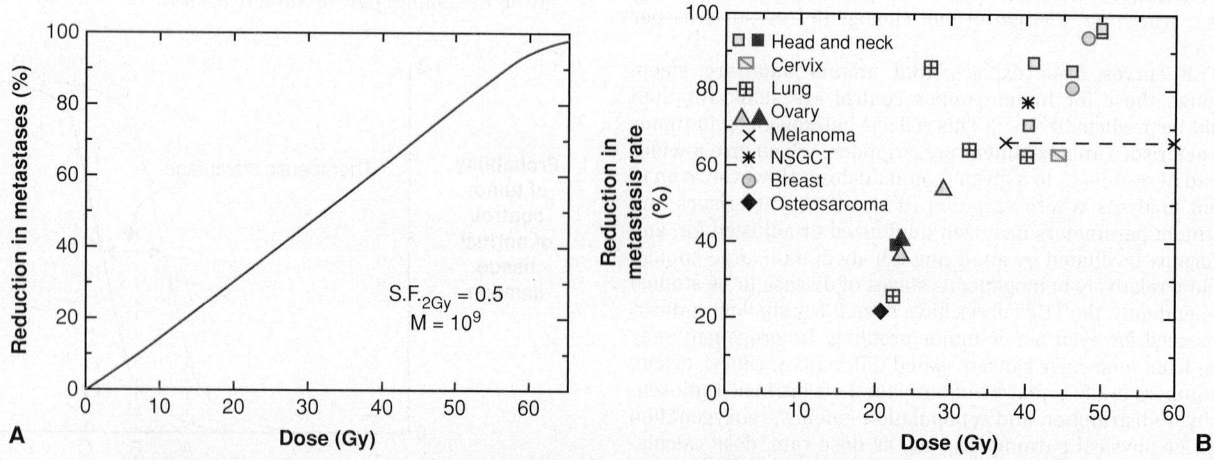

FIGURE 2.21. Percentage control rate as a function of dose for subclinical metastases. **A:** Modeling on the basis of a uniform distribution of the logarithm of numbers of metastatic tumor cells per patient ranging between 1 and 10^9. An SF_{2Gy} value of 0.5 was used. The intercept of this theoretic curve is displaced slightly from zero because of the random statistical chance that any cell will survive any dose of radiation. In addition, at high doses, the probability of sterilizing all tumor cells approaches 100% asymptotically for the same reason. **B:** Percentage reductions in recurrence as a function of dose from reports in the literature for various tumor types. Solid symbols represent data from prospective randomized trials. Other data are retrospective comparisons between control rates with and without elective irradiation. (From Withers HR, Peters LJ, Taylor JMG. Dose-response relationship for radiation therapy of subclinical disease. *Int J Radiat Oncol Biol Phys* 1995;31:353.)

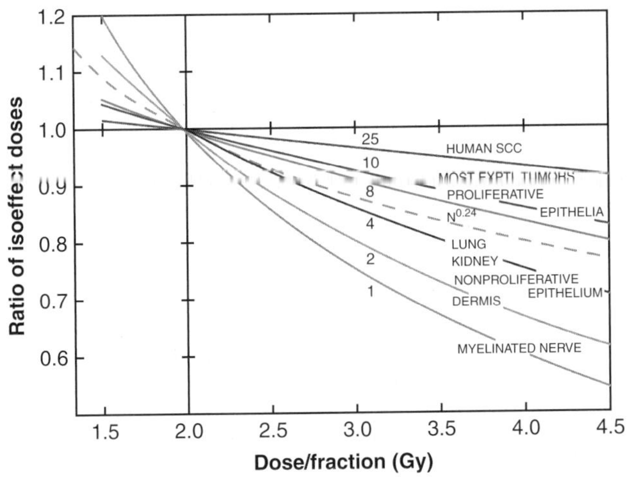

FIGURE 2.22. Isoeffect curves relating total dose to dose per fraction, with total dose being expressed as a ratio of that necessary in 2-Gy fractions (i.e., the $LQED_{2Gy}$). α/β ratios (in Gray) are shown on the curves. Although the α/β ratios are not yet established accurately or even precisely for most normal tissues, especially late-responding ones (Table 2.2), the likely order of fractionation sensitivities is as shown. The broken line traces the change in dose, as it would have been predicted by a factor $N^{0.24}$ in the NSD formula. Phenomena other than repair of sublethal injury, specifically repopulation, are not accounted for by these curves. (From Withers HR. Contrarian concepts in the progress of radiotherapy. *Radiat Res* 1989;119:395.)

early-responding tissues.[189] Regardless of the mechanism, late-responding tissues are spared more than acute-responding tissues by dose fractionation—that is, the dose for an isoeffect increases more rapidly in late-responding tissues as dose per fraction is reduced.

The slopes of the isoeffect curves in Figures 2.18 and 2.22 reflect the shape of the dose-survival or dose-function curves for responses in various tissues. Those in Figure 2.22 are constructed using the LQ formula (see later discussion) to correct the total dose (normalized to 1) to that which would be given if the dose per fraction were a standard 2 Gy. Shown for comparison is a plot based on the NSD formula[190] where the correction for time is ignored—that is, where $D = NSD \times N^{0.24}$.

In terms of the LQ cell survival model, late effects tissues have a low α/β ratio,[112,188,191] describing a curvier curve than that for acute-responding tissues (Fig. 2.13). Thus, low dose per fraction spares late- more than acute-responding tissues. Examples of α/β values for tissues are shown in Table 2.2.

Some specific clinical implications of the differences in fractionation response between acute- and late-responding tissues are as follows:

1. Large dose fractions are relatively more harmful for late-responding tissues. If two different fractionation regimens are used—one with large and the other with small doses per fraction—that achieve the same acute reactions, late responses will be more severe from the large dose per fraction regimen. This has been observed in many clinical studies.[112,165,192–194]
2. Because the therapeutic differential between late-responding tissues and acute-responding tumors increases with decreasing dose per fraction, a therapeutic gain should result from use of the smallest practical dose per fraction.[195] For example, if two fractions of 1.15 Gy achieve the same effect in a late-responding tissue as one fraction of 2 Gy yet two fractions of only 1.05 Gy achieve the same tumor control rate, the therapeutic gain would be 1.15/1.05 = 1.1. Thus, hyperfractionation using two fractions of 1.15 Gy to replace one fraction of 2 Gy would increase the biologically effective tumor dose by 10% with no increase in late complications, although acute-responding normal tissues will also receive an increased biologic dose.
3. To maximize the potential therapeutic gain from hyperfractionation, repair of SLD in late-responding tissues must be complete, implying fractionation intervals of at least 6 hours.[167,189] For the spinal cord, a longer interval seems needed.[80,189,196,197–198]
4. The relative biologic efficiency (RBE) for high LET radiations is greater at low doses than high doses for late effects because the sparing effect from fractionated x-ray doses is lost[188] (Fig. 2.13).

Linear Quadratic Formula for Calculating Isoeffect Relationships

It is possible to use the LQ response formula to change the size of dose per fraction (within limits)[165]:

$$D_{new}/D_{ref} = (\alpha/\beta + d_{ref})/(\alpha/\beta + d_{new}),$$

where D_{new} is the new total dose for a change in size of dose per fraction to d_{new}; D_{ref} is the previous total dose in fractions of d_{ref}; and α/β is for the tissue in question, all doses being expressed in Gray. For example, if d_{new} were 4 Gy and d_{ref} were 2 Gy, the ratio of total doses to achieve the same effects in a tissue with an α/β value of 2 Gy would be 0.66. For a tissue with an α/β value of 10 Gy, it would be 0.85. This calculation was used to derive the data in Figure 2.22.

The following caveats apply to this use of the LQ isoeffect formula:

1. The LQ response model does not apply equally well at all dose levels. It fits experimental data well over a limited dose range (e.g., 2 to 8 Gy); however, its validity and precision above[161] or below[199] that range is in doubt.
2. Using uncertain values for α/β ratios have more of an effect in late-responding tissues and carry more risk. There is little difference in isoeffect curves for different dose per fraction regimens delivered to tissues with α/β values of 10 Gy or more, whereas the difference is much larger for tissues with α/β values of 1 and 2 Gy (Fig. 2.22).
3. Dose corrections are most affected at low doses per fraction, where the LQ response model is poorly validated. Using the isoeffect formula presented earlier, or the curves in Figure 2.22, compare the ratios of isoeffect doses for a tissue characterized by an α/β value of 2 Gy when the dose per fraction is changed from 2 to 1 Gy (a 33% increase) and from 2 to 3 Gy (a 20% decrease).
4. The basic LQ model has no time parameter. This is not so important for late-responding tissues that turnover slowly as it is for tumors and acute-responding tissues. Factors can be added for incomplete repair, reoxygenation, and redistribution[184] and to account for the time to initiation of proliferation (kickoff time) and the impact of proliferation on overall response,[200] although the values are uncertain.

For these reasons, the LQ formula or curve should be used cautiously.

Influence of Regeneration (Repopulation)

Normal Tissues

The influence of overall duration of therapy on fractionation responses comes largely from large differences in the time of onset and kinetics of regeneration (repopulation) among various normal and neoplastic tissues (Fig. 2.3). This is why a constant exponent for overall treatment time in an isoeffect formula without regard to tissue type is a dangerous simplification with no biologic foundation. For example, early regeneration of intestinal mucosa or bone marrow makes a major contribution to the net response if a treatment regimen is spread out over several weeks, whereas it provides little or no benefit to spinal cord, kidney, or dermis. A constant exponent of <1 also implies a greater effect on isoeffect dose when values for T are small, whereas the major contribution of regeneration occurs when T values are large (e.g., 10 to 60 days).

Tumors

Such as with acute-responding normal tissues, tumors accelerate their growth in response to injury. Some clinical implications of tumor regeneration for curative RT are as follows:

1. Protracting treatment longer than necessary will likely be a disadvantage. For example, using 1.8 Gy rather than 2-Gy fractions given five times per week extends overall treatment time by about 10% and should be reserved for situations in which acute responses are likely to limit the rate of dose accumulation or where there may be substantial inhomogeneities in dose distribution. Inhomogeneity can lead to double trouble, with areas receiving a high total dose also receiving high doses per fraction. The increase in physical dose has an added biologic component that will compromise later-responding tissues (Fig. 2.23).
2. If a break in treatment is necessary because of acute toxicity, it should be kept as short as is tolerable.
3. Planned split-course therapy is inadvisable unless it is part of an accelerated treatment protocol that ultimately shortens the overall treatment duration (discussed later).
4. Breaks in therapy for nonmedical reasons (machine breakdown, holidays) may merit "catch-up" treatments in patients being treated for cure—for example, by treating twice on some remaining day.
5. Obviously, rapidly growing tumors must be treated rapidly. However, it is reasonable to accelerate treatment of tumors with a high proliferative index, regardless of their growth rate, because they are likely to reduce their rate of cell loss and regenerate earlier and faster during treatment. In fact, treatment should never be unnecessarily protracted (consistent with other considerations), because it is difficult to predict the accelerated repopulation response of individual tumors.

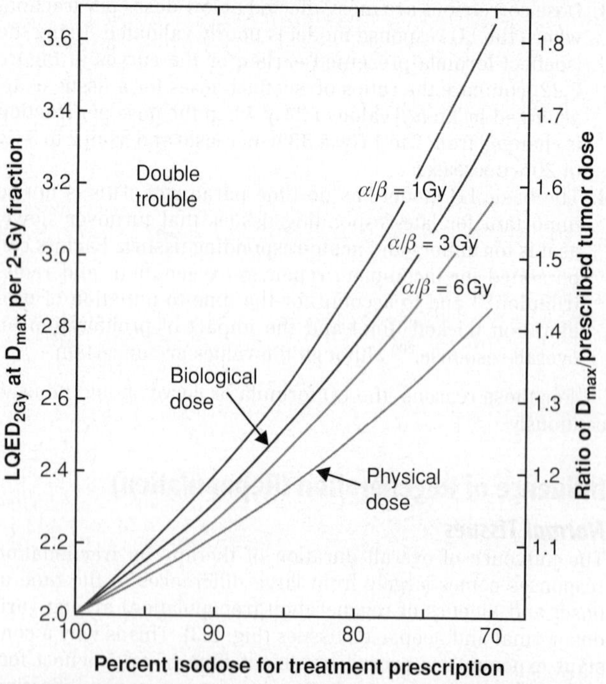

FIGURE 2.23. Influence of dose heterogeneity on physical and biologic doses as a function of the isodose line chosen for defining the tumor dose and of α/β ratio of the tissue located at D_{max}. The divergence of biologic and physical doses reflects the change in biologic dose that results from change in dose per fraction that derives from the heterogeneity of dose distribution. The lower the α/β ratio, the greater the divergence between biologic and physical doses. This "double trouble" is not reflected in physics isodose distributions and may explain not only a spurious volume effect but also may contribute to low values of tolerance doses that have appeared in the literature from time to time.

MODIFICATION OF DOSE FRACTIONATION PATTERNS

Standard RT regimens of about 2 Gy per day 5 days per week were developed empirically over the decades and serve as a good overall regimen for dose fractionation. However, it should be obvious that this may not be the best for all clinical situations and that it is certainly inappropriate in some (e.g., in obviously rapidly growing tumors[75,78,99]).

Some biologic factors relevant to modified dose fractionation are as follows:

1. Tissues differ in their response to multiple dose fractions (Figs. 2.14, 2.18, and 2.22) and tissue-related factors have to be taken into account.
2. Acute-responding normal tissues have an enormous capacity for repopulation (Fig. 2.3).
3. Tumors can show accelerated repopulation (Figs. 2.5, 2.6, and 2.7). Although there is probably great variability from tumor to tumor, on average, the lag time before its onset is longer and its rate slower than for acute-responding normal tissues.
4. Cell cycle redistribution to asynchrony between dose fractions produces a net sensitization in proliferative tissues but not in nonproliferative, late-responding tissues.
5. Hypoxia affects tumor responses to a lesser extent at low doses; however, the kinetics of reoxygenation are probably rapid in relation to the duration of most RT regimens, and it may be a factor only if single or a few large doses are used.
6. Slow-responding tissues "repair" better than acute-responding tissues.
7. Repopulation in normal tissues, and possibly in tumors, may occur rapidly during any treatment break.
8. The lag time to the onset of repopulation may be shortened to a limited extent by causing injury faster—for example, by increasing dose intensity or by concomitant chemotherapy.
9. Some tumors behave similar to late-responding tissues and have a low α/β ratio and proliferate slowly.
10. True "stem" cells and CSCs may be relatively quiescent and have different characteristics from the bulk of the normal tissue and tumor. For example, hematopoietic stem cells have a low α/β ratio[201] even though most bone marrow responses including lethality have a high α/β ratio. As a result, the target population for an end point has to be carefully considered.

Hypofractionation

Many clinical and experimental animal studies have shown that increasing the size of dose fractions increases the severity of late responses in relation to acute responses. Classically trained radiation oncologists typically associate high dose fractions with increased vascular injury and chronic inflammation, and fear severe late effects that can drastically affect patient quality of life and even be deadly. However, there are advantages in hypofractionation that may outweigh the biologic disadvantages in some circumstances, although these should be carefully evaluated in advance of treatment.

Logistic considerations have driven attempts to hypofractionate since the early days of RT, with little success outside of palliation. These are still important today. The advances in physics, particularly those related to the use of IMRT to minimize the dose to normal tissues and reduce tumor margins, along with CT scanning and gating techniques for precision positioning and to account for body motion, make compelling arguments for revisiting hypofractionation for certain conditions. From the radiobiologic perspective, if the fractionation response of the tumor is similar to that of late-responding normal tissues, increasing the size of dose fractions (hypofractionation) should not provide much of a therapeutic disadvantage, and decreasing the overall treatment time may help counter accelerated tumor repopulation, although this would not be expected in tumors with low α/β ratios; therefore, these advantages are mutually exclusive. Disadvantages include an increased risk of geographic miss and "cold spots" that will be discussed later. In addition, it is an oversimplification to state that any tissue or tumor has an α/β ratio. Every tissue contains multiple structures and different cell types, each with their own response to changing size of dose fractions. Using IMRT to minimize dose to critical normal tissue structures that could be affected by high dose fractions or accelerated treatment may be critical for successful hypofractionated treatments.

The use of single and high dose fractions has had some clinical success, outside of the phase III clinical trials that tested modestly accelerated RT in head and neck SCC in the 1970s,[202] which will be discussed later. Leksell[203] introduced sterotactic radiosurgery in the late 1960s at the Karolinska Institute to treat inaccessible cerebral lesions and in particular small arteriovenous malformations with single-dose treatments. This was followed by the use of linear accelerators to give single stereotactic radiosurgery doses or a small number of fractions as stereotactic radiotherapy (SRT), and these have proved clinically effective in treating a variety of benign and malignant brain diseases.[204] SRT has been extended to extracranial sites in the form of SBRT and its extension, stereotactic ablative radiotherapy (SABR), which uses a small number of high dose fractions, such as three fractions of 15 to 20 Gy. Although SABR is relatively new, the finding that it dramatically improves outcome in medically inoperable early-stage non–small cell lung cancer patients[5,205] and in patients with liver and other metastases[18] has generated much interest in applying it more widely. These findings, together with reports of excellent outcomes from high dose rate afterloading brachytherapy,[206] have prompted a re-evaluation of how traditional radiobiologic attitudes apply to these new clinical procedures.[207]

Stereotactic delivery of IR with IMRT is practically required for hypofractionation because it allows dose to a target to be chosen and delivered with a steep falloff to surrounding normal tissues. Tumor margins can be decreased so that less normal tissue receives high radiation doses, although the integral dose to the rest of the body is generally greater.[208] This contrasts with the homogeneous fields that tend to be used in more classical treatments. Relatively nonhomogeneous dose distributions result from IMRT, although this may be positively exploited by generating "hot spots" within targets where they are thought of most value (dose painting), although this currently has more theoretical value than practical application.

The dose falloff and inhomogeneity may have a biologic advantage in generating gradients of cytokines and chemokines that spatially organize infiltrating cells. The more-focused beam and sharp dose falloff may generate more "danger" signals for tumor immunity and more abscopal effects, which could assist in combating micrometastatic disease.[29,72,209,210] In fact, the preliminary data suggest that high single doses of ablative RT may not be optimal for the generation tumor-specific immunity and that moderately high hypofractionated doses may be superior in this respect[72] [Schaue, in press, 2011]. Proof of this would require clinical studies to be performed with different radiation protocols. Another possible advantage of high dose fractions or single radiation doses may be that they are more cytotoxic for microvasculature than 2 Gy, as was suggested by Fuks and Kolesnick,[24] although Tsai et al.[144] in murine prostate tumors showed that fractionated protocols can cause vascular loss not dissimilar to that of high single doses a few weeks after RT.

It is important to consider the aim of the hypofractionated therapy. Conventional RT aims to maintain normal tissue function. Hypofractionation can be applied in situations where there is no advantage to be gained from conventional fractionation; however, the aim should be the same, and it must be remembered that acute toxicity may be increased and tumor cure compromised by less reoxygenation. It may therefore be best to limit fraction sizes to <6 Gy, total time to at least 1 week, and the total dose to that predicted by the LQ model to be safe. If there is a gain to be had by exploiting differences in α/β ratios between tumor and late-responding normal tissue, hypofractionation may be a mistake, even allowing for improved technology.

As an example, if we assume α/β ratios of 10 Gy and 3 Gy for tumor and critical late-responding normal tissue, respectively, and change a treatment of 66 Gy in 2-Gy fractions to a 4-Gy regimen, the isoeffective total dose for the late-responding tissue would be 0.71 of 70 Gy (49.7 Gy). However, to keep tumor control rate constant would require only 0.86 of 70 Gy (60.4 Gy). By giving 49.7 Gy, the tumor would be relatively underdosed, receiving only 83% (0.71/0.86) of the equivalent of 70 Gy in 2-Gy fractions. To maintain the biologic effect on the tumor, a total of 60.4 Gy should be given, and the biologic dose to the late-responding tissues would be 20% (0.86/0.71) too high. Obviously, the therapeutic ratio will be reduced regardless of whether the change in total dose was aimed at an isoeffect for late responses (49.7 Gy) or for isocontrol rate for the tumor (60.4 Gy).

SABR, by contrast, has a very different aim. Using the LQ formula, 3 × 20 Gy is equivalent to around 275 Gy in 2-Gy fractions to late-responding tissues with an α/β ratio of 3 Gy[207]; clearly, this is a dose that would not be given conventionally, and this calculation in part reflects the inappropriateness of using the LQ model above 7-Gy dose sizes. However, no calculation is needed to know that 3 × 20 Gy is an ablative regimen. SABR doses do appear to be well tolerated in the limited situations where they have been employed, with the caveat that there are not sufficient patients treated in this fashion to allow long-term effects to be properly assessed. As well, the radiobiologic underpinnings of this technique still have to be fully evaluated.

Under any circumstances, SABR will cause both vascular and parenchymal cell loss. Critical questions to be asked relate to the site irradiated and the volume involved and what can be tolerated. Radiobiologic advantages of high dose to a small volume may include allowing angiogenesis and stem cell migration from surrounding normal tissue to effect better normal tissue recovery and limit the development of normal tissue hypoxia. On the other hand, serially organized parenchymal structures such as nerves and bronchioles will be compromised more than structures where FSUs are organized in parallel, which is why SABR doses have to be moderated for tumors that are centrally located in the lung. In the lung, loss of peripheral tissue function in small areas is not clinically important because there is ample residual lung function. This is not the case for all tissues. Site and volume appear to be the main constraints that must be applied for ablative therapy, although the dose-volume relationships are not known for most sites, and it is unlikely that dose-volume histograms can be relied on for guidance.

Accelerated Treatment

Accelerated treatment may be defined as a shortening of the overall treatment duration without a comparable reduction in total dose. However, in practice, lower doses in fraction sizes >2 Gy are generally given (e.g., 50 to 55 Gy in 3 to 4 weeks), with the continuous hyperfractionated accelerated radiotherapy (CHART) regimen being an exception with 1.5 Gy three times per day, 7 days per week. The aim of accelerated treatment is to minimize tumor growth or regeneration during therapy. The importance of accelerated repopulation during tumor treatment can be visualized by thinking that two to three doublings of surviving clonogens should add about the same (four- to eightfold) increment in tumor cell burden as a one-step increase in T-stage. The difficulty is to avoid excess toxicity in acute-responding normal tissues by reducing the benefit normally derived from its repopulation. Using larger doses per fraction would accelerate treatment; however, this is not advised in curative therapy unless under specific circumstances, as discussed earlier. In practice, accelerated regimens should use conventional or even reduced doses per fraction given more frequently than usual (i.e., six or more times per week).

There are numerous ways to increase the intensity of dose accumulation from the "standard" of 2 Gy, five times per week (a regimen that is already accelerated 10% in relation to 1.8-Gy fractions):

1. *Multiple standard 2-Gy fractions per day:* This type of regimen has been given in a continuous course lasting <2 weeks with good local control rates but a high frequency of severe complications.[211]
2. *Relative hypofractionation:* About 50 Gy given in 15 fractions in 3 weeks or 20 fractions in 4 weeks[134,172] are standard in a number of centers.
3. *Concomitant boosting:* The boost dose to a reduced volume is given "concomitantly" with the treatment of the initial larger volume rather than as a sequel, as would be standard in a shrinking-field procedure.[103] The boost is given as a second dose in the 1 day, with an interfraction interval of at least 6 hours, on several days, preferably during the later part of treatment when normal tissue regeneration is in full progress.
4. *CHART:* With CHART, 51 to 54 Gy is given as 1.4- or 1.5-Gy fractions, three times daily at 6-hour intervals for 12 consecutive days.[80,197] In a large prospective, randomized CHART trial, tumor control rates were increased with acceptable acute morbidity. Some permanent sequelae (e.g., xerostomia, fibrosis) were reduced, although myelopathy was more likely when the spinal cord was treated three times per day.
5. *Split-course accelerated treatment:* Head and neck tumors were given about 38 Gy over about 10 days as two fractions of 1.6 Gy per day; after a break of 12 to 14 days, an additional 28 Gy (approximately) was delivered, with the total treatment lasting about 6 weeks.[47,104] The results were better than in historic controls.
6. *Brachytherapy:* This form of accelerated RT will be discussed separately.
7. *Other:* A meta-analysis of randomized trials treating mostly cancer of the oropharynx and larynx and comparing conventional RT with accelerated RT with or without total dose reduction showed increased survival benefit of 2% without dose reduction and 1.7% with dose reduction at 5 years ($p = 0.02$).[202]

Because of the lag time before its onset, accelerated tumor regrowth has its greatest effect late in a standard regimen. Therefore, even a 1-week shortening could be advantageous (Figs. 2.5 and 2.6). However, excessive shortening to less than the lag time (e.g., to <3 to 4 weeks in head and neck cancer) is unlikely to improve tumor control rates, especially if the total dose is reduced to maintain acceptable acute toxicity.

Patients most suited to accelerated regimens are those with tumors that are rapidly growing or have a high potential for rapid regrowth—for example, those with a high proliferative index or a high cell loss factor. It may become possible to predict which tumors will repopulate early and quickly.[80,82,84] One sign may be rapid regression. In principle, all tumors should be treated in an overall time that is as short as possible and consistent with acceptable acute morbidity; however, caution should be taken to avoid self-defeating reductions in total dose below standard levels and gaps in treatment because of severe acute toxicity that can be counterproductive.

Although modifying and individualizing fractionation patterns may improve the outcome for some patients, accelerated tumor growth, repopulation in acute-responding tissues, and differences in response between late-responding normal tissues and tumors have important implications for everyday conventional treatment.[79] For example, RT, at least for head and neck cancers, should not be completed on a Monday after a weekend break because this is a 3-day extension. Likewise, a course of curative therapy should not start on a Friday. In general, breaks in treatment (public holidays, patient demands, etc.) should be countered by delivering more than five fractions in at least one of the weeks of treatment without resorting to large fractions. Chemotherapy given over several weeks before the start of RT may also initiate accelerated repopulation and compromise the chance for local tumor control. Such neoadjuvant therapy might be more effective if given during or after RT, at a time when surviving tumor clonogens are actively proliferating. Obviously, treatment of metastases may affect these decisions.

Hyperfractionation

Hyperfractionation is defined as the use of smaller-than-standard doses per fraction. It can be achieved without extending the overall treatment duration by treating once a day for 6 or 7 days per week but is usually achieved by giving two fractions per day for 5 days per week. Its aim is to increase the therapeutic differential between late-responding normal tissues and acute-responding tumors. It does this primarily by exploiting differences in their response to dose fractionation, although historically it was introduced to exploit the self-sensitizing effect of cell cycle redistribution present in the tumor but absent in late-responding normal tissues. Another rationale is that the OER is lower at low doses. When two fractions are given per day, the interfraction interval should be as long as possible, although preferably not less than 6 hours, and longer if CNS tissue is involved because repair there may continue for more than 12 hours. Hyperfractionation may not be an advantage in the treatment of slowly proliferating tumors because, as with slowly proliferating normal tissues, their α/β ratio may be low.

Clinical evidence suggests that to achieve comparable toxicity in fibrovascular tissues, one fraction of 2 Gy per day should be replaced with two fractions of about 1.2 Gy. For comparison, the dose per fraction necessary for an isoeffect in acute-responding tissues (and most tumors) would be about 1.05 Gy. Assuming that the isoeffect dose for late-responding tissues was increased by 20% and that it was increased for tumor by only 5%, the therapeutic differential would be increased by $1.2/1.05 = 1.14$. Therefore, if two fractions of 1.2 Gy per day replaced one fraction of 2 Gy per day, the acute responses of normal tissues and cytotoxicity for tumors would be increased as if the dose had been increased by 14%, whereas late responses would be unaltered. Coincidentally, if the overall treatment time were unchanged, the "biologic" rate of treatment of the tumor and acute-responding normal tissues would also be accelerated by 14%. Hyperfractionation has improved tumor control rates but also increases acute toxicity. A meta-analysis of randomized trials treating mostly cancer of the oropharynx and larynx and comparing conventional RT with hyperfractionated radiotherapy with or without total dose reduction showed increased survival benefit of 8% at 5 years.

Low Dose Rate Irradiation

Low dose rate continuous irradiation has the same biologic advantages as hyperfractionation. Additionally:

1. Proliferative cells may be delayed in their progression through the division cycle,[123,138] in particular in late G2 phase. Such a skewed redistribution could self-sensitize proliferative tissues and tumors without affecting late-responding normal tissues.
2. The overall duration of therapy is shortened.
3. The high-dose regions near the radioactive sources have a high probability of being completely sterilized of tumor cells. However, when the logarithmic nature of cell killing

is considered, this is not as great an advantage as it may seem. For example, radiation "cautery" of 50% of the tumor cells represents a gain that is equivalent to about 2 to 2.5 Gy of a standard multifraction regimen.

4. The volume of normal tissue receiving a high dose is minimized. Not only is the total dose beyond the treatment volume lower, the dose rate is as well, boosting further the sparing of late-responding tissues. This can be considered an inverse double-trouble effect, or a double advantage.
5. Potential biologic disadvantages are the relatively rapid falloff in dose beyond the treatment volume and the unintentional "cold spots" resulting from seed misplacement or movement. These could decrease the probability of tumor eradication if the tumor lay beyond the specified minimum tumor isodose (geographic miss).

In contrast to low dose rate brachytherapy, the advantages of high dose rate, high dose per fraction brachytherapy come from improved logistics and staff protection, as well as because normal tissues can be tolerably displaced from the high-dose field. Its biologic disadvantages may be loss of therapeutic differential between late effects tissues and tumors, reduced influence of cell cycle redistribution and delay, and increased influence of tumor hypoxia.

Permanent implants of low dose rate radioisotopes with long half-lives (e.g., ^{125}I) also have radiobiologic disadvantages. Late-responding normal tissues may accumulate high doses, and if a set total dose is to be delivered over a relatively long time, the initial dose rate may have to be so low as to facilitate "escape" of CSCs. As with high dose rate brachytherapy, other considerations may overwhelm these radiobiologic disadvantages.

Optimal Dose Rate

A change in dose rate, even between relatively high dose rates such as 10 Gy per minute (600 Gy per hour) to 1 Gy per minute (60 Gy per hour), can affect the response of tissues by allowing more SLD repair. However, sparing of late-responding tissues is most pronounced with the lower dose rates that are more characteristic of brachytherapy, between about 10 and 0.1 Gy per hour. However, in acute-responding tissues, and presumably also in a proportion of tumors, repopulation may be more important than repair at very low dose rates.

In late-responding tissues, such as rat spinal cord and lung,[212] a large dose rate effect is seen with change from 4 to 2 Gy per hour. Technical factors in such experiments make investigation of lower dose rates difficult; however, if 2 Gy per hour data are compared with multifraction data, the potential for substantial sparing with a further decrease in dose rate below 2 Gy per hour is indicated.[189,198] Such a large sparing effect of the reduced dose rate is to be expected in late-responding tissues for the same reasons as hyperfractionation spares such tissues.

Low Dose Rate Total Body Irradiation

Because proliferative bone marrow populations and leukemia[206] cells are characterized by a high α/β ratio (Table 2.2), it is reasonable to prepare patients for bone marrow transplantation using either multiple small dose fractions or continuous low dose rate exposure. Between about 1 and 7 Gy per hour has been chosen for various continuous total body irradiation regimens, which is where biologic effectiveness changes rapidly and even lower dose rates may provide better therapeutic differential.[212,213] Because the time to deliver the dose at such low dose rates is so long, many transplant centers give multifraction exposures. In general, low doses per fraction and low dose rates provide the best therapeutic differentials, provided the overall treatment duration is kept short in relation to the growth rate of the leukemic and normal stem cells.

Spatial Dose Considerations

Geographic Underdosage of Tumor

The impact of geographic underdosage (cold spots) of areas within tumor on the TCP depends on the number of CSCs in that area and the extent of the underdosage. The likely decline in TCP can be modeled with the assumption that the CSCs are distributed uniformly throughout the clinical tumor volume and are of uniform radiosensitivity. This is unlikely to be correct; however, the exercise is still instructive. Each tumor can be regarded as being composed of a large number of "tumorlets," each receiving a specified, although variable, dose. The overall TCP can be estimated by summing the TCPs for all the tumorlets. As illustrated in Figure 2.24, this TCP will decrease more the greater the number of underdosed tumorlets (volume) and the larger the decrement in dose. Dose homogeneity and the radiosensitivity of the tumor clonogens will be important. (Note that physical dose inhomogeneities are amplified in "biologic" dose to an extent that will depend on the α/β ratio.)

Figure 2.24 traces the decline in TCP as a function of volume of tumor underdosed and the magnitude of the underdosage. The magnitude of the underdose is shown as multiples of D_{10}, the dose that would reduce the number of surviving clonogens to 10% of the initial number—about 7 Gy for a standard regimen of 2 Gy fractions. Thus, from Figure 2.24 it can be seen that a 7 Gy ($1 \times D_{10}$) underdosage to 10% of the tumor would reduce TCP from 90% to 83%, whereas a 14 Gy underdosage to only 5% of the tumor would reduce TCP from 90% to 55%. The extent of underdosage is more important than the volume underdosed.

Theoretical dose-volume histograms are presented in Figure 2.25. The smallest deviation from 100% dose to 100% tumor is outlined by a-e, showing 5% of the tumor being underdosed by about 5% ($0.5 \times D_{10}$). Underdosage by 10% ($1 \times D_{10}$), 15% ($1.5 \times D_{10}$), or 20% ($2 \times D_{10}$) in a 70-Gy regimen is shown by b-e, c-e, and d-e, respectively. The impact on TCP of the four levels of underdosage depicted by the dose-volume histograms in Figure 2.25 can be read from Figure 2.24. Assuming that 70 Gy in 2-Gy fractions yields a TCP of 90%, then the effect of underdosing 5% of the tumor by 5% ($0.5 \times D_{10}$), 10% ($1 \times D_{10}$), 15% ($1.5 \times D_{10}$), or 20% ($2 \times D_{10}$) would be a decline in TCP by 1%, 3.5%, 12.5%, and 35%, respectively (Fig. 2.24).

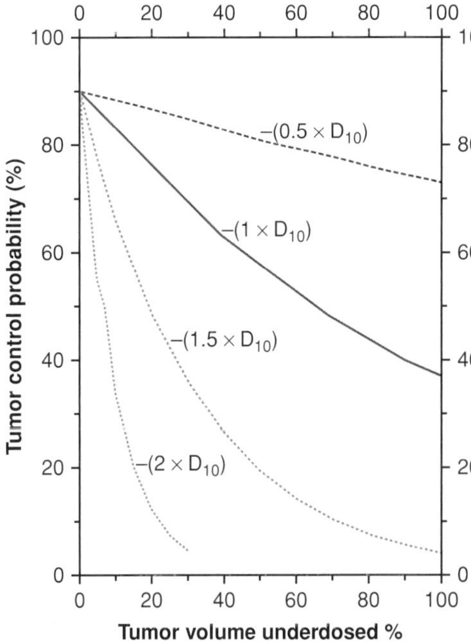

FIGURE 2.24. Effect of varying degrees of underdosage (in terms of D_{10} values) on tumor control probability (TCP) as a function of tumor volume underdosed. Note that the most important determinant is the magnitude of the underdosage.

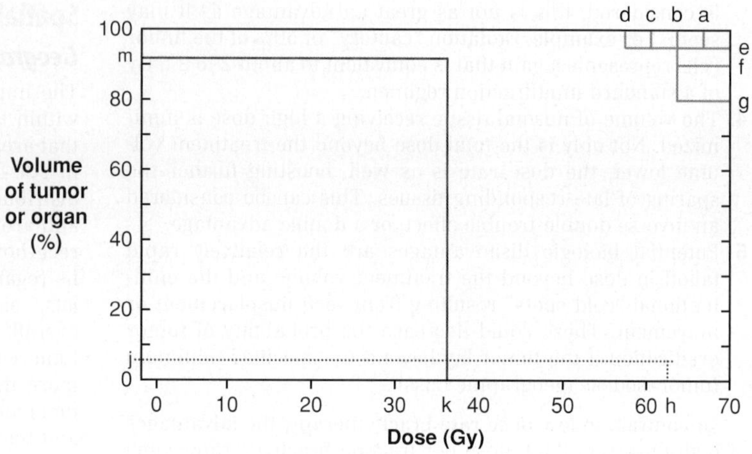

FIGURE 2.25. Multiple theoretical dose-volume histograms (DVH). By reference to Figure 2.24, the impact on TCP of indentations in the upper right corner of the DVH can be estimated (see text). The underdosage (a-e, b-e, c-e, d-e) is the most important determinant of TCP. The histogram h-j depicts a dangerous DVH for an organ with serially arranged FSUs such as spinal cord but benign for lung, liver, kidney, and so forth. Histogram k-m depicts danger for liver, lung, and kidney, although not for spinal cord.

It is obvious that most of the dose-volume histogram is irrelevant to TCP, but that small increments in the indentation along the x-axis in the upper right-hand corner may be critical, signifying that moderate to large reductions in dose to even small volumes are dangerous.

The dose-volume histograms b-e, b-f, and b-g in Figure 2.25 illustrate a 10% underdosage to 5%, 10%, and 20% of the tumor, respectively. From Figure 2.24, it can be seen that this 10% underdosage would decrease the calculated TCP by 3.5%, 7%, and 14%, respectively, much less of a loss than associated with the smaller indentations along the x-axis.

Clearly, the extent of underdosage is a more important determinant of TCP than the volume of tumor underdosed. Thus, the indentation along the x-axis of the upper right corner of the tumor dose-volume histogram in Figure 2.25 is more ominous than the indentation in the y-axis when considering TCP.

Geographic Overdosage of Tumor

Small areas of elevated dose, or hot spots (e.g., in ≤30% of the tumor) produce a negligible change in overall TCP, especially if the TCP from the homogeneous dose is already high (Fig. 2.26). Obviously, the larger the volume of tumor included in the overdosed region, the greater the potential for an increase in TCP, especially if the TCP from the homogeneously lower dose was already low (lower curves, Fig. 2.26). In general, raising the dose to the tumor by dose-painting subvolumes offers little advantage, whereas elevating the dose to the whole tumor could be of great value. For example, an escalation of dose to 30% of the tumor by 1 × D_{10} could raise the TCP from 10% to nearly 18%, whereas the same increment to the whole tumor could raise the TCP from 10% to 80%.

A significant advantage would only derive from introducing small hot spots in subvolumes within an otherwise homogeneous tumor dose distribution if the hot spots accurately targeted areas of substantially and consistently greater radioresistance (e.g., a nidus of hypoxic cells, or a CSC niche). A tumor with such a radioresistant nidus would not be cured by a relatively low homogeneous dose. At present, there are no proven ways of localizing tumor foci that are consistently radioresistant. Thus, with current levels of understanding and technical expertise, the largest and most certain benefits are likely to be achieved if the dose to the whole tumor is escalated. This is illustrated by the increasing slope of the curves in Figure 2.26 as the volume receiving the higher dose approaches 100%.

Effective Uniform Dose

The effects of inhomogeneous dose distribution on TCP can be quantified by the equivalent uniform dose (EUD).[214] An EUD produces a constant probability of tumor control for different volumes of tumor under- or overdosed. In Figures 2.24 and 2.26, a horizontal line for any chosen TCP would join EUDs for various volumes exposed to doses differing by various multiples of D_{10}, the relevant EUD value being the homogeneous dose that produced that TCP.

Dose-Volume Histograms for Normal Tissues

Heterogeneity of dose in the exposed volume will produce different levels of injury, although the net pathophysiologic outcome is dictated by the structure and function of the organ. An organ such as spinal cord with its FSUs arranged in series can be injured by a high dose to even a small volume (Fig. 2.25, h–j) but not by a low dose to a large volume (k-m). However, a large dose to a small volume (h-i) is of little consequence in an organ with a large "reserve" volume of FSUs. Conversely, a relatively low dose to a large volume (e.g., k-m), which may be of little consequence to spinal cord, could be devastating if applied to lung, liver, or kidney. Thus, dose-volume histogram configurations must be viewed against an understanding of the structure and physiology of the specific tissue, as discussed earlier.

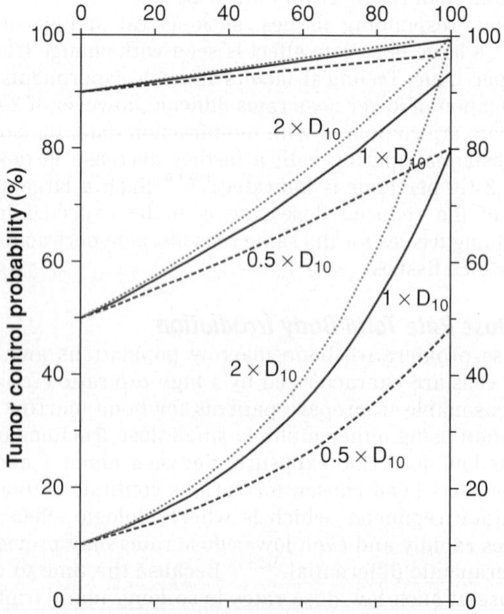

FIGURE 2.26. Modeling of the effect on tumor control probability (TCP) of increasing dose to increasing proportions of the tumor. Small hot spots are not very useful, especially if TCP is already high. The closer to 100% of the tumor being "overdosed," the steeper the TCP curve.

QUALITY OF RADIATION

Linear Energy Transfer

The rate at which a charged particle, such as an electron or proton, deposits its energy along its track is described as its LET; the heavier the particle, the higher its LET. Thus, electrons have a predominantly low LET, protons a slightly higher LET, neutrons an even higher LET, and heavily charged particles the highest LET of clinically used radiations.

The rate of energy transfer increases as particles slow, which means that LET is only an average value that is little more than a useful guide to the radiation therapist. As the LET of a beam increases, so does its biologic efficiency, although the increase is most rapid and peaks around 100 to 150 kv/μm. This is thought to represent where ionization events are spaced so that they are most likely to hit both strands of DNA. It then decreases per unit of measured physical dose with further increase in LET (an "overkill" phenomenon). As LET increases, OER decreases inversely with biologic effectiveness, and the impact of variations in cell cycle-related radiosensitivity become less.[113] At high LET, single-hit, nonrepairable cell killing increases relative to that from accumulation of sublethal injury; thus, the survival curve for neutrons or heavily charged particles is essentially linear over at least the first decade of cell killing, and there is little sparing from dose fractionation, reducing the differential in fractionation response between late-responding and acute-responding tissues.[188]

Relative Biologic Efficiency

RBE is a ratio of doses from two beams to produce the same effect:

RBE = dose (standard beam)/dose (test beam).

RBE is usually used to compare high and low LET radiations; however, it has wider applicability for comparing the effectiveness of treatment approaches such as high- and low dose rate x-irradiation. Initially, the standard photon beam was 250 kVp x-rays, but now, at least from the viewpoint of RT, it is ^{60}Co (250 kVp x-rays are about 15% more efficient than ^{60}Co in killing mammalian cells). It is not widely appreciated that even at relatively high dose rates, photon beam effectiveness varies with dose rate and also that this is an important determinant of RBE. Furthermore, it can only be measured accurately if the same effect is achieved by both radiations. The conditions of RBE measurements must, therefore, be explicitly and precisely stated.

Neutrons

Neutrons deposit energy in a tissue through collisions with nuclei (mainly of hydrogen) rather than with electrons, as occurs with photon beams. Although neutrons are uncharged, they eject protons from the nucleus; therefore, the cellular injury they produce is through free radicals formed from ion pairs—the same basic mechanism as that for x-rays. The difference is that the column of ionization produced by the proton ejected from the nucleus by the neutron is much denser than that produced by an electron ejected by a photon. Because of the density of resulting free radicals, neutrons are more likely than x-rays to cause irreparable single-lethal-hit injury to DNA.

The high density of ionization from neutron irradiation also results in a reduced OER. If the OER is 2.6 for x-rays and 1.6 for neutrons, the ratio, which has been called the *hypoxic gain factor,* would be 2.6/1.6 = 1.6. In other words, if a course of neutrons is given that produces normal tissue sequelae equivalent to those from 66 Gy of x-rays given in 2-Gy fractions, the biologic effect of the neutrons on a completely hypoxic tumor would be equivalent to that from (1.6 × 66 Gy) = 106 Gy of x-rays. Of course, not all tumor cells are hypoxic; thus, the therapeutic gain factor is lower than 1.6 and will depend on the percentage of hypoxic cells and, in a multifraction regimen, the extent of reoxygenation.[215]

The response of cells to neutrons is less influenced by position in the cell cycle than is the case with x-rays. Therefore, the RBE is greater for cells in x-ray–resistant than x-ray–sensitive phases of the cell cycle. This may affect the therapeutic gain or loss from using neutrons. For example, if a tumor were to consist entirely of cells in an x-ray–resistant phase of the cell cycle, for which the RBE were 5, and if the critical normal tissue were to have an RBE of 3, then the therapeutic gain factor would be 5/3 = 1.66.

Because single-hit nonrepairable events are greater with neutrons, cell survival rate is more nearly exponential over a wider dose range, and steeper, than for x-rays. In terms of the LQ survival curve formula, neutrons have a very high α/β value (e.g., 30 to 100 Gy). Therefore, dose fractionation is of less significance in neutron therapy than in x-ray RT.

Neutrons may have a therapeutic advantage for poorly reoxygenating, poorly redistributing, intrinsically x-ray–resistant, rapidly growing, and rapidly repopulating tumors. Predictive assays would be needed to identify such tumors prospectively, which would also permit more selective modification of x-ray regimens.[215]

ACKNOWLEDGMENTS

Jan Haas and Natalia Mackenzie helped in the preparation of this manuscript.

SELECTED REFERENCES

A full list of references for this chapter is available online.

1. Alper T, Howard-Flanders P. Role of oxygen in modifying the radiosensitivity of E. coli B. *Nature* 1956;178:978.
3. Banuelos CA, Banath JP, Kim JY, et al. GammaH2AX expression in tumors exposed to cisplatin and fractionated irradiation. *Clin Cancer Res* 2009;15:3344.
4. Puck TT, Marcus PI. Action of x-rays on mammalian cells. *J Exp Med* 1956;103:653.
6. Dewey WC, Ling CC Meyn RE. Radiation-induced apoptosis: relevance to radiotherapy. *Int J Radiat Oncol Biol Phys* 1995;33:781.
7. Kerr JF, Wyllie AH, Currie AR. Apoptosis: a basic biological phenomenon with wide-ranging implications in tissue kinetics. *Br J Cancer* 1972;26:239.
10. Kemp CJ, Sun S, Gurley KE. p53 induction and apoptosis in response to radio- and chemotherapy in vivo is tumor-type-dependent. *Cancer Res* 2001;61:327.
11. Hallahan DE, Haimovitz-Friedman A, Kufe DW, et al. The role of cytokines in radiation oncology. In: DeVita VT, Hellman S, Rosenberg SA, eds. *Important advances in oncology.* Philadelphia: Lippincott, 1993:71–80.
15. Rodemann HP, Binder A, Burger A, et al. The underlying cellular mechanism of fibrosis. *Kidney Int Suppl* 1996;54:S32.
18. Kavanagh BD, Schefter TE, Cardenes HR, et al. Interim analysis of a prospective phase I/II trial of SBRT for liver metastases. *Acta Oncologica* 2006;45:848.
19. Potten CS, Merritt A, Hickman J, et al. Characterization of radiation-induced apoptosis in the small intestine and its biological implications. *Int J Radiat Biol* 1994;65:71.
23. Stephens LC, Ang KK, Schultheiss TE, et al. Target cell and mode of radiation injury in rhesus salivary glands. *Radiother Oncol* 1986;7:165.
24. Fuks Z, Kolesnick R. Engaging the vascular component of the tumor response. *Cancer Cell* 2005;8:89.
26. Rotolo JA, Kolesnick R, Fuks Z. Timing of lethality from gastrointestinal syndrome in mice revisited. *Int J Radiat Oncol Biol Phys* 2009;73:6.
28. McBride WH, Chiang C-S, Olson JL, et al. A sense of danger from radiation. *Radiat Res* 2004;162:1.
29. Schaue D, McBride WH. Links between innate immunity and normal tissue radiobiology. *Radiat Res* 2010;173:406.
31. Hong JH, Chiang CS, Tsao CY, et al. Rapid induction of cytokine gene expression in the lung after single and fractionated doses of radiation. *Int J Radiat Oncol* 1999;75:1421.
32. Demaria S, Bhardwaj N, McBride WH, et al. Combining radiotherapy and immunotherapy: a revived partnership. *Int J Radiat Oncol Biol Phys* 2005;63:655.
33. Formenti SC, Demaria S. Systemic effects of local radiotherapy. *Lancet Oncol* 2009;10:718.
38. Chiang CS, Hong JH, Stalder A, et al. Delayed molecular responses to brain irradiation. *Int J Radiat Biol* 1997,72.45.
40. Anscher MS. Targeting the TGF-beta1 pathway to prevent normal tissue injury after cancer therapy. *Oncologist* 2010;15:350.
43. Withers HR, Mason KA, Thames HD Jr. Late radiation response of kidney assayed by tubule-cell survival. *Br J Radiol* 1986;59:587.
45. Withers HR. Recovery and repopulation in vivo by mouse skin epithelial cells during fractionated irradiation. *Radiat Res* 1967;32:227.
49. Neta R. Modulation of radiation damage by cytokines. *Stem Cells* 1997;15(Suppl 2): 87.
51. Farrell CL, Bready JV, Rex KL, et al. Keratinocyte growth factor protects mice from chemotherapy and radiation-induced gastrointestinal injury and mortality. *Cancer Res* 1998;58:933.
54. Mason KA, Withers HR, Chiang CS. Late effects of radiation on the lumbar spinal cord of guinea pigs: re-treatment tolerance. *Int J Radiat Oncol Biol Phys* 1993;26:643.
55. Landuyt W, Fowler J, Ruifrok A, et al. Kinetics of repair in the spinal cord of the rat. *Radiother Oncol* 1997;45:55.

56. Ang KK, Jiang GL, Feng Y, et al. Extent and kinetics of recovery of occult spinal cord injury. *Int J Radiat Oncol Biol Phys* 2001;50:1013.
57. Stewart FA, Oussoren Y, Van Tinteren H, et al. Loss of reirradiation tolerance in the kidney with increasing time after single or fractionated partial tolerance doses. *Int J Radiat Biol* 1994;66:169.
58. Withers HR. The 4Rs of radiotherapy. In: Lett JT, Adler H, eds. *Advances in radiation biology,* vol. 5. New York: Academic Press, 1975:241.
59. Malaise EP, Fertil B, Chavaudra N, et al. Distribution of radiation sensitivities for human tumor cells of specific histological types: comparison of in vitro to in vivo data. *Int J Radiat Oncol Biol Phys* 1986;12:617.
61. Lim E, Vaillant F, Wu D, et al. Aberrant luminal progenitors as the candidate target population for basal tumor development in BRCA1 mutation carriers. *Nat Med* 2009;15:907.
62. Pajonk F, Vlashi E, McBride WH. Radiation resistance of cancer stem cells: the 4 R's of radiobiology revisited. *Stem Cells* 2010;28:639.
63. Nichols AC, Faquin WC, Westra WH, et al. HPV-16 infection predicts treatment outcome in oropharyngeal squamous cell carcinoma. *Otolaryngol Head Neck Surg* 2009;140:228.
65. Meyn RE, Stephens LC, Hunter NR, et al. Reemergence of apoptotic cells between fractionated doses in irradiated murine tumors. *Int J Radiat Oncol Biol Phys* 1994;30:619.
66. McBride WH, Dougherty GJ. Radiotherapy for genes that cause cancer. *Nat Med* 1995;1:1215.
68. Thames HD, Bentzen SM, Turesson I, et al. Time-dose factors in radiotherapy: a review of the human data. *Radiother Oncol* 1990;19:219.
69. Brenner DJ, Hall EJ. Fractionation and protraction for radiotherapy of prostate carcinoma. *Int J Radiat Oncol Biol Phys* 1999;43:1095.
70. Bentzen SM, Agrawal RK, Aird EG, et al. The UK Standardisation of Breast Radiotherapy (START) Trial A of radiotherapy hypofractionation for treatment of early breast cancer: a randomised trial. *Lancet* 2008;9:331.
72. Dewan MZ, Galloway AE, Kawashima N, et al. Fractionated but not single-dose radiotherapy induces an immune-mediated abscopal effect when combined with anti-CTLA-4 antibody. *Clin Cancer Res* 2009;15:5379.
80. Dische S, Saunders MI. Continuous, hyperfractionated, accelerated radiotherapy (CHART). *Br J Cancer* 1989;59:325.
87. Hermens AF, Barendsen GW. Changes of cell proliferation characteristics in a rat rhabdomyosarcoma before and after x-irradiation. *Eur J Cancer* 1969;5:173.
95. Maciejewski B, Withers HR, Taylor JM, et al. Dose fractionation and regeneration in radiotherapy for cancer of the oral cavity and oropharynx: tumor dose-response and repopulation. *Int J Radiat Oncol Biol Phys* 1989;16:831.
103. Knee R, Fields RS, Peters LJ. Concomitant boost radiotherapy for advanced squamous cell carcinoma of the head and neck. *Radiother Oncol* 1985;4:1.
105. King C. Stereotactic body radiotherapy for prostate cancer: current results of a phase II trial. *Front Radiat Ther Oncol* 2011;43:428.
106. Hryniuk W. Will increases in dose intensity improve outcome. *Proc Am J Med* 1995;99:69S.
108. Kim JJ, Tannock IF. Repopulation of cancer cells during therapy: an important cause of treatment failure. *Nat Rev Cancer* 2005;5:516.
109. Terasima T, Tolmach LJ. Changes in the x-ray sensitivity of HeLa cells during the division cycle. *Nature* 1961;190:1210.
110. Elkind MM, Sutton H. X-ray damage and recovery in mammalian cells in culture. *Nature* 1959;184:1293.
111. Withers HR. Cell cycle redistribution as a factor in multifraction irradiation. *Radiology* 1975;114:199.
112. Thames HD Jr, Withers HR, Peters LJ, et al. Changes in early and late radiation responses with altered dose fractionation: implications for dose-survival relationships. *Int J Radiat Oncol Biol Phys* 1982;8:219.
114. Calabrese C, Poppleton H, Kocak M, et al. A perivascular niche for brain tumor stem cells. *Cancer Cell* 2007;11:69.
115. Gilbertson RJ, Rich JN. Making a tumour's bed: glioblastoma stem cells and the vascular niche. *Nat Rev Cancer* 2007;7:733.
116. Vlashi E, Kim K, Lagadec C, et al. In vivo imaging, tracking, and targeting of cancer stem cells. *J Natl Cancer Inst* 2009;101:350.
121. Deschner EE, Gray LH. Influence of oxygen tension on x-ray-induced chromosomal damage in Ehrlich ascites tumor cells irradiated in vitro and in vivo. *Radiat Res* 1959;11:115.
123. Hall EJ. Radiation dose-rate: a factor of importance in radiobiology and radiotherapy. *Br J Radiol* 1972;45:81.
124. Brown JM, Giaccia AJ. Tumour hypoxia: the picture has changed in the 1990s. *Int J Radiat Biol* 1994;65:95.
125. Jain RK. Barriers to drug delivery in solid tumors. *Sci Am* 1994;271:58.
126. Vaupel P, Schlenger K, Hoeckel M. Blood flow and tissue oxygenation of human tumors: an update. *Adv Exp Med Biol* 1992;317:139.
129. Powers WE, Tolmach LJ. A multicomponent x-ray survival curve for mouse lymphosarcoma cells irradiated in vivo. *Nature* 1963;197:710.
130. Olive PL. DNA damage and repair in individual cells: applications of the comet assay in radiobiology. *Int J Radiat Biol* 1999;75:395.
134. Henk JM, Kunkler PB, Smith CW. Radiotherapy and hyperbaric oxygen in head and neck cancer. Final report of first controlled clinical trial. *Lancet* 1977;2:101.
136. Henke M, Laszig R, Rube C, et al. Erythropoietin to treat head and neck cancer patients with anaemia undergoing radiotherapy: randomised, double-blind, placebo-controlled trial. *Lancet* 2003;362:1255.
137. Phillips TM, Kim K, Vlashi E, et al. Effects of recombinant erythropoietin on breast cancer-initiating cells. *Neoplasia* 2007;9:1122.
139. Hockel M, Schlenger K, Hockel S, et al. Hypoxic cervical cancers with low apoptotic index are highly aggressive. *Cancer Res* 1999;59:4525.
140. Graeber TG, Osmanian C, Jacks T, et al. Hypoxia-mediated selection of cells with diminished apoptotic potential in solid tumours. *Nature* 1996;379:88.
141. Chen FH, Chiang CS, Wang CC, et al. Radiotherapy decreases vascular density and causes hypoxia with macrophage aggregation in TRAMP-C1 prostate tumors. *Clin Cancer Res* 2009;15:1721.
142. Milas L. Tumor bed effect in murine tumors: relationship to tumor take and tumor macrophage content. *Radiat Res* 1990;123:232.
143. Ahn GO, Tseng D, Liao CH, et al. Inhibition of Mac-1 (CD11b/CD18) enhances tumor response to radiation by reducing myeloid cell recruitment. *Proc Natl Acad Sci U S A.* 2010;107:8363.
144. Tsai CS, Chen FH, Wang CC, et al. Macrophages from irradiated tumors express higher levels of iNOS, arginase-I and COX-2, and promote tumor growth. *Int J Radiat Oncol Biol Phys* 2007;68:499.
145. Ten Hagen TL, Eggermont AM. Changing the pathophysiology of solid tumours: the potential of TNF and other vasoactive agents. *Int J Hyperthermia* 2006;22:241.
146. Chan N, Koritzinsky M, Zhao H, et al. Chronic hypoxia decreases synthesis of homologous recombination proteins to offset chemoresistance and radioresistance. *Cancer Res* 2008;68:605.
148. Lyng H, Sundfor K, Rofstad EK. Changes in tumor oxygen tension during radiotherapy of uterine cervical cancer: relationships to changes in vascular density, cell density, and frequency of mitosis and apoptosis. *Int J Radiat Oncol Biol Phys* 2000;46:935.
150. Catcheside DG, Lea DE, Thoday JM. Types of chromosome structural change induced by the irradiation of Tradescantia microspores. *J Genet* 1946;47:113.
152. Joiner MC, Marples B, Lambin P, et al. Low-dose hypersensitivity: current status and possible mechanisms. *Int J Radiat Oncol Biol Phys* 2001;49:379.
153. Baverstock K. Radiation-induced genomic instability: a paradigm-breaking phenomenon and its relevance to environmentally induced cancer. *Mutat Res* 2000;454:89.
154. Little JB. Repair of potentially-lethal radiation damage in mammalian cells: enhancement by conditioned medium from stationary cultures. *Int J Radiat Biol Relat Stud Phys Chem Med* 1971;20:87.
155. Mothersill C, Seymour C. Radiation-induced bystander effects: past history and future directions. *Radiat Res* 2001;155:759.
156. Read J. The effect of ionizing irradiations on the broad bean root: X. The dependence on the x-ray sensitivity of dissolved oxygen. *Br J Radiol* 1952;25:89.
160. Douglas BG, Fowler JF. The effect of multiple small doses of x rays on skin reactions in the mouse and a basic interpretation. *Radiat Res* 1976; 66:401.
161. McBride WH, Schaue D. Radiation biology of SBRT: Is there a new biology involved? In: Ahmed MM, Pollack A, eds. *Hypofractionation. Scientific concepts and clinical experiences.* Ellicott City, MD: LumiText, 2011:3.
162. Brenner DJ. The linear-quadratic model is an appropriate methodology for determining isoeffective doses at large doses per fraction. *Semin Radiat Oncol* 2008; 18:234.
178. Withers HR, Peters LJ, Taylor JM. Dose-response relationship for radiation therapy of subclinical disease. *Int J Radiat Oncol Biol Phys* 1995;31:353.
179. Strandquist M. A study of the cumulative effects of fractionated x-ray treatment based on the experience at the Radiumhemmet with the treatment of 280 cases of carcinoma of the skin and lip. *Acta Radiol* 1944;55(Suppl):300.
184. Brenner DJ, Hlatky LR, Hahnfeldt PJ, et al. A convenient extension of the linear-quadratic model to include redistribution and reoxygenation. *Int J Radiat Oncol Biol Phys* 1995;32:379.
190. Ellis F. Nominal standard dose and the ret. *Br J Radiol* 1971;44:101.
196. Ang KK, Price RE, Stephens LC, et al. The tolerance of primate spinal cord to re-irradiation. *Int J Radiat Oncol Biol Phys* 1993;25:459.
197. Saunders MI, Dische S, Grosch EJ, et al. Experience with CHART. *Int J Radiat Oncol Biol Phys* 1991;21:871.
200. Fowler JF. The eighteenth Douglas Lea lecture. 40 years of radiobiology: its impact on radiotherapy. *Phys Med Biol* 1984;29:97.
201. Down JD, Boudewijn A, van Os R, et al. Variations in radiation sensitivity and repair among different hematopoietic stem cell subsets following fractionated irradiation. *Blood* 1995;86:122.
202. Bourhis J, Overgaard J, Audry H, et al. Hyperfractionated or accelerated radiotherapy in head and neck cancer: a meta-analysis. *Lancet* 2006;368:843.
203. Leksell L. Stereotactic radiosurgery. *J Neurol Neurosurg Psych* 1983;46:797.
204. Hazard LJ, Jensen RL, Shrieve DC. Role of stereotactic radiosurgery in the treatment of brain metastases. *Am J Clin Oncol* 2005;28:403.
205. Fakiris AJ, McGarry RC, Yiannoutsos CT, et al. Stereotactic body radiation therapy for early-stage non-small-cell lung carcinoma: four-year results of a prospective phase II study. *Int J Radiat Oncol Biol Phys* 2009;75:677.
206. Martinez AA, Demanes J, Vargas C, et al. High-dose-rate prostate brachytherapy: an excellent accelerated-hypofractionated treatment for favorable prostate cancer. *Am J Clin Oncol* 2010;33:481.
207. Fowler JF, Tome WA, Fenwick JD, et al. A challenge to traditional radiation oncology. *Int J Radiat Oncol Biol Phys* 2004;60:1241.
214. Niemierko A. Reporting and analyzing dose distributions: a concept of equivalent uniform dose. *Med Phys* 1997;24:103.

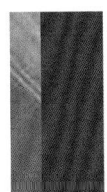

Chapter 3 Molecular Cancer and Radiation Biology

Michael Baumann, Nils Cordes, Mechthild Krause, and Daniel Zips

During the last three decades molecular cancer research has become a rapidly growing branch of the biomedical sciences. Many advances in our understanding of cancer are closely related to innovations in biotechnology—for example, techniques to knock out or to knock in a specific gene of interest, experimental maneuvers to manipulate temporal and spatial gene expression, the development of high-throughput methods to study the entire genome and proteome of cancer cells, and a vastly growing methodology to specifically interfere with signal transduction. This chapter provides an introductory overview of molecular cancer and radiation biology.

Cell biology approaches contribute to modern radiobiology and help to better understand effects of ionizing radiation on cells, tumors, and normal tissues. Knowledge in molecular cancer biology is important for clinical decision making in oncology and the development of novel biology-driven strategies in the multidisciplinary clinical environment.[1,2] *Molecular pathology* of tumors increasingly supplements classic histopathology and immunohistochemistry, thereby providing the basis for improved treatment stratification in oncology.[3,4] *Molecular pathophysiology* describes mechanisms leading to a characteristic microenvironment of tumors or the mechanisms that eventually lead to the manifestation of radiation sequelae in normal tissues.[5] *Molecular imaging* has become important not only for staging but also for biologic characterization of tumors and for determination of target volumes in radiation oncology, including new approaches such as dose painting.[6–8] *Molecular targeting* in radiotherapy may either increase the tumor response or protect normal tissues, thereby enhancing the therapeutic gain of the treatment.[9–10,11]

Compared to other fields of oncology, radiotherapy appears to be particularly promising to integrate molecular targeting approaches.[11] First, the radiobiologic mechanisms of the response of tumors and normal tissues to radiotherapy are well characterized, and the molecular pathways involved in these responses are increasingly known. Second, similar to conventional chemotherapeutic drugs, the novel drugs developed so far are not curative in themselves. In contrast, radiotherapy in itself is extremely efficient in eradicating cancer stem cells, and recurrences often occur from only one or a few surviving cancer stem cells.[12,13–14] Thus, even if novel drugs have only the potential to kill a limited number of cancer stem cells, this might be sufficient to increase local control when combined with radiotherapy. The same argument applies when these drugs increase the radiosensitivity of tumor cells or when normal tissues are specifically protected. Third, in contrast to systemic chemotherapy, radiotherapy can be modulated in dose, time, and space. This allows individual tailoring of the effects of combined treatments in consideration of the spatial distribution of cancer stem cell burden as well as with consideration of normal tissues. Preclinical data and early clinical results corroborate these arguments[15–19] and support further translational research on biologically enhanced radiotherapy.

PRINCIPLES OF MOLECULAR CANCER BIOLOGY

The majority of human cancers arise from single somatic cells as a result of a stepwise evolutionary process of accumulation of multiple genetic and epigenetic aberrations.[20] Genetic changes include point mutation, deletion, insertion, gene amplification, chromosomal instability, loss of heterozygosity, and translocation. Silencing of tumor suppressor genes by promoter hypermethylation, histone modifications, and microRNA (noncoding RNA) expression represents important epigenetic mechanisms of tumorigenesis.[21,22] Infection with oncogenic viruses might contribute to the development of human cancer, for example, human papilloma viruses in cervical or head and neck cancer, hepatitis B viruses in hepatocellular carcinoma, and human immunodeficiency viruses in Kaposi's sarcoma.[23,24] The hostile micromilieu in solid tumors, particularly hypoxia, further promotes progressive genomic alterations and clonal selection.[25] Consequently, cells gain advantage in proliferation and survival, which eventually results in malignant transformation, a prerequisite for the development of cancer and metastatic spread.

Conceptually, two classes of cancer genes can be distinguished. First, *oncogenes* are activated in cancer cells by genetic alterations resulting in a gain of function. Mutations in proto-oncogenes acting in a dominant fashion (i.e., a genetic alteration in one of the alleles) are sufficient for gene activation. Typical oncogene functions are stimulation of cell proliferation (e.g., by activation of Ras) and increase in cell survival (e.g., by activation of PI3K/Akt signaling). Disorders in the second class of cancer genes, *tumor suppressor genes,* cause a loss of function. Mutations in one allele of a tumor suppressor gene are recessive because they can be functionally compensated by the second, nonmutated (wild-type) allele. While some cancers can be attributed to single genetic alterations, most sporadic solid tumors exhibit a wide range of disorders in numerous cancer genes. Simplified mathematical modeling of the increasing incidence of common cancers as a function of age suggests that four to seven somatic gene alterations are required for carcinogenesis.[20,26] A typical example for multistep tumorigenesis is the adenoma–carcinoma sequence in colorectal cancer.[27]

Inherited cancer predisposition can be divided into the rare group of inherited cancer syndromes and familial cancers (strong predisposition) and the more frequent group of predisposition without evident family clustering (weak predisposition).[28] The first group includes syndromes caused by germline mutations affecting DNA repair, genomic stability, and cell cycle control, for example, *TP53* (Li–Fraumeni syndrome), nucleotide excision repair genes (xeroderma pigmentosum), *ATM* (ataxia telangiectasia), DNA mismatch repair genes (hereditary nonpolyposis colorectal cancer), and *BRCA 1/2* (familial breast cancer). An example of a familial cancer syndrome related to oncogene activation is neurofibromatosis type I, in which the mutated *NF1* gene results in activation of the Ras oncogene.[28] Germline mutations causing inactivation of the cell–cell adhesion molecule E-cadherin can be found, for example, in familial diffuse gastric carcinoma.[29]

The essential molecular biology of cancer can be summarized by a simplified concept based on a small number of underlying principles. In their seminal articles, Hanahan and Weinberg[30,31] described these principles shared by most human tumor types as the "*six hallmarks of cancer*" (Table 3.1). These six hallmarks are the consequence of specific genetic alterations in important oncogenes and tumor suppressor genes.

The Hallmarks of Cancer

Cancer is characterized by the loss of growth control due to acquired capabilities of autonomy of growth signaling,

TABLE 3.1 THE SIX HALLMARKS OF CANCER WITH INVOLVED ONCOGENIC AND TUMOR-SUPPRESSIVE MOLECULES (SELECTION)

Hallmark	*Involved Oncogenic and Tumor-Suppressive Molecules (Selection)*
Loss of growth control	
1. Self-sufficiency in growth signals	p53, TGF-β, RTKs, Ras, pRB, cyclin D, cdk4, p16/ARF, p27, Akt, PTEN, cytokine
2. Insensitivity to antigrowth signals	Receptors, JAK/STAT, APC, β-catenin, myc
3. Resistance to apoptosis	Caspase 8, FLIP, Bcl-2, Apaf-1, HSPs, IAPs, Akt, PTEN
4. Induction and sustaining of angiogenesis	VEGF, PDGF, FGF, TSP-1, angiostatin, endostatin
5. Tissue invasion and metastasis	MMPs, integrins, E-cadherin
6. Limitless replicative potential	p53, pRB, telomerase

Adapted from Hanahan D, Weinberg RA. The hallmarks of cancer. *Cell* 2000;100:57–70.

deteriorations in the cell cycle regulation, insensitivity to growth-inhibitory signals, evasion of apoptotic cell death, induction of neoangiogenesis, and activation of invasive growth and metastasis.[30,31] Normal cell division is tightly regulated by stimulatory and inhibitory growth signals. Growth signaling involves interaction of diffusible growth factors or cytokines with transmembrane receptors, as well as regulation of growth by components of the extracellular matrix and by cell–cell interactions. Once a resting cell receives a sufficient growth stimulus, it enters the cell cycle by passing the restriction point and four distinct phases of cytokinesis and mitogenesis: gap-1 (G1), DNA synthesis (S), gap-2 (G2), and mitosis (M).[32] Passage through the restriction point and entry into S and M (G1/S and G2/M checkpoints) are governed by several proto-oncogenes and tumor suppressor genes. Each phase of the cell cycle is regulated by specific complexes of cyclins (cyclins A to E) and their respective partners, the cyclin-dependent kinases (cdks). Important complexes are cyclin D/cdk4 and cyclin D/cdk6 (restriction point, G1), cyclin E/cdk2 (G1/S), cyclin A/cdk2 (S, G2), and cyclinB/cdk1 (M). There is increasing evidence that many functions of the cyclins are compensatorily covered among the cyclin family, that is, in the absence of one cyclin, other cyclins are able to act in different cell cycle phases.[33,34] Cyclins are directly upregulated by growth factors and indirectly via c-myc and Ras. Several cyclin/cdk complexes phosphorylate the retinoblastoma protein (pRB), facilitating the G1/S transition, as well as blocking differentiation. The activity of the cdks is regulated by phosphorylation and dephosphorylation events, as well as by interaction with various inhibitory molecules belonging to the INK4 (p15, p16, p18, and p19) and Cip1/Kip1 (p21, p27, and p57) families. The proteins p15 and p21 are related to two important tumor suppressors, the antiproliferative factor transforming growth factor-β (TGF-β) and p53, respectively.

Self-Sufficiency in Growth Signals

Mitogenic signals from growth factors, cytokines, extracellular matrix, and cell–cell adhesion molecules are transferred into the cell by different classes of transmembrane receptors.[30,31] Malignant cells acquire the capability to escape from the tightly regulated dependence on extracellular growth signals. The molecular mechanisms include overexpression of growth factors as well as growth factor receptors (autocrine and paracrine stimulation), receptor mutations leading to constitutive receptor activation without ligand binding, and molecular aberrations in the intracellular signal transduction pathways.

Receptor tyrosine kinases (RTKs) represent a group of oncogenic, transmembrane receptors consisting of an extracellular ligand-binding domain, a transmembrane part, and an intracellular catalytic domain with tyrosine kinase activity.[35] On ligand binding and receptor homo/heterodimerization, the protein kinase is subsequently activated, resulting in phosphorylation of tyrosine residues of the receptor itself (autophosphorylation) or target proteins. Depending on the cellular context, this triggers an intracellular signaling cascade that eventually leads to proliferation, survival, differentiation, and migration. Among the known human RTKs are the epidermal growth factor receptors (EGFRs), the platelet-derived growth factor receptors (PDGFRs), the vascular endothelial growth factor receptors (VEGFRs), the fibroblast growth factor receptors, the ephrin receptors, and tyrosine kinase receptor. The *EGFR family* consists of four distinct members (EGFR/ErbB-1, HER2/ErbB-2, HER3/ErbB-3, and HER4/ErbB-4).[36] The receptor ligands, such as epidermal growth factor, tumor growth factor-α, and neuroregulin-1, as well as their cognate receptors, are abundantly expressed in a large variety of human cancers, including lung, breast, head and neck, and gliomas, and have been related to poor prognosis. This finding led to the recognition of the EGFRs as important targets for cancer therapy. Mechanisms underlying the increased activation of the EGFR pathway in cancer cells include gene amplification and activating mutations, for example, EGFRvIII, a constitutively ligand-independent EGFR mutant.[36]

RTK-Initiated Signal Transduction

The extracellular signals received by the RTKs are translated into a large variety of different cellular responses by a cascade of molecular processes, that is, signal transduction.[35] This RTK signaling involves several distinct molecular pathways that are often deregulated in cancer cells. Prime examples of such deregulated pathways are the Ras/RAF/mitogen-activated protein kinase (MAPK) pathway, the phosphoinositide 3′ kinase (PI3K)/Akt pathway, the jak/stat molecules, and protein kinase C. Cooperative and mutual cross-talk between the different transduction pathways forms a complex signaling network.

An important signal transduction route that has been extensively studied in EGFR signaling represents the Ras/Raf/MAPK pathway. The *Ras proteins* (H-Ras, K-Ras4A, K-Ras4B, and N-Ras) are GTPases and are attached in their active state (GTP bound) to the inner surface of the cell membrane. The Ras proto-oncogene, predominantly K-Ras, is mutated in about one-third of human cancers. Activating mutations are frequent in adenocarcinomas of the pancreas (up to 90%), colorectum (about 50%), and the lung (about 30%).[37] The processing and membrane attachment of the functional Ras are governed by farnesyltransferases, which are the molecular target for specific pharmaceutical inhibitors of activated Ras.[38] EGFR activation channels via the Grb2/SOS complex to the Ras molecule. Activated Ras binds to *Raf,* facilitating its function as a serine/threonine kinase. Constitutively activated Raf proteins as a result of genetic alterations in the Raf genes have been shown in a large variety of human malignancies.[39] Raf associates with MEK1/2 kinases, which in turn activate *MAPKs.* Activated MAPKs are subsequently translocated to the nucleus and initiate transcription by the activation of several transcription factors, for example, Elk-1. Consequently, gene expression is changed, and proliferative processes are triggered.

In addition to Raf, activated Ras has an effect on various downstream molecules, including *PI3K.*[40] Following either direct activation by RTKs or indirect Raf-mediated activation, this group of kinases phosphorylates the 3′-OH group of the inositol ring in inositol phospholipids. Signaling mediator molecules of PI3K include phosphoinositide-dependent kinase 1, Akt, protein kinase C, and subsequently the nuclear transcription factor NFκB. The cellular responses on activation of the PI3K pathway are cell-type specific and include changes in gene expression, cell cycle progression, survival, and apoptosis. The last has been linked to PKB/Akt negatively controlling apoptosis-regulating molecules, such as Bad, caspase 9, Fas ligand, cAMP responsive element–binding protein, and IκB kinase. The tumor suppressor protein *PTEN* negatively regulates the PI3K/Akt pathway. Akt overexpression or hyperactivity and PTEN mutations are found in numerous human malignancies.[41] Akt phosphorylates, the molecular target of rapamycin, a compound that exhibits anticancer activity.[42]

Cytokine Receptors

A large number of growth-stimulating hormones, growth factors, and cytokines such as the interleukins, erythropoietin, and prolactin bind to the class of cytokine receptors that are structurally different from the previously described RTKs.[43] The intracellular signaling in response to cytokine receptor activation includes the *JAK* and *STAT* kinases. In addition to the cytokine receptors, many RTKs can activate the JAK/STAT pathway. In malignant cells the autonomy of growth signaling can be associated with mutations in cytokine receptors (e.g., in the erythropoietin receptor) and constitutively upregulated activity of the JAK/STAT pathway in hematopoietic malignancies. STAT activation may result from transformation of tyrosine kinases such as v-src, v-Abl, and Bcr/Abl by viral oncoproteins from human T-cell lymphotropic virus or Epstein–Barr virus.[44]

Wnt Signaling

Wnt proteins are diffusible growth factors that bind to specific surface receptors (Frizzeled) and trigger distinct intracellular pathways leading to cell growth.[45] Wnt signaling involves the tumor suppressor protein adenomatous polyposis coli (*APC*) and regulates by phosphorylation the steady-state levels of cytosolic β-catenin. An increased level of β-catenin facilitates its transit into the nucleus, activation of transcription factors, and subsequently transcription of β-catenin target genes, including c-myc, c-jun, and cyclin D1. The aberrant activation of Wnt signaling caused by mutations in the β-catenin and APC genes are typical findings in colon cancer and melanoma but also have been identified in a large variety of other human cancers. Wnt signaling has been shown to play an important role in tumorigenesis and in cancer stem cell self-renewal and differentiation and thus provides a promising target for anticancer treatment.[46]

Cytoplasmic, nonreceptor kinases are often activated in malignant disease. For example, the *Bcr/Abl* fusion protein kinase resulting from the translocation t(9;22) is a typical molecular finding in chronic myeloid leukemia and represents the molecular target for small-molecule inhibitors such as imatinib.[47] This drug also inhibits *c-KIT,* a cytoplasmic tyrosine kinase that has been shown to be activated by mutation in gastrointestinal stroma tumors, thus providing another molecular targeting approach.[48]

Transcription factors bind to the DNA and activate the expression of specific genes. Oncogenic transcription factors are overactive in most human cancers and contribute to the autonomy of growth signaling. Based on their mechanism of activation, three groups can be separated.[49] First are the *steroid receptors,* which are found in hormone-sensitive breast or prostate cancer. The second group of transcription factors resides in the nucleus, is governed by kinase signals, and consists of various members, including *myc, activator protein 1* (AP-1), and *E2F.* Myc transcription factors are induced in cancer by different mechanisms, including translocation and gene amplification. For example, c-myc is activated by the chromosomal translocation t (8;14), which brings the c-myc gene under the control of the immunoglobulin G enhancer, resulting in a constitutive c-myc expression in 80% of Burkitt lymphomas. N-myc and L-myc amplifications are found in neuroblastoma and small cell lung cancer, respectively. AP-1, consisting of JUN, FOS, ATF, and MAF, can exhibit oncogenic or antioncogenic effects depending on the cellular context.[50] The third group of oncogenic transcription factors—the latent transcription factors—is activated by ligand–receptor interactions and includes the STATs (see previous discussion), the WNT–β-catenin pathway (see previous discussion), NFκB, and the molecules Notch and Hedgehog. NFκB levels have been shown to be constitutively active in lymphomas, leukemias, and breast and colon cancer.[49]

Loss of Cell Cycle Control

Retinoblastoma Tumor Suppressor Protein (pRB)

The retinoblastoma protein is an important regulator of cell cycling and cell differentiation.[51] Loss of pRB function is often found in malignant cells and leads to an uncontrolled G1/S transition, genomic instability, and loss of differentiation. Hypophosphorylated pRB binds to several proteins, including the E2F transcription factors and histone deacetylases. These proteins are released on phosphorylation of pRB, for example, by cyclin D/cdk4, cyclin E/cdk2, and cyclin A/cdk2 complexes, and contribute to cell cycle transition and/or to inhibition of terminal differentiation. As a result, the cell is switched from a quiescent phenotype toward a proliferative state. Released E2F activates transcription of genes required for DNA synthesis such as dihydrofolate reductase, thymidylate reductase, and DNA polymerase. Loss of pRB function can result from mutation or inactivation by oncogenic viral proteins such as human papillomavirus (HPV) E7. Somatic mutations in the RB gene have been detected in a variety of epithelial and mesenchymal malignancies.[51] Loss of cell cycle control by impairment of the pRB pathway can also result from overexpression of cyclin D, activating mutations and amplification of cdk4, and loss of p16 (INK4), leading to a constitutive expression of E2F target genes.[51] Loss of function in the pRB pathway contributes to genomic instability by E2F-mediated overexpression of MAD2, an important component of the mitotic checkpoint.[52] The encoding RB gene was the first characterized tumor suppressor gene involved in retinoblastoma, a rare childhood tumor. Retinoblastoma is a typical example for the two-hit model of tumor induction.[26] The first hit, that is, mutation in one RB allele, is either a germline (inherited form, often bilateral) or an acquired somatic mutation (sporadic form, mostly unilateral). An acquired somatic mutation in the other RB allele causes the inactivation of the pRB and consequently tumorigenesis.

TP53 tumor suppressor gene is inactivated in the majority of cancers and has been associated with poor prognosis in some cancers.[53] Wild-type p53 binds to specific DNA sequences and activates transcription of numerous genes, including *MDM2, GADD45, p21*$^{CIP-1}$, *cyclin D,* and the proapoptotic BAX. On the other hand, p53 can negatively regulate gene transcription (e.g., for genes such as *myc, cyclin A, MDR1,* and the antiapoptotic *Bcl-2*).[54] The role of p53 for the radiation response is discussed later in this chapter. Loss of p53 function has numerous biologic consequences, including loss of cell cycle arrest at the G1/S-phase checkpoint after genotoxic stress, inhibition of apoptosis, and differentiation.[54] Furthermore, loss of p53 function seems to be critical for chromosomal stability, as p53 is involved in DNA repair, recombination, and replication. Inactivation of the TP53 gene is the most common genetic alteration in human cancer. More than 80% of the p53 alterations result from missense mutations in the DNA-binding domain.[55] The obvious predominance of specific missense mutations in human tumors with the presence of a full-length protein suggests an additional role of mutant p53 as an oncogenic protein with gain-of-function and dominant-negative properties. In addition to mutations, p53 function can be compromised by aberration of its negative regulator MDM2 or by viral proteins HPV E6/E7.[56] While most of the *TP53* mutations are sporadic, a high proportion of patients with Li–Fraumeni syndrome, a rare cancer syndrome with a spectrum of carcinomas and sarcomas at early age, carry germline mutations.

Insensitivity to Growth-Inhibitory Signals

TGF-β regulates multiple cell functions, such as proliferation, extracellular matrix synthesis, angiogenesis, immune response, apoptosis, and differentiation.[57] The TGF-β family (TGF-β1 to 5) belongs to the superfamily of peptide hormones. The different TGF-β isoforms bind to specific cell surface receptors (TβRI to TβRV). TGF-β–mediated growth inhibition is associated with activation and repression of target gene transcription. Genes of proproliferative kinases such as cdks are repressed, whereas genes of the major cyclin-dependent kinase inhibitors p15 and p21 are transcriptionally activated. Ligand binding to TβRV stimulates serine/threonine-specific phosphatases, which

TABLE 3.2 TYPES OF RADIATION-INDUCED CELL DEATH AND THEIR CHARACTERISTICS

Type of Cell Death	Important Morphologic Characteristics	Important Molecular Mechanisms
Mitotic catastrophe	During or after mitosis, missegregation of chromosomes, cell fusion, micronuclei, giant cell formation	Lethal chromosome damage, caspase independent
Apoptosis	Chromatin condensation, nuclear fragmentation, blebbing of cell membrane	Damage to DNA, and/or membranes, and/or alterations of intracellular signaling, caspase dependent (intrinsic pathway via caspase 9)
Senescence	Metabolically active but nondividing, functionally differentiated cells	Damage to DNA and/or alterations of intracellular signaling, generally p53-dependent terminal growth arrest, increased senescence-associated β galactosidase
Autophagy	Partial chromatin condensation, cell membrane blebbing, increased number of autophagic vesicles	Protein degradation characterized by double-membrane vesicles in the cytoplasm, possibly related to DNA protein kinase (DNA-PK) activity
Necrosis	Increased vacuolation, swelling of organelles and cells, rupture of cell membranes, formation of necrotic mass	Unregulated traumatic cell destruction; after irradiation as consequence of, e.g., mitotic catastrophe or vascular damage

Adapted from Brown JM, Wouters BG. Apoptosis, p53, and tumor cell sensitivity to anticancer agents. *Cancer Res* 1999;59:1391–1399, and Okada H, Mak TW. Pathways of apoptotic and non-apoptotic death in tumour cells. *Nat Rev Cancer* 2004;4:592–603.[90,236]

inhibit proliferation by dephosphorylation of pRB. Alteration of TGF-β signaling in tumors, for example, by mutations and transcriptional silencing leads to insensitivity to inhibitory ligands.

Resistance to Apoptosis

Under physiologic conditions, tissue homeostasis results from the balance of cell division and cell loss. This balance is disturbed in most tumors by an increased cell division rate due to the molecular mechanisms previously described and by an inappropriate rate of cell death, such as by senescence and apoptosis[53,58] (Table 3.2). Apoptosis is a complex, multistep process involving numerous molecules, including adapter proteins, members of the *Bcl-2* family, and cysteine-aspartate proteases (*caspases*).[59] The last are divided into initiator (apical) caspases (caspases 1, 2, 4, 5, 8 to 10, 12) and effector (executioner) caspases (caspases 3, 6, 7, 11, 13). Caspases activate specific substrates by proteolytic cleavage. The activity of caspases is regulated by heat-shock proteins and inhibitor of apoptosis proteins. The executive phase of the apoptotic program includes the release of cytochrome C from mitochondria after membrane depolarization, formation of the apoptosome complex (Apaf-1, pro–caspase 9, cytochrome C), and activation of effector caspases, leading subsequently to morphologic changes (e.g., DNA condensation and fragmentation). Initiator caspases are activated by two major pathways—the extrinsic, receptor-mediated pathway and the intrinsic, mitochondria-mediated pathway. The extrinsic apoptotic signaling starts from binding of death ligands, such as Fas, tumor necrosis factor (TNF), and *TRAIL*, to their corresponding cell-surface receptors. Subsequently, a cell type–specific intracellular program is executed, including caspases, and members of the Bcl-2 family (*Bax, Bid, Bak*) eventually trigger the release of cytochrome C (type II) or directly activate effector caspase 3 (type I). The intrinsic, mitochondria-mediated pathway is triggered in response to cellular stress, such as DNA damage, chemotherapy, ionizing radiation, growth factor withdrawal, and kinase inhibition. While the acquired capability to escape from apoptosis is a prerequisite for tumorigenesis, it does not necessarily correlate with resistance to cancer treatment.[53]

An important mediator between the recognition of DNA alterations and apoptosis is the tumor suppressor p53.[54] On DNA damage, p53 is stabilized and induces cell cycle arrest (see previous discussion), senescence, or apoptosis. Promotion of apoptosis by p53 results from transcriptional repression of antiapoptotic proteins (e.g., Bcl-2 and *survivin*) and activation of the proapoptotic proteins, including *Bax, PUMA,* and *NOXA*. Of importance, the apoptotic pathways are closely linked to protein kinase signaling. Thus, protein kinases such as MAPK and PI3K/Akt (see previous discussion) are able to modulate the balance between death and survival stimuli in the cell in a context-dependent manner. Given the complex regulation of apoptosis, it is not surprising that a large variety of molecular alterations can result in an escape of cancer cells from this type of cell death.[60] For instance, the extrinsic pathway is affected by downregulation of caspase 8 activity by promoter methylation, mutation, and upregulation of the negative regulator *FLIP*. Many tumor cells show a deregulated intrinsic, mitochondria-related apoptotic pathway caused by an imbalance of expression levels of proaptoptotic and antiapoptotic proteins of the Bcl-2 family. Abnormal expression levels of inhibitor of apoptosis proteins (Apaf-1) and heat-shock proteins result in an impaired execution phase of apoptosis in cancer cells. Moreover, important mediators and regulators of the apoptotic program, such as p53, PI3K/Akt, PTEN, and MAPK are often functionally deregulated. While it is well established that the escape from apoptosis represents an important and possibly essential step in tumorigenesis, the importance of this phenomenon for therapy resistance and outcome prediction and as a potential target to improve conventional cancer therapies remains unclear.[53,60]

Limitless Replicative Potential

Loss of growth control and resistance to cell death are not sufficient for the development of macroscopic tumors.[31] Normal cells have the capacity for a finite number of cell divisions, that is, a limited replicative potential. Thereafter cells either stop proliferating and enter the process of senescence, that is, a viable but nonproliferative state, or they die. During tumorigenesis, some premalignant cells become immortal by circumventing senescence, that is, by acquiring a capability of limitless replicative potential.[31] Of importance, malignant tumors consist of heterogeneous populations differing in their replicative potential. While most cancer cells have a limited replicative potential, a small subpopulation (i.e., cancer stem cells) have an infinite replicative capacity to reconstitute the tumor.[61] Thus, this subpopulation represents the target for curative cancer therapy, that is, all of these stem cells have to be inactivated by therapy to achieve cure. It remains to be clarified whether cancer stem cells represent a distinct tumor cell subpopulation or whether all cancer cells have a stem cell potential and can switch between different stages in response to stress or environmental conditions.

The molecular mechanisms underlying the escape from senescence and other modes of cell death include loss of tumor suppressor proteins such as p53 and pRB as well as telomere maintenance.[31] Telomeres are chromatin segments located at the ends of the chromosomes that protect these regions from recombination and degradation.[62] As telomeres are incompletely replicated, they become progressively shorter during each cell division, subsequently resulting in loss of chromosomal protection, which in turn triggers senescence. Cancer cells generally have shorter telomeres than normal cells but are able to perpetuate their replicative potential by expressing telomerase, a complex including DNA polymerase, which reconstitutes the telomeres.[62]

Induction and Sustaining Angiogenesis

To grow beyond microscopically sized cell aggregates of 1 to 2 mm, tumors depend on angiogenesis. Proliferating cells require appropriate oxygen and nutrient supply, which is physiologically limited to a distance of 100 to 200 μm from the next blood vessel. Therefore, malignant cells must induce and sustain their own vascular system to form tumors and metastases.[63] The process of the *angiogenic switch* during tumorigenesis (i.e., the transition from the avascular phase to the vascular stage) is governed by different molecular changes in tumor cells and in cells of the surrounding stroma. The major event of the angiogenic switch is that proangiogenic factors—mostly growth factors such as VEGFs, fibroblast growth factors, and PDGFs—outbalance antiangiogenic factors, such as thrombospondin (*TSP-1*), *angiostatin,* and *endostatin.* The driving forces toward the imbalance of angiogenic factors in tumors include activation of oncogenes; for example, Ras and myc activation results in VEGF upregulation and TSP-1 repression.[64,65] The loss of function in tumor suppressor proteins also contributes to the angiogenic switch by transcriptional regulation of angiogenic factors. For example, p53 upregulates TSP-1 and downregulates VEGF gene expression.[30] Hypoxia promotes tumor angiogenesis via the hypoxia inducible factor 1, which transcriptionally regulates many angiogenic molecules.[66,67] As originally proposed by Folkman,[68] effective targeting of molecules and pathways involved in angiogenesis has been shown to exhibit anticancer activity.[69]

Tissue Invasion and Metastasis

Locoregional and distant spread of tumor cells requires detachment from the primary tumor, invasion into surrounding tissues, intravasation into blood or lymphatic vessels, adhesion to endothelial cells at distant sites, extravasation, and eventually colonization in distant organs. The acquired capability of cancer cells to grow invasively and to metastasize is associated with multiple genetic and biochemical alterations of the cell–cell and cell–matrix interactions. Tissue invasion and metastasis require, at different steps, contrary capabilities—for example, detachment from the primary tumor versus adhesion at the metastatic site—suggesting that rapid adaptations, genetic instability, and clonal selection play an important role. Gene expression profiling revealed metastatic signatures in primary tumors but also host polymorphisms, resulting in a genetically determined individual disposition to develop metastases.[70,71] The often-observed nonrandom pattern of metastasis in different types of cancer led to the "seed and soil" hypothesis describing the complex interplay between cancer cells and environmental factors.[72] Experimental data suggest that bone marrow–derived endothelial progenitor cells exhibit preconditioning functions for metastases; that is, they reside in tumor-specific metastatic sites before the colonization with tumor cells and prepare the optimal environment for tumor cell homing.[73]

Many physiologic functions of the cell, such as proliferation, migration, survival, and differentiation, are regulated by interactions with neighboring cells and with molecules of the extracellular matrix (ECM). The ECM consists of a large variety of different components, including collagens, fibronectins, laminins, tenascin, proteoglycans, matrix proteases, and their specific inhibitors. Altered composition of the ECM is a typical finding in malignant tissues. For example, tenascin overexpression was found in the stroma of breast cancer, colon carcinoma, and glioma.[74] It has been suggested that, due to the antiadhesive properties of tenascin, this change in the ECM facilitates detachment of cancer cells and subsequently tissue invasion and metastasis. *Matrix proteases* are important for ECM turnover and enable tumor cells to degrade extracellular barriers, a prerequisite for tissue invasion and metastasis.[75] The different classes of matrix proteases include serine proteases (plasminogen activator, plasmin, and elastase), cysteine proteases (cathepsins), and matrix metalloproteinases (collagenases, stromelysins). The last are released from the cells in an inactive form and activated by binding to zinc ions. The activity of the matrix proteases, and thereby the ECM turnover rate, is also determined by inhibitors of the proteases such as tissue inhibitors of metalloproteases or plasminogen activator inhibitor. It has been shown that tissue invasion and metastasis in various types of cancer are associated with increased expression of matrix proteases and decreased activity of their inhibitors compared with normal cells.[76]

Cell–cell and cell–matrix interactions are mediated by different adhesion molecules, including integrins, cadherins, immunoglobulin-like cell adhesion molecules, and the hyaluronan receptor CD44.[77] Not only do these molecules exert structural functions, but they also are essential for signal transduction. *Integrins* represent a class of heterodimeric transmembrane ECM receptors.[78] At least 24 integrin receptors are formed by 18 α and 8 β subunits with overlapping binding affinity to ECM components and functions. Further diversity in the integrins results from posttranslational modification such as alternative splicing. Intracellular signal transduction on binding of integrins to ECM components includes activation of the focal adhesion kinase and subsequent association with PI3K, which is required for focal adhesion kinase-promoted cell migration and survival. Other signaling partners of integrins include ILK, protein kinase C, Rho family of small G proteins, and cytoplasmic kinases (src, Abl), which contribute to activation of MAPK/JNK and subsequently stimulate proliferation and migration.

Besides the ability to bind ECM proteins such as fibronectin, collagen, or laminin, some integrins recognize members of the disintegrin and metalloproteinase (ADAM) family or counter receptors on neighboring cells such as immunoglobulin-type receptors like intercellular cell adhesion molecules or vascular cell adhesion molecules.[79] Cross-talk between integrin signaling, growth factor signaling, and tumor suppressor proteins such as PTEN and p53 have been described. The capability of tissue invasion and metastatic spread has been associated with altered integrin function in tumors.[80] In general, cancer cells show a more pronounced variability in integrin combinations, an abnormal expression pattern, and aberrant spatial expression compared with nonmalignant cells, facilitating interaction with ECM of different composition and thereby permitting cancer cell survival and proliferation at distant sites. Alternative splicing of the hyaluronan receptor *CD44* results in a complex, cell type–specific expression pattern that has been demonstrated to be altered in many tumors and metastasis.[81] *E-Cadherin* is a glycoprotein expressed at the cell surface and intracellularly linked to the cytoskeleton via catenin proteins. In addition, E-cadherin is connected to multiple intracellular signaling pathways. The function of E-cadherin as a tumor suppressor was established from experimental and clinical observations that a loss of function (e.g., by mutation, promoter methylation, increased proteolytic degradation by matrix metalloproteinases, increased endocytotic degradation induced by phosphorylation) is a frequent finding in human cancers and is associated with an invasive and metastatic phenotype.[82] The multifunctional immunoglobulin-like cell adhesion molecules are expressed in a large variety of cell types. Some members of this superfamily, such as NCAM, CEA, Mel-CAM, and L1, are involved in tumorigenesis, metastasis, and invasion.[77]

MOLECULAR RADIATION BIOLOGY

Target Molecules of Radiation Damage

Radiation effects may occur as direct ionizations in an organic molecule or indirectly via free radical processes. As cells consist mostly of water, most ionizations produced by irradiation occur in water molecules. Within only 10^{-10} seconds, radiolysis of water leads, among other entities, to $e^{-}aq$, H·, and OH·. About 60% to 70% of cellular DNA damage produced by ionizing radiation is caused by OH·.[83] The radiation-induced reactive oxygen species (ROS) undergo further reactions—for

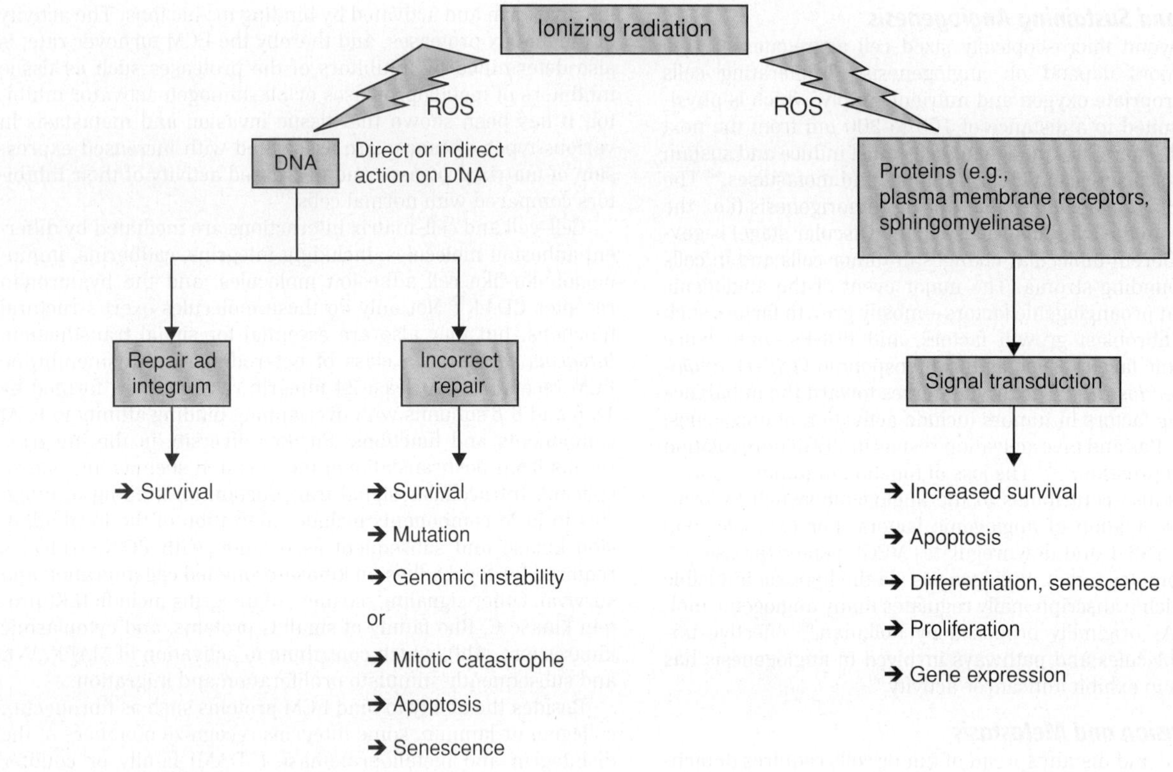

FIGURE 3.1. Simplified illustration of biologic effects of ionizing radiation mediated via DNA and non-DNA target molecules. ROS, reactive oxygen species.

example, production of H_2O_2 from two hydroxyl radicals. Aerobes have evolved antioxidant defenses to protect themselves against the oxygen-derived species generated *in vivo* or from external sources. These defenses include enzymes (such as superoxide dismutases, catalase, and glutathione peroxidase), low–molecular mass agents (such as α-tocopherol and ascorbic acid), and proteins that bind metal ions in forms unable to catalyze the generation of free radicals. In contrast to those defensive mechanisms, the oxygen molecule has a high affinity to free radicals, which may give rise to further cascades of radical production and thereby to the fixation of free radical damage to important macromolecules of the cell (e.g., DNA). This is one explanation of the oxygen effect of radiation damage, that is, the fact that well-oxygenated cells are more radiosensitive than hypoxic cells.[84,85]

By far the most important target for the biologic effects of ionizing radiation is the DNA (Fig. 3.1). This is obvious for the induction of mutations but has also been consistently demonstrated for the killing of cells in a number of different experiments. Irradiation of the cytoplasm of cells with short-range α-particles only leads to cell kill at very high doses, whereas 1,000-fold lower doses to the nucleus are sufficient to kill the cell.[86] Radioactive isotopes with short-range emission effectively kill cells when incorporated into the DNA but not when predominantly incorporated in cell membranes.[87] Modification of radiation-induced cell kill by different measures, including hypoxia, high–linear energy transfer radiation, or hyperthermia is linked closely with a change in the induction and repair of DNA double-strand breaks. Exposure of cells to about 1 Gy causes approximately 3,500 DNA injuries, 1,500 to 2,500 of which are damaged bases, 1,000 single-strand breaks (SSBs), 40 double-strand breaks (DSBs), and an estimated 100 to 200 local multiple-damaged sites, where one or several DSBs occur in close proximity to SSBs and base damage.[88] It will be shown later that most radiation-induced DNA damage is recognized and very efficiently repaired by the cell.

Besides effects on DNA, ionizing radiation also evokes biologically important responses on proteins (e.g., transmembrane receptors) and on lipids (e.g., ceramides) (Fig. 3.1). Radiation-induced activation of receptors will be discussed later. Ionizing irradiation induces rapid sphingomyelin hydrolysis by acid sphingomyelinase to generate ceramide, an inductor of apoptosis.[89]

Biologic Consequences of Irradiation

The effects of ionizing radiation on cellular target molecules may lead to various functional consequences. These functional effects can be broadly categorized into cell death, repair, cell cycle effects, altered gene expression, modification of signal transduction, mutagenesis, and genomic instability (Fig. 3.2). These categories are not exclusive.

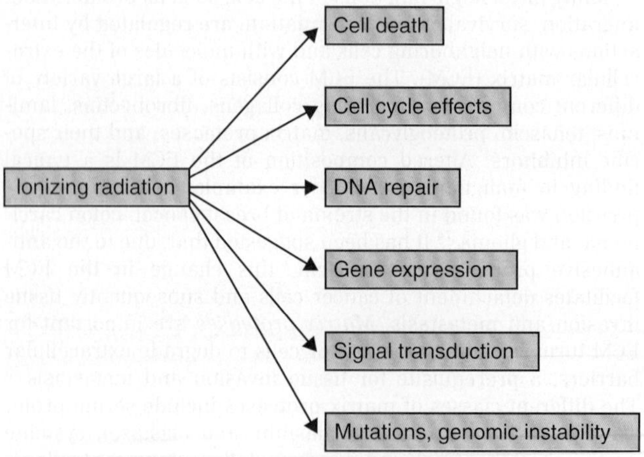

FIGURE 3.2. Functional effects of ionizing radiation on cells. The categories are not exclusive.

Cell Death

Among the functional consequences of ionizing radiation, cell death is the most important one for radiation oncology. Cells can die in several ways[90]—by apoptosis, mitotic catastrophe, senescence, necrosis, and autophagy (Table 3.2). Most important for the effect of radiotherapy of solid tumors is *mitotic catastrophe,* which is caused by lethal chromosome damage.[91] After irradiation, cells can pass through one or few mitotic cycles before missegregation of chromosomes or cell fusion leads to the loss of their replicative potential (or clonogenicity). Often micronuclei, containing nonrepaired chromosome fragments, can be detected. Those micronuclei, and hence essential genetic information, will be lost during the following cell cycle, which results in cell death. Frequent multinucleate giant cells reflect a radiation-induced failure of cytoplasmatic separation on cell division.

Neoplastic hematopoietic or lymphatic cells often die from radiation-induced *apoptosis* via the intrinsic, caspase 9–dependent pathway. Two different forms of radiation-induced apoptosis can be distinguished—early or premitotic versus late or postmitotic.[92] Early apoptosis is p53 dependent, occurs within few hours after irradiation before the cells enter mitosis, and is primarily a consequence of DNA damage. Early apoptosis represents a distinct mode of radiation-induced cell death. In contrast, secondary apoptosis occurs after mitosis and is one of several possible manifestations of radiation-induced lethal chromosome aberrations. In most cancers, particularly in solid tumors, apoptosis appears not to be the main mechanism of radiation-induced cell death.[53] No clear evidence exists that either apoptotic index or levels of p53, Bcl-2, or other Bcl-2 family members are predictive of the response of solid tumors to radiotherapy. For example, overexpression of Bcl-2 was shown to significantly decrease the apoptotic fraction in response to irradiation. However, this did not translate into a change of clonogenic cell survival after irradiation.[93]

Radiation-induced *senescence* plays an important role for development of normal tissue damage—for example, fibrosis[94]—but occurs also in response to nonlethal stress as in tumor cells.[95] Cells survive and are metabolically active but lose their replicative potential. *Necrosis* is an unregulated process of cell destruction by the release of intracellular components. This is usually the consequence of pathophysiologic conditions such as ischemia and inflammation.[90] So far no distinct pathway has been described that directly leads to cellular necrosis after clinically relevant doses of irradiation. However, it is well known that tumors often show massive necrosis after neoadjuvant radiotherapy or radiochemotherapy, which in some tumors correlates with improved prognosis.[96,97] It is likely that this radiation-induced induction of necrosis is explained by several factors, including mitotic catastrophe of tumor cells and the effects of irradiation on tumor vessels leading to changes in the microenvironment, which consequently cause cell death.

Autophagy is a form of nonapoptotic and nonnecrotic cell death that is related to lysosomal degradation of proteins and cell organelles that are then utilized for the production of new cells.[90] This mode of programmed cell death is triggered by growth factor withdrawal, differentiation, and developmental stimuli. Although the molecular regulation is not completely understood, recent data suggest that a high rate of autophagy contributes to radiation resistance[98] and that autophagy is regulated through different hypoxia-dependent pathways, thereby facilitating survival during metabolic stress.[99]

Recognition of Radiation-Induced DNA Damage

DNA damage, in particular DSBs, is sensed by different proteins that trigger an ataxia telangiectasia mutated (ATM)–dependent or, in some cases, ataxia telangiectasia and Rad3-related (ATR)–dependent signaling cascade[100] (Fig. 3.3). ATM activation requires the telomeric protein TRF2 and the MRN complex consisting of Rad50, meiotic recombination protein 11 (Mre11), Nijmegen breakage syndrome protein 1 (NBS1), mediator of

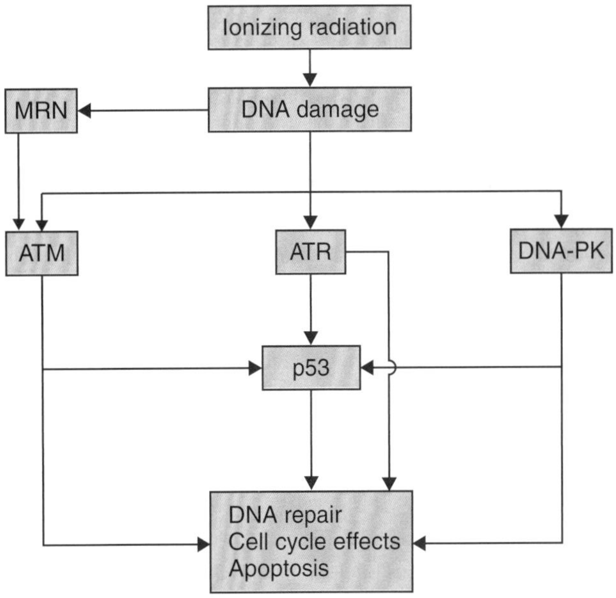

FIGURE 3.3. Simplified pathways of radiation-induced DNA damage recognition. ATM, ataxia telangiectasia–mutated; ATR, ataxia telangiectasia and Rad3–related; MRN, Mrc 11, Rad50, NB51 complex; PK, protein kinase.

DNA damage checkpoint protein-1 (MDC1), and 53BP1.[101] In addition to proper activation of downstream DNA-repair proteins, histone H2AX molecules need to be phosphorylated in the vicinity of the DSB. All of these proteins assemble at the site of the breaks and presumably control the choice of one of several repair pathways. In addition to its role in repair, ATM is involved in the regulation of multiple cell cycle checkpoints (G1/S, S, G2/M) after DNA damage.[102] ATM, ATR, and DNA-dependent kinase-catalytic subunit (DNA-PK_{CS}) phosphorylate p53 and a number of proteins involved in cell cycle delay, apoptosis, and induction of DNA repair. ATR appears to be important for sensing ultraviolet-related and other types of bulky lesions, as well as damage that induces a replication block, while ATM seems to be the sensor for DSB induced by ionizing radiation.[100] ATR may serve in some cases as a backup for ATM.

DNA Repair

Genome integrity is essential to the survival of cells and organisms. It is estimated that about 10^4 DNA lesions occur in a single human cell every day.[103] Most of the damage is caused by endogenous sources such as oxygen free radicals, replicative errors, and spontaneous desaminations. To cope with the plethora of permanent damage initially, a repair system was developed during evolution that also acts on external challenges such as radiation or chemical DNA damage. To enable repair of massive DNA damage, the cells stop proliferation. This may prevent replication or segregation of damaged genetic material. If repair is not possible, the cells either die or, in case of survival, may propagate mutated DNA (Fig. 3.2). When the DNA replication machinery meets damaged DNA, replication may continue despite the damage by translesion synthesis, which requires DNA polymerase with low fidelity. Different mechanisms are involved in DNA repair.[100,104]

Base Excision Repair

The mechanism of base excision repair (BER) is responsible for the repair of various kinds of base damage (abasic sites, oxidized bases, deaminated bases, and alkylated bases) and SSB. Base damages and SSB are the most frequent types of DNA damage after irradiation.[105,106] The major BER pathway is the short-patch pathway, which involves excision of only one base. The minor pathway—the long-patch repair—excises 2 to 10 nucleotides. In the short-patch pathway, DNA glycosylases recognize damaged bases and excise them from DNA. Apurinic/apyrimidinic endonuclease 1 (APE1 synonyms: HAP-1, redox effector factor 1) hydrolyzes the phosphodiester bond 5′ to the abasic site. Alternatively, an AP-lyase cleaves the 3′ sugar-phosphate bond. In both cases, the sugar residue is removed by either a 5′- or a 3′-phosphodiesterase. Polymerase β (Pol-β) incorporates a single nucleotide into the gap, and, finally, the nick in the DNA is sealed by DNA ligase III, which interacts with Pol-β. In this process, x-ray repair cross-complementing protein (XRCC1) interacts with several enzymes in this pathway and regulates their activity.[107] For the long-patch repair, the nick produced by AP-endonuclease or AP-lyase is extended to a gap 2 to 10 nucleotides by either a 5′- or a 3′-exonuclease, that is, exonuclease function of polymerase δ or ε (Pol-δ or ε), or by removal of a flap end by flap-end endonuclease-1 (Fen-1). Pol δ or ε and associated replication factors (proliferating cell nuclear antigen and replication factor C) then fill the gap. After the synthesis, DNA ligase I or, less frequently, ligase III, seals the nick.[108]

DSB Repair

Spontaneous DSBs occur either on topoisomerase failure during recombination and are forced by replication errors or are due to thermodynamic fluctuation. In germ cells, DSBs are produced during meiotic crossover in T and B lymphocytes during a sik-specific DNA recombination of *v*ariable diversity and joining genes (VDJ) on maturation of T cell receptors and antibodies. Radiation-induced DSBs are, despite their relatively low induction frequency (40 per Gy per cell), biologically much more important than base damage and SSB. Two major pathways—homologous recombination (HR) and nonhomologous end joining (NHEJ)—have evolved to repair DSB[109,110] (Fig. 3.4).

Whereas NHEJ occurs in all phases of the cell cycle, HR is particularly important in the S/G2 transition of the cell cycle.

HR is a slow, high-fidelity repair pathway. Regions of DNA homology—usually the sister chromatid—are used as the template. During HR, activated ATM recruits endonucleases that process broken ends, which ultimately creates single-stranded 3′ ends. For the processing, the MRN complex is required. In concert with BRCA1, BRCA2, and Rad51 paralogues (XRCC2, XRCC3, Rad51B, Rad51C, Rad51D, Rad52, Rad54), the Rad51 protein binds to single-stranded DNA with the aid of replication protein A and searches for a homologous sequence on the sister chromatid. On strand invasion, Rad51 enables the formation of a temporary triple helix. Once the complementary strands have paired, the 3′ end of the damaged DNA will be elongated by polymerases (not yet identified) beyond the position of the former DSB. When the 3′ single strand of the second end of the DSB also invades the structure, a quadruple-helix is formed called a *Holliday junction,* which can be extended in both directions. After the gap has been safely bridged (usually about 50 base pairs will be copied), the Holliday junction is resolved, and the remaining nicks are sealed by a DNA ligase (not yet identified).

NHEJ is a fast but error-prone, and thus potentially mutagenic, repair pathway that rejoins DNA ends, usually after removal of a limited number of base pairs. NHEJ is initiated by the Ku70/Ku80 heterodimer, which binds to DNA ends and recruits the DNA-PK_{CS}. DNA-PK_{CS} can phosphorylate a variety of repair proteins such as Ku, x-ray cross-complementation protein 4 (XRCC-4), Artemis, p53, or replication protein A. However, only the autophosphorylation has been identified as being essential for repair. Artemis, in concert with DNA-PK_{CS}, trims the DSB ends for subsequent processing. After release of DNA-PK_{CS} from the DNA, the end will be bridged by the complex

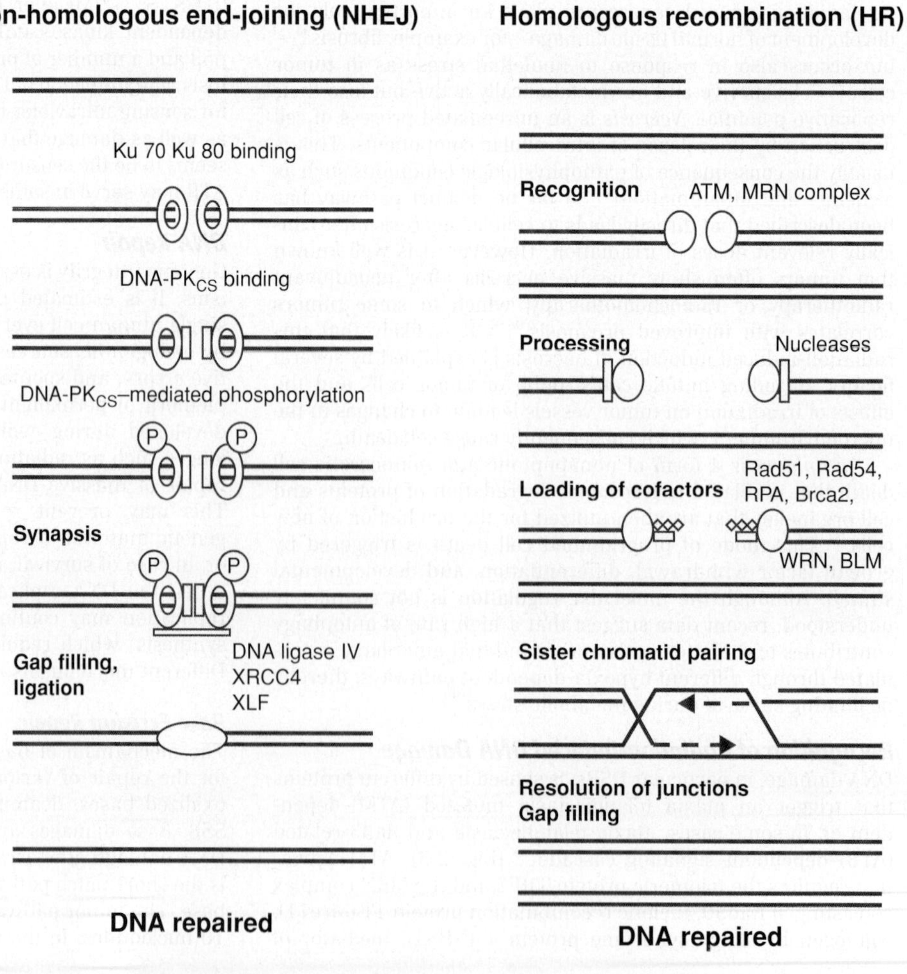

FIGURE 3.4. Mechanisms of DNA double-strand break repair in mammalian cells.

of ligase IV/XRCC-4/XRCC-4-like factor (XLF), which also performs the final ligation step. It has been observed that NHEJ can, to some extent, occur in the absence of several core proteins. This gave raise to the idea of a backup pathway that only operates when the DNA-PK–dependent NHEJ fails.[111] Recent data suggest that, besides the genuine repair proteins, the tumor suppressor p53 is involved in controlling the repair. P53 appears to suppress both HR and NHEJ in case error-free repair is not possible and thereby reduces the mutagenic risk of error-prone repair.[112]

Despite our molecular knowledge about DSB repair, the impact of the chromatin organization on DSB induction and repair has only recently been recognized.[113,114,115,116] Chromatin is organized as euchromatin and heterochromatin, representing loose and condensed DNA areas, respectively. While DSBs in euchromatin are easily accessible for repair proteins, DSBs in heterochromatic DNA regions need to be moved to less condensed areas for efficient repair.[114,116] Key molecules involved in this differential chromatin-dependent processes are ATM in association with heterochromatic marker proteins like KAP-1 and 53BP-1 and certain types of histones.[113,115]

Radiation-Induced Cell Cycle Delay

It has long been recognized that radiation-induced DNA damage is associated with delay in the cell cycle, which has been interpreted as allowing additional time for the cells to repair. Most recent findings show that DSBs can be found in all cell cycle phases, suggesting incomplete repair before entering the next phase. For example, tracking of radiation-induced γH2AX foci, representing DSBs, revealed transfer of DSBs induced in the G1 cell cycle phase to daughter cells.[117]

G1 Phase

The G1 cell cycle checkpoint prevents damaged DNA from being replicated and is the best understood checkpoint in mammalian cells.[118] Radiation-induced G1 phase cell cycle arrest is regulated by p53 (Fig. 3.5). Loss of p53 function, which is found in the majority of tumors, leads to a lack of G1-phase arrest. Instead, these cells exert a dose-dependent blockage in the G2 and M phases of the cell cycle. Central to the G1 checkpoint is the accumulation and activation of the p53 protein, which is controlled by the ATM and ATR kinases. These kinases, together with DNA-PK, are activated by and recruited to radiation-induced DNA lesions. Physiologically, p53 expression levels are low due to interaction with its negative regulator MDM2, which targets p53 for nuclear export and proteasome-mediated degradation in the cytoplasm.[119] Following radiation-induced DNA damage, ATM activates the downstream cell cycle checkpoint kinase Chk2 by phosphorylation at position Thr68,[120] which in turn phosphorylates amino acid residue Ser20 of p53. This results in a pronounced tetramerization, activity, and stability. The p53-Ser20 phosphorylation inhibits p53/MDM2 interaction, resulting in p53 accumulation. Moreover, ATM exerts p53 stability by directly phosphorylating MDM2 on Ser395.[121] Although it allows maintenance of MDM2/p53 interaction, this event prevents p53 nuclear export to the cytoplasm for degradation. *In vitro* studies showed Ser20 phosphorylation of p53 by the ATR-related cell cycle checkpoint–dependent kinase Chk1.[122] Transcriptional transactivation activity is mediated via Ser15 phosphorylation of p53.[123] Both ATM and ATR are able to directly phosphorylate this residue in response to irradiation. P53 target genes include several genes that are involved in the DNA damage response (e.g., MDM2, GADD45a, $p21^{Cip1}$). Accumulation of the cyclin-dependent kinase inhibitor $p21^{Cip1}$ blocks G1/S-phase progression by binding to the cyclinE/cdk2 complex, reducing cdk2 activity, which has an important function in phosphorylation of pRB.

S Phase

After irradiation, the rate of DNA synthesis is decreased via ATM- and NBS1-dependent pathways.[124] Radiation-induced DNA

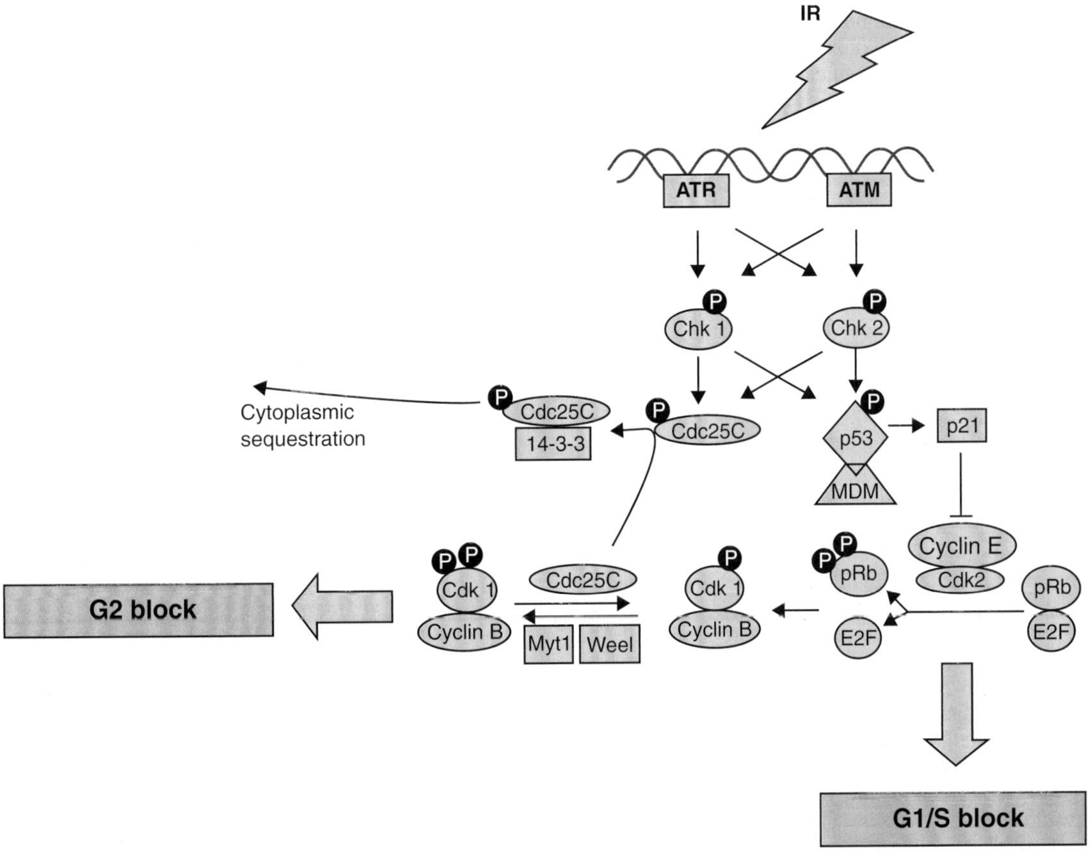

FIGURE 3.5. Pathways involved in radiation-induced G1/S and G2 cell cycle blocks. ATR, ataxia telangiectasia and Rad3–related; ATM, ataxia telangiectasia–mutated; IR, ionizing radiation.

damage activates ATM for Thr68 phosphorylation of Chk2.[125] Activated Chk2 targets CDC25A phosphatase for ubiquitination. As a result of CDC25A degradation, inhibitory phosphorylations of Cdk2 reside at Thr14 and Tyr15. The Cdk2/cyclin E and Cdk2/cyclin A complexes remain inactive, which prevents completion of DNA synthesis and G2 entry. Alternatively, radiation-activated ATM phosphorylates several downstream substrates, including BRCA1 at Ser1387, NBS1 at Ser343, and SMC1 at Ser957 and Ser966.[125,126] ATR phosphorylates the cell cycle checkpoint kinase Chk1 at Ser317 and Ser345. Subsequently, Chk1 phosphorylates CDC25A, which results in cytoplasmic sequestration and thereby in inhibition of S–G2 transition.[127]

G2 Phase

In contrast to the G1 checkpoint, all mammalian cells, normal or transformed, undergo cell cycle arrest in G2 after radiation-induced damage.[128] The G2 cell cycle checkpoint is the essential final determinant allowing cells to divide. The entry into mitosis is regulated by the activity of the cyclin-dependent kinase Cdk1[129] (Fig. 3.5). Phosphorylation of Thr14 and Tyr15 of Cdk1 blocks cell cycling into G2. These phosphorylations are removed by the phosphatase CDC25C. After irradiation, ATR and ATM activate the downstream checkpoint kinases Chk1 and Chk2, which phosphorylate CDC25C at Ser216.[130] This results in binding of 14-3-3 proteins. The CDC25C/14-3-3 protein complex is translocated into the cytoplasm for sequestration. As a consequence of this CDC25C degradation, Cdk1 remains phosphorylated, thereby preventing entry into mitosis. ATM appears to be more dominant at the early stage of G2/M checkpoint activation, whereas ATR seems to contribute mainly to sustained checkpoint events.[131]

Radiation-Induced Gene Expression

Radiation may modify gene expression.[132] Many of the transcriptionally activated proteins have been shown to be centrally involved in the pathogenesis of radiation damage or to modulate the effect of radiation on tumor cells. Early responses may occur within hours after irradiation and involve mostly transcription factors such as the proto-oncogenes jun, fos, junB, and early growth response gene 1 (Egr1).[133] Sustained activation of early radiation response genes such as NFκB may contribute to late radiation damage.[134] Other examples of radiation-induced genes that may occur early and/or late after irradiation include TGF-*β*, TNF-*α*, bFGF, PDGF, and interleukin 1 (IL-1).

Induction of *jun* is partly mediated by protein kinase C[133] and by reactive oxygen intermediates.[135] In addition to transcriptional activation, prolongation of the half-life of jun has also been observed.[136] Jun and fos form a heterodimer that represents the transcription factor *AP-1*. This transcription factor is a central regulator of cell proliferation, differentiation, and death.[137] For example, activation of AP-1 results in transcriptional suppression of MAPK phosphatases.[138] Furthermore, AP-1 appears to be an important regulator of the transcription of other radiation-induced genes, such as in the early transcription of TGF-*β*.[139] Redox-dependent DNA-binding activity of AP-1 is regulated by the DNA repair protein Ref-1.[140]

Gene expression and DNA-binding activity of *NFκB* are induced soon after ionizing radiation.[141] NFκB is a sequence-specific DNA-binding protein complex that binds to DNA as a dimer. Five mammalian proteins have been identified that belong to this family: NFκB1 (p50 and its precursor p105), NFκB2 (p52 and its precursor p100), c-Rel, RelA (p65), and RelB.[142] The most frequently occurring dimer is p50/p65. In the nonactivated state, this dimer is retained in the cytoplasm by binding to its inhibitor IκB (inhibitor of NFκB). On activation of the NFκB pathway, IκB is phosphorylated by a kinase complex named IκB kinase (*IKK*), consisting of the three subunits—*α*, *β*, and *γ*. According to its multiple functions, NFκB can also be activated by a variety of agents, like membrane receptors such as TNFR or Toll-like receptors and oxidative stress. Radiation-induced activation of NFκB is mediated by IKK.[143] This response does not depend on a nuclear signal, as it also occurs in enucleated cells.[144] However, it has been shown that ATM is required for chronic activation of the transcription factor NFκB.[145] NFκB acts in an antiapoptotic way and mediates radioresistance.[146]

Radiation exposure induces immediate and sustained *TGFβ1* gene expression, as well as activation of this cytokine.[147] On transcriptional activation TGF-*β* is produced as an inactive latent form and secreted. Latent TGF-*β* is stored in the extracellular matrix and proteolytically activated in irradiated tissues.[148] Active TGF-*β*1 binds and activates the TGF-*β*1 type I receptor, resulting in TGF-*β*1–dependent gene expression, inducing, for example, p21, p27, collagen, and TIMP.[11,139] This is most likely responsible for the cellular effects of TGF-*β*, such as modulation of proliferation, differentiation, and radiation sensitivity of fibroblasts, and for the biochemical events (e.g., collagen deposition, characteristic of radiation-induced fibrosis). In addition, TGF-*β* secreted by tumor cells on irradiation might contribute to the development of radiation-induced fibrosis.[149] Intervention of TGF-*β*–mediated effects (e.g., by TGF-*β*1–neutralizing antibodies and superoxide dismutase) offers a promising strategy to prevent radiation-induced fibrosis. Aside from fibrosis, TGF-*β* has been demonstrated to reduce latency, promote aggressive tumor growth, and increase estrogen receptor–negative breast cancers.[150] Moreover, the radiosensitivity of cancer cells can be enhanced by TGF-*β*–directed treatments.[151,152]

TNF-α belongs to the group of proinflammatory cytokines involved in radiation-induced normal tissue damage, such as pneumonitis and lung fibrosis. Immediately after irradiation, TNF-*α* is transcriptionally upregulated and released by the bronchiolar epithelium. TNF-*α* enhances phagocytosis and cytotoxicity by neutrophilic granulocytes and modulates the expression of other cytokines such as IL-1 and IL-6.[153] Experimental data show that also tumor lines, particularly pediatric sarcomas, may produce large quantities of bioactive TNF-*α* after irradiation. This may be of potential importance for tumor response and for normal tissue reactions after radiotherapy.[154]

Induction of genes by ionizing radiation has been experimentally exploited for therapy. For example, the early-response gene Egr1 was inserted upstream to TNF-*α*, which may act as a radiosensitizer. This provides a strategy for spatial and temporal control of the biologic effect by radiotherapy.[132,155]

Radiation Effects on Signal Transduction

Ionizing radiation may activate intracellular signaling.[156] The general mechanisms of activation involve the dose-dependent production of ROS and reactive nitrogen species (RNS), which stimulate, for example, cytoplasmic protein kinases, phosphatases, and cell membrane receptors or disturb, for example, lipid and protein metabolism.[157] Many signaling pathways are simultaneously activated in a dose- and cell type–dependent manner, which may contribute to different radiation responses in different cell types. Cooperative and mutual cross-talk occurs between parallel and upstream and downstream signaling routes.[158] Examples of important intracellular signaling pathways and their modulation by ionizing radiation are discussed in the following paragraphs.

EGFR-Mediated Signaling

The EGFR family belongs to the group of RTKs and consists of four different single receptors (EGFR/ErbB-1, HER2/ErbB-2, HER3/ErbB-3, and HER4/ErbB-4) that are dimerized after ligand binding to the extracellular domain.[159] In addition to activation through its natural ligands such as EGF, TGF-*α*, or amphiregulin and transactivation by cell adhesion molecules like integrins or immunoglobulin-like receptors,[160] ionizing radiation is able to stimulate EGFR.[161] Radiation doses of 1 to 2 Gy activate the EGFR and its downstream signaling cascades with similar efficiency as physiologic EGF concentrations of 0.1 to 1 nM. Radiation-dependent production of ROS/RNS seems to play a critical role in EGFR activation and downstream signaling via MAPK.[157,162] It was shown that protein tyrosine phosphatases contain ROS/RNS–sensitive cysteine residues at a site essential for phosphatase activity. Thus, the radiation-dependent activation of EGFR is likely to be controlled by ROS/RNS–regulated protein phosphatases. In addition, paracrine and autocrine activation of the EGFR can also result from radiation-induced release of TGF-α from irradiated cells or by release of growth factors stored in the extracellular matrix as result of activation of matrix-degrading proteases.[163–165]

EGFR signaling via Ras-Raf-MAPK after irradiation has been implicated in increased proliferation,[166] which corresponds to observations that EGFR overexpression is associated with repopulation during fractionated irradiation.[167,168–169] In addition, EGFR-dependent signaling via PI3K/Akt has been associated with increased cellular survival and cell cycle progression.[170,171] Another EGFR downstream pathway represents the c-Src–mediated activation of STAT3. STAT3 is involved in the TGF-α–mediated autocrine growth[172] and contributes to the regulation of angiogenesis by production of VEGF.[173] After radiation-induced activation, the EGFR is internalized and may function as a nuclear transcription factor.[174] In addition, internalized EGFR can activate DNA-PK. Pharmacologic inhibitors can block EGFR signaling at different levels and thereby influence several mechanisms of radioresistance, such as DNA repair, repopulation, antiapoptotic signaling, and tumor hypoxia.[18] The specific mutational status of the cells—for example, Ras mutations[164,175]—and the class of drugs[176,177] may critically modify effects of EGFR inhibition on radiation response. The concept of EGFR inhibition to improve outcome of radiotherapy has been proven recently in a phase III clinical trial.[17] However, considerable intertumoral heterogeneity has been observed, which is mechanistically only partly understood.[19] An important variant of the EGFR for radiation oncology is the constitutively active, truncated EGFRvIII, which is coexpressed with EGFR in a significant proportion of solid tumors.[178] EGFRvIII lacks the ability of EGF binding due to a deletion of the NH_2-terminal domain but, like wild-type EGFR, can be activated by irradiation.[179] Evidence suggests that EGFRvIII has altered signaling properties compared to normal EGF receptor and represents a cancer cell–specific target.[178] Experimental data indicate that activation of EGFRvIII leads to more-pronounced cytoprotective responses to radiation than wild-type EGFR.[179]

Ras Signaling

Mutant, constitutively active Ras, an important component of the MAPK pathway, has been found in many types of human cancers. Farnesyltransferase inhibitors (FTIs) can effectively block Ras-mediated signal transduction.[180] Application of FTI renders cells more sensitive to ionizing radiation. Combination of FTI with radiotherapy is under preclinical and clinical investigation.[38,181]

PDGF-Mediated Signaling

Radiation-induced autocrine and paracrine PDGF signaling plays an important role in fibroblast and endothelial cell activation and proliferation *in vitro*.[182] Combination of irradiation with PGDFR tyrosine kinase inhibitors resulted in decreased clonogenic survival of endothelial cells and fibroblasts *in vitro*.[182] Recent data suggest that inhibition of PDGFR signaling may attenuate development of radiation-induced pulmonary fibrosis.[183]

VEGFR-Mediated Signaling

Transmembrane receptors for VEGF and related ligands include VEGFR-1 (Flt-1), VEGFR-2 (KDR/Flk-1), VEGFR-3 (Flt-4), neuropilin-1, and neuropilin-2.[184] On irradiation, VEGF is upregulated via the EGFR/STAT signaling and released by tumor cells and exerts, via VEGFR/PI3K/Akt signaling, prosurvival stimuli on tumor and endothelial cells.[185] Upregulated VEGFR expression has been found after ionizing irradiation.[186,187] Besides normalizing the tumor micromilieu,[188] inhibition of radiation-induced VEGF/VEGFR signaling represents the rationale for combining anti-VEGF strategies with radiotherapy, which is under preclinical and clinical investigation.[189]

Cyclooxygenase-Mediated Signaling

The rate-limiting enzyme in the synthesis of prostaglandins is cyclooxygenase (COX). Two isoforms exist, COX-1 and COX-2. COX-2 is typically not expressed or is expressed at relatively low levels in normal tissues but overexpressed in 40% to 80% of cancers of the lung, colon, head and neck, breast, prostate, brain, and pancreas.[190] Among other stimuli, irradiation has been shown to upregulate expression of COX-2 in tumors and normal tissues.[191,192] COX-2 expression correlates with worse outcome after radiotherapy in patients.[193,194] Specific inhibition of COX-2 has been demonstrated to enhance radiation responses of tumor cells *in vivo* and *in vitro*.[195] Several mechanisms, including reduced angiogenesis, increased apoptosis, and immune responses, have been implicated in the radiosensitizing effects of COX-2 inhibitors. Recent experimental data suggest that inhibition of DNA repair by COX-2 inhibitors via downregulation of Ku70, and thereby inhibition of $DNA\text{-}PK_{CS}$, contributes significantly to the radiosensitizing effects.[196] Furthermore, COX-2 inhibitors appear to attenuate radiation gene expression via inhibition of NFκB.[196] Ongoing early clinical trials in combination with radiotherapy indicate feasibility of this approach,[197,198] although conflicting data exist[199] and efficacy at least for combination with radiochemotherapy in unselected non–small cell lung cancer patients may be questionable.[200]

Integrin-Mediated Signaling

Interactions between cells and ECM proteins are facilitated mainly by the integrin family of cell adhesion molecules.[201] Besides the influence of growth factors and cytokines, these interactions add a further facet to the network of microenvironmental factors that modulate the cellular behavior on exposure to ionizing radiation (Fig. 3.6). Chemotherapeutic compounds, as well as ionizing radiation, showed less cytotoxic efficacy in cells adherent to ECM compared to cells growing in suspension or on plastic surfaces.[202] Resistance-promoting effects by integrin-mediated adhesion to ECM were found in cell lines from solid tumors of the lung,[203,204] breast,[205] liver,[206] colon, pancreas,[202,207,208] ovary,[209] prostate,[210] brain,[211] and leukemia cells.[212] Certain integrins seem to communicate increased radiation and drug resistance, which is cooperatively influenced by RTKs like EGFR.[213] For example, $\alpha5\beta1$ integrin, the "classic" fibronectin receptor, acts as a major antagonist of cell death induced by doxorubicin or melphalan in multiple myeloma,[214] by paclitaxel in breast cancer or small cell and non–small cell lung cancer,[215,216] or by cisplatin or mitomycin C in non–small cell lung cancer.[215] Additional studies underscored the important role of $\beta1$ integrins in promoting resistance against ionizing radiation on the basis of signaling events via the adaptor proteins paxillin and p130Cas to the survival-regulating protein kinase JNK.[217,218] Further regulatory cytoplasmic cascades downstream of $\beta1$ integrins that exert survival advantage on treatment with genotoxic agents included regulation of the Akt1/FoxO cascade by the adaptor protein PINCH1,[219] the proapoptotic proteins Bim and Bax,[220,221] and the antiapoptotic Bcl-2–like proteins or Bcl-2/Bax.[212] In addition to regulating cell survival, cell–matrix interactions affect radiation-induced cell cycle arrest, that is, adhesion of cells to matrix proteins prolongs the G1 and G2 cell cycle blockage in parallel with enhanced activation of DNA repair pathways involving the checkpoint kinases Chk1, Chk2, and Cdk1, p53, and diverse cyclins.[215,222–224]

Following radiation exposure, the expression of several integrin subunits, including $\beta1$, $\beta3$, $\alpha5$, and αv, is upregulated in human skin and lung fibroblasts,[202] endothelial cells, and keratinocytes,[225] as well as in tumor cells of the colon,

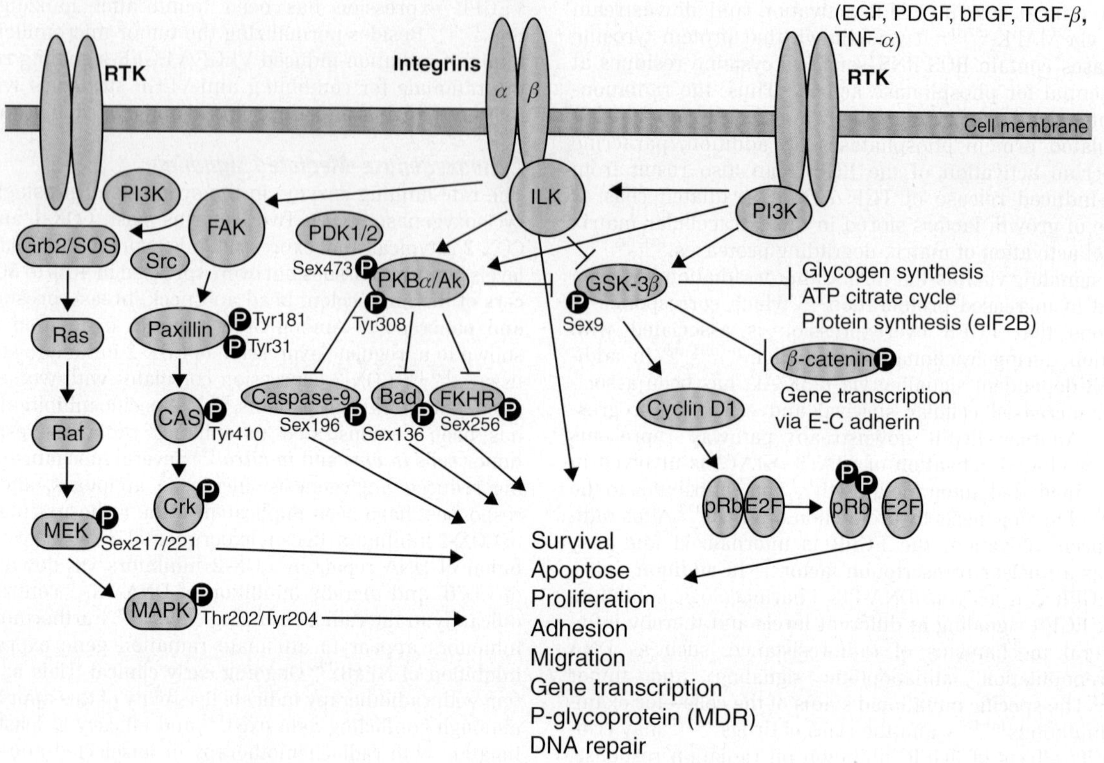

FIGURE 3.6. Cross-talk between receptor tyrosine kinase (RTK) and integrin-mediated signaling.

hematopoietic cells,[226] prostate,[227] lung,[228] brain,[229] and melanomas.[202] Generally, integrin-mediated adhesion to matrix proteins confers chemoresistance and radioresistance.[212,213,230]

Mutagenesis and Genomic Instability

Cells may survive radiation despite unrepaired or misrepaired DNA damage, that is, with mutations or chromosomal aberrations. These may remain silent or result in radiation-related secondary primary cancers or, as germline mutations, cause hereditary disease.[231–233] In addition to directly induced mutations, radiation may induce a heritable, genome-wide process of instability (i.e., genomic instability) that leads to an enhanced frequency of genetic changes occurring among the progeny of the original irradiated cell, which is transmissible over many generations of cell replication.[234] Whereas most mutations induced directly by radiation involve loss of large parts of the tested gene, leading to a loss of heterozygosity, most mutations resulting from radiation-induced genomic instability involve point mutations and small deletions.[234,235] While some studies, particularly on thyroid cancer in children after the Chernobyl fallout, suggest a nonrandom pattern of chromosomal damage, generally no fingerprint alterations have been identified that would unequivocally indicate radiation-induced cancer.[233]

SELECTED REFERENCES

A full list of references for this chapter is available online.

1. Baumann M. Keynote comment: radiotherapy in the age of molecular oncology. *Lancet Oncol* 2006;7:786–787.
2. Okunieff P, Chen Y, Maguire DJ, et al. Molecular markers of radiation-related normal tissue toxicity. *Cancer Metastasis Rev* 2008;27:363–374.
3. Bentzen SM. Preventing or reducing late side effects of radiation therapy: radiobiology meets molecular pathology. *Nat Rev Cancer* 2006;6:702–713.
4. Grade M, Becker H, Ghadimi BM. The impact of molecular pathology in oncology: the clinician's perspective. *Cell Oncol* 2004;26:275–278.
5. Vaupel P. Tumor microenvironmental physiology and its implications for radiation oncology. *Semin Radiat Oncol* 2004;14:198–206.
6. Bentzen SM, Gregoire V. Molecular imaging–based dose painting: a novel paradigm for radiation therapy prescription. *Semin Radiat Oncol* 2011;21:101–110.
7. Coleman CN. Linking radiation oncology and imaging through molecular biology (or now that therapy and diagnosis have separated, it's time to get together again!). *Radiology* 2003;228:29–35.
8. Bussink J, Kaanders JH, van der Graaf WT, et al. PET-CT for radiotherapy treatment planning and response monitoring in solid tumors. *Nat Rev Clin Oncol* 2011; 8:233–242.
9. Wilson GD, Bentzen SM, Harari PM. Biologic basis for combining drugs with radiation. *Semin Radiat Oncol* 2006;16:2–9.
10. Begg AC, Stewart FA, Vens C. Strategies to improve radiotherapy with targeted drugs. *Nat Rev Cancer* 2011;11:239–253.
13. Baumann M, Krause M, Hill R. Exploring the role of cancer stem cells in radioresistance. *Nat Rev Cancer* 2008;8:545–554.
14. Baumann M, Krause M, Thames H, Trott K, Zips D. Cancer stem cells and radiotherapy. *Int J Radiat Biol* 2009:1–12.
15. Ma BB, Bristow RG, Kim J, et al. Combined-modality treatment of solid tumors using radiotherapy and molecular targeted agents. *J Clin Oncol* 2003;21:2760–2776.
16. Bonner JA, Harari PM, Giralt JL. Cetuximab (Erbitux TM) prolongs survival in patients with locally advanced squamous cell carcinoma of the head and neck: a phase III study of high dose radiation therapy with and without cetuximab. *Proc Am Soc Clin Oncol* 2004;22:abstract 5507.
17. Bonner JA, Harari PM, Giralt J, et al. Radiotherapy plus cetuximab for locoregionally advanced head and neck cancer: 5-year survival data from a phase 3 randomised trial, and relation between cetuximab-induced rash and survival. *Lancet Oncol* 2010;11:21–28.
18. Baumann M, Krause M, Dikomey E, et al. EGFR-targeted anti-cancer drugs in radiotherapy: preclinical evaluation of mechanisms. *Radiother Oncol* 2007; 83:238–248.
19. Krause M, Gurtner K, Deuse Y, et al. Heterogeneity of tumour response to combined radiotherapy and EGFR inhibitors: differences between antibodies and TK inhibitors. *Int J Radiat Biol* 2009;85:943–954.
20. Sarasin A. An overview of the mechanisms of mutagenesis and carcinogenesis. *Mutat Res* 2003;544:99–106.
22. Sharma S, Kelly TK, Jones PA. Epigenetics in cancer. Carcinogenesis 2010; 31:27–36.
23. Chen R, Aaltonen LM, Vaheri A. Human papillomavirus type 16 in head and neck carcinogenesis. *Rev Med Virol* 2005;15:351–363.
25. Vaupel P, Harrison L. Tumor hypoxia: causative factors, compensatory mechanisms, and cellular response. *Oncologist* 2004;9(Suppl 5):4–9.
30. Hanahan D, Weinberg RA. The hallmarks of cancer. *Cell* 2000;100:57–70.
31. Hanahan D, Weinberg RA. Hallmarks of cancer: the next generation. *Cell* 2011; 144:646–674.
32. Vermeulen K, Van Bockstaele DR, Berneman ZN. The cell cycle: a review of regulation, deregulation and therapeutic targets in cancer. *Cell Prolif* 2003;36:131–149.
35. Blume-Jensen P, Hunter T. Oncogenic kinase signalling. *Nature* 2001;411:355–365.
36. Yarden Y, Sliwkowski MX. Untangling the ErbB signalling network. *Nat Rev Mol Cell Biol* 2001;2:127–137.
38. Brunner TB, Hahn SM, Gupta AK, et al.. Farnesyltransferase inhibitors: an overview of the results of preclinical and clinical investigations. *Cancer Res* 2003;63:5656–5668.

39. Beeram M, Patnaik A, Rowinsky EK. Raf: a strategic target for therapeutic development against cancer. *J Clin Oncol* 2005;23:6771–6790.
40. Fresno Vara JA, Casado E, de Castro J, et al. PI3K/Akt signalling pathway and cancer. *Cancer Treat Rev* 2004;30:193–204.
41. Sansal I, Sellers WR. The biology and clinical relevance of the PTEN tumor suppressor pathway. *J Clin Oncol* 2004;22:2954–2963.
42. Bjornsti MA, Houghton PJ. The TOR pathway: a target for cancer therapy. *Nat Rev Cancer* 2004;4:335–348.
45. Karim R, Tse G, Putti T, et al. The significance of the Wnt pathway in the pathology of human cancers. *Pathology* 2004;36:120–128.
46. Wend P, Holland JD, Ziebold U, et al. Wnt signaling in stem and cancer stem cells. *Semin Cell Dev Biol* 2010;21:855–863.
51. Knudsen ES, Knudsen KE. Tailoring to RB: tumour suppressor status and therapeutic response. *Nat Rev Cancer* 2008;8:714–724.
53. Brown JM, Attardi LD. The role of apoptosis in cancer development and treatment response. *Nat Rev Cancer* 2005;5:231–237.
56. Petitjean A, Achatz MI, Borresen-Dale AL, et al. TP53 mutations in human cancers: functional selection and impact on cancer prognosis and outcomes. *Oncogene* 2007;26:2157–2165.
57. Meulmeester E, Ten Dijke P. The dynamic roles of TGF-beta in cancer. *J Pathol* 2011;223:205–218.
58. Collado M, Serrano M. Senescence in tumours: evidence from mice and humans. *Nat Rev Cancer* 2010;10:51–57.
61. Clarke MF, Dick JE, Dirks PB, et al. Cancer stem cells—perspectives on current status and future directions: AACR Workshop on Cancer Stem Cells. *Cancer Res* 2006;66:9339–9344.
63. Folkman J. Role of angiogenesis in tumor growth and metastasis. *Semin Oncol* 2002;29:15–18.
66. Bergers G, Benjamin LE. Tumorigenesis and the angiogenic switch. *Nat Rev Cancer* 2003;3:401–410.
68. Folkman J. Tumor angiogenesis: therapeutic implications. *N Engl J Med* 1971;285:1182–1186.
69. Gaur P, Bose D, Samuel S, Ellis LM. Targeting tumor angiogenesis. *Semin Oncol* 2009;36:S12–S19.
70. Hunter K. Host genetics influence tumour metastasis. *Nat Rev Cancer* 2006;6:141–146.
71. Albini A, Mirisola V, Pfeffer U. Metastasis signatures: genes regulating tumor–microenvironment interactions predict metastatic behavior. *Cancer Metastasis Rev* 2008;27:75–83.
76. Bourboulia D, Stetler-Stevenson WG. Matrix metalloproteinases (MMPs) and tissue inhibitors of metalloproteinases (TIMPs): positive and negative regulators in tumor cell adhesion. *Semin Cancer Biol* 2010;20:161–168.
77. Cavallaro U, Christofori G. Cell adhesion and signalling by cadherins and Ig-CAMs in cancer. *Nat Rev Cancer* 2004;4:118–132.
79. Danen EH. Integrins: regulators of tissue function and cancer progression. *Curr Pharm Des* 2005;11:881–891.
81. Herrlich P, Morrison H, Sleeman J, et al. CD44 acts both as a growth- and invasiveness-promoting molecule and as a tumor-suppressing cofactor. *Ann N Y Acad Sci* 2000;910:106–118; discussion 118–120.
84. Wright EA, Howard-Flanders P. The influence of oxygen on the radiosensitivity of mammalian tissues. *Acta Radiol* 1957;48:26–32.
85. Gray LH, Conger AD, Ebert M, et al. The concentration of oxygen dissolved in tissues at the time of irradiation as a factor in radiotherapy. *Br J Radiol* 1953;26:638–648.
86. Munro TR, Gilbert CW. The relation between tumour lethal doses and the radiosensitivity of tumour cells. *Br J Radiol* 1961;34:246–251.
88. Ward JF. DNA damage produced by ionizing radiation in mammalian cells: identities, mechanisms of formation, and reparability. *Prog Nucleic Acid Res Mol Biol* 1988;35:95–125.
90. Okada H, Mak TW. Pathways of apoptotic and non-apoptotic death in tumour cells. *Nat Rev Cancer* 2004;4:592–603.
91. Eriksson D, Stigbrand T. Radiation-induced cell death mechanisms. *Tumour Biol* 2010;31:363–372.
94. Rodemann HP, Bamberg M. Cellular basis of radiation-induced fibrosis. *Radiother Oncol* 1995;35:83–90.
95. Ewald JA, Desotelle JA, Wilding G, et al. Therapy-induced senescence in cancer. *J Natl Cancer Inst* 2010;102:1536–1546.
98. Chaachouay H, Ohneseit P, Toulany M, et al. Autophagy contributes to resistance of tumor cells to ionizing radiation. *Radiother Oncol* 2011;99:287–292.
99. Rouschop KM, Wouters BG. Regulation of autophagy through multiple independent hypoxic signaling pathways. *Curr Mol Med* 2009;9:417–424.
102. Khanna KK, Lavin MF, Jackson SP, et al. ATM, a central controller of cellular responses to DNA damage. *Cell Death Differ* 2001;8:1052–1065.
104. Helleday T, Lo J, van Gent DC, et al. DNA double-strand break repair: from mechanistic understanding to cancer treatment. *DNA Repair* (Amst) 2007;6:923–935.
105. Fortini P, Dogliotti E. Base damage and single-strand break repair: mechanisms and functional significance of short- and long-patch repair subpathways. *DNA Repair* (Amst) 2007;6:398–409.
106. Wilson DM 3rd, Bohr VA. The mechanics of base excision repair, and its relationship to aging and disease. *DNA Repair* (Amst) 2007;6:544–559.
109. Mladenov E, Iliakis G. Induction and repair of DNA double strand breaks: the increasing spectrum of non-homologous end joining pathways. *Mutat Res* 2011; 711:61–72.
110. Barker CA, Powell SN. Enhancing radiotherapy through a greater understanding of homologous recombination. *Semin Radiat Oncol* 2010;20:267–273.
111. Iliakis G. Backup pathways of NHEJ in cells of higher eukaryotes: cell cycle dependence. *Radiother Oncol* 2009;92:310–315.
113. Storch K, Eke I, Borgmann K, et al. Three-dimensional cell growth confers radioresistance by chromatin density modification. *Cancer Res* 2010;70:3925–3934.
115. Goodarzi AA, Noon AT, Deckbar D, et al. ATM signaling facilitates repair of DNA double-strand breaks associated with heterochromatin. *Mol Cell* 2008;31:167–177.
117. Deckbar D, Jeggo PA, Lobrich M. Understanding the limitations of radiation-induced cell cycle checkpoints. *Crit Rev Biochem Mol Biol* 2011;46:271–283.
124. Taylor AM, Groom A, Byrd PJ. Ataxia-telangiectasia–like disorder (ATLD)—its clinical presentation and molecular basis. *DNA Repair* (Amst) 2004;3:1219–1225.
125. Falck J, Mailand N, Syljuasen RG, et al. The ATM-Chk2-Cdc25A checkpoint pathway guards against radioresistant DNA synthesis. *Nature* 2001;410:842–847.
132. Kufe D, Weichselbaum R. Radiation therapy: activation for gene transcription and the development of genetic radiotherapy—therapeutic strategies in oncology. *Cancer Biol Ther* 2003;2:326–329.
139. Martin M, Lefaix J, Delanian S. TGF-beta1 and radiation fibrosis: a master switch and a specific therapeutic target? *Int J Radiat Oncol Biol Phys* 2000;47: 277–290.
142. Senftleben U, Karin M. The IKK/NF-kappaB pathway. *Crit Care Med* 2002;30: S18–S26.
148. Barcellos-Hoff MH. Integrative radiation carcinogenesis: interactions between cell and tissue responses to DNA damage. *Semin Cancer Biol* 2005;15:138–148.
149. Yarnold J, Brotons MC. Pathogenetic mechanisms in radiation fibrosis. *Radiother Oncol* 2010;97:149–161.
150. Nguyen TD, Panis X, Froissart D, et al. Analysis of late complications after rapid hyperfractionated radiotherapy in advanced head and neck cancers. *Int J Radiat Oncol Biol Phys* 1988;14:23–25.
155. Weichselbaum RR, Kufe DW, Hellman S, et al. Radiation-induced tumour necrosis factor-alpha expression: clinical application of transcriptional and physical targeting of gene therapy. *Lancet Oncol* 2002;3:665–671.
156. Schmidt-Ullrich RK, Dent P, Grant S, et al. Signal transduction and cellular radiation responses. *Radiat Res* 2000;153:245–257.
159. Hynes NE, Lane HA. ERBB receptors and cancer: the complexity of targeted inhibitors. *Nat Rev Cancer* 2005;5:341–354.
161. Schmidt-Ullrich RK, Valerie K, Fogleman PB, et al. Radiation-induced autophosphorylation of epidermal growth factor receptor in human malignant mammary and squamous epithelial cells. *Radiat Res* 1996;145:81–85.
168. Eriksen JG, Steiniche T, Askaa J, et al. The prognostic value of epidermal growth factor receptor is related to tumor differentiation and the overall treatment time of radiotherapy in squamous cell carcinomas of the head and neck. *Int J Radiat Oncol Biol Phys* 2004;58:561–566.
169. Bentzen SM, Atasoy BM, Daley FM, et al. Epidermal growth factor receptor expression in pretreatment biopsies from head and neck squamous cell carcinoma as a predictive factor for a benefit from accelerated radiation therapy in a randomized controlled trial. *J Clin Oncol* 2005;23:5560–5567.
170. Mendelsohn J, Baselga J. The EGF receptor family as targets for cancer therapy. *Oncogene* 2000;19:6550–6565.
171. Marmor MD, Skaria KB, Yarden Y. Signal transduction and oncogenesis by ErbB/HER receptors. *Int J Radiat Oncol Biol Phys* 2004;58:903–913.
174. Lin SY, Makino K, Xia W, et al. Nuclear localization of EGF receptor and its potential new role as a transcription factor. *Nat Cell Biol* 2001;3:802–808.
175. Toulany M, Dittmann K, Baumann M, Rodemann HP. Radiosensitization of Ras-mutated human tumor cells in vitro by the specific EGF receptor antagonist BIBX1382BS. *Radiother Oncol* 2005;74:117–129.
176. Krause M, Schutze C, Petersen C, et al. Different classes of EGFR inhibitors may have different potential to improve local tumour control after fractionated irradiation: a study on C225 in FaDu hSCC. *Radiother Oncol* 2005;74:109–115.
177. Gurtner K, Deuse Y, Butof R, et al. Diverse effects of combined radiotherapy and EGFR inhibition with antibodies or TK inhibitors on local tumour control and correlation with EGFR gene expression. *Radiother Oncol* 2011;99:323–330.
179. Lammering G, Hewit TH, Valerie K, et al. EGFRvIII-mediated radioresistance through a strong cytoprotective response. *Oncogene* 2003;22:5545–5553.
180. McKenna WG, Muschel RJ, Gupta AK, et al. The RAS signal transduction pathway and its role in radiation sensitivity. *Oncogene* 2003;22:5866–5875.
184. Cross MJ, Dixelius J, Matsumoto T, et al. VEGF–receptor signal transduction. *Trends Biochem Sci* 2003;28:488–494.
185. Wachsberger P, Burd R, Dicker AP. Tumor response to ionizing radiation combined with antiangiogenesis or vascular targeting agents: exploring mechanisms of interaction. *Clin Cancer Res* 2003;9:1957–1971.
189. O'Reilly MS. Radiation combined with antiangiogenic and antivascular agents. *Semin Radiat Oncol* 2006;16:45–50.
190. Milas L. Cyclooxygenase-2 (COX-2) enzyme inhibitors and radiotherapy: preclinical basis. *Am J Clin Oncol* 2003;26:S66–S69.
192. Jaal J, Dorr W. Radiation induced inflammatory changes in the mouse bladder: the role of cyclooxygenase-2. *J Urol* 2006;175:1529–1533.
193. Khor LY, Bae K, Pollack A, et al. COX-2 expression predicts prostate-cancer outcome: analysis of data from the RTOG 92-02 trial. *Lancet Oncol* 2007;8:912–920.
195. Petersen C, Petersen S, Milas L, et al. Enhancement of intrinsic tumor cell radiosensitivity induced by a selective cyclooxygenase-2 inhibitor. *Clin Cancer Res* 2000; 6:2513–2520.
201. Hynes RO. Integrins: bidirectional, allosteric signaling machines. *Cell* 2002;110: 673–687.
212. Damiano JS, Cress AE, Hazlehurst LA, et al. Cell adhesion mediated drug resistance (CAM-DR): role of integrins and resistance to apoptosis in human myeloma cell lines. *Blood* 1999;93:1658–1667.
214. Hazlehurst LA, Dalton WS. Mechanisms associated with cell adhesion mediated drug resistance (CAM-DR) in hematopoietic malignancies. *Cancer Metastasis Rev* 2001;20:43–50.
217. Cordes N, Seidler J, Durzok R, et al. beta1-integrin–mediated signaling essentially contributes to cell survival after radiation-induced genotoxic injury. *Oncogene* 2006;25:1378–1390.
220. Hazlehurst LA, Damiano JS, Buyuksal I, et al. Adhesion to fibronectin via beta1 integrins regulates p27kip1 levels and contributes to cell adhesion mediated drug resistance (CAM-DR). *Oncogene* 2000;19:4319–4327.
229. Cordes N, Hansmeier B, Beinke C, et al. Irradiation differentially affects substratum-dependent survival, adhesion, and invasion of glioblastoma cell lines. *Br J Cancer* 2003;89:2122–2132.
231. Allan JM, Travis LB. Mechanisms of therapy-related carcinogenesis. *Nat Rev Cancer* 2005;5:943–955.
232. Hall EJ. Intensity-modulated radiation therapy, protons, and the risk of second cancers. *Int J Radiat Oncol Biol Phys* 2006;65:1–7.
233. Trott KR, Rosemann M. Molecular mechanisms of radiation carcinogenesis and the linear, non-threshold dose response model of radiation risk estimation. *Radiat Environ Biophys* 2000;39:79–87.
234. Little JB. Induction of genetic instability by ionizing radiation. *C R Acad Sci III* 1999;322:127–134.
236. Brown JM, Wouters BG. Apoptosis, p53, and tumor cell sensitivity to anticancer agents. *Cancer Res* 1999;59:1391–1399.

Chapter 4
Molecular Pathophysiology of Tumors

Rakesh K. Jain and Dan G. Duda

A solid tumor is an organlike structure containing neoplastic and stromal cells nourished by the tumor vasculature composed of endothelial cells, basement membrane, and perivascular cells. All of these components are embedded in an extracellular matrix (Fig. 4.1). The interactions between these cells, their surrounding matrix, and their local microenvironment influence the expression of various genes. The products encoded by these genes, in turn, control the pathophysiologic characteristics of the tumor. The tumor pathophysiology affects tumor growth, invasion, and metastasis, as well as the response to radiation and other therapies. In this chapter, we will discuss various pathophysiologic parameters that characterize the vascular and extravascular compartments of a tumor as well as the molecular players involved in the formation and function of these compartments. Finally, we will point out some clinical implications of the findings and present a future perspective.

VASCULAR COMPARTMENT

Neoplastic cells, similar to normal cells, need oxygen and other nutrients for their survival and growth. Every reproductively intact normal cell in our body is located within 100 to 200 μm from a blood capillary so that it can receive adequate levels of oxygen and other nutrients by the process of diffusion. Likewise, cells undergoing neoplastic transformation depend on nearby capillaries for growth. These preneoplastic (i.e., dysplastic or hyperplastic) cells can grow as spherical or ellipsoidal cellular aggregates. However, once the size of the cellular aggregate reaches the diffusion limit for critical nutrients, the aggregate may become dormant. Indeed, human tumors may remain dormant for a number of years despite active cell proliferation because of a balance between proliferation and cell death. However, once they have access to new blood vessels, the tumor may grow and metastasize. What triggers the growth of new vessels? What molecular and cellular players are involved? How do these vessels compare with normal vessels with respect to their structure and function?

Angiogenesis

The fact that the vascular system is associated with tumor growth in animals and humans has been known for more than a century.[1] Ide et al.[2] and Algire and Chalkley[3] provided powerful insight into the neovascularization of transplanted tumors using transparent window techniques (for reviews on this subject, see [4,5]). In 1968 Rijhsinghani et al.[6] and Ehrmann and Knoth[7] suggested the possibility that tumors produce an "angiogenic" substance. In 1971, Folkman[8,9] proposed the hypothesis that blocking angiogenesis should block tumor growth and metastasis. In 1978, Gullino[10] demonstrated that a tissue acquires angiogenic capacity during neoplastic transformation and proposed that antiangiogenesis approaches be used to prevent cancer. Both of these hypotheses have been validated in a number of preclinical studies.[11,12] A wide range of antiangiogenic strategies are currently being evaluated in the clinic to prevent or treat a large number of diseases, including cancer.[11] Most importantly, antiangiogenic strategies have yielded overall survival benefits in patients with advanced colorectal cancer, non–small-cell lung cancer, renal cell cancer, hepatocellular carcinoma, and gastrointestinal stromal tumors and have shown increased response rates and progression-free survival benefits in advanced breast, medullary thyroid, and ovarian cancer; pancreatic neuroendocrine tumors (pNETs); and glioblastoma.[13–21,22] This has led so far to U.S. Food and Drug Administration (FDA) approval for eight antiangiogenic drugs in the treatment of these diseases (Table 4.1).

The net balance between pro- and antiangiogenic factors governs both normal and pathologic angiogenic processes.[11] This balance is spatially and temporally regulated under physiologic conditions so that the "angiogenic switch" is "on" when needed (e.g., during embryonic development, wound healing, formation of corpus luteum) and "off" otherwise. During neoplastic transformation and tumor progression, this regulation is deranged, which results in ectopically formed blood vessels to support the growing mass.[11]

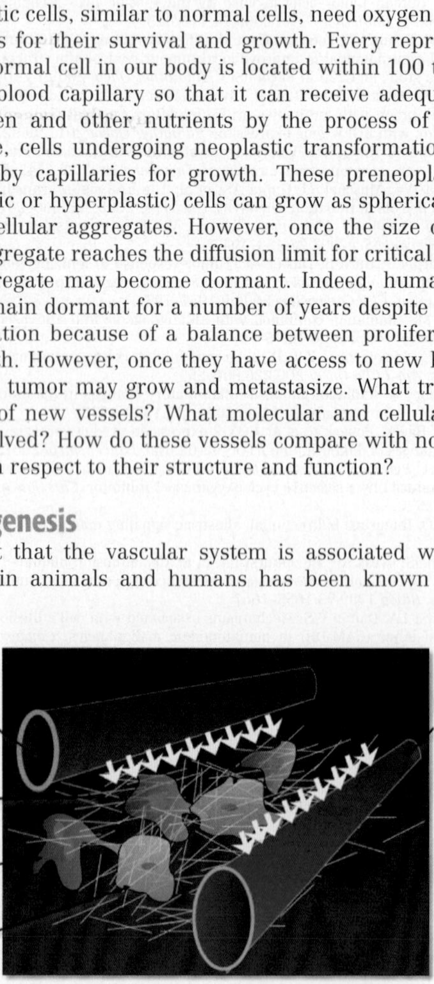

FIGURE 4.1. Schematic representation of a solid tumor–an organlike structure. The key components include cancer cells, host cells, and blood vasculature made of endothelial and perivascular cells–all embedded in a matrix bathed in interstitial fluid. The lymphatic vasculature, present in most normal tissues, is often lacking or is dysfunctional in solid tumors.

Cellular Mechanisms

Several cellular mechanisms have been described in the vascularization of tumors: (a) co-option, (b) intussusception, (c) sprouting (angiogenesis), (d) vasculogenesis from endothelial precursors, (e) cancer cell lining of vessels (vascular mimicry), or (f) transdifferentiation to the endothelial cell (Fig. 4.2).[11] Tumor cells can co-opt and grow around the existing vessels to form "perivascular" cuffs. However, as stated earlier, these cuffs cannot grow beyond the diffusion limit of critical nutrients, and they actually may cause the collapse of the vessels as a result of the growth pressure (referred to as "solid stress").[23,24,25] Alternatively, an existing vessel may enlarge in response to the growth factors released by tumors, and an interstitial tissue column may grow in the enlarged lumen and partition the lumen to form an expanded vascular network. This mode of intussusceptive microvascular growth has been observed during tumor growth, wound healing, and gene therapy.[26,27]

"Sprouting" angiogenesis is the most widely studied mechanism of vessel formation. During sprouting angiogenesis, the existing vessels become leaky in response to growth factors released by cancer or stromal cells; the basement membrane and the interstitial matrix dissolve; the pericytes dissociate from the vessel; endothelial cells (ECs) migrate and proliferate to form an array/sprout; a lumen is formed in the sprout (referred to as canalization); branches and loops are formed by confluence and anastomoses of sprouts to permit blood flow; and, finally, these

TABLE 4.1 FDA-APPROVED ANTI-ANGIOGENIC DRUGS

Drug	Approved Indication	Improvement in RR* (%)	Improvement in PFS* (months)	Improvement in OS* (months)
Bevacizumab	Metastatic colorectal cancer (with chemotherapy)	10	4.4	4.7
		0	1.4	1.4
		7.8	2.8	2.5
		14.1	2.6	2.1
	Metastatic non-squamous NSCLC (with chemotherapy)	20	1.7	2.0
		10.3–14.0	0.4–0.6	NS
	Metastatic breast cancer (with chemotherapy)	15.7	5.9	NS
		9–18	0.8–1.9	NS
		11.8–13.4	1.2–2.9	NS
		9.9	2.1	NS
	Recurrent GBM (monotherapy)		Currently only phase 2 data reported	
	Metastatic RCC (with IFNα)	18	4.8	NS
		12.4	3.3	NS
Sunitinib	Metastatic RCC	35	6.0	4.6
	GIST	6.8	4.5	NS
	PNET	9.3	4.8	?
Sorafenib	Metastatic RCC	8	2.7	NS
	Unresectable HCC	1	NS	2.8
	Unresectable HCC	2	1.4	2.3
Pazopanib	Metastatic RCC	27	5.0	N/A
	Advanced soft tissue sarcoma	6.0	3.0	NS
Vandetanib	Advanced medullary thyroid cancer	43	6.2	N/A
Axitinib	Advanced RCC	10	2.0	N/A
Regorafenib	Chemo-refractory metastatic colorectal cancer	0.6	0.2	1.4
Aflibercept	Chemo-refractory metastatic colorectal cancer	8.7	2.2	1.4

Updated from Carmeliet & Jain, *Nature* (2011).

immature vessels are invested in basement membrane and pericytes. During physiologic angiogenesis, these vessels differentiate into mature arterioles, capillaries, and venules, whereas in tumors they may remain immature.[5,11,28]

During mammalian embryonic development, a primitive vascular plexus is formed from angioblasts or endothelial precursor cells (EPCs) by a process referred to as vasculogenesis. Distinct signals specify arterial or venous differentiation.[29] Several studies showed that circulating EPCs mobilized from the bone marrow or peripheral blood also can contribute to postnatal vasculogenesis in tumors and other tissues.[30] Although debated, the repair of healthy adult vessels or the

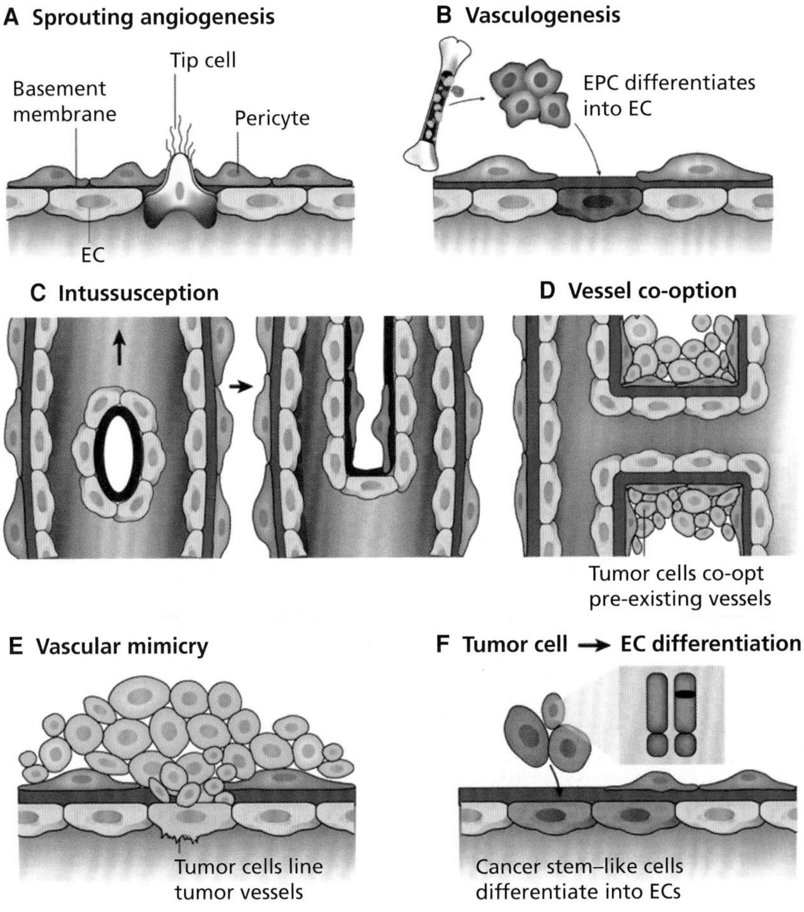

FIGURE 4.2. Modes of vessel formation in solid tumors. There are several known methods of blood vessel formation in normal tissues and tumors. **A–C:** Vessel formation can occur by sprouting angiogenesis **(A)**, by the recruitment of bone marrow–derived and/or vascular wall–resident endothelial progenitor cells (EPCs) that differentiate into endothelial cells (ECs; **B**), or by a process of vessel splitting known as intussusception **(C)**. **D–F:** Tumor cells can co-opt pre-existing vessels **(D)**, or tumor vessels can be lined by cancer cells (vascular mimicry; **E**) or by endothelial cells, with cytogenetic abnormalities in their chromosomes, derived from putative cancer stem cells **(F)**. Unlike normal tissues, which use sprouting angiogenesis, vasculogenesis, and intussusception **(A–C)**, tumors can use all six modes of vessel formation **(A–F)**. (Reproduced from Carmeliet P, Jain RK. Molecular mechanisms and clinical applications of angiogenesis. *Nature* 2011;473:298–307, with permission.)

expansion of pathologic vessels can be aided by the recruitment of bone marrow–derived cells (BMDCs) and/or EPCs to the vascular wall.[31] The progenitor cells then become incorporated into the endothelial lining in a process known as postnatal vasculogenesis. Collateral vessels, which bring bulk flow to ischemic tissues during revascularization, enlarge in size by distinct mechanisms, such as the attraction and activation of myeloid cells.[31,32] However, this process appears to be of rather limited importance in tumor neovascularization.[33–37]

Tissues can also become vascularized by other mechanisms, but the relevance of these processes is not well understood. For example, tumor cells can line vessels—a phenomenon known as vascular mimicry. Putative cancer stemlike cells can even generate tumor endothelium.[38,39–41]

The challenge now is to discern the relative contribution of each of these mechanisms of new vessel formation in tumors to optimize antiangiogenic treatment of cancer.[16,41,42]

Molecular Mechanisms

Various pro- and antiangiogenic molecules orchestrate different steps in vessel formation. Vascular endothelial growth factor (VEGF) is, perhaps, the most critical angiogenic molecule.

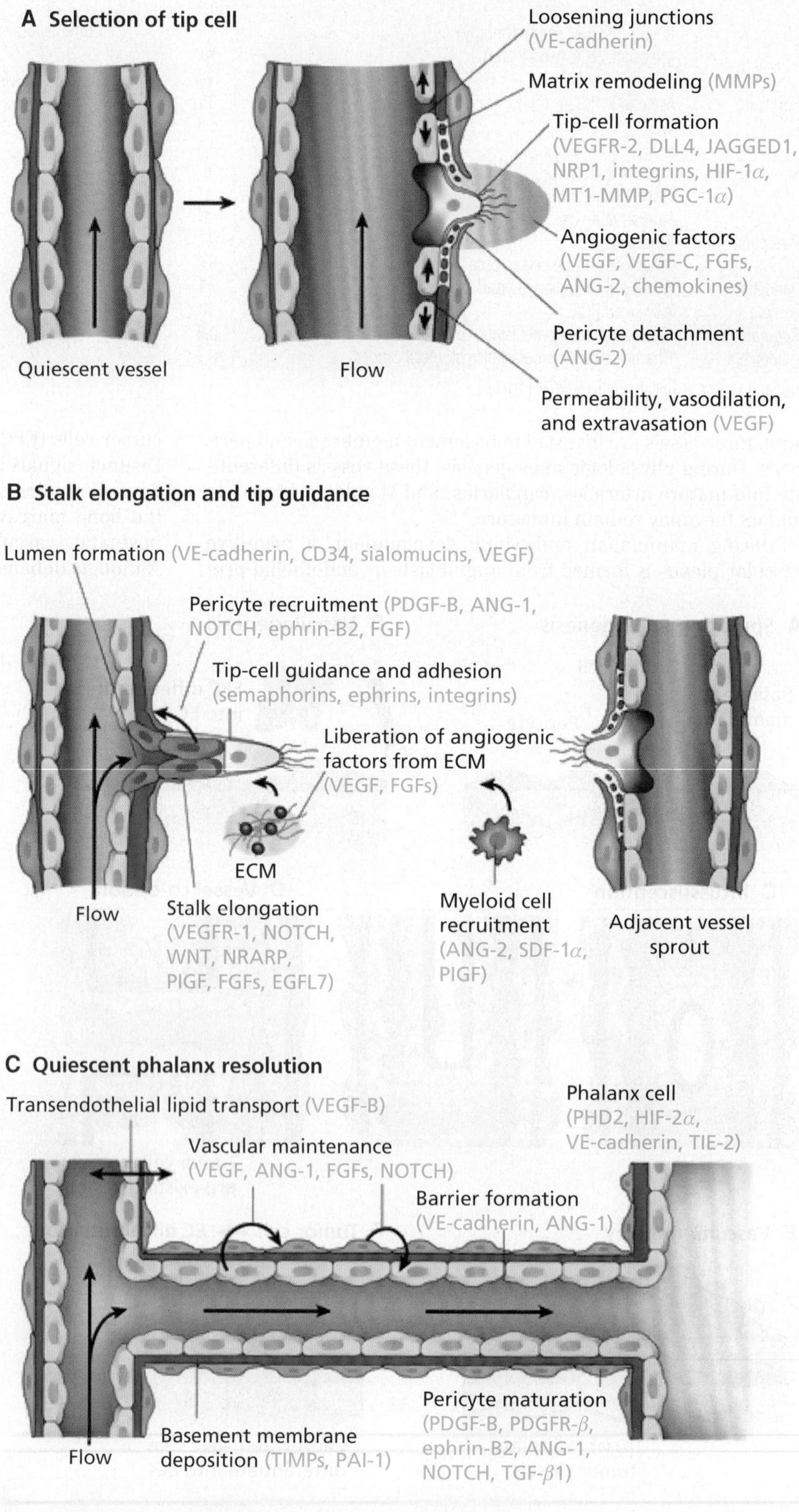

FIGURE 4.3. Molecular basis of vessel branching. The consecutive steps of blood vessel branching are shown, with the key molecular players involved denoted in parentheses. **A:** After stimulation with angiogenic factors, the quiescent vessel dilates and an endothelial-cell tip cell is selected (DLL4 and JAGGED1) to ensure branch formation. Tip-cell formation requires degradation of the basement membrane, pericyte detachment, and loosening of endothelial cell junctions. Increased permeability permits extravasation of plasma proteins (such as fibrinogen and fibronectin) to deposit a provisional matrix layer, and proteases remodel pre-existing interstitial matrix, all enabling cell migration. For simplicity, only the basement membrane between endothelial cells and pericytes is depicted, but in reality, both pericytes and endothelial cells are embedded in this basement membrane. **B:** Tip cells navigate in response to guidance signals (such as semaphorins and ephrins) and adhere to the extracellular matrix (mediated by integrins) to migrate. Stalk cells behind the tip cell proliferate, elongate, and form a lumen, and sprouts fuse to establish a perfused neovessel. Proliferating stalk cells attract pericytes and deposit basement membranes to become stabilized. Recruited myeloid cells such as tumor-associated macrophages (TAMs) and TIE-2–expressing monocytes (TEMs) can produce proangiogenic factors or proteolytically liberate angiogenic growth factors from the extracellular matrix. **C:** After fusion of neighboring branches, lumen formation allows perfusion of the neovessel, which resumes quiescence by promoting a phalanx phenotype, re-establishment of junctions, deposition of basement membrane, maturation of pericytes, and production of vascular maintenance signals. Other factors promote transendothelial lipid transport. (Reproduced from Carmeliet P, Jain RK. Molecular mechanisms and clinical applications of angiogenesis. *Nature* 2011;473:298–307, with permission.)

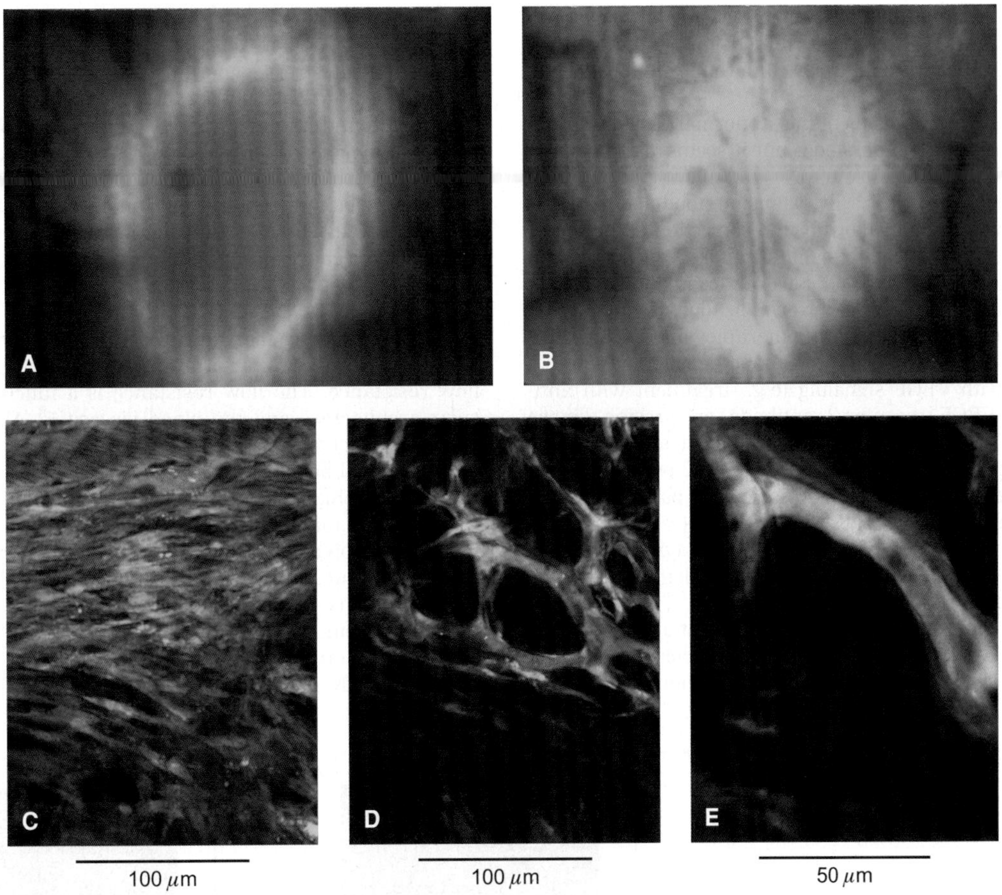

FIGURE 4.4. Tumor induction of host promoter activity in stromal cells. The expression of vascular endothelial growth factor (VEGF) in host cells can be examined using transgenic mice expressing green fluorescent protein (GFP) under the control of the VEGF promoter. **A:** A murine mammary carcinoma xenograft shows host cell VEGF expression mainly at the periphery of the tumor after 1 week. **B:** After 2 weeks, the VEGF-expressing host cells have infiltrated the tumor. (From Fukumura D, Xavier R, Sugiura T, et al. Tumor induction of VEGF promoter activity in stromal cells. *Cell* 1998;94:715–725, with permission). **C:** A GFP-expressing layer of host cells can be seen at the tumor–host interface. **D, E:** The VEGF-expressing host cells colocalize with the angiogenic tumor vessels. (From Brown EB, Campbell RB, Tsuzuki Y, et al. *In vivo* measurement of gene expression, angiogenesis and physiological function in tumors using multiphoton laser scanning microscopy. *Nat Med* 2001;7:866–870, with permission.)

Originally discovered in 1983 as the vascular permeability factor by Dvorak et al. and cloned in 1989 by Ferrara et al., VEGF increases vascular permeability, promotes migration and proliferation of ECs, serves as an EC survival factor, and is known to up-regulate leukocyte adhesion molecules on ECs.[43–44,45] During tumor progression, the variety and concentration of angiogenic molecules produced by a tumor can increase. Thus, if VEGF were blocked, tumor growth might continue as a result of the action of other angiogenic molecules (e.g., basic fibroblast growth factor [bFGF], interleukin-8 [IL-8], stromal cell–derived factor 1α [SDF1α]).[42,46,47] Other positive regulators include angiopoietins that are involved in blood vessel maturation;[48] various proteases involved in extracellular matrix remodeling and growth factor release;[11,28] and organ-specific angiogenic stimulators such as endocrine gland VEGF[45] (Fig. 4.3).

Angiogenesis inhibitors include soluble receptors of various proangiogenic ligands as well as molecules that down-regulate stimulator expression (e.g., interferons), interfere with stimulator release, or block binding of stimulators to their receptors (e.g., platelet factor 4). Thrombospondins are among the first and best characterized endogenous inhibitors that interfere with the growth, adhesion, migration, and survival of ECs. Other endogenous inhibitors include fragments of various plasma or matrix proteins, for example, angiostatin—fragment of plasminogen;[49] endostatin—fragment of collagen XVIII;[50] and tumstatin—fragment of collagen IV.[51]

The generation of pro- and antiangiogenic molecules can be triggered by injury, metabolic stress (e.g., low partial pressure of oxygen [Po_2], low pH, or hypoglycemia), mechanical stress (e.g., shear stress, solid stress), immune/inflammatory responses (e.g., immune/inflammatory cells that have infiltrated the tissue), and genetic mutations (e.g., activation of oncogenes or deletion of suppressor genes that control the production of angiogenesis regulators).[52–55,56–57] These molecules can emanate from cancer cells, endothelial cells, stromal cells, blood, and extracellular matrix[58,59,60] (Fig. 4.4). Because the host cells differ among organs, angiogenesis depends on host–tumor interactions.[59,61–64,65] Furthermore, because the tumor microenvironment is likely to change during tumor growth, regression, and relapse after treatment, profiles of pro- and antiangiogenic molecules are likely to change with time and space.[66–75] The challenge now is to develop a unified theoretic framework to describe the temporal and spatial profiles of this increasing number of angiogenesis regulators to develop effective therapeutic strategies.[42,76]

Vascular Architecture

In normal tissue, blood flows in a closed circuit from an artery to an arteriole to capillaries to venules to a vein. Although the tumor vasculature originates from these host vessels and the mechanisms of angiogenesis are similar, its organization may be completely different depending on the tumor type, its location, and whether it is growing, regressing, or relapsing.[77,78–79] In general, tumor vessels are dilated, saccular, tortuous, and chaotic in their patterns of interconnection. For example, whereas the normal vasculature is characterized by dichotomous branching, the tumor vasculature has many trifurcations and branches with uneven diameters.[80,81] The fractal dimensions and minimum path lengths of tumor vasculature are different from those of the normal host vasculature.[78,79,82]

The molecular mechanisms of this abnormal vascular architecture are not entirely understood, but it seems reasonable to hypothesize that an imbalance of pro- and antiangiogenic molecules is a key contributor.[11,83] By extension, modulation of this angiogenic imbalance may allow for the correction of the tumor vascular abnormalities, leaving behind a more structurally and functionally normal vascular bed. Several observations support this "normalization" hypothesis.[83] Normalization of tumor xenograft vasculature is observed during therapies that lower VEGF (e.g., hormone withdrawal from a hormone-dependent tumor[84]), that interfere with VEGF signaling (e.g., treatment with anti-VEGF or anti-VEGF receptor-2 antibody or tyrosine kinase inhibitor[85,86,87–90]) (Fig. 4.5), or that mimic an antiangiogenic cocktail (e.g., trastuzumab treatment of a HER2 overexpressing tumor[70]). Emerging clinical data from cancer patients treated with bevacizumab, an anti-VEGF antibody, or pan-vascular endothelial growth factor receptor (VEGFR) tyrosine kinase inhibitors AZD2171 (cediranib) or sunitinib lend even more compelling support to this hypothesis.[16,41,66,67,69,71,72,73,75,83,91,92] More crucially, the extent of vascular normalization directly correlates with the survival of patients with recurrent glioblastoma.[92] Moreover, the patients whose tumor blood flow increased most after cediranib treatment had the longest overall survival.[93,94]

Mechanical stress generated by proliferating tumor cells also may lead to partially compressed or totally collapsed vessels often found in tumors.[23,95] Decompression of blood vessels by depleting cells or matrix supports this mechanical hypothesis.[24,25,96] Perhaps the combination of both molecular and mechanical factors renders the tumor vasculature abnormal; thus, both must be taken into account when designing novel strategies for cancer treatment.

Blood Flow and Microcirculation

Blood flow in a vascular network—whether normal or abnormal—is governed by arteriovenous pressure difference and flow resistance. The flow resistance is a function of the vascular architecture and the blood viscosity.[97] Abnormalities in both the vasculature and blood viscosity increase the resistance to blood flow in tumors.[80,81,98–100] As a result, overall perfusion rates (blood flow rate per unit volume) in tumors are lower than in many normal tissues.[101–103]

Macroscopically and microscopically, tumor blood flow is temporally and spatially heterogeneous. Macroscopically, four spatial regions can be recognized in a tumor: an avascular necrotic region, a seminecrotic region, a stabilized microcirculation region, and an advancing front[12,104] (Fig. 4.6A). Microscopically, in normal tissues red blood cell (RBC) velocity is

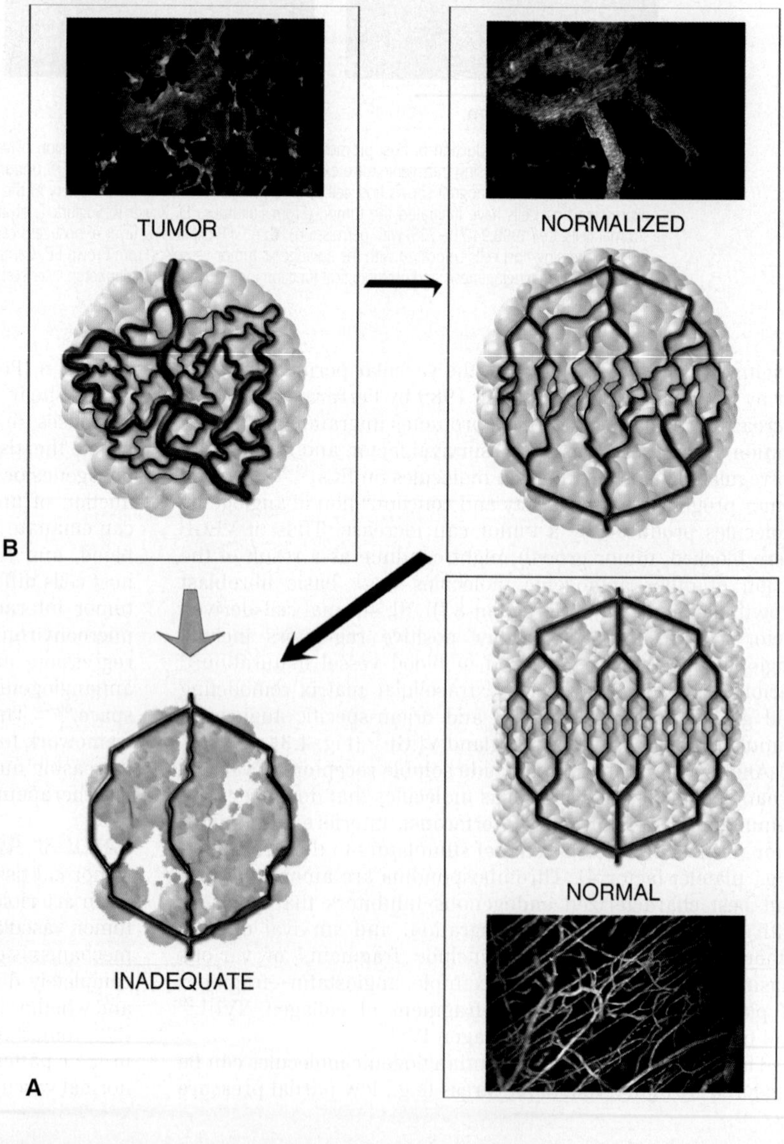

FIGURE 4.5. Normalization of tumor vasculature. **A:** Normal vessels are well organized with even diameters. **B:** In contrast, tumor vessels are tortuous with increased vessel diameter, length, density, and permeability. **C:** Antiangiogenic therapies "normalize" the tumor vascular network and ultimately may reduce the vasculature to the point that it provides inadequate support for tumor growth. (From Jain RK. Normalizing tumor vasculature with anti-angiogenic therapy: a new paradigm for combination therapy. *Nat Med* 2001;7:987–989; and Tong RT, et al. Vascular normalization by vascular endothelial growth factor receptor 2 blockade induces a pressure gradient across the vasculature and improves drug penetration in tumors. *Cancer Res* 2004;64:3731–3736, with permission.)

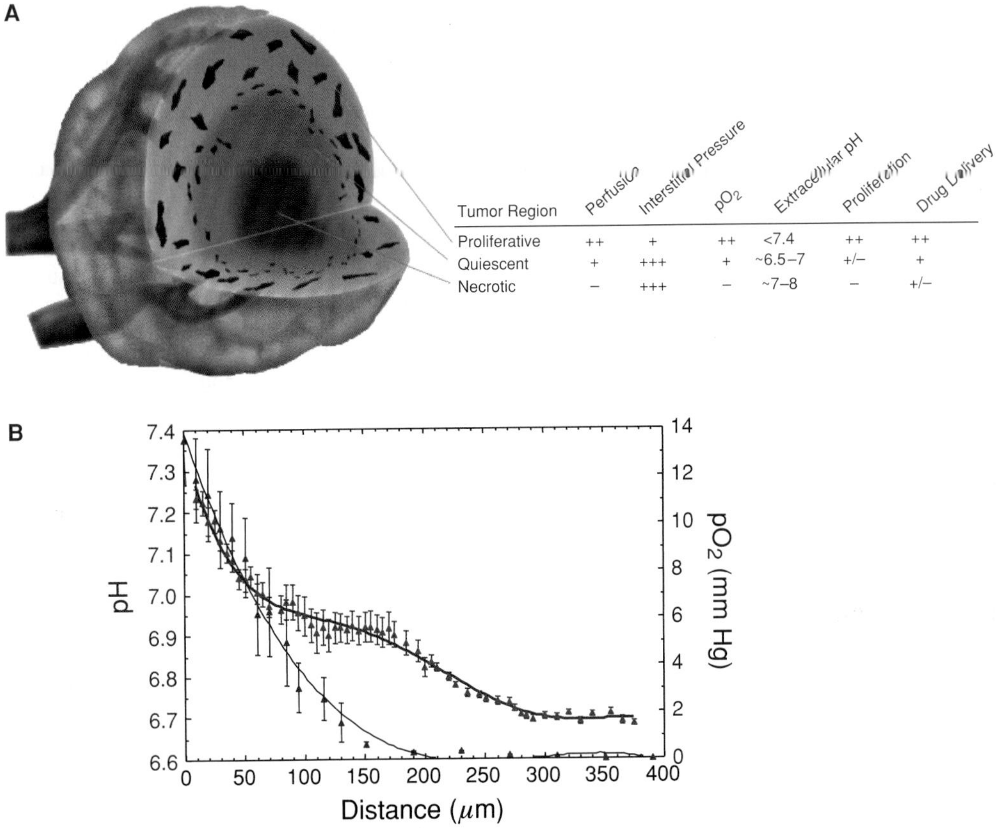

FIGURE 4.6. The tumor microenvironment is heterogeneous with proliferative, quiescent, and necrotic regions. **A:** These regions can be characterized in terms of various physiologic parameters. Decreasing magnitude of these parameters is indicated as + + +, + +, +, +/–, and – in the adjoining table. (From Jain RK, Forbes NS. Commentary–can engineered bacteria help control cancer? *Proc Natl Acad Sci U S A* 2001;98:14748–14750, with permission.) **B:** pH and Po_2 as a function of distance from a blood vessel in a tumor. The tumor environment becomes progressively more hypoxic and acidic farther away from a blood vessel. (From Helmlinger G, Yuan F, Dellian M, et al. Interstitial pH and Po_2 gradients in solid tumors in vivo: high-resolution measurements reveal a lack of correlation. *Nat Med* 1997;3:177–182, with permission.)

dependent on vessel diameter, but there is no such dependence in most tumors.[61,65,105] Furthermore, the average RBC velocity may be an order of magnitude lower in some tumors compared to the host tissue.[65] In a given tumor vessel, blood flow fluctuates with time and can even reverse its direction.[104,105–106]

In addition to the elevated geometric and viscous (rheologic) resistance, other molecular and mechanical factors contribute to this spatial and temporal heterogeneity. These include imbalance between pro- and antiangiogenic molecules,[105] solid stress generated by proliferating cancer cells,[23,24,25,95,96] vascular remodeling by intussusception, and coupling between luminal and interstitial fluid pressure via hyperpermeability of tumor vessels.[78,108–110] As discussed later, this heterogeneity contributes to both acute and chronic hypoxia in tumors—a potential cause of resistance to radiation and other therapies and increased metastatic potential.

Considerable effort has gone into modulating tumor blood flow to improve cancer treatment. This has been difficult to achieve reproducibly because the tumor vasculature consists of both vessels co-opted from the pre-existing host vasculature and vessels resulting from the angiogenic response of host vessels to cancer cells. The former are invested in normal contractile perivascular cells, whereas the latter either lack perivascular cells or are abnormally invested.[111–113] As a result, efforts to increase tumor blood flow and the delivery of cytotoxins, by pharmacologic or physical agents, have not always been successful.[97,114] In contrast, efforts to "starve" tumors by decreasing or shutting down tumor blood flow by "stealing" blood away from the passive component of the tumor vasculature by vasodilators[114] as well as by vascular targeting or intravascular coagulation have shown promise in experimental systems.[115] It also appears that judiciously applied antiangiogenic therapy may "normalize" the abnormal tumor vasculature and the resulting "normalized" vessels might be more responsive to vasoactive agents[12,16,41,83,116] (Fig. 4.5).

Vascular Permeability

Once a bloodborne molecule has reached an exchange vessel, its extravasation occurs by diffusion, convection, and, to some extent, presumably transcytosis.[117] The diffusive permeability of a molecule depends on the size, shape, charge, and flexibility of the molecule as well as the size, shape, charge, and dynamics of the transvascular transport pathway. In normal vessels, these pathways include diffusion through the EC membrane (for lipophilic solutes), trans-EC diffusion, interendothelial junctions (<7 nm), open or closed fenestrations (<10 nm), and transendothelial channels (including vesicles or vesicovacuolar organelles [VVOs]).[118] Some of these pathways may be lined with glycocalyx on ECs, thus effectively reducing the size of the pathway. A basement membrane may retard further the movement of molecules. Ultrastructural studies show widened interendothelial junctions; an increased number of fenestrations, vesicles, and VVOs in tumor vessels; and a lack of normal basement membrane and pericytes.[43,63,118,119–120]

In concert with these ultrastructural findings, both vascular permeability to solutes and water permeability (referred to as hydraulic conductivity) of tumors, in general, are significantly higher than that of various normal tissues.[65,100,121–124] Furthermore, unlike normal vessels, tumor vessels lack selectivity for the size of extravasating molecules.[125] However, positively charged molecules have a higher affinity for the negatively charged angiogenic tumor vessels.[126] Despite increased overall permeability, not all blood vessels of a tumor are leaky. Even the leaky vessels have a finite pore size that is tumor dependent, and ultrastructural studies show that the larger pore size in tumors represents wide interendothelial junctions.[63,120] Not only do the vascular permeability and pore size vary from one tumor to the next, but also within the same tumor they vary both spatially and temporally as well as during tumor growth, regression, and relapse.[63,70,84]

The local microenvironment plays an important role in controlling vascular permeability. For example, a human glioma (HGL21) is fairly leaky when grown subcutaneously in immunodeficient mice, but it exhibits blood–brain barrier properties in the cranial window.[65] Such site-dependent differences for other tumors have been observed in other orthotopic sites.[61,64,127] One possible explanation is that the host–tumor interactions control the production and secretion of cytokines associated with permeability increase (e.g., VEGF) and decrease (e.g., angiopoietin 1).[12,28,48,90,128] A better understanding of the molecular mechanisms of permeability regulation in tumors is likely to yield strategies for improved delivery of molecular medicine to tumors.[129]

Movement of Cells Across Vessel Walls

Both cancer cells and immune cells frequently move across the walls of blood vessels—the former in the process of metastasis and the latter during immune response or cell-based immunotherapy. Both transendothelial and periendothelial pathways have been proposed as a route for intravasation and extravasation of cells. Very little is known about intravasation, except that a tumor may shed more than a million cells per gram per day and most of these are not clonogenic, and that some may be shed as fragments along with stromal cells.[103,130–132] More is known about the molecular and cellular mechanisms of extravasation.[133–135] A cell within a blood vessel may continue to move with the flowing blood, collide with the vessel wall, adhere transiently or stably, and finally extravasate. These interactions are governed by both local hydrodynamic forces and adhesive forces. The former are determined by the vessel diameter and fluid velocity, and the latter by the expression, strength, and kinetics of binding between adhesion molecules and by the surface area of contact.[133,136,137–140] Deformability of cells affects both types of forces.[141]

Rolling of endogenous leukocytes is generally low in tumor vessels, whereas stable adhesion (≥30 seconds) is comparable between normal and tumor vessels.[142] However, both rolling and stable adhesion are nearly zero in angiogenic vessels induced in collagen gels by bFGF or VEGF, two of the most potent angiogenic factors. Whether the latter is due to a low flux of leukocytes into angiogenic vessels and/or down-regulation of adhesion molecules in these immature vessels is currently not known. Age may also play an important role in leukocyte–endothelial interactions.[143]

Further insight into the biology of cells that adhere to tumor vessels comes from studies on the localization of IL-2–activated natural killer (A-NK) cells in normal and tumor tissues in mice using positron emission tomography.[144,145] Immediately following systemic injection, these cells localized primarily in the lungs, whereas a nondetectable number of cells arrived in the tumor.[144] Increased rigidity caused by IL-2 activation may contribute to the mechanical entrapment of these cells in the lung microcirculation.[146,147] Constitutive expression of certain adhesion molecules in the lung vasculature also may facilitate their localization in the lungs.[133] One approach to reducing lung entrapment is to reduce the rigidity of these cells.[141,145] Alternatively, entrapment in lung vasculature can be circumvented by injecting A-NK cells directly into the blood supply of tumors. In this case, A-NK cells, both xenogeneic and syngeneic, adhered to some blood vessels in three different tumor models[145,148,149] via CD18 and very late antigen-4 (VLA-4) on the A-NK cells and intercellular adhesion molecule-1 (ICAM-1), vascular cell adhesion molecule-1 (VCAM-1), and E-selectin on the activated endothelium of angiogenic vessels.[44,150,151]

These molecules can be up-regulated by a number of cytokines, including tumor necrosis factor-α (TNF-α) and a protein of 90 kD molecular weight (p90); secreted by some neoplastic cells;[44,137] and down-regulated by others, for example, transforming growth factor-β (TGF-β) also, presumably, secreted by cancer cells.[62,152] Surprisingly, the proangiogenic VEGF also can up-regulate these molecules, whereas another proangiogenic molecule, bFGF, can down-regulate these molecules.[44,59,86,153] The challenge now is to decrease nonspecific entrapment of immune cells in normal vessels and to increase their delivery to tumor vessels to improve various cell-based therapies, including gene therapy. Judicious doses of anti-VEGF agents that "normalize" tumor vasculature can potentially realize this goal.[154,155]

EXTRAVASCULAR COMPARTMENT

Composition and Origin

The extravascular compartment of a solid tumor consists of neoplastic cells (parenchyma) and host cells (e.g., inflammatory cells, fibroblasts) residing in an interstitial subcompartment bathed by the interstitial fluid (Fig. 4.1). Depending on the tumor type and its stage of differentiation, neoplastic cells may be dispersed in the matrix as individual cells (e.g., lymphomas, melanomas) or as clumps or nests (e.g., carcinomas). More than 80% of tumors are carcinomas arising from epithelial cells. The remaining 20% include sarcomas arising from mesenchymal cells (e.g., bone or muscle cells), lymphomas arising from lymphoid tissue, leukemias arising from hematopoietic cells, and hemangiomas arising from endothelial cells. In a poorly differentiated carcinoma, the cancer cells may be loosely packed in clumps, whereas in a well-differentiated carcinoma, the cells may be connected with intercellular junctions and tightly packed in a nest enveloped by a basement membrane. With tumor progression, cancer cells may invade the basement membrane and spread to other regions.[43]

Unlike cancer cells, host cells must migrate into the tumor from normal tissue. Inflammatory cells may enter the tumor via blood vessels or may infiltrate from the adjacent tissue.[131] Other host cells, such as fibroblasts, may proliferate and migrate from the adjacent connective tissue[28,58,60,156,157] or from primary tumor to the metastatic site.[131] Increasingly, infiltrating host cells are being recognized as critical modulators of the tumorigenic process. For example, mesenchymal cells generically termed carcinoma-associated fibroblasts have been shown to promote tumor growth, metastasis, and angiogenesis, potentially through the secretion of stromal cell–derived factor-1α.[131,158–161] Furthermore, tumor-associated immune/inflammatory cells such as tumor-associated macrophages (TAMs), Tie2-expressing monocytes (TEMs), or Gr-1+ myeloid-derived suppressor cells (MDSCs) have been linked to both cancer immunosurveillance and suppression as well as to tumor promotion.[54,159,162,163,164] The challenge now is to establish approaches for skewing the TAMs toward a phenotype that promotes antitumor immune responses in cancer patients.[54]

The interstitial compartment of a tumor is bounded by the walls of the blood vessels on one side and by the membranes of cancer and stromal cells on the other. In normal tissues, the blood vessels are surrounded by a basement membrane, which is defective in tumors (see the Vascular Permeability section).[28,83] In addition, functional lymphatics may be confined to the tumor margin (see the Lymphatic Transport section).[165,166] Similar to normal tissues, the interstitial space of tumors is composed of a collagen and elastin fiber network that provides structural support to the tissue. Interdispersed in this cross-linked structure are the interstitial fluid and macromolecular constituents (polysaccharides hyaluronan and proteoglycans [PGs]), which form a hydrophilic gel.

Compared with our understanding of blood vessel formation, our understanding of stroma generation is minimal. Dvorak has proposed that the extravasated plasma protein fibrinogen, a key component of the tumor interstitial fluid (TIF), clots to form fibrin, which serves as a major component of the provisional stroma.[43] This provisional stroma eventually is replaced by more mature connective tissue stroma. The TIF also contains several proteins including fibronectin, vitronectin, osteopontin, thrombospondin, decorin, and tenascin. These proteins are present in both free and bound forms and contain the amino acid sequence arg-gly-asp (RGD). The RGD sequence provides a binding site for adhesion that assists in the migration of various cells, including stromal cells. In addition to extravasating from the leaky tumor vessels, these proteins, along with collagen and various PGs, also are synthesized by the stromal cells, albeit in a form that is different from that in the plasma or normal tissues.[43] TIF also may contain various growth factors that facilitate stroma formation. For example, *in vitro* studies suggest that platelet-derived growth factor-β is involved in the recruitment of fibroblasts to tumors, and TGF-β controls the production of collagen and other matrix molecules in tumors.[28,167] With the increasing interest in using the fragments of matrix constituents for controlling angiogenesis, our understanding of the molecular and cellular mechanisms of stroma generation in tumors is likely to increase.[156]

Interstitial Transport

Once a molecule has extravasated, its movement through the interstitial space occurs by diffusion and convection.[118] Diffusion is proportional to the concentration gradient in the interstitium, and convection is proportional to the interstitial fluid velocity, which, in turn, is proportional to the pressure gradient in the interstitium. Just as the interstitial diffusion coefficient, D (cm^2/s), relates the diffusive flux to the concentration gradient, the interstitial hydraulic conductivity, K ($cm^2/mm\ Hg \cdot s$), relates the interstitial velocity to the pressure gradient.[118] Values of these transport coefficients are governed by the structure and composition of the interstitial compartment as well as by the physicochemical properties of the solute molecule.[126,168,169–172]

The value of K (interstitial hydraulic conductivity) for a human colon carcinoma xenograft (LS174 T), measured using two different methods,[173,174] was found to be higher than that of a hepatoma,[172] which, in turn, was higher than that of the normal liver. Using fluorescence recovery after photobleaching, the diffusion coefficient (D) of various molecules in tumors was found to be about one-third that in water[175] and higher than the values in the host tissue.[169] Collagen content and structure have a significant effect on D in tumors.[171,173,176] This is surprising because hyaluronan and proteoglycans, and not collagen, account for most of the resistance to transport in normal tissues. Because collagen is produced by the host-derived cells (e.g., fibroblasts), the penetrability of macromolecules into a tumor will depend on the host–tumor interaction. Thus, agents that interfere with collagen synthesis and/or organization (e.g., relaxin, bacterial collagenase, losartan) may increase interstitial transport in tumors.[168,177,178]

The time constant for a molecule with diffusion coefficient D to diffuse across a distance L is approximately $L^2/4D$. For diffusion of IgG (immunoglobulin G) in tumors, this time constant is on the order of 1 hour for a 100-μm distance, days for a 1-mm distance, and months for a 1-cm distance. So for a 1-mm tumor, diffusional transport across the tumor would take days, and for a 1-cm tumor, it would take months. If the central vessels have collapsed completely as a result of cellular proliferation[23,24,96] and interstitial matrix rearrangement, the reduced delivery of macromolecules by blood flow would make diffusion the primary mechanism of delivery to this hypoxic center. Binding may further retard the transport in tumors.[175,179,180] The role of binding is illustrated clearly by comparing the rate of fluorescence recovery of a photobleached spot in tumor tissue injected with a nonspecific versus specific IgG. In addition to the heterogeneity of D in tumors, the most unexpected result of these photobleaching studies was the large extent (30% to 40%) of nonspecific binding.[175] These results collectively suggest that the interstitial compartment of a tumor can be a formidable barrier to the uniform delivery of therapeutic macromolecules (e.g., antibodies, genes using viruses, nano-therapeutics) in tumors, and strategies are needed to overcome this barrier.[117,126,177,178,181]

Lymphatic Transport

In most normal tissues, extravasated plasma and macromolecules are taken up by the lymphatics and returned to the central circulation. Although it is widely accepted that lymphatic vessels are present in the tumor margin and the peritumoral tissue, the hotly debated issue for nearly a century has been whether anatomically defined lymphatic vessels are present within solid tumors and, if so, whether they function.[166,182] Currently available immunohistochemical markers stain for structures in some tumors that resemble lymphatic vessels. However, because many of these markers lack specificity,[165,166,183] it is not clear whether they stain functional lymphatic vessels, endothelial cells from remnant lymphatic vessels, or some other structures or cell types (e.g., preferential fluid channels[173]). It is likely that the stress induced by proliferating cancer cells compresses and impairs lymphatic vessels that are co-opted or formed in a tumor[23,24] and/or lymphatic valves are impaired by tumor growth.[184] The impaired lymphatic vessels, in turn, may contribute to the interstitial hypertension characteristic of animal and human tumors (see the Interstitial Hypertension section). In addition, invasion of the functional peritumoral lymphatics is considered to be a poor prognostic factor for a number of tumors, and lymphatic metastasis is a major cause of morbidity and mortality.

Our understanding of the mechanisms of lymphangiogenesis lags behind our understanding of the mechanisms of angiogenesis. However, considerable progress has recently been made toward identifying molecular players responsible for lymphangiogenesis. VEGF-C, acting through VEGFR-3, appears to play a central role in tumor-associated lymphangiogenesis. Several experimental[185–186,187–189] and clinical[190] studies have demonstrated a positive correlation between VEGF-C expression and peritumoral lymphatic vessel density, lymphatic metastasis, and, in some cases, poor clinical outcomes. Like in vascular angiogenesis, other positive and negative regulators, such as VEGF,[191,192] VEGF-D,[186] hepatocyte growth factor, platelet-derived growth factor-BB, and angiopoietins are involved in lymphangiogenesis.[11,190] Furthermore, mechanisms analogous to co-option, intussusception, sprouting, and vasculogenesis may operate in lymphatic growth[11] (see the Angiogenesis: Cellular Mechanisms section). Similar to organ-specific angiogenic molecules (e.g., EG-VEGF)[45] and blood vascular endothelial precursor cells,[30,193] there may be organ-specific lymphangiogenic molecules and lymphatic endothelial precursor cells that contribute to tumor-associated lymphangiogenesis.[194] Moreover, the proteolytic processing of lymphangiogenesis molecules, as well as the phenotype and function of the resulting lymphatics, may depend on the tumor type as well as on the host organ in which the tumor is growing.[28,86,165,190]

The precise roles for these lymphangiogenic molecules in the induction of lymphatic metastasis are imperfectly understood. Recent data demonstrate that tumor VEGF-C overexpression induces peritumoral lymphatic hyperplasia through activation of VEGFR-3. Consequently, lymph fluid volumetric flow increases.[185] This results in increased tumor cell delivery to lymph nodes and a higher rate of lymphatic metastasis[185] (Fig. 4.7). It remains unclear how VEGF-C overexpression impacts tumor cell entry into lymphatic vessels; however, an attractive hypothesis is that the increased lymphatic surface

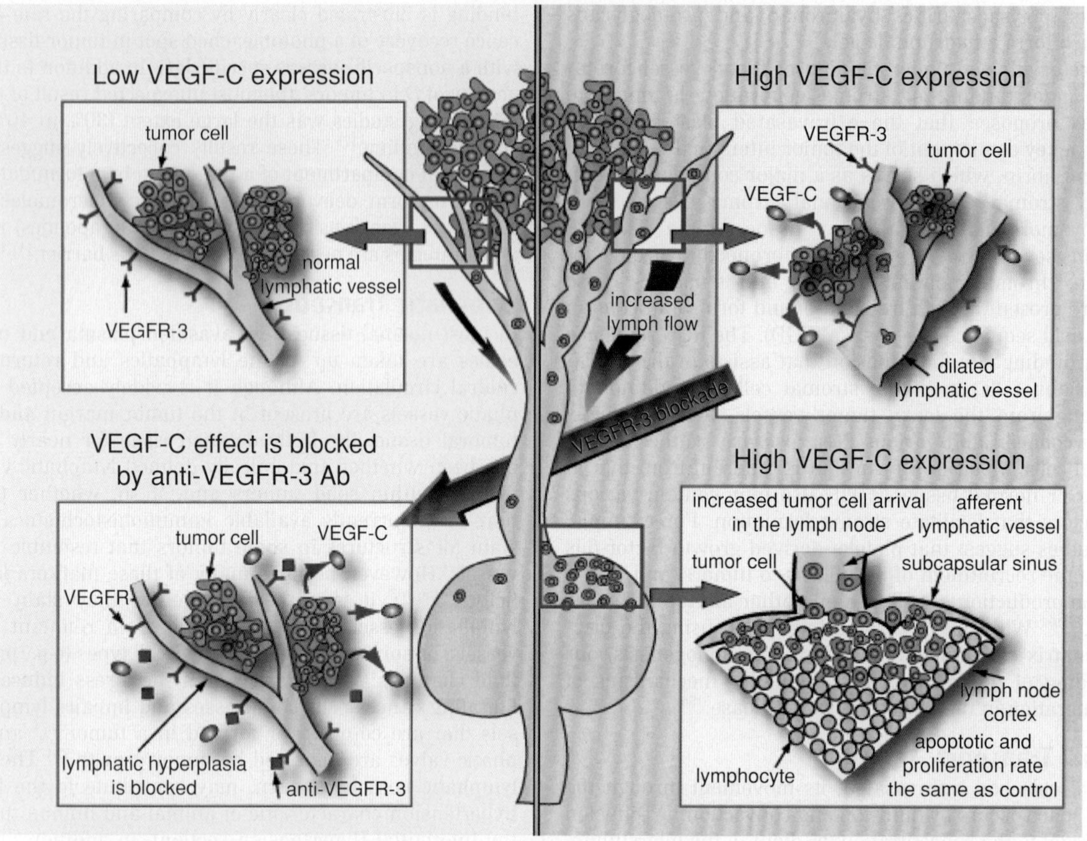

FIGURE 4.7. Schematic of lymphatics in low (*left*) versus high (*right*) vascular endothelial growth factor-C (VEGF-C)–expressing tumors. VEGF-C secreted from tumor cells stimulates vascular endothelial growth factor receptor-3 (VEGFR-3) expressed in lymphatic endothelial cells, inducing peritumor lymphatic hyperplasia (*top right*). An increase in lymphatic surface area may increase the opportunity for tumor cell entry into lymphatic vessels. Augmented lymph flow enhances tumor cell delivery to draining lymph nodes (*bottom right*). In the absence of VEGF-C overexpression, peritumor lymphatic hyperplasia is less pronounced and fewer tumor cells are delivered to draining lymph nodes (*left*). Anti-VEGF-C/anti-VEGFR-3 treatment inhibits VEGF-C–induced lymphatic hyperplasia and tumor cell delivery to draining lymph nodes (*bottom left*). (From Hoshida T, Isaka N, Hagendoorn J, et al. Imaging steps of lymphatic metastasis reveals that vascular endothelial growth factor-C increases metastasis by increasing delivery of cancer cells to lymph nodes: therapeutic implications. *Cancer Res* 2006;66:8065–8075, with permission.)

area simply increases the probability of tumor cell entry and dissemination. Alternatively, VEGF-C may stimulate the release of a chemotactic factor that recruits tumor cells into lymphatic vessels. Of potential clinical importance, VEGFR-3 blockade was shown to inhibit VEGF-C–induced lymphatic hyperplasia, tumor cell delivery to draining lymph nodes, and lymphatic metastasis when treatment was started at the time of tumor initiation. However, lymphatic metastases were not significantly reduced if VEGFR-3 blockade was started after tumor cell seeding of draining lymph nodes.[185,195] These data suggest that anti-VEGFR-3 therapy may be effective in preventing, but not treating, lymphatic metastases—the more common clinical imperative—except in cases where a significant fraction of vascular endothelial cells and/or cancer cells express VEGFR-3. The challenge now is to identify alternative strategies for treating lymphatic metastases, either through combination therapy (e.g., anti-VEGFR-2/anti-VEGFR-3) or modulation of other pathways.

Mechanical signals that trigger the lymphangiogenic switch are unknown. Because lymphatic vessels help maintain the balance of fluid in tissues, hydrostatic pressure is a likely trigger.[195,197] Whether the lymphatic hyperplasia seen in tumor margins is, in part, a response to the elevated hydrostatic pressure in tumors and whether the newly formed lymphatics remain open and relieve this pressure is an open question. Techniques such as microlymphangiography,[4,165,166,185,188,198,199] fluorescence photobleaching lymph flow quantitation,[182,185,198,200–202] and optical frequency domain imaging (OFDI)[203] will allow us to answer these important questions.

Interstitial Hypertension

Unlike normal tissues, where the interstitial fluid pressure (IFP) is around 0 mm Hg, both animal and human tumors exhibit interstitial hypertension.[69,71,73,118,166,174,204,205,206,207–211,212,213–215] The tumor IFP begins to increase as soon as the host vessels become leaky in response to angiogenic molecules such as VEGF.[216] Thus, IFP can be lowered by inhibiting the VEGF pathway using blocking antibodies.[69,71,72,73,88,217] The IFP increases with tumor size in some tumors[204,206,210] and remains independent of tumor size in others.[211]

Three mechanisms contribute to the interstitial hypertension in tumors. In normal tissues, lymphatics maintain fluid homeostasis; thus, the lack of functional lymphatics within tumors is a key contributor. Indeed, DiResta et al. have shown that one could lower the IFP by placing "artificial lymphatics" in tumors.[218] The second contributor is the leaky nature of tumor vessels. As a result, the hydrostatic and oncotic (colloid osmotic) pressures become almost equal between the intravascular and extravascular space.[82,88,205,219] At least two pieces of evidence support this hypothesis. First, lowering permeability by blocking VEGF signaling lowers IFP.[71,88,217] Second, IFP goes up and down with the microvascular pressure within seconds.[220–222] The two mechanisms described so far can only explain hypertension up to 20 to 30 mm Hg—the microvascular pressure of most exchange vessels in our body—but IFPs as high as 94 mm Hg have been measured in human tumors.[214] Because the microvascular pressure (MVP) is the driving force for IFP in tumors, these tumors must have a high MVP. Indeed, this is the case.[205] There are two possible explanations for the elevated MVP in tumors: (a) the tumor vessels have reduced arterial resistance so that the MVP becomes closer to arterial pressure, and/or (b) the tumor vessels have increased venous resistance as a result of compression and tortuosity so that the whole vascular network is under hypertension. Indirect evidence for the latter comes from the decrease in IFP following decompression of tumor vessels by drug-induced apoptosis of perivascular cancer cells.[24,96]

The elevated pressure can compromise the tumor microcirculation and delivery of therapeutics in three ways. First, reduced transmural pressure gradients resulting from equilibrium between MVP and IFP reduce convection across tumor vessels and thus compromise the transport of macromolecules.[82,88,97,205,221] Second, because IFP is nearly uniform throughout a tumor and drops precipitously in the tumor margin, the interstitial fluid "oozes" out of the tumor into the surrounding normal tissue, carrying macromolecules with it.[15,35,130] Finally, transmural coupling between IFP and MVP as a result of high permeability of tumor vessels can lead to blood flow stasis in tumors without physically occluding the vessels.[108–110] Thus, decreasing vascular leakiness might restore the transmural pressure gradients and potentially resume/re-establish blood flow in the nonperfused regions of tumors. Some direct and indirect antiangiogenic therapies may "normalize" the tumor vasculature through this mechanism[12,16,41,67,70,71,83,116,223] (Tables 4.2 and 4.3 and Fig. 4.5).

Metabolic Environment

Hypoxia

A key function of the vasculature is to provide adequate levels of nutrients to the parenchymal cells and to remove waste products. Based on the anatomy of the capillary bed and a mathematical model of oxygen diffusion and consumption, the Nobel laureate August Krogh introduced the concept of a diffusion limit for oxygen of 100 to 200 μm nearly a century ago.[224] This unit of tissue—a single capillary surrounded by a 100 to 200 μm radius cylinder—is referred to as a Krogh cylinder in physiology. Nearly 50 years later, Thomlinson and Gray identified similar "cords" in human lung cancer and found necrotic cells beyond 180 μm away from blood vessels, presumably due to a lack of oxygen.[225] This is referred to as *chronic hypoxia* or *diffusion-limited hypoxia.* Although various hypoxia markers and microelectrodes have suggested these gradients, the first direct measurements of these perivascular Po_2 gradients, as well as perivascular pH gradients, became possible only with the development of phosphorescence quenching microscopy[23,226] (Fig. 4.6B).

As discussed earlier, blood flow in tumor vessels is intermittent, and, thus, some regions of a tumor are periodically starved for oxygen. The resulting hypoxia is referred to as *acute hypoxia* or *perfusion-limited hypoxia.* A necessary consequence of intermittent blood flow is the resumption of blood flow after shutdown, and the resulting production of free

TABLE 4.2 STUDIES REPORTING ANTIANGIOGENIC THERAPY–INDUCED IMPROVEMENT IN TUMOR OXYGENATION

Antiangiogenic Therapy	*Tumor Model*	*Effect on Oxygenation*	*Time Window of Improved Oxygenation*
Antibody Therapy			
Bevacizumab	Melanoma, breast carcinoma, ovarian carcinoma	↑	2–4 days after start of therapy
Bevacizumab	GBM	↑	Up to 5 days
DC101	GBM	↑	2–8 days after start of therapy
Anti-PlGF Ab	Pancreatic carcinoma	No change	
TKI Therapy			
Sunitinib	Squamous carcinoma	↑	O_2 measured 4 days after start of therapy
Semaxanib	Melanoma	↑	O_2 measured 3 days after start of therapy
PI-103 (PI3 K inhibitor)	Fibrosarcoma, squamous carcinoma	↑	O_2 measured 10 days after start of therapy
Gefitinib (EGFR inhibitor)	Fibrosarcoma, squamous carcinoma	↑	O_2 measured 10 days after start of therapy
Erlotinib (EGFR inhibitor)	Squamous carcinoma, NSCLC	↑	O_2 measured 5 days after start of therapy
Endocrine Therapy			
Castration (androgen depletion)	Shionogi carcinoma	↑	O_2 measured 21 days after start of therapy
Metronomic Chemotherapy			
Low-dose gemcitabine	Pancreatic carcinoma	↑	O_2 measured 28 days after start of therapy
Other Therapies			
FTIs (Ras inhibitors)	Prostate carcinoma, bladder carcinoma, glioma, fibrosarcoma, squamous carcinoma	↑	O_2 increased up to 7–10 days
Nelfinavir (AKT inhibitor)	Fibrosarcoma, squamous carcinoma	↑	O_2 measured 10 days after start of therapy
TNP-470	Breast carcinoma	↑	O_2 measured 9 days after start of therapy
Suramin	GBM	↑	O_2 measured 5–6 weeks after start of therapy
Thalidomide	Liver carcinoma	↑	O_2 increased from day 2–4 after start of therapy
Thalidomide	Fibrosarcoma	↑	O_2 increased from day 2–3 after start of therapy
Genetic Models			
VEGF$^{-/-}$ (myeloid cells)	Lung carcinoma	↑	
nNOS$^{-/-}$ (tumor cells)	Glioblastoma	↑	
$\alpha_v\beta_3/\alpha_v\beta_5$ integrin-FAK-Rho knockdown (tumor cells)	Glioblastoma	↑	
SEMA3 A overexpression (transgene delivery)	Insulinoma	↑	O_2 increased after 4 weeks
Rgs5$^{-/-}$ (stroma)	Insulinoma	↑	
PHD2$^{-/-}$ (stroma or EC specific)	Melanoma, pancreatic carcinoma	↑	
IFN-β overexpression (transgene delivery)	Glioblastoma, neuroblastoma	↑	

GBM, glioblastoma multiforme; PlGF, placental growth factor; TKI, tyrosine kinase inhibitor; PI3 K, phosphoinostide-3-kinase; EGFR, epidermal growth factor receptor; NSCLC, non–small-cell lung cancer; FTI, farnesyl transferase inhibitor; VEGF, vascular endothelial growth factor; nNOS, neuronal nitric oxide synthase; FAK, focal adhesion kinase; PHD, prolyl hydroxylase domain protein; EC, endothelial cell; IFN, interferon.

Reproduced with permission from Goel S, Duda DG, Xu L, et al. Normalization of the vasculature for treatment of cancer and other diseases. *Physiol Rev* 2011;91(3):1071–1121.

TABLE 4.3 STUDIES REPORTING THE IMPACT OF ANTIANGIOGENIC/VASCULAR NORMALIZATION STRATEGIES UPON DELIVERY OF THERAPEUTIC COMPOUNDS/SYSTEMICALLY ADMINISTERED MOLECULES INTO TUMORS

Systemically Administered Molecule	*Normalization Strategy*	*Tumor Model(s)*	*Effect on Delivery*
Conventional Cytotoxics			
Irinotecan	A4.6.1	Colon carcinoma	↑
Topotecan, etoposide	Bevacizumab	Neuroblastoma	↑
Temozolomide	Sunitinib	Glioma	↑[a]
Cyclophosphamide, cisplatin	TNP-470	Lung carcinoma	↑
Temozolomide	TNP-470	Glioma	↓
Cyclophosphamide	Thalidomide	Liver carcinoma	↑
Doxorubicin	PDGF-D overexpression	Breast carcinoma	↑
Topotecan	IFN-β overexpression	Neuroblastoma	↑
Doxorubicin	Anti-TGF-β antibody or overexpression sTβrII	Breast carcinoma	↑
Nanoparticles			
Liposomal doxorubicin	Anti-TGF-β antibody or overexpression sTβrII	Breast carcinoma	↑
Antibodies			
Nonspecific IgG, anti-E-cadherin Ab	Axitinib	Lung carcinoma, pancreatic tumor	↑ (per vessel)
Viral Particles			
Oncolytic virus	Cilengitide	GBM	↑
Other Molecules			
BSA	DC101	Breast carcinoma, colon carcinoma	↑
FDG	Bevacizumab	Rectal carcinoma	↑ (per vessel)[b]

PDGF, platelet-derived growth factor; IFN, interferon; TGF, transforming growth factor; GBM, glomerular basement membrane; BSA, bovine serum albumin; FDG, fluorodeoxyglucose;

[a]Increased delivery of temozolomide noted with sunitinib 20 mg/kg, but not at 60 mg/kg.

[b]Study performed in human subjects.

Reproduced with permission from Goel S, Duda DG, Xu L, et al. Normalization of the vasculature for treatment of cancer and other diseases. *Physiol Rev* 2011;91(3):1071–1121.

radicals can lead to *ischemia-reperfusion injury* or *reoxygenation injury;* thus, applying additional selection pressure on cancer cells can cause them to become more locally aggressive, metastatic, and resistant to therapy.[227]

Low pH

Another consequence of the abnormal microcirculation of the tumor is low extracellular pH. There are at least two sources of H^+ ions in tumors—lactic acid and carbonic acid.[228] The former results from glycolysis, and the latter results from conversion of CO_2 and H_2O via carbonic anhydrase. However, the intracellular pH of cancer cells remains neutral or alkaline (≥7.2) despite the acidic extracellular pH. Because carbonic anhydrase-9 and various glucose transporters (GLUT-1, -3) and enzymes in the glycolytic pathway are up-regulated by hypoxia,[227] one would expect low extracellular pH and hypoxia to track each other and to colocalize with regions of low blood flow. It is surprising that there is a lack of spatial correlation among these parameters—a discovery made possible by recent developments in optical techniques that permit the simultaneous high-resolution mapping of multiple physiologic parameters.[23] A potential explanation for this lack of concordance is that some perfused tumor vessels carry hypoxic blood.[23] Thus, although they may not be able to deliver enough oxygen to the surrounding cells, they may be able to carry away the waste products (e.g., lactic acid).

Therapeutic Consequences

The presence of molecular oxygen during irradiation can "fix" biologic (e.g., DNA) free radicals, making radiation-induced damage irreparable (oxygen fixation hypothesis). Thus, hypoxia reduces the radiation sensitivity of neoplastic and normal cells both *in vitro* and *in vivo*. Similarly, hypoxia can compromise the efficacy of some chemotherapeutics. Independently, hypoxia can increase the metastatic potential of cancer cells.[227] Therefore, for nearly half a century considerable preclinical and clinical effort has been focused on alleviating hypoxia through a multitude of interventions such as improving tumor perfusion with mild hyperthermia or drugs, increasing oxygen content of the blood via hyperbaric oxygenation, and increasing hemoglobin/hematocrit by transfusion or exogenous erythropoietin. Unfortunately, the clinical outcomes have not met expectations. Although early studies suggested a marked benefit of transfusion in anemic cervical cancer patients undergoing definitive radiotherapy, careful analysis suggests that these studies are confounded by selection biases that preclude the conclusion that anemia correction by transfusion impacts outcome.[229,230] Furthermore, erythropoietin (or analog) treatment showed encouraging survival results in anemic cancer patients receiving nonplatinum chemotherapy and in anemic lung cancer patients receiving chemotherapy.[231,232] However, subsequent trials in anemic head and neck cancer patients and mainly nonanemic metastatic breast cancer patients actually suggested outcomes may be impaired by erythropoietic agents.[233,234] There are multiple possible reasons such interventions have yielded mixed results. These include the inability to increase tumor Po_2 as markedly as systemic Po_2,[235] the inability to increase Po_2 in all areas of a tumor to optimal levels due to abnormal vasculature,[82,116] and undesired "off-target" effects of interventions (e.g., immunosuppression with transfusion[236–238]). Furthermore, tumors may reoxygenate during radiation therapy with standard fractionation, potentially minimizing the impact of providing additional oxygen to the target tissue.

Similarly, low extracellular pH can adversely (or favorably) affect the uptake and cytotoxicity of some therapeutics. The pH gradient difference between tumor and normal tissue may offer a tumor-specific target for weak acid chemotherapeutics for the treatment of cancer.[239,240] The development of specific drugs that exploit this pH difference and strategies to modulate pH in tumors have not yet reached the clinic but are anticipated.[227]

Two broad strategies targeting the unique tumor metabolic environment are emerging: (a) exploit hypoxia to activate drugs or attract tumoricidal anaerobic bacteria and (b) dissect hypoxia-induced pathways to identify novel targets for drug development. The first strategy has led to the development of drugs such as tirapazamine and to renewed interest in bacteriolytic therapy;[241] both approaches are in clinical trials, but promising data are yet to emerge[242] (see Trial Identifier NCT00358397 at ClinicalTrials.gov). The second strategy has revealed several molecular players in the physiologic and pathophysiologic response to hypoxia.[227,243,244] The balance between hypoxia-induced apoptosis/necrosis on one hand and the increased resistance to cell death mediated by various hypoxia-induced pathways on the other determines whether a tumor can survive and even grow under hypoxic conditions. Ultimately, hypoxia selects for tumor cells that are more malignant, more invasive, and genetically unstable, rendering them resistant to various therapies. Therefore, certain players in the hypoxia-induced pathways now are being targeted in the development of diagnostic and therapeutic agents. Hypoxia-induced pathways include genes involved in oxygen delivery,

Box 4.1

Hypoxia and Epigenetic Regulation of Angiogenesis

The prolyl hydroxylase domain (PHD) proteins PHD1–3 are oxygen-sensing enzymes that hydroxylate the hypoxia-inducible factor (HIF) proteins HIF-1α and HIF-2α when sufficient oxygen is available. Once hydroxylated, HIFs are targeted for proteasomal degradation.[268] Under hypoxia, PHDs become inactive, and HIFs initiate broad transcriptional responses to increase the oxygen supply by angiogenesis, through the up-regulation of angiogenic factors such as vascular endothelial growth factor (VEGF).[269] HIFs are also activated in nonhypoxic conditions by oncogenes and growth factors, allowing tumor cells to stimulate angiogenesis before they become deprived of oxygen. In general, HIF-1α promotes vessel sprouting, whereas HIF-2α mediates vascular maintenance.[269] Reduced HIF-1α levels in mice impair embryonic vascular development, revascularization of ischemic tissues, and angiogenesis in injured tissues and tumors.[269] The use of HIF-1α inhibitors to block tumor or ocular angiogenesis has therefore received attention. Conversely, *Hif1 α* gene transfer in mice or activation of HIF-1α by pharmacologic blockade of PHDs promotes ischemic tissue revascularization.

HIF-1α also regulates tumor angiogenesis indirectly, by releasing chemoattractants such as stromal cell–derived factor 1α (SDF-1α) to recruit proangiogenic bone marrow–derived cells (BMDCs).[270] Gene silencing of Phd2 in mouse tumor cells enhances vessel growth by similar mechanisms. Hypoxia also regulates the polarization and proangiogenic activity of tumor-associated macrophages (TAMs) by means of HIF-1α and HIF-2α with different effects.[268] That hypoxia and inflammation are closely intertwined is illustrated by the finding that signaling by HIF-1α and nuclear factor-κB cross-activate each other. In certain cases, hypoxic up-regulation of VEGF occurs independently of HIF-1α and is mediated by the metabolic regulator peroxisome proliferator-activated receptor gamma coactivator (PGC)-1α in preparation for oxidative metabolism once the ischemic tissue is revascularized.[271] Because HIF signaling contributes to acquired resistance against anti-VEGF therapy, the combined blockade of VEGF and HIF-1α is being explored as a cancer treatment strategy.

There is increasing evidence for epigenetic control of angiogenesis, particularly by noncoding microRNAs (miRNAs),[272] which induce messenger RNA degradation or block translation. Because miRNAs target multiple genes, they are well positioned to regulate complex processes such as angiogenesis. Endothelial cells express several miRNAs that are induced by hypoxia or VEGF. Most of those stimulate angiogenesis by hijacking proangiogenic cascades while suppressing angiostatic pathways.[273] The expression of miR-126 is induced by the mechanosensitive transcription factor KLF2A and integrates the mechanosensory stimulus of blood flow to shape the vascular system.[274] Endothelial cell–specific loss of DICER, an exonuclease involved in miRNA biogenesis, impairs pathologic angiogenesis. Angiogenic miRNAs seem to offer significant pro- or antiangiogenic potential.

Reproduced with permission from Carmeliet P, Jain RK. Molecular mechanisms and clinical applications of angiogenesis. *Nature* 2011; 473:298–307.

glycolysis and glucose uptake, pH control, stress-response pathways, growth factor signaling, angiogenesis, transcription, apoptosis, growth inhibition, and invasion and metastasis (Fig. 4.3 and Box 4.1).[11,243]

Of the various molecular players involved in sensing and responding to hypoxia, hypoxia-inducible factor-1 a (HIF-1α) has received the most attention. This transcription factor is up-regulated in a number of human tumors.[243,245] Regulated by proline and asparagine hydroxylases, HIF-1α activates genes involved in an array of physiologic responses including angiogenesis, vasodilation, glycolysis, and RBC production by binding to the hypoxia-response element (HRE). Although HIF-1α is an attractive therapeutic target, its pleiotropic action may prove to be a major challenge for clinical exploitation. For example, teratomas arising from HIF-1α(–/–) embryonic cells grow more rapidly despite lower levels of VEGF and angiogenesis.[246] This counterintuitive finding may be a result of the ability of HIF-1α(–/–) cells to survive under hypoxic conditions, instead of undergoing apoptosis.[60] HIF-1α has also been shown to play an important role in determining tumor radioresponsiveness through the regulation of multiple, and sometimes opposing, processes.[247] Under some circumstances, HIF-1α inhibition *reduces* tumor cell radiosensitivity by protecting hypoxic cells from radiation-induced apoptosis and enhancing clonogenic survival potentially through reductions in adenosine triphosphate metabolism, cellular proliferation, and p53 activation.[247] Furthermore, HIF-1α serves a key function in inflammatory cell energy metabolism, and its inhibition results in profound immunodeficiency.[248] Consequently, molecular therapies that target HIF-1α or HRE, as well as more selective therapies that target key downstream effectors of HIF-1α, are under intensive investigation for cancer detection and treatment.[227,243,249]

CLINICAL IMPLICATIONS

Two major problems currently plague the nonsurgical treatment of malignant solid tumors. First, physiologic barriers within tumors impede the delivery of therapeutics and oxygen (a key radiation sensitizer) at effective concentrations to all cancer cells.[41,83,250] Second, inherent or acquired resistance resulting from genetic and epigenetic mechanisms reduces the effectiveness of conventional as well as novel therapies.[251] Can we take advantage of the unique pathophysiology of tumors to overcome these problems for better management of cancer? As discussed next, recent clinical data offer some hope.

Prognostic/Predictive Biomarker Implications

Multiple indices of tumor pathophysiology have been evaluated as potential predictors of treatment outcome including vessel density (reviewed in [42,252]), oxygen level (reviewed in[243,253]), interstitial pressure,[42,212,214,230] and blood or urine circulating molecules[73,91] (reviewed in[42]). Vessel density can be evaluated in biopsies and is measured either in "hot spots" (i.e., regions of most active angiogenesis) or in the tissue as a whole. The former presumably provides a measure of a tumor's aggressiveness, and the latter reflects the status of global oxygenation. Most studies to date show that poor outcome of radiation therapy correlates with high vessel density in "hot spots" and/or low overall microvessel density. There are, however, several studies showing a lack of correlation or an opposite correlation. This discrepancy may be the result of the morphometric techniques used or of differences in tumor types or treatment schedules.

The oxygen level in a tumor also has a potential prognostic value, and it can be directly measured with microelectrodes. Alternatively, immunohistochemical analysis of tumor tissue for endogenous or exogenous hypoxic markers (e.g., HIF-1α, glucose transporter-1, carbonic anhydrase-9, pimonidazole) can be used as a surrogate for tumor oxygenation status. However, immunohistochemical assessments of hypoxia do not necessarily correlate with oxygen status measured directly with microelectrodes.[254] A concerted effort is under way to assess hypoxia using novel, noninvasive imaging techniques.[255,256] Several studies have shown that tumor hypoxia is a predictor of a poor outcome of radiation therapy when used alone or in combination with other therapies. These findings are consistent with *in vitro* and *in vivo* preclinical studies showing the adverse effect of hypoxia on radiation responses.

Because the IFP is a reflection of the global physiology of tumors, a correlation between tumor IFP and the response to radiation therapy has been suggested. One cervical cancer study has shown that elevated tumor IFP can, indeed, independently predict a poor outcome of radiation therapy.[230] Further studies are needed to evaluate the prognostic significance of IFP in tumors. However, one potential application of the steep rise of pressure at the tumor periphery is improved localization of tumors before their removal.

Finally, circulating biomarkers may provide information about tumor pathophysiology and its changes after treatment. Of note, some of the emerging biomarkers—such as circulating collagen IV or soluble VEGFR-1—may represent biomarkers of vascular normalization and, if validated, could be useful in treatment decisions.[91,92]

Although each of these approaches has advantages, key disadvantages include their invasiveness and their potential for sampling error. With rapid developments in the field of noninvasive imaging, it is likely that the measurement of various physiologic and molecular parameters in tumors will become more refined and convenient for patients. Examples of such imaging approaches include blood oxygen level–dependent magnetic resonance imaging (BOLD MRI), electron paramagnetic resonance spectroscopy/imaging, and [^{18}F]-misonidazole positron emission tomography (FMISO-PET).[255–256,257–259] The promise of such imaging approaches has just started to be realized. FMISO-PET has been evaluated in a substudy of patients with stage III or IV squamous cell carcinoma of the head and neck randomized to concurrent radiotherapy with either tirapazamine and cisplatin or infusional fluorouracil and cisplatin. Pretreatment FMISO-PET–detected hypoxia was associated with a higher risk of locoregional recurrence among patients who did not receive the tirapazamine-containing regimen compared to patients who did receive tirapazamine.[259] This study suggests that FMISO-PET can provide clinically meaningful information about tumor physiology and simultaneously provides evidence that tirapazamine acts by specifically targeting hypoxic tumor cells. Such progress will continue and physiologic/molecular profiles of patients' tumors will yield improved and better-tailored therapies for individual patients.

Therapeutic Implications

Given the physiologic barriers to the delivery and effectiveness of various therapeutics, a strategy that is gaining increasing interest is targeting the tumor vasculature. This strategy has the advantage of targeting ECs that are easily accessible to a bloodborne drug and are presumably genetically stable. In addition, each EC supports multiple cancer cells, thus providing "therapeutic amplification." However, the inability to target *all* ECs in a tumor can reduce the effectiveness of antivascular therapy. Similarly, the dependence of ECs on multiple angiogenic molecules can limit the effectiveness of various antiangiogenic therapies when used alone.[41,83] These challenges may explain why currently available antiangiogenic agents, although demonstrating biologic activity, are unable to provide durable tumor control when used as monotherapy.

Although of limited utility when used alone, the judicious combination of antiangiogenic therapies with conventional cytotoxic therapies has led to improved tumor control in mice and lengthened survival in certain types of human tumors[14,16,17,240,260–263] (see Table 4.1). For example, in two human tumor xenograft models, a VEGFR-2–blocking antibody decreased the dose of fractionated radiation required to control 50% of tumors (TCD_{50}) by 11 to 27 Gy without modifying in-field skin reactions.[240] Thus, to maximize clinical gains, these agents must be employed in combination with radiation and chemotherapy. The challenge now is to

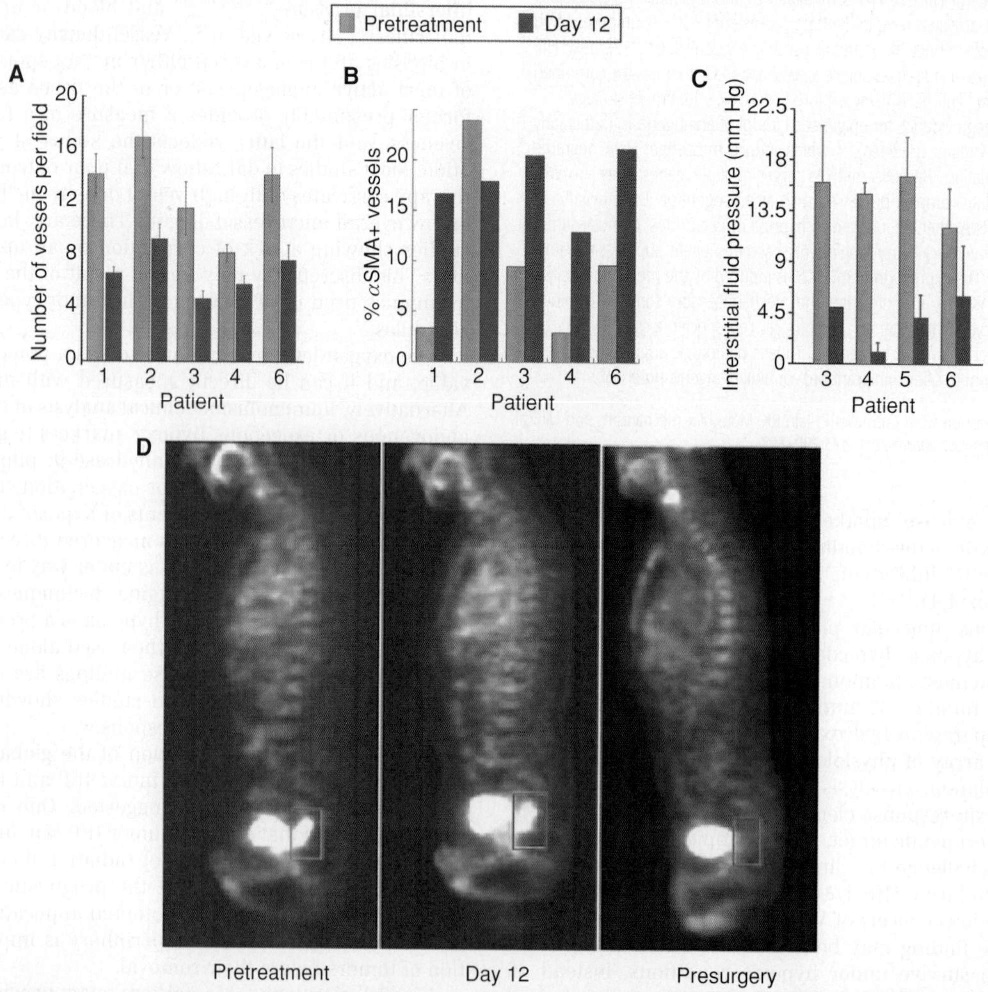

FIGURE 4.8. Vascular "normalization" in rectal cancer patients following treatment with the anti–vascular endothelial growth factor (VEGF) antibody, bevacizumab. **A–C:** Tumor vessel "normalization" following a single injection of bevacizumab is suggested by the reduction of tumor microvessel density **(A)**, by the increase in fraction of tumor vessels with pericyte coverage **(B)**, and by the drop in interstitial fluid pressure **(C)**. **D:** Positron emission tomography reveals no change in 18-fluorodeoxyglucose (FDG) uptake after a single dose of bevacizumab and complete resolution of FDG uptake following neoadjuvant chemoradiation (bevacizumab, 5-fluorouracil, pelvic external-beam radiation therapy). The stability of FDG uptake following bevacizumab monotherapy, despite marked reductions in microvessel density, suggests the efficiency of residual tumor blood vessels after bevacizumab treatment is improved. (From Willett CG, Boucher Y, di Tomaso E, et al. Direct evidence that the VEGF-specific antibody bevacizumab has antivascular effects in human rectal cancer. *Nat Med* 2004;145–147, with permission.)

optimally combine these therapies in patients. Destruction of tumor vasculature by antiangiogenic agents should antagonize chemo- and radiotherapy by compromising the delivery of therapeutics and oxygen, respectively. However, judiciously applied antiangiogenic therapy can prune inefficient tumor vessels and render the remaining vasculature more efficient (Fig. 4.5).[12,41,83,116,223] This "normalization" of tumor vasculature has been demonstrated in various preclinical models (reviewed in[41,83]) and in rectal cancer, hepatocellular carcinoma, ovarian carcinoma, and glioblastoma patients[66,67,69,71,73,75] (Fig. 4.8). Vascular "normalization" should result in improved delivery of cytotoxic chemotherapy and radiosensitizing oxygen, thereby improving tumor control. This principle has been rigorously tested in animal models[83,89,260,264–266] and confirmatory data on the impact of vascular "normalization" on patient outcomes await mature results of ongoing and future clinical trials.

ACKNOWLEDGMENTS

This chapter is an update of the chapter published in the fifth edition of *Principles and Practice of Radiation Oncology* and based on a review article by Carmeliet and Jain, *Nature* 2011.[11] The work summarized here was supported by continuous support from the National Cancer Institute since 1980 to RKJ. We want to acknowledge the support through grants P01CA80124, R01CA115767, R01CA85140, R01CA126642, and Federal Share/NCI Proton Beam Program Income (RKJ), and R21CA139168, R01CA159258, and Federal Share/NCI Proton Beam Program Income (DGD), as well as the National Foundation for Cancer Research Grant and Department of Defense Breast Cancer Research Innovator Award W81XWH-10-1-0016 (RKJ), and the American Cancer Society Research Grant RSG-11-073-01-TBG (DGD).

DISCLOSURE

R.K.J. has research grants from Dyax, MedImmune, and Roche; serves as a consultant to Noxxon Pharmaceuticals; serves on the Scientific Advisory Board of Enlight and SynDevRx; serves on the Board of Directors of XTuit; serves on the Board of Trustees of H&Q Healthcare Investors and H&Q Life Sciences Investors; and has equity in Enlight, SynDevRx and XTuit Pharmaceuticals.

SELECTED REFERENCES

A full list of references for this chapter is available online.

3. Algire GH, Chalkley HW. Vascular reactions of normal and malignant tissues in vivo. I. Vascular reactions of mice to wounds and to normal and neoplastic transplants. *J Natl Cancer Inst* 1945;6:73–85.
5. Jain RK, Munn LL, Fukumura D. Dissecting tumour pathophysiology using intravital microscopy. *Nat Rev Cancer* 2002;2(4):266–276.
8. Folkman J. Tumor angiogenesis: therapeutic implications. *N Engl J Med* 1971;285(21):1182–1186.
9. Folkman J. Angiogenesis: an organizing principle for drug discovery? *Nat Rev Drug Discov* 2007;6(4):273–286.
10. Gullino PM. Angiogenesis and oncogenesis. *J Natl Cancer Inst* 1978;61(3):639–643.
11. Carmeliet P, Jain RK. Molecular mechanisms and clinical applications of angiogenesis. *Nature* 2011;473:298–307.
12. Jain RK. Normalizing tumor vasculature with anti-angiogenic therapy: a new paradigm for combination therapy. *Nat Med* 2001;7(9):987–989.
13. Demetri GD, van Oosterom AT, Garrett CR, et al. Efficacy and safety of sunitinib in patients with advanced gastrointestinal stromal tumour after failure of imatinib: a randomised controlled trial. *Lancet* 2006;368(9544):1329–1338.
14. Hurwitz H, Fehrenbacher L, Novotny W, et al. Bevacizumab plus irinotecan, fluorouracil, and leucovorin for metastatic colorectal cancer. *N Engl J Med* 2004;350(23):2335–2342.
15. Llovet J, Ricci S, Mazzaferro V, et al. Sorafenib in advanced hepatocellular carcinoma. *N Engl J Med* 2008;359(4):378–390.
16. Jain RK, Duda DG, Clark JW, et al. Lessons from phase III clinical trials on anti-VEGF therapy for cancer. *Nat Clin Pract Oncol* 2006;3(1):24–40.
17. Sandler A, Gray R, Perry MC, et al. Paclitaxel-carboplatin alone or with bevacizumab for non-small-cell lung cancer. *N Engl J Med* 2006;355(24):2542–2550.
18. Miller K, Wang M, Gralow J, et al. Paclitaxel plus bevacizumab versus paclitaxel alone for metastatic breast cancer. *N Engl J Med* 2007;357(26):2666–2676.
19. Motzer RJ, Hutson TE, Tomczak P, et al. Sunitinib versus interferon alfa in metastatic renal-cell carcinoma. *N Engl J Med* 2007;356(2):115–124.
20. Cloughesy TF, Prados MD, Wen PY, et al. A phase II, randomized, non-comparative clinical trial of the effect of bevacizumab alone or in combination with irinotecan (CPT-11) on 6-month progression free survival in recurrent, treatment-refractory glioblastoma. *J Clin Oncol* 2008;26S:abstract 2010b.
21. Raymond E, Dahan L, Raoul JL, et al. Sunitinib malate for the treatment of pancreatic neuroendocrine tumors. *N Engl J Med* 2011;364(6):501–513.
23. Helmlinger G, Netti PA, Lichtenbeld HC, et al. Solid stress inhibits the growth of multicellular tumor spheroids. *Nat Biotechnol* 1997;15(8):778–783.
24. Padera TP, Stoll BR, Tooredman JB, et al. Pathology: cancer cells compress intratumour vessels. *Nature* 2004;427(6976):695.
28. Jain RK. Molecular regulation of vessel maturation. *Nat Med* 2003;9(6):685–693.
33. Duda DG, Cohen KS, Kozin SV, et al. Evidence for incorporation of bone marrow-derived endothelial cells into perfused blood vessels in tumors. *Blood* 2006;107(7):2774–2776.
34. Kozin SV, Kamoun W, Huang Y, et al. Recruitment of myeloid but not endothelial precursor cells facilitates tumor re-growth after local irradiation. *Cancer Res* 2010;70(14):5679–5685.
36. Peters BA, Diaz LA, Polyak K, et al. Contribution of bone marrow-derived endothelial cells to human tumor vasculature. *Nat Med* 2005;11(3):261–262.
37. Kozin SV, Duda DG, Munn LL, et al. Is vasculogenesis crucial for the regrowth of irradiated tumours? *Nat Rev Cancer* 2011;11(7):532.
38. Ricci-Vitiani L, Pallini R, Biffoni M, et al. Tumour vascularization via endothelial differentiation of glioblastoma stem-like cells. *Nature* 2010;468:824–828.
41. Carmeliet P, Jain RK. Principles and mechanisms of vessel normalization for cancer and other angiogenic diseases. *Nature Rev Drug Discov* 2011;10(6):417–427.
43. Dvorak HF. Vascular permeability factor/vascular endothelial growth factor: a critical cytokine in tumor angiogenesis and a potential target for diagnosis and therapy. *J Clin Oncol* 2002;20(21):4368–4380.
44. Melder RJ, Koenig GC, Witwer BP, et al. During angiogenesis, vascular endothelial growth factor and basic fibroblast growth factor regulate natural killer cell adhesion to tumor endothelium. *Nat Med* 1996;2(9):992–997.
47. Yoshiji H, Harris SR, Thorgeirsson UP. Vascular endothelial growth factor is essential for initial but not continued in vivo growth of human breast carcinoma cells. *Cancer Res* 1997;57(18):3924–3928.
52. Fukumura D, Xu L, Chen Y, et al. Hypoxia and acidosis independently up-regulate vascular endothelial growth factor transcription in brain tumors *in vivo*. *Cancer Res* 2001;61:6020–6024.
53. Hanahan D, Weinberg RA. Hallmarks of cancer: the next generation. *Cell* 2011;144(5):646–674.
54. Huang Y, Snuderl M, Jain RK. Polarization of tumor-associated macrophages: a novel strategy for vascular normalization and antitumor immunity. *Cancer Cell* 2011;19(1):1–2.
55. Jain RK, Duda DG. Role of bone marrow-derived cells in tumor angiogenesis and treatment. *Cancer Cell* 2003;3(6):515–516.
58. Fukumura D, Xavier R, Sugiura T, et al. Tumor induction of VEGF promoter activity in stromal cells. *Cell* 1998;94(6):715–725.
60. Brown EB, Campbell RB, Tsuzuki Y, et al. In vivo measurement of gene expression, angiogenesis and physiological function in tumors using multiphoton laser scanning microscopy. *Nat Med* 2001;7(7):864–868.
61. Fukumura D, Yuan F, Monsky WL, et al. Effect of host microenvironment on the microcirculation of human colon adenocarcinoma. *Am J Pathol* 1997;151(3):679–688.
62. Gohongi T, Fukumura D, Boucher Y, et al. Tumor-host interactions in the gallbladder suppress distal angiogenesis and tumor growth: involvement of transforming growth factor beta1. *Nat Med* 1999;5(10):1203–1208.
63. Hobbs SK, Monsky WL, Yuan F, et al. Regulation of transport pathways in tumor vessels: role of tumor type and microenvironment. *Proc Natl Acad Sci U S A* 1998;95(8):4607–4612.
64. Monsky WL, Carreira CM, Tsuzuki Y, et al. Role of host microenvironment in angiogenesis and microvascular functions in human breast cancer xenografts: mammary fat pad vs. cranial tumors. *Clin Cancer Res* 2002;8:1008–1013.
67. Batchelor TT, Sorensen AG, di Tomaso E, et al. AZD2171, a pan-VEGF receptor tyrosine kinase inhibitor, normalizes tumor vasculature and alleviates edema in glioblastoma patients. *Cancer Cell* 2007;11(1):83–95.
70. Izumi Y, Xu L, di Tomaso E, et al. Tumour biology: herceptin acts as an anti-angiogenic cocktail. *Nature* 2002;416(6878):279–280.
71. Willett CG, Boucher Y, di Tomaso E, et al. Direct evidence that the VEGF-specific antibody bevacizumab has antivascular effects in human rectal cancer. *Nat Med* 2004;10(2):145–147.
73. Willett CG, Duda DG, di Tomaso E, et al. Efficacy, safety, and biomarkers of neoadjuvant bevacizumab, radiation therapy, and fluorouracil in rectal cancer: a multidisciplinary phase II study. *J Clin Oncol* 2009;27(18):3020–3026.
76. Zhu AX, Duda DG, Sahani DV, et al. HCC and angiogenesis: possible targets and future directions. *Nat Rev Clin Oncol* 2011;8(5):292–301.
77. Baish JW, Stylianopoulos T, Lanning RM, et al. Scaling rules for diffusive drug delivery in tumor and normal tissues. *Proc Natl Acad Sci U S A* 2011;108(5):1799–1803.
83. Goel S, Duda DG, Xu L, et al. Normalization of the vasculature for treatment of cancer and other diseases. *Physiol Rev* 2011;91(3):1071–1121.
84. Jain RK, Safabakhsh N, Sckell A, et al. Endothelial cell death, angiogenesis, and microvascular function after castration in an androgen-dependent tumor: role of vascular endothelial growth factor. *Proc Natl Acad Sci U S A* 1998;95(18):10820–10825.
85. Chae S-S, Kamoun W, Farrar C, et al. Angiopoietin-2 interferes with anti-VEGFR-2-induced vessel normalization and survival benefit in mice bearing gliomas. *Clin Cancer Res* 2010;16:3618–3627.
87. Kamoun WS, Ley CD, Farrar CT, et al. Edema control by cediranib, a vascular endothelial growth factor receptor-targeted kinase inhibitor, prolongs survival despite persistent brain tumor growth in mice. *J Clin Oncol* 2009;27(15):2542–2552.
88. Tong RT, Boucher Y, Kozin SV, et al. Vascular normalization by vascular endothelial growth factor receptor 2 blockade induces a pressure gradient across the vasculature and improves drug penetration in tumors. *Cancer Res* 2004;64(11):3731–3736.
89. Winkler F, Kozin SV, Tong R, et al. Kinetics of vascular normalization by VEGFR2 blockade governs brain tumor response to radiation: role of oxygenation, angiopoietin-1 and matrix metalloproteinases. *Cancer Cell* 2004;6:553–563.
90. Yuan F, Chen Y, Dellian M, et al. Time-dependent vascular regression and permeability changes in established human tumor xenografts induced by an anti-vascular endothelial growth factor/vascular permeability factor antibody. *Proc Natl Acad Sci U S A* 1996;93(25):14765–14770.
91. Duda DG, Willett CG, Ancukiewicz M, et al. Plasma soluble VEGFR-1 is a potential dual biomarker of response and toxicity for bevacizumab with chemoradiation in locally advanced rectal cancer. *Oncologist* 2010;15(6):577–583.
92. Sorensen AG, Batchelor TT, Zhang WT, et al. A "vascular normalization index" as potential mechanistic biomarker to predict survival after a single dose of cediranib in recurrent glioblastoma patients. *Cancer Res* 2009;69(13):5296–5300.

93. Sorensen AG, Emblem KE, Polaskova P, et al. Increased survival of glioblastoma patients who respond to anti-angiogenic therapy with elevated blood perfusion. *Cancer Res* 2012;72:402–407.
94. Gerstner ER, Emblem KE, Chi AS, et al. Effects of cediranib, a VEGF signaling inhibitor, in combination with chemoradiation on tumor blood flow and survival in newly diagnosed glioblastoma. *J Clin Oncol* 2012;30 (suppl; abstr 2009).
96. Griffon-Etienne G, Boucher Y, Brekken C, et al. Taxane-induced apoptosis decompresses blood vessels and lowers interstitial fluid pressure in solid tumors: clinical implications. *Cancer Res* 1999;59(15):3776–3782.
97. Jain RK. Determinants of tumor blood flow: a review. *Cancer Res* 1988;48:2641–2658.
102. Vaupel P, Kallinowski F, Okunieff P. Blood flow, oxygen and nutrient supply, and metabolic microenvironment of human tumors: a review. *Cancer Res* 1989;49(23):6449–6465.
104. Endrich B, Reinhold HS, Gross JF, et al. Tissue perfusion inhomogeneity during early tumor growth in rats. *J Natl Cancer Inst* 1979;62(2):387–395.
112. Kashiwagi S, Izumi Y, Gohongi T, et al. NO mediates mural cell recruitment and vessel morphogenesis in murine melanomas and tissue-engineered blood vessels. *J Clin Invest* 2005;115(7):1816–1827.
115. Heath VL, Bicknell R. Anticancer strategies involving the vasculature. *Nat Rev Clin Oncol* 2009;6(7):395–404.
116. Jain RK. Normalization of tumor vasculature: an emerging concept in antiangiogenic therapy. *Science* 2005;307(5706):58–62.
118. Jain RK. Transport of molecules across tumor vasculature. *Cancer Metastasis Rev* 1987;6:559–594.
129. Weis SM, Cheresh DA. Pathophysiological consequences of VEGF-induced vascular permeability. *Nature* 2005;437(7058):497–504.
131. Duda DG, Duyverman AM, Kohno M, et al. Malignant cells facilitate lung metastasis by bringing their own soil. *Proc Natl Acad Sci U S A* 2010;107(50):21677–21682.
136. Hiratsuka S, Goel S, Kamoun WS, et al. Endothelial focal adhesion kinase mediates cancer cell homing to discrete regions of the lungs via E-selectin upregulation. *Proc Natl Acad Sci U S A* 2011;108(9):3725–3730.
142. Fukumura D, Salehi HA, Witwer B, et al. Tumor necrosis factor alpha-induced leukocyte adhesion in normal and tumor vessels: effect of tumor type, transplantation site, and host strain. *Cancer Res* 1995;55(21):4824–4829.
154. Hamzah J, Jugold M, Kiessling F, et al. Vascular normalization in Rgs5-deficient tumours promotes immune destruction. *Nature* 2008;453(7193):410–414.
155. Huang Y, Yuan J, Righi E, et al. Vascular normalizing doses of antiangiogenic treatment reprogram the immunosuppressive tumor microenvironment and enhance immunotherapy. *Proc Natl Acad Sci USA* 2012;doi:10.1073/pnas.1215397109.
159. Hiratsuka S, Duda DG, Huang Y, et al. C-X-C receptor type 4 promotes metastasis by activating p38 mitogen-activated protein kinase in myeloid differentiation antigen (Gr-1)-positive cells. *Proc Natl Acad Sci U S A* 2011;108(1):302–307.
162. de Visser KE, Eichten A, Coussens LM. Paradoxical roles of the immune system during cancer development. *Nat Rev Cancer* 2006;6(1):24–37.
164. Rolny C, Mazzone M, Tugues S, et al. HRG inhibits tumor growth and metastasis by inducing macrophage polarization and vessel normalization through downregulation of PlGF. *Cancer Cell* 2011;19(1):31–44.
166. Padera TP, Kadambi A, di Tomaso E, et al. Lymphatic metastasis in the absence of functional intratumor lymphatics. *Science* 2002;296(5574):1883–1886.
168. Brown EB, McKee T, diTomaso E, et al. Dynamic imaging of collagen and its modulation in tumors in vivo using second-harmonic generation. *Nat Med* 2003;9(6):796–800.
174. Znati CA, Rosenstein M, Mckee TD, et al. Irradiation reduces interstitial fluid transport and increases the collagen content in tumors. *Clin Cancer Res* 2003;9:5508–5513.
178. Diop-Frimpong B, Chauhan VP, Krane S, et al. Losartan inhibits collagen I synthesis and improves the distribution and efficacy of nanotherapeutics in tumors. *Proc Natl Acad Sci U S A* 2011;108(7):2909–2914.
179. Baxter LT, Jain RK. Transport of fluid and macromolecules in tumors. IV. A microscopic model of the perivascular distribution. *Microvasc Res* 1991;41(2):252–272.
181. Olive KP, Jacobetz MA, Davidson CJ, et al. Inhibition of Hedgehog signaling enhances delivery of chemotherapy in a mouse model of pancreatic cancer. *Science* 2009;324(5933):1457–1461.
185. Hoshida T, Isaka N, Hagendoorn J, et al. Imaging steps of lymphatic metastasis reveals that vascular endothelial growth factor-C increases metastasis by increasing delivery of cancer cells to lymph nodes: therapeutic implications. *Cancer Res* 2006;66(16):8065–8075.
186. Tammela T, Alitalo K. Lymphangiogenesis: molecular mechanisms and future promise. *Cell* 2010;140(4):460–476.
191. Cursiefen C, Chen L, Borges LP, et al. VEGF-A stimulates lymphangiogenesis and hemangiogenesis in inflammatory neovascularization via macrophage recruitment. *J Clin Invest* 2004;113(7):1040–1050.
192. Nagy JA, Vasile E, Feng D, et al. Vascular permeability factor/vascular endothelial growth factor induces lymphangiogenesis as well as angiogenesis. *J Exp Med* 2002;196(11):1497–1506.
198. Hagendoorn J, Padera TP, Kashiwagi S, et al. Endothelial nitric oxide synthase regulates microlymphatic flow via collecting lymphatics. *Circ Res* 2004;95(2):204–209.
198. Jeltsch M, Kaipainen A, Joukov V, et al. Hyperplasia of lymphatic vessels in VEGF-C transgenic mice. *Science* 1997;276(5317):1423–1425.
204. Boucher Y, Baxter LT, Jain RK. Interstitial pressure gradients in tissue-isolated and subcutaneous tumors: implications for therapy. *Cancer Res* 1990;50(15):4478–4484.
206. Boucher Y, Kirkwood JM, Opacic D, et al. Interstitial hypertension in superficial metastatic melanomas in humans. *Cancer Res* 1991;51(24):6691–6694.
212. Milosevic M, Fyles A, Hedley D, et al. Interstitial fluid pressure predicts survival in patients with cervix cancer independent of clinical prognostic factors and tumor oxygen measurements. *Cancer Res* 2001;61(17):6400–6405.
217. Lee CG, Heijn M, diTomasso E, et al. Anti-vascular endothelial growth factor treatment augments tumor radiation response under normoxic or hypoxic conditions. *Cancer Res* 2000;60:5565–5570.
223. Jain RK. Taming vessels to treat cancer. *Sci Am* 2008;298:56–63.
240. Kozin SV, Boucher Y, Hicklin DJ, et al. Vascular endothelial growth factor receptor-2-blocking antibody potentiates radiation-induced long-term control of human tumor xenografts. *Cancer Res* 2001;61:39–44.
243. Semenza GL. Oxygen sensing, homeostasis, and disease. *N Engl J Med* 2011; 365(6):537–547.
244. Mazzone M, Dettori D, Leite de Oliveira R, et al. Heterozygous deficiency of PHD2 restores tumor oxygenation and inhibits metastasis via endothelial normalization. *Cell* 2009;136(5):839–851.
246. Carmeliet P, Dor Y, Herbert JM, et al. Role of HIF-1alpha in hypoxia-mediated apoptosis, cell proliferation and tumour angiogenesis. *Nature* 1998;394(6692): 485–490.
248. Cramer T, Yamanishi Y, Clausen BE, et al. HIF-1alpha is essential for myeloid cell-mediated inflammation. *Cell* 2003;112(5):645–657.
251. McCormick F. New-age drug meets resistance. *Nature* 2001;412(6844):281–282.
255. Serganova I, Humm J, Ling C, et al. Tumor hypoxia imaging. *Clin Cancer Res* 2006;12(18):5260–5264.
256. Sorensen AG, Batchelor TT, Wen PY, et al. Response criteria for glioma. *Nat Clin Pract Oncol* 2008;5(11):634–644.
267. Helmlinger G, Yuan F, Dellian M, et al. Interstitial pH and pO2 gradients in solid tumors in vivo: high-resolution measurements reveal a lack of correlation. *Nat Med* 1997;3(2):177–182.
270. Du R, Lu KV, Petritsch C, et al. HIF1alpha induces the recruitment of bone marrow-derived vascular modulatory cells to regulate tumor angiogenesis and invasion. *Cancer Cell* 2008;13(3):206–220.
271. Arany Z, Foo SY, Ma Y, et al. HIF-independent regulation of VEGF and angiogenesis by the transcriptional coactivator PGC-1alpha. *Nature* 2008;451(7181): 1008–1012.

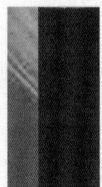

Chapter 5
Smart Radiotherapy

C. Norman Coleman, Eric J. Bernhard, Jacek Capala, Bhadrasain Vikram, and James A. Deye

When assigned this chapter title, "Smart Radiotherapy," we were challenged as to the best approach. Looking through the previous edition, there was no precedent for a chapter with this name. Was there to be a companion chapter or chapters of "So-So Radiotherapy" or "Oy-Vay Radiotherapy"? Although one could perhaps all-too-readily envision examples, we decided that the most positive approach would be to enhance what will be an excellent and complete textbook by top quality experts by providing some of the new areas of research that might impact clinical radiation therapy over the next 5 years from our perspective in the National Cancer Institute (NCI), Division of Cancer Treatment and Diagnosis, Radiation Research Program. We anticipate that the radiation biology chapter will include molecular aspects of radiation therapy and the basic aspects of tumor microenvironment, the physics chapter will discuss particle therapy including protons and carbon ions, and the clinical chapters will include molecular characterization of tumors, the use of molecular imaging, and the current studies with molecular targeted agents.

So, taking a broad view, what is likely to impact radiation oncology practice and thinking over the next 5 or so years? The technology of radiation therapy is growing in complexity and cost so that clinical utilization and possibly reimbursement will require definite or at least reasonable proof of principle. Bringing the spectacular particle-therapy treatment plans seen on a computer screen to accurate and reproducible delivery to the patient requires understanding the pitfalls of dose distribution. Conceivably, new accelerator design may provide innovative and less-expensive technology and also a range of particles beyond protons. The rapid advance in cancer biology and the availability of many new molecular-targeted agents will require more rapid clinical trials, with the randomized phase II trial becoming a major tool, potentially using new clinical trial design techniques.[1] The tumor microenvironment, long a province of radiation biology and radiation therapy, has enormous potential as a therapeutic target for cell killing and also for immune modulation. The threat of radiological terrorism has led to new investment in agents to mitigate radiation injury. This is research and development support above and beyond the NCI and National Institutes of Health funding allocation and may also have applications in cancer care. Nanotechnology and smaller biological delivery vehicles are bringing targeted systemic radiotherapy to a new level of possibility.

Cells know that they are irradiated, and as the "bystander effect" field has demonstrated, they not only respond but they tell their neighbors and progeny. Thus, the changing phenotype of the survivors might be utilized for treatment. Finally, on the macro level, the incidences of the noncommunicable diseases, cancer and heart disease, are already exceeding infectious diseases[2,3] as a cause of morbidity, mortality, and economic disaster in developing countries. Smart and socially responsible radiotherapy needs to aim to reach the patients who can afford and access the very sophisticated expert centers and also those patients struggling to obtain care—albeit symptom relief or curative treatment—in an underserved community in the developing and developed world.

In that any textbook is somewhat out of date by the time it goes from writing to printing, rapidly changing research fields will be obsolescent almost from the time the chapter is written. Our aim in this chapter is to address the topics from a mostly conceptual viewpoint, including a few key references and examples. We are hopeful that these topics will provide the reader with a sense of optimism of the potential advances and contributions radiation oncology, biology, and physics and models of social outreach can make to innovative, effective, and far-reaching improvements in cancer care.

TUMOR MICROENVIRONMENT

The efficacy of radiotherapy is in part determined by tumor microenvironmental factors, including the extent of tumor oxygenation, the tumor pH, and the interaction of tumor cells with host stroma and with inflammatory cells. Tumors contain areas of poor vascular perfusion, low pH, and oxygen, which may provide regions in which the delivery and activity of cytotoxic therapies is attenuated.[4] Resistance to therapy in these regions may be due to the effects of low oxygen, low pH, limited drug delivery presence of resistant cell niches,[5] or a combination of all four. The tumor microenvironment influences, and is in turn influenced by, the interaction of tumor cells with host stroma and with inflammatory cells. In addition, certain tumor environments may select for more aggressive or resistant tumor clonogens.[6]

Changes in the tumor microenvironment occur during radiotherapy.[7] Fractionated radiotherapy results in reoxygenation of the tumor due to elimination of well-oxygenated cells, thus increasing oxygen delivery to the previously hypoxic areas. Conversely, high-dose single fractions (over 13 Gy) have been shown to result in destruction of both tumor cells and vascular endothelium.[8] How and under what circumstances radiation-induced vascular injury impacts tumor responses continues to be a topic of investigation and is relevant to the current use of large fraction stereotactic radiosurgery or therapy.[9,10,11,12]

Tumor Hypoxia

Perhaps the best-studied example of tumor microenvironment effects on cancer cell survival is tumor oxygenation. It is known that radiation under atmospheric oxygen conditions enhances killing by a factor of 2 to 3 compared to irradiation under anoxic conditions, which has been termed the oxygen enhancement ratio[13] (as reviewed by Horsman et al.[7]). In the clinical setting, hypoxia affects outcome after radiotherapy.[14–15,16] But hypoxia has also been shown to be a poor prognostic factor after chemotherapy[17] and surgery.[18,19] These findings were attributed to chronic hypoxia induced under controlled culture conditions or oxygen levels measured with electrodes or immunohistochemical staining. Overcoming hypoxia by targeting hypoxic regions in tumors has proven difficult. Recent advances in noninvasive tumor hypoxia imaging may come into play in the future, allowing precise definition of hypoxic tumors and tumor subregions through imaging with positron emission tomography (PET), magnetic resonance imaging (MRI), or electron paramagnetic resonance oxygen imaging.[20–23]

More recent studies have shown that acute fluctuations in tumor oxygenation ("transient" or "cycling" hypoxia) interspersed with periods of reoxygenation may be even more effective in promoting tumor survival and progression than chronic hypoxia.[7] Defining whether intermittent or chronic hypoxia is more radiobiologically important is at present an open question; however, it is likely that both contribute to resistance. It is clear that cycling hypoxia may complicate efforts to identify and target radiobiologically important hypoxic regions within tumors using approaches such as radiation dose painting to hypoxic tumor subregions.[24] Regions of cycling hypoxia may be more difficult to image using current methods, such as nitroimidazole markers, which are better suited to detecting chronic hypoxia. Developments in imaging with MRI and electron paramagnetic resonance may facilitate real-time detection of hypoxic transients in the future.

Hypoxic Cell Sensitizers and Cytotoxins

There are two chemical approaches used to reduce the impact of hypoxic cells on radiotherapy response: radiosensitization and hypoxic cell cytotoxins. The nitroimidazole hypoxic cell sensitizer, nimorazole, used with radiotherapy has shown promising results in patients with hypoxic tumors.[25,26] However, testing and adoption of this drug in countries other than Denmark have been slow at least in part due to a lack of patent protection for the drug (an issue that may be relevant to the use of chemotherapeutic agents as radiation sensitizers). General adoption of this treatment could, in theory, improve outcome in certain tumors such as head and neck squamous cell carcinomas. An alternative approach of using hypoxic cell cytotoxins has also been tested. Tirapazamine (TPZ, 3-amino-1,2,4-benzotriazine-1, 4-dioxide) undergoes reduction under hypoxia to form a highly reactive radical that causes DNA damage leading to cell killing.[27] Under normoxic conditions the reduction of TPZ is reversed, thus providing the specificity of cytotoxicity for hypoxic tissues.[28,29] Despite promising early results, a recent phase III trial of TPZ in combination with chemoradiotherapy failed to demonstrate an improvement in failure-free survival, time to locoregional failure, or quality of life among patients with head and neck cancers.[30] The reasons for this failure are the subject of debate,[31,32] and the future of this compound is at present unclear. Development of new generation hypoxic cell cytotoxins with greater preclinical efficacy than TPZ is under way.[32]

The identification and selective treatment of hypoxic tumors is likely, in the future, to enhance the results of radiotherapy. The failure to select patients with hypoxic tumors in past studies may have led to the negative results with many of the approaches tested to date, but novel imaging methods to identify hypoxia and new generation hypoxic cytotoxins and sensitizers will benefit this approach.

Tumor Angiogenesis

Normal angiogenesis is a highly regulated process involving endothelial cells with differing functions (tip, stalk, and phalanx cells) under tight regulation of oxygen sensors (prolyl-hydroxylase-2 [PHD-2]), growth and maturation factors (vascular endothelial growth factor [VEGF], angiopoetins), and transmembrane receptors (Notch family) (reviewed in Carmeliet et al.[33]). Small changes or imbalance in the expression of these regulators can have a significant impact on vascular development and lead to the formation of abnormal tumor vessels that are inefficient in the transport of nutrients, oxygen, and metabolic wastes. Limited perfusion and convection also reduce the efficacy of chemotherapeutic delivery. Vascular endothelium largely comprises host cells, and these cells, unlike tumor cells, are genetically stable and thus an attractive target. Antiangiogenic agents reduce or cut off tumor vascular flow by selective targeting of tumor vessel growth by blocking VEGF signaling. Targeting the tumor vasculature was originally proposed by Judah Folkman.[34] It is now clear, however, that this approach is complicated by the fact that development, structure, and the potential for recovery of tumor vasculature after treatment are influenced by bone marrow–derived progenitor cells in addition to the tumor and other stromal elements.[35] In addition, where tumor cell–derived vascular channeling (vasculogenic mimicry) plays a role in tumor circulation,[36–38] the effects of antiangiogenic strategies that target host vascular endothelial cells may not be as effective. The activity of cilengitide, an inhibitor of integrin binding to extracellular matrix, as an antiangiogenic agent[39] is of particular interest in this regard. The resistance of glioblastomas to other antiangiogenic therapies may be related to their potential for vasculogenic mimicry.[38,40] As cilengitide targets integrins rather than endothelial cells per se, it might be active against vessel structures derived from tumor rather than host endothelial cells.

VEGF can be induced in response to radiation, and inhibition of VEGF can increase tumor control after radiation in preclinical models.[41] VEGF receptor inhibition reduces endothelial cell proliferation *in vitro* after irradiation and also reduces microvessel density in irradiated tumors.[42] Clinical trials have suggested a potential benefit in combining radiation and antiangiogenic therapy in rectal cancer and sarcoma.[43,44] However, the toxicity of bevacizumab in combination with radiotherapy has been of concern in some tumors.[45]

Tumor Vessel Normalization

Vascular normalization is a term coined to denote transient changes observed in tumor vessels after VEGF inhibition with DC101, a VEGF receptor-2 antibody.[46] Other antiangiogenic approaches have shown similar effects on tumor vasculature. Methylselenocysteine, which has antiangiogenic activity, has been shown to induce a more mature morphology in FaDu xenograft tumor vessels, accompanied by enhanced perfusion and a fourfold increase in doxorubicin delivery to treated tumors.[47] Normalization appears morphologically as a reduction in the chaotic branching and tortuosity of tumor vessels and is accompanied by a reduction in tumor hypoxia and enhanced radiosensitivity. The effects of vascular normalization may also involve reduction of tumor interstitial fluid pressure. High tumor interstitial fluid pressure has been shown to impact survival after irradiation and may also be influenced by the tumor stroma.[48] Tong et al.[49] have shown that blocking VEGF signaling by DC101 results in decreased interstitial fluid pressure in tumor xenografts in mice. Although the normalization period offers an opportunity for improved response to radiation and chemotherapy, the period of normalization obtained with direct targeting of VEGF signaling in preclinical studies lasts less than a week, followed by vascular insufficiency due to strong antiangiogenic activity of these inhibitors. In addition, vascular normalization may not occur in all tumors and has not been observed in all studies (reviewed in Horsman and Siemann[50]).

In the clinical setting, vascular normalization has been proposed as a predictive marker in patients undergoing cediranib treatment for recurrent glioblastoma.[51] Elevated blood perfusion after cediranib treatment has recently been associated with increased survival in these patients.[52]

More durable normalization of tumor vasculature might be clinically achievable through growth factor or oncogenic signaling inhibition. Studies have shown changes in vascular morphology, function, and maturation accompanied by decreased tumor hypoxia after inhibition targeting epidermal growth factor (EGF) receptor, RAS, phosphoinositide (PI) 3-kinase, or AKT in human tumor xenografts and spontaneous mouse tumors that last up to two weeks.[53] Others have shown showed that blocking EGF signaling increased tumor uptake of cisplatin at the same time that enhanced vascular function and oxygenation were seen in tumor xenografts.[54] Signaling inhibition in these studies decreased, but did not eliminate, VEGF production by tumors, which might account for the effects seen and their duration.

Other approaches to altering tumor vasculature are being investigated. Inhibition of $\alpha(v)\beta(3)/\alpha(v)\beta(5)$ integrin has been reported to cause effects similar to signaling inhibition on tumor vascular morphology.[55] Using another approach, investigators showed that shutting off NOS1 production by U87 glioblastoma tumors restored a nitric oxide gradient around the tumor vessels. This was accompanied by a normalized phenotype with less tortuous and more abundant vessels that had increased perivascular cell coverage.[56] Hypoxia in these tumors was reduced and their response to radiation increased as measured both by relative tumor volume and survival endpoints. Modulation of host PHD-2 can affect tumor vascular structure and maturity.[57] Inhibitors of PHD-2, such as DMOG, might be developed for clinical application.

Inhibition of Vasculogenesis

Vasculogenesis, unlike angiogenesis, recruits cells from distant sites, including the bone marrow, to participate in the formation of new blood vessels (reviewed in Patenaude et al.[58]). The process is thought to be an important contributor to the tumor vasculature, although the precise contribution of the different recruited cell types is still a matter of debate.[35] The CD11b positive, matrix metalloproteinase-9 (MMP-9) expressing myeloid cells appear to be central to this process.[59] A neutralizing antibody to CD11b inhibited the recruitment of myeloid cells to tumors and prolonged radiation-induced regrowth delay. Additionally, mice with reduced CD11b expression showed enhanced xenograft radiosensitivity.[60] Stromal derived factor-1 (SDF-1) and the chemokine receptor CXCR4 also contribute to recruitment of endothelial cell precursors and could be targeted. Inhibition of the CXCR4/SDF-1 interaction reduced bone marrow–derived progenitor cell recruitment into irradiated glioblastoma orthotopic xenografts and slowed tumor regrowth.[61] An inhibitor of SDF-1, AMD3100, is in clinical use for stem cell mobilization and could be quickly adopted for this purpose. Inhibition of tumor vasculogenesis may be an important future approach to block tumor vascular recovery after treatment.

Antivascular Therapy

Selectively destroying tumor vasculature with vascular disrupting agents (VDA) is an approach that seeks to kill tumors by shutting off their blood supplies (reviewed in McKeage and Baguley[62]). This approach, however, acts primarily on the tumor core and does not eradicate host vessels that border the tumor and are in proximity of normal host vasculature. Tumor cells at the host–tumor interface can remain viable after this treatment to repopulate the tumor. Furthermore, vascular disruption could generate areas of hypoxia that still contain viable tumor cells, thereby selecting for more resistant clones.[6] Combining VDA treatment with a cytotoxic modality could overcome this problem. The effects of VDAs both alone and in combination with antiangiogenics, chemotherapy, radiation, or other modalities, have been examined in a number of preclinical studies (reviewed by Horsman and Siemann[50]). VDAs are currently in phase II to III clinical trials alone or in combination with cytotoxic chemotherapies.[62–64]

Tumor Stroma and Extracellular Matrix

The tumor stromal compartment, including the extracellular matrix, host fibroblasts, and immune cells, is known to contribute to tumor progression and survival.[65,66] In certain tumors, like pancreatic cancers, activation of quiescent stromal cells, known as stellate cells, to myofibroblast-like cells involved in extracellular matrix production contributes significantly to tumor progression.[67] Activated fibroblasts deposit collagens, leading to changes in stromal rigidity. This mechanism for stromal-induced tumor promotion includes intercellular signaling initiation via integrins to prosurvival pathways, including PI3-kinase.[68] Stroma-mediated change in tumor tensile properties is thought to contribute to tumor progression.[69]

There are multiple points at which stromal changes can be inhibited, including inhibition of fibroblast or stellate cell activation by angiotensin-converting enzyme (ACE) inhibitors or other antifibrogenic compounds such as halofuginone.[70] Signaling by the cytokine tumor growth factor-β (TGF-β) strongly promotes fibrosis, both in response to tumor growth and in normal tissues in response to treatment with radiation. Direct inhibition of TGF-β in tumors can interrupt or mitigate desmoplasia and reduce tumor growth.[71] Angiotensin-II (Ang II) can promote stellate cell growth under pathologic conditions, and ACE inhibitors act in part through blocking Ang II.[72] Angiotensin-(1-7), an endogenous 7 amino-acid peptide antagonist of Ang II, has been shown to reduce TGF-β expression, block proliferation of cancer-associated fibroblasts, and inhibit tumor growth.[73] Inhibition of Hedgehog pathway signaling results in transient enhancement of vascular perfusion and gemcitabine delivery to spontaneous pancreatic cancer in a mouse model.[74] This model shares a high degree of stromal cell activation and poor vascular perfusion with human pancreatic ductal adenocarcinomas. In these tumors, the downstream Gli transcription factor is activated in the tumor stromal cells, resulting in a desmoplastic reaction. Inhibition of Hedgehog signaling to the Smoothened receptor blocks activation of Gli and thereby reduces the activation and proliferation of the stromal compartment.

Integrin binding and signaling have been identified as a potential target for cancer treatment, as these receptors are involved in both tumor growth and angiogenesis (reviewed in Desgrosellier and Cheresh[39]). Cilengitide is a pentapeptide mimic of the RGD binding site that blocks α(v)β3 and α(v)β(5), binding to extracellular matrix components.[75] In addition to its antiangiogenic activity, it inhibits focal adhesion kinase signaling.[76] Cilengitide is well tolerated and has some antitumor activity as a single agent.[77] It has been shown to be active in combination with radiation in several, but not in all reports.[78–80] However, questions remain about potential normal tissue toxicity in combined modality treatment because integrin signaling is required for normal cell function and survival.[79] In this regard, cilengitide was shown to aggravate experimental liver fibrosis in an animal model.[81] Despite this, clinical trial results combining cilengitide with temozolomide and radiation have been encouraging[82] when compared to historical controls. The primary focus of cilengitide studies has been on glioblastoma, but other tumor targets including melanoma and breast and pancreatic cancers are being tested for sensitivity to this agent.[78,83,84]

Targeting Stem Cells

The cancer stem cells (CSCs) model is currently used to as a framework for understanding cancer proliferation, growth and treatment resistance (reviewed in Bednar and Simeone[85]). CSCs are thought to be a subset of cells at the peak of a developmental chain within a tumor with the capacity for unlimited self-renewal and were first identified in breast cancer as cells that were surface marker CD44+/CD24− and capable of tumor initiation.[86] These cells give rise to more differentiated daughter cells with less replicative and tumorigenic potential that make up the bulk of the tumor cell population. The CSC may be more quiescent than the general population of cells in a tumor and relatively resistant to cytotoxic therapy.[87] Some studies have identified perivascular niches for these cells (reviewed in Borovski et al.[88]) and the conditions that promote their colonization and survival,[5] but the identification of both the stem cells and their niches in a disorganized and dynamic tumor environment remains challenging.[89] The perivascular niche and, in particular, the endothelial cells may both aid in tissue repair and promote tumor growth by secreting "angiocrine factors."[90] Targeting these factors could be an approach to cancer treatment. Disruption of the perivascular niche with vascular disrupting agents or antiangiogenics might also reduce CSC numbers.

The pericyte component of the tumor vasculature is another potential therapeutic target. Interferon-β treatment has been shown to decrease CD34+ cancer stem cells in a U87 orthotopic glioblastoma tumor model. Examination of the perivascular niches in which these stem cells are found showed increased numbers of pericytes. The increase in pericytes is hypothesized to block interactions of glioma stem cells with the vascular endothelium and also, perhaps, reduce their exposure to growth factors,[90] thus reducing stem cell frequency in these tumors.[91] The potential for CSCs as targets and potential biomarkers for radiotherapy has recently been reviewed by Krause et al.[92]

Immunological and Inflammatory Responses

Immune responses can both be modulated by and contribute to radiotherapy treatment responses (reviewed in Shiao and Coussens[93]). Although whole-body radiotherapy is immunosuppressive, localized treatment may boost immune reactivity toward a tumor by enhancing antigen presentation. This may be particularly true in the case of high-dose hypofractionated, but not single dose, delivery, as discussed below.[94] Irradiation can promote tumor cytokine release, as well as increasing class I antigen expression and intercellular and matrix cell surface adhesion molecules including ICAM-1 E-selectin and VCAM-1.[93] Manipulations of the immune system and tumor infiltrating cells are also being tested as therapeutic approaches. In the future, radiotherapy may be combined as an adjuvant to vaccination to promote antitumor immune responses.[95] As mentioned above, inhibition of CD11b monocytes can inhibit tumor revascularization.[60] Conversely, tumor hypoxia itself may have an immunosuppressive effect.[96] Tumor-associated macrophages (type M2) are known to influence both progression and metastasis. Their presence is associated with poor prognosis.[97,98] Modulating the differentiation of macrophage precursors to shift the balance toward effector (type I) macrophages may prove to be additional strategy for intervention.

Recent work indicates a novel potential target within the tumor stroma, fibroblast activation protein, which has the potential to enhance innate antitumor immune responses. In a transgenic mouse model the elimination (through genetic manipulation) of fibroblasts and pericytes expressing fibroblast activation protein enhanced antitumor immune responses. Activation of tumor-infiltrating T cells and the resulting increase in interferon-γ and tumor necrosis factor-α (TNF-α) promoted the antitumor immune response in a transgenic mouse model.[99] A possible pharmacologic approach to elimination of these activated fibroblasts is by inhibition of the matrix enzyme lysyl oxidase-like-2 (LOXL-2). Inhibition of this enzyme using a monoclonal antibody decreased desmoplasia and both primary and metastatic tumor growth[100]; small molecule inhibitors of

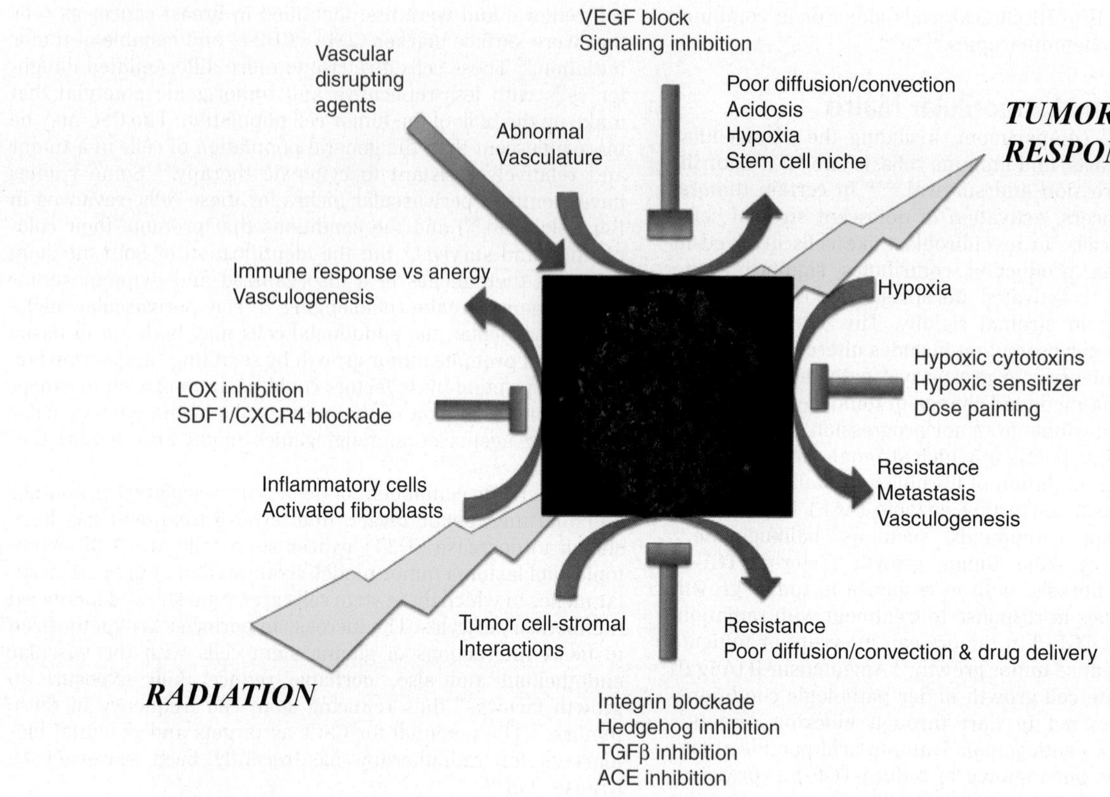

FIGURE 5.1. The tumor response to radiation is influenced by a number of interacting microenvironmental factors, which may in the future serve as targets for clinical intervention. Micrograph of human a tumor xenograft stained for nuclei (*blue*), vasculature (*green*), and hypoxia (*red*). (Courtesy of Professor A. van der Kogel.)

this enzyme also exist. Targeting lysyl oxidase (LOX), which has been shown to promote tumor growth in orthotopic and spontaneous mouse tumor models, might also be a means of inhibiting tumor growth (Fig. 5.1).[68]

Summary of Microenvironment

It is not possible to predict exactly how radiotherapy will evolve in its utilization of knowledge regarding the tumor microenvironment and host–tumor interactions. What appears clear is that increasing emphasis will be placed on these factors. Targeting changes specific to the microenvironment has the advantage of being largely tumor specific and potentially less toxic than cytocidal therapies. Future developments may allow for hypoxic tumor region dose painting. Alternatively, hypoxia targeting drugs may finally reach clinical maturity. Inhibition of hypoxia in tumors may also arise from strategies that revert tumor vasculature to a more normal morphology and function. This strategy has the added advantage of reducing hypoxia selection for aggressive tumor clones and enhancing chemotherapy delivery. The impact of the immune response on tumors, and in turn the effects of different radiotherapeutic interventions on immunity, may soon be exploited. Findings relating to the impact of host stromal elements on tumor cell radiation survival through direct intercellular signaling, autocrine stimulation, or mechanical force may also soon reveal new targets and interventions applicable to radiotherapy.

Combining agents that alter the tumor environment with radiotherapy requires strong preclinical data demonstrating at least additive effect and acceptable toxicities. Careful preclinical testing, including normal tissue response evaluation, may avoid subsequent problems in many instances. Having markers, and imaging, that detect the targets of interventions, such as hypoxia, cancer-associated fibroblasts, or immune infiltrating cells, and that can be used to assess intervention-mediated changes in the environment will be critical to fully exploiting this approach.

INNOVATIVE TARGETING

Molecular Imaging

To date, advances in radiotherapy (RT) have followed progress in nuclear and particle physics, computer sciences, and imaging technology combined with clinically relevant modifications of fractionation schemes resulting from radiobiological research at the laboratory and clinical levels. Because of the physical limitations of radiation dose delivery, further technical improvements are likely to provide only incremental benefits. Moreover, even the most advanced approaches to treatment planning, including sophisticated modeling response of normal and neoplastic tissues to radiation, in general, do not consider the specific characteristics of individual tumors, let alone nonoperable metastatic lesions. For these reasons, further increases in tumor control will require a better understanding of the mechanisms involved in cellular responses to radiation and their possible activation in individual tumors.

One cannot overemphasize the role of molecular imaging in the future of RT striving to individualize treatments, optimize responses, avoid toxicity and minimize the costs. Imaging of the molecular and biochemical features of cancer and their changes in response to therapeutic intervention can be sequentially repeated, allowing implementation of adoptive radiation therapy. Thereby, radiotherapy may extend the notion of personalized medicine from the current treatment planning stage to adoptive RT with molecular imaging, providing tools to monitor the effect of the therapy on the main tumor characteristics. For example, new more general markers of sustained proliferative signaling will be utilized including ^{18}F-FDHT,[101] ^{18}F-FLT,[102] and growth factor receptor–specific tracers such as ^{18}F-Affibody.[103] Replicative potential will be visualized by direct telomerase imaging.[104] Tumor-promoting, chronic inflammation can be observed by 18-fluorodeoxyglucose (^{18}F-FDG)[105] or NK1[106] imaging. FDG-, FLT-, RDG-, and MMP-targeted radiotracers[107] could be potentially used to observe changes of invasiveness and metastatic potential. RGD imaging of α(v)β(3)-intergin expression[108] will provide data on changes in neoangiogenesis. Induction of apoptosis will be monitored by ^{18}F-ML10 imaging.[109] FDG will provide data on the deregulated cellular energetics. As discussed in the preceding section on tumor microenvironment, hypoxia creates resistance to radiation and induces an aggressive cancer phenotype.[110] Therefore, the hypoxic parts of the tumor need to be exposed to a higher radiation dose or hypoxia-target agents. In the future, the presence of tumor hypoxia may be an indicator for the concomitant use of agents that target hypoxic pathways, a number of which are in development. Multiparametric analysis of tumor response and online adjustment of the RT based on the response of individual tumor will allow optimizing the treatment with carefully done clinical trials to assess the efficacy of the technological and biological intervention.[111]

Nuclear Medicine

Systemic targeted radiotherapy is an evolving and promising modality of cancer treatment. It provides a unique means to efficiently eradicate disseminated tumors cells and small metastases before they are detectable by currently available methods. The key characteristic of systemic targeted radiotherapy is its specificity. Using tumor-homing characteristics of a radioactive compound or conjugating therapeutic radionuclei with a tumor-targeting molecule (antibody, antibody fragment, or peptide), it can deliver higher amounts of a radionuclide to cancer cells than to normal tissue. A number of antigens and receptors present on the tumor cell surface, including CD20, CD45, PSMA, mucin-1 (MUC1), HER2, EGFR, TNF as well as VEGF, and α(v)β(3) abundant on the vascular endothelial cells within newly developed blood vessels have been advocated as potential targets for radioimmunotherapy (RIT) in patients.[112]

There are two different approaches that have been introduced into clinical practice, including the use of direct conjugation of radioisotope tagged to mAb or pretargeting of the tumor. In the first case, the patient receives a diagnostic dose of an antibody labeled with radionuclide compatible with appropriate imaging modality (single-photon emission computed tomography [SPECT] or PET). If the conjugate is stable and there is sufficient localization of an antibody at the site of disease, the patient can be injected with a therapeutic dose capable of inducing cytoreductive and potentially curative effects. This approach, however, has some limitations. First, radiation dose delivered to solid tumors might be insufficient due to poor penetration of the large size radioimmunoconjugate. Moreover, rather long serum half-life of mAbs together with long decay time of the radioisotope increase the radiation exposure to normal organs and can contribute to bone marrow toxicity.

In a pretargeting approach, the radionuclide is administrated separately from the antibody vehicle. There are two strategies: one involves the administration of radioactive biotin for selective localization on antibody streptavidin conjugates. This approach takes advantage of the rapid pharmacokinetics of the small biotin molecule and the high affinity of avidin-biotin binding.[113] Alternatively, chelators of radioactive metals and multispecific antibodies that are capable of simultaneously binding to a tumor-associated antigen and a metal chelator could be used.[114]

Advances in imaging and radiation transport will allow new approaches to radionuclide therapy treatment planning. By administration of a dosimetric (trace-labeled) dose and determination of the patient's residence time (a measure of how long the radionuclide is retained in the body), the therapeutic dose can be precisely adjusted to maximize the therapeutic effect and minimize toxicity. The paradigm of a targeted drug with a patient-specific dose may become more routine as targeted therapies are further developed along with better assays to directly measure drug levels. For the present, whole-body dosimetry is routinely applied for RIT, but in the near future the patient-specific maximally tolerated therapeutic radiation dose will be used to maximize efficacy while minimizing organ and bone marrow toxicity.[111]

Nanotechnology

In the future, the clinical application of nanotechnology might revolutionize cancer treatment. Multifunctional nanoparticles allow simultaneous targeted delivery of diagnostic and therapeutic agents to the tumor tissue, giving rise to a new, fast growing field of theragnostics that combines the modalities of diagnosis and therapy.[115]

Gold Nanoparticles

Over the past two decades, radiation dose enhancement by high atomic number elements such as iodine has been explored for cancer radiotherapy.[116] As a small-molecule radiation dose enhancer (smRDE), iododeoxyuridine (IUdR) has been used due to its facile incorporation into cellular DNA.[116,117] The subsequent external irradiation of high-energy photons on the IUdR-containing target cells can trigger the secondary emission of photoelectric radiation (i.e., Auger/secondary electron emission or x-ray fluorescence).[118] The resulting triggered emission from smRDE can cleave the nuclear DNA double strands that can induce the radio-sensitized cell death.[119] In this smRDE-mediated radiotherapy, several advantages have been demonstrated. The triggered emission from smRDEs generally decays in several millimeters, which is a typical length scale of a cell so that the resulting cytotoxicity is highly dependent on the cellular location of smRDEs. Therefore, only the smRDEs located inside the target cells can deliver high toxicity upon radiation while their off-target toxicity is reduced by virtue of their being outside the cells.[120]

Although such smRDEs can improve the radiotherapeutic efficacy with reduced side effects, safe and effective delivery of smRDE to target tissue remains one of the major drawbacks to clinical applications.[120] As iodine-attached tumor-targeting antibodies were used to improve their biodistribution, their targeting and therapeutic efficacies were not satisfied due to the rapid dehalogenation mechanism in DNA as well as the heterogeneity and limited expression of target receptors on cancer cells.[121] Furthermore, the prolonged treatments with high doses of iodine compounds should be avoided due to their toxic side effects to the host organs.

These limitations might be circumvented by development of a nano-encased RDE (nanoRDE) platform, based on functionalizable polymer-modified nanoparticles. NanoRDE platforms can demonstrate several advantages. First, the biodistribution of nanoRDE can be highly improved by the "enhanced permeation and retention" effect in solid tumor tissue, which allows for the selective accumulation of nanoRDE at diseased sites (passive targeting).[122,123] Second, high amounts of nanoRDE can be readily internalized in target cells by endocytic pathways, which are known as a completely different cellular internalization mechanism from that of small molecules.[124] In addition, the subsequent acidic endosomal environments can be used as a trigger for the pH-sensitive release of additional chemotherapeutic agents.[125]

In conventional chemotherapy, the rapid developments of multidrug-resistant characteristics in cancer cells cause a critical problem in clinical cancer treatments.[95] As such, it is obvious that a combinational therapy is highly favorable for the complete remission of cancers rather than a single-type treatment. To this end, anticancer drug-conjugated nanoRDE would be "smart combined modality therapy" as a multimodal delivery platform for *both* radio- and chemotherapy.

Gold nanoparticles have been tested for improvement of both chemotherapy[126] and radiotherapy.[127] The TNF-α PEG-colloidal gold nanoparticle, CYT-6091 (Citimmune, Gaithersburg, MD), has been shown to selectively traffic to tumor tissue. This agent has been evaluated for its ability to selectively deliver TNF-α to tumors in clinical trials. Gold nanoparticles are available in a broad range of sizes.

In addition to its properties as a nano carrier, colloidal gold, being a high-Z element, may also increase the radiation dose delivered specifically to the target cells. In this system, gold nanoparticles (AuNPs) are used as inorganic nanoRDEs for radiotherapy as well as a delivery platform for chemotherapeutic agents. Due to the K-edge of gold at 80.7 keV, x-ray radiation with the energy level of Au K-edge can trigger the secondary emission of photoelectric radiation from AuNPs.[128,129] The resulting radiation can induce the degradation of target molecules by ionization and can interact with surrounding water molecules to produce reactive oxygen species that can damage the target molecules.[130] As such, AuNP-sensitized degradations of plasmid DNA[131] and human proteins[132] upon x-ray radiation have been demonstrated in *in vitro* model systems. Additionally, when AuNP-containing tumor cells were irradiated, increased apoptotic cell death was detected due to the continuous stress on cytosolic organelles.[133] Furthermore, enhanced *in vivo* efficacy of AuNPs upon radiotherapy was also observed in human cancer-bearing mouse models.[134] However, these AuNPs have shown very poor pharmacokinetic results due in part to their limited surface functionality as a bare colloidal particle.

Recently, AuNPs have been used in a wide range of biological applications due to their biocompatibility and well-known surface chemistry. Using the known reactions, AuNPs can be readily modified with thiol-end-capped polymers[135] that can significantly alter the pharmacokinetics.[136,137] This functional polymer can be prepared by highly controllable reversible addition-fragmentation chain-transfer radical polymerization, which allows for copolymerization of a wide range of monomers.[138]

As the gold K-edge is at 80.7 keV and the enhancement is optimal in the photoelectric-dominated x-ray spectrum, irradiation conditions could be optimized by using monoenergetic x-rays. Finally, gold can be easily activated with thermal neutrons to emit 411 keV γ-rays, which could provide a means for monitoring their biodistribution by SPECT.

Liposomes

Another alternative approach would be using radiation as a trigger releasing or activating drugs delivered to the tumor prior to irradiation. One option could provide radiosensitive liposomes. Liposomes have been explored as viable carriers for targeting, imaging, and delivery of payload of drugs for decades.[139] However, practical applications of liposomes are limited due to poor understanding of *in vivo* interactions, factors affecting biodistribution, and lack of modalities for controlled disruption of liposomes at optimal time within a limited volume.[140,141] To date, various triggering modalities such as local hyperthermia, pH-triggered, tissue-associated enzyme-triggered, and radiation-triggered drug release have been developed.[139] Among these, electromagnetic radiation-triggered release of liposomal drugs appears a promising approach and includes strategically designed phospholipid molecules to initiate light-induced trigger. These liposomes are based on the principle of photopolymerization of lipids,[142] photosensitization by membrane anchored hydrophobic probes,[143] or photoisomerization[144] of photo-reactive lipids. However, none of the formulations developed so far have been successful for *in vivo* applications, presumably due to the lack of adequate photon energy produced by the radiation source(s) or inability of radiation to penetrate into biological tissues (Fig. 5.2).

Radiation-Activated Photodynamic Therapy

Photodynamic therapy (PDT) is increasingly being recognized as an attractive and useful tool in the treatment of many diverse human diseases, including macular degeneration, several dermatological disorders, and oncology.[145] PDT utilizes photosensitizers that can be preferentially localized in malignant tissues.

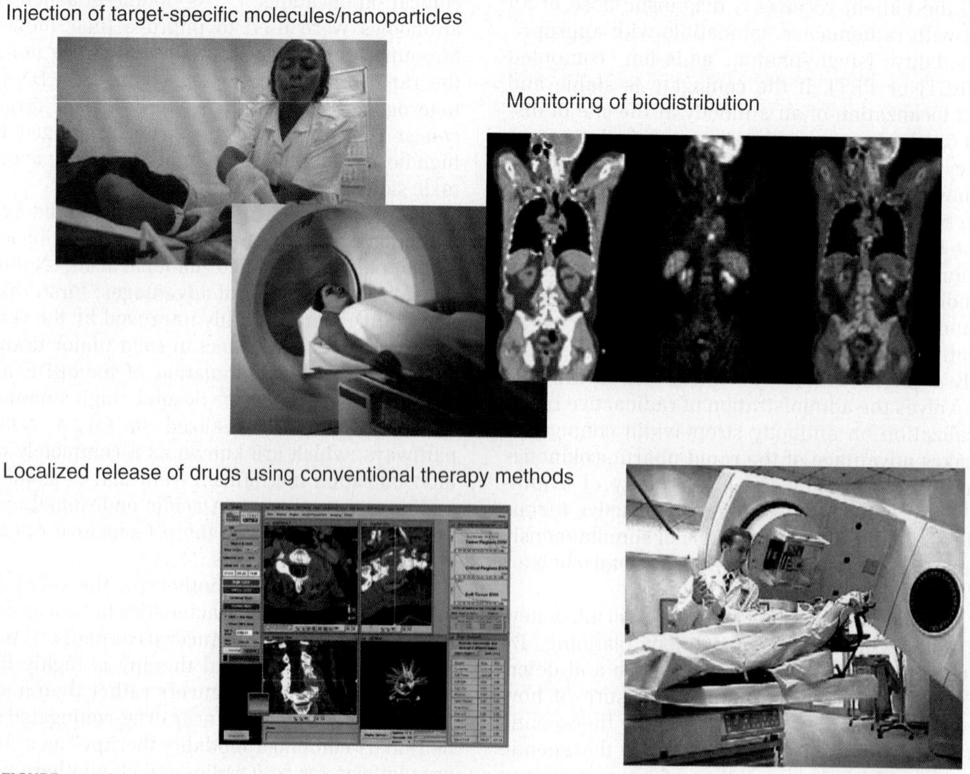

FIGURE 5.2. Three examples of combining nanotechnology with radiation therapy. **A:** Radiation triggers drug release from liposomes. **B:** Radiation prompts nanoscintilators to emit light that interacts with photosensitizes to produce toxic reactive oxygen species (photodynamic therapy). **C:** Nanoparticles are used to deliver chemical elements with a high atomic number that, after being internalized by tumor cells, enhance the effectiveness of x-rays.

The interaction of the photosensitizer and light results in the generation of cytotoxic species, including singlet oxygen ($^1O_2$), free radicals, and peroxides, which attack key structural entities within the targeted cells. These very toxic species are characterized by a short lifetime (<0.04 microseconds) and a short radius of action. Therefore, the damaged area is essentially confined to tissue that both contains the photosensitizer and is exposed to light.

Relative to current treatments, such as surgery, radiation therapy, and chemotherapy, PDT is also comparatively noninvasive, can be more accurately targeted, and is not subject to the total-dose limitations associated with radiotherapy; in addition the healing process typically results in little or no scarring.[146] Despite these advantages, PDT has not yet gained general clinical acceptance. The photosensitizers that have been approved for routine PDT treatment absorb light in the visible spectral regions below 700 nm, thus preventing access to deeper residing tumors. As a result, even with the advent of more sophisticated light delivery systems, the clinical application of PDT is limited to superficial solid tumors, endoscopically accessible regions, or skin lesions. The development of photosensitizers with absorbance in the near-infrared region, which would help overcome the limitation on the penetration depth, is an active area of research. There is also still need for isometrically pure photosensitizers. Improving the efficiency of $^1O_2$ production in the tissue microenvironment would allow reduction of the concentration of the photosensitizer necessary to treat the tumor. Finally, it would be helpful to develop better molecular targeting in order to improve the selectivity of the photosensitizers for the diseased tissue.

The combination of radiotherapy with photodynamic therapy, exploiting the tissue penetration of ionizing x-ray radiation and the cell-level targeting of PDT, might provide a novel approach to overcome the problems with penetration depth and might help with the delivery and targeting of photosensitizing agents. It has already been observed that under certain conditions, some photosensitizers act as radiosensitizers. The combination of Photofrin®, a U.S. Food and Drug Administration–approved photosensitizer, with radiation therapy led to significant enhancements in cytotoxic and apoptotic death of cancer cells.[147,148] However, the molecular mechanism for this effect is still unknown.

More recently, there has been interest in developing a nanoparticle-based photosensitizer delivery system for a combination of PDT with radiation therapy. Chen and Zhang[149] proposed using scintillating nanoparticles conjugated to photosensitizers; in response to irradiation with deeply penetrating x-rays, these nanoscintillators would produce light capable of activating the attached photosensitizers, thereby producing toxic amounts of free radicals in any desired location of the body. These nanoparticles would overcome the limitations imposed on current PDT and expand its application to deeply located tumors. In addition, it might be possible to conjugate molecules for receptor mediated internalization to the nanoparticles as well, ensuring delivery to the intracellular space; perhaps delivery could even be targeted to vulnerable subcellular structures.

Several doped nanoparticles ($LaF_3:Ce^{3+}$, $LuF_3:Ce^{3+}$, $CaF_2:Mn^{2+}$, $CaF_2:Eu^{2+}$, $BaFBr:Eu^{2+}$) and semiconductor nanoparticles (ZnO, ZnS, and TiO_2) are potential light sources for use in a nanoparticle-PDT system. The emission spectra of these nanoparticles can be matched perfectly to the absorption spectra of Photofrin, fullerenes, and TiO_2 nanoparticles. For example, $BaFBr:Eu^{2+}:Mn^{2+}$ nanoparticles excited by x-ray have three emission bands, one peaking at approximately 400, 500, and 640 nm, respectively. The emission spectrum of these nanoparticles is well matched to the absorption spectrum of hematoporphyrin. Another example is the x-ray luminescence spectrum of $LaF_3:Ce^{3+}$ nanoparticles with maximum emission at 350 nm, tailing to 500 nm. This emission spectrum matches the absorption spectra of most photosensitizers as well. If successful, this approach could lower the external radiation doses necessary to control cancer and, thereby, minimize the side effects while enhancing the benefits of radiation therapy.

NORMAL TISSUE COUNTERMEASURES

Research in normal tissue radiation biology received a substantial boost following the threat of radiological and nuclear terrorism that arose following the September 11, 2001, terrorist attacks. Scientists from academia and the government conceptualized a research plan that distinguished normal tissue modifiers into three time phases: (a) protectors that are administered before radiation, (b) mitigators that are used following radiation but before the damage has been fully manifest, and (c) treatment that is given for established radiation injury.[150] Some agents may function in more than one role. An advantage to developing drugs for terrorism-related use compared to clinical oncology is that tumor protection is not a concern; however, a challenge is to have a compound for a basically healthy population that is sufficiently nontoxic, which would be less of a problem for use in oncology. The program Medical Countermeasures against Radiological and Nuclear Threats was established in the National Institute of Allergy and Infectious Diseases (NIAID),[151] which has a research program built largely around six to eight Centers for Medical Countermeasure against Radiation. This effort had underpinnings from a long-standing and still ongoing program at the Armed Forces Radiobiology Research Institute.[152]

The radiological or nuclear incident research plan[153] includes the broad categories of (a) medical countermeasures (MCM), which are drugs or biologics developed as radiation mitigators; (b) biomarkers that can quantify an individual's radiation dose as a guide to treatment; and (c) agents that serve to reduce the exposure to internalized radionuclides by blocking uptake or enhancing excretion. The medical consequences of interest are those that result from a total body exposure (or significant partial body exposure) of a dose that can produce the acute radiation syndrome (ARS).[154] ARS is subdivided into organ syndromes based on the dose at which the syndrome is encountered and begins to result in mortality. The sequence from lower to higher doses is hematopoietic, gastrointestinal, dermatologic, and cardiovascular or neurological. However, there is an overlap in that sublethal damage to the gastrointestinal or dermatological systems can impact the outcome of hematological syndrome, and also that biomarkers produced by radiation even in the lower dose range can reflect a response by multiple organs, all of which sense and respond to the radiation. Consequently, while the treatment is often targeted to an organ (e.g., bone marrow cytokines for ARS, hematological syndrome), the physiological changes and overall management should recognize the multiorgan nature of the damage.[154] Table 5.1 includes the overall mission space for development of medical countermeasures.

A key underlying principle of the entire radiological or nuclear medical response program is that it is built on solid scientific underpinnings. There is continuity from the basic research programs of low-dose biology in the Department of Energy, Office of Science, to the NCI with its cancer-related doses, to the NIAID, which studies mechanisms *in vitro* and *in vivo,* to the Biodefense Research and Development Authority,[155] which supports advanced product development. In that a radiological or nuclear incident will be a "no-notice," and for nuclear a large-scale incident, the requirement for a medical countermeasure to be useful is that it is effective up to 24 hours after radiation.[155–158] What is not often appreciated is the concept of latency between exposure and clinical manifestation. To that end, there are two terms used to convey the concept that there may be a latency period between acute radiation exposure and clinical manifestation: acute radiation

TABLE 5.1 RADIATION COUNTERMEASURE MISSION SPACE FOR THE NATIONAL INSTITUTE OF ALLERGY AND INFECTIOUS DISEASES (NIAID) AND BIODEFENSE ADVANCED RESEARCH AND DEVELOPMENT AUTHORITY (BARDA) PROGRAMS

Acute Radiation Syndrome (ARS)	
Delayed Effect of Acute Radiation Exposure:	***Radionuclide Threats:***
Hematopoietic ARS:	Am-241
• Neutropenia	Co-60
• Thrombocytopenia	Cs-137
• Anemia	I-131
• Lymphopenia	Ir-192
Gastrointestinal ARS	Po-210
Central nervous system injury	Pu-238/239
Cutaneous injury	Sr-90
Lung injury	U-235
Kidney injury	
Combined radiation injury	
Biodosimetry Methods and Devices	***Late Effects:***
	Carcinogenesis
	Cardiovascular disease
	Cataractogenesis

From refs. 151, 155, 156, Courtesy of Bert Maidment, NIAID.

syndrome and delayed effect of acute radiation exposure. There are, indeed, ongoing chronic and progressive processes that produce late effects many years later. The potential mechanisms of action being addressed in the NIAID portfolio (Maidment, personal communication) include:

Mechanisms of action for medical countermeasures:
- Antioxidants
- Anti-inflammatories
- Antiapoptotics
- Growth factors and cytokines
- Cell-based therapies
- Others

Radionuclides to decrease internal exposure:
- Blocking agents
- Decorporation agents
- Enhancement of mucociliary clearance

Given the expense of product development from initial investment through to drug licensure, when possible the MCM and biomarker diagnostic program utilizes a "dual utility" approach. A drug that has a "day job" in additional to its use in a catastrophic event will not only be more cost-effective but will also be one that is likely to be available and for which the medical community will have experience using. The deployment efforts developed by the Office of the Assistant Secretary for Preparedness and Response includes a variety of approaches that would increase drug availability for no-notice incidents including vendor-managed, user-managed, and distributor-managed inventories. Dual utility would include the potential for using both biomarkers of radiation injury and radiation mitigators for cancer care. To that end, a path has been proposed, which assesses the potential that a mitigator could have the undesirable property of tumor protection.[159] Figure 5.3 presents a decision-tree for radiation mitigators and protectors.

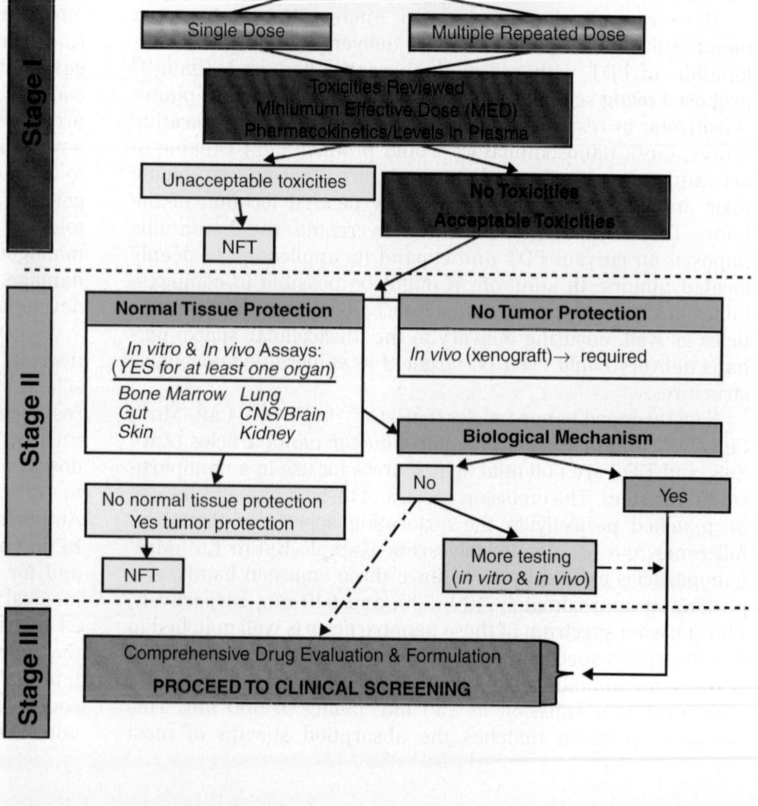

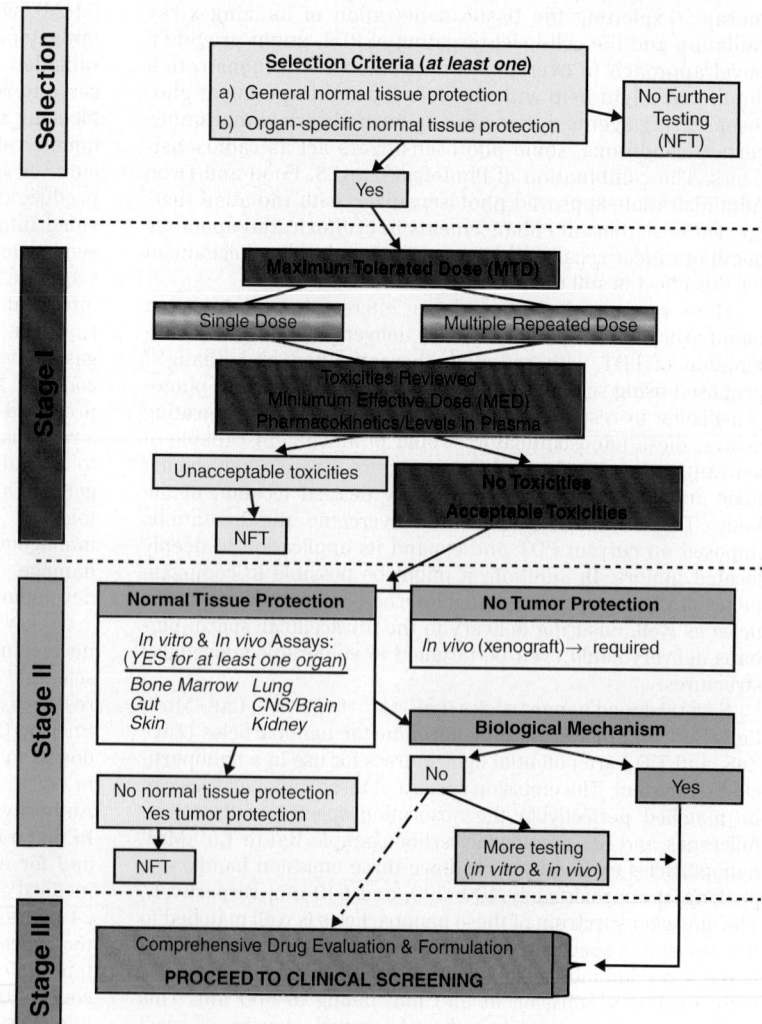

FIGURE 5.3. Decision tree for studying radiation mitigators and protectors for use in clinical radiation therapy. (From Ryan JL, Krishnan S, Movsas B, et al. Decreasing the adverse effects of cancer therapy: an NCI workshop on the preclinical development of radiation injury mitigators/protectors. *Radiat Res* 2011;176(5):688–691, with permission.)

NOVEL APPLICATIONS OF FRACTIONATED RADIATION

A number of research groups, including those at the NCI, have been exploring the use of radiation "as a drug," in which the dose size and fractionation of radiation would be employed to be used with other modalities in cancer treatment. There is extensive data beyond the scope of this chapter studying the cellular and molecular effects of radiation ranging from the low-dose studies (<0.1 Gy) from the Department of Energy Low Dose Program, to the typical fraction size used in radiation oncology (moderate dose) to large single doses now being used as part of stereotactic radiation therapy and radiosurgery (>15 Gy). Two potential future applications of fractionated radiation will be presented to introduce the concept: the enhancement of the immune response and the induction of a phenotype that can be targeted with systemic molecular therapeutics.

Radiation as a Component of Immunotherapy

Chakraborty et al.[160,161] showed that radiation can up-regulate surface changes on cells and render them susceptible to immune cell killing. This approach has been used in a clinical trial of fractionated radiation plus vaccine for prostate cancer,[162] and an immune response has been observed. The impact of these changes in immune response on tumor outcome remains to be proven[163] and regimens optimized.

Dewan et al.[94] have studied fractionated radiation in conjunction with 9H10, a drug that enhances the immune response through blockade of CTLA-4 receptor in order to overcome immune tolerance. They explored three radiotherapy regimens of 20 Gy × 1, 8 Gy × 3, and 6 Gy × 5 with varying drug schedules. Both fractionated regimens synergized with the immune modulator for enhancing local tumor effect. They also observed an abscopal effect on an unirradiated contralateral tumor with the 8 Gy × 3 being superior to the 6 Gy × 5.[94] Although there is much work yet to be done to harness immunotherapy and to define a role for radiation in enhancing the immune response, the observation that fractionated radiation may enhance local and systemic immune response opens up new potential applications for focal and fractionated radiation.

Radiation as a "Drug"

Two novel conceptual approaches to cancer treatment potentially involve radiation therapy. Luo et al.[164] have added to the "hallmarks of cancer" model of Hannahan and Weinberg[165] by adding nononcogene addiction targets to oncogene addiction. Figure 5.4, adapted from Luo et al., shows the six oncogene addiction pathways proposed by Hannahan and Weinberg in 2000 and the additional nononcogene pathways that result from the molecular anomalies in the cancer cell. The authors have added "radiation-induced" stress as it has the ability to physically target the stress response and produce all six of the nononcogene pathways. The term we have used for radiation therapy to induce or stimulate a specific molecular and cellular response is *focused biology*.

A second concept is that of synthetic lethality,[166] in which the presence of a mutated pathway in a tumor may render the cell susceptible to killing by the inhibition of a second pathway on which the cell is dependent by virtue of the first mutation. There is extensive research in synthetic lethality, but for this chapter the possibility of using radiation in this context will be noted. Tsai et al.[167] used DNA microarrays to study the effects of 10 Gy as a single dose or as fractionated radiation, 2 Gy × 5, in three tumor cell lines—breast, prostate, and brain—*in vitro* and *in vivo*. There is a substantially different gene expression pattern with fractionation compared to single dose, with immune response genes being a pathway significantly up-regulated with fractionation. Fractionated radiation made the

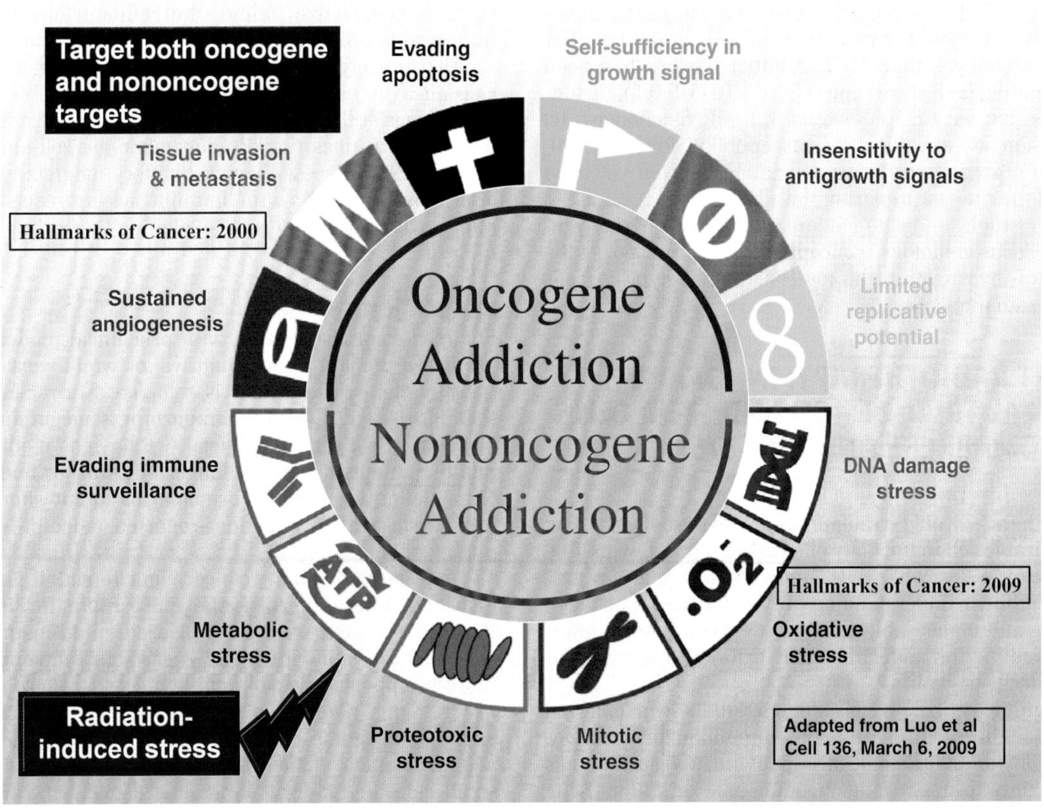

FIGURE 5.4. Oncogene and nononcogene addiction. (Adapted from Luo J, Solimini NL, Elledge SJ. Principles of cancer therapy: oncogene and non-oncogene addiction. *Cell* 2009;138(4):807–807.)

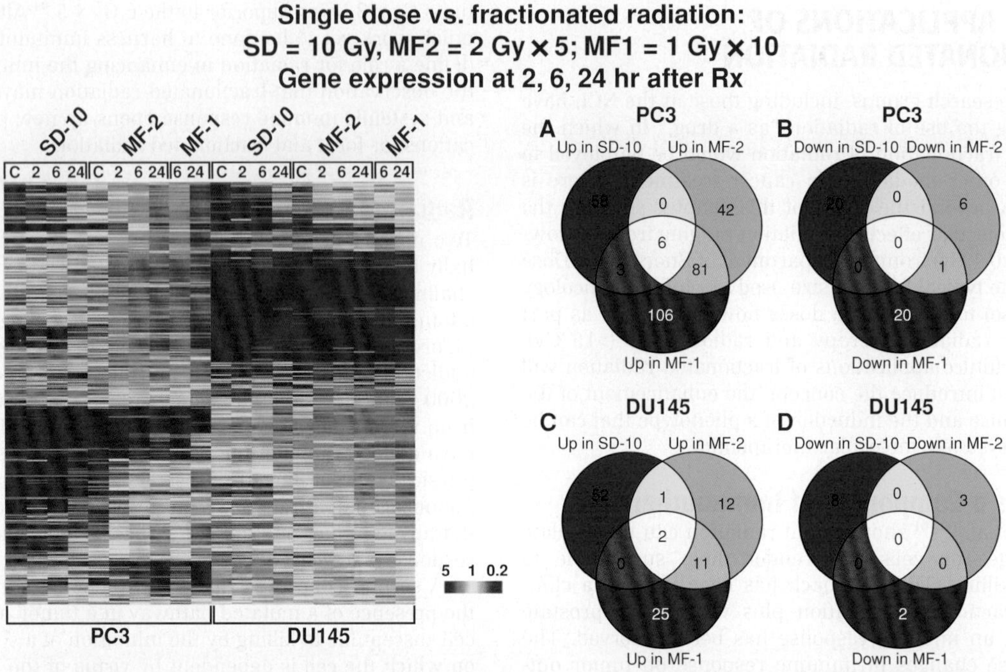

FIGURE 5.5. Single dose (SD) or multiple fractions (MF) produce different gene induction patterns in PC3 and DU145 prostate cancer cells. (From John-Aryankalayil M, Palayoor ST, Cerna D, et al. Fractionated radiation therapy can induce a molecular profile for therapeutic targeting. *Radiat Res* 2010;174(4):446–458, with permission.)

cell lines somewhat more alike (one of the hypotheses tested), and there was substantial difference of tumors treated *in vivo* versus *in vitro,* which might reflect the effects of radiation as well as the presence of a number of cell types within a tumor.

John-Aryankalayil et al.[168] have further studied the molecular changes in prostate cancer cells exposed to 10 Gy as a single dose (SD) or multiple fractions (MF) using 2 Gy × 5 (MF2) and 1 Gy × 10 (MF1). Figure 5.5 shows that the gene profiles are markedly different between SD and MF and that MF1 induces more changes than MF2. Additional work has been done investigating (a) 5 Gy SD and 0.5 Gy × 10 (MF 0.5), including cell lines that vary in p53 status, (b) miRNA changes, (c) proteomic changes, and (d) drug susceptibility following MF compared to preradiation. This information had not yet been published at the time of preparing this chapter.

The above studies indicate potential unique use of the radiation in the "focused biology" concept and also emphasizes the importance of investigating the molecular phenotype in cells that survive radiation.

SMART RADIOTHERAPY: INNOVATIVE CLINICAL TRIAL DESIGN AND STEM CELLS AS BIOMARKERS AND TARGETS

General

Smart radiotherapy would irradiate to a lethal dose to each and every undesirable cell in the body of a cancer patient, with little or no dose to the desirable cells. Implementing that strategy will require a better understanding of the differences between the desirable and undesirable cells and exploiting those differences for targeting the undesirables by external irradiation or radioactive drugs or both.

It is becoming technically feasible to irradiate from external sources any site in the human body with millimeter accuracy, but our inability to image small clusters of the undesirable cells limits our ability to destroy them. Better markers identifying the undesirable cells such as cancer stem cells, and better tools to image them must be developed. Current imaging methods can only display centimeter-size clusters for irradiating, which high doses can cause too much collateral damage.

A radioactive drug, as discussed above, consists of a radioactive "payload" attached to a molecule that can find, attach to, or enter the undesirable cells. This strategy shares some of the advantages and disadvantages (e.g., pharmacokinetic, pharmacodynamic) of all drug-based approaches. In rare cases, such as radioactive iodine, the radionuclide itself finds the undesirable cells because they are avid for iodine.

Alternatively, smart radiotherapy may alter the undesirable cells in a manner that makes them susceptible to killing by other drugs or the body's own immune mechanisms. Irradiation, even when it does not kill, does alter the cell and perhaps its progeny. As discussed above, better understanding of those alterations and of how the immune system reacts to them may offer novel opportunities for exploiting those changes to kill the undesirable cells.

Smart Clinical Trials

Smart clinical trials begin with preclinical models that better predict in the laboratory what will or won't work in the radiotherapy clinic. The reader is referred to a recent publication that addressed some of the important issues in that regard.[169]

A smart cancer clinical trial will have as its objective helping the patients live either longer or better or both. Therefore, for a definitive trial the principal endpoint should be either overall survival or a patient-reported outcome reflecting the quality of life.[170]

In designing a smart cancer clinical trial, it is important to focus on where there is the most room for improvement. Benchmark data from NCI-sponsored, multi-institutional trials can be most valuable in that regard. In the context of radiotherapy, opportunities abound in diseases where the local control remains poor after radiotherapy or radiochemotherapy (e.g., glioblastoma, local advanced human papilloma virus-negative cancer of the head and neck, locally advanced non–small cell lung cancer, pancreatic cancer, and hepatocellular carcinoma),[171] where morbid surgery is necessary due to infrequent pathological complete responses after radiotherapy or radiochemotherapy (e.g., sarcomas, rectal cancer) and where short- or long-term adverse effects are common. In diseases where distant metastases claim the lives of many patients, novel radiotherapeutic approaches to prevent or eradicate those metastases are needed, as discussed earlier.

Some new techniques of radiotherapy are intended to decrease the dose of radiation to the organs at risk. Examples include intensity-modulated radiation therapy (IMRT) and proton therapy. Smart clinical trials to evaluate these techniques must be adequately powered to not only demonstrate that toxicity was decreased but also that tumor control was not compromised. These new techniques carry a greater risk than conventional techniques of missing a part of the tumor due to inadequate quality assurance, patient or organ motion, or other factors.[172] Tools for *in vivo* dosimetry that can demonstrate in near real time that the planned dose distribution was actually realized in a patient do not yet exist. The ability to visualize the radiation deposition in near real time would help evaluate novel techniques without waiting years, even decades, for the clinical outcomes. For the foreseeable future, however, there is no alternative to well-controlled clinical trials in order to determine whether those new techniques live up to their *in silico* expectations. A recently published randomized clinical trial,[173] for example, showed that in protecting the parotid glands by IMRT, the tumor control may have been compromised.

Targeted Depletion of Host Cells

The principal focus in radiation oncology has been the targeted depletion of malignant cells. Some recent studies, however, suggest that the targeted depletion of some other kinds of cells may be helpful in treating not only cancers but also some other diseases. Adoptive cell therapy, for example, relies on autologous or engineered lymphocytes to treat malignant melanoma and perhaps some other kinds of cancers. Irradiating the patient prior to the infusion of those lymphocytes appears to markedly increase the odds of durable complete remission of metastatic melanoma, possibly by depleting some host lymphocytes and thereby facilitating proliferation of the infused lymphocytes.[174] The technique of irradiation employed (total body irradiation) was, however, rather crude. A better understanding of which host cells should be targeted for depletion (e.g., regulatory T cells) may further increase the effectiveness of irradiation without the morbidity of total body irradiation. Another possible explanation is the alteration by irradiation of the gut microbiome, leading to a more robust immunological response against the malignant cells.[175]

It has been shown in animals that targeted depletion of the host hepatocytes by irradiation prior to infusing donor hepatocytes facilitated engraftment and proliferation of the latter, enabling them to generate a "new" functioning liver.[176,177] Recently, a clinical trial began to evaluate this strategy in children awaiting liver transplantation. This strategy may be potentially applicable in many other diseases such as diabetes and neurodegenerative diseases.

Learning Health Care Systems

Radiation oncology is arguably the most computerized specialty in medicine. Not only does almost every patient have an electronic medical record, but thanks to the NCI-supported infrastructure multi-institutional clinical trials, a great deal of standardization and harmonization has been accomplished during the past decade in our ability to digitally exchange dosimetry and imaging data. That can facilitate the creation of large national, even global, databases that can be mined for generating and testing hypotheses and, with the development of the appropriate tools, provide decision support for both practitioners and patients, such as determining the "correct" target volume for a patient and the optimum field arrangement for a patient.

A significant step in this direction was recently undertaken by the Quantitative Analysis of Normal Tissue Effects in the Clinic working group.[178,179] This review provides dose, volume, and outcome information for many organs and has, in turn, encouraged others to convert these tables and guidelines into computable models[180] that integrate population-based data with patient-specific information in order to provide optimized therapy for the individual patient. Complementary efforts have been proposed[181] to create atlases of the incidence of complications to provide systematic information to facilitate analysis and meta-analysis of the safe limits of radiotherapy. Similar efforts are being developed in Europe by the Maastro Clinic's prediction efforts.[182]

ENSURING SMART THERAPY

Quality assurance (QA) demands on radiotherapy have always been based on best estimates of the key fault points in the treatment delivery as derived from clinical experience. However, by their very nature, clinical trials or *avant garde* treatments employ techniques that may not be in routine use and thus it is difficult, if not impossible, to arrive at such experience-based quality-control requirements. In addition, new modalities and treatment methods are becoming very complex and idiosyncratic to the institution that employs them. Proton therapy is a good example of this, because each facility has very unique beam delivery characteristics, patient imaging, and immobilization, which significantly impact the dosimetry both in and out of field. This adds to the difficulty of trying to specify prescriptive QA processes and argues strongly for outcomes-based QA metrics.

The integration of a learning health care system into clinical trials can lead to smarter, more efficient, and quality-adaptive trial methods. Rather than demanding prescriptive quality standards, which are based on best guesses of the critical factors that might compromise the science of a particular trial, adaptive QA would monitor, in an almost real-time manner, dosimetry compliance criteria and patient morbidity to discover outlier facilities that deserve further scrutiny of their planning and delivery methods. Such monitoring will be even better adapted to the treatment if one begins to capture parameters from the actual radiation delivery. These realities were captured in a recent NCI workshop that examined the challenges and opportunities for optimizing radiotherapy quality assurance in clinical trials.[159] The workshop resulted in four recommendations:

1. Develop a tiered (and more efficient) system for radiotherapy QA and tailor intensity of QA to clinical trial objectives. Tiers include (i) general credentialing, (ii) trial specific credentialing, and (iii) individual case review;
2. Establish a case QA repository;
3. Develop an evidence base for clinical trial QA and introduce innovative prospective trial designs to evaluate radiotherapy QA in clinical trials; and
4. Explore the feasibility of consolidating clinical trial QA in the United States.

Further, modern "smart" methods of radiotherapy, such as internal emitters and ion therapy, highlight the fact that dose is but a surrogate for biological effect and thus we need to move to more robust methods of ensuring comparable data from multiple sites. Such methods may include biodosimetric parameters as reflected by *in vivo* imaging, molecular characterization of tissues or fluids, as well as morbidity outcomes.[183]

In recognition of the importance of imaging to the response assessment of therapy, a program was initiated in 2008 under announcement PAR08-225 by the Cancer Imaging and Radiation Research Programs of the NCI titled Quantitative Imaging for the Evaluation of Responses to Cancer Therapies. This has resulted in a network of funded U01 applicants whose mission is to "improve the role of quantitative imaging for clinical decision making in oncology by the development and validation of data acquisition, analysis methods, and tools to tailor treatment to individual patients and to predict or monitor the response to drug or radiation therapy."[184]

HEALTH DISPARITIES: REACHING THOSE IN NEED WORLDWIDE

Smart radiotherapy, in the authors' opinion, includes but is also beyond the application of the latest technology and biology. It includes innovative and creative means of bringing the advances in cancer treatment to the many underserved in both developing and developed countries.

The incidence and prevalence of noncommunicable diseases (NCD) are greater than communicable diseases and growing.[3] This is not to imply that communicable diseases such as AIDS, tuberculosis, and diarrheal diseases are not of critical importance, and it is recognized that some cancers are related to viral infections, such as the human papilloma virus; however, there are also many people suffering from diseases such as heart disease, cancer, and respiratory diseases that have environmental, dietary, and lifestyle issues. Indeed, in September 2011 the United Nations highlighted the need to address NCDs diseases.[2]

This chapter concludes that smart radiotherapy plays a role for the community practitioner supporting and potentially working with existing programs, including those from the International Atomic Energy Agency[185] and those established by the NCI.[186,187] These social issues have potential research components, including implementation science,[188] creative economics,[189] and developing collaborative networks[190] and possibly unique career paths for sustainable mentor-mentee relationships (Cancer Expert Corps, personal communication). Addressing cancer in low- and middle-income countries is a charge and challenge from the Institute of Medicine[191] that truly requires smart approaches.

CONCLUSIONS

The opportunities exist for novel approaches to cancer care in all aspects of radiation oncology, including basic science, physics of dose delivery such as novel tumor targeting, innovative technology linked with imaging, health policy, and societal contributions. Perhaps the assigned chapter title, SMART radiotherapy, was meant to be an acronym? With the complexity of the cancer process and the multiple capabilities of radiation, there are many possibilities, such as this one:

*S*cience-focused clinical care based on cancer, molecular, cellular, and tissue biology,
*M*ultidimensional approach to all radiation issues facing society, including cancer treatment, prevention, and potential risk from radiation exposure,
*A*ccess to care for all, including the underserved for whom radiation oncologists (often called clinical oncologists) are the primary oncology care provider,
*R*esponsible implementation of technology so that we control our destiny based on data,
*T*raining and mentoring to ensure a broadly based, societal conscious next generation of clinicians, scientists, and educators.

The limitations on us, with the rising cost of health care and plateau in research funding, require creative thinking so that the physical and biological capabilities of radiation therapy are available to all who may obtain meaningful benefits. Smart is good!

SELECTED REFERENCES

A full list of references for this chapter is available online.

1. Kim ES, Herbst RS, Wistuba II, et al. The BATTLE trial: personalizing therapy for lung cancer. *Cancer Discovery* 2011;1(1):44–53.
3. WHO-Report. World Health Organization global status report on non-communicable diseases. Available at: http://whqlibdoc.who.int/publications/2011/9789240686458_eng.pdf.
4. Tredan O, Galmarini CM, Patel K, et al. Drug resistance and the solid tumor microenvironment. *J Natl Cancer Inst* 2007;99(19):1441–1454.
5. Mohyeldin A, Garzon-Muvdi T, Quinones-Hinojosa A. Oxygen in stem cell biology: a critical component of the stem cell niche. *Cell Stem Cell* 2010;7(2):150–161.
6. Graeber TG, Osmanian C, Jacks T, et al. Hypoxia-mediated selection of cells with diminished apoptotic potential in solid tumours. *Nature* 1996;379(6560):88–91.
10. Ogawa K, Boucher Y, Kashiwagi S, et al. Influence of tumor cell and stroma sensitivity on tumor response to radiation. *Cancer Res* 2007;67(9):4016–4021.
12. Garcia-Barros M, Thin TH, Maj J, et al. Impact of stromal sensitivity on radiation response of tumors implanted in SCID hosts revisited. *Cancer Res* 2010;70(20):8179–8186.
16. Nordsmark M, Bentzen SM, Rudat V, et al. Prognostic value of tumor oxygenation in 397 head and neck tumors after primary radiation therapy. An international multi-center study. *Radiother Oncol* 2005;77(1):18–24.
24. Lin Z, Mechalakos J, Nehmeh S, et al. The influence of changes in tumor hypoxia on dose-painting treatment plans based on 18F-FMISO positron emission tomography. *Int J Radiat Oncol Biol Phys* 2008;70(4):1219–1228.
32. Hicks KO, Siim BG, Jaiswal JK, et al. Pharmacokinetic/pharmacodynamic modeling identifies SN30000 and SN29751 as tirapazamine analogues with improved tissue penetration and hypoxic cell killing in tumors. *Clin Cancer Res* 2010;16(20):4946–4957.
35. Ahn GO, Brown JM. Role of endothelial progenitors and other bone marrow-derived cells in the development of the tumor vasculature. *Angiogenesis* 2009;12(2):159–164.
37. Wang R, Chadalavada K, Wilshire J, et al. Glioblastoma stem-like cells give rise to tumour endothelium. *Nature* 2010;468(7325):829–833.
48. Rofstad EK, Ruud EB, Mathiesen B, et al. Associations between radiocurability and interstitial fluid pressure in human tumor xenografts without hypoxic tissue. *Clin Cancer Res* 2010;16(3):936–945.
53. Qayum N, Muschel RJ, Im JH, et al. Tumor vascular changes mediated by inhibition of oncogenic signaling. *Cancer Res* 2009;69(15):6347–6354.
58. Patenaude A, Parker J, Karsan A. Involvement of endothelial progenitor cells in tumor vascularization. *Microvasc Res* 2010;79(3):217–223.
61. Kioi M, Vogel H, Schultz G, et al. Inhibition of vasculogenesis, but not angiogenesis, prevents the recurrence of glioblastoma after irradiation in mice. *J Clin Invest* 2010;120(3):694–705.
65. Tsai KK, Stuart J, Chuang YY, et al. Low-dose radiation-induced senescent stromal fibroblasts render nearby breast cancer cells radioresistant. *Radiat Res* 2009;172(3):306–313.
87. Prestegarden L, Enger PO. Cancer stem cells in the central nervous system—a critical review. *Cancer Res* 2010;70(21):8255–8258.
89. LaBarge MA. The difficulty of targeting cancer stem cell niches. *Clin Cancer Res* 2010;16(12):3121–3129.
92. Krause M, Yaromina A, Eicheler W, et al. Cancer stem cells: targets and potential biomarkers for radiotherapy. *Clin Cancer Res* 2011;17(23):7224–7229.
94. Dewan MZ, Galloway AE, Kawashima N, et al. Fractionated but not single-dose radiotherapy induces an immune-mediated abscopal effect when combined with anti-CTLA-4 antibody. *Clin Cancer Res* 2009;15(17):5379–5388.
108. Zannetti A, Del Vecchio S, Iommelli F, et al. Imaging of alpha(v)beta(3) expression by a bifunctional chimeric RGD peptide not cross-reacting with alpha(v)beta(5). *Clin Cancer Res* 2009;15(16):5224–5233.
111. He B, Wahl RL, Du Y, et al. Comparison of residence time estimation methods for radioimmunotherapy dosimetry and treatment planning—Monte Carlo simulation studies. *IEEE Trans Med Imaging* 2008;27(4):521–530.
112. Steiner M, Neri D. Antibody-radionuclide conjugates for cancer therapy: historical considerations and new trends. *Clin Cancer Res* 2011;17(20):6406–6416.
113. Zhang M, Zhang Z, Garmestani K, et al. Pretarget radiotherapy with an anti-CD25 antibody-streptavidin fusion protein was effective in therapy of leukemia/lymphoma xenografts. *Proc Natl Acad Sci USA* 2003;100(4):1891–1895.
114. Karacay H, Sharkey RM, McBride WJ, et al. Pretargeting for cancer radioimmunotherapy with bispecific antibodies: role of the bispecific antibody's valency for the tumor target antigen. *Bioconjug Chem* 2002;13(5):1054–1070.
115. Kelkar SS, Reineke TM. Theranostics: combining imaging and therapy. *Bioconjug Chem* 2011;22(10):1879–1903.
123. Peer D, Karp JM, Hong S, et al. Nanocarriers as an emerging platform for cancer therapy. *Nat Nanotechnol* 2007;2(12):751–760.
127. Hainfeld JF, Slatkin DN, Smilowitz HM. The use of gold nanoparticles to enhance radiotherapy in mice. *Phys Med Biol* 2004;49(18):N309–N315.
129. Carter JD, Cheng NN, Qu Y, et al. Nanoscale energy deposition by x-ray absorbing nanostructures. *J Phys Chem B* 2007;111(40):11622–11625.
133. Chang M-Y, Shiau A-L, Chen Y-H, et al. Increased apoptotic potential and dose-enhancing effect of gold nanoparticles in combination with single-dose clinical electron beams on tumor-bearing mice. *Cancer Sci* 2008;99(7):1479–1484.
146. Brown SB, Brown EA, Walker I. The present and future role of photodynamic therapy in cancer treatment. *Lancet Oncol* 2004;5(8):497–508.
149. Chen W, Zhang J. Using nanoparticles to enable simultaneous radiation and photodynamic therapies for cancer treatment. *J Nanosci Nanotechnol* 2006;6(4):1159–1166.
150. Stone HB, Moulder JE, Coleman CN, et al. Models for evaluating agents intended for the prophylaxis, mitigation and treatment of radiation injuries—report of the NCI workshop, December 3–4, 2003. *Radiat Res* 2004;162(6):711–728.
154. DiCarlo AL, Maher C, Hick JL, et al. Radiation injury after a nuclear detonation: medical consequences and the need for scarce resources allocation. *Disaster Med Public Health Preparedness* 2011;5:S32–S44.
156. Grace MB, Cliffer KD, Moyer BR, et al. The US government's medical countermeasure portfolio management for nuclear and radiological emergencies: synergy from interagency cooperation. *Health Physics* 2011;101(3):238–247.
159. Ryan JL, Krishnan S, Movsas B, et al. Decreasing the adverse effects of cancer therapy: an NCI workshop on the preclinical development of radiation injury mitigators/protectors. *Radiat Res* 2011;176(5):688–691.

161. Chakraborty M, Abrams SI, Coleman CN, et al. External beam radiation of tumors alters phenotype of tumor cells to render them susceptible to vaccine-mediated T-cell killing. *Cancer Res* 2004;64(12):4328–4337.
164. Luo J, Solimini NL, Elledge SJ. Principles of cancer therapy: oncogene and non-oncogene addiction (vol 136, pg 823, 2009). *Cell* 2009;138(4):807.
168. John-Aryankalayil M, Palayoor ST, Cerna D, et al. Fractionated radiation therapy can induce a molecular profile for therapeutic targeting. *Radiat Res* 2010;174(4):446–458.
169. Harrington KJ, Billingham LJ, Brunner TB, et al. Guidelines for preclinical and early phase clinical assessment of novel radiosensitisers. *Br J Cancer* 2011;105(5):628–639.
172. Ibbott GS, Followill DS, Molineu HA, et al. Challenges in credentialing institutions and participants in advanced technology multi-institutional clinical trials. *Int J Radiat Oncol Biol Phys* 2008;71(1 Suppl):S71–S75.
176. Guha C, Parashar B, Deb NJ, et al. Normal hepatocytes correct serum bilirubin after repopulation of Gunn rat liver subjected to irradiation/partial resection. *Hepatology* 2002;36(2):354–362.
179. Bentzen SM, Constine LS, Deasy JO, et al. Quantitative analyses of normal tissue effects in the clinic (QUANTEC): an introduction to the scientific issues. *Int J Radiat Oncol Biol Phys* 2010;76(3 Suppl):S3–S9.
183. Jeraj R, Cao Y, Ten Haken RK, et al. Imaging for assessment of radiation-induced normal tissue effects. *Int J Radiat Oncol Biol Phys* 2010;76(3):S140–S144.
185. Programme for Action for Cancer Therapy (PACT) from the International Atomic Energy Agency. 2011. Available at: http://cancer.iaea.org/wherewework.asp.
187. Cancer DCTD. Available at: http://rrp.cancer.gov/initiatives/cdrp/index.htm
189. Kerr DJ, Midgley R. Can we treat cancer for a dollar a day? guidelines for low-income countries. *N Engl J Med* 2010;363(9):801–803
190. Kerry VB, Auld S, Farmer P. Global Health. An international service corps for health—an unconventional prescription for diplomacy.. *N Engl J Med* 2010;363(13):1199–1201.
191. Institute of Medicine Report. Cancer control in low and middle income countries. Available at: http://iom.edu/Activities/Disease/LowMiddleCancerCare.aspx.

Part B Medical Radiation Physics

Chapter 6
Principles of Radiologic Physics and Dosimetry

James A. Purdy

A solid foundation in the principles of radiologic physics, dosimetry, and treatment planning is essential for the practice of modern-day radiation oncology. This chapter discusses the basic concepts in radiation physics, radiation therapy treatment machines, and the dosimetry parameters used for photon external beam treatment planning and dose/monitor unit calculations methods. As this textbook is aimed at practicing radiation oncologists and physician residents, these topics are not treated in the detail required for medical physicists. More details on these topics can be found in the medical physics textbooks listed in the references.[1–5]

ATOMIC AND NUCLEAR STRUCTURE

The *atom* may be thought of as consisting of a centrally located core, the *nucleus,* surrounded by small orbiting particles called *electrons.* The overall dimension of an atom is about 10^{-10} m, and the nucleus is about 10^{-14} m. An electron has a rest mass (m_e) of 9.109×10^{-31} kg and has a negative electrical charge equal to 1.602×10^{-19} coulomb (C). Most of the mass of the atom is contained in the nucleus, making it extremely dense (10^{15} kg/m^3). The nucleus is composed of two kinds of particles—*protons* and *neutrons,* known collectively as *nucleons.* A proton has a rest mass (m_p) of 1.673×10^{-27} kg and has a positive electrical charge equal in magnitude to the charge of the electron (1.602×10^{-19} C). Collectively, the protons constitute the electrical charge of the nucleus. A neutron is slightly more massive than a proton ($m_n = 1.675 \times 10^{-27}$ kg) and has no electrical charge.

Units used to describe atomic processes include the *atomic mass unit* (*amu*) for mass, *nanometer* (*nm*) for distance, *electron volt* (*eV*) for energy, and *electronic charge* (*e*) for electrical charge. The amu is defined as 1/12 the mass of the neutral carbon-12 atom. Thus, 1 amu = 1.660×10^{-27} kg. In terms of amu, a proton's rest mass is equal to 1.00727 amu, a neutron's rest mass is equal to 1.00866 amu, and an electron's rest mass is equal to 0.000548 amu. The electron volt (eV) is defined as the kinetic energy acquired by an electron accelerated through a potential difference (voltage) of 1 volt (V). One electron volt is equal to 1.6×10^{-19} joule (J) of energy. One writes 1,000 electron volts (keV) as 10^3 eV, and 1 million electron volts (MeV) as 10^6 eV. The nanometer is defined as equal to 10^{-9} m, and the electronic unit of charge is defined as equal to 1.602×10^{-19} C.

The planetary model of the atom is attributed to Niels Bohr, who in 1913 theorized that the hydrogen atom consisted of an electron orbiting around a nucleus of equal and opposite charge. He extended his theory to multielectron atoms, requiring the electrons surrounding a nucleus to be arranged in distinct, concentric shells or energy levels as shown in Figure 6.1. Energy is released when an electron moves to an orbit closer to the nucleus, and energy is required to move an electron into a higher orbit. Historically, the shells are labeled, from innermost outward, by the letters *K, L, M,* and so forth. There are a maximum number of electrons that can be accommodated in each shell: 2 in the first shell, 8 in the second, 18 in the third, and so on. The maximum number of electrons allowed in each shell is given by $2n^2$, where n is an integer specific to each shell and is called the *principal quantum number.* Other properties of the electron also have discrete values specified by quantum numbers. These include the electron's angular momentum as it orbits the nucleus, denoted by quantum number l ($l = 0, 1, \ldots, n - 1$); its spin about its axis, denoted by s ($s = \pm 1/2$); and its magnetic moment, denoted by m_l ($m_l = 0, \pm 1, \ldots, \pm l$). Thus, each electron in an atom has an associated set of quantum numbers (n, l, s, m_l). This is the basis of the *Pauli exclusion principle,* which states that no two electrons can have the same set of quantum numbers within a particular atom.

Modern physics has replaced the simplistic orbiting electron model of Bohr with a complex quantum mechanical model of diffuse electron clouds that represent probability functions of the electron's position. However, for an understanding of radiologic physics, the simple Bohr model of a nucleus composed of protons and neutrons and surrounded by orbiting electrons in distinct orbits (energy levels) is sufficient.

The atom of an *element* is specified by its *atomic number,* denoted by the symbol Z, and its *mass number,* denoted by the symbol A. The atomic number is equal to the number of protons in the nucleus, and the mass number is equal to the number of nucleons (protons and neutrons) in the nucleus. Hence, A minus Z is equal to the number of neutrons, denoted by the symbol N, within the nucleus. In addition, each element has an associated chemical symbol (e.g., Co for cobalt). When these definitions are used, the standard notation to specify an atom is $^{A}_{Z}X$, as illustrated by $^{60}_{70}Co$, which is a radioactive isotope of the element cobalt that has an atomic number of 27 (i.e., 27 protons) and a mass number of 60 (i.e., 60 nucleons, or 27 protons and 33 neutrons).

Isotopes of an element (e.g., $^{58}_{27}Co$, $^{59}_{27}Co$, and $^{60}_{27}Co$) have the same atomic number but different numbers of neutrons and therefore different mass numbers. Isotopes have the same chemical properties but have different physical properties. Atoms such as $^{60}_{27}Co$ and $^{60}_{28}Ni$, which have the same mass number but different numbers of protons and neutrons, are called *isobars.* Atoms such as $^{57}_{27}Co$ and $^{56}_{26}Fe$, which have the same number of neutrons but different atomic and mass numbers, are called *isotones.*

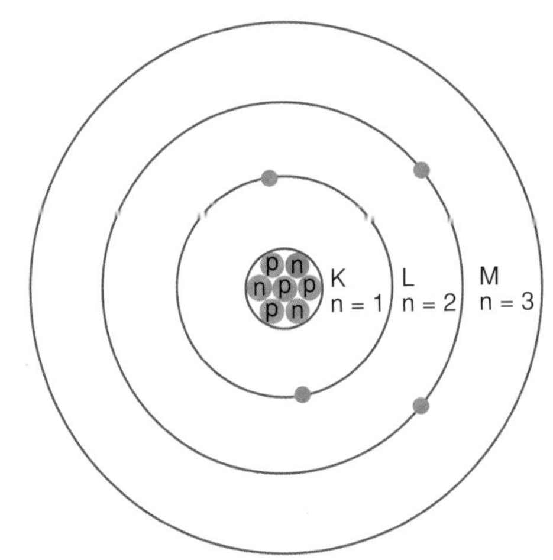

FIGURE 6.1. Schematic drawing of the Bohr model of the atom. The nucleus contains protons (p) and neutrons (n). Electrons revolve around the nucleus in specific orbits having discrete energy levels. By convention, the orbits (energy levels) are assigned either quantum numbers (n = 1, 2, 3, ...) or letters (K, L, M,...).

Every atom has a characteristic atomic mass A_m (sometimes referred to as atomic weight). The *gram-atomic mass* of an isotope is the amount of isotope in grams that is numerically equaled to the isotope's atomic mass. For example, 1 g-atomic mass of carbon-12 is 12 g. One gram-atomic mass contains 6.0228×10^{23} atoms, a constant that is called *Avogadro's number* (N_A). Useful parameters that can be calculated using Avogadro's number are as follows:

Number of atoms/gram = N_A/A_m

Number of electrons/gram = $(N_A Z)/A_m$

Number of grams/atom = A_m/N_A

The closer the electrons are to the nucleus, the more tightly bound they are to the nucleus. This results from the attraction between the negatively charged electrons and the positively charged nucleus and is referred to as the *Coulomb* or *electrostatic force*. To move an electron from an inner shell to an outer shell (*excitation*) or to remove it completely from the atom (*ionization*), energy must be supplied. The energy required to remove an electron completely from an atom is called the *binding energy* for the electron. Binding energies are considered negative because energy must be supplied to remove the electron from its orbit. Atomic shells often are described in terms of binding energy, as shown in Figure 6.2 for the tungsten atom. The binding energies for the K, L, and M shells are −69,500, −11,000, and −2,500 eV, respectively. The electrons in the outermost shells are called *valence electrons* and have a binding energy of only a few electron volts because they are very loosely bound. These electrons determine the atom's chemical properties.

ELECTROMAGNETIC RADIATION

Electromagnetic radiation can be represented by a varying electric and magnetic field that is conveniently described using a sine-wave model. The sine wave is characterized by two parameters: the *frequency*, represented by the Greek letter υ, and the *wavelength*, represented by the Greek letter λ. The wavelength is the distance from one crest of the sine wave to another; the frequency is the number of complete cycles or oscillations per second and is measured in *hertz* (Hz). The product of the frequency and wavelength is the speed with which the wave is propagated, which in a vacuum is the speed of light ($c = 3 \times 10^8$ m/sec).

Electromagnetic radiation wavelengths extend from approximately 10^7 to 10^{-13} m. The frequencies associated with these radiations are approximately 10^1 to 10^{21} Hz. the electromagnetic spectrum shown in Figure 6.3 includes the radio and television bands; radar and microwaves; the infrared, visible, and ultraviolet regions; and x-rays and cosmic rays.

Quantum physics allows electromagnetic radiation to be represented as waves and also as particles, called *photons*. This is referred to as the *wave–particle duality of nature*. The photon energy is directly proportional to the classic wave frequency and is related to it through a constant of proportionality known as *Planck's constant* (h), which has a numerical value of 6.625×10^{-34} J-sec. The relationship between energy, E, and frequency, υ, is given by the following equation:

$$E = h\upsilon$$

The relationship between photon energy and photon wavelength is given by the following equation:

$$E = hc/\lambda$$

in which c is the speed of light in a vacuum. These relationships show that as the wavelength becomes shorter or the frequency becomes larger, the energy of the photon becomes greater.

X-RAYS

Wilhelm Conrad Röentgen discovered *x-rays* on November 8, 1895.[6] He observed that a paper screen coated with fluorescent

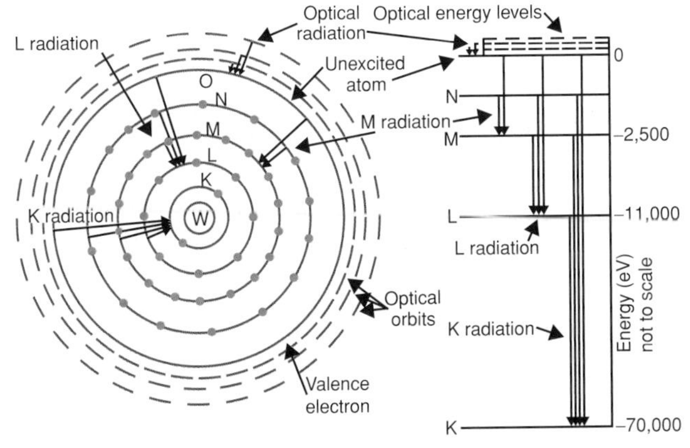

FIGURE 6.2. Schematic drawing of tungsten atom showing electron configuration and energy levels. (From Johns HE, Cunningham JR. *The physics of radiology*, 4th ed. Springfield, IL: Charles C Thomas; 1983.)

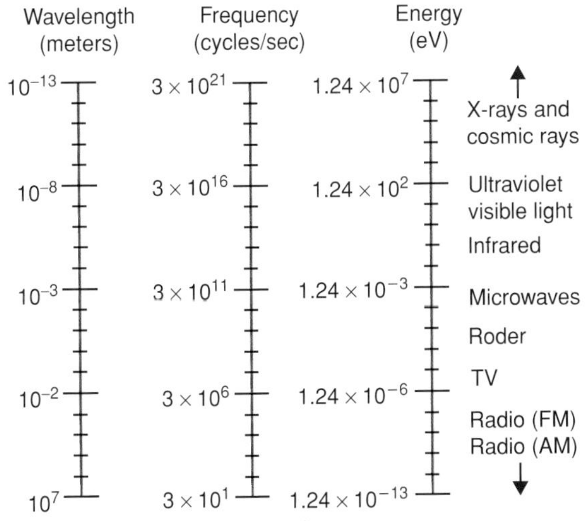

FIGURE 6.3. Electromagnetic spectrum extending over several orders of magnitude, with values of wavelength and frequency, and identifying values in some of the more common regions of the spectrum.

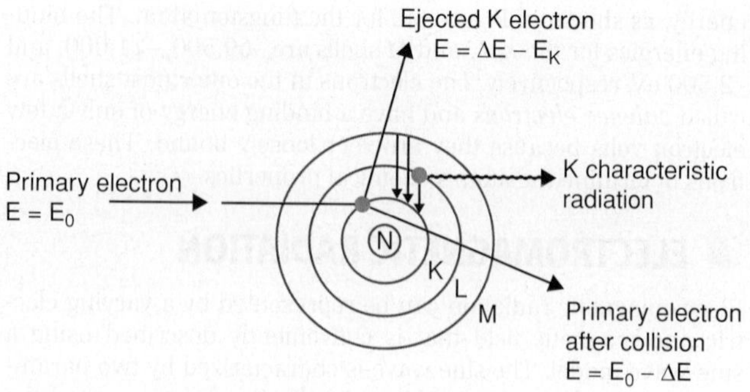

FIGURE 6.4. Schematic diagram illustrating characteristic x-ray production.

material glowed when placed in the vicinity of a tube of gas at low pressure through which electricity was being passed. We now know that the x-rays were produced where the electron beam struck the anode. Energetic electrons that impinge on matter interact with either the orbital electrons or the nuclei of target atoms. The kinetic energy of the electrons then is converted into thermal energy or electromagnetic energy (in the form of x-rays).

The impinging electron's kinetic energy is converted into thermal energy through interaction with an outer-shell electron of a target atom, which raises it to a higher energy level (referred to as *excitation*). The excited electron then returns to the normal energy level with the emission of low-energy electromagnetic radiation (*infrared*).

If the impinging electron's kinetic energy is high enough, the interaction can free an orbital electron (referred to as *ionization*), which then can result in the production of electromagnetic radiation (*characteristic x-rays*) when an outer orbital electron moves to the electron vacancy produced via ionization (Fig. 6.4). The characteristic x-ray energy is equal to the difference in the binding energies of the two orbital electrons involved. Occasionally, this excess energy is transferred directly to another orbital electron, causing it to be emitted from the atom. Such electrons are called *Auger electrons*.

The impinging electron also can lose its kinetic energy via a process called *bremsstrahlung* (braking radiation), which occurs when the incident electron interacts with the electric field of the nucleus (rather than the orbiting electrons) and is deflected and loses energy. This loss of energy reappears in the form of an x-ray photon. The impinging electron can lose any amount of its kinetic energy in the bremsstrahlung process. Thus, the x-radiation produced via the bremsstrahlung process is characterized by having a continuous range of energy values, unlike characteristic x-rays, which have only discrete energy values. A bremsstrahlung spectrum (i.e., a graph of x-ray intensity vs. energy) is shown in Figure 6.5. Superimposed on the continuous bremsstrahlung x-ray spectrum are the characteristic x-rays. The maximum energy of a bremsstrahlung x-ray is numerically equal to the maximum energy of the incident electrons. The direction of emission of the bremsstrahlung x-ray depends on the energy of the incident electron, with higher-energy electrons producing more-forward-directed x-rays.

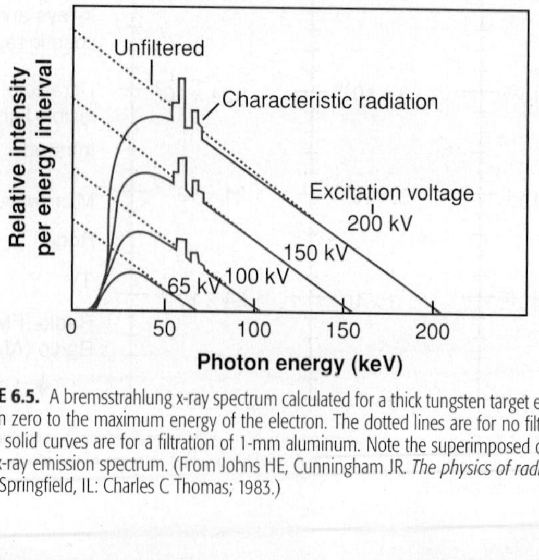

FIGURE 6.5. A bremsstrahlung x-ray spectrum calculated for a thick tungsten target extending from zero to the maximum energy of the electron. The dotted lines are for no filtration, and the solid curves are for a filtration of 1-mm aluminum. Note the superimposed characteristic x-ray emission spectrum. (From Johns HE, Cunningham JR. *The physics of radiology,* 4th ed. Springfield, IL: Charles C Thomas; 1983.)

RADIOACTIVITY

In 1896 Henri Becquerel conducted experiments in which he wrapped a photographic plate in black paper to keep out the light and then placed pieces of various elements against the wrapped plate.[7] He discovered that the mineral pitchblende emitted x-rays. Other elements—such as thorium, actinium, and two new elements (polonium and radium) discovered by Pierre and Marie Curie[8]—also emitted x-rays. Further experiments showed that the radioactive elements emitted three types of radiation: *α-particles,* having a positive electrical charge; *β-particles,* having a negative charge; and high-energy *γ-rays,* having no charge at all. We now know that an α-particle is a helium nucleus, β-particles are electrons, and γ-rays are electromagnetic radiation that is similar to x-rays except that it originates from within the nucleus of the atom.

Many other elementary particles have since been discovered and are important topics of current physics research, but they are not germane to our discussion of radiation oncology physics. Properties of the particles relevant to radiation therapy are listed in Table 6.1.

The radioactive decay processes are related to the forces involved. Huge electrostatic (Coulomb) forces of repulsion exist between the positively charged and closely spaced protons in a nucleus. However, a nuclear force of attraction (called the *strong nuclear force*) exists among the neutrons and protons, binding them together to form the nucleus. The strong nuclear force is much more complicated than the *electrostatic* (*Coulomb*) *force* and is still not completely understood. However, it is known that the strong nuclear force between nucleons depends on the distance between them and is effective only over a very short distance, whereas the electrostatic force decreases with the square of the distance. The strong nuclear force easily overcomes the repelling electrostatic force as long as the protons are very close together. However, for a large nucleus, the strong nuclear force binding the nucleons together may be weaker on opposite sides of the nucleus than the repelling electrostatic force. Therefore, a large nucleus is not as stable as a smaller nucleus.

Because neutrons interact through the attractive strong nuclear force and not the repelling electrostatic force, they can be considered stabilizing particles for the nucleus. For example, in light nuclei, only an equal number of neutrons and protons are required, but in heavier nuclei, the number of neutrons

TABLE 6.1 PARTICLES OF INTEREST IN RADIATION THERAPY

Particle	*Symbol*	*Charge*	*Mass*
Photon	hν, γ	0	0
Electron	e, e–, β^-	–1	0.000549 amu
Positron	e^+, β^+	+1	0.000549 amu
Proton	p, ${}^1_1H$	+1	1.007277 amu
Neutron	n, ${}^1_0n$	0	1.008665 amu
Alpha particle	α, ${}^4_2He^{++}$	+2	4.002604 amu
Neutrino	ν	0	<1/2,000 m_0
Pi mesons	π^+, π^-	+1, –1	273 m_0
	π^0	0	264 m_0
Mu mesons	μ^+, μ^-	+1, –1	207 m_0
K mesons	K^+, K^-	+1, –1	967 m_0
	K^0	0	973 m_0

1 amu = 1.66043×10^{-27} kg. m_0, rest mass of an electron, 9.1091×10^{-31} kg.

must be about 1.5 times greater than the number of protons to counteract the repelling electrostatic forces of the protons. A nuclide having too many more protons than neutrons is said to have an unfavorable *N*-to-*Z* ratio and thus undergoes *radioactive decay* to reach a stable configuration.

The *decay constant* of a radioactive nucleus is defined as the fraction of the total number of atoms that decay per unit of time and is denoted by the symbol λ. The decay process can be represented mathematically. If N_0 radioactive nuclei are initially present in a particular sample, the number of radioactive nuclei, *N*, remaining at a particular time, *t*, is given by the following equation:

$$N = N_0^{e-\lambda t}$$

Activity, which describes the radioactivity of a sample and is denoted by the symbol *A*, is defined as the total number of disintegrations per unit of time interval and is given by the following relationship:

$$A = \frac{\Delta N}{\Delta t} = -\lambda N$$

This decay-constant equation can be expressed in terms of activity:

$$A = A_0^{e-\lambda t}$$

where *A* is the activity at time *t* and A_0 is the initial activity. The *curie* (Ci), a unit of activity, is equal to 3.7×10^{10} disintegrations per second, the approximate number of decays per second by 1 g of ^{226}Ra. The *becquerel* (Bq), the special name in the International System of Units (SI) for the measure of activity, is equal to one disintegration per second (Table 6.2).

The *half-life* of a radioactive nuclide is the time required for the number of atoms in a particular sample to decrease by one-half. The half-life, $T_{1/2}$, is related to the decay constant by the following equation:

$$T_{1/2} = \frac{0.693}{\lambda}$$

The *average life*, T_a, of a radioactive nuclide is related to the decay constant and the half-life by the following equation:

$$T_a = \frac{1}{\lambda} = 1.44\, T_{1/2}$$

The average life represents the time period that a hypothetical source would need—if it retained its original activity for that time period and then suddenly decayed to zero activity—to produce the same number of disintegrations as produced over an infinite time period by the source if it decayed exponentially.

Gamma decay occurs when a nucleus undergoes a transition from a higher to a lower energy level. In this process, a high-energy photon, called a *γ-ray*, is emitted. These γ-rays are identical to the x-rays emitted by excited atoms, except that γ-rays originate from within the nucleus and x-rays originate from outside the nucleus. Half-lives for γ decay are usually very short, typically 10^{-15} second.

TABLE 6.2 INTERNATIONAL SYSTEM OF UNITS (SI UNITS) FOR RADIATION THERAPY

Quantity	*SI Unit (Special Name)*	*Non-SI Unit*	*Conversion Factor*
Exposure	C kg^{-1}	roentgen (R)	1 C $kg^{-1} \approx$ 3,876 R
Absorbed dose, kerma	J kg^{-1} (gray [Gy])	rad	1 Gy = 100 rad
Dose equivalent	J kg^{-1} (sievert [Sv])	rem	1 Sv = 100 rem
Activity	s^{-1} (becquerel [Bq])	curie	1 Bq = 2.7×10^{-11} Ci

Closely related to γ decay is the process called *internal conversion*. Instead of emitting a γ-ray, the excess energy from the excited nucleus is transferred to an electron in one of the inner atomic shells, causing ejection of the electron from the atom with emission of characteristic x-rays. The probability of internal conversion occurring increases as the atomic number increases.

In *β decay*, a neutron within the nucleus is converted into a proton, and an electron and an *antineutrino* are emitted, or a proton is converted into a neutron, and a *positron* and a *neutrino* are emitted:

β^- decay: $n \rightarrow p + \beta^- + \bar{v}$

β^+ decay: $p \rightarrow n + \beta^+ + v$

The positron was discovered in cosmic ray experiments in 1932. It is a positively charged particle with the same mass and spin as the electron and is considered the antiparticle of the electron. The neutrino and its antiparticle, the antineutrino, are massless particles (or at least have a very small mass) having no charge that carry opposite spins and account for the conservation of energy and continuous energy spectrum observed for β decay. Particle–antiparticle pairs interact by annihilating each other, converting all their mass into electromagnetic energy (two γ-ray photons, each of 0.51 MeV). In β decay, the emitted particles may vary in the kinetic energy they possess, which is rarely > 3MeV. Half-lives for β decay are long compared with γ decay half-lives, varying from seconds to years. The forces responsible for the β decay processes are weak compared with both the *strong nuclear force* and the *electrostatic force* among the nucleons. Accordingly, the force responsible for β decay is referred to as the *weak nuclear force*.

Electron capture is an alternative to *positron decay*. In this process, an electron, usually in the *K* shell, is captured within the nucleus and combined with a proton to create a neutron. Electron capture most often is followed by γ decay to release any excess nuclear energy.

Alpha decay occurs in nuclides with atomic number >82 and where the ratio of neutrons to protons is low, thus resulting in the repulsive Coulomb force of the protons overcoming the attractive strong nuclear force. The emitted α-particle is a helium nucleus (two protons and two neutrons). The kinetic energy for a particular α decay is monoenergetic (i.e., the transition may be to an excited energy state with subsequent γ emission) and often 4 to 5 MeV. Half-lives range from 10^{-3} to 10^{10} years. The radioactive decay of radium to radon is an example of α decay, where the *Q* term represents the total energy release in the transition (called *transition energy*). For example,

$$^{226}_{88}Ra \rightarrow\, ^{222}_{86}Rn + \,^{4}_{2}\alpha + \gamma + Q$$

The most recent version of the periodic table of the elements shows a grouping of 118 elements (elements 117 and 118 have not yet been observed but are included to show their expected positions). Only the first 92 occur naturally; the remaining ones have been produced artificially. In general, the elements with high atomic number tend to be radioactive; in fact, all but one of the elements with atomic number >82 (lead) are radioactive; only $^{209}_{83}Bi$ is stable.

The naturally occurring radioactive elements have been grouped into three radioactive series called the *uranium series*, the *actinium series*, and the *thorium series*, all of which terminate with a stable isotope of lead. The uranium series provides an example of radioactive nuclides undergoing successive transformations through α and β decay in which the parent nuclide produces a radioactive product called the *daughter nuclide*.

When the half-life of the parent nuclide is longer than the half-life of the daughter nuclide, an equilibrium condition exists. When this occurs, the ratio of the activity of the daughter nuclide to the activity of the parent nuclide becomes constant, and the apparent decay rate of the daughter nuclide is

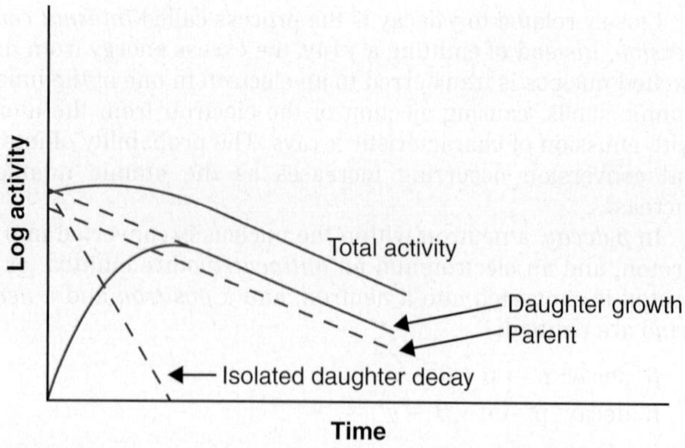

FIGURE 6.6. Transient equilibrium. Shown is a semilog plot of activity versus time for parent and daughter radionuclides illustrating conditions of transient equilibrium that may be achieved when the parent nuclide's half-life is not much greater than the half-life of the daughter nuclide. Once equilibrium is established, the daughter activity exceeds the parent activity, and both decay with the half-life of the parent.

controlled by the parent nuclide's decay rate. Two types of radioactive equilibrium conditions are defined: *transient equilibrium* and *secular equilibrium*. Transient equilibrium is established when the parent nuclide's half-life is not much greater than the daughter nuclide's half-life (Fig. 6.6). In secular equilibrium, the half-life of the parent nuclide is much greater than that of the daughter nuclide (Fig. 6.7). The two types of equilibrium are described mathematically by the following equations, in which A_P and A_D represent the activity of the parent and daughter nuclides, respectively:

$$\text{Transient equilibrium: } \frac{A_D}{A_P} = \frac{\lambda_D}{\lambda_D - \lambda_P}$$

$$\text{Secular equilibrium: } A_D = A_P$$

INTERACTION OF PHOTONS WITH MATTER

As stated previously, x-rays and γ-rays may be considered as bundles of energy called *photons*. If an x-ray photon enters a thin layer of matter, it is possible that it will pass through without interaction, or it may interact (usually with the atomic electrons, but sometimes with the atomic nuclei) in one of five different ways (*coherent scattering, photoelectric effect, Compton scattering, pair production,* and *photodisentegration*). The probability that a photon will interact when it traverses through

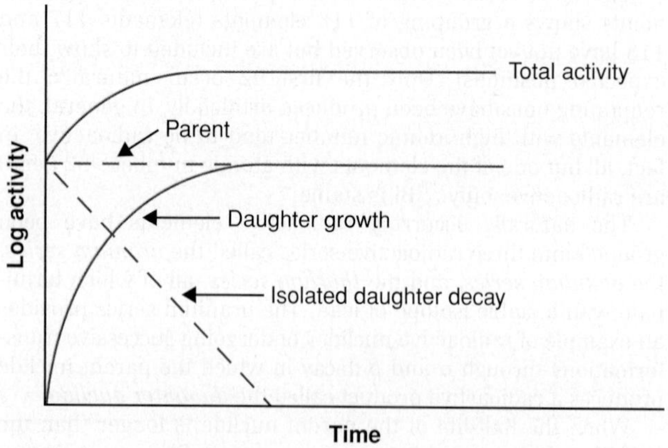

FIGURE 6.7. Secular equilibrium. Shown is a semilog plot of activity versus time for parent and daughter radionuclides illustrating conditions of secular equilibrium that may be achieved when the parent nuclide's half-life is much greater than the half-life of the daughter nuclide. Once secular equilibrium is established, activities of both parent and daughter are equal.

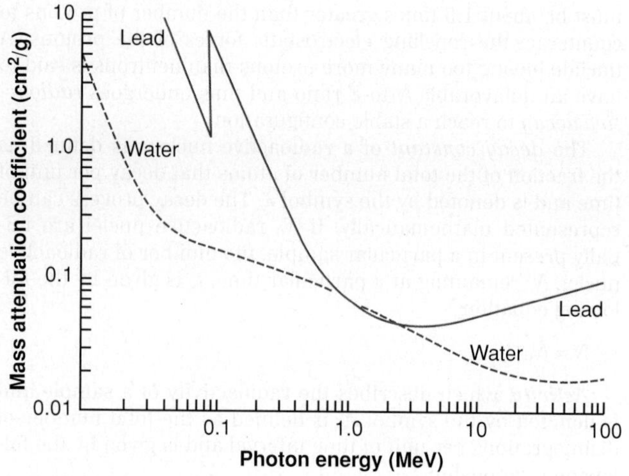

FIGURE 6.8. Mass attenuation coefficient for lead and water. Note sharp discontinuities, which are called *absorption edges*. (From Johns HE, Cunningham JR. *The physics of radiology*, 4th ed. Springfield, IL: Charles C Thomas; 1983.)

a given thickness of material is the product of the individual interaction probabilities for each of these processes. The attenuation process can be described mathematically by the following equation:

$$N = N_0 e^{-\mu x}$$

where N_0 is the number of photons in the beam impinging on an absorber of thickness x, e is the base of the natural logarithms, and μ is the linear attenuation coefficient. The quantity μ is actually the sum of the individual attenuation coefficients for the five processes. Its numerical value depends on the energy of the photon and the type of attenuating material.

There are a variety of tabulated attenuation coefficients, including the *linear attenuation coefficient* (μ), the *mass attenuation coefficient* (μ/ρ), the *mass energy-transfer coefficient* (μ_t/ρ), and the *mass energy-absorption coefficient* (μ_{en}/ρ). Each type of coefficient is intended for use in the solution of different types of attenuation or energy-absorption problems; division by ρ, the physical density of the medium, makes the coefficient medium independent. Figure 6.8 shows the mass attenuation coefficient for lead and water as a function of incident photon energy. The discontinuities where the attenuation coefficient suddenly increases are called *absorption edges* and occur at photon energies just equal to the binding energy of a specific electron shell.

The thickness of material that reduces the number of photons transmitted to one-half the incident number is termed the *half-value layer* (*HVL*). The HVL is related to the linear attenuation coefficient by the following equation:

$$\text{HVL} = \frac{0.693}{\mu}$$

This parameter is used to describe the *quality* or *penetrability* of the radiation and is discussed later in this chapter.

Coherent or Classical Scattering

If the photon energy is low enough that the quantum effects of the interaction are unimportant and the bound electron(s) can be regarded as essentially "free," the interaction corresponds to the "classical scattering" situation (called *coherent scattering*), in which the incident electrical field accelerates one or more orbital electrons and causes them to radiate. There are two types of coherent scattering: *Thomson scattering,* in which a single orbital electron is involved, and *Rayleigh scattering,* in which the orbital electrons act as a single group. In coherent scattering, no energy is transferred; only the direction

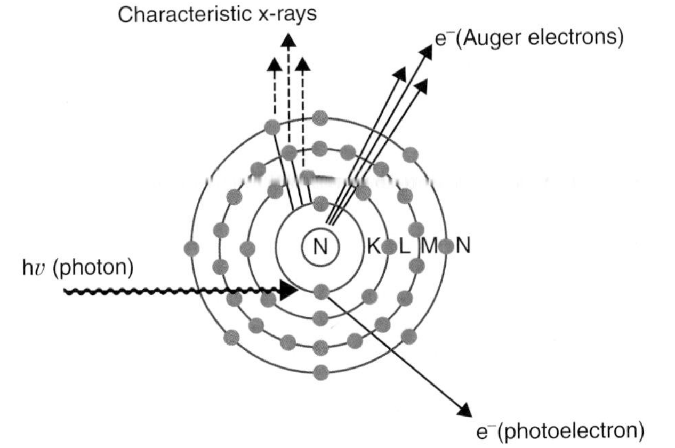

FIGURE 6.9. Photoelectric effect. In this type of photon interaction, the incident photon disappears, and an electron is ejected with kinetic energy equal to the incident photon's energy minus the binding energy of the electron. Characteristic x-rays and Auger electrons are emitted as the atom's electrons cascade to fill the vacancy created by the ejected electron.

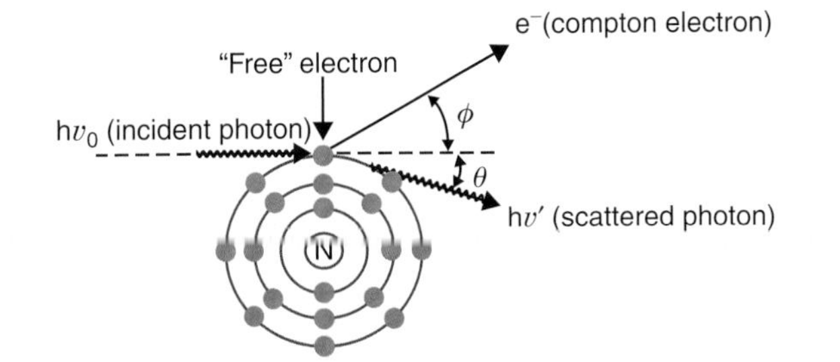

FIGURE 6.10. Compton effect. In this type of photon interaction, the incident photon interacts with one of the atom's outer electrons, and the energy is shared between the ejected electron and a scattered photon.

of the incident photon is changed. The coherent mass attenuation coefficient is denoted by σ_{coh}/ρ.

Photoelectric Effect

In the *photoelectric effect,* the total energy of the photon is transferred to an orbital electron, usually close to the nucleus, and the photon disappears. The electron then is ejected from the atom with an energy equal to the energy of the photon minus the binding energy of the electron (Fig. 6.9). The direction in which the electron is emitted depends on the energy of the incident photon. For the low-energy photons (e.g., 50 keV) the photoelectron is ejected at a large angle with respect to the incoming photon's direction, increasing in the forward direction as the photon's energy increases. After ejection of the electron, the neutral atom becomes a positively charged ion with a vacancy in an inner shell that must be filled. The atom returns to a stable condition by filling the vacancy with a nearby, less tightly bound electron farther out from the nucleus, and characteristic x-rays or an Auger electron is emitted.

The probability that a given photon will interact by means of the photoelectric process (denoted by τ/ρ) is a function of both the photon's energy and the atomic number of the target atom. For the process to occur, the incident photon must have energy greater than the binding energy of the involved orbital electron. In general, the probability per electron that a photon will undergo a photoelectric interaction is inversely proportional to the third power of the photon's energy and directly proportional to the third power of the atomic number of the target atom.

Compton Scattering

In *Compton scattering,* the incident photon interacts with a loosely bound orbital electron in which part of the photon's energy is transferred to the electron as kinetic energy and the remaining energy is carried away by another photon (Fig. 6.10). The binding energy of the electron is insignificant compared with the incident photon's energy and thus can be ignored. The energy of the Compton-scattered photon is equal to the difference between the energy of the incident photon and the energy transferred to the electron. If the incoming photon's energy is low (e.g., 100 keV), very little energy is transferred to the electron. As the photon's energy increases, a greater proportion of the energy is transferred to the electron, so the scattered photon necessarily retains a smaller proportion of the incident energy. The photon may be scattered at any angle with respect to the direction of the incident photon, but the Compton electron is confined to angles between 0 and 90 deg with respect to the direction of the incident photon. If the incoming photon's energy is low, the distribution of the scattered photons is isotropic (equal in all directions). The scatter angles decrease for photons and electrons as the incident photon's energy increases (e.g., at megavoltage photon energies, both are scattered predominantly in the forward direction).

As a result of conservation of energy and momentum, the energies of the incident photon, $h\upsilon_0$, the scattered photon, $h\upsilon'$, and the scattered electron, E, are given by the following relationships:

$$E = h\upsilon_0 \frac{\alpha(1 - \cos\theta)}{1 + \alpha(1 - \cos\theta)}$$

$$h\upsilon' = h\upsilon_0 \frac{1}{1 + \alpha(1 - \cos\theta)}$$

$$\cot(\varphi) = (1 + \alpha)\tan(\theta/2)$$

where $\alpha = h\upsilon_0/m_0c^2$, and m_0c^2 is the rest energy of the electron (0.511 MeV). If $h\upsilon_0$ is expressed in MeV, then $\alpha = h\upsilon_0/0.511$.

The probability that a photon will interact with a target atom via the Compton process (σ_c/ρ) depends on the energy of the incoming photon, generally decreasing as the energy of the photon is increased. The probability of a Compton interaction is nearly independent of the atomic number of the absorber and is directly proportional to the number of electrons per gram.

Pair Production

Pair production (Fig. 6.11) is possible only with photons having energies >1.02 MeV. When such an energetic photon approaches closely enough to the nucleus of the target atom, the incident photon energy may be converted directly into an electron–positron pair. Energy possessed by the photon in

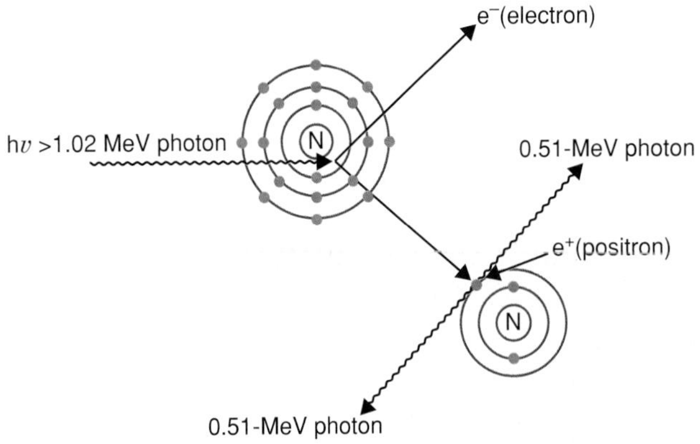

FIGURE 6.11. Pair production. In this type of photon interaction, the incident photon interacts with the electromagnetic field of the nucleus. The incident photon disappears, and two energetic electrons (a positron and a negatron) are produced. Two annihilation photons of energy 0.511 MeV then are produced when the positron interacts with its antiparticle, another electron.

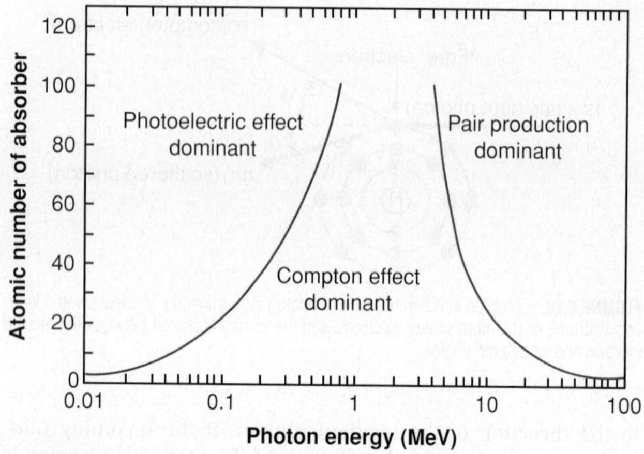

FIGURE 6.12. Relative importance of the three principal modes of interaction as a function of photon energy and atomic number of absorber. (From Hendee WR, Ritenour ER. *Medical imaging physics,* 3rd ed. St. Louis: Mosby-Year Book; 1992.)

excess of 1.02 MeV appears as kinetic energy, which may be distributed in any proportion between the electron and the positron. When the positron comes to rest, it combines with an electron, and both particles then undergo mutual annihilation, with the appearance of two photons with energy of 0.511 MeV traveling in opposite directions. The probability of pair production (π/ρ) occurring increases rapidly with incident photon energy above the 1.02-MeV threshold and is proportional to Z^2 per atom, Z per electron, and approximately Z per gram.

Photodisintegration

In *photodisintegration,* a high-energy photon interacts with the nucleus of an atom, totally disrupting the nucleus, with the emission of one or more nucleons. It typically occurs at photon energies much higher than those encountered in radiation therapy. However, it is important to account for this in designing shielding around high-energy accelerators, as this interaction is a source of low-energy neutrons.

Relative Importance of Interaction Processes

Figure 6.12 illustrates the relative importance of the photoelectric, Compton, and pair-production processes—the three principal modes of interactions pertinent to radiation therapy—as a function of energy and atomic number of the absorber. For example, for an absorber with an atomic number approximately equal to that of tissue (Z = 7) and for monoenergetic photons, the photoelectric effect is the dominant interaction below about 30 keV. Above 30 keV, the Compton effect becomes dominant and remains so until approximately 24 MeV, at which point pair production becomes the dominant interaction. The total mass attenuation coefficient accounting for all the photon interactions discussed is given by the sum of the individual coefficients:

$$\mu_{en}/\rho = \sigma_{coh}/\rho + \tau/\rho + \sigma_c/\rho + \pi/\rho$$

INTERACTION OF PARTICLES WITH MATTER

Electrons

An electron loses its kinetic energy when traversing matter via interactions that can be either *elastic,* in which no kinetic energy is lost, or *inelastic,* in which some portion of the kinetic energy is changed into some other form of energy. Elastic collisions occur with either atomic electrons or with atomic nuclei and are characterized by a change in direction of the incident electron with no loss of kinetic energy. Inelastic collisions can occur with atomic electrons, resulting in *ionizations* and *excitations* of atoms, or inelastic collisions with atomic nuclei, which result in the production of bremsstrahlung x-rays (*radiative losses*). In the case of ionization, it is possible for the ejected electron to acquire enough kinetic energy to cause additional ionizations of its own. These electrons are called *secondary electrons* or *δ rays,* and they can go on to produce additional ionizations and excitations. The typical energy loss in tissue for a therapeutic electron beam, averaged over its entire range, is about 2 MeV/cm in water.

The complete description of the energy and depth of penetration of the moving electrons at any point in the medium is complicated by the fact that the electrons are very much lighter than the atomic nuclei. As a result, the electron can lose a very large fraction of its energy in a single process and thus can be deflected by very large angles. This means that even if the electron beam is monoenergetic when first impinging on a medium, there will be a large variation among all the moving electrons as to where in the medium each will stop. This is referred to as *range straggling.*

Protons and Light Ions

Protons traverse relatively straight paths through matter, slowing down continuously by interactions with atomic electrons and with atomic nuclei. This results in depth–dose characteristics that show an approximately constant absorbed dose value over most of the beam range until near the end of the proton's range, where a very sharp increase in dose occurs (called the *Bragg peak*), as shown in Figure 6.13. Dose at the peak is approximately four times the dose at the surface, and the distal width of the peak is on the order of 1 cm, depending on beam energy and beam energy spread. Depth–dose characteristics customized for individual patients can be generated by superposition of multiple proton beams having different energies. This technique creates a *spread-out Bragg peak* that covers the target volume and decreases sharply to zero dose a few millimeters beyond the target. The relative biologic effectiveness (RBE) of proton beams is similar to that of other low-linear-energy transfer radiation, such as photon and electron beams. Pagnetti et al.[9] measured RBE equal to 1.0 in the plateau region and 1.1 in the center of the Bragg peak for a 250-MeV beam. Therefore, the clinical response established for photon and electron treatments is considered applicable to proton treatments.

Neutrons

Neutrons, like photons, are uncharged and thus are an indirectly ionizing radiation, which are exponentially attenuated by matter. The interactions are through processes that are primarily nuclear. They include elastic scattering with nuclei that make up the body's tissues (hydrogen, oxygen, carbon, nitrogen, etc.). Neutron interactions result in recoil protons and charged nuclear fragments that have relatively low energy. The RBEs of these resultant particles are not fully known, thereby complicating the understanding of the relationship between clinical response and absorbed dose.

RADIATION THERAPY TREATMENT MACHINES

Kilovoltage Units

Before 1951, most radiation treatment units were kilovoltage x-ray machines capable of producing photon beams having only limited penetrability. Today, this type of machine is still used in some clinics for the treatment of skin cancer. In these machines, the electrons are accelerated by an electric field produced from a high voltage generated in a transformer that is applied directly between the filament (cathode) and the x-ray target (anode). A schematic diagram of a radiation therapy

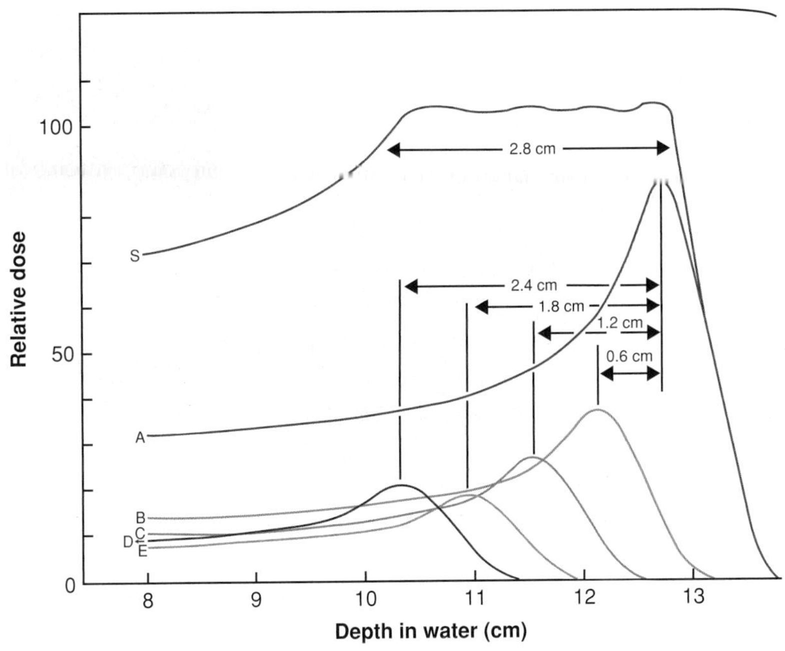

FIGURE 6.13. Drawing illustrating the way in which the Bragg peak for a proton beam can be spread out. Curve A is the depth–dose distribution for the primary beam of 160-MeV protons at the Harvard cyclotron. Beams of lower intensity and shorter range, as illustrated by curves B to E, can be added to give a composite curve, S, which results in a uniform dose of >2.8 cm. (From Hall EJ. *Radiobiology for the radiologist,* 4th ed. Philadelphia: JB Lippincott; 1994.)

Overview and Basic Science of Radiation Oncology

x-ray tube is shown in Figure 6.14. The potential difference (kVp) is variable on these machines, and metal filters can be added to absorb the lower-energy photons preferentially, changing the penetrability of the beam. The combination of variable kVp and different filtration provides the capability of generating multiple x-ray beams. The degree of penetrability is used to categorize the units as *contact, superficial,* and *orthovoltage* (deep-therapy) x-ray machines. A more detailed review of these type of treatment machine is provided by Biggs et al.[10]

Contact Units

A contact x-ray machine typically operates at potentials of 40 to 50 kVp and at a tube current of 2 to 5 milliamperes (mA). Attached cones are used for a source–skin distance (SSD) of typically 2 cm or less. Filters of 0.5- to 1.0-mm aluminum are used to give a typical HVL of 0.6-mm aluminum. The x-ray tube is rod shaped with an extremely thin mica–beryllium window, having an inherent filtration of 0.03-mm-aluminum equivalence, and the radiation is emitted axially. The primary radiation therapy application of a contact x-ray unit is for endocavitary irradiation of selected small rectal carcinomas.[11,12]

Superficial Units

A superficial unit is an x-ray machine that operates at potentials of 50 to 150 kVp and 5 to 10 mA. Added thickness of filtration (1-mm Al to 1-mm Al + 0.25-mm Cu) produces HVLs of 1.0 to 8.0 mm of aluminum. Attached cones typically are used; lead masks are used to define irregular fields. The SSD is typically 15 or 20 cm. These machines are used primarily to treat skin lesions.

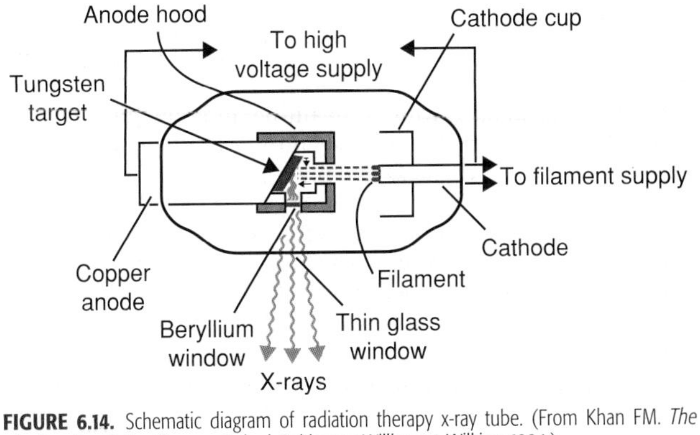

FIGURE 6.14. Schematic diagram of radiation therapy x-ray tube. (From Khan FM. *The physics of radiation therapy,* 3rd ed. Baltimore: Williams & Wilkins; 1994.)

Orthovoltage (Deep-Therapy) Units

Orthovoltage x-ray machines operate at potentials between 150 and 500 kV, with most operating between 200 and 300 kV, and with tube currents of 10 to 20 mA. HVLs of 1 to 4 mm of copper are common with the use of added filters, such as the *Thoraeus filter,* a combination of thin sheets of tin, copper, and aluminum arranged so that the highest–atomic number sheet is always closest to the x-ray target, ensuring that the higher-energy characteristic x-rays are absorbed by the lower-*Z* metal. Treatment fields usually are defined using detachable cones. The SSD is typically 50 cm. Very few of these types of machines are still in clinical use.

Supervoltage and Megavoltage Photon and Electron Beam Treatment Units

X-ray treatment machines operated in the range of 500 to 1,000 kV were designated as *supervoltage therapy* machines.[13] The *resonant transformer x-ray machine* is an example of this type of kilovoltage machine. X-ray treatment machines that can produce beams 1 MV or greater have been designated as *megavoltage therapy* machines. One of the first megavoltage machines was the *Van de Graaff generator,* which operated at 1 to 2 MV. Another early type of megavoltage machine was the *betatron,* first developed in 1941 by Kerst.[14] Betatrons used in radiation oncology produced x-ray beams with energies of >40 MV. All of these early machines are now obsolete and no longer in clinical use. Details on the history and development of these early accelerators used in radiation therapy can be found in the textbook by Karzmark et al.[15]

Cobalt-60 Teletherapy

The first *cobalt-60* (^{60}Co) *teletherapy* machine was loaded with its ^{60}Co source in August 1951 in the Saskatoon Cancer Clinic, Saskatoon, Canada, and the first patient was treated on November 8 of that year.[16,17] A detailed review of ^{60}Co teletherapy machines is provided by Glasgow.[18] The advantages of a ^{60}Co teletherapy machine are its relative constancy of beam output, predictability of decay because of a well-defined half-life, and lack of day-to-day small-output fluctuations typically found in electrical machines. Disadvantages include the need for source replacement approximately every 4 to 5 years, poor field flatness for large fields and large penumbra, and lower depth dose compared with high-energy photons generated by medical linear accelerators and discussed later. These types of machines became a mainstay for radiation therapy for nearly three decades but are rarely used in U.S. clinics today. Isocentric units with source-to-axis distance (SAD) of 80 or 100 cm were designed with maximum field sizes of 40 × 40 cm at the machine isocenter for the 100-cm SAD machine. Source activities vary from about 5,000 to 13,000 Ci in 1.5- to 2.0-cm-diameter sources and yield exposure rates from 150 to 250 R/min at 1 m. The radiation consists of 1.17- and 1.33-MeV γ-rays having a $d_{1/2}$ in tissue (the depth at which the dose has been reduced to 50% of the maximum dose value) of about 10 cm.

Gamma Knife

A second type of treatment machine that makes use of ^{60}Co sources is the Elekta *Gamma Knife* (Elekta AB, Stockholm, Sweden), which is a dedicated stereotactic radiosurgical device that was developed in 1968 by Dr. Lars Leksell,[19] a Swedish neurosurgeon. This machine made it possible to deliver a single, large dose of highly conformal radiation (γ-rays) precisely to a number of intracranial sites using multiple fixed ^{60}Co sources aimed at a center point. The Gamma Knife has three basic components—a spherical source housing, four collimator helmets, and a couch with electronic controls. The source housing (models U, B, and C) contains 201 ^{60}Co sources distributed in a quasihemispherical arrangement. The γ-rays from each source converge to the *unit center point* (*UCP*), which is 40 cm away from each source. The UCP is analogous to the isocenter of a teletherapy machine and is the location where the target volume must be positioned during a treatment. This is accomplished by the three-axis coordinate system on the Leksell stereotactic frame. Each source has an activity of approximately 30 Ci when newly installed, and the 201 sources combined provide a dose rate of approximately 300 cGy/min at the UCP. Along the path to the UCP, the radiation beam from each source is collimated twice—once by a primary collimator and then by one of four secondary collimator helmets. For each helmet, 201 tungsten collimators define specified circular apertures (4, 8, 14, or 18 mm projected at the UCP). To conform the radiation dose to the shape of the target in the patent, various combinations of aperture diameters, aperture blocking (*plugging*), irradiation times, and head positions are used. A specific combination of these four parameters defines what is referred to as a *shot* in Gamma Knife terminology. Hundreds of thousands of patients have been treated using this type of treatment machine.

More recently Elekta introduced a new model, the Gamma Knife Perfexion (Fig. 6.15), which is a major change in design from the previous models, with several advanced features, including an enlarged internal patient cavity for extended access to peripheral cranial anatomy. Unlike the earlier models, the Perfexion moves the entire patient on the couch to each stereotactic x, y, and z coordinate. The sources are arranged radially and divided into eight moving sectors with 24 sources each. Each sector is independently selectable, thereby providing various sector combinations for aperture size or blocking at each shot position during treatment. With the introduction of its associated Extend System accessory, the Perfexion has an increased reach to allow treatments to the upper cervical spine.

Linear Accelerators

The first microwave electron linear accelerator (8 MV) for medical use became operational in 1953 at the Radiation Research Center of the Medical Research Council at Hammersmith

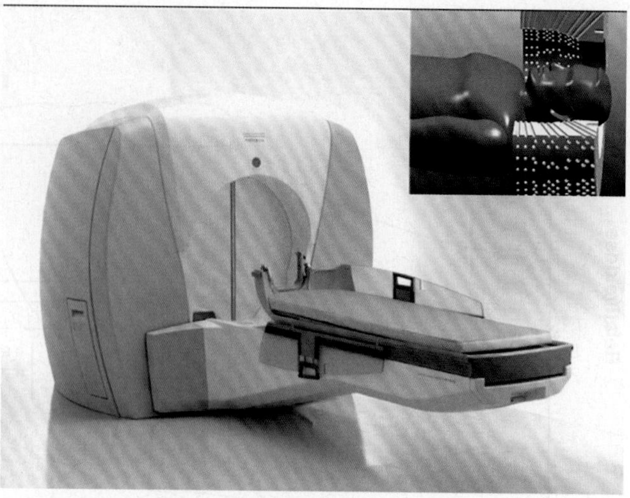

FIGURE 6.15. Elekta *Gamma Knife* (Elekta AB, Stockholm, Sweden) is a dedicated stereotactic radiosurgical device first developed in 1968 by Dr. Lars Leksell, a Swedish neurosurgeon, to provide highly accurate radiation ablative treatment of intracranial targets. Shown is the latest model, the Gamma Knife Perfexion, which broadens both the techniques and the scope of treatments, including the ability to treat lesions in the upper cervical spine.

Hospital in London.[20] The design for an isocentric gantry mount for the accelerator first was conceived by P. Howard-Flanders.[21] Shortly thereafter, Ginzton et al.[22] at Stanford University developed a 6-MV isocentric medical linear accelerator (*linac*). Since then there have been continued advances in accelerator design and construction, and today medical linear accelerators account for most of the operational megavoltage treatment units in clinical use.[15,23]

Figure 6.16 is a block diagram of a high-energy, bent-beam medical linear accelerator showing the major components. The linac uses electromagnetic waves of frequencies in the *S-band* microwave region (2,856 megahertz [MHz]) to generate an electric field. The microwave radiation is propagated through a device called an *accelerator structure,* and the electrons injected into the structure are accelerated by the electric field in a straight line. The accelerator structure consists of a stack of cylindrical metal cavities having an axial hole through which the accelerated electrons pass. The accelerator structure's electric field produced by the microwaves can be either a *traveling wave* or *standing wave* design. In a traveling wave design, the electrons travel with the electric field as the field propagates through the structure with time, somewhat in the manner of a surfboarder riding the crest of an ocean wave. In a standing wave accelerator, the reflected microwave power is used to produce a standing wave electric field. In that case, the microwave power is coupled into the accelerator structure by side-coupling cavities rather than through the accelerator structure's axial cavity apertures.

The accelerator structure in low-energy (4 to 6 MV) linacs most often is mounted vertically in the treatment head collinear along with the components associated with producing, controlling, and monitoring the x-ray beam (Fig. 6.17, left). High-energy (15 to 18 MV) linacs use a horizontally mounted accelerator structure with a beam-bending magnet system (Fig. 6.17, right). Accelerator structure technology now makes possible multiple high–dose rate photon beams of widely separated energies.

Other important components of a linac are the modulator, microwave power sources, electron gun, and the beam-handling components. The *modulator* is the source of pulsed direct current (DC) power, which is needed for the production of *microwave power.* Pulsed DC power is also supplied to the *electron gun* (a hot-wire filament that serves as the source of the accelerated electrons). The electrons are bunched before acceleration by a device called a *buncher.* The electron beam thus

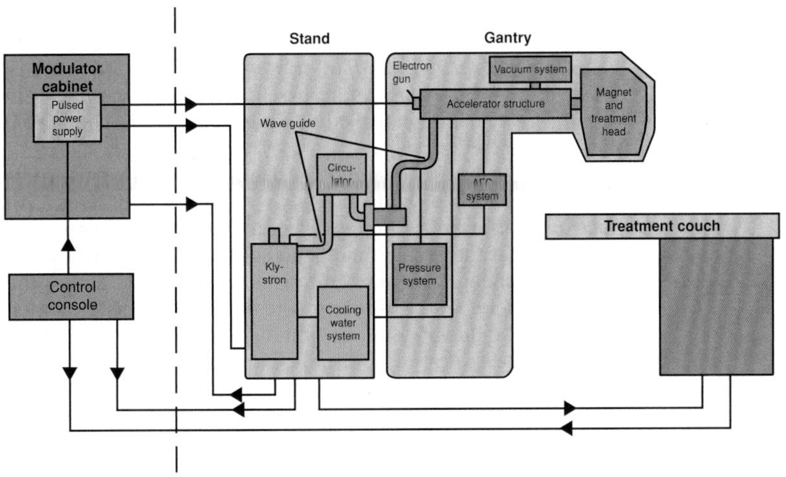

FIGURE 6.16. Schematic block diagram showing major components of a high-energy bent-beam medical linear accelerator. (Courtesy of Varian Associates, Palo Alto, CA.)

consists of pulses of bunched electrons in the form of a narrow pencil beam. The *magnetron* is a device that serves both as the source of the microwaves and as a power amplifier. The *klystron* is a device used to amplify the microwave power that is generated from a separate microwave source (*RF driver*). The microwave power coming from the magnetron or klystron is transported to the accelerator structure by a metallic pipe called a *waveguide*. A device called the *circulator* is used to isolate the klystron/magnetron from the reflected microwave power.

Other important components in a linac are located in the treatment head. These include the *x-ray target, fixed primary collimator, scattering foils, flattening filter, monitor ion chamber, movable secondary collimator jaws, light field localizer,* and *optical distance indicator.* In addition, the treatment head contains a significant amount of shielding material to minimize leakage radiation.

At the exit window of the accelerator structure, the high-energy electrons emerge in the form of a pencil beam of about 2 to 3 mm in diameter. In a low-energy (4 to 6 MeV) linac, the accelerated electrons proceed in a straight line and strike an x-ray target when in photon mode, producing bremsstrahlung x-rays. In high-energy linacs, because the accelerator structure is much longer and is placed horizontally or at some angle with respect to the horizontal, the electrons must be bent through a suitable angle, usually 90 or 270 deg between the accelerator structure and the target. This is enabled by the beam transport system, which consists of an *achromatic focusing and bending magnet,* as well as *steering* and *focusing coils.*

The *primary collimator* is a fixed collimator located just below the x-ray target and is used to collimate the x-ray beam in the direction of the patient treatment and reduces the leakage radiation from the x-ray source. The angular distribution of the bremsstrahlung x-rays produced by megavoltage electrons incident on a target is forward peaked. To make the x-ray beam intensity uniform across the field, a conical metal *flattening filter* is inserted in the beam. Filters are constructed of lead, tungsten, uranium, steel, and aluminum (or some combination of these), depending on x-ray energy. The flattened x-ray beam then passes through a *monitor ionization chamber.* In most cases, this system consists of several transmission-type parallel-plate ionization chambers, which cover the entire beam. These ion chambers are used to monitor the field symmetry, dose rate, and integrated dose per monitor unit.

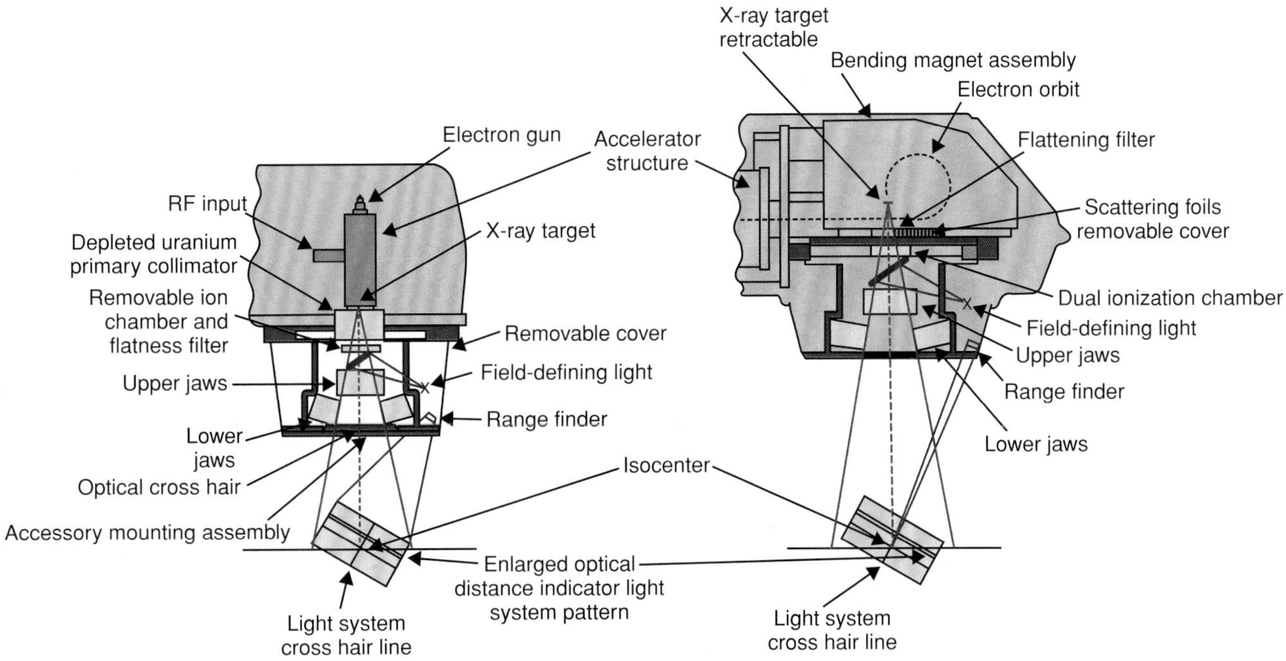

FIGURE 6.17. Schematic cutaway diagram of treatment heads for low-energy, straight-beam (left) and high-energy, bent-beam (right) medical linear accelerators. (Courtesy of Varian Associates, Palo Alto, CA.)

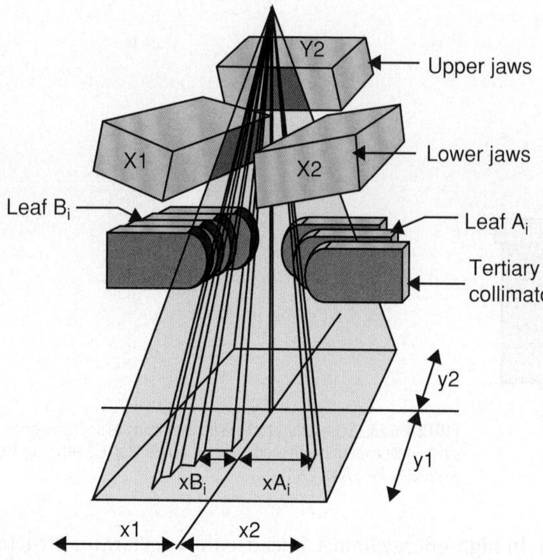

FIGURE 6.18. Schematic illustrating the geometry of a multileaf collimator for Varian linear accelerators. The *x*-direction is the field width across each leaf pair, and the *y*-direction is the field length. (Courtesy of Varian Associates, Palo Alto, CA.)

After passing through the monitor chamber, the beam can be further collimated by continuously movable x-ray collimators, consisting of two pairs of lead or tungsten jaws, which provide rectangular field sizes ranging from 0 to typically 40 × 40 cm at a distance of 100 cm. The field size is defined by a *light localizer* and a *mirror assembly. Independent jaw* capability is now common. This flexibility allows simplified patient positioning and improved safety by avoiding overlapping field abutments without the necessity of using heavy beam-splitting blocks.[24] Independent jaw technology in conjunction with computer control of the dose rate can be used to create a wedge-shaped isodose pattern.[25]

Most modern medical accelerators now come with *multileaf collimator* (*MLC*) systems (Fig. 6.18).[26,27] The leaf settings for each field are computer controlled. Modern treatment planning systems have the ability to configure MLC shaped fields, and the patient's MLC configuration files are sent via a local area network to the linac's MLC computer. Most important, computer-controlled MLC systems are used to create optimized modulated beam fluence. This form of therapy is referred to as *intensity-modulated radiation therapy* (*IMRT*) and is delivered at fixed gantry angles by (a) delivering multiple field segments (called *segmental MLC* [*SMLC*] or *step-and-shoot IMRT*) or (b) having the leaf pairs move across the field at a varying rate with the x-ray beam on (called *dynamic MLC* [*DMLC*] or *sliding window IMRT*).[28]

In the electron mode, the accelerator's beam current is reduced 1,000-fold and the x-ray target is retracted. An *electron-scattering foil* is moved into place on the beam centerline so that the accelerated pencil electron beam strikes it in order to broaden the beam and produce a flat field across the treatment field. The scattering foil typically consists of dual lead foils. The thickness of the first foil ensures that most of the electrons are scattered with only a minimum of bremsstrahlung x-rays. The second foil is generally thicker in the central region and is used to flatten the field. The bremsstrahlung produced appears as x-ray contamination of the electron beam and is usually <5% of the maximum dose. An *electron applicator* is mounted below the movable collimator jaws to provide the final field collimation. A schematic diagram of all the treatment head subsystems for both x-ray and electron beams is shown in Figure 6.19.

More recently, conventional medical linacs have integrated advanced imaging systems having *cone beam computed tomography* (*CBCT*) capability. Such linacs are referred to as *image-guided radiation therapy* (*IGRT*) linacs. The first commercial CBCT IGRT linac was the *Elekta Synergy* (Elekta).[29,30] The other medical linac manufacturers have also embraced the IGRT concept and have produced their own version of an IGRT linac—for example, *Varian Trilogy* and *TrueBeam* (Varian Medical Systems, Palo Alto, CA) and Siemens *ARTÍSTE* (Siemens Medical Solutions USA, Malvern, PA). The Synergy IGRT system (referred to as XVI) consists of a retractable kilovolt x-ray source, an amorphous silicon flat-panel imager mounted on the linear accelerator perpendicular to the radiation beam direction, and a software module for processing the data and tools for registering the images (Fig. 6.20). The XVI system provides for planar, motion, and volumetric imaging capabilities. Registration software is provided to compare the daily patient setup image with the stored prescription computed tomography (CT)–planning image, after which table adjustments can be made prior to treating the patient.

More recently, manufacturers of medical linacs and their associated planning systems have introduced features that provide rotational IMRT capability—for example, Elekta VMAT[31]

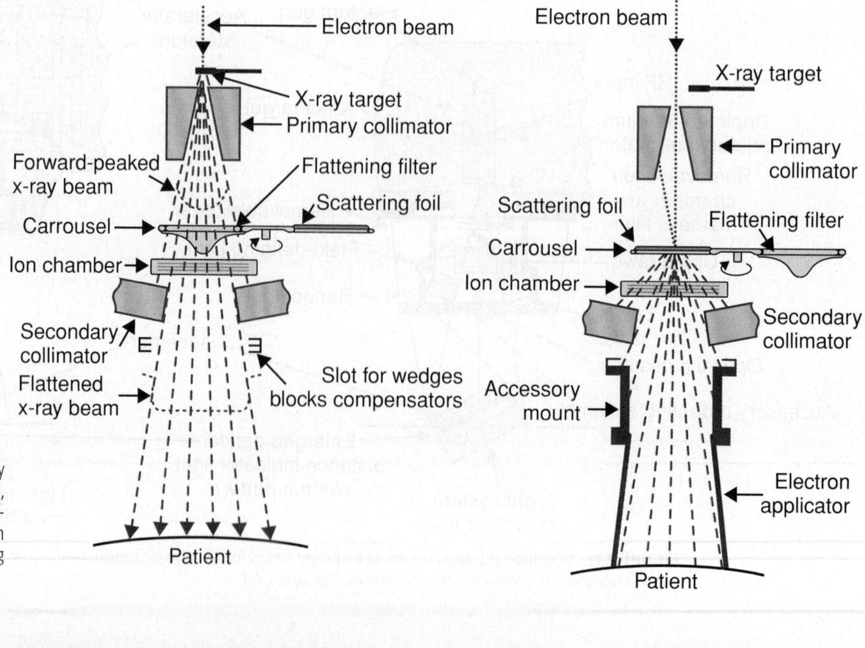

FIGURE 6.19. Schematic diagram of beam subsystems for x-ray beam **(A)** and electron beam therapy **(B)**. (From Karzmark CJ, Morton RJ. *A primer on theory and operation of linear accelerators in radiation therapy.* Rockville, MD: Department of Health and Human Services, Public Health Service, Food and Drug Administration, Bureau of Radiological Health; 1997.)

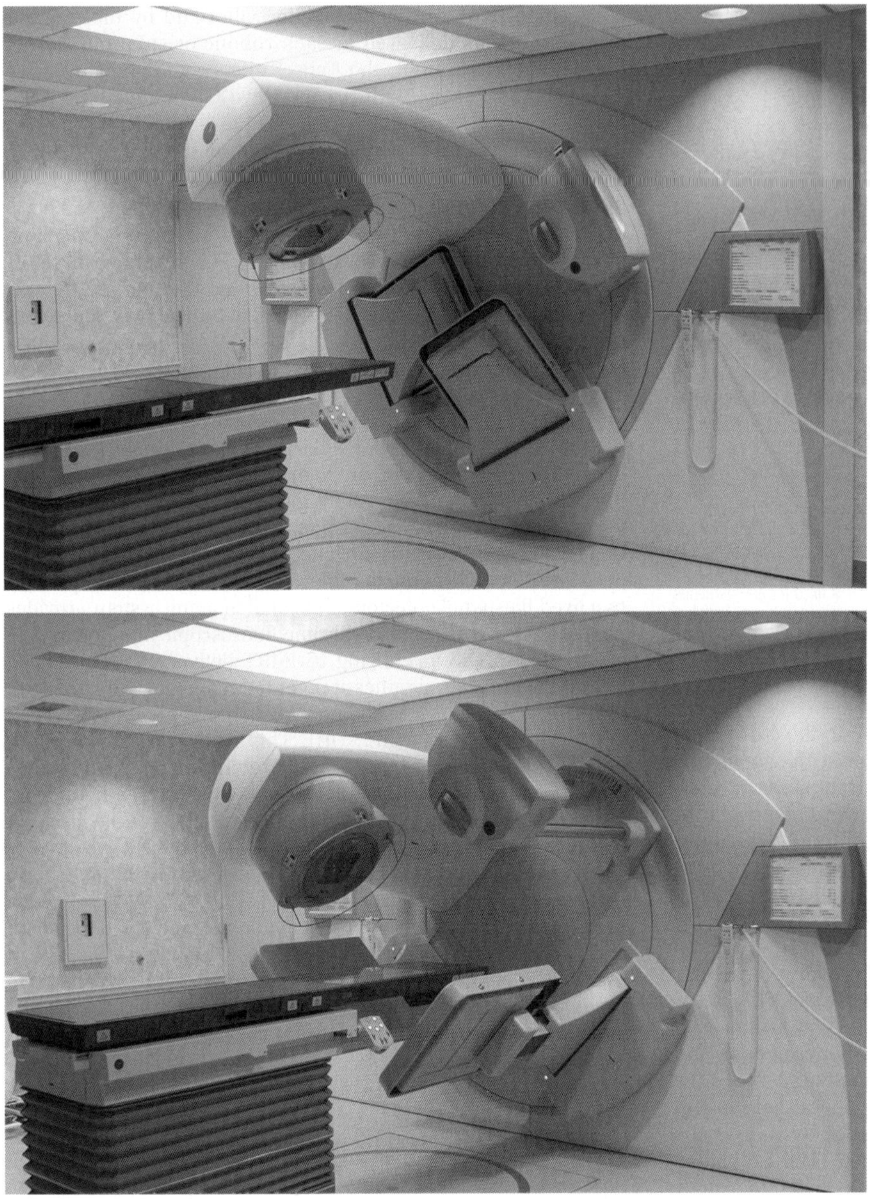

FIGURE 6.20. Elekta Synergy installed at the University of California, Davis. The unit consists of a conventional multimodality medical linac with a retractable kilovolt x-ray source, an amorphous silicon flat-panel imager mounted on the linear accelerator perpendicular to the radiation beam direction, and a software module (referred to as the XVI system). Top: The x-ray source, with the amorphous silicon flat panels retracted. Bottom: With the panels extended.

and Varian RapidArc.[32] The linac-based rotational IMRT concept was first proposed by Yu[33,34] and called intensity modulated arc therapy (IMAT), but planning software was not commercially available at that time. Rotational IMRT approaches on conventional linacs may provide even more conformal dose distributions delivered in a shorter treatment time compared with SMLC- or DMLC-IMRT approaches that use only a limited number of gantry directions. In addition, plan optimization is simpler since it eliminates the planner's iterative choices of beam number and direction. The conventional MLC approach for rotational IMRT is likely to improve IMRT plan quality and delivery efficiency,[32] although this remains somewhat controversial,[35,36] and more users will need to report their rotational IMRT experiences over the next few years.

Microtrons

The microtron, whose concept is credited to Veksler,[37] is an electron accelerator that combines the basic principles of the electron linear accelerator and the cyclotron. By using magnets to recirculate the electron beam through a microwave accelerator cavity (or cavities) one or more times, it is possible to achieve a high beam energy with a low-energy accelerating section. After each orbit in the magnet, the electron bunch must arrive in phase with the accelerator microwave field. Thus, the magnet system acts as an energy spectrometer, limiting the electron energy acceptance to a narrow energy width and consequently limiting to some extent the beam current.

This concept was developed further by Schwinger,[38] who proposed the *racetrack microtron*. It uses two D-shaped magnet pole pieces that are separated by a fixed distance, between which is a linac accelerator structure. A 50-MeV unit was developed for radiation therapy applications by the Swedish firm Scanditronics (Uppsala, Sweden) and was one of the first modern intensity-modulated radiation therapy delivery systems described in the literature.[39] Only two of this type of microtron were installed in the United States, and both have been replaced.

Tomotherapy

Helical tomotherapy was first proposed by Mackie et al.[40] and is now commercially available as the TomoTherapy HI-ART system (Accuray, Madison, WI).[41] A short, in-line, 6-MV linac (Siemens Oncology Systems, Concord, CA) rotates on a ring gantry at a source–axis distance of 85 cm. Figure 6.21 shows the unit installed at the University of California, Davis. The intensity-modulated radiation therapy treatment is delivered

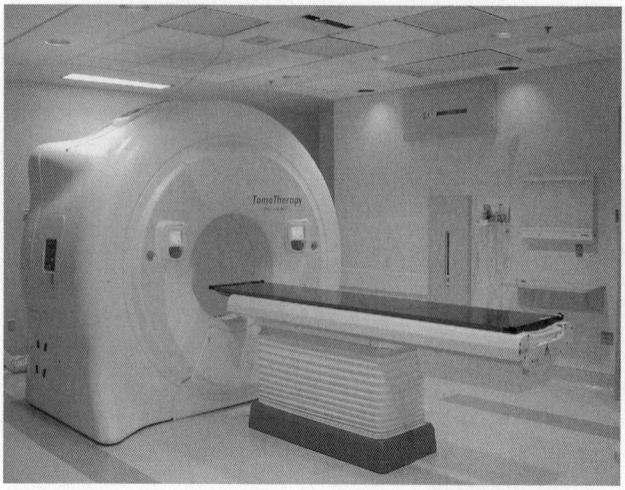

FIGURE 6.21. TomoTherapy HI-ART system installed at the University of California, Davis. A short, in-line 6-MV linac rotates on a ring gantry. Intensity-modulated radiation therapy treatment is delivered while the patient-support couch is translated through the gantry bore in the same way as a helical computed tomography study is conducted. The width of the beam in the patient-translated direction is defined by a pair of jaws that is fixed for any particular patient treatment, and laterally the treatment beam is modulated by a 64-leaf binary multileaf collimator.

while the patient-support couch is translated in the *y*-direction (toward the gantry) through the gantry bore in the same way as a helical CT study is conducted. Thus, in the patient's reference frame, the treatment beam is angled inward along a helix, with the midpoint of the fan beam passing through the center of the bore. Similar to helical CT, the treatment beam *pitch* is defined as the distance traveled by the couch per gantry rotation divided by the field width in the *y*-direction (typically between 0.2 and 0.5). The width of the beam in the *y*-direction is defined by a pair of jaws that is fixed for any particular patient treatment to one of three selectable values (1, 2.5, or 5 cm). Laterally, the treatment beam is modulated by a 64-leaf binary MLC, whose leaves transition rapidly between open and closed states. Each leaf has a projected width of 6.25 mm at the bore center, for a maximum possible open lateral field length of 40 cm. Intensity modulation is accomplished by varying the fraction of time different leaves are opened. The individual modulation pattern can change with angle (divided into exactly 51 projections over a full revolution). During the treatment, the gantry rotates at a constant velocity with a period ranging between 10 and 60 seconds/rotation. The extent to which a treatment beam projection is modulated is characterized through what is called the *modulation factor,* defined as the ratio of the maximum leaf open time to the average leaf open time for the projection. Pitch and maximum permissible modulation factor are new parameters that need to be specified by the treatment planner. Highly modulated treatments achieve greater conformality but inevitably take longer to deliver. A helical MVCT image is acquired using the on-board xenon CT detector system and the 6-MV linac (detuned to 3.6 MV) with the leave fully opened when the patient-support couch is translated in the *y*-direction through the gantry bore. Registration software is provided to compare the daily patient setup image with the stored prescription CT planning image.

CyberKnife

The use of a small X-band (~10,000 MHz) linear accelerator mounted on an industrial robotic arm was first developed for radiosurgery.[42,43] The robotic arm provides the capability for aiming a narrowly collimated x-ray beam with any orientation relative to the target volume. The system uses two ceiling-mounted diagnostic x-ray sources and amorphous silicon image detectors mounted flush to the floor. The treatment is specified by the trajectory of the robot and by the number of monitor units delivered at each robotic orientation. During the patient's treatment, the CyberKnife system correlates live radiographic images with preoperative CT or magnetic resonance imaging (MRI) scans in real time to determine patient and tumor position repeatedly over the course of treatment.

New and Evolving Photon Treatment Machines

There are several other new photon beam treatment machine designs that show significant promise. For example, the four-dimensional IGRT system proposed by Kamino et al. has a unique, gimbaled x-ray head design that allows the linear accelerator head to be pivoted.[44] By easily allowing noncoplanar beams without couch rotations, new degrees of freedom are made available for IMRT optimization, and even more conformal dose distributions may be possible.

The Vero (Brainlab AG, Feldkirchen, Germany) for stereotactic radiosurgery/stereotactic body radiotherapy was recently introduced, which uses a rotating ring gantry to which a megavolt x-ray treatment head is mounted on orthogonal gimbals.[45] Image guidance systems include an electronic portal imaging device (EPID) and two fixed kilovolt x-ray tubes combined with two fixed flat-panel detectors. This dual imaging system provides planar images, CBCT, and real-time fluoroscopic monitoring.

Another highly promising IG-IMRT delivery system on the horizon, which has significant potential to improve the ability to localize and track soft tissue tumors, is the Renaissance System 1000 (ViewRay, Cleveland, OH). This device utilizes a multi-headed ^{60}Co rotational IMRT system with MR image guidance and has the ability to image continually during treatment even while the beam is on. In addition to the Renaissance, research continues in the development of a MRI-linac hybrid system.[46]

Several investigators have also pointed out the utility of very high energy (VHE) electron beams (150 to 250 MeV).[47,48] Such high-energy beams are not yet available, and so only beam simulation software has been used to demonstrate the use of multi-VHE beams from opposed directions and the ability to modulated VHE beam intensity.[47,48] Such machines are clearly some time away, but these early studies show promise.

Proton, Light-Ion, and Neutron Beam Treatment Units

The first use of proton beams for radiation therapy is credited to Wilson,[49] who in 1946 pointed out the superior depth–dose characteristics provided by protons. Details on the history and development of proton beam radiation therapy (PBRT) machines are provided by Breuer and Smith[50] and Delaney and Kooy.[51] PBRT is seeing increasing interest worldwide because its depth–dose characteristics show advantages over those of photon beams.[52]

In most existing or proposed proton and light-ion particle treatment facilities, either a *cyclotron* or a *synchrotron* is used to accelerate proton beams to sufficient energy (200 to 250 MeV) and beam intensity.

Cyclotron

The cyclotron (Fig. 6.22) was invented by Ernest Lawrence of the University of California in 1929. It accelerates charged particles such as protons, deuterons, and light ions using a high-frequency, alternating voltage (potential difference) applied across two conducting D-shaped evacuated half-cylinders (Ds). A fixed magnetic field, perpendicular to the top of the two Ds, forces the charged particles to travel in a circular path. The charged particles accelerate only when passing through the gap between the two Ds. The beam spirals out to the edge of the container as the particle speeds increase. At this point, the particle speed approaches the speed of light. Proton beam energies of 200 to 250 MeV are considered adequate for most radiation therapy applications. Beam intensity from the accelerator must

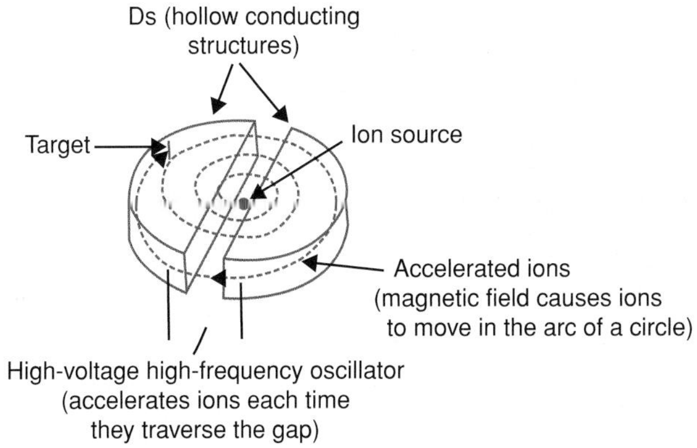

FIGURE 6.22. Schematic drawing showing principles of cyclotron operation. This machine is used for accelerating positive ions and is used clinically to produce proton and neutron beams. Metal half-disks (Ds) have an evacuated center through which the protons can travel. The protons are accelerated by an oscillating electric field operating between the half-disks. A magnetic field perpendicular to the plane of the half-disks confines the charged particles in the half-disks.

be adequate to overcome losses in the beam delivery system and provide tolerable treatment times.

Synchrocyclotron and Synchrotron

A *synchrocyclotron* varies either the magnetic field or the frequency of the applied electric field; a *synchrotron* varies both. By increasing these parameters appropriately as the particles gain energy, one can hold their path constant as they are accelerated. This allows the vacuum container for the particles to be a large, thin torus. In reality it is easier to use some straight sections and some bent sections using multiple bend magnets, thus creating the shape of a rounded-corner polygon. The proton beam facility at Loma Linda University Medical Center (Loma Linda, CA) is an example of this type of accelerator.[53]

The synchrotron has the advantage of simple energy variability, whereas the cyclotron produces continuous beams with a fixed energy and higher beam intensity, making their design somewhat simpler. Beam-spreading mechanisms obtain suitable field sizes for radiation therapy by passive modulation (scattering foil) systems or by dynamic pencil-beam spot-scanning systems,[53] which allow dose conformation not only at the distal edge of the tumor, but also at the proximal edge. Hall[54] pointed out that there is significant neutron leakage radiation for proton treatment machines that use a scattering foil and recommended moving to the pencil-beam scanning systems.

There are at least 9 modern PBRT facilities specifically designed for radiation therapy already operating in the United States and approximately 10 more either in development or scheduled to open over the next few years.

There are only a few active clinical facilities for light-ion radiation therapy (primarily carbon ion).[52,55] Two are operational in Japan, with a third coming on line soon and a fourth soon to begin construction. Heidelberg, Germany, has the first clinical center with multiple-ion capabilities from protons to carbon, including the first gantry for carbon beams; two more are currently under construction in Germany. The Centro Nazionale di Adroterapia Oncologica (National Center for Oncological Hadrontherapy) in Pavia, Italy, was scheduled to begin treatments in 2011. In addition, facilities are under construction in France and Austria.

Light-ion radiation therapy requires beams at much higher energies than proton therapy. For example, a proton beam of 150 MeV can penetrate 16 cm in water. To achieve the same penetration with carbon ions, energy of 3,000 MeV or 250 MeV/per nucleon is needed. Synchrotrons are the only available sources for such high-energy ion beams, and they are large, complex machines requiring large facilities and similarly large capital expenditures.

Interest in light-ion radiation therapy is due to its combination of two important physical advantages: (a) its depth–dose characteristics and (b) high linear energy transfer (LET) in the Bragg peak region of the beam. For its depth characteristics, the ratio of the Bragg peak dose to the entrance region dose is even larger than for protons. In addition, unlike proton beam therapy, there is a large increase in the radiation LET in the Bragg peak region of the beam. The combination of these two characteristics results in a potentially unique advantage—a high LET region that can be closely conformed to the target volume.

New and Evolving Proton Treatment Machines

New technologies for the delivery of PBRT are emerging. Single-gantry systems are being designed and manufactured, including the MEVION S250 Proton Therapy System (Mevion Medical Systems, Littleton, MA; formerly Still River Systems) shown in Figure 6.23. This system uses a superconducting synchrocyclotron that is gantry mounted and incorporates image-guidance and robotic patient positioning. The first unit was scheduled to be installed at Washington University (St. Louis, MO) in late 2011.

In addition, Varian recently announced their single-room PBRT system, which uses superconducting cyclotron technology and can be expanded into a multiroom facility when needed.

A more futuristic design concept has been reported by Caporaso et al.[56] This system is being codeveloped by Compact Particle Acceleration Corp (Livermore, CA) and TomoTherapy (Madison, WI). The design is based on *dielectric wall accelerator* (*DWA*) technology (under development by the Lawrence

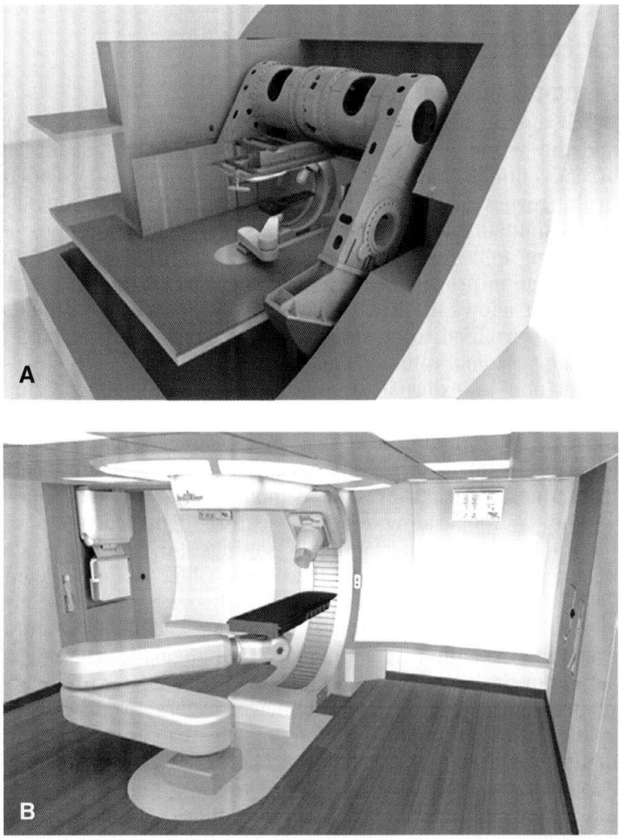

FIGURE 6.23. Rendering of next-generation proton therapy system (MEVION S250 Proton Therapy System, Mevion Medical Systems, Littleton, MA; formerly Still River Systems). **(A)** Outer gantry holds the proton accelerator in the center, pointing directly to the isocenter. Accelerator is a 250-MeV cyclotron specifically designed (uses superconducting magnets) for proton therapy (with intensity-modulated proton therapy capabilities, high dose rate, high reliability, and easy maintenance). **(B)** Treatment room depicting inner gantry and six-degree-of-freedom robotic couch.

Livermore National Laboratory, Livermore, CA[56]). The goal is to make a PBRT linac so compact that it can be installed in a conventional linac treatment room. This will require an average accelerating gradient of approximately 100 MV/m to yield a linac on the order of 2 m in length. If successful, the DWA PBRT machine would produce a 200-MeV proton beam composed of individual pulses that could be varied in intensity, energy, and spot width. While the DWA is still largely at a research level of development, the realization of a compact, image-guided PBRT system that can provide rotational intensity-modulated proton therapy and be sited in a treatment room not much larger than for a conventional linac would likely be a real "game changer" for radiation therapy.

Neutron Therapy Treatment Machines

Modern neutron therapy machines use cyclotrons to accelerate protons or deuterons to energies of about 50 MeV to produce neutron beams with depth–dose characteristics equivalent to those of about 6-MV x-rays. The p,Be (protons accelerated to strike a beryllium target) reaction is used most commonly because protons are much easier to bend around the gantry of an isocentric unit, and thus the cyclotron can be much smaller and thus less expensive. The only exception is the superconducting cyclotron installed at Harper Hospital (Detroit, MI), which uses the d,Be (deuterions strike beryllium target) reaction.[57] With superconducting technology, the entire cyclotron is small enough to be rotated around the patient on isocentric rings, thus eliminating the need for bending the deuteron beam around a rotating gantry. In addition, the neutron yield for the d,Be reaction is about five times that for the p,Be reaction. More details on the history and development of neutron beam therapy machines are provided in the review by Maughan and Yudelev.[58]

SIMULATORS

Conventional Simulator

Details on the development of the *radiation therapy simulator* and the selection, acceptance testing, and quality assurance of conventional radiation therapy simulators are provided in the review article by Van Dyk and Munro.[59] The conventional simulator mimics the functions and allowed motions of a therapy unit and uses a diagnostic x-ray tube to simulate the radiation properties of the treatment beam (Fig. 6.24). A simulator allows the beam direction and the treatment fields to be determined to encompass the projection of the target volume. Radiographic visualization of internal structures in relation to external landmarks allows special shielding devices (Cerrobend blocks) to be constructed to help minimize the dose to normal critical structures. Gantry arms are rigid enough to support heavy shielding blocks and simulated electron cones. Couch widths are similar to therapy-unit couch widths, and operating consoles feature digital displays of parameters and programmable settings for source-to-axis distance, gantry angles, and field sizes. Older models of conventional simulators were equipped with an x-ray fluoroscopy system consisting of an image intensifier and video camera system to expedite field setup and beam angulations. Modern simulator design has replace the image intensifier with amorphous silicon technology. The new imagers produce high spatial- and contrast-resolution images that approach film quality, facilitating the concept of filmless radiation oncology departments, and provide CBCT capability. While this feature allows volumetric imaging on a conventional simulator, they are still rapidly being replaced with CT simulators.

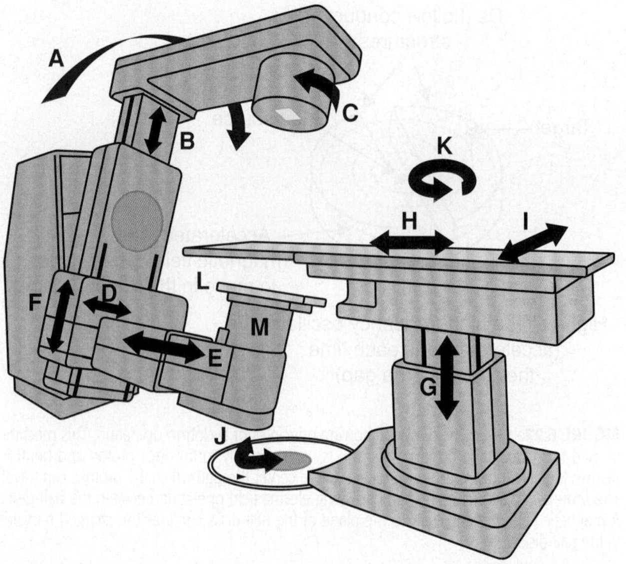

FIGURE 6.24. The basic components and motions of a radiation therapy simulator: **A:** Gantry rotation. **B:** Source–axis distance. **C:** Collimator rotation. **D:** Image intensifier (lateral). **E:** Image intensifier (longitudinal). **F:** Image intensifier (radial). **G:** Patient table (vertical). **H:** Patient table (longitudinal). **I:** Patient table (lateral). **J:** Patient table rotation about isocenter. **K:** Patient table rotation about pedestal. **L:** Film cassette. **M:** Image intensifier. Motions not shown include field-size delineation, radiation beam diaphragms, and source–tray distance. (From Van Dyk J, Mah K. Simulators and CT scanners. In: Williams JR, Thwaites DI, eds. *Radiotherapy physics.* New York: Oxford Medical Publications; 1993.)

CT Simulators

In the 1980s and early 1990s, research led to the integration of a diagnostic CT scanner with what was essentially a three-dimensional (3D) treatment-planning system, which led to the concept of *virtual simulation.*[60–62] Such a system is now referred to as a *CT simulator* and consists of a CT scanner, a flat-tabletop patient position–alignment system, including an orthogonal laser system, and a digital interface (DICOM) to a planning system that is equipped with virtual simulation software (Fig. 6.25). Simulation software provides many advanced image manipulation and viewing features, including *beam's-eye view* display, which allows the anatomy to be viewed from the perspective of the radiation beams and allows field shaping to be done electronically at the graphics display station, and the generation of *digitally reconstructed radiographs.* Modern CT simulation systems incorporate large-bore CT scanners especially designed for radiation oncology, with multislice capability, high-quality laser patient positioning/marking systems, and sophisticated virtual simulation software features. Details of the virtual simulation process are discussed in some detail in Chapter 9. More details on CT simulation can be found in the review article by Van Dyk and Taylor[63] and articles by Mutic et al.[64,65]

New and Evolving Simulation Machines

The most significant development now occurring with simulators is the continued integration of functional imaging with anatomic imaging in the simulation/planning process. Already commercially available are a magnetic resonance simulator and a large-bore positron emission tomography CT simulator, both with features specifically designed for radiation oncology. While not yet common in radiation oncology departments, it is very likely that multimodality imaging simulation systems will become common within the next decade and include full four-dimensional capabilities to address cases involving significant internal motion.

QUALITY OF RADIATION

The penetrability of an x-ray beam, referred to as the *quality* of the beam, is completely specified by its spectral distribution curve (i.e., the relative intensities of photons of various energies), which is the result of fluctuations of tube potential, the bremsstrahlung radiation process, characteristic radiation, and

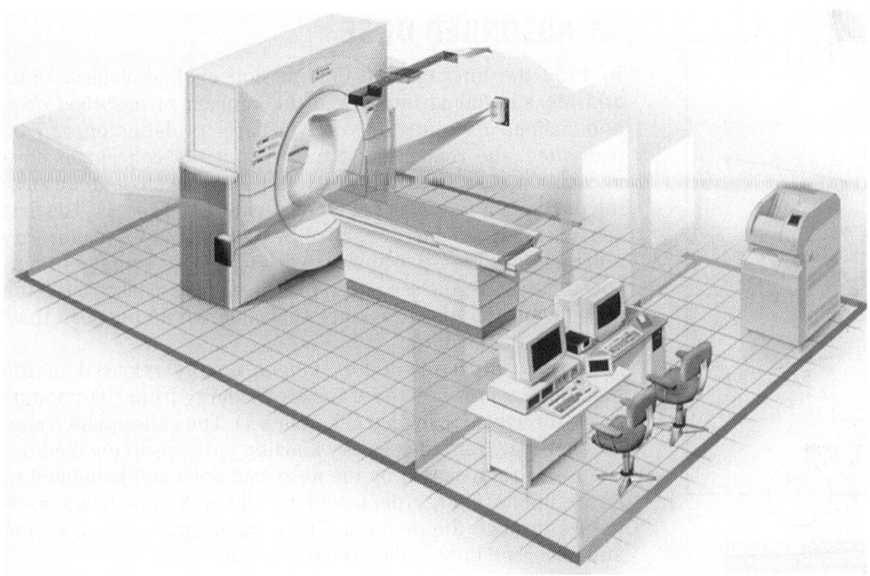

FIGURE 6.25. Typical computed tomography simulation suite showing the scanner, flat tabletop, orthogonal laser system, virtual simulation workstation, and hardcopy output device.

multiple interactions of the incident electrons and the x-ray target. The distribution of the photon energies, including the peak photon energy, in the continuous spectrum is governed solely by the x-ray tube potential. However, the energy of the characteristic photons increases with increasing atomic number of the target element. All other factors being equal, the radiation intensity is proportional to the atomic number of the target element.

Spectral distribution of an x-ray beam can be modified by placing absorbing materials of various thicknesses (i.e., filters) in the beam. In general, a filter removes relatively more low-energy photons than high-energy photons, although photons of all energies are removed to some extent. For radiation in the orthovoltage region (except for the absorption edge effect), the lower the energy of the photons, the larger is the total mass attenuation coefficient and therefore the greater is the likelihood that the photon will be absorbed. Thus, the beam emerges from the filter with a larger percentage of high-energy photons than it had on entering the filter. The beam has a greater penetration power and is said to have been "*hardened*" by the filter. The quality of an x-ray beam improves with increasing tube potential and with increasing thickness and atomic number of the filter.

A specification of beam quality based entirely on a spectral distribution is too cumbersome for radiation therapy. The usual method of specifying beam quality in superficial and orthovoltage therapy is to list the HVL and the accelerating potential. For megavoltage beams, only the maximum energy of the electrons striking the x-ray target typically is used. The *homogeneity coefficient* denotes how homogeneous an x-ray beam is with respect to its photon energies. It is defined as the ratio of the first HVL to the second HVL. As the filtration is increased, the exposure rate decreases; therefore, there is a practical limit of filter thickness in orthovoltage therapy with a given combination of kilovolts, milliamperes, and treatment distance. In certain situations, it is convenient to express the quality of the x-ray beam in terms of an "equivalent energy," which can be derived from knowledge of the HVL. The type of x-ray beam that is used in radiation therapy is always heterogeneous; however, the x-ray beam can be considered to have an *equivalent energy* of a monoenergetic x-ray beam that has a HVL equal to the measured HVL of the heterogeneous beam.

RADIATION EXPOSURE

In 1928 at the Second International Congress of Radiology, the ionization of air, called *exposure,* was adopted as the measurable effect of radiation of a photon beam.[66] As the beam passes through a material, it creates ion pairs via the ionization process. In air, these ion pairs have some mobility and can be collected by applying an electric field across the air. The number of ion pairs collected is a measure of the quantity of radiation passing through the air.

The *roentgen* (R), the unit for exposure, also was defined at the 1928 Congress. The definition has been modified slightly by subsequent congresses, but the basic concept remains the same. The roentgen is that amount of x- or γ-radiation that causes the associated corpuscular emission per 0.001293 g of air to produce, in air, ions carrying one electrostatic unit of charge of either sign. The value 0.001293 g is the mass of 1 cm^3 of air at 0°C and 760 mm Hg pressure; "associated corpuscular emission" refers to the Compton and pair-production electrons set in motion by the interactions between the incident photons and the air molecules. By conversion of units, the roentgen can be expressed as follows:

$$1 \text{ R} = 2.58 \times 10^{-4} \text{ C/kg of air}$$

With the advent of SI units, the roentgen no longer is used as a special name for a radiation unit, and the SI unit for exposure is coulombs per kilogram (C/kg), which is equivalent to approximately 3,876 R (Table 6.2).

The condition of electronic equilibrium must exist for the definition of the roentgen to be satisfied (Fig. 6.26). According to the definition, the electrons produced in a specified volume must spend all of their energies by ionization in air, and the total charge must be measured. However, because some electrons produced inside the specified volume create ion pairs outside the volume and some electrons produced outside the volume contribute ionization inside the specified volume, the gain and loss of ion pairs must be the same for the definition of the roentgen to be satisfied.

The free-air ionization chamber is used to measure exposure directly in roentgens.[1] It is designed to collect all the ions produced in a defined volume by the radiation beam and is used primarily by standards laboratories. Free-air chambers are bulky and too complicated to use for routine measurements. Instead, small ionization chambers called *thimble chambers* are typically used to measure exposure. The chamber gives a measure of the ionization produced, which then is converted to exposure in roentgens by use of an *exposure calibration factor,* N_x, traceable to the National Institute of Standards and Technology (Gaithersburg, MD). Thimble chambers are designed for use at specific energies; the thickness of

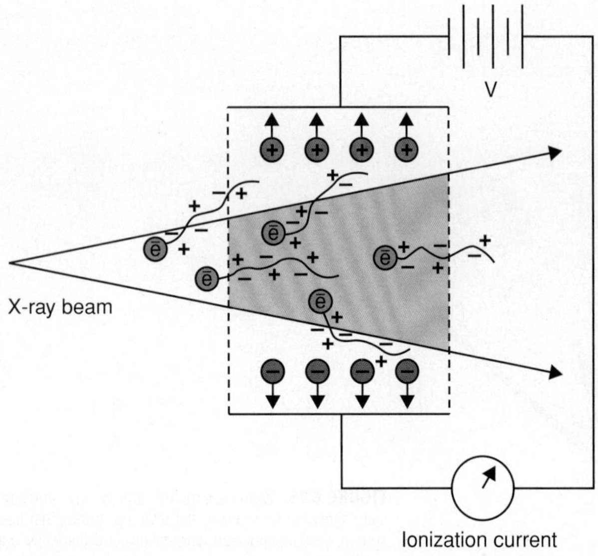

FIGURE 6.26. Schematic illustrating electronic equilibrium. (From Khan FM. *The physics of radiation therapy*, 3rd ed. Baltimore: Williams & Wilkins; 1994.)

the chamber wall is equal to the maximum electron range (electronic equilibrium established). If they are used at higher energies, at which the electron range is greater, an added wall thickness or *buildup cap* must be used.

To determine the exposure rate from an x-ray or γ-ray machine, an exposure-calibrated thimble chamber (with appropriate wall thickness) and connected to an *electrometer* is placed at beam center, in air, at right angles to the beam's central axis and at the point where the exposure rate is to be specified. The field size for which the exposure rate is to be measured is set, and the radiation machine is turned on for a specified time, *T,* to achieve a reading, *M,* on the connected electrometer. The reading is corrected for *temperature and atmospheric pressure, timer error, stem effect,* and *ion-recombination effects.* The therapy machine exposure rate, $\dot{X}$, is given in roentgens per minute by the following equation:

$$\dot{X} = \frac{M \cdot N_x \cdot C_{tp} \cdot C_{st} \cdot C_s}{T + \alpha}$$

where M is the raw ionization chamber reading, N_x is the exposure calibration factor obtained from a standards laboratory, C_{tp} is the temperature and pressure correction factor, C_{st} is the stem effect correction factor, C_s is the ion-recombination correction factor, T is timer (minutes) or monitor unit setting, and α is the timer error. The temperature-pressure correction factor C_{tp} is given by the following equation:

$$C_{tp} = \left(\frac{t + 273.16}{295.16}\right)\left(\frac{760}{p}\right)$$

The timer error α is given by the following equation:

$$\frac{M_1}{T + \alpha} = \frac{M_2}{T + n\alpha}$$

where M_1 is the instrument reading for a single long exposure of *T,* M_2 is the instrument reading for *n* short exposures of total time *T,* and α is the timer error (monitor end effect for linacs) for a single exposure.[67]

Beyond 3 MeV, the roentgen cannot be measured accurately, and thus calibrations of radiation therapy machines at these higher energies are performed using an exposure-calibrated ionization chamber such as a Bragg–Gray cavity, and the ionization readings are converted to absorbed dose as discussed in the following section.

ABSORBED DOSE

In 1953 the International Commission on Radiological Units and Measurements introduced the concept of *absorbed dose* and defined its unit, the *rad.*[66] Before its definition can be presented, the reader must understand the concept of dose absorption. As a beam of radiation passes through an absorbing medium, it interacts with it in a two-stage process. The first step occurs when energy carried by the photons—the indirectly ionizing particles—is transformed into kinetic energy of high-speed electrons; the second step occurs as these electrons—the directly ionizing particles—are slowed down and deposit their energy in the medium.

Kerma, an acronym for "kinetic energy released in the medium," represents the transfer of energy from the photons to the directly ionizing particles (step 1). The subsequent transfer of energy from the directly ionizing particles to the medium (step 2) is represented by the absorbed dose and is defined in terms of the energy deposited by the radiation beam as it passes through the medium. The relationship between kerma and absorbed dose is illustrated in Figure 6.27.

The *rad* represents the absorption of 0.01 J/kg of the absorbing material (1 rad = 0.01 J/kg). The rad now has been replaced with the SI unit for absorbed dose (1 J/kg) given the special name of *gray (Gy)* (Table 6.2). By conversion of units, the gray can be expressed as follows:

1 Gy = 1 J/kg = 100 cGy = 100 rad

Determination of Absorbed Dose

It is difficult to measure absorbed dose directly, but two direct methods—*calorimetry* and *Fricke dosimetry*—are available in some laboratories. Neither method is particularly practical nor widely used, and the reader is referred to the literature for more details.[68] Instead, a simpler, indirect method using an

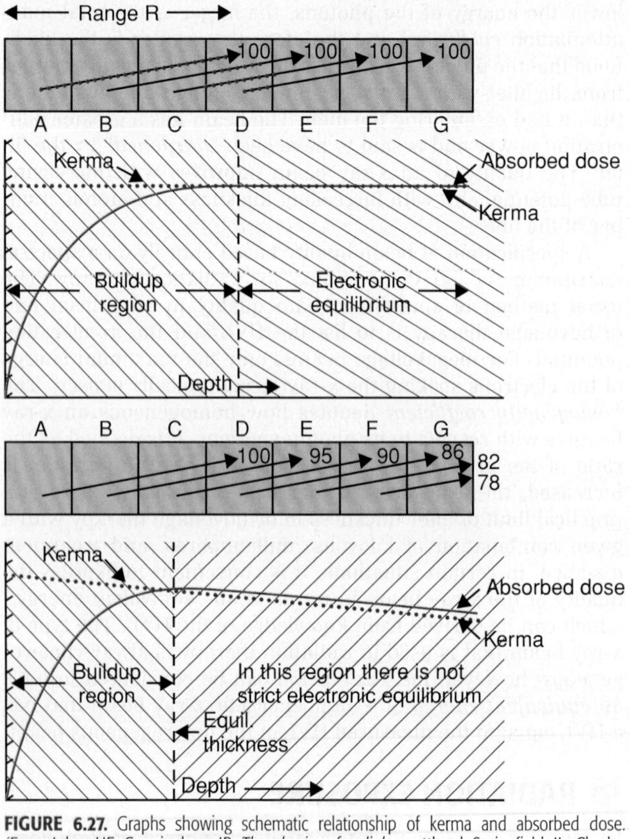

FIGURE 6.27. Graphs showing schematic relationship of kerma and absorbed dose. (From Johns HE, Cunningham JR. *The physics of radiology*, 4th ed. Springfield, IL: Charles C Thomas; 1983.)

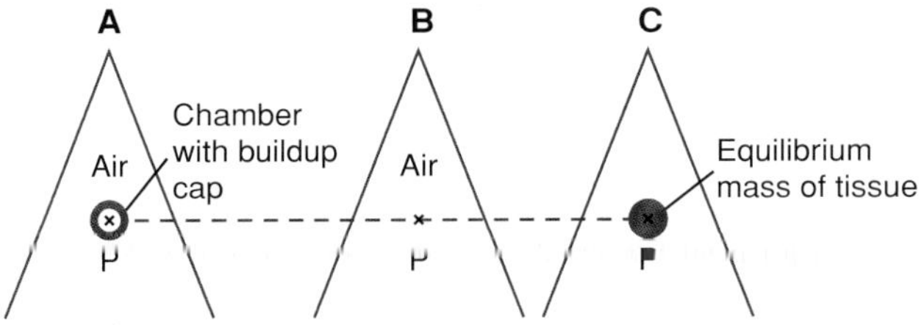

FIGURE 6.28. Schematic illustrating ionization measurement in air to determine dose in free space. (From Khan FM. *The physics of radiation therapy,* 2 nd ed. Baltimore: Williams & Wilkins; 1994.)

exposure-calibrated ionization chamber is used to determine absorbed dose.

Absorbed Dose Calculation from Exposure Measurement

For photon energies of ^{60}Co and lower, an ionization chamber having an exposure calibration factor assigned by an appropriate national calibration facility (e.g., a dosimetry calibration laboratory accredited by the National Institute of Standards and Technology or the American Association of Physicists in Medicine [AAPM; College Park, MD]) can be used to measure exposure in air as described in the section Radiation Exposure. Absorbed dose then can be calculated from the exposure as explained here. The energy deposited in a fixed mass of air from a known exposure can be calculated because it is known that an exposure of 1 R creates a finite number of ion pairs per unit mass of air (i.e., 1.61×10^{15} ion pairs per kilogram of air) and that the mean energy required to create an ion pair in air (denoted by *W*) is equal to 33.97 eV per ion pair. When these values are used, the relationship between the exposure, *X*, and the dose to air, D_{air}, is given by the following expression:

$$D_{air}\,(\text{Gy}) = \left(8.76\frac{\text{Gy}}{\text{R}}\right) \cdot X\,(\text{R})$$

The *dose in free space,* D_{fs}, is defined as the dose at the center of a small mass of phantom-like material just large enough to provide electronic equilibrium (Fig. 6.28) and can be derived from D_{air} using the ratio of the mass energy absorption coefficients (u_{en}/ρ) and an attenuation correction factor, A_{eq}, that accounts for the photon attenuation in the small mass of phantom-like material:

$$D_{fs} = \left[0.873\,\frac{(\mu_{en}/\rho)_{med}}{(\mu_{en}/\rho)_{air}}\right] \cdot X \cdot A_{eq}$$

The term in brackets is called the *f-factor* or the *roentgen-to-rad conversion factor* and is represented as f_{med}, giving the dose in free space as follows:

$$D_{fs} = f_{med} \cdot X \cdot A_{eq}$$

Values of f_{med} are shown in Figure 6.29 over the energy range commonly used in radiation therapy. Notice that the *f*-factor is a function of the medium and the energy of the photon beam. Typical values of A_{eq} are 0.989 and 1.00 for ^{60}Co and 250-kV energies, respectively.

An in-air calibration procedure is performed as follows. The calibrated ion chamber (with wall thick enough to ensure electronic equilibrium) is placed in air with its sensitive volume on the central axis of the beam and its stem at right angles to the beam direction. The center of the chamber most often is placed at a distance from the source (or target) equal to the nominal SSD of the machine plus the buildup depth. A standard field size is set, usually 10 × 10 cm, using either movable collimators or the standard treatment applicator. An exposure is made for a known time or number of monitor units. The ionization chamber reading is converted to units of Gy/min at the depth of the maximum dose within a phantom, d_{med}, using the following equation:

$$\dot{D}_{med} = \frac{M \cdot N_x \cdot C_{tp} \cdot C_{st} \cdot C_s \cdot A_{eq} \cdot f_{med} \cdot \text{TAR}(d_{max})}{T + \alpha}$$

where *M*, N_x, C_{tp}, C_{st}, C_s, A_{eq}, f_{med}, *T*, and α are used as defined earlier. The term TAR(d_{max}) represents the tissue–air ratio at the depth of maximum dose (i.e., the *backscatter* or *peakscatter factor*) and converts the dose in free space to the dose in a phantom at the depth of maximum dose. This parameter is

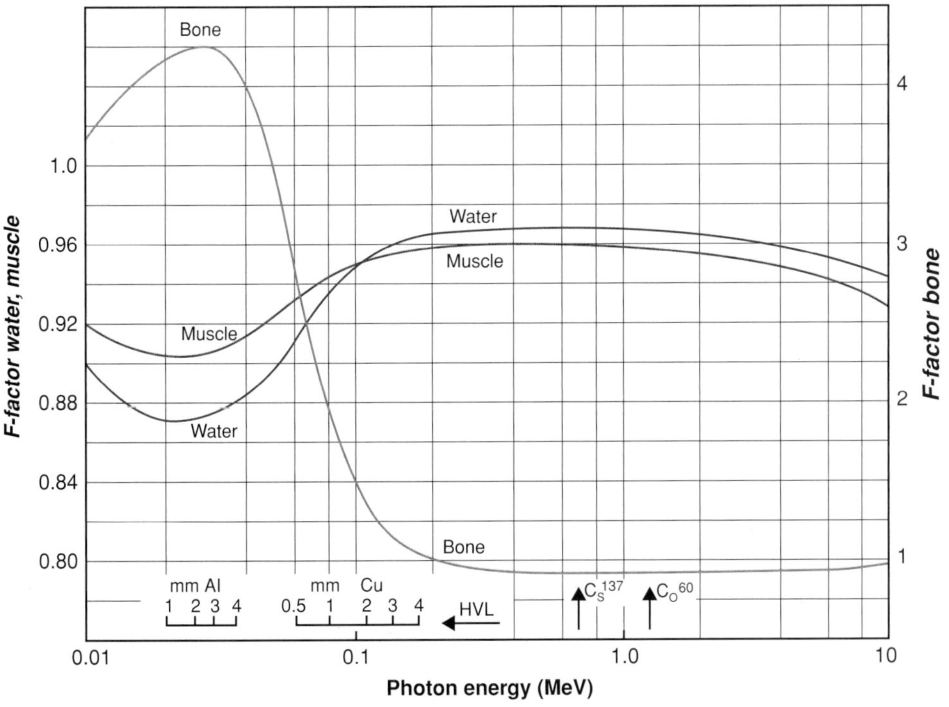

FIGURE 6.29. The roentgen-to-rad conversion factor for bone, muscle, and water as a function of photon energy. (From Johns HE, Cunningham JR. *The physics of radiology,* 4th ed. Springfield, IL: Charles C Thomas; 1983.)

discussed in more detail later. The preceding equation can be rewritten as follows:

$$\dot{D}_{\text{med}} = \dot{X} \cdot f_{\text{med}} \cdot A_{\text{eq}} \cdot \text{TAR}(d_{\text{max}})$$

and

$$\dot{D}_{\text{med}} = \dot{D}_{\text{fs}} \cdot \text{TAR}(d_{\text{max}})$$

This method is also valid when the measurements are made with the exposure-calibrated ion chamber embedded within a medium, such as a water phantom. In that case, the TAR(d_{max}) term is not included in the calculation, and the A_{eq} factor is replaced by a displacement factor, A_m. The numerical value of A_m is very close to that of A_{eq}, and for exposure measurements made within a water phantom, the dose rate is given by the following expression:

$$\dot{D}_{\text{med}} = \dot{X} \cdot f_{\text{med}} \cdot A_{\text{m}}$$

Absorbed Dose Calculation from Bragg–Gray Cavity Ionization Measurement

For energies above the level of ^{60}Co, exposure calibration factors are not available from the standards laboratories because of measurement limitations. In 1983, the AAPM introduced a protocol for the calibration of high-energy photon and electron beams that was based on *Bragg–Gray cavity theory* and allowed one to calculate dose directly from ion chamber measurements in a medium for energies above the level of ^{60}Co.[69] The protocol updated physical parameters and procedures for calibration and measurement and accounted for the different phantom materials (e.g., plastic and water) used for calibration and differences in ion chamber design and construction. The protocol introduced the *cavity-gas calibration factor,* N_{gas}, which is related to the ion chamber's ^{60}Co exposure-calibration factor, N_x, and is used in conjunction with restricted stopping-power ratios, $\bar{L}/\rho$, for the radiation beam in question to convert the ionization reading to absorbed dose using the following expression:

$$D_{\text{med}} = M \cdot N_{\text{gas}} \cdot (\bar{L}/\rho)^{\text{med}}_{\text{gas}} \cdot P_{\text{ion}} \cdot P_{\text{repl}} \cdot P_{\text{wall}}$$

where M is the raw ionization chamber reading per monitor unit corrected for temperature and pressure, P_{ion} is the ion recombination correction factor, P_{repl} is a correction factor for replacement of phantom material by the ionization chamber, and P_{wall} is a correction factor to account for ionization chamber wall composition.

In 1999, the AAPM published a new protocol (TG-51) for the calibration of high-energy photon and electron beams.[70] This protocol uses ion chambers with absorbed-dose-to-water calibration factors, $N^{\text{Co-60}}_{\text{D-W}}$, which are traceable to national primary standards via the ^{60}Co standard. The absorbed dose to water D^Q_W at the point of measurement of the ion chamber placed under reference conditions is given by the following equation:

$$D^Q_{\text{W}} = M \cdot k_Q \cdot N^{\text{Co-60}}_{\text{D,W}}$$

where Q is the beam quality of the clinical beam, M is the fully corrected ion chamber reading, and k_Q is the *quality conversion factor* that converts the calibration factor for a ^{60}Co beam to that for a beam of quality Q. The protocol is designed to be a simplification of the AAPM's TG-21 protocol in the sense that large tables of stopping-power ratios and mass-energy absorption coefficients are no longer needed, and the user does not need to calculate any theoretical dosimetry factors.[71–73]

Other Dosimetry Methods

Thermoluminescence Dosimetry

Certain crystalline materials exhibit a phenomenon known as *thermoluminescence.* When a crystal capable of thermoluminescence is irradiated, a small portion of the energy absorbed is stored in the structure of the crystal lattice. If the material is heated, the energy is released in the form of visible light. Several thermoluminescent phosphors are available, but lithium fluoride, with an effective atomic number of 8.2, is the most commonly used.

The physical theory of thermoluminescence dosimetry can be explained as follows. In the individual atom, electrons occupy discrete energy levels. However, in the crystal lattice, the electronic energy levels are perturbed by mutual interactions between atoms, giving rise to energy bands, so-called *allowed energy bands* and *forbidden energy bands.* Impurities in the crystal create energy traps in the forbidden bands, allowing metastable states to exist; for example, when the phosphor is irradiated, some of the electrons in the valence band (ground state) receive sufficient energy to be raised to the conduction band. If there is an instantaneous emission of light, the phenomenon is called *fluorescence.* If an electron in the trap requires energy to get out of the trap and return to the valence band, the emission of light is called *phosphorescence.* If the emission of light is slow at room temperature but can be sped up with heating, the process is called *thermoluminescence.*

Thermoluminescence dosimeters must be calibrated before they can be used for measuring an unknown dose. Because the response of the thermoluminescent material is affected by its radiation and thermal histories, the material must be annealed to remove residual effects. The standard preirradiation annealing procedure for lithium fluoride is 1 hour of heating at 400°C and 24 hours at 80°C. More details can be found in the review article by DeWerd et al.[74]

Film Dosimetry

When an x-ray film is exposed to ionizing radiation, the exposed silver bromide crystals form a latent image. In the film development process, the affected crystals cause a darkening of the film, and the unaffected crystals leave the film clear. The degree of blackening of the film is proportional to the energy absorbed and is measured by determining the optical density with a densitometer. The optical density is defined as follows:

$$\text{OD} = \log(I_0/I_T)$$

where I_0 is the amount of light detected without the film in place and I_T is the amount of light detected with the film in place. For radiation dosimetry, the net optical density is obtained by subtracting the densitometric reading for the base fog (clear portion of the film) from the measured optical density. Most films are exposed to yield an optical density between 1.3 and 1.7 for optimal viewing.

A plot of net optical density as a function of radiation exposure or dose is called the *sensitometric curve* or the *Hunter–Driffield (H-D) curve.* If the curve is nonlinear, appropriate corrections must be applied to convert net optical density to absorbed dose.

The use of film is a relatively straightforward method of dosimetry for electron beams, but it must be done with extreme care in photon dosimetry. The problem is that the photoelectric effect depends on Z^3 ($Z_{silver} = 47$), and the film emulsion strongly absorbs radiation below 100 kV. A concise review of radiographic film dosimetry can be found in the article by Das.[75]

Radiochromic Film Dosimetry

Radiochromic film consists of a thin (7 to 23 mm), radiosensitive, colorless leuco dye bonded to a 100-mm-thick Mylar base. Radiochromic films are colorless before irradiation and turn deep blue when irradiated without physical, chemical, or thermal processing. The film is approximately tissue equivalent, integrates simultaneously at all measurement points, and has a high spatial resolution (>1,200 lines/mm). It shows a stable, reproducible response if protected from ultraviolet light, unstable temperatures, and humidity. Because radiochromic dye is an aromatic hydrocarbon, like plastic scintillators, it has an energy response superior to that of diodes and comparable with thermoluminescence dosimetry. Interest in radiochromic film as a quantitative dosimeter has been stimulated by the appearance of a fourfold-more-sensitive film (model MD-55), which extends its response down to the 5-Gy level. More details on radiochromic film dosimetry are given in the article by Soares et al.[76]

Diode Dosimetry

Semiconductor diodes offer many advantages for clinical dosimetry, including high sensitivity, real-time read-out, robustness, and independence of air pressure. Most semiconductor diodes are made from silicon, which is either *n* type (silicon doped with group V material, such as phosphorus) or *p* type (silicon doped with group III material, such as boron). To form a diode detector, a *p-n* junction must be created.

The physical theory of semiconductor dosimetry can be explained as follows. During irradiation, electron–hole pairs are created both within and outside the depletion region in the body of the diode detector. The charge carriers are swept across the depletion region and collected rapidly under the action of the electric field that exists across it. In this way, a current is generated, flowing in the reverse direction to normal diode current flow, which can be measured and related to absorbed dose.

Dosimetry diodes are operated without an external reverse bias voltage and connected via cable to a simple electrometer. Details on their use for *in vivo* dosimetry are provided in AAPM Report 87.[77] Calibration of diodes typically is performed by comparison of readings against an ion chamber in a standard setup to establish a diode calibration factor for absorbed dose to water and the establishment of a series of correction factors to account for calibration differences when measurements are performed under various experimental conditions. Typical concerns are energy dependence, temperature sensitivity, directional dependence, and radiation damage. Each radiation therapy center should establish the responses of their diodes under the various conditions encountered and monitor them as the cumulative dose to the diodes increases. Frequency of checks should be adjusted according to the frequency of use of the diodes and the variability encountered. More details on diode dosimetry are given in the article by Zhu and Saini.[78]

Metal Oxide Semiconductor-Field Effect Transistor Dosimetry

Metal oxide semiconductor-field effect transistors represent another example of a semiconductor dosimeter. Originally developed for space dosimetry, the operation is based on the buildup of charge in the silicon oxide transistor gate created by ionizing radiation. The reader is referred to the article by Cygler and Scalchi[79] for more details on this type of dosimeter.

Polymer-Gel Dosimetry

Gel dosimetry is based on quantifying the effects of radiation-induced chemical changes occurring within some volume of material filled with an aqueous gel matrix. The degree of chemical change in the gel is related to dose. The dose-dependent changes are determined by imaging techniques, including magnetic resonance imaging, CT, and optical CT. Hence, gel dosimetry has the potential to provide full 3D dosimetry throughout the volume of the irradiated gel dosimeter.

For example, one form of this method exploits the radiation-induced free-radical chain polymerization of acrylic monomers dispersed in an aqueous gel. When irradiated, discrete, microscopic regions of cross-linked polymer are formed, the concentration of which is proportional to radiation dose. The water proton nuclear magnetic resonance relaxation rates in the gel are strongly affected by local changes in the polymer molecular structure and dynamics; thus, the distribution of

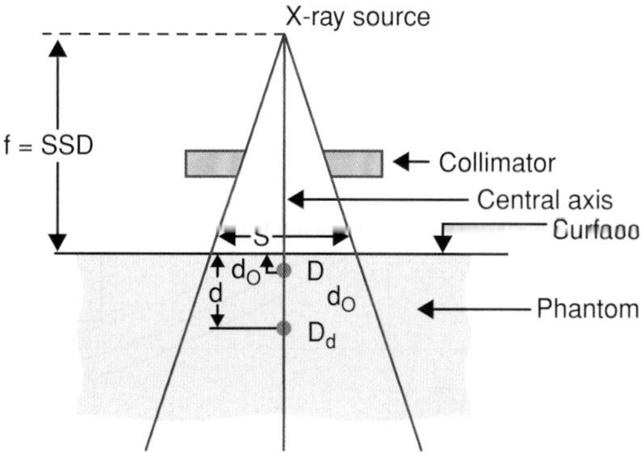

FIGURE 6.30. Schematic drawing illustrating definition of percentage depth dose, where *d* is any depth and d_0 is the reference depth, usually d_{max}.

radiation dose may be visualized and quantified with high resolution using MRI. Because the polymer microparticles scatter light, the dose distribution also can also be visualized in the transparent gel as a dose-dependent 3D optical turbidity and read by optical CT.

Unfortunately, gel dosimetry, while having the potential for tissue-equivalent 3D dosimetry for a little over two decades, has not come into common clinical use, as it as proven too difficult to use in the clinic setting.[80] Research continues in gel dosimetry, as there is clearly a need for a robust 3D high-resolution dosimetry system.[80,81]

DOSIMETRY PARAMETERS

Percentage Depth Dose

Percentage depth dose (*PDD*) can be understood by reference to Figure 6.30. It is the ratio, expressed as a percentage, of the absorbed dose on the central axis at depth d to the absorbed dose at the reference point d_0. Percentage depth dose is given by

$$\mathrm{PDD}(d, d_0, S, f, E) = \frac{D_d}{D_{d0}} \times 100$$

The functional symbols have been inserted in the expression to make it clear that the PDD is affected by a number of parameters, including d, d_0, field dimension S, source-to-surface distance f, and radiation beam energy (or quality) E. S refers to the side length of a square beam at a specified reference depth. Nonsquare beams may be designated by their equivalent square. Field shape and added beam collimation also can affect the central axis depth–dose distribution. Photon-beam PDD increases with increasing energy, SSD, and field size. Figure 6.31 shows that the depth of the 50th percentile increases from approximately 14 cm for 4-MV x-rays to nearly 23 cm for 25-MV x-rays. The depth of maximum dose varies from about 1 cm for 4-MV x-rays to >3.5 cm for 25-MV x-rays.

The PDD for one SSD is related to the PDD at a second SSD by the following equation:

$$\mathrm{PDD}(d, S, f_2) = \mathrm{PDD}(d, S, f_1)\left(\frac{f_1 + d}{f_2 d} \cdot \frac{f_2 + d_{max}}{f_1 + d_{max}}\right)^2$$

The term in the brackets is called the *Mayneord F-factor.*[82]

Tissue–Air Ratio

The tissue–air ratio (TAR) is defined as the ratio of the absorbed dose D_d at a given point in the phantom by the absorbed dose in free space, D_{fs}, that would be measured at the same point but in the absence of the phantom, if all other conditions of the

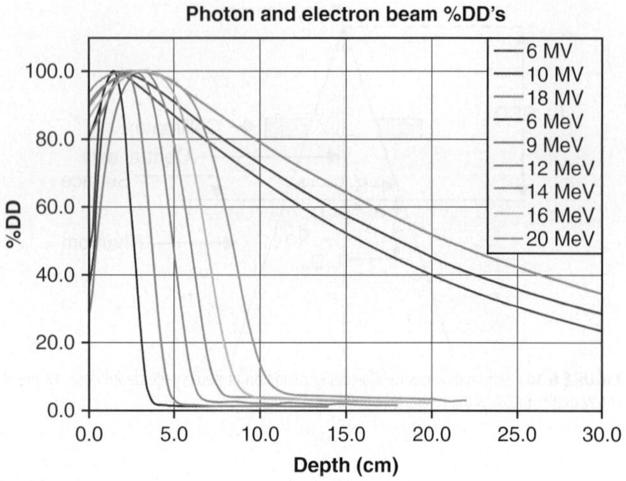

FIGURE 6.31. Examples of central axis percentage depth dose (DD) for megavoltage x-ray beams ranging from ^{60}Co to 18-MV x-rays and 6- to 20-MeV electron beams.

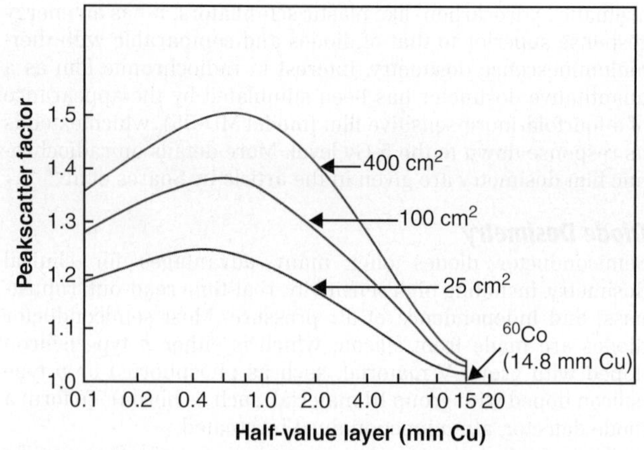

FIGURE 6.33. Variation of peakscatter factor with beam quality (half-value layer). (From Johns HE, Cunningham JR. *The physics of radiology*, 4th ed. Springfield, IL: Charles C Thomas; 1983.)

irradiation (e.g., collimator, distance from the source) are equal (Fig. 6.32). The TAR is expressed as follows:

$$\text{TAR}(d, S_d, E) = \frac{D_d}{D_{fs}}$$

where d is depth, E is radiation beam energy, and S_d is the beam dimension measured at depth d. TAR depends on depth, field size, and beam quality, but for all practical purposes it is independent of the distance from the source.

The TAR at the depth of maximum dose is called the *peakscatter factor.* It is perhaps better known as the backscatter factor, but because of the finite depth d_0, this tends to be misleading. Figure 6.33 shows the peakscatter factors for various field sizes and beam qualities.

Tissue–Phantom Ratio and Tissue–Maximum Ratio

The concepts of tissue–phantom ratio (TPR) and tissue–maximum ratio (TMR) were proposed for high-energy radiation as alternatives to TAR in response to arguments raised against the use of in-air measurement for a photon beam with a maximum energy >3 MeV.[83,84] As originally defined, TPR is given by the ratio of two doses:

$$\text{TPR}(d, d_r, S_d, E) = \frac{D_d}{D_{d_r}}$$

where D_{d_r} is the dose at a specified point on the central axis in a phantom with a fixed reference depth, d_r, of tissue-equivalent material overlying the point; D_d is the dose in the phantom at the same spatial point as before but with an arbitrary depth, d, of overlying material; and S_d is the beam width at the level of measurement (Fig. 6.34). In each instance, underlying material is sufficient to provide for full backscatter. There is no general agreement about the magnitude of the reference depth to be used for this quantity, particularly for high energies. The TPR is intended to be analogous to the TAR but has an advantage because the reference dose, D_{d_r}, is directly measurable over the entire range of x-rays and γ-rays in use, eliminating problems in obtaining a value for the dose in free space when the depth for electronic buildup is great.

The original TMR definition is similar to the definition of TPR, except that the reference depth, d_r, is the depth of maximum dose. However, the depth of maximum dose for megavoltage x-ray beams varies significantly with field size and also is a function of SSD. Thus, the definition of TMR creates a measurement problem because a variable d_r is required and the TMR depends on SSD. A modification by Khan et al.[85] proposed that the reference depth, d_r, must be equal to or greater than the largest depth of maximum dose.

Purdy[86] reported on the relationships between the central axis percentage depth dose and the TPR, TMR, and TAR. This work suggested that the degree to which the TPR and TMR are independent of distance from the radiation source depends largely on the linac's collimator/flattening-filter scatter component of the beam.

Scatter–Air Ratio and Scatter–Maximum Ratio

The scatter-air ratio (SAR) can be thought of as the scatter component of the TAR.[87] It is defined as follows:

$$\text{SAR}(d, S_d, E) = \text{TAR}(d, S_d, E) = \text{TAR}(d, 0, E)$$

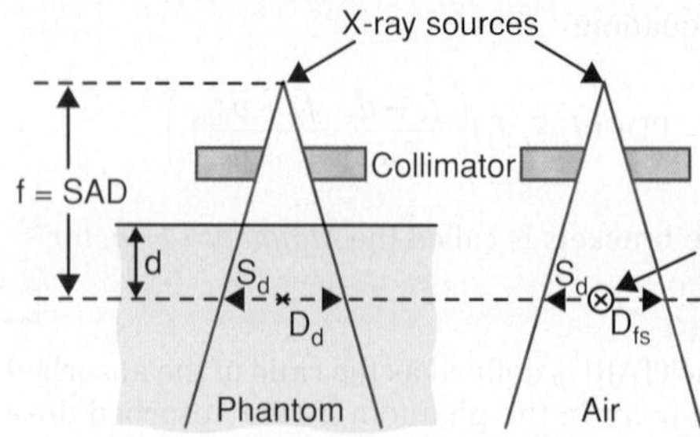

FIGURE 6.32. Schematic drawing illustrating the definition of tissue–air ratio, where d is the thickness of overlying material.

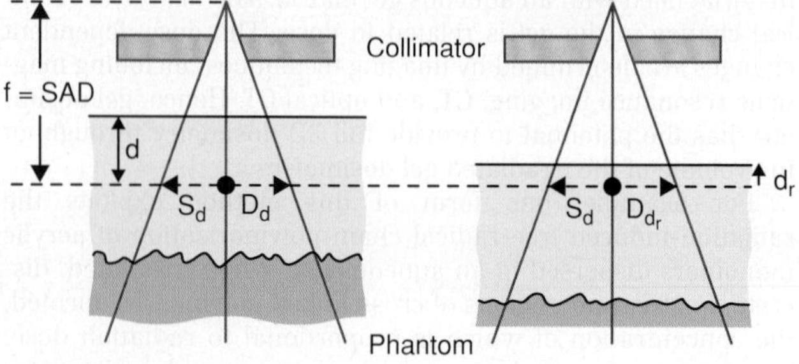

FIGURE 6.34. Schematic drawing illustrating the definition of tissue–phantom ratio and tissue–maximum ratio, where d is the thickness of overlying material and d_r is the reference thickness.

SAR is the difference between the TAR for a field of finite area and the TAR for a zero-area field size. The zero-area TAR is a mathematical abstraction obtained by extrapolation of the TAR values measured for finite field sizes.

Similarly, the scatter-maximum ratio (SMR), the scatter component of the TMR, is defined as follows:

$$\text{SMR}(d, S_d, E) = \text{TMR}(d, S_d, E) \cdot \frac{S_p(S_d, E)}{S_p(S_0, E)} - \text{TMR}(d, 0, E)$$

where S_p is a phantom scatter correction factor, which takes into account changes in scatter radiation originating in the phantom at the reference depth as the field size is changed.[85]

Output Factor

The output factor for a given field size is defined as the ratio of the dose rate at the depth of maximum dose for a given field size to that for the reference field size (usually 10 × 10 cm) at its d_{max}. The output factor varies with field size (Fig. 6.35) as a result of two distinct phenomena. As the collimator jaws are opened, the primary dose, D_p, at d_{max} on the central ray per monitor unit increases as a result of a larger number of primary x-ray photons scattered out of the flattening filter. In addition, the scatter dose, $D_s(d_{max}, r)$, at the measurement point per unit D_p increases as the scattering volume irradiated by primary photons increases with increasing collimated field size. These two components can vary independently of one another if nonstandard treatment distances or extensive secondary blocking is used.

Khan et al.[85] described a method for separating the overall output factor, $S_{c,p}$, into two components. One is the collimator scatter factor, $S_c(r_c)$, which is a function only of the collimator opening, r_c, projected to isocenter. The other is the phantom scatter factor, $S_p(r)$, which is a function only of the cross-sectional area or effective field size, r, irradiated at the treatment distance. They demonstrate that

$$S_{c,p}(r) = S_c(r_c) \cdot S_p(r)$$

In practice, the total and collimator scatter factors both are measured and the phantom scatter factor is calculated using the relationship listed previously. $S_c(r_c)$ is measured in air using an ion chamber fitted with an equilibrium-thickness buildup cap and given by the ratio of the reading for the given collimator opening to the reading for a reference field (typically 10 × 10 cm) collimator opening. The overall output factor is measured in-phantom using the standard treatment distance and is given by the reading relative to that for a 10 × 10 cm field size. By carefully extrapolating this measured ratio to zero-field size, one obtains the zero-field-size phantom scatter factor, $S_p(0)$. If a small-ion chamber is positioned axially in the beam, it is possible to measure $S_{c,p}$ for field sizes as small as 1 × 1 cm. Because of the loss of lateral secondary electron equilibrium encountered near the edges of high-energy photon beams, S_p deviates significantly from unity. Consistent separation of primary and scatter dose components significantly improves the accuracy of dose predictions for irregular field calculations, especially near block edges and the resultant dose falloff resulting from lateral electron disequilibrium, and under blocks, overcoming many of the dose-modeling problems presented by use of extensive customized blocking.

Isodose Curves

An isodose curve represents points of equal dose. A set of these curves, normally given in 10% increments normalized to the dose at the reference depth, can be plotted on a chart (i.e., isodose chart) to give a visual representation of the dose distribution in a single plane (Fig. 6.36). Beam parameters, such as source size, flattening filter, field size, and SSD, play important roles in the shape of the isodose curve.

Dose Profiles

A dose profile is a representation of the dose in an irradiated volume as a function of spatial position along a single line. Dose profiles are particularly well suited to the description of field flatness and penumbra. The data most often are given as ratios of doses normalized to the dose on the central axis

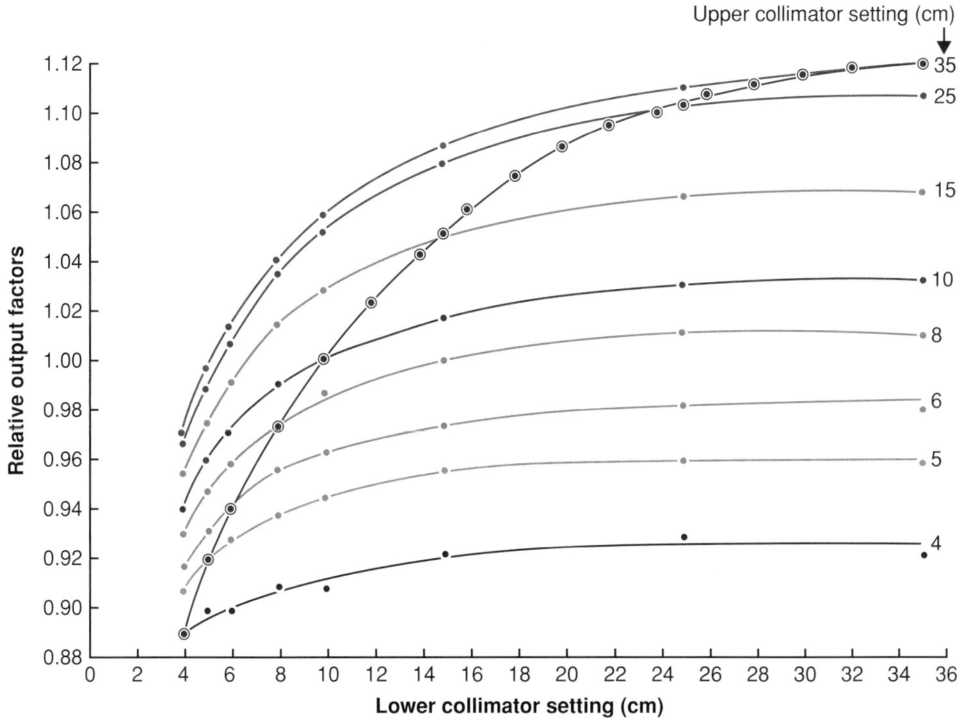

FIGURE 6.35. Example of output factor as a function of lower and upper collimator settings for a medical linear accelerator 18-MV x-ray beam.

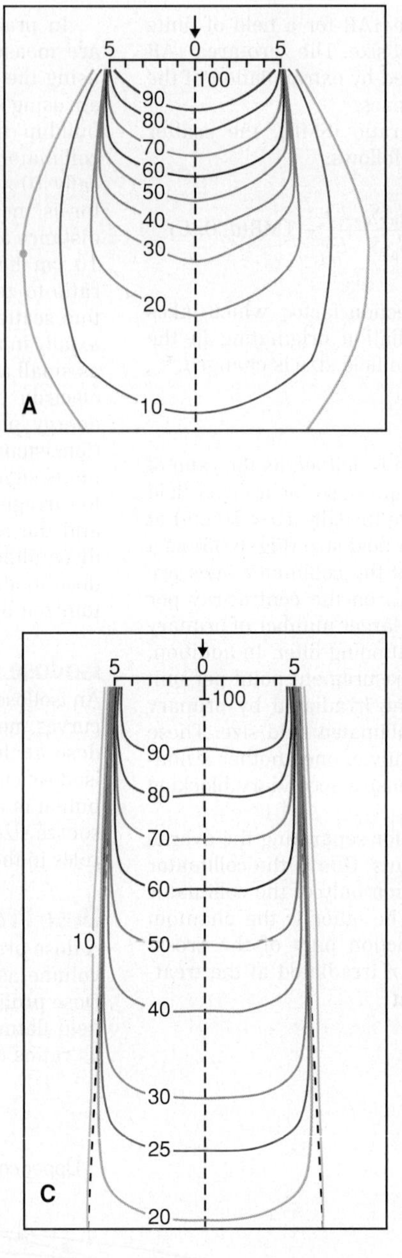

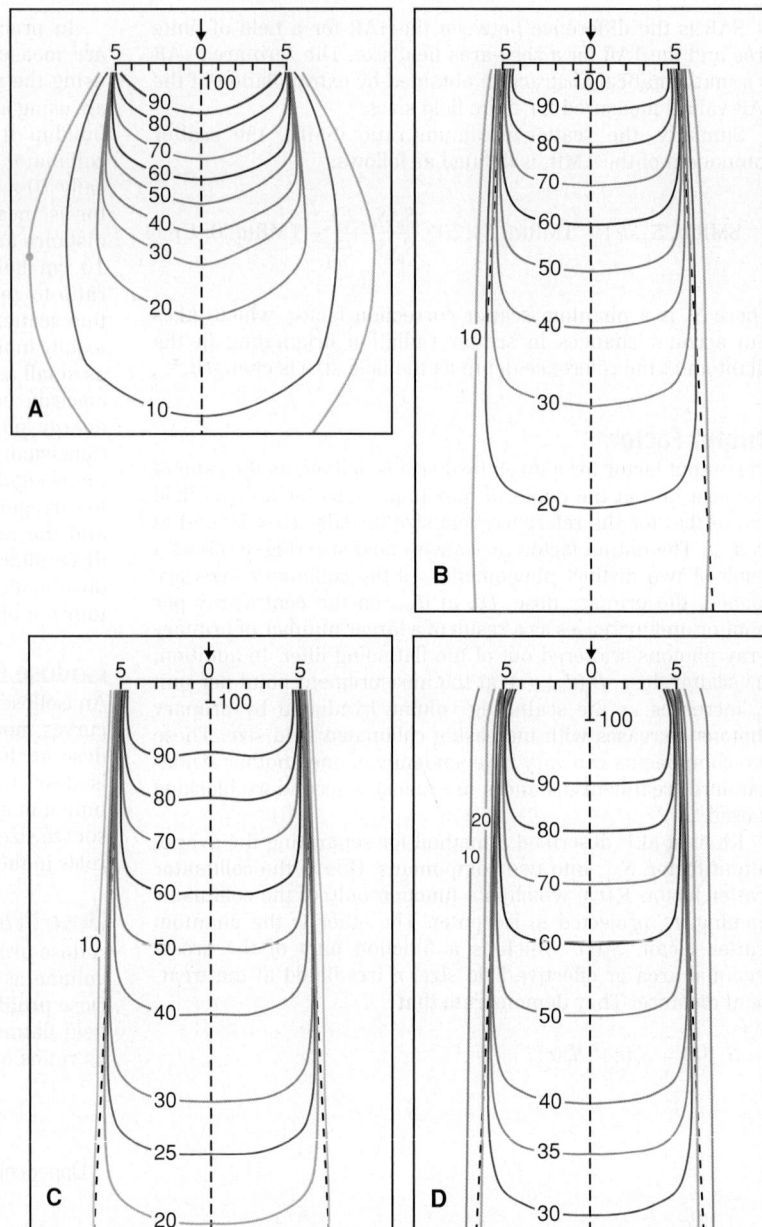

FIGURE 6.36. Isodose distributions for different quality radiations. **A:** 200 kVp, source–skin distance (SSD) = 50 cm, half-value layer (HVL) = 1 mm Cu, field size = 10 × 10 cm. **B:** ^{60}Co, SSD = 80 cm, field size = 10 × 10 cm. **C:** 4-MV x-rays, SSD = 100 cm, field size = 10 × 10 cm. **D:** 10-MV x-rays, SSD = 100 cm, field size = 10 × 10 cm. (From Khan FM. *The physics of radiation therapy*, 3rd ed. Baltimore: Williams & Wilkins; 1994.)

(Fig. 6.37). The profiles, called *off-axis factors* or *off-center ratios*, may be measured in air (i.e., with only a buildup cap) or in a phantom at selected depths. The in-air off-axis factor gives only the variation in primary beam intensity; the in-phantom off-center ratio shows the added effect of phantom scatter.

Wedge Filter

Wedge filters, first introduced by Ellis and Miller,[88] generally are constructed of brass, steel, or lead. When placed in the beam they progressively decrease intensity across the field, causing the isodose distribution to have a planned asymmetry.

The wedge angle is defined as the angle the isodose curve subtends with a line perpendicular to the central axis at a specific depth and for a specified field size. Current practice is to use a depth of 10 cm. Past definitions were based on the 50th-percentile isodose curve and, more recently, the 80th-percentile isodose curve. The wedge angle is a function of field size and depth. The wedge factor is defined as the ratio of the dose measured in a tissue-equivalent phantom at the depth of maximum buildup on the central axis with the wedge in place to the dose at the same point with the wedge removed.

Wedge isodose curves can be normalized in different ways, as shown in Figure 6.38. The wedged isodose distribution on the left side of the figure has been normalized to 100% at d_{max} on the central axis with the wedge in place; on the right, the normalization is done without the wedge in place. Thus, it is imperative that the normalization and the use of the wedge factor should be clearly understood before wedges are used clinically.

Beam hardening occurs when a wedge is inserted into the radiation beam. The PDD, therefore, can be considerably increased at depth. Differences in PDD of nearly 7% have been reported for a 4-MV x-ray, 60-deg wedge field, compared with the open field at a depth of 12 cm, and there have been reports of as much as a 3% difference between the 60-deg wedge field and the open field for a 25-MV x-ray beam.[89,90]

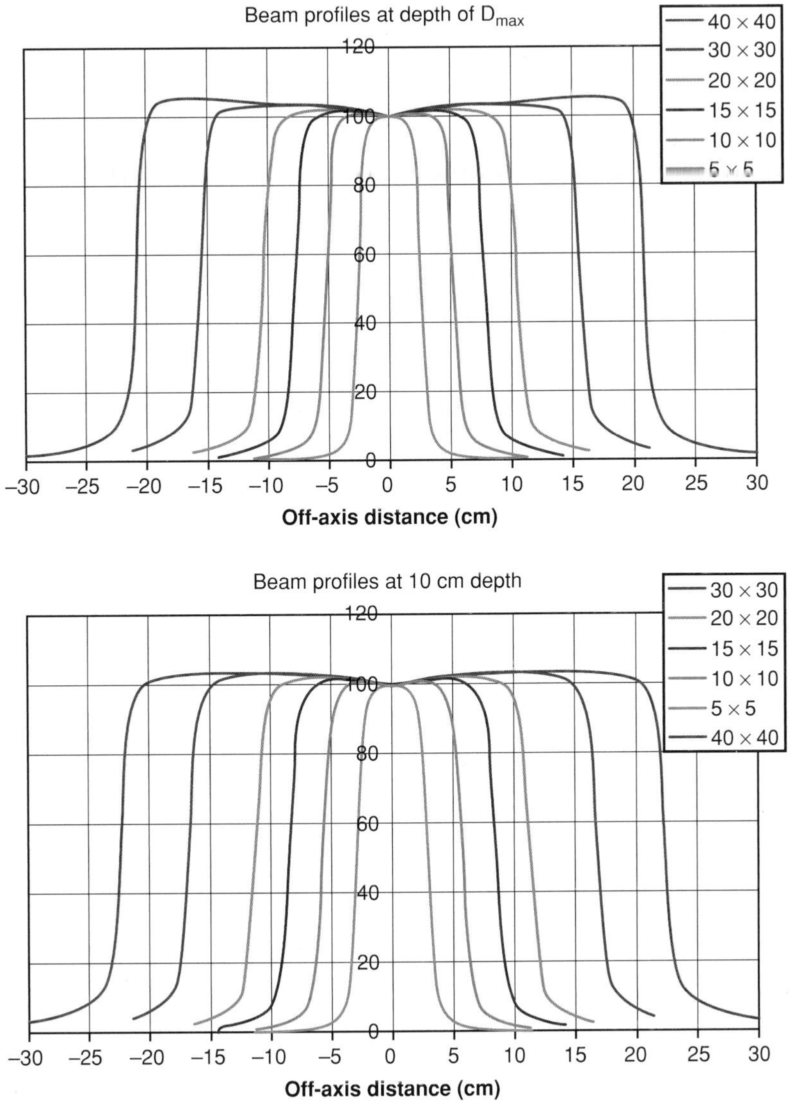

FIGURE 6.37. Example of dose profiles for an 18-MV linear accelerator x-ray beam measured at depths of 3 and 10 cm.

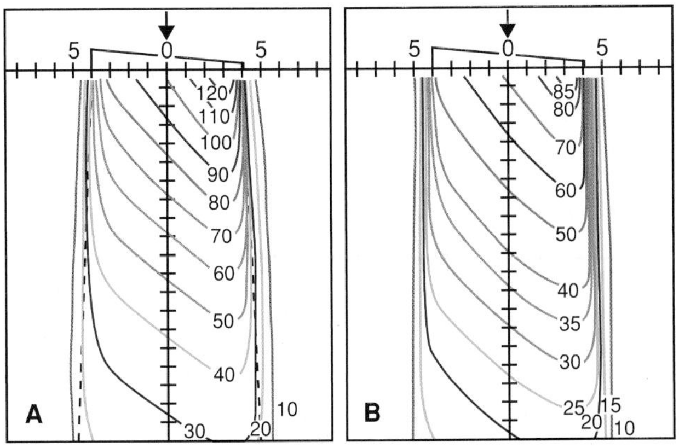

FIGURE 6.38. Isodose curves for a wedge filter. **A:** Normalized to D_{max}. **B:** Normalized to D_{max} without the wedge. ^{60}Co, wedge angle = 45 deg, field size = 8 × 10 cm, source–skin distance = 80 cm. (From Khan FM. *The physics of radiation therapy,* 3rd ed. Baltimore: Williams & Wilkins; 1994.)

REFERENCES

1. Khan FM. *The physics of radiation therapy.* 4th ed. Philadelphia: Lippincott Williams & Wilkins; 2010.
2. Podgorsak EB. *Radiation physics for medical physicists,* 2nd ed. Berlin: Springer; 2010.
3. Van Dyk J, ed. *The modern technology of radiation oncology.* Madison, WI: Medical Physics Publishing; 1999.
4. Williams JR, Thwaites DI. *Radiotherapy physics: in practice,* 2nd ed. Oxford: Oxford University Press; 2000.
5. Van Dyk J, ed. *The modern technology of radiation oncology,* Vol. 2. Madison, WI: Medical Physics Publishing; 2005.
6. Roentgen WC. A new kind of rays [in German]. *Sitzungber Phys Med Ges (Wurzburg)* 1895;137.
7. Becquerel H. Emission de radiations nouvilles par l'uranium métallique. *C R Acad Sci Paris* 1896;122:1086.
8. Curie P, Curie M, Belmont MG. Sur une nouvelle substance fortement radio-active, contenue dans la pechblende. *C R Hebdomadaires Séances Acad Sci Paris* 1898;127:1215.
9. Paganetti H, Niemierko A, Ancukiewicz M, et al. Relative biological effectiveness (RBE) values for proton beam therapy. *Int J Radiat Oncol Biol Phys* 2002;53(2):407–421.
10. Biggs P, Ma C-M, Doppke K, et al. Kilovoltage x-rays. In: Van Dyk J, ed. *The modern technology of radiation oncology.* Madison, WI: Medical Physics Publishing; 1999:287–312.
11. Aumock A, Birnbaum EH, Fleshman JW, et al. Treatment of rectal adenocarcinoma with endocavitary and external beam radiotherapy: results for 199 patients with localized tumors. *Int J Radiat Oncol Biol Phys* 2001;51(2):363–370.

12. Purdy JA, Prasad SC, Walz BJ, et al. Radiation protection considerations for endocavitary. *Int J Radiat Oncol Biol Phys* 1985;11:2177–2181.
13. Schulz MD. The supervoltage story. *Am J. Roentgenol Radium Ther Nucl Med* 1975;124:541–559.
14. Kerst DW. The betatron. *Radiology* 1943;40:120–127.
15. Karzmark CJ, Nunan CS, Tanabe E. *Medical electron accelerators.* New York: McGraw-Hill; 1993.
16. Johns HE, Bates IM, Watson TA. 1000 curie cobalt units for radiation therapy. I. The Saskatchewan cobalt-60 unit. *Br J Radiol* 1952;25:296.
17. Green DT, Errington RF. Design of a cobalt 60 beam therapy unit. *Br J Radiol* 1952;25:309.
18. Glasgow GP. Cobalt-60 teletherapy. In: Van Dyk J, ed. *The modern technology of radiation oncology.* Madison, WI: Medical Physics Publishing; 1999:313–348.
19. Leksell L. Cerebral radiosurgery: I. Gammathalamotomy in two cases of intractable pain *Acta Chir Scand* 1968;134:585–595.
20. Miller CW. Traveling-wave linear accelerator for x-ray therapy. *Nature* 1953; 171:297–298.
21. Howard-Flanders P. The development of the linear accelerator as a clinical instrument. *Acta Radiol* 1954;116:649–655.
22. Ginzton EL, Mallory KB, Kaplan HS. The Stanford medical linear accelerator. I. Design and development. *Stanford Med Bull* 1957;15:123–140.
23. Podgorsak EB, Metcalfe P, Van Dyk J. Medical accelerators. In: Van Dyk J, ed. *The modern technology of radiation oncology.* Madison, WI: Medical Physics Publishing; 1999:349–435.
24. Klein EE, Taylor M, Michaletz-Lorenz M, et al. A mono-isocentric technique for breast and regional nodal therapy using dual asymmetric jaws. *Int J Radiat Oncol Biol Phys* 1994;28:753–760.
25. Leavitt DD, Martin M, Moeller JH, et al. Dynamic wedge field techniques through computer-controlled collimator motion and dose delivery. *Med Phys* 1990;17: 87–91.
26. American Association of Physicists in Medicine. *Report 72: Basic applications of multileaf collimators: Report of Task Group 50 of the Radiation Therapy Committee.* Madison, WI: Medical Physics Publishing; 2001.
27. Klein EE, Harms WB, Low DA, et al. Clinical implementation of a commercial multileaf collimator: dosimetry, networking, simulation, and quality assurance. *Int J Radiat Oncol Biol Phys* 1995;33:1195–1208.
28. Intensity Modulated Radiation Therapy Collaborative Working Group. NCI IMRT Collaborative Working Group: Intensity modulated radiation therapy: current status and issues of interest. *Int J Radiat Oncol Biol Phys* 2001;51(4): 880–914.
29. Jaffray DA, Drake DG, Moreau M, et al. A radiographic and tomographic imaging system integrated into a medical linear accelerator for localization of bone and soft-tissue targets. *Int J Radiat Oncol Biol Phys* 1999;45:773–789.
30. Jaffray DA, Siewerdsen JH, Wong JW, et al. Flat-panel cone-beam computed tomography for image-guided radiation therapy. *Int J Radiat Oncol Biol Phys* 2002;53(5):1337–1349.
31. Rao M, Yang W, Chen F, et al. Comparison of Elekta VMAT with helical tomotherapy and fixed field IMRT: plan quality, delivery efficiency and accuracy. *Med Phys* 2010;37(3):1350–1359.
32. Ling CC, Zhang P, Archambault Y, et al. Commissioning and quality assurance of RapidArc radiotherapy delivery system. *Int J Radiat Oncol Biol Phys* 2008; 72(2):575–581.
33. Yu CX. Intensity modulated arc therapy with dynamic multileaf collimation: an alternative to tomotherapy. *Phys Med Biol* 1995;40(9):1435–1449.
34. Yu CX, Tang G. Intensity-modulated arc therapy: principles, technologies and clinical implementation. *Phys Med Biol* 2011;56(5):R31–R54.
35. Ling CC, Archambault Y, Bocanek J, et al. Scylla and Charybdis: longer beam-on time or lesser conformality—the dilemma of tomotherapy. *Int J Radiat Oncol Biol Phys* 2009;75(1):8–9.
36. Mehta M, Hoban P, Mackie TR. Commissioning and quality assurance of RapidArc radiotherapy delivery system: in regard to Ling et al. (*Int J Radiat Oncol Biol Phys* 2008;72;575–581): absence of data does not constitute proof; the proof is in tasting the pudding. *Int J Radiat Oncol Biol Phys* 2009;75(1):4–6.
37. Veksler VJ. A new method for acceleration of relativistic particles [in Russian]. *Dokl Akad Nauk SSSR* 1944;43:329.
38. Schwinger J. On the classical radiation of accelerated electrons. *Phys Rev* 1949; 75:1912–1925.
39. Brahme A. Design principles and clinical possibilities with a new generation of radiation therapy equipment. *Acta Oncol* 1987;26:403–412.
40. Mackie TR, Holmes T, Swerdloff S, et al. Tomotherapy: a new concept for the delivery of dynamic conformal radiotherapy. *Med Phys* 1993;20(6):1709–1719.
41. Jeraj R, Mackie TR, Balog J, et al. Radiation characteristics of helical tomotherapy. *Med Phys* 2004;31(2):396–404.
42. Adler JR, Chang SD, Murphy MJ, et al. The CyberKnife: a frameless robotic system for radiosurgery. *Stereotactic Functional Neurosurg*1997;69:124–128.
43. Adler JR, Murphy MJ, Chang SD, et al. Image-guided robotic radiosurgery. *Neurosurgery* 1999;44:1299–1307.
44. Kamino Y, Takayama K, Kokubo M, et al. Development of a four-dimensional image-guided radiotherapy system with a gimbaled x-ray head. *Int J Radiat Oncol Biol Phys* 2006;66(1):271–278.
45. Depuydt T, Verellen D, Haas O, et al. Geometric accuracy of a novel gimbals based radiation therapy tumor tracking system. *Radiother Oncol* 2011;98(3):365–372.
46. Kirkby C, Stanescu T, Rathee S, et al. Patient dosimetry for hybrid MRI-radiotherapy systems. *Med Phys* 2008;35(3):1019–1027.
47. DesRosiers C, Moskvin V, Bielajew AF, et al. 150–250 MeV electron beams in radiation therapy. *Phys Med Biol* 2000;45:1781–1805.
48. Fuchs T, Szymanowski H, Oelfke U, et al. Treatment planning for laser-accelerated very-high energy electrons. *Phys Med Biol* 2009;54:3315–3328.
49. Wilson RW. Radiological use of fast protons. *Radiology* 1946;47:487–491.
50. Breuer H, Smit BJ. *Proton therapy and radiosurgery.* Berlin: Springer-Verlag; 2000.
51. Delaney TF, Kooy HM. *Proton and charged particle radiotherapy.* Philadelphia: Lippincott Williams & Wilkins; 2008.
52. Schulz-Ertner D, Jakel O, Schlegel W. Radiation therapy with charged particles. *Sem Radiat Oncol* 2006;16(4):249–259.
53. Coutrakon G, Bauman M, Lesyna D, et al. A prototype beam delivery system for the proton medical accelerator at Loma Linda. *Med Phys* 1991;18((6)):1093–1099.
54. Hall EJ. Intensity-modulated radiation therapy, protons, and the risk of second cancer. *Int J Radiat Oncol Biol Phys* 2006;65(1):1–7.
55. Henning W, Shank C, eds. *Accelerators for America's future.* Washington, DC: U.S. Department of Energy; 2010.
56. Caporaso GJ, Mackie TR, Sampayan S, et al. A compact linac for intensity modulated proton therapy based on a dielectric wall accelerator. *Phys Med* 2008; 24(2):98–101.
57. Maughan RL, Powers WE. A superconducting cyclotron for neutron radiation therapy. *Med Phys* 1994;21(6):779–785.
58. Maughan RL, Yudelev M. Neutron therapy. In: Van Dyk J, ed. *The modern technology of radiation oncology.* Madison, WI: Medical Physics Publishing; 1999: 871–917.
59. Van Dyk J, Munro PN. Simulators. In: Van Dyk J, ed. *The modern technology of radiation oncology.* Madison, WI: Medical Physics Publishing; 1999:95–129.
60. Nishidai T, Nagata Y, Takahashi M, et al. CT simulator: A new 3-D planning and simulation system for radiotherapy. I. Description of system. *Int J Radiat Oncol Biol Phys* 1990;18:499–504.
61. Perez CA, Purdy JA, Harms WB, et al. Design of a fully integrated three-dimensional computed tomography simulator and preliminary clinical evaluation. *Int J Radiat Oncol Biol Phys* 1994;30(4):887–897.
62. Sherouse GW, Bourland JD, Reynolds K, et al. Virtual simulation in the clinical setting: some practical considerations. *Int J Radiat Oncol Biol Phys* 1990;19(4):1059–1065.
63. Van Dyk J, Taylor JS. CT simulators. In: Van Dyk J, ed. *The modern technology of radiation oncology.* Madison, WI: Medical Physics Publishing; 1999:131–168.
64. Mutic S, Palta JR, Butker EK, et al. Quality assurance for computed-tomography simulators and the computed-tomography-simulation process: Report of the AAPM Radiation Therapy Committee Task Group No. 66. *Med Phys* 2003;30 (10):2762–2792.
65. Mutic S, Purdy JA, Michalski JM, et al. The simulation process in the determination and definition of the treatment volume and treatment planning. In: Levitt SH, Purdy JA, Perez CA, et al., eds. *Technical basis of radiation therapy.* Berlin: Springer; 2006:107–133.
66. Almond P. A historical perspective: a brief history of dosimetry, calibration protocols, and the need for accuracy. In: Rogers DWO, Cygler JE, eds. *Clinical dosimetry measurements in radiotherapy.* Madison, WI: Medical Physics Publishing; 2009:1×27.
67. Orton CG, Seibert JB. The measurement of teletherapy unit timer errors. *Phys Med Biol* 1972;17:198.
68. Kron T. Dose measuring tools. In: Van Dyk J, ed. *The modern technology of radiation oncology.* Madison, WI: Medical Physics Publishing; 1999:753–821.
69. American Association of Physicists in Medicine, Task Group 21, Radiation Therapy Committee. A protocol for the determination of absorbed dose from high-energy photon and electron beams. *Med Phys* 1983;10:741–771.
70. Almond PR, Biggs PJ, Coursey BM, et al. AAPM's TG-51 protocol for clinical reference dosimetry of high-energy photon and electron beams. *Med Phys* 1999;26:1847–1870.
71. Huq MS, Andreo P. Reference dosimetry in clinical high-energy photon beams: comparison of the AAPM TG-51 and AAPM TG-21 dosimetry protocols. *Med Phys* 2001;28(1):46–54.
72. Huq MS, Andreo P, Song H. Comparison of the IAEA TRS-398 and AAPM TG-51 absorbed dose to water protocols in the dosimetry of high-energy photon and electron beams. *Phys Med Biol* 2001;46(11):2985–3006.
73. Huq MS, Song H. Reference dosimetry in clinical high-energy electron beams: comparison of the AAPM TG-51 and AAPM TG-21 dosimetry protocols. *Med Phys* 2001;28(10):2077–2087.
74. DeWerd LA, Bartol LJ, Davis SD. Thermoluminescent dosimetry. In: Rogers DWO, Cygler JE, eds. *Clinical dosimetry measurements in radiotherapy.* Madison, WI: Medical Physics Publishing; 2009:815–840.
75. Das IJ. Radiographic Film. In: Rogers DWO, Cygler JE, eds. *Clinical dosimetry measurements in radiotherapy.* Madison, WI: Medical Physics Publishing; 2009:865–890.
76. Soares CG, Trichter S, Devic S. Radiochromic film. In: Rogers DWO, Cygler JE, eds. *Clinical dosimetry measurements in radiotherapy.* Madison, WI: Medical Physics Publishing; 2009:759–813.
77. American Association of Physicists in Medicine. *Report 87. Diode in Vivo Dosimetry for Patients Receiving External Beam Radiation Therapy: Report of Task Group 62 of the Radiation Therapy Committee.* Madison, WI: Medical Physics Publishing; 2005.
78. Zhu TC, Saini AS. Diode dosimetry for megavoltage electron and photon beams. In: Rogers DWO, Cygler JE, eds. *Clinical dosimetry measurements in radiotherapy.* Madison, WI: Medical Physics Publishing; 2009:913–939.
79. Cygler JE, Scalchi P. MOSFET dosimetry in radiotherapy. In: Rogers DWO, Cygler JE, eds. *Clinical dosimetry measurements in radiotherapy.* Madison, WI: Medical Physics Publishing; 2009:941–977.
80. Baldock C, De Deene Y, Doran S, et al. Polymer gel dosimetry. *Phys Med Biol* 2010(55):R1–R51.
81. Schreiner LJ, Olding T. Gel dosimetry. In: Rogers DWO, Cygler JE, eds. *Clinical dosimetry measurements in radiotherapy.* Madison, WI: Medical Physics Publishing; 2009:979–1025.
82. Burns JE. Conversion of depth doses from one FSD to another. *Br J Radiol* 1958;31:643.
83. Holt JD, Laughlin JS, Moroney JP. The extension of the concept of tissue-air (TAR) to high energy x-ray beams. *Radiology* 1970;96:437–446.
84. Karzmark CJ, Deubert A, Loevinger R. Tissue-phantom ratios—an aid to treatment planning. *Br J Radiol* 1965;38:158-159.
85. Khan FM, Sewchand W, Lee J, et al. Revision of tissue-maximum ratio and scatter-maximum ratio concepts for cobalt 60 and higher energy x-ray beams. *Med Phys* 1980;7:230–237.
86. Purdy JA. Relationship between tissue-phantom ratio and percentage depth dose. *Med Phys* 1977;4:66.
87. Cunningham JR. Scatter-air ratios. *Phys Med Biol* 1972;17:42–51.
88. Ellis F, Miller H. The use of wedge filters in deep x-ray therapy. *Br J Radiol* 1944;17:90.
89. Abrath FG, Purdy JA. Wedge design and dosimetry for 25-MV x rays. *Radiology* 1980;136:757–762.
90. Sewchand W, Khan FM, Williamson J. Variations in depth-dose data between open and wedge fields for 4-MV x rays. *Radiology* 1978;127:789–792.

Chapter 7
Photon External-Beam Dosimetry and Treatment Planning

James A. Purdy and Eric E. Klein

The radiation oncologist, when planning the treatment of a patient with cancer, is faced with the problem of prescribing a treatment regimen with a radiation dose that is large enough potentially to cure or control the disease, but does not cause serious normal tissue complications. This task is a difficult one because tumor control and normal tissue effect responses for most disease sites are typically steep functions of radiation dose; that is, a small change in the dose delivered (±5%) can result in a dramatic change in the local response of the tissue (±20%).[1,2,3] Moreover, the prescribed curative doses are often, by necessity, very close to the doses tolerated by the normal tissues. Thus, for optimum treatment, the radiation dose must be planned and delivered with a high degree of precision.

One can readily compute the dose distribution resulting from photons, electrons, protons, or a mixture of these radiation beams impinging on a regularly shaped, flat-surface, homogeneous unit-density phantom. However, the patient presents a much more complicated situation because of irregularly shaped topography and having tissues of varying densities and atomic composition (called *heterogeneities*). In addition, beam modifiers, such as wedges, compensating filters, or bolus, are sometimes inserted into the radiation beam, further complicating the calculation of the absorbed dose.

In this chapter, several aspects of photon external-beam treatment planning and dosimetry are reviewed, including methods used for dose/monitor unit calculations, correction for the effects of the patient's irregular surface and internal heterogeneities on the calculated photon dose distribution, isodose distributions for combined fields, field junctions, field shaping and design of treatment aids, and related clinical dosimetry issues.

DOSE CALCULATION METHODS

For purposes of discussion, it is convenient to characterize photon beam dose calculation methods as either *correction based* or *model based*.[4] In the former method, the dose at a given point is calculated using measured central-axis data, for example, percent depth dose (PDD), tissue-air ratios (TARs), tissue-maximum ratios (TMRs), tissue-phantom ratios (TPRs), and off-axis ratios (OARs). These quantities are measured under reference conditions (i.e., in a homogeneous water phantom with a flat surface normal to the incident radiation beam at a standard distance from the x-ray source). Hence, specific correction factors (CFs) are used in planning the treatment of real patients to account for varying patient surfaces, tissue heterogeneities, irregular field shapes, and any beam modifiers used.

In the model-based algorithms, the dose distribution is computed in a phantom or patient from more of a first-principles approach accounting for lateral transport of radiation, beam energy, geometry, beam modifiers, patient surface topography, and electron density distribution, rather than correcting parameterized dose distributions measured in a water phantom. These models utilize convolution energy deposition kernels that describe the distribution of dose about a single primary photon interaction site, and provide much more accurate results even for complex heterogeneous geometries. Both methods are discussed in the following sections and more details on model-based photon dose calculation algorithms can be found in the references listed.[4,5]

Correction-Based Dose Calculation Methods

Using the notation of Khan et al.,[6] the dose at a point (D_P) at a depth d of overlying tissue on the central ray for an irregularly shaped field is given by:

$$D_P = D_{ref} \cdot S_c(r_c) \cdot S_p(r_d) \cdot TF \cdot WF \left(\frac{SCD}{SAD}\right)^2 \cdot TMR(d,\ r_d)$$

where S_c denotes the *collimator scatter factor*, *Sp* the *phantom scatter factor*, and *TMR* the tissue-maximum ratio. *TF* and *WF* denote the tray and wedge factors, respectively, and are defined as the ratio of the central ray dose with the tray or wedge filter in place relative to the dose in the open-beam geometry. The collimated field size is denoted by r_c and is usually described as the square field size equivalent to the rectangular collimator opening projected to isocenter. The effective field size is denoted by r_d and is specified to the isocenter distance (*SAD*). The inverse-square law factor accounts for the difference in distances from the source-to-point of dose calculation relative to the source to calibration point distance (*SCD*). Note that when isocentric calibration is used, this factor is unity. Also, note that collimator-defined field size is used for lookup of the collimator scatter factor, S_c, whereas effective field size projected to isocenter is used for lookup of the *TMR* value and the phantom scatter factor, *Sp*. By separately accounting for the effect of collimator opening on the primary dose component and the influence of cross-sectional area of tissue irradiated, most of the difficulties in accurately calculating a dose in the presence of extensive blocking are overcome. Details on determining the effective field size for an irregularly shaped field, taking into account both the primary and scatter dose components, will be discussed in a later section.

Correction for Varying Patient Topography (Air Gaps)

In the previous equation, it is assumed that the beam is normally incident on a unit-density uniform phantom. The following CF methods can be applied to the equation to account for the nonnormal beam incidence caused by the patient's varying surface.[7]

Air Gap CF: Ratio of Tissue-Air Ratio Method

In the ratio of TAR or TPR method, the surface (along a ray line) directly above point A (source-to-skin distance [SSD] = S′) is unaltered, so the primary component to the dose distribution at this point is unchanged (and the scatter component is also assumed to be unaltered) (see Fig. 7.1). Thus, the dose at point A can be considered as unaltered by patient shape. However, for point B, where there are considerable variations in the patient's topography, both the primary and scatter components of the radiation beam are altered. The CF may be determined using two TARs or TPRs as follows:

$$CF = \frac{T(d - h, s_d)}{T(d, s_d)}$$

where h = air gap.

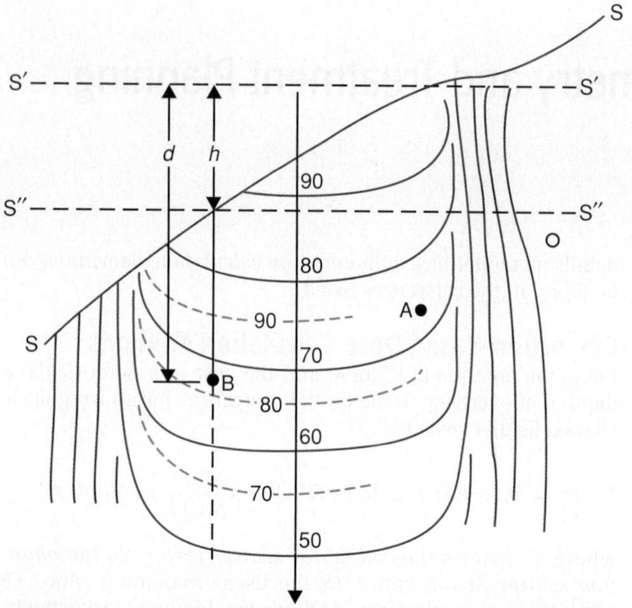

FIGURE 7.1. Schematic drawing illustrating tissue-air ratio and effective source-to-skin distance (SSD) methods for the correction of isodose curves under a sloping surface (*solid lines* for SSD = S″; *dashed lines* for SSD = S″). (From International Commission of Radiation Units and Measurements. *Report 24: Determination of absorbed dose in a patient irradiated by beams of × or gamma rays in radiotherapy procedures.* Washington, DC: International Commission of Radiation Units and Measurements, 1976.)

Air Gap CF: Effective Source-Skin Ratio Method

In the effective SSD method, the isodose chart to be used is placed on the patient's contour representation, positioning the central axis at the distance for which the curve was measured (Fig. 7.1). It then is shifted down along the ray line for the length of the air gap, h, resulting in SSD = S″. The PDD value at point B is read and modified by an inverse-square calculation to account for the effective change in the peak dose. The CF can be expressed as follows:

$$CF = \frac{P(d-h, d_O, S, f, E)}{P(d, d_O, S, f, E)} \cdot \left(\frac{f + d_O}{f + h + d_O}\right)^2$$

Correction for Tissue Heterogeneities

The following CF methods can be used to account for the tissue heterogeneities found within the patient.

Tissue Heterogeneities CF: Ratio of Tissue-Air Ratio Method

The ratio of TAR (RTAR) method of correction for inhomogeneities is given by:

$$CF = \frac{T(d_{eff}, S_d)}{T(d, S_d)}$$

where the numerator is the TAR for the equivalent water thickness, d_{eff}, and the denominator is the TAR for the actual thickness, *d*, of tissue between the point of calculation and the surface along a ray passing through the point. S_d is the dimension of the beam cross-section at the depth of calculation. The RTAR method accounts for the field size and depth of calculation. It does not account for the position of the point of calculation with respect to the heterogeneity. It also does not take into account the shape of the inhomogeneity; instead, it assumes that it extends the full width of the beam and has a constant thickness (i.e., referred to as *slab geometry*).

Tissue Heterogeneities CF: Power Law TAR Method

The *power law TAR method* was proposed by Batho[8] and generalized by Young and Gaylord.[9] This method, sometimes called the *Batho method,* attempts to account for the nature of the inhomogeneity and its position relative to the point of calculation. However, it does not account for the extent or shape of the inhomogeneity. The correction factor for the point P is given by:

$$CF = \left(\frac{T(d_2, S_d)}{T(d_1, S_d)}\right)^{\rho_2 - 1}$$

where d_1 and d_2 refer to the distances from point P to the near and far side of the non–water-equivalent material, respectively; S_d is the beam dimension at the depth of P; and ρ_2 is the relative electron density of the inhomogeneity with respect to water.

Sontag and Cunningham[10] derived a more general form of this correction factor, which can be applied to a case in which the effective atomic number of the inhomogeneity is different from that of water and the point of interest lies within the inhomogeneity. The correction factor in this situation is given by:

$$CF = \frac{T(d_2, S_d)^{(\rho_b - 1)}}{T(d_1, S_d)^{(\rho_b - \rho_a)}} \times \frac{(\mu_{en}/\rho)_a}{(\mu_{en}/\rho)_b}$$

where ρ_a is the density of the material in which point P lies at a depth d below the surface and ρ_b is the density of an overlying material of thickness $(d_2 - d_1)$; $(\mu_{en}/\rho)_a$ and $(\mu_{en}/\rho)_b$ are the mass energy absorption coefficients for the medium *a* and *b*.

Model-Based Dose Calculation Methods

Advanced three-dimensional dose calculation algorithms, such as the convolution/superposition algorithm and Monte Carlo, should now be considered the standard of practice.[4,5,11–13] These models provide accurate results even for complex heterogeneous geometries.

Convolution/Superposition Dose Calculation Algorithm

The convolution/superposition dose calculation algorithm is based on the following equation[4]:

$$D(\vec{r}) = \iint \iint T_E(\vec{s}) h(E, \vec{r} - \vec{s}) d^3 s dE$$

where *D* represents the dose at some point $\vec{r}$, $T_E(\vec{s})$ represents the total energy released by primary photon interactions per unit mass (or TERMA), and $h(E, \vec{r} - \vec{s})$ is the *point-spread function* (also called *dose spread array, differential pencil beam,* and *energy deposition kernal*). The point-spread function represents the fraction of the energy deposited (per unit volume) at point $\vec{s}$ that is subsequently transported to the calculation point, $\vec{r}$. Hence, the dose at point $\vec{r}$ is computed by integrating over all space the contributions from photons and electrons produced at all other points in the phantom or patient.

Ahnesjö et al.[14] showed that the point-spread function, $h(E, \vec{r} - \vec{s})$, changes only slightly as a function of energy, and thus, can be replaced by $h(\vec{r} - \vec{s})$ (defined as the average point-spread function weighted by the spectral components of the beam), reducing the basic convolution four-dimensional integral to a three-dimensional integral over all space. Point-spread functions for monoenergetic photons are generally precomputed using Monte Carlo methods.[14] The energy dependence of the TERMA, $T_E(\vec{s})$, can be expressed by applying the inverse-square law and exponential attenuation to the photon fluence at the surface of the phantom or patient.

The three-dimensional integral is typically evaluated in a two-step process. The first step takes into account the properties of the accelerator (including the finite source size, primary collimator, flattening filter, collimator jaws, multileaf collimators, and any beam-modifying devices used for the treatment, such as wedges, alloy blocks, and compensating filters) to compute the energy fluence at the phantom or patient surface. The second step of the calculation takes into account the inverse-square law and exponential attenuation to this incident fluence to determine the TERMA, $T_E(\vec{s})$, at each point within the phantom or patient and convolve the result with the point-spread function, $h(\vec{r} - \vec{s})$.

The convolution equation is strictly valid only for homogeneous media (i.e., $h(\vec{s})$ must be spatially invariant). To account for the effects of tissue heterogeneities, all physical distances in the convolution integral are replaced with radiologic distances, that is, the physical distance multiplied by the average density along the line in question.[11,14] Hence, the convolution/superposition algorithm accounts for the effects of heterogeneities anywhere in the vicinity of the calculation point in three dimensions. In contrast, most correction factor–based dose-calculation techniques require only a simple one-dimensional evaluation of radiologic path length, and can thus account for the effects of only those tissue heterogeneities that lie along a ray connecting the radiation source to the calculation point.

Several investigators have tested the convolution/superposition algorithm against measurements and Monte Carlo–generated data for complex phantom geometries including both homogeneous and heterogeneous phantoms and found that the convolution/superposition model gave accurate results, even in parts of the buildup region and penumbra.[15,16]

Monte Carlo Method

Monte Carlo is, in principle, the only method capable of computing the dose distribution accurately for all situations encountered in radiation therapy, including being able to accurately predict the dose near interfaces of materials with very dissimilar atomic number, such as near metal prostheses, or different densities such as tumors in lung tissue.[17] The Monte Carlo method uses the known cross-sections for electron and photon interactions in matter and follows individual photons and the associated electrons set in motion through the entire heterogeneous phantom or patient. By calculating the trajectories and interactions of a very large number of photons and electrons, one can accurately model the dose distribution. Recently, several Monte Carlo codes have been developed for radiotherapy treatment planning,[13,18] many of which have been implemented commercially. The reader is referred to the American Association of Physicists in Medicine (AAPM) Task Group (TG) 105 Report, which summarizes commercial use of Monte Carlo for radiation therapy treatment planning.[12] The reader is also referred to the review article by Siebers et al. for even more details on Monte Carlo calculation for external-beam radiation therapy.[17]

Dose Calculation Algorithms and Tissue Heterogeneities

In 2004, the AAPM published Report 85 (Task Group 65) on tissue inhomogeneity corrections for megavoltage photon beams.[19] The task group recommended an accuracy goal for tissue heterogeneity corrections of 2% in order to achieve an overall 3% accuracy in dose delivery. The AAPM report recommended heterogeneity corrections be applied to plans and prescriptions, with the condition that the algorithm used for calculations be reviewed and rigorously tested by the medical physicist. A brief summary of the site-specific recommendations follows. For the head and neck region, a one-dimensional path correction algorithm for point-dose estimations beyond mandible and ear cavities was thought to be reasonable. However, for soft tissue regions and volumes that are adjacent to these heterogeneities, superposition/convolution or Monte Carlo algorithms should be used. For the larynx, specifically, if the target volume was adjacent to the air cavity or severe case of disease in the anterior commissure, then the superposition/convolution or Monte Carlo algorithms should be used. For treatment of lung cancer, for interest points well beyond the lung interface, one-dimensional path corrections were thought to be reasonable. However, accounting for doses at tumor–lung interfaces, the superposition/convolution or Monte Carlo algorithms should be used. Also, the report recommended that photon energies of 12 MV or less should be used for treatment of lung cancer in order to minimize nonequilibrium conditions that exist with higher energies. For breast cancer treatment (particularly if the dose of interest of the target volume is considered to be chest wall), it is recommended that calculations be performed with superposition/convolution or Monte Carlo. However, for simple intact breast planning, one-dimensional algorithms were adequate. For the upper gastrointestinal tract, one-dimensional corrections were adequate. However, one should be leery if barium contrast is used as it can erroneously impact the dose calculation due to its high-Z. In terms of the pelvis and prostate, one-dimensional corrections were quite reasonable except in the presence of high-Z implanted hip prostheses. (Note, the dosimetric considerations for patients with hip prostheses undergoing pelvic irradiation are discussed in a later section). The study by Frank et al.[20] provides a clear method for safely transitioning clinical use from one based on planning that assumes a homogeneous unit-density patient to one using a heterogeneous patient model.

Recently the Radiological Physics Center published the results of a study comparing measured results of irradiated lung phantoms having various geometries with dose calculations for similar conditions using commercial treatment planning systems. They found significant differences if algorithms less sophisticated than the superposition/convolution-type algorithms were used.[21]

MONITOR UNIT CALCULATION METHODS

Monitor unit (MU) calculations refer to determining the linac MU setting per field to deliver the prescribed dose taking into account the tumor depth, treatment distance, multileaf collimator setting or secondary blocking configuration, and primary collimator opening. This is accomplished by using the various dosimetric quantities described in the preceding chapter to relate the dose corresponding to an arbitrary set of treatment parameters to the reference calibration geometry where the output of the machine is specified in terms of cGy/MU. The reference source to calibration point distance, field size, and depth of output specification are denoted by the symbols SCD, r_{cal}, and d_{cal}, respectively. For a fixed *SSD* calibration geometry:

$$SCD = SAD\ (source\text{–}axis\ distance) + d_{max}$$

$$r_{cal} = 10\ cm \times 10\ cm$$

$$d_{cal} = d_{max}$$

Normal incidence and open-beam geometry (i.e., absence of trays or any beam-modifying filters) are specified.

For treatment machines calibrated isocentrically, the point of MU specification is located at distance SAD rather than at distance SAD + d_{max} as stated previously. For isocentric calibration, SCD = SAD.

The linac is calibrated by adjusting the sensitivity of its internal monitor transmission ion chamber so that 1 MU equals 1 cGy for the reference calibration geometry condition. Several reports providing more details on monitor unit calculations and their verification are listed in the references.[22–24]

MU Calculation for Fixed Fields

When the patient is to be treated isocentrically, the point of dose prescription is located at the isocenter regardless of the target depth. Using the notation of Khan et al.,[6] the MU needed to deliver a prescribed tumor dose to isocenter (TD_{iso}) for a depth d of overlying tissue on the central ray is given by:

$$MU = \frac{TD_{iso}}{TMR(d, r_d) \cdot S_c(r_c) \cdot S_p(r_d) \cdot TF \cdot WF \left(\dfrac{SCD}{SAD}\right)^2}$$

where *TF* and *WF* denote the tray and wedge factors, respectively. They are defined as the ratio of the central ray dose with the tray or wedge filter in place relative to the dose in the open-beam geometry. The collimated field size is denoted by r_c and is usually described as the square field size equivalent to the rectangular collimator opening projected to isocenter. The effective field size is denoted by r_d and is always specified to the isocenter distance (*SAD*). The inverse-square law factor accounts for the difference in distances from the source-to-point of dose prescription relative to the point of MU specification. When isocentric calibration is used, this factor is unity. Note that collimator-defined field size is used for lookup of the collimator scatter factor, S_c, whereas effective field size projected to isocenter is used for lookup of *TMR* and the phantom scatter factor, S_p. By separately accounting for the effect of collimator opening on the primary dose component and the influence of cross-sectional area of tissue irradiated, most of the difficulties in accurately delivering a dose in the presence of extensive blocking are overcome.

When a fixed distance between the target and entry skin surface (SSD) is used to treat the patient, a dose-calculation formalism based on PDD is used rather than one based on isocentric dose ratios. When a dose *TD* is to be delivered to depth *d*, MUs are given by:

$$MU = \frac{TD \cdot 100}{PDD(SSD, d, r) \cdot S_c(r_c) \cdot S_p(r) \cdot TF \cdot WF \left(\frac{SCD}{SSD + d_{max}} \right)^2}$$

The field size (or its equivalent square) on the skin surface at central axis is denoted by *r* and is used for lookup of both *PDD* and S_p. The collimated field size r_c at the isocenter must be used for lookup of S_c. When an extended treatment distance is used, the collimated field size at isocenter differs significantly from that at the skin surface of the patient. Note that PDD is a function of SSD, depth, and effective field size. Collimator scatter factors measured at SAD are valid over a wide range of extended treatment distances.[6]

When this dose calculation formalism for highly extended treatment distances such as encountered in administering total-body irradiation is used, care must be taken to verify the validity of inverse-square law at these distances. It is recommended that such setups always be verified by ion chamber measurement at the extended distance. Because of the large scatter contribution to effective primary dose originating from the flattening filter and other components in the treatment head, the virtual source of radiation may be as much as 2 cm proximal to the target of the accelerator.

The TAR system of dose calculation is a widely used alternative to the Khan formalism. It is simply an extension of the familiar TAR and backscatter factor concepts, as used in ^{60}Co and orthovoltage dosimetry, to the megavoltage photon energy range. The needed dosimetry parameters are determined from ion chamber measurements (both in-phantom and in-air) like those performed for ^{60}Co, but now using a much larger buildup cap (radius thickness = d_{max}). Thus, the megavoltage peakscatter factor, *PSF(r)*, for an effective field size *r* is simply the ratio of the two ion chamber readings as shown here.

$$PSF(r) = \frac{\text{ionization at depth } d_{max} \text{ in phantom}}{\text{ionization with build} - \text{up cap in air at same point in space}}$$

And the megavoltage beam dose rate (Gy/MU) in free space, $\dot{D}_{fs}$, is given by:

$$\dot{D}_{fs}(SAD + d_{max}, r_c) = \frac{\dot{D}(SSD, r_c, d_{max})}{PSF(r_c)}$$

where the numerator is the measured d_{max} dose at distance SSD = SAD + d_{max} and collimator setting r_c. Implementation of this system requires a table of $\dot{D}_{fs}$ $(SAD + d_{max}, r_c)$ values for each collimator opening and a table of PSF versus effective field size. Then, dose at d_{max} per MU for any distance, effective field size, and collimator opening can be calculated easily.

When the patient is to be treated isocentrically, the MU needed to deliver a prescribed isocenter dose (ID) to a depth d on the central axis is given by:

$$MU = \frac{ID}{TAR(d, r_d) \cdot \dot{D}_{fs}(SAD + d_{max}, r_c) \cdot TF \cdot WF \cdot \left(\frac{SCD}{SAD} \right)^2}$$

If the treatment is fixed SSD, the MU needed to deliver a prescribed dose (TD) to a depth d on the central ray is given by:

$$MU = \frac{TD \times 100}{PDD(d, r) \cdot \dot{D}_{fs}(SAD + d_{max}, r_c) \cdot PSF(r) \cdot TF \cdot WF \cdot \left(\frac{SCD}{SSD + d_{max}} \right)^2}$$

All MU calculation formalisms require some means of estimating the square field size, *r*, that is equivalent, in terms of scattering characteristics, to an arbitrary rectangular field of width *a* and length *b*. Perhaps the most widely used rectangular equivalency principle is the "A/P" rule. It states that a square and a rectangle are equivalent if they have the same area/perimeter ratio; that is:

$$r = \frac{2(a \times b)}{(a + b)}$$

Another widely used approach to reducing rectangular estimates of effective field size to square field sizes is the equivalent square table published in the *British Journal of Radiology*.[25] Estimating the effective field size equivalent to an irregular field is best handled via irregular field calculations as discussed later in this chapter.[26,27]

MU Calculations for Asymmetric X-Ray Collimators

Asymmetric x-ray collimators (also referred to as independent jaws) allow independent movement of an individual jaw and may be available for one jaw pair or both pairs. Because MU calculations and treatment planning methods generally rely on symmetric jaw data, the dosimetric effects for asymmetric jaws must be fully documented before being implemented in the clinic. Several investigators have examined the effects of asymmetric jaws on *PDD*, collimator scatter, and isodose distributions.[28,29] Monitor unit calculations for asymmetric jaws are only slightly more complex than for symmetric jaws.[22] Typically, one simply applies an *off-axis ratio (OAR)* or *off-center ratio (OCR)* correction factor that depends only on the distance from the machine's central axis to the center of the independently collimated open field.[30,31] *PDD* is only minimally affected, but isodose curve shape can be altered and must be investigated for the particular treatment unit. Calculations for asymmetric wedge fields follow similar procedures by simply incorporating a wedge OAR or OCR.[29,32]

MU Calculations for Multileaf Collimator

Multileaf collimators (MLCs) have nearly completely replaced conventional alloy field shaping for photon beams in most clinics around the world. Several investigators have examined the effects of the Varian MLC design (tertiary system) on PDD, collimator scatter, and isodose distributions.[33] The effects due to field area shaped by this type of MLC on *PDD* and beam output parameters are similar to those resulting from Cerrobend field shaping. Thus, the dose/MU calculation methods discussed previously apply by simply using the equivalent area defined by the MLC. The collimator scatter factor and the dose in free space are determined using the x-ray collimator jaw settings, with an off-axis factor applied for any asymmetric jaw settings.

It should be noted, however, that for MLC systems that replace one of the collimating jaws, the MLC field shape can be a determining factor in selecting the appropriate output factor.[34] For example, in the case of the Elekta linacs (Elekta AB, Crawley, United Kingdom), in which the lower jaws are replaced by the MLC system, the calculation takes into consideration the collective blocked area that is created by both the MLC leaves and the lower backup diaphragms.[35] For an MLC system that replaces the upper jaw (e.g., Siemens linac, Siemens Medical Solutions USA, Inc., Malvern, PA), Das et al.[36] describe a method that relies on the blocked area for determining all the calculation parameters (mainly output, percent depth dose, and scatter factor).

Hence, because of MLC design differences and the fact that vendors are continuing to modify/improve MLC designs, the authors caution that when a new linac is installed, the impact of the MLC on the institution's MU calculation procedure should be fully documented before clinical use. The reader is also encouraged to review the AAPM Task Group 50 Report, which provides more detail on various MLC types and discusses quality assurance (QA) and MU calculations.[37]

MU Calculations for Irregular Fields

For large, irregularly shaped fields and at points off the central axis, it is necessary to take account of the off-axis change in intensity (relative to the central axis) of the beam, the variation of the SSD within the field of treatment, the influence of the primary collimator on the output factor, and the scatter contribution to the dose. Changes in the beam quality as a function of position in the radiation field also should be considered.[38,39]

The general method used for irregular-field calculations consists of summation at each point of interest of the primary and scatter irradiation, with allowance for the off-axis change in intensity (off-axis factor) and SSD.[26,27] The MUs required to deliver a specified tumor dose at an arbitrary point in an irregular field (Fig. 7.2) can be calculated as follows:

$$MU = \frac{TD}{[TAR(d,0) + \overline{SAR}(d)] \cdot \dot{D}_{fs}(SSD + d_{max}, r_c) \cdot TF \cdot OAF \left(\frac{SSD + d_{max}}{SSD + g + d}\right)^2}$$

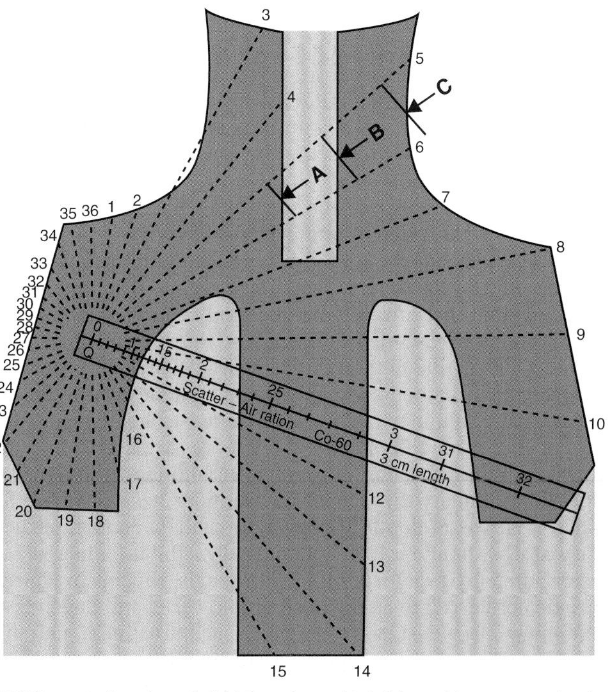

FIGURE 7.2. Outline of mantle field illustrating method of determining scatter-to-air ratio, used for irregular-field dose calculations. (From Cundiff JH, Cunningham JR, Golden R, et al. A method for the calculation of dose in the radiation treatment of Hodgkin's disease. *Am J Roentgenol* 1973;117:30–34.)

where the parameters used are:

- TAR(d, 0) = zero-field size TAR at depth d
- SAR(d) = average SAR for point in question at depth d determined using the Clarkson technique
- D_{fs} = Gy/MU in a small mass of tissue, in air, on the central axis at normal SSD + d_{max} for the collimated field size
- SSD = nominal SSD for treatment constraints
- d_{max} = depth of dose maximum
- TF = blocking tray attenuation factor
- g = vertical distance between skin surface over point in question and nominal
- SSD = (beam vertical)
- d = vertical depth, skin surface to point in question
- OAF = in-air off-axis factor

Computer implementations vary, but typically include using the expanded field size at a depth for the SAR calculation, determining the off-axis factor using the distance from the central axis to the slant projection of the point of calculation to the SSD plane along a ray from the source, and determining the zero-area TAR using the slant depth along a ray going from the source to the point of calculation. It is generally accepted that the off-axis factor should be multiplied by the sum of the zero-area TAR and the SAR as originally proposed.

Beam quality is a function of position in the field for beams generated by linear accelerators.[38,39] The TAR_0 may be expressed as a function of position in the beam so that changes in beam quality can be incorporated into calculations, and it can be related to the half-value layer (HVL) of water by the following equation:

$$TAR(d, 0, r) = e\left[\frac{-0.693(d - d_{max})}{HVL(r)}\right]$$

where d is the depth of the point of reference, d_{max} is the depth of maximum dose, r is the radial distance from the central axis of the beam to the point of calculation, e is the base of the natural logarithm, and $HVL(r)$ is the beam quality expressed as the HVL measured in water.

MU Calculations for Rotation Therapy

The classic method for MU calculations for rotation therapy is given by the following equation:

$$MU = \frac{ID}{TAR_{avg} \cdot \dot{D}_{fs}\left(\frac{SCD}{SAD}\right)^2}$$

and the MU per degree setting is given by:

$$MU/deg = \frac{monitor\ unit\ setting}{degrees\ of\ rotation}$$

where the symbols have the previous meaning and TAR_{avg} is an average TAR (averaged over radii [depth in the patient] at selected angular intervals, such as 10 or 20 degrees).

Most recently, manufacturers of linacs and their associated planning systems have introduced features that provide rotational intensity modulated radiation therapy (IMRT) capability[40,41] (e.g., Elekta VMAT[42] and Varian RapidArc[43]). The linac-based rotational IMRT concept was first proposed by Yu[44,45] and called *intensity modulated arc therapy (IMAT)*, but planning software was not commercially available at that time. Rotational IMRT approaches on conventional linacs may provide even more conformal dose distributions delivered in a shorter treatment time, compared with *SMLC-IMRT (step and shoot)* or *DMLC-IMRT (dynamic)* approaches that use only a limited number of gantry directions. In addition, plan optimization is simpler because it eliminates the planner's iterative choices of beam number and direction. The conventional MLC approach for rotational IMRT is likely to improve IMRT plan quality and delivery efficiency,[43] although this remains somewhat controversial at present[46,47] and more users will need to report their rotational IMRT experiences over the next few years. Monitor unit calculations for this more complex form of rotational therapy are generated via advanced treatment planning systems having this capability. All are techniques in which the MLC shape changes during a rotation therapy, and depending on the specific linac, other parameters, such as dose rate, may also change. This advanced type of treatment delivery is currently checked via phantom measurements rather than manual calculations prior to the patient's treatment.

It is apparent that the simple MU manual calculations methods described here are no longer adequate for the complex technologies in use today. Modern computer plans utilize dose weight points of interest, which classical MU calculation methods may not address; in addition, geometries that include the presence of heterogeneities, added tertiary devices such as MLCs and asymmetric jaws, and beam intensity modulation can all be problematic for manual check calculations. For example, when the dose weight point is within a small volume of mass surrounded by low-density tissue (e.g., a coin lesion in lung) or one that is at the border of a chest wall and lung (as in a postmastectomy patient), MU calculations cannot easily be confirmed by simple hand-calculated MU methods, and one must rely on the planning system for calculations such as these, emphasizing the importance of fully testing such system prior to clinical use. Dedicated commercial software for MU verification is now available, for example, RadCalc (LifeLine Software Inc, Austin, TX) based on the work of Kung et al.[48] and IMSure (Standard Imaging, Middleton, WI) based on the work of Yang et al.[49] Obviously such systems must also be validated by the physics user prior to clinical use.

CLINICAL PHOTON BEAM DOSIMETRY

Percent Depth Dose and Single-Field Isodose Charts

The central-axis PDD expresses the penetrability of a radiation beam. Table 7.1 summarizes beam characteristics for x-ray and γ-ray beams typically used in radiation therapy and lists the depth at which the dose is maximum (100%) and the 10-cm depth PDD value. Representative PDD curves are shown in Figure 7.3 for conventional SSDs. As a rule of thumb, an 18-MV, 6-MV, and ^{60}Co photon beam loses approximately 2%, 3.5%, and 4.5% per centimeter, respectively, beyond the depth of

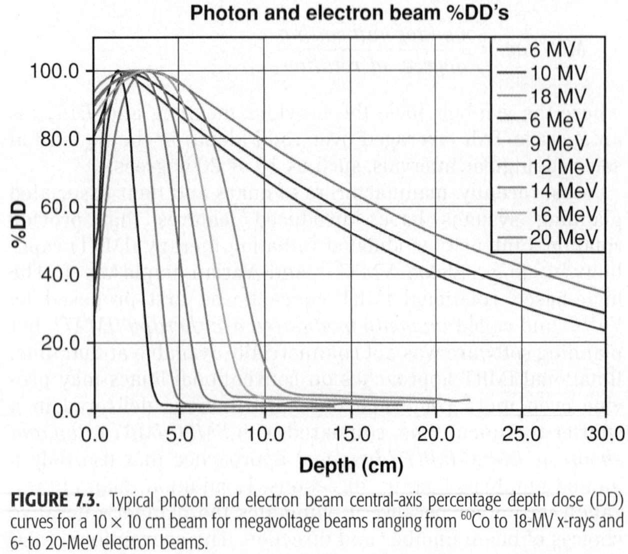

FIGURE 7.3. Typical photon and electron beam central-axis percentage depth dose (DD) curves for a 10 × 10 cm beam for megavoltage beams ranging from ^{60}Co to 18-MV x-rays and 6- to 20-MeV electron beams.

TABLE 7.1 BEAM CHARACTERISTICS FOR PHOTON BEAM ENERGIES OF INTEREST IN RADIATION THERAPY

200 kVp, 2-mm Cu HVL, SSD = 50 cm
- Depth of maximum dose = surface
- Rapid fall-off with depth due to (a) low energy and (b) short SSD
- Sharp beam edge due to small focal spot
- Significant dose outside beam boundaries due to Compton scattered radiation at low energies

^{60}CO, SSD = 80 cm
- Depth of maximum dose = 0.5 cm
- Increased penetration (10 cm PDD = 55%)
- Beam edge not as well defined–penumbra due to source size
- Dose outside beam low because most scattering is in forward direction
- Isodose curvature increases as the field size increases

4-MV x-ray, SSD = 80 cm
- Depth of maximum dose = 1–1.2 cm
- Penetration slightly greater than cobalt (10 cm PDD = 61%)
- Penumbra smaller
- "Horns" (beam intensity off-axis) due to flattening filter design ≈14%

6-MV x-ray, SSD = 100 cm
- Depth of maximum dose = 1.5 cm
- Slightly more penetration than ^{60}Co and 4 MV (10 cm PDD = 67%)
- Small penumbra
- Horns (beam intensity off-axis) due to flattening filter design ≈9%

15–18-MV x-ray, SSD = 100 cm
- Depth of maximum dose = 3–3.5 cm
- Much greater penetration (10 cm PDD = 80%)
- Small penumbra
- Horns (beam intensity off-axis) due to flattening filter design ≈5%
- Exit dose often higher than entrance dose

HVL, half-value layer; SSD, source-to-skin distance; PDD, percentage depth dose.

maximum dose, d_{max} (values are for a 10 × 10 cm field, 100-cm SSD). There is no agreement as to what is the single optimal x-ray beam energy; instead, institutional bias or radiation oncologist training typically influences its selection, and it is usually treatment site specific. As pointed out in Chapter 5, most modern linacs are multimodality, and provide a range of photon and electron beam energies ranging from 4 to 25 MV, with 6- and 15 or 18-MV x-ray beams the most common.

Isodose charts provide much more information about the radiation beam characteristics than do central-axis PDD data alone. However, even isodose charts are limited in that they represent the dose distribution in only one plane (typically the one containing the beam's central axis) and are usually available only for square or rectangular fields. Isodose charts are usually measured in a water phantom with the radiation beam directed perpendicular to the phantom's flat surface. Isodose curves show the relative uniformity of the beams across the field at various depths, and also provide a graphical depiction of the width of the beam's penumbra region. ^{60}Co teletherapy units exhibit a relatively large penumbra, and their isodose distributions are more rounded than those from linac x-ray beams. This is due to the relatively large source size (typically 1 to 2 cm in diameter vs. only a few millimeters for linacs). Linac beam penumbra width does increase slightly as a function of energy and if unfocused MLC leaves are used, but is still much less than that for ^{60}Co units. In addition to the smaller penumbra, linac x-ray isodose distributions have relatively flat isodose curves at depth. However, at shallow depths, particularly at d_{max}, linac x-ray beams typically exhibit an increase in beam intensity away from the central axis; this beam characteristic is referred to as the dose profile *horns* and depends on flattening filter design. In general, each treatment unit has unique radiation beam characteristics, and thus, isodose distributions must be measured, or at least verified, for each specific treatment unit.

Another important point to understand is how the radiation field size is defined. The radiation field size dimensions refer to

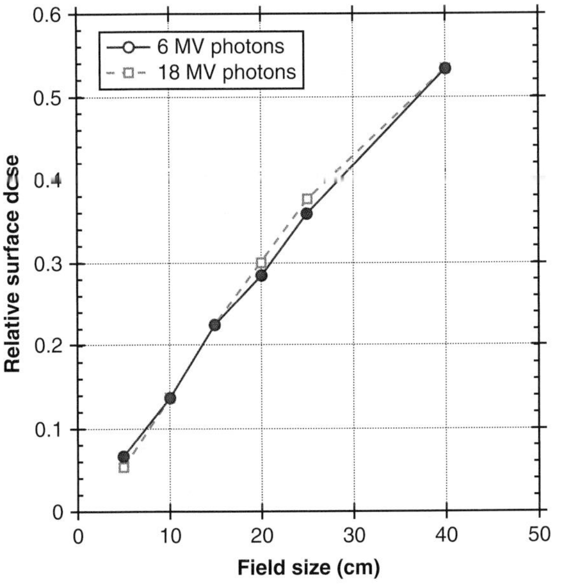

FIGURE 7.4. Relative surface dose versus field size with blocking tray in place for 6- and 18-MV photons. (From Klein EE, Purdy JA. Entrance and exit dose regions for Clinac-2100 C. *Int J Radiat Oncol Biol Phys* 1993;27:429–435.)

the distance perpendicular to the beam's direction of incidence that corresponds to the 50% isodose at the beam's edge. It is defined at the skin surface for SSD treatments, and at the SAD for isocentric treatments.

Depth-Dose Buildup Region

When a photon beam strikes the tissue surface, electrons are set in motion, causing the dose to increase with depth until the maximum dose is achieved at depth d_{max}. As the energy of the photon beam increases, the thickness of the buildup region is increased. The subcutaneous tissue-sparing effects of higher-energy x-rays, combined with their great penetrability, make them well suited for treating deep lesions. In general, the dose to the surface and in the buildup region for megavoltage photon beams generally increases with increasing field size and with the insertion of blocking trays made of plastic or other type material in the beam (Fig. 7.4). The blocking trays should be at least 20 cm above the skin surface because skin doses are significantly increased for lesser distances. Copper, lead, or lead glass filters beneath the blocking tray can be used to remove the undesired lower-energy electrons that contribute to skin dose, but this is nowadays rarely done routinely in the clinic.[50,51]

As the angle of the incident radiation beam becomes more oblique, the surface dose increases, and d_{max} moves toward the surface (Fig. 7.5). This is primarily due to more secondary electrons' contribution from the media below the surface along the oblique path of the beam.[52]

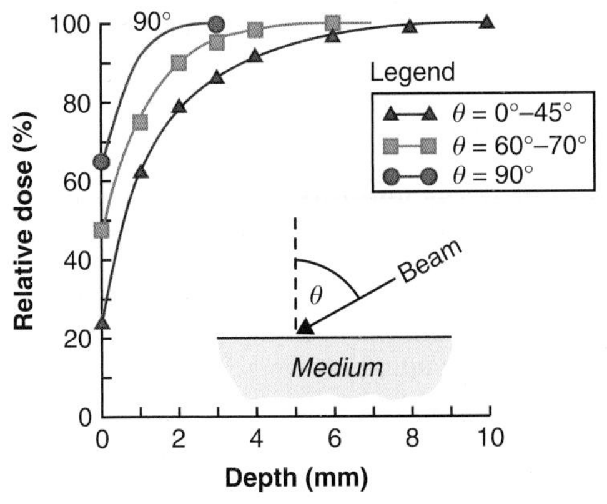

FIGURE 7.5. The variation of surface dose and depth of maximum dose as a function of the angle of incidence of the x-ray beam with the surface (4 MV, 10 × 10 cm).

Depth Dose/Exit Dose Region

The skin and superficial tissue on the side of the patient from which the beam exits receive a reduced dose if there is insufficient backscatter material present. The amount of dose reduction is a function of x-ray beam energy, field size, and the thickness of tissue that the beam has penetrated reaching the exit surface. For a 6-MV beam, a 15% reduction in dose with little dependency on field size has been reported,[50] and for 18-MV beams, an 11% reduction in exit dose was measured.[53] In general, the addition of a thickness of tissue-equivalent material on the exit side equivalent in thickness to approximately two-thirds of the d_{max} depth is sufficient to provide full dose to the build-down region on the exit side. Figure 7.6 shows the effects

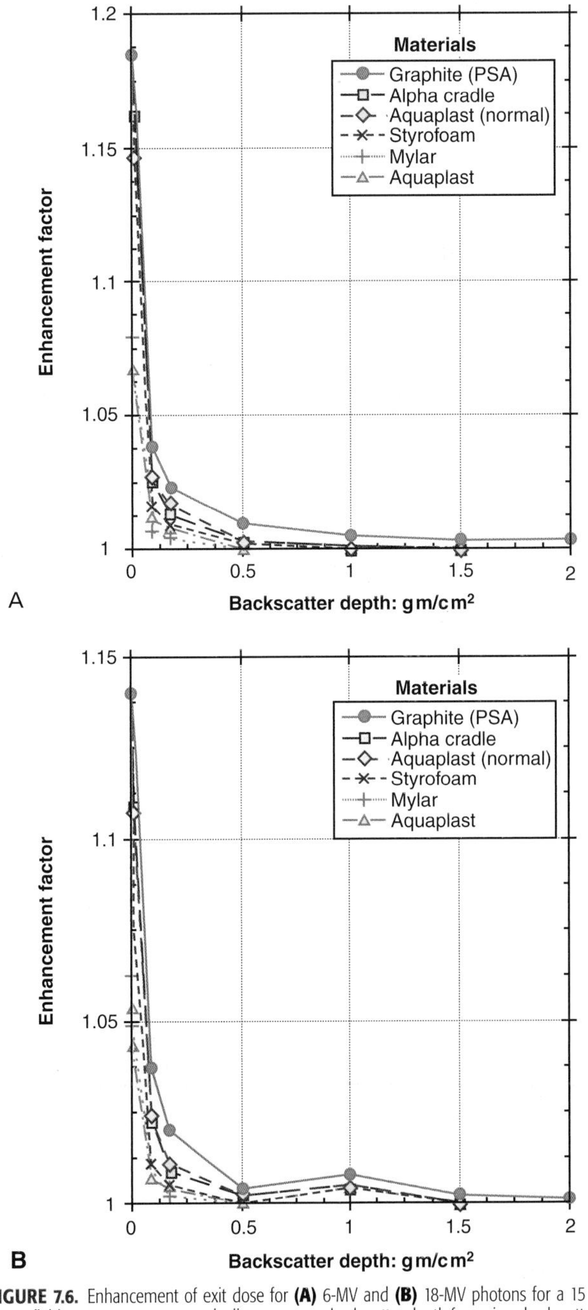

FIGURE 7.6. Enhancement of exit dose for **(A)** 6-MV and **(B)** 18-MV photons for a 15 × 15 cm field at 100-cm source-to-axis distance versus backscatter depth for various backscattering materials. (From Klein EE, Purdy JA. Entrance and exit dose regions for Clinac-2100 C. *Int J Radiat Oncol Biol Phys* 1993;27:429–435.)

of various backscattering media when placed directly behind the exit surface.

Tissue Heterogeneities and Tissue Interface Dosimetry

The presence of tissue heterogeneities, such as air cavities, lungs, bony structures, and prostheses, can greatly impact the calculated dose distribution. The change in dose is due to the perturbation of the transport of primary and scattered photons and that of the secondary electrons set in motion from photon interactions. Depending on the energy of the photon beam and the shape, size, and constituents of the inhomogeneities, the resultant change in dose can be large.

Perturbation of photon transport is more noticeable for lower-energy beams. There is usually an increase in transmission, and therefore dose, when the beam traverses a low-density inhomogeneity. The reverse applies when the inhomogeneity has a density higher than that of water. However, the change in dose is complicated by the concomitant decrease or increase in the scatter dose. For a modest lung thickness of 10 cm, there will be about a 15% increase in the dose to the lung for a ^{60}Co or 6-MV x-ray beam, but only about 5% for an 18-MV x-ray beam.[54]

When there is a net imbalance of electrons leaving and entering the region near an inhomogeneity (interfaces of different media), the condition of electron equilibrium is disrupted. The dose distribution in the patient in such transition zones depends on radiation field size (scatter influence), distance between interfaces (e.g., air cavities), differences between physical densities and atomic number of the interfacing media, and the size and shape of the different media. Because electrons have finite travel, the resultant change in dose is usually local to the vicinity of the inhomogeneity but may be quite large. The effects are more noticeable for the higher photon energy beams due to the increased energy and range of the scattered electrons. Near the edge of the lungs and air cavities, the reduction in dose can be larger than 15%.[55]

For inhomogeneities with density larger than water, there will be an increase in dose locally due to the generation of more electrons. However, most dense inhomogeneities have atomic numbers higher than that of water so that the resultant dose perturbation is further compounded by the perturbation of the multiple coulomb scattering of the electrons. Near the interface between a bony structure and waterlike tissue, large hot and cold dose spots can be present. Several benchmark measurements have been reported for various geometries simulating clinical situations and are discussed briefly in the following sections.

Air Cavities

Air cavities that appear in various locations of the body, most particularly in the head and neck region, pose a problem due to loss of equilibrium at the air–tissue boundaries internal to the patient. Epp et al.[56] reported that for cobalt beams, a reduction in dose of approximately 12% was found for a typical larynx air cavity, which recovered within 5 mm in the new buildup region. The loss was due to a lack of forward scattered electrons. Epp et al.[57] reported that for a 10-MV x-ray beam, a 14.5% loss was measured at the distal interface of the air cavity with a buildup curve that plateaued within 20 mm of the interface. Klein et al.[58] measured distributions about air cavities for 4-MV and 15-MV x-ray beams in both the distal and proximal regions. The combined dose distribution in a parallel-opposed fashion showed a 10% loss at the interfaces for both beam energies.

Lung Tissue

Although the problem of reestablishing equilibrium for lung interfaces is not as severe as with air cavities, a transition zone region at the lung–tissue interface still exists over the range of typical clinical photon beam energies. Rice et al. measured responses within various simulated lung media for 4-MV and 15-MV x-rays using a parallel-plate ion chamber and a phantom constructed of solid water and simulated lung material (average lung material density, $\rho = 0.31$ g/cm^3; some additional measurements made with materials having densities of 0.015 g/cm^3 and 0.18 g/cm^3).[59] Figure 7.7 shows the results in terms of measured CFs for the 15-MV beam. A considerable buildup curve was observed (10% change in CF) for small fields (5×5 cm^2) for the 15-MV beam, which began in the distal region of the lung and plateaued about 5 cm beyond the simulated lung interface.

Bone–Soft Tissue Interfaces

Das et al.[60] measured dose perturbation factors (DPFs) proximal and distal for simulated bone–tissue interface regions using a parallel-plate chamber for both 6- and 24-MV x-ray beams. They reported DPFs of 1.1 for the 6-MV beam and 1.07 for the 24-MV beam at the proximal interface. At the distal interface, a DPF of 1.07 was measured for the 24-MV beam, whereas the 6-MV beam exhibited a DPF of 0.95, resulting in a new buildup region in soft tissue. Note, both buildup and build-down regions dissipate within a few millimeters from the interfaces and the perturbations are independent of thickness and lateral extent of the bone or radiation field size.

Metal Prostheses

Das and associates measured DPFs following a 10.5-mm-thick stainless steel layer simulating a hip prosthesis geometry.[60] They reported a DPF of 1.19 for 24-MV photons, but only 1.03 for 6-MV photons; on the proximal side, they reported a DPF of 1.30 due to the backscattered electrons that was independent of energy, field size, or lateral extent of the steel. These interface effects dissipated within a few millimeters in polystyrene. Other reports dealing with dosimetry perturbations due to metal objects are included in the references.[61,62]

Niroomand-Rad et al. reported on dose perturbation effects at the tissue–titanium alloy implant interfaces in patients with head and neck cancer treated with 6-MV and 10-MV photon beams.[63] They found at the upper surface (toward the source) of the tissue–dental implant interface DPFs of 1.22 and 1.20 for the 6-MV and 10-MV photon beams, respectively. At the lower interface, dose reduction was approximately −13.5% and −9.5% for the 6-MV and 10-MV beams, respectively.

The most complete information currently available on hip prosthesis dosimetry is found in AAPM Report 81 (TG 63).[64] The report provides the current state of scientific understanding and clinical dosimetry in use for patients with high-Z hip prostheses undergoing radiation therapy. Beam arrangements that avoid the prosthesis should always be a first consideration. If this cannot be done, valuable information is available in Report 81, including values for different prostheses' electron density, approximate attenuation of the beam passing through the prosthesis, and possible dose increase to the hip bone. It should also be noted that some of the data provided and recommendations are also applicable to patients having other implanted high-Z prosthetic devices such as pins and humeral head replacements.

Silicone–Soft Tissue Interfaces

Klein and Kuske reported on interface perturbations with silicon breast prostheses.[65] Such prostheses have a density similar to breast tissue but have a different atomic number. They observed a 6% enhancement at the proximal interface and a 9% loss at the distal interface.

Wedge Filter Dosimetry

When a wedge filter is inserted into the beam, the dose distribution is angled at some specified depth to some desired angle relative to the incident beam direction over the entire transverse

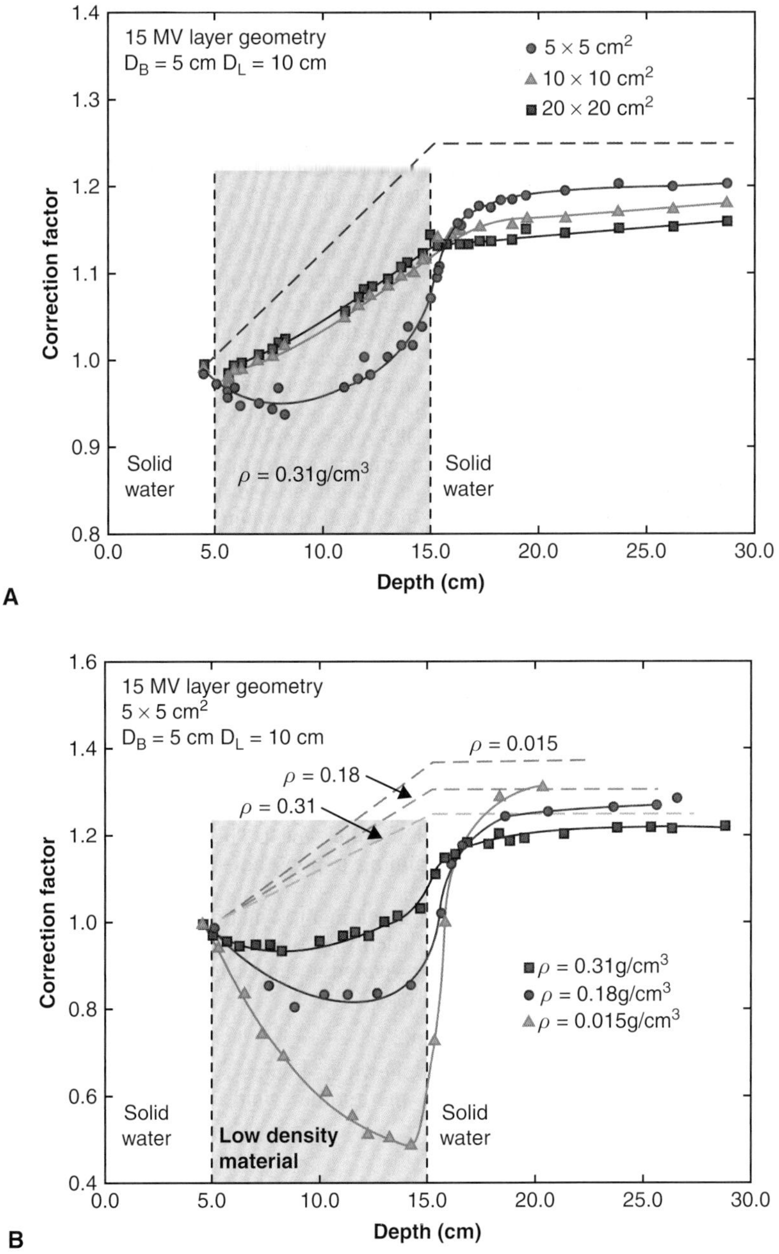

FIGURE 7.7. A: Dose correction factors as a function of depth for a transition zone geometry that simulates a lung–tissue interface for three different field sizes and a lung thickness of 10 cm for 15-MV x-rays. The modification to the primary dose only on the central axis (shown by the *dashed curve*) is independent of field size. **B:** Dose correction factors as a function of depth for a transition zone geometry that simulates a lung–tissue interface for three different densities, a 5 × 5 cm field, and a lung thickness of 10 cm for 15-MV x-rays. The modification to the primary dose only on the central axis is shown by the *dashed curve.* (From Rice RK, Mijnheer BJ, Chin LM. Benchmark measurements for lung dose corrections for x-ray beams. *Int J Radiat Oncol Biol Phys* 1988;15:399–409.)

dimension of the radiation beam (Fig. 7.8). For cobalt units, the depth of the 50% isodose usually is selected for specification of the wedge angle, whereas for high-energy linacs, higher-percentile isodose curves, such as the 80% curve, or the isodose curves at a specific depth (10 cm) are used to define the wedge angle.

Linacs are typically equipped with multiple wedges that may be used with an allowed range of field sizes. Although linac wedges can be designed for any desired *wedge angle,* 15-, 30-, 45-, and 60-degree wedges are the most common.

Some linacs (Elekta AB, Sweden) feature a single wedge, referred to as a *universal wedge,* located in the treatment head, and the desired wedged dose distribution is obtained by the proper combination of wedged and unwedged treatment. A simple approximate model for combining open and wedged fields was first proposed by Tatcher,[66] in which the effective wedge angle θ_E, resulting by the addition of a wedged and unwedged beam, is equal to the nominal wedge angle θ_W for the wedged beam, weighted by the fraction of wedged field B:

$$B = \theta_E/\theta_W$$

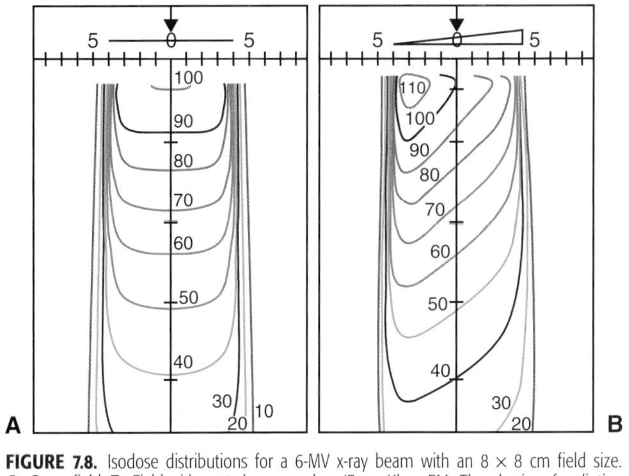

FIGURE 7.8. Isodose distributions for a 6-MV x-ray beam with an 8 × 8 cm field size. **A:** Open field. **B:** Field with a 45-degree wedge. (From Khan FM. *The physics of radiation therapy,* 2nd ed. Baltimore: Williams & Wilkins, 1994.)

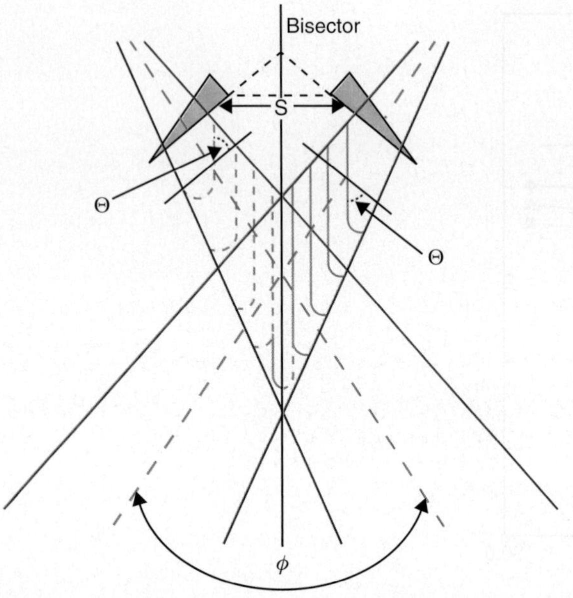

FIGURE 7.9. Parameters of the wedge beams: ϕ is the wedge angle, θ is the hinge angle, and *S* is separation. Isodose curves for each wedge field are parallel to the bisector. (From Khan FM. *The physics of radiation therapy,* 2nd ed. Baltimore: Williams & Wilkins, 1994.)

The Philips Medical Systems Division[67] proposed a slightly different method as follows:

$$B = tan(\theta_E)/tan(\theta_W)$$

Petti and Siddon[68] investigated both methods and showed that these are approximations to an exact theoretical solution, which is given by:

$$B = f/([tan(\theta_W)/tan(\theta_E)] + f - 1)$$

Most importantly, their investigations showed that Tatcher's approximation is good only for values of θ_W less than 45 degrees, and thus is inadequate for accelerators such as Elekta, which use a 60-degree motorized universal wedge. They did show that for the field sizes studied (up to 20 × 20 cm), the Philips relationship was valid to within 3 degrees.

The wedged isodose curves can be normalized in two different ways. In some older systems, the wedge dose distributions have the wedge factor (i.e., the ratio of the measured central-axis dose rate with and without the wedge in place) incorporated into the wedged isodose distribution. More commonly, the wedge isodose curves are normalized to 100% at d_{max}, and a separate *wedge factor* is used to calculate the actual treatment MUs or time. McCullough et al.[69] noted that wedge factors measured at d_{max} usually are accurate to within 2% for depths up to 10 cm, but at greater depths can be inaccurate to 5% or more. The inclusion (or noninclusion) of the wedge factor is an extremely important point to understand because serious error in dose delivered to the patient can occur if used improperly.

Sewchand et al.[70] and Abrath and Purdy[71] pointed out that beam hardening results when a wedge is inserted into the radiation beam. The PDD, therefore, can be considerably increased at depth. Differences reported were nearly 7% for a 4-MV 60-degree wedge field PDD from the open field PDDs at 12-cm depth, and a 3% difference in depth-dose values between the wedge field and the open field for a 60-degree wedge using 25-MV x-rays was reported.

Modern computer-controlled medical linacs now have software features that allow the user to create a wedge-shaped dose distribution by moving one collimator jaw across the field in conjunction with adjustment of the dose rate over the course of the daily single-field treatment.[72] This technology provides superior dose distributions and eliminates the previously mentioned beam-hardening problem seen in physical wedges. This feature can deliver a greater number of wedge angles, and over larger field sizes, including asymmetric field sizes (30 cm in the wedge direction, with 20 cm toward the wedge "heel," and 10 cm toward the wedge "toe"). The increased number of angles enhances planning options but also complicates commissioning and QA.[73]

When the patient's treatment is planned, wedged fields are commonly arranged such that the angle between the beams, the *hinge angle (θ),* is related to the wedge angle (ϕ) by the following relationship (Fig. 7.9):

$$\theta = 90 \text{ degrees} - \phi/2$$

For example, as shown in Figure 7.10, 45-degree wedge fields orthogonal to one another yield a uniform dose distribution.

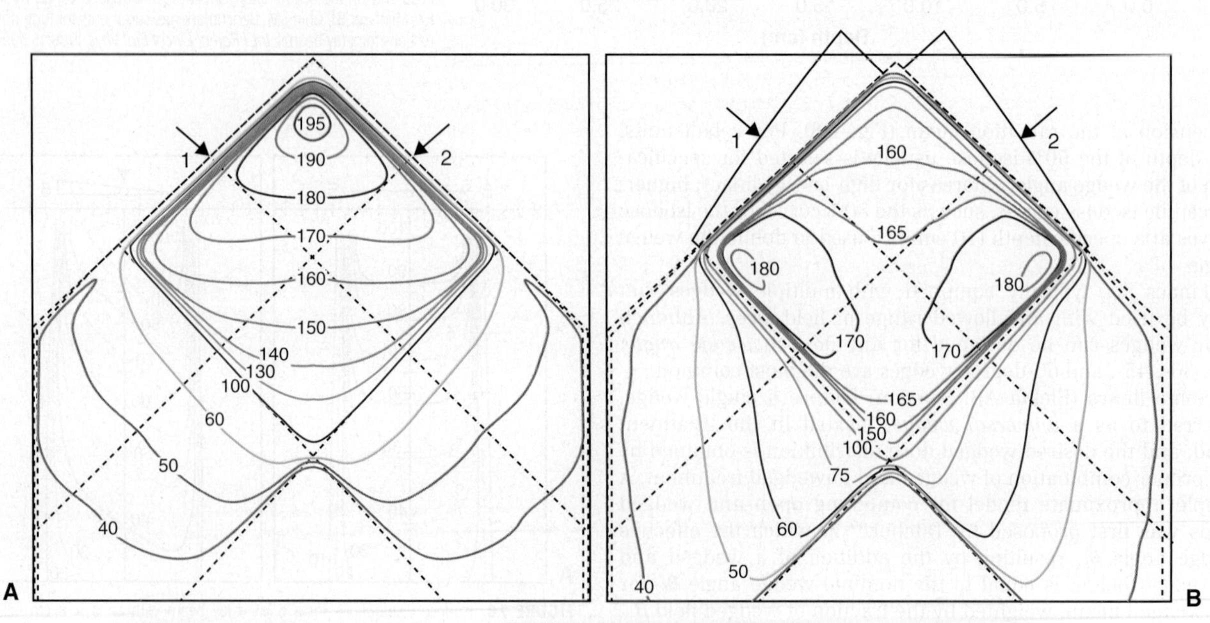

FIGURE 7.10. Isodose distribution for two angled beams. **A:** Without wedges. **B:** With wedges. Both: 4 MV; field size, 10 × 10 cm; source-to-skin distance, 100 cm; wedge angle, 45 degrees. (From Khan FM. *The physics of radiation therapy,* 2nd ed. Baltimore: Williams & Wilkins, 1994.)

TREATMENT PLANNING: COMBINATION OF TREATMENT FIELDS

Parallel-Opposed Fields

When only two unmodified x-ray beams are used in radiation therapy, they usually are parallel-opposed beams (i.e., directed toward each other from opposite sides of the anatomic site with the central axes coinciding). Figure 7.11 presents the normalized relative axis dose profiles from parallel-opposed photon beams for a 10 × 10 cm field at an SSD of 100 cm and for patient diameters of 15 to 30 cm in 5-cm increments. The weight of a beam denotes a numeric value assigned to the beam at some normalization point. For SSD beams, the weight specifies the relative dose assigned to the beam at d_{max}, and for isocentric beams, at isocenter. The beams shown are weighted 1 to 1 (i.e., assigned equal value 100% at d_{max}), and the dose profiles have been normalized to the cumulative midline PDD.

The maximum patient diameter easily treated with parallel-opposed beams for a midplane tumor requiring 50 Gy or less with low-energy megavoltage beams is approximately 18 cm. For "thicker" patients, higher x-ray energies produce improved dose profiles with less dose variation along the central axis without resorting to more complex multibeam arrangements.

For some treatment sites, the underdosing achieved near the skin surface with very–high-energy, parallel-opposed x-ray beams is a highly advantageous feature, but in others it may be desirable to achieve a higher dose nearer to the skin. With very–high-energy x-ray beams traversing small anatomic thicknesses, the exit dose can exceed the entry dose, and the exact dose distribution in the regions beneath the entry and exit surfaces from parallel-opposed high-energy x-ray beams must be carefully evaluated to consider properly the contribution from both entrance and exit components.

Unequal beam weightings are advantageous if the target volume is not midline. Figure 7.12 shows normalized central-axis dose profiles for other weightings, such as 2 to 1 and 3 to 1. The greater the unequal weighting, the greater will be the shift of the higher-dose region toward one surface and away

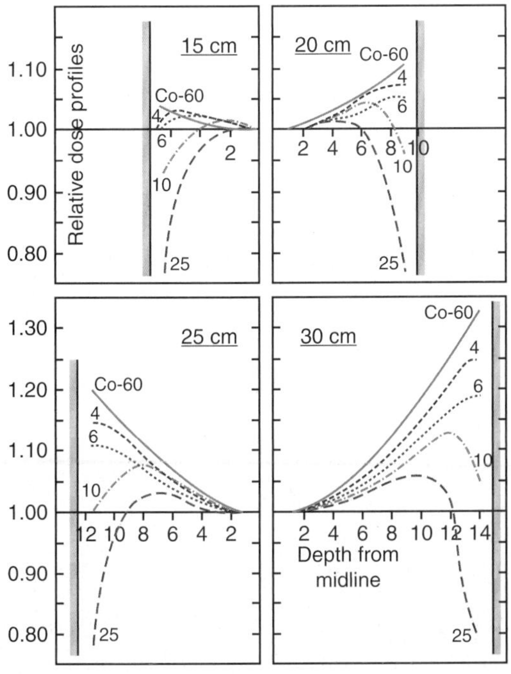

FIGURE 7.11. Relative central-axis dose profiles as a function of x-ray energy (^{60}Co or 4, 6, 10, and 25 MV) and patient thickness (15, 20, 25, and 30 cm). The parallel-opposed beams are equally weighted, and the profiles are normalized to unity at midline. Because of symmetry, only half of each profile is shown.

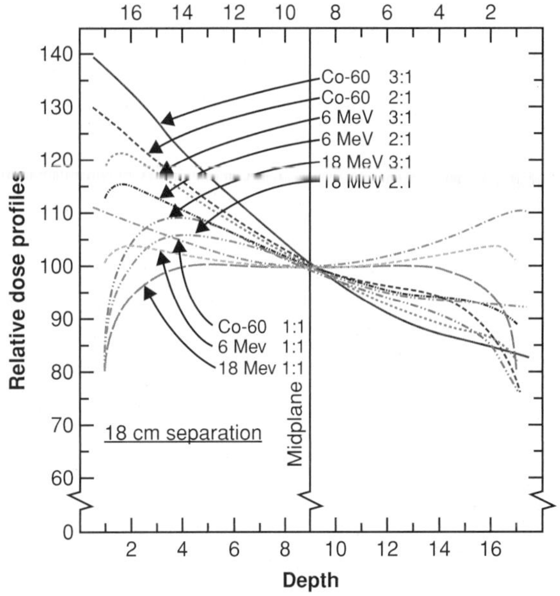

FIGURE 7.12. Dose profiles achieved with unequal weightings of parallel-opposed photon beams; profiles are normalized to unity at midline.

from midline. Although in some anatomic sites unequal weighting may be advantageous, special attention must be directed to the anatomic structures in the high-dose volume.

Multiple-Beam Arrangements

Figure 7.13 shows three commonly used coaxial three-field beam arrangements. A direct anterior field with two anterior oblique fields can be used to generate a high-dose region where the three fields overlap, whereas a low-dose region exists beyond this intersection point. For example, if this arrangement is used for treating the mediastinum, the spinal cord might be included in the anterior beam but spared by the anterior oblique beams. Moving the anterior oblique fields laterally to form a parallel-opposed pair yields a rectangular isodose region with a more uniform dose gradient; however, the magnitude of the dose gradient is determined by the relative weighting of the beams and the thickness of tissue traversed. An anterior field with two symmetrically placed posterior oblique beams yields elongated isodose curves. The degree of elongation is determined by the relative thickness of tissue each beam traverses to the point of intersection and by the relative weights of the beams. Three-field arrangements are often useful for treating tumors lateral to the midline of a patient.

Three-field nonaxial (noncoplanar) arrangements are readily achieved with linacs by rotating the table and gantry. A common technique for treating pituitary tumors uses two lateral fields and a vertex field with the beam entering through the top of the head. Astrocytomas often are treated with parallel-opposed lateral fields and a frontal field entering through the forehead. A 90-degree couch rotation is used with the gantry rotated laterally for the vertex or frontal fields. The lateral fields are also rotated by collimator to ensure the "heels" of the wedges are in the plane of the vertex/frontal field trajectory.

Four-field techniques typically are used in such sites as the abdomen or the pelvis. In most instances, the arrangements consist of pairs of parallel-opposed fields, with a common intersecting point, which yield a "boxlike" isodose distribution. Figure 7.14 compares the dose distributions achieved with a four-field "box technique" for 6- and 18-MV x-ray beams. The central dose distribution is similar for all beam energies, but the greater penetrability of the higher-energy beams yields a lower dose to the region outside the box. Variations in the dose gradient are achieved by differential weighting of each pair of beams.

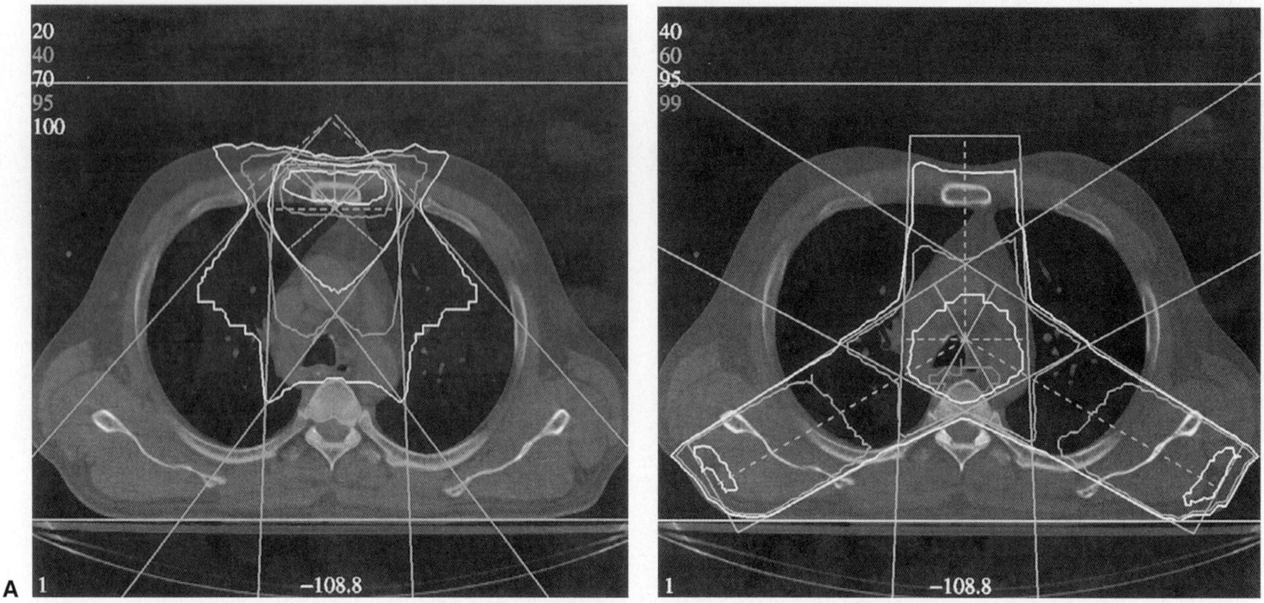

FIGURE 7.13. Three-field coaxial beam arrangements: Dose distribution for two different beam arrangements using 6-MV x-ray beams, 8 × 10 cm field size, 100-cm source-to-skin distance. Isodose curves have been renormalized to show the 100% line almost encompassing the target volume. **A:** Anterior field with two anterior oblique fields at 40 degrees off the midline, all equally weighted. **B:** Anterior field with a weight of 0.8 with two equally weighted (1) posterior oblique fields separated by 120 degrees.

Figure 7.15 shows other possible four-beam arrangements. Angulation of the beams yields a diamond-shaped dose distribution. A butterfly-shaped distribution is achieved if each pair of beams has a point of intersection lying on a common line but separated by a few centimeters.

Treatments involving more than four gantry angles, historically required with orthovoltage x-ray units to treat deep, midline lesions, were originally rarely used with high-energy megavoltage therapy units. However, with the broad introduction of *three-dimensional conformal radiation therapy (3DCRT)* and *IMRT*, there has been an increase in multibeam treatments such as the 3DCRT six-field technique commonly used for the treatment of prostate carcinoma[74] and the nine-field technique commonly used for head and neck cancer IMRT treatments.[75]

More recently, these multibeam arrangements are further refined by adding segments of field with the same beam angle to either improve dose homogeneity or to intentionally generate an inhomogeneous dose distribution (e.g., the simultaneous integrated boost technique).[76]

Rotation Therapy

Rotational (or *arc*) *therapy* techniques, in which the treatment is delivered while the gantry (and thus the radiation beam) rotates around the patient, can be thought of as an infinite extension of the multiple-field techniques already described. This technique is most useful when applied to small, symmetric, deep-seated tumors, and usually is limited to field sizes less than approximately 10 cm in width for the treatment of

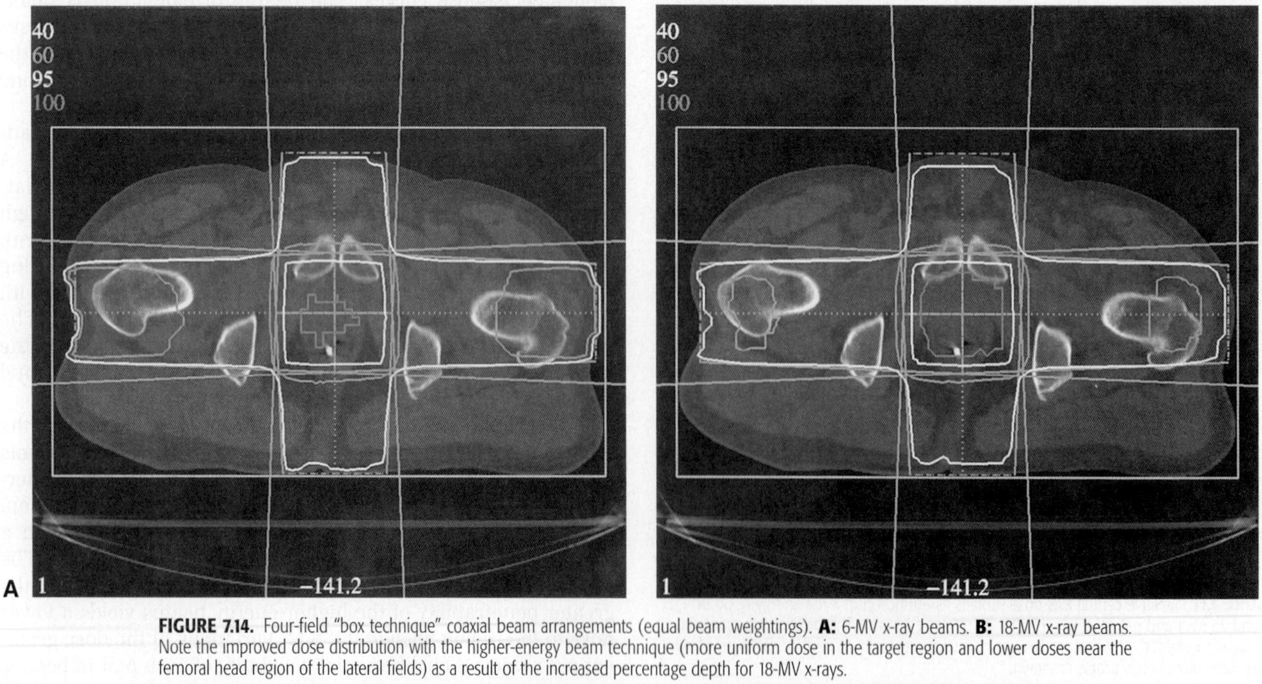

FIGURE 7.14. Four-field "box technique" coaxial beam arrangements (equal beam weightings). **A:** 6-MV x-ray beams. **B:** 18-MV x-ray beams. Note the improved dose distribution with the higher-energy beam technique (more uniform dose in the target region and lower doses near the femoral head region of the lateral fields) as a result of the increased percentage depth for 18-MV x-rays.

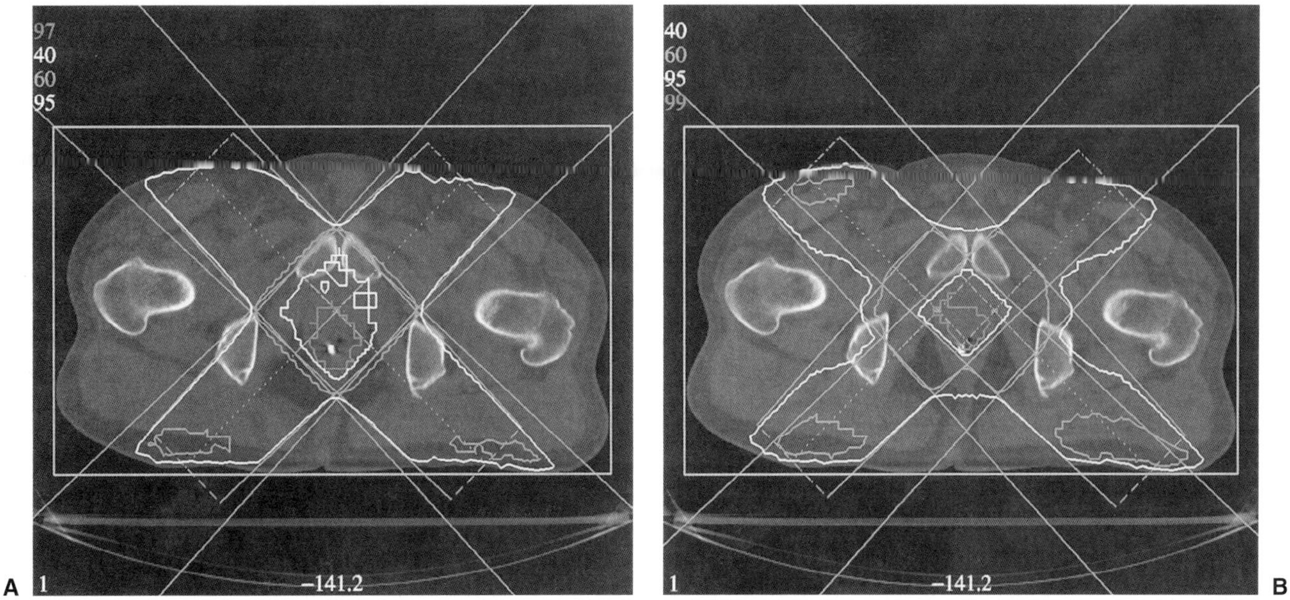

FIGURE 7.15. Four-field "oblique technique" coaxial beam arrangements (6-MV x-rays, equal beam weightings). **A:** With common isocenter resulting in a diamond-shaped dose distribution. **B:** Each beam pair intersecting at two different points on a common line resulting in a butterfly-shaped isodose distribution.

centrally located lesions (i.e., there is approximately an equal amount of tissue in all directions around the lesion).

Dose distributions generated by rotational techniques are not very sensitive to the energy of the photon beam. Figure 7.16 illustrates this fact, showing the dose distribution achieved using a 6-MV x-ray beam, and also the distribution using an 18-MV x-ray beam. There is a little less elongation in the direction of the shorter dimension of the patient's anatomy for the 18-MV beam, and the dose distribution in the periphery is slightly lower.

In arc therapy techniques, one or more sectors of a 360-degree rotation are skipped to reduce the dose to critical normal structures. When a sector is skipped, the high-dose region is shifted away from the skipped region. Therefore, the isocenter must be moved toward the skipped sector; this technique is referred to as *past-pointing,* as illustrated in Figure 7.17.

The prostate, bladder, cervix, and pituitary are clinical sites that have been treated, either initially or for boost doses, with rotational or arc therapy techniques. Although the dose distributions achieved by rotation or arc therapy yield high target-volume doses, these techniques normally result in a greater volume of normal tissue being irradiated (albeit at low doses) than fixed, multiple-field techniques.

As previously indicated, modern-day rotational therapy is now delivered by a variety of techniques (e.g., tomotherapy, RapidArc, VMAT). A new technology now being implemented on linacs and one that is likely to significantly impact modern-day rotational therapy is referred to as *flattening filter free (FFF);* that is, the flattening filter is not present during irradiation. The FFF feature allows dose rates up to 2,400 MUs per minute, thus greatly improving efficiency in dose delivery, which is particularly important for patients receiving treatments where very

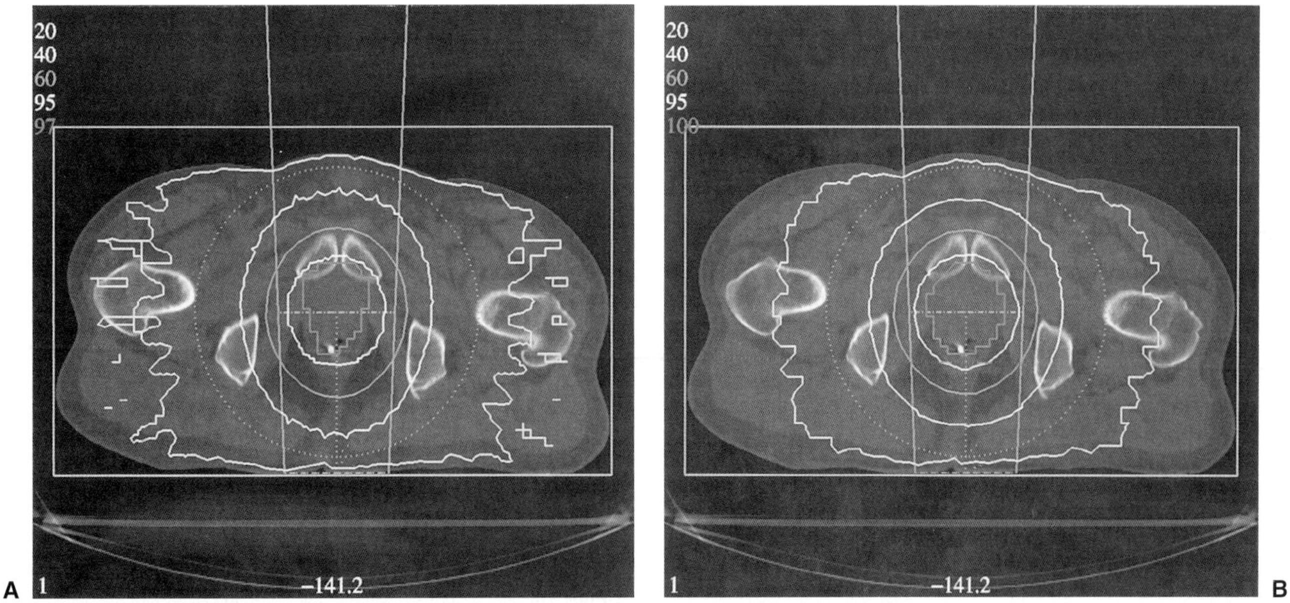

FIGURE 7.16. A 360-degree rotational therapy technique. **A:** 6-MV x-ray beams. **B:** 18-MV x-ray beams. Note that there is little difference in the dose distribution when using a higher-energy beam as a result of the offsetting effects of increased percentage depth versus higher exit dose.

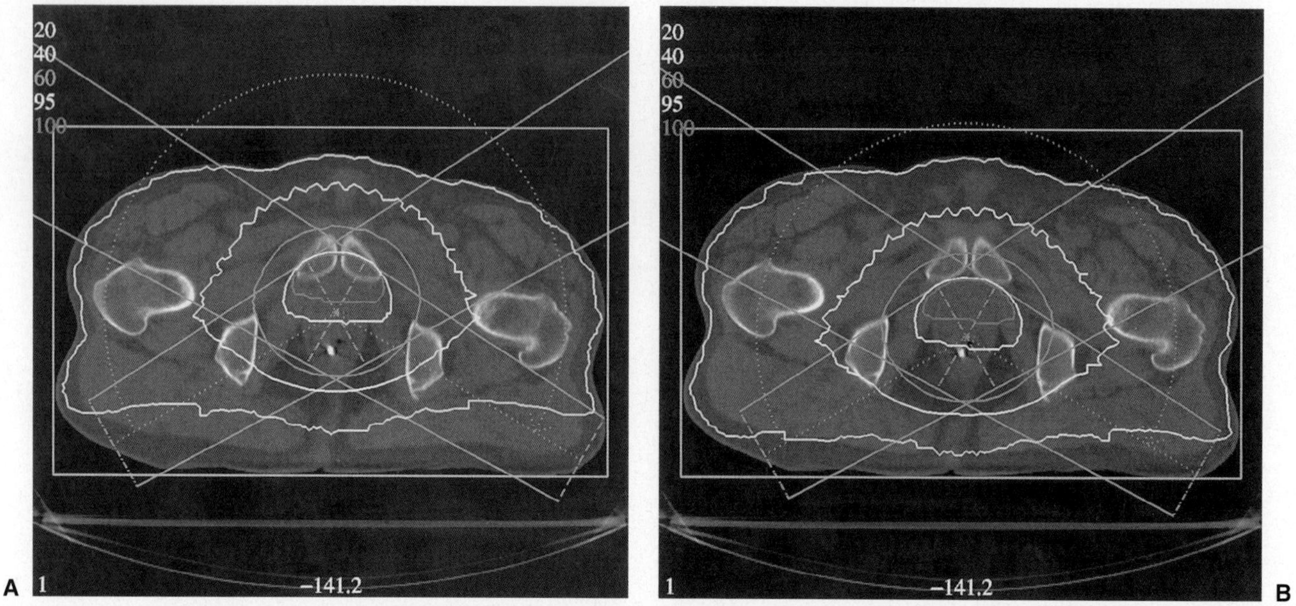

FIGURE 7.17. Arc therapy technique for 6-MV x-rays. **A:** 240-degree arc. Note that when a sector of the full 360-degree rotation is skipped, the high-dose isodose curves are shifted away from the skipped sector. **B:** 240-degree arc, but patient positioned so that isocenter is 2 cm lower toward the skipped sector (this technique is called *past-pointing*). Note high-dose isodose curves now encompass the target volume.

high daily doses are delivered, such as stereotactic body radiation therapy (SBRT).[77] The reader is referred to the reviews by Georg et al. regarding the current status and future perspective of FFF beams.[78]

FIELD SHAPING

A major constraint in the treatment of cancer using radiation is the limitation in the dose that can be delivered to the tumor because of the dose tolerance of the tissue (critical organs) surrounding or near the target volume. Shielding normal tissue and critical organs has allowed the radiation oncologist to increase the dose to the tumor volume while maintaining the dose to critical organs below some tolerance level. The frequently used tolerance doses for these organs are not absolute and depend on a number of clinical and treatment factors. Depending on the predominantly serial or parallel organization of the organ at risk, a large dose can sometimes be given to fractional volumes of organs with a parallel structure (liver, kidneys, lungs).[79,80] Shielding is usually accomplished using collimator jaws (with the asymmetric feature) and multileaf collimators, in which the beam aperture (field shape) is customized for individual patients. Use of low–melting-point alloy blocks is rapidly being replaced with the MLC technology.

MLC and Associated Dosimetry

Asymmetric Collimator Jaws

Field shaping and abutted field radiation therapy techniques have been made even more versatile with the asymmetric jaw feature found on modern-day linacs. This feature allows each set of jaws to open and close independently of each other (Fig. 7.18). The collimator jaw provides greater attenuation than the MLC leaf or alloy block, thus providing an advantage (which is readily apparent on portal films) in reducing the dose to blocked regions.

Depth-dose characteristics for asymmetric fields are similar to those of symmetric fields as long as the degree of asymmetry is not too extreme. Clinical sites where asymmetric jaws are typically used include breast (Fig. 7.19), head and neck, craniospinal, and prostate. In addition, the use of asymmetric jaws as beam splitters, for field reductions, and with MLCs is helpful for most sites. Several authors have reported on the use of asymmetric jaws to match supraclavicular and tangential fields for breast irradiation.[81–83] Such technology allows a single setup point for all of the treatment fields, including the posterior axillary field. The Y-jaws can beam split the caudal and cephalic regions for the supraclavicular and tangential beams, respectively, and the X-jaws are used to shield the ipsilateral lung and contralateral breast. Hence, a common match plane with one common isocenter can be used for all portals, eliminating the need to move the patient between portals, thus reducing overall patient setup time by almost a factor of two. In addition, the increased attenuation by the jaws reduces the dose to the contralateral breast and lung.[84] A technique for matching lateral head and neck fields and the supraclavicular field using asymmetric jaws was described by Sohn et al.[85]

Multileaf Collimation

Multileaf collimation, first introduced in Japan in the 1960s,[86] has now gained widespread acceptance and has replaced alloy blocking as the standard of practice for field shaping in

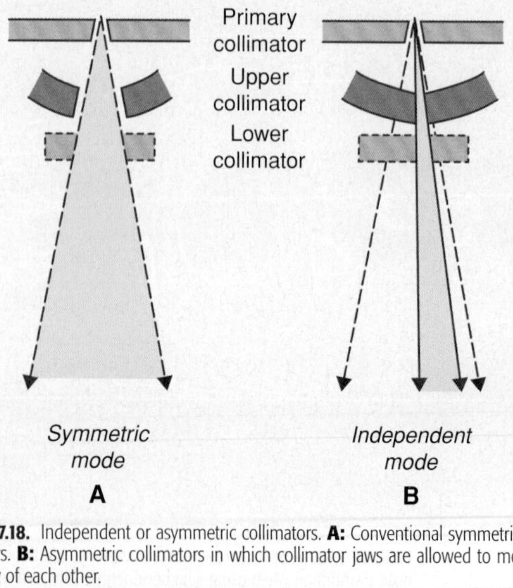

FIGURE 7.18. Independent or asymmetric collimators. **A:** Conventional symmetric pairs of collimators. **B:** Asymmetric collimators in which collimator jaws are allowed to move independently of each other.

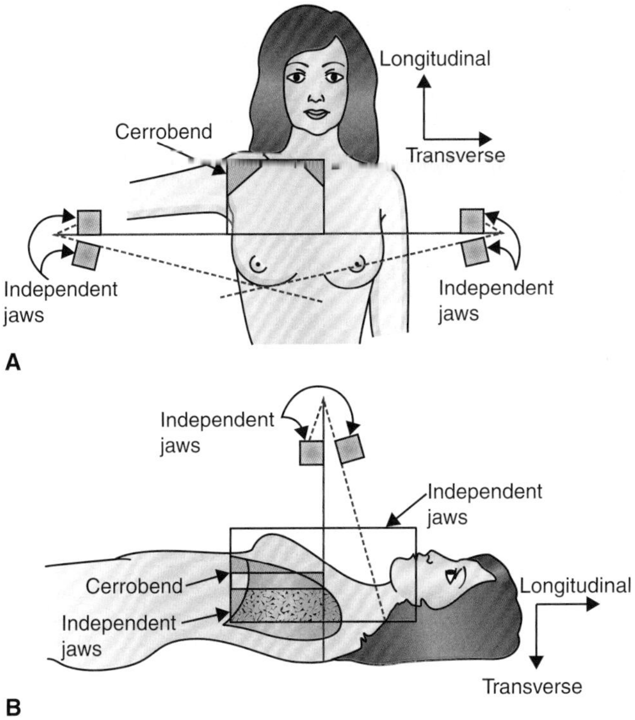

FIGURE 7.19. Treatment technique for breast cancer using independent collimators. (From Klein EE, Taylor M, Michaletz-Lorenz M, et al. A mono isocentric technique for breast and regional nodal therapy using dual asymmetric jaws. *Int J Radiat Oncol Biol Phys* 1994;28:753–760.)

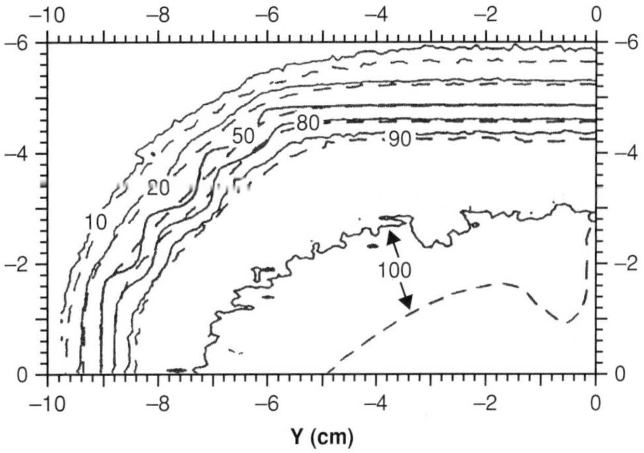

FIGURE 7.20. Comparison of beam's-eye-view isodose curves at 10-cm depth for multileaf collimator (*solid line*) and Cerrobend-shaped (*dashed line*) beam apertures for 18-MV photons. (From Klein EE, Harms WB, Low DA, et al. Clinical implementation of a commercial multileaf collimator: dosimetry, networking, simulation, and quality assurance. *Int J Radiat Oncol Biol Phys* 1995;33:1195–1208.)

modern radiation therapy clinics. The different manufacturers' MLC systems vary with respect to MLC location, leaf design, and field size coverage. The leaves are typically carried on two opposed carriages that transport the leaves in unison. The leaves have individual controls that are computer assigned and positioned. Initially, most commercial MLC systems were designed to serve as a block replacement, but now provide for dynamic IMRT delivery as well.

Elekta first introduced its MLC system in the late 1980s.[87] Their current MLC system replaces the upper photon collimator jaws, and therefore, the maximum field size can open to a full 40 × 40 cm. The MLC system is augmented by parallel diaphragms, which increase the leaf's attenuation by an additional two HVLs.

The Varian MLC system is considered a tertiary system placed below the photon collimator jaws. The latest Varian MLC (non-SRS) is a 120-leaf (60 on each side) system, in which the middle 20 cm consists of 0.5-cm-wide leaves, while the outer 20-cm leaves still project to 1.0-cm widths. This set of leaves projects to 16.0 cm in length at isocenter, and the leaf span range (maximum–minimum positions on the same carriage) is limited to 14.5 cm. The leaves move perpendicular to the beam's central axis. The distance from the x-ray target to the bottom of the leaves (on the central axis) is 54.0 cm. The leaves fan away from the central axis so that their sides are divergent with the beam's fan lines. The leaves are interdigitated by a tongue-and-groove design. The reader is referred to the references for details of the Siemens MLC system in which the lower collimating jaws are replaced with a double-focused leaf system.[36]

For the Varian MLC system, leaf transmission values of 1.5% to 2.0% for a 6-MV beam and 1.5% to 5% for an 18-MV beam have been reported.[33,88] These values are lower than those found for alloy blocks (3.5%), but higher than those for collimator jaw transmission (that being <1.0%). Transmission through abutted (closed) leaf pairs was as high as 28% for 18-MV photons on the central axis. The abutment transmission decreased as a function of off-axis distance to as low as 12%.

Figure 7.20 shows a comparison of MLCs and alloy blocks regarding penumbra. The discrete steps of the MLC systems introduce undulations in the isodose lines. This effect causes an apparent increase in penumbra with wave patterns after the undulations. Single, focused MLC systems have a slightly larger penumbra than do alloy shields and have an even larger difference in comparison with collimator jaws. Boyer et al. found the penumbra (80% to 20% isodose lines) generated by leaf ends to be wider than those generated by upper collimator jaws by 1.0 to 1.5 mm, and 1.0 to 2.5 mm compared with the lower jaws, depending on energy and field size.[89] Powlis and associates compared multileaf collimation and alloy field shaping and found few differences.[90] LoSasso and Kutcher found similar results and concluded that geometric accuracy is even improved with MLCs.[91]

The penumbras measured for the leaf sides are comparable with those found for upper jaws due to their divergent nature. The penumbra increase and stair-stepping effect are most prominent at d_{max}. The effects diminish at depth due to the influence of scattered electrons and photons as the scatter-to-primary ratio increases with depth. Adding an opposed beam leads to further smoothing of the undulations and penumbra differences become less significant. For multibeam arrangements, the differences in dose distribution between MLC and alloy shields are negligible.

Two methods for designing the optimal MLC configurations to fit the treatment plan's field apertures have evolved: (a) configuring the MLC based on a digitized film image using a dedicated MLC workstation (with or without automated optimization), and (b) configuring the MLC using treatment planning system software. The main limitation in optimizing the MLC leaf settings to conform to the shaped field is the discrete leaf steps. Most field shapes require only minor adjustment of collimator angle to achieve minimal discrepancy between the desired and resultant field shape. The criteria for optimizing the MLC leaf settings are governed by placing the most leaf ends tangent to the field and also maintaining the same internal area as originally prescribed. MLC shaping systems typically provide an option to place the leaf ends entirely outside the field (exterior), entirely within the field (interior), or crossing the field at midleaf (leaf-center insertion). The last is the most widely used criterion because the desired field area is more closely maintained. However, this choice leads to regions in which some treatment areas are shielded and some normal tissues are irradiated. Zhu et al. reported on a variable insertion technique in which leaves are placed only far enough into the field to cause the 50%

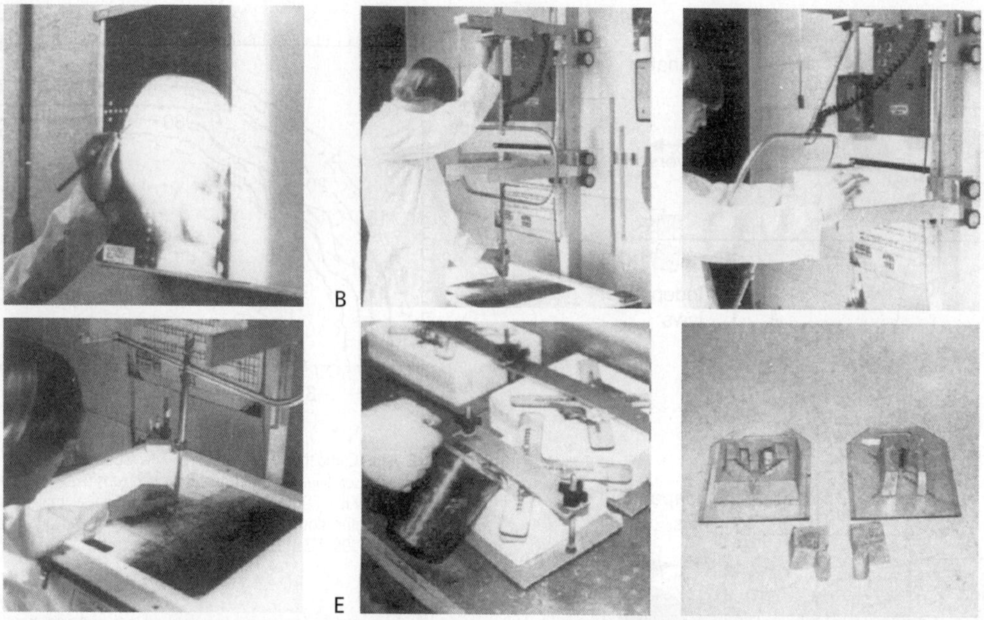

FIGURE 7.21. Composite photographs illustrating the low–melting-point alloy shielding block design and fabrication process. **A:** Physician defining the treatment volume on the x-ray simulator radiograph. **B:** Physics technician adjusting the source-to-skin distance and skin-to-film distance of a hot-wire cutter to emulate simulator geometry. **C:** Proper-thickness foam block aligned to the central axis of the cutter. **D:** Foam mold cut with hot-wire cutter. **E:** Foam pieces aligned and held in place using a special clamping device. Molten alloy is poured into the mold and allowed to harden. **F:** Examples of typical shielding blocks cast using this system. (From Purdy JA. Secondary field shaping. In: Wright AE, Boyer AL, eds. *Advances in radiation therapy treatment planning.* New York: American Institute of Physics, 1983.)

isodose contour to undulate outside and up to the desired contour.[92] LoSasso et al. reported on a method in which each leaf is inserted such that the treatment area covered by the leaf equals the normal tissue area that is not spared.[93] Brahme also demonstrated optimal choices for choosing a collimator angle to optimize leaf direction, depending on whether the field shape is convex or concave.[94] Du et al. reported on a method that defines optimal leaf positioning in combination with optimal collimator angulation.[95] Typically, the optimal direction for the leaf motion is along the narrower axis. For a simple ellipse the optimal leaf direction is parallel to the short axis. Reports on the effects of tissue heterogeneities on penumbra and resultant field definition indicate that the penumbra in lung increases (especially for 18-MV photons), whereas in bone, it decreases for both alloy blocks and MLCs.[33]

As indicated previously, because MLC systems are still evolving, a careful evaluation of the effect of MLCs on monitor unit calculations must be performed before clinical use. Extensive testing over the clinical range of field sizes and shapes should be undertaken before the MLC system is used clinically.

Low-Melting Alloy Blocks

Although alloy blocks are rapidly disappearing from clinical use, a short section is included in this chapter for completeness. The Lipowitz metal (Cerrobend) shielding block system was introduced by Powers et al.[96] Lipowitz metal consists of 13.3% tin, 50% bismuth, 26.7% lead, and 10% cadmium. The physical density at 20°C is 9.4 g/cm^3, compared with 11.3 g/cm^3 for lead. The block fabrication procedure is illustrated in Figure 7.21, and more details on using this form of field shaping can be found in the review article by Leavitt and Gibbs.[97]

Specific doses to critical organs may be limited by using either a full-thickness block, usually five HVLs (3.125% transmission) or six HVLs (1.562% transmission), or a partial transmission shield, such as a single HVL (50% transmission) of shielding material. The actual dose delivered under the shielded area is usually greater than these stated transmission levels because of scatter radiation beneath the blocks from adjacent unshielded portions of the field. The scatter component of the dose increases with depth as more radiation scatters into the shielded volume beneath the block. Thus, the dose to the blocked area is a function of block material, thickness (and width), field size, and energy. Figure 7.22 shows the attenuation of Lipowitz metal of x-rays produced at 2, 4, 10, and 18 MeV and ^{60}Co γ-rays.[98] Alloy blocks made from the standard thickness (7.6 cm) of foam molds reduce the primary beam intensity to 5% of its unattenuated value. Increasing the block thickness usually is not worthwhile because it makes the block

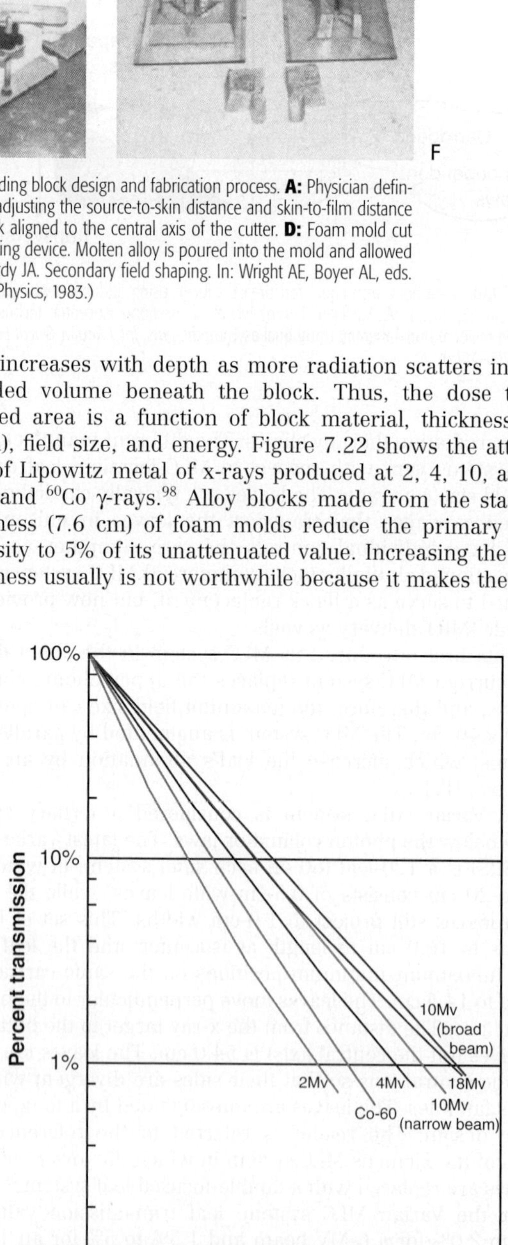

FIGURE 7.22. Attenuation in Lipowitz metal of x-rays produced at 2, 4, 10, and 18 MV and γ-rays from ^{60}Co. (From Huen A, Findley DO, Skov DD. Attenuation in Lipowitz's metal of x-rays produced at 2, 4, 10, and 18 MV and gamma rays from cobalt-60. *Med Phys* 1979;6:147.)

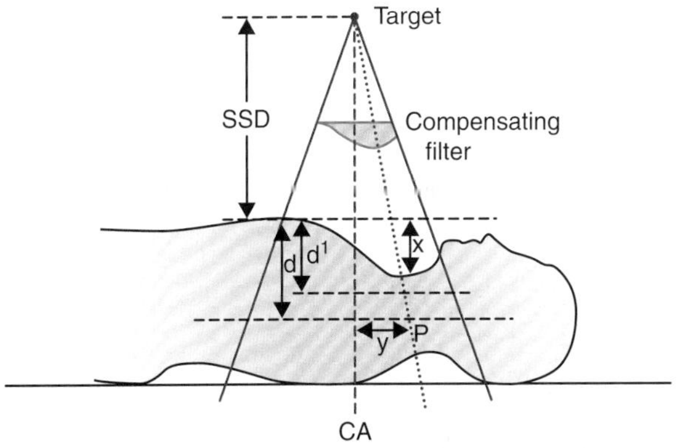

FIGURE 7.23. Schematic illustrating typical geometry used in the design of a compensator filter to account for patient's irregularly shaped surface. SSD, source-to-skin distance; CA, central axis.

heavier, whereas the scatter radiation contributes an equal or greater share of the dose under the blocks.

Due to the advent of multileaf collimation, metal blocks for photon beams are rarely used, as multileaf collimation afforded there to be no room for entry between treatment fields. In addition, the construction of blocks was time consuming and expensive. Also, the materials themselves, as they were heated, gave off potentially toxic air, particularly due to the lead and cadmium. The one advantage of blocks is that they provide smooth boundaries by having a continuous shape around the field and incur no field size limitation. However, the weight of the blocks can be excessive, sometimes up to 15 pounds, leading to the potential for injury to therapists and patients should they be mishandled.

COMPENSATING FILTERS

The compensating filter, introduced by Ellis et al.,[99] counteracts the effects caused by variations in patient surface curvature while still preserving the desirable skin-sparing feature of megavoltage photon beams. This is accomplished by placing the custom-designed compensating filter in the beam, sufficiently "upstream" from the patient's surface, as illustrated in Figure 7.23. Several different compensator systems have been used in the clinic.[100] However, the use of physical compensators to account for patient surface curvature is almost nonexistent in clinics today due to the advent of IMRT. But one particular IMRT delivery method does use a physical compensator, which is designed from the planning system and often constructed from a third-party vendor to deliver a modulated field.[101]

BOLUS

Tissue-equivalent material placed directly on the patient's skin surface to reduce the skin sparing of megavoltage photon beams is referred to as *bolus*. A tissue-equivalent bolus should have electron density, physical density, and atomic number similar to those of tissue or water and be pliable so that it conforms to the skin surface contour. Inexpensive, nearly tissue-equivalent materials used as a bolus in radiation therapy include slabs of paraffin wax, rice bags filled with soda, gauze coated with petrolatum, and synthetic-based substances, such as Super-Flab or Super Stuff.[102]

Thin slabs of bolus that follow the surface contour increase the dose to the skin beneath the bolus with a maximum reduction when the bolus thickness is approximately equal to the d_{max} depth for the photon beam. In addition, adding bolus to fill a tissue deficit may smooth an irregular surface. A bolus also can be shaped to alter the dose distribution as well, but normally wedges are used to alter the dose distribution for megavoltage photon beams to retain skin sparing.

PATIENT POSITIONING, REGISTRATION, AND IMMOBILIZATION

Ensuring accurate daily positioning of the patient in the treatment position and reduction of patient movement during treatment is essential to deliver the prescribed dose and achieve the planned dose distribution. The reproducibility achievable in the daily positioning of a patient for treatment depends on several factors other than the anatomic site under treatment, including the patient's age, general health, and weight. In general, obese patients and small children are the most difficult to position.

The fields to be treated typically are delineated in the computed tomography (CT) simulation process using either visible skin markings or skin markings visible only under an ultraviolet light. In some instances, external tattoos are applied. These markings are used in positioning a patient on the treatment machine using the machine's field localization light and distance indicator and the laser alignment lights mounted in the treatment room that project transverse, coronal, and sagittal light lines (or dots) on the patient's skin surface.

It is vital that the rigidity of the mask maintain consistency over the course of treatment. In the last 10 years the normal method of aligning the patient for treatment relied on the marks on a patient before placing a mask on. Therefore, the systems that interface with the mobilization systems and the treatment couch need to also be rigid and registered. As of now, patients are set up to treatment coordinates once they are fit on to the mobilization systems.

Numerous patient restraint and repositioning devices have been designed and used in treating specific anatomic sites. For example, the disposable foam plastic head holder provides stability for the head when the patient is in the supine position. If the patient is treated in the prone position, a face-down stabilizer can be used. This device has a foam rubber lining covered by disposable paper with an opening provided for the patient's eyes, nose, and mouth. It allows comfort and stability as well as air access for the patient during treatment in the prone position.

A vacuum-form body immobilization system is commercially available. This system consists of a vacuum pump and an outer rubber bag filled with plastic minispheres. The rubber bag containing the minispheres is positioned to support the patient's treatment position. A vacuum is then applied, causing the minispheres to come together to form a firm, solid support molded to the patient's shape. The bite block (Fig. 7.24) is another device used as an aid in patient repositioning in the treatment of head and neck cancer. With this device, the patient, in the treatment position, bites into a specially prepared dental impression material layered on a fork that is attached to a supporting device. When the material hardens, the impression of the teeth is recorded. The bite-block fork is connected to a support arm, which is attached to the treatment couch, and may be used either with or without scales for registration.

Thermal plastic masks are now widely used in the United States (Fig. 7.25). A plastic sheet is placed in warm water and draped over the site, and hardens on cooling.[103] The use of thermal plastic masks allows treatments with few skin marks made on the patient because most of the reference lines can be placed on the mask. Treatments can be given through the mask; however, there is some loss of skin sparing. When skin sparing is critical, the mask may be cut out to match the treatment portal, although some of the structural rigidity is lost.

Custom molds constructed from polyurethane formed to patient contours have gained widespread use as aids in immobilization and repositioning (Fig. 7.26). The constituent chemicals for the polyurethane foam are mixed in liquid form and allowed to expand and harden around the patient while the patient is in the treatment position. These molds are used for treatment of Hodgkin's disease with the mantle irradiation

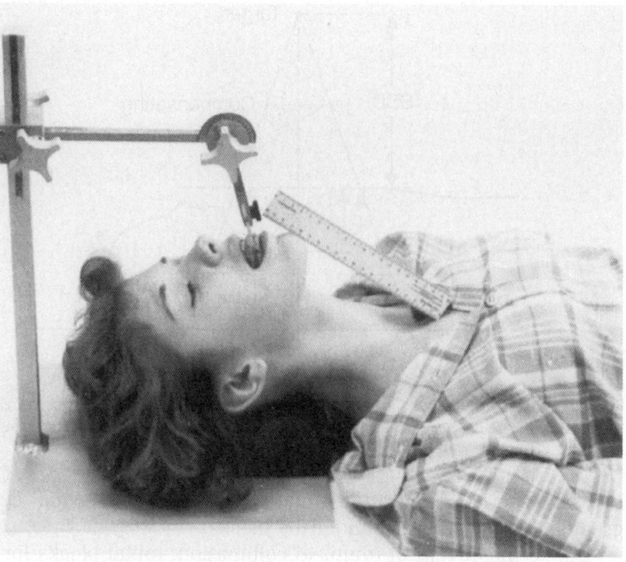

FIGURE 7.24. Example of a bite-block registration and immobilization system used in treatment of head and neck cancer. (Courtesy of Radiation Products Design, Buffalo, MN.)

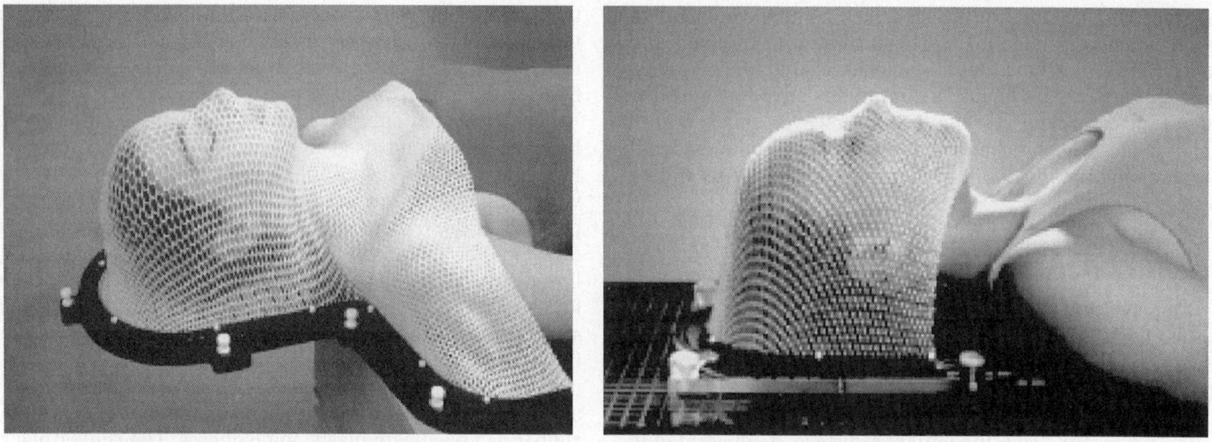

FIGURE 7.25. Example of a registration and immobilization system (thermal plastic mask) used in treatment of head and neck cancer.

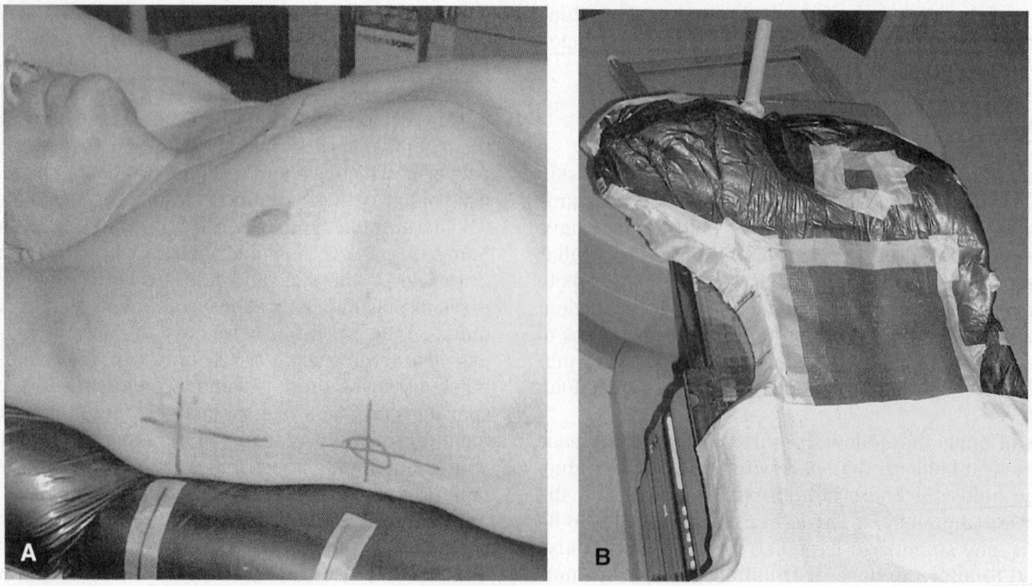

FIGURE 7.26. Examples of registration and immobilization systems (foam mold) used in treatment of the thorax. **A:** Mold is registered to table and the patient is registered to the mold by fiducial markings. **B:** Mold with cutout area to allow clear access to the treatment area, and built-in handgrip.

technique, in patients with cancer of the thorax or prostate, and for extremity repositioning/immobilization. Johnson et al.[104] reported on the effect on surface dose caused by the mold for ^{60}Co, 6- and 18-MV photon beams. Also, when concerned about surface dose effects caused by immobilization devices, one should not neglect understanding the effects also caused by carbon fiber couch inserts.[105]

A bite-block system or a thermal plastic face mask system is commonly used to immobilize patients with head and neck tumors. Patients immobilized with the bite-block system typically require a larger number of adjustments than when more effective systems like the thermal face mask are used. Also, patients may prefer the face mask because most of the reference marks are on the mask rather than on the skin. However, the final assessment of accuracy and reproducibility of the daily treatment is obtained by radiographic imaging of the area treated because there is the possibility of patient movement within the mask, especially if significant tumor shrinkage or weight loss has taken place.

SEPARATION OF ADJACENT X-RAY FIELDS

Field Junctions

Different techniques for matching adjacent fields are illustrated in Figure 7.27. A commonly used gap calculation method for adjacent radiation fields is illustrated in Figure 7.28A. The separation between adjacent field edges necessary to produce junction doses similar to central-axis doses follows from the similar triangles formed by the half-field length and SSD in each field. The field edge is defined by the dose at the edge that is 50% of the dose at d_{max}. For two contiguous fields of lengths L_1 and L_2, the separation, S, of these two fields at the skin surface can be calculated using the following expression:

$$S = \frac{1}{2}L_1\left(\frac{d}{SSD}\right) + \frac{1}{2}L_2\left(\frac{d}{SSD}\right)$$

A slight modification of this formula is needed when sloping surfaces are involved, as shown in Figure 7.28B.[106] Typically, the skin gap location is moved a number of times to reduce the hot and cold spots that arise with this technique. Figure 7.29 illustrates the dose distribution for three different field separations.[107]

Beam divergence may be eliminated by using a "beam splitter," created using a five- or six-HVL block over one-half of the treatment field. The central axes of the adjacent fields, where there is no divergence, are then matched. As previously discussed, this is a useful method on linacs with the asymmetric jaws feature. Match-line wedges or penumbra generators that generate a broad penumbra for linac beams have been reported but have not found widespread use.[108] Here the intent is to broaden the narrow penumbra of the linacs so that it is not so difficult to

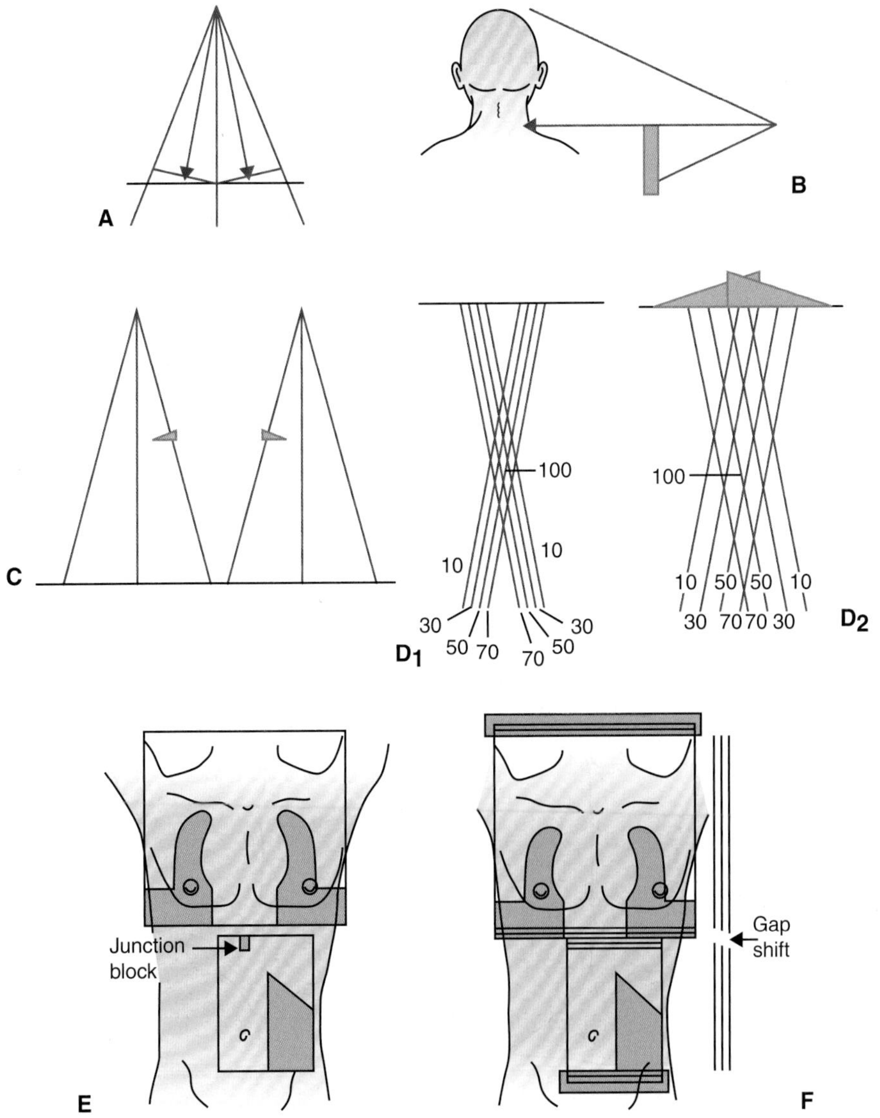

FIGURE 7.27. Different techniques for matching adjacent fields. **A:** Beam's central rays are angled slightly away from one another so that the diverging beams are parallel. **B:** Half-beam block to eliminate divergence. **C:** Penumbra generators (small wedges) to increase width of penumbra, as illustrated in **D₁** and **D₂**. **E:** Junction block over spinal cord. **F:** Moving gap technique. (From Bentel GC, ed. *Radiation therapy planning,* 2nd ed. New York: McGraw-Hill, 1996.)

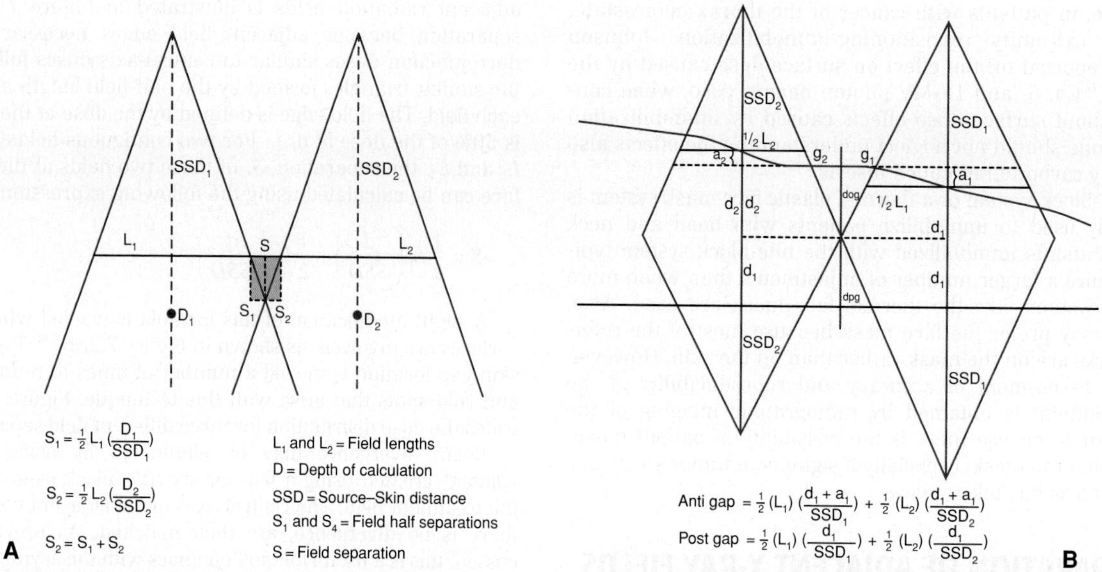

FIGURE 7.28. A: Standard formula for calculating the gap at the skin surface for a given depth using similar triangles. **B:** Modified formula for calculating the gap for matching four fields on a sloping surface. (From Keys RA, Grigsby PW. Gapping fields on sloping surfaces. *Int J Radiat Oncol Biol Phys* 1990;18:1183–1190.)

match the 50% isodose levels. The resulting dose distributions are similar to those obtained with a moving gap technique. Finally, there are several reports of edge-matching techniques based on the mathematical relationships between adjacent beams and the allowed angles of the gantry, collimators, and couch.[109]

Orthogonal Field Junctions

Figure 7.30 illustrates the geometry of matching abutting orthogonal photon beams. Such techniques are necessary, particularly in the head and neck region where the spinal cord can be in an area of beam overlap, in the treatment of medulloblastoma

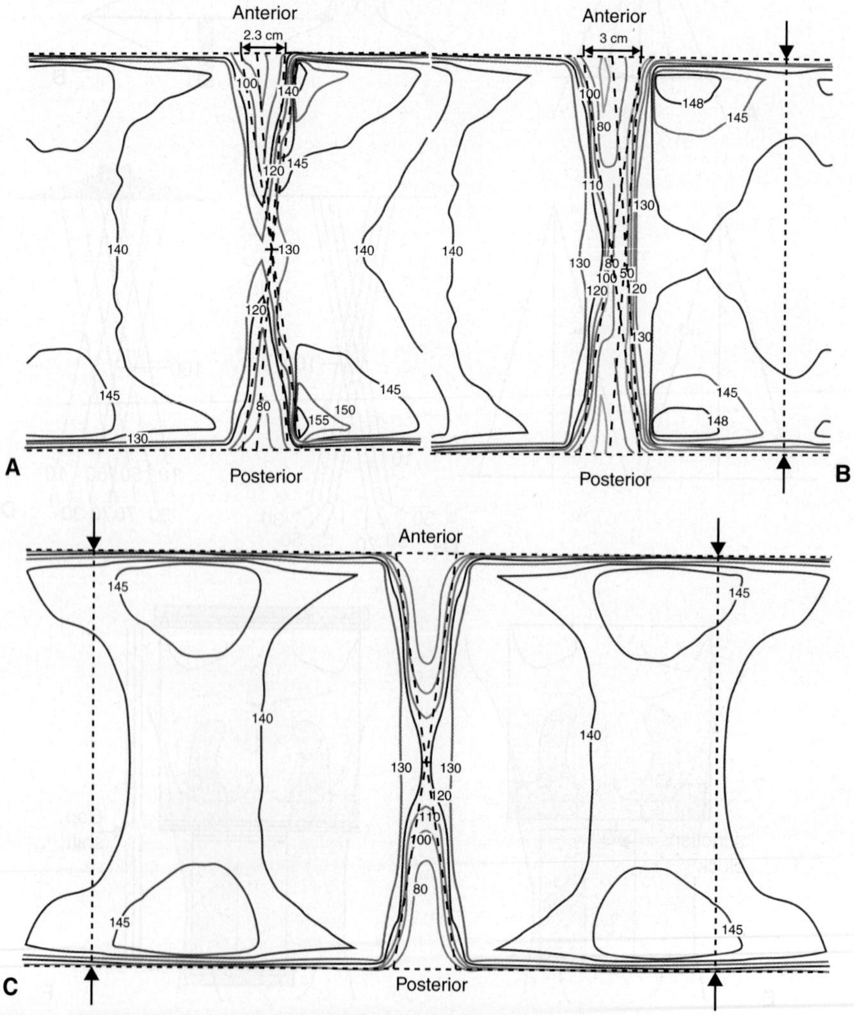

FIGURE 7.29. Dose distribution for geometric separation of fields with all four beams intersecting at midpoint. Adjacent field sizes: 30 × 30 cm and 15 × 15 cm; source-to-skin distance (SSD), 100 cm; anteroposterior thickness, 20 cm; 4-MV x-ray beams. **A:** Field separation at surface is 2.3 cm. A three-field overlap exists in this case because the fields have different sizes but the same SSD. **B:** The adjacent field separation increased to eliminate three-field overlap on the surface. **C:** Field separation adjusted to 2.7 cm to eliminate three-field overlap at the cord at 15 cm depth from anterior. (From Khan FM. *The physics of radiation therapy,* 2nd ed. Baltimore: Williams & Wilkins, 1994.)

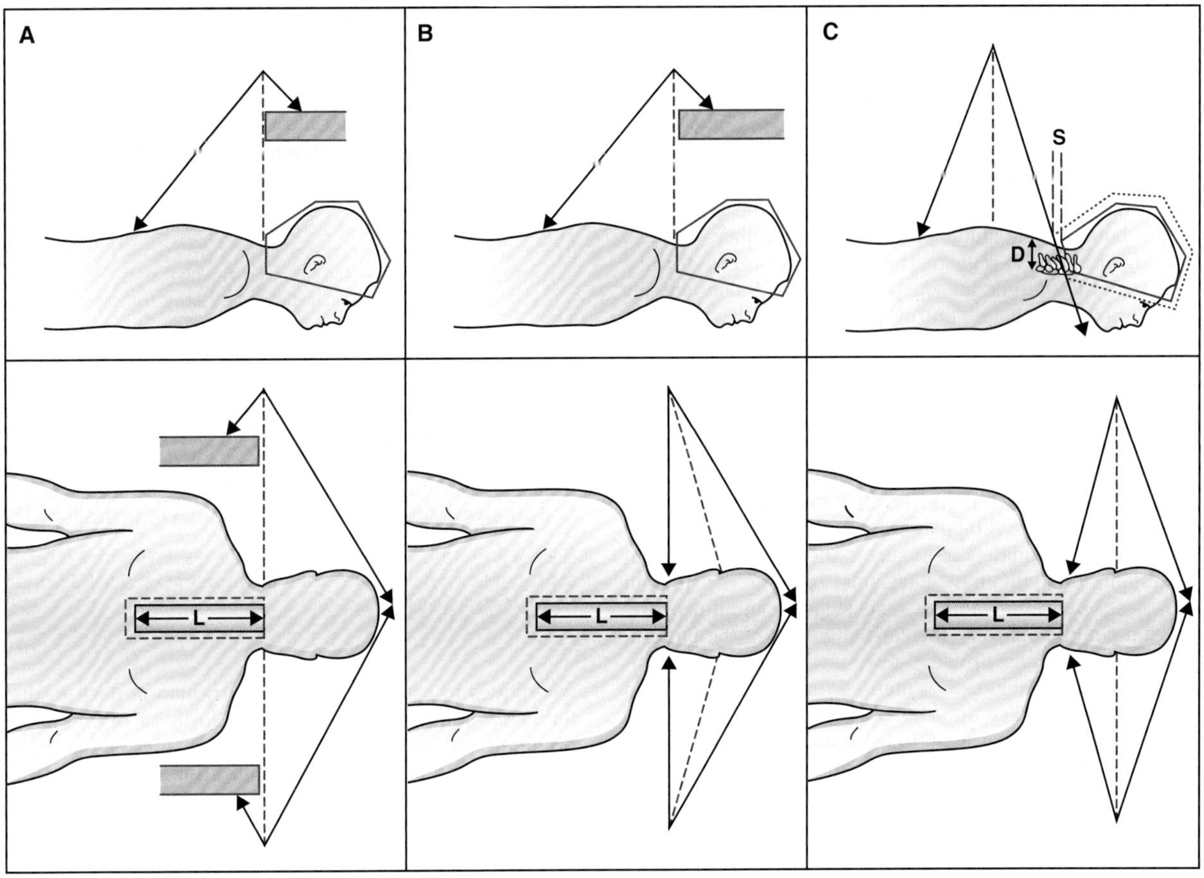

FIGURE 7.30. Some solutions for the problem of overlap for orthogonal fields. **A:** A beam splitter, a shield that blocks half of the field, is used on the lateral and posterior fields and on the spinal cord portal to match the nondivergent edges of the beams. **B:** The divergence in the lateral beams may also be removed by angling the lateral beams so that their caudal edges match. Because most therapy units cannot be angled like this, the couch is rotated through small angles in opposite directions to achieve the same effect. **C:** A gap technique allows the posterior and lateral field to be matched at depth using a gap *S* on the skin surface. The *dashed lines* indicate projected field edges at depth *D*, where the orthogonal fields meet. (From Williamson TJ. A technique for matching orthogonal megavoltage fields. *Int J Radiat Oncol Biol Phys* 1979;5:111.)

with multiple spinal portals and lateral brain portals. A common method of avoiding overlap is to use a half-block, as previously discussed, so that abutting anterior and lateral field edges are perpendicular to the gantry axis. In head and neck cancer, a notch in the posterior corner of the lateral oral cavity portal is commonly used to ensure overlap avoidance of the spinal cord when midline cord blocks cannot be used on anteroposterior portals irradiating the lower neck and matched to the oral cavity portals. Other techniques rotate the couch about a vertical axis to compensate for the divergence of the lateral field.[110] The angle of rotation is given by:

$$\tan \theta^{-1} = \left(\frac{\frac{1}{2}\text{field width}}{\text{SAD}} \right)$$

Another technique is to leave a gap, *S*, on the anterior neck surface between the posterior field of length *L* and lateral field edges.[111] *S* can be calculated using the following formula where d is the depth of the spine beneath the posterior field:

$$S = \frac{1}{2}(L)\left(\frac{\text{d}}{\text{SAD}}\right)$$

The potential for the occurrence of radiation myelopathy resulting from a potentially excessive dose from misaligned overlapping fields is always a concern when central nervous system tumors are treated. Craniospinal irradiation is well established as a standard method of treating suprasellar dysgerminoma, pineal tumors, medulloblastomas, and other tumors involving the central nervous system. Uniform treatment of the entire craniospinal target volume is possible using separate parallel-opposed lateral cranial portals rotated so that their inferior borders match with the superior border of the spinal portal, which is treated with either one or two fields, depending on the length of the spine to be treated.[112] Two junctional moves are typically made at one-third and two-thirds of the total dose. The spinal field central axis is shifted away from the brain by 0.5 cm and the field size length reduced by 0.5 cm with corresponding increases in the length of the cranial field, so that a match exists between the inferior border of the brain portal and the superior border of the spine portal. To achieve the match, a collimator rotation for the whole-brain portals must be done for an angle given by the following relationship:

$$\tan \theta^{-1} = \left(\frac{\frac{1}{2}\,\textit{spinal field length}}{\textit{SAD}} \right)$$

In addition, in order to eliminate the divergence between the cranial portal and spinal portal, the table is rotated through a floor angle given by the following relationship:

$$\tan \alpha^{-1} = \left(\frac{\frac{1}{2}\,\textit{cranial field length}}{\textit{SAD}} \right)$$

RADIATION THERAPY PATIENTS WITH CARDIAC PACEMAKERS

As the population ages, the likelihood of encountering patients with either a pacemaker or an implantable cardioverter–defibrillator (ICD) who require radiation therapy for chest and lower neck neoplasms has become commonplace. Pacemakers are electrical devices that may stimulate either the atria, ventricles, or both (single-chamber and dual-chamber models, respectively) in order to regulate the heart's natural rhythm.[113] ICDs are generally larger than pacemakers, and also actively shock the heart to help control life-threatening, irregular heartbeats, especially those that could cause sudden cardiac arrest; most new ICDs can act as both pacemakers and defibrillators.[114] Modern pacemakers and ICDs incorporate complementary metal oxide semiconductor (CMOS) circuitry into their generator units (encompassing a sealed lithium battery pack and circuitry only). Several groups have shown that these modern devices are much more sensitive to radiation than the older models that utilized bipolar transistor circuitry.[115–117]

To safely and adequately treat such patients, it is important to understand the potential effects of radiation therapy on these devices' operation and to take steps to minimize any actions that could jeopardize the cardiac health of the patient. The AAPM TG 34 Report provides a list of widely accepted clinical management guidelines.[118] Potential interactions between a functioning pacemaker and the radiation therapy environment fall into two categories: (a) electromagnetic noise interference (EMI) created by the treatment machine in the course of producing high-energy photon and electron beams, and (b) damage due to radiation. Most experts now believe category 1 is no longer a source of concern. However, dose and dose rate are very much a concern.[115,117] Modern pacemakers are radiosensitive and have a significant probability of failing catastrophically at radiation doses well below normal tissue tolerance and, therefore, should never be irradiated by the direct beam. Also, several authors have shown that recommended maximum doses obtained from manufacturers have not proven to be reliable and vary greatly among manufacturers.[119] A recent review by Hudson et al. provides the latest information and points out that radiation-induced device malfunctions are rare, and death associated with that malfunction is even more uncommon.[119] However, they conclude that the adequacy of published guidelines is not supported by hard data. They recommend that it is important to consider all aspects of radiation therapy treatment, not just accumulated dose. These include the effect of backscatter, dose rate, fractionation, and potential EMI with new technologies such as IMRT and respiratory gating. They recommend that each radiation oncology department employ their own policy for the management of patients with pacemakers and ICDs, potentially based on an updated standard national or international guideline similar to that released by the AAPM in 1994 (Table 7.2).

TABLE 7.2 MANAGEMENT GUIDELINES FOR RADIATION THERAPY PATIENTS WITH CARDIAC PACEMAKERS

1. Pacemaker-implanted patients should never be treated with a betatron.
2. Have the patient's coronary and pacemaker status evaluated by a cardiologist before and soon after completion of therapy.
3. Always keep the pacemaker outside the machine-collimated radiation beam, both during treatment and when taking portal films.
4. Carefully observe the patient during the first therapy session to verify that no transient malfunctions are occurring and during subsequent treatments if magnetron or klystron misfiring (sparking) occurs.
5. Before treatment, estimate and record the dose (from scatter) to be received by the pacemaker. The total accumulated dose should not exceed approximately 2 Gy.
6. If treatment within these guidelines is not possible, the physician should consider having the pacemaker either temporarily or permanently moved before irradiation.
7. If a patient has an automatic implantable cardioverter–defibrillator (AICD), the physicist should follow the same steps as one would for pacemakers in contacting the manufacturer and simultaneously ascertaining the dose expected to the AICD. If there is no manufacturer information concerning radiation effects to the ACID, a conservative threshold of 100 cGy should be considered.

Modified from Marbach JR, Sontag MR, Van Dyk J, et al. Management of radiation oncology patients with implanted cardiac pacemakers: report of AAPM Task Group No. 34. *Med Phys* 1994;21(1):85–90.

FETAL DOSE

Radiation therapy is standard treatment for several malignancies (e.g., Hodgkin lymphoma, breast cancer) in which the population of women is often of childbearing age. The issues are complex, and the patient along with the radiation oncologist must evaluate treatment risk to the fetus in such cases. Radiation effects to the fetus are not fully understood and cannot be comfortably predicted for each individual case. If the decision is to irradiate, the dose levels outside the treatment fields should be quantified, and every effort should be made to lower the dose to the fetus. This may require changes in irradiation technique (i.e., modified mantle fields), elimination of double-exposure portal images, and the addition of special patient shields. The AAPM TG 36 Report provides data and techniques to estimate and reduce radiation dose to the fetus for beam energies ranging from ^{60}Co to 18 MV.[120] Before the pregnant patient is treated, the pregnancy stage should be known to estimate the size and location of the fetus throughout the treatment. Dose-estimation points should be selected that allow estimation of dose throughout the fetus (e.g., fundus, symphysis pubis, and umbilicus).

Two methods can be used to reduce the dose to the fetus, namely, modification of treatment techniques and the use of special shields. Modifications include changing field angle (avoiding placement of the gantry close to the fetus, i.e., treatment of a posterior field with the patient lying prone on a false tabletop), reducing field size, choosing a different radiation energy (avoiding ^{60}Co because of high leakage or energies of >10 MV because of neutrons), and using tertiary collimation to define the field edge nearest to the fetus. When shields are designed, the shielding device must allow for treatment fields above the diaphragm and on the lower extremities. Safety to the patient and personnel is a primary consideration in shield design. As part of the management of a pregnant patient, the treatment planning tasks listed in Table 7.3 should be performed to ensure that the dose to the fetus is kept to a minimum.[120]

It should be noted that the aforementioned AAPM TG Report was based on treatment machines that predated modern MLCs. One study showed that the use of tertiary MLC systems such as those found on Varian linacs actually reduced fetal dose during irradiation of a pregnant patient.[121] The leaf and carriage system provided some absorption, and if the MLC leaves were oriented in direction along the plane of concern, such as typically when a patient with Hodgkin's disease is treated (i.e., leaves oriented along the length of the table), the reduction difference when compared to having no MLCs was on the order of 2.5 to 3.

GONADAL DOSE

Many of the reports used to estimate peripheral dose and fetal dose apply to dose estimations to both testes and ovaries.[122,123] Simultaneously, there have been studies to determine the genetically significant dose (GSD) as it applies to peripheral radiotherapy dosage to ovaries and testes. Niroomand-Rad and Cumberlin[124] combined measured data and GSD data to determine the GSD for particular treatment techniques that deliver peripheral dose to ovaries and testes. They summarized that

TABLE 7.3 TREATMENT-PLANNING TASKS TO ENSURE THAT DOSE TO THE FETUS IS KEPT TO A MINIMUM

1. Complete all planning as though the patient were not pregnant.
2. Consider modifications of the plan that would minimize the fetal dose (e.g., changing field size and angle, using a different energy).
3. Estimate dose to fetus without shielding using a phantom or data from the AAPM report.[120]
4. Design and construct special shielding if necessary; four or five HVLs of lead usually suffice.
5. Measure dose to fetus in a phantom during simulated treatment with shielding in place.
6. Document the treatment plan and discuss the treatment with all personnel involved with the treatment.
7. Check all aspects of safety, including the load-bearing limits of the couch and support and movement of the shields, to ensure that there will be no injury to the patient or to personnel. The setup of each field should be photographed for documentation.
8. Monitor fetal size and location throughout the course of therapy and update estimates of fetal dose if necessary.
9. Document the completion of treatment by estimating the total dose to the fetus due to the radiation therapy.

Modified from Stovall M, Blackwell CR, Cundiff J, et al. Fetal dose from radiotherapy with photon beams: report of AAPM Radiation Therapy Committee Task Group No. 36. *Med Phys* 1995;22:63–82.

GSDs from conventional therapies are minimal. However, there are circumstances, such as treatment of seminoma, when it is necessary to use a testicular shield to surround the testes to reduce head scatter and leakage, and some internal scatter.[125]

SELECTED REFERENCES

A full list of references for this chapter is available online.

2. Herring DF. The consequences of dose response curves for tumor control and normal tissue injury on the precision necessary in patient management. *Laryngos* 1975;85:119–125.
4. Mackie RT, Liu HH, McCullough EC. Treatment planning algorithms: model-based photon dose calculations. In: Khan FM, ed. *Treatment planning in radiation oncology*, 2nd ed. Philadelphia: Lippincott Williams & Wilkins, 2007:63–77.
5. Ahnesjö A, Aspradakis MM. Dose calculations for external photon beams in radiotherapy. *Phys Med Biol* 1999;44:R99–R155.
6. Khan FM, Sewchand W, Lee J, et al. Revision of tissue-maximum ratio and scatter-maximum ratio concepts for cobalt 60 and higher energy x-ray beams. *Med Phys* 1980;7:230–237.
7. International Commission on Radiation Units and Measurements. *ICRU Report 24: determination of absorbed dose in a patient irradiated by beams of X or gamma rays in radiotherapy procedures.* Washington, DC: International Commission on Radiation Units and Measurements, 1976.
8. Batho HF. Lung corrections in Cobalt 60 beam therapy. *J Can Assoc Radiol* 1964; 15:79–83.
9. Young MEJ, Gaylord JD. Experimental tests of corrections for tissue inhomogeneities in radiotherapy. *Br J Radiol* 1970;43:349–355.
10. Sontag MR, Cunningham JR. Corrections to absorbed dose calculations for tissue inhomogeneities. *Med Phys* 1977;4:431–436.
11. Mackie TR, Scrimger JW, Battista JJ. A convolution method of calculating dose for 15-MV x-rays. *Med Phys* 1985;12:188–196.
12. Chetty IJ, Curran B, Cygler JE, et al. Report of the AAPM Task Group No. 105: issues associated with clinical implementation of Monte Carlo-based photon and electron external beam treatment planning. *Med Phys* 2007;34(12):4818–4853.
13. Verhaegen F, Seuntjens J. Monte Carlo modelling of external radiotherapy photon beams (Topical Review). *Phys Med Biol* 2003;48(21):R107–R164.
14. Ahnesjö A, Andreo P, Brahme A. Calculation and application of point spread functions for treatment planning with high energy photon beams. *Acta Oncol* 1987;26:49–56.
16. Ahnesjö A. Collapsed cone convolution of radiant energy for photon dose calculation in heterogeneous media. *Med Phys* 1989;16:577–592.
17. Siebers JV, Keall PJ, Kawrakow I. Monte Carlo dose calculations for external beam radiation therapy. In: Dyk JV, ed. *The modern technology of radiation oncology—a compendium for medical physicists and radiation oncologists,* vol 2. Madison, WI: Medical Physics Publishing, 2005:91–130.
18. Cygler JE, Daskalov GM, Chan GH, et al. Evaluation of the first commercial Monte Carlo dose calculation engine for electron beam treatment planning. *Med Phys* 2004;31(1):142–153.
19. American Association of Physicists in Medicine. *Report 85: tissue inhomogeneity corrections for megavoltage photon beams: report of Task Group 65 of the Radiation Therapy Committee.* Madison, WI: Medical Physics Publishing, 2004.
20. Frank SJ, Forster KM, Stevens CW, et al. Treatment planning for lung cancer: traditional homogeneous point-dose prescription compared with heterogeneity-corrected dose-volume prescription. *Int J Radiat Oncol Biol Phys* 2003;56(5): 1308–1318.
21. Davidson SE, Popple RA, Ibbott GS, et al. Heterogeneity dose calculation accuracy in IMRT: study of the commercial treatment planning systems using an anthropomorphic thorax phantom. *Med Phys* 2008;35:5434–5439.
22. Gibbons JP, ed. *Monitor unit calculations for external photon and electron beams.* Madison, WI: Advanced Medical Publishing, 2000.
23. Georg D, Huekelom S, Venselaar J. Formalisms for MU calculations, ESTRO booklet 3 versus NCS report 12. *Radiother Oncol* 2001;60(3):319–328.
24. Stern RL, Heaton R, Fraser MW, et al. Verification of monitor unit calculations for non-IMRT clinical radiotherapy: report of AAPM Task Group 114. *Med Phys* 2011;38(1):504–530.
25. Central axis depth dose data for use in radiotherapy. *Br J Radiol* 1996;25(Suppl).
26. Cundiff JH, Cunningham JR, Golden R, et al. A method for the calculation of dose in the radiation treatment of Hodgkin's disease. *Am J Roentgenol* 1973;117:30–44.
27. Cunningham JR. Scatter-air ratios. *Phys Med Biol* 1972;17:42–51.
29. Rosenberg I, Chu JC, Saxena V. Calculation of monitor units for a linear accelerator with asymmetric jaws. *Med Phys* 1995;22:55–61.
30. Slessinger ED, Gerber RG, Harms WB, et al. Independent collimator dosimetry for a dual photon energy linear accelerator. *Int J Radiat Oncol Biol Phys* 1993;27(3):681–687.
31. Palta JR, Ayyangar KM, Suntharalingam N. Dosimetric characteristics of a 6 MV photon beam from a linear accelerator with asymmetric collimator jaws. *Int J Radiat Oncol Biol Phys* 1988;14:383–387.
33. Klein EE, Harms WB, Low DA, et al. Clinical implementation of a commercial multileaf collimator: dosimetry, networking, simulation, and quality assurance. *Int J Radiat Oncol Biol Phys* 1995;33:1195–1208.
34. Palta JR, Yeung DK, Frouhar V. Dosimetric considerations for a multileaf collimator system. *Med Phys* 1996;23(7):1219–1224.
35. Jordan TJ, Williams PC. The design and performance characteristics of a multileaf collimator. *Phys Med Biol* 1994;39:231–251.
36. Das IJ, Desobry GE, McNeeley SW, et al. Beam characteristics of a retrofitted double-focused multileaf collimator. *Med Phys* 1998;25(9):1676–1684.
37. Boyer A, Biggs P, Galvin J, et al. AAPM report 72: basic applications of multileaf collimators, report of Task Group 50. Published for the American Association of Physicists in Medicine. Madison, WI: Medical Physics Publishing, 2001.
38. Hanson WF, Berkley LW. Calculative technique to correct for the change in linear accelerator beam energy at off-axis points. *Med Phys* 1980;7(2):147–150.
40. Otto K. Volumetric modulated arc therapy: IMRT in a single gantry arc. *Med Phys* 2008;35(1):310–317.
41. Bedford JL, Warrington AP. Commissioning of volumetric modulated arc therapy (VMAT). *Int J Radiat Oncol Biol Phys* 2009;73(2):537–545.
42. Rao M, Yang W, Chen F, et al. Comparison of Elekta VMAT with helical tomotherapy and fixed field IMRT: plan quality, delivery efficiency and accuracy. *Med Phys* 2010;37(3):1350–1359.
43. Ling CC, Zhang P, Archambault Y, et al. Commissioning and quality assurance of RapidArc radiotherapy delivery system. *Int J Radiat Oncol Biol Phys* 2008; 72(2):575–581.
45. Yu CX, Tang G. Intensity-modulated arc therapy: principles, technologies and clinical implementation. *Phys Med Biol* 2011;56(5):R31–R54.
47. Mehta M, Hoban P, Mackie TR. Commissioning and quality assurance of RapidArc radiotherapy delivery system: in regard to Ling et al. (*Int J Radiat Oncol Biol Phys* 2008;72:575–581): absence of data does not constitute proof; the proof is in tasting the pudding. *Int J Radiat Oncol Biol Phys* 2009;75(1):4–6.
48. Kung JH, Chen GTY, Kuchnir FK. A monitor unit verification calculation in intensity modulated radiotherapy as a dosimetry quality assurance. *Med Phys* 2000;27(10):2226–2230.
49. Yang Y, Xing L, Li JG, et al. Independent dosimetric calculation with inclusion of head scatter and MLC transmission for IMRT. *Med Phys* 2003;30(11):2937–2947.
50. Purdy JA. Buildup/surface dose and exit dose measurements for 6-MV linear accelerator. *Med Phys* 1986;13:259.
52. Gerbi BJ, Meigooni A, Khan FM. Dose buildup for obliquely incident photon beams. *Med Phys* 1987;14:393–399.
53. Klein EE, Purdy JA. Entrance and exit dose regions for Clinac-2100 C. *Int J Radiat Oncol Biol Phys* 1993;27:429–435.
54. Cunningham JR. Tissue inhomogeneity corrections in photon-beam treatment planning. In: C.G. Orton, ed. *Progress in medical physics,* vol 1. New York: Plenum Press, 1982:103–131.
55. Kornelsen RO, Young MEJ. Changes in the dose-profile of a 10 MV x-ray beam within and beyond low density material. *Med Phys* 1982;9:114–116.
56. Epp ER, Lougheed MN, McKay JW. Ionization build-up in upper respiratory air passages during teletherapy units with cobalt-60 irradiation. *Br J Radiol* 1958;31:361.
57. Epp ER, Boyer AL, Doppke KP. Underdosing of lesions resulting from lack of electronic equilibrium in upper respiratory air cavities irradiated by 10 MV x-ray beams. *Int J Radiat Oncol Biol Phys* 1977;2:613.
59. Rice RK, Mijnheer BJ, Chin LM. Benchmark measurements for lung dose corrections for x-ray beams. *Int J Radiat Oncol Biol Phys* 1988;15:399–409.
60. Das IJ, Kase KR, Meigooni AS, et al. Validity of transition-zone dosimetry at high atomic number interfaces in megavoltage photon beams. *Med Phys* 1990; 17(1):10–16.
61. Sibata CH, Mota HC, Hoggins PD, et al. Influence of hip prostheses on high energy photon dose distribution. *Int J Radiat Oncol Biol Phys* 1990;18:455–461.
62. Thatcher M. Perturbation of Cobalt 60 radiation doses by metal objects implanted during oral and maxillofacial surgery. *J Oral Maxillofac Surg* 1984;42:108–110.
63. Niroomand-Rad A, Razavi R, Thobejane S, et al. Radiation dose perturbation at tissue-titanium dental interfaces in head and neck cancer patients. *Int J Radiat Oncol Biol Phys* 1996;34(2):475–480.
64. Reft C, Alecu R, Das IJ, et al. Dosimetric considerations for patients with HIP prostheses undergoing pelvic irradiation. Report of the AAPM Radiation Therapy Committee Task Group 63. *Med Phys* 2003;30(6):1162–1182.
65. Klein EE, Kuske RR. Changes in photon dosimetry due to breast prosthesis. *Int J Radiat Oncol Biol Phys* 1993;25(3):541–549.
66. Tatcher M. A method for varying effective angle of wedge filters. *Radiology* 1970; 97:132.
68. Petti PL, Siddon RL. Effective wedge angles with a universal wedge. *Phys Med Biol* 1985;30(9):985–991.
69. McCullough EC, Gortney J, Blackwell CR. A depth dependence determination of the wedge transmission factor for 4-10 MV photon beams. *Med Phys* 1988; 15:621–623.
70. Sewchand W, Khan FM, Williamson J. Variations in depth-dose data between open and wedge fields for 4-MV x rays. *Radiology* 1978;127:789–792.
71. Abrath FG, Purdy JA. Wedge design and dosimetry for 25-MV x rays. *Radiology* 1980;136:757–762.

72. Leavitt DD, Martin M, Moeller JH, et al. Dynamic wedge field techniques through computer-controlled collimator motion and dose delivery. *Med Phys* 1990;17: 87–91.
73. Klein EE, Low DA, Meigooni AS, et al. Dosimetry and clinical implementation of dynamic wedge. *Int J Radiat Oncol Biol Phys* 1995;31:583–592.
78. Georg D, Knöös T, McClean B. Current status and future perspective of flattening filter free photon beams. *Med Phys* 2011;38(3):1280–1293.
79. Emami B, Lyman J, Brown A, et al. Tolerance of normal tissue to therapeutic irradiation. *Int J Radiat Oncol Biol Phys* 1991;21:109–122.
80. Marks LB, Ten Haken RK, Martel MK. Guest editor's introduction to QUANTEC: a users guide. *Int J Radiat Oncol Biol Phys* 2010;76(3, Suppl 1):S1–S2.
81. Rosenow UF, Valentine ES, Davis LW. A technique for treating local breast cancer using a single set-up point and asymmetric collimation. *Int J Radiat Oncol Biol Phys* 1990;19:183–188.
83. Klein EE, Taylor M, Michaletz-Lorenz M, et al. A mono-isocentric technique for breast and regional nodal therapy using dual asymmetric jaws. *Int J Radiat Oncol Biol Phys* 1994;28:753–760.
85. Sohn JW, Suh JH, Pohar S. A method for delivering accurate and uniform radiation dosages to the head and neck with asymmetric collimators and a single isocenter. *Int J Radiat Oncol Biol Phys* 1995;32:809–814.
86. Takahaski S. Conformation radiotherapy-rotation techniques as applied to radiography and radiotherapy of cancer. *Acta Radiol Suppl* 1965;242: 1–142.
87. Hounsell AR, Sharrock PJ, Moore CJ, et al. Computer-assisted generation of multileaf collimator settings for conformation therapy. *Br J Radiol* 1992;65: 321–326.
89. Boyer AL, Ochran TG, Nyerick CE, et al. Clinical dosimetry for implementation of a multileaf collimator. *Med Phys* 1992;19(5):1255–1261.
90. Powlis WD, Smith AR, Cheng E, et al. Initiation of multileaf collimator conformal radiation therapy. *Int J Radiat Oncol Biol Phys* 1993;25:171–179.
91. LoSasso T, Kutcher GJ. Multi-leaf collimation vs. Cerrobend blocks: analysis of geometric accuracy. *Int J Radiat Oncol Biol Phys* 1995;32:499–506.
92. Zhu Y, Boyer AL, Desorby GE. Dose distributions of x-ray fields as shaped with multileaf collimators. *Phys Med Biol* 1992;37:163–173.
93. LoSasso T, Chui CS, Kutcher GJ. The use of a multi-leaf collimator for conformal radiotherapy of carcinomas of the prostate and nasopharynx. *Int J Radiat Oncol Biol Phys* 1993;25:161–170.
94. Brahme A. Optimization of stationary and moving beam radiation therapy techniques. *Radiother Oncol* 1988;12:129–140.
95. Du MN, Yu CX, Symons M, et al. A multi-leaf collimator prescription preparation system for conventional radiotherapy. *Int J Radiat Oncol Biol Phys* 1995;32: 513–520.
96. Powers WE, Kinzie JJ, Demidecki AJ, et al. A new system of field shaping for external-beam radiation therapy. *Radiology* 1973;108:407–411.
97. Leavitt DD, Gibbs FA Jr. Field shaping. In: Purdy JA, ed. *Advances in radiation oncology physics: dosimetry, treatment planning, and brachytherapy.* New York: American Institute of Physics, 1992:500–523.
98. Huen A, Findley DO, Skov DD. Attenuation in Lipowitz's metal of x-rays produced at 2, 4, 10, and 18 MV and gamma rays from cobalt-60. *Med Phys* 1979;6:147–148.
99. Ellis F, Hall EJ, Oliver R. A compensator for variations in tissue thickness for high energy beams. *Br J Radiol* 1959;32:421–422.
101. Chang SX, Cullip TJ, Deschesne KM, et al. Compensators: an alternative IMRT delivery technique. *J Appl Clin Med Phys* 2004;5(3):15–36.
102. Humphries SM, Boyd K, Cornish P, et al. Comparison of super stuff and paraffin wax bolus in radiation therapy of irregular surfaces. *Med Dosimetry* 1996; 21(3):155–157.
104. Johnson MW, Griggs MA, Sharma SC. A comparison of surface doses for two immobilizing systems. *Med Dosimetry* 1995;20(3):191–194.
105. Higgins DM, Whitehurst P, Morgan AM. The effect of carbon fiber couch inserts on surface dose with beam size variation. *Med Dosimetry* 2001;26(3): 251–254.
106. Keys R, Grigsby PW. Gapping fields on sloping surfaces. *Int J Radiat Oncol Biol Phys* 1990;18:1183–1190.
107. Johnson JM, Khan FM. Dosimetric effects of abutting extended source to surface distance electron fields with photon fields in the treatment of head and neck cancers. *Int J Radiat Oncol Biol Phys* 1994;28:741–747.
108. Fraass BA, Tepper JE, Glatstein E, et al. Clinical use of a match line wedge for adjacent megavoltage radiation field matching. *Int J Radiat Oncol Biol Phys* 1983;9:209–216.
109. Christopherson D, Courlas GJ, Jette D. Field matching in radiotherapy. *Med Phys* 1984;3:369.
110. Siddon RL, Tonnesen GL, Svensson GK. Three-field techniques for breast treatment using a rotatable half-beam block. *Int J Radiat Oncol Biol Phys* 1981; 7:1473–1477.
111. Williamson TJ. A technique for matching orthogonal megavoltage fields. *Int J Radiat Oncol Biol Phys* 1979;5:111.
112. Lim MLF. A study of four methods of junction change in the treatment of medulloblastoma. *Am Assoc Med Dosim J* 1985;10:17–24.
115. Hurkmans CW, Scheepers E, Springorum BGF, et al. Influence of radiotherapy on the latest generation of implantable cardioverter-defibrillators. *Int J Radiat Oncol Biol Phys* 2005;63(1):282.
118. Marbach JR, Sontag MR, Van Dyk J, et al. Management of radiation oncology patients with implanted cardiac pacemakers: report of AAPM Task Group No. 34. *Med Phys* 1994;21(1):85–90.
119. Hudson F, Coulshed D, D'Souza E, et al. Effect of radiation therapy on the latest generation of pacemakers and implantable cardioverter defibrillators: a systematic review. *J Med Imaging Radiat Oncol* 2010;54(1):53–61.
120. Stovall M, Blackwell CR, Cundiff J, et al. Fetal dose from radiotherapy with photon beams: report of AAPM Radiation Therapy Committee Task Group No. 36. *Med Phys* 1995;22:63–82.
122. Francois P, Beurtheret C, Dutreix A. Calculation of the dose delivered to organs outside the radiation beams. *Med Phys* 1988;15(6):879–883.
123. van der Giessen PH. A simple and generally applicable method to estimate the peripheral dose in radiation teletherapy with high energy x-rays or gamma radiation. *Int J Radiat Oncol Biol Phys* 1996;35(5):1059–1068.
124. Niroomand-Rad A, Cumberlin RL. Measured dose to ovaries and testes from Hodgkin's fields and determination of genetically significant dose. *Int J Radiat Oncol Biol Phys* 1993;25(4):745–751.
125. Fraass BA, Kinsella TJ, Harrington ES, et al. Peripheral dose to the testes: the design and clinical use of a practical and effective gonadal shield. *Int J Radiat Oncol Biol Phys* 1985;11(3):609–616.

Chapter 8
Electron-Beam Therapy Dosimetry, Treatment Planning, and Techniques

Eric E. Klein and Rojano Kashani

Megavoltage-photon–based radiation therapy treatment of shallow tumor volumes is complicated by the buildup and radiation transport properties of megavoltage beams. These beams are capable of treating both shallow and deep tumors; however, when treating shallow tumors, the radiation beams transit through the entire patient, exposing distal normal tissues. Megavoltage electron beams have the property of a finite range and therefore do not deliver significant radiation doses to distal depths. Electron-beam therapy is therefore suitable for shallow tumors (<5 cm deep), such as head and neck cancers, skin and lip cancers, chest wall irradiation for breast cancer, and boost dose to nodes. Electrons will typically provide dose uniformity in these target volumes, with minimal dose to distal organs. In fact, G.H. Fletcher[1] had gone as far as saying, "there is no alternative treatment to electron-beam therapy." Even the strongest proponents of photon or proton therapy acknowledge that electron therapy is necessary to complete any radiotherapy program.

In 1976, Tapley[2] published one of the earlier comprehensive treatises on electron radiation therapy, in which she states, "There is no practical way for every radiation therapy department, either in hospitals or private offices, to be equipped with all modalities of irradiation beams. Ideally, electron beams should be available for those clinical situations where electrons are indispensable or very clearly superior." Electrons are now used at most radiation therapy centers. It still might be advantageous to refer patients to regional centers for special treatment techniques utilizing electrons.

Since the late 1970s, there have been three developments in electron-beam radiation therapy technology that have improved significantly our ability to deliver electron therapy. First, the advent of computed tomography (CT)-based treatment planning allowed for coverage of the planning target volume (PTV) by the therapeutic dose and the dose to normal tissues and structures to be more accurately assessed. Use of CT provides a physical description of the anatomy, which is required for accurate dose calculations.[3,4] Second, the development of the electron pencil-beam algorithms (PBAs) and their implementation into treatment-planning systems in the early 1980s provided a mechanism for accurately calculating dose.[5,6]

More recently, the use of Monte Carlo calculations has moved development to commercial platforms.[7] They have demonstrated high degrees of accuracy, especially with the presence of inhomogeneties. Third, manufacturers have refined the quality of their electron beams (i.e., depth dose, off-axis uniformity, and penumbral width) by providing dual-scattering foil systems and electron applicators. Klein et al.[8] describe dosimetric improvement with the most recent Varian electron-beam delivery system. Presently, the differences in the electron-beam dose characteristics of various radiation therapy machines from different vendors are minimal. More recently, Kashani et al.[9] described electron-beam characteristics of a new configured beam line in the Varian TrueBeam machine.

Electron-beam therapy is advantageous because it delivers a reasonably uniform dose from the surface to a specific depth, after which dose falls off rapidly, eventually to a near-zero value. The depth of treatment is controlled by selecting the appropriate energy and, when necessary, the bolus thickness. Using electron beams with energies up to 20 MeV allows disease within approximately 6 cm of the surface to be treated effectively, sparing distal normal tissues.

Electron-beam therapy is useful in treating cancer of the skin and lips, upper respiratory and digestive tract, head and neck,[10,11] breast, and a variety of other sites.[2,12,13] Treatment sites of the skin include the eyelids, nose, ear,[14] scalp,[2,15] and more widely spread diseases of the limbs (e.g., melanoma and lymphoma)[16] or total skin (e.g., mycosis fungoides).[17,18] Treatment sites of the upper respiratory and digestive tract include the floor of mouth, soft palate, retromolar trigone, and salivary glands.[10,19] Treatments of the breast include chest wall irradiation following mastectomy[2,20,21]; nodal irradiation, often internal mammary chain (IMC) and occasionally axillary; and boost to the surgical bed following mastectomy or lumpectomy.[22] Current techniques of using tangential photon adjunct fields abutting supraclavicular and posterior axillary fields are difficult enough without the addition of treating a separate medial breast internal mammary field with a mixture of photon and electrons. Other sites of electron-beam therapy include the retina,[23] orbit,[24] paraspinal muscles,[3,25] pancreas and other abdominal structures (intraoperative therapy),[26] vulva,[27] and cervix (intracavitary irradiation).[28]

The purpose of this chapter is to discuss the treatment and treatment-planning techniques necessary to deliver the most effective electron-beam therapy. This requires a basic knowledge of dose distribution in water, dose in the heterogeneous patient, treatment-planning tools and principles, and special techniques using electron beams.

DOSE DISTRIBUTION IN WATER

To appreciate the clinical use of electron beams, their dose distributions in water must be understood. Understanding the properties of depth dose, off-axis ratios (OARs), and two-dimensional (2D) isodose contour plots will clarify the concept of dose distribution in water. As well, an understanding of the dependence of the dose distribution on incident energy, field size, and source-to-surface distance (SSD) is required. It is assumed that the dose distribution for a specified energy, field size, and SSD is machine dependent. Applicator design may have a minor influence on dose distributions.

Depth Dose

This section discusses percentage of dose (values are normalized to 100% at the depth of dose maximum, R_{100}) versus depth in water. Central-axis depth dose implies that the electron field is symmetric about the central axis, and the focus initially will be on square fields. Electron depth dose varies with field size; however, once the field reaches a certain size, side-scatter equilibrium is achieved, and further increasing the size has an insignificant effect on depth dose.[29,30] In the energy range of up to 20 MeV, a 10 by 10 cm^2 field size typically will achieve side-scatter equilibrium on central axis. The energy dependence of depth dose is illustrated in Figure 8.1, where central-axis depth dose is plotted for a 10 by 10 cm^2 field for energies in the range of 7 to 18 MeV. The family of curves illustrates how the dosimetric characteristics vary with the incident electron energy:

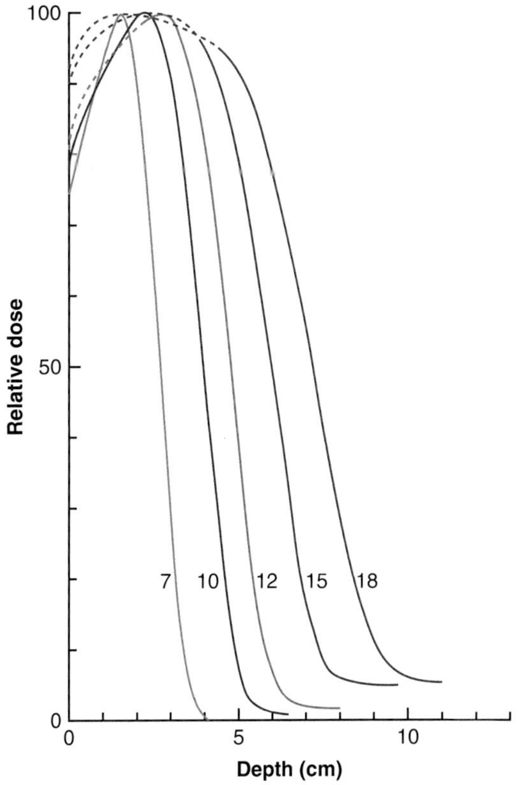

FIGURE 8.1. Energy dependence of depth dose. Plot of relative dose (%) versus depth for a 10 by 10 cm^2 field size for 7- to 18-MeV beams on a Siemens Mevatron 77 radiation therapy unit (source-to-surface distance, or SSD = 100 cm). (From Meyer JA, Palta JR, Hogstrom KR. Demonstration of relatively new electron dosimetry measurement techniques on the Mevatron 80. *Med Phys* 1984;11:670–677, with permission.)

1. Surface dose (D_s) increases from approximately 75% to 95% as energy increases. The slow increase in dose from the surface to the depth of maximum dose (R_{100}) occurs as a result of electrons undergoing multiple Coulomb scattering in water.[29]
2. Depth of distal 90% (R_{90}), often the therapeutic prescription depth, increases as energy increases.
3. The practical range (R_p) (maximum penetration) of the electrons increases as energy increases.
4. X-ray dose attributable to bremsstrahlung that lies beyond the electron dose component is characterized by its value (D_x) and is taken from the PDD curve 10 cm beyond the practical range (R_p). D_x increases as energy increases. Machines are designed to provide Rx values less than 5%.
5. The R_{100} depth (dmax) can vary irregularly with depth and model of electron treatment machine; its dependence is insignificant for treatment planning, although it is significant to the medical physicist for constructing percent depth–dose data and in beam calibration.

Table 8.1 gives dosimetric parameters for a modern (Triology, Varian) linear accelerator.

Depth dose has a significant dependence on field size, which varies with incident electron energy. The primary reason for the field-size dependence is loss of side-scatter equilibrium,

TABLE 8.1 VARIAN TRILOGY MEASURED ELECTRON DEPTHS (R_P, R_{50}) AND CALCULATED ENERGIES (E_P, E_0)

Nominal Energy	*Measured E_o (MeV)*	*Measured E_p (MeV)*	*R_{90}: Depth of 90% (cm)*	*R_{50}: Depth of 50% (cm)*	*R_p (cm)*	*Dx (%)*
6	5.55	6.08	1.53	2.38	2.95	0.1
9	8.41	8.84	2.69	3.61	4.33	0.3
12	11.77	12.23	3.85	5.05	6.02	0.9
16	15.63	16.02	5.10	6.71	7.900	1.6
20	19.62	20.78	6.14	8.42	10.25	2.1

E_0: Average energy at the surface, where $E_0 = 2.33 \times R_{50}$.

E_p: Most probable electron energy at the surface, where $E_p = C_1 + C_2 R_p = C_3 R_p^2$; where C1, C2, and C3 are constants, with C1 = 0.22 MeV, C2 = 1.98 MeV cm^1, and C3 = 0.01025 MeV cm^2.

which has been discussed in detail by Hogstrom[29] and Kahn et al.[30] Figure 8.2, which shows the field-size dependence of percentage depth dose at 9 and 20 MeV, clearly illustrates that it is a greater issue at higher energies. Loss of side-scatter equilibrium, which begins first at the deeper depths, results in R_{90} shifting toward the surface as field size decreases. As the field size gets even smaller, the maximum dose decreases, and when it is normalized to 100%, the relative dose at the surface, D_s, increases. In addition, the effects on the distal portion of the depth–dose curve are greater. The most clinically significant effect is the decrease in R_{90} with decreasing field size, which can require a greater energy than initially proposed for treatment using very small fields (<5 cm).

Depth–dose variations with SSD are usually minimal. Differences in the depth dose resulting from inverse square effect are small because electrons do not penetrate that deep (≤6 cm in the therapeutic region) and because the significant growth of penumbra width with SSD restricts the SSD in clinical practice to typically 115 cm or less. The primary effect of inverse square is that R_{90} penetrates a few millimeters deeper at extended SSD at the higher energies, as illustrated in Figure 8.3. In relatively few cases (e.g., when the electron beam has a large component of collimator-scattered electrons), the variation in depth dose with SSD can become more significant. In such cases, the collimator-scattered electrons are scattered out of the beam, resulting in a depth dose with a lower D_s and greater R_{90}.[31]

For rectangular fields, Hogstrom[32] derived and others have confirmed[31,33] that percentage of depth dose can be calculated by taking the geometric mean of the percentage of depth doses for a square field of length dimension (*L*) and one of width dimension (*W*). That is:

$$\%D(d; LxW) = \sqrt{\%D(d; LxL) \cdot \%D(d; WxW)} \quad (1)$$

If the square field, percentage of depth–dose curves do not have a common R_{100}, then the result of equation 1 must be normalized such that its maximum equals 100%. This method is referred to as the square-root method.

In some instances (e.g., intraoperative, intraoral, or intravaginal cones), circular fields are used. In such cases, it will be necessary to measure the dose distributions independent of those determined for square or rectangular fields.

Usually, a collimating insert is placed inside an electron applicator to form an irregular-shaped field, occasionally blocking the central axis. In this instance, central-axis depth dose makes little sense, and the term *central-field depth dose* should be used, providing that the field has an axis of symmetry. In cases where the insert is irregular, the depth dose can be approximated using a rectangular-shaped field that approximates the irregular-shaped field.[34] In highly irregular-shaped fields, the dose distribution should be calculated using an appropriate dose algorithm in a three-dimensional (3D) treatment-planning system. For very small fields, irregular or otherwise, it

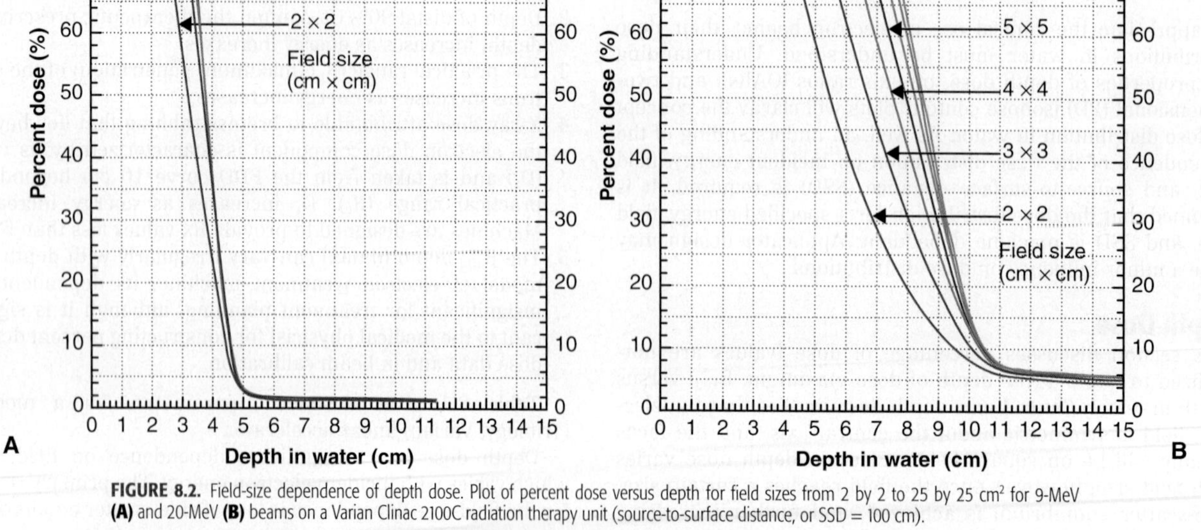

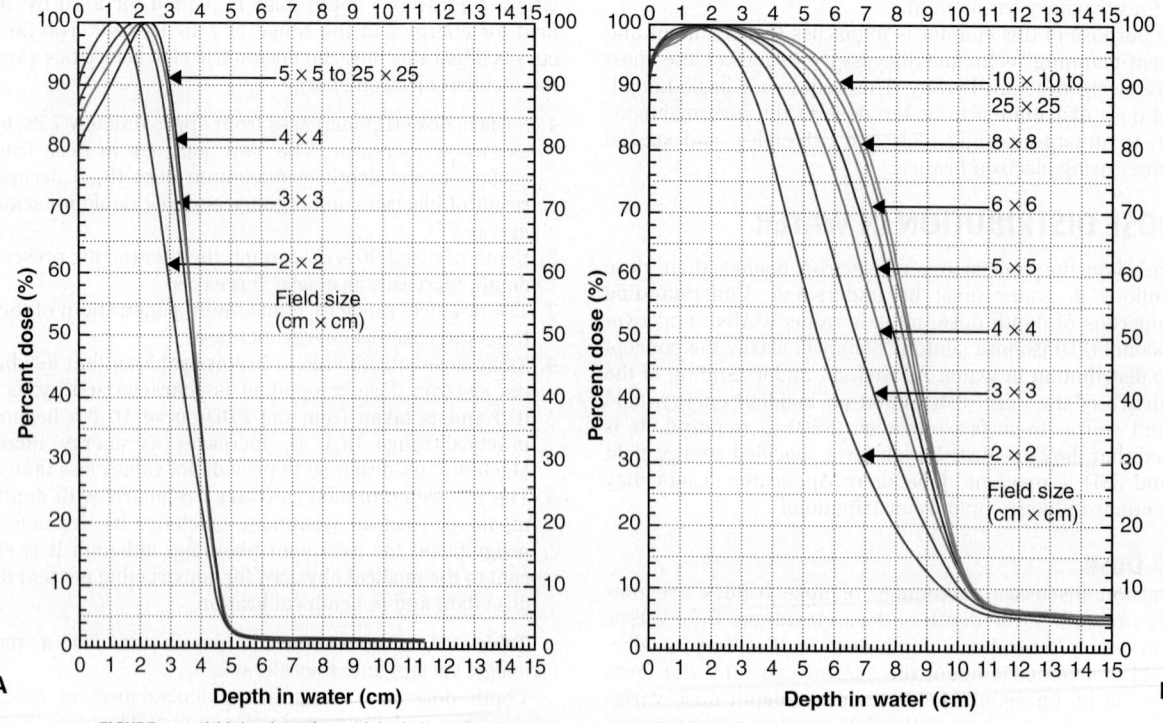

FIGURE 8.2. Field-size dependence of depth dose. Plot of percent dose versus depth for field sizes from 2 by 2 to 25 by 25 cm² for 9-MeV **(A)** and 20-MeV **(B)** beams on a Varian Clinac 2100C radiation therapy unit (source-to-surface distance, or SSD = 100 cm).

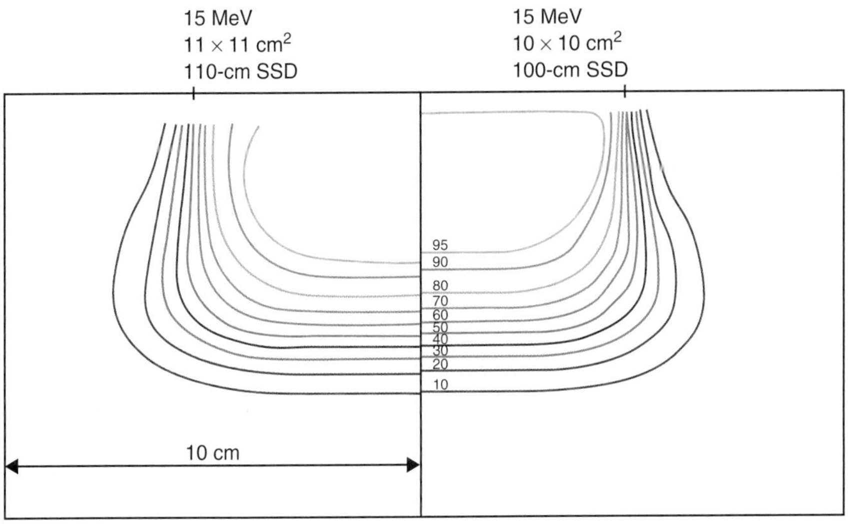

FIGURE 8.3. Source-to-surface distance (SSD) dependence of depth dose. Comparison of isodose plots for 15-MeV beam, 10 by 10 cm^2 at 100-cm SSD with 11 by 11 cm^2 field at 110-cm SSD. (From Hogstrom KR. Clinical electron-beam dosimetry: basic dosimetry data. In: Purdy JA, ed. *Advances in radiation oncology physics: dosimetry, treatment planning, and brachytherapy.* Woodbury: American Institute of Physics, 1991:390–429, with permission.)

is highly recommended that PPD measurements be performed to properly determine prescriptive choices (i.e, R_{90}).

Off-Axis Dose

Dose profiles in the dimensions perpendicular to the central axis can be described by OARs. The OAR is defined as the ratio of dose at an off-axis position to that on the central axis at the same depth. OARs measured in water are used to assess off-axis beam quality, which is characterized by flatness and symmetry in the uniform portion of the beam and by its falloff in the region of the penumbra (e.g., 90% to 10%, or 80% to 20%, respectively).

Manufacturers should be able to provide electron beams with a symmetry specification of 2% for opposing points in the beam and a flatness specification of ±3% of the *central-axis value* along the major axes (±4% along diagonals). The American Association of Physicists in Medicine (AAPM) Task Group 25 recommended that flatness and symmetry should be evaluated along major axes (lines containing central axis and perpendicular to the collimator edges) and along diagonal axes.[30] Task Group 25 also recommended that flatness and symmetry be evaluated at depths near the surface and therapeutic depth. Practically, this is performed at R_{100}.

Flatness and symmetry are evaluated inside the penumbra, which usually is ensured by setting the boundaries of evaluation 2 cm inside the collimating edge ($2\sqrt{2}$ cm along diagonals). When physicists acceptance-test a treatment machine, and during subsequent annual reviews, they use the AAPM Task Group 142 recommendations of 2% symmetry and 5% flatness.[35] This is usually performed for each energy with an average-size applicator but should be tested for each applicator during acceptance. Subsequently, the profiles acquired during acceptance should be reviewed monthly and be consistent to within 1% of the acceptance values. Figure 8.4 shows the result for a typical accelerator performance evaluation.[36]

Penumbra of electron beams is predetermined by the design of the beam flattening system, the air gap between the final collimator, and the scatter of electrons in water. Penumbra—a function of depth—is the root mean square addition of two penumbral components: one the result of the air gap and one the result of scatter in the water.[6] This dependence is complex but can be appreciated qualitatively by the illustration in Figure 8.5, which compares isodose plots for normal (100 cm) and extended (110 cm) SSD at 6 and 16 MeV, respectively. These data show that penumbra grows in a nonlinear fashion with depth, that air gap is more significant at the lower energies, and that scatter in water dominates at the higher energies. Fortunately, the complex dependence of penumbra can be modeled accurately in treatment-planning systems using the pencil-beam or more sophisticated dose algorithms.[29,32,34,37]

Isodose Plots

Combining depth dose with OARs results in the 3D dose distribution, and the properties of the 3D dose distribution can be appreciated by viewing 2D isodose contour plots in a plane containing the central axis and a major axis. Examples of these plots for a 15 by 15 cm^2 field are illustrated in Figure 8.5. As field width decreases or increases, the penumbra shape changes insignificantly because it is most significantly

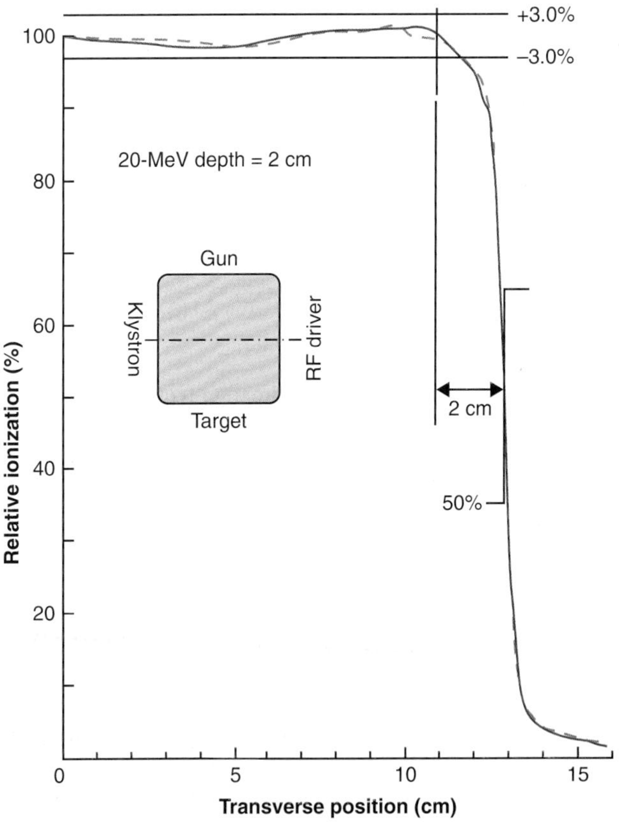

FIGURE 8.4. Beam uniformity verification. Plot of off-axis ratios versus position along a major axis. Data having a negative position (*dashed curve*) is reflected about central axis for comparison with data having a positive position (*solid curve*). Data measured at a depth of 2 cm in water at 100-cm SSD for a 20-MeV beam (Varian Clinac 2100C, 25 by 25 cm^2 open applicator).

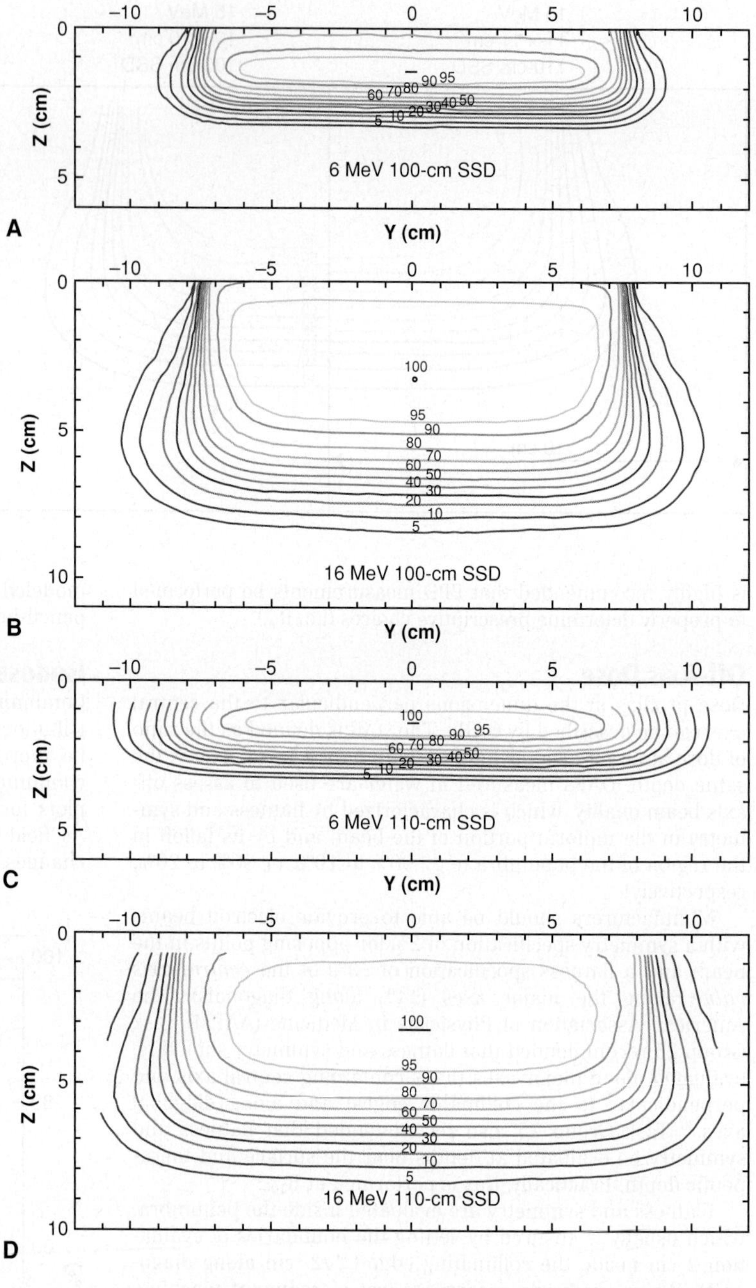

FIGURE 8.5. Variation of dose distribution with energy and SSD. Isodose plots (5% to 100%) in water for open 15 by 15 cm^2 applicator and for 6 MeV, 100-cm SSD **(A)**; 16 MeV, 100-cm SSD **(B)**; 6 MeV, 110-cm SSD **(C)**; and 16 MeV, 110-cm SSD **(D)** (Varian Clinac 2100C).

influenced by air gaps and by collimation type. Collimating on the skin, for example, reduces penumbra significantly.

Data required for isodose contours are acquired for an inclusive spread of field sizes at each energy. Two-dimensional isodose contour plots and data are useful for manual treatment planning, input data required by dose algorithms, verification of dose calculated by a treatment-planning system, and quality assurance standards.[29,30,38]

DOSE IN THE HETEROGENEOUS PATIENT

For most clinical circumstances, the ideal irradiation condition is for the electron beam to be incident normal to a flat surface with underlying homogeneous soft tissues. The dose distribution for this condition, similar to that for a water phantom described previously, contains a reasonably uniform dose inside the penumbra from the surface to R_{90}, and it has the sharpest possible falloff laterally and with depth. As the angle of incidence deviates from normal, as the surface becomes irregular, and as internal heterogeneous tissues (e.g., air, lung, and bone) become present, the qualities of the dose distribution degrade.[39] Internal heterogeneities can change the depth of beam penetration as a result of differences in the rate of energy loss, which can result in PTV underdose and critical structure overdose. Both irregular surfaces and internal heterogeneities create changes in side-scatter equilibrium, producing volumes of increased dose (hot spots) and decreased dose (cold spots), potentially leading to an increased dose to critical structures and decreased dose to the PTV.[3,39] These pertubations can be reduced or eliminated by modifying the treatment technique.

Irregular Surfaces

Two geometries that illustrate the effects on the dose distribution caused by an irregular patient surface are the sloped skin surface and the stepped skin surface. Figure 8.6 illustrates changes in the depth–dose curve as a result of nonnormal incidence of an electron beam onto a flat surface. Compared with normal incidence, the nonnormal incident electron beam, central-axis, depth–dose curve shows the following: (a) an increased surface dose, (b) an increased maximum dose, (c) a decreased penetration of the therapeutic dose (R_{90}), and (d) an increased range of penetration.[30,40] These changes can be

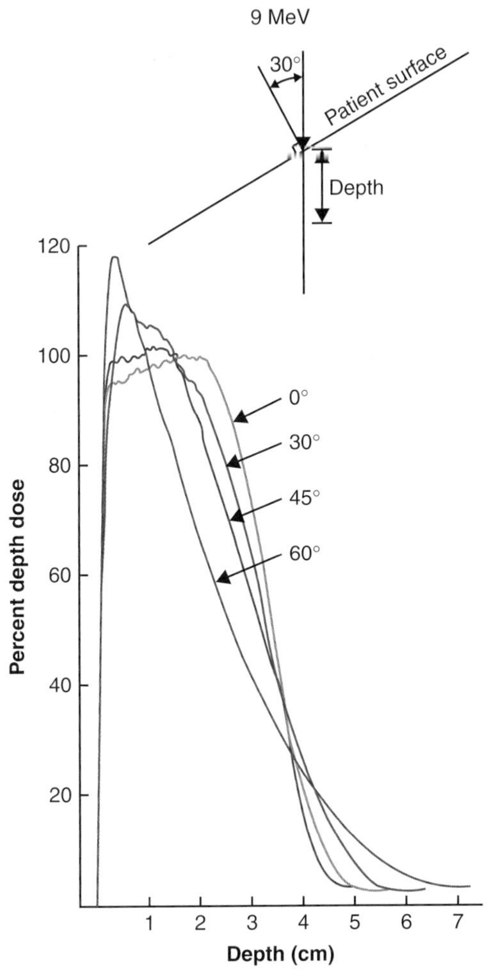

FIGURE 8.6. Effect of angle of incidence on depth dose. Dose versus depth for a 9-MeV beam incident on water angled 0 degrees to 60 degrees from the normal. (From Ekstrand KE, Dixon RL. The problem of obliquely incident beams in electron-beam treatment planning. *Med Phys* 1982;9:276–278, with permission.)

clinically significant, particularly at angles of incidence greater than 30 degrees from the normal. Such conditions can occur when irradiating curved patient surfaces with large fields (e.g., chest wall, limbs, neck, and scalp). In addition, it should be appreciated that the depth of R_{90} is specified along the central axis of the beam, and if the depth is taken perpendicular to the surface, then the depth is further reduced (approximately) by a factor cos (ϕ), where ϕ is the deviation of the incident angle from the normal.

Any time a sharp gradient (stepped surface) occurs on the patient's surface, side-scatter equilibrium will be lost, resulting in a cold spot beneath the proximal surface and a hot spot beneath the distal surface.[32,39,41,42] This can occur as a result of a sharp bolus edge, surgical defects, or within normal anatomy. For example, in the use of a uniform thickness bolus that partially covers a field, a 90-degree step can result in hot or cold spots as great as 20%, as illustrated in Figure 8.7. In such a case, the bolus should be tapered as much as possible. The results of a 45-degree tapered bolus in Figure 8.7 show a reduction in the hot spot but, more significantly, an increased coverage of the 90% isodose contour. The nose is a protrusion that creates a cold spot beneath itself, often the location of the tumor.[5,33,39] The ear canal (Fig. 8.8) and surgical voids, which are characterized by a depression in the patient's surface, can result in hot spots in excess of 50%, depending on void dimension and beam energy.[43,44] Such depressions normally should be filled with some type of bolus material. Normal anatomy contains many irregular surface depressions and protrusions (e.g., the ear canal and the nose, respectively) and should be accounted for by accurate treatment planning.

Air Cavities

The influence of an internal air cavity is illustrated in Figure 8.9, which compares isodose contours beneath an air cavity to those without the air cavity. Results show that (a) the isodose contours in the shadow of air are shifted distally, (b) the dose beneath the air cavity increases as a result of loss of side-scatter equilibrium, and (c) the influence of the air increases laterally with depth. Internal air cavities of clinical interest primarily occur in treatment of the head and neck (e.g., nasal passages, ethmoid sinuses, maxillary sinuses, larynx, and mastoids).[32,39]

Another significant effect is the reduction in dose in unit density tissue lateral to an air cavity. Electrons scattering from the unit density tissue into the air are not replaced because air is unable to scatter an equal amount back into the unit density tissue. Frequently, nose tumors can spread into the septum, in which case bolus should be used to eliminate or reduce underdosing.

Lung

In lung, electrons can penetrate three to four times farther than in unit density tissue. This is demonstrated in Figure 8.10, where isodose contours from a typical electron chest wall treatment are compared with those in which the lung is assumed unit density. Assuming a given dose of 50 Gy, the 40% isodose contour corresponds to 20 Gy, approximately the threshold for pneumonitis, if significant lung volume is irradiated. Ignoring the low density of lung would grossly underestimate the volume of lung receiving more than 20 Gy.[32]

This effect increases with energy. For example, increasing the beam energy from 9 to 12 MeV results in an additional 1.5 cm of penetration in waterlike tissue (electrons lose energy at a rate of approximately 2 MeV per centimeter in water), and this corresponds to as much as 6.0 cm in lung (assuming a lung density of 25%). Consider the patient whose chest wall thickness requires an energy of 10 MeV for treatment and that 12 MeV must be selected. This results in as much as 4 cm in depth of needless irradiation in lung, unless 1 cm of bolus is used to effectively lower the energy incident on the patient to 10 MeV.

Care must be taken when irradiating targets where the lung is immediately distal, such as with entire chest wall irradiation.

Bone

Interactions of electrons with bone are complex and interesting. The influence of bone is illustrated in Figure 8.11, which compares isodose contours beneath hard bone to those without the bone. The results show that:

1. The isodose contours in the shadow of the bone are shifted proximally,
2. Dose outside (inside) the bone–water interface increases (decreases) by approximately 5% as a result of loss of side-scatter equilibrium, and
3. The lateral dimension of the region having its dose perturbed by the bone increases with depth.

Actual bones are not uniformly dense throughout their cross-section, and in most cases their edges are not parallel to the incident beam. Both differences decrease the influence of bone in generating inhomogeneity in the patient's dose distribution. Dense bones that significantly affect the dose distribution include the mandible, bones of the skull (e.g., frontal bone and zygoma in orbit treatment or temporal bone in treatment of parotid), clavicles, and vertebral processes (e.g., craniospinal irradiation).

One might ask, what is the clinical significance of the increase in dose in or around bone due to increased scatter? The

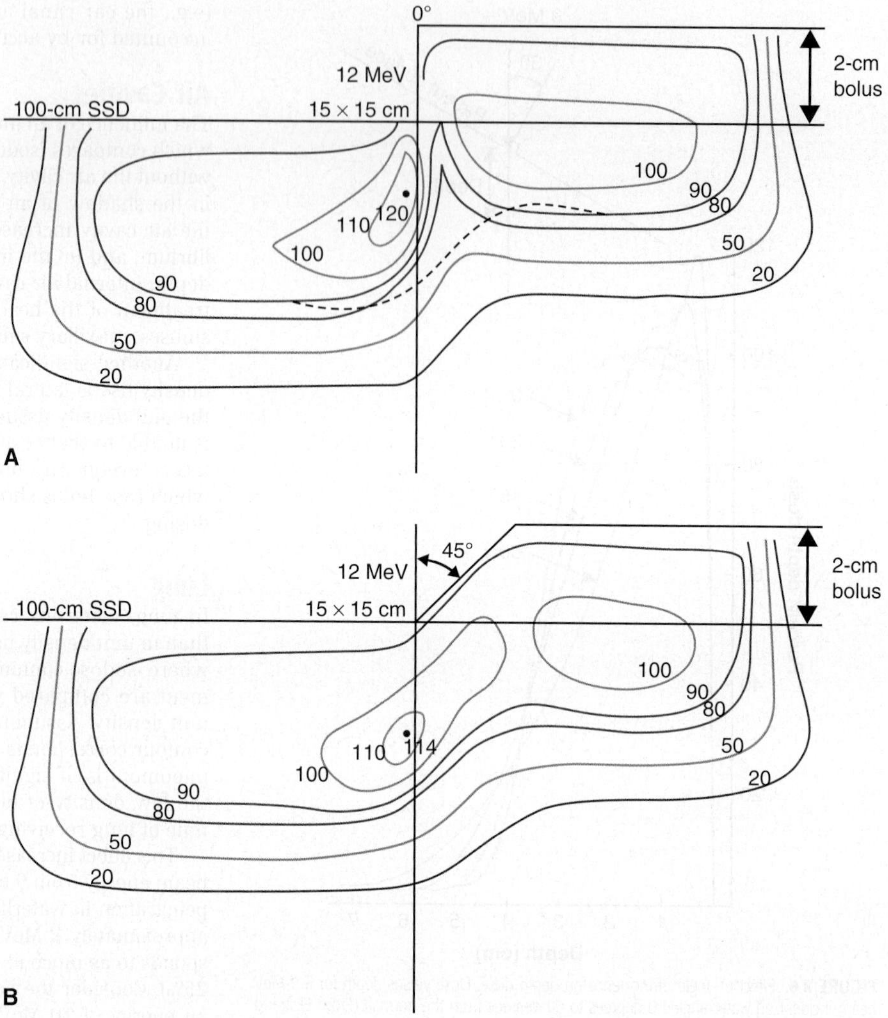

FIGURE 8.7. Effect of irregular patient surface on dose distribution. Plot of isodose contours for a 12-MeV, 15 by 15 cm^2 beam incident on water at 100-cm source-to-surface distance (SSD) having a stepped surface resulting from a 2-cm slab of bolus **(A)** and a beveled edge (45 degree) on the stepped surface **(B)**. The dashed line in the top figure shows the location of the 90% isodose contour in the bottom one. (From Hogstrom KR. Treatment planning in electron-beam therapy. In: Vaeth JM, Meyer JL, eds. *Frontiers of radiation therapy and oncology vol. 25: the role of high energy electrons in the treatment of cancer.* Basel: S. Karger AG, 1991:30–52, with permission.)

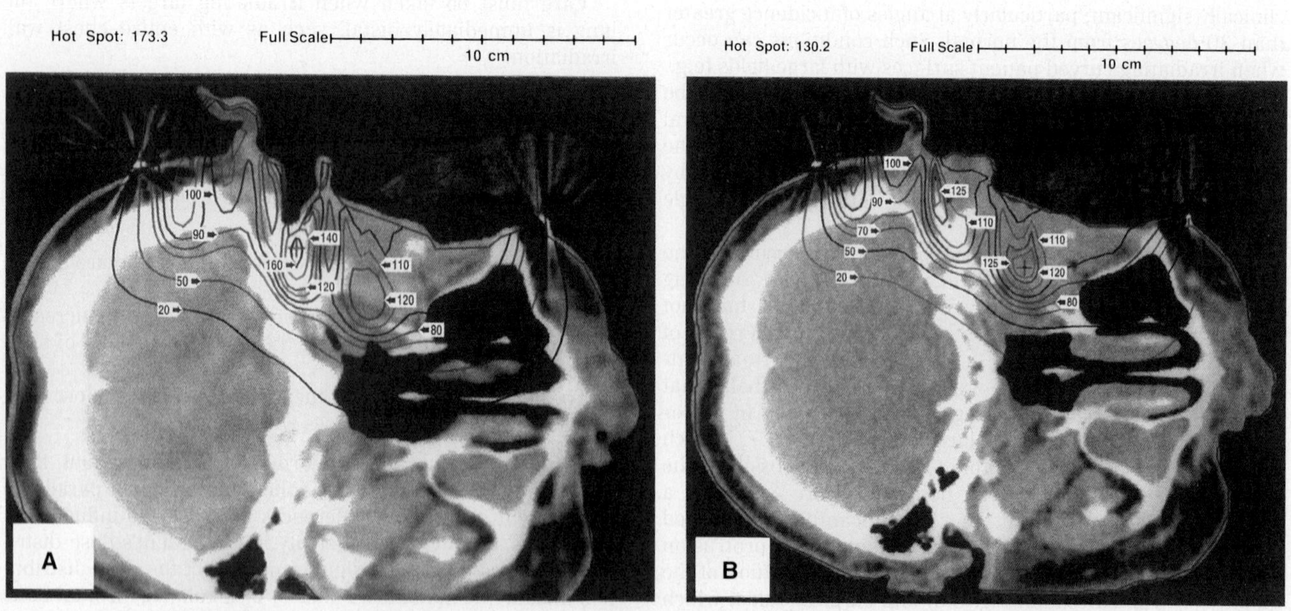

FIGURE 8.8. Impact of irregular surface anatomy on dose distribution. A 15-MeV electron beam irradiates the left side of a patient treated for dermal squamous carcinoma with perineural invasion. A beeswax bolus protects the posterior cranial fossa and the maxillary sinus. Isodose contours, expressed as a percentage of given dose, show how the ear canal results in an unacceptable hot spot of 160% to the middle ear **(A)** and how filling the ear canal with bolus (saline solution) eliminates that hot spot **(B)**. The residual hot spot of 125% is a result of the external ear. (From Morrison WH, Wong PF, Starkschall G, et al. Water bolus for electron irradiation of the ear canal. *Int J Radiat Oncol Biol Phys* 1995;33:479–483, with permission.)

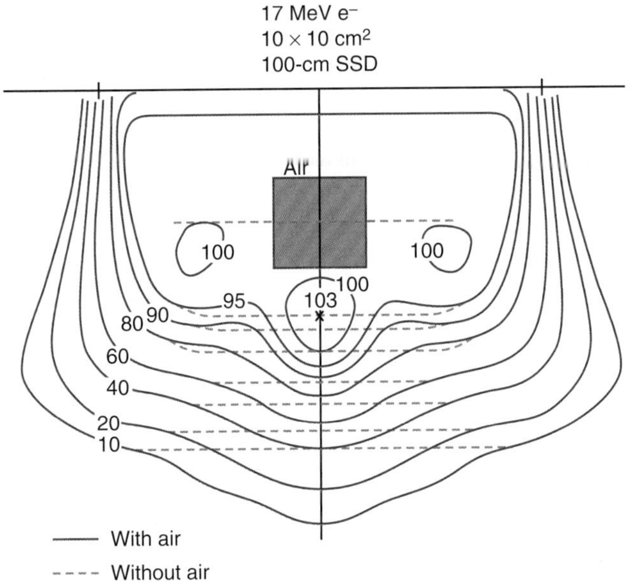

FIGURE 8.9. Effect of internal air cavity on underlying dose distribution. Dose calculated by the pencil-beam algorithm (PBA) for a 2 by 2 cm^2 cylinder of air located 2 cm below the surface in water is compared to that in its absence. (From Hogstrom KR. Dosimetry of electron heterogeneities. In: Wright AE, Boyer AL, eds. *Advances in radiation therapy treatment planning.* New York: American Institute of Physics, 1983:223–243, with permission.)

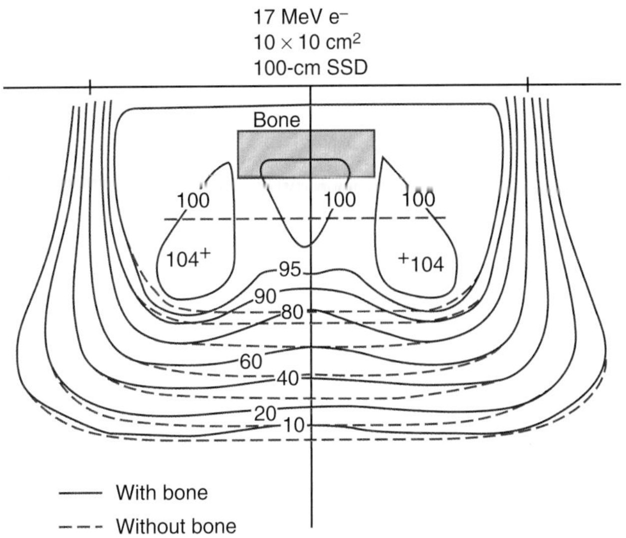

FIGURE 8.11. Effect of hard bone on underlying dose distribution. Dose calculated by the pencil-beam algorithm (PBA) for a 3 by 1 cm^2 cylinder of hard bone substitute located 1 cm below the surface in water is compared to that in its absence. (From Hogstrom KR. Dosimetry of electron heterogeneities. In: Wright AE, Boyer AL, eds. *Advances in radiation therapy treatment planning.* New York: American Institute of Physics, 1983:223–243, with permission.)

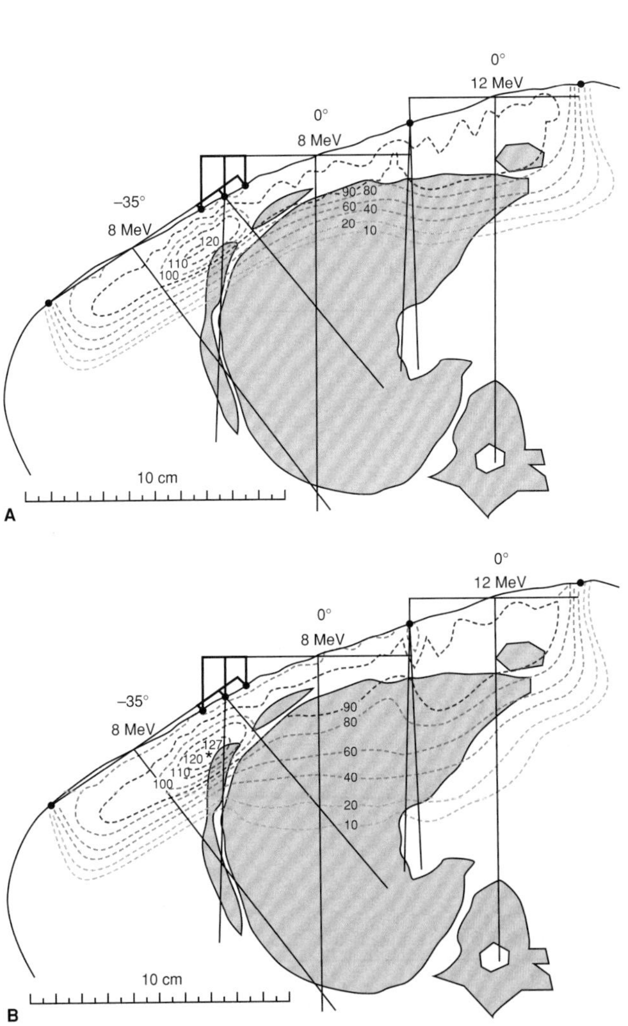

FIGURE 8.10. Effect of lung on dose distribution underlying chest wall. Comparison of dose calculated by the pencil-beam algorithm (PBA) for 8-MeV chest wall irradiation, assuming patient is water **(A)** and heterogeneous anatomy **(B)** based on computed tomography data.

maximum dose increase expected as a result of backscattered electrons is 5%, and the maximum dose increase expected inside bone and in adjacent exit tissues is approximately 7%.[45] These increases represent maximum dose estimates because actual bones are not as dense through and through as are the bone substitute in which these data were taken. These estimates of the increased dose are not expected to be clinically significant. In fact, untoward effects in or around bone that can be attributed to dosimetry have not been observed in patients treated with electron-beam therapy.

DOSE PRESCRIPTION AND CALCULATION OF MONITOR UNITS

Dose Prescription

It is recommended that dose be prescribed to given dose or 90% of given dose. Intermediate or lower prescription (95%, 85%, 80%) can be prescribed if the energy (typically stepped in 3 to 4 MeV increments) choices are too coarse to maintain a single baseline prescription recipe. Given dose is defined as the maximum central-axis dose in a water phantom at the SSD of the patient for the energy, applicator, and field size identical to that used for patient treatment. If the field shape is irregular, then the field size is taken to be a rectangular field representative of the irregular field shape. The most representative rectangular field is not well defined; however, Hogstrom et al.[37] have provided one methodology for determining its estimate.

It is recommended that dose be prescribed to given dose or a percentage of it and not to a point in the patient. It is quite possible that a dose prescription point in the patient could be in a region of increased or decreased dose because of tissue heterogeneity or irregular surface, which could result in PTV underdose or overdose, respectively.

Calculation of Monitor Units

Monitor units can be determined by

$$MU = \frac{D_{prescribed}/\%D}{O(E, C, LxW, SSD)}, \tag{2}$$

where $D_{prescribed}$ is the prescribed dose, $\%D$ is the percentage of given dose to which dose is prescribed (e.g., 90%), and

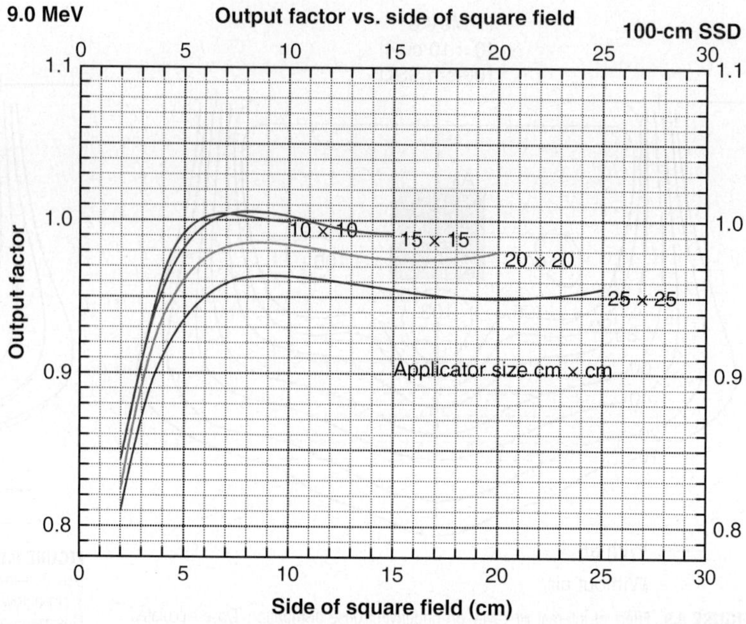

FIGURE 8.12. Field-size dependence of output (dose/monitor unit). Plot of output factor (cGy/MU) versus side of square field from 2 by 2 cm^2 to the open applicator for four applicators and for the 9-MeV beam of a Varian Clinac 2100C.

O(E, C, LxW, SSD) is the output (dose per monitor unit) for a beam of energy *E*, applicator *C*, field size *LxW*, and *SSD*. To use this methodology, the medical physicist must measure dose output as a function of square field size and SSD for each energy-applicator combination at the time of commissioning the accelerator. Output for rectangular fields can be determined using the square-root method of Mills et al.[14,46] and Shiu et al.[31]:

$$O(E, C, LxW, SSD) = [O(E, C, LxL, SSD) \cdot O(E, C, WxW, SSD)]^{1/2} \quad (3)$$

Output for rectangular fields also can be determined using an equivalent square method[30,33,47,48]; however, Biggs et al.[47] recommend limiting this method to an aspect ratio (*L:W*) of 2:1. The square-root method is not limited to the aspect ratio, and Shiu et al.[31] have shown it to be more accurate. Figure 8.12 illustrates beam output data at 9 MeV for four common applicators used on the Varian Clinac 2100C (Varian Medical Systems, Palo Alto, CA) at 100 cm SSD.

Output at extended SSD can be determined by either the air-gap method or the effective-source method.[30] The effective-source method is covered in detail by Khan.[48] The air-gap method has a sounder physical basis. Although both methods give similar answers, only the air-gap method will be covered here.[33] Output at extended SSD is given by the product of output at the nominal SSD (SSD_0), the air-gap factor (fair), and an inverse square term,

$$O(E, C, LxW, SSD) = O(E, C, LxW, SSD_0)\, f_{air}\,(E, LxW, SSD) \times \left(\frac{SSD_o + R_{100}}{SSD + R_{100}}\right) \quad (4)$$

f_{air} is determined by measuring dose output for square fields at the extended SSD and then solving equation 4. For rectangular fields, the air-gap factor is determined using the square-root method[31]:

$$f_{air}(E, LxW, SSD) = \sqrt{f_{air}(E, LxL, SSD) \cdot f_{air}(E, WxW, SSD)} \quad (5)$$

As f_{air} is assumed independent of applicator, the dose output needs to be measured only for the smallest applicator that contains the square field size. Figure 8.13 plots the square field air-gap factors for the 9-MeV beam of the Varian Clinac 2100C for SSD from 100 to 120 cm. For a more detailed explanation of dose output and sample calculations of monitor units for electron beams, refer to Hogstrom et al.[34] Another practical option is to fix incremented SSDs to be used clinically (i.e., 100, 105, 110, 115 cm) and establish tabular outputs for each energy/applicator SSD combination.

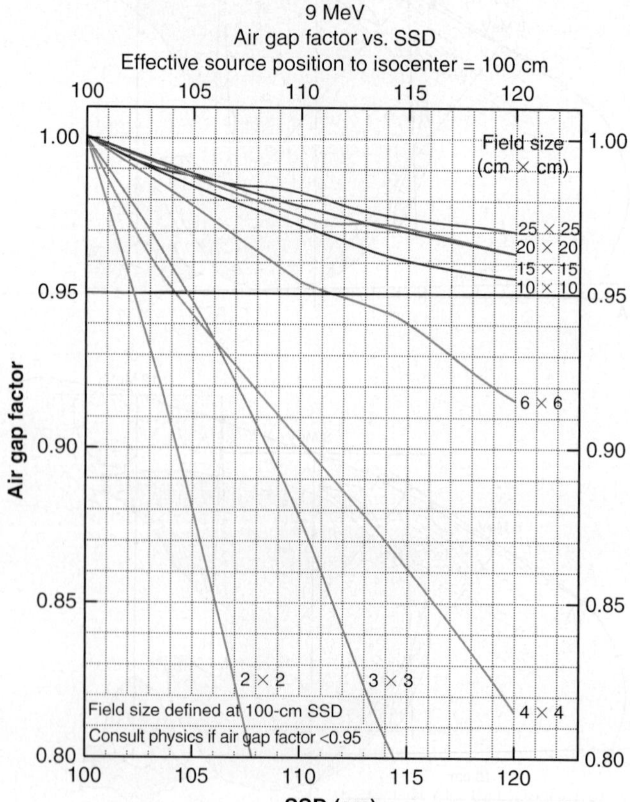

FIGURE 8.13. Dependence of air-gap factors on source-to-surface distance (SSD) and field size. Plot of f_{air} versus SSD for field sizes ranging from 2 by 2 to 25 by 25 cm^2 and for the 9-MeV beam (Varian Clinac 2100C).

CALCULATION OF DOSE IN PATIENT

Standards for Patient Dose Calculations

Sound treatment-planning decisions require accurate dose calculation in the patient. Therefore, the following recommendations are made for electron-beam treatment planning. First, dose should be calculated in the full three dimensions to allow for evaluation of dose homogeneity in the PTV, coverage of the PTV by the 90% isodose contour, and dose to critical structures. Second, the dose algorithm should account for patient heterogeneity. Failure to properly account for patient heterogeneity can result in failure to appreciate dose heterogeneity, PTV underdose, or normal-tissue overdose.[5,39,49] Third, the dose algorithm should be accurate, and for those conditions for which this is not the case, physicians and physicists should discuss the proper interpretation of the dose calculations.

To expand on the final recommendation, a dose algorithm must meet certain criteria to be most effective in the clinic.[50] First, it should be accurate to within 4% in regions of low-dose gradients or within 2 mm in regions of high-dose gradient (e.g., penumbra or depth-dose falloff region).[38,51] Second, the dose algorithm should be commissioned easily by a qualified medical physicist. Third, the accuracy of the dose algorithm should be well documented. Since 1981, the PBA has best met this requirement. Presently, several new, more accurate algorithms, both analytical and Monte Carlo–based, are being implemented into commercial treatment-planning systems and will replace or supplement the PBA in due time.[52] Regardless of the algorithm, it is the medical physicist's responsibility to commission the algorithm, to understand its accuracy, and to train medical dosimetrists and radiation oncologists in its use and limitations.

Dose Algorithms

For the past 20 years, the standard methodology for dose calculation in the patient has been the PBA. As computing power increased, it was possible to implement the algorithms into 3D format.[53] Detailed instructions for commissioning the dose algorithm and documentation of its accuracy have been published.[5,6,50] The PBA has been shown to be quite accurate in water at standard and extended SSD, correctly predicting the changes in penumbra.[29,32,34] It is also quite accurate in predicting changes in dose resulting from oblique incidence and irregular surfaces.[5,50] Regarding internal heterogeneities, it correctly predicts the penetration in lung and the growth of the penumbra width in lung[50]; however, it tends to underestimate the dose in lung near the mediastinum as a result of its central axis approximation.[50] In bone, it correctly predicts the shortening of the dose penetration behind the bone, and it slightly underestimates (<5%) the magnitude of the hot and cold spots under the edge of a thick hard bone such as the mandible.[5] The PBA does not predict the increased dose (<5%) resulting from backscatter at the proximal tissue–bone interface, nor does it predict the increased dose (>7%) in bone resulting from increased scatter. The PBA underestimates the hot and cold spots under the air–tissue interfaces.[5,50]

New dose algorithms that are accurate to 4% or better are becoming available in commercial treatment-planning systems. Many of these algorithms have been reviewed by Hogstrom and Steadham.[50] One of these is the pencil-beam redefinition algorithm (PBRA), whose commissioning is similar to that of the conventional PBA, although its accuracy is significantly improved.[54–56] Figure 8.14 illustrates the improvement of the PBRA.

Many of the newer algorithms are based on Monte Carlo methods, which allow them to be quite accurate.[57–61] Cygler et al.[52] published a report on the first commercial system using Monte Carlo–based electron calculations, demonstrating excellent results. Ding et al.[62] demonstrated outstanding results for a macro–Monte Carlo algorithm, along with a companion report showing superior results for Monte Carlo compared with PBA.[63]

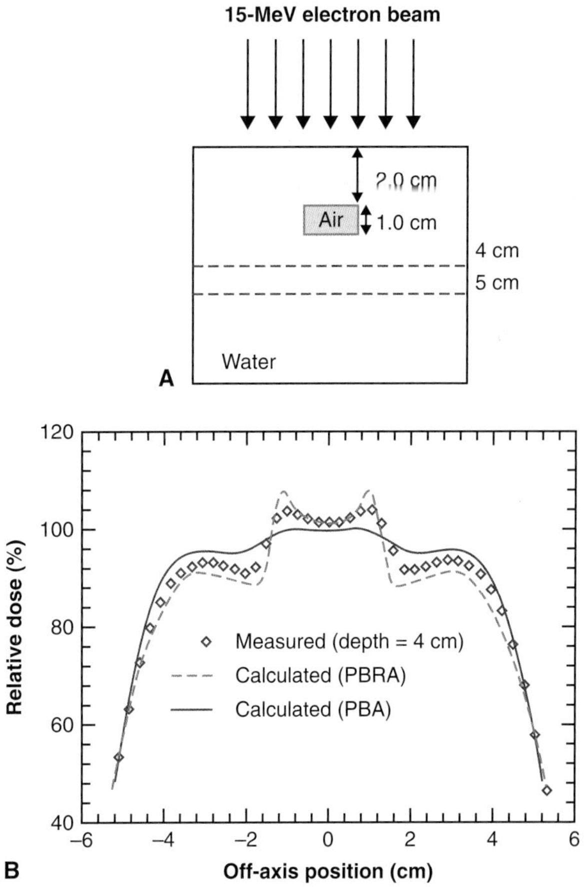

FIGURE 8.14. Evaluation of accuracy of dose algorithms below air cavity. **A:** Dose is measured distal to an internal air cavity. **B:** Measured dose profile at a depth of 4 cm is compared to that calculated by the pencil-beam algorithm and the pencil-beam redefinition algorithm. PBA, pencil-beam algorithm; PRBA, pencil-beam redefinition algorithm. (From Shiu AS, Hogstrom KR. Pencil-beam redefinition algorithm for electron dose distributions. *Med Phys* 1991;18:7–18, with permission.)

TREATMENT-PLANNING PRINCIPLES, TOOLS, AND METHODS

Electron therapy usually is restricted to a PTV that is within 6 cm distal from the patient's surface. Electrons may be used alone or in conjunction with photon beams. In the case of the former, the objective of the treatment planner is usually to select the appropriate beam direction, energy, and field size to provide as uniform a dose as possible to the PTV while delivering minimal dose to normal tissue and structures. To optimize dose homogeneity, the beam direction should be as close to normal incidence to the patient surface as practical. Once beam direction is specified, the selection of energy and field-size specification follows. Figure 8.15 compares the isodose contours in water with the beam edges and R_{90}. Electrons are unique in that the uniform region of dose lies inside the 90% isodose contour. Dose in the patient outside the 90% isodose contour falls off rapidly. However, the patient anatomy can differ significantly from water so that effects resulting from patient heterogeneity make the resulting treatment plan unacceptable, according to the original prescription. In addition, the PTV can be at a variable depth beneath the surface so that a single beam energy is inadequate. The treatment plan can be improved by utilization of special treatment aids such as skin

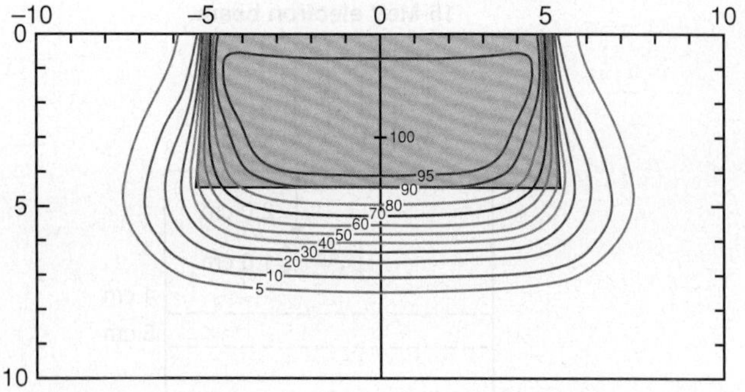

FIGURE 8.15. Plot of isodose curves for a 15-MeV, 10 by 10 cm^2 electron beam in water (source-to-surface distance, or SSD = 100 cm). Note the shape of the 90% isodose contour with respect to the shaded area, which is framed by the diverging field edges and the R_{90} depth.

or internal collimation, bolus, field abutment, or other special techniques.

Selection of Energy

The energy of the incident electron beam should be selected so that the distal surface of the 90% (of given dose) dose surface encompasses the PTV and that critical structures lie beyond the maximum penetration of the electrons or at an acceptable dose level. For planning purposes, a general rule is the following:

$$E_{p,0}(MeV) \sim 3.3 \cdot R_{90}(cm), \quad (6)$$

where $E_{p,0}$ is the most probable incident electron energy in MeV. The energy should be selected such that R_{90} just exceeds the maximum depth of the PTV. This approximation is true in water for field sizes large enough to have side-scatter equilibrium on the central axis. For small field sizes that do not have side-scatter equilibrium, R_{90} will be less, thus a higher energy might be required. As well, heterogeneous tissue (e.g., bone or air) can affect the penetration, requiring greater or lesser energy, respectively.

Similarly, for planning purposes, a general rule is the following:

$$E_{p,0}(MeV) = 2 \cdot R_p(cm), \quad (7)$$

where R_p is the practical range in centimeters of the electron beam (32). The treatment planner can select an energy such that R_p is less than the minimal depth of a critical structure. This approximation has no field-size limitation; however, as before, heterogeneous tissue (e.g., bone, lung, or air) can affect the penetration, allowing greater or lesser energy.

As an example of how to use these general rules, consider irradiating the posterior cervical nodes of the neck with electrons to spare the spinal cord because its dose is already near tolerance. If the maximum depth of the nodes is 3 cm and the minimum depth of the spinal cord is 6 cm, then equations 6 and 7 indicate that the minimum energy to cover the PTV is 9.9 MeV and the maximum energy that protects the spinal cord is 12 MeV, respectively. Hence, beam energies in the range of 10 to 12 MeV should be acceptable. In all cases, the energy of the beam should be confirmed by performing a 3D dose calculation for the planned treatment using a CT representation of the patient. Bolus may be strategically used to tune the beam penetration either globally or in discrete areas and ideally should be placed at the time of the CT.

Design of Electron Collimation

Electron collimation consists of multiple collimating components; however, the electron field shape usually is defined by an applicator's collimating insert and/or skin collimation. Custom electron collimators are constructed from lead or low–melting-point lead alloy (Lipowitz metal). The lead thickness in millimeters required to stop the primary electrons equals one-half the incident most probable energy of the electron beam in MeV.[29,30] To account for small variations in thickness resulting from the lead-sheet manufacturing process, a 1-mm surplus can be added. That is:

$$t_{Pb}(mm) = 0.5 \cdot E_{p,0}\ (MeV) + 1 \quad (8)$$

For example, an 18-MeV beam requires 10 mm of lead. Lipowitz metal comprised mostly of lead along with bismuth has density 20% less lead; therefore, its thickness should be increased by 20%. For example, an 18-MeV beam requires 12 mm of Lipowitz metal. Lipowitz metal collimating inserts usually are fabricated at a constant thickness—namely, that sufficient for the greatest energy on the treatment machine. For a machine whose maximum energy is 20 MeV, the Lipowitz metal thickness should be a minimum of 13 mm.

Skin Collimation

The closer the field-defining collimator is to the patient, the sharper the beam's penumbra; hence, skin collimation provides the sharpest possible penumbra. Because of the significant effort often required to fabricate skin collimation, its use is restricted to applications for which it has the greatest benefit, for example: (a) small-field treatments, (b) providing maximal protection to adjacent critical structures, (c) reducing penumbra beneath a bolus, (d) reducing penumbra when treating at an extended air gap, (e) reducing penumbra in electron arc therapy, and (f) where patient motion may be an issue. Proper use of skin collimation requires that it be in contact with the skin surface and that it extend sufficiently inwardly and outwardly to intercept the penumbra from upstream collimation.

Skin collimation thickness is usually available in units of 0.0625-inch lead sheets and normally is taken to be the minimum thickness necessary to shield the maximum. The maximum possible dose beneath the skin collimation occurs at the skin surface with no air gap between the two.[30,33] The transmitted dose, which is the result of bremsstrahlung photons from the incident beam and those generated by electrons stopping in the lead, is slightly greater than that with no lead present. It is recommended that a table of measured dose under the lead, as a function of lead thickness, is available for each beam energy.[29] As the air gap between the lead and the patient increases, the transmitted dose to the patient decreases. These values can be measured at the time of beam commissioning. If not, and for cases where precise determination of dose beneath a block is critical, in vivo dosimetry (e.g., thermoluminescent dosimetry) should be used.

In designing the shape of the aperture of a collimating insert, due consideration is made for the penumbra. Typically, there is approximately a 1-cm margin between the projected edge of the collimator and outer boundary of target volume when both are projected to the isocenter. This margin varies with energy, depth, and air gap, and it only can be appreciated by utilization of isodose curves (Figs. 8.5 and 8.15). Again, the adequacy of the margin between the aperture and PTV should be confirmed by performing a 3D dose calculation for the planned treatment using a CT representation of the patient.

The utility of skin collimation for small-field treatments is illustrated in Figure 8.16. A 6-MeV, 3 by 3 cm^2 field with a 10-cm air gap (collimator to surface) is essentially all penumbra, resulting in an unsatisfactory dose distribution. However, by opening the collimator to 6 by 6 cm^2 and then forming the 3 by 3 cm^2 field using skin collimation, the dose distribution becomes clinically satisfactory. This application is used for treatment of the eyelid, nose, and other small target volumes.

In the presence of skin collimation, the depth dose is approximated by that for the field size on the skin surface (i.e., that defined by the skin collimator). In contrast, the dose output is approximated by that for the field-size incident on the skin collimation (i.e., that defined by the applicator cutout). For the example in Figure 8.16, the depth dose is taken to be that

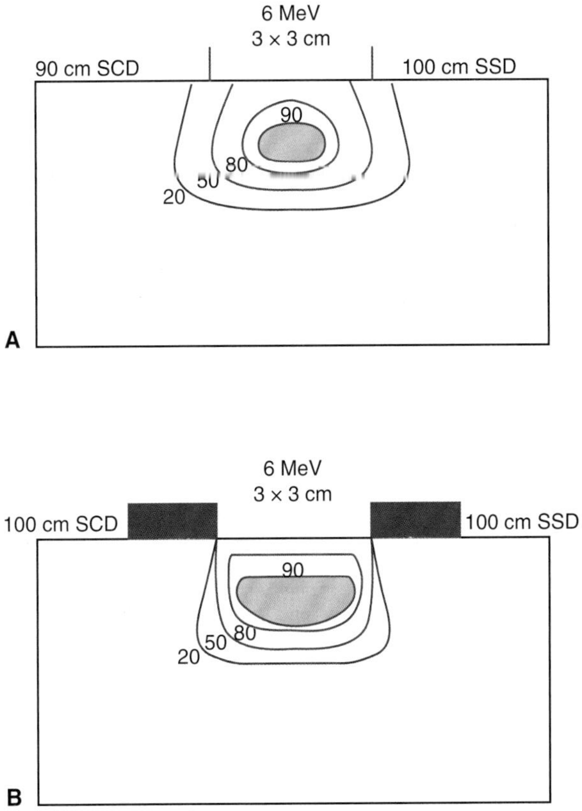

FIGURE 8.16. Impact of skin collimation for small electron fields. Isodose plots are compared for results of a computer simulation of a 6-MeV electron beam in water for a 3 by 3 cm^2 field formed by an applicator insert 10 cm above the patient **(A)** and a 3 by 3 cm^2 field formed by collimation at the surface with a 6 by 6 cm^2 applicator insert 10 cm above the patient **(B)**. (From Hogstrom, KR. Clinical electron-beam dosimetry: basic dosimetry data. In: Purdy JA, ed. *Advances in radiation oncology physics: dosimetry, treatment planning, and brachytherapy.* Woodbury: American Institute of Physics, 1991:390–429, with permission.)

of the 3 by 3 cm^2 field; the dose output is taken to be that of the 6 by 6 cm^2 field. This simple approximation slightly overestimates dose output, if the depths of maximum dose for the two field sizes differ. In such a case, the output of the larger field is multiplied by the depth–dose factor of the larger field at the depth of maximum dose of the smaller field.[34]

Multileaf Collimation

Using existing photon multileaf collimators (MLCs) to modulate electron beams has been shown to be somewhat feasible, although a report by Klein et al.[64] showed that an SSD of 70 cm was necessary to provide clinical acceptable fields using the photon MLC. This is because of the dispersion of the electrons in air. They performed a feasibility study of using existing photon MLC to modulate electron beams, which was shown to be somewhat feasible. An important aspect from that work demonstrated that when using existing photon MLC to produce narrow electron-beam segments, the large generated penumbra could be an advantage in terms of beam matching.

The other possibility is not to use the existing photon MLC but rather to have a tertiary electron MLC system that is closer to the patient, thereby narrowing the penumbra that is produced when the MLC is far from the patient. Lee et al.[65] found that replacing air with helium in the treatment head made a significant impact in predicted dose distributions. Karlsson et al.[66] demonstrated that penumbra, effective source position, field shape, and matching could be optimized by replacing air with helium in the treatment head below the MLC leaves and by shifting the position of the scattering foils, monitor chamber, and MLC position.

Bolus

Bolus is an essential tool for the delivery of optimal electron radiation therapy. Electron bolus is defined as water- or near water-equivalent material that normally is placed either in direct contact with the patient's skin surface, close to the patient's skin surface, or inside a body cavity. This material is designed to provide extra scattering or energy degradation of the electron beam. Its purpose usually is to shape the dose distribution to conform to the target volume or to provide a more uniform dose inside the target volume.[29,32] More specifically, electron bolus has three primary applications:

1. To shape the coverage of the treatment volume in the depth direction to conform as closely as possible to the target volume while avoiding critical structures,
2. To increase dose to the patient's external surface, and
3. To serve as a missing tissue compensator for surface irregularities and internal air cavities.

In the second application, bolus is being used to either eliminate or decrease the adverse effects of patient heterogeneities on the dose distribution, which can result in a geographic miss at depth, dose nonuniformity within the target volume, and excessive dose-to-distal critical structures.[29,32]

Because dose typically is prescribed to 90% to 100% of the given dose, it is often desirable to increase surface dose to 90% or higher when treating with low-energy electrons. To accomplish this, a higher energy beam is selected and a uniformly thick bolus is placed on or near the skin surface. The surface dose of the higher energy electron beam is greater, and the bolus places the skin at a deeper depth, further increasing the surface dose. The energy–bolus thickness combination is selected to place R_{90} at the prescription depth while increasing the surface dose (D_s) to near 90%. To assist in usage of this technique, a table that allows selection of the optimal energy–bolus thickness combination is recommended. Table 8.2 illustrates a sample for the five electron-beam energies of a typical radiation therapy machine.

Two bolus methods are used for this function. One places flexible sheet material (e.g., Superflab) directly on the skin surface. This material is approximately water equivalent and comes in thickness increments of 0.3 to 4 cm. It is particularly useful for chest wall irradiation, both for fixed-beam and arced-beam therapies. In some treatments, the bolus is used for only a portion of the field, in which case care must be taken to ensure the edge of the bolus is tapered to reduce the magnitude of the hot or cold spot created by the surface irregularity (such as is seen in Fig. 8.7).[29,32]

For highly irregular or sensitive skin surfaces, which often are encountered in head and neck or postsurgical irradiations,

TABLE 8.2 VALUES OF SURFACE DOSE AND THERAPEUTIC DEPTH FOR VARIOUS ENERGY–BOLUS COMBINATIONS

Superflab Thickness (cm)	*0.0*	*0.3*	*0.5*	*1.0*	*1.5*	*2.0*
Energy: 6 MeV						
D_s (%)	72	79	83	93	100	–
R_{90} (cm)	2.0	1.7	1.5	1.0	0.5	–
Energy: 9 MeV						
D_s (%)	78	83	85	89	95	99
R_{90} (cm)	3.0	2.7	2.5	2.0	1.5	1.0
Energy: 12 MeV						
D_s (%)	83	88	89	91	94	96
R_{90} (cm)	4.0	3.7	3.5	3.0	2.5	2.0
Energy: 16 MeV						
D_s (%)	87	92	93	96	97	98
R_{90} (cm)	5.0	4.7	4.5	4.0	3.5	3.0
Energy: 20 MeV						
D_s (%)	91	96	97	98	99	100
R_{90} (cm)	6.1	5.8	5.6	5.1	4.6	4.1

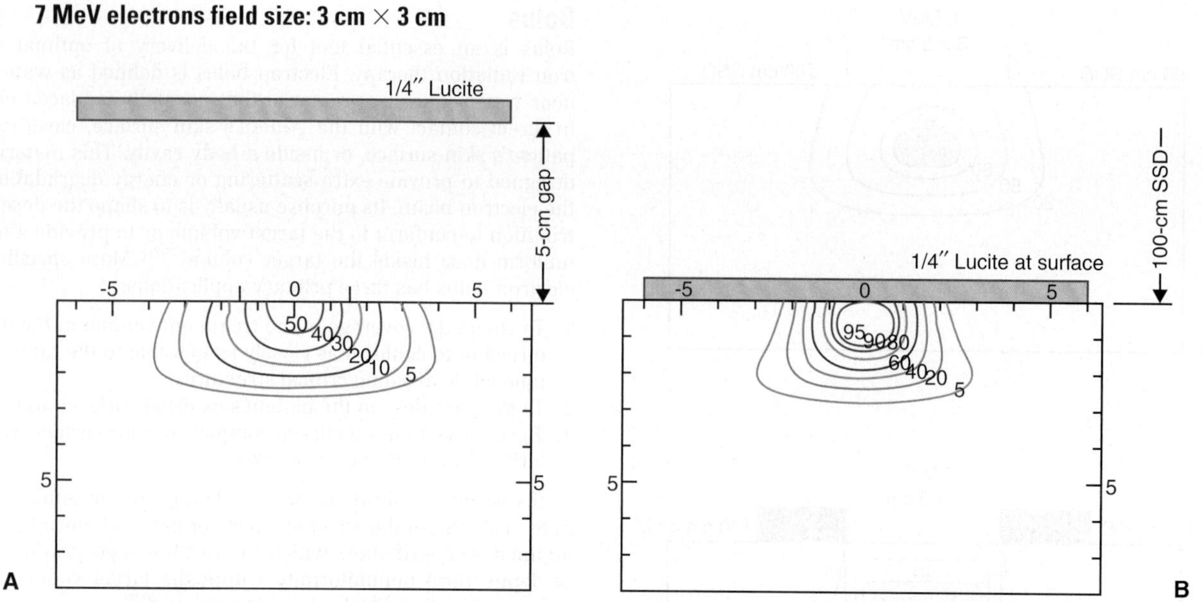

FIGURE 8.17. Proper location of slab bolus. Constant thickness (slab) bolus is used to increase surface dose and to fine tune electron-beam penetration (Table 8.2). Its location is important for irradiation by a small field (3 by 3 cm^2) and low energy (7-MeV) electron beam. **A:** If a 0.25-inch polymethylmethacrylate (PMMA) plate is located 5 cm above the patient, electrons are scattered away from the field resulting in needless broadening of the penumbra and a decrease in given dose of approximately 50% (given dose without the bolus is 100%). **B:** Placing the 0.25-inch PMMA plate on the surface preserves both the given dose and beam penumbra.

it is advantageous to have a rigid bolus sheet (often referred to as a scatter plate because it not only degrades the energy of the electron beam but also scatters the beam) close to but not necessarily in direct contact with the patient.[32] For such cases, standard thicknesses of polymethylmethacrylate (PMMA) (0.125 to 0.25 inches) are placed perpendicular to the beam, as illustrated in Figure 8.17. To restore a sharp penumbra, skin collimation usually is recommended with use of the scatter-plate bolus method. Rules for using skin collimation with the bolus have been discussed by Hogstrom.[32] It is important that the bolus be in contact or close to the patient because too large of an air gap can create an exceedingly large penumbra. This is

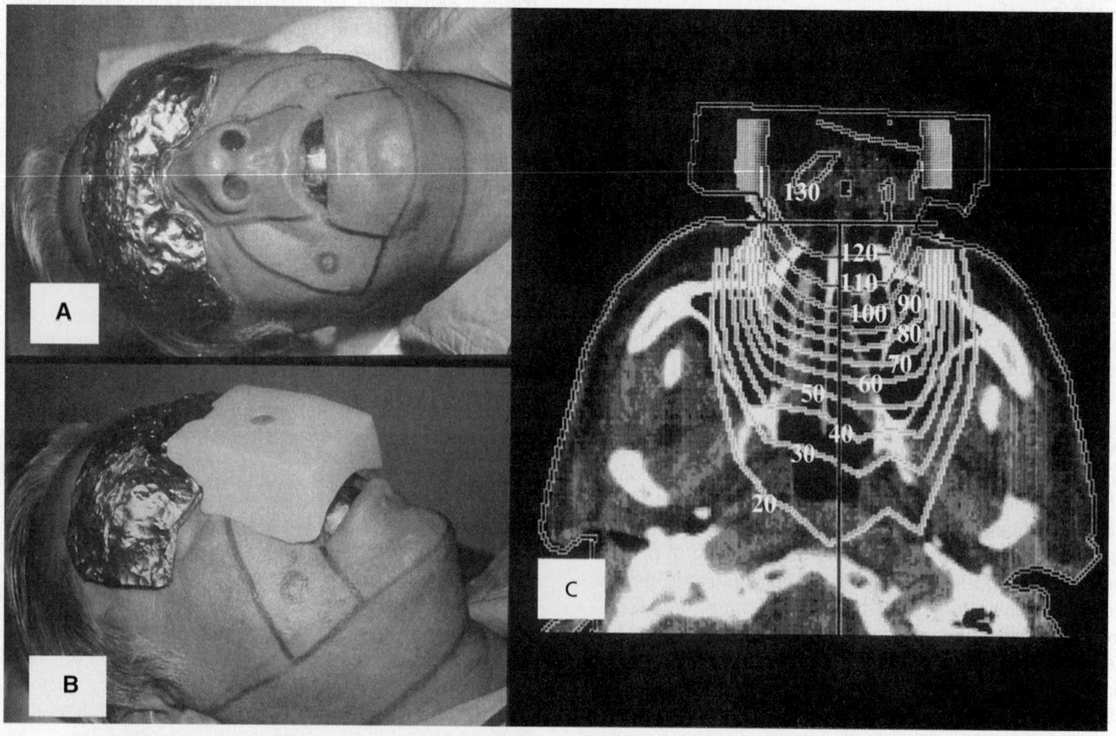

FIGURE 8.18. Utility of bolus to remove dose inhomogeneity caused by surface irregularity of nose. **A:** Bolus in nasal air passages prevents cold spots in the septum. (In addition, note the skin collimation used to restore penumbra under nose bolus and the intraoral stent used to protect the tongue.) **B:** Wax bolus surrounding the nose eliminates irregular patient surface. **C:** Isodose curves superimposed on a transverse computed tomography scan illustrate how the bolus makes the patient more like a water phantom, resulting in a homogeneous dose distribution characteristic of that in a water phantom. The patient dose is delivered 12-MeV electrons: ^{60}Co photons = 4:1. (Note that the surface dose is lower than that shown because the treatment-planning system calculated the photon dose assuming the bolus was in place during its delivery, which is not the case.) (From Hogstrom KR. Treatment planning in electron-beam therapy. In: Vaeth JM, Meyer JL, eds. *Frontiers of radiation therapy and oncology vol. 25: the role of high energy electrons in the treatment of cancer.* Basel: S. Karger AG, 1991:30–52, with permission.)

demonstrated in Figure 8.17, where a 5-cm air gap results in a 50% decrease in the given dose because of the bolus scattering electrons away from the field.

Bolus is considered part of the beam; however, it also can be considered part of the patient, effectively shortening the SSD. For uniform bolus thickness (t), it is recommended to adjust the dose output for inverse square.[34] That is:

$$O_{bolus} = O \cdot \left[\frac{SSD + t + R_{100}}{SSD + R_{100}} \right]^2 \qquad (9)$$

Various methods exist for using bolus to remove surface irregularities, which result in volumes of overdose and underdose resulting from scatter inequilibrium if ignored.[4,32] One method involves fabrication of a beeswax bolus onto a positive cast of the patient, as is used for treatment of carcinoma of the nose (Fig. 8.18). In this case, the bolus is used to surround the protrusion of the nose with scatter material. In other applications, air cavities, such as the ear canal[43] (Fig. 8.8), or surgical defects are filled with a saline solution, water-filled bags, paraffin wax, or bolus material customized to fit the defect. In each of these applications, the philosophy is to make the patient as much like a flat-surfaced water phantom as possible.

A more sophisticated use of bolus is to design custom bolus for the purpose of electron conformal therapy. In this application, the bolus usually is designed to conform the 90% isodose line to the PTV while minimizing dose to nearby critical structures and maintaining dose uniformity as much as possible within the 90% dose contour. Proper design of custom bolus requires use of a 3D treatment-planning system[67] that utilizes bolus design operators[68] and a 3D PBA.[53] The methodology of bolus design to optimize target coverage and critical structure searing is seen in Figure 8.19. Perkins et al.[20] have demonstrated the use of custom bolus for chest wall irradiation in the cases of highly distorted anatomy and of a chest wall recurrence (Fig. 8.20), and Kudchadker et al.[69] have demonstrated its use in head and neck treatment. Low et al.[25] have shown its utilization for sparing spinal cord, lung, and kidney in treatment of the paraspinal muscles.

It is recommended that the intent of bolus be verified by measurement or calculation. Bolus used to increase skin dose can be verified by performing in vivo dosimetry measurements (e.g., using thermoluminescent dosimetry). Complex bolus

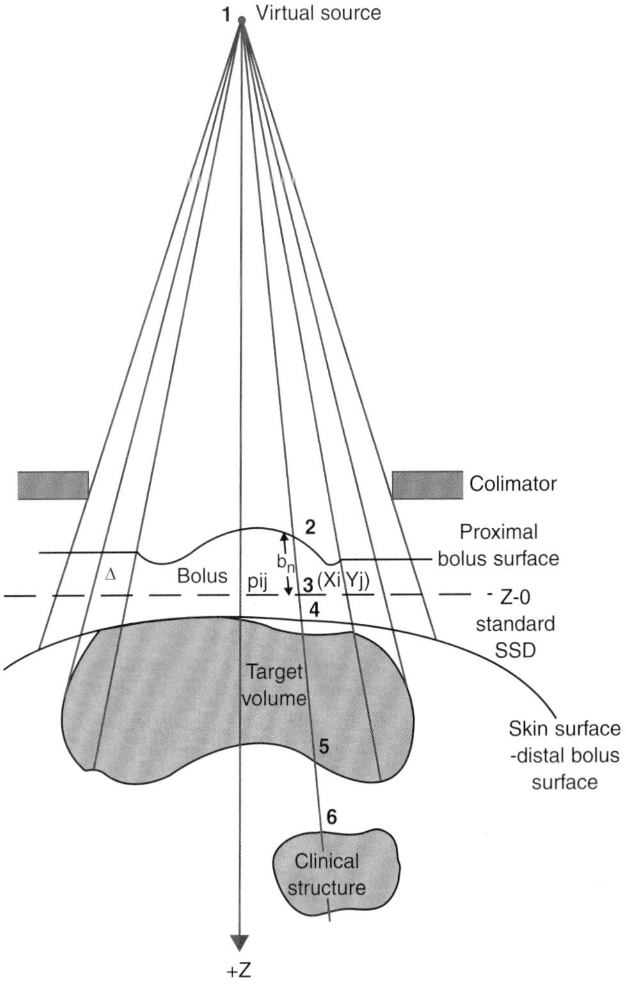

FIGURE 8.19. Schematic representation of the patient contour, target volume, and compensating bolus designed to optimize the coverage of the target while minimizing the dose to the underlying critical structure. (From Low DA, Starkschall G, Bujnowski SW, et al. Electron bolus design for radiation therapy treatment planning: bolus design algorithms. *Med Phys* 1992;19:115–124, with permission.)

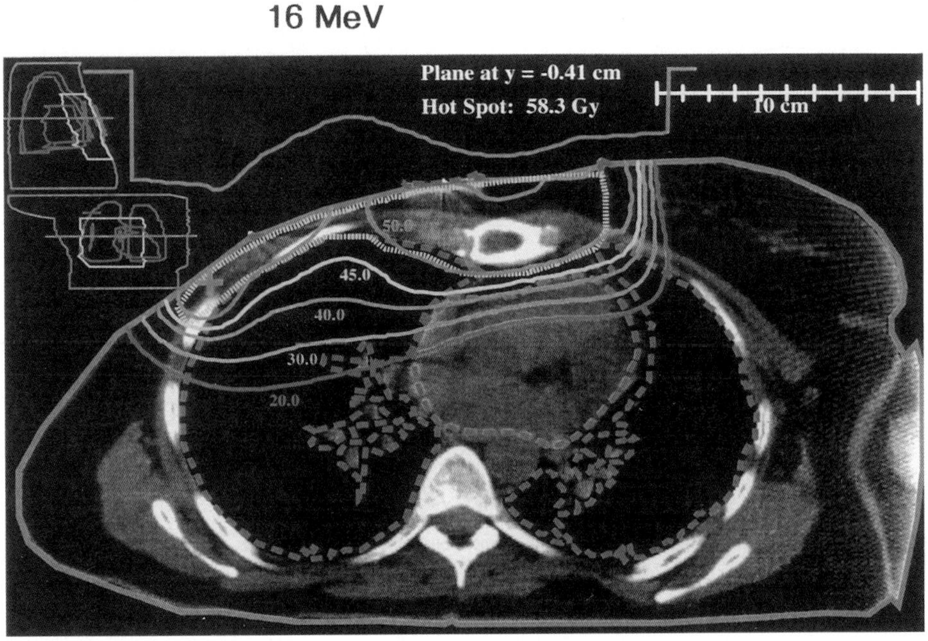

FIGURE 8.20. Conformal electron therapy using variable thickness bolus. Bolus is used to shape the 90% isodose surface (45 Gy) to the distal surface of the chest wall in treating a chest wall occurrence, optimally sparing lung. (From Perkins GH, McNeese MD, Antolak JA, et al. A custom three-dimensional electron bolus technique for optimization of postmastectomy irradiation. *Int J Radiat Oncol Biol Phys* 2001;51:1142–1151, with permission.)

shapes, as used to remove surface irregularities or for electron conformal therapy, can be verified by CT scanning the patient with the bolus in place.[20,25] The dose distribution then can be recalculated using the electron dose algorithm in a treatment-planning system.

This method of electron conformal therapy may be facilitated by a commercial vendor that can create the custom bolus from treatment plan machinist coordinates.[70]

Internal Shielding

Internal shields stops electrons that enter the body before they reach critical structures and deposit any significant dose. Examples of clinical utilization of internal shielding are intraoral blocks protecting salivary glands during head and neck treatments[2]; eye blocks protecting the lens in irradiation of the eyelid,[71] orbit, or retina; and sheets of lead used to protect internal structures during intraoperative therapy.

There are two important concepts to remember in the use of internal shielding. First, the collimator must be sufficiently thick to stop the energy of the electrons in the beam at depth. Electron-beam energy is reduced by 2 MeV per centimeter in unit density tissue; hence, the energy of a 12-MeV beam at a depth of 2 cm is 8 MeV. The thickness of lead required to stop 8-MeV electrons is 4 mm (8 MeV · 0.5 mm/MeV).

One application where ensuring that collimation is sufficiently thick that has been sometimes overlooked is the use of internal eye shields. Shiu et al.[71] showed that x-ray eye shields constructed of plastic-coated lead and designed to shield the eyes from kilovoltage x-rays did not stop 6-MeV electrons, resulting in penetration of approximately 50% of the given dose. However, electron eye shields constructed of enamel-coated tungsten can stop electrons with energies as great as 9 MeV (Fig. 8.21). By using higher density tungsten (ρ = 19.3 g/cm^3) instead of lead (ρ = 11.5 g/cm^3), the eye shields remain sufficiently thin to fit under the eyelid. If only x-ray eye shields are available, bolus should be placed on top of the eye and eye shield to ensure that the electron energy is reduced sufficiently so that electrons do not penetrate the eye shield.

Second, electrons backscattered from lead at a lead–tissue interface increase dose, the increase ranging from approximately 20% at 20 MeV to 60% at 4 MeV, where the energy is the average energy of electrons incident on the lead.[30,72] Das and Bushe[73] published a comprehensive data set demonstrating the range for backscatter electrons as a function of energy, on the order of a few millimeters, and increases as a function of energy. Inserting two half-value layers of bolus between the lead and the tissue usually reduces the dose to upstream tissue to a clinically acceptable value. The thickness of one half-value layer ranges from approximately 1 cm at 10 MeV to 0.5 cm at 3 MeV.[30,74] Intraoral lead stents are coated routinely with acrylic,[28] and a material such as dental wax can be applied easily to lead sheets placed between the mucosa and gums. Eye shields, however, only have clearance for 1 to 2 mm of coating; hence, backscatter dose to the eyelids is an important consideration in treatment management.[71] When determining lead thickness for an internal shielding at a particular depth, one must first determine the energy of the electron beam at that location. The energy of the electron beam on the surface is $E_{o,p}$ typically close to the "console selected" energy. As electrons lose energy by 2 MeV per centimeter, one can determine the remaining energy of any depth. For example, 12 MeV beams at surface would be approximate 6 MeV after 3 cm.

Field Abutment

The purpose of field abutment usually is to enlarge the radiation field or to change the beam energy or modality. In either case, beam uniformity requires that three criteria be met. First, the beams must abut along the entire border.[29,30,32,75] If the edges of the two beams coincide exactly (Fig. 8.22A), then the two

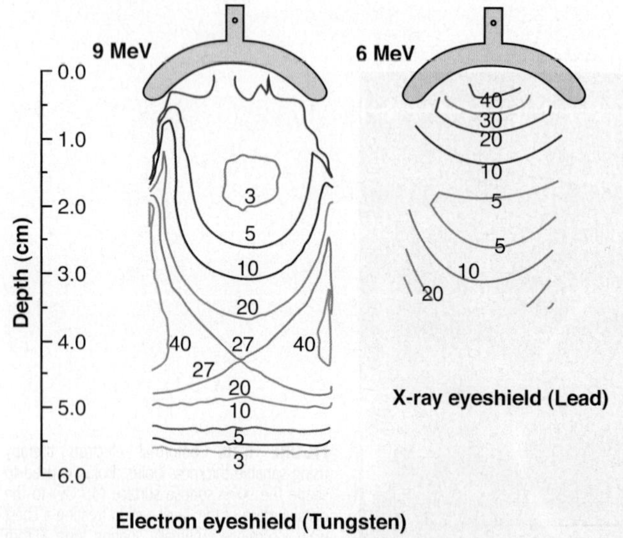

FIGURE 8.21. Electron eye shields. The dose distribution under tungsten electron eye shields demonstrates its ability to stop 9-MeV electrons. The dose distribution under a lead x-ray eye shield shows its inability to stop 6-MeV electrons. (From Shiu AS, Tung SS, Gastorf RJ, et al. Dosimetric evaluation of lead and tungsten eye shields in electron-beam treatment. *Int J Radiat Oncol Biol Phys* 1996;35:599–604, with permission.)

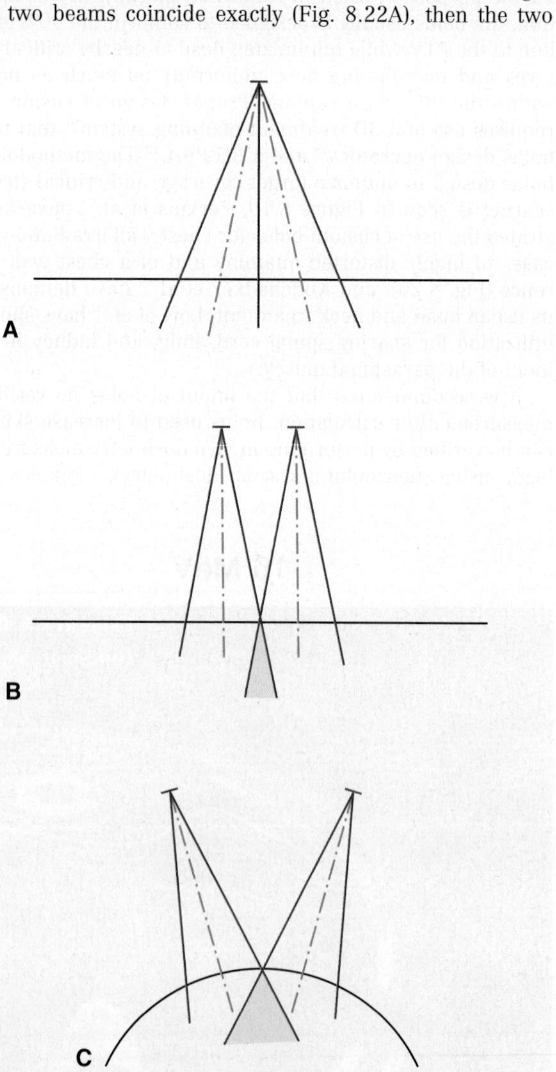

FIGURE 8.22. Comparison of abutment geometries. **A:** Common edge is created by having diverging central axes. **B:** Parallel central axes result in overlapping edges. **C:** Converging central axes result in the greatest overlap. (From ICRU Report 35. *Radiation dosimetry: electron beams with energies between 1 and 50 MeV.* Bethesda, MD: International Commission on Radiation Units and Measurement, 1984, with permission.)

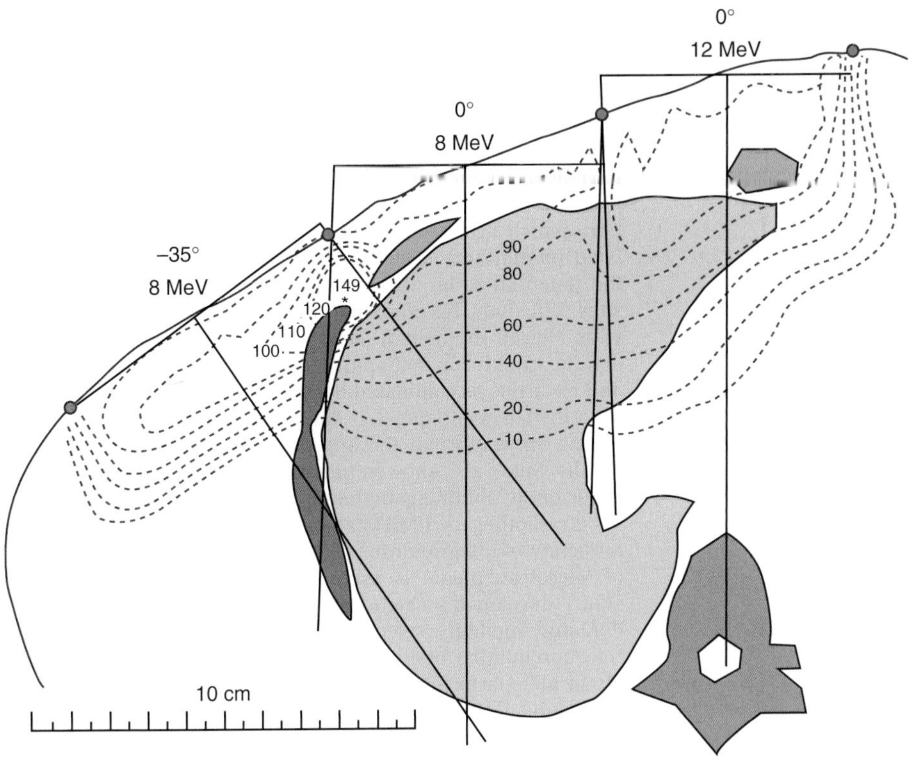

FIGURE 8.23. Clinical example of abutting electron fields in chest wall treatment. Dose homogeneity is acceptable at the border of internal mammary chain (IMC) and medial chest wall fields because central axes are parallel and field widths are small. Dose homogeneity is unacceptable at the border of medial and lateral chest wall fields because central axes are converging (Fig. 8.10B). Dose homogeneity is improved at border of medial and lateral chest wall fields by delivering equal doses with the match line being moved 1 cm twice during treatment.

beams will be equivalent to a single beam and optimal uniformity will be achieved. If the central axes of the two beams are parallel (Fig. 8.22B), then the diverging beam edges will overlap, creating a cold spot upstream and a hot spot downstream of the region of intersection. This is least significant for narrow fields, as encountered in irradiation of the cervical nodes of the neck or abutting the internal mammary and medial chest wall fields. If the central axes are converging (Fig. 8.22C), then there is an even greater amount of overlap. This is the case for abutting lateral and medial chest wall fields. In such cases, feathering the beam edge ±1 cm can reduce the dose heterogeneity. This is illustrated in Figure 8.23 for a standard postmastectomy chest wall irradiation using electrons.

The second criterium is that the beam penumbra must be matched. This is the case for the two spinal fields referred to earlier; however, it is not the case in general, particularly in abutting electron to photon fields. In such cases, either one or both of the field edges must be feathered. Third, it is best that the penumbra be somewhat broad. This reduces the impact of misalignment on the uniformity of dose in the abutted region. Harms and Purdy[49] demonstrated the influence of SSD energy and match bolus on match-line dosimetry. Figure 8.24 displays dose homogeneity for abutted 12 MeV fields depending on gap. In addition, the matching of electron and photo fields is a planning challenge, as two differing penumbra are abutted. Johnson and Khan[76] performed a study of matched electron/photon fields as a function of energy and SSD. Figure 8.25 demonstrates match-line profiles for a typical head and neck field match.

Mixed-Beam Therapy

Electron beams frequently are mixed with photon beams to create an appropriate treatment. The mixed beams can irradiate a common volume of tissue, or they can be abutted. In the former case, an electron field may be added to a primarily photon-beam treatment, or a photon field may be added to a primarily electron-beam treatment. For example, electron boosts are used to deliver localized dose to the surgical site following photon breast irradiation, to treat the postcervical nodes once spinal cord tolerance is reached, and to reduce spinal cord dose (e.g., in lymphoma treatment).[77] In some head and neck treatments, the photon beam is a surrogate to the electron beam, being used to reduce skin dose and to increase dose penetration while still sparing the contralateral salivary gland.[2,10] With the future availability of intensity-modulated photon and modulated electron therapy, the effectiveness of mixed-beam therapy can be expected to increase in breast and head and neck radiation therapy.

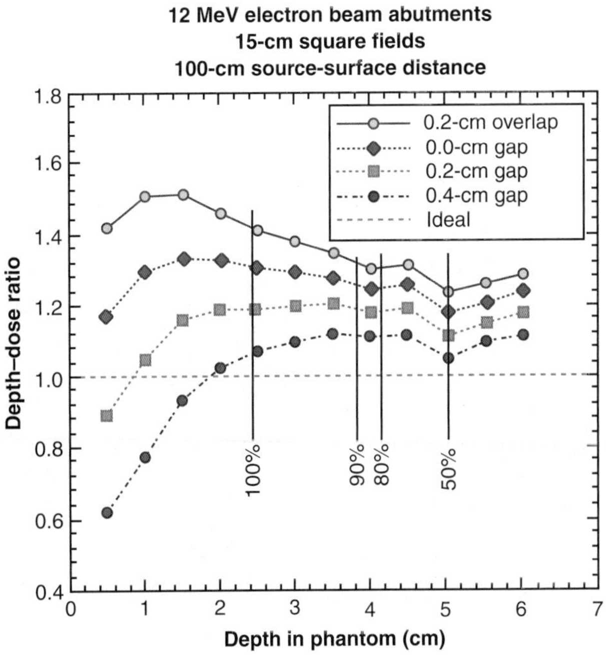

FIGURE 8.24. Graph depicting dose homogeneity for abutted 12-MeV electron fields for a series of gaps. (From Harms WB, Purdy JA. Abutment of high energy electron fields. *Int J Radiat Oncol Biol Phys* 1991;20(4):853–858, with permission.)

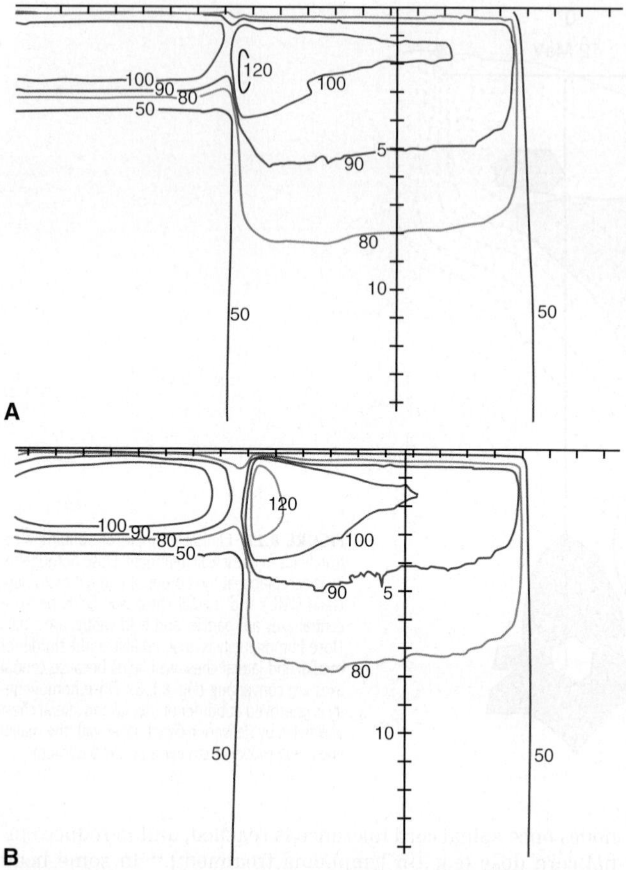

FIGURE 8.25. Isodose curves in a plane perpendicular to the junction line between abutting photon and electron fields. 9-MeV electron beam; field size equals 10 by 10 cm^2; 6-MV photon beam; source-to-surface distance (SSD) equals 100 cm. **A:** Electron beam at standard SSD of 100 cm. **B:** Electron beam at extended SSD of 120 cm. (From Johnson JM, Khan FM. Dosimetric effects of abutting extended source to surface distance electron fields with photon fields in the treatment of head and neck cancers. *Int J Radiat Oncol Biol Phys* 1994;28(3):741–747, with permission.)

Abutted mixed beams are used when separate portions of the anatomy can benefit from the two individually. The most common application of this process is the utilization of electron fields for irradiation of the IMC, supraclavicular, or axillary lymph nodes as part of breast or chest wall irradiation.[2] Matching of tangential photon fields and IMC electron fields is complex because of surface irregularities and heterogeneities. Careful treatment planning must be performed, especially if prescriptive decisions for electron energy and dosage are predicated on the resultant dose distribution. Figure 8.26 displays a tangential photon IMC electron field initial plan with a plan performed with partially wide tangent, a technique suggested to remove the field abutment dilemma.[78] This technique is also used for irradiating the total scalp or for craniospinal irradiation, which are described later. The use of combined modulated photon and electron fields has been reported. This has the potential to be an ideal therapy for particular treatment sites. Thus far, this combined therapy has been demonstrated with Microtron (helium head) machines. Early publications demonstrated conventional (nonmodulated) use of photons and electrons as collimated by MLC. Zackrisson and Karlsson[79] described a technique for matching of electron and photon beams for conformal therapy of target volumes at moderate depths. Mu et al.[80] showed that mixed photon and electron was superior in obtaining planning goals versus intensity-modulated radiotherapy (IMRT) alone. One essential aspect was the reduction of integral dose. The same computer-controlled MLC of Microtron model is used for photons and electrons. Das et al.[81] developed an algorithm using automated beam orientation and modality selection for optimal beam arrangement selection in IMRT of mixed photon and electron beams. Finally, Ma et al.[82] performed a comparative study on tangential photon beams, IMRT, and modulated electron radiotherapy (MERT) for breast cancer treatment.

SPECIALIZED ELECTRON TECHNIQUES

Although electron-beam therapy is used less frequently than is photon-beam therapy, it remains an essential modality. To fully use electron-beam therapy, there must be access to comprehensive electron treatment and treatment-planning techniques. This includes specialized electron techniques, which, in the present context, are defined as those that are seldom required and that use a complex treatment geometry, special treatment delivery hardware, or special treatment-planning software. It is not recommended that all radiation therapy facilities offer all techniques; however, radiation oncologists should be aware of these techniques and should be able to refer patients to a regional center for those that are impractical in smaller settings. This recommendation is based on the significant time, resources, and costs of implementing, maintaining, and providing some of the more complex special electron procedures.

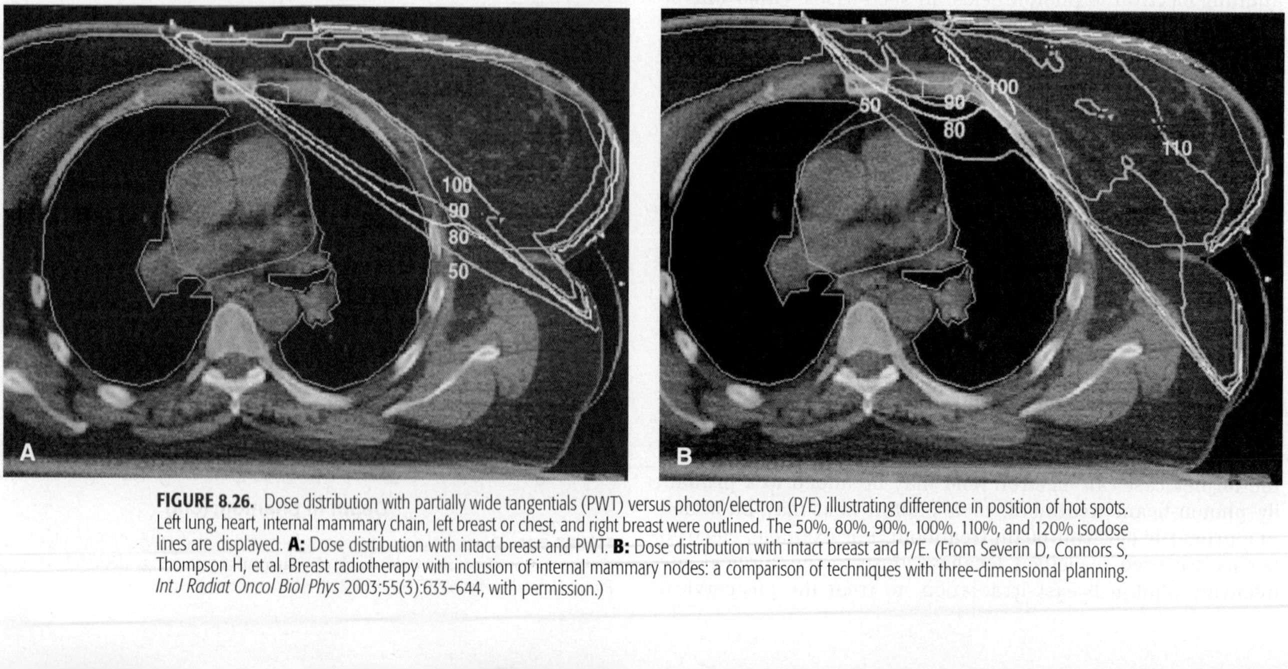

FIGURE 8.26. Dose distribution with partially wide tangentials (PWT) versus photon/electron (P/E) illustrating difference in position of hot spots. Left lung, heart, internal mammary chain, left breast or chest, and right breast were outlined. The 50%, 80%, 90%, 100%, 110%, and 120% isodose lines are displayed. **A:** Dose distribution with intact breast and PWT. **B:** Dose distribution with intact breast and P/E. (From Severin D, Connors S, Thompson H, et al. Breast radiotherapy with inclusion of internal mammary nodes: a comparison of techniques with three-dimensional planning. *Int J Radiat Oncol Biol Phys* 2003;55(3):633–644, with permission.)

The American College of Medical Physics has reviewed the manpower effort and cost associated with several special procedures, which include electron arc therapy, intraoperative electron therapy, and total-skin electron irradiation.[83]

Four types of special techniques are discussed here. First, the treatment of internal tissues is exemplified by intraoperative radiation therapy and intracavitary radiation therapy. Second, the utilization of abutted electron and photon fields is exemplified by craniospinal and total-scalp treatment techniques. Third, the treatment of superficial tissues for a cylindric geometry is exemplified by the total-limb and total-skin treatment techniques. Fourth, an alternative to fixed-beam therapy of the chest wall is exemplified by arc therapy.

Intracavitary Irradiation

Applicators of appropriate design can be used for intracavitary electron irradiation, which delivers an improved dose distribution over that traditionally delivered using orthovoltage x-rays. Intracavitary irradiation most frequently is used to boost the primary site while sparing nearby normal tissues. Intracavitary irradiation has been a choice for intraoral, transvaginal, and intraoperative treatments. Wang[19] showed the benefit of intraoral cones for boosting the oral lesions of the floor of the mouth, soft palate, tongue, and retromolar trigone while sparing mandible, teeth, gum, and salivary glands. McGinnis et al.[28] reported using a transvaginal applicator to boost carcinoma of the cervix with electrons, reducing bulk tumor to subsequently allow intracavitary brachytherapy. Intraoperative radiation therapy can be used in many sites[13]; however, it is used primarily for abdominal sites. Merrick et al.[26] reviewed the experience in the United States of using intraoperative radiotherapy for treatment of pancreatic, biliary, and gastric carcinomas.

The criteria for intracavitary electron irradiation are similar regardless of site. A treatment applicator is necessary so that healthy tissue can be restrained from intercepting electrons irradiating the tumor. The applicator wall must be sufficiently thick to stop electrons from escaping to outside tissue while being thin enough not to interfere with tumor access. Guidelines for accomplishing this for intraoperative applicators have been discussed by Hogstrom et al.[84] Another issue is how to ensure accurate alignment while maintaining patient safety with an applicator. Appropriate cone positioning requires having a method for looking down the cone to view the tumor. Proper alignment of the applicator after inserting it into the patient requires methods for docking it to the machine. For soft docking, the applicator is not physically attached to the machine[84,85] (Fig. 8.27). For hard docking, the applicator is physically attached to the machine, and there are methods for its breaking away under stress.[28,86]

Treatment planning for intracavitary cones typically is done manually because it is not possible to CT scan the patient in the treatment position or under operating room conditions. The electron energy and cone size are selected to match measured isodose distributions to the dimensions of the clinical target volume. Examples of dose distributions for intraoperative applicators are shown in Figure 8.28.[87] These examples show two characteristics of such applicators. First, for the larger diameter applicators, scatter off the wall of the applicator can lead to hot spots near the applicator's periphery. Second, ends of the applicator often are beveled to make it easy to establish contact when the anatomic plane is not perpendicular to the direction of approach (i.e., the central axis of the beam). Note how the depth of the 90% isodose contour beneath the surface decreases from 3.6 cm at 0-degrees incidence to 3.0 cm at 30-degrees incidence, as a result of the effects described earlier.

Total-Scalp Irradiation

Total-scalp irradiation is sometimes necessary in the management of malignancies (e.g., cutaneous lymphoma, melanoma,

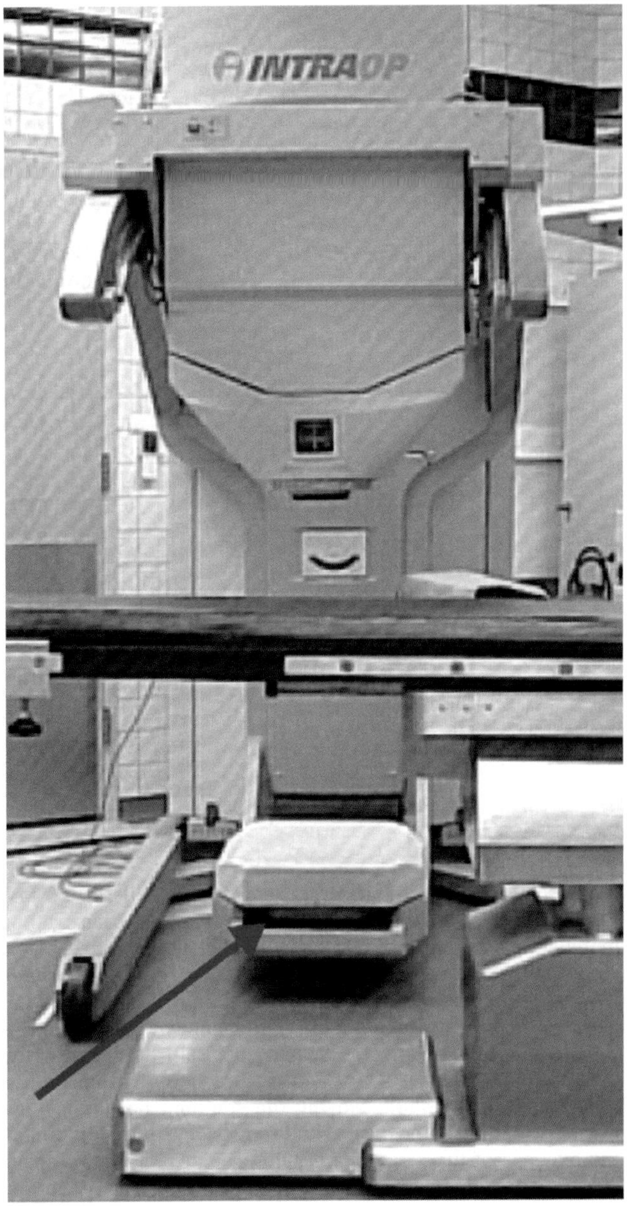

FIGURE 8.27. Intraoperative electron radiation therapy accelerator. View of the Mobetron self-shielded mobile intraoperative radiation therapy unit by IntraOp Medical Corporation. (From Beddar AS, Biggs PJ, Chang S, et al. Intraoperative radiation therapy using mobile electron linear accelerators. AAPM Radiation Therapy Committee Task Group No. 72, Report No. 92, 2006, with permission.)

and angiosarcoma) that present with widespread involvement of the scalp and forehead.[2,15] Electron-beam therapy is a practical means of achieving the therapeutic goal of delivering a uniform dose to the scalp with minimal dose to underlying brain. For many years, total-scalp irradiation was achieved by patching multiple electron fields.[2,88] Although effective, the treatment was tedious as a result of the large number of fields, their requirement for skin collimation, and the need to move the abutment border to improve dose homogeneity.[88] Akazawa[89] from the University of California–San Francisco reported a simpler technique that abuts lateral electron fields to parallel opposed photon fields, the latter of which treats the rind of the scalp while avoiding brain tissue. Tung et al.[15] modified the abutment scheme to account for beam divergence and demonstrated improved dose uniformity by comparing 3D dose calculations with in vivo dose measurements. Figure 8.29 illustrates the abutment scheme. The outer edge of the electron field overlaps the inner edge of the 6-MV x-ray field by

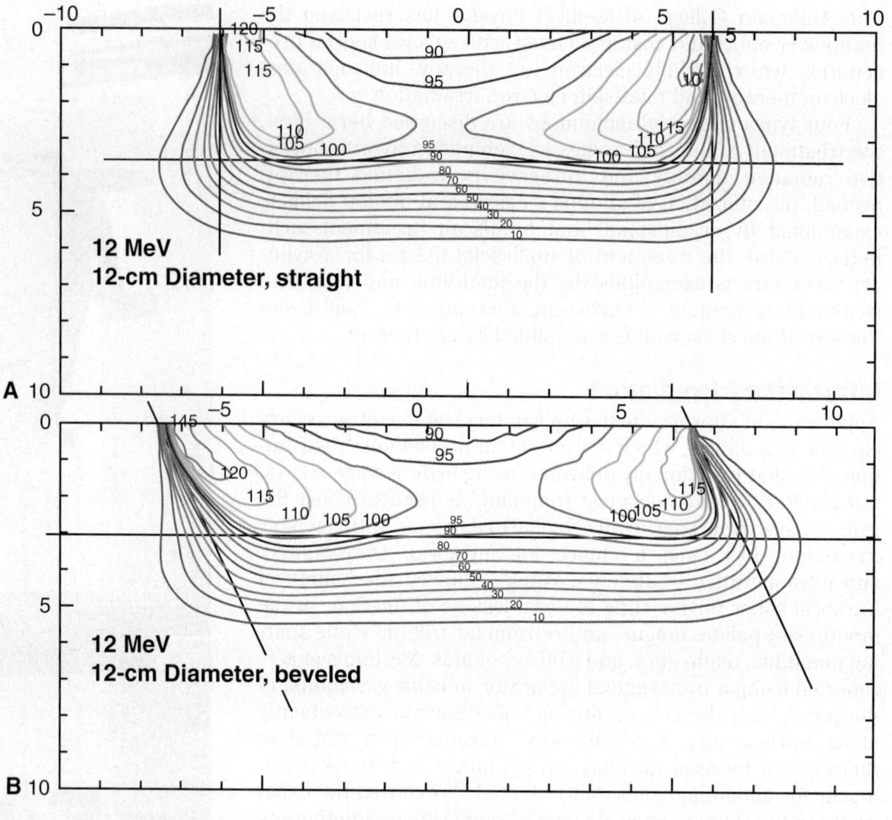

FIGURE 8.28. Isodose plots illustrating typical intraoperative dose distributions at 12 MeV. **A:** 12-cm diameter cone, normal incidence. **B:** 30-degree beveled, 12-cm diameter cone. Note the decreased depth of the 90% dose beneath the surface for the beam 30 degrees from normal incidence relative to that for normal incidence. (From Nyerick CE, Ochran TG, Boyer AL, et al. Dosimetry characteristics of metallic cones for intraoperative radiation therapy. *Int J Radiat Oncol Biol Phys* 1991;21:501–510, with permission.)

3 mm to account for the divergence of the contralateral 6-MV x-ray field. Because the electron and x-ray penumbras are not matched, their common border is moved 1 cm toward beam center halfway through treatment to improve dose homogeneity. Figure 8.30 shows the dose distribution in a transverse CT plane, which illustrates the dose homogeneity achieved in the region of abutment and the sparing of brain tissue. Initially, the common border is set at approximately 0.5 cm inside the inner table of the skull. Moving the common border farther toward the inner table of the skull reduces brain irradiation at the expense of the x-ray beam being replaced by an electron beam that would begin to graze the skull. As discussed earlier, grazing radiation penetrates less deeply, possibly underdosing the scalp in this region. Also noticeable in Figure 8.30 is a 6-mm thick wax bolus, which increases surface dose for both the electron and x-ray fields. Although this technique is straightforward to plan and implement, concern of hot spots along to the midline superior brain tissue along the plane is a concern.

Walker et al.[90] described a six-field electron-beam technique for treatment of mycosis fungoides of the scalp. This technique of overlapping beams was verified with thermoluminescent dosimetry measurements. The dose prescriptions were 20 and 30 Gy for the two patients in this study. Yaparpalvi et al.[91]

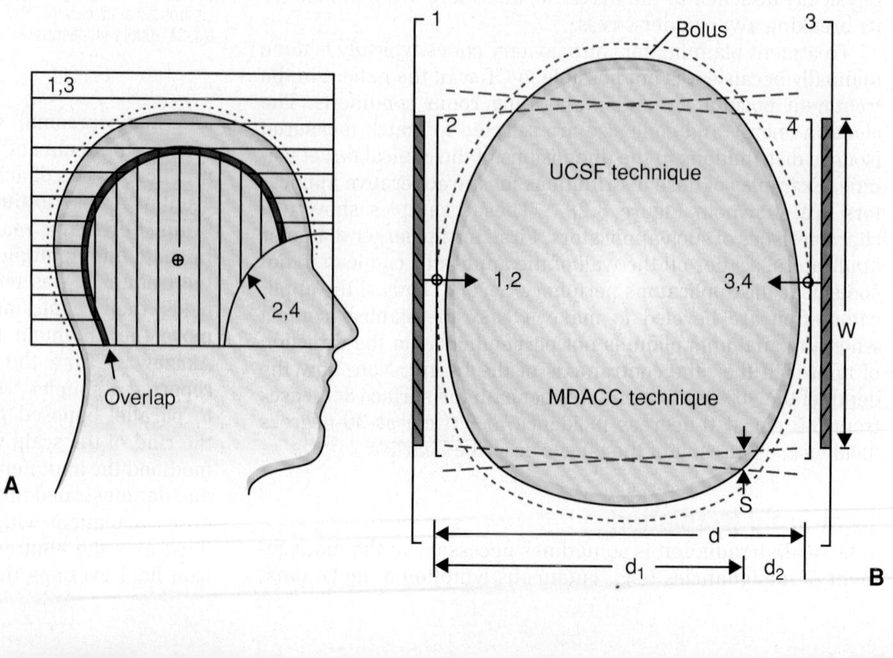

FIGURE 8.29. Abutment scheme for total-scalp irradiation (x-ray fields, 1,3; electron fields, 2,4). **A:** The electron field edge, placed just inside the skull, overlaps the edge of the ipsilateral x-ray field by approximately 3 mm to account for divergence of the edge of the contralateral x-ray field. Halfway through treatment, the field edges are moved 1 cm to improve dose homogeneity in the region of abutment. **B:** The need for the 3-mm overlap (MD Anderson Cancer Center [MDACC] technique) is better appreciated viewing the divergent edges of all fields in a transverse plane. (From Tung SS, Shiu AS, Starkschall G, et al. Dosimetric evaluation of total scalp irradiation using a lateral electron-photon technique. *Int J Radiat Oncol Biol Phys* 1993;27:153–160, with permission.)

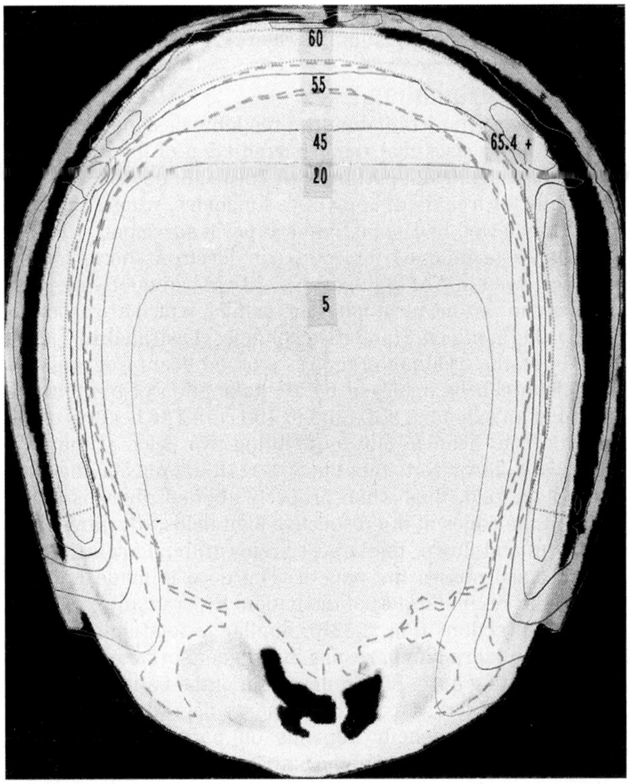

FIGURE 8.30. Dose distribution in a transverse computed tomography plane, illustrating the homogeneity of dose in the abutment region and the degree of brain sparing with this technique. Isodose values in Gray. (From Tung SS, Shiu AS, Starkschall G, et al. Dosimetric evaluation of total scalp irradiation using a lateral electron-photon technique. *Int J Radiat Oncol Biol Phys* 1993;27:153–160, with permission.)

developed a technique for scalp irradiation that used a single posterior-superior field with concentric circles that varied in electron energy. This interesting technique was not confirmed with anthropomorphic phantom dosimetry studies. Peters[92] described use of an electron reflector to improve dose uniformity to the scalp during total-skin electron therapy.

Total-Limb Irradiation

It may be advantageous to irradiate the superficial anatomy of a limb for management of cancer (e.g., melanoma, lymphoma, Kaposi's sarcoma). If the depth beneath the surface is 2 cm or less, electrons offer a uniform dose while sparing deep tissues and structures. This technique has been described by Wooden et al.[16] for the treatment of the lower calf of a patient with Kaposi's sarcoma. Illustrated in Figure 8.31, six equally spaced 5-MeV electron beams are used to irradiate a 9-cm diameter cylinder. Each beam is sufficiently wide so that the entire circle falls within the uniform portion of each beam. Tangential radiation to the surface of the cylinder delivers a greater dose as a result of oblique incidence, which is partially offset by the inverse square effect. Additionally, the tangential radiation penetrates less deeply. The utilization of six or more beams begins to simulate 360-degree arc therapy (which is not feasible due to collisions). The resulting dose distribution illustrates three interesting characteristics. First, the average maximum dose along each radius is approximately 2.5 times the given dose of each of the six fields. Second, 90% of the average maximum dose penetrates 8 to 10 mm, reduced from the value of 15 mm for a single beam incident normally on a flat surface (Fig. 8.32). Third, the surface dose has increased to 90% or greater of average maximum dose compared with approximately 70% of the given dose for a single beam incident normally on a flat surface. This is the result of the self-bolusing effect of tangential electron radiation.

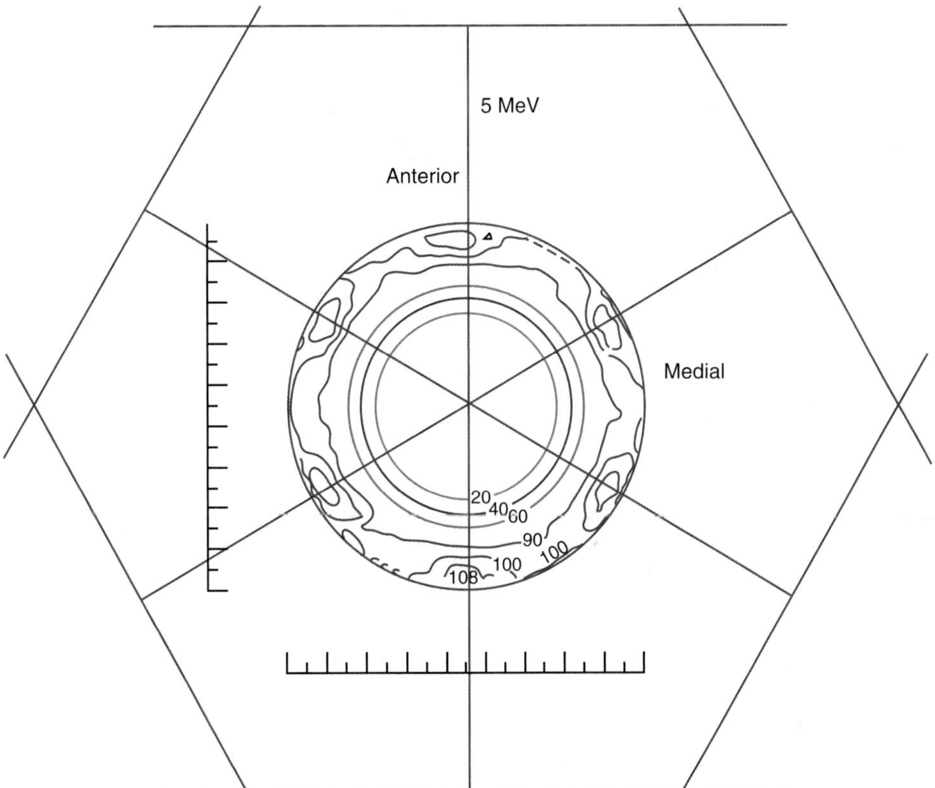

FIGURE 8.31. Dose distribution for total-limb irradiation. Six equally spaced 17-cm wide, 5-MeV electron beams are used to irradiate a 9-cm diameter cylinder. 100% equals 2.55 times the given dose from a single field. (From Wooden KK, Hogstrom KR, Blum P, et al. Whole-limb irradiation of the lower calf using a six-field electron technique. *Med Dosim* 1996;21:211–218, with permission.)

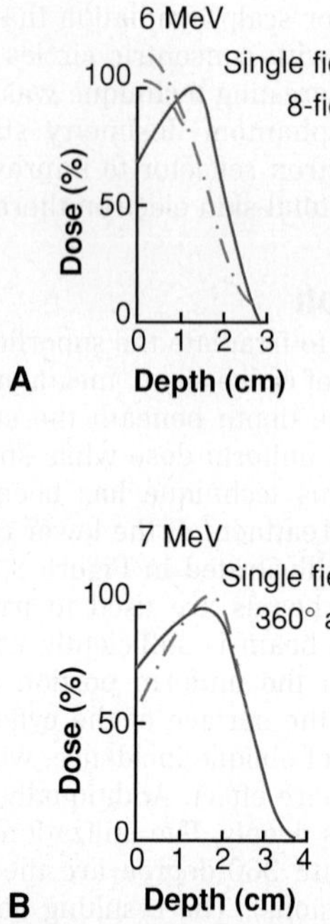

FIGURE 8.32. Treating circular anatomy with multiple beams spaced over 360 degrees. Depth dose along a radial axis depends on the field width. **A:** Depth dose for a broad, 6-MeV beam, resulting from an 8-field technique around a 20-cm diameter water cylinder, is governed by grazing radiation, typical of total-skin and total-limb irradiation. **B:** Depth dose for a narrow, 7-MeV beam, resulting from rotating around a 20-cm diameter water cylinder, is governed by focusing of the radiation toward isocenter, typical of arc electron therapy.

The dosimetric characteristics should be carefully evaluated using one's treatment-planning system.

Total-Skin Irradiation

Total-skin electron irradiation is a modality designed for management of diseases that require irradiation of the entire skin surface or a significant portion of it. The technique is used most frequently for treatment of mycosis fungoides, whose management is reviewed by Hoppe,[17] and Kaposi's sarcoma.

Multiple techniques for total-skin electron therapy have been reviewed in AAPM Report No. 23.[18] The underlying principles of the various techniques are similar, which are exemplified by the modified Stanford technique, illustrated in Figure 8.33. First, the treatment requires a broad beam from right to left, which can be achieved by a combination of treating the patient at an extended SSD (300 to 400 cm). The beam is made uniform from head to foot by abutting two fields at the 50% OAR (Fig. 8.33A). (Note that the 50% OAR lies outside the edge of the light field, thus when properly abutted, there is a gap between the edges of the respective light fields.) By aiming the beams up and down, the largest bremsstrahlung contribution (central axis) misses the patient. The dose is made uniform around the circumference of the patient by irradiating from six different directions (Fig. 8.33B). Similar to total-limb irradiation, tangential radiation results in a higher surface dose and a less penetrating dose. Placed upstream of the patient is a plastic screen that serves as both an energy degrader and a scatterer. Dose homogeneity depends on patient position, and reproducing the positions of the Stanford technique (Fig. 8.33C) is important. Despite efforts to create a homogeneous dose,

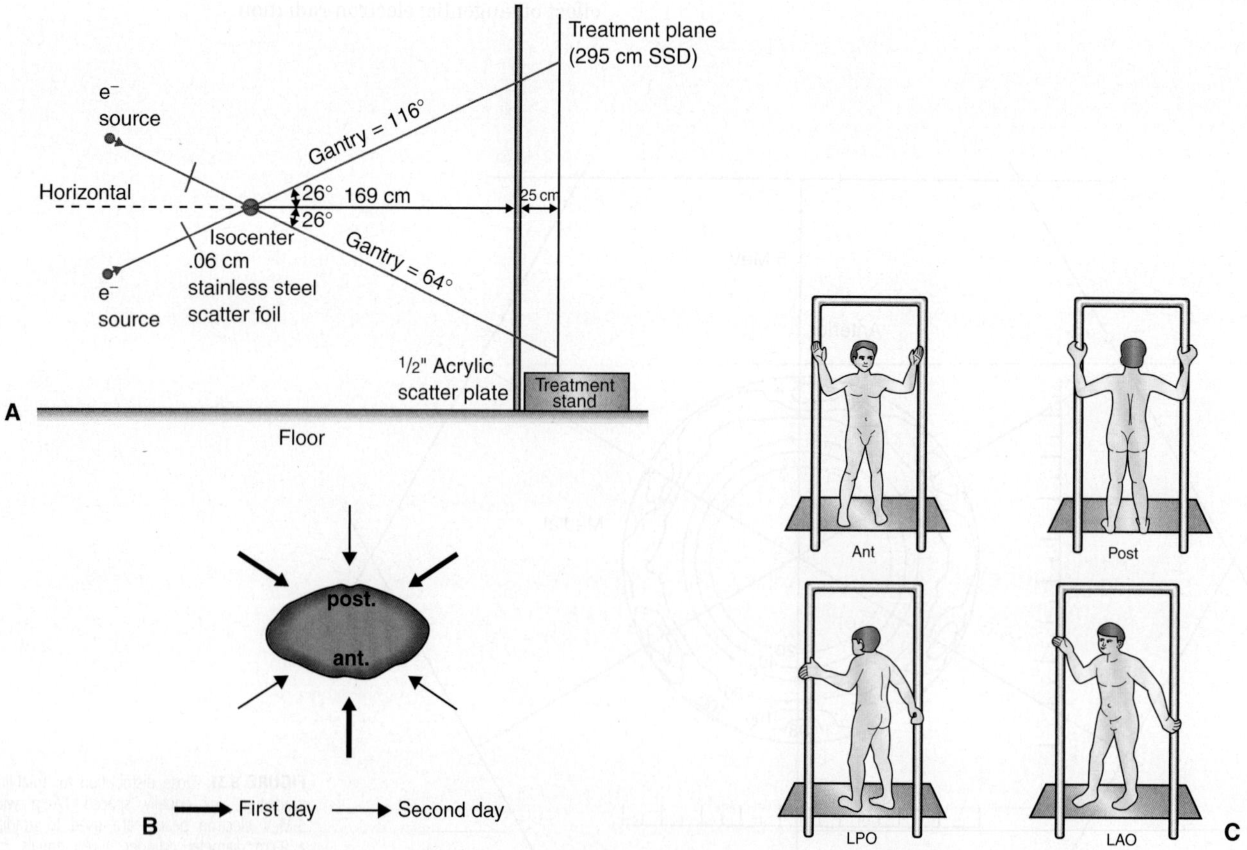

FIGURE 8.33. Schematic of modified Stanford technique. Side view of setup shows the relative position of patient plane, scatter plate, isocenter, and gantry angles **(A)**. Six beam directions **(B)** are achieved by placing the patient in six patient positions **(C)**. (From Almond PR. Total skin electron irradiation technique and dosimetry. In: Kereiakes JG, Elson HR, Born CG, eds. *Radiation oncology physics 1986.* New York: American Institute of Physics, 1987:296–332; and Karzmark CJ, Anderson J, Fessenden P, et al. *AAPM Report No. 23, total skin electron therapy: technique and dosimetry.* New York: American Institute of Physics, 1987, with permission.)

there always will be areas that are underdosed (e.g., top of scalp, sole of feet, perineum, and under the breast or under the panniculus of obese individuals). These areas and sometimes tumorous lesions require separate treatment and boosting, respectively. In contrast, fingers, feet, and toes typically receive excess dose and are shielded for a portion of the treatment. In vivo measurement of patient dose on an individual basis is important when making decisions on prescriptions for supplemental treatments.

Implementation of this technique is complex. It requires an external patient stand with a plastic diffuser, an external scattering foil to broaden the beam, special dosimetry equipment for quality assurance and calibration, special shields for selected parts of the patient, and access to in vivo dosimetry.[93] It is also necessary for the radiation therapy accelerator to have a high–dose rate mode and interlocks for electron energy, gantry angle, and x-ray jaws. Implementation of this technique has been estimated at 105 hours.[83] An institution must have a warranted patient population requiring this technique.

Electron Arc Therapy

Electron arc therapy is a useful technique for treating postmastectomy chest wall.[21] It is used in lieu of parallel-opposed tangential photon irradiation. It is more useful in "barrel-chested" women, where tangential beams can irradiate too much lung. It is also difficult to achieve homogeneous dose in the region where the medial tangential beam used for the chest wall abuts the anterior beam used for the IMC. In such cases, treating both areas with only opposed tangent photon beams irradiates too much lung. In such cases, electron arc therapy is a viable option. This can be particularly important in patients with bilateral disease.

The treatment geometry and dosimetry for arc therapy are unique. There are three levels of collimation in electron arc therapy: the primary x-ray collimators, a shaped secondary cerrobend insert, and skin collimation (Fig. 8.34). The secondary collimator typically projects a 5- to 6-cm beam width at isocenter. There is typically a large air gap between the secondary collimating insert and the patient, resulting in a large penumbra; also in addition, the finite width of the field results in a broad edge at the end of the arc. The sharpness of the penumbra is restored utilizing skin collimation. This requires that the edge of the field of the secondary collimator extends well beyond the edge of the field defined by skin collimation. In the plane of rotation, this is achieved by rotating approximately 15 degrees beyond the treatment field edge (Fig. 8.35).

As discussed previously, depth dose for an arced beam differs from that for a fixed beam (Fig. 8.27B); the surface dose is significantly less, and the dose falloff becomes slightly sharper. Consequently, bolus may be required to deliver adequate dose superficially. Another consequence of arcing is that a constant width of the secondary collimator results in dose inhomogeneity in the cephalocaudal direction. The radius of curvature of the patient with respect to the accelerator isocentric axis is typically less superiorly, as the neck is approached. If the radius of curvature is less, then the skin is farther from the electron source (i.e., a greater SSD). Contrary to fixed-beam therapy, the dose to that region increases rather than decreases as a result of focusing of the electron fluence toward isocenter; however, by reducing the collimator width, the dose can be made more uniform.

The treatment-planning process for arc therapy requires patient CT scanning, delineation of PTV, selection of isocenter location, specification of electron arc boundaries, energy and slab bolus selection, design of secondary collimator, and calculation of dose and monitor units. Figure 8.36 shows a typical dose distribution that can be achieved using arc therapy for irradiation MERT of the IMC and chest wall. Physics commissioning to initiate this procedure is on the order of 4 to 6 weeks.

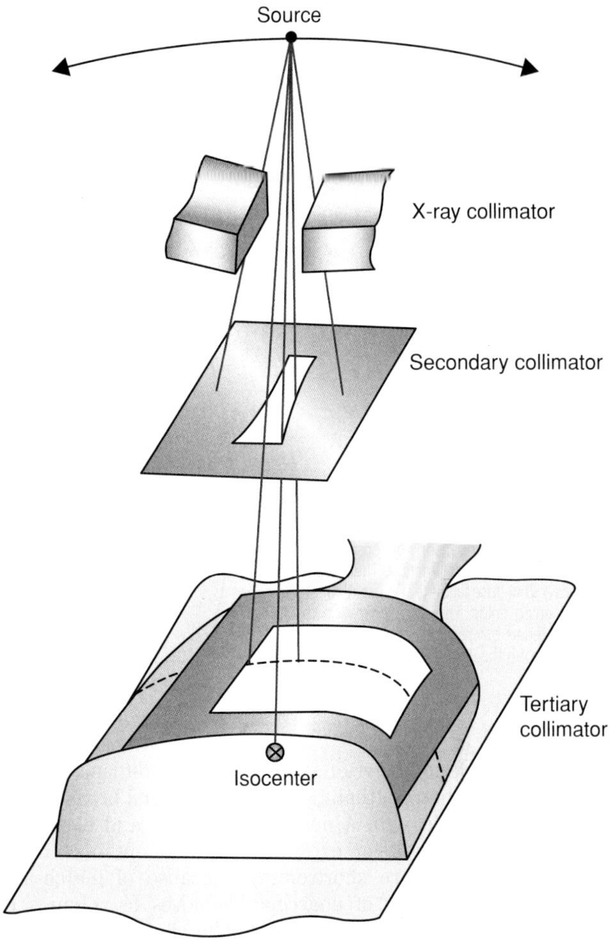

FIGURE 8.34. Schematic of treatment geometry for electron arc therapy. Skin collimation is required because of the large air gap between secondary collimator and patient, which is needed to allow rotation of the gantry around the patient.

Electron radiotherapy has not advanced beyond conventional therapy because of the labor-intensive (cutouts and bolus) tasks to shape and modulate beams, limited conformity in the depth direction, limited lateral conformity, no inverse planning, and no dynamic beam delivery. If these were overcome via an automated method, the conformation of dose distributions to shallow tumors might greatly improve—hence the advent of MERT. There is a definitive niche for MERT to complement a photon IMRT program. MERT will be able to achieve lateral dose conformity by intensity modulation (such as photon IMRT) and dose conformity along the depth direction using energy modulation (unique to electron beams). In addition, MERT may increase dose uniformity in the target both laterally and along the depth direction, reduce high or moderate concomitant dose to distal organs (e.g., lung, heart, and contralateral breast for breast treatments), and improve skin coverage or sparing when combined with photon IMRT.[82,94]

Disease sites such as postmastectomy chest wall, and mycosis fungoides or any cutaneous manifestation of lymphoma of the scalp, and so forth are likely best suited for modulated electrons, either with or without photons, or perhaps a combination of both. However, the inherent collimation systems in modern accelerators were optimized for megavoltage photons and are not conducive to electron-beam delivery (in lieu of extended applicators), nor do commercial treatment-planning systems model electrons collimated without applicators.

As an example of targeted sites that would be improved with MERT, treatment to the chest wall stands out. Current techniques of using tangential photon adjunct fields abutting

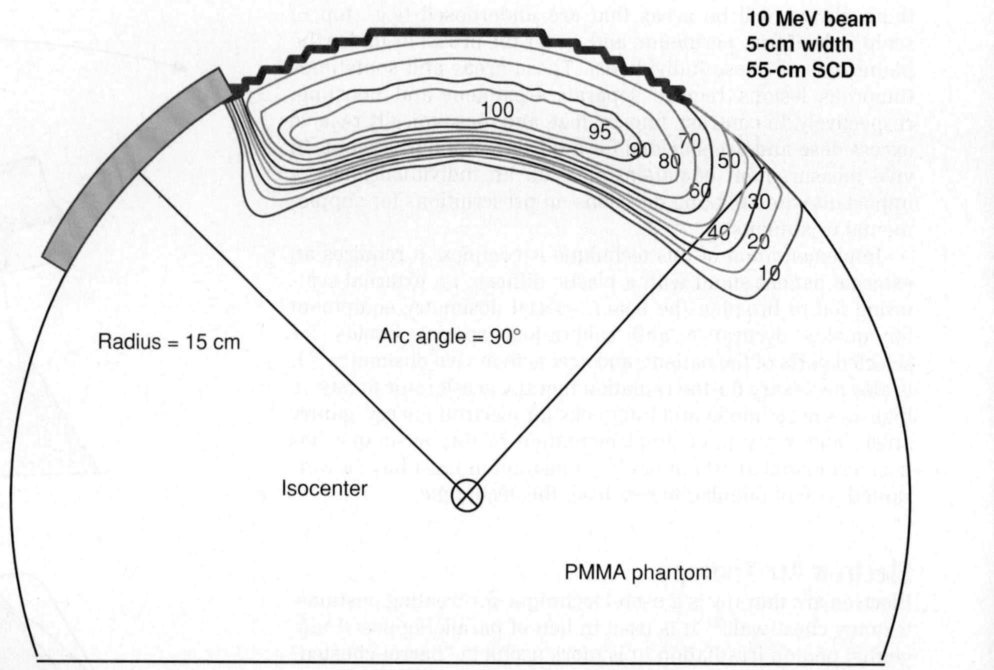

FIGURE 8.35. Comparison of dose distribution with and without skin collimation. The uncollimated edge has a slow dose falloff that is useful for abutting to other arced fields. The skin collimation restores the beam edge but requires rotating the beam 15 degrees beyond the edge of the skin collimator.

supraclavicular and posterior axillary fields are difficult enough without the addition of treating a separate medial breast internal mammary field with a mixture of photon and electrons. Although there has been extensive work to optimize these techniques,[95] there are shortcomings because of match-line problems and delivery of unacceptable doses to volumes of heart, lung, and contralateral breast. The clinical side effects can be edema, fibrosis, heart disease, and pneumonitis. Delivery by tangential photon beams to the chest wall is also not ideal because of the heterogeneous dose delivered in the secondary electron buildup region of the breast. Bolus may be used; however, this unfortunately reduces skin sparing. Electron arc therapy was developed in the 1980s to address the limitations of tangential photon-beam treatments,[96] although it was extremely time-consuming to implement.

Many centers have used photon IMRT to improve dose conformity; however, the fundamental limitations because of megavoltage photon beams, such as excess distal dose and the buildup dose, are still challenges. MERT has been proposed as an alternative, particularly for postmastectomy patients.[62,82] The principal advantage is the rapid distal dose falloff. In principle, electron beams are well suited for these shallow targets, as they will spare distal regions, such as lung and heart.

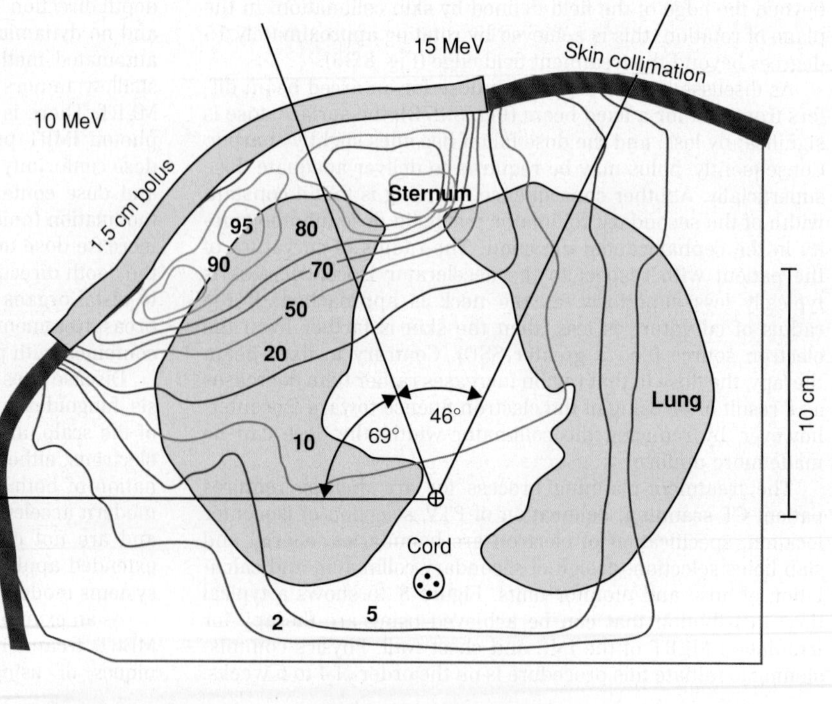

FIGURE 8.36. Typical dose distribution achieved by arc electron therapy. Note the different energies used for the internal mammary chain (IMC) and chest wall fields, the exact abutment of the IMC and chest wall fields, the rotation 15 degrees beyond the skin edges of the skin collimator, and the use of bolus to increase the surface dose. (From Hogstrom KR, Kurup RG, Shiu AS, et al. A two-dimensional pencil-beam algorithm for calculation of arc electron dose distributions. *Phys Med Biol* 1989;34:315–341, with permission.)

Optimization is another important aspect for a MERT program. Many people have come up with inverse planning techniques for photons and even more recently for electrons. Al-Yahya et al.[97] came up with a method of optimizing electron-beam planning for a few leaf-electron collimator (FLEC). Planning was performed via Monte Carlo calculations and optimization using simulated annealing—a powerful mathematical tool that is the basis for inverse planning. FLEC consists of four motor-driven trimmer bars at the end of an applicator that creates rectangular shapes. The report claims potential treatment times of 15 minutes or less. Very comprehensive work by Lee et al.[65] described a Monte Carlo optimization scheme for modulated electron-beam radiotherapy based on a stop and shoot technique. One of the most challenging things in both calculating and optimizing is the leaf scatter, where distributions could vary up to 20% depending on leaf positions. Lee et al.[65] performed MLC planning accomplished by calculating composite distributions for electron beamlets as collimated by tertiary electron MLC. Scatter and leakage contributions were included in the final dose calculation. An inverse planning dose optimization engine designed weights for each beamlet. The particle generation and absorption within the MLC leaves created demanding calculations but were necessary for accurate organ-at-risk calculations. Therefore, modeling of leaf scatter and transmissions is vital for accurate dose calculations. It is key that a multiple source model be developed. Publications describing the use of photon MLCs to modulate electrons have promoted an effective method to reform conformal electron therapy.[98–100]

SUMMARY

Electron-beam therapy remains an important modality to the practice of radiation therapy. As discussed earlier, its effective use requires knowledge of the unique properties of electron-beam dose distributions, the impact of the patient on the dose distribution, and the basic principles for good practice. It requires access to and the proper use of comprehensive treatment planning and delivery tools. It also requires access to special techniques that offer unique treatment solutions for a limited number but broad range of patient conditions.

Electron therapy can be expected to become more sophisticated in the future as the enthusiasm for MERT grows. Advances in electron dose calculations, methods for electron-beam optimization, and availability of MLCs for electrons will enable the practice of combined intensity-modulated photon and energy-modulated electron therapy. This will advance both electron conformal and mixed-beam therapy.

REFERENCES

1. Fletcher GH. Introduction. In: Tapley N, ed. *Clinical applications of the electron beam.* New York: John Wiley and Sons, 1976:1.
2. Tapley ND, ed. *Clinical applications of the electron beam.* New York: John Wiley and Sons, 1976.
3. Hogstrom KR, Fields RS. Use of CT in electron beam treatment planning: current and future development. In: Ling CC, Rogers CC, Morton RJ, eds. *Computed tomography in radiation therapy.* New York: Raven Press, 1983:241–252.
4. Hogstrom KR. Implementation of CT treatment planning. In: Wright AE, Boyer AL, eds. *Advances in radiation therapy treatment planning.* New York: American Institute of Physics, 1983:268–281.
5. Hogstrom KR, Mills MD, Meyer JA, et al. Dosimetric evaluation of a pencil-beam algorithm for electrons employing a two-dimensional heterogeneity correction. *Int J Radiat Oncol Biol Phys* 1984;10:561–569.
6. Hogstrom KR. Evaluation of electron pencil beam dose calculations. In: Kereiakes JG, Elson HR, Born CG, eds. *Radiation oncology physics 1986.* New York: American Institute of Physics, 1987:532–557.
7. Popple RA, Weinber R, Antolak JA, et al. Comprehensive evaluation of a commercial macro Monte Carlo electron dose calculation implementation using a standard verification data set. *Med Phys* 2006;33(6):1540–1551.
8. Klein EE, Low DA, Purdy JA. Dosimetric changes with the new scattering foil applicator system on a C12100 C. *Int J Radiat Oncol Biol Phys* 1995;32:483–490.
9. Kashani R, Santanam L, Moore K, et al. Electron beam dosimetric characteristics for the Varian TrueBeam [abstract]. *Med Phys* 2011;38:3662.
10. Fields RS, Hogstrom KR. Optimization of electron-photon mixed beam planning. In: *Proceedings of the Eighth International Conference on the Use of Computers in Radiation Therapy.* Silver Spring, MD: IEEE Computer Society Press, 1984:248–254.
11. Million RR, Parson JT, Bova FJ, et al. Electron beam: the management of head and neck cancer. In: Vaeth JM, Meyer JL, eds. *Frontiers of radiation therapy and oncology vol. 25: The role of high energy electrons in the treatment of cancer.* Basel: S. Karger AG, 1991:107–127.
12. Kun LE. Electron beam therapy in children. In: Vaeth JM, Meyer JL, eds. *Frontiers of radiation therapy and oncology vol. 25: the role of high energy electrons in the treatment of cancer.* Basel: S. Karger AG, 1991:201–206.
13. Vaeth JM, Meyer JL, eds. *Frontiers of radiation therapy and oncology vol. 25: the role of high energy electrons in the treatment of cancer.* Basel: S. Karger AG, 1991.
14. Mills MD, Hogstrom KR, Fields RS. Determination of electron beam output factors for a 20-MeV linear accelerator. *Med Phys* 1985;12:473–476.
15. Tung SS, Shiu AS, Starkschall G, et al. Dosimetric evaluation of total scalp irradiation using a lateral electron-photon technique. *Int J Radiat Oncol Biol Phys* 1993;27:153–160.
16. Wooden KK, Hogstrom KR, Blum P, et al. Whole-limb irradiation of the lower calf using a six-field electron technique. *Med Dosim* 1996;21:211–218.
17. Hoppe RT. Total skin electron beam therapy in the management of mycosis fungoides. In: Vaeth JM, Meyer JL, eds. *Frontiers of radiation therapy and oncology vol. 25: the role of high energy electrons in the treatment of cancer.* Basel: S. Karger AG, 1991:80–89.
18. Karzmark CJ, Anderson J, Fessenden P, et al. *AAPM Report No. 23, total skin electron therapy: technique and dosimetry.* New York: American Institute of Physics, 1987.
19. Wang CC. Intraoral cone for carcinoma of the oral cavity. In: Vaeth JM, Meyer JL, eds. *Frontiers of radiation therapy and oncology vol. 25: the role of high energy electrons in the treatment of cancer.* Basel: S. Karger AG, 1991:128–131.
20. Perkins GH, McNeese MD, Antolak JA, et al. A custom three-dimensional electron bolus technique for optimization of postmastectomy irradiation. *Int J Radiat Oncol Biol Phys* 2001;51:1142–1151.
21. Stewart JR, Leavitt DD, Prows J. Electron arc therapy of the chest wall for breast cancer: rationale, dosimetry, and clinical aspects. In: Vaeth JM, Meyer JL, eds. *Frontiers of radiation therapy and oncology vol. 25: The role of high energy electrons in the treatment of cancer.* Basel: S. Karger AG, 1991:134–150.
22. Recht A, Triedman SA, Harris JR. The "boost" in the treatment of early-stage breast cancer: electrons versus interstitial implants. In: Vaeth JM, Meyer JL, eds. *Frontiers of radiation therapy and oncology vol. 25: the role of high energy electrons in the treatment of cancer.* Basel: S. Karger AG, 1991:169–179.
23. Kirsner SM, Hogstrom KR, Kurup RG, et al. Dosimetric evaluation in heterogeneous tissue of anterior electron beam irradiation for treatment of retinoblastoma. *Med Phys* 1987;14:772–779.
24. Donaldson SS, Findley DO. Treatment of orbital lymphoid tumors with electron beams. In: Vaeth JM, Meyer JL, eds. *Frontiers of radiation therapy and oncology vol. 25: the role of high energy electrons in the treatment of cancer.* Basel: S. Karger AG, 1991:187–200.
25. Low DA, Starkschall G, Sherman NE, et al. Computer-aided design and fabrication of an electron bolus for treatment of the paraspinal muscles. *Int J Radiat Oncol Biol Phys* 1995;33:1127–1138.
26. Merrick HW III, Dobelbower RR Jr, Konski AA. Intraoperative radiation therapy for pancreatic, biliary and gastric carcinoma: the US experience. In: Vaeth JM, Meyer JL, eds. *Frontiers of radiation therapy and oncology vol. 25: the role of high energy electrons in the treatment of cancer.* Basel: S. Karger AG, 1991: 246–257.
27. Perez CA. Management of vulvar cancer. In: Vaeth JM, Meyer JL, eds. *Frontiers of radiation therapy and oncology vol. 25: the role of high energy electrons in the treatment of cancer.* Basel: S. Karger AG, 1991:183–186.
28. McGinnis WL, Bischof CJ, Latourette HB. Transvaginal cone electron beam technique for a Varian 18 MeV linear accelerator. *Int J Radiat Oncol Biol Phys* 1979;5:123–125.
29. Hogstrom KR. Clinical electron beam dosimetry: basic dosimetry data. In: Purdy JA, ed. *Advances in radiation oncology physics: dosimetry, treatment planning, and brachytherapy.* Woodbury: American Institute of Physics, 1991:390–429.
30. Khan FM, Doppke KP, Hogstrom KR, et al. Clinical electron-beam dosimetry: report of AAPM Radiation Therapy Committee Task Group No. 25. *Med Phys* 1991;18:73–109.
31. Shiu AS, Tung SS, Nyerick CE, et al. Comprehensive analysis of electron beam central axis dose for a radiation therapy linear accelerator. *Med Phys* 1994;21: 559–566.
32. Hogstrom KR. Treatment planning in electron beam therapy. In: Vaeth JM, Meyer JL, eds. *Frontiers of radiation therapy and oncology vol. 25: the role of high energy electrons in the treatment of cancer.* Basel: S. Karger AG, 1991:30–52.
33. Meyer JA, Palta JR, Hogstrom KR. Demonstration of relatively new electron dosimetry measurement techniques on the Mevatron 80. *Med Phys* 1984;11: 670–677.
34. Hogstrom, KR, Steadham RE, Wong PF, et al. Monitor unit calculations for electron beams. In: Gibbons JP, ed. *Monitor unit calculations for external photon and electron beams.* Madison, WI: Advanced Medical Publishing, 2000:113–126.
35. Klein EE, Hanley J, Bayouth J, et al. Task Group 142 report: quality assurance of medical accelerators. *Med Phys* 2009;36(9):4197–4212.
36. Kutcher GJ, Coia L, Gillin M, et al. Comprehensive QA for radiation oncology: report of AAPM Radiation Therapy Committee Task Group 40. *Med Phys* 1994;21(4):581–618.
37. Hogstrom KR, Horton JL, Kutcher GJ, et al. *ACMP Task Group Report: survey of physics resources for radiation oncology special procedures.* Reston, VA: American College of Medical Physics, 1998.
38. Fraass B, Doppke K, Hunt M, et al. American Association of Physicists in Medicine Radiation Therapy Committee Task Group 53: quality assurance for clinical radiotherapy treatment planning [review]. *Med Phys* 1998;25(10):1773–1829.
39. Hogstrom KR. Dosimetry of electron heterogeneities. In: Wright AE, Boyer AL, eds. *Advances in radiation therapy treatment planning.* New York: American Institute of Physics, 1983:223–243.
40. Ekstrand KE, Dixon RL. The problem of obliquely incident beams in electron-beam treatment planning. *Med Phys* 1982;9:276–278.
41. Boyd RA, Hogstrom KR, Antolak JA, et al. A measured data set for evaluating electron-beam dose algorithms. *Med Phys* 2001;28:950–958.

42. Shiu AS, Tung S, Hogstrom KR, et al. Verification data for electron beam dose algorithms. *Med Phys* 1992;19:623–636.
43. Morrison WH, Wong PF, Starkschall G, et al. Water bolus for electron irradiation of the ear canal. *Int J Radiat Oncol Biol Phys* 1995;33:479–483.
44. Perry DJ, Holt JG. A model for calculating the effects of small inhomogeneities on electron beam dose distributions. *Med Phys* 1980;7:207–215.
45. Shiu AS, Hogstrom KR. Dose in bone and tissue near bone-tissue interface from electron beam. *Int J Radiat Oncol Biol Phys* 1991;21:695–702.
46. Mills MD, Hogstrom KR, Almond PR. Prediction of electron beam output factors. *Med Phys* 1982;9:60–68.
47. Biggs PJ, Boyer AL, Doppke KP. Electron dosimetry of irregular fields on Clinac-18. *Int J Radiat Oncol Biol Phys* 1979;5:433–440.
48. Khan FM. *The physics of radiation therapy,* 4th ed. Baltimore: Lippincott Williams & Wilkins, 2009.
49. Harms WB, Purdy JA. Abutment of high energy electron fields. *Int J Radiat Oncol Biol Phys* 1991;20(4):853–858.
50. Hogstrom KR, Steadham RE. Electron beam dose computation. In: Palta JR, Mackie TR, eds. *Teletherapy: present and future.* Madison, WI: Advanced Medical Publishing, 1996:137–174.
51. Craig T, Brochu D, Van Dyk J. A quality assurance phantom for three-dimentional radiation treatment planning. *Int J Radiat Oncol Biol Phys* 1999;44(4):955–966.
52. Cygler JE, Daskalov GM, Chan GH, et al. Evaluation of the first commercial Monte Carlo dose calculation engine for electron beam treatment planning. *Med Phys* 2004;31(1):142–153.
53. Starkschall G, Shiu AS, Bujnowski SW, et al. Effect of dimensionality of heterogeneity corrections on the implementation of a three-dimensional electron pencil-beam algorithm. *Phys Med Biol* 1991;36:207–227.
54. Boyd RA, Hogstrom KR, Rosen II. Effect of using an initial polyenergetic spectrum with the pencil-beam redefinition algorithm for electron-dose calculations in water. *Med Phys* 1998;25:2176–2185.
55. Boyd RA, Hogstrom KR, Starkschall G. Electron pencil-beam redefinition algorithm dose calculations in the presence of heterogeneities. *Med Phys* 2001;28:2096–2104.
56. Shiu AS, Hogstrom KR. Pencil-beam redefinition algorithm for electron dose distributions. *Med Phys* 1991;18:7–18.
57. Faddegon B, Balogh J, Mackenzie R, et al. Clinical considerations of Monte Carlo for electron radiotherapy treatment planning. *Radiat Phys Chem* 1998;53:217–227.
58. Jiang SB, Kapur A, Ma CM. Electron beam modeling and commissioning for Monte Carlo treatment planning. *Med Phys* 2000;27(1):180–191.
59. Ma CM, Mok E, Kapur A, et al. Clinical implementation of a Monte Carlo treatment planning system. *Med Phys* 1999;26(10):2133–2143.
60. Neuenschwander H, Born EJ. A macro Monte-Carlo method for electron-beam dose calculations. *Phys Med Biol* 1992;37(1):107–125.
61. Neuenschwander H, Mackie TR, Reckwerdt PJ. MMC—a high-performance Monte Carlo code for electron beam treatment planning. *Phys Med Biol* 1995;40(l):543–574.
62. Ding GX, Duggan DM, Coffey CW, et al. First macro Monte Carlo based commercial dose calculation module for electron beam treatment planning—new issues for clinical consideration. *Phys Med Biol* 2006;51(11):2781–2799.
63. Ding GX, Cygler JE, Yu CW, et al. A comparison of electron beam dose calculation accuracy between treatment planning systems using either a pencil beam or a Monte Carlo algorithm. *Int J Radiat Oncol Biol Phys* 2005;63(2):622–633.
64. Klein EE, Li Z, Low DA. A feasibility study of multileaf collimated electrons with a scattering foil based accelerator. *Radiother Oncol* 1996;41:189–196.
65. Lee MC, Jiang SB, Ma CM. Monte Carlo and experimental investigations of multileaf collimated electron beams for modulated electron radiation therapy. *Med Phys* 2000;27(12):2708–2718.
66. Karlsson MG, Karlsson M, Ma CM. Treatment head design for multileaf collimated high-energy electrons. *Med Phys* 1999;26(10):2161–2167.
67. Starkschall G, Antolak JA, Hogstrom KR. Electron beam bolus for 3-D conformal radiation therapy. In: Purdy JA, Emami B, eds. *3-D radiation treatment planning and conformal therapy, proceedings of an international symposium.* Madison, WI: Medical Physics Publishing, 1995:265–282.
68. Low DA, Starkschall G, Bujnowski SW, et al. Electron bolus design for radiation therapy treatment planning: bolus design algorithms. *Med Phys* 1992;19:115–124.
69. Kudchadker RJ, Hogstrom KR, Garden AS, et al. Electron conformal radiation therapy using bolus and intensity modulation. *Int J Radiat Oncol Biol Phys* 2002;53:1023–1037.
70. Zeidan OA, Chauhan BD, Estabrook WW, et al. Image-guided bolus electron conformal therapy—a case study. *J Appl Clin Med Phys* 2010;12(1):3311.
71. Shiu AS, Tung SS, Gastorf RJ, et al. Dosimetric evaluation of lead and tungsten eye shields in electron beam treatment. *Int J Radiat Oncol Biol Phys* 1996;35:599–604.
72. Klevenhagen SC, Lambert GD, Arbabi A. Backscattering in electron beam therapy for energies between 3 and 35 MeV. *Phys Med Biol* 1982;27:363–373.
73. Das IJ, Bushe HS. Backscattering and transmission through a high Z interface as a measure of electron beam energy. *Med Phys* 1994;21(2):315–319.
74. Lambert GD, Klevenhagen SC. Penetration of backscattered electrons in polystyrene for energies between 1 and 25 MeV. *Phys Med Biol* 1982;27:721–725.
75. ICRU Report 35. *Radiation dosimetry: electron beams with energies between 1 and 50 MeV.* Bethesda, MD: International Commission on Radiation Units and Measurement, 1984.
76. Johnson JM, Khan FM. Dosimetric effects of abutting extended source to surface distance electron fields with photon fields in the treatment of head and neck cancers. *Int J Radiat Oncol Biol Phys* 1994;28(3):741–747.
77. Mills MD, Fuller LM, Zagars GK, et al. Spinal cord dose reduction using an anterior 13 MeV electron field situated between a split anterior ^{60}Co supraclavicular field. *Int J Radiat Oncol Biol Phys* 1987;13:1571–1575.
78. Severin D, Connors S, Thompson H, et al. Breast radiotherapy with inclusion of internal mammary nodes: a comparison of techniques with three-dimensional planning. *Int J Radiat Oncol Biol Phys* 2003;55(3):633–644.
79. Zackrisson B, Karlsson M. Matching of electron beams for conformal therapy of target volumes at moderate depths. *Radiother Oncol* 1996;39(3):261–270.
80. Mu X, Olofsson L, Karlsson M, et al. Can photon IMRT be improved by combination with mixed electron and photon techniques? *Acta Oncol* 2004;43(8):727–735.
81. Das SK, Bell M, Marks LB, et al. A preliminary study of the role of modulated electron beams in intensity modulated radiotherapy, using automated beam orientation and modality selection. *Int J Radiat Oncol Biol Phys* 2004;59(2):602–617.
82. Ma CM, Ding M, Li JS, et al. A comparative dosimetric study on tangential photon beams, intensity-modulated radiation therapy (IMRT) and modulated electron radiotherapy (MERT) for breast cancer treatment. *Phys Med Biol* 2003;48(7):909–924.
83. Mills MD. Analysis and practical use: the Abt Study of Medical Physicist Work Values for Radiation Oncology Physics Services—round II. *J Am Coll Radiol* 2005;2(9):782–789.
84. Hogstrom KR, Boyer AL, Shiu AS, et al. Design of metallic electron beam cones for an intraoperative therapy linear accelerator. *Int J Radiat Oncol Biol Phys* 1990;18:1223–1232.
85. Beddar AS, Biggs PJ, Chang S, et al. Intraoperative radiation therapy using mobile electron linear accelerators. AAPM Radiation Therapy Committee Task Group No. 72, Report No. 92, 2006.
86. Biggs PJ, Wang CC. Breakaway safety feature for an intra-oral cone system. *Int J Radiat Oncol Biol Phys* 1984;10:1117–1119.
87. Nyerick CE, Ochran TG, Boyer AL, et al. Dosimetry characteristics of metallic cones for intraoperative radiation therapy. *Int J Radiat Oncol Biol Phys* 1991;21:501–510.
88. Able CM, Mills MD, McNeese MD, et al. Evaluation of a total scalp electron irradiation technique. *Int J Radiat Oncol Biol Phys* 1991;21:1063–1072.
89. Akazawa C. Treatment of the scalp using photon and electron beams. *Med Dosim* 1989;14:129–131.
90. Walker C, Wadd NJ, Lucraft HH. Novel solutions to the problems encountered in electron irradiation to the surface of the head. *Br J Radiol* 1999;72(860):787–791.
91. Yaparpalvi R, Fontenla DP, Beitler JJ. Improved dose homogeneity in scalp irradiation using a single set-up point and different energy electron beams. *Br J Radiol* 2002;75(896):670–677.
92. Peters VG. Use of an electron reflector to improve dose uniformity at the vertex during total skin electron therapy. *Int J Radiat Oncol Biol Phys* 2000;46(4):1065–1069.
93. Almond PR. Total skin electron irradiation technique and dosimetry. In: Kereiakes JG, Elson HR, Born CG, eds. *Radiation oncology physics 1986.* New York: American Institute of Physics, 1987:296–332.
94. Alexander A, Soisson E, Hijal T, et al. Comparison of modulated electron radiotherapy to conventional electron boost irradiation and volumetric modulated photon arc therapy for treatment of tumour bed boost in breast cancer. *Radiothera Oncol* 2011;100(2):253–258. Epub 2011 Jul 6.
95. Jin JY, Klein EE, Kong FM, et al. An improved internal mammary irradiation technique in radiation treatment of locally advanced breast cancers. *J Appl Clin Med Phys* 2005;6(1):84–93.
96. Gaffney DK, Leavitt DD, Tsodikov A, et al. Electron arc irradiation of the postmastectomy chest wall with CT treatment planning: 20-year experience. *Int J Radiat Oncol Biol Phys* 2001;51(4):994–1001.
97. Al-Yahya K, Hristov D, Verhaegen F, et al. Monte Carlo based modulated electron beam treatment planning using a few-leaf electron collimator—feasibility study. *Phys Med Biol* 2005;50(5):847–857.
98. Klein EE, Vicic M, Ma CM, et al. Validation of calculations for electrons modulated with conventional photon multileaf collimators. *Phys Med Biol* 2008;53(5):1183–1208.
99. Klein EE, Mamalui-Hunter M, Low DA. Delivery of modulated electron beams with conventional photon multi-leaf collimators. *Phys Med Biol* 2009;54(2):327–339.
100. Surucu M, Klein EE, Mamalui-Hunter M, et al. Planning tools for modulated electron radiotherapy. *Med Phys* 2010;37(5):2215–2224.

Chapter 9
Conformal Radiation Therapy Physics, Treatment Planning, and Clinical Aspects

James A. Purdy

Modern anatomic imaging technologies, such as x-ray computed tomography (CT) and magnetic resonance imaging (MRI), provide a fully three-dimensional model of the cancer patient's anatomy, which is often complemented with functional imaging, such as positron emission tomography (PET) or magnetic resonance spectroscopy. Such advanced imaging allows the radiation oncologist to more accurately identify tumor volumes and their relationship with other critical normal organs. Powerful x-ray CT-simulation and three-dimensional treatment-planning systems (3DTPS) have been commercially available since the early 1990s, and three-dimensional conformal radiation therapy (3DCRT) is now firmly in place as the standard of practice.[1–3] In addition, advances in radiation treatment-delivery technology continue, and medical linear accelerators now come equipped with sophisticated computer-controlled multileaf collimator systems (MLCs) and integrated volumetric imaging systems that provide beam aperture and/or beam-intensity modulation capabilities that allow precise shaping and positioning of the patient's dose distributions.[3,4]

Conformal treatment plans generally use an increased number of radiation beams that are shaped to conform to the target volume. To improve the conformality of the dose distribution, conventional beam modifiers (e.g., wedges, partial transmission blocks, and/or compensating filters) are sometimes used. This "*forward planning*" approach used for 3DCRT (Fig. 9.1) is rapidly giving way to an "*inverse planning*" approach referred to as *intensity-modulated radiation therapy* (IMRT) (Fig. 9.2), which can achieve even greater conformity by optimally modulating the individual beamlets that make up the radiation beams.[5,6] IMRT dose distributions can be created to conform much more closely to the target volume, particularly for those volumes having complex/concave shapes, and also shaped to avoid critical normal tissues in the irradiated volume. This increased conformality results in IMRT treatments being much more sensitive to geometric uncertainties than the two-dimensional or forward-planned 3DCRT approaches and has spurred the development of treatment machines integrated with advanced volumetric imaging capabilities,[2,3,7,8] which is again pushing the frontiers in conformal radiation therapy (CRT) practice from IMRT to what is now referred to as *image-guided IMRT*, or simply *image-guided radiation therapy* (IGRT).[2–4] Of course, the concept of image guidance is not revolutionary and really should be viewed as an evolutionary component in the development of CRT. In the past, many systems and/or processes have been developed to help better localize the patient for treatment (and hence conform the dose), including dedicated x-ray simulators, megavoltage radiographic port films, electronic portal imaging devices, implanted radiopaque markers, ultrasound imaging systems, and optical surface-tracking systems.[9,10] Even the early isocentric cobalt-60 teletherapy machines in the 1960s came equipped with a kilovolt x-ray tube attached to the beam stop.

This chapter will review the critical components that make up the CRT planning and delivery process, focusing mainly on the forward-planned 3DCRT process. However, it should be understood that most of concepts and tasks discussed apply equally well to IMRT and IGRT, particularly with regard to target volume definition, plan evaluation, and many aspects of clinical quality assurance (QA). In addition, the reader should understand that the use of the terms two-dimensional (*2D*), three-dimensional (*3D*), and even four-dimensional (*4D*)[11] as descriptors for the CRT planning and delivery process refers to a process and tools used and not merely to beam arrangements. For example, 3D treatment planning certainly does not require the use of "noncoplanar" beams—a common

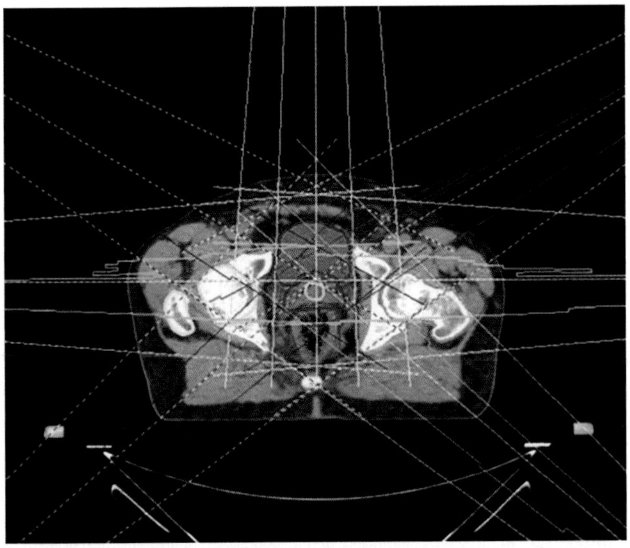

FIGURE 9.1. Three-dimensional conformal radiation therapy (3DCRT), considered a "forward planning" CRT approach that uses an increased number of radiation beams that are shaped to conform to the target volume. To improve the conformality of the dose distribution, beam modifiers (e.g., wedges, partial transmission blocks, and/or compensating filters) are sometimes used. Shown is a prostate seven-field coplanar beam arrangement.

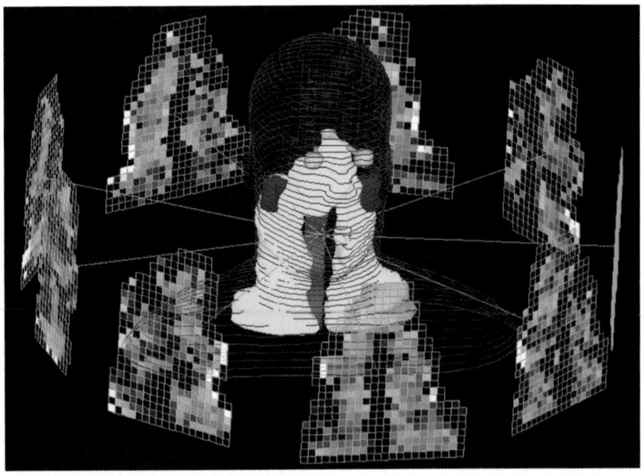

FIGURE 9.2. Intensity-modulated radiation therapy (IMRT) is considered an "inverse planning" conformal radiation therapy approach that can achieve even greater conformity than three-dimensional conformal radiation therapy by optimally modulating the individual beamlets that make up the radiation beams. IMRT dose distributions can be created to conform much more closely to the target volume, particularly for those volumes having complex/concave shapes, and also shaped to avoid critical normal tissues in the irradiated volume.

misconception—but does require the ability to plan and visualize volumetric dose distributions for such beam arrangements. Even today, newer tools are being developed that allow 4D, image-based CRT planning, that is, target volume segmentation and dose calculation in the presence of moving organs and target volumes. Thus, the reader will be able to appreciate the CRT approach much more fully if it is viewed as a constantly evolving planning and treatment delivery workflow process using ever-advancing computer software and technology.

HISTORICAL DEVELOPMENT OF CONFORMAL RADIATION THERAPY AND 3D TREATMENT-PLANNING SYSTEMS

Conformational treatment methods were pioneered in the 1950s and 1960s by several groups, including Takahashi in Japan,[12] Proimos[13] and Trump, Wright, et al. in the United States,[14] and Green et al. in Great Britain.[15] Work continued into the 1970s, when several groups actually implemented computer-controlled radiation therapy, including a project of the Joint Center for Radiation Therapy in Boston led by Bjarngard and Kijewski[16] and the Tracking Cobalt Project led by Davy et al.[17] at the Royal Free Hospital in London.

Sterling et al.[18,19] are credited with the first 3D approach to treatment planning (dose calculation and display). They demonstrated a technique by which a computer-generated film loop gave the illusion of a 3D view of the patient's relevant anatomic features and the calculated isodose distribution (2D color washes) throughout a treatment volume. However, this effort did not result in a practical 3DTPS and was viewed as simply a demonstration project. The Rhode Island Hospital/Brown University group made the first real step in implementing a clinically usable 3DTPS based on a new type of display, called *beam's-eye view* (BEV), which simulated the treatment planner's viewing point from the perspective of the radiation source looking out along the axis of the radiation beam, similar to that obtained when viewing a simulation radiograph.[20,21]

The advent of CT spurred further development of 3D planning systems. In 1983, Goitein and coworkers reported on their system,[22,23] which took advantage of CT and increased minicomputer capabilities. The system produced high-quality color BEV displays and could display radiographic images computed from the digital CT data; such computed radiographs are now called *digitally reconstructed radiographs* (DRRs). By the latter half of the 1980s, several other academic groups had developed 3D planning systems having powerful new features.[24–27]

In the 1990s, the commercial availability of 3DTPSs led to widespread adoption of 3D planning and CRT as the standard of practice. One of the keys to this development was a series of research contracts funded by the National Cancer Institute (NCI) in the 1980s and 1990s to evaluate the potential of 3D planning and to make recommendations to the NCI for future research in this area.[28] Each of the research contracts funded a collaborative working group (CWG). The participating institutions in each CWG are shown in Table 9.1. Their charge was to evaluate various aspects of this new planning process and develop new software tools needed. The CWGs were composed of physicists, clinicians, and computer scientists. Many important developments and/or refinements in 3D planning came from these NCI research CWGs, particularly planning-evaluation software tools such as *dose–volume histograms* (DVHs),[29,30] *electronic view-box,*[31] and biologic effect models such as *tumor control probability* (TCP) and *normal tissue complication probability* (NTCP) models.[32] Even IMRT has benefited from the CWG approach, as a consensus statement was developed in 2001 that helped clarify many issues and pointed to important research areas regarding that form of CRT.[33]

TABLE 9.1 NATIONAL CANCER INSTITUTE RESEARCH CONTRACTS IN SUPPORT OF THREE-DIMENSIONAL RADIATION THERAPY TREATMENT PLANNING

Evaluation of Treatment Planning for Heavy Particles (1982–1986)
Lawrence Berkeley Laboratory and University of California
Massachusetts General Hospital, Harvard University
M.D. Anderson Cancer Center, University of Texas
University of Pennsylvania School of Medicine and Fox Chase Cancer Center
Evaluation of Treatment Planning for External-Beam Photons (1984–1987)
Massachusetts General Hospital, Harvard University
Memorial Sloan-Kettering Cancer Center
University of Pennsylvania School of Medicine and Fox Chase Cancer Center
Washington University in St. Louis
Evaluation of Treatment Planning for External-Beam Electrons (1986–1989)
M.D. Anderson Cancer Center, University of Texas
University of Michigan
Washington University in St. Louis
Development of Radiation Therapy Treatment Planning Software Tools (1989–1994)
University of North Carolina
University of Washington
Washington University in St. Louis

VOLUME SPECIFICATION FOR CONFORMAL RADIATION THERAPY

The International Commission on Radiation Units and Measurements (ICRU) first addressed the issue of consistent volume and dose specification in radiation therapy with the publication of ICRU Report 29 in 1978.[34] That report defined the *target volume* as *the volume containing those tissues that are to be irradiated to a specified absorbed dose according to a specified time–dose pattern* (Fig. 9.3A). It is interesting to note that this report (even though published in the 2D era) attempted to address spatial uncertainties by pointing out that the size and shape of a target volume may change during the course of a treatment and that one should take into account the following parameters when describing the target volume:

1. Expected movements (e.g., caused by breathing) of those tissues that contain the target volume relative to anatomic reference points (e.g., skin markings, suprasternal notch).
2. Expected variation in shape and size of the target volume during a course of treatment (e.g., urinary bladder, stomach).
3. Inaccuracies or variations in treatment setup during the course of treatment.

However, the report did not address the issues of coordinate systems (e.g., patient vs. treatment machine), and no attempt was made to define and explicitly separate the margins for the different types of uncertainties.

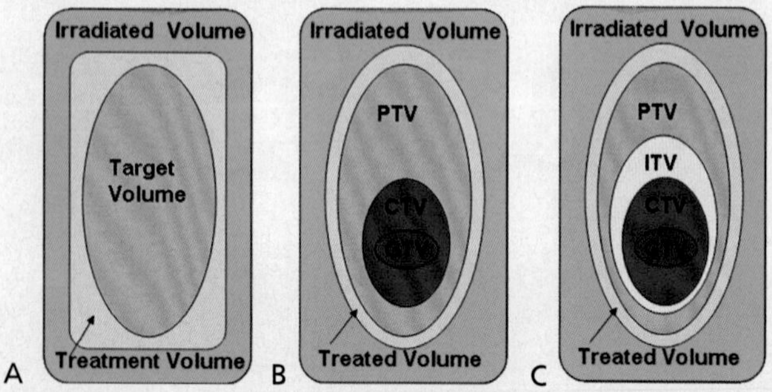

FIGURE 9.3. A: Schematic illustration of the boundaries of the volumes defined by International Commission on Radiation Units and Measures (ICRU) Report 29: target volume, treatment volume, and irradiated volume. **B:** Boundaries of the volumes defined by ICRU Report 50: gross tumor volume (GTV), clinical target volume (CTV), planning target volume (PTV), treated volume, and irradiated volume. **C:** Boundaries of the volumes defined by ICRU Report 62: GTV, CTV, internal target volume (ITV), PTV, treated volume, and irradiated volume.

In addition to the target volume, ICRU Report 29 defined two other volumes: (a) the *treatment volume* and (b) the *irradiated volume.* These volumes were not based on anatomy, but instead were based on the dose distribution. The treatment volume was defined as *the volume enclosed by the isodose surface representing the minimal target dose,* and the irradiated volume was defined as *the volume that receives a dose considered significant in relation to normal tissue tolerance* (e.g., 50% isodose surface).

Report 29 defined *organs at risk* (OAR) as *especially radiosensitive organs in or near the target volume whose presence influences treatment planning and/or prescribed dose.* The report also recognized the importance of tissues outside the target area that received a dose higher than 100% of the specified target dose. This was defined as a *hot spot* and was considered clinically meaningful only if the corresponding isodose curve enclosed an area of at least 2 cm^2 in a section.

In retrospect, ICRU Report 29 recommendations were well suited for the technology of the 1970s and 1980s, that is, using a conventional simulator to generate a planning radiograph for designing beam portals based on bony and soft tissue landmarks for standardized beam arrangement techniques applied to whole classes of comparable patients. Several generations of radiation oncologists were trained using this nomenclature and method, and the ICRU recommendation for reporting dose and volumes helped advance radiation oncology.

In 1993, the ICRU updated its recommendations for specifying dose/volume in Report 50, which were well suited for conformal therapy.[35] The target volume definition was separated into three distinct volumes: (a) visible tumor, that is, *gross tumor volume* (GTV), (b) a volume to account for uncertainties in microscopic tumor spread, that is, *clinical target volume* (CTV), and (c) a volume to account for geometric and other uncertainties, that is, *planning target volume* (PTV), as illustrated in Figure 9.3B.

The GTV and CTV are anatomic-clinical concepts that should be defined before a choice of treatment modality and technique is made. Labels or subscripts with the GTV nomenclature can be used to distinguish between primary disease and other areas of macroscopic tumor involvement such as involved lymph nodes that are visible on imaging studies (e.g., $GTV_{primary}$ and GTV_{nodal}, or GTV-T and GTV-N). Similarly, the GTV together with this surrounding volume of local subclinical involvement that defines the CTV can be denoted as CTV-T. Note that even if the GTV has been removed by radical surgery, the volume can be designated as CTV-T. In specifying the CTV, the physician must consider not only microextensions of the disease near the GTV, but also the natural avenues of spread for the particular disease and site, including lymph node, perivascular, and perineural extensions. These may be designated CTV-N (and, if necessary, CTV-N1, CTV-N2, etc.).

The *PTV* is defined by specifying the margins that must be added around the CTV to manage the effects of organ, tumor and patient movements, inaccuracies in beam and patient setup, and any other uncertainties. The PTV is a static, geometric concept used for treatment planning and for specification of dose. Its size and shape depend primarily on that of the GTV/CTV and the effects caused by internal motions of organs and the tumor, technical aspects of treatment technique (e.g., patient fixation). The PTV can be considered a 3D envelope in which the tumor and any microscopic extensions reside and move. Once the PTV is defined, appropriate beam sizes to account for penumbra and beam arrangements must be selected to ensure the desired dose coverage of the PTV. Note that multiple PTVs may be defined for a patient's radiation therapy treatment. For example, it is common practice to plan a higher dose to the PTV enclosing the GTV and a lower dose to the PTV containing the CTV. Such planning volumes are typically subscripted using the dose level prescribed; for example, PTVs for 66 Gy and 54 Gy can be represented as PTV_{66} and PTV_{54}, respectively.

ICRU Report 50 essentially retained the definition of the two dose volumes defined in ICRU Report 29, changing the treatment volume name to *treated volume* and refining the definition as *the volume enclosed by an isodose surface, selected and specified by the radiation oncologist as being appropriate to achieve the purpose of treatment* (e.g., tumor eradication, palliation), and the irradiated volume as that *tissue volume that receives a dose that is considered significant in relation to normal tissue tolerance.*

Report 50 refined the definition of organs at risk as *normal tissues whose radiation sensitivity may significantly influence treatment planning and/or prescribed dose.* The report did state that any possible movement of the organ at risk during treatment, as well as uncertainties in the setup during the whole treatment course, must be considered, but did not provide a method to do so.

The hot spot definition was modified to be *a volume outside the PTV that received a dose larger than 100% of the specified PTV dose.* This was considered clinically meaningful only if the minimum diameter exceeded 15 mm (note: previously it had been 2 cm^2). However, if the hot spot occurs in a small organ, such as the optic nerve, a dimension smaller than the recommended 15 mm should be considered.

As previously stated, Report 50 was well suited to conformal therapy, and it stimulated broad interest in the radiation oncology community. However, irradiation techniques continued to evolve (e.g., IMRT), and advances in imaging procedures (e.g., PET, MRI) provided even more information on functionality, the location, shape, and limits of tumor/target volumes, and organs at risk. In response to these developments, the ICRU in 1999 published Report 62,[36] which expanded on some of the definitions and concepts of Report 50 and took into account the consequences of the technical and clinical progress referred to previously. However, it should be clearly understood that Report 62 was intended to complement the recommendations contained in Report 50 and not to replace it.

ICRU Report 62 refined the definition of PTV by introducing the concept of an *internal margin* to take into account variations in size, shape, and position of the CTV in reference to the patient's coordinate system using anatomic reference points, as well as the concept of a *setup margin* to take into account all uncertainties in patient–beam positioning in reference to the treatment machine coordinate system. Identification of these two types of margins is needed, as they compensate for different types of uncertainties and refer to different coordinate systems. Internal margin uncertainties are due to physiologic variations (e.g., filling of rectum, movements due to respiration) and are difficult or almost impossible to control from a practical viewpoint. Setup margin uncertainties are related largely to technical factors that can be dealt with by more accurate setup and immobilization of the patient and improved mechanical stability of the machine. However, exactly how these margins should be combined is still not clear. This point will be discussed further in a later section, but for now it is necessary to understand that the selection of an overall margin and delineation of the border of the PTV typically involves a compromise that requires the experience and the judgment of the radiation oncologist and the treatment-planning team.

ICRU Report 62 defines the volume formed by the CTV and the internal margin as the *internal target volume* (ITV) (Fig. 9.3C). The ITV represents the movements of the CTV referenced to the patient coordinate system and is specified in relation to internal and external reference points, which preferably should be rigidly related to each other through bony structures. In cases not involving significant internal organ motion, the radiation oncologist can simply ignore having to explicitly define the ITV and use only the GTV, CTV, and PTV concepts. However, in cases involving significant motion, such as often is the case with lung cancer, the ITV concept has proven useful and should be used.[37]

TABLE 9.2 SUMMARY OF THE INTERNATIONAL COMMISSION ON RADIATION UNITS AND MEASUREMENTS (ICRU) NOMENCLATURE FOR VOLUMES (1970s TO PRESENT)

ICRU Report 29: 1970s–1993	*ICRU Report 50: 1993–Present*	*ICRU Report 62: 1999–Present*	*ICRU Report 83: 2010–Present*
Target volume	GTV CTV PTV	GTV CTV ITV PTV	GTV CTV ITV PTV
Treatment volume Irradiated volume Organ at risk	Treated volume Irradiated volume Organ at risk	Treated volume Irradiated volume Organ at risk PRV	Treated volume Irradiated volume Organ at risk PRV RVR
Hot spot (area outside target that receives dose >100% of specified target dose; at least 2 cm^2 in a section)	Hot spot (volume outside PTV that receives dose >100% of specified PTV dose; >15 mm diameter)	Hot spot (volume outside PTV that receives dose >100% of specified PTV dose; 15 mm diameter)	High dose to RVR
Dose heterogeneity (no value given)	Dose heterogeneity (+7 to −5% of prescribed dose)	Dose heterogeneity (+7 to −5% of prescribed dose)	Not specified

CTV, clinical target volume; GTV, gross tumor volume; ITV, internal target volume; PRV, planning risk volume; PTV, planning target volume; RVR, remaining volume at risk.

ICRU Report 62 refined the definition of the two dose volumes defined ICRU Report 50 as follows:

> *The treated volume is the tissue volume that (according to the approved treatment plan) is planned to receive at least a dose selected and specified by radiation oncology team as being appropriate to achieve the purpose of the treatment, e.g., tumor eradication or palliation, within the bounds of acceptable complications.*

The irradiated volume is the *tissue volume that receives a dose that is considered significant in relation to normal tissue tolerance.*

Report 62 refined the definition of organs at risk as *normal tissues (e.g., spinal cord) whose radiation sensitivity may significantly influence treatment planning and/or prescribed dose.* The report also included a discussion regarding a system of classifying organs at risk as "serial," "parallel," or "serial-parallel." Report 62 also addressed what was perhaps the most criticized limitation of Report 50, which was that it did not provide a method to account for organ-at-risk movements and changes in shape and/or size, as well as setup uncertainties. To account for such spatial uncertainties, Report 62 introduced the concept of the *planning organ at risk volume* (PRV), in which a margin is added around the organ at risk to compensate for that organ's geometric uncertainties. The PRV margin around the organ at risk is analogous to the PTV margin around the CTV. The introduction of the PRV concept is timely, as its use is even more important for those conformal therapy cases involving IMRT because of the increased sensitivity of this type treatment to geometric uncertainties. For example, it is common practice to add a 0.5-cm rind around the spinal cord contour. Note that the PTV and the PRV may overlap, and often do so, which implies searching for a compromise in weighting the importance of each in the planning process. A summary of the ICRU volume nomenclature recommendations per report is presented in Table 9.2.

CONFORMAL RADIATION THERAPY PLANNING PROCESS

As previously stated, CRT treatment planning and delivery should be looked at as a process and the tools used. This process is summarized in Table 9.3 and includes (a) establishing the patient's treatment position, constructing a patient repositioning immobilization device when needed, and obtaining a volumetric image data set of the patient in treatment position; (b) contouring target volume(s) and organs at risk using the volumetric planning image data set; (c) specifying a prescription dose for the PTV and dose–volume constraints for any OARs; (d1) for 3DCRT forward planning, determining beam orientation and designing beam apertures and computing a 3D dose distribution according to the dose prescription; (d2) for IMRT inverse planning, setting up initial beam orientations and entering optimization parameters (i.e., dose–volume constraints for PTV[s] and all regions of interest) and initiating the TPS optimization process,

TABLE 9.3 CONFORMAL RADIATION THERAPY PROCESS

1. Patient treatment position, immobilization, and planning imaging
   - Position patient in proposed treatment position.
   - Fabricate immobilization devices.
   - Place radiopaque markers, and mark repositioning lines on patient and immobilization devices.
   - Obtain topograms to check patient alignment.
   - Perform volumetric computed tomography (CT) scan of patient in treatment position.
   - Make illustrative photographs to assist in repositioning the patient at the treatment couch.
   - Transfer CT images to three-dimensional treatment-planning system (3DTPS).
   - Perform imaging studies (e.g., magnetic resonance imaging, positron emission tomography/CT, etc.) as requested by treating physician, and transfer image data to 3DTPS.
2. Delineation of tumor/target volumes and organs at risk
   - Physician contours target volume(s).
   - Physician or dosimetrist contours organs at risk.
3. Dose prescription
   - Physician provides prescription dose for planning target volume (PTV) and dose–volume constraints for organs at risk.

4a. Forward planning (three-dimensional conformal radiation therapy)
   - Set up initial beam configuration and design field shapes; wedges/bolus/no beam modifiers; beam weights.
   - Compute 3D dose matrix.
   - Compute treatment machine monitor units.

4b. Inverse planning (intensity-modulated radiation therapy [IMRT])
   - Set up initial beam configuration.
   - Enter desired dose–volume constraints for PTV(s) and all regions of interest.
   - Initiate treatment-planning system optimization process, which generates beam fluences, resulting dose distribution, monitor units, and leaf motion files.

5. Plan evaluation and improvement
   - Evaluate plan (dose–volume histograms, planar isodose display, 3D isodose display) and modify until plan is found to be acceptable by treating physician.
   - Transfer patient's plan to patient's chart (Electronic Medical Record) and treatment machine verify and record (V&R) system.
6. Plan implementation and treatment verification
   - Physicist performs second check of treatment plan and transfer of data to V&R system.
   - For IMRT plans, perform phantom dosimetric verification.
   - Verify patient position and isocenter placement on treatment machine using orthogonal portal electronic portal imaging devices (EPIDs) vs. digitally reconstructed radiograph (DRRs) or using on-board CT vs. planning CT.
   - For 3DCRT, check field shapes by comparing treatment field DRRs with treatment beam EPIDs.
   - Capture treatment machine settings in V&R system.
   - Check first-day treatment with diode measurements.
   - Perform periodic imaging verification checks during treatment (e.g., orthogonal EPIDs/DRRs or beam EPIDs/DRRs, cone beam CT/planning CT).

which generates beam fluences, resulting dose distribution, monitor units, and leaf motion files; (e) evaluating the treatment plan and, if needed, modifying the plan (e.g., beam orientations, apertures, beam weights, etc.) until an acceptable plan is approved by the radiation oncologist; and (f) implementing the approved plan on the treatment machine and verifying the patient's treatment using appropriate QA procedures throughout the treatment. All of these tasks make up the CRT process and are discussed in the ensuing sections.

Patient Treatment Position and Immobilization, and Planning of Imaging

In the initial part of the CRT process (preplanning), the proposed treatment position of the patient is determined, and the immobilization device to be used during simulation/treatment is selected. In should be clearly understood that repositioning patients and accounting for internal organ movement for fractionated radiation therapy in order to accurately reproduce the planned dose distribution remain difficult technical aspects of the CRT process. Errors may occur if patients are inadequately immobilized, with resultant treatment fields inaccurately aligned from treatment to treatment (interfraction). In addition, patients and/or their tumor volume may also move during treatment (intrafraction) because of either inadequate immobilization or physiologic activity. Accounting for all of the uncertainties in the CRT planning and delivery process remains a challenge for radiation oncology, and research and development is ongoing.

Determining the treatment position of the patient and constructing the immobilization device are done in a dedicated radiation therapy CT-simulator facility. A radiation therapy CT-simulator consists of a diagnostic-quality CT scanner, laser patient positioning/marking system, virtual simulation 3D treatment-planning software, as well as various digital display systems for viewing the DRRs.[38,39] The CT scanner is used to acquire a volumetric planning CT scan of a patient in treatment position. The use of intravenous or other contrast to help delineate target volumes needs to be considered during simulation in some cases. CT topograms should be generated first and reviewed prior to acquiring the planning scan to ensure that patient alignment is correct, with adjustments to be made if needed. Radiopaque markers can be placed on the patient's skin and the immobilization device to serve as fiducial marks to assist in any coordinate transformation needed as a result of 3D planning and eventual plan implementation. An example of a typical immobilization repositioning system used for patients undergoing radiation therapy for head and neck (H&N) cancer is shown in Figure 9.4.

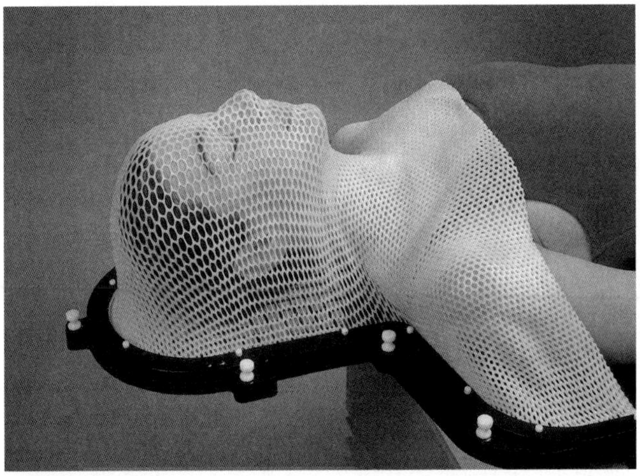

FIGURE 9.4. Example of immobilization repositioning system used for patients undergoing radiation therapy for head and neck cancer. It should be clearly understood that being able to accurately reposition the patient and account for internal organ movement in order to accurately deliver the planned dose distribution is one of the most important steps in the conformal therapy process. (Courtesy of MEDTECH, Inc., Orange City, IA.)

Planning CT scan protocols are tumor site dependent and typically range from 2 to 5 mm in slice thickness and 50 to 200 slices. In general, a 3-mm slice thickness provides adequate-quality DRR. In some sites, such as those of H&N cancer, slice thicknesses of 1 mm are often needed for delineation of very small volumes, such as the optic chiasm and the optic nerves. The same holds true for optimal reconstruction of the position of any implanted markers used, such as in prostate cancer radiation therapy.

The planning CT data set is typically transferred to a 3DTPS via a computer network. The planning CT data set provides an accurate geometric model of the patient, as well as the electron density information needed for the calculation of the 3D dose distribution that takes into account tissue heterogeneities.

Delineation of Tumor/Target Volumes and Organs at Risk

Delineation of tumor/target volume and organs at risk contours using the volumetric CT data set is typically performed by the radiation oncologist and the medical dosimetrist working as a team. The CT data are displayed at the 3DTPS workstation (Fig. 9.5), and contours are drawn manually by the radiation oncologist/dosimetrist, most often using a computer mouse or stylus on a slice-by-slice basis. Some OARs with distinct boundaries (e.g., skin, lung) can be contoured automatically, with only minor editing required; others (e.g., brachial plexus) require the hands-on effort of the radiation oncologist.[40] With modern 3DTPS image segmentation software, contouring generally takes 0.5 to 1 hour, depending on the disease site. However, for some complex sites, such as H&N cancer, where many OARs and complex tumor/target volumes are the norm, this task can take several hours.

CT is still the principal source of imaging data used for defining the GTV for most sites, but this imaging modality presents several potential pitfalls. First, when contouring the GTV, it is essential that the appropriate CT window and level settings be used in order to determine the maximum dimension of what is considered potential gross disease (Fig. 9.6). Second, for those treatment sites in which there is considerable organ motion, such as for tumors in the thorax, CT images do not correctly represent either the time-averaged position of the tumor or its shape, and hence newer 4D CT technology must be used.[41–43] This can be understood by appreciating the fact that single or few-slice CT simulators rely almost exclusively on the use of fast spiral CT technology and thus acquire data essentially in 2D and combine them to construct a 3D matrix. This has the effect of capturing the tumor cross-section images at particular positions in the breathing cycle. If the tumor motion is significant, different, and possibly noncontiguous, transverse sections of the tumor could be imaged at different points of the breathing cycle, leading to volume uncertainties. The interpolation process in spiral CT technology adds further to the uncertainty. As a result, the 3D reconstruction of the GTV from temporally variant 2D images often results in a poor representation of the tumor and its motion. Currently, 4D CT technology has become the standard for CT simulators, making it possible to capture images in each phase of the respiratory cycle.[44,45] In addition, other technologies and methodologies to explicitly help manage the movements induced by the respiratory motion (to the order of <5 mm during treatment preparation and delivery) continue to be developed, including respiratory-gated techniques, respiration-synchronized techniques, breath-hold techniques, and forced shallow-breathing methods.[46]

Delineating the CTV is even more difficult and must be done by the radiation oncologist based on clinical experience (and/or the use of published CTV atlases for certain clinical sites) because current imaging techniques cannot be used to directly detect subclinical tumor involvement. This field has seen a virtual explosion in the use of multimodality imaging over the last

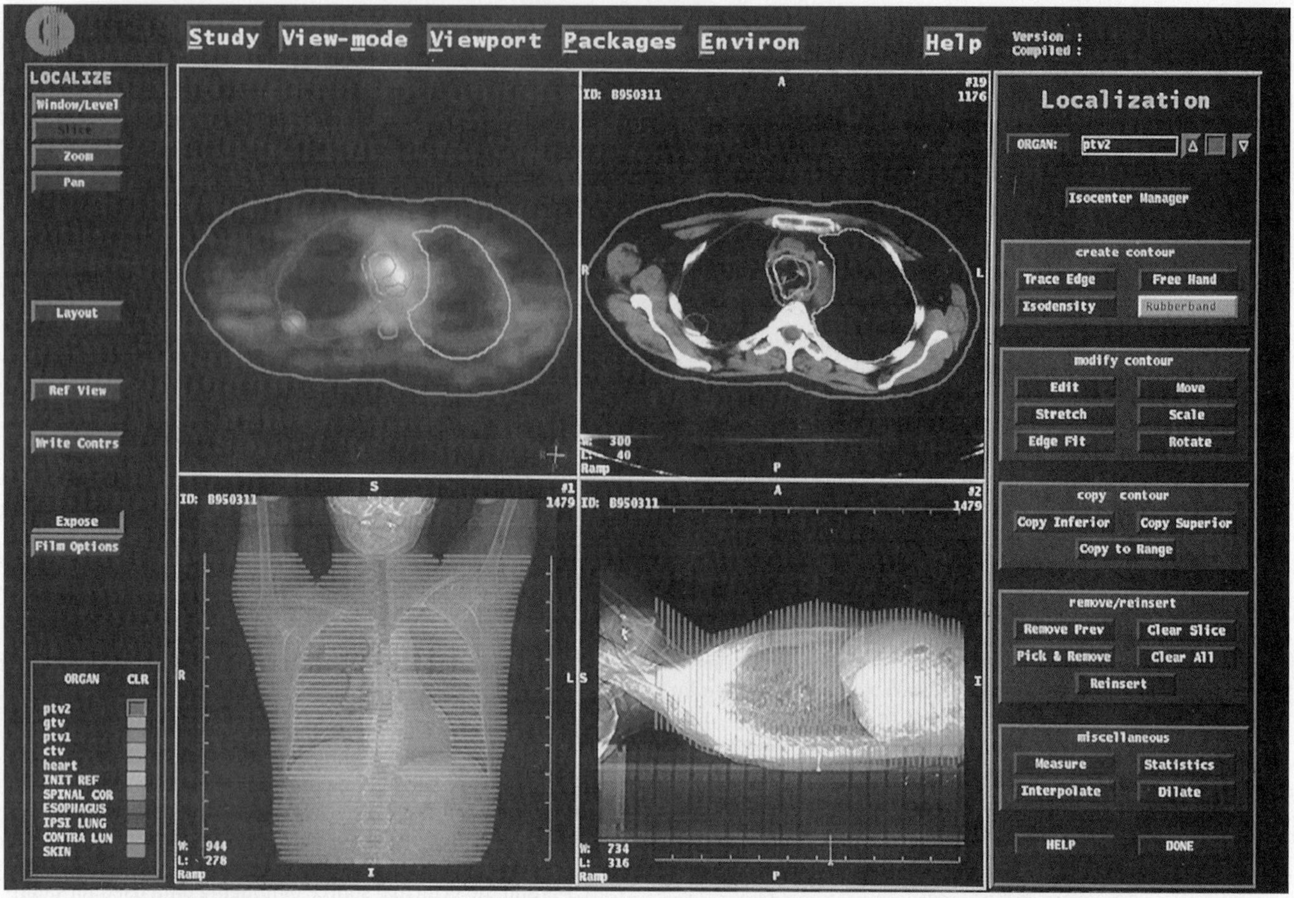

FIGURE 9.5. Advanced image-segmentation software provides tools for radiation oncologists and treatment planners to determine critical structures and tumor and target volumes for three-dimensional planning. Computed tomography (CT) data are displayed, and contours are drawn by the treatment planner/radiation oncologist around the tumor, target, and normal tissues on a slice-by-slice basis, as seen in upper right panel. At the same time, planar images from both anteroposterior and lateral projections are displayed in bottom right and left panels. Upper left panel shows positron emission tomography scan data with overlying contours after image registration with the CT data.

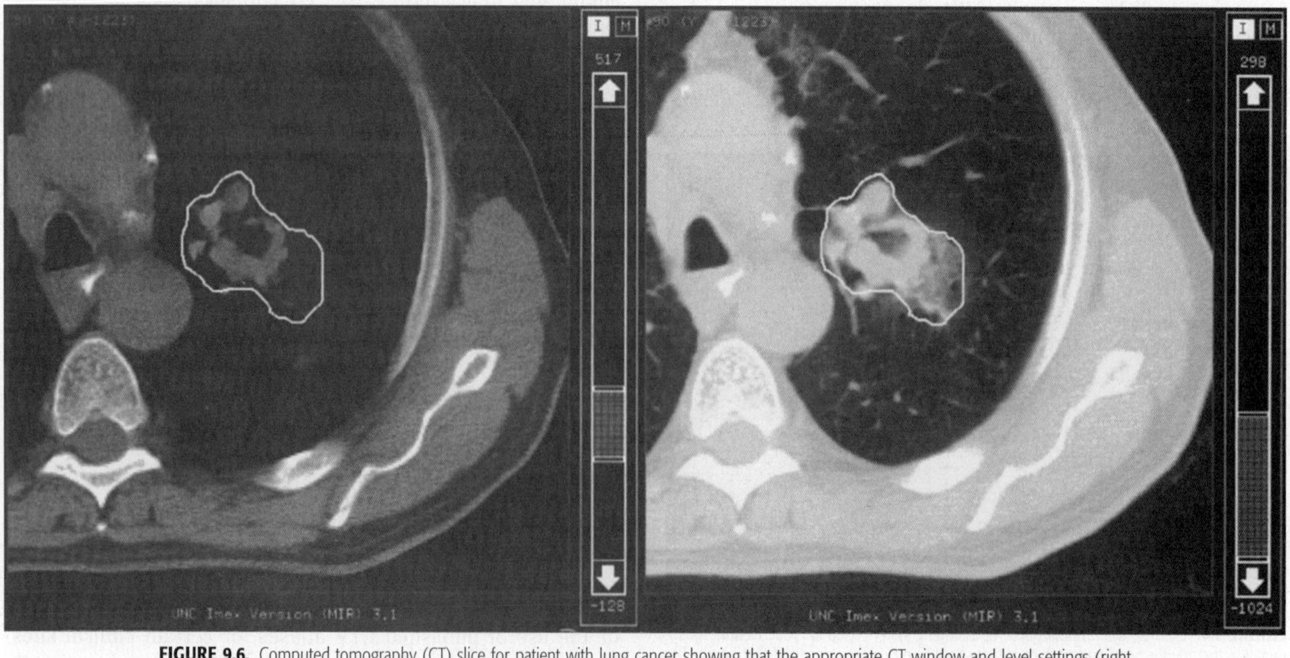

FIGURE 9.6. Computed tomography (CT) slice for patient with lung cancer showing that the appropriate CT window and level settings (right frame) must be used to determine the maximum dimensions of the gross tumor volume (GTV). Note that a much smaller GTV would have been contoured with the settings used in the left frame. (From Purdy JA. Advances in three-dimensional treatment planning and conformal dose delivery. *Semin Oncol* 1997;24:655–672.)

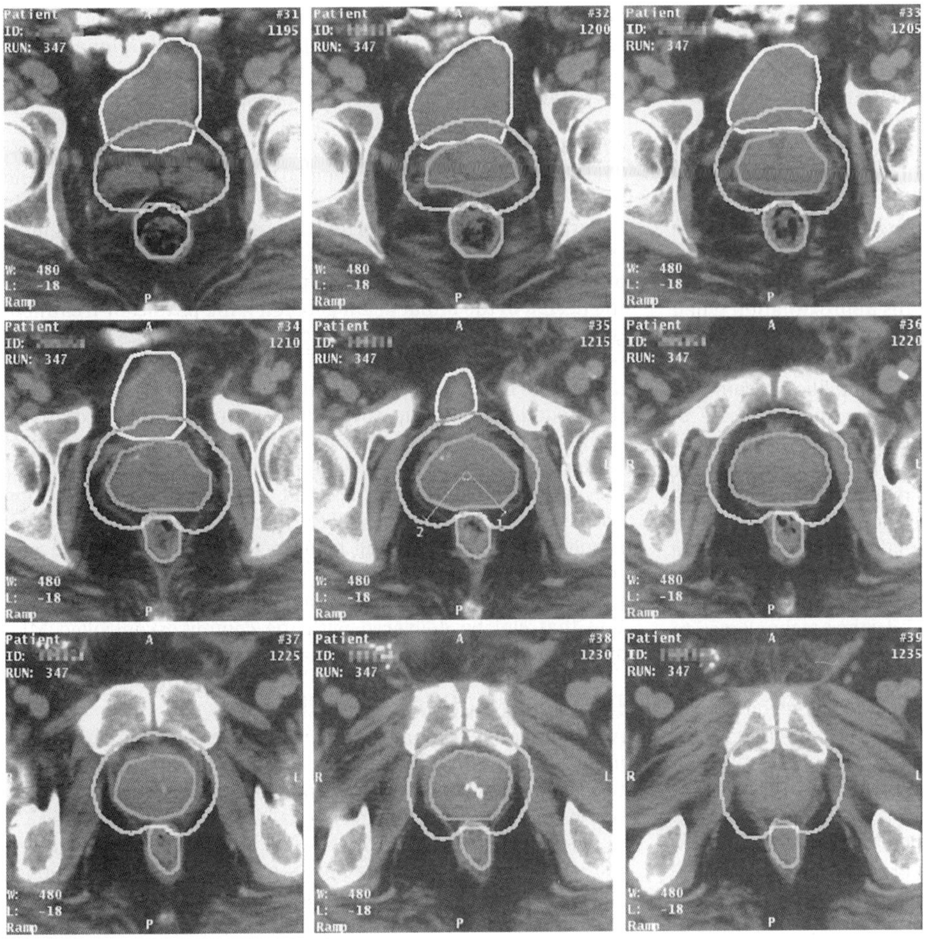

FIGURE 9.7. Computed tomography images of patient with prostate cancer showing the contour outlines for the gross tumor volume (GTV), planning target volume (PTV), bladder, and rectum. The physician made the decision that no additional margin around the prostate for the clinical target volume (CTV) was required (i.e., CTV = GTV). Note that a nonuniform margin around the GTV/CTV was used to define the PTV in the region of the rectum (see middle frame). Also note the additional PTV contours needed to cap the GTV/CTV (upper left and lower right frames). (From Purdy JA. Three-dimensional treatment planning and conformal dose delivery: a physicist's perspective. In: Mittal BB, Purdy JA, Ang KK, eds. *Advances in radiation therapy.* Boston: Kluwer Academic Publishers, 1998:1–33.)

decade, and radiation oncologists have developed considerable imaging expertise in order to accurately define GTVs and be able to define nonimaged CTVs. However, the need for a higher level of image-based cross-sectional anatomy training in this field is well recognized.[47]

The PTV margin is specified by the radiation oncologist, often in consultation with the radiation oncology physicist and/or therapist. In most occasions, it is based on published clinical experience, that is, not calculated based on measurements performed by the department for a particular treatment machine/technique and team. Van Herk and colleagues reported extensively on the influence of systematic and random errors/variations on the required margins to account for setup error and organ motion and developed margin recipes for calculating individualized (for a department, machine, and team) margins as given by the following equation[48,49]:

$$\text{PTV margin} = 2.5\Sigma + 0.7\sigma,$$

where Σ is the standard deviation of the systematic errors and σ is the standard deviation of the random errors.

When defining the PTV, the radiation oncologist should account for the asymmetric nature of positional uncertainties (Fig. 9.7). For example, it is recognized that prostate organ motion and daily setup errors may be anisotropic (side-to-side or rotational shifts of the position of the patients are likely to have a different result compared to movement in the antero-posterior direction). Thus, the PTV margin around a CTV generally should not be uniform.

Typically, when the beam portal is defined, additional margin beyond the PTV is typically required to obtain dose coverage because of beam penumbra and treatment technique. This emphasizes that treatment portal margins in relation to the PTV must be set according to the dosimetric characteristics of the beams being used. Typically, a 5-mm margin (portal edge to PTV) is a good starting point, which can be increased if needed, but one must be knowledgeable about the characteristics of the actual beams used to make this starting-point determination. An additional point to understand is that in the case of coplanar treatment techniques, the margins required across the plane of treatment and the margins orthogonal (say superior–inferior) to this plane will be different. To clarify this point, consider a pelvic four-field axial technique as an example. Portions of the lateral aspects of the PTV that are in the low-dose regions (near the penumbra) of the anterior–posterior and posterior–anterior fields will be in the high-dose regions (well away from the beam penumbra) of the lateral fields. However, the superior and inferior aspects of the PTV will always be in the same low-dose regions of all four fields, so there will be no dose filling from any of the fields. Thus, a larger portal margin in the inferior–superior dimension is needed to ensure that the prescription isodose resulting from all beams contains the PTV, while the lateral and anterior–posterior portal margins for each field may be reduced due to the other beams filling in the dose. The same holds true for the portals of the boost fields used in the so-called "integrated boost technique," in which the beams used for treating the large volume fill up the dose in the buildup region of the boost volume. Last, the size of the margins will also be affected by the relative beam weighting. Hence, making hard rules about margin sizes is impossible and requires some planning iteration to find the right mix of beam margins.

When a PTV overlaps with a contoured normal structure, it is important to be explicit as to which volume the overlapping voxels are assigned for optimization purposes and for DVH calculations. Planning systems should allow the overlapping voxels to be included in both volumes for plan evaluation and reporting purposes. This ensures that the clinician is aware of the potential for the high-dose region to include part of the normal structure as well as the PTV when reviewing the DVHs.

In addition, most 3DTPS cannot accurately account for a PTV contour that extends outside the skin surface, resulting in a DVH that does not reflect clinical reality due to the lack of dose generated in air and in the buildup region just below the skin. In those cases, the best solution is to delineate the PTV 5 mm below the skin surface. This will also help reduce acute skin reactions by preventing the optimization process from increasing the skin dose to excessive levels. In all cases, however, the treating physician should be aware of this approximation when setting or approving actual field margins.

All of the issues discussed in this section point out the fact that the PTV/PRV concept is a useful tool that simplifies accounting for geometric uncertainties. However, its use does give rise to several dilemmas. Particularly important is the loss of actual tumor and normal organ volume information reported for researchers developing TCP and NTCP models. Although it does not appear possible to totally eliminate the PTV concept at this time, it does appear possible to use smaller margins for some sites if more frequent imaging or other technical innovation is used to reduce geometric uncertainties. For example, for prostate cancer, the use of daily imaging and other technologies to relocate the target volume in reference to the machine isocenter does allow for a smaller margin for the PTV.[10,50] However, one must still be prudent in the amount of margin reduction for the prostate PTV when using these technologies. The different methods include various tradeoffs ranging from treatment machine control, which is not dependent on the patient, to systems that are completely dependent on the patient. Again, regardless of which technique is used to reduce the overall PTV margin, one must be prudent in the amount of margin reduction.

Dose Prescription

Dose prescription is the responsibility of the radiation oncologist, generally using institutional protocols based on evidence published in the literature combined with institutional experience. Typically, the CRT prescription is specified as a dose at or near the center of the PTV or (particularly for IMRT) as a dose covering a certain percentage of the PTV—for example, $D_{95\%}$, a dose that covers 95% of the PTV. Because the resulting dose distribution can be quite different depending on the dose prescription methodology, it is imperative that publications provide a clear and unambiguous description of the dose specification for the radiation treatment results being reported. The ICRU recently updated their recommendations for dose specification, and these will be discussed in a later section.[51]

Conformal Planning

For 3D CRT planning, beams can be arranged and beam apertures shaped with MLC leaves or shielding blocks to help conform the prescribed dose to the PTV and avoid OARs using BEV displays. This "forward planning" approach to CRT has now been supplemented—but not replaced—by an "inverse planning" approach as used for IMRT, which can achieve even greater conformity and OAR dose avoidance.

Forward Planning: 3DCRT

Design of the beam arrangement is the next step in the planning process for 3DCRT. The ability to orient beams in 3D allows one to develop treatment plans that use noncoplanar beams. However, when noncoplanar beam arrangements are used, care must be taken to avoid the selection of gantry and couch angles that results in table/gantry collisions or a conflict with other treatment room restrictions. The *BEV* and the *DRR display*,[23,52] as shown in Figure 9.8, allows the planner to easily view the target volume and the organs at risk so that shielding blocks or MLC apertures can be drawn using a computer mouse or, as available with most current 3DTPS software versions, automatically generated with a chosen margin around the selected volume. DRRs also provide planar reference images that can be used in facilitating the plan implementation and treatment verification phases of CRT.

Inverse Planning: IMRT

The major differences between 3DCRT forward planning and IMRT inverse planning is the use of a computer optimization program that requires a formal description of the requirements using a mathematical *objective function* and constraints that are used by the program to find the solution. For example, after the design of the initial beam geometry, the physician/treatment planner puts into the TPS the desired dose–volume constraints for the PTVs and all OARs. The TPS optimization algorithm then divides each beam into many small *beamlets* (i.e., pencil beams that together make up the IMRT beam) and then iteratively alters the beamlet intensities until the 3D dose distribution best conforms to the a priori–specified dose–volume objectives. After the optimal beam intensities and resulting dose distribution have been determined, the TPS then calculates the MLC leaf sequence motions that will achieve this dose distribution and the dose recalculated. Typically there may be some differences in the optimized dose distribution and the final dose distribution that can be delivered with the computer-controlled MLC system, but this difference is usually acceptable.

Dose Distribution Calculation

A rectilinear coordinate system affixed to the patient 3D CT image set is typically used for calculating the dose distribution. This "patient or CT system" coordinate system typically has its x-axis along the horizontal axis of the transverse CT images, the y-axis along the vertical axis, and the z-axis along the couch motion. Contour points are specified as a sequence of points having x, y, z coordinates in this system. The center of each voxel in the 3D CT image matrix is computed relative to the same coordinate system and is used to look up the relative electron density values that are related to the CT numbers (see later discussion). The selection of grid spacing for the 3D dose matrix is an important consideration regarding dose computational accuracy, calculation speed, and computer hardware requirements. Drzymala et al.[30] pointed out that a 2% dose accuracy or 2-mm isodose positional accuracy can generally be achieved with a grid spacing of 5 mm. However, in regions of high-dose gradients, a finer grid is typically needed, which creates larger computer files and increases the 3DTPS memory and mass storage requirements.

The reader should also understand that CT numbers are not used directly in photon dose calculations. Instead, the CT numbers are correlated with the electron density of the corresponding tissues at each voxel relative to the electron density of water.[53] This is because Compton scattering is the dominant mode of interaction for the type of photon beam used in radiation therapy (cobalt-60 through 25-MV x-rays), and the absorption and scattering of photons in tissue depends primarily on the electron density of the tissue. Errors in CT numbers can result in inaccurate dose calculations. Generally, however, errors of 10% or less in electron density (CT numbers) will not result in significant errors in the dose distribution.[53]

Details on specific dose calculation algorithms are discussed in a separate chapter, and so only issues pertinent to the CRT planning process are discussed in this section. In the past, dose calculation algorithms were traditionally based on parametrizing dose distributions measured in water phantoms under standard conditions and applying correction factors to the beam representations for the nonuniform surface contour of the patient or the obliquity of the beam, tissue heterogeneities, and beam modifiers such as blocks, wedges, and compensator. However, more-advanced models, such as the superposition/convolution method, have been developed for CRT planning.[53] It is my opinion that heterogeneity-corrected 3D treatment

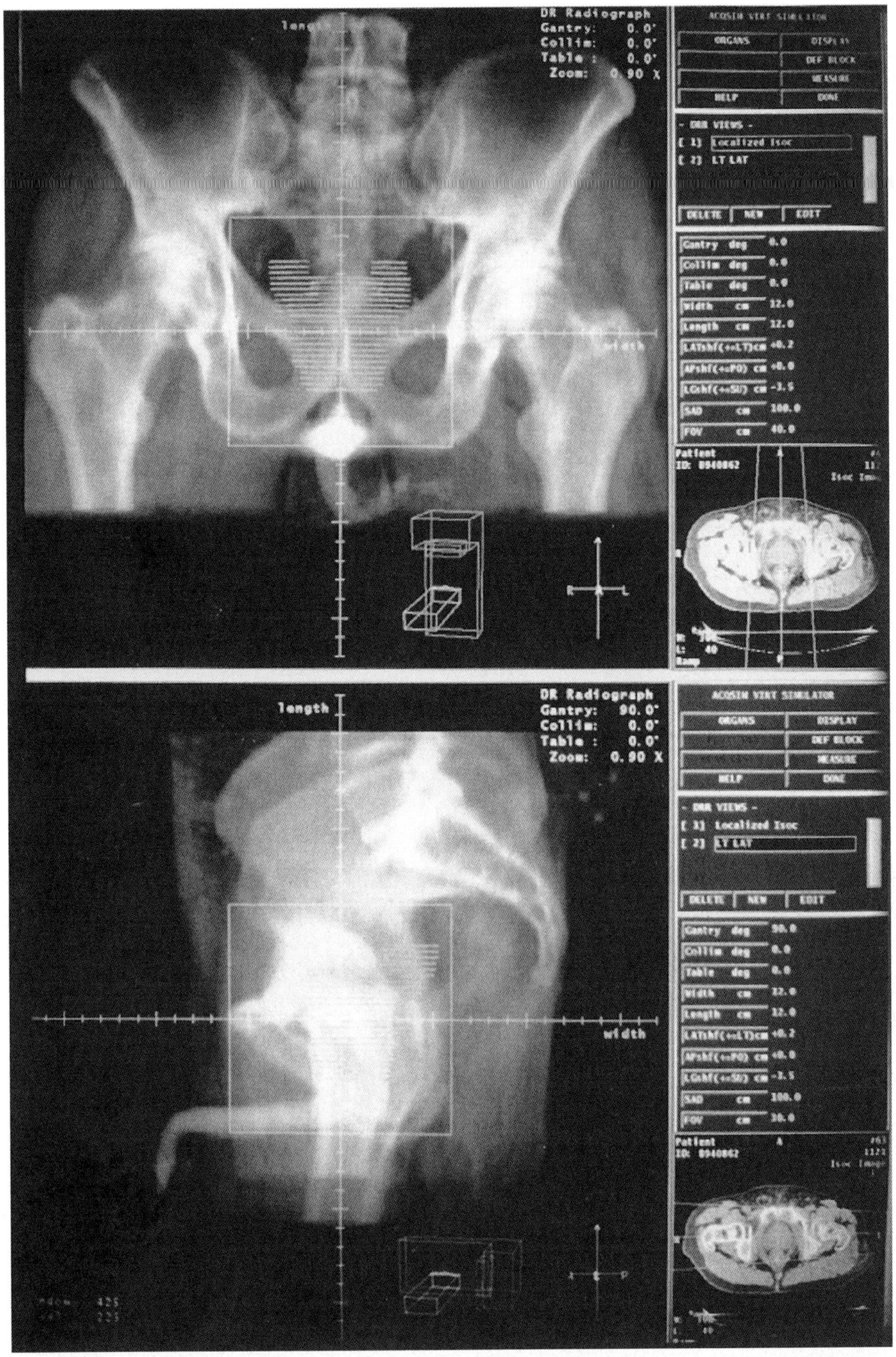

FIGURE 9.8. Beam's-eye-view (BEV) and digitally reconstructed radiograph (DRR) display of three-dimensional radiation therapy treatment planning for a prostate cancer patient. BEV display is useful in identifying best gantry, collimator, and couch angles at which to irradiate the target and avoid irradiating adjacent normal structures by interactively moving patient and treatment beam. Critical structures and target volumes are outlined on the patient's serial computed tomography sections. Contours are seen in perspective, as though the observer's eye is at the radiation source looking out along the axis of the radiation beam. The beam shape is defined by multileaf collimator (MLC). (From Purdy JA. Advances in three-dimensional treatment planning and conformal dose delivery. *Semin Oncol* 1997;24:655–672.)

plans generated using such advanced algorithms should be standard of practice today for CRT planning. The study by Frank et al.[54] provides a clear method for safely transitioning from a clinical experience based on planning assuming a homogeneous unit density patient to a heterogeneous patient model.

Plan Evaluation and Improvement

The 3DCRT plan evaluation/improvement process involves an iterative, interactive approach. Typically, the initial beam arrangement has been selected based primarily on clinical experience using BEV displays. The generated dose distribution is reviewed by the planner/physician, and the beam arrangement is then modified based on the review of DVHs (Fig. 9.9) and multilevel 2D displays showing isodose lines superimposed on CT images (Fig. 9.10); sometimes the display is in the form of a *color wash,* that is, a spectrum of colors superimposed on the anatomic information.

Another powerful display feature in a 3DTPS is the "*room-view*" or *room's-eye-view* (*REV*), in which the planner can simulate any arbitrary viewing location within the treatment room.[26,55] The REV display is used to display "*dose clouds*" along with rendered PTVs and OARs. Hot or cold spots that occur in the volumes of interest are clearly seen, as shown in Figure 9.11. Another valuable REV display is the so-called "*skin view,*" in which the beam aperture projection can be clearly seen on the skin of the (virtual) patient (Fig. 9.12).

The planned dose distribution approved by the radiation oncologist is most often one in which a uniform dose is delivered to the target volume (e.g., +7% and −5% of the prescribed dose) with doses to critical structures held below tolerance levels,[56–59] as well within the constraints for the absolute maximum dose, a median dose, or a volume (e.g., V_{20Gy}) that has been specified by the radiation oncologist.

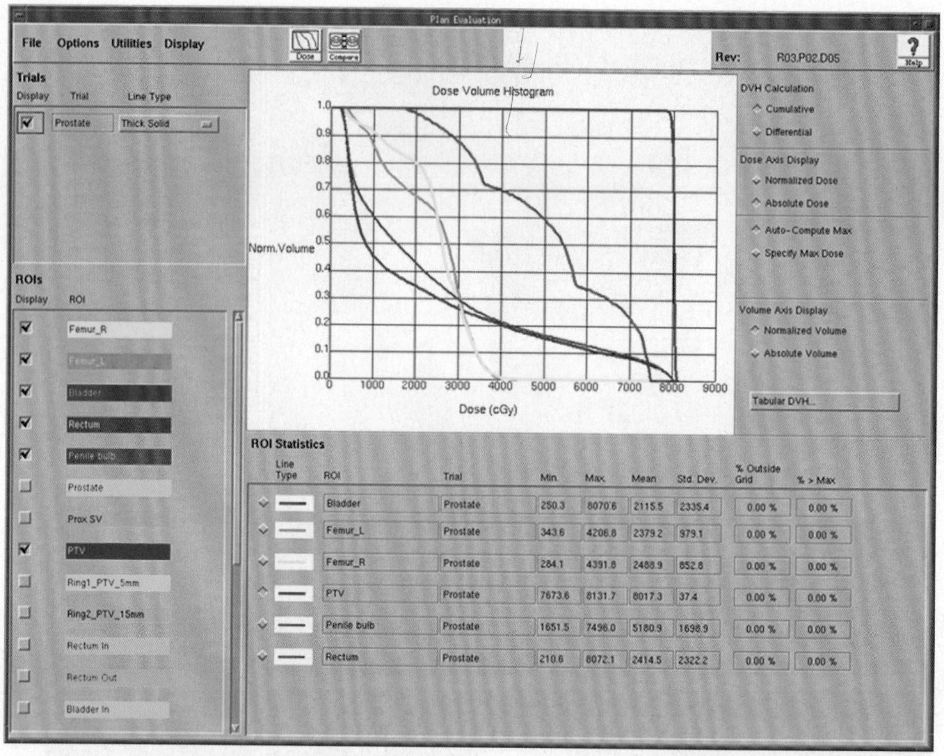

FIGURE 9.9. Example of a treatment-planning system display (Pinnacle, Philips Medical Systems, Highland Heights, OH), showing the cumulative dose volume histograms for a typical prostate cancer patient's plan: the prostate PTV (*red*) and multiple OARs (penile bulb, *magenta;* right femur, *yellow;* left femur, *orange;* rectum, *brown;* bladder, *blue*); also shown are associated dose statistics for the various defined volumes.

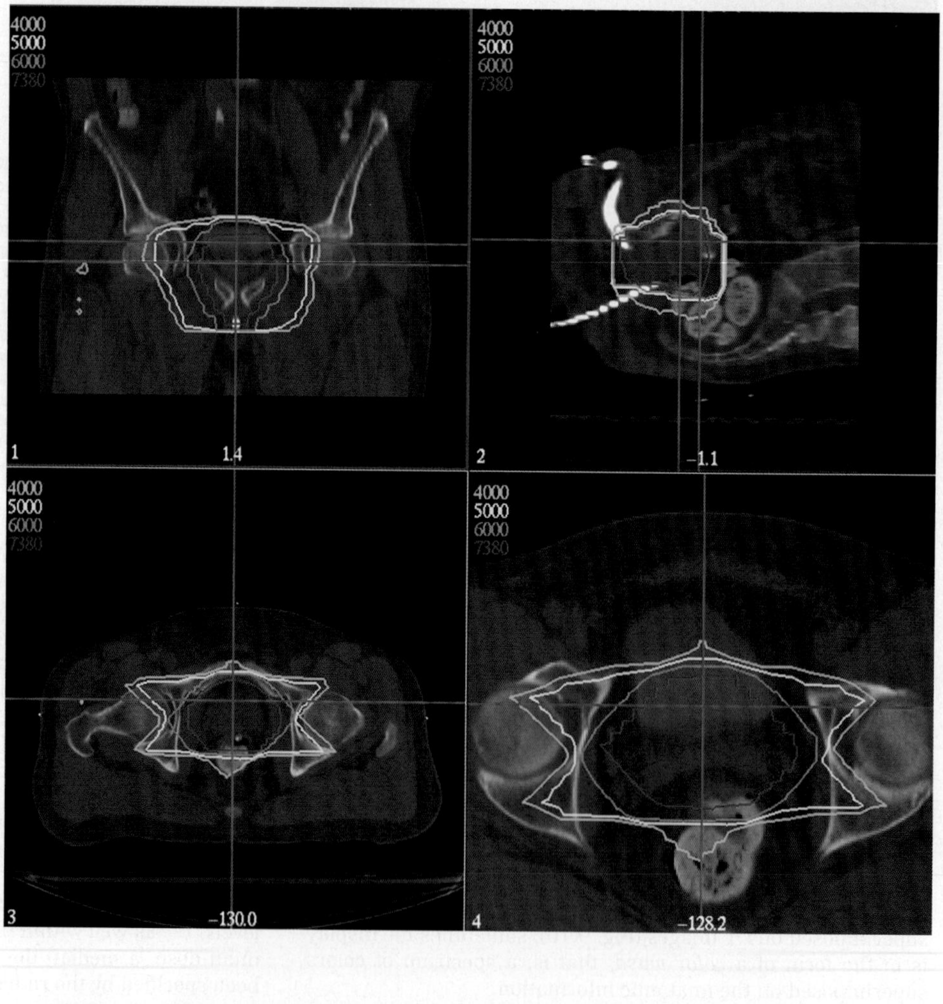

FIGURE 9.10. Dose distribution displays for a patient with prostate cancer showing coronal, sagittal, and two-axial computed tomography (CT) sections with superimposed color-coded isodose lines (73.8, 60, 50, and 40 Gy). Vertical and horizontal lines displayed on each CT section indicate the positions of each section. Evaluating volumetric three-dimensional dose distributions using only this type of two-dimensional display is difficult and time-consuming.

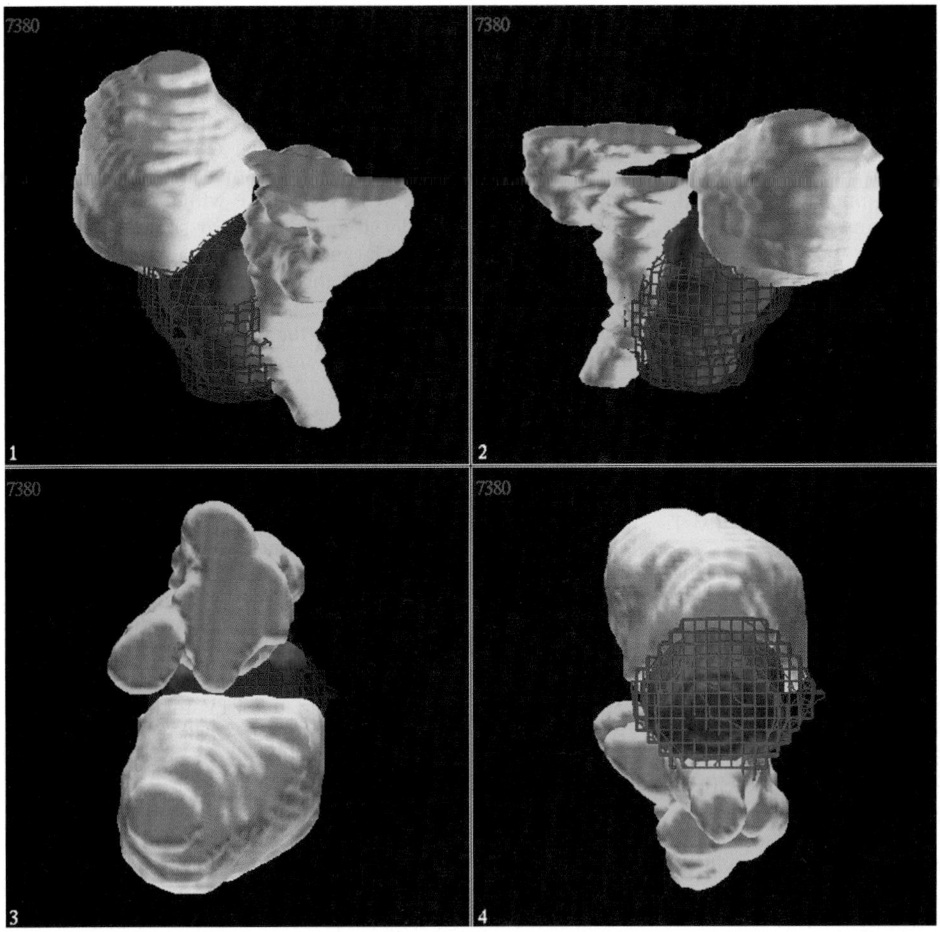

FIGURE 9.11. Room's-eye-view (REV) three-dimensional (3D) isodose surface display with real-time interactivity is a valuable tool for evaluation of 3D dose distributions in terms of adequate coverage of target volumes and sparing of critical structures. The REV display enables radiation oncologists to view target volume or normal tissue volume with superimposed isodose surfaces or "dose clouds" from any arbitrary viewing angle. Shown is a four-panel REV display of the 73.8-Gy isodose volume, the prostate planning target volume (PTV), bladder, and rectum of a patient with prostate cancer treated with a six-field technique. The location of the PTV region not covered by the specified dose level is easily discernible using the REV display.

Plan Implementation and Treatment Verification

Once the treatment plan has been designed, evaluated, and approved, documentation for plan implementation must be generated. Documentation includes beam parameter settings transferred to the treatment machine verify and record (V&R) system, including multileaf collimator parameters communicated over a network to the treatment machine's computer system that controls the MLC system, DRR generation, and transfer to the machine's image database.

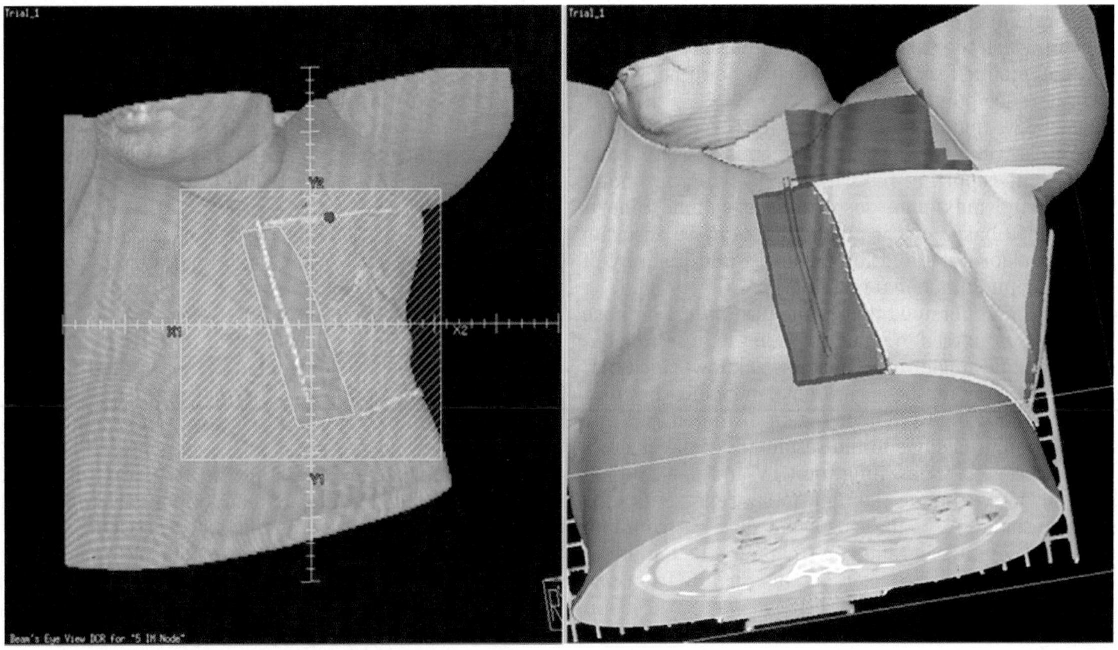

FIGURE 9.12. Room's-eye-view (REV) display showing simulated skin surface for a breast cancer patient undergoing radiation therapy using tangential, supraclavicular, and internal mammary fields. Beam aperture projection can be clearly seen on the skin of the (virtual) patient.

In the initial period of implementing CRT techniques (or of implementing nonconventional beam arrangements) in the clinic, a verification simulation procedure is commonly done to confirm the geometric validity and accuracy of the 3D treatment plan. DRRs generated by the 3DTPS are used for comparison with the verification simulation radiographs to confirm the correctness of the beam orientations in the physical implementation. When a beam orientation cannot be simulated, orthogonal radiographs may be taken and compared with similar DRRs to ensure correct isocenter positioning. The optical distance indicator is also useful in assessing the correctness of the setup of a particular beam. Documentation provides the depth of isocenter below the skin surface on the central ray of the beam, which can then be compared with the isocenter depth measured on the simulator or treatment machine after the beam is set up using the couch and gantry positions specified by the treatment plan. Currently, however, many modern radiotherapy departments no longer have a functional conventional simulator in clinical use, and many of these types of checks are done on the treatment machine prior to first treatment.

QA checks used to confirm the validity and accuracy of the CRT plan typically include an independent check of the plan and monitor unit calculation by a physicist, isocenter placement check on the treatment machine using orthogonal radiographs, or, in some occasions a cone beam computed tomography comparison with the planning CT. Depending on the irradiated site and the departmental protocol, field aperture check using portal films or electronic portal images, and diode or metal oxide semiconductor field-effect transistor (MOSFET) in vivo dosimetry check, can be performed as well. Most important, careful scrutiny must be given to the input of data into the V&R system to assure that it is correct. These checks will be discussed in more detail in a separate section.

Dose Reporting and Dose Prescription

ICRU Reports 50 and 62 define a series of doses, including the minimum, maximum, mean dose, and *ICRU reference dose* (defined at the *ICRU reference point*) for reporting dose relevant to CRT. The *ICRU reference point* for a particular treatment plan should be chosen based on the following criteria: It should be (a) clinically relevant and defined in an unambiguous way, (b) located where the dose can be accurately determined, and (c) located in a region where there are no steep dose gradients. In general, this point should be in the central part of the PTV. In cases in which the treatment beams intersect at a given point, it is recommended that the intersection point be chosen as the ICRU reference point.

ICRU Report 83[51] updates the previous ICRU recommendation on CRT dose reporting and recommends moving from single-spatial-point reporting (i.e., the ICRU reference point dose, minimum and maximum dose) to dose–volume reporting. This is justified based on the availability of more accurate dose-calculation algorithms and the advances and ubiquity of modern-day anatomic/functional imaging.

It also should be understood that in the past *minimum dose* and *maximum dose* referred to point doses in the dose calculation grid assigned to a single voxel. It is now acknowledged that the minimum dose may not be accurately determined because it is often located in a high-gradient region at the edge of the PTV, making it highly sensitive to the resolution of the calculation and the accuracy of delineating the CTV and determining the PTV. Moreover, treatment planning today represents only one single representation of the calculated dose distribution, while over the full course of a radiation treatment the minimum and maximum dose points are likely to shift slightly from one day to another. For all those reasons, ICRU Report 83[51] recommends discontinuing the use of maximum dose and minimum dose and instead recommends for dose reporting the use of the *near-maximum* (corresponding to $D_{2\%}$) and the *near-minimum* ($D_{98\%}$). In addition, the *median dose,* specified by $D_{50\%}$, should be reported, as it is considered to best correspond the previously defined dose at the ICRU reference point.

The maximum dose as specified by a single calculation point (D_{max} or $D_{0\%}$) has often been reported for serial-like organs or structures. Previously such a reported maximum dose was considered relevant only if the involved organ had a minimum diameter of at least 15 mm, while an even smaller dimension was considered appropriate for some organs, such as eye, optical nerve, or larynx.[35] The ICRU acknowledged that the minimum diameter for the maximum dose region in a structure is not always easy to establish and hence recommend that $D_{2\%}$ be reported. However, the ICRU pointed out that care should be taken in a change from maximum dose to the near-maximum dose, $D_{2\%}$.

With regard to dose homogeneity, ICRU Report 50 recommends that the dose coverage of the PTV be kept within specific limits, namely +7% and −5% of the prescribed dose.[35] However, this level of dose homogeneity might not be achieved in all cases (particularly for current IMRT techniques), and ICRU Report 50 explicitly states that if this degree of homogeneity cannot be achieved, it is the responsibility of the radiation oncologist to decide whether the dose heterogeneity is acceptable, pointing out that in those parts of the PTV where the highest malignant cell concentration may be expected, that is, the GTV, a higher dose might even be an advantage. Similarly, a slight underdose to the PTV might be required (particularly if in close proximity to an OAR) or result for lung tumors surrounded by low-density lung tissue as a result of electronic disequilibrium.

Noted that ICRU Reports 50 and 62 do not make strict recommendations regarding dose prescription; instead, the ICRU states "the radiation oncologist should have the freedom to prescribe the parameters in his/her own way, mainly using what is current practice to produce an expected clinical outcome of the treatment."[35] For dose reporting, however, it is recommended to also state the prescribed dose if the actual prescription was not done accordingly.

It is now recognized that there is a large variability among institutional results in IMRT planning and reporting.[60,61] Studies strongly support the ICRU Report 83 recommendation to move away from single-spatial-point prescription/reporting to dose–volume prescription/reporting. In addition, the American Society of Radiation Oncology (ASTRO) has gone even further and recommends that specific details of the inverse treatment planning and image-guided treatment processes be recorded using (a) an *IMRT Treatment Planning Directive,* (b) a *Treatment Goal Summary,* (c) an *Image Guidance Summary,* and (d) a *Motion Management Summary.*[62] I strongly encourage manufacturers of radiation oncology electronic medical record systems (e.g., Elekta-Impac MOSAIQ and Varian ARIA) to quickly incorporate these templates into their user interfaces, allowing physicians to enter their IMRT prescriptions in a more robust and unambiguous manner.

Dose–Volume Histograms

The large amount of dosimetric data that must be analyzed when a CRT plan is evaluated has prompted the development of methods of condensing and presenting the data in more easily understandable formats. One such data reduction tool is the *dose volume histogram.*[29,30] Two types of DVHs, *differential* and *cumulative,* are available in CRT planning, with the latter now widely used in plan evaluation for assessing PTV(s) coverage and dose to OARs, as displayed in Figure 9.13. However, it must be clearly understood that the DVH does not provide any spatial information and thus can only complement and not replace spatial dose-distribution display tools such as isodose displays.

The *differential DVH* (*dDVH*), as shown in Figure 9.13A, is essentially a plot of the frequency distribution of the individual

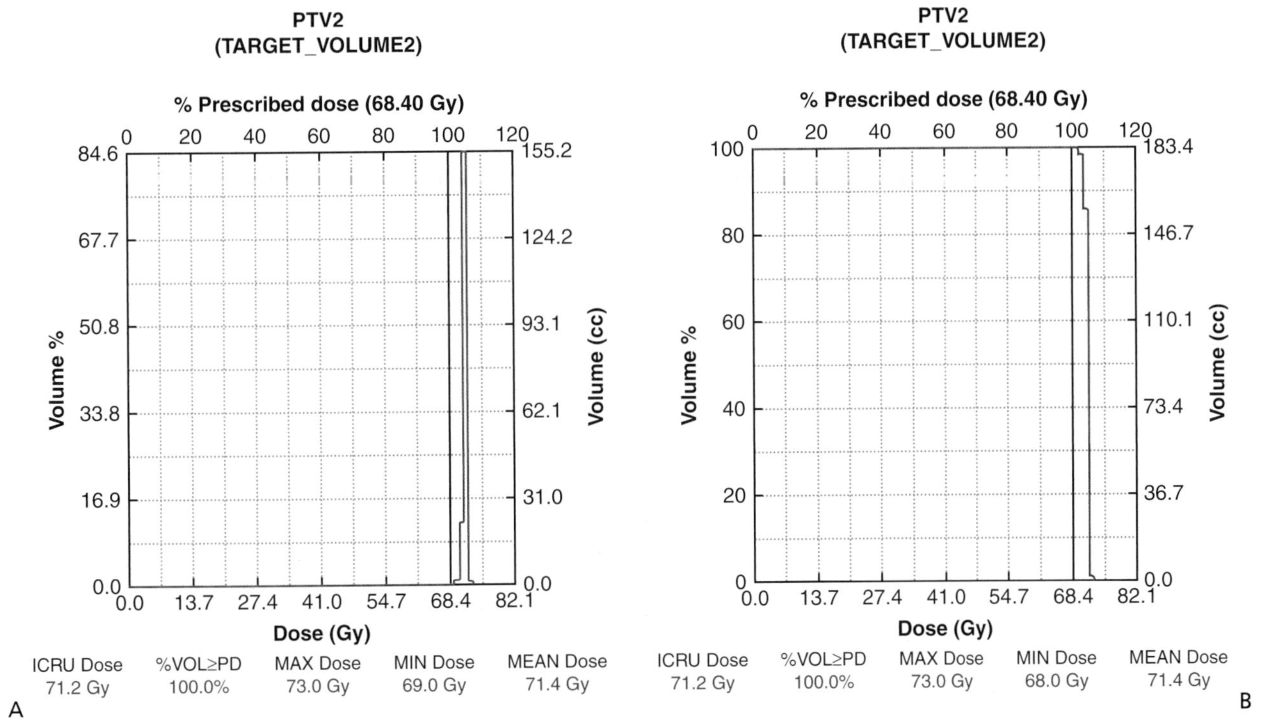

FIGURE 9.13. A: The differential dose–volume histogram (dDVH) for a specified target volume (PTV2)—the volume is subdivided into individual elements (called voxels) and tagged according to dose received as determined from the three-dimensional dose grid. Voxels are then grouped according to each specified dose bin value without regard to their spatial location. A plot of the number of voxels in each bin (*y*-axis) versus the bin dose range (*x*-axis) is by definition a dDVH. **B:** The corresponding cumulative DVH (cDVH) is generated by summing for each dose bin all of the voxels of the PTV2 dDVH to the right of each dose bin; the *y*-axis gives the volume, or percentage of volume, that receives a dose equal to or greater than the indicated dose on the *x*-axis.

dose distribution elements (called *dose voxels*) obtained from the dose grid. Typically, the grid size is small enough so that the dose can be assumed to be constant within each voxel. The volume's dose distribution is then divided into *dose bins,* and the voxels are grouped according to their dose bin value without regard to their spatial location. A plot of the number of voxels in each bin (y-axis) versus the bin dose range (x-axis) is by definition a differential DVH. The size of the dose bin used determines the height of each bin of the dDVH. For example, if the bin widths were increased, the heights of the histogram bins would increase because more voxels would fall into any given bin. Thus, it should be clearly understood that the detailed shape of a differential DVH depends on the dose bin size used, even though the underlying dose–volume data are the same.

A *cumulative DVH* (*cDVH*), as shown in Figure 9.13B, is a plot in which each bin represents the volume, or percentage of volume (y-axis), that receives a dose equal to or greater than the indicated dose on the x-axis. The cDVH is generated by summing all of the voxels of the corresponding dDVH to the right of each dose. The volume value for the first bin (dose origin) is the full volume of the structure because the total volume receives at least zero dose, and the volume for the last bin is that which receives the maximum dose. Note that in the literature, the "c" in the cDVH is generally dropped, leaving just DVH.

Explicit values of dose–volume parameters can be extracted from the DVH data and are called *dose–volume statistics* or simply *dose statistics*. Examples for target volumes include maximum dose, minimum dose, mean dose, and percentage volume receiving greater than or equal to the prescription dose; for OARs, they typically include maximum point dose, mean dose, and percentage volume receiving greater than or equal to an established tolerance dose. As previously stated, ICRU Report 83[51] recommends replacing the *minimum dose* and *maximum dose* point doses with *near-maximum* (corresponding to $D_{2\%}$) and *near-minimum* ($D_{98\%}$).[51]

Biologic Models for Dose–Volume Response

Evaluation of the quality of a treatment plan (i.e., is plan A better than plan B?) is difficult and at best a qualitative procedure. For example, it is not clear what degree of dose uniformity within the PTV is optimum, as dose levels can now be significantly escalated using CRT techniques; nor is it always clear which plan is best if the two DVHs for a specific OAR cross each other (i.e., difficulty in weighting importance of dose vs. volume).

Researchers have developed biophysical models that attempt to translate the dose–volume information into estimates of biologic response—*tumor control probability* (*TCP*) and *normal tissue complication probability* (*NTCP*) models.[58,59,63] Most authors agree that the TCP and NTCP models developed thus far are not accurate enough such that the absolute values can be used to predict clinical outcome; however, they are used to compare rival plans and as such help to rank plan quality. In any case, such biologic indices should be used clinically only when their utility has been firmly established for well-defined clinical conditions. ICRU Report 83 is clear in stating that if biologically based metrics are to be reported, the assumptions used in the models, their parameters, and the model itself must be unambiguously specified.[51]

Tumor Control Probability

TCP plotted as a function of dose has a classic sigmoid shape, having zero control at some low dose to control at some high dose. Rather than attempt to review in detail the various models, here I discuss some relevant issues. Readers are referred to the article by Moiseenko et al. for more details.[64] Simple phenomenological TCP models can be represented by the logistic function as follows:

$$\mathrm{TCP} = \frac{1}{1 + \left(\dfrac{D_{50\%}}{D}\right)^{4\gamma_{50\%}}}$$

where $D_{50\%}$ is the dose at which the TCP is 50%, $\gamma_{50\%}$ is the slope of the dose–response curve at 50% tumor control, and D is the dose administered.[65] Note that the use of the logistic function assumes an approximate uniform cell response and a uniform dose distribution.

For a nonuniform dose distribution, the total tumor volume is reduced to smaller volumes having "uniform" doses within each subvolume element v_i. The TCP value for each volume element, TCP(v, D), can be inferred from the TCP for uniform irradiation of the entire tumor volume, TCP(1, D), using the following equation:

$$\text{TCP}(v, D) = \text{TCP}(1, D)^v$$

Thus, the TCP for the tumor receiving an inhomogeneous dose is given by the product of the individual volume element TCPs as follows:

$$\text{TCP} = \prod_{i=1}^{N} \text{TCP}(v_i, D_i)$$

Here TCP(v_i, D_i) is the TCP for the ith volume element receiving dose D_i, and N is the total number of tumor volume elements. Recall that the validity of this equation is highly dependent on the validity of the assumptions that the individual tumor volume elements are uniformly distributed throughout the tumor volume and are equally radiosensitive.

Normal Tissue Complication Probability

There are mainly two different approaches used in radiation therapy in modeling NTCP: the *empiric model* introduced by Lyman and Wolbarst[66,67] and *functional models* that introduced concepts of *serial* and *parallel* tissue organization and *functional subunits* (*FSUs*).[65,68–70]

The *Lyman NTCP model* can be expressed in terms of an error function of dose (D) and volume (v) as follows:

$$\text{NTCP}(D, v) = \frac{1}{\sqrt{2\pi}} \int_{-\infty}^{t} \exp(-t^2/2)dt,$$

where

$$t = [D - D_{50}(v)]/[m \cdot D_{50}(v)],$$

with v equal to the partial volume (V/V_{ref}) and the tolerance dose volume dependence given by the following power-law relationship:

$$D_{50}(v) = D_{50}(1) \cdot v^{-n}$$

$D_{50}(1)$ is the tolerance dose for 50% complications for uniform whole-organ irradiation, and $D_{50}(v)$ is the 50% tolerance dose for uniform partial-organ irradiation to the fractional volume v. The arbitrary variables m and n are found by fitting tolerance doses for uniform whole and uniform partial-organ irradiation, where m characterizes the gradient (slope) of the dose–response function at D_{50} and n characterizes the effect of volume. When n is near unity, the volume effect is large; conversely, when n is near zero, the volume effect is small. When NTCP is plotted against dose, the NTCP equation demonstrates a sigmoid shape.

Two methods are used to extend this model to nonuniform organ irradiation. The *interpolation method*, proposed by Lyman and Wolbarst,[67] modifies the DVH to one in which the whole organ receives an effective uniform dose, D_{eff}, that is less than or equal to the maximum organ dose. The second method, called the *effective volume method*, proposed by Kutcher and Burman,[71] modifies the DVH to one in which a fraction of the organ, v_{eff}, receives the maximum organ dose. The Lyman model coupled with the Kutcher–Burman DVH reduction scheme (now called the Lyman–Kutcher–Burman model) is the most widely used NTCP model.[63]

Other NTCP models include two developed by Niemierko and Goitein—the *critical element model*, used for serial-like organs,[72] and the *critical volume model*, for parallel-like organs.[73] These are similar in form to that of Lyman and Wolbarst[66] but include additional terms to better account for the radiosensitivity of the FSUs.

Equivalent Uniform Dose

Equivalent uniform dose (EUD) is a concept first introduced by Niemierko[74] for use in evaluating and reporting inhomogeneous dose distributions and later redefined by the following equation[75]:

$$\text{EUD} = \left(\sum_i v_i D_i^a \right)^{1/a},$$

where v_i is the volume of the dose-volume bin with a dose D_i, and the exponent a is a complication-specific parameter.

The EUD concept assumes that any two dose distributions are equivalent if they cause the same radiobiologic effect and appears well suited for use in evaluating competing conformal plans. However, McGary et al. pointed out that there are conditions in which EUD is not adequate as a single parameter to report or analyze inhomogeneous dose distributions—for example, when the minimum dose is significantly lower than the mean dose.[76–78]

MANAGEMENT OF CONFORMAL RADIATION THERAPY DATA

To accurately perform the steps involved in CRT, several forms of patient imaging and other data must be acquired, displayed, manipulated, and stored. Typically, patient image data acquired from several imaging subsystems must be communicated to a TPS to permit these images to be used for treatment planning. Several software components also must be integrated so that the output of one processing step can be made available for use as input to the next step. Daily IGRT imaging is also putting large demands on data storage, and the need for more robust image processing tools is evident. These issues in data management in CRT are complex and continue to be somewhat problematic, although some progress is being made through the Integrating the Healthcare Enterprise in Radiation Oncology effort initiated by ASTRO.[79]

This issue is just part of larger informatics issues facing radiation oncology. There is an explosion in the types and volume of data that must be made available for scientific query. Difficulty in accessing the data in practical ways has become a critical limitation to investigators in the field and to its advancement. Unfortunately, the commercially available radiation oncology information systems are not yet adequate to meet this challenge. The great volume and diversity of the data have rendered their storage, management, and processing extremely problematic, resulting in situations in which important data and information are inefficiently disseminated and sometimes lost. In the busy clinic, failure to manage critical information may compromise patient safety. Here, a major issue is the lack of integration of the radiation oncology electronic medical record (EMR), based in systems such as Elekta-Impac MOSAIQ or Varian ARIA, with the electronic hospital record (EHR), based in systems such as those provided by Epic (Verona, WI). In most cases, we must resort to hybrid charting systems (ad hoc combinations of EMR, her, and paper charting), which entails risks and gives rise to a dangerous situation. Immediate and focused efforts in achieving these integrations and improving the radiation oncology informatics infrastructure are urgently needed.

QUALITY ASSURANCE FOR CONFORMAL RADIATION THERAPY

It is most important to realize that a QA program for CRT is an interdisciplinary effort involving radiation oncologists, radiation physicists, dosimetrists, radiation therapists, clinical engineers, and information technology specialists and that the efforts of each group often overlap substantially. To be effective, it is also essential to have the full support of the department chair and hospital administration.

While in general, radiation therapy has a long, successful history of QA, most authors have come to realize that the current approach (which relies heavily on prescriptive QA tests, tolerances, and frequencies as provided by consensus expert groups from national/international professional/scientific organizations) is likely inadequate by itself for more advanced modalities such as CRT.[80–82]

For example, today's imaged-guided CRT planning and delivery processes have become much more complex and much less intuitive. These complexities, coupled with the inadequate informatics infrastructure and outdated national QA guidelines, have created enormous QA challenges. Communication among members of the planning team, including physician, resident, simulation therapist, dosimetrist, physicist, and treating therapist, is often rushed, cryptic, and complicated by the lack of integration of the radiation oncology EMR (e.g., Elekta-Impac MOSAIQ) with the hospital's EHR (e.g., Epic software). In fact, in most cases, one must resort to a hybrid charting system (ad hoc combinations of EMR, EHR, and paper charts), which is a dangerous situation. In addition, multiple imaging modalities are often used to define target volumes, and now 4D imaging is being implemented clinically, all complicating the processing of the information. CRT plan data, transferred over a network to the V&R system and computer-controlled linac systems, carry complex specifications for treatment, including positioning of MLC leaves, sometimes variable dose rates, collimator rotation, gantry angles, and, in some instances, a moving treatment table or gantry or both. In some cases, different vendor software systems are used, and interoperability is not always robust. This continuing increasing complexity of devices and systems is clearly problematic for a totally prescriptive QA approach, and it results in increased time demands on staff and groups where there are already shortages. Recent *New York Times* articles[81] have brought needed attention to this issue and spurred national organizations to work to improve the current QA situation.[83,84]

While it is believed that the prescriptive QA approach is valid and valuable for much of the CRT technology and procedures currently in place, new and different approaches need to be developed in parallel.[85,86] These must be risk/evidence based and process oriented rather than device and procedure oriented; they likely need to be multidisciplinary in nature, resource and risk optimized, and flexible enough to cope with current and anticipated changes in technology.[87] Such process-oriented QA includes risk-based analysis, process mapping, application of failure modes and effects analysis (FMEA), and fault tree analysis (FTA), including analyses of human actions and responses.[88]

That said, radiation oncology departments must do all that they can now to ensure that processes for safe planning and delivery of CRT are in place and appropriately resourced. Table 9.4 provides a list of guiding principles to help a department prioritize QA efforts for improving patient safety and quality for CRT. This list is a compilation of pertinent key recommendations made by several national and international groups.[80,83,89–93]

Quality Assurance: Treatment-Planning System

The complexity of 3DTPSs continues to increase to better facilitate the accurate delivery of CRT. In a number of instances, the TPS is an integral component of the treatment machine.

TABLE 9.4 GUIDING PRINCIPLES FOR CONFORMAL RADIATION THERAPY QUALITY ASSURANCE PROGRAM

1. Establish a safety-conscious culture within the department and ensure that the processes for safe delivery of conformal radiation therapy (CRT) are in place and appropriately resourced. To that end, perform the following:
   a. Establish a formal covenant and commitment to safety. The radiation therapy team should work under a radiation safety covenant, and each member of the team should pledge a commitment to protect the safety of each and every patient.
   b. Make sure it is clear that each member of the treatment team has the right and the responsibility to declare a "time out" if he or she has concerns or questions about the plan or course of treatment for a patient.
   c. Make sure that the quality assurance (QA) program is properly resourced.
2. Seek practice accreditation by the appropriate national body; e.g., American College of Radiology (ACR)/American Society for Radiation Oncology (ASTRO).
3. Participate in external dosimetric audits such as provided by the Radiological Physics Center (RPC) annual External Reference Dosimetry Audit.
4. Expand the use of checklists in CRT treatment planning and treatment delivery.
5. Implement a formal policy that ensures that CRT policy and procedures (P&Ps), including checklists, are in place and are regularly updated and reviewed on an annual basis (require documentation that this is actually done).
6. Conduct periodic reviews of staffing levels to ensure that the staffing and skills mix are appropriate for the numbers of patients treated and the complexity of treatments delivered.
7. Implement a Clinical Operations Committee (COC), with supervisor representatives from each group, to address any problematic issues in the clinic and to help ensure that good communication exists among all groups involved in the CRT treatment process.
8. Conduct town hall meetings (with QA program being a major focus) with department faculty/staff at least quarterly to help ensure good communication exists among all groups involved in the treatment process.
9. Maintain training records for all staff involved in radiation therapy. They should be detailed and specific to particular procedures, i.e., an internal form of CRT credentialing.
10. Maintain funding to support training and continuing education, particularly when new CRT techniques are introduced.
11. Introduction of new CRT techniques always needs to be carefully planned with thorough risk assessment, review of staffing levels and skills required, and development of pertinent P&Ps. All staff involved in the process should undergo specific training in the new treatment technique or process prior to clinical use.
12. Working environment, particularly in two areas–treatment machine console and treatment planning–needs to be conducive to safety and designed such that it ensures that staff can work without inappropriate interruptions.
13. Prescriptive QA program should be in place but continually evaluated to ensure that each specific test adds value and that those that do not add the required value are eliminated.
14. Perform systematic risk analysis and improvement using industrial engineering-based tools such as process mapping, failure modes and effects analysis (FMEA), and fault tree analysis (FTA) for all advanced treatment modalities.
15. Implement a treatment table registration system (CT-simulator and treatment machines) so that all patient/immobilization device positions on the table can be registered.
16. Use treatment planning/delivery systems tolerance tables for specific procedures, and monitor setup variability (i.e., any therapist overrides of treatment couch, gantry, collimator position, etc., settings in order to treat patient).
17. Perform on-treatment verification imaging as needed, but be mindful of imaging dose, and look for ways to become more efficient.
18. Perform *in vivo* dosimetry (e.g., diode checks) at the beginning of treatment for all 3DCRT patients when physically possible.
19. Conduct weekly peer review chart rounds (review prescription, verification images, dose distribution, and other pertinent documentation, e.g., signed consent, pathology, etc).
20. Conduct weekly peer review Planning Conference to review CRT plans. Review of GTV, CTV, and PTV contours, DRRs, and dose distributions helps to develop a consistent approach in implementing ICRU 50/62/83 methodology.
21. Implement a treatment-planning workflow monitoring software system.
22. Implement a software system for reporting and analyzing errors and near-misses, with feedback to the staff at town hall meetings.
23. Strive to have the right balance between accountability and openness in the department's incident-reporting culture.
24. Department should strongly endorse a national/international incident reporting system for radiotherapy incidents.

Hence, this results in having more than one planning system in the department, thus increasing QA complexity. Rigorous acceptance and commissioning of the TPS is essential to ensure it is functioning accurately before it is used clinically; in this respect, it is no different than other medical devices. Full details on acceptance, commissioning, and periodic QA tests are available elsewhere.[94–101]

The accuracy of dose calculations must be thoroughly examined during the 3DTPS commissioning process. Periodic checks of calculations versus measured dose are also essential due to possible data corruptions in the TPS itself and to how well treatment machine parameters such as flatness and symmetry are maintained. It should be appreciated that the 3DTPS can never be fully tested, nor can the manufacturer assure the user that the system is "bug free." Rather, the system should be tested over a range of parameters that are typical of those used in the clinic. For example, tests should include (a) consistency of input/output data, (b) monitor units calculations, (c) relative dose distributions, (d) graphical data, including BEV and field aperture display, and (e) plan evaluation tools such as DVHs and DRRs. The test procedures and results should be fully documented, as they will provide the basic test data to which the periodic QA tests can be compared.

Quality Assurance: Patient Positioning and Immobilization and Imaging Data Acquisition

CT, MRI, PET, and ultrasound imaging are used, depending on disease site, for acquiring imaging data to determine patient external contours and target and organs-at-risk volumes. Hence, there are a number of additional QA demands placed on imaging units that are specific to CRT treatment planning.[39] Since the patient needs to be repositioned reproducibly on the treatment machine, special patient positioning-immobilization devices are needed. Such devices should be constructed so that they can be attached in similar manner to the treatment machine couch and the CT, MR, or PET imaging system couches used in obtaining the planning imaging data. These devices should not only attach and lock to all couches, but they also should do so in a configurable manner to allow indexing of the devices to the treatment couch for daily reproducibility.

In some instances the composition of these devices is also important; for example, low–atomic number materials are necessary for CT scanners. In addition, patient motion can distort MRI and CT images, which can cause changes in the electron densities used for dose calculation that are derived from CT. Furthermore, the position of the patient in the CT scanning ring can lead to errors in the CT numbers that are used to derive the linear attenuation coefficients of the patient.

Geometric accuracy of all imaging modalities used for planning must be checked. This can be accomplished by imaging suitably designed phantoms on the various machines and comparing the results with the known values. Special care should be given to MRI units, which may suffer from appreciable spatial distortions. If a PET-CT is used, special attention should be paid to the physical alignment of the table couch and both imaging rings. If images from CT, MR, and/or PET are registered and fused, a QA program must be implemented to ensure that the inherent algorithm used and departmental procedures are able to produce accurate composite images for planning.[102,103] Finally, for CT, it is necessary to obtain or confirm the relationship between CT number and electron density.

The transfer of image data routinely occurs directly via a computer network but should be checked on a regular basis. Vigilance is also necessary to eliminate any systematic errors; for example, an error in the specification of a scan diameter can lead to geometric distortions of the image.

Quality Assurance: Volume(s) Delineation

Target volume delineation is viewed by many experts in the field as being the weakest link in the entire CRT workflow chain. A high variation continues to be seen in all studies evaluating consistency of delineation of target volumes and organs at risk among physicians.[104–109] This can be explained by a lack of generally accepted guidelines for volume delineation and also, most likely, insufficient training of radiation oncology residents in modern cross-sectional imaging. It is clear that errors/inconsistencies in volume delineation can seriously undermine the goals of CRT. One approach toward solving this difficult issue is to adopt guidelines and consensus volumes based on the delineation performed by a number of experts in the field.[108,110] Both the Radiation Therapy Oncology Group and the European Society of Therapeutic Radiation Oncology have placed high priority on this approach and now offer more online guidelines for several sites.

It is also possible to improperly define an OAR due to faulty or incomplete CT procedures. For example, the base of the brain may be better defined on the CT slice if sagittal reconstructions are also available while contouring. In addition, if contrast is used, density overrides may be needed before treatment planning is performed to avoid the erroneous effects of the high-Z media. Related to this is the situation that occurs when high-Z materials like hip prostheses are found within the patient and density overrides are required to account for artifacts.

Quality Assurance: Designing Beams

MLC leaf settings or block apertures and beam orientation displays must be confirmed prior to clinical use and checked after any software modification. In addition, it is possible to define beam orientations that are physically impossible to set up, and this process requires use of clinical judgment by the dosimetrist generating the treatment plan. Thus, the ability to physically set up a particular beam orientation must be reviewed and verified, particularly for beam orientations involving couch rotation. In such cases, tests might have to be performed to verify clearance between the treatment machine gantry and the patient or the gantry and the treatment couch before finalizing the treatment plan.

Quality Assurance: Plan Evaluation

The fidelity of the 3DTPS plan evaluation tools (i.e., dose distribution displays, DVHs, hard copy, etc.) depends upon many factors in addition to just the accuracy of the dose calculation algorithm, and thus they should be regularly checked. For example, nonlinearities in graphical display and/or plotting systems can lead to distortions in the displayed patient anatomy and the overlying dose distributions. Hence, it is good practice to have fixed length scales displayed/printed in order to be able to check the geometric accuracy of the plan output. Furthermore, the dose distribution calculations can be sensitive to the grid size, and DVHs can additionally be sensitive to the dose bin size.[111]

As mentioned earlier, plan evaluation is becoming more cumbersome as treatment techniques are becoming more complex. This loss of direct "clinical feeling" of the adequacy of a treatment plan is problematic. Plan evaluation using DVHs, planar isodoses, and room's-eye views of dose surfaces is made more robust if the department adopts a evidence-based list of dose–volume constraints for target volumes and organs at risk and documents reasons when compliance is not followed.

Quality Assurance: Treatment Plan Review

All CRT treatment plans should be reviewed, signed, and dated by the treatment planner. The treating physician should of course also review, approve, and sign the treatment plan. In addition, all plans should be independently checked prior to initiation of radiation therapy by a physicist who was not involved directly in the production of the plan. The independent plan check should assure that setup instructions have been properly recorded—for example, field size, gantry angle, and so on. In addition, beam normalization points (normally at isocenter) can be problematic if near nontissue medium or under or near an MLC leaf edge and hence should be moved to a more suitable location. The number of monitor units to realize the dose prescription is typically obtained directly from the 3DTPS. These values must be independently checked either by hand calculations or, more typically, independent computer calculations. An action level should be established based upon the accuracy of the computer algorithm and independent dose calculation procedure. Obviously, any monitor unit (MU) check system must be tested prior to clinical use and following any change or software upgrade. The American Association of Physicists in Medicine Task Group 114 report provides valuable information on the verification of MU calculations for non-IMRT radiotherapy treatments.[112]

Note that IMRT plans require additional checks, including review of optimization parameters, minimum gap size, minimum MU/segment, and maximum doses in and outside of the target. In addition, in the United States the patient's plan must undergo phantom measurement checks on the intended treatment machine to verify both point dose and spatial dose distribution agreement.

Quality Assurance: Planning Conference

One of the most important components of a CRT QA program is the establishment of a weekly planning QA conference that is attended by radiation oncologists, medical physicists, radiation therapists, and dosimetrists. This is in addition to the normal new-patient chart rounds conference, at which the patient's pertinent medical history, physical, pathology, and diagnostic imaging findings along with the tumor staging and proposed plan of treatment, including the prescription, are presented by the attending radiation oncologists or residents. In a planning QA conference, the group can review the CRT plans using a high-resolution, large-screen video projector connected to the 3DTP network. GTV, CTV, and PTV contours, DRRs, and dose distributions can all be reviewed very efficiently. This type of planning conference helps the staff to develop a very consistent approach in implementing ICRU 50/62/83 methodology for specifying volumes and provides a very effective peer review mechanism for a CRT clinical program.

Quality Assurance: Plan Implementation and Treatment Verification

If a clinic is in the initial phases of implementing CRT techniques or if experienced users implement new CRT modalities using nonconventional beam orientations, a verification simulation procedure is recommended to confirm the correctness of the beam orientations. It is important to check that all treatment plan parameters are properly implemented. This can be best accomplished by having the treatment planning team available (or on call) during this procedure so that any detected ambiguities or problems can be addressed immediately. When a beam orientation cannot be simulated, electronic portal imaging devices (EPIDs) can be used to obtain orthogonal images for comparison with similar DRRs to ensure correct isocenter positioning. Today, even more-advanced on-board imaging and other data localization systems (i.e., ultrasound, video surfacing, static kilovolt imaging, kilovolt cone beam CT, megavolt helical CT, and megavolt cone beam CT) are available.[10,50] Clearly written policy and procedures (P&Ps) should be in place with regard to (a) localization procedures, (b) therapist instructions and tolerance criteria to move (or not move) a patient, (c) whether post imaging is required when a move is made, (d) subsequent reviews by physicians, and (e) the process for peer review of verification images. Special care should be taken to ensure that all beam-modifying devices are correctly positioned. Although errors in MLC settings or block fabrication/mounting should be observed when reviewing the portal images, wedge or compensator misalignment is much more problematic and may only be revealed by careful observation during patient setup.

The optical distance indicator is also useful in assessing the correctness of the setup of a particular beam. Documentation provides a depth of isocenter below the skin surface on the central ray of the beam, which can then be compared with the isocenter depth measured on the simulator or treatment machine after the beam is set up using the couch and gantry positions specified by the treatment plan.

A V&R system should be used to assure that the same parameters (within tolerance limits) are used each day. Such systems are valuable for the verification and recording of at least the following parameters: (a) monitor units, (b) energy, (c) mode, (d) collimator settings (including independent jaws and multileaf collimator), (e) collimator angle, (f) gantry angle, (g) table position, and (h) wedge number and orientation. However, V&R systems must be used with care since they can give the user a false sense of security. For example, if a setup error is made on the first day and the machine geometry parameters are captured, the system will faithfully verify this erroneous setting from day to day. To reduce the chance of this occurring, the patient should be carefully set up according to the treatment plan (best if there is a direct electronic transfer of plan parameters to the V&R system) and a robust P&P for approval of patient treatment position should be in place; upon approval, the parameters are captured with the V&R system. As vendor implementation of Digital Imaging and Communications in Medicine data exchange has matured significantly, the direct transfer of data from the TPS to the V&R system has undoubtedly reduced such errors; however, a careful check of patient position is still recommended.

Thermoluminescent dosimeters (TLDs), diodes, and MOSFET detectors are often used for in-vivo dosimetry. Diodes or MOSFETS are most used for dose checks at the beginning of treatment for all non-IMRT patients. TLDs are typically used for checking multiple dose locations for unusual treatment conditions or for critical structures in or near the treatment volume. In addition, implantable dosimeters are now being used for real-time dosimetry.[113] Recently, exit portal dosimetry using EPIDs has been used to provide full-field information, even for IMRT fields.[114,115]

SUMMARY

I strongly believe that the use of 3D treatment planning and CRT has had (and will continue to have) a major impact on the practice of radiation therapy. Phase I/II and III CRT dose-escalation studies in several disease sites have been conducted (or are underway) by the Radiation Therapy Oncology Group under cooperative agreement with the National Cancer Institute.[116] In addition, there are many other individual institutional studies that have shown the benefits of 3D planning and conformal therapy, particularly for prostate cancer, head and neck cancer, and lung cancer, as documented in the literature.[117] Patients identified to benefit most from 3D planning and CRT are those with tumors in sites with complex anatomy, irregularly shaped tumor volumes, tumors adjacent to radiation-sensitive normal structures, and undergoing small-volume or high-dose treatments. However, as with any major technical advance in radiation oncology, CRT use must be supported with enhanced quality assurance from all members of the treatment team.

REFERENCES

1. Purdy JA. 3-D radiation treatment planning: a new era. In: Meyer JL, Purdy JA, eds. *3-D conformal radiotherapy: a new era in the irradiation of cancer.* Basel: Karger; 1996:1–16.
2. Purdy JA. From new frontiers to new standards of practice: advances in radiotherapy planning and delivery. In: Meyer JL, ed. *IMRT, IGRT, SBRT.* Basel: Karger; 2007:18–39.
3. Purdy JA. Advances in the planning and delivery of radiotherapy: new expectations, new standards of care. In: Meyer JL, ed. *IMRT, IGRT, SBRT,* 2nd ed. Basel: Karger; 2011:1–28.

4. Bortfeld T, Schmidt-Ullrich R, De Neve W, et al. *Image-guided IMRT.* Berlin: Springer; 2006.
5. Purdy JA. Intensity-modulated radiation therapy. *Int J Radiat Oncol Biol Phys* 1996;35(4):845–846.
6. Webb S. *Intensity-modulated radiation therapy.* Bristol: Institute of Physics Publishing; 2000.
7. Jaffray DA, Drake DG, Moreau M, et al. A radiographic and tomographic imaging system integrated into a medical linear accelerator for localization of bone and soft-tissue targets. *Int J Radiat Oncol Biol Phys* 1999;45:773–789.
8. Jaffray DA, Siewerdsen JH, Wong JW, et al. Flat-panel cone-beam computed tomography for image-guided radiation therapy. *Int J Radiat Oncol Biol Phys* 2002;53(5):1337–1349.
9. Ling CC, York E, Fuks Z. From IMRT to IGRT: frontierland or neverland? *Radiother Oncol* 2006;78:119–122.
10. Dawson LA, Balter JM. Interventions to reduce organ motion effects in radiation delivery. *Semin Radiat Oncol* 2004;14(1):76–80.
11. Keall PJ. 4-dimensional computed tomography imaging and treatment planning. *Semin Radiat Oncol* 2004;14(1):81–90.
12. Takahaski S. Conformation radiotherapy-rotation techniques as applied to radiography and radiotherapy of cancer. *Acta Radiol Suppl* 1965;242:1–142.
13. Proimos BS. Synchronous field shaping in rotational megavoltage therapy. *Radiology* 1960;74:753–757.
14. Trump JG, Wright KA, Smedal MI, et al. Synchronous field shaping and protection in 2-million-volt rotational therapy. *Radiology* 1961;76:275–283.
15. Green A, Jennings WA, Christie HM. Rotational roentgen therapy in the horizontal plane. *Acta Radiol* 1960;31:275–320.
16. Bjarngard BE, Kijewski PK. Computer-controlled radiation therapy. In: *Proceedings 2nd Annual Symposium on Computer Applications in Medical Care.* Long Beach, CA; 1978.
17. Davy TJ, Brace J. Dynamic 3-D treatment using a computer-controlled cobalt unit. *Br J Radiol* 1979;53:612–616.
18. Sterling TD, Knowlton KC, Weinkam JJ, et al. Dynamic display of radiotherapy plans using computer-produced films. *Radiology* 1973;107:689–691.
19. Sterling TD, Perry H, Katz L. Automation of radiation treatment planning V. Calculation and visualization of the total treatment volume. *Br J Radiol* 1965; 38:906–913.
20. McShan DL, Silverman A, Lanza D, et al. A computerized three-dimensional treatment planning system utilizing interactive color graphics. *Br J Radiol* 1979; 52:478–481.
21. Reinstein LE, McShan D, Webber BM, et al. A computer-assisted three-dimensional treatment planning system. *Radiology* 1978;127:259–264.
22. Goitein M, Abrams M. Multi-dimensional treatment planning: I. Delineation of anatomy. *Int J Radiat Oncol Biol Phys* 1983;9:777–787.
23. Goitein M, Abrams M, Rowell D, et al. Multi-dimensional treatment planning: II. Beam's eye view, back projection, and projection through CT sections. *Int J Radiat Oncol Biol Phys* 1983;9:789–797.
24. Fraass BA, McShan DL. 3-D treatment planning. I. Overview of a clinical planning system. In: *Proceedings of the 9th International Conference on the Use of Computers in Radiation Therapy.* Scheveningen, Netherlands; 1987.
25. Mohan R, Barest G, Brewster LJ, et al. A comprehensive three-dimensional radiation treatment planning system. *Int J Radiat Oncol Biol Phys* 1988;15:481–495.
26. Purdy JA, Wong JW, Harms WB, et al. Three dimensional radiation treatment planning system. In: *Proceedings of the 9th International Conference on the Use of Computers in Radiation Therapy.* Scheveningen, Netherlands; 1987.
27. Sherouse GW, Mosher CE, Novins K, et al. Virtual simulation: concept and implementation, in the use of computers in radiation therapy. In: *Proceedings of the 9th International Conference on the Use of Computers in Radiation Therapy.* Scheveningen, Netherlands; 1987.
28. Smith AF, Purdy JA. Editors' note. *Int J Radiat Oncol Biol Phys* 1991;21(1):1.
29. Drzymala RE, Holman MD, Yan D, et al. Integrated software tools for the evaluation of radiotherapy treatment plans. *Int J Radiat Oncol Biol Phys* 1994;30(4): 909–919.
30. Drzymala RE, Mohan R, Brewster L, et al. Dose–volume histograms. *Int J Radiat Oncol Biol Phys* 1991;21(1):71–78.
31. Bosch WR, Low DA, Gerber RL, et al. The electronic viewbox: a software tool for radiation therapy treatment verification. *Int J Radiat Oncol Biol Phys* 1995;31(1):135–142.
32. Goitein M. The probability of controlling an inhomogeneously irradiated tumor. In: Goitein M, Lyman J, Maor M, et al., eds. *Report of the working groups on the evaluation of treatment planning for particle beam radiotherapy.* Bethesda, MD: National Cancer Institute; 1987.
33. IMRT Collaborative Working Group. Intensity modulated radiation therapy: current status and issues of interest. *Int J Radiat Oncol Biol Phys* 2001;51(4):880–914.
34. International Commission on Radiation Units and Measurements. *Report 29: Dose Specification for reporting external beam therapy with photons and electrons.* Washington, DC: International Commission on Radiation Units and Measurements; 1978.
35. International Commission on Radiation Units and Measurements. *Report 50: Prescribing, recording, and reporting photon beam therapy.* Bethesda, MD: International Commission on Radiation Units and Measurements; 1993.
36. International Commission on Radiation Units and Measurements. *Report 62: Prescribing, recording, and reporting photon beam therapy (Supplement to ICRU Report 50).* Bethesda, MD: International Commission on Radiation Units and Measurements; 1999.
37. Jin J-Y, Ajlouni M, Chen Q, et al.. A technique of using gated-CT images to determine internal target volume (ITV) for fractionated stereotactic lung radiotherapy. *Radiother Oncol* 2006;78(2):177–184.
38. Perez CA, Purdy JA, Harms WB, et al. Design of a fully integrated three-dimensional computed tomography simulator and preliminary clinical evaluation. *Int J Radiat Oncol Biol Phys* 1994;30(4):887–897.
39. Mutic S, Palta JR, Butker EK, et al. Quality assurance for computed-tomography simulators and the computed-tomography-simulation process: Report of the AAPM Radiation Therapy Committee Task Group No. 66. *Med Phys* 2003; 30(10):2762–2792.
40. Hall WH, Guiou M, Lee NY, et al. Development and validation of a standardized method for contouring the brachial plexus: preliminary dosimetric analysis among patients treated with IMRT for head-and-neck cancer. *Int J Radiat Oncol Biol Phys.* 2008;72(5):1362–1367.
41. Caldwell CB, Mah K, Skinner M, et al. Can PET provide the 3D extent of tumor motion for individualized internal target volumes? A phantom study of the limitations of CT and the promise of PET. *Int J Radiat Oncol Biol Phys* 2003;55(5):1381–1393.
42. Chen GTY, Kung JH, Beaudette KP. Artifacts in computed tomography scanning of moving objects. *Semin Radiat Oncol* 2004;14(1):19–26.
43. Rietzel E, Chen GT, Choi NC, et al. Four-dimensional image-based treatment planning: Target volume segmentation and dose calculation in the presence of respiratory motion. *Int J Radiat Oncol Biol Phys* 61(5):1535–1550.
44. Rietzel E, Pan T, Chen GT. Four-dimensional computed tomography: image formation and clinical protocol. *Med Phys* 2005;32(4):874–889.
45. Qi XS, White J, Rabinovitch R, et al. Respiratory organ motion and dosimetric impact on breast and nodal irradiation. *Int J Radiat Oncol Biol Phys* 2010; 78(2):609–617.
46. Bortfeld T, Jiang S, Rietzel E. Effects of motion on the total dose distribution. *Semin Radiat Oncol.* 2004;14(1):41–51.
47. Chino JP, Lee WR, Madden R, et al. Teaching the anatomy of oncology: evaluating the impact of a dedicated oncoanatomy course. *Int J Radiat Oncol Biol Phys* 2011;79(3):853–859.
48. van Herk M. Errors and margins in radiotherapy. *Semin Radiat Oncol* 2004; 14(1):52–64.
49. van Herk M, Remeijer P, Lebesque JV. Inclusion of geometric uncertainties in treatment plan evaluations. *Int J Radiat Oncol Biol Phys* 2002;52(5):1407–1422.
50. Keall P. Locating and targeting moving tumors with radiation beams. In: Meyer JL, ed. *IMRT, IGRT, SBRT,* 2nd ed. Basel: Karger; 2011:118–131.
51. International Commission on Radiation Units and Measurements. Report 83: Prescribing, Recording, and reporting photon-beam intensity-modulated radiation therapy (IMRT). *J ICRU* 2010;10(1):1–106.
52. Sherouse GW, Novins K, Chaney EL. Computation of digitally reconstructed radiographs for use in radiotherapy treatment design. *Int J Radiat Oncol Biol Phys* 1990;18(3):651–658.
53. Mackie RT, Liu HH, McCullough EC. Treatment planning algorithms: model-based photon dose calculations. In: Khan FM, ed. *Treatment planning in radiation oncology,* 2nd ed. Philadelphia: Lippincott Williams & Wilkins; 2007:63–77.
54. Frank SJ, Forster KM, Stevens CW, et al. Treatment planning for lung cancer: Traditional homogeneous point-dose prescription compared with heterogeneity-corrected dose-volume prescription. *Int J Radiat Oncol Biol Phys* 2003;56(5): 1308–1318.
55. Purdy JA, Harms WB, Matthews JW, et al. Advances in 3-dimensional radiation treatment planning systems: room-view display with real time interactivity. *Int J Radiat Oncol Biol Phys* 1993;27(4):933–944.
56. Emami B, Lyman J, Brown A, et al. Tolerance of normal tissue to therapeutic irradiation. *Int J Radiat Oncol Biol Phys* 1991;21:109–122.
57. Milano MT, Constine LS, Okunieff P. Normal tissue tolerance dose metrics for radiation therapy of major organs. *Semin Radiat Oncol* 2007;17(2):131.
58. Marks LB, Ten Haken RK, Martel MK. Guest Editor's Introduction to QUANTEC: A Users Guide. *Int J Radiat Oncol Biol Phys* 2010;76(3, Suppl 1):S1–S2.
59. Marks LB, Yorke ED, Jackson A, et al. Use of normal tissue complication probability models in the clinic. *Int J Radiat Oncol Biol Phys* 2010;76(3, Suppl 1):S10–S19.
60. Das IJ, Chang C-W, Chopra KL, et al. Intensity-modulated radiation therapy dose prescription, recording, and delivery: patterns of variability among institutions and treatment planning systems. *J Natl Cancer Inst* 2008;100(5):300–307.
61. Willins J, Kachnic L. Clinically relevant standards for intensity-modulated radiation therapy dose prescription. *J Natl Cancer Inst* 2008;100(5):288–290.
62. Holmes T, Das R, Low D, et al. American Society for Radiation Oncology recommendations for documenting intensity-modulated radiation therapy treatments. *Int J Radiat Oncol Biol Phys* 2009;74(5):1311–1318.
63. Bentzen SM, Constine LS, Deasy JO, et al. Quantitative Analyses of Normal Tissue Effects in the Clinic (QUANTEC): an introduction to the scientific issues. *Int J Radiat Oncol Biol Phys* 2010;76(3, Suppl 1):S3–S9.
64. Moiseenko V, Deasy JO, Van Dyk J. Radiobiological modeling for treatment planning. In: Van Dyk J, ed. *The modern technology of radiation oncology,* Vol. 2. Madison, WI: Medical Physics Publishing; 2005:185–220.
65. Schultheiss TE, Orton CG, Peck RA. Models in radiotherapy: volume effects. *Med Phys* 1983;10:410–415.
66. Lyman JT, Wolbarst AB. Optimization of radiation therapy. III. A method of assessing complication probabilities from dose-volume histograms. *Int J Radiat Oncol Biol Phys* 1987;13:103–109.
67. Lyman JT, Wolbarst AB. Optimization of radiation therapy. IV. A dose-volume histogram reduction algorithm. *Int J Radiat Oncol Biol Phys* 1989;17(2):433–436.
68. Källman P, Lind BK, Brahme A. An algorithm for maximizing the probability of complication free tumor control in radiation therapy. *Int J Radiat Oncol Biol Phys* 1992;37:871–890.
69. Olsen DR, Kambestad BK, Kristoffersen DT. Calculation of radiation induced complication probabilities for brain, liver and kidney, and the use of a reliability model to estimate critical volume fractions. *Br J Radiol* 1994;67:1218–1225.
70. Withers HR, Taylor JMG, Maciejewski B. Treatment volume and tissue tolerance. *Int J Radiat Oncol Biol Phys* 1988;14:751–759.
71. Kutcher G, Berman C. Calculation of complication probability factors for non-uniform tissue irradiation: the effective volume method. *Int J Radiat Oncol Biol Phys* 1989;16:1623–1630.
72. Niemierko A, Goitein M. Calculation of normal tissue complication probability and dose-volume histogram reduction schemes for tissues with a critical element architecture. *Radiother Oncol* 1991;20:166–176.
73. Niemierko A, Goitein M. Modeling of normal tissue response to radiation: the critical volume module. *Int J Radiat Oncol Biol Phys* 1993;25:135–145.
74. Niemierko A. Reporting and analyzing dose distributions: a concept of equivalent uniform dose. *Med Phys* 1997;24(1):103–110.
75. Niemierko A. A generalized concept of equivalent uniform dose (EUD) [Abstract]. *Med Phys* 1999;26:1100.
76. McGary JE, Grant W, Woo SY, et al. Comment on "Reporting and analyzing dose distributions: A concept of equivalent uniform dose" [*Med. Phys.* 24, 103–109 (1997)]. *Med Phys* 1997;24(8):1323–1324.
77. McGary JE, Grant W, Woo SY. Applying the equivalent uniform dose formulation based on the linear-quadratic model to inhomogeneous tumor dose distributions: caution for analyzing and reporting. *J Appl Clin Med Phys* 2000;1(4):126–137.
78. Niemierko A. Response to Comment on "Reporting and analyzing dose distributions: A concept of equivalent uniform dose" [*Med. Phys.* 24, 1323–1324 (1997)]. *Med Phys* 1997;24(8):1325–1327.
79. Abdel-Wahab M, Rengan R, Curran B, et al. Integrating the healthcare enterprise in radiation oncology plug and play—the future of radiation oncology? *Int J Radiat Oncol Biol Phys* 76(2):333–336.

80. Kutcher GJ, Coia L, Gillin M, et al. Comprehensive QA for radiation oncology: report of AAPM Radiation Therapy Committee Task Group 40. *Med Phys* 1994;21(4):581–618.
81. Bogdanovitch W. Radiation offers new cures, and ways to do harm. *New York Times* 24 Jan 2010. Available at: http://www.nytimes.com/2010/01/24/health/24radiation.html.
82. Williamson JF, Dunscombe PB, Sharpe MB, et al. Quality assurance needs for modern image-based radiotherapy: recommendations from 2007 interorganizational symposium on "Quality Assurance of Radiation Therapy: Challenges of Advanced Technology." *Int J Radiat Oncol Biol Phys* 2008;71(1, Suppl 1):S2–S12.
83. Klein EE, Hanley J, Bayouth J, et al. Task Group 142 report: quality assurance of medical accelerators. *Med Phys* 2009;36(9):4197–4212.
84. ASTRO. Press release: ASTRO reaffirms commitment to quality, issues progress report on patient safety plan; 2011. Available at: http://www.astro.org/News-and-Media/News-Releases/2011/Target-Safely,-a-six-point-patient-protection-plan-developed-in-January-2010,-to-improve-the-safety-and-quality-of-radiation.aspx.
85. Pawlicki T, Mundt AJ. Quality in radiation oncology. *Med Phys* 2007;34(5):1529–1534.
86. Ford EC, Gaudette R, Myers L, et al. Evaluation of safety in a radiation oncology setting using failure mode and effects analysis. *Int J Radiat Oncol Biol Phys* 2009;74(3):852–858.
87. Pawlicki T, Dunscombe PB, Mundt AJ, et al., eds. *Quality and safety in radiotherapy.* New York: Taylor & Francis; 2011.
88. Rath F. Tools for developing a quality management program: proactive tools (process mapping, value stream mapping, fault tree analysis, and failure mode and effects analysis). *Int J Radiat Oncol Biol Phys* 2008;71(1, Suppl 1):S187–S190.
89. American College of Radiology. *Practice guidelines and technical standards.* Reston, VA: American College of Radiology; 2010.
90. International Atomic Energy Agency. *Safety Report Series No. 17: Lessons learned from accidental exposures in radiotherapy.* Vienna: International Atomic Energy Agency; 2000.
91. International Atomic Energy Agency. *Comprehensive audits of radiotherapy practices: a tool for quality improvement.* Vienna: International Atomic Energy Agency; 2007.
92. Royal College of Radiologists, Society and College of Radiographers, Institute of Physics and Engineering in Medicine, National Patient Safety Agency, British Institute of Radiology. *Towards safer radiotherapy.* London: Royal College of Radiologists; 2008.
93. Hendee WR, Herman MG. Improving patient safety in radiation oncology. *Med Phys* 2011;38(1):78–82.
94. Fraass B, Doppke K, Hunt M, et al. AAPM Radiation Therapy Committee Task Group 53: Quality assurance for clinical radiotherapy treatment planning. *Med Phys* 1998;25:1773–1829.
95. Jacky J, White CP. Testing a 3-D radiation therapy planning program. *Int J Radiat Oncol Biol Phys* 1990;18:253–261.
96. Van Dyk J, Barnett RB, Cygler JE, et al. Commissioning and quality assurance of treatment planning computers. *Int J Radiat Oncol Biol Phys* 1993;26(2):261–273.
97. Van Dyk J. Quality assurance of radiation therapy planning systems: current status and remaining challenges. *Int J Radiat Oncol Biol Phys* 2008;71(1, Suppl 1):S23–S27.
98. International Atomic Energy Agency. *Commissioning and quality assurance of computerized planning systems for radiation treatment of cancer.* Vienna: International Atomic Energy Agency; 2004.
99. Ezzell GA, Burmeister JW, Dogan N, et al. IMRT commissioning: multiple institution planning and dosimetry comparisons, a report from AAPM Task Group 119. *Med Phys* 2009;36(11):5359–5373.
100. Bruinvis IAD, Keus RB, Lenglet WJM, et al. *Quality assurance of 3-D treatment planning systems for external photon and electron beams: Report 15 of The Netherlands Commission on Radiation Dosimetry.* Delft, Netherlands; 2006.
101. Mijnheer B, Olszewska A, Fiorino C, et al. *Quality assurance of treatment planning systems: practical examples of non-IMRT photon beams. ESTRO Booklet No. 7.* Brussels; 2004.
102. Lavely WC, Scarfone C, Cevikalp H, et al. Phantom validation of coregistration of PET and CT for image-guided radiotherapy. *Med Phys* 2004;31(5):1083–1092.
103. Mutic S, Dempsey JF, Bosch WR, et al. Multimodality image registration quality assurance for conformal three-dimensional treatment planning. *Int J Radiat Oncol Biol Phys* 2001;51(1):244–260.
104. Gregoire V, Coche E, Cosnard G, et al. Selection and delineation of lymph node target volumes in head and neck conformal radiotherapy. Proposal for standardizing terminology and procedure based on the surgical experience. *Radiother Oncol* 2000;56(2):135–150.
105. Gregoire V, Levendag P, Ang KK, et al. CT-based delineation of lymph node levels and related CTVs in the node-negative neck: DAHANCA, EORTC, GORTEC, NCIC, RTOG consensus guidelines. *Radiother Oncol* 2003;69(3):227–236.
106. Matzinger O, Gerber E, Bernstein Z, et al. EORTC-ROG expert opinion: radiotherapy volume and treatment guidelines for neoadjuvant radiation of adenocarcinomas of the gastroesophageal junction and the stomach. *Radiother Oncol* 2009;92:164–175.
107. Poortmans PMP, Ataman F, Bernard Davis J, et al. Guidelines for target volume definition in post-operative radiotherapy for prostate cancer, on behalf of the EORTC Radiation Oncology Group. *Radiother Oncol* 2007;82:121–127.
108. Symon Z, Tsvang L, Wygoda M, et al. An interobserver study of prostatic fossa clinical target volume delineation in clinical practice: are regions of recurrence adequately targeted? *Am J Clin Oncol* 2011;34(2):145–149.
109. van Mourik AM, Elkhuizen PHM, Minkema D, et al. Multiinstitutional study on target volume delineation variation in breast radiotherapy in the presence of guidelines. *Radiother Oncol* 2010;94(3):286–291.
110. Miralbell R, Vees H, Lozano J, et al. Endorectal MRI assessment of local relapse after surgery for prostate cancer: A model to define treatment field guidelines for adjuvant radiotherapy in patients at high risk for local failure. *Int J Radiat Oncol Biol Phys* 2007;67(2):356–361.
111. Henriquez FC, Castrillon SV. Confidence intervals in dose volume histogram computation. *Med Phys* 2010;37(4):1545–1553.
112. Stern RL, Heaton R, Fraser MW, et al. Verification of monitor unit calculations for non-IMRT clinical radiotherapy: Report of AAPM Task Group 114. *Med Phys* 2011;38(1):504–530.
113. Black RD, Scarantino CW, Mann GG, et al. An analysis of an implantable dosimeter system for external beam therapy. *Int J Radiat Oncol Biol Phys* 2005;63(1):290.
114. Kruse JJ. On the insensitivity of single field planar dosimetry to IMRT inaccuracies. *Med Phys* 2010;37(6):2516–2524.
115. Mans A, Wendling M, McDermott LN, et al. Catching errors with in vivo EPID dosimetry. *Med Phys* 2010;37(6):2638–2644.
116. RTOG. Image-Guided Radiation Therapy Committee. *Int. J. Radiat Oncol Biol. Phys.* 2001;51(3, Suppl 2):60.
117. Meyer JL, ed. *IMRT, IGRT, SBRT,* 2nd ed. Basel: Karger; 2011.

Chapter 10

Intensity-Modulated Radiation Treatment Techniques and Clinical Applications

K.S. Clifford Chao, Radhe Mohan, Timothy D. Marinetti, and Lei Dong

The previous edition of this chapter included literature reports through 2006. At that time intensity-modulated radiation therapy (IMRT) was still something of a novelty; 5 years later it is safe to say that the technique has become the *de facto* standard practice for many tumors. IMRT's coming of age is described in thorough terms in the 2010 International Commission on Radiation Units (ICRU) report (hereafter ICRU 83), which spans 106 pages with over 350 references.[1] Readers new to the field will find this report an excellent synthetic introduction to IMRT; experienced practitioners should also note that it contains new reporting guidelines for clinical treatments.

The use of ionizing radiation for diagnosis and treatment goes back over a century; for a wonderfully concise review see Bernier et al.[2] An enduring clinical problem has been to achieve high levels of irradiation at the tumor site without causing extremely toxic or even fatal consequences in normal tissues in the path of the treatment beam. Advances in technology—especially fast, affordable computers—opened the prospect of true three-dimensional (3D) tailoring of radiation fluence with equipment and a planning timescale usable in the clinic. Since its introduction into clinical use,[3–4,5] IMRT has generated widespread interest. IMRT optimally assigns nonuniform intensities (i.e., weights) to tiny subdivisions of beams, which have been called rays or "beamlets." The ability to optimally manipulate the intensities of individual rays within each beam permits greatly increased control over the radiation fluence, enabling custom design of optimum dose distributions. These improved dose distributions potentially may lead to improved tumor control and reduced normal tissue toxicity. For example, tumors of the head and neck often require concave-shaped treatment volumes to spare closely adjacent sensitive critical structures (e.g., brainstem, spinal cord). Such fluence distributions are easily done with IMRT but may be difficult or impossible by other techniques, including three-dimensional conformal radiation therapy (3DCRT). This is illustrated in Figure 10.1, which is taken from ICRU 83.

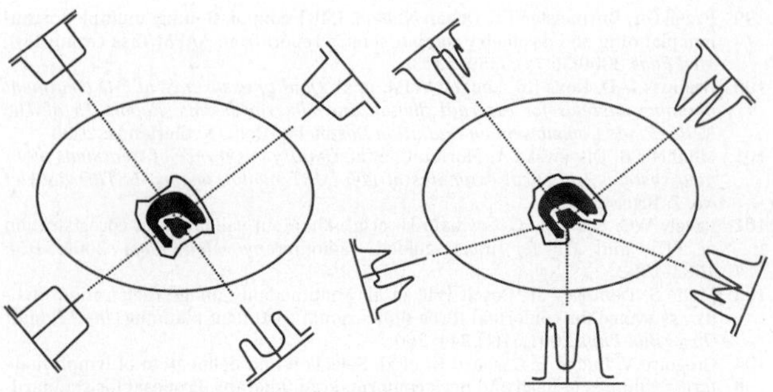

FIGURE 10.1. Comparison of conformal radiation therapy (CRT) (*left*) and intensity-modulated radiation therapy (IMRT) (*right*). The ability for CRT to alter isodose lines was limited to shaping of field boundaries with multileaf collimators (MLCs) or blocks, the use of wedges or compensators for missing tissues, and the use of central blocks for shielding critical structures. The IMRT beams can have highly nonuniform beam intensities (fluences) and are capable of producing a more concave-shaped absorbed-dose distribution. With neither conformal therapy nor IMRT can the planning organ at risk volume (PRV) always be completely avoided, but with IMRT the concave isodose curve that includes the planning target volume (PTV) better avoids the PRV. The black region indicates the PTV, the gray region indicates a PRV, and the line surrounding the PTV is a typical isodose contour. (Reprinted from ICRU Report 83: prescribing, recording, and reporting photon-beam intensity-modulated radiation therapy [IMRT]. *J ICRU* 2010;10[1]:1–106, with permission.)

IMRT requires setting the relative intensities of tens of thousands of rays which make up an intensity-modulated treatment plan. This task cannot be accomplished manually and requires the use of specialized computer-aided optimization methods. The optimum beamlet intensities are determined using a systematic iterative process during which the computer sequentially generates intensity-modulated plans one by one, evaluates each of them according to user-selected criteria ("desired objectives"), and makes incremental changes in the ray intensities based on the deviation from the desired objectives. The quality of an intensity-modulated treatment plan produced in this manner depends on a number of factors. These include the mathematical function and parameters used by the optimization process to evaluate and compare competing treatment plans; the mathematics and algorithms of optimization; the number, orientation, and energy of radiation beams; margins assigned to the planning target volume (PTV) and to normal structures; dose-calculation algorithms; and so on. We will discuss many of these in this chapter.

The 2010 ICRU 83 report has some important conceptual changes. The previous ICRU reports for photon therapy (No. 50 in 1993 and its supplement, No. 62, in 1999) defined a reference point within the treatment volume, one that was easily located with anatomic landmarks and where dosage could be accurately measured. The prescription dose was something of an ideal to be sought. However, with IMRT, treatment ***volumes*** are more relevant, and doses are given and bounds set within those volumes. Also, the prescription dose itself is now taken to be the final result of treatment planning by the physicists and radiation oncologists. With literally thousands of degrees of freedom available to the planner, the dosage to a single point is no longer adequate to describe or evaluate a plan.

ICRU 83 cites the increase in the clinical impact and use of IMRT in the recent past: "In a survey performed in 2003 in the USA, among 168 radiation oncologists randomly selected, one-third was using IMRT. In 2005, a similar survey showed that more than two-thirds of radiation oncologists were using some form of IMRT, mainly for increased normal-tissue sparing or target-dose escalation".[1,6,7] Another noteworthy metric is the number of research reports in the peer-reviewed literature concerning IMRT. A scan of the Web of Science database showed full papers with IMRT in the title as numbering <50 per year through 2001. It reached 100 in 2005 and has plateaued at about 140 for the years 2009–2011. One presumes the flattening of the publication rate has more to do with the fiscal woes plaguing the industrial countries since 2008 than a loss of interest in IMRT.

IMRT RATIONALE

The term *IMRT* is used to mean much more than its literal meaning might suggest. Strictly speaking, the use of wedges and conventional compensators for surface curvature is also intensity modulation. In this chapter, IMRT is a form of 3DCRT in which a *computer-aided optimization process is used to determine customized nonuniform fluence distributions to attain certain specified dosimetric and clinical objectives.*

Viewed in this light, IMRT is intimately tied to 3D imaging. As ICRU 83 states: "Three-dimensional CRT, in general, and IMRT, in particular, increase the need for accurate anatomic delineation. This requires an adequate specification of the tumor location and a thorough knowledge of the processes of likely infiltration and spread".[1]

IMRT has many potential advantages. It can be used to produce dose distributions that are far more conformal than those possible with standard 3DCRT. Dose distributions within the PTV, in theory, can be made more homogeneous, and, if so desired, a sharper fall-off of dose at the PTV boundary can be achieved. Experience with current IMRT systems has led to an impression among many that IMRT inherently produces inhomogeneous dose distribution within the target volume. Inhomogeneity commonly observed is the result of the overriding need to partially or wholly protect one or more critical organs. In other words, the dose distributions tend to be more heterogeneous because the homogeneity criterion is made less important than the normal structure avoidance criterion. If all things were equal, the IMRT plan always should produce more homogeneous dose distribution than a plan made with uniform beams. A sharper fall-off of dose at the PTV boundary, in turn, means that the volume of normal tissues exposed to high doses may be reduced significantly. These factors may allow escalation of tumor dose, reduction of normal tissue dose, or both, hopefully leading to an improved outcome, including lower morbidity. A lower rate of complications also may mean lower cost of patient care following the treatment. In addition, IMRT has the potential to be more efficient with regard to treatment planning and delivery than standard 3DCRT, although gains in this direction are being realized rather slowly. The treatment design process is relatively insensitive to the choice of planning parameters, such as beam direction.[8–10] There are no secondary field-shaping devices other than the computer-controlled multileaf collimator (MLC). Furthermore, large fields and boosts can be integrated into a single treatment plan, and, in many cases, electrons can be dispensed with, permitting the use of the same integrated boost plan for the entire course of treatment.[11,12] An integrated boost treatment may offer an additional radiobiologic advantage[13] in terms of lower dose per fraction to normal tissues while delivering higher dose per fraction to the target volume. Higher dose per fraction also reduces the number of fractions and hence lowers the cost and burden to the patient for a treatment course. IMRT also offers the potential of adaptive therapy—revision of the treatment plan according to imaging of tumor reduction and organ movement during the course of radiation therapy. Mechalakos et al. present a case study where weekly cone beam computed tomography (CBCT) was used to track treatment of a recurrent neck mass from a nasopharyngeal cancer.[14]

IMRT Limitations and Risks

We should recognize, however, that IMRT has limitations. There are many dose distributions (or dose–volume combinations) that are simply not physically achievable. Furthermore, our knowledge about what is clinically optimal and achievable and how best to define clinical and dosimetric objectives of IMRT is often limited. Moreover, the best solution may elude us because of the limitations of the mathematical formalism used or because of the practical limits of computer speed and the time required for finding it.

Uncertainties of various types (e.g., those related to daily, or interfraction, positioning; displacement and distortions of internal anatomy; intrafraction motion; and changes in physical and radiobiologic characteristics of tumors and normal tissues during the course of treatment) may limit the applicability and efficacy of IMRT. Dosimetry characteristics of a delivery device, such as radiation scattering and transmission through the MLC leaves, introduce some limitations in the accuracy and deliverability of IMRT fluence distributions. In addition, the limited spatial and temporal coverage and overall accuracy of current IMRT dosimetric verification systems, based principally on radiographic and radiochromic film, diminish the confidence in the delivered dose. Furthermore, most current dose-calculation models are limited in their accuracy, especially for the small, complex shapes required for IMRT. It is quite conceivable that inaccuracies in dose calculations may yield a solution different from the one derived if dose calculations were accurate. However, the most important factor that may limit the immediate success of IMRT is the inadequacy of imaging technology to define the true extent of the tumor, its extensions, and radiobiologic characteristics as well as geometric, dose-response, and functional characteristics of normal tissues.

We also should be aware of the risks of IMRT. The effect of large fraction sizes used in integral boost IMRT on tissues embedded within the gross tumor volume is uncertain and may present an increased risk of injury.[15] There also may be an increased risk that improper use of spatial margins, coupled with the high degree of conformality with IMRT, may lead to geographic misses of the disease and recurrences, especially for disease sites where positioning and motion uncertainties play a large role or where there are significant changes in anatomy and radiobiology during the course of radiotherapy. Similarly, high doses in close proximity to normal critical structures may pose a greater risk of normal tissue injury. In addition, IMRT dose distributions are unusual and highly complex, and existing experience is too limited to interpret them properly and evaluate their efficacy. Finally, while IMRT can spare specific tissues compared to conventional radiation therapy, the use of many more beams and irradiation angles means that a larger volume of normal tissue is being exposed, albeit at lower accumulated doses. This may lead to unforeseen sequelae.

IMRT—An Unconventional Paradigm

The application, process, and dose distributions of IMRT are significantly different from those of conventional two-dimensional (2D) CRT or 3DCRT. This means the traditional methods of specification and fractionation of treatments, evaluation of treatment plans, and reporting of results are limited and new methods need to be introduced.

The traditional 3DCRT process involves "forward planning," in which beam parameters (directions, apertures and their margins, beam weights, beam modifiers) are specified and dose distributions are computed. The treatment plan is evaluated by a human being, and, if necessary, beam parameters are modified to achieve a satisfactory dose distribution. In IMRT, an inverse process ("inverse planning") is used in which the desired dosimetric and clinical objectives are stated mathematically (in the form of an "objective function").[9,16–18] The term *inverse planning* should not be confused with the mathematical operation of matrix inversion. In the present context the word *inverse* is used to distinguish it from forward planning for conventional 3DCRT. As ICRU 83 concisely notes:

> The word "inverse" is used in reference to the established body of mathematical inverse problem-solving techniques, which start at the final or desired result and work backwards to establish the best way to achieve it. So-called inverse treatment planning starts by describing a goal, *i.e.*, a series of descriptors characterizing the desired absorbed-dose distribution within the tumor, with additional descriptors designed to spare normal tissues.

The inverse-planning process works iteratively to determine beam shapes and fluence patterns to achieve an optimal or acceptable absorbed-dose distribution. The IMRT optimization software iteratively adjusts beam parameters with the aim of obtaining the best possible approximation of the desired dose distribution. In each optimization iteration, the optimization software computes the value of the objective function (i.e., the IMRT plan score) to judge the overall quality of each of a large number of plans to choose the optimum one. However, it must be kept in mind that limitations of planning time may preclude full exploration of all the degrees of freedom (there can be many thousands), so whether the optimization is done by a variant of gradient or stochastic methods, the computed solution may not be the true global one. Final review by the radiation oncologist of any plan, of course, is required.

IMRT is most conformal and most efficient when all target volumes (gross disease, subclinical extensions, and electively treated nodes) are treated simultaneously using different fraction sizes. Such a treatment strategy has been called the simultaneous integrated boost.[15,19] This is in contrast to conventional radiotherapy in which the same fraction size (typically 1.8 or 2 Gy) is used for all target volumes with successive reductions in field sizes to protect critical normal structures and to limit the dose to electively treated and subclinical disease regions.

Alternative IMRT Approaches

During the past 15 years, a variety of techniques have been explored for designing and delivering optimized IMRT.[4,5,8,15,20–49] Many of these are implemented in commercial IMRT systems. The most significant differences among the various approaches are in terms of the mechanisms they use for the delivery of nonuniform fluences. Although the merits of each often are speculated, the superiority of any of the approaches is difficult to assess because there have been no systematic comparisons of clinical treatment plans.

Of the various approaches proposed, two dominant but significantly different methods have emerged. Mackie et al.[34] proposed an approach called *tomotherapy* in which intensity-modulated photon therapy is delivered using a rotating slit beam. A temporally modulated slit MLC is used to rapidly move leaves in or out of the slit. Like a CT unit, the radiation source and the collimator continuously revolve around the patient. The patient is translated either stepwise between successive rotations (serial tomotherapy) or continuously during rotation (helical tomotherapy). For helical tomotherapy, the system looks like a conventional CT scanner and includes a megavoltage portal detector to provide for the tomographic reconstruction of the delivered dose distribution.

A commercial slit collimator (called *MIMiC*) of the type proposed by Mackie et al.[34] has been designed and built by the NOMOS Corporation (North American Scientific, Chatsworth, CA). It has been incorporated into the company's serial tomotherapy system, known as Peacock, for planning and rotational delivery of intensity-modulated treatments.[26,27] Figure 10.2 shows an original "binary" collimator built by NOMOS and as mounted on a linac. The figure also shows a modern tomotherapy machine.

In the second approach, implemented first into clinical use at Memorial Sloan-Kettering Cancer Center,[4,5,35,37,44,45,50] a standard MLC is used to deliver the optimized fluence distribution in either dynamic mode (defined as the leaves moving while the radiation is on) or static mode (i.e., "step-and-shoot" mode, defined as sequential delivery of radiation subportals that combine to deliver the desired fluence distribution), to deliver a set of intensity-modulated fields incident from fixed-gantry angles (see Fig. 10.3). These techniques are gaining wide acceptance rapidly. Every major commercial treatment-planning system manufacturer has implemented one or both of these.

A third approach, called *intensity-modulated arc therapy* or IMAT, developed by Yu,[49] uses a combination of dynamic multileaf

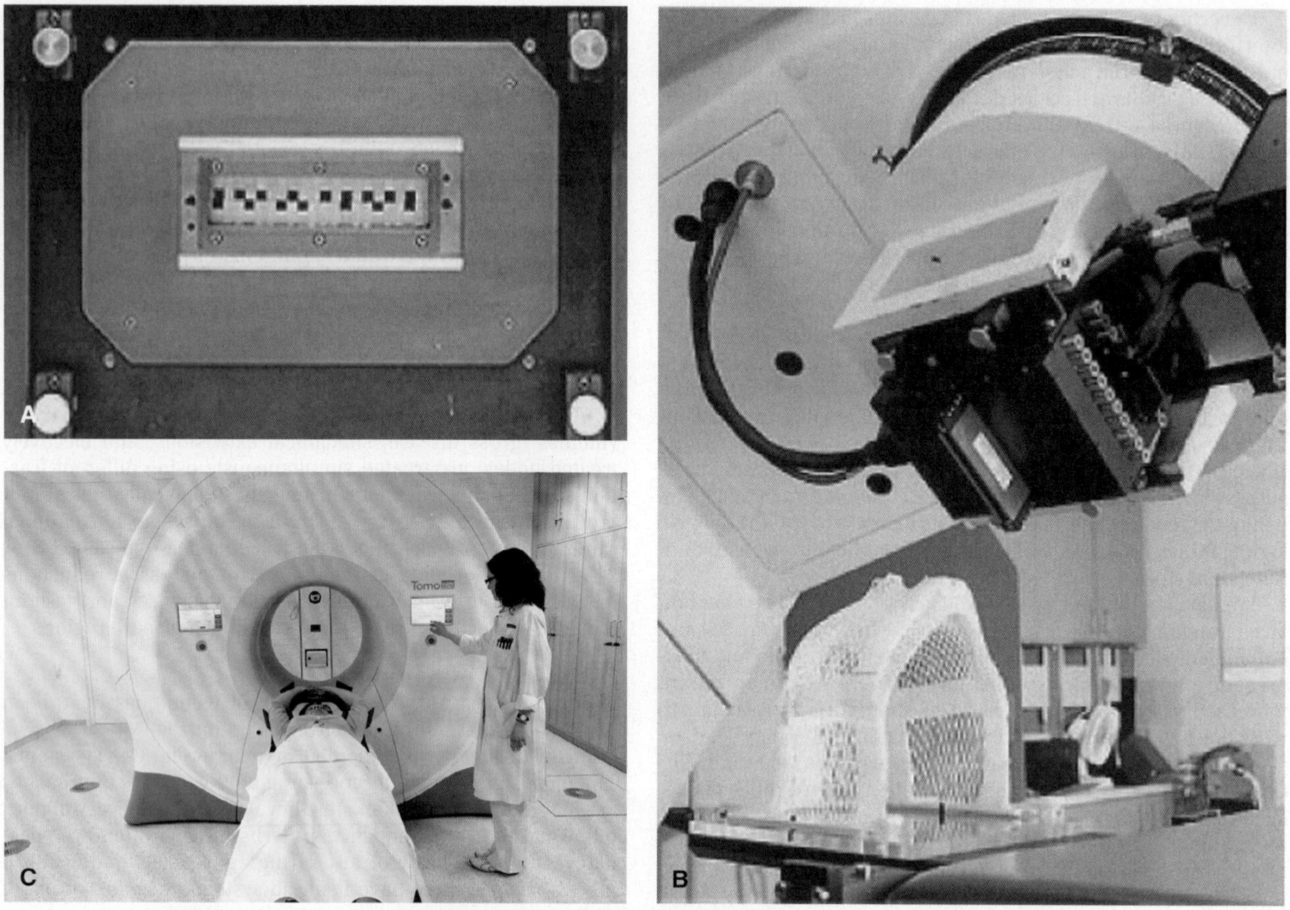

FIGURE 10.2. Commercial serial tomotherapy delivery hardware mounted on a conventional linear accelerator. **A:** View looking into the collimator toward the radiation source. A leaf pattern is shown that highlights the system's capability for delivering complex fluence patterns. **B:** The multileaf collimator mounted to a conventional linear accelerator. **C:** Modern tomotherapy TomoHD® machine. (C used with permission by Accuray, Incorporated, Madison, WI.)

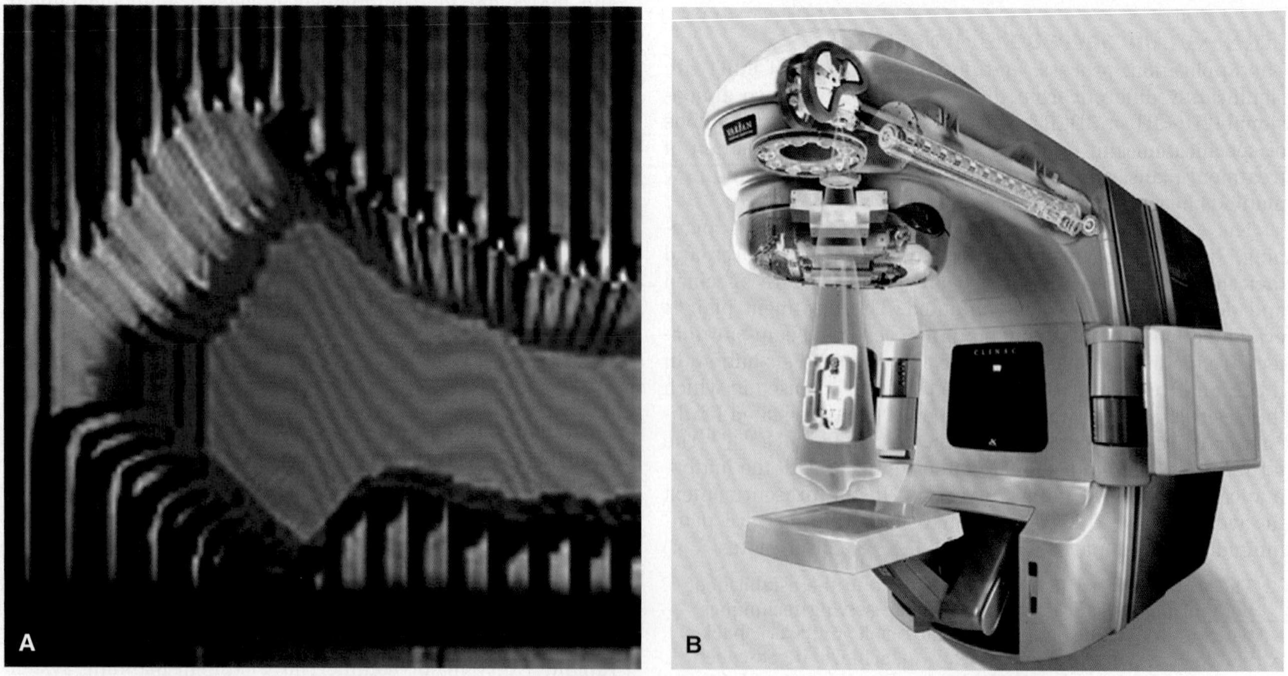

FIGURE 10.3. **A:** A typical multileaf collimator used for delivery of intensity-modulated radiation therapy looking toward the radiation source. In the dynamic mode, the leaves move back and forth or sweep across the field continuously to form the sequence of required field shapes while the beam is on. In the static or step-and-shoot mode, the beam is turned off when the leaves move to form the required field shapes. **B:** Cutaway diagram of linac head, Varian Clinac®. (Courtesy of Varian Medical Systems, Palo Alto, CA.)

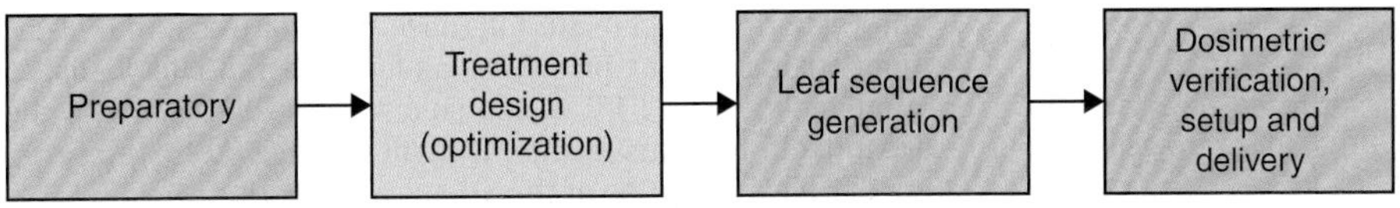

FIGURE 10.4. Overview of a typical intensity-modulated radiation therapy planning and delivery process.

collimation and arc therapy. The shape of the field formed by the MLC changes continuously during gantry rotation. Multiple superimposing arcs are used, and the field shape for a specific gantry angle changes from one arc to the next appropriately so that the cumulative fluence distribution of all arcs is equal to the desired distribution. Arc therapy is discussed in a recent review of various intensity-modulated techniques.[51]

In addition to these approaches, the University of Michigan has used the so-called multisegment approach in which each of a number of beams is divided into multiple segments.[52] One segment for each beam frames the entire target while the others spare one or more normal structures. Each segment is uniform in intensity. The weights of segments of all beams are optimized to produce the desired treatment plan. The treatments are delivered as a sequence of multiple uniform field segments. A similar approach previously was proposed by Mohan et al.[53] In almost all of these significantly different treatment-delivery approaches, the underlying principles of optimization are similar, although the specifics may be quite different.

THE IMRT PROCESS OVERVIEW

As mentioned previously, there are significant differences in 3DCRT and IMRT concepts and processes. However, there are also many similarities. In particular, IMRT relies on many of the same imaging, dose calculations, plan evaluation, quality assurance (QA), and delivery tools as 3DCRT.

The IMRT planning, QA, and delivery phases of the dynamic or static MLC process are summarized in Figure 10.4. Figure 10.5 shows the steps in each phase of the IMRT optimization process. The tomotherapy process is similar, except that the

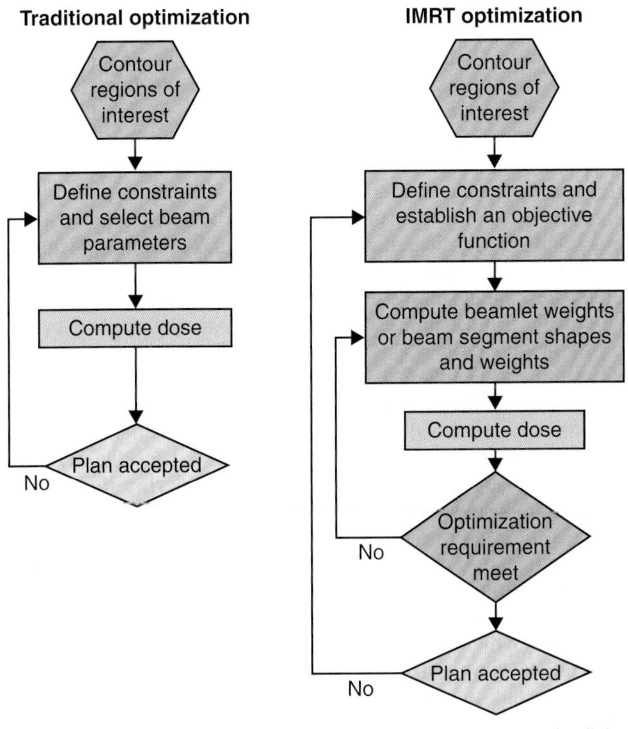

FIGURE 10.5. Comparison between traditional (*left*) and intensity-modulated radiation therapy (IMRT) (*right*) optimization processes. (Reprinted from ICRU Report 83: prescribing, recording, and reporting photon-beam intensity-modulated radiation therapy [IMRT]. *J ICRU* 2010;10[1]:1–106, with permission.)

fixed-beam angle selection is replaced by selection of the slice thickness and, for serial tomotherapy, the gantry rotation angles.

In the preparatory phase of the IMRT process, volumes of interest (such as tumors and normal organs) are delineated on 3D CT images,[54] often with assistance from other coregistered imaging modalities. The second imaging technique most often used is magnetic resonance imaging (MRI); the latter has an advantage over CT in that it can provide both structural and physiologic information.[55] Other imaging modalities such as positron emission tomography (PET) use intrinsic or externally added molecular markers to visualize specific metabolic processes or cellular phenotypes.[56–60] Also, the desired objectives in the form of an objective function, its parameter values, and the IMRT fractionation strategy are specified, and beam configuration is defined. Typically the objective function[61] assigns a weighted "cost" to the square of the difference between the desired 3D fluence distribution and that calculated at a given iteration. The software attempts to minimize the costs—maximizing dosage to the tumor volume and minimizing exposure of normal tissues.

In the treatment-plan optimization phase, an iterative process is used to adjust and set the intensities of rays of each beam (or portion of the arc) so that the resulting intensity distributions yield the best approximation of the desired objectives. The IMRT plan then is evaluated to ensure that the tradeoffs made by the optimization system are acceptable. If further improvement is deemed necessary and possible, the objective function parameters are modified and the optimization process is repeated until a satisfactory treatment plan is achieved.

In the leaf sequence-generation phase, the intensity distributions are converted into sequences of leaf positions. It is conceivable that certain dose distributions cannot be delivered as a result of the leakage characteristics of the delivery devices. Therefore, in most treatment-planning systems, the leaf sequences are used in a reverse process to calculate the dose distributions they are expected to deliver. These dose distributions, called the *deliverable dose distributions,* are evaluated for clinical adequacy. If necessary, objective function parameters are further adjusted to produce an intensity distribution that leads to a deliverable dose distribution that meets the desired objectives. This is the practice in most systems. However, in some systems, the leaf sequence-generation process is incorporated into the IMRT plan optimization loop so that the optimized and deliverable dose distributions are identical. More details on this are given later in this chapter.

The leaf sequences then are transmitted to the treatment machine and used to verify that the dose distribution that will be delivered to the patient is correct and accurate. The patient then is set up in the usual fashion and treated. In general, the entire treatment is delivered remotely without the need to reenter the treatment room in between fields.

PREPARATORY AND IMRT PLANNING PHASES

This section discusses each of the steps of the preparatory and IMRT plan design phases. For reasons of clarity, the order in which these steps are discussed is not the same as the order in which they occur as shown in Figure 10.5. Figure 10.6 sketches the quality assurance process.

Imaging and Volumes of Interest

ICRU 83 presents updated definitions for the assorted volumes that will form the skeleton of the treatment plan.[1] Conceptually,

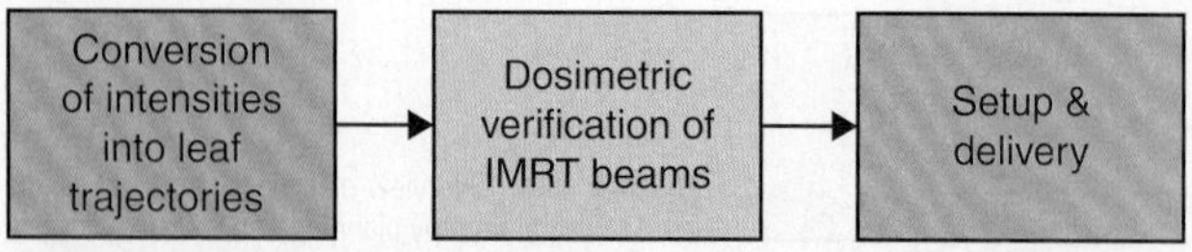

FIGURE 10.6. Intensity-modulated radiation therapy (IMRT) process: Quality Assurance (QA) and delivery phase.

the volumes contain three types of tissue: (a) malignant lesion, (b) otherwise normal tissue near the tumor that is already or likely to be infiltrated by microscopic disease, and (c) more distant normal tissue and organs. The quoted definitions that follow are from ICRU 83.

- *Gross tumor volume (GTV):* "The GTV is the gross demonstrable extent and location of the tumor. The GTV may consist of a primary tumor (primary tumor GTV or GTV-T), metastatic regional node(s) (nodal GTV or GTV-N), or distant metastasis (metastatic GTV, or GTV-M)".[1] They note that in some cases it may not be possible to differentiate expanding primary lesions from nearby metastatic disease. The GTV for IMRT is always defined from anatomic images, usually CT with or without MRI, and increasingly supplemented by PET.
- *Clinical target volume (CTV):* "The CTV is a volume of tissue that contains a demonstrable GTV and/or subclinical malignant disease with a certain probability of occurrence considered relevant for therapy. There is no general consensus on what probability is considered relevant for therapy, but typically a probability of occult disease higher than from 5% to 10% is assumed to require treatment".[1] The volumes outside the GTV encompassed by the CTV will depend a great deal on the particular tumor (e.g., with high or low propensity for lymph node extension). In the past, the CTV was effectively the GTV (including affected nodes) plus a 1- to 2-cm margin. The current definition stresses more the physiologic criteria based on the specifics of disease spread for each tumor. Gregroire et al. have compiled studies on CTV margins into a book.[62] In postoperative situations, following an R0 or R1 resection, there is no gross tumor so only the CTV need be defined. Readers are strongly encouraged to consult ICRU 83 for details.
- *Planning target volume (PTV):* "The PTV is a geometrical concept introduced for treatment planning and evaluation. It is the recommended tool to shape absorbed-dose distributions to ensure that the prescribed absorbed dose will actually be delivered to all parts of the CTV with a clinically acceptable probability, despite geometrical uncertainties such as organ motion and setup variations".[1]
- *Organ at risk (OAR):* "The OAR or critical normal structures are tissues that if irradiated could suffer significant morbidity and thus might influence the treatment planning and/or the absorbed-dose prescription. In principle, all non-target tissues could be OARs. However, normal tissues considered as OARs typically depend on the location of the CTV and/or the prescribed absorbed dose".[1] All normal tissue exposed to radiation during treatment is at risk, but the OAR is generally taken to be rather more specific—structures in the immediate vicinity of the PTV, sparing of which may demand specific recontouring of the CTV or PTV. Historically, OARs have been loosely grouped into "serial" or "parallel" organs or a combination of the two, following the work of Withers et al. using the concept of functional subunits in each organ.[64,65] Serial organs, such as the spinal cord, can suffer unacceptable damage if only a small portion is irradiated, whereas parallel organs, such as the liver, can suffer loss of a portion without total loss of function.
- *Planning organ at risk volume (PRV):* "As is the case with the PTV, uncertainties and variations in the position of the OAR during treatment must be considered to avoid serious complications. For this reason, margins have to be added to the OARs to compensate for these uncertainties and variations, using similar principles as for the PTV. This leads, in analogy with the PTV, to the concept of PRV".[1] As with the OAR itself, margins in the PRV will be affected by the serial or parallel attributes of the adjacent tissues.
- *Remaining volume at risk (RVR):* "The RVR is operationally defined by the difference between the volume enclosed by the external contour of the patient and that of the CTVs and OARs on the slices that have been imaged".[1] Definition of an RVR and its inclusion in the treatment plan (at least in the form of dose constraints) is essential in IMRT. Without such limits, the optimization software could craft excellent dose distributions for the CTV and OAR but cause toxic irradiation levels in otherwise uncontoured tissues.
- *Treated volume (TV):* "The TV is the volume of tissue enclosed within a specific isodose envelope, with the absorbed dose specified by the radiation oncology team as appropriate to achieve tumor eradication or palliation, within the bounds of acceptable complications".[1] The TV is what is physically deliverable given limitations of beam collimation and homogeneity and, more importantly, the risks of treatment-associated morbidity acceptable to the oncologist and the patient. ICRU 83 proposes that, in conformity with its proposal for proton therapy, the TV be defined as the dosage received by 98% of the PTV. This serves as a measure of the minimum absorbed dose, and is also referred to as $D_{near\ minimum}$. In an analogous manner, a $D_{near\ maximum}$ is defined as $D_{2\%}$, the dose received by 2% of the PTV receiving the highest fluence. Readers are referred to Section 3 of ICRU 83.

It should be noted that the GTV, CTV, and OAR represent volumes based on anatomic and physiologic judgments on the location of malignant growths or normal tissues in danger from metastatic spread and/or treatment-induced toxicity. These are independent of the particular irradiation protocol employed (i.e., 3DCRT, IMRT, or particle beams). The PTV, PRV, and TV are intimately tied to the specific radiation therapy used.

Beam Configurations

Systems Using Fixed Intensity-Modulated Fields

The beam configuration can have a significant impact on the quality of an optimized IMRT plan. It may be argued that, because of the greater control over dose distributions afforded by optimized intensity modulation, the fine-tuning of beam angles may not be as important for IMRT as it is for standard radiotherapy. However, optimization of beam angles may find paths least obstructed by critical normal tissues, thus facilitating the achievement of desired distribution with a minimum of compromise.

Beam-angle optimization, however, is not a trivial problem. There have been some attempts to solve this problem,[66–67,68] and advances in mathematical operations research applied to the problem have been reviewed recently.[69] To appreciate the magnitude of the problem, consider the following example. If the angle range is divided into 5-degree steps, nearly 60,000 combinations would need to be tested for three beams, nearly 14 million combinations for five beams, nearly 1.5 billion combinations for seven beams, and so on. Considering the magnitude of the search space, none of the optimization methods is likely to be able to demonstrate a significant improvement in treatment plans, let alone find a truly optimum combination when the number of beams is five or more. Furthermore, the beam-angle optimization problem is known to have multiple minima,[70] which means that fast gradient-based optimization techniques may fail. Stochastic methods,[71,72] in principle, should avoid the local minimum problem but may present excessive computing time demands. These should prove less of a problem in the near future, especially with the use of dedicated parallel processors, which can drastically reduce computation time. For a review see Pratx and Xing.[73]

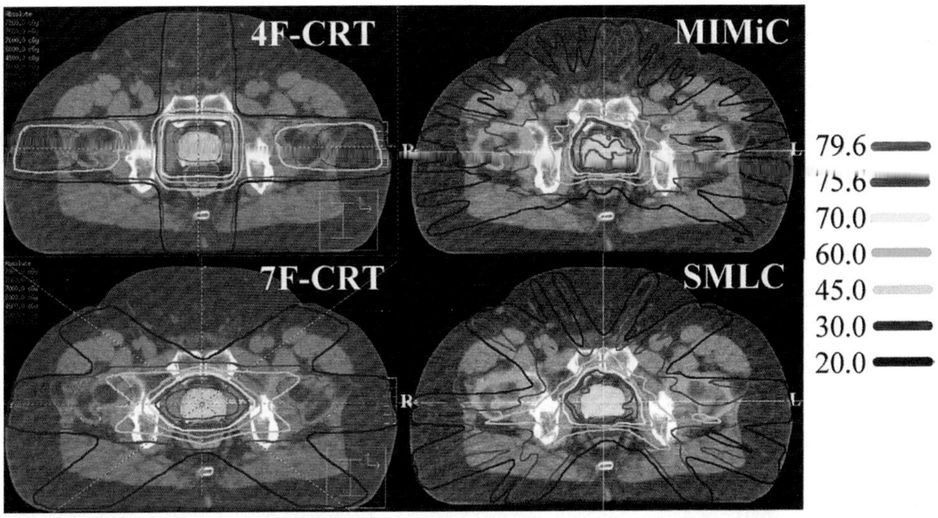

FIGURE 10.7. Typical isodose distributions for treating prostate cancer from (*1*) a four-field three-dimensional conformal radiation therapy (3DCRT) plan; (*2*) a seven-field 3DCRT plan; (*3*) an intensity-modulated radiation therapy (IMRT) plan delivered by serial tomotherapy using MIMiC (NOMOS Corp, Sewicky, PA); and (*4*) a 10-field step-and-shoot segmental multileaf collimator (SMLC) plan. (Reprinted from Chao et al. *Practical essentials of IMRT,* 2nd edition. Philadelphia: Lippincott Williams & Wilkins, 2005, with permission.)

Another question that may be asked is how many beams are optimal. In principle, a larger number of beams would provide a larger number of parameters to adjust and therefore a greater opportunity to achieve desired dose distributions. (Thus, in theory, a rotational beam would be the ultimate.) However, for fixed-beam IMRT, it may be desirable to minimize the number of beams to reduce the time and effort required for planning, QA, dosimetric verification, and delivery of treatments. Fewer intensity-modulated beams would be needed if beam angles were optimized than if the beams were placed at equiangular steps. Calculations by Webb[9] indicate that seven or nine fields give adequate conformal dose distributions for both serial tomography and fixed-gantry IMRT.

Figure 10.7 compares prostate treatment plans employing different numbers of fields using 3DCRT, serial tomography, and step-and-shoot IMRT. Consistent with published experience, the plan quality improves but the incremental improvement diminishes with increasing number of beams. Optimum nonuniform placement of beams can further improve dose distribution. Figure 10.8A, B shows a head and neck IMRT case for two different beam angles. The patient, treated with the beam configuration shown in Figure 10.8A, developed significant mucositis at the early phase of treatment. This was consistent with the "horn" in dose distribution shown by the arrow. Revising the beam-angle arrangement as shown in Figure 10.8C led to improved dose distribution, shown in Figure 10.8D.

In general, it is most advantageous to place beams so that they are maximally avoiding each other and the opposing beams with the stipulation that directions that overlap significant obstructions, such as heavily attenuating bars in the treatment couch, be avoided. For simplicity, beams often are constrained to lie in the same transverse plane. However, noncoplanar beams will provide an additional degree of freedom and potentially an additional gain in the quality of treatments. It should be noted that the beam configurations used for 3DCRT may not be optimal for IMRT.[74]

Although reducing the number of beams is a desirable goal for IMRT delivered with several fixed-gantry angles and dynamic MLC, it should not be the overriding consideration. IMRT can be planned and delivered automatically in times not significantly different from the times for much simpler conventional treatments. Therefore, the delivery times for six to 20 beams may be quite acceptable. Keep in mind, however, that some of the current linear accelerators are limited in their ability to accurately deliver a large number of intensity-modulated beams each with a very small number of monitor units.[75]

Systems Using Rotating Slit (Tomotherapy) Approach

Tomotherapy delivery has substantial differences from fixed-portal IMRT. Mackie has published a historical review of tomotherapy, intertwined as it is with his career.[76] The linear accelerator rotates during delivery, and the beam is modulated during rotation. Typically, the modulation is subdivided into small gantry angle ranges (e.g., 5 degrees) and the beam is independently modulated at each gantry angle. Each leaf is used to deliver a single rotating pencil. The pencil-beam modulation is conducted for each leaf by opening that leaf for a fraction of the gantry range consistent with the fractional fluence to be delivered from that gantry angle. For example, for a 5-degree-angle-range bin, if a leaf is to deliver 50% fluence, the leaf will be open for 2.5 degrees over the 5-degree range. Because of geometric constraints of modulating the radiation fan beams, only one or two thin planes can be treated with each rotation. The Peacock system,[26] for instance, uses two banks of opposing leaves projecting to 1.7 or 3.4 cm, depending on user-selected mechanical stops. This delivers modulated beams to two abutting, independently modulated planes. The helical tomotherapy unit uses a single leaf bank with a backup collimator that allows the radiation field width to be continuously adjusted. Narrower leaf widths provide higher spatial resolution for modulation but require more treatment arcs and consequently more delivery time. The current TomoHD MLC uses tungsten leaves 10 cm thick (in beam direction) and with a width of 0.625 cm. Leaves are driven pneumatically and switch in 20 msec.

Aperture Margins

IMRT has the inherent capacity to reduce margins attributable to the beam penumbra. When a photon beam traverses the body, it is scattered, depositing dose not only along the path of each ray of the beam but also at points away from it. The electrons knocked out by the incident photons travel laterally to points in the neighborhood of each ray, depositing dose along the way. Near the middle of a uniform beam, outgoing electrons are offset by incoming electrons and equilibrium exists. However, at and just inside the boundaries of the beam, there are no incoming electrons to balance electrons flowing out of the beam. Therefore, a "lateral electronic disequilibrium" exists that leads to a dose deficit inside the boundaries of beams. For lower-energy beams and at large depths, scattered photons significantly contribute to this effect also. The conventional approach to overcome this deficiency is to add a margin for the "beam penumbra" to the PTV so that the tumor dose is maintained at the required level.

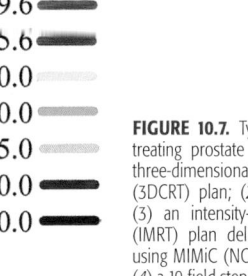

For IMRT plans, there is another method to counterbalance the dose deficit. The intensity of rays just inside the beam

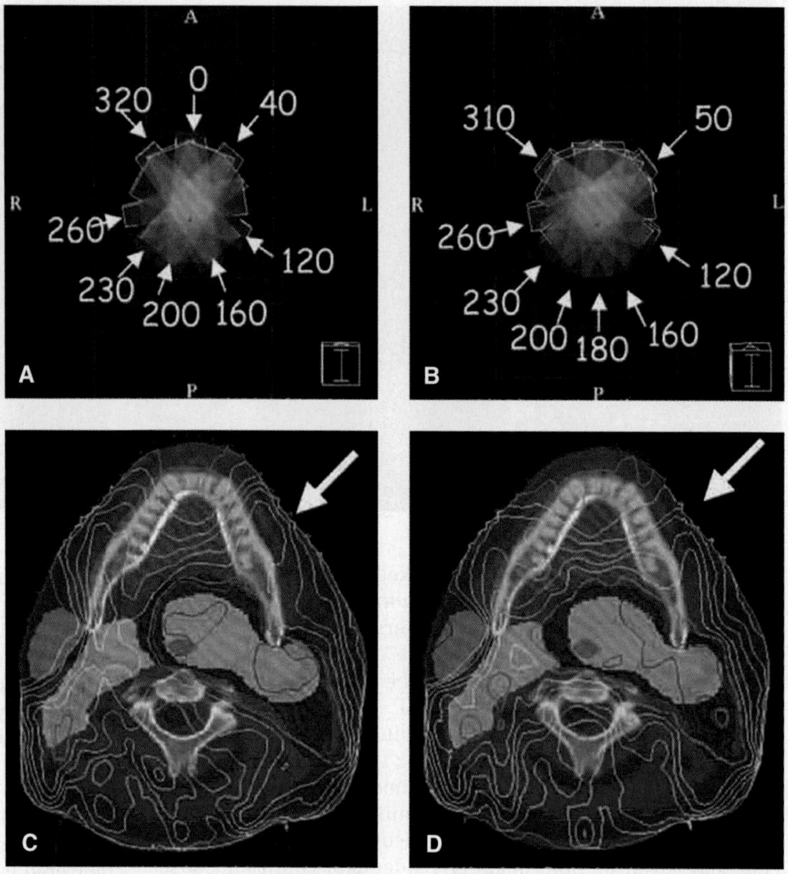

FIGURE 10.8. A patient with carcinoma of the base of the tongue was treated with intensity-modulated radiation therapy. **A** and **B** depict the beam angle arrangement and the resulting isodose distribution. Arrow on **(C)** indicated a "horn" of high dose to the left oral tongue and buccal mucosa. Rearrangement of anterior beam placement as shown in **(B)** led to improvement of dose distribution to the normal mucosa of the left anterior oral cavity **(D)**.

boundary may be increased. Because some of the increased energy must also flow out, a very large increase would be required if the margin for the penumbra were set to zero or to a very small value. Therefore, an increase in boundary fluence alone is not enough. A combination of an increased fluence and the addition of a margin, albeit a much smaller one, is a better solution. This reduction in margin can be exploited quite usefully to reduce the volume of normal tissues exposed to high doses of radiation with a corresponding reduction in toxicity and a further potential for dose escalation.

The beam–boundary-sharpening and margin-reduction feature of IMRT can be taken advantage of only if the dose-computation method is able to adequately take into account the lateral transport of radiation[77] and if the intensity matrix grid size is sufficiently small. Initially, dose distribution for a given configuration of beams is computed by taking lateral transport into consideration. In each optimization iteration, the intensity distribution first is designed ignoring lateral transport. At the end of the iteration, the dose distribution is recalculated, thereby incorporating the effects of field-shaping devices on lateral transport and revealing the resulting deviations from the anticipated dose distribution. In the next iteration, ray intensities are adjusted further to rectify the deviations, and so on.[50,78] Carrasco et al. compared several dose-computation algorithms in lung phantoms.[77]

A schematic example shown in Figure 10.9 illustrates the issues involved. Figure 10.9A shows a normal organ overlapping the target volume. The target volume is being irradiated by two parallel-opposed beams. It is desired that the dose to the region of overlap be 60% of the target dose. If more dose is delivered, damage to the normal organ may result; but lower than the desired dose may cause local failure. If the role of lateral transport in optimization is ignored, the intensity resulting from the optimization process is essentially a step function, as shown in Figure 10.9B (solid curve). The corresponding dose distribution (the dotted curve) shows a dose deficit inside the high-dose target volume as well as the outside edge of the region of overlap and an excess of dose in the region of overlap adjacent to the high-dose volume. If lateral transport is incorporated by adjusting fluence, the fluence and dose patterns shown in Figure 10.9C result. Fluence is increased at both boundaries. It also is increased in the high-dose side of the interface with the overlap region and decreased on the lower-dose side. The dose is now much closer to the desired dose. Comparing Figures 10.9B and 10.9C, it also appears that a modest increase in fluence just inside the boundary does not lead to a perceptible increase in dose outside the beam boundary. This is presumably the result of the fact that the excess dose flowing out of the target periphery is deposited in a much larger volume of tissue. A reduction of margins attributable to penumbra by as much as 8 mm has been found to be feasible for prostate treatments.[50,78]

IMRT Fractionation

In principle, conventional fractionation strategies can be used to design IMRT plans as well. For example, in a strategy similar to the conventional 1.8-Gy to 2-Gy/fx schedule, a major portion of the dose could be delivered in the initial phase using uniform fields designed with standard 3D conformal methods followed by an IMRT boost. Alternatively, separate IMRT plans could be designed for both the initial large-field treatment and the boost treatment. It may be intuitively obvious that, if a large portion of the dose already has been delivered using large fields, it may be very difficult, if not impossible, to achieve a high level of dose conformation with the remaining fractions in the IMRT-boost phase.[15] As indicated earlier in this chapter, IMRT may be most conformal if all target volumes (gross disease, subclinical extensions, and electively treated nodes) are treated simultaneously using different fraction sizes.[15] Such a treatment strategy has been called the

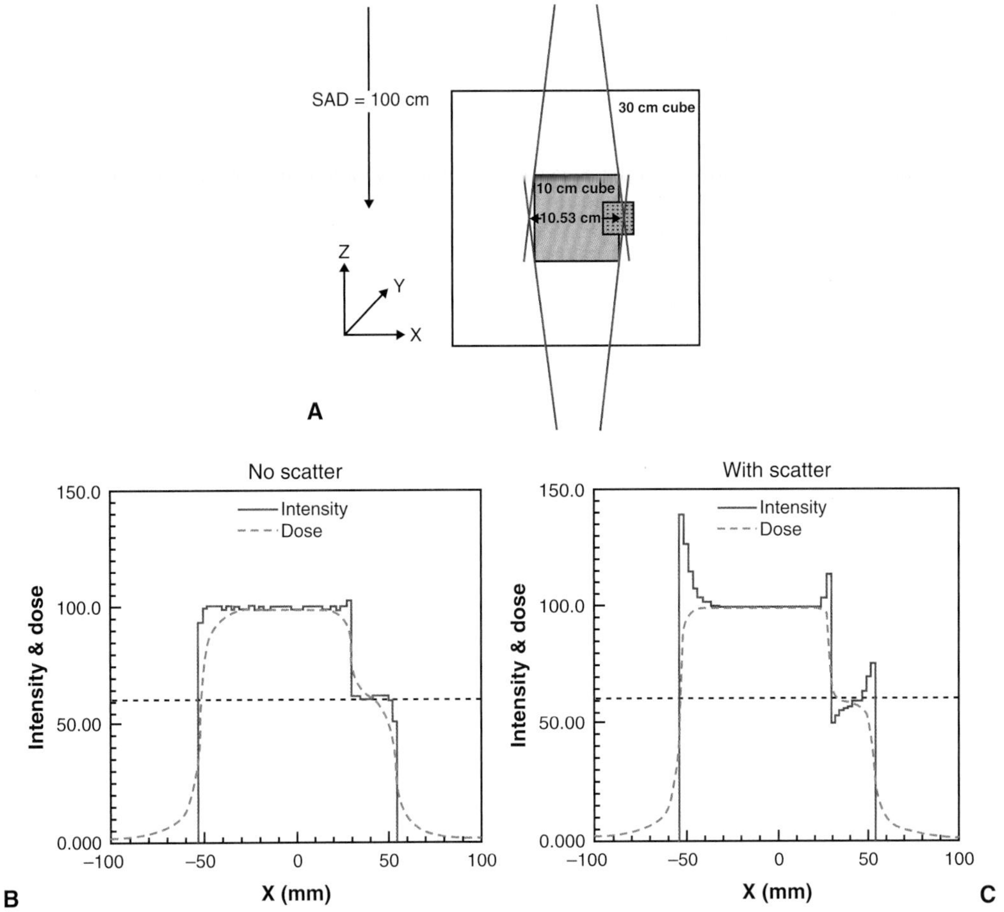

FIGURE 10.9. A schematic example illustrating the sharpening of penumbra with intensity-modulated radiation therapy.

simultaneous integrated boost (SIB).[11,12,15,19] Mackie et al. had also indicated the possibilities for irradiation boost in their first paper on serial tomography.[79] The SIB IMRT strategy not only produces superior dose distributions but also is an easier, more efficient, and perhaps less error-prone way of planning and delivering IMRT because it involves the use of the same plan for the entire course of treatment. Furthermore, in many cases, there is no need for electron fields, and the nodal volumes can be included in the IMRT fields; thus, the perennial problem of field matching[80] encountered in the treatment of many sites is thereby avoided.

Because each of the target regions receives different doses per fraction in the SIB IMRT strategy, prescribed nominal (physical) dose and dose per fraction must be adjusted appropriately. The adjusted nominal dose and fraction size for each target region depend on the number of IMRT fractions. The fraction sizes may be estimated using an isoeffect relationship based on the linear-quadratic model and the values of its parameters (such as α/β ratios, tumor doubling time).

The effect of the modified fractionation on acute and late toxicity of normal tissues both outside and within the volumes to be treated also should be considered. Because of the improved conformality of IMRT plans, dose to normal tissues outside the target volume is typically lower than for conventional treatment plans. In addition, if the number of fractions is greater than the number of fractions used to deliver large fields in conventional therapy, the dose per fraction to normal tissues is lower. Therefore, the biologically effective dose would be lower still. However, normal tissues embedded within or adjacent to the target volumes would receive high doses per fraction and may be at higher risk. Isoeffect formulae for normal tissues also may be derived to estimate the effect of a particular fractionation strategy (see ICRU 83, pp. 36–38). These formalisms would need to incorporate regeneration and change in sensitivity over the treatment course.

The values of parameters for the computation of altered fractionation may, in theory, be obtained from published studies. Studies by Maciejewski et al.[81] and Withers et al.[82–84] for example, have yielded important information for estimating tumor parameters for head and neck carcinoma. In general, the data available are limited. Furthermore, there is considerable uncertainty in the data, and there are concerns about the validity of numerous assumptions in the linear-quadratic model and the isoeffect formalism, especially with regard to normal tissues. (For an early review of the linear-quadratic model see Fowler[85]). Much of the accumulated data on normal tissue complications comes from clinical experience in the era of wide-field radiation therapy, so the dosage limits reported from such studies may not be immediately applicable to IMRT. Nevertheless, various investigators have carried out the necessary calculations and adopted SIB IMRT fractionation strategies. Continued investigations and clinical trials are needed to develop more reliable time-dose fractionation models, to produce better estimates of their parameters, and to evaluate alternate SIB IMRT fractionation strategies for all sites.[13] The following are some examples of IMRT fractionation strategies that have been used for IMRT of head and neck cancers.

In the Radiation Therapy Oncology Group H-0022 protocol for early-stage oropharyngeal cancer, 30 daily fractions (5 per week × 6 weeks) are used to simultaneously deliver 66 Gy (2.2. Gy per fraction) to the PTV, 60 Gy (2 Gy per fraction) to the high-risk subclinical disease ("levels II–IV bilaterally, Ib ipsilaterally, and level V and retropharyngeal nodes if the jugular nodes were involved"), and 54 Gy (1.8 Gy per fraction) to subclinical disease. These are biologically equivalent to 70, 60, and 50 Gy, respectively, if given in 2 Gy per fraction. For normal structures, brainstem, spinal cord, and mandible are maintained below 54, 45, and 70 Gy, respectively. The mean dose to the parotid glands is maintained below 26 Gy and/or 50% of one of the parotids is maintained below 30 Gy and/or at least 20 mL of the combined volume of both parotids is constrained to receive no more than 20 Gy. Sixty-nine patients were accrued at 14 institutions. Treatment-associated xerostomia improved following therapy, in contrast to regular radiation therapy. High locoregional control was achieved with stringent adherence to protocol guidelines.[86]

The SIB strategy at Virginia Commonwealth University involves a dose-escalation protocol in which primary nominal dose levels of 68.1, 70.8, and 73.8 Gy, given in 30 fractions (biologically equivalent to 74, 79, and 85 Gy, respectively, if given in 2 Gy per fraction), are used.[87] Simultaneously, the subclinical disease and electively treated nodes were prescribed 60 and 54 Gy, respectively (biologically equivalent to 60 and 50 Gy, respectively, if given in 2 Gy fractions). Spinal cord and brainstem are maintained below 45 and 55 Gy, respectively, and an attempt is made to allow no more than 50% of at least one parotid to receive higher than 26 Gy.

At the Mallinckrodt Institute of Radiology, the SIB strategy for definitive IMRT prescribes 70 Gy in 35 fractions in 2 Gy per fraction to the volume of gross disease with margins. The adjacent soft tissue and nodal volumes at high risk were treated to 63 Gy in 1.8 Gy per fraction and simultaneously 56 Gy in 1.6 Gy per fraction to the elective nodal regions. This regimen has been shown to be well tolerated when combined with concurrent chemotherapy.[78]

The most conservative normal tissue constraints for head and neck sites based on the most recent RTOG protocols (1016, 1008, 0920, and 0912) are: optic nerve and chiasm <30 Gy; eyes <30 Gy; brainstem <48–52 Gy to any 0.03 cc volume; brain <60 Gy to any 0.03 cc volume; spinal cord <45–48 Gy to any 0.03 cc volume; ipsilateral cochlea <50 Gy; parotid glands <26 Gy and at least 20 cc volume <20 Gy; submandibular glands mean <39 Gy; mandible <60 Gy; cervical esophagus mean <35 Gy; pharynx mean <40–45 Gy (for details, see www.rtog.org). Other workers[88–90] have determined dose levels to the pharyngeal constrictors above which severe dysphagia will occur: V65 Gy >30%, V55 Gy >80%, and a mean dose >60 Gy were predictive of feeding tube dependence.

Optimization of Intensity Maps

The optimization of ray intensities may be carried out using one of several mathematical formalisms and algorithms, also termed *optimization engines*.[69] Each method has its strengths and weaknesses. The choice depends in part on the nature of the objective function and in part on individual preference. Although the details are complex, the basic principles are not difficult to comprehend. Each ray of each beam is traced from the source of radiation through the patient. Only the rays that pass through the target volume need to be traced (plus through a small margin assigned to ensure that the lateral loss of scattered radiation does not compromise the treatment). Others are set to a weight of zero.

The patient's 3D image is divided into voxels. The dose at every voxel in the patient is calculated for an initial set of ray weights. The resulting dose distribution is used to compute the "score" of the treatment plan (i.e., the value of the objective function that mathematically states the clinical objectives of the intended treatment).

The ray-tracing process identifies the tumor and normal tissue voxels that lie along the path of the ray. The effect of a small change in a ray weight on the score then is calculated. If the increase in ray weight would result in favorable consequences for the patient, the weight is increased, and vice versa. Mathematically speaking, the ray weight is changed by an amount proportional to the gradient of the score with respect to the ray weight. Realizing that the improvement in the plan at each point comes from rays from many beams and that each ray affects many points, only a small change in ray weight may be permitted at a time. This process is repeated for each ray. At the end of each complete cycle (an iteration), a small improvement in the treatment plan results. The new pattern of ray intensities then is used to calculate a new dose distribution and the new score of the plan, which then is used as the basis of further improvement in the next iteration. The iterative process continues until no further improvement takes place, the optimization process is assumed to have converged, and the optimum plan is assumed to have been achieved.

Many current optimization systems use variations of gradient techniques to optimize IMRT plans. These calculations are prodigious given the thousands of free parameters in variation—it was only with the advent of powerful and affordable computers that such calculations could become clinically realistic. Direct aperture optimization has been proposed as an alternative that reduces the parameter space and eliminates nonphysical dose distributions at the start; for a review see Broderick.[91] The use of gradient techniques assumes that there is a single extremum (a minimum or a maximum, depending on the form of the objective function). This is indeed the case for objective functions based on variance of dose and when only ray weights are optimized. For other cases, it would be necessary to determine whether multiple extrema exist and whether such multiple extrema have an impact on the quality of the solution found. Multiple extrema have been found to exist when beam directions are optimized or when dose–response-based objective functions are used to optimize weights of uniform beams.[53,92,93] One can expect that multiple minima also exist when dose–response-based objective functions are used to optimize IMRT plans. Using simple schematic examples, it also has been shown that multiple minima exist when dose–volume-based objectives are used.[94] Although this may be the case in theory, the existence of multiple minima has not been found to be a serious impediment in dose–volume-based or dose–response-based optimization using gradient techniques. In fact, in a study of dose–volume-based IMRT optimization, Wu and Mohan[95] found that, starting from vastly different initial intensities, the solutions converged to nearly the same plans. The reasons for this have been speculated but not conclusively proven and need to be investigated further.

If multiple minima are discovered to be a factor, then some form of stochastic optimization technique may need to be considered. At the simplest, one may use a random search technique in conjunction with one of the gradient techniques. A more sophisticated stochastic technique is "simulated annealing" or its variation, the "fast simulated annealing".[8,46,53,92] These techniques allow the optimization process to escape from the local minima traps. Other forms of stochastic approaches, such as "genetic algorithms," also have been proposed.[96] In principle, the simulated annealing technique and other stochastic approaches can find the global minimum, but, practically, there is no guarantee that the absolute optimum has been found, only that the best among the solutions examined has been found. (This, of course, is true for gradient techniques as well.) Stochastic techniques tend to be extremely slow and should be used in routine work only if it is established that they are necessary. Nevertheless, some commercial systems have implemented the simulated annealing approach for IMRT optimization.[3] Also, as noted earlier, rapid advances in parallel processing using off-the-shelf components can dramatically reduce computation times.[73] In 2005, Xu and Mueller reported an order of magnitude decrease in the time to process a CT image on a PC when equipped with a dedicated graphics board.[97]

OBJECTIVE FUNCTIONS

Dose-Based Objective Functions

A simple example of an objective function is the criteria stated in terms of the sum of the squares of the differences of desired dose and computed dose at each point within each of the volumes of interest. That is,

$$S = \sum_i (D_{T,0} - D_{Ti})^2 + \sum_n \sum_j p_n \times H(D_{n,0} - D_{n,j}) \times (D_{n,0} - D_{n,j})^2 \quad (1)$$

This type of objective function is called the *quadratic* or *variance* objective function. The optimization process attempts to minimize the treatment plan score S. $D_{T,0}$ in expression Eq. (1) is the desired dose to the target volume and $D_{n,0}$ is the tolerance dose of the nth normal structure. $D_{T,i}$ is the computed dose at the ith voxel of the target and $D_{n,j}$ is the computed dose at the jth voxel of the nth normal structure. For normal organs, the function $H(D_{n,j} - D_{n,0})$ is a Heaviside step function defined as follows:

$$\begin{aligned} H(D_{n,j} - D_{n,0}) &= 0 \quad \text{for} \quad D_{n,j} \le D_{n,0} \quad \text{and} \\ &= 1 \quad \text{for} \quad D_{n,j} > D_{n,0} \end{aligned} \quad (2)$$

In other words, so long as the dose in a normal tissue voxel does not exceed the tolerance limit, the voxel does not contribute to the score function. The quantity p_n is the "relative penalty" for exceeding the tolerance dose.

Dose–Volume-Based Objective Functions

Purely dose-based criteria, such as the one previously described, are not sufficient. In general, the response of the tumor and normal tissues is a function of not only radiation dose but also (to varying degrees depending on the tissue type) the volume subjected to each level of dose. Currently, dose–volume-based objective functions are the most widely used clinically. Dose–volume-based objective functions are expressed in terms of the limits on the volumes of each structure that may be allowed to receive a certain dose or higher. ICRU 83 sets its IMRT reporting guidelines in terms of dose–volume criteria, and dose–volume histograms (DVHs) are a mandatory part of treatment planning.

A practical scheme to incorporate dose–volume-based objectives has been suggested by Bortfeld et al.[98] It is explained in Figure 10.10 using a simple schematic example of one organ at risk. The dose–volume constraint is specified as $V(>D_1) < V_1$. In other words, the volume receiving dose greater than D_1 should be less than V_1. To implement such a constraint into the objective function, we seek another dose value D_2 so that in the current dose–volume histogram $V(D_2) = V_1$. The objective function component for this OAR then may be written as:

$$p_n \cdot \sum_j H(D_2 - D_j) \cdot H(D_j - D_1) \cdot (D_j - D_1)^2 \quad (3)$$

That is, only the points with dose values between D_1 and D_2 contribute to the score. Therefore, they are the only ones penalized.

For the target volumes, two types of dose–volume criteria may be specified to limit both the hot and cold spots. For instance, for the desired target dose of 80 Gy, we may specify V (>85 Gy) ≤ 5% and V (>79 Gy) ≥ 95%. In other words, the volume of the target receiving dose >85 Gy should be no more than 5%, and the volume of target receiving 79 Gy or higher should be at least 95%. Dose-based criteria can be considered as a subset of the dose–volume criteria in which the volume is set to an extreme value (0% or 100%, as appropriate). Dose–volume criteria provide more flexibility for the optimization process and greater control over dose distributions. The reason is that dose-based optimization penalizes all the points above the dose limit, whereas the dose–volume-based optimization penalizes only the subset of points within the lower end of range of dose values above the dose limit. For the example of Figure 10.10A, the dose–volume-based optimization process attempts to bring only the points between D_1 and D_2 into compliance with the constraint. In contrast, the dose-based optimization process attempts to constrain all of the points above D_1. Furthermore, dose–volume criteria are highly "degenerate" functions of dose distributions (i.e., there is a very large number of dose distributions that correspond to the same dose–volume constraint). Therefore, the optimization system has a large solution space to choose from, making it easier to find a better solution.

Limitations of Dose–Volume-Based Objective Functions

Dose–volume-based criteria have been demonstrated to have limitations. To illustrate one such limitation, consider the example in Figure 10.10B of a normal structure for which a constraint has been specified that no more than 25% of the volume is to receive 50 Gy or higher. All three DVHs shown meet this criteria. However, the DVH represented by the solid curve clearly causes the least damage. One can argue that we can overcome this limitation by specifying multiple dose–volume constraints or even the entire DVH. However, as illustrated in Figure 10.10C, this would be too limiting. Multiple DVHs could lead to an equivalent injury to a particular organ, but each DVH may produce a different effect on other organs and the tumor. When this happens, DVHs usually cross each other, as shown in Figure 10.10C. Only one of them is optimum so far as the tumor and other organs are concerned.

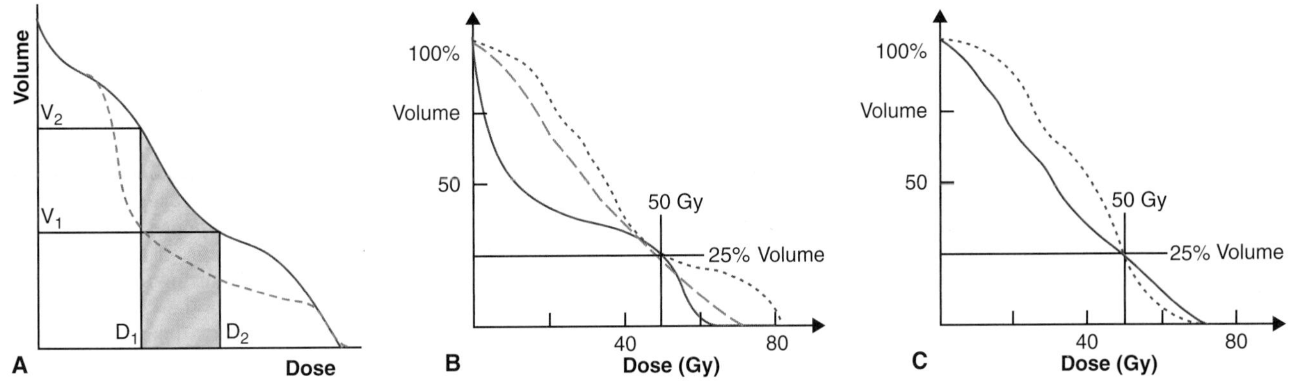

FIGURE 10.10. A: Incorporation of dose–volume constraints in intensity-modulated radiation therapy optimization. (Adapted from Wu Q, Mohan R. Multiple local minima in IMRT optimization based on dose-volume criteria. *Med Phys* 2002;29[7]:1514–1527.) **B, C:** Limitations of dose–volume-based criteria (see text).

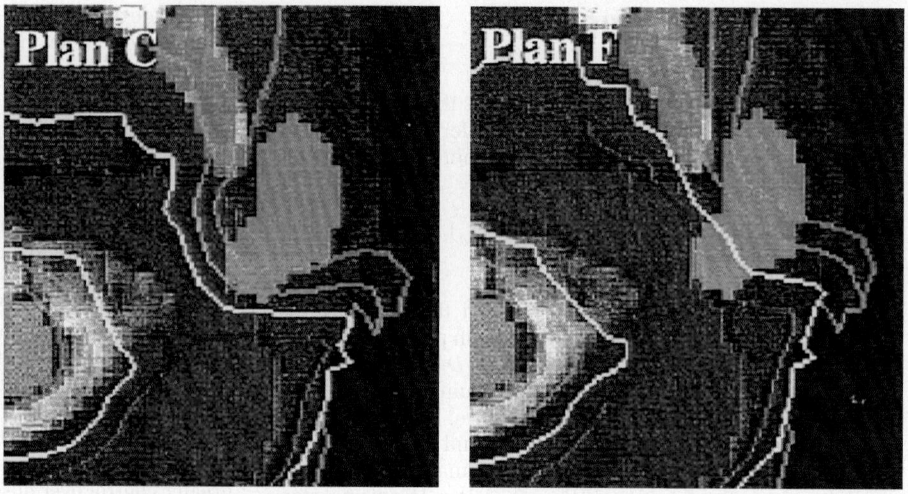

FIGURE 10.11. Effect of adjusting dose-prescription parameters on the resulting treatment plan. The parotid gland and target are shown in green and blue, respectively. Plan C emphasizes parotid sparing, and plan F emphasizes tumor coverage. (Interested readers should view the full set of six plans as presented in the original paper. From Chao KS, Low DA, Perez CA, et al. Intensity-modulated radiation therapy in head and neck cancers: the Mallinckrodt experience. *Int J Cancer* 2000;90[2]:92–103.)

To overcome the limitations of dose–volume-based criteria, they may be supplemented with biologic (or dose–response-based) criteria, for instance, in terms of such indices as tumor control probability (TCP), normal tissue complication probabilities (NTCPs), and equivalent uniform dose (EUD).[77] Dose–response-based objective functions are the subject of ongoing investigations.[53,99] The ICRU currently includes NTCP and EUD projections in its Level 3 reporting (i.e., still investigative). The report (see p. 51) notes that most of the tissue tolerance data go back to the period before 3D imaging, but they do cite newer prospective studies involving 3DCRT or IMRT.[100,101]

Objective Function Parameters

The desired IMRT dose distributions are specified in terms of parameters of the objective function. In Eq. (1), for instance, the parameters of the objective function are the desired dose limits $D_{T,0}$ and $D_{n,0}$ for target and normal structures, respectively, and the relative importance (or penalty) factors p_n for deviating from desired dose limits. Most often, the objective functions are specified in terms of one or more "soft" dose–volume constraints for each volume of interest, one for each constraint. That is, if the computed dose deviates from the desired value, the plan is not rejected, but it is assessed a penalty. The optimization software computes a "subscore" corresponding to each constraint. The subscore value depends on the deviation of dose distribution from the desired dose distributions and the penalty factor. The overall score of an IMRT plan is an accumulation of subscores of individual volumes of interest. The IMRT optimization system uses the IMRT plan score to arrive at the optimum plan according to the specified objective function. The optimized solution involves trade-offs that balance specified normal tissue objectives against each other and against tumor objectives. An IMRT treatment-planning system should provide parameters that allow the treatment planner to adjust the trade-off for each critical structure in a straightforward manner. An example of this is shown in Figure 10.11, where a head and neck target volume nearly abuts the parotid gland.[102] Two of six plans are shown—Plans C and F use parameters that emphasize parotid-gland sparing and tumor coverage, respectively. This is an excellent example of the flexibility of moving the steep dose gradient in and out of the target volume.

The plan considered to be the best by the computer may not be judged the best (or even good enough) by the treatment planner. Parameters are adjusted by trial and error to obtain a satisfactory plan. A confounding factor is that a change in a parameter of one volume of interest affects not only its own subscore and DVH but also the subscores and DVHs of other structures in a complicated manner. For a complex IMRT problem, in which there may be several dozen parameters, their adjustment is an extremely difficult task. The trial-and-error approach used currently is time consuming and leads to suboptimal results. Future research based on artificial intelligence techniques may provide a systematic means of determining optimum parameter values.

Treatment Plan Evaluation

IMRT dose distributions tend to be highly conformal but complex and unconventional. Traditional methods of evaluation and reporting may be too limited for such dose distributions. In principle, the target dose distributions for IMRT should be more homogeneous than for 3DCRT. In practice, the opposite is the case, due in part to the competing demands of sparing of normal tissues and in part to the inadequacy of objective functions. Dose distributions in normal structures as well are, in general, more nonuniform than for 3DCRT.

In the current practice of radiotherapy, treatment plans are evaluated using dose and dose–volume parameters including such quantities as dose to a point in the volume of interest, minimum dose, maximum dose, minimum dose to a specified fractional volume, or the volume of the structure receiving a specified dose or higher. Monitor units (MUs) are set to deliver the prescribed dose to a specified point or to an isodose line (or surface) just enclosing the target volume. For some sites and techniques (e.g., stereotactic radiosurgery of brain tumors), an index of conformality (the ratio of volume occupied by the prescription isodose surface and the volume of the target) is used for plan evaluation. Cumulative dose and dose–volume data are reported as a part of the patient's chart and used for correlation with outcome.

Because of the unconventional nature of IMRT dose distributions, especially the high degree of dose heterogeneity and fluctuations in dose as a function of position in volumes of interest, indices such as dose to a point, minimum dose, or maximum dose may not correlate well with dose response. Instead, dose to a specified fractional volume is more appropriate, and this is the approach taken by ICRU 83. ICRU reporting now specifies a $D_{98\%}$ or $D_{\text{near minimum}}$ (dose to at least 98% of the PTV) and a corresponding $D_{2\%}$ (dose received by the most heavily irradiated 2% of the PTV).[1]

Limitations of dose and dose–volume plan evaluation parameters have been articulated in the literature.[103] These limitations become more significant for the complex dose distributions of IMRT. It has been argued that biophysical dose-response indices, which summarize complex dose distributions using a single clinically relevant index in each volume of interest, may be more appropriate. Currently, indices such as TCP, NTCPs, and biologically EUD often are computed and recorded but rarely are used for routine plan evaluation. This is because of the unreliability of published dose-response data and weaknesses of models to compute these indices. This is, in turn, the result of the various sources of uncertainty both in the quantification of response and in doses delivered to the structures. Levegrun et al.[104] analyzed data from patients with prostate cancer treated at Memorial Sloan-Kettering Cancer Center and concluded that the biopsy-based response did not correlate with minimum tumor dose, EUD, or TCP. Instead, they found the mean dose to be a very good predictor of response. They attributed this observation to large treatment margins for PTV, substantial target motion, and relatively homogeneous dose distributions. As functional imaging (e.g., PET and nanoparticle optical probes) becomes more widespread, treatment will become more adaptive, with planning readjusted to reflect tumor regression or persistence. Recently, Moeller et al. reported a prospective study using 18-fluorodeoxyglucose (FDG)-PET to assess tumor response in head and neck cancers.[60] PET was seen to be superior to CT in the subset of patients with high-risk disease.

GENERATION OF LEAF SEQUENCES

Fixed Intensity-Modulated Fields

For the IMRT mode using multiple fixed fields, the plan optimization process produces nonuniform intensity distributions (see Fig. 10.12) for each set of fields. In principle, such intensity distributions can be delivered using custom-fabricated compensators made of lead alloys to attenuate the appropriate amount of radiation along each ray of the beam. Such devices would have to be produced using computerized milling machines. In addition, to use them it would be necessary for the operator (radiation therapist) to enter the treatment room to insert the device for each field. This process would be highly labor intensive and impractical considering that a large number of beams often may be needed for optimum intensity-modulated treatments.

The most efficient means of delivering fixed-field IMRT is the standard MLC in dynamic mode using such methods as the "sliding-window" technique or the step-and-shoot technique. In either case, leaf position sequences as a function of MUs need to be generated. The MLC leaves are made of approximately 5- or 6-cm-thick tungsten and are typically 0.5 or 1 cm wide (projected to isocenter). MLCs with leaves of a width as small as 1 mm have been introduced. Smaller leaf width may be of greater value for IMRT than for standard 3DCRT. For the former, the leaf width affects the dose delivered to the entire slice, whereas for the latter, it affects only the shape of the boundary. A smaller leaf width undoubtedly would produce more conformal dose distributions, but the electromechanical complexity and cost of the device would increase. Because of the smearing caused by finite-sized radiation sources, lateral secondary electron transport, and the use of multiple fields, and because of motion and positioning uncertainties, an acceptable leaf width may not need to be very small. The minimum desirable leaf width would depend on numerous factors including shapes and locations of volumes of interest, dose gradients desired, and number and orientations of beams. Although the issue of leaf width has been debated for quite some time, there are no definitive studies to guide the choice of the most suitable width.

MLCs transmit only 0.5% to 2% of incident radiation (except through small interleaf gaps and the rounded ends of some MLCs). However, as discussed later in this chapter, because intensity-modulated treatments require a substantially larger number of MUs than do the conventional uniform field treatments, the cumulative effective transmission may be considerably larger.

Leaf Sequence Generation–Sliding-Window Technique

In the sliding-window method, the gap formed by each pair of opposing leaves is swept across the target volume under computer control while the radiation is on. The gap opening and its speed are optimally adjusted. Because the dose rate of the treatment machine might fluctuate slightly, the motion is indexed to MUs rather than time. The basic principle is that as the gap slides across a point, the radiation received by the point is proportional to the number of MUs delivered during the time the tip of the leading leaf goes past the point and exposes it until the tip of the trailing leaf moves in to block it again. (The point also receives additional radiation transmitted through or scattered from the leaves, which must be accounted for. See

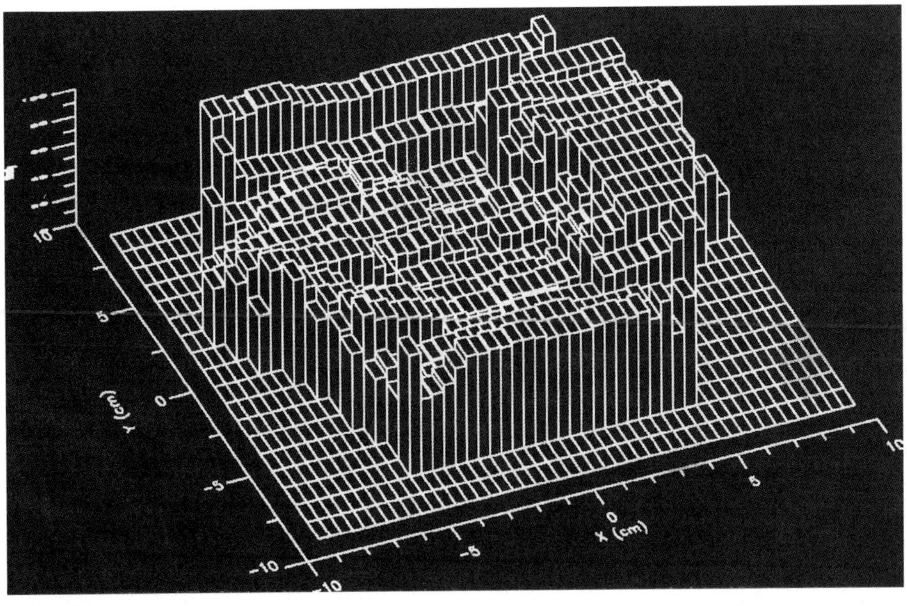

FIGURE 10.12. Intensity profile of the left lateral beam of an intensity-modulated radiation therapy plan designed for the treatment of the cervix. Intensity distribution in a plane through the isocenter and normal to the direction of the beam is plotted. The grid size along the y-axis is 1 cm, corresponding to the width of multileaf collimator leaves. Each intensity curve along the x-axis corresponds to one pair of opposing leaves.

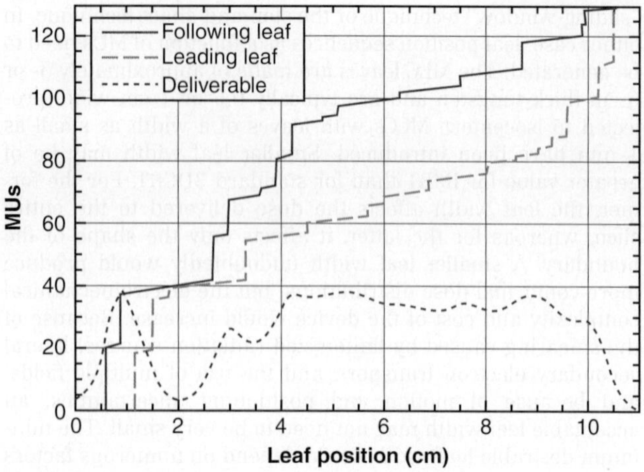

FIGURE 10.13. A typical trajectory of one of the pairs of leaves used to deliver intensity-modulated beam profiles of the type shown in Fig. 10.12. Intensity-modulated radiation therapy optimization based on deliverable dose distributions using the sliding-window technique. Positions of the leading and following leaves are plotted as a function of monitor units (MUs). The gap formed by the pair of leaves moves from left to right. Its width and speed are adjusted by the computer to allow a predetermined amount of radiation to reach each point within the field. Note that the fluence is the differences in MUs for the left leaf and the right leaf.

later discussion in this chapter.) The setting of the gap opening and its speed for each pair at any instant are determined by a technique first introduced by Convery and Rosenbloom[105] and refined and studied further by Bortfeld et al.,[23] Spirou and Chui,[40,41] Stein et al.,[42] Svensson et al.,[106] and others.[44,107] Knowledge of the maximum leaf speed is taken advantage of to maximize the gap between the opposing pair of leaves and, therefore, to minimize the treatment time. The number of leaves participating in the delivery of a beam depends on the projected size of the target volume. The data describing leaf trajectories, produced by the leaf sequence-generation process, are in the form of a table of positions of leaves versus the corresponding MUs (depicted graphically in Fig. 10.13).

Leaf Sequence Generation–Step-and-Shoot and Multisegment Techniques

With the step-and-shoot technique (as well as for multisegment technique), the fixed-gantry radiation beam is composed of multiple static MLC segments, with each segment having its own aperture shape and weight or monitor (MU) settings. The leaf sequence-generation algorithms take the optimized intensity pattern as the input and decompose it into multiple segments, each to be shaped as an aperture formed by the MLC. Fluence intensity throughout each MLC segment is relatively uniform. The summation of all static segments yields the required intensity-modulated dose distributions. Ideally, the segments are sorted to minimize the MLC leaf travel time between the segments. Note that such sorting is neither necessary nor possible for the sliding-window technique.

The first step of the leaf sequence-generation process is the discretization of the continuous intensity distribution into a limited number of intensity levels. These intensity levels then are converted into leaf sequences using one of several methods described in the literature. Bortfeld et al.,[23] for example, have proposed a method in which each row of intensity is handled separately, similar to the sliding-window algorithm. The advantage is that the total number of MUs is small but at the cost of possibly large numbers of segments. Xia and Verhey[108] proposed the so-called areal algorithm. Instead of dividing the intensities into levels of equal steps, they divided them into levels in powers of 2 to reduce the number of steps and to gain efficiency. Wu et al.[99] proposed a technique called the *K-means clustering* in which the intensity levels are grouped together based on their values and the user-specified error tolerance levels. The intensity levels are not equally spaced and can be arbitrary.

Unlike the sliding-window algorithm, the maximum leaf speed is not important for the step-and-shoot and multisegment techniques. Similarly, while the number of segments is not an issue for the sliding-window techniques, it could affect the step-and-shoot delivery efficiency significantly. For the former, the only penalty of the large number of segments is the size of computer storage, whereas for the latter it leads to inefficiency because the beam is off during the transition between the segments. Furthermore, for some linear accelerators, there is an overhead time associated with each segment.

Que[109] compared several step-and-shoot algorithms and found that the algorithm used by Xia and Verhey[108] frequently, but not always, produces the least number of segments. Other investigators have reported methods to minimize the number of segments as well. The algorithm of Dai and Zhu[110] checks numerous candidates for each segment, and the candidate that would result in a residual intensity matrix with the least complexity is selected. If more than one candidate exists with the same complexity, the one with the largest size is chosen. Langer et al.[111] reported a technique based on the integer programming that can minimize the number of segments under the constraints that the MUs do not exceed a certain limit. It was found that the technique produces considerably fewer segments than the algorithms of Bortfeld et al.[8,98] and Xia and Verhey[108] for the same or fewer MUs.

Monitor Units of IMRT Beams

Based on methods similar to those previously described, software systems have been developed to convert intensity distributions to leaf trajectories. The input to this software is the intensity distribution for each field in terms of MUs or, to be more precise, "effective" MUs. Effective MUs are fractions of MUs transmitted through the intensity modulation or compensation device. The intensity distribution-to-leaf trajectory conversion software not only produces trajectories but also computes actual MU settings for each beam as a natural by-product of the conversion process. Trajectories of leaves and the MUs for each beam are transmitted to the computer-controlled radiation treatment machine for dosimetric verification and the delivery of treatment.

It is important to note that the relationship between the prescribed dose and MUs required for delivering each of the intensity-modulated beams is highly complex and not obvious. There is no practical way to calculate MUs by hand as is done for traditional treatments as an independent check of the predicted MU values. To ensure patient safety and to satisfy the requirements of the independent check, some systems have implemented independent software for a second MU calculation. Others have adopted the policy to measure the dose or dose distribution for each of the beams before the first treatment.

Impact of MLC Characteristics

ICRU 83 notes that the tolerances for MLC operation must be more stringent than even those required for beam blockage in 3DCRT. This stems from the steep dose gradients made possible by and employed with IMRT. Slippage of leaf position would cause a cumulative degradation of the dose distribution actually delivered. Leakage through closed leaves may also pose a problem for which consideration in planning must be taken.[112] Adjustments to leaf trajectories are required to account for the various effects associated with MLC characteristics, including the rounded leaf tips, tongue-and-groove leaf design, interleaf and intraleaf transmission, leaf scatter, and collimator scatter upstream from the MLC. The accuracy of dose delivered and the agreement between calculated and measured dose distributions depend on the adequate accounting of these effects. Approximate empirical corrections are applied for these effects by algorithms and software that convert optimized intensity distributions into leaf trajectories.

MLCs have an interlocking tongue-and-groove leaf design to minimize interleaf leakage. However, there is a difference in interleaf leakage and leakage through the leaves. This difference can become significant for beams that require a large number of MUs and in portions of the beams that receive large fractions of their dose through leakage. Currently, this effect is ignored, although the use of Monte Carlo techniques to account for it is being investigated.[113,114]

In addition, there are circumstances during creation of intensity profiles when a thin strip of the irradiated medium is shielded by the tongue of one leaf pair or the groove of the adjacent leaf pair rather than being completely exposed or completely blocked. van Santvoort and Heijmen[43] have demonstrated that this leads to an underdosage in the thin strip. They, and subsequently Webb et al.,[48] also showed that this effect could be removed by the use of leaf motion-synchronizing techniques. However, such techniques result in an increase in the number of MUs. Furthermore, this effect is not considered to be of significant clinical consequence because of the smearing caused by multiple fields and the positioning and motion uncertainties. Using different collimator angles for each field can reduce this effect further.

Depending on the complexity (the frequency and amplitudes of peaks and valleys) of the intensity pattern, points within the field aperture may receive a substantial portion of the dose as a result of radiation transmitted through or scattered from the leaves when the points are in the shadow of the leaves. Points outside the leaf aperture receive their entire dose through these "indirect" sources. The complexity of intensity distributions produced by the IMRT optimization process depends on a combination of several clinical factors including the shapes, sizes, and relative locations of tumor and normal tissues; required tumor dose; dose homogeneity; and dose–volume limits of normal tissues. Intensity distributions for head and neck cases, for example, tend to be considerably more complex than for prostate cases. For beams with highly complex intensity patterns, the average window width to deliver the treatment tends to be small and, for the same dose received by the tumor, the treatment time (i.e., the number of MUs) is long. Consequently, the contribution of radiation transmitted through and scattered from the leaves may form a significant fraction of the total dose delivered. Because these contributions are accounted for approximately, the uncertainty in dose delivered is increased. In addition, the differences between interleaf and intraleaf transmissions may no longer be negligible. Another consequence of complex intensity patterns is that the lower limit of the deliverable intensity is high.

The deliverable dose distributions may be significantly different from the original optimized ones. There are different ways to overcome the difficulties resulting from the differences in desired and deliverable dose distributions. For example, if the deliverable dose to a particular normal structure is higher than the original optimized dose, the planner could modify the objective function to demand an appropriately lower dose. Alternatively, the optimization loop could include a pass-through leaf sequence generation and calculation of deliverable dose distributions. The optimizer then adjusts ray weights based on deliverable dose distributions rather than the idealized ones. This scheme has been investigated by Siebers et al.[115]

QA FOR INTENSITY-MODULATED TREATMENTS

A number of QA steps unique to IMRT are needed to ensure the accuracy and safety of treatments. These include QA of the MLC in dynamic mode, dosimetric verification for each dynamic beam as well as for the composite treatment plans, portal imaging, treatment verification, *in vivo* dosimetry, and reduction in uncertainty associated with daily positioning and internal organ motion during irradiation. In recognition of the special demands of IMRT, the American Association of Physicists in Medicine (AAPM) recently commissioned Task Force 142 to recommend new QA guidelines and these have been published.[116]

When using conventional 3DCRT, MLC leaf position calibration errors influence the accuracy of the radiation distribution at the portal boundary. Because of PTV and beam penumbra margins, small errors in leaf calibration will have a minimal effect on the target volume dose. The accepted leaf calibration accuracy is 2 mm, but this is too large[1] because in IMRT the MLCs are used to generate inhomogeneous fluence distributions. In the sliding-window technique, for instance, this is done by adjusting the velocity and width of leaf gaps during radiation delivery. If the MLC calibration is inaccurate, the delivered dose distribution will be in error. The error is a function of the ratio of leaf calibration error to the sliding-window width. For example, a 1-mm imprecision in the gap would result in a 10% error in dose if a uniform field were to be delivered using a sliding window of 1 cm. For step-and-shoot delivery, magnitudes of dose errors are greater (owing to the steep dose gradients near the MLC leaf edges), but they are confined to the subfield edges. Thus, it is important that the manufacturers of MLCs used for IMRT ensure that the leaves can be positioned with accuracy of better than 0.25 mm, and the physicists must ensure through routine QA procedures that such precise positioning is achieved and maintained. It is interesting that integral dose error is similar for both the step-and-shoot and sliding-window techniques, but the distribution of the error is different.

Because MLC leaf calibration and the accuracy of MLC operations influence the delivered dose distribution, new, more rigorous MLC QA procedures have been developed. Chui et al.,[117] LoSasso and Chui,[118] and Ling et al.,[5] among others, have developed QA procedures specifically for MLCs used in dynamic mode. Periodic QA checks must ensure that the leaves of the MLC do indeed move to their designated positions at the specified values of MUs. Moreover, to ensure safe and accurate delivery of treatments with an MLC, the manufacturers must include redundant and independent sensors for the leaves of the MLC. Furthermore, in the event of treatment field interruption and resumption, there should be no perceptible change in dose delivered.

Another aspect of QA important for IMRT is the daily positioning uncertainty and motion during irradiation. IMRT is a highly conformal and highly precise form of radiotherapy frequently used to escalate dose. Dose distributions may have steep dose gradients between the target and the neighboring normal structures. Furthermore, margins may be much smaller than in conventional treatments. Patient positioning and immobilization requirements are more stringent than ever to ensure that the target volumes are covered adequately and the normal tissues are spared adequately. In fact, special immobilization devices and techniques are being developed to reproducibly and accurately position the target volume and normal anatomy. Many of these devices already are available commercially (e.g., rectal inserts to improve positioning for prostate IMRT).

Similarly, motion during treatment, mainly as a consequence of respiration, also can be a serious problem for IMRT of sites in the thorax and abdomen. Because IMRT is delivered dynamically, the moving target volume may move in and out of the instantaneous field of radiation. Some portions of the target volume may get more than the planned dose, whereas others may get less. A way to minimize effects of respiratory motion would be to use "gated treatments" in which radiation and leaf motion are turned on only during a specific, reproducible portion of the respiratory cycle or in an interval during which the patient's breath is voluntarily, or involuntarily, held.[119] New methodologies, typically employing CT imaging, are being used to synchronize patient breathing motion with the irradiation beam.[120–122]

DOSIMETRIC VERIFICATION OF INTENSITY-MODULATED TREATMENTS

To implement a new treatment technology into routine clinical use, there are usually three distinct but closely related phases: *Acceptance tests:* This is the initial set of tests that ensures the hardware and software meet the factory- or customer-provided specifications. Usually, but not always, the written specifications contain the necessary instructions or guidelines for these tests (in order to avoid legal ambiguity in the measurements). It is also a good opportunity for the users to establish some performance baselines, especially for the hardware purchased. *Commissioning tests:* The IMRT commissioning is a process to implement IMRT treatments using the customer's hardware and beam data. Various groups have studied the general guidelines for commissioning a treatment-planning system, and the AAPM issued a new report on IMRT commissioning in 2009.[123] The process usually starts with collection of essential beam data for beam modeling. The parameters of the dose-calculation algorithm are then tuned to provide the best performance for the user's beam. Additional tests should be performed to evaluate the limitations of the treatment-planning system and a solution or a work-around should be found if the problem is clearly identified. Then IMRT phantom measurements should be performed to test the accuracy of the delivery system and data connectivity. If the accuracy is judged to be acceptable, the system can be released to the clinic after the necessary user training and procedural implementations. It is recommended that a small (interdisciplinary) focus group should be assigned to lead the IMRT implementation in the clinic. The "train-the-trainer" approach has proven to be effective in translating new technology into routine clinical practice.

Ongoing QA: After the system is released to the clinic, it is important to establish a routine QA program. The performance of various steps involved in performing IMRT treatments needs to be tracked so that the quality of the treatments can be maintained. The ongoing QA program can be separated into patient-specific QA and equipment QA, which will be described in more detail in the following section.

Patient- and Equipment-Specific QA

Because of the complexity of irregular field shapes, small-field dosimetry, and time-dependent deliverable leaf sequences, it is recommended by the AAPM and ASTRO that patient-specific QA should be performed as a part of the IMRT management process and a requirement for billing for IMRT services. Figure 10.14 shows the general categories of patient- and equipment-specific QA, which are detailed in the following.

Patient setup, although not specific to IMRT dosimetry, is considered a key step in ensuring accurate IMRT treatments. A variety of image-guided localization techniques have been proposed for use with IMRT treatments, from simple orthogonal portal films to the beam's eye view portal film with IMRT intensity pattern overlays,[124] imaging of implanted fiducials,[125,126] daily ultrasound-guided localization,[127–129] and to the most integrated tomotherapy solutions.[130] The detailed discussion of these specific image-guided procedures is out of the scope of this chapter, but QA in patient positioning remains an important issue for IMRT. A somewhat related problem of organ motion due to breathing has been discussed earlier. Several recent studies have examined the use of cone beam CT for patient setup or respiratory gating.[131–134] The implementation of patient-specific QA depends highly on each institution. For

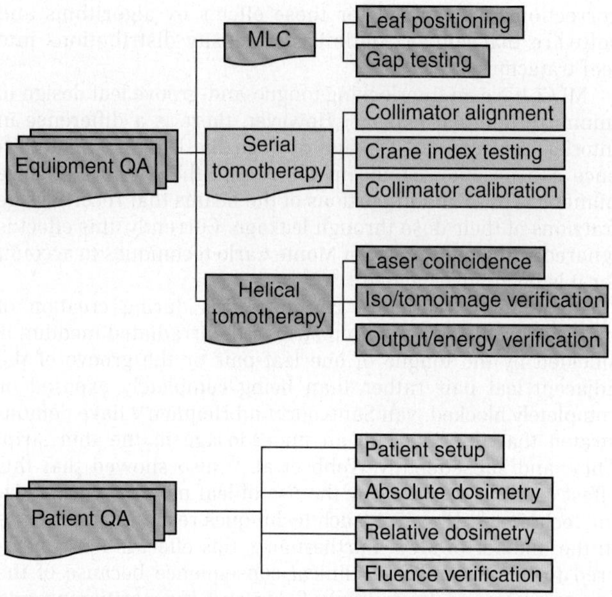

FIGURE 10.14. Overview of intensity-modulated radiation therapy quality assurance (QA) includes patient-specific and equipment-specific procedures. MLC, multileaf collimator.

example, dosimetric measurements of MU settings can be verified for each beam individually (usually in a flat [slab] phantom geometry) or for the composite treatment plan (usually in a specially designed phantom, but it is also possible to use the simple slab phantom setup). Unlike single-beam verification in which the single-beam dose distribution can be significantly different from the original patient plan, the advantage of measuring the composite treatment plan in a phantom (regardless of the shape of the phantom) is that the composite dose distribution or the dose "pattern" generated in a phantom is usually similar to those in the original patient plan. This can be useful in selecting the measurement points or in visualizing potential dose errors. Absolute dosimetry is usually referred to as "MU verification" for IMRT. The traditional manual process for MU verification is virtually impossible to perform because of the large number of fields involved and the irregular shape and size of the treatment segments. Attempts have been made to verify MU settings in an IMRT plan using alternative calculation methods.[135] However, these alternative calculation methods cannot predict the uncertainties during the actual delivery at the treatment machines and are also subject to limitations and approximations in their dose-calculation models. The most reliable and practical technique currently for IMRT MU verification is still the ion chamber-based point dose measurement in a phantom. Absolute dose measurement in a phantom is usually performed through a process called the *hybrid phantom plan.* In this plan, all beam angles and deliverable intensity patterns for a patient plan are transferred to the phantom, and doses in the phantom are computed for QA. The basic assumption in this process is that if the dose calculated in the phantom agrees with the measurement in the phantom, then the dose delivered to the patient agrees with the dose calculated in the patient. Relative dosimetry is usually performed using radiographic films or 2D array detectors. The process is similar to absolute dose measurement using the hybrid phantom plan technique. For film dosimetry, it is important to convert film density into relative dose using a film calibration process. Because of the additional dimensionality, it becomes difficult to define good numerical criteria for evaluating relative 2D/3D measurements. Various numerical indicators (such as the distance to agreement, and gamma, or normalized agreement test) were proposed. In particular, the concept of gamma, combining the dose difference and distance to agreement, is appealing in evaluating 2D or 3D dose distributions. For clinical applications,

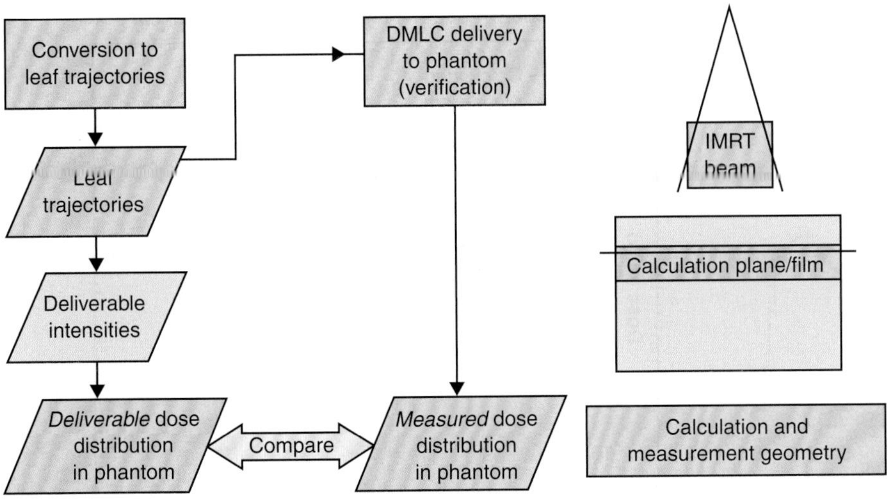

FIGURE 10.15. Diagram illustrating dosimetric verification of individual intensity-modulated radiation therapy fields. DMLC, dynamic multileaf collimator; IMRT, intensity-modulated radiation therapy.

the most reliable and practical way to evaluate 2D distribution is to overlay the measurement isodose lines with the calculated ones. Special attention should be paid to the low-dose regions near critical structures in the original patient plan. Attention should also be paid to the systematic shifts of isodose lines, which may reveal if the isocenter or any reference setup point may be off. The relative dosimetry verification for IMRT should be performed in conjunction with the absolute dose verification for IMRT. It would be useful if the relative dose distribution can be normalized to the absolute dose measurement point, which converts the relative dose measurement into absolute dose distributions.

Two-dimensional fluence verification of intensity patterns gained popularity with the invention of 2D array detectors and the necessary software.[135–137] Fluence verification usually is performed for each IMRT beam at a fixed-gantry angle with or without a flat phantom geometry. The purpose of fluence verification is to make sure the intensity patterns created in each IMRT plan can be faithfully delivered under ideal conditions (2D, beam's eye view). Fluence verification should be combined with other patient-specific and equipment QAs to make sure that IMRT treatments are executed accurately.

Figure 10.14 also illustrates equipment-specific QA procedures. In general, IMRT QA is a subset of general equipment QA processes. The technology of IMRT and techniques for QA are also evolving. It is strongly suggested that users of IMRT should attempt to attend national meetings and technology conferences or training courses so that their knowledge about the use of IMRT can be updated regularly.

IMRT has been variously termed as *opaque, unintuitive,* and *nontransparent,* partly because it is delivered using dynamic techniques. Many are skeptical about whether the dose distribution displayed on an IMRT plan is, in fact, delivered. Furthermore, because of the complexity of computations involved, there is no practical way to verify the MU settings by hand calculations, as is done for conventional treatments. Moreover, because of the inherent nonuniformity of IMRT fields, it is important to know the dose accurately at every point within the beam. One way to check if the intended dose would be delivered to the patient at the time of the treatment is to conduct dosimetric verification measurements.

Two broad categories of IMRT treatment-plan verification approaches have been developed for MLC-based IMRT. First, the dose distribution from radiation fields is independently measured and evaluated. This often is accomplished by using a flat homogeneous water-equivalent phantom and irradiating each field independently. The film-measured dose distributions are compared against calculations conducted by the treatment-planning system under the same geometric conditions. The process is explained in Figure 10.15. For calculation of dose distributions, each field is transferred to a treatment plan with a flat homogeneous phantom. A typical example for a sliding-window intensity-modulated beam dosimetric verification is shown in Figure 10.16. This technique has the advantage that discrepancies between the planned and delivered dose can be attributed to individual radiation portals. However, the total integrated dose distribution is not checked.

The second method uses a phantom that is irradiated by all beam portals, allowing the evaluation of the total dose distribution delivered.[138,139] Typically, ionization chambers and radiographic film are the dosimeters used for these measurements. Although ionization chambers can be benchmark-quality dosimeters, they suffer from volume averaging and are inefficient for measuring multiple points. Because of the complexity of the dose distributions being measured, a 2D dosimeter is required for thorough evaluations of nonuniform dose distribution. Quantitative radiographic film measurements require careful dose calibrations using independently measured sensitometric curves. The film optical densities are measured and converted to absolute dose using film calibration data and compared with the predictions of the treatment-planning system.[44]

In vivo dosimetry commonly is used to verify the dose delivered by conformal therapy radiation fields. The complex fluence distribution of IMRT fields makes quantitative use of *in vivo* dosimetry, specifically the use of skin surface–mounted dosimeters, difficult.

Film, thermoluminescent dosimeters, and diodes may not be sufficiently accurate; are laborious to use; and, in the case of thermoluminescent dosimeters and diodes, are incapable of providing detailed information. In the long run, the most efficient way to verify fixed intensity-modulated fields is expected to be with real-time 2D dosimetry systems using appropriately calibrated electronic portal imaging devices (EPIDs). A general review of EPIDs has appeared recently.[140] Such devices could be used for dosimetric verification of IMRT beams before treatment delivery and for exit dosimetry using transmitted portal dose images (PDIs). For electronic portal imaging devices to be used for pretreatment dosimetric verification and exit dosimetry, they must operate in the integration mode to capture the transmitted radiation over the entire exposure of each beam. The result is a PDI that can be compared with an intensity-modulated digitally reconstructed PDI. For pretreatment dosimetric verification of a given beam, a PDI may be created using a 3D treatment-planning system to compute dose deposited in the electronic portal imaging device detector. For exit dosimetry, the PDI may be calculated using the 3D CT image of the patient. In either case, for accurate dosimetric verification, the effect of scattered radiation and the variation in response of

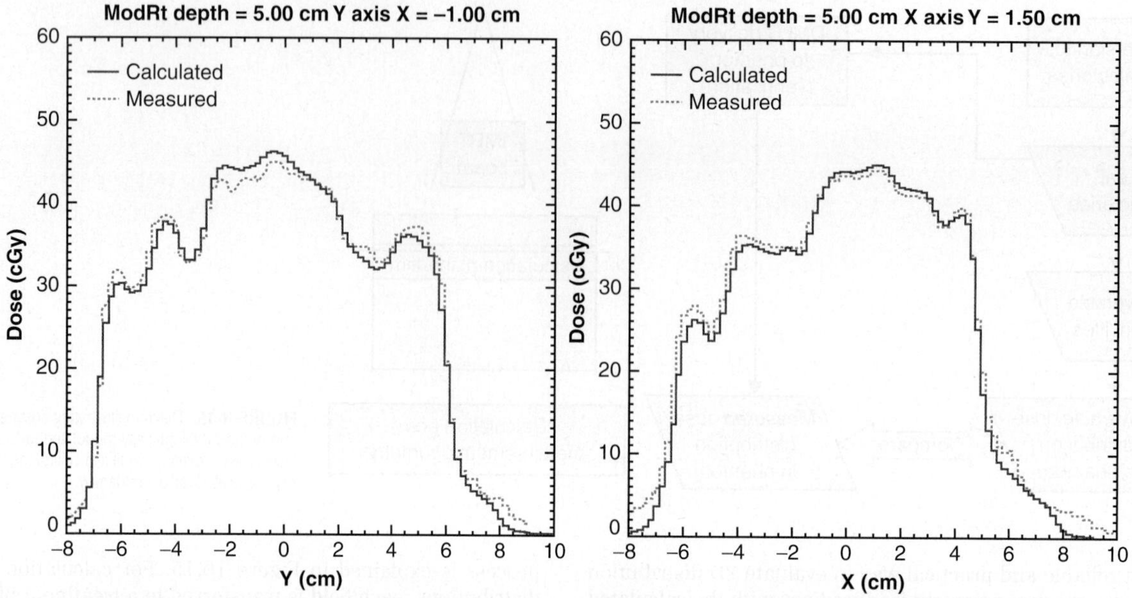

FIGURE 10.16. Dosimetric verification example comparing measured and calculated dose profiles of a right-lateral field generated with sliding-window technique for the intensity-modulated radiation therapy of gynecologic cancer.

the detector with energy must be included. The former effect can be taken into account with dose-spread kernel superposition methods, but both can be accounted for using Monte Carlo techniques.

TREATMENT SETUP AND DELIVERY

Fixed-Gantry Intensity-Modulated Fields

As for conventional radiotherapy, for IMRT techniques using fixed intensity-modulated fields, it is necessary to verify the patient alignment using portal images with beams used for actual treatment before the delivery of the first treatment and then periodically thereafter. However, no beam apertures are required for IMRT. Therefore, special fields for portal imaging with apertures are created in which the shape of each aperture is defined by the terminal positions of the leading leaf tips and the starting positions of the trailing leaf tips.

Intensity-modulated treatments may be delivered remotely or automatically under computer control. The treatment machine computer may automatically set up the various components of the machine and switch on the radiation beam. For the sliding-window technique, it moves leaves during irradiation in the sequence specified in the leaf motion dataset. In the step-and-shoot mode, the radiation pauses while the leaves move. At the completion of the first field, the computer sets the machine for the next field and again goes through its leaf motion sequence and irradiation. This process is repeated until all fields are delivered. The treatment times may vary somewhat and depend on the number of fields involved and the complexity of the fluence distribution. Current time estimates range from 5 to 20 minutes, excluding patient setup.[4,5,44]

SETUP AND IMRT DELIVERY WITH SERIAL TOMOTHERAPY

Current delivery of serial tomotherapy is concisely described in a recent review.[141] A new-generation serial treatment machine with multiple photon heads as well as an electron source has been described by Achterberg and Müller.[142] Because there are no specific beam directions or portals associated with serial tomotherapy beam delivery, the treatment QA concentrates on patient positioning and immobilization. The add-on multileaf collimator (MIMiC) is relatively heavy and its removal is time consuming, so portal films often are acquired with the MIMiC in place. This limits the portal fields to a roughly 3.4 × 20 cm² field size. Therefore, the imaging of useful, immobile, bony anatomic landmarks is critical for each port film, meaning that the selection of the portal film locations is critical to the accurate determination of patient-treated indices, but the digitally reconstructed radiograph that is used to compare against the portal film must be simulated at the same relative couch position as the portal film is acquired. Typically, anteroposterior and lateral films are acquired, and if the target is longer than 10 cm and is in a location where patient structures are flexible (e.g., in the neck), portal films may be required at multiple couch positions to ensure the patient is in the correct orientation throughout the length of treatment.

Treatments are conducted by placing the patient on the couch and aligning the patient to the linear accelerator in the standard fashion. Once the patient is aligned (to a point analogous to isocenter for conventional treatments), the couch translation device (called *CRANE*) coordinates are set to zero and the couch is moved to the location of the first index. This position is determined by the treatment-planning system. The gantry is rotated to the starting arc position, and the patient treatment plan is loaded onto the MIMiC control computer. The linear accelerator is operated in normal arc mode, and the MIMiC control computer determines if the treatment can proceed. If the gantry speed is within acceptable limits, the MLC leaves are opened in their programmed sequence. The MIMiC communicates with the linear accelerator using the conventional door interlock. If the MIMiC control computer determines the treatment should not continue, the door interlock circuit is interrupted and the linear accelerator ceases operation just as if the door had been opened (the door interlock fault is tripped on the accelerator). Once the arc is delivered, the therapist enters the room to move the CRANE to the next couch position and reprograms the MIMiC control computer by following the screen prompts.

TOMOTHERAPY VERSUS FIXED-GANTRY IMRT

The physical and operational differences between tomotherapy and fixed-gantry IMRT lead to trade-offs when considering each system. The rotational beams used in tomotherapy could be a significant advantage until robust beam configuration optimization tools are developed, particularly those involving noncoplanar beams.

For serial tomotherapy delivery, one of the difficulties is the requirement of precisely moving the patient between successive arc deliveries (couch indexes). The dose-delivery error made for an incorrect junction move is similar to the errors in abutting conventional fields. Studies have shown that the maximum dose error is 25% mm^{-1} in the abutment region for errors in couch index movement or intrajunction patient motion.[143] When conventional fields are abutted, feathering often is used to reduce the risk of systematic dose errors. A similar technique has been suggested for distributing the abutment regions for serial tomotherapy[144] by creating multiple treatment plans with modified target volumes to force a redistribution of indexes.

Even when perfectly abutted, there are dose heterogeneities within the abutment region caused by the divergent radiation fields, especially when arcs of less than 360 degrees are used. Low et al.[143] studied the abutment region dose distributions for arcs ranging from 180 degrees to 340 degrees and determined that the tumor doses can have significant cold spots when short arcs are used. These become more severe when the longer leaf setting (1.7 cm) is used. The accuracy of the treatment-planning system in predicting these heterogeneities was not evaluated, but the system tends to underestimate the severity of the heterogeneities. Although the divergence in the radiation beams is still present in helical tomotherapy, the helical path of the field edge distributes the diverging distribution such that dose errors caused by inaccuracies in couch motion, or by patient movement, are significantly smaller than with serial tomotherapy.

One of the advantages of fixed-gantry IMRT is the availability of noncoplanar directions. The commercial hardware device used to precisely move the couch between successive indexes also is produced in a model that attaches directly to the couch, allowing for couch rotations. Although limited noncoplanar dose delivery is possible when using serial tomotherapy, especially when treating the brain, this has not been widely adopted.

Gating for serial tomotherapy is impractical because of the use of conventional linear accelerators and the lack of shared information between the MLC and the linear accelerator control computers. Breath-hold techniques are also impractical because of the relatively long time to rotate the linear accelerator gantry. Because of the potentially large abutment-region dosimetry errors, it is important to consider the immobilization accuracy of targets and critical structures when selecting targets for serial tomotherapy. Gating for helical tomotherapy is possible by pausing the radiation beam and the couch motion when the gating circuitry dictates that no treatment should be delivered. However, there will be a delay in restarting the treatment after the gating signal has been restarted while waiting for the gantry to return to its position when the gating signal was interrupted.

Because the dose is delivered over many indexes or gantry rotations, there are many more MUs used when treating with tomotherapy than for conventional 3DCRT or MLC-based IMRT. The ratio of MUs can be as high as 10:1 even when compared with MLC-based IMRT.[145] This increase in MUs leads to increases in whole-body dose that may yield a significant increase in secondary radiation-induced malignancies. The solution to this is to improve the linear accelerator head shielding, the source of most of the whole-body dose in tomotherapy.

Another limitation of tomotherapy is the lack of electron beams. Electron beams (including energy and intensity-modulated electron beams), by themselves or in combination with intensity-modulated photon beams, currently are employed in the treatment of both breast and skin cancers.

A major advantage of helical tomotherapy is that it is a dedicated IMRT device. However, MLC-based IMRT is likely to compete as a delivery mode resulting in part from the limitations of tomotherapy discussed earlier. Furthermore, the large base of MLC-mounted linear accelerators will mean that the adoption of tomotherapy for significant numbers of IMRT patient treatments will take many years.

SPECIAL REQUIREMENTS OF FACILITY DESIGN FOR IMRT

The room-shielding design characteristics for IMRT delivery are different than those for conventional radiotherapy. Shielding requirements are determined separately for primary and scattered radiation barriers and for tomotherapy and MLC-based IMRT. For MLC-based IMRT, the total integrated radiation fluence remains similar to that used in conformal therapy, so no change in primary barrier thicknesses is expected. However, the increase in MUs of about a factor of 3 is expected to increase the required secondary shielding barrier attenuation, at least until the linear accelerator manufacturers improve the head leakage characteristics. For serial tomotherapy without a beam stopper, the same primary barrier is struck for each couch index, indicating that an increase in primary barrier thickness may be required. However, the use of a rotating beam, and the relatively small angle subtended by the MIMiC, reduces the effective use factor to the point that it almost exactly cancels the number of times the beam strikes the primary barrier. Increases in secondary shielding, however, may be greater than for IMRT because the total number of MUs is significantly greater.

CLINICAL EXPERIENCE WITH IMRT

IMRT of Head and Neck Cancer

The first report of the application of IMRT to head and neck neoplasms was from Baylor College. Kuppersmith et al.[146] reported a decrease in dose to the parotid glands to <30 Gy in 28 patients treated with IMRT using serial tomotherapy. They also found the incidence of acute toxicity to be drastically lower than with conventional radiation therapy. Later, Butler et al.[147] implemented the "simultaneous modulated accelerated radiation therapy"[148] technique, an equivalent of the SIB technique, and found that 19 out of 20 patients treated had complete response with acceptable toxicity. Low et al.[149] have described the application of the serial tomotherapy technique and QA practices for head and neck treatments at Washington University in St. Louis. Preliminary results of the use of these techniques for 17 patients were reported by Chao et al.[101] and showed that the tumor control is promising with no severe adverse acute side effects. A subsequent prospective clinical study conducted by Chao et al.[150] also showed that the sparing of parotid glands translated into objective and subjective improvement of both xerostomia and quality-of-life scores in patients with head and neck cancers treated with IMRT.

In another study, Chao et al.[151] also reported the dosimetric advantage of IMRT treatment in patients with oropharyngeal carcinoma (260 with primary tumors in the tonsil and 170 with primary tumors at the base of the tongue). No adverse impact on local control or disease-free survival (DFS) was seen, but there was a significant reduction of late salivary toxicity. Fixed-field IMRT and serial tomography gave superior GTV coverage and lower parotid doses compared to conventional RT in nasopharyngeal cancer.[152] Groups at Memorial Sloan-Kettering[153] and UCSF[154] found similar results for nasopharyngeal patients. IMRT likewise showed promise for oral and oropharyngeal caner[155] and in dose escalation studies of head and neck squamous cell carcinoma.[12,87] Examples of target delineation for nasopharyngeal and hypopharyngeal cancer are shown in Figures 10.17 and 10.18, respectively.

Since the early part of the past decade, IMRT usage in head and neck cancers has become ubiquitous. The Web of Science database records 135 papers with "head and neck" and "IMRT" in the title from 2002 through 2011. Of these, 102 appeared in

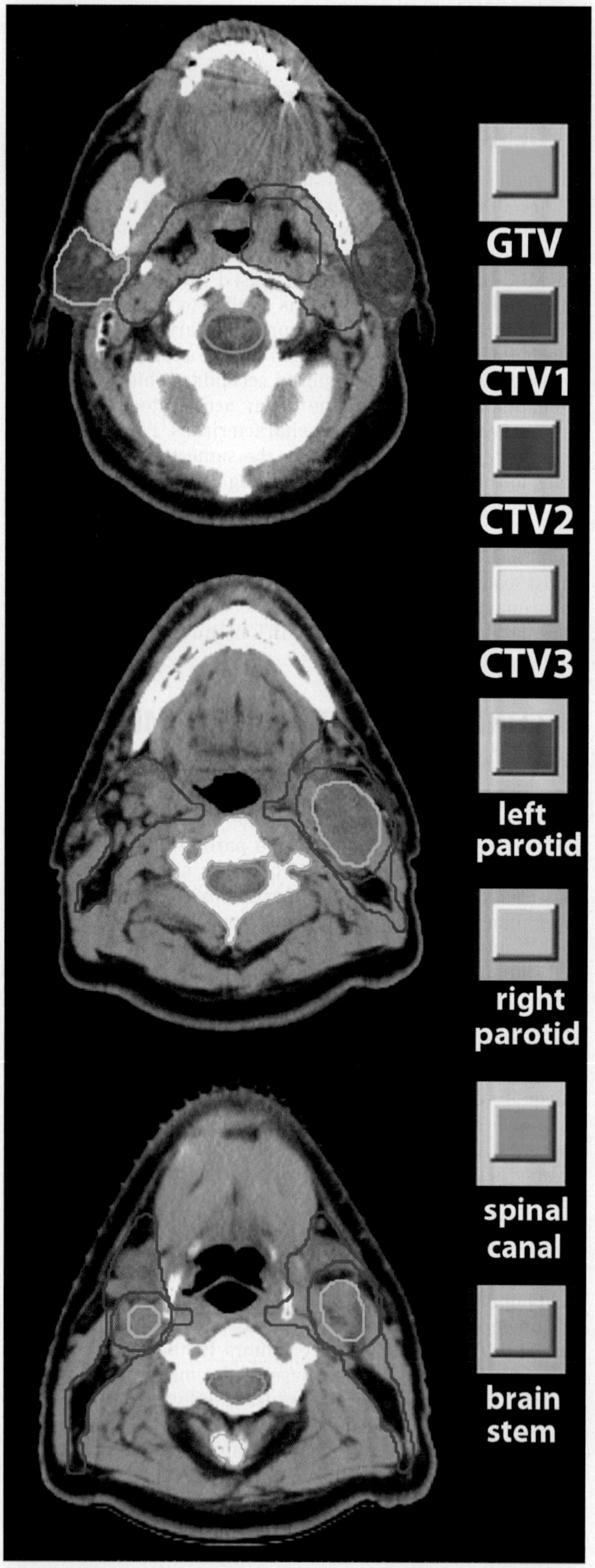

FIGURE 10.17. Intensity-modulated radiation therapy (IMRT) target delineation for stage T2N2 nasopharyngeal cancer. Three axial slices are shown.

or after 2006. Recent review articles pertaining to head and neck cancers include the following: Lee and Terezakis[156] in 2008 and Maingon et al.[157] in 2010. Lu and Yao found improved quality of life and survival benefit in IMRT treatment of nasopharyngeal cancer.[158] Reviews focused on quality-of-life issues include Scott-Brown et al.[159] and Tribius and Bergelt;[160] swallowing issues are reviewed by Roe et al.[161] Early work by Chao et al.[150,151] showed significant reduction in salivary gland toxicity in the IMRT-treated patients. Nutting et al.[162] reported the results from a head-to-head phase III trial of IMRT versus conventional radiation therapy in patients with pharyngeal squamous cell carcinoma (T1–4, N0–3, M0). The IMRT arm showed significantly less grade 2 (or worse) xerostomia compared to radiation therapy: at 12 months, 74% for radiation therapy versus 38% for IMRT; at 24 months, 83% for radiation therapy versus 29% for IMRT. At 24 months, no significant differences were seen in other toxicities or in local control or overall survival.

This raises a question—given the increased complexity and cost in equipment and physician time for IMRT compared to conventional radiation therapy, is the improvement in quality of life alone worth the cost? This was the *raison d'être* for the study by Tribus and Bergelt.[160] The answer is obviously yes for the patient. More to the point, what possibilities are there for improvement of outcome in survival and locoregional control? IMRT by itself is still radiation therapy—the photon sources do not have the coherence of an optical laser, so there are beam-edge effects and also beam scattering from the MLC leaves and within the patient's body as the depth increases. This puts limits on the dose gradients that can actually be achieved, and if OAR sparing is to occur it will mean less homogeneous doses to the GTV. There are several ways to approach this problem:

1. Better imaging during a course of treatment. Changes in tumor size and/or location during treatment will require imaging to adjust the IMRT plan. Various promising imaging modalities useful for radiation oncology were reviewed by Apisarnthanarax and Chao;[57] more recently Moeller et al.[60] reported on a prospective trial using FDG-PET and CT imaging in head and neck cancer. Cone beam CT has also been reviewed recently.[163]
2. Accelerated fractionation. Here one makes use of the radiobiologic advantages of IMRT[13] to perform dose escalation to tumor while constraining the dose to critical normal tissue. Ling et al. have discussed the effects of dose rate in terms of the widely used linear-quadratic model.[164] Chakraborty et al.[165,166] observed 95% disease-free survival in 20 patients with squamous cell carcinomas at various head and neck sites, but the SIB group treated at a higher dose did have more acute toxicities.
3. Combined-modality treatment. Combined chemotherapy and radiation treatment is the current approach for locally advanced head and neck squamous cell carcinoma.[167] Chemoradiation for locally advanced head and neck disease has also been reviewed by Seiwert et al.[168] Traditionally cisplatinum compounds have been used, but attention is turning to antiangiogenesis agents and epidermal growth factor receptor inhibitors. Similar themes were expressed in the 2008 Southwest Oncology Group report.[169] Riesterer et al. discuss the last decade of work on chemosensitization with molecular signaling agents followed by radiation.[170]

Thus far, we have only considered photon irradiation since that is what is used in the overwhelming majority of external radiation treatments. New technologies, in particular beams of charged heavy ions (protons or carbon), show promise due to their highly depth-dependent energy deposition profile (the spread-out Bragg peak). Thariat et al. recently published a concise review of these and other techniques as applied to head and neck cancers.[171] Heavy ion beam therapy is very costly and available only at a few centers, so in the immediate future it will likely be limited to those cases such as malignancies close to the eyes or optic chiasm where photon beams cause unacceptable vision loss.

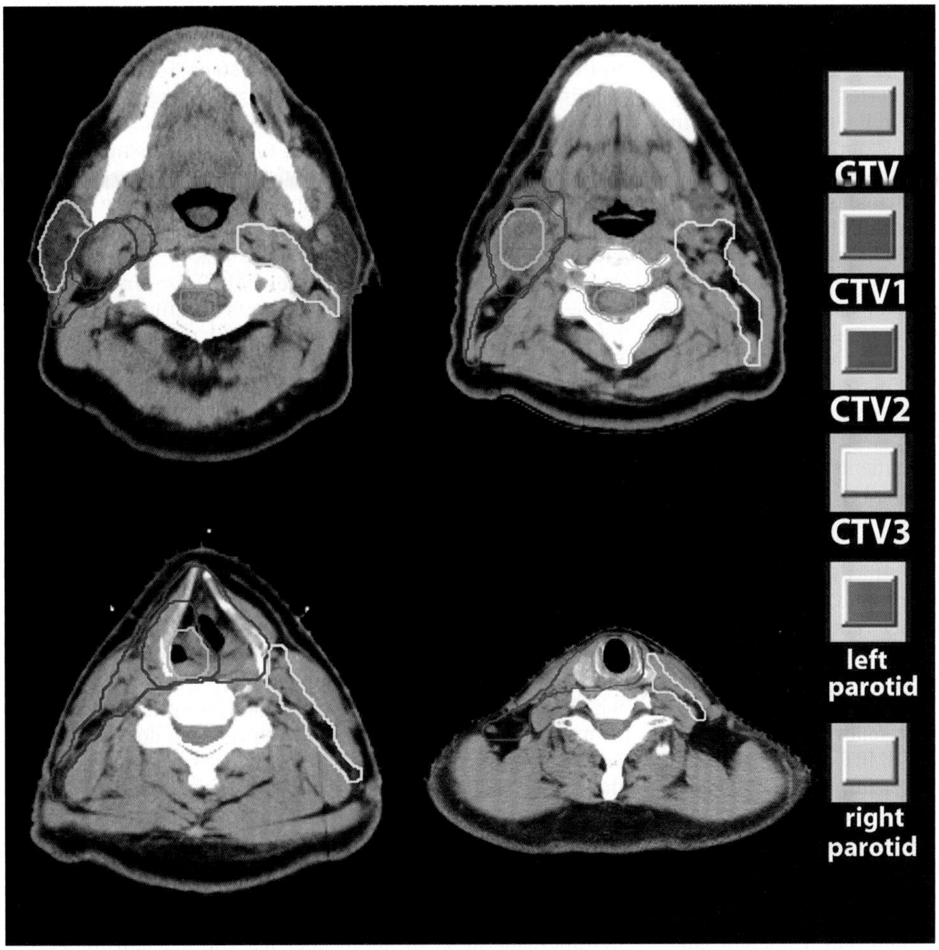

FIGURE 10.18. Intensity-modulated radiation therapy (IMRT) target delineation for stage T2N1 hypopharyngeal cancer. Four axial slices are shown; the spinal canal is contoured in orange.

IMRT of Prostate Cancer

The prostate is another organ with closely associated nerves and other structures (seminal vesicles, urethra, bladder, and rectal wall), the impairment of which can cause important quality-of-life issues. The prostate was in fact one of the first targets of IMRT in the work of Ling et al. at Memorial Sloan-Kettering.[4,5]

Studies involving hundreds of patients followed: in 2000, Zelefsky et al.[172] demonstrated superior target coverage with IMRT compared to conventional RT and 3DCRT; in 2002 they reported a larger study showing the feasibility of high-dose IMRT with reduced acute toxicities[173]:

A total of 772 patients were treated: 698 to 81.0 Gy and 74 to 86.4 Gy. Acute grade 2 rectal toxicity was seen in 35 (4.5%), but none at grade 3 or above. Acute grade 2 urinary symptoms developed in 217 patients (28%), but only 1 patient with grade 3 problems. Late rectal bleeding (grade 2) was experienced by 11 patients (1.5%). PSA relapse-free survival rates (3-year actuarial) were 92%, 86%, and 81% for the favorable, intermediate, and high-risk groups, respectively. This early work was extended by other workers,[174,175] and the field has been extensively reviewed.[176–178]

As with head and neck and other organ sites, concurrent chemotherapy is being used both to sensitize malignant cells for radiation treatment and to eradicate micrometastatic disease. This is used for patients at high risk, with aggressive cancers refractory to hormonal treatment or irradiation alone. For a recent review, see Sanfilippo et al.,[179] who reported on a phase I/II trial in 22 patients with locally advanced hormone-ablated disease (T1–3). Paclitaxel was given biweekly, with four-field 3DCRT starting at 63 Gy and escalating to 66.6, 70.2, and 73.8 Gy. Acute toxicities included diarrhea (mostly grade 1 and 2, but with grade 3 in four patients); at 38 months, 21 (95%) were alive. But six of 22 (27%) had developed relapsed disease. Tucker et al.[180,181] analyzed Radiation Therapy Oncology Group (RTOG) 9406 data to obtain Lyman NTCP parameters and the linear-quadratic α/β ratio for late rectal toxicity in prostate-irradiated patients.

The treatment of prostate cancer has been greatly impacted by advances in magnetic resonance, both standard MRI and magnetic resonance spectroscopic imaging (MRSI). This growing field has been extensively reviewed; for two recent articles, see Sciarra et al.[182] and Mazaheri et al.180.[183] MRI and MRSI are noninvasive imaging modalities that depend on the resonant absorption of radiofrequency energy by nuclei with magnetic moments (normally protons, and also 31-P). The exact resonant behavior of each nucleus depends on the total magnetic field at its location, and this in turn is a combination of the external field of the instrument and the internal magnetic variations caused by the molecular structure in which the nucleus exists. Tumor tissues can be distinguished from normal tissues by differences in the intrinsic nuclear spin relaxation times (T1 and T2), and this can be used to accentuate (or eliminate) their magnetic resonance signals. Thus, magnetic resonance can often "see" details of the prostate tumor that are not observable on a CT scan. MRI can be used for much more precise tumor target delineation for IMRT than would otherwise be possible, and this has had significant clinical impact.

IMRT of Intracranial Malignancies

With FDG-PET and/or MRI, tumors within the brain can be visualized more clearly than on CT. Given the desire to avoid extensive neurologic damage, IMRT is expected to offer some advantages in sparing normal tissues and possibly improving the often bleak prognosis of central nervous system cancer patients. For example, Gutierrez et al. reported a planning study with tomotherapy to provide an integrated boost to whole-brain irradiation in an effort to spare the hippocampus.[184]

Iuchi et al.[185] from Japan published a retrospective report on 25 patients with malignant astrocytomas (World Health Organization grade III and IV) treated with IMRT using a hypofractionated regimen of 48 to 68 Gy in eight fractions. Thirteen patients were treated to 68 Gy and 12 patients received doses of 48 to 65 Gy. The IMRT group was compared to 60 patients treated with conventional techniques to doses of 40 to 60 Gy using 2 Gy daily fractions. The 2-year overall survival was significantly improved (p = .043) in patients treated with hypofractionated IMRT (55.6%) compared to those patients treated with conventional techniques (19.4%).

Huang et al.[186] reported on 15 patients with pediatric medulloblastoma treated with conventional craniospinal radiotherapy followed by a boost to the posterior fossa using IMRT. IMRT delivered much lower doses of radiation to the auditory apparatus while maintaining full doses to the desired target volume. Their findings suggested that, despite receiving higher doses of cisplatin and despite receiving radiotherapy before cisplatin therapy, IMRT can significantly decrease the rate of hearing loss in children treated for medulloblastoma.

Glioblastoma multiforme (GBM) has a very poor outcome, with a median survival of 9 to 11 months following resection.[187] Floyd et al.[188] used hypofractionated IMRT tomotherapy to treat 20 patients with primary disease. Fifty Gy in 10 daily fractions was given with 30 Gy (10 fx) to surrounding edema. Time to disease progression was 7 months, so no gain in survival was seen, but the treatment time was reduced from 6 to 2 weeks. Stupp et al.[189] studied outcomes in GBM patients after resection who were treated with RT with or without adjuvant temozolomide: the chemoradiation group had a median survival of 14.6 months compared to 12.1 months with RT alone. A review of temozolomide therapy for brain tumors was recently done by Koukourakis et al.[190] Amelio et al.[191] have recently reviewed the use of IMRT, including hypofractionation, in the treatment of glioblastoma. They concluded that there is clinical advantage with IMRT because higher doses can be given in shorter times without increasing toxicity.

IMRT of Breast Cancer

RT for breast cancer poses challenges, in particular large differences in tissue thickness in the radiation field and the close proximity of the lung apex and the heart, coupled with target motion during the breathing cycle. Taylor et al.[192] reviewed excess mortality due to cardiac damage in patients treated from 1950 through 1990, when cardiac doses of up to 14 to 17 Gy were given. In addition, part of the radiation field contains the skin boundary between tissue and air. Because air scatters much less of the x-ray fluence, there can be significant dose inhomogeneities and overdosing of the skin ("skin flash"). Commercial systems are now available that can autocontour the volume of breast tissue within conventionally designed tangential photon portals and then use an inverse-planning algorithm to optimize dose homogeneity within these tangential portals. However, most commercial inverse planning systems could not handle the "skin flash" appropriately. Due to setup uncertainties and breathing motion, a portion of the breast (target) tissue may move outside the skin line as indicated by the treatment-planning CT images of the patient. The traditional IMRT technique to overcome target motion uncertainty is to expand the PTV and optimize the dose coverage to the entire PTV. However, this strategy may not work because a portion of the PTV will be expanded into the air, which does not have the necessary mass to absorb the dose. Some treatment-planning systems ignore the regions outside the skin contour entirely. Therefore, it may be necessary to add "virtual" tissues in the PTV for the inverse-planning system. Sometimes it may require users to manually open certain IMRT segments to take care of the skin flash effect.

Nevertheless, there has been interest in using IMRT for left-sided breast cancers in order to spare myocardium from the high-dose region of the radiotherapy fields. The Guerrero Urbano and Nutting IMRT review includes a concise summary of early work through about 2002.[193] No robust data regarding clinical outcomes after IMRT for breast cancer exist; however, a variety of dosimetric studies[194–198,199,200] have suggested reductions in lung and myocardium doses when IMRT is compared to conventional radiotherapeutic techniques. Hurkmans et al.[201] used an NTCP model to estimate the NTCP for cardiac and lung complications due to radiotherapy and found that IMRT did decrease the NTCP for late cardiac toxicity compared to more conventional radiotherapy techniques but had a minimal effect on the NTCP for radiation pneumonitis.

Hong et al.[196] reported a dosimetric study of IMRT in 10 cases of intact breast cancer showing significant reduction of dose to the coronary arteries, ipsilateral lung, and surrounding soft tissues. It simultaneously improved dose homogeneity throughout the target volume. Li et al.[197] described a combined electron and IMRT technique for breast cancer treatment, which led to improvement over the conventional treatment technique using tangential fields with reduced dose to the ipsilateral lung and the heart. Other studies[195,200] also confirmed that IMRT reduces the high-dose volume in tangential breast irradiation significantly and enables more complete cardiac sparing without compromising PTV coverage in some patients. Furthermore, IMRT creates a possibility to improve field matching in case of multiple field irradiations of the breast and lymph nodes.[200,202,203] In addition, IMRT for tangential breast radiation therapy was found to be an effective and efficient method to achieve uniform dose throughout the breast. Preliminary findings reveal minimal or no acute skin reactions for patients with different breast sizes in 32 patients with early-stage breast cancer.[202] Taylor et al.[204] reviewed results of RT of breast cancer patients in 2006 and found that use of more modern planning had significantly reduced mean heart doses to 2.3 Gy but that a small part of the heart still received more than 20 Gy in left-sided irradiation.

IMRT of Gynecologic Cancer

In regard to the targeting of pelvic lymphatics with IMRT, Taylor et al.[205] mapped the pelvic lymphatics of 20 patients using MRI with the administration of iron oxide particles and found that a modified CTV margin of 7 mm around the iliac vessels resulted in adequate coverage of the pelvic lymphatics.

Ahamad et al.[206] analyzed the normal tissue-sparing effects of IMRT in the treatment of the pelvis after hysterectomy in patients with gynecologic cancers and found that although more small bowel, bladder, and rectum could be spared with IMRT compared to conventional radiotherapeutic techniques, these benefits rapidly diminished with even small expansions of the target volumes. D'Souza et al.[207] used the same dataset of patients as Ahamad et al.[206] and found that IMRT may allow higher doses of radiation (54 Gy) to be delivered safely to the node-bearing regions of the pelvis and the vaginal apex compared to conventional techniques that administer 50.4 Gy. Gielda et al.[148] reported on a small study of gynecologic cancer patients ineligible for brachytherapy who were treated with tomotherapy in an attempt to reduce toxicity to bowel and femoral heads.

Salema et al.[208] reported on 13 patients treated with extended field pelvic and para-aortic radiotherapy using IMRT and found that two patients experienced grade 3 or higher toxicity. Both of these patients received concurrent cisplatin-based chemotherapy.

Portelance et al.[209] reported dosimetric comparison between 3DCRT and IMRT for 10 patients with cervical cancer. They demonstrated that, with similar target coverage, normal tissue sparing was superior with IMRT. Mundt et al.[210] reported the clinical experience of 40 patients with gynecologic malignancy who underwent IMRT to the pelvis. Compared with 35 historic control patients who were treated with conventional techniques, patients treated with IMRT experienced fewer acute gastrointestinal (GI) symptoms than those treated with conventional whole-pelvic radiotherapy. The ability of IMRT to deliver local control while reducing grade ≥2 bowel toxicity was shown in a recent report by Portelance et al.[211] from the multi-institutional RTOG 0418 cervical cancer trial. Ring et al.[212] did a study on 36 patients with FIGO (International Federation of Gynecology and Obstetrics) stage IB2 to IIIB cervical cancer. They were treated with extended-field RT with concurrent cisplatin to target suspicious pelvic or para-aortic lymph nodes or excessive local pelvic tumor burden. At 32 months, 24 patients were disease free and an additional eight were still alive but with disease.

IMRT of Gastrointestinal Cancer

Pancreatic cancer remains a disease with a poor prognosis. In 1995 Lillemoe[213] reviewed then-current disease management. By this time mortality from surgical resection had been reduced to 2% or 3%, but the weighted-average 5-year overall survival was still only about 22%. In 2011, Showalter et al.[214] reanalyzed the data from RTOG 9704 on the results of surgical resection and adjuvant chemoradiation. Interpolating their Figure 2, one can estimate 5-year overall survival as about 28% for node negative and 19% for one to three positive nodes—not significantly different in 15 years.

Crane et al.[215] attempted a dose-escalation study with RT and gemcitabine in unresectable pancreatic cancer patients but had to discontinue due to dose-limiting toxicity.

Ben-Josef et al.[216] reported on 15 patients with pancreatic cancer treated with concurrent capecitabine and IMRT (45 to 55 Gy) and reported that only one patient had grade 3 GI toxicity, specifically GI ulceration, which responded to medical management.

Brown et al.[217] performed a dosimetric analysis of 15 patients with pancreatic cancer and compared 3DCRT, IMRT with sequential boost, and IMRT with integrated boost and found that IMRT with integrated boost allowed dose escalation up to 64.8 Gy to the primary tumor. More recently, Yovino et al.[218] reported that IMRT produced a statistically significant reduction in upper and lower GI toxicity compared to 3DCRT in chemoradiation treatment following RTOG 9704 guidelines.

IMRT for gastrointestinal cancers (including pancreas) was recently reviewed by Bockbrader and Kim[219] from the radiobiologic and dosimetric as well as clinical outcomes viewpoint. Meyer et al.[220] gave the rationale for IMRT with PET/CT in anorectal cancers as to reduce radiation-associated morbidity. They also present some clinical data.

Guerrero Urbano et al.[221] performed a dosimetric evaluation in five patients with locally advanced rectal cancer and found that IMRT with simultaneous integrated boost theoretically reduced the radiation dose to the small bowel compared to 3D conformal techniques. Milano et al.[222] reported on 17 patients with squamous cell carcinomas of the anal canal treated with IMRT with whole-pelvic radiation does of 45 Gy followed by boost to the anal canal. Thirteen patients received concurrent 5-fluorouracil and mitomycin-C chemotherapy. Treatment was well tolerated with no grade 3 or higher nonhematologic toxicity and no required treatment breaks from skin or GI toxicity. However, one patient receiving mitomycin-C chemotherapy did experience grade 4 hematologic toxicity. Three patients who did not achieve a complete response required abdominoperineal resection and colostomy. With a mean follow-up of 20.3 months, there were no other local failures.

Milano et al.[223] also reported on seven patients with gastric cancer treated with IMRT to a dose of 50.4 Gy. No patient experienced grade 3 toxicity. The treated IMRT plans were compared to conventional anteroposterior/posteroanterior and three-field plans, and the IMRT plans were found to provide better coverage of the target volumes compared to conventional techniques, with better sparing of the liver and kidneys.

IMRT of Lung Cancer

Because of concerns regarding respiratory motion in radiotherapy of lung cancer, the use of IMRT in lung cancer requires some method to account for tumor and organ motion during treatment planning and delivery; these techniques include both respiratory gating[120] and four-dimensional CT planning.[224] Starkschall et al.[225] recently reported direct 4D CT measurements of interfraction GTV movement during free breathing and concluded that breath-hold gating provides reproducible tumor localization. With cone beam CT or orthovoltage x-ray, the appropriate margins are 0.3 cm for implanted fiducials and 0.8 cm for bony landmarks.

The poor local control rates of conventional radiotherapy doses in the treatment of lung cancer[226] have led to much interest in using IMRT to allow for dose escalation to improve local control. Holloway et al.[227] reported the initial results of five patients with unresectable stage II and III non–small-cell carcinoma treated on a phase I dose-escalation trial using induction chemotherapy followed by IMRT to a dose of 84 Gy using 2.4 Gy daily fractions. PET CT was used to define target volumes. One patient developed lethal radiation pneumonitis and the trial was halted. Murshed et al.[228] performed a dosimetric analysis of 41 patients initially treated with 3DCRT to a dose of 63 Gy. IMRT plans were then generated using these patients' initial planning CT scans, and IMRT was found to decrease the volume of lung irradiated to both 10 and 20 Gy. Target coverage was improved with IMRT, and the volumes of heart and esophagus irradiated were also reduced. Figures 10.19 and 10.20 illustrate MLC portals and IMRT treatment plans for lung cancer.

Grills et al.[229] performed a dosimetric comparison of four radiotherapy techniques in 18 patients with stage I–IIB lung cancer. The study compared IMRT, optimized multiple-beam 3DCRT, two- to three-beam 3DCRT, and traditional wide-field radiotherapy with elective nodal irradiation. This study found that IMRT and optimized 3DCRT resulted in similar doses of radiotherapy to normal tissues in node-negative patients; however, in node-positive patients, IMRT resulted in a 15% decrease in the volume of lung treated to 20 Gy ($V_{20\ GY}$) and a 30% decrease in the NTCP for radiation pneumonitis. In 2010, Liao et al.[230] reported the outcomes of 409 non–small-cell lung carcinoma patients treated at MD Anderson. Three hundred and eighteen patients received CT/3DCRT and 91 received 4D CT/IMRT to a median dose of 63 Gy. The mean lung dose was slightly higher for the IMRT group (24.9 Gy compared to 22.1), but the mean and 95% confidence interval range was lower for IMRT (34.4% ± 1.2% vs. 37.0% ± 1.1%). When corrected for factors such as smoking status, histology, and nodal status, the hazard ratio for IMRT to 3DCRT was significantly less than one, as was that for toxicity (grade 3 pneumonitis), while distant metastases were similar. Thus, IMRT gave similar or better results in terms of survival and local control while reducing treatment toxicity. Vogelius et al.[231,232] pose a cautionary warning—their dosimetric modeling showed that when RT is used in combination with chemotherapy, the larger volume exposed to lower radiation doses in IMRT could pose problems with pneumonitis as compared to 3DCRT or proton therapy. They propose inclusion of chemotherapy in radiation planning as an equivalent radiation dose in the tissue volume.

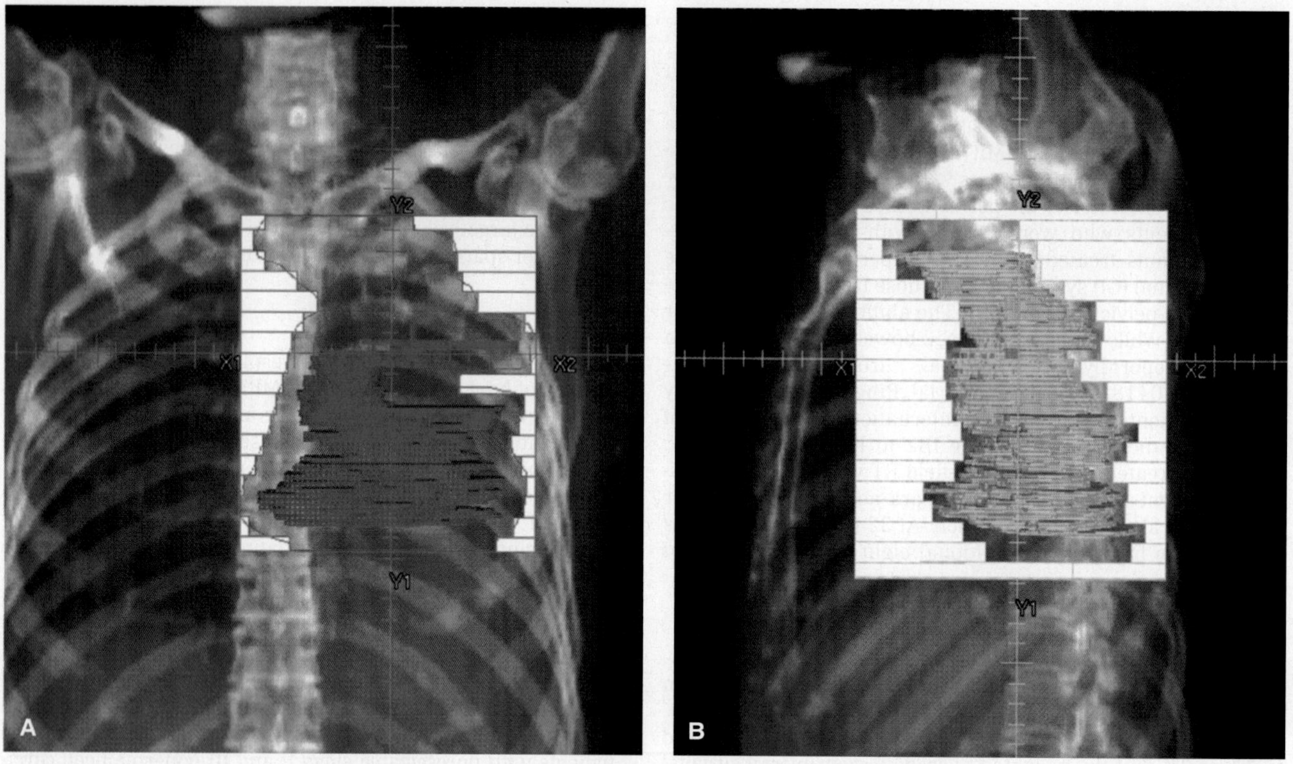

FIGURE 10.19. Illustration of anterior-posterior **(A)** and oblique **(B)** multileaf collimator configuration.

IMRT Experience with Other Cancer Sites

In addition to strong data supporting the use of IMRT in head and neck and prostate cancer, there are a number of preliminary studies reporting the feasibility and outcomes of IMRT in other cancers; many of these reports are theoretical dosimetric studies. Theoretically improved dosimetry alone probably does not serve as sufficient justification for the routine use of IMRT in these cases, and in the absence of robust clinical data regarding actual treatment outcomes, IMRT in these settings should be considered investigational.

In closing, IMRT clearly results in improved radiation dose distributions in a variety of cancers. In some cases, the superior dosimetry of IMRT has resulted in improved clinical outcomes for patients; however, the scientific evidence documenting these clinical improvements lags far behind the data documenting improved dosimetry. Many patients present with disease for which the likelihood of cure is remote, but for whom reduction of tumor burden with fewer debilitating toxicities will be an attractive option. Reduction in treatment morbidity is an immediately realizable benefit of IMRT. Improvement of survival will

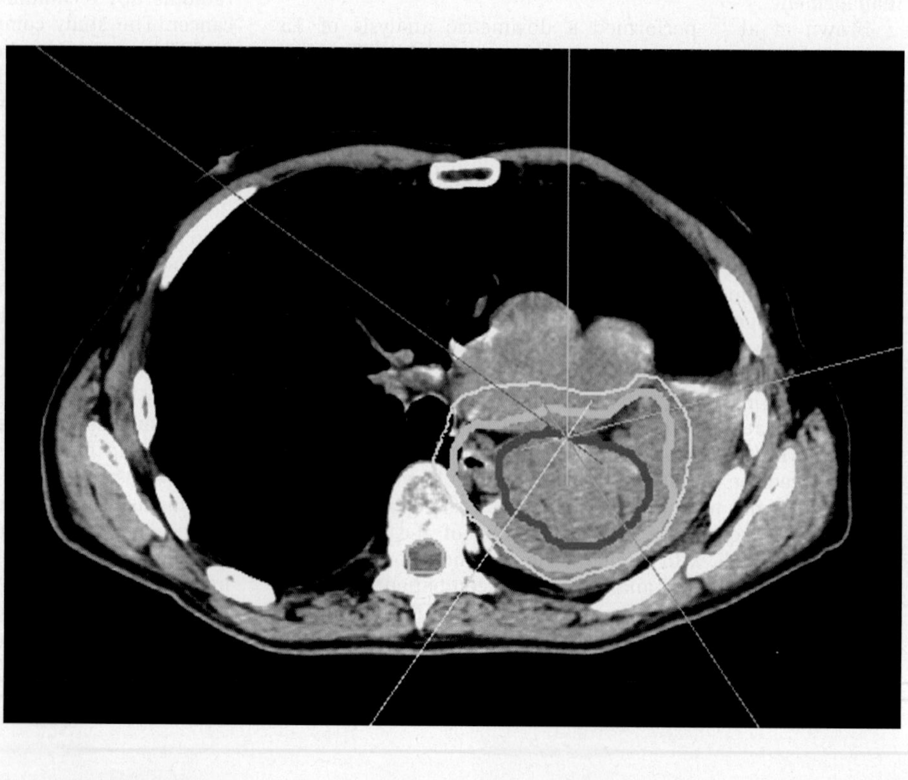

FIGURE 10.20. Intensity-modulated radiation therapy (IMRT) plan for locally advanced non–small-cell lung cancer. Inner red line is the gross tumor volume (GTV); clinical tumor volume (CTV) is shown as a light blue aqua contour, which includes nodal regions to left of the GTV. The outermost yellow contour is the 60 Gy isodose line.

require better ability to image the biologic activity of malignancies, and this is an area of very active research. It is incumbent on radiation oncologists to continue to document improved clinical outcomes with IMRT in the peer-reviewed literature if we wish to justify the use of this expensive technology to our communities in an era of skyrocketing medical costs.

SELECTED REFERENCES

A full list of references for this chapter is available online.

1. ICRU. ICRU report 83: prescribing, recording, and reporting photon-beam intensity-modulated radiation therapy (IMRT). *J ICRU* 2010;10(1):1–106.
2. Bernier J, Hall EJ, Giaccia A. Timeline - radiation oncology: a century of achievements. *Nat Rev Cancer* 2004;4(9):737–747.
3. Carol MP. Peacock (TM) - a system for planning and rotational delivery of intensity-modulated fields. *Int J Imag Syst Technol* 1995;6(1):56–61.
4. Ling CC, Burman C, Chui CS, et al. Conformal radiation treatment of prostate cancer using inversely-planned intensity-modulated photon beams produced with dynamic multileaf collimation. *Int J Radiat Oncol Biol Phys* 1996;35(4):721–730.
8. Bortfeld T, Schlegel W. Optimization of beam orientations in radiation therapy: some theoretical considerations. *Phys Med Biol* 1993;38(2):291–304.
9. Webb S. Optimizing the planning of intensity-modulated radiotherapy. *Phys Med Biol* 1994;39(12):2229–2246.
10. Sodertrom S, Brahme A. Optimization of the dose delivery in a few field techniques using radiobiological objective functions. *Med Phys* 1993;20(4):1201–1210.
12. Lauve A, Morris M, Schmidt-Ullrich R, et al. Simultaneous integrated boost intensity-modulated radiotherapy for locally advanced head-and-neck squamous cell carcinomas: II–clinical results. *Int J Radiat Oncol Biol Phys* 2004;60(2):374–387.
13. Orlandi E, Palazzi M, Pignoli E, et al. Radiobiological basis and clinical results of the simultaneous integrated boost (SIB) in intensity modulated radiotherapy (IMRT) for head and neck cancer: a review. *Crit Rev Oncol Hematol* 2010;73(2):111–125.
14. Mechalakos J, Lee N, Hunt M, et al. The effect of significant tumor reduction on the dose distribution in intensity modulated radiation therapy for head-and-neck cancer: a case study. *Med Dosim* 2009;34(3):250–255.
19. Allison RR, Gay HA, Mota HC, et al. Image-guided radiation therapy: current and future directions. *Future Oncol (London, England)* 2006;2(4):477–492.
36. Mohan R, Ling CC, Stein J, et al. The number of beams in intensity-modulated treatments: in response to Drs. Soderstrom and Brahme. *Int J Radiat Oncol Biol Phys* 1996;34(3):758–759.
51. Jin JY, Wen N, Ren L, et al. Advances in treatment techniques arc-based and other intensity modulated therapies. *Cancer J* 2011;17(3):166–176.
55. Bradbury M, Hricak H. Molecular MR imaging in oncology. *Magn Reson Imag Clin N Am* 2005;13:225–240.
57. Apisarnthanarax S, Chao KSC. Current imaging paradigms in radiation oncology. *Radiat Res* 2005;163(1):1–25.
58. Frank SJ, Chao KSC, Schwartz DL, et al. Technology insight: PET and PET/CT in head and neck tumor staging and radiation therapy planning. *Nat Clin Pract Oncol* 2005;2(10):526–533.
59. Cheebsumon P, Yaqub M, van Velden FHP, et al. Impact of (18)F FDG PET imaging parameters on automatic tumour delineation: need for improved tumour delineation methodology. *Eur J Nucl Med Mol Imaging* 2011;38(12):2136–2144.
68. Webb S. The physical basis of IMRT and inverse planning. *Br J Radiol* 2003; 76(910):678–689.
69. Ehrgott M, Guler C, Hamacher HW, et al. Mathematical optimization in intensity modulated radiation therapy. *Ann Operations Res* 2010;175(1):309–365.
76. Mackie TR. History of tomotherapy. *Phys Med Biol* 2006;51(13):R427–R453.
85. Fowler JF. The linear-quadratic formula and progress in fractionated radiotherapy. *Br J Radiol* 1989;62(740):679–694.
140. van Etmpt W, McDermott L, Nijsten S, et al. A literature review of electronic portal imaging for radiotherapy dosimetry. *Radiother Oncol* 2008;88(3):289–309.
141. Bailat CJ, Baechler S, Moeckli R, et al. The concept and challenges of TomoTherapy accelerators. *Rep Prog Phys* 2011;74(8).
146. Kuppersmith RB, Greco SC, Teh BS, et al. Intensity-modulated radiotherapy: first results with this new technology on neoplasms of the head and neck. *Ear Nose Throat J* 1999;78(4):238, 241–236, 248 passim.
147. Butler EB, Teh BS, Grant WH, 3rd, et al. Smart (simultaneous modulated accelerated radiation therapy) boost: a new accelerated fractionation schedule for the treatment of head and neck cancer with intensity modulated radiotherapy. *Int J Radiat Oncol Biol Phys* 1999;45(1):21–32.
148. Gielda BT, Shah AP, Marsh JC, et al. Helical tomotherapy delivery of an IMRT boost in lieu of interstitial brachytherapy in the setting of gynecologic malignancy: feasibility and dosimetric comparison. *Med Dosim* 2011;36(2):206–212.
149. Low DA, Chao KS, Mutic S, et al. Quality assurance of serial tomotherapy for head and neck patient treatments. *Int J Radiat Oncol Biol Phys* 1998;42(3):681–692.
150. Chao KS, Deasy JO, Markman J, et al. A prospective study of salivary function sparing in patients with head-and-neck cancers receiving intensity-modulated or three-dimensional radiation therapy: initial results. *Int J Radiat Oncol Biol Phys* 2001;49(4):907–916.
151. Chao KS, Majhail N, Huang CJ, et al. Intensity-modulated radiation therapy reduces late salivary toxicity without compromising tumor control in patients with oropharyngeal carcinoma: a comparison with conventional techniques. *Radiother Oncol* 2001;61(3):275–280.
152. Cheng JC, Chao KS, Low D. Comparison of intensity modulated radiation therapy (IMRT) treatment techniques for nasopharyngeal carcinoma. *Int J Cancer* 2001;96(2):126–131.
153. Hunt MA, Zelefsky MJ, Wolden S, et al. Treatment planning and delivery of intensity-modulated radiation therapy for primary nasopharynx cancer. *Int J Radiat Oncol Biol Phys* 2001;49(3):623–632.
154. Lee N, Xia P, Quivey JM, et al. Intensity-modulated radiotherapy in the treatment of nasopharyngeal carcinoma: an update of the UCSF experience. *Int J Radiat Oncol Biol Phys* 2002;53(1):12–22.
155. Claus F, Duthoy W, Boterberg T, et al. Intensity modulated radiation therapy for oropharyngeal and oral cavity tumors: clinical use and experience. *Oral Oncol* 2002;38(6):597–604.
156. Lee NY, Terezakis SA. Intensity-modulated radiation therapy. *J Surg Oncol* 2008; 97(8):691–696.
157. Maingon P, Marchesi V, Crehange G. Intensity modulated radiation therapy. *Bull Cancer* 2010;97(7):759–768.
158. Lu HM, Yao M. The current status of intensity-modulated radiation therapy in the treatment of nasopharyngeal carcinoma. *Cancer Treat Rev* 2008;34(1):27–36.
159. Scott-Brown M, Miah A, Harrington K, et al. Evidence-based review: quality of life following head and neck intensity-modulated radiotherapy. *Radiother Oncol* 2010;97(2):249–257.
160. Tribius S, Bergelt C. Intensity-modulated radiotherapy versus conventional and 3D conformal radiotherapy in patients with head and neck cancer: is there a worthwhile quality of life gain? *Cancer Treat Rev* 2011;37(7):511–519.
161. Roe JWG, Carding PN, Dwivedi RC, et al. Swallowing outcomes following intensity modulated radiation therapy (IMRT) for head & neck cancer - a systematic review. *Oral Oncol* 2010;46(10):727–733.
162. Nutting CM, Morden JP, Harrington KJ, et al. Parotid-sparing intensity modulated versus conventional radiotherapy in head and neck cancer (PARSPORT): a phase 3 multicentre randomised controlled trial. *Lancet Oncol* 2011;12(2):127–136.
163. Boda-Heggemann J, Lohr F, Wenz F, et al. kV cone-beam CT-based IGRT: a clinical review. *Strahlenther Onkol* 2011;187(5):284–291.
164. Ling CC, Gerweck LE, Zaider M, et al. Dose-rate effects in external beam radiotherapy redux. *Radiother Oncol* 2010;95(3):261–268.
166. Chakraborty S, Ghoshal S, Patil V, et al. Acute toxicities experienced during simultaneous integrated boost intensity-modulated radiotherapy in head and neck cancers - experience from a North Indian regional cancer centre. *Clin Oncol* 2009;21(9):676–686.
167. Wirth LJ, Posner MR. Recent advances in combined modality therapy for locally advanced head and neck cancer. *Curr Cancer Drug Targets* 2007;7(7):674–680.
168. Seiwert TY, Salama JK, Vokes EE. The chemoradiation paradigm in head and neck cancer. *Nat Clin Pract Oncol* 2007;4(3):156–171.
169. Okunieff P, Kachnic LA, Constine LS, et al. Report from the Radiation Therapy Committee of the Southwest Oncology Group (SWOG): Research Objectives Workshop 2008. *Clin Cancer Res* 2009;15(18):5663–5670.
170. Riesterer O, Milas L, Ang KK. Combining molecular therapeutics with radiotherapy for head and neck cancer. *J Surg Oncol* 2008;97(8):708–711.
171. Thariat J, Bolle S, Demizu Y, et al. New techniques in radiation therapy for head and neck cancer: IMRT, CyberKnife, protons, and carbon ions. Improved effectiveness and safety? Impact on survival? *Anticancer Drugs* 2011;22(7):596–606.
173. Zelefsky MJ, Fuks Z, Hunt M, et al. High-dose intensity modulated radiation therapy for prostate cancer: early toxicity and biochemical outcome in 772 patients. *Int J Radiat Oncol Biol Phys* 2002;53(5):1111–1116.
176. Guckenberger M, Flentje M. Intensity-modulated radiotherapy (IMRT) of localized prostate cancer - a review and future perspectives. *Strahlenther Onkol* 2007;183(2):57–62.
177. Hatano K, Araki H, Sakai M, et al. Current status of intensity-modulated radiation therapy (IMRT). *Int J Clin Oncol* 2007;12(6):408–415.
178. Shridhar R, Bolton S, Joiner MC, et al. Dose escalation using a hypofractionated, intensity-modulated radiation therapy boost for localized prostate cancer: preliminary results addressing concerns of high or low alpha/beta ratio. *Clin Genitourinary Cancer* 2009;7(3):E52–E57.
179. Sanfilippo N, Hardee ME, Wallach J. Review of chemoradiotherapy for high-risk prostate cancer. *Rev Recent Clin Trials* 2011;6(1):64–68.
181. Tucker SL, Thames HD, Michalski JM, et al. Estimation of alpha/beta for late rectal toxicity based on RTOG 94-06. *Int J Radiat Oncol Biol Phys* 2011;81(2):600–605.
182. Sciarra A, Barentsz J, Bjartell A, et al. Advances in magnetic resonance imaging: how they are changing the management of prostate cancer. *Eur Urol* 2011;59(6):962–977.
183. Mazaheri Y, Shukla-Dave A, Muellner A, et al. MRI of the prostate: clinical relevance and emerging applications. *J Magn Reson Imaging* 2011;33(2):258–274.
184. Gutierrez AN, Westerly DC, Tome WA, et al. Whole brain radiotherapy with hippocampal avoidance and simultaneously integrated brain metastases boost: a planning study. *Int J Radiat Oncol Biol Phys* 2007;69(2):589–597.
185. Iuchi T, Hatano K, Narita Y, et al. Hypofractionated high-dose irradiation for the treatment of malignant astrocytomas using simultaneous integrated boost technique by IMRT. *Int J Radiat Oncol Biol Phys* 2006;64(5):1317–1324.
186. Huang E, Teh BS, Strother DR, et al. Intensity-modulated radiation therapy for pediatric medulloblastoma: early report on the reduction of ototoxicity. *Int J Radiat Oncol Biol Phys* 2002;52(3):599–605.
188. Floyd NS, Woo SY, Teh BS, et al. Hypofractionated intensity-modulated radiotherapy for primary glioblastoma multiforme. *Int J Radiat Oncol Biol Phys* 2004;58(3):721–726.
189. Stupp R, Mason WP, van den Bent MJ, et al. Radiotherapy plus concomitant and adjuvant temozolomide for glioblastoma. *N Engl J Med* 2005;352(10):987–996.
190. Koukourakis GV, Kouloulias V, Zacharias G, et al. Temozolomide with radiation therapy in high grade brain gliomas: pharmaceuticals considerations and efficacy; a review article. *Molecules* 2009;14(4):1561–1577.
191. Amelio D, Lorentini S, Schwarz M, et al. Intensity-modulated radiation therapy in newly diagnosed glioblastoma: a systematic review on clinical and technical issues. *Radiother Oncol* 2010;97(3):361–369.
192. Taylor CW, Nisbet A, McGale P, et al. Cardiac exposures in breast cancer radiotherapy: 1950s-1990s. *Int J Radiat Oncol Biol Phys* 2007;69(5):1484–1495.
193. Guerrero Urbano MTG, Nutting CM. Clinical use of intensity-modulated radiotherapy: part II. *Br J Radiol* 2004;77(915):177–182.
194. Cho BC, Schwarz M, Mijnheer BJ, et al. Simplified intensity-modulated radiotherapy using pre-defined segments to reduce cardiac complications in left-sided breast cancer. *Radiother Oncol* 2004;70(3):231–241.
195. Evans PM, Donovan EM, Partridge M, et al. The delivery of intensity modulated radiotherapy to the breast using multiple static fields. *Radiother Oncol* 2000;57(1):79–89.
196. Hong L, Hunt M, Chui C, et al. Intensity-modulated tangential beam irradiation of the intact breast. *Int J Radiat Oncol Biol Phys* 1999;44(5):1155–1164.
197. Li JG, Williams SS, Goffinet DR, et al. Breast-conserving radiation therapy using combined electron and intensity-modulated radiotherapy technique. *Radiother Oncol* 2000;56(1):65–71.

198. Remouchamps VM, Vicini FA, Sharpe MB, et al. Significant reductions in heart and lung doses using deep inspiration breath hold with active breathing control and intensity-modulated radiation therapy for patients treated with locoregional breast irradiation. *Int J Radiat Oncol Biol Phys* 2003;55(2):392–406.
200. van Asselen B, Raaijmakers CP, Hofman P, et al. An improved breast irradiation technique using three-dimensional geometrical information and intensity modulation. *Radiother Oncol* 2001;58(3):341–347.
201. Hurkmans CW, Cho BC, Damen E, et al. Reduction of cardiac and lung complication probabilities after breast irradiation using conformal radiotherapy with or without intensity modulation. *Radiother Oncol* 2002;62(2):163–171.
203. Landau D, Adams EJ, Webb S, et al. Cardiac avoidance in breast radiotherapy: a comparison of simple shielding techniques with intensity-modulated radiotherapy. *Radiother Oncol* 2001;60(3):247–255.
204. Taylor CW, Povall JM, McGale P, et al. Cardiac dose from tangential breast cancer radiotherapy in the year 2006. *Int J Radiat Oncol Biol Phys* 2008;72(2):501–507.
205. Taylor A, Rockall AG, Reznek RH, et al. Mapping pelvic lymph nodes: guidelines for delineation in intensity-modulated radiotherapy. *Int J Radiat Oncol Biol Phys* 2005;63(5):1604–1612.
206. Ahamad A, D'Souza W, Salehpour M, et al. Intensity-modulated radiation therapy after hysterectomy: comparison with conventional treatment and sensitivity of the normal-tissue-sparing effect to margin size. *Int J Radiat Oncol Biol Phys* 2005;62(4):1117–1124.
207. D'Souza WD, Ahamad AA, Iyer RB, et al. Feasibility of dose escalation using intensity-modulated radiotherapy in posthysterectomy cervical carcinoma. *Int J Radiat Oncol Biol Phys* 2005;61(4):1062–1070.
208. Salama JK, Mundt AJ, Roeske J, et al. Preliminary outcome and toxicity report of extended-field, intensity-modulated radiation therapy for gynecologic malignancies. *Int J Radiat Oncol Biol Phys* 2006;65(4):1170–1176.
209. Portelance L, Chao KS, Grigsby PW, et al. Intensity-modulated radiation therapy (IMRT) reduces small bowel, rectum, and bladder doses in patients with cervical cancer receiving pelvic and para-aortic irradiation. *Int J Radiat Oncol Biol Phys* 2001;51(1):261–266.
210. Mundt AJ, Lujan AE, Rotmensch J, et al. Intensity-modulated whole pelvic radiotherapy in women with gynecologic malignancies. *Int J Radiat Oncol Biol Phys* 2002;52(5):1330–1337.
211. Portelance L, Moughan J, Jhingran A, et al. A phase II multi-institutional study of postoperative pelvic intensity modulated radiation therapy (IMRT) with weekly cisplatin in patients with cervical carcinoma: two year efficacy results of the RTOG 0418. *Int J Radiat Oncol Biol Phys* 2011;81(2):S3 (abstr.).
212. Ring KL, Young JL, Dunlap NE, et al. Extended-field radiation therapy with whole pelvis radiotherapy and cisplatin chemosensitization in the treatment of IB2-IIIB cervical carcinoma: a retrospective review. *Am J Obstet Gynecol* 2009;201(1):6.
214. Showalter TN, Winter KA, Berger AC, et al. The influence of total nodes examined, number of positive nodes, and lymph node ratio on survival after surgical resection and adjuvant chemoradiation for pancreatic cancer: a secondary analysis of RTOG 9704. *Int J Radiat Oncol Biol Phys* 2011;81(5):1328–1335.
215. Crane CH, Antolak JA, Rosen, II, et al. Phase I study of concomitant gemcitabine and IMRT for patients with unresectable adenocarcinoma of the pancreatic head. *Int J Gastrointest Cancer* 2001;30(3):123–132.
216. Ben-Josef E, Shields AF, Vaishampayan U, et al. Intensity-modulated radiotherapy (IMRT) and concurrent capecitabine for pancreatic cancer. *Int J Radiat Oncol Biol Phys* 2004;59(2):454–459.
217. Brown MW, Ning H, Arora B, et al. A dosimetric analysis of dose escalation using two intensity-modulated radiation therapy techniques in locally advanced pancreatic carcinoma. *Int J Radiat Oncol Biol Phys* 2006;65(1):274–283.
218. Yovino S, Poppe M, Jabbour S, et al. Intensity-modulated radiation therapy significantly improves acute gastrointestinal toxicity in pancreatic and ampullary cancers. *Int J Radiat Oncol Biol Phys* 2011;79(1):158–162.
219. Bockbrader M, Kim E. Role of intensity-modulated radiation therapy in gastrointestinal cancer. *Exp Rev Anticancer Ther* 2009;9(5):637–647.
220. Meyer JJ, Willett CG, Czito BG. Emerging role of intensity-modulated radiation therapy in anorectal cancer. *Exp Rev Anticancer Ther* 2008;8(4):585–593.
221. Guerrero Urbano MT, Henrys AJ, Adams EJ, et al. Intensity-modulated radiotherapy in patients with locally advanced rectal cancer reduces volume of bowel treated to high dose levels. *Int J Radiat Oncol Biol Phys* 2006;65(3):907–916.
222. Milano MT, Jani AB, Farrey KJ, et al. Intensity-modulated radiation therapy (IMRT) in the treatment of anal cancer: toxicity and clinical outcome. *Int J Radiat Oncol Biol Phys* 2005;63(2):354–361.
224. Alasti H, Cho YB, Vandermeer AD, et al. A novel four-dimensional radiotherapy method for lung cancer: imaging, treatment planning and delivery. *Phys Med Biol* 2006;51(12):3251–3267.
225. Starkschall G, Balter P, Britton K, et al. Interfractional reproducibility of lung tumor location using various methods of respiratory motion mitigation. *Int J Radiat Oncol Biol Phys* 2011;79(2):596–601.
226. Byhardt RW, Scott C, Sause WT, et al. Response, toxicity, failure patterns, and survival in five Radiation Therapy Oncology Group (RTOG) trials of sequential and/or concurrent chemotherapy and radiotherapy for locally advanced non-small-cell carcinoma of the lung. *Int J Radiat Oncol Biol Phys* 1998;42(3):469–478.
227. Holloway CL, Robinson D, Murray B, et al. Results of a phase I study to dose escalate using intensity modulated radiotherapy guided by combined PET/CT imaging with induction chemotherapy for patients with non-small cell lung cancer. *Radiother Oncol* 2004;73(3):285–287.
228. Murshed H, Liu HH, Liao Z, et al. Dose and volume reduction for normal lung using intensity-modulated radiotherapy for advanced-stage non-small-cell lung cancer. *Int J Radiat Oncol Biol Phys* 2004;58(4):1258–1267.
229. Grills IS, Yan D, Martinez AA, et al. Potential for reduced toxicity and dose escalation in the treatment of inoperable non-small-cell lung cancer: a comparison of intensity-modulated radiation therapy (IMRT), 3D conformal radiation, and elective nodal irradiation. *Int J Radiat Oncol Biol Phys* 2003;57(3):875–890.
230. Liao ZX, Komaki RR, Thames HD Jr, et al. Influence of technologic advances on outcomes in patients with unresectable, locally advanced non-small-cell lung cancer receiving concomitant chemoradiotherapy. *Int J Radiat Oncol Biol Phys* 2010;76(3):775–781.
231. Vogelius IR, Westerly DC, Aznar MC, et al. Estimated radiation pneumonitis risk after photon versus proton therapy alone or combined with chemotherapy for lung cancer. *Acta Oncol* 2011;50(6):772–776.
232. Vogelius IS, Westerly DC, Cannon GM, et al. Intensity-modulated radiotherapy might increase pneumonitis risk relative to three-dimensional conformal radiotherapy in patients receiving combined chemotherapy and radiotherapy: a modeling study of dose dumping. *Int J Radiat Oncol Biol Phys* 2011;80(3):893–899.

Chapter 11
Image-Guided Radiation Therapy

Loren K. Mell, William Y. Song, Todd Pawlicki, and Arno J. Mundt

Image-guided radiation therapy (IGRT) consists of a panoply of technological applications with the common purpose of maximizing target and normal tissue localization for radiotherapy. The exact subset of applications that defines IGRT is somewhat controversial. Proposed definitions of IGRT have ranged from narrow ("external beam radiation therapy with positional verification using imaging prior to each treatment fraction"[1]) to broad ("any use of imaging to aid in decisions in the radiotherapy process"[2]), the former risking the exclusion of techniques as *avant garde* as adaptive four-dimensional (4D) positron emission tomography (PET), and the latter risking the inclusion of techniques as banal as a staging chest x-ray. The American College of Radiology and American Society of Radiation Oncology practice guideline defines IGRT as "a procedure that refines the delivery of therapeutic radiation by applying image-based target relocalization to allow proper patient repositioning for the purpose of ensuring accurate treatment and minimizing the volume of normal tissue exposed to ionizing radiation,"[3] while Greco and Ling[4] defined IGRT more broadly as "the use of imaging for detection and diagnosis, delineation of target and organs at risk (OARs), determining biological attributes, dose distribution design, dose delivery assurance, and deciphering treatment response," a so-called six-dimensional definition. For the purposes of this chapter, the authors also favor a broader perspective and define IGRT as the use of innovative imaging modalities to augment target and normal tissue localization for radiotherapy planning and delivery. This encompasses a wide range of imaging techniques used for delineation, adjusting for motion or positional uncertainty, and adapting treatment to response. Exploring IGRT in its many facets leaves one simultaneously awed by the pace and extent of technological achievements, yet daunted by the task of critically assessing their tangible benefits to patients.

RATIONALE FOR IMAGE-GUIDED RADIATION THERAPY

Increasing the accuracy and precision of radiotherapy delivery has always been a therapeutic goal. *Inaccuracy* refers to systematic errors that, on average, bias the treatment delivery with respect to the true target location. Systematic errors can originate, for example, from improper target delineation, poorly representative simulation, dissociation between skin marks and internal anatomy, or predictable organ motions (e.g., periodicity of a lung tumor). *Imprecision,* on the other hand, refers to stochastic (random) errors that introduce variance in the spatial location of treatment around the true target. Stochastic errors can originate, for example, from inevitable fluctuations in daily setup and from unpredictable target motions (e.g., uterine anteversion or retroversion). Insufficient compensation for these uncertainties leads to target underdosing and overdosing of nearby OARs, whereas overcompensation for uncertainties leads to unnecessary irradiation of normal tissue and constraints in treatment planning. This creates a tradeoff between tumor control probability (TCP) and normal tissue complication probability (NTCP) and emphasizes the role of minimizing uncertainties to enhance the therapeutic ratio of radiation.

Uncertainty in target delineation is a well-documented problem.[5,6] Even among experts, reproducibly defining targets is a challenge, as both intra- and interobserver variation contribute to ambiguity in target localization, and existing guidelines for target delineation are predominantly based on qualitative judgments. Furthermore, while computed tomography (CT) and magnetic resonance imaging (MRI) have become standard for 3D planning, functional imaging techniques—particularly PET—have been increasingly incorporated into treatment planning[7] to facilitate demarcation of tumor borders and characterize subregions of targets with different physiologic properties. Quantitative imaging can help raise consistency in target delineation, while automated segmentation and deformable image registration software are becoming increasingly available to facilitate and standardize treatment planning.

The use of conformal and hypofractionated radiotherapy techniques, with prolonged treatment times and steeper dose gradients, accentuates the effects of uncertainties related to target localization and the need for IGRT to compensate for them. Toxicity is often an important barrier to treatment intensification, including radiation dose escalation and intensive combined modality therapy. By mitigating toxicity, IGRT may permit implementation of more intensive, but isotoxic, treatment approaches. Furthermore, as therapies continue to improve tumor control, the importance of reducing late and chronic effects of radiotherapy becomes increasingly imperative to maximize patients' quality of life. Determining the functional relation between IGRT, changes in tumor and OAR dose, and changes in clinical outcomes (e.g., TCP and NTCP models) are of critical importance in evaluating the effectiveness of IGRT techniques compared to standard approaches. There is a rapidly growing need for validated models to estimate the impact of IGRT on *cumulative* dose distributions and the corresponding effects of cumulative dose on TCP and NTCP.

Conventional radiotherapy techniques are limited due to motion and changes of both tumor and normal tissues occurring between (*inter*fraction) or during (*intra*fraction) treatment. In many situations, the treatment model based on a static initial simulation is inadequate, necessitating adaptation of the initial plan. In particular, changes that occur in response to therapy could be indicative of a more or less favorable prognosis, in which case modifications to the treatment strategy could be considered. Theoretically, adaptive radiotherapy can take place either between fractions (offline) or while the patient is in the treatment position (online). Innovative strategies to monitor and optimize therapy throughout the treatment course, such as 4D PET-CT, in-room MRI, and fast online adaptive replanning, ideally will advance the quality of radiotherapy for current and future generations.

IMAGE-GUIDED TARGET AND NORMAL TISSUE DELINEATION

Positron Emission Tomography

PET has revolutionized the staging and treatment of cancer. PET scanning involves the systemic administration of a tracer labeled with a radioactive isotope, which emits positrons as it decays. The tracer accumulates in a region of interest and the emitted positron annihilates with a local negatron, releasing two 511 keV photons that propagate in 180 degrees opposite directions. The scanner is equipped with parallel mounted sensors that can detect and determine the spatial location of these annihilation events and, therefore, the regions of increased radiotracer accumulation. Most modern treatment planning systems offer tools to facilitate image registration and fusion with the planning CT to aid target delineation. Commercial software systems that incorporate deformable image registration can aid delineation by accommodating changes in patient anatomy and positioning between scans and segmenting target volumes based on quantitative methods (Fig. 11.1).[6,8]

F18-Fluorodeoxyglucose

The most widely used tracer is F18-fluorodeoxyglucose (^{18}F-FDG), which is taken into cells by active transport, then phosphorylated by hexokinase, trapping the molecule intracellularly. ^{18}F decays to ^{18}O, and the molecule enters the

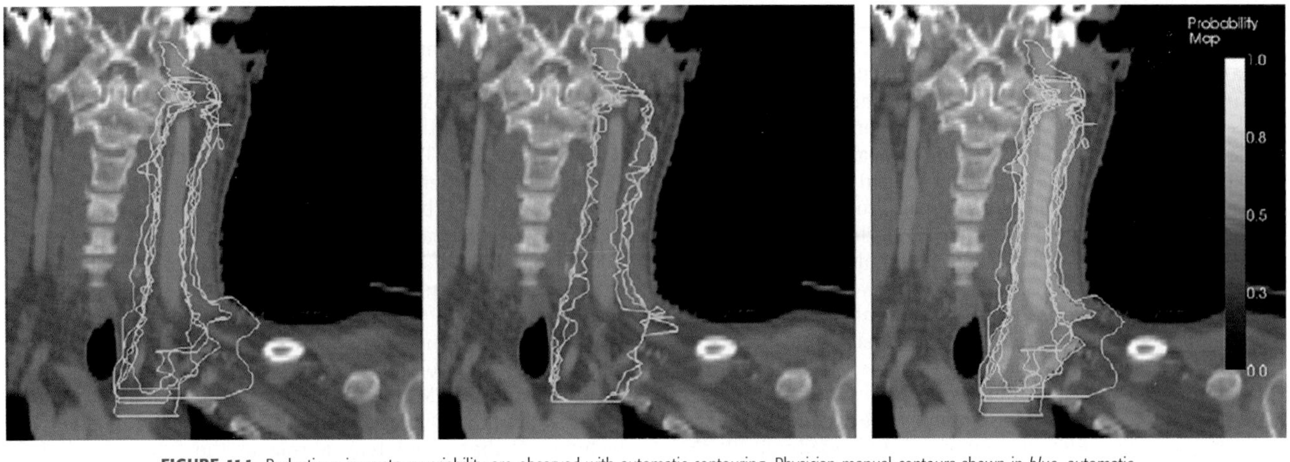

FIGURE 11.1. Reductions in contour variability are observed with automatic contouring. Physician manual contours shown in *blue,* automatic contours modified by physicians shown in *purple,* and manual contours using Simultaneous Truth and Performance Level Estimation algorithm shown in *brown.* (From Stapleford LJ, Lawson JD, Perkins C, et al. Evaluation of automatic atlas-based lymph node segmentation for head-and-neck cancer. *Int J Radiat Oncol Biol Phys* 2010;77:959–966, with permission from Elsevier.)

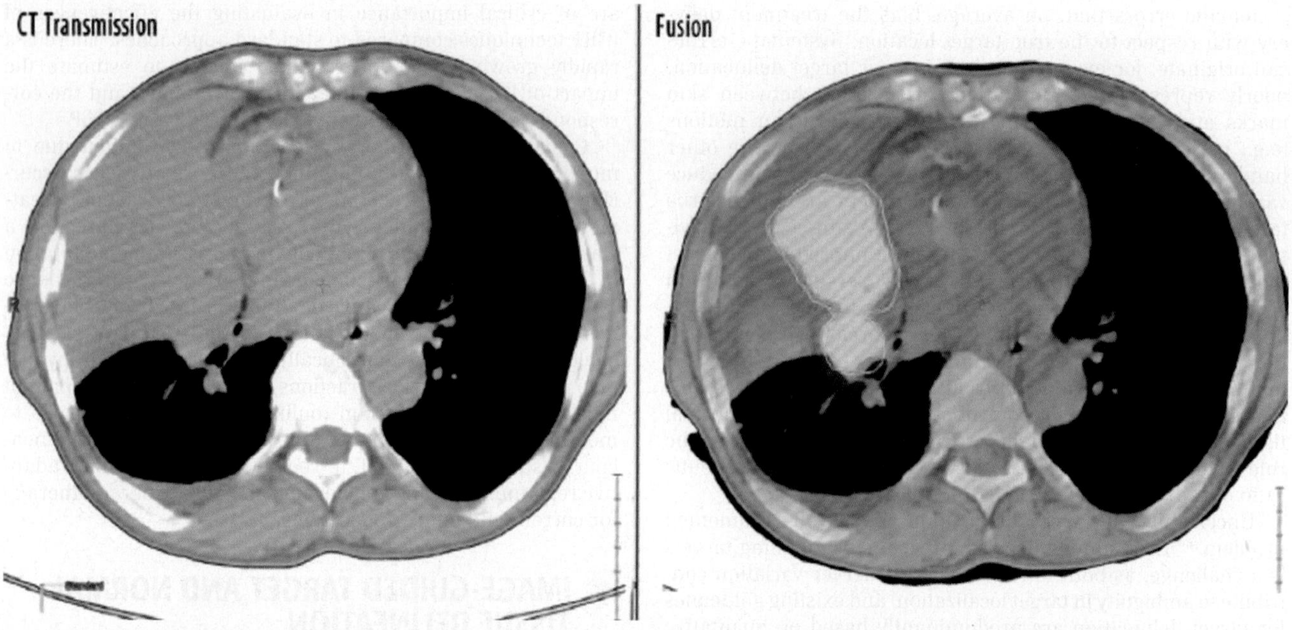

FIGURE 11.2. Fluorodeoxyglucose (FDG) positron emission tomography–computed tomography (PET-CT) scan in a patient with a right middle lobe lung carcinoma. On CT[MB15] (*left*), the limits of the tumor are obscured by postobstructive pneumonia and atelectasis. On the fused scan (*right*), the tumor is intensely FDG avid and more easily differentiated. (From Spratt DE, Diaz R, McElmurray J, et al. Impact of FDG PET/CT on delineation of the gross tumor volume for radiation planning in non-small-cell lung cancer. *Clin Nucl Med* 2010;35:237-243, with permission.)

glycolytic pathway, but the metabolism of FDG is slow relative to normal glucose, accounting for the high relative accumulation in metabolically active cells, including inflammatory tissue, neurons, brown fat, bone marrow, gastrointestinal (GI) epithelium, and tumors.[9] Studies in many different types of cancer have found that FDG-PET improves staging,[10–11,12,13,14] leading to more appropriate risk-adapted management. Other studies have found that increased FDG uptake within tumors prior to or following treatment confers an adverse prognosis,[15,16,17] indicating subsets of patients suitable for alternative treatment strategies.

Multiple studies have investigated the role of FDG-PET in radiotherapy planning for lung cancer.[18–23] FDG-PET imaging alters treatment volumes in approximately 40% to 60% of non–small cell lung cancer (NSCLC) patients[19,21,23,24]; it appears to aid targeting for mesothelioma as well.[25] It is valuable both for detection of occult nodal involvement and for distinguishing tumor from atelectasis,[19,26] which can be difficult to detect on CT alone (Fig. 11.2). Vanuytsel et al.[21] found that FDG PET-CT altered treatment volumes in 45 of 73 (62%) lymph node–positive patients staged by mediastinoscopy; in 16 the volume was enlarged, and in 29 it was contracted. Results of the Radiation Therapy Oncology Group's (RTOG) study RTOG-0515, a phase II trial with 52 NSCLC patients, were recently reported[22]; incorporation of FDG PET-CT led to alterations in nodal volumes in 51% of the 47 evaluable patients and in general led to smaller tumor gross tumor volumes (GTV) and mean lung dose. There is no definite consensus on how PET-guided volumes should be delineated, although PET does appear to improve interobserver target definitions.[18] Yu et al.[24] reported that the optimal standardized uptake value (SUV) threshold correlating with pathologic specimens was 31% ± 11%. However, recent studies in both phantoms and patients indicate that gradient-based methods may be a more accurate and consistent technique for target volume contouring.[8,27]

Studies of FDG PET in head and neck cancer (HNC) have similarly found that planning volumes are frequently altered after incorporating PET imaging.[23,28–35] In a study of 40 HNC patients, Paulino et al.[30] compared IMRT plans based on FDG PET to those based on CT. In 25% of patients, CT-based plans were suboptimal in covering the PET-delineated GTV. In a prospective analysis of 20 patients, Schwartz et al.[32] found that IMRT plans could be optimized with FDG PET-CT to improve parotid and laryngeal sparing and allow dose escalation up to 81 Gy. A study from Memorial Sloan-Kettering Cancer Center found significant differences in target volumes drawn with and without PET or MRI guidance, indicating complementary information comes from multiple sources, including CT and physical examination, and is necessary to optimally tailor target delineation for each patient.[33] GTVs delineated by FDG PET appear to be significantly smaller than those delineated on CT alone.[33–35] Some concerns exist regarding the technical aspects of PET-guided radiation therapy (RT) in HNC, including difficulties in establishing optimal image registration[36] and large variability in target definition.[37] Recent studies indicate that automated techniques to guide delineation in HNC can improve consistency,[6,38,39] however, target delineation is still highly dependent on both segmentation and reconstruction methods, emphasizing the importance of clarifying and standardizing methodologies across institutions.[40,41]

FDG PET for target delineation has been extensively studied in both esophageal[14,42,43–47] and rectal[48,49–52] cancers. Hong et al.[44] studied 25 esophageal cancer patients undergoing FDG PET-CT for radiotherapy planning; PET influenced target delineation in 21 patients (84%), with changes classified as major in 9 (34%). However, Muijs et al.[14] reviewed 30 studies spanning 1,222 patients and found no conclusive evidence supporting the necessity of PET for radiotherapy planning. It is clear that PET is helpful in determining lymph node status and detecting occult metastases, but whether it is superior to other modalities for GTV delineation remains unclear. If used to delineate GTV, a threshold of 2.5 for either absolute SUV or SUV relative to liver uptake has been proposed.[47] As for rectal cancer, Braendengen et al.[48] compared GTV delineation with MRI versus FDG PET-CT in 77 patients; PET-guided volumes were smaller than MRI volumes, but PET-guidance appeared to complement data from MRI and led to alteration of management in 15% of patients. Dynamic FDG PET-CT is also an emerging technique[50] that could play a role in the future for image-guided target delineation for rectal and other cancers.

Researchers at Washington University have extensively studied FDG PET for cervical cancer.[53–55] PET-guided targeting for cervical cancer patients with involved para-aortic lymph nodes can facilitate safe dose escalation to 60 Gy along with intensity-modulated radiation therapy (IMRT).[53] Serial changes in cervical tumor volume during brachytherapy[54] and external beam RT[55] have been documented, but it is unclear yet how treatment should be adapted in the face of poor response. Lin et al.[56] reported that FDG PET-based brachytherapy planning significantly optimized GTV coverage without increasing bladder or rectal dose. Liang et al.[57] analyzed 10 patients treated with FDG PET-guided bone marrow–sparing IMRT for pelvic malignancies in a prospective trial. IMRT plans significantly reduced dose to active bone marrow, and this approach was feasible and well tolerated. Related work by Rose et al.[58] has indicated that dose to metabolically active bone marrow subregions identified by FDG PET is a significant predictor of hematologic toxicity.

Studies of FDG PET for radiation planning in other disease sites have found mixed results. It has potential utility in contouring lumpectomy cavities in breast cancer,[59] involved nodal or involved field radiation therapy for lymphoma[60,61] and GTV for pancreatic cancer,[62] but less apparent utility in treating sarcoma.[63] Application of FDG PET in central nervous system (CNS) tumors is limited by high background uptake of FDG by normal brain cells, whereas its utility in prostate cancer is limited by relatively lower uptake of FDG in tumor cells. Douglas et al.[64] successfully used FDG PET in 40 patients for dose escalation in malignant glioma, however, no improvement in patient outcomes was observed. As discussed below, other PET tracers have been more extensively studied in these diseases.

Other Positron Emission Tomography Tracers

Although most studies to date have focused on FDG, many other radiotracers have been studied, including ^{18}F-thymidine (FLT), ^{18}F-misonidazole (MISO), ^{18}F-azomycin arabinoside (FAZA), ^{18}F-fluoroethyl-L-tyrosine (FET), ^{18}F-choline, ^{11}C-choline, ^{11}C-methionine (MET), ^{11}C-acetate, and ^{60}Cu(II)-diacetyl-bis(N^4-methylosemicarbazone) (^{60}Cu-ATSM). ^{15}O and ^{13}N—labeled H_2O, CO_2, O_2, or NH_3—molecules have also been used to measure blood flow, apoptosis, or hypoxia with PET.[65–67] New tracers are continually being developed and tested. For further discussion of novel molecular imaging applications, refer to several reviews.[65,66–68,69]

Background uptake of MET in neural tissue is low, making it useful for image-guided planning of brain tumors. Grosu et al.[70] analyzed 39 patients with glioblastoma multiforme (GBM); in 29 patients (74%), MET uptake extended (up to 4.5 cm) beyond the tumor identified by MRI. MET also appears to improve GTV delineation for skull-base meningiomas.[71] A limitation of MET PET, however, is the short half-life of ^{11}C (20 minutes). FET leads to different GTV compared to MRI alone[72] but appears to be comparable to MET (Fig. 11.3),[73] with the advantage of a longer isotope half-life. Milker-Zabel et al.[74] evaluated ^{68}Ga-(0)-D-Phe (1)-Tyr (221)-octreotide (DOTATOC) PET in 26 meningiomas patients. This technique takes advantage of high expression of the somatostatin type 2 receptor, which binds DOTATOC. In 19 patients, DOTATOC PET significantly influenced target design. Gehler et al.[75] found similar results, with DOTATOC PET-CT significantly influencing target volumes in 17 of 26 patients.

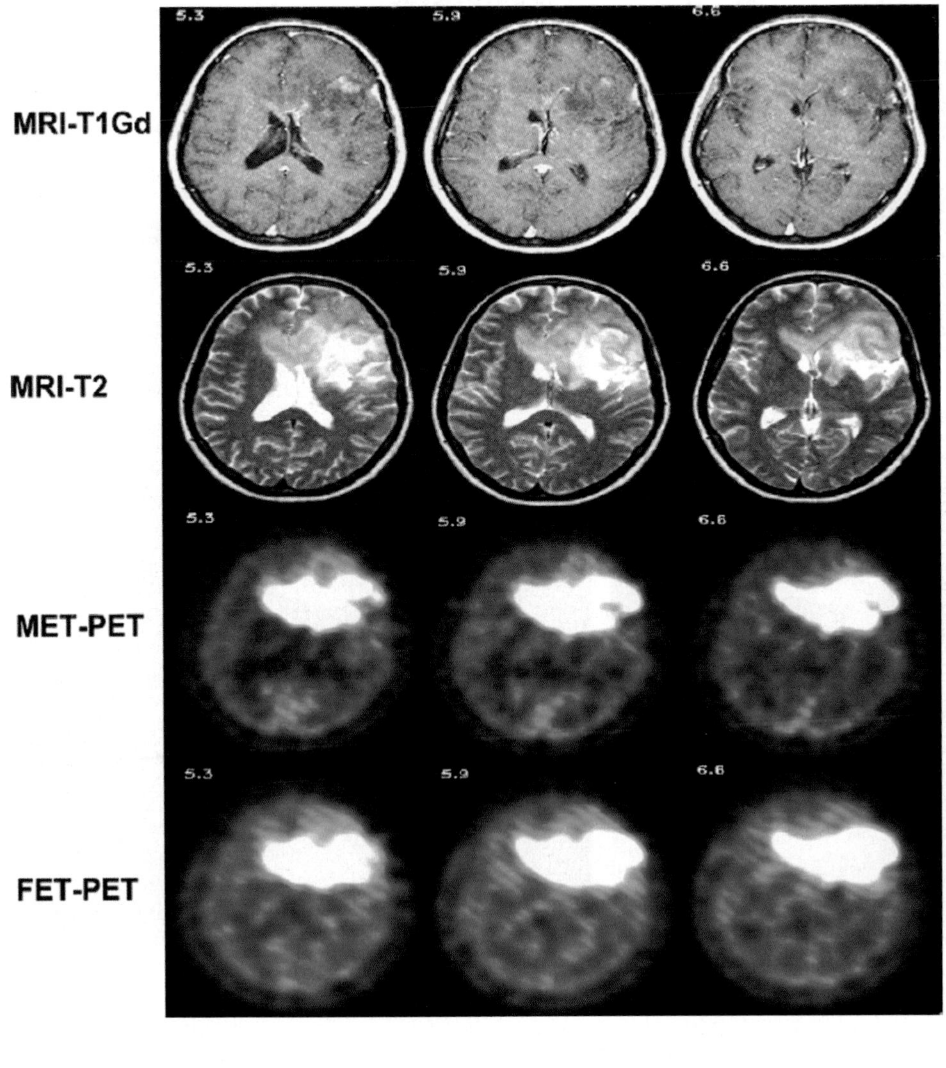

FIGURE 11.3. Comparison of magnetic resonance imaging, L-(methyl-11C)methionine positron emission tomography (PET_, and O-(2-[18F]fluoroethyl)-L-tyrosine PET for a patient with grade III astrocytoma. (From Grosu AL, Astner ST, Riedel E, et al. An interindividual comparison of O-(2-[18F]fluoroethyl)-L-tyrosine (FET)- and L-[methyl-11C]methionine (MET)-PET in patients with brain gliomas and metastases. *Int J Radiat Oncol Biol Phys* 2011;81:1049–1058, with permission from Elsevier.)

Several investigators have explored PET-guided RT using MISO[76,77] and FAZA.[78] The Trans-Tasman Radiation Oncology Group correlated hypoxia identified on MISO PET with outcomes in 45 stage III or IV HNC patients undergoing chemoradiotherapy, with or without the hypoxic cytotoxin tirapazamine.[77] Baseline hypoxia and residual hypoxia (detected on MISO PET scans at week 4 or 5 of treatment) were correlated with higher rates of locoregional failure. Four of six patients with residual hypoxia recurred locally compared to 4 of 23 patients without residual hypoxia. ^{60}Cu-ATSM has attracted attention for hypoxia imaging due to its potential biokinetic advantages and better resolution. ^{60}Cu-ATSM PET-guided hypoxia imaging has been investigated in HNC and cervical cancer.[79,80] In a pilot study in 14 cervical cancer patients, ^{60}Cu-ATSM appeared to provide good prognostic discrimination; 5 of 5 patients with hypoxic tumors developed recurrence versus 3 of 9 with normoxic tumors.[80]

Both ^{11}C-choline and ^{18}F-choline have been studied in prostate cancer[81,82]; however, the utility of this approach in routine settings is unclear. SUV at 60% of the maximum value appears to correlate well with histopathologic specimens as a threshold for contouring dominant intraprostatic lesions.[81] FLT PET has shown utility in some settings, such as esophageal cancer, where its positive predictive value for involved nodes may be higher than for FDG PET.[51] In a study of five NSCLC patients undergoing serial baseline and on-treatment FLT PET, reductions in FLT uptake within both tumor and bone marrow were observed.[83] However, its value for tumor and nodal delineation in rectal cancer and HNC appears more limited.[84,85]

In summary, a wide body of literature supports the utility of PET for image-guided treatment planning. Further research efforts are needed to standardize approaches and determine the impact of PET-guided planning on patient outcomes.

Magnetic Resonance Imaging

The utility of MRI in RT planning, particularly for CNS, HNC, and pelvic malignancies, is well known.[86–94] In addition, MR simulators and MRI-only planning approaches are becoming more widely available (Fig. 11.4).[95] Increasingly, quantitative MRI techniques have been used to improve RT planning. For example, functional MRI (fMRI) has been used to reduce radiation dose to normal functioning brain during planning for CNS tumors.[96–100] Aoyama et al.[99] evaluated the use of magnetoencephalography and anisotropic diffusion weighted MRI to plan 20 patients, 15 of whom had arteriovenous malformation (AVM). In 15 patients, targets were modified with significant reduction in the volume of sensitive regions receiving more than 15 Gy. Fast imaging employing steady-state acquisition can facilitate visualization of the trigeminal nerve during radiosurgery planning.[101,102] The ^{1}H MR spectroscopy (MRS) has also been used to guide planning in gliomas.[103,104] Underdosing of ^{1}H MRS-delineated metabolically active areas has been associated with worse outcomes in GBM.[104]

In patients with prostate cancer, van Lin et al.[105] have reported the feasibility of escalating doses to 90 Gy to dominant intraprostatic lesions identified by ^{1}H MRS. MR lymphography with intravenous ferumoxtran-10 has also been used to identify pathologic nodal involvement in prostate cancer (Fig. 11.5).[106,107]

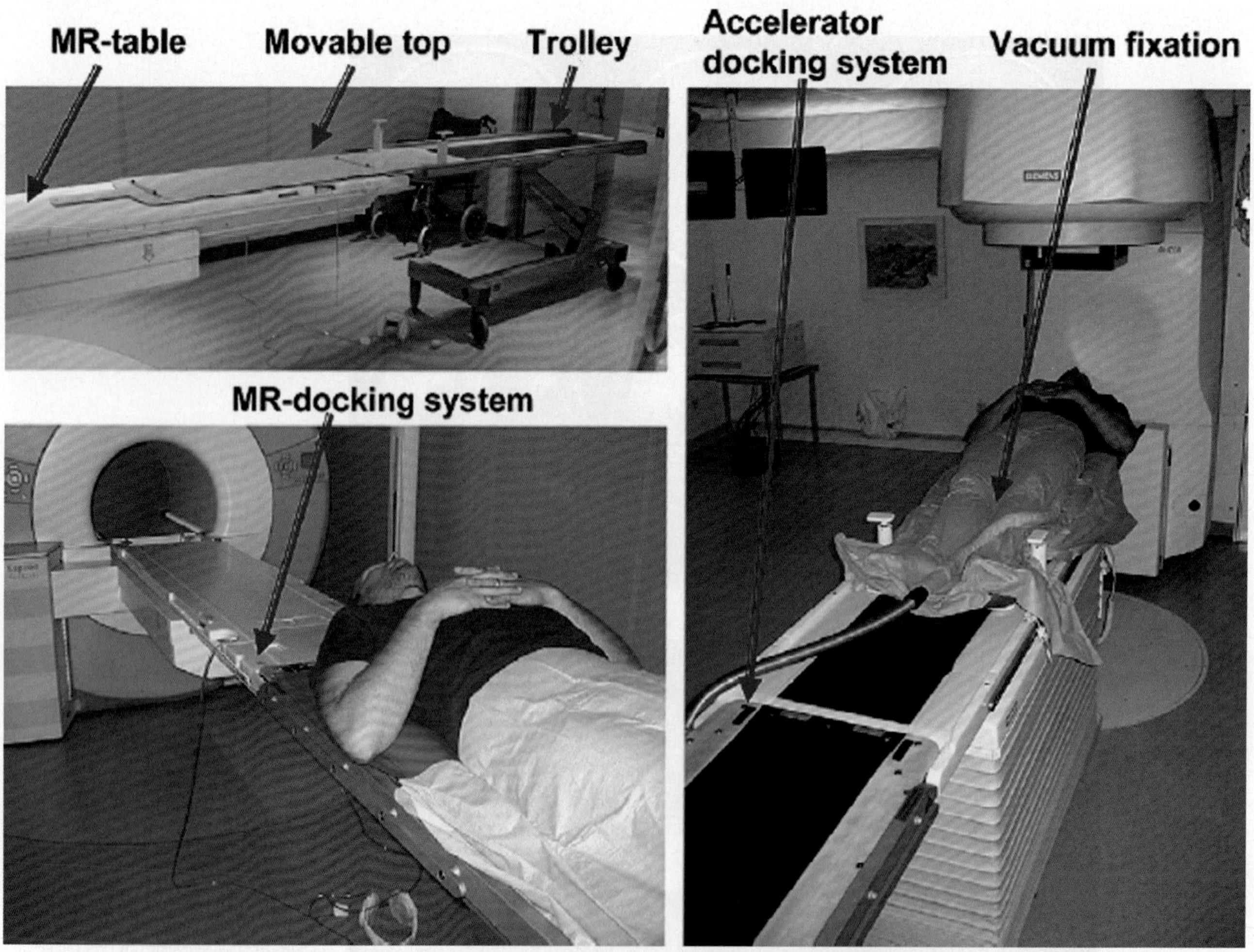

FIGURE 11.4. Integration of magnetic resonance (MR) imaging and radiotherapy, with trolley solution and specialized docking device for smooth transfer between MR and linear accelerator. (From Karlsson M, Karlsson MG, Nyholm T, et al. Dedicated magnetic resonance imaging in the radiotherapy clinic. *Int J Radiat Oncol Biol Phys* 2009;74:644–651, with permission from Elsevier.)

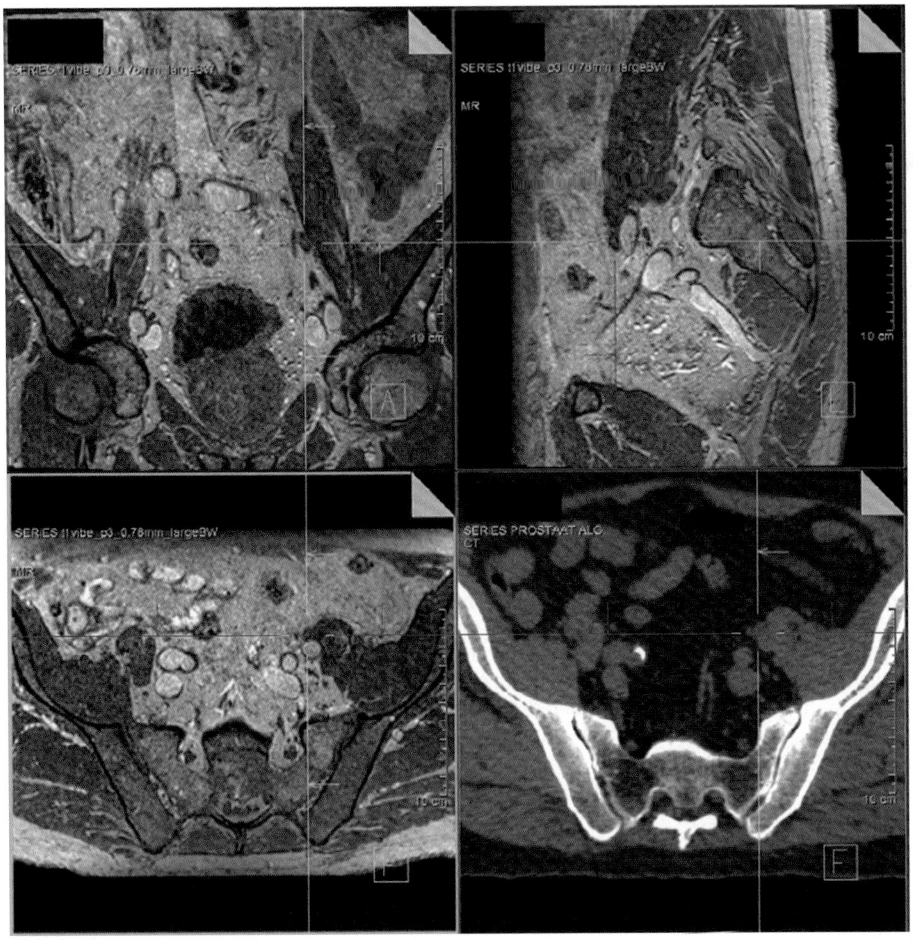

FIGURE 11.5. Fusion of magnetic resonance (MR) lymphography (*upper right* and *left* and *lower left*) and computed tomography (CT) (*lower right*). With the help of MR lymphography, the node identified on CT is identified as pathologic. (From Meijer HJ, van Lin EN, Debats OA, et al. High occurrence of aberrant lymph node spread on magnetic resonance lymphography in prostate cancer patients with a biochemical recurrence after radical prostatectomy. *Int J Radiat Oncol Biol Phys* 2012;82(4):1405–1410; with permission from Elsevier.)

In a study of 47 patients treated with salvage RT for rising post-prostatectomy prostate-specific antigen (PSA), 79% were found to have at least one aberrant positive lymph node, including 10 of 18 (61%) with a PSA less than 1.0 ng/mL. MR lymphography may therefore be useful in helping to define nodal boost volumes in prostate cancer.

Dynamic contrast-enhanced (DCE) MRI has been investigated for RT planning in a variety of tumors including HNC, lung, rectal, and cervical cancers.[108–110,111] Mayr et al.[111] studied 102 cervical cancer patients treated with DCE MRI. Patients with a low total volume of tumor voxels with low DCE signal had significantly worse tumor control and disease-specific survival. Liang et al.[112] used an MRI technique called iterative decomposition of water and fat with echo asymmetry and least-squares estimation to study fractional changes in fat content of pelvic bone marrow during pelvic chemoradiotherapy (Fig. 11.6). Conversion of bone marrow from low fat, high cellularity to high fat, low cellularity during RT is readily observed, enabling noninvasive quantitative methods to analyze the impact of local changes in radiation dose.

In summary, novel and quantitative or functional MRI techniques have been increasingly implemented for RT planning.

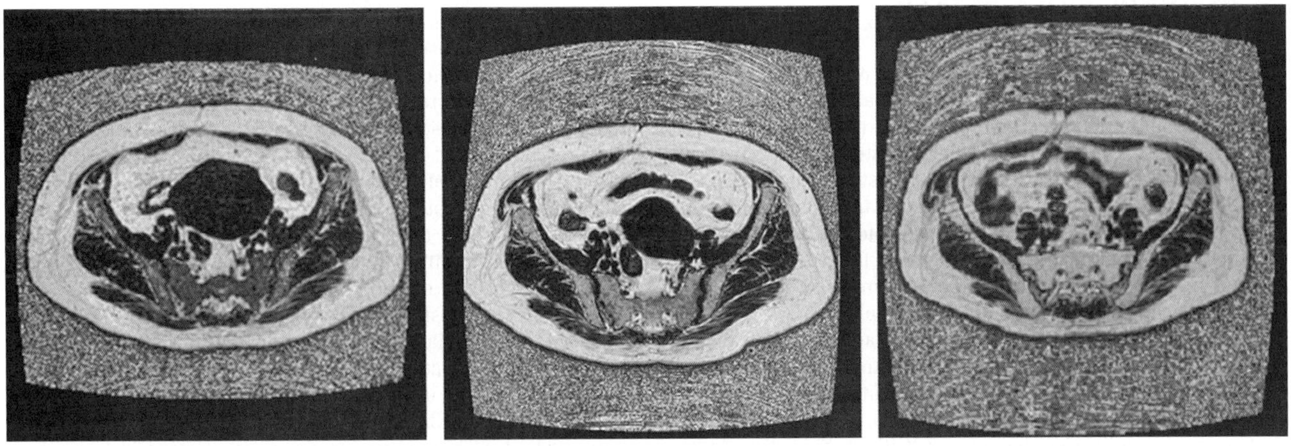

FIGURE 11.6. Axial iterative decomposition of water and fat with echo asymmetry and least-squares estimation magnetic resonance imaging scans of the pelvis in a gynecologic cancer patient undergoing chemoradiotherapy. Scans were acquired at baseline (*left*), midtreatment (*middle*), and posttreatment (*right*) and show a steady increase in fraction of fat relative to water within the pelvic bones, indicated by conversion to progressively higher signal.

Ongoing research is seeking to define the clinical benefits of MRI-based IGRT techniques.

Single Photon Emission Computed Tomography

Single photon emission computed tomography (SPECT) is a relatively inexpensive functional imaging technique, with a wide range of potential tracers. Although PET is generally more quantitatively accurate than SPECT in determining *in vivo* radioactivity distribution,[69] SPECT tracers often have a longer half-lives and release less energy, leading to favorable dosimetry and utility for studying slower biological processes.[69] Nonetheless, SPECT appears to have more limited utilization than PET in RT planning.[7]

Several studies of ^{111}In-capromab pendetide radioimmunoscintigraphy (RIS) have found it useful in planning both external beam RT[113,114–115] and brachytherapy[116,117] for prostate cancer. Jani et al.[114] reported that RIS influenced RT volumes and decision making in a significant proportion of patients undergoing postprostatectomy salvage RT. Of 54 evaluable patients, 18.5% had treatment plans altered by RIS, including 4 who were not offered RT based on the RIS findings. In a multivariate analysis of 107 patients (53 planned with RIS), RIS was associated with an improved 3-year biochemical failure-free survival (bFFS).[115] A similar analysis of 82 patients undergoing RIS for salvage therapy, however, did not reveal a clear benefit of RIS.[118] Ellis et al.[116] treated 80 low-intermediate risk prostate cancer patients with RIS-assisted brachytherapy. Regions of the prostate showing increased RIS uptake were prescribed 150% of the standard dose. The overall 4-year biochemical failure-free survival was 97.4%.

Other applications of SPECT-guided treatment planning have been studied, including ^{123}IMT (^{123}I-alpha-methyl-L-tyrosine) SPECT for gliomas[119–121] and meta-^{123}iodo-benzylguanidine scans for neuroblastoma.[122] Krengli et al.[121] studied 21 patients with high-grade gliomas using fused ^{99m}Tc-MIBI SPECT and MRI. Similar to findings of Grosu et al.,[119] target volumes were significantly augmented by SPECT, with an average increase of 33% over MRI alone, particularly in resected cases.

SPECT has also been used to guide normal tissue avoidance. In patients with NSCLC, Christian et al.[123] used ^{99m}Tc SPECT to identify functional lung to avoid using inverse RT planning, and showed the V20 of functioning lung could be reduced without compromising target coverage. Roeske et al.[124] used ^{99m}Tc SPECT to identify active bone marrow subregions to reduce hematologic toxicity in patients receiving pelvic chemoradiotherapy.

IN-ROOM IMAGE-GUIDED RADIOTHERAPY TECHNIQUES

Numerous studies have found that motion and setup errors for various disease sites can be quite substantial,[125] leading to inaccurate or suboptimal treatment plans and potentially poorer tumor control.[126–129,130] For example, in a study of 127 prostate cancer patients treated *without* daily prostate localization, de Crevoisier et al.[130] found that significant rectal distension resulting in anterior displacement of the prostate at simulation was an independent risk factor for biochemical failure. Strategies to address motion have included wide margins, elaborate immobilization techniques, resimulation and replanning, and portal radiography. IGRT approaches take advantage of more frequent and sophisticated imaging to setup the patient and localize the target with greater accuracy, ostensibly improving treatment delivery and allowing reduction of margins.

This section will describe various IGRT technologies developed to address both interfraction and intrafraction motion. Particular attention is devoted to clinical applications of in-room IGRT technologies and data supporting their use. Although some of these technologies have been available for many years, others have only recently been introduced, yet appear to have been adopted rapidly by clinicians.[131] Many others are still under development and have not yet been implemented clinically.

Ultrasound

Ultrasound (US) is one of the most common IGRT approaches in practice, particularly for prostate cancer.[131] It involves emission of high-frequency sound waves to produce images of internal anatomy, consisting of a transducer encased in a probe applied to the skin surface, reflecting sound waves back as echoes when a change in impedance is encountered due to density differences between tissues. The time an echo takes to return is used to calculate the depth of the tissue interface. Image information is obtained along the beamline of the probe, with a complete image created by sweeping across the region of interest. Although three operational modes are available, B (brightness) mode is the primary one used. Readers interested in a more complete description are referred elsewhere.[132]

Several US products are currently available. All have a system to map the image coordinate system to both the linear accelerator (LINAC) coordinate system and the simulation images. This can be achieved either by tracking the position of a stereotactic arm or using an infrared imaging system to detect the probe position. The target location can be determined in the room prior to treatment, with the necessary shifts conducted to bring the anatomy into position. A widely used US system is the B-mode acquisition and targeting (BAT) transabdominal system (NOMOS, North American Scientific, Chatsworth, CA). The probe is registered to a stereotactic arm on the LINAC gantry, allowing its position to be tracked. Prior to treatment, transverse and sagittal images are generated and the target and normal tissue contours from the planning CT scan are overlaid on the US images. If the target is displaced, the CT structures are maneuvered on a touch screen and the necessary 3D couch shifts are calculated. Another system is SonArray (Varian Medical Systems, Palo Alto, CA), which combines US localization with an optical guidance system to track the position of the probe in the treatment room.[133,134] A similar system is available from BrainLab (Heimstetten, Germany). The I-Beam system (Computerized Medical Systems Inc, St. Louis, MO) uses a machine vision pattern recognition technique to calibrate the probe relative to the gantry. Clarity (Elekta, Stockholm, Sweden) incorporates structure-based tissue matching and segmentation tools to facilitate contouring.

At experienced centers, the additional time required to implement US-based IGRT is reported to be 5 minutes or less.[135,136] Additional time may be necessary, however, when the technology is first adopted or if moves need to be checked online by a physician. Increased skin-to-prostate distances, increased thickness of tissue anterior to the bladder, and less prostate gland present superior to the symphysis can reduce image quality.[137] However, reproducibility and image quality are generally reported to be high for prostate localization.[137–139] Probe-induced prostate motion is also a consideration, as displacements up to 1 cm have been observed,[140] although generally the magnitude of displacements is 3 mm or less.[133,135,138,140,141]

Numerous investigators have compared US systems versus conventional setup techniques (i.e., external skin markers) for prostate localization.[133–135,136,137,138,139,140,141–144,145] In a review of nine series, Kuban et al.[145] reported that shifts from the initial setup were greatest in the anterior-posterior (AP) direction, with standard deviations in the AP, superior-inferior (SI), and right-left (RL) directions ranged from 2.7 to 6.4 mm, 2.8 to 7.3 mm, and 2.1 to 4.6 mm, respectively, with maximum values of 29.8, 30.3, and 34.9 mm, respectively. Several investigators have evaluated shifts in prostate patients undergoing daily portal imaging,[138,140] removing the impact of patient setup uncertainty. In a study of 35 patients using BAT, Little et al.[140] reported mean shifts of −1.3, −1.6, and −0.89 mm in the AP, SI, and RL directions, respectively. Trichter and Ennis[138] reported that the margins necessary to encompass the prostate at the 95% confidence level using daily portal imaging alone (without US) were 9.2, 14.6, and 10.2 mm in the RL, SI, and AP directions, primarily due to organ motion rather than setup error.

Although US-based localization accounts for interfraction organ motion, it does not address intrafraction motion. However, the magnitude of such motion in patients with prostate cancer appears to be small. In a study of 20 patients undergoing pre- and posttherapy US, Huang et al.[146] noted mean shifts of 0.2 ± 1.3 mm, 0.1 ± 1 mm, and 0.01 ± 0.4 mm, in the AP, SI, and RL directions, respectively. Trichter and Ennis[138] similarly noted small mean intrafraction shifts using pre- and posttherapy US; however, large *maximum* shifts of 8.1, 20.4, and 8.3 mm in the AP, SI, and RL directions, respectively, were noted.

Several authors have compared prostate localization with CT[136,145,147,148] and implanted fiducial markers (144,149,150). Lattanzi et al.[136] found average disagreements between the modalities were small: −0.09 mm (AP), −0.03 mm (SI), and −0.16 mm (RL). O'Daniel et al.[148] compared four target alignment techniques: skin marks, bony registration, US, and in-room CT. Direct alignment with US and CT provided better target coverage compared to the other methods. Scarbrough et al.[150] compared US with fiducial markers in 40 patients and found that US was associated with significantly greater systematic and random errors than fiducials. Similarly, Gayou and Miften[151] found that US was associated with a higher percentage of shifts greater than 5 mm compared to cone beam CT (CBCT).

Limited data exist regarding the impact of US IGRT on patient outcomes. Indirect support is garnered, however, from the excellent outcome of prostate cancer patients treated using daily US guidance.[152,153–154] Kupelian et al.[152] reported on 100 patients undergoing short-course IMRT, using daily BAT. Margins around the target were 4 mm posteriorly, 8 mm laterally, and 5 mm in other directions. With a median follow-up of 66 months, the 5-year bFFS was 85%, with 5% of patients developing grade 2 or 3 rectal sequelae. Similarly, Zerini et al.[153] treated 25 low- to intermediate-risk patients to 70 Gy in 30 fractions with daily BAT. With a mean follow-up of 45 months, one patient had biochemical relapse and no patients developed grade 3 or higher late rectal toxicity.

Jani et al.[155] evaluated acute toxicity in patients treated with (n = 50) versus without (n = 49) daily BAT, reporting that patients treated using BAT experienced less rectal toxicity. They also separately analyzed late sequelae in patients treated with and without BAT.[156] Although less toxicity was observed in patients treated with BAT, there was no significant correlation between BAT usage and toxicity on multivariate analysis. Bohrer et al.[157] also reported that patients treated using BAT had less rectal toxicity compared to patients treated prior to BAT implementation. However, no differences in bladder toxicity or PSA control were seen between the two groups. US may also be useful in the post-prostatectomy setting.[158,159] Chinnaiyan et al.[159] evaluated SonArray in six post-prostatectomy patients. The average shifts from the initial setup were 5 ± 4 mm, 3 ± 4 mm, and 3 ± 3 mm, in the AP, SI, and RL directions, respectively.

Fewer studies have reported on the utility of US in other tumor sites. US can be useful to confirm bladder volume and position in gynecologic patients undergoing pelvic RT, which is known to be volatile.[160] In intracavitary brachytherapy planning, US is a valuable tool for both detection and prevention of perforations.[161,162] Several investigators have also recently evaluated US-based IGRT to define and verify position of the lumpectomy boost cavity in breast cancer.[163,164] Boda-Heggeman et al.[165] used US guidance for frameless stereotactic radiosurgery (SRS) for liver metastases, using active breathing control to reduce tumor motion. Fuss et al.[166] evaluated US-based IGRT in 62 patients with upper abdominal malignancies, predominantly pancreatic cancer. The mean shifts in the AP, SI, and RL directions were 6 ± 5.31 mm, 6 ± 6.7 mm, and 4.9 ± 4.35 mm, respectively. Meeks et al.[167] performed US-guided extracranial SRS in 16 patients. Single-fraction doses ranging from 12.5 to 24.0 Gy were delivered without significant acute complications. US-guided extracranial SRS appears safe for treatment of GI malignancies as well.[168–170] For example, in a series of 10 gallbladder cancer patients treated to a median dose of 59 Gy with daily US localization, all but one experienced grade 2 or less acute toxicity.[168]

As newer IGRT approaches are introduced in the clinic, the future role of US remains unclear. Declining utilization was noted in a recent survey.[131] Nonetheless, an advantage of US is that it does not involve additional ionizing radiation, making it likely that it will always play a role in clinical practice.

Video and Surface Imaging

Video-based techniques for patient positioning have been used for over 25 years. Connor et al.[171] described a close-circuit television camera and monitor system plus a videodisc recorder, which reduced positional errors to less than 1 mm. The recorder stored a reference image of each treatment setup and was superimposed, in reverse color, on the live camera image. Investigators at the University of Chicago developed an online video "subtraction" setup system, consisting of wall- and ceiling-mounted charge-coupled device cameras linked to a computer equipped with a frame grabber.[172,173] After optimal positioning, a reference image is obtained and, on subsequent days, is subtracted in real time from live video images. Subtraction images are displayed on an in-room monitor and used to interactively realign the patient. Milliken et al.[172] reported high levels of accuracy in both 2D and 3D repositioning using this system. Johnson et al.[173] performed a clinical study of this system in five HNC patients undergoing twice daily RT. Conventional setup was used in the morning, with the video used simply to record the final patient position. In the afternoon, patients were first aligned with conventional techniques and then live subtraction images were used for setup correction. Although the standard deviation of setup error using room lasers was σ = 3.9 mm, it was reduced by 56% (σ = 1.7 mm) using video setup. The entire process generally required approximately 1 minute.

Several investigators have evaluated video-based setup techniques in breast cancer patients. Baroni et al.[174] developed a video system based on optoelectronics and close-range photogrammetry that captures in real time the position of markers on the patient that are used to monitor and adjust the patient position. Bert et al.[175] investigated a commercial stereovision surface imaging system (AlignRT, Vision RT Ltd, London, UK) for setup of partial-breast irradiation patients, which uses close-range photogrammetry to generate a 3D image of the patient's surface. The resultant image is compared to an image generated at simulation or of the patient's external surface generated from a CT dataset. Phantom studies found that the system was capable of identifying translational shifts and rotations of less than 0.1 degree. The AlignRT system is currently being used clinically in the treatment of breast cancer patients undergoing adjuvant whole breast RT (Fig. 11.7).[176]

A novel use of the AlignRT system is in the setup and monitoring of patient positioning for those undergoing cranial SRS using minimal immobilization. Cerviño et al.[177] used AlignRT to monitor positioning in patients immobilized with only a head mold that leaves the face exposed. Using anthropomorphic head phantoms and volunteers, the motion inside the head mold was small and could be accurately detected by real-time surface imaging. These investigators recently presented their initial experience using this approach in 23 patients undergoing SRS.[178] The average setup time for both surface imaging and CBCT was 26 minutes, with surface imaging requiring on average 14 minutes. The mean time from initial setup on the table through the last delivery was 40 minutes. Overall, eight

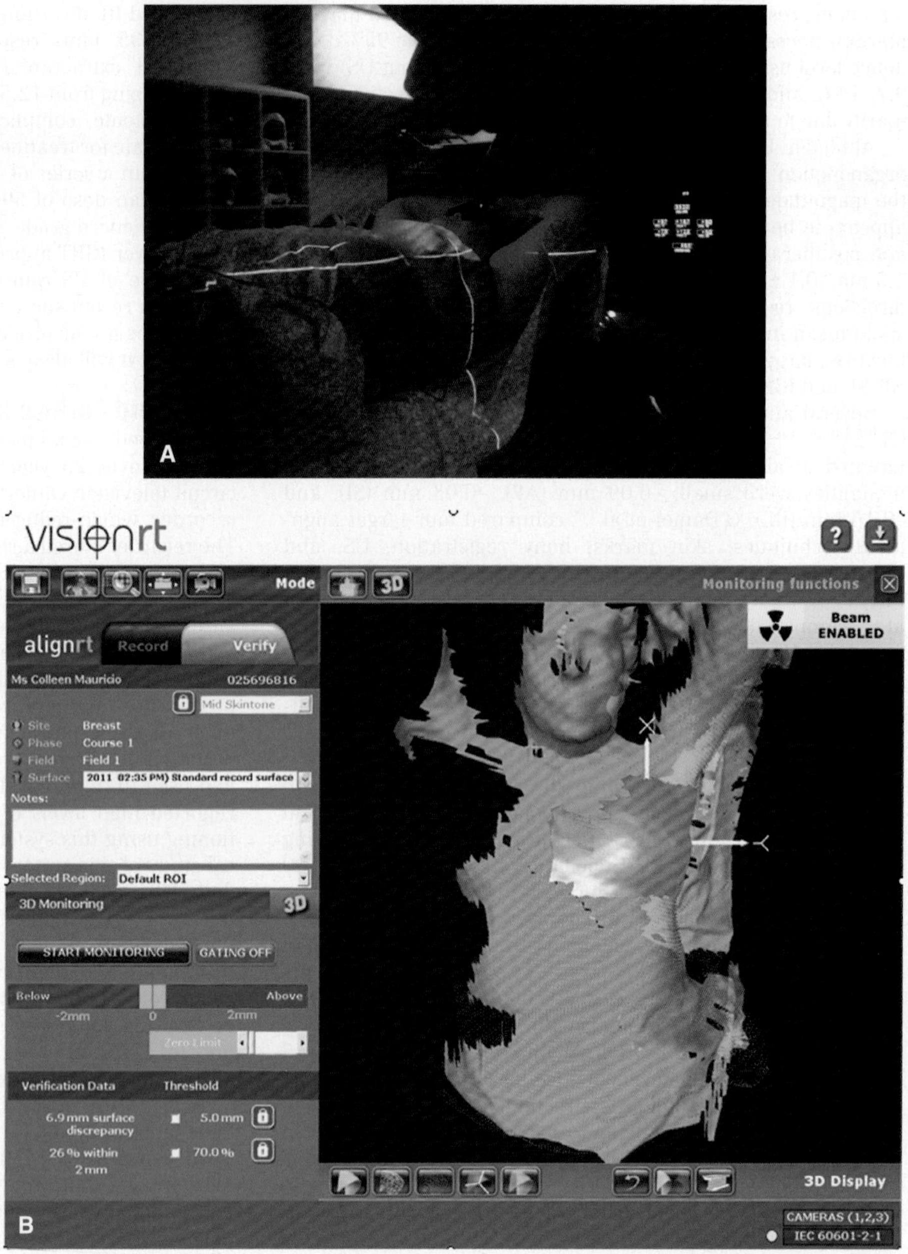

FIGURE 11.7. AlignRT for breast cancer. **A:** Alignment of patient surface to planning computed tomography using video cameras. **B:** Surface monitoring showing the region of interest of the breast in *pink* and the tolerance level displayed on the left in *dark blue.*

patients (35%) required repositioning during treatment. Others have similarly used video surface imaging in patients undergoing cranial radiosurgery.[179]

Li et al.[180] and Djajaputra and Li[181] developed a real-time video-guided IMRT approach in breast cancer patients using a camera capable of capturing full-frame 3D surface images through a single snapshot. Patient setup parameters are determined semiautomatically, and the IMRT leaf segments are modified in real time. Unlike other video approaches, this system compensates for changes in surface topology by modifying the treatment plan rather than adjusting the patient position. This system is also being applied to patients undergoing fractionated stereotactic RT.[182]

Overall, video and surface imaging approaches are among the least commonly used IGRT technologies in the clinic today, with only 3.2% of responding physicians reporting its use on a recent survey performed in the United States.[131] As new commercial systems and new applications are introduced (e.g., real-time positioning monitoring for frameless radiosurgery), utilization of such technologies may increase in the future.

Planar Imaging

Planar imaging approaches, which include both megavoltage (MV) and kilovoltage (kV), are the most common in-room IGRT approaches used today. In a national survey from 2009, the percentage of respondents using megavolt- and kilovolt-planar systems were 63% and 58%, respectively.[131] These systems were used in nearly all disease sites, particularly CNS tumors and prostate cancer (together with implanted fiducial markers). MV-planar systems were adopted earlier, with the majority of users (53%) having implemented them by 2004. The adoption of kilovolt-planar–based systems occurred later, with the majority of users (54%) having adopted them by 2006.

Electronic Portal Imaging Devices

Electronic portal imaging devices (EPIDs) provide a means of generating an electronic image of a treatment field with the patient on the treatment table. Similar to conventional portal imaging, EPIDs produce images using the therapeutic (MV) beam. However, EPIDs overcome many of the limitations of conventional port films, including delays due to image processing. Moreover, EPID images can be digitally processed for better visualization of the relevant anatomy and stored for offline review. Numerous EPIDs have been introduced including video-based, liquid ion chamber, and solid-state systems. Most commercial systems in use today are based on flat-panel amorphous silicon (aSi) detectors. With this method, a scintillator first converts x-rays to visible light. A photodiode array then converts the light to electrons, which in turn activate pixels in a layer of aSi. The pixels are then read out in successive rows, processed, and displayed on a computer screen for viewing. Clinical studies illustrating the benefits of EPID-based IGRT approaches initially appeared in the early 1990s,[183–184,185] and since then it has been studied in many disease sites.[186–192] Readers interested in an overview of EPID technologies are referred elsewhere.[193,194]

Concerns over increased workload and excess dose have increased interest in on offline EPID approaches. One approach is the so-called shrinking action level strategy.[195] Initially, EPID images are obtained on a given number (N_{max}) of consecutive days. The 3D setup deviation is calculated offline, and the length of the deviation vector is compared to a predetermined "action level." If exceeded, a setup correction is performed at the next session. The feasibility of this approach was demonstrated in a multi-institutional prostate cancer trial.[196] Favorable results have also been reported in lung cancer[197] and HNC.[198] An alternative approach is the "no action level" strategy, whereby the mean setup error over a fixed number of fractions is calculated and always corrected for.[199]

EPID is useful for prostate localization in conjunction with implanted seed markers.[200,201] Pouliot et al.[202] presented an overview of the prostate seed marker protocol developed at University of California–San Francisco (UCSF) using EPID. Prior to simulation, three gold markers were inserted (two laterally on each side of the prostate and one in the apex). A planning CT scan was performed, the location of each marker was contoured, and a digitally reconstructed radiograph (DRR) was generated. Prior to treatment, a lateral EPID image was obtained to assess SI and AP shifts, requiring approximately 0.02 Gy of dose. Comparison of the center of mass of the markers with their expected position on the DRR was used to evaluate the need for repositioning. If shifts were greater than 3 mm, the couch was adjusted. Most investigators report excellent marker visualization,[200–201,202,203,204] particularly when gold markers are used with a minimum diameter of 0.9 mm.[201] At least two gold markers are typically visible,[203] and high reproducibility has been reported using this approach.[204,205] Although marker migration is a potential concern, several investigators have reported minimal migration of implanted markers.[200–201,202,203,204] Kupelian et al.[206] evaluated seed marker position throughout the course of treatment in 56 prostate cancer patients. Of 2,037 alignments, the average directional variation of all intermarker distances was –0.31 ± 1.41 mm. Only two markers (1%) showed frequent changes in position, most likely caused by prostate deformation. Of note, others have reported marker movement in patients undergoing hormonal therapy as the prostate involutes.[207]

Limited data exist for EPID and implanted markers in other tumor sites.[208] EPID has been compared with CBCT nongenitourinary (GU) sites, with some studies reporting superior setup accuracy with CBCT.[209–211] Topolnjak et al.[210] compared the two modalities in 20 breast cancer patients undergoing adjuvant RT, noting that EPID underestimated the bony anatomy setup error by 20% to 50%.

Several investigators have reported outcomes of patients treated with EPID-based IGRT. Nichol et al.[212] treated 140 stage T1 or T2 prostate cancer patients to 75.6 Gy with daily EPID setup corrections based on bony anatomy. Overall, late grade 2 or higher GI and GU toxicities were noted in 2% and 1% of patients, respectively. Others have reported favorable results using EPID and the shrinking action level approach.[213] Ost et al.[214] compared acute GI and GU toxicity in 196 prostate cancer patients treated with postoperative salvage RT. Overall, patient position was corrected using EPID (prior to 2006, n = 116) or CBCT (after 2006, n = 80). Patients treated with CBCT verification had less grade 1 or 2 GU toxicity compared to those treated using EPID. No differences were seen in GI or high grade GU toxicity between the two groups.

EPID has long been among the most common in-room IGRT technologies used clinically. In the national IGRT survey,[131] EPID was the most commonly used IGRT technology across nearly all disease sites. With the proliferation of newer technologies, notably CBCT, however, its use may decrease in the future.

CyberKnife

CyberKnife (Accuray Inc, Sunnyvale, CA) consists of a compact X-band 6 MV linear accelerator coupled to a multijointed robotic manipulator with 6 degrees of freedom (Fig. 11.8).[215] The current generation of CyberKnife technology consists of two precisely calibrated diagnostic x-ray tubes fixed to the ceiling of the treatment vault and two nearly orthogonal aSi flat-panel detectors. After coarse alignment, projected images from the cameras are automatically registered with the DRRs from the planning CT. Changes in target position are relayed to the robotic arm, which adjusts pointing of the treatment beam. During treatment, the robotic arm moves through a sequence of positions (nodes). At each node, a pair of images is obtained, the patient position is determined, and adjustments are made.

CyberKnife was initially based on tracking the skeletal anatomy of the skull and upper spine, limiting treatment to tumors of the brain, head and neck, and upper spine. Subsequently, the ability to track implanted fiducial markers was introduced, allowing treatment of lower spinal tumors with submillimeter precision.[216] More recently, software has been developed that obviates the need for implanted fiducials in spine patients and enables respiratory tracking.

Several preclinical studies have been published reporting high levels of accuracy of CyberKnife. Murphy and Cox[217] noted a mechanical accuracy of the beams of 0.7 mm with a calibration accuracy of plus or minus 0.5 mm along each axis. Yu et al.[218] reported submillimeter accuracy in a phantom study using fiducial markers. Many clinical studies have described favorable outcomes for patients treated with CyberKnife, including adenoma,[219,220] schwannoma,[221] glioma,[222,223] brain metastases,[224] meningioma,[225] trigeminal neuralgia,[226,227] AVM,[228] and tumors abutting the optic nerves or chiasm.[229,230]

A provocative use of the CyberKnife is for pediatric brain tumors. CyberKnife avoids the need for a rigid head frame and, in select children, general anesthesia. Moreover, frameless treatment can be fractionated. Investigators at Baylor University reported promising results with the CyberKnife in infants[231] and the general pediatric population.[232] Giller et al.[232] treated 21 children (median age, 6 years) with CNS tumors, with a median dose of 18.8 Gy primarily delivered in a single fraction. At a median follow-up of 18 months, 10 children had evidence of decreased tumor size or stable disease on follow-up imaging.

Many studies have focused on CyberKnife for spinal lesions (Table 11.1).[233,234–237,238,239,240,241–244,245,246,247,248] Dodd et al.[233] treated 51 patients with 55 benign intradural extramedullary spinal tumors, with a median dose of 19.6 Gy delivered primarily in 1 or 2 fractions. All patients with more than 2 years of follow-up had either stable or smaller tumors on repeat imaging. Most patients had stable or improved symptoms. One developed a spinal cord injury 8 months following treatment. Investigators at the University of Pittsburgh reported on 125 primarily malignant spinal lesions (115 patients) treated to a median dose of 14 Gy in 3 to 5 fractions (Fig. 11.9).[238] At a median follow-up of 18 months, no patient developed new symptoms or had evidence of RT sequelae, despite the fact that 68% had received prior RT. Of 79 patients presenting with pain, 74 (94%) noted improvement. Others have reported

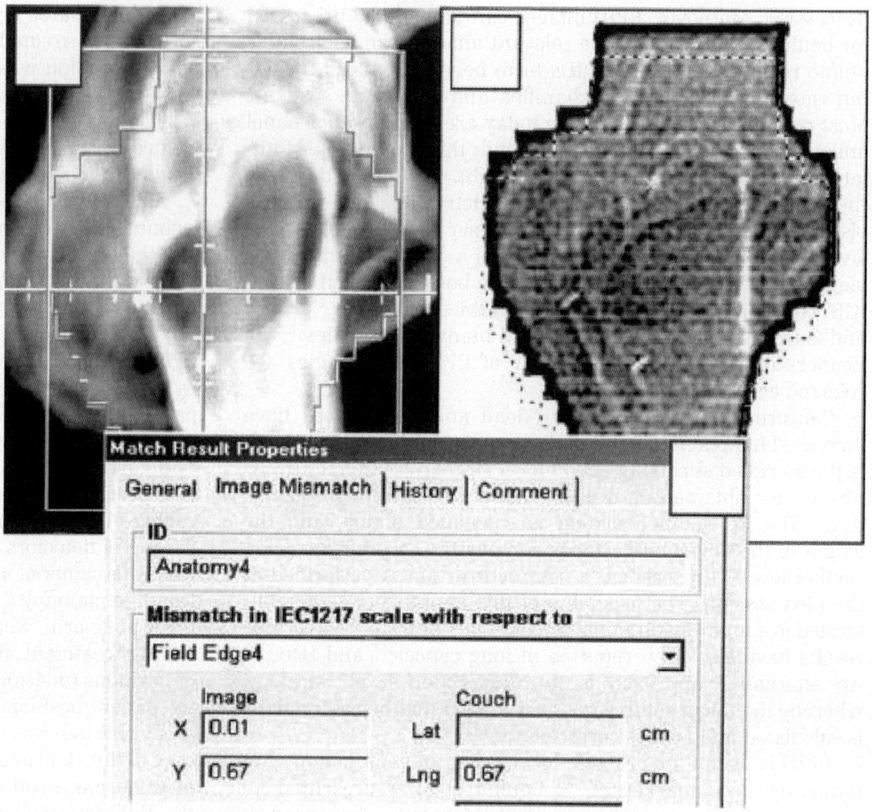

FIGURE 11.8. CyberKnife radiosurgery system. Two amorphous silicon x-ray detectors are positioned orthogonally to the treatment couch. (From Gerszten PC, Ozhasoglu C, Burton SA, et al. Cyberknife frameless stereotactic radiosurgery for spinal lesions: clinical experience in 125 cases. *Neurosurgery* 2004;55:89–99, with permission.)

TABLE 11.1 OUTCOMES FROM SELECTED SERIES OF SPINAL TUMORS TREATED WITH CYBERKNIFE

Author (Reference)	*Patients/Lesions*	*Tumor Histology*	*Median Dose, Gy (Range)*	*Number of Fractions*	*Median Follow-Up, Months*	*Outcomes and Complications*
Dodd et al. (233)	51/55	Various benign	19.6 (16–30)	1–5	36	100% LC[a] 25%–50% improved pain 1 late spinal cord injury
Ryu et al. (234)	16/16	Various benign and malignant	11–25	1–5	≥6	100% LC No complications
Sinclair et al. (235)	15/15	AVM	20.5[b] (20–25)	2–5	27.9	86%[c] with decreased volume. No new symptoms or hemorrhage
Gerszten et al. (236)	18/18	Sacral tumors (94% malignant)	15 (12–20)	1	6	100% LC. No new neurologic symptoms
Gerszten et al. (237)	26/26	Various metastatic	18 (16–20)	1	16	All patients underwent kyphoplasty, 92% had improved pain
Gerszten et al. (238)	115/125	108 metastases, 17 benign	14 (12–20)	1	18	No new neurologic symptoms, 94%[d] with improved pain
Bhatnagar et al. (239)	44/59	Various benign	16 (10–31)	1 (95%)	8	96% LC[e]
Gibbs et al. (247)	74/102	Various metastatic	NS (14–25)	1–5	9 (mean)	84% symptomatic improvement; 1-year survival 46%; 3 with radiation myelopathy
Gagnon et al. (245)	200/274	Various benign and malignant	No prior RT: 26.4 Prior RT: 21.1	3 (mean)	12	Reduced pain scores and increased mental quality of life; no late complications.
Kufeld et al. (241)	36/39	Meningioma and schwannoma	14 (12–15)	1	18	100% LC; 42% pain reduction; no complications
Chang et al. (249)	129/167	Various metastatic	16–39	1–5	6	91% pain relief
Patel et al. (240)	117/154	Various metastatic	16 (12–20)	1	8	Re-treatment: whole vertebral body (WB) 11% vs. partial (PB) 19%. 2-year survival: WB 21% vs. PB 29%. Local progression: WB 20% vs. PB 35%
Tsai et al. (244)	69/127	Various metastatic	15.5 (10–30)	1–5	10	97% LC; Reduced pain scores and functional disability; 27% acute nausea

LC, local control; AVM, arteriovenous malformation; RT, radiation therapy; NS, not stated.
[a]Of 28 patients with more than 2 years of follow-up. [b]Mean dose.
[c]Of 7 patients with more than 3 years of follow-up. [d]Of 79 patients presenting with pain.
[e]Of patients with follow-up imaging (includes nonspinal extracranial tumors).

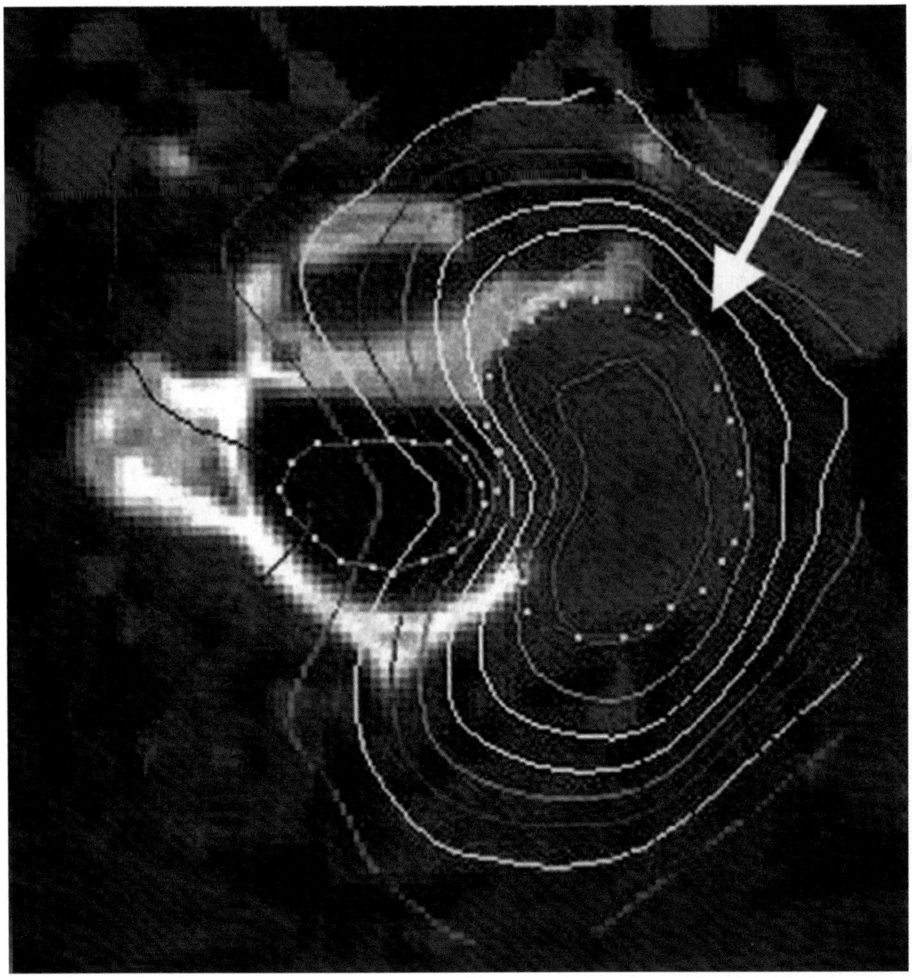

FIGURE 11.9. X-ray with isodose lines of a treatment plan for a renal cell metastasis to C5 in a 70-year-old woman (*arrow*). The patient had severe pain that recurred after initial external beam irradiation. The tumor was treated with 14 Gy to the 80% isodose line in a single fraction (*orange line*). Notice the conformality of the isodose lines around the spinal cord. The patient had significant pain relief within 1 month of treatment. (From Gerszten PC, Ozhasoglu C, Burton SA, et al. Cyberknife frameless stereotactic radiosurgery for spinal lesions: clinical experience in 125 cases. *Neurosurgery* 2004;55:89–99, with permission.)

similarly promising results in patients with benign and malignant spinal tumors.[235–249]

Recently, CyberKnife has been used to treat extracraniospinal sites.[250–258] However, outcome data remain limited. King et al.[252] treated 41 low-risk prostate cancer patients, prescribing 36.25 Gy in 5 fractions of 7.25 Gy. At a median follow-up of 33 months, two patients developed grade 3 GU toxicity and no patients developed grade 3 or higher GI toxicity. Less rectal toxicity was observed with an every-other-day approach versus 5 consecutive days (0% vs. 38%; P = .0035). At last follow-up, all patients remained biochemically controlled. Of 32 patients with 1-year minimum follow-up, 25 (78%) achieved a PSA nadir of 0.4 ng/mL or less.

Several investigators have explored the use of CyberKnife in patients with lung cancer.[251,254] Nuyttens et al.[251] treated 20 patients with lung tumors in whom fiducial markers had been implanted for tumor tracking. A system of light-emitting diodes placed on the patient's abdomen was used to monitor the location of fiducials with respect to respiratory motion and provide feedback to the robotic arm of the CyberKnife for tracking. Four-dimensional CT simulation scans were acquired, and patients were treated with hypofractionated radiation (36 to 60 Gy in 3 fractions). With a median follow-up of 4 months, no local failures were observed.

Novalis

The Novalis system (BrainLab Inc, Westchester, IL) consists of a 6 MV linear accelerator equipped with a micro-multileaf collimator (MLC). Infrared camera and stereoscopic kilovoltage x-ray imaging technologies are used for patient positioning. Two 80 to 100 kV x-ray tubes mounted in the floor of the treatment room are used to acquire images of internal anatomy (e.g., the vertebral bodies), which are automatically compared with the DRRs from the planning CT scan. The cameras are used to detect the positions of sensors on the patient's skin, which are automatically compared with their position at simulation to determine necessary couch shifts.

In an analysis of the positional accuracy of the Novalis system, simulated infrared marker shifts revealed that positioning errors of the planned isocenter were 0.6 ± 0.3, 0.5 ± 0.2, and 0.7 ± 0.2 mm along the lateral, longitudinal, and vertical axes, respectively.[259] Simulated target shifts indicated that positioning errors of the planned isocenter were 0.6 ± 0.3, 0.7 ± 0.2, and 0.5 ± 0.2 mm along the three axes. Others studies have similarly reported submillimeter accuracy with the Novalis system.[260]

Various investigators have reported outcomes of patients with intracranial tumors and conditions treated with Novalis.[261,262–268] In a series of 32 trigeminal neuralgia patients, Chen et al.[261] found good-to-excellent pain relief in 78%. Pedroso et al.[263] treated 44 cranial AVM patients to a median dose of 15 Gy in a single fraction. The obliteration rate was 53%. Three patients (7%) bled following treatment; however, none developed significant late sequelae.

Others have reported on the use of Novalis in spinal tumors.[269–272] Investigators at Henry Ford Hospital treated 10 spinal metastases with external beam RT (25 Gy in 10 fractions) followed by a 6 to 8 Gy SRS boost on a Novalis unit (Fig. 11.10).[271] All patients presenting with pain experienced significant relief. No acute or chronic sequelae were noted at a median follow-up of 6 months. These same investigators reported their experience with SRS alone (10 to 16 Gy) in 49 patients with 61 spinal metastases.[272] Complete and partial pain relief was noted in 85% of

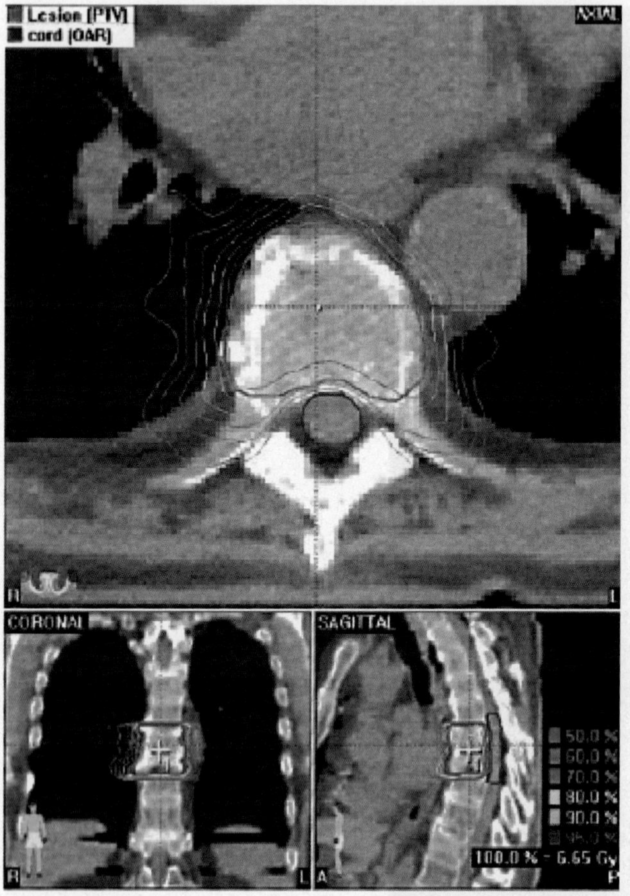

FIGURE 11.10. An intensity-modulated stereotactic spinal radiosurgery plan in a patient treated on a Novalis unit. The patient had multiple myeloma involving the seventh and eighth thoracic vertebral bodies. (From Ryu S, Yin FF, Rock J, et al. Image-guided and intensity-modulated radiosurgery for patients with spinal metastasis. *Cancer* 2003;97:2013–2018, with permission.)

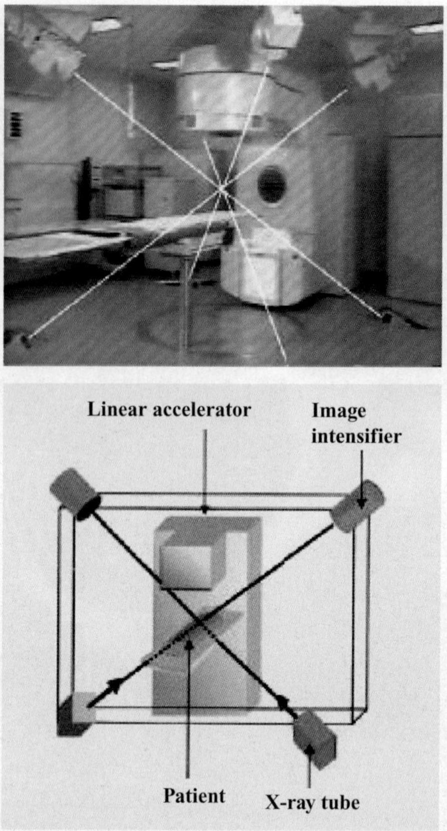

FIGURE 11.11. The real-time tumor-tracking radiation therapy (RTRT) system. (From Harada T, Shirato H, Ogura S, et al. Real-time tumor-tracking radiation therapy for lung carcinoma by the aid of insertion of a gold marker using broncho-fiberoscopy. *Cancer* 2002;95:1720–1727, with permission.)

patients. Others have reported similarly promising results in malignant and benign spinal tumors.[269,270]

The Novalis system is being increasingly used in other tumor sites.[273–274,275–279] Ryu et al.[277] treated 13 HNC tumors with either SRS (12 to 18 Gy in 1 fraction) or hypofractionated RT (30 to 36 Gy in 6 fractions). Six patients achieved a complete and three a partial response. Soete et al.[278] reported short-term outcomes of prostate cancer patients treated with hypofractionated RT (56 Gy in 3.5 Gy daily fractions). Acute grade 2 rectal and bladder toxicity was noted in 12% and 29% of patients, respectively, with no grade 3 or higher toxicities. In a separate study, Soete et al.[279] noted significant improvements in positioning of prostate cancer patients using Novalis compared to conventional setup techniques. Setup errors of 5 mm or more occurred in 2% to 14% of patient positionings, versus 28% to 53% with conventional positionings.

Real-Time Tumor Tracking

The real-time tumor-tracking radiation treatment (RTRT) system (Mitsubishi Electronics Co Ltd, Tokyo, Japan) consists of four sets of diagnostic x-ray tubes and imagers (Fig. 11.11).[280] Each x-ray unit has a 1.5 MHU x-ray tube with a fixed collimator mounted in the floor with a corresponding imager mounted in the ceiling. During treatment, two of the four x-ray systems are selected to track an implanted fiducial marker using motion-tracking software.[281] The treatment beam is gated to irradiate when the position of the marker coincides with its planned position.

Phantom experiments demonstrate that the RTRT system is highly accurate, with geometric accuracy better than 1.5 mm for moving targets up to a speed of 40 mm per second. Dose due to the diagnostic x-ray monitoring ranges from 0.01% to 1% of the target dose measured in a chest phantom.[280] A 4D RTRT system has also been developed.[282]

Investigators at Hokkaido University in Japan have presented a number of clinical studies using the RTRT system.[280–293] In an early report, Shirato et al.[280] described the treatment of 14 patients with a variety of tumors, including lung, bladder, prostate, liver and rectal cancers. All patients were treated with tight planning target volume (PTV) margins (<10 mm). At a median follow-up of 6 months, no local or marginal recurrences were noted. These investigators and others have explored the RTRT system in tumors of the lung,[281,286,289–291] prostate,[283,285] GI tract,[287,293,294] and female genital tract.[288,290] In a study of 18 lung cancer patients, Harada et al.[281] placed gold markers via bronchofiberoscopy under video guidance. Markers were shown to be stable in 65% of tumors throughout treatment. All patients received 35 to 40 Gy in 4 fractions, with tight (5 mm) margins around the tumor. At a median follow-up of 9 months, all were locally controlled, with only one patient developing symptomatic pneumonitis.

Hashimoto et al.[287] treated 20 GI patients (14 esophagus, 2 stomach, and 4 duodenum) with the RTRT system. Markers were placed either intraoperatively or via endoscopy and tight (5 mm) margins were used. At a median follow-up of 10 months, no grade 3 or higher late toxicities were noted. Ahn et al.[294] used the RTRT system in three unresectable pancreatic cancer patients. All received intraoperative electrons and external beam RT. None developed grade 2 or higher acute toxicity. At a median follow-up of 3 months, three partial responses and one stable disease were noted. The RTRT system is discussed further in the section "Respiratory Gating" below.

University of Michigan System

Investigators at the University of Michigan developed an IGRT system for high-dose irradiation of intrahepatic tumors comprising a racetrack microtron and diagnostic x-ray tubes mounted on the floor and ceiling of the treatment room.[295] An in-room shielded control booth allows direct visual contact of the patient during kilovoltage imaging. This system was designed for use in conjunction with an active breathing control (ABC) apparatus to reduce tumor motion due to respiration. In a feasibility study, daily orthogonal images were obtained under ABC and aligned to the planning CT, using the diaphragm for SI alignment and the vertebral bodies for LR and AP alignment.[296] Overall, 171 of 262 (65%) fractions required repositioning. Setup errors were reduced from 3.8 mm (AP), 6.7 mm (SI), and 4.0 mm (RL) to 2.3 mm (AP), 3.5 mm (SI), and 2.1 mm (RL). Treatment time was 25 to 30 minutes, with breath holds of up to 35 seconds.

In a review of the 128 patients with unresectable intrahepatic tumors treated with high-dose conformal RT and hepatic artery floxuridine, Ben-Josef et al.[297] reported a median survival of 15.8 months, which was significantly improved over historical controls. Grade 3 and 4 toxicities were noted in 21% and 9% of patients, respectively. However, outcomes of patients treated with or without online setup corrections were not compared, so the direct effect of IGRT on patient outcome is not clear.

Prototype Gantry-Mounted Systems

Investigators at Tohoku University in Japan have modified a commercial linear accelerator to include x-ray generators (mounted on the gantry at plus or minus 45 degrees from the beam axis) opposite two sets of aSi flat panel sensors with images obtained at 15 frames per second (Fig. 11.12).[298] In a subsequent study, Takai et al.[299] used this system to image a gold seed on a rotating disc and a seed implanted in a metastatic lung tumor and reported excellent visualization of both. This system was combined with a dynamic MLC approach, potentially allowing tracking and continuously irradiating a moving target.

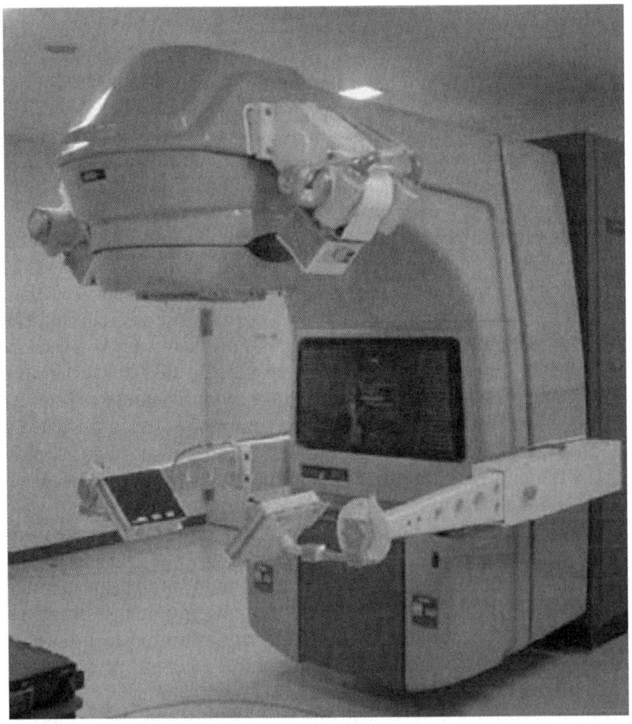

FIGURE 11.12. The prototype gantry-mounted image-guided radiation therapy (IGRT) system developed by Takai et al. at Tohoku University in Japan. (From Takai Y, Mitsuya M, Nemoto K, et al. Development of a new linear accelerator mounted with dual x-ray flouroscopy using amorphous silicon flat panel x-ray sensors to detect a gold seed in a tumor at real treatment position [abstr]. *Int J Radiat Oncol Biol Phys* 2001;51[Suppl]:381, with permission.)

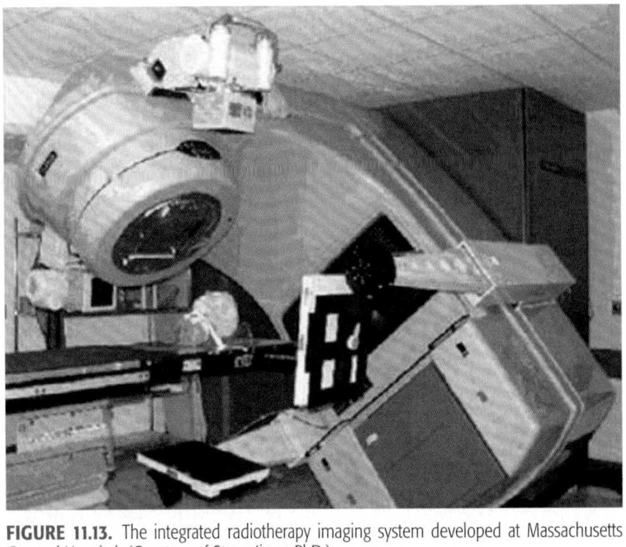

FIGURE 11.13. The integrated radiotherapy imaging system developed at Massachusetts General Hospital. (Courtesy of Steve Jiang, PhD.)

Inter- and intrafractional prostate organ motion has been evaluated using this system in eight patients with implanted gold markers.[299] After alignment using skin marks, images were obtained and isocenter shifts were calculated. Images were also obtained prior to every field with corrections of intrafractional displacements greater than 1 mm. The mean magnitudes of interfractional displacements were 1.76, 3.14, and 3.78 mm in the LR, SI, and AP directions, respectively. Corresponding intrafractional displacements were 0.45, 1.08, and 1.45 mm, respectively. Of 214 fractions, 84 (39%) required intrafractional corrections.

An integrated radiotherapy imaging system (IRIS) comprising two gantry-mounted diagnostic x-ray units mounted on either side of the machine head opposite two aSi flat panel detectors has been developed at Massachusetts General Hospital (Fig. 11.13).[300] The system co-rotates with the gantry, maintaining relative positions between the megavoltage and kilovoltage x-ray beams. It is also integrated with the pulsing of the LINAC to limit the amount of megavoltage noise during imaging. Each flat panel has an active area of 39.7 cm by 29.8 cm. To accommodate larger coverage for cone-beam CT acquisition (see "Volumetric Imaging" below), the panels are able to slide 13.2 cm along their long axes from their home position. Unlike commercially available systems, the dual-imager IRIS provides a *stereoscopic* view of the tumor, allowing assessment of the 3D trajectory of tumor motion. To date, no clinical studies have been published using this system.

Commercial Gantry-Mounted Systems

Two commercially gantry-mounted planar imaging systems are currently available: the Varian On-Board Imaging (OBI) system (Varian Medical Systems, Palo Alto, CA) and the Elekta Synergy (Elekta Oncology Systems, Norcross, GA). Both produce high-resolution diagnostic quality x-ray images of the patient in treatment position with considerably less dose than EPID. The Varian OBI system consists of an x-ray tube opposed to an aSi flat panel detector, both mounted to the LINAC gantry orthogonal to the treatment beam axis. The x-ray tube and aSi detector panel can be retracted from the imaging position via robotic arms (Fig. 11.14). The x-ray tube produces 40 to 150 kV x-rays with an image size of 40 by 30 cm^2. Images are acquired at 7.5 frames per second at 0.195 mm per pixel and 15.0 frames per second at 0.390 mm per pixel.

Fox et al.[301] presented an overview of OBI software and hardware and a performance evaluation of the automated image registration algorithm. In phantom verification tests, the registration algorithm was capable of detecting known

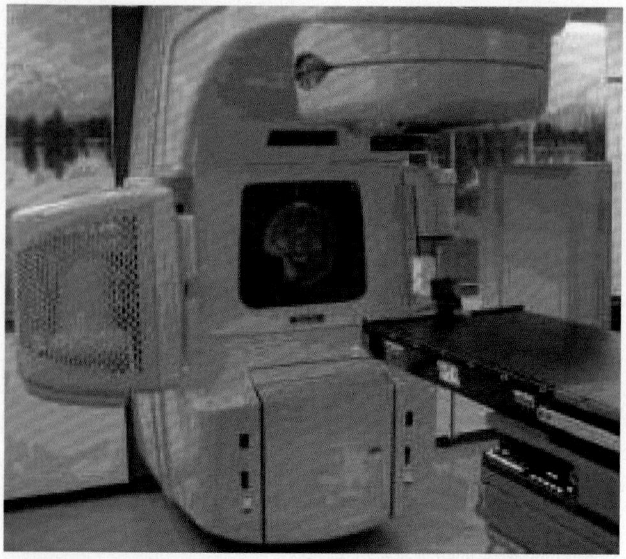

FIGURE 11.14. The Varian On-Board Imaging (OBI) system. (From Fox T, Huntzinger C, Johnstone P, et al. Performance evaluation of an automated image registration algorithm using an integrated kilovoltage imaging and guidance system. *J Appl Clin Med Phys* 2006;7:97–104, with permission.)

translations and rotations with an accuracy of less than 1.4 mm for a 3D vector offset (0.4 mm, 1.1 mm, and 0.8 mm in the lateral, longitudinal, and vertical dimensions, respectively). Earlier work demonstrated that the isocenter stability of the LINAC with the OBI arms extended is less than 1 mm.[302]

The Elekta Synergy system consists of an x-ray tube opposed to an aSi flat panel detector, both mounted to the LINAC gantry orthogonal to the treatment beam axis. Similar to the Varian system, the x-ray tube and aSi detector panel can be retracted via mechanical arms. The x-ray tube produces 60 to 150 kV x-rays with an image size of 41 by 41 cm^2. Modern day LINAC-based kilovolt imaging systems were originally developed by investigators at the William Beaumont Hospital (Fig. 11.15). A full description of their original system is provided by Jaffray et al.[303]

Commercial gantry kilovoltage planar systems are becoming increasing used clinically in the radiation oncology community.[131] Lawson et al.[304] presented their early clinical experience using the OBI system in 117 patients (2,088 sessions) with a wide variety of tumors. Overall, the great majority of alignments

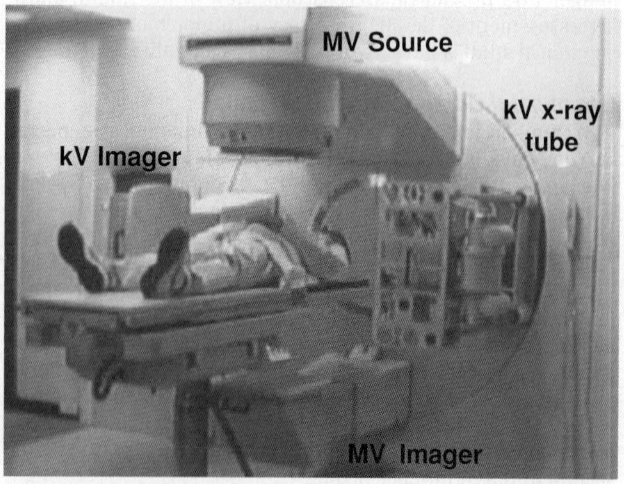

FIGURE 11.15. A modified Elekta linear accelerator (LINAC) with dual kilovoltage and megavoltage imaging capability. (From Jaffray SA, Drake DG, Moreau M, et al. A radiographic and tomographic imaging system integrated into a medical linear accelerator for localization of bone and soft-tissue targets. *Int J Radiat Oncol Biol Phys* 1999;45:773–789, with permission from Elsevier.)

based on either bones or implanted fiducial markers were small; however, 10% of lateral, longitudinal, and vertical shifts were 0.8 cm or more, 0.6 cm, and 0.7 cm, respectively. Median vector shifts varied between anatomic sites: 0.42 cm (HNC), 0.40 cm (brain), 0.59 (prostate), and 0.73 cm (breast). Pisani et al.[305] evaluated the accuracy of online setup errors using a kilovoltage and megavoltage dual-beam imaging system mounted on an Elekta SL-20 linear accelerator. Inter- and intraobserver variability was less with kilovoltage imaging in most cases.

Perkins et al.[306] presented the outcome of 13 GI tumor patients undergoing IMRT and concomitant chemotherapy with daily online setup corrections based on bony landmarks or surgical clips using the OBI system. Of 276 fractions, average isocenter shifts were 0.30 ± 0.42 cm (vertical), 0.33 ± 0.34 cm (longitudinal), and 0.35 ± 0.39 cm (lateral). Maximum corresponding shifts were 4.0, 2.3, and 2.4 cm, respectively. Grade 2 or higher acute nausea and diarrhea were noted in five and two patients, respectively. At a median follow-up of 6 months, 21% had disease regression and 71% stable disease. Investigators at Karolinska University reported on OBI in prostate cancer patients with implanted gold markers.[307] Shifts were determined by comparing daily orthogonal films of the patient on the treatment couch with reference DRRs at simulation, using a 2D matching algorithm with couch movements made remotely. The entire process added less than 1 minute to the treatment.

Others have presented their initial experiences using OBI in patients with prostate,[308] pancreas,[309,310] HNC,[311,312] and gynecologic cancers.[313–330] This system has also been used in patients undergoing SRS,[314] stereotactic body RT (SBRT),[315] and intracavitary brachytherapy.[316] An intriguing use of OBI is the daily localization of select normal tissues. Willis et al.[317] used daily OBI for verifying the location of kidneys in patients undergoing abdominal irradiation. In that study, kidneys were well visualized in 60% of the images. Ability to visualize the kidneys depended on multiple factors, including the relative anterior-posterior patient and kidney separation, axial profile of the kidneys, and relative contrast between the kidneys and surrounding structures.

Volumetric Imaging

In the IGRT survey, 59% of practicing radiation oncologists reported using volumetric imaging approaches clinically, most commonly in HNC, lung, GI, and prostate cancers.[131] Compared to other in-room IGRT approaches, volumetric IGRT technologies had been adopted more recently, with the majority of users having adopted them only since 2007.

Fusion of Computed Tomography and Linear Accelerator

The fusion of CT and LINAC (FOCAL) system comprises a Mitsubishi EXL-15DP linear accelerator (Mitsubishi Electric, Tokyo, Japan), a high-speed DX/I General Electric CT scanner (GE Medical Systems, Tokyo, Japan), and conventional x-ray simulator (Fig. 11.16). Developed at the National Defense Medical College in Japan, this system was designed primarily for stereotactic irradiation of lung tumors.[318] The gantry axes of the LINAC, CT scanner, and simulator are all coaxial, and the table can be rotated in three directions, allowing imaging with the CT scanner and simulator and treatment with the LINAC. Accuracy of the matching of the LINAC isocenter with the CT image is 0.5 mm or less.

Uematsu et al.[318–321] published a series of reports on the utility of FOCAL. Lung cancer patients are immobilized supine and instructed to perform shallow breathing, often with the aid of an oxygen mask. The position and motion of the lung tumor are first evaluated using planar x-rays. The table is then rotated to the CT and serial thin-slice scans are performed at 4 seconds per slice to ensure capturing of the full extent of tumor motion. The target volume is determined, the plan generated, and the table is rotated to the LINAC for treatment. Using this approach, Uematsu et al.[319] treated 50 stage I or II lung cancer

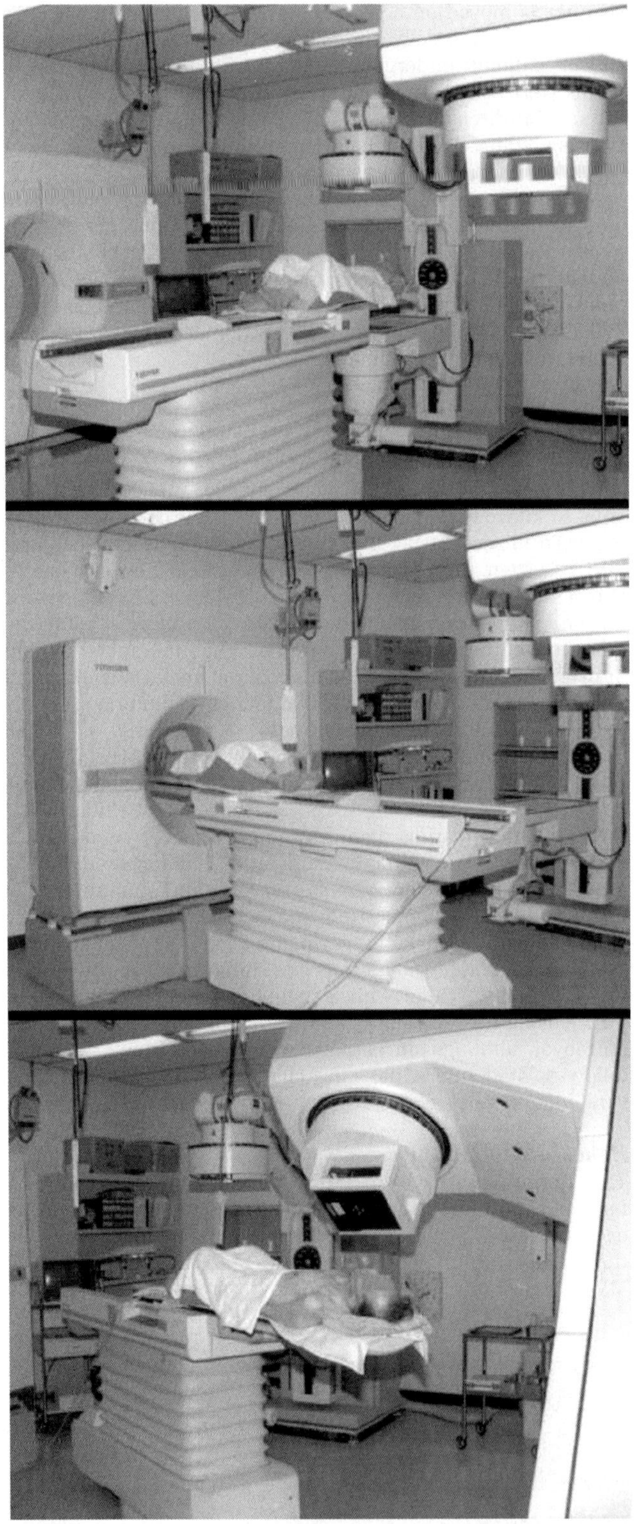

FIGURE 11.16. Fusion of computed tomography (CT) and linear accelerator (LINAC) unit (*top*). The table is rotated to the x-ray simulator to monitor respiratory motion, then to the CT for scanning (*middle*), and finally to the LINAC for treatment (*bottom*). (From Uematsu M, Shioda A, Suda A, et al. Intrafractional tumor position stability during computed tomography (CT)-guided frameless stereotactic radiation therapy for lung or liver cancers with a fusion of CT and linear accelerator (FOCAL) unit. *Int J Radiat Oncol Biol Phys* 2000;48:443–448, with permission from Elsevier.)

patients, primarily with 50 to 60 Gy in 5 to 10 fractions. At a median follow-up of 36 months, local control was 94%. No adverse sequelae were noted, apart from minor bone fractures and temporary pleural pain in two and six patients, respectively.

In a separate study, FOCAL was used to evaluate intrafraction tumor stability in 38 lung and 12 liver tumor patients.[320] Overall, no intrafraction movements greater than 10 mm were noted, and 68% of lesions had clinically negligible changes in position (0 to 5 mm). The percentage of upper lung, lower lung, and liver tumors with 5 mm or less movements were 100%, 50%, and 25%, respectively. However, in addition to coaching all patients on shallow breathing, abdominal belts were used in select patients to further reduce motion.

Memorial Sloan-Kettering Cancer Center System

Investigators at Memorial Sloan-Kettering Cancer Center (MSKCC) have constructed a treatment system consisting of a conventional CT scanner (Phillips Medical Systems, Milpitas, CA) and a Clinac 2100EX linear accelerator (Varian Medical Systems, Palo Alto, CA).[322,323] The CT scanner couch and LINAC table are aligned, permitting a smooth transfer to the LINAC after the CT is performed. In an initial report, Yenice et al.[322] described the treatment of paraspinal patients with this system. Patients were first immobilized in a stereotactic body frame, using pressures points on select skeletal structures. A planning CT scan was then performed and an IMRT plan generated. A CT scan in the treatment room was then obtained and automatically registered using bony landmarks and surgical hardware to the planning CT scan. Prior to treatment, a second registration was performed using fiducial markers on the frame and patient. The entire process required approximately 60 to 85 minutes for the initial fraction. Overall 3D accuracy of the system was 1.3 ± 0.8 mm.

The outcome of 35 paraspinal tumor patients (14 primary, 21 metastatic) undergoing IMRT using the MSKCC system has been presented.[323] Overall, 24 (68%) had received prior RT. A planning margin of 10 mm was used, except at the spinal cord interface where 5 mm was used. The median prescribed dose was 20 Gy in 5 fractions. At a median follow-up of 11 months, the 2-year local control for primary and metastatic tumors was 75% and 81%, respectively. Of 30 patients with more than 3 months follow-up, 90% experienced excellent palliation. No patient developed late RT-related sequelae. In their latest report focusing on previously irradiated patients,[324] daily CT myelograms were performed to improve localization of the spinal cord and cauda equina.

Recently, investigators at MSKCC published a study of patients with extracranial metastases treated with either single fraction or hypofractionated SBRT regimens.[325] The 3-year actuarial local progression-free survival for the entire group was 44%. However, lesions that were treated with high-dose single fraction sizes (≥24 Gy) had a local progression-free survival of 88%, compared to 21% in lesions treated with lower single fraction doses (<24 Gy) and 17% in those undergoing hypofractionated RT.

Computed Tomography on Rails

The initial CT-on-rails system was developed at the University of Yamanashi in Japan. It consists of a linear accelerator, a CT scanner, and a common treatment couch, with the LINAC and the CT gantries positioned at opposite ends of the patient couch.[326] This system minimizes patient movement and displacement by moving the gantry of the CT scanner instead of the couch within the gantry. The basis of this system is the Smart Gantry system (GE Medical Systems, Tokyo, Japan), which comprises one middle and two side rails. The side rails ensure controlled horizontal gantry movement, whereas the middle rail guides the gantry forward and backward in the direction of scanning. Kuriyama et al.[326] reported that the positional accuracy of the common couch was 0.2, 0.18, and 0.39 mm in the lateral, longitudinal, and vertical directions, respectively. The scan-position accuracy of the CT gantry was less than 0.4 mm in all three axes.

In a series of reports, Onishi et al.[327,328] described the utility of the CT-on-rails system in patients with unresected lung cancer. Twenty-two stages I to IIIB patients were treated using voluntary breath hold and self-directed beam control. Patients were able to turn the beam on or off using a hand-held switch.[327] Using fluoroscopy, a comfortable degree of breath hold was identified, which maintained tumor position. Tumor position was found to be highly reproducible, with average positional differences of 2.2, 1.4, and 1.3 mm in the SI, AP, and RL positions, respectively, between the daily and planning CT scans. In a separate report, they treated 35 stage I lung cancer patients with 60 Gy in 10 fractions.[328] At a median follow-up of 13 months, 94% of tumors were locally controlled. Five patients developed mild (grade 1 or 2) late respiratory symptoms.

Recently, several investigators have published experiences using commercial CT-on-rails systems. Investigators at M.D. Anderson Cancer Center used Varian ExaCT Targeting System (Varian Medical Systems, Palo Alto, CA), which integrates a high-speed CT scanner on rails (GE Medical Systems, Milwaukee, WI) with a Varian dual-energy LINAC equipped with a 120 MLC.[329,330] The couch base is rotated to position the patient for either treatment or scanning, without the need to transfer onto the CT couch. Court et al.[331] reviewed the accuracy of this system and noted that the largest single uncertainty was the couch position on the CT side after a rotation (0.5 mm in the lateral direction). All other sources of uncertainty, including the difference in couch sag between the CT and LINAC, were less than 0.3 mm.

Chang et al.[330] treated 15 patients with spine metastases with IMRT on a phase I clinical trial using ExaCT. All patients were immobilized in a stereotactic body frame and received 30 Gy in 5 fractions, with a maximum cord dose of 10 Gy. On average, the duration of the daily procedure was 1.5 hours. At a median follow-up of 9 months, no patient developed significant RT-related sequelae. These investigators reported the outcome of 63 patients with 74 spine lesions treated using CT-on-rails on the phase I trial and a subsequent phase II trial.[332] At a median follow-up of 21.3 months, the 1-year local progression-free survival was 82%, with 52% of patients pain free at 12 months. No patient developed late grade 3 or higher neurologic sequelae. Favorable results have similarly been reported using this approach in patients with renal cell spine metastases[333] and those undergoing reirradiation.[334]

Others have reported their experiences using the Siemens Primatom CT-on-rails (Siemens Oncology Systems, Concord, CA). This system consists of a Somatom CT scanner and a Primus linear accelerator in the same vault sharing a common table or couch (Fig. 11.17).[335–338] As with other systems, the CT scanner is moved on a pair of horizontal rails. Wong et al.[335] used Primatom to deliver the boost treatments in 108 prostate cancer patients undergoing IMRT. Overall, isocenter adjustments were common. The percentage of adjustments in the AP, SI, and LR directions were 54%, 27%, and 34%, respectively. Corresponding shifts of 1 cm or greater were noted in 15%, 4%, and 5% of patients, respectively.

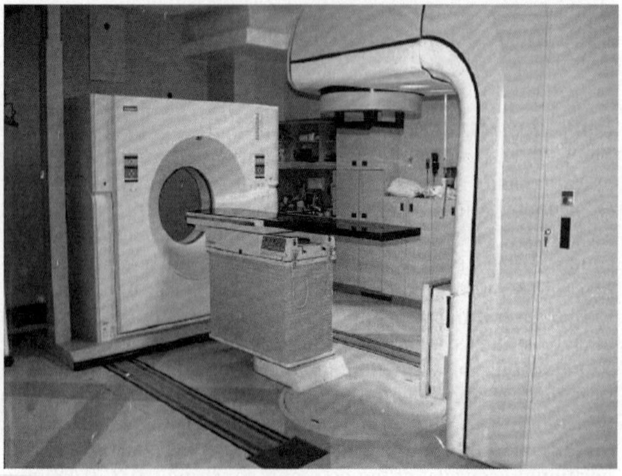

FIGURE 11.17. The Siemens Primatom computed tomography-on-rails system. (From Wong JR, Grimm L, Uematsu M, et al. Image-guided radiotherapy for prostate cancer by CT-linear accelerator combination: prostate movements and dosimetric considerations. *Int J Radiat Oncol Biol Phys* 2005;61:561–569, with permission from Elsevier.)

Ma and Paskalev[339] provided an excellent review of in-room CT systems and techniques. The future of such systems remains unclear given the increasing availability of other commercial volumetric imaging systems, including on-board CBCT and helical tomotherapy.[340] However, the value and possible applications of high-quality in-room conventional CT images remains an interesting area for clinical research.

Megavoltage Systems

Early Megavoltage Computed Tomography Systems

The underlying principle of megavoltage CT (MVCT) is analogous to kilovoltage CT, namely an x-ray source and detectors are used to reconstruct 2D images into 3D datasets. The first MVCT system was developed in 1982, consisting of a modified 4 MV linear accelerator with a detector array mounted on the LINAC gantry.[341] In addition to the appeal of using the megavoltage beam for imaging, MVCT has the added benefit of producing images free of the streaking artifacts common in kilovoltage CT, secondary to dental fillings or hip prostheses.

More recently, investigators at the University of Tokyo mounted a small detector on the gantry of a 6 MV LINAC in order to generate MVCT images in lung tumor patients undergoing SRS.[342,343] All patients were instructed to maintain shallow breathing during planning and treatment to minimize organ motion. Moreover, at simulation, tumor motion was assessed by fluoroscopy, and, if greater than 1 cm, an oxygen mask and a belt compressing the chest and abdomen were used. Immediately prior to treatment, a MVCT was obtained on the treatment table and appropriate shifts are made. In a series of 14 patients treated with a median single fraction dose of 20 Gy using this approach, the overall local control was 95%. Moreover, although all patients with greater than 3 months follow-up had interstitial lung changes, only one developed symptomatic pneumonitis.

Helical Tomotherapy

The Tomotherapy system (Tomotherapy Inc., Madison, WI) has a 6 MV LINAC and a detector array mounted opposite each other on a ring gantry that continuously rotates while the couch is translated through the gantry (Fig. 11.18).[344,345] MVCT imaging on the Tomotherapy system is performed by

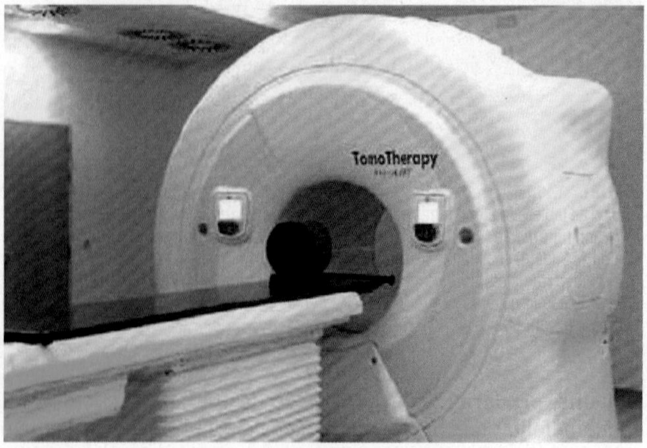

FIGURE 11.18. The helical Tomotherapy system. (From Tomsej M. The Tomotherapy Hi-Art System for sophisticated IMRT and IGRT with helical delivery: recent developments and clinical applications. *Cancer Radiother* 2006;10:288–295, with permission from Elsevier.)

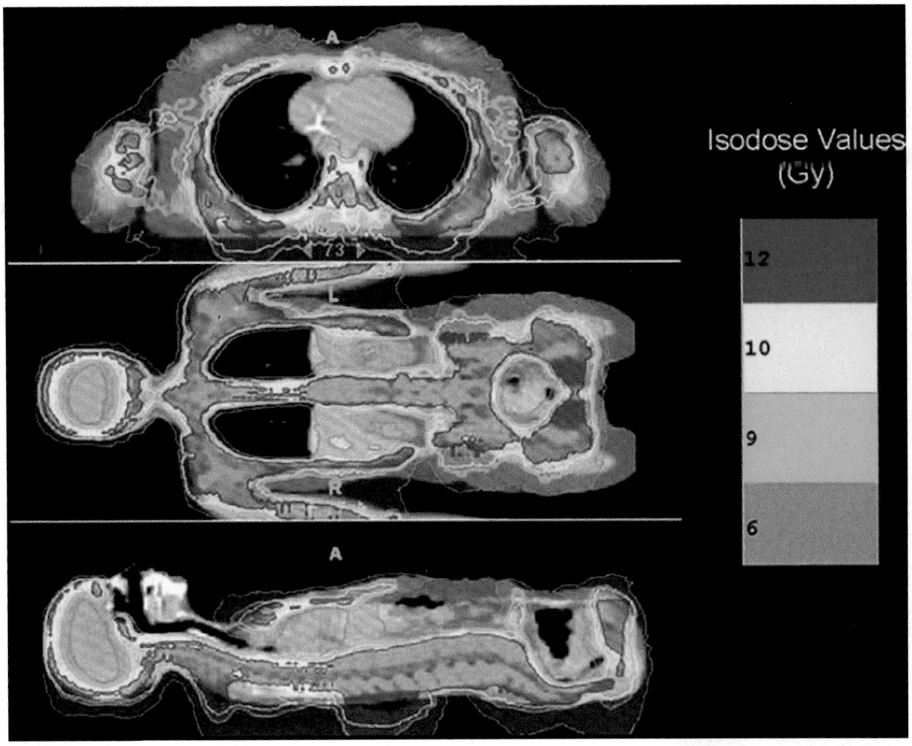

FIGURE 11.19. Color wash showing dose distribution for a 20-year-old female patient treated with targeted total body irradiation using Tomotherapy. The target structure is skeletal bone. Relative sparing of the brain, oral cavity, thyroid, lungs, heart, soft tissue, and gastrointestinal tract is seen. (From Wong JYC, Rosenthal K, Liu A, et al. Image guided total marrow irradiation (TMI) using helical Tomotherapy in patients with multiple myeloma and acute leukemia undergoing hematopoietic cell transplantation. *Int J Radiat Oncol Biol Phys* 2009;73:273–279, with permission from Elsevier.)

reducing the nominal energy of the incident electron beam to 3.5 MeV.[346] Three acquisition modes are available (fine, normal, and coarse).

Investigators at the University of Wisconsin evaluated Tomotherapy MVCT imaging for optimizing setup in eight dogs undergoing RT.[347] Prior to treatment, a MVCT scan was obtained and aligned with the planning kilovoltage CT scan in the transverse and sagittal planes. MVCT images were of sufficient quality for verification of treatment setup in all eight animals, although soft tissue contrast was inferior to that of the kilovoltage CT scans. Both the primary tumor and adjacent bony landmarks were used for alignment. The entire process took approximately 5 to 12 minutes, including 3 minutes for image acquisition.

Mahan et al.[348] reported on Tomotherapy for optimizing patient setup in eight patients undergoing reirradiation of spinal metastases. The mean retreatment dose was 28 Gy, with the maximum cord dose of 27% to 56% of the prescribed dose. Prior to treatment, MVCT images were acquired and autofused with the planning CT scan, allowing calculation of couch translations. The range of interfraction displacement was as great as 1.5 cm, with standard deviations of ± 4 mm (AP), ± 4.3 (SI), and ± 4.1 (RL). At a median follow-up of 15.2 months, all eight patients responded (two partial, six complete). None developed an in-field recurrence or significant late toxicity. Others have reported the value of daily setup verification using the Tomotherapy system in other sites, notably lung cancer.[349,350]

A concern with the use of the Tomotherapy system for daily setup verification is image quality. Although less of a concern when bony landmarks are used, this is important when alignment is based solely on soft tissues. Song et al.[351] evaluated the feasibility of Tomotherapy for daily prostate localization. MVCT images were acquired and compared to the planning kilovoltage CT images in five patients. Of note, prostate volumes were smaller and more consistent on kilovoltage CT scans. Moreover, inter- and intraobserver contouring uncertainty was greater for MVCT. Daily alignment can be improved in prostate patients, however, with implanted fiducials, which are well visualized on the Tomotherapy system.[352]

Tomotherapy is a popular IGRT treatment approach, with multiple dosimetric studies supporting its potential benefits.[353,354–360] Multiple investigators have reported favorable results using the Tomotherapy system for HNC[361] and CNS,[362] pediatric,[363] GI,[364] gynecologic,[365] and GU[366] tumors. An intriguing use of Tomotherapy is in the delivery of total marrow irradiation in place of total body irradiation in leukemia patients undergoing allogeneic stem cell transplantation (Fig. 11.19).[367]

Megavoltage Cone-Beam Computed Tomography Systems

Megavoltage CBCT imaging is accomplished by first generating a series of 2D projections around the patient with the megavoltage beam and a detector.[368] A 3D dataset is then reconstructed using the Feldkamp algorithm,[369] in a process analogous to conventional CT imaging, whereby an x-ray source and a detector are mounted on a rotating gantry. However, whereas a conventional CT system uses a 1D linear detector array, the CBCT system uses a 2D array.

Multiple investigators have evaluated the utility of megavoltage CBCT,[370,371–373,374,375] with the largest published experience from UCSF.[370,374,375–376] Pouliot et al.[374] described patient alignment and dose verification using a 6-MV Primus linear accelerator (Siemens Oncology Systems, Concord, CA) operating in arc mode equipped with an aSi flat-panel EPID. Megavoltage CBCT scans were generated using an anthropomorphic head phantom, frozen sheep or pig cadaver heads, and HNC patients, requiring doses of 0.05 to 0.15 Gy. Acquisition and processing times were both on the order of 90 seconds. Megavoltage CBCT and conventional CT datasets were registered with millimeter and degree accuracy.

Morin et al.[370] evaluated the potential benefits of megavoltage CBCT imaging in HNC, lung, and pelvic cancer patients treated on a prospective clinical trial. In a locally advanced HNC patient, megavoltage CBCT detected a misalignment of the vertebral bodies and spinal cord in the neck not seen on portal imaging (Fig. 11.20). Megavoltage CBCT has also been found to complement treatment planning in patients with implanted metallic objects.[377]

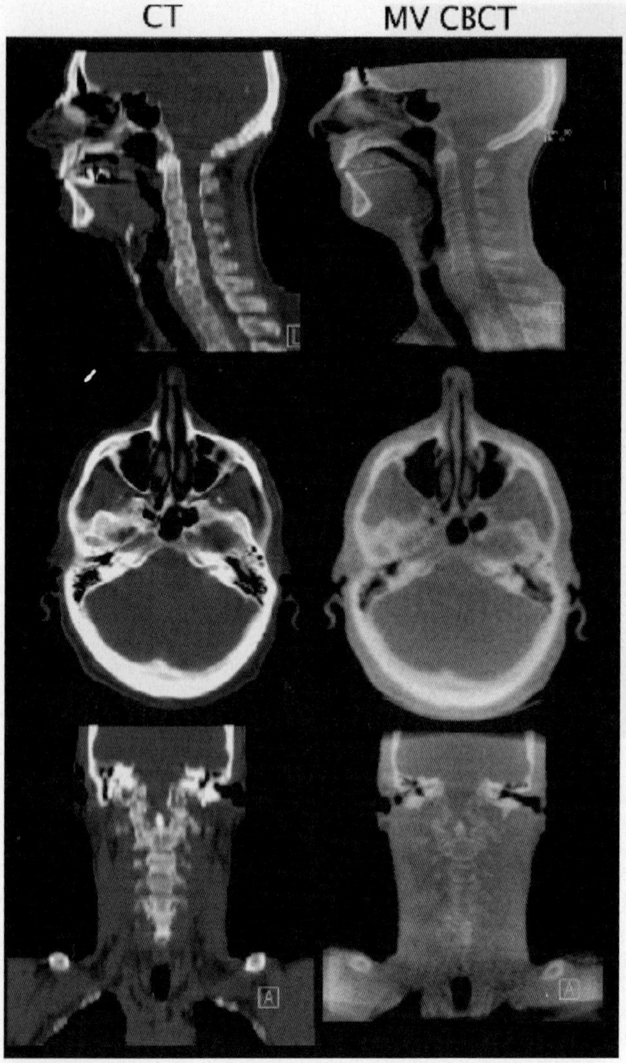

FIGURE 11.20. Comparison of a kilovoltage computed tomography (CT) scan (*left*) with a megavoltage cone-beam CT (*right*) of a head-and-neck cancer patient. The window level of both images was adjusted to provide the best soft-tissue contrast. (From Morin O, Gillis A, Chen J, et al. Megavoltage cone-beam CT: system description and clinical applications. *Med Dosim* 2006;31:51–61, with permission from Elsevier.)

Outcomes of patients specifically undergoing megavoltage CBCT imaging during treatment are limited. Swamy et al.[378] evaluated the use of dose-escalated IMRT treatment in 12 intact prostate cancer patients. Following implantation of fiducials, patients underwent megavoltage CBCT daily to localize the prostate. At a mean follow-up of 12.2 months, 92% of patients were biochemically controlled. Only one patient developed grade 2 proctitis following treatment; no grade 3 or higher toxicities were seen.

Kilovoltage Systems

Mobile Fluoroscopic C-Arm Systems

Several groups have reported on kilovoltage CBCT scanning using a mobile fluoroscopic C-arm imager.[378–380] Swamy et al.[378,380] modified a commercial mobile isocentric fluoroscopic C-arm (Power-Mobil, Siemens Medical Solutions, Erlangen, Germany), replacing the standard image intensifier with an aSi flat-panel detector. A projection set of 100 to 1,000 images are obtained while the C-arm rotates around the patient in a 180-degree arc. Similar to megavoltage CBCT imaging, kilovoltage CBCT images are reconstructed using the Feldkamp algorithm, modified due to the limited projection arc.[381] Similar units have been developed at other centers.[382]

The feasibility of using kilovoltage CBCT imaging produced by a mobile C-arm system in patients with prostate and HNC to improve setup and target localization has been presented.[378] Patients underwent kilovoltage CBCT imaging weekly and the images were assessed offline. Overall, the imaging procedure was performed in less than 5 minutes with less dose than conventional CT. Although spatial resolution was good, image quality was not ideal (e.g., differentiation of the prostate from the rectum in the area of the prostate-rectum interface was poor). In sites prone to respiratory-induced motion, image quality can be improved by correlating the CBCT acquisition with breathing.[380]

Gantry-Mounted Cone-Beam Computed Tomography Systems

Most major linear accelerator vendors currently offer gantry-mounted kilovoltage CBCT solutions. The Elekta Synergy and Varian OBI systems consist of kilovoltage x-ray tubes mounted opposite flat panel detectors orthogonal to the treatment beam on retractable arms.[383,384] In collaboration with investigators at the University of Heidelberg, Siemens is developing an "in-line" system that places the diagnostic x-ray tube at 180 degrees to the megavoltage source (Fig. 11.21).[385,386] All three systems acquire kilovoltage projections during a 360-degree gantry rotation, which are reconstructed into a 3D dataset.[387]

The initial prototype (and its corresponding commercial counterpart) of the Elekta kilovoltage CBCT system has been presented in reports from William Beaumont Hospital.[388,389] In a phantom study in prostate cancer, kilovoltage CBCT was found to achieve a setup accuracy of 1 mm or less in the LR, AP, and SI directions. Setup error was reduced in nearly all cases and was generally within ± 1.5 mm. The entire image-guided process required 23 to 35 minutes. Others have presented their experiences using the Elekta kilovoltage CBCT system.[390–394] In 20 patients with various tumors, McBain et al.[390] noted sufficient image quality in all patients, including those in whom full gantry rotations were not possible (extremity and breast tumor patients). In general, soft tissue delineation was sufficient to allow assessment of the target and normal tissues. However, prostate images were not sufficiently distinct to allow organ contouring, compensation for small (<3 mm) movements, or for verification of small PTV margins.

Guckenberger et al.[391] compared the utility of the Elekta kilovoltage CBCT system with EPID in terms of setup accuracy in 24 patients with a variety of tumors. Kilovoltage CBCT was found to add little in the assessment of translational errors. Translational errors detected with either approach differed by less than 1 mm in 70.7% and less than 2 mm in 93.2% of measurements. However, CBCT was superior in the detection of rotational errors. Rotational errors greater than 2 degrees were noted in 3.7%, 26.4%, and 12.4% of pelvic cancers, thoracic cancers, and HNC, respectively. Such rotational errors led to poorer target coverage and increased normal tissue dose in cases with elongated targets in close proximity to normal tissues. Several authors have presented their experience using the Varian kilovoltage CBCT system in the treatment of a variety of tumors including neuroblastoma[395] and bladder cancer.[396]

Thilmann et al.[386] evaluated the utility of the in-line kilovoltage CBCT system developed in collaboration with Siemens. In a study of various tumor sites, bony landmarks were easily visualized on all images, allowing table shifts to be automatically calculated. Soft tissue contrast was acceptable except in one morbidly obese patient. Using an action level of 2 mm, setup corrections were performed in four of six patients. Approximately 10 to 12 minutes were required to perform imaging, reconstruction, analysis, and positional corrections.

No detailed clinical outcome studies are yet available in patients treated using kilovoltage CBCT for either setup or target localization. However, Groh et al.[397] compared the performance of megavoltage and kilovoltage CBCT technologies.

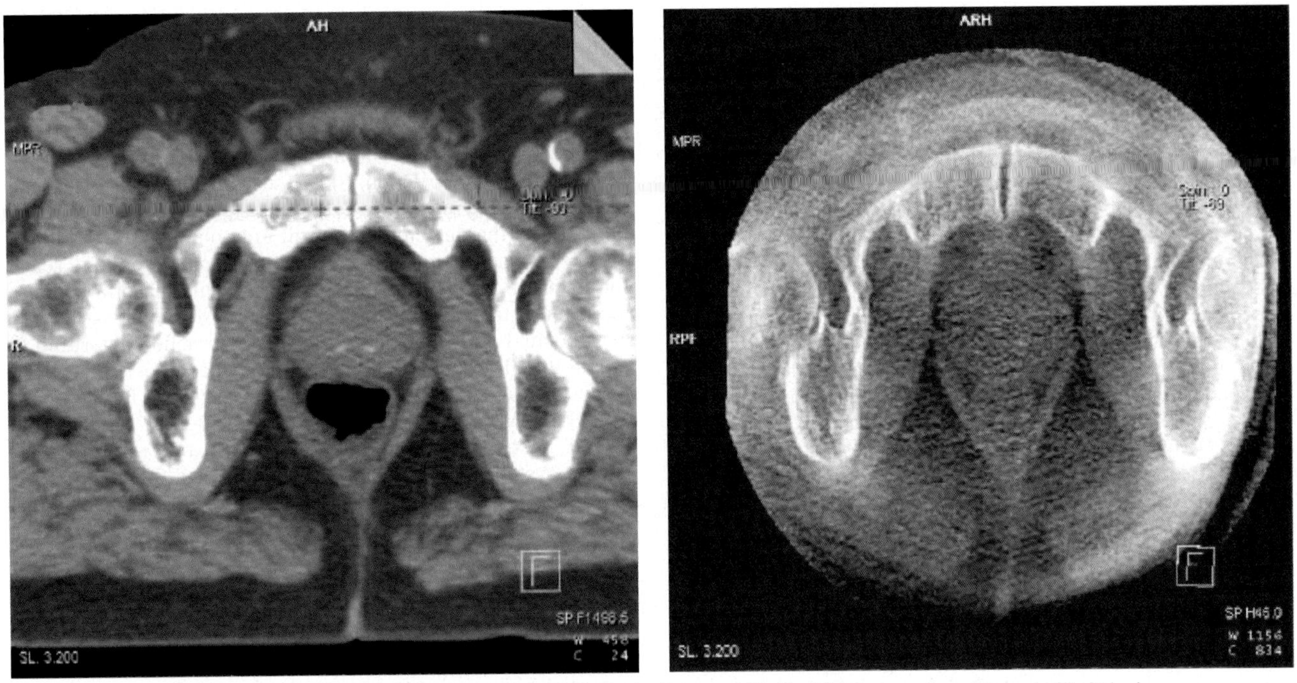

FIGURE 11.21. Comparison of a conventional computed tomography (CT) scan (*left*) with a kilovoltage cone-beam CT scan (*right*) obtained using a mobile fluoroscopic C-arm imager in a patient with prostate cancer. (From Sorensen SP, Chow PE, Kriminiski S, et al. Image-guided radiotherapy using a mobile kilovoltage x-ray device. *Med Dosim* 2006;31:40–50, with permission from Elsevier.)

Megavoltage CBCT was found to offer an advantage in terms of simplicity of mechanical integration with a linear accelerator. In contrast, kilovoltage CBCT was found to be superior in terms of imaging of soft tissue structures and the signal-to-noise ratio per unit dose.

In the coming years, numerous advancements are expected in kilovoltage CBCT technology. One area of active research is digital tomosynthesis (DTS), a method of reconstructing 3D slices from 2D cone beam x-ray projections data acquired with limited source angulation (e.g., 40 degrees). Unlike conventional kilovoltage CBCT approaches, DTS requires less scan time and results in less radiation exposure to the patient. Investigators from Duke University recently illustrated the ability to generate high-quality images using the DTS approach in patients with prostate, HNC, and liver tumors.[398]

Electromagnetic Localization Systems

Electromagnetic localization systems are typically based on a magnetic dipole source and one or more sensors to detect a magnetic field created by the dipole. The dipole source is excited by a radiofrequency (RF) signal that creates a magnetic field. Overall, the system operates such that when the RF signal is removed, a capacitor is discharged, resulting in an oscillating magnetic dipole. A transponder is an electric device used to wirelessly transmit and receive electrical signals. The dipole sources in clinical electromagnetic systems are generally referred to as transponders. Each transponder is similar in size to a gold fiducial marker. The transponders are permanently implanted within the tissue to be treated. To date, the only commercial system is supplied by Calypso Medical Technologies, Inc. (Seattle, WA). An excellent review of this technology and its clinical use in IGRT is given by Litzenberg.[399] The benefits of electromagnetic tracking systems are: (a) transponders can be implanted directly into the target, (b) nonionizing radiation is used, and (c) real-time positional determination is possible during the treatment fraction.

Particular attention has been focused on the use of the Calypso system for prostate cancer patients undergoing definitive RT.[400–404] Kupelian et al.[400] reported a multi-institutional study of 35 patients undergoing prostate localization and continuous monitoring during treatment. An average initial displacement (from setup skin marks) exceeding 5 mm was seen in more than 75% of sessions analyzed. Displacement of 3 mm or move and 5 mm or more for 30 seconds or longer occurred during 41% and 15% of sessions, respectively. The percentage of fractions in an individual patient with displacements of 3 mm or more varied considerably (3% to 87%). In a study of 28 patients with implanted Calypso transponders, Rajendran et al.[401] noted that the average number of treatment days with shifts beyond 0.5 cm in the vertical, longitudinal, and lateral directions were 62%, 35%, and 38%, respectively. No outcome comparisons have been performed of prostate cancer patients treated with and without the Calypso system; hence, the clinical importance of this intrafraction displacement remains unclear.

Less attention has been focused on the use of the Calypso system in other tumor sites. Shinohara et al.[405] recently evaluated the potential of using the Calypso system in five patients with locally advanced pancreatic cancer. Overall, the markers were well tolerated, with minimal migration noted, except in one patient who expulsed a single transponder. The mean initial shifts (from the setup markers) were 4.5 mm, 6.4 mm, and 3.9 mm in the x, y, and z directions, respectively. Mean intrafraction motion was significant in all directions: superior (7.2 mm), inferior (11.9 mm), anterior (4.9 mm), posterior (2.9 mm), left (2.2 mm), and right (3.1 mm).

Few in-room IGRT systems provide the ability to perform continuous monitoring of target position. Thus, particularly in sites in which intrafraction motion is a concern, the use of the Calypso system remains appealing.

Emerging In-Room Imaging Technologies

Increasing interest has focused on the combining treatment devices with advanced imaging modalities to create novel in-room IGRT platforms. These platforms can incorporate functional and high-resolution imaging to facilitate better setup and target delineation than is possible with CT-based techniques. Such technologies may provide the possibility for improved adaptive RT techniques in the future.

Magnetic Resonance–Linear Accelerator Systems

MRI provides superior soft-tissue resolution compared to CT. Because linear accelerators are the dominant radiation delivery device in developed radiotherapy programs, in-room MR-LINAC systems are being developed, but to date no commercial systems are available. An early proposal for an integrated MR-LINAC was from the University Medical Center Utrecht.[406] This system was designed as a 1.5-T MRI scanner with diagnostic quality imaging integrated with a 6-MV LINAC. More recently, simultaneous MRI and megavoltage transmission images were acquired with the imaging systems without interfering with each other.[407] The first operational prototype system reported in the literature was at the Cross Cancer Institute.[408] This prototype used a fixed gantry 6-MV LINAC in conjunction with a 0.2-T MRI system and fully operational MRIs were acquired during LINAC beam-on. There are issues with MR-LINAC systems such as magnetic interference at the LINAC due to the MR fringe fields, beam losses with the electron gun and RF noise from MLC motors. However, these are active areas of research and do not appear to be insurmountable hurdles toward the clinical implementation of MR-LINAC systems.[409–411]

Magnetic Resonance–Cobalt Systems

Due to some of the technical issues limiting MR-LINAC systems, MR-cobalt systems have also been developed.[412] MR-cobalt systems consist of one or more high-dose-rate cobalt sources, an MRI system, and MLCs for IMRT (the same issues exist with RF noise from MLC motors as for MR-LINAC systems). A commercial cobalt-MR system has been developed by ViewRay Inc. (Oakwood Village, OH) and utilizes a 0.35-T MR, 3 KCi cobalt sources and three double-focused MLCs (Fig. 11.22).

As with MR-LINAC systems, the dose distributions can be significantly affected by high magnetic fields. The effect is a significant increase in dose at tissue air boundaries, due to returning electrons in the presence of magnetic fields, known as the electron return effect. The magnitude of this effect depends on the strength of the magnetic field. It has been demonstrated that this effect is minimal for lower magnetic fields of about 0.2 T.[413] Therefore, it is advantageous to use the lowest possible magnetic field strength while still obtaining MR images with sufficient spatial resolution.

On-Board Single-Photon Emission Computed Tomography Imaging Systems

SPECT imaging uses a radiotracer attached to a biologically active molecule, which is injected into the patient. The energy of γ-ray emission depends on the radionuclide used in the procedure. A gamma camera is used in SPECT imaging to create 3D images. The gamma camera collects γ-rays that are emitted from within the patient. An image of the radionuclide location within the patient is generated from the data collected by the gamma camera. The aspects making up the gamma camera are the collimator, detector crystal, photomultiplier tube array, and reconstruction algorithm such as filtered back projection or iterative reconstruction. SPECT uses collimation (e.g., lead block containing many tiny holes that is positioned between the patient and the detector) to permit only photons of essentially parallel trajectory to pass through the collimator and reach the detector. Given knowledge of the orientation of a collimator's holes, the original path of a detected photon is linearly extrapolated and thus used in the reconstruction algorithm to create the 3D image. Simulation studies have been performed to determine the potential localization accuracy for on-board SPECT-LINAC systems. It was determined that conventional SPECT systems were too cumbersome, and realization of such a system would be better accomplished using a smaller gamma camera with a limited imaging region that would also be mobile to move it closer to the patient and to enhance the spatial resolution.[414]

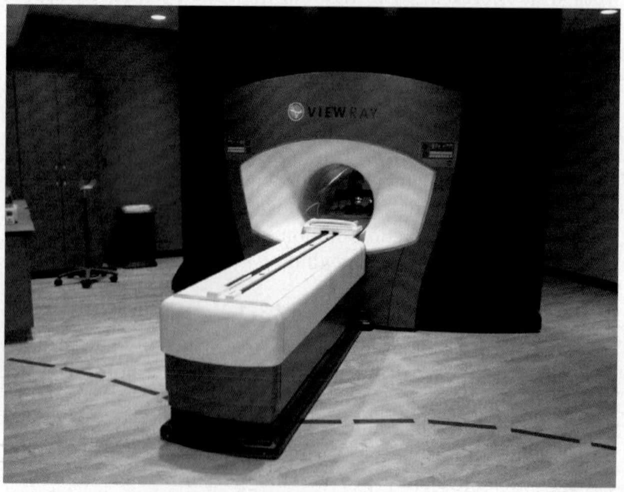

FIGURE 11.22. Viewray cobalt magnetic resonance system. (Courtesy of Timothy Sokolich.)

Proton–Positron Emission Tomography Systems

PET, similar to SPECT, is an imaging technique in which a radionuclide is synthetically introduced into a molecule of potential biological relevance and administered to a patient. However, the physics of photon emission is different from that for SPECT. In PET, the photons emitted from the radiotracer are coincident, that is, nearly back to back. Locating the source of an annihilation event is a method known as coincident detection. PET systems have similar components as SPECT systems (e.g., detectors, photomultiplier tube, collimators, and a reconstruction algorithm), except that a PET camera is constructed so that opposing detectors are used. Each annihilation event is presumed to have occurred at some point along an imaginary line between the two. This information is registered in the reconstruction algorithm. Coincidence detection is a very efficient technique and contributes to PET's superior sampling rates and sensitivity compared to SPECT.

During proton therapy, inelastic reactions between the treatment protons and nuclei of the tissues in the patient produce small amounts of short-lived positron-emitting isotopes. PET imaging has been suggested as a method to determine the geometric accuracy of the treatment delivery. The threshold of inelastic nuclear reactions leading to tissue positron activation is in the energy range of 15 to 20 MeV. The distal activity falloff is not exactly matched to the dose falloff at the end of the proton range. Nonetheless, a clinical study was completed to investigate proton-PET IGRT for offline proton treatment verification.[415] This pilot study was followed by further development of this approach to include efficient analytical models to accurately predict the expected PET images based on the treatment plan.[416] Furthermore, mobile PET scanners have been investigated to provide a low-cost solution for in-room PET imaging, which also has the advantage of increasing the imaging sensitivity partly due to lower biological washout.[417]

FOUR-DIMENSIONAL IMAGING AND MOTION MANAGEMENT

Respiratory Motion

Respiratory-induced organ motion presents a significant challenge. Particularly for tumors in the thorax and upper abdomen, movements can be greater than 3 cm if the motion is not actively controlled (Fig. 11.23).[285,418] Respiratory motion can result in imaging artifacts on both the planning CT and the CBCT used for treatment guidance. If left uncorrected, this can lead to target delineation and beam placement uncertainties that compromise the overall effectiveness of the treatment. There are numerous

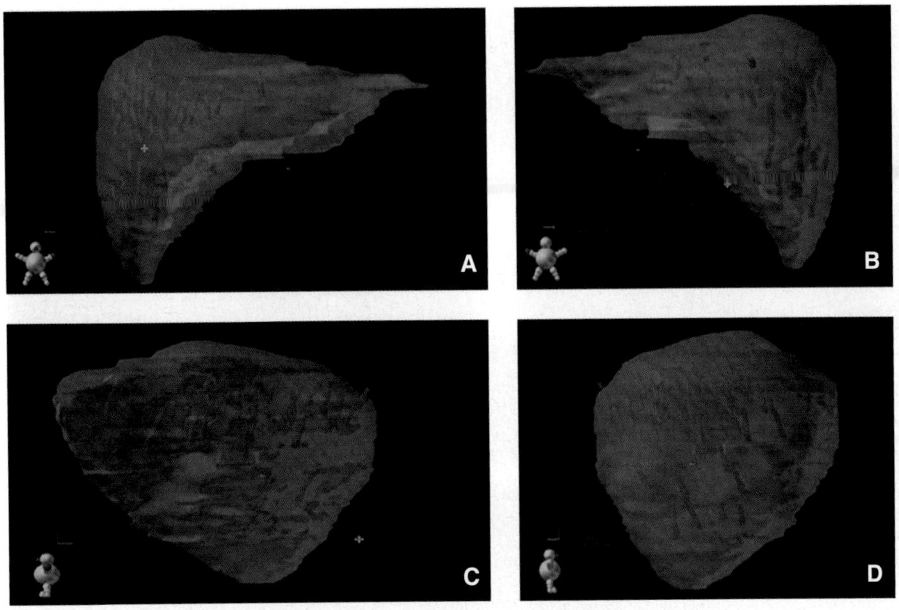

FIGURE 11.23. Tumor trajectories in 20 liver cancer patients, measured using a total of 49 implanted markers during cone-beam computed tomography acquisition: **(A)** Anterior-to-posterior, **(B)** Posterior-to-anterior, **(C)** Left-to-right, and **(D)** Right-to-left projection view. An average motion of up to 3.0 ± 0.4 cm was observed for a patient, in 1 fraction.

ways to compensate for motion and minimize its impact on the treatment integrity, including 4D imaging, 4D target delineation, increased planning margins, voluntary breath-hold and shallow breathing, abdominal compression, respiratory gating, and real-time tumor tracking. Although most of these approaches have been in clinical use in various forms, each has pros and cons that need to be weighed for use in an individual clinic.

Four-Dimensional Imaging

Four-dimensional imaging refers to the acquisition of spatial motion information over time. This can be done with CT,[419,420] PET,[421] or MRI.[422] All have all been successfully used for RT planning. Only 4D CT has seen widespread use in the past decade, although 4D PET is gaining more interest, especially used in combination with 4D CT.[423,424] The need for 4D CT is nicely illustrated in Figure 11.24. As can be seen, without 4D imaging, significant and unpredictable artifacts can render tumor visualization difficult. Depending on the scanning speed relative to the tumor motion speed, artifacts appear in different ways.[425] If the scan speed is much *slower* than the tumor speed, a smeared image is captured. If the scan speed is much *faster*, tumor position and shape are captured at an arbitrary breathing phase. If the scan and tumor speeds are *comparable*, which is the case in Figure 11.2 and in most currently available CT scanners, the tumor position and shape are heavily distorted. Based on an experiment and computer simulations, it was found that distortions along the axis of motion could result in either a lengthening or shortening of the target. In addition to shape distortion, the center of the imaged target can be displaced by as much as the amplitude of the motion.[425]

To overcome these problems, a respiratory-correlated or 4D CT is performed. The idea behind 4D CT is that at every position of interest along the patient's long axis, images are oversampled and each image is tagged with breathing phase information (Fig. 11.25). The instantaneous breathing phase information can be obtained through the real-time position management (RPM) system,[426] (GateCT, VisionRT, London, UK),[427] spirometry,[428] and pressure belts,[429] among others. After the scan is done, images are sorted based on the corresponding breathing phase or amplitude signals. Many 3D CT sets are thus obtained, each corresponding to a particular breathing phase, and together they constitute a 4D CT set covering the whole breathing cycle. Four-dimensional CT decreases motion-induced artifacts and accurately assesses the extent of intrafraction motion. Downsides to 4D CT include the increased time for image acquisition and increased dose to the patient from multiple CT scans. An excellent review of 4D CT scanning was presented by Keall.[430]

Four-Dimensional Target Delineation and Planning

There are several approaches to internal target volume (ITV) delineation of moving lung tumors.[431–437] Lagerwaard et al.[432] used multiple "slow" CT scans to define the ITV, showing that this volume provided better target coverage than a free-breathing CT-derived ITV with isotropic margins. This method is old and limited, however, by the presence of motion-induced artifacts in 3D CT that hamper accurate target delineation. Breath-hold or forced shallow breathing during a 3D CT acquisition can theoretically minimize the motion-induced artifacts.[433] However, such approaches may not be well tolerated in many patients, particularly those with poor pulmonary function. More sophisticated methods to improve target delineation are based on 4D CT imaging.

Various investigators have proposed numerous 4D CT-based techniques, which can largely be classified into four categories: (a) maximum intensity projection (MIP)-based ITV delineation,[434–436] (b) using two extrema phases with a margin,[434] (c) time-weighted mean tumor position with a margin,[437] and (d) using all 10 phases to create composite volume.[434,436] The MIP-based ITV technique is popular due to the simple and rapid construction of the ITV, based on a single 3D image. It has been shown to have good agreement with the "two extrema phases" and "all 10 phases" techniques.[435] Wolthaus et al.[437] have found, however, that the MIP-based ITV technique can overtreat normal tissues by up to 33% compared with a mean tumor position approach. In addition, Muirhead et al.[436] have found that, although the MIP-based ITV technique is safe in most cases, compared with the all 10 phases technique as a gold standard, there are still special cases when the tumor is at or near the diaphragm, the MIP-based ITV technique would lead to underestimation of the actual ITV. This occurs because the tumor is similar in electron density with the diaphragm and other surrounding healthy tissues, such that when an MIP is generated, one cannot distinguish the borders between the overlapping tumor and its similar-density surroundings (Fig. 11.26). Therefore, the MIP-based ITV technique should not be entrusted in all situations, and the all 10 phases technique may be preferable in cases of doubt.

For liver cancers, the authors discourage the use of the MIP-base ITV technique, because the electron density of the

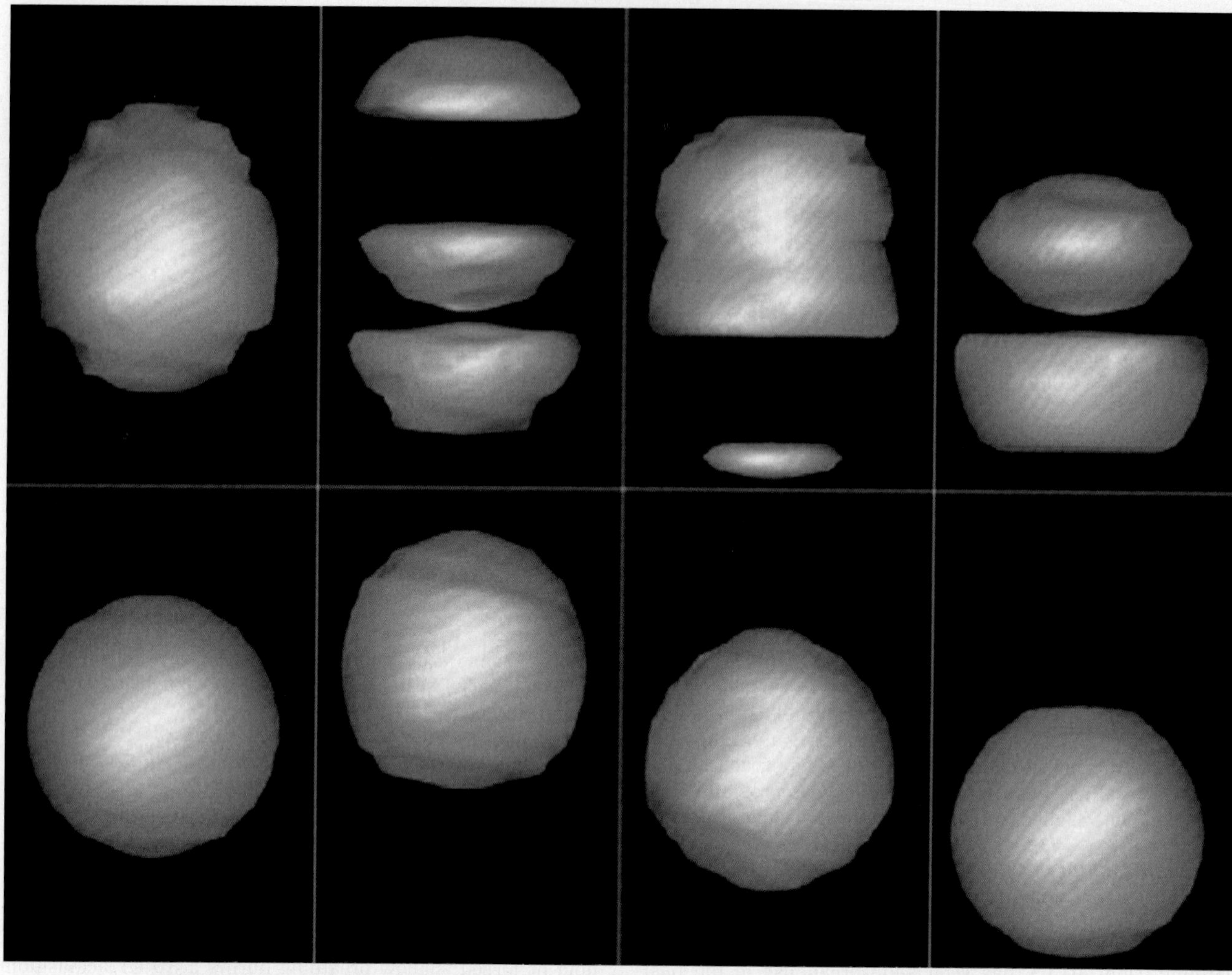

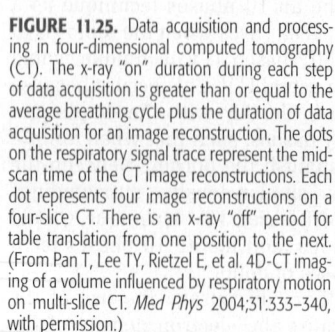

FIGURE 11.24. Computed tomography (CT) images of a spherical object in periodic motion in the axial direction. *Top row:* artifacts obtained in helical CT. Such artifacts depend on the relative phase between CT data acquisition and object motion. To evaluate different artifacts, CT scans were started at different phases. The *right image* shows the disconnected top and bottom of the sphere. *Bottom row:* On the *left* is a CT scan of the static object. The other images show three positions of the moving sphere as imaged by four-dimensional CT. Only small residual artifacts (on the surface) remain on the images at different positions of the motion cycle. (From Rietzel E, Pan T, Chen GT. Four-dimensional computed tomography image formation and clinical protocol. *Med Phys* 2005;32:874–889, with permission).

liver tumor is generally lower than the surrounding normal liver tissue. Thus, the MIP image underestimates the ITV volume. The remedy for this is to use the minimum intensity projection (MinIP) instead. In terms of planning and dose calculations, the authors recommend using the average intensity projection images over a MIP, MinIP, or free-breathing CT images, due to the fact that it more closely represents the time-averaged anatomy of the patient than the other images. To be most accurate, 4D planning (Fig. 11.27) is desired (i.e., calculating dose on each 4D CT phase image and accumulating the dose using a deformable dose tracking technique).[438,439] However, full implementation of the 4D planning approach is

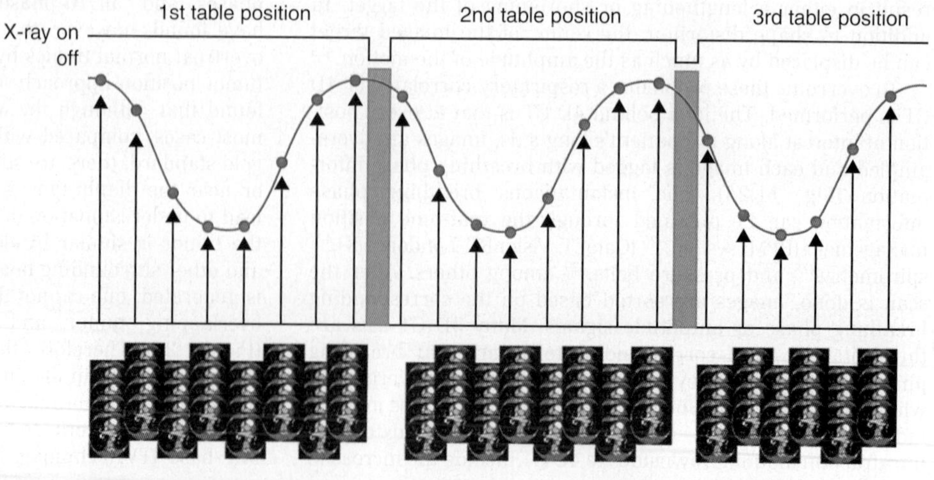

FIGURE 11.25. Data acquisition and processing in four-dimensional computed tomography (CT). The x-ray "on" duration during each step of data acquisition is greater than or equal to the average breathing cycle plus the duration of data acquisition for an image reconstruction. The dots on the respiratory signal trace represent the mid-scan time of the CT image reconstructions. Each dot represents four image reconstructions on a four-slice CT. There is an x-ray "off" period for table translation from one position to the next. (From Pan T, Lee TY, Rietzel E, et al. 4D-CT imaging of a volume influenced by respiratory motion on multi-slice CT. *Med Phys* 2004;31:333–340, with permission.)

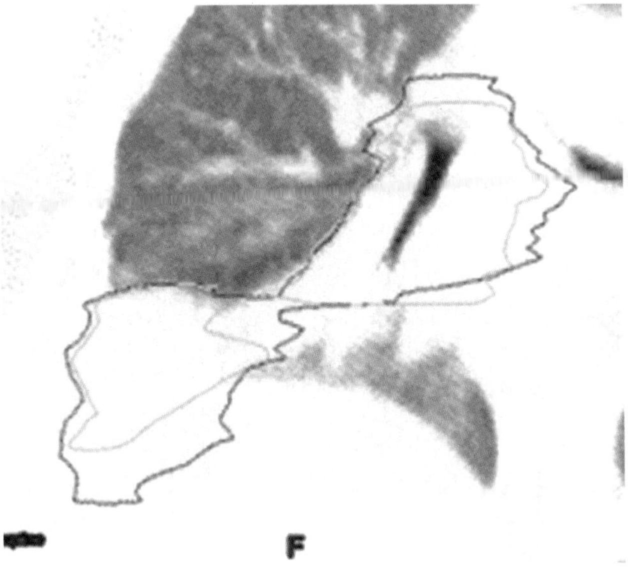

FIGURE 11.26. An example difference in the internal target volumes generated based on the maximum intensity projection (*blue*) and the 10-phase four-dimensional computed tomography (*purple*) images, when the tumor is adjacent to the diaphragmatic tissue of similar density. (From Muirhead R, McNee SG, Featherstone C, et al. Use of maximum intensity projections (MIPs) for target outlining in 4DCT radiotherapy planning. *J Thoracic Oncol* 2008;3:1433–1438, with permission.)

currently limited due to the computational resources needed to perform the increased number of dose calculations and deformable image registrations. If computational burden is not an issue, then a fully integrated 4D IMRT optimization based on the 4D CT phase images and 4D dose accumulations would be the best approach.[440]

The ways to treat a moving tumor can largely be classified into five categories[441]: (a) motion-encompassing, (b) respiratory gating, (c) breath-hold, (d) forced shallow breathing with abdominal compression, and (e) real-time tumor tracking. Motion-encompassing methods refer to treating the entire ITV, without intervention to minimize the treatment volume, in a patient's natural breathing state. Once the ITV is delineated, the beam portal can be made large enough to adequately cover the volume during the planning stage. During treatment, it is necessary to monitor the patient to ensure that the patient breathes consistently without any drifts or sudden change in the amplitude. One should also be aware that presently most linear accelerator systems do not offer 4D imaging for patient

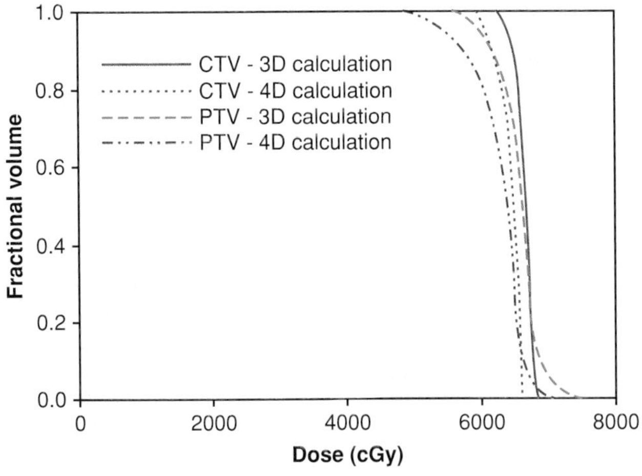

FIGURE 11.27. Dose–volume histograms for target volumes for two patients, showing three-dimensional and four-dimensional dose calculations. (From Starkschall G, Britton K, McAleer, et al. Potential dosimetric benefits of four-dimensional radiation treatment planning. *Int J Radiat Oncol Biol Phys* 2009;73:1560–1565, with permission from Elsevier.)

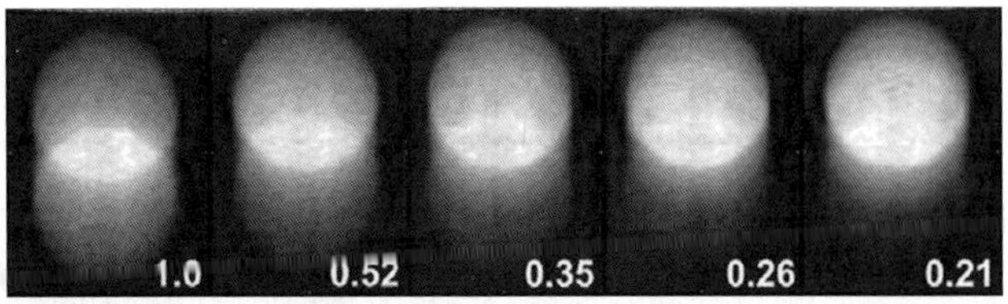

FIGURE 11.28. Three-dimensional cone-beam computed tomography (3D CBCT) images of five simulated respiratory profiles. The ratio of time spent in inspiration to expiration is indicated on the bottom right corner of each 3D CBCT. (From Vergalasova I, Maurer J, Yin FF. Potential underestimation of the internal target volume (ITV) from free-breathing CBCT. *Med Phys* 2011;38:4689–4699, with permission.)

setup (e.g., 4D CBCT).[442,443] Therefore, adequate training to properly recognize the motion-induced blurring effects in 3D CBCT is critical to the image registration accuracy and the overall treatment effectiveness. Figure 11.28 illustrates blurring of the 3D CBCT images that can result due to breathing pattern (i.e., inspiration-to-expiration duration ratio).[444]

Respiratory Gating

There are two main approaches to respiratory gating—internal[445,446] and external[176,433,447]—although a combination is also possible.[448,449] Internal gating utilizes internal tumor motion surrogates such as implanted fiducial markers or marker-less imaging of internal anatomy, whereas external gating uses external respiratory surrogates such as markers placed on the surface of the patient's abdomen, a compression belt, or spirometer signals.

The only internal gating system currently in clinical use is the RTRT system.[281] Its major strength is its precise and real-time localization of the tumor position during treatment. Implanted markers are often good surrogates for tumor position, and marker migration is usually not an issue, particularly if multiple markers are used. Major weaknesses include its invasiveness and the high imaging dose required for fluoroscopic tracking.

The RPM system (Varian Medical Systems, Palo Alto, CA) can be viewed as representative of external gating systems. This system consists of a lightweight plastic block with two or six passive infrared reflective markers placed on the patient's anterior abdominal surface and monitored by a charge-coupled–device video camera mounted on the treatment room wall. The surrogate signal is the abdominal surface motion. Both amplitude and phase gating are allowed. During treatment, a periodicity filter checks the regularity of the breathing waveform and disables the beam when the waveform becomes irregular, such as with patient motion or coughing, and re-enables the beam after establishing breathing is again regular. The RPM system is also used during simulation to acquire the patient's geometry in the gating window and to set up the gating window.

Major strengths of external gating are that it is noninvasive, relatively easy to use, and well tolerated by patients. Moreover, it does not require any radiation dose for imaging. However, it should be noted that tracking the external marker is not equivalent to tracking the tumor, and blindly trusting the external surrogate can result in errors.[448] In particular, the relation between the tumor motion and the surrogate signal may change over time, inter- and intrafractionally.

BrainLab (Westchester, IL) has a U.S. Food and Drug Administration–cleared respiratory gating device called ExacTrac Gating/Novalis Gating.[449] This device uses external markers for gating the radiation beam, however, it uses x-ray imaging to determine the internal anatomy position and to verify its reproducibility during treatment. By updating the correlation between the internal and external signals in a reasonable frequency, x-ray exposure to the patient is minimized, while the external gating signal accuracy is maintained.

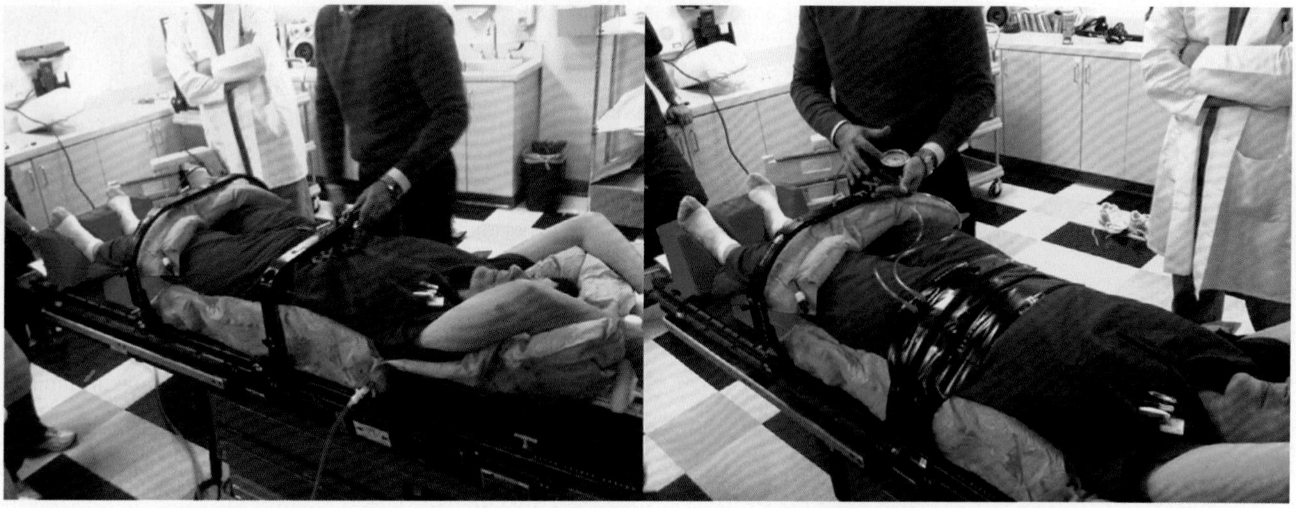

FIGURE 11.29. Examples of abdominal compression devices on the market: a plastic plate (*left*) and a pressure belt (*right*).

Breath-hold and deep inspiration breath-hold techniques[450–453] are attractive options for patients who are capable of repeatedly holding for greater than 15 seconds due to reduced setup uncertainty (and hence, planning margins). The technique is useful for thoracic and upper abdominal targets as well as left-sided breast cancers, due to heart sparing. Setup reproducibility is challenging, due to the different levels of inspiration that are possible. Breathing coaching is helpful, and a monitoring device is essential. Any of the monitoring techniques involving internal and external signals (discussed earlier) can be used, including the spirometer,[450] ABC device,[450–452] RPM,[449,450] and AlignRT surface tracking system.[454]

Forced shallow breathing in combination with abdominal compression devices is an effective technique for controlling the motion in upper abdominal tumors and inferior lung tumors.[452,455–457] This was originally developed by Lax et al.[455] and has since been replicated around the world. Eccles et al.[456] has thoroughly analyzed the impact of the abdominal compression on the liver motion of 60 patients using cine MRI. They have found that more than 90% of patients showed reduction in motion along at least one direction and that more than 40% of patients showed greater than 3-mm motion reduction. However, this technique can be quite uncomfortable and even painful for some patients, and thus the level of compression should be balanced between patient comfort and a reasonable motion reduction (Fig. 11.29). Also, due to the difficulty in reproducibly positioning the abdominal compression device, couch indexed positioning and the subsequent imaging is essential at each treatment fraction. The technique is most appropriate for SBRT for early-stage lung and liver tumors without mediastinal involvement or nodal disease.

Tumor Tracking

Tumor tracking is perhaps the most ideal—and most technologically intense—strategy, as real-time tumor localization, fast processing and relay of information, and corresponding repositioning of the beam all need to be dynamically seamlessly integrated.[458–473] Compared to the motion "freezing" methods, tumor tracking techniques are associated with higher delivery efficiency and less residual target motion. These factors may be particularly important to SBRT of thoracic and abdominal tumor sites, where a large dose is delivered during a single or a few relatively lengthy treatment sessions. However, there are a number of technical hurdles before this approach becomes clinically feasible, including treatment planning and the accurate response of the MLC to tumor positions measured in real time. The actual tumor movement as well as its relation to surrounding critical structures during the treatment cannot be known at the time of treatment planning. Therefore, planning can only be done based on some kind of average patient geometry

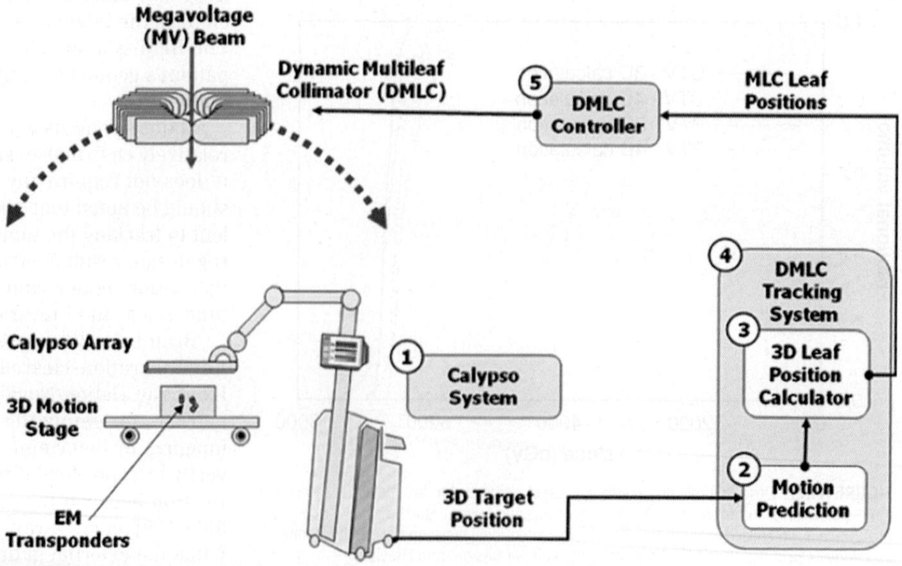

FIGURE 11.30. Flowchart of electromagnetically guided real-time dynamic multileaf collimator tracking. (From Keall PJ, Sawant A, Cho B, et al. Electromagnetic-guided dynamic multileaf collimator tracking enables motion management for intensity-modulated arc therapy. *Int J Radiat Oncol Biol Phys* 2011;79:312–320, with permission from Elsevier.)

information or at best on 4D CT simulation data, and an adaptive scheme must be used throughout the treatment course.

As mentioned earlier, tumor tracking is presently not in widespread clinical use. Most studies carried out so far are still at an investigational stage for linear accelerator–based approaches, except for a few specialized commercial systems.[461,466] There are a number of ways one can obtain the real-time 3D position information of the tumor including: (a) markerless imaging,[445,446,472] (b) marker-guided imaging,[281,462,463,467–469] and (c) using implantable magnetic transponders.[465,470,473] Of these approaches, the use of implantable magnetic transponders is most promising due to lack of x-ray exposure, minimal system latency, and relative ease with which the system can be integrated in the clinical linear accelerator-based systems. The same argument in terms of x-ray exposure also applies to MRI-guided tumor tracking[472]; however, MRI implementation requires a whole new design to interface with linear accelerators. System latency is also a complex issue, due to the need to process the images and provide near real-time 3D tumor position information. Figure 11.30 illustrates a flowchart of a possible tumor tracking strategy with dynamic MLC (DMLC), based on the real-time 3D position information provided by the magnetic transponders (Calypso, Seattle, WA).

ADAPTIVE RADIOTHERAPY

Radiation therapy has traditionally involved generating a static plan, based on a single snapshot of the patient's anatomy, which is then delivered over a number of weeks. Modern IGRT technologies can transform this static process into a dynamic one, whereby plans are continuously altered throughout the treatment course or even during a single fraction. In many ways, altering the treatment plan during treatment is not new; for example, patients are often replanned due to weight loss or rapid tumor response. What is different is the speed and sophistication with which IGRT enables this process.

The term *adaptive radiation therapy* (ART) was first coined by Yan et al.[474] in 1997. This was around the time that David Jaffray at the same institution (William Beaumont Hospital, Royal Oak, MI) was working on the integration of CBCT with a linear accelerator to enable in-room *soft-tissue* imaging before, during, or after treatment.[475] Thus, the concept of ART was proposed based on the idea that advancements in in-room imaging technologies would make the process of target localization and definition more precise.

The optimal level of adaptation is a broad question, and it is unlikely that a global solution exists for all situations. An intriguing approach is to use the knowledge of patient setup and organ motion information to decide the prescribed "safe dose" (i.e., isotoxicity) to be delivered for *each patient*, rather than prescribing the same dose for all patients because normal tissue tolerance is usually what limits the prescription dose. Song et al.[476] evaluated the maximum dose that can be delivered while keeping the same rectal NTCP level (i.e., iso-NTCP dose escalation) using various IGRT approaches (Fig. 11.31). It was found that the possible dose escalation levels were highly patient dependent, even if the same target localization approaches were used, and that image registration based on soft tissues provided the least discrepancy among patients.

This level of adaptation was proven to be clinically feasible.[477,478] Their approach was as follows. Based on the planning CT simulation, an initial treatment plan is generated with a 1-cm CTV–PTV margin. Each of the first 4 days of therapy, daily EPID and CT scans are acquired immediately before or after treatment. Confidence-limited PTV margins are generated based on each patient's setup inaccuracies and internal organ motion. Rectal and bladder constraints are used to determine the individual patient's total dose, ranging from 70.2 to 79.2 Gy. Using this isotoxicity ART strategy, they found no statistically different rectal toxicity rates across the prescription dose ranges. This was the first clinical evidence that an *individualized* prescription is possible indicating benefits of image-guided ART.

Deutschmann et al.[479] further used online aperture adaptation to reduce planning margins in 39 prostate cancer patients, after correcting for interfraction shifts based on implanted fiducials. They found that this approach was feasible, and correcting for intrafraction 6-degree rotations could allow reduced planning margins to 3 mm. Intrafraction motion based on pretreatment kilovoltage planar imaging versus last beam EPID images showed RL rotations up to 26.9 degrees (mean, 2.5 degrees) and 3D translations up to 10.2 mm (mean, 3.0 mm).

The need to adapt to changes in the patient anatomy (tumor(s) or normal tissues) is not limited to prostate cancer. Multiple investigators have reported significant morphologic changes in tumors or normal tissues in a wide variety of tumor sites, including HNC,[480,481] lung cancer,[482,483] and gynecologic tumors.[484] Barker et al.[480] noted a mean volume reduction of the GTV of 0.2 cm^3/day in HNC patients treated on a CT-on-rails system. Of note, the parotid gland volume decreased by 0.19 cm^3/day and

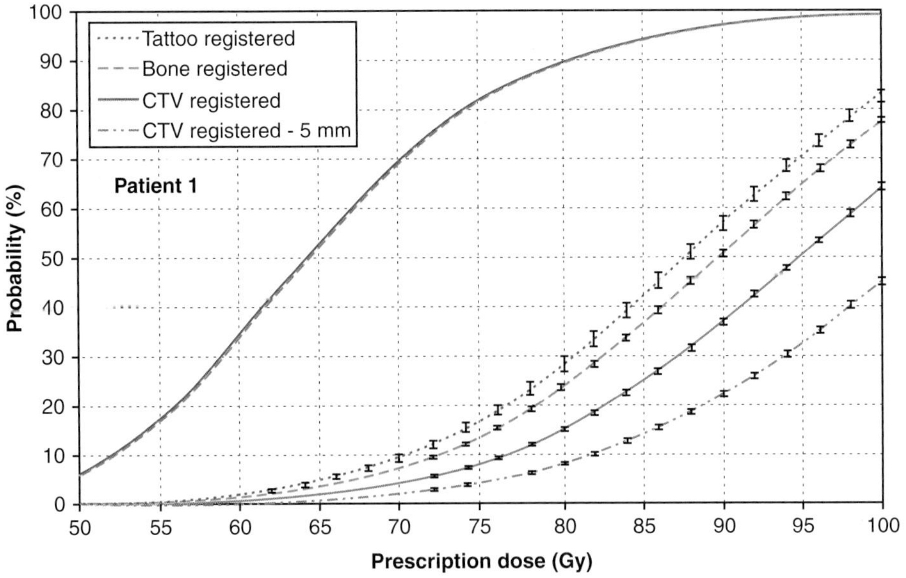

FIGURE 11.31. Tumor control probability (TCP) and rectum normal tissue complication probability (NTCP) curves for prostate cancer patients, from 50 to 100 Gy in 2-Gy per-fraction increments, for the three image-guided adaptive registration techniques: tattoo, bone, clinical target volume (CTV) registered, and CTV-registered with margin reduced to 5 mm. TCP curves are on the *left* and NTCP curves are on the *right*. Error bars are standard deviations. (From Song WY, Schaly B, Bauman G, et al. Image-guided adaptive radiation therapy (IGART): radiobiological and dose escalation considerations for localized carcinoma of the prostate. *Med Phys* 2005;32:2193–2220, with permission.)

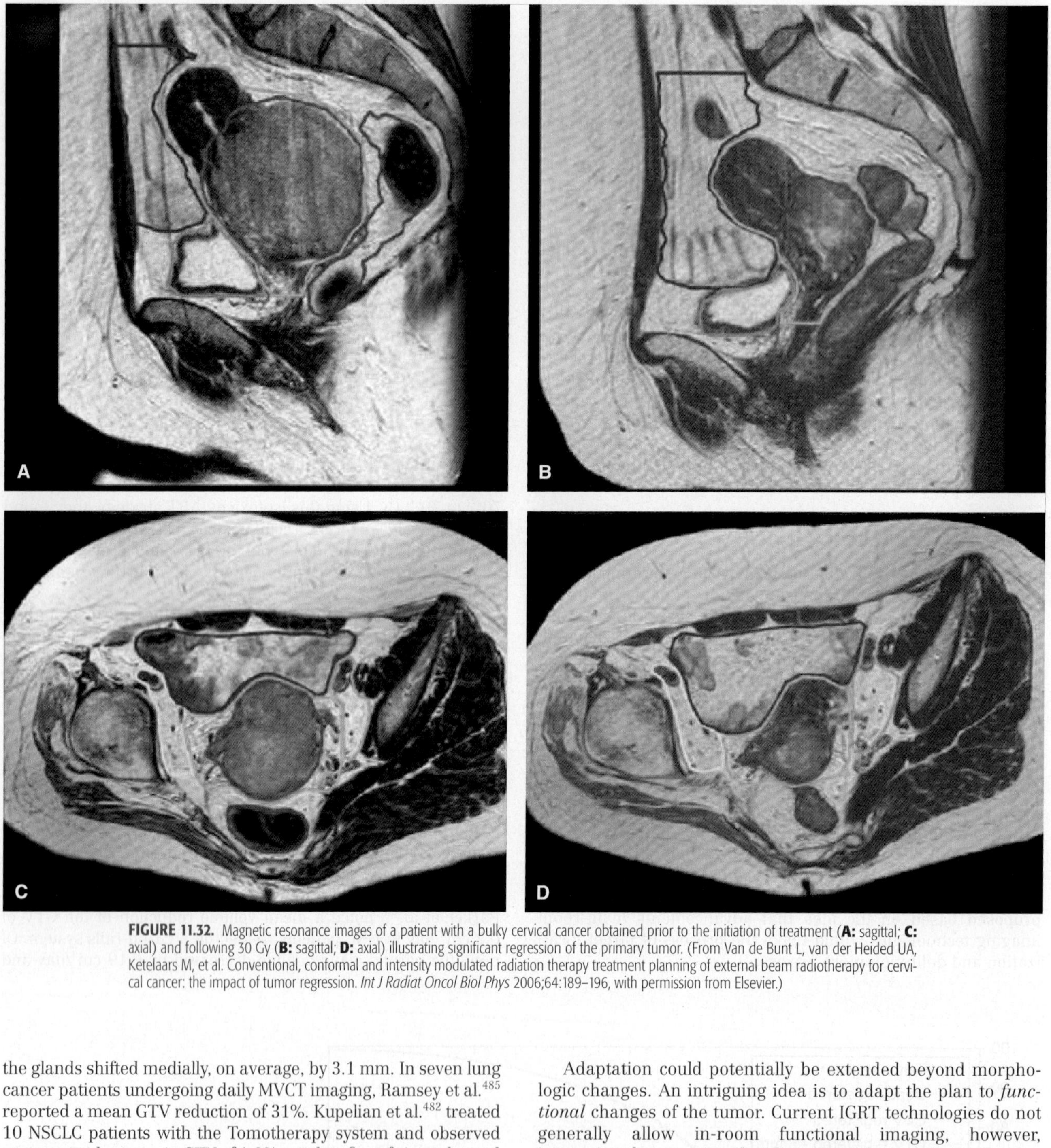

FIGURE 11.32. Magnetic resonance images of a patient with a bulky cervical cancer obtained prior to the initiation of treatment (**A:** sagittal; **C:** axial) and following 30 Gy (**B:** sagittal; **D:** axial) illustrating significant regression of the primary tumor. (From Van de Bunt L, van der Heided UA, Ketelaars M, et al. Conventional, conformal and intensity modulated radiation therapy treatment planning of external beam radiotherapy for cervical cancer: the impact of tumor regression. *Int J Radiat Oncol Biol Phys* 2006;64:189–196, with permission from Elsevier.)

the glands shifted medially, on average, by 3.1 mm. In seven lung cancer patients undergoing daily MVCT imaging, Ramsey et al.[485] reported a mean GTV reduction of 31%. Kupelian et al.[482] treated 10 NSCLC patients with the Tomotherapy system and observed an average decrease in GTV of 1.2% per day; five of six replanned cases demonstrated small increases in tumor dose delivery. Van de Bunt et al.[484] reported an average reduction in the GTV of 46% in 14 cervical cancers reimaged with MRI after the delivery of 30 Gy (Fig. 11.32).

Several investigators have reported that adapting to morphologic changes may improve treatment delivery. Ramsey et al.[485] found that the lung V20 would be decreased from 23% to 17% by adapting to reductions in the GTV in lung cancer patients, corresponding to 17% less reduction in lung perfusion. Hansen et al.[481] evaluated the impact of replanning in a cohort of 13 HNC patients with either significant weight loss or tumor response during IMRT (Fig. 11.33). Compared to replanning, *not* replanning significantly decreased dose to the target volume and increased doses to normal tissues (spinal cord and brainstem). The doses to 95% of the PTVGTV and the PTVCTV decreased by up to 6.3 Gy and 7.4 Gy, respectively.

Adaptation could potentially be extended beyond morphologic changes. An intriguing idea is to adapt the plan to *functional* changes of the tumor. Current IGRT technologies do not generally allow in-room functional imaging, however, increasing data suggest that functional changes in tumors are correlated with outcome.[17,486] For example, Wieder et al.[486] examined changes in tumor ^{18}FDG avidity in patients undergoing preoperative chemoradiotherapy for esophageal carcinoma (Fig. 11.34). In 27 patients undergoing midtreatment ^{18}FDG PET, a decline in SUV greater than 30% was associated with improved 2-year overall survival and histopathologic response. Whether adapting the plan (e.g., intensifying treatment in patients with suboptimal metabolic changes) would improve patient outcomes remains unclear.

From a technical standpoint, a major concern is *how* exactly to adapt to changes in the tumor or normal tissues during treatment. Although it may be trivial to occasionally replan a limited number of patients *offline,* frequent replannings of many patients are labor and time intensive, especially if *online* replanning is necessary. New software tools, approaches, and fast and reliable computing are needed. This is currently an

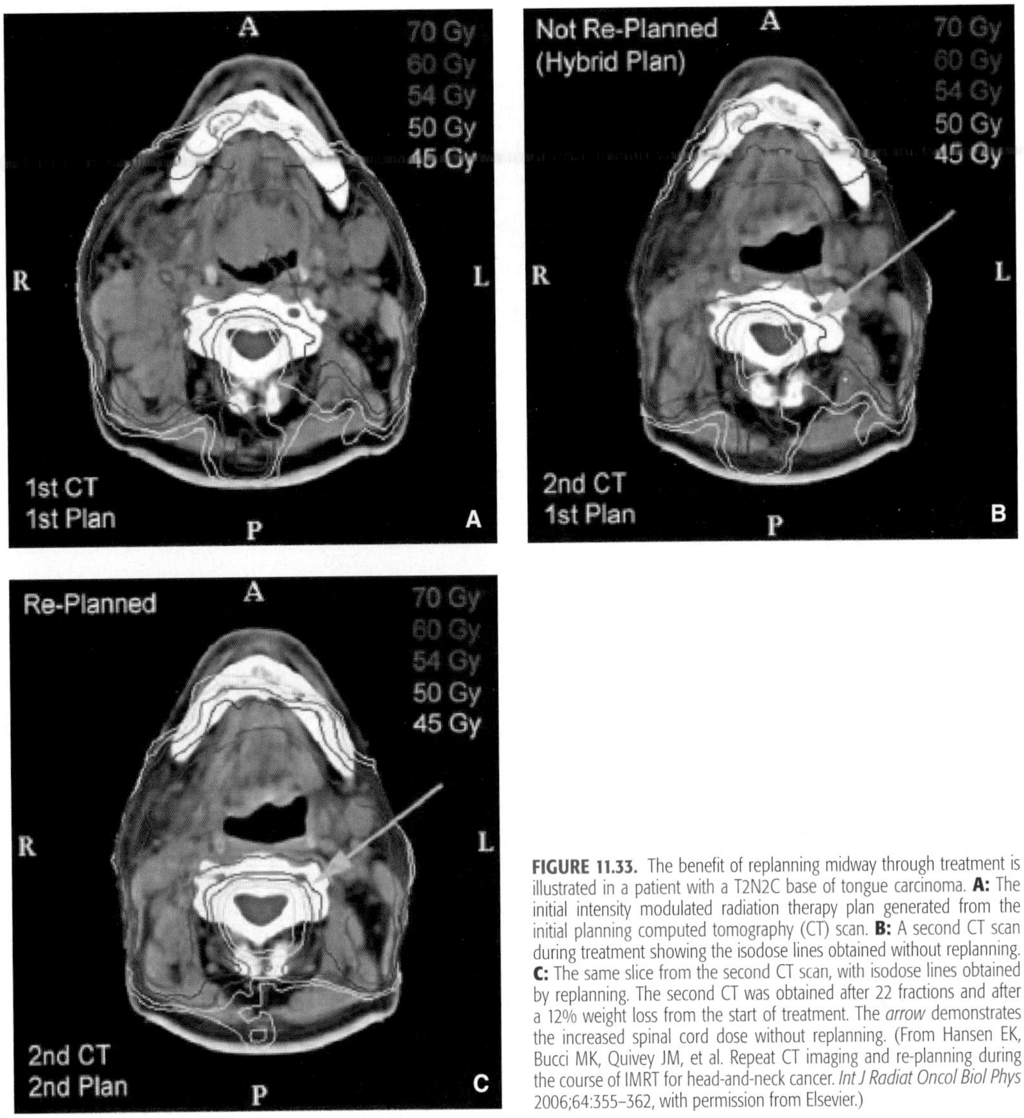

FIGURE 11.33. The benefit of replanning midway through treatment is illustrated in a patient with a T2N2C base of tongue carcinoma. **A:** The initial intensity modulated radiation therapy plan generated from the initial planning computed tomography (CT) scan. **B:** A second CT scan during treatment showing the isodose lines obtained without replanning. **C:** The same slice from the second CT scan, with isodose lines obtained by replanning. The second CT was obtained after 22 fractions and after a 12% weight loss from the start of treatment. The *arrow* demonstrates the increased spinal cord dose without replanning. (From Hansen EK, Bucci MK, Quivey JM, et al. Repeat CT imaging and re-planning during the course of IMRT for head-and-neck cancer. *Int J Radiat Oncol Biol Phys* 2006;64:355–362, with permission from Elsevier.)

active area of research. Researchers at the University of California–San Diego have explored the potential to perform online replanning utilizing the vast computational capability of the graphics card technology (Fig. 11.35).[487–495] Graphics processing unit (GPU) cards were originally developed for the gaming industry, where a fast display of large graphics data is necessary to enhance the quality of the gaming experience. By developing new algorithms with mathematical structures suitable for GPU parallelization, it is possible to dramatically improve the computational efficiency of the traditionally computationally intense tasks in RT such as dose calculations,[487,491,493,495] inverse planning reoptimizations,[489,493] CT reconstructions,[490,494] and deformable image registrations for fast contour mapping.[489] Of note, Gu et al.[487,493] have shown that a full 3D-dose calculation based on finite-size pencil beam algorithm achieved a speed up of 200 to 400 times, taking less than 1 second for typical IMRT plans. Men et al.[488,492] found that, for a typical nine-field prostate IMRT plan with 5-by-5 mm^2 beamlet size and 2.5-by-2.5-by-2.5 mm^3 voxel size, reoptimization would only take 2.8 seconds. Park et al.[494] found that for a filtered back-projection reconstruction of a typical 3D CBCT, volume can be done in a real-time fashion (i.e., as soon as the scan is done), while Gu et al.[489] found that a daemons deformable image registration of a typical 3D CBCT volume can be completed in 7 to 11 seconds.

Another computational acceleration approach is the utilization of Cloud computing for RT applications, pioneered by Meng et al.[496] and Wang et al.[497] at Stanford University. Cloud computing is a recent advancement in supercomputing technology where the end user only needs Internet access and he or she requests computations to a large network of computers (nodes) that are not visible to the end user. The task is divided up and handled in a parallel computing manner, automatically. The larger the number of nodes used, the faster the computations. Because this system does not require the computers to be physically located near the user, and they can be accessed from anywhere with an Internet connection, the potential for their use in ART applications irrespective of the location of the clinic is tremendous. The technology is new and research in RT is in its infancy; but the potential benefits remain to be seen.

Even if computational issues are completely resolved and online replanning can be technically implemented, many questions still remain to be answered before various ART strategies can be introduced into clinical practice. For example, how often should new plans be generated? Once? Weekly? Daily? Another question is whether altering the target volume would *adversely* impact tumor control. In the study by Hansen et al.[481], attempts were made to "maintain the size of the original GTV in the second plan without extending it beyond the skin contour or into adjacent normal structures," ensuring irradiation of potential

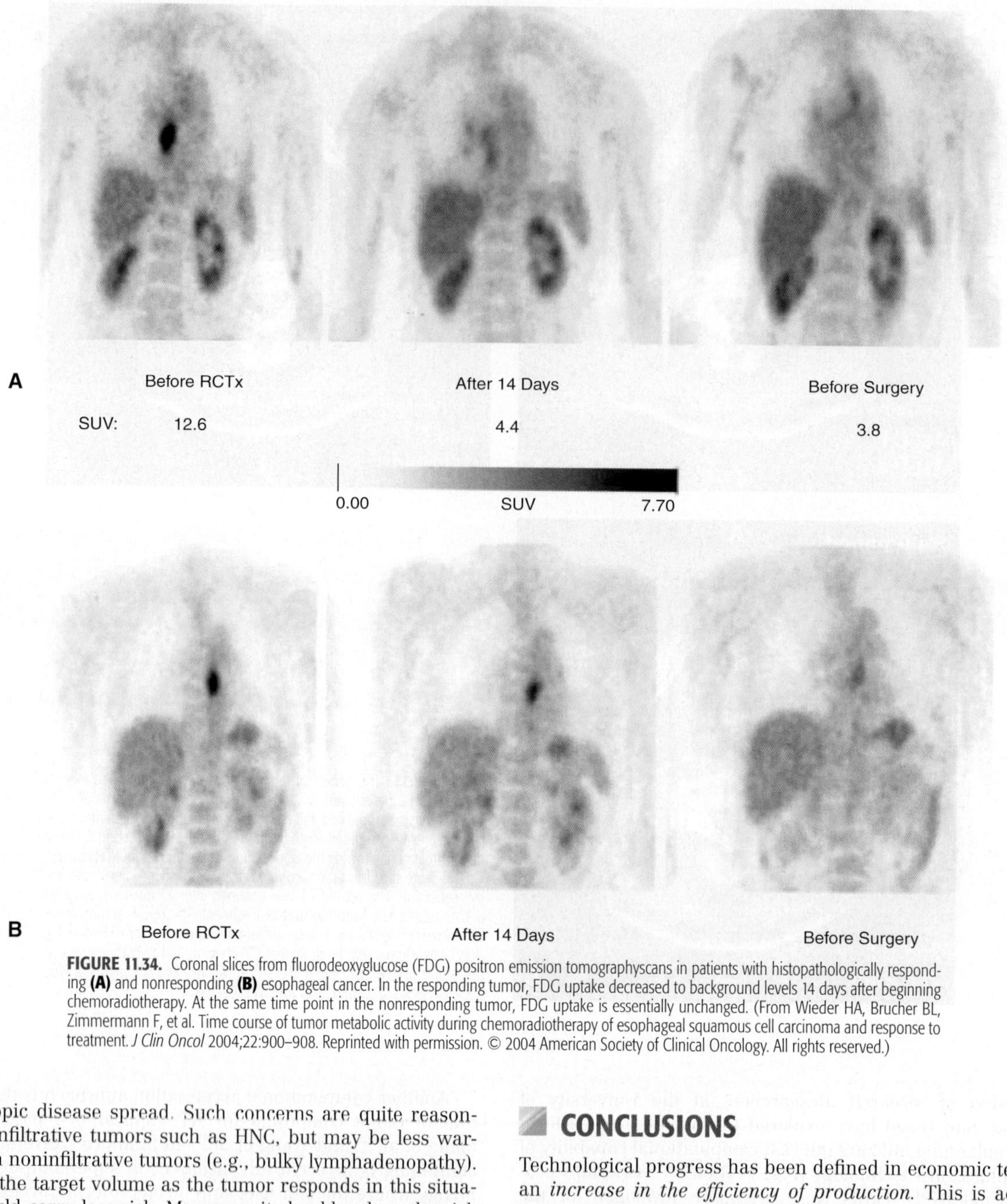

FIGURE 11.34. Coronal slices from fluorodeoxyglucose (FDG) positron emission tomographyscans in patients with histopathologically responding **(A)** and nonresponding **(B)** esophageal cancer. In the responding tumor, FDG uptake decreased to background levels 14 days after beginning chemoradiotherapy. At the same time point in the nonresponding tumor, FDG uptake is essentially unchanged. (From Wieder HA, Brucher BL, Zimmermann F, et al. Time course of tumor metabolic activity during chemoradiotherapy of esophageal squamous cell carcinoma and response to treatment. *J Clin Oncol* 2004;22:900–908. Reprinted with permission. © 2004 American Society of Clinical Oncology. All rights reserved.)

microscopic disease spread. Such concerns are quite reasonable in infiltrative tumors such as HNC, but may be less warranted in noninfiltrative tumors (e.g., bulky lymphadenopathy). Altering the target volume as the tumor responds in this situation should carry less risk. Moreover, it should reduce the risk of toxicity and allow the delivery of higher, more effective doses. The answer to these and other questions should be resolved through prospective clinical trials.

CONCLUSIONS

Technological progress has been defined in economic terms as an *increase in the efficiency of production.* This is achieved by producing more output for a given set of inputs, or alternately, requiring fewer inputs to produce a given output. In medicine, technological progress might be defined similarly—as an *increase in the efficiency of medical services*—where

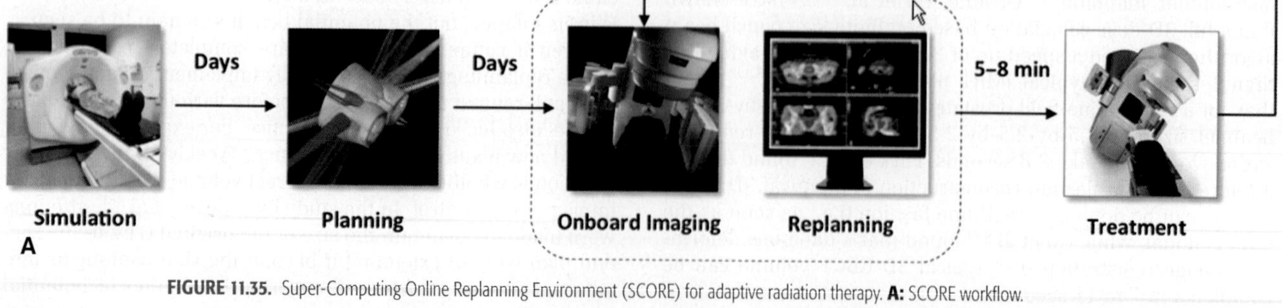

FIGURE 11.35. Super-Computing Online Replanning Environment (SCORE) for adaptive radiation therapy. **A:** SCORE workflow.

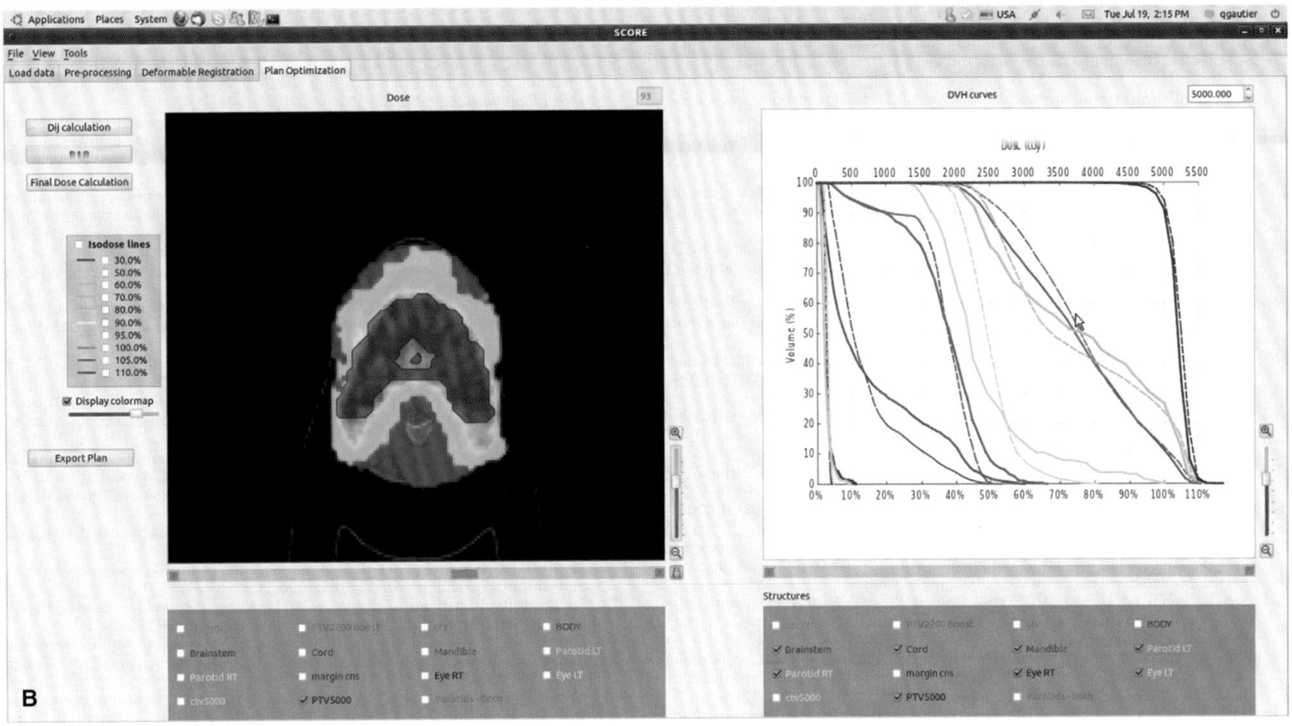

FIGURE 11.35. *(continued)* **B:** Reoptimized dose distribution (*left*) and calculated dose-volume histograms (*right*) for a head and neck cancer patient undergoing SCORE simulation. The SCORE plan is generated then exported back to the treatment planning system for verification before treatment. (Courtesy of Xun Jia and Steve Jiang.)

improved patient outcomes ("outputs") are achieved for less cost ("inputs"), and medical costs may include both economic resources and adverse events. When therapeutic outcomes are achieved for less toxicity, technological progress is tantamount to an increase in the therapeutic ratio. An ongoing challenge for the field of radiation oncology is to develop, test, and implement new technologies that meet this definition of progress.

SELECTED REFERENCES

A full list of references for this chapter is available online.

3. ACR–ASTRO Practice Guideline For Image-Guided Radiation Therapy (IGRT). American College of Radiology. http://www.acr.org/SecondaryMainMenuCategories/quality_safety/guidelines/ro/IGRT.aspx.
6. Stapleford LJ, Lawson JD, Perkins C, et al. Evaluation of automatic atlas-based lymph node segmentation for head-and-neck cancer. *Int J Radiat Oncol Biol Phys* 2010;77:959–966.
7. Simpson DR, Lawson JD, Nath SK, Rose BS, Mundt AJ, Mell LK. Utilization of advanced imaging technologies for target delineation in radiation oncology. *J Am Coll Radiol* 2009;6:876-883.
8. Werner-Wasik M, Nelson AD, Choi W, et al. What is the best way to contour lung tumors on PET scans? Multiobserver validation of a gradient-based method using a NSCLC digital PET phantom. *Int J Radiat Oncol Biol Phys* 2012;82(3):1164–1171.
9. Plathow C, Weber WA. Tumor cell metabolism imaging. *J Nucl Med* 2008;49(Suppl 2):43S-63S.
10. MacManus MP, Hicks RJ, Matthews JP, et al. High rate of detection of unsuspected distant metastases by PET in apparent stage III non-small-cell lung cancer: implications for radical radiation therapy. *Int J Radiat Oncol Biol Phys* 2001;50:287–293.
11. Pieterman RM, van Putten JW, Meuzelaar JJ, et al. Preoperative staging of non-small-cell lung cancer with positron-emission tomography. *N Engl J Med* 2000;343:254–261.
14. Muijs CT, Beukema JC, Pruim J, et al. A systematic review on the role of FDG-PET/CT in tumour delineation and radiotherapy planning in patients with esophageal cancer. *Radiother Oncol* 2010;97:165–171.
15. Schoder H, Noy A, Gonen M, et al. Intensity of 18-fluorodeoxyglucose uptake in positron emission tomography distinguishes between indolent and aggressive non-Hodgkin's lymphoma. *J Clin Oncol* 2005;23:4643–4651.
17. Schwarz JK, Siegel BA, Dehdashti F, et al. Metabolic response on posttherapy FDG-PET predicts patterns of failure after radiotherapy for cervical cancer. *Int J Radiat Oncol Biol Phys* 2012;83(1):185–190.
21. Vanuytsel LJ, Vansteenkiste JF, Stroobants SG, et al. The impact of (18)F-fluoro-2-deoxy-D-glucose positron emission tomography (FDG-PET) lymph node staging on the radiation treatment volumes in patients with non-small cell lung cancer. *Radiother Oncol* 2000;55:317–324.
22. Bradley J, Bae K, Choi N, et al. A phase II comparative study of gross tumor volume definition with or without PET/CT fusion in dosimetric planning for non-small-cell lung cancer (NSCLC): primary analysis of Radiation Therapy Oncology Group (RTOG) 0515. *Int J Radiat Oncol Biol Phys* 2012;82:435–441.e1.
23. Grosu AL, Piert M, Weber WA, et al. Positron emission tomography for radiation treatment planning. *Strahlenther Onkol* 2005;181:483–499.
42. Leong T, Everitt C, Yuen K, et al. A prospective study to evaluate the impact of FDG-PET on CT-based radiotherapy treatment planning for oesophageal cancer. *Radiother Oncol* 2006;78:254–261.
48. Braendengen M, Hansson K, Radu C, et al. Delineation of gross tumor volume (GTV) for radiation treatment planning of locally advanced rectal cancer using information from MRI or FDG-PET/CT: a prospective study. *Int J Radiat Oncol Biol Phys* 2011;81:e439–e445.
61. Hutchings M, Loft A, Hansen M, et al. Clinical impact of FDG-PET/CT in the planning of radiotherapy for early-stage Hodgkin lymphoma. *Eur J Haematol* 2007;78:206–212.
65. Schöder H, Ong SC. Fundamentals of molecular imaging: rationale and applications with relevance for radiation oncology. *Semin Nucl Med* 2008;38:119–128.
69. Wahl RL, Herman JM, Ford E. The promise and pitfalls of positron emission tomography and single-photon emission computed tomography molecular imaging-guided radiation therapy. *Semin Radiat Oncol* 2011;21:88–100.
77. Rischin D, Hicks RJ, Fisher R, et al. Prognostic significance of [18F]-misonidazole positron emission tomography-detected tumor hypoxia in patients with advanced head and neck cancer randomly assigned to chemoradiation with or without tirapazamine: a substudy of Trans-Tasman Radiation Oncology Group Study 98.02. *J Clin Oncol* 2006;24:2098–2104.
95. Karlsson M, Karlsson MG, Nyholm T, et al. Dedicated magnetic resonance imaging in the radiotherapy clinic. *Int J Radiat Oncol Biol Phys* 2009;74:644–651.
99. Aoyama H, Kamada K, Shirato H, et al. Integration of functional brain information into stereotactic irradiation treatment planning using magnetoencephalography and magnetic resonance axonography. *Int J Radiat Oncol Biol Phys* 2004;58:1177–1183.
106. Meijer HJ, van Lin EN, Debats OA, et al. High occurrence of aberrant lymph node spread on magnetic resonance lymphography in prostate cancer patients with a biochemical recurrence after radical prostatectomy. *Int J Radiat Oncol Biol Phys* 2012;82(4):1405–1410.
111. Mayr NA, Huang Z, Wang JZ, et al. Characterizing tumor heterogeneity with functional imaging and quantifying high-risk tumor volume for early prediction of treatment outcome: cervical cancer as a model. *Int J Radiat Oncol Biol Phys* 2012;83(3):972–979.
115. Jani AB, Blend MJ, Hamilton R, et al. Radioimmunoscintigraphy for post-prostatectomy radiotherapy: analysis of toxicity and biochemical control. *J Nucl Med* 2004;45:1315–1322.
130. de Crevoisier R, Tucker SL, Dong L, et al. Increased risk of biochemical and local failure in patients with distended rectum on the planning CT for prostate cancer radiotherapy. *Int J Radiat Oncol Biol Phys* 2005;62:965–973.
131. Simpson DR, Lawson JD, Nath SK, et al. A survey of image-guided radiation therapy use in the United States. *Cancer* 2010;116:3953–3960.
136. Lattanzi J, McNeeley S, Hanlon A, et al. Ultrasound-based stereotactic guidance of precision conformal external beam radiation therapy in clinical localized prostate cancer. *Urology* 2000;55:73–78.
138. Trichter F, Ennis RD. Prostate localization using transabdominal ultrasound imaging. *Int J Radiat Oncol Biol Phys* 2003;56:1225–1233.
140. Little DJ, Dong L, Levy LB, et al. Use of portal images and BAT ultrasonography to measure setup error and organ motion for prostate IMRT: implications for treatment margins. *Int J Radiat Oncol Biol Phys* 2003;56:1218–1224.

145. Kuban DA, Dong L, Cheung R, et al. Ultrasound-based localization. *Semin Radiat Oncol* 2005;15:180–191.
146. Huang E, Dong L, Chandra A, et al. Intrafraction prostate motion during IMRT for prostate cancer. *Int J Radiat Oncol Biol Phys* 2002;53:261–268.
150. Scarbrough TJ, Golden NM, Ting JY, et al. Comparison of ultrasound and implanted seed marker prostate localization methods: implications for image-guided radiotherapy. *Int J Radiat Oncol Biol Phys* 2006;65:378–387.
152. Kupelian PA, Thakkar VV, Khuntia D, et al. Hypofractionated intensity-modulated radiotherapy (70 Gy at 2.5 Gy per fraction) for localized prostate cancer: long-term outcomes. *Int J Radiat Oncol Biol Phys* 2005;63:1463–1468.
155. Jani AB, Gratzle J, Muresan E, et al. Analysis of acute toxicity with the use of transabdominal ultrasonography for prostate positioning during intensity modulated radiotherapy. *Urology* 2005;65:504–508.
157. Bohrer M, Schroder P, Welzel G, et al. Reduced rectal toxicity with ultrasound-based image guided radiotherapy using BAT (B-mode acquisition and targeting system) for prostate cancer. *Strahlenther Onkol* 2008;184:674–678.
166. Fuss M, Salter BJ, Cavanagh SX, et al. Daily ultrasound-based image-guided targeting for radiotherapy of upper abdominal malignancies. *Int J Radiat Oncol Biol Phys* 2004;59:1245–1256.
167. Meeks SL, Buatti JM, Bouchet LG, et al. Ultrasound-guided extracranial radiosurgery: technique and application. *Int J Radiat Oncol Biol Phys* 2003;55:1092–1101.
178. Cerviño LI, Detorie N, Taylor M, et al. Initial clinical experience with a frameless and maskless stereotactic radiosurgery treatment. *Pract Radiat Oncol* 2012; 2:54–62.
185. Michalski JM, Graham MV, Bosch WR, et al. Prospective clinical evaluation of a electronic portal imaging device. *Int J Radiat Oncol Biol Phys* 1996;34:943–951.
190. Herman MG. Clinical use of electronic portal imaging. *Sem Radiat Oncol* 2005; 15:157–167.
202. Pouliot J, Aubin M, Langen KM, et al. (Non)-migration of radiopaque markers used for on-line localization of the prostate with an electronic portal imaging device. *Int J Radiat Oncol Biol Phys* 2003;56:862–866.
204. Schallenkamp JM, Herman MG, Kruse JJ, et al. Prostate position relative to pelvic bony anatomy based on intraprostatic gold markers and electronic portal imaging. *Int J Radiat Oncol Biol Phys* 2005;63:800–811.
206. Kupelian PA, Willoughby TR, Meeks SL, et al. Intraprostatic fiducials for localization of the prostate gland: monitoring inter-marker distances during radiation therapy to test for marker stability. *Int J Radiat Oncol Biol Phys* 2005;62:1291–1296.
212. Nichol A, Chung P, Lockwood G, et al. A phase II study of localized prostate cancer treated to 75.6 Gy with 3D conformal radiotherapy. *Radiother Oncol* 2005;76:11–17.
213. Peeters STH, Heemsbergen WD, van Putten WLJ, et al. Acute and late complications after radiotherapy for prostate cancer: results of a multicenter randomized trial comparing 68 Gy to 78 Gy. *Int J Radiat Oncol Biol Phys* 2005;61:1019–1034.
225. Colombo F, Casentini L, Cavedon C, et al. CyberKnife radiosurgery for benign meningiomas: short-term results in 199 patients. *Neurosurgery* 2009;64:A7–A13.
232. Giller CA, Berger BD, Pistenmaa DA, et al. Robotically guided radiosurgery for children. *Pediatr Blood Cancer* 2005;45:304–331.
233. Dodd RL, Ryu MR, Kamnerdsupaphon P, et al. Cyberknife radiosurgery for benign intradural extramedullary spinal tumors. *Neurosurgery* 2006;58:674–685.
238. Gerszten PC, Ozhasoglu C, Burton SA, et al. Cyberknife frameless stereotactic radiosurgery for spinal lesions: clinical experience in 125 cases. *Neurosurgery* 2004;55:89–99.
240. Patel VB, Wegner RE, Heron DE, et al. Comparison of whole versus partial vertebral body stereotactic body radiation therapy for spinal metastases. *Technol Cancer Res Treat* 2012;11:105–115.
245. Gagnon GJ, Nasr NM, Liao JJ, et al. Treatment of spinal tumors using CyberKnife fractionated stereotactic radiosurgery: pain and quality-of-life assessment after treatment in 200 patients. *Neurosurgery* 2009;64:297–306.
247. Gibbs IC, Kamnerdsupaphon P, Ryu MR, et al. Image-guided robotic radiosurgery for spinal metastases. *Radiother Oncol* 2007;82:185–190.
252. King CR, Brooks JD, Gill H, et al. Stereotactic body radiosurgery for localized prostate cancer: interim results of a prospective phase II clinical trial. *Int J Radiat Oncol Biol Phys* 2009;73:1043–1048.
257. Roh KW, Jang JS, Kim MS, et al. Fractionated stereotactic radiotherapy as reirradiation for locally recurrent head and neck cancer. *Int J Radiat Oncol Biol Phys* 2009;74:1348–1355.
261. Chen JC, Girvigian M, Greathouse H, et al. Treatment of trigeminal neuralgia with linear accelerator radiosurgery: initial results. *J Neurosurg* 2004;101:346–350.
271. Ryu S, Yin FF, Rock J, et al. Image-guided and intensity-modulated radiosurgery for patients with spinal metastasis. *Cancer* 2003;97:2013–2018.
273. Ernst-Stecken A, Lambrecht U, Mueller R, et al. Hypofractionated stereotactic radiotherapy for primary and secondary intrapulmonary tumors: first results of a phase I/II study. *Strahlenther Onkol* 2006;182:696–702.
274. Videtic GM, Stephans K, Reddy C, et al. Intensity-modulated radiotherapy-based stereotactic body radiotherapy for medically inoperable early-stage lung cancer: excellent local control. *Int J Radiat Oncol Biol Phys* 2010;77:344–349.
281. Harada T, Shirato H, Ogura S, et al. Real-time tumor-tracking radiation therapy for lung carcinoma by the aid of insertion of a gold marker using bronchofiberoscopy. *Cancer* 2002;95:1720–1727.
290. Shimizu S, Shirato H, Ogura S, et al. Detection of lung tumor movement in real-time tumor-tracking radiotherapy. *Int J Radiat Oncol Biol Phys* 2001;51:304–310.
295. Balter J, Brock K, Litzenberg DW, et al. Daily targeting of intrahepatic tumors for radiotherapy. *Int J Radiat Oncol Biol Phys* 2002;52:266–271.
297. Ben-Josef E, Normolle D, Ensminger WD, et al. Phase II trial of high-dose conformal radiation therapy with concurrent hepatic artery floxurdine for unresectable intra-hepatic malignancies. *J Clin Oncol* 2005;23:8739–8747.
301. Fox T, Huntzinger C, Johnstone P, et al. Performance evaluation of an automated image registration algorithm using an integrated kilovoltage imaging and guidance system. *J Appl Clin Med Phys* 2006;7:97–104.
304. Lawson JD, Fox T, Elder E, et al. Early clinical experience with kilovoltage image-guided radiation therapy for interfraction motion management. *Med Dosim* 2008;33:268–274.
309. Jayachandran P, Minn AY, Van Dam J, et al. Interfractional uncertainty in the treatment of pancreatic cancer with radiation. *Int J Radiat Oncol Biol Phys* 2010; 76:603–607.
319. Uematsu M, Shioda A, Suda A, et al. Computed tomography-guided frameless stereotactic radiotherapy for stage I non-small cell lung cancer: a 5-year experience. *Int J Radiat Oncol Biol Phys* 2001;51:666–670.
322. Yenice KM, Lovelock DM, Hunt MA, et al. CT image-guided intensity-modulated therapy for paraspinal tumors using stereotactic immobilization. *Int J Radiat Oncol Biol Phys* 2003;55:583–593.
325. Zelefsky MJ, Greco C, Motzer R, et al. Tumor control outcomes after hypofractionated and single-dose stereotactic image-guided intensity-modulated radiotherapy for extracranial metastases from renal cell carcinoma. *Int J Radiat Oncol Biol Phys* 2012;82(5):1744–1748.
328. Onishi H, Kuriyama K, Komiyama T, et al. Clinical outcomes of stereotactic radiotherapy for stage I non-small cell lung cancer using a novel irradiation technique: patient self-controlled breath-hold and beam switching using a combination linear accelerator and CT scanner. *Lung Cancer* 2004;45:45–55.
334. Garg AK, Wang XS, Shiu AS, et al. Prospective evaluation of spinal reirradiation by using stereotactic body radiation therapy. *Cancer* 2011;117:3509–3516.
348. Mahan SL, Ramsey CR, Scaperoth DD, et al. Evaluation of image-guided helical tomotherapy for the re-treatment of spinal metastasis. *Int J Radiat Oncol Biol Phys* 2005;63:1576–1583.
353. Hui SK, Kapatoes J, Fowler J, et al. Feasibility study of helical tomotherapy for total body or total marrow irradiation. *Med Phys* 2005;32:3214–3224.
364. Engels B, Tournel K, Everaert H, et al. Phase II study of preoperative helical tomotherapy with a simultaneous integrated boost for rectal cancer. *Int J Radiat Oncol Biol Phys* 2012;83(1):142–148.
367. Wong JYC, Rosenthal K, Liu A, et al. Image guided total marrow irradiation (TMI) using helical tomotherapy in patients with multiple myeloma and acute leukemia undergoing hematopoietic cell transplantation. *Int J Radiat Oncol Biol Phys* 2009;73:273–279.
368. Jaffray DA. Emergent technologies for 3-dimensional image-guided radiation delivery. *Sem Radiat Oncol* 2005;15:208–216.
370. Morin O, Gillis A, Chen J, et al. Megavoltage cone-beam CT: system description and clinical applications. *Med Dosim* 2006;31:51–61.
374. Pouliot J, Bani-Hashemi A, Chen J, et al. Low-dose megavoltage cone-beam CT for radiation therapy. *Int J Radiat Oncol Biol Phys* 2005;61(2):552–650.
389. Letourneau D, Martinez AA, Lockman D, et al. Assessment of residual error for online cone-beam XT-guided treatment of prostate cancer patients. *Int J Radiat Oncol Biol Phys* 2005;62:1239–1246.
393. Ho KF, Marchant T, Moore C, et al. Monitoring dosimetric impact of weight loss with kilovoltage (kV) cone beam CT (CBCT) during parotid-sparing IMRT and concurrent chemotherapy. *Int J Radiat Oncol Biol Phys* 2012;82:e375–e382.
398. Godfrey DJ, Yin FF, Oldham M, et al. Digital tomosynthesis with an on-board kilovoltage imaging device. *Int J Radiat Oncol Biol Phys* 2006;65:8–15.
400. Kupelian P, Willoughby T, Mahadevan A, et al. Multi-institutional clinical experience with the Calypso system in localization and continuous, real-time monitoring of the prostate gland during external radiotherapy. *Int J Radiat Oncol Biol Phys* 2007;67:1088–1098.
405. Shinohara ET, Kassaee A, Mitra N, et al. Feasibility of electromagnetic transponder use to monitor inter- and intrafractional motion in locally advanced pancreatic cancer patients. *Int J Radiat Oncol Biol Phys* 2012;83(2):566–573.
406. Lagendijk JJ, Raaymakers BW, Raaijmakers AJ, et al. MRI/Linac integration. *Radiother Oncol* 2008;86:25–29.
407. Raaymakers BW, de Boer JC, Knox C, et al. Integrated MV portal imaging with a 1.5 T MRI Linac. *Phys Med Biol* 2011;56:N207–N214.
423. Nehmeh SA, Erdi YE. Respiratory motion in positron emission tomography/computed tomography: a review. *Semin Nuc Med* 2008;38:167–176.
430. Keall P. 4-Dimensional computed tomography imaging and treatment planning. *Semin Radiat Oncol* 2004;14:81–90.
434. Rietzel E, Liu AK, Doppke KP, et al. Design of 4D treatment planning target volumes. *Int J Radiat Oncol Biol Phys* 2006;66:287–295.
437. Wolthaus JW, Sonke JJ, van Herk M, et al. Comparison of different strategies to use four-dimensional computed tomography in treatment planning for lung cancer patients. *Int J Radiat Oncol Biol Phys* 2008;70:1229–1238.
450. Mageras GS, Yorke E. Deep inspiration breath hold and respiratory gating strategies for reducing organ motion in radiation treatment. *Semin Radiat Oncol* 2004; 14:65–75.
456. Eccles CL, Patel R, Simeonov AK, et al. Comparison of liver tumor motion with and without abdominal compression using cine-magnetic resonance imaging. *Int J Radiat Oncol Biol Phys* 2011;79:602–608.
458. Jiang SB. Radiotherapy of mobile tumors. *Semin Radiat Oncol* 2006;16:239–248.
474. Yan D, Vicini F, Wong J, et al. Adaptive radiation therapy. *Phys Med Biol* 1997;42:123–132.
479. Deutschmann H, Kametriser G, Steininger P, et al. First clinical release of an online, adaptive, aperture-based image-guided radiotherapy strategy in intensity-modulated radiotherapy to correct for inter- and intrafractional rotations of the prostate. *Int J Radiat Oncol Biol Phys* 2012;83(5):1624–1632.
480. Barker JL, Garden AS, Ang KK, et al. Quantification of volumetric and geometric changes during fractionated radiotherapy for head-and-neck cancer using an integrated CT/linear accelerator system. *Int J Radiat Oncol Biol Phys* 2004;59:960–970.
481. Hansen EK, Bucci MK, Quivey JM, et al. Repeat CT imaging and re-planning during the course of IMRT for head-and-neck cancer. *Int J Radiat Oncol Biol Phys* 2006;64:355–362.
484. Van de Bunt L, van der Heided UA, Ketelaars M, et al. Conventional, conformal and intensity modulated radiation therapy treatment planning of external beam radiotherapy for cervical cancer: the impact of tumor regression. *Int J Radiat Oncol Biol Phys* 2006;64:189–196.
485. Ramsey CR, Langen KM, Kupelian PA, et al. A technique for adaptive image-guided helical tomotherapy for lung cancer. *Int J Radiat Oncol Biol Phys* 2006; 64:1237–1244.
486. Wieder HA, Brucher BL, Zimmermann F, et al. Time course of tumor metabolic activity during chemoradiotherapy of esophageal squamous cell carcinoma and response to treatment. *J Clin Oncol* 2004;22:900–908.
487. Gu X, Choi DJ, Men C, et al. GPU-based ultra-fast dose calculation using a finite pencil beam model. *Phys Med Biol* 2009;54:6287–6297.
488. Men C, Gu X, Choi DJ, et al. GPU-based ultrafast IMRT plan optimization. *Phys Med Biol* 2009;54:6565–6573.

SECTION II TECHNIQUES, MODALITIES, AND MODIFIERS IN RADIATION ONCOLOGY

Chapter 12
Altered Fractionation Schedules

Anesa Ahamad

This chapter discusses radiotherapy fractionation schedules that are different from the conventional fractionation in the United States of 1.8- to 2-Gy doses given once daily, Monday through Friday. The first section addresses background radiobiology. The second section reports outcomes of clinical studies. New results of pure hypofractionated radiotherapy for prostate and breast cancer have been added to this edition. Hypofractionated radiation schedules with highly conformal stereotactic body radiotherapy techniques or brachytherapy are discussed elsewhere in this book. Regimens are classified as either *hyperfractionated* or *accelerated*. In *hyperfractionation,* the total dose is increased, the size of dose per fraction is significantly reduced, the number of dose fractions is increased, and overall time is relatively unchanged. In *accelerated fractionation,* overall time is significantly reduced.

BACKGROUND RADIOBIOLOGY

Perhaps the most important consequence of altering a fractionation schedule is the sensitive change in late effects as the dose per fraction changes.[1] Acute reactions are more sensitive to changes in the rate of dose accumulation.

The classic descriptions of early and late reactions are couched in terms of target cell killing. This characterization is on firmer ground with acute effects, for which direct connections can be made between depletion of identified cell populations and measurable injury, than with late effects, for which such identification is more problematic[2] (see also Chapter 2 of this book). Despite this shortcoming, the conventional understanding of the potential advantages of alternative fractionation strategies is framed within the target cell concept.

Time–Dose Parameters

The time–dose parameters that determine normal tissue tolerance are total dose, overall duration of treatment, size of dose per fraction, and frequency of dose fractions. The last two determine the rate of dose accumulation, sometimes referred to as the *weekly dose rate.* The intensity of acute reactions in epithelial and other tissues organized into stem cell, maturation, and functional compartments (e.g., bone marrow) reflects the balance between the rate of cell killing by irradiation and the rate of regeneration of surviving stem cells. This balance depends primarily on the rate of dose accumulation. The fraction size is also a factor in determining the severity of acute reactions (large fractions being more damaging gray unit–for–gray unit than small ones) but to a lesser extent than is the case for late reactions. After an acute reaction has peaked (e.g., moist desquamation of the skin or confluent mucositis of the mucosa has occurred), further stem cell killing cannot produce an increase in *intensity* of the acute reaction but manifests as an increased time to heal the reaction. If sufficient stem cells do not survive to repopulate tissues, acute reactions may progress into a *consequential* late injury.[3]

The conventional view is that late reactions occur in tissues characterized by slow cellular turnover, such as mature connective tissues and the parenchymal cells of various organs. Because cellular depletion in such tissues does not manifest until after a typical course of radiation therapy is completed, the rate of dose accumulation and overall duration of treatment would be of minor significance in determining the severity of late reactions. Therefore, late reactions would depend primarily on total dose, size of dose per fraction, and interfraction interval.

There are difficulties with this simplified description. For example, there is evidence that the frequency of some late reactions correlates with the level of acute reactions, possibly through an influence of the rate of dose accumulation.[4–5,6] In addition, there is evidence that late effects can be modified by pharmacologic intervention. For example, amifostine administration protects lung tissue and the esophageal mucosa in the treatment of lung cancer,[7] and other agents have been shown to affect the development of radiation-induced nephritis (captopril) and fibrosis (pentoxifylline and vitamin E).

Size of Dose per Fraction and Length of Interfraction Interval

The influence of fraction size on radiation therapy outcome is manifest through the slope of the response to multifractionated doses, and this is a reflection of the *repair capacity* of the target cells. The experimental literature was reviewed,[8] and the results shown in Figure 2.18 (Chapter 2) indicate that changes in isoeffect doses for late effects with changing dose per fraction (solid curves) are steeper than for acute effects (dashed curves). The significance of this is that if tumors are similar to acutely responding normal tissues in their sensitivity to changing fraction size, then a gain in the therapeutic ratio can be realized by significantly reducing the fraction sizes and escalating the total dose (hyperfractionation). These results are independent of any mathematical models and rest instead on the data shown in Figure 2.18. It is, however, convenient to be able to quantify the fractionation sensitivity, and this is most easily done using the linear-quadratic (LQ) model, assuming that the target cell hypothesis is correct and that the LQ model correctly describes the target-cell survival curves. Given these conditions, the ratio α/β of the parameters of the LQ model is a quantitative measure of this sensitivity to changes in fraction size[8]: low ratios signify high fractionation sensitivity, and high ratios signify low fractionation sensitivity. Low ratios imply relatively large changes in isoeffective dose when dose per fraction is changed, and the converse is true for high values. The implication is that the tolerance dose for late effects can be increased more by the use of smaller fraction sizes than the tolerance dose for tumors and acute effects (hyperfractionation). The α/β ratios for some animal normal tissues are set out in Table 2.1 in Chapter 2 and for human tissues and tumors in Table 12.1.

In general, the estimated values of α/β for early and late reactions in human normal tissues are consistent with results from experimental animals. With regard to tumors, squamous cell carcinomas of the head and neck, cervix, and skin and non–small cell lung cancers (NSCLCs) are characterized by high α/β ratios, in agreement with rodent models. However, data from melanomas and liposarcomas suggest somewhat lower α/β ratios for these tumor types. The α/β ratio for breast adenocarcinomas may be lower than those for other carcinomas listed in Table 12.1.[9] The situation is different with prostate tumors, which contain unusually small fractions of cycling cells.[10] Prostate tumors might not respond to changes in fractionation in the same way as other cancers[11,12] and respond to changes in fractionation more like a late-responding normal tissue. In mathematical terms, the α/β ratio for prostate cancer

TABLE 12.1 ESTIMATES OF α/β FOR HUMAN TISSUES AND TUMORS

Tissue/Tumor	*Reference*	*Estimate/Bound of α/β in Gy (95% CI)*
Acutely Responding		
Skin		
Desquamation (time ≤29 days)	Turesson and Thames[6]	11.2 (8.5–17.6)
Erythema	Turesson and Thames[6]	8.8 (6.9–11.6)
	Bentzen et al.[148]	12.3 (2–23)
Mucous membrane–ulcer	Rezvani et al.[149]	15 (0–45.2)
Lung–acute	Cox[150]	>8.8
Late Responding		
Supraglottic larynx–late sequelae	Maciejewski et al.[151]	3.8 (0.8–14)
Larynx–cartilage necrosis	Henk and James[152]	~3.4
	Horiot et al.[153]	≤4.4
	Fletcher et al.[154]	
	Stell and Morrison[155]	≤4.2
Larynx–pharynx	Taylor et al.[156]	7.8 (3–∞)
	Rezvani et al.[149]	3.5 (1.1–5.9)
Oropharynx–late sequelae	Horiot et al.[157]	~4.5
Skin		
Subcutaneous fibrosis	Bentzen et al.[158]	1.9 (0.8–3)
Telangiectasia	Turesson and Thames[6]	3.9 (2.7–4.8)
	Bentzen et al.[158]	3.7 (0.2–4.7)
	Bentzen and Overgaard[159]	2.8 (0–8.1)
Mucosal ulceration (consequential effects)	Withers et al.[160]	21.3 (5.2–∞)
Shoulder–impaired movement	Bentzen et al.[161]	3.5 (0.7–6.2)
Rib–fracture	Overgaard[162]	1.8–2.8
Bone–exposure/necrosis	Withers et al.[160]	0.8 (0–2.4)
Lung		
Pneumonitis	Cox[150]	≤3.8
Computed tomography density	van Dyk et al.[163]	3.3 (0.5–6.5)
Spinal cord–myelopathy	Dische et al.[164]	≤3.3
Brachial plexus–plexopathy	Powell et al.[165]	≤5.3
Bowel–stricture/perforation	Bennett,[166] Edsmyr et al.[80]	2.2 ≤α/β≤8
Tumors		
Tonsil	Withers et al.[160]	14.7 (4.4–∞)
Vocal cord	Harrison et al.[167]	>9.9
Larynx	Rezvani et al.[168]	T2[a]: 18 (0–42), T3[a]: 13 (3–23)
Oral cavity/oropharynx	Maciejewski et al.[169]	~25
	Byhardt et al.[170]	>6.5
	Cox et al.[171]	~10.3
	Handa et al.[172]	>7
Lung–non-small cell carcinomas	Cox et al.[171]	50–90
Cervix	Watson et al.[173]	>13.9
Skin	Trott et al.[174]	8.5 (4.5–11.3)
Prostate	Brenner et al.[14]	1.2 (0.03–4.1)
	Brenner and Hall[175]	1.5 (0.8–2.2)
	Fowler et al.[176]	1.5 (1.3–1.8)
	King and Fowler[177]	1.8–2.8
Melanoma	Bentzen et al.[161]	0.6 (0–2.5)[b]
Liposarcoma	Thames and Suit[178]	0.4 (0–5.4)[b]

CI, confidence interval.

[a]American Joint Committee on Cancer staging system.

[b]Lower confidence limit is negative but is listed as 0 because a negative α/β has no biologic meaning.

Modified from Thames HD, Hendry JH. *Fractionation in radiotherapy*. London: Taylor & Francis, 1987.

is low, in the range 1 to 3 Gy, which is comparable to that for late sequelae.[13–16] The radiobiology of prostate cancer appears to favor large fractions, with evidence emerging from hypofractionated high-dose-rate (HDR) brachytherapy.[17]

The arguments presented here really relate to the α/β value for prostate cancer *in relation to the α/β value for the relevant late-responding normal tissue.* There is good evidence both from animal[11,18–22] and from human[5,23,24–25] studies that for late rectal sequelae a value of α/β of >4 Gy is higher than for most other late sequelae. If the α/β value for prostate cancer is actually less than that for the surrounding late-responding normal tissue, hypofractionation (by external beam or HDR) at the appropriate dose would be expected to yield increased tumor control for a given level of late complications or decreased late complications for a given level of tumor control.

Whereas hypofractionation in a curative setting may result in unacceptable late effects,[26,27] reports of hypofractionation for prostate cancer reveal minimal long-term urologic or bowel morbidity even with the much poorer dose distributions than are now routine, such as a 6-fraction 6-Gy protocol from London[28] and a 15-fraction 3.1-Gy protocol from the Christie Hospital, Manchester, United Kingdom.[16] Clinical trials of prostate cancer hypofractionation have been started using intensity-modulated radiation therapy (IMRT). In those studies that have reported on potential late sequelae, there is little indication of any unexpected late sequelae after median follow-up periods of 31,[29] 48,[30] 66,[31] 68,[32] and 97 months.[28] Early results of randomized trials of prostate hypofractionation are given in the second section of this chapter and Table 12.5.

Repair Kinetics

To realize an increase in tolerance of late-responding tissues through dose fractionation, the time interval between the dose fractions needs to be adequate to allow repair to approach completion. If doses are too closely spaced, injury will accumulate between dose fractions, and successive doses will become increasingly more damaging. This emphasizes the importance of *repair kinetics,* which is quantified by the half-time for repair. Of the tissues in experimental models in which repair kinetics have been studied, half-times for repair tend to be longest (1 to several hours) in the skin, kidney, and spinal cord, shortest (approximately 1/2 hour) in the jejunal mucosa, and intermediate in the lung and colon.[2,33–34,35–42] The exact values vary according to the experimental protocol, and considerable overlap exists in the confidence limits of repair half-time. The important point is to ensure an adequate interfraction interval during hyperfractionation.

Repair kinetics is of particular importance in determining the response of the spinal cord to fractionation schedules of more than one daily fraction. In rats, experimental data showed that repair is best described by a biexponential function in which the slower component has a half-time of 3.8 hours.[43] This would imply that any fractionation schedule using more than one fraction per day is associated with some degree of incomplete repair in the spinal cord. A clinical report of radiation myelopathy occurring in four patients whose spinal cords received 45 to 48 Gy in 28 fractions of 1.5 Gy three times a day with a 6-hour interval over 9 consecutive days supports this observation,[44] although incomplete repair cannot fully account for the observed frequency of injury.[45] Two reports from the Radiation Therapy Oncology Group (RTOG)[46,47] showed an increased rate of other late complications in patients treated on hyperfractionated protocols when the mean interval was <4.5 hours. For clinical practice, it is prudent to account for the potential compounding effect of incomplete repair. A minimum 6-hour interval between dose fractions is adequate.[48]

Data on repair kinetics in human normal tissues are extremely sparse, but, as indicated earlier, some evidence suggests that interfraction recovery may be slower in humans than in rodents. Bentzen et al.[49] analyzed late complications in the Continuous, Hyperfractionated, Accelerated Radiation Therapy (CHART) randomized trial, and their findings are in agreement with this picture. Estimated repair half-times, with 95% confidence intervals, were 4.9 hours (3.2, 6.4) for laryngeal edema, 3.8 hours (2.5, 4.6) for skin telangiectasia, and

4.4 hours (3.8, 4.9) for subcutaneous fibrosis. These results are consistent with observations from two other randomized altered fractionation trials: European Organization for Research and Treatment of Cancer (EORTC) 22791 and EORTC 22851.[50,51] Six hours should be regarded as the minimum interfraction interval for twice-daily fractionation.

Overall Time

The intensity of acute reactions is determined primarily by the rate of dose accumulation (weekly dose rate). Acute reactions represent a deficit in the balance between the rate of cell killing by radiation and cell regeneration from surviving stem cells. After the stem cell population is depleted the acute reaction peaks, and further depopulation produces no apparent increase in severity of the reaction. This means that the peak intensity of acute reactions is influenced more by the rate of dose accumulation than by the total dose, after a certain threshold of total dose has been reached.

Conversely, the time taken to heal depends on total dose, provided that the weekly dose rate exceeds the regenerative ability of the surviving stem cells. This is because healing is a function of the absolute number of stem cells surviving the course of treatment, and the higher the total dose, the lower is the number of stem cells surviving. Although most classic late radiation sequelae (e.g., spinal cord injury) show little or no dependence on overall time, overall time may be of significance for another set of late effects: consequential late effects that are attributed to severe and prolonged epithelial denudation rather than to direct radiation injury of the mesenchymal tissues normally associated with late reactions.[3,52–55]

The cure rates of many cancers (particularly squamous cell carcinomas) are also highly dependent on overall treatment time, with decrease in tumor control with longer treatment times. This has been interpreted in terms of accelerated regeneration of tumor clonogens.[56] After a variable lag period, surviving tumor clonogens regenerate rapidly during fractionated radiation therapy to the extent that each additional day of treatment requires approximately 0.6 Gy, on average, to offset clonogenic cell regeneration, again suggesting a clonogenic cell doubling time of 3.5 to 5 days. This is illustrated in Figure 2.6 in Chapter 2.[57–59]

Other evidence has been adduced for accelerated regeneration of surviving tumor cells after therapeutic intervention.[60] The majority of recurrences of squamous cell carcinomas of the head and neck occur within 2 years of treatment.[61] This would have required approximately 30 volume doublings of nonsterilized tumor clonogens, and the median doubling time must have been about 6 days.[43] Comparison of split-course treatment with continuous-course treatment suggests that 0.5 Gy per day is required to compensate for treatment interruption. Assuming that 2 to 3 Gy in 2-Gy fractions is necessary to reduce the surviving fractions of clonogenic cells by 50%, four to six doublings must occur during the 3-week treatment split, yielding a clonogenic cell doubling time of 3.5 to 5 days. Therefore, after initiation of radiotherapy, surviving clonogens in squamous cell carcinomas of the head and neck can regenerate with doubling times as short as 3 to 5 days.

Conversely, reduction of the overall treatment time may increase the probability of local tumor control. Molecular marker profiles (TP53, E-cadherin, KI-67, and EGFR) may aid in the selection of patients likely to benefit from reduction in overall treatment time.[62]

Isoeffect Formulas

The effect of changes of dose fractionation schedule on the total dose required to produce a certain level of biologic effect is approximated by isoeffect curves or formulas. The first clinical isoeffect curve was produced by Strandqvist.[63] This was followed by other studies,[64–66,67] culminating in the nominal standard dose formula of Ellis[68]: $D = N^{0.24} \times T^{0.11}$, where D is the dose, N is the number of dose fractions, and T is the overall time. None of these explicitly included dose per fraction.

In the early 1980s, it was pointed out that the different exponents for early and late effects could be interpreted in terms of survival curves for different target cell populations[8] in which the curves for late effects were "curvier" than those for acute effects. The consequence of this is that isoeffect doses for various late effects in normal tissues are more sensitive to changes in dose per fraction than are corresponding doses for acute effects. With the widespread use of the LQ model to quantify the fractionation sensitivity, the following model has gained in popularity: $D_1 = D_2(\alpha/\beta + d_2)/(\alpha/\beta + d_1)$, where D_2 is the reference total dose given in fractions of size d_2, and it is desired to calculate the total dose D_1 in fractions of size d_1 that would be isoeffective. This basic formula assumes complete repair between dose fractions, and no time factor is incorporated in it (see Chapter 2 for a detailed discussion). Thus, the basic formula may be used only when dose fractions are spaced widely enough apart to ensure complete repair and when either the endpoint is time independent (as with most late reactions) or the two schedules being compared involve the same overall time–dosing intensity.

Whereas the LQ-based isoeffect model is internally consistent for a wide range of tissue types and endpoints, clinical application of the model for derivation of new fractionation schedules is limited by at least two factors. First, there is the lack of precision of estimates of α/β. Even in closely controlled animal systems, estimates of α/β show large confidence intervals (Table 2.1 in Chapter 2). The α/β ratios of human data are consistent with the experimentally determined α/β ratios but have very wide confidence bounds (see Table 12.1). Second, as discussed earlier, the severity of complications can be modulated by various agents, including growth factors, radioprotectors, and pharmacologic agents, and current isoeffect concepts will doubtlessly have to be modified as the results of future studies become available. *The bottom line is that no isoeffect formula is sufficiently reliable to preempt clinical judgment, and, in the final analysis, each new fractionation schedule must be tested clinically to establish its safety.*

Rationale for Hyperfractionation

The basic rationale of hyperfractionation is that the use of small-dose fractions allows higher total doses to be administered within the tolerance of late-responding normal tissues, and this translates into a higher biologically effective dose to the tumor. For this rationale to hold, the α/β ratio for tumor cells must be greater than that for the dose-limiting normal tissue. Acutely responding tissues as a class have higher α/β ratios than late-responding normal tissues. Because of the kinetic similarity between tumors and acutely responding normal tissues, it may be predicted that tumors (with possible exceptions, such as the prostate) also tend to have large α/β ratios. Other rationales for hyperfractionation are radiosensitization through redistribution and lesser dependence on oxygen effect. The greater the number of dose fractions, the greater is the chance that cells would be in a more radiosensitive phase at the time of the next fraction. With small fractional doses, the influence of tumor cell hypoxia is reduced on two counts. First, the proportion of hypoxic cells needs to be higher to increase significantly the surviving fraction and, second, the oxygen enhancement ratio is lower.[69]

Hyperfractionation has been tested in more than 20 randomized trials, and these are summarized in the data presented in Table 12.2.

Rationale for Accelerated Fractionation

The rationale for accelerated fractionation is that reduction in overall treatment time decreases the opportunity for tumor

TABLE 12.2 DATA OF PHASE III CLINICAL TRIALS ADDRESSING HYPERFRACTIONATION

Tumor Site and Type	Number of Patients	Dose/ Fx (Gy)	Fx/day	Total Dose (Gy)	Overall Time (wk)	Tumor Response	Side Effects	Reference
Head and Neck Carcinomas								
Oropharynx, stage III–IV	98	1.1 2.0	2 1	70.4 66.0	6.5 6.5	Tumor response: 84% vs. 64% ($p = .02$) 3.5-yr OS: 27% vs. 8% ($p = .03$)	Earlier onset of acute reactions with HF Late complications: no details	Pinto et al.[73]
Oropharynx, T2–3, N0–1	356	1.15 2.0	2 1	80.5 70.0	7.0 7.0	5-yr LRC: 59% vs. 40% ($p = .02$). Improved local control of T3 tumors.	More acute mucositis with HF No difference in late complication rate	Horiot et al.[51] Horiot[72]
Various sites, T3–4, N0, or any T, N+	331	1.45 2.55	2 1	58.0 51.0	4.0 4.0	5-yr LRC: 45% vs. 37% ($p = .01$) 5-yr OS: 40% vs. 30% ($p = .01$)	More acute mucositis with HF 5-yr grade 3–4 late toxicity: 8% vs. 14% ($p = .31$)	Cummings et al.[74]
Various sites, stage III–IV, stage II of tongue base, hypopharynx	1,073	1.2 1.8* 1.6 2.0	2 1–2 2 1	81.6 72.0 67.2 70.0	6.0 7.0 6.0 7.0	LRC: higher with HF and CB ($p = .045$ and 0.05) DFS: trend in favor of HF and CB ($p = .067$ and 0.054) but no difference in OS	More acute mucositis with all altered fractionations No difference in late complication rate	Fu et al.[71]
Bladder Cancer (TCC)								
T2–4	168	1.0 2.0	3 1	84.0 64.0	8.0 8.0	Survival: higher with HF with a RH of 1.52 (95% CI: 1.10–2.09) OS benefit persists at 10 yr	Trend for increase in bowel injury requiring surgical treatment	Naslund et al.[81]
Non-Small Cell Lung Cancer								
Stage II–III (surgically unresectable)	458	1.2 2.0	2 1	69.6 60.0	5.8 6.0	No significant difference in median or 5-yr survival (induction chemotherapy arm yielded better OS)	Late toxicity not presented in detail	Sause et al.[82]
Stage III (RTOG 9410); arm A, neoadjuvant chemotherapy; arms B and C, concurrent chemotherapy	610	A: 2.0 B: 2.0 C: 1.2	1 1 2	60.0 60 69.6	6.0 6.0 5.8	No significant difference in median survival between arms B and C; improved 5-yr survival for concurrent chemotherapy	Acute grade 3–5 nonhematologic toxic effects were higher with concurrent than sequential therapy, but late toxic effects were similar	Curran et al.[83]
Brainstem Tumors								
Age, 3–21 yr	130	1.17 1.80	2 1	70.2 54.0	6.0 6.0	No significant difference in time to disease progression and overall survival	Morbidity similar in both arms	Mandell et al.[84]
Cranial Radiation for Treatment of High-Risk Acute Lymphoblastic Leukemia								
Children treated on two consecutive protocols for high-risk ALL	369	0.9 1.8	2 1	18.0 18.0	2.0 2.0	8-yr EFS 72% ± 3% vs. 80% ± 3% ($p = .06$), OS 78% ± 3% vs. 85% ± 3% ($p = .06$); CNS HF may compromise antileukemic efficacy	Provides no benefit in terms of cognitive late effects No difference in intelligence, academic achievement, visuospatial reasoning, or verbal learning Children on HF arm exhibited a modest advantage for visual memory ($p \leq 0.05$)	Weber et al.,[86] LeClerc et al.[85]
Children with Rhabdomyosarcoma								
Children enrolled into the Intergroup RMS Study IV with group III RMS	490	1.1 1.8	2 1	59.4 50.4	5.5 5.5	No difference in 5-yr FFS or OS between HF and SF	Analysis by intention to treat; high noncompliance analysis by actual treatment also shows no difference; higher acute toxicity with HF	Donaldson et al.[87]
Unresected Brain Metastases (Hyperfractionation Versus Accelerated Hypofractionation)								
RTOG 9104; patients with measurable brain metastasis and KPS at least 70; AHF versus AF	429	1.6 3.0	2 1	54.4 30.0	3.5 2.0	No difference in 1-yr OS: 19% in AF vs. 16% in AHF	Grade III or IV toxicity was equivalent in both arms	Murray et al.[88]
Prophylactic Cranial Irradiation for Limited-Stage Small Cell Lung Cancer in Complete Remission After Chemotherapy and Thoracic Radiotherapy								
Standard or higher total dose using either conventional or accelerated hyperfractionated radiotherapy	720	2.5 2.0 1.5	1 1 2	25 36.0 36	2.0 3.5 3	No difference in incidence of brain metastases; significant increase in mortality after higher-dose PCI	Slightly higher acute toxicity in the higher-dose arm but greater serious adverse events in the standard-dose group	Le Péchoux et al.[89]

The outcome data given *x*% vs. *y*% imply that *x* is the experimental-arm result. AF, accelerated fractionation; AHF, accelerated hyperfractionation; ALL, acute lymphoblastic leukemia; CI, confidence interval; CNS, central nervous system; DFS, disease-free survival; EFS, event-free survival, FFS, failure-free survival; Fx, fraction(s); Gy, Gray; HF, hyperfractionation; KPS, Karnofsky performance score; LC, local control; LRC, locoregional control; MST, median survival time; N+, nodal stage; NSCLC, non–small cell lung cancer; OS, overall survival; PCI, prophylactic cranial irradiation; TCC, transitional cell carcinoma; RMS, rhabdomyosarcoma; SF, standard fractionation; T, tumor stage; wk, week.

TABLE 12.3 DATA OF PHASE III CLINICAL TRIALS ADDRESSING PURE ACCELERATED FRACTIONATION

Tumor Site and Type	Number of Patients	Dose/Fx (Gy)	Fx/d (Ti, hr)	Total Dose (Gy)	Overall Time (wk)	Tumor Response	Side Effects	Reference
Inoperable non–small cell lung cancer	204	2.0 2.0	2 1	60 ± Carbo 60 ± Carbo	3.0 6.0	No significant difference in median survival time and 2-yr OS	Esophageal toxicity significantly greater in AF	Ball et al.[90]
Various head and neck carcinomas, stage III–IV	82	2.0 2.0	2 (≥6) 1	66.0 66.0	3.4 6.8	CR: 35% vs. 29% (p = .18) No difference in 3-yr relapse-free survival	Grade 3–4 reactions: 27 vs. 8 (p = .00005) Grade 4 late toxicity: 8 vs. 2 (p = .10)	Jackson et al.[91]
Various head and neck carcinomas, T2-4, N0-1	100	1.8–2.0 1.8–2.0	1 1	~70.0 ~70.0	5.0 7.0	3-yr LC: 82% vs. 37% ($p \le 0.0001$) and 3-yr OS: 78% vs. 32% ($p \le .0001$)	Severe mucositis: 62% vs. 26% Late complications: 10% vs. 0%	Skladowski et al.[92]
Various head and neck carcinomas, all stages	1,485	2.0 2.0	1 1	~66.0 ~66.0	6.0 7.0	5-yr LRC: 66% vs. 57% (p = .01). 5-yr DFS: 72% vs. 65% (p = .04); no difference in OS	More acute mucositis with AF No difference in late complication rate	Overgaard et al.[94]
Larynx carcinomas, T1-3, N0	395	2.0 2.0	1–2 (≥6) 1	66.0 66.0	5.5 6.5	LRC: higher with AF (p = .03).	More acute reactions with AF; no difference in late complications except for telangiectasia	Hliniak et al.[95]
Nasopharynx cancer	416	1.8–1.9 1.8–1.9 2.0	1 1 1	74–76 74–76 +Cis/5-FU 70–76	6.0 6.0 7.0	LR 16.7% vs. 13.6% vs. 27.3% ($p \le 0.05$) 5-yr OS 53.6% vs. 57.6% vs. 43.8% ($p \le 0.05$) Acceleration had a similar improvement as concurrent chemotherapy	Acute reactions higher with acceleration	Wang et al.[93]

The outcome data given as *x*% vs. *y*% imply that *x* is the experimental-arm result. AF, accelerated fractionation; Carbo, carboplatin; Cis, cisplatin; CR, complete response; DFS, disease-free survival; Fx, fraction(s); 5-FU, 5-flourouracil; Gy, gray; hr, hours; LC, local control; LR, local recurrence; LRC, local-regional control; OS, overall survival; Ti, inter-fraction interval time; wk, week.

cell regeneration during treatment and therefore increases the probability of tumor control for a given total dose. Because overall treatment time has little influence on the probability of late normal tissue injury, a therapeutic gain should be realized, provided the size of dose per fraction is not increased and the interval between dose fractions is sufficient for complete repair to take place.

When the overall duration of treatment is markedly reduced, it is necessary to reduce total dose to prevent excessively severe acute reactions. A therapeutic gain is then realized only if the reduction in dose is less than the dose equivalent of blocked regeneration of tumor cells due to shortened time.

Strategies to accelerate radiation can be divided into two categories: (a) *pure accelerated fractionation* regimens, with reduced overall treatment time without concurrent changes in the fraction size or total dose (examples are given in Table 12.3); and (b) *hybrid accelerated fractionation*, with reduced overall treatment time in conjunction with changes in other parameter(s), such as the fraction size, total dose, and time distribution. Four forms of hybrid accelerated fractionation were designed, and the regimes tested in randomized clinical trials are given in Table 12.4. The categories are further described as follows (Fig. 12.3):

Type A: There is drastic reduction of the overall time, with substantial decrease in the total dose.

Type B: Duration of treatment is more modestly reduced, with total dose kept in the same range, and there is a break in treatment.

Type C: Duration of treatment is more modestly reduced, with total dose kept in the same range, with a concomitant boost phase.

CLINICAL STUDIES

This section summarizes the results of hyperfractionated (HF) radiotherapy trials and accelerated fractionation (AF) radiotherapy trials. A new subsection summarizes results of pure hypofractionated radiotherapy (fraction size of >2 Gy). There is also a summary of combined altered fractionation with concurrent chemotherapy; critical fractionation issues to consider when IMRT is used; common clinically practiced fractionation schedules; and future directions in combining molecular targeting with altered fractionation. Hypofractionated radiation schedules with highly conformal stereotactic body radiotherapy techniques or brachytherapy are discussed elsewhere in this book.

Results of Hyperfractionated Radiotherapy Trials

The key findings of hyperfractionated radiotherapy include the following:

- HF is better than standard fractionation in locoregional control of intermediate to locally advanced head and neck carcinoma. This was also associated with an improvement in survival in three trials.[56]
- Reducing the fraction size from 2 Gy to 1.1 to 1.2 Gy permits a 7% to 17% total radiation dose escalation without increase in late complications. This supports the existence of differential fractionation sensitivity (variable α/β ratios) between human late-responding normal tissues and head and neck carcinomas.
- There is significant survival benefit at 5 years with hyperfractionated radiotherapy on meta-analysis versus 2% with accelerated radiotherapy for head and neck cancer.

Altered fractionation radiotherapy improves survival in patients with head and neck squamous cell carcinoma.[70] Comparison of the different types of altered radiotherapy suggests that hyperfractionation provides the greatest benefit. An individual patient data meta-analysis was conducted to see the effect of altered fractionation radiotherapy. It revealed a significant absolute survival benefit of 3.4% at 5 years with altered fractionation radiotherapy (hazard ratio [HR] = 0.92, 95%

TABLE 12.4 DATA OF PHASE III CLINICAL TRIALS ADDRESSING HYBRID ACCELERATED FRACTIONATION

Tumor Site and Type	*Number of Patients*	*Dose/Fx (Gy)*	*Fx/d (Ti, hr)*	*Total Dose (Gy)*	*Overall Time (wk)*	*Tumor Response*	*Side Effects*	*Reference*
Accelerated Fractionation with Total Dose Reduction (Type A)								
Various head and neck carcinomas, mainly stage II–IV	918	1.5 2.0	3 (6) 1	54.0 66.0	2.0 6.5	No difference in LRC, disease-free interval, and OS	More acute mucositis but less epidermis, telangiectasia, mucosal ulceration, and edema with AF	Dische et al.[97]
Various head and neck carcinomas, stage III-IV	350	1.8 2.0	2 (≥6) 1	59.4 70.0	3.5 7.0	5-yr LRC: 52% vs. 47% ($p = .30$) 5-yr DFS: 41% vs. 35% ($p = .32$) 5-yr DSS: 46% vs. 40% ($p = .40$)	More severe acute mucositis ($p = .00008$) but reduced incidence of grade ≥2 late soft tissue effects ($p \leq .05$) with AF (except for mucosal late effect)	Poulsen et al.[98]
All sites of head and neck carcinomas; oropharynx 75%; T4 70%	268	2.0 2.0	2 1	~63.0 70.0	3.3 7.0	2-yr LRC: 58% vs. 34% ($p \leq 0.01$) No difference in OS	Grade 3–4 mucositis: 83% vs. 28% ($p \leq .01$) Similar late toxicity	Bourhis et al.[99]
Postoperative head and neck	70	1.4 2.0	3 (6) 1	46.2 60.0	2.0 6.0	3-yr LRC: 88 ± 4% vs. 57% ± 9% ($p = .01$) OS: 60 ± 10% vs. 46 ± 9% ($p = .29$)	More rapid and more severe mucositis; fibrosis and edema more frequent after accelerated	Awwad et al.[100]
RTOG 9104; patients with measurable brain metastasis and KPS at least 70; AHF vs. AF	429	3.0 1.6	1 2	30.0 54.4	2.0 3.5	No difference in 1-yr OS: 19% in AF vs. 16% in AHF	Grade III or IV toxicity was equivalent in both arms	Murray et al.[88]
Locally advanced non–small cell lung cancer	563	1.5 2.0 split course	3 (6) 1	54.0 60.0	2.0 6.0	2-yr OS: 29% vs. 20% ($p = .008$) Lower risk of local progression ($p = .033$)	No difference in short- or long-term morbidity	Saunders et al.[103]
Stage IIIA and B non–small cell lung cancer	141	1.5 2.0	3 1	57.6 60.0	2.5 6.5	Trend suggesting a survival advantage in MS 20.3 vs. 14.9 mo ($p = .28$); 2-yr OS 44% vs. 34%, 3-yr OS 24% vs. 14%	Study included induction CT closed prematurely because concurrent CRT now seems more effective; 388 patients were needed	Belani et al.[104]
Locally advanced non–small cell lung cancer CHARTWEL (CHART weekend less)	406	1.5 2.0	3 (6) 1	60.0 60.0	2.5 6.0	No difference in 2, 3, and 5 yr (31%, 22%, and 11%) vs. CF (32%, 18%, and 7%; HR = 0.92, 95% CI = 0.75–1.13, $p = .43$)	Acute dysphagia and radiologic pneumonitis were more pronounced after CHARTWEL	Baumann et al.[105]
Split-Course (Type B) and Concomitant Boost (Type C) Accelerated Fractionation								
Various head and neck carcinomas, T2–4, N0-1	500	1.6 2.0 split course	3 1	72.0 70.0	5.0 7.0	5-yr LRC: 59% vs. 46% ($p = .02$) Trend for higher 5-yr DFS ($p = .08$) but no difference in OS ($p = .96$)	More severe acute mucositis and higher incidence of severe late morbidity ($p \leq .001$) with AF	Horiot et al.[50]
Various head and neck carcinomas, stage III–IV, stage II of tongue base, hypopharynx	1,073	1.8[a] 1.20 1.60 split course 2.0	1–2 2 2 1	72.0 81.6 67.2 70.0	6.0 7.0 6.0 7.0	LRC: higher with CB and HF ($p = .05$ and .045) DFS: strong trend in favor of CB and HF ($p = .054$ and .067) but no difference in OS	More acute mucositis with all altered fractionations No difference in late complication rate	Fu et al.[71]
Unresectable epidermoid tumors of oropharynx	192	2.0 1.6 split course 2[b]	1 2 1	66–70 64–67.2 66–70	6.5–7 5.5 6.5–7	Concurrent chemotherapy almost doubled the 5-yr overall survival, relapse-free survival, and locoregional control rates but did not reach statistical significance	SF had less severe mucositis than AFS or SF chemo; concurrent chemotherapy showed slightly more subcutaneous and mucosal G3+ late side effects	Fallai et al.[106]
T2-3, N0-1 bladder tumors	229	1.8 (a.m.), 2 (p.m.) split course 2.0	2 1	60.8 64.0	5.0 6.5	No difference in 3- or 5-yr DFS and OS 5-yr OS 37% vs. 40%	More acute bowel reactions with AF	Horwich et al.[107]

(continued)

TABLE 12.4 (CONTINUED)

Tumor Site and Type	*Number of Patients*	*Dose/Fx (Gy)*	*Fx/d (Ti, hr)*	*Total Dose (Gy)*	*Overall Time (wk)*	*Tumor Response*	*Side Effects*	*Reference*
Various head and neck carcinomas, high-risk surgical-pathologic features	151	1.8 1.8	1–2 1	63.0 63.0	5.0 7.0	A trend for higher LRC (p = .11) and OS (p = .08) with CB Cumulative time was a significant prognostic factor for LRC (p = .005) and OS (p = .03)	More acute mucositis with CB No difference in late complication rate	Ang et al.[101]
High-risk features (pT4, + margins, pN >1, perineural/lymphovascular invasion, extracapsular extension, subglottic extension) after surgery	226		1–2 1	64.0 60.0	5.0 6.0	No difference in OS and LRC but trend for improved LRC among patients who had delayed RT	More acute mucositis with CB	Sanguineti et al.[102]
Accelerated hyperfractionation								
Glioblastoma multiforme	231	1.6 1.8	2 1	70.4 ± DMFO 59.4 ± DMFO	4.4 6.5	No difference in PFS (p = .32) and OS (p = .48)	Cerebral necrosis was not observed; morbidity more common in the DFMO arms	Prados et al.[111]

The outcome data given as *x*% vs. *y*% imply that *x* is the experimental-arm result. There are three types of hybrid accelerated: accelerated with dose reduction (A), accelerated with split course (B), and accelerated with concomitant boost (C). AF, accelerated fractionation; AFS, accelerated hyperfractionated split course; AHF, accelerated hyperfractionated; CB, concomitant boost; CHART, Continuous, Hyperfractionated, Accelerated Radiation Therapy; CI, confidence interval; CRT, concurrent chemoradiation; CT, chemoradiation; DFS, disease-free survival; DMFO, difluoromethylornithine; DSS, disease-specific survival; EFS, event-free survival; Fx, fraction(s); Gy, Gray; HF, hyperfractionation; hr, hours; KPS, Karnofsky performance score; LRC, local-regional control; MS, median survival; OS, overall survival; PFS, progression-free survival; RTOG, Radiation Therapy Oncology Group; SF, standard fractionation; SF chemo, standard fraction plus concomitant chemotherapy; Ti, inter-fraction interval time; wk, week.
[a]Boost dose given in 1.5-Gy fractions. [b]Third arm with concurrent chemotherapy.

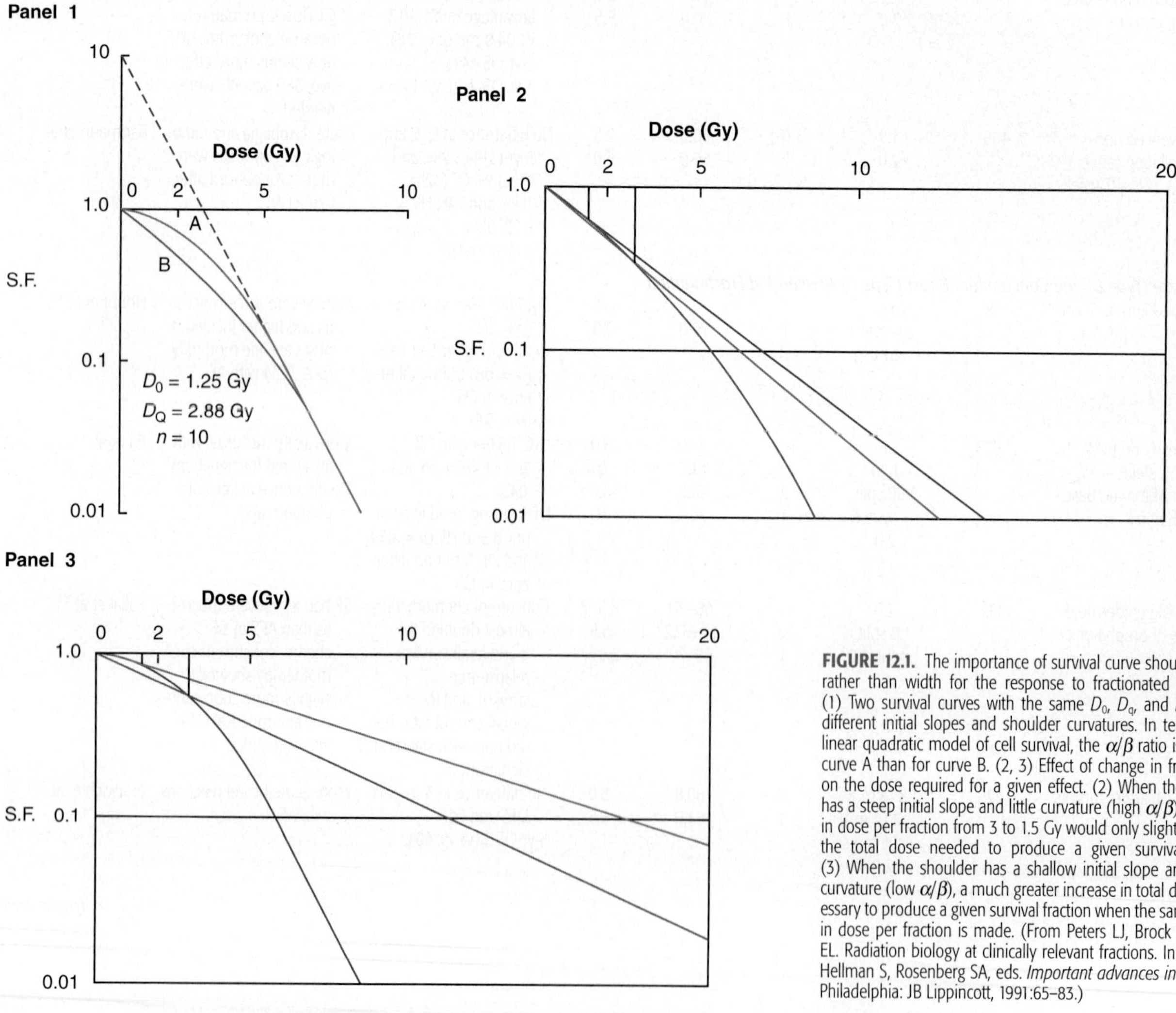

FIGURE 12.1. The importance of survival curve shoulder *shape* rather than width for the response to fractionated irradiation. (1) Two survival curves with the same D_0, D_q, and n but with different initial slopes and shoulder curvatures. In terms of the linear quadratic model of cell survival, the α/β ratio is lower for curve A than for curve B. (2, 3) Effect of change in fraction size on the dose required for a given effect. (2) When the shoulder has a steep initial slope and little curvature (high α/β), a change in dose per fraction from 3 to 1.5 Gy would only slightly increase the total dose needed to produce a given survival fraction. (3) When the shoulder has a shallow initial slope and marked curvature (low α/β), a much greater increase in total dose is necessary to produce a given survival fraction when the same change in dose per fraction is made. (From Peters LJ, Brock WA, Travis EL. Radiation biology at clinically relevant fractions. In: DeVita V, Hellman S, Rosenberg SA, eds. *Important advances in oncology.* Philadelphia: JB Lippincott, 1991:65–83.)

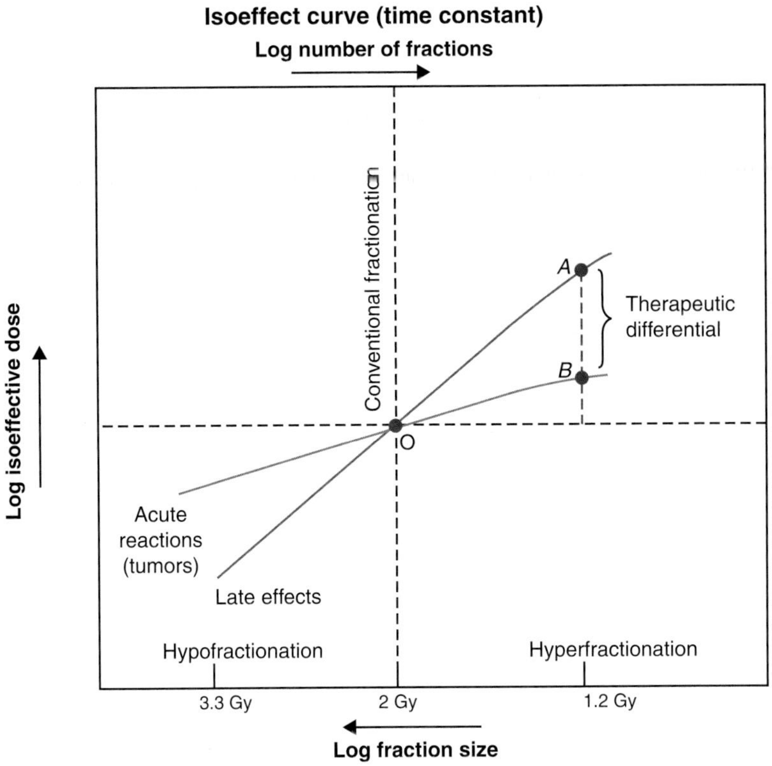

FIGURE 12.2. Effect of change in size of dose fraction (with overall time held constant) on the total dose necessary to produce a given level of acute and late effects. The curves are normalized to the "conventional" 2 Gy per fraction. Changes in fraction size have a relatively greater effect on the isoeffective doses for late reactions than for acute reactions and for the response of tumors with high α/β ratios. Consequently, by reducing the dose per fraction—for example, from 2 to 1.2 Gy—the total dose for equivalent late effects can be increased from *O* to *A*, which is greater than the increase (*O* to *B*) required to achieve an equivalent tumor response. The increment in dose from *B* to *A* represents the therapeutic differential achieved by hyperfractionation.

confidence interval [CI] = 0.86 to 0.97; $p = .003$) among 6515 patients with nonmetastatic head and neck squamous cell carcinomas in 15 randomized trials comparing conventional radiotherapy with altered fractionation. Significant survival benefit at 5 years with hyperfractionated radiotherapy was 8%, with accelerated radiotherapy was 2% (without total dose reduction), and was 1.7% (with total dose reduction; $p = .02$). Locoregional control was better with altered fractionation (6.4% at 5 years; $p < .0001$), with particularly effect improved local control and less benefit for nodal control. The benefit was significantly higher in the youngest patients, <50 years old.

Table 12.2 summarizes reported prospective, randomized trials addressing hyperfractionation for the treatment of patients with head and neck, bladder, lung, and brainstem tumors, whole-brain radiotherapy for pediatric acute lymphoblastic leukemia, whole-brain radiotherapy for brain metastases or prophylactic whole-brain radiotherapy, and rhabdomyosarcoma. The most striking results are from trials in head and neck squamous cell carcinoma (HNSCC), for which hyperfractionation was accompanied by an increase in dose.

Head and Neck

In all four head and neck trials[51,71–74] HF allowed a higher total dose to be delivered, which produced improved locoregional control by 8% to 20%. In three of these trials, HF improved overall survival by 10% to 19%. In all four studies, HF produced more severe acute mucositis but no increase in late morbidity. A Brazilian Group[73] tested HF of 70.4 Gy at 1.1 Gy twice daily and showed improved local response by 20% and 3.5-year overall survival from 8% to 27%. The EORTC

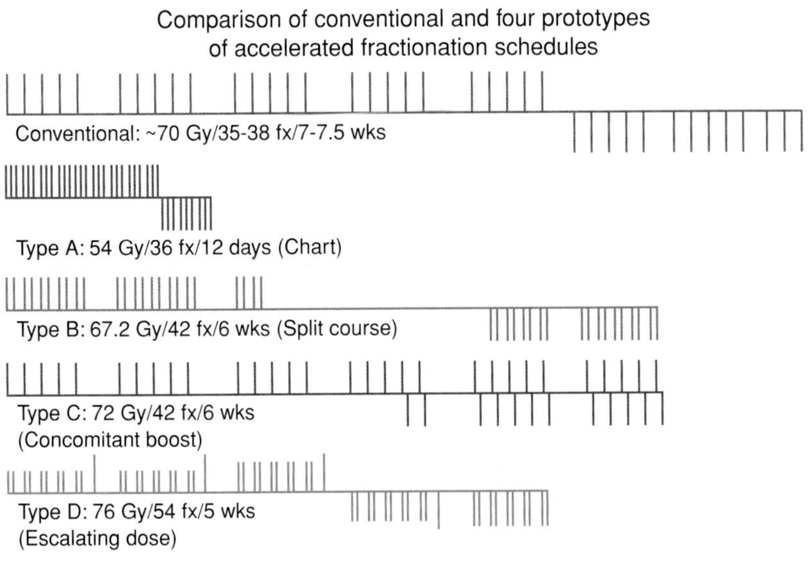

FIGURE 12.3. Conventional and accelerated fractionation schedules. For each regimen, the large-field treatment is depicted by the bars above the horizontal line and the boost-field irradiation by the bars below the line. The dotted bars represent treatment omitted in the lower ranges of total dose. fx, fraction.

tested 80.5 Gy HF at 1.15 Gy per fraction twice per day for 7 weeks.[51] The 10-Gy increase in dose improved locoregional control from 38% to 56% and overall survival.[57,72] The Princess Margaret Hospital (Toronto, Canada) tested 58 Gy at 1.45 Gy twice per day over 4 weeks versus 51 Gy at 2.55 Gy per fraction once daily (a standard fractionation at that institute).[74] The 7-Gy increase in dose improved locoregional control from 37% to 45% and improved 5-year overall survival from 30% to 40%.

The RTOG 9003 trial[71] tested 81.6 Gy at 1.2 Gy per fraction HF twice per day over 6 weeks versus 70 Gy at 2 Gy per fraction versus two AF regimes (a continuous and a split-course accelerated regime), as shown in Tables 12.2 and 12.4. HF improved locoregional control from 46% to 54.4% (similar to the improvement by AF with the concomitant boost arm of the trial). This trial gives strong evidence that total dose and treatment duration are important to outcome. Locoregional control was significantly improved by an increase of the total dose without changing overall time using HF or by accelerated overall treatment time without changing total dose using concomitant boost fractionation.

Meta-analysis of hyperfractionated and accelerated radiotherapy in unresected locally advanced squamous cell carcinoma of the head and neck showed a substantial prolongation of median survival (14.2 months; $p < .001$) for hyperfractionated compared to conventional radiotherapy.[75] Of the four hyperfractionation trials,[51,71,73] one from Barcelona[76] has been criticized for questionable quality.[77] All four trials showed a statistically significant survival benefit. Studies testing HF without dose escalation did not show a survival advantage.[78,79] HF is a useful tool to enable dose escalation without an increase of severe late toxicity.

Bladder Cancer

In the study by Edsmyr et al.,[80] T2–4 bladder tumors were randomized to either three 1-Gy daily fractions 4 hours apart with interfraction intervals to 84 Gy, or a single daily fraction of 2 Gy to total dose of 64 Gy, both given in a split course over 8 weeks. Cystoscopic complete response rate increased from 36% to 65% by HF ($p < .001$), and the 5-year survival rate also significantly increased. However, severe late complications were higher in the hyperfractionated arm, indicating that the dose chosen might not be equivalent for late normal tissue injury. An updated analysis revealed that the survival benefit persisted for 10 years, but there was a trend for higher bowel complications requiring surgery in the HF group.[81]

Non–Small Cell Lung Cancer

The joint Intergroup trial[82] of the RTOG, the Eastern Cooperative Oncology Group (ECOG), and the Southwest Oncology Group compared induction chemotherapy (cisplatin and vinblastine) plus 60 Gy in 2-Gy fractions or HF (69.6 Gy in 1.2-Gy fractions) with conventional fractionation (60 Gy in 2-Gy fractions). HF, although slightly better, did not significantly improve survival over the standard fractionation.

Two concurrent regimens with standard or hyperfractionated radiotherapy were tested as part of three arms of RTOG 9410, a phase III trial. Six hundred ten patients had either neoadjuvant cisplatin and vinblastine or the same chemotherapy concurrent with 60-Gy standard fractionation versus concurrent cisplatin and etoposide with hyperfractionated radiotherapy with 69.6 Gy delivered as 1.2-Gy twice-daily fractions. Median survival times were 14.6, 17.0, and 15.6 months, respectively. Five-year survival was statistically significantly higher for patients treated with the concurrent regimen with once-daily radiotherapy (TRT) compared with the sequential treatment (5-year survival: sequential, arm 1, 10% [20 patients], 95% CI = 7% to 15%; concurrent, arm 2, 16% [31 patients], 95% CI = 11% to 22%, $p = .046$; concurrent, arm 3, 13% [22 patients], 95% CI = 9% to 18%). Late toxic effects were similar.[83]

Childhood Brainstem Tumor

The trial of the Pediatric Oncology Group[84] compared the efficacy of 70.2 Gy given as 1.17 Gy per fraction versus 54 Gy in 1.8-Gy fractions, both in combination with 100 mg/m^2 cisplatin. This study showed no difference in the median time to disease progression, median time to death, or survival rates at 1 and 2 years, with no significant difference in toxicity.

Cranial Radiation Therapy for High-Risk Acute Lymphoblastic Leukemia

To test whether hyperfractionated (twice daily) therapy can reduce incidence and severity of late toxicities associated with 18-Gy prophylactic cranial radiotherapy, 369 children on two consecutive Dana-Farber Cancer Institute Consortium protocols were randomized to 18 Gy delivered in ten 1.8-Gy fractions once daily over 2 weeks versus 18 Gy delivered in twenty 0.9-Gy fractions. No benefit was seen in terms of cognitive late effects, and the results suggested that HF may compromise antileukemic efficacy.[85,86]

Group III Rhabdomyosarcoma

A study of 490 children with group III rhabdomyosarcoma (RMS) who were randomized to hyperfractionated radiotherapy (HFRT; 59.4 Gy in fifty-four 1.1-Gy twice-daily fractions) versus conventionally fractionated radiotherapy (CFRT) to 50.4 Gy in the Intergroup RMS Study IV showed that HFRT did not improve local/regional control, failure-free survival, or overall survival compared with CFRT and that HFRT actually produced more acute toxicity.[87] Unlike studies in HNSCC showing positive results with dose-escalated HFRT, an escalation of dose by 9.5 Gy did not improve outcome for RMS.

Unresected Brain Metastasis

RTOG 9104 compared 1-year survival and acute toxicity rates between an accelerated hyperfractionated radiotherapy (1.6 Gy twice a day) to a total dose of 54.4 Gy and an accelerated hypofractionated arm of 30 Gy in 10 daily fractions in patients with unresected brain metastasis. Of 429 analyzable patients, the median survival time was 4.5 months in both arms. The 1-year survival rate was 19% in the hypofractionated arm versus 16% in the hyperfractionated arm. Grade III or IV toxicity was equivalent in both arms. In spite of an escalated dose, HF was of no benefit.[88]

Prophylactic Cranial Irradiation for Limited-Stage Small Cell Lung Cancer

To test whether higher-dose prophylactic cranial irradiation (PCI) would reduce brain metastases, 720 patients with limited-stage small cell lung cancer (SCLC) who were in complete remission after chemotherapy and thoracic radiotherapy were randomized to standard 25 Gy in 10 daily versus 36 Gy either as 18 daily 2-Gy fractions or accelerated hyperfractionated as 24 twice-daily 1.5-Gy fractions in 16 days. There was no significant difference in the 2-year incidence of brain metastases and a lower overall survival in the higher-dose group. PCI at 25 Gy was recommended as the standard of care in limited-stage SCLC.[89]

Results of Accelerated Radiotherapy Trials

Key findings of AF regimens include the following:

- Modest acceleration by 1 week by delivering six fractions of 2 Gy per week or a concomitant boost regimen without dose reduction or treatment break yields superior locoregional control of head and neck carcinomas without increase in late toxicity but without clear impact on survival. Acceleration by more than 3 weeks with a 10% total dose reduction (<6 to 7 Gy) also improves the locoregional control without demonstrable increase in late complications. However, a further 5% to 8% total dose reduction abrogates the gain in tumor control but appears to reduce the severity of some late normal tissue complications, such as fibrosis and edema.

- Mucositis per se or its consequential late toxicity prevents delivery of more than 12 Gy per week when given in two fractions of 2 Gy per day for 5 days a week or daily fractions throughout weekends to a total dose of 66 to 70 Gy (pure acceleration).
- Acceleration achieves significantly improved local control for well-differentiated tumors and advanced primary mucosal site tumors but may be of little benefit to advanced nodal disease and poorly differentiated tumors. This supports the existence of the accelerated proliferation phenomenon in mucosa-derived tumor cells.

The trials are classified into either pure accelerated, with same total dose, or hybrid accelerated, of which there are three types: (a) accelerated with dose reduction, (b) accelerated with split course, and (c) accelerated with concomitant boost.

Pure Accelerated Fractionation

Table 12.3 summarizes the radiation regimens and outcomes of six reported randomized trials of pure AF for the treatment of patients with NSCLC lung and head and neck carcinoma.

Non–Small Cell Lung Cancer

A study of 204 patients randomized them to 60 Gy in 3 weeks versus 60 Gy in 6 weeks, both with and without concurrent carboplatin.[90] The results showed no survival advantage with either AF or concurrent carboplatin. The study showed that 60 Gy in 3 weeks induced a significantly greater esophagitis than did 60 Gy in 6 weeks.

Head and Neck Cancer

The first two HNSCC studies shown in Table 12.3[91,92] induced unacceptable toxicity, leading to early termination, and these two fractionations have been abandoned. However, two of the other three trials showed positive results,[93,94] whereas one[95] showed no benefit and similar late toxicity.

The Polish Cooperative Group compared 66 Gy given in 33 fractions over 38 days (two fractions every Thursday) as compared with a conventional regimen of 66 Gy given in 33 fractions over 45 days. In the study, 395 patients with T1-3, N0, M0 glottic and supraglottic laryngeal cancer were randomized. There was no difference in terms of locoregional control ($p = .37$).[95]

The Danish trial, one of the largest trials of altered fractionation,[94] accrued 1,485 patients with larynx, oropharynx, and oral cavity carcinomas of all stages. Six versus 7 weeks of treatment was achieved by giving a sixth fraction each week. Overall 5-year locoregional control rates improved (70% vs. 60%; $p = .0005$). The benefit of shortening treatment time was seen for primary tumor control (76% vs. 64%; $p = .0001$) but not for neck-node control. Acceleration from 7 to 6 weeks improved voice preservation in laryngeal cancer (80% vs. 68%; $p = .007$) and improved disease-specific survival (73% vs. 66%; $p = .01$) but not overall survival. Multivariate analysis of 754 larynx cancers showed that AF was beneficial in tumors that were moderately and well differentiated, with no benefit for those that were poorly differentiated. This effect suggests that the mechanism of repopulation in the primary tumor may be similar to the response in the original normal mucosa and in its functional mechanism of regeneration. This capacity to respond to the trauma of irradiation is more likely to exist in well-differentiated tumors, and the process may be facilitated by signaling from the surrounding normal mucosa. Accelerated proliferation may, therefore, be a response of the primary tumor and not the nodal metastases.[96]

Nasopharynx

Pure acceleration for nasopharynx cancer was tested in Guangxi, China. In the study, 416 patients were randomized to three arms: all had 7,400 to 7,600 cGy given as AF six fractions per week versus AF with concurrent cisplatin and 5-fluorouacil (AFC) versus the conventional five 2-Gy fractions per week. The local recurrence rates were 16.7% in the AF group, 13.6% in the AFC group, and 27.3% in the conventional fractionated group ($p < .05$). The 5-year survival rates were 53.6%, 57.6%, and 43.8% ($p < .05$), respectively. The interesting finding was that acceleration had a similar effect as concurrent chemotherapy with acceleration for nasopharynx cancer.[93]

Hybrid Accelerated Fractionation

Table 12.4 summarizes the details of regimens and outcomes of reported prospective, randomized trials addressing the role of types A to C hybrid accelerated fractionation (Fig. 12.4).

Type A

AF regimens (with dose reduction) were addressed in trials shown in Table 12.4, including a trial in HNSCC (definitive and postoperative), brain metastases, and NSCLC. It includes trials by the British Medical Research Council (MRC), the Trans-Tasman Radiation Oncology Group (TROG), the French Radiotherapy Oncology Group for Head and Neck Cancer (GORTEC), and ECOG.

Head and Neck

As shown in Table 12.4, two trials for HNSCC—the MRC CHART[97] and TROG regimens[98]—did not yield improvement in locoregional control and disease-free and overall survival rates. In contrast, the GORTEC regimen[99] for locally advanced head and neck carcinoma, with a 3.5-week acceleration and

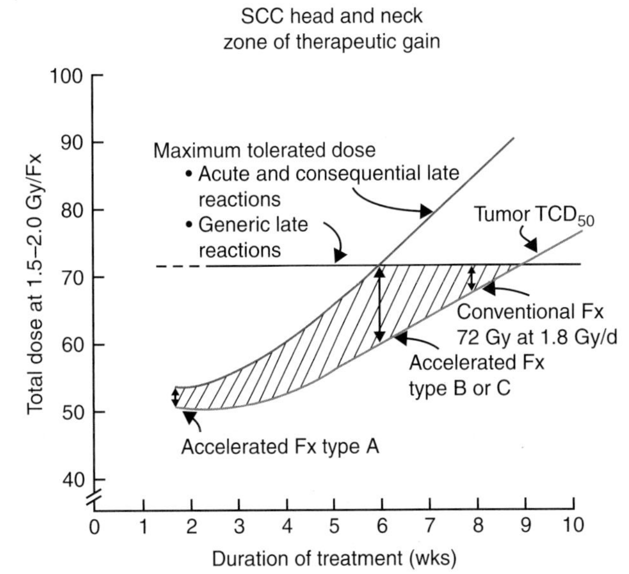

FIGURE 12.4. Zone of therapeutic gain in squamous cell carcinomas of the head and neck for different accelerated fractionation schedules. Type A is 54 Gy in 36 fractions over 12 days, type B is 67.2 Gy in 42 fractions over 42 days, and type C is 72 Gy in 42 fractions over 40 days. For explanation, see text. (From Peters LJ, Brock WA, Travis EL. Radiation biology at clinically relevant fractions. In: DeVita V, Hellman S, Rosenberg SA, eds. *Important advances in oncology.* Philadelphia: JB Lippincott, 1991:65–83.)

only 7-Gy (10%) dose reduction, significantly improved the locoregional control, with no gain in the overall survival rate.

Based on the potential for accelerated proliferation after surgery, Awwad et al.[100] in Cairo explored acceleration in postoperative radiotherapy of locally advanced HNSCC. Seventy patients with T2/N1-2 or T3-4/any N squamous cell carcinoma of the oral cavity, larynx, and hypopharynx were randomized to accelerated hyperfractionation of 46.2 Gy in 12 days versus conventional 60 Gy per 6 weeks. The 3-year locoregional control rate was better with accelerated treatment (88% ± 4%) versus conventional group (57% ± 9%; $p = .01$), with no difference in survival (60% ± 10% vs. 46% ± 9%; $p = .29$). As expected, acute mucositis was more severe in the accelerated group, and fibrosis and edema also tended to be more frequent; this finding contrasts with the results in two postoperative studies of type C (concomitant boost) described later and in Table 12.4.[101,102]

Non–Small Cell Lung Cancer

One randomized, controlled trial showed that CHART improves survival over standard radiotherapy of 60 Gy in 30 fractions in patients with locally advanced, unresectable stage III NSCLC. This MRC trial[103] showed that CHART with a 4-week acceleration and 6-Gy (10%) dose reduction decreased the risk for local progression and improved the overall survival significantly without increasing short- and long-term morbidity. These patients are now routinely given concurrent chemotherapy. However, in some countries, selected patients who are not fit for chemotherapy or patients who prefer radiotherapy only may be considered for CHART. The ECOG tested accelerated radiotherapy after induction chemotherapy (two cycles of carboplatin plus paclitaxel) in stage IIIA and B NSCLC. Acceleration was achieved with 57.6 Gy (1.5 Gy three times a day for 2.5 weeks) versus conventional 64 Gy (2 Gy per day). Of 141 patients enrolled, 83% were randomly assigned—60 accelerated and 59 conventional. The median survival was 20.3 and 14.9, respectively ($p = .28$). With the acceptance that concurrent chemoradiation is more effective than sequential treatment, this trial closed early.[104]

Further acceleration to 2.5 weeks was tested in a trial of CHARTWEL (CHART weekend less), in which 406 patients with NSCLC were randomized to receive three-dimensional planned radiotherapy to 60 Gy/40 fractions/2.5 weeks (CHARTWEL) or 66 Gy/33 fractions/6.5 weeks (conventional fractionation [CF]). Overall survival (OS; primary endpoint) at 2, 3, and 5 years was not significantly different after CHARTWEL (31%, 22%, and 11%) versus CF (32%, 18%, and 7%; HR = 0.92, 95% CI = 0.75 to 1.13, $p = .43$). Local tumor control rates and distant metastases did not significantly differ.[105]

Split-Course Accelerated Fractionation Regimen (Type B)

Split-course AF regimens (type B) are also shown in Table 12.4. This was addressed by EORTC[50] and RTOG,[71] by a study from Florence, Italy,[106] of patients with locally advanced head and neck carcinomas, and by the Royal Marsden NHS Trust, Institute of Cancer Research, London, for bladder cancer.[107] The EORTC regimen consisted of 28.8 Gy over 7 days, followed by a 2-week break, then 43.2 Gy over 11 days to a cumulative dose of 72 Gy in 45 fractions over 5 weeks. Although the 2-week acceleration improved locoregional control, it produced twice as many grade 3 to 4 acute morbidities, more late toxicity ($p < .001$), seven cases of permanent peripheral neuropathy, and two cases of myelopathy. This regimen has been abandoned.

The RTOG split regimen was comparable to that of the Massachusetts General Hospital study:[108] two fractions of 1.6 Gy per day to a total dose of 67.2 Gy in 6 weeks, including a 2-week break in treatment after 38.4 Gy, with the standard 70 Gy in 7 weeks. This 1-week acceleration with a 3.8-Gy (5%) dose reduction increased acute mucositis without improving the locoregional control rate (69), with the concomitant boost and hyperfractionation arm being superior. Fallai et al.[106] reported an Italian multicenter randomized trial that treated 192 patients with advanced carcinoma of the oropharynx with conventional radiotherapy (arm A: 66 to 70 Gy in 33 to 35 fractions for 5 days a week over 6.5 to 7 weeks) versus accelerated split-course radiotherapy (arm B: 64 to 67.2 Gy in two fractions of 1.6 Gy for 5 days a week with 2-week split at 38.4 Gy) versus concomitant chemoradiation (arm C: same radiotherapy as arm A plus concomitant carboplatin and 5-fluorouracil). Although the results did not reach statistical significance, chemoradiation almost doubled the 5-year overall survival (21%, 21%, and 40% for arms A, B, and C, respectively) and relapse-free survival (15%, 17%, and 36% for arms A, B, and C, respectively). There was a slight trend toward better 5-year locoregional control ($p = .07$) for the combined arm: patients without locoregional relapse in arm C, 21%, 18%, and 48% for arms A, B, and C, respectively. The occurrence of persistent G3 xerostomia was comparable in the three treatment arms

The Royal Marsden study in London evaluated the efficacy and toxicity of an AF regimen to treat T2 or T3, N0 or N1 muscle-invasive bladder cancer. The 229 patients were randomized into two groups and given 60.8 Gy in 32 fractions over 5 weeks with a 1-week treatment gap after the first 12 fractions versus 64 Gy in 32 fractions over 6.5 weeks. Acceleration was achieved by two fractions per day of 1.8 and 2.0 Gy. RTOG grade 2 or 3 bowel toxicity in the accelerated arm was 44% versus 26% in the conventional arm (p trend = .001), with no difference is acute grade 2 or 3 bladder toxicity or late RTOG grade 2 toxicity equivalent. There was no significant difference in disease-free survival and overall survival at 3 and 5 years.[107]

Concomitant Boost Accelerated Fractionation Regimen (Type C)

Concomitant boost AF regimen (type C) was also addressed by the RTOG[71]; this regimen was designed at the MD Anderson Cancer Center[109] and administers 54 Gy of wide-field irradiation in 1.8-Gy fractions over 6 weeks and 18 Gy of boost dose given in 1.5-Gy fractions as second daily fractions during the last 2.5 weeks. This regimen was found to improve the locoregional control rate, with a strong trend for a higher disease-free survival rate and with more severe mucositis but no detectable increase in late complications.

Concomitant boost-type fractionation was also tested for postoperative radiation therapy in two phase III trials.[102,110] Ang et al.[110] randomized patients with high-risk pathologic features to 63 Gy given in 35 fractions over either 5 weeks (daily fractions for 3 weeks and then two fractions per day for 2 weeks) or 7 weeks. This study showed that the cumulative time of the combined treatment was a significant determinant of locoregional control and overall survival. Concomitant boost partially offsets the detrimental effect of a delay in initiating radiation therapy beyond 6 weeks after surgery without inducing a detectable increase in late complications. These findings were confirmed by Sanguineti et al.[102] in Genoa, Italy, who randomized patients from four institutions with one or more high-risk features after surgery to conventional 60 Gy in 6 weeks versus 64 Gy in 5 weeks with twice-daily treatment in the first and last weeks of treatment. Once again, there was no difference in outcome between the two arms; however, there was a trend for improved locoregional control for patients who had a delay in starting radiotherapy and who were treated with AF compared with those with a delay who were treated with CF (HR = 0.5; 95% = 0.2 to 1.1). Acceleration does not seem worthwhile postoperatively for carcinoma of the head and neck, although it might be an option for patients who delay starting radiotherapy.

A phase III trial in patients with glioblastoma multiforme assessed the role of a combined accelerated, hyperfractionated regimen with a 2-week reduction of therapy duration and a dose increment of 11 Gy (18%).[111] This radiation regimen, with or without difluoromethylornithine, was found to yield no better progression-free and overall survival rates.

Pure Hypofractionated Radiotherapy for Breast and Prostate Cancer

Although 2.0-Gy fraction size is considered standard, hypofractionation has long been the common practice in countries such as the United Kingdom and Canada, where a lower total dose using fewer, larger fractions (hypofractionation) is often used. Data are now available from hypofractionated trials in breast and prostate cancer. These are summarized in Table 12.5.

The UK Standardisation of Breast Radiotherapy Trial B of radiotherapy hypofractionation for adjuvant whole-breast

TABLE 12.5 DATA OF PHASE III CLINICAL TRIALS ADDRESSING PURE HYPOFRACTIONATION: BREAST CANCER AND PROSTATE CANCER

Tumor Site and Type	*Number of Patients*	*Dose/Fx (Gy)*	*Fx/d*	*Total Dose (Gy)*	*Overall Time (wk)*	*Tumor Control*	*Side Effects*	*Reference*
Early breast cancer (pT1-3a, pN0-1, M0)	2,215	2.67 2.0	1 1	40 50.0	3 5	No difference in LRC	Lower rates of late adverse effects after 40 Gy hypofractionated	Bentzen et al.[112]
Early breast cancer (pT1-3a, pN0-1, M0)	2,236	3.2 3.0 2.0	1 1 1	41.6 39.0 50	5 5 5	No difference in LRC	Lower rates of late adverse effects after 39 Gy hypofractionated	Bentzen et al.[113]
Early breast cancer with clear margins, nodes negative	1,234	2.67 2.0	1 1	42.5 50	3 5	No difference in LRC	No difference in adverse effects after hypofractionation	Whelan et al.[114]
Prostate adenocarcinoma T1/T2, PSA < 40	936	2.625 2	1 1	52.5 66		At 5 yr, the composite of biochemical or clinical failure probability was 52.95% in the conventional arm and 59.95% in the hypofractionated arm (difference 90% CI = 12.6%–1.4%), favoring the conventional arm by 7.0%; no difference in 2-yr postradiotherapy biopsy or in overall survival	Acute toxicity was 4.4% higher in the hypofractionated arm (11.4%) vs. the conventional arm of 7% (95% CI = 8.1%–0.6%); late toxicity was similarly low in both arms (3.2%)	Lukka et. al.[32]
Prostate adenocarcinoma, stage T1-3 intermediate to high risk	100	2.7 2.0	1 1	70.2 76	5.2 7.6	Efficacy not reported	Little difference in acute toxicity but slight increase in GI toxicity during weeks 2, 3, and 4 with hypofractionation	Pollack et. al.[116]
Prostate adenocarcinoma, localized stage	91	[3× 13 Fx] + [4.5× 4 Fx] 2	1 1	57 74	3.5 7.5	Efficacy not reported	Lower grade 2 GU acute toxicity with hypofractionation: 19.1% vs. 47.7% (*p* = .003); lower median duration of overall GI acute toxicity with hypofractionation: 3 vs. 6 wk (*p* = .017)	Norkus et. al.[117]
Prostate adenocarcinoma, T1/T2, N0, M0 (any risk)	217	2.75 2	1 1	55 64	4 6.5	The biochemical relapse-free, but not overall, survival at 90 mo was significantly better with the hypofractionated (53%) than with the conventional (34%) schedule	Urgency of defecation and significantly worse individual and total GI symptom scores at 1 mo in the hypofractionated vs. the conventional schedule; however genitourinary symptoms were worse at 4 yr for conventional schedule	Yeoh et al.[118]
Localized prostate adenocarcinoma	457	3 3 2	60 57 74			No yet reported	Hypofractionated radiotherapy seems equally well tolerated as conventionally fractionated treatment at 2 yr; grade 2 or worse bowel toxicity at 2 yr: 74-Gy group: 4.3% (95% CI = 1.6–9.2); 60-Gy group: 3%–6% (1.2–8.3); 57-Gy group: 1.4% (0.2–5.0); grade 2 or worse bladder toxicity: 74-Gy group: 2.2% (0.5–6.2), 60-Gy group: 2.2% (0.5–6.3); 57-Gy group: 0.0% (0.0–2.6)	Dearnaley et al.[119]

The outcome data given as *x*% vs. *y*% imply that *x* is the experimental-arm result. CI, confidence interval; d, day; Fx, fraction(s); GI, gastrointestinal; GU, genitourinary; Gy, Gray; LRC, local-regional control N, nodal stage; T, tumor stage; wk, week.

irradiation in early breast cancer was a randomized trial of 50 Gy in 25 fractions of 2.0 Gy over 5 weeks versus 40 Gy in 15 fractions of 2.67 Gy over 3 weeks.[112] Two thousand two hundred fifteen women with pT1-3a, pN0-1, M0 breast cancer were followed for a median of 6.0 years (IQR 5.0 to 6.2). Treatment with 40 Gy in 15 fractions produced the same rates of local-regional tumor relapse and late adverse effects as that with 50 Gy in 25 fractions. The rate of local-regional tumor relapse at 5 years was 2.2% (95% CI = 1.3 to 3.1) in the 40-Gy group and 3.3% (95% CI = 2.2 to 4.5) in the 50-Gy group, representing an absolute difference of –0.7% (95% CI = –1.7% to 0.9%). The rates of late adverse effects were lower after 40-Gy than after 50-Gy treatment by photographic and patient self-assessments.

The UK Standardisation of Breast Radiotherapy Trial A tested two dose levels of a 13-fraction schedule against the standard regimen with the aim of measuring the sensitivity of normal and malignant tissues to fraction size.[113] Two thousand two hundred thirty-six women with early breast cancer (pT1-3a, pN0-1, M0) were randomized to receive after primary surgery standard 50 Gy in 25 fractions versus 41.6 Gy or 39 Gy in 13 fractions of 3.2 Gy or 3.0 Gy over the same 5 weeks. After a median follow-up of 5.1 years (IQR 4.4 to 6.0) the rate of local-regional tumor relapse at 5 years was 3.6% (95% CI 2.2 = 5.1) after 50 Gy, 3.5% (95% CI 2.1 = 4.3) after 41.6 Gy, and 5.2% (95% CI 3.5 = 6.9) after 39 Gy. There was a lower rate of late adverse effects after 39 Gy than with 50 Gy, with an HR for late change in breast appearance (photographic) of 0.69 (95% CI = 0.52 to 0.91, p = .01). From a planned meta-analysis with the pilot trial, the adjusted estimate of α/β value for tumor control was 4.6 Gy (95% CI = 1.1 to 8.1) and for late change in breast appearance (photographic) was 3.4 Gy (95% CI = 2.3 to 4.5).

A Canadian study of a hypofractionated accelerated schedule of whole-breast irradiation of 42.5 Gy in 16 fractions in 3-week versus a standard dose of 50.0 Gy in 25 fractions showed that it was as effective as a 5-week schedule in 1,234 women with invasive breast cancer after breast-conserving surgery, with clear resection margins and negative axillary lymph nodes.[114] At 10 years the risk of local recurrence was similar: 6.7% with standard fractionation versus 6.2% with hypofractionated regimen (absolute difference, 0.5 percentage points; 95% CI = –2.5 to 3.5). The rate of women with a good or excellent cosmetic outcome was also similar.

The data from the foregoing three trials show that for early breast cancer, a lower total dose in a smaller number of fractions could offer similar rates of tumor control and normal tissue damage as the standard fractionation schedule of 50 Gy in 25 fractions.

However, it remains controversial whether these results apply to all subgroups of patients. The American Society for Radiation Oncology therefore developed an evidence-based guideline to provide direction for clinical practice.[115]

Data were considered sufficient to support the use of hypofractionated whole-breast irradiation for patients with early-stage breast cancer who were of age 50 years or older, had disease stage pT1-2, pN0, did not receive chemotherapy, and were treated with a radiation dose homogeneity within ±7% in the central axis plane. They recommended that the heart should be excluded from the primary treatment fields but could not agree on the appropriateness of a tumor bed boost in these patients.

Early results for hypofractionated prostate cancer are somewhat mixed, as given in Table 12.5. A clear consensus would be challenging to derive because most trials compared a hypofractionated regimen against doses that are lower than 75.6 to 81 Gy, which is now commonly used, and most trials did not use contemporary intensity-modulated and image-guided radiotherapy techniques.

In 2005 a Canadian study deduced that it could not exclude the possibility that a hypofractionated radiation regimen might be inferior to the standard regimen. Nine hundred thirty-six early-stage (T1 or T2) prostate cancer patients were treated to 66 Gy in 33 fractions versus 52.5 Gy in 20 fractions. At 5.7 years median follow-up, biochemical or clinical failure probability was 52.95% versus 59.95% favoring the conventional arm. Acute toxicity was slightly higher in the hypofractionated arm, but late toxicity was similar in both arms.[32]

A randomized trial at the Fox Chase Cancer Center found that there was a slight but significant increase in gastrointestinal toxicity during weeks 2, 3, and 4 with hypofractionation. The acute toxicity was reported on the first 100 men enrolled. The study compared 76 Gy in 38 fractions to 70.2 Gy in 26 fractions using intensity-modulated radiotherapy. There were no differences in overall maximum acute gastrointestinal (GI) or genitourinary (GU) toxicity acutely. However, GI toxicity was slightly increased during weeks 2, 3, and 4 with hypofractionation. Efficacy was not reported.[116]

Conversely, a smaller study of only 91 patients in Lithuania that was reported quite early (minimum follow-up of 3 months) suggested that a hypofractionated of schedule of 57 Gy in 17 fractions for 3.5 weeks (13 fractions of 3 Gy plus four fractions of 4.5 Gy) may induce even lower acute toxicity compared 74 Gy in 37 fractions in patients with prostate cancer. Although there were acute grade 3 or 4 toxicities, grade 2 GU acute toxicity was 19.1% in the hypofractionated arm versus 47.7% (chi-squared test, p = .003). The median duration of overall GI acute toxicity was also shorter with hypofractionation—3 compared to 6 weeks with CFRT (median test, p = .017).[117]

Even more interesting are the findings of a larger study of 217 patients with longer follow-up of median 90 months (range, 3 to 138) in Australia that found a therapeutic advantage of hypofractionation for prostate cancer. This study found better biochemical relapse-free, but not overall, survival at 90 months with the hypofractionated (53%) than with the conventional (34%) schedule. Multivariate analyses revealed that conventional fractionation was an independent prognostic factor for inferior biochemical failure and genitourinary symptoms at 4 years. A two-dimensional computed tomography method was used to compare 55 Gy in 20 fractions to 64 Gy in 32 fractions. It is difficult to reconcile the results with results of contemporary doses and techniques.[118]

The pending efficacy results of a trial in the United Kingdom is very important: intensity-modulated radiotherapy was used, and it is the largest study (457 patients) that used >70 Gy as the control arm.[119] They used a higher dose (60 Gy in 20 fractions) of hypofractionated radiotherapy than the Canadian study (52.5 Gy in 20 fractions) and the Australian study (55 Gy in 20 fractions). It was tested against conventionally fractionated 74 Gy in 37 fractions and was found to be equally well tolerated at 2 years.

The Combination of Altered Fractionation with Concurrent Chemotherapy

In a meta-analysis conducted at the Institute Gustave-Roussy (Villejuif, France) an absolute benefit of 3% (from 36% to 39%; HR = 0.92; 95% CI = 0.87 to 0.97; p = .004) was observed at 5 years in favor of the altered fractionation regimens.[120] In light of the data in support of the superiority of altered fractionation to standard radiotherapy alone and findings of improved local control and survival with the addition of concurrent chemotherapy to radiotherapy in several randomized studies[121,122–123] and two recent meta-analyses,[124,125] at least 11 studies reported on investigation of addition of chemotherapy to altered fractionation (Table 12.6). These studies did not explore chemotherapy results with varying fractionation regimes, except for one study,[29,126] which tested the addition of chemotherapy to

TABLE 12.6 PHASE III TRIALS ADDRESSING CONCURRENT CHEMOTHERAPY AND ALTERED FRACTIONATION IN PATIENTS WITH HEAD AND NECK CANCER

Reference	*Tumor Site and Stage*	*Number of Patients*	*Therapy Regimen*	*Tumor Response*	*Complications*
Accelerated Fractionation Plus Chemotherapy					
Dobrowsky and Naude[128]	Various sites T1-4, N0-3	239	V-CHART: 55.3 Gy/17 d (2.5 Gy on d 1, then 1.65 Gy, b.i.d., on d 2–17) V-CHART + MMC: 20 mg/m^2 on d 5 CF: 70 Gy/7 wk	V-CHART + MMC yielded higher LRC ($p < .05$) and survival ($p \leq .03$) than V-CHART and CF	V-CHART induced more mucositis than CF but not intensified by MMC Late toxicity not reported
Staar et al.[129]	Stage III–IV unresectable oropharynx and hypopharynx	240	69.9 Gy/5.5 wk + carboplatin (70 mg/m^2/d) and 5-FU (600 mg/m^2/d) for 5 d ×2 69.9 Gy/5.5 wk (1.8 Gy every day for 3.5 wk, then b.i.d., 1.8 Gy + 1.5 Gy, for 2 wk)	2-yr OS: 48% vs. 39% ($p = .11$) 2-yr LRC 51% vs. 45% ($p = .14$) Patients receiving G-CSF had worse LRC ($p = .007$)	Grade 3–4 mucositis: 68% vs. 52% ($p = .01$) Grade 3–4 vomiting: 8.2% vs. 1.6% ($p = .02$) Late swallowing problems and feeding tube dependency: 51% vs. 25% ($p = .02$)
Bourhis et al.[99]	Various sites Advanced inoperable	109	62–64 Gy/5 wk + Cis (100 mg/m^2 on d 1, 16, 32) and 5-FU (1 g/m^2/d on d 1–5, 31–35) 62–64 Gy/3 wk	Not reported yet	Early cessation due to higher treatment-related deaths in the combined arm
Wang et al.[93]	Nasopharynx cancer	416	74–76 Gy in 6 wk (6 fractions/wk) + Cis/5-FU 74–76 Gy in 6 wk (6 fractions/wk) 70–76 Gy in 7 wk	LRC 13.6% vs. 16.7% vs. 27.3% ($p < .05$), 5-yr OS 57.6% vs. 53.6% vs. 43.8% ($p < .05$); acceleration had a similar improvement as concurrent chemotherapy	Acute reactions higher with acceleration
Alternating Chemoradiation Versus Partly Accelerated Radiotherapy in Locally Advanced Squamous Cell Carcinoma of the Head and Neck					
Corvo et al.[130]	Unfavorable stage II or stage III–IV	136	1 wk Cis (20 mg/m^2/d + 5-FU 200 mg/m^2)/d for 5 d alternated with three 2-wk courses of 20 Gy 2 Gy/d, 5 d/wk (60 Gy) vs. 75 Gy/40 CB in 6 wk	3-yr OS: 37% vs. 29%; 3-yr PFS: 35% vs. 27% 3-yr LRC: 32% vs. 27%	Acute skin and late mucosal and skin toxicities significantly less with chemoradiation, but radiotherapy dose was 15 Gy or less
Split-Course Accelerated Fractionation Plus Chemotherapy					
Denham et al.[4]	Various sites T2-4, N0-3	122	RT: 70 Gy/47 d in 1.25 Gy b.i.d. (7–10/d break after 40 Gy) + Cis and 5-FU wk 1 and 6 RT alone: 75 Gy/42 d in 1.25 Gy, b.i.d.	3-yr LRC: 70% vs. 44% ($p = .01$) 3-yr RFS: 61% vs. 41% ($p = .07$) 3-yr OS: 55% vs. 34% ($p = .07$)	Similar mucositis; increased internal feeding and sepsis Similar late complications
Byhardt et al.[170]	Various sites, stage III–IV	270	70.2 Gy/51 d plus Cis, 5-FU, and leucovorin 70.2 Gy/51 d (23.4 Gy in 1.8-Gy fractions, b.i.d., for 3 cycles with 10-d break)	3-yr LRC: 36% vs. 17%, ($p < .004$) 3-yr OS: 48% vs. 24% ($p < .0003$)	Grade 3–4 acute mucositis: 38% vs. 16% ($p < .001$) Serious late side effects: 10% vs. 6.4% (NS)
Chemoradiation with Split-Course Prolonged Radiotherapy					
Adelstein et al.[126]	Stage III or IV unresectable disease	295	30 Gy at 2 Gy/d with concurrent 5-FU and Cis wk 1–3, 5-wk break with chemotherapy followed by 30–40 Gy/wk 8–11 vs. 70 Gy at 2 Gy/d plus Cis on d 1, 22, and 43 vs. (3) 70 Gy at 2 Gy/d alone	3-yr projected OS: 27% vs. 37% vs. 23%. Median survival: 13.8 vs. 19.1 vs. 12.6 mo; no difference between arms 1 and 3 3-yr DSS 41% vs. 51% vs. 33%; arm 2 was better ($p = .01$)	Grade 3 or worse toxicity: 77% vs. 89% vs. 52% ($p < .001$)
Hyperfractionation Plus Chemotherapy					
Denham et al.[54]	Various sites, stage III–IV	130	77 Gy/7 wk + Cis (6 mg/m^2/d) 77 Gy/7 wk (1.1 Gy, b.i.d.).	5-yr LRPFS: 50% vs. 36% ($p = .04$) 5-yr PFS: 46% vs. 25% ($p = .007$) 5-yr DMFS: 86% vs. 57% ($p = .001$) 5-yr OS: 46% vs. 25%. ($p = .008$)	No significant difference in acute morbidity (except for leucopenia, $p = .006$) or late toxicity
Hugeunin et al.[133]	Squamous cell carcinomas of the head and neck	224	74.4 Gy; 1.2 Gy b.i.d. + Cis 20 mg/m^2 (on 5 d wk 1 and 5) 74.4 Gy; 1.2 Gy b.i.d.	Failure-free rate at 2.5 yr was 45% and 33%; LRC was significantly improved, log-rank test ($p < .039$)	Late toxicity was comparable
Hyperfractionated Accelerated Chemoradiation with Concurrent Chemotherapy Versus Dose-Escalated Hyperfractionated Accelerated Radiation Therapy Alone in Locally Advanced Head and Neck Cancer					
Budach et al.[75]	Various sites, stage III–IV	384	70.6 Gy in 6 wk (30 Gy, 2 Gy/d + 40.6 at 1.4 Gy b.i.d.) + 5-FU (600 mg/m^2) + mitomycin (10 mg/m^2 77.6 Gy (14 Gy at 2 Gy/d + 1.4 Gy b.i.d.): dose-escalated radiotherapy	5-yr LRC 49.9% vs. 37.4% ($p = .001$) 5-yr OS: 28.6% vs. 23.7% ($p = .023$)	Maximum acute mucositis, moist desquamation, and erythema were higher in dose-escalated radiotherapy; no differences in late reactions

b.i.d., twice-a-day irradiation; CB, concomitant boost; CF, conventional fractionation; Cis, cisplatin; DMFS, distant metastasis–free survival; DSS, disease-specific survival; 5-FU, 5-flourouracil; LC, local control; LRC, locoregional control; LRPFS, locoregional progression-free survival; MMC, mitomycin-C; NS, not significant; OS, overall survival; PFS, progression-free survival; G-CSF, granulocyte colony–stimulating factor; RFS, relapse-free survival; V-CHART, Vienna variation of Continuous Hyperfractionated Accelerated Radiation Therapy.

radiation in patients with unresectable squamous cell HNSCC by adding chemotherapy to either standard fractionation or a complicated prolonged split-course regime.

Key Findings of Combined Altered Fractionation with Concurrent Chemotherapy

Although the magnitude of its effect was less marked for survival indices than for local-regional control, the addition of chemotherapy to altered fractionation regimens results in a clear improvement compared with hyperfractionated or accelerated regimens alone; however, the effect on late toxicity of normal tissues is not fully known.

In nasopharynx cancer, the benefit of concurrent chemotherapy is similar to that of acceleration without chemotherapy. The potential biologic interactions between chemotherapy and radiotherapy by the addition of radiation can be summarized as follows[127]:

1. Shift of cell survival curves toward higher cell-killing levels and lower cell-surviving fractions for a given dose of irradiation
2. Cooperation to prevent the emergence of resistant clones
3. A decrease in tumor mass and reoxygenation
4. Specific toxicity for hypoxic cells
5. Selective toxicity depending on cell-cycle phase
6. Cytokinetic cooperation
7. Inhibition of DNA repair
8. Increased apoptosis

Table 12.6 summarizes the results of randomized studies investigating the efficacy of concurrent chemotherapy regimens with altered fractionation.

Acceleration Versus Chemoradiation or with Chemotherapy

An Austrian three-arm trial tested the addition of mitomycin C (MMC) on day 5 of treatment to the Vienna variation of Continuous, Hyperfractionated, Accelerated Radiation Therapy (V-CHART): 55.3 Gy in 17 days. The three arms were 70 Gy of conventional fractionation alone versus V-CHART and versus V-CHART with concurrent MMC on day 5 (V-CHART plus MMC).[128] Two hundred thirty-nine patients were randomized. Locoregional tumor control was 31% after conventional fractionation, 32% after V-CHART, and 48% after V-CHART plus MMC, respectively ($p < .05$). Overall crude survival was 24% after conventional fractionation, 31% after V-CHART, and 41% after V-CHART plus MMC, respectively ($p < .05$). Therefore, reducing the treatment time from 7 weeks to 17 consecutive days and dose of radiotherapy from 70 to 55.3 Gy produced identical results, whereas the addition of MMC on day 5 to the accelerated fractionated treatment produced a significant improvement in local tumor control and survival. This supports an argument for adding chemotherapy to AF.

A German Cooperative Group compared a concomitant boost radiation regimen with or without carboplatin and 5-fluorouracil.[129] The addition of chemotherapy produced a trend for better locoregional control and survival rates, but it induced a significantly higher incidence of chronic dysphagia, resulting in feeding-tube dependence (51% vs. 25%). A secondary randomization to receive or not receive granulocyte colony–stimulating factor to reduce mucositis produced the startling finding that *the administration of granulocyte colony–stimulating factor significantly reduced the probability of locoregional control in both treatment arms.*

The French Cooperative Group GORTEC tested the combination of 62 to 64 Gy given in 5 weeks with cisplatin and 5-fluorouracil but terminated the trial prematurely due to unacceptable toxicity.[74] The nasopharynx trial from China gave a very interesting finding that accelerated radiotherapy provides the same benefit as adding concurrent chemotherapy; this was discussed earlier in the section on accelerated radiotherapy.[25]

Alternating chemoradiotherapy was studied in Italy by Corvo et al.[130] and compared with high-dose accelerated radiotherapy. The 136 patients with unfavorable stage II or stage III-IV head and neck carcinoma were randomized to alternating cisplatin and 5-fluorouracil with three 2-week courses of radiotherapy (20 Gy at 2 Gy per day: 60 Gy vs. 75 Gy at 40 fractions in 6 weeks) using a concomitant boost technique. At 60 months there were no differences in overall survival, progression-free survival, or locoregional control.

Split-course altered fractionation with or without concurrent chemotherapy was tested in two trials. Both added cisplatin and 5-fluorouracil to split-course AF schedules (70 Gy in 42 to 51 days).[123,131] Both showed that a chemotherapy regime improved locoregional control versus altered fractionation alone. However, a split-course accelerated regimen is now known to be no more effective than standard fractionation. The locoregional control improved, with an 18% to 26% increase in late effects. The larger trial showed improved overall survival.

Adelstein et al.[126] reported on the Head and Neck Intergroup's trial to test the addition of chemotherapy to radiation in patients with unresectable squamous cell HNSCC by adding chemotherapy to either standard fractionation or a prolonged split-course regime. The 295 patients were randomized into three arms: 70 Gy at 2 Gy per day (radiation [RT] only) versus the same radiation therapy with concurrent bolus cisplatin (RT + chemotherapy [C]) versus a third arm: split-course radiotherapy with chemotherapy during the break in radiotherapy (split RT + C) from week 9. They did not meet the accrual goal. Grade 3 or worse toxicity occurred in 52% of patients in the RT-only arm, 89% in the RT + C arm ($p < .0001$), and 77% in the split RT + C arm ($p < .001$). The 3-year projected overall survival for patients in the RT-only arm was 23%, compared with 37% for the RT + C arm ($p = .014$) and 27% for the split RT + C arm (p = not significant). The addition of concurrent high-dose, single-agent cisplatin to conventional radiation significantly improves survival and increases toxicity; however, multiagent chemotherapy did not offset the loss of efficacy resulting from prolongation by split-course radiation.

Concurrent Chemotherapy in Addition to Hyperfractionated Radiotherapy

A randomized trial by Jeremic et al.[132] tested the addition of low-dose daily cisplatin to 77 Gy at 1.1 Gy per fraction twice daily over 7 weeks. Daily cisplatin improved the results of HF radiation, with better locoregional progression-free survival (50% vs. 36%; $p = .04$), 5-year progression-free survival (46% vs. 25%; $p = .007$), 5-year distant metastases–free survival (86% vs. 57%; $p = .001$), and 5-year overall survival (46% vs. 25%; $p = .008$). This was a true therapeutic gain because there was no difference in late side effects.

A study conducted in Zurich reported similar results.[133] The 224 patients with squamous cell carcinomas were randomized to two cycles of concurrent cisplatin 20 mg/m^2 on 5 days of weeks 1 and 5 with HF radiotherapy (median dose, 74.4 Gy; 1.2 Gy twice daily) versus the same radiotherapy. Locoregional control and distant disease–free survival were significantly improved with cisplatin (log-rank test; $p = .039$ and .011, respectively) with no difference in overall survival and similar late toxicity. The therapeutic index of HF radiotherapy was improved by concomitant cisplatin.

A third trial, reported by the German Cancer Society with an even greater number of patients, confirmed this outcome, using a nonplatinum regime with HF accelerated radiation versus dose-escalated HF accelerated radiation.[134] The 84 patients with stage III (6%) and IV (94%) oropharyngeal (59.4%), hypopharyngeal (32.3%), and oral cavity (8.3%) cancer were randomized to concurrent chemotherapy and HF accelerated radiation therapy to 70.6 Gy in 6 weeks versus HF accelerated radiation therapy alone to 77.6 Gy. Chemotherapy was 5-fluoroucil (600 mg/m^2, 120-hour continuous infusion) days 1 through 5 and mitomycin (10 mg/m^2) on days 5 and 36. At 5 years, the locoregional control was 49.9% versus 37.4% (p = .001), and overall survival was 28.6% versus and 23.7% (p = .023), respectively. Progression-free and metastases-free rates were 29.3% and 51.9% versus 26.6% and 54.7%, respectively (p = .009 and .575, respectively). There were no differences in late reactions. They concluded that concurrent chemotherapy with HF accelerated radiotherapy to 70.6 Gy is superior to dose-escalated HF radiotherapy to 77.6 Gy, with less acute reactions and equivalent late reactions, indicating an improvement of the therapeutic ratio.[134]

Results of Radiation Therapy Oncology Group Trial of Concurrent Chemotherapy to Select Fractionation Schedules

The RTOG conducted a randomized trial to determine whether accelerated fractionation improves the outcome of concurrent cisplatin chemotherapy (i.e., whether the benefit of altered fractionation remains true in the setting of concurrent chemotherapy).[135] Acceleration of radiotherapy did not improve outcome in the setting of concurrent cisplatin chemotherapy. Seven hundred forty-three patients with stage III or IV squamous cell carcinoma of the oral cavity, oropharynx, hypopharynx, or larynx were randomized into two arms: *standard radiation* (70 Gy in 35 fractions once daily over 7 weeks [SFX]) with three cycles of concurrent cisplatin (100 mg/m^2 given every 3 weeks during radiotherapy) versus accelerated *fractionation with concomitant boost* 72 Gy in 42 fractions in 6.5 weeks (AFX-C) with *two cycles* of the same chemotherapy. Seven hundred twenty-one cases were analyzable (360 for AFX-C; 361 for SFX). Two arms were balanced by site, stage, performance status, and age. At analysis, 418 patients were alive with median follow-up of 4.8 (0.3 to 6.5) years. First analysis of this trial showed that, when combined with concurrent cisplatin, AFX-C did not improve outcome or increase late toxicity. No differences were observed in OS (5-year: 59% vs. 56%; HR = 0.90, CI= 0.72 to 1.13; p = .18), disease-free survival (45% vs. 44%; p = .42), local-regional failure (31% vs. 28%; p = .76), or metastasis (18% vs. 22%; p = .06). There were also no differences in the overall grade 3–4 acute mucositis (33% vs. 40%) and worst grade 3–4 late toxicity (26% vs. 21%). Feeding tube rates were 22% and 25% pretreatment, 67% and 69% at therapy end, 28 and 29% at 1 year, respectively, but declined later to 5% to 15%. When analyzed for the effect of radiotherapy duration and cisplatin dose, they both affected survival significantly. Cisplatin improved OS more by reducing local-regional progression, but it also increased toxicity. The effect of AFX-C approximated the third cisplatin dose, suggesting that cisplatin acted, in part, by inhibiting clonogen repopulation.

This finding suggests that for patients undergoing standard fractionation who are unable to have their full planned concurrent chemotherapy, acceleration of the remaining course of radiotherapy may be of benefit. This may be achieved by treating two fractions per day on one of their treatment days each week.

As a continuous variable, each day of radiotherapy delay in RTOG 0129 was associated with compromised OS, progression-free survival, and local-regional progression by 5%, 4%, and 4% (p = .001, .006, and .02), respectively.[136]

Critical Fractionation Issues to Consider When Intensity-Modulated Radiation Treatment Is Used

There is great diversity in IMRT fractionation. A survey of international practice of IMRT fractionation showed that among 14 international centers, 12 different dose fractionations were practiced: conventional daily 2 Gy/fraction was used in 3 of 14 centers with concurrent chemotherapy, whereas 11 of 14 centers used altered fractionation, including a 6–fractions/week Danish Head and Neck Cancer Group regime in 3 centers, ≤2.2 Gy/fraction in 3 centers, dose-escalated hypofractionation (≥2.3 Gy/fraction) in 4 centers, hyperfractionation in 1 center, continuous acceleration in 1 center, and concomitant boost in 1 center. Reasons for fractionation practice included (a) dose escalation, (b) total irradiated volume, (c) number of target volumes, (d) synchronous systemic treatment, (e) shorter overall treatment time, (f) resources availability, (g) longer time on treatment couch, (h) variable gross tumor volume margins, (i) confidence in treatment setup, (j) late tissue toxicity, and (k) use of lower neck anterior fields.[137]

The new era of high-precision radiation therapy brings two major advantages: improved coverage of tumor volumes by the prescribed dose without the use of multiple matched fields, and increased sparing of normal tissues, such as parotid gland, spinal cord, brainstem, brain, and optic using IMRT. However, there are two important fractionation issues to be considered:

- If a single plan is used, all targets are treated in the same overall number of fractions. This may result in treating secondary targets to a lower dose per fraction. This has to be corrected by alteration of the total dose to the secondary targets to avoid the potentially serious disadvantage of delivering a lower biologically effective dose.
- IMRT may allow an increased dose to be delivered if the dose-limiting toxicity can be spared by organ avoidance. This may be delivered as additional fractions with prolongation of the duration of treatment or by giving more than one fraction per day. Alternatively, the dose per fraction may be increased and the total escalated dose delivered in the same or shortened treatment time.

Potential Delivery of Lower Biologically Effective Dose to Targets and Lower Probability of Cure

Classic non-IMRT techniques for HNSCC deliver doses at a fixed dose per fraction to all targets. A large initial field delivers an initial dose to the entire volume, and the field is reduced sequentially to boost additional regions to a higher dose (shrinking-field technique). For example, a classic head and neck three-field plan uses opposed lateral photon fields and abutting electron fields to deliver 50 Gy at 2 Gy per fraction to gross disease at the primary site and nodes, elective nodal regions, and regions around the tumor that may contain microscopic tumor cells. Smaller fields are then used to deliver an additional 16 to 20 Gy in 8 to 10 fractions to boost the gross tumor and nodal disease to 66 to 70 Gy, depending on the size of the gross tumor. A posterior electron field may be added to bring the dose adjacent to the gross nodal tumor to 56 to 60 Gy. This type of fractionation is used especially with concurrent chemotherapy. This contrasts with IMRT, with which the dose prescribed to various portions of the treatment volume is delivered simultaneously. Each fraction delivers a specific constant dose per fraction throughout the treatment to each target. All targets are treated in the same number of fractions. For example, 70 Gy in 35 fractions prescribed to the gross tumor will deliver 2 Gy per fraction to this volume. The 56 and 50 Gy prescribed to secondary target volumes will also be delivered in 35 fractions in 7 weeks using IMRT at a 1.6 and 1.43 dose per fraction over 7 weeks, respectively. The biologically effective dose to 56 and

TABLE 12.7 COMMONLY USED FRACTIONATION REGIMES FOR HEAD AND NECK CANCER

Dose/Fractionation	GTVs (Gy)	Intermediate Risk Target Volume (Gy)	Low Risk Target Volume Suspicious of Microscopic Disease (Gy)
United States: IMRT[a]			
70/33 Fx; s.i.d. with chemotherapy	70 Gy	60–63	57–60
Concomitant Boost			
72 Gy/42 Fx b.i.d. for 10–12 d	72	57–63	54
66/30 Fx s.i.d.	66	60	54
Without chemotherapy postoperative			
60–66/30 FX s.i.d.	66	56–57	54
Canada (PMH): IMRT[a]			
70 Gy/35 Fx s.i.d.	70	63	56
60 Gy/25 Fx	60	56	50
T2, N0 larynx small, T1–2 oropharynx			
64 Gy/40 Fx; b.i.d.	64	56	46
T3, T4 with low-volume nodal disease			
Postoperative boost			
66 Gy/33 Fx; s.i.d.	66	60	56
60 Gy/30 Fx; s.i.d.	60	60	54
51 Gy/20 Fx			
T1a, N0, M0 glottic cancer			
Manchester (United Kingdom; Christie Hospital)			
50–52.5/16 Fx for small volume (5–6 cm) larynx			
55 Gy in 20 Fx for modest volumes up to 10 cm long			
Postoperative 50 Gy/20 Fx with chemotherapy			
50–52.5 Gy/20 Fx without chemotherapy			
Denmark			
70 Gy/35 Fx; 6 Fx/wk			

The biologically isoeffective dose for tumor control to targets in the third and fourth columns with IMRT takes into consideration the effect of reduced dose per fraction and the effect of prolonged overall treatment time. b.i.d., twice a day; Fx, fraction; Gy, Gray; GTVs, gross tumor volumes; IMRT, intensity-modulated radiotherapy; N, nodal stage; PMH, princess margaret hospital; s.i.d., once per day; T, tumor stage; wk, week.
[a]Single-phase treatment schedule.

50 Gy in 35 fractions in 7 weeks is lower using IMRT because of the effect of the smaller dose per fraction and longer treatment time. This must be compensated for by increasing the total dose to the elective and intermediate dose targets, as suggested in Table 12.7.

Prospect for Improving the Therapeutic Ratio by Dose Escalations to Targets Without Increased Dose to Normal Tissues

The experience and conclusions of altered fractionation studies are based entirely on results of traditional radiotherapy techniques and conventional conformal techniques. These techniques deliver the boost dose to a much larger volume of tissue of normal tissues, which inevitably receive the full boost dose. However, IMRT delivers much reduced doses to normal structures with potential for less toxicity. For example, IMRT produced significant reduction in incidence and severity of xerostomia with parotid-sparing head and neck.[138,139–140] However, a further advantage of IMRT may be its potential for dose escalation. Preclinical comparative dosimetry studies suggested that dose escalation may be feasible using simultaneous boosts to tumor subvolumes.[141] Further work is ongoing to explore whether the boost volume may be localized using metabolic or hypoxic imaging.[142]

Common Standard Clinical Practice

An analysis by the Meta-analysis of Chemotherapy on Head and Neck Cancer Collaborative Group revealed that concurrent chemoradiation yielded a larger survival benefit than that achieved with altered fractionation regimens.[125] This benefit is seen predominantly in more locally advanced (i.e., stage IV) HNSCC, and concurrent chemoradiation is often recommended for patients with large T3 or T4 tumors or with N2-3 nodes usually given with standard fractionation.

Because accelerated regimens seem to preferentially benefit local control at the primary site and not nodal control, it is reasonable to choose altered fractionation for patients with T2, exophytic T3, or N0-1 disease who are not routinely given chemotherapy and those with more advanced locoregional tumor who are unfit to receive chemotherapy.[143]

In much of the United States and Europe, standard fractionation remains 2 Gy per day. However, there is considerable variation in common practice, and despite the results of randomized studies, institutions tend to adhere to dose fractionation schedules with which they are experienced. Examples of commonly used schedules in Manchester (United Kingdom), Canada, Denmark, and the United States are shown in Table 12.7.

FUTURE DIRECTIONS: COMBINING THE GAINS OF MOLECULAR IMAGING AND MOLECULAR TARGETING WITH ALTERED FRACTIONATION

Advances in the understanding of tumor biology have opened exciting new opportunities to develop specific molecularly targeted strategies to selectively enhance tumor response to radiation. For example, epidermal growth factor receptor (EGFR) overexpression is a strong independent prognostic indicator for overall survival and disease-free survival and a robust predictor for locoregional relapse but not for distant metastasis in patients with advanced HNSCCs.[71] This suggests that EGFR immunohistochemistry should be considered for selecting patients for more aggressive combined therapies.[109]

Promising preclinical and earlier phase clinical results support the use of EGFR blockade in combination with radiation for advanced HNSCC.[144] A phase III multinational trial confirmed that radiosensitization following molecular inhibition of EGFR signaling improves outcome. Cetuximab, a monoclonal antibody against the EGFR, when added to high-dose radiation in patients with locoregionally advanced HNSCC produced improved locoregional control and reduced mortality without increasing the common toxic effects. Four hundred twenty-four patients were randomized to receive either radiation alone for 6 to 7 weeks (RT) or radiation plus weekly cetuximab 400 mg/m^2 (RT + C). The median duration of locoregional control was 24.4 months in the RT + C arm versus 14.9 months in the RT-only arm (hazard ratio for locoregional progression or death, 0.68; $p = .005$). At median follow-up of 54.0 months, the median overall survival was 49.0 months in the RT + C arm versus 29.3 months in the RT-only arm (hazard ratio for death, 0.74; $p = .03$). Cetuximab significantly prolonged progression-free survival (hazard ratio for disease progression or death, 0.70; $p = .006$). With the exception of acneiform rash and infusion reactions, the incidence of grade 3 or greater toxic effects, including mucositis, did not differ significantly between the two groups.[145,146] However, further exploration did not show a benefit of adding cetuximab to chemotherapy plus altered fractionation. RTOG 0522 trial was a randomized trial of concurrent accelerated radiation and cisplatin versus concurrent accelerated radiation, cisplatin, and cetuximab in 940 study patients with stage III-IV cancer of the oropharynx, larynx, and hypopharynx. The initial results showed that the addition of cetuximab to the radiation–cisplatin platform did not improve progression-free or overall survival and was associated with higher rates of mucositis and cetuximab-induced skin reactions.[147]

ACKNOWLEDGMENT

I gratefully acknowledge the editorial assistance of Sharon A. Salenius, M.P.H., Executive Director, Research and Education, 21st Century Oncology (Fort Myers, FL).

SELECTED REFERENCES

A full list of references for this chapter is available online.

2. Thames HD, Hendry JH. *Fractionation in radiotherapy.* London: Taylor & Francis; 1987.
6. Turesson I, Thames HD. Repair capacity and kinetics of human skin during fractionated radiotherapy: erythema, desquamation, and telangiectasia after 3 and 5 year's follow-up. *Radiother Oncol* 1989;15(2):169–188.
8. Thames HD Jr, Withers HR, Peters LJ, et al. Changes in early and late radiation responses with altered dose fractionation: implications for dose–survival relationships. *Int J Radiat Oncol Biol Phys* 1982;8(2):219–26.
24. Dorr W, Hendry JH. Consequential late effects in normal tissues. *Radiother Oncol* 2001;61(3):223–231.
25. Wang CJ, Leung SW, Chen HC, et al. The correlation of acute toxicity and late rectal injury in radiotherapy for cervical carcinoma: evidence suggestive of consequential late effect (CQLE). *Int J Radiat Oncol Biol Phys* 1998;40(1):85–91.
26. Cox JD. Large-dose fractionation (hypofractionation). *Cancer* 1985;55(9, Suppl): 2105–2111.
27. Peters LJ, Withers HR. Morbidity from large dose fractions in radiotherapy. *Br J Radiol* 1980;53(626):170–171.
28. Collins CD, Lloyd-Davies RW, Swan AV. Radical external beam radiotherapy for localised carcinoma of the prostate using a hypofractionation technique. *Clin Oncol* 1991;3(3):127–132.
29. Akimoto T, Muramatsu H, Takahashi M, et al. Rectal bleeding after hypofractionated radiotherapy for prostate cancer: correlation between clinical and dosimetric parameters and the incidence of grade 2 or worse rectal bleeding. *Int J Radiat Oncol Biol Phys* 2004;60(4):1033–1039.
31. Kupelian PA, Thakkar VV, Khuntia D, et al. Hypofractionated intensity-modulated radiotherapy (70 Gy at 2.5 Gy per fraction) for localized prostate cancer: long-term outcomes. *Int J Radiat Oncol Biol Phys* 2005;63(5):1463–1468.
32. Lukka H, Hayter C, Julian JA, et al. Randomized trial comparing two fractionation schedules for patients with localized prostate cancer. *J Clin Oncol* 2005;23(25):6132–6138.
33. Ang KK, Thames HD Jr, van der Kogel AJ, et al. Is the rate of repair of radiation-induced sublethal damage in rat spinal cord dependent on the size of dose per fraction? *Int J Radiat Oncol Biol Phys* 1987;13(4):557–562.
34. Ang KK, Xu FX, Landuyt W, van der Schueren E. The kinetics and capacity of repair of sublethal damage in mouse lip mucosa during fractionated irradiations. *Int J Radiat Oncol Biol Phys* 1985;11(11):1977–1983.
43. Ang KK, Jiang GL, Guttenberger R, et al. Impact of spinal cord repair kinetics on the practice of altered fractionation schedules. *Radiother Oncol* 1992;25(4):287–294.
46. Cox JD, Pajak TF, Marcial VA, et al. ASTRO plenary: interfraction interval is a major determinant of late effects, with hyperfractionated radiation therapy of carcinomas of upper respiratory and digestive tracts: results from Radiation Therapy Oncology Group protocol 8313. *Int J Radiat Oncol Biol Phys* 1991;20(6): 1191–1195.
48. Thames HD, Peters LJ, Ang KK. Time–dose considerations for normal-tissue tolerance. *Front Radiat Ther Oncol* 1989;23:113–130.
49. Bentzen SM, Saunders MI, Dische S. Repair halftimes estimated from observations of treatment-related morbidity after CHART or conventional radiotherapy in head and neck cancer. *Radiother Oncol* 1999;53(3):219–226.
50. Horiot JC, Bontemps P, van den Bogaert W, et al. Accelerated fractionation (AF) compared to conventional fractionation (CF) improves loco-regional control in the radiotherapy of advanced head and neck cancers: results of the EORTC 22851 randomized trial. *Radiother Oncol* 1997;44(2):111–121.
51. Horiot JC, Le Fur R, N'Guyen T, et al. Hyperfractionation versus conventional fractionation in oropharyngeal carcinoma: final analysis of a randomized trial of the EORTC cooperative group of radiotherapy. *Radiother Oncol* 1992;25(4):231–241.
56. Withers HR, Taylor JM, Maciejewski B. The hazard of accelerated tumor clonogen repopulation during radiotherapy. *Acta Oncol* 1988;27(2):131–146.
57. Bentzen SM, Thames HD. Clinical evidence for tumor clonogen regeneration: interpretations of the data. *Radiother Oncol* 1991;22(3):161–166.
58. Dubben HH. Local control, TCD50 and dose–time prescription habits in radiotherapy of head and neck tumours. *Radiother Oncol* 1994;32(3):197–200.
59. Thames HD, Bentzen SM. Time factor for tonsillar carcinoma. *Int J Radiat Oncol Biol Phys* 1995;33(3):755–758.
62. Eriksen JG, Buffa FM, Alsner J, et al. Molecular profiles as predictive marker for the effect of overall treatment time of radiotherapy in supraglottic larynx squamous cell carcinomas. *Radiother Oncol* 2004;72(3):275–282.
63. Strandqvist M. Studien uber die kumulative wirkung der rontgenstrahlen bei fraktionierung. *Acta Radiol* 1944;55(Suppl):1.
67. Fowler JF, Stern BE. Fractionation and dose-rate. II. Dose–time relationships in radiotherapy and the validity of cell survival curve models. *Br J Radiol* 1963;36: 163–173.
68. Ellis F. Nominal standard dose and the ret. *Br J Radiol* 1971;44(518):101–108.
70. Baujat B, Bourhis J, Blanchard P, et al. Hyperfractionated or accelerated radiotherapy for head and neck cancer. *Cochrane Database Syst Rev* 2010(12): CD002026.
71. Fu KK, Pajak TF, Trotti A, et al. A Radiation Therapy Oncology Group (RTOG) phase III randomized study to compare hyperfractionation and two variants of accelerated fractionation to standard fractionation radiotherapy for head and neck squamous cell carcinomas: first report of RTOG 9003. *Int J Radiat Oncol Biol Phys* 2000;48(1):7–16.
72. Horiot JC. Controlled clinical trials of hyperfractionated and accelerated radiotherapy in otorhinolaryngologic cancers [in French]. *Bull Acad Natl Med* 1998;182(6):1247–1260.
73. Pinto LH, Canary PC, Araujo CM, et al. Prospective randomized trial comparing hyperfractionated versus conventional radiotherapy in stages III and IV oropharyngeal carcinoma. *Int J Radiat Oncol Biol Phys* 1991;21(3):557–562.
74. Cummings B, O'Sullivan B, Keane T. 5-year results of a 4 week/twice daily radiation schedule: the Toronto Trial. *Radiother Oncol* 2000;56:S8.
75. Budach W, Hehr T, Budach V, et al. A meta-analysis of hyperfractionated and accelerated radiotherapy and combined chemotherapy and radiotherapy regimens in unresected locally advanced squamous cell carcinoma of the head and neck. *BMC Cancer* 2006;6:28.
76. Sanchiz F, Milla A, Torner J, et al. Single fraction per day versus two fractions per day versus radiochemotherapy in the treatment of head and neck cancer. *Int J Radiat Oncol Biol Phys* 1990;19(6):1347–1350.
77. Bourhis J, Lapeyre M, Tortochaux J, et al. Very accelerated versus conventional radiotherapy in HNSCC: results of the GORTEC 94–02 randomized trial. *Int J Radiat Oncol Biol Phys* 2000;51(Suppl 1):39.
79. Willers H, Liertz-Petersen C, Dubben HH, et al. Outcome of hyperfractionated radiation therapy in randomized clinical trials. *Int J Radiat Oncol Biol Phys* 1998;40(1):257–259.
80. Edsmyr F, Andersson L, Esposti PL, et al. Irradiation therapy with multiple small fractions per day in urinary bladder cancer. *Radiother Oncol* 1985;4(3):197–203.
81. Naslund I, Nilsson B, Littbrand B. Hyperfractionated radiotherapy of bladder cancer. A ten-year follow-up of a randomized clinical trial. *Acta Oncol* 1994;33(4):397–402.
82. Sause W, Kolesar P, Taylor SI, et al. Final results of phase III trial in regionally advanced unresectable non–small cell lung cancer: Radiation Therapy Oncology Group, Eastern Cooperative Oncology Group, and Southwest Oncology Group. *Chest* 2000;117(2):358–364.
84. Mandell LR, Kadota R, Freeman C, et al. There is no role for hyperfractionated radiotherapy in the management of children with newly diagnosed diffuse intrinsic brainstem tumors: results of a Pediatric Oncology Group phase III trial comparing conventional vs. hyperfractionated radiotherapy. *Int J Radiat Oncol Biol Phys* 1999;43(5):959–964.
85. LeClerc JM, Billett AL, Gelber RD, et al. Treatment of childhood acute lymphoblastic leukemia: results of Dana-Farber ALL Consortium Protocol 87–01. *J Clin Oncol* 2002;20(1):237–246.
86. Waber DP, Silverman LB, Catania L, et al. Outcomes of a randomized trial of hyperfractionated cranial radiation therapy for treatment of high-risk acute lymphoblastic leukemia: therapeutic efficacy and neurotoxicity. *J Clin Oncol* 2004;22(13):2701–2707.
87. Donaldson SS, Meza J, Breneman JC, et al. Results from the IRS-IV randomized trial of hyperfractionated radiotherapy in children with rhabdomyosarcoma—a report from the IRSG. *Int J Radiat Oncol Biol Phys* 2001;51(3):718–728.
88. Murray KJ, Scott C, Greenberg HM, et al. A randomized phase III study of accelerated hyperfractionation versus standard in patients with unresected brain metastases: a report of the Radiation Therapy Oncology Group (RTOG) 9104. *Int J Radiat Oncol Biol Phys* 1997;39(3):571–574.
89. Le Pechoux C, Dunant A, Senan S, et al. Standard-dose versus higher-dose prophylactic cranial irradiation (PCI) in patients with limited-stage small-cell lung cancer in complete remission after chemotherapy and thoracic radiotherapy (PCI 99–01, EORTC 22003–08004, RTOG 0212, and IFCT 99–01): a randomised clinical trial. *Lancet Oncol* 2009;10(5):467–474.
90. Ball D, Bishop J, Smith J, et al. A randomised phase III study of accelerated or standard fraction radiotherapy with or without concurrent carboplatin in inoperable non–small cell lung cancer: final report of an Australian multi-centre trial. *Radiother Oncol* 1999;52(2):129–136.
91. Jackson SM, Weir LM, Hay JH, et al. A randomised trial of accelerated versus conventional radiotherapy in head and neck cancer. *Radiother Oncol* 1997;43(1):39–46.
92. Skladowski K, Maciejewski B, Golen M, et al. Randomized clinical trial on 7-day-continuous accelerated irradiation (CAIR) of head and neck cancer—report on 3-year tumour control and normal tissue toxicity. *Radiother Oncol* 2000;55(2):101–110.
93. Wang RS, Liu WQ, Li J, et al. Accelerated fractionated radiotherapy with concurrent chemotherapy in advanced nasopharyngeal carcinoma [in Chinese]. *Ai Zheng* 2003;22(9):982–984.
94. Overgaard J, Hansen HS, Grau C. The DAHANCA 6 and 7 trial: a randomized multicenter study of 5 versus 6 fractions per week of conventional radiotherapy of squamous cell carcinoma (SCC) of the head and neck. *Radiother Oncol* 2000;56:S4.
95. Hliniak A, Gwiazdowska B, Szutkowski Z. Radiotherapy of the laryngeal cancer: the estimation of the therapeutic gain and the enhancement of toxicity by the one-week shortening of the treatment time. Results of the randomized phase III multicenter trial. *Radiother Oncol* 2000;56:S5.
96. Overgaard J, Hansen HS, Specht L, et al. Five compared with six fractions per week of conventional radiotherapy of squamous-cell carcinoma of head and neck: DAHANCA 6 and 7 randomised controlled trial. *Lancet* 2003;362(9388):933–940.
97. Saunders MI, Rojas AM, Parmar MK, Dische S. Mature results of a randomized trial of accelerated hyperfractionated versus conventional radiotherapy in head-and-neck cancer. *Int J Radiat Oncol Biol Phys* 2010;77(1):3–8.
98. Poulsen MG, Denham JW, Peters LJ, et al. A randomised trial of accelerated and conventional radiotherapy for stage III and IV squamous carcinoma of the head and neck: a Trans-Tasman Radiation Oncology Group Study. *Radiother Oncol* 2001;60(2):113–122.
99. Bourhis J, Lapeyre M, Tortochaux J, et al. Preliminary results of the GORTEC 96–01 randomized trial, comparing very accelerated radiotherapy versus concomitant radio-chemotherapy for locally inoperable HNSCC. *Int J Radiat Oncol Biol Phys* 2001;51(3, Suppl 1):39.
100. Awwad HK, Lotayef M, Shouman T, et al. Accelerated hyperfractionation (AHF) compared to conventional fractionation (CF) in the postoperative radiotherapy of locally advanced head and neck cancer: influence of proliferation. *Br J Cancer* 2002;86(4):517–523.

101. Ang KK, Trotti A, Brown BW, et al. Randomized trial addressing risk features and time factors of surgery plus radiotherapy in advanced head-and-neck cancer. *Int J Radiat Oncol Biol Phys* 2001;51(3):571–578.
102. Sanguineti G, Richetti A, Bignardi M, et al. Accelerated versus conventional fractionated postoperative radiotherapy for advanced head and neck cancer: results of a multicenter Phase III study. *Int J Radiat Oncol Biol Phys* 2005;61(3): 762–771.
103. Saunders M, Dische S, Barrett A, et al. Continuous, hyperfractionated, accelerated radiotherapy (CHART) versus conventional radiotherapy in non–small cell lung cancer: mature data from the randomised multicentre trial. CHART Steering committee. *Radiother Oncol* 1999;52(2):137–148.
104. Belani CP, Wang W, Johnson DH, et al. Phase III study of the Eastern Cooperative Oncology Group (ECOG 2597): induction chemotherapy followed by either standard thoracic radiotherapy or hyperfractionated accelerated radiotherapy for patients with unresectable stage IIIA and B non–small-cell lung cancer. *J Clin Oncol* 2005;23(16):3760–3767.
105. Baumann M, Herrmann T, Koch R, et al. Final results of the randomized phase III CHARTWEL-trial (ARO 97–1) comparing hyperfractionated-accelerated versus conventionally fractionated radiotherapy in non–small cell lung cancer (NSCLC). *Radiother Oncol* 2011;100(1):76–85.
106. Fallai C, Bolner A, Signor M, et al. Long-term results of conventional radiotherapy versus accelerated hyperfractionated radiotherapy versus concomitant radiotherapy and chemotherapy in locoregionally advanced carcinoma of the oropharynx. *Tumori* 2006;92(1):41–54.
111. Prados MD, Wara WM, Sneed PK, et al. Phase III trial of accelerated hyperfractionation with or without difluromethylornithine (DFMO) versus standard fractionated radiotherapy with or without DFMO for newly diagnosed patients with glioblastoma multiforme. *Int J Radiat Oncol Biol Phys* 2001;49(1):71–77.
112. Bentzen SM, Agrawal RK, Aird EG, et al. The UK Standardisation of Breast Radiotherapy (START) Trial B of radiotherapy hypofractionation for treatment of early breast cancer: a randomised trial. *Lancet* 2008;371(9618):1098–1107.
113. Bentzen SM, Agrawal RK, Aird EG, et al. The UK Standardisation of Breast Radiotherapy (START) Trial A of radiotherapy hypofractionation for treatment of early breast cancer: a randomised trial. *Lancet Oncol* 2008;9(4):331–341.
114. Whelan TJ, Pignol JP, Levine MN, et al. Long-term results of hypofractionated radiation therapy for breast cancer. *N Engl J Med* 2010;362(6):513–520.
115. Smith BD, Bentzen SM, Correa CR, et al. Fractionation for whole breast irradiation: an American Society for Radiation Oncology (ASTRO) evidence-based guideline. *Int J Radiat Oncol Biol Phys* 2011;81(1):59–68.
116. Pollack A, Hanlon AL, Horwitz EM, et al. Dosimetry and preliminary acute toxicity in the first 100 men treated for prostate cancer on a randomized hypofractionation dose escalation trial. *Int J Radiat Oncol Biol Phys* 2006;64(2): 518–526.
117. Norkus D, Miller A, Kurtinaitis J, et al. A randomized trial comparing hypofractionated and conventionally fractionated three-dimensional external-beam radiotherapy for localized prostate adenocarcinoma: a report on acute toxicity. *Strahlenther Onkol* 2009;185(11):715–721.
118. Yeoh EE, Botten RJ, Butters J, et al. Hypofractionated versus conventionally fractionated radiotherapy for prostate carcinoma: final results of phase III randomized trial. *Int J Radiat Oncol Biol Phys* 2011;81(5):1271–1278.
119. Dearnaley D, Syndikus I, Sumo G, et al. Conventional versus hypofractionated high-dose intensity-modulated radiotherapy for prostate cancer: preliminary safety results from the CHHiP randomised controlled trial. *Lancet Oncol* 2012;13(1):43–54.
120. Bourhis J, Audry H, Overgaard J, et al. Meta-analysis of conventional versus altered fractionated radiotherapy in head and neck squamous cell carcinoma (HNSCC): final analysis. *Int J Radiat Oncol Biol Phys* 2004;60(1, Suppl):S190–S191.
122. Merlano M, Benasso M, Corvo R, et al. Five-year update of a randomized trial of alternating radiotherapy and chemotherapy compared with radiotherapy alone in treatment of unresectable squamous cell carcinoma of the head and neck. *J Natl Cancer Inst* 1996;88(9):583–589.
123. Wendt TG, Grabenbauer GG, Rodel CM, et al. Simultaneous radiochemotherapy versus radiotherapy alone in advanced head and neck cancer: a randomized multicenter study. *J Clin Oncol* 1998;16(4):1318–1324.
124. El-Sayed S, Nelson N. Adjuvant and adjunctive chemotherapy in the management of squamous cell carcinoma of the head and neck region. A meta-analysis of prospective and randomized trials. *J Clin Oncol* 1996;14(3):838–847.
125. Pignon JP, Bourhis J, Domenge C, et al. Chemotherapy added to locoregional treatment for head and neck squamous-cell carcinoma: three meta-analyses of updated individual data. MACH-NC Collaborative Group. Meta-Analysis of Chemotherapy on Head and Neck Cancer. *Lancet* 2000;355(9208):949–955.
126. Adelstein DJ, Li Y, Adams GL, et al. An intergroup phase III comparison of standard radiation therapy and two schedules of concurrent chemoradiotherapy in patients with unresectable squamous cell head and neck cancer. *J Clin Oncol* 2003;21(1):92–98.
127. Bernier J. Alteration of radiotherapy fractionation and concurrent chemotherapy: a new frontier in head and neck oncology? *Nat Clin Pract* 2005;2(6): 305–314.
129. Staar S, Rudat V, Stuetzer H, et al. Intensified hyperfractionated accelerated radiotherapy limits the additional benefit of simultaneous chemotherapy—results of a multicentric randomized German trial in advanced head-and-neck cancer. *Int J Radiat Oncol Biol Phys* 2001;50(5):1161–1171.
130. Corvo R, Benasso M, Sanguineti GL, et al. Alternating chemoradiotherapy versus partly accelerated radiotherapy in locally advanced squamous cell carcinoma of the head and neck: results from a phase III randomized trial. *Cancer* 2001;92(11):2856–2867.
131. Brizel DM, Albers ME, Fisher SR, et al. Hyperfractionated irradiation with or without concurrent chemotherapy for locally advanced head and neck cancer. *N Engl J Med* 1998;338(25):1798–1804.
132. Jeremic B, Shibamoto Y, Milicic B, et al. Hyperfractionated radiation therapy with or without concurrent low-dose daily cisplatin in locally advanced squamous cell carcinoma of the head and neck: a prospective randomized trial. *J Clin Oncol* 2000;18(7):1458–1464.
133. Huguenin P, Beer KT, Allal A, et al. Concomitant cisplatin significantly improves locoregional control in advanced head and neck cancers treated with hyperfractionated radiotherapy. *J Clin Oncol* 2004;22(23):4665–4673.
134. Budach V, Stuschke M, Budach W, et al. Hyperfractionated accelerated chemoradiation with concurrent fluorouracil–mitomycin is more effective than dose-escalated hyperfractionated accelerated radiation therapy alone in locally advanced head and neck cancer: final results of the radiotherapy cooperative clinical trials group of the German Cancer Society 95–06 Prospective Randomized Trial. *J Clin Oncol* 2005;23(6):1125–1135.
135. Ang K, Pajak TF, Wheeler R, et al. A phase III trial to test accelerated versus standard fractionation in combination with concurrent cisplatin for head and neck carcinomas (RTOG 0129): report of efficacy and toxicity. *Int J Radiat Oncol Biol Phys* 2010;77(1):1–2.
136. Ang K, Zhang Q, Wheeler R, et al. A phase III trial (RTOG 0129) of two radiation–cisplatin regimens for head and neck carcinomas (HNC): impact of radiation and cisplatin intensity on outcome. *J Clin Oncol* 2010;28(15, Suppl):5507.
137. Ho KF, Fowler JF, Sykes AJ, et al. IMRT dose fractionation for head and neck cancer: variation in current approaches will make standardisation difficult. *Acta Oncol* 2009;48(3):431–439.
138. Lin A, Kim HM, Terrell JE, et al. Quality of life after parotid-sparing IMRT for head-and-neck cancer: a prospective longitudinal study. *Int J Radiat Oncol Biol Phys* 2003;57(1):61–70.
147. Ang K, Zhang QE, Rosenthal D, et al. A randomized phase III trial (RTOG 0522) of concurrent accelerated radiation plus cisplatin with or without cetuximab for stage III–IV head and neck squamous cell carcinomas (HNC). *J Clin Oncol* 2011;29(15, Suppl):5500.

Chapter 13
Late Effects and QUANTEC

John P. Kirkpatrick, Michael T. Milano, Louis S. Constine, Zeljko Vujaskovic, and Lawrence B. Marks

The modern era of cancer therapy is predicated on the safe intensification of radiation, chemotherapy, and biologic adjuvants. This has resulted in a markedly increased survivorship, which now exceeds 64% overall, and for some malignancies, such as breast and prostate cancer, is much higher. Malignancies resistant to therapy may demand an aggressive treatment approach that often resides at the limit of, or even exceeds, normal tissue tolerance to some "acceptable" degree. Clearly, the potential to ameliorate or prevent such normal tissue damage, or to manage and rehabilitate affected patients, requires an understanding of tissue tolerance to therapy. Because "late effects" manifest months or years after cessation of treatment, therapeutic decisions intended to obviate such effects can be based only on the probability, not the certainty, that such effects will develop. In making such decisions, the balance between efficacy and potential for toxicity should be considered, as well as the influence of host, disease, and treatment-related risk factors.

Historically, radiation therapy fields and doses were selected empirically, based largely on physicians' clinical experience and judgment. They understood that these empiric guidelines were imprecise and did not completely reflect the underlying anatomy, physiology, molecular biology, and dose distributions. The introduction of three-dimensional (3D) treatment planning offered the promise of quantitative correlates of doses/volumes with clinical outcomes. This promise was partly delivered. When 3D dosimetric information became widely available, guidelines were needed to help physicians predict

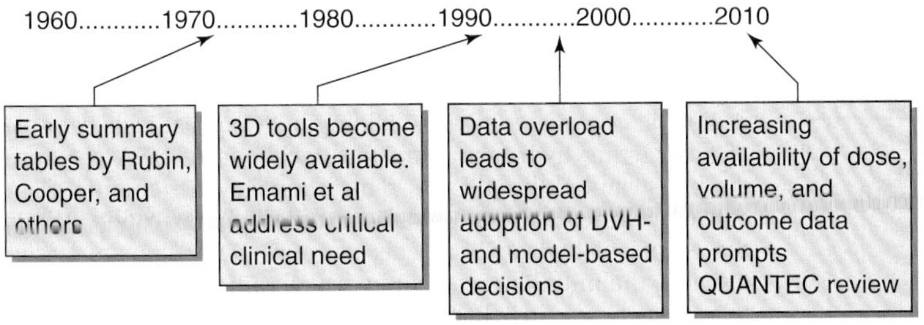

FIGURE 13.1. Key events in the development of dose–volume and normal tissue toxicity relationships in radiation oncology.

the relative safety of proposed treatment plans, although only limited data were available.

In 1991, investigators pooled their clinical experience, judgment, and information regarding partial organ tolerance doses and produced the "Emami paper".[1] As discussed later, this paper clearly stated the uncertainties and limitations in its recommendations, and it is rightly admired for addressing a critical clinical need. Over the past two decades, numerous studies have reported associations between dosimetric parameters and normal tissue outcomes. In 2007, a joint task force of physicists and physicians was formed, with the support of the American Society for Therapeutic Radiology and Oncology (ASTRO) and the American Association of Physicists in Medicine (AAPM), to summarize the available data in a format useful to clinicians and to update/refine the estimates provided by Emami et al.

The resulting QUANTEC reviews[2] (quantitative analysis of normal tissue effects in the clinic), published in a special issue of the *International Journal of Radiation Oncology, Biology and Physics* in March 2010, are summarized in this chapter.

HISTORICAL BACKGROUND

The relationship between dose–volume parameters and outcome has been the focus of numerous investigators for decades. A brief summary of historical landmarks is provided to follow, along with our opinion regarding the key contributions and shortcomings of these reviews (Fig. 13.1 and Table 13.1).

THE INCORPORATION OF 3D DOSE–VOLUME INFORMATION INTO CLINICAL GUIDELINES

The pre-Emami reports[3] were novel in that there were no tools available (to either the authors or clinicians) to accurately quantify the fraction of various organs that were being irradiated. Thus, the dose/volume/outcome information presented consisted largely of estimates based on expert opinion. Similarly, clinicians needed to estimate the partial volumes of different organs that were being irradiated in their patients in order to apply the provided information.

In the late 1980s and early 1990s, 3D planning systems were providing clinicians with a plethora of information. However, systematic dose/volume/outcome data to guide clinical decisions based on this information were limited. There was an urgent need for clinicians to have some guidance in making clinical dose–volume decisions. The report by Emami et al.[1] met this critical need. This report was, and remains, a landmark summary of decades worth of data for a wide variety of organs, supplemented with expert opinion where data were lacking. This article remains a required reading for all trainees in our field.

During the 1990s and 2000s, a large number of studies related dose–volume data to clinical outcomes. The QUANTEC review was an attempt to refine the guidelines based on the available 3D dose/volume/outcome data.

DOSE–VOLUME HISTOGRAMS AND ASSOCIATED FIGURES OF MERIT

Three-dimensional dose–volume data can be difficult for clinicians to readily digest. Visualizing isodose distributions is challenging, and comparing competing distributions is almost impossible. Therefore, dose–volume histograms (DVHs; essentially two-dimensional [2D] representations of the 3D data) were embraced as a rapid way to summarize the dose distribution. Note that DVHs discard information regarding the spatial character of dose as well as (usually) variations in fraction size. However, DVHs can also be challenging for clinicians to consider and compare. Therefore, it has become attractive to extract "figures of merit" from the DVH, such as the V_x (the percent of an organ receiving $\geq x$ Gy). Thus, DVHs and their associated figures of merit are necessary tools to enable clinicians to readily apply 3D information clinically. They are excellent tools but obviously have their shortcomings.

MODEL-BASED ESTIMATES OF OUTCOMES

The Emami et al. report systematically used the same DVH-based construct across many organs, for example, the $TD_{5/5}$ and $TD_{50/5}$ for the uniform irradiation of one-third, two-thirds, and the whole volume of an organ. This uniform approach enabled the application of "single unifying models" of dose/volume/outcome across organs. For example, the dose/volume/outcome estimates from Emami et al. were used by Lyman et al.,[4] Kutcher et al.,[5] and Burman et al.[6] to generate a set of organ-specific model parameters. Such a uniform approach is attractive to modelers and busy clinicians.

During the last two decades, many clinical dose/volume/outcome reports computed parameters for these "unifying models" (e.g., Ten Haken et al.[7–8,9]). Other investigators have suggested alternative models that appeared to be better suited to specific organs (*vide infra*).

The dose/volume/outcome data available for the QUANTEC review were not of a uniform format. Outcomes across organs were correlated with a diverse array of dose–volume metrics (e.g., threshold volumes [V_x],

TABLE 13.1 HISTORICAL OVERVIEW OF SUMMARIES OF DOSE/VOLUME/OUTCOME INFORMATION

Report	*Key Contributions*	*Key Shortcomings*
Rubin, 1975[3]	Introduced the concept of $TD_{5/5}$ and $TD_{50/5}$	Minimal dose–volume data
Emami, 1991[1]	Concise summary addressing most clinically meaningful endpoints in a uniform manner Based on available data and expert opinion	Dose–volume relationship based on limited data and, thus, much expert opinion
QUANTEC, 2010[2]	Driven largely by the available 3D dose/volume/outcome data. Systematic review addressing many challenges such as organ delineation and confounding factors such as chemotherapy	Because dose/volume/outcome data on all meaningful clinical outcomes are *not* available, the summary is not able to guide all clinical practice

TABLE 13.2 COMPARISON OF THE CHARACTER/CONTENT OF EMAMI ET AL AND QUANTEC

Characteristic	*Emami et al.*[1]	*QUANTEC*[2]
Number of organs	26	16
3D data available	Minimal	More/moderate (18-year interval)
Format dose–volume limits	Uniform $TD_{5/5}$ and $TD_{50/5}$ for one-third, two-thirds, whole organ	Nonuniform
Endpoints	Specific, complete	Specific, incomplete
Expert opinion	Dominant	Much less
Impact of chemotherapy	Not explicitly discussed	Addressed individually for each organ

threshold doses [D_x], mean doses). Therefore, the QUANTEC review included model-based parameters for just a few organs, and not always in a systematic fashion.

MAJOR DIFFERENCES BETWEEN THE QUANTEC AND EMAMI REVIEWS

Emami et al.[1] provided information for 26 organs, judged necessary to support protocols for "three dimensional treatment planning for high energy photons (RFP #NCI-CM-36716-21)." Conversely, the QUANTEC review was focused on organs for which the steering committee thought that there were meaningful dose/volume/outcome data (Table 13.2).

Emami et al. addressed a wide variety of clinical outcomes and thus provided the reader with a set of dose–volume parameters for *essentially* all clinical situations. Conversely, the QUANTEC review was focused on endpoints where there were dose/volume/outcome data. In this regard, the Emami tables are more complete. For example, consider the QUANTEC summary for the small bowel. A volume restriction is provided for the endpoint of acute grade ≥3 toxicity. No guidance is provided for late small bowel injury, as the authors did not believe that there was meaningful dose/volume/outcome data for late injury. This is a shortcoming of the QUANTEC review as it is not "complete." When evaluating a proposed 3D treatment plan, one obviously must consider both acute and late injury.

Emami et al. presented information in a systematic/uniform manner, facilitating interorgan comparisons and model-based parameter estimates. The QUANTEC review presented dose/volume/outcome data in the diverse manner in which they were available in the literature.

MOLECULAR MECHANISMS OF LATE RADIATION DAMAGE

The design of optimal radiation treatment plans and identification of therapeutic strategies to prevent radiation-induced damage would benefit from an understanding of the underlying late effects from ionizing radiation. Both of these issues are further complicated by the variability in sensitivity to radiation observed across disease types and between patients, as well as the current absence of identifiable factors that predict a propensity for radiation-induced toxicity.[10–13] While the initial damage done to the DNA, proteins, and membrane lipids of cells by exposure to ionizing radiation is well known, the mechanisms behind the sustained changes in gene expression and signaling pathways that contribute to latent and permanent tissue injury are less clear. This section will focus on the established mechanisms of radiation-induced tissue injury and identify areas in which further efforts are needed to determine the mechanisms driving tissue injury and prognostic markers for the development of radiation injury.

Early Cellular Effects of Radiation

Exposure to ionizing radiation causes direct DNA damage through linear energy transfer as well as indirect damage by radiolytic cleavage of water, yielding hydroxyl radicals capable of abstracting hydrogen from the backbone of DNA to cause double-stranded breaks.[14,15] This damage to genomic DNA causes cell death by apoptosis or mitotic catastrophe. While the ability of hydroxyl radicals to cause DNA damage is significant, the initial increase in hydroxyl radical and other reactive oxygen species (ROS) attributable to radiation exposure is negligible compared to the baseline presence of ROS in the cell.[15] Within a few hours of radiation exposure, however, the cell responds by increasing ROS production, creating a cellular environment capable of exacerbating the initial injury by causing oxidative damage to proteins and lipids.[16] This is thought to occur via ROS-mediated activation of mitochondria-dependent and -independent metabolic enzymes, including nitric oxide synthases (NOSs) and oxidoreductase enzymes.

Sources of Reactive Oxygen Species

NADPH Oxidases

Nicotinamide adenine dinucleotide phosphate (NADPH) oxidases are a family of broadly distributed oxidoreductase enzymes. Membrane-associated NADPH oxidases are the primary source of ROS in nonphagocytic cells.[17] Under normal conditions, NADPH oxidase–derived superoxide anion is a mediator of maintenance and smooth muscle tone of the vasculature.[18] When these enzymes are induced to begin pathologic overproduction of ROS, however, they can contribute to the development of oxidative stress, resulting in cell damage and disruption of signaling pathways.[19] Nox4, a hydrogen peroxide–producing isoform, is of particular interest, as overproduction of hydrogen peroxide by Nox4 has been shown to be a necessary element of tumor growth factor-β1 (TGF-β1)–mediated cell death.[20]

Mitochondria

Under normal conditions, electrons from the electron transport chain can leak into the mitochondrial matrix and react with oxygen to form superoxide anion.[21] Following radiation, Leach et al. observed that mitochondria in squamous carcinoma cells undergo a permeability transition, causing release of high levels of ROS into the cytoplasm.[22] They further showed that inhibition of this transition not only attenuates the increase in cytoplasmic free radicals but also prevents radiation-induced activation of mitogen-activated protein (MAP) kinase, suggesting a causal link between mitochondrial ROS/reactive nitrogen species (RNS) generation and a large group of signal transduction pathways. The role of mitochondrial-generated ROS/RNS in radiation injury is further supported by the radioprotective effect of Mn porphyrin superoxide dismutase (SOD) mimetics, which accumulate preferentially within the mitochondria.[23]

Augmentation of Reactive Oxygen Species from Other Sources

Superoxide anion from any source can react with nitric oxide to form peroxynitrite (ONOO–), itself a powerful oxidizing species capable of reacting with other molecules and cellular elements to perpetuate free radical overproduction and cause oxidative damage to the cell.[24]

Free Radicals and the Tissue Response to Radiation

When the increase in ROS production exceeds the antioxidant capacity of the cell, the intracellular environment becomes strongly oxidizing. This change results in altered gene expression as a part of the response to oxidative damage to genomic DNA, modification of redox-sensitive protein activity, and membrane lipid oxidation.[25] All of these insults can affect the structure, function, and signaling capacity of the cell. Of particular importance to the radiation response is the persistent up-regulation of transcription factors, including hypoxia-inducible factor-1α (HIF-1α) and nuclear factor κB (NFκB), and cytokines, including TGF-β, which contributes to the development of radiation-induced tissue injury.[16,26] These molecules all contribute to the vascular changes, inflammation, and cell death observed in response to radiation, but their roles in complex signalling pathways suggest that early changes in the activity of these molecules may also contribute to the disease process of latent injury. The role of ROS in radiation-induced tissue injury has been confirmed by the finding that SOD overexpression and the use of SOD mimetics can mitigate tissue injury following ionizing radiation exposure.[11,23,27–29,30]

The Role of Inflammation in the Response to Radiation

Although the manifestations of radiation injury can be divided into early and late effects, irradiated tissues show a dynamic population of different inflammatory cell types throughout the "latency" period, suggesting that, on a cellular level, radiation injury is an ongoing disease process.[31] Localization of inflammatory cells is mediated by vascular adhesion markers, and preferentially blocking intercellular adhesion molecule-1 (ICAM-1) does indeed reduce the inflammatory response to radiation in the lungs of C57BL/6 mice.[32,33] The resulting reduction in inflammation was, however, not sufficient to suppress development of latent pulmonary damage, suggesting that there are other mechanisms at work during this latent period that contribute to disease processes.[32] With the changing inflammatory cell populations come changes in cytokine activity, specifically interleukins, tumor necrosis factor-α (TNF-α), TGF-β, monocyte chemoattractant protein-1 (MCP-1), and keratinocyte chemoattractant (KC).[31,34,35] Expression of interleukin-1 (IL-1) messenger RNA (mRNA), together with a two-part up-regulation of TGF-β expression, is known to coincide with the development of fibrosis in C57BL/6J mice, suggesting that the inflammatory response does indeed contribute to the development of latent tissue injury.[36] This idea is further supported by the finding that early inhibition of TGF-β reduces radiation-induced pulmonary fibrosis and improves lung function.[37,38–39] Further studies indicate that administration of exogenous SOD following thoracic radiation reduced the early up-regulation of IL-1, TNF-α, and TGF-β and extended post-radiation survival.[40] The apparent link between ROS, inflammatory signaling, and latent injury development suggests that early changes in ROS production do affect delayed tissue damage through ongoing perturbations of signaling pathways.

Radiation-Induced Vascular Changes

Exposure to ionizing radiation causes damage to endothelial cells and vascular structural elements, causing increased vascular permeability.[41] This vascular dysfunction results in edema as well as decreased perfusion, which can lead to development of hypoxic regions within the affected tissues.[42] Hypoxia exacerbates the initial injury by increasing recruitment of inflammatory cells that, in the process of undergoing the respiratory burst, produce ROS and increase tissue hypoxia by consuming the available oxygen.[43] Hypoxia also results in activation of HIFs. HIF-1α is an ROS-stabilized transcription factor that, under hypoxic conditions, forms a heterodimer with HIF-1β. This heterodimer is translocated to the nucleus where it binds the hypoxia response element (HRE), inducing transcription of genes involved in migration proliferation, apoptosis, and angiogenesis.[44] This element of the hypoxia response contributes to endothelial cell damage, increasing vascular permeability and, as a result, leakage of fibrin into the extracellular matrix.

Vascular endothelial growth factor (VEGF) is an HIF-mediated growth factor. Under hypoxic conditions, VEGF expression is increased, resulting in aberrant vascular network formation, which leads to irregular perfusion.[45] The resulting cycles of hypoperfusion and reperfusion contribute to oxidative stress, further damaging tissue.[38]

Macrophage accumulation further contributes to the self-perpetuating nature of radiation-induced tissue injury. Accumulation of macrophages is known to occur in areas of low perfusion and inadequate supply of oxygen and is observed in tissues following radiation exposure.[46,47] When activated, these cells produce HIF-1α in order to initiate angiogenesis to correct low perfusion.[47] This response on the part of macrophages increases the level of oxidative stress, continuing the spread of damage through inappropriate continuation of wound-healing mechanisms.

Possible Metabolic Changes

Carbonic anhydrase-9 (CA-9) is commonly used as a hypoxia marker because CA-9 transcription is dependent on HIF-1α. Because carbonic anhydrases act to catalyze the conversion of metabolically produced carbon dioxide to bicarbonate,[48] this increase in CA-9 suggests that cells may also be undergoing a metabolic shift in response to their hypoxic environments. The observed changes in mitochondrial activity would support altered metabolism in postradiation cells, but further work is necessary to determine the nature of such a change.

Implications

Exposure to ionizing radiation disrupts DNA, causing cell death, but it also causes increased production of ROS in viable cells. The oxidizing environment that results from ROS production exceeding the antioxidant capacity of the cell causes further damage by disrupting cell function and signaling pathways. This disturbance results in changes in vascular integrity, an ongoing inflammatory response, and aberrant angiogenesis. Because overproduction of ROS is self-perpetuating, these effects are amplified, increasing the area and severity of damage.

Though many of the mechanisms through which ROS production affects the development of late radiation effects remain unclear, it is likely that these early changes initiate disease processes that progress over time to cause the observed late injury.

SUMMARY BY ORGAN SYSTEM

To provide a consistent summary of the extensive information in the individual organ reviews, the following outline is utilized:

1. Clinical Significance
2. Endpoints
3. Challenges Defining Volumes
4. Dose/Volume/Toxicity Data
5. Factors Affecting Risk
6. Mathematic/Biologic Models
7. Special Situations
8. Recommended Dose–Volume Limits
9. Future Studies
10. Toxicity Scoring Criteria

Note that the brief summaries for each review do not substitute for reading and understanding the original papers and, as necessary, the underlying literature. In addition, the dose–volume limits described in the QUANTEC reviews are intended to supplement, not supplant, clinical judgment.

CENTRAL NERVOUS SYSTEM

Brain

Clinical Significance. The acute and late effects of radiotherapy on the brain are common and represent a significant source of morbidity.[49] In particular, patients with tumor-related neurocognitive dysfunction may exhibit exacerbated deficits after radiotherapy. In addition, the radiation fields used to treat the upper aerodigestive tract (e.g., sinuses and pharynx) often include a portion of the brain.

Endpoints. The acute side effects of radiation therapy (RT) to the brain include nausea, vomiting, and headache; seizures, visual disturbances, and vertigo are less common.[49] These symptoms are typically transient and generally respond well to medication. The endpoints for assessing long-term radiation-induced complications are typically radiation necrosis or asymptomatic radiologic changes as seen on serial magnetic resonance imaging (MRI) scans.[49] Other measures have included steroid usage, preservation of performance status, and neurocognitive function.[50,51–52]

Challenges Defining Volumes. Contouring the entire brain is straightforward, and with appropriate immobilization, there is little intra- or interfraction motion. However, delineation of subregions (e.g., the border between the brainstem and thalamus) and functional segments (e.g., Broca area) of the brain is challenging, and the utility of defining such areas has not yet been proven.[49]

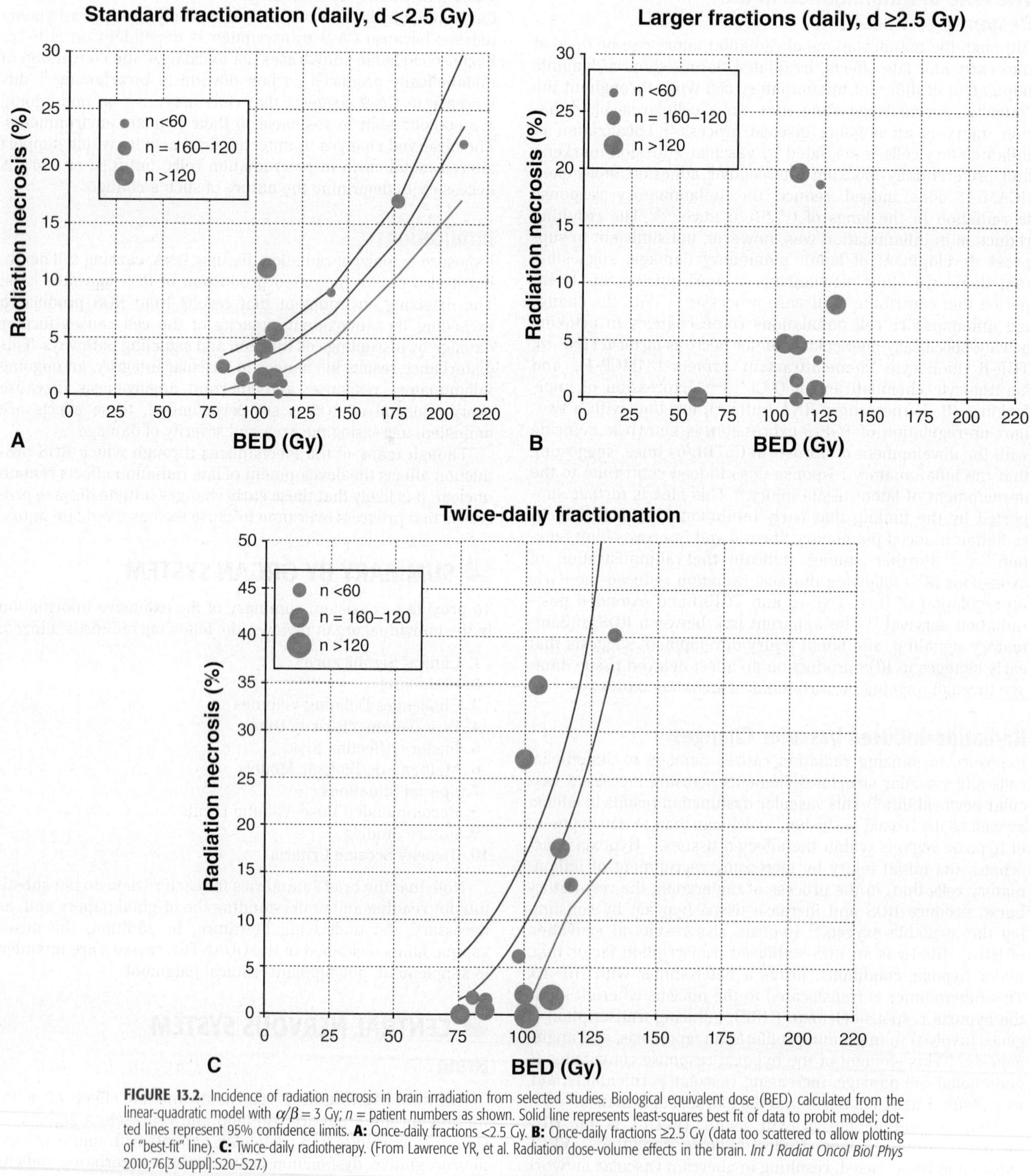

FIGURE 13.2. Incidence of radiation necrosis in brain irradiation from selected studies. Biological equivalent dose (BED) calculated from the linear-quadratic model with $\alpha/\beta = 3$ Gy; *n* = patient numbers as shown. Solid line represents least-squares best fit of data to probit model; dotted lines represent 95% confidence limits. **A:** Once-daily fractions <2.5 Gy. **B:** Once-daily fractions ≥2.5 Gy (data too scattered to allow plotting of "best-fit" line). **C:** Twice-daily radiotherapy. (From Lawrence YR, et al. Radiation dose-volume effects in the brain. *Int J Radiat Oncol Biol Phys* 2010;76[3 Suppl]:S20–S27.)

Dose/Volume/Toxicity Data. For fractionated radiotherapy to the brain, the relationship between dose and radiation necrosis for partial brain irradiation is shown in Figure 13.2 for various fractionation schemes.[53–60] Lawrence et al. compared different fractionation schemes by calculating the biologically effective dose (BED),[61] with an α/β ratio of 3 Gy.[49] For standard fractionation, a dose–response relationship appears to exist, such that an incidence of side effects of 5% and 10% occur at a BED of 120 Gy_3 (range, 100 to 140) and 150 Gy_3 (range, 140 to 170), respectively (corresponding to 72 Gy [range 60 to 84] and 90 Gy [range, 84 to 102] in 2-Gy fractions). For twice-daily fractionation, a steep increase in toxicity is apparent when the BED exceeds 80 Gy. For daily large fraction sizes (>2.5 Gy), the incidence and severity of toxicity are unpredictable. Lawrence et al. caution against overinterpreting this analysis given the heterogeneity of the data pool (i.e., different target volumes, endpoints, sample sizes, and brain regions).

In children, whole-brain radiotherapy appears associated with neurocognitive decline. With central nervous system prophylaxis for acute lymphoblastic leukemia, the addition of 24-Gy radiation to the whole brain (to a chemotherapy regimen) is associated with a median 13-point intelligence quotient reduction at 5 years after radiotherapy, as well as poorer academic performance and greater psychological distress.[62] Reported toxicities have been lower when 14 to 18 Gy was used.[63–65] In medulloblastoma, the post-RT intelligence quotients were 10 to 15 points higher for a total whole-brain dose of 23.4 Gy versus 36 Gy.[66,67] In adults, the neurocognitive effects of whole-brain irradiation are less clear.

In stereotactic radiosurgery (SRS) of brain lesions, normal tissue toxicity appears to be a function of dose, volume, and location in the brain. The Radiation Therapy Oncology Group (RTOG) conducted a dose-escalation study (RTOG 9005) of radiosurgery to recurrent brain metastases and primary tumors in patients who previously received whole- or partial-brain irradiation.[68] The goal of this study was to determine the maximal tolerated dose as a function of maximum diameter of the lesion. Unacceptable toxicity was defined as acute irreversible severe neurologic symptoms, requiring inpatient or outpatient medications, any life-threatening neurologic toxicity, or death. This study found a maximum tolerated prescription dose to the tumor margin of ≥24 Gy, 18 Gy, and 15 Gy for tumors with a maximal diameter of ≤2.0 cm, 2.1 to 3.0 cm, and 3.1 to 4.0 cm, respectively. The rates of acute and late unacceptable toxicities in patients treated at these doses were 0% and 10%, 0% and 14%, and 0% and 20%, respectively. The dose limits appear to be validated by the results of the RTOG 9508, a randomized study of SRS + whole-brain radiation therapy (WBRT) versus WBRT alone in 333 patients with brain metastases.[50] Using the dose constraints developed in RTOG 90-05, this study found a 3% and 6% rate of grade 3 and 4 acute and late toxicities, respectively, in the group of 167 patients receiving radiosurgery.

The results of dose–volume studies of the development of "radionecrosis" following single-fraction radiosurgery are shown in Table 13.3.[49,69–78] While a common element in many of these studies is the volume receiving a dose of 10 or 12 Gy or more (V_{10} or V_{12}, respectively), there is a broad variation in the crude rate of radionecrosis as a function of volume irradiated. This is likely due to difference in the definition of *radionecrosis,* the location irradiated, the proximity to and sparing of critical structures, and the length and intensity of clinical follow-up.

These results suggest that the rate of complications increases rapidly as the V_{12} increases beyond 5 to 10 cm^3. Note, however, that V_{12} will far exceed these limits for lesions 2 cm or greater in mean diameter when the RTOG guidelines are utilized. For example, assume that spherical lesions 1, 2, 3, and 4 cm in diameter are treated under the RTOG guidelines with single-fraction radiosurgery with the plans yielding V_{12}'s of six, five,

TABLE 13.3 SELECTED STUDIES OF RADIONECROSIS IN PATIENTS RECEIVING BRAIN STEREOTACTIC RADIOSURGERY

Reference	*Diagnosis*	*n*	*Mean D_{min}, Gy (Range)*	*Overall Incidence of RN*	*Subgroup*	*Incidence of RN in Subgroup*	*Primary Predictor of Toxicity*	*Other Risk Factors*
Lax and Karlsson[74]	AVM	823	?	5%			Average dose in 20 cm^3	
Voges et al.[78]	Mixed	133	15.0 (7.0–25.0)	12.8%	V_{10} <10 mL	0%	V_{10}	Location
					V_{10} >10 mL	23.7%		
Flickinger et al.[71]	AVM	307	20.9 (12–30)	10.7%			V_{12}	Location
Miyawaki et al.[75]	AVM	73	16 (10–22)	14%	Tx volume: <1 mL	0%	Tx volume	Dose, prior brain insult
					1–3.9 mL	15%		
					4–13.9 mL	14%		
					>14 mL	27%		
Chin et al.[70]	Mixed	243	20 (10–30)	7%			V_{10}	Repeated radiosurgery, glioma
Nakamura et al.[76]	Mixed	749	18 (16–19)[a]	?	Rx volume:	0%	Rx volume	
					0.05–0.66 mL	3%		
					0.67–3 mL	7%		
					3.1–8.6 mL	9%		
					8.7–95.1 mL			
Barker et al.[69]	AVM	1,250	10.5 (4–65)	4.1%			Dose and volume combined	Age, location
Friedman et al.[72]	AVM	269	?	4.7%			V_{12}	
Varlotto et al.[77]	Brain metastases	137	16 (12–25)	11.4%	Tx volume:	3.7%	Volume	
					<2 mL	16%		
					>2 mL			
Korytko et al.[73]	Tumor	129	17.3 (11–25)	30%	V_{12}:	23%	V_{12}	Location, previous WBRT, male
					0–5 mL	20%		
					5–10 mL	54%		
					10–15 mL	57%		
					>15 mL			

[a]Range refers to 25th to 75th quartile.

RN, radionecrosis; AVM, arteriovenous malformation; V_{10}, volume receiving 10 Gy, V_{12}, volume receiving 12 Gy; Tx, treatment; Rx, prescription; WBRT, whole-brain radiotherapy.

Adapted from Lawrence YR, et al. Radiation dose-volume effects in the brain. *Int J Radiat Oncol Biol Phys* 2010;76(3 Suppl):S20–S27.

four, and three times the lesion volume, respectively. Then, the calculated V_{12}'s are 3, 21, 57, and 101 cm^3, respectively.

The location of the lesion is important as the severity of expressed damage is greater in the more eloquent parts of the brain. For example, for a V_{12} of 10 cm^3, Flickinger et al.[71] found a <5% symptomatic postradiosurgery injury for arteriovenous malformations (AVMs) in the frontal, temporal, and parietal lobes versus >20% for AVMs in the brainstem, thalamus, and basal ganglia.

Factors Affecting Risk. Younger age is associated with a higher risk of neurocognitive decline in children undergoing cranial irradiation.[79,80] Other risk factors include female gender, neurofibromatosis-1 (NF-1) mutation, extent of surgical resection, hydrocephalus, concomitant chemotherapy (especially methotrexate), location, and volume of brain irradiated.[81] No evidence has shown that children are at particular risk of radiation necrosis,[82,83] however.

Mathematic/Biologic Models. While the linear-quadratic model appears useful in comparing dose/fraction for conventionally fractioned radiotherapy schemes, its utility at high doses per fraction (≥8 Gy) is controversial. In general, quantitative dose/volume/clinical toxicity relationships have not been established for neurocognitive function in partial brain irradiation. The apparent increased risk of radionecrosis in twice-daily partial brain irradiation suggests that the time constant for repair of radiation-induced damage may be longer than the typical interfraction interval, but this has not been modeled for this specific system.

Special Situations. Reirradiation of the whole brain is frequently performed in the setting of recurrent, multiple brain metastases. A meta-analysis of whole-brain reirradiation (interval between courses, 3 to 55 months) found no cases of necrosis when the total radiation dose was <100 Gy (normalized to 2 Gy/fraction with an α/β ratio = 2 Gy).[84] In primary central nervous system lymphoma, whole-brain radiotherapy has been associated with an atypically high risk of cognitive decline, especially in those >60 years old.[85,86] The heightened sensitivity of this population to irradiation might be explained by the tumor's highly diffuse, angiocentric growth pattern and that most patients receive high-dose methotrexate, a potent neurotoxin. As a result, up-front full-dose RT is now often avoided in elderly patients with this disease. A lower radiation dose of 23.4 Gy delivered in 1.8-Gy daily fractions appears to be associated with minimal cognitive toxicity, even in older patients.[87]

Recommended Dose–Volume Limit.[49] For partial-brain irradiation at a conventional dose per fraction, there is a predicted 5% and 10% risk of symptomatic radiation necrosis at a BED of 120 Gy_3 (range, 100 to 140) and 150 Gy_3 (range, 140 to 170), respectively, which corresponds to 72 Gy (range 60 to 84 Gy) and 90 Gy (range 84 to 102 Gy) for 2-Gy daily fractions. This is a less conservative estimate than the 5% risk of radionecrosis for one-third of the brain irradiated to 60 Gy in the Emami paper.[1] The authors stress that for most cancers, there is no clinical indication for partial-brain dose above 60 Gy and that, in some scenarios, an incidence of 1% to 5% radiation necrosis at 5 years would be unacceptably high. The brain appears especially sensitive to fraction sizes >2 Gy and, surprisingly, twice-daily irradiation.

For radiosurgery, the available data suggest that it is prudent to minimize the volume of normal brain receiving >12 Gy in a single fraction and to consider both target diameter and anatomic location when prescribing dose. However, the QUANTEC authors admit that "the substantial variation between the reported treatment parameters and outcomes from different centers has prevented [more] precise toxicity risk predictions."

Future Studies. Key questions that would benefit from systematic study include:

1. What is the dose/volume/location/clinical toxicity relationship for brain metastases and other common lesions treated with single-fraction SRS?
2. What is the rate of local and distant failure for the aforementioned sets of patients as a function of prescribed dose?
3. How does the gross tumor volume (GTV) to planning target volume (PTV) expansion influence the incidence of normal tissue toxicity and failure rates in single-fraction SRS?
4. How is the incidence of normal tissue toxicity affected by previous large-field irradiation to the brain, particularly the combination of WBRT and SRS in the treatment of brain metastases?
5. How do systemic treatments affect the incidence of normal tissue toxicity?
6. What is the time interval for repair of radiation-induced damage in the brain?

Toxicity Scoring Criteria. Studies of brain radiotherapy should report detailed dosimetric and outcome data, including neurocognitive and neurologic dysfunction (e.g., per the Common Terminology Criteria for Adverse Events, version 4.0 [CTCAE v. 4.088]), the prescription dose, dose/fraction, target volume, V_{12}, anatomic location treated, and clinical outcome data (e.g., adverse events, patterns of failure).

Optic Apparatus

Clinical Significance. The optic nerves and chiasm frequently receive a substantial dose during therapeutic irradiation of brain, base of skull, and head and neck targets, and the optic apparatus is frequently the dose-limiting structure in these cases. While rare, damage to the optic apparatus can produce devastating and, at present, irreversible visual deficits.[88]

Endpoints. The primary endpoint for radiation-induced optic neuropathy (RION) is visual impairment, defined by visual acuity and the size/extent of visual fields.[89] Of course, damage to the lens (development of cataracts), retina (retinitis), and lacrimal apparatus and trigeminal nerve (dry eye syndrome) can also produce impaired vision.[90] While toxicity may be objectively scored using CTCAE version 4[91] and late effects of normal tissues, subjective, objective, medical management and analytical evaluation of injury (LENT-SOMA) criteria,[92,93] it is important to obtain a comprehensive ophthalmologic examination of patients with suspected RION.

Challenges Defining Volumes. The optic nerve originates roughly at the posterior center of the globe and is bracketed by the rectus muscles as it tracks posteriorly through the orbit to pass through the optic notch, just medially to the anterior clinoid process. The optic nerves join and decussate to form the optic chiasm, an X-shaped structure that sits just superiorly to the sella turcica with the center immediately anterior to the pituitary stalk.[94] The optic nerves and chiasm are thin (<5 mm diameter) and visualization is best performed using thin-cut (≤3 mm) T1- or T2-weighted magnetic resonance imaging. Contouring the optic nerves/chiasm is challenging, and it is important to ensure that these structures are drawn in continuity (i.e., there is not a gap in the contours). Appropriate contouring of these structures is facilitated by visualizing this region in multiple planes and using fused imaging modalities (e.g., utilizing the magnetic resonance images in the axial and coronal planes to track the optic nerves/chiasm and sagittal computed tomography [CT] views to see the sella turcica).

Dose/Volume/Toxicity Data. The data for the incidence of RION with conventional fractionation for selected studies[95–96,97–102] are summarized in Figure 13.3. The risk of RION

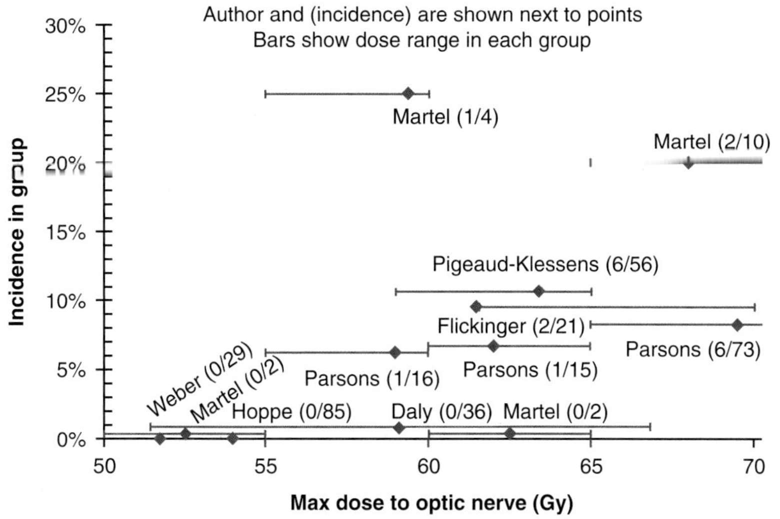

FIGURE 13.3. Incidence of radiation-induced optic neuropathy (RION) in selected studies.[95–96,97–102] Points offset from 0% to 1% were shifted to clearly show range bars. The single patients in the studies by Parsons et al.[95] and Martel et al.[96] with events in the 55–60 Gy range were treated to 59 Gy and 59.5 Gy, respectively. (From Mayo C, et al. Radiation dose-volume effects of optic nerves and chiasm. *Int J Radiat Oncol Biol Phys* 2010;76[3 Suppl]:S28–S35.)

appears to rise steeply past 60 Gy. None of the patients in the study by Parsons et al.[95] with a maximum point dose (D_{max}) to the optic nerves/chiasm <59 Gy developed RION. In the study by Martel et al.,[96] the average maximum chiasm and nerve dose was 53.7 Gy (range 28 to 70 Gy) and 56.8 Gy (range 0 to 80.5 Gy) for patients without RION. The optic nerves had received a D_{max} of 64 Gy with 25% of the volume receiving >60 Gy for patients with moderate to severe complications. Jiang et al.[97] reported no incidence of ipsilateral RION for a dose <56 Gy and a <5% incidence at 10 years for a dose <60 Gy at ~2.5 Gy/fraction.

The risk of RION appears to be related to the fraction size. Parsons et al.[95] reported 15-year actuarial rates of RION for total doses of 60 to <70 Gy of 50% versus 11% at ≥1.9 versus <1.9 Gy dose/fraction, respectively. No patients treated twice daily with 1.2 Gy/fraction developed RION. At total doses of 70 to 83 Gy, the incidence was 33% versus 11% for ≥1.9 versus <1.9 Gy/fraction and 12% for 1.2 Gy twice-daily fractions. Bhandare et al.[103] noted reductions in RION rates for twice-versus once-daily treatment.

Results from proton treatments appear consistent with those utilizing photons.[102,104–106] Note that the proton doses are reported as cobalt gray equivalent (CGE), reflecting their greater biologic effect, and that photons were often used in combination with protons. Most proton series have reported a very low incidence of RION, and in the few cases of reported RION, a threshold dose in the range of 55 to 60 CGE has been observed, consistent with the photon experience. As with photons, many patients exceeding this threshold did not develop RION. Wenkel et al.,[106] Noel et al.,[104] Weber et al.,[102] and Nishimura et al.[105] used a D_{max} constraint to the optic structures of 54, 55, 56, and 60 CGE, respectively.

Because of the small size of the optic nerves/chiasm and steep dose gradients in radiosurgery, most studies of RION involving SRS use the D_{max} to the optic nerves/chiasm as the critical dose metric.[88] As shown in Table 13.2, single-fraction SRS studies describe a range of threshold D_{max} for RION. In analyzing their early experience with radiosurgery, Tishler et al.[107] reported RION at D_{max} as low as 9.7 Gy and recommended 8 Gy as the dose limit for the optic nerves/chiasm in SRS. Stafford et al.[108] found RION in four of 215 patients receiving a median D_{max} of 10 Gy. The D_{max} in the patients ranged from 0.4 to 16 Gy, and three of the four had received previous external beam radiotherapy to this area. They estimated a 1.7%, 1.8%, 0%, and 6.9% incidence of RION for D_{max} of <8, 8 to 10, 10 to 12, and >12 Gy, respectively.

Conversely, Pollock et al.[109] observed no cases of RION in 62 patients with nonfunctioning pituitary adenomas receiving a median D_{max} of 9.5 +/− 1.7 Gy to the optic apparatus during single-fraction SRS, using a 12 Gy D_{max} as the dose constraint for the optic apparatus. From a study of 50 patients with benign base-of-skull tumors treated with single-fraction SRS and a median follow-up of 40 months, Leber et al.[110] estimated a 0%, 27%, and 78% risk of RION for D_{max} of <10, 10 to <15, and ≥15 Gy, respectively. No data for dose–volume and RION were available for hypofractionated stereotactic radiotherapy (4 to 8 Gy/fraction).[88]

Factors Affecting Risk. There appears to be an increased risk of RION with increasing age.[95] Parsons et al.[95] reported that none of the 38 patients in the 20- to 50-year-old range developed RION, even though the reported optic nerve doses were >60 Gy for 58% and >70 Gy for 26%. In contrast, for patients with doses >60 Gy, the incidence was 26% and 56% for the 50- to 70- versus >70-year-old age groups. RION in children is poorly characterized, but treatment of the developing optic apparatus should be approached cautiously. Reports on the effect of other factors such as adjuvant chemotherapy, diabetes mellitus, and hypertension have been inconsistent. Minimal data are available on reirradiation of the optic apparatus and the effect of the interval between courses on RION. Flickinger et al.[111] found that one of 10 patients undergoing reirradiation of the optic apparatus developed RION—the affected received an initial 40 Gy, and after a 7.5-year interval, an additional 46 Gy, both at 2 Gy/fraction.

Mathematic/Biologic Models. The original Lyman-Kutcher-Burman normal tissue complication probability volumetric modeling[4] estimated TD_{50} = 65 Gy, n = 0.25, and m = 0.14. The dose–response data from Jiang et al.[97] (1.5–2.2 Gy/fraction) suggests TD_{50} ≈72 to 75 Gy. Martel et al.[96] and Brizel et al.[112] estimated TD_{50} at 72 and 70 Gy, respectively. Extrapolation of the Parsons dose–response data[95] suggests that TD_{50} exceeds 70 Gy.

Special Situations. There is a suggestion that RION may occur at lower doses in patients with pituitary tumors, as complications at doses as low as 46 Gy at 1.8 Gy/fraction have been reported.[100,113,114] Mackley et al.[100] and van den Bergh et al.[113] constrained the optic structure D_{max} to 46 and 45 Gy, respectively. The RION latency also appeared shorter in patients with pituitary tumors. The average latency was 10.5 and 31 months (range 5 to 168 months) in patients with pituitary targets and nonpituitary targets, respectively.[100,114]

Recommended Dose–Volume Limits. The estimate by Emami et al.[1] of a 5% risk of blindness within 5 years of treatment for a dose of 50 Gy appears inaccurate. The QUANTEC review[88] suggests that the incidence of RION was unusual (<2%) for D_{max} <55 Gy, particularly for fraction sizes <2 Gy. The risk increases (3% to 7%) in the region of 55 to 60 Gy and becomes more substantial (>7% to 20%) for doses >60 Gy when dose per fraction of 1.8 to 2.0 Gy is used. The patients with RION treated in the 55 to 60 Gy range were typically treated to doses in the very high end of that range (i.e., 59 Gy). For particles, most investigators found that the incidence of RION was low for a D_{max} <54 CGE. One exception to this range was for pituitary tumors, in which investigators used a constraint of D_{max} <46 to 48 Gy for 1.8 Gy/fraction.

The aforementioned studies suggest that the incidence of RION in single-fraction radiosurgery is rare for D_{max} <8 Gy, increases in the range of 8 to 12 Gy D_{max}, and becomes >10% when D_{max} exceeds 12 Gy. Though the QUANTEC paper presents isoeffect curves for RION over a range of 2 to 12 Gy/fraction using various radiobiologic models, the authors emphasize that there are no data in the hypofractionated range and caution that the curves should not be used to predict toxicity in this regime.

Future Studies. In addition to reporting detailed dose–volume data for patients with and without RION receiving radiation to the optic apparatus, investigators must consistently, completely, and accurately contour the optic apparatus.

Toxicity Scoring Criteria. Visual deficits should be scored using the CTCAE v. 4.0.[37]

Brainstem

Clinical Significance. As with the optic apparatus, irradiation of the brain, base of skull, and neck can deliver a significant dose to the brainstem, which is frequently the dose-limiting structure.

Endpoints. Radiation-induced damage to the brainstem may be manifest as specific cranial neuropathies; focal motor, sensory, or balance deficits; or mild to life-threatening global dysfunction. This is reflected in the CTCAE,[91] which scores brainstem-related toxicity on the basis of symptoms. The study of radiation-induced brainstem injury is challenging because (a) the reported incidence of injury is low, (b) survival time is short for many patients, (c) formal grading of brainstem effects is subjective and is often characterized categorically (i.e., "yes–no") for cranial neuropathy, and (d) for patients with intracranial tumors, it is often difficult to distinguish between side effects and disease progression.[115]

Challenges Defining Volumes. Contouring the brainstem on axial MRI is usually straightforward, although it requires special attention to the superior extent and interfaces at the cerebral and cerebellar peduncles where the borders are indistinct. Coronal and sagittal views, in addition to axial images, are frequently helpful in visualizing the brainstem and its interfaces. The adult brainstem volume is on the order of 35 ± 8 mL.[116]

Dose/Volume/Toxicity Data. Studies of potential radiation-induced brainstem toxicity in conventionally fractionated partial-brain, base-of-skull, or neck irradiation variably report crude radiographic and functional toxicities over typically short follow-up periods.[99,102,104–106,117–126] Reported toxicities attributable to radiation of the brainstem and dose constraints are presented in Table 13.4. Uy et al.[126] reported brainstem necrosis in one of 40 adult meningioma patients treated with intensity-modulated radiation therapy (IMRT). For this patient, the D_{max} was 55.6 Gy, and the absolute volume of brainstem that exceeded 54 Gy was 4.7 mL. Jian et al.[121] noted a grade 1 neurologic deficit in three of 48 patients with nasopharyngeal cancer treated with 1.2 Gy twice-daily photons to 74.4 Gy and concomitant chemotherapy.

In the largest study, Debus et al.[117,118] reported on 367 patients with base-of-skull tumors with a combination of conformal photon and proton radiation therapy. Nineteen late brainstem-related toxicities were observed, including three deaths. On univariate analysis, significant predictors of toxicity were D_{max} >64 CGE, V_{50} CGE >5.9 mL, V_{55} CGE >2.7 mL, V_{60} CGE >0.9 mL, two or more skull-based surgeries, diabetes, and high blood pressure. On multivariate analysis only V_{60} >0.9 mL, two or more skull-based surgeries, and diabetes were predictive. In a study of 46 patients with recurrent base-of-skull meningiomas, treated to a median brainstem D_{max} of 58.0 CGE, Wenkel et al.[106] found that one patient developed brainstem injury at a dose that exceeded an unspecified constraint value by 10%. Two others with neurologic toxicities had brainstem doses that exceeded the constraints as shown in Table 13.4.

In pediatric patients with brainstem glioma (treated with opposed lateral fields that encompassed the majority of the brainstem), no toxicity was reported at doses of 54 to 60 Gy at 2 Gy/fraction, 75.6 Gy at 1.26 Gy twice daily,[119] or 78 Gy at 1 Gy twice daily.[123] The primary limitation of these studies was

TABLE 13.4 SELECTED STUDIES OF RADIATION-INDUCED BRAINSTEM TOXICITY WITH CONVENTIONAL FRACTIONATION OR HYPERFRACTIONATION

Reference	*Patients/Disease*	*Modality*	*Dose Constraint*	*Radiation-Induced Brainstem Toxicity*
Jian et al.[121]	48 Adults/nasopharyngeal cavity	Photons	V_{65} <3 mL V_{60} <5 mL	3 Grade 1 neurologic toxicities
Hoppe et al.[120]	85 Adults/nasal cavity and/or paranasal sinus	Photons	D_{max} <50 Gy	
Daly et al.[99]	36 Adults/nasal cavity and/or paranasal sinus cavity	Photons	$D_{1\%}$ <54 Gy	
Schoenfeld et al.[125]	100 Adults/pharynx or larynx	Photons	V_{55} <0.1 mL	
Uy et al.[126]	40 Adults/intracranial meningioma	Photons	Unknown	1 BS necrosis @ D_{max} 55.6 Gy, V_{54} 4.7 mL
Merchant et al.[122]	68 Children/infratentorial ependymoma	Photons	No separate brainstem constraint	1 BS necrosis @ D_{mean} 59 Gy
Freeman et al.[119]	136 Children/brainstem glioma	Photons	Prescribed 54–60 Gy at 2 Gy once daily or 75.6 Gy at 1.26 Gy twice daily	None reported
Packer et al.[123,124]	98 Children/brainstem glioma	Photons	Prescribed 72 or 78 Gy total @ 1 Gy twice daily	One treatment-related death at 72 Gy total @ 1 Gy twice daily and concurrent β-IFN
Weber et al.[102]	29 Adults/chordoma, chondrosarcoma	Protons	Surface ≤ 63 CGE Center ≤54 CGE	None reported
Nishimura et al.[105]	14 Adults/olfactory neuroblastoma	Protons	Surface <64 CGE Center <53 CGE	None reported
Noel[104]	45 Adults/BOS tumors	Photons + protons	Surface ≤63CGE Center ≤54CGE	
DeBus[117,118]	367 Adults/BOS tumors	Photons + protons	Surface ≤64CGE Center ≤53CGE	19 BS toxicities, including 3 deaths
Wenkel[106]	46 Adults/BOS meningiomas	Photons + protons	Surface ≤ 64CGE Center ≤53CGE	1 BS injury, 2 neurologic toxicities

CGE, cobalt gray equivalents; BOS, base of skull; BS, brainstem; β-IFN = recombinant β-interferon.

the short median survival, <12 months. Of 32 patients treated to 72 Gy twice daily in combination with recombinant β-interferon, there was at least one treatment-related death.[124]

Most pediatric protocols for central nervous system tumors recommend doses >54 Gy, and separate brainstem dose constraints are often absent. Merchant et al. studied 68 patients with infratentorial ependymoma treated with surgery and conformal RT (54 to 59.4 Gy).[122] In patients with full recovery, a considerable portion of the brainstem received over 60 Gy (V_{60} = 7.8 ± 1.4 mL). There was no difference in brainstem recovery based on absolute or percent volume of the brainstem that received more than 54 Gy. Differences in these values for patients without full recovery were not statistically significant. One patient died with autopsy-confirmed residual tumor and focal areas of brainstem necrosis. The mean brainstem dose was 59 Gy, and he also exhibited severe perioperative morbidity after two surgeries.

A limited number of studies report brainstem toxicity in single-fraction SRS or hypofractionated stereotactic radiotherapy (HFSRT).[127,128–131] A broad range of prescription isodose levels and dose metrics are reported, making it difficult to develop a predictive dose–volume model for brainstem toxicity.[115] In the study with the largest number of patients, Foote et al.[127] analyzed the outcome in 149 vestibular schwannoma patients treated with SRS between 1988 and 1998; 41 were treated before 1994, when radiosurgery was primarily based on CT imaging, and 108 after 1994, when planning was MRI based. Large single-fraction doses (10 to 22.5 Gy) were used. Their analysis revealed a "learning curve," with a 5% and 2% actuarial 2-year rate of facial and trigeminal neuropathies, respectively, for patients treated after 1994 compared with 29% for both neuropathies for the earlier patients. This study found a significant increase, with a 2-year actuarial rate of facial and trigeminal neuropathies of 29% and 7% for patients treated before and after 1994, respectively. The authors ascribe this difference to the use of MRI rather than CT-based imaging and lower prescription doses in the latter years. A univariate analysis showed an incidence of cranial nerve neuropathy of 2% for <12.5 Gy versus 24% for >12.5 Gy (p <.0003). On multivariate analysis, the prescription dose >12.5 Gy, prior surgery, and treatment prior to 1994 were significant variables.

Mathematic/Biologic Models. The Emami review estimates a 5-year, 5% rate of complications, defined in that study as "necrosis/infarct," at 50, 53, and 60 Gy delivered to the whole, two-thirds of, and one-third of the brainstem, respectively.[1] The corresponding Lyman-Kutcher-Berman (LKB) parameters for calculation of the normal tissue complication probability (NTCP) were n = 0.16, m = 0.14, and a tolerance dose for 50% probability of these complications (TD_{50}) equal to 65 Gy.[26] These estimates and model parameters appear overly conservative. For example, the LKB model estimates a 12% risk of severe complications for 54 Gy to the whole brainstem or a 3% risk of complications when the proton dose constraints (Table 13.4) are utilized. The clinical data would suggest that a larger TD_{50}, smaller m, or larger m values might produce more reasonable estimates of toxicity. For example, an LKB model with a larger TD_{50} (72 Gy) or smaller m (0.1) would reduce the predicted risks to <5% or <1%, respectively. However, there are insufficient existing dose/volume/complication data to generate a more accurate model estimate at this time.

Recommended Dose–Volume Limits. The QUANTEC study concludes that the entire brainstem may be treated to 54 Gy using conventional fractionation with limited risk of severe or permanent neurologic effects.[115,122] While the precise dose–volume relationship is unclear, partial volumes of the brainstem (1 to 10 mL) may be irradiated to a maximum dose of 59 Gy for dose fractions ≤2 Gy. The risk appears to increase markedly at doses >64 Gy. In radiosurgery, it appears that a maximum brainstem dose of 12.5 to 13 Gy is associated with a low (<5%) risk of cranial neuropathy in patients with vestibular schwannomas treated with single-fraction SRS. The risk appears to increase rapidly when the marginal prescription dose is >15 Gy or when the target volume exceeds 4 mL.[115,127,132] However, doses of 15 to 20 Gy have been used to treat brainstem metastases with a low reported rate of complications, potentially because of the limited survival time for these patients.[129,133]

Future Studies. Uniform, complete reporting of patient-specific dose/volume/outcome data for patients with and without complications are required.

Toxicity Scoring Criteria. Patients should undergo a complete history and physical examination at regular intervals with particular attention to the neurologic exam. Toxicity should be scored and reported using the CTCAE v. 4.0.[91]

Auditory Apparatus

Clinical Significance. Radiation therapy to brain tumors and head and neck cancers may damage the cochlea and/or acoustic nerve, leading to sensorineural hearing loss (SNHL) and compromised quality of life.[134]

Endpoints. SNHL following conventionally fractionated radiotherapy is typically measured by a decrease in the bone conduction threshold at 0.5 to 4 kHz,[134] the primary range for human speech, using pure-tone audiometry (PTA). While the technique is well established and standardized, a broad range of specific audiometric parameters are used to characterize SNHL, including the frequency (range) used for testing, the threshold chosen for a clinically significant change in the bone conduction threshold (BCT, 10 to 20 dB), and the control/standard used for comparison. In stereotactic radiosurgery, SRS, or HFSRT, hearing status is more commonly evaluated using the Gardner-Robertson scale, which is based on both PTA and speech discrimination. Hearing loss after SRS/HFSRT may be characterized by changes in Gardner-Robertson hearing grade or retention of serviceable hearing (i.e., functional hearing with the aid of a hearing aid) or any measurable hearing. In addition, the length of follow-up will influence reported hearing loss, as deficits may develop more rapidly following single-fraction SRS than HFSRT, and hearing loss increases over time in both situations.

Challenges Defining Volumes. Contouring of the acoustic nerve and brainstem is best accomplished on high-resolution, contrast-enhanced T1-weighted and fast imaging with steady-state precession MRI. The cochlea and associated bony anatomy are better delineated on fine-cut (≤1 mm slice thickness) CT scans. Both the acoustic nerve and cochlea are small structures, and the dose gradient at the latter structure is often quite steep. Moreover, the acoustic nerve anatomy is distorted by the tumor, significantly increasing its apparent diameter. Thus, the dose to these structures is typically characterized by an average or maximum dose, rather than a dose–volume distribution. In many studies, the primary dose metric was the dose to the acoustic neuroma, rather than the normal tissue structures per se, which is not unreasonable as the dose to the tumor appears to be correlated with the dose received by the acoustic nerve.[45]

Dose/Volume/Toxicity Data. SNHL at key frequencies following radiotherapy for head and neck cancer with conventionally fractionated radiotherapy[134–135,136–139,140,141] is summarized in Figure 13.4. Pan et al.[135] prospectively studied the BCT in 31 patients after unilateral RT with standard fractionation using changes seen in the contralateral ear as standard (0.25 to 8 kHz). Changes in BCT >10 dB were rarely observed unless

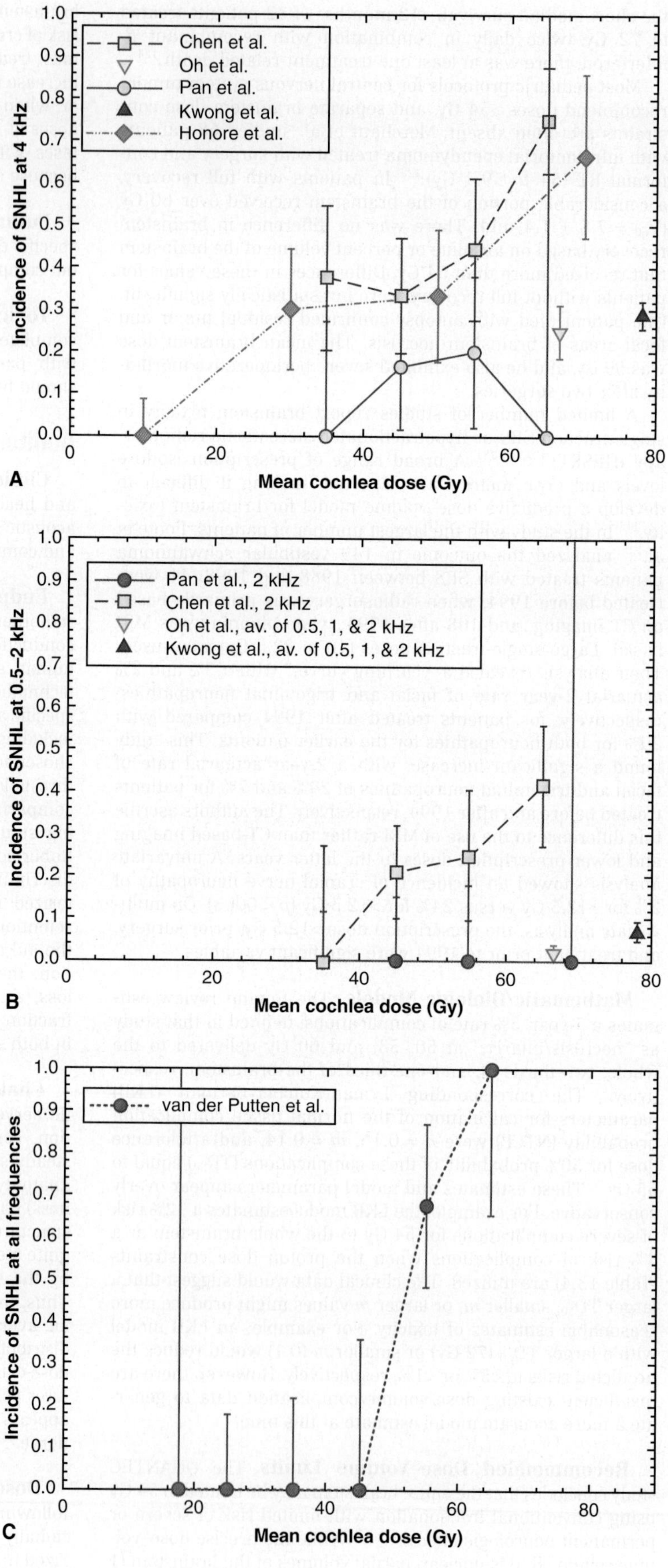

FIGURE 13.4. Mean dose response for sensorineural hearing loss (SNHL) at **(A)** 4 kHz,[135,136–137,139,140] **(B)** 0.5–2 kHz,[135,136–137,139] and **(C)** all frequencies[141] (0.25–12 kHz). (From Bhandare N, et al. Radiation therapy and hearing loss. *Int J Radiat Oncol Biol Phys* 2010;76[3 Suppl]:S50–S57.)

TABLE 13.5 HEARING PRESERVATION IN STEREOTACTIC RADIOSURGERY AND RADIOTHERAPY

Reference	*Technique: Number of Patients*	*Treatment Dose, Gy*	*Mean/Median Follow-Up, Months (Range)*	*Tumor Control,%*	*Rate of Hearing Preservation,%*
Hirsch and Noren[149]	SRS: 126	18–25	56	86	26
Noren et al.[153]	SRS: 254 (NF2: 61)	18–20 10–15	(12–204)	Unilateral: 94 NF2: 84	22 (moderate vs. severe hearing loss: 55% vs. 23%)
Foote et al.[148]	SRS: 36	16–20	(2.5–36)	100	42 ± 17 at 2 years
Flickinger et al.[147]	SRS: 273 (CT vs. MRI planned: 118 vs. 155)	12–20		CT: 44 MRI: 32	CT: 39 MRI : 68
Kondziolka et al.[150]	SRS: 162	12–20 Mean: 16.6	(6–102) (60% > 60)	94	47–51
Lunsford et al.[151]	SRS: 402	Earlier in the series: 17 Later in the series: 12–14	36	93	Earlier in the series: 39 Later in the series: 68
Flickinger et al.[146]	SRS: 190	11–18 Median: 13	30 (Max: 80)	91 at 5 years	74
Andrews et al.[142]	SRS: 64 (NF2: 5) FSRT: 46 (NF2: 10)	SRS: 12 FSRT: 50 (2 Gy/fx)	SRS: 30 ± 17 SRT: 30 ± 24	SRS: 98 SRT: 97	SRS: 33 SRT: 81
Combs et al.[143]	FSRT: 106	57.6 Gy (1.8 Gy/fx)	49 (3–172)	94% @ 3 years 93% @ 5 years	94 @ 5 years
Williams[154]	HFSRT: 125	Tumors <3 cm: 25/5 fxs Tumors ≥ 3 cm: 30/10 fxs	22 (12–68)	100	64
Meijer et al.[152]	SRS: 12 HFSRT: 25	SRS: 10–12 HFSRT: 20–25	25 (12–61)	–	91

SRS, stereotactic radiosurgery; NF2, neurofibromatosis type 2; CT, computed tomography; MRI, magnetic resonance imaging; FSRT, fractionated stereotactic radiotherapy; fx, fraction; HFSRT, hypofractionated stereotactic radiotherapy.

the corresponding difference in mean cochlear dose was >45 Gy. The dose to the contralateral cochlea ranged from 0.5 to 31.3 Gy (mean, 4.2 Gy). Honore et al.[140] retrospectively estimated mean cochlear doses in 20 patients treated with radiation therapy for head-and-neck cancer.[142–144] A dose–response relationship was observed at 4 kHz, but not at other frequencies.

Chen et al.[136] retrospectively studied 22 patients treated with RT for nasopharyngeal cancer (with fraction sizes from 1.6 to 2.3 Gy and concurrent/adjuvant chemotherapy) and studied BCT 12 to 79 months post-RT. A significant increase in hearing loss (change in BCT of >20 dB at one frequency or >10 dB at two consecutive frequencies) was observed for all frequencies (0.5 to 4 kHz) when the mean dose received by the cochlea exceeded 48 Gy. Van der Putten et al.[141] retrospectively evaluated changes in BCT after head and neck radiotherapy in 21 patients with unilateral parotid tumors (fraction sizes 1.8 to 3.0 Gy). Using the contralateral ear as a control, SNHL, defined as a >15 db difference in BCT at three or more frequencies between 0.25 and 12 kHz, was seen when mean doses received by the cochlea were >50 Gy. Oh[139] prospectively studied changes in BCT (0.25 to 4 kHz) post-RT in 25 patients with nasopharyngeal cancer (fraction size 2 Gy). In that study, inner ear doses were high (63 to 70 Gy), and hearing loss (a >15 db decrease in BCT from baseline) correlated with total dose received by the inner ear.

Table 13.5 summarizes the reported incidence of hearing loss for single-fraction SRS and fractionated stereotactic radiotherapy (FSRT) in the treatment of vestibular schwannomas.[142,143,145–154] The range of hearing loss reported is broad, in part due to the variation in the definition of hearing preservation and the length of follow-up. Nonetheless, several studies suggest that there is a relationship between the volume/length of acoustic nerve irradiated and/or the dose to the nerve and cochlea with hearing loss. In a study of 82 patients treated to a marginal dose of 12 Gy in single-fraction SRS, Massager et al.[155] found that increased intracanalicular tumor volume (<100 vs. ≥100 mm^3) and volume-averaged intracanalicular dose were significant predictors of increased hearing loss. Pollock et al. reported that hearing preservation was more likely when tumors <3 cm versus >3 cm in diameter were treated with single-fraction SRS.[156]

Niranjan et al.[157] found that the dose extending beyond the intracanalicular tumor volume and the prescription dose were the most important factors adversely affecting hearing. In that study, serviceable hearing was preserved in 100% of patients treated with a marginal tumor dose of ≤14 Gy in single-fraction SRS versus 20% in those receiving >14 Gy. Similarly, Kondziolka et al. and Lunsford et al. reported significantly improved hearing preservation rates when the marginal dose was reduced from 16 to 20 Gy to 12 to 14 Gy.[150,151]

Several studies suggest that the rate of hearing preservation is improved with FSRT versus single-fraction SRS.[142–144] However, there is an issue of selection bias in that patients are frequently selected for fractionated treatment because their hearing is good. Meijer et al.[152] found no significant difference in hearing preservation in acoustic neuroma patients treated with four to five fractions of 5 Gy HFSRT vs. 10 to 12.5 Gy single-fraction SRS (61% vs. 75%), though trigeminal nerve preservation was significantly higher with HFSRT (98% vs. 92%).

Factors Affecting Risk. While the mean total dose to the cochlea during fractionated radiation therapy to the head and neck and to the acoustic nerve in SRS for vestibular schwannomas is a dominant factor in affecting hearing loss postradiotherapy (see earlier), the effects of fraction size and twice- versus once-daily treatment are not well characterized. Cisplatin, administered during or after radiotherapy, may exacerbate SNHL.[136,158,159]

Mathematic/Biologic Models. The results of SNHL in conventionally fractionated radiotherapy of head and neck cancers have been fit using multivariate regression models, as discussed in the QUANTEC paper.[134]

Special Situations. The QUANTEC analysis applies only to adult patients; hearing loss after radiotherapy may be more problematic in pediatric patients, particularly in combination with chemotherapy.[160] In patients with neurofibromatosis type 2, treatment of vestibular schwannomas by SRS appears to result in increased hearing loss, as well as poorer tumor control, compared to patients with sporadic tumors.[161–163]

Recommended Dose–Volume Limits. For conventionally fractionated RT, the mean dose to the cochlea should be limited to ≤45 Gy (or more conservatively ≤35 Gy) to minimize the risk for SNHL.[134] Because a threshold for SNHL has not been established, the dose to the cochlea should be kept as low as possible to prevent hearing loss. To minimize hearing loss while maintaining adequate control of vestibular schwannomas, the QUANTEC authors recommend a marginal dose of 12 to 14 Gy for single-fraction SRS.[127,134,164] Though data for hypofractionated regimens are quite limited, the authors speculate that a total dose of 21 to 30 Gy, presumably delivered in three 7-Gy, five 5-Gy, or ten 3-Gy fractions, would provide an acceptable balance of hearing preservation and tumor control.[134]

Future Studies. The effects of concurrent chemotherapy in radiotherapy for head and neck cancer, of acoustic nerve length irradiated and fractionation in vestibular schwannomas, and of the absolute dose to the cochlea in all settings would benefit from prospective, multi-institutional studies.

Toxicity Scoring Criteria. An audiometric evaluation should be performed for both ears immediately before radiotherapy and biannually thereafter. The QUANTEC authors recommend that a "clinically significant hearing loss" should be defined as an increase in the threshold of 10 dB in postradiotherapy BCT or a decline of 10% in a speech discrimination evaluation.[134]

Spinal Cord

Clinical Significance. Although the spinal cord proper is from the base of the skull through the top of the lumbar spine, individual nerves continue down the spinal canal to the level of the pelvis. Thus, portions of the spinal cord and canal are often included in radiotherapy fields during treatment of malignancies involving the neck, thorax, abdomen, and pelvis.[165] In addition, metastatic disease to the bony spine is encountered in ~40% of all cancer patients,[166] and this disease is often treated with radiotherapy. Though rare, radiation-induced spinal cord injury (i.e., myelopathy) can be severe, resulting in pain, paresthesias, sensory deficits, paralysis, Brown-Sequard syndrome, and bowel/bladder incontinence.[167]

Endpoints. Myelopathy is defined as a grade 2 or higher myelitis, per CTCAE v. 4.0.[91] Under this definition, asymptomatic changes in the cord detected radiographically and mild signs/symptoms, such as the Babinski sign or L'hermitte syndrome, would not be classified as myelopathy. Consequently, a diagnosis of myelopathy is based on the appearance of signs/symptoms of sensory or motor deficits, loss of function, or pain, now frequently confirmed by magnetic resonance imaging. Radiation myelopathy rarely occurs less than 6 months after completion of radiotherapy and, in most cases, appears within 3 years.[168]

Challenges Defining Volumes. In conventional external-beam RT, the field generally encompasses the entire circumference of the cord, vertebral body, and spinal nerve roots and precise organ definition is not critical apart from correctly identifying the level of the involved cord. Delineation of the cord in radiosurgery is unsettled, with various studies contouring the critical organ in the axial plane as the spinal cord, the spinal cord expanded 2 to 3 mm, the thecal sac and its contents, or the entire spinal canal.[169] As the volume receiving a high dose often extends superiorly and inferiorly to the target, several studies expand the critical organ volume above and below the target volume. For example, RTOG protocol 0631, a study of

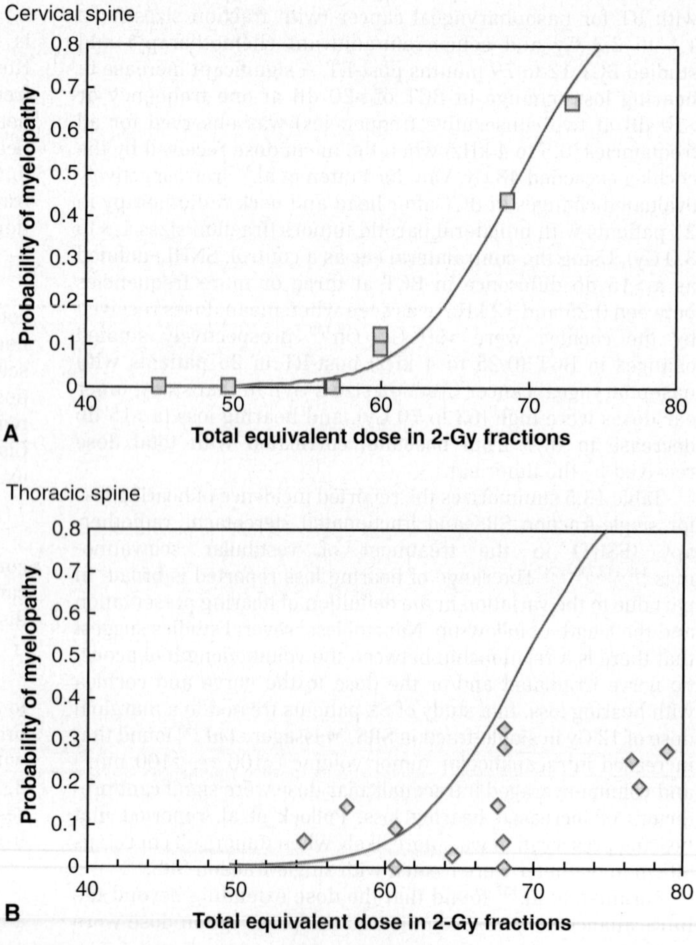

FIGURE 13.5. Incidence of transverse myelopathy from selected studies. **A:** Cervical cord: data for selected studies[168,171–174] shown by □ with probability of myelopathy corrected for estimated survival and solid line fit to these data by the method of Schultheiss. **B:** Thoracic cord: data for selected studies[175–186] shown by ◊ with probability of myelopathy corrected for estimated survival. Solid line is the best fit to the cervical cord data, as thoracic cord data were insufficient to permit an adequate fit. (Adapted from Schultheiss TE. The radiation dose-response of the human spinal cord. *Int J Radiat Oncol Biol Phys* 2008;71(5):1455–1459.)

image-guided radiosurgery of spine metastases, defines the cord as the unexpanded cord itself visualized in MRI and extends the volume of the partial spinal cord 5 to 6 mm above and below the target volume.

Dose/Volume/Toxicity Data. Schultheiss[165,170] compiled and analyzed published reports of radiation myelopathy in 335 and 1,946 patients receiving radiotherapy to the full-circumference, previously unirradiated cervical[168,171–174] and thoracic[175–186] spines, respectively (Fig. 13.5A,B). While a small number of these patients received relatively high doses per fraction, none was treated using stereotactic techniques to exclude a portion of the circumference of the cord. Note that the dose to the cord is the prescribed dose reported in those studies; typically, dosimetric data were not available to calculate the true cord dose. As discussed later, the rate of myelopathy appears very low below total doses of 50 Gy for conventional radiation delivered at 2 Gy per fraction.

Published reports of radiation myelopathy from radiosurgery to the spine are summarized in Table 13.6.[187–194] Of the

TABLE 13.6 TRANSVERSE MYELOPATHY IN STEREOTACTIC RADIOSURGERY (SRS) OF THE SPINE

Reference	*Cases of Myelopathy/ Total Patients*	*Total Dose (Gy)*	*Dose/Fraction (Gy)*	*Dose to Cord (Gy)*	*BED to Cord (Gy_3)*	*Proportion of Patients Previously Irradiated to Involved Segment of Spine*
Gibbs et al.[190]	6/1,075	12.5–25	5–25	D_{max}: 3–28	Range: 24–121 Gy_3	>55%
		25	***12.5***	***D_{max}: 26.2***	***D_{max}: 141***	
		20	***12.5***	***D_{max}: 29.9***	***D_{max}: 81***	
		21	***10.5***	***D_{max}: 19.2***	***D_{max}: 46***	
		24	***8***	***D_{max}: 13.9***	***D_{max}: 129***	
		20	***10***	***D_{max}: 10***	***D_{max}: 33***	
		20	***20***	***D_{max}: 8.5***	***D_{max}: 43***	
Ryu et al.[195]	1/86[a]	<10–18	<10–18	Mean ± SD D_{max}: 12.2 ± 2.5 D_{10}: 8.6 ± 2.1 Maximum D_{max}: 19.2 D_{10}:13	Mean ± SD D_{max}: 62 ± 4.6 D_{10}: 33 ± 3.6 Maximum D_{max}: 142 D_{10}: 69	0%
		18[b]	18	Mean ± SD D_{max}: 13.8 ± 2.2 D_{10}: 9.8 ± 1.5	Mean ± SD D_{max}: 77 ± 3.8 D_{10}: 42 ± 2.3	
		16	***16***	***D_{max}: 14.8*** ***D_1: 13.0*** ***D_{10}: 9.6***	***D_{max}: 88*** ***D_1: 69*** ***D_{10}: 40***	
Gwak et al.[191]	2/9	21–44	3–5	Median D_{max}: 32.9 D_{25}: 11.0 Range D_{max}: 11–37 D_{25}: 1.2–24	Median D_{max}: 106 D_{25}: 21 Range D_{max}: 19–172 D_{25}: 1–88	33%
		30	***10***	***D_{max}: 35.2*** ***D_{25}: 15.5***	***D_{max}:172*** ***D_{25}: 42***	
		33	***11***	***D_{max}: 32.9*** ***D_{25}: 24.0***	***D_{max}: 153*** ***D_{25}: 88***	
Benzil et al.[187]	3/31	Median: 10 ***100*** ***12*** ***20***	Median: 5 ***50*** ***12*** ***5***	Median: 6.0	Median: 12	Unknown
Sahgal et al.[194]	0/38	24	8	Median $D_{0.1\ mL}$: 10.5 $D_{1\ mL}$: 7.4	Median $D_{0.1\ mL}$: 23 $D_{1\ mL}$: 14	62%
Sahgal et al.[193]	0/16	21	7	Median D_{max}: 20.9 $D_{1\ mL}$: 13.8 Range D_{max}: 4.3–23 $D_{1\ mL}$: 2.8–19	Median $D_{1\ mL}$: 22 Range $D_{1\ mL}$: 6–54	6%
Chang et al.[188]	0/63	30 pts: 30 Gy 33 pts: 27 Gy	30 pts: 6 Gy 33 pts: 9 Gy	30 pts: <10 33 pts: <9	30 pts: <16.7 33 pts: <18	56%
Gerzsten et al.[189]	0/50	19	19	Mean D_{max}: 10 Range D_{max}: 6.5–13	Mean D_{max}: 21 Range D_{max}: 11–32	96%
Nelson et al.[192]	0/32	Median: 18	Median: 7	Mean ± SD D_{max}: 14.4 ± 2.3 D_{10}: 11.5 ± 2.1 Maximum D_{max}: 19.2 D_{10}: 15.2	Mean ± SD D_{max}: 46.0 ± 13.2 D_{10}: 31.2 ± 8.1 Maximum D_{max}: 78.3 D_{10}: 46.5	58%

After Kirkpatrick JP, van der Kogel AJ, Schultheiss TE. Radiation dose-volume effects in the spinal cord. *Int J Radiat Oncol Biol Phys* 2010;76(3 Suppl):S42–S49.

exactly 1,400 cases of spinal radiosurgery presented in the published literature, there are only 12 reported instances of radiation-induced myelopathy, equaling a crude rate of 0.8%. Because the survival is generally short for most of these patients, this may be an underestimate of the true rate of injury. Given the small number of reported cases of myelopathy, as well as the variation in published dosimetric parameters, it is not feasible to construct a quantitative model for the risk of myelopathy as a function of cord dose in spinal radiosurgery. In fact, most of the cases of myelopathy involved cord doses well within the range of doses *not* associated with myelopathy, as discussed later.

Factors Affecting Risk. Animal studies suggest that the immature spine is somewhat more susceptible to radiation-induced complications and the time to manifestation of damage is shorter.[196,197–199] Though the literature on radiation-induced myelopathy in children is sparse, care should be exercised in irradiating a child's spine because of the increased sensitivity of the developing central nervous system and bone to ionizing radiation.[200] There are a handful of reports of myelopathy at relatively low radiation doses to the spine post-chemotherapy.[201–204] Many chemotherapeutic agents are directly neurotoxic[205] and should be used with caution during irradiation of the central nervous system.[206]

Mathematic/Biologic Models. Schultheiss[170] calculated the risk of myelopathy as a function of dose using a probability distribution model, using the data for cervical and thoracic spinal cord myelopathy adjusted for estimated overall survival. A good fit to the combined cervical and thoracic cord data was not possible, and separate analyses were performed. For the cervical cord data, D_{50} = 69.4 Gy and α/β ratio = 0.87 Gy provided a reasonable fit of the data, as shown in Figure 13.5. The 95% confidence interval was 66.4 to 72.6 Gy for D_{50} and 0.54 to 1.19 Gy for α/β ratio. At 2 Gy per fraction, the calculated probability of myelopathy is 0.03% at a total dose of 45 Gy and 0.2% at 50 Gy. Because of the dispersion of the thoracic data, it was not possible to obtain a good fit to those data. As shown in Figure 13.5b, the data points for the thoracic cord generally lie to the right of the dose–response curve generated from the cervical cord. This suggests that the thoracic cord may be less radiation sensitive than the cervical cord.

At the high doses per fraction encountered in radiosurgery, the applicability of the linear-quadratic model is controversial and the biologically equivalent doses presented in Table 13.6 should be used solely for making rough comparisons of the different dose regimens. In particular, data obtained at a low dose per fraction should not be extrapolated to regimens employing doses of 10 Gy or more per fraction.[165,207] Applying the Schultheiss model[170] to spinal radiosurgery appears to overestimate the risk of myelopathy. For example, using the α/β ratio of 0.87 Gy, the model yields an estimated risk of myelopathy of 0.8%, 13.6%, 50%, and 73% for 12, 13, 13.7, and 14 Gy, respectively, delivered in a single fraction. In contrast, Ryu et al.[195] found only one case of myelopathy in 86 patients treated with single-fraction spine radiosurgery at a mean cord D_{max} of 12.2 Gy (± 2.5 Gy standard deviation) and no cases in the subset of 39 lesions prescribed 18 Gy and treated to a mean cord D_{max} of 13.8 Gy. Note that the Medin et al.[208] study of single-fraction irradiation of the swine spinal cord shows a steep dose–response curve with a median effective D_{max} of 20 Gy.

Special Situations. The need to reirradiate previously treated cord is often encountered in the setting of recurrent spine metastases following spinal irradiation or new spine lesions within a previously treated lung, pancreas, or esophageal field. In evaluating reirradiation of the spinal cord, the dose regimen for each course, the volume and region (re)irradiated, and the time interval between the courses of radiation therapy must be considered.[209] Animal studies support a time-dependent model of repair for radiation damage to the spinal cord.[196,210–214] For example, Ang et al.[196] treated the thoracic and cervical spines of rhesus monkeys to 44 Gy and then reirradiated these animals with an additional 57 Gy at 1 to 2 years or 66 Gy at 2 to 3 years, yielding aggregate doses of 101 and 110 Gy, respectively. Of 45 animals evaluated, four developed myelopathy by the end of the observation period. The reirradiation tolerance model developed from these and similar data[210] estimates a recovery of 34 Gy (76%), 38 Gy (85%), and 45 Gy (101%) at 1, 2, and 3 years, respectively. Under conservative assumptions, an overall recovery of 26 Gy (61%) was calculated.

Table 13.7 summarizes published reports involving reirradiation of the spinal cord in humans using both conventional and full-circumference external-beam radiotherapy.[209,215–227] For purposes of comparing different regimens, an α/β ratio of 3 Gy was used to calculate the biologically equivalent dose in Gy_3. In all of these studies, the median interval between courses was at least 6 months, and only a small number of cases were treated at intervals <6 months. Note that few cases of myelopathy are reported despite large cumulative doses, with essentially no cases of myelopathy observed for cumulative doses <60 Gy in 2 Gy equivalent doses. These observations are consistent with the predictions of postradiotherapy repair observed in the animal models.

As discussed earlier, radiosurgery at a high dose per fraction is increasingly employed in the treatment of spinal lesions. Though reports of toxicity are rare, the follow-up time is short and patient numbers small. Prudence should be observed when prescribing the dose and every reasonable effort made to limit the dose to the cord by immobilization, image guidance, and attention to patient comfort. Estimates of toxicity based on conventional fractionation should not be applied to such treatments without further careful study.

Recommended Dose–Volume Limits. With conventional fractionation of 2 Gy per day including the full cord cross-section, total doses of 50 Gy, 60 Gy, and ~69 Gy are associated with a 0.2%, 6%, and 50% rate of myelopathy. The level of acceptable risk will depend on the clinical scenario; that is, a 5% risk of myelopathy may be acceptable in treatment of a primary spinal cord tumor but not in irradiation of a lung lesion. For reirradiation of the full cord cross-section at 2 Gy per daily fraction after prior conventionally fractionated treatment, cord tolerance appears to increase at least 25% 6 months after the initial course of RT. In spine radiosurgery, a maximum cord dose of 13 Gy in a single fraction or 20 Gy in three fractions appears associated with a <1% risk of myelopathy. In comparison, Sahgal et al.[228] recommend a *de novo* single-fraction maximum point dose to the thecal sac of 10 Gy to avoid myelopathy entirely, and RTOG protocol 0631 specifies a cord D_{10} and $D_{0.35mL}$ of 10 Gy and D_{max} of 14 Gy for the involved spine.

Future Studies. A model of dose/volume/outcome for spinal cord toxicity will require that more extensive and detailed data be collected over many years, including data on entire cohorts of patients treated with radiotherapy and radiosurgery, not just those with myelopathy. Dosimetric parameters to be collected should include D_{max}, D_1, D_{10}, D_{50}, $D_{0.1mL}$, $D_{0.35mL}$, and $D_{1\,mL}$, and the volume of the involved segment of the spinal cord, as well as the prescribed total dose, dose per fraction, involved spinal level(s), portion of the vertebral body irradiated, irradiation technique, and patient characteristics/demographics. In addition, preclinical studies identifying the fundamental mechanisms of radiation-induced toxicity would be valuable.

Toxicity Scoring Criteria. Toxicity should be scored and reported using CTCAE v. 4.0.[91]

TABLE 13.7 TRANSVERSE MYELOPATHY IN REIRRADIATION OF THE SPINE

Reference	*Cases of Myelopathy/ Total Patients*	*Median F/U (Months)*	*BED, Initial Course (Gy_3) Median (Range)*	*BED, Reirradiation (Gy_3) Median (Range)*	*Interval Between Courses (Months) Median (Range)*	*Total BED (Gy_3) Median (Range)*	*2-Gy Dose Equivalent, $\alpha/\beta = 3$ Gy Median (Range)*
Wright et al.[227]	0/37	8	60 (10–101)	16 (5–50)	19 (2–125)	79 (21–117)	47 (13–70)
Langendijk et al.[219]	0/34	–	–	–	–	<100	<60
Nieder et al.[209,216,221]	0/15	30	70 (34–83)	50 (38–83)	30 (6–96)	115 (91–166)	69 (54–100)
Schiff et al.[224]	4/54	4[a]	60	37	10 (1–51)	97	58
	4		*All 60*	*73[b] (29–115)*	*9 (5–21)*	*133 (109–175)*	*80 (65–105)*
Ryu et al.[223]	0/1	60	75	72	144	147	88
Kuo et al.[218]	0/1	8	75	42	37	117	70
Bauman et al.[215]	0/2	>3–9	(40–56)	(18–35)	(8–20)	(58–91)	(35–57)
Sminia et al.[225]	0/8	–	56 (29–78)	42 (36–83)	30 (4–152)	106 (65–159)	64 (39–96)
Magrini et al.[220]	0/5	168	47 (32–47)	55 (33–67)	24 (12–36)	94 (80–113)	57 (48–68)
Rades et al.[222]	0/62	12	29 (29–47)	29 (29–47)	6 (2–40)	69 (59–77)	41 (35–46)
Jackson and Ball[217]	0/6	15	All 73	36 (32–39)	15	106 (103–109)	63 (62–65)
Wong et al.[226]	11/-[c]	*11*	*72 (28–96)*	*42 (14–86)*	*11 (2–71)*	*115 (100–138)*	*69 (60–83)*

[a]Overall survival.

[b]One patient received two courses of reirradiation; another received three courses.

[c]Total number of patients not reported.

After Kirkpatrick JP, van der Kogel AJ, Schultheiss TE. Radiation dose-volume effects in the spinal cord. *Int J Radiat Oncol Biol Phys* 2010;76(3 Suppl):S42–S49.

NECK

Larynx and Pharynx

Clinical Significance. Radiation therapy is often utilized as the primary treatment of early-stage laryngeal cancers in an effort to preserve speech and swallowing. However, radiation-induced progressive edema and associated fibrosis can lead to long-term problems with phonation and swallowing.[229] Irradiation of the pharynx and larynx, particularly in combination with concurrent chemotherapy, can produce severe dysphagia, compromising nutrition, protection of the airway, and quality of life.

Endpoints. The critical larynx-specific endpoints examined were laryngeal edema and vocal function.[230] Dysphagia, resulting from laryngeal and/or pharyngeal dysfunction, may be assessed by instrument-based swallowing studies,[231] by observer-based criteria (e.g., CTCAE v. 4.0[91]), or by patient-reported quality-of-life questionnaires.

Challenges Defining Volumes. Phonation and swallowing are complex processes involving multiple anatomic structures in close proximity to one another. The relative importance of various normal tissue structures affecting vocal function and swallowing is controversial. In studying vocal dysfunction, doses to the epiglottis, base of tongue, lateral pharyngeal walls, pre-epiglottic space, aryepiglottic folds, false vocal cords, upper esophageal sphincter, and cricoid cartilage have been considered.[230,232,233] Radiation-induced dysphagia has been correlated with the dose to the pharyngeal constrictor muscles and specific points in the supraglottic and glottic larynx.[232,234–237] Precise identification of these structures for treatment planning requires a high-resolution, contrast-enhanced CT scan.

Dose/Volume/Toxicity Data. On multivariate analysis, Sanguineti et al.[233] found that the mean laryngeal dose or percentage of volume receiving >50 Gy and neck stage were the only independent predictors of grade 2 or greater laryngeal edema. Vocal function is usually well preserved after radiotherapy for stage T1 laryngeal cancer[230] (typically 60 to 66 Gy). Less information is available regarding voice quality after treatment of more locally advanced laryngeal cancers. However, Dornfeld et al.[232] found a strong correlation between speech quality and the doses delivered to the aryepiglottic folds, pre-epiglottic space, false vocal cords, and lateral pharyngeal walls at the level of the false vocal cords. In particular, a steep decrease in vocal function was observed when the dose to these structures exceeded 66 Gy.

In a prospective study using intensity-modulated radiotherapy to reduce dysphagia in patients undergoing chemoradiation, Feng et al.[235] observed a strong correlation between the mean doses and the dysphagia endpoints (Fig. 13.6). Aspiration was observed when the mean dose to the pharyngeal constrictors was >60 Gy and the dose–volume threshold for the pharyngeal constrictor volume receiving ≥40, ≥50, ≥60, and ≥65 Gy was 90%, 80%, 70%, and >50%, respectively. For aspiration to occur, the glottic/supraglottic larynx dose–volume threshold was >50% of volume receiving ≥50 Gy. In a retrospective study of conventional radiotherapy, Jensen et al.[236] found that doses <60 Gy to the supraglottic area, larynx, and upper esophageal sphincter were associated with a low risk of aspiration. Dornfeld et al.[232] found that swallowing difficulties increased progressively with radiation doses >50 Gy to the aryepiglottic folds, false vocal cords, and lateral pharyngeal walls near the false cord. Levendag et al.[237] reported that a median dose of 50 Gy to the superior and middle pharyngeal constrictor muscles predicted a 20% probability of dysphagia and that this increased significantly beyond a mean dose of 55 Gy.

Factors Affecting Risk. The addition of concurrent chemotherapy to high-dose RT at least doubles the risk of laryngeal edema and dysfunction.[230] Severe laryngeal dysfunction secondary to tumor will often persist following radiotherapy, and a laryngectomy may be preferred to chemoradiation in this setting.

Mathematic/Biologic Models. Rancati et al.[238] fit dose–volume data for grade 2 to 3 laryngeal edema using the Lyman-Kutcher-Burman model and the logit model with the

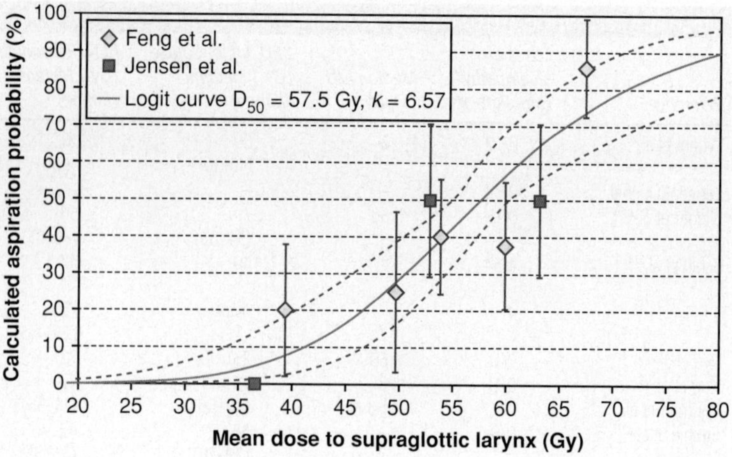

FIGURE 13.6. Probability of aspiration (proxy for dysphagia) versus larynx dose for selected studies.[235,236] Solid line fit of logit model to combined data; dotted lines represent 68% confidence area. (From Rancati T, et al. Radiation dose-volume effects in the larynx and pharynx. *Int J Radiat Oncol Biol Phys* 2010;76[3 Suppl]:S64–S69.)

dose–volume histogram reduced to the equivalent uniform dose (EUD). Both models fit the clinical data well. The best fit parameters for the Lyman-Kutcher-Burman model were n = 0.45 ± 0.28, m = 0.16 ± 0.05, and TD_{50} = 46.3 ± 1.8 Gy. Based on these findings, the investigators suggested an EUD of <30 to 35 Gy to reduce the risk of grade 2 to 3 laryngeal edema. The Feng et al. study[235] suggests that a 50% normal tissue complication probability is observed at mean doses of 50 to 60 Gy to the pharyngeal constrictors and the larynx (Fig. 13.6).

Special Situations. Pretherapy vocal and swallowing function should be considered when assessing the functional response to radiation therapy of the larynx and pharynx.[239]

Recommended Dose–Volume Limits. To minimize the risk of laryngeal edema, the QUANTEC authors recommend limiting the mean noninvolved larynx dose to 40 to 45 Gy and the maximal dose to <63 to 66 Gy, if possible, according to the tumor extent.[230] Minimizing the volume of the pharyngeal constrictors and larynx receiving >60 Gy and reducing, when possible, the volume receiving >50 Gy is associated with reduced dysphagia/aspiration.[230] Of course, the impact of any such dose reduction on tumor control must be considered, given the uncertainties in target delineation.

Future Studies and Toxicity Scoring Criteria. Prospective studies that include pretherapy assessments of vocal and swallowing function should be conducted to correlate observer-rated scores such as the CTCAE v. 4.0 system,[91] patient-reported quality scores, and objective swallowing.[230] Such studies should focus on patients receiving concurrent chemoradiation, as this population is at the greatest risk of laryngeal/pharyngeal toxicity. While CTCAE-based scoring is simple and widely utilized, objective measurement by a speech pathologist is often necessary to quantify swallowing dysfunction following radiotherapy.

Salivary Glands

Clinical Significance. In radiotherapy of head and neck tumors, the parotid, submandibular, and minor salivary glands often receive substantial doses of radiation. Reduced salivary production is a common toxicity and adversely affects the patient's quality of life. Inadequate salivary function leads to multiple problems, including poor dental hygiene, a propensity to oral infections, sleep disturbances, pain, and difficulty chewing and swallowing.[240] The majority of stimulated salivary production comes from the parotid glands, while resting (unstimulated) salivary production is due primarily to the submandibular, sublingual, and numerous small oral salivary glands.[241]

Endpoints. Xerostomia (dry mouth secondary to inadequate saliva production) can be assessed based on the patient's symptoms (altered taste or sensation of dryness) and/or quantitative saliva production.

Challenges Defining Volumes. Parotid and submandibular salivary glands can be adequately delineated on contrast-enhanced CT scans. However, during irradiation, parotid glands typically shrink during RT, potentially resulting in decreased gland sparing. For example, Robar et al.[242] found that while the medial position of the parotid gland was stable over a course of radiation therapy, the lateral borders shrank ~1 mm/week, yielding total displacements of 4 to 6 mm.

Dose/Volume/Toxicity Data. A variety of dose–volume parameters have been correlated with salivary endpoints, including subjective xerostomia and objective stimulated/unstimulated salivary flow. In particular, mean parotid gland dose[242–245] appears associated with whole-mouth or individual gland salivary production. Table 13.8 summarizes the reported dose–volume predictors for salivary flow, the incidence of complications, and salivary function recovery. Minimal reduction in flow is observed at mean doses <10 to 15 Gy, decreases gradually over the range of 20 to 40 Gy, and is markedly reduced above 40 Gy.[243,247] The risk of xerostomia is reduced when at least one parotid gland or submandibular gland is spared.[248] In the study by Portaluri et al., [249] patients receiving <30 Gy to the contralateral parotid reported either no or mild subjective xerostomia.

Some recovery of salivary function occurs over time, with the dose required to obtain an equivalent reduction in salivary flow increasing at longer follow-up times (Fig. 13.7).[245,248,250–253] The whole-mouth or ipsilateral salivary measurement-based tissue dose required for a 50% response (TD_{50}) tends to be lower than the scintigraphy-based TD_{50}, yielding a higher TD_{50} compared with those derived from salivary flow data. The wide variation in the reported TD_{50} values may be the result of several factors, including variations in dose distributions, salivary measurement methods, segmentation, and inherent tissue sensitivity.

Factors Affecting Risk. Patient factors (e.g., gender and age) and the use of chemotherapy have typically not correlated with xerostomia risk. However, pretreatment salivary function and medications affecting salivary function can influence the risk of xerostomia.[240]

Mathematic/Biologic Models. As noted earlier, there is a wide variation in the observed dose/volume/toxicity relationship, depending on the patient population, treatment technique, and endpoint selected. Thus, models predicting the risk of xerostomia as a function of dose–volume parameters have

TABLE 13.8 DOSIMETRIC PREDICTORS OF XEROSTOMIA

Reference	*Patients (n)/Follow-Up*	*Total Prescribed Target Dose (Gy)*^{a}	*Dose–Volume Parameters* *Unstimulated*	*Dose–Volume Parameters* *Stimulated*
Eisbruch et al.[246]	88/1–12 months	58–72	Mean dose ≤22–25 Gy^b V15 <66% V30 <43% V45 <26%	Mean dose ≤25–26 Gy^c V15 <67% V30 <45% V45 <24%
Maes et al.[245]	39/1–4 months	66–70	–	Mean dose ≤20 Gy^d
Blanco et al.[243]	55/6 months 29/12 months	50–71	Mean dose <25.8 Gy	–
Li et al.[244]	142/1–24 months	60–75	Mean dose <25–30 Gy	Mean dose <25–30 Gy

V_x = percentage of gland volume receiving >*x* Gy.

^{a}Treated at 1.5–2.0 Gy per fraction.

^{b}24 Gy at 1 and 3 months, 22 Gy at 6 months, and 25 Gy at 12 months; threshold dose defined as mean dose above which saliva production appeared to abruptly approach zero.

^{c}26 Gy at 1, 3, and 6 months, 25 Gy at 12 months; threshold dose defined as mean dose above which saliva production appeared to abruptly approach zero.

^{d}Corresponds to probability of 70% that loss of salivary excretion fraction was <50%.

yielded a broad range of parameters.[240,243,247,252,255,256] Because the glands seem to respond independently to irradiation, the function of the parotid glands should be modeled separately. Attempts to predict the effect of fraction size on toxicity using the linear-quadratic model have returned low to high α/β ratios, perhaps because the different endpoints examined represent acute versus late effects.[240]

Special Situations. Submandibular gland sparing appears to reduce the risk of both stimulated and unstimulated xerostomia.[248] The mean dose to the oral cavity (which contains minor salivary glands) has been found to be an independent risk factor in some studies[254] but not others,[257] probably because of differences in technique. Although quantitative data are admittedly sparse, amifostine has been shown to increase the functional tolerance of the parotid and submandibular glands to therapeutic radiation.[258]

Recommended Dose–Volume Limits. Severe xerostomia (long-term salivary function <25% of baseline) can usually be avoided if at least one parotid gland receives a mean dose of less than about 20 Gy or if both glands receive a mean dose of less than approximately 25 Gy. In patients with head and neck cancer treated with IMRT, the mean dose to each parotid gland should be kept as low as possible, taking into account the

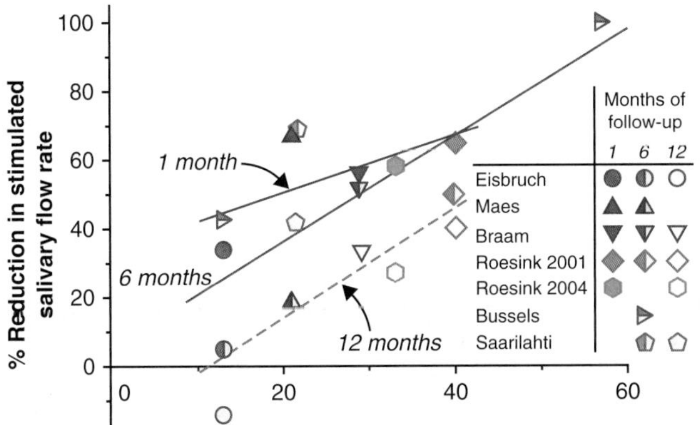

FIGURE 13.7. Mean percentage of reduction in stimulated salivary flow rate versus mean parotid gland dose for selected studies[245,248,250–253,254] using different follow-up durations. Nominal follow-up intervals of 1, 6, and 12 months represent ranges of 1 to 1.5, 6 to 7, and 12 months, respectively. Lines represent least-squares fit of data for each nominal follow-up interval. (From Deasy JO, et al. Radiotherapy dose-volume effects on salivary gland function. *Int J Radiat Oncol Biol Phys* 2010;76[3 Suppl]:S58–S63.)

desired target coverage. Similarly, keeping the dose to the submandibular glands to modest levels (<35 Gy) may reduce the severity of xerostomia.[240]

Future Studies. Key questions on radiation-induced salivary gland dysfunction and xerostomia include:

1. Does partially sparing the submandibular glands or salivary minor glands have a positive impact on quality of life (QOL)?
2. Is the (arbitrary) 25% salivary threshold the best quantitative measure with respect to QOL?
3. Should parotid gland shrinkage during RT explicitly be accounted for in functional predictions?
4. How should submandibular sparing be incorporated into predictive salivary function models?
5. How does oral cavity sparing quantitatively affect xerostomia?
6. Does the radioprotector amifostine provide a clinically significant benefit for whole-mouth salivary function?

Toxicity Scoring Criteria. The QUANTEC authors recommend that an observer-based system (e.g., CTACAE v. 4.0) be supplemented by a validated quality-of life instrument (e.g., the xerostomia questionnaire[254]) and/or quantitative salivary measurements.

CHEST

Lung

Clinical Significance. The lung's primary function is the exchange of oxygen for carbon dioxide. Radiation-associated lung injury is one of the most common side effects seen in clinical oncology, and its risk limits the dose of radiation that can be used for treatment of thoracic tumors.

Endpoints. Radiation damage to the lung can result in symptomatic pneumonitis and fibrosis. Symptomatic radiation pneumonitis is characterized by dyspnea, cough, and occasionally a low-grade fever, typically occurring several weeks to months after radiation. Long-term lung fibrosis can lead to respiratory insufficiency. It is often challenging to distinguish radiation-related pulmonary symptoms from comorbid illnesses (e.g., exacerbation of chronic obstructive pulmonary disease, infection, cardiac events).[259] Objective reductions in the lungs' ability to move and exchange gas can be measured by formal pulmonary function tests (PFTs). The various endpoints shown in Table 13.9 are arbitrarily segregated by their manifestation (clinical vs. subclinical) and whether they reflect regional or global lung function.

TABLE 13.9 ENDPOINTS FOR RADIATION-INDUCED LUNG INJURY

	Geographic Distribution	
Manifestation	*Regional*	*Global*
Clinical	Symptomatic bronchial stenosis	Respiratory symptoms (dyspnea, cough)
Subclinical	Radiologic abnormalities (computed tomography, perfusion/ventilation scans)	Pulmonary function tests, exercise testing results

Challenges Defining Volumes. Because the lungs move and their volume changes with respiration, there are inherent inaccuracies when defining the lung volume. As the mass of the lung is relatively constant during respiration and its density must decline with increased lung volumes, one could consider using dose–mass histograms rather than DVHs. To our knowledge, this approach has not been widely applied. Due to this variation in volumes with respiration, it is very likely that the dose/volume/outcome data are dependent on the type (if any) of respiratory control. The vast majority of dose/volume/outcome data are derived from free-breathing scans/treatment. These may not apply to patients being treated under, for example, breath-hold techniques. Further, there are uncertainties in defining the lung borders in the vicinity of the central airways. Variable inclusion of the conducting airways in the "defined lung" can influence interpatient/institutional comparisons.

Dose/Volume/Toxicity Data. Several parameters have been shown to be associated with the risk of radiation pneumonitis, including V_5 to V_{70}, mean lung dose (MLD), and model-based parameters.[9,260] These dosimetric parameters are mutually correlated, accounting for the fact that in most studies examining a range of V_x's, many appear statistically significant.[261–276] Figure 13.8 summarizes the studies discussed here.

A normal tissue complication probability (NTCP) analysis from the Netherlands, in collaboration with the University of Michigan, suggests that using the MLD (linear function) is more predictive than using V_x (step function).[270] However, V_{13} tended to be more predictive in situations where the MLD exceeded 20 Gy or V_{13} exceeded 50%. The TD_{50} values in this study were an MLD of 30.8 Gy, V_{13} >77%, and V_{20} >65%, similar to the MLD of 31.8 Gy reported in an earlier multi-institutional study.[267] From a study at the Memorial Sloan-Kettering Cancer Center (MSKCC),[276] a mean lung dose of ~26 Gy, V_{13} of >80% to the ipsilateral lung, or V_{40} of >32% to the lower lung results in a 50% risk of developing late complications. A mean lung dose of ~12 Gy or a V_{13} of >40% to the ipsilateral lung results in a 5% late complication risk. A V_{13} of 36% to the lower lung, 42% to the total lung, or 62% to the ipsilateral lung results in a 20% risk of developing late grade 3 or higher complications.

Another study from MSKCC of patients treated with radiation alone reported a significantly increased risk of grade 3 or higher pulmonary toxicity, 38% for V_{25} >30% versus 4% for V_{25} <30% (p = .04).[261] In subsequent studies from this same group, significant variables for predicting grade 3 or higher pulmonary toxicity include mean lung dose, the range of V_5 to V_{40} of

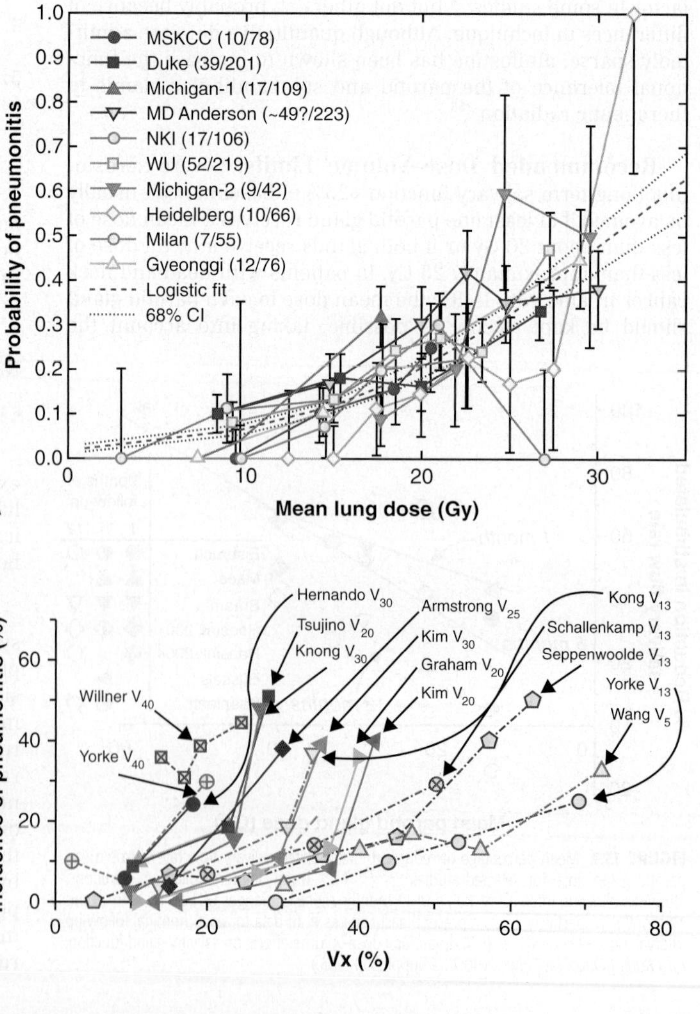

FIGURE 13.8. The rate of radiation pneumonitis after fractionated partial lung radiotherapy as a function of **(A)** mean lung dose (MLD) and **(B)** lung volume receiving *x* Gy (V_x). **(A)** MLD: Confidence intervals (bars) represent ± 1 standard deviation. Results from Memorial Sloan-Kettering Cancer Center (MSKCC),[275] Radiation Therapy Oncology Group (RTOG) grade 3 or higher pulmonary toxicity at 6 months; Duke,[264] Common Terminology Criteria for Adverse Events (CTCAE) grade 1 or higher at 6 months; Michigan,[277] Southwest Oncology Group (SWOG) grade 2 or higher at 6 months; M.D. Anderson Cancer Center,[272] CTCAE grade 3 or higher, 1 year actuarial–includes concurrent chemotherapy patients; Netherlands Cancer Institute (NKI),[278] SWOG grade 2 or higher at 6 months; Washington University (WU),[265] SWOG grade 2 or higher; Michigan,[279] SWOG grade 1 or higher; Heidelberg,[280] RTOG acute grade 1 or higher; Milan,[281] SWOG grade 2 or higher, no time limit, patients without chronic obstructive pulmonary disease, includes induction chemotherapy patients; Gyeonggi,[266] RTOG grade 3 or higher at 6 months, includes concurrent chemotherapy patients. Dashed line is best fit of these data fit to the logistic expression of the form [f/(1 + f)], where f = exp(b0 + b1 * MLD). Best-fit values (95% confidence intervals) are b0 = −3.87 (−3.33, −4.49) and b1 = 0.126 (0.100, 0.153), corresponding to TD_{50} = 30.75 (28.7, 33.9) Gy and γ_{50} = 0.969 (0.833, 1.122), where γ_{50} represents the increase in response (measured as percentage) per 1% increase in dose around the 50% dose–response level. **(B)** V_x. Data from Yorke,[275] Willner,[273] Hernando,[364] Tsujino,[282] Kong,[277] Armstrong,[283] Kim,[266] Graham,[260] Seppenwoolde,[270] Wang,[272] and Schallenkamp.[269] Some of the above data were modified or derived from the original publications, as described in Marks et al.[284] (From Marks LB, et al. Radiation dose-volume effects in the lung. *Int J Radiat Oncol Biol Phys* 2010;76[3 Suppl]:S70–S76.)

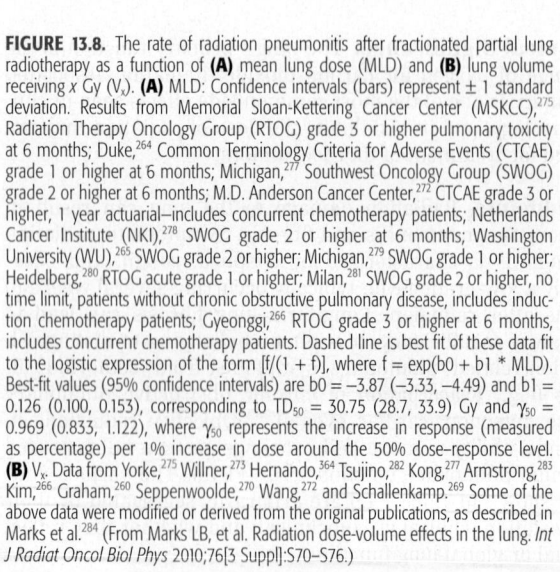

total lung, V_5 to V_{40} of ipsilateral lung, and V_5 to V_{50} of lower lung.[275,276] The range of V_5 to V_{20} ipsilateral lung was most predictive.

Washington University was another of the early investigators to show the risk of pneumonitis significantly correlates with the V_{20}; the 2-year incidence of grade 2 or higher radiation pneumonitis was 36%, 13%, 7%, and 0% with a V_{20} of >40%, 32% to 40%, 22% to 31%, and <22% ($p = .0013$), respectively.[260] In another study by Washington University, radiation pneumonitis was significantly correlated with V_5 to V_{80}, with peak significance in the V_5 to V_{15} and V_{70} to V_{75} ranges; radiation pneumonitis was also significantly correlated with the dose delivered to 5% to 100% of the lung (D_5 to D_{100}), with peak significance in the D_{30} to D_{40} and V_{90} to V_{95} ranges.[265]

A study from Duke, in which 18% of patients received concurrent chemoradiotherapy, found that a V_{30} of >18% versus <18% was associated with a risk of grade 1 or higher radiation pneumonitis of 24 versus 6% ($p = .0003$).[264] MLDs of <10, 10 to 20, 21 to 30, and >30 Gy were associated with risks of 10%, 16%, 27%, and 44%, respectively. A Japanese study of patients treated with platinum-based chemoradiotherapy found a 6-month risk of grade 2 or higher radiation pneumonitis to be 85%, 51%, 18.3%, and 8.7% ($p < .0001$) with a V_{20} of ≥31%, 26% to 30%, 21% to 25%, and ≤20%, respectively.[282] In a University of Michigan study, a 10% risk for grade 2 or higher pneumonitis and fibrosis was associated with a V_{20} of >30% and an MLD of >20 Gy. These thresholds provided a positive predictive value of 50% to 71% and a negative predictive value of 85% to 89%.[277] In a study from M.D. Anderson Cancer Center (MDACC), the mean lung dose and V_5 to V_{65} were highly correlated with risk of pneumonitis, and V_5 was the most significant factor in a multivariate analysis.[272] For a V_5 ≤42% versus >42%, the risk of grade 3 or higher pneumonitis at 1 year was 3% versus 38% ($p = .001$). In a Mayo Clinic study, V_{10} to V_{13} was most predictive of radiation pneumonitis; a V_{10} = 32% to 43%, V_{13} = 29% to 39%, V_{15} = 27% to 34%, and V_{20} = 21% to 31% resulted in a 10% to 20% risk of pneumonitis.

Several dose-escalation studies have used V_{20}, V_{eff}, and/or NTCP to stratify the risk of toxicity as a function of dose.[285–288] In the RTOG 93-11 dose-escalation study,[285] patients with a V_{20} of <25% experienced a 7% to 16% 18-month actuarial rate of grade 3 or higher late lung toxicity with prescribed doses of 70.9 to 90.3 Gy; the absolute risk of grade 2 or higher late lung toxicity was 30% to 45%, with one fatal lung complication at the 90.3 Gy dose level. Patients with a V_{20} of 25% to 36% treated to doses of 70.9 to 77.4 Gy experienced 15% grade 3 or higher late toxicity at 18 months and an 40% to 60% risk of grade 2 or higher late lung toxicity. D_{15} was the most predictive variable for radiation pneumonitis.[262]

Factors Affecting Risk. The effect of dose to regions of the lung was investigated in a Dutch study,[278] dividing the lung into central and peripheral; ipsilateral and contralateral; caudal and cranial; and anterior and posterior subvolumes. The mean regional doses to the posterior, caudal, ipsilateral, central, and peripheral lung subvolumes were significantly correlated with the incidence of steroid-requiring radiation pneumonitis. In a similar study from MSKCC, the risk of radiation pneumonitis was better correlated with the radiation dose to the inferior, as opposed to the superior, aspect of the lung.[276]

Tumor location within the chest may also be a factor affecting risk of pneumonitis. In the study from Washington University,[265] inferior tumor location was the most significant predictor of radiation pneumonitis. Tumor location was not a strong correlate with radiation pneumonitis in RTOG 93-11, perhaps attributable, in part, to differences in treatment (with RTOG 93-11 treating smaller volumes to higher doses) and differences in tumor size and location (the RTOG 93-11 tumors tended to be smaller and more superiorly located).[262] Using a combined dataset of patients from RTOG 93-11 and Washington University, tumor location and MLD were significant predictors of toxicity.

Mathematic/Biologic Models. Most of the aforementioned studies used NTCP models to fit the toxicity data. In the QUANTEC analysis,[284] a fit of the data for radiation pneumonitis as a function of MLD to the logistic expression (see Fig. 13.7) yields a predicted TD_{50} = 30.8 Gy (95% confidence interval [CI], 28.7 to 33.9 Gy) and γ_{50} = 0.97 (0.83 to 1.12). The latter parameter represents the percent increase in radiation increase in response per 1% increase in dose at the 50% dose–response level. A fit using the probit response function (equivalent to a fit of the Lyman model with $n = 1$) yields TD_{50} = 31.4 Gy (95% CI, 29.0 to 34.7 Gy) and m = 0.45 (0.39 to 0.51), with the result essentially identical to that of the logistic fit in the region occupied by the data.

Special Situations. IMRT provides unique dose distributions for some patients with advanced-stage non–small-cell lung cancer,[289] potentially reducing the risk of normal tissue injury. Investigators at MDACC compared rates of lung toxicity in their patients treated with IMRT versus 3D planning and noted a reduction in toxicity with the use of IMRT.[290] A V_5 >70% was associated with a 21% risk of grade 3 or higher pneumonitis versus a 2% risk with V_5 ≤70% ($p = .017$). Similarly, a study from MSKCC found a low rate of clinical lung injury in patients with non–small-cell cancer treated with IMRT.[291]

In a study from Dana Farber,[292] in which patients received thoracic IMRT after pneumonectomy for mesothelioma, six of 13 patients developed fatal pneumonitis. The median V_{20}, V_5, and MLD for patients who developed pneumonitis was 17.6%, 98.6%, and 15.2 Gy, respectively, versus 10.9%, 90%, and 12.9 Gy for those who did not develop pneumonitis. While these differences were not significant, the severity of the toxicities suggests caution in treating patients to large volumes after a pneumonectomy. In a study from Duke,[293] one of 13 patients treated with IMRT for mesothelioma died from pneumonitis, and two others developed symptomatic pneumonitis. The median V_{20}, V_5, and MLD for patients developing pneumonitis were 2.3%, 92%, and 7.9 Gy, respectively, versus 0.2%, 66%, and 7.5 Gy for those who did not develop pneumonitis and 6.9%, 92%, and 11.4 Gy for the patient who developed fatal pneumonitis. In a study of mesothelioma patients treated at MDACC,[294] six of 63 died from pulmonary-related causes (including two patients with fatal pneumonitis). The V_{20} was significant on univariate and multivariate analyses ($p = .017$), with V_{20} >7% corresponding to a 42-fold increase in the risk of pulmonary death.

Stereotactic body radiotherapy (SBRT) generally involves a few large fractions (e.g., three 18-Gy or five 10-Gy fractions) given over 5 to 20 days.[295–296,297] Typically, the high-dose volumes in SBRT are small and dose gradients steep, minimizing dose to surrounding critical structures. However, because multiple beams are used, large volumes of lung receive low to medium doses.[297] Consequently, the dose–volume characteristics of lung SBRT are quite different from those of conventional RT and deserve special consideration. Radiation pneumonitis is relatively uncommon after SBRT, usually <10%[296,298,299] but as high as 25% in one study.[300] Bronchial injury/stenosis, an unusual complication with conventional dose fractionation,[301] has been associated with SBRT to perihilar/central tumors.[296]

Recommended Dose–Volume Limits. Individual studies note a dose–response relationship for radiation pneumonitis based on a variety of metrics. However, the QUANTEC analysis[284] of the pooled data shows that there is no specific threshold for pneumonitis, with risks increasing gradually as dose increases. Since many dose–volume parameters of the lung (i.e., V_5 through V_{30}, MLD) are correlated with each other, there likely is not an "optimal" parameter. For patients with non–small-cell lung cancer, it is prudent to limit the V_{20} to <30% to 35%, and the mean lung dose to <20 to 23 Gy, in order to reduce the risk of pneumonitis to <20%. In patients irradiated after pneumonectomy for mesothelioma, it is prudent to limit the V_5 to below 60%, V_{20} to <4% to 10%, and the mean lung dose to <8 Gy.

Future Studies. Radiation-induced pneumonitis appears more commonly in patients with lower versus upper lobe tumors and may be better correlated with radiation doses to the lower versus upper lung. The cause of this correlation is presently unknown and requires further investigation, though it may be related to heart irradiation. Additional work is needed to better understand the impact of clinical factors (e.g., preradiotherapy functional status, tobacco use) and systemic agents (e.g., chemotherapy) on the risk of lung injury. Studies aimed at determining and exploiting the ability of biomarkers such as TGF-β (measured before and/or during lung radiotherapy) on radiation pneumonitis would be valuable.

Toxicity Scoring Criteria. The LENT-SOMA system should be used for scoring toxicity as it explicitly captures symptomatic, functional, and radiographic endpoints. A global score can be generated, but the granular data should be recorded and maintained.

Heart

Clinical Significance. The heart is a muscular organ typically located in the left hemithorax, which, via continuous rhythmic contraction, pumps blood throughout the blood vessels. The functional and structural complexity of the heart places it at risk for a spectrum of radiation and chemotherapy injuries that can manifest months to years following therapy.[302]

Endpoints. All components of the heart and pericardium are susceptible to radiation damage. Radiation-induced cardiac injury includes pericarditis, congestive heart failure, restrictive cardiomyopathy, valvular insufficiency and stenosis, coronary artery disease, ischemia, and infarction.

Challenges Defining Volumes. The substructures of the heart, as well as the intersection/border of the heart, great vessels, liver, diaphragm, and stomach, can be challenging to delineate on CT imaging. The heart moves during the respiratory and cardiac cycles, with different regions moving to different degrees. The uncertainties that accompany these anatomic/physiologic realities must be considered when contouring targets and normal tissue structures and when interpreting DVHs.

Dose/Volume/Toxicity Data. Multiple studies show an increased risk of cardiac morbidity following left- versus right-sided thoracic radiation in patients undergoing treatment for breast cancer. It is generally recognized that reducing the dose prescribed to the mediastinum and reducing the volume of heart in the radiation field reduce the risk of late toxicity.[303–304,305] Recent studies from Duke demonstrated that an increased percentage of the left ventricle irradiated correlates with a greater risk of cardiac perfusion defects.[306–307,308] Even over the range of low dose exposure (~8 to 20 Gy) to small volumes of the cardiac apex, an increased risk of heart disease has been reported.[309]

A study from Stockholm used normal tissue complication probability modeling to predict the risk of late heart toxicity in women treated for breast cancer.[310] The models predicted a TD_{50} of 52 Gy for dose to the myocardium. A 5% risk of excess cardiac mortality at 15 years was associated with a myocardial dose of ~30 Gy, V_{33} >60%, V_{38} >33%, *or* V_{42} >20%. Calculations using the whole-heart volume (as opposed to myocardium) yielded equivalent results.

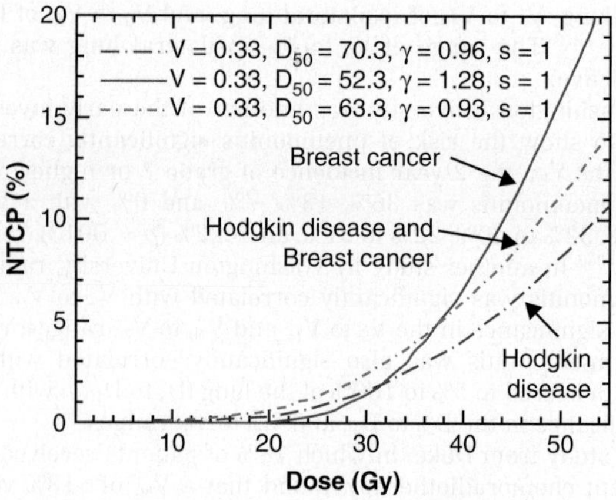

FIGURE 13.9. Dose–response curves for long-term cardiac mortality in patients with Hodgkin disease (HD) and breast cancer treated with thoracic radiotherapy. NTCP = normal tissue complication probability, defined in that study as the excessive risk of ischemic heart disease. Curves were obtained by fitting data from breast cancer trials, a cohort of patients with Hodgkin disease, and the combined dataset. Plotted curves correspond to uniform irradiation of one-third of the heart volume. (From Eriksson F, et al. Long-term cardiac mortality following radiation therapy for Hodgkin's disease: analysis with the relative seriality model. *Radiother Oncol* 2000;55[2]:153–162.)

The same group from Stockholm used a similar analysis to assess cardiac risk in Hodgkin disease patients.[311] Patients were stratified based on a V_{38} >35% versus <35%. The excess mortality risk at 15 years was 7.9% and 4.7%, respectively. The TD_{50} was calculated to be 70 Gy. Heart doses of 42 and 53 Gy resulted in a 5% and 10% risk of cardiac complications, respectively. The corresponding values in the breast cancer patients were 37 Gy and 44 Gy, respectively (lower threshold doses and steeper gradient). The differences in complication probabilities and TD_{50} between the breast cancer and Hodgkin disease cohorts (Fig. 13.9) suggest that radiation exposure to different portions of heart results in differences in cardiac risk, though there may be other confounding variables (i.e., patient age at treatment, overlapping breast cancer and cardiac disease risk factors, etc.).

A study from MDACC described the risk of pericardial effusions in patients treated for esophageal cancer.[312] A mean dose >26 Gy and relative volumes of the pericardium treated at doses greater than 3 to 50 Gy (V_3 to V_{50}) showed the greatest risk, with the association strongest at V_{30}. For V_{30} <46% versus >46%, the rate of pericardial effusion was 73% versus 13% (p = .001) 18 months postradiation. For a mean pericardium dose <26 Gy versus >26 Gy, the rate of pericardial effusion was 73% versus 13% (p = .001). A study from the University of Michigan[313] also demonstrated that a mean dose >27 Gy and a maximum dose of 47 Gy correlated with risk of pericardial effusion. However, only patients treated with 3.5-Gy fractions developed pericardial effusions.

The incidence of valvular disease has been related to mediastinal radiation doses >30 Gy and younger age at irradiation.[314] Subclinical valvular disease has been detected at 2 to 20+ years postradiation, but it appears to take much longer for clinical symptoms to become apparent (median interval 22 years from radiation to symptoms). For patients treated for Hodgkin lymphoma more than 10 years prior with radiation, aortic disease, usually consisting of mixed stenosis and regurgitation, is more common than mitral and right-sided valvular disease.[314,315]

Factors Affecting Risk and Special Situations. Anthracycline chemotherapy can exacerbate radiation-elated cardiac toxicity. In Hodgkin disease patients, radiation exposure, in conjunction with anthracyclines, may impair ejection fraction and increase risk of myocardial infarction, congestive heart failure, and valvular disorders. A Dutch study[316] of 1,474 Hodgkin lymphoma survivors showed that risks of myocardial infarction and congestive heart failure were significantly increased, with standard incidence ratios of 3.6 and 4.9, respectively, for these survivors versus the general population. Mediastinal radiation alone increases the risks of myocardial infarction, angina pectoris, congestive heart failure, and valvular disorders (two- to sevenfold). The addition of anthracyclines further elevated the risks of congestive heart failure and valvular disorders, with hazard ratios of 2.81 and 2.10, respectively. The 25-year cumulative incidence of congestive heart failure following combined radiation and anthracycline chemotherapy was 7.9%.

Other risk factors for cardiac disease, particularly coronary artery disease, also must be considered. For example, a University of Rochester study[317] assessed the risk of coronary artery disease in survivors of Hodgkin lymphoma and also the prevalence of cardiac risk factors. The relative risk of cardiac death was 3.1 for males versus 1.8 for females. Other risk factors were more common than in the general population; among patients with Hodgkin lymphoma experiencing morbid cardiac events, 72% smoked, 72% were male, 78% had hypercholesterolemia, 61% were obese, 28% had a positive family history, 33% had hypertension, and 6% had diabetes.

Mathematic/Biologic Models. There are no well-accepted models for cardiac toxicities. Nevertheless, several authors have computed model parameters for various cardiac endpoints, as summarized in the QUANTEC review.[302]

Recommended Dose–Volume Limits. A heart V_{30} to V_{40} of ~30% to 35% is associated with a ~5% excess risk of cardiac death at ~15 years. A heart V_{30} of >45% and a mean cardiac dose of >26 Gy are associated with a higher risk of pericarditis. In patients with breast and lung cancer, it is recommended that the irradiated heart volume be minimized as much as possible without compromising target coverage. In patients with lymphoma, the whole heart should be limited to 30 Gy if treated with radiation alone and to 15 Gy for patients also receiving anthracycline chemotherapy. Although there is no direct evidence that eliminating traditional cardiac risk factors alters the natural history of radiation-associated cardiac disease, it seems prudent to minimize such factors.[302,318,319]

Future Studies. Issues that would benefit from further systematic study are the effects of radiation on specific subvolumes of the heart, the impact of modern radiotherapy techniques on cardiac toxicity, the relationship between heart irradiation and baseline cardiovascular risk factors on the development of cardiac disease, the effect of hypofractionation encountered in thoracic stereotactic body radiotherapy, and the global physiologic effects of thoracic radiotherapy (e.g., interactions between simultaneous heart and lung irradiation.)[302]

Toxicity Scoring Criteria. The QUANTEC authors recommend that the LENT-SOMA system[93,320] be considered to describe cardiac toxicity, as it explicitly includes clinical, radiologic, and functional assessments of cardiac dysfunction.

Esophagus

Clinical Significance. Acute esophagitis is very common and often severe in patients receiving radiation for intrathoracic malignancies (e.g., primary lung cancer and esophageal cancer). Patients with severe esophagitis may require a feeding tube and/or treatment interruptions.

Endpoints. Because most patients with thoracic cancers have a poor prognosis, acute toxicity may be considered more clinically relevant than late injury. Late esophageal complications include dysphagia, stricture, dysmotility, odynophagia, and rarely necrosis or fistula.

Challenges Defining Volumes. The esophagus can be challenging to visualize on axial imaging, and the use of dilute oral contrast can assist in its identification. Also, the esophagus often has folds such that its external contour as seen on an axial image may not accurately represent its true circumference. Indeed, in CT imaging the circumference of the esophagus appears highly variable on different axial levels, when in fact the esophagus has a relatively uniform circumference. One study has suggested that the dosimetric parameters that apply this prior anatomic knowledge are better predictors of acute and late esophageal injury than are traditional dosimetric parameters.[321]

Dose/Volume/Toxicity Data. A variety of dose–volume parameters have been associated with the incidence of esophagitis.[312,322–329] While a continuous dose–response curve for acute esophagitis is observed based on a range of dosimetric parameters, as shown in Figure 13.10, there is no consensus as to the optimal dosimetric predictors of acute or late esophageal injury.

In a series from Washington University, grade 3 to 5 esophageal toxicity (acute and late) was associated with a maximal dose (D_{max}) of >58 Gy, a mean dose of >34 Gy, and the administration of concurrent chemotherapy.[328] The V_{55} was not significant. A study from China reported that maximal dose >60 Gy, as well as the use of concurrent chemotherapy, was a significant factor for esophageal toxicity (acute and late).[327] In a study from Duke, V_{50}, the surface dose receiving ≥50 Gy (S_{50}), the length of esophagus receiving >50 to 60 Gy, and a circumferential D_{max} >80 Gy were significant predictors of late esophageal toxicity.[326] A V_{50} >32% or an S_{50} >32% resulted in crude rates of ~30% late esophageal toxicity versus 7% below these thresholds. With >3.2 cm of the esophagus receiving >50 Gy, late toxicity occurred in ~30%, versus 4% in those with <3.2 cm receiving >50 Gy (p = .008).

In another study from Duke, grade 1 or higher late toxicity was correlated with several dose parameters: the entire circumference receiving ≥50 Gy and ≥55 Gy; 75% of the circumference receiving ≥70 Gy; and maximal percentage of circumference receiving ≥60 to 80 Gy.[322] The rate of grade 1 or higher late toxicity was ~5% in patients with a V_{50} to V_{70} of 0% to 30% versus ~25% in those with a V_{70} of 31% to 64% and ~10% in those with a V_{50} >60% (nonsignificant). Acute esophageal toxicity was

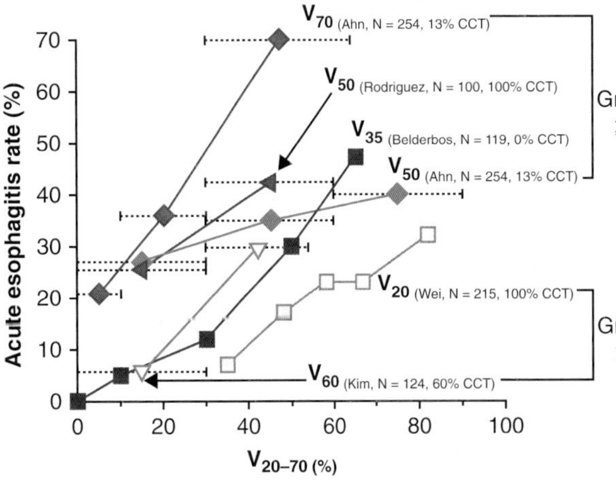

FIGURE 13.10. Incidence of acute esophagitis according to V_x (volume receiving more than x Gy) for selected studies. x-Axis values estimated from range of doses reported. Datasets annotated as follows: V_{dose} (investigator, number of patients, percentage with concurrent chemotherapy [CCT]). (From Werner-Wasik M, et al. Predictors of severe esophagitis include use of concurrent chemotherapy, but not the length of irradiated esophagus: a multivariate analysis of patients with lung cancer treated with nonoperative therapy. *Int J Radiat Oncol Biol Phys* 2000;48[3]:689–696.)

the greatest predictor of late toxicity. In two studies, most of the patients who developed late grade 3 or higher toxicity had developed acute grade 3 or higher toxicity, though roughly 25% to 40% of patients who developed grade 3 or higher late toxicity had only grade 0 to 2 acute esophageal toxicity.[327,328]

Factors Affecting Risk. Greater rates of acute esophagitis have been observed with more aggressive radiotherapy regimens (e.g., hyperfractionation, concurrent boost), the addition of concurrent chemotherapy, increasing age, and several other clinical factors (e.g., pre-existing dysphagia and increasing nodal stage). The incidence of grade 3 or higher acute esophagitis is ~1% for patients treated with once-daily radiotherapy alone versus as high as 49% with concurrent gemcitabine. Several studies have assessed the putative radioprotector amifostine. Three single-institution phase III studies suggested a benefit for amifostine in reducing the rate of grade 2 or higher esophagitis, but this result was not confirmed in a large cooperative group phase III randomized trial (RTOG trial 9801).[330–333]

Mathematic/Biologic Models. Using data on grade 2 or higher acute esophagitis, two studies obtained relatively consistent estimates of Lyman-Kutcher-Burman model parameters, including TD_{50} of 47 to 51 Gy.[7,323] Note that these parameters differ significantly from those derived from the Emami data,[4] which examined a more clinically severe endpoint (stricture and perforation).

Special Situations. Esophageal toxicity data for hypofractionated treatments in stereotactic body radiotherapy to central thoracic lesions are quite limited,[334] and long-term data in this and other altered fractionation settings (e.g., accelerated fraction and concomitant boosts) have not been comprehensively reported.[335]

Recommended Dose–Volume Limits. Given the available data, there are no strict dose–volume limits for the esophagus. Several parameters are associated with the risk of adverse events, and clinicians can apply these data as seems reasonable for the clinical situation. Unfortunately, the anatomic reality for many patients with locally advanced non–small-cell lung cancer is that the PTV (and certainly the GTV) is often immediately adjacent to the esophagus, and thus, it is not possible to limit the doses as desired without compromising target coverage. The ongoing phase III intergroup trial, RTOG 0617, has recommended (but has not mandated) that the mean dose to the esophagus be kept to <34 Gy.

Future Studies. IMRT may provide increased flexibility in sparing the esophagus during lung irradiation, and outcome as function of dose–volume should be systematically studied for this treatment technique. As in other organ systems, detailed outcome and dosimetric data should be reported, based on clearly defined methods of contouring the target and organs at risk.

Toxicity Scoring Criteria. Esophageal toxicities should be scored using the CTCAE v. 4.0.[37]

ABDOMEN/PELVIS

Liver

Clinical Significance. The liver is a vital organ, involved in the metabolism of ingested nutrients, detoxification, protein synthesis, bile production, glycogen storage, and red blood cell decomposition. The liver may be incidentally irradiated during radiation therapy of abdominal or thoracic tumors and will be irradiated in patients undergoing partial hepatic radiation for liver metastases or hepatocellular carcinoma. There is no effective treatment to reverse the process of radiation-induced liver disease (RILD); therefore, prophylaxis and prevention are best. Anticoagulants, paracentesis, and diuretics can be used to mitigate symptoms, while liver transplantation is required for frank radiation hepatopathy.

Endpoints. RILD generally presents as vague to intense right upper abdominal pain followed by abdominal swelling due to hepatomegaly and ascites, resulting in weight gain. Anicteric ascites often develops 2 to 4 months after irradiation; chemoradiation-induced liver disease may occur more rapidly (e.g., 1 to 4 weeks post radiation therapy in a bone marrow transplantation setting). Other sequelae of RILD include elevation of liver enzymes, jaundice, asterixis (tremor), encephalopathy, or coma.

The basic pathophysiologic sequelae of classic RILD is central vein thrombosis at the lobular level, which results in retrograde congestion leading to hemorrhage and secondary alterations in surrounding hepatocytes. This often occurs between 2 weeks and 3 months after therapy. Severe acute hepatic changes often progress to fibrosis or cirrhosis and liver failure.

Nonclassic RILD implies dramatic elevations of liver transaminases (greater than five times the upper limit) or decline in liver function in the absence of classic RILD. The underlying pathology of nonclassic RILD is unclear.[336]

Challenges Defining Volumes. The liver is readily identified on CT and MRI. For radiation planning, it must be recognized that the liver moves with the respiratory cycle.[336]

Dose/Volume/Toxicity Data. The liver parenchyma is composed of innumerable, redundant, parallel functional subunits, which allows the liver to potentially tolerate focal injury without clinical sequelae if adequate normal liver parenchyma can be spared.

In a study of 79 patients treated with liver radiotherapy at the University of Michigan, nine of 33 patients who received whole-liver radiotherapy developed late radiation toxicity versus none of 46 who underwent partial liver radiation.[337] Several studies have explored partial liver radiation in more detail, many of which used mean liver dose as a dose–volume metric (Table 13.10). In a series from Taipei, patients with irradiated hepatocellular carcinoma who developed late liver toxicity had received a mean hepatic dose of 25 Gy (vs. 20 Gy in patients without toxicity, $p = .02$).[346] In a Korean study of 105 patients with hepatocellular carcinoma, the mean dose and V_{20} to V_{40} parameters to total liver and normal liver (total liver minus GTV) were investigated.[345] The total liver V_{30} was the only significant parameter ($p < .001$). Grade 2 or higher liver toxicity was observed in only 2.4% of patients with a total liver V_{30} of ~60% and 55% of patients with a total liver V_{30} of >60% ($p < .001$).

Factors Affecting Risk and Mathematic/Biologic Models. A wide variety of agents have been reported to elevate liver enzymes: nitrosoureas (BCNU), methotrexate, and some combinations of chemotherapy agents such as cyclophosphamide, doxorubicin, vincristine, and prednisone (CHOP) and proMace-MOPP (prednisone, methotrexate, doxorubicin, cyclophosphamide, etoposide, and MOPP). In bone marrow transplantation, preparatory regimens can be toxic.

As described earlier, the dose to partial liver volumes can impact the risk of RILD. Several studies have used NTCP modeling to help predict risks. In a study from University of Michigan, no late liver toxicity was observed with a mean liver dose <31 Gy, with normal tissue complication probability models being optimized with a TD_{50} of 43 Gy and TD_5 of 31 Gy for whole-liver radiation; the risk of complications was strongly dependent on volume of liver irradiated.[338] Other risk factors for late toxicity included primary hepatobiliary carcinoma (as

TABLE 13.10 RADIATION-INDUCED LIVER DISEASE IN PARTIAL LIVER IRRADIATION

Reference	*n/% C-P A*	*Diagnosis*	*Dose Fractionation*	*Crude Rate of RILD*	*Mean Normal Liver Dose in Patients with vs. without RILD*
Michigan[338,339]	203/100%	PLC + LMC	1.5 Gy bid	9%	37 vs. 31.3 Gy
Taipei[340]	89/76%	HCC	1.8–3 Gy qd	19%	23 vs. 19 Gy
Shanghai[341,342]	109/85%	PLC	4–6 Gy qd	16%	24.9 vs. 19.9 Gy
Guangdong[343]	94/46%	HCC	4–8 Gy qd	17%	Not stated
S. Korea (Seong et al.)[344]	158/74%	HCC	1.8 Gy qd	7%	Not stated
S. Korea (Kim et al.)[345]	105/81%	HCC	2.0 Gy qd	12%	25.4 vs. 19.1 Gy

% C-P A, percent of patients with baseline Child-Pugh A score (in all studies, patients were either A or B); RILD, radiation-induced liver disease; PLC, primary liver cancer; LMC, metastatic disease to the liver; bid, twice-daily treatment; HCC, hepatocellular carcinoma; qd, once-daily treatment.

After Pan CC, et al. Radiation-associated liver injury. *Int J Radiat Oncol Biol Phys* 2010;76(3 Suppl):S94–S100.

opposed to metastatic disease), use of bromodeoxyuridine chemotherapy (as opposed to fluorodeoxyuridine), and male gender. The normal tissue complication probability models predict a TD_5 in excess of 80 Gy if less than one-third of the liver is irradiated. With irradiation of two-thirds of the liver, the TD_5 is on the order of 50 Gy and TD_{50} on the order of 60 Gy.

In the series of hepatocellular carcinoma patients from Taipei (discussed earlier),[346] the TD_{50} for whole-liver, two-thirds liver, and one-third liver radiation was modeled to be approximately 43 Gy, 50 Gy, and 67 Gy, respectively. The TD_5 for whole-liver, two-thirds liver, and one-third liver radiation was modeled to be approximately 25 Gy, 28 Gy, and 38 Gy, respectively. The volume effect of liver radiation was less in this series. In another study from the same group, the mean liver dose and hepatitis B virus positivity were significant predictors of radiation toxicity; with NTCP modeling, the TD_{50} was ~50 Gy.[340]

The data from Asia differs from that in the West, perhaps reflecting differences in the treated malignancy (mostly metastases in the West vs. primary liver cancer in Asia, which often occurs in the setting of liver cirrhosis), as shown in Figure 13.11. In addition, radiation fractionation, concurrent therapies delivered with radiation, and the fact that the majority of patients with hepatocellular carcinoma from Asia have hepatitis B viral infections may impact liver tolerance.[336] Poor preexisting liver function is also predictive of poorer tolerance to radiation.[336]

Special Situations. The hypofractionated delivery of radiation, using novel techniques such as SBRT and/or image-guided radiation therapy (IGRT), for primary and metastatic liver lesions presents a unique situation in which small volumes of normal liver receive very high doses of radiation per fraction. In a collaborative phase I study, the University of Colorado and Indiana University enrolled 18 patients with one to three liver metastases treated with three fractions of SBRT.[347] No patients developed grade 2 or higher toxicity. Late radiographic changes of well-circumscribed hypodense lesions were commonly seen, corresponding to the 30-Gy dose distribution. In a follow-up analysis, including an additional 18 patients treated in a phase II study of three fractions of 20 Gy, one patient developed subcutaneous tissue breakdown; no radiation-related liver toxicity occurred.[348] In a subsequent study, in which ≥700 mL of normal liver was required to receive <15 Gy in three fractions, no patient experienced RILD.[349]

Princess Margaret Hospital treated 41 patients with primary hepatocellular or intrahepatic biliary cancer in a phase I study of 24 to 60 Gy in six fractions.[350] Using normal tissue complication modeling, patients were stratified into three different dose-escalation groups, based on the effective liver volume to be irradiated. Acute (<3 months) elevation of liver enzymes occurred in 24%, acute grade 3 nausea occurred in 7%, and acute transient biliary obstruction occurred in 5% of patients. In contrast, among 68 patients with liver metastases treated similarly with SBRT, two patients (3%) developed grade 3 liver enzyme changes, but no RILD or other grade 3 or higher liver toxicity was reported.[351]

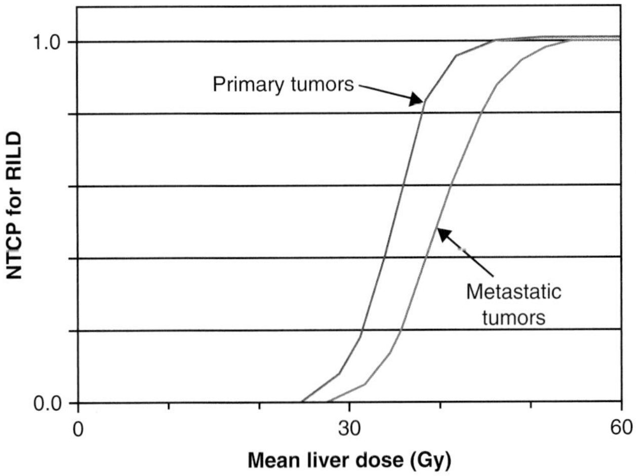

FIGURE 13.11. Mean liver dose, corrected with linear-quadratic modeling for 2-Gy fractions versus Lyman normal tissue complication probability (NTCP) of classic radiation-induced liver disease (RILD) for primary and metastatic liver cancer. (From Pan CC, et al. Radiation-associated liver injury. *Int J Radiat Oncol Biol Phys* 2010;76[3 Suppl]:S94–S100.)

Recommended Dose–Volume Limits. For patients with liver metastases undergoing partial-volume liver radiation, the risk of radiation-induced liver toxicity appears to be more dependent upon the volume of liver irradiated. Partial volumes of liver can tolerate relatively high doses. Liver tolerances, however, are lower for patients with primary liver cancer (who are more apt to have underlying liver disease). For whole-liver radiation, doses ≤28 to 30 Gy in 2-Gy fractions (28 Gy for liver metastases and 30 Gy for primary liver cancer) and ≤21 Gy in 3-Gy fractions are recommended. For partial-liver radiation, treated with standard fractionation, the mean dose to normal liver (liver minus GTV) is suggested to be <30 Gy for liver metastases and <28 Gy for primary liver cancer.

Future Studies. Studies that better correlate dose–volume parameters with long-term clinical/objective outcomes are needed. The impact of treatment-related (including fractional dose and systemic therapies) and host-related variables should be better defined.

Toxicity Scoring Criteria. The CTCAE v. 3.0 grades hepatobiliary toxicity according to clinical criteria of jaundice, asterixis, and encephalopathy or coma for grades 2, 3, and 4, respectively. The much more commonly occurring alteration in liver enzymes, in the absence of symptomatic manifestations, is classified under the CTCAE metabolic/laboratory category of elevations of alanine aminotransferase (ALT) and aspartate aminotransferase (AST). The use of CTCAE criteria for elevations of AST and ALT and other metabolic effects is advisable to promote consistency of reporting.

Small Bowel/Stomach

Clinical Significance. The stomach and small bowel aid in the digestion and absorption of food and nutrients. Symptoms from radiation-related late toxicities include dyspepsia, gastric ulceration, diarrhea, bowel obstruction, and ulceration, fistula, or perforation.[352]

Endpoints. Nausea and vomiting can occur immediately or within hours after RT to the stomach or small bowel. The radiosensitivity of the gastric mucosa is reflected in the early depression of hydrochloric acid and pepsin secretion after modest radiation doses of 15 to 20 Gy. Although some recovery of cellular structure occurs, suppression can continue for 6 months to many years after irradiation. Usually, at total doses at or above 50 Gy, cellular and functional recovery is never complete. Ulcers are the most common complication of gastric irradiation and present clinically with dyspepsia, significant pain, and sometimes hemorrhage. An ulcer in this anatomic setting can lead to hemorrhage and perforation, which, although rare, can be fatal. Ulcerations have been described as typically antral, perhaps because of placement of radiation therapy fields, and develop as early as 2 to 12 months after treatment. Pyloric obstruction may be a late development due to fibrosis after ulcer healing.

The early onset of malabsorption of fat and hypermotility after modest doses of radiation illustrates the radiosensitivity of the small intestine. Usually, recovery at dose levels below 40 to 45 Gy occurs, although some persistence of small bowel dysfunction and mesenteric cramping may be noted. Surgical intervention and adhesions can precipitate a more serious course of events. Higher doses result in diarrhea, malabsorption of fat, and leakage of albumin into the bowel. If an obliterative arteritis develops, the risk of infarction and perforation remains despite recovery. The underlying lesion is one of ulceration and segmental enteritis that can lead to stenosis of the bowel lumen, with varying degrees of obstruction during the chronic period.

Challenges Defining Volumes. The stomach and small bowel are well visualized, particularly with the use of intravenous contrast and/or oral contrast. The stomach and small bowel position can be variable, and it is therefore recommended that patients avoid large meals or carbonated beverages prior to simulation and treatment.

Dose/Volume/Toxicity Data. Because stomach and small bowel are mobile and distensible, determining accurate dose–volume (or dose–surface) constraints is challenging. Late radiation-induced stomach injury has been reported to occur with increasing frequency with increasing doses. In a study from Walter Reed, the rates of gastric ulceration were 4% and 16% after treatment of <50 versus >50 Gy, respectively. Similarly, the rates of perforation were 2% and 14% in the same dose cohorts, respectively. Overall, the dose of approximately 50 Gy to the stomach is associated with about a 2% to 6% incidence of severe late injury. The volume effect for late stomach injury is not well defined. For late small bowel toxicity, doses of approximately 50 Gy are associated with obstruction/perforation rates that are approximately 2% to 9%.

There is a paucity of good quantitative data on dose–volume metrics that predict for gastric or bowel late toxicity. Nevertheless, there are data that demonstrate a volume effect. The risk of bowel obstruction among patients with rectal cancer whose fields extended to L1 or L2 was 30% versus 9% in those treated with pelvis-only fields.[353] The University of Michigan investigated gastric and duodenal bleeding after radiation of patients with liver tumors.[354] Normal tissue complication modeling was consistent with a dose threshold (~60 Gy) for bleeding without a large volume effect.

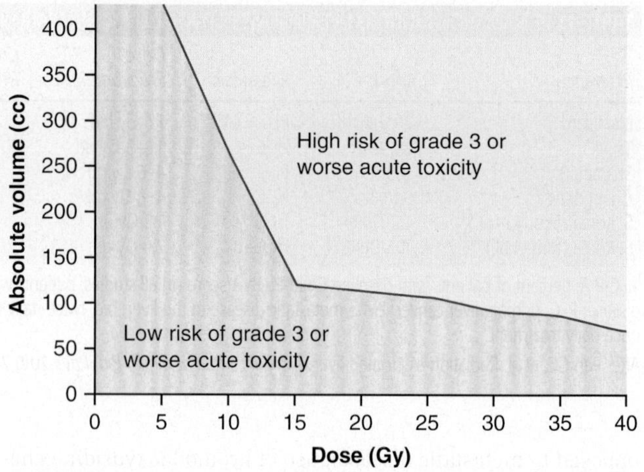

FIGURE 13.12. Graphic representation of the Baglan–Robertson[356,357] threshold model for acute small bowel toxicity. "Low risk" implies <10% and "high risk" >40% grade 3 toxicity. Absolute volume is based on contouring individual bowel loops, not the entire peritoneal space. (From Kavanagh BD, et al. Radiation dose-volume effects in the stomach and small bowel. *Int J Radiat Oncol Biol Phys* 2010;76[3 Suppl]:S101–S107.)

Factors Affecting Risk. Factors affecting risk of late toxicity include total dose (with doses in excess of 40 to 50 Gy increasing the risk of late complications), fractional dose, prior abdominal surgery (which increases the risk of bowel obstruction), and concurrent chemotherapy use. In the European Organisation for Research and Treatment of Cancer (EORTC) Hodgkin lymphoma study, the rate of complications was 3% without prior abdominal surgery versus 12% with prior abdominal surgery.[355]

Mathematic/Biologic Models. The University of Michigan analyzed gastric bleeding among patients treated with radiation for liver tumors.[354] Variables significantly impacting bleeding risk included NTCP, mean dose to stomach, and presence of cirrhosis. Data from William Beaumont Hospital has suggested that the volume of bowel exposed to radiation doses of >5 to 40 Gy correlates with risk of acute grade 3 toxicity; their studies[356,357] and others have shown small bowel V_{15} to be highly significant ($p < .0001$).[358] The model results are graphically depicted in Figure 13.12. Using NTCP modeling for patients undergoing preoperative radiation for rectal cancer, IMRT has been shown to reduce the anticipated rate of grade 2 or higher diarrhea from 40% to 27% (with further reductions if IGRT is also used).[352]

Special Situations. High-grade small bowel mucositis, ulceration, and perforation, as well as acute gastroparesis, have been reported in patients undergoing hypofractionated SBRT for pancreatic malignancies,[359] though the reported rate of such grade 3 to 4 toxicities (albeit in a patient population with poor survival) has been relatively low in U.S. studies.[360–362] Among patients undergoing three- to five-fraction SBRT for liver metastases, bowel toxicity has been reported to occur with maximal doses to the bowel of >30 Gy.[336]

Recommended Dose–Volume Limits. Using the entire potential small bowel space, it is suggested that the small bowel exposed to V_{45} to V_{50} should be <195 mL to reduce acute toxicity (not discussed earlier)[352,363]; while using the visualized loops of bowel, it is recommended that the V_{15} should be <120 mL.[352,356] While these dose constraints were derived from acute toxicity data, they do provide guidelines that should help minimize risk of late toxicity as well. For the stomach, it is recommended to maintain the dose to the whole stomach to <45 Gy; a maximum point dose might be an important predictor of toxicity, but more data are needed to confirm this hypothesis.

Future Studies. More detailed dose–volume effects for late bowel toxicity are needed, particularly for altered fractionation (i.e., SBRT). As many gastrointestinal cancers are treated with chemotherapy, data on the impact of chemotherapy on acute and late stomach and bowel toxicity are needed.

Toxicity Scoring Criteria. The CTCAE v. 4.0 is used to grade gastric and small bowel toxicity.[91]

Kidneys

Clinical Significance. The kidney functions to remove wastes; regulate electrolytes; produce erythropoietin, which stimulates red blood cell production; and modulate blood pressure through the renin-angiotensin pathway as well as through fluid/electrolyte balance. Radiation nephropathy is an uncommonly reported toxicity, not because kidneys are radioresistant, but because clinicians carefully respect renal tolerance doses.

Endpoints. Five distinct clinical syndromes may overlap in symptoms, signs, and time sequence: acute radiation nephropathy, chronic radiation nephropathy, benign hypertension, malignant hypertension, and hyperreninemic hypertension secondary to a scarred encapsulated kidney (Goldblatt kidney). The signs (i.e., decreased glomerular filtration rate) and symptoms of radiation nephropathy are not distinguishable from other causes of renal damage, and these should be excluded. Acute (within 6 months) radiation-induced kidney injury is generally subclinical. Urinary findings consist of microscopic hematuria, proteinuria, and urinary casts. Blood alterations in β_2-microglobulin correlate linearly with both inulin and creatinine clearance and with later elevations of blood urea nitrogen (BUN). There is a 6- to 12-month latency period before the clinical expression of acute radiation nephropathy. In this subacute phase, the signs and symptoms include dyspnea, headaches, ankle edema, lassitude, anemia, hypertension, albuminuria, papilledema, elevated blood urea, and urinary abnormalities (granular and hyalin casts, red blood cells). Death may occur from chronic uremia or left ventricular failure, pulmonary edema, pleural effusion, and hepatic congestion. Chronic radiation nephropathy and hypertension do not develop until after 12 to 18 months. When chronic nephropathy is severe, death may result.

Challenges Defining Volumes. The kidneys are readily defined on contrast and noncontrast CT imaging. Ideally, the "functional" kidney parenchyma as opposed to the collecting system should be contoured.

Dose/Volume/Toxicity Data. Several studies have investigated whole-kidney dose tolerance, either after whole-abdominal radiation or total-body irradiation (generally delivered with lower fractional doses). Renal toxicity can occur after bilateral kidney doses ≥10 Gy, and the risk is quite high (50% to 80%) after 20 Gy. Thus, the kidneys have a relatively low threshold for damage. The dose–volume effect on the kidneys has been long recognized, even prior to the planning CT era, because kidneys are well visualized on plain simulation films. From these studies, when greater than half of the kidney receives doses >20 to 30 Gy, or greater than one-third receives >30 to 40 Gy, patients are at increased risk of developing renal atrophy, decreased kidney function, and hypertension.[1,364–365,366]

There is little published on dose–volume parameters to predict late renal toxicity, in part because clinicians make an effort to minimize the volume of kidney exceeding the accepted tolerance dose. Low doses, 10 to 15 Gy, to large volumes of kidney increase the risk of nephrotoxicity,[77,367,368] while smaller volumes of kidney with doses exceeding ~20 to 25 Gy can result in late renal toxicity.[77,367,369,370] In a series from Heidelberg, normal tissue complication modeling was used to estimate the risk of late complications.[369] A median dose of ~17.5 to 21.5 Gy and 22 to 26 Gy corresponded to a 5% and 50% late complication risk (anemia, azotemia, hypertension, and edema), respectively. In another German study, reduced kidney function, as measured by scintigraphy changes, was analyzed as a function of dose and volume.[367] After irradiation of 10% to 30%, 30% to 60%, and 60% to 100% of the kidney volume to 20 Gy, the incidence of reduced activity was <10%, ~40%, and >70%, respectively. After irradiation of 10% to 30%, 30% to 60%, and 60% to 100% of the kidney volume to 30 Gy, the incidence of reduced activity was ~35%, >90%, and >98%, respectively. In a Dutch study of patients with gastric cancer (treated with concurrent radiation and cisplatin or capecitabine), the left kidney V_{20} of ≥64% and mean left kidney dose of ≥30 Gy were associated with a significant decrease in left kidney function as compared to the right.[370]

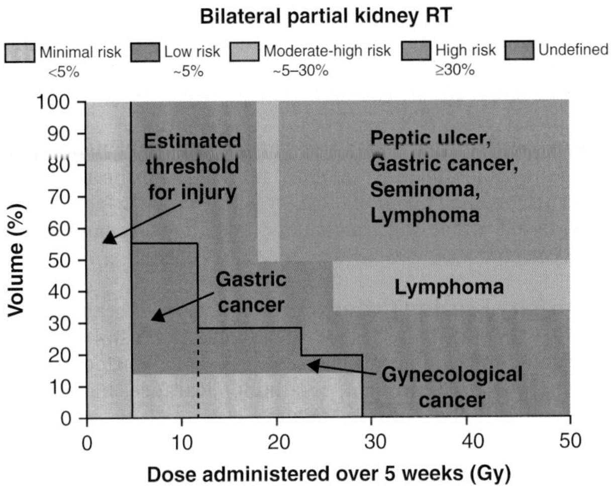

FIGURE 13.13. Schematic diagram of bilateral kidney dose–volume histogram from selected studies, represented as regions associated with minimal (<5%), low (~5%), moderate to high (~5% to 30%), high (>30%), or undefined estimated risk of toxicity. Clinical situation that yielded risk estimates for each region is also indicated. Actual risks are patient and plan specific and are associated with substantial uncertainty. (Adapted from Dawson LA, et al. Radiation-associated kidney injury. *Int J Radiat Oncol Biol Phys* 2010;76[3 Suppl]:S108–S115.)

Recognizing the limitations described earlier, the QUANTEC study summarized the toxicity data for bilateral kidney irradiation in Figure 13.13.

Factors Affecting Risk. A variety of agents have been implicated as toxic or as radiosensitizers (i.e., retinoic acid, cisplatin, BCNU, actinomycin D), administered either singly or in combination chemotherapy. Of note, angiotensin-converting enzyme (ACE) inhibitors and angiotensin II receptor blockers have been shown to delay the progression of radiation injury in the experimental setting.[371] Total-body irradiation (TBI) dose rates (≤6 cGy/minute versus ≥10 cGy/minute) have been shown to significantly impact risk of renal toxicity.[372] Patient-related factors may include underlying renal insufficiency, diabetes, hypertension, liver disease, heart disease, and smoking.[373]

Special Situations. Several reports have described the use of SBRT in the treatment of medically unresectable kidney cancer and/or in patients with only one functioning kidney. With limited follow-up, SBRT with high dose (≥10 Gy) has been reportedly well tolerated.[373]

Recommended Dose–Volume Limits.[373] For whole (bilateral) kidney radiation, doses <10 Gy delivered over five to six fractions (at a <6 cGy/minute dose rate) and <15 to 18 Gy for radiation delivered over ≥5 weeks are recommended. For partial-kidney radiation, the volume of kidneys receiving

>20 Gy predicts risk of renal toxicity. The recommendation for partial-kidney radiation is to maximally spare the kidneys and maintain a mean dose of <18 Gy to both kidneys, or maintain a V_6 <30% if one kidney cannot be adequately spared.

Future Studies. Studies are needed to better define partial kidney tolerance to radiation, investigating the impact of underlying kidney function, dose–volume exposure (accounting for regional variation), fractionated dose delivery, and radiation protectors.

Toxicity Scoring Criteria. The CTCAE v. 4.0 can be used to grade renal toxicity.[91] Severity of injury can also be graded according to the glomerular filtration rate, serial urine protein, serum blood urea nitrogen, creatinine clearance, blood pressure, and symptoms of renal failure.

Rectum

Clinical Significance. The rectum is the terminal portion of the large intestines that functions as a temporary storage for feces, as well as providing the urge to defecate. A portion of the rectum is irradiated in patients undergoing radiation for prostate cancer, gynecologic cancers, and other pelvic tumors (such as sarcomas).

Endpoints. Acute rectal toxicity includes diarrhea or loose stools, tenesmus, proctitis, and rectal urgency and/or frequency. The most common late radiation-related rectal complication is bleeding. Rectal ulceration and fistula are much less common. Other late injuries include stricture and decreased rectal compliance, which can result in frequent small stool and/or tenesmus. The anus is also at risk of late complications including stricture and laxity, leading to fecal incontinence.

Challenges Defining Volumes. The rectum extends from the rectosigmoid junction to the anus, with the inferior extent variably defined as the level of the anal verge the ischial tuberosities or 2 cm below the ischial tuberosities, or above the anus (the most inferior 3 cm of the intestines). The rectum should be segmented from above the anal verge to the turn into the sigmoid colon, though the superior and inferior borders of the rectum are not always easy to define on CT imaging, and definition of the cranial and caudal extents is variable.[374] The rectum is mobile and distensible, and therefore its position and volume can vary between and during radiation fractions.

The percentage of rectum or rectal wall receiving a given dose can be somewhat subjective (i.e., based on how much of the rectum is segmented); using the absolute volume of rectum[375] or rectal wall is less subjective, though defining the rectal wall is not standardized. William Beaumont Hospital demonstrated that the rectal volume as well as rectal wall V_{50} to V_{70} values predict late toxicity, with the rectal wall being more predictive of grade 2 to 3 late effects; acute toxicity is also predictive of late toxicity.[376] MDACC has also shown the rectal wall to be better predictive of late rectal bleeding.[377]

Review of Dose/Volume/Toxicity Data. Abundant dosimetric data have shown a correlation of risk with rectal volume and surface/rectal wall doses among patients undergoing radiation for prostate cancer. Figure 13.14 summarizes many of the studies discussed here.

MSKCC has shown a significant difference in the DVHs between patients who developed rectal bleeding versus those who did not after conformal radiation for prostate cancer.[378] The percent rectum exposed to 62% and 102% of the prescription dose (70.2 or 75.6 Gy) was significant; the rectal wall being encompassed by the 50% isodose line, higher maximal dose to the rectum, and smaller rectal volume were also significantly adverse risk factors.[378,387] In a recent study of 1,571 patients treated at MSKCC, the use of IMRT and the lack of acute rectal toxicity predicted for lower risk of late rectal toxicity.[388]

In a randomized trial of 70 Gy versus 78 Gy from MDACC in the treatment of early- to intermediate-risk early-stage prostate cancer, the risk of grade 2 or higher late rectal complications was significantly greater with a rectal V_{70} ≥25% versus V_{70} <25% (46 vs. 16%, p = .001).[389] A retrospective analysis from MDACC showed that the risk is a continuous function of dose and volume, with suggested cut-off points for lowering the complication risk: V_{60} ≤41%, V_{70} ≤26%, V_{76} ≤16% or 3.8 mL, and V_{78} ≤5% or 1.4 mL.[379] At 6 years, the risk of grade 2 or higher late rectal complications was 54% for patients with a rectal V_{70} ≥26% versus 13% for a V_{70} <26%.

Among patients treated in the Dutch randomized trial of 68 versus 78 Gy for prostate cancer,[390] the mean anal dose (as well as V_5 to V_{60}) significantly predicted the rate of grade 2 or higher gastrointestinal toxicity (at 4 years, 16% vs. 31% for a mean dose of <19 Gy versus >52 Gy).[391] The mean dose (as well as V_5 to V_{70}) also predicted the risk for use of incontinence pads (at

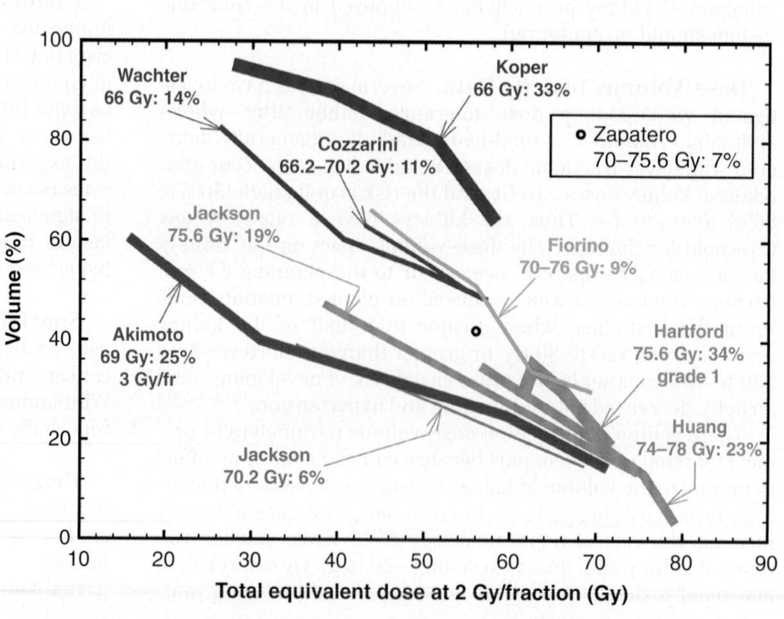

FIGURE 13.14. Dose–volume histogram thresholds for grade 2 or higher rectal toxicity from selected studies.[378,379,380,381,382–386] Thicker lines indicate higher rates of overall toxicity (percentages are indicated on the figure along with the physical prescription dose). Threshold doses are expressed as the total equivalent dose delivered in 2-Gy fractions, adjusted using the linear-quadratic model with $\alpha/\beta = 3$ Gy. The associated equivalent prescription doses are coded by color spectrum from lowest (blue) to highest (red). Volumes shown in the graph are based on the full length of the anatomic rectum. Note that these curves converge in the high dose range, implying that doses in this range are more consistently associated with rectal toxicity. (From Michalski JM, et al. Radiation dose-volume effects in radiation-induced rectal injury. *Int J Radiat Oncol Biol Phys* 2010;76[3 Suppl]:S123–S129.)

5 years, <5% vs. >20% for a mean dose <28 Gy vs. >46 Gy). The anorectal V_{65} (as well as V_{55} to V_{60}) was significantly predictive of rectal bleeding (4-year risk <1% and >10% for a V_{65} <23% vs. >29%).[391] Several other studies have shown that the volume of rectum receiving >50 to 70 Gy has been shown to significantly correlate with late rectal toxicity.[380,381,392,393] From a 1998 Dutch study, recommendations for the volume of rectal wall (vs. rectal volume) exceeding 65 Gy, 70 Gy, and 75 Gy are <40%, <30%, and <5%, respectively.[394] Data from the Cleveland Clinic[375] and William Beaumont Hospital[376] showed a significantly increased risk of grade 2 or higher rectal toxicity with rectal or rectal wall V_{70} to V_{78} of ≥15 mL versus <15 mL (~20% to >30% vs. ~5% to 10%).[376]

Women undergoing radiation for gynecologic malignancies are also susceptible to rectal toxicity. From historical data, the incidence of severe proctitis in patients with cancer of the cervix is dependent on the prescribed point A dose, with a <4% incidence with doses of <80 Gy, a 7% to 8% incidence after 80 to 95 Gy, and a 13% incidence for doses of ≥95 Gy.[395,396] With modern radiation delivery, particularly with IMRT planning, the rate of severe gastrointestinal toxicity is low. In a University of Chicago series of 183 patients treated with conventional radiation and brachytherapy, 9% developed grade 1 to 2 rectal toxicity and 7% developed grade 3 toxicity; a history of diabetes, point A dose, and the pelvic external-beam radiotherapy dose were most significantly correlated with rectal toxicity. Among patients experiencing diarrhea or loose stools after pelvic radiotherapy, rectal toxicity becomes difficult to differentiate from small bowel toxicity. In another report from the University of Chicago, of 50 women treated with pelvic IMRT for gynecologic malignancies, acute gastrointestinal toxicity was correlated with small bowel dose (see above), but not rectum receiving 25% to 110% of the prescription.[244] However, the rectum was constrained to receive <40 Gy to >40% with a maximum dose of 49 Gy.

Factors Affecting Risk. Several patient-related variables, such as history of diabetes and/or vascular disease, inflammatory disease, and age, may impact the risk of late toxicity.[390,397,398] Prior abdominal surgery is also relevant.[399] From 1,010 prostate cancer patients enrolled in the RTOG 94-06, cardiovascular disease was significantly (p = .015) associated with a higher rate of late rectal toxicity, while diabetes, hypertension, rectal volume, rectal length, neoadjuvant hormone therapy, and prescribed dose per fraction (1.8 vs. 2 Gy) were not significant factors.

Mathematic/Biologic Models. Rectal toxicity has been modeled using the Lyman-Kutcher-Burman NTCP model, mostly from patients treated with 3D conformal radiation. Most data are suggestive of a small volume effect, meaning that small volumes receiving high dose are most predictive for late effects.[374] The TD_{50} of grade 2 or higher late rectal toxicity is estimated to be around 77 to 79 Gy (with 95% CIs of ~74 to 82 Gy).[374] From the largest study to date of 1,010 patients enrolled in the RTOG 94-06, the TD_{50} was 79 Gy; the fit based on dose-wall histogram data was not significantly different. Equivalent uniform dose has also been modeled as a predictor of late rectal toxicity.[400]

Special Situations. Stereotactic body radiotherapy for prostate cancer is under investigation. In one study 67 patients were treated with 7.25 Gy × 5, in which rectal DVH goals were $V_{18.1\%}$ <50%, $V_{29\%}$ <20%, $V_{32.6\%}$ <10%, and $V_{36.3\%}$ <5%.[401] Grade 3, 2, and 1 rectal toxicities were seen in 0%, 2%, and 12.5% of patients, respectively. Persistent rectal bleeding was not observed. In another study, after SBRT (9.5 Gy × 4), acute grade 1 to 2 and 3 rectal toxicity occurred in 33% and 0% of patients, respectively, and late grade 1 to 2 and 3 acute genitourinary toxicity occurred in 8% and 0%, respectively.[402] For patients treated with permanent interstitial brachytherapy[403,404] or afterloaded high-dose-rate brachytherapy[405] for prostate cancer (either as monotherapy or as a boost), the dose–volume exposure of rectum has been correlated with late rectal toxicity. Combined external-beam radiation and brachytherapy may lower the threshold for rectal toxicity after prostate brachytherapy.[406]

Recommended Dose–Volume Limits. For patients undergoing radiation therapy in which the rectum is irradiated, it is recommended to limit the rectal V_{50}, V_{60}, V_{65}, V_{70}, and V_{75} to less than 50%, 35%, 25%, 20%, and 15%, respectively. While the data supporting these dose constraints primarily are from prostate cancer patients treated with conventional radiotherapy, studies of patients undergoing IMRT for prostate cancer suggest similar dose constraints.[407]

Future Studies. Future studies should be directed at achieving accurate dose–volume distributions for the rectum, which is a mobile, distensible structure, and correlating these dosimetric characteristics with toxicity. More robust data are needed for hypofractionated radiation delivery to the rectum, as with SBRT or HDR brachytherapy, as well as with low-dose brachytherapy and combined modality approaches.

Toxicity Scoring Criteria. The CTCAE v. 4.0[91] or RTOG scoring criteria can be used to grade rectal toxicity.

Urinary Bladder

Clinical Significance. The bladder is a highly distensible organ that collects urine. Symptoms from late radiation-related toxicities include increased urinary frequency, hematuria, and dysuria. Necrosis, contracted bladder, and hemorrhage are less common, severe effects. Perhaps late bladder toxicity is underreported due to its long latency as well as toxicity being attributed to more common causes.

Endpoints. Bladder injury can be broadly classified as focal damage (e.g., bleeding) or more global injury (e.g., reduced bladder capacity with secondary urinary frequency). Acute side effects from incidental bladder irradiation are common and include urinary frequency, urgency, and dysuria (symptoms that may also reflect acute urethral toxicity). Late effects attributable to global injury include dysuria, frequency, urgency, contracture, spasm, reduced flow, and incontinence. In contrast, late effects arising from focal injury include hematuria, fistula, obstruction, ulceration, and necrosis.

Challenges Defining Volumes. The bladder is a mobile and distensible structure, depending upon the volume of urine within the bladder. Postvoid residuals may vary due to variable emptying and constant filling. In contouring the bladder, either the volume of the bladder and contents or the bladder wall alone can be segmented (with the latter more representative of a surface).

Dose/Volume/Toxicity Data. Because the bladder is mobile and distensible, determining accurate dose–volume (or dose–surface) constraints is challenging. Detailed dose–volume (or dose–surface) constraints have not been published, in part due to the complexities of assigning dose–volume or dose–surface metrics to a mobile, distensible structure. Whole-bladder tolerances have been mostly studied in patients with urinary bladder cancer, while partial bladder tolerances have been mostly studied in patients with genitourinary (mostly prostate) and gynecologic cancers.[408]

For whole-bladder irradiation, doses in excess of 60 Gy, particularly with fraction sizes >2 Gy and/or accelerated radiation regimens, result in a significant risk of grade 3 or higher late toxicity. Risks are lower when the whole bladder receives 45 to 55 Gy followed by a boost to >60 Gy to a portion of the bladder, though toxicity risk has not been correlated to dose–volume metrics. With prostate cancer treated to high doses (≥72 Gy), the inferior portion of the bladder (e.g., trigone area) also receives ≥70 Gy. This tends to be well tolerated with respect to bladder toxicity. Arguably, the urinary toxicity that does develop after radiation is due in part to the prostatic urethra receiving suprathreshold doses.

Factors Affecting Risk. Prior pelvic surgery can result in increased risk of bladder toxicity as a direct result of bladder or urethral trauma and/or denervation of the bladder, which can cause urinary hesitancy or retention, resulting in overflow incontinence.[408] Patients receiving anticoagulants may be at greater risk of hematuria. Cytoxan, independently or with radiation, can cause chronic hemorrhagic cystitis, incontinence, contractions, and vesicoureteral reflux. Radiation-sensitizing chemotherapy may increase risk of acute and late bladder toxicity, though data supporting this are lacking.

Mathematic/Biologic Models. Quantitative mathematic modeling of bladder toxicity is lacking.

Special Situations. Stereotactic body radiotherapy for prostate cancer is an emerging investigative approach. In one study, after SBRT (7.25 Gy × 5), grade 1 to 2 genitourinary toxicity occurred in 28% and grade 3 toxicity was reported in 3% of patients (two patients required cystoscopies and dilatation procedures for dysuria[401]). Urinary incontinence, complete obstruction, or persistent hematuria was not observed. In another study, after SBRT (9.5 Gy × 4), acute grade 1 to 2 and 3 acute genitourinary toxicity occurred in 71% and 0% of patients, respectively, and grade 1 to 2 and 3 late acute genitourinary toxicity occurred in 11% and 5%, respectively; grade 3 toxicity included temporary urinary catheterization and intermittent self-catheterization.[402]

Recommended Dose–Volume Limits. For whole-bladder radiation, the reported risks of grade 3 or higher toxicity in doses of 50 to 60 Gy range from ≤5% to 40%. This variation is likely attributable to the challenges of correlating toxicity with dose delivered to a mobile structure, which is even more problematic when correlating partial volume exposures to toxicity. With the caveat of these issues, bladder constraints of ~15%, 25%, 35%, and 50% receiving ≥80 Gy, ≥75 Gy, ≥70 Gy, and ≥65 Gy, respectively, as recommended in the RTOG 0415 study of prostate cancer, are suggested. The protocol advises an empty bladder at the time of simulation and treatment; the bladder is segmented from the base to the dome.

Future Studies. Studies that incorporate the changing size and shape of the bladder may provide a better understanding of the dose–volume tolerance of the bladder. Incorporating day-to-day variation with adaptive planning DVHs and/or use of deformable modeling would be informative. More detailed studies are needed to assess regional variation in radiation susceptibility (i.e., trigone vs. dome).

Toxicity Scoring Criteria. The CTCAE v. 4.0 or RTOG scoring criteria can be used to grade genitourinary toxicity.

Penile Bulb

Clinical Significance. Radiation dose to the penile bulb can affect erectile function, as a direct result either of damage to this structure or of damage to surrounding structures, whose radiation-induced damage is correlated with the dose exposure of the penile bulb. The most common scenario in which the penile bulb is irradiated is in the treatment of prostate cancer. IMRT is often used to minimize the dose to the penile bulb.[409,410]

Endpoints. Erectile dysfunction reported by the patient can be the result of treatment or other confounding factors including age, medications (particularly hormonal therapy), or comorbid conditions (e.g., diabetes, peripheral vascular disease, hypertension). Objective diagnostic tests can be performed to help establish the etiology of erectile dysfunction; these include nocturnal penile tumescence, somatosensory evoked potentials, bulbocavernous reflex latency, penile electromyography, color duplex Doppler ultrasound, dynamic infusion cavernosometry, and pharmacologic testing.

Challenges Defining Volumes. The anatomy of the pelvic floor is challenging to visualize on CT or MRI and hence definition of the penile bulb is somewhat subjective. The QUANTEC authors recommend defining the penile bulb as the most proximal portion of the penis sitting immediately caudal to the prostate.[411]

Dose/Volume/Toxicity Data. Several studies have investigated dose–volume parameters to predict risk of erectile dysfunction. In several studies, no correlation was discerned for penile bulb dose and erectile function.[409,412,413] In one study attempts were made to reduce the dose to the penile bulb (mean dose of 25 Gy), and thus, few patients received high dose to the penile bulb.[409] In another study of 70 patients, no correlation was found for mean dose or maximal dose to the penile bulb, penile crura, or superiormost 1 cm of the penile crura; DVHs were also compared and found to be similar.[413]

In a small (21 patients), early study from University of California, San Francisco, patients receiving a D_{70} of <40%, 40% to 70%, and >70% to the penile bulb had a 0%, 80%, and 100% risk, respectively, of experiencing radiation-induced impotence.[414] In a study (29 patients) from Thomas Jefferson University, several dose–volume metrics were analyzed; a D_{30} >67 Gy, D_{45} >63 Gy, D_{60} >42 Gy, and D_{75} >20 Gy to the proximal penis were correlated with increased erectile dysfunction as well as decreased ejaculatory function.[415] In a study from Royal Marsden Hospital, a D_{90} >50 Gy to the penile bulb was associated with significantly worse erectile function, while D_{15}, D_{30}, and D_{50} showed a similar (albeit not significant) trend toward increased doses in impotent versus intermediately potent versus potent patients.[416] The largest study (158 patients) to date to investigate penile bulb dose is an analysis of the RTOG 9406 dose-escalation study.[417] A median dose of ≥52.5 Gy was associated with a greater risk of impotence (50% vs. 25% at 5 years).

Factors Affecting Risk. The etiology of erectile dysfunction following radiation is likely multifactorial. In additional to radiation effects, pretreatment erectile function, diabetes, smoking history, and a history of hypertension have been implicated as important factors affecting risk, though the data to date have been somewhat conflicting.[416]

Special Situations. Hormonal therapy, which is commonly used in patients with early-stage intermediate- to high-risk prostate cancer or advanced-stage prostate cancer, in and of itself can result in erectile dysfunction. However, the interaction (if any) of hormonal therapy and dose–volume delivery to the penile bulb is not well established.[411] Proton therapy is a well-established treatment approach for prostate cancer and is becoming more widely utilized as more proton centers are developed. While proton therapy can reportedly lower penile bulb dose, the impact on erectile dysfunction is unknown.[418] Proton therapy may reduce postradiation testosterone suppression.[419] Interstitial brachytherapy (either with high–dose-rate sources using afterloaded catheters or with permanent low–dose-rate seeds) is a standard radiation modality as well. Data correlating erectile function with penile bulb dose from brachytherapy are sparse. In one study, there was no correlation between the penile bulb dose and postbrachytherapy erectile dysfunction.[420] Stereotactic body radiotherapy for prostate cancer is an emerging investigative approach. The impact of hypofractionated SBRT on erectile dysfunction or the dose–volume parameters predictive of risk after prostate SBRT are not well studied. In one small study of 32 patients, penile bulb dose did not correlate with erectile dysfunction.[421]

Recommended Dose–Volume Limits. Based on published data for photon external-beam radiation, the QUANTEC authors recommend keeping the mean dose to 95% of the penile bulb below 50 Gy, and limiting D_{70} and D_{90} to 70 Gy and 50 Gy, respectively.[411]

Future Studies. Studies should be directed at better anatomic definition of the putative anatomic sites impacted by erectile dysfunction and rigorous prospective correlation of dose–volume parameters with erectile dysfunction.

Toxicity Scoring Criteria. Pre- and posttreatment assessment of erectile dysfunction should be performed using the International Index of Erectile Function Scale.[411]

COMPOSITE SUMMARY OF DOSE/VOLUME/OUTCOME DATA

Table 13.11 summarizes the dose/volume/outcome findings in the QUANTEC reviews. Note that clinicians must understand the clinical situations from which the QUANTEC recommendations were derived, and there is no substitute for reading the original QUANTEC papers. At the same time, clinical judgment as applied to a specific patient is essential. In addition to the QUANTEC papers, the Emami paper continues to play an important role in estimating normal tissue toxicity during radiotherapy. Finally, as more comprehensive dose/volume/outcome data are developed—particularly in combination with emerging and evolving chemotherapy regimens—the radiation oncologist will need to continually and critically keep abreast of the clinical literature on normal tissue toxicity.

CLINICAL APPLICATION, LIMITATIONS, AND IMPLICATIONS OF QUANTEC

Implications for Understanding the Underlying Mechanisms of Radiation-Induced Normal Tissue Injury

The consistent structure of the Emami dose–volume limits, and the application of that information to predictive models, may be taken to imply a uniform mechanism of radiation-induced injury. The diversity of the structure of the information obtained in the QUANTEC review suggests a more diverse mechanism of radiation-induced injury. An interorgan comparison of dose–response functions from the QUANTEC review is interesting (Fig. 13.15) and may have implications for our understanding of radiation-induced normal tissue injury.

1. There are marked variations in the dose–response curves for different organs, suggesting that there are different mechanisms for radiation-induced injury in different organs and/or that the endpoints selected for the different organs reflect a varied type of injury.
2. Organs that are classically considered structured in series (e.g., spinal cord, optic nerve, and small bowel, analogous to electrical circuits in series) have steep dose–response curves at doses beyond an apparent critical threshold. This is expected based on our understanding of the structure/anatomy of the series of organs: damage to a functional subunit can render the entire structure dysfunctional.

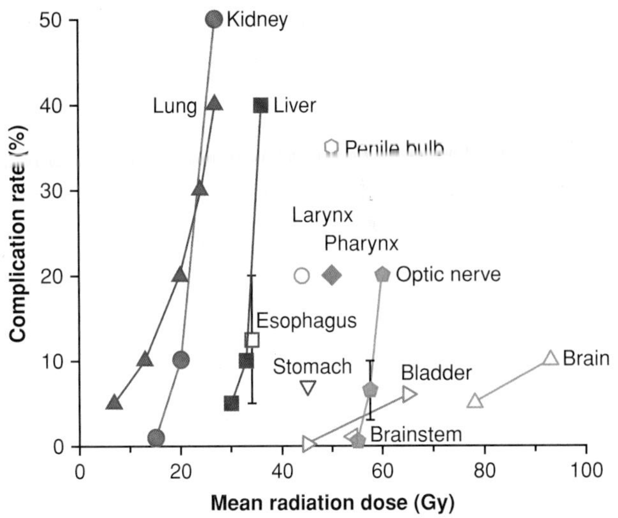

FIGURE 13.15. Composite diagram of normal tissue complication rates versus mean radiation dose.

3. Several neural structures exhibit a similar threshold dose for injury: ≈55 to 60 Gy (corresponding to a BED of ≈100 for an α/β ratio of 3 Gy) for brain, brainstem, optic nerve, and spinal cord. This suggests that there may be a common mechanism of injury in these structures. Because all of these organs are dependent on the vasculature, it is tempting to implicate vascular injury as the common target for these organs.
4. Organs that are classically considered structured in parallel (e.g., lung, liver, parotid, and kidney, analogous to electrical circuits) experience injury at far lower doses and have more gradual dose–response curves compared to series organs. The presence of injury at lower doses suggests that a different mechanism of injury is occurring in these organs as compared to series organs. It appears that these organs each have critical components that are more sensitive to the radiation than are the critical components within the neuronal tissues. It is thus tempting to conclude that subunits such as hepatocytes, nephrons, and alveoli are relatively radiation sensitive.
5. During heterogeneous organ irradiation, the predictive value of mean organ dose in some parallel-structured organs is interesting but counterintuitive. Consider the lung. Relatively uniform fractionated whole-lung doses as high as 15 to 23 Gy have a very low risk of symptomatic pneumonitis. Thus, the lung's "functional subunit" must generally be able to tolerate these doses. However, heterogeneous lung irradiation to a mean lung dose of ≈15 to 23 Gy is associated with a 10% to 25% risk of symptomatic pneumonitis. Thus, during heterogeneous lung irradiation, it is likely that the mean dose is merely a surrogate for the percent of lung exposed to various other doses of radiation. The same may be true in other parallel organs as well.

CONCLUSIONS

The QUANTEC effort is one further step in our field's decades-long effort to better quantify the relationship between dose–volume parameters and clinical outcomes. As the scope of the QUANTEC review was largely limited to organ systems with meaningful dose/volume/outcome data, the review, by itself, is an incomplete tool to guide clinical care. Consistent and clear reporting of dose/volume/outcome data[423] will enable further refinements in clinical guidelines and will hopefully improve patient care.

TABLE 13.11 QUANTEC SUMMARY: CLINICAL DOSE/VOLUME/OUTCOME DATA

Organ	*Volume Segmented*	*Irradiation Type (Partial Organ unless Otherwise Stated)*[a]	*Endpoint*	*Dose (Gy), or Dose–Volume Parameters*[a]		*Rate (%)*	*Notes on Dose–Volume Parameters*
Brain	Whole organ	3DCRT	Symptomatic necrosis	D_{max}	<60	<3	Data at 72 and 90 Gy extrapolated from BED models
	Whole organ	3DCRT	Symptomatic necrosis	D_{max}	72	5	
	Whole organ	3DCRT	Symptomatic necrosis	D_{max}	90	10	
	Whole organ	SRS (single fraction)	Symptomatic necrosis	V_{12}	<5–10 mL	<20	Rapid rise when V_{12} >5–10 mL
Brain stem	Whole organ	Whole organ	Permanent cranial neuropathy or necrosis	D_{max}	<54	<5	
	Whole organ	3DCRT	Permanent cranial neuropathy or necrosis	$D_{1-10\ mL}$	≤59	<5	
	Whole organ	3DCRT	Permanent cranial neuropathy or necrosis	D_{max}	<64	<5	Point dose << 1 mL
	Whole organ	SRS (single fraction)	Permanent cranial neuropathy or necrosis	D_{max}	<12.5	<5	For patients with acoustic tumors
Optic nerve/ chiasm	Whole organ	3DCRT	Optic neuropathy	D_{max}	<55	<3	Given the small size, 3DCRT often covers the whole circumference of the organ[b]
	Whole organ	3DCRT	Optic neuropathy	D_{max}	= 55–60	3–7	
	Whole organ	3DCRT	Optic neuropathy	D_{max}	>60	>7–20	
	Whole organ	SRS (single fraction)	Optic neuropathy	D_{max}	<12	<10	
Spinal cord	Partial organ	3DCRT	Myelopathy	D_{max}	50	0.2	Including full cord cross-section
	Partial organ	3DCRT	Myelopathy	D_{max}	60	6	
	Partial organ	3DCRT	Myelopathy	D_{max}	69	50	
	Partial organ	SRS (single fraction)	Myelopathy	D_{max}	13	1	Partial cord cross-section irradiated
	Partial organ	SRS (hypofraction)	Myelopathy	D_{max}	20	1	3 fractions, partial cord cross-section irradiated
Cochlea	Whole organ	3DCRT	Sensory neural hearing loss	Mean dose	≤45	<30%	Mean dose to cochlea, hearing at 4 kHz
	Whole organ	SRS (single fraction)	Sensory neural hearing loss	Prescription dose	≤14	<25%	Serviceable hearing
Parotid	Bilateral whole parotid glands	3DCRT	Long-term parotid salivary function reduced to <25% of pre-RT level	Mean dose	<25	<20%	For combined parotid glands[c]
	Unilateral whole parotid gland	3DCRT	Long-term parotid salivary function reduced to <25% of pre-RT level	Mean dose	<20	<20%	For single parotid gland. At least one parotid gland spared to <20 Gy[c]
	Bilateral whole parotid glands	3DCRT	Long-term parotid salivary function reduced to <25% of pre-RT level	Mean dose	<39	<50%	For combined parotid glands[c]
Pharynx	Pharyngeal constrictors	Whole organ	Symptomatic dysphagia and aspiration	Mean dose	<50	<20	Based on Section B4 of paper
Larynx	Whole organ	3DCRT	Vocal dysfunction	D_{max}	<66	<20	With chemotherapy
	Whole organ	3DCRT	Aspiration	Mean dose	<50	<30	With chemotherapy
	Whole organ	3DCRT	Edema	Mean dose	<44	<20	Without chemotherapy, based on single study in patients without larynx cancer[a]
	Whole organ	3DCRT	Edema	V_{50}	<27%	<20	
Lung	Whole organ	3DCRT	Symptomatic pneumonitis	V_{20}	≤30%	<20	For combined lung. Gradual dose response
	Whole organ	3DCRT	Symptomatic pneumonitis	Mean dose	7	5	Excludes purposeful whole-lung irradiation
	Whole organ	3DCRT	Symptomatic pneumonitis	Mean dose	13	10	
	Whole organ	3DCRT	Symptomatic pneumonitis	Mean dose	20	20	
	Whole organ	3DCRT	Symptomatic pneumonitis	Mean dose	24	30	
	Whole organ	3DCRT	Symptomatic pneumonitis	Mean dose	27	40	
Esophagus	Whole organ	3DCRT	Grade 3 or higher acute esophagitis	Mean dose	<34	5–20	Based on RTOG and several studies
	Whole organ	3DCRT	Grade 2 or higher acute esophagitis	V_{35}	<50%	<30	A variety of alternate threshold doses have been implicated. Appears to be a dose–volume response
	Whole organ	3DCRT	Grade 2 or higher acute esophagitis	V_{50}	<40%	<30	
	Whole organ	3DCRT	Grade 2 or higher acute esophagitis	V_{70}	<20%	<30	
Heart	Pericardium	3DCRT	Pericarditis	Mean dose	<26	<15	Based on single study
	Pericardium	3DCRT	Pericarditis	V_{30}	<46%	<15	
	Whole organ	3DCRT	Long-term cardiac mortality	V_{25}	<10%	<1	Overly safe risk estimates based on model predictions

TABLE 13.11 (CONTINUED)

Organ	*Volume Segmented*	*Irradiation Type (Partial Organ unless Otherwise Stated)*[a]	*Endpoint*	*Dose (Gy), or Dose–Volume Parameters*[a]		*Rate (%)*	*Notes on Dose–Volume Parameters*
Liver	Whole liver–GTV	3DCRT or whole organ	Classic RILD	Mean dose	<30–32	<5	Excluding patients with pre-existing liver disease or hepatocellular carcinoma, as tolerance doses are lower in these patients
	Whole liver–GTV	3DCRT	Classic RILD	Mean dose	<42	<50	
	Whole liver–GTV	3DCRT or whole organ	Classic RILD	Mean dose	<28	<5	In patients with Child-Pugh A pre-existing liver disease or hepatocellular carcinoma, excluding hepatitis B reactivation as an endpoint
	Whole liver–GTV	3DCRT	Classic RILD	Mean dose	<36	<50	
	Whole liver–GTV	SBRT (hypofraction)	Classic RILD	Mean dose	<13 <18	<5 <5	3 Fractions, for primary liver cancer 6 Fractions, for primary liver cancer
	Whole liver–GTV	SBRT (hypofraction)	Classic RILD	Mean dose	<15 <20	<5 <5	3 Fractions, for liver metastases 6 Fractions, for liver metastases
	>700 mL of normal liver	SBRT (hypofraction)	Classic RILD		<15	< 5	Critical volume based, in 3–5 fractions
Kidney	Bilateral whole kidney[d]	Bilateral whole organ or 3DCRT	Clinically relevant renal dysfunction	Mean dose	<15–18	<5	
	Bilateral whole kidney[d]	Bilateral whole organ	Clinically relevant renal dysfunction	Mean dose	<28	<50	
	Bilateral whole kidney	3DCRT	Clinically relevant renal dysfunction	V_{12} V_{20} V_{23} V_{28}	<55% <32% <30% <20%	<5	For combined kidney
Stomach	Whole organ	Whole organ	Ulceration	D_{max}	<45	<7	
Small bowel	Individual small bowel loops	3DCRT	Grade 3 or higher acute toxicity[e]	V_{15}	<120 mL	<10	Volume based on segmentation of the individual loops of bowel, not the entire potential space within the peritoneal cavity
	Entire potential space within peritoneal cavity	3DCRT	Grade 3 or higher acute toxicity[e]	V_{45}	<195 mL	<10	Volume based on the entire potential space within the peritoneal cavity
Rectum	Whole organ	3DCRT	Grade 2 or higher late rectal toxicity, Grade 3 or higher late rectal toxicity	V_{50}	<50%	<15 <10	Prostate cancer treatment
	Whole organ	3DCRT	Grade 2 or higher late rectal toxicity, Grade 3 or higher late rectal toxicity	V_{60}	<35%	<15 <10	
	Whole organ	3DCRT	Grade 2 or higher late rectal toxicity, Grade 3 or higher late rectal toxicity	V_{65}	<25%	<15 <10	
	Whole organ	3DCRT	Grade 2 or higher late rectal toxicity, Grade 3 or higher late rectal toxicity	V_{70}	<20%	<15 <10	
	Whole organ	3DCRT	Grade 2 or higher late rectal toxicity, Grade 3 or higher late rectal toxicity	V_{75}	<15%	<15 <10	
Bladder	Whole organ	3DCRT	Grade 3 or higher late RTOG	D_{max}	<65	<6	Bladder cancer treatment. Variations in bladder size/shape/location during RT hamper ability to generate accurate data.
	Whole organ	3DCRT	Grade 3 or higher late RTOG	V_{65} V_{70} V_{75} V_{80}	≤50% ≤35% ≤25% ≤15%		Prostate cancer treatment. Based on current RTOG 0415 recommendation

(continued)

TABLE 13.11 (CONTINUED)

Organ	Volume Segmented	Irradiation Type (Partial Organ unless Otherwise Stated)[a]	Endpoint	Dose (Gy), or Dose–Volume Parameters[a]		Rate (%)	Notes on Dose–Volume Parameters
Penile bulb	Whole organ	3DCRT	Severe erectile dysfunction	Mean dose to 95% of gland	<50	<35	
	Whole organ	3DCRT	Severe erectile dysfunction	D_{90}	<50	<35	
	Whole organ	3DCRT	Severe erectile dysfunction	D_{60-70}	<70	<55	

Clinically, these data should be applied with caution. Clinicians are strongly advised to use the individual QUANTEC articles to check the applicability of these limits to the clinical situation at hand. These endpoints largely do not reflect modern IMRT.

3DCRT, three-dimensional conformal radiotherapy; SRS, stereotactic radiosurgery; D_x, minimum dose received by the "hottest" *x*% (or x mL) of the organ; RILD, radiation-induced liver disease (characterized by anicteric hepatomegaly and ascites, typically occurring between 2 weeks and 3 months after therapy; classic RILD also involves elevated alkaline phosphatase, more than twice the upper limit of normal or baseline value); RTOG, Radiation Therapy Oncology Group; SBRT, stereotactic body radiotherapy.

[a]All at standard fractionation (i.e., 1.8–2.0 Gy per daily fraction) unless otherwise noted.

[b]For optic nerve, the cases of neuropathy in the 55–60 Gy range received ~59 Gy (see optic nerve paper for details). Excludes patients with pituitary tumors where the tolerance may be reduced.

[c]Severe xerostomia is related to additional factors including the doses to the submandibular glands.

[d]Nontraumatic brain injury. [e]With combined chemotherapy.

Adapted from Marks et al.[422] based on the literature summarized in the QUANTEC reviews[49,88,115,134,165,230,240,284,302,335,336,352,373,374,408,411] (unless otherwise noted).

ACKNOWLEDGMENTS

Supported in part by grants from the National Institutes of Health CA69579 (L.B.M.) and the Lance Armstrong Foundation (L.B.M.). Parts of this chapter were adapted from Rubin et al., *ALERT: Adverse Late Effects of Radiation Therapy.*

SELECTED REFERENCES

A full list of references for this chapter is available online.

1. Emami B, et al. Tolerance of normal tissue to therapeutic irradiation. *Int J Radiat Oncol Biol Phys* 1991;21(1):109–122.
2. Marks LB, Ten Haken RK, Martel MK. Guest editor's introduction to QUANTEC: a users guide. *Int J Radiat Oncol Biol Phys* 2010;76(3 Suppl):S1–S2.
6. Lyman JT. Complication probability as assessed from dose-volume histograms. *Radiat Res Suppl* 1985;8:S13–S19.
9. Ten Haken RK, et al. Use of Veff and iso-NTCP in the implementation of dose escalation protocols. *Int J Radiat Oncol Biol Phys* 1993;27(3):689–695.
15. Ward JF. The complexity of DNA damage: relevance to biological consequences. *Int J Radiat Biol* 1994;66(5):427–432.
25. Mikkelsen RB, Wardman P. Biological chemistry of reactive oxygen and nitrogen and radiation-induced signal transduction mechanisms. *Oncogene* 2003;22(37): 5734–5754.
30. Vujaskovic Z, et al. A small molecular weight catalytic metalloporphyrin antioxidant with superoxide dismutase (SOD) mimetic properties protects lungs from radiation-induced injury. *Free Radic Biol Med* 2002;33(6):857–863.
37. Anscher MS, et al. Small molecular inhibitor of transforming growth factor-beta protects against development of radiation-induced lung injury. *Int J Radiat Oncol Biol Phys* 2008;71(3):829–837.
42. Vujaskovic Z, et al. Radiation-induced hypoxia may perpetuate late normal tissue injury. *Int J Radiat Oncol Biol Phys* 2001;50(4):851–855.
48. Olive PL, et al. Carbonic anhydrase 9 as an endogenous marker for hypoxic cells in cervical cancer. *Cancer Res* 2001;61(24):8924–8929.
49. Lawrence YR, et al. Radiation dose-volume effects in the brain. *Int J Radiat Oncol Biol Phys* 2010;76(3 Suppl):S20–S27.
50. Andrews DW, et al. Whole brain radiation therapy with or without stereotactic radiosurgery boost for patients with one to three brain metastases: phase III results of the RTOG 9508 randomised trial. *Lancet* 2004;363(9422):1665–1672.
57. Shaw E, et al. Prospective randomized trial of low- versus high-dose radiation therapy in adults with supratentorial low-grade glioma: initial report of a North Central Cancer Treatment Group/Radiation Therapy Oncology Group/Eastern Cooperative Oncology Group study. *J Clin Oncol* 2002;20(9):2267–2276.
61. Fowler JF. The linear-quadratic formula and progress in fractionated radiotherapy. *Br J Radiol* 1989;62(740):679–694.
68. Shaw E, et al. Single dose radiosurgical treatment of recurrent previously irradiated primary brain tumors and brain metastases: final report of RTOG protocol 90-05. *Int J Radiat Oncol Biol Phys* 2000;47(2):291–298.
71. Flickinger JC, et al. Complications from arteriovenous malformation radiosurgery: multivariate analysis and risk modeling. *Int J Radiat Oncol Biol Phys* 1997;38(3):485–490.
88. Mayo C, et al. Radiation dose-volume effects of optic nerves and chiasm. *Int J Radiat Oncol Biol Phys* 2010;76(3 Suppl):S28–S35.
91. Program, C.T.E. *Common Terminology Criteria for Adverse Events (CTCAE) Version 4.0.* Available at: http://evs.nci.nih.gov/ftp1/CTCAE. Accessed January 16, 2011.
92. Pavy JJ, et al. EORTC Late Effects Working Group. Late Effects toxicity scoring: the SOMA scale. *Int J Radiat Oncol Biol Phys* 1995;31(5):1043–1047.
93. Rubin P, et al. RTOG Late Effects Working Group. Overview. Late Effects of Normal Tissues (LENT) scoring system. *Int J Radiat Oncol Biol Phys* 1995;31(5):1041–1042.
95. Parsons JT, et al. Radiation optic neuropathy after megavoltage external-beam irradiation: analysis of time-dose factors. *Int J Radiat Oncol Biol Phys* 1994;30(4): 755–763.
96. Martel MK, et al. Dose-volume complication analysis for visual pathway structures of patients with advanced paranasal sinus tumors. *Int J Radiat Oncol Biol Phys* 1997;38(2):273–284.
115. Mayo C, Yorke E, Merchant TE. Radiation associated brainstem injury. *Int J Radiat Oncol Biol Phys* 2010;76(3 Suppl):S36–S41.
122. Merchant TE, et al. Factors associated with neurological recovery of brainstem function following postoperative conformal radiation therapy for infratentorial ependymoma. *Int J Radiat Oncol Biol Phys* 2010;76(2):496–503.
127. Foote KD, et al. Analysis of risk factors associated with radiosurgery for vestibular schwannoma. *J Neurosurg* 2001;95(3):440–449.
134. Bhandare N, et al. Radiation therapy and hearing loss. *Int J Radiat Oncol Biol Phys* 2010;76(3 Suppl):S50–S57.
135. Pan CC, et al. Prospective study of inner ear radiation dose and hearing loss in head-and-neck cancer patients. *Int J Radiat Oncol Biol Phys* 2005;61(5):1393–1402.
140. Honore HB, et al. Sensori-neural hearing loss after radiotherapy for nasopharyngeal carcinoma: individualized risk estimation. *Radiother Oncol* 2002;65(1):9–16.
165. Kirkpatrick JP, van der Kogel AJ, Schultheiss TE. Radiation dose-volume effects in the spinal cord. *Int J Radiat Oncol Biol Phys* 2010;76(3 Suppl):S42–S49.
167. Schultheiss TE, et al. Radiation response of the central nervous system. *Int J Radiat Oncol Biol Phys* 1995;31(5):1093–1112.
169. Sahgal A, Larson DA, Chang EL. Stereotactic body radiosurgery for spinal metastases: a critical review. *Int J Radiat Oncol Biol Phys* 2008;71(3):652–665.
190. Gibbs IC, et al. Delayed radiation-induced myelopathy after spinal radiosurgery. *Neurosurgery* 2009;64(2 Suppl):A67–A72.
195. Ryu S, et al. Partial volume tolerance of the spinal cord and complications of single-dose radiosurgery. *Cancer* 2007;109(3):628–636.
196. Ang KK, et al. The tolerance of primate spinal cord to re-irradiation. *Int J Radiat Oncol Biol Phys* 1993;25(3):459–464.
208. Medin PM, et al. Spinal cord tolerance to single-fraction partial-volume irradiation: a swine model. *Int J Radiat Oncol Biol Phys* 2011;79(1):226–232.
221. Nieder C, et al. Update of human spinal cord reirradiation tolerance based on additional data from 38 patients. *Int J Radiat Oncol Biol Phys* 2006;66(5):1446–1449.
230. Rancati T, et al. Radiation dose-volume effects in the larynx and pharynx. *Int J Radiat Oncol Biol Phys* 2010;76(3 Suppl):S64–S69.
235. Feng FY, et al. Intensity-modulated radiotherapy of head and neck cancer aiming to reduce dysphagia: early dose-effect relationships for the swallowing structures. *Int J Radiat Oncol Biol Phys* 2007;68(5):1289–1298.
240. Deasy JO, et al. Radiotherapy dose-volume effects on salivary gland function. *Int J Radiat Oncol Biol Phys* 2010;76(3 Suppl):S58–S63.
254. Eisbruch A, et al. Xerostomia and its predictors following parotid-sparing irradiation of head-and-neck cancer. *Int J Radiat Oncol Biol Phys* 2001;50(3):695–704.
262. Bradley JD, et al. A nomogram to predict radiation pneumonitis, derived from a combined analysis of RTOG 9311 and institutional data. *Int J Radiat Oncol Biol Phys* 2007;69(4):985–992.
275. Yorke ED, et al. Correlation of dosimetric factors and radiation pneumonitis for non-small-cell lung cancer patients in a recently completed dose escalation study. *Int J Radiat Oncol Biol Phys* 2005;63(3):672–682.
284. Marks LB, et al. Radiation dose-volume effects in the lung. *Int J Radiat Oncol Biol Phys* 2010;76(3 Suppl):S70–S76.
297. Timmerman RD, Park C, Kavanagh BD. The North American experience with stereotactic body radiation therapy in non-small cell lung cancer. *J Thorac Oncol* 2007;2(7 Suppl 3):S101–S112.
302. Gagliardi G, et al. Radiation dose-volume effects in the heart. *Int J Radiat Oncol Biol Phys* 2010;76(3 Suppl):S77–S85.
305. Hancock SL, Tucker MA, Hoppe RT. Factors affecting late mortality from heart disease after treatment of Hodgkin's disease. *JAMA* 1993;270(16):1949–1955.
308. Marks LB, et al. The incidence and functional consequences of RT-associated cardiac perfusion defects. *Int J Radiat Oncol Biol Phys* 2005;63(1):214–223.
311. Eriksson F, et al. Long-term cardiac mortality following radiation therapy for Hodgkin's disease: analysis with the relative seriality model. *Radiother Oncol* 2000;55(2):153–162.
318. Jones LW, et al. Early breast cancer therapy and cardiovascular injury. *J Am Coll Cardiol* 2007;50(15):1435–1441.

335. Werner-Wasik M, et al. Radiation dose-volume effects in the esophagus. *Int J Radiat Oncol Biol Phys* 2010;76(3 Suppl):S86–S93.
336. Pan CC, et al. Radiation-associated liver injury. *Int J Radiat Oncol Biol Phys* 2010;76(3 Suppl):S94–S100.
337. Lawrence TS, et al. The use of 3-D dose volume analysis to predict radiation hepatitis. *Int J Radiat Oncol Biol Phys* 1992;23(4):781–788.
339. Jackson A, et al. Analysis of clinical complication data for radiation hepatitis using a parallel architecture model. *Int J Radiat Oncol Biol Phys* 1995;31(4):883–891.
349. Rusthoven KE, et al. Multi-institutional phase I/II trial of stereotactic body radiation therapy for liver metastases. *J Clin Oncol* 2009;27(10):1572–1578.
352. Kavanagh BD, et al. Radiation dose-volume effects in the stomach and small bowel. *Int J Radiat Oncol Biol Phys* 2010;76(3 Suppl):S101–S107.
366. Willett CG, et al. Renal complications secondary to radiation treatment of upper abdominal malignancies. *Int J Radiat Oncol Biol Phys* 1986;12(9):1601–1604.
373. Dawson LA, et al. Radiation-associated kidney injury. *Int J Radiat Oncol Biol Phys* 2010;76(3 Suppl):S108–S115.
374. Michalski JM, et al. Radiation dose-volume effects in radiation-induced rectal injury. *Int J Radiat Oncol Biol Phys* 2010;76(3 Suppl):S123–S129.
408. Viswanathan AN, et al. Radiation dose-volume effects of the urinary bladder. *Int J Radiat Oncol Biol Phys* 2010;76(3 Suppl):S116–S122.
411. Roach M 3rd, et al. Radiation dose-volume effects and the penile bulb. *Int J Radiat Oncol Biol Phys* 2010;76(3 Suppl):S130–S134.
417. Roach M, et al. Penile bulb dose and impotence after three-dimensional conformal radiotherapy for prostate cancer on RTOG 9406: findings from a prospective, multi-institutional, phase I/II dose-escalation study. *Int J Radiat Oncol Biol Phys* 2004;60(5):1351–1356.
422. Marks LB, et al. Use of normal tissue complication probability models in the clinic. *Int J Radiat Oncol Biol Phys* 2010;76(3 Suppl):S10–S19.

Chapter 14
Methodology of Clinical Trials

Yaacov Richard Lawrence, James J. Dignam, and Maria Werner-Wasik

In this chapter, we discuss the design, conduct, and analysis of oncology clinical trials, pointing out particular areas of interest to radiation oncology and reviewing some recent ideas in clinical trials and related research studies. This chapter provides a brief and essentially nontechnical sketch of the main concepts and current research areas, and we refer the reader to comprehensive texts on clinical trial conduct in oncology for further details. Excellent recent texts, such as *Handbook of Statistics in Clinical Oncology, Clinical Trials in Oncology,* and *Oncology Clinical Trials: Successful Design, Conduct and Analysis* provide the fundamentals, as well as up-to-date discussion of new challenges and active research in statistical methods for oncology clinical trials.[1–3]

Clinical trials enable physicians to advance medical care in a safe, scientific, and ethical manner. Formally defined, clinical trials are a set of procedures in medical research conducted to allow safety and efficacy data to be collected for health interventions.[4] A more detailed definition for our purposes would describe a clinical trial as a prospective study that includes an active intervention, carried out in a well-defined patient cohort and producing interpretable information about the action of the intervention.[5] Although in some ways similar to a well-designed laboratory experiment, the involvement of living human subjects demands adherence to strict ethical principles while also adding to the complexity of interpretation of the results. The past 60 years have witnessed an unprecedented appreciation of the importance of clinical trials and a consequent surge in the number of clinical trials performed. In the field of radiation oncology alone, according to a PubMed search, 376 clinical trials were published in 2010, of which 65 were phase III trials.

Over the course of less than a century, the evidence on which medicine is practiced has evolved from being entirely empirical to being a highly regulated scientific process based on vigorously designed clinical trials tightly overseen by numerous scientific and governmental agencies. Cardinal chapters in the history of clinical trial design and implementation include the following:

- 1747—James Lind's work on the effect of citrus fruits in the prevention of scurvy among sailors in the Royal Navy
- 1863—Austin Flint's use of a placebo group for comparison with an experimental treatment in the treatment of rheumatic fever
- 1947—Nuremberg Code, a result of the appreciation that much of the medical experimentation performed by physicians in Nazi Germany was both ethically wrong and scientifically uninterpretable
- 1948—The first double blind trial, performed by the British Medical Research Council to assess the value of streptomycin in the treatment of tuberculosis
- 1964—Declaration of Helsinki developed by the World Medical Association, ethical guidelines, which continue to be updated, for the performance of clinical trials
- 2000—Creation of the ClinicalTrials.gov Web site, a registry of clinical trials under the auspices of the National Institutes of Health (NIH)

The performance of high-quality cancer clinical trials involves the cooperation of multiple bodies, so-called stakeholders, including cancer patients and their families, physicians (who accrue the patients), their operating environment (academic institution or practice), the research team (who runs the trial on a day-to-day basis), sponsors (who oversee and fund the trial), independent monitors (to ensure the correct performance of the research team), government regulatory agencies, contract research organizations (CROs, which may carry out specific aspect of the trial such as auditing), and medical insurance companies. Modern clinical trials may require involvement of translational scientists, and clinical psychologists, as well as experts in quality of life, cost-effectiveness, and other disciplines. The complexity of clinical trials adds to the regulatory work involved. For instance, a multi-institutional federally sponsored clinical trial protocol will require the approval of at least three different research ethics oversight committees (institutional review boards [IRBs]) within the group coordinating the trial, at each institution that opens the trial to accrue patients, and at the sponsor.

Although many phase I and phase II trials are carried out by investigators within a single institution, many larger phase II and most phase III trials are generally multi-institutional. Thus, clinical trial investigator networks have emerged as essential players in the performance of large phase II and III clinical trials. The U.S. National Cancer Institute–sponsored Cancer Cooperative Group Program is an example,[6] as are similar groups such as the European Organisation for Research and Treatment of Cancer (EORTC). One cooperative group, the Radiation Therapy Oncology Group (RTOG), founded by Simon Kramer in 1968, is dedicated to trials involving radiation therapy, has activated 460 protocols, and has accrued approximately 90,000 patients to its trials. Early studies sought to answer questions regarding radiation dose and fractionation. As cancer therapy became multimodal, the group addressed questions relating to combining systemic chemotherapy with radiation therapy. Most recent trials seek to combine targeted agents with contemporary radiation therapy techniques.[6]

Clinical trials are extremely expensive to perform, with costs continuing to rise as a result of both increased regulatory oversight and greater trial complexity. It has been estimated that implementation of the European Union's Clinical Trials Directive (laws and regulations related to implementation of good clinical practice in the conduct of clinical trials) led to a doubling of the cost of running noncommercial cancer trials in the United Kingdom.[7] Large phase III trials can cost in excess of $100 million; as a result, clinical trials are frequently financed by the pharmaceutical industry. An unfortunate consequence is that clinical trials are rarely performed on established generic drugs, where there is little commercial interest in establishing new indications. Conversely, the performance of rigorous clinical trials contributes significantly to the costs involved in the development of new pharmaceutical agents, which are subsequently reflected in the commercial pricing of the product.

OVERVIEW OF ETHICAL CONSIDERATIONS

Medical ethics are based on the principles of autonomy (the patient's right to refuse or choose treatment), beneficence (a practitioner should act in the best interest of the patient), nonmaleficence (first, do no harm), justice (fairness and equality), dignity, and honesty. Without due diligence, physicians may infringe on these principles when encouraging patient participation in clinical trials. Are the physicians confident that the proposed treatment is beneficial and not harmful? Are the potential subjects fully aware of the implications of participation? Do all segments of the population have equivalent chance to participate and receive potentially better treatment? Despite the universal acceptance of these principles, there have been numerous examples of grossly unethical research being performed in the Western world within living memory. Documents seeking to address these issues include the Nuremberg Code, the declaration of Helsinki, and the Belmont Report. Emanuel et al.[8] have listed seven requirements that provide a systematic and coherent framework for determining whether clinical research is ethical (Table 14.1).

Ethical principles themselves and the creation of guidelines are insufficient to ensure the ethical conduct of medical research. Physicians within Nazi Germany performed atrocities despite the existence of German guidelines published in 1931,[9] reflecting the need for legislation. The International Conference on Harmonisation of Technical Requirements for Registration of Pharmaceuticals for Human Use (ICH) brought together the regulatory authorities of Europe, Japan, and the United States and experts from the pharmaceutical industry to regulate scientific and technical aspects of pharmaceutical product registration. The ICH guidelines are legally binding in many countries (although not the United States) and are updated every few years, reflecting the increasing sophistication of the field. An example of a recent addition is the introduction of data and safety monitoring committees (DSMCs), which are independent groups of experts who monitor patient safety and treatment efficacy data in ongoing clinical trials. Another recent advance is the requirement for the registration of clinical trials at sites such as ClinicalTrials.gov. Such registration both improves transparency concerning what clinical trials have been and are being performed and empowers patients to find relevant clinical trials.

TABLE 14.1 COHERENT FRAMEWORK FOR DETERMINING WHETHER CLINICAL RESEARCH IS ETHICAL

Characteristic	*Description*
Value	Will the research enhance medical science?
Scientific validity	Is the research methodologically rigorous?
Fair subject selection	Scientific objectives, not vulnerability or privilege, should determine subject inclusion within the trial.
Favorable risk-benefit ratio	Risks must be minimized and potential benefits enhanced from both an individual's and society's perspective.
Independent review	Unaffiliated individuals must review and approve the research prior to initiation.
Informed consent	Individuals should be informed about the research and provide their voluntary consent.
Respect for enrolled subjects	Subjects should have their privacy protected, the opportunity to withdraw, and have their well-being monitored.

Based on Emanuel EJ, Wendler D, Grady C. What makes clinical research ethical? *JAMA* 2000;283:2701–2711.

OVERVIEW OF TRADITIONAL CLINICAL TRIAL DEVELOPMENT PHASES

Traditionally, a new anticancer agent is tested in a three-step process, starting with a small dose finding trial (phase I), followed by a pilot efficacy trial (phase II), and culminating with a large comparative randomized trial (phase III). This development paradigm was created and established in the era of cytotoxic chemotherapies and continues to be used today in the era of often less-toxic (and possibly not dose-dependent) targeted therapies, with some adaptations and innovations that we discuss later. Here we review the traditional paradigm without technical details, which can be found in many excellent sources for clinical trial design and conduct.[2,5]

Phase I

The main objective of the phase I trial is to determine the maximum tolerable dose of an agent to be subsequently used in testing for efficacy. Although initially developed in the setting of drug testing, this concept has been adapted to test radiation alone and combined drug/radiation regimens. The basic conceptual approach is that of sequential dose increases, or escalation, in small patient cohorts until the treatment-related adverse event rate reaches a predetermined level or unexpected toxicity is seen. This stepwise testing in phase I trials determines what is known as the maximum tolerated dose (MTD), which is putatively the most effective level at which to evaluate efficacy.

The key parameters to be defined at the outset of a phase I trial include patient eligibility criteria, starting dose and schedule of dose escalation (which should frame the expected MTD), events comprising the adverse event/toxicity response and the expected MTD, and finally the escalation design plan.[10] By far, the dominant design has been the so-called 3+3 approach, where cohorts of three patients are exposed to a given dose, and based on the outcomes in that cohort, either de-escalation, escalation, or additional enrollment takes place. There are a large number of other designs, one of which may be particularly suited for radiation therapy trials, as we discuss shortly. It should be appreciated that the MTD is a relative concept that can change over time. For example, hematologic toxicity may be less dose limiting today than it was before the development of bone marrow stimulators such as erythropoietin and filgrastim.

Phase II

The primary purpose of the phase II trial is to determine the response rate of the treatment, seeking early evidence of clinical activity. An important secondary purpose is to gather more robust adverse event information at the established dose. The primary efficacy end point of the phase II trial has traditionally been tumor response; however, duration of response, progression-free survival (PFS), and site-specific activity such as locoregional control are all relevant and increasingly used. Measures of patient survival are usually secondary end points in phase II trials because of the limited sample size and follow-up duration of these trials. In general, phase II trials usually are not designed to provide definitive evidence that the test treatment is superior to current options. In fact, phase II trials have traditionally been single-arm studies comparing against a benchmark historical response rate. Reliance on this nonconcurrent external control rate can be problematic.[11–13] Furthermore, patient selection factors can influence the results—for example, overall response rates in single-institution phase II trials can be significantly higher than in multicenter studies or subsequent phase III controlled trials.[14] Randomized phase II trials have historically had a role in multiarm trials aimed at selecting the best treatment(s) to take forward for further testing.[15] More recently, they have become favored as a means of providing more reliable pilot efficacy data.[16] However, the preferred approach is changing as described later.

Phase III

Phase III trials are randomized comparisons between a new treatment regimen that has already shown promise in phase I/II trials and the current best standard of care (i.e., the control). Randomization offers a critical advantage over nonrandomized studies. Specifically, randomization balances the distribution of prognostic factors between treatment arms and ensures that treatment is assigned independent of these factors, thereby minimizing or eliminating these effects when comparing outcomes by treatment. When randomization is combined with treatment blinding of patients, researchers, or both, then even subjective outcomes can be assessed with minimal bias. Additionally, in multicenter studies, randomization can balance any systematic bias of the treating physicians or institutions.

Phase III trials can address one of several types of primary questions. For example, a study can be designed to determine if standard treatment is better than best supportive care. More often, phase III studies are designed to compare a new treatment with the current standard treatment. Phase III studies can also compare two or three different regimens with each other, as well as with standard treatment. Finally, a trial may be designed to demonstrate that a given treatment option is not worse than another by more than a tolerable margin. These "equivalence" trials, more accurately referred to as noninferiority trials, play an important role in development of less invasive or less burdensome treatment regimens.

The primary end point of a phase III trial is most typically overall survival (time to death from any cause); however, other important clinical end points such as disease-free survival (DFS) are increasingly justified. Because these trials aim to definitively demonstrate benefit with respect to these end points, the number of participants and follow-up period required for phase III trials is much longer than in phase II trials. Important secondary end points can include locoregional control and other site-specific failure end points, adverse event profiles, and quality of life measures.

Phase IV

Phase IV trials are also known as a postmarketing surveillance trials. These trials involve the safety surveillance of a drug after it receives regulatory approval for standard use. The safety surveillance is designed to detect any rare or long-term adverse effects over a much larger patient population and longer time period than was possible during the phase I–III clinical trials.

UNIQUE FEATURE OF CLINICAL TRIALS IN RADIATION ONCOLOGY

Therapeutic clinical trials in radiation oncology typically involve the introduction of new technologies (e.g., the use of stereotactic body radiation for a new indication) or more frequently the novel combination of radiation therapy with a systemic agent. There are unique challenges—both biologic and clinical—that characterize clinical trials in radiation oncology compared to those not involving radiation.

Response rate is frequently used in early-phase medical oncology trials to indicate activity; however, considering radiation therapy itself is highly effective at shrinking tumors, this end point is not useful in radiation trials. A more appropriate "activity" end point for radiation trials may be PFS, although this itself is often difficult to objectively assess. Modern imaging end points (such as fluorodeoxyglucose [FDG] uptake) show promise as early readouts of activity but still require vigorous validation for individual disease sites. Furthermore, efficacy and toxicity end points in radiation trials depend on multiple biologic factors, including size of the target, proximity of tumor to sensitive normal tissues, accuracy of target volume definition, degree of patient immobilization, dose of radiation, and fractionation scheme. Consequently, quality-assurance measures are an essential feature of radiation trials, especially in the multi-institutional setting.[17] Inadequate quality assurance and lack of consistency in radiation delivery have led to the conclusions obtained from large, expensive clinical trials being questioned.[18–24] As a recent example, in RTOG 9704, which evaluated postoperative adjuvant chemoradiation treatment of pancreatic cancer, subtle protocol violations in target definition influenced both toxicity and survival.[25]

In medical oncology trials, adverse events typically occur during or within days of completing treatment. In contrast, toxicity following radiation therapy follows a biphasic course, early (within 3 months of starting treatment) and late (months to years later). Late toxicity is typically irreversible and hence important in determining the tolerability of an experimental treatment. Utilizing long-term toxicity as the primary end point in clinical trials is not practical; however, it nonetheless is imperative to collect and report robust information on long-term outcomes from radiation therapy trials. In fact, even in phase I radiation therapy trials, the follow-up period can be significantly longer than for those evaluating chemotherapy. A recent approach to dose escalation in phase I trials that considers late toxicities when deciding whether to advance to the next dosing level is discussed later.[26]

A further difference relates to the population studied. In medical oncology early-phase trials, participants have often received several lines of treatment and lack further therapeutic options. In contrast, patients in phase I radiation trials typically receive full-dose radiation treatment, and subjects may be treatment naïve. Furthermore, phase I trials in medical oncology are frequently "first in human" experience for the agent; toxicity is unpredictable and pharmacokinetic studies essential. Conversely, most multimodality phase I trials in radiation oncology involve systemic agents that have already been through extensive clinical testing; systemic toxicity is known and pharmacokinetic studies unnecessary. The purpose of the trial is to define the extent of local toxicity within the radiation field; consequently, radiation oncology phase I trials are organ specific. A recent study demonstrated that in reality, radiation phase I trials rarely utilize first in human agents, are associated with qualitatively predictable toxicity, and are comparatively safe.[27] Examples of contemporary trial design in radiation oncology are provided in Table 14.2.

STATISTICAL ISSUES IN CLINICAL TRIAL DESIGN

Patient Population Definition and Stratification

A key issue in a clinical trial is a well-defined patient population to which the potential therapy applies. This is typically defined in terms of traditional disease characteristics reflecting putative prognosis, such as stage or its components. Increasingly, tumor

TABLE 14.2 EXAMPLES OF CLINICAL TRIAL DESIGNS FROM THE RADIATION THERAPY ONCOLOGY GROUP[a]

Study Title	*Type of Trial*	*Primary Trial Question(s)*
RTOG 0227: Phase I/II Study of Pre-Irradiation Chemotherapy with Methotrexate, Rituximab, and Temozolomide and Post-Irradiation Temozolomide for Primary Central Nervous System Lymphoma	Phase I "3 + 3" dose finding, followed by phase II single arm	To assess the maximum tolerated dose of the triple drug combination when administered prior to twice daily fractionated whole-brain radiation therapy in patients with primary central nervous system lymphoma
RTOG 0813: Seamless Phase I/II Study of Stereotactic Lung Radiotherapy (SBRT) for Early Stage, Centrally Located, Non-Small Cell Lung Cancer (NSCLC) in Medically Inoperable Patients	Phase I time to event continual reassessment (TiTe-CRM), followed by phase II single arm	To test the safety of stereotactic body radiation therapy (SBRT) at different dose levels with patients who have a centrally located early-stage lung cancer
RTOG 0926: A Phase II Protocol for Patients with Stage T1 Bladder Cancer to Evaluate Selective Bladder Preserving Treatment by Radiation Therapy Concurrent with Cisplatin Chemotherapy Following a Thorough Transurethral Surgical Re-Staging	Phase II pilot efficacy: single arm	To evaluate the efficacy of a nonoperative approach to early-stage disease, with primary end point being "rate of freedom from radical cystectomy at 3 years"
RTOG 1119: Phase II randomized study of whole brain radiotherapy in combination with concurrent lapatinib in patients with brain metastasis from HER2 positive breast cancer, a collaborative study of RTOG and KROG	Phase II pilot efficacy: two-arm randomized design	To determine if there is a sufficient evidence of improved 12-week complete response rate with the addition of lapatinib to whole-brain radiation therapy to warrant a phase III trial.
RTOG 0825: Phase III Double-Blind Placebo-Controlled Trial of Conventional Concurrent Chemoradiation and Adjuvant Temozolomide Plus Bevacizumab Versus Conventional Concurrent Chemoradiation and Adjuvant Temozolomide in Patients with Newly Diagnosed Glioblastoma	Phase III superiority comparison	To determine whether the addition of bevacizumab to temozolomide and radiation improves efficacy as measured by progression-free and/or overall survival
RTOG 1016: Phase III Trial of Radiotherapy Plus Cetuximab Versus Chemoradiotherapy in HPV-Associated Oropharynx Cancer	Phase III noninferiority comparison	To determine whether substitution of cisplatin with cetuximab will result in comparable 5-yr overall survival in HPV-associated oropharynx cancer

[a]Trial protocols can be found at http://www.rtog.org/ClinicalTrials/ProtocolTable.aspx.

pathology or marker features may be included. In any case, these must be unambiguously defined. Because factors defining eligibility are often critically related to prognosis, any randomized comparative study may use a stratified randomization approach to ensure equal representation of prognostic risk among treatment arms. Stratification factors need to be limited to a reasonable number because the total number of strata equals the product of the number of categories for each. For example, in a recently completed RTOG prostate cancer trial, stratification factors consisted of two levels of prostate-specific antigen (PSA) (<4 vs. 4 to 20), three cell differentiation categories (well, moderate, poor), and nodal status (N0 versus NX). The possible combinations of these variables create $2 \times 3 \times 2 = 12$ strata within which treatments are to be balanced in allocation.

Randomization

Randomization is used differently in various phases of development but serves a similar purpose, which is to render treatment groups similar with respect to factors other than treatment that can influence outcomes. In phase I trials, there typically are not comparative groups, although there are situations where parallel cohorts of patients are being evaluated. Thus, randomization into cohorts ensures that these groups can be compared later for response biomarkers or other factors of interest. In phase II trials, randomization has been used in two similar but distinct ways. First, so-called selection designs have been used to help decide which of several potential candidate treatments to take forward to further definitive testing.[15] In these trials, interest is not in statistically significant differences between treatments but rather is in the ability to nominally rank candidates in terms of best potential efficacy. It can be shown that this approach has high probability of identifying the most likely superior arm, although at the cost of false-positive findings, particularly if misused.[28] A second and more recent role of randomization in phase II trials is to provide evidence, albeit at a less stringent criteria, that a test treatment is indeed promising.[16] In phase III, randomization is critical for definitive unbiased evaluation.

With regard to implementation, randomization assignments can be simple or, more commonly, implemented using blocking or dynamic approaches with respect to balancing treatment arms by key factors, such as stratification variables mentioned earlier. Several proven methods are available.[5]

It is important to note that investigators must protect against practices that can erode or nullify the benefits of randomization. First, any breach of the random assignment process has an irreparable effect on the validity of the trial. Second, a large number (or differential number per treatment arm) of patient withdrawals can make the validity of the comparison suspect. Similarly, differential follow-up and consequently ascertainment of patient status between treatment arms can bias the treatment effect estimate. Third, bias in assessment of outcomes can have a major impact on the estimated treatment effect; thus, objective outcome measures and blinding of treatment assignment become important. Treatment assignment blinding is not feasible for radiotherapy and most chemotherapy regimens but can be used for many agents. In either case, and in particular for studies that cannot be blinded (among patients or caregivers), unambiguous, objectively defined end points are essential. In cases where determination of the end point involves possible observer subjectivity, such as when reading a diagnostic scan to determine disease progression, keeping assessors unaware of treatment assignment may be necessary.

End Points

In clinical trials, end points must be unambiguously defined, be assessable and reproducible, and reflect the action of the intervention. Typically, there is a single primary end point in a clinical trial; however, there may be numerous secondary end points.

Traditionally, in phase II cancer trials, treatment activity has been defined in terms of reduction in tumor burden. The most recent criteria for measuring activity are known as the Response Evaluation Criteria in Solid Tumors (RECIST).[29] The criteria require the identification of target and nontarget lesions at baseline and their largest single dimensions. Categories of response are then defined—for example, complete response (CR), or disappearance of all target and nontarget lesions and no new lesions; partial response (PR), or 30% or greater decrease in the sum of the longest diameter of all target lesions, no progression of nontarget lesions, and no new lesions; and progressive disease (PD), or 20% or greater increase in target lesions, progression of nontarget lesions, or the occurrence of new lesions. A patient not satisfying either response or progression criteria is classified as having stable disease. Those achieving either a CR or PR are typically defined as objective responders, and the proportion of patients responding is then the primary end point of interest. Although widely used, there has long been concern that response defined this way is an inadequate substitute for more clinically relevant and objective end points such as survival time. In one study, fewer than 25% of agents that produced tumor response were eventually found to extend survival in comparative trials,[30] whereas another suggested that tumor response is a reasonable surrogate for survival extension.[31] Additional problems with the use of response rates in phase II trials include subjectivity and lack of reproducible assessments.[32]

As mentioned earlier, response is not as frequently used when radiation therapy is the test question, and in any case, other discrete binary end points can readily be used. For example, the proportion free from a given event (i.e., proportion alive, proportion recurrence-free, etc.) at a fixed time landmark such as 2 years is a common and straightforward end point.

A more informative end point that is used in many phase II and most phase III trials is the elapsed time from trial entry until occurrence of some event. The most straightforward of these is overall survival time, or time to death from any cause. This simple end point does not depend on adjudication of cause of death and its attendant complexities and naturally corrects for both favorable and unfavorable consequences of treatment. Although it can be verified or even ascertained from public records because of its simplicity, active follow-up per protocol remains of paramount importance. Cause-specific survival end points may also be considered; however, as mentioned, assigning cause of death is not simple, and one must account for "other cause" deaths and whether these have any relationship to treatment. In addition, whenever cause-specific deaths or other site-specific failure end points are used, methods for appropriately dealing with competing risks are required.[33,34]

Other commonly used time-to-event end points include DFS (time to recurrence or death from any cause) or PFS (time to disease progression, possibly determined via imaging or other assessments at regular intervals), although definitions of these are not standardized (e.g., see Hudis et al.[35]), and the specific failure events comprising given end points should be carefully specified. The main advantage of using DFS or PFS is the more rapid rate of events, leading to a smaller required sample size. In many cancer types, benefit with respect to these end points does not necessarily imply subsequent lengthened survival, although they may still represent clinical benefit for patients. For other disease settings (e.g., adjuvant therapy in colon cancer), DFS is a reliable and well-accepted primary end point that is strongly correlated with survival.[36] This raises the topic of so-called surrogate end points, which are end points on which treatment benefits can be reliably measured. Various biomarkers and clinical end points have been studied and proposed as surrogate end points in clinical trials. Prentice[37] specified criteria that a surrogate end point must fulfill if it is used to substitute for a clinical end point: the therapeutic intervention must exert benefit on both the surrogate and the clinical end point; the surrogate and clinical end point must be associated; and the effect of intervention on surrogate end point must mediate the clinical effect. An example of a widely studied surrogate marker is PSA, applied either as a static measure or as dynamic measures (PSA velocity; PSA doubling time; time to PSA nadir, particularly useful after radiation therapy of the intact prostate) to assess time to biochemical failure in patients with nonmetastatic adenocarcinoma of the prostate.[38,39] This continues to be a developing area, and there remain many caveats and cautions regarding surrogate end points in clinical trials.[40]

Statistical Power and Sample Size

The overarching design consideration in clinical trials is to obtain sufficient information about an intervention so that a reliable decision can be made regarding its further development or use. In the classical (e.g., frequentist) statistical hypothesis testing paradigm, one sets up a null hypothesis of no treatment effect and an alternative hypothesis (which one hopes to validate) indicating a treatment effect. The type II or β error equals the probability that a statistical test fails to produce a decision in favor of a treatment effect when in fact the treatment is superior in the population. The complement of this probability $(1 - \beta)$ is referred to as *statistical power* and equals the probability of correctly deciding in favor of a treatment benefit. Statistical power depends on the other principal parameters considered when planning the trial, specifically the probability of incorrectly finding in favor of a difference when none exists (type I or alpha error, usually set to 0.05 or 0.01 by convention), the a priori specification of a treatment effect that is considered both realistic and clinically material, and of course the sample size. It is imperative that trials be designed to achieve adequate statistical power; typically, 0.80 to 0.90 is desirable so as not to obtain equivocal findings concerning the potential worth of new treatments under consideration. Studies with low statistical power can cause delay or even abandonment of the development of promising treatments, as well as waste valuable resources, not least of which is the participation and goodwill of patients.[41] In contrast, a "negative" trial that does not find the test treatment to be superior, if adequately powered, is informative in that resources can be directed into other more promising alternatives.

Thus, sample size to satisfy the power desired for the specified effect of interest is the key calculation in phase II and III clinical trials. (Phase I trials do not rely on hypothesis-driven sample size calculations, and the sample size derives from the specific design used.) The specific sample size calculation depends on the end point, and technical details will not be provided here; however, the two most common types of end points can be summarized as follows.

For a discrete binary end point in a phase II trial—for example, responded or did not respond—sample size calculations are straightforwardly performed using formulas for comparison of proportions. In a single-arm study, one aims to compare the observed response rate for the new agent to some historical response proportion, p_0, or the response rate achievable with standard therapy in the target population. The main objective is to determine whether there is sufficient evidence to conclude that the response rate for the new regimen is greater than p_0. We designate p_A as a response rate which, if true, would be clinically material. We test the null hypothesis, $H_0 : p = p_0$, against the alternative hypothesis $H_A : p = p_A$. The values of p_0 and p_A and (and more importantly the difference), along with the sample size, will determine the power of the study. Note that to detect a small improvement (say, $\leq$10%) requires a large sample size. For example, to detect an improvement from a historical value of 20% to 30% with 85% power, more than 120 subjects are required. In addition, the value for both p_0 and p_A must be realistic; it is of little value to design and carry out a study to detect an effect size $p_A - p_0$ that is unlikely to be realized, simply because it is compatible with the number of patients that can be recruited.

For two-arm randomized phase II trials with discrete end points, the previous discussion is simply redefined in terms of two-sample comparisons of proportions, and the sample size is consequently much larger. Table 14.3 shows some sample size requirements for various response differences, illustrating the influence of the effect size and power on the number required. Finally, if the end point is a fixed time landmark, such as proportion event free or alive at 1 year, then the estimates of the proportions may be derived from survival analysis methods to appropriately account for losses to follow-up.

In many randomized phase II and nearly all phase III trials, the time from randomization until occurrence of the event is of principal interest rather than the event status at some fixed time landmark. In larger phase II and phase III trials, recruitment may take place over a lengthy interval, with each patient having a different follow-up duration, and the use of follow-up time per patient is more efficient than waiting until all patients

TABLE 14.3 SAMPLE SIZE FOR A TWO-ARM COMPARATIVE (1:1 ALLOCATION) TRIAL WITH A BINARY END POINT[a]

P_1	*Improvement in Response Rate ($P_2 - P_1$) in Group 2*									
⇓	*0.05*	*0.10*	*0.15*	*0.20*	*0.25*	*0.30*	*0.35*	*0.40*	*0.45*	*0.50*
0.05	1,240[b]	412	226	148	108	84	66	54	46	38
	946[c]	318	176	116	86	66	54	44	36	32
0.10	1,912	570	292	184	128	96	76	60	50	42
	1,448	436	224	142	100	76	60	48	40	34
0.15	2,500	708	348	212	146	106	82	66	52	44
	1,888	538	266	164	114	84	64	52	42	36
0.20	3,004	822	394	238	158	114	88	68	54	44
	2,264	626	302	182	124	90	68	54	44	38
0.25	3,424	918	432	254	168	120	90	70	56	46
	2,578	696	330	196	130	94	72	56	46	38
0.30	3,760	990	460	268	176	124	92	72	56	44
	2,828	750	350	206	136	96	74	56	46	38
0.35	4,012	1,044	478	276	178	126	92	70	54	44
	3,018	790	364	212	138	98	74	56	44	36
0.40	4,180	1,074	488	278	178	124	90	68	52	42
	3,142	814	372	214	138	96	72	54	42	34
0.45	4,264	1,086	488	276	176	120	88	66	50	38
	3,206	822	372	212	136	94	68	52	40	32
0.50	4,264	1,074	478	268	168	114	82	60	46	34
	3,206	814	364	206	130	90	64	48	36	28

[a]Table entries are the total number of patients required, shown for two different levels of power for a response proportion P_1 in group 1 and $P_1 + P_2$ in group 2. For example, for group 1, response proportion = 0.10, and for group 2, response proportion = 0.30 ($P_2 - P_1 = 0.20$); 184 patients are needed (92 per arm) for 90% power.

[b]First row: $\alpha = 0.05$ and $\beta = 0.10$ (power = 90%).

[c]Second row: $\alpha = 0.05$ and $\beta = 0.20$ (power = 80%).

TABLE 14.4 SAMPLE SIZE FOR A TWO-ARM COMPARATIVE (1:1 ALLOCATION) TRIAL WITH A TIME-TO-EVENT END POINT[a]

Reduction in Hazard of Failure for New Treatment	*Control Group Event-Free at 5 Year*					*Number of Events Required*
	0.500	*0.600*	*0.700*	*0.800*	*0.900*	
25%	S(5) = 0.595	0.682	0.765	0.846	0.924	386
	Pts = 850	1,072	1,440	2,174	4,372	
33%	0.630	0.711	0.788	0.862	0.932	198
	452	572	768	1,162	2,340	
40%	0.660	0.736	0.807	0.875	0.939	126
	300	380	510	774	1,558	
50%	0.707	0.775	0.837	0.894	0.949	72
	180	226	306	464	934	

[a]Table entries show the 5-year survival in the experimental treatment group [S(5)] and the total number of patients needed (Pts) for the hazard reduction owing to the new treatment on the left-hand column and the 5-year survival in the standard treatment group (middle columns, top; assuming 80% power, two-sided $\alpha = 0.05$). The approximate number of patients shown here is based on Freedman's formula.[43] The actual number of patients required for the trial to obtain results in some specified time period will depend on the rate at which patients can be accrued and possibly other factors. The right-most column shows the number of failure *events* required, which is determined only by the hazard reduction and is thus the same for different absolute failure proportion reductions.

have reached some fixed time. The treatment effect measure is then specified in terms of failure *hazards*, which can be thought of as failure rates per unit of time. Hypotheses are thus usually formulated in terms of the hazard ratio (HR) as H_0 : $\lambda_A/\lambda_B = HR = 1.0$, where λ_A and λ_B are the hazards for treatments A and B, versus the alternative, H_A : $HR < 1.0$, for some value of the HR that represents a clinically important difference in outcomes. Under the assumption that this ratio is relatively constant over time, a given HR can be converted to an absolute difference between groups in proportions remaining event free at a specific follow-up time. For example, a new/standard HR equal to 0.75, or a 25% reduction in failure rate in the experimental group relative to the standard group, may translate into an absolute difference in the proportion of patients remaining free from the event between groups of 4.6% at 5 years, if the standard group 5-year survival percentage is 80% (Table 14.4).

From the specification of difference of interest or effect size, then, the sample size in terms of number of *events* required to detect this difference with desired statistical power and significance level is determined. Depending on the anticipated accrual rate and the prognosis (e.g., rapidity of failure events) in the control treatment group, the number of *patients* required can then be approximated. The number of events required depends strongly on the HR, becoming dramatically larger as the HR approaches 1.0 (Table 14.4). The number of patients required and total duration of the trial depend on the rate of patient accrual and the failure rate in the control group, both of which contribute to the determination of how rapidly the requisite events will be observed. The accrual rate is typically estimated from previous experience and may also involve querying investigators to project the accrual rate per unit of time. Similarly, the failure rate for patients under standard therapy is derived from available data. The final computations are straightforward but generally require computer programs,[42] although under certain assumptions can be approximated.[43] Sample size methods have been extended to take into account other factors that will influence power, such as patients withdrawing from treatment (dropout), switching from the assigned treatment to the other group (crossover), or deviating from protocol treatment (noncompliance).[44–46]

Interim Analysis and Stopping Rules

Primarily for ethical considerations but also to make the best use of resources, interim analysis plans are used in all phases of clinical trials. These plans provide for early decision making in a trial regarding continuation, disclosure of findings, or modification of the trial while preserving integrity of the study with respect to power and type I error control described earlier. These methods are needed because with repeated hypothesis tests, the probability of at least one test resulting in an erroneous rejection of the null hypothesis increases.

Phase I trials have stopping rules that are integral to the design, in that termination of enrollment to a given dose is based on observed cumulative adverse event rates at a given time. We refer to a review of the designs for more details.[1]

Phase II trials more formally incorporate stopping rules, usually restricted to futility stopping, or discontinuation when results do not appear promising. For trials with discrete end points such as tumor response, this is accomplished through multistage study designs, whereby a cohort of patients is enrolled and assessed for response, and if a specific minimum response proportion is observed, the trial continues to full accrual or otherwise discontinues enrollment. The most commonly used designs are those proposed by Simon,[47] although there are other similar approaches.[2] In trials with a time-to-event end point, futility rules similar to those for phase III trials (discussed next) can be used to discontinue after a period of follow-up if results appear unpromising. Early stopping of single-arm phase II trials for extraordinary efficacy is unusual but certainly not prohibited.

Phase III trials use repeated testing strategies derived from an area of statistics known as group sequential methods.[48] Briefly, the primary hypothesis is evaluated at predefined increments (typically three to five looks) of the total information (usually in the form of failure events) needed for definitive analysis. The individual tests are designed to (a) protect against spurious early stopping owing to the unstable nature of "early" results and (b) correct for the effect of repeated testing on type I error, which can also lead to spurious declaration of treatment effects that may not be reliable. Commonly used approaches include the Haybittle-Peto approach, for which each test through the penultimate look requires a constant highly significant result, such as $p < 0.0001$, in order to stop,[49,50] and the O'Brien-Fleming approach and its subsequent approaches,[51] in which the required significance level decreases over the looks, becoming less extreme as more information accumulates. There are many variations and extensions of the latter approach, with different properties and advantages in special circumstances. In addition to efficacy monitoring rules, phase III trials increasingly also incorporate formal futility stopping rules, although methods such as conditional power calculations have been available and used for some time.[52,53] Futility stopping rules similarly involve setting a boundary such that when the test statistic falls beyond it, one considers stopping because the new treatment will not ultimately prevail. Stopping for futility is a complex decision requiring careful consideration,[54] and methods continue to be studied and developed.[55,56]

Definitive Analysis and Secondary Analyses

When a trial reaches maturity either as planned or earlier as a result of the monitoring plan, then definitive analysis takes place. Prior to this, it not conventional or recommended to disclose any results from the trial,[57] and this policy is adhered to in National Cancer Institute (NCI) cooperative group trials.

A critical aspect of clinical trial analysis is the definition of the analyzed cohort. The concept of analysis by *intention to treat* is often cited; however, the definition of this term can sometimes be unclear, thus it is best to explicitly describe which patients are included.[58] In the strictest sense, the intention-to-treat cohort includes all patients randomized, regardless of eligibility, adherence to assigned treatment, or any other post-randomization deviations from protocol. However, it is often the case that patients found ineligible for the trial after randomization owing to being incorrectly staged or for other reasons are excluded from the primary analysis, and this practice (used with caution) is sometimes advocated, as it allows for evaluation of the therapy in the population for whom it was intended.[2] A rarely acceptable practice involves exclusion of patients who did not or could not comply with assigned therapy regimens or received nonprotocol therapy or other post-randomization conditions. Such exclusions can easily lead to biased comparisons, and in general, any post-hoc analysis of treatment benefit by dose received is fraught with interpretational difficulties and should be avoided in primary analysis.[59]

Primary analysis methods follow naturally from a well-written protocol (see later discussion) and thus should be straightforward. Given that major journals increasingly require that study protocols be provided at the time of publication, and that regulatory agencies and public sponsors do likewise, it behooves the trialist to outline the analysis plan in the protocol and then carry it out at study conclusion. This does not suggest that additional analyses cannot be carried out but that having a framework for the planned analysis adds credibility to the findings.

Secondary prognostic factor analysis using statistical models or other techniques often follows primary analysis of phase III trials. Of particular interest is whether there are particularly responsive or nonresponsive subsets of patients in an attempt to render the findings more relevant to practice. The modeling process—which entails deciding what factors to include, determining the correct way to represent a given factor (i.e., in categories, on a continuous scale, etc.), consideration of interrelationships (e.g., interactions) among factors, and many other issues—can be complex, and it should be recognized that these analyses will be largely viewed as exploratory. Although possibly worth exploring, true differential effects of treatment by other factors usually require a large sample size, unless the effects are very large.[60] A comprehensive review of current modeling methods applied to oncology data is provided by Schumacher et al.[61]

PRACTICAL ISSUES IN THE DESIGN, CONDUCT, AND REPORTING OF CLINICAL TRIALS

Protocol Document and Study Conduct

The goal of a clinical trial is to answer a well-formulated question that will change clinical practice. To achieve that, the investigators must know the current state of knowledge on the studied disease; clearly describe the eligibility criteria of the studied population; understand the number of patients who will be eligible in their institution/cooperative group; choose simple and achievable end points; establish statistical assumptions based on thorough review of pre-existing data; and collaborate with a biostatistician to decide on study design, sample size, and power.

The clinical trial protocol document must contain the title, investigator and sponsor names, phase (I, II, or III), protocol synopsis, background knowledge, study design and schema, objectives, methodology, subject selection criteria, registration procedures, treatment plan, dosing modifications, adverse events reporting, data and safety monitoring plan, study calendar, outcome measures, data reporting, statistical considerations, and the informed consent.[62]

Choosing the right study end points is crucial, because it needs to reflect the primary goal of the trial. Any number of end points may be of suitable scientific and clinical value, although if there is interest in regulatory approval, then obviously the end point must reflect the requirements of those parties involved. Overall survival largely remains the gold standard for a registration trial designed to gain marketing approval. However, survival length may be affected by effective salvage therapies or by patients "crossing over" to the other study arm. End points such as DFS and PFS have been used for either expedited drug approval or regular approval, depending on the disease site.[63] If end points subject to assessment bias are to be used (e.g., PFS or tumor response), then appropriate bias reduction measures are needed. One approach to circumvent this problem is an independent review panel—such as radiologists reviewing baseline and follow-up images to quantify tumor responses and note the moment of tumor progression—consisting of experts not associated with the trial and unaware of the arm to which the patient was enrolled. One must also consider validity of modern end points even under unbiased review. For example, the phenomena of pseudoprogression and pseudoresponse have made imaging-based end points—including overall radiographic response and PFS—problematic.[64]

Successful completion of a clinical trial requires constant attention to its practical aspects. Sufficient personnel are necessary to ensure the smooth running of the study and safety of the participating subjects. Clinical research nurses, clinical research associates, data managers, and investigational pharmacists are crucial components of the research team.[65] Of particular importance is careful and immediate recording and attribution of all adverse events. Severe adverse events have to be reported promptly to appropriate regulatory agencies (the IRB in the institution where the study is open, the U.S. Food and Drug Administration [FDA], and others) and to the study sponsor. Because most protocols have amendments added during their lifetime and new toxicities are reported from other studies, the research protocol commonly evolves over several successive versions. As a result, new versions of consent forms must be created as well, and IRB approval may again be required. It is imperative that patients enrolled to the study sign the most current version of the consent form. All prescribed follow-up tests (imaging, blood work, etc.) have to be scheduled ahead of time and must coincide with the study calendar. Departures from any the procedures are scored as protocol deviations during periodic audits and will impact adversely on the study's validity. Additionally, designated independent medical monitors are assigned to high-risk trials (such as most single-institution investigator-initiated trials) to continuously review any reported events, which are later evaluated periodically by the institutional DSMC.

Data and Safety Monitoring Committees

The decision to alter a clinical trial in progress, including discontinuation of accrual and/or treatment, depending on its current state, and to release findings early is typically vested in an independent DSMC. In addition to evaluating according to the monitoring rules described earlier, the DSMC considers the information available from the trial as well as external information that bears on treatment for the disease under study. Specifically, it should be noted that the early stopping rules described previously are meant to serve as guidelines, and there may at any decision point be additional considerations that must be taken into account.[66] The policies and procedures for NCI-sponsored cooperative group trials provide a good overview of DSMC structure and function.[67]

Trial Reporting

Once a study is completed and the data are fully analyzed, its results should be reported promptly. Publication of the results of a trial in a scientific journal represents culmination of investigator efforts and allows wide distribution of the findings. However, lack of precise requirements of reporting may lead to inaccurate or biased results presentation. The Consolidated Standards of Reporting Trials (CONSORT) statement is used worldwide to improve the quality of reporting of randomized controlled trials.[68] It provides a 25-item checklist of all required elements and a flow diagram to ensure accounting of all enrolled patients. Many journals require authors to follow CONSORT guidelines because "diligent adherence by authors to the checklist items facilitates clarity, completeness, and transparency of reporting."[68] The International Committee of Medical Journal Editors (ICMJE) similarly publishes guidelines on uniform requirements for manuscripts submitted to biomedical journals.[69] There have also been calls for improvements in reporting of phase I and II trials.[70,71] In addition to quality with respect to content, a full disclosure of any financial conflict of interest by the investigators to the readers is necessary as well. Redundant publications (repeating the same results in several journals) are discouraged, and there is an obligation to publish negative studies. Study of the publication rate of cancer cooperative group trials regardless of findings shows that there is room for improvement with respect to a responsible approach to clinical trial conduct.[72]

In the United States, reporting requirements are trending toward an expansion to more "open access" sources, based on mandates arising from recently enacted legislation. ClinicalTrials.gov is the largest clinical trials database in the world, run by the National Library of Medicine at NIH. Initially including information only on NIH-sponsored studies, the database now contains studies sponsored by the pharmaceutical companies and demands "basic results" information not later than 1 year after the study's primary completion date. The requirements for results reporting was prompted by removal of several drugs from the market because of earlier unrealized toxicity—knowledge about which was obscured by lack of publication or other public documentation.

RECENT APPROACHES TO CLINICAL TRIAL DESIGN

An Alternative Phase I Design for Radiation Oncology Trials

As mentioned earlier, phase I trials in radiation therapy present a unique challenge in that toxicities may occur long after treatment and need to be incorporated into dose evaluation. Traditional stepwise designs do not accommodate this; therefore, the time-to-event continual reassessment method (TITE-CRM), an extension of the continual reassessment method (CRM),[73] was developed that incorporates the time-to-event (i.e., time-to-toxicity) information for each patient.[26,74] In the TITE-CRM approach, a dose-response model is first posited that identifies the starting dose and range to be considered, along with a time frame for events occurring anywhere up to T time units from administration of therapy. Rather than waiting for each cohort of patients to be followed for this length of time, however, one can enter new patients at, say, half-month intervals. As in the original CRM, the first patient is assigned to a dose level on the basis of prior information or, as in the modified CRM, to the lowest candidate dose. At the time the next patients are to be enrolled, the observed toxicities and follow-up times of patients already entered are used to form an updated estimate of the β parameter that defines the dose-response curve, and the dose level for the next patients is selected according to the usual CRM or modified CRM criteria. In simulation studies, the TITE-CRM produced results comparable to its CRM counterpart while significantly reducing the average duration of the trial. However, the TITE-CRM method was associated with slightly more toxicities, particularly in situations where events tend to occur near the end of the observation period, because escalation to the next dose may have already occurred before toxicities were observed.[74] Another problematic issue is rapid accrual, where premature escalation of dose may be indicated. A recent review and suggested modifications may make this approach even more suitable for radiation oncology trials.[75]

Alternative Phase II Trial Designs

As indicated earlier, the value of traditional single-arm phase II trials has been called into question in terms of providing a reliable basis for further pursuit of promising treatments. The currently favored design is a randomized phase II trial with a standard of care comparison group.[12,16,76] This approach and the goal of accelerating development has led to consideration enhancements to the phase II design, including adaptive randomization, where one favors enrollment to the arm(s) that seem to be prevailing while reducing probability of enrollment on other arms, and even dropping some treatment arms. This is an idea with a long history[77]; however, recent innovations in computing and bayesian methods, as well as a newfound interest in accelerated development, have brought it to wider use in some settings.[78] In some instances, it may offer advantages but must be weighed against simpler approaches with similar or even greater efficiency.[79]

Changes in therapeutic approaches also suggest design changes. Because primarily cytostatic agents (i.e., most biologic drugs) are not expected to necessarily result in tumor response in the traditional sense, there is a need to consider alternative phase II designs based on end points other than response rates. For trials enrolling patients who have failed prior therapy, Mick et al.[80] propose a method that uses each patient as his or her own control, comparing the time to progression (possibly censored) under the new agent with the time to progression under prior therapy. Rosner et al.[81] propose a randomized discontinuation design to evaluate cytostatic drugs in which all patients are initially treated with the experimental agent. After a specified interval, responders remain on drug and those who progress discontinue, whereas those patients with stable disease are randomized to either continued active treatment or placebo. This randomized comparison allows one to assess whether the drug is truly slowing the rate of growth of the tumor, as opposed to the investigators having simply selected patients with slow-growing tumors. Because patients with stable disease form a more homogeneous subgroup, this design also requires a smaller sample size than would a trial that randomized all patients at entry. It is important to note that the purpose of this design is to determine whether the drug is active in an explanatory sense. Whether the percentage of patients exhibiting stable disease is high or low has bearing on the efficiency of the approach, because in the latter case, the total sample size required may be quite large and any demonstration of activity in the randomized component would only be relevant to a small subset of the population. Korn et al.[82] point out other caveats with this design. For example, patients may find it unattractive to potentially discontinue a treatment that they perceive to be helping their disease.

Using Biomarkers as Inclusion Criteria

It is increasingly understood that the response of tumors to targeted agents highly depends on their molecular subtype. Consequently, trials increasingly screen for molecular characteristics of tumors to use as eligibility criteria or, at a minimum, stratification factors. For example, recent and currently accruing RTOG brain tumor trials stratify patients according to whether or not the *MGMT* gene is methylated, whereas head and neck cancer trials require human papillomavirus (HPV) status to be determined at entry. When studies enroll sufficient numbers of patients, then treatment by marker synergisms, referred to statistically as interaction effects, can be investigated. Robust evaluation of true differential benefit according to markers requires that treatments be randomized; thus, randomized phase II and phase III trials are ideal settings for developing tailored treatments.

In many instances, potentially responsive subsets of patients may be small and may also be identified after trials have initiated enrollment. For instance, anaplastic lymphoma kinase (ALK) inhibitors are highly effective, although only in the 3% to 5% of lung cancers that have *ALK* gene rearrangements. It may simply not be feasible to perform separate phase III trials for each lung cancer subtype. One possible alternative is "adaptive randomized" trial designs in which the data gathered as the trial progresses is used to change some aspect of the trial as it progresses. Some recent examples are the Biomarker-integrated Approaches of Targeted Therapy for Lung Cancer Elimination (BATTLE) trial in lung cancer[83] and the I-SPY trials in breast cancer.[84] However, there are limitations and challenges to these complex trial designs. For example, to be able to acquire information rapidly enough to undertake weighted randomization favoring more promising arms or to eliminate nonresponsive arms, surrogate end points such as "disease control rate at 8 weeks" must be used. It is not clear whether such short-term end points are relevant to radiation oncology where local control is very frequently achieved.

Several recent papers in the clinical literature have provided excellent reviews of the opportunities and challenges involved in incorporating modern molecular medicine into clinical trial design.[85,86]

MOVING BEYOND CLINICAL TRIALS

Comparative Effectiveness Research

The randomized phase III clinical trial is considered the most robust method of comparing the efficacy of a new treatment with the standard of care. Grading systems for evaluating clinical evidence universally place randomized controlled trials above observational trials.[87] More recently, this hierarchical approach to scientific evidence has been attacked;[17] criticisms include the high fiscal cost of clinical trials, the length of time that it takes to obtain a conclusion (by which time the results are frequently no longer relevant because the standard of care has changed), and the large number of trials with negative results.

A specific criticism relates to clinical protocols that typically allow enrollment of only the fittest patients who lack comorbidities and have good performance status—criteria that subsequently limit the generalizability of the results. For example, studies have shown that older patients are excluded unnecessarily out of concern for potential adverse events.[88–90] There have indeed long been calls for simpler and more inclusive eligibility criteria.[91]

In some sense, the desire to reduce exclusivity and broaden trial enrollment to more closely match the population is antithetical to "personalized medicine" and more focused trials, as mentioned previously. However, there are some ways in which the two concepts can possibly work in concert. Larger trials that can robustly support subset analysis according to biologic, clinical, and health history/behavior factors can at once be more inclusive and address questions regarding particularly responsive subgroups.

Another response to the criticism of phase III trials has been a reappreciation of the importance of population-based retrospective studies as a way to measure a treatment's effectiveness in the "real world." Even more useful are well-designed prospective cohort studies, such as Cancer of the Prostate Strategic Urologic Research Endeavor (CaPSURE), which will provide information both on factors driving treatment choice and the effects of specific intervention strategies for which randomized trial evidence is currently lacking.[92] Another key strategy is conducting trials in parallel with concurrent registries of patients treated according to physician and patient choice and/or common convention, such as the Trial Assigning Individualized Options for Treatment (Rx), or TAILORx.[93] In this trial, 7,000 women with breast cancer are screened using a molecular profiling tool. For those with profiles in the range where the utility of the tool is uncertain, randomization between hormonal therapy alone and hormonal therapy plus chemotherapy is performed. Patients obtaining scores below or above this range are registered to accurately record treatment choices and ensure that good follow-up data is obtained. This trial will both serve to determine the utility of the profiling tool in the uncertain range and provide high-quality data on the validity of treatment decisions based on it.

Meta-analysis

A formal quantitative means of combining evidence from multiple clinical trials is by meta-analysis—a widely used analytic tool in many areas of social and medical science. Meta-analysis refers to a process whereby data from independent studies are combined to form a quantitative summary estimate of a given effect.

Meta-analyses are considered by some to be a level I evidence source along with large randomized clinical trials. A meta-analysis combines results of several studies, all of which ask a similar research question but may be individually too small to have enough statistical power to definitively answer the question. Performing a systematic analysis of data from all identified randomized trials can define a modest yet real advantage associated with a new therapeutic approach. To address the likelihood of publication bias (i.e., a greater representation of trials with positive results appearing in the literature), the meta-analysis should include unpublished studies as well, although their quality may be sometimes doubtful because of lack of peer review. The choice of trials to be included is critical, because analyzing trials with disparate patient populations or treatment methods may lead to erroneous conclusions. Despite some limitations, meta-analyses can be influential in guiding treatment practice. For example, a meta-analysis of sequential versus concurrent chemotherapy combined with thoracic radiotherapy in stage III non–small cell lung cancer[94] confirmed the concurrent approach to be superior in overall survival and contributed to its validity as standard therapy. An excellent example of the methods and data summaries used in meta-analysis in oncology can be found in the reports of the Early Breast Cancer Trialists' Collaborative Group.[95,96]

CONCLUSIONS

Advances in molecular biology over the previous two decades have led to an explosion in the number of new anticancer agents being developed, as well as a rapid increase in the number of clinical trials performed, with resulting improvements in the overall survival and quality of life of cancer patients. In parallel, however, the escalating costs of conducting trials, their increasing complexity, and the ever-expanding regulatory requirements have placed an undue burden on all involved, which has strained the available resources. Inadequate harmonization between countries preventing the straightforward conduct of international trials is another source of inefficiency, sometimes leading to unnecessary duplication of efforts between American and European cooperative groups. Furthermore, the imbalance of funding between academic-sponsored (e.g., NCI) versus pharmaceutical company–sponsored studies may lead to competition for available patients. The public's and physicians' awareness and understanding of the importance of clinical trial enrollment need to be improved; likewise, enhancing diverse socioeconomic and ethnic groups' access to trials is essential.

Contemporary efforts to make electronic clinical trials management systems widespread and unified, to have tissue specimens and data banks accessible to all researchers, and the study results readily available to the public will facilitate the optimal utilization of these precious resources and, most importantly, lead to meaningful improvements in the care of cancer patients.

ACKNOWLEDGMENTS

Some content was modified from previous editions of this chapter. The current authors gratefully acknowledge author contributions from the previous edition.

REFERENCES

1. Crowley J, Ankerst D. *Handbook of statistics in clinical oncology.* New York: Chapman & Hall/CRC, 2006.
2. Green S, Benedetti J, Smith A. *Clinical trials in oncology.* Chapman & Hall/CRC, 2012.
3. Kelly K, Halabi S. *Oncology clinical trials: successful design, conduct and analysis.* New York: Demos Medical, 2009.
4. Unknown. *Wikipedia.* Available at: http://en.wikipedia.org/wiki/Clinical_trial.
5. Piantadosi S. *Clinical trials: a methodologic perspective.* John Wiley & Sons, 2005.
6. National Cancer Institute. *NCI's Clinical Trials Cooperative Group Program.* Available at: http://www.cancer.gov/cancertopics/factsheet/NCI/clinical-trials-cooperative-group.
7. Hearn J, Sullivan R. The impact of the 'Clinical Trials' directive on the cost and conduct of non-commercial cancer trials in the UK. *Eur J Cancer* 2007;43:8–13.
8. Emanuel EJ, Wendler D, Grady C. What makes clinical research ethical? *JAMA* 2000;83:2701–2711.
9. Wendler D. The ethics of clinical research. In: Zalta EN, ed. *The Stanford encyclopedia of philosophy,* 2009. Available at: http://plato.stanford.edu/cgi-bin/encyclopedia/archinfo.cgi?entry=clinical-research.
10. Piantadosi S. Principles of clinical trial design. *Semin Oncol* 1988;15:423–433.
11. Ratain MJ, Sargent DJ. Optimising the design of phase II oncology trials: the importance of randomisation. *Eur J Cancer* 2009;45:275–280.
12. Mandrekar SJ, Sargent DJ. Randomized phase II trials: time for a new era in clinical trial design. *J Thorac Oncol* 2010;5:932–934.
13. Tang H, Foster NR, Grothey A, et al. Comparison of error rates in single-arm versus randomized phase II cancer clinical trials. *J Clin Oncol* 2010;28:1936–1941.
14. Leventhal BG. An overview of clinical trials in oncology. *Semin Oncol* 1988;15:414–422.
15. Simon R, Wittes RE, Ellenberg SS. Randomized phase II clinical trials. *Cancer Treat Rep* 1985;69:1375–1381.
16. Rubinstein LV, Korn EL, Freidlin B, et al. Design issues of randomized phase II trials and a proposal for phase II screening trials. *J Clin Oncol* 2005;23:7199–7206.
17. Vogelbaum MA. The future of clinical research beyond phase III trials. *Clin Neurosurg* 2009;56:37–39.
18. FitzGerald TJ, Urie M, Ulin K, et al. Processes for quality improvements in radiation oncology clinical trials. *Int J Radiat Oncol Biol Phys* 2008;71:S76.
19. Justin EB, Joachim Y. Quality of radiotherapy reporting in randomized controlled trials of Hodgkin's lymphoma and non-Hodgkin's lymphoma: a systematic review. *Int J Radiat Oncol Biol Phys* 2009;73:492–498.
20. Morris SL, Beasley M, Leslie M. Chemotherapy for pancreatic cancer. *N Engl J Med* 2004;350:2713–2715; author reply 2713–2715.
21. Bydder S, Spry N. Chemotherapy for pancreatic cancer. *N Engl J Med* 2004;350:2713–2715; author reply 2713–2715.
22. Crane CH, Ben-Josef E, Small W Jr. Chemotherapy for pancreatic cancer. *N Engl J Med* 2004;350:2713–2715; author reply 2713–2715.
23. Rischin D, Peters L, Fisher R, et al. Tirapazamine, cisplatin, and radiation versus fluorouracil, cisplatin, and radiation in patients with locally advanced head and neck cancer: a randomized phase II trial of the Trans-Tasman Radiation Oncology Group (TROG 98.02). *J Clin Oncol* 2005;23:79.
24. Weiner MA, Leventhal B, Brecher ML, et al. Randomized study of intensive MOPP-ABVD with or without low-dose total-nodal radiation therapy in the treatment of stages IIB, IIIA2, IIIB, and IV Hodgkin's disease in pediatric patients: a Pediatric Oncology Group study. *J Clin Oncol* 1997;15:2769–2779.
25. Abrams RA, Winter KA, Regine WF, et al. Failure to adhere to protocol specified radiation therapy guidelines was associated with decreased survival in RTOG 9704-A phase III trial of adjuvant chemotherapy and chemoradiotherapy for patients with resected adenocarcinoma of the pancreas. *Int J Radiat Oncol Biol Phys* 2012;82(2):809–816.
26. Normolle D, Lawrence T. Designing dose-escalation trials with late-onset toxicities using the time-to-event continual reassessment method. *J Clin Oncol* 2006;24:4426–4433.
27. Glass C, Den R, Dicker AP, et al. *Toxicity of phase I radiation oncology trials: worldwide experience, abstract #1605. American Society for Therapeutic Radiation Oncology (ASTRO) 52nd Annual Meeting,* October 31–November 4, 2010, San Diego, CA.
28. Liu PY, LeBlanc M, Desai M. False positive rates of randomized phase II designs. *Control Clin Trials* 1999;20:343–352.
29. Therasse P, Arbuck SG, Eisenhauer EA, et al. New guidelines to evaluate the response to treatment in solid tumors. European Organization for Research and Treatment of Cancer, National Cancer Institute of the United States, National Cancer Institute of Canada. *J Natl Cancer Inst* 2000;92:205–216.
30. Chen TT, Chute JP, Feigal E, et al. A model to select chemotherapy regimens for phase III trials for extensive-stage small-cell lung cancer. *J Natl Cancer Inst* 2000;92:1601–1607.
31. Buyse M, Thirion P, Carlson RW, et al. Relation between tumour response to first-line chemotherapy and survival in advanced colorectal cancer: a meta-analysis. Meta-Analysis Group in Cancer. *Lancet* 2000;356:373–378.
32. Moertel CG. Improving the efficiency of clinical trials: a medical perspective. *Stat Med* 1984;3:455–468.
33. Gaynor JJ, Feuer EJ, Tan CC, et al. On the use of cause-specific failure and conditional failure probabilities: examples from clinical oncology data. *J Am Stat Assoc* 1993:400–409.
34. Dignam JJ, Kocherginsky MN. Choice and interpretation of statistical tests used when competing risks are present. *J Clin Oncol* 2008;26:4027–4034.
35. Hudis CA, Barlow WE, Costantino JP, et al. Proposal for standardized definitions for efficacy end points in adjuvant breast cancer trials: the STEEP system. *J Clin Oncol* 2007;25:2127–2132.
36. Sargent DJ, Wieand HS, Haller DG, et al. Disease-free survival versus overall survival as a primary end point for adjuvant colon cancer studies: individual patient data from 20,898 patients on 18 randomized trials. *J Clin Oncol* 2005;23:8664–8670.
37. Prentice RL. Surrogate endpoints in clinical trials: definition and operational criteria. *Stat Med* 1989;8:431–440.
38. Buyyounouski MK, Hanlon AL, Horwitz EM, et al. Interval to biochemical failure highly prognostic for distant metastasis and prostate cancer-specific mortality after radiotherapy. *Int J Radiat Oncol Biol Phys* 2008;70:59–66.
39. Denham JW, Steigler A, Wilcox C, et al. Time to biochemical failure and prostate-specific antigen doubling time as surrogates for prostate cancer-specific mortality: evidence from the TROG 96.01 randomised controlled trial. *Lancet Oncol* 2008;9:1058–1068.
40. Schatzkin A, Gail M. The promise and peril of surrogate end points in cancer research. *Nat Rev Cancer* 2002;2:19–27.
41. Halpern SD, Karlawish JH, Berlin JA. The continuing unethical conduct of underpowered clinical trials. *JAMA* 2002;288:358–362.
42. Shuster J. Power and sample size for phase III clinical trials of survival. *Handbook of statistics in clinical oncology.* New York: Chapman & Hall/CRC, 2006: 207–226.
43. Freedman LS. Tables of the number of patients required in clinical trials using the logrank test. *Stat Med* 1982;1:121–129.
44. Ahnn S, Anderson SJ. Sample size determination in complex clinical trials comparing more than two groups for survival endpoints. *Stat Med* 1998;17:2525–2534.
45. Lachin JM, Foulkes MA. Evaluation of sample size and power for analyses of survival with allowance for nonuniform patient entry, losses to follow-up, noncompliance, and stratification. *Biometrics* 1986;42:507–519.
46. Shih JH. Sample size calculation for complex clinical trials with survival endpoints. *Control Clin Trials* 1995;16:395–407.
47. Simon R. Optimal two-stage designs for phase II clinical trials. *Control Clin Trials* 1989;10:1–10.
48. Jennison C, Turnbull BW. *Group sequential methods with applications to clinical trials.* London: Chapman & Hall/CRC, 2000.
49. Haybittle JL. Repeated assessment of results in clinical trials of cancer treatment. *Br J Radiol* 1971;44:793–797.
50. Peto R, Pike MC, Armitage P, et al. Design and analysis of randomized clinical trials requiring prolonged observation of each patient. II. Analysis and examples. *Br J Cancer* 1977;35:1–39.
51. Fleming TR, Harrington DP, O'Brien PC. Designs for group sequential tests. *Control Clin Trials* 1984;5:348–361.
52. Halperin M, Lan KK, Ware JH, et al. An aid to data monitoring in long-term clinical trials. *Control Clin Trials* 1982;3:311–323.
53. Lan KK, Wittes J. The B-value: a tool for monitoring data. *Biometrics* 1988;44: 579–585.
54. Dignam JJ, Bryant J, Wieand HS, et al. Early stopping of a clinical trial when there is evidence of no treatment benefit: protocol B-14 of the National Surgical Adjuvant Breast and Bowel Project. *Control Clin Trials* 1998;19:575–588.
55. Freidlin B, Korn EL, Gray R. A general inefficacy interim monitoring rule for randomized clinical trials. *Clin Trials* 2010;7:197–208.
56. Freidlin B, Korn EL. A comment on futility monitoring. *Control Clin Trials* 2002; 23:355–366.
57. Fleming TR, Sharples K, McCall J, et al. Maintaining confidentiality of interim data to enhance trial integrity and credibility. *Clin Trials* 2008;5:157–167.
58. Gail MH. Eligibility exclusions, losses to follow-up, removal of randomized patients, and uncounted events in cancer clinical trials. *Cancer Treat Rep* 1985;69:1107–1113.
59. Redmond C, Fisher B, Wieand HS. The methodologic dilemma in retrospectively correlating the amount of chemotherapy received in adjuvant therapy protocols with disease-free survival. *Cancer Treat Rep* 1983;67:519–526.

60. Schmoor C, Sauerbrei W, Schumacher M. Sample size considerations for the evaluation of prognostic factors in survival analysis. *Stat Med* 2000;19:441–452.
61. Schwarzer G, Schumacher M, Sauerbrei W, et al. Prognostic factor studies. In: Crowley J, Ankerst DP eds. *Handbook of Statistics in Clinical Oncology,* 2nd ed. New York: Chapman & Hall, 2005:289–333.
62. Grant N, Sacatos M, Kelly K. The trials and tribulations of writing an investigator initiated clinical study. In: Kelly K, Halabi S, eds. *Oncology clinical trials: successful design, conduct and analysis.* New York: Demos Medical, 2009:119–130.
63. FDA. Guidance for industry: clinical trial endpoints for the approval of cancer drugs and biologics. Available at: http://www.fda.gov/downloads/drugs/GuidanceComplianceRegulatoryInformation/Guidances/UCM071590.pdf. Accessed November 9, 2011.
64. Brandsma D, Stalpers L, Taal W, et al. Clinical features, mechanisms, and management of pseudoprogression in malignant gliomas. *Lancet Oncol* 2008;9:453–461.
65. De Pourcq F. Defining the roles and responsibilities of study personnel. In: Kelly K, Halabi S, eds. *Oncology clinical trials: successful design, conduct and analysis.* New York: Demos Medical, 2009:321–326.
66. Lan KK, Lachin JM, Bautista O. Over-ruling a group sequential boundary—a stopping rule versus a guideline. *Stat Med* 2003;22:3347–3355.
67. Smith MA, Ungerleider RS, Korn EL, et al. Role of independent data-monitoring committees in randomized clinical trials sponsored by the National Cancer Institute. *J Clin Oncol* 1997;15:2736–2743.
68. Schulz KF, Altman DG, Moher D. CONSORT 2010 statement: updated guidelines for reporting parallel group randomised trials. *BMJ;*340:c332.
69. International Committee of Medical Journal Editors (ICMJE). Uniform requirements for manuscripts submitted to biomedical journals: writing and editing for biomedical publication. *Haematologica* 2004;89:264.
70. Mariani L, Marubini E. Content and quality of currently published phase II cancer trials. *J Clin Oncol* 2000;18:429–436.
71. Zohar S, Lian Q, Levy V, et al. Quality assessment of phase I dose-finding cancer trials: proposal of a checklist. *Clin Trials* 2008;5:478–485.
72. Krzyzanowska MK, Pintilie M, Tannock IF. Factors associated with failure to publish large randomized trials presented at an oncology meeting. *JAMA* 2003;290:495–501.
73. O'Quigley J, Pepe M, Fisher L. Continual reassessment method: a practical design for phase 1 clinical trials in cancer. *Biometrics* 1990;46:33–48.
74. Cheung YK, Chappell R. Sequential designs for phase I clinical trials with late-onset toxicities. *Biometrics* 2000;56:1177–1182.
75. Polley MY. Practical modifications to the time-to-event continual reassessment method for phase I cancer trials with fast patient accrual and late-onset toxicities. *Stat Med* 2011;30:2130–2143.
76. Cannistra SA. Phase II trials in *Journal of Clinical Oncology. J Clin Oncol* 2009; 27:3073–3076.
77. Zelen M. Play the winner rule and the controlled clinical trial. *J Am Stat Assoc* 1969; 64:131–146.
78. Biswas S, Liu DD, Lee JJ, et al. Bayesian clinical trials at the University of Texas M.D. Anderson Cancer Center. *Clin Trials* 2009;6:205–216.
79. Korn EL, Freidlin B. Outcome—adaptive randomization: is it useful? *J Clin Oncol* 2011;29:771–776.
80. Mick R, Crowley JJ, Carroll RJ. Phase II clinical trial design for noncytotoxic anticancer agents for which time to disease progression is the primary endpoint. *Control Clin Trials* 2000;21:343–359.
81. Rosner GL, Stadler W, Ratain MJ. Randomized discontinuation design: application to cytostatic antineoplastic agents. *J Clin Oncol* 2002;20:4478–4484
82. Korn EL, Arbuck SG, Pluda JM, et al. Clinical trial designs for cytostatic agents: are new approaches needed? *J Clin Oncol* 2001;19:265–272.
83. Kim ES, Herbst RS, Wistuba II, et al. The BATTLE trial: personalizing therapy for lung cancer. *Cancer Discov* 2011;1:44–53.
84. Barker AD, Sigman CC, Kelloff GJ, et al. I-SPY 2: an adaptive breast cancer trial design in the setting of neoadjuvant chemotherapy. *Clin Pharmacol Ther* 2009;86:97–100.
85. Freidlin B, McShane LM, Korn EL. Randomized clinical trials with biomarkers: design issues. *J Natl Cancer Inst* 2010;102:152–160.
86. Simon R. The use of genomics in clinical trial design. *Clin Cancer Res* 2008; 14:5984–5993.
87. Harbour R, Miller J. A new system for grading recommendations in evidence based guidelines. *BMJ* 2001;323:334–336.
88. Hutchins LF, Unger JM, Crowley JJ, et al. Underrepresentation of patients 65 years of age or older in cancer-treatment trials. *N Engl J Med* 1999;341:2061–2067.
89. Kumar A, Soares HP, Balducci L, et al. Treatment tolerance and efficacy in geriatric oncology: a systematic review of phase III randomized trials conducted by five National Cancer Institute–sponsored cooperative groups. *J Clin Oncol* 2007;25:1272–1276.
90. Lewis JH, Kilgore ML, Goldman DP, et al. Participation of patients 65 years of age or older in cancer clinical trials. *J Clin Oncol* 2003;21:1383–1389.
91. George SL. Reducing patient eligibility criteria in cancer clinical trials. *J Clin Oncol* 1996;14:1364–1370.
92. Lubeck DP, Litwin MS, Henning JM, et al. The CaPSURE database: a methodology for clinical practice and research in prostate cancer. CaPSURE Research Panel. Cancer of the Prostate Strategic Urologic Research Endeavor. *Urology* 1996;48:773–777.
93. Sparano JA. TAILORx: trial assigning individualized options for treatment (Rx). *Clin Breast Cancer* 2006;7:347–350.
94. Auperin A, Le Pechoux C, Rolland E, et al. Meta-analysis of concomitant versus sequential radiochemotherapy in locally advanced non-small-cell lung cancer. *J Clin Oncol* 2010;28:2181–2190.
95. Clarke M, Collins R, Darby S, et al. Effects of radiotherapy and of differences in the extent of surgery for early breast cancer on local recurrence and 15-year survival: an overview of the randomised trials. *Lancet* 2005;366:2087–2106.
96. Davies C, Godwin J, Gray R, et al. Relevance of breast cancer hormone receptors and other factors to the efficacy of adjuvant tamoxifen: patient-level meta-analysis of randomised trials. *Lancet* 2011;378:771–784.

Chapter 15
Total-Body and Hemibody Irradiation

Kenneth B. Roberts, Zhe Chen, and Stuart Seropian

Historically, total-body irradiation (TBI) has been used without stem cell support for palliation of radiation-sensitive disease such as chronic lymphocytic leukemia (CLL) or follicular lymphomas. TBI is mainly performed in the context of hematopoietic transplantation for its cytoxic and immunologic effects. Normal bone marrow tolerance for radiation is exceeded, and the patient's hematopoietic system is reconstituted by the stem cell transplantation procedure. Donor cells may come from another human or from the patient's pool of stem cells, referred to as allogeneic or autologous transplantation, respectively. In the case of donor stem cells from an identical twin, the term syngeneic transplantation is appropriate. Hemibody irradiation (HBI) has a different therapeutic goal, which is generally for palliation of diffuse metastatic disease. Stem cell support is not required.

TOTAL-BODY IRRADIATION

Historical Use of TBI without Stem Cell Rescue

Total-body irradiation has been used as a form of systemic therapy for various malignant diseases since the beginning of the 20th century.[1] However, the usefulness of TBI without hematopoietic stem cell rescue is limited because the median lethal dose of whole-body radiation exposure given as a single fraction is approximately 4 Gy in humans. Given the radiosensitivity of chronic lymphocytic leukemia or low grade, advanced-stage non-Hodgkin lymphoma, TBI was an effective palliative modality using doses as low as 0.025 to 0.15 Gy several times a week, titrating total dose to clinical response.[2,3] Because of myelosuppression—especially thrombocytopenia—the standard recommendation was to allow a 4- to 8-week treatment break after each cumulative 0.5 Gy of TBI.[4,5] Johnson reported in the 1970s that one-third of patients with chronic lymphocytic leukemia attained complete remission with low-dose TBI alone, and slightly more did so when alkylating chemotherapy was added.[5] These results were not supported by a Eastern Cooperative Oncology Group phase III trial, however,[6] and the role for TBI without stem cell rescue has diminished further with advances in cytotoxic chemotherapy since the 1960s, as well as with the recent availability of anti-CD20 antibody therapies, including radioimmunoconjugates.

TBI in Stem Cell Transplantation

The conditioning regimen for hematopoietic stem cell transplantation has several functions. One is cytotoxicity: to contribute to the eradication of any residual cancer. Another important function of the conditioning regimen is immunosuppression so that the host does not reject the allogeneic donor stem cells. TBI in the broad range of 2 to 15 Gy in conjunction with chemotherapy serves these functions well.

Radiobiologic Effects on Normal Hematopoietic System

Successful hematopoietic stem cell engraftment requires (a) eradication of the recipient bone marrow, (b) immunosuppression to prevent rejection of donor marrow in the case of an allotransplant, and (c) relative sparing of the recipient's bone marrow stromal cells. The reported D_0 values of bone marrow stem cells usually range from 0.5 to 1.4 Gy, indicating intrinsic radiosensitivity.[7,8] Although conventional wisdom assumes that recipient marrow cells must be removed to leave space for donor cells in stem cell microenvironmental conditions to favor the donor cells in a competitive repopulation, this concept has been challenged. In fact, mixed bone marrow chimerism resulting from a less cytotoxic nonmyeloablative transplantation may be acceptable or even desirable.

Immunosuppression in the setting of allogeneic bone marrow transplantation is necessary to avoid rejection of donor marrow, and TBI is a very efficient immunosuppressant. In animal work by Storb and colleagues, equivalent doses of fractionated TBI were significantly less effective than single-dose TBI to condition DLA-identical littermate dogs before bone marrow transplantation.[9,10] Their conclusion was that there was significant repair of DNA damage by lymphoid cells during interfraction intervals. In a murine model, Salomon et al. looked at three TBI schemas from schedules that had been proposed for human TBI (8.5 Gy single-dose TBI, 2 Gy times 6 fractions of TBI, and 1.2 Gy times 12 fractions of hyperfractionated TBI).[11] In terms of the immunosuppressive effects, the results favored single-dose TBI. A marked initial shoulder on the dose–survival curve has been reported for T-lymphocyte precursors[12] and for a human lymphoblastoid cell line.[13] There is a marked fractionation sensitivity of the immunosuppressive effect of TBI, leading one to conclude that fractionated TBI would lead to more graft rejections than the same dose delivered in a single fraction. Clinical data confirm these findings, in that fractionated TBI programs using total doses of 13 to 15 Gy are roughly equivalent to the efficacy of 10-Gy single-dose TBI.

If bone marrow stromal cells and their progenitors (fibroblast colony-forming cells) are damaged, delayed engraftment or even graft failure may follow.[14] Progenitors of human bone marrow stromal cells have been found to have a D_0 of 1.46 Gy.[15] They are also sensitive to dose rate effects and fractionation; thus, fractionated TBI spares bone marrow stromal cells and their progenitors better than does single-dose TBI.[16]

Radiobiologic Effects on Leukemia

In the setting of stem cell transplantation procedures, TBI achieves significant leukemia cell killing and, in conjunction with chemotherapy and graft-versus-leukemia (GVL) effect, leads to eradication of malignant clones in a significant portion of cases. The use of the D_0 value gives a rough indication of the radiosensitivity of various cell populations; most D_0 values for both animal and human leukemias cell lines range from 0.8 to 1.5 Gy,[17–18,19-20] although extreme values range from 0.3 to >5 Gy. Leukemic cell lines frequently show a minimal initial shoulder in radiation cell survival curves, leading to the hypothesis that fractionation (or reduced dose rate exposure) should have only a minor effect on cell survival. Split-dose radiation experiments lend further support to this hypothesis. Greater repair capacity is seen with more differentiated leukemias or lymphocytes (e.g., B- or T-cell phenotypes).

Graft-Versus-Leukemia/Tumor Effects

Allogeneic stem cell transplantation is largely an immunologic therapy. Allogeneic hematopoietic cells must be matched with the recipient for the majority of the major histocompatibility antigens to avoid rejection and minimize graft-versus-host disease, but minor human leukocyte antigen (HLA) differences facilitate a graft-versus-leukemia effect that enhances transplantation efficacy. Early studies demonstrated improved leukemia control with allogeneic bone marrow cells as compared to syngeneic (identical twin) donor cells. Further evidence for the graft-versus-leukemia effect derives from the efficacy of donor lymphocyte infusions after relapse of leukemia following allotransplant. In general with allogeneic transplantation, it is necessary to modulate the immune reconstitution during engraftment (e.g., using cyclosporine) to produce a graft-versus-leukemia effect while minimizing graft-versus-host disease.

Graft-Versus-Host Disease

Despite HLA matching, allogeneic stem cell transplantation is limited by graft-versus-host disease (GVHD). GVHD results from the activation and proliferation of mature donor T cells that recognize recipient alloantigens presented as peptide molecules by antigen-presenting cells (APCs). In the setting of allogeneic transplantation, despite HLA matching, a repertoire of peptides displayed on recipient cells can be recognized as minor histocompatibility antigens by donor T cells due to the polymorphisms in genes outside the HLA system.[21] The activation of donor T cells after contact with specialized APCs leads to differentiation to effector cells that produce cytokines such as interferon-gamma and tumor necrosis factor, as well as mediate cytotoxicity against normal recipient organs. Acute GVHD includes clinical damage to skin, gastrointestinal tract, and liver, but other organs can also be involved. Later GVHD may present as a chronic form with more varied clinical symptoms similar to rheumatologic or connective tissue diseases.

Despite the prophylactic use of immunosuppressive agents such as cyclosporine, tacrolimus, methotrexate, prednisone, or mycophenolate mofetil, more than half of the recipients undergoing HLA-matched sibling hematopoietic transplants develop some degree of GVHD.[22,23] Advanced forms of graft-versus-host disease require augmented immunosuppression, typically with high doses of corticosteroids, which place patients at higher risk for posttransplant infections.[24] GVHD can be mitigated by T-cell depletion of the donor cells during the transplant procedure, but this then leads to an increased risk for infections, as well as to concerns that the desirable graft-versus-leukemia effects are diminished or lost. Nevertheless, there have been some clinical success with T cell–depleted allogeneic transplants in reducing GVHD, which typically relies on TBI-based myeloablative conditioning regimens.[25,26]

Recent laboratory work has focused on identifying T-cell subsets in the donor product that may be responsible for GVHD and differentiating them from T-cell populations that retain the important ability to mediate graft-versus-tumor effects and to reconstitute T-cell immunity to various viral and fungal pathogens such as cytomegalovirus, Epstein-Barr virus, *Candida albicans,* influenza, and varicella-zoster virus. So-called naive T cells appear to mediate GVHD and in humans have distinct cell surface antigens of CD45RA and CD62L.[27,28] Selective depletion of naive T cells with specific retention of memory T-cell subsets in murine experimental models of allogeneic transplantation have successfully reduced GVHD while retaining graft-versus-leukemia effects.[29–32,33] This observation has led to current investigations of selective T-cell depletion of CD45RA cells in the donor product along with fludarabine and TBI myeloablative conditioning. The hope is that T-cell populations including natural killer (NK) cells, NK/T cells, and central memory T cells will be retained to mediate important immunologic mechanisms of leukemia, tumor, and pathogen kill that improve the therapeutic ratio of transplantation.

TBI Dose-Limiting Toxicity—Pneumonitis and Other Late Effects

Early in the history of TBI, grade 4–5 solid-organ toxicities were found to be a major limitation, prompting a movement away from low-dose-rate, single-fraction TBI to fractionated regimens and non-TBI regimens. Studies in mice and humans show that the toxicities of TBI can be improved further by fractionating the radiation, as well as delivering by radiation at low dose rate. There is a high interfraction repair capacity of normal lung tissue. Thames and Hendry reported a low α/β value (3 to 6 Gy) for lung.[34] This has been confirmed with both animal and human data.[35–37] Sampath et al. estimated the α/β ratio for lung to be 2.8 Gy based on statistical modeling from 20 reports of clinical TBI in a total of 1,090 patients.[38] The lung-sparing effect for fractionation has been shown to be important down to roughly 1 Gy.[39] This dose roughly corresponds to the lowest fraction size in some hyperfractionated TBI schedules.[40] The marked lung-sparing effect of fractionation or of a decrease in dose rate has been confirmed by the work of Penney showing a progressive sparing of the lung with increased fractionation for both early pneumonitis and late fibrosis.[41] The rate of lung repair between fractions was reviewed by Travis, indicating the presence of two significantly different repair rates corresponding to a fast-repair half-time of 0.40 hour and a slow half-time of 4.01 hours.[42] The slow-repair component needs to be kept in mind when designing TBI schedules that include two or three fractions per day.[37]

The reduction of the risk of pneumonitis by fractionation is supported by a randomized clinical trial comparing low-dose-rate, single-fraction TBI (9.2 or 10 Gy) with low-dose-rate, fractionated TBI (12 Gy in six fractions over 3 days) for patients with acute myelogenous leukemia in first remission, which showed a significant improvement in event-free survival with fractionation, mainly because of a reduction in early mortality. Interstitial pneumonitis in these patients was decreased from 26% to 15% with fractionation.[43] Other studies confirmed that fractionated TBI regimens markedly reduce the incidence of idiopathic interstitial pneumonitis[44,45–46] to less than 20% without increasing the rate of tumor recurrence. Within a range of conventional fraction sizes of 1.5 to 2 Gy given once or twice daily, no significant increase in the incidence of interstitial pneumonitis was noted up to total doses as high as 15 Gy.[44,47,48] Nevertheless, total dose delivered to the lung is a key determinant of pneumonitis risk.[49,50]

Another radiobiologic approach to reduce the incidence of interstitial pneumonitis has been to lower the radiation dose rate—in essence a kind of continuous fractionation. Empirically this was found to be efficacious,[51,52] but treatment times of 2 to 3 hours or more are impractical for most radiotherapy departments. Moreover, such long treatment times are poorly tolerated by patients. Fractionated TBI appears to be a better way of exploiting the potential advantages inherent in the different radiobiologic properties of tumor cells and the lung. Within the context of fractionated TBI schemes, instantaneous dose rates of 0.05 to 0.18 Gy/min have been generally used, often determined by the available output of linear accelerators at extended treatment distances. It is unclear whether higher instantaneous dose rates are detrimental, despite theoretical concerns in this regard. One small study that compared dose rates of 0.075 versus 0.15 Gy/min in context of a TBI prescription of 12 Gy in six fractions reported a pneumonitis risk of 13% versus 43%, respectively, although there were many confounding covariates.[53] Other studies have not shown that dose rate is an important predictor of pneumonitis from fractionated TBI, but rather that total dose to the lung is the more critical determinant.[38]

Clinical Myeloablative Stem Cell Transplantation

Bone marrow or stem cell transplantation was conceived as a method of rescuing patients from the lethal effects of dose-intensive chemoradiotherapy. TBI has been a central part of allogeneic transplantation for leukemias ever since the pioneering work of Thomas and associates beginning in the late 1950s. A single dose of 9.2 Gy at a low dose rate of 0.07 Gy/min was required to obtain a consistent and sustained engraftment of allogeneic marrow in experimental animals. Consequently, a dose of 10 Gy at a dose rate of 0.07 to 0.10 Gy/min using cobalt teletherapy was used in humans.

The premise that TBI had to be given as a single fraction was challenged in the late 1970s when Peters et al. demonstrated the marked sensitivity of most normal tissues to altered fractionation and dose rate with minimal effects on bone marrow progenitors and leukemic cells.[52,54] It was concluded that with the same total dose an improved therapeutic ratio would be expected from a reduction in the dose rate of single-fraction TBI or by TBI fractionation. Calculations of various fractionation schemes and dose rates have been published based on the linear quadratic model.[55–57] O'Donoghue calculated that for very low dose rate TBI to be equivalent radiobiologically to the more common fractionated TBI schedules, an unreasonable radiation time of 20 to 24 hours would be necessary.[57] With concepts of both radiobiology and practicality in mind, a large variety of fractionated TBI schedules have been used. After a generation of clinical investigation, no one regimen is clearly superior to another; so many confounding variables exist (including TBI technique, disease and patient heterogeneity, chemotherapy, supportive care, and immunosuppression) that it is impossible to clearly demonstrate the superiority of a particular regimen. At present, most myeloablative TBI programs use a twice- or three-times-daily fractionation scheme over 3 to 4 days to deliver a total dose of 12 to 15 Gy.

Chemotherapy Used with TBI

Chemotherapy agents used in conjunction with TBI include cyclophosphamide, etoposide, and cytosine arabinoside, with cyclophosphamide at 120 mg/kg over 2 days being the most common based on early work from E. Donnall Thomas and colleagues in Seattle. Programs adding other agents have been used primarily in high-risk transplant settings, but cyclophosphamide remains a backbone, given its effectiveness in immunosuppression and cytotoxicity. Reduced-intensity or nonmyeloablative transplant regimens using low-dose TBI that have been developed in recent years have often used fludarabine or pentostatin in place of cyclophosphamide.[58,59] Chemotherapy and TBI are given sequentially rather than concurrently to avoid any potential increase in normal tissue toxicity. Whether chemotherapy should be given before or after TBI is unclear, and in the absence of clinical data showing which is best, logistic issues are the main consideration. Typically, TBI over 3 to 4 days is best delivered during the regular work week, when the full technical support staff is available. TBI may be better tolerated if given first when the patient is less fatigued and not sick from the effects of chemotherapy. The risk of nosocomial infections may be marginally lower when the patient travels to the radiotherapy department before becoming neutropenic later in the conditioning course. Alternatively, TBI at the end of the preparative regimen allows the stem cell transplant to proceed immediately thereafter; unlike chemotherapy, there is no washout period for elimination of the cytotoxic agent that would otherwise be harmful to the stem cells, thus saving a day or so of expected neutropenia while awaiting engraftment.

Non-TBI Conditioning Regimens

Although the evolution of TBI has led to significant reduction in toxicities, the initial concern about risk for fatal radiation pneumonitis lead to the development of non-TBI regimens. Santos at Johns Hopkins was the first to administer busulfan in place of radiotherapy in the busulfan–cyclophosphamide (BuCy) regimen.[60] Subsequently, a reduction in the cyclophosphamide dose (BuCy2) reduced toxicity without an apparent compromise in efficacy, and this regimen was established as a standard alternative to TBI-based conditioning.[61,62–63]

There have been numerous comparisons of the BuCy conditioning regimen and TBI-based conditioning, including five prospective randomized studies, several meta-analyses, and registry review studies with large patient numbers.[64–69,70,71,72–73,74–75] A French randomized clinical trial compared BuCy to cyclophosphamide-TBI before allogeneic bone marrow transplantation for adult acute myeloid leukemia (AML) in first remission.[65] The results showed that cyclophosphamide-TBI was superior for disease-free survival, relapse, and transplant mortality. A similar randomized study by the Nordic Bone Marrow Transplant Group also showed superior survival and lower morbidity with TBI-based conditioning.[64] In contrast, in chronic myeloid leukemia (CML) in chronic phase, the Seattle group demonstrated that BuCy was better tolerated and associated with a survival and relapse probability that was comparable to that of cyclophosphamide-TBI.[67] In 2001 Socie et al. reviewed the pooled outcome of all patients in the aforementioned four randomized studies with a mean follow-up of 7 years.[71] The probability for cure was statistically similar for both CML and AML, although a nonsignificant advantage for TBI in patients with AML was suggested. Long-term complications occurred equally following both types of conditioning, except that a higher risk of cataracts with TBI and irreversible alopecia with busulfan were noted. Registry reviews and meta-analyses typically show similar results for either regimen, with a possible advantage for TBI-based conditioning in AML and a higher risk of veno-occlusive disease of the liver in association with busulfan use.[63,72–73,74–75]

Studies on either side of the question have held very few variables constant, making the data almost impossible to interpret. Advances in the safe delivery of busulfan with pharmacokinetic monitoring and an intravenous formulation have further reduced the differences noted between conditioning regimens. The choice of conditioning regimen prior to transplantation depends upon a variety of factors that include the type of transplantation (allogeneic or autologous), the disease type, patient treatment history and condition, and the status of disease.

Toxicity Concerns Related to Choice of Conditioning Regimens

As TBI techniques have evolved, the risk of pneumonitis has become similar between TBI and non-TBI regimens. However, radiation factors are critical to keeping this risk of pneumonitis and other end-organ damage to a minimum. Not only attention to total dose, fractionation, and dose rate is important, but also dose homogeneity, organ dose reduction, and prior exposures, particularly from other cytotoxic therapies, must be considered. Prior thoracic radiotherapy is a risk factor for fatal pneumonitis (32% risk after TBI in patients with prior chest radiation doses >20 Gy in one study) and would be a reason to avoid myeloablative TBI.[76] Prior chemotherapy exposures must also enter the equation in choosing a transplant conditioning regimen. One contemporary series of myeloablative transplants documented a distinctly high rate of pneumonitis in 33% of patients, in which the number of prior chemotherapy regimens was a significant risk factor for lung toxicity.[77] (This study may have also highlighted the pitfalls of poor lung-dose homogeneity from the use of lateral TBI fields in adults using low-megavoltage photons in the 4- to 6-MV range, in spite of lung dose compensation.)

Historically, a significantly higher risk of hepatic veno-occlusive disease, hemorrhagic cystitis, and seizures has been associated with BuCy compared with TBI-based regimens.[64,70,78–80] Advances in pharmacokinetic monitoring of busulfan blood levels and the advent of an intravenous formulation of the drug have been associated with reductions in hepatic toxicity and improved tolerability, even in older patient populations.[81,82] A once-daily regimen of intravenous busulfan combined with the purine analogue fludarabine was associated with improved outcome compared to the BuCy2 regimen in a retrospective comparison.[83]

A relative advantage in using TBI for stem cell transplantation is that the dose delivery throughout the body is highly controllable. In contrast to chemotherapy, dose distribution is independent of such factors as blood supply, and there are no concerns about agent activation, metabolism, excretion, or dose modifications based on liver or kidney function. TBI may also reach chemotherapy sanctuary sites, which is of particular concern, for example, in patients at risk for or with central nervous system (CNS) involvement.

Historically, radiation oncologists have aimed to deliver a relatively homogeneous dose of TBI throughout the whole body, given the concern that leukemias are systemically distributed. Whether this is always an important goal is unclear, because microscopic disease burden during remission may not be uniform throughout the body. Some TBI programs use photon energies greater than 20 MV, which may theoretically deliver higher marrow doses due to increased pair production and higher bone absorption.[84] Many correct for skin-sparing effects of megavoltage irradiation, for instance, with use of beam spoilers, although this is probably not necessary for low-energy photons in the absence of leukemia cutis or a trophism for skin involvement such as in monocytic leukemias. Where there is concern for a higher burden of disease, boost radiation fields may be added to TBI. Augmented doses of radiation may be delivered to the head in the setting of CNS relapse or prophylaxis or to the testes in males with ALL, as examples.

Clinical Data Regarding TBI Dose and Fractionation Schedule

A randomized study from Seattle in the setting of AML compared single-dose TBI (10 Gy) to a fractionated schedule (2 Gy times six fractions). The last update of this trial showed significant superiority of the fractionated scheme in terms of event-free survival.[85] Investigators from France[86] and Italy[87] reported that dose rate did not influence the relapse rate. Another Seattle randomized trial of AML in first remission compared fractionated TBI doses of 12 Gy with 15.75 Gy, showing a decreased relapse rate from 35% to 12% but at the expense of a significant increase in therapy-related mortality, resulting in no survival advantage to a higher radiation dose.[47] In short, in the setting of AML, (a) fractionated TBI appears superior to 10-Gy, single-dose TBI in terms of leukemia-free survival, and (b) dose rate has little impact on leukemia-free survival.

In contrast, a significant dose rate effect has been found for CML in chronic phase treated with allotransplant. A higher dose rate correlated with a decreased relapse rate.[87,88] In addition, a multi-institutional, nonrandomized French study of 180 patients with CML showed that TBI fractionation was associated with an increase in relapse rate.[89] In a French trial comparing busulfan/cyclophosphamide and cyclophosphamide/TBI, the actuarial risk of relapse was 11.1% after single-dose TBI (10 Gy) and 31% after fractionated TBI.[69] The same trend is seen for patients receiving T cell–depleted marrow. In summary, a decrease in dose rate for single-fraction schemes or TBI fractionation in CML in chronic phase may lead to reduced leukemic cell killing.[16]

For ALL there is a paucity of clinical data regarding the optimal dose fractionation schedule for TBI. In a series from the City of Hope Medical Center, there was no significant difference in relapse rate between single-dose (10 Gy) and hyperfractionated TBI (1.2 Gy times 11 fractions over 4 days).[90] A multicenter French study, however, showed a high likelihood of relapse for patients who received fractionated TBI with GVHD prophylaxis mainly via T-cell depletion.[91] Together with elimination of GVHD, T-cell depletion also results in the loss of the GVL effect, which may unmask the known differences in antileukemic efficacy of TBI schedules that otherwise might be obscured by the combined efficacy of the conventional chemotherapy–irradiation–GVL association.[92] In fact, there is evidence of both a dose-rate effect (less relapse with dose rates >14 cGy per minute) and fractionation effect (more relapse with fractionation), suggesting a repair capacity of some leukemic cells.[16] A retrospective study from the Center for International Blood and Marrow

Transplant Research and the City of Hope Medical Center reported improvement in outcome of patients with ALL in second remission when the dose of TBI exceeded 13 Gy.[93]

Nonmyeloablative or Reduced-Intensity Stem Cell Transplantation

In the last decade, growing recognition of the immunotherapeutic potential of allografts led to a reconsideration of the need for the high-dose myeloablative conditioning regimens traditionally administered prior to transplantation. Pioneering work of Storb and others in canine models established that highly immunosuppressive but nonmyeloablative regimens could establish stable mixed hematopoietic chimerism in major histocompatibility complex–matched littermates using one-sixth of the usual ablative dose of TBI in combination with postgrafting immunosuppressive drugs.[9,94] Subsequently, numerous clinical trials have established that a spectrum of subablative conditioning regimens of varying intensity may allow engraftment of donor cells with reduction in regimen-related toxicity, permitting transplantation of patients traditionally excluded from allografting because of age or medical condition.[59,95–99] In essence, allogeneic reduced-intensity transplantation is a form of immunotherapy. The primary purpose of the nonmyeloablative preparatory regimen is to suppress the patient's immune system sufficiently to allow the engraftment of donor cells with minimum host toxicity. The graft-versus-tumor effect leads to eradication of tumor cells.

Common to these regimens is sufficient immunosuppression to overcome host resistance to engraftment using either antimetabolites such as fludarabine, TBI, or both in combination with other agents. Other factors, such as patient age, HLA disparity with the donor, tumor burden, and prior therapy, may also affect the degree of engraftment. A series of clinical studies by the Seattle transplant group, for example, demonstrated that a single 2-Gy fraction of TBI in combination with postgrafting cyclosporine and mycophenolate is sufficient to achieve a high rate of donor engraftment in patients with a prior history of autologous stem cell transplantation, but additional immunosuppression in the form of fludarabine is necessary to ensure engraftment in less heavily pretreated patients or patients receiving unrelated donor grafts.

Reduced-intensity transplants now account for approximately 25% of all allotransplants being performed. Efficacy is difficult to evaluate in the absence of randomized trials, but reduced-intensity conditioning regimens have allowed for an expanded use of transplants in high-risk populations. As an example, elderly patients with acute leukemias in first remission have long-term survival rates of greater than 40% with nonmyeloablative transplants, which is a remarkable achievement compared to historical experience, in which very few patients would have been expected to survive.[100] Toxicity is significantly lower than with traditional myeloablative transplants. The Seattle group reported a 1-year non–relapse-related mortality of allotransplants of 30% for ablative regimens compared to 16% for reduced-intensity conditioning regimens ($p = .04$).[101] Certainly based on first principles, the toxicity of a single dose of 2 Gy of TBI should be minimal. Most transplant centers delivering this dose of TBI would dispense with the complexities of lung blocks, as well as with compensating filters to optimize dose homogeneity. Intensity-modulated radiotherapy is being investigated for total-body irradiation.[102–111] In one form using helical tomotherapy, whole-body marrow and lymphoid compartments are targeted while other organs are relatively spared from radiation exposures. The hypothesis is that the whole body does not need to be uniformly treated. Moreover, in the application of reduced-intensity transplantation, the important targets for radiotherapy may be the marrow to kill residual malignant cells felt to be in higher density in that hematopoietic compartment and the lymphoid tissues to effect immunosuppression. Of course, malignant cells may be in circulation or elsewhere in the body; statistical modeling of circulating cells suggests that a reasonable radiation dose may still be expected to be delivered to the blood pool with tomotherapy.[112] However, one warning for this approach comes from an older clinical trial of single-fraction TBI with varying lung blocking, which showed that excessive lung shielding may reduce leukemia control.[113] Nevertheless, there are early data employing total marrow and lymphoid irradiation (TMLI). A protocol at the City of Hope Medical Center combined fludarabine, melphalan, and TMLI to 12 Gy in eight fractions over 4 days. Dose to the brain, lungs, heart, intestines, kidneys, and bladder are specifically reduced. In a cohort of 33 patients with a variety of high-risk hematologic malignancies, this form of tomotherapy was found to be feasible and reduced median lung doses to 5.7 Gy compared to the expected 8 to 9 Gy with conventional techniques. Acute mucositis was still a significant problem, and the 1-year event-free survival rate was 72%.[114] Further trials need to sort out whether this is a better method of using radiotherapy for hematopoietic transplantation.[115]

Total-Body Irradiation Technique and Dosimetry

Basic Requirements

Given the concern that leukemias are systemically distributed, TBI techniques have been designed historically to deliver a relatively homogeneous dose throughout the whole body. Because the large variations in body geometry and tissue density, the requirement on whole-body dose uniformity has been stated typically as within a specified window, for example, ±10%, of a prescribed dose, except in regions where additional local dose tailoring is planned for the protection of critical organs, such as the lungs, and/or for intensifying target cell kill, such as in bone marrow and lymphocytes, as dictated by clinical presentations. To ensure that a planned dose distribution is accurately delivered to TBI patients, all TBI techniques must undergo a rigorous and comprehensive dosimetric characterization. In the context of general radiotherapy, the International Commission of Radiation Units and Measurements has recommended an overall accuracy in dose delivery of ±5% based on analysis of dose–response data and evaluation of errors in dose delivery. For TBI and HBI, there is evidence that a 5% change in lung dose could result in 20% change in the incidence of radiation pneumonitis, a complication that is usually fatal for whole-lung irradiation.[50,116] Therefore, the basic dosimetry of TBI and HBI techniques should be performed as precise as readily achievable.[117] Accurate dosimetry coupled with an effective quality assurance program will ensure not only safe delivery of TBI treatments, but also accurate dosimetry data for meaningful dose–response analysis. Because some clinical procedures, such as bone marrow transplantation, require TBI at a specified time within a comprehensive drug and radiation treatment protocol, once a patient begins a course of TBI the timing of successive fractions becomes critical to the outcome of the procedure. It is imperative to plan a backup TBI system either within the same institution or in a nearby radiation therapy department when establishing a TBI program. When the primary system is down, a fully commissioned backup TBI system can complete the remaining treatment.

Total-Body Irradiation Techniques

Many techniques have been described in the literature for effective irradiation of the whole body, and, indeed, improvements in both the irradiation technique and physical dosimetry are still being reported.[118–124] Much of the early clinical experience with TBI and HBI procedures was obtained at centers with facilities designed specifically for large-field irradiation.[125] Although a few dedicated systems still exist, current TBI procedures are largely performed with techniques established on

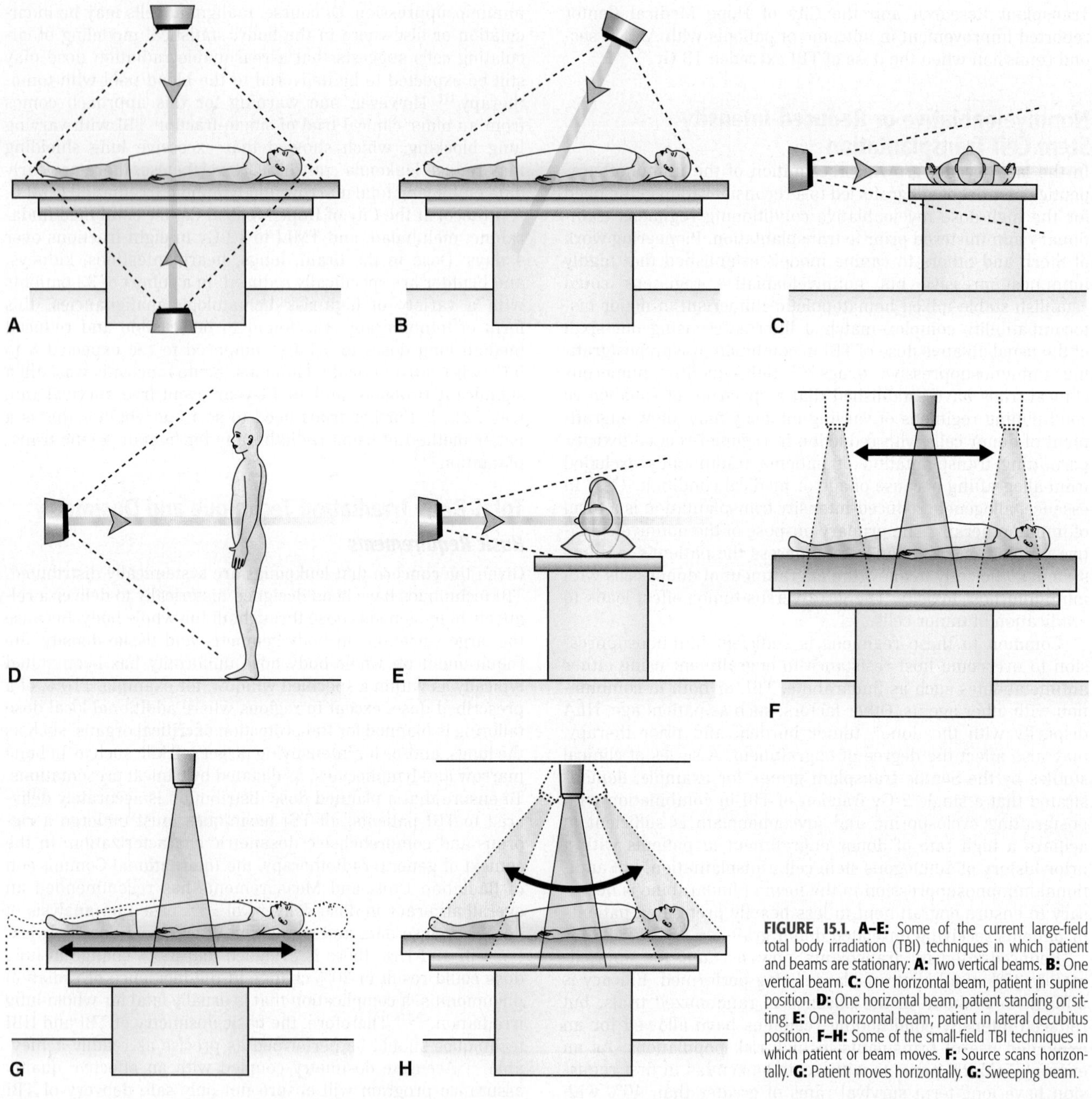

FIGURE 15.1. A–E: Some of the current large-field total body irradiation (TBI) techniques in which patient and beams are stationary: **A:** Two vertical beams. **B:** One vertical beam. **C:** One horizontal beam, patient in supine position. **D:** One horizontal beam, patient standing or sitting. **E:** One horizontal beam; patient in lateral decubitus position. **F–H:** Some of the small-field TBI techniques in which patient or beam moves. **F:** Source scans horizontally. **G:** Patient moves horizontally. **G:** Sweeping beam.

linear accelerators that are used for conventional radiotherapy. Common to these TBI techniques is the use of radiation fields that are larger than the maximum field size (~40 by 40 cm^2) available at standard source-to-surface distance (SSD) treatment distance (~100 cm) by treating TBI patients at extended SSD of 200 to 600 cm. For treatment rooms larger enough to accommodate SSD of 5 m or greater, a single square field at maximum collimator opening will be sufficient to completely encompass patients of typical height placed along the diagonal of the field (Fig. 15.1 A–E). At shorter SSDs, multiple abutting fields are necessary (Fig. 15.1 F–H), and the irradiation of the whole body can be achieved by translating the radiation field[126] or the patient[127] or by sweeping the radiation field over a stationary patient.[128] For these irradiation techniques, patients are typically treated with two parallel-opposed fields. When a single radiation source is used, this can be accomplished by rotating the patient 180 degrees along the patient's longitudinal axis between the two irradiations. In a dedicated system with two radiation sources mounted opposite to each other, the treatment can be accomplished by irradiating the two fields simultaneously without changing the patient's position. Various patient positions, ranging from sitting or standing upright to lying horizontally in supine or lateral decubitus positions,[129,130] have been used in these techniques (Fig. 15.1). The technique using a single large field encompassing the entire patient at extended SSD is by far the simplest and the most prevalent TBI technique used today. The treatment is typically delivered with a horizontal field directed toward the primary shielding wall. It eliminates the dosimetry complications occurring in the junctions of multiple abutting fields. It also alleviates the concern that cells circulating through the body may potentially receive a reduced dose when abutting fields are delivered sequentially.

Recently, with the introduction of intensity-modulated radiation therapy (IMRT) and advanced IMRT delivery systems such as volumetric modulated arc therapy (VMAT) on conventional linear accelerators and spiral tomotherapy on dedicated treatment units, the possibility of delivering TBI-type of treatments at SSDs of conventional radiotherapy has been explored by several research groups.[122–124] In addition to obviating the need of using extended SSD, these new techniques open the possibility of designing and delivering customized dose distributions throughout the whole body. Their ability to seamlessly deliver integrated boost dose to total marrow and/or lymphatic system while keeping doses to uninvolved critical organs low has the potential to further improve the therapeutic ratio of TBI treatment. Only limited clinical experience has been reported.[131] More carefully designed and controlled clinical testing of these new techniques is needed to fully establish its clinical utility and efficacy.

Dosimetric Characterization of Total-Body Irradiation Techniques

Once an irradiation technique is chosen, a careful characterization of the dosimetric properties of the technique should be performed by a qualified medical physicist. The dosimetric data needed to model the treatment planning system for accurate planning of TBI for individual patients should be carefully measured and validated. The technical issues and method of radiation dosimetry for TBI has been reviewed in several rep orts.[125,132,133] In particular, the report of American Association of Physicists in Medicine (AAPM) Task Group 29 (TG-29) on the physical aspects of total and half-body photon irradiation provides a comprehensive discussion on dosimetry issues and techniques specific to large-field TBI.[125] It is a good resource for medical physicists charged to commission a large-field TBI technique.

Since the publication of TG-29 report, the reference dosimetry protocol for external beams at standard treatment SSD, known as the TG-21 protocol, has been updated by a new calibration protocol (TG-51). For photon beams at standard SSD, the TG-51 protocol produces similar results as the TG-21 protocol. However, the TG-51 protocol cannot be applied directly for large fields at extended SSD as encountered in TBI. AAPM has established a working group on dosimetry calibration protocol for beams that are not compliant with TG-51. This working group is charged to develop standardized procedures for calibration of noncompliant beams, among other assignments. In the meantime, the calibration of a TBI beam can be established with direct traceability to TG-51 by using an approach similar to that proposed by Curran et al.[134] In this approach, the photo source of the TBI beam is calibrated first under the TG-51 reference condition at standard SSD. The dose per unit beam-on time at a reference point of the TBI beam under TBI treatment condition is then related to the dose per unit beam-on time of the same photon source at the TG-51 reference point by a correction factor that accounts for the TBI setup geometry and scattering conditions. This correction factor, as well as the relative dose factors that characterize the spatial distribution of the TBI beam, such as the percentage depth dose (PDD) or tissue maximum ratio (TMR) along the central axis, can be measured directly under the TBI treatment conditions using a phantom with size similar to that of a typical patient. In-phantom off-axis beam profiles at various depths, especially along the diagonal near the corners of the field, should also be measured at TBI treatment distance to evaluate the dose variation across the radiation beam. Independent verification of the TBI calibration should be performed after the initial commissioning. The modeling of treatment planning system should also be verified on an anthropomorphic phantom.[135–138] A thermoluminescent dosimeter calibrated on an independent linear accelerator can be used to verify TBI calibration and doses at other points of interest. Ion chamber and film may be used to assess dose distributions.[139]

Skin Surface Dose

Although skin sparing is often a desirable feature of megavoltage irradiation in conventional radiotherapy, for TBI it may be desirable to have skin surface receive close to full prescription dose, as leukemia may circulate through or infiltrate the skin. When needed, the skin dose can be increased by using either bolus placed on the skin or a beam spoiler positioned between the source and the patient.[140] In the latter technique, a large plastic screen (e.g., 2-cm-thick acrylic plastic sheet or acrylic resin) covering the whole body is placed approximately 10 cm from the patient. As the photons of TBI beam pass through the beam spoiler, scattered electrons are produced, which deposit most of their energy at shallow depths near the skin surface. The use of a beam spoiler alters the depth–dose characteristics of the TBI beam in the buildup region. The magnitude of this modifying effect depends on the photon energy of the TBI beam, the composition and thickness of the scatter screen, and the distance between the screen and patient. It should be carefully evaluated as part of the commissioning task for the TBI technique. The dosimetric effect of the beam spoiler can be treated separately or included in the TBI beam calibration. When the beam spoiler is included in the calibration, choice of the calibration depth becomes an important consideration. Calibration measurements performed at a depth of 5 cm or greater decrease the influence of beam spoiler–generated electrons significantly.

Dose Rate

As discussed in preceding sections, the rate of TBI dose delivery could have an impact on the biologic effects of TBI, depending on the disease.[141] Many clinical protocols require low-dose-rate treatment at the rate of 0.05 to 0.10 Gy/min.[125] Modern linear accelerators offer a wide range of dose rates, for example, from 1 to 6 Gy/min in steps of 1 Gy/min, to the depth of maximum buildup at standard SSD. At extended SSD, the nominal dose rate will be smaller due to inverse-square falloff of photon fluence with SSD. The dose rate at the TBI treatment distance is dependent on the combination of SSD and the nominal dose rate programmed at the linear accelerator (LINAC) console. If a given combination of SSD and nominal LINAC dose rate does not produce a desired dose rate at TBI patient, a custom-made attenuator can be placed in the beam path to help achieve a desired dose rate. TBI calibration and dosimetry characterization should be performed with the desired treatment dose rate to ensure accurate dose delivery.[125]

Patient Positioning

Because treatment times may last up to 30 or 40 minutes for each fraction of a fractionated TBI protocol (even longer for single-fraction protocols), patients must be placed in a comfortable and reproducible position. When a pair of parallel-opposed fields is used, irradiation along the anterior-posterior/posterior-anterior (AP/PA) direction is generally preferred, as the body thickness in the AP/PA direction is usually smaller than in the lateral direction, which would result in better dose uniformity along the beam path for a given photon energy. As depicted in Figure 15.1, this may be accomplished with patient lying in the supine/prone position under the vertical beam arrangement or with the patient lying on the side in decubitus position when a horizontally directed beam is used. Irradiation with patient lying in supine position using a horizontally directed beam is feasible for patients with small lateral separations, such as pediatric patients, or when a high-energy photon beam is employed. Because of clinical problems associated with patient fatigue and orthostatic hypotension, special patient stands are used in some institutions to facilitate upright patient positioning.

Treatment Planning

The calculation of radiation beam-on time for a prescribed dose and treatment planning for TBI are often performed with a specialized in-house program or by manual computation. This is because most commercial treatment planning systems designed and commissioned using standard data sets for conventional radiotherapy do not automatically apply to TBI configurations.

Some new versions of commercial treatment planning systems can be adapted for isodose planning of TBI at extended SSD by using depth doses, beam profiles, and other parameters measured directly under the TBI condition. For example, a special TBI beam model was successfully commissioned on the Theraplan Plus 3D system and used in routine TBI treatment planning at Yale. Others have commissioned and evaluated an extended SSD photon model on the Pinnacle[3] planning system for TBI.[142] Newer techniques for total marrow and/or lymphatic irradiation using tomotherapy or VMAT at standard treatment distance can take advantage of the beam models already commissioned in an existing treatment planning system, although the dosimetric accuracy must undergo a careful validation for irradiating large and complex target volumes demanded by TBI/total marrow irradiation (TMI).

In addition to TBI beam characteristics, an accurate description of patient geometry is needed for patient-specific treatment planning. The external body contour of a TBI patient in treatment position could be reconstructed from the measurements of body thickness at representative anatomic points judiciously distributed over the patient body. Recently, computed tomography (CT) scan of the whole body became feasible. It provides the best description of patient geometry and is required for the new IMRT-based TBI/TMI techniques. For conventional extended SSD TBI techniques using two parallel-opposed beams, dose variation over the patient body arises primarily from (a) photon attenuation along the beam path, (b) changing body contour across the patient, and (c) variations in tissue density.

The dose variation caused by photon attenuation along the beam path is dependent on both the beam energy and the body thickness. It decreases with decreasing body thickness and increasing photon energy. Because the body is typically thinner in the anterior–posterior direction, treating patients using the AP/PA technique with higher photon energy will improve dose uniformity along the beam path. Using lateral opposed beams will usually result in greater dose variation compared to AP/PA treatments, especially for adult patients. The dose variation caused by changing body contour may be reduced by using a missing-tissue compensator or tissue-equivalent bolus material placed directly on the patient. The ability to compute isodose distribution across the body is highly desirable for compensator design. A missing-tissue compensator for TBI is typically constructed to even out the variation of body thickness along the head-to-toe direction. Such a one-dimensional compensator can be constructed manually using multiple thin copper (or other material) plates. Because the compensator is usually mounted at the head of the linear accelerator, small variations in the placement of compensating plates will be magnified at the extended SSD distance. Care must be exercised in constructing these compensators. For example, when compensating plates are used for the head and neck region, mounting the compensator too far inferiorly could result in underdose to the shoulders. In addition, careful alignment of patient to the planned position becomes important to achieve the desired missing-tissue compensation.

Dose variation caused by tissue heterogeneity in the thoracic region requires special attention because the lungs are a critical dose-limiting structure in TBI. Without compensation for air density, particularly for AP/PA treatments, dose inhomogeneity can exceed the prescribed dose by 10% to 24%, depending on the energy of beams used.[125] To reduce lung toxicity, correction for lung air density using lung blocks is commonly used to reduce the dose to whole lung. The use of lung blocks increases the complexity of the TBI procedure, and accurate repositioning of lung blocks can be a challenge for fractionated treatments. Several techniques have been reported to increase the repositioning accuracy of lung blocks.[143–145] At Yale, individualized thin lung blocks (with ~85% photon transmission) are mounted close to the patient on an acrylic resin tray using a hook-and-loop fastener system that allows easy repositioning of lung blocks for each fraction (Fig. 15.2C, D). Verification of correct lung block positioning is carried out by using a customized online electronic portal imaging. For the lateral technique, the arm can be used to shield the lungs, thereby improving dose homogeneity. Care must be taken to cover the lung with the arm. For pediatric patients, the arm may not be large enough laterally to cover the entire lung.

Dose Description and Reporting

Because there is no standard treatment technique for TBI and HBI, significant differences in dose distributions can exist with different treatment methods. Two institutions can prescribe the same dose at some selected prescription point, but dose to other points could vary considerably if different treatment techniques are used. Without supplemental information on the dose distribution, it would be difficult to assess the clinical effectiveness of different TBI programs based on the reported prescription dose alone.

To facilitate treatment comparison among institutions, various methods for prescribing the dose for TBI treatments have been reported.[146,147] One method uses a single-point prescription dose supplemented with the specified limits of highest and lowest dose levels acceptable for any point within the body. In addition, dose limits are also set for certain specific tissues such as the lungs. An example of such a TBI prescription is given in AAPM TG-29, which uses the midpoint at the level of the umbilicus as the prescription point. A prescription would be read as follows: "The dose to the midpoint at the level of the umbilicus is 14 Gy to be delivered in eight fractions with two fractions on each day separated by at least 6 hours. All points in the body should receive doses within the limits of −5% and +10% of prescription dose. The dose to lung should be no more than 85% of the prescription dose." When reporting TBI experience, the actual value of the corresponding dose-prescription descriptors achieved by the treatment plan should be provided. When CT-based TBI treatment planning is available, a dose–volume histogram of the target volume and critical organs should be reported.

Quality Assurance

To improve the dosimetric accuracy and consistency, periodic check of TBI calibration and beam characteristics should be performed as a part of an ongoing quality assurance program. Each patient's treatment plan, including the design of customized tissue compensation filter when used, should be checked by an independent physicist. In addition, *in vivo* dosimetry verification of the treatment plan should be performed on the first fraction for all TBI patients. Changes in patient body shape (e.g., due to weight loss between the time of simulation and treatment delivery) and in positioning can alter the dose distributions. Adjustment of radiation beam-on time and of tissue compensation filter may be needed for the subsequent treatments based on the *in vivo* verification (assuming the accuracy and confidence of *in vivo* measurement have already been established). Thermoluminescent dosimeters and diode detectors are typical choices for *in vivo* monitoring of doses delivered to patients.[138,139] These detectors should be calibrated in the TBI beam under the treatment condition prior to commencing the patient treatment. A diode dosimetry system with multiple diode detectors is especially convenient for this type of measurements because they allow simultaneous measurement of doses at multiple anatomic sites in nearly real time. At Yale, *in vivo* dose verification is performed using such a system for each patient on the first treatment fraction. Adjustments made to the treatment plan are verified in the following treatment fraction when necessary.

Lung (and Other Organ) Dose Attenuation

Many transplant centers use lung blocks during TBI in order to correct for the dosimetric effects of lung density or to specifically

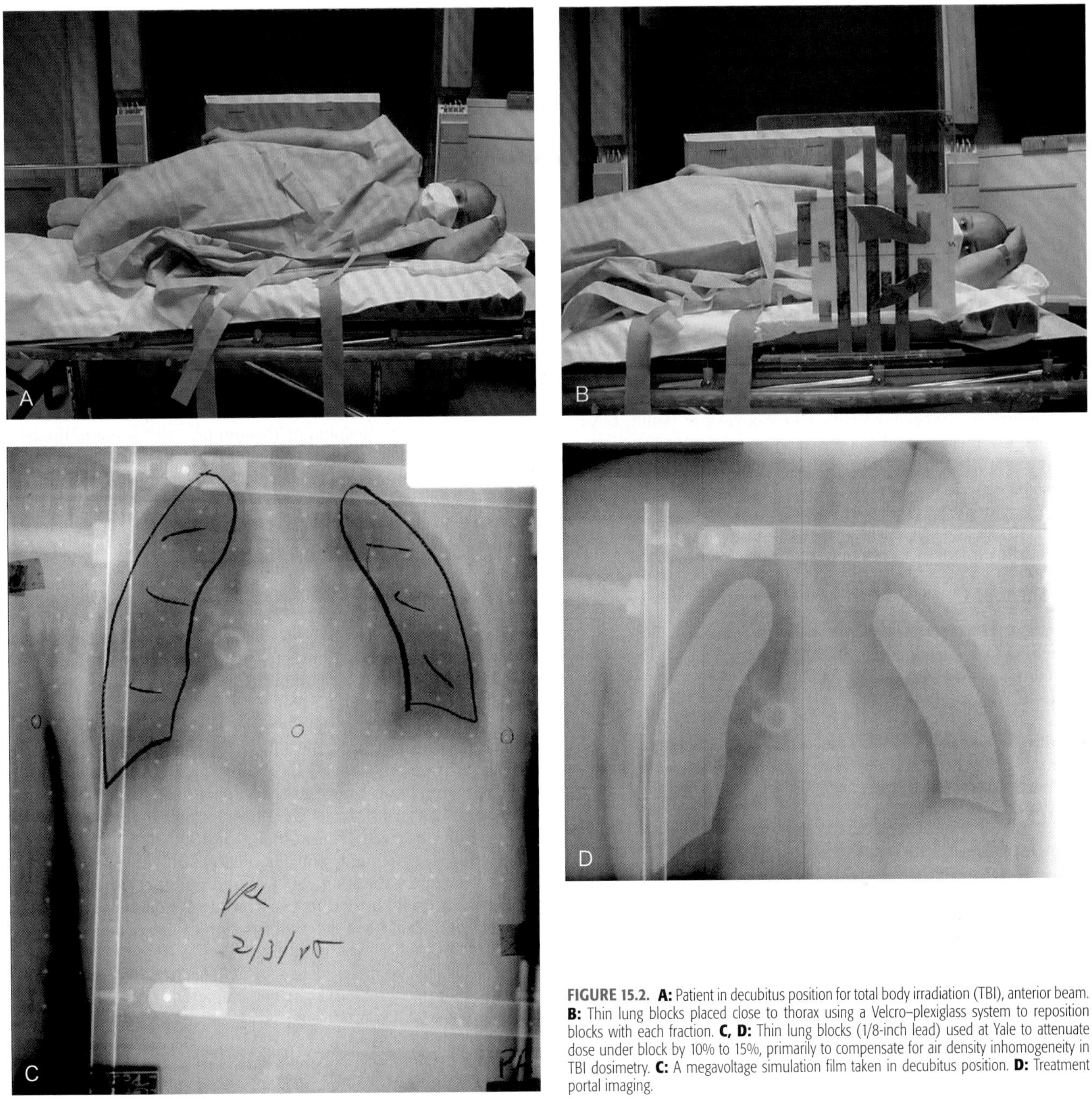

FIGURE 15.2. **A:** Patient in decubitus position for total body irradiation (TBI), anterior beam. **B:** Thin lung blocks placed close to thorax using a Velcro–plexiglass system to reposition blocks with each fraction. **C, D:** Thin lung blocks (1/8-inch lead) used at Yale to attenuate dose under block by 10% to 15%, primarily to compensate for air density inhomogeneity in TBI dosimetry. **C:** A megavoltage simulation film taken in decubitus position. **D:** Treatment portal imaging.

reduce the dose to a majority of lung tissue, thereby reducing the risk for pneumonitis. This is particularly important in patients who have baseline lung dysfunction.[148] Lung shielding will clearly reduce the risk of pneumonitis, all other factors being equal.[38] Overcompensation, however, risks an increase in leukemia recurrence.[113] Specifically, a study from the Institut Gustave-Roussy delivering 10 Gy as a single fraction of TBI over 4 hours, showing a higher incidence of relapse in patients whose lung dose is limited by lung blocks to 6 instead of 8 Gy.[113] The technique at Yale uses 1/8-inch lead filters that attenuate the dose by 10% to 15%, in essence a slight overcorrection for the dosimetric effects of pulmonary air density[149] (see Figure 15.2). The Memorial Sloan Kettering Cancer Center group uses 1–half-value layer (HVL) shielding,[45] with the use of electron boosts of the chest wall under the lung blocks. There are considerable dosimetric problems with this technique: treatments are planned in supine position but delivered standing; there are overlap issues of photon and electron fields; there is surface contour variability, especially from breast tissue in women; and there is still delivery of unwanted radiation dose to some limited volume of lungs. The Institut Gustave-Roussy reported no clinical benefit to electron boosts to chest wall under such lung blocks.[150] The Johns Hopkins group reported using thick (7 HVL) blocks for just one fraction of their TBI course over several days.[151] The Seattle group uses 1- or 2-HVL blocks for half of the TBI fractions without a chest wall boost. Other transplant groups, such as at the one at the University of Minnesota, have reported using partial transmission blocks to the liver and kidneys to reduce the risk of hepatic veno-occlusive disease or nephropathy.[152,153] When TBI is used for nonneoplastic diseases (e.g., aplastic anemia), for which the main objective is immunosuppression, one may also consider shielding radiosensitive structures such as the gonads or eyes (i.e., the lens).[154]

Boosting of Selected Organs with TBI

A relative advantage of TBI is the treatment of chemotherapy sanctuary sites, of particular concern in patients at high risk for CNS relapse. Theoretically, regions of the body where there is a higher burden of disease at the time of transplant may be boosted with additional radiation fields to supplement TBI. In selected patients with lymphoblastic leukemia, CNS preventative therapy includes cranial radiation. When such patients are determined at diagnosis to be best managed with an allogeneic transplant, it is reasonable to defer prophylactic cranial radiation until the time of TBI. Augmented doses of radiation may be delivered to the head, bringing the cumulative cranial dose to 14–18 Gy (a current standard in children and many adults with ALL). Higher total doses to the head and perhaps the spine can be contemplated in patients being managed for CNS leukemia. Boost doses to the head using lateral fields may be given in 1.8- to 2.0-Gy fractions. Caution is necessary for additional CNS boost treatments when patients received prior cranial irradiation due to toxicity concerns. Similarly, the testes in males with ALL may be boosted to a cumulative dose of 16 to 18 Gy. The scrotum may be treated with *en face* electrons of appropriate energy (or orthovoltage x-rays in young boys). Because the incremental toxicity of such testicular irradiation is low regardless of fraction size and the fact that some programs have not observed testicular relapses after TBI, dose prescriptions for testicular boosting vary from 0 to 4 Gy. Boost treatments to the spleen in CML or to chloromas in AML are theoretically attractive although not of proven benefit.[155,156]

Complications

Low-Dose Total-Body Irradiation

With low-dose TBI historically given for CLL and low-grade lymphomas, the principal side effect is thrombocytopenia, usually occurring after cumulative doses exceeding 1 to 1.5 Gy.[1,157] Nausea and vomiting are sometimes observed, controllable by standard antiemetics. When used with alkylating agent chemotherapy, a significant risk of acute leukemia or myelodysplasia has been observed, on the order of 8% to 9% at 15 years of follow-up.[158]

High-Dose Total-Body Irradiation

Side effects from TBI used with stem cell transplantation have complex interactions with cytotoxic drugs and other supportive care or immunosuppressive agents. In addition, graft-versus-host disease has its own set of toxicities, which have complex interactions with the conditioning regimen. Infectious complications also have a significant role in transplant-related toxicities. Isolating what toxicities are strictly related to TBI is not straightforward; nevertheless, the randomized trials from the Seattle group comparing 12 versus 15 Gy showed that non–transplant-related mortality increases with higher radiation doses.[47,48]

Acute Toxicity. Nausea, vomiting, and diarrhea are the most common early side effects when a single fraction of 8- to 10-Gy TBI is given.[52,159,160] These side effects also can be caused by cytotoxic drugs if given prior to TBI. Xerostomia, headaches, fevers, and hypertension were historically reported in roughly half of patients receiving single-fraction TBI.[161] The use of fractionated or low-dose-rate TBI reduces the incidence, as well as the severity, of these and other side effects; moreover, fever and hypertension are rarely seen with fractionated TBI.[46,160] Patients also develop a dry mouth, a reduction in tear formation, and oral and esophageal mucositis within 10 days. Reversible alopecia develops at approximately 2 weeks in all patients.[52] One side effect that is unique to TBI is parotitis, which usually occurs after the first day of irradiation and subsides within 24 to 48 hours, is very common with single-fraction radiotherapy, but occurs in less than 10% of cases with fractionated regimens.[160–161,162]

Nausea may be controlled with the use of serotonin receptor-3 antagonists, as shown in several small randomized trials.[163,164,165,166] Mucositis that results from both radiation and chemotherapy may be ameliorated by good dental hygiene[167] along with a variety of topical agents showing variable effects on reduced analgesic needs. Regardless, supportive care with parenteral nutrition and narcotics is common. These adjunctive agents that have been studied include topical chlorhexidine digluconate,[168,169] calcium phosphate slurry,[170] sulcralfate,[171] and clarithromycin.[172] Amifostine was studied in one trial of allogeneic stem cell transplantation, showing a reduction in duration of mucositis, with fewer severe infections but no effects on hepatic or renal toxicity or hematopoietic engraftment.[173] Recombinant human keratinocyte growth factor was found to reduce mucositis after TBI and intensive chemotherapy, resulting in reduced narcotic and parenteral nutrition usage in one autologous transplant study.[174]

Delayed Toxicity

Lung. Interstitial pneumonitis is the major dose-limiting toxicity for TBI and upper HBI. The radiobiology of lung tolerance has been extensively studied.[37,175] Published experience from the Princess Margaret Hospital in Toronto provides some of the best data regarding lung tolerance. A cohort of 245 patients with metastatic solid tumors received a variety of single-fraction upper HBI doses up to 10 Gy at dose rates of 0.3 to 0.8 Gy/min. The actuarial incidence of acute radiation pneumonitis, defined as the sudden onset roughly 16 weeks after irradiation of cough, dyspnea, and opacities visible on chest radiographs, was strikingly dose dependent. When doses were corrected for density heterogeneity, producing an upward estimation of the doses actually received by the lungs, analysis yielded the sigmoid-shaped curve shown in Figure 15.3. On the basis of heterogeneity-corrected data, the incidence of pneumonitis is estimated to be negligible for single doses, less than about 7.5 Gy.[116]

Pneumonitis in the BMT setting has a multifactorial etiology, reflecting not only the effects of radiation, but also the effects of chemotherapy, GVHD, lung injury from tumor, baseline lung function, opportunistic infections, patient age, and other risk factors.[38,49,176] Cyclophosphamide is almost universally given with TBI. The addition of other drugs is based on institutional treatment policies. Many anticancer drugs are known to injure the lung. BMT conditioning regimens that do not use TBI (which tend to use high-dose busulfan in place of radiation) in fact have rates of interstitial pneumonitis similar to those of regimens including TBI. GVHD may cause lung injury directly, and the drugs used to control GVH may also cause pulmonary toxicity.[177] T cell–depleted transplants tend to have lower risk for pneumonitis.[178]

Liver. Hepatic veno-occlusive disease of the liver (VOD) has been recently renamed sinusoidal obstructive syndrome (SOS), given the recognition that this clinical problem principally seen in myeloablative transplants is an endothelial injury to hepatic sinusoids and that hepatocyte injury and hepatic thrombosis are

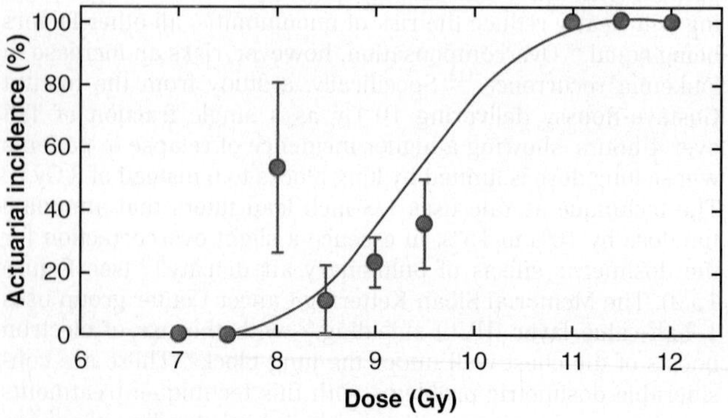

FIGURE 15.3. Incidence of radiation pneumonitis in patients receiving single-dose, whole-lung irradiation at dose rates of 0.3 to 0.8 cGy/min. Doses are corrected for tissue-air heterogeneity. (Data are from Van Dyk et al.[116])

secondary late-stage effects.[179–181] This syndrome, accounting for significant morbidity and mortality in high-dose transplant regimens, is characterized by painful hepatic enlargement, ascites, jaundice, encephalopathy, and weight gain in 10% to 40% of patients.[80,160,181,182] This disease, which needs to be distinguished from cholestatic drug injury and acute graft-versus-host disease, is best diagnosed by transvenous hepatic biopsy, in which an elevated hepatic venous pressure gradient is documented, along with characteristic histology showing hepatic sinusoidal and central vein fibrosis and accompanying hepatocyte necrosis. SOS/VOD is a result of toxic injury to hepatic sinusoids caused by a variety of agents or their metabolites included in myeloablative conditioning regimens. Cyclophosphamide metabolites, high-dose TBI (>14 Gy), busulfan, gemtuzumab, and preexisting or concomitant liver disease have been associated with increased risk.[183] Radiobiologically, hepatocytes respond to dose fractionation (or dose rate) in a manner similar to late-responding tissue, with large variations of the isoeffect dose when fraction size (or dose rate) is modified.[34,184] An α/β ratio of 1 to 2 Gy has been estimated.[185]

Clinically in the transplant setting, the incidence of SOS/VOD has been minimized by fractionating TBI and keeping total doses to less than 13.2 Gy. The Seattle group reported considerably more SOS/VOD after 10-Gy, single-fraction TBI than after 12-Gy, fractionated TBI in a randomized trial.[43] A nonrandomized retrospective study found that fractionated TBI resulted in less SOS/VOD disease but with borderline significance.[186] Barrett showed a decrease in the incidence of SOS/VOD with a lower dose rate.[187] Others showed that modifications of chemotherapy dosing and scheduling based on individual pharmacodynamics may also lower the risk.[64,181] Replacement of cyclophosphamide with fludarabine in combination with busulfan resulted in a low risk of SOS/VOD.[188] Other prevention strategies for SOS/VOD include the administration of low–molecular weight heparins and ursodiol as part of the pretransplant supportive care regimen.[181] In one well-designed clinical trial, ursodiol prevented cholestatic liver injury and graft-versus-host disease but had no effect on SOS/VOD.[189] Treatment is mainly supportive care, but there is some limited evidence that defibrotide, a single-stranded polydeoxyribonucleotide drug with antithrombotic and anti-ischemic properties, may be helpful.[190]

Lens. There is a high intrinsic radiation sensitivity of the lens. Schenken and Hagemann derived an α/β ratio of 1.2 Gy (0.6 to 2.1 Gy), suggesting a high fractionation or dose-rate sensitivity for cataract induction.[191] In the first Seattle experience, greater than 75% of patients developed cataracts after 5 years after single-dose TBI.[162] The introduction of fractionated TBI in the 1980s has significantly reduced this risk. Ozsahin et al. calculated a difference in the 5-year estimated cataract incidence between single-dose TBI (39%) and fractionated TBI (13%) and also showed a beneficial effect of lower dose rate.[192] Bray et al. reported a 63% cataract induction rate from TBI, but that risk was lower with fractionation TBI.[193] Tichelli et al. reported that the probability of requiring cataract surgery was 85% after single-dose TBI and 20% after fractionated TBI.[194] This was confirmed in the Seattle long-term analysis, showing that fractionated TBI was much less toxic to the lens than a single-dose regimen.[195] Steroid therapy is an independent risk factor for cataract formation after bone marrow transplantation, even in the absence of TBI. Lens shielding during TBI is not recommended because of the risk of retro-ocular relapse of leukemia but is a consideration in aplastic anemia and other nonneoplastic disease managed with stem cell transplantation.

Kidney. Renal toxicity has been underreported as a major late complication of bone marrow transplantation. A report by Tarbell et al. in 1988 showed a 35% rate of renal dysfunction in ALL patients receiving transplants.[196] However, a more contemporary report places this risk at 17%, influenced by the use of TBI, cyclosporine for immunosuppression, and presence of significant GVHD.[197] Calculations α/β ratio for kidney in a variety of animal and human systems consistently show relatively low values indicative of fractionation and dose-rate radiosensitivity.[198–200] A protracted value of the half-time for repair for late damage of 2.10 hours (1.90 to 2.31 hours) was found by von Rongen et al.[201] Because transplant patients often also receive various nephrotoxic drugs (etoposide, teniposide, amphotericin B, aminoglycoside antibiotics) before, during, and after intensive cytoreductive therapy, the contribution of TBI to renal dysfunction is not clearly established.[202] Graft-versus-host disease also has complex interactions with radiation dose in determining the risk of transplant-related nephritis.[203] Helenglass et al. reported a trial comparing cyclophosphamide/TBI with melphalan/TBI. The benefit obtained by melphalan in reducing the relapse rate was offset by its nephrotoxic effect.[204] Other studies suggest that use of TBI and chronic GVHD are risk factors for posttransplant chronic kidney disease.[197,205] Some transplant programs used partial transmission blocks over the kidneys or limitations of the total dose, suggesting that kidney doses greater than 12 Gy are associated with increased risks of nephropathy.[153,206] There is no standard recommendation in this regard, however.

Growth, Gonadal, and Endocrine Effects. Almost all children who undergo bone marrow transplantation with TBI experience decreased growth velocity, which is less with fractionated than single-dose TBI.[207,208] Growth hormone deficiency may be detected in 34% of adults who received TBI in their childhood.[209] Other endocrine effects in this setting include Leydig cell dysfunction in 23% and primary hypothyroidism in 34% of cases.[209] High-dose TBI produces primary gonadal failure in almost all patients, but recovery may occur in females.[208] In children, puberty is usually delayed but can be induced by appropriate hormone replacement.[210,211] Thyroid dysfunction is reported in as many as 43% of patients after TBI.[207,212] Subclinical hypothyroidism is the most common picture, with raised thyroid-stimulating hormone and normal thyroxine levels. The incidence of thyroid dysfunction is lower when hyperfractionated TBI is used.[213]

Secondary Cancers. The risk for development of a second tumor 15 years after intensive chemoirradiation and stem cell transplantation is estimated to be approximately 13% to 20%.[210,211,214,215–220] This risk for a secondary malignancy is approximately four times higher than for the general population.[220] The largest series of secondary malignancy from combined registries of the International Bone and Marrow Transplant Research Centers and the Fred Hutchinson Cancer Research Center observed 189 solid cancers among 28,874 transplant patients, more than 6,000 of whom had survived greater than 5 years.[221] Two-thirds of this cohort received radiotherapy as part of the conditioning, which was a major determinant for a secondary cancer along with chronic immunosuppression. Patients less than 30 years of age at the time of treatment had a ninefold increased risk for non–squamous cell cancers over those who did not receive radiotherapy. Chronic GVHD and male age increased the risk for squamous cell cancers. Other studies documented an increased risk for skin cancers and oral cavity cancers, the latter related to chronic lichenoid oral lesions and the historical use of azathioprine for GVHD immunosuppression.[222] Common posttransplant non–squamous cell cancers include melanoma, cervical or uterine cancer, thyroid cancer, breast cancer, and gliomas.[220] Higher TBI doses were associated with increased risk of solid cancers in one study[214] but has not been observed in others.[221] Myelodysplastic syndrome and acute myelogenous leukemia are the most common secondary tumors in patients treated for lymphoid malignancies. Patients who are older, who experienced acute GVHD treated with anti–thymocyte globulin or anti-CD3 antibodies, or who receive TBI are at greatest risk.[210,216–219] Some lymphoproliferative disorders that occur after allotransplantation are associated with Epstein-Barr virus and may be successfully managed with anti–B cell antibodies,[223,224] adoptive immunotherapy,[225–227] or donor lymphocyte transfusions.[226]

HEMIBODY IRRADIATION

Hemibody irradiation has been used for many years to palliate widely metastatic solid tumors, often very late in the course of the disease.[228–230] As the field of medical oncology has developed a larger array of systemic therapies for disseminated cancers, this form of radiotherapy has been less frequently employed.

Applications

Patients with osseous metastases tend to have multiple sites of disease, with multiple areas of pain developing over the course of their illness in up to 75% of patients.[231] The pain relief produced by single-fraction HBI for skeletal metastases involving several sites is fast, with nearly 50% of all responding patients doing so within 48 hours and 80% within 1 week after treatment.[232,233] More than 70% of treated patients experience pain relief, as documented in a number of studies, including various Radiation Therapy Oncology Group (RTOG) trials from the 1980s.[231,232,234–236] The duration of pain relief persists for at least 50% of the patient's remaining life.[228,232] The most effective HBI doses found by the RTOG study are 6 Gy for upper HBI and 8 Gy for lower and middle HBI. Doses beyond these levels do not appear to increase pain relief or its duration or give a faster response.[232]

When treatment of the other half of the body is indicated, it is advisable to wait 6 to 8 weeks to allow a sufficient recovery of blood cells and irradiated marrow to take place.[228] Planned sequential upper and lower HBI 6 to 8 weeks apart has been used to treat multiple myeloma, malignant lymphoma, and other widely disseminated tumors.[228,237–241] HBI appears to be capable of delaying the progression of existing asymptomatic metastasis and the clinical development of new metastases,[231,237,238,242] which eliminates or reduces the need for patients to spend a substantial portion of their remaining lives commuting to treatment centers. At least for multiple myeloma, however, a randomized trial did not support routine use of hemibody radiotherapy.[241]

Technique

The physical considerations for HBI are similar to those for TBI as already discussed; however, the field size required for HBI is much smaller than that for TBI, and HBI can often be delivered on a conventional linear accelerator, albeit using extended distances. By convention, sub–total-body irradiation is usually divided into upper HBI, lower HBI, and middle HBI.[232,243] An arbitrary line at the bottom of L4 is commonly used to separate upper and lower HBI,[243] although this may be modified based on individual circumstances. Treatment is delivered using anteroposterior parallel-opposed fields. The patient is positioned with a vertical beam allowing coverage of the hemibody, and the treatment table is lowered to the appropriate level or to the floor. Shielding of previously irradiated areas or other body regions to reduce toxicity, such as the salivary glands and the lungs, may be employed. The dose is prescribed to the midplane of the patient at the central axis of the beam.

Complications

In general, HBI is well tolerated. The most common side effects associated with single-dose HBI are nausea and vomiting, mainly when the abdomen is included within the fields. These occur shortly after radiation administration and last a few hours.[228,232,233] Premedication with steroids and antiemetics is required. Because these patients are frequently anorectic or cachectic from their underlying illness, dehydration and need for intravenous fluids is common with HBI, and hospitalization for supportive care may be desirable.[243] Fractionated HBI makes therapy more acutely tolerable, similar to the experience with TBI.[244] Diarrhea occurs commonly when a significant volume of the intestines is irradiated and may last for several days. The severity of this side effect can be reduced by limiting the dose to the abdomen to 6 Gy.[232] The risk of pneumonitis is very low if the single-fraction dose to the whole lungs is limited to 7 Gy (uncorrected for air density). If 8 Gy is delivered to the upper body, partial transmission lung blocks to limit the lung dose at 6 to 7 Gy is recommended. Hematologic recovery usually occurs in 4 to 6 weeks.

SELECTED REFERENCES

A full list of references for this chapter is available online.

1. Mendenhall NP, Noyes WD, Million RR. Total body irradiation for stage II-IV non-Hodgkin's lymphoma: ten-year follow-up. *J Clin Oncol* 1989;7:67–74.
9. Storb R, Raff RF, Appelbaum FR, et al. Fractionated versus single-dose total body irradiation at low and high dose rates to condition canine littermates for DLA-identical marrow grafts. *Blood* 1994;83:3384–3389.
10. Storb R, Raff RF, Appelbaum FR, et al. Comparison of fractionated to single-dose total body irradiation in conditioning canine littermates for DLA-identical marrow grafts. *Blood* 1989;74:1139–1143.
17. Cosset JM, Socie G, Girinsky T, et al. Radiobiological and clinical bases for total body irradiation in the leukemias and lymphomas. *Semin Radiat Oncol* 1995;5: 301–315.
18. O'Donoghue JA, Wheldon TE, Gregor A. The implications of *in-vitro* radiation-survival curves for the optimal scheduling of total-body irradiation with bone marrow rescue in the treatment of leukaemia. *Br J Radiol* 1987;60:279–283.
22. Chao NJ, Chen BJ. Prophylaxis and treatment of acute graft-versus-host disease. *Semin Hematol* 2006;43:32–41.
26. Jakubowski AA, Small TN, Young JW, et al. T cell depleted stem-cell transplantation for adults with hematologic malignancies: sustained engraftment of HLA-matched related donor grafts without the use of antithymocyte globulin. *Blood* 2007;110: 4552–4559.
28. Anderson BE, McNiff J, Yan J, et al. Memory CD4+ T cells do not induce graft-versus-host disease. *J Clin Invest* 2003;112:101–108.
33. Zheng H, Matte-Martone C, Jain D, et al. Central memory CD8+ T cells induce graft-versus-host disease and mediate graft-versus-leukemia. *J Immunol* 2009;182: 5938–5948.
40. Shank B, Chu FC, Dinsmore R, et al. Hyperfractionated total body irradiation for bone marrow transplantation. Results in seventy leukemia patients with allogeneic transplants. *Int J Radiat Oncol Biol Phys* 1983;9:1607–1611.
43. Deeg HJ, Sullivan KM, Buckner CD, et al. Marrow transplantation for acute nonlymphoblastic leukemia in first remission: toxicity and long-term follow-up of patients conditioned with single dose or fractionated total body irradiation. *Bone Marrow Transplant* 1986;1:151–157.
44. Phillips GL, Herzig RH, Lazarus HM, et al. Treatment of resistant malignant lymphoma with cyclophosphamide, total body irradiation, and transplantation of cryopreserved autologous marrow. *N Engl J Med* 1984;310:1557–1561.
47. Clift RA, Buckner CD, Appelbaum FR, et al. Allogeneic marrow transplantation in patients with acute myeloid leukemia in first remission: a randomized trial of two irradiation regimens. *Blood* 1990;76:1867–1871.
48. Clift RA, Buckner CD, Appelbaum FR, et al. Allogeneic marrow transplantation in patients with chronic myeloid leukemia in the chronic phase: a randomized trial of two irradiation regimens. *Blood* 1991;77:1660–1665.
58. Miller KB, Roberts TF, Chan G, et al. A novel reduced intensity regimen for allogeneic hematopoietic stem cell transplantation associated with a reduced incidence of graft-versus-host disease. *Bone Marrow Transplant* 2004;33:881–889.
59. McSweeney PA, Niederwieser D, Shizuru JA, et al. Hematopoietic cell transplantation in older patients with hematologic malignancies: replacing high-dose cytotoxic therapy with graft-versus-tumor effects. *Blood* 2001;97:3390–3400.
60. Santos GW, Tutschka PJ, Brookmeyer R, et al. Marrow transplantation for acute nonlymphocytic leukemia after treatment with busulfan and cyclophosphamide. *N Engl J Med* 1983;309:1347–1353.
61. Tutschka PJ, Copelan EA, Klein JP. Bone marrow transplantation for leukemia following a new busulfan and cyclophosphamide regimen. *Blood* 1987;70:1382–1388.
64. Ringden O, Ruutu T, Remberger M, et al. A randomized trial comparing busulfan with total body irradiation as conditioning in allogeneic marrow transplant recipients with leukemia: a report from the Nordic Bone Marrow Transplantation Group. *Blood* 1994;83:2723–2730.
65. Blaise D, Maraninchi D, Archimbaud E, et al. Allogeneic bone marrow transplantation for acute myeloid leukemia in first remission: a randomized trial of a busulfan-cytoxan versus cytoxan-total body irradiation as preparative regimen: a report from the Group d'Etudes de la Greffe de Moelle Osseuse. *Blood* 1992;79:2578–2582.
66. Blaise D, Maraninchi D, Michallet M, et al. Long-term follow-up of a randomized trial comparing the combination of cyclophosphamide with total body irradiation or busulfan as conditioning regimen for patients receiving HLA-identical marrow grafts for acute myeloblastic leukemia in first complete remission [2]. *Blood* 2001;97:3669–3671.
67. Clift RA, Buckner CD, Thomas ED, et al. Marrow transplantation for chronic myeloid leukemia: a randomized study comparing cyclophosphamide and total body irradiation with busulfan and cyclophosphamide. *Blood* 1994;84:2036–2043.
68. Blume KG, Kopecky KJ, Henslee-Downey JP, et al. A prospective randomized comparison of total body irradiation-etoposide versus busulfan-cyclophosphamide as preparatory regimens for bone marrow transplantation in patients with leukemia who were not in first remission: a Southwest Oncology Group study. *Blood* 1993;81:2187–2193.

69. Devergie A, Blaise D, Attal M, et al. Allogeneic bone marrow transplantation for chronic myeloid leukemia in first chronic phase: a randomized trial of busulfan-cytoxan versus cytoxan-total body irradiation as preparative regimen: a report from the French Society of Bone Marrow Graft (SFGM). *Blood* 1995;85:2263–2268.
71. Socie G, Clift RA, Blaise D, et al. Busulfan plus cyclophosphamide compared with total-body irradiation plus cyclophosphamide before marrow transplantation for myeloid leukemia: long-term follow-up of 4 randomized studies. *Blood* 2001;98:3569–3574.
74. Uberti JP, Agovi MA, Tarima S, et al. Comparative analysis of BU and CY versus CY and TBI in full intensity unrelated marrow donor transplantation for AML, CML and myelodysplasia. *Bone Marrow Transplant* 2011;46:34–43.
75. Shi-Xia X, Xian-Hua T, Hai-Qin X, et al. Total body irradiation plus cyclophosphamide versus busulphan with cyclophosphamide as conditioning regimen for patients with leukemia undergoing allogeneic stem cell transplantation: a meta-analysis. *Leuk Lymphoma* 2010;51:50–60.
76. Van der Jagt RH, Appelbaum FR, Petersen FB, et al. Busulfan and cyclophosphamide as a preparative regimen for bone marrow transplantation in patients with prior chest radiotherapy. *Bone Marrow Transplant* 1991;8:211–215.
77. Kelsey CR, Horwitz ME, Chino JP, et al. Severe pulmonary toxicity after myeloablative conditioning using total body irradiation: an assessment of risk factors. *Int J Radiat Oncol Biol Phys* 2011;81:812–818.
83. Andersson BS, de Lima M, Thall PF, et al. Once daily i.v. busulfan and fludarabine (i.v. Bu-Flu) compares favorably with i.v. busulfan and cyclophosphamide (i.v. BuCy2) as pretransplant conditioning therapy in AML/MDS. *Biol Blood Marrow Transplant* 2008;14:672–684.
84. Bradley J, Reft C, Goldman S, et al. High-energy total body irradiation as preparation for bone marrow transplantation in leukemia patients: treatment technique and related complications. *Int J Radiat Oncol Biol Phys* 1998;40:391–396.
86. Ozsahin M, Pene F, Touboul E, et al. Total-body irradiation before bone marrow transplantation. Results of two randomized instantaneous dose rates in 157 patients. *Cancer* 1992;69:2853–2865.
87. Scarpati D, Frassoni F, Vitale V, et al. Total body irradiation in acute myeloid leukemia and chronic myelogenous leukemia: influence of dose and dose-rate on leukemia relapse. *Int J Radiat Oncol Biol Phys* 1989;17:547–552.
93. Marks DI, Forman SJ, Blume KG, et al. A comparison of cyclophosphamide and total body irradiation with etoposide and total body irradiation as conditioning regimens for patients undergoing sibling allografting for acute lymphoblastic leukemia in first or second complete remission. *Biol Blood Marrow Transplant* 2006;12:438–453.
94. Storb R, Yu C, Wagner JL, et al. Stable mixed hematopoietic chimerism in DLA-identical littermate dogs given sublethal total body irradiation before and pharmacological immunosuppression after marrow transplantation. *Blood* 1997;89:3048–3054.
100. Niederwieser D, Gentilini C, Hegenbart U, et al. Allogeneic hematopoietic cell transplantation (HCT) following reduced-intensity conditioning in patients with acute leukemias. *Crit Rev Oncol Hematol* 2005;56:275–281.
101. Diaconescu R, Flowers CR, Storer B, et al. Morbidity and mortality with nonmyeloablative compared with myeloablative conditioning before hematopoietic cell transplantation from HLA-matched related donors. *Blood* 2004;104:1550–1558.
109. Wong J, Rosenthal J, Liu A, et al. Image-guided total-marrow irradiation using helical tomotherapy in patients with multiple myeloma and acute leukemia undergoing hematopoietic cell transplantation. *Int J Radiat Oncol Biol Phys* 2009;73:273–279.
112. Molloy JA. Statistical analysis of dose heterogeneity in circulating blood: Implications for sequential methods of total body irradiation. *Med Phys* 2010;37:5568–5578.
113. Girinsky T, Socie G, Ammarguellat H, et al. Consequences of two different doses to the lungs during a single dose of total body irradiation: results of a randomized study on 85 patients. *Int J Radiat Oncol Biol Phys* 1994;30:821–824.
114. Rosenthal J, Wong J, Stein A, et al. Phase 1/2 trial of total marrow and lymph node irradiation to augment reduced-intensity transplantation for advanced hematologic malignancies. *Blood* 2011;117:309–315.
115. Giralt S. TMLI: A better TBI or more of the same? *Blood* 2011;117:9.
116. Van Dyk J, Keane TJ, Kan S, et al. Radiation pneumonitis following large single dose irradiation: a re-evaluation based on absolute dose to lung. *Int J Radiat Oncol Biol Phys* 1981;7:461–467.
117. Van Dyk J. Magna-field irradiation: physical considerations. *Int J Radiat Oncol Biol Phys* 1983;9:1913–1918.
125. Van Dyk J, Galvin JM, Glasgow GP. *The physical aspects of total and half body photon irradiation: a report of Task Group 29 Radiation Therapy Committee.* College Park, MD: American Association of Physicists in Medicine; 1986.
140. Shank B. Techniques of magna-field irradiation. *Int J Radiat Oncol Biol Phys* 1983;9:1925–1931.
148. Singh AK, Karimpour SE, Savani BN, et al. Pretransplant pulmonary function tests predict risk of mortality following fractionated total body irradiation and allogeneic peripheral blood stem cell transplant. *Int J Radiat Oncol Biol Phys* 2006;66:520–527.
149. Dutreix J, Janoray P, Bridier A, et al. Biologic and anatomic problems of lung shielding in whole-body irradiation. *J Natl Cancer Inst* 1986;76:1333–1335.
155. Gratwohl A, Hermans J, von Biezen A, et al. No advantage for patients who receive splenic irradiation before bone marrow transplantation for chronic myeloid leukaemia: results of a prospective randomized study. *Bone Marrow Transplant* 1992;10:147–152.
156. Dusenbery KE, Howells WB, Arthur DC, et al. Extramedullary leukemia in children with newly diagnosed acute myeloid leukemia: a report from the Children's Cancer Group. *J Pediatr Hematol Oncol* 2003;25:760–768.
162. Deeg HJ. Acute and delayed toxicities of total body irradiation. Seattle Marrow Transplant Team. *Int J Radiat Oncol Biol Phys* 1983;9:1933–1939.
164. Spitzer TR, Bryson JC, Cirenza E, et al. Randomized double-blind, placebo-controlled evaluation of oral ondansetron in the prevention of nausea and vomiting associated with fractionated total body irradiation. *J Clin Oncol* 1994;12:2432–2438.
166. Okamoto S, Takahashi S, Tanosaki R, et al. Granisetron in the prevention of vomiting induced by conditioning for stem cell transplantation: a prospective randomized study. *Bone Marrow Transplant* 1996;17:679–683.
174. Spielberger R, Stiff P, Bensinger W, et al. Palifermin for oral mucositis after intensive therapy for hematologic cancers. *N Engl J Med* 2004;351:2590–2598.
183. McDonald GB. Hepatobiliary complications of hematopoietic cell transplantation, 40 years on. *Hepatology* 2010;51:1450–1460.
195. Benyunes MC, Sullivan KM, Deeg HJ, et al. Cataracts after bone marrow transplantation: long-term follow-up of adults treated with fractionated total body irradiation. *Int J Radiat Oncol Biol Phys* 1995;32:661–670.
197. Ellis MJ, Parikh CR, Inrig JK, et al. Chronic kidney disease after hematopoietic cell transplantation: a systematic review. *Am J Transplant* 2008;8:2378–2390.
214. Curtis RE, Rowlings PA, Deeg HJ, et al. Solid cancers after bone marrow transplantation. *N Engl J Med* 1997;336:897–904.
221. Rizzo JD, Curtis RE, Socie G, et al. Solid cancers after allogeneic hematopoietic cell transplantation. *Blood* 2009;113:1175–1183.
231. Poulter CA, Cosmatos D, Rubin P, et al. A report of RTOG 8206: a phase III study of whether the addition of single dose hemibody irradiation to standard fractionated local field irradiation is more effective than local field irradiation alone in the treatment of symptomatic osseous metastases. *Int J Radiat Oncol Biol Phys* 1992;23:207–214.
232. Salazar OM, Rubin P, Hendrickson FR, et al. Single-dose half-body irradiation for palliation of multiple bone metastases from solid tumors. Final Radiation Therapy Oncology Group report. *Cancer* 1986;58:29–36.
244. Salazar OM, DaMotta NW, Bridgman SM, et al. Fractionated half-body irradiation for pain palliation in widely metastatic cancers: comparison with single dose. *Int J Radiat Oncol Biol Phys* 1996;36:49–60.

Chapter 16
Stereotactic Radiosurgery and Radiotherapy

John C. Flickinger and Ajay Niranjan

Stereotactic radiosurgery and radiotherapy are techniques to administer precisely directed, high-dose irradiation that tightly conforms to an intracranial target to create a desired radiobiologic response while minimizing radiation dose to surrounding normal tissue. These techniques exploit the fact that the radiation tolerance of normal tissue is volume dependent. With these techniques the complication risks for any radiation dose delivered are reduced by minimizing or eliminating the margin of normal tissue otherwise included in the radiation treatment volume with conventional radiotherapy techniques. In the case of radiosurgery, all of the irradiation is done in a single session or fraction, while in stereotactic radiotherapy, more than one fraction of irradiation is administered. Table 16.1 lists the key requirements for successful stereotactic irradiation. Advances in imaging, computers, and treatment planning in the last two decades have led to the development of a variety of different stereotactic radiosurgery/radiotherapy techniques and their wider applications. Successful clinical experience with intracranial radiosurgery for a variety of applications has led to a re-examination of radiobiology and exploration of both fractionated approaches and extracranial applications. Margin reduction with radiosurgery and fractionated stereotactic irradiation techniques makes target definition accuracy more critical. Drawing contours from different imaging techniques or by different physicians are approaches to reduce target definition error (Fig. 16.1).

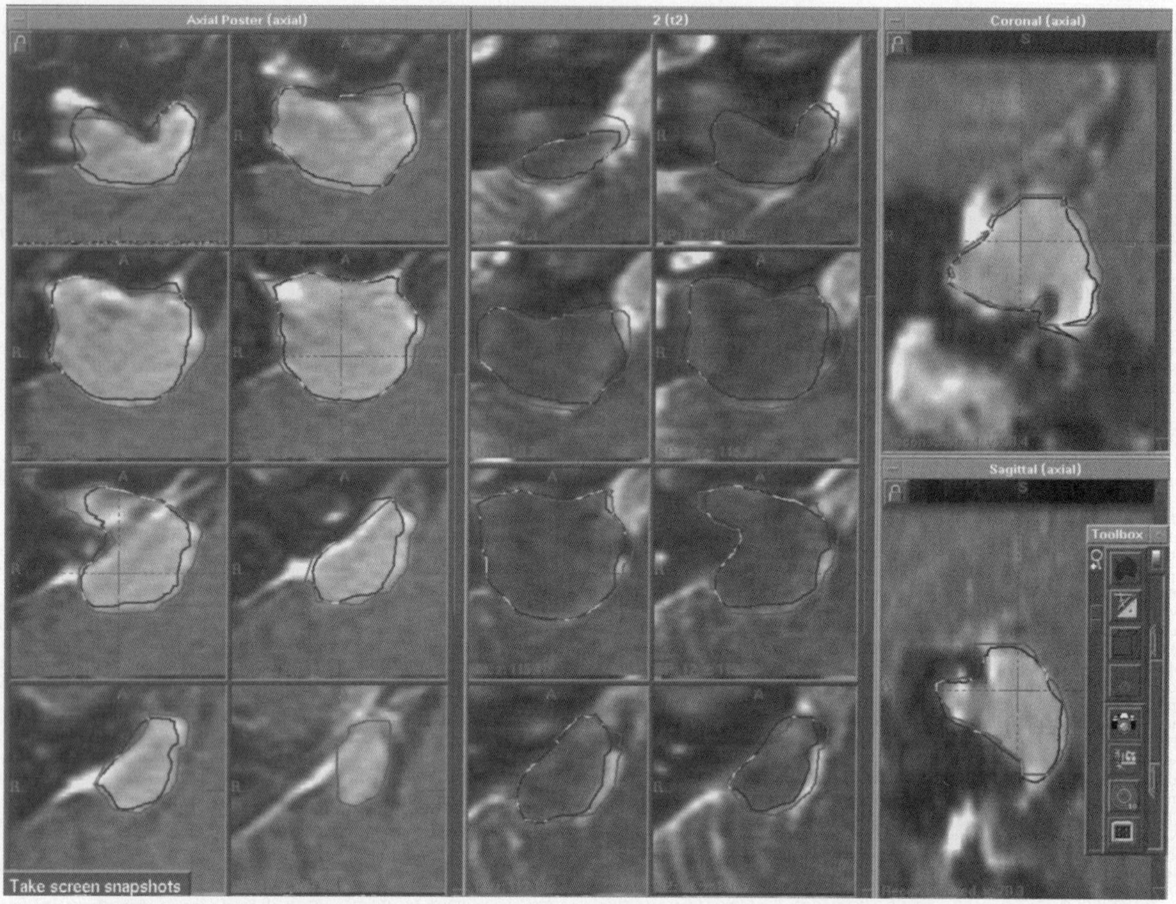

FIGURE 16.1. Comparisons of acoustic schwannoma contours drawn from T1-contrast magnetic resonance (MR) images (eight axial images on the left side, with coronal and sagittal images on the right side) with contours drawn from T2 MR images (the darker eight axial images in the center). T1 contours can sometimes slightly overestimate extension into the internal auditory canal and unnecessarily include adjacent blood vessels.

TERMINOLOGY

Stereotactic refers to using a precise three-dimensional mapping technique to guide a procedure. The terminology used in stereotactic irradiation can be confusing. The term *radiosurgery* or *stereotactic radiosurgery* (SRS) is used for stereotactically guided conformal irradiation of a defined target volume in a single session. Radiosurgery or SRS can be delivered with Gamma Knife (Elekta Inc., Norcross, GA) modified LINAC radiosurgery systems (including CyberKnife [Accuray Inc., Sunnyvale, CA] and image-guided radiotherapy systems), tomotherapy, or proton beam systems. The term *stereotactic radiation therapy* (SRT) refers to stereotactically guided delivery of highly conformal radiation to a defined target volume in multiple fractions, typically using noninvasive positioning techniques. The term *fractionated stereotactic radiosurgery* (FSR) is limited to stereotactically guided high-dose conformal radiation administered to a precisely defined target volume in two to five sessions. Although it would have been less confusing to refer to this as *hypofractionated* SRT and reserve the term *radiosurgery* for single-fraction irradiation, the terminology is already in use. Adding intensity-modulated radiation therapy (IMRT) to the nomenclature can further complicate or confuse the terminology. Any radiation treatment plan that uses individual treatment beams that irradiate only part of the target at a time is IMRT. Strictly speaking, multiple isocenter radiosurgery (of a single target volume) meets the criteria for IMRT or stereotactic IMRT (SIMRT), but the term *SIMRT* is usually only used when multileaf collimators are employed. The terminology is useful to distinguish when the same linear accelerator is equipped either to treat with fixed circular collimators for radiosurgery (SRS or SRT mode) or to deliver IMRT using multileaf collimators (SIMRT mode).

TABLE 16.1 KEY REQUIREMENTS FOR OPTIMAL STEREOTACTIC IRRADIATION

Requirement	*Rationale*
Small target/treatment volume	Reducing the volume of normal and target tissue irradiated to high doses improves tolerance
Sharply defined target	Can be treated with little or no extra margin of surrounding normal tissue and/or without unintentional underdosage of the target (marginal miss)
Accurate radiation delivery	No margin of normal tissue needed for setup error and/or reduced chance of underdosing target
High conformality	Reduces the treatment volume to match the target volume
Sensitive structures excluded from target	Dose-limiting structures (such as optic chiasm, spinal cord) should be able to be defined and excluded from the target volume to limit the risk of radiation injury

RADIOBIOLOGIC CONSIDERATIONS

Prior to the introduction of radiosurgery, essentially all clinical irradiation was administered with radiation dose fractions between 1.2 and 3 Gy for intracranial targets. Extracranial targets were usually treated with 1.2- to 4-Gy fractions, with 6- to 8-Gy fractions used occasionally for treatment of bone metastases or malignant melanoma. Before the rapid adaption of radiosurgery into the clinic in the late 1980s, most radiation oncologists and radiation biologists believed that fractionating radiation treatment lessens the relative risk of injury to normal tissue compared with tumor in essentially all circumstances. Radiobiologic analysis of a limited number of malignant tumors in cell culture and clinical experience with conventionally fractionated radiotherapy of fast-growing malignant tumors established this radiobiologic dogma. Increasing the fractionation of radiotherapy for slow-growing benign tumors may not necessarily improve the balance between tumor control and radiation complication. Slow-growing benign tumors are difficult to study in either cell culture or animal models, so the effect of fractionation has not been well delineated. Stereotactic radiosurgery allowed clinicians to administer high single doses of radiation to intracranial targets with relative safety, thereby leading to a new appreciation of the underlying radiobiology. Laboratory studies suggest that the radiation response for the high-dose single fractions used in radiosurgery is predominantly related to the supporting endothelial cells.[1] Pathology studies of benign and malignant tumors treated by radiosurgery also support a vascular response.[2]

Analysis of clinical data from radiosurgery to delineate dose–response relationships and define radiobiologic parameters is fraught with difficulties. Typical radiosurgery treatment plans use inhomogeneous dose distributions with the prescription isodose covering anywhere from 90% to 100% of the target volume. The absolute minimum dose to the target typically is 5% to 30% lower than the prescription dose. Contours of the same tumor/target volume or critical structures may vary slightly from one clinician to another. Using the linear-quadratic formula to extrapolate from experience with conventional radiotherapy with low-dose fractions to high-dose single fractions for radiosurgery appears problematic. Using single-fraction radiosurgery dose–response curves for arteriovenous malformation (AVM) obliteration and radiation injury to brain parenchyma and cranial nerves to calculate α/β ratios yields values of −30 to −60 rather than 2 to 3 as expected from conventional fractionated radiotherapy data.[3,4] Comparing dose responses for fractionated SRT to radiosurgery is hampered by limited data with dose–response curves that have insufficient slopes for accurate comparison.

RADIOSURGICAL TECHNIQUES

Radiosurgery was originally envisioned to treat intracranial lesions by delivering a high dose of ionizing radiation in a single treatment session using multiple beams precisely collimated to the target inside the cranium. Advances in both imaging and computer technologies resulted in wider applications of radiosurgery. There are now a variety of different radiosurgery and SRT techniques available for intracranial and extracranial use.

Gamma Knife Radiosurgery

After prior experience with stereotactic treatment using orthovoltage radiotherapy and proton beam irradiation, Leksell and Larson created the first prototype of the gamma knife in 1967. The gamma knife uses a relatively hemispherical array of multiple fixed cobalt-60 beams (201 in most models) that are sharply collimated to create small, relatively spherical treatment volumes of varied diameter with sharp dose falloff. The earlier model originally was referred to as the *U-style* and contained cobalt sources arranged in a hemispherical array, including sources at the pole of the hemisphere. These units present challenging loading and reloading issues with the cobalt-60 sources, particularly with radiation protection. To eliminate this problem, the B-unit (Elekta, Inc., Norcross, GA) (after Bergen, Norway, the first site) was redesigned so that sources were arranged in an annular section of a hemisphere, similar to the Northern Hemisphere with the Arctic Circle excluded. In 1999, the model C version of the gamma knife was introduced with the option to use robotic positioning to set treatment coordinates. This expedites execution of multiple-isocenter treatment plans. Manual positioning is still needed for some targets far from the center of the head. The model 4-C, introduced in 2005, was equipped with enhancements designed to improve workflow, increase accuracy, and provide integrated imaging capabilities. The Perfexion model introduced in 2006 uses a larger patient aperture and internally mounted secondary collimators. Because of the larger patient aperture, it is able to treat all intracranial and even cervical spine targets quickly and efficiently with robotic positioning.

Rotating Gamma System

A radiosurgery device called the *rotating gamma system* (RGS) was developed in China. The rotating gamma system (OUR International Inc., Shenzen, China) employs 30 cobalt-60 radiation sources in a revolving hemispherical shell. The secondary collimator is a coaxial hemispheric shell with six groups of five different collimators to produce spherical treatment volumes of different diameter. The experience with this system is somewhat limited.

Proton Radiosurgery

The chief advantage of charged proton radiosurgery is that the beams stop at a depth related to the beam's energy. Electron beams also use charged particles but lack the sharp beam edge of the proton beam. The lack of an exit dose and the sharp beam profile of protons allow target irradiation with lower integral doses than are delivered with photon (LINAC x-ray or cobalt-60 gamma) irradiation. An unmodified proton beam irradiation deposits increased energy in the last couple of millimeters of the path length. This area of increased ionization, where cell killing is even higher because of an increased radiobiologic effect, is termed the *Bragg peak* or *Bragg-Gray peak*. To allow homogeneous irradiation of targets greater than a millimeter or two, the Bragg peak is normally modulated or spread out throughout the target, essentially eliminating its effect. The first treatment of a malignant tumor by irradiation with a proton beam Bragg peak was carried out in 1957 and followed by functional neurosurgery for advanced Parkinson's disease in 1958. Presently, proton beam irradiation is available at a limited number of centers because of the high cost of equipment and maintenance. If technical improvements and increased competition lead to continued cost reductions, proton beam irradiation will become increasingly used because of its dosimetric advantages.

LINAC Radiosurgery

The pioneering work of many researchers in the 1980s led to the gradual modifications of linear accelerators (LINACs) designed for conventional radiotherapy to be used for radiosurgery. LINAC technologies were modified by incorporating improved guiding (stereotactic) devices and methods to measure and improve accuracy of various components. Unmodified LINACs for conventional radiotherapy tend to deviate from alignment with the isocenter at different gantry angles. Most early LINAC-based radiosurgery techniques used multiple radiation arcs with circular secondary collimators to create spherical dose distributions for stereotactically defined three-dimensional targets. Improved hardware and advanced dose-planning software have been developed to enhance conformity. These include beam shaping with micromultileaf collimators and intensity modulation with inverse treatment-planning algorithms. Many LINAC-based systems such as XKnife (Radionics Inc., Burlington, MA), Novalis (BrainLAB, Heimstetten, Germany), the Peacock System (NOMOS Corp., Sewickley, PA), and CyberKnife (Accuray Inc., Sunnyvale, CA) are commercially available. The Peacock system uses inverse planning and multileaf wedge-generated intensity-modulated beams to obtain target conformity. The CyberKnife combines a miniaturized LINAC mounted on an industrial robot with a system for target tracking and beam realignment. This system uses a 6-MeV LINAC with different-sized circular collimators attached to a six-axis robotic manipulator. Stereotactic frames are not normally used for targeting. CyberKnife plans use multiple fixed-beam positions and multiple isocenters. Before the radiation is delivered from any beam position, the target position is tracked using an integrated x-ray image processing system, consisting of two orthogonal diagnostic x-ray cameras and an optical tracking system. During treatment, the image processing system acquires x-ray images of the patient's body multiple times throughout the treatment, while stealth tracking software compares the actual images with the target images to correct alignment of the beam.

Tomotherapy

Tomotherapy, literally "slice" therapy, is a new form of radiotherapy that modifies the design of a diagnostic computerized tomography (CT) scan into a treatment delivery machine, thereby combining the precision of CT imaging with the radiation treatment. This is done by adding a LINAC megavoltage treatment beam to the rotating x-ray source and moving table design of the diagnostic CT unit, which normally uses only a kilovoltage diagnostic x-ray beam. Unlike traditional radiation therapy systems with a slow-moving external gantry designed for positioning individual beams onto the tumor from a few different directions, tomotherapy rapidly rotates the beam around the patient (and inside the housing of the unit), thus allowing the beam to enter the patient from many different angles in succession. Beam intensity modulation (IMRT) is possible through the use of a multileaf collimator system. The inclusion of CT imaging technology within the tomotherapy unit allows precise localization of the target before and during treatment.

LINAC Image-Guided Radiotherapy

The combination of diagnostic three-dimensional imaging with highly conformal treatment delivery in a single unit to maintain accuracy is the basis of various treatment techniques and processes collectively known as *image-guided radiation therapy* (IGRT). Although tomotherapy (which is also a type of IGRT) accomplishes this by modifying a CT unit into a megavoltage radiotherapy machine, most other IGRT techniques add CT imaging capability to a LINAC radiotherapy unit equipped for stereotactic and IMRT use. Because any patient movement between image acquisition and treatment delivery (or during treatment delivery) can introduce error, these IGRT systems use noninvasive immobilization devices and patient position tracking systems. Several manufacturers currently offer IGRT using LINAC technology capable of delivering SRS and radiotherapy, including the Trilogy (Varian Medical Systems, Inc.) and the SynergyS (Elekta, Inc.) equipped with cone-beam CT imaging capability.

NORMAL TISSUE TOLERANCE IN SRS AND SRT

Radiosensitivity

Estimating the risks of a proposed treatment plan with various doses is an essential part of treatment planning and dose prescription for SRS and SRT. The ability of normal tissue to tolerate radiation without injury depends on the radiation dose administered, the volume of tissue irradiated, the sensitivity of the tissue affected, history of any prior radiation treatment to the region, and any individual variation in radiation sensitivity between different people. At present, with the exception of patients with known increased radiation sensitivity, such as those with ataxia telangiectasia, there is usually no information available to modify treatment plans for individual differences in radiosensitivity. Prior fractionated radiotherapy appears to have limited effects on the risks of developing parenchymal edema and neurologic sequelae after radiosurgery but has been observed to affect optic nerve tolerance.

Location Effects

Analysis of postradiosurgery injury reactions in AVM patients revealed no difference in the likelihood of postradiosurgery injury imaging changes (increased signal developing in surrounding brain on long relaxation time or T2-weighted images) in different regions of the brain.[3,5] Dramatic differences were seen in the rates of developing neurologic sequelae between different regions of the brain (as shown in Fig. 16.2).

Radiation Therapy Oncology Group (RTOG) Dose-Escalation Studies

The RTOG Radiosurgery Dose-Escalation Study established tolerance doses for radiosurgery of recurrent brain metastases and high-grade gliomas not involving the brainstem.[6] They administered radiosurgery to 156 patients with brain metastases or primary brain tumors that recurred or progressed after conventional radiotherapy following a dose-escalation

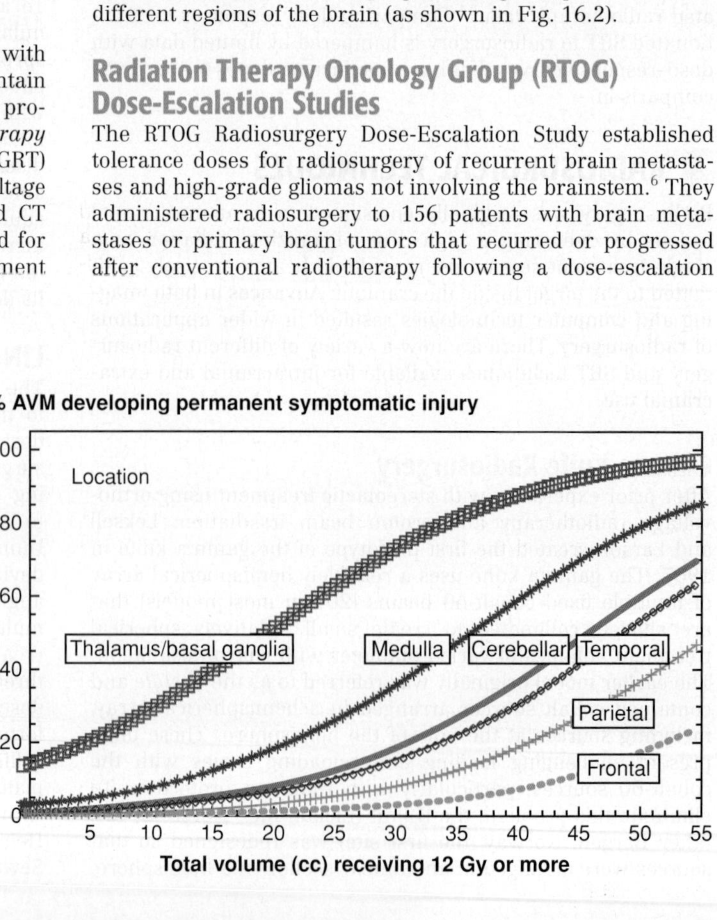

FIGURE 16.2. Effect of location on the risk of developing permanent symptomatic neurologic injury following arteriovenous malformation (AVM) radiosurgery.

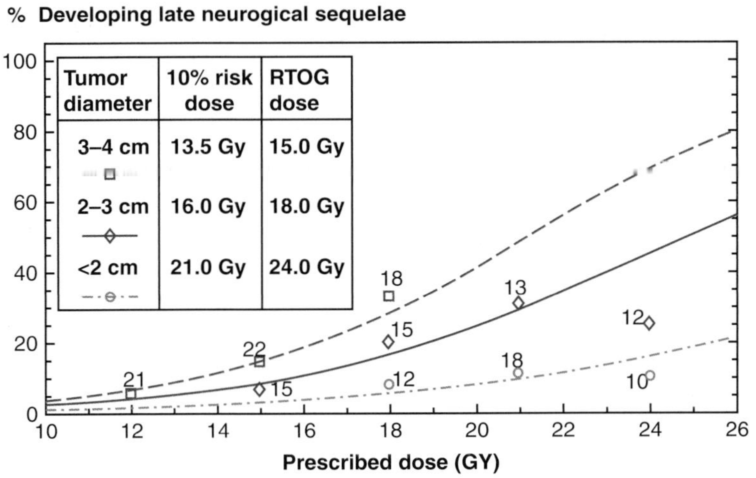

FIGURE 16.3. Phase I Radiation Therapy Oncology Group (RTOG) dose-escalation data for radiosurgery of recurrent brain metastases and glioblastoma fit to logistic dose–response curves. The numbers at each data point indicate the number of patients in each dose/diameter group.[6]

protocol. Starting with initial doses of 18, 15, and 12 Gy for diameters <20, 21 to 30, and 31 to 40 mm, respectively, they escalated prescription doses in 3-Gy intervals until irreversible toxicity was seen in >20% of patients within 3 months. The exception was with tumors <20 mm in diameter where dose-limiting toxicity was not reached and investigators were reluctant to escalate above 24 to 27 Gy. The recommended tolerance doses from that protocol were 24, 18, and 15 Gy for diameters of <20 mm, 21 to 30, and 31 to 40 mm, respectively. The data with longer follow-up beyond 3 months to assess late toxicity were fitted to individual logistic dose–response curves shown in Figure 16.3. These tolerance doses have been widely used as dose guidelines for radiosurgery of malignant tumors, often with interpolation for tumors close to 20 and 30 mm in diameter (e.g., 20 Gy for 18- to 22-mm-diameter and 16.5 Gy for 28- to 32-mm-diameter treatment volumes).

Optic Nerve Tolerance for Radiosurgery

The first analysis of optic nerve tolerance to radiosurgery—a combined Harvard and University of Pittsburgh study of patients with cavernous sinus meningiomas, craniopharyngioma, and pituitary adenomas—recommended 8 Gy as a safe maximum dose limit for the optic nerves/chiasm.[7] The lowest optic chiasm dose at which optic neuropathy developed in that study was reported as being 9.7 Gy. Optic nerve/chiasm doses were estimated from isodose distributions overlaid on CT images, unlike the present day when the entire optic system is usually outlined on detailed magnetic resonance (MR) images and maximum doses are assessed from dose–volume histograms. It is highly likely that the true maximum doses to the optic system were higher and laid in portions of the nerve that were poorly visualized.

Stafford et al.[8] reported a later analysis of four cases of optic neuropathy occurring out of 215 Mayo Clinic radiosurgery patients with a median dose of 10 Gy to the optic chiasm. One case developed after an optic nerve/chiasm dose of 12.8 Gy with radiosurgery alone, at which the risk level appeared to be approximately 3%. The other cases developed in patients with prior fractionated radiotherapy (7 Gy after 58.8 Gy, 9 Gy after 45 Gy, and two procedures delivering 9 and later 12 Gy to the optic system after 50.4 Gy).

Leber et al.[9] analyzed optic nerve injury risks in 50 patients with 24- to 60-month follow-up (median, 40 months) who underwent gamma knife radiosurgery for benign skull-base tumors. Their risks of optic neuropathy were 0% with <10 Gy, 27% with 10 to 15 Gy, and 78% with >15 Gy. They found no cavernous sinus nerve injury with doses of 5 to 30 Gy.

Considering these data and published risks of optic neuropathy for conventional fractionated radiotherapy, α/β ratios in the range of 0 to 1 seem reasonable for estimating fractionated radiotherapy dose equivalents for radiosurgery doses for the optic nerve and probably other cranial nerves.

Tolerance of Other Cranial Nerves

From clinical experience with fractionated conventional radiosurgery and radiosurgery, it appears that special sensory nerves (optic and auditory) are the most radiosensitive, followed by somatic sensory nerves (trigeminal) and finally the motor nerves (cranial nerves II, IV, VI, VII, and IX through XII). After acoustic schwannoma radiosurgery to doses of 12 to 13 Gy, FSR to 18 Gy in three fractions, or SRT to 45 to 50 Gy in 25 to 28 fractions, decreased hearing develops in 30% to 50% of patients, facial numbness in 2% to 3%, and facial weakness in ≤0.5%. Radiosurgery with present techniques for meningiomas involving the cavernous sinus is associated with a risk of trigeminal neuropathy in approximately 3% of patients, with radiation injuries to cranial nerves III, IV, or VI more uncommon.[5,10–13]

Spinal Cord Tolerance

The tolerance of the spinal cord to SRS or SRT depends on the volume of spinal cord irradiated, the distribution of that radiation (e.g., maximum dose), the dose of radiation previously administered to the spinal cord, and the time interval between initial radiation and retreatment. Spinal cord tolerance to SRS or SRT has not been well defined because of a fortunate paucity of radiation injury reactions in clinical experience so far. Gerszten et al.[14] reported on 125 patients who underwent CyberKnife spine radiosurgery (17 benign and 108 metastatic cases). Seventy-eight lesions had previously received external-beam radiotherapy. Treatment volumes varied from 0.3 to 232 mL, with a mean of 27.8 mL. Prescription doses varied between 12 and 20 Gy (mean, 14 Gy) to an 80% isodose treatment volume. Spinal cord volumes receiving >8 Gy varied from 0.0 to 1.7 mL (mean, 0.2 mL). They identified no acute radiation toxicity or new neurologic deficits after a median follow-up of 18 months (range, 9 to 30 months). Benzil et al.[15] reported the New York Medical College experience with spine radiosurgery in 31 patients using a Novalis LINAC unit. Two patients who received biologic equivalent doses of >60 Gy developed radiculitis.

CLINICAL USES OF SRS AND SRT

Table 16.2 lists the most commonly used indications for radiosurgery, with representative references. Except for functional radiosurgery, there are varied levels of experience with SRT for each of these indications.

TABLE 16.2 COMMON INDICATIONS FOR RADIOSURGERY OR HYPOFRACTIONATED STEREOTACTIC RADIOTHERAPY

Indication	*Experience*	*Value*	*References*
Functional			
a. Trigeminal neuralgia	a. Extensive	1. Less numbness than rhizotomy	a. 16,17
b. Unilateral tremor	b. Moderate	2. In poor candidates for deep brain stimulation	b. 1,18–20
Vascular			
a. AVM	a. Extensive	a. High	a. 14,21–23
b. Cavernous	b. Moderate	b. Controversial	b. 24–26
Benign tumors: schwannoma, pituitary adenoma, meningioma, and others	Extensive	High tumor control, acceptable morbidity for selected small tumors	10–12,26–29,30,30,31–56
Brain metastases	Extensive	Control rates equal to or higher than those for surgery for small metastases	57,58
Primary malignant brain tumors	Extensive for GBM; limited with other uses	Initial SRS appears ineffective for GBM; helpful for recurrent tumors, possibly initial pilocytic, neurocytoma	59–67
Spinal metastases	Moderate	High for recurrent tumors; no phase III comparison with conventional XRT for initial treatment	68,69

AVM, arteriovenous malformation; GBM, glioblastoma multiforme; SRS, stereotactic radiosurgery; XRT, radiotherapy.

Functional Radiosurgery

The most widely used functional application for radiosurgery is in the management of typical trigeminal neuralgia refractory to medical therapy.[3,4,16,17,70] Atypical or constant pain does not respond. Other alternatives for managing typical trigeminal neuralgia are medication, open surgery with microvascular decompression, and rhizotomy procedures using glycerol injection, balloon compression, or radiofrequency injury to the nerve. Typically, 4-mm collimators are used for radiosurgery to a maximum dose of 80 Gy. Response rates reach approximately 85%, typically 1 week to 4 months after the procedure, but can develop as late as 6 months later. Approximately 50% of typical trigeminal neuralgia patients remain pain-free and off medication 5 years following radiosurgery. A typical radiosurgery plan for trigeminal neuralgia is shown in Figure 16.4.

A small destructive lesion in the ventralis intermedius nucleus of the thalamus can be created either invasively with a needle equipped with a radiofrequency generator or noninvasively with radiosurgery using 4-mm-diameter collimators and a maximum dose of 130 Gy to alleviate medically refractory unilateral tremor in patients with essential tremor and/or Parkinson's disease.[1,18–20] Nondestructive management through insertion of a deep brain stimulator is preferred in most patients, but not all patients are acceptable candidates. Limited experiences with radiosurgery of the globus pallidus (pallidotomy) to attempt to alleviate more generalized parkinsonian symptoms have not been as favorable.[71–73] There is favorable limited experience with bilateral radiosurgical capsulotomy for managing severe, refractory obsessive-compulsive disorder.[74] Radiosurgery to hypothalamic hamartomas may help control refractory gelastic seizures.[52,75] The use of radiosurgery as an alternative to extensive surgery in medically refractory mesial temporal lobe epilepsy shows promise and continues to be investigated.[55]

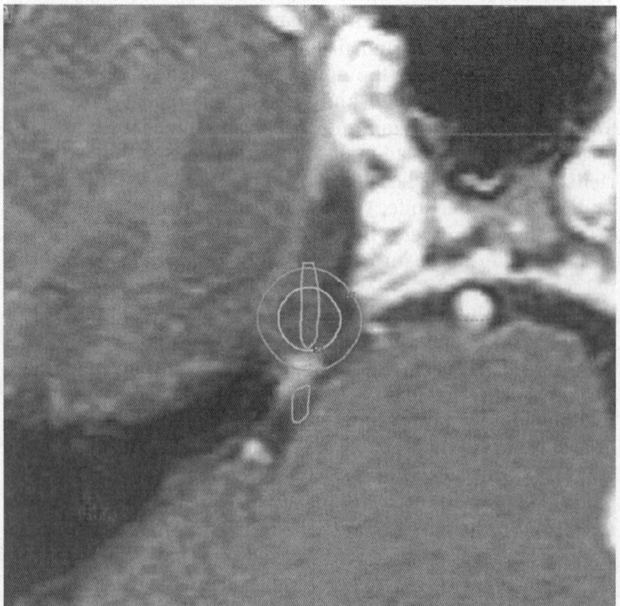

FIGURE 16.4. Typical radiosurgery plan for right trigeminal neuralgia. The right trigeminal nerve is outlined in white. The 30% and 50% isodose volumes from treating a single isocenter with 4-mm-diameter collimators with a gamma unit are shown. A maximum dose of 80 Gy will deliver 40 Gy to the 50% isodose volume and 16 Gy to the 20% volume.

Vascular Malformations

Untreated intracranial AVMs have a bleeding risk of approximately 3% per year, or higher if prior bleeds have occurred.[41,44] This results in an average of 1% of untreated AVM patients dying each year from hemorrhage. Management options include observation, surgical resection, embolization, and radiosurgery. Radiosurgery can dramatically reduce the risk of hemorrhage. Radiosurgery obliterates the AVM nidus in approximately 75% of patients within 3 years of the procedure.[4,59,76] Individual obliteration rates vary from 50% to 88% depending on marginal dose administered, as shown in the dose–response curve illustrated in Figure 16.5.

Although AVM obliteration rates appear to be optimized with marginal doses of approximately 23 Gy, lower doses are selected for most patients to minimize complications. The risk of neurologic sequelae from radiosurgery averages approximately 3% but varies with treatment volume, dose, and location (Fig. 16.2). The risk of hemorrhage while waiting for complete obliteration to develop seems unaltered.[44] All of these risks and benefits of radiosurgery need to be considered together to optimize management of individual AVM patients.

When an AVM nidus fails to completely obliterate by 3 years after radiosurgery, irradiation can be repeated with acceptable morbidity.[45] Although some residual radiation injury effect would be expected within the previously irradiated, unobliterated AVM nidus vasculature, retreatment appears to require similar, if not higher, doses to achieve similar rates of complete obliteration as initial radiosurgery.[45]

Management of large AVMs is presently difficult because radiosurgery may be associated with high complication risks and low obliteration rates. Recent improvements in embolization with liquid glue (ev3, Inc., Plymouth, MN) or polymer can sometimes help reduce the target volume but adds to the total risks of the overall management.[77] Another promising approach is staged radiosurgery, in which large AVMs are treated in two

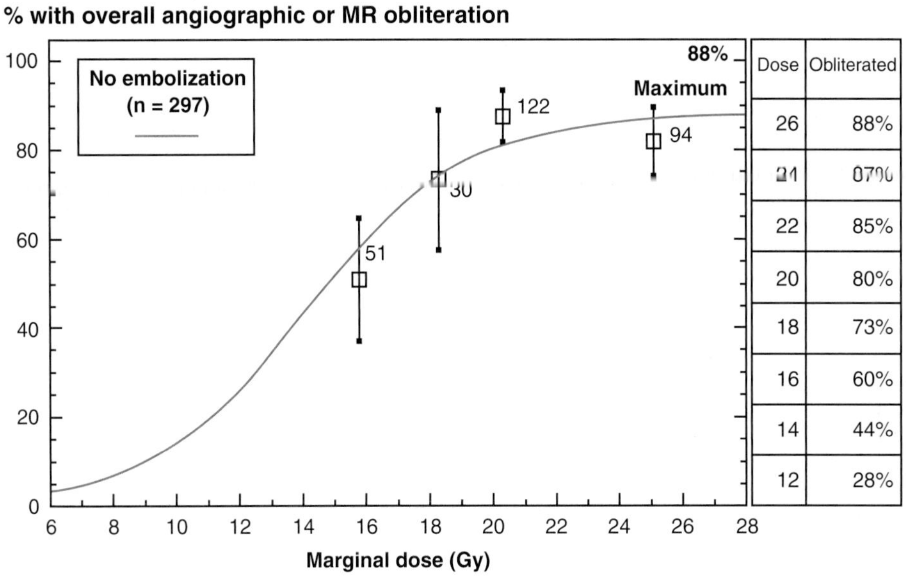

FIGURE 16.5. Dose response for obliteration of arteriovenous malformation after radiosurgery from 297 patients treated at University of Pittsburgh without embolization.[4] MR, magnetic resonance.

or three sections separated by 4- to 6-month intervals to reduce acute toxicity. Whether there is any benefit to fractionating stereotactic irradiation of AVMs is presently unclear.[78]

Cavernous malformations do not show detectable flow on angiography but nevertheless are vascular lesions with annual hemorrhage risks of 0.5% per year with no prior bleed, 4.5% with one prior hemorrhage, and approximately 32% per year after a history of two or more hemorrhages.[77,79–82] Lower pressures in these lesions lead to smaller bleeds than are typically seen with AVM. Repeated bleeds from brainstem cavernous malformations can cause considerable neurologic morbidity. Symptomatic, surgically accessible lesions should be resected. Radiosurgery of brainstem cavernous malformations with a history of two or more prior hemorrhages appears to reduce the risk of subsequent bleeds to approximately 1% per year with acceptable morbidity.[76,81,83–85]

Benign Tumors

Most small benign intracranial tumors are well managed with radiosurgery, FSR, or SRT. Radiosurgery control rates are high with radiosurgery, with prescription doses on the order of 12 to 14 Gy.[10–12,26–29,57] Kondziolka et al.[86] evaluated long-term tumor control in 285 consecutive patients who underwent radiosurgery for benign intracranial tumors between 1987 and 1992, with a median follow-up period of 10 years. This included 157 patients with vestibular schwannomas, 10 with other cranial nerve schwannomas, 85 with meningiomas, 28 with pituitary adenomas, and five with craniopharyngiomas. Forty-four percent of the patients had prior surgical resection and 5% had prior fractionated radiotherapy. They found that 95% of the 285 patients had imaging-defined local tumor control (63% had tumor regression and 32% had no further tumor growth). The crude tumor control was 95% (271/285 patients) with a 15-year actuarial tumor control rate of 93.7%. In 5% of the patients, delayed tumor growth was identified. Resection was performed after radiosurgery in 13 patients (5%) for tumor growth.

Vestibular Schwannomas

Vestibular schwannomas, also known as *acoustic neuromas,* are benign tumors arising from Schwann cells. They are associated with loss of genetic information on chromosome 22.[36] Vestibular schwannomas either occur on one side as spontaneous mutations or bilaterally as the hallmark of type 2 neurofibromatosis (NF-2). Vestibular schwannomas usually arise within the internal auditory canal and later extend intracranially into the cerebellar pontine angle. Because these tumors lack the ability to invade bone, the portion of tumor outside the canal in the cerebellar pontine angle eventually grows into a globular extension that is larger than the intracanalicular portion (Fig. 16.1). The differential diagnosis of a cerebellar pontine angle tumor includes vestibular schwannoma (90%), meningioma (close to 10%), cholesteatomas, facial or trigeminal schwannoma, and rare primary or metastatic malignant tumors. Cerebellar pontine angle meningiomas (which can be managed similarly to vestibular schwannomas) also may involve the internal auditory canal but are usually distinguished by a broad, flat, dural attachment that is lacking in vestibular schwannomas.

Observation and surgical resection were essentially the only management strategies offered to acoustic schwannoma patients until favorable experiences with gamma knife radiosurgery were reported in the 1980s. Observation may be appropriate in selected NF-2 patients and some elderly patients with small, minimally symptomatic vestibular schwannomas, but early intervention appears to be the best strategy for long-term hearing preservation for most patients.[87,88] Surgery appears to be the best initial strategy in patients with vestibular schwannomas large enough to cause symptomatic brainstem compression with obstructive hydrocephalus. For small to medium vestibular schwannomas, tumor control rates with radiosurgery or SRT are comparable to those of surgical resection.[30,30,31–52]

Early radiosurgery series including patients treated during the 1980s with higher doses (14 to 18 Gy) and less conformal treatment plans had higher rates of postradiosurgery cranial neuropathies (15% to 20% trigeminal and/or facial and 67% with a drop in their Gardner-Robertson hearing level).[72] This led some groups to pursue SRT for vestibular schwannomas, while others pursued radiosurgery with refined techniques and lower doses. Both approaches led to improved results.[30,30,31–52] The University of Pittsburgh reported on 313 previously untreated unilateral acoustic schwannoma patients who underwent gamma knife radiosurgery doses of 12 to 13 Gy between February 1991 and February 2001.[16] Median follow-up was 24 months, maximum follow-up was 115 months, and 36 patients had >60 months of follow-up. The actuarial clinical tumor control rate, free of surgical intervention, was 98.6% at 7 years. One patient's growing tumor was subsequently completely resected. The only other failure required a partial resection because of an enlarging adjacent subarachnoid cyst, despite control of the irradiated tumor. The 7-year actuarial rates for unchanged facial strength, unchanged facial sensation, unchanged hearing level, and useful hearing preservation were 100%, 95.6%, 70.3%, and 78.6%, respectively. Eight patients developed new trigeminal neuropathy, six of whom developed numbness (7-year actuarial rate = 2.5%), and the other two developed new typical trigeminal neuralgia (7-year actuarial rate = 1.9%). The risk of developing postradiosurgery trigeminal neuropathy was associated with increasing tumor volume ($p = .038$). Similar results with low-dose radiosurgery of vestibular schwannomas were reported by Iwai et al.,[58] Paek et al.,[42] Muacevic et al.,[35] and Rowe et al.[56]

Various fractionation schemes (18 Gy/3, 20 Gy/4 to 5, 25 Gy/5, 45 to 50 Gy/25, and 54 Gy/30) have been used with vestibular schwannoma with minor differences in results. After accounting for length and quality of follow-up, treatment results seem similar to those of radiosurgery with 12 to 13 Gy, but an advantage for fractionation cannot be excluded entirely.[13] Combs et al.[11] from Heidelberg reported seemingly better useful hearing preservation (94%) in 106 acoustic schwannoma patients managed with fractionated stereotactic radiation therapy (FSRT) to a median dose of 57.6 Gy with 1.8-Gy fractions. They reported 98% actuarial hearing preservation for non–NF-2 patients compared to 68% for NF-2 patients. These numbers were based on telephone questioning rather than audiograms, making comparison to radiosurgery series difficult. Their 5-year actuarial tumor control rate was 93%, and postradiation trigeminal and facial neuropathy rates were 3.4% and 2.3%, respectively. The University of California, Los Angeles, also reported unusually good hearing preservation (93%) for their experience with 50 unilateral acoustic schwannoma patients irradiated to 54 Gy in 30 fractions to a 90% isodose treatment volume including a 1- to 3-mm margin around gross tumor.[89] All tumors were controlled with a median follow-up of 36 months (range, 6 to 74 months). They defined useful hearing preservation as the ability to talk on the telephone and listen with the affected ear. New facial numbness developed in one patient (2%) and facial weakness also developed in one patient (2%) after radiotherapy.

Andrews et al.[90] analyzed the Jefferson vestibular schwannoma experience, comparing 69 radiosurgery patients with 50 SRT patients who received 50 Gy in 25 fractions. Their first 25 vestibular schwannoma patients were treated using a linear accelerator, and later radiosurgery patients were treated with gamma knife radiosurgery. The authors had similar facial and trigeminal neuropathy rates for the radiosurgery and fractionated radiotherapy groups but the rate of hearing loss was significantly higher in their radiosurgery group. There were only a small number of patients with serviceable (useful) hearing in each group prior to irradiation (12 in the radiosurgery and 21 in the FSRT groups) and follow-up was limited. Meijer et al.,[31] from Amsterdam, also reported a single-institution comparison of radiosurgery (LINAC to 10 or 12.5 Gy) and SRT (20 Gy/4 to 5 fractions) for vestibular schwannoma. They selected 49 edentulous patients (mean age, 63 years) for radiosurgery and 80 patients (mean age, 43 years) with intact dentition for SRT. They found a higher rate of trigeminal neuropathy following radiosurgery (8%) than SRT (2%) at 5 years ($p = .048$), but similar hearing loss with radiosurgery (25%) than SRT (39% FSRT; $p > .05$), similar but higher than usual rates of new facial neuropathy (7% radiosurgery vs. 3% FSRT; $p > .05$), and similar 5-year actuarial tumor control rates (100% with radiosurgery vs. 94% with SRT).

Nonacoustic Schwannomas

Schwannomas may occasionally involve other cranial nerves, particularly V, VII, and XI through XII in the jugular foramen. Tumor control rates are similar, but postradiosurgery neuropathies seem less common as somatic sensory and particularly motor nerves seem less sensitive to radiation injury than special sensory nerves like VIII.[53–56]

Meningiomas

Radiosurgery and SRS are both excellent management options for most small benign meningiomas, with in-field tumor control rates well above 90%, as has been seen with most other benign tumors.[69,86] Marginal recurrence rates as high as 25% may develop because of the tight margins used for radiosurgery or SRT treatment volumes limited to small recurrences or residual tumor after resection of large parasagittal meningiomas.[10,26,87,91,92] Marginal recurrences are far less of a problem with unresected (and usually unbiopsied) meningiomas. A University of Pittsburgh study.[69] analyzed 219 imaging-diagnosed meningiomas (unbiopsied) managed with gamma knife radiosurgery to a prescription dose of 8.9 to 20 Gy (median, 14 Gy) and treatment volumes of 0.47 to 56.5 mL (median, 5.0 mL), with 2 to 164 months of follow-up (median, 29 months). Tumors progressed in seven patients; two of the tumors proved to be different ones (metastatic nasopharyngeal adenoid cystic carcinoma and chondrosarcoma). Another patient with local control of the lesion developed a subsequent brain metastasis, changing the diagnosis of the first lesion to the same. The actuarial tumor control rate was 93.2% at both 5 and 10 years. The actuarial rate of identifying a diagnosis other than meningioma was at both 5 and 10 years. No pretreatment variables, including dose, correlated with tumor control in univariate or multivariate analysis. The actuarial rate for developing any postradiosurgical injury reaction was 8.8% at 5 and 10 years. The risk of postradiosurgery sequelae was lower (5.3%) after 1991 (with stereotactic MR imaging and lower doses; $p = .0104$).

Atypical and malignant (anaplastic) meningiomas have higher rates of local and marginal recurrence after therapeutic intervention. Complete surgical resection is advocated whenever possible, followed by a full course of conventional radiotherapy with at least 1-cm margins around the tumor volume. Radiosurgery has been recommended to improve local control of unresectable tumor.[6,92–94] Malik et al.[84] reported 5-year actuarial control rates of 87% for typical meningiomas, 49% for atypical meningiomas, and 0% for malignant meningiomas in the Sheffield gamma knife experience. Harris et al.[24] reported on the Pittsburgh gamma knife experience in 12 malignant and 18 atypical meningiomas. Their 5-year local tumor control was 72% for malignant and 83% for atypical meningiomas; however, 10-year actuarial survival rates were only 59% and 0%, respectively. Katz et al.[60] could not substantiate that either accelerated fractionated radiotherapy or a radiosurgery boost improved tumor control or survival in their analysis of 27 atypical and nine malignant meningioma patients managed at the University of Florida.

Pituitary Adenoma

Management of pituitary adenomas requires a multidisciplinary approach to properly select which patients are suitable for different approaches with medical therapy, surgery, fractionated radiotherapy, and radiosurgery, or combinations of these. Most patients with visual compromise, particularly with a hemianopsia or greater, will do better with initial surgical decompression. Prolactinomas are usually initially managed with medical therapy.[50] Most other small pituitary adenomas, where the target volume can be separated from the optic nerves, are reasonable candidates for radiosurgery.[10,27–29]

Sheehan et al.[94] performed a review of 35 peer-reviewed reports of radiosurgery for pituitary adenoma that included 1,621 patients. Most studies reported >90% control of tumor size (range, 68% to 100%). The weighted average tumor control rate for all published series (encompassing 1,283 patients) was 96%. In eight published series with mean or median patient follow-up periods of ≥4 years, tumor growth control rates varied from 83% to 100%.

Twenty-two series have published radiosurgery results for 314 Cushing's disease patients. The mean radiosurgical prescription (margin) doses for these series varied from 15 to 32 Gy. In those series with at least 10 patients and a median follow-up of 2 years, endocrinologic remission rates range from 17% to 83%. Many of the patients in older series were treated in the pre-CT and MR imaging era of radiosurgery, sometimes as many as four times before their Cushing's disease went into remission.

Malignant Tumors

Brain Metastases

Brain metastases are the most common and best studied of the indications for radiosurgery.[30] Early clinical investigations found impressive tumor control with radiosurgery for brain metastases that progressed after prior whole-brain radiotherapy (WBXRT). The RTOG phase I dose-escalation trial in recurrent brain tumors to some degree standardized dose prescription for brain metastasis radiosurgery.[4] Because of the success of radiosurgery in controlling brain metastases after whole-brain radiotherapy and the high rate of eventual local tumor progression in brain metastases after conventional WBXRT, radiosurgery has been increasingly used in initial management of brain metastases.[4] The subsequent phase III randomized trial, RTOG 95-08, established that radiosurgery immediately following standard WBXRT (37.5 Gy in 15 fractions) improves local control and quality of life for patients with one to three brain metastases while also improving overall survival for patients with solitary metastasis, all compared with patients initially managed with WBXRT only.[95]

Although RTOG 95-08 established the role of radiosurgery after WBXRT in managing one to three brain metastases, questions remained about managing brain metastases with radiosurgery alone, preserving full-dose WBXRT as an option for later managing cases with subsequent progression. Aoyama et al.[21] recently published the outcome of a prospective randomized controlled trial to evaluate whether initial WBXRT provides better outcomes when added to SRS compared to using SRS alone. The 11-hospital study done by Aoyama et al.[21] randomized 132 patients with one to four brain metastases <3 cm in diameter to radiosurgery either with or without initial WBXRT. They found that the median survival time and the 1-year actuarial survival rates were not significantly different with or without WBXRT. The 1-year brain tumor "recurrence rate" (corresponding to the development of additional brain metastases) was higher in the SRS-alone group compared with the patient group that received both WBXRT and SRS. Earlier retrospective studies had similar observations. The most common primary site in these studies was lung. Separate analyses of radiosurgery of brain metastases of different histologies with and without WBXRT found that WBXRT reduced subsequent development of brain metastases in lung cancer patients but not patients with melanoma or renal cell carcinoma. Administering initial WBXRT and waiting a month before radiosurgery for subsequent tumor shrinkage is a reasonable strategy for limiting radiation injury reactions and/or improving tumor control for brain metastases >3 cm in diameter and for brainstem metastases >2 cm in diameter.

There is no clear limit as to how many metastases and what total volume of metastases can or should be treated by radiosurgery. RTOG 95-08 was limited to one to three metastases, while the trial of Aoyama et al.[21] and a smaller University of Pittsburgh trial included patients with up to four brain metastases.[96] Bhatnagar et al.[97] analyzed 205 patients who underwent radiosurgery for four to 18 brain metastases (median, five). They reported a median survival of 8 months after radiosurgery and found that survival correlated with the total volume of metastases, age, and RTOG-RPA class, but not the total number of brain metastases. Presently, many centers use WBXRT alone to initially manage patients with five or more metastases and subsequently consider radiosurgery for patients who are unable to be withdrawn from steroid medication and for patients whose brain metastases progress after WBXRT.

Glioblastomas

During the late 1980s and 1990s, many centers that had been using brachytherapy for recurrent high-grade gliomas and as boosts after conventional radiotherapy switched to radiosurgery.[30,98] Although retrospective series appeared to show that initial brachytherapy or radiosurgery boosts after conventional radiotherapy improved survival of glioblastoma patients, prospective randomized trials of both modalities used prior to conventional radiotherapy of glioblastoma patients were negative.[30,98] Radiosurgery appears to be a reasonable option for small, well-circumscribed, high-grade gliomas that recur after prior conventional large-field radiotherapy and chemotherapy.

Radiosurgery of Spinal Metastases

Radiosurgery has been used to treat spinal tumors, mostly metastases, either as initial treatment or for recurrence after prior fractionated radiotherapy.[14,15,20,22] By limiting spinal cord radiation dose with radiosurgery techniques, higher doses can be safely given to the tumor target volume with the hope of achieving greater local tumor control and higher response rates. Spinal cord tolerance in the experience of Gerszten et al.[14] with 125 CyberKnife spine radiosurgery procedures in 17 benign and 108 metastatic cases was previously discussed in this chapter. Gerszten et al.[20] separately reported results for single-fraction CyberKnife radiosurgery of 68 breast carcinoma metastases to the spine in 50 patients after 6 to 48 months of follow-up (median, 16 months). Pain was the most common indication for radiosurgery (in 57 lesions). Radiosurgery was delivered for radiographic tumor progression, as a postsurgical boost, and for a progressive neurologic deficit in one case each. Radiosurgery was used as primary management in eight patients. Target volumes varied from 0.8 to 197 mL (mean, 27.7 mL). Maximum tumor doses were 15 to 22.5 Gy (mean, 19 Gy). No radiation-induced toxicity occurred during the follow-up period (6 to 48 months). CyberKnife radiosurgery achieved long-term pain improvement in 55 of the 57 patients (96%) who were treated primarily for pain. Long-term radiographic tumor control was seen in all patients who underwent primary radiosurgery as well as those treated for radiographic tumor progression after radiotherapy or as a postsurgical treatment. Similar results were seen in separate reports for spine radiosurgery of melanoma metastases.[22] Randomized trials are needed to prove that SRS or hypofractionated SRT improve results compared with conventionally fractionated radiotherapy or IMRT with conventional immobilization.[99]

Stereotactic Irradiation of Lung Tumors

Hypofractionated SRT has been used for treatment of small, medically inoperable non–small cell lung cancer primary tumors and to manage lung metastases in patients with limited metastatic disease.[75,100,101] Beitler et al.[102] reported the Staten Island experience with SRT using five fractions of 8 Gy each in 75 patients (67 SRS alone and eight with SRS boost after conventional radiotherapy) with 1 to 92 months of follow-up (median, 17 months). Treatment volumes varied from 0.26 to 1197 mL, with a median of 26.8 mL. Complete responses developed in seven patients, tumor shrinkage in 25, stable disease in 22, and tumor progression in nine; 12 lacked follow-up. Radiation pneumonitis was reported in two patients. Patients with tumors <65 mL had a median survival of 26 months compared with 10 months for those with tumors >65 mL.

Ernst-Stecken et al.[12] reported results with hypofractionated stereotactic irradiation of 39 primary or secondary lung tumors in 21 patients. They delivered five fractions of either 7 Gy ($n = 21$) or 8 Gy ($n = 18$) to median tumor volumes of 2.9 mL (0.15 to 67.9 mL) using planning target volumes of 7.2 to 124.0 mL (median, 25.8 mL). They reported complete remission in 51%, partial in 33%, no change in 3%, and progressive disease in 13%. Most patients experienced grade 1 toxicity; none developed grade 2 or 4, but one patient developed grade 3 dyspnea 6 months after SRT.

Schefter et al.[91] reported a phase I/II dose-escalation study of stereotactic body radiotherapy for lung metastases in 25 patients. Using 5-mm radial and 10-mm cranial-caudal margins, they administered three fractions of 16, 18, or 20 Gy while restricting the percentage of normal lung receiving >15 Gy to under 35%. Fourteen patients were in the phase I part of the study: six at 48 Gy, four at 54 Gy, and four at 60 Gy. Afterward, 14 patients were enrolled in the phase II part and received 60 Gy in three fractions, but follow-up was insufficient to report toxicity. Dose-limiting toxicity, defined as higher than grade 3 lung, esophageal, or spinal toxicity occurring in any single patient, never developed in this study. Grade 1 to 2 esophagitis developed in three-fourths of the patients in the lowest-dose group only. Grade 1 dermatitis developed in one=fourth of the patients receiving 18 Gy × 3 and in one-fourth of the patients with 20 Gy × 3. Grade 1 pain developed in one-fourth of the patients within each dose level.

Miscellaneous Uses

Radiosurgery and hypofractionated SRT have been used as a substitute for brachytherapy in the management of recurrent head and neck tumors.[73,100] Liver metastases can also be irradiated with these techniques.[92] Hypofractionated prostate SRT is also being explored.[63,82]

REFERENCES

1. Garcia-Barros M, Paris F, Cordon-Cardo C, et al. Tumor response to radiotherapy regulated by endothelial cell apoptosis. *Science* 2003;300:1155–1159.
2. Szeifert GT, Massager N, DeVriendt D, et al. Observations of intracranial neoplasms treated with gamma knife radiosurgery. *J Neurosurg* 2002;97:623–626.
3. Flickinger JC, Kondziolka D, Pollock BE, et al. Complications from arteriovenous malformation radiosurgery: multivariate analysis and risk modeling. *Int J Radiat Oncol Biol Phys* 1997;38:485–490.
4. Flickinger JF, Kondziolka D, Maitz AH, et al. An analysis of the dose-response for arteriovenous malformation radiosurgery and other factors affecting obliteration. *Radiother Oncol* 2002;63:347–354.
5. Flickinger JC, Kondziolka D, Lunsford LD, et al. Development of a model to predict permanent symptomatic postradiosurgery injury for arteriovenous malformation patients. Arteriovenous Malformation Radiosurgery Study Group. *Int J Radiat Oncol Biol Phys* 2000; 46:1143–1148.
6. Shaw E, Scott C, Souhami L, et al. Single dose radiosurgical treatment of recurrent previously irradiated primary brain tumors and brain metastases: final report of RTOG protocol 90–05. *Int J Radiat Oncol Biol Phys* 2000;47: 291–298.
7. Tishler RB, Loeffler JS, Lunsford LD, et al. Tolerance of cranial nerves of the cavernous sinus to radiosurgery. *Int J Radiat Oncol Biol Phys* 1993;27: 215–221.
8. Stafford SL, Pollock BE, Leavitt JA, et al. A study on the radiation tolerance of the optic nerves and chiasm after stereotactic radiosurgery. *Int J Radiat Oncol Biol Phys* 2003;55:1177–1181.
9. Leber KA, Bergloff J, Pendl G. Dose-response tolerance of the visual pathways and cranial nerves of the cavernous sinus to stereotactic radiosurgery. *J Neurosurg* 1998;88:43–50.
10. Combs SE, Thilmann C, Edler L, et al. Efficacy of fractionated stereotactic reirradiation in recurrent gliomas: long-term results in 172 patients treated in a single institution. *J Clin Oncol* 2005;23:8863–8869.
11. Combs SE, Volk S, Schulz-Ertner D, et al. Management of acoustic neuromas with fractionated stereotactic radiotherapy (FSRT): long-term results in 106 patients treated in a single institution. *Int J Radiat Oncol Biol Phys* 2005;63:75–81.
12. Ernst-Stecken A, Lambrecht U, Mueller R, et al. Hypofractionated stereotactic radiotherapy for primary and secondary intrapulmonary tumors: first results of a phase i/ii study. *Strahlenther Onkol* 2006;182:696–702.
13. Flickinger JC, Kondziolka D, Lunsford L. Fractionation of radiation treatment in acoustics. Rationale and evidence in comparison to radiosurgery. *Neurochirurgie* 2004;50:421–426.
14. Gerszten PC, Ozhasoglu C, Burton SA, et al. CyberKnife frameless stereotactic radiosurgery for spinal lesions: clinical experience in 125 cases. *Neurosurgery* 2004;55:89–98.
15. Benzil DL, Saboori M, Mogilner AY, et al. Safety and efficacy of stereotactic radiosurgery for tumors of the spine. *J Neurosurg* 2004;101(Suppl 3):413–418.
16. Flickinger JC, Kondziolka D, Niranjan A, et al. Acoustic neuroma radiosurgery with marginal tumor doses of 12 to 13 Gy. *Int J Radiat Oncol Biol Phys* 2004; 60:225–230.
17. Florio F, Lauriola W, Nardella M, et al. Endovascular treatment of intracranial arterio-venous malformations with Onyx embolization: preliminary experience. *Radiol Med (Torino)* 2003;106:512–520.
18. Foote KD, Friedman WA, Buatti JM, et al. Analysis of risk factors associated with radiosurgery for vestibular schwannoma. *J Neurosurg* 2001;95(Suppl): 440–449.
19. Friedman DP, Goldman HW, Flanders AE, et al. Stereotactic radiosurgical pallidotomy and thalamotomy with the gamma knife: MR imaging findings with clinical correlation–preliminary experience. *Radiology* 1999;212:143–150.
20. Gerszten PC, Burton SA, Ozhasoglu C, et al. Stereotactic radiosurgery for spinal metastases from renal cell carcinoma. *J Neurosurg Spine* 2005;3:288–295.
21. Aoyama H, Shirato H, Tago M, et al. Stereotactic radiosurgery plus whole-brain radiation therapy vs stereotactic radiosurgery alone for treatment of brain metastases: a randomized controlled trial. *JAMA* 2006;295:2483–2491.
22. Gerszten PC, Burton SA, Quinn AE, et al. Radiosurgery for the treatment of spinal melanoma metastases. *Stereotact Funct Neurosurg* 2005;83:213–221.
23. Hadjipanayis CG, Kondziolka D, Flickinger JC, et al. The role of stereotactic radiosurgery for low-grade astrocytomas. *Neurosurg Focus* 2003;14:1–7.
24. Harris AE, Lee JY, Omalu B, et al. The effect of radiosurgery during management of aggressive meningiomas. *Surg Neurol* 2003;60:298–305.
25. Hasegawa T, Kondziolka D, Spiro R, et al. Repeat radiosurgery for refractory trigeminal neuralgia. *Neurosurgery* 2002;50:494–502.
26. Hasegawa T, McInerney J, Kondziolka D, et al. Long-term results after stereotactic radiosurgery for patients with cavernous malformations. *Neurosurgery* 2002;50:1190–1198.
27. Henson CF, Goldman HW, Rosenwasser RH, et al. Glycerol rhizotomy versus gamma knife radiosurgery for the treatment of trigeminal neuralgia: an analysis of patients treated at one institution. *Int J Radiat Oncol Biol Phys* 2005;63: 82–90.
28. Hsieh PC, Chandler JP, Bhangoo S, et al. Adjuvant gamma knife stereotactic radiosurgery at the time of tumor progression potentially improves survival for patients with glioblastoma multiforme. *Neurosurgery* 2005;57:684–692.
29. Huang YC, Tseng CK, Chang CN, et al. LINAC radiosurgery for intracranial cavernous malformation:10-year experience. *Clin Neurol Neurosurg* 2006;108: 750–756.
30. Mehta MP, Tsao MN, Whelan TJ, et al. The American Society for Therapeutic Radiology and Oncology (ASTRO) evidence–based review of the role of radiosurgery for brain metastases. *Int J Radiat Oncol Biol Phys* 2005;63:37–46.
31. Meijer OW, Vandertop WP, Baayen JC, et al. Single-fraction vs. fractionated linac-based stereotactic radiosurgery for vestibular schwannoma: a single-institution study. *Int J Radiat Oncol Biol Phys* 2003;56:1390–1396.
32. Mingione V, Yen CP, Vance ML, et al. Gamma surgery in the treatment of nonsecretory pituitary macroadenoma. *J Neurosurg* 2006;104:876–883.
33. Modha A, Gutin PH. Diagnosis and treatment of atypical and anaplastic meningiomas: a review. *Neurosurgery* 2005;57:538–550.
34. Morita A, Coffey RJ, Foote RL, et al. Risk of injury to cranial nerves after gamma knife radiosurgery for skull base meningiomas: experience in 88 patients. *J Neurosurg* 1999;90:42–49.
35. Muacevic A, Jess-Hempen A, Tonn JC, et al. Results of outpatient gamma knife radiosurgery for primary therapy of acoustic neuromas. *Acta Neurochir Suppl* 2004;91:75–78.
36. Narod SA, Parry DM, Parboosingh J, et al. Neurofibromatosis type 2 appears to be a genetically homogeneous disease. *Am J Hum Genet* 1992;51:486–496.
37. Nicolato A, Foroni R, Alessandrini F, et al. The role of Gamma Knife radiosurgery in the management of cavernous sinus meningiomas. *Int J Radiat Oncol Biol Phys* 2002;53:992–1000.
38. Niranjan A, Jawahar A, Kondziolka D, et al. A comparison of surgical approaches for the management of tremor: radiofrequency thalamotomy, gamma knife thalamotomy and thalamic stimulation. *Stereotact Funct Neurosurg* 1999;72: 178–184.
39. Ohye C, Shibazaki T, Sato S. Gamma knife thalamotomy for movement disorders: evaluation of the thalamic lesion and clinical results. *J Neurosurg* 2005; 102(Suppl):234–240.
40. Okun MS, Stover NP, Subramanian T, et al. Complications of gamma knife surgery for Parkinson disease. *Arch Neurol* 2001;58:1995–2002.
41. Ondra SL, Troupp H, George ED, et al. The natural history of symptomatic arteriovenous malformations of the brain: a 24-year follow-up assessment. *J Neurosurg* 1990;73:387–391.
42. Paek SH, Chung HT, Jeong SS, et al. Hearing preservation after gamma knife stereotactic radiosurgery of vestibular schwannoma. *Cancer* 2005;104: 580–590.
43. Pan L, Wang EM, Zhang N, et al. Long-term results of Leksell gamma knife surgery for trigeminal schwannomas. *J Neurosurg* 2005;102(Suppl):220–224.
44. Pollock BE, Flickinger JC, Lunsford LD, et al. Factors that affect the hemorrhage risk of arteriovenous malformations. *Stroke* 1996;27:1–6.
45. Pollock BE, Flickinger JC, Lunsford LD, et al. Hemorrhage risk after radiosurgery for arteriovenous malformations. *Neurosurgery* 1996;38.
46. Pollock BE, Garces YI, Stafford SL, et al. Stereotactic radiosurgery for cavernous malformations. *J Neurosurg* 2000;93:987–991.
47. Pollock BE, Kondziolka D, Flickinger JC, et al. Preservation of cranial nerve function after radiosurgery for nonacoustic schwannomas. *Neurosurgery* 1993;33: 597–601.
48. Pollock BE, Lunsford LD, Kondziolka D, et al. Outcome analysis of acoustic neuroma management: a comparison of microsurgery and stereotactic radiosurgery. *Neurosurgery* 1995;36:215–225.
49. Pollock BE, Stafford SL. Results of stereotactic radiosurgery for patients with imaging defined cavernous sinus meningiomas. *Int J Radiat Oncol Biol Phys* 2005;62:1427–1431.
50. Pouratian N, Sheehan J, Jagannathan J, et al. Gamma knife radiosurgery for medically and surgically refractory prolactinomas. *Neurosurgery* 2006;59: 255–266.

51. Rades D, Schild SE. Value of postoperative stereotactic radiosurgery and conventional radiotherapy for incompletely resected typical neurocytomas. *Cancer* 2006;106:1140–1143.
52. Regis J, Hayashi M, Eupierre LP, et al. Gamma knife surgery for epilepsy related to hypothalamic hamartomas. *Acta Neurochir Suppl* 2004;91:33–50.
53. Regis J, Metellus P, Hayashi M, et al. Prospective controlled trial of gamma knife surgery for essential trigeminal neuralgia. *J Neurosurg* 2006;104:913–924.
54. Regis J, Pellet W, Delsanti C, et al. Functional outcome after gamma knife surgery or microsurgery for vestibular schwannomas. *J Neurosurg* 2002;97:1091–1100
55. Regis J, Rey M, Bartolomei F, et al. Gamma knife surgery in mesial temporal lobe epilepsy: a prospective multicenter study. *Epilepsia* 2004;45:504–515.
56. Rowe JG, Radatz MW, Walton L, et al. Gamma knife stereotactic radiosurgery for unilateral acoustic neuromas. *J Neurol Neurosurg Psychiatr* 2003;74: 1536–1542.
57. Inoue HK. Low-dose radiosurgery for large vestibular schwannomas: long-term results of functional preservation. *J Neurosurg* 2005;102(Suppl):111–113.
58. Iwai Y, Yamanaka K, Shiotani M, et al. Radiosurgery for acoustic neuromas: results of low-dose treatment. *Neurosurgery* 2003;53:282–288.
59. Karlsson B, Lindquist C, Steiner L. Prediction of obliteration after gamma knife surgery for cerebral arteriovenous malformations. *Neurosurgery* 1997;40:425–430.
60. Katz TS, Amdur RJ, Yachnis AT, et al. Pushing the limits of radiotherapy for atypical and malignant meningioma. *Am J Clin Oncol* 2005;28:70–74.
61. Kim DS, Park YG, Choi JU, et al. An analysis of the natural history of cavernous malformations. *Surg Neurol* 1997;48:9–17.
62. Kim MS, Pyo SY, Jeong YG, et al. Gamma knife surgery for intracranial cavernous hemangioma. *J Neurosurg* 2005;102(Suppl):102–106.
63. King CR, Lehmann J, Adler JR, et al. CyberKnife radiotherapy for localized prostate cancer: rationale and technical feasibility. *Technol Cancer Res Treat* 2003; 2:25–30.
64. Kondziolka D, Flickinger JC, Perez B. Judicious resection and/or radiosurgery for parasagittal meningiomas: outcomes from a multicenter review. Gamma Knife Meningioma Study Group. *Neurosurgery* 1998;43:405–413.
65. Kondziolka D, Levy EI, Niranjan A, et al. Long term outcomes after meningioma radiosurgery: physician and patient perspectives. *J Neurosurg* 1999;91:44–50.
66. Kondziolka D, Lunsford LD, Flickinger JC, et al. Reduction of hemorrhage risk after stereotactic radiosurgery for cavernous malformations. *J Neurosurg* 1995;83:825–831.
67. Kondziolka D, Lunsford LD, Flickinger JC. Stereotactic radiosurgery for the treatment of trigeminal neuralgia. *Clin J Pain* 2002;18:42–47.
68. Flickinger JC, Kondziolka D, Lunsford LD. Radiobiological analysis of tissue responses following radiosurgery. *Technol Cancer Res Treat* 2003;2:87–92.
69. Flickinger JC, Kondziolka D, Maitz AH, et al. Gamma knife radiosurgery of imaging-diagnosed intracranial meningioma. *Int J Radiat Oncol Biol Phys* 2003; 56:801–806
70. Flickinger JC, Pollock BE, Kondziolka D, et al. Does increased nerve length within the treatment volume improve trigeminal neuralgia radiosurgery? A prospective double-blind, randomized study. *Int J Radiat Oncol Biol Phys* 2001;51:449–454.
71. Kondziolka D, Lunsford LD, Kestle JR. The natural history of cerebral cavernous malformations. *J Neurosurg* 1995;83:820–824.
72. Kondziolka D, Lunsford LD, McLaughlin MR, et al. Long-term outcomes after radiosurgery for acoustic neuromas. *N Engl J Med* 1998;339:1426–1433.
73. Kondziolka D, Lunsford LD. Stereotactic radiosurgery for squamous cell carcinoma of the nasopharynx. *Laryngoscope* 1991;101:519–522.
74. Lippitz BE, Mindus P, Meyerson BA, et al. Lesion topography and outcome after thermocapsulotomy or gamma knife capsulotomy for obsessive-compulsive disorder: relevance of the right hemisphere. *Neurosurgery* 1999;44:452–460.
75. Unger F, Schrottner O, Feichtinger M, et al. Stereotactic radiosurgery for hypothalamic hamartomas. *Acta Neurochir Suppl* 2002;84:57–63.
76. Maruyama K, Kawahara N, Shin M, et al. The risk of hemorrhage after radiosurgery for cerebral arteriovenous malformations. *N Engl J Med* 2005;352:146–153.
77. Maesawa S, Flickinger JC, Kondziolka D, et al. Repeated radiosurgery for incompletely obliterated arteriovenous malformations. *J Neurosurg* 2000;92:961–970.
78. Sirin S, Kondziolka D, Niranjan A, et al. Prospective staged volume radiosurgery for large arteriovenous malformations: indications and outcomes in otherwise untreatable patients. *Neurosurgery* 2006;58:17–27.
79. Liscak R, Vladyka V, Simonova G, et al. Gamma knife surgery of brain cavernous hemangiomas. *J Neurosurg* 2005;102(Suppl):207–213.
80. Liu KD, Chung WY, Wu HM, et al. Gamma knife surgery for cavernous hemangiomas: an analysis of 125 patients. *J Neurosurg* 2005;102(Suppl):81–86.
81. Mabanta SR, Buatti JM, Friedman WA, et al. Linear accelerator radiosurgery for nonacoustic schwannomas. *Int J Radiat Oncol Biol Phys* 1999;43:545–548.
82. Madsen BL, Hsi RA, Pham HT, et al. Intrafractional stability of the prostate using a stereotactic radiotherapy technique. *Int J Radiat Oncol Biol Phys* 2003;57:1285–1291.
83. Mahajan A, McCutcheon IE, Suki D, et al. Case-control study of stereotactic radiosurgery for recurrent glioblastoma multiforme. *J Neurosurg* 2005;103: 210–217.
84. Malik I, Rowe JG, Walton L, et al. The use of stereotactic radiosurgery in the management of meningiomas. *Br J Neurosurg* 2005;19:13–20.
85. Martin JM, Katati M, Lopez E, et al. Linear accelerator radiosurgery in treatment of central neurocytomas. *Acta Neurochir (Wien)* 2003;145:749–754.
86. Kondziolka D, Nathoo N, Flickinger JC, et al. Long-term results after radiosurgery for benign intracranial tumors. *Neurosurgery* 2003;53:815–822.
87. Sakamoto T, Shirato H, Takeichi N, et al. Annual rate of hearing loss falls after fractionated stereotactic irradiation for vestibular schwannoma. *Radiother Oncol* 2001;60:45–48.
88. Shirato H, Sakamoto T, Sawamura Y, et al. Comparison between observation policy and fractionated stereotactic radiotherapy (SRT) as an initial management for vestibular schwannoma. *Int J Radiat Oncol Biol Phys* 1999;44:545–550.
89. Lin VY, Stewart C, Grebenyuk J, et al. Unilateral acoustic neuromas: long-term hearing results in patients managed with fractionated stereotactic radiotherapy, hearing preservation surgery, and expectantly. *Laryngoscope* 2005;115:292–296.
90. Andrews DW, Suarez O, Goldman HW, et al. Stereotactic radiosurgery and fractionated stereotactic radiotherapy for the treatment of acoustic schwannomas: comparative observations of 125 patients treated at one institution. *Int J Radiat Oncol Biol Phys* 2001;50:1265–1278.
91. Schefter TE, Kavanagh BD, Raben D, et al. A phase I/II trial of stereotactic body radiation therapy (SBRT) for lung metastases: Initial report of dose escalation and early toxicity. *Int J Radiat Oncol Biol Phys* 2006;66(4 Suppl):S120.
92. Schefter TE, Kavanagh BD, Raben D, et al. A phase I/II trial of stereotactic body radiation therapy (SBRT) for lung metastases: Initial report of dose escalation and early toxicity. *Int J Radiat Oncol Biol Phys* 2006;66(4 Suppl):S120.
93. Selch MT, Pedroso A, Lee SP, et al. Stereotactic radiotherapy for the treatment of acoustic neuromas. *J Neurosurg* 2004;101(Suppl 3):362–372.
94. Sheehan JP, Niranjan A, Sheehan JM, et al. Stereotactic radiosurgery for pituitary adenomas: an intermediate review of its safety, efficacy, and role in the neurosurgical treatment armamentarium. *J Neurosurg* 2005;102:678–691.
95. Andrews DW, Scott CB, Sperduto PW, et al. Whole brain radiation therapy with or without stereotactic radiosurgery boost for patients with one to three brain metastases: phase III results of the RTOG 9508 randomized trial. *Lancet* 2004;363:1665–1672.
96. Kondziolka D, Patel A, Lunsford LD, et al. Stereotactic radiosurgery plus whole brain radiotherapy versus radiotherapy alone for patients with multiple brain metastases. *Int J Radiat Oncol Biol Phys* 1999;45:427–434.
97. Bhatnagar AK, Flickinger JC, Kondziolka D, et al. Stereotactic radiosurgery for four or more intracranial metastases. *Int J Radiat Oncol Biol Phys* 2006; 64(3):898–903.
98. Souhami L, Seiferheld W, Brachman D, et al. Randomized comparison of stereotactic radiosurgery followed by conventional radiotherapy with carmustine to conventional radiotherapy with carmustine for patients with glioblastoma multiforme: report of Radiation Therapy Oncology Group 93-05 protocol. *Int J Radiat Oncol Biol Phys* 2004;60:853–860.
99. Bilsky MH, Yamada Y, Yenice KM, et al. Intensity-modulated stereotactic radiotherapy of paraspinal tumors: a preliminary report. *Neurosurgery* 2004;54: 823–831.
100. Voynov G, Heron DE, Burton S, et al. Frameless stereotactic radiosurgery for recurrent head and neck carcinoma. *Technol Cancer Res Treat* 2006;5:529–535.
101. Weber DC, Chan AW, Bussiere MR, et al. Proton beam radiosurgery for vestibular schwannoma: tumor control and cranial nerve toxicity. *Neurosurgery* 2003;53:577–586.
102. Beitler JJ, Badine EA, El-Sayah D, et al. Stereotactic body radiation therapy for nonmetastatic lung cancer: an analysis of 75 patients treated over 5 years. *Int J Radiat Oncol Biol Phys* 2006;65:100–106.
103. Aiba T, Tanaka R, Koike T, et al. Natural history of intracranial cavernous malformations. *J Neurosurg* 1995;83:56–59.
104. Bush DA, McAllister CJ, Loredo LN, et al. Fractionated proton beam radiotherapy for acoustic neuroma. *Neurosurgery* 2002;50:270–273.
105. Chang SD, Gibbs IC, Sakamoto GT, et al. Staged stereotactic irradiation for acoustic neuroma. *Neurosurgery* 2005;56:1254–1263.
106. Niranjan A. Gamma knife thalamotomy for disabling tremor. *Arch Neurol* 2002; 59:1660.
107. Kupersmith MJ, Kalish H, Epstein F, et al. Natural history of brainstem cavernous malformations. *Neurosurgery* 2001;48:47–53.
108. Lax I, Karlsson B. Prediction of complications in gamma knife radiosurgery of arteriovenous malformation. *Acta Oncol* 1996;35:49–55.
109. Lederman G, Lowry J, Wertheim S, et al. Acoustic neuroma: potential benefits of fractionated stereotactic radiosurgery. *Stereot Funct Neurosurg* 1997;69(1–4 Pt 2): 175–182.
110. Lee JY, Niranjan A, McInerney J, et al. Stereotactic radiosurgery providing long-term tumor control of cavernous sinus meningiomas. *J Neurosurg* 2002; 97(1):65–72.
111. McDermott MW, Berger MS, Kunwar S, et al. Stereotactic radiosurgery and interstitial brachytherapy for glial neoplasms. *J Neurooncol* 2004;69:83–100.
112. Tyler-Kabara E, Kondziolka D, Flickinger JC, et al. Stereotactic radiosurgery for residual neurocytoma. Report of four cases. *J Neurosurg* 2001;95:879–882.
113. Williams JA. Fractionated stereotactic radiotherapy for acoustic neuromas. *Int J Radiat Oncol Biol Phys* 2002;54:500–504.
114. Wowra B, Muacevic A, Jess-Hempen A, et al. Outpatient gamma knife surgery for vestibular schwannoma: definition of the therapeutic profile based on a 10-year experience. *J Neurosurg* 2005;102(Suppl):114–118.
115. Young RF, Jacques S, Mark R, et al. Gamma knife thalamotomy for treatment of tremor: long-term results. *J Neurosurg* 2000;93(Suppl 3):128–135.
116. Young RF, Vermeulen S, Posewitz A, et al. Pallidotomy with the gamma knife: a positive experience. *Stereotact Funct Neurosurg* 1998;70(Suppl 1):218–228.
117. Zabel A, Debus J, Thilmann C, et al. Management of benign cranial nonacoustic schwannomas by fractionated stereotactic radiotherapy. *Int J Cancer* 2001;96:356–362.

Chapter 17
Stereotactic Irradiation of Tumors Outside the Central Nervous System

Brian D. Kavanagh, Jeffrey D. Bradley, and Robert D. Timmerman

Departing from the established traditions of conventionally fractionated external beam radiotherapy, in the late 1980s and early 1990s investigators in the United States, Sweden, and Japan began to explore the use of extremely brief hypofractionated radiation treatment regimens for spine, lung, liver, and selected other malignant extracranial tumors.[1–3] In essence these clinical researchers were modifying techniques proven clinically valuable in the context of cranial and spine stereotactic radiosurgery in an effort to exploit the efficiency and biological potency of high–dose-per-fraction irradiation.[4] This idea was soon appreciated for its clinical promise by other researchers in numerous countries across the world.

Pioneers in the field initially used customized ancillary equipment constructed in their own institutions to immobilize patients and to adapt ordinary linear accelerators for the task of precise internal tumor targeting. Now, however, the administration of high-dose, tightly focused external beam radiation therapy is greatly facilitated by a wide assortment of commercially available systems that immobilize patients, address the problem of respiratory motion during treatment, and ensure accurate treatment with the use of image guidance. The newest generation of linear accelerators from several manufacturers is either exclusively dedicated to cranial or extracranial stereotactic radiotherapy or is equipped with a built-in package of features that provide an easy means of administering this type of treatment.

Stereotactic body radiation therapy (SBRT) is the term applied in the United States by the American Society of Therapeutic Radiology and Oncology (ASTRO) for the management and delivery of image-guided high-dose radiation therapy with tumor-ablative intent within a course of treatment that does not exceed 5 fractions.[5] Other descriptive terms have been occasionally applied to describe what is officially called SBRT, including the acronym SABR, an abbreviation for *s*tereotactic *ab*lative *r*adiotherapy.[6]

BIOLOGICAL AND ONCOLOGICAL RATIONALE FOR SBRT

The appeal of SBRT is based on the nonlinear relation between radiation dose and cytotoxic effect, whereby one or a few large individual doses of radiation therapy have substantially more cell-killing effect than the same dose of radiation given in smaller individual doses. Traditionally, the expected relation between radiation dose and tumor cell kill has been commonly estimated by the well-known linear-quadratic (LQ) model of radiation dose response, often relied on for the purpose of comparing the biological potency of different schedules of conventionally fractionated radiation therapy. In the range of dose per fraction used in SBRT, however, there has been an emerging appreciation that the LQ model overestimates the potency of fraction sizes on the order of 8 to 10 Gy or higher.

A variety of alternative mathematical models have been proposed to account for the observed inaccuracy of the LQ model for doses in this range. For example, Guerrero and Li[7] have proposed a modification of Curtis's[8] lethal-potentially lethal model that accounts for ongoing repair processes occurring during the time of an individual radiation treatment, thus predicting lower cytotoxicity from high doses administered over time intervals resembling typical clinical treatment times. Experimental data modeling cranial radiosurgery offer support for this concept.[9] Alternatively, Park et al.[10] have offered the universal survival curve formalism, which combines the LQ model for doses in the range used in conventional fractionation with a multitarget model for doses in the range used for SBRT. This piecewise function effectively achieves the same key mathematical result as other departures from the LQ model applied to SBRT, namely a more linear slope in the relation between dose and log cell kill in the high dose region.

In the special case of prostate cancer, the rationale for evaluating SBRT for prostate cancer also includes a fundamentally different consideration. Here, applying the LQ model-based assumptions and interpretation, the α/β ratio for prostate cancer has been estimated to be very low, likely in the range of 1.5 to 3.0 Gy.[11,12] If this estimate of α/β ratio for prostate cancer is correct, then higher doses per fraction should provide a more favorable therapeutic ratio than a conventionally fractionated regimen. Accumulating evidence from randomized clinical trials comparing conventional daily fractions of 2 Gy with hypofractionated regimens using fractions sized on the order of 3 Gy per day offer strong support for this hypothesis and the safety of using this approach.[13–15] Clinical reports involving SBRT for prostate cancer have involved doses that are higher than 3 Gy and are discussed later in the chapter.

None of the aforementioned models of high–dose-per-fraction tumor cell–killing effects explicitly incorporate a mechanism of tumor cell kill that might be of equal or greater importance than tumor DNA damage-based injury, namely the antiangiogenic effect of endothelial cell apoptosis occurring above an apparent threshold dose on the order of 8 to 10 Gy. First observed preclinically and reported by Garcia-Barros et al.,[16] clinical evidence indirectly supporting the importance of this mechanism includes measures of an increase in serum markers of apoptosis post-SBRT.[17] Other similar threshold effects, which do not occur until the dose per fraction exceeds a minimum "unconventional" level, have been observed, suggesting new ways in which SBRT might be further exploited.[18–20]

Beyond its uses as primary therapy for selected early-stage cancers, SBRT has also been used as a noninvasive and efficient means of eradicating discrete metastatic tumors, and the argument for this application can be built on numerous overlapping lines of evidence or conceptual theories of cancer growth and dissemination or cytotoxic abscopal effects: (a) the empiric or phenomenological, (b) the patterns-of-failure concept, (c) the theory of oligometastases, (d) a lethal burden variation of the Norton-Simon hypothesis, or (e) immunological enhancement.[21]

The most straightforward argument for SBRT in the setting of isolated sites of metastatic disease is what might be termed an empiric or phenomenological rationale. There have been numerous reports of patients enjoying a high rate of 3- to 5-year survival following various forms of aggressive local treatment (e.g., surgical resection, radiofrequency ablation, cryotherapy) for limited metastases in the liver or lung from an assortment of solid tumor types. On one level, then, SBRT is a valid, noninvasive substitute for other local modalities if it provides similar efficacy and the same or less toxicity.

The indications for SBRT in the setting of metastatic disease might be alternatively couched in terms of a patterns-of-failure model. A traditional example of a patterns-of-failure approach would be combined modality therapy for lymphomas, where systemic treatment with chemotherapy is combined with involved field radiotherapy to the sites of disease that were grossly evident at the time of diagnosis, indicating that they contain the highest number of clonogenic cells and are thus least likely to be completely eliminated by the chemotherapy. A patterns-of-failure analysis by Rusthoven et al.,[22] involving patients who received chemotherapy for metastatic non–small cell lung cancer, reveals a similar result: patients are most likely to manifest tumor recurrence in sites initially involved prior to chemotherapy, opening an opportunity for SBRT to sites of residual disease following some form of systemic therapy to be given with this goal in mind. An earlier analysis by Mehta et al.[23] yielded very similar observations.

Yet another argument that has been advanced in support SBRT in this setting is the theory of oligometastases. As articulated by Hellman and Weichselbaum,[24] this viewpoint considers that there seems to be a subgroup of patients with metastatic disease that is intermediate between completely absent and widely metastatic. For such patients the entire systemic disease burden is then entirely contained within the finite number of individual sites of gross disease recognized by the pertinent imaging studies. This condition would reflect an intermediate point in the natural history of that individual's cancer; therefore, these patients might be cured if their limited numbers of metastatic sites are eradicated. Among the many studies lending support to this theory would be the report by Stinauer et al.[25] involving patients treated with SBRT for metastases from melanoma or renal cell carcinoma, where there was significantly longer survival for patients with oligometastatic disease, there defined as three or fewer sites, than for patients with more extensive disease.

The theory of oligometastases may be extended beyond subdividing patients according to the integer number of detectable lesions present and, instead, toward characterizing prognosis according to a continuous rather than discrete metric of disease burden. In one sense this approach is a variation of the Norton-Simon hypothesis, as applied to the whole host rather than simply tumor cell kinetics. This conjecture arose from experimental observations in animal models where the number of cancer cells within the host increases from beneath the threshold of detectability, through a phase of rapid growth, and onward toward a plateau level that is lethal to the host.[26] This observation was translated into clinical trials by postulating that traditional DNA-targeted chemotherapy is expected to render the greatest degree of cytotoxicity to cancer cells in the rapid phase of growth, when there is higher mitotic activity that renders DNA more vulnerable. Trials testing dose-dense chemotherapy were designed to exploit the enhanced chemosensitivity of rapidly growing cancer cells with the use of frequent dosing schedules that capture tumors repeatedly at relatively smaller volume, without allowing time for regrowth into relatively less sensitive, near-lethal tumor volumes.[27]

An example of evidence in support of the concept of a clinical lethal burden of disease, as measured by a continuous rather than discrete metric, includes the observations of Lee et al.,[28] who used a positron emission tomography scan-based method of quantifying the metabolically active tumor burden in patients with lung cancer and observed that it independently predicted overall survival. SBRT given to a patient with metastatic disease could, in principle, have favorable effects that align with the tenets of the Norton-Simon hypothesis. First, the SBRT might reduce the patient's total burden of disease in such a way that the remaining cancer within the patient's body enters into a state of relatively higher growth fraction and is thus more susceptible to cytotoxic systemic agents. Second, the SBRT could prevent or delay the condition of lethal systemic tumor burden that is fatal to the patient.[29]

A fifth consideration that has emerged in recent years is the possibility that high–dose-per-fraction radiation therapy influences immune system responses in a manner that can be exploited for favorable therapeutic effect. Preclinical studies have demonstrated that high–dose-per-fraction ionizing radiation can induce antigen presentation within the tumor stroma.[30] Furthermore, antibody-mediated induction of T cell activity can be combined with high–dose-per-fraction ionizing radiation to enhance not only the effect on the irradiated tumor but also to create an abscopal effect whereby tumor implants remote from the irradiated site regress.[31] Findings such as these suggest ideas for new investigations into the combination of SBRT and immunomodulatory agents for patients with metastatic disease.

There is overlap among all of these perspectives, and it would be impossible to prove the exclusive validity of any one above another. Improved disease-free and overall survival following the use of SBRT to metastatic sites of disease would support any of these theories. Nevertheless, it is very important to consider the larger context of cancer treatment in which SBRT is applied for metastatic disease, and these theories can serve to frame the clinical or investigational objectives when SBRT is applied as a treatment for metastatic disease, either alone or in combination with a systemic agent.

STEREOTACTIC BODY RADIATION THERAPY GUIDELINES, PHYSICS OVERVIEW, AND SAFETY CONSIDERATIONS

ASTRO and the American College of Radiology (ACR) have published guidelines that characterize the personnel qualifications and responsibilities, documentation, quality control, and clinical operations recommended for the safe and proper administration of SBRT and follow-up care for patients treated.[5] The ASTRO-ACR guidelines advise that the following components should be in place within and institution's SBRT program:

1. Qualified personnel:
   a. Board-certified radiation oncologist
   b. Qualified medical physicist
   c. Licensed radiation therapist
   d. Other support staff as indicated (dosimetrists, oncology nurses, and so forth);
2. Ongoing machine quality assurance program;
3. Documentation in accordance with the *ACR Practice Guideline for Communication: Radiation Oncology;*
4. Quality control of treatment accessories;
5. Quality control of planning and treatment images;
6. Quality control of treatment planning system;
7. Simulation and treatment systems that account for systematic and random errors associated with setup and target motion in a manner that is based on actual measurement of organ motion and setup uncertainty.

The American Association of Physicist in Medicine Task Group 101 (TG101) moved forward from the ASTRO-ACR guidelines to generate a report that considers additional important nuances in the planning and treatment delivery of SBRT.[32] Included within the TG101 report are discussions of potential imaging artifacts and their impact on treatment planning, the challenges of small field dosimetry, and the importance of using an acceptable dose calculation algorithm, among other issues.

Proper patient repositioning, target localization, and management of breathing-related motion are essential for SBRT. A variety of patient immobilization devices are available, including several types of body frames with external fiducial markers. So-called frameless systems incorporate ultrasound, kilovolt-range imaging, or near real-time computed tomography (CT) scanning to verify the location of internal targets relative to the beams to be used. Because SBRT treatment sessions are lengthier than conventional external beam treatments, patient comfort is an important issue.

Techniques, Modalities, and Modifiers in Radiation Oncology

Breathing-related motion control devices and systems fall into three general categories: (a) dampening, (b) gating, and (c) tracking or "chasing." Respiratory dampening techniques include systems of abdominal compression intended to diminish one of the largest contributors to breathing-related motion, namely diaphragmatic excursion, by obliging the inspiratory–expiratory lung motion pattern to involve more intracostal expansion and shallower breathing overall. Also included in this category are the systems employing breath-holding maneuvers to stabilize the tumor in a reproducible stage of the respiratory cycle (e.g., deep inspiration). Gating systems for SBRT, as for any radiotherapy application, follow the respiratory cycle using a surrogate indicator for respiratory motion, for example, chest wall motion, and employ an electronic beam activation trigger allowing irradiation to occur only during a specified range of expected tumor locations. Tracking or "chasing" systems move the radiation beam or patient to follow the movement of the tumor.

Regardless of the system employed, the procedure of treatment planning must include the same consideration for respiratory motion management to be used during treatment. Despite available motion control equipment, some positional uncertainty will remain. The planning target volume (PTV) margins used to account for this residual motion of the gross tumor volume (GTV) will typically range from 5 to 10 mm.

The word *stereotactic* has heretofore usually implied that some sort of external reference markers indexed to internal structures facilitate internal target relocalization, but the definition has expanded to include systems of image-guided radiation therapy (IGRT) that relate the position of internal targets to a three-dimensional coordinate geometry registered to the treatment machine without the use of external markers on the patient. SBRT always involves some form of IGRT to guide for treatment delivery.

Most reports describing SBRT published to date have employed high-energy photons (x-rays) as the source of therapeutic radiation, although other particles can also be used. There is no absolute standard for the combination of beam or arc angles ideal for any given clinical situation, and each case can present unique challenges. In general to achieve a tightly focused high-dose distribution within the PTV and rapid dose falloff outside the PTV, a combination of multiple (often 10 or more) noncoplanar beams or multiple arcs are required. Intensity modulation across the individual beams or arc segments can be incorporated within SBRT.

As part of ASTRO's Target Safely campaign, the Multidisciplinary Quality Assurance Subcommittee of the Clinical Affairs and Quality Committee of ASTRO commissioned a white paper on the topic of cranial radiosurgery and SBRT titled "Quality and Safety Considerations in Stereotactic Radiosurgery and Stereotactic Body Radiation Therapy."[33] Of particular importance within the white paper are sections emphasizing the importance of creating a proactive culture of safety with procedural checkpoints and error analysis mechanisms.

CLINICAL EXPERIENCE WITH STEREOTACTIC BODY RADIATION THERAPY IN SELECTED SITES

Liver

The two major reasons for considering SBRT for hepatocellular cancer (HCC) is that underlying severe liver disease often renders patients medically inoperable and that other nonsurgical therapies have generally achieved at best rather modest success in that setting. The natural history of untreated HCC has been reported to involve a median survival in the range of 3 to 8 months,[34–36] and so a safe and effective therapy is needed in this setting.

The earliest observations following SBRT for HCC were reported by a group at Karolinska Hospital,[2] and more recent formal prospective studies have followed. The Princess Margaret Hospital group utilized a 6-fraction regimen in a prospective phase I study in patients with HCC (n = 31) or intrahepatic cholangiocarcinoma (n = 10).[37] Prescription doses were selected according to a normal tissue complication probability (NTCP) model based on conventionally fractionated radiotherapy to the liver. The median dose to the tumor was 36 Gy (range, 24 to 54 Gy). The NTCP model overestimated the chance of radiation-induced liver disease, and it is possible that the dose could have been escalated to a higher level in most cases. Nevertheless, in this group of heavily pretreated patients (over 60% had had at least one prior therapy for HCC), a remarkable median survival of 12 months was observed.

Méndez Romero et al.[38] at Erasmus University Medical Center treated eight patients with 11 separate lesions of HCC in 3 to 5 fractions to a dose of 25.0 to 37.5 Gy. A 1-year survival of 75% was observed. Choi et al.[39] at the Catholic University of Korea treated 23 patients with 32 individual lesions in a 3-fraction regimen to a median dose of 36 Gy (range, 30 to 39 Gy). No patient experienced severe toxicity, although follow-up was limited (median 11 months). Interestingly, in a subsequent analysis of predictors for decline in liver function after SBRT, on multivariate analysis the only predictor for a decrease in Child-Pugh classification (CPC) from baseline level was the volume of normal liver receiving 18 Gy or more (V18). The rate of negative impact on CPC rose sharply when the V18 exceeded 800 cc.[40] This latter observation favors a model of SBRT effect on normal liver in line with a critical volume model, whereby it is important to preserve a certain minimum level of function by sparing an adequate volume of normal liver from receiving a dose above a certain threshold.

The group from the Korea Institute of Radiological and Medical Sciences treated a prospectively registered cohort of 38 patients with inoperable HCC with SBRT, all of whom had failed prior transarterial chemoembolization.[41] The median tumor volume was 40.5 cc (range, 11 to 464). The SBRT dose was 33 to 57 Gy in 3 or 4 fractions. Minimal grade 3 toxicity (<3%) was observed, and the 2-year overall survival was 61%.

Cardenes et al.[42] from Indiana University and the University of Colorado reported a multi-institutional phase I dose escalation study of SBRT given in 3 fractions for HCC. Eligibility requirements were CPC-A or -B, medical or technical inoperability, and three or fewer lesions of cumulative tumor diameter 6 cm or less. The study enrolled 17 patients with 25 individual lesions. Dose was escalated from 36 to 48 Gy (16 Gy per fraction) in CPC-A patients without dose-limiting toxicity; however, two patients with CPC-B status at baseline developed grade 3 hepatic toxicity at the 42 Gy (14 Gy per fraction) dose level. Consequently, the dose for CPC-B patients was reduced to 40 Gy in 5 fractions. There were no local failures within the treated volume, and six patients proceeded to liver transplantation. The 2-year overall survival for the entire group was 60%.

The Indiana University group has separately reported their single institution experience involving a total of 60 patients: 34 CPC-A, 25 CPC-B, and 1 CPC-C.[43] The median number of fractions, dose per fraction, and total dose, was 3, 14 Gy, and 44 Gy, respectively, for those with CPC-A cirrhosis and 5, 8 Gy, and 40 Gy, respectively, for those with CPC-B. With a median follow-up time of 27 months, the 2-year local control rate was 90%. Two-year overall survival was 67%. SBRT served as a bridge to liver transplant for 23 patients who underwent transplant at a median time of 7 months following SBRT. A progression in CPC was observed in 20% of patients within 3 months of treatment.

Outcomes following SBRT for liver metastases have also been reported by numerous groups[44–51] and are summarized in Table 17.1. Regimens of 1 to 5 fractions have been employed, and total doses up to 60 Gy to the planning target volume have been administered. Taken together, the results show good survival outcomes achieved in heavily pretreated

TABLE 17.1 STEREOTACTIC BODY RADIATION THERAPY FOR LIVER METASTASES

Institution (Ref.)	*Patients/Lesions*	*SBRT Dose and Fractionation*	*Results*
Heidelberg (44)	37/60	11–21 Gy × 1	18 months LC: Low dose (<16): 0% High dose (>16): 81%
Würzburg (45)	39/51	7 Gy × 4 10 Gy × 3 12.5 Gy × 3 26 Gy × 1	2 year LC: Low dose (28–30): 58% High dose (others): 82%
Aarhus-Copenhagen (46)	44/not stated	10 Gy × 3	2 year LC: 79% All pts CRC 3 ulcers with intestinal dose >30 Gy
Erasmus (47)	17/34	10 Gy × 3 12.5 Gy × 3	54% 15 pts CRC; 1 late portal hypertension in multiply treated patient
Colorado/multi-institutional (48)	47/63	12–20 Gy × 3	2-year LC: ≤3 cm: 100% >3 cm: 75%
Princess Margaret Hospital (49)	68/141	Variable, NTCP-based Median 7 Gy × 6	1-year LC: 71% Better for higher dose, smaller volume
Stanford (50)	19/35	18–30 Gy × 1	1-year LC: 77% Combined with 7 patients with primarily liver cancer; maximum tolerated dose not reached
University of Texas–Southwestern (51)	26/35	6–12 Gy × 5	2-year LC 56%, 89%, 100% for total dose 30, 50, 60 Gy, respectively

PTV, planning target volume; LC, local control; OS, overall survival; CRC, colorectal cancer; NTCP, normal tissue complication probability.

individuals and a trend toward improved local control with increasing dose.

Chang et al.[52] reported a pooled analysis from three institutions with the use of liver SBRT for liver metastases from colorectal primary cancers. The combined experience from Stanford, Princess Margaret Hospital, and the University of Colorado included 65 patients with a total of 102 individual liver metastases from colorectal cancer treated. More than half of the patients had had at least one prior systemic therapy regimen, and over 40% of the patients had had two or more prior systemic regimens. The analysis indicated that to achieve durable local control of treated lesion, a 3-fraction total dose on the order of 48 Gy is needed. Sustained local control after SBRT was closely associated with improved survival on multivariate analysis ($P = .06$).

Technical issues and posttreatment imaging follow-up considerations unique to liver SBRT have been included in these reports and in review papers.[53,54] Briefly, target delineation and image guidance can be difficult, because liver metastases are not well visualized on CT scans or in-room volumetric imaging used for IGRT. In many centers, radiopaque fiducial markers are place in or near the metastases to facilitate IGRT. In all centers, the planning target volume is an expansion of the gross tumor volume in consideration of the setup and intrafraction motion to be expected with the particular setup and delivery system employed. Typically the margin used to expand a GTV into a PTV is on the order of 5 mm axially and 5 to 10 mm craniocaudally.

The Colorado group first applied the critical volume approach to normal liver dose constraints in their initial phase I study[55] and subsequent phase II study. Noted above in relation to the observations of the Catholic University of Korea in their treatment of primary liver tumors, the critical volume model liver SBRT is an adaptation of the early work of Yeas and Kalend.[56] Applicable for organs of radiobiologically parallel structure, the crux of this application is to work backward, in a sense, from an estimate of how much volume of the organ is essential and must be protected from functional ablation. The estimate for liver that at least 700 cm³ should receive less than 15 Gy during a 3-fraction SBRT course was derived from a combination of prior reports of outcomes after partial hepatectomy documenting approximate minimum volumes required and estimates of the effects of that dose of radiation extrapolated from prior reports of conventionally fractionated treatment.

One feature of the normal tissue effect of liver SBRT consistently observed within the first few months after SBRT is a zone of hypodensity observed on follow-up CT scans corresponding to the volume that received approximately 30 Gy.[55] This phenomenon, first described by Herfarth et al.[57] following single-dose liver SBRT, is likely related to local veno-occlusive effects.[58] There is no known clinical consequence associated with the finding, but it can cloud the assessment of tumor response within the first few months after liver SBRT.

CASE STUDY

Liver Stereotactic Body Radiation Therapy

A 45-year-old female had been diagnosed with stage IV breast cancer 2 years previously. Biopsy-proven liver metastases were present at the time of diagnosis. Numerous systemic agents had been given, most recently gemcitabine and trastuzumab. Although all other measurable or assessable sites of disease were stable or regressing, a mass in the liver had progressed from 2.5-by-2.9 cm to 6.0-by-4.2 cm within the past 3 months. Because the patient was tolerating the regimen well and apparently having a response in most sites, she was offered SBRT in an effort to eradicate tumor in the liver.

The lesion diameter (>6 cm) rendered the patient ineligible for an ongoing phase II trial of SBRT for liver metastases, and the dose given was lower than the protocol doses (Fig. 17.1). The 53 cm³ GTV was expanded by 5 mm radially and 10 mm in the superior-inferior direction to generate the PTV. The dose distribution shown was administered in 3 fractions within 1 week using multiple dynamic conformal arcs and a controlled breath-holding device. The nominal prescription dose was 45 Gy. The maximum point dose was 59 Gy, and the equivalent uniform dose was 54 Gy. The volume of normal liver receiving less than 15 Gy was 1,800 cm³. The portion of the right kidney receiving above 15 Gy was 13%. Follow-up scans at 6 months and 10 months show a Herfarth type 2 reaction with hyperdensity in the treated normal liver.[57] There is also volume loss in the nearby normal liver parenchyma surrounding the lesion, a phenomenon that has also been described elsewhere.[58] The lesion remained controlled for the duration of the patient's life; she eventually died of complications related to central nervous system metastases.

Lung

Medically inoperable early-stage lung cancer has historically provided a substantial management challenge. Conventionally fractionated radiotherapy has yielded generally unsatisfactory outcomes with high rates of local failure and 3-year survivals in the range of approximately 30%. For this reason, medically

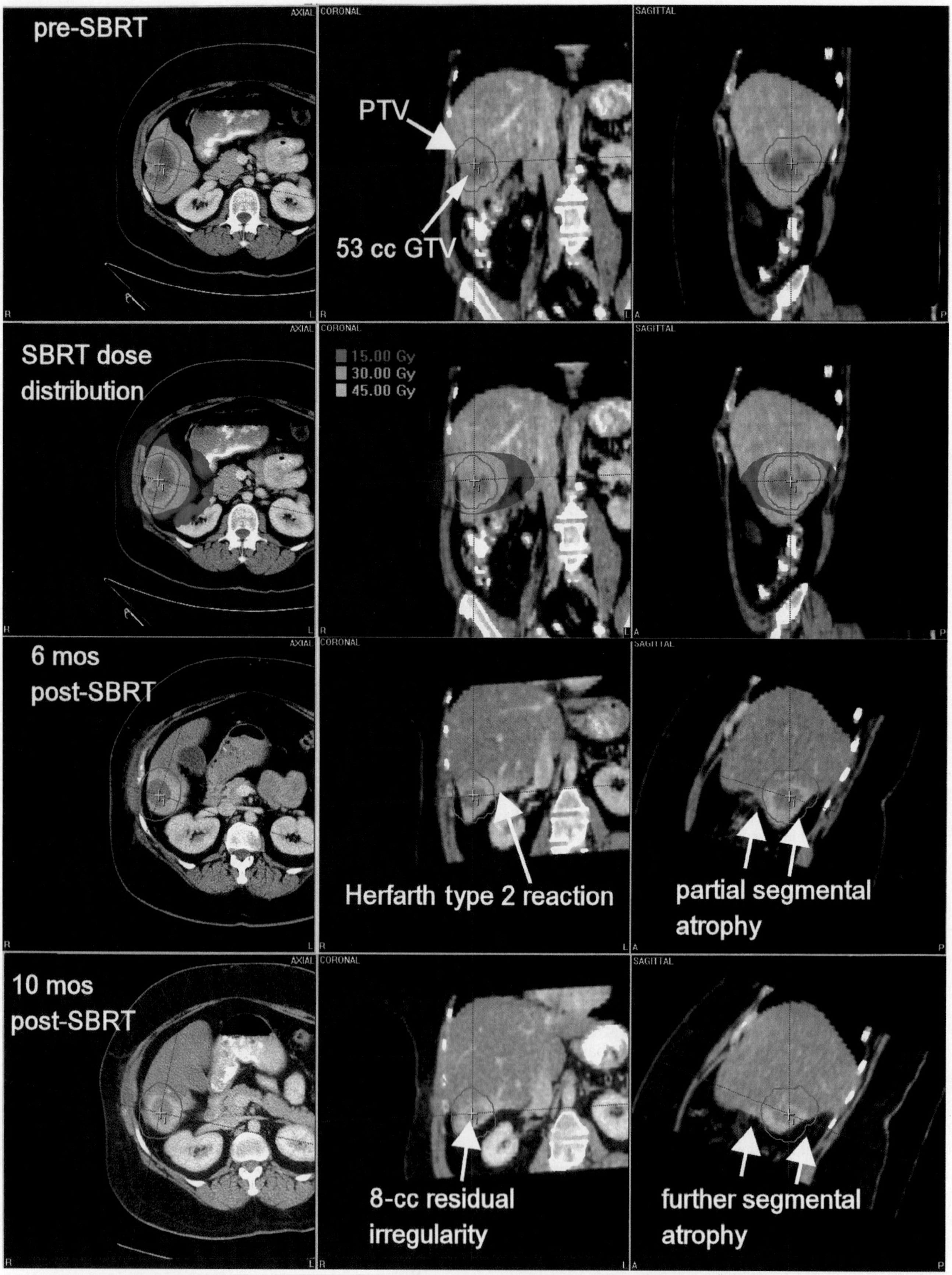

FIGURE 17.1. Example of liver stereotactic body radiation therapy (SBRT). *Top panel:* Pre-SBRT planning computed tomography images with *thin arrow* pointing to the gross tumor volume (GTV) and *wide arrow* showing the planning target volume (PTV), which is outlined. *Second panel:* SBRT composite dose distribution. *Third panel:* Images obtained 6 months post-SBRT illustrating a Herfarth type 2 reaction in adjacent parenchyma and partial segmental atrophy. *Bottom panel:* Shows images 10 months post-SBRT, indicating continued tumor regression as the ablated liver volume continues to recede.

TABLE 17.2 MAJOR PROSPECTIVE STUDIES OF STEREOTACTIC BODY RADIATION THERAPY FOR MEDICALLY INOPERABLE NON–SMALL CELL LUNG CANCER

Institution (Reference)	*Number of Patients*	*SBRT Dose and Fractionation*	*3-Year Results*
Indiana University (61)	70	60–66 Gy/3 fractions	LC 88%, OS 43%
Nordic Group (62)	57	45 Gy/3 fractions	LC 92%, OS 60%
RTOG (63)	55	54 Gy/3 fractions	LC 98%, OS 56%
University of Torino (64)	62	45 Gy/3 fractions	LC 88%, OS 57%

RTOG, Radiation Therapy Oncology Group; LC, local control; OS, overall survival.

inoperable early-stage lung cancer was the first clinical indication for which SBRT was studied in prospective clinical trials. Following the early exploratory studies of lung SBRT for stage I non–small cell lung cancer at the Karolinska Hospital in Stockholm[59] and National Medical Defense Hospital in Saitama,[60] numerous formal prospective studies of SBRT for medically inoperable non–small cell lung cancer have been now been reported. Table 17.2 lists the major prospective studies (N = 50 or more) with a minimum median follow-up of 24 months at the time of reporting, along with local control and overall survival at 3 years.[61–64] The consistent observation is that 3-year survival on the order of 50% to 60% has been achieved, a noteworthy improvement relative to conventionally fractionated radiotherapy.

One important observation from the Indiana University studies was that although the treatment was generally well tolerated, tumor location near large airways in the vicinity of the pulmonary hilum (called the zone of the proximal bronchial tree) was associated with a markedly higher risk of toxicity. For this reason, in the Radiation Therapy Oncology Group's (RTOG) study RTOG-0236 of SBRT for medically inoperable non–small cell lung cancer, patients with tumors located in the zone of the proximal bronchial tree were excluded.[63] The RTOG has launched a separate dose-escalation study (ROTG-0813) in which tumors near the proximal bronchial tree are treated. Both RTOG and the Japanese Clinical Oncology Group have completed enrollment to studies that expand the use of SBRT to patients with early-stage lung cancer who are medically operable.

Although many retrospective studies of lung SBRT contain a mixture of both primary and metastatic lesions, a few prospective studies exclusively focused on SBRT for lung metastases have been reported. In the University of Colorado phase I SBRT trial for lung metastases,[65] eligible patients had one to three pulmonary metastases from a solid tumor, cumulative tumor diameter less than 7 cm, and adequate pulmonary function (forced expiatory volume in the first second of expiration [FEV_1] >1.0 L). The PTV was typically constructed from the GTV by adding a 5-mm radial and 10-mm craniocaudal margin. The first cohort received 48 Gy to the PTV in 3 fractions. The SBRT dose was escalated in subsequent cohorts up to a preselected maximum of 60 Gy in 3 fractions. The percentage of normal lung receiving more than 15 Gy (V15) was restricted to less than 35%. Dose-limiting toxicity (DLT) included acute grade 3 lung or esophageal toxicity or any acute grade 4 toxicity. No patient experienced a DLT, and the SBRT dose was escalated to 60 Gy in 3 fractions without reaching a maximum tolerated dose. No consistent significant effects on pulmonary functions tests were noted.

The phase II study of SBRT for lung metastases the Colorado study group included 38 patients with 63 lesions.[66] Most had received at least one prior systemic regimen for metastatic disease, and approximately one-third had received two or more prior regimens. The incidence of any grade 3 toxicity was 8% (3/38), and no grade 4 toxicity was seen. Symptomatic pneumonitis occurred in one patient (2.6%). For 50 lesions assessable for local control, the median follow-up was 15.4 months. The median gross tumor volume was 4.2 cc. The actuarial 2-year local control was 96%. Median overall survival was 19 months.

CASE STUDY

Lung Stereotactic Body Radiation Therapy

A 74-year-old female had undergone wedge resection for a pT1N0M0 non–small cell cancer of the right lung 7 years previously. She had a right pneumonectomy 3 years later as salvage treatment for a locoregional recurrence. She was later observed to have developed a left lung nodule on a surveillance chest x-ray, and needle biopsy proved it to be a non–small cell lung cancer, presumed to be a second primary. Staging studies revealed no other sites of disease. She was given systemic therapy and enjoyed a transient minor response and then regrowth of the lesion (Fig. 17.2).

The patient used supplemental oxygen, 2 L/min at bedtime and occasionally during the day. She was offered SBRT as potentially curative therapy for a new T1N0M0 lung cancer. The 4 cm^3 GTV was expanded by 5 mm radially and 10 mm in the superior-inferior direction to generate the 29 cm^3 PTV. The dose distribution shown was administered in 3 fractions within 1 week using multiple dynamic conformal arcs. The patient did not comfortably tolerate a breath-holding technique because of her supplemental oxygen requirements; therefore, an abdominal compression technique was used during simulation and treatment. The nominal prescription dose was 60 Gy. The maximum point dose was 79 Gy, and the equivalent uniform dose was 72 Gy. The portion of normal lung receiving less than 15 Gy was 12.7%. The lesion remained controlled for the duration of the patient's life; she died of unrelated causes more than 2 years after SBRT.

Spine

The earliest investigation into what would now be termed spine SBRT was that of Hamilton et al.,[1,67] who used a rigid immobilization with a device surgically attached to the spinal column. Conservative doses in the range of 8 to 10 Gy were given in 1 fraction to nine patients with recurrent lesions in the spine following prior conventional radiotherapy. Spinal cord doses were very low using this technique (0.5 to 3.2 Gy). Limited follow-up suggested a favorable clinical effect in some patients, and no complications were observed. More recently, less invasive techniques have been investigated.

Ryu et al.[68] at the Henry Ford Hospital initially studied the treatment of spine metastases with initial fractionated radiotherapy followed by a spinal radiosurgery boost (6 to 8 Gy), observing prompt relief of pain in nearly all 10 treated patients. In a subsequent study of single fraction spinal radiosurgery alone (10 to 16 Gy), this group observed complete or partial pain relief in 85% of the 49 patients treated.[69] Perhaps even more importantly, pain relief was rapid after SBRT, sometimes within hours of treatment.

Chang et al.[70,71] at the M.D. Anderson Cancer Center performed a prospective phase I dose escalation study in treating spinal metastases and later updated their institutional experience. The equipment used included a "CT on rails" that allowed for imaging immediately to guide patient repositioning. Sixty-three cancer patients underwent near-simultaneous CT-guided SBRT. Spinal magnetic resonance imaging was conducted at baseline and at each follow-up visit. The median tumor volume of 74 spinal metastatic lesions was 37.4 cc. Approximately half the patients received 30 Gy in 5 fractions, and the other half received 27 Gy in 3 fractions. A conservative constraint of 9 to 10 Gy maximum dose to the spinal cord was applied. No neuropathy or myelopathy was observed during a median follow-up period of nearly 2 years. The actuarial 1-year tumor progression-free rate was 84%. The investigators noted two characteristic patterns of failure: (a) recurrence in the bone

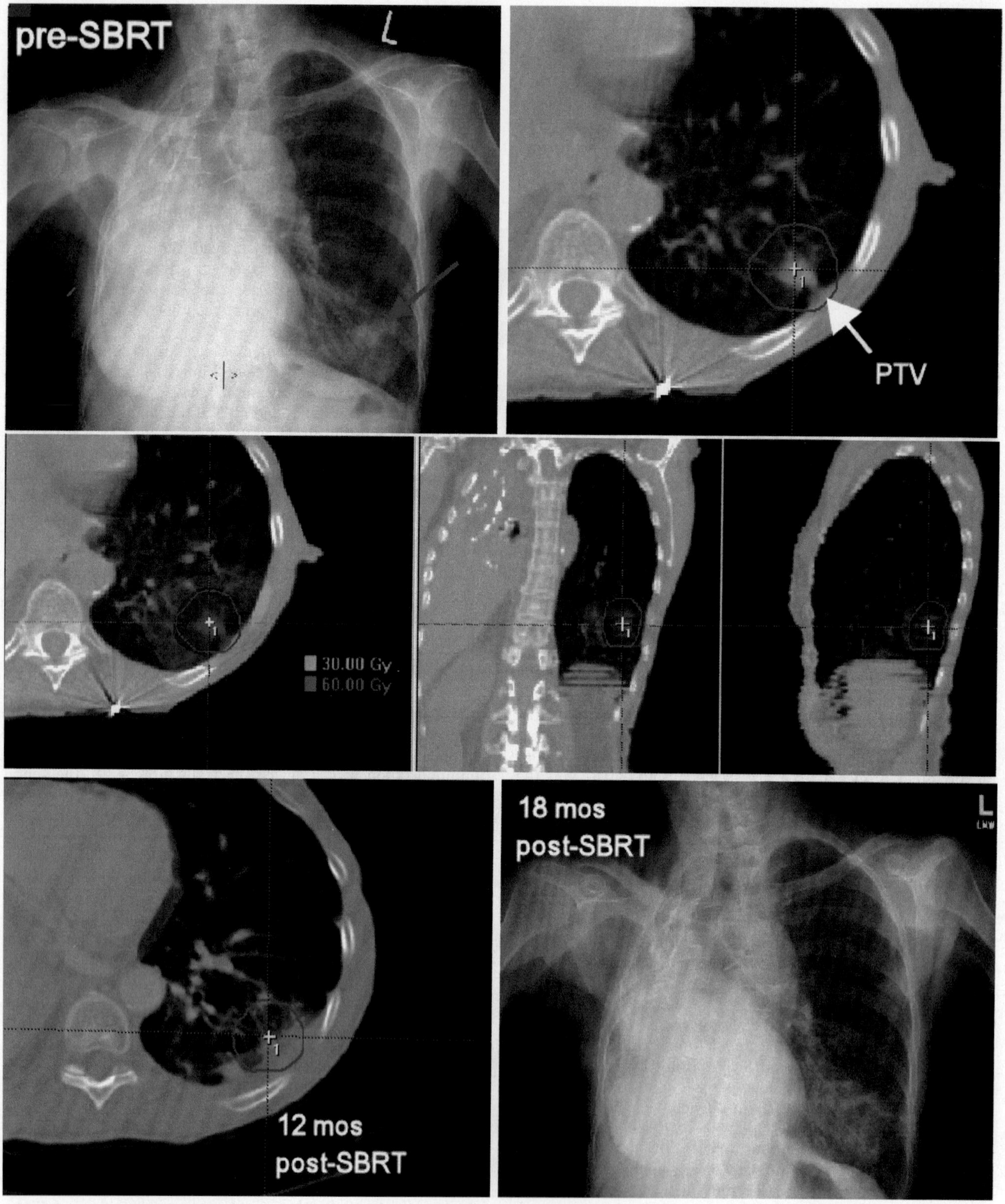

FIGURE 17.2. Example of lung stereotactic body radiation therapy (SBRT). *Top panel:* Pre-SBRT chest x-ray showing the left lung nodule (*red arrow*) and axial planning computed tomography (CT) image with *white arrow* pointing to the planning target volume (PTV), which is outlined. *Middle panel:* SBRT composite dose distribution shown in axial, coronal, and sagittal perspectives. *Bottom panel:* Follow-up CT scan axial image obtained 12 months post-SBRT illustrating stable patchy fibrosis in the high dose region (*left*) and chest x-ray obtained 12 months post-SBRT, indicating minimal residual haziness in the region treated.

adjacent to the site of previous treatment, and (b) recurrence in the epidural space adjacent to the spinal cord. A low rate of any grade 3 toxicity was observed.

Similar observations of good tumor control and minimal toxicity have been reported from other centers.[72–76] The largest is from Gerszten et al.[74] of the University of Pittsburgh, who analyzed a cohort of 500 cases of spinal metastases. The maximum intratumoral dose ranged from 12.5 to 25 Gy (mean, 20). Tumor volume ranged from 0.20 to 264 mL (mean, 46). Durable pain reduction was achieved in 86% of patients, and durable tumor control was demonstrated for approximately 90% of the lesions treated. The vast majority of patients with a progressive neurologic deficit before treatment experienced at least some clinical improvement.

Regarding normal tissue toxicities, the Memorial Sloan-Kettering Cancer Center group reported that post-SBRT vertebral fracture is common when there is metastatic lytic disease involving more than 40% of the vertebral body and location at or below T10.[77] The M.D. Anderson Cancer Center group also analyzed the risk of fracture after spine SBRT and noted that fractures were more common among patients of age over 55 years, those with a pre-existing fracture, and pain at the time of treatment,[78] suggesting that patients at very high risk might appropriately be considered for prophylactic vertebral stabilization or augmentation procedures. Fortunately, spinal cord toxicity has only rarely been observed after SBRT. Case-control comparisons offer some suggestions of parameters that might elevate the risk, but the paucity of events evaluable make it difficult to draw firm conclusions.[79,80] Constraints used to guide spine SBRT have included maximum point dose to the cord in the range of 10 to 14 Gy and limiting the volume of adjacent spinal cord receiving more than 10 Gy in a single fraction to 10% or less.

Prostate Cancer

The first publication on SBRT for prostate cancer was the work of Madsen et al.,[81] who recently updated their observations.[82] In a prospective trial, 40 patients with low-risk cancer (Gleason score ≤6 and prostate-specific antigen [PSA] ≤10 ng/mL) were treated to a dose of 33.5 Gy in 5 daily fractions The median age was 69 years (range, 50 to 82), and the median follow-up period was 5 years. The overall 5-year Phoenix definition (nadir plus 2 ng/mL) biochemical relapse-free survival rate was 93%. No patients died of prostate cancer. Late grade 3 genitourinary toxicity was rare, occurring in only one patient, and no late grade 3 or higher gastrointestinal was observed.

The groups at Winthrop University and the University of California–San Francisco have also reported trials of SBRT for early-stage prostate cancer.[83,84] Using doses of 35 to 38 Gy in 4 or 5 fractions, both groups reported similarly low rates of grade 3 or higher toxicity of any kind (<1% in aggregate between the studies) after a median follow-up of 1 year. King et al.[85] from Stanford University recently updated a prospective trial in which 67 patients with clinically localized low-risk prostate cancer were treated with SBRT to a dose of 36.25 Gy, administered in 5 fractions. The 4-year biochemical relapse-free survival was 94%, and no grade 3 or higher rectal toxicity was observed. There were only two cases (3%) of grade 3 or higher bladder toxicity, both of which were believed to have been caused or exacerbated by procedures performed for dysuria (cystoscopies or dilatation).

A separate recently published analysis combined a subset of the Stanford patients with a cohort of patients treated in an identical manner at a community center in Naples, Florida, all of whom had a minimum of 5 years of follow-up after SBRT.[86] The 5-year biochemical relapse-free survival was 93%, and no severe treatment-related toxicity was observed. Another prospective trial conducted at several Harvard-affiliated centers involved a very similar regimen of 5 fractions of 7.25 to 7.5 Gy for low-risk prostate cancer.[87] At a median follow-up of 44.5 months, the outcomes essentially replicated the Stanford-Naples experience, with a 3-year biochemical relapse-free survival of 98% and a 2% and 4% chance of grade 3 urinary or rectal toxicity, respectively.

Boike et al.[88] from the University of Texas–Southwestern have completed a dose escalation for prostate SBRT, aiming for a more aggressive regimen potentially suitable for patients with intermediate or high-risk disease. In a prospective phase I trial, it was shown that with careful attention to the rectal and bladder doses, it was possible to administer safely a dose of 50 Gy in 5 fractions, with an observed risk of 2% and 4% for grade 3 or higher rectal and genitor-urinary toxicity, respectively. The maximum tolerated dose was not reached in this trial, and the 50 Gy in 5-fraction regimen was selected for continuation in an ongoing prospective phase II trial.

Pancreas Cancer

A major challenge in the application of concurrent chemotherapy and conventionally fractionated radiotherapy is the high rate of nonhematologic toxicity. Recent North American cooperative group studies involving various chemotherapy regimens and conventionally fractionated radiotherapy to a dose of 50.4 Gy given in 28 fractions have been associated with rates of grade 3 or higher nonhematologic toxicity in the range of 29% to 79%.[89–92] SBRT would be an appealing alternative if equivalent survival could be achieved with lower rates of toxicity related to the reduction of the volume of normal tissue exposed to a high dose of radiation.

SBRT regimens for pancreas cancer have included treatments given in 1 to 5 fractions. The relation of risk of toxicity to the volume of normal tissue receiving a high dose is illustrated by the Danish cooperative group study. Here, a dose of 45 Gy in 3 fractions to a volume that included generous margins around the gross tumor volume, such that the median volume receiving more than 30 Gy, was 136 cc.[93] The toxicity from this high-volume treatment was unacceptably high.

More recent studies have incorporated tighter planning margins around the primary tumor and achieved reduction in toxicity and improvement in survival. The Stanford experience included 55 patients treated with a single 25 Gy fraction to the gross tumor volume plus 3-mm margin, with gemcitabine (GEM) given for 1 cycle prior to and 4 to 6 cycles after SBRT.[94] A median survival of 13 months was observed. The San Bartolo Hospital group gave 30 Gy in 3 fractions to a similar target volume, again with GEM given before and after SBRT, and observed an 11-month median survival.[95] The Beth Israel Deaconess group used a dose of 24 to 36 Gy in 3 fractions, with the GEM given after SBRT for 6 cycles, and observed a 14-month median survival.[96] The incidence of grade 3 or higher SBRT-related toxicity was very low for each study. In the San Bartolo Hospital and Beth Israel Deaconess studies, the rates of grade 3 or higher nonhematologic toxicity were 0% and 14%, respectively.

The Stanford group analyzed potential dosimetric factors that predicted for a risk of duodenal toxicity after single fraction SBRT for pancreatic cancer.[97] Among 73 patients evaluable, 6 patients experienced grade 2 toxicity and 6 experienced grade 3 or 4 toxicity. Numerous interrelated metrics proved to be able to distinguish groups of lower versus higher risk of toxicity. For example, the volume of duodenum receiving a dose of 15 Gy or higher (V15) was significant: for V15 9.1 cc or more, the rate of toxicity was 52%, whereas for V15 less than 9.1 cc, the rate was 11% ($P = .002$).

CONCLUSIONS

SBRT has emerged as a versatile strategy with a wide range of applications for many different types and stages of cancer. As with any form of radiation therapy, careful attention to matters of patient selection and technical quality assurance is essential for the effective and safe implementation of SBRT. Future advances will refine our understanding of the biological mechanisms and optimal integration and sequencing of SBRT with other anticancer therapies.

REFERENCES

1. Hamilton AJ, Lulu BA, Fosmire H, et al. Preliminary clinical experience with linear accelerator-based spinal stereotactic radiosurgery. *Neurosurgery* 1995;36:311–319.
2. Blomgren H, Lax I, Naslund I, et al. Stereotactic high dose fraction radiation therapy of extracranial tumors using an accelerator. Clinical experience of the first thirty-one patients. *Acta Oncol* 1995;34:861–870.

3. Uematsu M, Shioda A, Tahara K, et al. Focal, high dose, and fractionated modified stereotactic radiation therapy for lung carcinoma patients: a preliminary experience. *Cancer* 1998;82:1062–1070.
4. Kavanagh BD, Timmerman RD. Stereotactic radiosurgery and stereotactic body radiation therapy: an overview of technical considerations and clinical applications. *Hematol Oncol Clin North Am* 2006;20:87–95.
5. Potters L, Kavanagh B, Galvin JM, et al. American Society for Therapeutic Radiology and Oncology (ASTRO) and American College of Radiology (ACR) practice guideline for the performance of stereotactic body radiation therapy. *Int J Radiat Oncol Biol Phys* 2010;76(2):326–332.
6. Loo BW, Chang JY, Dawson LA, et al. Stereotactic ablative radiotherapy: what's in a name? *Pract Rad Oncol* 2011;1:38–39.
7. Guerrero M, Li X. Extending the linear–quadratic model for large fraction doses pertinent to stereotactic radiotherapy. *Phys Med Biol* 2004;49:4825–4835.
8. Curtis SB. Lethal and potentially lethal lesions induced by radiation—a unified repair model. *Radiat Res* 1986;106:252–270.
9. Benedict SH, Lin PS, Zwicker RD, et al. The biological effectiveness of intermittent irradiation as a function of overall treatment time: development of correction factors for LINAC-based stereotactic radiotherapy. *Int J Radiat Oncol Biol Phys* 1997;37:765–769.
10. Park C, Papiez L, Zhang S, et al. Universal survival curve and single fraction equivalent dose: useful tools in understanding potency of ablative radiotherapy. *Int J Radiat Oncol Biol Phys* 2008;70:847–852.
11. Brenner DJ, Hall EJ. Fractionation and protraction for radiotherapy of prostate carcinoma. *Int J Radiat Oncol Biol Phys* 1999;43:1095–1101.
12. Williams SG, Taylor JM, Liu N, et al. Use of individual fraction size data from 3756 patients to directly determine the alpha/beta ratio of prostate cancer. *Int J Radiat Oncol Biol Phys* 2007;68:24–33.
13. Arcangeli G, Saracino B, Gomellini S, et al. A prospective phase III randomized trial of hypofractionation versus conventional fractionation in patients with high-risk prostate cancer. *Int J Radiat Oncol Biol Phys* 2010;78:11–18.
14. Yeoh EE, Botten RJ, Butters J, et al. Hypofractionated versus conventionally fractionated radiotherapy for prostate carcinoma: final results of phase III randomized trial. *Int J Radiat Oncol Biol Phys* 2011;81:1271–1278.
15. Dearnaley D, Syndikus I, Sumo G, et al. Conventional versus hypofractionated high-dose intensity-modulated radiotherapy for prostate cancer: preliminary safety results from the CHHiP randomised controlled trial. *Lancet Oncol* 2012;13:43–54.
16. Garcia-Barros M, Paris F, Cordon-Cardo C, et al. Tumor response to radiotherapy regulated by endothelial cell apoptosis. *Science* 2003;300(5622):1155–1159.
17. Zhang L, Kavanagh B, Thorburn A, et al. Preclinical and clinical estimates of a cancer's basal apoptotic rate predict for the amount of apoptosis induced by subsequent pro-apoptotic stimuli. *Clin Cancer Res* 2010;16:4478–4489.
18. Lee Y, Auh SL, Wang Y, et al. Therapeutic effects of ablative radiation on local tumor require CD8+ T cells: changing strategies for cancer treatment. *Blood* 2009;114:589–595.
19. Kim DW, Huamani J, Niermann KJ, et al. Noninvasive assessment of tumor vasculature response to radiation-mediated, vasculature-targeted therapy using quantified power Doppler sonography: implications for improvement of therapy schedules. *J Ultrasound Med* 2006;25:1507–1517.
20. DeRose P, Thorpe PE, Gerber DE. Development of bavituximab, a vascular targeting agent with immune-modulating properties, for lung cancer treatment. *Immunotherapy* 2011;3:933–944.
21. Timmerman RD, Bizekis CS, Pass HI, et al. Local surgical, ablative, and radiation treatment of metastases. *CA Cancer J Clin* 2009;59:145–170.
22. Rusthoven K, Hammerman SF, Kavanagh BD, et al. Is there a role for consolidative stereotactic body radiation therapy following first-line systemic therapy for metastatic lung cancer? A patterns-of-failure analysis. *Acta Oncol* 2009;48: 578–583.
23. Mehta N, Mauer AM, Hellman S. Analysis of further disease progression in metastatic non-small cell lung cancer: implications for locoregional treatment. *Int J Oncol* 2004;25:1677–1683.
24. Hellman S, Weichselbaum RR. Oligometastases. *J Clin Oncol* 1995;13:8–10.
25. Stinauer MA, Kavanagh BD, Schefter TE, et al. Stereotactic body radiation therapy for melanoma and renal cell carcinoma: impact of single fraction equivalent dose on local control. *Radiat Oncol* 2011;6(1):34.
26. Norton L, Simon R, Brereton HD, et al. Predicting the course of Gompertzian growth. *Nature* 1976;264(5586):542–545.
27. Fornier M, Norton L. Dose-dense adjuvant chemotherapy for primary breast cancer. *Breast Cancer Res* 2005;7(2):64–69.
28. Lee P, Weerasuriya DK, Lavori PW, et al. Metabolic tumor volume predicts for disease progression and death in lung cancer. *Int J Radiat Oncol Biol Phys* 2007;69: 328–333.
29. Kavanagh BD, Kelly KA, Kane M. The promise of stereotactic body radiation therapy in a new era of oncology. *Front Radiat Ther Oncol* 2007;40:340–351.
30. Zhang B, Bowerman NA, Salama JK, et al.: Induced sensitization of tumor stroma leads to eradication of established cancer by T cells. *J Exp Med* 2007;204:49–55.
31. Dewan MZ, Galloway AE, Kawashima N, et al. Fractionated but not single-dose radiotherapy induces an immune-mediated abscopal effect when combined with anti-CTLA-4 antibody. *Clin Cancer Res* 2009;15:5379–5388.
32. Benedict SH, Yenice KM, Followill D, et al. Stereotactic body radiation therapy: the report of AAPM Task Group 101. *Med Phys* 2010;37:4078–4101.
33. Solberg TD, Balter JM, Benedict SH, et al. Quality and safety considerations in stereotactic radiosurgery and stereotactic body radiation therapy: executive summary. *Pract Radiat Oncol* 2012;2:2–9.
34. Yeung YP, Lo CM, Liu CL, et al. Natural history of untreated nonsurgical hepatocellular carcinoma. *J Gastroenterol* 2005;100:1995–2004.
35. Ruzzenente A, Capra F, Pachera S, et al. Is liver resection justified in advanced hepatocellular carcinoma? Results of an observational study in 464 patients. *J Gastrointest Surg* 2009;13:1313–1320.
36. Meng M, Cui Y, She B, et al. Transcatheter arterial chemoembolization in combination with radiotherapy for unresectable hepatocellular carcinoma: a systematic review and meta-analysis. *Radiother Oncol* 2009;92:184–194.
37. Tse RV, Hawkins M, Lockwood G, et al. Phase I study of individualized stereotactic body radiotherapy for hepatocellular carcinoma and intrahepatic cholangiocarcinoma. *J Clin Oncol* 2008;26:657–664.
38. Méndez Romero A, Wunderink W, Hussain SM, et al. Stereotactic body radiation therapy for primary and metastatic liver tumors: a single institution phase i-ii study. *Acta Oncol* 2006;45(7):831–837.
39. Choi BO, Choi BI, Jang HS, et al. Stereotactic body radiation therapy with or without transarterial chemoembolization for patients with primary hepatocellular carcinoma: preliminary analysis. *BMC Cancer* 2008;8:351.
40. Son SH, Choi BO, Ryu MR, et al. Stereotactic body radiotherapy for patients with unresectable primary hepatocellular carcinoma: dose-volumetric parameters predicting the hepatic complication. *Int J Radiat Oncol Biol Phys* 2010;78:1073–1080.
41. Seo YS, Kim M-S, Yoo S, et al. Preliminary result of stereotactic body radiotherapy as a local salvage treatment for inoperable hepatocellular carcinoma. *J Surg Oncol* 2010;102:209–214.
42. Cardenes HR, Price TR, Perkins SM, et al. Phase I feasibility trial of stereotactic body radiation therapy for primary hepatocellular carcinoma. *Clin Transl Oncol* 2010;12:218–225.
43. Andolino DL, Johnson CS, Maluccio M, et al. Stereotactic body radiotherapy for primary hepatocellular carcinoma. *Int J Radiat Oncol Biol Phys* 2011;81: e447–e453.
44. Herfarth KK, Debus J, Wannenmacher. Stereotactic radiation therapy of liver metastases: Update of the initial phase-I/II trial. *Front Radiat Ther Oncol* 2004;38: 100–105.
45. Wulf J, Guckenberger M, Haedinger U, et al. Stereotactic radiotherapy of primary liver cancer and hepatic metastases. *Acta Oncol* 2006;45:838–847.
46. Hoyer M, Roed H, Traberg-Hansen A, et al. Phase II study on stereotactic body radiotherapy of colorectal metastases. *Acta Oncol* 2006;45:823–830.
47. van der Pool AE, Mendez-Romero A, Wunderink W, et al. Stereotactic body radiation therapy for colorectal liver metastases. *Br J Surg* 2010;97:377–382.
48. Rusthoven K, Kavanagh BD, Cardenes H, et al. Mature results of a multi-institutional phase I/II trial of stereotactic body radiation therapy for liver metastases. *J Clin Oncol* 2009;27:1572–1578.
49. Lee MT, Kim JJ, Dinniwell R, et al. Phase I study of individualized stereotactic body radiotherapy of liver metastases. *J Clin Oncol* 2009;27:1585–1591.
50. Goodman KA, Wiegner EA, Maturen KE, et al. Dose-escalation study of single-fraction stereotactic body radiotherapy for liver malignancies. *Int J Radiat Oncol Biol Phys* 2010;78:486–493.
51. Rule W, Timmerman R, Tong L, et al. Phase I dose-escalation study of stereotactic body radiotherapy in patients with hepatic metastases. *Ann Surg Oncol* 2011; 18:1081–1087.
52. Chang DT, Swaminath A, Kozak M, et al. Stereotactic body radiotherapy for colorectal liver metastases: a pooled analysis. *Cancer* 2011;117:4060–4069.
53. Schefter TE, Kavanagh BD. Radiation therapy for liver metastases. *Sem Rad Oncol* 2011;21:264–270.
54. Høyer M, Swaminath A, Bydder S, et al. Radiotherapy for liver metastases: a review of evidence. *Int J Radiat Oncol Biol Phy.* 2012;82:1047–1057.
55. Schefter TE, Kavanagh BD, Timmerman RD, et al. A phase I trial of stereotactic body radiation therapy (SBRT) for liver metastases. *Int J Radiat Oncol Biol Phys* 2005;62:1371–1378.
56. Yeas RJ, Kalend A. Local stem cell depletion model for radiation myelitis. *Int J Radiat Oncol Biol Phys* 1988;14:1247–1259.
57. Herfarth KK, Hof H, Bahner ML, et al. Assessment of focal liver reaction by multiphasic CT after stereotactic single-dose radiotherapy of liver tumors. *Int J Radiat Oncol Biol Phys* 2003;57:444–451.
58. Olsen CC, Welsh J, Kavanagh BD, et al. Microscopic and macroscopic tumor and parenchymal effects of liver stereotactic body radiotherapy. *Int J Radiat Oncol Biol Phys* 2009;73(5):1414–1424.
59. Blomgren, H, Lax, I, Goranson, H, et al. Radiosurgery for tumors in the body: clinical experience using a new method. *J Radiosurg* 1998;1:63–74.
60. Uematsu M, Shioda A, Tahara K, et al. Focal, high dose, and fractionated modified stereotactic radiation therapy for lung carcinoma patients: a preliminary experience. *Cancer* 1998;82:1062–1070.
61. Fakiris AJ, McGarry RC, Yiannoutsos CT, et al. Stereotactic body radiation therapy for early-stage non-small-cell lung carcinoma: four-year results of a prospective phase II study. *Int J Radiat Oncol Biol Phys* 2009;75:677–682.
62. Baumann P, Nyman J, Hoyer M, et al. Outcome in a prospective phase II trial of medically inoperable stage I non–small-cell lung cancer patients treated with stereotactic body radiotherapy. *J Clin Oncol* 2009;27:3290–3296.
63. Timmerman R, Paulus R, Galvin J, et al. Stereotactic body radiation therapy for inoperable early stage lung cancer. *JAMA* 2010;303:1070–1076.
64. Ricardi U, Filippi AR, Guarneri A, et al. Stereotactic body radiation therapy for early stage non-small cell lung cancer: results of a prospective trial. *Lung Cancer* 2010;68(1):72–77.
65. Schefter TE, Kavanagh BD, Raben D, et al. A phase I/II trial of stereotactic body radiation therapy (SBRT) for lung metastases: initial report of dose escalation and early toxicity. *Int J Radiat Oncol Biol Phys* 2006;66(4S): S120–S127.
66. Rusthoven K, Kavanagh BD, Burri SH, et al. Multi-institutional phase I/II trial of stereotactic body radiation therapy for lung metastases. *J Clin Oncol* 2009;27: 1579–1584.
67. Hamilton AJ, Lulu BA, Fosmire H, et al. LINAC-based spinal stereotactic radiosurgery. *Stereotact Funct Neurosurg* 1996;66:1–9.
68. Ryu S, Fang Yin F, Rock J, et al. Image-guided and intensity-modulated radiosurgery for patients with spinal metastasis. *Cancer* 2003;97(8):2013–2018.
69. Ryu S, Rock J, Rosenblum M, et al. Patterns of failure after single-dose radiosurgery for spinal metastasis. *J Neurosurg* 2004;101(Suppl 3):402–405.
70. Chang EL, Shiu AS, Lii MF, et al. Phase I clinical evaluation of near-simultaneous computed tomographic image-guided stereotactic body radiotherapy for spinal metastases. *Int J Radiat Oncol Biol Phys* 2004;59:1288–1294.
71. Chang EL, Shiu AS, Mendel E, et al. Phase I/II study of stereotactic body radiotherapy for spinal metastasis and its pattern of failure. *J Neurosurg Spine* 2007; 7:151–160.
72. Nelson JW, Yoo DS, Sampson JH, et al. Stereotactic body radiotherapy for lesions of the spine and paraspinal regions. *Int J Radiat Oncol Biol Phys* 2009;73(5): 1369–1375.
73. De Salles AA, Pedroso AG, Medin P, et al. Spinal lesions treated with Novalis shaped beam intensity-modulated radiosurgery and stereotactic radiotherapy. *J Neurosurg* 2004;101(S3):435–440.
74. Gerszten PC, Burton SA, Ozhasoglu C, et al. Radiosurgery for spinal metastases: clinical experience in 500 cases from a single institution. *Spine* 2007;32:193–199.
75. Gibbs IC, Kamnerdsupaphon P, Ryu MR, et al. Image-guided robotic radiosurgery for spinal metastases. *Radiother Oncol* 2007;82:185–190.
76. Yamada Y, Bilsky MH, Lovelock DM, et al. High-dose, single fraction image-guided intensity-modulated radiotherapy for metastatic spinal lesions. *Int J Radiat Oncol Biol Phys* 2008;71:484–490.

77. Rose PS, Laufer I, Boland PJ, et al. Risk of fracture after single fraction image-guided intensity-modulated radiation therapy to spinal metastases. *J Clin Oncol* 2009;27(30):5075–5079.
78. Boehling NS, Grosshans DR, Allen PK. Vertebral compression fracture risk after stereotactic body radiotherapy for spinal metastases. *J Neurosurg Spine* 2012;16(4):379–386.
79. Sahgal A, Ma L, Gibbs I, et al. Spinal cord tolerance for stereotactic body radiotherapy. *Int J Radiat Oncol Biol Phys* 2010;77:548–553.
80. Sahgal A, Ma L, Weinberg V, et al. Reirradiation human spinal cord tolerance for stereotactic body radiotherapy. *Int J Radiat Oncol Biol Phys* 2012;82:107–116.
81. Madsen BL, His RA, Pham HT, et al. Stereotactic hypofractionated accurate radiotherapy of the prostate (SHARP), 33.4 Gy in five fractions for localized disease: first clinical trial results. *Int J Radiat Oncol Biol Phys* 2007;67:1099–1105.
82. Pham HT, Song G, Badiozamani K, et al. Five-year outcome of stereotactic hypofractionated accurate radiotherapy of the prostate (SHARP) for patients with low-risk prostate cancer. *Int J Radiat Oncol Biol Phys* 2010;78:S58.
83. Katz A, Santoro M, Ashley R, et al. Stereotactic body radiotherapy for organ-confined prostate cancer. *BMC Urol* 2010;10:1.
84. Jabbari S, Weinberg VK, Kaprealian T, et al. Stereotactic body radiotherapy as monotherapy or post-external beam radiotherapy boost for prostate cancer: technique, early toxicity, and PSA response. *Int J Radiat Oncol Biol Phys* 2012;82:228–234.
85. King CR, Brooks JD, Harcharan G, et al. Long-term outcomes from a prospective trail of stereotactic body radiotherapy for low-risk prostate cancer. *Int J Radiat Oncol Biol Phys* 2012;82(2):877–882.
86. Freeman DE, King CR. Stereotactic body radiotherapy for low-risk prostate cancer: five-year outcomes. *Rad Oncol* 2011;6:3.
87. McBride SM, Wong DS, Dombrowski JJ, et al. Hypofractionated stereotactic body radiotherapy in low-risk prostate adenocarcinoma: preliminary results of a multi-institutional phase 1 feasibility trial. *Cancer* 2012;118(15):3681–3690.
88. Boike TP, Lotan Y, Chinsoo Cho L, et al. Phase I dose-escalation study of stereotactic body radiation therapy for low-and intermediate-risk prostate cancer. *J Clin Oncol* 2011;29:2020–2026.
89. Rich TA, Harrision J, Abrams R, et al. Phase II study of external irradiation and weekly paclitaxel for nonmetastatic, unresectable pancreatic cancer: RTOG-98–12. *Am J Clin Oncol* 2004;27:51–56.
90. Rich TA, Myerson RJ, Harris J, et al. A randomized phase II trial of weekly gemcitabine (G), paclitaxel (P), and external irradiation followed by the farnesyl transferase inhibitor R115777 (NSC#702818) for locally advanced pancreatic cancer (RTOG 0020). *Proceedings of the ASCO Gastrointestinal Cancers Symposium*, San Francisco, CA, 2006, Abstract 121. Available at: www.asco.org/ascov2/Meetings/Abstracts?&vmview=abst_detail_view&confID=41&abstractID=43.
91. Crane CH, Winter K, Regine WF, et al. Phase II study of bevacizumab with concurrent capecitabine and radiation followed by maintenance gemcitabine and bevacizumab for locally advanced pancreatic cancer: Radiation Therapy Oncology Group RTOG 0411. *J Clin Oncol* 2009;27:4096–4102.
92. Loerher PJ Sr, Feng Y, Cardenes H, et al. Gemcitabine alone versus gemcitabine plus radiotherapy in patients with locally advanced pancreatic cancer: an Eastern Cooperative Oncology Group trial. *J Clin Oncol* 2011;29:4105–4112.
93. Hoyer M, Roed H, Sengelov L, et al. Phase II study on stereotactic radiotherapy of locally advanced pancreatic carcinoma. *Radiother Oncol* 2005;76(1):48–53.
94. Schellenberg D, Quon A, Minn AY, et al. ^{18}Fluorodeoxyglucose PET is prognostic of progression-free and overall survival in locally advanced pancreas cancer treated with stereotactic radiotherapy. *Int J Radiat Oncol Biol Phys* 2010;77(5):1420–1425.
95. Polistina F, Constantin G, Cassamissima F, et al. Unresectable locally advanced pancreatic cancer: a multimodal treatment using neoadjuvant chemoradiotherapy (gemcitabine plus stereotactic radiosurgery) and subsequent surgical exploration. *Ann Surg Oncol* 2010;17:2092–2101.
96. Mahadevan A, Jain S, Goldstein M, et al. Stereotactic body radiotherapy and gemcitabine for locally advanced pancreatic cancer. *Int J Radiat Oncol Biol Phys* 2010;78(3):735–742.
97. Murphy JD, Christman-Skieller C, Kim J, et al. A dosimetric model of duodenal toxicity after stereotactic body radiotherapy for pancreatic cancer. *Int J Radiat Oncol Biol Phys* 2010;78(5):1420–1426.

Chapter 18
Intraoperative Radiotherapy

Timothy J. Kinsella

Intraoperative radiotherapy (IORT) involves the delivery of radiation during surgery using various types of radiation sources/technologies, including intraoperative electron radiation therapy (IOERT), high-dose-rate brachytherapy (HDR-IORT), and electronic brachytherapy/low-kilovoltage x-rays (KV-IORT). The major advantage of IORT is the potential for delivery of higher effective radiation doses to a tumor or, more ideally, to the bed of a grossly resected tumor, while limiting the radiation dose to adjacent, dose-limiting, normal tissues or organs. This normal tissue sparing is accomplished by the dosimetric features of these different IORT technologies and by surgical approaches and/or customized lead shielding to exclude/limit normal tissues during IORT. Although IORT may be used alone following resection of certain primary or recurrent cancers, it is more often (and ideally) combined with external beam radiotherapy (EBRT), typically administered preoperatively with or without concurrent chemotherapy. Indeed, based on clinical IORT data generated over the last three decades, one can conclude that the acute and late normal tissue toxicities and local tumor control rates are quite acceptable in patients with a variety of solid cancers treated with curative intent combining EBRT (± chemotherapy) with gross total resection and IORT. Effective use of IORT requires a multidisciplinary approach, including close cooperation with surgical oncology, medical physics, and surgical nursing personnel. However, despite encouraging clinical data and more widespread use of IORT throughout the world over the last decade, level 1 evidence based on large phase III trials is lacking, with the possible exception of its use in the treatment of breast cancer.

This chapter begins with an overview of the radiobiology of IORT, based largely on comprehensive preclinical experiments using canine models that established normal tissue and organ-specific guidelines, principally for IOERT ± EBRT. Using American foxhounds and beagles as models, acute and late normal tissues responses to IOERT ± EBRT were categorized using experimental designs that mimicked thoracic and abdominal cavity surgeries where IOERT was anticipated to be used clinically. Next, the physics and technical applications of IORT are described with details regarding the specific uses of IOERT, HDR-IORT, and KV-IORT. Finally, a summary of the available clinical IORT data is presented for some tumor sites where IORT has shown efficacy as a component of multimodality treatment. A discussion of potential future clinical uses of IORT is also presented in this final section.

RADIOBIOLOGY PRINCIPLES AND EXPERIMENTAL STUDIES OF IORT

Radiobiologic Modeling for the Determination of Equivalent Single-Fraction IORT Doses

The principal advantage of IORT is the ability to maximally exclude adjacent normal tissues by surgical mobilization and/or the use of customized lead wafer shielding in the cases of IOERT and HDR-IORT. However, the clinical application of IORT to treat minimal gross (R_2 resection) or suspected microscopic residual disease (R_1 resection) in a resected tumor bed necessitates inclusion of partial volumes of adjacent normal tissues or organs based on tumor location, tumor size, and extent of infiltration of adjacent normal tissues, including regional lymph node basins. Based on typical *in vitro* clonogenic studies and *in vivo* small animal studies, where large single doses of 5 to 20 Gy have often been used, it is evident that IORT doses of 15 to 25 Gy could provide a theoretical disadvantage with respect to IORT-related tumor cell kill (or local control) versus normal tissue toxicities.[1,2]

Typically, the radiation dose–response curve for acute reacting normal tissues, such as gastrointestinal epithelium and bone marrow, is very steep, and a small change in the radiation dose near the tissue tolerance level can result in a significant risk of toxicity. In contrast, the radiation dose–response curve for late-reacting normal tissues, such as heart muscle, peripheral nerve, large arterial blood vessels, and bone, is less steep and correlates directly with the volume of tissue included within the irradiated field. Extrapolating from the linear-quadratic model using clonogenic survival data, one can extrapolate the shape of the radiation survival curve for tumor and normal tissues using the α/β ratio. A late-reacting normal tissue has a low α/β ratio (usually <5 Gy), whereas acute-reacting normal tissues, as well as most solid tumors, have α/β ratio of greater than 7 Gy. Using these α/β ratios, one can estimate the single-fraction IORT dose (compared to conventional fractionated EBRT) to control tumor while limiting specific normal tissue toxicities. For example, for a squamous cell carcinoma with minimal residual disease following surgery, an EBRT dose of 60 Gy using 2-Gy fractions (D_{2Gy} = 60) is required, and the α/β ratio for squamous cell carcinoma cells is 10 Gy. We can use the formula

$$D_{IORT} = ½[(\alpha/\beta)^2 + 4D_{2Gy}(\alpha/\beta + 2)^{0.5} - \alpha/\beta]$$

to calculate the equivalent D_{IORT} to be 22.3 Gy, which is supported by multiple single-institution IORT clinical studies that included patients with recurrent or locally advanced head and neck cancers.[3] Similarly, such an equivalent IORT dose can be calculated for a late-reacting normal tissue, such as peripheral nerve, using D_{2Gy} = 70 and α/β ratio = 2 Gy. The calculated D_{IORT} is 16 Gy, which is again supported by experimental canine and human clinical data.[4–6]

Although the D_{IORT} calculation has some clinical utility, as these two examples illustrate, many other clinical variables are not factored into the calculation, such as prior or recent EBRT ± chemotherapy; the inclusion of multiple types and volumes of acute- and late-reacting normal tissues within the IORT field; and other patient-specific comorbidities, for example, cardiovascular disease, diabetes, and connective tissue disease. Indeed, in patients treated with preoperative or postoperative EBRT ± chemotherapy, the IORT boost dose calculation should include these additional treatment effects, particularly with regard to both acute- and late-reacting normal tissues. There are experimental canine data, specifically from the beagle dog model, to assist in the $D_{IORT\ boost}$ calculation, which is often in the 10- to 15-Gy range. In addition, from a radiobiologic perspective, it is recognized that tumor cell hypoxia is the major factor determining tumor radioresponse, as other biologic factors, such as repair, reoxygenation, and repopulation, are not operative with single-fraction treatment.

Another radiobiologic effect that is not included within the D_{IORT} calculation for normal tissue toxicity is the risk of a radiation-induced cancer. Radiation-induced cancers are typically a late effect, often occurring a decade or more after radiation therapy. For an IORT-induced cancer, the cancer should arise within the IORT field and should have a different histology than the original primary. In the canine studies of normal tissue tolerance to varying IORT doses, long-term follow-up (up to 5 years) demonstrated IORT-induced sarcomas of bone and soft tissue, evident at autopsy, in up to 20% to 25% of animals receiving greater than 25 Gy.[7] No IORT-induced cancers have been reported in humans, although many IORT-treated patients have very aggressive primary or recurrent cancers and often die from progressive metastatic disease within 1 to 2 years after IORT without autopsy evaluation of the IORT volume. Because IORT is being used for some pediatric oncology cases, it will be especially important to follow these patients closely for the potential risk of an IORT-induced cancer as a late effect.

Experimental Studies of IOERT with or without EBRT to Establish Normal Tissue Tolerance Guidelines

Comprehensive studies of acute and late normal tissue responses to IOERT ± EBRT were performed using two canine models. The American foxhound model was principally used for IOERT studies at the National Cancer Institute (NCI), whereas a beagle dog model was used for IOERT ± EBRT studies at Colorado State University (CSU). Both canine species are large enough to allow surgical procedures in the thoracic and abdominal cavities that mimic surgeries for human cancers for which IORT may be applied. The goal of these studies was to establish dose guidelines of IOERT alone (NCI) and IOERT ± EBRT (CSU) to reduce acute and late normal tissue toxicities in selected intact and surgically manipulated tissues that mimicked clinical situations in which IOERT might be used. After IOERT ± EBRT, dogs were closely followed clinically and by various sequential diagnostic studies for up to 5 years. All dogs were subjected to complete autopsy with detailed histologic analyses of irradiated tissues.

A description of the NCI IOERT studies is presented in Table 18.1. A more comprehensive overview of these studies is summarized in two reviews.[8,9] A total of 13 sites or target tissues were studied using escalating IOERT doses and a fixed IOERT volume based on the target site. In total, these NCI studies involved 227 dogs, with 196 receiving IOERT and 31 receiving sham IOERT (0 Gy). At CSU, adult beagles were randomized to receive IOERT alone (5 × 8 cm field; 6 MeV; dose range 17.5 to 55 Gy); EBRT alone (5 × 10 cm field; 6-MV photons; dose range 60, 70, and 80 Gy in 30 fractions of 2, 2.33, and 2.67 Gy, respectively); or initial EBRT (5 × 10 cm field; 6-MV photons; dose 50 Gy in 25 fractions of 2 Gy) followed by IOERT (5 × 8 cm field; 6 MeV; dose range 10 to 45.5 Gy). A summary of the clinical and pathologic data regarding normal tissue tolerance from these collective NCI and CSU canine studies are presented in Table 18.2 and briefly described below.

Vascular Tissues

Because the vasculature determines, in large measure, the viability and functionality of all normal tissue systems, an understanding of the tolerance thresholds of IORT on blood vessels is critically important. Intact large vessels (aorta, vena cava) appear to tolerate large single IOERT doses without significant clinical sequelae, based on serial follow-up radiographic studies for up to 5 years.[10] At autopsy, no pathologic changes were found following a 20-Gy dose, and only mild to moderate subintimal fibrosis was found after 30- and 40-Gy doses, respectively. However, the combination of 50-Gy EBRT and >20-Gy IOERT resulted in an IOERT dose-related luminal narrowing with thrombus formation and moderate mural fibrosis pathologically, with up to 2 years of follow-up.[11] To evaluate the IORT tolerance of intraoperatively mandated vascular repairs and anastomoses, a transection and end-to-end reanastomosis of the infrarenal abdominal aorta was performed, followed by IOERT doses of 20 to 45 Gy.[10] Pathologically, moderate medial wall fibrosis was found at doses greater than 30 Gy. Although anastomotic integrity was maintained at all doses, follow-up arteriograms showed anastomotic occlusion at doses greater than 30 Gy within 6 to 12 months. However, occlusion was sufficiently slow to allow formation of arterial collaterals around the occlusion, preventing any clinical or pathologic signs of ischemia distal to the anastomosis. At 45 Gy, development of a late arteriovenous fistula at the anastomotic site in one dog suggested the potential for IORT dose-limiting, clinically relevant, toxicity.

The tolerance of vascular grafts to IORT was investigated in beagles, for which a segmental resection of the infrarenal aorta was performed with reconstruction using a polyfluorotetraethlene graft.[12] IOERT up to 30 Gy was immediately delivered

TABLE 18.1 NATIONAL CANCER INSTITUTE INTRAOPERATIVE ELECTRON RADIATION THERAPY STUDIES OF NORMAL TISSUE TOLERANCE

Sites	*Surgical Procedure*	*IOERT Field; Electron Energy (MeV)*	*Dose Range (Gy): Number Treated*
Retroperitoneal soft tissues, aorta, vena cava, left ureter, lower pole left kidney	LAP; exposure to unilateral retroperitoneum	4 × 15 cm; 11	0:4; 20:4; 30:4; 40:4; 50:4
Aortic anastomosis and small bowel suture line	LAP; transection and reanastomosis of aorta; Roux-en-y with blind loop	4 × 15 cm; 11	0:1; 20:1; 30:1; 45:1
Aortic anastomosis	LAP; transection and reanastomosis	4 × 15 cm; 11	0:1; 20:4; 30:3; 45:3
Small bowel suture line; retroperitoneal soft tissues	LAP; Roux-en-y with small bowel blind loop	4 × 15 cm; 11	0:1; 20:5; 30:5; 45:5
Intact extrahepatic bile duct	LAP; mobilization of biliary tree	5-cm circle; 11	0:1; 20:3; 30:2; 45:2
Extrahepatic bile duct with jejunal anastomosis	LAP; biliary-jejunal anastomosis	5-cm circle; 11	0:2; 20:3; 30:2; 45:2
Trigone of bladder	LAP; cystotomy	5-cm circle; 12	0:3; 20:3; 25:3; 30:3; 35:3; 40:7
Arterial vascular graft to infrarenal aorta	LAP; segmental resection and immediate grafting	4 × 15 cm; 9	0:6; 20:8; 25:8; 30:8
Peripheral nerve; lumbosacral plexus (L4-L5)	LAP; exposure of unilateral lumbosacral plexus	9-cm circle; 11	0:3; 10:4; 15:4; 20:8; 25:4; 30:3; 35:3; 40:4; 50:2
Spinal cord	LAP; exposure of retroperitoneum over lumbar spine	4 × 15 cm; 11	0:3; 20:7; 25:7; 30:8
Right upper lobe lung and mediastinum including right atrium	Right thoracotomy	5-cm circle; 9	0:3; 20:7; 30:7; 40:7
Left bronchial stump, pulmonary artery and vein, left atrium	Left pneumonectomy	5-cm circle; 13	0:3; 20:4; 30:4; 40:4
Esophagus	Right thoracotomy and mobilization of esophagus	6-cm circle; 9	0:1; 20:7; 30:5

IOERT, intraoperative electron radiation therapy; LAP, laparatomy.

following the prosthetic grafting, and half of the dogs were randomized to receive postoperative EBRT to 36 Gy in 10 fractions over 4 weeks. Arterial graft occlusion occurred acutely in both treatment groups but was correctable by thrombectomy. During clinical follow-up, most dogs receiving ≥30-Gy IOERT ± EBRT developed late graft occlusion (within 12 months) but again showed evidence of progressive collateralization by arteriography, preventing distal ischemia–related complications.

Gastrointestinal Tissues

Due to its rapidly proliferating mucosa and rich blood supply, the small and large intestines are among the most radiosensitive normal tissues. As such, the intestine needs to be surgically mobilized and excluded from IORT portals. NCI investigators assessed the IORT tolerance of small intestinal suture lines where a jejunal blind loop was created surgically and intestinal continuity maintained by distal jejunojejunostomy.[13] The IOERT field encompassed the suture line and the full thickness of the intestinal wall, and doses of 20 to 45 Gy were delivered. No immediate histologic changes were seen, and no clinical evidence of suture line dehiscence was found with 5 years of follow-up. However, internal interloop fistulae occurred following 45 Gy. Thus, whereas acute IOERT tolerance of a defunctionalized bowel loop was acceptable to 45 Gy, chronic complications suggest a maximum of 30 Gy. However, functional small and large bowel showed clinical and pathologic manifestations of ulceration, stricture, and perforations following doses as low as 15 to 20 Gy.

Hepatobiliary Tissues

Bile duct tolerance to IOERT was studied at the NCI using a 5-cm IORT portal to the subhepatic space, which encompassed

TABLE 18.2 TOLERANCE DOSES TO INTRAOPERATIVE RADIOTHERAPY IN CANINE MODELS

System	*Organ*	*Maximum Tolerated IORT Dose (Gy)*	*Maximum Follow-up Period (Months)*	*Comments*
Cardiothoracic	Aorta	30	60	Threshold for fibrosis, patency to 60 Gy
	Vena cava	30	60	Threshold for fibrosis, patency to 60 Gy
	Arterial anastomosis	30	36	Threshold for stenotic occlusion
	Arterial graft	30	24	Threshold for occlusion
	Heart	30	60	Threshold for fibrosis, no clinical effects to 40 Gy
	Tracheobronchus	30	60	Threshold for fibrosis, no clinical effects to 40 Gy
	Bronchial suture line	40	60	Intact to 40 Gy, bronchovascular fistulae at 20 Gy
	Lung	20	60	Threshold for fibrotic pneumonitis, no clinical effects to 40 Gy
	Esophagus	20	60	Ulceration and stricture with full-thickness exposure, no sequelae to 40 Gy partial thickness
Gastrointestinal	Duodenum	18	6	Threshold for ulceration, obstruction, or perforation
	Small intestine diverted loop	45	60	Defunctionalized bowel loop, no clinical effects, fibrosis at ≥20 Gy
Hepatobiliary-pancreatic	Bile duct	20	60	Threshold for fibrosis and stenosis
	Bile duct anastomosis	<20	12	Dehiscence at all doses ≥20 Gy
Urinary	Kidney	15	60	Threshold for tubular loss
	Ureter	30	60	Threshold for fibrosis and stenosis
	Bladder	30	60	Threshold for ureterovesical junction stenosis, normal contractility to 40 Gy
Nervous	Peripheral nerve	15	60	Threshold for motor neuropathy

IORT, intraoperative radiotherapy.
Adapted from Sindelar WF, Kinsella TJ. Normal tissue tolerance to intraoperative radiotherapy. *Surg Oncol Clin North Am* 2003;12(4):925–942.

the extrahepatic bile duct.[14] When using a dose range of 20 to 45 Gy, no acute complications were noted, but progressive and IOERT dose-related chemical evidence of partial biliary obstruction was seen within 2 to 8 months of follow-up. Frank biliary cirrhosis developed in one-half of dogs receiving 30 Gy or more that were followed for a minimum of 12 months. The tolerance of biliary-enteric anastomoses was also studied using a similar IOERT dose range. After laparotomy and formation of a jejunal biliary loop, the bile duct was transected and anastomosed to the jejunal loop, followed by immediate IOERT to the anastomotic site. All animals developed acute complications within several weeks, with either anastomotic disruption or subacute anastomotic obstruction, resulting in cholangitis or bile duct necrosis. Thus, although the intact bile duct may tolerate doses of up to 20 Gy, a bile duct anastomosis cannot be included within an IORT field.

Urinary Tract Tissues

In the IOERT study involving the intact unilateral retroperitoneum,[10] a 12-cm segment of ureter, as well as the inferior pole of one kidney, were irradiated to IOERT doses as high as 50 Gy. Dogs were followed clinically with renal function testing and radiographic pyelography. The kidney showed dose-related fibrosis and hyalinization. Acute obstructive nephropathy secondary to ureteral obstruction was evident with 50 Gy, whereas subacute obstructive nephropathy was evident at 2 to 3 months of follow-up in the 40-Gy dogs and at 6 to 12 months following 30 Gy. In the 20 Gy–treated dogs, no clinical or pathologic changes in the irradiated ureter were evident. A CSU study showed that shorter (≤4 cm) segments of ureter would tolerate doses of 30 Gy.[15] Typically, the ureter can be surgically mobilized and excluded from the IORT field, but segments at high risk of residual microscopic disease may be included, and prophylactic ureteral stenting may reduce the risk of narrowing/obstruction as a subacute complication.

Bladder tolerance to IOERT was studied using the foxhound model at the NCI.[16,17] Following laparotomy and cystotomy, a 5-cm circular IORT portal, including the trigone and both ureteral orifices, was treated with doses of 20 to 40 Gy. Dogs were then followed for up to 5 years with clinical evaluation, kidney function tests, intravenous pyelography, and cystometry. Although no acute complications were noted, some dogs who received 25 Gy or greater developed fibrotic strictures at the ureterovesical junction within 2 years, which became more frequent at 5 years in the ≥30 Gy–treated dogs. Whereas pathologic changes of fibrosis and microvascular changes in the bladder wall were evident at 30 Gy or greater, follow-up cystometric studies showed little difference in post-IOERT bladder contractility from baseline at all IOERT doses.

Cardiothoracic Tissues

In the NCI studies of IOERT to the canine mediastinum, atrial appendages of the heart received doses up to 40 Gy.[18,19] Dense fibrosis of the myocardium was found pathologically following IOERT doses of 30 Gy or greater, with early (within 1 month) medial hyaline degeneration followed by radiation vasculopathy and infarction within 12 months. However, due to the limited irradiated volume of cardiac muscle, no clinical signs of cardiac failure were evident with up to 5 years of follow-up.

Segments of the trachea and main stem bronchi also received IOERT of 20 to 40 Gy in the NCI mediastinal IOERT studies.[18,19] Pathologic changes of fibrosis in the tracheobronchial wall were evident at doses of 30 Gy or greater, with infrequent development of chondronecrosis of the tracheal rings at doses of less than 40 Gy; however, most animals showed no clinical respiratory symptoms. In addition, the canine pneumonectomy study found normal healing of the bronchial stump following IOERT to 20 to 40 Gy, and no clinical sequelae were observed through 5 years of follow-up.[20] However, when limited amounts of lung tissue received IOERT, acute confluent pneumonitis progressing to interstitial fibrosis and pulmonary arteriolar sclerosis developed at all doses within 12 months.[18,20]

IOERT tolerance of the esophagus was also evaluated in the NCI mediastinal studies, with both full-thickness and partial-thickness (<50% of circumference) treatment.[18,19] Clinical examinations, barium swallows, and esophagoscopies were performed for up to 2 years following doses to 30 Gy for full-thickness irradiation and to 40 Gy for partial-thickness irradiation. With full-thickness esophageal IOERT, all animals receiving 20 Gy or more showed acute clinical toxicity with signs of dysphagia and weight loss. Acute, but transient, inflammatory changes to esophageal mucosa were found at 20 Gy, but progressive severe inflammatory changes leading to ulceration and stricture by 2 to 3 months were found following 30 Gy. With partial esophageal wall IOERT, no severe clinical or radiographic sequelae occurred at doses up to 40 Gy, with dose-related fibrosis but no mucosal ulcers or strictures.

Nervous Tissue

Whereas peripheral nerves were traditionally considered to be relatively radioresistant, clinical IORT trials at the NCI reported a significantly increased risk of lumbosacral neuropathy following IOERT + EBRT in patients with localized but technically resectable retroperitoneal sarcomas.[5,21] In this clinical trial, patients were randomized to receive postoperative EBRT alone (initial 40 Gy, followed by a 14- to 16-Gy boost) or IOERT (20 Gy using multiple abutting fields based on tumor bed size/location) followed by postoperative EBRT (36 Gy). Subacute (within 1 to 3 months) and late (>6 months) clinical motor and/or sensory neuropathies to the lower trunk and/or lower extremity were found in 9 of 15 patients randomized to IOERT + EBRT and in 1 of 20 patients randomized to postoperative EBRT alone ($p < .01$).[22]

To further establish the tolerance of peripheral nerve trunks to IORT, a series of studies was conducted at the NCI and CSU.[4–6,22–24] In the initial NCI study using foxhounds, the lumbosacral plexus was surgically exposed and IOERT doses of 20 to 75 Gy were delivered.[5] Hind limb motor changes developed in 90% of treated dogs within 12 months, ranging in severity from slight motor strength weakness to complete motor paralysis, with an approximately inverse relationship between IOERT dose and the time to onset and severity of neurologic signs. However, no threshold dose for neuropathy was found, even with the use of nerve conduction times as a measure. Pathologically, loss of large nerve fibers and perineural fibrosis with radiation vasculopathy in perineural connective tissue were seen. A follow-up NCI trial attempted to establish a threshold dose for IORT-induced neuropathy in the lumbar-sacral plexus.[4] No animal receiving IOERT doses of up to 15 Gy developed clinical neuropathy by exam and nerve conduction testing for more than 3 years following IOERT, whereas all animals receiving 20 Gy developed hind leg paresis with lower nerve conduction testing within 12 months. With up to 5 years of follow-up, dogs treated with IORT doses of up to 15 Gy showed continued lack of neurotoxicity.[22]

Studies assessing lumbar nerve injury following IOERT alone, EBRT alone, and combined IOERT plus EBRT were performed at CSU using a beagle dog model.[6,23,24] Similar neurologic and nerve conduction testing as used in the NCI studies were performed for up to 2 years of follow-up. Although no neurologic complications were found using EBRT alone, dose- and time-related neuropathy was seen in IOERT alone– and in IOERT + EBRT–treated dogs with an IOERT dose threshold of 15 Gy. Radiation-induced changes to Schwann cells and nerve vasculature were found, similar to the NCI findings, and ultrastructural studies suggested microvascular damage causing regional hypoxia and subsequent nerve fiber loss. Thus, peripheral nerve appears to be a dose-limiting tissue for IOERT, in contrast to the relative radioresistance of peripheral nerves to EBRT.

IORT-Induced Malignancies

As mentioned previously, radiation-induced malignancies are infrequent following conventionally fractionated EBRT and are most commonly seen several to many years after the successful treatment of childhood cancers. Although IORT-induced cancers have not been reported in humans, the canine data support a potential risk in humans. Again, an IORT-induced cancer should fulfill several criteria, including occurring within the IORT field, developing after an appropriate latency period (e.g., a few years in canines), and being histologically confirmed and of a histologic type that develops infrequently in the particular dog species.

In studies of IOERT-related toxicity to bone at CSU, a 21% incidence of osteosarcoma was noted, with at least 4 years of follow-up following IOERT alone to greater than 25 Gy with or without EBRT.[25] In dogs treated with EBRT alone for spontaneous soft tissue tumors, a 3% incidence of osteosarcoma within the EBRT volume was seen. IOERT-induced tumors were also seen in the NCI canine trials.[7,26] Among 59 animals followed for 2 or more years, 12 tumors were pathologically confirmed at complete necropsy. Three tumors did not meet the criteria for being radiation induced, including 2 benign fibrous tumors and a mammary carcinoma. The 9 IORT-related tumors included a bladder rhabdomyosarcoma, a soft tissue malignant fibrous histiocytoma, and 7 sarcomas of bone or cartilage. In dogs receiving >25-Gy IOERT, the overall incidence of radiation-induced neoplasms was 25%, consistent with the CSU data.

In summary, the validity of the canine tissue tolerance models as described in this section and Table 18.2 as representative of the human tissue response to IORT is supported by clinical IORT data from human trials. Although the tolerance to IORT-induced acute and late toxicities can vary considerably between tissues, doses up to 20 Gy are generally tolerated. The general principle providing the rationale for IORT should always be practiced, that is, maximize the radiation dose to the tumor or, ideally, the bed of a grossly resected tumor while minimizing dose exposure to adjacent normal tissues.

PHYSICS AND TECHNICAL ASPECTS OF IORT

Definition of Techniques

IORT involves the use of a single fraction of radiation therapy delivered while the patient is under anesthesia. Three different technologies can be used to deliver IORT, including electrons (IOERT), high-dose brachytherapy with iridium-192 (^{192}Ir; HDR-IORT), and low-kV x-rays (KV-IORT). IOERT is delivered by a linear accelerator electron beam in the 6- to 15-MeV dose range. Although the use of a conventional linear accelerator in the radiation oncology department was the standard for IOERT delivery in the 1970s and early 1980s, the subsequent development of mobile linear accelerators that are transported to the operating room (OR), or the installation of a dedicated accelerator in an OR, improved the efficiency and use of IOERT, no longer requiring the patient to be transported under anesthesia. At present, there are three commercial mobile linear accelerators designed for IOERT, including the Mobetron (4- to 12-MeV electrons; IntraOp Medical, Sunnyvale, CA), the Novac 7 (4- to 10-MeV electrons; NRT SpA, Rome, Italy), and the LIAC (4- to 10-MeV electrons; Sordina SpA, Saonara, Italy). HDR-IORT uses a high-dose-rate afterloader with ^{192}Ir that decays via β or electron capture, and the daughter isotopes are short lived, emitting γ-rays of various energies. The β decay is absorbed by the source capsule, and the average photon energy emitted is 370 keV with a 74-day half-life. HDR-IORT is feasible only after a near gross total resection, as the maximum depth of coverage is typically 0.5 cm deep from the surface of the resected tumor bed. Several ^{192}Ir HDR remote afterloaders are commercially marketed by Nucleotron (Veenendaal, Netherlands) and by Varian Medical Systems (Crowley, United Kingdom). A shielded OR is required for HDR-IORT. Over the last decade, mobile IORT devices using low-kV x-rays (KV-IORT) have been developed. Low-kV x-rays (20 to 50 kV) have the advantage of a steep dose gradient, not requiring specially shielded ORs, but have a major disadvantage in that the target (tumor bed) should ideally be spherical in shape with a maximum tissue treatment radius of 1 to 2 cm. Two commercial low-KV-IORT devices are available, including the Zeiss Intrabeam (Zeiss Surgical, Oberkochen, Germany) and the Xoft S700 Axxent System (Zoft, Medford, MA).

IOERT: Physics and Technical Applications

With the development of mobile linear accelerators as described earlier, no permanent OR shielding is required, unlike a fixed OR-based linear accelerator, because the maximum electron beam energy is 12 MeV or less and these mobile linear accelerators are designed without bending magnets. In addition, neutron contamination is not a problem for OR personnel or patients. The Mobetron has a fixed beam stopper, whereas the Novac 7 and LIAC accelerators are equipped with mobile beam stoppers. The 90% depth dose in water ranges from 1.1 cm for 4-MeV electrons to 3.5 cm for 12-MeV electrons. A variety of applicator shapes (e.g., circular, rectangular) and sizes are available from the manufacturers. However, to commission a machine for IORT, a minimum set of dosimetry measurements is required for each applicator and each electron energy including percentage depth dose, beam profiles in two orthogonal planes, isodose curves in two orthogonal planes, and applicator ratios. The applicator ratios are compared to a reference applicator for which the accelerator output is calibrated.

Quality assurance (QA) procedures for mobile IOERT linear accelerators are outlined in detail in the reports of the American Association of Physicists in Medicine (AAPM) Radiation Therapy Task Groups 48 and 72.[27,28] Because any malfunction of these mobile accelerators could result in a patient not receiving the scheduled IOERT treatment or in having a patient's surgery delayed, a high level of QA requires calibration of all electron energies early on the day of surgery, in addition to a rigorous process of periodic checks similar to the QA for a standard linear accelerator. Unique factors to the mobile IOERT linear accelerators are the lack of adjustable collimators and bending magnets. QA checks are necessary of the alignment of the soft docking system as used in the Mobetron and of a hard docking system for the two other mobile accelerators. Although *in vivo* dosimetry using TLDs or silicon diodes is not feasible for placement in a sterile surgical resection bed during IOERT, offline procedures such as the use of radiochromic films or real-time methods such as the use of metal oxide semiconductor field effect transistors are being applied to breast cancer[29,30] IORT and may be applied to other tumor sites.

Mobile IOERT accelerators, however, have limited mobility, requiring the patient and OR table to be moved to the accelerator in the OR and sometimes requiring a change in the patient's position. The use of special OR tables with fine movement capabilities superiorly, inferiorly, laterally, and pitch and roll positioning, as well as Trendelenburg and reverse Trendelenburg movements, makes IOERT patient positioning and docking much easier and faster. The soft docking process required for the Mobetron is facilitated by a set of lasers in the accelerator head. The hard docking system used with the Novac 7 and LIAC accelerators involves a two-part applicator. Once the appropriate field size and applicator shape are determined, the superior part of the applicator is fixed to the linear accelerator head and then physically mated with the inferior part, which is in contact with the target (tumor bed). Once aligned, a rigid interlocking of the two parts is made prior to IOERT delivery. Typically, the process of soft or hard docking requires less than 10 to 15 minutes.

However, prior to docking, a detailed determination of the IOERT treatment volume is required, involving close collaboration between the surgical oncologist and the radiation oncologist. Typically, surgical sutures or clips are placed by the surgeon to better visualize the tumor bed, and at least a 1-cm margin is added. Next, the size, shape, and degree of bevel for the suitable applicator are determined, as well as determining whether one or more IOERT fields are necessary to cover the tumor bed. Although the IOERT applicators can function as a normal tissue retractor, additional surgical packing is often required to further exclude certain normal tissues, for example, bowel. In the clinical situation in which sensitive normal tissues cannot be physically displaced from the IOERT field secondary shielding using sterilized lead sheets can be placed with appropriate thickness to attenuate 90% or more of the dose. Lead shielding is also essential to prevent any dose overlap, if multiple IOERT fields are required to cover the tumor bed with at least 1-cm margins. Finally, to reduce the accumulation of serous fluid in the tumor bed during IOERT (which would attenuate the dose), placement of suction adjacent to the IOERT applicator is recommended.

HDR-IORT: Physics and Technical Applications

HDR-IORT involves the use of an ^{192}Ir HDR afterloader to deliver a large single fraction of brachytherapy to a grossly resected tumor bed with necessary retraction and physical shielding of adjacent normal tissues, similar to the guidelines for IOERT as described. Because of the high activity of ^{192}Ir afforded by computer-controlled remoter afterloading, HDR-IORT treatment times of 30 to 60 minutes can be accomplished, based on the target (tumor bed) size. The desired dose distribution is generated by superimposing a large number of single-source radiation distributions at different locations and different dwell times. Two AAPM publications from Task Group 43 summarize in detail the dose calculations for ^{192}Ir in air and water.[31,32] A recent review of HDR-IORT is also recommended.[33]

Construction of an HDR-IORT dedicated facility requires a shielded OR equipped with door interlocks, room radiation monitors, and additional adjacent space for the OR team (surgeon, radiation oncologist, nurses) to remain sterile during HDR-IORT, should any emergency reentry be needed. Anesthesia and surgical monitoring via video cameras must also be available in this adjacent OR space. Ideally, construction of a HDR-IORT facility in the hospital OR complex allows for most efficient use of OR personnel and equipment. The QA program for HDR-IORT follows guidelines outlined by AAPM task groups.[34] Typically, a series of QA checks is performed 24 hours prior to each HDR-IORT procedure and involves determination of source positioning and source strength, verification of proper functioning of room radiation monitors, and checking of equipment for use in the event of emergency source retraction.

For HDR-IORT, the applicator must be rigid enough to secure the afterloader catheters in a fixed and reproducible position while also conforming to the tumor bed contour. The applicator design must provide adequate thickness to maintain a 0.5-cm distance between the source plane and the treatment surface.[33] Prior to HDR-IORT delivery, the radiation oncologist must confirm that the applicator is in direct contact with the tissue surface throughout the entire target area, as a separation of only 0.5 cm can reduce dose delivery by up to 30%. Treatment planning for HDR-IORT is greatly facilitated by creating a plan atlas of clinically anticipated tumor volumes.[35] Plans incorporating optimized dwell times enhance efficiency and reduce risks of error. However, a plan atlas cannot anticipate the need to spare an adjacent normal tissue in certain patients, but customized lead wafers of 0.3 cm thickness can be used at the applicator–tissue interface.

KV-IORT: Physics and Technical Applications

The Zeiss Intrabeam has a miniature x-ray source at the end of a 10-cm-long, 3-mm-wide probe, where electrons are accelerated at a gold target in the probe tip, resulting in a nearly isotronic distribution of low-kV x-rays in the 30- to 50-kV range. Because these x-rays are of such low energy, no special shielding is required in a standard OR, which normally has adequate shielding for the intraoperative use of diagnostic radiology equipment. The Intrabeam is small, lightweight, designed with a floor stand, and can be easily accommodated in a standard OR. A dose rate of 2 Gy/min at 1 cm in water from the center of the target is possible with a 50-kV setting. However, the dose decreases in tissue as the inverse cube of the distance. It has an extended lifetime of over 10 years.

The Xoft S700 Axxent System is an electronic brachytherapy apparatus with a Wolfram target that operates at x-ray energies of 20 to 50 kV. As with the Intrabeam, the 50-kV energy is most commonly used. A miniature x-ray tube is located within a flexible, disposable sheath, which permits water cooling of the x-ray tube. The Xoft source is more adaptable in the OR compared to the Intrabeam source and has a higher depth–dose rate of 0.6 Gy/min at 3 cm in water. In addition, because of heavier filtration, the dose falls off less slowly in tissue than the Intrabeam source. However, the typical Xoft source lifetime is only 2.5 hours, and it has been used clinically for a much shorter time period (3 years), compared to more than a decade for Intrabeam.

A recent comprehensive review of these two KV-IORT systems is available.[36] Both units are potentially suited for IORT treatment of breast cancer, either as a boost or as definitive treatment, although most of the current clinical data involve the use of the Intrabeam. Both manufacturers are expanding the clinical use of their respective low-kV IORT systems to superficial skin tumors and vaginal applications for endometrial cancers. The main applicators for the Intrabeam are spherical, with diameters ranging from 1.5 to 5 cm, and are composed of solid biodegradable material with a 2.8-mm central cavity where the source is placed. A homogeneous surface dose is generated with the addition of an aluminum flattening filter for applicators greater than 3.5 cm in diameter. The Xoft system uses inflatable balloons, similar to MammoSite (Hologic, Bedford, MA) for breast irradiation, with spherical or ellipsoidal balloon shapes. The balloon sizes vary from 3 to 6 cm for spherical balloons and 5 × 7 cm and 6 × 7 cm for ellipsoidal balloons. Both systems have a number of safety features to alert the user to the emission of x-rays and allow monitoring of the output dose. QA procedures involving pretreatment checks, monthly checks, and yearly checks were recently reviewed.[36]

Comparison of IORT Technical Applications

A comprehensive comparison of the technical applications of the three IORT approaches was recently published.[37] The potential advantages of IOERT compared to HDR-IORT include better dose homogeneity, faster treatment times, requirement for less OR shielding, and, the ability to treat gross residual disease based on depth–dose characteristics. Potential disadvantages include surface dose of less than 90% with 6- to 9-MeV electrons (compensated with the use of bolus) and difficulty in treating anatomic areas such as the low pelvis, abdominal side walls, retropubic areas, subdiaphragmatic areas, thoracic side walls, and skull base. Low-kV IORT requires a small target (tumor) volume, where the depth in tissue at risk is 0.5 to 1.0 cm or less from the surface of the applicator.

CLINICAL RESULTS OF IORT WITH OR WITHOUT EBRT: AN OVERVIEW

A comprehensive review of the clinical experience of IORT ± EBRT (± chemotherapy) is beyond the scope of this chapter, and the reader is referred to a recently published textbook of IORT in which the clinical data by tumor site are presented in detail.[38] In addition, some of the IORT clinical data are discussed in this textbook in chapters devoted to specific cancers and tumor sites. The general conclusions from these mostly nonrandomized studies in selected cancers will be discussed here, in addition to a brief overview of the limited clinical data from a few prospective, randomized trials. A general conclusion is that IORT, as a component of a multidisciplinary approach for typically locally advanced primary and recurrent cancers, is feasible and appears to improve local control, as well as overall survival in some cancers, with acceptable acute and late toxicities based on the normal tissue tolerance guidelines previously presented (Table 18.2). The clinical use of IORT in a larger number of institutions across the world over the last 10 to 15 years has been aided by improvements in IORT technology as described in the last section. The more widespread use and the promising nonrandomized, generally single-institution, clinical data, as well as data from a few prospective, randomized trials, will, it is hoped, facilitate the design and implementation of prospective, randomized trials in specific tumor sites in the next decade.

Colorectal Cancer

The clinical experience with the use of IOERT and HDR-IORT as part of a multidisciplinary approach to locally advanced colorectal cancer was recently summarized.[39] More than 900 patients have been treated with IOERT and 59 patients with HDR-IORT, usually following preoperative combined-modality treatment with EBRT (45 to 54 Gy) and concomitant infusional 5-fluorouracil (5-FU). These data are derived from multiple, nonrandomized, single-institution studies in the United States and Europe. No randomized, prospective studies are available or ongoing. Most patients had clinical T4 or tethered T3 lesions in these IORT studies, making direct comparison to large prospective, randomized trials, such as the German Rectal Cancer Study, difficult, because, certainly, the clinical T4 lesions would not be included in the phase III trial. The 3- to 5-year local control rates for IORT-treated patients were, respectively, 85% to 90% for R_0 patients and 50% to 75% for R_1/R_2 resections, with a 5% to 10% risk of grade 2 or 3 normal tissue toxicities to peripheral nerve or ureter. The 3- to 5-year disease-free survivals were in the 50% to 60% range for R_0 patients but dropped to 25% to 35% for R_2 patients. Thus, these data suggest some benefit to IORT in these clinically tethered T3 and T4 patients, but systemic relapse remains a major problem.

A similar general conclusion can be reached for the use of IORT in patients with recurrent colorectal cancer, based on a recent summary of the literature.[40] For this patient group, many will have already received EBRT ± 5-FU-based chemotherapy at the time of presentation, making the use of further EBRT (± chemotherapy) somewhat limited. The largest experience with IOERT in this patient group is from the Mayo Clinic. In a group of 140 patients with prior EBRT, the subsequent use of 30-Gy preoperative EBRT followed by IOERT (10 to 20 Gy based on extent of resection) resulted in a 3-year local control rate of 70% and overall survival rate of 30%. Again, no randomized, prospective data are available to more accurately assess the role of IORT in this patient group, but the single-institution data are encouraging.[40]

Gastric Cancer

The clinical data regarding the integration of IORT as a component of combined-modality treatment of resectable gastric cancer were recently summarized in detail.[41] Three randomized prospective trials of IOERT have been reported. In 1988, M. Abe from Kyoto University, Japan, reported a trial in which more than 200 patients with stage I-IV stomach cancer (using the Japanese Surgical Staging System) were randomized to surgery alone versus surgery + IOERT (28 to 35 Gy).[42] A non-statistically significant trend toward improved 5-year overall survival was seen in stage II-IV patients. However, two smaller phase 3 studies did not show a survival benefit. At the National Cancer Institute, 40 stage III and IV (American Joint Committee on Cancer) patients were randomized to surgery + IORT (20 Gy) versus surgery + EBRT (50 Gy), whereas at the University of Freiburg (Freiburg, Germany), 115 patients were randomized to surgery versus surgery + IORT (28 Gy).[43,44] Data from other single-institution, nonrandomized studies suggest a benefit to IORT or IORT + EBRT compared to surgery alone (summarized by Martinez-Monge et al.[41]). The present standard of care for locally advanced (node positive and/or margin positive) gastric cancer includes postoperative chemoradiation or perioperative chemotherapy alone, based on recent phase 3 trial experience.[45,46] Thus, any future trial testing the integration of IORT in locally advanced gastric cancer must include these approaches.

Pancreatic Cancer

The results of many single-institution, nonrandomized clinical trials in patients with pancreas cancer were recently summarized.[47] For patients found to have localized but technically unresectable disease, the use of IORT ± EBRT ± chemotherapy is associated with better long-term epigastric pain control but with no effect on median or overall survival. In patients with resectable pancreatic cancer, the combination of preoperative EBRT (± chemotherapy) followed by IORT appears to increase local control and overall survival modestly. Any future trials of IORT in pancreatic cancer will require the integration of more effective systemic therapy.

Sarcomas

IORT has played a role in the management of adult soft tissue sarcomas arising in the retroperitoneum, trunk, and extremities as a component of combined-modality treatment. IORT has also been used in the treatment of some primary bone sarcomas in adolescents. Both IOERT and HDR-IORT techniques have been used.

Retroperitoneal soft tissue sarcomas, although rare, are an appropriate tumor for using IORT because these tumors are typically large (>10 to 15 cm) and locally invasive, making wide excisions with negative margins very difficult to achieve. A comprehensive review of the IORT studies in retroperitoneal sarcomas was recently published.[48] In the only randomized, prospective trial, a small group of 35 patients with technically resectable retroperitoneal sarcomas were randomized to receive postoperative EBRT (50 to 55 Gy; control group; 20 patients) or IOERT (20 Gy to multiple abutting fields) plus reduced-dose postoperative EBRT (30 to 35 Gy; study group; 15 patients).[21] With a minimum follow-up of 5 years, in-field local recurrences occurred in 20% of the study group and in 80% of the controls ($p < .001$). However, there were no differences in overall survival or risk of distant metastases, which were correlated primarily with pathologic stage. Differences in the type of acute and late normal tissue complications were found with significantly increased gastrointestinal toxicities in the control group and significantly increased peripheral nerve toxicities in the study group. Multiple nonrandomized, single-institution studies support an improved local control rate with less peripheral nerve toxicities using IOERT doses of 15 Gy or less.[48] Two institutions have published their experience using combinations of EBRT and HDR-IORT for primary or locally recurrent retroperitoneal sarcomas. A prospective, nonrandomized trial at Memorial Sloan-Kettering Cancer Center (MSKCC) included 32 patients (12 with primary disease and 20 with recurrent disease) who each received 14 Gy at 0.5 cm deep to the resected tumor bed using HDR-IORT. The MSKCC group reported a 5-year local control rate of 74% and 54% and a 5-year overall survival rate of 55% and 30%, respectively, in the primary and recurrent tumor patient groups.[49] A second series of 46 patients with primary or recurrent retroperitoneal sarcomas from the Curie Cancer Center in France received 20-Gy HDR-IORT following a gross total resection (30 patients with R_0 resection and 16 patients with R_1 resection). These patients experienced actuarial 5-year overall survival and local recurrence survival rates of 55% and 51%, respectively.[50]

The IORT literature for extremity and truncal soft tissue sarcomas was recently summarized.[51] Although local recurrence risks using surgery and EBRT (either preoperative or postoperative) are low (5% to 8%) with R_0 resections, patients with positive margins or gross residual disease require higher EBRT doses, with an increased risk of acute and late normal tissue toxicities. For these patients, IOERT or HDR-IORT treatments have been used as a treatment boost while maintaining the EBRT dose at 45 to 50 Gy. In general, local control is excellent (≥85%), and normal tissue complications and functional outcomes are acceptable.[52]

The more limited experience with IORT in bone sarcomas was also recently reviewed.[53] Typically, IOERT has been used for marginally resected Ewing's sarcomas and osteosarcomas in adolescents at centers in Germany, Spain, and Japan. Although local control is excellent in these high-risk patients, the risks of late normal tissue complications, including IORT-induced second cancers, are of concern, and long-term follow-up is needed before an endorsement of the role of IORT in these patient groups can be made.

Breast Cancer

IORT is playing a major role in the curative treatment of early-stage breast cancer throughout the world, as recently reviewed.[54] Based on several prior single-institution, nonrandomized studies,[54] two large phase III studies have been designed for patients with early-stage disease to test the concept of IORT as full-dose, single-dose partial breast irradiation treatment compared to standard, conventionally fractionated whole-breast radiation therapy (WBRT). In addition, the concept of using IORT as a boost followed by WBRT for patients with adverse pathologic features is being evaluated by the European Group of the International Society of Intraoperative Radiotherapy (ISIORT Europe). A brief description of the two large phase III studies of definitive IORT and the ongoing single arm IORT boost study is given later. A more detailed discussion of these trials is provided in the chapter of this book on breast cancer.

The Targeted Intraoperative Radiotherapy Trial enrolled and randomized more than 2,200 early-stage (T1, T2; N0) breast cancer patients with invasive ductal carcinoma without evidence of lobular carcinoma and older than 45 years of age to single-fraction, orthovoltage IORT to 20 Gy (surface dose) or conventionally fractionated WBRT to 50 Gy.[55] Only in the case of specific risk factors was the IORT complemented with WBRT. The first interim analysis, published in June 2010, with a median follow-up of 2 years, reported a similar local recurrence risk at 4 years (1.2% in IORT arm vs. 0.95% in the WBRT arm) and similar normal tissue complication rates (3.3% with IORT vs. 3.9% with WBRT).[55] Although encouraging, longer follow-up is needed before definitive conclusions may be drawn.

The Electron Intraoperative Treatment Trial compared IOERT to 24 Gy to the 90% isodose line to the use of WBRT. The Novac 7 and LIAC mobile electron machines were used.[56] This trial has reached its anticipated accrual of approximately 650 patients on each arm, and the first interim analysis will soon be published. However, a single-arm study of IORT to 21 Gy was reported by Veronesi et al.[57] from Milan, Italy, on 574 early-stage breast cancer patients. In this study, a 1.05% rate of in-breast recurrence was found, with a median follow-up of 20 months. Again, these preliminary data are encouraging for the use of IORT as a single-dose, partial-breast irradiation treatment.

Since 2005, the ISIORT Europe Group of six institutions has enrolled more than 1,200 patients to a single-arm study of an IOERT boost to 10 Gy to the 90% isodose line prior to WBRT to 50 Gy.[58] At least 60% of patients had at least one adverse prognostic factor for developing a local recurrence, including a tumor size of greater than 2 cm, high-grade histology, young age (<45 years), and/or positive lymph nodes. With a median follow-up of 6 years, a 1.2% local recurrence rate was found. Thus, IORT may also be used as an effective boost treatment combined with WBRT for higher-risk patients.

Other Cancer Types

The clinical data regarding the use of IORT for lung cancers, head and neck cancers, CNS malignancies, and pediatric cancers were recently reviewed in detail,[38] and the reader is referred to chapters in this textbook on specific tumor sites for additional information. No prospective, randomized trials of IORT for these cancers are available or in development.

REFERENCES

1. Hall EJ, Marchese M, Hei TK, et al. Radiation response characteristics of human cells in vitro. *Radiat Res* 1988;114(3):415–424.
2. Thames HD, Suit HD. Tumor radioresponsiveness versus fractionation sensitivity. *Int J Radiat Oncol Biol Phys* 1986;12(4):687–691.
3. Hu K, Yom S, Kaplan M, et al. Head and neck cancer. In: Gunderson L, Willett C, Calvo F, et al., eds. *Intraoperative irradiation: techniques and results*, 2nd ed. Totowa, NJ: Humana Press; 2011:163–168.
4. Kinsella TJ, DeLuca AM, Barnes M, et al. Threshold dose for peripheral neuropathy following intraoperative radiotherapy (IORT) in a large animal model. *Int J Radiat Oncol Biol Phys* 1991;20(4):697–701.
5. Kinsella TJ, Sindelar WF, DeLuca AM, et al. Tolerance of peripheral nerve to intraoperative radiotherapy (IORT): clinical and experimental studies. *Int J Radiat Oncol Biol Phys* 1985;11(9):1579–1585.
6. LeCouteur RA, Gillette EL, Powers BE, et al. Peripheral neuropathies following experimental intraoperative radiation therapy (IORT). *Int J Radiat Oncol Biol Phys* 1989;17(3):583–590.
7. Barnes M, Duray P, DeLuca A, et al. Tumor induction following intraoperative radiotherapy: late results of the National Cancer Institute canine trials. *Int J Radiat Oncol Biol Phys* 1990;19(3):651–660.
8. Sindelar WF, Kinsella TJ. Normal tissue tolerance to intraoperative radiotherapy. *Surg Oncol Clin N Am* 2003;12(4):925–942.
9. Vujaskovic Z, Willett CG, Tepper J, et al. Normal tissue tolerance to IOERT, EBRT, or both: animal and clinical studies. In: Gunderson L, Willett CG, Calvo F, et al., eds. *Intraoperative irradiation: techniques and results*, 2nd ed. Totowa, NJ: Humana Press, 2011:119–138.
10. Sindelar WF, Tepper JE, Kinsella TJ, et al. Late effects of intraoperative radiation therapy on retroperitoneal tissues, intestine, and bile duct in a large animal model. *Int J Radiat Oncol Biol Phys* 1994;29(4):781–788.
11. Gillette EL, Powers BE, McChesney SL, et al.. Response of aorta and branch arteries to experimental intraoperative irradiation. *Int J Radiat Oncol Biol Phys* 1989;17(6):1247–1255.
12. Johnstone PA, Sprague M, DeLuca AM, et al. Effects of intraoperative radiotherapy on vascular grafts in a canine model. *Int J Radiat Oncol Biol Phys* 1994; 29(5):1015–1025.
13. Tepper JE, Sindelar W, Travis EL, et al.. Tolerance of canine anastomoses to intraoperative radiation therapy. *Int J Radiat Oncol Biol Phys* 1983;9(7):987–992.
14. Sindelar WF, Tepper J, Travis EL. Tolerance of bile duct to intraoperative irradiation. *Surgery* 1982;92(3):533–540.
15. Gillette EL, Gillette S, Powers BE. Studies at Colorado State University of normal tissue tolerance of beagles to IOERT, EBRT or a combination. In: Gunderson L, Willett CG, Calvo F, et al., eds. *Intraoperative irradiation: techniques and results*, 1st ed. Totowa, NJ: Humana Press; 1999:147–163.
16. DeLuca AM, Johnstone PA, Ollayos CW, et al. Tolerance of the bladder to intraoperative radiation in a canine model: a five-year follow-up. *Int J Radiat Oncol Biol Phys* 1994;30(2):339–345.
17. Kinsella TJ, Sindelar WF, DeLuca AM, et al. Tolerance of the canine bladder to intraoperative radiation therapy: an experimental study. *Int J Radiat Oncol Biol Phys* 1988; 14(5):939–946.
18. Barnes M, Pass H, DeLuca A, et al. Response of the mediastinal and thoracic viscera of the dog to intraoperative radiation therapy (IORT). *Int J Radiat Oncol Biol Phys* 1987;13(3):371–378.
19. Tochner ZA, Pass HI, Sindelar WF, et al. Long term tolerance of thoracic organs to intraoperative radiotherapy. *Int J Radiat Oncol Biol Phys* 1992;22(1):65–69.
20. Pass HI, Sindelar WF, Kinsella TJ, et al. Delivery of intraoperative radiation therapy after pneumonectomy: experimental observations and early clinical results. *Ann Thorac Surg* 1987;44(1):14–20.
21. Sindelar WF, Kinsella TJ, Chen PW, et al. Intraoperative radiotherapy in retroperitoneal sarcomas. Final results of a prospective, randomized, clinical trial. *Arch Surg* 1993;128(4):402–410.
22. Johnstone PA, DeLuca AM, Bacher JD, et al. Clinical toxicity of peripheral nerve to intraoperative radiotherapy in a canine model. *Int J Radiat Oncol Biol Phys* 1995;32(4): 1031–1034.
23. Vujaskovic Z, Gillette SM, Powers BE, et al. Intraoperative radiation (IORT) injury to sciatic nerve in a large animal model. *Radiother Oncol* 1994;30(2):133–139.
24. Vujaskovic Z, Gillette SM, Powers BE, et al. Ultrastructural morphometric analysis of peripheral nerves after intraoperative irradiation. *Int J Radiat Biol* 1995;68(1): 71–76.

25. Gillette SM, Gillette EL, Powers BE, et al. Radiation-induced osteosarcoma in dogs after external beam or intraoperative radiation therapy. *Cancer Res* 1990;50 (1):54–57.
26. Johnstone PA, Laskin WB, DeLuca AM, et al. Tumors in dogs exposed to experimental intraoperative radiotherapy. *Int J Radiat Oncol Biol Phys* 1996;34(4): 853–857.
27. Beddar AS, Biggs PJ, Chang S, et al. Intraoperative radiation therapy using mobile electron linear accelerators: report of AAPM Radiation Therapy Committee Task Group No. 72. *Med Phys* 2006;33(5):1476–1489.
28. Palta JR, Biggs PJ, Hazle JD, et al. Intraoperative electron beam radiation therapy: technique, dosimetry, and dose specification: report of task force 48 of the Radiation Therapy Committee, American Association of Physicists in Medicine. *Int J Radiat Oncol Biol Phys* 1995;33(3):725–746.
29. Ciocca M, Orecchia R, Garibaldi C, et al. *In vivo* dosimetry using radiochromic films during intraoperative electron beam radiation therapy in early-stage breast cancer. *Radiother Oncol* 2003;69(3):285–289.
30. Consorti R, Petrucci A, Fortunato F, et al. In vivo dosimetry with MOSFETs: dosimetric characterization and first clinical results in intraoperative radiotherapy. *Int J Radiat Oncol Biol Phys* 2005;63(3):952–960.
31. Nath R, Anderson LL, Luxton G, et al. Dosimetry of interstitial brachytherapy sources: recommendations of the AAPM Radiation Therapy Committee Task Group No. 43. American Association of Physicists in Medicine. *Med Phys* 1995;22 (2):209–234.
32. Rivard MJ, Butler WM, DeWerd LA, et al. Supplement to the 2004 update of the AAPM Task Group No. 43 Report. *Med Phys* 2007;34(6):2187–2205.
33. Furhang EE, Sillanpaa JK, Hu KS, et al. HDR-IORT: physics and techniques. In: Gunderson L, Willett CG, Calvo F, et al., eds. *Intraoperative irradiation: techniques and results,* 2nd ed. Totowa, NJ: Humana Press, 2011:73–84.
34. Kutcher GJ, Coia L, Gillin M, et al. Comprehensive QA for radiation oncology: report of AAPM Radiation Therapy Committee Task Group 40. *Med Phys* 1994; 21(4):581–618.
35. Anderson LL, Hoffman MR, Harrington PJ, et al. Atlas generation for intraoperative high dose rate brachytherapy. *J Brachyther Int* 1997;13:333–340.
36. Kraus-Tiefenbacher U, Biggs PJ, Vaidya J, et al. Electronic brachytherapy/low KV-IORT: physics and techniques. In: Gunderson L, Willett CG, Calvo F, et al., eds. *Intraoperative irradiation: techniques and results,* 2nd ed. Totowa, NJ: Humana Press, 2011:85–98.
37. Nag S, Willett CG, Gunderson L, et al. IORT with electron-beam, high-dose-rate brachytherapy or low-KV/electronic brachytherapy: methodological comparisons. In: Gunderson L, Willett CG, Calvo F, et al., eds. *Intraoperative irradiation: techniques and results,* 2nd ed. Totowa, NJ: Humana Press, 2011:99–115.
38. Gunderson L, Willett CG, Calvo F, et al., eds. *Intraoperative irradiation: techniques and results,* 2nd ed. Totowa, NJ: Humana Press, 2011: Part IV, 139–518.
39. Nils D, Arvold ND, Hong TS, et al. Primary colorectal cancer. In: Gunderson L, Willett CG, Calvo F, et al., eds. *Intraoperative irradiation: techniques and results,* 2nd ed. Totowa, NJ: Humana Press, 2011:297–322.
40. Haddock MG, Nelson H, Valentini V, et al. Recurrent colorectal cancer. In: Gunderson L, Willett CG, Calvo F, et al., eds. *Intraoperative irradiation: techniques and results,* 2nd ed. Totowa, NJ: Humana Press, 2011:323–351.
41. Martinez-Monge R, Gaztanaga M, Alvarez-Cienfuegos J, et al. Gastric cancer. In: Gunderson L, Willett CG, Calvo F, et al., eds. *Intraoperative irradiation: techniques and results,* 2nd ed. Totowa, NJ: Humana Press, 2011:223–248.
42. Abe M, Takahashi M, Ono K, et al. Japan gastric trials in intraoperative radiation therapy. *Int J Radiat Oncol Biol Phys* 1988;15(6):1431–1433.
43. Kramling HJ, Willich N, Cramer C, et al. Early results of IORT in the treatment of gastric cancer. *Front Radiat Ther Oncol* 1997;31:157–160.
44. Sindelar WF, Kinsella TJ, Tepper JE, et al. Randomized trial of intraoperative radiotherapy in carcinoma of the stomach. *Am J Surg* 1993;165(1):178–186; discussion 186–177.
45. Cunningham D, Allum WH, Stenning SP, et al. Perioperative chemotherapy versus surgery alone for resectable gastroesophageal cancer. *N Engl J Med* 2006; 355(1):11–20.
46. Macdonald JS, Smalley SR, Benedetti J, et al. Chemoradiotherapy after surgery compared with surgery alone for adenocarcinoma of the stomach or gastroesophageal junction. *N Engl J Med* 2001;345(10):725–730.
47. Miller RC, Valentini V, Moss A, et al. Pancreas cancer. In: Gunderson L, Willett CG, Calvo F, et al., eds. *Intraoperative irradiation: techniques and results,* 2nd ed. Totowa, NJ: Humana Press, 2011:249–271.
48. Czito B, Donohue J, Willett CG, et al. Retroperitoneal sarcomas. In: Gunderson LL, Willett CG, Calvo F, et al., eds. *Intraoperative irradiation: techniques and results,* 2nd ed. Totowa, NJ: Humana Press, 2011:353–386.
49. Alektiar KM, Hu K, Anderson L, et al. High-dose-rate intraoperative radiation therapy (HDR-IORT) for retroperitoneal sarcomas. *Int J Radiat Oncol Biol Phys* 1 2000;47(1):157–163.
50. Dziewirski W, Rutkowski P, Nowecki ZI, et al. Surgery combined with intraoperative brachytherapy in the treatment of retroperitoneal sarcomas. *Ann Surg Oncol* 2006;13(2):245–252.
51. Petersen IA, Krempien R, Beauchamp C, et al. Extremity and trunk soft-tissue sarcomas. In: Gunderson LL, Willett CG, Calvo F, et al., eds. *Intraoperative irradiation: techniques and results,* 2nd ed. Totowa, NJ: Humana Press, 2011: 387–405.
52. Kunos C, Colussi V, Getty P, et al. Intraoperative electron radiotherapy for extremity sarcomas does not increase acute or late morbidity. *Clin Orthop Relat Res* 2006:247–252.
53. Calvo F, Sierrasesumaga L, Patino A, et al. Bone sarcomas. In: Gunderson LL, Willett CG, Calvo F, et al., eds. *Intraoperative irradiation: techniques and results,* 2nd ed. Totowa, NJ: Humana Press, 2011:407–429.
54. Sedlmayer F, DuBois J-B, Reitsamer R, et al. Breast cancer. In: Gunderson LL, Willett CG, Calvo F, et al., eds. *Intraoperative irradiation: techniques and results,* 2nd ed. Totowa, NJ: Humana Press, 2011:189–200.
55. Vaidya JS, Joseph DJ, Tobias JS, et al. Targeted intraoperative radiotherapy versus whole breast radiotherapy for breast cancer (TARGIT-A trial): an international, prospective, randomised, non-inferiority phase 3 trial. *Lancet* 2010;376(9735): 91–102.
56. Intra M, Leonardi C, Luini A, et al. Full-dose intraoperative radiotherapy with electrons in breast surgery: broadening the indications. *Arch Surg* 2005;140(10): 936–939.
57. Veronesi U, Orecchia R, Luini A, et al. Full-dose intraoperative radiotherapy with electrons during breast-conserving surgery: experience with 590 cases. *Ann Surg* 2005;242(1):101–106.
58. Sedlmayer F, Fastner G, Merz F, et al. IORT with electrons as boost strategy during breast conserving therapy in limited stage breast cancer: results of an ISIORT pooled analysis. *Strahlenther Onkol* 2007;183(Spec No 2):32–34.

Chapter 19
Proton Therapy

Nancy Price Mendenhall and Zuofeng Li

The burgeoning interest in proton therapy is related to its potential to improve the therapeutic ratio for many malignancies treated with radiation. This chapter will touch on the rationale, evolving technology, potential applications, efficacy, toxicity, comparative effectiveness, and economic challenges associated with proton therapy.

RATIONALE

Therapeutic Ratio

With any medical intervention there is an optimum balance between the potential to benefit and the potential to harm the patient, called the therapeutic ratio. In radiation oncology, it is the balance between radiation effects on the tumor and radiation effects on normal, nontargeted tissues. This ratio informs every physician and patient decision, but different priorities may mandate different decisions in different clinical situations. For example, in a patient with an advanced paranasal sinus tumor adjacent to the optic nerves and chiasm, one physician might recommend a treatment that minimizes the risk of optic nerve damage at the price of a lower probability of tumor control, while another physician might recommend a treatment with a greater risk of optic nerve damage to provide a greater probability of tumor control. In another example, the potential risks of low-dose radiation exposure to a large volume of the brain tissue may be of greater concern to the parents of a young child than to an elderly patient with a short life expectancy. In evaluating new radiation modalities, the first question is whether there exists a potential to improve the therapeutic ratio.

The Impact of Dose Distribution on the Therapeutic Ratio

A number of factors influence radiation effects, and thus the therapeutic ratio, including total dose, dose intensity (the overall time or number of fractions in which a dose is given), relative biologic effectiveness (RBE), and modifying factors such as chemotherapy, patient age, and comorbidities. But none of these factors is as important as dose distribution—the relative dose to the target compared with the dose to nontargeted normal tissues—because radiation therapy is a nonspecific therapy that affects both normal and cancerous cells. A constant principle in radiation oncology is that the higher or more intense the radiation dose, the greater the probability of tumor control. The risk of treatment-related toxicity is similarly related to the dose and dose intensity to normal tissue, as well as to the volume of the normal tissue exposed to various radiation dose levels. This principle has been demonstrated in many malignancies (i.e., prostate, breast, head and neck) but may not always be apparent when tumoricidal doses cannot be delivered to the target because of excessive risks to normal tissues or when adequate tools for measuring toxicity are not available.

The primary barrier to maximizing local tumor control through dose escalation or intensification is the risk of damaging normal tissues either by delivering too high a dose or exposing too much of the normal tissue to radiation. Whereas tumor control is a dichotomized end point, toxicity occurs as a spectrum of end points over a long period of time in a variety of tissues and can be difficult to measure. When toxicities are easily defined, are functionally significant, and occur early, the risk of the radiation complication is often prioritized over the probability of cure, leading to a low therapeutic ratio because of low disease control rates. Conversely, when toxicities are ill-defined, are difficult to measure, or occur late, disease control will be prioritized. In most clinical settings, there is an opportunity for improvement of the therapeutic ratio by increasing disease control or by reducing toxicity. The most direct means of improving the therapeutic ratio is by reducing the radiation dose to nontargeted tissues, which both reduces toxicity and facilitates dose escalation for increased tumor control: herein lies the rationale for proton therapy.

The Problem with X-Rays and the Promise and Challenge of Protons

Most x-rays from an external beam pass through the patient without effect, but some are absorbed as they randomly interact with subatomic particles along their path, initiating a cascade of biochemical reactions that result in cell injury or cell death. X-rays thus leave a track of tissue damage from the skin-surface entrance to the skin-surface exit, much like the track of a bullet. With accumulating x-ray absorptions, the dose deposited along the beam path is attenuated as the number of x-rays available for interactions decreases. This pattern of radiation dose deposition with x-ray-based external-beam radiotherapy (EBRT; Fig. 19.1) is particularly problematic because the dose to tissues along the beam entrance path is always higher than the dose to the target. In addition, along the exit path of the beam, more normal tissues are exposed to doses of radiation only slightly less than the dose to the target. *Thus, most of the radiation dose with x-ray-based therapy is deposited in the patient outside of the target.*

Many elegant strategies have been developed for offsetting this basic problem (i.e., multiple fields, four-field box, stereotactic radiosurgery and stereotactic radiation therapy [SRT], three-dimensional conformal radiation therapy [3DCRT], intensity-modulated radiation therapy [IMRT], tomotherapy, arc therapy, robotic radiosurgery, etc.), but even with these technologies, radiation to nontargeted tissues is primarily redistributed, rather than reduced, and more radiation dose is deposited outside, versus inside, the target. Because the total dose to a given tissue is one of the key determinants of toxicity, certain toxicities are reduced when using these sophisticated techniques. Nevertheless, it is likely that other toxicities, influenced by the volume of tissue exposed to radiation, will increase by these integral dose redistribution methods as greater volumes of normal tissue are exposed to radiation. Some of the effects related to low-dose exposure to larger volumes of tissue may require more time for clinical manifestation (second malignancies), and some injuries may require more subtle measurement tools for detection (neurocognitive testing), leading to an early underestimation of toxicity with these sophisticated methods.

The pattern of dose deposition with protons differs significantly from that of x-rays. A proton is simply a hydrogen atom that has lost its electron. It has a mass of approximately 1,800 times that of an electron and carries a positive charge. As protons traverse matter, they lose energy primarily through interactions with atomic electrons. Due to the significantly larger mass of protons relative to electrons, protons lose only a small portion of their energy in each interaction (in contrast to x-rays) and experience only small directional changes.

As protons traverse matter, the rate of energy loss in electronic interactions is described by the linear stopping power,

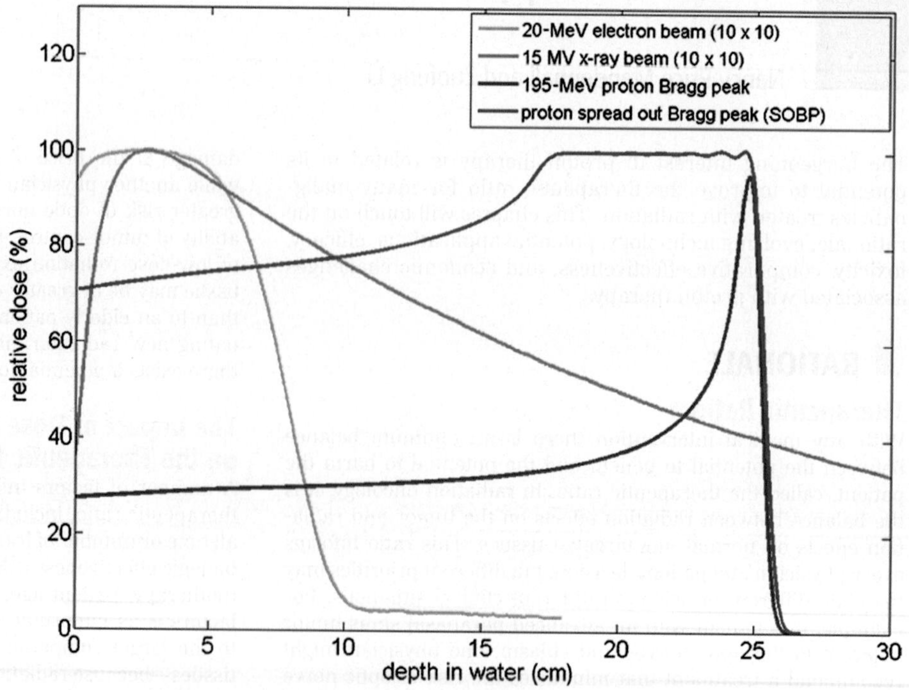

FIGURE 19.1. The shape of the depth-dose curves for electrons (tan), photons/x-rays (orange), a pristine proton Bragg peak (purple), and a spread-out Bragg peak (blue), composed of multiple pristine Bragg peaks, differs significantly. Compared to photons or electrons, the entrance dose with protons is constant and reduced relative to the target dose and there is no exit dose. The dose fall-off at the end of the proton range is much sharper than for electrons. In summary, with photons, most of the radiation energy is deposited outside of the target, whereas with protons, most of the radiation energy is deposited inside the target.

S(E), defined as *dE/dx*, where *dE* is the mean energy lost by a proton in electronic collisions over a distance of *dx* in media. A more commonly used function is the mass stopping power, s = S(E)/ρ, which denotes the energy loss *dE* when protons travel through a distance of *dx* in a media of density ρ.[1]

Linear energy transfer, or LET, is a closely related concept to stopping power. Whereas stopping power indicates energy lost by the protons, LET denotes the energy transferred to a medium as the protons traverse it. LET therefore represents the density of energy deposition in media and is directly related to the local RBE of the radiation, similar to its significance in other radiation modalities. At higher energies (e.g., along the entrance path), protons have a small stopping power and low LET values; their LET values increase sharply by up to two orders of magnitude as the proton's energy decreases just before coming to a complete stop. This phenomenon creates the Bragg peak of radiation dose deposition characteristic of a proton beam, with a small, nearly constant, dose along the entrance path followed by a sharp peak in dose deposition immediately before the protons stop in media. In addition, the LET values rise sharply, corresponding to a sharp increase in RBE values near the end of a proton beam range. Much work has been done to determine *in vitro* and *in vivo* proton beam RBE values.[2] For clinical applications of protons, it is currently recommended that an RBE multiplicative value of 1.10 should be applied to the physical dose.[1] Currently, this RBE factor is applied uniformly to the physical dose distribution, without explicitly accounting for the increased RBE values near the end of a proton beam range. There is a rapid rise in RBE during the last several mm^3 of the proton range, so that the actual RBE-corrected dose at the very end of the range may exceed the physical dose by up to 25%, thus producing an RBE value up to 1.3 at the very end of the proton range. RBE effects are much more significant in heavier ions like carbon due to their significant variations along beam paths; nascent carbon ion treatment-planning systems are attempting to account for these variations in RBE along the carbon beam path.[4]

In addition to energy loss through electronic collisions, high-energy protons also experience nuclear interactions in media. Such interactions, from the perspective of clinical proton therapy, remove protons from the initial proton fluence and produce secondary protons and heavier particles, such as deuterons, tritons, ^3He, and α; these particles contribute only a small percentage of the dose along the beam path.[5] Although negligible, most of the dose from the neutrons produced in these nuclear interactions is deposited downstream from the stopping point of the proton beam, beyond the Bragg peak. The neutrons produced by protons within the patient, as well as those produced in the beam delivery mechanical components, have been under intense investigation for their potential secondary cancer-inducing effects. Hall[6] raised concern that such scattered neutrons may increase the incidence of secondary tumors in patients treated with historical proton therapy systems, similar to the transition from conventional 3DCRT to IMRT.[7] Much research has been performed estimating secondary cancer risks from contemporary proton therapy systems using either scattering-beam techniques or scanning-beam techniques. A review of literature on this subject finds consistent advantages of proton therapy over photon therapy techniques in the form of reduced secondary cancer risks in the treatment of medulloblastoma, prostate cancer, and liver cancer.[8]

Accordingly, the rationale and promise of protons, compared with x-rays, lie in the significant reduction in dose to nontargeted tissues along the entrance path and the absence of exit dose. This reduction in dose (physical and RBE dose) to normal tissues should translate into a lower risk of complications for a given target dose and probability of tumor control (i.e., an improved therapeutic ratio compared with x-rays). A lower risk of complications could be leveraged for dose escalation or intensification to yield higher disease control in certain settings or for hypofractionation to reduce costs or increase tumor control in other settings.

TECHNOLOGY

Beam Production and Transport

Protons are produced either from hydrogen gas obtained from electrolysis of deionized water or from commercially available high-purity hydrogen gas. Application of a high-voltage electric current to the hydrogen gas strips the electrons off the hydrogen atoms, leaving positively charged protons. The protons are then accelerated to energy applicable for clinical proton therapy with either a cyclotron or a synchrotron (Fig. 19.2). Energies on the order of 250 MeV are required for penetrating approximately 32 cm into tissue. Cyclotrons produce a continuous beam of nearly monoenergetic and unidirectional protons. The beam must then be degraded to meet specific requirements for each treatment field in each patient. This process takes place shortly after the beam exits the cyclotron in a device composed of a material of variable thickness with a low atomic number known as the "energy degrader." The proton beam exiting the energy degrader will have an energy spread centered around the desired final beam energy and direction variations that reduce the quality of the final treatment beam. An energy selection system (ESS), consisting of energy slits, bending magnets, and focusing magnets, is then used to eliminate protons with excessive energy or deviations in angular direction. Cyclotrons can produce a large proton beam current of up to 300 nA and thus deliver proton therapy at a high dose rate using the traditional double-scattering technique.

Synchrotrons, however, produce proton beams of selectable energy, thereby eliminating the need for the energy degrader and energy selection devices. A proton pulse exiting a preaccelerator, with energy typically up to 7 MeV, is injected into the ring-shaped accelerator. Each complete circuit of the proton pulse through the accelerator ring structure incrementally increases the proton pulse energy. When the desired beam energy is reached, the proton pulse is extracted from the accelerator. The time segment between pulses depends on the final energy required of the proton beam, ranging from subseconds to several seconds for the highest beam energy. The pulsed nature of the beam introduces additional complexity in certain treatment delivery scenarios, such as gated treatment of mobile targets and intensity-modulated proton therapy (IMPT).[9] Beam currents from synchrotrons are typically much lower than with cyclotrons, thus limiting the maximum dose rates that can be used for patient treatment, especially for larger field sizes. The maximum dose rate available from a commercially available synchrotron-based proton therapy system for a 25 × 25-cm^2 field has been specified at 0.8 Gy per minute.[10] The elimination of the energy degrader and selection system removes a major source of radiation production in the accelerator vault. A synchrotron vault is therefore accessible immediately after the beam is stopped for maintenance, whereas for a cyclotron vault, approximately 30 minutes is necessary to allow the activated parts of the accelerator and ESS to "cool down" before maintenance can be performed, or longer if access to internal parts of the cyclotron is required. The shielding requirements for cyclotrons are higher than for synchrotrons as well due to the high radiation produced by the ESS. However, the overall footprint of a cyclotron vault, including the additional shielding required, is actually similar to or smaller than that of a synchrotron vault because of the smaller physical dimensions of cyclotrons.

The proton beam, whether exiting the ESS for a cyclotron-based system or exiting the accelerator for a synchrotron-based system, is transported to the treatment room(s) via the beam transport system. Maintenance of beam focusing, centering, spot size, and divergence throughout the beam transport system

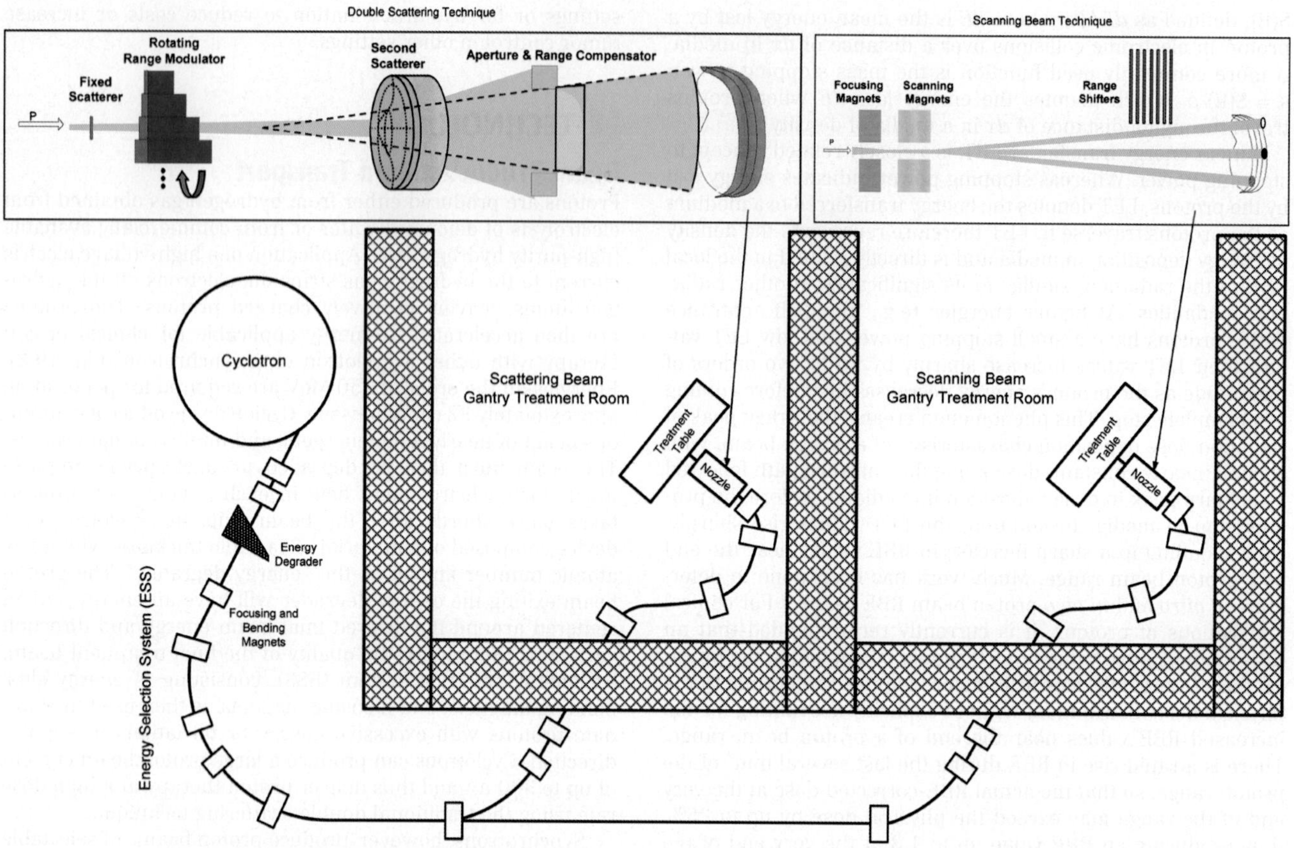

FIGURE 19.2. Proton therapy system with cyclotron, energy selection system, beam line, gantry, and nozzle. Scattering is illustrated in the nozzle on the left and scanning in the nozzle on the right.

is critical to maintaining a high-quality proton beam for treatment delivery. Paganetti et al.[11] performed Monte Carlo calculations of the dosimetric effect of proton beam energy spread, spot size, and angular energy spread on the shape of the Bragg peak. They found that small deviations in these parameters from their nominal values will result in a widening of the Bragg peak and increased entrance doses. Beam transport systems in clinical proton facilities therefore include bending and focusing magnets and beam profile monitors so that the proton beam quality may be monitored and adjusted ("tuned") as it is transported through the beam transport system.

Recent progress in accelerating and control technologies has led to new designs of proton therapy systems in the form of single-treatment-room systems with small cyclotrons that may be mounted on a gantry, as well as dielectric wall accelerators (DWAs) and laser-accelerated accelerators.[12] Single-room proton therapy systems are currently available from a number of commercial vendors, each with its own strengths and weaknesses, although none was in clinical operation at the time this chapter was written. DWA and laser-accelerated systems are currently under development. One of the primary drivers for development of these single-room proton therapy solutions is facility cost reduction.

Beam Delivery

The proton beam exiting the transport system (Fig. 19.2) is a pencil-shaped beam with minimal energy and direction spread. The beam has a small spot size in its lateral direction and a narrow Bragg peak dose in its depth direction. Two basic techniques have been developed to convert this narrow pencil beam into a dose distribution suitable for treatment of a 3D target, broadly categorized into the "scattering technique" and the "scanning technique." These techniques are implemented in the proton treatment "nozzle," or treatment head.

The scattering technique aims to produce a dose distribution with a flat lateral profile, similar to what is achieved in linear accelerator–produced 3D conformal x-ray beams, but a depth dose with a low entrance dose and a plateau region, followed by the sharp fall-off of doses to zero. The depth-dose curve, with a plateau of adequate width to cover the full thickness of the target, is produced by summing a number of Bragg peaks, each with progressively reduced maximum energy and range in the patient. The weights of the individual Bragg peaks are optimized to achieve a flat top region of the depth-dose curve. A constant energy proton beam may be used for such treatments, with range-reducing materials inserted into the beam path to create subsequent Bragg peaks of reduced ranges. Range modulation wheels consisting of variable thicknesses of "acrylic glass" (polymerized methyl methacrylate) or graphite steps are traditionally used for this purpose.[11] The proton beam travels through the variable-thickness steps, with each step creating a Bragg peak of a precalibrated range. The widths and thicknesses of the modulation wheels are calibrated to achieve a flat depth dose, or "spread-out Bragg peak" (SOBP). The width of the SOBP is controlled by turning the beam off when a prescribed width is reached. Alternatively, a "ridge filter" may be used to create an SOBP,[13] with the advantage of eliminating sensitivity to organ motion in the formation of the SOBP but the added complexity that each ridge filter is designed to achieve a single SOBP width.

The scattering technique produces a large, flat lateral dose profile through physical scattering filters in the proton beam path.[11] Either a single scattering filter may be used, creating a wide beam with a Gaussian dose profile (single scattering beam), or a second scattering filter can be added into the beam that flattens the beam to create a flat lateral dose profile (double scattering beam). Apertures fabricated out of brass or other metal are used to confine the treatment field to the target. A tissue-equivalent range compensator (or bolus) is designed to adjust the beam range throughout the field to conform to the distal profile of the target.[14]

In the scanning technique, as the pencil beam exits the transport system, it is magnetically steered in the lateral directions to deliver dose to a large treatment field.[10,15–17] The proton beam intensity may be modulated as the beam is moved across the field, resulting in the modulated scanning beam technique, or IMPT, delivery. Current implementation of IMPT uses the so-called spot scanning technique, in which the beam spot is moved to a location within the target and the prescribed dose delivered to the spot, before it is moved to the next spot to deliver its prescribed dose. In the beam axis direction, IMPT treatments are delivered using the layer-stacking technique. A pencil beam with a pristine peak is scanned through the deepest layer of the target to deliver the intensity-modulated dose distribution for the layer before a range shifter—effectively an energy degrader of predetermined thickness—is inserted into the beam path to deliver dose to a depth immediately proximal to the deepest layer. Doses to each subsequent layer are delivered by inserting additional range shifters. The size of the spot, represented by the sigma of the Gaussian function describing the pencil-beam profile, is a critical parameter of the pencil beam. Smaller beam sigma values allow intricate sculpting of the intensity-modulated dose distribution, at the cost of increased control system complexity and delivery time; larger beam sigma values result in greater lateral penumbra of the delivered dose distribution and reduce the dose gradient achievable at interface regions of target and critical organs.

Similar to the interplay effect reported for IMRT,[18–21] scanning techniques are sensitive to organ motion because moving the pencil beam across the treatment field for dose delivery to a given layer and inserting range shifters for dose delivery to subsequent layers are time consuming. Additional motion mitigation measures, such as breath holding, gated therapy, and abdominal compression, may be necessary to minimize the dosimetric effects of organ motion.

Treatment Planning

Treatment planning for proton therapy requires a volumetric patient computed tomography (CT) scan dataset. The CT Hounsfield Unit numbers are converted to proton stopping-power values for calculating the proton range required for the treatment field.[22,23] Unlike the relatively reliable conversion of CT numbers to relative electron density for photon dose calculations, errors and uncertainties in the conversion of CT numbers to proton stopping power in proton dose calculations translate linearly into proton range calculation uncertainties and errors. In clinical practice, these uncertainties are handled during the treatment planning process by bracketing the intended SOBP with a distal margin beyond the target and a proximal margin before the target in the range calculation of each treatment field.[24] Other considerations in determining the values for distal and proximal margins include target motion, daily setup errors, beam delivery uncertainties, and uncertainties in patient anatomy and physiology changes throughout treatment that could affect the water-equivalent depth of the target. In the lateral direction of the beam's eye view (BEV) of a proton field, planning target volume (PTV) margins are necessary to accommodate setup errors and target movements, identical to their usage in x-ray treatments. It is therefore worth noting that the concept of PTV, as defined in the various International Commission on Radiation Units and Measurements (ICRU) reports,[1,25,26] does not strictly apply to proton therapy. Generally, a PTV expansion, with either uniform or nonuniform margins, is used for x-ray planning, which accommodates maximum target motion and setup error in each of the patient axes (longitudinal, lateral, and anterior/posterior). In contrast to x-ray planning, the PTV for proton therapy is specific for each treatment field. Lateral margins are identical to traditional definitions, but the distal and proximal margins along the beam axis are calculated to account for proton-specific uncertainties. The lower entrance dose and absence of exit dose of a proton beam afford proton therapy practitioners the additional flexibility to select beam angles where lateral target motion and setup error are minimal; thus, the PTV expansion margin may be less for a given proton beam than would be required in IMRT to accommodate for uncertainties for all beam angles. State-of-the-art proton therapy dose calculations use pencil-beam algorithms,[27–30] which model proton interaction and scattering in various heterogeneous media of the beam path, including the nozzle, range compensators, and the patient. Monte Carlo calculations have been used to study the accuracy of such dose calculation algorithms, with results indicating errors near tissue interfaces, particularly near interfaces of media differing significantly in density and composition, such as air cavity and bone in head and neck treatments.[31–33] A number of fast Monte Carlo calculation algorithms have been proposed to improve proton therapy dose calculation accuracy,[34–36] although none is currently available from commercial treatment-planning system vendors.

POTENTIAL PROTON THERAPY APPLICATIONS

Many publications have reported significant differences in dose distribution with proton treatment plans compared with x-ray-based treatment plans in a wide range of malignancies and benign lesions throughout the body, including the eye,[37] brain,[38,39] sinonasal structures,[40,41] oropharynx, nasopharynx, skull base, lung,[42,43] lymphoma,[44,45] pancreas,[46] esophagus,[47] bladder, rectum, pediatric malignancies, prostate,[48,49] cervix,[50] breast,[51,52] sarcomas, and standard target volumes such as pelvic lymph nodes[53] and craniospinal irradiation.[54] In all cases there is a striking advantage with protons for reduction in the volume of nontargeted normal tissue receiving low- to medium-range radiation doses. In some cases, there is also a reduction in the volume of nontargeted tissue receiving moderate- to high-dose irradiation. With double-scattered proton delivery modes currently in common usage, the target dose homogeneity and conformality index can sometimes, but not always, be inferior to that of IMRT. With scanned proton delivery modes, IMPT plans generally have not only significant reductions in low and moderate integral doses but also improved dose homogeneity and conformality indexes when compared with IMRT. Each case within each tumor type is different, and until comparative plans are performed, it may not be clear whether protons will be helpful or whether IMPT would be useful. At this stage in the development of proton therapy, there are no clear class solutions to treatment planning. In addition, the full potential for dose distribution improvements with protons has not been realized because of uncertainties in both treatment-planning algorithms and delivery modes. Strategies for motion management and quality assurance necessary to implement advanced proton delivery modes into routine practice are not fully developed. Finally, the clinical impact of some patterns of dose distribution improvements achievable with proton therapy may not be anticipated at this time and/or may require time, careful trial design, and special assessments to define.

Currently, proton therapy is a rare medical resource best used in situations where outcomes with commonly available radiation strategies present opportunities for improvement in the therapeutic ratio via improvements in dose distributions. Listed in Figures 19.3 through 19.10 are eight clinical settings that exemplify particular kinds of opportunities for proton therapy. The proton plans are all double-scattered mode, as few practices today are able to deliver IMPT. The first two examples (Figs. 19.3 and 19.4) represent opportunities where reductions in relatively high doses to critical structures make it possible to

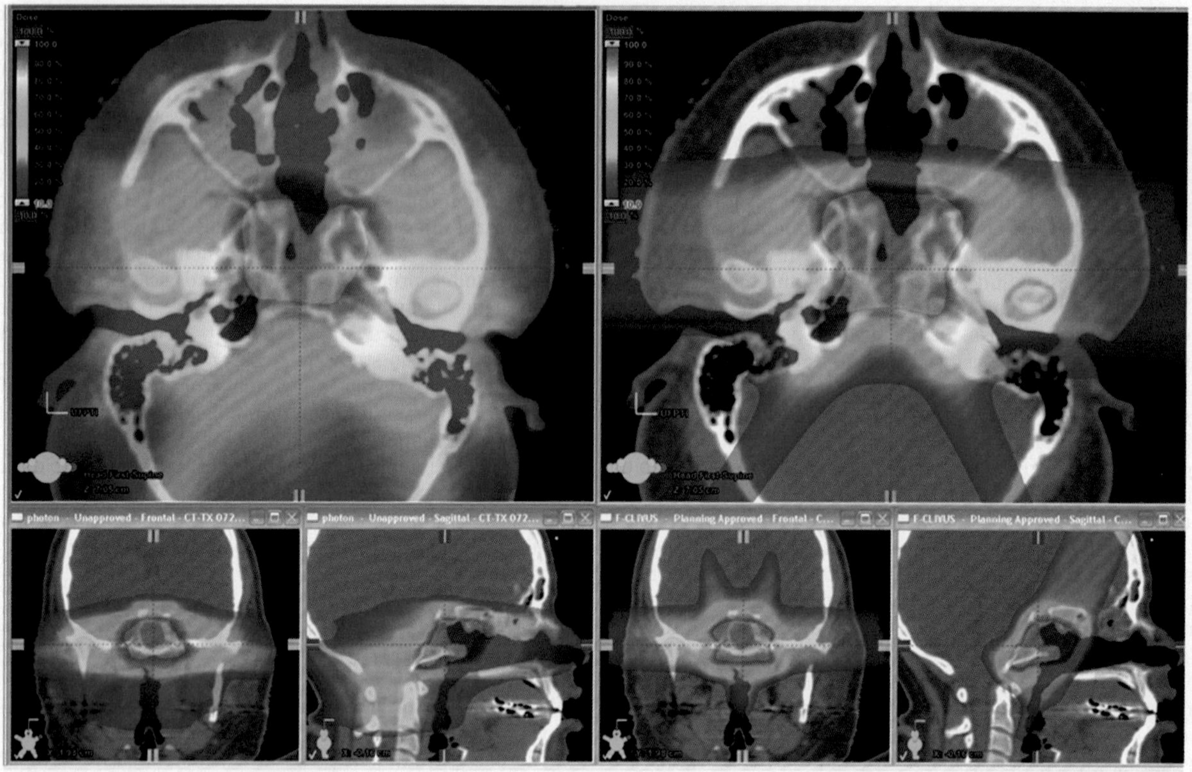

IMRT Proton

FIGURE 19.3. Axial and sagittal planes from intensity-modulated radiation therapy (IMRT) plans are shown on the left and proton plans on the right for a skull-base sarcoma. In this particular case, the major advantage to the proton plan over the IMRT plan is the sharp gradient between the target and brainstem achievable with the proton plan. The maximum and mean relative doses to the brainstem are 71% and 42% with IMRT compared to 59% and 11% with protons, respectively. The lower maximum and mean relative doses to the brainstem permit delivery of a higher dose to the clivus sarcoma target. In addition, there is a substantial reduction in low-dose exposure to nontargeted tissue such as the posterior fossa, spinal cord, and nasal cavity, which might result in more acute tolerance of treatment or fewer late neurocognitive sequelae.

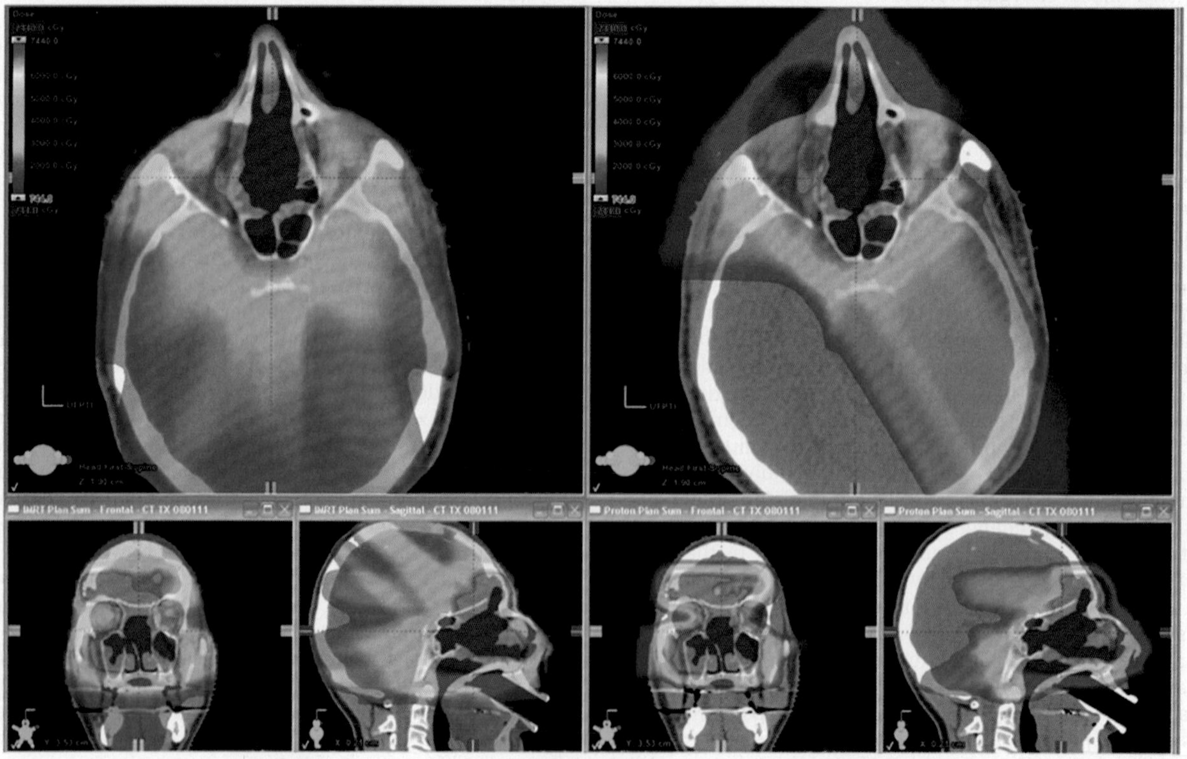

IMRT Proton

FIGURE 19.4. Axial and sagittal planes from intensity-modulated radiation therapy (IMRT) plans are shown on the left and proton plans on the right for a paranasal sinus tumor. In this particular case, the major advantages to the proton plan compared to the IMRT plan are reductions in mean dose to the chiasm (4,356 to 3,590 cGy [relative biologic effectiveness, RBE]), the right optic nerve (5,237 to 4,228 cGy [RBE]), and the brainstem (3,698 to 2,743 cGy [RBE]). Target coverage was more homogeneous with proton therapy as well. When 100% of the prescribed dose of 75 Gy/cGy (RBE) was delivered to at least 90% of the target volume with each plan, mean and maximum doses were, respectively, 7,860 cGy (RBE) and 8,680 cGy (RBE) with protons and 8,096 cGy and 9,463 cGy with IMRT.

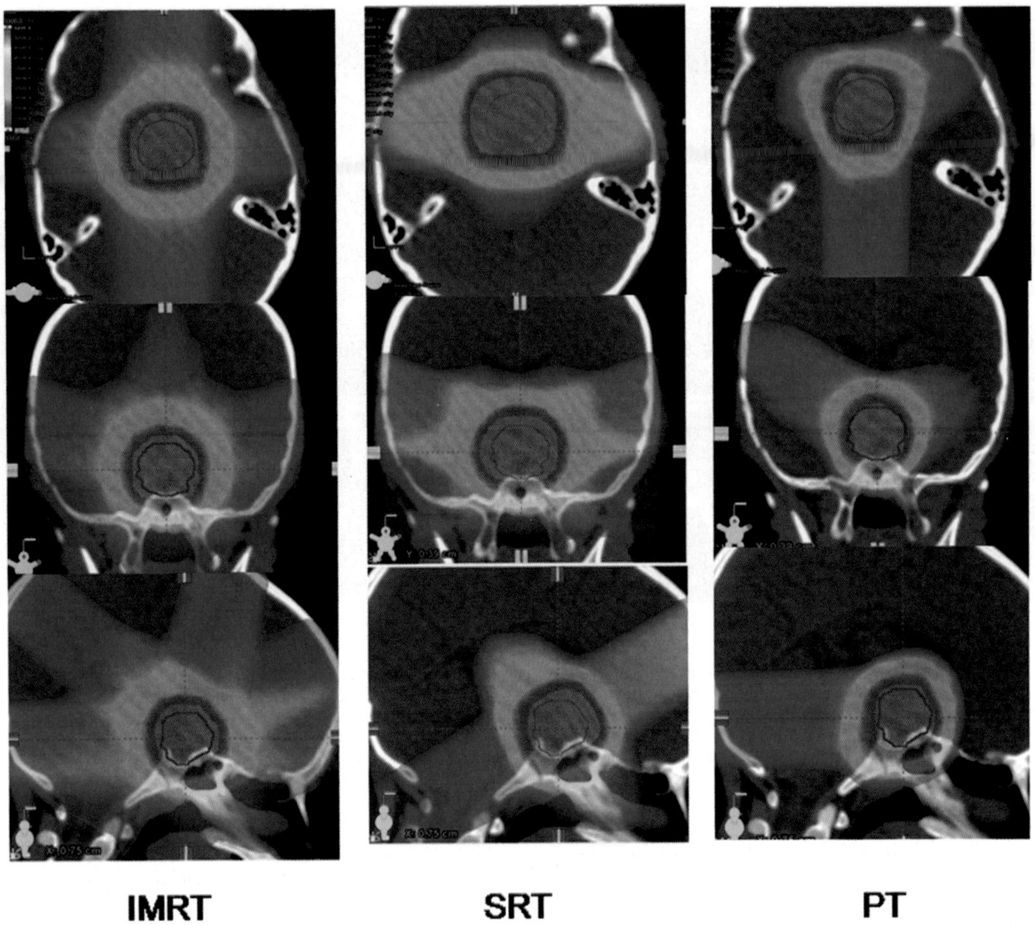

FIGURE 19.5. Axial and coronal planes are shown from intensity-modulated radiation therapy (IMRT) plans (*left*), stereotactic radiation therapy (SRT) plans (*center*), and proton therapy plans (*right*) for a small craniopharyngioma. As apparent, the volume of tissue exposed to low- and intermediate-dose irradiation is reduced with the proton plan. Mean body and mean brain dose excluding the planning target volume (PTV) are 233 cGy and 888 cGy with IMRT, 215 cGy and 810 cGy with SRT, and 63 cGy (relative biologic effectiveness [RBE]) and 358 cGy (RBE) with protons, respectively. The mean right temporal lobe dose is 904 cGy with IMRT, 1,090 cGy with SRT, and 297 cGy (RBE) with protons. The mean left temporal dose is 951 cGy with IMRT, 1,200 cGy with SRT, and 370 cGy (RBE) with protons. The mean left hippocampal dose is 2,749 cGy with IMRT, 3,299 cGy with SRT, and 815 cGy (RBE) with protons. The mean right cochlear dose is 807 cGy with IMRT, 388 cGy with SRT, and 7 cGy (RBE) with protons. The mean left cochlear dose is 792 cGy with IMRT, 887 cGy with SRT, and 5 cGy (RBE) with protons.

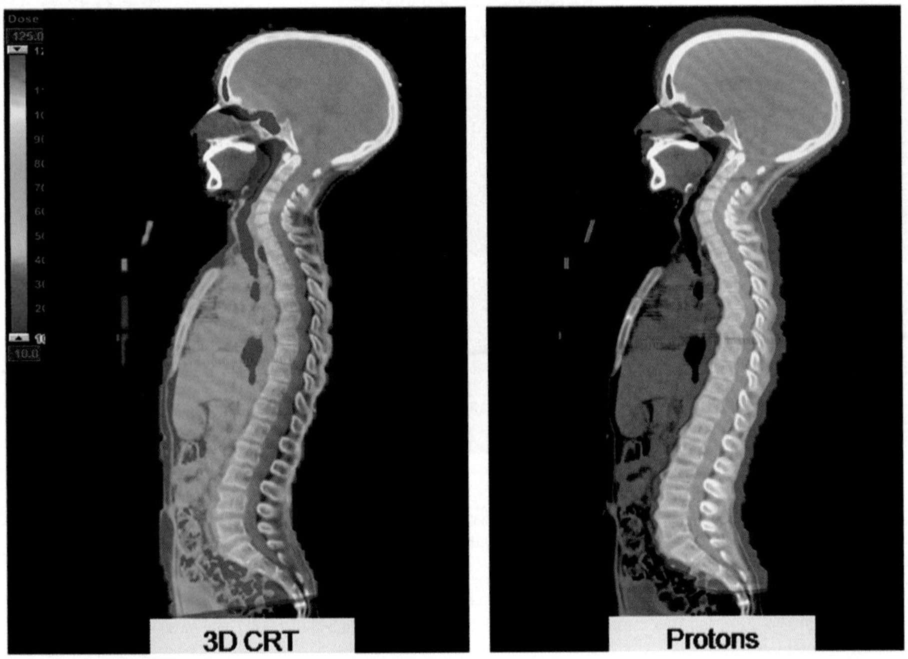

FIGURE 19.6. Sagittal planes from three-dimensional conformal radiation therapy (3DCRT) plans are shown on the left and proton plans on the right for craniospinal axis irradiation necessary in a variety of brain tumors, most of which occur in young patients at risk for late effects. As apparent in the figure, the risks for functional and neoplastic effects in the thyroid, heart, lungs, breast, gut, and gonads from photon therapy can be avoided with proton therapy because of the lack of an exit dose. The total-body V_{10} and total body integral dose are 37.2% and 0.223 Gy-m^3 with 3DCRT compared with 28.7% and 0.185 Gy-m^3 with proton therapy, respectively.

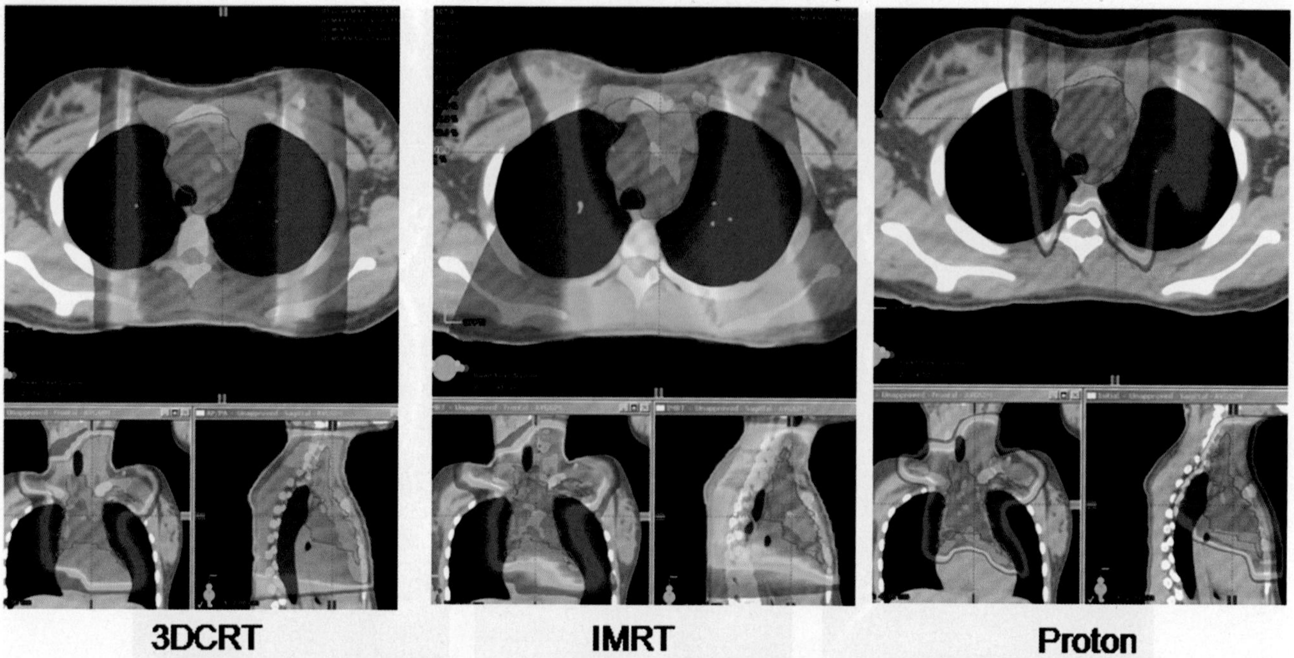

FIGURE 19.7. Axial, coronal, and sagittal planes are shown for three-dimensional conformal radiation therapy (3DCRT; *left*), intensity-modulated radiation therapy (IMRT; *center*), and proton therapy (*right*) for a female patient with neck and mediastinal involvement by Hodgkin lymphoma. As apparent, the proton therapy plans expose a smaller volume of nontargeted tissue (particularly heart, lung, spinal cord, and breast) to radiation than either photon plan. Lung V_4 and V_{20} are 59% and 25% with 3DCRT, 62% and 9% with IMRT, and 32% and 16% with proton therapy, respectively. Heart V_4 and V_{20} are 79% and 54% with 3DCRT, 76% and 26% with IMRT, and 40% and 26% with proton therapy, respectively.

deliver a sufficiently high target dose with proton therapy to make disease control possible in cases not often cured with photon therapy. The next three examples (Figs. 19.5 through 19.7) are opportunities to reduce early functional and potentially fatal late toxicities with proton therapy by reducing the volume of tissue exposed to low and moderate radiation doses. Figures 19.8 and 19.9 represent opportunities to increase the effectiveness of combined modality therapy by increasing dose or dose intensity of either chemotherapy and/or radiation therapy made feasible through reducing moderate-dose irradiation to critical structures subject to acute toxicity. The last example (Fig. 19.10) represents an opportunity to improve the therapeutic ratio in a tumor generally considered to be well treated with sophisticated x-ray techniques; in this case, a small reduction in

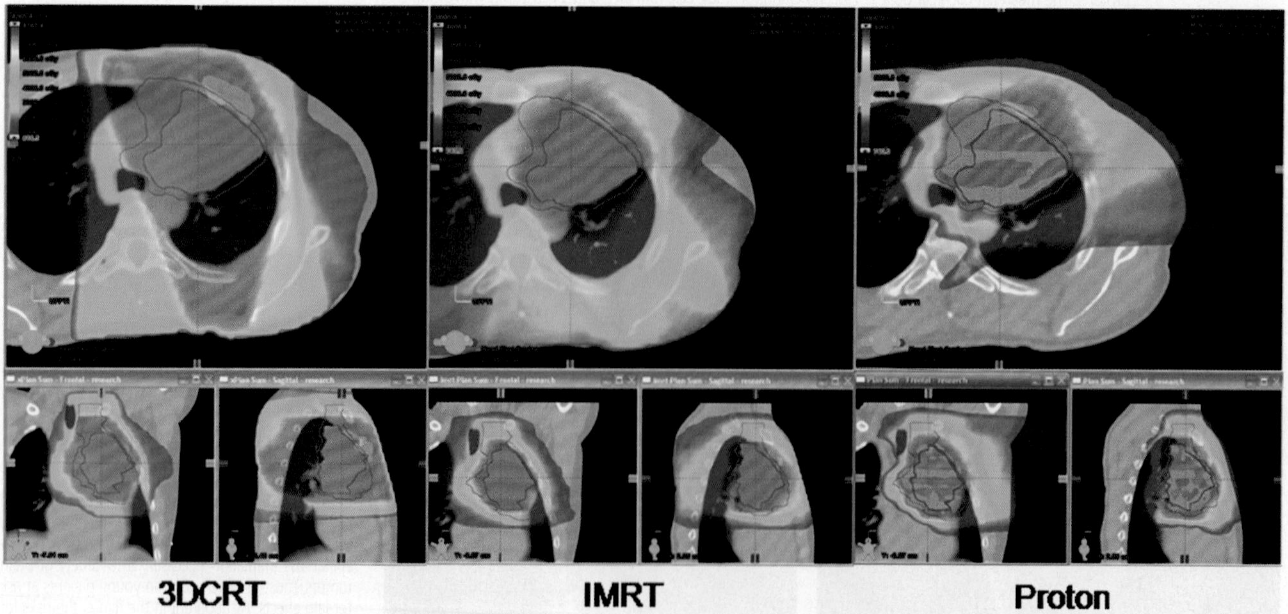

FIGURE 19.8. Axial, coronal, and sagittal planes are shown for three-dimensional conformal radiation therapy (3DCRT; *left*), intensity-modulated radiation therapy (IMRT; *center*) and proton therapy (*right*) for a patient with lung cancer. As apparent, both the IMRT and proton therapy plans reduce the volume of nontargeted tissue receiving high-dose irradiation. The proton therapy plan further reduces the volume of nontargeted tissue receiving low- and intermediate-dose irradiation compared to both the 3DCRT and IMRT plans. The 3DCRT, IMRT, and proton therapy plans respectively produced mean lung doses of 1,170 cGy, 1,424 cGy, and 819 cGy (relative biologic effectiveness [RBE]); lung V_5 of 36%, 50%, and 21%; lung V_{10} of 27%, 37%, and 18%; lung V_{20} of 23%, 22%, and 13%; mean heart doses of 1,156 cGy, 714 cGy, and 548 cGy (RBE); and mean esophageal doses of 3,401 cGy, 2,617 cGy, and 2,171 cGy (RBE).

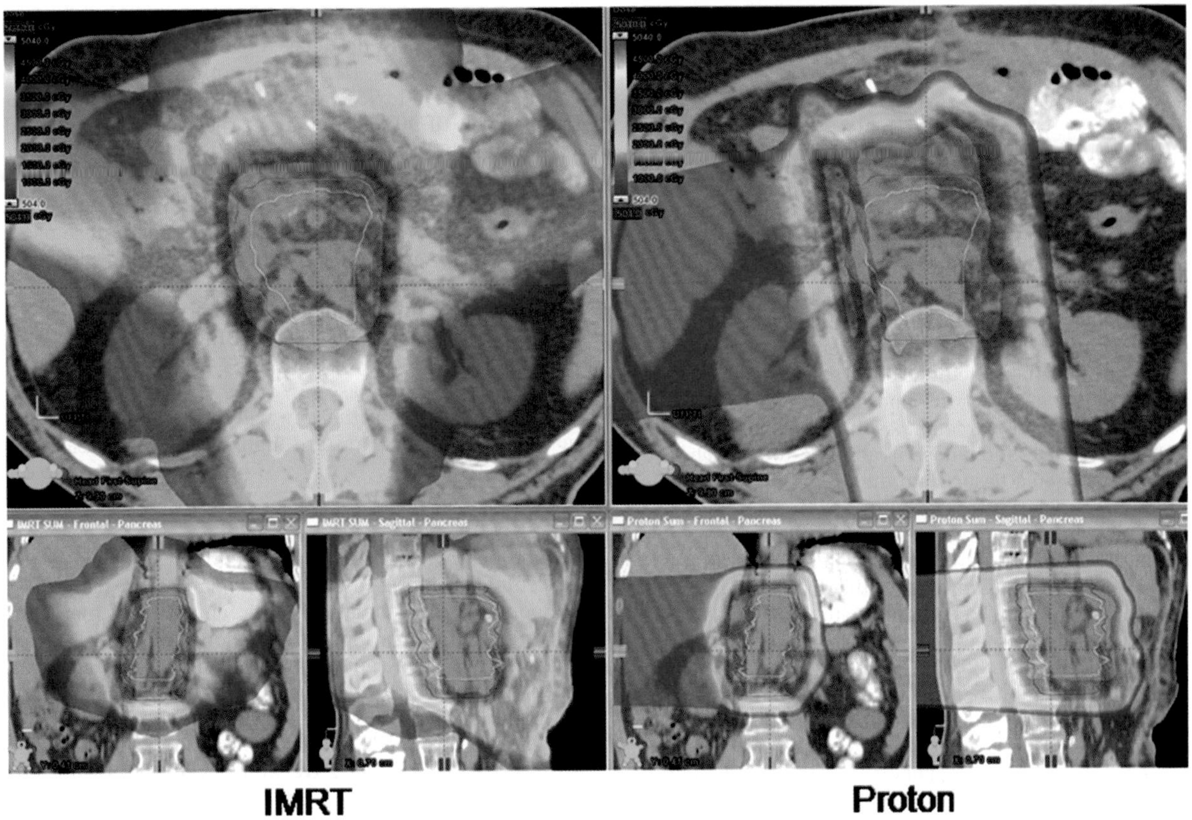

FIGURE 19.9. Axial, coronal, and sagittal planes of intensity-modulated radiation therapy (IMRT; *left*) and proton therapy (*right*) plans for a carcinoma of the pancreatic head. As apparent, there is much less low to intermediate dose to the bowel, kidney, and liver with the proton plan. Mean doses with IMRT and proton therapy are 1,174 cGy and 760 cGy (relative biologic effectiveness [RBE]) to the liver and 1,705 cGy and 443 cGy (RBE) to the small bowel, respectively. While mean right and left kidney doses are similar for the IMRT and proton therapy plans, over 40% of the left kidney tissue is unirradiated with the proton therapy plan.

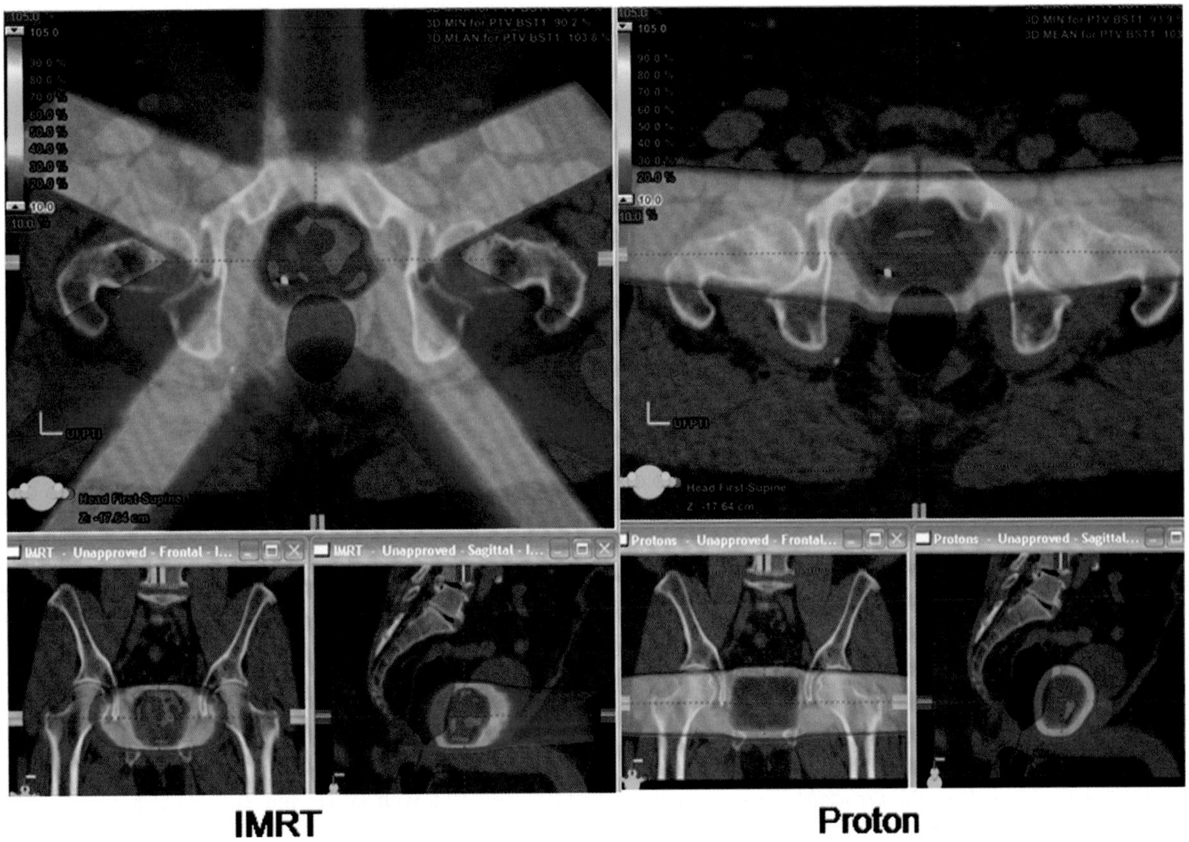

FIGURE 19.10. Axial, coronal, and sagittal planes of intensity-modulated radiation therapy (IMRT; *left*) and proton therapy (*right*) plans for prostate cancer. The five-field IMRT plan appears more conformal than the two-field double-scatter proton therapy plan; however, the proton therapy plan exposes a much smaller volume of nontargeted tissue to radiation. The rectal wall V_{30}, V_{40}, and V_{50} are 29%, 23%, and 17% with the IMRT plan compared to 18%, 16%, and 14% with the proton therapy plan, respectively.

toxicity can be leveraged to facilitate hypofractionation, which may both enhance disease control and reduce health care costs without increasing toxicity.

Skull-Base Sarcomas

Skull-base sarcomas frequently are not amenable to complete resection and require very high radiation doses for disease control. Their adjacency to the brainstem, optic chiasm, and optic nerves often precludes delivery of optimal tumor doses for fear of fatal or severe functional radiation injuries. Proton therapy in these cases can achieve dose distributions that often permit the delivery of potentially curative doses of radiation to the tumor with minimal risk of brainstem necrosis or blindness, and may offer the patient the only realistic chance of cure. Figure 19.3 demonstrates IMRT and proton plans in a patient with skull-base chondrosarcoma. As apparent in Figure 19.3, the IMRT plan delivers low-dose irradiation to a much larger volume of nontargeted tissue than the proton plan, in particular, to the nose, posterior fossa, brainstem, and spinal cord.

The relative minimum dose received by 98% of the volume ($D_{98\%}$), the relative maximum dose received by 2% of the volume ($D_{2\%}$), and the relative mean dose to the spinal cord are 62%, 56%, and 61% with IMRT compared with 16%, 15%, and 1% with proton therapy, respectively. For the brainstem, the $D_{98\%}$, $D_{2\%}$, and mean doses are 20%, 66%, and 42% with IMRT compared with 0%, 39%, and 10% with proton therapy, respectively. The significant reduction in relative dose to the brainstem and spinal cord permits the delivery of higher doses to the tumor with proton therapy. In other skull-base sarcomas, the benefits from proton therapy may differ or differ in degree. With the currently available double-scatter mode of proton delivery, "patch" fields are often required (as in this case) to avoid critical structures at the expense of a considerable increase in planning and delivery complexity to minimize dose inhomogeneities within the target. In essence, separate small fields (which cover parts of the target volume from optimal angles to avoid critical structures) are "patched" together to cover the entire target, somewhat similar to IMRT. In the aforementioned case, $D_{98\%}$, $D_{2\%}$, and mean target doses are 96%, 106%, and 104% with IMRT compared with 94%, 118%, and 110% with proton therapy, respectively. Care must be taken to avoid placing potential hot spots in critical structures. In the future, scanning-mode proton therapy will eliminate the need for patch fields and reduce the need for apertures and compensators, providing increased dose homogeneity within the target.

It is highly likely that the benefits of proton therapy in skull-base tumors will increase with the availability of IMPT. In addition, future improved treatment-planning systems may also more accurately estimate the actual dose inhomogeneity at tissue interfaces and other heterogeneities, including possible surgical hardware in the base of the skull. The dosimetric validation of treatment-planning systems in these complex anatomic regions is difficult and the use of Monte Carlo calculations can be helpful.[32]

Paranasal Sinus Tumors

Paranasal sinus tumors frequently extend into the orbit or anterior cranial fossa adjacent to critical optic structures, such as the chiasm, optic nerves, retinae, lacrimal glands, cornea, and lens. With photon-based therapy, it is often difficult to deliver adequate doses to the entire tumor target without injury to at least one of the critical optic structures. The physician must choose between prioritizing tumor control and preserving vision. Figure 19.4 shows a comparison of IMRT and proton plans in a patient with a paranasal sinus tumor. Both plans were specified to deliver the *prescribed dose to at least 90% of the target volume*. Compared to the proton plan, the IMRT plan exposes a much larger volume of nontargeted tissue to low-dose radiation, which includes the right temporal lobe, posterior fossa, oral cavity, and supratentorial brain. In addition, the IMRT plan produces a less homogeneous dose within the target with $D_{98\%}$, $D_{2\%}$, and mean doses of 82%, 118%, and 109% compared to 93%, 112%, and 106% with proton therapy, respectively. If 90% of the target receives the prescribed dose of 75 Gy/cobalt gray equivalent (CGE), likely necessary to control such tumors, the target dose ranges from approximately 61.5 to 88.5 Gy with a mean dose of 88.5 Gy with IMRT and from 69.8 (RBE) to 84 Gy (RBE) with a mean dose of 79.5 Gy (RBE) with protons. There is relative sparing of most of the optic structures with proton therapy with mean doses to the chiasm, right optic nerve, left optic nerve, and brainstem of 44 and 36 Gy (RBE), 53 and 43 Gy (RBE), 44 and 36 Gy (RBE), and 43 and 29 Gy (RBE) with the IMRT and proton plans, respectively. As with skull-base sarcomas, the benefits and degree of benefits with proton therapy will vary among different paranasal sinus tumors and are highly likely to increase with the availability of IMPT.

Craniopharyngioma

Craniopharyngioma is usually diagnosed in children and adolescents. Its suprasellar location places the temporal lobes, hippocampi, hypothalamus, optic chiasm, and nerves at risk for radiation injury. Figure 19.5 shows IMRT, SRT, and proton plans in an adolescent patient. All three plans achieve target coverage goals of 95% of the prescribed dose (54 Gy) to 100% of the target and 100% of the prescribed dose to at least 95% of the target. Mean body and mean brain doses excluding the PTV are, respectively, 4% (2.2 Gy) and 17% (9.2 Gy) with IMRT, 4% (2.2 Gy) and 15% (8.1 Gy) with SRT, and 1% (0.5 Gy [RBE]) and 6% (3.2 Gy [RBE]) with proton therapy. The relative mean doses with IMRT, SRT, and proton therapy for the following structures are right temporal lobe—17%, 20%, and 8%; left temporal lobe—18%, 22%, and 10%; left hippocampus—50%, 61%, and 16%; right cochlea—16%, 7%, and 0%; and left cochlea—14%, 16%, and 1%, respectively. These reductions in dose to nontargeted brain tissues with proton therapy are likely to result in reduced loss in neurocognitive and auditory function.

Craniospinal Axis Irradiation

Craniospinal axis irradiation is required in most medulloblastomas and occasionally in other brain tumors, such as advanced or metastatic germ cell tumors, primitive neuroectodermal tumors (PNETs), and ependymomas. Most patients with these tumors are young and at risk for late effects of radiation. As shown in Figure 19.6, the exit dose from photon therapy exposes the thyroid, heart, lung, gut, and gonads to functional and neoplastic risks that can be avoided with proton therapy. The total-body V_{10} and total-body integral dose are, respectively, 37.2% and 0.223 Gy-m^3 with 3DCRT compared with 28.7% and 0.185 Gy-m^3 with proton therapy, a reduction likely to result in a lower risk of second malignancy.

Lymphomas

Lymphomas frequently involve the mediastinum but typically require only a moderate dose of radiation therapy in conjunction with chemotherapy for disease control. Unfortunately, even low to moderate radiation doses place the patient at risk for late cardiac injury and second cancers, particularly breast cancers. Figure 19.7 shows a comparison of 3DCRT, IMRT, and proton therapy plans in a young woman with Hodgkin lymphoma. The proton plan shows a significant reduction in the volume of heart, lung, breast, spinal cord, and other soft tissues exposed to low-dose irradiation. Mean relative lung dose, lung V_4, and lung V_{20} are 48%, 59%, and 25% with 3DCRT; 43%, 62%, and 10% with IMRT; and 27%, 31%, and 16% with proton therapy, respectively. Mean relative cardiac dose, cardiac V_4, and cardiac V_{20} are 72%, 79%, and 54% with 3DCRT; 57%, 76%, and 26% with IMRT; and 37%, 40%, and 26% with proton therapy, respectively. These reductions are likely to result in lower risks of late cardiac injury and second malignancy.

Lung Cancers

Lung cancers typically are diagnosed at an advanced stage and occur in patients with underlying lung damage. Consequently, concern for protection of unaffected lung tissue often mandates compromise in the tumor dose. Figure 19.8 shows IMRT and proton plans in a patient with stage III lung cancer. As apparent, a smaller volume of nontargeted lung tissue, spinal cord, esophagus, and heart is exposed to radiation with proton therapy. The mean relative lung dose was 23% with 3DCRT, 19% with IMRT, and 11% with proton therapy. Lung V_4 and V_{20} were 40% and 23% with 3DCRT, 54% and 22% with IMRT, and 22% and 13% with proton therapy, respectively. The mean relative heart dose was 15% with 3DCRT, 9% with IMRT, and 7% with proton therapy. The relative mean esophagus dose was 45% with 3DCRT, 35% with IMRT, and 28.7% with protons. In this case, the proton plan lowers the risk of acute (potentially fatal) pneumonitis and acute esophagitis, likely impacting the delivery of chemotherapy, as well as the cardiac exposure, likely correlating with greater chance of survival.

Pancreatic Cancers

Pancreatic cancers have an extremely low therapeutic ratio with radiation alone or combined with surgery and chemotherapy. The disease is frequently localized for a window of time before spreading, providing a potential opportunity to improve the overall outcome by intensifying local therapy. Figure 19.9 shows IMRT and proton therapy plans for a patient with cancer in the head of the pancreas. As apparent, there is much less low to intermediate dose to the bowel, kidney, and liver with the proton therapy plan. Mean relative doses with IMRT and proton therapy are 23% and 15% to the liver and 34% and 9% to the small bowel, respectively. While mean right and left kidney doses are similar for the IMRT and proton therapy plans, over 40% of the left kidney tissue is unirradiated with the proton therapy plan. This savings in normal-tissue exposure may be leveraged to permit either radiation or chemotherapy dose escalation or intensification, potentially increasing the opportunity for complete surgical resection, cure, or both.

Prostate Cancer

Prostate cancer results with IMRT are generally excellent, but dose-escalation trials from the M.D. Anderson Cancer Center (Houston, TX)[55] show that the volumes of rectum and rectal wall receiving low- to moderate-dose radiation with x-ray-based therapy are significantly associated with the incidence of gastrointestinal toxicity. Dosimetry studies[48] show that the low to moderate doses delivered to the rectum with proton therapy are less than with IMRT. Figure 19.10 shows a five-field IMRT plan and a two-field double-scattered proton plan for a patient with low-risk prostate cancer. Rectal wall V_{30}, V_{40}, and V_{50} were 29%, 23%, and 17% with IMRT compared with 18%, 16%, and 14% with proton therapy, respectively, potentially providing a lower risk of rectal injury (see discussion regarding clinical significance later).

CLINICAL EVIDENCE FOR PROTON THERAPY

Efficacy and Toxicity

Despite the existence of only a few facilities with technology capable of proton delivery to most cancers, the efficacy of proton therapy has already been demonstrated in a variety of malignancies and benign lesions including representative series in eye cancers[56–60]; base of skull sarcomas[61,62]; brain and spinal cord tumors[63,64]; paranasal sinus tumors[65,66]; oropharyngeal carcinoma[67]; esophageal cancer[68]; early- and advanced-stage lung cancer[69,70]; low-, intermediate-, and high-risk prostate cancer[71–73]; Hodgkin and other lymphomas[74,75]; sarcomas[76]; a variety of pediatric malignancies[77–81]; hepatocellular carcinoma[82]; pancreatic cancer[83]; cervical cancer[84]; and benign lesions like acoustic neuroma, vestibular schwannoma, arteriovenous malformations (AVMs), age-related macular degeneration, pituitary adenomas, craniopharyngiomas, and meningioma.[85,86] In general, toxicity rates reported with proton therapy appear to be low; however, comparisons with contemporary x-ray-based therapies are often difficult because of the absence of controlled studies, small patient numbers, patient selection, lack of appropriate comparative groups, and variable criteria for toxicity assessment.

Comparative Effectiveness

In most clinical situations, level 1 evidence of comparative effectiveness is desirable; however, it has been difficult to conduct randomized controlled trials in proton therapy. While there may be small differences in relative biologic effectiveness with proton therapy compared to photon therapy, laboratory and clinical data suggest that these differences are quite small. Therefore, the basic difference between protons and photons is simply the difference in entrance dose and exit dose to nontargeted tissues. The essence of a randomized controlled clinical trial of proton therapy and x-ray-based therapy would be the question of whether low to intermediate doses to nontargeted tissue would result in measureable good or harm to a patient. The nature of this question raises some ethical concerns. In addition, there are practical issues: patients may not choose to enroll in such a trial, particularly if they must travel to one of the few currently available proton facilities to face randomization between proton and photon therapy. Finally, the numbers of patients and resources required for randomized controlled trials raise concerns regarding the best use of currently available proton therapy facilities, specifically whether more questions could be answered using the same time frame, number of patients, and level of resources with a series of well-designed sequential studies aimed at optimizing proton therapy through dose escalation or hypofractionation. For a variety of ethical and practical reasons, there are currently no completed prospective randomized comparative-effectiveness trials between proton therapy and other radiation modalities, although two are under way. One randomized trial between proton therapy and IMRT in stage III lung cancer is ongoing as collaboration between the M.D. Anderson Cancer Center and Massachusetts General Hospital (Boston, MA). A second trial at the University of Heidelberg (Germany) in skull-base sarcomas randomizes patients to either proton therapy or carbon ion therapy.[87]

When there is a compelling dosimetric advantage to proton therapy, or strongly suggestive level 2 and 3 clinical evidence, level 1 evidence of an increased therapeutic ratio may not be necessary. Examples of clinical situations in which level 1 evidence may not be necessary include base-of-skull and paranasal sinus tumors, pediatric and young adult cancers, and eye malignancies.

The therapeutic ratio in paranasal sinus tumors with conventional x-ray-based radiation therapy has been low, with either low cure rates[88] or high visual toxicity rates,[89] which suggests physician prioritization of toxicity avoidance in the first scenario and tumor control in the second. Dosimetry studies comparing proton therapy and IMRT in patients with paranasal sinus tumors have suggested a substantial benefit in dose distribution from proton therapy[40,90] that could lead to clinical benefits. Reports of the clinical experience with proton therapy for paranasal tumors from Massachusetts General Hospital suggest a notably higher therapeutic ratio, with both high disease control rates and low toxicity rates,[65,66] than previously reported.[88,89] Such remarkable improvements in the therapeutic ratio for proton therapy compared with contemporary x-ray-based experiences may obviate the need for a controlled trial. Similarly, excellent disease control rates have been achieved in skull-base sarcomas at Massachusetts General Hospital with proton therapy dose regimens that are not feasible with photon-based therapy, likely obviating the desire for level 1 clinical evidence for proton therapy.

In pediatric cancer survivors, an increased risk of second malignancies has been associated with radiation doses as low as 4 to 15 Gy.[91,92] Similar doses are believed to be associated with increased late cardiac injury.[93] In addition, elegant dose-modeling studies at St. Jude Children's Hospital (Memphis, TN) have suggested no threshold dose for radiation injury in the childhood brain.[94] Thousands of children and many years of follow-up would be required to assess the results of a hypothetical controlled trial of proton therapy and conventional radiation to determine whether the reduction in low-dose exposure to the brain and total body with proton therapy would indeed result in a lower incidence of second malignancies or late cardiac injury. In the process, many children would intentionally be exposed to low-dose radiation in nontargeted tissues in the brain, likely resulting in permanent decreased neurocognitive function. Therefore, most clinicians consider the dosimetric evidence of significant reduction in the volume of tissue exposed to low- and moderate-dose irradiation sufficiently compelling to obviate the need for a controlled trial of proton therapy in children. Similar arguments follow for Hodgkin lymphoma, another malignancy occurring in relatively young patients. Hodgkin lymphoma has a high cure rate and long life expectancy but also high risks for second malignancy and late cardiac injury.[44,45]

There is substantial experience with proton therapy for choroidal and uveal melanomas. Several large retrospective comparative studies of long-term outcomes using various strategies for choroidal or uveal melanoma have provided solid level 2 evidence of the benefits from proton therapy[57] with respect to disease control and preservation of vision, likely making a controlled trial unnecessary.

The area of greatest controversy is prostate cancer. More than 10,000 men with prostate cancer have been treated with proton therapy or a combination of proton therapy and photon therapy with excellent results. Disease control rates appear comparable to outcomes with photon therapy given with the same dose-fractionation schedules[72]; however, toxicity, particularly rectal toxicity, appears to be lower with proton therapy than with photon therapy at the same dose-fractionation schedules.[71–73] While dose-escalation trials in prostate cancer have typically demonstrated a significant rise in toxicity with higher doses,[55,95,96] when protons were used for approximately one-third of the dose in one dose-escalation trial,[73] there was no significant increase in grade 3 toxicity with the higher doses, and toxicity rates for both dose levels appeared to be lower than reported with contemporary photon dose-escalation trials. A Radiation Therapy Oncology Group (RTOG) study of 3DCRT in localized prostate cancer[97] found that increasing both the daily dose to 2 Gy and the total dose to 78 Gy resulted in a higher risk of grade 2 or higher gastrointestinal toxicity than observed with regimens of 79.2 Gy or less delivered in 1.8-Gy once-daily fractions or 74 Gy delivered in once-daily fractions of 2 Gy. The rate of grade 3 or higher gastrointestinal toxicity with 78 Gy delivered in 2-Gy fractions was 4% when the prostate only was treated and 7% when the prostate and part of the seminal vesicles were treated. In contrast, with proton therapy on three prospective trials at a single institution, a grade 3 toxicity rate of <1% was observed with doses of 78 Gy (RBE) delivered in once-daily 2-Gy (RBE) fractions,[71] suggesting that even small reductions in the volume of rectum exposed to moderate radiation doses may impact the rate of radiation toxicity and that, in the case of prostate cancer, these relatively small toxicity reductions may facilitate the delivery of hypofractionated regimens, which could reduce health care costs and potentially increase disease control.[98] Because increased toxicity observed with dose escalation and hypofractionation (or dose intensification) with photons[55,95–97] has not been observed thus far in the proton experiences,[71,73] there is speculation that the potential benefits from proton therapy in prostate cancer may be increasingly apparent with either dose-escalated or hypofractionated regimens. One driver of interest in comparative effectiveness has been economic concern—proton therapy appears more expensive than photon therapy. Differential potential for safe hypofractionation of the treatment regimen might reverse the economic concerns regarding the cost-effectiveness of proton therapy and photon therapy.

ECONOMICS

Many factors must be accounted for in comparing the costliness and cost-effectiveness of different radiation technologies. Some of these include facility and equipment costs, operating and maintenance costs, patient throughput, and the global and individual financial impact of clinical outcomes. The perspectives of the patient, the providing physician and institution, the payor, and the nation on these factors may differ.

Current proton therapy equipment and facilities are up to 10-fold more expensive than current conventional radiation therapy facilities capable of treating a similar patient volume. In addition, operating costs are higher by one- to threefold. However, there are substantial differences between patient throughput in conventional radiation and proton facilities that must be accounted for in any financial comparison.

Conventional radiation therapy business models are based on treating a single—or slightly extended—shift each day, 5 days a week. The equipment generally depreciates over 7 to 10 years and replacement occurs when equipment begins to fail, becomes technically obsolescent, or is less promising than an alternative technology. When capacity with a single shift is exceeded, most facilities choose to add another treatment machine rather than add another shift of personnel. It is possible that many conventional radiation facilities are underutilized, replaced prematurely, or both; however, either economic considerations or equipment durability issues continue to support the single-shift model of conventional radiation therapy delivery and the 7- to 10-year replacement schedules.

In contrast, most proton therapy facilities operate two shifts a day and equipment is sufficiently robust to last 20 or more years. The Harvard cyclotron was in use for over 40 years and closed primarily because of the availability of a new gantry-based clinical facility. The Loma Linda University (Loma Linda, CA) synchrotron and most of its gantries have been in continuous operation for over 20 years. Proton therapy equipment appears to be substantially more durable than linear accelerators. Patient mix in conventional radiation therapy and proton therapy facilities may differ, but there does not appear to be a significant difference in time required for treatment of a given clinical condition. Thus, the actual patient throughput (for a given patient mix) in a proton facility may be substantially higher than typical for a conventional radiation therapy facility, perhaps double the patients per day (because of double shifts) for two to six times as many years of operation, leading to a four- to 12-fold increased throughput with proton facilities compared to photon facilities. Proton therapy throughput may be further enhanced if hypofractionation is more feasible with proton therapy than with x-rays. (As discussed earlier, proton therapy has been delivered to early-stage prostate cancer patients in 8 weeks with the same or less toxicity as a 9-week course of IMRT.[71,97,99])

While initial capital costs and operational costs of proton facilities are substantially higher than conventional radiation facilities, long-term patient throughput with a proton facility may more than offset the initial capital costs and increased operational costs. If patient outcomes are also improved with proton therapy, as the rationale and early data in some tumor sites suggest, there will be additional savings related to reduced costs associated with treatment toxicity and disease recurrences. Accordingly, a blanket statement comparing cost-effectiveness of proton therapy and photon therapy based solely on initial capital costs of equipment is naïve and misleading.

Nevertheless, a shift to proton therapy requires a paradigm shift in philosophy about profit: it will not be a rapid "return on investment" but rather a benefit realized over time by way of increased throughput and improved outcomes. Daily operations must be focused not on work completion within a shift, but on maximal utilization of beam time, which implies focused attention on preventative maintenance, facility staffing, patient expectations, and program culture.

CONCLUSIONS

Proton therapy offers the promise of reduced toxicity to patients compared with photon therapy by reducing the radiation dose to nontargeted tissues. Reduced toxicity may be leveraged to increase disease control through dose escalation or intensification (hypofractionation). Hypofractionation may result in lower health care costs, as well as increased disease control and reduced toxicity. Additional research is needed to optimize treatment planning and delivery of proton therapy, to document and maximize its potential clinical benefits, and to understand its full impact on health care economics.

REFERENCES

1. DeLuca P, Wambersie A, Whitmore G. Prescribing, recording, and reporting proton-beam therapy (ICRU Report 78). *J ICRU* 2007;7.
2. Paganetti H, Niemierko A, Ancukiewicz M, et al. Relative biological effectiveness (RBE) values for proton beam therapy. *Int J Radiat Oncol Biol Phys* 2002;53: 407–421.
3. Paganetti H, Goitein M. Radiobiological significance of beamline dependent proton energy distributions in a spread-out Bragg peak. *Med Phys* 2000;27:1119–1126.
4. Combs SE, Bohl J, Elsasser T, et al. Radiobiological evaluation and correlation with the local effect model (LEM) of carbon ion radiation therapy and temozolomide in glioblastoma cell lines. *Int J Radiat Biol* 2009;85:126–137.
5. Paganetti H. Nuclear interactions in proton therapy: dose and relative biological effect distributions originating from primary and secondary particles. *Phys Med Biol* 2002;47:747–764.
6. Hall EJ. Intensity-modulated radiation therapy, protons, and the risk of second cancers. *Int J Radiat Oncol Biol Phys* 2006;65:1–7.
7. Hall EJ, Wuu CS. Radiation-induced second cancers: the Impact of 3D-CRT and IMRT. *Int J Radiat Oncol Biol Phys* 2003;56:83–88.
8. Newhauser WD, Durante M. Assessing the risk of second malignancies after modern radiotherapy. *Nat Rev Cancer* 2011;11:438–448.
9. Tsunashima Y, Vedam S, Dong L, et al. The precision of respiratory-gated delivery of synchrotron-based pulsed beam proton therapy. *Phys Med Biol* 2010;55:7633–7647.
10. Smith A, Gillin M, Bues M, et al. The M. D. Anderson proton therapy system. *Med Phys* 2009;36:4068–4083.
11. Paganetti H, Jiang H, Lee SY, et al. Accurate Monte Carlo simulations for nozzle design, commissioning and quality assurance for a proton radiation therapy facility. *Med Phys* 2004;31:2107–2118.
12. Schippers JM, Lomax AJ. Emerging technologies in proton therapy. *Acta Oncol* 2011;50:838–850.
13. Akagi T, Higashi A, Tsugami H, et al. Ridge filter design for proton therapy at Hyogo Ion Beam Medical Center. *Phys Med Biol* 2003;48:N301–N312.
14. Urie M, Goitein M, Wagner M. Compensating for heterogeneities in proton radiation therapy. *Phys Med Biol* 1984;29:553–566.
15. Pedroni E, Bacher R, Blattmann H, et al. The 200-MeV proton therapy project at the Paul Scherrer Institute: conceptual design and practical realization. *Med Phys* 1995;22:37–53.
16. Pedroni E, Bearpark R, Bohringer T, et al. The PSI Gantry 2: a second generation proton scanning gantry. *Z Med Phys* 2004;14:25–34.
17. Kooy HM, Clasie BM, Lu HM, et al. A case study in proton pencil-beam scanning delivery. *Int J Radiat Oncol Biol Phys* 2010;76:624–630.
18. Yu CX, Jaffray DA, Wong JW. The effects of intra-fraction organ motion on the delivery of dynamic intensity modulation. *Phys Med Biol* 1998;43:91–104.
19. Bortfeld T, Jokivarsi K, Goitein M, et al. Effects of intra-fraction motion on IMRT dose delivery: statistical analysis and simulation. *Phys Med Biol* 2002;47:2203–2220.
20. Paganetti H, Jiang H, Adams JA, et al. Monte Carlo simulations with time-dependent geometries to investigate effects of organ motion with high temporal resolution. *Int J Radiat Oncol Biol Phys* 2004;60:942–950.
21. Zenklusen SM, Pedroni E, Meer D. A study on repainting strategies for treating moderately moving targets with proton pencil beam scanning at the new Gantry 2 at PSI. *Phys Med Biol* 2010;55:5103–5121.
22. Schneider U, Pedroni E, Lomax A. The calibration of CT Hounsfield units for radiotherapy treatment planning. *Phys MedBiol* 1996;41:111–124.
23. Szymanowski H, Oelfke U. CT calibration for two-dimensional scaling of proton pencil beams. *Phys Med Biol* 2003;48:861–874.
24. Moyers MF, Miller DW, Bush DA, et al. Methodologies and tools for proton beam design for lung tumors. *Int J Radiat Oncol Biol Phys* 2001;49:1429–1438.
25. Measurements ICoRUa. *Prescribing, recording, and reporting proton-beam therapy (ICRU Report 50)*. Bethesda, MD, 1993, Contract No.: 50.
26. Measurements ICoRUa. *Prescribing, recording, and reporting photon beam therapy (ICRU Report 62)*. Bethesda, MD, 1999, Contract No.: 62.
27. Schaffner B, Pedroni E, Lomax A. Dose calculation models for proton treatment planning using a dynamic beam delivery system: an attempt to include density heterogeneity effects in the analytical dose calculation. *Phys Med Biol* 1999;44: 27–41.
28. Szymanowski H, Oelfke U. Two-dimensional pencil beam scaling: an improved proton dose algorithm for heterogeneous media. *Phys Med Biol* 2002;47: 3313–3330.
29. Bortfeld T. An analytical approximation of the Bragg curve for therapeutic proton beams. *Med Phys* 1997;24:2024–2033.
30. Hong L, Goitein M, Bucciolini M, et al. A pencil beam algorithm for proton dose calculations. *Phys Med Biol* 1996;41:1305–1330.
31. Ciangaru G, Polf JC, Bues M, et al. Benchmarking analytical calculations of proton doses in heterogeneous matter. *Med Phys* 2005;32:3511–3523.
32. Paganetti H, Jiang H, Parodi K, et al. Clinical implementation of full Monte Carlo dose calculation in proton beam therapy. *Phys Med Biol* 2008;53:4825–4853.
33. Newhauser W, Fontenot J, Zheng Y, et al. Monte Carlo simulations for configuring and testing an analytical proton dose-calculation algorithm. *Phys Med Biol* 2007; 52:4569–4584.
34. Fippel M, Soukup M. A Monte Carlo dose calculation algorithm for proton therapy. *Med Phys* 2004;31:2263–2273.
35. Yepes P, Randeniya S, Taddei PJ, et al. Monte Carlo fast dose calculator for proton radiotherapy: application to a voxelized geometry representing a patient with prostate cancer. *Phys Med Biol* 2009;54:N21–N28.
36. Hotta K, Kohno R, Takada Y, et al. Improved dose-calculation accuracy in proton treatment planning using a simplified Monte Carlo method verified with three-dimensional measurements in an anthropomorphic phantom. *Phys Med Biol* 2010;55:3545–3556.
37. Weber DC, Bogner J, Verwey J, et al. Proton beam radiotherapy versus fractionated stereotactic radiotherapy for uveal melanomas: a comparative study. *Int J Radiat Oncol Biol Phys* 2005;63:373–384.
38. Beltran C, Roca M, Merchant TE. On the benefits and risks of proton therapy in pediatric craniopharyngioma. *Int J Radiat Oncol Biol Phys* 2012;82(2)e281–e287.
39. Boehling NS, Grosshans DR, Bluett JB, et al. Dosimetric comparison of three-dimensional conformal proton radiotherapy, intensity-modulated proton therapy, and intensity-modulated radiotherapy for treatment of pediatric craniopharyngiomas. *Int J Radiat Oncol Biol Phys* 2012;82(2):643–652.
40. Chera BS, Malyapa R, Louis D, et al. Proton therapy for maxillary sinus carcinoma. *Am J Clin Oncol* 2009;32:296–303.
41. Mock U, Georg D, Bogner J, et al. Treatment planning comparison of conventional, 3D conformal, and intensity-modulated photon (IMRT) and proton therapy for paranasal sinus carcinoma. *Int J Radiat Oncol Biol Phys* 2004;58:147–154.
42. Chang JY, Zhang X, Wang X, et al. Significant reduction of normal tissue dose by proton radiotherapy compared with three-dimensional conformal or intensity-modulated radiation therapy in stage I or stage III non-small-cell lung cancer. *Int J Radiat Oncol Biol Phys* 2006;65:1087–1096.
43. Zhang X, Li Y, Pan X, et al. Intensity-modulated proton therapy reduces the dose to normal tissue compared with intensity-modulated radiation therapy or passive scattering proton therapy and enables individualized radical radiotherapy for extensive stage IIIB non-small-cell lung cancer: a virtual clinical study. *Int J Radiat Oncol Biol Phys* 2010;77:357–366.
44. Hoppe BS, Flampouri S, Su Z, et al. Consolidative involved-node proton therapy for stage IA-IIIB mediastinal hodgkin lymphoma: preliminary dosimetric outcomes from a phase II study. *Int J Radiat Oncol Biol Phys* 2012;83(1)260–267.
45. Chera BS, Rodriguez C, Morris CG, et al. Dosimetric comparison of three different involved nodal irradiation techniques for stage II Hodgkin's lymphoma patients: conventional radiotherapy, intensity-modulated radiotherapy, and three-dimensional proton radiotherapy. *Int J Radiat Oncol Biol Phys* 2009;75:1173–1180.
46. Bouchard M, Amos RA, Briere TM, et al. Dose escalation with proton or photon radiation treatment for pancreatic cancer. *Radiother Oncol* 2009;92:238–243.
47. Welsh J, Gomez D, Palmer MB, et al. Intensity-modulated proton therapy further reduces normal tissue exposure during definitive therapy for locally advanced distal esophageal tumors: a dosimetric study. *Int J Radiat Oncol Biol Phys* 2011; 81(5):1336–1342.
48. Vargas C, Fryer A, Mahajan C, et al. Dose-volume comparison of proton therapy and intensity-modulated radiotherapy for prostate cancer. *Int J Radiat Oncol Biol Phys* 2008;70:744–751.
49. Fontenot JD, Lee AK, Newhauser WD. Risk of secondary malignant neoplasms from proton therapy and intensity-modulated x-ray therapy for early-stage prostate cancer. *Int J Radiat Oncol Biol Phys* 2009;74:616–622.
50. Slater JD, Slater JM, Wahlen S. The potential for proton beam therapy in locally advanced carcinoma of the cervix. *Int J Radiat Oncol Biol Phys* 1992;22:343–347.
51. Moon SH, Shin KH, Kim TH, et al. Dosimetric comparison of four different external beam partial breast irradiation techniques: three-dimensional conformal radiotherapy, intensity-modulated radiotherapy, helical tomotherapy, and proton beam therapy. *Radiother Oncol* 2009;90:66–73.
52. Ares C, Khan S, Macartain AM, et al. Postoperative proton radiotherapy for localized and locoregional breast cancer: potential for clinically relevant improvements? *Int J Radiat Oncol Biol Phys* 2009;76:685–697.
53. Chera BS, Vargas C, Morris CG, et al. Dosimetric study of pelvic proton radiotherapy for high-risk prostate cancer. *Int J Radiat Oncol Biol Phys* 2009;75: 994–1002.
54. Krejcarek SC, Grant PE, Henson JW, et al. Physiologic and radiographic evidence of the distal edge of the proton beam in craniospinal irradiation. *Int J Radiat Oncol Biol Phys* 2007;68:646–649.
55. Kuban DA, Tucker SL, Dong L, et al. Long-term results of the M. D. Anderson randomized dose-escalation trial for prostate cancer. *Int J Radiat Oncol Biol Phys* 2008;70:67–74.
56. Caujolle JP, Mammar H, Chamorey E, et al. Proton beam radiotherapy for uveal melanomas at nice teaching hospital: 16 years' experience. *Int J Radiat Oncol Biol Phys* 2010;78:98–103.
57. Char DH, Kroll S, Phillips TL, et al. Late radiation failures after iodine 125 brachytherapy for uveal melanoma compared with charged-particle (proton or helium ion) therapy. *Ophthalmology* 2002;109:1850–1854.

58. Damato B, Kacperek A, Chopra M, et al. Proton beam radiotherapy of choroidal melanoma: the Liverpool-Clatterbridge experience. *Int J Radiat Oncol Biol Phys* 2005;62:1405–1411.
59. Wilson MW, Hungerford JL. Comparison of episcleral plaque and proton beam radiation therapy for the treatment of choroidal melanoma. *Ophthalmology* 1999;106:1579–1587.
60. Char DH, Quivey JM, Castro JR, et al. Helium ions versus iodine 125 brachytherapy in the management of uveal melanoma. A prospective, randomized, dynamically balanced trial. *Ophthalmology* 1993;100:1547–1554.
61. Munzenrider JE, Liebsch NJ. Proton therapy for tumors of the skull base. *Strahlenther Onkol* 1999;175:57–63.
62. Weber DC, Rutz HP, Pedroni ES, et al. Results of spot-scanning proton radiation therapy for chordoma and chondrosarcoma of the skull base: the Paul Scherrer Institut experience. *Int J Radiat Oncol Biol Phys* 2005;63:401–409.
63. Mizumoto M, Tsuboi K, Igaki H, et al. Phase I/II trial of hyperfractionated concomitant boost proton radiotherapy for supratentorial glioblastoma multiforme. *Int J Radiat Oncol Biol Phys* 2010;77:98–105.
64. Kahn J, Loeffler JS, Niemierko A, et al. Long-term outcomes of patients with spinal cord gliomas treated by modern conformal radiation techniques. *Int J Radiat Oncol Biol Phys* 2011;81:232–238.
65. Chan AW, Liebsch NJ. Proton radiation therapy for head and neck cancer. *J Surg Oncol* 2008;97:697–700.
66. Weber DC, Chan AW, Lessell S, et al. Visual outcome of accelerated fractionated radiation for advanced sinonasal malignancies employing photons/protons. *Radiother Oncol* 2006;81:243–249.
67. Slater JD, Yonemoto LT, Mantik DW, et al. Proton radiation for treatment of cancer of the oropharynx: early experience at Loma Linda University Medical Center using a concomitant boost technique. *Int J Radiat Oncol Biol Phys* 2005;62: 494–500.
68. Mizumoto M, Sugahara S, Okumura T, et al. Hyperfractionated concomitant boost proton beam therapy for esophageal carcinoma. *Int J Radiat Oncol Biol Phys* 2011;81(4):e601–e606.
69. Chang JY, Komaki R, Lu C, et al. Phase 2 study of high-dose proton therapy with concurrent chemotherapy for unresectable stage III nonsmall cell lung cancer. *Cancer* 2011.
70. Bush DA, Slater JD, Shin BB, et al. Hypofractionated proton beam radiotherapy for stage I lung cancer. *Chest* 2004;126:1198–1203.
71. Mendenhall NP, Li Z, Hoppe BS, et al. Early outcomes from three prospective trials of image-guided proton therapy for prostate cancer. *Int J Radiat Oncol Biol Phys* 2012;82(1):213–221.
72. Slater JD, Rossi CJ Jr, Yonemoto LT, et al. Proton therapy for prostate cancer: the initial Loma Linda University experience. *Int J Radiat Oncol Biol Phys* 2004;59: 348–352.
73. Zietman AL, Bae K, Slater JD, et al. Randomized trial comparing conventional-dose with high-dose conformal radiation therapy in early-stage adenocarcinoma of the prostate: long-term results from proton radiation oncology group/American College of Radiology 95-09. *J Clin Oncol* 2010;28:1106–1111.
74. Li J, Dabaja B, Reed V, et al. Rationale for and preliminary results of proton beam therapy for mediastinal lymphoma. *Int J Radiat Oncol Biol Phys* 2011;81:167–174.
75. Hoppe BS, Flampouri S, Li Z, et al. Cardiac sparing with proton therapy in consolidative radiation therapy for Hodgkin lymphoma. *Leuk Lymphoma* 2010;51: 1559–1562.
76. Delaney TF, Liebsch NJ, Pedlow FX, et al. Phase II study of high-dose photon/proton radiotherapy in the management of spine sarcomas. *Int J Radiat Oncol Biol Phys* 2009;74:732–739.
77. MacDonald SM, Safai S, Trofimov A, et al. Proton radiotherapy for childhood ependymoma: initial clinical outcomes and dose comparisons. *Int J Radiat Oncol Biol Phys* 2008;71:979–986.
78. MacDonald SM, Trofimov A, Safai S, et al. Proton radiotherapy for pediatric central nervous system germ cell tumors: early clinical outcomes. *Int J Radiat Oncol Biol Phys* 2011;79:121–129.
79. Timmermann B, Schuck A, Niggli F, et al. Spot-scanning proton therapy for malignant soft tissue tumors in childhood: first experiences at the Paul Scherrer Institute. *Int J Radiat Oncol Biol Phys* 2007;67:497–504.
80. Yock T, Schneider R, Friedmann A, et al. Proton radiotherapy for orbital rhabdomyosarcoma: clinical outcome and a dosimetric comparison with photons. *Int J Radiat Oncol Biol Phys* 2005;63:1161–1168.
81. Habrand JL, Schneider R, Alapetite C, et al. Proton therapy in pediatric skull base and cervical canal low-grade bone malignancies. *Int J Radiat Oncol Biol Phys* 2008;71:672–675.
82. Mizumoto M, Okumura T, Hashimoto T, et al. Proton beam therapy for hepatocellular carcinoma: a comparison of three treatment protocols. *Int J Radiat Oncol Biol Phys* 2011;81(4):1039–1045.
83. Hong TS, Ryan DP, Blaszkowsky LS, et al. Phase I study of preoperative short-course chemoradiation with proton beam therapy and capecitabine for resectable pancreatic ductal adenocarcinoma of the head. *Int J Radiat Oncol Biol Phys* 2011;79:151–157.
84. Kagei K, Tokuuye K, Okumura T, et al. Long-term results of proton beam therapy for carcinoma of the uterine cervix. *Int J Radiat Oncol Biol Phys* 2003;55:1265–1271.
85. Zambarakji HJ, Lane AM, Ezra E, et al. Proton beam irradiation for neovascular age-related macular degeneration. *Ophthalmology* 2006;113:2012–2019.
86. Noel G, Bollet MA, Calugaru V, et al. Functional outcome of patients with benign meningioma treated by 3D conformal irradiation with a combination of photons and protons. *Int J Radiat Oncol Biol Phys* 2005;62:1412–1422.
87. Nikoghosyan AV, Karapanagiotou-Schenkel I, Munter MW, et al. Randomised trial of proton vs. carbon ion radiation therapy in patients with chordoma of the skull base, clinical phase III study HIT-1-Study. *BMC Cancer* 2010;10:607.
88. Hoppe BS, Nelson CJ, Gomez DR, et al. Unresectable carcinoma of the paranasal sinuses: outcomes and toxicities. *Int J Radiat Oncol Biol Phys* 2008;72:763–769.
89. Mendenhall WM, Amdur RJ, Morris CG, et al. Carcinoma of the nasal cavity and paranasal sinuses. *Laryngoscope* 2009;119:899–906.
90. Lomax AJ, Goitein M, Adams J. Intensity modulation in radiotherapy: photons versus protons in the paranasal sinus. *Radiother Oncol* 2003;66:11–18.
91. Travis LB, Hill DA, Dores GM, et al. Breast cancer following radiotherapy and chemotherapy among young women with Hodgkin disease. *JAMA* 2003;290:465–475.
92. van den Belt-Dusebout AW, Aleman BM, Besseling G, et al. Roles of radiation dose and chemotherapy in the etiology of stomach cancer as a second malignancy. *Int J Radiat Oncol Biol Phys* 2009;75:1420–1429.
93. Mulrooney DA, Yeazel MW, Kawashima T, et al. Cardiac outcomes in a cohort of adult survivors of childhood and adolescent cancer: retrospective analysis of the Childhood Cancer Survivor Study cohort. *BMJ* 2009;339:b4606.
94. Merchant TE, Kiehna EN, Li C, et al. Radiation dosimetry predicts IQ after conformal radiation therapy in pediatric patients with localized ependymoma. *Int J Radiat Oncol Biol Phys* 2005;63:1546–1554.
95. Peeters ST, Heemsbergen WD, Koper PC, et al. Dose-response in radiotherapy for localized prostate cancer: results of the Dutch multicenter randomized phase III trial comparing 68 Gy of radiotherapy with 78 Gy. *J Clin Oncol* 2006;24: 1990–1996.
96. Dearnaley DP, Sydes MR, Graham JD, et al. Escalated-dose versus standard-dose conformal radiotherapy in prostate cancer: first results from the MRC RT01 randomised controlled trial. *Lancet Oncol* 2007;8:475–487.
97. Michalski JM, Bae K, Roach M, et al. Long-term toxicity following 3D conformal radiation therapy for prostate cancer from the RTOG 9406 phase I/II dose escalation study. *Int J Radiat Oncol Biol Phys* 2010;76:14–22.
98. Arcangeli G, Saracino B, Gomellini S, et al. A prospective phase III randomized trial of hypofractionation versus conventional fractionation in patients with high-risk prostate cancer. *Int J Radiat Oncol Biol Phys* 2010;78:11–18.
99. Zelefsky MJ, Levin EJ, Hunt M, et al. Incidence of late rectal and urinary toxicities after three-dimensional conformal radiotherapy and intensity-modulated radiotherapy for localized prostate cancer. *Int J Radiat Oncol Biol Phys* 2008; 70:1124–1129.

Chapter 20
Carbon Ions

Pascal Pommier, Stephanie E. Combs, and Tadashi Kamada

PRESENT STATUS AND PERSPECTIVE FOR CARBON IONS

Carbon ion therapy is an innovative radiotherapy modality that is mostly dedicated to cancers considered as unresectable and radioresistant to photons. Its radiobiologic properties combine the advantages of the high-dose distribution conformity of protons for deep tumors (superior to photons and neutrons) and the higher biologic effectiveness (compared to photons and protons) of high linear energy transfer (LET) particles such as neutrons. Moreover, the combination of the biologic and ballistic properties of carbon ions greatly reduces the treatment period compared with photon or proton radiotherapy.

Lawrence Berkeley Laboratory

The use of charged particles (protons and ions) for clinical applications was first proposed in 1946 by R. R. Wilson.[1] A decade later, the Lawrence Berkeley Laboratory (LBL) in California started patient irradiation. The LBL began with protons in 1954 and then with light ions. From 1957 through 1974, helium and higher particles were used in more than 2,000 patients. From 1974 through 1992, the year of closure of the center, neon ions were primarily used in 433 patients. Few patients were treated with carbon ions at the LBL. Miscellaneous cancer types were treated with neon ions, mainly base of skull tumors with several pathologic types, including chordoma, chondrosarcoma, meningioma, and adenoid cystic carcinomas (ACCs), as well as osteosarcomas, sacral chordoma, glioblastoma, cholangiocarcinoma, head and neck squamous cell carcinoma, and prostate cancer. Despite severe limitations in terms of beam application (fixed horizontal beam only), quality of imaging modalities available at that time, and limited periods for clinical applications (30% of the Bevalac running time), the LBL experience permitted first to report a high local tumor control in radioresistant tumors, especially with neon particles, and to demonstrate the feasibility and the safety of high LET particle therapy.[2–6]

National Institute of Radiological Sciences

The heavy ion radiotherapy project in Japan started in 1984. A unique double-synchrotron ring heavy ion accelerator system dedicated to the project was designed and constructed. It system consists of two ion sources, a radiofrequency quadrupole (RFQ) linear accelerator, an Alvarez linear accelerator, two synchrotron rings, a high-energy beam transport system, and an irradiation system. It was completed in October 1993 at the National Institute of Radiological Sciences (NIRS) in Chiba, Japan, and was named the heavy ion medical accelerator in Chiba (HIMAC). At NIRS, there are three treatment rooms with fixed vertical and horizontal beam lines. The accelerated energy of the vertical carbon ion beam is 290 MeV per nucleon or 350 MeV per nucleon, and that of the horizontal beam is 290 MeV per nucleon or 400 MeV per nucleon. The range of the 290-MeV per nucleon carbon ion beam is approximately 15 cm in water, that of the 350-MeV per nucleon beam is 20 cm, and that of the 400-MeV per nucleon carbon ion beam is 25 cm. Maximum field size is 15 cm by 15 cm.[7] To produce uniform irradiation fields, a passive beam delivery system is employed with a pair of wobbler magnets and a scatterer. The range shifter is applied for adjusting the residual range of carbon ions in the patient and the ridge filter to spread out the Bragg peak in the depth-dose distribution of carbon ions. After commissioning of the system, including preclinical biologic study, in June 1994, NIRS started heavy ion radiotherapy using carbon ion beams generated by HIMAC.[8]

Since 1994, clinical studies to develop safe and secure irradiation technologies such as respiration gating and optimized dose fractionation for various cancers have been conducted. All carbon therapies have been performed as prospective phase I/II and II clinical trials in an attempt to identify tumor sites suitable for this treatment, including radioresistant tumors, and to determine optimal dose fractionation, especially for hypofractionation in common cancers. In the phase I/II studies to confirm the safety of carbon ion therapy and to obtain a clue to an antitumor effect, the number of fractions and treatment period were fixed for each disease, and the total dose was gradually increased by 5% to 10%. When the recommended doses were determined in the phase I/II studies, they were incorporated into the phase II studies. At NIRS, more than 6,000 patients have been treated with carbon ion beams for past 17 years, and the clinical efficacy of carbon ion therapy has been demonstrated for many malignant diseases.

In 2011, a new medical facility opened at HIMAC that uses the existing synchrotron. It comprises three rooms: two with a robotic arm–controlled patient table for fixed horizontal and vertical scanning irradiation ports and the third one equipped with a lightweight rotating gantry with the superconducting magnets. NIRS completed installation of scanning equipment and commissioning of the system at one room with fixed beam lines and started a clinical trial in May 2011.

Present Status and Perspective for Carbon Ions in Japan

At present, five carbon ion therapy facilities are operating around the world, with three of them in Japan. In 1984, the Japanese government embarked on a program of carbon ion therapy at the first facility in Chiba. Clinical studies that began in 1994 have shown promising outcomes in general and have led to the development of the other carbon ion therapy facilities in Japan.

The second center, the Hyogo Ion Beam Medical Center in Hyogo, Japan, was established in 2001—the world's first ion beam facility providing both proton and carbon ion beams. By the end of September 2010, 2,735 patients were treated at Hyogo, including 915 patients receiving carbon ion therapy. Its lower energy (320 MeV per nucleon) and smaller field size (10 cm by 10 cm) for carbon ion beam compared with HIMAC restricted indications of carbon ion therapy for smaller and shallower tumors.

The third Japanese carbon ion therapy facility was completed in March 2010 at Gunma University Heavy Ion Medical Center. It is a concise carbon ion therapy accelerator complex almost one-third the size and construction cost of HIMAC with the same performance.

The fourth facility, SAGA HIMAT (heavy ion medical accelerator in Tosu), a concise Gunma-type system located in the southern part of Japan, is under construction and will begin treating patients in 2013. The fifth is at planning stage in Kanagawa prefecture near Tokyo and will start its operation in 2015.

Gesellschaft für Schwerionenforschung

In Germany, carbon ion research and treatment was made possible at a basically preclinical research institution. Beginning in 1997 at Gesellschaft für Schwerionenforschung (GSI) in Darmstadt, Germany, patients were treated with carbon ions by the Department of Radiation Oncology in Heidelberg, Germany. Within the research context of GSI, three beam time blocks per year were provided for patient treatment. As a collaborative effort consisting of clinicians, biologists, physicists, and engineers from the University Hospital of Heidelberg, the German Cancer Research Center (DKFZ) in Heidelberg, Germany, the Forschungszentrum Rossendorf in Dresden, and the Biophysics Group at GSI, patient treatment could be realized accompanied by extensive preclinical research.

For beam delivery provided by a synchrotron, the intensity-modulated raster scanning technique was developed, and biologic dose calculation was refined using the local effect model (LEM) developed by Kraft and Scholz.[9–11] Clinical efficacy of this approach was shown and validated in more than 600 patients with special focus on radioresistant tumors such as chordomas and chondrosarcomas of the skull base, ACCs, and high-grade meningiomas.

Heidelberg Ion Therapy Center

In Europe, the only center treating patients with carbon ion radiotherapy is the Heidelberg Ion Therapy Center (HIT) in Heidelberg, Germany. The center is equipped with a synchrotron, providing different particle species for three treatment rooms. Two rooms are equipped with a horizontal beam line; in the third room, the world's first carbon ion gantry has been realized. Since November 2009, the center has been in clinical operation offering particle treatment for approximately 1,300 patients per year. The center is directly connected to the existing Department of Radiation Oncology to allow for a streamlined work flow, and patients can be treated as both inpatients and outpatients.[12,13] The center delivers particle treatments via active raster scanning; as well, treatment planning and biologic plan optimization has been adopted from the work performed previously at GSI.[14]

Uptake of clinical routine is based on the indications treated at GSI, focusing on skull base chordomas, chondrosarcomas, and ACCs.[12] Subsequently, several clinical studies on varying indications started recruiting with different treatment concepts, including a randomized trial of carbon ion versus proton radiotherapy.[15–17]

Perspective for Carbon Ions in Europe, the United States, and Asia

To date, HIT is the only facility in Germany treating with carbon ions. Facilities in Marburg and Kiel, Germany, have been built but have not taken up clinical routine. In Europe, the National Centre for Oncological Treatment (CNAO) in Pavia, Italy, is a center equipped for proton and carbon ion treatments that started taking up clinical service in mid-2011. In Austria, the carbon facility (MedAUSTRON) at Wiener Neustadt is under construction and will offer proton and carbon ion treatments. The creation of a carbon ion clinical facility (the ETOILE project) in France is under discussion.

In Asia, a radiotherapy facility including photons, protons, and carbon ion beams is under construction in Shanghai.

More than 50 years after the world's first carbon ion therapy in Berkeley, there is a growing interest within the radiotherapy community to again invest in that domain.

TECHNICAL ASPECTS: PRESENT STATUS AND PERSPECTIVE

Beam Delivery

The current passive beam delivery system used in Chiba is a quite reliable and robust system and has had proven stable performance at HIMAC since 1994. A respiratory-gated irradiation technique was also put into practical use for the treatment of moving targets with the passive beam delivery system.[18] The similar systems are adopted at Hyogo and Gunma University.

A scanning irradiation method, which uses "narrow" pencil beams of carbon ions to cover a target volume by superimposing the spot beams of carbon ions slice by slice has been developed and applied at GSI and then at HIT. The new facilities at HIMAC Pavia and in Germany and Austria are (or will be) equipped with this system. Compared to passive methods, the scanning irradiation techniques permit a more conformal irradiation of the target volume, especially with a better sparing of the normal tissue located in the beam channel entrance (i.e., skin). Therefore, the technique is more appropriate for the treatment of complex-shaped lesions that cannot be adequately irradiated by the passive beams. The scanning also eliminates the need for constructing compensation filters as well as patient-specific collimators.

Gantry

To date, no gantry is available for treatment with carbon ions, whereas gantries are standard in proton therapy, primarily owing to the immense constructions required for building such a gantry to accommodate the large size and weight of the necessary magnets for beam delivery. However, to provide optimal dose distributions, especially for paraspinal tumors and tumors of the gastrointestinal tract, the use of horizontal beams is limiting treatments in these patients.

The world's first carbon ion gantry was designed and constructed at HIT (with a total weight of more than 600 tons of steel, about 420 tons precisely turning around the patient, and a length of 25 m and diameter of 13 m). Clinical operation of the gantry is anticipated for mid-2012.

A lightweight rotating gantry using superconducting magnets has been designed and should be installed in the new HIMAC facility.

Gating and Tracking

To reduce the enlargement of irradiated volume with respiration, a respiratory-gated irradiation technique was developed for carbon ion therapy at HIMAC. In this technique, the irradiation-gate signal is generated only when the target is located at the designed position and the synchrotron can extract a beam. Thus, one of the key technologies for respiratory-gated irradiation is the beam-extraction method from the synchrotron according to the gate signal. For this purpose, the radio frequency–knockout (RF-KO) slow-extraction method, which utilizes a transverse beam heating by an RF-field tuned with a wave number of a horizontal betatron oscillation, was developed[19] as well as the respiratory-gated irradiation system.[18] In this system, the respiration signal is generated by observation of movement of light-emitting diode set on the surface of the patient's body through a position-sensitive detector. The respiratory-gated irradiation system has been utilized primarily for treatment of liver and lung tumors since 1996 and has been very effective for reduction of fraction number in these tumors moving along with respiration.

Treatment of moving organs with ions applied with the raster scanning technique confront the physicist and clinician with novel challenges. Because of the interplay effect of the scanning beam and the moving target, substantial over- and underdosage within the target volume is generated; therefore, it cannot be precisely calculated and guaranteed that the planned dose will be applied homogeneously.[20] Thus, effective compensation mechanisms are necessary for the treatment of moving targets.

Several approaches for moving target irradiation are under investigation: monitoring breathing motion and using the information for gating strategies (irradiating during set gating windows) can significantly reduce interaction.[20] Another approach is the rescanning technique: the volume is not scanned by the beam with the whole calculated dose (i.e., particle number); the volume is scanned several times, and the particles (or dose) are divided onto the scanning runs. With this concept, a more homogeneous spread of the particles and dose over the volume can be achieved, with increasing homogeneity with the number of scanning runs.[21] A sophisticated concept is monitoring organ motion and making the beam follow the movement of the target volume; this requires fast communication between the beam-scanning system and the monitoring setup to provide real-time tracking of the volume.[20]

The concepts presented are under evaluation; potentially, the technique used may depend on the tumor type or anatomic region treated. Additionally, target volume concepts might help to compensate for some minor organ movement. However, using only compensatory target volumes, such as internal target volumes (ITVs) used in photon radiotherapy, will not suffice.[20] Variation of spot scanning size and reduction of grid size can help to compensate organ motion as well. It is most likely that a combination of several approaches—that is, specific target volume, modification of spot size, and perhaps gating—will provide optimal and clinically applicable dose distributions.

Beam Imaging

As a by-product of particle radiotherapy, β^+ activity is generated and can be monitored using conventional positron emission tomography (PET) scanners to in vivo monitoring of dose delivery. Several centers offering particle therapy have established this possibility.

At GSI, an online PET imager was built into the treatment cave, allowing for online monitoring of b^+ activity during each fraction and enabling later correlation with the planned and calculated treatment plan for passive beam delivery centers, such as Massachusetts General Hospital in Boston or centers in Japan.

Promising experience in PET imaging of proton and carbon ion therapy has been obtained for more than 50 patients monitored after passive proton treatments in the United States and Japan, and more than 400 patients have been monitored during scanned carbon ion beam irradiation at GSI. At the GSI pilot project, the value of PET for improving the accuracy of the semiempirical computed tomography (CT)-range calibration curve employed by the treatment planning system, as well as for detecting and quantifying deviations between planned and actual treatment delivery owing to patient misalignments or anatomic changes over the course of fractionated therapy, could be demonstrated.[22] At HIT, a commercial PET/CT scanner has been installed in a dedicated room adjacent to the treatment area, and clinical evaluation is ongoing within a prospective trial.

CARBON ION RADIOBIOLOGIC PROPERTIES: RATIONALE FOR PATIENT SELECTION

Carbon ions for clinical applications are characterized by two main properties: (a) a depth-dose distribution with a sharp maximal energy deposition at a definite depth (the Bragg peak) related to the beam incidence energy, with almost no dose deposited beyond this peak (Fig. 20.1) and (b) a biologic efficiency increasing at the end of the beam's range within the Bragg peak.

Although not demonstrated by large prospective randomized clinical trials, the potential clinical gains achievable by these ballistic advantages led to the definition of several "standard" indications for proton therapy (i.e., base of skull chordoma and chondrosarcoma, eye melanoma, selected pediatric brain tumors).[23,24]

Dose Distribution: Bragg Peak and Spread-Out Bragg Peak

Although similar, there are some notable differences between the dose-depth distribution of protons and carbon ions that may have clinical impacts (the presence of a "fragmentation tail" for carbon ions owing to nuclear interactions, allowing high-quality PET imaging) and a very narrow penumbra for carbon ions compared to protons.[24]

Similarly to protons, carbon ion beams are spread out to conform to the target, resulting in the spread-out Bragg peak (SOBP) after a low dose "plateau" within the entrance channel beyond the target (Figs. 20.2 and 20.3). This can be achieved using several techniques, mainly with passive scattering, but also with more advanced techniques (e.g., pencil beam with wobbling or uniform scanning) has to achieve a lower dose deposit within the normal tissue in the entrance of the beam (proximally to the tumor volume) while optimizing the distal dose distribution and therefore a higher dose distribution conformation.

Treatment Plan Intercomparisons

There have been several publications based on comparative dosimetric analyses of dose distribution outcomes with photon intensity-modulated radiation therapy (IMRT) versus particle therapy (protons and/or carbon ions) with passive or active beam delivery. The general conclusion of publications dealing with protons is that similar dose distribution can be achieved with the target volume for all techniques but that particle therapy permits lowering of the dose delivered to the surrounding critical normal tissues even for large target volumes.[25–28]

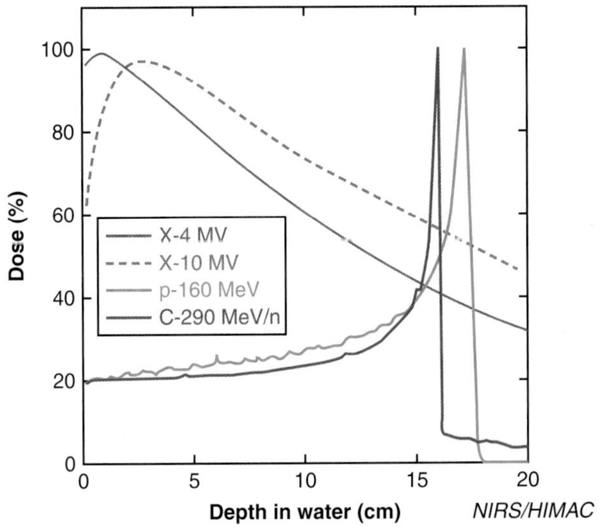

FIGURE 20.1. Bragg peak (protons versus carbon ions versus photons)

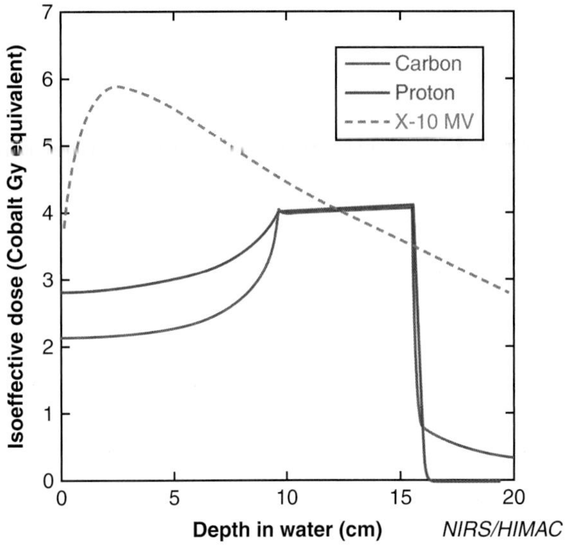

FIGURE 20.2. Spread-out Bragg peak (protons versus carbon ions versus photons).

Few treatment planning studies with carbon ions have been published thus far. For similar and strict constraints to critical organs at risk, Schulz-Ertner et al.[29] have demonstrated that carbon ions alone or a combination of carbon ions and photon IMRT was superior to photon IMRT alone for spinal chordomas and ACC with infiltration of the skull base.[29,30] Amirul et al.[31] have noted a dosimetric benefit both for tumor coverage and OAR preservation for selected head and neck tumors.

Integral Dose

Another advantage of particle beams is that fewer fields are required to achieve an acceptable dose distribution for difficult

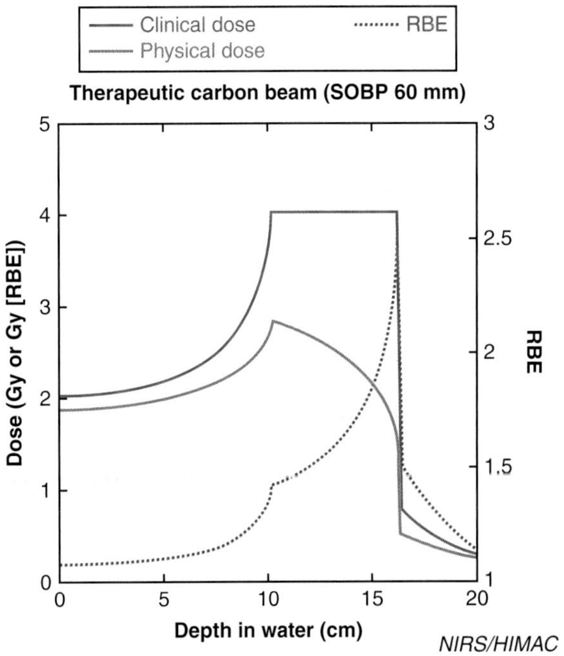

FIGURE 20.3. Design of a carbon ion spread-out Bragg peak (SOBP). The high LET region of the carbon ion beam is located in the distal part of the Bragg peak, and the SOBP becomes a weighted function of several Bragg peaks at various energies, which results in a dilution of the dose-average LET in the target volume. Therefore, the physical dose (Gray) has to be decreased as the relative biologic efficiency (RBE) value rises so as to have a flat biologically effective dose across the SOBP.

cases, which leads to a dramatic decrease of the integral dose (and potentially a lower incidence of radio-induced cancer, especially in pediatric indications) compared to intensity-modulated x-ray therapy (IMXT).[32]

Biologic Effectiveness and Equivalent Biologic Rate

As with neutrons, carbon ion interactions are characterized by a high LET that provides for a given physical dose for a higher biologic effect compared to low LET irradiation modalities (photons and protons). Therefore, the dose delivered with high LET particles is prescribed in Gray equivalents (GyE) or cobalt Gray equivalents (CGE) equal to the measured physical dose in Gray multiplied by a relative biologic efficiency (RBE) factor. The RBE is the ratio of the dose of radiation required to produce a certain biologic effect with photons relative to the dose required to produce the same effect with another form of ionizing radiation (such as protons and light ions).

Interestingly for clinical applications, this higher biologic efficiency, which may lead to a higher tumor control probability (TCP) for radioresistant tumors but may also increase the normal tissue complication probability (NTCP), is limited to the Bragg peak (thus to the SOBP). Within the "entrance" channel where the main proportion of organs at risk should be, there is no additional biologic effect.

The RBE of carbon ions is difficult to calculate; for dose-reporting purposes, a value of three is often utilized based on neutron experience. However, several other parameters should be taken into account, such as dose per fraction, fractionation, tissue type, target volume, and pO_2 value at each point in the irradiated volume as well as the variation in RBE along the SOBP (higher at the distal part than at the proximal part)[24] (Fig. 20.3). In NIRS, the LET dependency is taken into account in the design of clinical dose distribution by choosing the 10% survival of the human salivary gland tumor cells as end points; this was evaluated through TCP analysis for non–small cell lung cancer.[33,34] The LEM, a generic model allowing for RBE-calculation in various tissue types and for various end points, has been developed and applied at GSI and is in use for biologic treatment planning at HIT.[9,10]

Dose Fractionation

The capacity for normal and cancer tissues to repair from sublethal radiation injury is sharply reduced with high LET radiation both for normal tissues and cancer cells. This leads to questioning the need for dose fractionation (applying a standard fractionation scheme with a low dose per fraction) justified in low LET therapy (photons and protons) by a higher kinetic of sublethal radiation injury repair for normal tissue versus radiosensitive tumors.

Experimental data with high LET particles did not find any differences in RBE values between tumor and normal cell lines in standard culture condition.[35,36] However, experiments conducted with fast neutrons and carbon ions have demonstrated that increasing the dose per fraction tends to lower the RBE of both the tumor and normal tissues but with a more important decrease for the normal tissue given a higher therapeutic ratio for short-course hypofractionation schemes with carbon ion radiotherapy.[35,37] At NIRS in Chiba, Japan, hypofractionated carbon ion radiotherapy has been investigated systematically for a variety of tumor entities, and it seems that a significant reduction of overall treatment time can be accomplished for many tumor entities without enhancing toxicity.[8]

Applications for Patient Selection and Radiotherapy Schemes

To summarize, the best indications for carbon ions based on their biologic advantages over low LET radiation (photons and protons) and poor dose-depth distribution (photons and neutron) are tumors that demonstrate low radiosensitivity when treated with photons, particularly if the tumor is surrounded by radiosensitive normal tissue.

Carbon ion biologic and physical properties also justify the use of a larger fraction dose than that used in conventional radiotherapy schemes with an impact on patient quality of life (shorter overall treatment time) as well as a major economical impact (reduction of the cost for the health insurance).

CLINICAL DATA

Primarily based on the clinical experience of NIRS and GSI, various clinical data are available to assess the efficacy and tolerance of carbon ion radiotherapy in miscellaneous tumor locations and pathologies.[8,23,24,38]

To date, medical data on carbon ion therapy rely on prospective phase I (dose-escalation and hypofractionation assessments) and phase II trials conducted in more than 7,000 patients, mostly at NIRS and GSI. The main clinical data are summarized for each tumor site in Tables 20.1 through 20.7.

Head and Neck Cancers (Table 20.1)

Carbon ion therapy has been applied in several tumor types for primary or recurrent cancers (unresectable or R1-R2 tumors) and in some selected cases as a second irradiation in phase I and II prospective studies.[39–49]

The most impressive data have been obtained for ACC, malignant mucosal melanoma, and sarcomas known as highly radioresistant tumors.[39,40,44–46,48,50]

When compared to NIRS historical data, a dose response was demonstrated for sarcoma in the NIRS experience in terms of 3-year local control (91.8% vs. 23.6% for 70.4 GyE vs. 57.6 or 64 GyE) and 3-year overall survival (74.1% vs. 42.9% for 70.4 GyE vs. 57.6 or 64 GyE).[44]

The comparison of the clinical outcome for locally advanced ACC treated within the same period by the Heidelberg radiotherapy team either with a combination of photon IMRT with a carbon ion boost (39 patients) (total median dose, 72 GyE) or with photon IMRT alone (29 patients) (median dose, 66 Gy) was in favor of carbon ion boost versus photons only with a 4-year locoregional control, disease-free survival, and overall survival rates of 77.5 versus 24.6 ($p = 0.08$), 53% versus 23% ($p = 0.19$), and 75.8 versus 77.9, respectively.[48]

Several prospective trials have been launched at HIT.[51,52]

Sarcoma (Soft Tissue and Osteosarcoma) and Chordomas (Tables 20.2 and 20.3)

The initial phase I trial (64 patients) conducted at NIRS from June 1996 to February 2000 has established a reference dose and fractionation of 70.4 GyE (16 fractions, 4 weeks).[53]

Since then, to August 2011, 495 patients (514 tumors) were entered in a phase II trial: 405 bone sarcoma/chordoma (chordoma in 177, chondrosarcoma in 81, osteosarcoma in 81, Ewing/primitive neuroectodermal tumor [PNET] in 28, miscellaneous in 38) and 109 soft tissue sarcomas (malignant fibrous histiocytoma [MFH] in 21, malignant peripheral nerve sheath tumor [MPNST] in 15, synovial sarcoma in 11, leiomyosarcoma in 11, miscellaneous in 51). The 2- and 5-year overall survival were 79% and 59%, respectively, and 2- and 5-year local control were 85% and 69%, respectively, with 2% of grade 3/4 skin/soft tissue late toxicity (toxicity primarily related to the tumor volume and its location that may be reduced by advanced beam delivery techniques).[54]

Sacral Chordoma

Carbon ion radiotherapy appears effective and safe in the management of patients with sacral chordoma. It offers a promising alternative to surgery with a high local control, similar, see superior to surgical procedures alone[55] or with adjuvant proton therapy[56] and a higher functional outcome with few or no severe toxicities regarding urinary and anorectal function.[54,57,58] The occurrence of severe neuropathy was related to the dose

TABLE 20.1 HEAD AND NECK CANCERS (ADENOID CYSTIC CARCINOMA, MUCOSAL MELANOMA, ADENOCARCINOMA, SARCOMA)

Author/Year	*Type of Study (Number of Patients)*	*Treatment*	*Median Follow-Up*	*Tumor Characteristics*	*OS*	*LC/DFS/LRFS*	*Toxicity (Late ≥Grade 3)*
Hasegawa et al. 2011[40]	Phase II 404 pts (4/1997–2/2011)	CIRT: 57.6 GyE (265 pts) or 64.0 GyE (142 pts) in 16 fractions/4 wk	NA	Unresectable or R2 ACC: 151 MM: 102 Adeno: 50	*5-y OS* All: 53% ACC: 72% MM: 35% Adeno: 62%	*5-y LC* All: 73% ACC: 74% MM: 79% Adeno: 77%	Grade 3: 0
Hasegawa et al. 2011[50]	Phase II 134 pts (4/1997–2/2010)	CIRT: 57.6 GyE or 64.0 GyE in 16 fractions/4 wk	42.5 mo	ACC 108: unresectable or recurrent or R2	5-y OS: 70% T1-3: 91% T4, recurrent or R2:67%	5y-LC: 80% T1-3: 96% T4, recurrent or R2: 78%	Grade 3: 0 Brain toxicity grade 2: 9%
Schulz-Ertner et al. 2005[48]	Phase I/II 29 pts (6/1995–12/2003)	X: 54 Gy (30 sessions of 1.8 Gy) C. boost: 18 GyE (6 sessions of 3 Gy)	16 mo (2–60)	R2; unresectable or recurrent ACC	2-y: 86.6 4-y: 75.8%	2-y LC:77.5% 4-y LC:77.5%	Mucositis grade 3: 2 pts Infection: 1 pt
Jingu et al. 2011[45]	Phase II 37 pts (4/2006–3/2009)	CIRT: 57.6 GyE, 16 fractions/4 wk + CT (DAV) (concurrent)	19 mo (31 pts)	MM Median GTV: 25.7 mL (2.0–137.1)	3-y OS: 81.1%	3-y LC: 65.3% 3-y MFS: 37.6%	Grade 3: 0
Jingu et al. 2011[44]	Phase II 27 pts (4/2001–2/2008)	CIRT: 70.4 GyE/16 fractions	37 mo	Unresectable bone and soft tissue sarcoma	3-y OS: 74.1%	3-y LC: 91.8%	Visual loss: 1 pt Bone grade 3: 4 pts

OS, overall survival; LC, local control; DFS, disease-free survival; LRFS, local relapse-free survival; pt(s), patient(s); CIRT, carbon ion radiotherapy; NA, not applicable; ACC, adenoid cystic carcinoma; MM, mucosal melanoma; Adeno, adenocarcinoma; X, photons; C. boost, carbon ions boost; CT, chemotherapy; DAV, dacarbazine (DTIC), nimustine hydrochloride (ACNU), and vincristine (VCR); GTV, gross tumor volume; MFS, metastatis-free survival.

level (>73.6 GyE). The application of particle radiotherapy for tumors adjacent to the gastrointestinal tract may be restricted because of the low tolerance of the intestine. In that situation, a surgical spacer may be placed before particle radiotherapy.[59] To note, a more than 10% of tumor volume increase at the end of the radiotherapy without further progression was described in 50% of cases.[60]

Osteosarcoma

Several series with protons and photons have demonstrated that high-dose irradiation may lead to a relatively high local control at 5 years (approximately 70%) in unresected or incompletely resected osteosarcoma, with a 5-year overall survival of 40% to 67%.[61,62]

Similar results have been reported by NIRS in a series of 78 patients with unresectable osteosarcoma of the trunk (median diameter of 9 cm)—a location known to have the worst prognosis[63,64]—treated exclusively with carbon ions, with a 5-year local control and overall survival of 61% to 32%.[65] Tumor volume was a major prognostic factor (5-year local control and overall survival of 87% and 46% for volume <500 cc).

A prospective study of nonresectable osteosarcoma has been launched at HIT.[66]

Base of Skull Chordoma and Chondrosarcoma

For base of skull chordoma and chondrosarcoma, similar results with a high local control rate have been reported.[23,67,68] A dose-response relationship has been observed by Mizoe et al.[67] and Schulz-Ertner et al.,[68] with 3- to 5-year local control of 60% and 100%, respectively, for dose less or more than 60 GyE. Postoperative carbon ion radiotherapy should improve the survival rate and quality of life of patients with skull base chordomas after surgical removal of the tumor around the brain stem and the optic nerve.[69]

TABLE 20.2 SKULL BASE (AND SPINAL) CHORDOMA AND CHONDROSARCOMA

Author/Year	*Type of Study (Number of Patients)*	*Treatment*	*Follow-Up*	*Tumor Characteristics*	*OS*	*LC/DFS/LRFS*	*Toxicity (Late ≥Grade 3)*
Mizoe et al. 2009[67]	33 pts (34 cases[a]) Phase I/II (6/1995–7/2003) Phase II (4/2010–6/2007)	16 fractions/4 wk 48.0: 5 pts 52.8: 3 pts 57.6: 7 pts 60.8 GyE: 5 pts 60.8 GyE: 14 pts	Mean 53 mo	Chordoma Skull base: 27 pts Paracervical spine: 7 pts Biopsy or 1 resection: 21 pts >2 resections: 13 pts CTV median 51 cc (2–328 cc)	5-y OS: 87.7% 10-y OS: 67%	5-y LC: 85.1% 10-y LC: 63.8% Dose 60.8, LC: 100%	Grade 3: 0 1 brain grade 2 toxicity (steroids)
Schulz-Ertner & Tsujii 2007[23]	Phase I/II (96 pts) 11/1998–7/2005	CIRT: 60 GyE (60–70 GyE) (20 fractions/3 wk)	Mean 31 mo (3–91)	*Base of skull chordoma* (gross tumor) Median PTV-HR: 80.3 cc (13.9–594.2) Primary: 59 pts; recurrent: 37 pts	3-y OS: 91,8% 5-y OS: 88,5%	3-y LC: 80,6% 5-y LC: 70% >60 GyE: 100% <60 GyE: 63%	Grade 3 optic nerve neuropathy: 4 pts Grade 3 necrosis of fat plomb: 1
Schulz-Ertner et al. 2007[68]	Phase I/II (54 pts) 11/1998–9/2005	CIRT: 60 GyE (57–70 GyE) (20 fractions/3 wk)	Median 33 mo (3–84)	*Skull base low-grade and intermediate-grade chondrosarcomas* R2 after surgery	5-y OS: 98.2%	(2 local recurrence) 3-y LC: 96.2% 4-y LC: 89.8%	Grade 3: 1 pt (nerve IV paresis)

OS, overall survival; LC, local control; DFS, disease-free survival; LRFS, local relapse-free survival; pt(s), patient(s); CTV, clinical target volume; CIRT, carbon ion radiotherapy; PTV-HR, high-risk planning target volume.

[a]One patient was treated twice for a marginal recurrence.

TABLE 20.3 UNRESECTABLE BONE/SOFT TISSUE SARCOMAS AND SACRAL CHORDOMA (HEAD AND NECK EXCLUDED)

Author/Year	Type of Study (Number of Patients)	Treatment	Median Follow-Up	Tumor Characteristics	OS	LC/DFS/LRFS	Toxicity (Late ≥Grade 3)
Kamada et al. 2002[53]	Phase I/II 57 pts (64 lesions) (6/1996–12/1999)	CIRT: 52.8–73.6 GyE, 16 fractions/4 wk	21 mo (2–60)	*Sarcoma* Median CTV: 559 cc (20–2,290)	5-y: 37%	5-y LC: 63%	Grade 3 skin/soft tissue toxicity: 6
Serisawa et al. 2009[71]	Phase I/II 24 pts (5/1997–2/2006)	CIRT: 52.8–73.6 GyE, 16 fractions/4 wk	36 mo (6–143)	*Unresectable retroperitoneal sarcoma* MFH: 6, lipoS: 3, MPNST: 3, Ewing/PNET: 2, miscellaneous: 10 Median CTV: 525 cm^3 (57–1,194)	2 y: 75% 5 y: 50%	2 y: 77% 5 y: 69%	No grade 3
Imai et al. 2011[54]	Retrospective 95 pts (1996–2007)	CIRT: 52.8–73.6 GyE (median 70.4 GyE), 16 fractions/4 wk	Median 42 mo (13–112)	*Medically unresectable sacral chordomas* Primary tumor: 84 Local recurrence > surgery: 11 Median CTV: 370 cc	5-y OS: 86%	5-y LC: 88%	2 pts (skin necrosis) 15 pts severe sciatic nerve toxicity (medication)
Imai et al. 2011[65]	Phase II 78 pts (2000–2011)	CIRT: 52.8–73.6 GyE (median 70.4 GyE), 16 fractions/4 wk	NA	*Unresectable osteosarcoma of the trunk* Mean tumor diameter: 9 cm (<500 cc: 28 pts)	*5-y OS* All: 32% <500 cc: 46% >500 cc:19%	5-y LC: 61% <500 cc: 87% >500 cc: 21%	NA

OS, overall survival; LC, local control; DFS, disease-free survival; LRFS, local relapse-free survival; pt(s), patient(s); CIRT, carbon ion radiotherapy; CTV, clinical target volume; MFH, malignant fibrous histiocytoma; lipoS, liposarcoma; MPNST, malignant peripheral nerve sheath tumor; PNET, primitive neuroectodermal tumor; NA, not applicable.

Combs et al.[70] published their experience in 17 young adults and children (5 to 21 years; median age 18 years) treated with carbon ions for a primary (14 patients) or a recurrent (3 patients) chordoma (10 patients) or chondrosarcoma (10 patients). With a median 49-month follow-up, no severe toxicity was observed, and only one patient experienced a recurrence marginal to the treated volume.

The potential advantages of carbon ions over protons in base of skull chordoma and chondrosarcoma are being assessed in a randomized trial conducted by the HIT team.[16,17]

Retroperitoneal Sarcoma

Despite the very high risk for severe toxicity in retroperitoneal sarcoma, the preliminary experience of NIRS, including 24 patients, demonstrated a high local control (77% and 69% at 2 and 5 years, respectively) and overall survival (75% and 50% at 2 and 5 years, respectively) without grade 3 toxicities.[71]

Meningioma (Table 20.4)

Results of carbon ions used as a boost (18 GyE) after photon therapy (50.4 Gy) has been reported in 10 patients by the Heidelberg team.[72] Compared to their own experience with high-dose photon therapy,[73] a trend for a higher local control and survival was reported. Similar results have also been reported by NIRS.[74]

A prospective protocol has been launched by HIT to evaluate a carbon ion boost applied to the macroscopic tumor in conjunction with photon radiotherapy in patients with atypical meningiomas after incomplete resection or biopsy.[75]

TABLE 20.4 BRAIN TUMORS: MENINGIOMA, ASTROCYTOMA, AND GLIOBLASTOMA

Author/Year	Type of Study (Number of Patients)	Treatment	Median Follow-Up	Tumor Characteristics	OS	LC/DFS/LRFS	Toxicity (Late ≥Grade 3)
Combs et al. 2010[72]	Phase II 10 pts (1999–2003)	XRT: 50.4 Gy (FSRT or IMRT) C boost: 18 GyE	NA	*Meningioma* Primary: 8 pts Reirradiation: 2	*Primary* 5-y OS: 75% 7-y OS: 63%	*Primary* 5-y LC: 86% 7-y LC: 72%	NA
Adeberg et al. 2011[73]	Phase II 85 pts (6/1985–10/2009)	XRT (FSRT or IMRT) + C boost *Total dose* Mean: 57.6 Gy (30–68.4 Gy), 1.8–3.0 Gy/fraction	Median 73 mo	*Meningioma* Atypical: 62 Malignant: 23 Postoperative: 60% Progression: 19% Primary: 8.3% Median PTV:156.0 mL	*5-y OS* Atypical: 81% Anaplastic: 53%	*5-y PFS* Atypical: 50% Anaplastic: 13%	NA
Hasegawa et al. 2011[77]	Phase I/II 14 pts (10/1994–2/2002)	46.2–50.4 GyE (9 pts) 55.2 GyE (5 pts) 24 fractions/6 wk	Mean 62 mo (10–152)	*Astrocytomas* WHO grade 2 diffuse	*Median OS* Dose ≤50.4 GyE: 28 mo Dose 55.2: NA	*Median PFS* Dose ≤50.4 GyE: 18 mo Dose 55.2: 91 mo	No grade ≥3
Mizoe et al. 2007[76]	Phase I/II 48 pts (10/1994–2/2002)	XRT: 50 Gy, 25 fractions/5 wk CRT: 16.8–24.8 GyE, 8 fractions/2 wk ACNU concurrent	NA	*Malignant gliomas* AA: 16 GBM: 32	*MST* AA: 35 mo GBM: 17 mo	*GBM (high dose)* Median PFS: 14 mo MST: 26 mo	No grade ≥3 Grade 2 brain toxicity: 4 pts

OS, overall survival; LC, local control; DFS, disease-free survival; LRFS, local relapse-free survival; pt(s), patient(s); XRT, X-ray radiotherapy; FSRT, fractionated stereotactic radiotherapy; IMRT, intensity-modulated radiotherapy; C boost, carbon ions boost; NA, not applicable; PTV, planning target volume; PFS, progression-free survival; WHO, World Health Organization; CRT, carbon ion radiotherapy; ACNU, nimustine hydrochloride; AA, anaplastic astrocytoma; GBM, glioblastoma multiforme; MST, median survival time.

Astrocytoma, Glioblastoma (Table 20.4)

A dose effect has been observed in a phase I/II series of 48 patients treated with a combination of photons, boost with carbon ion (dose escalation), and concomitant chemotherapy.[76] NIRS also reported their experience in 14 diffuse grade 2 astrocytoma patients treated with exclusive carbon ion therapy, also reporting a high local control for high carbon ion dose and no severe toxicities.[77]

Two prospective randomized protocols are ongoing at HIT for glioblastoma: (a) a randomized phase II trial evaluating a carbon ion boost applied after combined radiochemotherapy with temozolomide versus a proton boost after radiochemotherapy with temozolomide in patients with primary glioblastoma[15] and (b) a phase I/II trial reirradiation using carbon ions compared to fractionated stereotactic radiotherapy (FSRT) in patients with recurrent gliomas.[78]

Reirradiation (Brain, Skull Base, Head and Neck, and Sacral Region)

Thanks to its ballistic and biologic properties, carbon ion therapy has been performed for reirradiation after local recurrence following photon (or carbon ion) therapy.

HIT reported their experience in patients with recurrent tumors of the brain, skull base, head and neck, and sacral region (mainly skull base chordoma).[42,79] Survival after reirradiation was 86% at 24 months and 43% at 60 months. For skull base tumors, local tumor control after reirradiation was 92% at 24 months and 64% at 36 months.[79]

Lung Cancer (Table 20.5)

Stage I non–small cell lung cancer has been a model for NIRS to assess the feasibility of dose escalation and hypofractionation with exclusive carbon ion therapy.[80]

From 1994 to 1999, phase I/II trials established two standard radiotherapy protocols, leading to more than 95% local control with a low severe toxicity (grade 3 pneumonitis in 2.7%): 90 GyE in 18 fractions over 6 weeks and 72 GyE in 9 fractions over 3 weeks.[81,82] The results of the later fractionation were confirmed in a phase II trial including 50 patients.[83] At the same time, another phase II trial validated another radiotherapy schedule using only 4 fractions with two levels of dose according to tumor size (52.8 and 60 GyE, respectively, for stage IA and IB).[84]

These results led to the initiation of a phase I/II single-fraction dose escalation protocol (from 28 to 50 GyE). This trial is in progress.

On multivariate analysis, overall survival outcomes obtained with carbon ions was significantly better when compared with conventional radiotherapy and similar to those obtained by stereotactic radiotherapy and protons.[85]

Liver (Table 20.6)

From 1995 to 2001, phase I dose escalation and hypofractionation studies (110 patients) have been conducted at NIRS,[86] resulting in a phase II study (47 patients) with 52.8 GyE delivered in four sessions (1 week).[87] A high local control was obtained (96% at 3 and 5 years) without severe toxicity (≥2 increase of the Child-Pugh score in 10%) but with a low overall survival related to the poor general status of these patients.

An even more hypofractionated scheme with only two fractions within a phase I and then a phase II study was developed (ongoing), showing a dose effect, and for the high-dose group (>40.8 GyE) a high local control rate (94.5% at 3 years) whatever the diameter of the tumor (100% for tumor >5 cm), and a low rate of severe toxicity (≥2 increase of the Child-Pugh score in 5% to 7%).[87,88] The compensatory enlargement in the nonirradiated liver observed after carbon ion radiotherapy may have contribute to the improvement of the prognosis.[89]

Taking into account the alternative therapies, the optimal candidates for carbon ion therapy would be Child-Pugh A or B liver function, tumor diameter more than 3 cm, and tumor adjacent to the porta hepatis (size and locations more difficult to treat with radiofrequency ablation or percutaneous ethanol injection).[88]

A phase I study is planned at HIT.[90]

Locally Recurrent Rectal Cancer (Table 20.6)

Phase I/II studies have been conducted at NIRS since 2001 (an ongoing phase II study delivering 73.6 GyE in 16 fractions) for postoperative locally recurrent rectal cancer (no previous radiotherapy). Although most patients had tumors considered to be unresectable, results in 140 patients (148 lesions), including

TABLE 20.5 STAGE I NON–SMALL CELL LUNG CANCER

Author/Year	*Type of Study*	*Treatment*	*Median Follow-Up*	*Tumor Characteristics*	*OS*	*LC/CSS/LRFS*	*Toxicity (Late ≥Grade 3)*
Miyamoto et al. 2003[82]	Phase I/II 47 pts (48 lesions) (10/1994–8/1998)	CIRT 59.4–95.4 GyE, 18 fractions/3 wk	37.5 mo	Mean tumor diameter: 2.92 cm (0.5–6) Mean PTV: 59.1 mL (4.8–290)	5 y: 42% 5-y CSS: 60%	5-y LC: 64%	0
	Phase I/II 34 pts (9/1997–2/1999)	CIRT 68.4–79.2 GyE, 9 fractions/ 3 wk		Mean tumor size: 3.57 cm (1.2–8) Mean PTV: 112.2 mL (16.9–467.4)		5-y LC: 84%	0
Miyamoto et al. 2007[83]	Phase II 50 pts (51 lesions) (4/1999–12/2000)	*CIRT* 72 GyE, 9 fractions/3 wk	59.2 mo (6–83)	Mean PTV: 117.5 mL (9.8–424.4) Mean tumor diameter: 2.96 cm (1–7)	5 y: 50%	5-y LC: 94.7%	Grade 3 pulmonary radiographic reactions: 15 Grade 3 skin toxicity: 1
Miyamoto et al. 2007[84]	Phase II 79 pts (80 lesions) (12/2000–11/2003)	*CIRT* Stage IA: 52.8 GyE, 4 fractions; IB: 60 GyE, 4 fractions	38.6 mo (2.5–72.2)	Mean PTV: 86.74 mL ± 50.71	5 y: 45% 5-y CSS: 68%	5-y LC: 90%	0
Yamamoto et al. 2011[80]	Phase I/II 131 pts (4/2003–8/2010)	*CIRT* Single fractionation 28–50 GyE	35.2 mo (1.6–68.4)	T1: 78 pts T2: 53 pts	5-y OS: 52.6%	*5-y LC* All: 80.5% T1: 82.8% T2: 78.4% CSS: 71.5%	Grade 3: 0% Late grade 2: 2 pts

OS, overall survival; LC, local control; CSS, cause-specific survival; LRFS, local relapse-free survival; pt(s), patient(s); CIRT, carbon ion radiotherapy; PTV, planning target volume.

TABLE 20.6 DIGESTIVE CANCERS (HEPATOCARCINOMA, RECURRENT RECTAL CANCER, PANCREATIC CANCER)

Author/Year	*Type of Study*	*Treatment (CIRT)*	*Median Follow-Up*	*Tumor Characteristics*	*OS*	*LC/DFS/LRFS*	*Toxicity*
Imada et al. 2010[89]	Phase I/II 64 pts (4/2000–3/2003)	52.8 GyE, 4 fractions/1 wk	39.6 mo (5.7–97.8)	*Hepatocarcinoma* Stage II: 36%, IIIA: 50%, IVA: 14% Tumor diameter: median 4 cm (1.2–12) Primary: 49% Recurrence: 51% <2 cm MPV: 18 Child-Pugh A: 77%, B: 23%	*5-y OS* Distance from MPV: <2 cm: 22.2% >2 cm: 34.8%	5-y LC: 94% Distance from MPV: <2 cm: 87.8% >2 cm: 95.7%	*Increase of Child-Pugh score ≥2* 10% (no grade 4)
Imada et al. 2011[87]	Phase I/II 117 pts (4/2003–4/2006)	32–38.8 GyE, 2 fractions	28.9 mo (6–84.4)	*Hepatocarcinoma* Tumor diameter: median 4.4 cm (1.4–14)	NA	*3-y LC* Dose >42.8: 94.5% Dose <42.8: 73.7%	*Increase of Child-Pugh score ≥2* Diameter <5 cm: 5% >5 cm: 7% (no grade 4)
Yamada et al. 2011[91]	Phase I/II 140 pts (4/2001–2/2010)	67.2–73.6 GyE, 16 fractions/4 wk 73.6 GyE: 118 pts	33.6 mo (8–105)	*Locally recurrent rectal cancer*	*3- and 5-y OS* 67.2 GyE: 36%–24% 70.4 GyE: 51.7%–27.5% 73.6 GyE: 73.5%–42.3%	*3- and 5-y LC* 70.4 GyE: 88.5% 73.6 GyE: 95.2%	Grade 3: 4 pts (no grade 4)
Shinoto et al. 2011[92]	Phase I 25 pts (10/2003–7/2010)	*Preoperative CIRT* 30.0–36.8 GyE	Median 13.9 mo (3.2–73.1)	*Resectable pancreatic cancer* 21: surgery	*5-y OS* All: 39% Postoperative: 48%	No local failure (postoperative) Metastases: 68%	Grades 3–4: 2 pts (unrelated to CIRT)
Shinoto et al. 2011[93]	Phase I 60 pts (4/2007–2/2011)	(a) 43.8 GyE (8 fractions) + Gem 400–1,000 mg/m² (b) 45.6–52.8 GyE (12 fractions/3 wk) + Gem 1,000	NA	*Locally advanced pancreatic cancer* Stage III: 54; IV: 6 pts	Median survival: 19 mo *2-y OS* All: 32% ≥45.6 GyE: 66%	*2-y LC* All: 26% ≥45.6 GyE: 47%	Grade 3: 1 pt

CIRT, carbon ion radiotherapy; OS, overall survival; LC, local control; DFS, disease-free survival; LRFS, local relapse-free survival; pt(s), patient(s); MPV, main portal vein; NA, not applicable; Gem, gemcitabine.

118 patients treated with the highest dose, were comparable to the best published surgical results.[91]

Preliminary results in 23 patients also demonstrated a high disease-free survival (51%) for carbon ions (70.4 GyE in 16 fractions) used as a second irradiation after local rectal cancer recurrence but with a grade 3 toxicity in 6 patients (peripherical neuropathy and infection).

Pancreatic Cancer (Table 20.6)

Carbon ion therapy has been assessed as a neoadjuvant therapy in radiographically resectable pancreatic cancer[92] within a phase I dose escalation study (30 to 36.8 GyE with eight fractions in 2 weeks). With a median follow-up time of 13.9 months (range, 3.2 to 73.1), there was no local failure in postoperative patients (21 of 25 patients); however, there was a high rate of metastases (68%). Two patients experienced a grade 3 to grade 4 toxicity unrelated to carbon ion radiotherapy.

NIRS also demonstrated the feasibility of carbon ion radiotherapy combined with gemcitabine in locally advanced pancreatic cancers, resulting in a low toxicity rate and a high local control and survival for the highest radiotherapy dose compared to historical data.[93]

Prostate Cancer (Table 20.7)

More than 1,300 patients have been treated with carbon ion beam for prostate cancer (primarily high and intermediate risk) at NIRS with two main fractionations (20 and 16 fractions).[94–96] A new trial with 12 fractions in 3 weeks is ongoing. Preliminary results may indicate a higher disease-free survival, especially in high-risk patients, when compared with standard alternative therapies.[97]

Miscellaneous

Several other tumors sites and pathology have been treated with carbon ions within phase I/II trials: locally advanced or

TABLE 20.7 PROSTATE CANCER

Author/Year	*Type of Study*	*Treatment*	*Median Follow-Up*	*Tumor Characteristics*	*OS*	*LC/DFS/LRFS*	*Toxicity (Late ≥Grade 3)*
Shimazaki et al. 2010[95]	Phase II 254 pts (2003–2009)	CIRT ± HT	NA	NA	NA	*8-y DFS* Low risk: 76% Intermediate risk: 91% High risk: 76%	NA
Tsuji et al. 2011[97]	Phase II 1,005 pts (2000–2011)	CIRT ± HT 63–66 GyE, 20 fractions: 466 pts 57.6 GyE, 16 fractions: 539 pts	≥12 mo	NA	5-y OS: 95.4%	5-y DFS: 90.6% T1-2 vs. T3: 94% vs. 84% PSA >20 vs. >20: 92% vs. 89% GS <6 vs. 7 vs. >8: 92% vs. 94% vs. 84%	NA

OS, overall survival; LC, local control; DFS, disease-free survival; LRFS, local relapse-free survival; pt(s), patient(s); CIRT, carbon ion radiotherapy; HT, Hormontherapy; NA, not applicable; PSA, prostate-specific antigen; GS, gleason score.

unfavorably located choroidal melanoma,[97] skin,[98] esophagus,[99] and cervix,[100,101] which need continued investigation to confirm therapeutic efficacy.

CONCLUSIONS AND PERSPECTIVES

The accumulated clinical experience has indicated that certain types of tumors, such as advanced radioresistant head and neck tumors (ACC, adenocarcinoma, and mucosal malignant melanoma), large skull base tumors, rectal cancer (postoperative pelvic recurrence), and sarcomas, can only be appropriately controlled and cured by carbon ion therapy with high probability.[44,46,53,65] It has been made clear that this therapy is capable of suppressing several types of tumors, such as peripheral-type non–small cell lung cancer, liver cancer, and prostate cancer, safely in a relatively short period of time through these clinical trials. Patients with such tumors can be remarkably healed by this therapy within a few days or weeks with minimal discomfort.

To date, no randomized clinical trial has shown the superiority of carbon ion beams to protons or photon radiotherapy. Therefore, in the future, not only evaluation of carbon ions alone in specific tumor types but also comparing to advanced photon techniques, such as IMRT, are required to exploit the full advantage of high LET particle therapy and to stratify patients for specific treatments.

REFERENCES

1. Wilson R. Radiological use of fast protons. *Radiology* 1946;47:487–491.
2. Castro JR, Linstadt DE, Bahary JP, et al. Experience in charged particle irradiation of tumors of the skull base: 1977–1992. *Int J Radiat Oncol Biol Phys* 1994;29:647–655.
3. Castro JR, Phillips TL, Prados M, et al. Neon heavy charged particle radiotherapy of glioblastoma of the brain. *Int J Radiat Oncol Biol Phys* 1997;38:257–261.
4. Linstadt DE, Castro JR, Phillips TL. Neon ion radiotherapy: results of the phase I/II clinical trial. *Int J Radiat Oncol Biol Phys* 1991;20:761–769.
5. Schoenthaler R, Castro JR, Petti PL, et al. Charged particle irradiation of sacral chordomas. *Int J Radiat Oncol Biol Phys* 1993;26:291–298.
6. Schoenthaler R, Castro JR, Halberg FE, et al. Definitive postoperative irradiation of bile duct carcinoma with charged particles and/or photons. *Int J Radiat Oncol Biol Phys* 1993;27:75–82.
7. Sato K, Yamada S, Ogawa K, et al. Performance of HIMAC. *Nucl Phys A* 1995;588:229–234.
8. Tsujii H, Mizoe JE, Kamada T, et al. Overview of clinical experiences on carbon ion radiotherapy at NIRS. *Radiother Oncol* 2004;73(Suppl 2):S41–S49.
9. Elsasser T, Kramer M, Scholz M. Accuracy of the local effect model for the prediction of biologic effects of carbon ion beams in vitro and in vivo. *Int J Radiat Oncol Biol Phys* 2008;71:866–872.
10. Elsasser T, Weyrather WK, Friedrich T, et al. Quantification of the relative biological effectiveness for ion beam radiotherapy: direct experimental comparison of proton and carbon ion beams and a novel approach for treatment planning. *Int J Radiat Oncol Biol Phys* 2010;78:1177–1183.
11. Weyrather WK, Ritter S, Scholz M, et al. RBE for carbon track-segment irradiation in cell lines of differing repair capacity. *Int J Radiat Biol* 1999;75:1357–1364.
12. Combs SE, Ellerbrock M, Haberer T, et al. Heidelberg Ion Therapy Center (HIT): Initial clinical experience in the first 80 patients. *Acta Oncol* 2010;49:1132–1140.
13. Combs SE, Jakel O, Haberer T, et al. Particle therapy at the Heidelberg Ion Therapy Center (HIT)—integrated research-driven university-hospital-based radiation oncology service in Heidelberg, Germany. *Radiother Oncol* 2010;95:41–44.
14. Rieken S, Habermehl D, Nikoghosyan A, et al. Assessment of early toxicity and response in patients treated with proton and carbon ion therapy at the Heidelberg Ion Therapy Center using the raster scanning technique. *Int J Radiat Oncol Biol Phys* 2011;81:e793–e801.
15. Combs SE, Kieser M, Rieken S, et al. Randomized phase II study evaluating a carbon ion boost applied after combined radiochemotherapy with temozolomide versus a proton boost after radiochemotherapy with temozolomide in patients with primary glioblastoma: the CLEOPATRA trial. *BMC Cancer* 2010;10:478.
16. Nikoghosyan AV, Rauch G, Munter MW, et al. Randomised trial of proton vs. carbon ion radiation therapy in patients with low and intermediate grade chondrosarcoma of the skull base, clinical phase III study. *BMC Cancer* 2010;10:606.
17. Nikoghosyan AV, Karapanagiotou-Schenkel I, Munter MW, et al. Randomised trial of proton vs. carbon ion radiation therapy in patients with chordoma of the skull base, clinical phase III study HIT-1-Study. *BMC Cancer* 2010;10:607.
18. Minohara S, Kanai T, Endo M, et al. Respiratory gated irradiation system for heavy-ion radiotherapy. *Int J Radiat Oncol Biol Phys* 2000;47:1097–1103.
19. Noda K, Kanazawa M, Itano A, et al. Slow beam extraction by a transverse RF field with AM and FM. *Nucl Instrum Meth A* 1996;374:269–277.
20. Bert C, Gemmel A, Saito N, et al. Gated irradiation with scanned particle beams. *Int J Radiat Oncol Biol Phys* 2009;73:1270–1275.
21. Furukawa T, Inaniwa T, Sato S, et al. Moving target irradiation with fast rescanning and gating in particle therapy. *Med Phys* 2010;37:4874–4879.
22. Parodi K, Saito N, Chaudhri N, et al. 4D in-beam positron emission tomography for verification of motion-compensated ion beam therapy. *Med Phys* 2009;36:4230–4243.
23. Schulz-Ertner D, Tsujii H. Particle radiation therapy using proton and heavier ion beams. *J Clin Oncol* 2007;25:953–964.
24. Suit H, DeLaney T, Goldberg S, et al. Proton vs carbon ion beams in the definitive radiation treatment of cancer patients. *Radiother Oncol* 2010;95:3–22.
25. Lee CT, Bilton SD, Famiglietti RM, et al. Treatment planning with protons for pediatric retinoblastoma, medulloblastoma, and pelvic sarcoma: how do protons compare with other conformal techniques? *Int J Radiat Oncol Biol Phys* 2005;63:362–372.
26. Lin R, Hug EB, Schaefer RA, et al. Conformal proton radiation therapy of the posterior fossa: a study comparing protons with three-dimensional planned photons in limiting dose to auditory structures. *Int J Radiat Oncol Biol Phys* 2000;48:1219–1226.
27. Miralbell R, Lomax A, Bortfeld T, et al. Potential role of proton therapy in the treatment of pediatric medulloblastoma/primitive neuroectodermal tumors: reduction of the supratentorial target volume. *Int J Radiat Oncol Biol Phys* 1997;38:477–484.
28. St Clair WH, Adams JA, Bues M, et al. Advantage of protons compared to conventional x-ray or IMRT in the treatment of a pediatric patient with medulloblastoma. *Int J Radiat Oncol Biol Phys* 2004;58:727–734.
29. Schulz-Ertner D, Nikoghosyan A, Didinger B, et al. Treatment planning intercomparison for spinal chordomas using intensity-modulated photon radiation therapy (IMRT) and carbon ions. *Phys Med Biol* 2003;48:2617–2631.
30. Schulz-Ertner D, Didinger B, Nikoghosyan A, et al. Optimization of radiation therapy for locally advanced adenoid cystic carcinomas with infiltration of the skull base using photon intensity-modulated radiation therapy (IMRT) and a carbon ion boost. *Strahlenther Onkol* 2003;179:345–351.
31. Amirul IM, Yanagi T, Mizoe JE, et al. Comparative study of dose distribution between carbon ion radiotherapy and photon radiotherapy for head and neck tumor. *Radiat Med* 2008;26:415–421.
32. Miralbell R, Lomax A, Cella L, et al. Potential reduction of the incidence of radiation-induced second cancers by using proton beams in the treatment of pediatric tumors. *Int J Radiat Oncol Biol Phys* 2002;54:824–829.
33. Kanai T, Endo M, Minohara S, et al. Biophysical characteristics of HIMAC clinical irradiation system for heavy-ion radiation therapy. *Int J Radiat Oncol Biol Phys* 1999;44:201–210.
34. Kanai T, Matsufuji N, Miyamoto T, et al. Examination of GyE system for HIMAC carbon therapy. *Int J Radiat Oncol Biol Phys* 2006;64:650–656.
35. Ando K, Kase Y. Biological characteristics of carbon-ion therapy. *Int J Radiat Biol* 2009;85:715–728.
36. Suzuki M, Kase Y, Yamaguchi H, et al. Relative biological effectiveness for cell-killing effect on various human cell lines irradiated with heavy-ion medical accelerator in Chiba (HIMAC) carbon-ion beams. *Int J Radiat Oncol Biol Phys* 2000;48:241–250.
37. Denekamp J, Waites T, Fowler JF. Predicting realistic RBE values for clinically relevant radiotherapy schedules. *Int J Radiat Biol* 1997;71:681–694.
38. Jensen AD, Munter MW, Debus J. Review of clinical experience with ion beam radiotherapy. *Br J Radiol* 2011;84(Spec No 1):S35–S47.
39. Hasegawa A, Jingu K, Mizoe J, et al. Carbon ion radiotherapy for malignant head-and-neck tumors invading the skull base. *Int J Radiat Oncol Biol Phys* 2010;78:S173.
40. Hasegawa A, Koto M, Takagi R, et al. Carbon ion radiotherapy for malignant head-and-neck tumors. Proceedings of NIRS-ETOILE 2nd Joint Symposium on Carbon Ion Radiotherapy, November 25–27, 2011, Centre ETOILE, Lyon, France.
41. Jensen AD, Nikoghosyan AV, Ecker S, et al. Carbon ion therapy for advanced sinonasal malignancies: feasibility and acute toxicity. *Radiat Oncol* 2011;6:30.
42. Jensen AD, Nikoghosyan A, Ellerbrock M, et al. Re-irradiation with scanned charged particle beams in recurrent tumours of the head and neck: acute toxicity and feasibility. *Radiother Oncol* 2011;101:383–387.
43. Jensen AD, Nikoghosyan AV, Ecker S, et al. Raster-scanned carbon ion therapy for malignant salivary gland tumors: acute toxicity and initial treatment response. *Radiat Oncol* 2011;6:149.
44. Jingu K, Tsujii H, Mizoe JE, et al. Carbon ion radiation therapy improves the prognosis of unresectable adult bone and soft-tissue sarcoma of the head and neck. *Int J Radiat Oncol Biol Phys* 2012;82(5):2125–2131.
45. Jingu K, Kishimoto R, Mizoe JE, et al. Malignant mucosal melanoma treated with carbon ion radiotherapy with concurrent chemotherapy: prognostic value of pretreatment apparent diffusion coefficient (ADC). *Radiother Oncol* 2011;98:68–73.
46. Mizoe JE, Tsujii H, Kamada T, et al. Dose escalation study of carbon ion radiotherapy for locally advanced head-and-neck cancer. *Int J Radiat Oncol Biol Phys* 2004;60:358–364.
47. Ramaekers BL, Pijls-Johannesma M, Joore MA, et al. Systematic review and meta-analysis of radiotherapy in various head and neck cancers: comparing photons, carbon-ions and protons. *Cancer Treat Rev* 2011;37:185–201.
48. Schulz-Ertner D, Nikoghosyan A, Didinger B, et al. Therapy strategies for locally advanced adenoid cystic carcinomas using modern radiation therapy techniques. *Cancer* 2005;104:338–344.
49. Thariat J, Bolle S, Demizu Y, et al. New techniques in radiation therapy for head and neck cancer: IMRT, CyberKnife, protons, and carbon ions. Improved effectiveness and safety? Impact on survival? *Anticancer Drugs* 2011;22:596–606.
50. Hasegawa A, Koto M, Takagi R, et al. Carbon ion radiotherapy for adenoid cystic carcinoma of the head and neck. *Int J Radiat Oncol Biol Phys* 2011;81:S77–S78.
51. Jensen AD, Nikoghosyan A, Windemuth-Kieselbach C, et al. Combined treatment of malignant salivary gland tumours with intensity-modulated radiation therapy (IMRT) and carbon ions: COSMIC. *BMC Cancer* 2010;10:546.
52. Jensen AD, Nikoghosyan A, Hinke A, et al. Combined treatment of adenoid cystic carcinoma with cetuximab and IMRT plus C12 heavy ion boost: ACCEPT [ACC, Erbitux(R) and particle therapy]. *BMC Cancer* 2011;11:70.
53. Kamada T, Tsujii H, Tsuji H, et al. Efficacy and safety of carbon ion radiotherapy in bone and soft tissue sarcomas. *J Clin Oncol* 2002;20:4466–4471.
54. Imai R, Kamada T, Sugahara S, et al. Carbon ion radiotherapy for sacral chordoma. *Br J Radiol* 2011;84(Spec No 1):S48–S54.
55. Fuchs B, Dickey ID, Yaszemski MJ, et al. Operative management of sacral chordoma. *J Bone Joint Surg Am* 2005;87:2211–2216.
56. Park L, Delaney TF, Liebsch NJ, et al. Sacral chordomas: impact of high-dose proton/photon-beam radiation therapy combined with or without surgery for primary versus recurrent tumor. *Int J Radiat Oncol Biol Phys* 2006;65:1514–1521.
57. Imai R, Kamada T, Tsuji H, et al. Effect of carbon ion radiotherapy for sacral chordoma: results of phase I-II and phase II clinical trials. *Int J Radiat Oncol Biol Phys* 2010;77:1470–1476.
58. Nishida Y, Kamada T, Imai R, et al. Clinical outcome of sacral chordoma with carbon ion radiotherapy compared with surgery. *Int J Radiat Oncol Biol Phys* 2011;79:110–116.
59. Takahashi M, Fukumoto T, Kusunoki N, et al. [Particle beam radiotherapy with a surgical spacer placement for unresectable sacral chordoma]. *Gan To Kagaku Ryoho* 2010;37:2804–2806.

60. Serizawa I, Imai R, Kamada T, et al. Changes in tumor volume of sacral chordoma after carbon ion radiotherapy. *J Comput Assist Tomogr* 2009;33:795–798.
61. Ciernik IF, Niemierko A, Harmon DC, et al. Proton-based radiotherapy for unresectable or incompletely resected osteosarcoma. *Cancer* 2011;117:4522–4530.
62. Oertel S, Blattmann C, Rieken S, et al. Radiotherapy in the treatment of primary osteosarcoma—a single center experience. *Tumori* 2010;96:582–588.
63. Bielack SS, Wulff B, Delling G, et al. Osteosarcoma of the trunk treated by multimodal therapy: experience of the Cooperative Osteosarcoma study group (COSS). *Med Pediatr Oncol* 1995;24:6–12.
64. Bielack SS, Kempf-Bielack B, Delling G, et al. Prognostic factors in high-grade osteosarcoma of the extremities or trunk: an analysis of 1,702 patients treated on neoadjuvant cooperative osteosarcoma study group protocols. *J Clin Oncol* 2002;20:776–790.
65. Imai R, Kamada T, Tsuji H, et al. Carbon ion radiotherapy for bone and soft tissue sarcomas. Proceedings of NIRS-ETOILE 2nd Joint Symposium on Carbon Ion Radiotherapy, November 25–27, 2011, Centre ETOILE, Lyon, France.
66. Blattmann C, Oertel S, Schulz-Ertner D, et al. Non-randomized therapy trial to determine the safety and efficacy of heavy ion radiotherapy in patients with non-resectable osteosarcoma. *BMC Cancer* 2010;10:96.
67. Mizoe JE, Hasegawa A, Takagi R, et al. Carbon ion radiotherapy for skull base chordoma. *Skull Base* 2009;19:219–224.
68. Schulz-Ertner D, Nikoghosyan A, Hof H, et al. Carbon ion radiotherapy of skull base chondrosarcomas. *Int J Radiat Oncol Biol Phys* 2007;67:171–177.
69. Takahashi S, Kawase T, Yoshida K, et al. Skull base chordomas: efficacy of surgery followed by carbon ion radiotherapy. *Acta Neurochir (Wien)* 2009;151:759–769.
70. Combs SE, Nikoghosyan A, Jaekel O, et al. Carbon ion radiotherapy for pediatric patients and young adults treated for tumors of the skull base. *Cancer* 2009; 115:1348–1355.
71. Serizawa I, Kagei K, Kamada T, et al. Carbon ion radiotherapy for unresectable retroperitoneal sarcomas. *Int J Radiat Oncol Biol Phys* 2009;75:1105–1110.
72. Combs SE, Hartmann C, Nikoghosyan A, et al. Carbon ion radiation therapy for high-risk meningiomas. *Radiother Oncol* 2010;95:54–59.
73. Adeberg S, Hartmann C, Welzel T, et al. Long-term outcome after radiotherapy in patients with atypical and malignant meningiomas—clinical results in 85 patients treated in a single institution leading to optimized guidelines for early radiation therapy. *Int J Radiat Oncol Biol Phys* 2012;83(3):859–864.
74. Koto M, Hasegawa A, Takagi R, et al. Carbon ion radiotherapy for skull base and paracervical tumors. Proceedings of NIRS-ETOILE 2nd Joint Symposium on Carbon Ion Radiotherapy, November 25–27, 2011, Centre ETOILE, Lyon, France.
75. Combs SE, Edler L, Burkholder I, et al. Treatment of patients with atypical meningiomas Simpson grade 4 and 5 with a carbon ion boost in combination with postoperative photon radiotherapy: the MARCIE trial. *BMC Cancer* 2010;10:615.
76. Mizoe JE, Tsujii H, Hasegawa A, et al. Phase I/II clinical trial of carbon ion radiotherapy for malignant gliomas: combined x-ray radiotherapy, chemotherapy, and carbon ion radiotherapy. *Int J Radiat Oncol Biol Phys* 2007;69:390–396.
77. Hasegawa A, Mizoe JE, Tsujii H, et al. Experience with carbon ion radiotherapy for WHO grade 2 diffuse astrocytomas. *Int J Radiat Oncol Biol Phys* 2012; 83(1):100–106.
78. Combs SE, Burkholder I, Edler L, et al. Randomised phase I/II study to evaluate carbon ion radiotherapy versus fractionated stereotactic radiotherapy in patients with recurrent or progressive gliomas: the CINDERELLA trial. *BMC Cancer* 2010; 10:533.
79. Combs SE, Kalbe A, Nikoghosyan A, et al. Carbon ion radiotherapy performed as re-irradiation using active beam delivery in patients with tumors of the brain, skull base and sacral region. *Radiother Oncol* 2011;98:63–67.
80. Yamamoto N, Baba M, Nakajima M, et al. Carbon ion radiotherapy in a hypofractionation regimen for stage I non small cell lung cancer. Proceedings of NIRS-ETOILE 2nd Joint Symposium on Carbon Ion Radiotherapy, November 25–27, 2011, Centre ETOILE, Lyon, France.
81. Koto M, Miyamoto T, Yamamoto N, et al. Local control and recurrence of stage I non-small cell lung cancer after carbon ion radiotherapy. *Radiother Oncol* 2004; 71:147–156.
82. Miyamoto T, Yamamoto N, Nishimura H, et al. Carbon ion radiotherapy for stage I non-small cell lung cancer. *Radiother Oncol* 2003;66:127–140.
83. Miyamoto T, Baba M, Yamamoto N, et al. Curative treatment of stage I non-small-cell lung cancer with carbon ion beams using a hypofractionated regimen. *Int J Radiat Oncol Biol Phys* 2007;67:750–758.
84. Miyamoto T, Baba M, Sugane T, et al. Carbon ion radiotherapy for stage I non-small cell lung cancer using a regimen of four fractions during 1 week. *J Thorac Oncol* 2007;2:916–926.
85. Grutters JP, Kessels AG, Pijls-Johannesma M, et al. Comparison of the effectiveness of radiotherapy with photons, protons and carbon-ions for non-small cell lung cancer: a meta-analysis. *Radiother Oncol* 2010;95:32–40.
86. Kato H, Tsujii H, Miyamoto T, et al. Results of the first prospective study of carbon ion radiotherapy for hepatocellular carcinoma with liver cirrhosis. *Int J Radiat Oncol Biol Phys* 2004;59:1468–1476.
87. Imada H, Yasuda S, Yamada S, et al. Carbon ion radiotherapy for liver cancer. Proceedings of NIRS-ETOILE 2nd Joint Symposium on Carbon Ion Radiotherapy, November 25–27, 2011, Centre ETOILE, Lyon, France.
88. Imada H, Kato H, Yasuda S, et al. Comparison of efficacy and toxicity of short-course carbon ion radiotherapy for hepatocellular carcinoma depending on their proximity to the porta hepatis. *Radiother Oncol* 2010;96:231–235.
89. Imada H, Kato H, Yasuda S, et al. Compensatory enlargement of the liver after treatment of hepatocellular carcinoma with carbon ion radiotherapy—relation to prognosis and liver function. *Radiother Oncol* 2010;96:236–242.
90. Combs SE, Habermehl D, Ganten T, et al. Phase I study evaluating the treatment of patients with hepatocellular carcinoma (HCC) with carbon ion radiotherapy: the PROMETHEUS-01 trial. *BMC Cancer* 2011;11:67.
91. Yamada S, Shinoto M, Endo S, et al. Carbon ion radiotherapy for patients with locally recurrent rectal cancer. Proceedings of NIRS-ETOILE 2nd Joint Symposium on Carbon Ion Radiotherapy, November 25–27, 2011, Centre ETOILE, Lyon, France.
92. Shinoto M, Yamada S, Yasuda S, et al. Efficacy and safety of short course carbon-ion radiotherapy for patients with preoperative pancreatic cancer. *Int J Radiat Oncol Biol Phys* 2011;81:S331.
93. Shinoto M, Yamada S, Yasuda S, et al. Carbon ion for pancreatic cancer. Proceedings of NIRS-ETOILE 2nd Joint Symposium on Carbon Ion Radiotherapy November 25–27, 2011, Centre ETOILE, Lyon, France.
94. Ishikawa H, Tsuji H, Kamada T, et al. Carbon ion radiation therapy for prostate cancer: results of a prospective phase II study. *Radiother Oncol* 2006;81: 57–64.
95. Shimazaki J, Tsuji H, Ishikawa H, et al. Carbon ion radiotherapy for treatment of prostate cancer and subsequent outcomes after biochemical failure. *Anticancer Res* 2010;30:5105–5111.
96. Tsuji H, Yanagi T, Ishikawa H, et al. Hypofractionated radiotherapy with carbon ion beams for prostate cancer. *Int J Radiat Oncol Biol Phys* 2005;63:1153–1160.
97. Tsuji H, Mizoguchi N, Toyama S, et al. Carbon ion radiotherapy for prostate cancer. Proceedings of NIRS-ETOILE 2nd Joint Symposium on Carbon Ion Radiotherapy, November 25–27, 2011, Centre ETOILE, Lyon, France.
98. Zhang H, Li S, Wang XH, et al. Results of carbon ion radiotherapy for skin carcinomas in 45 patients. *Br J Dermatol* 2012;166(5):1100–1106.
99. Akutsu Y, Yasuda S, Nagata M, et al. A phase I/II clinical trial of preoperative short-course carbon-ion radiotherapy for patients with squamous cell carcinoma of the esophagus. *J Surg Oncol* 2012;105(8):750–755.
100. Kato S, Ohno T, Tsujii H, et al. Dose escalation study of carbon ion radiotherapy for locally advanced carcinoma of the uterine cervix. *Int J Radiat Oncol Biol Phys* 2006;65:388–397.
101. Suzuki Y, Oka K, Ohno T, et al. Prognostic impact of mitotic index of proliferating cell populations in cervical cancer patients treated with carbon ion beam. *Cancer* 2009;115:1875–1882.

Chapter 21
Methods of Immobilization and Stabilization

Joshua Evans, Edwin Crandley, Bruce Libby, and Stanley Benedict

OVERVIEW OF EXTERNAL BEAM IMMOBILIZATION AND STABILIZATION

Rationale for Patient Immobilization and Stabilization

Accurate delivery of the prescribed treatment is critical to achieve a successful outcome in radiotherapy. There are many sources of uncertainty in the radiation therapy delivery process that can result in a geometric miss of the intended target volume. A geometric miss of the intended target volume will not only decrease the probability of tumor control, but will also increase the volume of normal tissue that is irradiated, which will increase the probability of a treatment-related complication. Geometric uncertainties may be broadly classified as mechanical inaccuracies, localization inaccuracies, and positioning inaccuracies. Mechanical inaccuracies include the coincidence of the light and radiation fields, mechanical stability of the couch, laser alignment, and correspondence of the simulation and treatment isocenters. Localization error relates to the difficult nature of defining the location and extent of the target volume during both planning and treatment delivery. Positioning uncertainties relates to errors in reproducing the patient's positioning from simulation to treatment delivery, the most undesirable result of which is the target volume moving out of and critical normal tissues moving into the treatment field.

The goal of daily patient setup is to reproduce the position at the time of simulation as best as possible; however, interfractional setup variations from day to day will inevitably occur. Intrafractional positioning uncertainty can also arise

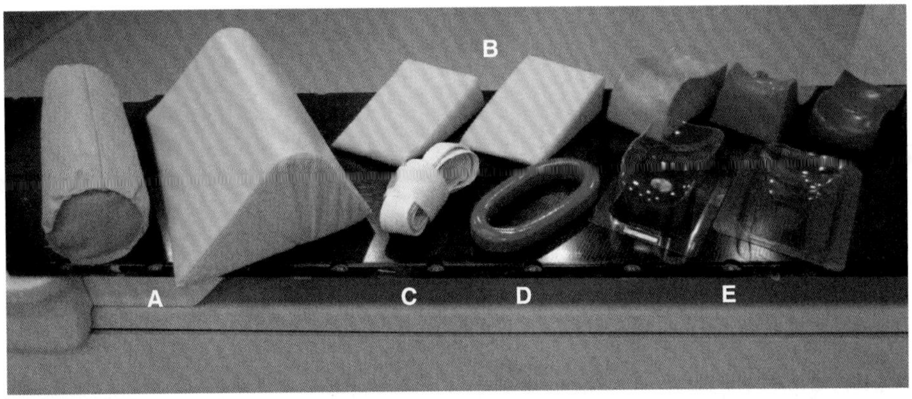

FIGURE 21.1. Simple devices are cost-effective and can reduce intrafraction positioning errors by increasing patient comfort. Shown here are rolls and wedges that can be placed under the knees **(A)** and wedges to support the arms and shoulders **(B)**. A simple strap **(C)** can be used to suppress the shoulders in head and neck patients, and grip rings **(D)** can be used for the patient to hold on to. Headrests **(E)** are available in a wide range of shapes and sizes.

from motion of the patient during treatment. Patients may fidget from being uncomfortable or anxious during the treatment delivery. Furthermore, organs can move internally with respect to bony anatomy, skin marks, and other soft tissues due to normal and unavoidable physiologic processes such as respiration, swallowing, and peristalsis. An early study by Haus and Marks[1] reported that approximately 30% of the localization errors they observed in their clinic were caused by patient motion. Dunscombe et al.[2] also concluded that observed field placement errors were largely due to patient motion.

The focus of this chapter is to describe devices and methods for patient immobilization and stabilization in radiotherapy. The goal of immobilization and stabilization techniques is to reduce positioning uncertainties from patient motion during each fraction (intrafraction error) and to also increase the reproducibility of the patient setup for each fraction (interfraction error). Immobilization devices can decrease the time needed for daily setup and target localization, thus increasing a clinic's throughput. Certain immobilization devices may also allow setup marks to be made directly on the device instead of the patient's skin, which can improve the patient's psychological well-being while under treatment. The immobilization system should be lightweight for ease of setup and transport, yet strong and durable so that the device does not break during the patient's course of treatment. Furthermore, the device should be made of materials that minimally affect the megavoltage treatment beam and do not cause computed tomography (CT) imaging artifacts that could impact three-dimensional (3D) visualization of the patient's anatomy.

The devices and techniques for patient immobilization and stabilization described in this chapter have been shown to improve interfraction setup reproducibility, as well as reduce intrafraction uncertainties. The overall accuracy of any immobilization system, however, is dependent on the skill and patience of the therapists forming the device at the time of simulation and setting the patient up on the treatment table for each fraction. Adequate training should be provided for each immobilization system employed in a given clinic, and adequate time should be scheduled for the therapist to properly set up and immobilize the patient. Furthermore, some patients will be more challenging to reproducibly align than others. A variety of devices and positions should be available for each treatment indication to help create a treatment position that maximizes both interfraction and intrafraction reproducibility for each patient. Finally, it must be noted that in some cases, even the most robust techniques for patient immobilization do not guarantee accurate daily localization of the tumor volume and should not be a substitute for image guidance when indicated. Tumors are well known to change position relative to other soft tissue anatomy, external marks, and bony anatomy. Thus, strategies for daily target localization, described elsewhere in this textbook, are also important and are intimately tied to patient immobilization.

Simple Immobilization Devices

Simple methods to reduce intrafraction positioning uncertainty due to patient motion have been in use for decades to ensure that the patient is comfortable. Figure 21.1 illustrates a variety of simple devices available that can be used to enhance the patient's comfort. For patients treated in a supine position, a wedge or roll underneath the knees can help to reduce stress on the lower back. For arms-down positioning, a ring for the patient to grip can increase comfort. For lung and liver treatments, it may be preferable to position the patient with the arms above the head. In these cases, the arms may be supported under the shoulder by foam wedges to help the patient attain a restful position. For some head and neck patients, the patient's shoulders may block the inferior portion of lateral treatment fields. In this case, a simple strap can be used to pull the shoulders down and out of the treatment fields. A headrest is almost always used with supine positioning to elevate the head and reduce strain on the neck. Standard sets of Timo and Silverman headrests come in a variety of shapes, sizes, and materials. For those not adequately accommodated by the standard set of headrests, several manufacturers offer customizable head cushions that can be molded to the patient's head contour. All of these devices are relatively inexpensive and reusable, and they can be covered and/or cleaned between uses.

Immobilization Features of a Dedicated Radiation Oncology CT Simulator

Simple devices incorporated during initial simulation can improve patient comfort and reduce intrafraction motion due to patient movement. However, they may not address day-to-day variations of overall patient setup and positioning accuracy. A major objective of a robust immobilization system is to reproduce the patient's anatomic geometry at the time of simulation for all subsequent treatment fractions. An example of a robust immobilization system to treat a patient with breast cancer is shown in Figure 21.2 to illustrate some of the desired features of a dedicated radiation oncology CT simulator. With this immobilization system, the patient lies supine with an ergonomic wedge under the knees. The arms are positioned above the head and out of the tangential treatment fields. A custom-formed, reusable vacuum-lock bag, described in more detail in the following body conformal section, helps to support the patient's arms, and a T-bar may be used for the patient to grip. The angled baseboard on which the vacuum-lock bag rests uses gravity to help the breasts fall into a more reproducible position and can be adjusted to minimize skin folds. This example of a breast setup, where one or both arms may be positioned above the head, highlights the advantage of a wide bore (e.g., >85-cm diameter) CT scanner for radiation oncology treatment simulation, as opposed to the more common 70-cm bore diameter, which may limit the options for positioning certain patients.

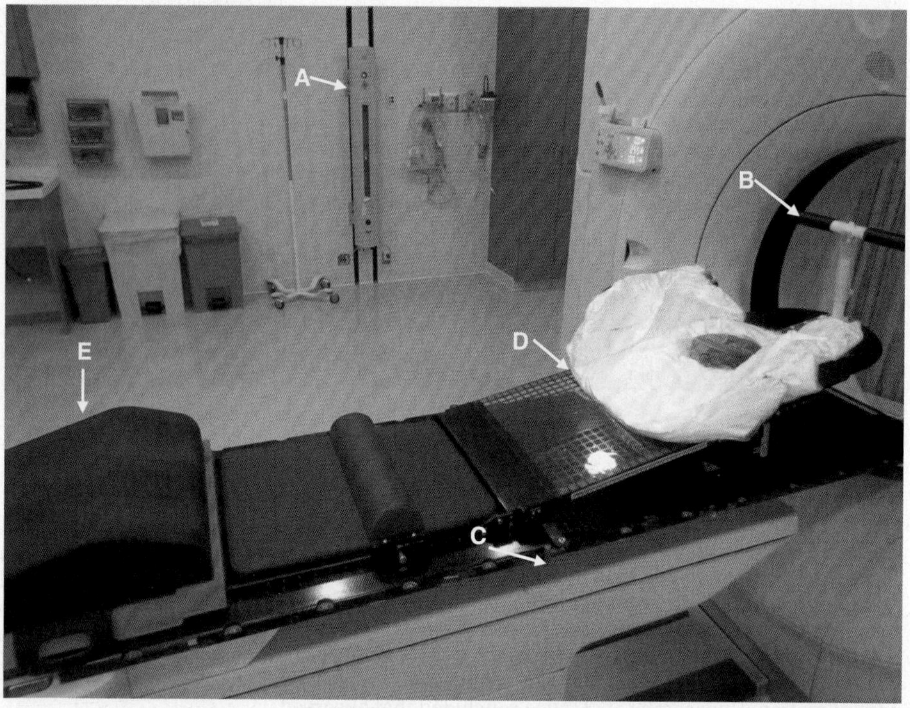

FIGURE 21.2. Immobilization system for a breast cancer patient in the simulator suite at the University of Virginia. Some key features of a dedicated radiation oncology CT simulator are an in-room laser system to mark the reference point position **(A)**, a wide patient bore (85-cm diameter) to allow more flexibility in patient positioning **(B)**, and an indexed flat couch-top overlay **(C)** to reproduce the geometry of the treatment table. An angled breast board **(D)** can improve patient comfort and provide optimal positioning of the breast for radiotherapy. An indexing bar is used to attach the breast board to the flat couch-top overlay. A vacuum lock mattress **(D)** and a T-bar **(B)** support the patient's arms above the head. An ergonomic knee support **(E)** can reduce stress on the lower back.

Flat couches are favored for radiation oncology treatments to accommodate a wide range of patient sizes, setup positions, and immobilization devices. Diagnostic CT scanners feature a curved couch for patient comfort; the geometry of a patient simulated on a curved diagnostic couch top will be challenging to reproduce on a flat treatment couch. Flat couch-top inserts are offered by numerous vendors to reproduce the couch geometry of the treatment unit. An important feature of a couch-top insert is the indexing system, which allows an assortment of immobilization devices to be rigidly affixed in concert to both the simulator and treatment tables with high accuracy. The indexing system improves the interfraction reproducibility of the patient setup and can also decrease the amount of time to set up a patient.

External marks placed either on the patient's skin or the immobilization devices are used for initial laser alignment on the treatment machine as a surrogate for the internal target anatomy. An in-room laser system in the CT simulator suite is a necessary feature to provide external references points that correlate to the internal reference point location. After the simulation CT scan is acquired, the isocenter is defined and the coordinates are transferred to the in-room laser system. The laser system and CT table are then moved to the defined setup point, and external setup marks can be made, thus correlating the position of an internal setup point to the external markings.

Head and Neck Immobilization Devices

Adequate immobilization is particularly critical in the treatment of head and neck (H&N) cancers, as the target is frequently located in close proximity to critical structures. Thermoplastic masks have replaced traditional plaster-casting methods in most clinics. Thermoplastic masks are heated to approximately 70°C in a water bath. At this temperature, the thermoplastic material becomes malleable and can be stretched and shaped to conform to the patient's face, head, and neck. The patient's head and neck is supported by a simple cushion like those previously described and illustrated in Figure 21.1. The mask is connected to a base plate, which is attached to the couch via the indexing system. Setup marks can be made directly onto the thermoplastic mask, eliminating the need for unsightly marks to be placed on the patient's face for the duration of the treatment.

Early work with thermoplastic mask immobilization for H&N cancer by Bentel et al.[3] showcased the efficacy of the thermoplastic mask in comparison to the traditional plaster three-strip immobilization technique. In terms of the rate of physician-requested shifts from port films, the thermoplastic mask had a frequency of 6.2%, compared to 16.1% for the plaster-casting method. However, this advantage was only observed when the mask was rigidly affixed to the couch, highlighting the importance of the couch indexing system.[3] Since then, numerous studies quantifying the accuracy of patient setup for H&N cancer have appeared in the literature. The bulk of these studies used two-dimensional portal imaging to quantify setup displacements, although studies using 3D cone-beam CT data are appearing more frequently as this technology becomes adopted by more clinics. Generally, systematic and random errors have been reported to have standard deviations ranging from 1 to 4 mm.[4–8] Based on a review of studies assessing setup errors using portal imaging, Hurkmans et al.[6] suggested that random and systematic errors of 2 mm or less should be a practically achievable goal for H&N patients, given current technology and methods.

Figure 21.3 illustrates the flexibility of patient positioning options with thermoplastic masks. Masks can encompass the head only or can extend inferiorly to cover the shoulders (Fig. 21.3A). Gilbeau et al.[5] compared the setup accuracy of the short and long thermoplastic masks in the treatment of head and neck cancer. Portal images were acquired for isocenters placed at the level of the head, neck, and shoulders. Their results show similar setup accuracy with the long and the short mask for the isocenters in the head and neck. For isocenter placement at the shoulder level, the use of the long mask resulted in a random setup error of approximately 1.0 mm, which was significantly less than the 2.3-mm error of the short mask ($p = 0.01$).[5] Thus, a long mask to immobilize the shoulders is recommended for patients receiving supraclavicular treatment in which the isocenter will be placed at the level of the shoulders. Thermoplastic systems can also accommodate prone or lateral setups when these may be indicated (Fig. 21.3B). Some commercially available base plates can be angled to allow for the patient to be set up with the neck in an extended or flexed position, which may be used to avoid critical structures such as the

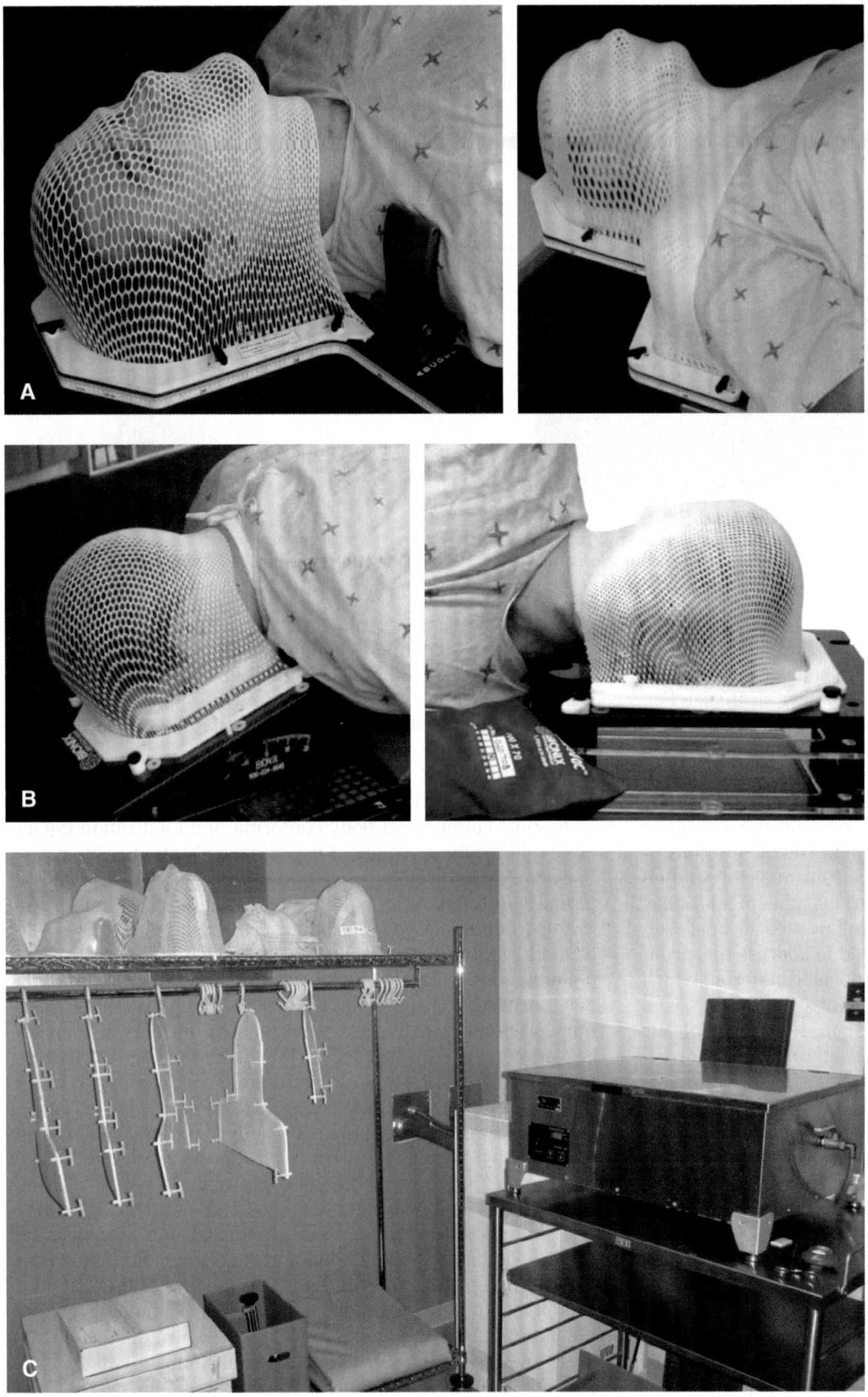

FIGURE 21.3. For treatment of targets in the head and neck, thermoplastic masks are routinely used for custom immobilization. **A:** Thermoplastic sheets are commercially available in short versions that cover only the head, as well as in longer versions that extend over the patient's shoulders. **B:** They can also be used to treat patients in the prone and lateral positions. **C:** Additional space is needed to accommodate the water bath used to warm the thermoplastic sheets. (A and B courtesy of Bionix Radiation Therapy, Toledo, OH.)

eyes. Neck extension can be used with prone positioning for craniospinal irradiation. For prone setup, a donut-shaped cushion supports the patient's face in the base plate, and the thermoplastic mask is formed around the posterior aspect of the head to hold the patient's face in the donut. A potential disadvantage of treatment with a flexed or extended neck position is the need for registration with different imaging modalities (e.g., positron emission tomography [PET]-CT or magnetic resonance [MR]-CT) in which the PET or MR were not performed in the patient treatment position.

Every clinic must consider space limitations when selecting particular immobilization and stabilization systems. Thermoplastic H&N systems necessitate more equipment and thus more space in the simulation suite. The water bath to heat the thermoplastic sheets for the long H&N masks can be large (Fig. 21.3C). For clinics with insufficient space to house a large water bath, smaller water baths are commercially available that will fit the short head-only masks. Furthermore, some commercially available base plates (e.g., VersaBoard, Bionix Radiation Therapy, Toledo, OH) incorporate shoulder suppression systems, which consist of rigid plastic panels to exert downward pressure on the shoulders. When a long thermoplastic mask is not indicated or not available, a base plate with shoulder suppression panels can help to keep the shoulders out of the beam

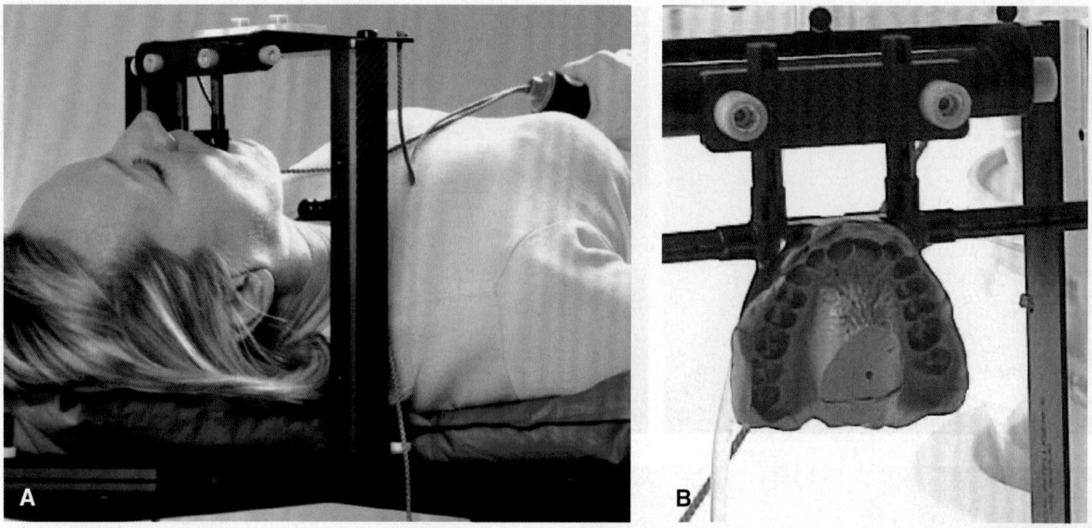

FIGURE 21.4. A: The Elekta HeadFIX is an example of a bite-block system that can provide an alternative method for immobilizing head and neck patients who are not able to tolerate a thermoplastic mask due to anxiety or claustrophobia. **B:** A custom dental mold is formed for each patient and is suctioned to the patient's hard palate. The dental mold is attached to a carbon fiber frame featuring a quick-release handle. (Courtesy of Elekta, Norcross, GA.)

path for lateral head and neck beams (Fig. 21.3A). In lieu of long thermoplastic masks or base plates with shoulder suppression panels, the patient can pull on a simple shoulder strap (see Fig. 21.1) to move the shoulders inferior and avoid unnecessary irradiation of the shoulders when opposed lateral beams are used to treat the neck.

Thermoplastic masks have been observed to shrink as they cool in the 24-hour period after formation, and this has been shown to lead to systematic setup errors if not taken into consideration.[9] Furthermore, a mask that has shrunk after the simulation process may be uncomfortable for the patient and may require resimulation and another treatment plan to be developed. Bionix Radiation Therapy attempted to address this problem with the Klarity Green line of thermoplastic material, which is designed to have reduced shrinkage coupled with increased rigidity. As with any immobilization system, the thermoplastic manufacturer's recommendations should be carefully followed, and adequate time should be allowed during simulation for the mask to harden properly to minimize the effect of shrinkage.

Thermoplastic masks are widely used for H&N treatment indications; however, they are not well tolerated by all patients, particularly patients with claustrophobia. For these patients, bite block systems that do not incorporate a mask may be an acceptable alternative. Elekta (Norcross, GA) offers a bite-block system, the HeadFIX, which is illustrated in Figure 21.4. A custom dental mold is formed to the patient's maxillary teeth, and a vacuum system creates suction of the mold to the hard palate. A custom cushion is placed under the patient's head, neck, and shoulders. The mouthpiece is attached to a carbon fiber frame, which is fixed to the treatment table's indexing system. The head is thus rigidly immobilized via the connection of the mouthpiece to the head frame. The carbon fiber design of the HeadFIX product allows for the use of in-room kilovoltage (kV) image guidance systems for target localization and the validation of setup accuracy. The mold can be quickly released from the frame if the patient feels discomfort. Setup accuracy has been shown to be similar to that of thermoplastic masks, on the order of 1 to 3 mm.[10,11] These stand-alone bite-block systems, however, require a high level of patient compliance and may not be suitable for patients with poor dentition or who are endentulous. Use of bite blocks formed with a patient's false teeth is highly discouraged and may result in inaccurate setups or breakage of the dentures. Custom-formed dental molds can also be incorporated in the conventional thermoplastic mask systems described earlier to provide an additional point of support for the patient. A custom bite block may also be formed with primary goals other than immobilization—for example, to separate the tongue from the roof of the mouth. This can be useful in treatment of sinus/nasal cavity tumors to decrease dose to the tongue and vice versa.

Body Conformal Immobilization Devices

Numerous commercial body conformal immobilization devices are available for a variety of treatment indications. One type of body conformal system uses a two-part foaming agent to form a permanent mold of the patient's body. One such system, Alpha Cradle (Smithers Medical Products, North Canton, OH), is illustrated in Figure 21.5A,B. Forms are available for treatment of patients with a variety of disease sites, including the head and neck, breast, thorax, abdomen, pelvis, and extremities. At the time of simulation the appropriate body form is chosen and is placed in a polyvinyl bag. The two-part chemical foaming agents are mixed together, initiating the chemical reaction that causes the foam to expand. The mixed foaming agent is then distributed evenly throughout the body form and sealed inside the polyvinyl bag. The patient is positioned inside the form as the foaming agent expands and conforms to the patient's body contour. The foam will continue to expand for approximately 10 to 15 minutes. During the foam expansion, the therapists will need to vigilantly guide the foam around the patient to prevent the foam from escaping the bag and moving into locations of least resistance that may contribute little to immobilization of the patient. As with any immobilization device, adequate training is needed to form a high-quality customized patient mold, and the manufacturer's instructions should be carefully followed. Chemical foaming agent systems generally require two therapists to form at the time of simulation, and the process can require approximately 30 minutes. Obviously, great care is needed to prevent any of the chemicals from having direct contact on the skin, as this may cause irritation.

Another class of body conformal systems, termed here "vacuum-lock bags," comprise a bag filled with plastic minispheres. These bags are available in a variety of sizes to accommodate different treatment sites and patient positioning. At the time of simulation, the bag is first conformed to the patient's body contour by pushing the minispheres to fill in around the patient. A vacuum pump is then connected to the bag, and the air is evacuated from the bag, causing the plastic minispheres to lock together to rigidly retain the device's shape. During the evacuation, the therapists maneuver the minispheres within the

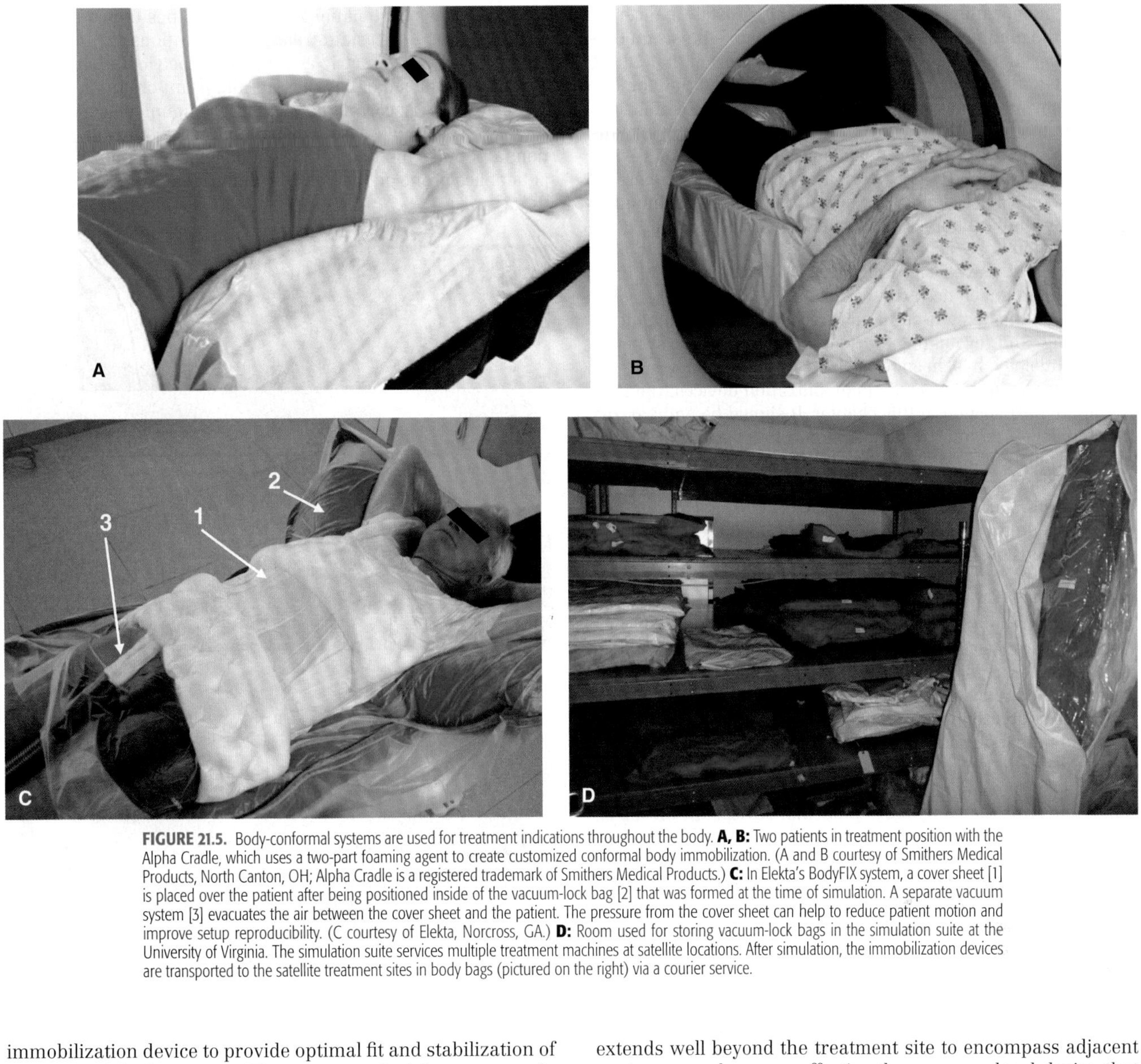

FIGURE 21.5. Body-conformal systems are used for treatment indications throughout the body. **A, B:** Two patients in treatment position with the Alpha Cradle, which uses a two-part foaming agent to create customized conformal body immobilization. (A and B courtesy of Smithers Medical Products, North Canton, OH; Alpha Cradle is a registered trademark of Smithers Medical Products.) **C:** In Elekta's BodyFIX system, a cover sheet [1] is placed over the patient after being positioned inside of the vacuum-lock bag [2] that was formed at the time of simulation. A separate vacuum system [3] evacuates the air between the cover sheet and the patient. The pressure from the cover sheet can help to reduce patient motion and improve setup reproducibility. (C courtesy of Elekta, Norcross, GA.) **D:** Room used for storing vacuum-lock bags in the simulation suite at the University of Virginia. The simulation suite services multiple treatment machines at satellite locations. After simulation, the immobilization devices are transported to the satellite treatment sites in body bags (pictured on the right) via a courier service.

immobilization device to provide optimal fit and stabilization of the patient's body contour. These vacuum-lock bags are made of a durable nylon material to resist tears or punctures and can be expected to retain their shape for 6 weeks or more. They are reusable and may require less time to generate a customized mold than the expanding foam systems. Another advantage of the vacuum-lock bag is that if during the simulation process the device is found not to provide the intended level of immobilization or is found to be uncomfortable for the patient, it can be reinflated and remolded to achieve the desired shape as many times as is necessary. The vacuum-lock systems, however, do require a time commitment to clean and remove any setup marks prior to use with subsequent patients. In addition, if a tear or puncture occurs during the course of treatment, a new vacuum-lock bag would need to be formed, and the simulation and treatment planning process may need to be repeated to deliver the remaining fractions. Each clinic should consider the benefits and drawbacks of each system. It is not uncommon to see both types of body conformal systems used within one institution.

Because body conformal devices are used to treat a wide range of sites throughout the entire body, careful thought should be given to each specific case to ensure that the treatment site is properly immobilized, the setup is reproducible from day to day, and the patient is able to maintain the position for the duration of each fraction. An immobilization device that extends well beyond the treatment site to encompass adjacent anatomy can be more effective than a more local device that focuses only on the treatment region. For example, Bentel et al.[12] showed that for Hodgkin lymphoma, a cradle that extends below the pelvis is more effective than a cradle that only includes the upper torso. Devices that extend around the patient also give the ability to make setup marks directly on the immobilization device for which to align the radiation isocenter. Aligning the beam to setup marks on the immobilization device can increase the daily setup reproducibility[13] by reducing the reliance on skin marks, which can be especially troublesome for larger or older patients, in whom the skin can be more mobile overtop the underlying anatomy. Marks can then be made on the patient to help align the patient within the immobilization device. Longer devices also allow for longer setup marks to be made in the superior–inferior direction, which can help to detect small rotational setup errors.

Early work by Bentel and colleagues at Duke University showed that immobilization with the Alpha Cradle expanding-foam system reduced the frequency of physician-requested setup corrections based on portal images for a variety of treatment indications, including Hodgkin lymphoma[12] and lung,[14] breast,[15] and prostate cancer.[13] It should be noted, however, that not all studies show a clear-cut advantage in setup accuracy with body conformal immobilization devices. For example, an early study by Song et al.[16] showed no statistical advantage of using immobilization in the treatment of prostate cancer in terms of the number of deviations greater than 5 mm as quantified on portal images. They did show, however, that obese patients tend to have larger setup errors,[16] highlighting the fact that certain subpopulations of patients may be more difficult to set up than others. The review of setup accuracy by Hurkmans et al.,[6] as assessed with portal imaging, provides a good review of the data up to 2001. This work concluded that with current patient setup, portal imaging, and immobilization techniques, systematic and random setup errors on the order of 2.5 to 3.5 mm should be achievable for treatments of the thorax, abdomen, and pelvis. The integration of cone-beam CT units into treatment machines is an excellent tool for assessing setup accuracy and is being used in an increasing number of studies comparing and evaluating various immobilization systems. This technology has been especially leveraged to study the setup accuracy of stereotactic immobilization devices, the subject of the next section in this chapter. It should be emphasized that the degree of interfraction setup accuracy achievable by a particular institution will depend on the skill and knowledge of the personnel involved in forming patient immobilization devices, setting up patients for daily treatments, making adjustments based on verification imaging, and the understanding of the limitations of each step of the process.

The Elekta BodyFIX is a unique immobilization system that uses a dual-vacuum system as shown in Figure 21.5C. For simulation, the patient is first placed in a vacuum-lock bag system. A thin plastic cover sheet is then placed over the patient, which is attached to the vacuum-lock bag via special adhesive strips. A vacuum pump is then used to evacuate the air under the cover sheet, creating a continuous pressure of up to 600 mbar. The additional pressure created by the cover-sheet vacuum system helps the patient settle into the vacuum-lock bag, which is molded to the patient and then evacuated with a second vacuum system to create the body-conformal device. For all subsequent treatment fractions, the pressure from the cover-sheet vacuum system ensures that the patient is reproducibly located in the vacuum-lock bag. The BodyFIX can provide a degree of abdominal compression on the vacuum sheet that is placed over the abdomen, which may help to decrease the respiratory excursion of certain tumors. Internal target motion management is discussed further in the section of this chapter on stereotactic immobilization. Patients in our clinic tolerate the BodyFIX dual-vacuum system very well, with infrequent complaints of claustrophobia or discomfort. If the patient feels that the pressure from the cover sheet is uncomfortable, the vacuum for the cover sheet can be turned down, or the vacuum-lock bag can be used by itself for certain indications.

Whole-body expanding-foam or vacuum-lock bag systems can provide excellent patient comfort and immobilization, but they are large devices, making the issue of space very relevant. Adequate space is required to store each patient's custom-formed device for up to 6 weeks or more while a patient is under treatment. At the Emily Couric Clinical Cancer Center at the University of Virginia (Charlottesville, VA), a dedicated room next to the simulation suite and large closets in each treatment room are used for storing patient body conformal immobilization devices (Fig. 21.5C). For clinics where one simulation suite is used to support multiple satellite clinics, such as at the University of Virginia, the logistics of transporting the immobilization device must also be considered. At the University of Virginia, a courier service is used to transport the large body-conformal devices in body bags from the simulation site to satellite treatment facilities. Each clinic must assess space availability when deciding which system to adopt in patient care.

PRONE POSITIONING AND IMMOBILIZATION

The body-conformal devices just described can help to provide reproducible patient setup from day to day for a wide range of disease sites. The patient is most often positioned supine in these devices. For certain treatment indications, a prone setup may provide a dosimetric advantage. In pelvic and abdominal irradiation, the small bowel is an important organ at risk, and acute toxicity is correlated with the amount of small bowel that receives a high dose. For patients receiving pelvic irradiation, a popular method is to use a belly board (Fig. 21.6A). The patient lies prone on the board with the stomach positioned over

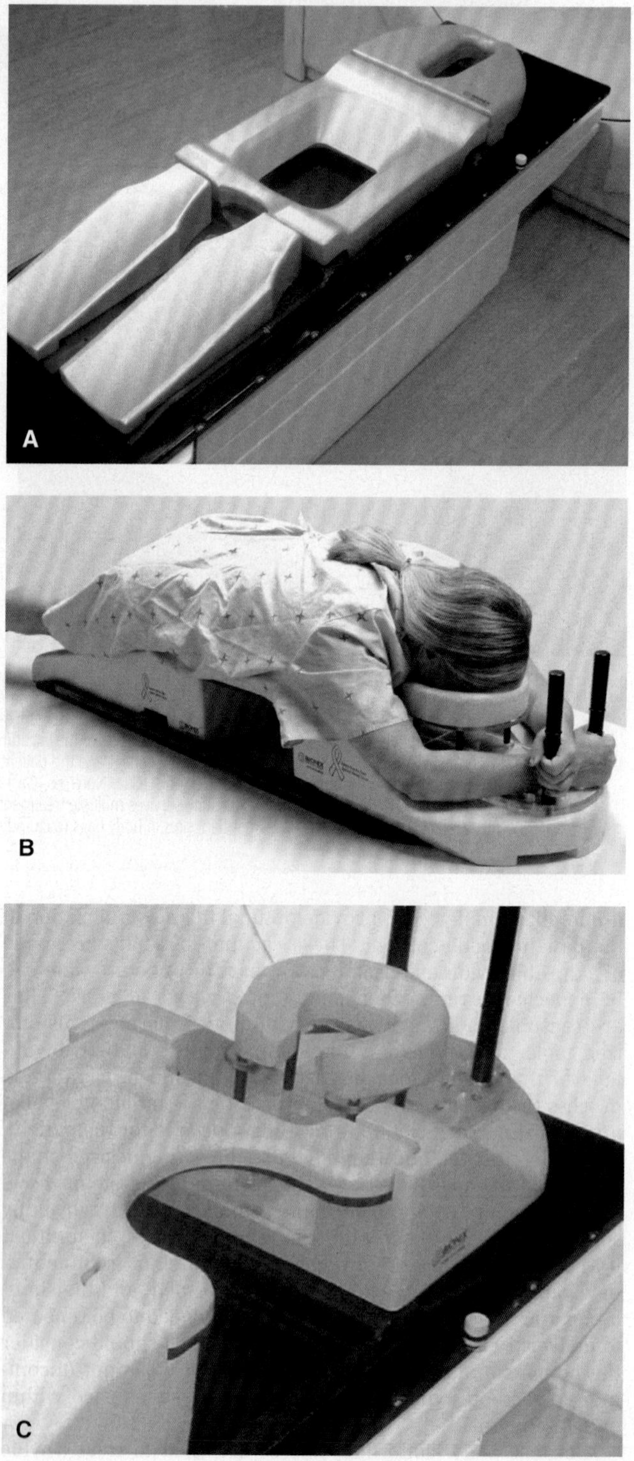

FIGURE 21.6. Immobilization devices specifically designed for prone positioning. **A:** A prone belly board can be used in treating targets in the pelvis. Gravity assists small bowel migration out of the treatment fields, which can reduce treatment-related toxicity. **B, C:** A prone breast board offered by Bionix Radiation Therapy can be advantageous for patients with large, pendulous breasts. The board features a cutout that is easily reversible for treatment of either breast. (Courtesy of Bionix Radiation Therapy, Toledo, OH.)

the cutout region. With the aid of gravity, the small bowel will fall into the board's cutout and can reduce the amount of bowel in the treatment fields. The use of a prone belly board has been demonstrated to reduce the volume of small bowel at all dose levels.[17–20] Even with intensity-modulated radiation therapy, the use of a belly-board technique has been shown to further reduce the small bowel dose.[18]

The magnitude of the small-bowel reduction with prone belly board positioning can be highly patient-dependent. Kim et al.[18] correlated the amount of small bowel at the 50% isodose level with a patient's age, weight, and gender. For example, this work showed a larger amount of small bowel (total volume in cubic centimeters) at the 50% isodose level for the subgroups of patients greater than 56 years old, female patients, and patients weighing less than 65 kg (143 lb). In contrast, Das et al. did not find any correlation with patient weight, age, gender, or whether radiation was delivered presurgery or postsurgery. It must also be noted that some investigators reported that the use of a belly board worsened the reproducibility of the patient setup.[17] For example, Martin et al.[19] reported having to reposition the patient based on portal imaging 68% of the time with a prone belly-board system, compared to 23% of the time with supine positioning. In contrast, Olofsen-Acht et al.[20] reported similar setup reproducibility between prone positioning with a belly board and patients in the supine position. Each patient should be assessed at the time of simulation for the efficacy of the belly-board method to displace small bowel, as well as the patient's ability to tolerate lying on the belly board itself.

Another site where prone positioning has been used is in the treatment of breast cancer patients. Figure 21.6B shows a patient positioned on a prone breast board offered by Bionix Radiation Therapy. The patient is positioned on the cushioned platform with her face resting in a donut-shaped cushion. The patient can hold the hand posts to help improve reproducibility and comfort. The prone positioning is most efficacious for patients with large, pendulous breasts, although it may also be an effective option for patients with severe arthritis that may be unable to hold their arms over their head.[21] Patients with large breasts tend to have larger tissue separation, larger treatment volumes, worse surface irregularity, and an accentuated inframammary fold. These characteristics can cause patients with large breasts to have higher reported rates of both acute and late toxicities such as high-grade dermatitis and fibrosis.[22,23]

The prone position has been shown to improve the dose homogeneity throughout the breast volume since the lateral tissue separation is minimized in the pendant geometry.[24,25] This improved dose homogeneity may decrease the rate of late toxicities such as fibrosis, which can lead to undesirable cosmetic consequences. Decreased tissue separation can decrease the entrance dose needed to provide target coverage and may decrease the overall hot spot for the treatment plan, particularly at the skin surface.[21] Improved dose homogeneity and decreased skin dose from prone positioning may also prove to be advantageous for hypofractionated breast regimens, where larger doses per fraction are delivered. Five-year follow-up data from Stegman et al.[21] showed that the prone position offers comparable local control to traditional supine positioning for whole-breast irradiation, with lower levels of toxicity. With the breast hanging in the prone setup, it may also be possible to reduce the dose to nearby normal tissues. The increased separation of the breast tissue from the chest wall has been shown to decrease the amount of irradiated lung in whole-breast irradiation.[26] Dose to the heart is more variable; for left-breast patients, most heart doses (20 to 30 Gy) are decreased in the prone position, although some patients did exhibit higher heart doses when prone.[26]

Large-breasted patients can also be very troublesome to reproducibly set up with supine positioning because the breast can lie in different positions from day to day. In the supine position, a ring or tube can be used to keep the pendulous breast from folding over. With the aid of gravity, daily setup can be more reproducible with the breast hanging in the prone position. There are, however, potential disadvantages to the prone setup for breast patients. The therapists have reduced visibility of the breast with which to align the treatment fields on a daily basis. Furthermore, the prone positioning may not be tolerable for elderly or obese patients. Finally, the prone position may not be logistically suitable for patients requiring regional nodal irradiation because the prone position would severely limit visual alignment of an anterior supraclavicular field.

Total Body Irradiation Immobilization

Several devices are available for clinical programs that include total body irradiation (TBI) with photons, generally in preparation for bone marrow transplantation. These devices can also be designed to rotate and also provide total skin irradiation for treatment of mycosis fungoides. Features of these systems generally include a beam spoiler, because a maximum dose at the skin entrance is preferred for TBI; strategies for applying partial lung blocks; and methods to keep the patient stable while standing for the treatments, which may take from 10 to 40 minutes, depending upon the treatment protocol. The major disadvantage for these systems is identifying storage in the treatment room; they are large and often take up vital space in the treatment area. It is important to note that these systems usually operate at a distance of about 5 m from the target, with the gantry at a horizontal angle (90 or 270 degrees). Figure 21.7 shows two representative TBI devices from Radiation Products Design (Albertville, MN) and Mick Radio-Nuclear Instruments (Mount Vernon, NY). Features such as a bicycle seat, handgrips, and shoulder stabilizers are used to help support the patient. Some TBI stands offer a harness that will provide an additional measure of security to prevent the patient from falling over in case the patient succumbs to fatigue and faints.

Dosimetric Effects of Immobilization Devices

Any material placed between the patient and the radiation source can modify characteristics of the treatment beam. Modern immobilization devices made of low-density materials have little impact on the depth–dose characteristics of megavoltage energy treatment beams. Electrons liberated within the immobilization device can, however, lead to a measurable increase in the patient's surface dose, that is, a bolusing effect. Clinical experience supports this effect and has shown that skin reactions are more frequent, and tend to occur earlier in the treatment course, when beams are delivered through an immobilization device.[27,28] The magnitude of the bolus effect depends on the composition, density, and thickness of the immobilization device.

For thermoplastic head and neck masks, the bolus effect is reduced when the masks are stretched more as the thickness of material in the beam's path is subsequently reduced. The clinician may also cut out parts of the mask to remove material in the beam path to reduce skin reactions. Care must be taken, however, to ensure that the integrity of the mask and its ability to provide rigid immobilization are not compromised. With proper skill and attention, thermoplastic masks with cutouts to improve skin sparing have been shown to achieve similar setup accuracy as unmodified masks.[7,29] For custom-made foam body-conformal systems, such as the Alpha Cradle, foam lying in the beam path can be shaved away to reduce the thickness along the beam path. Reusable vacuum-lock bags are commercially available with treatment beam portals for standard beam arrangements to avoid bolusing.

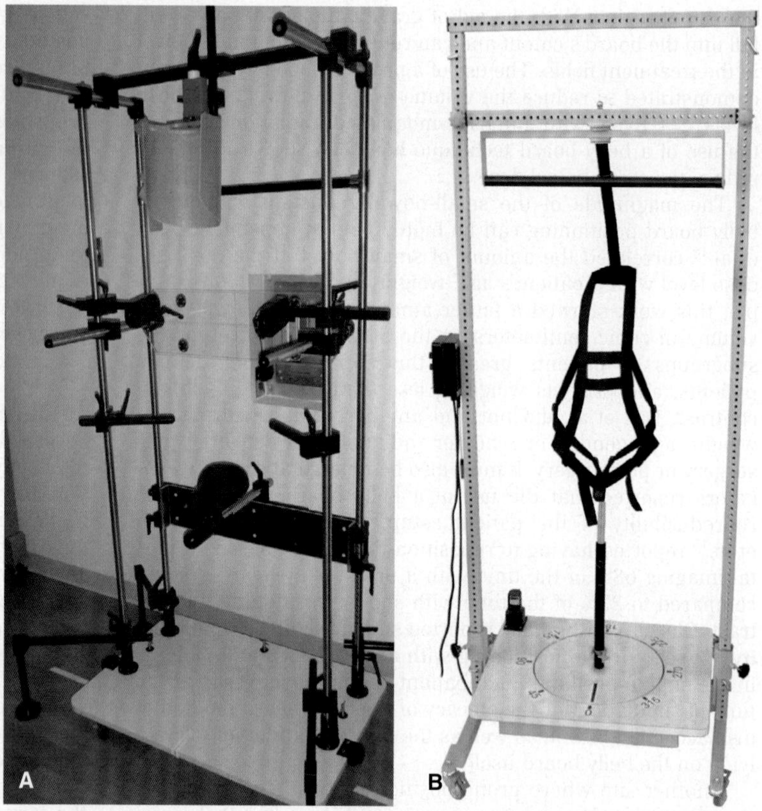

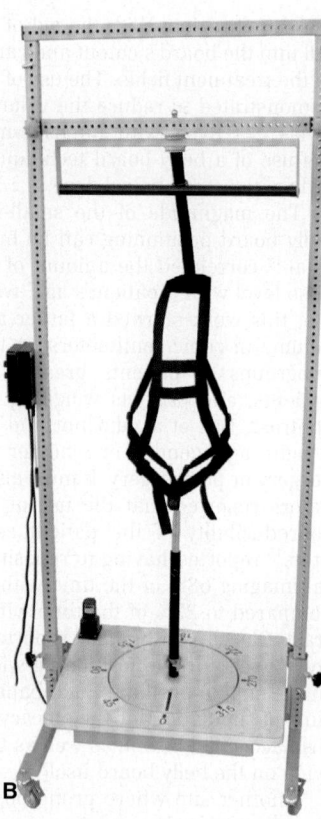

FIGURE 21.7. A stand is commonly used to help position patients for total body irradiation (TBI) with photons and electrons. **A:** Common features of TBI stands include hand grips and a seat to help support the patient. **B:** Harness used to prevent the patient from falling in the case of fatigue and/or fainting. (B courtesy of RPD, Albertville, MN.)

ADOPTION OF STEREOTACTIC IMMOBILIZATION AND STABILIZATION

Hypofractionated stereotactic techniques enable the radiation oncologist to deliver high-dose conformal radiation therapy with a sharp dose falloff to both intracranial and extracranial targets. Here, we describe radiation therapy delivered as a single high-dose fraction as stereotactic radiosurgery (SRS) and therapy delivered over a small number of high-dose fractions stereotactic radiotherapy (SRT). The target volume may be in close proximity to critical structures, such as the spinal cord, optic structures, esophagus, or great vessels, with dose limitations that must be respected in order to prevent significant, often irreversible, and potentially lethal radiation-induced toxicity. To be executed safely, a reproducible, stable, and comfortable setup is necessary to ensure target coverage, avoidance of adjacent organs at risk, and patient tolerance of the treatment.

Delivering a high dose to the target volume in only a few fractions increases the requirements for precise delivery of the radiation. In hypofractionated stereotactic radiotherapy, interfractional and intrafractional variation must be diligently accounted for. Improvements in patient immobilization and localization, particularly with advances in image guidance, can help to decrease interfractional variation in patient setup. Intrafraction target motion occurs in lung and liver tumors due to normal physiologic processes such as respiration, and numerous strategies to minimize this motion are discussed later in this section. Longer treatment times associated with hypofractionated SRT may also lead to decreased intrafractional treatment accuracy.[30] Intrafraction error from patient movement within the device during treatment can be decreased by improving the comfort and stability of the immobilization system. As with all immobilization methods and devices, patients with poorer performance status may have worse interfractional setup reproducibility and more intrafraction motion within the immobilization device.[31]

Invasive Cranial Immobilization Devices

Invasive cranial stereotactic radiation therapy frames use metal pins that are driven into the skull and attached to a frame, usually via metal posts. Generally, two long posts are placed anterior and two shorts posts are placed posterior. Some systems use a curved front piece on the frame to allow for intubation during treatment. The patient then undergoes imaging (either CT or magnetic resonance imaging [MRI], depending on the compatibility of the device) with a fiducial system attached to the frame to provide stereotactic coordinates of the tumor location within the frame. A treatment plan is then developed. At time of treatment, the head frame is connected to either a floor-mounted stand or the treatment table to provide rigid cranial immobilization. A device-specific stereotactic localizer system is then used to set up to the isocenter, and treatment is delivered, usually in a single fraction. The primary advantage of the invasive, frame-based, nonrelocatable stereotactic head frame is the rigid immobilization it provides, with accuracy generally reported on the range of less than 1 mm.[32,33]

The Leksell Stereotactic Coordinate Frame G (Elekta; Fig. 21.8) can be used to deliver intracranial stereotactic radiosurgery on Gamma Knife (Elekta) or linear accelerator platforms. The frame is attached to four adjustable posts, and four self-tapping screws are driven into the skull to fix the device to the head. A CT or MRI indicator is then attached to the frame, and treatment planning imaging is obtained. At the time of patient setup on the treatment machine, the head ring is attached to the couch for rigid immobilization and is shifted into position based on the stereotactic coordinates determined from the planning imaging. A phantom study on the Gamma Knife system using GafChromic film (Ashland, Wayne, NJ) found the mean overall accuracy (± standard deviation) of an irradiation position defined by MRI to be 0.21 ± 0.32 and 0.15 ± 0.26 mm in the x and y axes, and 0.06 ± 0.09 and 0.04 ± 0.09 mm in the x and y axes when using a CT-based target definition.[32]

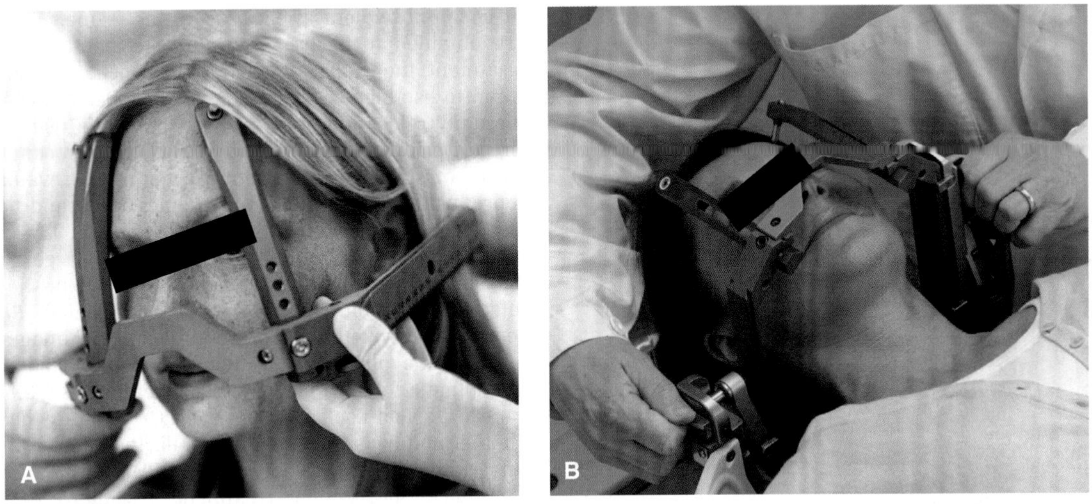

FIGURE 21.8. A: The Leksell Coordinate Frame G is fixed to the patient's head via four self-tapping screws. **B:** At the time of treatment delivery, the frame is attached to the treatment table. (Courtesy of Elekta, Norcross, GA.)

The Brown-Roberts-Wells (BRW) frame system (Integra Radionics, Burlington, MA) is commercially available for use with linear accelerator (linac)-based radiosurgery head rings for the delivery of linac-based SRS. To achieve cranial immobilization, a ring is rigidly fixed to the patient's head. The frame is connected to four posts, which are then fixated to the skull by four pins. The BRW localizer frame, which features a set of vertical and diagonal indicators rods to facilitate stereotactic location within the image set, is then attached. Both CT- and MRI-compatible indicator rods are available. At the time of radiation delivery, the ring and BRW frame are attached with an adapter to the treatment couch or to a floor-mounted stand for stereotactic localization. Ramakrishna et al.[34] used stereoscopic kV x-ray imaging to evaluate setup accuracy and intrafraction motion using the BRW system. The mean deviation between frame-based and image-guided positioning was 1.0 ± 0.5 mm, and the mean intrafraction deviation was 0.4 ± 0.3 mm.

A disadvantage of these invasive, nonrelocatable devices is that they are for the most part limited to single-fraction radiosurgery, which requires ring placement, image acquisition, radiation therapy treatment planning, quality assurance, and treatment delivery to occur in the same day. The patient will have the frame placed early in the morning and will have to wait several hours with the frame in place before treatment can be completed. An alternative to single-fraction radiosurgery with an invasive immobilization device is the TALON removable head frame system designed by Best Nomos (Pittsburgh, PA).

The TALON system is a relocatable invasive stereotactic head frame that uses two self-tapping titanium screws, which are inserted into the patient's skull at the vertex. The detachable TALON assembly is then attached to the screws implanted in the skull for patient positioning on imaging and treatment tables. Salter et al.[35] evaluated repositioning accuracy of the system with CT imaging and reported a mean isocenter deviation of 0.99 ± 0.28 mm in patients treated with SRS and a mean isocenter deviation of 1.38 ± 0.48 mm in patients treated over 6 weeks. This immobilization system requires the placement of two screws into the skull that must remain in place for the duration of therapy but allows more time for treatment planning after simulation CT/MRI, as well as the ability to perform multifraction radiotherapy.

Noninvasive Cranial Immobilization Devices: Frame Based

Invasive cranial immobilization devices have been successfully used for many years to deliver SRS, but use of these systems requires placement of screws into the patient's head, which carries the risk of bleeding and infection and requires the use of premedication and dedicated nursing support.[34] The compressed treatment planning time required for nonrelocatable systems may also be less desirable in certain scenarios. Several varieties of noninvasive, relocatable, frame-based solutions for cranial immobilization have been developed that can provide accurate and reproducible immobilization of the head without the use of screws driven into the skull. Similar to the invasive systems, a stereotactic fiducial-based localizer system can be attached to the ring at the time of image acquisition for treatment planning. The stereotactic localizer is then used for setup to the isocenter on the treatment machine. The ring is attached to either a floor-mounted device or the couch at the time of treatment delivery. These devices are capable of providing reproducible and stable setups for the delivery of multiple fractions of radiation therapy. They also allow more time for treatment planning after simulation and do not carry the risks associated with invasive fixation of the frame to the skull. Similar to the previously described invasive systems, the noninvasive, relocatable head ring systems are capable of providing excellent setup reproducibility and stability to limit intrafraction motion.

The Stereoadapter 5000 noninvasive stereotactic localizer and immobilization device is commercially available through Sandstrom Trade and Technology (Welland, Canada). This device is mounted to the patient's head with two earplugs and a nasal bridge support. The ear plugs are inserted into the external auditory canals bilaterally, and the nasal support is lowered until it rests on the nasal bridge. The earplugs are secured in place by tightening the nasal screw. Two side arms are first attached to a connector plate and then attached to a vertex stabilizer. A band is then fastened against the occiput to provide additional stabilization of the frame. Measurements obtained from the millimeter scales on the Stereoadapter components are recorded and used for reproducing the setup in future applications of the device. The device is compatible with both MRI and CT imaging and uses an xyz Cartesian coordinate system for target localization. Kalapurkal et al.[36] evaluated setup reproducibility of this immobilization system using portal images coregistered with the CT scout image and reported mean isocenter shifts of 1.0 ± 0.7, 0.8 ± 0.8, and 1.7 ± 1.0 mm in the x, y, and z axes, respectively.

The Brainlab Non-Invasive Mask System (Brainlab, Munich, Germany; Fig. 21.9) uses a U-shaped frame, two vertical posts, a three-piece thermoplastic mask, and an optional bite-block attachment for noninvasive rigid cranial immobilization. At the time of simulation, the three thermoplastic shells are custom

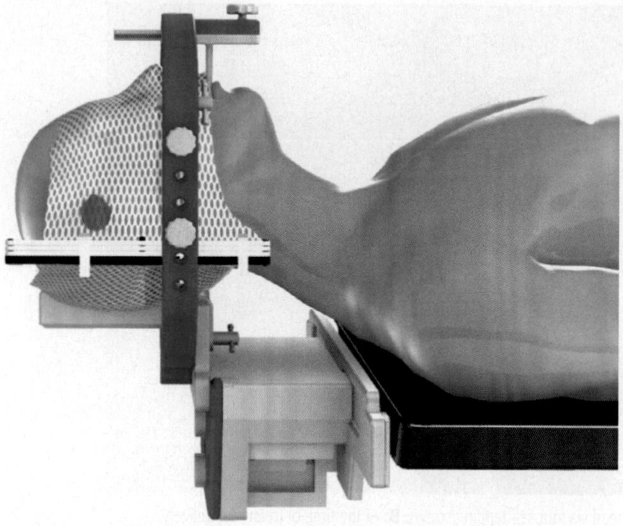

FIGURE 21.9. The Brainlab noninvasive mask system uses three pieces of thermoplastic material custom molded to the patient's head and attached to vertical posts on either side of the patient's head. These posts are then attached to a U-shaped frame, which is attached to the treatment couch, thus providing rigid immobilization of the head. A stereotactic localizer box may be used for target localization. (Courtesy of Brainlab, Munich, Germany.)

shaped to the anterior and posterior aspects of the patient's head. The shells are fastened to the vertical posts, which are attached to the head ring. The ring is attached to the CT couch by an adapter, and a stereotactic localizer device can then be attached. An optional bite plate can be connected to the anterior aspect of the frame to provide additional points of support to the patient. Ali et al.[37] evaluated the setup accuracy of the Brainlab mask system with onboard kV imaging and reported mean shifts of 0.7 ± 2.0, 1.6 ± 2.6, and 0.1 ± 2.2 mm in the *x*, *y*, and *z* dimensions, respectively. Bednarz et al.[38] also evaluated setup accuracy with pretreatment kV imaging and found a mean 3D displacement from isocenter of 3.17 ± 1.9 mm. Hong et al.[33] evaluated the Brainlab mask system with a dental bar using pretreatment kV imaging and reported mean deviations of 0.3 ± 0.8, 0.1 ± 1.4, and 0.0 ± 0.9 mm in the *x*, *y*, and *z* dimensions, respectively. They reported intrafractional motion of 0.4 ± 1.0, 0.0 ± 1.3, and 0.1 ± 0.8 mm in the *x*, *y*, and *z* axes, respectively. Ramakrishna et al.[34] evaluated intrafraction motion with the Brainlab system using posttreatment kV imaging and reported a mean intrafraction shift of 0.7 ± 0.5 mm.

Masi et al.[39] evaluated the setup accuracy and intrafraction motion of a frame-based thermoplastic mask system with and without the use of a bite block. All patients underwent frame-guided setup followed by cone-beam CT (CBCT), and mean overall shifts based on bony anatomy were 2.9 ± 1.3 mm with a bite block and 3.2 ± 1.5 mm without a bite block ($p = .15$). Mean intrafraction motion measured with CBCT did not differ between the patients treated with and without a bite block and was found to be 0.2 ± 0.55, 0.1 ± 0.61, and 0.3 ± 0.55 mm in the *x*, *y*, and *z* dimensions, respectively.

The Gill-Thomas-Cosman (GTC) Relocatable Head Ring (Integra, Plainsboro, NJ) is a frame-based, noninvasive, relocatable cranial immobilization device that is compatible with the BRW localizer coordinate system. Two custom devices are used: a mold of the patient's upper dentition that is mounted to the head ring anteriorly, and a patient-specific headrest that is mounted to the ring posteriorly. A Velcro strap is connected to the headrest posteriorly and connects to each side of the ring anteriorly. The straps are marked at time of simulation to allow for setup reproducibility. Measurements are then obtained with the XKnife Depth Helmet (Integra), a clear plastic device with holes that is placed over the ring. A rod with millimeter scale is inserted into each hole, and a measurement is taken. At each subsequent application of the frame, measurements are obtained to ensure accurate placement. At the time of treatment, the ring is attached to the couch or a floor-mounted stand to establish rigid immobilization. Das et al.[40] measured the daily relocation error of the GTC frame using the Depth Helmet prior to each fraction and found a mean radial displacement of 1.03 ± 0.34 mm. Burton et al.[41] evaluated setup reproducibility with the Depth Helmet and found that 97% of displacement vectors were within 2.5 mm and 92% of displacement vectors were within 2 mm, with the largest mean displacement in a single dimension of 0.4 mm in the superior–inferior direction. Kumar et al.[42] evaluated daily setup reproducibility with daily pretreatment portal imaging coregistered to the planning CT digitally reconstructed radiograph and found a total 3D mean displacement of 1.8 ± 0.8 mm.

The Tarbell-Loeffler-Cosman (TLC) pediatric head ring is another noninvasive cranial immobilization device offered from Integra that is compatible with the BRW coordinate system for stereotactic localization. Treatment of pediatric patients often requires the use of general anesthesia with intubation, and this device is designed to allow access to the airway during treatment. Rigid fixation is achieved with a face mask that is molded around the eyes and nasal bridge and connected to an adjustable occipital head cup. Lateral ear bars provide support but are not involved in fixation of the frame to the patient's head. After placement of the device on the patient's head, the XKnife Depth Helmet can be used to confirm accurate ring positioning. The system can then be attached to the treatment couch with an adapter or to a floor-mounted stand for treatment delivery.

The Elekta eXtend frame system (Fig. 21.10) is a relocatable, noninvasive cranial immobilization device for fractionated stereotactic radiotherapy. Similar to the previously described HeadFIX system, a dental imprint is obtained, and a custom dental mold is placed in the mouth with suction to the hard palate. The mouthpiece is then connected to a carbon fiber frame that is attached to the treatment couch, immobilizing the patient. A vacuum device is connected to the mouthpiece to generate the suction of the dental block to the hard palate. Prior to treatment, the repositioning check tool (RCT) is used to confirm that the patient's head is accurately relocated within the frame. As can be seen in Figure 21.10B, the RCT consists of a plastic box that is rigidly affixed to the frame. Through holes in the RCT box, a spring-loaded digital gauge is placed to measure the distance between the frame and the patient's head, which is compared to values measured on the first day of treatment.[43] Ruschin et al.[43] reported on the setup accuracy of the eXtend frame using the repositioning check tool, as well as intrafraction motion with the system. The mean 3D setup error was 0.8 mm in patients treated on a linear accelerator and 1.3 mm in patients treated on Gamma Knife Perfexion. The mean intrafraction motion was measured at 0.4 ± 0.3 mm. They concluded that the RCT was adequate to confirm accurate frame positioning, and that the system provided excellent immobilization for fractionated intracranial radiosurgery. Sayer et al.[44] reported on their initial experience of four patients treated with the eXtend frame system with Gamma Knife Perfexion, and the mean radial positioning error for all patients was between 0.33 and 0.84 mm.

Noninvasive Cranial Immobilization Devices: Frameless

Frame-based systems are able to provide rigid and accurate patient setups by defining the tumor's stereotactic location within the frame, which can be reproduced daily at treatment delivery with the use of a stereotactic coordinate reference device and the in-room laser system. An alternative strategy is to use a thermoplastic mask with daily pretreatment image guidance to improve interfractional accuracy in patient positioning. Another option for frameless intracranial SRS is to use optically guided fiducial markers as a surrogate for daily

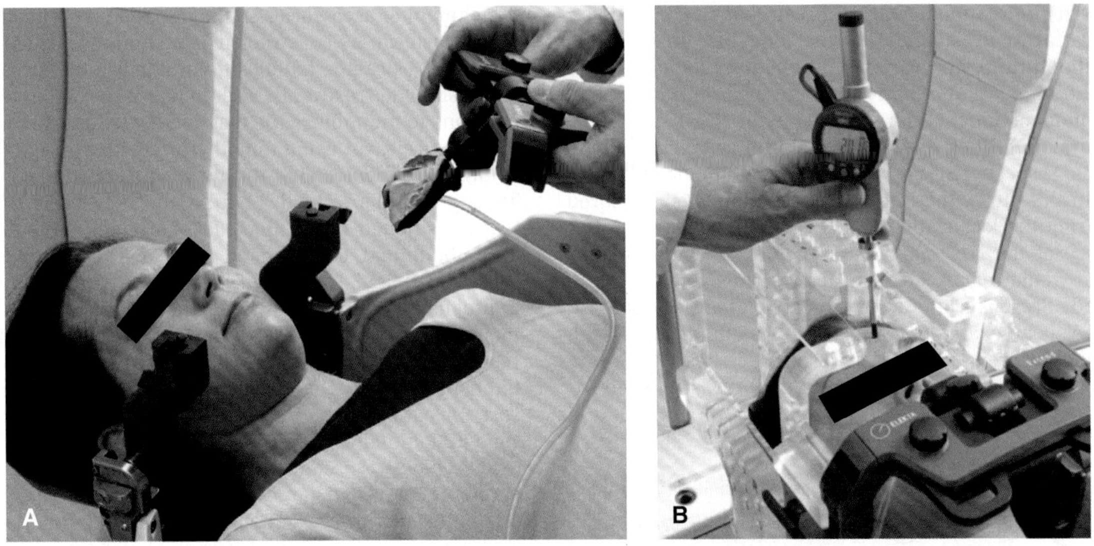

FIGURE 21.10. The Elekta eXtend is a relocatable immobilization device designed for fractionated stereotactic radiotherapy. **A:** A custom mold of the maxillary dentition is fixated to the hard palate with suction and then attached to a carbon fiber frame to provide rigid immobilization to the couch. **B:** Setup accuracy is assessed with the repositioning check tool prior to the delivery of each treatment. (Courtesy of Elekta, Norcross, GA.)

target localization and to monitor patient motion in real time. Tryggestad et al.[45] evaluated four frameless, thermoplastic mask-based immobilization systems with CBCT to determine whether they would be adequate for image-guided intracranial radiosurgery. They reported mean interfraction deviation of 2.1 to 2.7 mm and mean intrafraction deviation of 0.7 to 1.1 mm for the four systems. They concluded that a frameless setup using a variety of thermoplastic masks in combination with image guidance to reduce interfractional setup error was acceptable for intracranial radiosurgery.

In 1997, researchers at the University of Florida (Gainesville, FL) reported on an institutionally developed, high-precision, frameless, optically guided stereotactic radiotherapy system that separated immobilization and localization.[46] The immobilization device consisted of a custom head holder posteriorly and a custom thermoplastic mask anteriorly extending from the forehead to the upper lip. A custom bite plate was fitted to the maxillary dentition, and a set of six infrared light-emitting diodes was attached to the plate for stereotactic localization with an infrared camera system. This system allowed for reproducible, noninvasive setup with the ability to perform real-time tracking of the infrared markers and thus patient motion. They reported that the bite plate could be positioned and repositioned within 0.5 ± 0.3 mm. Peng et al.[47] evaluated the accuracy of a frameless immobilization system using a thermoplastic mask and bite block with optically guided fiducials by setting up patients using the SonArray system (Varian, Palo Alto, CA) and then acquiring CBCT. They reported a mean setup error of 1.2 ± 0.7 mm.

Invasive Extracranial Immobilization Devices

In 1995, Hamilton et al.[48] from the University of Arizona (Tucson, AZ) published their preliminary clinical experience with linear accelerator–based SRS of the spine in five patients. They developed a spinal stereotactic frame consisting of a rigid box with two semicircular metal arches. Clamps were placed and secured transcutaneously to the spinous processes one to two vertebral levels above and below the target volume under local or general anesthesia, usually through a 2-cm incision. Rigid immobilization of the spine was achieved by attaching the clamps to the semicircular metal arches on the stereotactic frame. After CT simulation and treatment planning, the frame was transferred to a modified linear accelerator and set up to coordinates derived from the planning CT. The patients were then treated with single-fraction SRS to doses ranging from 8 to 10 Gy. Although this device was important in demonstrating the feasibility of extracranial stereotactic radiation therapy, techniques for stereotactic body radiotherapy (SBRT) immobilization have migrated to noninvasive systems.

Noninvasive Extracranial Immobilization Devices

SBRT immobilization systems are generally customizable devices and include thermoplastic molds, conformal body molds, and stereotactic body frames. Stereotactic localizer frames may be used in daily setup. Due to the highly mobile nature of extracranial targets, however, pretreatment image-guided localization is recommended by the American Association of Physicists in Medicine (AAPM) Task Group 101 for patients being treated with SBRT.[49]

The Elekta BodyFIX is an example of a body-conformal system used in SBRT. It has a dual-vacuum design and is available in multiple sizes to accommodate a variety of patient body types and target locations for SBRT. As described in the preceding section and illustrated in Figure 21.5C, the BodyFIX system includes a bead-filled vacuum-lock mattress, base plate, thin, clear plastic cover sheet, and a dual-vacuum pump. This system accommodates a stereotactic localizer box to be attached to the base plate or the linear accelerator couch. At the time of simulation, the patient is positioned in the bag, and the clear plastic cover sheet is placed over the patient's body and attached to the bag. The vacuum is then attached to evacuate the air between the patient and the cover sheet. As the air is evacuating, the therapists mold the vacuum-lock bag to the posterior and lateral aspects of the patient's body. Once a satisfactory setup is achieved, any remaining air is evacuated from the mattress and the minispheres lock into place, creating a customized, reusable, rigid body mold. The unique negative pressure created by the cover sheet and vacuum of the BodyFIX provides additional immobilization of the patient during treatment delivery. A study of repositioning accuracy of the BodyFIX system revealed rotational error around the x, y, and z axes of 0.9 ± 0.7, 0.8 ± 0.7, and 1.8 ± 1.6 deg, respectively.[50] Under the assumption of a rigid-body relationship of the target and bony anatomy, mean deviation was 2.9 ± 3.3, 2.3 ± 2.5, and 3.2 ± 2.7 mm in the x, y, and z dimensions, respectively, and the median and mean vectors of target isocenter deviation were 4.9 and 5.7 ± 3.7 mm, respectively. A study of 126 patients treated with SBRT for lung tumors used pretreatment and posttreatment CBCT to determine intrafractional stability of the BodyFIX system and reported the intrafraction variation of mean tumor position to be 2.7 ± 2.6 mm.[51] Han et al.[52] found the mean intrafractional tumor motion of lung tumors treated with SBRT using the BodyFIX system to be 0.8, 1.5, and 0.9 mm in the *x*, *y*, and *z* dimensions, respectively, with a mean overall tumor motion of 2.3 mm. In this study, the intrafraction motion was measured by comparing the localization CBCT to a CBCT obtained after the delivery of the coplanar beams (before any noncoplanar beams that would require a couch kick were delivered).

The Body Pro-Lok from Civco Medical Solutions (Kalona, IA; Fig. 21.11A) is an example of a modular system for SBRT with the capability of treating a variety of disease sites. The entire length of the lightweight carbon fiber platform is indexed for attachment of accessories so that a patient-specific immobilization device can be constructed. Attachments include headrests, forehead restraints, handles to immobilize the arms above the head, shoulder restraints, abdominal compression devices, and cushions to immobilize the feet and legs. Gutierrez et al.[53] evaluated this system using tomotherapy with pretreatment megavoltage CT to determine the mean interfractional setup error. Twenty patients treated for liver and lung tumors with SBRT were positioned in the Body Pro-Lok with a vacuum cushion and abdominal compression device. The mean localization error was 0.9 ± 3.1, 1.2 ± 5.5, and 6.5 ± 2.6 mm in the *x*, *y*, and *z* dimensions, respectively, and the mean composite displacement vector was 8.2 ± 2.0 mm. Civco also offers an inflatable respiratory belt system (Fig. 21.11A inset) to achieve abdominal compression. The belt can be inflated to a tolerable pressure for patients who experience too much discomfort with the rigid abdominal compression panel.

The Elekta Stereotactic Body Frame (SBF; Fig. 21.11B) has a reference system for reproducible isocenter localization. It can be used with a vacuum cushion and abdominal compression device as described by Murray et al.[54] Intrafractional variation in mean tumor position using the SBF system was evaluated with pretreatment and posttreatment CBCT and reported to be 1.5 ± 1.1 mm.[51] Purdie et al.[30] evaluated interfraction and intrafraction tumor movement with the SBF in 28 lung cancer patients treated with SBRT. Patients were positioned in the SBF with a full-body vacuum-lock bag, and an abdominal compression device was used with tumors demonstrating motion greater than 10 mm at time of simulation. They found the systematic setup error in the *x*, *y*, and *z* dimensions to be 4.3, 3.7, and 6.1 mm, respectively, and 5.0 mm overall. The reproducibility of intrafraction target position was evaluated by comparing the planning CT to a midtreatment or posttreatment CBCT, with a mean and median time interval of 34 minutes between localization CBCT and mid/end of treatment CBCT. The mean 3D tumor position compared to the planning CT was 2.2 ± 1.2 mm with imaging performed within 34 minutes of target localization and 5.3 ± 3 mm when performed more than 34 minutes after target localization ($p < .01$), highlighting the effect that longer treatment times can increase the intrafractional error. This device has been used in multiple institutions and international protocols but is no longer commercially available from Elekta.

Another example of a modular SBRT immobilization system is the Bionix Radiation Therapy Omni V SBRT positioning system (Fig. 21.11C), which uses a lightweight, radiolucent indexing T-Form Treatment Base with a vacuum-lock cushion. A variety of additional structures can be attached, including an abdominal compression device, thigh and foot positioners, and an upper-arm support. An external fiducial arch is available for attachment to the treatment base for setup and localization.

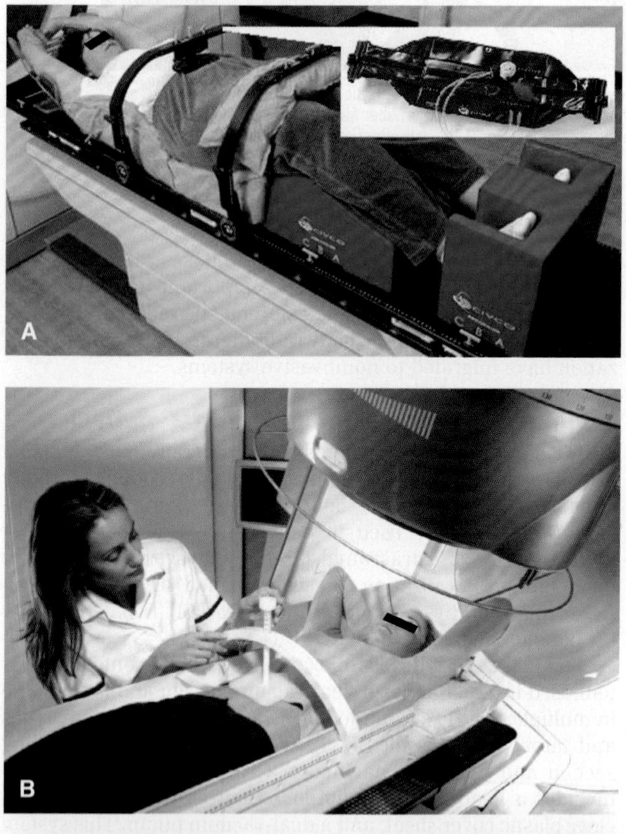

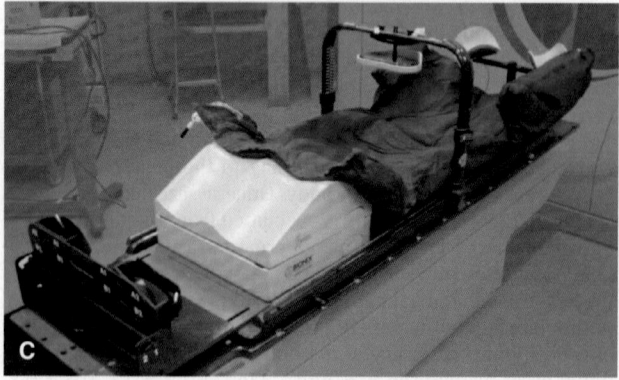

FIGURE 21.11. A: The Body-Pro Lok is a modular immobilization system that can be used for stereotactic body radiotherapy. Multiple attachments are available to build a device customized to the needs of each patient. This particular setup uses an abdominal compression plate. (A courtesy of Civco Medical Solutions, Kalona, IA.) **B:** The Stereotactic Body Frame has a reference system that runs along the length of the device. (B courtesy of Elekta, Norcross, GA.) **C:** The Omni V is another modular system with a variety of options to provide customized patient immobilization. (C courtesy of Bionix Radiation Therapy, Toledo, OH.)

Immobilization and Internal Motion Management

In addition to intrafractional error due to patient movement within the immobilization device, internal target motion due to breathing must be accounted for in SBRT, particularly in treatment of lung and liver tumors. The AAPM Task Group 101 recommended that all patients with tumors in the thorax or abdomen who will be treated with SBRT undergo tumor motion assessment.[49]

The AAPM Task Group 76 report[55] addressed the management of respiratory motion in radiation therapy. As detailed in this report, which describes the results of a variety of studies evaluating lung tumor motion, mean tumor motion is greatest in the superior–inferior (*y* axis) dimension, particularly in tumors of the lower lobes. The mean tumor motion values in the *x*, *y*, and *z* dimensions were 2.4 to 7.3, 3.9 to 12.5, and 2.4 to 4.9 mm, respectively. Superior–inferior (*y* axis) motion ranged from 4.3 to 7.5 mm for upper- and middle-lobe tumors and from 9.5 to 18.5 mm for lower-lobe tumors. Seppenwoolde et al.[56] evaluated lung tumor motion with peritumoral fiducial markers and fluoroscopy. They found the mean amplitude of motion in the superior–inferior dimension to be greater for lower-lobe/nonfixed tumors compared to upper-lobe or fixed tumors (12 ± 6 vs. 2 ± 2 mm, $p = .005$). Baba et al.[57] measured lung tumor motion with fluoroscopy and found the superior–inferior mean amplitude of tumor motion to be 9.2 ± 7.1 mm for all tumor locations, 14.2 ± 6.9 mm for lower lung field tumors, and 4.8 ± 3.3 mm for upper lung field tumors.

The AAPM Task Group 76 report[55] also summarizes the findings from various reports of liver motion. The mean liver motion in the superior–inferior dimension was 10 to 25 mm with shallow breathing and 37 to 55 mm with deep breathing. Case et al.[58] demonstrated a mean amplitude of liver motion in free-breathing patients with no internal motion control to be 1.4, 9.0, and 5.1 mm in the *x*, *y*, and *z* axes, respectively. In a study of 16 patients with 30 tumors, Eccles et al.[59] found the mean free-breathing liver motion by fluoroscopy to range from 22 to 40 mm. A study of liver tumor motion in 20 patients by Kitamura et al.[60] using peritumoral fiducial markers showed mean amplitudes of tumor motion of 4 ± 4, 9 ± 5, and 5 ± 3 mm in the *x*, *y*, and *z* dimensions, respectively. Statistically significant differences in tumor motion in right-lobe tumors compared to left-lobe tumors in the *x* axis (5 ± 4 vs. 2 ± 1 mm, $p = .01$) and *z* axis (6 ± 3 vs. 3 ± 2 mm, $p = .01$) were found but not in the superior–inferior dimension. In a study of liver and lower-lobe lung tumor motion using four-dimensional (4D) CT in 10 patients, mean overall tumor motion with no motion control was 13.6 mm.[61]

Multiple strategies have been developed to account for internal target motion, including deep inspiration breath hold, active breathing control, respiratory gating, real-time tumor tracking, and abdominal compression devices. Abdominal compression devices are patient immobilization accessories designed to control respiratory excursion. This technique may also be referred to as forced shallow breathing. Abdominal compression devices typically consist of a plate attached to an arch by a screw, which is attached to a stereotactic body frame or treatment couch. The plate is placed a few centimeters below the xiphoid process, and the screw is tightened until the desired amount of internal motion control is achieved. The screw is marked so that it can be reproducibly tightened for the setup of subsequent treatment fractions. The arch should also have an indexed position on the stereotactic body frame or treatment couch for reproducible setup in the superior–inferior direction. Abdominal compression devices are available from a variety of companies, including Civco Medical Solutions for use on the Pro-Lok immobilization system, and from Bionix Radiation Therapy for use on the Omni V system.

A study of motion with four-dimensional (4D) CT in 10 patients with liver and lower-lobe lung tumors showed a decrease in mean overall tumor motion from 13.6 mm with free breathing to 8.3 mm with medium abdominal compression force and 7.2 mm with high abdominal compression force.[61] High abdominal compression was defined as the mean force to limit respiratory excursion of the tumor to less than 1 cm over 10 breathing cycles (90.7 ± 27.1 N), and medium compression was defined as 50% of this force (47.6 ± 16.0 N). Medium compression reduced respiratory motion to less than 1 cm in three patients, and high compression reduced tumor motion to less than 1 cm in all patients. Negoro et al.[62] studied lung tumor motion in 18 patients treated with SBRT and found the mean tumor motion in the superior–inferior dimension measured with fluoroscopy to decrease from 12.3 mm to 7.0 mm (range 2 to 11 mm) with the use of abdominal compression. The mean amplitude of liver motion measured during free breathing with CBCT has been shown to change respectively from 1.4, 9.0, and 5.1 mm in the *x*, *y*, and *z* dimensions to 2.2, 6.7, and 3.3 mm in the *x*, *y*, and *z* dimensions when an abdominal compression device was added.[58] The mean amplitude for liver motion measured with fluoroscopy was shown to decrease from 40 mm with free breathing to 11 mm with the use of an abdominal compression device.[59] Liver tumor motion measured with fiducial markers and fluoroscopy showed a decrease in median excursion of 62% in the superior–inferior dimension and 38% in the anterior–posterior dimension with the use of an abdominal compression device when compared to free breathing.[63] However, the addition of an abdominal compression device increased excursion in the left–right dimension by 15% (maximum 1.6 mm). Table 21.1 is a summary of immobilization devices discussed in this chapter.

IMMOBILIZATION METHODS IN BRACHYTHERAPY

Historically, the focus in brachytherapy has been on immobilization of the applicator, leaving the patient to move freely. For example, manufacturers such as Nucletron and Varian sell brachytherapy stands that clamp onto the applicator. Although advancement in design has made these stands CT and MR compatible, the patient can still move and possibly change the position of the applicator with respect to the organ that is to be treated. In addition, patient flow issues can cause difficulties in brachytherapy treatments. An applicator typically is placed in the patient in an operating room. The patient is then moved to either the radiology or radiation oncology department for imaging and then to the brachytherapy suite for treatment. Each time the patient is moved, the applicator can become displaced from the optimal position. In addition, for treatments that are delivered over several days, such as interstitial implants, the patient is moved to a room in the hospital between treatments.

Immobilization for Genitourinary Treatment

Brachytherapy treatment is common for prostate cancer for men and various gynecologic malignancies for women. Figure 21.12B illustrates an ultrasound probe mounted in a stepper that is used to localize the prostate during low-dose-rate (seed implant) or high-dose-rate brachytherapy treatments.[64] It has been well established that insertion of needles into the prostate for brachytherapy treatment can cause both motion and deformation of the prostate.[65] The stabilizing needle (Fig. 21.12A) is designed to reduce the amount of prostate movement from the insertion of the needles used to deposit seeds throughout the prostate. Stabilizing needles are commercially available, for example, from RPD (Albertville, MN), as well as the Mick Radio-Nuclear Instruments Morgenstern Stabilizing Needle. Immobilization of the prostate is accomplished by deploying a side barb into the prostate tissue. The stabilizing needle is then secured with a "lock spring" to the proximal side of the implantation template. Two stabilizing needles are used in the periphery of the prostate to provide adequate stabilization.

The issue of applicator immobilization for brachytherapy of gynecologic malignancies has been known for many years. Maintenance of the relative position of the applicator to the target and normal tissue, such as bladder and rectum, can determine the quality of the outcome. Vaginal packing and waistbands have commonly been used to immobilize the applicator but are physician dependent and may often be unsatisfactory.[66] An early study measured the displacement of tandem and ovoid applicators of up to 5 mm due to movement of the patient from simulation to the treatment room and then back to simulation.[67] This movement caused a change in dose of up to 10% to point A and 9% and 17% to the rectal and bladder points, respectively. More recently, a comparison of immobilization methods for vaginal cuff brachytherapy was undertaken, showing that even when the cylinder insertion was performed by the same physician with the same immobilization

TABLE 21.1 IMMOBILIZATION DEVICE SUMMARY

Device Name	*Description*	*Pros*	*Cons*	*Typical Sites*	*Reusable?*	*Indexed?*	*Relative Cost*
Timo and Silverman headrests	Foam and plastic headrests with various sizes for a range of body habitus	Inexpensive and reusable	Not custom formed	H&N, craniospinal, thoracic, abdominal, pretty much all supine patients	Yes	Some clip to baseplate, which is indexed to the couch; others do not clip to the couch	$
Thermoplastic masks	Thermoplastic mask material is warmed in a water bath until pliable and then stretched over the patient's face to create a customized device.	Accurate, custom-formed immobilization; can cut out treatment portals to reduce bolusing	Potential for mask shrinkage; patient anxiety or claustrophobia; bolusing effect	H&N, craniospinal	No	Yes; clip to baseplate	$$
Elekta HeadFIX	Bite block for image-guided treatment; advantageous for claustrophobic patients	Noninvasive, relocatable; does not require thermoplastic mask material to be tightly molded to patient's face	Requires operator skill to create custom maxillary dentition molds; may not be best option for patients with poor dentition	H&N	Frame, yes; bite block, no	Yes; stereotactic	$$$
Elekta eXtend	Relocatable bite-block system designed for fractionated stereotactic radiotherapy	Noninvasive, relocatable; does not require thermoplastic mask material to be tightly molded to patient's face; allows for fractionated SRS; high degree of patient setup accuracy.	Requires operator skill to create custom maxillary dentition molds; may not be best option for patients with poor dentition	Intracranial and some extracranial in neck	Frame, yes; bite block, no	No	$$$
Invasive, nonrelocatable intracranial stereotactic immobilization devices	Frame is attached to the patient's skull with four screws; used for single-fraction radiosurgery	Excellent accuracy in patient repositioning	Typically requires sedation; risk of infection and bleeding; patient discomfort	Intracranial	Frame, yes; skull screws, can be sterilized and re-used	Rigidly attached directly to treatment machine (Gamma Knife), table, or floor-mounted stand	$$$
Noninvasive, relocatable intracranial mask based immobilization; e.g., Brainlab noninvasive mask system	Three thermoplastic shells custom molded to patient's head and face, which are attached to U-shaped frame via two posts on either side of the patient's head	Does not require placement of screws into the patient's skull; allows for fractionated SRS; high degree of patient setup accuracy	Thermoplastic mask may be undesirable in certain patients, such as those with claustrophobia or anxiety	Intracranial	Frame and posts, yes; thermoplastic mask, no	Attach to treatment table	$$$
Noninvasive, relocatable mask-less intracranial stereotactic immobilization	Variety of frame-based, noninvasive techniques for reproducible immobilization of the head; may be used for single-fraction and fractionated SRS	Do not require placement of screws in to the patient's skull; allows for fractionated SRS; no thermoplastic mask required; high degree of setup accuracy	May require bite block in some systems; some systems require additional time for setup verification (e.g., Depth Helmet)	Intracranial	Frame, yes; custom headrests and bite blocks, no	Attach to treatment table or floor-mounted stand	$$$
Alpha Cradle	Expanding foam device custom molded to patient body contour	Rigid immobilization for wide range of body sites	One-time use; one shot to achieve adequate and comfortable immobilization	Thorax, abdomen, pelvis, extremities	No	Potentially; an indexing bar can be used to make indentations in the bottom of the bag for later setup with the indexing bar	$$
Vacuum-lock bags	Nylon bag filled with plastic minispheres; upon evacuation minispheres lock together to form a custom mold of the patient body contour	Reusable; can quickly reinflate and re-form during simulation if necessary	Punctures, tears, or loss of vacuum may necessitate resimulation of the patient	Thorax, abdomen, pelvis, extremities	Yes	Potentially; an indexing bar can be used to make indentations in the bottom of the bag for later setup with the indexing bar	$$

TABLE 21.1 (CONTINUED)

Device Name	Description	Pros	Cons	Typical Sites	Reusable?	Indexed?	Relative Cost
Elekta BodyFIX	Vacuum-lock bag with plastic cover sheet; dual-vacuum system for increased immobilization	Reusable; cover sheet may provide abdominal compression	Some patients may find cover sheet uncomfortable	Thorax, abdomen, pelvis	Vacuum-lock bag; yes; cover sheet, no	Potentially; an indexing bar can be used to make indentations in the bottom of the bag for later setup with the indexing bar	$$$
Prone breast board	Prone breast board can improve dosimetry for patients with large, pendulous breasts	Separates target tissue from chest wall to minimize skin folds and lung dose	May not be tolerated by all patients; poor visualization of treatment field alignment; not suitable for regional nodal irradiation	Breast	Yes	Yes	$$
Prone belly board	Prone board to help the small bowel fall out of the treatment fields	Displacement of bowel out of treatment field can reduce toxicity	May not be tolerated by all patients; variability in bowel sparing	Pelvis	Yes	Yes	$$
Modular stereotactic body immobilization systems; e.g., Elekta Stereotactic Body Frame; Civco Body-Pro Lok; Bionix Radiation Therapy Omni V	Indexed base board with a wide range of attachments for immobilization, localization and motion management	Flexibility to treat variety of disease sites with SBRT; attachment of devices for abdominal compression	More room for storage; more time for setup and indexing of attachments	Spine, lung, liver, abdomen, pelvis, neck	Yes	Yes	$$$

H&N, head and neck; SBRT, stereotactic body radiotherapy; SRS, stereotactic radiosurgery.

method and identical patient setup position, variations occurred in the cylinder geometry between simulation and subsequent insertions.[68] The magnitude of the deviation was smaller for stand-type applicator immobilization as opposed to a skirt-type system. It has been shown that the angle of the applicator in vaginal brachytherapy can have a large effect on the normal tissue (bowel) dose and that the applicator should be held in a horizontal position.[69] In addition, as vaginal cuff brachytherapy has migrated from a single-applicator insertion for low-dose-rate brachytherapy to multiple-applicator insertions used in high-dose-rate (HDR) treatments, the positional variation of the applicator geometry has been documented, along with variations in the dose to the normal tissue.[70] Furthermore, because of the steeper dose gradient around HDR sources, the variation of the applicator position magnifies the variation of the dose.

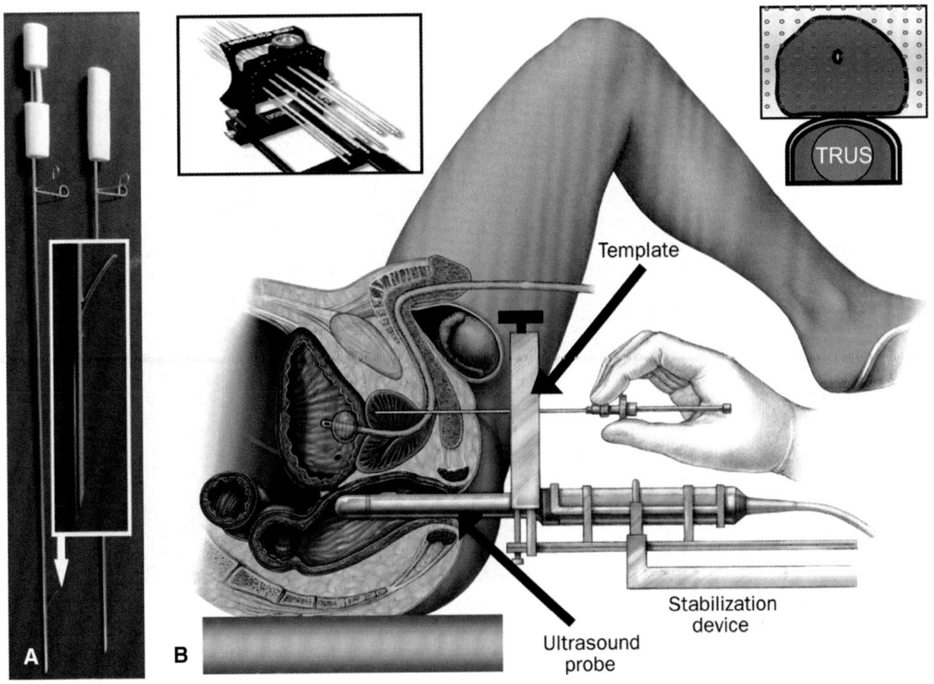

FIGURE 21.12. A: Stabilizing needles used in prostate brachytherapy. Note the barb (inset) that is deployed in the prostate. **B:** Diagram illustrating the prostate brachytherapy implantation procedure using transrectal ultrasound for prostate visualization and a template for guiding the needle loading process. (B reproduced from Pisansky TM, Gold DG, Furutani KM, et al. High-dose-rate brachytherapy in the curative treatment of patients with localized prostate cancer. *Mayo Clin Proc* 2008;83:1364–1382; courtesy of Elsevier; copyright 2008.)

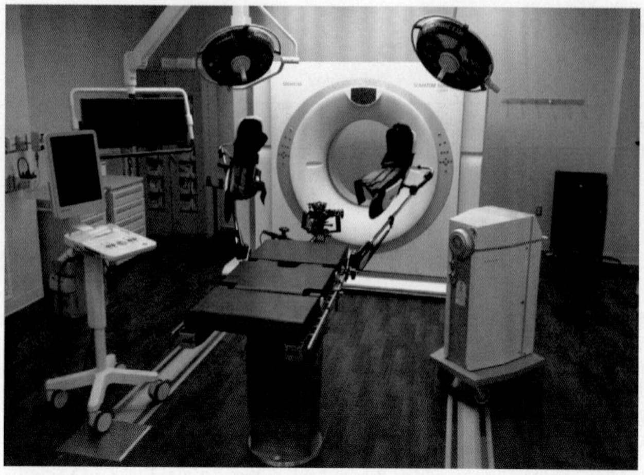

FIGURE 21.13. The brachytherapy suite at the Emily Couric Cancer Center (Charlottesville, VA) features a CT on rails for image guidance, showing the rails on either side of the table on the floor along which the CT scanner translates over the patient. The room is equipped with high-quality operating room lights and has full anesthesia capabilities. The operating room table allows for numerous attachments to be mounted; illustrated here are leg stirrups for placement of the legs in the dorsal lithotomy position and a transrectal ultrasound stepper. Note the high-dose-rate afterloader to the right side of the table.

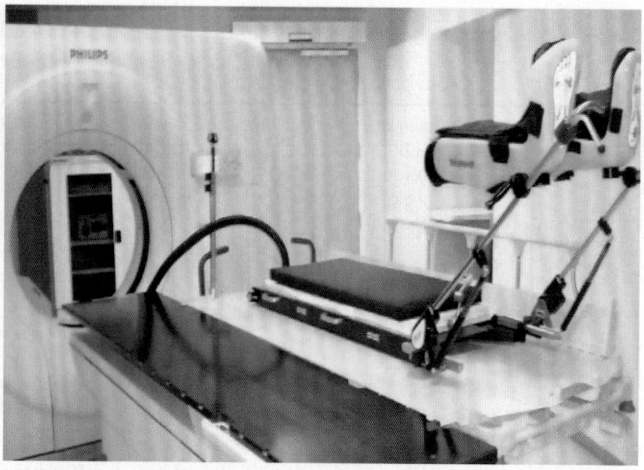

FIGURE 21.14. The Zephyr patient transport system used to minimize patient movement during brachytherapy scanning, planning, and treatment. (Courtesy of Diacor, Salt Lake City, Utah.)

The ideal situation to mitigate motion in brachytherapy would be to scan, plan, and treat in a single room without having to move the patient from the treatment position. The development of integrated brachytherapy suites, such as the Nucletron Integrated Brachytherapy Unit (Elekta) or the Varian Acuity Suite, allows for the placement of applicators, imaging, and treatment all in the same room. These suites use an in-room cone-beam CT system for image guidance. At the University of Virginia the image-guided brachytherapy suite (Fig. 21.13) features a CT-on-rails for in-room patient imaging and 3D treatment planning. Contrary to conventional CT, in which the patient translates through the scanner, in this setup the scanner itself translates over the patient while he or she is immobilized on the table. The image-guided suite at the University of Virginia is also designed to accommodate a full anesthesia team. With in-room imaging capabilities, if the imaging study shows that the applicator is not optimally placed, it can be readily adjusted. Furthermore, in-room imaging allows for real-time treatment planning with the patient in the treatment position. Treatment can then be delivered with confidence that the patient position does not change between planning and treatment.

Unfortunately, most facilities lack the ability to perform volumetric CT imaging and HDR brachytherapy treatments within the same dedicated room. In lieu of a dedicated image-guided suite, one strategy to decrease displacement of the applicator is to minimize movement of the patient after applicator placement. The Zephyr Patient Transport System (Diacor, Salt Lake City, Utah), shown in Figure 21.14, is designed to minimize applicator motion when the patient is moved between different rooms during the course of a brachytherapy treatment. The patient is kept in the same position on the transport system to allow for CT scanning and subsequent treatment. The Zephyr system uses air-bearing technology to easily move patients from the transport bed to the CT or treatment couches. This system has the potential to minimize logistical and applicator movement issues of patient transport for departments without a dedicated image-guided brachytherapy suite.[71]

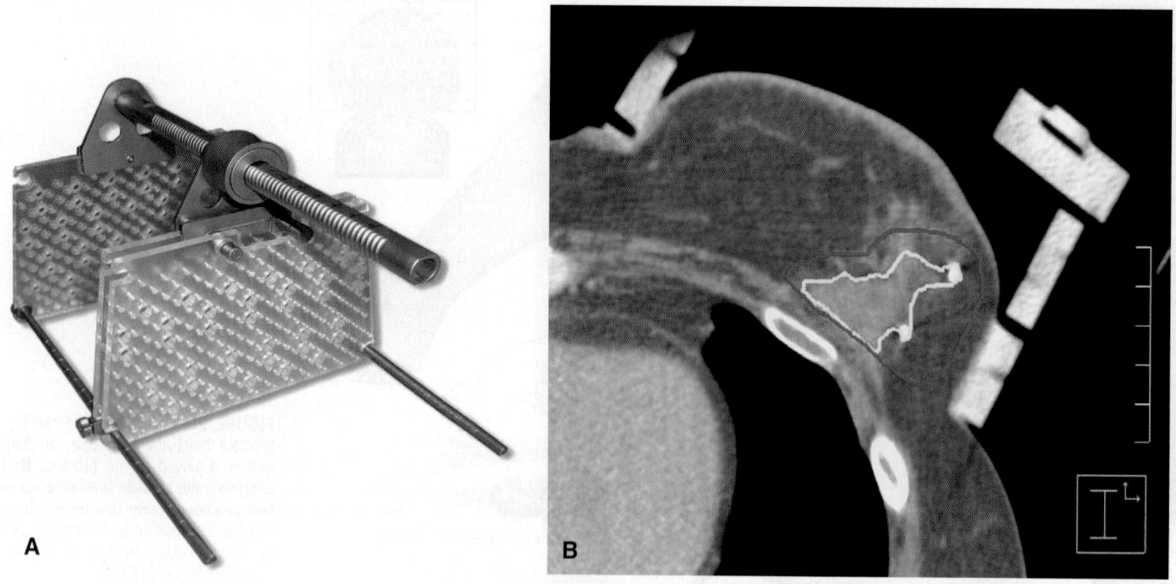

FIGURE 21.15. The advanced breast bridge system **(A)** used for interstitial catheter placement and a CT scan **(B)** showing a breast bridge along with the demarcated lumpectomy cavity (*yellow*). (A courtesy of Varian. B reproduced from Major T, Fröhlich G, Lövey K, et al. Dosimetric experience with accelerated partial breast irradiation using image-guided interstitial brachytherapy. *Radiother Oncol* 2009;90:48–55; courtesy of Elsevier, copyright 2009.)

Immobilization for Breast Brachytherapy

The use of brachytherapy to treat breast cancer has become more common since the introduction of balloon-based catheter systems, such as the MammoSite (Hologic, Bedford, MA) or the Contura (SenoRx, Irvine, CA), along with the related SAVI applicator (Cianna, Medical, Aliso Viejo, CA). Traditionally, breast irradiation has been delivered over 5 to 7 weeks to the whole breast after the tumor has been removed. Implanted catheters or balloons have allowed the use of accelerated regimens decreasing this time to 5 treatment days.[72,73] These implanted devices are simpler to administer compared to the

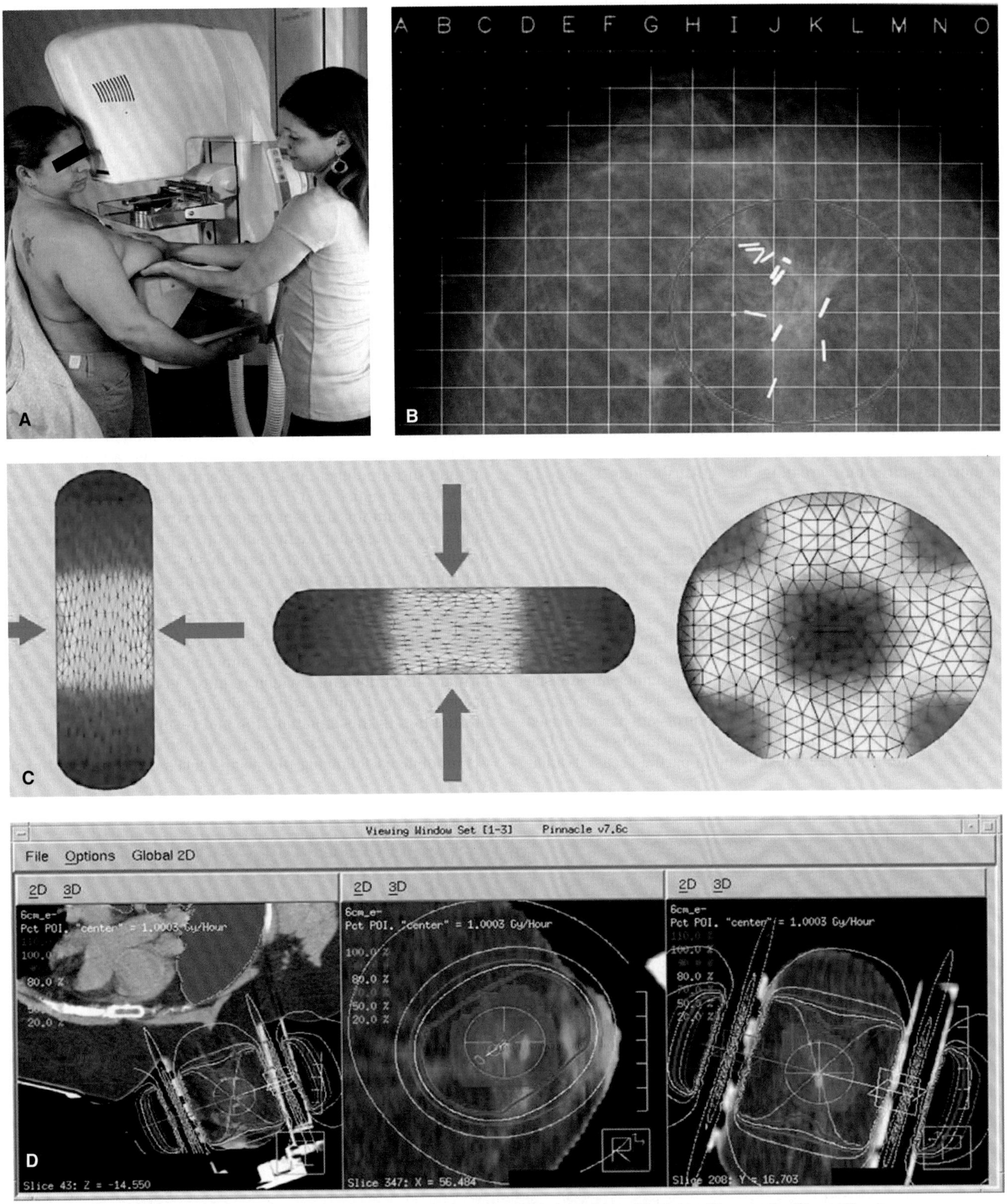

FIGURE 21.16. AccuBoost noninvasive image-guided breast brachytherapy. The breast is immobilized with mild compression **(A)** and a kilovoltage image is obtained for tumor bed targeting and appropriate applicator selection **(B)**. **C:** Schematic demonstrating breast compression and treatment in a parallel-opposed fashion sequentially along two orthogonal axes. **D:** Three-dimensional dose distribution covering the tumor bed using parallel-opposed applicators along a single-compression axis. (Reproduced from Hepel J, Wazer DE. A comparison of brachytherapy techniques for partial breast irradiation. *Brachytherapy*. Philadelphia: Elsevier, 2011; courtesy of Elsevier, copyright 2011.)

more complicated interstitial implants, in which catheters were placed through the breast tissue to treat the lumpectomy cavity.[74,75] The implanted balloon or SAVI applicators, along with the interstitial implants, are used to only treat the lumpectomy cavity, which is known as partial-breast irradiation (PBI). Partial-breast irradiation can also be accomplished with external beam radiation. The arrangement of beams to treat the lumpectomy cavity, however, is much more complicated than the normal tangential arrangement for whole-breast irradiation. Breast bridges, such as the one manufactured by Varian shown in Figure 21.15, made the interstitial placement of catheters more reproducible between patients, as opposed to freehand placement.[75]

A more recent development for noninvasive breast brachytherapy (NIBB), as opposed to the insertion of catheters or balloons that can lead to infection, is the AccuBoost (Tyngsboro, MA) system, which immobilizes the breast for imaging and subsequent high-dose-rate brachytherapy treatment.[76] NIBB using the AccuBoost system consists of a three-step process. In the first step, the breast is immobilized between two mammographic paddles, achieving a stable position for imaging and treatment. This immobilization of the breast aids in the delivery of the partial-breast irradiation without the uncertainties that can arise from delineating the target with a CT scan. In addition, respiratory motion and daily setup errors can also affect the treatment if external beam radiation is used for the PBI. After the mammogram has been performed, the lumpectomy cavity is delineated, typically using radiopaque clips placed at the time of surgery. The brachytherapy treatment is then delivered in a parallel-opposed technique from each orthogonal direction, creating dose distributions shown in Figure 21.16.[77]

IMMOBILIZATION STRATEGIES FOR INTRAOPERATIVE RADIOTHERAPY

In intraoperative radiotherapy (IORT), a single high-dose fraction of radiation is delivered directly to the tumor bed immediately following surgical resection. The dose delivery occurs in the operating room while the patient is still under anesthesia. There is growing evidence that many low-risk breast cancer patients can achieve comparable local control with partial-breast irradiation as with traditional whole-breast radiotherapy.[72] Use of smaller volumes of irradiated tissue in partial-breast irradiation allows for treatment courses to be delivered on an accelerated schedule. The potential to deliver a therapeutic dose in a shorter period of time can increase patient convenience and expand access to treatment for those with transportation limitations. IORT, which delivers a highly localized dose, is well suited for partial-breast irradiation candidates, and hence most of the clinical experience with IORT is in the treatment of low-risk breast cancer. The advantages of IORT are lower rates of toxicity because less normal tissue is irradiated, and enhanced patient convenience because a therapeutic dose can be delivered during the surgical procedure.[78] IORT is being used as both sole therapy[79,80] and as an upfront boost with external beam whole-breast therapy to follow.[81] Reitsamer et al.[78] present an excellent overview of the rationale and methodology of IORT.

Both electrons and low-kVp photons are being used to deliver IORT. The TARGIT trial uses a 50-kVp x-ray source that is placed directly in the lumpectomy cavity following excision of the tumor.[79] The x-ray source is housed in a spherical applicator to provide separation between the source and the target tissue. An alternative delivery method uses a mobile linac to deliver the dose to the target tissue with electrons. The current commercially available accelerators designed for IORT are capable of producing electrons with energies up to 12 MeV, giving therapeutic ranges of up to roughly 3 cm in tissue. When using a linear accelerator–based delivery method for electron IORT, a collimator cone must be placed on the target tissue and then aligned with the electron beam exiting the linac.

One mobile accelerator system, the Mobetron (IntraOp Medical Corporation, Sunnyvale, CA), has an interesting method to immobilize and stabilize the irradiation geometry, illustrated in Figure 21.17. Following excision of the tumor, the tissue surrounding the lumpectomy cavity that is to be irradiated is sewn together by the surgeon. A metal shield is placed downstream of the target tissue to protect the thoracic wall and underlying lung tissue. The appropriate-diameter collimator cone is chosen and placed by the physician directly over the target tissue. The linac is then rolled into place to be connected to the collimator cone. For most mobile accelerator systems, the linac must then be rigidly connected to the cone, a process termed "hard docking," which requires great care and skill to properly align the linac while maintaining the physician's cone positioning. In this situation, the end result is that the cone is attached to the linac itself. For the Mobetron system, the cone is immobilized following physician placement via a rigid arm

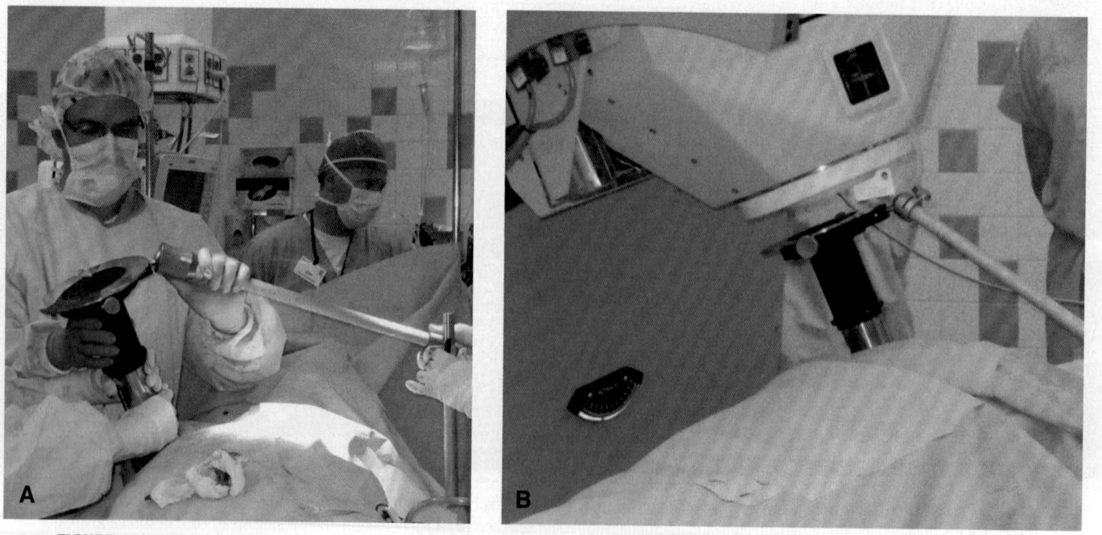

FIGURE 21.17. **A:** For intraoperative radiotherapy with the Mobetron system, the cone is placed by the physician directly over the target tissue following lumpectomy. The cone is fastened to the surgical table by a rigid arm. **B:** The linear accelerator is then positioned above the cone and automatically aligned using laser guidance with the mirror on the cone. (Courtesy of IntraOp Medical Corporation, Sunnyvale, CA.)

clamped to the surgical table. A unique feature of the Mobetron is the "soft-docking" system in which an internal laser-guided system uses a mirror on the top of the cone to precisely align the radiation beam; the linac never actually contacts the collimating cone. The entire procedure is performed while the patient is under anesthesia.

THE EVOLUTION OF PATIENT IMMOBILIZATION

Radiation therapy strategies to immobilize patients have been developed since it was introduced as a treatment modality more than 100 years ago. In this chapter we presented a wide array of simple devices that have continued to be used for decades, albeit with new designs and materials that make their use more comfortable, convenient, and sanitary for patients and therapists. We also presented highly specialized systems that may be used in the most sophisticated of radiation therapy treatment modalities that address specific concerns of image guidance and highly conformal treatments with high doses, such as stereotactic radiation therapy, brachytherapy, and intraoperative therapy. The common theme in current radiation therapy immobilization has been patient comfort in concert with an effective and safe approach to localize the target during the actual treatment in accordance with the simulation and the ability to verify the patient positioning prior to treatment with image guidance. Image-guided radiation therapy (IGRT) and immobilization are interlinked, and IGRT will likely play an increasing role with every type of treatment in the future. It is therefore not surprising that the commercial radiation therapy industry will continue to focus on providing safe and effective immobilization that is compatible in both CT and MRI.

Furthermore, the importance of patient and applicator immobilization has begun to be migrated to brachytherapy treatments, especially with the development of image-guided brachytherapy, analogous to IGRT, in which the patient has the applicator placed, simulation is performed, and the patient is treated with minimal motion of the patient or applicator. The advances that have been made in immobilization devices for external beam radiation, such as CT and MR compatibility, are finding increased use in brachytherapy. Integrated brachytherapy suites, which can combine imaging and treatment modalities, are becoming increasingly common.

In conclusion, effective radiation treatment is dependent on both proper localization of the tumor and proper immobilization of the patient. As radiation therapy has evolved, so have the strategies for immobilization of the patient. Image-guided radiation therapy, including hypofractionated stereotactic body radiation therapy, as well as image-guided brachytherapy, require that the patient be comfortably immobilized to ensure that the radiation is properly delivered to the tumor. This is especially necessary as the dose per fraction is increased, which could lead to serious complications should the normal tissue surrounding the tumor receive excessive dose due to poor localization and immobilization.

REFERENCES

1. Haus AG, Marks JE. Detection and evaluation of localization errors in patient radiation therapy. *Invest Radiol* 1973;8(6):384–391.
2. Dunscombe PB, et al. The investigation and rectification of field placement errors in the delivery of complex head and neck fields. *Int J Radiat Oncol Biol Phys* 1993;26(1):155–161.
3. Bentel GC, et al. Comparison of two head and neck immobilization systems. *Int J Radiat Oncol Biol Phys* 1997;38(4):867–873.
4. Engelsman M, et al. Intra- and interfractional patient motion for a variety of immobilization devices. *Med Phys* 2005;32(11):3468–3474.
5. Gilbeau L, et al. Comparison of setup accuracy of three different thermoplastic masks for the treatment of brain and head and neck tumors. *Radiother Oncol* 2001;58(2):155–162.
6. Hurkmans CW, et al. Set-up verification using portal imaging; review of current clinical practice. *Radiother Oncol* 2001;58(2):105–120.
7. Velec M, et al. Cone-beam CT assessment of interfraction and intrafraction setup error of two head-and-neck cancer thermoplastic masks. *Int J Radiat Oncol Biol Phys* 2010;76(3):949–955.
8. Verhey LJ, et al. Precise positioning of patients for radiation therapy. *Int J Radiat Oncol Biol Phys* 1982;8(2):289–294.
9. Tsai JS, et al. A non-invasive immobilization system and related quality assurance for dynamic intensity modulated radiation therapy of intracranial and head and neck disease. *Int J Radiat Oncol Biol Phys* 1999;43(2):455–467.
10. Olch AJ, Lavey RS. Reproducibility and treatment planning advantages of a carbon fiber relocatable head fixation system. *Radiother Oncol* 2002;65(3):165–168.
11. Sweeney R, et al. Repositioning accuracy: comparison of a noninvasive head holder with thermoplastic mask for fractionated radiotherapy and a case report. *Int J Radiat Oncol Biol Phys* 1998;41(2):475–483.
12. Bentel GC, et al. Comparison of two repositioning devices used during radiation therapy for Hodgkin's disease. *Int J Radiat Oncol Biol Phys* 1997;38(4):791–795.
13. Bentel GC, et al. The effectiveness of immobilization during prostate irradiation. *Int J Radiat Oncol Biol Phys* 1995;31(1):143–148.
14. Bentel GC, Marks LB, Krishnamurthy R. Impact of cradle immobilization on setup reproducibility during external beam radiation therapy for lung cancer. *Int J Radiat Oncol Biol Phys* 1997;38(3):527–531.
15. Carter DL, Marks LB, Bentel GC. Impact of setup variability on incidental lung irradiation during tangential breast treatment. *Int J Radiat Oncol Biol Phys* 1997;38(1):109–115.
16. Song PY, et al. A comparison of four patient immobilization devices in the treatment of prostate cancer patients with three dimensional conformal radiotherapy. *Int J Radiat Oncol Biol Phys* 1996;34(1):213–219.
17. Das IJ, et al. Efficacy of a belly board device with CT-simulation in reducing small bowel volume within pelvic irradiation fields. *Int J Radiat Oncol Biol Phys* 1997;39(1):67–76.
18. Kim JY, et al. Intensity-modulated radiotherapy with a belly board for rectal cancer. *Int J Colorectal Dis* 2007;22(4):373–379.
19. Martin J, et al. Treatment with a belly-board device significantly reduces the volume of small bowel irradiated and results in low acute toxicity in adjuvant radiotherapy for gynecologic cancer: results of a prospective study. *Radiother Oncol* 2005;74(3):267–274.
20. Olofsen-van Acht M, et al. Reduction of irradiated small bowel volume and accurate patient positioning by use of a bellyboard device in pelvic radiotherapy of gynecological cancer patients. *Radiother Oncol* 2001;59(1):87–93.
21. Stegman LD, et al. Long-term clinical outcomes of whole-breast irradiation delivered in the prone position. *Int J Radiat Oncol Biol Phys* 2007;68(1):73–81.
22. Moody AM, et al. The influence of breast size on late radiation effects and association with radiotherapy dose inhomogeneity. *Radiother Oncol* 1994;33(2):106–112.
23. Taylor ME, et al. Factors influencing cosmetic results after conservation therapy for breast cancer. *Int J Radiat Oncol Biol Phys* 1995;31(4):753–764.
24. Algan O, et al. Use of the prone position in radiation treatment for women with early stage breast cancer. *Int J Radiat Oncol Biol Phys* 1998;40(5):1137–1140.
25. Merchant TE, McCormick B. Prone position breast irradiation. *Int J Radiat Oncol Biol Phys* 1994;30(1):197–203.
26. Griem KL, et al. Three-dimensional photon dosimetry: a comparison of treatment of the intact breast in the supine and prone position. *Int J Radiat Oncol Biol Phys* 2003;57(3):891–899.
27. Hadley SW, Kelly R, Lam K. Effects of immobilization mask material on surface dose. *J Appl Clin Med Phys* 2005;6(1):1–7.
28. Mellenberg DE. Dose behind various immobilization and beam-modifying devices. *Int J Radiat Oncol Biol Phys* 1995;32(4):1193–1197.
29. Weltens C, et al. Comparison of plastic and Orfit masks for patient head fixation during radiotherapy: precision and costs. *Int J Radiat Oncol Biol Phys* 1995;33(2):499–507.
30. Purdie TG, et al. Cone-beam computed tomography for on-line image guidance of lung stereotactic radiotherapy: localization, verification, and intrafraction tumor position. *Int J Radiat Oncol Biol Phys* 2007;68(1):243–252.
31. Li W, et al. Effect of immobilization and performance status on intrafraction motion for stereotactic lung radiotherapy: analysis of 133 patients. *Int J Radiat Oncol Biol Phys* 2011;81(5):1568–1575.
32. Heck B, et al. Accuracy and stability of positioning in radiosurgery: long-term results of the Gamma Knife system. *Med Phys* 2007;34(4):1487–1495.
33. Hong LX, et al. Clinical experiences with onboard imager KV images for linear accelerator-based stereotactic radiosurgery and radiotherapy setup. *Int J Radiat Oncol Biol Phys* 2009;73(2):556–561.
34. Ramakrishna N, et al. A clinical comparison of patient setup and intra-fraction motion using frame-based radiosurgery versus a frameless image-guided radiosurgery system for intracranial lesions. *Radiother Oncol* 2010;95(1):109–115.
35. Salter BJ, et al. The TALON removable head frame system for stereotactic radiosurgery/radiotherapy: measurement of the repositioning accuracy. *Int J Radiat Oncol Biol Phys* 2001;51(2):555–562.
36. Kalapurakal JA, et al. Repositioning accuracy with the Laitinen frame for fractionated stereotactic radiation therapy in adult and pediatric brain tumors: preliminary report. *Radiology* 2001;218(1):157–161.
37. Ali I, et al. Evaluation of the setup accuracy of a stereotactic radiotherapy head immobilization mask system using kV on-board imaging. *J Appl Clin Med Phys* 2010;11(3):3192.
38. Bednarz G, et al. Report on a randomized trial comparing two forms of immobilization of the head for fractionated stereotactic radiotherapy. *Med Phys* 2009;36(1):12–17.
39. Masi L, et al. Cone beam CT image guidance for intracranial stereotactic treatments: comparison with a frame guided set-up. *Int J Radiat Oncol Biol Phys* 2008;71(3):926–933.
40. Das S, et al. Accuracy of relocation, evaluation of geometric uncertainties and clinical target volume (CTV) to planning target volume (PTV) margin in fractionated stereotactic radiotherapy for intracranial tumors using relocatable Gill-Thomas-Cosman (GTC) frame. *J Appl Clin Med Phys* 2010;12(2):3260.
41. Burton KE, et al. Accuracy of a relocatable stereotactic radiotherapy head frame evaluated by use of a depth helmet. *Clin Oncol (R Coll Radiol)* 2002;14(1):31–39.
42. Kumar S, et al. Treatment accuracy of fractionated stereotactic radiotherapy. *Radiother Oncol* 2005;74(1):53–59.
43. Ruschin M, et al. Performance of a novel repositioning head frame for gamma knife perfexion and image-guided linac-based intracranial stereotactic radiotherapy. *Int J Radiat Oncol Biol Phys* 2010;78(1):306–313.

44. Sayer FT, et al. Initial experience with the eXtend System: a relocatable frame system for multiple-session gamma knife radiosurgery. *World Neurosurg* 2011;75(5-6): 665–672.
45. Tryggestad E, et al. Inter- and intrafraction patient positioning uncertainties for intracranial radiotherapy: a study of four frameless, thermoplastic mask-based immobilization strategies using daily cone-beam CT. *Int J Radiat Oncol Biol Phys* 2011;80(1):281–290.
46. Bova FJ, et al. The University of Florida frameless high-precision stereotactic radiotherapy system. *Int J Radiat Oncol Biol Phys* 1997;38(4):875–882.
47. Peng LC, et al. Quality assessment of frameless fractionated stereotactic radiotherapy using cone beam computed tomography. *Int J Radiat Oncol Biol Phys* 2010;78(5):1586–1593.
48. Hamilton AJ, et al. Preliminary clinical experience with linear accelerator-based spinal stereotactic radiosurgery. *Neurosurgery* 1995;36(2):311–319.
49. Benedict SH, et al. Stereotactic body radiation therapy: the report of AAPM Task Group 101. *Med Phys* 2010;37(8):4078–4101.
50. Fuss M, et al. Repositioning accuracy of a commercially available double-vacuum whole body immobilization system for stereotactic body radiation therapy. *Technol Cancer Res Treat* 2004;3(1):59–67.
51. Shah C, et al. Intrafraction variation of mean tumor position during image-guided hypofractionated stereotactic body radiotherapy for lung cancer. *Int J Radiat Oncol Biol Phys* 2012;82(5)1636–1641.
52. Han K, et al. A comparison of two immobilization systems for stereotactic body radiation therapy of lung tumors. *Radiother Oncol* 2010;95(1):103–108.
53. Gutierrez AN, et al. Clinical evaluation of an immbolization system for stereotactic body radiotherapy using helical tomotherapy. *Med Dosim* 2011;36(2): 126–129.
54. Murray B, Forster K, Timmerman R. Frame-based immobilization and targeting for stereotactic body radiation therapy. *Med Dosim* 2007;32(2):86–91.
55. Keall PJ, et al. The management of respiratory motion in radiation oncology report of AAPM Task Group 76. *Med Phys* 2006;33(10):3874–3900.
56. Seppenwoolde Y, et al. Precise and real-time measurement of 3D tumor motion in lung due to breathing and heartbeat, measured during radiotherapy. *Int J Radiat Oncol Biol Phys* 2002;53(4):822–834.
57. Baba F, et al. Stereotactic body radiotherapy for stage I lung cancer and small lung metastasis: evaluation of an immobilization system for suppression of respiratory tumor movement and preliminary results. *Radiat Oncol* 2009;4:15.
58. Case RB, et al. Inter- and intrafraction variability in liver position in non-breath-hold stereotactic body radiotherapy. *Int J Radiat Oncol Biol Phys* 2009;75(1): 302–308.
59. Eccles CL, et al. Interfraction liver shape variability and impact on GTV position during liver stereotactic radiotherapy using abdominal compression. *Int J Radiat Oncol Biol Phys* 2011;80(3):938–946.
60. Kitamura K, et al. Tumor location, cirrhosis, and surgical history contribute to tumor movement in the liver, as measured during stereotactic irradiation using a real-time tumor-tracking radiotherapy system. *Int J Radiat Oncol Biol Phys* 2003; 56(1):221–228.
61. Heinzerling JH, et al. Four-dimensional computed tomography scan analysis of tumor and organ motion at varying levels of abdominal compression during stereotactic treatment of lung and liver. *Int J Radiat Oncol Biol Phys* 2008;70(5): 1571–1578.
62. Negoro Y, et al. The effectiveness of an immobilization device in conformal radiotherapy for lung tumor: reduction of respiratory tumor movement and evaluation of the daily setup accuracy. *Int J Radiat Oncol Biol Phys* 2001;50(4):889–898.
63. Wunderink W, et al. Reduction of respiratory liver tumor motion by abdominal compression in stereotactic body frame, analyzed by tracking fiducial markers implanted in liver. *Int J Radiat Oncol Biol Phys* 2008;71(3):907–915.
64. Kanikowski M, et al. Permanent implants in the treatment of prostate cancer. *Rep Pract Oncol Radiother* 2008;13(3):150–167.
65. Stone NN, et al. Prostate gland motion and deformation caused by needle placement during brachytherapy. *Brachytherapy* 2002;1(3):154–160.
66. Nag S, et al. Proposed guidelines for image-based intracavitary brachytherapy for cervical carcinoma: report from Image-Guided Brachytherapy Working Group. *Int J Radiat Oncol Biol Phys* 2004;60(4):1160–1172.
67. Pham HT, et al. Changes in high-dose-rate tandem and ovoid applicator positions during treatment in an unfixed brachytherapy system. *Radiology* 1998;206(2): 525–531.
68. Yaparpalvi R, et al. Skirt vs. stand applicator immobilization system in vaginal cylinder HDR brachytherapy. *Brachytherapy* 2008;7(2):152.
69. Hoskin PJ, Bownes P, Summers A. The influence of applicator angle on dosimetry in vaginal vault brachytherapy. *Br J Radiol* 2002;75(891):234–237.
70. Datta NR, et al. Variations of intracavitary applicator geometry during multiple HDR brachytherapy insertions in carcinoma cervix and its influence on reporting as per ICRU report 38. *Radiother Oncol* 2001;60(1):15–24.
71. Nag S. Zephyr—a novel "airchusion" patient transportation system for transferring brachytherapy patients for imaging and treatment while minimizing risk of applicator displacement. *Brachytherapy* 2011;10:S97–S98.
72. Arthur DW, Vicini FA. Accelerated partial breast irradiation as a part of breast conservation therapy. *J Clin Oncol* 2005;23(8):1726–1735.
73. Arthur DW, et al. Accelerated partial breast irradiation: an updated report from the American Brachytherapy Society. *Brachytherapy* 2003;2(2):124–130.
74. Baglan KL, et al. The use of high-dose-rate brachytherapy alone after lumpectomy in patients with early-stage breast cancer treated with breast-conserving therapy. *Int J Radiat Oncol Biol Phys* 2001;50(4):1003–1011.
75. Major T, et al. Dosimetric experience with accelerated partial breast irradiation using image-guided interstitial brachytherapy. *Radiother Oncol* 2009;90(1): 48–55.
76. Sioshansi S, et al. Dose modeling of noninvasive image-guided breast brachytherapy in comparison to electron beam boost and three-dimensional conformal accelerated partial breast irradiation. *Int J Radiat Oncol Biol Phys* 2011;80(2): 410–416.
77. Hepel J, Wazer DE. A comparison of brachytherapy techniques for partial breast irradiation. *Brachytherapy* 2012;11(2)163–175.
78. Reitsamer R, et al. Concepts and techniques of intraoperative radiotherapy (IORT) for breast cancer. *Breast Cancer* 2008;15(1):40–46.
79. Vaidya JS, et al. The novel technique of delivering targeted intraoperative radiotherapy (Targit) for early breast cancer. *Eur J Surg Oncol* 2002;28(4):447–454.
80. Veronesi U, et al. Full-dose intraoperative radiotherapy with electrons during breast-conserving surgery: experience with 590 cases. *Ann Surg* 2005;242(1):101–106.
81. Reitsamer R, et al. The Salzburg concept of intraoperative radiotherapy for breast cancer: results and considerations. *Int J Cancer* 2006;118(11):2882–2887.

Chapter 22
Physics and Biology of Brachytherapy

Jeffrey F. Williamson, X. Allen Li, and David J. Brenner

Brachytherapy (BT) (*brachy* is Greek for "short distance") consists of placing sealed radioactive sources very close to or in contact with the target tissue. Because the absorbed dose falls off rapidly with increasing distance from the sources, high doses may be delivered safely to a localized target region over a short time. This chapter reviews the properties and applications of commonly used sealed radionuclides and sources; the basic biologic principles governing clinical response to BT; methods of dose calculation and source-strength specification; and principles of implant design and dose specification for interstitial and intracavitary BT.

BASIC TERMINOLOGY

Implantation techniques may be classified in terms of surgical approach to the target volume (interstitial, intracavitary, translumінal, or mold techniques); the means of controlling the dose delivered (temporary or permanent implants); the source loading technology (preloaded, manually afterloaded, or remotely afterloaded); and the dose rate (low, medium, or high).

Intracavitary insertion consists of positioning applicators (bearing the radioactive sources) into a body cavity in close proximity to the target tissue. Intracavitary BT is used most widely for treatment of localized gynecologic malignancies. All intracavitary implants are *temporary implants;* they are left in the patient for a specified time to deliver the prescribed dose. With a few exceptions, during temporary implantation, the patient must be confined to a controlled, if not shielded, area in the hospital to manage the radiation safety hazard posed by the large ambient exposure rates around the implant.

Interstitial brachytherapy consists of surgically implanting small radioactive sources directly into the target tissues. A *permanent* interstitial implant remains in place indefinitely and is not removable; the initial source strength is chosen so that the prescribed dose is fully delivered only when the implanted radioactivity has decayed to a negligible level.

Surface-dose applications (sometimes called plesiocurie therapy or mold therapy) consist of an applicator containing an array of radioactive sources, usually designed to deliver a uniform dose distribution, that is placed on the skin or mucosal surface immediately adjacent to the target tissue.

Transluminal brachytherapy consists of inserting a single line source into a body lumen to treat its surface and adjacent tissues.

Until the early 1960s, radioactive sources (needles for interstitial therapy or preloaded applicators for intracavitary therapy) were implanted directly into the patient. Radiation exposure to the brachytherapist and operating room staff was reduced significantly with the advent of *afterloading* technology.[1,2] *Manual afterloading* consists of implanting nonradioactive tubes or intracavitary applicators into the patient. Following transport of the patient to his or her room, sources are manipulated into the applicators by means of forceps and other handheld tools. Exposure to staff responsible for source loading and the care of BT patients can be greatly reduced or eliminated by use of a *remote afterloading system,* which consists of a pneumatically driven or motor-driven source transport system for robotically transferring radioactive material between a shielded safe and each treatment applicator.

According to Report No. 38 of the International Commission on Radiation Units and Measurements (ICRU),[3] *low–dose-rate (LDR)* implants deliver doses at the rate of 40 to 200 cGy/hour (0.4 to 2 Gy/hour), requiring treatment times of 24 to 144 hours, during which the patient is confined to an inpatient treatment room. At the other extreme, *high–dose-rate (HDR)* BT uses dose rates in excess of 0.2 Gy/minute (12 Gy/hour). In fact, modern HDR remote afterloaders deliver instantaneous dose rates as high as 0.12 Gy/second (430 Gy/hour) at a distance of 1 cm, resulting in treatment times of a few minutes. Such treatments must be delivered in heavily shielded vaults using remote afterloading devices, but allow fractionated BT to be delivered on an outpatient basis. Medium dose-rate delivery, defined as the 2- to 12-Gy/hour range, rarely is used. Although not recognized by ICRU Report No. 38, the ultra-low–dose-rate range (0.01 to 0.3 Gy/hour) is of great importance; it is the dose-rate domain used in permanent implants with ^{125}I and ^{103}Pd seeds.

PROPERTIES OF BRACHYTHERAPY SOURCES AND RADIONUCLIDES

The clinical utility of any radionuclide depends on physical properties such as half-life, radiation output per unit activity specific activity (Ci/g), and photon energy. In addition, the methods of producing the radionuclide and its physical or chemical form strongly influence cost-effectiveness, safety, and toxicity. Detailed properties of BT radionuclides are listed in Table 22.1.

Photon Spectrum and Dosimetric Characteristics of Brachytherapy Sources

The dose delivered with a BT procedure depends on the individual source strengths, source arrangement, and implant duration, tissue composition, as well as the dosimetric characteristics of the implanted sources. These dosimetric characteristics are described by specifying the distribution of dose rates per unit strength about the source, often in terms of an "away-and-along" table[4] in Cartesian coordinates or in terms of the Task Group 43 protocol[5] described later in this chapter. The single-source dose distribution is of central importance to treatment planning because commercial computer planning systems estimate dose distribution from the spatial coordinates of the implanted sources using the principle of superposition. The source-superposition algorithm estimates the contribution of each source, given its tip-and-end coordinates and the single-source dose-rate array, to each point of interest. These contribution estimates are summed to estimate the total dose rate at each point. Often, total dose rates are calculated over a two-dimensional (2D) grid of points and are represented as isodose-rate curves.

For conventional BT, for which the therapeutically relevant distance range is 3 to 20 mm, only photons (γ-rays or characteristic x-rays) with energies in excess of 15 keV (kiloelectron

TABLE 22.1 PHYSICAL PROPERTIES AND USES OF BRACHYTHERAPY RADIONUCLIDES

Element	*Isotope*	*Energy (MeV)*	*Half-Life*	*HVL-Lead (mm)*	*Exposure Rate Constant[a]* Γ_δ	*Source Form*	*Clinical Application*
Obsolete Sealed Sources of Historical Significance							
Radium	^{226}Ra	0.83 (average)	1,626 years	16	8.25[b] 7.71[c]	Tubes and needles	LDR intracavitary and interstitial
Radon	^{222}Rn	0.83 (average)	3.83 days	16	8.25[b]	Gas encapsulated in gold tubing	Permanent interstitial Temporary molds
Currently Used Sealed Sources							
Cesium	^{137}Cs	0.662	30 years	6.5	3.26	Tubes and needles	LDR intracavitary and interstitial
Cesium	^{131}Cs	0.030	9.69 days	0.030	0.64	Seeds	LDR permanent implants
Iridium	^{192}Ir	0.397 (average)	73.8 days	6	4.69	Seeds in nylon ribbon; metal wires Encapsulated source on cable	LDR temporary interstitial Intravascular brachytherapy; cardiac HDR interstitial and intracavitary Intravascular brachytherapy: peripheral
Cobalt	^{60}Co	1.25	5.26 years	11	13.07	Encapsulated spheres	HDR intracavitary
Iodine	^{125}I	0.028	59.6 days	0.025	1.45	Seeds	Permanent interstitial
Palladium	^{103}Pd	0.020	17 days	0.013	1.48	Seeds	Permanent interstitial
Gold	^{198}Au	0.412	2.7 days	6	2.35	Seeds	Permanent interstitial
Strontium/Yttrium	^{90}Sr–^{90}Y	2.24 β_{max}	28.9 years	–	–	Plaque Seeds	Treatment of superficial ocular lesions Intravascular brachytherapy
Developmental Sealed Sources							
Americium	^{241}Am	0.060	432 years	0.12	0.12	Tubes	LDR intracavitary
Ytterbium	^{169}Yb	0.093	32 days	0.48	1.80	Seeds	HDR interstitial
Californium	^{252}Cf	2.4 (average) neutron	2.65 years	–	–	Tubes	High-LET LDR intracavitary
Samarium	^{145}Sm	0.043	340 days	0.060	0.885	Seeds	LDR temporary interstitial

HVL, half-value layer; LDR, low dose rate; HDR, high dose rate; LET, linear energy transfer.

[a]No filtration in units of $R \cdot cm^2 \cdot mCi^{-1} \cdot h^{-1}$.

[b]0.5 mm platinum filtration; units of $R \cdot cm^2 \cdot mg^{-1} \cdot h^{-1}$.

[c]1.0 mm platinum filtration; units of $R \cdot cm^2 \cdot mg^{-1} \cdot h^{-1}$.

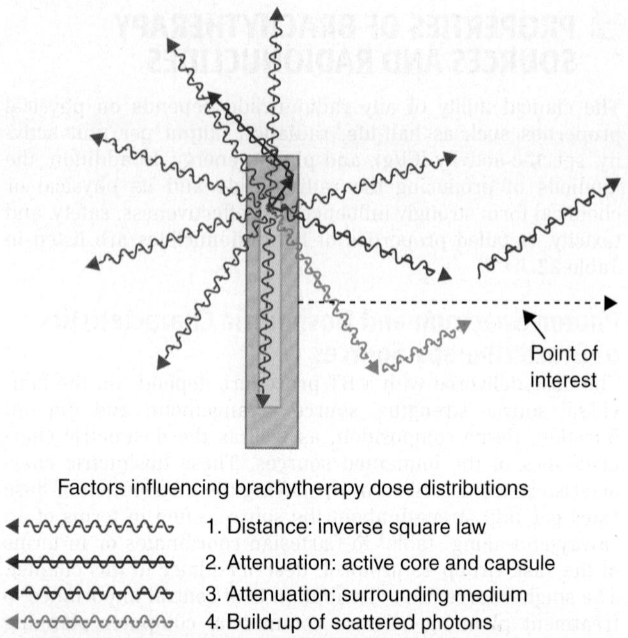
Point of interest
Factors influencing brachytherapy dose distributions
1. Distance: inverse square law
2. Attenuation: active core and capsule
3. Attenuation: surrounding medium
4. Build-up of scattered photons

FIGURE 22.1. Typical cylindrical brachytherapy source, consisting of an active core (inner cylinder within which radioactivity is uniformly distributed) and the surrounding encapsulation (usually stainless steel or titanium for modern sources). The four principal factors influencing the relative dose distribution include (1) distance, (2) attenuation and scattering in source structure, (3) attenuation by surrounding medium, and (4) accumulation of scattering in surrounding medium.

volts) contribute to the therapeutic effect. In general, four factors influence the single-source dose distribution for photon-emitting sources: (a) distance (inverse-square law), (b) absorption and scattering in the source core and encapsulation, (c) photon attenuation, and (d) scattering in the surrounding medium (Fig. 22.1). Encapsulation prevents radioactive material from leaking out of the source and absorbs nonpenetrating radiation (β-rays, α-rays, and low-energy photons), which would otherwise give rise to high surface doses while contributing nothing to the therapeutic effect.

Each voxel of radioactive core material shown in Figure 22.1 can be assumed to be an isotropic point source (Fig. 22.2). Because of the straight-line emission of photons with equal likelihood in all directions, photon intensity or fluence, $\Phi(r)$, at any point is proportional to the inverse square of its distance, r:

$$\Phi(r) = \frac{\text{no. incident photons}}{\text{unit area irradiated}} = \frac{\text{no. photons emitted}}{4\pi r^2} \propto \text{dose}(r) \propto \text{exposure}(r) \qquad (1)$$

assuming that attenuation and scattering can be neglected.

As a result of this purely geometric effect, the absorbed doses $D(r_1)$ and $D(r_2)$ at the two distances r_1 and r_2 (Fig. 22.2) are related by:

$$\frac{D(r_1)}{D(r_2)} = \frac{\Phi(r_1)}{\Phi(r_2)} = \left(\frac{r_2}{r_1}\right)^2 \qquad (2)$$

This fundamental law applies exactly to each point of the radioactive core of the source shown in Figure 22.1 assuming that there is no attenuation and scattering of photons by the surrounding medium. However, Eq. (2) will not accurately describe the "collective" dose fall-off arising from the combined action of the point sources distributed throughout the core,

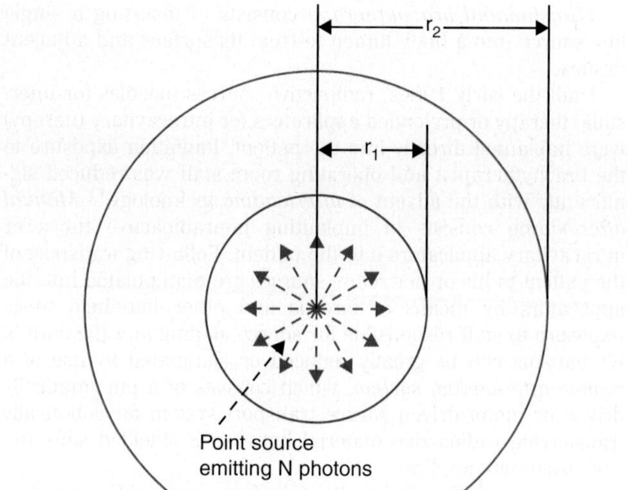
r2
r1
Point source
emitting N photons

FIGURE 22.2. An *isotropic point source* of activity, A. To illustrate the derivation of inverse-square law, the source is surrounded by vacuum and placed at the center of two concentric spherical surfaces of radii r_1 and r_2. By definition, an *isotropic point source* has no extension and radiates photons with equal likelihood in all directions in straight-line paths.

unless both r_1 and r_2 are large relative to the active source dimensions. Of the four factors influencing the dose distribution (Fig. 22.1), inverse-square law is by far the most important. For a pure isotropic point source, dose will decrease by a factor of 100 between the distances of 0.5 and 5 cm. The influence of the remaining factors over the same distance range rarely exceeds a factor of 2 or 3. Consequently, most of the clinical characteristics of implants (e.g., the heterogeneous dose distribution within the target tissue and rapid fall-off of dose outside the implanted volume) can be accounted for by applying inverse-square law to each pointlike element of radioactivity within the implant. Control of intersource spacing and positioning relative to the target and dose-limiting tissues is the most challenging issue in delivering BT.

Although inverse-square law dominates the dose distribution, the surrounding medium and the source structure do significantly affect the dose distribution (Fig. 22.1). The source core and surrounding capsule reduce dose at the point of interest through absorption and scattering of primary photons. Primary photons contributing dose to points located near the longitudinal source axis (cylindrical axis of the source or axis of rotation) must traverse longer path lengths of capsule and core material and therefore experience more attenuation than photons contributing dose to equidistant points on the transverse source axis (plane perpendicular to the longitudinal source axis that bisects its active core). At a fixed distance from the source center, the dose near the longitudinal axis is usually smaller than on the transverse axis. This phenomenon is known as *oblique filtration* and is the main cause of dose *anisotropy* (variation of dose as a function of polar angle at each fixed distance relative to the source center) characteristic of extended BT sources. Because BT sources are cylindrically symmetric, the dose distribution will be equatorially isotropic (constancy of dose as a function of azimuthal angle for each fixed polar angle and distance).

The tissue-equivalent medium surrounding the source affects the dose distribution in two important and competing ways (factors (3) and (4) of Fig. 22.1). At each point of interest, the intervening medium reduces the dose distribution by attenuating primary photons (deflecting them from their straight-line trajectories). At the same time, photons are being emitted in all directions from the source and interacting with the medium by means of Compton scattering and photoelectric

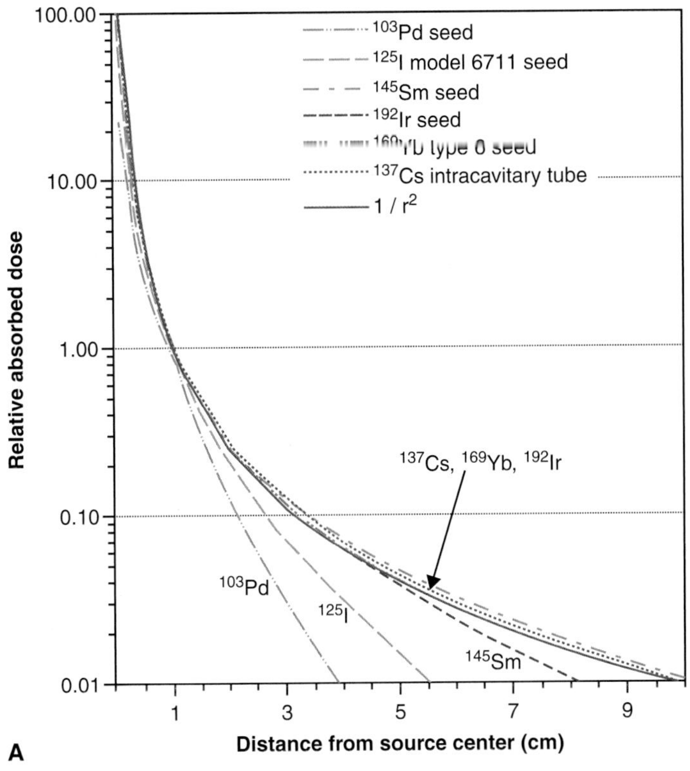

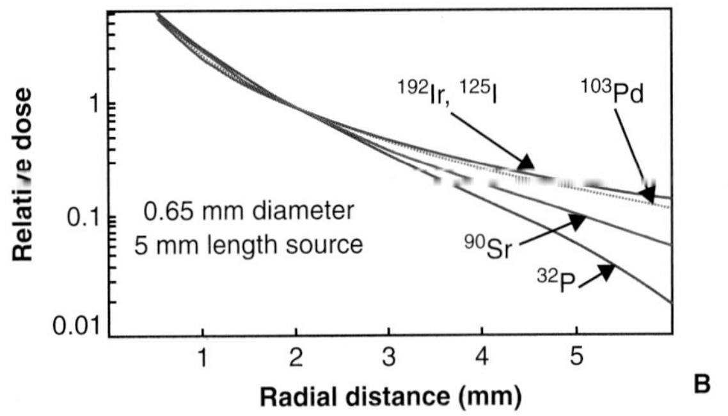

FIGURE 22.3. **A:** Variation of dose as a function of distance for point sources of ^{60}Co, ^{226}Ra, ^{137}Cs, ^{198}Au, ^{192}Ir, and ^{125}I. The results are normalized to 100% at 1-cm distances. The function ($1/r^2$) is plotted for comparison. **B:** Relative dose (normalized to 1.0 at 1 mm) versus distance for various cylindric sources (0.65 mm diameter and 5 mm long) over the 1- to 5-mm distance range. (From Amols HI, Zaider M, Weinberger J, et al. Dosimetric considerations for catheter-based beta and gamma emitters in the therapy of neointimal hyperplasia in human coronary arteries. *Int J Radiat Oncol Biol Phys* 1996;36:913–921, with permission from Elsevier.)

absorption. Thus, each volume element of tissue is effectively radiating scattered photons in all directions, many of which contribute to dose at the point of interest. This mechanism, known as scattered-photon buildup, enhances the dose. The overall influence of the surrounding medium is the combined effect of these two competing processes: photon attenuation and scattered-photon buildup. In contrast to external-beam therapy, in which the scattering volume is limited to a narrow cone, scattered photons dominate BT dose distributions at distances >2 cm. Photon scattering is the main source of complexity in BT dose measurement and algorithm development.

Figure 22.3 demonstrates that the relative dose versus distance from the source is nearly independent of its photon energy so long as the average photon energy is >200 keV. In this energy range, dose deviates from inverse-square law by <5% over the 1- to 5-cm distance range. All of the "radium substitute" isotopes, including ^{137}Cs, ^{192}Ir, and ^{198}Au, fall into this energy range. This behavior, which greatly simplifies BT dosimetry, is the result of equilibrium between primary photon attenuation and buildup of scattered photons. Only for low-energy sources (e.g., ^{103}Pd and ^{125}I) does the depth-dose curve significantly deviate from inverse-square law. Because photon absorption rather than Compton scattering dominates energy deposition below 40 keV, scatter buildup is unable to compensate for loss of dose resulting from attenuation.

For radium-substitute radionuclides, Figure 22.4A,B shows that the absolute dose rate (cGy/hour to fat or water tissue per mgRaEq or unit air-kerma strength [S_K]) and the relative dose distribution are nearly independent of both energy and composition of the surrounding medium above 100 keV. Compton scattering, which dominates photon absorption and scattering above 100 keV, depends mainly on electron density (electrons/g) of the medium, which is nearly constant for all biologic materials. Below this energy range, absolute and relative dose distributions vary significantly with energy and composition (atomic number) of the surrounding medium. Implanting an ^{125}I seed in fat medium (effective atomic number of $Z_{eff} = 6$) will deliver about half the absorbed dose at 1 cm, compared to the expected dose in water ($Z_{eff} = 7.5$). This is because energy absorption per unit mass from photo-effect interactions is proportional to the cube of the atomic number (Z^3_{eff}) of the medium. Despite the significant impact of tissue composition heterogeneities on low-energy seed BT dose delivery, current treatment planning and dose measurement practices assume that patients are composed of uniform homogeneous water media.

Figure 22.4B demonstrates that the inverse-square law actually underestimates relative dose at 5 cm by as much as a factor of 2 in the 60- to 100-keV energy range. In this narrow energy range, called the intermediate low-energy range, photoelectric effect is negligible, whereas Compton scattering transfers most of the colliding primary photon energy to the scattered photon rather than to the Compton electron. As a result of this imbalance between energy absorption and photon scattering, buildup of scattered photons overcompensates for loss of dose as a result of primary photon attenuation out to distances of 4 to 6 cm.

Above the 100-keV threshold, the photon-energy spectrum is much less important to optimizing BT dose-rate distributions than in external-beam therapy. Because artificial BT radionuclides in this energy range (^{60}Co, ^{137}Cs, ^{192}Ir, ^{198}Au) have dose-rate distributions nearly identical to those of ^{226}Ra in the 1- to 5-cm distance range, they are referred to as radium substitutes.

Figure 22.4C demonstrates that although photon energy is a relatively unimportant determinant of tissue dosimetry, it significantly influences the cost, weight, and thickness of shielding required to protect critical anatomic structures in the patient and personnel involved in patient care. The half-value layer (HVL) in lead varies from 0.5 mm for a 100-keV source to 12 mm for ^{60}Co BT sources. Thus, for classical radium-equivalent BT, a radionuclide with a mean energy of about 100 to 200 keV is optimal. The major benefit of ^{125}I and ^{103}Pd BT sources is the ability to provide complete protection by thin lead foils (0.1 to 0.2 mm), greatly reducing exposure to physicians during the implant procedure and allowing permanent-implant patients to be released from medical confinement without posing a radiation safety hazard to the general public. Recently, interest has been expressed in using radionuclides in the intermediate low-energy range (60 to 120 keV).[6,7–8] Tissue dose distributions are still

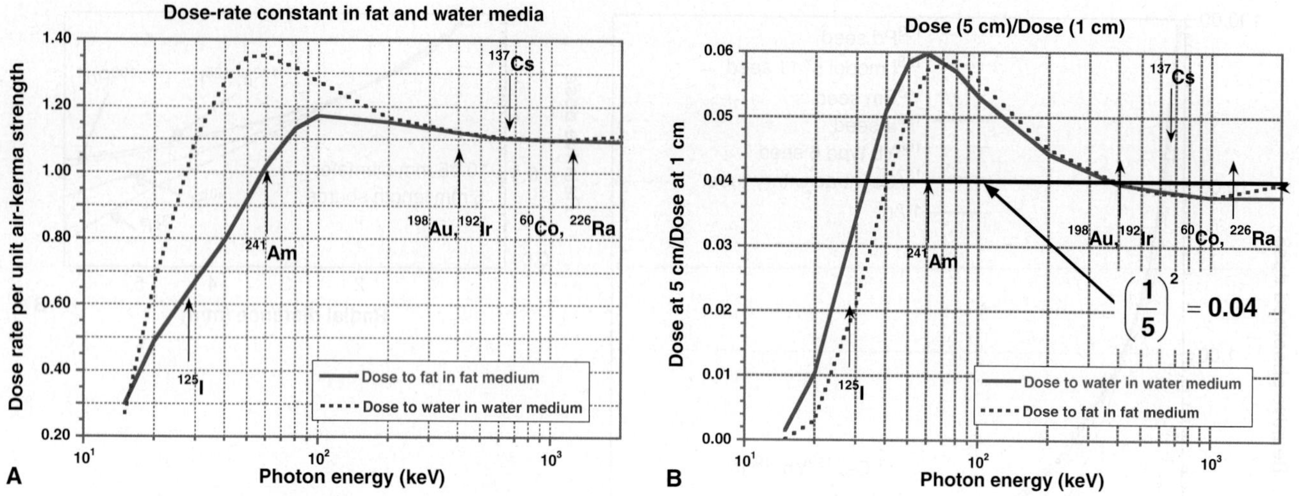

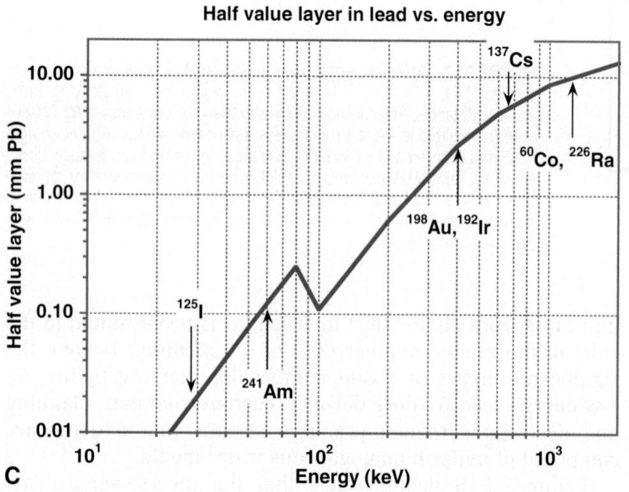

FIGURE 22.4. Variation of dosimetric properties of monoenergetic point sources as a function of photon energy. The location (in terms of average energy) of commonly used radionuclides is indicated by the labeled vertical arrows. **A:** Absolute dose rate per unit source strength in fat and water media at 1-cm distance. Source strength is specified in terms of output in air. **B:** Dose at 5 cm as a fraction of dose at 1 cm in fat and water media. The effect of inverse-square law, $(1/5)^2 = 0.04$, is shown for comparison as a heavy black line. **C:** Half-value layer in lead, the thickness (mm) in lead required to reduce primary dose by a factor of 2.

approximately radium equivalent in this energy range, and thin layers of lead provide significant sparing of dose-limiting normal tissues near the implanted volume.

Sources for Low-Dose-Rate Intracavitary Brachytherapy

Since the 1930s, sources for classical LDR intracavitary BT have taken the form of "tubes" having a physical length of 2 to 2.5 cm and an external diameter of about 3 mm. For treatment systems influenced by the Manchester[9] and M.D. Anderson[10] treatment techniques, active lengths of 1.3 to 1.5 cm are typical. Radionuclides for intracavitary applications should have a half-life long enough to support a 5- to 10-year working life without large variations in prescription dose rate so that the high cost of these reusable sources can be amortized over a large number of patient treatments. The average photon energy should be at least 60 to 100 keV, as the dose fall-off for lower-energy sources (e.g., ^{125}I) is too rapid to adequately treat the target volume periphery (2 to 5 cm from the applicator center) without overtreating the mucosal surfaces in contact with the applicator system.

Radium 226 Sources

Radium 226, a naturally occurring radionuclide, was the first radionuclide isolated, intensively investigated, and used in clinical BT. The unit of activity, the curie (Ci), originally was defined as the rate of disintegration within 1 g of ^{226}Ra. Radium 226 has a complex decay scheme, consisting of a cascade of transformations from one daughter product to another, ending with a stable isotope of lead, $^{206}_{82}$Pb. Radium decays to gaseous ^{222}Rn with a half-life of 1,626 years. Approximately 75 γ-rays are emitted by radium and its decay products, ranging in energy from about 0.05 to 2.4 MeV, giving an average energy of about 0.8 MeV. The maximum β-ray energy is about 3.26 MeV. The exposure-weighted average energy of ^{226}Ra is 1.25 MeV when its photon spectrum is filtered by 0.5 mm of platinum. Nearly all ^{226}Ra BT sources are filtered by at least 0.5 mm Pt, which reduces the surface dose contributed by β particles to a negligible level.

Clinical ^{226}Ra sources consisted of discrete cells of radium salt (radium sulfate plus filler) placed in needles or tubes with platinum walls of thickness of 0.5 and 1.0 mm, respectively. Intracavitary radium tubes were usually 22 mm long, containing 5 to 30 mg of radium (S_K = 30 to 200 μGy·m^2·h^{-1}), with active lengths of 15 mm. For interstitial BT, the full-, half-, and quarter-intensity needles popularized by the Manchester LDR implant system typically contain 0.66 mg, 0.33 mg, or 0.165 mg of radium per centimeter of active length, respectively.

The clinical use of radium has disappeared and is now only of historic interest. The potential for damaged sources to leak radioactive salts or emit radon gas (^{222}Rn) is the major reason for its decline, as well as the exposure hazard to interstitial BT practitioners.[11] Another factor is the high cost of extracting radium from pitchblende ore in comparison with the cost of radium-substitute sources. Finally, the safe disposal of spent ^{226}Ra sources is a significant financial liability. However, because of its many years of therapeutic use, several widely used quantities for source-strength specification and prescription of intracavitary treatment are derived from the early experience with ^{226}Ra.

Cesium 137 Sources

Cesium 137, a fission byproduct, is a popular radium substitute because of its 30-year half-life. Its single γ-ray (0.66 MeV) is less penetrating (HVL_{Pb} = 0.65 cm) than the γ-rays from radium (HVL_{Pb} = 1.4 cm) or ^{60}Co (HVL_{Pb} = 1.1 cm). Because ^{137}Cs decays to solid barium 137, ^{137}Cs sources have virtually replaced ^{226}Ra intracavitary tubes in LDR gynecologic applications.

Cesium 137 BT sources were introduced in the early 1960s.[12,13] Recently marketed sources (e.g., the Amersham model CDCS-J tube [Amersham, UK] and 3M model 6500 intracavitary tube [St. Paul, MN]) consist of radioactive cesium distributed within an insoluble glass or ceramic matrix,[4] which produces far less radiochemical hazard from ruptured sources than does the radon gas or cesium salts. These sources are encapsulated in stainless-steel sheaths with wall thicknesses of 0.5 to 1.0 mm, active lengths of 13.5 to 15 mm, diameters of 2.6 to 3.1 mm, and total lengths of about 20 mm. Figure 22.5 shows that cesium and radium sources produce nearly identical transverse-axis dose-rate distributions when their active lengths and source strengths are the same. However, the ^{226}Ra tube isodose curves exhibit significant retraction along the longitudinal source axis as a result of oblique filtration of ^{226}Ra γ-rays through the dense ($\rho = 21$ g·cm^{-3}) 1-mm-thick platinum capsule. In contrast, lightly filtered ^{137}Cs tubes produce nearly elliptical isodose curves. Consequently, vaginal applicator systems containing modern ^{137}Cs sources with their axes positioned perpendicular to the coronal patient plane (e.g., the Fletcher colpostat) always will give rise to higher bladder and rectal doses than when loaded with ^{226}Ra tubes.[14]

Many other ^{137}Cs source designs have been used over the last 20 years including spherical steel-encapsulated ^{137}Cs pellets for the Selectron-composable source-train remote afterloader.[15] For preoperative treatment of endometrial cancer[16] or definitive treatment of medically inoperable endometrial cancer, afterloading sources with nominal strengths of 72 μGy·m^2·h^{-1}, external diameters of about 1.2 mm, and lengths of 12 mm attached to the end of long metal stems (Heyman-Simon sources) were widely used up to the present time. However, all of these

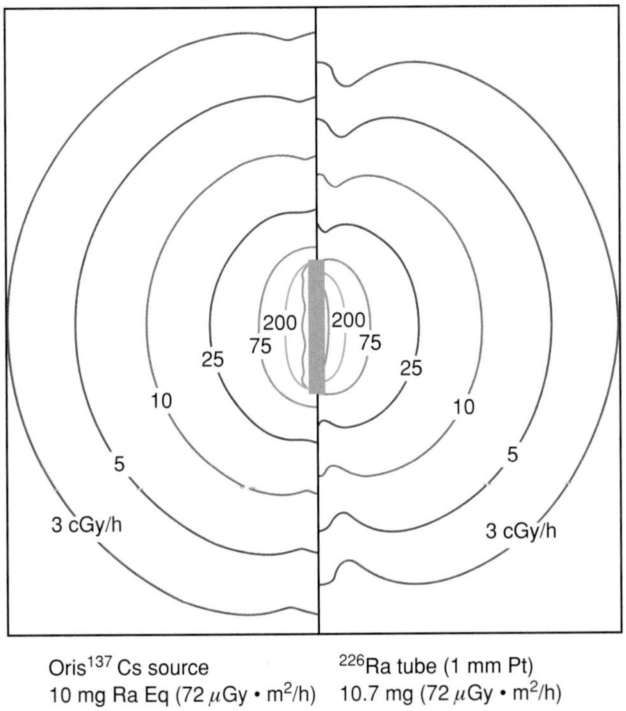

FIGURE 22.5. Comparison of isodose curves for a modern steel-clad ^{137}Cs source (*left*) containing radioactive ceramic pellets[14] and a ^{226}Ra tube (*right*) consisting of a $RaSO_4$ core encapsulated in 1-mm-thick Pt. Both sources have an air-kerma strength of 72 μGy · m^2 · h^{-1} (10 mgRaEq).

^{137}Cs source configurations have disappeared from the market, reflecting the widespread conversion of LDR intracavitary BT to HDR techniques. As of this writing, only intracavitary tubes are commercially available from two manufacturers: Isotope Product Laboratories (Valencia, CA)[17] and Bebig-IBt (Berlin, Germany).[18]

Experimental Intracavitary Brachytherapy Radionuclides

Californium 252 is a unique radionuclide that decays by α-emission with a half-life of 2.65 years and emits neutrons by spontaneous fission with average energies of 2.1 to 2.3 MeV. Depending on the distance from the source, one-half to two-thirds of the total dose is the result of the neutron component. Assuming a relative biologic effectiveness (RBE) of 6 for the neutron component, approximately 90% of the biologically effective dose derives from the neutron component. The radiobiologic rationale for using ^{252}Cf, especially in treating bulky gynecologic malignancies, is that the high linear energy transfer (LET) neutron component more effectively depopulates the tumor's radioresistant hypoxic core, thereby improving local control, while the rapid dose fall-off maintains an acceptable level of late complications.[19] Californium 252 sources require carefully designed radiation protection and source handling procedures to reduce radiation exposure hazards to an acceptable level, due to the high neutron quality factor of 10 to 20 that is assumed by radiation protection standards.[20] Afterloading tube sources, suitable for use in LDR intracavitary BT, are fabricated at Oak Ridge National Laboratories (Oak Ridge, TN).[21]

Ytterbium 169[7] and americium 241[6] are examples of so-called intermediate low-energy photon emitters, giving rise to 60-keV and 100-keV photons, respectively. The emitted photon energy is low enough that relatively thin lead foils can be used to shield personnel and dose-limiting tissues in the patient but high enough that the resultant dose distributions in tissue remain approximately radium equivalent.[22] Because relatively thin lead sheets can be used to shield critical structures (e.g., 0.4-mm-thick lead for 50% dose reduction from ^{169}Yb), customized rectal and bladder shielding can be more easily fabricated. Ytterbium 169 seeds[7] (100-keV mean energy, 32-day half-life) have been investigated as a possible substitute for ^{192}Ir in interstitial implants[23] and for intracavitary treatment. In addition, ^{169}Yb has an extremely high specific activity. An HDR ^{169}Yb source and an associated single-stepping source remote afterloading system has recently been approved for sale.[8]

Sources for Low-Dose-Rate Temporary Interstitial Brachytherapy

The main additional requirement for radionuclides used in temporary interstitial BT is a specific activity sufficient to support fabrication of miniaturized sources (<2 mm external diameter) so as to minimize trauma to the implanted tissues. Current interstitial implantation techniques favor disposable sources containing short-lived radionuclides that support afterloading and customization of active length.

Nonafterloading ("Preloaded") Sources: Radium and Cesium Needles

Radium 226 needles were the mainstay of interstitial BT until about 1970. These sources had external diameters of 1.5 to 2 mm, active lengths ranging from 3 mm to 4.5 cm, and Pt-Ir alloy encapsulation ranging from 0.5 to 0.65 mm in thickness. Because needle implantation can result in large exposures to the radiation oncologist's fingers, as well as whole-body exposure to operating room and implant imaging staff, interstitial implantation of ^{226}Ra nor ^{137}Cs needles has been abandoned.

Afterloading Interstitial Sources: ^{192}Ir Ribbons and Wires

Temporary interstitial BT experienced a renaissance in the 1960s because of the introduction of ^{192}Ir.[11] This useful radionuclide is produced by bombarding nonradioactive ^{191}Ir (available in relatively pure form) with thermal neutrons in a

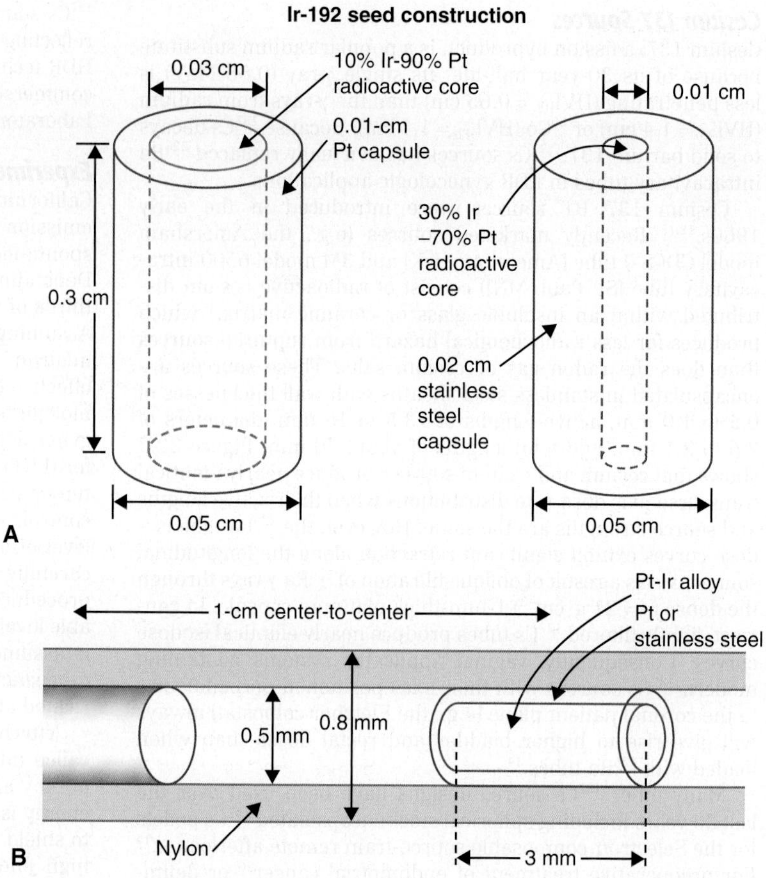

FIGURE 22.6. A: Construction and dimensions (in mm) of the two types of commercially available ^{192}Ir seeds. (A from Williamson JF. The accuracy of the line and point dose approximation in Ir-192 dosimetry. *Int J Radiat Oncol Biol Phys* 1986;12:409, with permission from Elsevier.) **B:** The 0.8-mm external diameter nylon carrier or ribbon in which the seeds are "encapsulated." (B from Anderson LL, Nath R, Weaver KA, et al. *Interstitial brachytherapy: physical, biological and clinical considerations.* New York: Raven, 1990.)

nuclear reactor. ^{191}Ir has an extremely large neutron-capture cross-section, and produces no significant contaminant radioisotopes. Because of these properties, very high specific activities can be achieved. Miniaturized interstitial sources can be fabricated relatively cheaply. The use of ^{192}Ir in BT was pioneered by Ulrich Henschke,[24] who developed a family of widely used afterloading techniques, and by Pierquin and Dutreix,[25] who developed the ^{192}Ir-based Paris interstitial system in the early 1960s.

Iridium 192 has a 73.8-day half-life and a complex decay scheme, dominated by β decay to ^{192}Pt, but also including some electron capture and β+ decay. Its photon spectrum includes characteristic x-rays and γ-rays ranging from 63 keV to 1.4 MeV and has an exposure-weighted average energy of 397 keV. Compared with higher-energy ^{137}Cs, the thicknesses of lead and concrete shielding can be reduced by 33% and 20%, respectively.[26] More important advantages of ^{192}Ir sources are compatibility with afterloading techniques, technical flexibility, and patient comfort.

In the United States, ^{192}Ir is available in the form of seeds, 0.5 mm in diameter and 3 mm long, for LDR BT (Fig. 22.6). Iridium seeds, encapsulated in a 0.8-mm-diameter nylon ribbon and spaced at 1-cm or 0.5-cm center-to-center intervals, are available in strengths of 1 to 150 μGy · m^2 · h^{-1} (0.1 to 20 mgRaEq). In Europe, ^{192}Ir is used in the form of a wire (0.3-mm or 0.6-mm outer diameter) consisting of an iridium-platinum radioactive core encased in a 0.1-mm sheath of platinum. In addition to eliminating radiation exposure hazards in the operating room, ^{192}Ir ribbons and wires can be trimmed to the appropriate active length for each catheter. Generally, ^{192}Ir ribbons or wires are used only for one to three patient procedures and then returned to the vendor for disposal.

Low-Energy Sources for Temporary Interstitial Brachytherapy

High-intensity ^{125}I sources[27] have been proposed for temporary interstitial implantation at classical dose rates. High-intensity model 6711 or 3631 A/M ^{125}I seeds now are used routinely as temporary interstitial sources for episcleral plaque treatment of intraocular choroidal melanoma.[28] By placing a 0.5-mm-thick gold shield over the episcleral plaque, tissues posterior to the eye are shielded, and radiation directed toward the tumor is partially collimated.[29] A disadvantage of high-intensity ^{125}I seed therapy is its high cost relative to ^{192}Ir seeds.

Sources for Permanent Interstitial Brachytherapy

There are two basic approaches to permanent implantation. Classical LDR permanent BT originally used ^{222}Rn seeds, and more recently ^{198}Au seeds, both of which have half-lives of a few days. To manage the radiation hazard as a result of the high-energy γ-rays emitted by these sources, the patient must be confined to the hospital until the source strength decays to a safe level (two to three half-lives or about 10 days). The contemporary approach to permanent implantation, ultra-low–dose-rate (ULDR) BT, uses longer-lived but low-energy photon emitters (e.g., ^{103}Pd and ^{125}I). The patient's tissues or a thin lead foil are sufficient to reduce ambient exposure rates to negligible levels, eliminating the need to hospitalize patients solely for radiation protection. During the implant procedure, low-energy photon sources markedly reduce radiation exposure to operating room personnel and to the radiation oncologist's hands.

Mathematics of Radioactive Decay

The phenomenon of exponential decay results in a reciprocal relationship between dose rate achieved and radionuclide half-life. The total activity, A(t), present in the implant after an interval of time t has elapsed after source insertion is given by Figure 22.7:

$$A(t) = A(0) \cdot e^{-\ln 2 \cdot t/T_{1/2}} \qquad (3)$$

where A(0) is the activity at the time of insertion, ln2 is the natural logarithm of 2 (equal to 0.693), and $T_{1/2}$ is the half-life

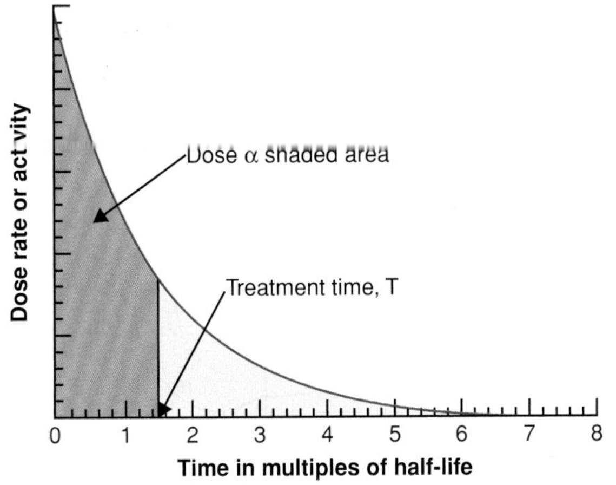

FIGURE 22.7. Illustration of exponential decay of source strength and dose rate. The area of the shaded region is the total dose administered to the patient over treatment time, T.

of the radionuclide. The quantity $\ln 2/T_{1/2}$, represented by the symbol λ, is called the decay constant. Eq. (3) is applicable to any measure of source strength (S_K, equivalent mass of radium, etc.). Because dose rate, $\dot{D}(t)$ at time t is proportional to activity, that is, $\dot{D}(t) \propto A(t)$, we can write:

$$\dot{D}(t) = \dot{D}(0) \cdot e^{-t \cdot \ln 2/T_{1/2}} \quad (4)$$

where $\dot{D}(0)$ is the dose rate at the time of source insertion. The total dose, D(T), accumulated over time interval T after source insertion is the shaded area under the curve of Figure 22.7 and can be obtained by integrating Eq. (4):

$$\begin{aligned} D(T) &= \dot{D}(0) \cdot \int_0^T e^{-t \cdot \ln 2/T_{1/2}} \cdot dt \\ &= \dot{D}(0) \cdot T_{1/2} \cdot 1.443 \cdot [1 - e^{-T \cdot 0.693/T_{1/2}}] \end{aligned} \quad (5)$$

The product $T_a = 1.443T_{1/2}$ is called the average life of the radionuclide and is the time required for all radioactive atoms to decay, assuming the rate of decay remains fixed at its initial value, A(0). Eq. (5) should be used to calculate the total dose delivered by any implant when the treatment time, T, is more than 5% of the half-life. For shorter treatment times (<4 days for ^{192}Ir or <3 days for ^{125}I), the approximate expression

$$D(T) = \dot{D}(0) \cdot T \quad (6)$$

is accurate within 2% and may be used.

For permanent implants, the total dose administered to the patient, D_{tot}, resulting from complete decay of the implant can be obtained from Eq. (5):

$$D_{tot} = \lim_{T \to \infty} D(T) = 1.443 \cdot T_{1/2} \cdot \dot{D}(0) = T_a \cdot \dot{D}(0) \quad (7)$$

This equation demonstrates that initial dose rate and radionuclide half-life are in reciprocal relationship with one another: the longer the half-life, the lower the dose rate will be. Typical total dose rates and total doses are given in Table 22.2 for commonly used permanent implant sources. These sources fall into two categories: short-lived radium substitute sources with initial dose rates within the classical LDR range and longer-lived low-energy sources with dose rates below the classical range (ULDR).

TABLE 22.2 TOTAL DOSE AND INITIAL DOSE RATES FOR PERMANENTLY IMPLANTED RADIONUCLIDES

Radionuclide	Mean Photon Energy	$T_{1/2}$	Typical Prescribed Dose	Initial Dose Rate
^{222}Rn	1.2 MeV	3.83 days	100 Gy	75 cGy · h^{-1}
^{198}Au	412 keV	2.70 days	100 Gy	107 cGy · h^{-1}
^{131}Cs	29 keV	9.7 days	115 Gy	34.2 cGy · h^{-1}
^{125}I	28 keV	59.6 days	145 Gy	7.0 cGy · h^{-1}
^{103}Pd	22 keV	17 days	125 Gy	21.2 cGy · h^{-1}

Classical Low-Dose-Rate Permanent Implant Sources: ^{198}Au

Seeds consisting of ^{222}Rn gas encapsulated in thin-walled gold tubes[30] were used for permanent implantation for many years. Institutions[31] that are still practicing classical LDR permanent interstitial BT use a reactor-produced radionuclide, ^{198}Au, which emits monoenergetic 412-keV γ-rays and has a half-life of 2.7 days. Its decay product is a nontoxic solid, thereby eliminating the contamination hazards associated with production and use of ^{222}Rn. ^{198}Au seed implantation is not widely practiced because of exposure hazards to operating room personnel (especially the brachytherapist), the need to confine the patient to the hospital for radiation protection reasons, and the logistic problems associated with maintaining an appropriate inventory of such short-lived sources.

Ultra-Low-Dose-Rate and Energy Permanent Implant Sources: ^{125}I and ^{103}Pd

The introduction of electron-capture decay radionuclides, which have moderately long half-lives (10 to 60 days) and emit cascades of low energy (20 to 40 keV) characteristic x-rays and γ-rays, reignited interest in permanent BT. The first practical K-capture source, the titanium-encapsulated ^{125}Iodine seed (half life: 59.6 days, mean energy: 28 keV), was developed by Donald C. Lawrence[32] in the early 1960s and its clinical applications first investigated in the late 1960s by Basil Hilaris and his colleagues[33–35] at Memorial Sloan-Kettering Hospital. Iodine 125 is produced by neutron activation in a specially equipped reactor designed to minimize activation of the contaminant radioisotope, ^{126}I. It produces a single 35-keV γ-ray. The captured K-shell electron produces a cascade of 27- to 32-keV characteristic x-rays. In addition, 93% of the γ-rays are internally converted, producing a second characteristic x-ray cascade. Thus, ^{125}I is an "x-ray emitter" because 95% of the useful primary photons are characteristic x-rays of atomic rather than nuclear origin.

Other important electron-capture radionuclides are ^{103}Pd (^{103}Palladium, 17-day half-life and 22-keV mean energy), commercially realized in 1987, and ^{131}Cs (^{131}Cesium, 9.6-day half-life and 29-keV mean energy), which was initially proposed by Henschke and Lawrence[36] but has only recently become available commercially.[37] The low-energy photons emitted by these sources dramatically reduce external exposure hazards: an 8-cm thickness of tissue reduces exposure 10-fold. Thin (0.2 mm) lead foils also produce almost complete shielding. Thus, there is usually no need to confine patients to the hospital solely for radiation safety reasons. As a result of the rapidly increasing popularity of transperineal ultrasound (TRUS)-guided permanent implant[38,39] for definitive treatment of low- and intermediate-risk prostate cancer,[40,41] approximately 25 different models of ^{125}I and ^{103}Pd sources have been introduced to the market since 1999 (see the American Association of Physicists in Medicine [AAPM] revised Task Group [TG] 43 Report[5,42] and the Joint AAPM/Radiological Physics Center [RPC] Source Registry[43] for a review of many of the available sources). Most of these interstitial seeds are encapsulated in thin (0.05- to 0.10-mm thick) titanium tubing (see Wang and Hertel[44] for an exception) with external dimensions of approximately 0.8 × 4.5 mm (Fig. 22.8). The widely used Model 6711 seed,[45] the only ^{125}I source available from 1983 to 1998, contains a 3-mm-long silver rod on which radioactive iodine is absorbed and is available in strengths of 0.5 to 7 $\mu Gy \cdot m^2 \cdot h^{-1}$ (0.5 to 5 mCi) (Fig. 22.8A, top). The silver rod is radio-opaque, so that the seeds can be visualized on orthogonal or stereoshift radiographs. Figure 22.8A (center) illustrates the more recent I-Seed ^{125}I source[46] product, which consists of radioactive iodine distributed in a low-density cylindrical annulus that fits over a gold rod used for radiographic localization.

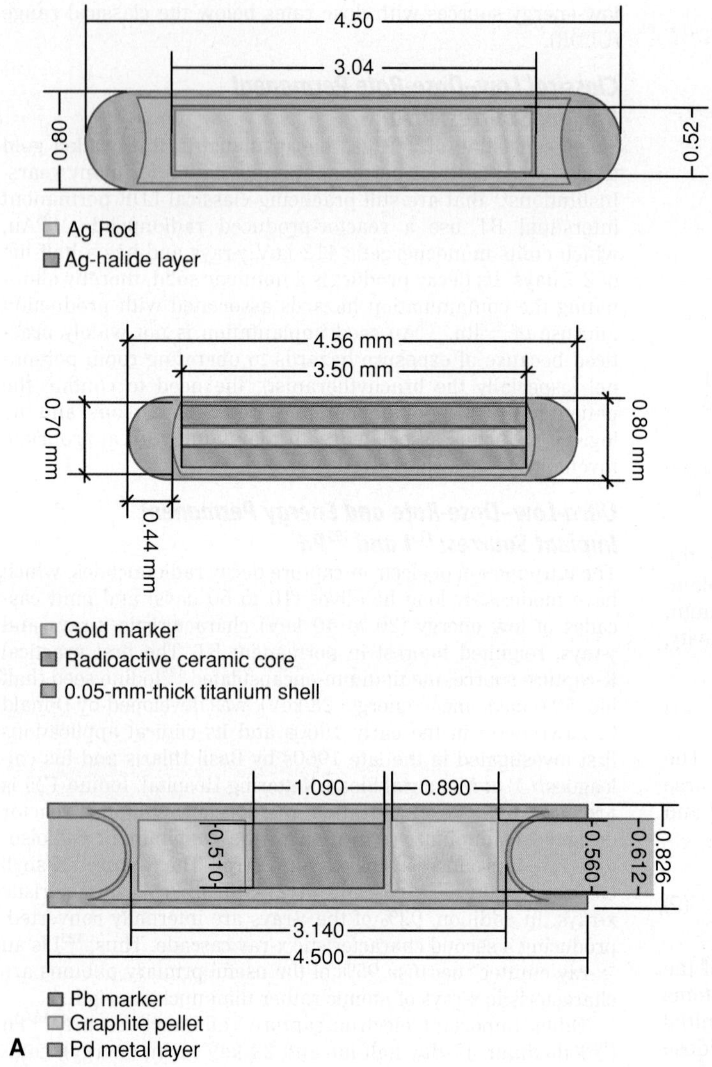

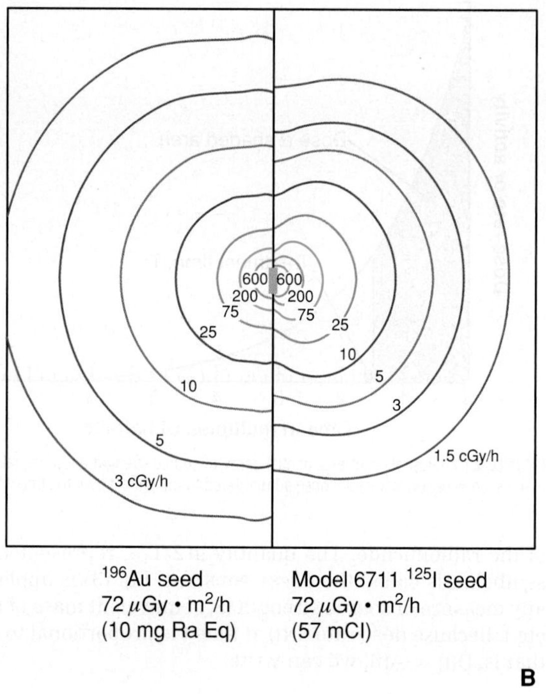

FIGURE 22.8. A: Design characteristics of the GE Healthcare (formerly Amersham and 3M) Model 6711 ^{125}I seed[50] (*top*), the Bebig IsoSeed (formerly Symmetra) Model I25.S06 ^{125}I seed[45] (*center*), and the Theragenics Model 200 ^{103}Pd seed[49] (*bottom*). **B:** Isodose curves for a ^{198}Au seed (*left half*) and Model 6711 ^{125}I seed (*right half*) both with air-kerma strengths of 72 μGy · m^2 · h^{-1} (equivalent to 35 mCi of ^{198}Au and 57 mCi of ^{125}I).

^{103}Pd decays by K-electron capture and emits characteristic x-rays of 21 keV. It has all of the radiation protection advantages of ^{125}I along with a significantly shorter half-life of 17 days. With this source, an implant can deliver 112 Gy (90% of prescribed dose) in approximately 8 weeks at an initial peripheral dose rate of 21 cGy/hour. The Model 200 seed (Fig. 22.8A bottom) was the only commercially available ^{103}Pd seed from 1988 to 1999. The radioactive palladium is distributed within a thin Pd metal coating of the two graphite pellets, which are encapsulated in Ti tubing of the same dimensions as ^{125}I seeds. Currently, there are at least four different ^{103}Pd seed models commercially available. The biologic rationale for using shorter-lived ^{103}Pd and ^{131}Cs interstitial sources is discussed later in the Biology section of this chapter.

Low-energy seed implantation poses a number of challenges. Their dose distributions are not radium equivalent (Fig. 22.8B), falling off more rapidly with distance. Dose estimation is inherently more complex, depending significantly on photon energy and composition of the surrounding medium (Fig. 22.4),[47,48] and is exquisitely sensitive to the internal seed geometry.[49,50] Because of shifts in calibration standards, large uncertainties in dose measurement, and questionable applicability of the classical dose calculation model, ^{125}I and ^{103}Pd dosimetry has been uncertain and variable over most of the clinical life of these products.[11] For example, between 1975 and 1999, the ^{125}I dose-rate constant was revised downward, in several steps, by nearly 50%.[11] Only with the development and validation of more sophisticated experimental and computation dosimetry techniques in the past 10 to 15 years can we claim to know low-energy seed dose-rate distributions with an uncertainty of 3% to 7%.[51] Because of the low dose rates used, low-energy seed implantation is effectively a different therapeutic modality than classical LDR BT. In addition, 20- to 30-keV photons have a significantly higher LET spectrum, which results in an RBE for ^{125}I of 1.3 to 1.5 in *in vitro* systems compared with unity for radium-substitute photon spectra.[52,53] Thus, classical LDR clinical experience cannot be used to guide therapeutic decision making for ^{125}I permanent implantation. Despite these limitations, low-energy source permanent implantation has been demonstrated to be a highly effective and convenient treatment for prostate cancer.[40,54]

Sources for High–Dose-Rate Brachytherapy

In contrast to inpatient-based LDR BT, HDR BT uses high-intensity sources to deliver discrete fractions ranging from 3 to 10 Gy in an outpatient setting. As described in more detail elsewhere in this text, a remote afterloading device must be used. A radionuclide with high specific activity (activity per unit mass; Ci/g) is needed so that treatment dose rates of at least 12 Gy/hour can be achieved without sacrificing the level of miniaturization needed to support intracavitary and interstitial BT. A source no larger than 1 mm diameter by 4 mm long with an exposure rate of at least 1 R/second at 1 cm is required.

TABLE 22.3 SPECIFIC ACTIVITIES AND MAXIMUM EXPOSURE RATES ACHIEVABLE FOR DIFFERENT RADIONUCLIDES

Radionuclide	Maximum Ci/g Possible	Fraction Practicably Achievable (%)	Exposure Rate[a] (R/s) at 1 cm from 1 mm × 4 mm Seed
^{226}Ra	0.98	100	0.04 R · cm² · s⁻¹
^{137}Cs	87	23	0.22 R · cm² · s⁻¹
^{60}Co	1,020[b]	49	50 R · cm² · s⁻¹
^{192}Ir	7,760[b]	35	248 R · cm² · s⁻¹
^{169}Yb	33,700[b]	14	51 R · cm² · s⁻¹

[a]Neglecting self-absorption.

[b]Reactor-produced by neutron activation: a flux = 10^{14} n·cm^{-2}·s^{-1} and 100% target purity are assumed.

The upper limit on specific activity of any substance, achieved when 100% of its atoms are radioactive, is a fundamental property that depends on its number of atoms per gram:

$$\text{atoms/g} = \left(\frac{\text{Avogadro's no. } (6.023 \times 10^{23} \text{ atoms/mole})}{\text{Atomic Weight}}\right) \quad (8)$$

For radionuclides produced by neutron activation, competition with radioactive decay precludes activating 100% of the target atoms. The theoretically achievable maximum Ci/g (Table 22.3) depends on the neutron capture cross-section of the target and the neutron flux in the reactor.[55] The extent to which this limit can be reached in practice depends on isotopic purity of the target, limits on reactor activation time, and the time required for shorter-lived contaminant radioisotopes to decay to an acceptable level. Finally, the exposure rate achieved by a small source (e.g., a 1 × 4-mm cylinder as shown in Table 22.3) depends on the chemical form (i.e., relative mass of nonradioactive atoms) of the source, its density, exposure-rate constant of the radionuclide, and photon self-absorption.

Table 22.3 shows that ^{226}Ra cannot support HDR BT and that ^{137}Cs is, at best, a marginal choice. Cobalt 60 (5.26-year half-life and γ-rays of 1.17 and 1.33 MeV) has been widely used as an intracavitary HDR source in the form of small spherical pellets. Based solely on specific activity considerations, ^{192}Ir is the optimal choice for HDR BT and is the most widely used radionuclide for this application. Sources with external diameters as small as 0.6 mm are now available for use in single-stepping source remote afterloading devices. In contrast to ^{60}Co, the lower-energy ^{192}Ir photons are shielded effectively by the scatter and leakage barriers present in most existing ^{60}Co teletherapy and linear accelerator vaults. Because of their short half-lives, ^{192}Ir HDR sources usually are replaced at quarterly intervals. Because of the relative ease with which its low-energy photons can be shielded, a ^{169}Yb source for HDR intraoperative and intravascular BT has been developed.[8]

BRACHYTHERAPY DOSIMETRY AND SOURCE-STRENGTH SPECIFICATION

Two eras of BT dosimetry can be distinguished. The *classical era* (1940–1980) encompassed the maturation of the classical BT systems, the transition from ^{226}Ra to artificial radionuclide sources, and the rise of modern BT. It began with the successful application of Bragg-Gray cavity theory[56] to the calibration of ^{226}Ra and other high-energy sources in terms of exposure,[57] which allowed BT to be quantified using the same system of units and quantities as the orthovoltage external-beam therapy of the day. Classical or semiempirical dose computation models are based on the dose distribution about an idealized point source. Dose rates around needle and tube sources were calculated by integrating the basic point source model over their extended radioactivity distributions. Because of the technical difficulties in measuring absorbed dose in the presence of steep dose gradients, BT treatment planning relied largely on calculated rather than measured dose distributions.

The modern or *quantitative* era of BT dosimetry began in the 1980s and continues to the present. Quantitative dosimetry relies on measurement of source-specific dose distributions by means of small thermoluminescent dosimeters (TLDs) or silicon diode dosimeters.[58] Alternatively, radiation transport calculations in the form of three-dimensional (3D) Monte Carlo simulations are accepted as an accurate and reliable source of clinically useful dosimetry data.[58] These technical developments were motivated by concerns that semiempirical dose calculation algorithms were not valid in the low-energy regimen of ^{125}I and ^{103}Pd sources. To clinically utilize dose measurements and Monte Carlo calculations, and empirical dose calculation formalism, the TG-43 protocol[5] was developed. Both the classical and quantitative dosimetry methods are based on the principle that BT source strength should be specified in terms of radiation output in free space.

Source-Strength Specification Quantities and Units

Brachytherapy calibration is an unnecessarily confusing topic due to the multitude of quantities that have been used to specify source strength throughout its history. Many of the historically obsolete but still widely used quantities (e.g., apparent activity and mgRaEq) were defined in terms of ^{226}Ra properties, the only BT radionuclide intensively studied until about 1940. Such quantities obscure the experimental origin of calibration measurements by describing output measurements in activity units. Finally, the BT literature has added to the lack of conceptual clarity by obscuring the important distinction between quantities and units. A *quantity* is a property of nature that is directly or indirectly measurable (e.g., kerma, equivalent mass of radium, length, time), whereas a *unit* is a selected sample of a quantity to which the magnitude unity (1.0) is assigned (e.g., gray, mgRaEq, meter, second). A quantity such as absorbed dose can have many units (e.g., rad, cGy, Gy, J/kg).

Regardless of the units and quantity chosen to describe a calibration, all photon-emitting sealed BT sources are calibrated in terms of output (kerma rate, dose rate, or exposure rate) in air at a specific reference point on the transverse bisector of the source. Much like superficial x-ray beam calibration, a calibrated ion chamber (Fig. 22.9) is used to measure the BT source output in a free-air geometry in which the source and chamber are suspended in air in a large room.

Air-Kerma Strength

In North America, photon-emitting source strength is specified in terms of air-kerma strength, denoted by S_K, a practice that was introduced by the AAPM in 1987.[59] The AAPM[5] currently defines S_K as the air-kerma rate, $\dot{K}_{\delta\text{air}}(d)$ at distance d, *in vacuo* and due to photons of energy greater than δ, multiplied by the square of this distance, d^2:

$$S_K = \dot{K}_{\delta,\text{air}}(d) \cdot d^2 \quad (9)$$

The distance d is the distance from the source center to the point of air-kerma rate specification (usually but not necessarily the point of measurement), which must be in the transverse plane of the source (the plane normal to the long axis of the source, which bisects its radioactivity distribution). S_K is independent of specification distance so long as d is large relative to the maximum linear dimension of the radioactivity distribution. $\dot{K}_{\delta\text{air}}(d)$ is usually inferred from transverse-plane air-kerma rate measurements performed in a free-air geometry (see Fig. 22.9) at distances large in relation to the maximum linear dimensions of the detector and source, typically on the order of 1 meter. The *in vacuo* qualifier (equivalent in meaning to "in free space") means that $\dot{K}_{\delta\text{air}}(d)$ must be specified as if the source and small mass of air, producing ionization at distance d, were immersed in a vacuum. Air-kerma rate measurements must be corrected for photon attenuation and scattering by the surrounding air as well as for scattering from nearby objects.

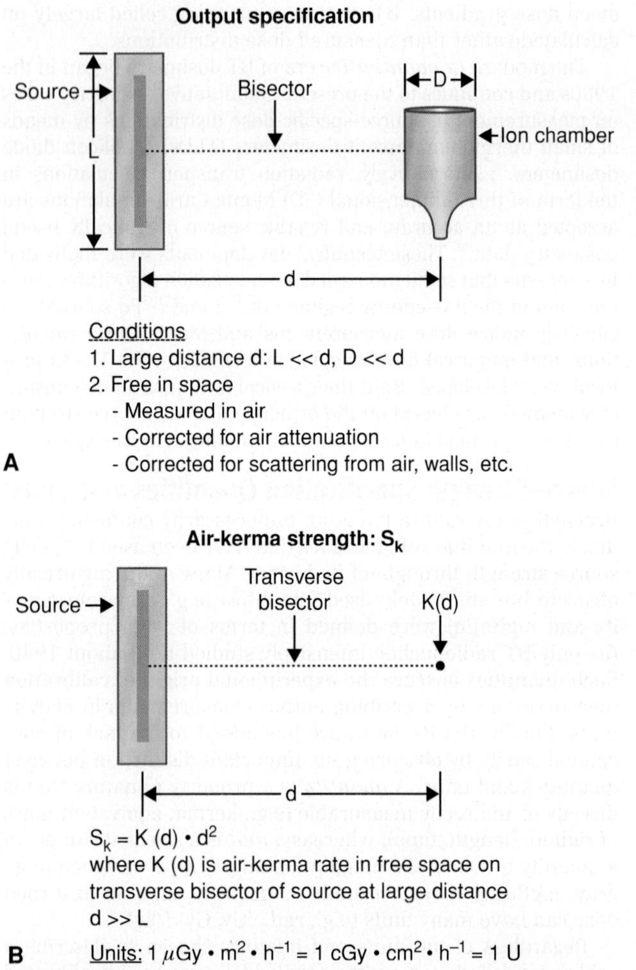
Output specification
Source
Bisector
D
Ion chamber
L
d
Conditions
1. Large distance d: L << d, D << d
2. Free in space
- Measured in air
- Corrected for air attenuation
- Corrected for scattering from air, walls, etc.
A
Air-kerma strength: S_k
Transverse bisector
K(d)
Source
d
S_k = K (d) • d²
where K (d) is air-kerma rate in free space on transverse bisector of source at large distance d >> L
B
Units: 1 μGy • m² • h⁻¹ = 1 cGy • cm² • h⁻¹ = 1 U

FIGURE 22.9. A: Illustration of a free-air geometry for measuring brachytherapy source strength in terms of a radiation output quantity such as air kerma. In practice, the source and cavity chamber are suspended in air in a large room and separated by a 20-cm to 100-cm distance (which must be large in relation to the detector and source dimensions). The measured air kerma must be corrected for photon scattering from walls, floor, and ceiling and for photon scattering and attenuation by the intervening air. **B:** Definition of air-kerma strength. For an actual source, the air-kerma rate must be measured at a distance, d, which is large in relation to the source dimensions.

The energy cutoff, δ, is intended to exclude low-energy contaminant photons (e.g., characteristic x-rays originating in the outer layers of steel or titanium source cladding[60]) that increase $\dot{K}_{\delta \text{air}}(d)$ without contributing significantly to dose at distances >0.1 cm in tissue. The value of δ is typically 5 keV for a low-energy photon-emitting BT source. The unit of air kerma strength is $\mu\text{Gy} \cdot \text{m}^2 \cdot \text{h}^{-1}$ and is often denoted in the literature by the symbol "U," where $1\ \text{U} = 1\ \text{cGy} \cdot \text{cm}^2 \cdot \text{h}^{-1} = 1\ \mu\text{Gy} \cdot \text{m}^2 \cdot \text{h}^{-1}$.

Air-kerma strength is numerically (but not dimensionally) equal to the quantity reference air-kerma rate, $\dot{K}_{ref}$, a very similar quantity defined by the ICRU[3,61] and used outside North America. $\dot{K}_{ref}$ is defined as the air-kerma rate in free space at a reference distance, l (taken to be 1 m), on the transverse axis; it has units of $\mu\text{Gy} \cdot \text{h}^{-1}$ at 1 m. Thus, $\dot{K}_{ref} = S_K/l^2$. The procedures for standardizing and measuring $\dot{K}_{ref}$ and S_K are identical.

The U.S. National Institute of Standards and Technology (NIST) maintains primary S_K standards for commercially available ^{137}Cs sources,[62] LDR ^{192}Ir seeds,[63] and all ^{103}Pd, ^{131}Cs, and ^{125}I seeds.[64] A *primary standard* is an instrument against which all other S_K measurement devices, called secondary or tertiary standards, must be intercompared. Such instruments are designed to permit inference of air-kerma values from the measured charge and instrument design using first principles. For ^{137}Cs and ^{192}Ir sources, the S_K standard is based on transverse-axis air-kerma measurements using spherical ion chambers with carbon walls—the same instruments used to maintain the ^{60}Co teletherapy air-kerma standard. For low-energy interstitial seeds, a special free-air chamber,[64] called the wide-angle free-air chamber (WAFAC), is used. Brachytherapy sources calibrated directly by the NIST standard or one of the AAPM-Accredited Dosimetry and Calibration Laboratories (ADCLs) are said to have *directly NIST traceable calibrations.* Sources that are calibrated against sources or ion chambers, which themselves have directly traceable NIST calibrations, are said to have *indirectly NIST-traceable* calibrations. For a more detailed description of air-kerma–based standards, measurement techniques, and traceability requirements, the reader is referred to a recent review by DeWerd.[65] The AAPM[66] recommends that individual clinics using BT sources maintain instrumentation able to make indirectly traceable calibration measurements for verification of vendor-supplied calibrations.

Kerma (kinetic energy released in the medium), K_x, is the ratio $\Delta E_{tr}/\Delta m$, where ΔE_{tr} is the total kinetic energy transferred to charged particles by photon interactions with atoms in small mass, Δm, of medium x.[67] For photons, ΔE_{tr} includes the initial kinetic energies of any secondary charged particles (e.g., Compton electrons, photoelectrons, and positrons) liberated by Compton, photoelectric, and pair production interactions. Kerma is defined only for indirectly ionizing radiations (e.g., photons and neutrons) and quantifies the transfer of energy from these radiation fields to matter. It takes the same units (cGy and Gy) as the related quantity absorbed dose. Although kerma can be specified in any medium x, usually air medium (x = air) is assumed for radiation metrology. K_{air} replaces the obsolete quantity exposure and is closely related to absorbed dose, D: the ratio, $\Delta E_{ab}/\Delta m$, where ΔE_{ab} is the energy imparted to Δm by the radiation field. Because the secondary electrons released by photon collisions may travel a significant distance before depositing their energy and may convert some of their kinetic energy to Bremsstrahlung radiation, D_{air} and K_{air} are not necessarily equal. When kerma remains relatively constant over the range of the secondary electrons, a special condition, secondary charged particle equilibrium (CPE), exists.[55,68] When the CPE is obtained, the rates of energy absorption and energy transfer are approximately equal, so that kerma closely approximates absorbed dose:

$$D_{air} = X \cdot \left(\frac{W}{e}\right) = K_{air} \cdot (1 - g) \qquad (10)$$

where X represents the quantity exposure. The quantity (W/e) is the average energy imparted to air per ion pair created and is a constant, independent of photon energy: (W/e) = 33.97 eV/ion pair = 33.97 J/C = 0.876 cGy/R.[69] The factor g is the fraction of kinetic energy transferred to the medium converted back to radiant energy (photons) by the Bremsstrahlung process; g is <0.001 at BT energies and usually is ignored, further simplifying Eq. (10). Virtually all BT dose calculation algorithms and dosimetric analyses assume that CPE is obtained and that dose, D, can be well approximated by kerma, K, everywhere. Although generally valid, CPE can be expected to break down in the presence of steep dose gradients near sources,[70] near metal–tissue interfaces,[71] and within the active elements of thin, bounded detectors.[72]

Activity

To define the obsolete quantities for describing source output, the quantity activity, A, must be introduced. It is defined as the rate of nuclear disintegration or transformation within a radioactive source. The contemporary unit of activity is the becquerel (1 Bq = 1 disintegration/second). We will freely use the more traditional but obsolete unit, the curie (1 Ci = 3.7×10^{10} disintegrations/s = 3.7×10^{10} Bq). A more convenient multiple of the curie, the millicurie, is defined as 1 mCi = 10^{-3} Ci = 3.7×10^7 disintegrations/second. Each disintegration represents the spontaneous transformation of an atom from one nuclear state to another. For most BT radioisotopes, such transformations of nuclear state give rise to photons in the form of unconverted γ-rays, annihilation photons, characteristic x-rays, and Bremsstrahlung photons. Activity is measured by counting the number of photons, β particles, or other particles emitted by an unencapsulated point source of the radionuclide by means of scintillation or proportional counters, from which its activity is inferred.[73] For sealed BT sources, A refers to activity contained inside the sealed source.

Activity, as defined in this strict sense, is no longer used in BT dosimetry. However, activity continues to serve as the basis for treatment specification and dosimetry of unsealed radiopharmaceuticals used for diagnosis and therapy. NIST maintains contained activity standards for a wide variety of radionuclides in aqueous solution.[74]

Relationship Between Activity and Exposure Rate

The activity, A, of radioactive nuclide-emitting photons and the exposure rate in free space, $\dot{X}_\delta(r)$, (in R/hour) at distance r (in centimeters) due to photons of energy greater than δ, are related by a fundamental quantity, the exposure rate constant, $(\Gamma_\delta)_X$, defined as follows[67]:

$$(\Gamma_\delta)_X = \frac{\dot{X}_\delta(r) \cdot r^2}{A} \tag{11}$$

$(\Gamma_\delta)_X$ has units of R cm^2 mCi^{-1} h^{-1} and is equal to the exposure rate in R/hour at 1 cm from a 1-mCi point source. It describes the rate at which air is ionized as a result of the emission of photons resulting from radioactive decay. The energy cutoff δ eliminates low-energy Bremsstrahlung and characteristic x-rays from consideration that are always absorbed within any practical source. The precise value of δ depends on the application; it usually is assumed to be about 10 keV. Because $(\Gamma_\delta)_X$ is defined in terms of an isotropic point source and exposure rates are corrected for air attenuation and scattering, inverse-square law applies exactly. Thus, $(\Gamma_\delta)_X$ is independent of the distance r used in Eq. (11).

$(\Gamma_\delta)_X$ depends only on the number and energy of the photons emitted per disintegration. Suppose there are N different photons emitted per disintegration with energies $E_1, E_2, \ldots E_N$ in units of MeV. Each time an atom decays, suppose P_i photons of energy E_i are emitted where i = 1,..., N. The list $\{E_i, P_i\}_{i=1}^N$ is the photon spectrum of the radionuclide. If the spectrum is known, then $(\Gamma_\delta)_X$ can be calculated by:

$$(\Gamma_\delta)_X = 193.7 \cdot \sum_{i=1}^{N} P_i \cdot E_i \cdot (\mu_{en}/\rho)_i^{air} \tag{12}$$

where $(\mu_{en}/\rho)_i^{air}$ is the mass energy absorption coefficient (in units of cm^2/g) for air at energy E_i. A detailed derivation of this fundamental relationship is given in a recently published review[22] and in a previous edition of this chapter.[75] The exposure-rate constant has been replaced by the air-kerma rate constant, $(\Gamma_\delta)_K$, by the ICRU.[67] $(\Gamma_\delta)_X$ is a fundamental property of the radionuclide's unencapsulated photon spectrum, applies only to an ideal point source, and neglects many significant properties of real sources such as self-absorption, filtration, and extension.[67]

^{226}Ra is an exception to this practice. First, radium source strength is specified by the quantity—mass of ^{226}Ra contained inside the source—denoted by M_{Ra}. M_{Ra} excludes the nonradioactive core components as well as radioactive decay products. Historically, M_{Ra} was introduced and widely used before the more general activity standards were available. Indeed, the unit curie originally was defined as the number of disintegrations produced by 1 g of ^{226}Ra. M_{Ra} standards were prepared by carefully weighing pure ^{226}Ra samples in an analytic balance. The first M_{Ra} standard was prepared by Marie Curie in 1913 and the currently used NIST standard was prepared by Hönigschmidt in 1934. To calibrate a user's source in M_{Ra}, its radiation output is compared with that of the NIST radium standard by means of an ion chamber. NIST no longer offers an M_{Ra} calibration service. In contrast to the other radionuclides, exposure-rate constant of ^{226}Ra—denoted by the special symbol $(\Gamma_\delta)_{Ra,t}$ in this chapter—is tabulated as a function of its effective capsule thickness, t, in millimeters of platinum. $(\Gamma_\delta)_{Ra,t}$ is normalized to the mass of radium contained in the source and has units of R cm^2 mg^{-1} h^{-1}.

Obsolete Quantities for Specifying Source Output

Because of the close association of early BT with ^{226}Ra, it is not surprising that the measured output of BT sources continues to be expressed as multiples of the output of a 1-mg radium needle. This quantity, equivalent mass of radium (M_{eq}), was introduced when artificial radioisotopes, such as ^{60}Co and ^{137}Cs, were developed as radium replacements. It allowed old implant and radium needle dosimetry tables, which gave dose per milligram-hour (mg-h) of ^{226}Ra, to be used without modification for these new sources. *M_{eq} is that mass of ^{226}Ra filtered by 0.5 mm Pt that has the same S_K as that of the given source.* Because M_{eq} is simply a statement of S_K relative to that of a hypothetic radium needle, the given source being quantified need not contain ^{226}Ra, be encapsulated in Pt, or have a wall thickness of 0.5 mm. Because K_{air} = X · (W/e) and $(\Gamma_\delta)_{Ra,0.5}$ = 8.25 R · cm^2 · mg^{-1} · h^{-1} for ^{226}Ra filtered by 0.5 mm Pt,[76] S_K and M_{eq} are related by:

$$\begin{aligned} S_K &= M_{eq} \cdot (\Gamma_\delta)_{Ra,0.5} \cdot (W/e) = M_{eq} \cdot 7.223 \\ M_{eq} &= \frac{S_K}{(\Gamma_\delta)_{Ra,0.5} \cdot (W/e)} = \frac{S_K}{7.223} \end{aligned} \tag{13}$$

where (W/e) = 33.97 eV/ion pair. M_{eq} continues to be widely used to specify strength of intracavitary and interstitial BT radium-substitute sources such as ^{137}Cs and ^{192}Ir.

Similar to the philosophy of M_{eq}, apparent activity, A_{app}, is a statement of source output relative to that of a hypothetic unfiltered point source. *A_{app} is the activity of a hypothetic unfiltered point source that has the same S_K as that of the given source:*

$$A_{app} = \frac{S_K}{(\Gamma_\delta)_X \cdot (W/e)} \tag{14}$$

Apparent activity in units of mCi continues to be widely used for specifying strength for permanent interstitial implants (e.g., ^{125}I and ^{103}Pd sources). In contrast to M_{eq}, which is based on the universally accepted $(\Gamma_\delta)_{Ra,0.5}$ value of 8.25 R · cm^2· mCi^{-1}· h^{-1}, no consensus as to $(\Gamma_\delta)_X$ values for the other radionuclides exists. Often different vendors will assume different $(\Gamma_\delta)_X$ values for the same radionuclide. Thus, A_{app} is an inherently ambiguous means of describing source strength. In an effort to reduce low-energy dose calculation errors associated with this ambiguity, the AAPM[5] recommends that the $(\Gamma_\delta)_X$ values of 1.476 and 1.45 R · cm^2 · mCi^{-1} · h^{-1} for ^{103}Pd and ^{125}I sources, respectively, be used universally for specification of A_{app}. Nearly all scientific societies involved in BT[3,66,77] recommend that M_{eq} and A_{app} be abandoned in favor of S_K for source ordering, dose calculation, and implant prescription.

Milligram-Hours and Integrated Reference Air-Kerma

In gynecologic intracavitary therapy, the quantities M_{Ra} and M_{eq} are used both to describe source loadings and to prescribe individual treatments. For prescribing therapy, these quantities, in units of milligrams of ^{226}Ra or mgRaEq, are integrated over treatment time yielding the so-called quantities mg-h and mgRaEq-h. As the product of total source strength and treatment time, mg-h and mgRaEq-h represent the total exposure or air-kerma accumulated at a distance of 1 m from the implant, under the assumptions that the implant is a point source and that tissue attenuation is negligible. The ICRU[3] recommends that mg-h be abandoned as a prescription or reporting quantity in favor of quantities defined in terms of air-kerma. The

American Brachytherapy Society (ABS) has proposed the quantity integrated reference air-kerma (IRAK), K_{ref}:

$$K_{ref} = \sum_{i=1}^{N} S_{K,i} \cdot t_i \quad (15)$$

where $S_{K,i}$ and t_i are the air-kerma strength and treatment time in hours, respectively, of the *i*th source. Thus, 1 unit of IRAK = 1 cGy · cm^2 = 1 μGy · m^2 = 1 U-h. A numerically identical quantity, total reference air kerma (TRAK), with units of μGy at 1 m, has been recommended by the ICRU.[3] IRAK and TRAK are related to mg-h and mgRaEq-h:

$$K_{ref} = \begin{cases} \text{mg-h} \times 6.754 & \text{for filtration } t = 1 \text{ mm Pt} \\ \text{mgRaEq-h} \times 7.227 & \text{for filtration } t = 0.5 \text{ mm Pt} \end{cases} \quad (16)$$

Intracavitary treatment systems[10] historically based on ^{226}Ra tubes (1-mm Pt encapsulation) typically use mg-h, whereas systems based on ^{137}Cs or other radium substitutes prescribe therapy in units of mgRaEq-h. Because of the difference in platinum filtration assumed by these two milligram-based quantities, numerically identical prescriptions can deliver quantities of IRAK that differ by 7%. Use of IRAK as an integrated output reporting quantity eliminates this 7% ambiguity that has confused comparison of different implant systems since the appearance of radium-substitute sources for BT.

Classical Dose Calculation Formalism: Isotropic Point Source

Consider an unencapsulated point source with an air-kerma strength of S_K, illustrated in Figure 22.10. Because this source has no extension, there is no attenuation of the emitted radiation by the source itself. Isotropy (Fig. 22.2) implies that photons are emitted with equal likelihood in all directions and travel in straight lines. In contrast, actual BT sources are encapsulated, have finite dimensions, and usually are cylindrically rather than spherically symmetric. The dose rate, $\dot{D}(r)$ (cGy/hour), at distance r (cm) in the water-equivalent medium surrounding the source is given by:

$$\dot{D}_{med}(r) = S_K \cdot \frac{\overline{(\mu_{en}/\rho)}^{med}_{air}}{r^2} \cdot T(r) \quad (17)$$

The inverse-square law term corrects for the difference in dose specification distance, r, and the 1-cm reference point assumed by the units of air-kerma strength. The quantity $\overline{(\mu_{en}/\rho)}^{med}_{air}$ is the ratio of mass-energy absorption coefficients in medium to that in air averaged over the photon spectrum in

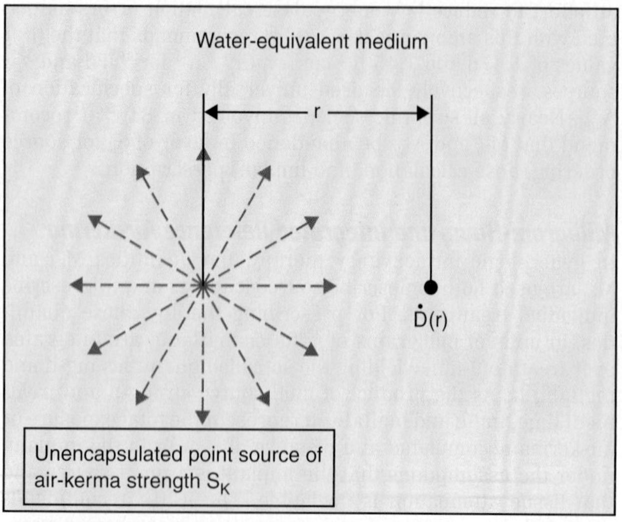

FIGURE 22.10. Unencapsulated point source of strength S_K immersed in an unbounded water-equivalent medium.

free space. This correction, equal to $\dot{K}_{med}/\dot{K}_{air}$ in free space, is a consequence of the fundamental relationship between particle fluence and dose.[22,75] It corrects for the efficiency with which the medium extracts energy from the emitted photons compared with air. For all radionuclides emitting photons with energies >200 keV, including all radium substitutes, $\overline{(\mu_{en}/\rho)}^{med}_{air}$ has the value 1.11 in water medium.

The last term of Eq. (17)—the kerma-to-dose conversion factor, T(r)—describes the net influence of primary photon attenuation and buildup of scattered photons in the surrounding medium. Sometimes this factor is termed the effective attenuation factor or the scatter-buildup factor.

$$T(r) = \frac{\text{Dose in medium}}{\text{Medium – kerma in free space}} = \left.\frac{\text{Exposure in medium}}{\text{Exposure in air}}\right\} \begin{matrix}\text{at distance r from a}\\ \text{point source}\end{matrix} \quad (18)$$

Figure 22.11 shows T(r) for several radium-substitute radionuclides as well as for a few low-energy radionuclides. For ^{226}Ra-equivalent radionuclides, T(r) deviates <5% from unity (1.00) out to distances, r, of 5 cm. Numerous tabulations of T(r) are available in the literature; those of Meisberger et al.,[78] Berger,[79] and Van Kleffens and Star[80] are among the best known. Most of these data are derived from theoretic photon transport calculations. The classical semiempirical model assumes that T(r) is a function only of the radionuclide photon spectrum and that a single dataset (e.g., for ^{192}Ir) can be used for all ^{192}Ir sources regardless of their construction.

By solving Eqs. (13) and (14) for S_K and substituting the results into Eq. (18), one can derive equations relating the dose rate at distance r to equivalent mass of radium and apparent activity for the same unfiltered point source:

$$\dot{D}_{med}(r) = M_{eq} \cdot \frac{(\Gamma_\delta)_{Ra,0.5} \cdot f_{med}}{r^2} \cdot T(r) \quad \text{Equivalent Mass of } ^{226}\text{Ra} \quad (a)$$

$$\dot{D}_{med}(r) = A_{app} \cdot \frac{(\Gamma_\delta)_X \cdot f_{med}}{r^2} \cdot T(r) \quad \text{Apparent Activity} \quad (b)$$

(19)

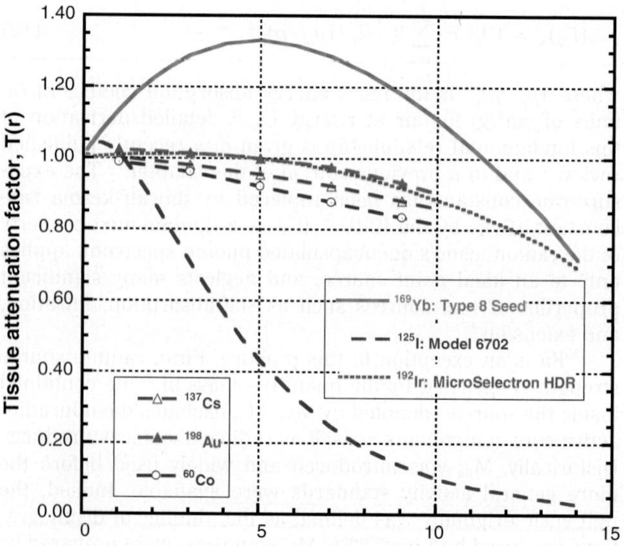

FIGURE 22.11. Photon attenuation and scatter factors, T(r), for a number of radium-equivalent radionuclides, as presented in the classic paper of Meisberger et al.,[192] and for several low-energy radionuclides. Meisberger et al. fit their data to a third-degree polynomial $T(r) = A + B \cdot r + C \cdot r^2 + D \cdot r^3$, which is widely used to represent T(r) in modern treatment-planning systems.

where f_{med} is the dose-to-exposure conversion factor given by:

$$f_{med} = \frac{D_{med}}{X} = (W/e) \cdot \left[\frac{(\mu_{en}/\rho)^{med}}{(\mu_{en}/\rho)^{air}} \right] \tag{20}$$
$$= 0.876 \frac{cGy}{R} \cdot \overline{(\mu_{en}/\rho)}^{med}_{air} \Big\} \text{ in free space}$$

For all ^{226}Ra substitutes (radionuclides with photon energies of more than 200 keV), f_{med} has the value 0.974 cGy · R^{-1} for water and 0.966 cGy · R^{-1} for muscle medium.[55]

Eqs. (17) and (19) give the dose rate, $\dot{D}_{med}(r)$, for a point source surrounded by an arbitrary medium that has been specified in terms of equivalent mass of radium, apparent activity, and S_K. Assuming that the same exposure rate constants, $(\Gamma_\delta)_{Ra,0.5}$ and $(\Gamma_\delta)_X$, were used to evaluate absorbed dose as were used to convert the measured air-kerma strength to M_{eq} and A_{app} via Eqs. (13) and (14), all three equations should give numerically identical dose rates. This demonstrates that Γ_δ is, in fact, a "dummy" constant that plays no physical role in the dosimetry of output-calibrated sealed sources because any arbitrary, but consistently used, value will yield identical dose-rate distributions. These unit conversions may not be performed by the same individual. For example, the vendor calibrates ^{125}I sources by intercomparing them with the NIST S_K standards. The vendor calculates A_{app} from the measured S_K by Eq. (14) using an assumed $(\Gamma_\delta)_X$ value and records the result on the source's calibration certificate. The hospital physicist, in calculating dose rates by Eq. (19), also must use an assumed $(\Gamma_\delta)_X$ value. If the physicist fails to use the same value as the vendor, significant dose calculation errors may result. Use of S_K for clinical source-strength specification eliminates these dummy constants, thereby eliminating errors resulting from inconsistent conventional choices.

Modeling of Source Anisotropy: The Anisotropy Factor

Despite its simplicity, the classical isotropic point-source model, Eq. (17), accurately predicts the transverse-axis dose-rate distributions of most actual radium-substitute sources. Simply by using an output quantity to calibrate the source, rather than contained activity, A, the influence of its internal structure (filtration and self-absorption) has been implicitly accounted for. Had true activity, A, instead of A_{app} been used in Eq. (19b), then the expression for $(\Gamma_\delta)_X$ (Eq. 12) would require correction for attenuation and scattering in the radioactive core and surrounding encapsulation. Any uncertainties in $\{E_i,P_i\}_{i=1}^{N}$ (which are large for many radionuclides) and filtration corrections would directly degrade dose calculation accuracy. In addition, fundamental activity measurements are technically difficult for the high-intensity sources used in BT. For this reason, contained activity does not play a role in photon BT dosimetry. In contrast, Eq. (17) infers dose rate from a quantity measured outside the source, which is not influenced significantly by knowledge of the unfiltered photon spectrum. The required quantities, $\overline{(\mu_{en}/\rho)}^{med}_{air}$ and T(r), are ratios and are therefore insensitive to errors in the assumed spectrum.

Practically all BT sources are cylindrical, giving rise to anisotropic dose distributions. In addition, some sources, especially those used in intracavitary BT, have active lengths that are comparable to typical calculation distances. Thus, the dose rate, $\dot{D}(r,\theta)$, around a BT source depends both on distance, r, and polar angle, θ (Fig. 22.8B). $\dot{D}(r,\theta)$ may deviate significantly from the transverse-axis dose rate, $\dot{D}(r,\pi/2)$, predicted by Eq. (17), especially near the long axis of the seed.

In the case of implants consisting of many randomly oriented seeds with active lengths less than the minimum distance of interest, Eq. (17) will accurately represent the multiple-seed dose distribution if an average correction for single-seed dose anisotropy is applied.[81] This correction factor, which the TG-43 protocol refers to as the "1-D anisotropy function," $\phi_{an}(r)$, is defined by averaging the dose at each fixed distance r with respect to solid angle Ω:

$$\phi_{an}(r) = \frac{\text{Average dose at r}}{\text{Transverse-axis dose at r}} = \frac{\int_{4\pi} \dot{D}(r,\theta) \cdot d\Omega}{4\pi \dot{D}(r,\pi/2)} = \frac{\int_0^\pi \dot{D}(r,\theta) \cdot \sin\theta \cdot d\theta}{2 \cdot \dot{D}(r,\pi/2)} \tag{21}$$

Often a distance-independent average value of $\phi_{an}(r)$, called the anisotropy constant, $\bar{\phi}_{an}$, is used. Incorporating this average correction into Eq. (17) leads to:

$$\dot{D}_{med}(r) = \frac{S_K \cdot \overline{(\mu_{en}/\rho)}^{med}_{air}}{r^2} \cdot T(r) \cdot \bar{\phi}_{an} \tag{22}$$

For radium-substitute sources, $\bar{\phi}_{an}$ was often evaluated by measuring relative photon fluence in air at relatively large distances (30 to 100 cm) using a NaI or GeLi scintillation detector.[45,82]

Eq. (22) implies that source strength should be increased by a constant fraction ranging from 2% (^{192}Ir seeds) to 10% (^{103}Pd seeds) to correct for polar anisotropy effects. Lindsay et al.[83] compared prostate implant 3D dose distributions derived from the isotropic point-source model, $\dot{D}(r)$, to those derived from the full 2D single-source dose calculation model, $\dot{D}(r,\theta)$. Based on voxel-by-voxel comparisons, they found that the isotropic point-source model introduced errors exceeding 10% of the D_{90} (see section on dose specification) in 8% and 33% of the target volume for the Model 6711 ^{125}I and Model 200 ^{103}Pd sources. Corbett et al.[84] found that large local dose-distribution differences, including 2D anisotropy effects, did not alter the dose–volume histogram (DVH): neither the V_{100} nor the margin between D_{100} and the prostate boundary were altered significantly. For volume implants consisting of parallel arrays of ^{192}Ir seeds, a similar finding has been reported.[81]

Dose Calculation for Extended Sources: The Sievert Integral Model

Dose distributions around larger sources, such as intracavitary tubes and interstitial needles, are calculated by partitioning the extended source into a set of point sources to which corrections for distance, oblique filtration, attenuation, and scattering are applied separately. By summing these point-source contributions, the dose at point P can be estimated. This class of algorithms, first described by Rolf Sievert in 1921,[85] is known as the Sievert integral algorithm, or more generally, the one-dimensional (1D) pathlength model.[22,86]

Assume that the source illustrated in Figure 22.12 has an air-kerma strength, S_K, and contained activity, A. The classical Sievert model approximates the cylindrical active core by a line of radioactivity positioned along its axis. The axial length of the core is called the active length, L. Oblique filtration is modeled by assuming that the capsule reduces dose by exponential attenuation using an effective filtration coefficient, μ'. The dose rate $\Delta\dot{D}(x,y)$ at point (x,y) from the incremental source ΔL, located at angle Γ is:

$$\Delta\dot{D}(x,y) = A \cdot \frac{\Delta L}{L} \cdot \frac{(\Gamma_\delta)_X \cdot f_{med}}{(x/\cos\theta)^2} \cdot T(x/\cos\theta) \cdot e^{-\mu' \cdot t/\cos\theta} \tag{23}$$

where $(\Gamma_\delta)_X$ is the exposure-rate constant of the unfiltered source material. Because $S_K = A \cdot (W/e) \cdot (\Gamma_\delta)_X \cdot e^{-\mu' t}$, Eq. (23) becomes:

$$\Delta\dot{D}(x,y) = S_K \cdot \frac{\Delta L}{L} \cdot e^{\mu' \cdot t} \cdot \frac{\overline{(\mu_{en}/\rho)}^{med}_{air}}{(x/\cos\theta)^2} \cdot T(x/\cos\theta) \cdot e^{-\mu' \cdot t/\cos\theta} \tag{24}$$

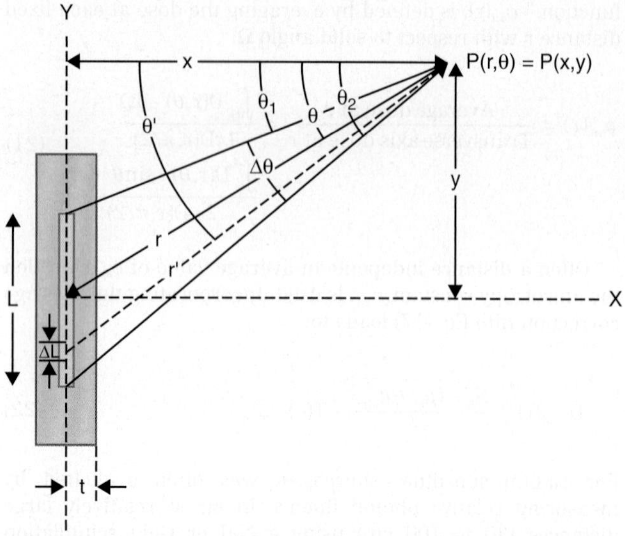

FIGURE 22.12. A typical encapsulated line source, illustrating calculation of dose rate at point P at (x,y) relative to the source center by the Sievert integral method. The active length and radial encapsulation thickness are denoted by L and t, respectively. The distances x and y are referred to as "distance away" and "distance along," respectively, in the literature.

By summing over all these incremental sources (i.e., integrating with respect to θ') and transforming to polar coordinates, we obtain the Sievert integral:

$$\dot{D}(r,\theta) = \frac{S_K \cdot \overline{(\mu_{en}/\rho)}_{air}^{med} \cdot e^{\mu' \cdot t}}{L \cdot r \cdot \cos\theta} \cdot \int_{\theta_1}^{\theta_2} e^{-\mu' t \cdot \sec\theta} \cdot T(x \cdot \sec\theta) \cdot d\theta \qquad (25)$$

The extra $e^{\mu' t}$ term outside the integral is needed to avoid global "double correction" for filtration.

Variants of Eq. (25) applicable to the regions near the source capsule ends are available. Numerous improvements to the basic model have been introduced over the years,[87,88] including modeling of photon absorption by the source core, extension to noncylindrical sources, generalization to radioactivity distributed over a volume,[4] extension to low-energy sources,[86] and treatment of applicator shielding and attenuation.[89,90]

The Sievert algorithm is widely used to model 2D dose distributions around ^{137}Cs tubes and needles for clinical treatment planning. Both experimental[91,92] and Monte Carlo studies[4,93] have demonstrated that the Sievert model accurately predicts dose-rate distributions in this energy range. When the filtration coefficient μ' is approximated[94] by the linear energy absorption coefficient μ_{en} (0.023 mm^{-1} for steel-clad ^{137}Cs sources), maximum errors are no larger than 5% to 8% and are much smaller (<3%) near the transverse axis. Published dose-rate distributions derived from the Sievert model, tabulated in terms of distances away and along, are available for several types of ^{137}Cs sources[4,93] and ^{226}Ra sources.[95] Williamson[86] showed that the classical Sievert integral gives rise to large errors (20% to 37% maximum error, 7% to 16% average error) when applied to lower-energy sources of ^{192}Ir, ^{169}Yb, and ^{125}I. Although accuracy can be improved by modifying the basic model,[86] classical semiempirical models should be used cautiously at photon energies below ^{137}Cs. Tabulated dose-rate distributions derived from direct measurement or Monte Carlo simulation are preferable for these sources.

If the encapsulation thickness is set to zero (t = 0) in Eq. (25), the Sievert integral reduces to a simple closed-form analytic expression:

$$\dot{D}(x,y) = S_K \cdot \overline{(\mu_{en}/\rho)}_{air}^{med} \cdot \frac{\Delta\theta}{L \cdot x} \qquad (26)$$

where $\Delta\theta$ is the angle, in radians, subtended by the active length, L, with respect to the point of interest (Fig. 22.12).

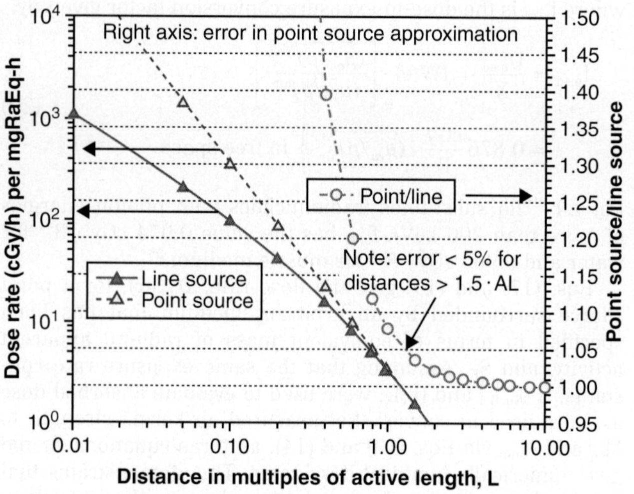

FIGURE 22.13. Error in the isotropic point source model relative to the line source model [Eq. (26)] as a function of transverse-axis distance expressed in multiples of active length.

When the interest point lies on the transverse axis (y = 0), then $\Delta\theta = 2 \cdot \tan^{-1}(L/2x)$, where $\tan^{-1}$ denotes the inverse tangent or arctan function in units of radians rather than degrees (180 degrees = π radians). This approximation is extremely useful as a manual calculation aid and is highly accurate near the transverse axis of lightly encapsulated ^{137}Cs sources.

Figure 22.13 shows that as the distance $r = \sqrt{(x^2 + y^2)}$ becomes large in relation to active length, L, Eq. (26) reduces to the point-source formula. For distances less than L (1.5 cm for intracavitary tubes), use of Eq. (17) will yield errors of at least 10%. For distances >1.5L (2 to 2.5 cm for gynecologic tubes), the point-source approximation is accurate within 5%.

Modern Quantitative Dosimetry

In contrast to classical dose calculation models, which assume that the parameters T(r) and $\overline{(\mu_{en}/\rho)}_{air}^{wat}$ depend only on the radionuclide used, quantitative dosimetry methods assume that dosimetry parameters are source-geometry specific and should be measured or calculated specifically for each type of source (i.e., commercially released source model). Classical approaches to BT dosimetry began to break down with the introduction of ^{125}I interstitial seeds in the early 1970s, as this 30-keV x-ray emitter clearly fell outside the scope of validated analytic models.[11] Although ^{125}I dose distributions derived from semiempirical models were published[96] and widely used, it was recognized[45] that internal seed structure could modulate the emitted photon spectrum and have significantly alter the absorbed dose distribution. The growing use of ^{125}I and the introduction of a primary exposure standard in 1985[97] motivated investigation of more quantitative dosimetry methods. For a more detailed review of ^{125}I dosimetry history, the reader is referred to Appendix C of the original TG-43 report.[98] Currently, both experimental methods and sophisticated computational dosimetry approaches are routinely used to derive such source-specific parameters. Both the classical and quantitative dosimetry approaches are based on the NIST air-kerma strength standards.

Experimental Brachytherapy Dosimetry

Clinical acceptance of measured dose rates in BT is a relatively recent phenomenon, beginning in the mid-1980s. Historically, this is due not only to the difficulties and labor intensity attending such measurements, but also to a consensus that dose measurement was so difficult and intrinsically inaccurate that even simplistic theoretic models were more reliable. Brachytherapy dose measurement does indeed place severe demands on detectors because the dose distributions are characterized by large dose gradients, a large range of dose rates, and relatively low photon energies. The most severe measurement artifact is the exquisite sensitivity of detector response to positioning errors; measurement of dose near a point source with 2% accuracy requires that the source-to-detector distance be specified with accuracy of 20, 50, 100, and 200 μm, respectively, at distances of 2, 5, 10, and 20 mm.

Commonly used dose detectors include thermoluminescent detectors (TLDs), small ion chambers, diode detectors, and silver-halide radiographic film. Radiochromic film[99] and plastic scintillator detectors[100,101] show promise as planar dose measurement systems. Three-dimensional dose measurement technologies under investigation include liquid scintillation cocktails[102] with dose distributions reconstructed by optical emission tomography and polymer gel dosimetry[103,104] using magnetic resonance imaging (MRI) to quantify the detector signal. One consideration in selecting a detector for BT dosimetry is minimizing energy-response artifacts, which arise from compositional differences between water and the detector and can result in variation of detector reading/unit dose in medium as the photon spectrum changes with position. Silicon diodes are useful detectors for measuring relative dose distributions around ultra-low-energy sources (e.g., ^{103}Pd and ^{125}I) because diode sensitivity is nearly independent of measurement point location,[105,106] but they are not recommended for higher-energy BT sources, as variations in sensitivity with position in the phantom as large as 15% for ^{137}Cs and 75% for ^{192}Ir have been reported.[107]

Among the established dosimetric techniques, LiF TLD dosimetry is considered to offer the best compromise between sensitivity, small size, and freedom from energy-response artifacts[58] and is currently considered to be standard of practice.[5] The acceptance of TLD dosimetry owes much to a 3-year (1987–1989) multi-institutional contract to perform a definitive review of low-energy seed dosimetry that was funded by the National Cancer Institute. The three institutions, collectively called the Interstitial Collaborative Working Group (ICWG), consisted of Memorial Sloan-Kettering, Yale, and University of California, San Francisco (UCSF), led by principal investigators Lowell Anderson, Ravinder Nath, and Keith Weaver, respectively.[108] Using TLD-100 thermoluminescent chips and powder capsules, embedded in machined solid-water phantoms, the ICWG developed procedures, including TLD dose calibration and energy-response correction, for making quantitative estimates of absolute dose rates in water. Each of the three ICWG investigator groups independently measured transverse-axis dose distributions for the ^{125}I and ^{192}Ir then available to validate their TLD measurement methodology.[108] This was followed by more complete 2D dose distributions about ^{125}I, ^{192}Ir, and ^{103}Pd BT sources then available.[105,109,110] The results showed good agreement among the different measurements and, overall, substantial differences between measured and classically computed dose rates for ^{125}I seeds (when normalized to the 194 Loftus air-kerma strength standard,[97] $S_{K,N85}$, then available), but good agreement between the classical and experimental approaches for ^{192}Ir. With careful correction for TLD linearity, perturbation of the photon field by the detectors, and relative energy response, absolute dose rate (cGy/hour in tissue per unit S_K) can be measured with a total uncertainty of 7% to 9% in the 1- to 5-cm distance range.[5,58]

Measured dose-rate distributions using TLD detectors are available for many common BT sources, including nearly all commercially available ^{125}I and ^{103}Pd sources (see the revised TG-43 Report[5] and a recent review article[58] for more comprehensive discussions); many ^{192}Ir sources for LDR, HDR, and pulsed dose rate (PDR) applications; and for many investigational sources. For radium-substitute sources, the measurements are in close agreement with the classical semiempirical models: isotropic point source and Sievert integral models.[4,22,86] For ^{125}I sources normalized to the $S_{K,N85}$ standard, measured dose rates were found to be 10% to 20% lower than those predicted by Eq. (17).[5,111] Better agreement[22] is observed between classical models and measurements when calibrations traceable to the 1999 WAFAC standard ($S_{K,N99}$)[64] are used. However, classical models such as the Sievert integral are not recommended for the low-energy source regimen as they poorly predict low-energy source anisotropy[96] and do not take into account modulation of the dose distribution by internal source geometry.

Computational Dosimetry Methods: Monte Carlo Photon Transport Simulation

Concurrently with the development of TLD dosimetry in the 1990s, other investigators were investigating the use of Monte Carlo photon-transport techniques as tools for quantitative evaluation of single-source dose distributions. Based on an accurate and detailed mathematical model of the internal structure of the source, photon histories can be generated and then evaluated to assess absorbed dose. Monte Carlo techniques are now accepted as a reliable and probably the most accurate source of BT dosimetry data.[5,58] As illustrated in Figure 22.14, this theoretical method uses a digital computer to randomly select a small number (10^5 to 10^7) of photon trajectories or "histories." A geometric model indicating the location of all media boundaries and photon sources must be available. By using probability distributions derived from total and differential cross-sections, a photon is randomly constructed by following each photon from birth through successive scattering events and, eventually, to absorption or escape from the system. At each decision point, random sampling is used to decide the fate of the photon. The process of randomly constructing photon trajectories is equivalent to selecting photon histories from the set of all those possible by random sampling. To statistically estimate the dose rate at a specified point, the dose contributed by each simulated collision is estimated and then averaged over all collisions. Monte Carlo simulation techniques are reviewed in more detail elsewhere.[58] Because particle histories can be accurately and efficiently constructed even in the presence of complex 3D geometries, approximation-free but statistically inexact solutions, derived from first principles, are possible for a wide range of geometrically complex but clinically relevant BT problems.

The dosimetric accuracy of Monte Carlo simulation has been confirmed across the entire energy spectrum from ^{125}I to ^{137}Cs. Agreement between Monte Carlo and TLD measurement ranges from 2% to 6%, both in homogeneous medium and in the presence of tissue and applicator heterogeneities.[7,48,107,112,113] In contrast to experimental methods, Monte Carlo accuracy is not limited by dosimeter artifacts such as energy response and volume averaging. Because the geometric model can be specified exactly, detector positioning error is not an issue in Monte Carlo. Recent analyses[5,51,58] have shown that the uncertainty (including all known systematic and random error sources) of Monte Carlo absolute dose-rate estimates on the transverse axis of ^{125}I seeds is 2.5% to 5% over the 1- to 5-cm distance range. Unlike dose measurements, Monte Carlo dose calculations cannot account for unsuspected deviations from the design specifications of the problem (e.g., a contaminant radionuclide in the source or an error in measuring its source strength).

Currently, the most important role of Monte Carlo simulation is calculation of reference-quality transverse-axis dose-rate distributions and anisotropy functions for low- and medium-energy BT sources. For low-energy interstitial seeds for routine clinical use, both experimental and Monte Carlo–based published dosimetry studies in peer-reviewed journal are required for developing AAPM-approved consensus datasets or posting the interstitial seed product on the Joint AAPM/RPC Source Registry.[5,114] Monte Carlo simulation is a useful alternative to dose measurement in many other applications such as characterizing the effects of applicator shielding materials[7,107] and tissue heterogeneities[48] on BT dose distributions;

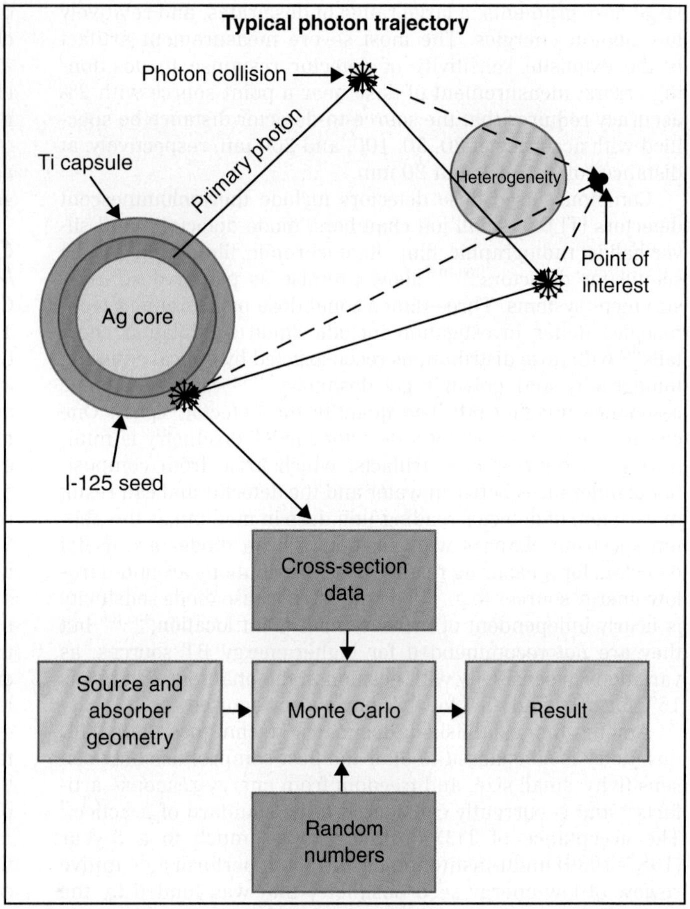

FIGURE 22.14. A: Two-dimensional representation of a typical photon history. The heavy solid lines illustrate the origin of the primary photon (randomly selected from the assumed distribution of radioactivity), and each successive collision, which is randomly selected from the competing collision mechanisms (photo-effect, Compton scattering, and coherent scattering), is based on their relative probabilities. The dashed lines illustrate the problem of estimation (i.e., calculating the probable contribution of each simulated collision to the point of interest). **B:** Functional diagram of a Monte Carlo code illustrating the required input data. Cross-section data include total attenuation coefficients, total cross-sections for each collision process, and differential cross-sections, which are used to randomly sample the distance between successive collisions, the interaction mechanism at each collision, and the angle and energy of the scattered photon leaving each collision, respectively. Sequences of random numbers are obtained from a "random number generator," a computer program designed to generate a pseudorandom sequence of numbers uniformly distributed between 0 and 1.

validating heuristic dose calculation algorithms;[115] and optimizing new source and applicator designs.[116]

Because Monte Carlo simulation statistical precision increases with the square root of computing time, the long computing time (several hours or even days) characteristic of general purpose codes has limited Monte Carlo–based treatment planning[117] to the experimental setting. However, due to advances in hardware and use of sophisticated variance reduction techniques,[118] this logistic barrier has been effectively overcome. At least one group[119] has reported single-processor calculation times on the order of a minute for clinical prostate seed implants. Even faster specialized BT codes have been introduced, including a fast correlated sampling code[120] and a planning code derived from EGSnrc.[121] Other groups have investigated deterministic transport solutions, mainly discrete ordinates codes[122] (also called "grid-based Boltzmann solvers" or GBBSs by some investigators) for more efficient but quantitatively accurate dose calculation for clinical treatments. Recently, Varian Medical Systems (Palo Alto, CA) has introduced a dose calculation engine based on the discrete ordinates method in its BrachyVision HDR planning system,[123] the first commercially available BT dose calculation engine based on a rigorous radiation transport simulation. Unlike current TG-43 clinical dose computations, Monte Carlo or deterministic transport solutions can account for the perturbing effect of multiple implanted sources on the single-source dose distributions, deviations in tissue composition from the assumed water medium, and the influence of applicator shielding and attenuation. These phenomena have been shown to introduce dose estimation as large as a factor of two. For more information on model-based dose calculation and its potential clinical impact, the reader is referred to a recent review by Rivard et al.[124]

AAPM Task Group 43 Report: A Table-Based Dose Calculation Formalism

An important milestone in modern BT dosimetry is the publication of the original AAPM Task Group 43 Report in 1995[98] and a substantially revised and expanded version in 2004.[5] The TG-43 approach consists of using measured and Monte Carlo–generated dose-rate distributions directly for clinical dose calculation aided by a standard table-lookup formalism. The revised TG-43 report and a more recent supplement[42] include the following:

1. A recommended dose calculation formalism for representing 2D and 1D dose distributions around interstitial sources specifically designed to use a sparse matrix of Monte Carlo or measured dose rates as its input.
2. A critically reviewed set of 2D dose distribution data for 16 ^{125}I ^{103}Pd seed models that satisfy the AAPM dosimetric prerequisites[114] as of July 2003. For each of these source types, a consensus dose distribution in TG-43 formalism format is recommended based on "merging" published Monte Carlo and experimental dosimetry datasets that met the standards laid out in Section V of the report.
3. A history of air-kerma strength primary standards,[64,97] which summarizes previous AAPM guidance,[125,126] including the impact of calibration shifts on the delivered-to-prescribed dose ratio.
4. Methodologic recommendations for obtaining TG-43 dosimetry parameters from TLD measurements or Monte Carlo simulations, including uncertainty analyses.
5. Guidance on clinical implementation of TG-43 report recommendations.

The TG-43 report recommends that treatment-planning software vendors accept the TG-43 formalism as the basis of

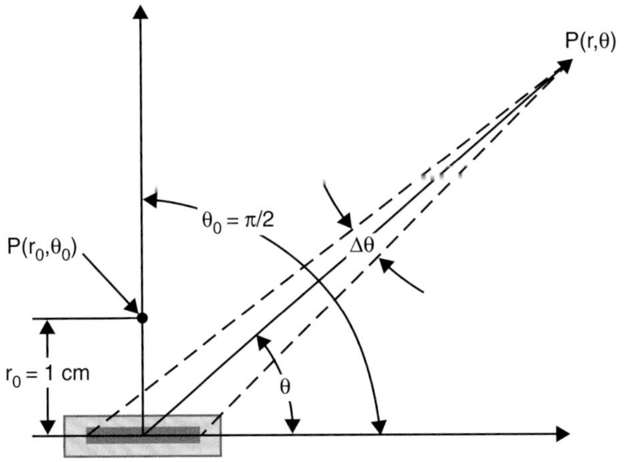

FIGURE 22.15. Illustration of Task Group Report 43 formalism for calculation of absorbed dose rate, $\dot{D}(r,\theta)$, at (r,θ), in a polar coordinate system centered about the source active core.

dose calculation or at least for data entry, allowing users to easily input the new data into their systems. With the introduction of the new WAFAC-based air-kerma strength standard by NIST and the growing number of low-energy interstitial BT sources commercially available, the radiotherapy community has embraced the TG-43 dose calculation formalism, described later, as well as many AAPM recommendations associated with TG-43 implementation. Most important among these are the AAPM dosimetric prerequisites for routine non-institutional review board–approved BT procedures.[114] Only low-energy sources with NIST-traceable S_K calibrations supported by annual intercomparisons among NIST, the ADCLs, and the vendor[127] and two independent Monte Carlo and experimental dosimetry studies published in the peer-reviewed literature will be posted on the AAPM/RPC website[43] or included in future TG-43 supplements. A similar dosimetry validation process is under development for higher-energy sources.[128]

Because changes in calibration standards and dosimetry parameters also alter prescribed-to-delivered dose ratios, radiation oncologists must embrace new dosimetry systems and source-strength standards that can have important implications for selection of prescribed dose, interpreting published outcome studies, and consistently reproducing their clinical experience through time. AAPM reports provide detailed discussions and recommendations on managing these changes. For example, in ^{125}I monotherapy for prostate cancer, the pre– TG-43 prescribed dose of 160 Gy is equivalent to 145 Gy using the TG-43 dosimetry parameters.[125] Managing the up to 10% variations in prescribed-to-administered dose ratios due to the complex dosimetric history of ^{103}Pd monotherapy is reviewed in a 2005 AAPM report.[126]

General Formalism for the Two-Dimensional Case

For a cylindrically symmetric source of strength S_K (Fig. 22.15), dose rate, $\dot{D}(r,\theta)$, at the point (r,θ) is calculated in the TG-43 formalism as follows:

$$\dot{D}(r,\theta) = S_K \cdot \Lambda \cdot \frac{G_L(r,\theta)}{G_L(r_0,\theta_0)} \cdot g_L(r) \cdot F(r,\theta) \tag{27}$$

where r denotes the distance (in cm) from the center of the active source to the point of interest, θ denotes the polar angle specifying the point of interest relative to the source longitudinal axis, r_0 denotes the reference distance (specified to be 1 cm), and θ_0 is the reference angle (90 degrees or $\pi/2$ radians) that defines the source transverse plane. For ^{125}I and ^{103}Pd sources, AAPM guidance[125,126] uses the symbols $S_{K,N99}$ to designate the 1999 WAFAC-based NIST standard[64] and $S_{K,N85}$ to designate the previous standard introduced by Loftus[97] in 1985. The other symbols in Eq. (27) denote the following quantities:

$G_L(r,\theta)$ is the line-source geometry function in units of cm^{-2}.
Λ is the dose-rate constant of the source type in units of $cGy \cdot h^{-1} \cdot U^{-1}$.
$F(r,\theta)$ is the dimensionless 2D anisotropy function that takes the value unity for θ_0 at all r.
$g(r)$ is the dimensionless radial dose function that takes the value unity at $r = r_0$.

The dose-rate constant in liquid-water medium is defined by:

$$\Lambda = \frac{\dot{D}(r_0,\theta_0)}{S_K} = \frac{\dot{D}(1\text{ cm}, 90°)}{S_K} \tag{28}$$

where $\dot{D}(r_0,\theta_0)$ is the measured dose rate at the reference point. Λ includes the effects of source geometry, spatial distribution of radioactivity, encapsulation, self-filtration in the source, and attenuation and scattering of photons in the surrounding medium. It also depends on the standardization measurements to which the S_K calibration of the source is traceable. For radium-substitute point sources, $\Lambda = \overline{(\mu_{en}/\rho)}^{med}_{air} \cdot T(r)$. During the era (1984–1999) of the $S_{K,N85}$ standard, Table 22.4 shows that the classical point-source model overestimated absolute doses by as much as 15% for ^{125}I sources relative to TLD measurements and Monte Carlo calculations. In 1999, the $S_{K,N85}$ standard was replaced by the WAFAC ($S_{K,N99}$), which required an upward adjustment of these values, bringing the classical and quantitative values closer together. The old and new dose calculations are in close agreement for ^{192}Ir and other radium substitutes. This table shows that for both ^{103}Pd and ^{125}I sources, average

TABLE 22.4 DOSE-RATE CONSTANTS FOR SELECTED INTERSTITIAL SEEDS

	Λ $(cGy\ h^{-1}\ U^{-1})^a$			
Source	*2004 TG-43*	*Classical Model*	*Quantitative*	*Author/Method*
Best Industries ^{192}Ir (Fe Clad)	–	1.12[78]	1.11	TLD: ICWG[108]
			1.11	MC: Williamson[111]
Nycomed-Amersham ^{125}I	0.965		0.877 $(S_{K,N85})^b$	MC: DLC-99[111]
(Model 6711)		1.04[45]	0.935 $(S_{K,N99})^c$	MC: DLC-146[341]
			0.879 $(S_{K,N85})^b$	TLD: ICWG[108]
			0.980 $(S_{K,N99})^c$	TLD: ICWG[108]
Theragenics I-Seed ^{125}I	1.012	1.029[342]	1.033^c	TLD[343]
(Model I25.S06)			0.991^c	MC: DLC-146[46]
Theragenics ^{103}Pd	0.686	0.683[49]	0.74 $(S_{K,T88})^d$	TLD: 1995 TG-43[98]
(Model 200)			0.68^c	TLD[344]
			0.691^c	MC: DLC-146[49]
North American Scientific ^{103}Pd	0.688	0.683[49]	0.68^c	TLD[345]
(MED 3633)			0.677^c	MC: DLC-99[346]

MC, Monte Carlo; TLD, measured by thermoluminescent dosimetry; DLC, Data Code Library indicating vintage of cross-section library.
^{a}All measured Λ include solid-to-liquid water conversion factors.
^{b}Denotes National Institute of Standards and Technology (NIST) 1985 standard, $S_{K,N85}$.
^{c}Normalized to NIST 1999 standard, $S_{K,N99}$.
^{d}Denotes original vendor-maintained standard implemented in 1988.

agreement between TLD and Monte Carlo is about 5%, well within the total uncertainty of these comparisons.[58]

The purpose of the geometry function, $G_X(r,\theta)$ (where the subscript x denotes point or line source), is to improve the accuracy with which dose rates can be estimated by interpolation from data tabulated at discrete points. Physically, $G_X(r,\theta)$ neglects scattering and attenuation and provides an effective inverse-square law correction based on an *approximate model* of the spatial radioactivity distribution within the source. Because the geometry function is used only to interpolate between tabulated dose-rate values at defined points, highly simplistic approximations yield sufficient accuracy for treatment planning.[5] To improve the accuracy of linear interpolation near the source, the AAPM protocol requires use of (r,θ) for 2D calculations and prefers $G_L(r,\theta)$ over $G_P(r,\theta)$ for 1D calculations. For small cylindrical seeds, $G_X(r,\theta)$ is approximated by a line source.

$$G_P(r,\theta) = r^{-2} \quad \text{point-source approximation}$$

$$G_L(r,\theta) = \begin{cases} \dfrac{\Delta\beta}{Lr\sin\theta} & \text{if } \theta \neq 0^\circ \\ (r^2 - L^2/4)^{-1} & \text{if } \theta = 0^\circ \end{cases} \quad \text{line-source approximation} \tag{29}$$

where $\Delta\beta = \theta_2 - \theta_1$ is the angle (in radians) subtended by the active source with respect to the point (r,θ). For sources where the radioactivity is distributed over or within a right-cylindrical volume or annulus, L can be taken as the length of this cylinder. For sources containing uniformly spaced multiple radioactive components, L should be taken as the effective length, L_{eff}, given by $L_{eff} = \Delta S \times (N)$, where N represents the number of discrete pellets contained in the source with a nominal pellet center-to-center spacing, ΔS.

The 2D anisotropy function $F(r,\theta)$ gives the angular variation of dose about the source at each distance as a result of self-filtration, oblique filtration of primary photons through the encapsulating material, and photon attenuation and scattering in the surrounding medium.

$$F(r,\theta) = \frac{\dot{D}(r,\theta)}{\dot{D}(r,\theta_0)} \frac{G_L(r,\theta_0)}{G_L(r,\theta)} \tag{30}$$

where the dose rates, $\dot{D}(r,\theta)$, are obtained by measurement or Monte Carlo simulation. The line-source geometry function is used to suppress the influence of inverse-square law on the angular dose distribution at short distances. Thus, $F(r,\theta)$ needs be tabulated only at a few distances, r, to facilitate accurate interpolation at all distances. Examples of anisotropy functions for various interstitial sources are illustrated in Figure 22.16 and Table 22.6.

The radial dose function, $g_X(r)$, accounts for the fall-off of dose along the transverse axis as a result of attenuation and scattering in the medium, capsule filtration, and self-absorption.

$$g_X(r) = \frac{\dot{D}(r,\theta_0)}{\dot{D}(r_0,\theta_0)} \frac{G_X(r_0,\theta_0)}{G_X(r,\theta_0)} \tag{31}$$

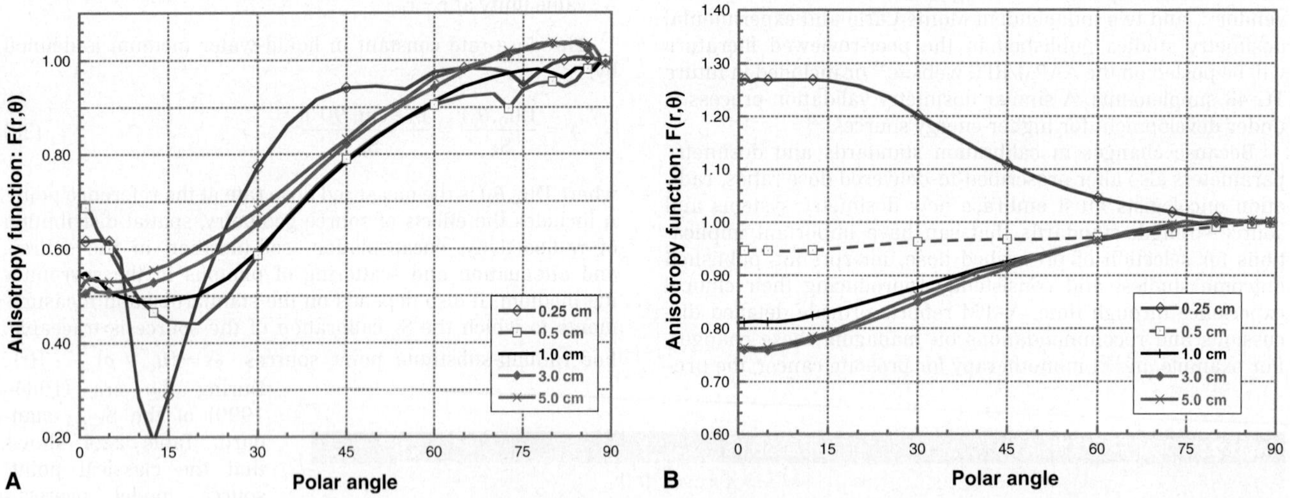

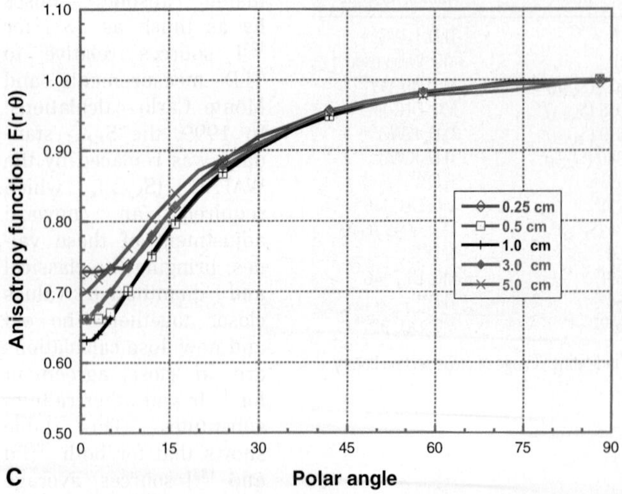

FIGURE 22.16. Examples of anisotropy functions evaluated for three different interstitial sources by the author's group. **A:** Theragenics Model 200 "light seed" ^{103}Pd source.[49] **B:** DRAXIMAGE Model LS-1 ^{125}I seed.[342] **C:** Nucletron MicroSelectron Model V2 high–dose-rate ^{192}Ir source.[347]

TABLE 22.5 LINE-SOURCE RADIAL DOSE FUNCTIONS FOR VARIOUS ^{125}I SEED SOURCES[a]

	Line Source Approximation					
r [cm]	Amersham 6702 L = 3.0 mm	Amersham 6711 L = 3.0 mm	Best 2301 L = 4.0 mm	NASI MED3631-A/M L = 4.2 mm	Bebig 125. S06 L = 3.5 mm	Imagyn 1S12501 L = 3.4 mm
0.10	1.020	1.055	1.033		*1.010*	*1.022*
0.15	**1.022**	1.078	1.029		**1.018**	*1.058*
0.25	**1.024**	1.082	1.027	*0.998*	*1.030*	*1.093*
0.50	1.030	1.071	1.028	*1.025*	*1.030*	1.080
0.75	1.020	**1.042**	1.030	*1.019*	**1.020**	**1.048**
1.00	1.000	1.000	1.000	1.000	1.000	1.000
1.50	0.935	0.908	0.938	0.954	0.937	0.907
2.00	0.861	0.814	0.866	0.836	0.857	0.808
3.00	0.697	0.632	0.707	0.676	0.689	0.618
4.00	0.553	0.496	0.555	0.523	0.538	0.463
5.00	0.425	0.364	0.427	0.395	0.409	0.348
6.00	0.322	0.270	0.320	0.293	0.313	0.253
7.00	0.241	0.199	0.248	0.211	0.232	0.193
8.00	0.179	0.148	0.187		0.176	0.149
9.00	0.134	0.109	0.142		0.134	0.100
10.00	0.0979	0.0803	0.103		0.0957	0.075

[a]Bold entries indicate interpolated values; italicized entries indicate extrapolated values.

From Rivard MJ, Coursey BM, DeWerd LA, et al. Update of AAPM Task Group No. 43 Report: a revised AAPM protocol for brachytherapy dose calculations. *Med Phys* 2004;31(3):633–674.

$g_X(r)$ is normalized to unity at 1 cm distance and is illustrated by Table 22.5. For 2D dose calculations, TG-43 recommends that X = L.

One-Dimensional Isotropic Source Approximation

Most commercial treatment-planning systems used for permanent implant dose computation support only 1D isotropic point-source calculations. Thus, the TG-43 formalism includes a 1D equation analogous to the classical isotropic point-source model, Eq. (22).

$$\dot{D}(r) = S_K \cdot \Lambda \cdot \frac{G_L(r,\theta_0)}{G_L(r_0,\theta_0)} \cdot g_L(r) \cdot \phi_{an}(r) \tag{32}$$

where $\phi_{an}(r)$ is the 1D anisotropy function defined by Eq. (21) and illustrated by Table 22.6.

INTERSTITIAL IMPLANTATION

The traditional implant systems (Manchester, Quimby, and Paris) that arose early in the 20th century were developed to guide the radiation oncologist in arranging and positioning radium needles within the surgically identified target volume. In contrast, the most frequently practiced implant procedure today, transperineal permanent implants of the prostate, uses image guidance to position the sources. In place of nomograms and classical system lookup tables, 3D computerized planning is used to prescribe dose and to optimize the implant geometry. However, even the most sophisticated commercially available dwell-weight optimization software used with single-stepping source remote afterloaders (see Chapters 23 and 24) requires the operator to specify the source and needle locations. To guide source positioning, we continue to rely on the classical systems of BT and their later variants.

Classical Systems for Interstitial Brachytherapy with Radium-Substitute Sources

The Manchester and Quimby systems were developed before the advent of computer-aided dosimetry in implant therapy, whereas the Paris system is based on multiplanar isodose distributions. All interstitial implant systems consist of the following components:

1. *Distribution rules:* Given a target volume, the distribution rules determine how to distribute the radioactive sources and applicators in and around the target volume.
2. *Dose specification and implant optimization criteria:* At the heart of each system is a dose specification criterion (i.e., a definition of prescribed dose). In the Manchester system,

TABLE 22.6 EXAMPLE OF A TABULATED 2D ANISOTROPY FUNCTION, $F(r,\theta)$ TABLE, ALONG WITH ITS ASSOCIATED 1D ANISOTROPY FUNCTION, $\phi_{an}(r)$, VALUES FOR A THERAGENICS I-SEED (MODEL 125.S06) ^{125}I SOURCE

Polar Angle	r [cm]							
θ (Degrees)	0.25	0.5	1	2	3	4	5	7
0	*0.302*	*0.429*	0.512	0.579	0.610	0.631	*0.619*	*0.604*
5	*0.352*	*0.436*	0.509	0.576	0.610	0.635	*0.651*	*0.689*
10	*0.440*	*0.476*	0.557	0.622	0.651	0.672	*0.689*	*0.721*
20	*0.746*	*0.686*	0.721	0.757	0.771	0.785	*0.790*	*0.807*
30	*0.886*	*0.820*	0.828	0.846	0.857	0.862	*0.867*	*0.874*
40	*0.943*	*0.897*	0.898	0.907	0.908	0.913	*0.918*	*0.912*
50	*0.969*	*0.946*	0.942	0.947	0.944	0.947	*0.949*	*0.946*
60	*0.984*	*0.974*	0.970	0.974	0.967	0.966	*0.967*	*0.976*
70	*0.994*	*0.989*	0.988	0.990	0.984	0.985	*0.987*	*0.994*
80	*0.998*	*0.998*	0.998	1.000	0.994	1.000	*0.993*	*0.999*
$\phi_{an}(r)$	*1.122*	*0.968*	0.939	0.939	0.938	0.940	*0.941*	*0.949*

Reproduced from Rivard MJ, Coursey BM, DeWerd LA, et al. Update of AAPM Task Group No. 43 Report: a revised AAPM protocol for brachytherapy dose calculations. *Med Phys* 2004;31(3):633–674.

TABLE 22.7 MANCHESTER SYSTEM RULES

Feature	*Paterson and Parker (Manchester System) Rules*
Dose and dose rate	6,000 R to 8,000 R in 6–8 days (1,000 R/day; 40 R/hour)
Dose specification criterion	Effective minimum dose is 10% above the absolute minimum dose in treatment plane or volume.
Dose gradient	Dose in treatment volume or plane varies by no more than ± 10% from stated dose except for localized hot spots.
	For double-plane implants with a separation >1 cm, dose is specified on interior plane 0.5 cm from implanted plane, resulting in 10% to 30% midplane cold spots. The single-plane mgRaEq-h is multiplied by a separation factor to obtain total double-plane mgRaEq-h.
Linear activity	Variable: 0.66 and 0.33 mgRaEq/cm
Source strength distribution: planar	Area < 25 cm^2: 2/3 periphery; 1/3 center
	25 < Area < 100 cm^2: 1/2 periphery; 1/2 center
	Area >100 cm^2: 1/3 periphery; 2/3 center
Source strength distribution: volume	Cylinder: belt : core : end : end = 4:2:1:1
	Sphere: belt : core = 6:2
	Cube: 1/8 of the activity in each face 2/8 of the activity in the core
Source implant pattern and spacing between sources	Constant uniform spacing: 1-cm separation between sources recommended. Smaller spacings must be used to satisfy distribution rules for small implants.
Crossing needles	Perpendicular to and at the active ends of the parallel needles; if placed beyond the active ends of the needles, should be double strength. Crossing needles used when possible.
	Planar implant: Target area effectively treated is reduced in length by 10% per uncrossed end.
	Volume implant: Target volume effectively treated is reduced by 7.5% per uncrossed end.
	1 uncrossed end : belt : core = 4:2:1
	2 uncrossed ends : belt : core = 4:2
Elongation corrections	Long : Short Dimension: 1.5:1 2:1 2.5:1 3:1 4:1
	Correction factors (Applied to mgRaEq-h, not area or volume)
	Planar 1.025 1.05 1.07 1.09 1.12
	Volume 1.03 1.06 1.10 1.15 1.23
Relation between implanted volume/area and treated (target) volume/area	Peripheral and crossing needles placed on the target volume boundaries. Active length determines target length.

for example, the prescribed dose is the modal dose in the volume bounded by the peripheral sources. The distribution rules and dose specification criterion together often reflect a compromise between mutually exclusive goals such as dose homogeneity, normal tissue sparing, number of catheters implanted, dosimetric margins around the target, and presence of high-dose regions outside the target.

3. *Dose calculation aids:* These devices are used to estimate the source strengths required to achieve the prescribed dose rate as defined by the system for source arrangements satisfying its distribution rules. Older systems (Manchester and Quimby) use tables that give dose delivered per mgRaEq-h as a function of treatment volume or area. The more recent Paris system makes extensive use of computerized treatment planning to relate absorbed dose to source strength and treatment time.

The Manchester System

The Manchester system was developed by Ralston Paterson (radiation oncologist) and Herbert Parker (physicist) in the 1930s[129–132] and often is called the Paterson-Parker (P-P) system. The P-P system remains relevant to today's practice

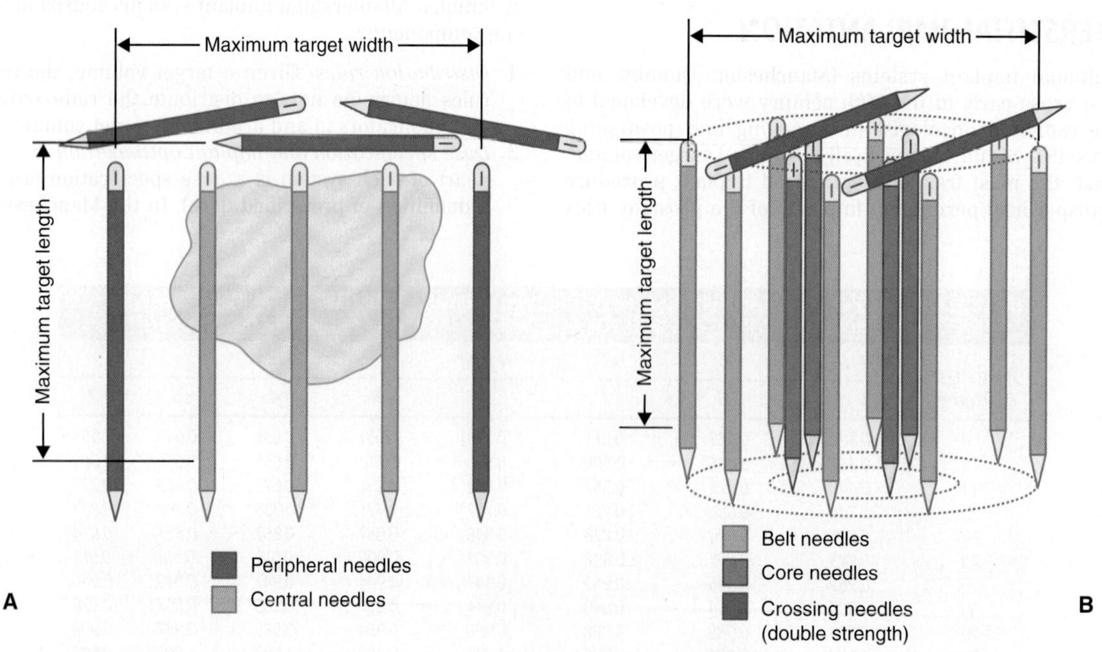

FIGURE 22.17. Relationship between target volume or area and peripheral needles (*solid color active regions*) and central needles (*hatched active regions*). Notice that peripheral needles always are placed on the boundary of the target region. **A:** A planar implant designed to treat a target area. **B:** A volume implant designed to treat a cylindrical target volume. The peripheral needles distributed on the cylindrical surface of the target are called *belt* needles, whereas those at right angles are called *end* or *crossing* needles. Because the inferior of these implants are uncrossed, the target volumes effectively treated are 7.5%–10% shorter than the active length of the belt or peripheral needles.

patterns: its distribution rules, anticipating the "peripheral loading technique," were designed to maximize dose homogeneity inside the implanted volume for volume implants and in the treatment plane (plane parallel to the needles at the treatment distance) for mold or planar implants (Fig. 22.17). Its volume and area lookup tables remain useful as QA tools for optimized HDR volume implants.

The P-P system rules preferentially concentrate radioactivity in the rind or periphery of the implant, compensating for the dose fall-off characteristic of a uniform-density implant, thereby improving dose uniformity. After deriving the optimal fraction of radioactivity to be implanted in the rind and core (4:2 ratio) using a radioactive fluid model, Parker coalesced the continuous radioactivity distribution into several concentric cylindrical surfaces and then further discretized these surfaces into individual needles. A more detailed discussion of the mathematical derivation of the Manchester system is given by Anderson and Presser.[133] Table 22.7 lists the rules of the Manchester system, and Table 22.8 lists the stated dose per mgRaEq-h and unit IRAK as a function-treated area or volume.

The P-P rules are designed to yield target area or volume dose distribution that deviates by no more than ± 10% of the stated dose, excluding cold spots in the corners and local hot-spots at distances <5 mm from the source centers. For planar implants, the target or treatment surface (Fig. 22.17) is that area bounded by the peripheral needles, which is parallel to and 5 mm from the needle plane. For volume implants, the target volume is that region bounded by the peripheral sources. The distribution rules assume that both planar and volume implants will be crossed at both ends by needles placed orthogonal to the predominant direction of insertion and at the level of the belt needle active tips. Fixed 1-cm needle spacing is recommended, with full-intensity sources placed on the periphery of planar implants and partial-strength needles used as central needles. For volume implants, these two groups of sources are called "belt" and "core" sources, respectively. The stated or prescribed dose is the modal dose in the target region and is approximately 10% higher than the minimum peripheral dose (minimum dose to the implanted volume or area) and 10% below the effective maximum dose.

In effect, single-plane interstitial implants with crossed ends treat a 1-cm-thick target volume with an area equal to that bounded by the peripheral sources. Thicker target volumes (>1 cm) must be treated by using two parallel planes of needles placed on the target volume boundaries (double-plane implant), with source strength arranged according to the single-plane rules. The mgRaEq-h is calculated from the 0.5-cm single-plane table, multiplied by the appropriate two-plane separation factor, and divided between the two planes. The dose actually is delivered to the inner plane 0.5 cm from each needle plane, resulting in midplane cold spots ranging from 10% to 30% for separations of 1.5 to 2.5 cm. Target volumes thicker than 2.5 cm must be treated by the volume implant system.

Volume implants can treat cylindrical, spherical, or cubic target volumes in which needles or seeds are arranged on concentric cylinders, concentric spheres, or parallel planes, using a 1-cm needle-to-needle spacing when possible. The target region is the volume encompassed by the peripheral sources. Regardless of implant size, 75% of the source strength should be placed in the rind and 25% in the core, with more specific rules for cylinder implants.

To apply the P-P system, the relationship between target volume, implanted volume (region enclosed by peripheral sources), and treated volume (region receiving 90% of the stated dose) must be appreciated for crossed and uncrossed end cases. The treated volume may be larger than the target volume but always

TABLE 22.8 MANCHESTER IMPLANT TABLES

Volume Implants			*Planar Implants*		
Volume (cm³)	*mgRaEq-h/1,000 'P-P' R*[a]	*Min Dose/IRAK*[b] *cGy/(μGy · m²)*	*Area (cm²)*	*mgRaEq-h/1,000 'P-P' Ra*	*Min Dose/IRAK*[b] *cGy/(μGy · m²)*
1	34	3.49	0	30	3.97
2	54	2.20	2	97	1.23
3	70	1.68	4	141	0.844
4	85	1.38	6	177	0.672
5	99	1.194	8	206	0.578
10	158	0.752	10	235	0.506
15	207	0.574	12	261	0.456
20	251	0.474	14	288	0.413
25	291	0.408	16	315	0.378
30	329	0.361	18	342	0.348
40	398	0.298	20	368	0.323
50	462	0.257	24	417	0.285
60	522	0.228	28	466	0.255
70	579	0.206	32	513	0.232
80	633	0.188	36	558	0.213
90	684	0.174	40	603	0.197
100	734	0.162	44	644	0.185
110	782	0.152	48	685	0.174
120	829	0.143	52	725	0.164
140	919	0.129	56	762	0.156
160	1,005	0.118	60	800	0.149
180	1,087	0.110	64	837	0.142
200	1,166	0.102	68	873	0.136
220	1,242	0.0958	72	908	0.131
240	1,316	0.0904	76	945	0.126
260	1,389	0.0857	80	981	0.121
280	1,459	0.0815	84	1,016	0.117
300	1,528	0.0779	88	1,052	0.113
320	1,595	0.0746	92	1,087	0.109
340	1,661	0.0716	96	1,122	0.106
360	1,725	0.0690	100	1,155	0.103
380	1,788	0.0665	120	1,307	0.0910
400	1,851	0.0643	140	1,463	0.0813
–	–	–	160	1,608	0.0740
–	–	–	180	1,746	0.0682
–	–	–	200	1,880	0.0633
–	–	–	220	2,008	0.0593
–	–	–	240	2,132	0.0558
–	–	–	260	2,256	0.0527
–	–	–	280	2,372	0.0502
–	–	–	300	2,495	0.0477

[a]Original Manchester values from Paterson R, Parker HM. A dosage system for interstitial radium therapy. *Br J Radiol* 1938;11:313–339.

[b]Modified from original values for Ir-192 assuming 860 cGy minimum peripheral dose per 1,000 'P-P' R and 7.227 μGy · m²/mgRaEq-h.

should contain the latter. When both ends are crossed, the active length (AL) required and target length (TL) are identical. For volume implants, AL should be at least 7.5% longer than TL for each uncrossed end. For planar implants, the required AL can be calculated as follows:

$$\begin{aligned}&\text{Two crossed ends} \quad \text{AL} = \text{TL planar and volume}\\&\text{One crossed end} \quad \text{AL} = \begin{cases}\text{TL}/0.90 & \text{planar}\\ \text{TL}/0.925 & \text{volume}\end{cases}\\&\text{No crossed ends} \quad \text{AL} = \begin{cases}\text{TL}/0.81 & \text{planar}\\ \text{TL}/0.85 & \text{volume}\end{cases}\end{aligned} \tag{33}$$

Conversely, given AL, the length of the treated volume always can be calculated by solving the appropriate Eq. (33) for TL. The area and volume used for looking up dose per mg Ra Eq-h from Table 22.8 should be calculated using the treated length. For example, for a single-plane implant with two uncrossed ends, width W and needles of active length AL, the area, A, used for table lookup is given by $A = W \times AL \times 0.81$.

To apply P-P tables to modern implants using ^{192}Ir wires or ribbons, several corrections must be applied. The 1938 P-P tables assumed a Γ value of 8.4, ignored attenuation and scattering, neglected oblique filtration, and specified treatment in terms of exposure rather than absorbed dose. For ^{226}Ra needles, an average correction of 0.90[95] was applied to the original P-P tables to estimate absorbed dose. Modifying these corrections for ^{137}Cs needles and ^{192}Ir seeds and adding an additional factor of 10% to convert from stated (modal target dose) to minimum target volume dose, we obtain the following equivalencies:

$$1\,\text{'P–P' R} = \begin{Bmatrix} 0.97\cdot\frac{8.25}{8.4} & 0.98 & 0.98 & 0.90\\ 0.97\cdot\frac{8.25}{8.4} & 1.00 & 0.98 & 0.90\\ 0.97\cdot\frac{8.25}{8.4} & 1.00 & 1.00 & 0.90\\ (\text{cGy/R})\cdot\left(\frac{\Gamma_{new}}{\Gamma_{old}}\right) & (\text{filtration}) & (\text{attenuation/buildup}) & \left(\frac{\text{min}}{\text{stated}}\,\text{dose}\right)\end{Bmatrix} = \begin{Bmatrix}0.82\text{ cGy radium needles}\\ 0.84\text{ cGy cesium needles}\\ 0.86\text{ cGy iridium ribbons}\\ \left(\frac{\text{Modern cGy}}{\text{'P–P' R}}\right)\end{Bmatrix} \tag{34}$$

Using the 0.90 cGy/P-P R conversion factor, Stovall and Shalek[95] found excellent agreement between computer calculations and the P-P tables for a variety of planar and cylindrical implants following the Manchester distribution rules. For single-plane implants, 90% of the stated dose in cGy covers 94% to 99% of the target area. For cubic arrays of seeds using fixed 1-cm spacing, agreement between the tables and computer calculations is excellent for larger treatment volumes (>100 cm^3)[134,135] but exhibits errors ranging from 10% to 40% for smaller arrays. These discrepancies probably result from deviations from the 4:2 activity ratio and use of a dose specification criterion incompatible with the Manchester system.

The classical implant systems are based on ^{192}Ir wires or interstitial needles, consisting of continuous distributions of radioactivity (i.e., line sources) with well-defined active lengths. To apply the classical systems to modern interstitial sources consisting of discrete seeds, the dosimetric equivalence between ribbons of discrete seed sources and line sources must be appreciated (Fig. 22.18). A ribbon consisting of N seeds with center-to-center separations, S, has a dose distribution that closely approximates that of a continuous line source of length, AL, and strength $(S_K)_{line}$:[81,136]

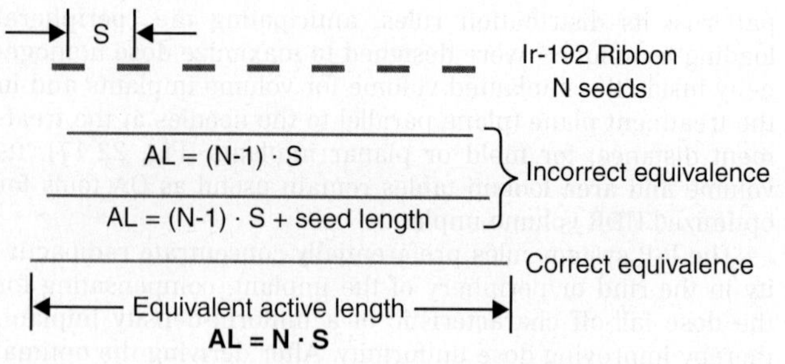

FIGURE 22.18. Relationship between a linear array of equally spaced discrete seeds and its dosimetrically equivalent line source. Both sources are assumed to have the same total strength. Common errors in defining this equivalence are illustrated.

$$\left.\begin{aligned}AL &= N\cdot S\\ (S_K)_{line} &= N\cdot (S_K)_{seed}\end{aligned}\right\} \tag{35}$$

This equivalence tends to break down at distances less than S/2: the cylindrical isodose curves break up into ellipsoidal shapes centered about each seed. In addition, the ribbon isodose curves undulate significantly at distances comparable with or less than the gap, S, between adjacent seeds, although on average the equivalence remains accurate.

Because the P-P system uses 1-cm interneedle spacing, the fraction of sources in the core (versus periphery) increases as volume increases. Thus, using uniform-strength ^{192}Ir ribbons and fixed spacing results in underloading the core for very small implants and overloading the core for very large implants, relative to the P-P distribution rules. In the latter case, the gap between minimum peripheral dose and central maximum dose widens. An alternative to the differential loading method is to vary the ribbon spacing with implant size, using smaller (<1 cm) spacing for very small implants and larger spacing (up to a limit of 1.5 cm) for larger implants, so that the relative number of central ribbons complies approximately with the P-P rules, allowing uniform seed strengths to be used. Two examples of this strategy are given in the next section.

To use the Manchester tables for verification of computerized dose calculations requires a method for objectively identifying the computer-generated isodose surface that corresponds to the minimum peripheral dose rate predicted by the Manchester system. For volume implants, mean central dose (MCD), a quantity proposed by the ICRU report on dose specification in interstitial BT, is useful[61] (Fig. 22.19). In the authors' experience, the maximum dose (110% of stated dose) of the Manchester system is closely approximated by MCD. Minimum peripheral dose and stated dose are given by 80% and 89%, respectively, of MCD. For planar implants, the minimum dose/MCD ratio varies from 55% to 70%, depending on catheter spacing, and is of limited value.

Manchester Volume Implant Example

A 5-cm-high by 5-cm-diameter cylindrical target volume is to be treated using ^{192}Ir ribbons with seed-to-seed and intercatheter spacings of 1 cm and 1.3 cm, respectively (Fig. 22.20). The followings describe steps to calculate (a) the minimum ribbon length needed, (b) the required ribbon arrangement, and (c) the strength/seed needed to deliver 45 cGy/hour to the P-P minimum dose specification volume.

a. There are two approaches: treating the ribbons as needles with uncrossed ends or treating the proximal and distal seeds of each ribbon as crossing sources. In the uncrossed end approach, Eq. (33) implies that

   $AL = \text{target length}/0.925^2 = 5\text{ cm}/0.85 = 5.9\text{ cm}$

   Eq. (35) implies that N = 6 seeds/ribbon are required.

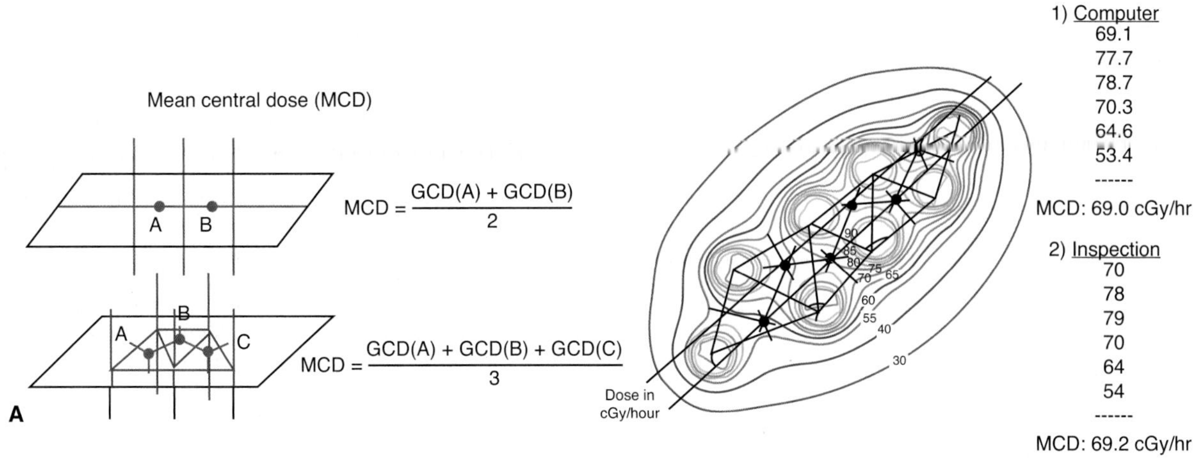

FIGURE 22.19. **A:** Calculation of mean central dose (MCD) as the arithmetic mean of the doses at mid-distance between each pair of adjacent sources for single-plane implants and the mean of the local minimum doses between each group of three adjacent sources in a multiple-plane implant. All local minimum doses are specified in the "central transverse" plane, which is normal to and bisects the source axes. **B:** Practical specification of MCD for a computer plan.

In the crossed-end approach, the first and last seeds must be placed at the target volume surfaces, again requiring 6 seeds/ribbon.

b. To satisfy the 1.3-cm ribbon-spacing requirement, 12 ribbons must be placed on the cylindrical target boundary, six ribbons must be placed on an inner cylindrical surface, and there should be one central ribbon. Treating the ends as uncrossed and assuming that the ribbons have uniform strengths, the belt-to-core ratio is 0.63:0.37, which is close to the P-P 4:2 ratio. Again, assuming all seeds have the same strength, Figure 22.20 shows that the required crossed-end ratios are also closely approximated. This illustrates that ribbon spacing can be manipulated to adhere to the P-P distribution rules with uniform strength sources.

c. Assuming the uncrossed end point of view:

$$TL = AL \times 0.85 = (1\text{ cm}) \times 0.85 = 5.1\text{ cm}$$

$$\text{Treated (lookup) Volume} = \pi \times (2.5)^2 \times 5.1 = 100.1\text{ cm}^3$$

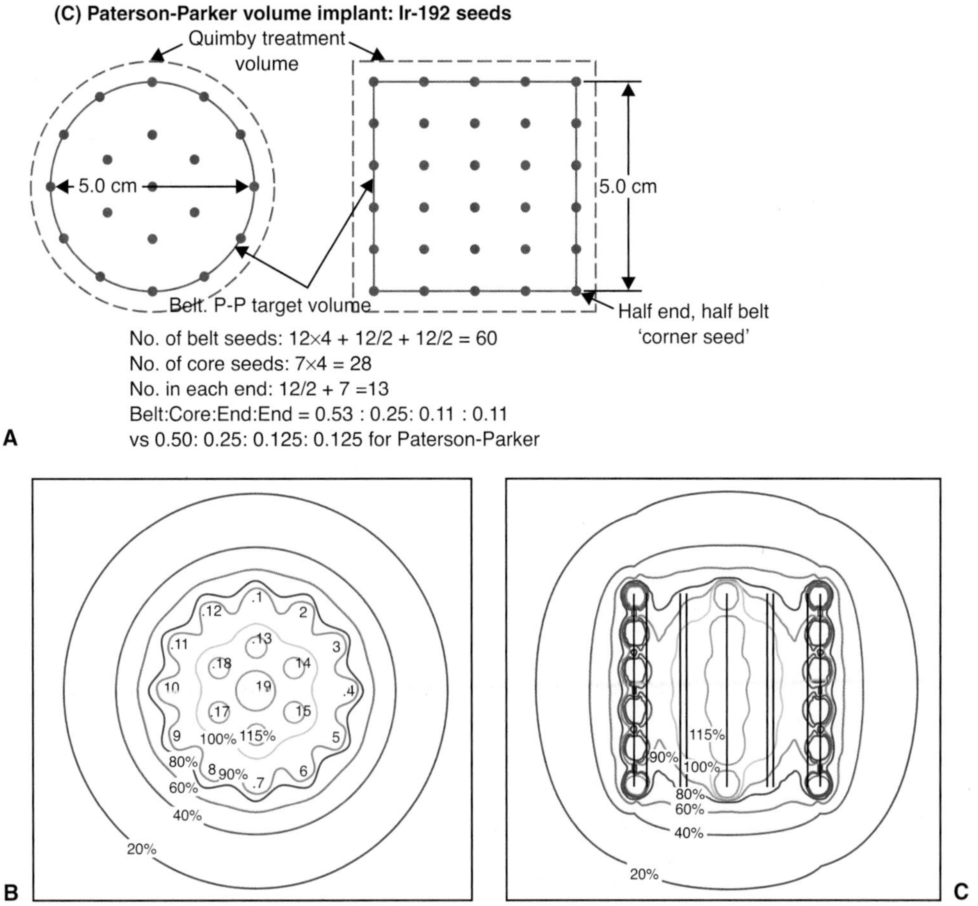

FIGURE 22.20. **A:** Cylindric volume implant, example (C), using uniform strength ^{192}Ir ribbons spaced at 1.3-cm intervals. Central transverse **(B)** and coronal **(C)** isodose curves are plotted normalized to the mean central dose (MCD) = 58.9 cGy/hour = 100%: 115% (68 cGy/hour), 100% (59 cGy/hour), 90% (53 cGy/hour), 80% (47 cGy/hour), 60% (35 cGy/hour), 40% (24 cGy/hour), 20% (12 cGy/hour). Note that 80% of MCD, 47 cGy/hour, agrees closely with the minimum peripheral dose rate of 45 cGy/hour predicted by the Paterson-Parker tables.

Hence:

$$\frac{734\ \text{mg-h}}{1000'\text{P} - \text{P}'\text{R}} = \frac{734\ \text{mg-h}}{860\ \text{cGy minimum dose}} = \frac{1\ \mu\text{Gy}\cdot\text{m}^2}{0.162\ \text{cGy}}$$

Differential Loading:

$$S_{K/\text{seed}} = \frac{45\ \text{cGy/h}}{0.162\ \text{cGy}} \cdot \times \begin{cases} \dfrac{2}{3} \cdot \dfrac{1\ \mu\text{Gy}\cdot\text{m}^2}{12\ \text{ribbons} \times 6\ \text{seeds/ribbon}} = 2.6\ \mu\text{Gy}\cdot\text{m}^2\cdot\text{h}^{-1}\ \text{periphery} \\ \dfrac{1}{3} \cdot \dfrac{1\ \mu\text{Gy}\cdot\text{m}^2}{7\ \text{ribbons} \times 6\ \text{seeds/ribbon}} = 2.2\ \mu\text{Gy}\cdot\text{m}^2\cdot\text{h}^{-1}\ \text{core} \end{cases}$$

Uniform Loading:

$$S_{K/\text{seed}} = \frac{45\ \text{cGy/h}}{0.162\ \text{cGy/h}} \cdot \frac{1\ \mu\text{Gy}\cdot\text{m}^2}{19\ \text{ribbons} \times 6\ \text{seeds/ribbon}} = 2.4\ \mu\text{Gy}\cdot\text{m}^2\cdot\text{h}^{-1}$$

The Quimby System

The Quimby system was developed by Edith Quimby et al.[137–139] at New York Memorial Hospital from 1920 to 1940. Unlike the Manchester system, equal linear intensity (mgRaEq/cm) needles are distributed uniformly (fixed spacing) in each implant. Like the Manchester system, the associated Quimby tables give the mgRaEq-h needed to deliver a stated exposure of 1,000 R as a function of target volume or area.

The so-called planar implant tables were intended for surface molds; none of the early Memorial publications suggest that it was used for single-plane interstitial implants. In part because Quimby's stated dose is the maximum dose in the treatment plane, Quimby planar implants deliver 30% to 40% less radiation (IRAK) per unit stated dose than an equivalent Manchester implant delivers. Rules for distributing radium needles (relationship to target-area boundaries, crossed ends, spacing, etc.) are not clearly described. Volume implant needle arrangements are similar to their Manchester counterparts; both systems recommend crossed ends and placing peripheral needles on or beyond the target volume boundaries. However, Quimby allows the needle spacing to vary with implant size and specifies dose as the absolute minimum to the target volume. The physical and mathematical origins of the widely cited Quimby volume implant table are obscure; the tables published in the 1951 edition of *Physical Foundations of Radiology*[138] deliver 25% to 90% more mgRaEq-h per unit dose than P-P volume implants of similar size. Because they are evenly spaced, uniform-strength sources approximate the Manchester distribution rules for medium-size volumes, and these differences are likely a result of differences in the definition of "minimum dose" used by the two systems. Although vague on the subject, Quimby appears to specify minimum dose at a point located 3 to 5 mm from the peripheral needles (and therefore outside the target volume) near their active tips.[139] This corresponds to a treatment volume (volume encompassed by prescription isodose surface) that is 6 to 10 mm larger in diameter than the implanted volume (used for table lookup) in each linear dimension. The Quimby planar and volume dose specification criteria are clearly inconsistent, and a detailed derivation of the associated tables is lacking. For these reasons, we do not recommend Quimby tables for clinical use.

The Paris System

The Paris system was developed in the early 1960s by Pierquin, Chassagne, Dutreix, and Marinello[140,141] and was motivated by the ^{192}Ir afterloading techniques developed by Henschke. Outside the United States, the Paris system is widely used for definitive BT of localized lesions in the head and neck, breast, and many other sites. An up-to-date summary of the system has been published by Gillin and Mourtada.[142]

The starting point of the Paris system is the definition of the target volume, which is described in terms of thickness T, length L, and width W. The system provides rules for constructing implants, which, if followed, guarantee that the target volume is completely covered by the prescription isodose surface (Table 22.9). The prescription dose level, called the "reference dose," is a fixed percentage (85%) of the basal dose (see Fig. 22.21), which closely resembles the more general concept of

TABLE 22.9 PARIS SYSTEM CHARACTERISTICS

Feature	*Paris System Rules*
Dose and dose rate	6,000 cGy to 7,000 cGy in 3–11 days (25 cGy/hour to 90 cGy/hour).
Dose specification criterion	Reference dose (prescribed dose) is 85% of the basal dose and encompasses the target volume when distribution rules are followed. Basal dose is the average of the minimum doses between pairs or groups of adjacent sources in the central transverse plane.
Dose gradient	Fixed 15% gradient between reference dose and basal dose. The "hyperdose sleeve" (region receiving at least twice the reference dose) diameter should be <8–10 mm.
Linear activity	Constant (4–14 μGy · m^2 · h^{-1}/cm) linear density Ir-192 wires used.
Source arrangement geometry for target volume of thickness, width, and length of T × W × L	Only single- and double-plane implants allowed. Spacing, S, and lateral margin (called "safety margin" for double-plane case), M, are fixed fractions of T and constant within a given implant. Active length, AL, is a fixed fraction of L, which varies with S. *Single plane:* $T \leq 12$ mm $S = 2 \times T$ (2 sources) $S = 1.67 \times T$ (3 sources) $M = 0.37 \times T$ $AL = (1.3 - 1.49) \times T$ *Double plane:* (square pattern): $S = 0.62 \times T$, $M = 0.27 \times T$, $AL = (1.37 - 1.62) \times L$ (triangle pattern): $S = 0.77 \times T$, $M = 0.15 \times T$, $AL = (1.33 - 1.49) \times L$
Source spacing, S, limits	Short sources (1–4 cm): 8 mm ≤ S ≤ 15 mm Long sources (≤10 cm): 15 mm ≤ S ≤ 22 mm
Crossing needles	Generally not used; AL = 1.45 × L to compensate for uncrossed ends. For oral cavity implants, hairpins are common, which approximate crossed ends.
Relation between target volume and implanted volume	W = distance between outermost sources + 2 × M L = AL/(1.3 – 1.62) $T = \begin{cases} S/1.67 & \text{Single plane} \\ S + 2 \times M & \text{Double plane: squares} \\ S \times \cos 30° + 2 \times M & \text{Double plane: triangles} \end{cases}$

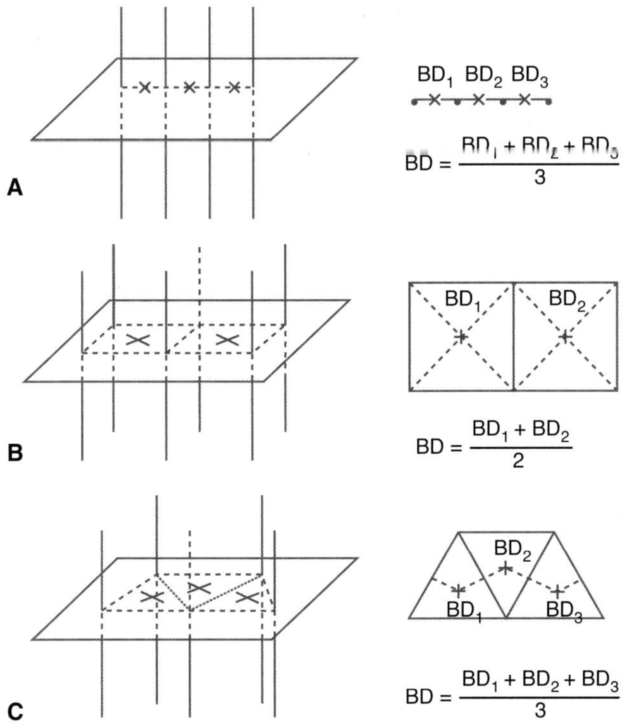

FIGURE 22.21. The three central plane configurations allowed by the Paris system: **(A)** single-plane implant, **(B)** double-plane implant using the pattern of squares, and **(C)** double-plane implant using the pattern of equilateral triangles. The calculation of basal dose rate at a point equidistant from each group of adjacent sources is illustrated for each configuration. (From Gillin MT, Albano KS, Erickson B. Classical systems II for planar and volume temporary interstitial implants: the Paris and other systems. In: Williamson JF, Thomadsen BR, Nath R, eds. *Brachytherapy physics.* Madison, WI: Medical Physics Publishing, 1995:232–343, with permission.)

mean central dose in Figure 22.19. ^{192}Ir wire sources are arranged in parallel rectilinear arrays with their centers located in the central plane, which is perpendicular to the sources. Adjacent sources must be equidistant from one another, resulting in single-plane implants with equal spacing and double-plane implants with groups of adjacent sources arranged in equilateral triangles or squares in the central plane (see Fig. 22.21). The linear density (μGy · m^2 · h^{-1}/cm) must be uniform and the same for all sources. Interneedle spacing scales with the thickness, T, of the target volume. The number of sources is determined largely by the relative shape of the target volume cross-sectional area, W × T. In contrast, the Manchester system uses fixed spacing and increases the number of sources as the cross-sectional area of the target volume increases.

Table 22.9 shows that the location of the peripheral sources relative to the treated volume (region encompassed by the reference isodose-rate surface, as shown in Fig. 22.22) differs from the Manchester system, which implants to the boundary of the treated tissue. In the transverse plane, the peripheral sources lie 2 to 4 mm (the lateral margin distance, M) inside the treatment surface, whereas longitudinally the AL extends 15% to 20% beyond the distal and proximal margins of the target volume. In practice, the margin, M, is treated as a safety margin, and the peripheral needles are implanted along the margins of the clinical target volume (CTV). The maximum thickness, T, of a target volume treatable in the Paris system is about 2.5 cm. An example of a double-plane implant arranged in squares is shown in Figure 22.23.

To apply the Paris system, the target thickness T must be known, which defines the spacing and determines whether single-plane or double-plane geometry is required. The number of sources and selection of a square or triangular arrangement are defined by the relative cross-sectional shape of the target volume in the central plane perpendicular to the sources. Finally, the active length is calculated. The source tip and end coordinates are reconstructed from orthogonal radiographs and the dose distribution and basal dose are calculated by computer for the actual implant geometry realized in the patient, not the idealized implant of clinical intention. This approach differs from the classical Manchester method, which bases dose prescription on the P-P table and, in general, ignores deviations of the actual implant geometry from the ideal. The Paris system addresses only single- and double-plane implants; large-volume implants for treating pelvic masses and brain tumors were not part of the original system. Extensions of Paris system principles to large-volume implants are discussed by Leung[143] and Gillin et al.[144]

Dose Specification in Interstitial Brachytherapy

Many of the differences between the Manchester, Paris, and Quimby systems can be attributed to fundamental differences in dose specification. Because of the high-dose gradients near the peripheral sources or the target volume boundary, reproducible

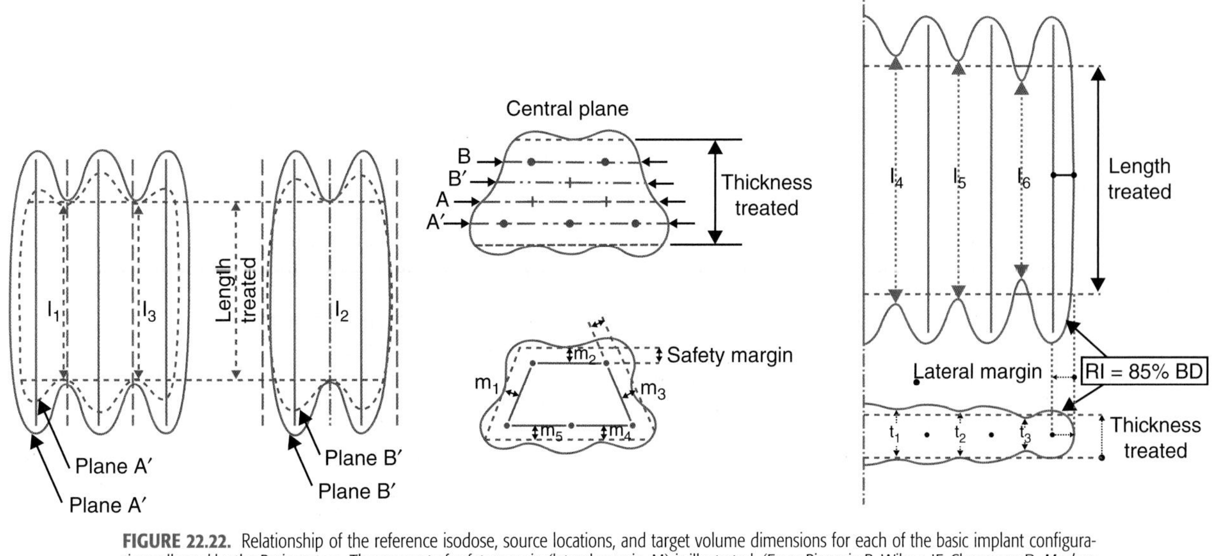

FIGURE 22.22. Relationship of the reference isodose, source locations, and target volume dimensions for each of the basic implant configurations allowed by the Paris system. The concept of safety margin (lateral margin, M) is illustrated. (From Pierquin B, Wilson JF, Chassange D. *Modern brachytherapy.* New York: Masson, 1987, with permission.)

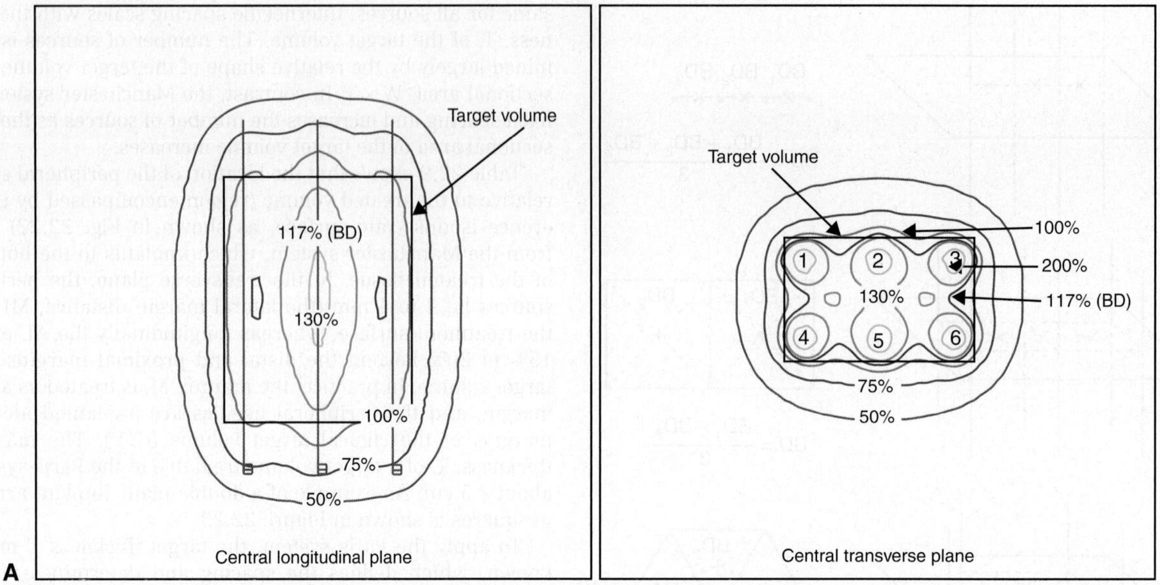

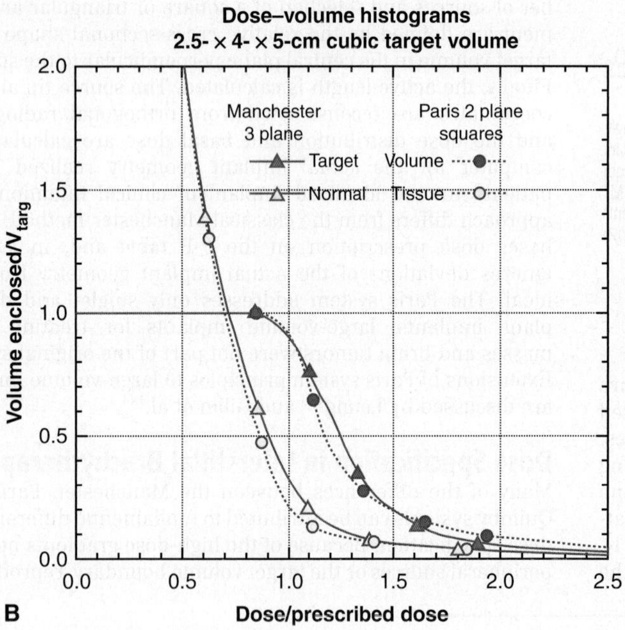

FIGURE 22.23. A: Isodose curves of a Paris system double-plane implant arranged "in squares" to treat a 2.5-cm × 4-cm × 5-cm target volume (*heavy lines*). The separation and active lengths of the ^{192}Ir wires are 1.6 cm and 7.3 cm, respectively. A linear strength of 6 μGy · m^2 · h^{-1}/cm gives reference (100%) and basal (117%) dose rates of 60 cGy/hour and 70.6 cGy/hour, respectively. **B:** Comparison of dose–volume histograms (DVHs) calculated separately for the 2.5-cm × 4-cm × 5-cm target volume and the tissue outside the target for the Paris implant shown and a Manchester implant consisting of three planes, 15 ^{192}Ir ribbons with six seeds each, and 1.25-cm spacing between planes and ribbons. Each graph shows volume of tissue (in multiples of volume of the target) receiving at least the specified dose (in multiples of prescribed dose). For the Paris and Manchester implants, respectively, prescribed dose is the calculated reference dose and minimum target dose predicted by the Paterson-Parker volume table. In both systems, the prescription isodose surface covers about 90% of the target. Surprisingly, both normal tissue sparing and dose homogeneity in the target are slightly better for the Paris implant.

specification of dose and evaluation of implant quality are difficult. Conversely, small differences in dose specification criteria can lead to large differences in treatment time or in the geometric relationship between implanted and treated volume. The term *dose specification* means objective identification of a spatial volume or location for evaluating absorbed dose for the purposes of prescription (defining the dose that the radiation oncologist intends to deliver), for describing the quantity of radiation actually delivered to the patient, or for reporting. The "specified dose" sometimes is called "reference dose." The dose that an implant actually delivers to the patient, based on postinsertion treatment planning, may differ significantly from the dose prescribed for a variety of reasons. For example, anatomic or technical constraints may preclude accurate positioning of sources at their intended locations, resulting in a partial geometric miss or underdose of the specified volume. Dose specification for reporting purposes usually refers to efforts to develop reproducible and system-independent specification schemes to promote comparison of different implantation systems so as to minimize patient-to-patient and operator-to-operator variability in level of treatment delivered. The ability to objectively compare different interstitial implant plans as to target volume coverage, normal tissue sparing, and dose homogeneity depends on dose specification. Several divergent and rather abstract approaches to dose specification have been developed and promoted by various national and international advisory groups; no single approach to dose specification has been widely accepted within the BT community.

Minimum Dose to an Anatomically Defined Target Volume

The minimum dose to the anatomically defined target volume harboring malignant cells is conceptually attractive because it is based on the intuitively satisfying premise that local tumor control will be determined by the minimum dose received by tumor cells. The ABS[145] recommends that minimum dose should be identified as accurately as possible by the best means available and should be used for dose prescription, evaluation, and reporting. In practice, minimum target dose specification is difficult to implement clinically for many implants.

In the prostate BT literature,[146] minimum target dose usually is called "minimum peripheral dose," or mPD, when used for implant preplanning prescription and D_{100} (see discussion on dose–volume histograms) when used for postimplant dose evaluation. When imaging studies showing the target volume in relation to the sources are not available, the ABS recommends approximate target localization by means of intraoperatively placed surgical clips, orthogonal planar imaging, or measurements relative to peripheral sources. A clear disadvantage of minimum dose specification is that the target volume surface lies within the zone of largest dose gradient. This can result in large patient-to-patient fluctuations in the central-to-specified dose ratio because of small variations in the peripheral source locations relative to the apparent target boundary or uncertainties in delineating the target volume. As discussed in the Permanent Implantation section later, reviews of CT-based prostate implant dose evaluations show that absolute minimum delivered doses (D_{100}) relative to the prescribed dose show large patient-to-patient variabilities and average 30% to 60%.[147,148] The minimum dose covering at least 99% (or 95%) of the target volume has been found to be much less sensitive to small changes in the peripheral seed locations or uncertainties in the target volume surface location.

Minimum Implant Dose Relative to Sources

Traditional treatment planning uses planar radiographs for 3D reconstruction of radioactive source positions, yielding accurate dose estimates relative to the sources but not relative to an anatomic target volume.[149] Thus, it is natural to prescribe treatment to a point or surface that has a fixed relationship to the peripheral sources. The minimum implant dose, or MID, is the minimum dose received by the so-called target volume defined relative to the implanted volume, the smallest regular geometric shape circumscribing the peripheral sources. Often this specification volume is taken to be that volume that is 2 to 5 mm larger in each linear dimension relative to the implanted volume, as in the Paris and Quimby systems. With the exception of image-guided prostate implants, MID is perhaps the most widely used specification approach and is the basis of the classical systems and the U.S. practice of selecting prescription isodose surfaces from 2D isodose curve plots. However, MID yields information about tumor coverage only to the extent that the radiation oncologist has implanted peripheral sources at known distances from the anatomic target volume boundaries. In addition, MID lies in the zone of maximum dose gradient and can be difficult to evaluate objectively for an implant of irregular shape, again leading to large patient-to-patient variations and variations in the central-to-prescribed dose ratio. The Paris and Manchester systems eliminate the possibility of subjective isodose selection by rigidly specifying dose rate by means of basal dose rate and implant tables, respectively.

Mean Central Dose

The ICRU report on dose specification in interstitial BT[61] emphasizes reporting mean central dose (MCD; see Fig. 22.19), although it recommends reporting the prescribed dose, the peripheral dose (minimum target dose), and a description of dose uniformity as well. MCD specifies dose in the low-gradient regions located between adjacent source locations in the central plane of the implant. Thus, MCD is relatively free of the variability inherent in minimum peripheral or target dose specification. It is a generalization of the Paris system basal dose. As a reporting parameter, MCD can be reproducibly estimated from 2D central transverse-plane isodoses and should be very useful for comparing implants performed using different clinical systems. However, for systems other than the Paris and Manchester systems (which rigidly specify how sources are to be arranged relative to the target volume), MCD does not have a known relationship to minimum peripheral or target dose. Thus, its value as a prescription parameter is limited.

Three-Dimensional Dose–Volume Histogram Representations

DVHs are 1D plots that describe the distribution of tissue volumes, V, irradiated by the implant with respect to dose, D. DVHs can be presented in either differential, $\Delta V(D)/\Delta D$, or cumulative, V(D), forms. DVH computation involves calculating dose over a fine 3D grid extending at least 2 cm beyond the peripheral seeds, dividing the dose axis into small bins of width ΔD, and then counting the number of voxels falling into each dose interval. The cumulative DVH gives the volume of tissue, V(D), receiving a dose of at least D.

DVHs can be evaluated for specific anatomic regions (e.g., target and normal tissue as illustrated by Fig. 22.23) or can be evaluated for tissue irradiated by the implant without regard to anatomic boundaries. For bounded volumes, V(D) is flat below the minimum dose received by the structure. When evaluated over unbounded space, V(D) steeply increases with decreasing dose and asymptotically approaches the central point-source DVH, $V_{point}(\dot{D}) = (4\pi/3) \cdot [S_K \cdot \Lambda/\dot{D}]^{3/2}$. The use of DVHs has enriched discussions of dose specification by focusing attention on describing the 3D dose distribution rather than on single parameters. However, in the absence of target volume and normal tissue geometry, DVHs in themselves do not solve the dose specification problem.

Because 3D anatomic models were often lacking until recently, several figures of merit (FOMs) derived from DVHs have been proposed that do not require an anatomically defined target volume. Such FOMs may be useful for ranking the quality of competing implant geometries in terms of uniformity and normal-tissue sparing or for optimally selecting a specification dose rate for a given implant geometry. An important contribution is the "natural" DVH introduced by Anderson.[150,151] The natural DVH is a plot $\Delta V(u)/\Delta u$ where $u = D^{-3/2}$. The natural DVH plots as a horizontal line for a central point source. It suppresses r^{-2} effects, which dominate the conventional V(D) plot, making its detailed implant geometry–specific structure more evident. Low and Williamson[152] introduced an alternative modified DVH, $R_p(D) = V_{impl}(D)/V_{point}(D)$. Both of these modified DVHs show a sharply defined peak centered about MCD, the width and height of which quantify the volume of tissue receiving an approximately uniform dose. Other useful quality measures include the uniformity index[153] and the dose nonuniformity ratio (DNR).[154] The DNR, usually plotted as a function of reference dose, D_r, is defined as the ratio of volume receiving a specified multiple of D_r (usually 1.25 or 1.5) to that receiving at least D_r.

Target volume–dependent DVH quality indices were introduced by Saw and Suntharalingam.[155] For single- and double-plane implants designed to cover specified cubic target volumes, respectively, they defined three indices as a function of reference dose D_r. The coverage index, $CI(D_r)$, is that fraction of the target tissue receiving a dose $\geq D_r$. The homogeneity index, $HI(D_r)$, is the fraction of target volume receiving doses between D_r and 1.5 D_r. The external volume index, $EI(D_r)$, is the volume of tissue outside the target volume, expressed in multiples of the target volume, receiving dose rates $\geq D_r$. When these indices are plotted (Fig. 22.24), the tradeoffs among these clinical end points are evident. If a prescription dose rate is selected to maximize dose homogeneity (i.e., maximize HI), then 85% to 95% coverage of the target must be accepted. To minimize irradiation of tissue outside the target, both target coverage and dose homogeneity must be compromised. Low and Williamson[152] suggested ranking competing implant geometries by specifying the HI achieved for the maximum reference dose level that yields a CI of unity. Zwicker and Schmidt-Ullrich[156] have applied this general approach to the problem of identifying optimal interplane separations in double-plane implants.

For TRUS-guided prostate implantation, DVH metrics such as D_{100}, D_{99}, and D_{90}, denoting the minimum doses administered to the highest dose volumes covering 100%, 99%, and 90% of the contoured CTV or PTV (planned target volume),

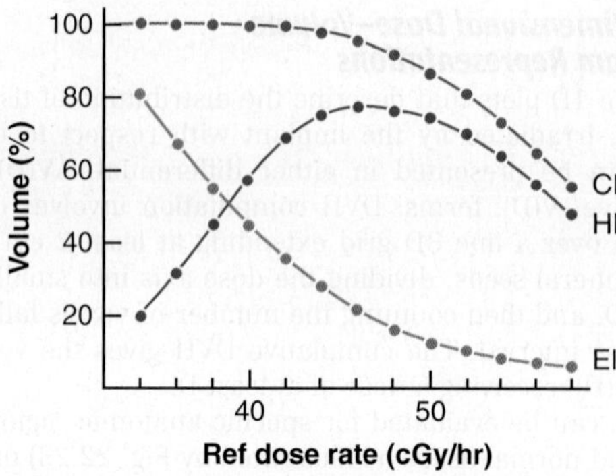

FIGURE 22.24. Plot of coverage index (CI), external index (EI), and homogeneity index (HI) as a function of reference dose rate for double-plane implant consisting of five ^{192}Ir ribbons with seven 1-mCi seeds in each plane and a 6-cm × 6-cm × 2.5-cm target volume. Ribbon and plane spacings of 1.5 cm were used. (From Saw CB, Suntharalingam N. Reference dose rates for single and double plane ^{192}Ir implants. *Med Phys* 1988;15:391, with permission.)

respectively, have become widely accepted as reporting parameters.[157] Volumetric indices, such as the V_{150}, V_{100}, and V_{90}, which denote the fraction of the CTV or PTV receiving at least 150%, 100%, and 90%, respectively, of the prescribed dose, are recommended to assess dose homogeneity and to assess adequacy with which the prescription has been fulfilled.

Permanent Implantation

In contrast to temporary implantation, in which treatment time is varied to control the total dose delivered, the dose delivered by a permanent implant is determined by the initial geometric arrangement of sources and S_K per source: once the patient is implanted, neither the total dose delivered nor the relative distribution can be modified easily. Up through the mid-1980s, manual planning and dose calculation tools were used widely to estimate the number and density of sources needed to deliver the prescribed dose or to intraoperatively correct for deviations between the planned and actual source locations. For radium-substitute sources (e.g., ^{198}Au), the Manchester, Laughlin,[134] or Shalek[135] tables and associated distribution rules have been used for this purpose.

Manual planning aids for radium-equivalent sources cannot be applied to low-energy seed (^{125}I and ^{103}Pd) implants because of the importance of tissue attenuation in this energy range. The influence of photon energy on the relationship between dose rate, $\dot{D}$ and implanted volume, V, is illustrated by Figure 22.25. Parker[129] recognized that this relationship can be described accurately by a power-law formula, of the form

$$\dot{D} = \alpha \cdot S_K \cdot V^{-\beta} \quad (36)$$

In fact, the original Manchester table (Table 22.8), converted to modern units and quantities, can be derived from Eq. (36) by setting $\alpha = 3.49$ and $\beta = 2/3$. Although ^{103}Pd and ^{125}I volume implants also can be described by the power-law formula, they have somewhat larger exponents, β, demonstrating that dose rate falls off faster with increasing volume than for radium-substitute sources.[158,159] The proportionality constants, α, are substantially lower, indicating that low-energy seed implants require higher source strengths to achieve a stated dose rate. The author-to-author

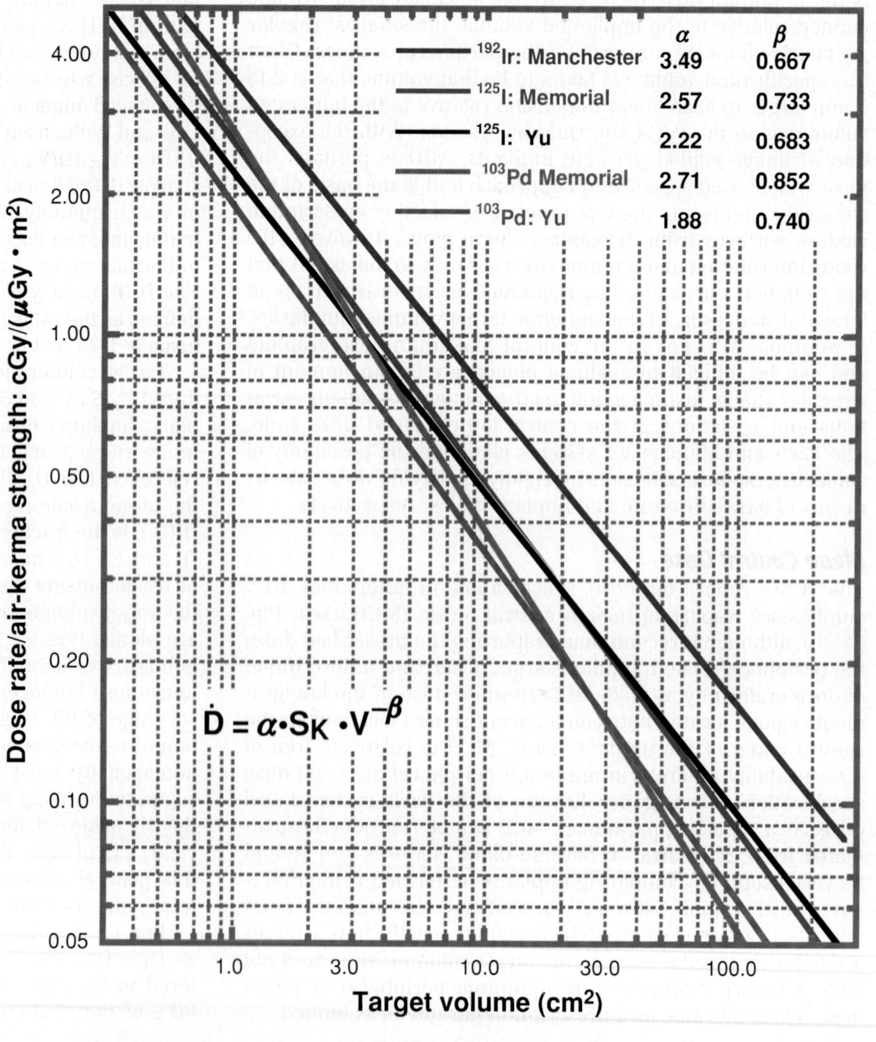

FIGURE 22.25. Comparison of reference dose rate per unit air-kerma strength versus volume of the target volume for Manchester volume implants and ^{103}Pd and ^{125}I permanent prostate implants. The inset gives the exponents and proportionality constants needed to describe these relationships in terms of a simple power-law equation [Eq. (36)]. The data in the figure are from Yu,[159] Memorial,[158] and Manchester.[129]

variations in α values for the same radionuclide are due, in part, to differences in dose specification and implant construction. Anderson's[158] analysis, based on the pre-TRUS era Memorial nomogram, assumes that dose is specified in terms of matched peripheral dose (MPD) and that all seeds are implanted 2 to 5 mm inside the target (prostate) boundary, whereas Yu[159] assumes that peripheral seeds are implanted on or outside the boundary and that minimum target dose is specified. Manual planning tools[159–162] are available for a variety of implant types, characterized by different underlying single-source dose-rate distributions, seed arrangements, dose specification criteria, and absolute prescribed doses, yielding estimated seed strengths that differ significantly from one another. Before using one of these methods for quality assurance checks or preplanning, readers should assess carefully its consistency with dose calculation and planning methods used in their clinical practices.

The best-known manual planning tool for permanent ^{125}I implantation is the Memorial dimension averaging method.[158,163] The associated nomogram was used for manual intraoperative planning of implants delivered by directly implanting seeds into the surgically exposed prostate. After surgical exposure of the target volume (prostate), the three orthogonal dimensions of target volume are measured, and the arithmetic mean of these measurements, or average diameter, d_a, in units of centimeter, is calculated. Next, the total apparent activity, A_{app} (in mCi units), to be implanted is calculated as follows:

$$A_{app} = \begin{cases} 5 \cdot d_a & d_a < 3 \text{ cm} \\ 1.34 \cdot d_a^{2.2} & d_a \geq 3 \text{ cm} \end{cases} \quad (37)$$

By means of a nomogram consisting of several juxtaposed logarithmic scales, the total number of seeds needed is estimated graphically given the strength per seed. Other nomogram scales were used to estimate the spacing between needles given the seed spacing along each needle track. The seeds are to be implanted inside the target volume boundary, such that peripheral needle-to-target boundary distance is <50% of the interneedle spacing. Anderson et al.[158] have extended the dimension-averaging nomogram to ^{103}Pd and reviewed the underlying assumptions of this method.

Eq. (37) is designed to deliver an MPD of 160 Gy over the life of the implant when d_a is more than 3 cm.[158] MPD is defined as the dose level whose corresponding 3D isodose surface encompasses a volume, V_E, equal to that of an ellipsoid having the same orthogonal dimensions as the originally measured target volume ($V_E = \pi d_x d_y d_z/6$). For a given implant, MPD is derived from the corresponding cumulative DVH, V(D), according to $V_E = V(\text{MPD})$. By design, the Memorial nomogram delivers significantly higher MPDs to target volumes with average dimensions <3 cm. Prescribed doses of 160 Gy delivered in the 1985–1999 era correspond to doses of 144 Gy when corrected for implementation of the WAFAC primary standard and Task Group 43 dosimetry parameters.[126] The MPD overestimates minimum target dose (mPD) because the prostate gland is rarely ellipsoidal and has small protrusions that may extend outside the MPD isodose surface. Likewise, small deviations of the peripheral seeds from their planned locations can alter dramatically the shape of the MPD isodose surface. One study[164] found that, on average, MPD was twice the D_{99} level (the dose ensuring 99% target coverage on postoperative CT imaging) and that only 69% to 89% of the target volume received a dose equal to or greater than MPD.

Modern Developments in Interstitial Brachytherapy

Computerized Treatment Planning

Three modern developments in BT planning and delivery technology have significantly influenced implant design and utilization of classical system rules: (a) computer isodose calculations, (b) dwell-weight optimization of single-stepping source remotely afterloaded implants, and (c) utilization of 3D imaging to define target volumes and to guide applicator insertion.

Computer isodose calculations for interstitial implants were introduced in the early 1960s[11] and, along with software for reconstructing implant geometry from radiographs, have been routinely available for about 35 years. In contrast to the older classical systems, which are based on idealized geometries, computer-assisted planning capability permits evaluation of the dose distribution for the implant geometry actually realized in the patient. Thus, the brachytherapist can compensate for deviations between the actual and intended implant geometries through selection of the prescription isodose or by modifying the catheter loadings or locations. In principle, dose calculation capability permits preprocedure customization of catheter spacings, loadings, and locations relative to the target boundary as an alternative to classical system distribution rules. Because manual forward planning is so time intensive, only a small number alternative plans can be compared in practice. However, use of computer dose calculation to design implants and to specify dose has displaced the tables and implant rules of classical systems in many U.S. centers. Khan[165] calls this approach the "computer system" and points out that, in fact, it does assume simple guidelines for distributing the sources. These include 1-cm intercatheter spacing, uniform loading, and implanting to the boundary of the tumor. Dose specification usually is based on the concept of MID, described earlier. Thus, even in the era of computerized dose calculation, distribution rules derived from one of the historical implant systems still have relevance.

Dwell-Weight Optimization

A major development of the last two decades is a pronounced shift from LDR manual afterloading techniques to HDR BT. Single-stepping HDR source remote afterloading (see Chapter 24 for a detailed treatment) allows the treatment time (dwell time) to be individually specified at each treatment (dwell) position in the catheter. This permits use of dwell-weight optimization as a tool for improving dose uniformity and target coverage within implants. In contrast to the classical systems, which assume that ribbons and needs are of uniform linear density, dwell-weight optimization supports far more elaborate nonuniform source-strength distributions than those envisioned by the Manchester system rules. The published experience, confined largely to Paris-like double-plane breast implants, demonstrates that geometric optimization[166] preferentially increases the dwell times at dwell positions near the catheter ends. The most striking finding is that optimization allows the active-to-target length (AL/TL) ratio to be reduced from 1.33–1.5 to 1.1–1.25.[167–169] In the transverse plane, target coverage remains unchanged, whereas dose homogeneity is improved modestly, depending on the figure of merit used to quantify this effect. When dose-point optimization (specifying dose constraints at dose calculation points throughout the treatment volume) is used, acceptable dose homogeneity results with even smaller AL/TL ratios, even when all peripheral dwell positions are placed inside the target volume (AL/TL = 1.0)[152,170] for idealized volume implants and clinical volume implants.[168] These early efforts did not address the practical problem of how to distribute dose-constraint points in clinical volume implants with irregular catheter spacings and how to select dwell positions to be activated in each catheter. Although dwell-weight optimization has the potential to reduce AL/TL ratios to near unity without sacrificing target coverage or dose homogeneity, the brachytherapist must rely on clinical experience or one of the classical systems to determine the catheter arrangement and locations relative to the target volume boundaries.

Image-Guided Brachytherapy and Image-Based Dose Reconstruction

The use of 3D imaging to preplan implants or intraoperatively guide catheter or seed insertion is growing rapidly. The most widely practiced form of image-guided BT is use of intraoperative TRUS to guide transperineal insertion of needles used to implant the prostate gland with low-energy seeds.[38,39] However, image-guided implant methodologies have been developed for HDR multicatheter interstitial[171] and balloon-applicator intracavitary[172] implants for accelerated partial breast irradiation following lumpectomy as well as HDR interstitial implantation for prostate cancer.[173] All of these approaches require delineation of the target volume and critical structure surfaces from 3D imaging studies. Then catheter or needle trajectories and, ultimately, seed or dwell position locations can be selected to improve target volume coverage while minimizing unnecessary dose to critical structures. The issues involved in utilizing image-guided and -based BT in HDR interstitial brachytherapy, including treatment planning, selection of imaging modality, and impact on clinical workflow, are covered in detail elsewhere.[174]

As practiced by most brachytherapists, image-guided, intraoperatively planned implants continue to rely on the operator's judgment for selecting source locations. These decisions are guided by a "loading approach," or set of guidelines that specify margins, seed locations relative to the target boundary, spacings, and approximate periphery-to-core loading ratios.[175,176] Dose calculations and DVH quality indices often are used to guide manual source position adjustments to improve target volume coverage, improve dose homogeneity, and select source strengths (or dwell times) and the prescription isodose.

An important advance upon standard dose-point optimization is anatomy-based optimization in which constraints and treatment goals are defined in terms of doses to CTV or normal tissues contoured from 3D imaging studies rather than surfaces defined relative to dwell positions. The simulated annealing HDR dwell-time optimization technique developed by Lessard and Pouliot[177] illustrates the general features of the various optimization approaches[178–181] that have been brought to bear on this problem (see Ezzell's[182] review for a highly readable introduction to BT optimization techniques). An objective or cost function mathematically measures the compliance of each candidate 3D dose distribution with the treatment goals and constraints specified by the physician. It consists of the sum of individual penalty factors, one for dose or dose-volume constraint for a specified structure, e.g., CTV, urethra, rectum, etc. Lower values imply greater success in meeting the specified treatment goals. The optimizer tries to find the set of dwell weights that minimizes the objective function. The inverse-planning technique of Lessard and Pouliot[177] reduces CTV dose heterogeneity (V_{150} of 29% vs. 50%) and urethral doses in clinical prostate implants compared to geometric optimization[183] and solves the problem of selecting active dwell positions and locations for dose-constraint points faced by the older dose-point optimization algorithms. While anatomy-based inverse planning does not optimize catheter trajectories, its proponents[184] argue that it reduces the dependence of implant quality on the number and accurate positioning of the catheters relative to the CTV boundary. If true, inverse planning could reduce the dependence of implant quality on operator skill and reduce the need to follow system-based needle insertion rules.

In summary, computerized dose calculation, dwell-weight optimization, and image-guided BT have made anatomy-based dose specification and higher quality implants a reality in some clinical settings. However, innovations still require users to conceptually plan implants in terms of specified source and needle distribution patterns, implant-target volume margins, and loading ratios. Specific rules borrowed from the classical systems (e.g., AL/TL ratios) may require significant modification when adapted to these modern technologies.

Permanent Implant Developments

The most important advance in permanent implantation in the last two decades is the rise of image-based and -guided techniques in prostate BT, currently its only widely practiced indication. The transperineal approach using intraoperative TRUS[38,185] typically consists[174] of (a) acquiring a preplanning TRUS examination or "volume" study 2 to 3 weeks before the scheduled implant, (b) inserting the needles using interactive real-time TRUS imaging, (c) followed by CT-based postprocedure planning 0 to 30 days after the procedure. During preplanning, the PTV often is defined as the contoured prostate gland plus a discretionary margin. Most brachytherapists practice some form of peripheral loading to improve uniformity and reduce dose to the urethra. For example, the modified uniform loading as defined by Butler[175] distributes about 75% of the source activity in the periphery and emphasizes insertion of peripheral needles on or near the PTV boundary. Typically, needle locations and seed strengths are manipulated to achieve a prescribed minimum target dose (mPD or $D_{100\%}$) of 145 Gy for ^{125}I monotherapy. For ^{103}Pd monotherapy, the ABS[186] recommends retaining the prescribed dose of 125 Gy (compared to 115 Gy used before 2000) following implementation of the NIST $S_{K,N99}$ standard and recently revised TG-43 parameters, based on the AAPM's most recent analysis[126] of ^{103}Pd prescribed-to-administered dose ratios due to changes in calibration standards and dosimetry practice.

Dose specification, for recording and reporting doses actually administered by a permanent implant, is based on postimplant dose evaluation.[146] Following the implant procedure, a CT exam is obtained; the prostate gland, rectum, and bladder are contoured; and the seed locations are identified from the transverse images. The choice of dose specification parameter for this purpose has been the subject of intense investigation. Based on analysis of both idealized and actual implants, Yu et al.[159] found that the postinsertion D_{100} was very sensitive to small random displacements of the seeds from their intended positions, which resulted in underdoses of 15% or more to small volumes in the target periphery. However, they found that the mPD of the idealized implant (no seed displacement) covered at least 90% of the target (i.e., $D_{90} \geq$ mPD and $V_{100} \geq$ 90%), even in the face of 6-mm seed displacements. Subsequent retrospective studies of patient implants (e.g., Merrick et al.[147]) have confirmed these findings. Two groups[187,188] found a correlation between prostate-specific antigen (PSA) relapse-free survival at 4 years and D_{90}. In particular, Potters et al.[187] found a D_{90} dose-response cutoff of 90% of the prescribed dose but could find no statistically significant cutoffs for D_{100} and V_{100}.

An important contemporary development is "intraoperative planning,"[174,189] in which TRUS-based planning (and postimplant dose evaluation as well, in some implementations) is performed during the procedure itself rather than on a volume study acquired weeks before. Intraoperative planning eliminates uncertainties from differences in planning and treatment anatomy due to probe positioning errors or impact of hormone ablation or external-beam therapy. An extension of intraoperative planning is dose-guided implantation[174,190] or "dynamic dose planning,"[191] in which intraoperative planning is repeated one or more times during the implantation procedure, thereby allowing optimized insertion of needles yet to be implanted to overcome errors in previously inserted sources.

INTRACAVITARY BRACHYTHERAPY

In contrast to the comparatively uniform dose distributions of interstitial BT, the unidirectional source arrangements used in gynecologic intracavitary BT give rise to dose distributions that fall off rapidly with distance from the applicator surface, producing large dose gradients across the target volume. Such large dose gradients make target volume–based dose specification difficult and give this treatment modality a highly empirical character. Numerous parameters have been used to prescribe, constrain, or report intracavitary therapy applications, including mg-h, mgRaEq-h, reference point doses (points A and B), bladder and rectal reference point doses, vaginal surface dose, treatment time, and the ICRU Report No. 38[3] 60-Gy reference volume. This section will emphasize the physical relationships among these parameters and their dependence on applicator characteristics. Systems for treating carcinoma of the cervix, the most intensively studied form of intracavitary therapy, will be reviewed. Our focus will be further restricted to applicator geometries and treatment systems (e.g., Fletcher and Washington University/Mallinckrodt systems) derived from the Manchester system. This limited focus is justified by the fact that Manchester- or Fletcher-style applicators continue to be the dominant choice across the world for both HDR and LDR treatments.

The Manchester Family of Intracavitary Therapy Systems

The Manchester system, developed in 1938 by Tod and Meredith,[9] has heavily influenced intracavitary treatment practice patterns throughout the world, especially in North America. The widely used Fletcher-Suit applicator system, the Fletcher loadings, and the point A and B reference points are all derived from the Manchester system. This system was the first to use applicators and loadings designed to satisfy specific dosimetric constraints.[9,192] It was the first system to use a radiation field quantity, exposure at point A, rather than mg-h, to specify treatment.

The Classical Manchester System

The original Manchester applicator system consisted of a rubber intrauterine tandem and two vaginal "ovoids," whose ellipsoidal shape was designed to conform to the isodose curves arising from ^{226}Ra tubes placed along their long axes. The applicators were designed for use with ^{226}Ra tubes 2.2 cm long with 1-mm platinum filtration and an active length between 1 and 1.5 cm. The small, medium, and large ovoid minimum diameters were 2, 2.5, and 3 cm, respectively, and are the same as Fletcher's small, medium, and large colpostats.[193] The preloaded ovoids contained no shielding and relied on extensive anterior and posterior packing to spare bladder and rectal tissue.

The reference point A (Fig. 22.26) originally was defined as the point "2 cm lateral to the center of the uterine canal and 2 cm from the mucous membrane of the lateral fornix in the plane of the uterus."[9] This seemingly arbitrary definition reflected the system developers' view that "radiation necrosis is not the result of direct effects of radiation on the bladder and rectum, but high dose effects in the area in medial edge of the broad ligament where the uterine vessels cross the ureter."[194] They believed the radiation tolerance of this area, termed *the paracervical triangle,* to be the limiting factor in the treatment of cervical cancer and used point A exposure to represent its average dose. In current practice, point A dose is used to approximate the average or minimum dose to the tumor. Point B, defined to be 5 cm from the patient's midline at the same level as point A, was intended to quantify the dose delivered to the obturator lymph nodes.

The Manchester ovoid dimensions and applicator loadings were designed to ensure that the point A dose rate, about 0.52 Gy/hour in modern units, remained constant for all allowed applicator loadings and combinations. The design also ensured that the vaginal loading contribution to point A was limited to 40% of the total dose. Small, medium, and large ovoids were loaded with 17.5, 20, and 22.5 mg of radium, respectively, to compensate for the greater source-to-point A treatment distances with the larger ovoids. Medium (4 cm long) and long (6 cm) tandems were loaded, os to fundus, with source trains consisting of 10- and 15-mg sources and 10-, 10-, and 15-mg sources, respectively, whereas the short tandem (used for cervical stump cancer) was loaded with a single 20-mg radium tube. With the exception of the short tandem, these loadings satisfied the dosimetric constraints within 2%. The point B dose, determined largely by inverse-square law, is approximately 9 Gy for every 4,000 mg-h administered.

Without external-beam treatment to the whole pelvis, a total point A exposure of 8,000 R (72.8 Gy) in 140 hours split between two applications was prescribed.[192] Because the point A dose rate is constant whether the application contains 60 mg of ^{226}Ra (small ovoids, medium tandem) or 80 mg (large ovoids, long tandem), delivery of a fixed point A dose amounts to using time, not milligram-hours, as the factor that terminates the treatment. In contrast to the Paris and Stockholm systems, which prescribed a fixed number of milligram-hours, equivalent Manchester treatment regimens can deliver from 8,400 to 11,200 mg-h—a variation of 33%.

As the size of an intracavitary application (i.e., colpostat diameter and tandem length) increases, the penetration or "lateral throw-off" of the dose distribution increases. As colpostat diameter increases from 2 to 3 cm, the vaginal surface dose decreases by 35% relative to the dose 2 cm from the applicator surface; this is simply a consequence of increasing

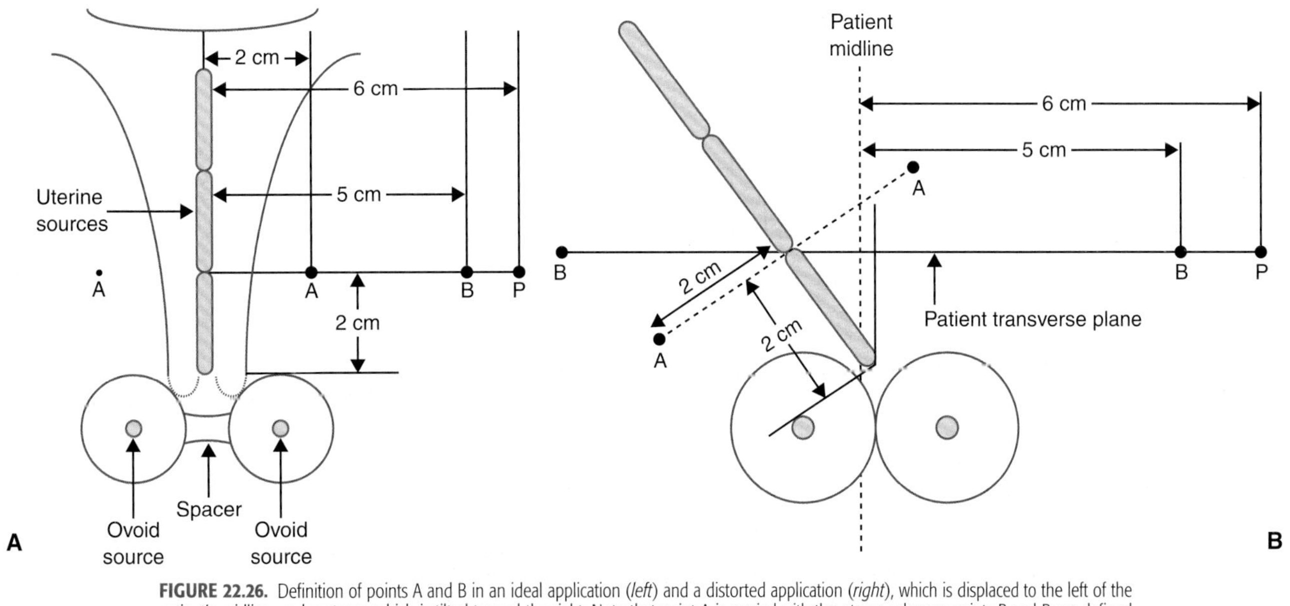

FIGURE 22.26. Definition of points A and B in an ideal application (*left*) and a distorted application (*right*), which is displaced to the left of the patient's midline, and a uterus, which is tilted toward the right. Note that point A is carried with the uterus, whereas points B and P are defined to be 5 and 6 cm, respectively, to the right and left of patient midline. Point P is used by the Mallinckrodt Institute of Radiology System to specify minimum dose to the pelvic lymph nodes. (Adapted from Meredith WJ. Dosage for cancer of cervix uteri. In: Meredith WJ, eds. *Radium dosage: The Manchester System,* 2nd ed. Edinburgh: E & S Livingston, 1967:42–50.)

the source-to-surface distance. Similarly, increasing the tandem length increases the point B contribution relative to the uterine cavity surface dose; the radioactivity near the ends of the long tandem contributes little to the surface dose (because of inverse-square law), whereas each tandem segment makes roughly equal contributions to points remote from the applicator. These physical principles underlie the practice of using the largest colpostats and longest tandem that the patient's anatomy can accommodate.[10,192]

Modern Fletcher-Suit Applicator Systems

The Fletcher applicator system (Fig. 22.27A) adhered to the basic Manchester design while incorporating many improvements including internal shielding. These shields are located on the medial aspects of the anterior and posterior colpostat faces (Fig. 22.27B) and consist of 180-degree and 150-degree disk-shaped 3- to 5-mm-thick tungsten sectors to shield the rectum and bladder, respectively.[193] The cylindrical colpostat body has a diameter of 2 cm that can be increased to 2.5 and 3 cm by use of small and large slip-on plastic caps, thereby retaining the Manchester ovoid dimensions. Afterloading capability was added to the Fletcher applicator by Suit et al.[2] The Fletcher loadings—15, 20, and 25 mg for small, medium, and large colpostats, respectively—are similar to those of the Manchester system, whereas tandem loadings are identical to their Manchester counterparts. Because of the similarity of Fletcher loadings (55 to 85 mg) to the Manchester loadings, point A dose rates are nearly independent of applicator dimensions.

The shielded Fletcher colpostat was designed to reduce dose to the bladder trigone and the anterior rectal wall without

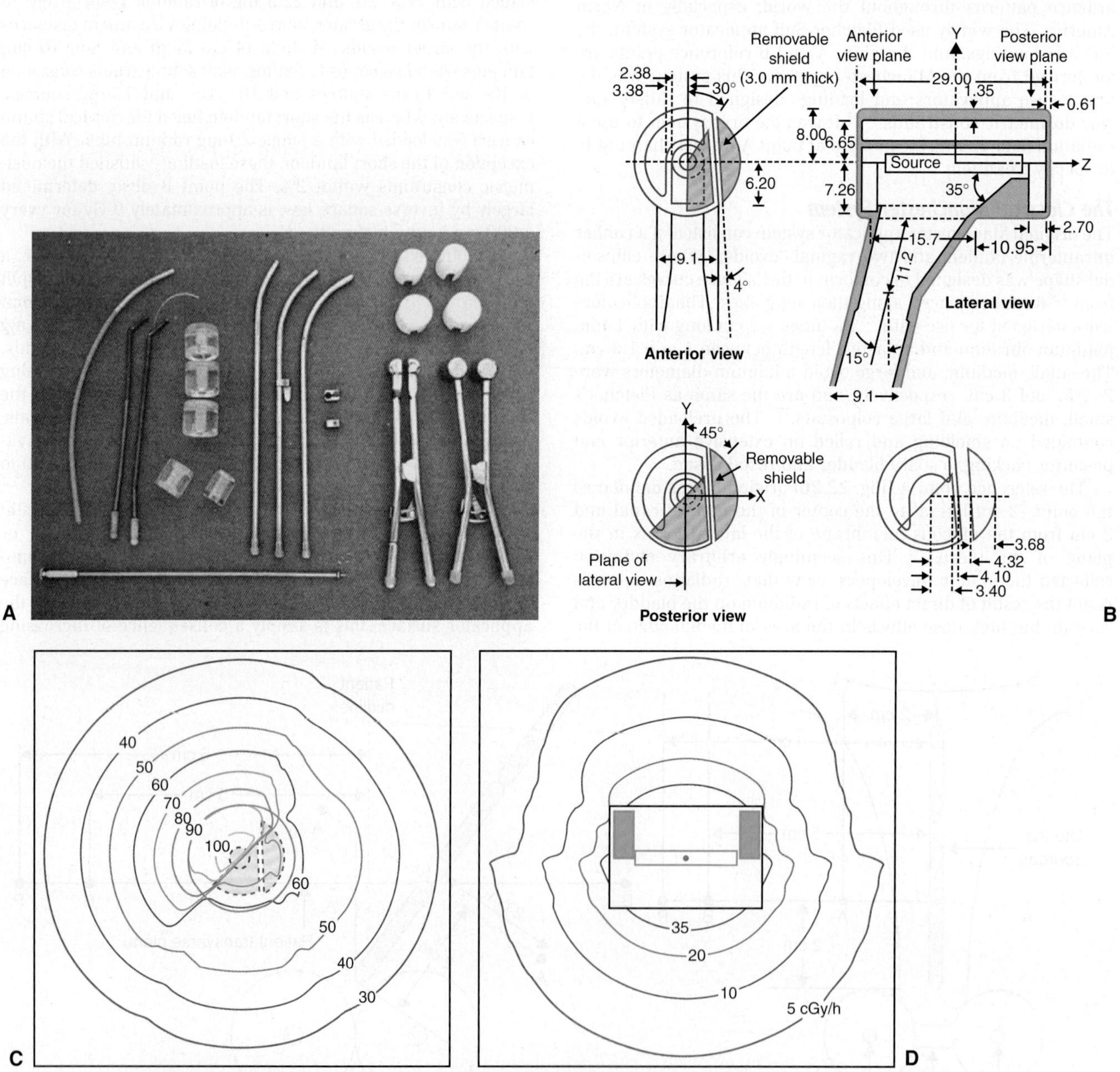

FIGURE 22.27. A: Fletcher-Suit applicator system. From left to right are tandem insert loaded with dummy sources, colpostat source holders, vaginal cylinder sleeves, three curvatures of intrauterine tandems, cervical collars, Delclos mini-colpostats, and round-handled Fletcher-Suit colpostats with small and medium caps. The tubelike instrument in the left foreground is a cervical localization seed implanter. (A from Fletcher GH, Hamberger AD. Squamous cell carcinoma of the uterine cervix: treatment techniques according to size of the cervical lesion and extension. In: Fletcher GD, eds. *Textbook of radiotherapy,* 3rd ed. Philadelphia: Lea & Febiger, 1980:732–772, with permission.) **B:** Three orthogonal views of the 3M Fletcher-Suit Delclos colpostat, consisting of a stainless steel body. The removable parts of the tungsten alloy shield, which allow conversion of the applicator to a shielded Delclos mini-colpostat, are inset into a nylon cap (not shown) with an outer diameter of 2 cm. Shown are isodose curves **(C)** in the coronal plane 10 mm from the posterior face of the applicator and **(D)** in the transverse plane of the colpostat for a 72 $\mu Gy \times m^2 \times h^{-1}$ ^{137}Cs tube. (B–D from Williamson JF. Dose calculations about shielded gynecological colpostats. *Int J Radiat Oncol Biol Phys* 1990;19:167–178, with permission from Elsevier.)

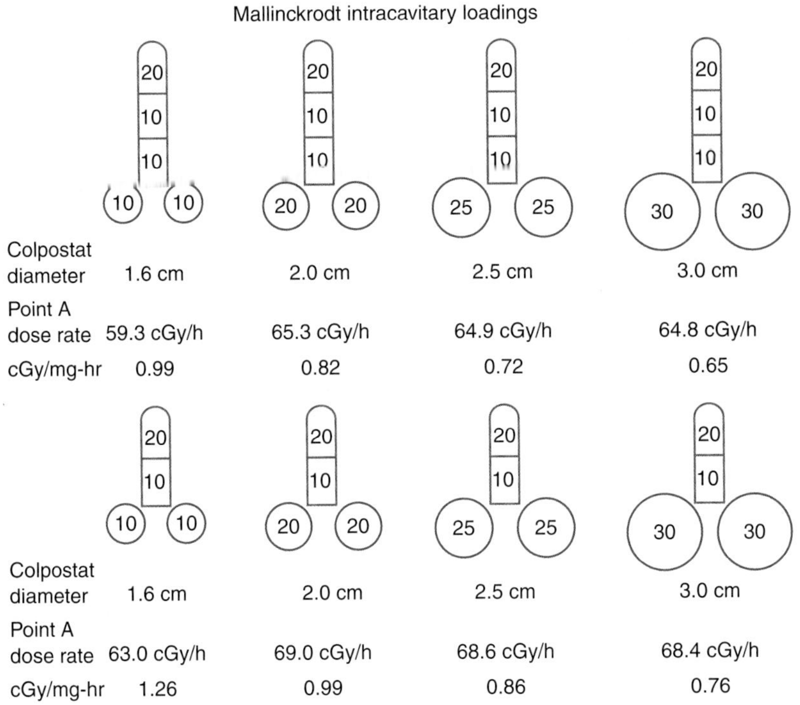

FIGURE 22.28. Mallinckrodt Institute of Radiology/Washington University (WU) applicator loadings used with Fletcher-Suit applicators for treatment of cervix carcinoma. Because the WU system uses Model 6500 3M ^{137}Cs tubes, equivalent mass of radium is used to specify loadings and mgRaEq-h, rather than mg-h, to prescribe intracavitary therapy. The point A dose rates assume the classical Manchester definition and average colpostat separations and tandem-colpostat alignments.

decreasing irradiation to the uterosacral and broad ligaments, thereby reducing the need for the extensive vaginal packing characteristic of Manchester insertions.[193] For a single colpostat (Fig. 22.27B–D), the maximum dose reduction varies from 40% to 50%.[14,195,196] When the effects of the intrauterine tandem and the contralateral colpostat are included, applicator shielding reduces midline rectal and bladder doses by 21% to 34% relative to conventional treatment-planning calculations, which ignore shielding and include only the effects of source encapsulation.[197] CT-based dose evaluation studies reveal that colpostat shielding modestly reduces rectal doses, reducing the rectal $D_{2\%}$ by 2% to 11%[198] and the D_{2mL} by 10%.[199] Modern versions of the shielded Fletcher colpostat for LDR BT include the LDR 3M Fletcher-Suit-Delclos (FSD)[14] and reproductions of the round-handled Fletcher-Suit[195] colpostats. For HDR BT, the Fletcher-Williamson[200] applicator duplicates the original Fletcher shielding configuration. Weeks and Montana[201] have designed a CT-compatible version with afterloadable shields and an aluminum body having the same dimensions as the FSD applicator.

Dose Specification in Intracavitary Brachytherapy

Point A Dose and Milligram-Hours

Two quantities are used widely to prescribe intracavitary BT: mg-h (or its modern equivalent, IRAK) is used in practices influenced by the M.D. Anderson Cancer Center system,[10,202,203] whereas some form of the Manchester point A dose specification is used by most other practitioners. Efforts to unify these two prescription practices by identifying a linear relationship between the two quantities are misguided[204] from the perspective of the Manchester system. The Manchester-like loadings specified by the Washington University/Mallinckrodt Institute of Radiology (WU) clearly show (Fig. 22.28) that despite a twofold variation in source strength loaded into the smallest versus the largest applicator system, the point A dose rate varies by only 15%. To deliver a fixed point A dose of 65 Gy with WU loadings, a constant total treatment time of approximately 100 hours is needed, resulting in delivery of mgRaEq-h ranging from 5,200 to 10,000 in any sample of patients characterized by a range of applicator sizes. Conversely, for fixed mgRaEq-h, prescription would result in a nearly twofold variation in total treatment time and point A dose.

The proportionality of point A dose and treatment time applies only to the classical (Manchester) definition of point A. Many radiation oncologists use a revised definition of point A (Fig. 22.29) that references its location to the cervical os (tandem collar, proximal aspect of the most caudal tandem source, or a gold seed implanted in the cervix) rather than to the lateral fornix. This practice obscures the relationship between point A and milligram-hour prescription philosophies. Potish and Gerbi's[204] study of 90 Fletcher applications demonstrates that the revised point A dose rates vary widely from patient to patient and are, on average, significantly higher than the classical Manchester value. Because point A is fixed to the tandem and the vertical tandem-to-colpostat displacement varies with each patient, the vaginal contribution to point A is highly variable. In contrast, classically defined point A dose rates are tightly grouped, are independent of the loading, and are in close agreement with the Tod-Meredith value. The vaginal contribution to classical point A is fixed by definition, whereas the intrauterine contribution is insensitive to colpostat-to-tandem displacement because of the parallel

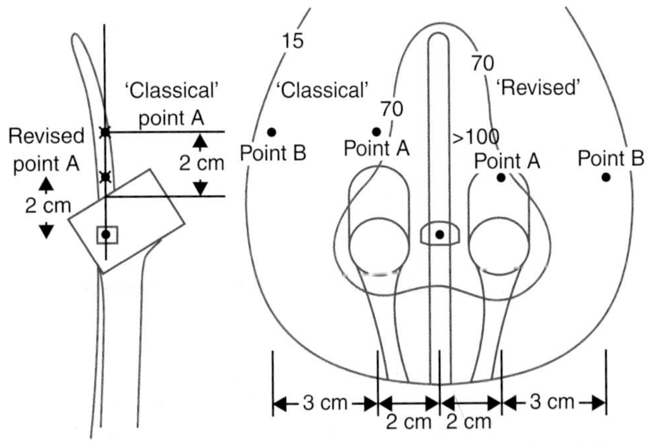

FIGURE 22.29. Radiographic definition of classical point A (2 cm above the cephalic-most aspect of the colpostat in the tilted coronal plane) and the revised point A (2 cm above the cervical collar top or center). Because the distance from the caudal-most intrauterine source tip to the colpostat center (tandem-to-colpostat displacement) varies from patient to patient, the vaginal contribution to revised point A is highly variable. The revised definition was suggested by Tod and Meredith in their 1953 article.[192] (From Potish RA, Gerbi BJ. Role of point A in the era of computerized dosimetry. *Radiology* 1986;158:827–831, with permission.)

tandem isodose curves. Thus, the revised point A definition does not have the physical significance of the classical quantity. Use of revised point A dose to prescribe therapy for "free-floating" tandem and colpostat insertions may introduce large patient-to-patient fluctuations in treatment times because of small, clinically insignificant variations in implant geometry.

The previous discussion is applicable only to the Fletcher applicator system with relative loadings approximating those of the Manchester system. As the intrauterine-to-vaginal loading ratio (1:1 for the Manchester system) increases, and the maximum width of the pear-shaped reference isodoses falls and the rectal dose increases,[205] appreciation of how loading influences isodose shape and normal-tissue doses is especially important in HDR BT as dwell-weight optimization invites deviation from classical loading rules. Using judiciously placed dose points to control the relative dimensions of the point A isodose surface, Mai et al.[206] were able to increase tapering near the cephalad aspect of the tandem, reduce the vaginal surface dose, and modestly reduce the rectal dose with only slight loss of the maximum width of the pear-shaped isodose. These considerations suggest that dose-point–driven optimization of the dwell-weight distribution should be accompanied by a geometric analysis of the point A isodose surface (see ICRU Report 38 discussion later in this chapter) so that changes to target coverage can be assessed at least approximately.

Other applicators in current use include the HDR tandem and ring applicator[207] and the LDR Henschke applicator.[1] The latter consists of hemispheric colpostats rigidly attached to the tandem with the vaginal source axes parallel to the intrauterine sources rather than transverse as in the Fletcher system. Henschke colpostats with internal shielding[208] are available. Delclos et al.[195] note that the Fletcher and Henschke applicators system do not yield equivalent dose distributions, especially with respect to normal tissue sparing. The vaginal ring applicator consists of a circular guide tube (usually 34 mm outer diameter) with its plane fixed rigidly normal to the tandem. It is placed up against the cervix and vaginal fornices with a donut-shaped cap attached, which increases the distance between the vaginal mucosa and the circular array of dwell positions (of which only the lateral dwell positions are activated) to 7 mm (compared to 10 to 15 mm for the Fletcher colpostat). Thus, the fraction of source strength loaded into the ring must be reduced to avoid overdosing the vaginal mucosa.[206,209] Although rectal and vaginal vault doses relative to the point A dose similar to that of the Fletcher system can be achieved through careful optimization, the lateral coverage (i.e., maximum coronal width of the point A isodose) is reduced.[206] Care must be taken in positioning the applicator system to avoid underdosing the gross tumor volume. Applicator geometry and loading practices should be changed only after extensive comparative evaluation of the old and new dose distributions to avoid dose distribution changes that would invalidate the evaluated clinical experience on which the brachytherapist's knowledge of dose response rests. Finally, for applicator systems that deviate from the classical Manchester geometry or relative loading rules, one cannot assume that point A dose is proportional to treatment time over all allowed variations of applicator sizes and loadings.

Volumetric Specification of Intracavitary Treatment: ICRU Report No. 38 Recommendations

The ICRU[3] introduced the concept of reference volume enclosed by the reference isodose surface for reporting and comparing intracavitary treatments performed in different centers regardless of the applicator system, insertion technique, and method of treatment prescription used. Specifically, ICRU Report No. 38 recommended that the reference volume be taken as the 60-Gy isodose surface, resulting from the addition of dose contributions from any external-beam whole-pelvis irradiation and all intracavitary insertions. The ICRU proposed that this pear-shaped reference volume (Fig. 22.30) be described in terms of

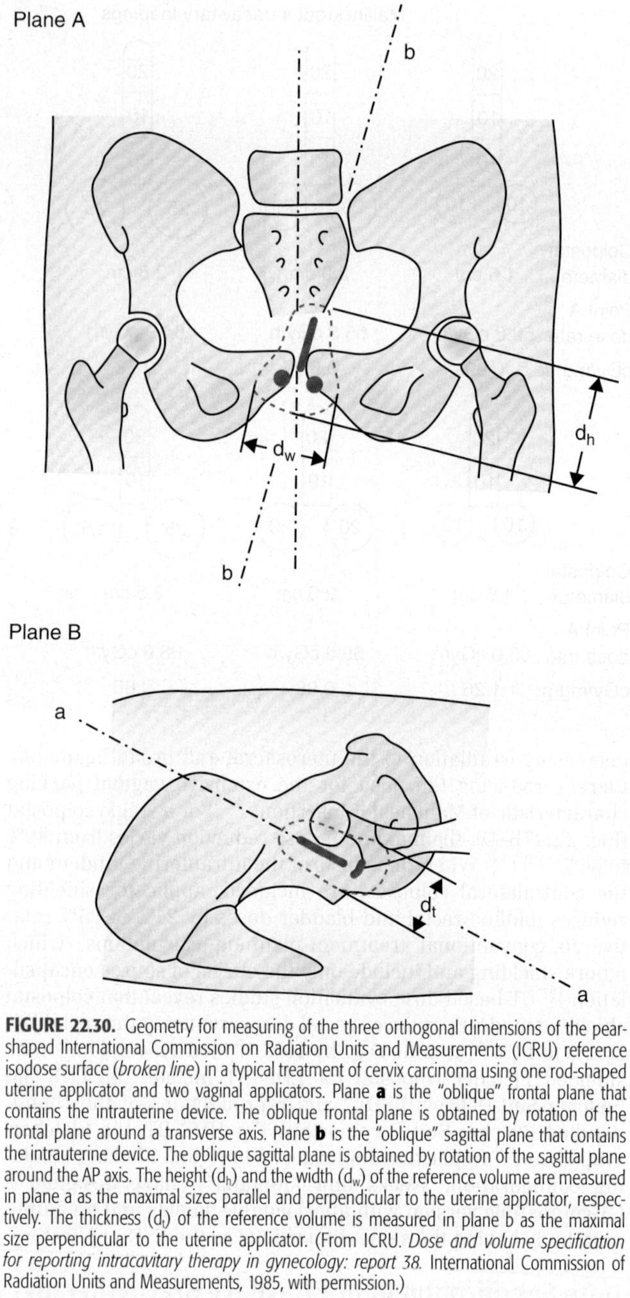

FIGURE 22.30. Geometry for measuring of the three orthogonal dimensions of the pear-shaped International Commission on Radiation Units and Measurements (ICRU) reference isodose surface (*broken line*) in a typical treatment of cervix carcinoma using one rod-shaped uterine applicator and two vaginal applicators. Plane **a** is the "oblique" frontal plane that contains the intrauterine device. The oblique frontal plane is obtained by rotation of the frontal plane around a transverse axis. Plane **b** is the "oblique" sagittal plane that contains the intrauterine device. The oblique sagittal plane is obtained by rotation of the sagittal plane around the AP axis. The height (d_h) and the width (d_w) of the reference volume are measured in plane a as the maximal sizes parallel and perpendicular to the uterine applicator, respectively. The thickness (d_t) of the reference volume is measured in plane b as the maximal size perpendicular to the uterine applicator. (From ICRU. *Dose and volume specification for reporting intracavitary therapy in gynecology: report 38.* International Commission of Radiation Units and Measurements, 1985, with permission.)

its three orthogonal maximal dimensions: height (d_h), width (d_w), and thickness (d_t), measured in the oblique coronal and sagittal planes containing the intrauterine sources. Figure 22.31 illustrates the bladder and rectal reference points recommended by the ICRU.

In contrast to point A dose and mgRaEq-h, the ICRU proposal is only a means of describing or reporting treatment. No guidance is given as to how to prescribe treatment, use these measurements to evaluate implant quality, or correlate reference volume dimensions with clinical outcome. The 60-Gy dose-level choice appears to have been motivated by the preoperative radiotherapy regimen popular within the French school of radiotherapy at the time.[210] Descriptions of institution-specific treatment techniques for early stage cervical cancer patients include rules for evaluating the 60-Gy reference volume dimensions and offsets relative to the applicator system for the allowed combinations of applicator dimensions and loadings.[210] Within North America, Potish et al.,[211,212] and later Eisbruch et al.,[213] found that the individual ICRU reference

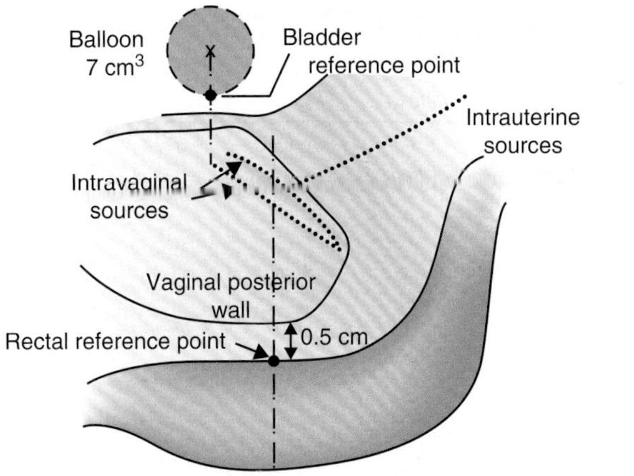

FIGURE 22.31. Reference points for bladder and rectal brachytherapy doses proposed by International Commission on Radiation Units and Measurements (ICRU) Report 38.[3]

volume dimensions and various geometric characteristics of Fletcher implants (e.g., colpostat separation and vertical and horizontal displacement of the tandem from the colpostat centers) were moderately well correlated. Other investigators[214–216] have proposed using the product of ICRU dimensions, $V_{ICRU} = d_t \times d_w \times d_h$, to estimate the relative volume contained within the reference isodose surface. Esche et al.[215] found that V_{ICRU} was directly proportional to mg-h, whereas Nath et al.[216] pointed out that V_{ICRU} increased steeply with increasing whole-pelvis dose. In a retrospective clinical study,[214] grade 3 rectal complications were correlated with high $d_t \times d_w \times d_h$ product, and severe bladder complications were associated with the combination of high bladder doses and large V_{ICRU} on a 2D scattergram. The rationale for studying the product of ICRU reference volume dimensions is the well-established correlation between the volume of tissue irradiated by external irradiation and clinical outcome.[217] In contrast to ICRU Report 38,[3] which defines reference isodose surface dimensions for a single fixed dose level, these studies treat ICRU reference volume dimensions as functions of total dose or intracavitary dose.

The ICRU reference volume concept appropriately emphasizes that volume of tissue irradiated, as well as dose, is an important predictor of clinical response to intracavitary irradiation. Wilkinson and Ramachandran[218] and Eisbruch et al.[213] used DVHs to study the correlation between volume enclosed by intracavitary isodose surfaces and other prescription parameters. The latter analyzed the volumetric characteristics of 204 intracavitary insertions in 128 patients with carcinoma of the cervix and demonstrated that intracavitary implants delivering the same mgRaEq-h have nearly identical DVHs over the dose range of clinical interest despite significant differences in geometry and loadings (Fig. 22.32). They also showed that the volume, V(D,M), enclosed by isodose surfaces can be estimated accurately from a modified power-law model requiring knowledge of only the intracavitary dose in cGy (D) and mgRaEq-h (M):

$$V(D,M) = \left[104.8 - 8.103\left(\frac{M}{D}\right) + 0.437\left(\frac{M}{D}\right)^2\right] \cdot \left(\frac{M}{D}\right)^{1.635} \quad (38)$$

The volume predicted by this simple model is accurate within ± 10% in 95% of the implants when M/D is more than 0.8, which corresponds to an intracavitary dose of 100 Gy for 8,000 mgRaEq-h of intracavitary therapy. In addition, the ratio of ICRU dimension product to the true volume given by DVH analysis, $d_t \times d_w \times d_h/V(D,M)$, varied widely from patient to patient and differed systematically from one implant type to another.

The consequences of Eq. (38) can be summarized as follows:

1. Volumetrically, an intracavitary implant behaves like a central point source: $V(D,M) \propto (M/D)^{3/2}$.

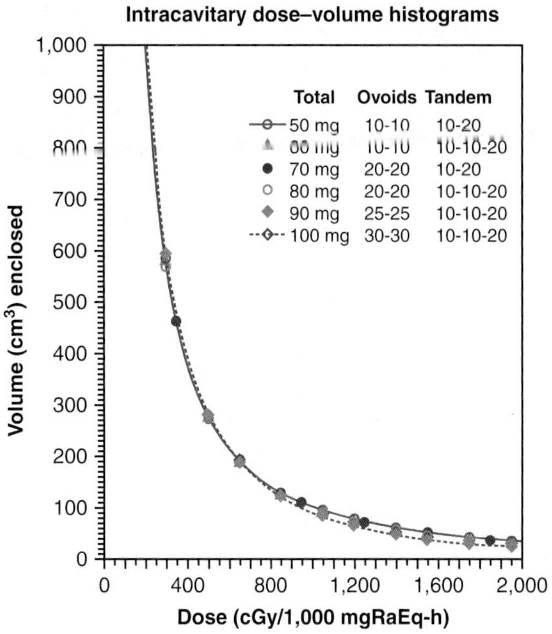

FIGURE 22.32. Dose–volume histograms for seven Washington University (WU) intracavitary insertions using 1.4-cm-active-length ^{137}Cs sources. The strength of each source was determined by the loading rules for WU schema C (20 Gy, whole pelvis plus 8,000 mgRaEq-h) and then was scaled down to 1,000 mgRaEq-h. Note that as the size of the insertion increases, the volume of tissue encompassed by the high-dose isosurfaces decreases. Point A doses ranged from 8.28 to 11.35 Gy.

2. Describing an implant in terms of volume contained within its isodose curves carries no more information content than a statement of mgRaEq-h or total reference air kerma.
3. The volume of tissue irradiated to a specified dose is closely related to total exposure given by the implant in terms of mgRaEq-h, TRAK, or IRAK.

Consequence (2) suggests that the correlation between clinical outcome, in terms of tumor control and complications and isodose surface volume, should be no better or worse than the correlation between clinical outcome and mgRaEq-h for a fixed external pelvis dose. Consequence (3) suggests a new and fundamental physical interpretation of mgRaEq-h or its derivative, total reference air kerma. Prescribing intracavitary BT by mgRaEq-h is equivalent to treating until each specified isodose surface achieves a fixed volume independent of the underlying implant geometry. Use of mgRaEq-h to constrain intracavitary treatment therefore limits the volume of tissue irradiated to high doses. This observation may help explain the clinical utility of mgRaEq-h as a dose specification parameter. Finally, the individual reference isodose dimensions, which are more strongly influenced by implant geometry than their product, clearly convey additional information about the spatial extension of the reference isodose surface in their respective planes and cannot be reduced to a statement of total exposure from the implant and may have additional prognostic significance.

Practical Systems for Intracavitary Prescription and Reporting

For Manchester-like loadings and applicators, if treatment were to be prescribed as a fixed number of mgRaEq-h or IRAK without regard to the diameter and length of the applicators, the treatment times and total point A doses would differ by the ratio of total source strengths in the applications. Small applications would have unacceptably high point A and vaginal vault surface doses and excessively long treatment times. In contrast, large applications treated to a fixed mgRaEq-h prescription would underdose these reference points. In contrast, the ICRU reference volume for fixed levels of whole pelvic

TABLE 22.10 SIMPLIFIED FLETCHER SYSTEM PRESCRIPTIONS

Treatment Scheme	Indications	External Beam		Intracavitary Maximum		Range: Smallest to Largest Insertion		
		Whole Pelvis	Split Field	mg-h[a]	Time (h)	Point A	Point B[b]	mg-h[a]
A	<1 cm tumor	0 Gy	0 Gy	6,000 4,000	72 48	59–63 Gy	17–22	6,600–10,000
B	IB/IIB 1–3 cm tumor	0	<40	5,400 3,600	72 48	56–59	57–60	6,600–9,000
C		20	<20	3,600 3,900	48 52	67–69	54–56	5,500–7,500
D	Endocervical tumor; Ib/IIb moderate bulk (3–6 cm) disease; IIB/IIIB bulky (>6 cm) tumor with good regression	40	<10[c]	3,250 3,250	48 48	81–90	63–64	5,280–6,500
E	Bulky disease with poor regression	50	0	2,500 2,500 or 5,000	48 48 or 72	81–94	62	5,000

[a]Radium tubes with 1-mm platinum filtration. [b]With maximum split field dose.
Adapted from Potish RA, Gerbi BJ. Cervical cancer intracavitary dose specification and prescription. *Radiology* 1987;165:555–560.

irradiation and mgRaEq-h would be independent of the loading because the mgRaEq-h is constant. Conversely, when the point A dose is held constant, the mgRaEq-h needed to deliver these doses will vary significantly, introducing corresponding variations in the volume of the ICRU reference isodose.

Clearly, no IRAK-based system would endorse such a naive approach. Actual mgRaEq-h–based systems use a combination of parameters. Physically, mgRaEq-h or IRAK controls the volume of tissue treated to high doses, and parameters such as time, colpostat surface dose, and point A are used to control doses at points near the applicator to ensure that surface tolerance is not exceeded and that the tumor is not undertreated. For each applicator combination and choice of external-beam dose, a compromise between volume of tissue treated and dose delivered near the applicator must be reached. For example, the Fletcher system[10,212] specifies both a maximum treatment time and maximum milligram-hour constraint for each combination of external-beam and intracavitary therapy (Table 22.10). Whichever constraint is reached first terminates the application. Small applications tend to be terminated by the maximum time constraint, which limits the milligram-hour and prevents tissues near the applicator from exceeding tolerance doses, whereas larger applications are terminated by the milligram-hour constraint, ensuring adequate dose to the tumor. Although the historical Fletcher system does not use point A dose either for prescription or reporting, the total point A dose is constant within 12% for allowed tandem and colpostat loadings within each treatment scheme (A–E) of Table 22.10. The reader should note that the Fletcher system is a complex, highly individualized treatment system that resists formulation in terms of a few rules. Table 22.10 is a highly condensed and simplified summary derived from the literature, not from observation of current M.D. Anderson Cancer Center practice patterns.

The Washington University/Mallinckrodt Institute of Radiology (WU) system for prescribing intracavitary therapy illustrates another empirical approach for ensuring adequate dose delivery to the tumor while limiting the volume of tissue treated to high doses. Like the Fletcher system, intracavitary BT prescriptions are stated in mgRaEq-h. Historically, the WU system used Manchester-like applicators and loadings preloaded with ^{226}Ra or ^{60}Co tubes, until the late 1950s when the Ter-Pogossian applicator was introduced. The system changed with the introduction of high-energy x-ray external-beam therapy in 1958, the adoption of the Fletcher-Suit applicator in 1965, and the acquisition of ^{137}Cs tubes in 1971.[203] Because of the long association of the WU system with artificial radionuclides, equivalent mass of radium rather than mass of radium is used to specify source strength; hence, 1 mgRaEq-h in the WU system is equivalent to 1.07 mg-h in the Fletcher system, which, in turn, is equivalent to an IRAK of 0.00723 mGy m^2.

Manchester-like applicator loadings (Fig. 22.28) currently are used for LDR applications, yielding an approximately constant point A dose rate of 65 cGy/hour. For HDR applications, the dwell weights are selected to duplicate the relative Manchester loadings and the IRAK per insertion is reduced to reflect the increased radiobiologic effectiveness of the HDR fractionation schedule relative to the LDR regimen. Classically defined point A doses are calculated for reporting purposes for all patients, although this quantity plays no role in prescribing therapy. Dose to the pelvic lymph nodes is calculated at point P, located 2 cm superior to the lateral fornix and 6 cm lateral to the patient's midline. Bladder and rectal reference points (Fig. 22.31) are defined according to ICRU Report No. 38.[3] The prescribed doses for the external-beam and intracavitary (delivered in two LDR insertions) components of treatment are listed in Table 22.11 as a function of extent and stage of disease. The mgRaEq-h prescription is divided equally between the vaginal and uterine components and is delivered exactly as prescribed only in the case of the standard 80-mgRaEq application (2 cm diameter colpostats and long tandem, loaded 20-10-10). For nonstandard loadings using mini-colpostats, the vaginal and intrauterine IRAK prescriptions are modified independently. When Delclos minicolpostats are used, vaginal IRAK is constrained by the vaginal vault surface dose limit, which for LDR is 150 Gy (including whole-pelvic dose and the dose from the ipsilateral colpostat but excluding dose from the tandem and contralateral colpostat.). For medium and large colpostats, the vaginal mgRaEq-h is increased by 16% and 28%, respectively, to compensate for their larger source-to-surface distances. When medium and short tandem loadings are used, the target IRAK prescription is modified by the ratio of the actual loading to the standard loading (80 mgRaEq-h).

Table 22.12 illustrates detailed application of the WU system to three applicator configurations for prescription schema C, listing total doses for point A, point P, and the vaginal mucosa along with the volumes of tissue enclosed by point A and ICRU 60-Gy reference isodose surfaces. The mgRaEq-h actually delivered by equivalent implants varies by a factor of 1.62, leading to a reference volume variation of 2.08. However, compared to fixed point A prescription 65 Gy, which would allow administered mgRaEq-h to vary by a factor of 2.31, the

TABLE 22.11 WASHINGTON UNIVERSITY PRESCRIPTIONS FOR CARCINOMA OF THE CERVIX

		External-Beam Treatment		*Intracavitary Treatment*		*Range: Smallest to Largest Insertion*		
Treatment Scheme	*Indication*	*Whole Pelvis (Gy)*	*Split Field (Gy)*	*Target mgRaEq-h*	*Maximum Vaginal Vault Dose (Gy)*	*Point A Dose (Gy)*	*Point P Dose (Gy)*	*mgRaEq-h*
A	IB <2 cm	0	45	7,000	150	58–60	56–60	5,580–7,980
B	IB 2–4 cm	10	40	7,500	150	71–72	61–66	5,580–8,550
C	IB/IIA/IIB/IIIA bulky (>4 cm) limited parametrial extension	20	30	8,000	150	84–86	61–67	5,600–9,100
D	IIB/IIB bulky extensive parametrial extension	20	40	8,000	150	84–86	71–77	5,600–9,100
E	IIB, IIIB, IV poor anatomy, poor regression	40	20	6,500	150	92–94	69–74	4,610–7,410

variation of irradiated volume is somewhat limited. These rules represent an empirically developed compromise between limiting volume of tissue treated and maintaining a tumoricidal dose contribution to the colpostat surface and to point A.

Table 22.11 shows that as tumor size increases and therapeutic emphasis shifts from intracavitary insertions to external-beam therapy, the point A dose increases, from 58 Gy for small IB lesions (schema A) to 94 Gy for stage IV lesions (schema E). The mgRaEq-h actually administered within a given treatment group may deviate from the target mgRaEq-h prescriptions by as much as −30% to +40% for very small and large insertions, respectively. Despite reliance on the mgRaEq-h prescription philosophy, treatment times are approximately constant and total point A doses are nearly independent of applicator size, the defining features of the Manchester system.

Summary Principles: Intracavitary Brachytherapy Dose Specification

The most widely used intracavitary BT systems in North America are based on Manchester-type loadings and applicators, in which the point A dose rate is approximately constant and independent of loading, leading to a linear relationship between point A dose and time, not mgRaEq-h. Practical mgRaEq-h systems use various dose specification parameters to constrain and guide treatment and are far more Manchester-like than the "strict" milligram-hour philosophy would suggest. These parameters have the following roles: (a) IRAK limits volume of tissue treated to a high dose, (b) point A dose ensures that tumor periphery receives adequate dose, (c) vaginal surface dose ensures that dose to mucosal surfaces in contact with the applicator system remains within tolerance, and (d) treatment time ensures indirect control of point A dose.

Although the traditional treatment specification quantities have clear physical meanings and interrelationships, these concepts can be applied to patient treatment only within a clinical system supported by a base of evaluated clinical experience. In current practice, implant placement is guided by direct visualization and palpation, and treatment prescription is guided by the radiation oncologist's knowledge of treatment outcome averaged over groups of uniformly treated patients with similar tumor size and location and medical condition. This implies that the implant system must be applied as a whole: mixing dose specification methods, insertion techniques, and normal-tissue dose-response relationships from different clinical systems is a dangerous practice that can lead to suboptimal or indeterminate clinical outcomes. For example, use of the WU-recommended rectal tolerance dose (75 to 80 Gy) to guide prescription in a system using higher whole-pelvic doses will not guarantee an acceptable level of complications. Second, because classical dose specification quantities incompletely describe the dose distribution, a radiation oncologist must be trained in all details of an intracavitary system to duplicate the results of its developers. Finally, for the clinical physicist, consistency of current dosimetric practice with past clinical experience may be more important than absolute dose computation accuracy or compliance with a practice standard external to the treatment system.

Image-Guided Intracavitary Brachytherapy

Classical intracavitary BT, with its empirically based rules, prescription practices, and feedback derived from patient follow-up to shape and position intracavitary dose distributions, demonstrates that even massive cervical cancers are potentially curable with concomitant chemoradiation therapy. In an effort to improve clinical outcomes in locally advanced cervical cancer and to reduce the incidence of local failure and late normal-tissue toxicity, many groups are investigating anatomy-based dose specification using 3D x-ray CT or magnetic resonance imaging (MRI) studies acquired with the applicator system in place. Early studies[219–221] consistently demonstrated that conventional orthogonal film-based reference points overestimate minimum doses to the cervix and underestimate maximum doses to critical structures by factors of 1.5 to 2.3 with large patient-to-patient variations. Because MRI has been shown to be far superior to CT for distinguishing tumor from normal cervical stroma[222] and for delineating surrounding critical structures, advisory groups[223,224] recommend using T2-weighted

TABLE 22.12 WASHINGTON UNIVERSITY SCHEMA C: 8,000 mg-h, 20 Gy WHOLE PELVIS, AND 30 Gy SPLIT PELVIS

Applicator	*Loading*	*Time*	*mgRaEq-h*	*Vaginal[a] Surface Dose*	*Total Point A Dose (Volume)*	*Total Point P Dose (Gy)*	*ICRU Volume (40 Gy)*
Small tandem	20, 10	× 100 hr =	3,000	152.3 Gy	83.5 Gy (85 cm^3)	61.0	165 cm^3
Mini ovoids	10 10	× 130 hr =	2,600				
			5,600				
Standard tandem	20, 10, 10	× 100 =	4,000	150.1 Gy	86.3 Gy (131 cm^3)	65.2	281 cm^3
2-cm colpostats	20 20	× 100 hr =	4,000				
			8,000				
Standard tandem	20, 10, 10	× 100 =	4,000	98.6 Gy	85.6 Gy (160 cm^3)	66.9 Gy	343 cm^3
3-cm colpostats	30 30	× 85 hr =	5,100				
			9,100				

ICRU, International Commission on Radiation Units and Measurements.

[a]On surface of single colpostat, neglecting other sources.

MRI studies acquired prior to initiating treatment and after each intracavitary insertion for BT planning and dose reconstruction. One such group, the gynecologic GEC-ESTRO Working Group, has proposed a widely accepted target volume nomenclature (high-risk, intermediate-risk, and low-risk CTVs)[223] and specific DVH parameters[225] for assessing the correlation between clinical outcome and the delivered dose distribution.

Early reports of image-based conformal therapy in locally advanced cervical cancer are promising. For example, use of intensity-modulated radiation therapy (IMRT) to replace traditional whole- and split-pelvis fields[226,227] suggests that grade 3/4 late toxicity is significantly reduced relative to historical controls without increasing local recurrence. The most extensively reported experience with MRI-based intracavitary BT planning (156 patients at Medical University of Vienna) achieved excellent 3-year local control rates of 86% to 100% (FIGO Ib to IIIb) with grade 2/4 late toxicities of 4% or less.[228] A robust dose-response relationship between high-risk CTV (HRCTV) D_{90} and D_{100} for large tumors[229] was demonstrated as well as a correlation between bladder and rectal DVH parameters (e.g., D_{2ml}) and major late complications.[230] Challenges to image-guided intracavitary therapy include substantial soft-tissue displacement and deformation due to applicator insertion and removal, tumor regression, and bladder and rectal filling variations (all ignored by clinical experiences cited earlier), making it difficult to meaningfully evaluate cumulative dose distributions. An important area of research is application of deformable image registration to account explicitly for the temporal sequence of deforming 3D anatomies needed to accurately characterize a multiple insertion course of intracavitary and external-beam therapy.[231] Using dose summation over weekly magnetic resonance image sets that had been contoured and nonrigidly registered, Lim et al.[232] demonstrated that 5-mm PTV expansion of the intermediate-risk CTV surface for the IMRT component of treatment was adequate for most patients, although large variations between planned and cumulative normal-tissue doses were observed for some patients. As IMRT is used to create more conformal external-beam dose distributions and to address peripheral HRCTV underdoses by the intracavitary treatment components, the need to accurately account for local tissue deformation will become more acute.[233]

THE RADIOBIOLOGY OF BRACHYTHERAPY

The development of high-strength remote-afterloading stepping sources and low-energy permanently implantable sources has resulted in clinical utilization of dose rates and dose-time-fractionation patterns that can differ radically from conventional LDR BT protocols. A clear understanding of the principles governing selection of dose-time-fractionation protocols in BT or combined external-beam radiation therapy (EBRT-BT) has become an essential clinical tool.

The highly conformal dose distribution characteristic of BT sources significantly reduces the exposed volume, and often, the maximum dose in adjacent normal tissues, compared to EBRT.[233,234] As well as diminishing late-responding normal-tissue complications, such dose sparing keeps early-responding normal tissue sequelae to acceptable levels, making the short treatment times commonly used in temporary-implant BT tolerable. This is in contrast to EBRT, where the risk of early-responding tissue sequelae requires treatment times to be prolonged for up to about 8 weeks, potentially reducing tumor control through repopulation. The short overall treatment times used in temporary implants are likely to contribute significantly to clinical efficacy and social-economical benefits for those tumor sites (e.g., cervix, head and neck, and lung) where long overall treatment time is associated with reduced local control.

Biophysical Modeling of Brachytherapy

Based on improved understanding of the radiobiologic principles of BT, biophysical models have been developed for predicting responses to alternative temporal dose-delivery schemes. In the 1970s, before the differential response of early- and late-responding tissues was understood, the most widespread approach for designing alternative fractionation schemes was the nominal standard dose (NSD) equation,[235] which was based on data from early-responding tissues only. By contrast, the currently used linear-quadratic (LQ) model unequivocally distinguishes between early and late responses and is based on mechanistic notions about how cells are killed by radiation. After several decades of investigation and use, the basic ideas and parameters in the LQ model have been well supported by clinical experience and outcome data.

The Linear-Quadratic Model and Its Mechanistic Basis

Central to the LQ approach is a biologic model of radiation action, which was spelled out in detail more than 50 years ago by Lea and Catcheside,[236,237] based on a mechanistic analysis of radiation-induced chromosome aberration induction. The application of the LQ formalism to radiation therapy has been reviewed by Thames and Hendry,[238] Dale,[239] Fowler,[240] and many others. The LQ model assumes that radiotherapeutic response is primarily related to cell survival (or survival of groups of cells). Although not the sole determinant of biologic response, there is now a wealth of evidence that cell killing (i.e., loss of reproductive integrity) is the dominant determinant of radiotherapeutic response, both for early- and late-responding end points.[238]

In the most basic LQ approach, cellular survival, S, from dose D given in a single acute exposure or fraction, is written as:

$$S(D) = \exp(-\alpha D - \beta D^2) \quad (39)$$

The mechanistic interpretation of Eq. (39) is that cell killing results from the interaction of two elementary damaged species, most often DNA double-strand breaks (DSB), to produce species that cause cell lethality, such as dicentric chromosomal aberrations. The first term in Eq. (39), which is linear in dose, describes production of two DSBs by the same ionizing radiation quantum (usually a charged particle), while the second term, quadratic in dose, describes production of multiple DSBs by two independent quanta. If the radiation is delivered over a protracted period rather than delivered acutely, the two DSBs may be formed at different times. Therefore, it is possible that the first may be repaired before it has a chance to interact with the second. This will not affect the first term in Eq. (39), because the two DSBs are formed simultaneously from a single particle track, but DSB repair during a prolonged exposure will result in a reduction of the second, quadratic term in Eq. (39) by a factor denoted by "G":[236,237]

$$S(D) = \exp(-\alpha D - G \cdot \beta D^2) \quad (40)$$

where, for acute exposures, $G \rightarrow 1$, and for very long exposures, $G \rightarrow 0$. In this context, "acute" and "long" are defined relative to the half-time (T_r) for DSB repair of sublethal damage. In general, G will depend on the detailed temporal distribution of dose delivery, as well as on T_r. For many simple cases, G can be calculated analytically. For example, for a permanent exponentially decaying implant, G can be approximated as $\lambda/(\mu + \lambda)$ where $\lambda = \ln 2/T_{1/2} = 0.693/T_{1/2}$ is the decay constant of the radionuclide, and μ (=$0.693/T_r$) is the sublethal damage repair rate. In the case of our two-DSB damage model, μ describes repair of single DSBs. Formulae for G for many other standard schemes also have been derived,[237,241] as has a general formalism for any possible protraction scheme.[242]

The LQ formalism, described by Eqs. (39) and (40), is not simply a convenient formula for fitting cellular survival curves, but can be derived from a variety of underlying mechanistic models via first-order time-dependent perturbation theory when the dose or dose rate is not too high, a constraint that includes most clinically and experimentally relevant doses and dose rates.[243] For example, the theory of dual radiation action[244] is only one of several different approaches to describe radiobiologic damage mechanistically. The approach devised by Lea and Catcheside[236,237] deals instead with the kinetics of damage development. Typical kinetic models track the temporal evolution of lesions as a cell gradually repairs or misrepairs initial damage.[245–247] Many different molecular mechanisms have been studied kinetically, such as pairwise misrepair of DNA DSBs, direct one-hit induction of lethal lesions, and saturable repair pathways in which the repair enzyme system can be overloaded.

Practical Applications of the LQ Model

Eq. (40) can be used either to design "equivalent" dose protraction protocols (i.e., design a regimen with the same tumor response, or the same late complications, as a "tried and tested" regimen) or to predict absolute radiotherapeutic responses. We will discuss both approaches here, although we will argue that designing equivalent protraction schemes is a considerably more robust procedure.

In order to design a new dose protraction protocol (labeled "2") that will have the same effect as a current protocol (labeled "1"), based on Eq. (40), we need to ensure the quantity ($\alpha D + G\beta D^2$) is equal for the two protocols; that is:

$$D_1(1 + G_1D_1/(\alpha/\beta)) = D_2(1 + G_2D_2/(\alpha/\beta)) \tag{41}$$

The quantity on either side of Eq. (41) is often called the biologically effective dose (BED),[240] so generating a new "equivalent" regimen amounts to matching its BED to that of the old regimen.

By contrast, to use the LQ model to calculate absolute tumor control probabilities (TCPs) or normal-tissue complication probabilities (NTCPs), we need additional models relating cellular survival (*S*) with TCP or with NTCP. The simplest approach, the Poisson statistics TCP,[248] equates TCP with the probability that after radiation treatment there are no remaining tumor stem cells capable of initiating tumor regrowth. Let us suppose that a dose, D, delivered in a given protraction pattern produces a stem-cell-survival probability, S. Let K be the initial number of potential stem cells in the tumor. Then, the probability that any given stem cell will be unable to initiate tumor regrowth is (1 – S). Thus, the TCP for the irradiated tumor is simply $(1 - S)^K$, which, for small values of S, can be approximated as:

$$TCP = \exp(-S \cdot K) \tag{42}$$

Thus, if cell survival, S, is described by Eq. (40), then

$$\begin{aligned} TCP(D) &= \exp(-K \cdot \exp[-\alpha D - G \cdot \beta D^2]) \\ &= \exp(-\exp[\ln K - \alpha D - G \cdot \beta D^2]) \end{aligned} \tag{43}$$

Eq. (43) may also be used to calculate NTCP, except that now the parameter K does not refer to the number of tumor cells that need to be sterilized, but rather to the number of groups of cells in the normal tissue ("tissue-rescuing units"),[249] whose destruction would result in the late complication.

A challenge faced by Poisson TCP models and similar approaches is their exquisite sensitivity to the parameter values assumed, particularly the K parameter. In contrast, using the LQ model to compare competing protraction regimens [Eq. (41) and its extensions described later] makes no assumptions about the relationship between surviving fraction and clinical outcome, therefore making them much less sensitive to the LQ parameter values.[250]

To improve the clinical utility of TCP or NTCP models, extensive efforts have been made to fit these models to clinical data, yielding tumor/tissue-specific model parameters, for example, for head and neck tumors,[251,252] breast tumors,[253,254] prostate cancer,[255,256] brain tumors,[257] rectal cancer,[258] and liver cancer.[259]

Use of the Linear-Quadratic Model in Brachytherapy

Quantifying the Rationale for Low-Dose-Rate Brachytherapy

It has long been known that lowering the dose rate generally reduces radiobiologic damage[260] because of increased opportunity to repair sublethal damage.[236,237] It also has been clear since the pioneering work of Coutard[261] that fractionating or protracting a radiotherapeutic exposure improves the "therapeutic ratio" (ratio of tumor control to complications). However, the exact link between these observations was not clearly made until the 1980s by Withers et al.[262,263]

To understand their insight, consider the isoeffect curves in Figure 22.33 representing "equivalent" schemes for either early- or late-responding end points as a function of treatment time. For higher dose rates, the dose reduction needed to match late effects is larger than the dose reduction needed to match tumor control. For any selected dose, increasing the dose rate will increase late effects much more than it will increase tumor control. Conversely, decreasing the dose rate will decrease late effects much more than it will decrease tumor control. Thus, the therapeutic ratio increases as the dose rate decreases.

These observations can be interpreted in terms of the α/β ratio[262] in the LQ Eq. (40). In terms of survival curves (Fig. 22.34), the α/β ratio essentially describes the degree of "curviness" of the acute survival curve. A small value of α/β means that the β (dose squared) term dominates cell killing at radiotherapeutic doses, resulting in a curvy survival curve (Fig. 22.34). A large value of α/β means the α (linear in dose) term dominates, resulting in a straighter semi-log survival curve. Now, as a first approximation, the dose-response relation for a fractionated (or LDR) regimen can be thought of as simply the result of multiple repeats of the initial part of the survival

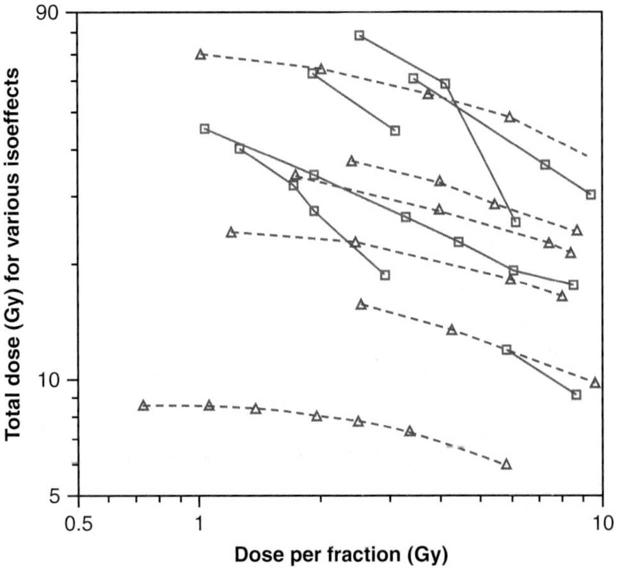

FIGURE 22.33. Isoeffect curves showing the total dose to produce a given end point, plotted against dose per fraction, a surrogate, in this context, for dose rate. The triangles, joined by dashed lines, refer to a variety of different early-responding end points (of which tumor control is an example), whereas the squares, joined by solid lines, refer to a variety of different late-responding sequelae. Note the generally steeper slopes of the solid lines, suggesting that late-responding tissues are more sensitive than early-responding tissues to changes in the protraction of a given radiation dose. (Adapted from Withers HR, Taylor JMG, Maciejewski B. The hazard of accelerated tumor clonogen repopulation during radiotherapy. *Acta Radiol* 1988;27:131–146.)

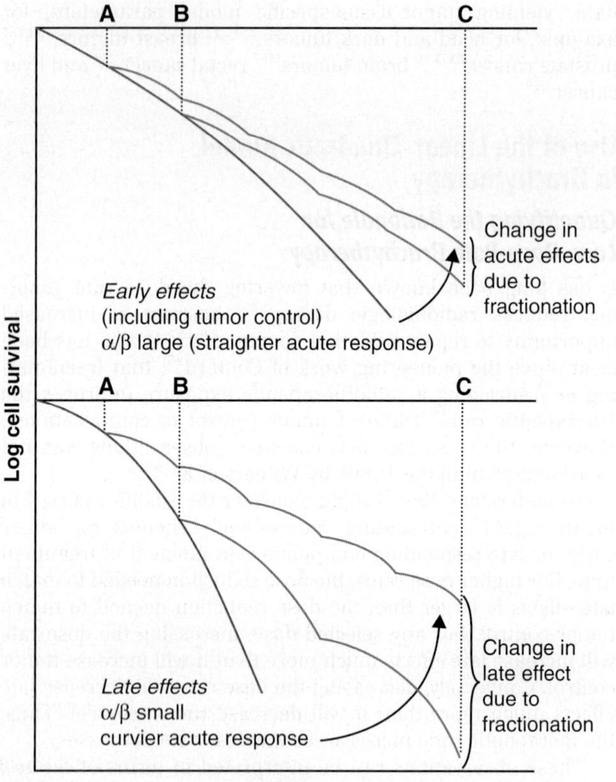

FIGURE 22.34. Illustration of the differing effects of protraction on early- and late-responding tissues, as elucidated by Thames et al.[262]

curve. It is clear that repeating the early part of a curvy survival curve many times will result in far more sparing than repeating the early part of a straighter survival curve.

Thus, late effects, which are very sensitive to changes in fractionation, are characterized by small values of α/β (a typical value is 3 Gy), and early effects (tumor control or early-responding normal sequelae) are characterized by large values of α/β, a typical value for most tumors being about 10 Gy. As clinical data from which α/β ratios can be derived have accumulated, the dichotomy between α/β ratios for early and late effects that has held up remarkably well. Consequently, when using the LQ model, it is essential to be clear about whether the calculation is designed to refer to early- or late-responding tissue, and to then use the appropriate α/β value. From Eq. (41), it is clear that use of different values of α/β will result in different predictions for the isoeffect dose.

Modeling the Effect of Treatment Time

For temporary implants or HDR, the effect of tumor cell repopulation is generally small, but this is not necessarily the case with longer permanent implants. By increasing the surviving fraction by a factor $\exp(\gamma T)$, where T is the overall treatment time, Eq. (40) can be modified to take into account repopulation as a function of T.[264] One can also take into account delay in the onset of accelerated repopulation, by replacing T with $(T - T_D)$, where T_D is the delay after the beginning of the treatment before tumor-cell proliferation begins.[240] With these two corrections, the surviving fraction becomes:

$$S = \exp(-\alpha D - G \cdot \beta D^2 + \gamma[T - T_D]) \qquad (44)$$

The parameter γ determines the speed of repopulation, and is given by $\gamma = 0.693/T_P$, where T_P is the effective doubling time of cells in the tumor. If we can ignore cell loss, T_P is the same as T_{POT}, which is the measurable[265] *in vitro* doubling time of the tumor cells.

If tumor repopulation is relevant, then, in order to design a new equivalent regimen, rather than matching the quantity $(\alpha D + G \cdot \beta D^2)$, we need to match $(\alpha D + G \cdot \beta D^2 - \gamma[T - T_D])$, and Eqs. (41) or (43) can be modified correspondingly.

Redistribution and Reoxygenation

Radiobiologic response is dominated by the four Rs: repair, repopulation, redistribution, and reoxygenation.[266] Eq. (40) describes repair, which is extended using Eq. (44) to include repopulation. The LQ model can be further extended to include the remaining two Rs[267] by treating redistribution of cells among the phases of the cell cycle and reoxygenation as a single phenomenon, termed resensitization, which occurs when a radiation exposure preferentially kills the more radiosensitive cells in a diverse population, leaving a cell population with decreased average radiosensitivity. Subsequent biologically driven changes then tend to gradually restore the original population average radiosensitivity. The resultant LQR model uses two additional adjustable parameters—an overall resensitization rate τ_S (analogous to sublethal damage repair rate) and overall resensitization amplitude $\frac{1}{2}\sigma^2$. The LQR model replaces the LQ Eq. (40) with:

$$S(D) = \exp(-\alpha D - G\beta D^2 + \tfrac{1}{2}\sigma^2 \hat{G} D^2). \qquad (45)$$

The new term, $\frac{1}{2}\sigma^2\hat{G}D^2$, is the product of $\frac{1}{2}\sigma^2$ (representing the average of the dominant resensitization effects over the heterogeneous tumor) while the factor $\hat{G}$ models the influence of fractionation on resensitization. In fact, $\hat{G}$ has exactly the same form as the sublethal damage repair function, G, except that μ is replaced by τ_S. In contrast to repair, resensitization tends to increase radiosensitivity as the overall time increases. For example, tumor cells in a resistant part of the cell cycle at the beginning of the treatment, and thus that were spared preferentially, may move to a more sensitive part of the cell cycle as the treatment progresses. While mechanistically driven, LQR is sufficiently simple that it can be used for isoeffect calculations in radiation therapy and supporting reasonable fits to relevant experimental data.[267]

If reoxygenation or repopulation are relevant, then, in order to design a new equivalent regimen, we need to match the quantity $(\alpha D + G\beta D^2 - \frac{1}{2}\sigma^2\hat{G}D^2)$ and Eqs. (41) or (43) can be modified correspondingly.

The Effects of Tumor Shrinkage

If the reference surface to which dose is prescribed diminishes in size as the tumor shrinks during the treatment, then the physical dose rate and total dose will increase as cells near the dose specification surface are closer to the implanted sources. This phenomenon has been described using the LQ formalism by Dale et al.[268,269] For permanent implants in tumors with long doubling times, tumor shrinkage may significantly enhance the clinical potential of longer-lived permanent implant radionuclides such as ^{125}I but would have much less effect for short-lived radionuclides such as ^{103}Pd or ^{131}Cs or for rapidly growing tumors. In fact, this is one argument against the use of long-lived nuclides for permanent-implant BT, in that the outcome may depend on shrinkage parameters that we are not able to predict.

Nonuniform Dose Distributions

The LQ model and many other radiobiologic models assume that an implant dose delivery can be approximated by a single uniformly administered prescribed dose, an assumption that ignores the highly nonuniform dose distributions produced by BT. Suppose the dose distribution over an organ or tumor is described by a DVH $\{D_i, v_i\}_{i=1}^{N}$, where v_i is the fractional volume of dose bin D_i. If the structure is a tumor, the biologic effect of this inhomogeneous dose distribution can be quantified by computing the overall surviving fraction S for the entire tumor target:

$$S(\{D_i, v_i\}) = \sum_{i=1}^{N} v_i S(D_i) = \sum_{i=1}^{N} \exp(-\alpha D_i - G_i \cdot \beta D_i^2) \quad (45)$$

where Eq. (40) has been used as an example. A more intuitive simple scalar metric for quantifying impact of such nonuniform dose is the equivalent uniform dose (EUD) concept proposed by Niemierko.[270] It is defined as the uniform dose that, if delivered with the same dose protraction regimen as the nonuniform dose distribution of interest, yields the same radiobiologic effect. In terms of BED and equivalent dose in 2 Gy fractions (D_{2Gy})s, EUD is given by:

$$EUD_{BED} = -\log[S(\{D_i, v_i\})]/\alpha$$

$$EUD_{2Gy} = \frac{-\log[S(\{D_i, v_i\})]}{\alpha(1 + 2/(\alpha/\beta))} \quad (46)$$

showing that EUD computation requires knowing the absolute value of α. To extend the concept of EUD to normal tissues, Mohan et al.[271] and then Niemierko[272] proposed a phenomenologic formula referred to as the generalized EUD or gEUD:

$$gEUD = \left(\sum_i v_i D_i^a\right)^{1/a}, \quad (47)$$

where v_i is the fractional organ volume receiving a dose D_i and a is a tissue-specific parameter that describes the volume effect. For $a \to -\infty$, gEUD approaches the minimum dose; thus, negative values of a are used for tumors. For $a \to +\infty$, gEUD approaches the maximum dose (serial organs). For $a = 1$, gEUD is equal to the arithmetic mean dose. For $a = 0$, gEUD is equal to the geometric mean dose. Unlike EUD, gEUD is a purely empirical model without a more mechanistic interpretation rooted in cell survival. However, the gEUD is often used as a plan comparison and optimization metric for EBRT and may be used for comparing different protraction schemes in BT because the same functional form can be applied to both target volumes and organs at risk (OARs) with a single parameter capturing (it is hoped) the dosimetric "essence" of the biologic response.

To compare different inhomogeneous dose distributions, TCP and NTCP can be computed by substituting Eq. (45) into the Poisson TCP model, Eq. (42), yielding

$$\begin{aligned} TCP(\{D_i, v_i\}) &= \exp\left(-K \cdot \sum_i v_i S(D_i)\right) \\ &= \prod_i [\exp(-K \cdot S(D_i))]^{v_i} \\ &= \exp(-K \cdot e^{-\alpha \cdot EUD_{BED}}) \end{aligned} \quad (48)$$

The second equation shows that inhomogeneous dose TCP, ($\{D_i, v_i\}$), is the product of exponentially scaled (by volume fraction, v_i) TCPs, each describing uniform tumor irradiation by dose bin D_i. The third equation shows that substituting EUD into the uniform dose TCP also reproduces TCP ($\{D_i, v_i\}$). Several authors[273,274] have extended this approach also to account for nonuniform distributions of target cells within the tumor and intertumoral radiosensitivity (α) variations over a patient population. Similar approaches have been proposed for NTCP models[275] based on the survival of functional subunits (FSUs). Many organs are best modeled by FSUs organized with a parallel architecture such that a complication results only when a sufficiently large number of FSUs are inactivated,[276] although serial architectures such as the spine can also be modeled.[273]

The Relative Effectiveness of Different Radioisotopes Used in Brachytherapy

As discussed earlier in this chapter, the mean photon energies of currently used BT radionuclides range from 398 keV (^{192}Ir) down to 21 keV (^{103}Pd). It is well established that biologic effectiveness varies with photon energy, as a result of different patterns of energy deposition produced by the different photon spectra.[277,278] It is possible, however, to estimate the RBE of these different isotopes directly from the energy deposition patterns—the subject matter of microdosimetry.[279] In this approach, the response per unit dose at low dose rates (or low doses), R_i, to a particular radiation, i, can be written as[280]:

$$R_i = \int w(y) \cdot d_i(y) \cdot dy \quad (49)$$

where y is the stochastic quantity, lineal energy,[279] defined as the energy deposited by a single photon track, divided by the average path length in the cellular target, and $d_i(y)$ is the dose-weighted probability that a photon will deposit lineal energy y in the target volume of interest. The quantity $d_i(y)$ often is referred to as the microdosimetric single-event spectrum. It can be measured using a low-pressure proportional counter or calculated.[279] The quantity w(y) describes the response of an individual cellular target to a lineal energy deposition, y. For sparsely ionizing radiations (e.g., photons and electrons), it is reasonable to assume that w(y) is proportional to y.[279] Thus, at low dose rates:

$$RBE_i \propto \int y \cdot d_i(y) \cdot dy \quad (50)$$

where $d_i(y)$ is the dose-averaged lineal energy. Based on this approach, RBE values have been estimated from measured or calculated microdosimetric spectra.[278,281] For example, Wuu et al.[278] report low–dose-rate RBE values relative to ^{60}Co of 1.3, 2.1, 2.1, and 2.3, respectively, for ^{192}Ir, ^{241}Am, ^{125}I, and ^{103}Pd. These values are comparable to those obtained experimentally. The approach outlined previously is applicable only to LDR BT, but it can be generalized to HDR regimens.[280] Incorporating the low–dose-rate RBE into the LQ equations is surprisingly easy,[282] requiring a simple modification of Eq. (41):

$$BED = D[RBE + G \cdot D/(\alpha/\beta)] \quad (51)$$

The LQ Model for Permanent Implants

To use the LQ model to predict the total dose that a permanent implant needs to deliver to a repopulating tumor with an effective doubling time of T_p, we need to match the quantity ($\alpha D + G \cdot \beta D^2 - \gamma[T - T_D]$) [see Eq. (44)] to an appropriate reference regimen. However, as shown by Dale,[283] the effective treatment time, T_{eff}, for a permanent implant is not infinite, but achieves a finite value when the dose rate becomes sufficiently low that the rate of cell kill equals the number of tumor cells created per unit time by repopulation, at which point the treatment is effectively over and any subsequent dose is wasted. This can be expressed by requiring that $\alpha(\partial BED(T_{eff})/\partial t) = \alpha\dot{D}_0 e^{-\lambda T_{eff}} \approx \gamma$, assuming that $G \approx 1$ at low dose rates and $TD \ll T_{eff}$. Thus:

$$T_{eff} = -\frac{1}{\lambda}\ln\left[\frac{0.693}{\alpha \dot{D}_0 T_{pot}}\right] = -\frac{1}{\lambda}\ln\left[\frac{\gamma}{\alpha \dot{D}_0}\right] \quad (52)$$

where λ is the radioactive decay constant of the particular nuclide used and T_{pot} is the potential doubling time of the tumor. At this time, T_{eff}, the dose that has been delivered, is not the total dose, D, but rather a smaller effective dose, given by:

$$D_{eff} = D(1 - e^{-\lambda T_{eff}}) \quad (53)$$

As an example, using reasonable parameters for prostate tumors, the effective dose for a 145-Gy ^{125}I permanent seed implant is actually 139 Gy, which is the value that would be used in LQ-based calculations.

The LQ model can be used to optimize the choice of radionuclide for a permanent implant.[284,285–286] The most common sources in current use are ^{125}I and ^{103}Pd (with half-lives of 59 and 17 days, respectively), although ^{131}Cs (half-life 10 days) is being increasingly considered.[287] The optimal radionuclide for a given tumor depends on its growth rate, α/β ratio, radiosensitivity (α), and DSB repair rate. Generally speaking, short-lived radionuclides are more advantageous for treating fast-growing tumors, while longer-lived radionuclides are more optimal for slow-growing tumors. However, short-lived radionuclides can effectively treat in addition, are less sensitive to the tumor properties and LQ parameter values assumed than is the case for long-lived radionuclides.

HDR Intracavitary Brachytherapy for Cervical Cancer

There has been a trend in the past few years toward increased use of HDR BT in some tumor sites, driven largely by the economic and logistical benefits of outpatient-based fractionated HDR BT. While sometimes delivered in a single fraction, more often three to 12 HDR fractions are used. In some situations, such as palliative or intraoperative BT, the therapeutic ratio between tumor control and late sequelae is not a primary consideration; but, in general for curative intent treatments, increasing the dose rate is likely to *decrease* the therapeutic advantage between tumor control and late sequelae. However, there are two curative applications (intracavitary implants for cancer of the uterine cervix and implant therapy for prostate cancer) where, for differing reasons, HDR BT is as effective, or potentially even more effective, compared to LDR BT.

The radiobiologic principles involved in converting LDR to HDR intracavitary insertions are illustrated schematically in Figure 22.35, which shows typical dose-response relationships for early- and late-responding tissues. As we have discussed, the dose-response relations for late effects are significantly "curvier" (smaller α/β ratio) than for early-responding tissues such as tumors, which have larger α/β ratios. Suppose that we want to replace an LDR treatment delivering dose D with an HDR treatment that gives identical tumor control. As illustrated in the left panel, we need to reduce the dose by a dose reduction factor, DRF (see left panel). From the right panel, however, it can be seen that this adjusted dose, DRF × D, will result in increased late effects compared to LDR. But now let us suppose that the LDR dose to OAR giving rise to the late effects is not the treatment dose D, but some lower dose (e.g., D/2). This is the case for cervical BT because the bladder and rectum are generally some significant distance from the cervical implant. From the right-hand panel in Figure 22.35, we see that if HDR preserves the LDR level of dose sparing (i.e., delivers dose DRF × D/2 to the OAR, where DRF matches tumor control), we will *not* get more late effects for HDR compared to LDR, but actually a similar late-effect probability because we are further up the survival curve. Indeed, if the rectal dose were an even smaller fraction of the treatment dose (say D/3, in Fig. 22.35), HDR would have even *fewer* late effects than the equivalent LDR regimen. In fact, if the cervical BT results in a dose to the bladder/rectum that is less than about three-fourths of the treatment dose, and then if the HDR dose is reduced to give equal tumor control compared with LDR, the HDR late effects should not be worse than the LDR late effects.[242,288]

Of course, there is another related factor to consider, which is that the short treatment time characteristic of HDR allows packing and retraction of the sensitive organs, which typically results in a 20% further decrease in the rectal/bladder dose compared to that achievable with LDR.[289] This gives an extra, physically based advantage to HDR, in addition to the biologic factors discussed here.

To summarize, radiobiologic considerations suggest that if the dose to the dose-limiting critical normal tissues (e.g., bladder and rectum) is less than about three-fourths of the prescribed dose, HDR BT (administered in five or more fractions to ensure adequate tumor reoxygenation) results in comparable (or fewer) late effects than LDR—for the same level of tumor control. These theoretical conclusions are supported by a number of clinical studies[290–296] showing that HDR and LDR for cervical BT produce similar rates of local control and late complications.

As BT is often combined with pelvic EBRT,[297] different time-dose patterns of EBRT and intracavitary BT should be taken into account to calculate the combined effects to tumor and OARs. For a given BT effective dose, BED_{BT}, the equivalent EBRT dose expressed in conventional fractionation of 2 Gy per day (EQD2) can be calculated as $EQD2 = BED_{BT}/(1 + 2/(\alpha/\beta))$. Also, the dose from EBRT has to be recalculated if a fractionation schedule different from 2 Gy per day is to be used. EQD2 values from EBRT and BT may be summed assuming that the volumes and points of interest of BT receive the stated EBRT dose. This estimate serves as a worst-case assumption for OARs and is reasonable for the BT target volume, which usually receives a uniform EBRT dose. More realistic calculations must consider the highly nonuniform dose delivery of BT and IMRT, as described in the next section.

Brachytherapy for Prostate Cancer

Optimized Dose Protraction for Prostate Cancer Brachytherapy

As discussed earlier, one of the main reasons for protracting any radiotherapeutic exposure is that protraction spares late responding normal tissues more than typical tumors; this strategy is supported by the generally lower α/β ratios found for late-responding normal tissues (3 Gy is typical) relative to tumors (10 Gy is typical). These different α/β ratios are thought to be due to the larger proportion of cycling cells in tumors compared with normal

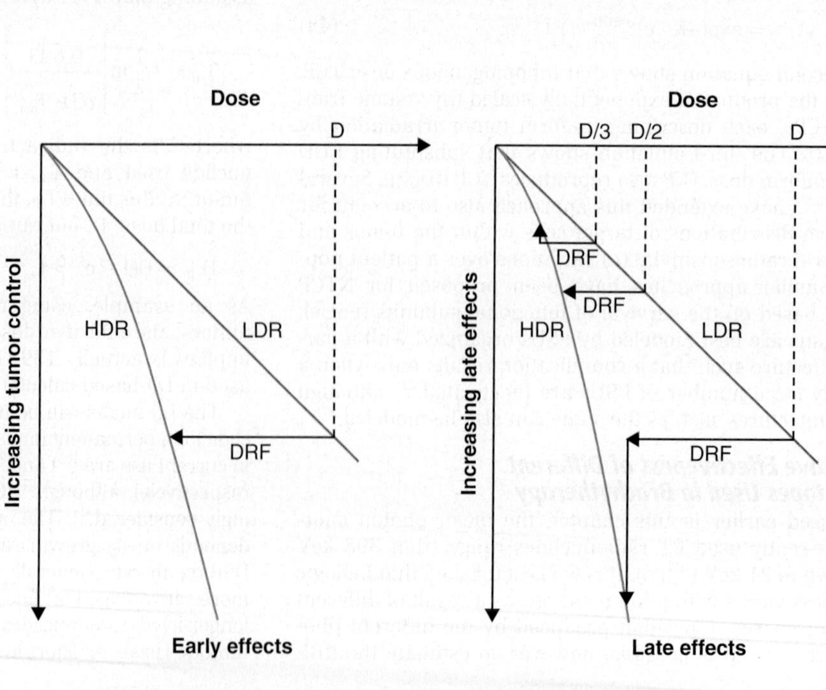

FIGURE 22.35. Illustration of the interplay between early and late effects for low-dose-rate (LDR) and high-dose-rate (HDR) brachytherapy for cervical cancer. DRF is the dose reduction factor that produces the same early effects (tumor control) for HDR as LDR. If D is the LDR giving rise to late effects, then reducing D by DRF for HDR will result in more late effects than at LDR. As the HDR dose to late-responding tissue is reduced by treatment planning, then reducing that dose by the factor DRF no longer produces worse late effects than at LDR.

tissues. Because prostate tumors contain unusually small fractions of cycling cells,[265] it has been hypothesized that they may have α/β ratios and responses to protraction more typical of late-responding normal tissues.[298,299] If so, much of the rationale for low dose rate, or highly fractionated regimens, would disappear.

A first estimate of α/β for prostate cancer was made in 1999[298] by comparing results from EBRT with those from permanent seed ^{125}I BT. Consistent with the theoretical hypotheses (see earlier), the estimated value of α/β was 1.5 Gy (95% confidence interval [CI]: 0.8 to 2.2 Gy), indeed comparable to α/β values for late-responding normal tissues and much smaller than those for most tumors.

Since this first estimate of α/β for prostate, there have been more than 20 further estimates.[256,300–305] These analyses have considered the impact of many potential biases and uncertainties, including the comparison of EBRT and permanent seed implant (which has much higher dose delivery uncertainties) outcomes; differences in dose inhomogeneity; RBE and overall time differences;[306] patient selection bias; differences in outcome endpoints; and[307] any or all of which could bias the α/β estimate. However, most of these analyses support the hypothesis that the α/β value for prostate cancer is indeed quite low, probably in the 1 to 4 Gy range, similar to those of most late-responding tissues. For example two studies each analyzed the results of more than 5,000 prostate cancer patients who received different external beam fractionation schedules, and derived estimated α/β values of 1.55 Gy[308] and 1.4 Gy[309] respectively. A review of all the studies concluded that the results are all reasonably consistent, the mean of all estimated values being 2.7 Gy.[310]

If the α/β value for prostate cancer is indeed similar to that for the surrounding late-responding normal tissue, HDR or hypofractionated external-beam therapy regimens could be employed to match conventional fractionated regimens with respect to tumor control and late sequelae while reducing early urinary sequelae[311] and improving cost-effectiveness and patient convenience.

The arguments presented here really relate to the α/β value for prostate cancer in relation to the α/β value for the relevant late-responding normal tissue. Brenner[312] reported an α/β value for Radiation Therapy Oncology Group (RTOG) grade 2 or higher late rectal toxicity of 5.4 ± 1.5 Gy based on an analysis of clinical data. Another recent analysis of RTOG 94-06 data suggested that the α/β value for grade 2 or higher late rectal toxicity was 4.8 Gy.[313] These α/β values, which are larger than that of most late-responding tissues, are higher than recent estimates of prostate tumor α/β ratio. This suggests that HDR prostate BT, as well as being logistically convenient, might actually improve the therapeutic outcome of prostate cancer BT.

HDR (or hypofractionation) in a curative setting, even when the dose is appropriately lowered, is a *prima facie* unsettling idea. However, there is now a significant body of clinical evidence suggesting that these approaches do not lead to increased early or late sequelae after prostate radiotherapy, either for EBRT or for BT, providing further evidence to support the underlying radiobiologic rationale. For EBRT, in those hypofractionation studies that have reported on late sequelae, to date there is little indication of any unexpected late sequelae after median follow-up periods of 48 to 97 months.[314–317] Indeed, two completed phase III trials have reported similar therapeutic ratios with a suggestion of an advantage for hypofractionation.[318,319] HDR has been used in prostate BT both as a monotherapy[320,321] and, more commonly, as a boost to external-beam radiotherapy.[322–325] In both cases, the results are promising with no evidence for excessive normal tissue complications. The American Brachytherapy Society has recently published consensus clinical and treatment planning guidance on HDR prostate brachytherapy.[326]

Comparing and Combining External-Beam Radiation Therapy with Brachytherapy for Prostate Cancer

BT (permanent-implant or HDR BT) is widely used in treatment of prostate cancer, either as sole therapy or as a boost in conjunction with EBRT. We can use the EUD formalism to compare the biologic effectiveness of various EBRT-BT combinations using the LQ model to account dose nonuniformity and dose-time fractionation effects at each voxel.[327] For typical DVHs, $\{D_i, v_i\}$, the surviving fraction for each modality is calculated by:

$$S(\{D_i, v_i\}) = \sum_{i=1}^{N} v_i e^{-\alpha D_i - G_i \cdot \beta D_i^2 + \gamma T_{eff}} \quad (54)$$

For EBRT and HDR BT treatment courses, delivering a total dose $D = nd$ of n fractions, T_{eff} is the number of treatment fractions multiplied by 1.4 (five fractions per week). Assuming each EBRT fraction is delivered over a short time relative to the repair half-time, $G = 1/n$. However, for each HDR BT fraction, the delivery time T_f (assumed to be 15 minutes in analysis to follow) is typically comparable to the repair half-time for prostate tumor cells,[327] necessitating a more complex sublethal damage repair correction[255,328]:

$$G = \frac{2}{n\mu T_f}\left[1 - \frac{1}{\mu T_f}(1 - e^{-\mu T_f})\right] \quad (55)$$

where μ and λ denote the sublethal damage repair rate and physical decay constant, respectively.

For permanent BT, the total dose D and effective treatment are given by Eqs. (53) and (52), respectively. The sublethal damage repair correction is given by[283,327]:

$$G = \frac{2\dot{D}_0^2}{D^2(\mu - \lambda)}\left[\frac{1}{2\lambda}(1 - e^{-2\lambda T_{eff}}) - \frac{1}{\mu + \lambda}(1 - e^{-(\mu+\lambda)T_{eff}})\right] \quad (56)$$

where $\dot{D}_0$ is the initial dose rate.

The overall surviving fraction S of a combined EBRT and BT regimen is given by:

$$S = S_{EBRT} \cdot S_{BT} \cdot e^{\gamma T'} \quad (57)$$

where S_{EBRT} and S_{BT} are estimated from Eq. (54) using typical DVHs and T′ is the time interval between the two treatments (T′ = 0 if the treatments are overlapped with each other). TCP may be calculated using Eq. (42). To quantify the combined-modality surviving fraction S in terms of EUD, relative to a reference EBRT regimen consisting of 2-Gy daily fractions, we compute:

$$EUD = \frac{-\log(S)}{\alpha + \beta d - 1.4\gamma/d} \quad (58)$$

Table 22.13 illustrates the combined-modality EUD evaluation, along with corresponding TCPs, for the RT regimens commonly used for localized high-risk prostate cancer. The results show that the permanent seed BT alone offers high-risk prostate cancer control rates intermediate to EBRT alone delivering conventional (70.2 Gy) and escalated (81 Gy) prescribed doses. An interesting observation is that combined treatments of EBRT and permanent/HDR BT support higher EUDs and

TABLE 22.13 COMPARING EBRT, BT, AND EBRT + BT BASED ON CALCULATED EUD AND TCP USING TWO SETS OF LQ PARAMETERS

Modalities	*Prescribed Dose[a] (Gy)*	*EUD[b] (Gy)*	*TCP[b] (%)*	*EUD[c] (Gy)*
EBRT alone	70.2	68	20	66
EBRT alone	81	78	87	77
^{125}I BT alone	145	71	43	71
^{103}Pd BT alone	124	74	69	77
EBRT + ^{125}I	45 (EBRT) + 108 (BT)	94	99	96
EBRT + ^{103}Pd	45 (EBRT) + 100 (BT)	103	100	104
EBRT + HDR	45 (EBRT) + 3 × 6 Gy (BT)	78	87	97

EBRT, external-beam radiation therapy; BT, brachytherapy; EUD, equivalent uniform dose; TCP, tumor control probability; LQ, linear-quadratic.

[a]For EBRT, 1.8-Gy fraction size assumed.

[b]LQ parameters:[256] $\alpha = 0.15$ Gy^{-1}, $\alpha/\beta = 3.1$ Gy, $T_r = 16$ minutes, $T_d = 42$ days, $K = 1.1 \times 10^7$.

[c]LQ parameters:[300] $\alpha = 0.039$ Gy^{-1}, $\alpha/\beta = 1.0$ Gy, $T_r = 1.9$ h and with repopulation effect ignored.

TABLE 22.14 PRESCRIBED BRACHYTHERAPY DOSE NEEDED TO ACHIEVE STATED CUMULATIVE EUD WHEN COMBINED WITH EBRT DOSE OF 46 Gy (2.0 Gy × 23)

Cumulative EUD[a]	*Permanent BT*		*HDR BT*			
	I-125	*Pd-103*	*2 Fractions*	*3 Fractions*	*4 Fractions*	*5 Fractions*
68 Gy	50 Gy	34 Gy	5.8 Gy × 2	4.5 Gy × 3	3.8 Gy × 4	3.2 Gy × 5
72 Gy	57 Gy	40 Gy	6.7 Gy × 2	5.2 Gy × 3	4.3 Gy × 4	3.7 Gy × 5
80 Gy	72 Gy	53 Gy	8.4 Gy × 2	6.5 Gy × 3	5.4 Gy × 4	4.7 Gy × 5
90 Gy	92 Gy	70 Gy	10.2 Gy × 2	8.1 Gy × 3	6.8 Gy × 4	5.9 Gy × 5
100 Gy	112 Gy	87 Gy	12.2 Gy × 2	9.5 Gy × 3	8.0 Gy × 4	7.0 Gy × 5
110 Gy	133 Gy	106 Gy	13.8 Gy × 2	10.8 Gy × 3	9.2 Gy × 4	8.0 Gy × 5

EUD, equivalent uniform dose; EBRT, external-beam radiation therapy.

[a]LQ parameters[256]: $\alpha = 0.15\ Gy^{-1}$, $\alpha/\beta = 3.1$ Gy, $T_r = 16$ minutes, $T_d = 42$ days, $K = 1.1 \times 10^7$.

TCPs, and therefore should lead to more disease control than either EBRT or BT monotherapy.

Table 22.14 demonstrates how the combined-modality LQ-EUD analysis can be applied to design brachytherapy dose prescription schedules. The prescribed BT dose needed to achieve cumulative EUDs ranging from 68 to 110 Gy for an ^{125}I, ^{103}Pd, or fractionated HDR implant when combined with an EBRT dose of 46 Gy is tabulated using the LQ parameter set b from Table 22.13. To achieve TCPs of 90% to 100%, cumulative EUDs in the range of 80 to 100 Gy must be delivered. It is gratifying to note that at the upper end of this EUD range, the predicted BT doses of 112 Gy, 87 Gy, and 9.5 Gy × 3 for ^{125}I, ^{103}Pd, and HDR BT, respectively, are close to those used in current clinical practice. The currently practiced multimodality regimen treatment (initial EBRT + permanent/HDR BT boost) is predicted to support superior tumor control than current monotherapy protocols. Hypofractionation with either EBRT or HDR BT can also improve EUD and TCP with significantly lower prescription doses. These radiobiologic tools may be useful in analyzing treatment outcomes or in designing clinical trials to explore new treatment regimens. However, caution needs to be exercised in using these results to modify clinical decisions. One must consider the radiation effects (e.g., EUD) not only on prostate but also on OARs. In addition, the results are sensitive to the LQ parameters used. For example, to achieve a specified EUD, the required EBRT prescribed doses for a fraction size of 4.0 Gy will vary by 10% as in the α/β ratio range of 1.5 to 3.1. Small uncertainties in the model parameters can lead to large EUD and TCP uncertainties if there are cold spots in the tumor and/or hot spots in normal tissue. For more detailed discussion of these issues, readers are referred to previous publications.[327,329,330]

Summary: Biophysical Outcome Models in Brachytherapy

This survey of biophysical models for predicting clinical outcomes from brachytherapy regimens shows that the basic linear-quadratic model is sufficiently supported by clinical experience to be used for developing equivalent fractionation regimens or for optimizing therapeutic ratios in many clinical settings. More sophisticated NTCP and TCP models, while not sufficiently robust for use in clinical planning, are able to semiquantitatively account for the LDR and HDR brachytherapy clinical outcomes in several sites in terms of underlying descriptive radiobiologic mechanisms.

CONCLUSIONS

This chapter has focused on several basic topics including the interplay between physical properties, single-source dosimetry, source-strength specification, classical interstitial and intracavitary brachytherapy systems and dose specification, and biologic effects and clinical utility of brachytherapy sources. Many topics usually covered in an introductory survey have been omitted. For a review of radiographic imaging and localization of brachytherapy sources, the reader is referred to more specialized recent reviews.[149,331] For discussions on quality assurance of manual and remote afterloading brachytherapy and treatment planning, the reader is referred to Chapters 23, 24, and 25 of this text as well as a number of excellent reviews[66,332–335] including appropriate chapters from *Brachytherapy Physics,* 2nd edition.[336] For a more systematic approach to brachytherapy quality management, including application of industrial engineering approaches, the textbook by Thomadsen[337] and the proceedings of recent ASTRO Symposium on quality assurance for technologically advanced radiation therapy[338] are recommended. For a discussion of brachytherapy licensing and regulatory issues, the review by Glasgow[339] is suggested. For more detailed discussions on applications of radiobiological models to clinical brachytherapy, the reader is referred to the many sources cited by this review.

SELECTED REFERENCES

A full list of references for this chapter is available online.

3. ICRU. *Dose and volume specification for reporting intracavitary therapy in gynecology: report 38.* Bethesda, MD: International Commission of Radiation Units and Measurements, 1985.
4. Williamson JF. Monte Carlo-based dose-rate tables for the Amersham CDCS.J and 3M model 6500 ^{137}Cs tubes. *Int J Radiat Oncol Biol Phys* 1998;41(4):959–970.
5. Rivard MJ, Coursey BM, DeWerd LA, et al. Update of AAPM Task Group No. 43 Report: a revised AAPM protocol for brachytherapy dose calculations. *Med Phys* 2004;31(3):633–674.
7. Perera H, Williamson JF, Li Z, et al. Dosimetric characteristics, air-kerma strength calibration and verification of Monte Carlo simulation for a new Ytterbium-169 brachytherapy source. *Int J Radiat Oncol Biol Phys* 1994;28:953–971.
8. Medich DC, Tries MA, Munro JJ 2nd. Monte Carlo characterization of an ytterbium-169 high dose rate brachytherapy source with analysis of statistical uncertainty. *Med Phys* 2006;33(1):163–172.
9. Tod MC, Meredith WJ. A dosage system for use in the treatment of cancer of the uterine cervix. *Br J Radiol* 1938;11:809–824.
10. Fletcher GH, Hamberger AD. Squamous cell carcinoma of the uterine cervix: treatment techniques according to size of the cervical lesion and extension. In: Fletcher GD, ed. *Textbook of radiotherapy,* 3rd ed. Philadelphia: Lea & Febiger, 1980:732–772.
11. Williamson JF. Brachytherapy technology and physics practice since 1950: a half-century of progress. *Phys Med Biol* 2006;51:R1–R23.
21. Rivard MJ. Dosimetry for Cf-252 neutron emitting brachytherapy sources: protocol, measurements, and calculations. *Med Phys* 1999;26(8):1503–1514.
22. Williamson JF. Semi-empirical dose-calculation models in brachytherapy. In: Thomadsen BR, Rivard MJ, Butler WM, eds. *Brachytherapy physics,* 2nd ed. Madison, WI: Medical Physics Publishing, 2005:201–232.
24. Henschke UK, Hilaris BS, Mahan GD. Afterloading in interstitial and intracavitary radiation therapy. *Am J Roentgenol* 1963;90:386–395.
28. Chiu-Tsao S-T. Episcleral eye plaques for treatment of intra-ocular malignancies and benign diseases. In: Thomadsen BR, Rivard MJ, Butler WM, eds. *Brachytherapy physics,* 2nd ed. Madison, WI: Medical Physics Publishing, 2005:673–706.
32. Lawrence DC, Sondhaus CA, Feder B, et al. Soft x-ray "seeds" for cancer therapy. *Radiology* 1966;86:143–143.
37. Murphy MK, Piper RK, Greenwood LR, et al. Evaluation of the new cesium-131 seed for use in low-energy x-ray brachytherapy. *Med Phys* 2004;31(6):1529–1538.
38. Holm HH, Juul N, Pederson JF. Transperineal Iodine-125 seed implantation in prostatic cancer guided by transrectal ultrasonography. *J Urol* 1983;130:283–286.
39. Blasko JC, Radge H, Schumacker D. Transperineal percutaneous Iodine-125 implantation for prostatic carcinoma using transrectal ultrasound and template guidance. *Endocuriether Hypertherm Oncol* 1987;3:131–139.
40. Grimm PD, Blasko JC, Sylvester JE, et al. 10-year biochemical (prostate-specific antigen) control of prostate cancer with (125)I brachytherapy. *Int J Radiat Oncol Biol Phys* 2001;51(1):31–40.
42. Rivard MJ, Butler WM, DeWerd LA, et al. Supplement to the 2004 update of the AAPM Task Group No. 43 report. *Med Phys* 2007;34(6):2187–2205.
43. Joint AAPM/RPC registry of brachytherapy sources meeting the AAPM dosimetric prerequisites. 2011. Available at: http://rpc.mdanderson.org/rpc./ Accessed October 11, 2011.
45. Ling CC, Yorke ED, Spiro IJ. Physical dosimetry of I-125 seeds of a new design for interstitial implant. *Int J Radiat Oncol Biol Phys* 1983;9:1747–1752.
49. Monroe JI, Williamson JF. Monte Carlo-aided dosimetry of the Theragenics TheraSeed® model 200 ^{103}Pd interstitial brachytherapy seed. *Med Phys* 2002; 29:609–621.
50. Williamson JF, Rivard MJ. Quantitative dosimetry methods for brachytherapy. In: Thomadsen BR, Rivard MJ, Butler WM, eds. *Brachytherapy physics,* 2nd ed. Madison, WI: Medical Physics Publishing, 2005:233–294.
51. DeWerd LA, Ibbott GS, Meigooni AS, et al. A dosimetric uncertainty analysis for photon-emitting brachytherapy sources: report of AAPM Task Group No. 138 and GEC-ESTRO. *Med Phys* 2011;38(2):782–801.
58. Williamson JF, Rivard MJ. Thermoluminescent detector and Monte Carlo techniques for reference-quality brachytherapy dosimetry. In: Rogers DWO, Cygler J, eds. *Clinical dosimetry measurements in radiotherapy (AAPM 2009 Summer School).* Madison, WI: Medical Physics Publishing, 2009:437–499.
61. ICRU. *Dose and volume specification for reporting interstitial therapy.* Report No. 58. Bethesda, MD: International Commission on Radiation Units and Measurements, 1997.
64. Seltzer SM, Lamperti PJ, Loevinger R, et al. New national air-kerma-strength standards for ^{125}I and ^{103}Pd brachytherapy seeds. *J Res Natl Inst Stand Technol* 2003;108:337–358.
65. DeWerd LA. Calibration of brachytherapy sources. In: Thomadsen BR, Rivard MJ, Butler WM, eds. *Brachytherapy physics,* 2nd ed. Madison, WI: Medical Physics Publishing, 2005:153–172.

66. Nath R, Anderson LL, Meli JA, et al. Code of practice for brachytherapy physics: report of the AAPM Radiation Therapy Committee Task Group No. 56. American Association of Physicists in Medicine. *Med Phys* 1997;24(10):1557–1598.
67. ICRU. *Fundamental quantities and units for ionizing radiation.* Report No. 58. Bethesda, MD: International Commission on Radiation Units and Measurements, 1998.
76. Attix FH, Ritz VH. A Determination of fhe gamma-ray emission of radium. *J Res Natl Bureau Standards* 1957;59:293–305.
78. Meisberger LL, Keller RJ, Shalek RJ. The effective attenuation in water of the γ-rays of gold-198, iridium-192, cesium-137, radium-226, and cobalt-60. *Radiology* 1968; 90:953–957.
86. Williamson JF. The Sievert integral revised: evaluation and extension to low energy brachytherapy sources. *Int J Radiat Oncol Biol Phys* 1996;36:1239–1250.
97. Loftus TP. Exposure standardization of Iodine-125 seeds used for brachytherapy. *J Res Natl Bureau Standards* 1984;89:295–303.
98. Nath R, Anderson LL, Luxton G, et al. Dosimetry of interstitial brachytherapy sources: recommendations of the AAPM Radiation Therapy Committee Task Group No. 43. *Med Phys* 1995;22(2):209–234.
107. Williamson JF, Perera H, Li Z, et al. Comparison of calculated and measured heterogeneity correction factors for ^{125}I, ^{137}Cs and ^{192}Ir brachytherapy sources near localized heterogeneities. *Med Phys* 1993;20:209–222.
108. Anderson LL, Nath R, Weaver KA, et al. *Interstitial brachytherapy: physical, biological and clinical considerations.* New York: Raven, 1990.
111. Williamson JF. Comparison of measured and calculated dose rates in water near I-125 and Ir-192 seeds. *Med Phys* 1991;28:776–786.
114. Williamson JF, Coursey BM, DeWerd LA, et al. Dosimetric prerequisites for routine clinical use of new low energy photon interstitial brachytherapy sources. *Med Phys* 1998;25(12):2269–2270.
119. Chibani O, Williamson JF. MCPI: a sub-minute Monte Carlo dose calculation engine for prostate implants. *Med Phys* 2005;32(12):3688–3698.
120. Sampson A, Le Y, Williamson JF. Fast patient-specific Monte Carlo brachytherapy dose calculations via the correlated sampling variance reduction technique. *Med Phys* 2012;39:1058–1069.
121. Taylor RE, Yegin G, Rogers DW. Benchmarking brachydose: voxel based EGSnrc Monte Carlo calculations of TG-43 dosimetry parameters. *Med Phys* 2007;34(2): 445–457.
123. Zourari K, Pantelis E, Moutsatsos A, et al. Dosimetric accuracy of a deterministic radiation transport based ^{192}Ir brachytherapy treatment planning system. Part I: single sources and bounded homogeneous geometries. *Med Phys* 2010;37(2):649–661.
124. Rivard MJ, Venselaar JLM, Beaulieu L. The evolution of brachytherapy treatment planning. *Med Phys* 2009;36(6):2136–2153.
125. Williamson JF, Coursey BM, DeWerd LA, et al. Guidance to users of Nycomed Amersham and North American Scientific, Inc. I-125 interstitial sources: dosimetry and calibration changes: recommendation of the American Association of Physicists in Medicine Radiation Therapy Committee Ad Hoc Subcommittee on Low-Energy Seed Dosimetry. *Med Phys* 1999;26:570–573.
126. Williamson JF, Butler W, Dewerd LA, et al. Recommendations of the American Association of Physicists in Medicine regarding the impact of implementing the 2004 task group 43 report on dose specification for ^{103}Pd and ^{125}I interstitial brachytherapy. *Med Phys* 2005;32(5):1424–1439.
127. DeWerd LA, Huq MS, Das IJ, et al. Procedures for establishing and maintaining consistent air-kerma strength standards for low-energy, photon-emitting brachytherapy sources: recommendations of the Calibration Laboratory Accreditation Subcommittee of the American Association of Physicists in Medicine. *Med Phys* 2004;31(3):675–681.
128. Li ZF, Das RK, DeWerd LA, et al. Dosimetric prerequisites for routine clinical use of photon emitting brachytherapy sources with average energy higher than 50 kev. *Med Phys* 2007;34(1):37–40.
129. Parker HM. A dosage system for interstitial radium therapy. II. Physical aspects. *Br J Radiol* 1938;11:252–266.
131. Paterson R, Parker HM. A dosage system for γ-ray therapy. *Br J Radiol* 1934;7: 592–632.
140. Dutriex A, Marinello G. The Paris system. In: Pierquin B, Wilson JF, Chassagne D, eds. *Modern brachytherapy.* New York: Masson, 1987:25–42.
142. Gillin MT, Mourtada F. Manchester planar and volume implants and the Paris system. In: Thomadsen BR, Rivard MJ, Butler WM, eds. *Brachytherapy physics,* 2nd ed. Madison, WI: Medical Physics Publishing, 2005:351–372.
146. Yu Y, Anderson LL, Li Z, et al. Prostate seed implant brachytherapy: report of the American Association of Physicists in Medicine Task Group No. 64. *Med Phys* 1999;26:2054–2076.
147. Merrick GS, Butler WM, Dorsey AT, et al. Potential role of various dosimetric quality indicators in prostate brachytherapy. *Int J Radiat Oncol Biol Phys* 1999; 44(3):717–724.
155. Saw CB, Suntharalingam N. Reference dose rates for single and double plane ^{192}Ir implants. *Med Phys* 1988;15:391–396.
157. Nath R, Bice WS, Butler WM, et al. AAPM recommendations on dose prescription and reporting methods for permanent interstitial brachytherapy for prostate cancer: report of Task Group 137. *Med Phys* 2009;36(11):5310–5322.
174. Williamson J, Cormack R. Three-dimensional conformal brachytherapy: current trends and future promise. In: Timmerman R, Xing L, eds. *Image guided and adaptive radiation therapy.* Philadelphia: Wolters Kluwer-Lippincott Williams & Wilkins, 2010:99–188.
175. Butler WM, Merrick GS, Lief JH. Comparison of seed loading approaches in prostate brachytherapy. *Med Phys* 2000;27:381–392.
177. Lessard E, Pouliot J. Inverse planning anatomy-based dose optimization for HDR-brachytherapy of the prostate using fast simulated annealing algorithm and dedicated objective function. *Med Phys* 2001;28:773–779.
182. Ezzell GA. Optimization in brachytherapy. In: Thomadsen BR, Rivard MJ, Butler WM, eds. *Brachytherapy physics,* 2nd ed. Madison, WI: Medical Physics Publishing, 2005:415–434.
187. Potters L, Cao Y, Calugaru E, et al. A comprehensive review of CT-based dosimetry parameters and biochemical control in patients treated with permanent prostate brachytherapy. *Int J Radiat Oncol Biol Phys* 2001;50:605–614.
189. Zelefsky MJ, Yamada Y, Cohen GN, et al. Intraoperative real-time planned conformal prostate brachytherapy: post-implantation dosimetric outcome and clinical implications. *Radiother Oncol* 2007;84(2):185–189.
191. Nag S, Ciezki JP, Cormack R, et al. Intraoperative planning and evaluation of permanent prostate brachytherapy: report of the American Brachytherapy Society. *Int J Radiat Oncol Biol Phys* 2001;51(5):1422–1430.
192. Tod M, Meredith WJ. Treatment of cancer of the cervix uteri: a revised Manchester method. *Br J Radiol* 1953;26:252–257.
193. Fletcher GH. Cervical radium applicators with screening in the direction of bladder and rectum. *Radiology* 1953;60:77–84.
194. Meredith WJ. Dosage for cancer of cervix uteri. In: Meredith WJ, ed. *Radium dosage: the Manchester system,* 2nd ed., Edinburgh: E. & S, Livingston, Ltd., 1967: 42–50.
204. Potish RA, Gerbi BJ. Role of point A in the era of computerized dosimetry. *Radiology* 1986;158:827–831.
213. Eisbruch A, Williamson JF, Dickson R, et al. Estimation of tissue volume irradiated by intracavitary implants. *Int J Radiat Oncol Biol Phys* 1993;25:733–344.
220. Gebara WJ, Weeks KJ, Hahn CA, et al. Computed axial tomography tandem and ovoids (CATTO) dosimetry: three-dimensional assessment of bladder and rectal doses. *Radiat Oncol Investig* 1998;6(6):268–275.
223. Haie-Meder C, Potter R, Van Limbergen E, et al. Recommendations from Gynaecological (GYN) GEC-ESTRO Working Group (I): concepts and terms in 3D image based 3D treatment planning in cervix cancer brachytherapy with emphasis on MRI assessment of GTV and CTV. *Radiother Oncol* 2005;74(3):235–245.
224. Nag S, Cardenes H, Chang S, et al. Proposed guidelines for image-based intracavitary brachytherapy for cervical carcinoma: report from Image-Guided Brachytherapy Working Group. *Int J Radiat Oncol Biol Phys* 2004;60(4):1160–1172.
225. Potter R, Haie-Meder C, Van Limbergen E, et al. Recommendations from gynaecological (GYN) GEC ESTRO working group (II): concepts and terms in 3D image-based treatment planning in cervix cancer brachytherapy-3D dose volume parameters and aspects of 3D image-based anatomy, radiation physics, radiobiology. *Radiother Oncol* 2006;78(1):67–77.
226. Kidd EA, Siegel BA, Dehdashti F, et al. Clinical outcomes of definitive intensity-modulated radiation therapy with fluorodeoxyglucose-positron emission tomography simulation in patients with locally advanced cervical cancer. *Int J Radiat Oncol Biol Phys* 2010;77(4):1085–1091.
228. Potter R, Georg P, Dimopoulos JCA, et al. Clinical outcome of protocol based image (MRI) guided adaptive brachytherapy combined with 3D conformal radiotherapy with or without chemotherapy in patients with locally advanced cervical cancer. *Radiother Oncol* 2011;100(1):116–123.
231. Christensen GE, Carlson B, Chao KS, et al. Image-based dose planning of intracavitary brachytherapy: registration of serial-imaging studies using deformable anatomic templates. *Int J Radiat Oncol Biol Phys* 2001;51(1):227–243.
241. Dale RG. The application of the linear-quadratic dose-effect equation to fractionated and protracted radiotherapy. *Br J Radiol* 1985;58:515–528.
242. Brenner DJ, Hall EJ. Fractionated high dose-rate versus low dose-rate brachytherapy of the cervix. I. General considerations based on radiobiology. *Br J Radiol* 1991;64:133–141.
256. Wang JZ, Guerrero M, Li XA. How low is the alpha/beta ratio for prostate cancer? *Int J Radiat Oncol Biol Phys* 2003;55(1):194–203.
260. Hall EJ, Bedford JS. Dose-rate: its effect on the survival of HeLa cells irradiated with gamma-rays. *Radiat Res* 1964;22:305–315.
267. Brenner DJ, Hlatky LR, Hahnfeldt PJ, et al. A convenient extension of the linear-quadratic model to include redistribution and reoxygenation. *Int J Radiat Oncol Biol Phys* 1995;32:379–390.
268. Dale RG, Jones B. The effect of tumour shrinkage on biologically effective dose, and possible implications for fractionated high dose rate brachytherapy. *Radiother Oncol* 1994;33:125–132.
270. Niemierko A. Reporting and analyzing dose distributions: a concept of equivalent uniform dose. *Med Phys* 1997;24(1):103–110.
271. Mohan R, Mageras GS, Baldwin B, et al. Clinically relevant optimization of 3-D conformal treatments. *Med Phys* 1992;19(4):933–944.
274. Webb S, Nahum AE. A model for calculating tumour control probability in radiotherapy including the effects of inhomogeneous distributions of dose and clonogenic cell density. *Phys Med Biol* 1993;38(6):653–666.
275. Yorke ED. Modeling the effects of inhomogeneous dose distributions in normal tissues. *Semin Radiat Oncol* 2001;11(3):197–209.
276. Jackson A, Kutcher GJ, Yorke ED. Probability of radiation-induced complications for normal tissues with parallel architecture subject to non-uniform irradiation. *Med Phys* 1993;20(3):613–625.
283. Dale RG. Radiobiological assessment of permanent implants using tumor repopulation factors in the linear-quadratic model. *Br J Radiol* 1989;62(735):241–244.
284. Armpilia CI, Dale RG, Coles IP, et al. The determination of radiobiologically optimized half-lives for radionuclides used in permanent brachytherapy implants. *Int J Radiat Oncol Biol Phys* 2003;55(2):378–385.
287. Bice WS, Prestidge BR, Kurtzman SM, et al. Recommendations for permanent prostate brachytherapy with (131)Cs: a consensus report from the Cesium Advisory Group. *Brachytherapy* 2008;7(4):290–296.
288. Brenner DJ, Huang Y-P, Hall EJ. Fractionated high dose-rate versus low dose-rate regimens for intracavitary brachytherapy of the cervix: equivalent regimens for combined brachytherapy and external irradiation. *Int J Radiat Oncol Biol Phys* 1991;21:1415–1423.
298. Brenner DJ, Hall EJ. Fractionation and protraction for radiotherapy of prostate carcinoma. *Int J Radiat Oncol Biol Phys* 1999;43(5):1095–1101.
300. Fowler J, Chappell R, Ritter M. Is alpha/beta for prostate tumors really low? *Int J Radiat Oncol Biol Phys* 2001;50(4):1021–1031.
306. Brenner DJ, Martinez AA, Edmundson GK, et al. Direct evidence that prostate tumors show high sensitivity to fractionation (low alpha/beta ratio), similar to late-responding normal tissue. *Int J Radiat Oncol Biol Phys* 2002;52(1):6–13.
309. Miralbell R, Roberts SA, Zubizarreta E, et al. Dose-fractionation sensitivity of prostate cancer deduced from radiotherapy outcomes of 5,969 patients in seven international institutional datasets: α/β = 1.4 (0.9-2.2) Gy. *Int J Radiat Oncol Biol Phys* 2011.
313. Tucker SL, Thames HD, Michalski JM, et al. Estimation of α/β for late rectal toxicity based on RTOG 94-06. *Int J Radiat Oncol Biol Phys* 2011;81(2):600–605.
327. Wang JZ, Li XA. Evaluation of external beam radiotherapy and brachytherapy for localized prostate cancer using equivalent uniform dose. *Med Phys* 2003; 30(1):34–40.
328. Dale RG. The application of the linear-quadratic dose-effect equation to fractionated and protracted radiotherapy. *Br J Radiol* 1985;58(690):515–528.
329. Haworth A, Ebert M, Waterhouse D, et al. Prostate implant evaluation using tumour control probability - the effect of input parameters. *Phys Medi Biol* 2004; 49(16):3649–3664.
330. Li XA, Wang JZ, Stewart RD, et al. Designing equivalent treatment regimens for prostate radiotherapy based on equivalent uniform dose. *Br J Radiol* 2008; 81(961):59–68.

Chapter 23
Clinical Applications of Brachytherapy: Low-Dose Rate and Pulsed-Dose Rate

Alexandra J. Stewart, Caroline L. Halloway, and Phillip M. Devlin

Brachytherapy was the first form of conformal radiation therapy, utilizing placement of radioactive sources within or very close to a tumor and allowing high cancer to normal tissue dose ratios. From the time that Roentgen discovered radiography, the effects of ionizing radiation on the skin were noticed. Those exposed to the early cathode ray tubes, both patients and radiographers, developed radiation dermatitis and hair loss. After the isolation of radium, Henri Bequerel and Pierre Curie reported radium burns similar to those experienced by the early x-ray users. Radium was first used to treat skin lesions and superficial tumors using boxes and tubes as applicators. From there, radium in metal needles or radon gas in glass seeds were placed in direct contact with tumors using surface applicators, intracavitary, and interstitial implants.[1] Source positioning within the tumor allowed high doses within the cancer with small volumes of normal tissue irradiated and sufficient dose at the margin between cancer and normal tissue to eradicate microscopic tumor foci. Early results were promising and revolutionized cancer treatment.

In the 1950s, the use of brachytherapy was widespread; however, at that time brachytherapy had a number of disadvantages. Classical radium needles were rigid with a wide outer diameter (≥1.5 mm).[2] Brachytherapists had to have a high level of surgical skill to site the needles accurately, to achieve good dosimetry and quickly, and to minimize their own and others' radiation exposure. Therefore, the emergence of teletherapy, with its advantages of decreased staff radiation exposure and radiation accessibility to more areas of the body with no dependence on surgical techniques, led to a decrease in the use of brachytherapy.

However, brachytherapy has experienced a revival due to the emergence of newer artificial high-activity isotopes, afterloading systems, and improved radiological imaging with more sophisticated dose planning techniques. Modern radiotherapy techniques have focused on dose escalation to the target and decreasing the dose to normal tissues. Brachytherapy can deliver both of these objectives in a highly conformal manner over a wide variety of disease sites. Factors such as patient convenience, for example, prostate brachytherapy requiring one or two hospital visits compared to 7 to 8 weeks with prostate external beam radiotherapy (EBRT), and high reimbursement in nonnationalized health care systems have also played a part in the resurgence of brachytherapy.

Early texts describe the important principles of brachytherapy as uniformity in cross section, depth, and opportunity (time).[2] These principles remain the cornerstone of modern brachytherapy practice, although modern techniques allow better assessment of these. CT and MRI scanning has enabled enhanced imaging in brachytherapy, allowing more accurate target definition, superior determination of applicator position, and improved evaluation of the position of normal tissues. In combination with computerized dosimetry, this has allowed better determination of the dosimetric coverage of a brachytherapy implant and an estimation of the subsequent risk of normal tissue toxicity.

DOSE RATE DEFINITIONS

Three categories of brachytherapy were defined in Report 38 of the International Commission on Radiation Units and Measurements[3]:

- Low-dose rate (LDR): a range of 0.4 to 2 Gy per hour. In clinical practice the usual range is 0.4 to 1 Gy per hour.
- Medium-dose rate (MDR): a range of 2 to 12 Gy per hour.
- High-dose rate (HDR): over 12 Gy per hour.

Permanent seed implants deliver a high total dose at a very low-dose rate (vLDR), usually at <0.4 Gy per hour. Pulsed-dose rate (PDR) brachytherapy was developed in an effort to simulate the radiobiological advantages and dosimetric properties of LDR, but with the advantages of computer optimization of dose, a stepping source, and remote afterloading usually achieved by HDR. A source with activity in the realm of one-tenth of HDR activity is used. Generally, the same total dose and total time as LDR are prescribed but the radiation is administered in a large number of small fractions, usually a pulse every 1 to 4 hours. There are indications that the toxicity of PDR can be the same as for LDR or HDR in clinical practice.[4,5] It also has the advantage of a single afterloaded source compared to an inventory of LDR sources of different strengths. This will become increasingly important as manufacture of traditional LDR sources ceases and disposal costs of existing LDR sources rise. Table 23.1 demonstrates the advantages and disadvantages of LDR and PDR brachytherapy.

TABLE 23.1 THE ADVANTAGES AND DISADVANTAGES OF LOW-DOSE RATE (LDR) AND PULSED-DOSE RATE (PDR) BRACHYTHERAPY

Advantages		*Disadvantages*	
LDR	*PDR*	*LDR*	*PDR*
>100 years of data	Source easily available	Often inpatient treatment with prolonged bed rest	One machine per patient used for 3–5 days
Standardized doses	Standard source strength	Radiation exposure to staff	More intense maintenance
Standardized treatment plans	Minimal staff exposure	Limited by available source strength	Requires more physician–physicist time in certain locations
Less source changes needed (depending on isotope used)	Dose optimization of normal tissues	Many LDR sources no longer being manufactured	More expensive than LDR[a]
Less shielding needed during treatment	Radiation free periods aid nursing care		Caution with conversion of dose from LDR to PDR especially as intervals increase
	No source inventory required		May require prolonged bed rest depending on implant location
	With short pulse intervals uses log held doses with known safety and efficacy		

[a]See ref. 251.

CLINICAL USES OF BRACHYTHERAPY ISOTOPES

Brachytherapy uses radioactive isotopes to deliver therapeutic doses of radiation (Table 23.2). The ideal radioisotope for brachytherapy should have a relatively short half-life in order to deliver the radiation in as short a time as possible and a high specific activity so that the source is small and therefore more versatile to implant. The emissions produced should have an adequate penetration to deliver the dose to the depth desired with rapid falloff to prevent damage to the surrounding normal tissue. Particular source characteristics such as half-life or specific activity can be tailored to the tumor and the surrounding organs at risk (OAR).

Temporary Implants

The first temporary isotope used was radium-226 (^{226}Ra), which was generally implanted in metal tubes with 1-mm platinum filtration. These were bulky, inflexible needles that were difficult to implant and resulted in a high radiation exposure to surrounding staff. Radium-226 also has an extremely long half-life for future disposal concerns. Cobalt-60 (^{60}Co) was one of the first artificial radionuclides used, available in interstitial needles and wires, but its usefulness for brachytherapy was limited by its low activity and short half-life, although it is used in afterloaders in the developing world with the advantage of decreased pressure on quality assurance and cost.[6,7] Cesium-137 (^{137}Cs) sealed into a ceramic or glass pellets was in use from the 1960s. From the 1970s, ^{137}Cs was the predominant isotope used worldwide for intracavitary gynecologic implants. However, production of this isotope ceased in 2002 and most departments wishing to continue using LDR-style dose and characteristics have switched to isotopes more suitable for remote afterloading, often using PDR techniques. Strontium-90 (^{90}Sr) is a pure beta-emitter; therefore, it is suitable for very superficial applications and commonly used for coronary brachytherapy and ophthalmic problems such as pterygium. It has a half-life of 28.1 years, so many departments are still using applicators purchased in the 1980s. Ruthenium-106 (^{106}Ru) is also a beta-emitter but with a much shorter half-life (1 year), lessening disposal concerns and making treatment delivery faster.

Iridium-192 (^{192}Ir) has been used since the 1960s in afterloading systems—both manual and remote. Its high specific activity makes it extremely suitable for remote afterloading due to the increased flexibility available with a smaller source. The small source size has enabled implants in areas where cesium sources would be too large, and the afterloading machine allows implants into much longer applicators, such as the esophagus and bronchus, than was easily attainable with manually afterloaded ^{192}Ir wires.

Permanent Implants

Radon-222 gas (^{222}Rn) sealed into glass seeds was used in the first permanent implants. This had a very short half-life and required harvesting from radium sources. Gold-198 (^{198}Au) was the first artificial isotope to be used in permanent implants. It matched the classical LDR dose rate of 0.3 to 1 Gy per hour but with such a short half-life did not overcome the logistical problems of ^{222}Rn (i.e., time and radiation protection). The newer artificial isotopes—iodine-125 (^{125}I), palladium-103 (^{103} Pd), and cesium-131 (^{131}Cs)—are all used in modern permanent vLDR implants. The isotope used can be chosen according to its individual characteristics, which may be desirable in different implants (e.g., slower dose delivery may decrease normal tissue toxicity or a tumor with a higher alpha/beta ratio may theoretically have more cell kill using an isotope with a shorter half-life). All three isotopes are almost completely shielded with 0.2 cm of lead foil, making radiation protection easier.

Clinical Suitability for Brachytherapy

Cancers with clinically and radiologically well-defined margins with a low risk of regional and metastatic spread are the most suitable for brachytherapy as a single modality. However, brachytherapy is becoming increasingly important when integrated with EBRT to give a highly localized boost. EBRT is used to sterilize a larger area of possible microscopic or nodal spread with brachytherapy used for areas of gross macroscopic or microscopic residual disease. This ensures that high doses are achieved within tumors while normal tissues are not taken beyond recognized organ tolerance levels. It also has the potential for highly conformal localized dose escalation to areas at high risk of tumor recurrence.

In EBRT the dosimetric goal is a homogeneous dose distribution with doses ranging from 95% to 107% of the prescribed dose.[8] In contrast, brachytherapy has an extremely heterogeneous dose distribution with isolated areas receiving in excess of 200% of the dose. The steep gradients are a consequence of the proximity of the clinical target volume (CTV) to the sources and decreasing dose with distance secondary to the inverse square law. The normal tissues benefit from the inherent heterogeneity of the brachytherapy dose. As the dose falls off with distance, the normal tissue experiences not only a reduced dose but also a reduced dose rate, which results in enhanced cell sparing. The sharp dose fall off with brachytherapy contrasts with the more gradual dose fall off seen with EBRT.

Brachytherapy can be given over a short duration (e.g., using LDR a radical head and neck treatment course can be administered over 5 to 6 days compared to 5 to 7 weeks for a conventional EBRT head and neck regime). Brachytherapy can also be used as a method of retreatment when a patient has received irradiation to normal tissue tolerance using EBRT. Using the principles described above of sharp dose falloff and highly conformal dosing, a clinically useful radiation dose can be administered while minimizing the risk of increased late toxicity resulting from reirradiation.

Brachytherapy can be used anywhere in the body that can be accessed for direct source placement. For many years, surface applicators and intracavitary gynecologic brachytherapy were the

TABLE 23.2 CHARACTERISTICS OF RADIOISOTOPES THAT CAN BE USED FOR BRACHYTHERAPY

	Isotope	*Half-Life*	*Principal Emission*	*Mean Photon Energy*	*Half Value Layer (mm of Lead)*
Temporary	Radium 226	1,602 years	Gamma	0.83 MeV[a]	14
	Cobalt-60	5.27 years	Gamma	1.25 MeV	10.2
	Caesium-137	30.07 years	Gamma	0.662 MeV	5.57
	Iridium-192	74.2 days	Gamma	0.38 MeV	2.5
	Strontium-90	28.78 years	Beta	0.54 MeV	0.14
	Phosphorus-32	14.26 days	Beta	1.7 MeV	Minimal[b]
Permanent	Radon-222	3.82 days	Gamma/Beta	5.59 MeV	Minimal[b]
	Gold-198	2.7 days	Gamma/Beta	0.412 MeV	2.68
	Iodine 125	59.6 days	Gamma	28 keV	0.025
	Palladium 103	17.0 days	Gamma	21 keV	0.004
	Caesium 131	9.6 days	Gamma	29 keV	Minimal[b]

[a]Radium-226 mean photon energy given with 0.5 mm platinum filtration, all others given with no filtration.

[b]The exact half value layer data could not be found for these isotopes.

Techniques, Modalities, and Modifiers in Radiation Oncology

predominant modes of brachytherapy. However, with the advent of modern surgical techniques and interventional radiology, many more areas of the body are now accessible to the brachytherapist. Brachytherapy applicators can be placed within tubular organs in the body, either under direct vision (e.g., cervix or vagina) or with the use of radiological or endoscopic guidance (e.g., bile ducts or esophagus).

Interstitial implants can be placed with or without image guidance (e.g., prostate implants using rectal ultrasound guidance and a template or a freehand extremity sarcoma implant). Interstitial implants can take the form of free seeds, seeds within linked strands, or catheters that will be loaded with the radioactive source. Of course, surface applicator techniques are still used, with the added benefits of modern imaging and dosimetry techniques to ensure target coverage.

LDR sources can be placed directly into the body; however, with higher activity sources and large implants, this can result in a high radiation exposure to the brachytherapist and operating room staff. To overcome this problem, afterloading techniques were developed. Initial techniques required applicator placement in the operating room and manual afterloading of sources in a shielded room at a later time. This has mainly been supplanted by remote afterloading techniques, where the patient has the applicators placed while in the operating room and is later connected to a remote afterloading machine in a shielded room. The sources will only enter the patient when all personnel are at a safe distance from the patient; this can be used for LDR and is essential for PDR.

When using LDR or PDR, it is important that the patient can be safely left in a room without direct supervision, because during the period of source excursion radiation dose to staff must be kept to a minimum. During an LDR implant, careful monitoring of the sources must be maintained to detect source displacement. During a PDR implant, the patient should be monitored for applicator displacement between pulses; this may be under direct vision or using radiological confirmation. Devices aiding local protection of OAR may be used (e.g., leaded gum shield during lip brachytherapy).

Target Definition

Many of the same definitions for delineation of treatment volumes in EBRT are used for brachytherapy.[8,9] There may be delineation of high-risk and low-risk areas if discrete areas of dose escalation are required within the CTV. The high-risk area has the highest risk of local recurrence, usually due to the presence of gross residual disease. An intermediate area may be defined that corresponds to areas where there was macroscopic tumor at the time of diagnosis that has regressed by the time of brachytherapy implant. The low-risk area includes potential microscopic spread (i.e., the traditionally defined CTV). In EBRT the planning target volume (PTV) traditionally consists of the CTV plus a margin that will allow for physiological movement and setup uncertainty. Generally, in brachytherapy these variations are minimized and therefore the PTV is usually the same as the CTV.

In a brachytherapy implant there will be *high-dose regions* around each source. Generally, the volume of the region receiving over 150% (V_{150}) of dose is reported.[3] *Low-dose regions* are those within the CTV receiving <90% of the prescribed dose. Due to the heterogeneity of dose in brachytherapy, the average dose within the prescribed volume is usually far higher than the prescribed dose at the reference isodose point on the periphery of the implant. This is tolerated due to the volume–effect relationship: very small normal tissue volumes (e.g., 1 to 2 cm^3) can tolerate very high radiation doses that larger volumes would not tolerate. The dose to organs at risk should be reported, either as a total dose or a ratio of volume. Methods such as the minimum dose received by the most irradiated 2 cm^3 (D2cc) of tissue or the volume receiving over 90% of the dose (V_{90}) or dose received by 90% of the CTV (D_{90}) are assessed.

RADIOBIOLOGIC CONSIDERATIONS

Radiobiological principles are important in the daily clinical use of all forms of brachytherapy. Brachytherapy was initially developed empirically with doses being determined by clinical effect. In the modern era, radiobiological modeling is used to predict the biological effect of varying dose prescriptions. The importance of radiobiology and its use within brachytherapy was emphasized by the move from LDR treatment to PDR and fractionated HDR treatment. Of course, it must be remembered that applicator and source placement remains the single most important factor in brachytherapy such that, in an implant with poor geometry, changing radiobiologic parameters, such as fractionation or dose rate, will not improve the outcome.

Factors contributing to the response of tissues to radiotherapy have been labeled the "4 Rs of radiotherapy"[10]: repair, reassortment, repopulation, and reoxygenation. The way in which these radiobiological characteristics relate clinically to the use of LDR and PDR either alone or in comparison to HDR follows.

Repair

Sublethally damaged cells are capable of repair if they are allowed sufficient time and if the cell contains all of the necessary DNA repair proteins and enzymes. If sublethally damaged cells are exposed to further irradiation before repair occurs, the damage may become lethal. Late-reacting normal tissues seem more capable of repair than tumor cells so, at a given therapeutic dose, tumor is preferentially killed over normal tissue. This is probably due to a loss of repair fidelity in addition to a lack of relevant repair proteins and enzymes in the tumor cell. The lower the dose rate of radiation that a cell is exposed to, the more likely it is that repair of normal tissues will occur within that cell before a second injury occurs.

The time course of LDR or PDR treatment over several days allows time for sublethal damage repair in normal tissues. In contrast, the short treatment time of HDR treatment prohibits this repair during the actual irradiation. Using PDR, generally the same total dose and total time as LDR are prescribed. If PDR is given at a pulse width of 10 minutes and a 1-hour pulse interval, the dose is equivalent to LDR 0.6 Gy per hour.[11,12] If the dose per pulse is small (≤0.5 Gy) and the normal tissue repair half-time is over 30 minutes, the differential effect to LDR is <10%. If the dose per pulse is over 2 Gy or the tissue repair half-time is under half an hour, this is not the case and the PDR effect becomes biologically closer to a highly fractionated HDR treatment, especially in close proximity to the source.[13] In this situation, a lower total PDR dose than LDR can be given in the same overall time to achieve equivalent clinical effect. Sometimes PDR is prescribed using an "extended office hours" schedule (i.e., 8 a.m. to 8 p.m.). This is done commonly to overcome regulatory issues where a physicist and physician must be present for every source excursion. One general rule when transferring PDR to LDR dose is not to exceed the overall dose rate that would be delivered by LDR in a day (e.g., at a dose rate of 0.5 Gy per hour, LDR delivers a total dose of 12 Gy per 24 hours), thus by using a daytime-only PDR schedule, providing a similar biological effect and normal tissue complication probability, the overall treatment time will commonly be slightly extended.[14]

Dose rate is a key factor in determining the biological effects of brachytherapy. In general, the effects of radiotherapy increase as the dose rate increases, predominantly due to a decrease in repair. It has been suggested that the total dose of LDR prescribed should be corrected for overall time of the implant,[15] although some investigators have found no difference in local control with the same total dose administered using a dose rate ranging from 0.005 to 0.0167 Gy per minute.[16] A randomized study in cervix carcinoma showed no difference in overall survival or local control for a dose rate of 0.4 versus 0.8 Gy per hour.[17,18] However, there was a significant increase in late complications in the higher dose rate group. A similar trend has also been seen in LDR brachytherapy for breast cancer and head and neck carcinoma.[19,20] Therefore, it is recommended that the LDR (and PDR equivalence) should be in the range of 0.3 to 1 Gy per hour due to the effects on late complications rather than local control. If the dose rate exceeds 1 Gy per hour, a reduction in the total dose can be calculated using the biologically equivalent dose (BED) equation (see Chapter 22).

Reassortment

In normal cells, proliferation occurs in a sequence of events termed the *cell cycle.*[21] There is a theoretical advantage of an improved effect on reassortment using LDR treatment because, during the overall treatment time, cells will pass out of the relatively radio-resistant cell cycle phases of late S and early G_2 into the more radio-sensitive phases of late G_2 and M. This has been shown *in vitro,*[22] but *in vivo* the effect of reassortment has not been shown to give a true advantage, possibly due to a disruption of the mechanisms of the cell cycle in cancer cells.[21]

Repopulation

In squamous cell carcinoma, studies have shown improved tumor control and increased survival when a radiotherapy course is given in the shortest overall time.[23–26] This may be because shorter treatment times allow less time for tumor cell repopulation or for accelerated repopulation to occur. The continuous administration of LDR and PDR probably prevents repopulation during treatment.

Reoxygenation

The response of cells to radiation is strongly dependent on oxygen. Radiation results in free-radical formation within a tumor, and oxygen reacts with these free radicals to make DNA damage irreparable. The effect of hypoxia on tumor control has been well documented with decreased survival in certain patients with a low initial hemoglobin levels.[27–29] There are two hypoxic cell populations within tumors: chronic and transient. As a tumor outgrows its blood supply, a proportion of cells will become necrotic. Viable cells near this necrotic zone will be chronically hypoxic. Transient hypoxia may occur over minutes to hours as small vessels within the tumor open and close or small tumor emboli intermittently block blood vessels. When using LDR and PDR, transient hypoxia may correct during the treatment time,[30] which is not possible during the short duration of HDR brachytherapy. If the brachytherapy is fractionated, tumor shrinkage and reoxygenation of areas of chronic hypoxia may occur between insertions.

MEASUREMENT OF BRACHYTHERAPY DOSE

Dosimetry systems aim to give the brachytherapist a set of guidelines to follow, which result in a prescribed dose being delivered to a patient in a predictable fashion. Initial brachytherapy dosimetry systems were developed for LDR implants using an empirical approach toward source placement and dose calculation. More modern techniques use computer programs to generate isodose distributions, which can then be analyzed in two dimensions, three dimensions, and volumetrically. In order to achieve the best ratio of cancer to normal tissue dose, the selection of an appropriate prescription point is essential. Applicator positioning is of primary importance, as differential loading cannot compensate for a poorly sited implant.

The Manchester dosimetry system was one of the first published dosimetry systems, with its origin dating from the 1930s.[31] Guidelines for the use of LDR wires and tubes are set out for surface molds, interstitial planar implants, and volume implants. However, it required a range of isotope activities to be available, and at that time the available radium sources in the United States had a more limited range of activity. Therefore, the Quimby system modified the Manchester system to allow uniform source strengths to be used throughout the implant.[32] The Paris dosimetry system developed guidelines in the 1970 s for modern LDR brachytherapy sources such as flexible ^{192}Ir wires.[33] It is difficult to achieve an implant that conforms exactly to the Paris rules without the use of a template (see Chapter 24).

Where LDR uses fixed source positions and strengths to calculate the dose at the prescription point, afterloading machines and computerized dosimetry systems allow optimization of source dwell times to customize dose delivery to the patient's individual anatomy and tumor volume. PDR takes advantage of this dose optimization in a way that LDR cannot. Optimization results in nonuniform source loadings that give greater dose uniformity and CTV coverage that is often similar to an idealized Manchester dosimetry system implant.[34] Prior to the introduction of computerized dosimetry, the dosimetry of an implant was based on the intended source position rather than the actual source position. This could be highly dependent on the expertise of the individual brachytherapist. Improved radiological imaging has allowed more accurate definition of the CTV and associated normal tissues, giving dose specification according to patient anatomy rather than applicator position. This is more likely to correlate with patient outcome than previous dosimetry systems. This may result in not only better tumor control but also decreased risk of late complications.

Now that computerized dosimetry is available, brachytherapists may be tempted to abandon knowledge of the previous dosimetric systems and place sources as they see fit, using the computer to calculate dose distribution. This approach risks overdosing part of the volume. There is a steep dose gradient around each wire and wide-spaced sources may form large high-dose regions and increase the risk of necrosis. In the same way, an isodose that covers the volume but is at a large distance from the sources may also cause necrosis in the vicinity of the sources. The maximum source separations and treatment thickness in the Paris system are useful rules to remember to decrease this risk. The principle of extending the sources beyond the target or crossing at the ends should also be remembered to overcome the inherent dose fall off at the end of the source. This can be achieved using optimization with PDR brachytherapy. The rules from individual systems should not be mixed, even if computerized dosimetry is used for dose calculation.

Brachytherapy dose delivery traditionally was thought not to be affected by alterations in the treatment position. Although this may be true for dose delivery to the target volume, the position of organs at risk in relation to the brachytherapy implant may be altered, thereby increasing the dose delivered (e.g., a patient undergoes simulation lying flat on a computed tomography [CT] scanner with a breast implant that falls laterally with gravity). On sitting up, this applicator may then fall more medially, potentially changing cardiac, lung, and skin doses.

CLINICAL SITES

There are areas where LDR techniques continue to predominate (e.g., vLDR prostate brachytherapy), areas where HDR techniques predominate (e.g., esophageal brachytherapy), and areas where the use of HDR and LDR (now moving to PDR) are generally equal (e.g., cervix cancer). The sections below present an overview of clinical uses for LDR and PDR with an emphasis on the brachytherapy dose rate rather than the treatment technique. Individual indications will be described in the site specific chapters.

Cervix Cancer

The use of LDR for cervix cancer treatment was first described with intracavitary implants in 1903 and with interstitial implants in 1913.[35] It has withstood technological innovations to remain an essential part of curative cervix cancer treatment.[36,37] for all but the very earliest stages of the disease. The use of LDR has many years of safety and efficacy data, and physicians can be confident in their choice of brachytherapy dose. These doses have been shown to be biologically equivalent using PDR as long as the rules governing pulse length and pulse interval are carefully followed.[14,38] In contrast, a wide variety of HDR dose and fractionation schemes are used,[39] with shorter follow-up data for efficacy and toxicity. Randomized clinical trials have shown the equivalence of HDR brachytherapy and LDR brachytherapy,[40] and some studies suggest a lower morbidity with HDR brachytherapy, which could possibly be due to the ability to optimize the dose away from normal tissues.[41,42]

Several trials demonstrated the superiority for chemoradiotherapy over radiotherapy alone in cervix cancer treatment.[43] All of these trials used LDR brachytherapy, and there are no prospective randomized safety data on the use of HDR brachytherapy and chemoradiotherapy. PDR brachytherapy utilizes the dose and scheduling of LDR and thus should have a similar efficacy profile while allowing the dose optimization capability of HDR, which may improve normal tissue toxicity. Studies have shown this to be the case in clinical practice.[44–46]

With the use of CT- and magnetic resonance imaging–based target volume and organ at risk definition, dose reporting in cervix cancer brachytherapy has changed from being point based to volume based.[47,48] This means that tumor coverage is improved and the doses to normal tissues can be decreased. This method relies on the use of dose optimization and thus moves away from LDR and toward PDR as an equivalent treatment modality. The longer time taken to deliver 1 overall fraction of PDR than HDR is important when optimizing dose away from normal tissues, and it is important to recognize that the dose delivered to normal tissues over the whole treatment time may differ from that predicted, up to 33% more.[49] A comprehensive description of this volume-based dosing is given in Chapter 25 (see Table 25.3). American Brachytherapy Society guidelines for the use of LDR and PDR in cervix cancer have recently been updated,[50] incorporating the volume-based dosimetry and updated quality control recommendations.

The applicator is generally placed under operative conditions. Review of preoperative imaging is essential to determine which applicator is most appropriate. The patient may require a general anesthetic, but spinal anesthesia (Fig. 23.1) has been shown to provide excellent analgesia, which can be maintained throughout the length of the implant using a spinal catheter.[51] Spinal anesthesia does not affect tumor oxygenation during an HDR implant,[52] thus it is unlikely to during the whole duration of an LDR or PDR implant. With the patient in the lithotomy position, examination under anesthesia confirms preoperative imaging findings. The cervix is then dilated and a uterine tandem is placed, preferably using ultrasound guidance.[53] A variety of commercial applicators are available for intracavitary brachytherapy (Fig. 23.2), with the tandem and ring applicator becoming increasingly popular for tumors <5 cm. For tumors over this size, the addition of interstitial needles into specialized applicators (e.g., the Vienna applicator)[54] is becoming more common because it has brought the ability to deliver interstitial brachytherapy to a wider group. Interstitial template applicators such as the Syed-Neblett[55] or the multiple site perineal applicator[56] applicator can be used to treat disease with lateral extension, although it is important to maintain a degree of central dose heterogeneity (in contrast to the heterogeneity preferred in interstitial implants in other areas of the body) to maintain the central cervix doses needed for cure (Fig. 23.3).[57] Customized vaginal molds can be used and are particularly prevalent in France,[58] offering truly customized brachytherapy dosing.

An LDR applicator is typically afterloaded once the patient returns to the shielded isolated patient room. The patient will undergo CT scanning and using PDR dose-optimized planning before dose delivery. When the patient is receiving the dose, she will be nursed lying flat with prophylaxis against venous thromboembolism. Typically, agents are given to slow bowel motility, and it may be preferable to follow a low-irritant fiber diet before and during the implant. A urinary catheter is maintained throughout treatment. Prophylactic antibiotics are not routinely required. Pain and discomfort may be managed by epidural or intravenous patient controlled analgesia. Care is taken to minimize exposure to the medical staff caring for the patient through the use of mobile shielding placed around the bed and by the training of the staff as to the time and distance radiation safety rules. Pregnant staff members are not allowed in the area so as to minimize risk of dose to fetus.

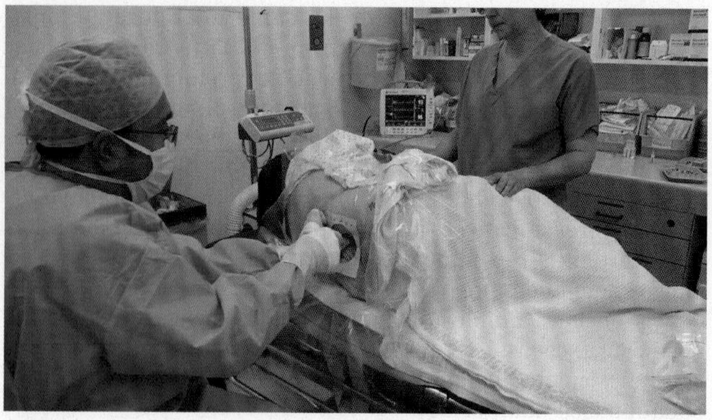

FIGURE 23.1. Administration of a spinal anesthetic prior to a pelvic brachytherapy procedure.

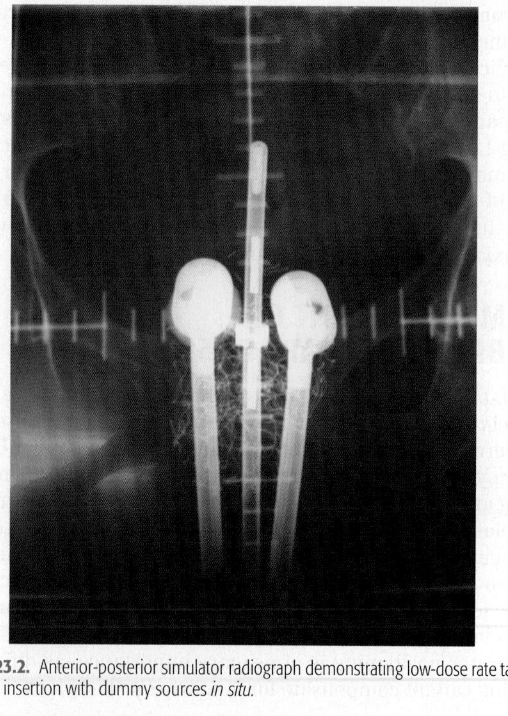

FIGURE 23.2. Anterior-posterior simulator radiograph demonstrating low-dose rate tandem and ovoid insertion with dummy sources *in situ*.

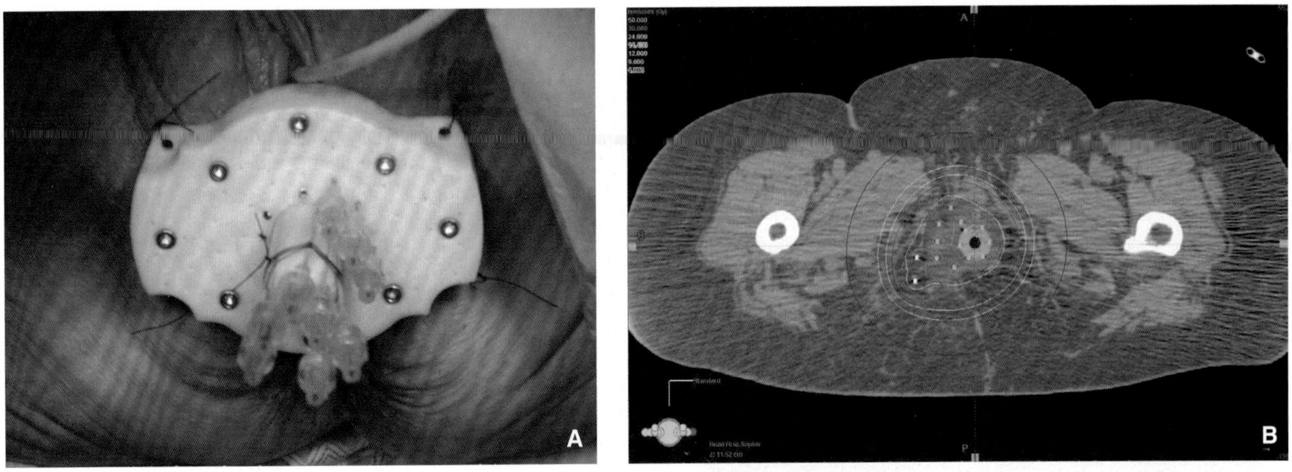

FIGURE 23.3. A: Low-dose rate (LDR) template interstitial implant for a vaginal vault recurrence of cervical carcinoma. **B:** Axial computed tomography slice demonstrating the target volume and dosimetry of an LDR vaginal vault template interstitial implant.

Endometrium

Endometrial carcinoma is the most common female pelvic malignancy in Western countries.[59,60] Brachytherapy for the management of endometrial carcinoma was first described by Heyman[61] in 1935, prior to the routine use of hysterectomy for uterine cancer. The majority of endometrial cancer patients now present at an early stage, and the use of radiation alone has evolved. The primary treatment for endometrial cancer is surgery (total abdominal hysterectomy and bilateral salpingo-oophorectomy) with or without adjuvant radiotherapy and chemotherapy based on the histology of the tumor and stage of presentation. As endometrial carcinoma is linked to obesity and hypertension, some patients have medical comorbidities that preclude surgery; for those, radiation therapy may be the definitive treatment of choice. In this group, treatment is delivered via intracavitary uterine brachytherapy, with or without EBRT.[62–64]

For definitive treatment, packing the uterus with capsules allows excellent coverage of the entire endometrial cavity that can be adapted to every patient's individual anatomy.[65,66] Standardized applicators may provide more straightforward and reproducible dosimetry. Double channel applicators such as the Rotte applicator[67] can be used with CT planning, and computerized optimization with HDR delivers a very similar dose to the serosa,[68] which could be replicated with PDR (Fig. 23.4). Various whole uterus prescription points have been described[69,70]; however, CT planning allows contouring of the outer contour of the uterus for volume-based dose prescription. A typical dose is 70to 80 Gy prescribed to the outer contour of the uterus alone or 35 to 50 Gy in combination with 30 to 45 Gy EBRT.[71]

Vaginal vault brachytherapy can be used in the adjuvant treatment of endometrial cancer and vaginal vault recurrence of endometrial carcinoma and also in other gynecologic malignancies such postoperative early-stage cervix cancer or early-stage vaginal cancer.[60,72–74] The target for adjuvant vaginal vault brachytherapy is the vaginal mucosa and the operative scar. Ninety percent of recurrences occur at the vaginal vault and 10% in the distal vagina[75]; therefore, in the majority of cases the upper third to half of the vagina is treated. This decreases the morbidity associated with treating the whole vagina, such as vaginal dryness or shortening.[71] Brachytherapy can be prescribed at the cylinder surface or at 5 mm into tissue, a depth that approximates the vaginal lymphatics.

Vaginal vault brachytherapy can be administered using a variety of different applicators. The commonly used single channel cylinder comes in a variety of widths chosen according to patient anatomy and comfort (Fig. 23.5). This may be a less favorable choice when using LDR as the lack of optimization leads to effects from source anisotropy. The vaginal apex is

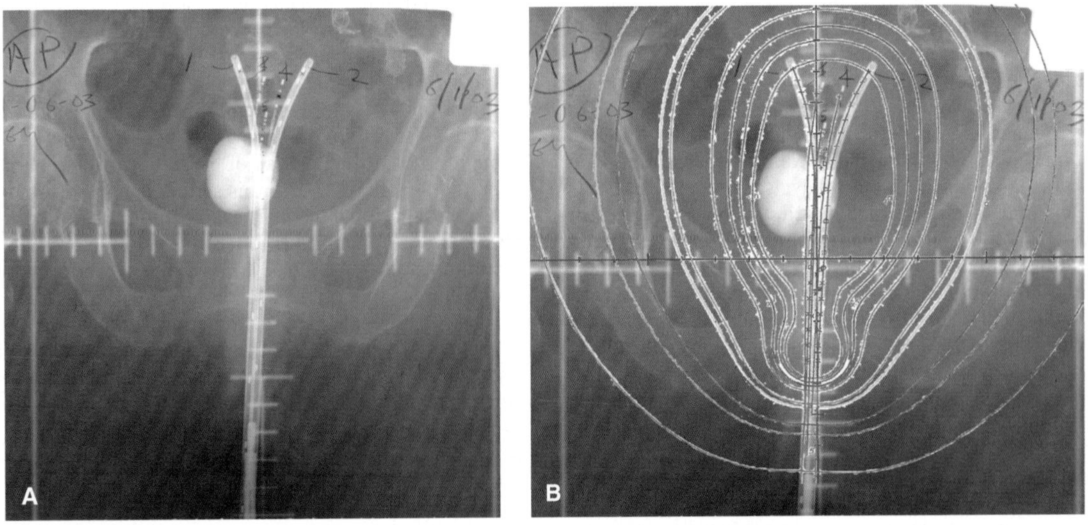

FIGURE 23.4. A: Double tandem Martinez applicator in place with three Heyman's capsules placed within the uterus. **B:** Anterior-posterior simulator radiograph demonstrating the brachytherapy insertion pictured in Figure 23.5, with isodose lines overlaid. (Courtesy of Dr Akila Viswanathan.)

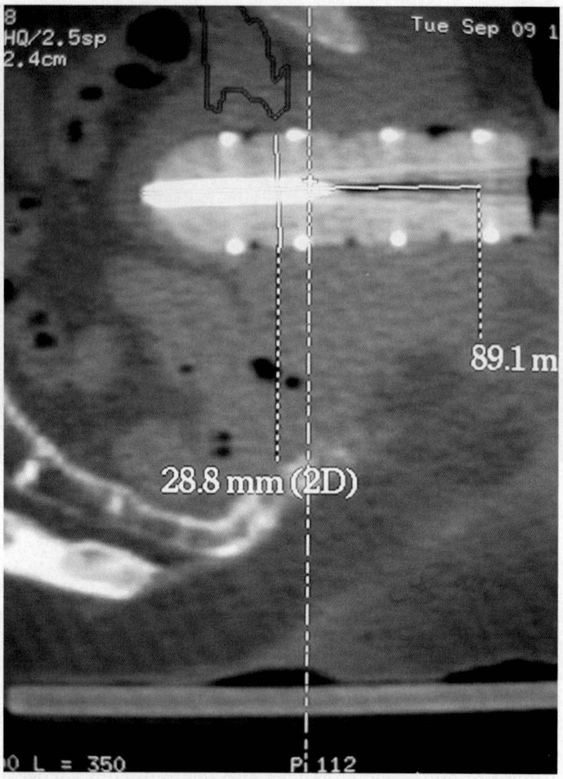

FIGURE 23.5. Lateral image of a digitally reconstructed radiograph demonstrating a vaginal cylinder *in situ* and its relationship to surrounding normal tissues.

located along the longitudinal axis of the source; therefore, the vaginal apex is exposed to the greatest effects of source anisotropy. It is important that planning systems contain modifications for source anisotropy. Li et al.[76] used Monte Carlo simulations to show that not accounting for anisotropy can result in underdosing by as much as 30% at the vaginal apex. The use of optimization with PDR to points off the cylinder apex can overcome this problem and may lead to decreased late toxicity.[77] Of course it must be considered that the doses we commonly prescribe for brachytherapy to the vaginal apex are those formulated using years of empirical dosing, and the received dose at the vaginal apex may have actually been much higher than the prescribed dose. If we now use the same prescribed dose but lower the actual dose received by the vaginal mucosa using methods such as optimization to the cylinder apex or anisotropy correction, it is possible that it could be detrimental to tumor control. Vaginal colpostats are an alternative applicator that delivers a dose more localized to the vaginal vault and less dose to the midlower vagina.

The use of pelvic radiotherapy in selected stage Ia and Ib patients (intermediate risk) has been examined in randomized trials[75,78–80] and a Cochrane meta-analysis.[81] Selected patients may have vaginal cylinder brachytherapy alone as adjuvant radiotherapy, which gives similar regional control rates to pelvic EBRT with significantly less toxicity.[82,83] Adjuvant primary vaginal vault irradiation has been shown to decrease the incidence of vaginal apex recurrence in endometrial cancer from 12% to 15% to as low as 0% in selected patients, although it has no impact on overall survival.[72,82] The dose for LDR vaginal vault alone is 50 Gy prescribed at 5 mm over 4 to 5 days or 0.5 Gy per hour and approximately 15 Gy when combined with 45 Gy EBRT.[71] The radiation dose received by the pelvic organs varies according to physiological variations (e.g., the bladder dose may vary according to the extent of bladder filling, which may also affect the amount of small bowel in the field).[84,85]

TABLE 23.3 INCLUSION CRITERIA FOR PROSTATE BRACHYTHERAPY

Selection Criteria for Prostate Brachytherapy
Patient Factors
Life expectancy >5 years
IPSS <15
Prostate volume <60 cm^3
No defect if previous TURP
Minimal pubic arch interference
Tumor Factors
Monotherapy: T1–T2b, Gleason score ≤7, PSA ≤15[a]
Boost therapy: ≥T2 c, Gleason score ≥7, PSA ≥10

IPSS, International Prostate Symptom Score; TURP, transurethral resection of prostate; PSA, prostate specific antigen.

[a]Gleason score 7 and PSA >10 may be considered for either monotherapy or boost therapy.

From refs. 114, and 252.

Prostate

Prostate brachytherapy has become part of the treatment paradigm in prostate cancer for all stages of localized disease (Table 23.3). It can be used as monotherapy or in combination with EBRT or hormone therapy for higher risk disease. The most common application for monotherapy is with LDR permanent seeds. When used as a boost, both LDR and HDR techniques are used as well as recent publications of PDR boost. Prostate brachytherapy is also being investigated as salvage therapy after external beam radiation[86] and is currently under investigation through the Radiation Therapy Oncology Group (RTOG) study RTOG-0526.

A transrectal ultrasound-guided transperineal technique is the most popular technique for implanting the prostate. Other modalities incorporating MRI[87] and MRI spectroscopy imaging have also been proposed.[88] The techniques for implanting ^{125}I and ^{103}Pd have been well described.[89–91] The patient criteria for selection include ability to undergo a general, spinal, or less commonly local anesthetic,[92] prostate volume <60 cm^3, favorable anatomy (minimal or no pubic arch interference, median lobe), and minimal obstructive uropathy. Significant transurethral resection of prostate defect is also a relative contraindication to a seed implant.[93] Tumor criteria depend on whether monotherapy or boost therapy is planned. Typically monotherapy is reserved for patients with so-called favorable risk disease (e.g., low-intermediate risk disease: T1 to T2b disease, Gleason score <7, prostate specific antigen <15 ng/mL) and boost therapy for patients with intermediate- and high-risk disease. The role of EBRT and hormone therapy in combination with LDR brachytherapy is unclear and under investigation. Adjuvant androgen deprivation therapy (ADT) is used for prostatic cytoreduction in patients who do not have ideal prostatic geometry.[94] Cytoreduction may be achieved with use of luteinizing hormone-releasing hormone agonists and antiandrogens or antiandrogen in combination with 5α-reductase inhibitors.[95] ADT is also considered in patients thought to be at higher risk of prostate cancer recurrence, however, the benefit of ADT in this setting is not well defined.[96–99]

In transperineal techniques, treatment planning can be done either as a preplan or intraoperatively. In the preplan technique, a volume study is acquired prior to the procedure and the prostate volume and pubic arch interference are assessed. Axial images (5 mm) of the prostate from the base to the apex are taken and then used for brachytherapy planning (Fig. 23.6). Sagittal imaging can be used to help identify the base and apex. Reproducibility of the prostate position on the day of insertion must be ensured in this technique. Intraoperative techniques are defined as intraoperative preplanning, interactive planning, and dynamic dose calculation. Intraoperative preplanning avoids two separate ultrasound studies and involves the creation of a plan at the time of the implant procedure. It, like preplanned techniques, does not account for deviations of needle position or

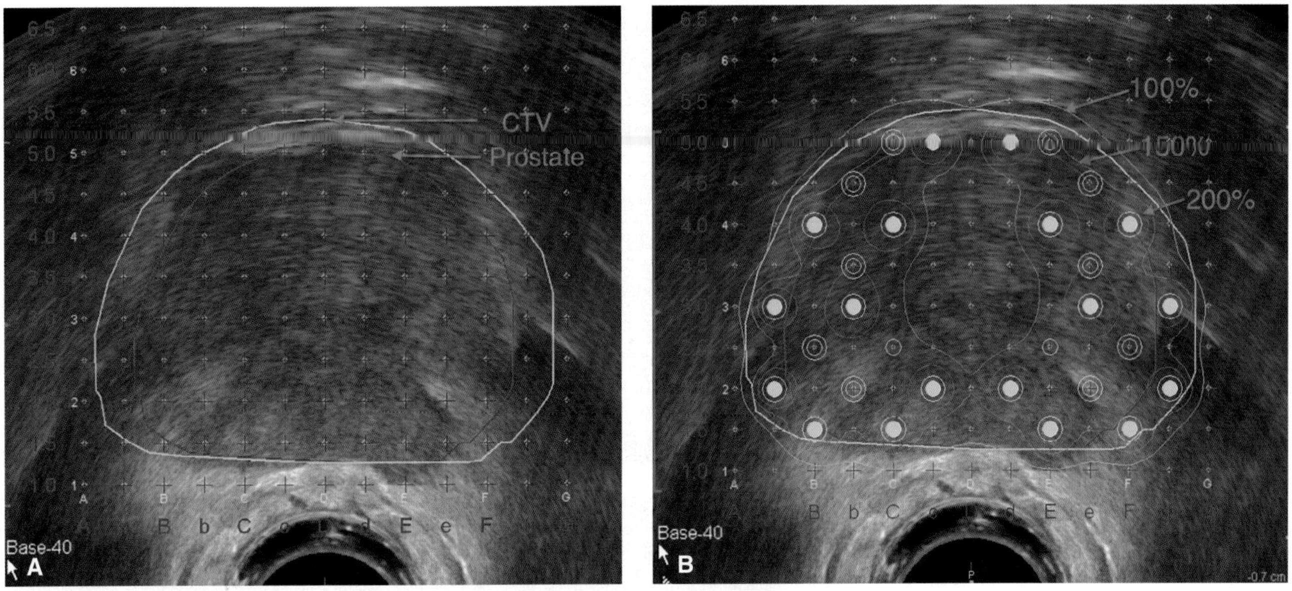

FIGURE 23.6. Prostate volume study with prostate and clinical target volume defined **(A)**, preplan with peripheral loading technique **(B)**.

prostate geometry changes from the preplan.[100] The time required for the implant tends to be more prolonged using this technique compared to the preoperative technique. Interactive planning allows for refinement of the treatment plan based on needle-position feedback and estimation of seed placement. Modifications can then be made to needle position or additional seeds can be added to optimize the plan. Dynamic dose calculation allows constant updating of the dose distribution based on the actual seed positions and takes into account changes in the prostate volume.[101,102]

Current permanent LDR techniques involve implanting ^{125}I or ^{103}Pd seeds. Cesium-131 is also approved for prostate brachytherapy and is used at some institutions. These isotopes have differing energies and half-lives and therefore initial dose rates (see Table 23.2). It had been postulated that ^{103}Pd compared with ^{125}I was more effective at treating dedifferentiated tumors as the dose rate is higher; however, studies evaluating clinical outcomes for patients with prostate cancer have shown no difference.[103–105] Studies evaluating the toxicity to OAR, including rectum, bladder, and sexual function, have shown no difference in acute or long-term toxicity or difference in sexual function.[106–108] There is a difference in the time for the International Prostate Symptom Score (IPSS) to return to the preimplant baseline, with ^{103}Pd returning to baseline faster.[109] Cesium-131 has not been studied as extensively. Commercially, ^{125}I and ^{103}Pd seeds are available as either loose or stranded seeds. Dosimetrically, the two are similar. The incidence of seed migration is decreased with stranded seeds as compared with that of loose seeds, with the greatest difference being in migration to the lung and perineum.[110]

The prescription dose for permanent LDR brachytherapy is dependent on the isotope and the indication for the implant, either monotherapy or as a boost. Table 23.4 describes the recommended doses for ^{125}I, ^{103}Pd, and ^{131}Cs when used as monotherapy or when combined with 40 to 50 Gy EBRT.[94,111,112] The prescription dose covers the entire prostate (CTV) and typically includes a margin. The dose for ^{131}Cs is still investigational.

TABLE 23.4 PRESCRIPTION DOSE FOR PERMANENT LOW-DOSE RATE BRACHYTHERAPY WHEN USED AS MONOTHERAPY OR AS A BOOST COMBINED WITH 40–50 Gy EXTERNAL BEAM RADIATION THERAPY

	Monotherapy (Gy)	*Boost (Gy)*
Iodine-125	145	110
Palladium-103	125	100
Cesium-131	115	85

In the preoperative technique, the dose to the target volume as well as the organs at risk are evaluated. Different loading techniques are used to achieve these goals based on the needle placement, spacing of seeds, and seed energy.[93] A peripheral loading technique is common to avoid excess dose to the urethra with ^{125}I, and a modified uniform loading is used with ^{103}Pd.[113] The source placement with ^{131}Cs has different guidelines from ^{125}I and ^{103}Pd, with needles placed farther from the urethra and rectum.[111] Good preimplantation dosimetry and toxicity levels correlate with a V_{100} >95% of CTV, D_{90} >100%, and V_{150} ≤50% of CTV, rectum D2cc less than reference prescription dose, D_{max} 150% of reference prescription dose, prostatic urethra D_{10} <150%, and D_{30} <130%.[102] Dose limits to structures such as the penile bulb and neurovascular bundles are under investigation.

Postimplant dose reporting in a structured quality assurance program is highly recommended and should include dose parameters to both the target as well as the OAR.[112,114] Timing of the postimplant imaging varies at different centers but ideally should relate to the time at which edema is at a minimum. Evaluation at either day 0 or day 30 is most common. Seed localization is crucial as is the contouring of the prostate and normal structures. CT-MRI fusion if possible allows for identification of both the seeds and accurate definition of the prostate, particularly at the apex and base, which tend to be difficult to delineate on CT (Fig. 23.7). Primary parameters to report and evaluate include the intended dose—D_{90}, D_{100}, V_{100}, V_{150}—to the prostate gland and rectal volume and dose and urethral doses. For patients with unacceptably cold implants, consideration for reimplantation should be given. There are no parameters at present for penile bulb and neurovascular bundles.

Studies have shown that prostate brachytherapy is associated with a "learning curve" effect.[115–117] As with any brachytherapy technique, outcomes and toxicities are dependent on where the radiation has been delivered. With permanent seed brachytherapy, there can be no dose optimization once the seeds are placed. A quality assurance process that enables closing the feedback loop for optimizing subsequent implants is therefore crucial. Peer review, assessments of dosimetry, toxicity and outcomes as well continuing education should be part of any prostate brachytherapy program.[118–122]

Under spinal or general anesthetic, the patient is positioned supine in the lithotomy position. If a preplan was used, the same couch angle and ultrasound probe angle must be reproduced. Contrast agent is typically injected into the bladder for

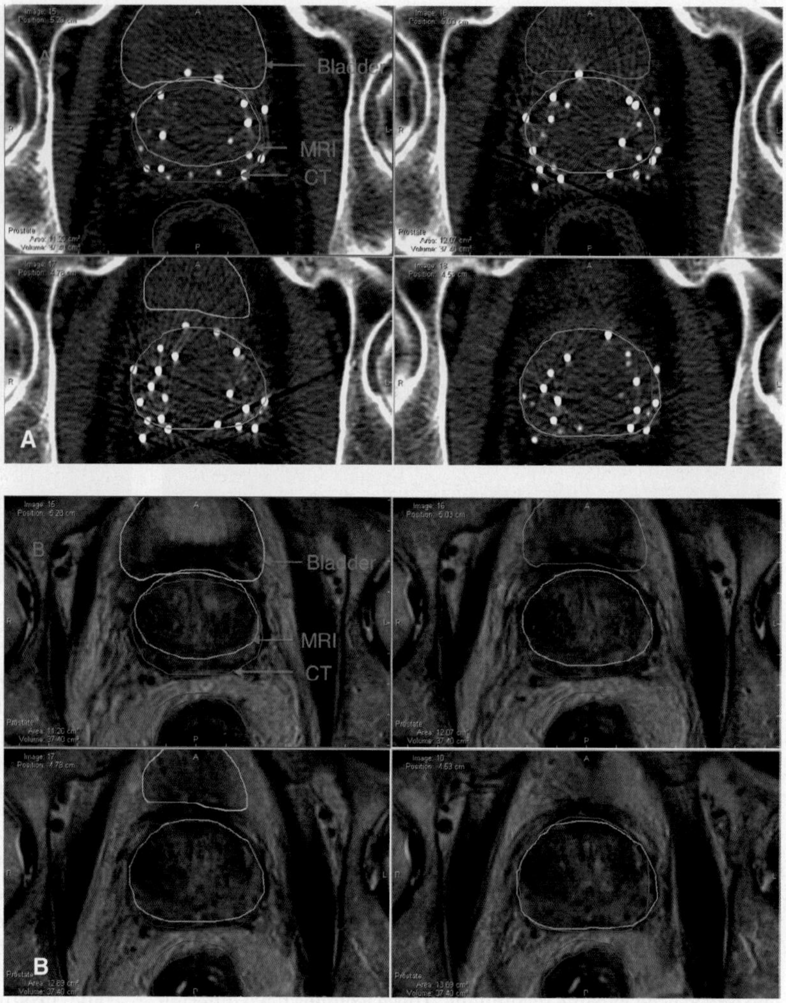

FIGURE 23.7. Prostate brachytherapy post plan with computed tomography and magnetic resonance (CT-MRI) fusion. The prostate volumes were drawn independently on the CT **(A)** and MRI **(B)** to show the difference in contours at the base of the prostate. The MRI images are better able to delineate the prostate, whereas the CT scan is better able to give information on the brachytherapy seed location.

visualization under fluoroscopy. Visualization of the urethra is essential and can be accomplished by injecting foamed Mucogel into the urethra during the procedure. Alternatively, a urethral catheter can be inserted and left in place during the implant; however, some clinicians avoid the latter technique to prevent changing the shape of the prostate. The prostate, bladder, seminal vesicles, and pubic arch are identified on ultrasound. The base and apex of the prostate gland are also identified. Preloaded needles are kept within a shielded vault or sleeve until the physician is ready to insert the individual needles. Each hollow-bore needle has a beveled edge and central stylet. Ultrasound images in both the axial and sagittal views (if available) guide the placement of the needle. Once the first needle is in the correct position (in three-dimensional coordinates), the retraction plane is set for positioning of the remaining needles. To drop the seeds within the prostate the central stylet is held securely in place and the outer needle is slowly pulled back along the stylet. On-demand fluoroscopy can be taken to check seed position relative to bony and organ anatomy. Additional seeds may be placed at the end of the procedure as required. Bladder irrigation and cystoscopy can be performed to evacuate migrated seeds in the bladder. Patients are conveniently discharged home the same day of the procedure.

In intermediate- to high-risk prostate cancer, brachytherapy in combination with EBRT has been evaluated with both LDR permanent seeds and HDR brachytherapy.[123–126] The same techniques used in HDR boost brachytherapy can be applied to temporary implants with LDR ^{192}Ir strands or PDR brachytherapy, with special attention to techniques that ensure the apparatus stays in place over the treatment time. PDR boost brachytherapy is not as extensively studied as HDR or permanent implants, but preliminary studies[127,128] show acceptable toxicity and tumor control with limited follow-up. In the Pieters et al.[128] study, the patients were treated with ≤1.2-Gy pulse at short time intervals ≤2.2 hours. The doses in their study are relatively low, with an equivalent dose in 2-Gy fractions between 68.8 and 74.4 Gy. They note that the tumor control at 5 years is comparable to many HDR studies and that there are large areas of prostate receiving >20% of the prescription dose because of the heterogeneous nature of brachytherapy. They recorded low rectal and urinary toxicity, and the IPSS returned to baseline by 12 weeks postbrachytherapy. Further dose escalation with PDR was felt to be worth pursuing because of the low rectal and urinary toxicity. Studies evaluating ^{192}Ir LDR for boost have also been done but are not commonly used.[129–131]

Penile Cancer

Penile cancer is rare in Western countries, representing only 1% of male malignancies. Squamous cell carcinoma is the predominant histology. Brachytherapy is used as an organ-sparing technique in T1, T2, and select T3 lesions (<4 cm) that do not involve the shaft of the penis.[132,133] Both surface mold techniques (lesions <5 mm)[134,135] and interstitial techniques (Fig. 23.8)[136–140] have been described. The 5-year local control with interstitial brachytherapy is 70% to 86% with penile preservation of 72% to 88%. Typical doses range from 50 to 65 Gy delivered in 4 to 7 days. Typically at least two planes are required as it is difficult to assess the depth of disease. Crook et al.[141] describe their implantation technique in detail for 75 cases implanted between 1989 and 2009 with both ^{192}Ir wire or seeds

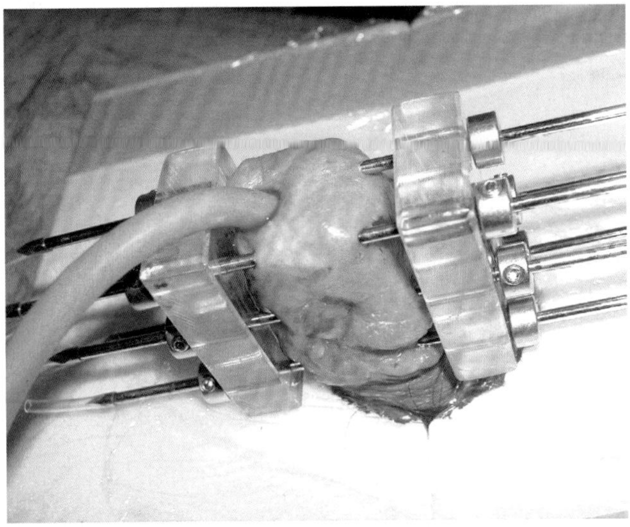

FIGURE 23.8. Low-dose rate interstitial multiplane penile implant.

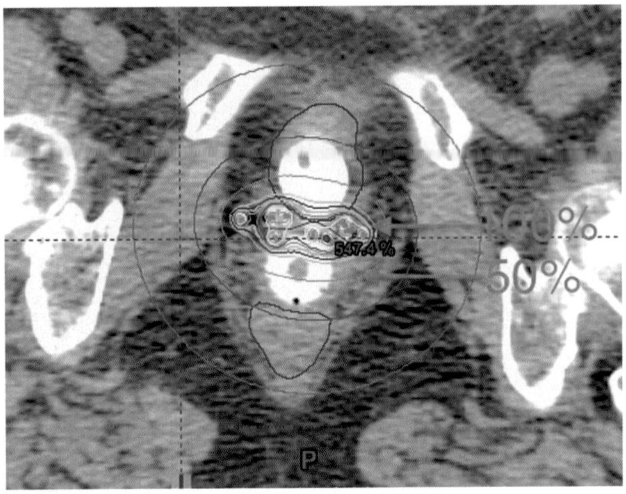

FIGURE 23.9. Low-dose rate interstitial multiplanar urethral implant.

and PDR techniques. The implants are based on the Paris system using rigid templates with spacing between 12 and 18 mm. Computerized dosimetry mimics the Paris system and allows for visualization of dose to the target and organs at risk. They prescribed 60 Gy at a dose rate of 0.5 to 0.65 Gy per hour with manually afterloaded ^{192}Ir or 0.5 to 0.55 Gy in hourly fractions when using PDR. Penile preservation was 88% at 5 years and 67% at 10 years with actuarial survival of 59% at 10 years and cause specific survival of 83.6%.[137] They reported a soft tissue necrosis rate of 12% and urethral stenosis rate of 9%. The soft tissue necrosis rate quoted in the literature ranges from 12% to 26% and increases with a dose >60 Gy, T3 disease, large volume implants (>30 cm^3), and more than two needle planes.[137–140,142] If conservative measures fail to manage soft tissue necrosis, hyperbaric oxygen therapy has shown success prior to resorting to surgical interventions such as debridement or amputation.[143] Urethral stenosis is reported in 10% to 45%[138–140,144,145] of cases and relates to the proximity of the needles to the urethra and the number of treatment planes. Using PDR brachytherapy allows manual optimization of dose around the urethra and may decrease the rate of stenosis. It is recommended that all men undergo circumcision prior to brachytherapy as this exposes the tumor, potentially removes disease allowing for a smaller implant, and decreases the risk of ulceration and necrosis to the foreskin.[139,141] Dose to the urethra and testes should be recorded. In men wishing to retain fertility, lead shielding can be placed around the testes.

Urethra

Brachytherapy may be used in the treatment of both male and female urethral cancers. Intraluminal, intracavitary, and interstitial techniques have been described. Intraluminal brachytherapy is limited to superficial lesions and involves a single catheter into the urethra.[146] Interstitial implants for the penile urethra are similar to penile implants. In treatment of the female urethra, an interstitial implant may be used in combination with a molded vaginal applicator[146] or alone (Fig. 23.9). The dose with LDR as a monotherapy is 60 to 70 Gy in 3 to 5 days (0.5 to 1 Gy per hour PDR) and 20 to 25 Gy if used as a boost. Milosevic et al.[147] published their experience of 34 patients who were treated with radiation. Twenty of these patients received brachytherapy (5 brachytherapy alone, 15 EBRT plus brachytherapy). The tumors treated with brachytherapy tended to be ≤4 cm, involved the distal urethra, and did not invade adjacent organs. The majority of the patients underwent volume implants. Patients who had brachytherapy as part of their treatment had better local control, with 7-year local relapse-free rates of 77% versus 32% with EBRT alone. There was no difference in cause-specific survival and 7-year actuarial overall survival (41%). The risk of vesicovaginal fistulas was reported as 15%.

Head and Neck

Brachytherapy can be used to treat head and neck cancers either as definitive treatment or as a boost following EBRT. Use of brachytherapy may avoid disfiguring or mutilating surgery and allow organ conservation. Brachytherapy can also be used as a method of reirradiation for localized recurrence.[148] There are many years of safety and efficacy data for LDR brachytherapy, and PDR appears to replicate these results.[149–151,152] Intensity-modulated radiation therapy (IMRT) is becoming increasing standard for head and neck cancer; however, there are indications that delivery of CT-planned optimized brachytherapy continues to deliver superior results over IMRT.[153,154] Aspects of plan quality that are important for local control and risk of toxicity are similar to interstitial implants elsewhere:quality index, volume gradient ratio, and tube distance.[155]

Patient selection is key for head and neck brachytherapy. Patients who are unfit for radical surgery may still be poor candidates for brachytherapy. PDR may allow the use of brachytherapy for patients with more complex nursing needs in whom LDR would have been contraindicated. It is important that the patient is fully assessed prior to brachytherapy. Dental assessment is essential, and tooth extractions may be required; and for implants encompassing the oral cavity, customized leaded mandibular shields decrease the risk of osteoradionecrosis. Feeding needs should be assessed, and where necessary nasogastric or percutaneous gastrostomy feeding tubes may be placed before the implant. For base of tongue implants, the patient should be prepared to have a tracheostomy, which can be reversed as soon as the postimplant edema subsides. The patient should be assessed regularly during the duration of the implant for displacement of the sources or applicators. Analgesia should be administered and mouth washes are often helpful.

The majority of head and neck implants are placed in an operative procedure by freehand technique in a multiplane implant (Fig. 23.10). These can be sited using a variety of techniques, with use of afterloading catheters being preferred in the modern era for radiation safety reasons.[156] Standard applicators such as the Rotterdam applicator, which can be sited under local anesthetic without image guidance, are also available (Fig. 23.11). Similar to other sites described below, interstitial ^{125}I seed implants can be used in cases of unresectable disease with favorable rates of control and toxicity.[157–159]

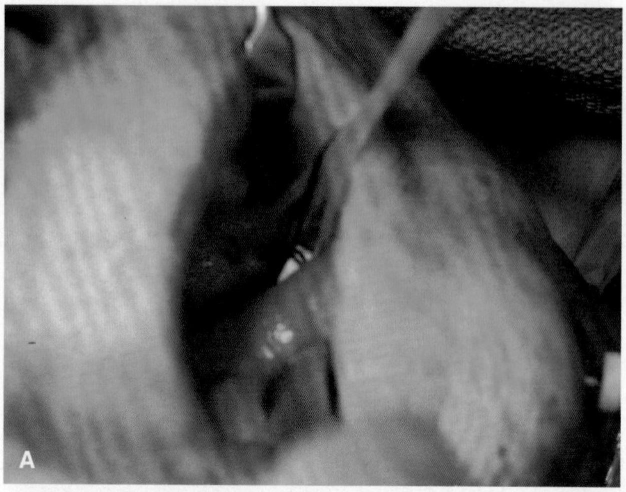

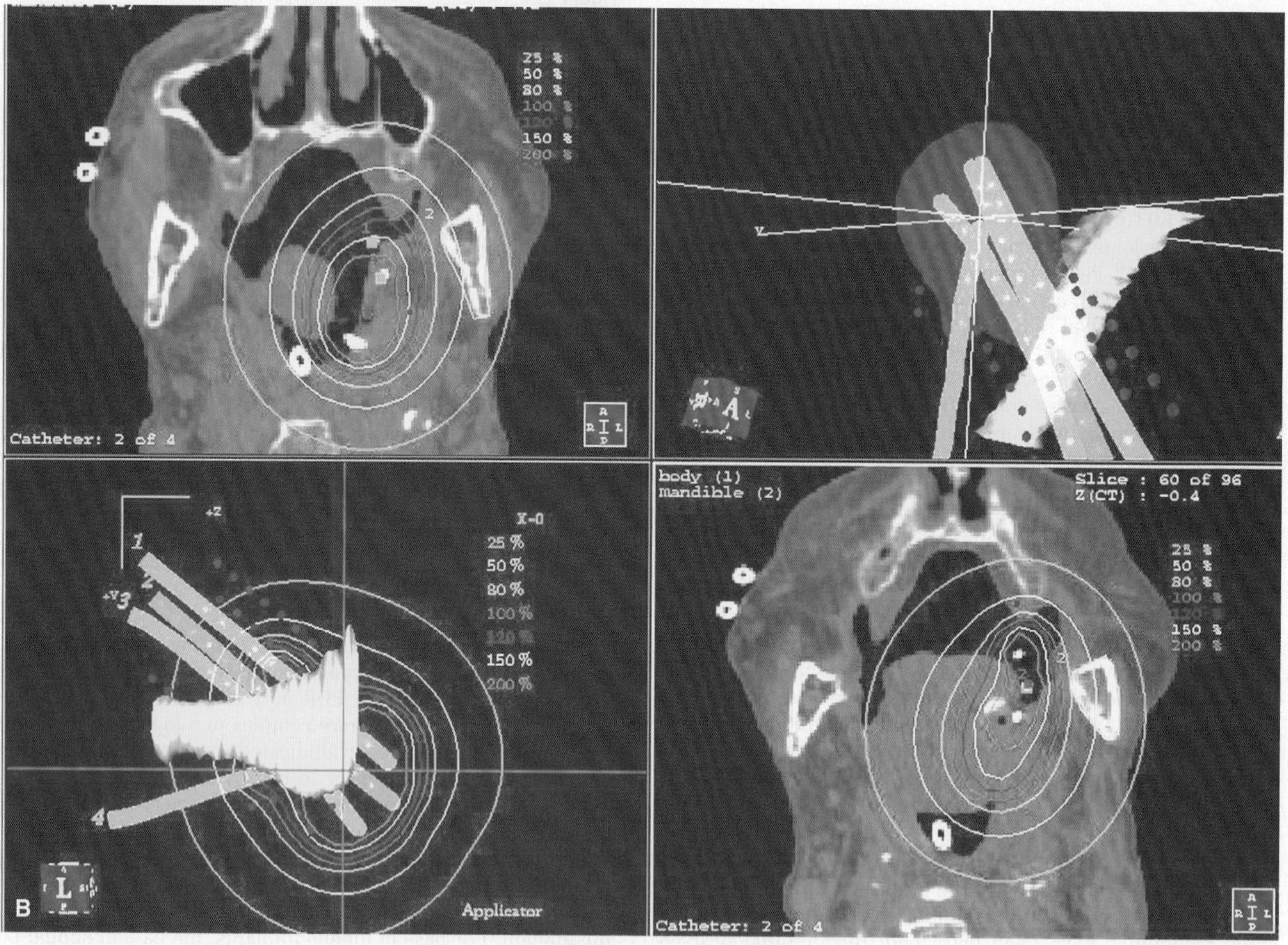

FIGURE 23.10. A: Catheters placed to deliver a brachytherapy boost to the pharynx. **B:** Three-dimensional computer optimized dosimetry of the pharynx implant.

Brachytherapy is indicated in the majority of lip cancers, either as the sole modality in tumors 0.5 to 5 cm or as a boost following EBRT in tumors over 5 cm. For very superficial tumors, a surface applicator may be appropriate (Fig. 23.12), thus preventing scars from puncture wounds. However, the majority of tumors require the placement of two or three interstitial catheters across the tumor (Fig. 23.13); these can be placed freehand under local anesthetic. Typical doses are 45 to 75 Gy at the 85% reference isodose (higher doses for larger tumors, although at the risk of decreased cosmesis). Local control rates with LDR are 90% to 95%.[156,160]

For oral tongue tumors, brachytherapy offers similar control rates to surgery with the benefit of organ and function preservation. Brachytherapy alone can be used for smaller lesions or as a boost for larger lesions. Interstitial implants are preferred, whare are placed under general anesthetic using a metal trocar and threading the afterloading catheters through these. Looped catheters were popular when using ^{192}Ir ribbons, but with optimized PDR it is difficult for the source to pass into the curved tube; therefore, individual button-ended catheters are preferred for source excursion (Fig. 23.14). To prevent a cold spot on the tongue, an extra spacer can maintain the catheter above the tongue or dose optimization can be used, taking care not to cause a localized hot spot. Mandibular shielding is preferred. A dose of 65 Gy is typical as sole treatment and 20 to 25 Gy as a boost.[161] Local control compares

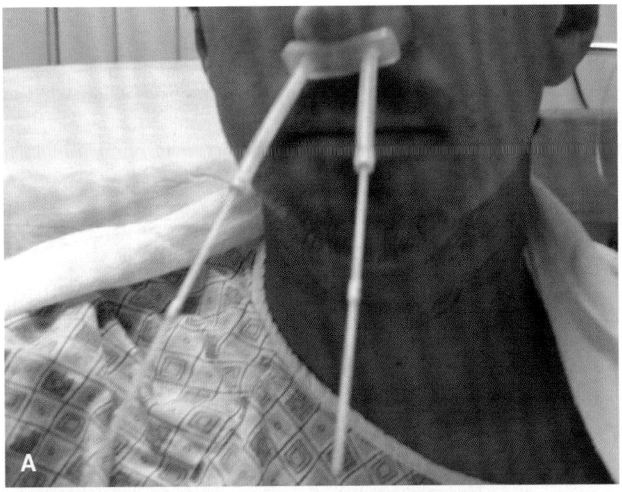

FIGURE 23.11. A: Patient with a Rotterdam applicator in situ within the nasopharynx. **B:** Three-dimensional dosimetry of the Rotterdam applicator, delivering computer optimized brachytherapy.

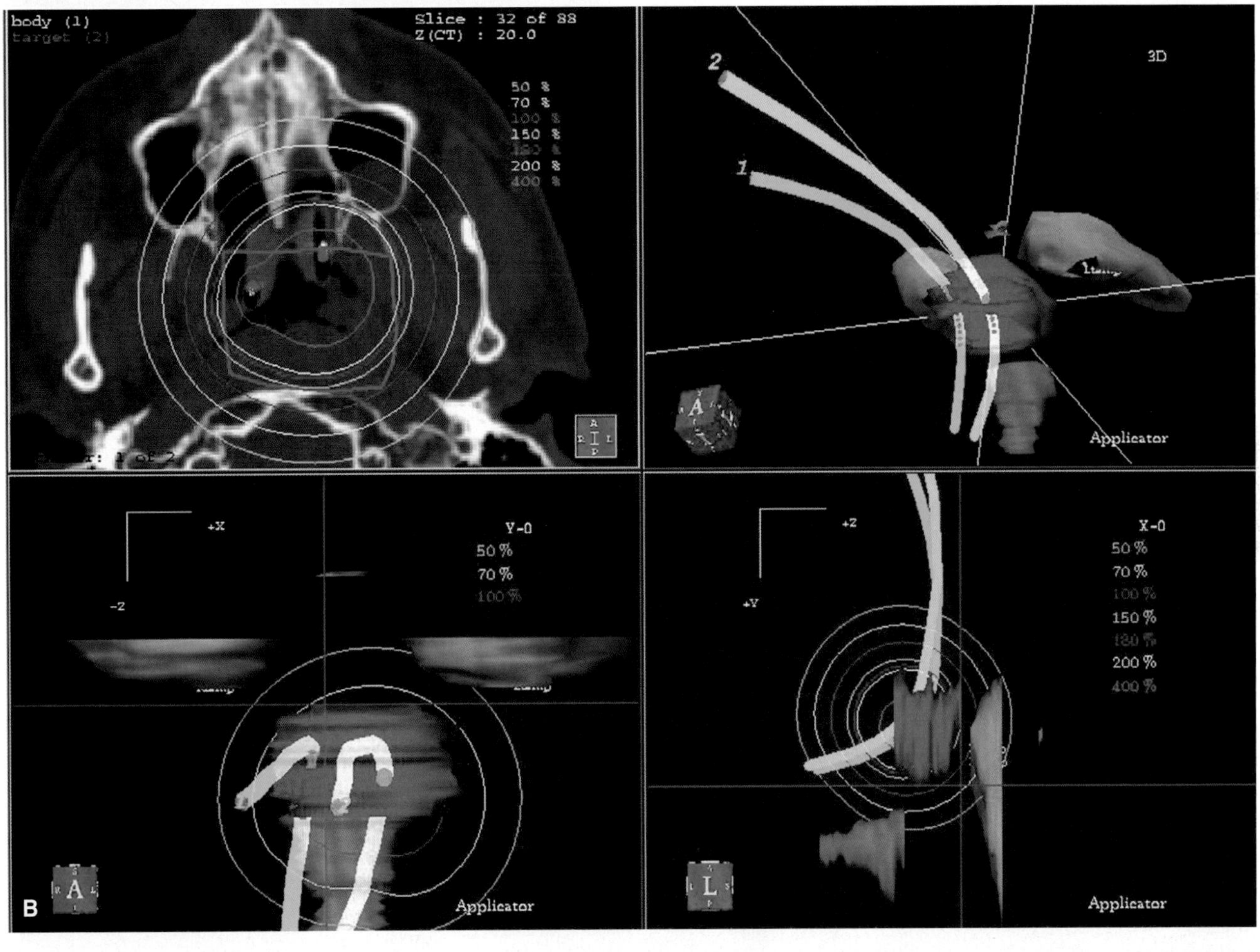

well to surgery, with small superficial tumors showing local control rates over 90%.[20]

Floor of mouth tumors are also best treated with interstitial implants with similar technique to tongue implants. Distance to the mandible is critical to prevent osteoradionecrosis. It may be preferable to perform surgery with reconstruction rather than risk late sequelae. Elective nodal dissection may be preferable to EBRT in advanced cases.[162] A dose of 65 Gy for sole treatment and 20 to 30 Gy boost is recommended, keeping overall treatment time as short as possible. Control rates range from 50% to 92% depending on tumor size, but bone necrosis is more common than other sites up to 30%.[156,162]

Oropharyngeal cancer traditionally present at an advanced stage due to its location in an area that is not visible with few pain fibers. Surgery can be very debilitating; therefore, EBRT and localized boost techniques are favored. A boost of 20 to 30 Gy is delivered using an interstitial implant. The implant is performed under general anesthetic with nasal intubation, and a covering tracheostomy is usually required. Hemorrhage may occur in implant removal, so it is important to remove the catheters under controlled conditions with venous access and surgical support. Local control rates up to 90% are reported with good rates of organ preservation.

Most nasopharyngeal tumors are inoperable due to their position at the base of the skull. However the nasopharynx is

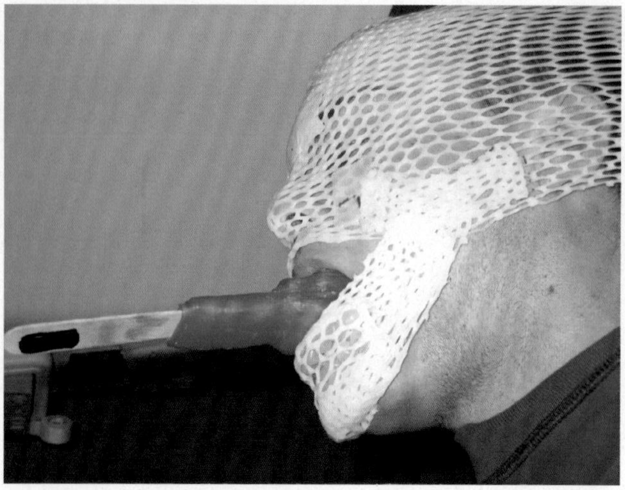

FIGURE 23.12. Surface applicator technique used to deliver a boost dose to a lower lip sarcoma following external beam radiation therapy. The wax mouth bite was used to displace the tongue and could be placed for every pulse of the pulsed-dose rate.

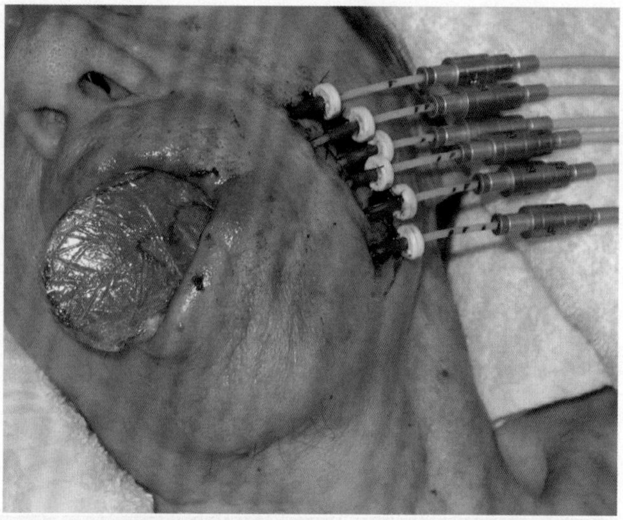

FIGURE 23.13. Multicatheter single-plane cheek implant. The metal gum shield can be placed for every pulse of the pulsed-dose rate.

easily accessible to brachytherapy catheters. These can be placed under topical anesthetic (e.g., using the Rotterdam applicator) or under direct vision using a Le Fort osteotomy. The main role of brachytherapy is as a localized boost or as a sole reirradiation technique, with typical doses of 12 to 20 Gy and 60 Gy, respectively. Local control is excellent even in reirradiation, where control rates of at least 50% are reported.[156]

Thoracic Seed Implants

Intraoperative permanent radioactive ^{125}I seed implantation can be used in the treatment of malignant thoracic tumors when resection margins are close or macroscopically or microscopically involved with tumor[163–178] or for palliation of inoperable disease.[179] The surgeon selects patients preoperatively when there is a concern of incomplete tumor resection or close or positive margins and refers to the brachytherapist. The patient is consented in advance for a permanent implant to be placed intraoperatively if required. Details of previous radiotherapy and chemotherapy treatment are carefully reviewed prior to surgery. The brachytherapy team is on call for the surgical procedure. Frozen-section analysis of margins may be needed to assess whether an implant is needed. Seeds are placed directly into a tumor as a volume implant or woven in a grid pattern in a planar implant. Volume implants require

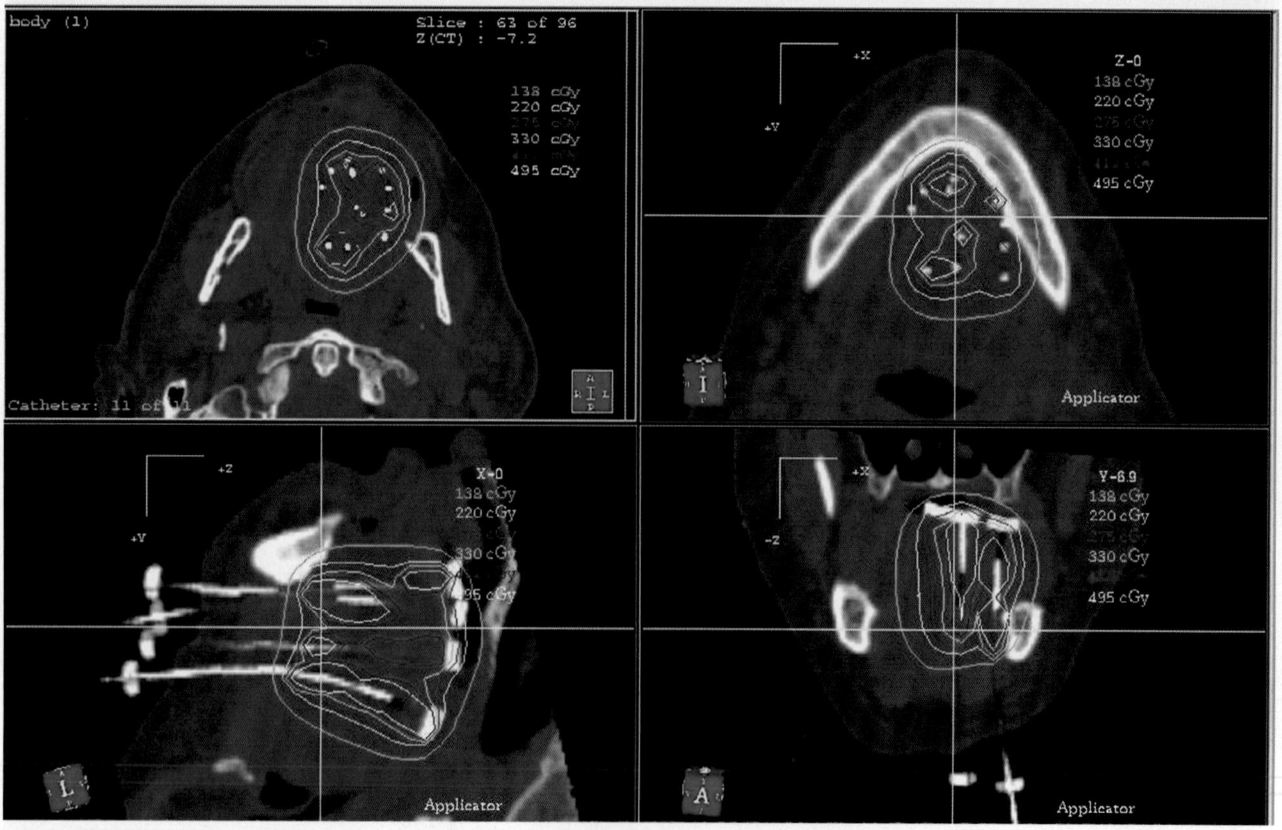

FIGURE 23.14. Tree-dimensional computer-optimized dosimetry of a tongue implant using button ended catheters.

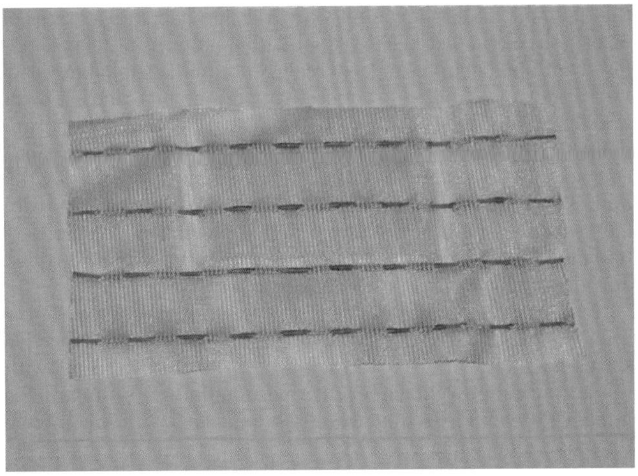

FIGURE 23.15. Premade seed mesh.

the use of an applicator or preloaded needles to deliver the seeds directly to the tumor. A planar implant can be ordered readymade in advance (Fig. 23.15), or custom made intraoperatively (Fig. 23.16).[180] Iodine-125 seeds set into Vicryl suture with 1-cm spacing between seeds can be woven into a mesh or sutured directly to the area at risk. The Vicryl suture and accompanying mesh degrades naturally after approximately 60 days, and at this point much of the dose has been delivered and the seeds are often held in position by local fibrotic reactions. The mesh can be used in open surgery thoracoscopically or utilizing a robotic system.[181] Seeds can be placed at equally spaced intervals into a layer of foam,[170,182] but this implant may be more difficult to suture in place, as the seeds are not easily visible and are therefore at risk of being displaced or damaged by the suture needle. Alternative seed placement devices may aid seed placement such as the customized suture gun (Fig. 23.17). Radiation exposure during the procedure to the implanting radiation oncologist and surgeon is very low[183] and well within occupational radiation exposure guidelines. When the implant has been sited, the operating room is surveyed for the presence of radiation. The patient is surveyed at the outer body surface over the implant, at 0.5 m and 1 m. In the immediate postoperative period, no change in patient care is required, subject to standard post-vLDR implant precautions of preventing exposure to children or pregnant women.[184]

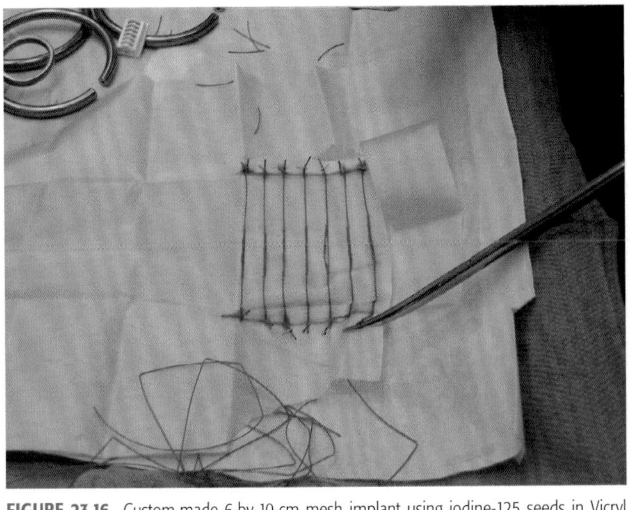

FIGURE 23.16. Custom-made 6-by-10-cm mesh implant using iodine-125 seeds in Vicryl carrier. The steel rings used to shield the isotope in transit can be seen at the *top left* of the picture.

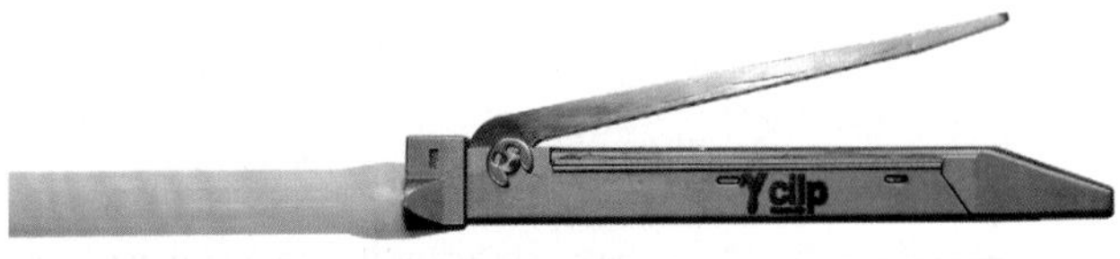

FIGURE 23.17. Seed staple gun.

For sublobar resection, the dose recommended is 100 Gy, at 5 mm from the mesh or 7 mm from the central axis of the implant. For incomplete resection of tumor or positive margins, the dose chosen will depend on many factors, such as adjacent structures or previous radiation, and the type of surgery performed must also be considered in case there is an increased risk of late normal tissue toxicity.[185] The curvature of the implant should also be assessed because, over a curved surface, dose penetration is asymmetric compared to a linear implant.[186] Isodoses on the concave side of a curvature are farther from the implant surface, potentially decreasing the dose delivered. The asymmetry increases with decreasing radii of curvature (Fig. 23.18). Interestingly, *in vitro* studies have shown that selected human lung cancer cell lines show a greater sensitivity to ^{125}I seed brachytherapy than HDR irradiation, an effect that was further potentiated with the use of radiosensitizers.[187]

Lobectomy is the standard of care for patients with operable stage I non–small cell lung cancer; however, intraoperative ^{125}I seed placement has been used in conjunction with sublobar resection in patients with lung cancer who are medically unfit for lobar resection.[168,171,172,174–178] Retrospective studies showed

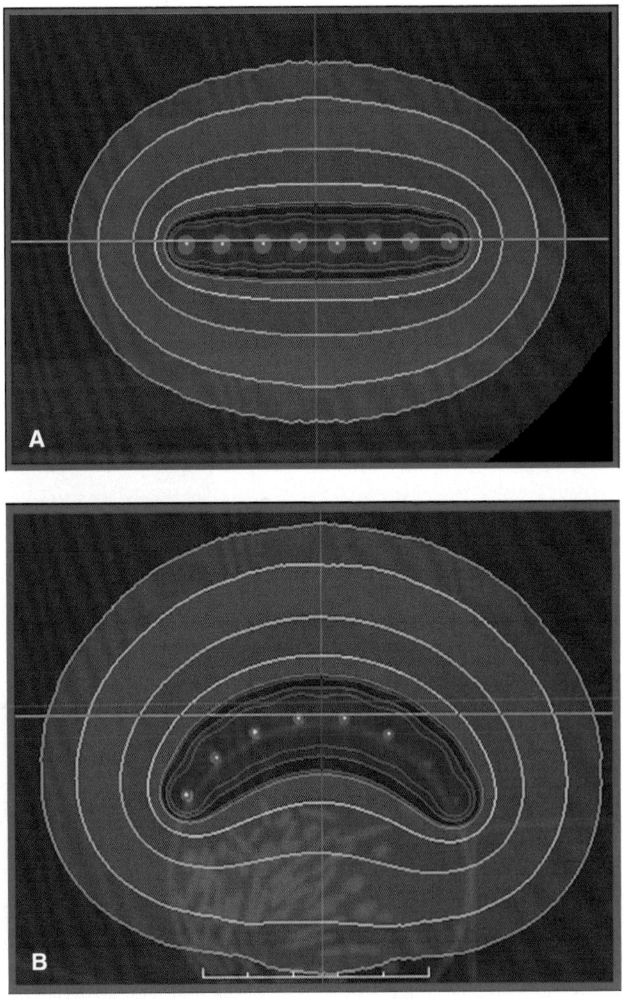

FIGURE 23.18. Effect of curvature on the dosimetry of a single planar mesh seed implant.

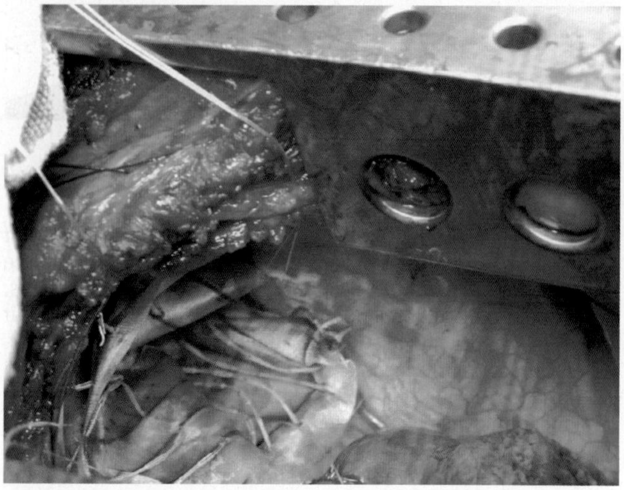

FIGURE 23.19. Intraoperative photograph of a custom-made mesh interstitial very low-dose rate brachytherapy implant placed at the apex of the thoracic cavity following resection of a Pancoast tumor with close resection margins. The surgically collapsed lung can be seen at the base of the image.

that patients undergoing sublobar resection had similar rates of disease-free and overall survival, but that patterns of relapse differed with higher rates of local recurrence in the sublobar resection group.[188] Thus, intraoperative permanent seed implant brachytherapy has been evaluated in a multi-institution randomized prospective trial by the American College of Surgeons Oncology Group (study Z4032).[189] Preliminary reports show no adverse pulmonary morbidity in patients who underwent sublobar resection and brachytherapy compared with sublobar resection alone.[190,191] Addition of the brachytherapy procedure added approximately 15 minutes to the anesthesia time.[175]

For intrathoracic tumors with incomplete resection or microscopic close margins, retrospective and prospective series have shown disease-free and overall survival rates with the addition of an intraoperative permanent seed implant are improved over those that would be expected with incomplete resection alone (Fig. 23.19).[163–166,169]

Breast

Breast-conserving surgery is a proven alternative to mastectomy in patients with early-stage breast cancer, offering equivalent disease-free and overall survival.[192–194] Adjuvant radiotherapy

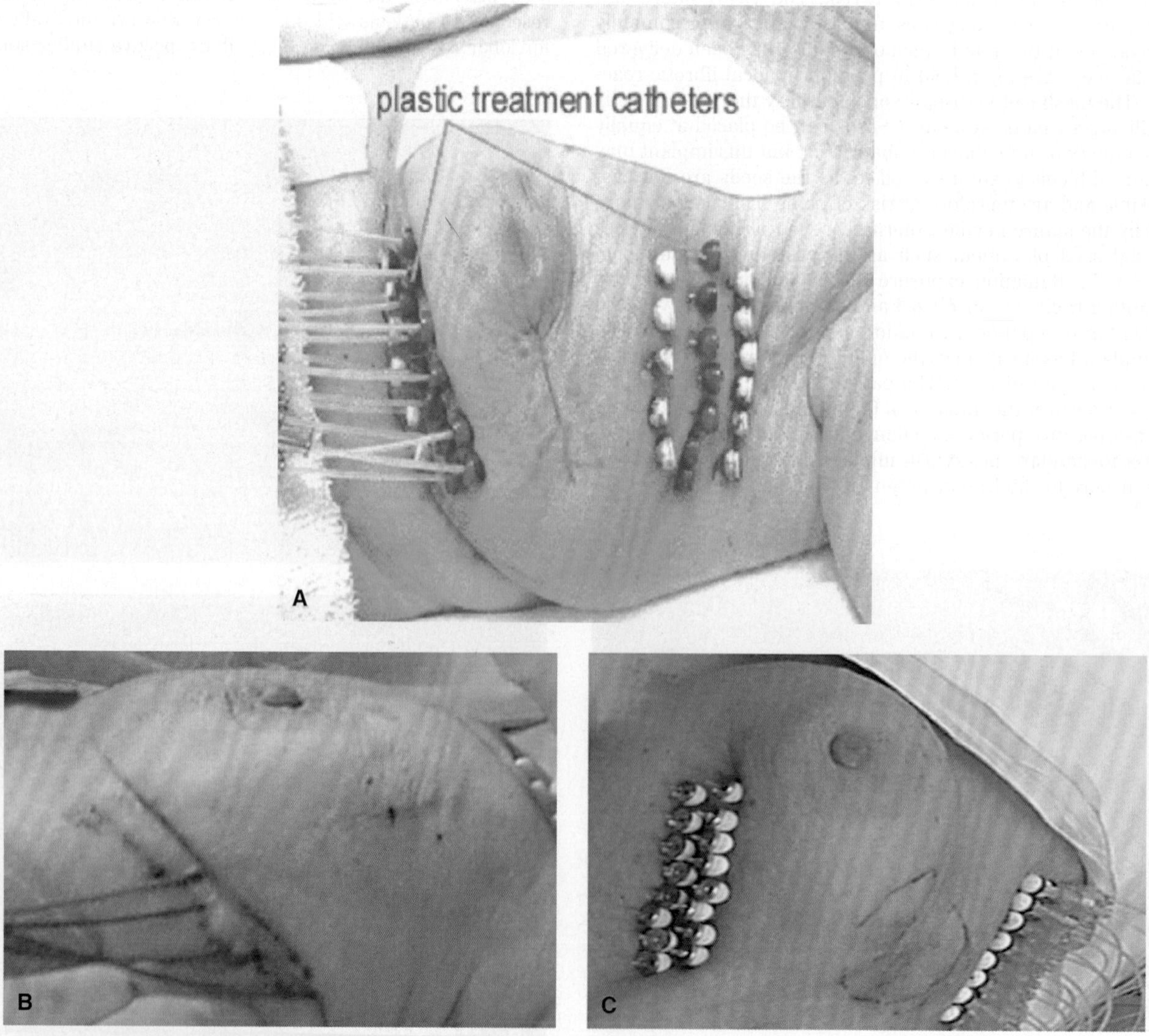

FIGURE 23.20. A: Interstitial template breast implant, which could be used for low-dose rate (LDR), pulsed-dose rate (PDR), or high-dose rate (HDR). **B,C:** Freehand breast implant, which could be used for LDR, PDR, or HDR. (From Kelley JR, et al. Breast brachytherapy. In: Devlin P, ed. *Brachytherapy: applications and techniques.* Philadelphia: Lippincott Williams & Wilkins, 2006, with permission.)

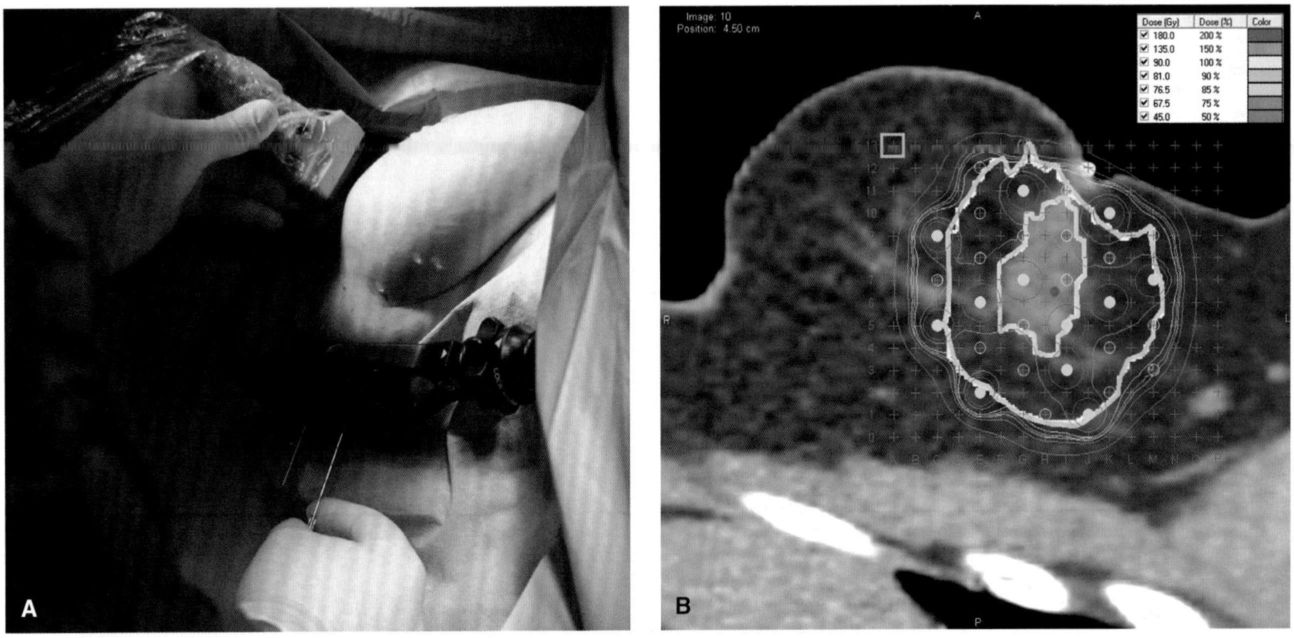

FIGURE 23.21. **A:** Intraoperative photograph demonstrating a template partial breast implant using iodine-125 seeds under ultrasound guidance. **B:** Sagittal computed tomography image to demonstrate the postoperative dosimetry of the implant. (Courtesy Dr Jean-Phillipe Pignol.)

is required because it results in a significant reduction in the risk of death due to breast cancer; unfortunately, this is offset by an increase in deaths due to other causes.[194] In the nonirradiated breast, recurrences tend to occur in the tumor bed with an elsewhere recurrence rate of up to 3.5%.[192,193,195,196] Therefore, partial breast irradiation (PBI) is being investigated as an alternative treatment for selected patients with early-stage breast cancer.

Postoperative PBI using brachytherapy was initially developed using interstitial implants. A number of needles or tubes are placed across the tumor bed usually under general anesthetic, either using a template or freehand (Fig. 23.20). The treatment volume is generally the tumor cavity plus a 1- to 2-cm margin. The dose is custom shaped to this treatment volume. The dose can be delivered using LDR or PDR brachytherapy, typically over 4 to 5 days. The large number of catheters in an interstitial implant allows more control over skin and chest wall doses than single catheter techniques, especially with PDR dose optimization. The dose within the tumor is more homogenous with many smaller hot spots compared with one large hot spot with single catheter techniques.[197]

Interstitial implants have been in use for over 10 years, and phase I or II studies describe excellent results.[198–204] The largest matched-pair analysis compared 199 interstitial catheter PBI patients treated between 1980 to 1997 to 199 whole breast radiation therapy (WBRT) patients randomly selected from 709 eligible controls.[198] Each brachytherapy patient was matched to a WBRT patient according to multiple prognostic factors such as age, tumor size, histological grade, and lymph node status. There was no significant difference in local recurrence, elsewhere failure, and disease-free or overall survival. There was a significantly lower incidence of contralateral breast cancer in the brachytherapy group.

Permanent interstitial seed implant has been described for PBI (Fig. 23.21).[205] Palladium-103 seeds were implanted using ultrasound guidance and a dose of 90 Gy was prescribed to the tumor cavity plus a 1.5-cm margin. In a group of 67 patients, no recurrences were seen at a median of 32 months follow-up with acceptable rates of toxicity and patient confidence. A radiobiologic dosimetric modeling study predicts that for PBI, using brachytherapy toxicity will be lower for a seed implant than for a multicatheter interstitial technique.[206]

Sarcoma

In the modern era, sarcoma surgery has become more refined, moving away from disfiguring, disabling surgery and toward a multidisciplinary approach combining surgery and EBRT and, in certain tumors, chemotherapy.[207,208] The use of LDR brachytherapy for soft tissue sarcoma (STS) was first described in 1963 using a variety of isotopes, including ^{222}Ra and ^{192}Ir.[209] Brachytherapy offers several advantages over EBRT: the catheters can be placed at the time of initial resection and loaded 5 days postoperatively, enabling the whole STS treatment to be completed within 10 to 14 days. Placement under direct vision allows accurate coverage of the resection cavity. There may be less hypoxia immediately postoperatively, enabling the radiotherapy to be more effective. The heterogeneity of dose delivery allows high doses to the tumor bed while minimizing the dose to surrounding normal tissues, thus minimizing toxicity.

The American Brachytherapy Society issued guidelines for the use of brachytherapy in patients with STS.[210] Table 23.5 presents a summary of the general principles for STS brachytherapy. Catheters are placed at the time of surgery, either using a single entry sealed end catheter (Fig. 23.22) or double

TABLE 23.5 GENERAL RECOMMENDATIONS FOR SOFT TISSUE SARCOMA BRACHYTHERAPY (INCORPORATING AMERICAN BRACHYTHERAPY SOCIETY GUIDELINES)

Discuss patient preoperatively in a multidisciplinary setting
Determine CTV by radiographic, surgical, and pathologic findings
Place catheters to encompass CTV, demarcate CTV with surgical clips if possible
Identify and demarcate normal structures that are at risk for complications
Cover tenuous wounds with well-vascularized flaps
Place microvascular anastomoses away from radiation target area
Use drains over catheters to act as a spacer to increase the distance of the wound from the implant
Use spacers (e.g., Gelfoam) to increase the distance between catheters and critical normal structures
Ensure catheters enter skin at least 1 cm from surgical incision
Space catheters at 1- to 1.5-cm intervals in parallel arrays
Secure catheters carefully, immobilizing extremity if necessary
Use computed tomography to determine the CTV and organs at risk
Do not load catheters until after day 5 postoperatively

CTV, clinical target volume.

From refs. 210 and 211.

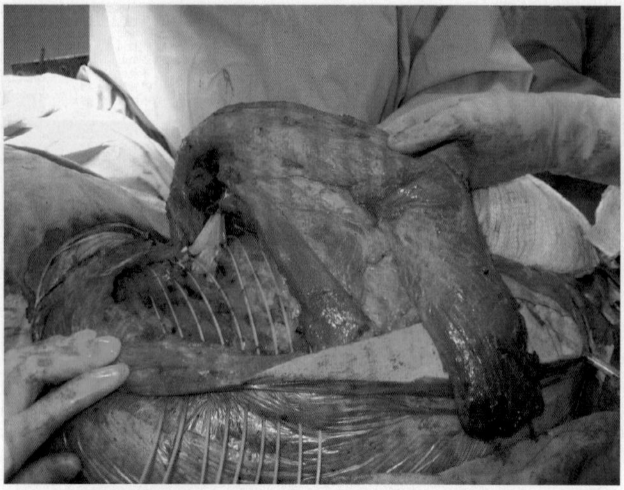

FIGURE 23.22. Intraoperative photograph of a multicatheter interstitial pulsed-dose rate brachytherapy implant following excision of a sarcoma of the upper back.

entry button-ended catheters. The catheter is secured with plastic buttons, which do not produce artifact in CT or MRI scanning. The catheters can then be used for afterloaded LDR ^{192}Ir strands or connected to an afterloading PDR machine. A mesh implant can also be used with a similar technique to that described in the thoracic vLDR section.[163] A typical radical LDR dose is 42 to 45 Gy,[211] PDR 45 to 60 Gy,[212] and mesh implant 100 to 150 Gy at 5 mm.[163] A typical boost dose is 15 Gy for LDR or PDR or 50 to 70 Gy for mesh implant.

Phase II trials showed the utility of LDR brachytherapy for postoperative STS treatment[166,213] and therefore a randomized phase III trial was conducted.[214] One hundres seventeen patients were randomized to brachytherapy or no brachytherapy following R0 or R1 resection, and patients were stratified by various factors, including size and grade. Five-year actuarial local control for all patients was 82% versus 69% (P = .04), but on subgroup analysis, no effect was seen in the patients with low-grade tumors. With longer follow-up of the high-grade tumors only, local control was 89% versus 66% (P = .0025) but no effect was seen on distant metastases or overall survival. Functional parameters were well maintained post-brachytherapy. PDR brachytherapy has been used in adults and children, either as a boost (for large tumors where compartmental surgery proved difficult) or as radical treatment.[212,215,216] Studies report excellent local control with good cosmetic results and acceptable toxicity comparable to results achieved with LDR. However, a retrospective study of adjuvant LDR brachytherapy to pre- or postoperative IMRT in primary extremity sarcoma showed 5-year local control with IMRT to be better than that for brachytherapy (92% vs. 81%; P = .04), despite the fact that the IMRT group had significantly higher rates of adverse features (e.g., tumors over 10 cm in size and close or positive surgical margins).

Surface Applicators

Brachytherapy surface applicators can be used to treat a variety of superficial targets using LDR or PDR. For curved or irregular surface or thicker lesions, a customized mold can be constructed, often using an acrylic or thermoplastic cast (Fig. 23.23). The brachytherapy catheters can be laid directly on to the mold or used with a spacer to ensure uniform catheter distribution. When used with computerized optimization, this surface applicator technique has been shown to give dose distributions that are more homogeneous than those for conventional electron techniques.[217] PDR carries the benefit of dose optimization, which allows the treatment depth to vary along different points of an individual catheter for lesions of varying thickness. Suitable superficial targets can also be treated

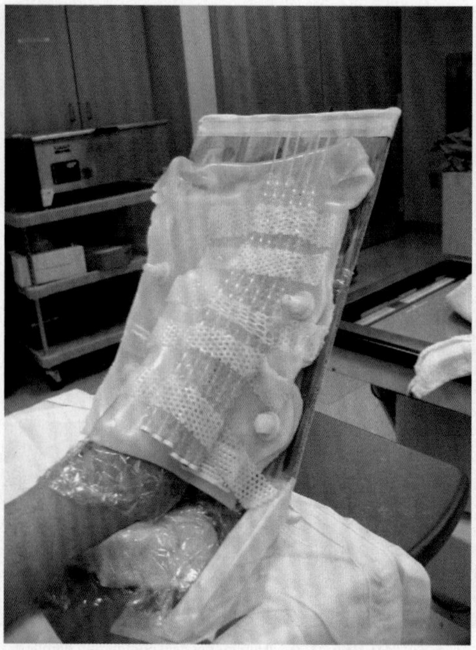

FIGURE 23.23. Surface applicator mold used to administer brachytherapy to the dorsum of the foot following incomplete excision of a soft tissue sarcoma.

with interstitial implants, which can give greater penetration of dose beneath the skin surface.

Surface applicator techniques have been used to treat primary tumors in both the radical and the palliative setting. When ^{90}Sr surface applicator brachytherapy was used at a dose of 20 Gy in 4 fractions by Fraunholtz et al.[218] to treat keloid scarring after surgical excision, the results were assessed by patient satisfaction questionnaires. Sixty-one percent of patients were extremely or mainly satisfied with the therapeutic outcome and 51% with the cosmetic outcome. With a median follow-up of over 5 years, 44% of keloids had recurred, with a significant increase in sternal lesion relapse (86%) (an area described by other investigators as a common site of keloid relapse[219,220]). Grade 3 skin toxicity occurred in 16% of the relapse-free group and 25% of the relapse group, although these skin changes may be indistinguishable from relapse in the latter group.

Surface applicator brachytherapy techniques have been used to treat locally recurrent breast cancer following previous chest wall irradiation. Using LDR, ^{192}Ir implanted into flexible silicone sheets delivered in 2 or 3 fractions at monthly intervals to administer a total dose of 65 Gy 2 to 4 mm below the skin surface, Delanian et al.[221] showed a complete regression of tumor in 9 of 11patients. The two patients who did not respond died from pulmonary lymphangitis 4 and 5 months after brachytherapy. One patient developed a necrotic ulcer in the skin, which healed after 8 weeks of symptomatic treatment. One patient died from respiratory failure that may have been related to cumulative pulmonary toxicity, which must be considered as a treatment complication. Some patients also received interstitial implants in the chest wall, which would have increased the dose at depth to the previously irradiated tissue and to the underlying lung.

Harms et al.[222] used PDR brachytherapy and flexible rubber surface applicator molds in 58 patients with local recurrence of breast cancer who had received previous breast or chest wall EBRT. A median dose of 40 Gy to the skin surface in 2 fractions was administered at a median time interval of 31 days. The local recurrence-free survival at 1 year was 96% for patients with microscopic disease at the time of brachytherapy and 89% for patients with macroscopic disease, 75% and 71%, respectively, at 3 years. Seven percent of patients developed

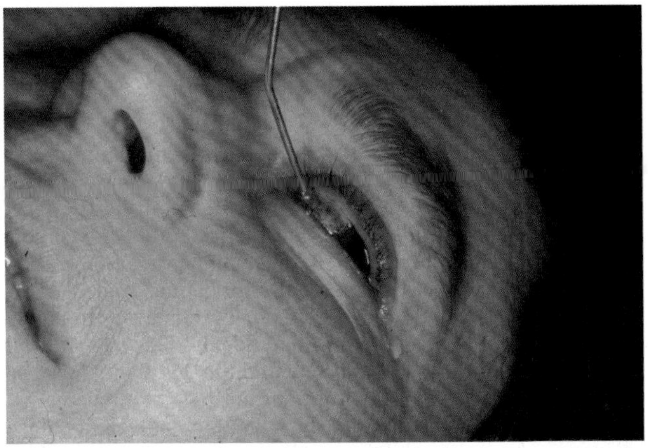

FIGURE 23.24. Patient receiving a strontium ophthalmic application. (Courtesy Dr Steve Whitaker.)

chronic ulcer, two of whom had undergone surgical treatment prior to reirradiation, and 50% of patients developed grade 3 telangiectasia in the treatment field. The skin toxicity was higher in this study, but this may have been a result of improved reporting of skin complications because the incidence of telangiectasia and fibrosis was not reported in the LDR study.

Ophthalmic Plaques

Ophthalmic brachytherapy applicators can be applied directly to the eye to deliver a highly localized dose with rapid falloff (Fig. 23.24). These deliver dose to the conjunctiva of the eye, most commonly for malignant tumors of the conjunctiva such as squamous carcinoma, melanoma, and lymphoma or to prevent recurrence of pterygium following surgical excision. Iodine-125 seeds are inserted into plaques formed of silicone rubber and gold and are then sutured to the sclera. Strontium-90 and ^{106}Ru are manufactured as curved applicators, ^{90}Sr as a fixed diameter applicator (typically 12 mm) (Fig. 23.25), and ^{106}Ru in a range of diameters. The eye is anesthetized with installation of local anesthetic eye drops. The applicator is soaked in an antiseptic solution, followed by double rinsing in sterile saline. Sterile lubricant is then applied to the active surface of the applicator to lessen trauma to the cornea and sclera. The applicator is then gently applied over the area of bare sclera, adjacent limbus, and affected cornea and held in place by the operator for short applications or sutured to the sclera for longer applications. Undue pressure must be avoided, as this increases trauma and reduces the distance from the applicator to the lens, which is the dose limiting normal tissue. If necessary, two treated fields can be overlapped if the area to be treated exceeds that of the active surface of the applicator, although this, inevitably, carries a risk of increased acute and chronic sequelae. After treatment, the patient wears an eye patch for 2 hours until the local anesthetic wears off. Some degree of conjunctivitis is common and if mild, can be treated with antibiotic eye drops. If moderate to severe, a steroid-containing eye drop should be used. Long-term sequelae are unusual but more likely with higher fraction size and higher total dose. Scleral ulceration is the most common complication in doses up to 52 Gy, with a small percentage of eyes developing symblepharon fusion of the eyelid to the globe. Surgical trauma also plays a part in these sequelae. A small percentage of eyes will develop radiation-induced cataracts, again at higher doses (>45 Gy).

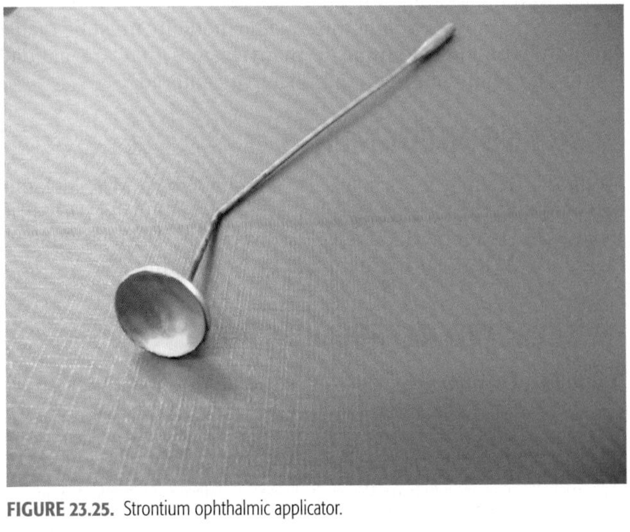

FIGURE 23.25. Strontium ophthalmic applicator.

The Collaborative Ocular Melanoma Study group conducted two randomized trials in North America examining the use of ^{125}I for choroidal melanoma. The study examining the use of ^{125}I brachytherapy versus enucleation for tumors of 3- to 8-mm depth demonstrated no difference in survival and similar rates of toxicity[223,224] for the two techniques, thus supporting the use of ^{125}I. The use of ^{103}Pd and ^{131}Cs seeds has also been investigated with promising dosimetric results.[225,226] Modern dosimetry planning is being employed to investigate whether side effects may be lessened with optimal planning techniques.[226–228]

Strictly speaking, ^{90}Sr delivers HDR brachytherapy (a beta-emitter) with a typical dose rate of 100 Gy per hour compared to ^{125}I (a gamma-emitter) with a dose rate of 0.5 to 1 Gy per hour. Thus, ^{90}Sr delivers a single fraction treatment dose over 2 to 3 hours, whereas ^{125}I delivers a treatment dose over 30 to 300 hours. The percentage depth dose in tissue falls from 100% at the surface to 4% at 4 mm, 1% at 6.5 mm, and 0.9% at 8 mm (corresponding to the anterior surface of the lens and equator and posterior surface of the lens, respectively). Van Ginderdeuren et al.[229] demonstrated a 90% 15-year tumor control rate for sclera melanoma using a ^{90}Sr applicator, with a proportion of the recurrences at the edges possibly due to the small applicator size, using doses of 450 to 800 Gy at the sclera. There was a 45% preservation of good vision, which was generally dependent on tumor position rather than dose delivered. Ruthenium-106 eye plaques can also be used and may become the beta-emitter of choice, as ^{90}Sr eye plaques gradually decay beyond useful dose delivery. They deliver similar results to ^{90}Sr and have even been used with thermotherapy to deliver improved outcomes.[230,231]

Pterygium is a benign proliferation of the conjunctiva over the cornea, occurring most commonly in areas with high sun exposure. Surgery can be performed for irritative symptoms, effects on vision, or cosmesis but carries a high recurrence rate. Locally applied ^{90}Sr has been used to decrease the rate of recurrence to as low as 0.5%,[232] using doses varying from 20 to 60 Gy in 1 to 6 fractions. The incidence of sclera complications is lower with fractionated treatment (4.5% vs. 1%). However, alternative treatments such as topical chemotherapy and conjunctival autografting are replacing ophthalmic plaque brachytherapy.[233,234] Brachytherapy should not be combined with topical chemotherapy due to the risk of scleral melting.

Strontium-90 has been used in the treatment of wet macular degeneration, visual impairment caused by neovascularization beneath the retinal pigment of the retina. Studies including brachytherapy have not shown conclusive results, with the possible side effect of radiation retinopathy; thus, this technique has been largely supplanted by the use of vascular endothelial growth factor inhibitors.[235] However, it may be of use in certain cases, particularly large areas.[236]

Anus

Squamous cell carcinoma of the anus is a rare cancer that is usually treated with chemoradiotherapy with good rates of sphincter preservation. The most common site of relapse is locally, and thus methods of local dose escalation have been explored. EBRT, preferably with chemotherapy, is necessary to treat the tumor, and wider nodal area then the tumor boost can be delivered using brachytherapy.[237] Interstitial brachytherapy implants typically consist of a single-plane catheter implant using a plastic perineal template curved around the anus. Catheter placement may be optimized by the use of advanced imaging techniques such as three-dimensional endoluminal ultrasound.[238,239] Papillon et al.[240] described an LDR boost using ^{192}Ir to deliver 20 to 30 Gy in 221 patients 2 months after completing EBRT. Local control rates were comparable to surgical techniques and 90% of patients with no evidence of relapse remained colostomy free. It has been suggested that, when using a split course technique, if treatment time is extended over 80 days, a brachytherapy boost may provide better local control than EBRT.[241] PDR techniques have been described with similar rates of disease control and toxicity to LDR.[242–244]

Central Nervous System

Although initial treatment for glioblastoma has improved over the past decade, most glioblastomas recur, the majority of these within 2 cm of the original tumor cavity. Because the majority of patients will have received 60 Gy to the tumor at the time of initial diagnosis, retreatment techniques may be limited; ^{125}I seeds can be used to deliver a conformal dose of reirradiation. At the time of recurrence, the surgeon will perform the maximal resection possible and implant ^{125}I seeds in the excision cavity at 0.5- to 1-cm intervals. This gives a highly localized boost, assuming the volume of disease residual is small because the dose falloff is rapid. The procedure appears to be well tolerated, and survival compares favorably to similar patients who did not receive brachytherapy.[245–247] The use of ^{125}I seeds at the time of initial radiotherapy has been investigated, but no difference was seen in randomized trials.[248,249] Thus, if a boost is required, this technique has generally been supplanted by stereotactic radiosurgery, which does not require a second invasive surgical procedure.

Iodine-125 seed placement has also been described in patients with paraspinal tumors with a low rate of toxicity and good local control rates.[167,173] The procedure was well tolerated and no myelitis was seen, despite cumulative cord doses of up to 167 Gy.

Customized yttrium-90 dural plaques have been used intraoperatively in patients with spinal or paraspinal sarcomas to deliver a high localized dose to the dura while minimizing the dose delivered to the underlying spinal cord (Fig. 23.26). Local control rates are promising, and there were no acute or late complications from brachytherapy.[250]

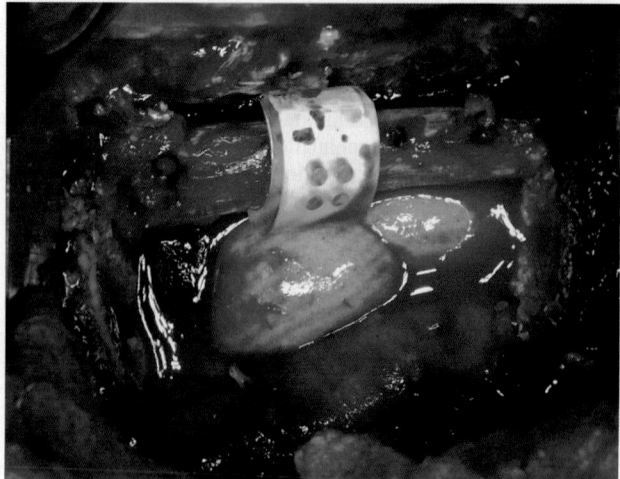

FIGURE 23.26. A dural plaque utilizes phosphorus-32 chemically bonded to a flexible polymeric film. The film is 0.5-mm thick and is backed by 4.5 mm of polycarbonate. Typical dose rates at time of treatment are in the 1.5 to 2.5 Gy per minute range.

CONCLUSIONS

The dosimetry of LDR brachytherapy treatment planning has evolved from estimation of dose delivered to accurate image-guided, computer-optimized determinations of dose. Exact knowledge of the position of organs at risk and of the conformation of target volumes combined with dose optimization achievable with PDR computerized afterloading source delivery allows the brachytherapist to tailor dose delivery to highly specific ideals and deliver with great fidelity. This has allowed improved prediction of late toxicity and the possibility for dose escalation in areas with a high tumor burden.

Brachytherapy is particularly suited to subvolume dose escalation due to its ability to deliver a highly localized dose with rapid dose falloff in the surrounding tissue. This could allow increased dose to subvolumes within a CTV without a corresponding increase in dose to surrounding normal tissues. It is important with the advent of these new techniques that the accepted methods of practice are constantly re-examined to ensure that the patient receives the optimum treatment with the lowest risk of complications in the future.

Dosimetry remains critically important within modern brachytherapy practice. Knowledge of the established dosimetry systems is critical to prevent late complications resulting from suboptimal catheter placement with reliance on computerized optimization to overcome this. Modern imaging techniques can provide three-dimensional information about a target volume and surrounding normal structures. It is important to generate methods of incorporating this new knowledge with existing practice.

LDR and PDR brachytherapy often require indwelling applicators or catheters that necessitate hospitalization for the duration of the brachytherapy course. Surgical procedures are often required to place the brachytherapy seeds and applicators. Special skill and training are required to perform brachytherapy, much of which is not generally a part of oncology training rotations. LDR brachytherapy may result in radiation exposure to medical staff, although remote afterloaders and PDR techniques minimize this exposure. Such a highly localized treatment can result in little or no dose to adjacent areas at risk of tumor spread, risking marginal misses and tumor recurrence if case selection is not carefully considered.

Brachytherapy also requires a high initial capital outlay. An adequate number of cases are required both to maintain the brachytherapist's skill and to justify the expenditure. The American Board of Radiology is conducting a pilot program of Focused Practice Recognition in Brachytherapy, encouraging brachytherapy to be practiced mostly by physicians with additional training and ongoing peer support or review. The choice of brachytherapy as a radiotherapeutic modality must be made carefully with consideration of many factors that are patient centered, tumor centered, and resource centered.

ACKNOWLEDGMENTS

We thank Dr. Robert Cormack, Dr. Juanita Crook, Mrs. Melanie Cunningham, Dr. George Dundas, Mr. Jorgen Hansen, Dr. Mira Keyes, Mr. Desmond O'Farrell, Dr. Howard Pai, Dr. Jean-Phillipe Pignol, Dr. Akila Viswanathan, and Dr. Steve Whittaker.

SELECTED REFERENCES

A full list of references for this chapter is available online.

3. International Commission on Radiation Units and Measurements. *Dose and volume specifications for reporting intracavitary therapy in gynecology* (report 38). Bethesda, MD: International Commission on Radiation Units and Measurements, 1985:1–23.
5. Swift PS, Purser P, Roberts LW, et al. Pulsed low dose rate brachytherapy for pelvic malignancies. *Int J Radiat Oncol Biol Phys* 1997;37:811–817.

11. Dale RG, Jones B. The clinical radiobiology of brachytherapy. *Br J Radiol* 1998; 71:465–483.
13. Fowler JF, van Limbergen EFM. Biological effect of pulsed dose rate brachytherapy with stepping sources if short half-times of repair are present in tissues. *Int J Radiat Oncol Biol Phys* 1997;37(4):877–883.
37. Georg D, Kirisits C, Hillbrand M, et al. Image-guided radiotherapy for cervix cancer: high-tech external beam therapy versus high-tech brachytherapy. *Int J Radiat Oncol Biol Phys* 2008;71(4):1272–1278.
38. Polo A. Pulsed dose rate brachytherapy. *Clin Transl Oncol* 2008;10:324–333.
43. Green J, Kirwan J, Tierney J, et al. Concomitant chemotherapy and radiation therapy for cancer of the uterine cervix. *Cochrane Database Syst Rev* 2005;3:CD002225.
47. Haie-Meder C, Potter R, Van Limbergen E, et al. Recommendations from the gynaecological (GYN) GEC ESTRO working group: concepts and terms in 3D image based 3D treatment planning in cervix cancer brachytherapy with emphasis on MRI assessment of GTV and CTV. *Radiother Oncol* 2005;74:235–245.
48. Potter R, Haie-Meder C, Van Limbergen E, et al. Recommendations from gynaecological (GYN) GEC ESTRO working group (II): concepts and terms in 3D image-based treatment planning in cervix cancer brachytherapy-3D dose volume parameters and aspects of 3D image-based anatomy, radiation physics, radiobiology. *Radiother Oncol* 2006;78:67–77.
50. Lee LJ, Das IJ, Higgins SA, et al. American Brachytherapy Society consensus guidelines for locally advanced carcinoma of the cervix. Part III: low-dose-rate and pulsed-dose-rate brachytherapy. *Brachytherapy* 2012;11:53–57.
51. Benrath J, Kozek-Langenecker S, Hüpfl M, et al. Anaesthesia for brachytherapy—5½ yr of experience in 1622 procedures. *Br J Anaesth* 2006;96(2):195–200.
71. Potter R, Gerbaulet A, Haie-Meder C. Endometrial cancer. In: Gerbaulet A, et al., eds. *The GEC ESTRO handbook of brachytherapy*. Leuven, Belgium: ESTRO, 2002: 365–402.
81. Kong A, Johnson N, Cornes P, et al. Adjuvant radiotherapy for stage I endometrial cancer. *Cochrane Database Syst Rev* 2007;2:CD00396.
93. Rosenthal SA, Bittner NH, Beyer DC, et al. American Society for Radiation Oncology (ASTRO) and American College of Radiology (ACR) practice guideline for the transperineal permanent brachytherapy of prostate cancer. *Int J Radiat Oncol Biol Phys* 2011;79(2):335–341.
94. Nag S, Beyer D, Friedland J, et al. American Brachytherapy Society (ABS) recommendations for transperineal permanent brachytherapy of prostate cancer. *Int J Radiat Oncol Biol Phys* 1999;44(4):789–799.
102. Nath R, Bice WS, Butler WM, et al. AAPM recommendations on dose prescription and reporting methods for permanent interstitial brachytherapy for prostate cancer: report of Task Group 137. *Med Phys* 2009;36(11):5310–5322.
111. Bice WS, Prestidge BR, Kurtzman SM, et al. Recommendations for permanent prostate brachytherapy with (131)Cs: a consensus report from the Cesium Advisory Group. *Brachytherapy* 2008;7(4):290–296.
114. Ash D, Flynn A, Battermann J, et al. ESTRO/EAU/EORTC recommendations on permanent seed implantation for localized prostate cancer. *Radiother Oncol* 2000;57(3):315–321.
141. Crook J, Jezioranski J, Cygler JE. Penile brachytherapy: technical aspects and postimplant issues. *Brachytherapy* 2010;9(2):151–158.
152. Mazeron JJ, Gerbaulet A, Simon JM, et al. How to optimize therapeutic ratio in brachytherapy of head and neck squamous cell carcinoma? *Acta Oncol* 1998; 37(6):583–591.
156. Han P, Hu KS, Shankar RA, et al. Head and neck brachytherapy. In: Devlin PM, ed. *Brachytherapy: applications and techniques*. Philadelphia: Lippincott Williams & Wilkins, 2007:49–92.
180. Stewart AJ, Mutyala S, Holloway CL, et al. Intra-operative seed placement for thoracic malignancy—a review of technique, indications and published literature. *Brachytherapy* 2009;8(3):63–69.
210. Nag S, Janjan N, Petersen I, et al. The American Brachytherapy Society recommendations for brachytherapy of soft tissue sarcomas. *Int J Radiat Oncol Biol Phys* 2001;49(4):1033–1043.
223. Collaborative Ocular Melanoma Study Group. The COMS randomized trial of iodine 125 brachytherapy for choroidal melanoma: V. Twelve-year mortality rates and prognostic factors: COMS report No. 28. *Arch Ophthalmol* 2006;124(12): 1684–1693.

Chapter 24
The Physics and Dosimetry of High–Dose-Rate Brachytherapy

Bruce Thomadsen and Rupak K. Das

NATURE OF HIGH–DOSE-RATE BRACHYTHERAPY

Conventional brachytherapy was developed very soon after the discovery of radium. The limited amount of radium that could be packed into the needles and tubes dictated the use of many sources to deliver a treatment dose through a target volume, and even with many sources, the delivery of the dose-required durations from 1 day to 1 week. For the most part, when new radionuclides became available, they matched the strength of the radium sources to facilitate application of the clinical experience gained through the decades of radium treatments. This conventional treatment format describes low–dose-rate (LDR) brachytherapy, as discussed in detail in Chapter 22.

Beginning around 1962, a new approach to brachytherapy developed. Using very intense, small sources (usually of ^{60}Co in the early machines and often three in number) on the ends of cables, a treatment unit would move the source through the volume to be treated, delivering the radiation in a relatively short time (<1 hour). The rapid treatment delivery gave these treatments the name high–dose-rate (HDR) brachytherapy. The original units most often oscillated the source through a catheter's treatment length, a method in common use until the modern generation of units developed in the early 1980s, described later. The treatments took so little time that the therapy proceeded on an outpatient basis. However, for reasons discussed later in this chapter, the treatment regimen usually entailed several fractions delivered over days or weeks.

The modern HDR units move a single source through the treatment volume in a stepwise fashion, moving at intervals, determined by the machine construction and the operator, to positions where the source pauses (dwell positions) for durations (dwell times) determined through optimization procedures.

Advantages and Disadvantages

Advantages of HDR brachytherapy over LDR include the following:

1. *Optimization.* The stepping-source design permits very fine control of the source position through the target volume. In most treatments, the determination of the dwell times comes from inverse planning, that is, specifying the doses desired at various locations and using some algorithm to calculate the dwell times that best fit the dose specifications. The map of how long the source dwells at each possible dwell position can be finely tailored to the geometry and needs of the particular patient because of the wide range of dwell times available. This process constitutes *optimization.* Although optimization is possible and frequently used with LDR applications, it forms a more natural part of the planning process with HDR brachytherapy.
2. *Immobilization and stability.* The relatively short duration of the HDR treatments allows better stability of many intracavitary treatment applicators during the treatment and, thus, higher precision in conforming the dose to the target. In addition to simply not giving much time for applicator motion, the applicator and the patient can both be immobilized with respect to the treatment table over the duration of the treatment. Such fixation is not possible with LDR brachytherapy because the patient would not tolerate the immobility for long periods. Interstitial cases may or may not exhibit better stability. The needles often tend to slide outward over the time that prostate implants remain in the patient, even with a template sutured to the patient that fixes the needles. In such a patient, the needles' positions require adjustment before each fraction but move very little during the treatment delivery. Performing the same treatment using LDR brachytherapy would include

needle movement during the long, slow delivery. On the other hand, head and neck implants with buttons anchoring the catheters at both ends may allow very little movement from the time of insertion through removal. Such cases would not find improvement in stability with HDR brachytherapy.

3. *Dose reduction to normal tissue.* Again, the short duration of HDR intracavitary treatments often allows displacement of normal tissue structure to a greater extent than with LDR treatments. This holds true for gynecologic and oral intracavitary cases but not for intraluminal applications, such as endoesophageal or endobronchial treatments. Most interstitial cases cannot make use of this feature since the needles or catheters fix all the tissues in place. Exceptions are mostly in the head, where the tongue sometimes can be moved away from the treatment site.
4. *Outpatient treatment.* Most HDR patients receive treatment as an outpatient. Exceptions include patients with indwelling needles such as prostate or gynecologic implants delivered in multiple fractions. Patients containing plastic catheters (i.e., not with sharp needle tips poking into flesh) almost always leave the hospital between fractions. All intracavitary treatments are on an outpatient basis. Outpatient treatments present many advantages over the inpatient treatments characteristic of LDR brachytherapy:
   - *Patient comfort.* Patients confined to a room during LDR treatments often feel closed in. Compounding the claustrophobic effects, radiation safety considerations limit the time nursing staff can spend with the patient (sometime very severely), leading patients to feel like a pariah.
   - *Patient health.* Many LDR brachytherapy applications require the patients to stay in bed, increasing the probability of thrombosis or bedsores. Although pneumatic socks greatly reduce the likelihood of thrombosis, aching muscles from immobility still create discomfort. In many cases, patients who could not tolerate protracted LDR treatments will be able to receive their treatments using HDR techniques.
   - *Economics.* The cost of staying in the hospital greatly exceeds that of outpatient treatment. Counterbalancing the cost of hospitalization, the costs of the HDR remote afterloading equipment far exceed those for LDR applications. However, the HDR equipment costs quickly become amortized with a modest patient load, whereas the hospitalization costs remain constant for each LDR brachytherapy patient.
5. *Less discomfort due to small size.* Because the encapsulated HDR source is only 1 mm or less in diameter, the gynecologic intrauterine tandem need only be 3 mm in diameter, compared with 7 mm for the standard LDR tandem. Another way of looking at this comparison is to recognize that the diameter of the HDR tandem equals the smallest-size dilator used to stretch the cervical os to accept the LDR tandem. Much of the pain and discomfort from a cervical cancer treatment comes during the dilation. Eliminating that step eliminates much of that pain. Some facilities use only light sedation for the HDR tandem insertion rather than a general anesthetic, as is common with LDR procedures.
6. *Elimination of delays.* When applications fail to follow a plan or when plans have to change due to a finding in the operating room during the procedure, HDR treatments can still proceed following localization with little, if any, delay. LDR treatments likely would require ordering new sources to match the new situation and a delay in treatment to await delivery. The HDR model eliminates extra charges accruing from multiple-source orders.
7. *Intraoperative procedures.* HDR brachytherapy allows treatment intraoperatively, with suitable shielding in the operating room. With the short duration for dose delivery, a surgeon can add placement of the applicator and treatment of the patient to surgery with little additional time.
8. *Radiation safety.* HDR brachytherapy eliminates radiation exposure to personnel.

Unfortunately, HDR brachytherapy carries with it the following disadvantages:

1. *Radiobiology.* Compared with low–dose-rate brachytherapy, HDR treatments have worse therapeutic ratios, that is, the amount of damage to tumor cells compared with damage to normal tissue cells for the same dose. The damage to both types of cells per unit dose increases with dose rate, but the increase is greater for normal cells. Just as with external-beam radiotherapy, which also is high–dose-rate delivery, fractionating the treatment mitigates this effect. Although LDR therapy usually entails a single session or two, most curative HDR regimens use three or more fractions. The next section discusses the radiobiology in greater detail.
2. *Error hazard.* The increased complexity of the procedures and the compressed time frame of delivery increase the probability of errors in the treatment compared with LDR therapy.
3. *Potential for very high radiation doses to patients and unit operators following failure of the source to retract.* The HDR source can deliver 7.4 Gy/min at 1 cm in the patient. If the source stops moving or separates from the drive cable, serious injury occurs in a short time.
4. *Resources.* HDR treatments demand more resources than LDR treatments:
   - *Personnel.* Because many HDR treatments proceed quickly from placement of the treatment appliance to delivery of the treatment, all of the persons involved with the treatment must be available at the same time or in relatively quick secession. That means that the facility must have sufficient staffing to release these persons on demand of the HDR brachytherapy cases.
   - *Economics.* The HDR afterloading equipment comes with a large initial investment (at the time of writing approximately $500,000 to $1,000,000), not including the significant costs of shielding the treatment room and the increased cost for all the treatment applicators and supplies.

Radiobiologic Dosimetry

Because of the radiobiologic disadvantage of HDR treatments, considerable care must be taken in planning the time course of the therapy regimen. The following discussion is intended as a supplement to that in the first two chapters of this book. One of the important tools for such planning is the linear-quadratic model for biologic response.

The Linear-Quadratic Model

The basis for the model for biological response to radiation stems from an approximation to the cell survival curves as shown in Figure 24.1.

Several models have been used over the years to describe the shape of the curve, each giving different insights into the interaction of the radiation and the organism irradiated. One of the more useful when investigating radiotherapy regimen is the linear-quadratic (LQ) model.[1–3]

This model approximates the cell survival, S, a function of dose, D, as

$$S = e^{-\alpha D - \beta D^2}. \tag{1}$$

Like any model, this equation fits the curves well over a particular range—in this case, the ranges of doses and dose rates used in radiotherapy—which makes it useful. It can also shed some light on biological underpinnings. However, the model should not be seen as a true and complete description and explanation of a complex biological phenomenon.

The curves shown apply to a single exposure of the cells over a short period of time at given dose rate. As can be seen, the

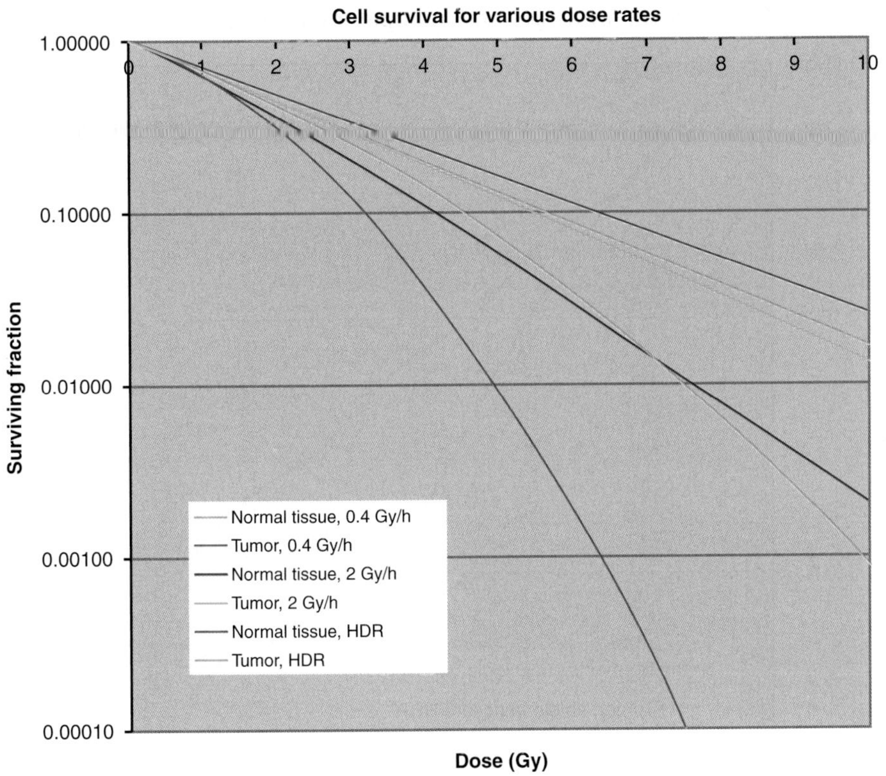

FIGURE 24.1. Typical cell survival curves with dose on the abscissa and surviving fraction on the ordinate, for three dose rates. The curves in the figure used α/β = 3 Gy for normal tissue, α/β = 10 Gy for the tumor, and α = 0.35 Gy^{-1} and μ = 1.5 h^{-1} for both types of tissue.

effect of dose rate markedly changes the survival of the cells. This discussion need only consider the two components of the exponent in Equation 1. Conceptually, the first term, αD, corresponds to damage to the cells when a single charged-particle track breaks both sides of a DNA molecule rung (e.g., both a guanine and a cytosine), referred to as a double-strand break. This form of killing the cells requires a double-strand break. The surviving fraction depends only on the dose, and the effect does not depend on the dose rate. The second term, βD^2, represents damage done when one charged-particle path breaks the bonds on one side of the DNA rung, say the guanine, and a different track breaks the other side (the cytosine). After the break on the first side, called a single-strand break, the DNA attempts repair. Because of the remaining cytosine on the opposite side, only a guanine will fit into the hole left on the damaged side. The nucleus contains many free guanine molecules, and one will be attracted to the opening and heal the wound. The repair takes place with a half-time of T_{bio}, which corresponds to a repair rate of

$$\mu = 0.693/T_{\text{bio}}. \tag{2}$$

Because the repair takes some time, there is a window in which the second break must take place for the entire rung to be removed. If the second hit takes place after repair of the first, the damage still only forms a single-strand break, and the opposite side must be hit again to form a double-side break. Because forming a double-strand break in this way requires two independent hits, the probability follows D^2. Because the second hit must occur before the repair of the first, the incidence of double-strand breaks depends on the dose rate. Frequently, calculations use a value for T_{bio} of 1.5 hours, although most normal tissues probably have a more complicated repair pattern, with a fast component of about 20 minutes and a longer one of about 2 hours.

The surviving fraction also depends on the values of α and β. These parameters are characteristic of the tissue being irradiated and the type of tissue injury being caused. The actual values are often not well known, and large variations in most tissues have been reported. However, in general, the values of α tend to be very similar for most tissues (within the uncertainties), with most of the variations being in the β term. Although the variations in the values determined for the two parameters tend to be large, smaller variation characterizes the ratio of α/β, the quantity most often given in the literature. For the most part, this ratio tends to be on the order of 2 to 3 for late effects in normal tissues and 5 to 20 for early effects. In general, tissues exhibiting less mitotic activity show lower values. Most tumors behave similarly to normal-tissue early effects but with a much wider range of values. Prostate cancer forms a notable exception, with an α/β between 1.5 and 2.

Figure 24.1 shows that as the dose rate increases, the fraction survival decreases for a given dose, and this effect is more marked for tissues with a low value for α/β. Thus, as stated earlier, compared with low–dose-rate brachytherapy, normal tissue has a comparative disadvantage for high–dose-rate brachytherapy. The usual approach to overcome the disadvantage fractionates the dose delivery. Figure 24.2 shows a survival curve with the dose delivered in several fractions. The pauses in the delivery allows repair of those single-strand breaks not converted into double-strand breaks by a second hit. Thus, at the beginning of each fraction the curve exhibits a new shoulder as the first single-strand breaks begin accumulating. The fractionation has no affect on the α term. Fractionation has a long history in external-beam radiotherapy, which, as noted, also is high–dose-rate delivery. Understanding the repair mechanism allows for a definition of what dose rates qualify as "high": a delivery duration that remains much less than T_{bio}, or about 30 minutes.

Surviving fraction does not depend directly on dose; instead, the whole exponent forms the independent variable. Because the α tends to be constant, it is often pulled out, leaving what is called the biologically effective dose (BED) or equivalently the effective radiation dose (ERD) as

$$\text{BED} = D + \frac{D^2}{\left(\dfrac{\alpha}{\beta}\right)} = D\left[1 + \frac{D}{\left(\dfrac{\alpha}{\beta}\right)}\right]. \tag{3}$$

For the fractionated, high–dose-rate irradiations, each new fraction starts the shape of the curve over but at the surviving

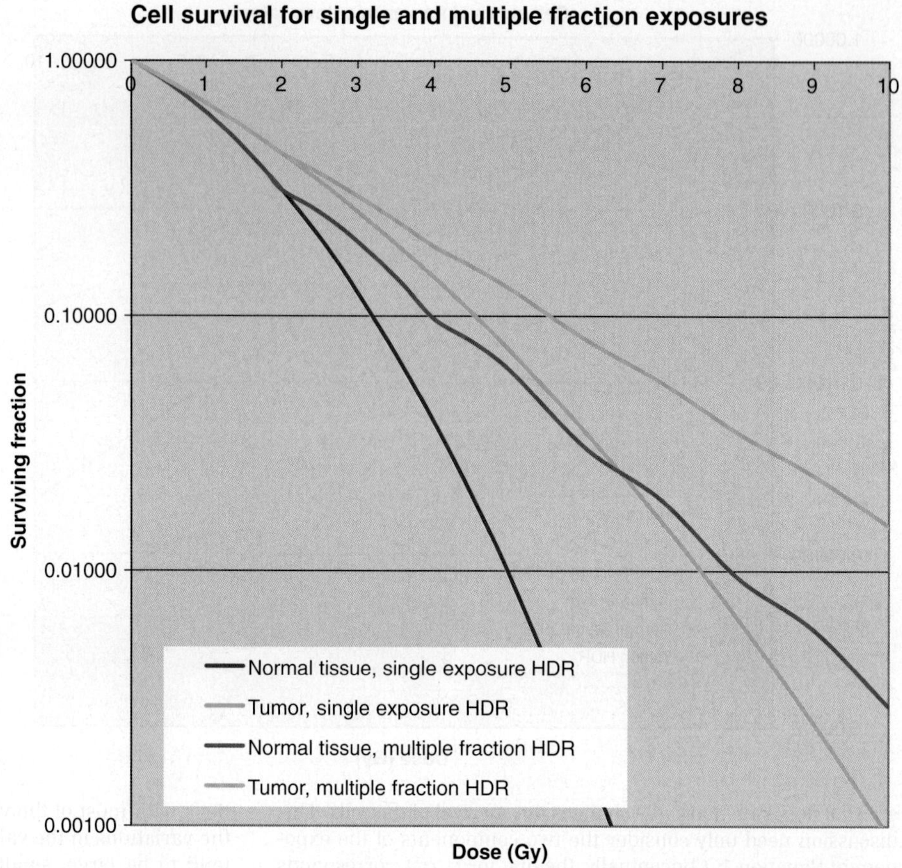

FIGURE 24.2. Survival curves illustrating the effects of fractionation. Again, the curves used $\alpha/\beta = 3$ Gy for normal tissue, $\alpha/\beta = 10$ Gy for the tumor, and $\alpha = 0.35\ \text{Gy}^{-1}$ and $\mu = 1.5\ \text{h}^{-1}$ for both types of tissue.

fraction level where it left off at the end of the previous fraction (in the absence of proliferation), and the equation becomes

$$\text{BED}_{\text{HDR}} = n\left[d\left(1 + \frac{d}{\left(\frac{\alpha}{\beta}\right)}\right)\right] = nd\left(1 + \frac{d}{\left(\frac{\alpha}{\beta}\right)}\right), \quad (4)$$

where n is the number of fractions and d is the dose per fraction.

The LDR situation becomes more complicated because repair takes place during the irradiation, reducing the effectiveness. In this case, BED becomes

$$\text{BED}_{\text{LDR}} = D\left(1 + \frac{2R}{\left(\frac{\alpha}{\beta}\right)\mu}\frac{1 - e^{-\mu T}}{\mu T}\right), \quad (5)$$

where T is the duration of the treatment and R is the dose rate. Because the BED depends on the α/β used, the convention when giving a value for BED requires that the units of gray carry a subscript specifying the α/β. For example, the BED of 10 Gy for late-responding tissue with an α/β of 3 might be stated as BED = 10 Gy_3.

In fact, the equations for both modalities also contain a term, not shown in the equations,

$$\frac{0.693T}{\alpha T_{\text{pot}}} \quad (6)$$

to account for cell repopulation over the total treatment duration. T_{pot} represents the potential cell doubling time. Most applications ignore this term because of the large uncertainties in the values for α and T_{pot}. In situations comparing the BED of low- and high-dose-rate application where the total duration of the therapy would be approximately the same, this omission probably causes no significant loss of information.

Conversion from Low- to High-Dose-Rate Brachytherapy

Often, when beginning an HDR brachytherapy program, the biggest questions relating to treatments become how many fractions to use and what dose per fraction. The larger the number of fractions, the better is the therapeutic effect, measured as the ratio of the damage to tumor cells to the damage to normal tissue cells. This ratio improves with each additional fraction, but the amount by which the ratio increases decreases with each added fraction. For example, going from four to five fractions improves the therapeutic ratio by 4%. Adding a sixth fraction improves the therapeutic ratio but only by another 3.5%. Each additional fraction carries with it costs in departmental resources (particularly the time of those persons involved) and inconvenience (and possibly discomfort) to the patient. Thus, selecting the number of fractions becomes a compromise. Most curative regimens use 5 or 6 fractions if applicator insertion procedures are involved and 8 to 12 fractions if the applicator can be left in place and the patient simply treated. Small-volume applications, such as vaginal cuff or most endobronchial treatments, may require only 3 or 4 fractions. After establishing the number of fractions, determining the dose per fraction comes next. One method that uses the LDR experience sets the BED equal for the two modalities and then solves for the dose per fraction:

$$\text{BED}_{\text{HDR}} = \text{BED}_{\text{LDR}} \quad (7a)$$

$$nd\left[1 + \frac{d}{\left(\frac{\alpha}{\beta}\right)}\right] = D_{LDR}\left\{1 + \left[\frac{2R}{\left(\frac{\alpha}{\beta}\right)\mu}\right] \bullet \left[\frac{1 - e^{-\mu T}}{\mu T}\right]\right\} \quad (7b)$$

$$d = \frac{-\left(\frac{\alpha}{\beta}\right) + \sqrt{\left(\frac{\alpha}{\beta}\right)^2 + \left(\frac{4D_{LDR}}{n}\right)\left(\frac{\alpha}{\beta}\right)\left[1 + \frac{2R}{\left(\frac{\alpha}{\beta}\right)}\left(\frac{1 - e^{-\mu T}}{\mu^2 T}\right)\right]}}{2} \quad (7c)$$

The absolute value for the dose per fraction depends on the ratio α/β, thus requiring another decision. Projecting d from the LDR experience, the normal-tissue toxicities could be held constant and an α/β of 3 used, or tumor cure could be the endpoint, suggesting an α/β of 10 (or a value of the particular type of tumor under treatment). Holding the late complications constant will lead to a BED for the tumor considerably less than was used with the LDR treatments, whereas attempting to achieve the same tumor control produces normal-tissue BED values much higher than those for the LDR regimen. For intracavitary treatments, the normal tissues sometimes can be held away from the applicator during the treatment delivery, for example, by keeping the rectal retractor in the vagina during a tandem and ovoid treatment. This would allow a dose based on equivalent tumor control. In interstitial applications, distance to the normal tissue in the implanted volume cannot be increased, but often with the improved optimization available with the HDR approach, high doses in the implant can be significantly reduced compared to conventional LDR implants, again allowing the dose based on tumor control. Seldom have HDR treatments produced more severe normal-tissue toxicities than those delivered at LDR. In general, the maximum significant dose, that is, the highest value of isodose surface that encompasses more than one catheter or needle track, should be kept to <150% of the prescription dose.

High–Dose-Rate Devices

Remote Afterloaders

A remote afterloader (RAL) is a computer-driven system that transports the radioactive source from a shielded safe into the applicator placed in the patient. On termination or interruption of the treatment, the source is driven back to its safe. The device may move the source by one of several methods, most commonly pneumatic or cable drives. A stepping-source RAL is a particular design of the treatment unit that consists of a single source at the end of a cable that moves the source through applicators placed in the treated volume. The treatment unit can treat implants consisting of many needles or catheters in the patient. Multiple catheters are often required to cover the target with uniform radiation doses. Each catheter or part of an applicator is connected to the RAL through a channel. The computer drives the cable so that the source moves from the safe through a given channel to the programmed dwell position for a specific dwell time. In any applicator, there may be many dwell positions. After treating all the positions in a given catheter (channel) the source is retracted to its safe and then driven to the next channel. There can be several dwell positions per centimeter in each channel, and the dwell time can vary from 0 to almost 1000 seconds in 0.1-second increments, thereby giving a high level of flexibility of dose delivery. All currently available HDR RALs use the stepping-source design. Four models of HDR RALs are available in the market, three in the United States: MicroSelectron (Nucletron, and Elekta Company, Veenendaal, Netherlands) and GammaMed and VariSource (both from Varian Medical Systems, Palo Alto, CA). In Europe, the Bebig MultiSource (Eckert & Ziegler BEBIG, Seneffe, Belgium) is also available. Figure 24.3 shows two of the units. Even though they may vary in details, all available HDR RALs consist of the same general components (Fig. 24.4): (a) shielded safe, (b) radioactive source, (c) source drive mechanism, (d) indexer, (e) transfer tube, (f) treatment control station, and (g) treatment control panel.

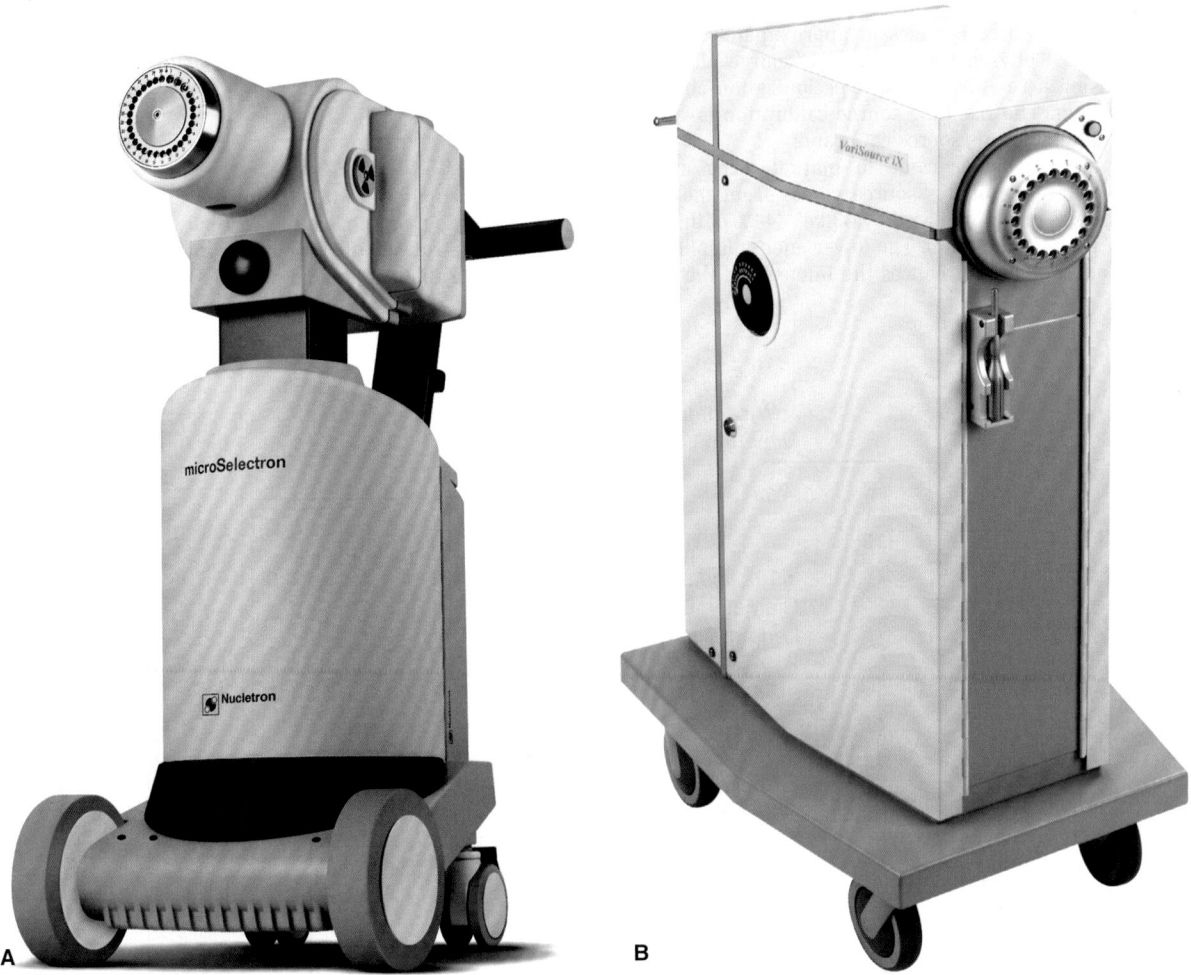

FIGURE 24.3. A: The Nucletron MicroSelectron. **B:** The Varian VariSource. (A, courtesy of Nucletron, an Elekta Company; B, courtesy of Varian Medical Systems.)

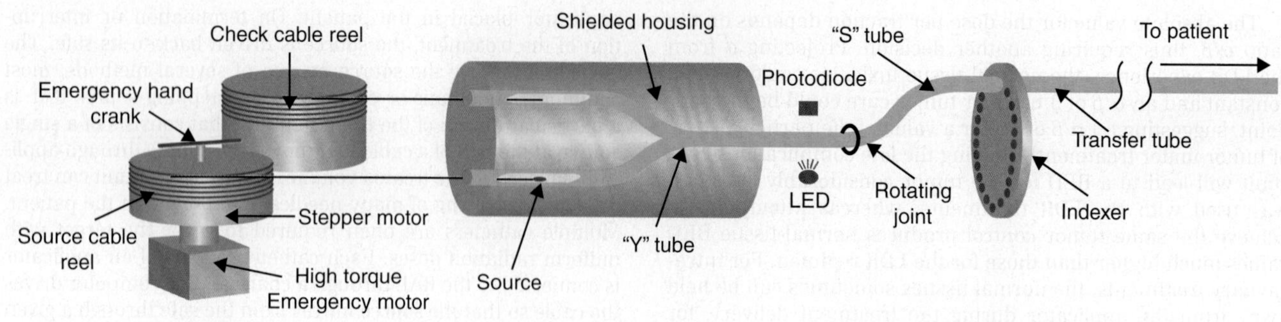

FIGURE 24.4. Components of a high–dose-rate brachytherapy remote afterloader. (Figure by Adam Uselmann after a draft by Liyong Lin.)

Sources

Whereas delivering the HDR brachytherapy requires an intense source, passing the source through needles placed through a tumor requires one of a small size. The radioactive source in an HDR RAL is usually 3 to 10 mm in length and <1 mm in diameter, fixed at the end of a steel cable. The Nucletron source is placed in a stainless steel capsule and welded to the cable, whereas the Varian source is placed in a hole drilled into the cable and closed by welding. Figure 24.5 shows diagrams of the sources. ^{192}Ir is now used for almost all HDR RALs; the Bebig unit offer the choice of ^{192}Ir or ^{60}Co. ^{192}Ir emits many photon energies, mostly between 110 and 704 keV, with an effective energy around 380 keV. A new source has an activity near 0.37 TBq (10 Ci, approximately 44 mGy m^2 h^{-1}). Because ^{192}Ir has a half-life of 74 days, the source should be replaced every 3 months to keep the treatment in the HDR radiobiologic regime (see later discussion). The potential advantage of using ^{60}Co is the 5.3-year half-life, extending the time between source changes to approximately 5 years. A trained medical physicist calibrates the source after each installation using a re-entrant, well-type ionization chamber, as discussed later. The resulting source calibration is verified against the manufacturer's source calibration.

Recently, an afterloader came to market using a ^{169}Yb source. The advantage of this source comes from the lower energy of its emissions, dominated by 63 keV (44% of the time) and 198 keV (36% of the time). The lower energy implies that shielding in any applicator reduces the intensity of the radiation to a greater extent than for ^{192}Ir and also opens the possibility of including shielding in smaller structures, such as an intrauterine tandem.

Applicators

An array of applicators for different treatment sites is marketed by each vendor. Each vendor designs its own applicators that can only be used with its transfer tubes and HDR RALs. Before an applicator is used clinically, tests should be performed to verify the functionality of the applicator. It should also be radiographed with dummy sources (ribbons) to verify agreement with the vendor's specifications. The length of each applicator, location of the dwell positions with respect to the applicator, and integrity of the applicators should be a part of the routine quality assurance (QA) program to ensure safe and precise delivery of the radiation treatment plan. Figure 24.6 shows a comparison between an HDR and a LDR intrauterine cervical tandem. The smaller diameter of the HDR applicator leads to greater patient comfort during the procedure. Because the high–dose-rate iridium source is much smaller than the low–dose-rate cesium tubes, high–dose-rate applicators have a smaller radius.

Pulsed Brachytherapy

Pulsed brachytherapy (also known as pulsed high–dose-rate brachytherapy or, not quite correctly but most commonly, pulsed dose-rate [PDR] brachytherapy), attempts to eliminate the unfavorable radiobiology of HDR brachytherapy while

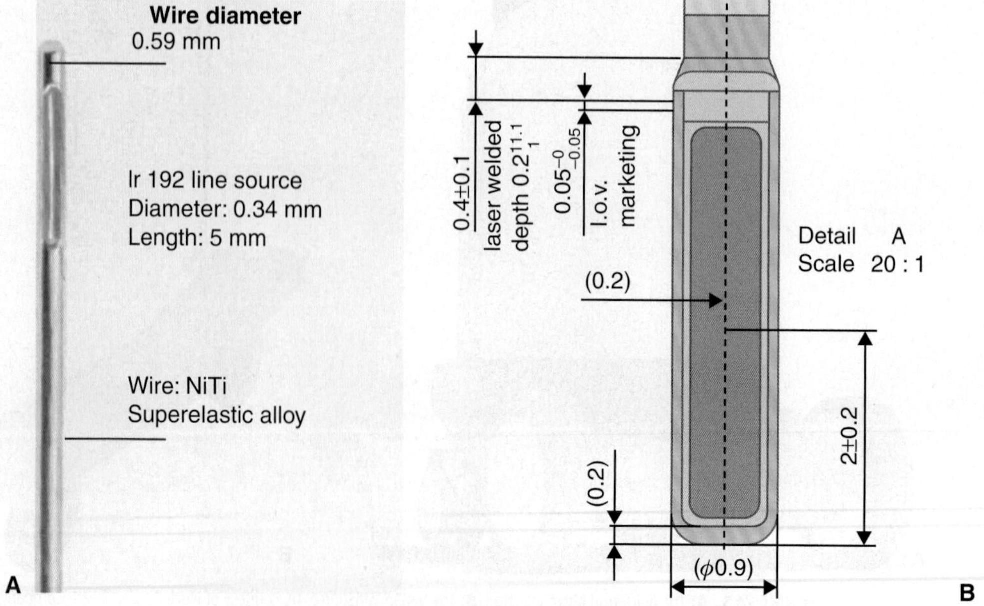

FIGURE 24.5. Diagrams of two HDR brachytherapy sources: for the VariSource **(A)** and for the MicroSelectron **(B)**. (A, courtesy of Varian Medical Systems, Palo Alto, CA; all rights reserved; B, courtesy of Nucletron, and Elekta Company, Veenendaal, Netherlands.)

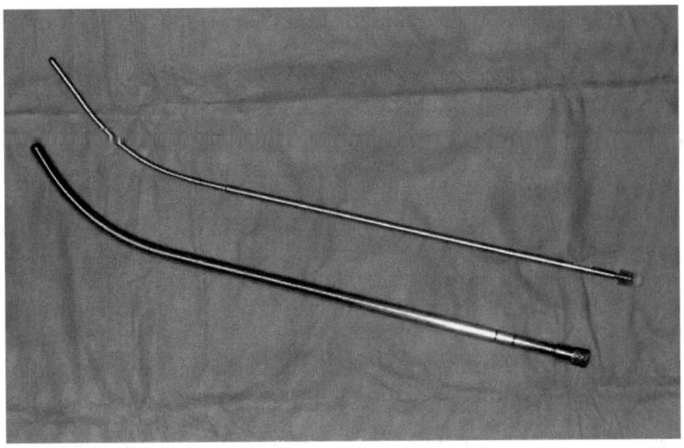

FIGURE 24.6. HDR (*top*) and LDR (*bottom*) intrauterine tandems.

maintaining the ability to optimize finely the dose distributions and eliminate the personnel exposure to radiation. The pulsed brachytherapy unit is the same as an HDR unit except the source is shorter and only about 1/10 as active. The treatment also follows the same pattern as an HDR treatment, except that the patient remains in the hospital, and instead of 10 fractions, the source runs through the treatment once each hour. These hourly treatment pulses last only a few minutes, but the overall duration usually covers 1 or 2 days. Thus, biologically, because each fraction comes before complete repair of sublethal cellular damage, the tissues experience the radiation as almost continuous, mimicking LDR brachytherapy.

Although this approach incorporates the biologic advantages of LDR treatments and the optimization advantage of HDR brachytherapy, it also has many of the disadvantages of both modalities, including (a) inpatient treatments, (b) lack of applicator stabilization, and (c) possibility of mechanical failures. Because the source treats the patient 24 times per day, and each treatment includes three or more catheters, the number of source transits becomes quite large and many times more than for a normal HDR regimen. Such frequent source use increases the likelihood of source failure during a treatment. Should a source become caught during transit, the dose to the patient could become quite large. Unlike HDR procedures, the operator does not sit at the control panel always ready to retrieve a stuck source. Limiting the activity of the source to 1/10 of the normal HDR source allows 10 times the response time for a stuck source before significant injury to the patient. The other reason for the low activity is that, with the treatment divided into so many small fractions, the dwell times become too short for the treatment unit to control with a very active source. In summary, pulsed brachytherapy presents opportunities to potentially improve brachytherapy, but it also comes with detriments. PDR brachytherapy is discussed in more detail in Chapter 23.

OPERATION

Personnel Roles

The report of Task Group 59 (TG-59) of the American Association of Physicists in Medicine discusses the roles of the members of the treatment team for high–dose-rate brachytherapy.[4] For the most part, the roles follow standard procedures for any brachytherapy, with the physician inserting the treatment appliance and prescribing the treatment; the nurse monitoring the patient's condition and welfare; therapists or radiographers performing the imaging for localization; and the physicist assuring the correct calibration of the source. Who performs some of the functional roles discussed in what follows varies by institution but needs clarification so all persons involved understand the distribution of responsibilities.

Daily Quality Assurance

The tests of the treatment unit at the beginning of the treatment day often fall to the medical physicist. However, in some facilities, a therapist or dosimetrist performs the actual tests, and the medical physicist reviews the results of the tests before the first treatment.

Treatment Planning Calculation

The report of TG-59 discusses options for entering the patient data into the dose-calculation computer and generating the treatment parameters (dwell positions and dwell times).[4] One model presented in that report had a dosimetrist running the program and a physicist monitoring the input to correct errors as they occur. Studies have shown that such supervision provides little protection against errors.[5] Either a physicist or a dosimetrist may perform the treatment plan generation.

Quality Assurance on the Treatment Plan

Regardless of who generates the treatment plan, a medical physicist should review the plan for appropriateness and correctness. The reviewing medical physicist should *not* be the same person who generated the plan, so in facilities with only one medical physicist, a dosimetrist should perform the planning.

Delivery of the Treatment

Several factors enter into considerations of who should staff the control panel during the treatment. In some states, regulations dictate that only therapists may deliver treatments and control treatment units. The regulations in most states and from the U.S. Nuclear Regulatory Commission are silent on the issue. At the time of writing, regulations almost uniformly require the attendance of a medical physicist at the treatment (or within unamplified voice communication of the unit operator). As a result, many facilities have the medical physicist operate in the unit during treatments. One important consideration is that at least one person in the control area during treatments must be ready and willing to enter the room and take appropriate actions in case the source becomes stuck in the patient.

Normal Procedures

When the afterloader receives a command from the treatment control panel to initiate a treatment, the source cable advances from the shielded safe through the Y tube and then the S tube to the first channel in the indexer and then along a path constrained by transfer tubes to the first treated dwell position in the applicator (see Fig. 24.4). The source dwells at that position for a predetermined duration. After completing that dwell it goes on to the subsequent dwell positions. Some units step as the source drives out (MicroSelectron and Gamma-Med), stopping first at the dwell position most proximal to the afterloader, whereas in the other (VariSource) the source travels first to the most distal dwell (toward the tip of the applicator) and a bit farther and then steps as the source returns toward the safe. Stepping on the outward drive obviates any concern about the effect of slack in the drive mechanism affecting the accuracy of the source position. The unit that steps on the way back into the unit includes correction for slack in the calibration of the source location. On completion of the treatment for the first channel, the source is retracted into the safe and redirected to travel to the second channel. The process is repeated for all the subsequent treatment channels. The programmed movement of the source is verified by means of an optical encoder or other device that compares the angular rotation of a stepper motor or cable length ejected or retracted with the number of pulses sent to the drive motor. This system is capable of detecting catheter obstruction or constriction as increased friction in the cable movement. Under certain fault conditions, such as if the stepper motor fails to retract the source, a high-torque direct current emergency motor will retract the source.

The confirmation of the source exit from and return to the safe is carried out by an opto-pair, consisting of a light-sensitive detector and an infrared light source, which detects the cable when its tip obstructs the light path. All the currently marketed afterloaders are also equipped with check cables, or "dummy sources." The check cable is an exact duplicate of the radioactive source along with its cable, except that it is not radioactive. Before the ejection of the radioactive source, the check cable is first ejected to check the integrity of the catheter system. After a noneventful check by this dry run with the dummy source, the radioactive source is then sent for treatment.

Emergency Procedures

Because HDR RALs are complicated devices containing very-high-activity radioactive sources, serious accidents can happen very quickly, thereby demanding many safety features and operational interlocks to prevent erroneous source movement or facilitate rapid operator response in the event of a system failure.

Door Interlock

Interlock switches prevent initiation of a treatment with the door open. Opening the door interrupts the treatment's progress. This safety feature protects the medical personnel from radiation exposure in the event someone enters the treatment room without the knowledge of the operator. If a door is opened inadvertently during the treatment, the treatment is interrupted and the source returns to the safe. The treatment can be resumed at the same point where it was interrupted by closing the door and pressing the start or the resume button at the control panel.

Emergency Switches

Numerous emergency off switches are located at convenient places and are easily accessible in case a situation arises. One is located on the control panel for the HDR operator. Another is located on the top of the remote afterloader treatment head. Vendors also install two or more switches in the walls of the treatment room. In the event a treatment is initiated with someone other than the patient in the treatment room, that person can stop the treatment and retract the source by pressing the emergency off button.

Emergency Crank

In the event of the failure of a source to retract normally, as well as the failure of the emergency motor, all HDR RALs have emergency cranks to retract the source cable. Using the crank requires the operator to enter the room with the source unshielded.

Emergency Service Instruments

If the radioactive source fails to retract after termination or interruption, pushing the emergency switch, or cranking the stepper motor manually, the immediate priority is to remove the source from the patient. Because the source is in contact with the patient, it can cause severe injury in a very short time. However, working at a greater distance, it is unlikely that the operator will receive a dose exceeding regulatory limits for 1 year, let alone one that would cause health problems. Once the source is removed from the patient and moved to the distance of even 1 m, the exposure rate drops drastically, and actions can then be taken to remove the patient from the room safely.

The safest approach to a source that will not retract by any of the methods is to remove the applicator from the patient as quickly as possible and place the applicator containing the source in a shielded container. If it is clear that the cable is caught in the transfer tube and not in the applicator per se, the applicator may be disconnected from the transfer tube and the patient removed from the treatment room. In some cases, this will be faster than removing the applicator. The reason to avoid disconnecting the applicator from the transfer tube is that a source may stay in the applicator if the source capsule shatters or come free from the cable. In that case, removing the applicator attached to the transfer tube keeps the system closed, whereas disconnecting the two opens a path for parts of a broken source to fall from the applicator into body cavities or crevices or roll onto the floor.

A situation might arise when the source needs to be detached manually from the treatment unit. Such a rare situation might occur if the unit with an unretractable source fell on a person and could not be moved by hand (perhaps by something else falling on the unit). The source could be close to the person but not inside. In this situation, the source cable should be cut from the unit and the source placed in the shielded container always present in the room. In cutting the source cable, it must be clear that the cut is *not* through the source capsule. For units with the capsule welded on the cable, the cut must be through the braided cable as opposed to the smooth steel capsule. For sources imbedded in the cable, a sufficient length of the cable must be seen to ensure that the cut occurs behind the source. Thus, emergency tools that must be present in the treatment room and always readily accessible include a wire cutter, a pair of forceps, and a shielded service container. The source should *never* be cut from the cable while the source is still in an applicator in the patient!

FACILITY DESIGN

The radioactive source in the high–dose-rate machine starts about at 10 Ci with an in-air equivalent dose rate at a distance of 1 m from the source of about 44 mSv/h. According to the rules and regulations of the Nuclear Regulatory Commission (NRC), the annual limit for radiation exposure to the public is 1 mSv and the annual occupational limit is 5 mSv. (The actual limit for occupational exposure is 50 mSv/y, but following the principle of maintaining exposures as low as is reasonable achievable, the NRC usually holds licensees to exposure 1/10 of the actual limit.) In addition to the annual limit, NRC requires that in an unrestricted area the dose equivalent rate should not be more than 0.02 mSv in any hour. Thus, the high–dose-rate machine needs to be housed in an adequately shielded room. To meet these requirements in an HDR suite, where the walls and the ceiling are at least 5 feet from the machine head, concrete walls of about 43 to 50 cm (or 4 to 5 cm of lead) are needed. For larger rooms the concrete wall thickness will be lower because the exposure rate is inversely proportional to the square of the distance from the radioactive source. The tenth-value layer thicknesses for ^{192}Ir are 1.6 cm and 15 cm of lead and concrete, respectively. For details on the procedures for calculating the thickness of barriers for a particular facility, see a health physics text such as that by Cember and Johnson,[6] McGinley,[7] or the report from the Nation Council on Radiation Units and Measurement.[8]

Imaging plays an important part in most brachytherapy, so consideration of required imaging modalities should enter into the room design. If the facility will perform a significant amount of gynecologic intracavitary insertions, fluoroscopic and radiographic equipment in the room saves a considerable amount of time and eliminates the motion inherent in moving the patient between rooms for imaging and treatment. Also for gynecological cases, ready access to magnetic resonance imaging should be considered. Having space and access for anesthesia in the room facilitates HDR brachytherapy for prostate cases.

All HDR brachytherapy rooms must have video and audio communication for monitoring the patient. Radiation detectors for monitoring the radiation levels in the room and indicating when the source is out of its shielding also are required.

QUALITY CONTROL OF THE REMOTE AFTERLOADING DEVICE

Several of the disadvantages of HDR brachytherapy concerned the probability of failure, either human or mechanical. Both aspects of the treatments require effective quality management. This section deals with quality assurance for the treatment unit. One report from the American Association of Physicists in medicine discusses this topic,[4] as do fundamental publications by Ezzell,[9,10] Chenery et al.,[11] Flynn,[12] Grigsby,[13] Jones,[14] and Meigooni et al.[15] Williamson et al.[16] assembled much of the important material into a chapter. For a fairly comprehensive discussion, the reader is directed to Thomadsen.[17]

As for any piece of radiotherapy equipment, the QA begins with acceptance testing and commissioning. Periodic QA includes tests performed with each new source (approximately quarterly for most units) and those at the beginning of each treatment day. Of all of these, the daily morning checks form the basic set of essential tests.

Morning Checks

Although the list of safety checks seems long, the evaluation need not consume a great deal of time. At our facility, the entire morning routine takes about 10 to 15 minutes. Most of the items could be tested in numerous manners, but only one set of techniques will be discussed here. Individual units may differ in the exact methods. The procedure in the list often assumes the successful completion of all of the items going before. Failure of *any* item requires evaluation by the physicist of the appropriateness of continuing with patient treatments in light of the particular failure. The morning checks focus on ensuring that the unit is operating safely and correctly.

Safety Checks

The following items should be considered in a safety check:

Communication equipment. See that the television and intercom systems function.

Catheter-attachment lock. Attach a transfer tube to one of the channels of the unit, but do not lock the transfer tube in place (often accomplished by the locking ring). Program the unit to send the source to a dwell position that would be in an applicator were one attached, and initiate a source run. A program time for a single dwell of about 20 seconds would allow execution of the tests to follow. The unit should detect that the transfer tube has not been locked in place and prevent the source run. Were a treatment to take place in this condition, the source cable could push the transfer tube out of the unit and never enter the applicator.

Applicator attachment. Keeping the same program, lock the transfer tube in place but still do *not* attach an applicator to the transfer tube. Again attempt to initiate a source run. The check cable run should detect the absence of an applicator and prevent sending out the source. Failure of the unit to detect this situation could lead to the source indicating that it treated a catheter when in reality the catheter was never attached. This test also checks that the unit will not send out a source if the pathway is blocked, because for most transfer tubes, the applicators push aside a blockage of the tube when they lock in place.

Door interlock. Lock an applicator into the transfer tube. For future tests it is convenient to use a needle in a well-type ionization chamber. Keeping the same program as in the previous tests and with the door to the room open, try to initiate a run. The unit should refuse to initiate the treatment and indicate that the door is open.

Source-out indicators. Close the door, and initiate the source run. Observe that the indication lamps operate. Most rooms have three beam-on indicator lamps: one connected to a treatment-unit microswitch that triggers when the source leaves its shielded housing, one that lights when the signal on the radiation detector in the room exceeds its trip level, and one from the on-board Geiger counter. Let the exposure continue for the next test.

Room monitor audio operation. Listen through the intercom for the sound of the room radiation monitor. It should make a mild but clearly audible sound. It should not be too loud, for that would disturb the patient. There is no regulation in most states or with the NRC that the in-room monitor provides any audible signal. The presence of such a signal would alert anyone who is in the room unintentionally when the source is out. Some practitioners feel that any such signal causes concern on the part of the patient. We have tried both situations and have found that patients do not mind the signal if they have been informed that it would occur. Continue the exposure.

Room monitor visual operation. Open the door to the room and observe the visual indicators on the room monitor. The room design should provide protection to a person in the doorway until the source retracts. At the same time as this test is performed, so is the next.

Hand-held monitor operation. Immediately on opening the door during the previous test, hold the hand-held monitor in the doorway and see whether it indicates the presence of radiation. The hand-held detector is to be carried upon entry to the treatment room any time after a source run. Alternatively, the detector could be tested with a dedicated check source at the beginning of each day. Performing the test along with the room monitor makes the treatment unit the dedicated check source.

Door interrupt. During the previous two tests, the unit should have been retracting the source, beginning from the opening of the door. The retraction should take no longer than 4 to 6 seconds to return the source to its shielded location.

Emergency stop. Close the door and reinitiate the exposure. Once the source reaches the dwell position, press the emergency off button. The unit must immediately retract the source and likely require a reset.

Treatment interrupt. Reinitiate the exposure and once the source again reaches the dwell position, press the treatment interrupt button. Again, the unit must immediately retract the source.

Timer termination. Reinitiate the exposure and let it continue until the elapsed duration equals the time set on the timer. At that time, the unit stops the exposure and retracts the source.

Dosimetry Checks

The thrust of the dosimetry checks focuses on the delivery of the correct dose to the proper location.

Source Positioning Accuracy

Proper treatment requires that the source occupy the position along the catheter corresponding to that used in the treatment plan. The uncertainty of the determination of the dwell positions on the treatment plan is discussed elsewhere in this chapter. Here, the issue becomes duplicating the dwell locations on the treatment plan during execution. A usual criterion for coincidence with the planned treatment dwells is 2 mm, although the HDR units are able to place the source in a given location within 1 mm. Precision <0.5 mm begins to be less reproducible. To direct the source to correct locations corresponding to each dwell position, the source controller requires the distance along the catheter corresponding to the first dwell position. The distance may refer to the length from some part of the unit (such as the front face, the point of catheter insertion, or a microswitch that tells the unit when the source enters the catheter), or it may be from some fictitious point (similar in concept to the effective source for electron beams). Verifying that the unit can place the center of the source at a specified distance becomes an important part of the morning QA.

Three methods for verifying the source placement accuracy will be discussed here, although many others exist. The first method makes an autoradiograph of the source. After taping a clear catheter to a piece of paper-jacketed film (e.g., XV-2 "ready pac"; Carestream, Woodbrige CT) and inserting the x-ray marker wire, mark the position of the first dwell marker on the film. (This method assumes the x-ray marker to be correct. Verification of that is discussed with tests following a source replacement.) This can be done by using pinpricks or pressing hard with a ballpoint pen. If one is using a pinprick, the lights in the room should be dimmed and the film processed immediately after exposure. A pinprick at a far distance from the source track gives an indication of the amount of signal due to light exposures. If one is using a pen, lines about 1 cm long with an end at the center of the marker help to see the actual position. Pen marks must be strong enough to etch the film through the jacket but not so strong as to tear the jacket. With either technique, marking both sides of the catheter makes determining the center of the marker on the film easier. It is a good idea to establish that the unit not only places the source at the correct location for the first dwell position but also keeps track of relative positions. To do this, also mark some additional dwell positions, such as dwell positions 5 and 10 cm from the first. Program the source to stop at the marked positions for about 2 seconds each for a source with a strength of 0.04 Gy m^2 h^{-1}. The times for other source strengths vary in inverse proportion. Deliver the exposure and process the film. The resultant image looks like a dark blot, where the centroid indicates the effective center of the source. This centroid should fall between the marks, plus or minus the allowed tolerance. The distance to the centroid of other marked dwell positions should be much better than the absolute tolerance for hitting the first dwell position. Many factors influence the results of this method and interpretation of the results. One is the effect of light exposing the film when using pinpricks. To assess the size of the exposure due to light, poke a hole in the film well away from the catheter path. After processing, the dark blot by this hole should remain less than half the diameter of the holes marking dwell positions. If the light-leak hole shows a blot about the same size as the actual test holes, then the test holes mostly just indicate room light and provide no information about source positioning. Figure 24.7 shows a typical test film.

Another method uses the ruler provided with the unit. Such a ruler provides a channel for the source to follow alongside a scale marked in the distance. Using any ruler requires a good television system able both to distinguish the source capsule clearly and resolve the markers on the ruler. The lighting of the ruler becomes an important variable. For one vendor's unit, a televised check of the source positions on a ruler forms a routine part of any treatment. For another, the ruler is just part of the unit QA equipment and requires a separate television system, such as that used to monitor the patient. To perform the check, attach the ruler as appropriate for the unit and program the source to a distance that shows on the rule. Watch on the video screen as the source moves into position. The tip of the source will be seen at some distance that should be farther than that distance programmed. From the distance of the tip, subtract the distance from the tip to the center of the source as shown in Figure 24.5.

A simpler and more precise method of verifying the positioning of the source follows the technique determined by DeWerd et al.[18] This procedure uses a well-type ionization chamber with a special insert that includes lead attenuators and plastic transmission disks and is shown in Figure 24.8. The lead attenuators reduce the signal from the source to approximately one-third its unshielded value, whereas the plastic discs have little affect. As the source passes through the needle centered in this insert, the measured signal appears as in Figure 24.9. The peaks occur when the source is centered on the plastic discs, and the greatest gradient occurs when half

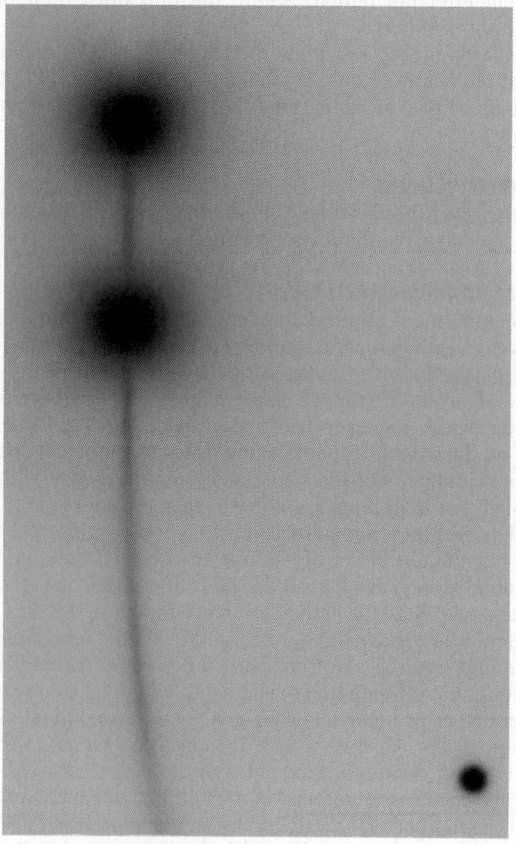

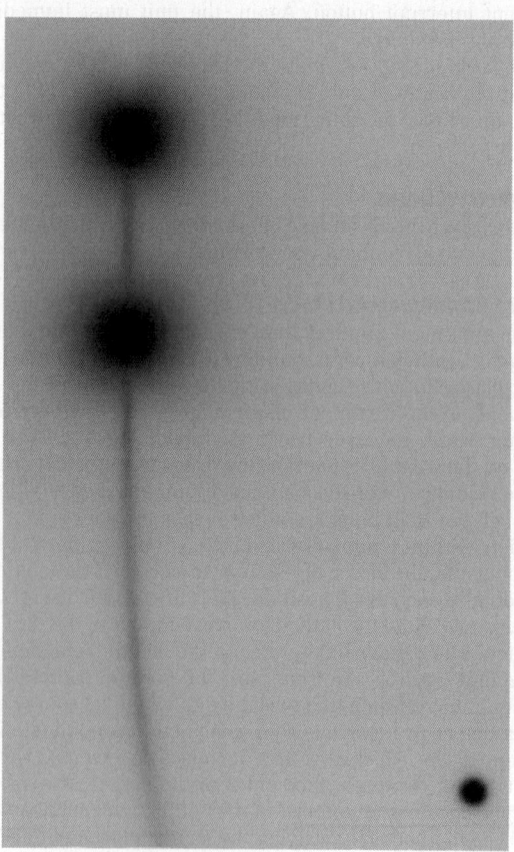

FIGURE 24.7. A typical image made to test the accuracy of the high–dose-rate unit source positioning.

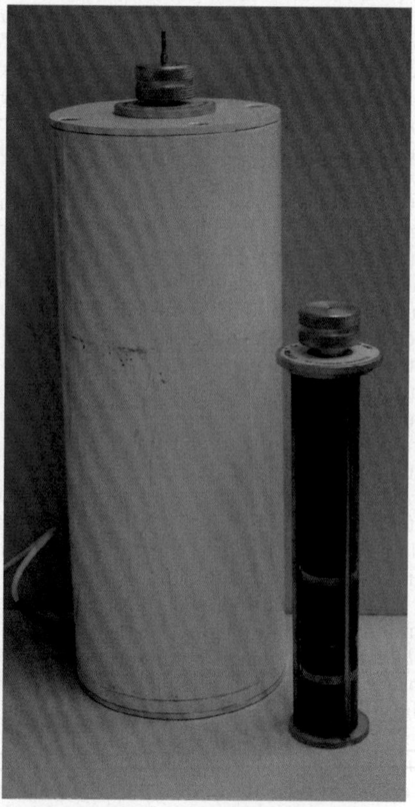

FIGURE 24.8. A special insert designed to assist in the evaluation of source positioning accuracy, with large lead cylinders separated by a plastic disc.

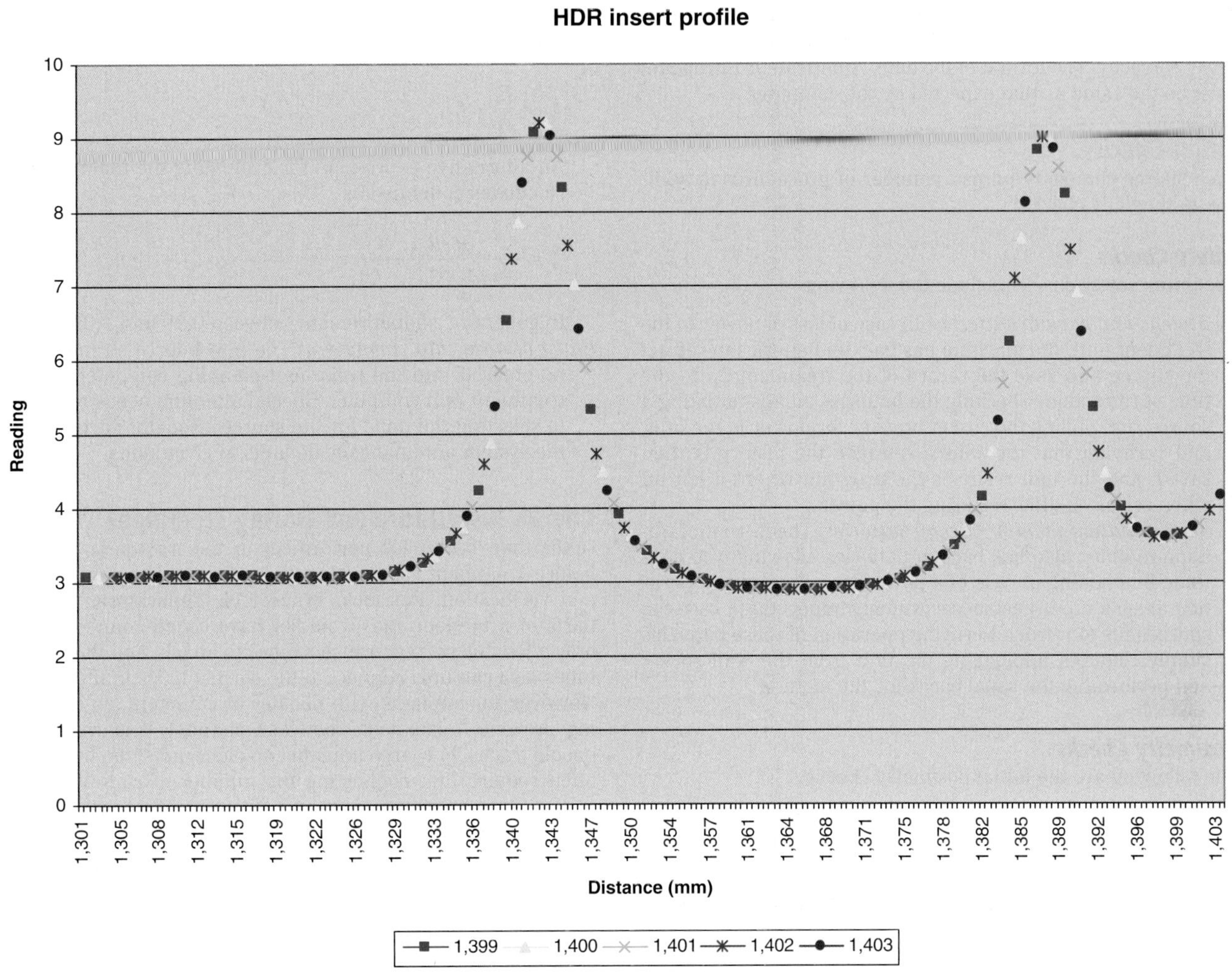

FIGURE 24.9. The signal produced as the source passes through the insert shown in Figure 24.8. Notice the high signal gradient that corresponds to the source centered on the plastic–lead interface.

the source is shielded and half is on the plastic. At these points, the signal depends critically on the precise position of the source, with the signal changing approximately 3.5%/mm. The signal at the plateau changes little over 2 mm. Dividing the current signal at the high-gradient point by that at the plateau removes any variations in the reading due to source decay, timer miscalibration, or atmospheric density. Thus, the ratio of signals gives a sensitive indication of whether the unit accurately places the source to the correct location. Making measurements at two high-gradient points and the peak assesses not only the correct placement of the source at the one point, but also the correct interval between. Use of this method requires measurement of the signal profile as a function of distance along the axis of the well chamber after initial verification of the source position using one of the other methods. Once put in place, this approach takes <1 minute. If the insert is left in the well chamber, the needle can be used for the safety checks, and this test can follow the safety checks without requiring re-entry into the room.

Dose Consistency

Correct dose delivery hinges on the proper operation of the timer controlling the exposure. The proper operation does *not* depend on the timer accurately keeping true clock time. The only important features of the timer are that it operates linearly and that its operation remains consistent over time. The daily QA generally needs only check two times to evaluate timer consistency and linearity, compared with the tests performed during the source exchange. The uncertainty in the measurement should be on the order of a few tenths of a second in order to check the shorter times.

One technique for checking the timer observes the reading produced in a radiation detector as a function of the timer settings. To evaluate the timer, the measurement system must respond linearly to radiation dose and the setup provide a stable and reproducible geometry. A well chamber, such as that used for calibration, performs this function well. Such measurements in a well chamber include the effects of source decay and the source transit time. For the most part, source decay seldom deviates from the expected but should be checked because there have been sources with contaminant radionuclides that produce an anomalous decay. Because the reading varies directly with the set exposure time, these readings can form a check of the timer. The chamber reading needs a baseline, for example, a reading taken immediately after the initial calibration of the source. The expected reading can be tabulated as a function of day by correcting the initial reading by the decay factor, $e^{-0.693t/73.8\text{ days}}$, where t is the time in days since the initial reading. The reading should remain within ±2% of the projected reading, values that also could be in the table. Deviations from the projected values indicate changes in the timer operation (linearity or consistency), changes in the unit's transit time, or anomalous decay. Further tests would be required to sort out the actual problem.

Source Strength Value

The value for the source strength at any time should be the same in the treatment-planning computer as in the treatment unit computer to within 0.5%. The date and time in the treatment unit must be correct for the unit to calculate the source decay correctly. The format of the date, American or European, must be the same as that expected by the computer.

Initial Checks

Each source change requires a number of procedures in addition to the daily checks.

Safety Checks

The initial safety checks include the following:

Treatment-unit backup batteries. In case of loss of power to the treatment unit, the machine has backup batteries to retract the source and save the record of the treatment up to the time of retraction. Checking the batteries entails initiating a source run, pulling the circuit breaker for power to the unit, and verifying that the source retracts; the history is then saved, and the unit resumes the program where it left off when restarted after restoring the power.

In-room radiation-monitor backup batteries. The in-room radiation monitor also has backup batteries allowing it to continue functioning in case of a power loss. Continued operation at such times becomes extremely important in case the source fails to retract. Verifying operation of these batteries simply requires unplugging the unit from the wall socket and performing the usual check for the monitor.

Dosimetry Checks

The following are the initial dosimetry checks:

Calibration. The accepted method for calibration of an HDR source uses a well-type ionization chamber that has been calibrated in terms of HDR source strength per unit current. The calibration factor for the same chamber will differ for low–dose-rate and high–dose-rate ^{192}Ir sources because of differences in source construction. The uncertainty in source-strength calibrations using such chambers usually runs around 1% from national standards plus an additional 5% in the national standard with respect to absolute measures of energy absorbed per unit mass. The source strength is in terms of air-kerma strength, S_K, with units of μGy m^2 h^{-1}, often called U for convenience.[19] This unit gives numbers that become very large, so sometimes units of mGy m^2 h^{-1} (called U_h) are used. Most treatment-planning computers accommodate at least one of these units; however, many practitioners still relate better to source strength converted into curies, derived simply by multiplying S_K by a constant that must be the same as that used by the manufacture in the treatment-planning program.

Timer linearity. The verification for timer linearity uses several readings, R_i, for various increasing times t_i taken in the well chamber. The free-running reading rate can be defined as

$$\dot{R} = \frac{R_{i+1} - R_i}{t_{i+1} - t_i} \quad (8)$$

and contains no effect from the source transit, which cancels during the subtractions. Taking approximately five readings covering the range of dwell times common in treatments gives four values for the free-running reading rate using adjacent times. These values should differ by <0.5%.

The transit time from the unit to the dwell position is hard to measure and is not important directly. What is important is that the transit time remains constant. An effective transit time can be defined as the time it would take to deliver the extra reading in the chamber due to the irradiation during the time the source moves into and then leaves the measurement dwell position, *if* the extra reading were delivered at the free-running reading rate. One expression for the effective transit time, t_ε, becomes

$$t_\varepsilon = \frac{R_i}{\dot{R}} - t_i. \quad (9)$$

An alternative expression for evaluating the timer linearity calculates ζ, defined as

$$\zeta = \frac{R_i/R_{i+1}}{(t_i - t_\varepsilon)/(t_{i+1} - t_\varepsilon)}. \quad (10)$$

In general, ζ should remain between 0.99 and 1.01.

Entry of data into computers. The new source strength must be entered into the treatment-planning computer and the treatment unit computer. Special attention needs to be paid to selecting the units for the source strength, particularly if the system automatically defaults to given units.

Checks Just Before and During Treatment

Other than the check performed on the treatment plan just before treatment, connecting the patient also requires care and verification. For most gynecologic applicators, the three parts of a tandem and ovoid set have coded connectors that only allow the correct transfer tubes to attach, and the transfer tubes also can only connect to the correct holes in the indexer. However, for implants with needles or catheters, no interlocking prevents mismatches between channels and catheter or needle tracks. For large implants on older units, the treatments often require first connecting the number of catheters equal to the number of channels and delivering the part of treatment that uses those channels. Those channels are then disconnected, and the next set of catheters is then connected to the indexers starting again with channel number 1. One of the most likely errors would be connecting a channel during the second set to a catheter from the first or vice versa. Newer treatment units often have enough channels to accommodate most large implants.

Also for interstitial implants, between fractions the catheters often move from the position they occupied during the imaging used for treatment planning. Immediately before treatment, the catheters must be returned to their original position, for example, by snugging the buttons on one side to the skin.

During the treatment, the operator needs to watch for movement by the patient that could affect the treatment and ensure that the source moves through its program.

Checks After Treatment

At the end of a treatment, the operator verifies complete source retraction by taking the following steps:

- Noting the completion of treatment as indicated by the control console
- Observing the radiation monitors in the room
- Measuring the radiation levels at the patient using the hand-held radiation detector
- Measuring the radiation levels at the treatment unit with the hand-held detector

The last reading should be in front of the unit in line with the source path out of the shielding container.

DOSIMETRY AND TREATMENT PLANNING

Time Course of Procedures

As with LDR brachytherapy, treatment planning for HDR cases may follow different patterns, based on the treatment approach. For example, treatments of cervical cancer using a tandem and ovoid usually have the physician place the treatment appliance, followed by localization imaging and then dosimetric calculations. Less likely than with LDR approach, there can still be planning first based on an idealized application, such as a surface application. Some treatment planning may be interactive, such as with prostate implants, where dosimetry following needle placement can direct subsequent needle placement. Despite this range of options, in most HDR cases the treatment plan generation follows applicator placement, and that model will be assumed in this discussion.

Differences Between Low- and High–Dose-Rate Brachytherapy Treatment Planning

HDR brachytherapy treatment planning differs from LDR brachytherapy in three ways. The first difference results from the time course of the treatments. In treatments of several sites, particularly most gynecologic applications and some methods for treatment of the prostate, the patient waits in the treatment position during the treatment plan generation. Most interstitial and intraluminal treatments differ little from the LDR varieties, with treatment plan generation performed with the patient elsewhere. For those cases with the patient waiting in the treatment position, time becomes an important factor. If the plan generation takes too long, the patient will begin moving with respect to the applicator even though both may be "immobilized." Additional problems with excessively long dosimetry sessions include patient discomfort (other than leading to movement) and cost of support staff such as anesthesiologists.

A second difference entails the quantities involved with the dose calculation. LDR applications often use source strength input by the user—for example, cesium sources used in a tandem and ovoid—and calculate resulting dose rates based on the source configuration. The problem in many cases, particularly in interstitial implants, becomes selecting the dose-rate isodose surface on which to base the treatment duration. The case may have many sources, possibly of various strengths, but only a single duration for all sources. High–dose-rate brachytherapy has one source strength and many different dwell times. In both cases, the dose calculation algorithm uses the product of the source strength and time at a given location as the basis for the resulting dose distribution.

The third difference concerns the role of quantities as input or output. As noted earlier, LDR calculations most often input the source strengths and calculate the resultant dose-rate distribution. Sometimes the treatment duration is also specified, generating a dose distribution. HDR brachytherapy planning usually reverses the process, starting with the dose pattern desired and working backward to the dwell-time distribution necessary to achieve that dose, a process termed reverse planning. A common part of reverse planning is *optimization*, a process to achieve a treatment plan that is "best" according to some criteria.

Optimization

The term *optimization* implies finding a plan that maximizes some aspects of the dose distribution. Many approaches actually only address finding a set of dwell times that deliver a specified dose to specified locations. Other approaches also try to control the dose distribution more finely and possibly limit the dose to specified organs at risk. The umbrella of optimization covers many disparate processes.

Optimization Approaches

Optimization in brachytherapy has taken many forms. The approaches fall into general categories, although considerable controversy surrounds the classifications. Ezzell[20] presents an excellent review of optimization. The discussion here can only brush the surface of the topic. One listing of the categories with examples follows.

Stochastic approaches to optimization start from a distribution of dwell times for the selected dwell positions. The starting dwell-time distribution may be arbitrary, but information on typical solutions can reduce the time to solution. Through the initial set of dwell times, the program calculates a value for an *objective function*. An objective function assigns a numerical value to the solution set that allows ranking the set according to quality. The objective function may be as simple as the difference between the value of dose calculated at a set of point and the dose desired. Objective functions (OFs) often become more complicated, as in the following equation:

$$\mathrm{OF} = w_{\mathrm{t}}(0.95D_{\mathrm{pre}} - D_{\mathrm{t,m}})_{D_{\mathrm{t,m}}<0.95D_{\mathrm{pre}}} + \sum_i w_{\mathrm{OAR},i}(\bar{D}_{\mathrm{OAR},i,\mathrm{calc}} - D_{\mathrm{OAR},i,\mathrm{limit}})^2_{\bar{D}_{\mathrm{OAR},i,\mathrm{calc}}>D_{\mathrm{OAR},i,\mathrm{limit}}} \quad (11)$$

In Equation 11, D_{pre} represents the prescription dose and $D_{\mathrm{t,m}}$ stand for the minimum dose in the planning target volume. In this example, the person running the optimization wants to evaluate whether the dwell time set results in part of the target receiving <95% of the prescribed dose, and, if so, to keep track of how much less. The second term considers the average doses ($\bar{D}$) to each of the organs at risk (OAR) and determines for each the amount over some limiting dose assigned for that organ. The objective function, OF, in this case is a penalty paid for the dwell-time distribution. The first term would be omitted as long as the minimum target dose equaled or exceeded 95% of the prescription dose, and the term for any of the organs at risk would be zero as long as the dose remained below the limiting value. The power of 2 in the exponent indicates tolerance of a little excess dose but imposes serious penalties for larger values. The weighting factors, w, allow a differentiation between the importance given to achieving the desired dose distribution and limiting the dose to a given organ at risk. In addition to the objective function, the dwell-time set might also be subject to *hard constraints* that would reject the set outright if the target dose fell to <90% of the prescribed dose or an organ at risk exceeded a different, maximum limit. Because the value of the OF increases as the dose distribution gets worse, the program tries to minimize this function. Keep in mind that this equation only illustrates the concepts and is not intended to serve as a model of a good objective function.

The methodology for finding the best set of dwell times differs among the stochastic approaches. In *simulated annealing*,[21–24] random changes, often sizable, are made form an arbitrary initial solution for the dwell times of some or all of the dwell positions. After the changes and recalculation of the objective function, the program holds on to the better of the two dwell-time sets. New random changes are made from the better set, and again the sets are compared using the objective function. As this process continues, the allowed changes become smaller and the objective function should improve as the process moves toward the solution—the set with the best objective function. The process as described can fall into a local minimum for the objective function, where any changes make the function worse, whereas somewhere distant to this local minimum lower values obtain. To avoid such traps, the program periodically allows big jumps in the dwell times to investigate completely different regions of dwell times. If the new region does not seem promising because the objective functions are worse, the program goes back to the better region.

Often, the value of the objective function changes little with fairly large changes in individual dwell times in the neighborhood of the optimal solution. Going from a close dwell-time set to the true optimum can require a considerable amount of computer time and often more than getting close in the first place. Most programs contain a criterion for stopping the process once the objective function finds an adequate solution instead of continuing to the true optimum.

Other stochastic approaches, such as the *genetic algorithm*,[25] use different search mechanisms, but the overall procedures tend to be similar.

A nonstochastic approach, *geometric optimization* solves for dwell times that would give the same doses to the vicinities around each of the dwell positions, based on several simplifying assumptions.[26] This approach recognizes that the dose near any dwell position results not only from the nearby dwell, but also from the sum of the contributions from all the other sources. This method first calculates how much dose would be deposited to a dwell position from all the other dwell positions and then weights the dwell time at that dwell position under consideration by the inverse of this dose. Thus, each dwell position needs only make up for the difference between the dose it already receives from the other positions and the dose desired. The first step sets the dwell weight, τ (the relative dwell time, normalized as described later), for dwell position i with the geometric contributions of the other positions, in the formalism of AAPM Task Group 43,[27] as

$$\tau_i = \left[\sum_{j \neq i} \frac{g(r_{i \leftarrow j}) \cdot \varphi(r_{i \leftarrow j})}{r^2_{i \leftarrow j}} \right]^{-1}, \tag{12}$$

where $r_{i \leftarrow j}$ is the distance between dwell positions i and j, $g(r_{i \leftarrow j})$ is the radial dose function, and $\phi(r_{i \leftarrow j})$ is the anisotropy factor. This equation assumes that the dose rate follows the inverse-square law (i.e., approximates the source as a point). Commercial versions of this algorithm usually ignore the radial-dose function, which remains within 2% of unity out to a distance of 5 cm for ^{192}Ir, and the anisotropy factor, which falls within 3.5% of 0.98 over that same range. The errors from these omissions and the point source approximation (inherent in the inverse-square relationship) remain smaller than errors that creep in later.

Determining the absolute dwell times then requires specifying the dose desired to a point or the average of several points. For the average dose to several points (indicated by q), the equation for the average dose to the points is

$$\bar{D}_{\text{initial pass}} = \frac{S_K \cdot \Lambda}{n} \sum_{q=n}^{1} \sum_{j=m}^{1} \frac{\tau_j \cdot g(r_{q \leftarrow j}) \cdot \varphi(r_{q \leftarrow j})}{r^2_{q \leftarrow i}}, \tag{13}$$

where S_K is the source strength in mGy m^2 h^{-1}, Λ is the dose rate constant in Gy cm^2/unit source strength, n is the number of dose points in the average, and m is the number of dwell positions, and t_j from Equation 12 serves as the initial estimate of the dwell time at position j.

Adjusting $\bar{D}_{\text{initial pass}}$ to become $D_{\text{prescribed}}$ requires scaling the dwell times. Letting each of the t_j be the time to deliver $D_{\text{prescribed}}$ and c be the scaling factor such that $t_j = c\tau_j$, then we have

$$c = \frac{\bar{D}_{\text{initial pass}}}{D_{\text{prescribed}}}. \tag{14}$$

This process assumed the equality of all the dwell times at the first step when calculating the dwell weights. Yet, when using the dwell weights in Equation 13 and then scaling them by a constant, each dwell time in the equation had individual values. Thus, the situation for which Equation 12 applies never obtains, compromising the uniformity of dose through the volume. The uniformity could improve by iterating the process, at the sacrifice of its very high speed. The process also assumes that the implant, and particularly the dwell positions, matches the target volume.

Adjacent dwell positions along the same catheter track can produce the greatest affect on the dwell weights, resulting in isodose surfaces that tend to follow the catheters rather than conform to the shape of the implanted volume as a whole. This is especially the case if the separation between dwell positions along a catheter is much less than the separation between catheters. To reduce this effect, a version of the algorithm neglects all other dwell positions along the same catheter track when calculating the dwell weights in a given catheter. This variation is called *volume optimization* because it tends to spread the doses throughout the implanted volume. The original version, which includes the contributions of all other dwell positions for the calculation of any dwell weight, is called *distance optimization* because the isodose surfaces tend to follow a catheter at a constant distance.

The analytic approach, also known as *point optimization* or *point-dose optimization,* attempts to solve algebraically for the set of dwell times that produce the desired dose distribution, as represented by a set of points, called *optimization points,* each with its own specified desired dose. In the most basic form, the specified doses and the dwell times establish a set of simultaneous equations of the form[28,29]

$$D_i = \sum_{j=1}^{m} C_{i,j} \cdot t_j, \tag{15}$$

where D_i is the dose specified to point i, m is the number of dwell positions, t_j is the dwell time at position j, and the $C_{i,j}$ are factors that give the dose contribution at i due to the source at position j, with the sum over all sources. The source strength at each source position forms a variable (unknown), and each dose-specification point yields an equation. Equal numbers of dwell times and dose points form a *determined* system with an exact solution. In more complex cases, there may be more optimization points than source positions, resulting in an *overdetermined* system (more equations than variables). This would be the situation in which optimization points were spread around the contour of a region of interest and scattered through the volume. Faced with this situation, one can vary the source strengths to minimize the square of the differences between the desired and calculated doses at the optimization points. At the other extreme, a case may have more source positions than optimization points (more variables than equations), resulting in an *underdetermined* system. This situation most often happens with large implants and a minimum of optimization points or complicated gynecologic applicators with only a few dose-control points. With this situation the source strengths have no well-defined values; many solutions would possibly exist with the same value for the square of the difference between the doses desired and those calculated. Distinguishing between the solutions requires some other criteria. One often is a minimization of the total dwell time, under the assumption that such would also minimize the integral dose to the patient.

Determined and overdetermined systems can (and often do) generate solutions with negative dwell times. Simply truncating the negative dwell times often results in a very unsatisfactory dose distribution. Avoiding this nonphysical situation also requires an additional criterion. One possible criterion minimizes the differences between adjacent source strengths. For m dwell positions, this term becomes

$$\delta_i = \sum_{j=1}^{n-1} (t_j - t_{j+1})^2. \tag{16}$$

Including this term in the optimization limits the fluctuations between adjacent sources. To deliver a dose to the target volume requires a net positive total dwell time, and so limiting the amount of difference between the dwell times eventually results in all positive times. An additional condition for underdetermined systems selects solutions that minimize the total radiation to the patient as a whole, which depends directly on the total source strength. The final optimization becomes minimizing the chi-squared value in

$$X^2 = \sum_{i=1}^{m} w_i \left(D_i - C_{ij} \sum_{j=1}^{n} t_j \right)^2 + v \sum_{j=1}^{n-1} (t_j - t_{j+1})^2 + u \sum_{j=1}^{n} t_j, \tag{17}$$

where, in addition to those quantities defined earlier, n is the number of dose points specified, w_i is the weighting given to the dose specification at point i (how much the operator wants the correct dose there), v represents the importance in minimizing the fluctuations between adjacent sources, and u represents the importance of minimizing the integral dose to the patient.

With a large number of optimization points or source positions, or both, the running of the program solving the equations becomes long, and approximations cut the calculation time greatly without significantly compromising the accuracy of the final dose distribution. By setting the dwell time

$$t_i = \sum_{k=1}^{p} a_k \cdot F_k(j-1), \tag{18}$$

where F is a fitting function, such as a polynomial or Fourier series of order p, and a_k is the coefficient for the kth element, and substituting that into the X^2 Equation 17, the optimization now need only solve for the fitting coefficients, presumably a much smaller set of values. An alternative approach to solving the equation follows Newton's method.[30,31]

Obviously, the selection of the optimization points becomes very important. The number of points must adequately describe the shape of the dose distribution desired. The dose distributions may satisfy the specifications established for the optimization points but leave portions of the target without dose specification points untreated. However, the points should avoid regions of large dose gradients because specification there can produce unexpected and inappropriate results.

In general, lower values for v in equation 17 allow better conformality of the dose distribution, and the optimum value often is that just sufficient to prevent negative dwell times. However, simply solving for the dose to specified points can produce an unwanted dose distribution, even when the points seem to follow normal guidelines. Thomadsen et al.[32] give an example similar to that in Figure 24.10. Here, the dose points mirror the basal dose points equidistant from the surrounding catheters. With a low value for v in the optimization equation, the simple solution places all of the source material in the center, bottom needle—not at all what was really desired. The situation could be avoided by limiting the dwell-time variations or using more dose points, particularly on the outside of the implant. Alternatively, performing a geometric optimization to obtain an approximate source distribution, followed by optimization on the points, also alleviates the problem.

The output of any optimization approach may leave the operator wanting to make modifications. One method commercially available works on the computer screen display of the dose distribution and allows the operator to "grab" a dose line on the display with the cursor and move the line to a desired location. These fine adjustments make changes that would be difficult to describe in the optimization routine's specifications. Most of the programs allow adjusting the impact of any change between changing all of the dwell times (scaling the distribution, making the whole larger or smaller) and changing a single dwell time (effecting very local changes). Even local changes, however, result in changes in image planes other than the one on which the change has made because the radiation carries the dose beyond the immediate locale.

Changes in the dose distribution to produce desired modifications can also produce unintended changes. Of particular concern would be expending the prescription isodose surface and inadvertently also expending the higher-dose surfaces, possibly into a significant volume. During any manipulation of the isodose surfaces, the display should also show the higher doses. Assuming that most of the manipulation occurs with the 100% surface, the 150% should also be on display.

Evaluation of Dose Distributions

Optimization calculations compute relative dose distributions and require only spatial dose information. After establishing the shape of the dose distribution, the entire distribution must be raised or lowered to give the correct absolute dose to a specified point or the average at a number of specified points. This process requires some evaluation of the dose distribution.

Other than visually examining the isodose distribution resulting from the optimization routine, there are some tools that provide quantitative assessments of various aspects. Thomadsen[17] provides a fuller discussion. Intracavitary evaluation mostly relies on visual interpretation, so the discussion below focuses on evaluation of the dose distribution for interstitial implants.

The *maximum significant dose* (MSD) refers to the highest-level isodose surface that encompasses more than one needle track. The dose very close to a needle track becomes very high, but the body seems to tolerate these small local volumes. The MSD provides a convenient criterion for when the high-dose

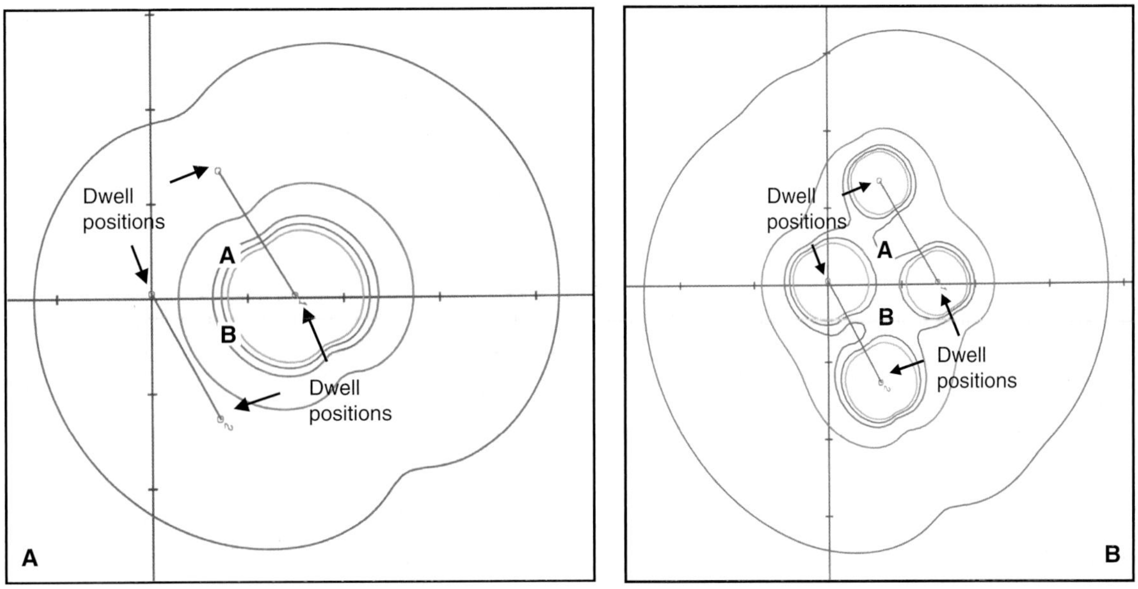

FIGURE 24.10. An example of potential optimization problem. **A:** The criterion was that the two optimization points (A and B) receive the same dose, which was satisfied by a single active dwell position. **B:** Adding constrains on the dwell-time variation solved the problem. (Example inspired by van der Laarse.[28])

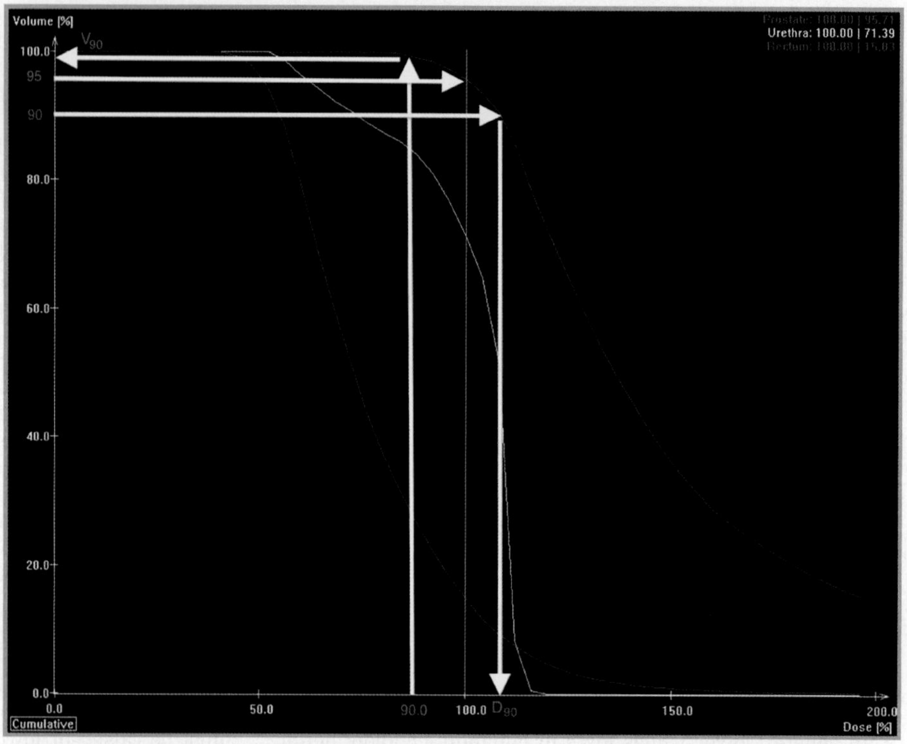

FIGURE 24.11. A dose–volume histogram (DVH) for a prostate implant. The vertical green line indicates that 95% of the prostate is to receive 100% of the prescribed dose. The fractional volume of the prostate receiving 90% of the prescribed dose, V_{90}, and the dose that covers 90% of the prostate, D_{90}, are also shown. This DVH also shows the volumes raised to specified fractions of the prescription dose for the rectum and bladder.

volumes become "significant" and likely to produce biologic consequences. For most implants, the MSD should remain <150% of the prescription dose, assuming that the prescription dose encompasses the target volume. For vary large volumes, the limiting value should decrease to about 125% of the prescription dose.

Figure 24.11 shows a typical volume–dose histogram for an implant. The histogram provides the basis for many of the analytical quantities. Ideally, the target structure curve should follow the 100% (or 1.00) level (top of the graph) from the low doses on the left through the target dose, indicating that the entire target receives at least the target dose. In practice, such coverage often becomes challenging. The volume of the target receiving at least a dose "x" is indicated by the symbol V_x, where the x can be either a percentage of the prescription dose or an absolute dose. Alternatively, sometime the quantity of interest is the dose received by a volume "y," indicated as D_y, where y can be either the fraction of the region of interest or an absolute volume. In this chapter (although not a very common practice) a preceding subscript indicates delimitations, such as confining the value to the planned target volume (PTV) or looking at the value through the entire universe ("total").

Competing treatment plans may have quite different features. Some quantities that can help condense some characteristics into values include the following. It should be noted that some of the quantities originally applied to the dose distribution in the absence of any regions of interest but have been adapted to the modern situation in which volume images provide a context for assessment and evaluation. Unless indicated, the volumes are the fraction of the whole region of interest (ROI).

High-dose volume (HDV)[33–35] is the volume of a region of interest raised to a dose significantly higher than the target dose, often higher by a factor of 1.5. Symbolically, we have

$$\mathrm{HDV} = {}_{\mathrm{ROI}}V_{150\%}. \tag{19}$$

Coverage index (CI)[35–37] is the fraction of the target volume receiving a dose equal to or greater that the target dose:

$$\mathrm{CI} = {}_{\mathrm{CTV}}V_{100\%} \tag{20}$$

Dose nonuniformity ratio (DNR)[35,36] is the ratio of the CTV high-dose volume to that taken to at least the target dose:

$$\mathrm{DNR} = {}_{\mathrm{CTV}}V_{150\%}/{}_{\mathrm{CTV}}V_{100\%}. \tag{21}$$

External volume index (EI)[35,36] is the volume of nontarget tissue receiving doses equal to or greater than the target dose, as a fraction of the target volume:

$$\mathrm{EI} = ({}_{\mathrm{total}}V_{100\%} - {}_{\mathrm{CTV}}V_{100\%})/{}_{\mathrm{CTV}}V. \tag{22}$$

In this case, all the volumes are absolute, for example, in cubic centimeters.

Relative dose homogeneity index (HI)[35,36] is the fraction of the target volume receiving a dose between the target dose and the high-dose level:

$$\mathrm{HI} = {}_{\mathrm{CTV}}V_{150\%} - {}_{\mathrm{CTV}}V_{100\%}. \tag{23}$$

Conformality number or *index* (CN)[38,39] is a measure of how well the dose distribution fits the target:

$$\mathrm{CN} = \frac{{}_{\mathrm{CTV}}V_{100\%}}{{}_{\mathrm{total}}V_{100\%}} \cdot \frac{{}_{\mathrm{CTV}}V_{100\%}}{{}_{\mathrm{CTV}}V}. \tag{24}$$

Here, again, all the volumes are absolute.

Each of these quantities tells a small part of the dose distribution's entire story. Each can help in the evaluation of a dose distribution, and all, taken together, give a better picture. However, none of the indices—even together—captures the complexity and nuances of the total dose distribution. Inspection of the results of the optimization remains a necessity.

Quality Control of Treatment Plan

The use of HDR brachytherapy in the definitive management of gynecologic cancer,[2] early-stage breast cancer,[40,41] and prostate cancer[42] has made the HDR RAL a very common treatment modality in most radiotherapy clinics. Treatment-planning systems for HDR RALs are now interfaced with multimodality images (computed tomography [CT], magnetic resonance imaging [MRI], and ultrasound) and sophisticated dose optimization software like inverse planning or interactive graphical optimizers, which enable the planner to maximize the dose uniformity while minimizing the implant volume needed to adequately cover the target volume and at the same time reduce the dose to the organs at risk. Such flexibility creates a challenge for the verification of the optimized calculations with practical manual calculation techniques. With the time constraint between HDR planning and the delivery of treatment while the patient is in the operating room, an efficient, precise, and easy method for checking the complex computer calculation is necessary for quality control of the treatment plan. Every institution should have an established quality control program that takes only a few minutes but at the same time gives a high probability of detecting significant errors, since the NRC considers a difference between the administered dose and calculated dose of 20% a reportable medical event.[43]

Simplistic models to verify computer calculations quickly have drawbacks because applicators or interstitial implants used in HDR treatments are complex in design, and simple point-dose or linear source calculations tends to fall apart in most circumstances.[16,44,45] Because all treatment-planning systems have the capability of generating dose–volume histograms, it is logical that volume-based QA should be the choice. Das et al.[46,47] addressed this possibility and provided an easy and quick calculation check for most HDR interstitial and intracavitary implants. Because HDR treatments are delivered through a wide variety of applicators, the study was divided into three categories:

1. Single-catheter system, which includes tandem and cylinders and vaginal cylinders, as well as MammoSite balloons
2. Two- and three-catheter systems, which include tandem and ovoid pairs or ovoid pairs only
3. Multicatheter system for interstitial implants

EXAMPLE APPLICATIONS

The following examples illustrate some of the aspects of the treatments that are unique for HDR applications. Other chapters discuss the actual therapies in more detail.

Cervical Cancer Brachytherapy

Intracavitary brachytherapy has been a major part of the treatment for cervical cancer for about 85 years, with a significant experience using HDR approaches since the mid-1980s. Of the advantages of HDR brachytherapy given earlier, several apply directly to these treatments, particularly the small size of the source and the concomitant smaller diameter of the intrauterine tandem, the greater stability of the treatment appliance and higher accuracy and relevance of the calculated dose distribution, and the ability to hold organs at risk away from the applicator and source track. Imaging plays a major role in these treatments, with the future likely seeing an increase in that role. Ultrasound often provides guidance during the placement of the intrauterine tandem, particularly when the tumor obliterates the external cervical os. Fluoroscopy provides guidance during placement of the appliance, assisting in the assessment of applicator geometry (e.g., evaluating the centering of the tandem with the ovoids in both the anteroposterior and the lateral projections) and the positions of the rectum and bladder. Most commonly, images after fluoroscopy indicate a satisfactory placement, and radiographic images are made for dosimetric localization and reconstruction.

Imaging for gynecologic brachytherapy is evolving very rapidly, particularly for HDR approaches.[48] Both the brachytherapy arm of the European Society for Therapeutic Radiology and Oncology (Groupe Européen de Curiethérapie [GEC-ESTRO])[49–51] and a group sponsored by several U.S. organizations, principally the Gynecological Oncology Group,[52] recommended moving toward image-based target prescriptions. Identifying the target, that is, tumor tissue in the uterus, requires MRI, the only form of imaging that also reliably differentiates the uterus from other pelvic tissues. The U.S. group felt that it was premature to prescribe the dose to the target identified on MRI because there was no information on what doses tumors had been receiving historically, and they believed that protocols should gather data on tumor doses based on conventional treatment approaches. GEC-ESTRO, on the other hand, proposed using the doses conventionally delivered to Manchester points A, approximately 85 Gy, including the external-beam contribution, as the dose to the identified clinical target volume.

Although only MRI identifies the target and the uterus, CT images the rectum and the bladder well. Although using CT localization does not permit as detailed target information as MRI, it does allow moderate target definition and does facilitate determining the doses to the organs at risk when using conventional treatment prescriptions.[53–55] Dose calculations based on either CT or MRI often indicate that the maximum dose to the bladder falls 2 to 4 cm superior to the conventional point indicated following Report 38 of the International Commission on Radiation Units and Measurement (ICRU)[56] and may be two to four times the dose to the conventional point. The ICRU-indicated rectal point differs less than the bladder point, with the true maximum falling between 1 and 3 cm superiorly and the true maximum dose being one to three times the conventional point.

The accuracy and precision of determining the dose matter much more in HDR intracavitary brachytherapy for the cervix than for LDR treatments for two reasons. The first concerns the precision of dose delivery. King et al.[57] demonstrated that the typical LDR tandem and ovoids move an average of 2 cm over the course of treatment. HDR tandems and ovoids move a maximum of 3 mm when not moving the patient.[45] Thus, the added precision of volume-imaged–based dose calculations would be lost in the general positional uncertainty of LDR intracavitary brachytherapy. In the second place, HDR applications not only can use the dosimetric accuracy, but they may require it. Because of the radiobiologic disadvantage of HDR brachytherapy, knowing the dose distribution with a high certainty is necessary to avoid complications.

Avoiding complications leads to several differences of the cervical applications with HDR compared to LDR brachytherapy. To prevent rectal complications, the dose to the rectum should remain <70% of the dose to the Manchester point A.[2] Treating with the rectal retractor in place usually accomplishes this goal. As noted under the advantages of HDR brachytherapy, patients would not tolerate such a practice over the long durations with LDR applications. Adding distance to the bladder generally uses copious packing anterior to the ovoids, taking care not to let the packing slip between the ovoid surface and the superior or lateral fornices. An unpublished 1988 review of LDR cervical cases at the University of Wisconsin found the beginning of late complications in the superior bowel (fistulae) at about 13 years after treatment and that the prevalence increased continually with time out. That problem with LDR treatments generated concern that the situation might be worse with HDR treatments due to the unfavorable radiobiology. Thus, in the early approach, the dose to the superior bowel was reduced by pulling the uterus low into the vagina during treatment and making the dose distribution more square than the LDR applications so that less unnecessary dose extended into the upper uterus and into the superior bowel.[2] The current practice at the University of Wisconsin is to leave the uterus in a neutral position and simply not use the first few dwell positions. Most commonly, the first dwell position used is 1 cm from dwell position number 1, but that varies with the extent of the disease and the patient's anatomy. Figure 24.12 shows radiographs of a typical case. Figure 24.13 compares a conventional LDR application with a HDR treatment,

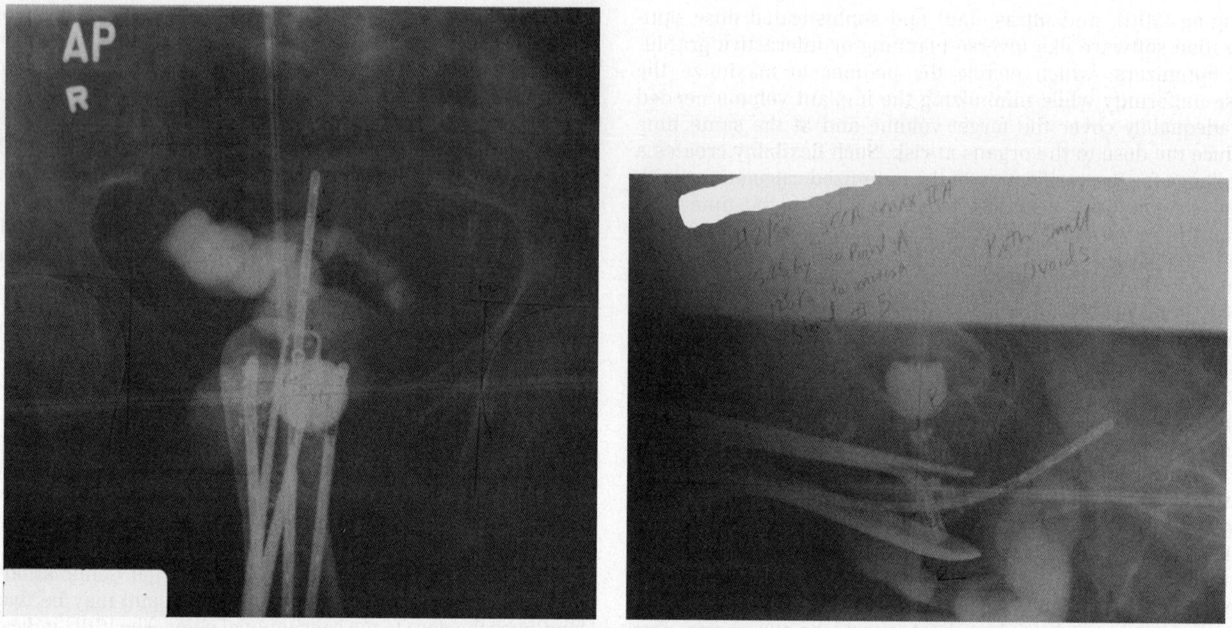

FIGURE 24.12. Radiographs of an HDR application using a tandem and ovoids for the treatment of cervical cancer, with a anteroposterior on the left and lateral on the right.

both normalized to point A, defined as per the American Brachytherapy Society.[58,61]

At Wisconsin, these cases use point-dose optimization. For a tandem and ovoid, the optimization starts 1 cm below the first dwell position used (which normally is 2 cm below the dwell position number 1) with optimization points 18 cm lateral to the tandem on both sides. Placing the points on both sides gives an average correcting for any twist of the tandem or varying contributions from the ovoids. The next points fall 1 cm inferior to the first at 2 cm lateral to the tandem, with subsequent points also 2 cm lateral and 1 cm inferior to the previous points until reaching the position of point A. Regardless of where the previous points were, optimization points are placed at point A and also 2 cm lateral to the next dwell position. Placing any more points along the tandem tends to interfere with the dose distribution around the ovoids. For the ovoids, optimization points are placed on the lateral ovoid surface ¼ cm posterior and anterior of the center.

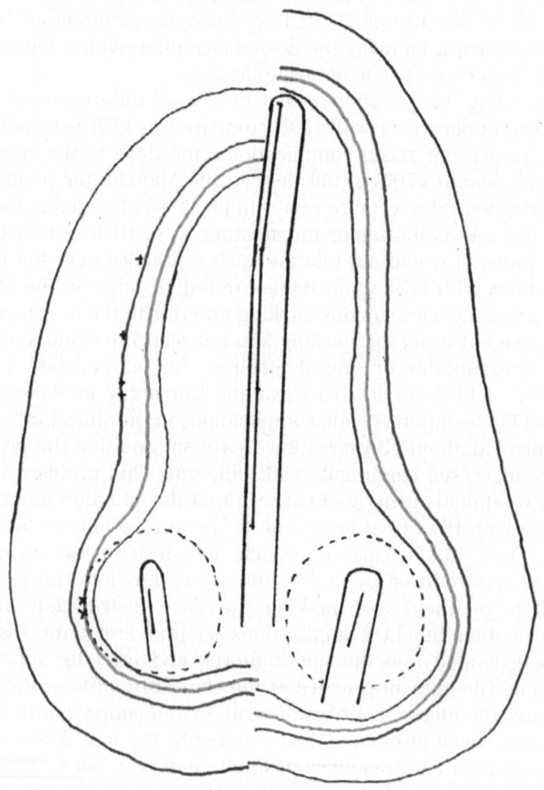

FIGURE 24.13. Comparison of an LDR (*left*) and an HDR (*right*) dose distribution for a tandem and ovoid application for cervical cancer. The HDR dose distribution also shows the locations of the optimization points.

The optimization process assumes that the anatomy follows the applicator because the dose distribution conforms to the treatment appliance. When MRI targeting becomes more widely available, the optimization process would be customized to the patient's disease and limited by the normal anatomy. At the time of writing, the expense and design of MRI and CTI compatible applicators prevent wide use, as do the limitations on access to, and the price of, MR imaging. All of these impediments should resolve in the very near future.

The absolute dose used may depend on the stage of disease, the number of fractions used, and concomitant other therapy, including external-beam therapy and chemotherapy. At Wisconsin, 26.25 Gy over five 5.25-Gy fractions serves for most patients; differences based on stage occur with the external-beam portion of the treatments. Orton et al.[62] cautioned not to exceed 7 Gy per fraction based on a survey of users, but it was unclear whether the users who had problems with the higher doses per fraction had calculated the biologic equivalency of the regimen on normal tissues.

Prostate Brachytherapy

Given the relatively new finding that the α/β for prostate may be lower than for normal, healthy tissue instead of considerably higher as with most tumors, the general rules for preserving organs at risk change markedly. As discussed earlier, normally slow delivery of the radiation, such as with LDR treatments, allows normal tissues to recover better than tumors, whereas HDR causes a greater increase in the damage to the normal tissues than to tumors. When the relative size of the α/β inverts, as in prostate cancer, the advantages also invert. High doses per fraction cause a greater increase in damage to the tumor cells with an α/β of 2 than the normal-tissue cells with an α/β of 3. This situation make HDR brachytherapy look attractive.[63]

Currently, the process for HDR treatments of the prostate follows the LDR model fairly closely. Ultrasound images provide guidance for the insertion of the catheters, although MRI guidance has also been reported and is likely to become more common in the future.[64–66] Generally, placement of the catheters follows a pattern such as four around the urethra and then at 1- to 1.5-cm intervals around the periphery of the gland. The square-hole pattern complicates placement at regular intervals, but the final dose distribution is relatively insensitive to the exact location of the catheters. Commercial software exists to guide the user in the placement of the catheters, but those experienced in prostate implants probably perform as well without computer assistance.

After placement, the optimization routine calculates dwell times to achieve the criteria specified for the patient. The resultant dose distribution may still require adjustment through graphical optimization. On approval of the plan, the operator connects the needles to the treatment unit using the transfer tubes. Because the needles have no inherent numbering, great care must be taken during this process to ensure correct correlation between the needles in the patient and those in the treatment plan.

The location of the first dwell position in the needles would have been determined previously. Radiographing the needles with the x-ray markers in place forms one of the simplest methods. If the treatment unit does not seek the end of the needle to establish the first dwell position, all needles must be tested for uniformity of length.

Treating multiple fractions with the same insertion requires verification of the needle depth. Between fractions the needles tend to work toward the surface and may need repositioning under ultrasound or fluoroscopic guidance. Marks on the needles where they enter a template also can serve as indicators of the needle for repositioning.

Breast Brachytherapy

Accelerated partial-breast irradiation (APBI) for breast cancer patients with HDR brachytherapy as monotherapy following lumpectomy has produced excellent local control rates and cosmesis.[46,67] Interstitial and intracavitary (catheter balloon) implants are commonly being used for this treatment modality. Usually within 8 weeks of lumpectomy and axillary nodal evaluation, the patient undergoes an interstitial implant with one of two methods: a prone, stereotactic, template method with digital mammographic guidance or a supine, ultrasound-guided technique, both under local anesthesia. Due to the perceived technical challenge of multi-catheter interstitial implants, alternative, intracavitary methods for APBI have been developed. One approach uses multiple catheters around the central catheter within a balloon that is placed within the lumpectomy cavity closed, often under ultrasound guidance, and inflated with saline or diluted contrast medium. Two such systems are the Contura (SenoRx, Bard Biopsy System, Tempe, AZ) and multi-catheter MammoSite (Hologic, Bedford, MA). An alternative is the SAVI device (Cienna Medical, Aliso Viejo, CA), that uses six to ten struts in a configuration that looks similar to an egg whisk to hold the tylectomy cavity open instead of a balloon. The struts also serve as the paths for the source travel. The multiple catheters of each of these devices allow some shaping of the dose distribution, but not comparable to that obtainable with the multi-catheter, interstitial implants. Imaging of the balloon for its integrity, as well as rotation of the multiple-catheter devices, should be performed before the initiation of each treatment.

ACKNOWLEDGMENTS

We thank Adam Uselmann and Liyong Lin for the artwork they contributed to this chapter.

REFERENCES

1. Dale RG. The application of the linear-quadratic dose-effect equation to fractionated and protracted radiotherapy. *Br J Radiol* 1985;58:515–528.
2. Stitt JA, Fowler JF, Thomadsen BR, et al. High dose rate intracavitary brachytherapy for carcinoma of the cervix: the Madison system: I. Clinical and radiobiological considerations. *Int J Radiat Oncol Biol Phys* 1992;24:335–348.
3. Stitt JA, Thomadsen BR, Fowler JF. High-dose-rate brachytherapy for cervical carcinoma. *Int J Radiat Oncol Biol Phys* 1992;24:574.
4. Kubo HD, Glasgow GP, Pethel TD, et al. High dose-rate brachytherapy treatment delivery: report of the AAPM Radiation Therapy Committee Task Group No. 59. *Med Phys* 1998;25:375–403.
5. Thomadsen B, Lin SW, Laemmrich P, et al. Analysis of treatment delivery errors in brachytherapy using formal risk analysis techniques. *Int J Radiat Oncol Biol Phys* 2003;57:1492–1508.
6. Cember H, Johnson T. *Introduction to health physics,* 4th ed. New York: McGraw-Hill Medical, 2009.
7. National Council on Radiation Units and Measurement, Report 151: *Structural Shielding Design and Evaluation for Megavoltage Radiotherapy Facilities.* Bethesda MD: author, 2005.
8. McGinley P. *Shielding techniques for radiation oncology facilities*, 2nd ed. Madison, WI: Medical Physics Publishing, 2002.
9. Ezzell GA. Acceptance testing and quality assurance for high dose-rate remote afterloading systems. In: Martinez AA, Orton, CG, Mould, RF, eds. *Brachytherapy HDR and LDR.* Columbia, MD: Nucletron Corporation, 1990:138–159.
10. Ezzell G. Quality assurance in HDR brachytherapy: physical and technical aspects. *Activity Selectron Brachytherapy J* 1991;5:59–62.
11. Chenery SG, Pla M, Podgorsak EB. Physical characteristics of the Selectron high dose rate intracavitary afterloader. *Br J Radiol* 1985;58:735–740.
12. Flynn A. Quality assurance checks on a microSelectron-HDR. *Activity Selectron Brachytherapy J* 1990;4:112–115.
13. Grigsby PW. Quality assurance of remote afterloading equipment at the Mallinckrodt Institute of Radiology. *Activity Selectron User's Newsl* 1989:1–15.
14. Jones C. Quality assurance in brachytherapy using the Selectron LDR/MDR and microSelectron-HDR. *Activity Selectron Brachytherapy J* 1990;4:48–52.
15. Meigooni A, Williamson J, Slessinger E. Practical quality assurance tests for positional and temporal accuracy of HDR remote afterloaders. *Endocuriether Hyperthermia Oncol* 9:46–48.
16. Williamson J, Ezzell G, Olch AJ, et al. Quality assurance for high dose rate brachytherapy. In: Nag S, ed. *High dose rate brachytherapy: a textbook.* Armonk, NY: Futura, 1994:147–212.
17. Thomadsen BR. *Achieving quality in brachytherapy.* London: Taylor and Francis, 1999.
18. DeWerd LA, Jursinic P, Kitchen R, et al. Quality assurance tool for high dose rate brachytherapy. *Med Phys* 1995;22:435–440.
19. Nath R, Anderson LL, Jones D, et al. *Specification of brachytherapy source strength: report of AAPM Task Group No. 32.* New York: American Institute of Physics, 1987.
20. Ezzell G. Optimization in brachytherapy. In: Thomadsen BR, Rivard MJ, Butler WM, eds. *Brachytherapy physics,* 2nd ed. Madison, WI: Medical Physics Publishing, 2005: 415–434.
21. Pouliot J, Kim Y, Lessard E, et al. Inverse planning for HDR prostate brachytherapy used to boost dominant intraprostatic lesions defined by magnetic resonance spectroscopy imaging. *Int J Radiat Oncol Biol Phys* 2004;59:1196–1207.
22. Pouliot J, Lessard E, Hsu I-C. Number of catheters in prostate high dose rate brachytherapy: the role of inverse planning. Presented at the Joint Brachytherapy Meeting GEC/ESTRO-ABS-GLAC, Barcelona, Spain, 2004.
23. Sloboda RS. Optimization of brachytherapy dose distributions by simulated annealing. *Med Phys* 1992;19:955–964.
24. Sloboda RS, Pearcey RG, Gillan SJ. Optimized low dose rate pellet configurations for intravaginal brachytherapy. *Int J Radiat Oncol Biol Phys* 1993;26:499–511.
25. Lahanas M, Baltas D, Zamboglou N. Anatomy-based three-dimensional dose optimization in brachytherapy using multiobjective genetic algorithms. *Med Phys* 1999;26:1904–1918.
26. Edmundson GK. Geometry based optimization for stepping source implants. In: Martinez AA, Orton CG, Mould RF, eds. *Brachytherapy HDR and LDR.* Columbia, MD: Nucletron Corporation, 1990:184–192.
27. Nath R, Anderson LL, Luxton G, et al. Dosimetry of interstitial brachytherapy sources: recommendations of the AAPM Radiation Therapy Committee Task Group No. 43. American Association of Physicists in Medicine. *Med Phys* 1995;22: 209–234.
28. van der Laarse R. Optimization of high dose rate brachytherapy. *Activity Selectron User's Newsl* 1989;2:14–15.
29. van der Laarse R, Edmundson GK, Luthmann RW, et al. Optimization of HDR brachytherapy dose distributions. *Activity Selectron User's Newsl* 1991;5: 94–101.
30. Holmes T, Mackie TR. A comparison of three inverse treatment planning algorithms. *Phys Med Biol* 1994;39:91–106.
31. Luenberger DG. *Linear and nonlinear programming,* 2nd ed. Reading, MA: Addison and Wesley, 1989.
32. Thomadsen B, Houdek P, van der Laarse R. Treatment planning and optimization. In: Nag S, ed. *High dose rate brachytherapy: a textbook.* Armonk, NY: Futura, 199:104–108.
33. Pierquin B, Dutreix A, Paine CH, et al. The Paris system in interstitial radiation therapy. *Acta Radiol Oncol Radiat Phys Biol* 1978;17:33–48.
34. Pierquin B, Chassagne D, Chahbazian C, et al. *Brachytherapy.* St. Louis, MO: Warren H. Green, 1978.
35. Saw CB, Suntharalingam N. Reference dose rates for single- and double-plane 192Ir implants. *Med Phys* 1988;15:391–396.
36. Saw CB, Suntharalingam N. Quantitative assessment of interstitial implants. *Int J Radiat Oncol Biol Phys* 1991;20:135–139.
37. Saw CB, Waterman FM, Ayyangar K, et al. Quantitative evaluation of planar 192Ir implants [Abstract]. *Med Phys* 1986;13–580.
38. van't Riet A, Mak AC, Moerland MA, et al. A conformation number to quantify the degree of conformality in brachytherapy and external beam irradiation: application to the prostate. *Int J Radiat Oncol Biol Phys* 1997;37:731–736.
39. Baltas D, Kolotas C, Geramani K, et al. A conformal index (COIN) to evaluate implant quality and dose specification in brachytherapy. *Int J Radiat Oncol Biol Phys* 1998;40:515–524.

40. Clarke DH, Vicini FA, Jacobs H, et al. High dose rate brachytherapy for breast cancer. In: Nag S, ed. *High dose rate brachythreapy: a textbook*. Armonk, NY: Futura, 1994:321–329.
41. Kuske R, Bolton J, Wilenzick R, et al. Brachytherapy as the sole method of breast irradiation in Tis, T1, T2, N0,1 breast cancer. *Int J Radiat Oncol Biol Phys* 1994; 30S1:245.
42. Martinez AA, Pataki I, Edmundson G, et al. Phase II prospective study of the use of conformal high-dose-rate brachytherapy as monotherapy for the treatment of favorable stage prostate cancer: a feasibility report. *Int J Radiat Oncol Biol Phys* 2001;49:61–69.
43. U.S. Nuclear Regulatory Commission. *Code of federal regulations—energy*, Title 10, Chapter 1, Part 35, *Medical use of by-product material*. Washington, DC: Government Printing Office, 2011.
44. Kubo HD, Chin RB. Simple mathematical formulas for quick-checking of single-catheter high dose rate brachytherapy treatment plans. *Endocuriether Hyperthermia Oncol* 1992;8:165–169.
45. Thomadsen BR, Shahabi S, Stitt JA, et al. High dose rate intracavitary brachytherapy for carcinoma of the cervix: the Madison system: II. Procedural and physical considerations. *Int J Radiat Oncol Biol Phys* 1992;24:349–357.
46. Das RK, Patel R, Shah H, et al. 3D CT-based high-dose-rate breast brachytherapy implants: treatment planning and quality assurance. *Int J Radiat Oncol Biol Phys* 2004;59:1224–1228.
47. Das RK, Bradley KA, Nelson IA, et al. Quality assurance of treatment plans for interstitial and intracavitary high-dose-rate brachytherapy. *Brachytherapy* 2006; 5:56–60.
48. Thomadsen BR. Volume imaging in gynecological brachytherapy. In: Thomadsen BR, Rivard MJ, Butler W, eds. *Brachytherapy physics*. 2nd ed. Madison, WI: Medical Physics Publishing, 2005:785–796.
49. Haie-Meder C, Potter R, Van Limbergen E, et al. Recommendations from Gynaecological (GYN) GEC-ESTRO Working Group (I): concepts and terms in 3D image based 3D treatment planning in cervix cancer brachytherapy with emphasis on MRI assessment of GTV and CTV. *Radiother Oncol* 2005;74:235–245.
50. Potter R, Haie-Meder C, Van Limbergen E, et al. Recommendations from gynaecological (GYN) GEC ESTRO working group (II): concepts and terms in 3D image-based treatment planning in cervix cancer brachytherapy-3D dose volume parameters and aspects of 3D image-based anatomy, radiation physics, radiobiology. *Radiother Oncol* 2006;78:67–77.
51. Lang S, Nulens A, Briot E, et al. Intercomparison of treatment concepts for MR image assisted brachytherapy of cervical carcinoma based on GYN GEC-ESTRO recommendations. *Radiother Oncol* 2006;78:185–193.
52. Nag S, Cardenes H, Chang S, et al. Proposed guidelines for image-based intracavitary brachytherapy for cervical carcinoma: report from Image-Guided Brachytherapy Working Group. *Int J Radiat Oncol Biol Phys* 2004;60:1160–1172.
53. Schoeppel SL, Fraass BA, Hopkins MP, et al. A CT-compatible version of the Fletcher system intracavitary applicator: clinical application and 3-dimensional treatment planning. *Int J Radiat Oncol Biol Phys* 1989;17:1103–1109.
54. Schoeppel SL, LaVigne ML, Martel MK, et al. Three-dimensional treatment planning of intracavitary gynecologic implants: analysis of ten cases and implications for dose specification. *Int J Radiat Oncol Biol Phys* 1994;28:277–283.
55. Viswanathan AN, Dimopoulos J, Kirisits C, et al. Computed tomography versus magnetic resonance imaging-based contouring in cervical cancer brachytherapy: results of a prospective trial and preliminary guidelines for standardized contours. *Int J Radiat Oncol Biol Phys* 2007;68:491–498.
56. International Commission on Radiation Units and Measures. *Report 38: Dose and volume specification for reporting intracavitary therapy in gynecology*. Bethesda, MD: Author, 1985.
57. King CC, Stockstill TF, Bloomer WD, et al. Point dose variations with time in brachytherapy for cervical carcinoma. *Med Phys* 1992;19:777.
58. Nag S, Chao C, Erickson B, et al. The American Brachytherapy Society recommendations for low-dose-rate brachytherapy for carcinoma of the cervix. *Int J Radiat Oncol Biol Phys* 2002;52:33–48.
59. Nag S, Erickson B, Thomadsen B, et al. The American Brachytherapy Society recommendations for high-dose-rate brachytherapy for carcinoma of the cervix. *Int J Radiat Oncol Biol Phys* 2000;48:201–211.
60. Viswanathan AN, Beriwal S, De Los Santos JF, et al. American Brachytherapy Society consensus guidelines for locally advanced carcinoma of the cervix. Part II: high-dose-rate brachytherapy. *Brachytherapy* 2012;11(1):47–52.
61. Viswanathan AN, Thomadsen B. American Brachytherapy Society consensus guidelines for locally advanced carcinoma of the cervix. Part I: general principles. *Brachytherapy* 2012;11(1):33–46.
62. Orton CG, Seyedsadr M, Somnay A. Comparison of high and low dose rate remote afterloading for cervix cancer and the importance of fractionation. *Int J Radiat Oncol Biol Phys* 1991;21:1425–1434.
63. Yamada Y, Rogers L, Demanes DJ, et al. American Brachytherapy Society consensus guidelines for high-dose-rate prostate brachytherapy. *Brachytherapy* 2012;11(1):20–32.
64. Cormack RA, Kooy H, Tempany CM, et al. A clinical method for real-time dosimetric guidance of transperineal 125I prostate implants using interventional magnetic resonance imaging. *Int J Radiat Oncol Biol Phys* 2000;46: 207–214.
65. D'Amico A, Cormack R, Kumar S, et al. Real-time magnetic resonance imaging-guided brachytherapy in the treatment of selected patients with clinically localized prostate cancer. *J Endourol* 2000;14:367–370.
66. Menard C, Susil RC, Choyke P, et al. MRI-guided HDR prostate brachytherapy in standard 1.5T scanner. *Int J Radiat Oncol Biol Phys* 2004;59:1414–1423.
67. Patel RR, Das RK. Image-guided breast brachytherapy: an alternative to whole-breast radiotherapy. *Lancet Oncol* 2006;7:407–415.

Chapter 25
Clinical Aspects and Applications of High–Dose-Rate Brachytherapy

Subir Nag and Granger R. Scruggs

Brachytherapy has the advantage of delivering a high radiation dose to the tumor while sparing the surrounding normal tissues. Brachytherapy procedures were initially performed by inserting radioactive material directly into the tumor ("hot" loading), thereby giving high radiation exposure to the physicians performing the procedure. Manually afterloaded techniques were introduced to increase accuracy and reduce the radiation hazards. In afterloaded techniques, hollow needles, catheters, or applicators are first inserted into the tumor then loaded with radioactive materials. The introduction of remote-controlled insertion of sources eliminated radiation exposure to visitors and medical personnel. In this technique, the patient is housed in a shielded room and the radiation therapist controls the treatment from outside the room. Hollow applicators, needles, or catheters are inserted into the tumor and connected by transfer tubes to the radioactive material, which is stored in a shielded safe within the high–dose-rate afterloader. The radiation source is driven through the transfer tubes and into the tumor by remote control.

Remote-controlled brachytherapy can be performed using low–dose-rate (LDR), medium–dose-rate (MDR), or high–dose-rate (HDR) techniques. Although the International Commission on Radiation Units and Measurements (ICRU) definition No. 38 of HDR is >12 Gy/hour,[1] the usual dose rate employed in current HDR brachytherapy units is about 100 to 300 Gy/hour. HDR has the added advantage that the treatments take only a few minutes, and therefore can be given on an outpatient basis with minimal risk of applicator movement and minimal patient discomfort. Additionally, use of a single-stepping source, as used in most modern HDR afterloaders, allows optimization of dose distribution by varying the dwell time at each dwell position. However, it should be emphasized that while optimization can improve the dose distribution, it should not be used to substitute for a poorly placed implant. Nag and Samsami[2] have provided examples of inappropriate optimization strategies that can lead to suboptimal dosimetry plans and clinical problems. HDR is normally given as a course of a number of fractionated HDR treatments, although it can be given as a single treatment, as in intraoperative HDR brachytherapy, if doses to the normal tissues can be sufficiently reduced by displacement or shielding. The advantages and disadvantages of HDR in comparison to LDR are enumerated in Table 25.1.

The previously mentioned advantages have led to increased use of HDR worldwide; however, training and expertise are required for proper administration of these treatments. Guidelines and recommendations for the use of HDR at various sites have been published by the American Brachytherapy Society (ABS), much of which is summarized in this chapter,[3–11] and the reader should refer to these publications for details. Controlled clinical trials are needed to critically evaluate the efficacy of these procedures.

TABLE 25.1 ADVANTAGES AND DISADVANTAGES OF HIGH-DOSE-RATE COMPARED WITH LOW-DOSE-RATE BRACHYTHERAPY

Advantages	*Disadvantages*
1. Radiation protection • HDR eliminates radiation exposure hazard for caregivers and visitors. Caregivers are able to provide optimal patient care without fear of radiation exposure. • HDR eliminates source preparation and transportation. • Because there is only one source, there is minimal risk of losing a radioactive source.	1. Radiobiologic • The short treatment times do not allow for the repair of sublethal damage in normal tissue or the redistribution of cells within the cell cycle or reoxygenation of the tumor cells; hence, multiple treatments are required.
2. Allows shorter treatment times • There is less patient discomfort because prolonged bed rest is eliminated. • It is possible to treat patients who may not tolerate long periods of isolation and those who are at high risk for pulmonary embolism due to prolonged bed rest. • There is less risk of applicator movement during therapy. • There are reduced hospitalization costs because outpatient therapy is possible. • HDR may allow greater displacement of nearby normal tissues (by packing or retraction), which could potentially reduce morbidity. • It is possible to treat a larger number of patients in institutions that have a high volume of brachytherapy patients but insufficient inpatient facilities (e.g., in some developing countries). • Allow intraoperative treatments, which are completed while patient is still in the operating room.	2. Limited experience • Few centers in the United States have long-term (>20 years) experience. • Until recently, standardized treatment guidelines were not available; however, the American Brachytherapy Society (ABS) has provided guidelines for HDR at various sites.[5–8,10,11]
3. HDR sources are of smaller diameter than the cesium sources that are used for intracavitary LDR. • This reduces the need for dilatation of the cervix and therefore reduces the need for heavy sedation or general anesthesia. • High-risk patients who are unable to tolerate general anesthesia can be more safely treated. • HDR allows for interstitial, intraluminal, and percutaneous insertions.	3. The economic disadvantage • The use of HDR brachytherapy as compared to manual afterloading techniques requires a large initial capital expenditure because the remote afterloaders cost about $400,000. • There are additional costs for a shielded room and personnel costs are higher as the procedures are more labor intensive.
4. HDR makes treatment dose distribution optimization possible. • Variations of the dwell times of a single-stepping source allow an almost infinite variation of the effective source strengths, and the source position allows for greater control of the dose distribution and potentially less morbidity.	4. Greater potential risks • Because a high activity source is used, there is greater potential harm if the machine malfunctions or if there is a calculation error. The short treatment times, compared to LDR, allow much less time to detect and correct errors.

HDR, high-dose-rate; LDR, low-dose-rate.

RADIOBIOLOGIC PRINCIPLES OF HIGH-DOSE-RATE BRACHYTHERAPY

Most radiation oncologists are familiar with LDR brachytherapy. LDR (at 30 to 50 cGy/hour) can be added to external-beam radiation therapy (EBRT) doses (at 2 Gy/day) to obtain equivalent total doses. HDR brachytherapy is distinct from LDR brachytherapy, and radiation oncologists who are accustomed to LDR techniques must realize that experience in LDR cannot be automatically translated into expertise in HDR. It is important to review the current literature and survey the experiences of centers that have been performing HDR. When converting from LDR to HDR, one must keep the other parameters (chemotherapy, EBRT field/dose, dose specification point, applicators, patient population, and so forth) the same, changing only the LDR to HDR.

Fractionation schemes for HDR are widely variable, and many radiation oncologists are not very familiar with the resultant biologic effects. Empirical methods such as the NSD (nominal standard dose), TDF (time-dose factor), or a dose reduction factor of 0.6 have been used in the past to convert HDR doses to LDR equivalent doses. The linear-quadratic (LQ) equation can be used to guide development of HDR doses and fractionation schedules.[12] However, the LQ mathematical calculations are tedious and may not be practical on a day-to-day basis. Hence, a simplified computer program was developed by Nag and Gupta[13] to obtain the isoeffective doses to be used for HDR. The clinician needs only to enter the EBRT total dose and dose/fraction, HDR dose, and the number of HDR fractions. The computer program will automatically calculate the isoeffective doses for tumor and normal tissue effects. Isoeffective doses are expressed in clinically familiar terms, as if given at 2 Gy per fraction (EQD_2), rather than as biologically equivalent doses (BEDs), which are unfamiliar to clinicians. Furthermore, a dose-modifying factor (DMF) is applied to the normal tissues to account for the fact that doses to normal tissues are different from the doses to the tumor, thus providing a more realistic equivalent normal tissue effect. This program can be used to determine HDR doses that are equivalent to LDR brachytherapy doses (EQD_2) used to treat various cancers. Alternatively, the program may be used to express the isoeffective dose of different HDR dose fractionation regimens. Although the LQ biomathematic model can be helpful in determining isoeffective doses, it has many limitations that must be kept in mind when using the program. The LQ model accounts for the repair of sublethal damage, but it does not account for reoxygenation of hypoxic cells, reassortment within the cell cycle, or repopulation of tumor cells. These factors are generally small under normal circumstances. However, large doses per fraction do not allow reoxygenation of hypoxic tumor cells or reassortment of tumors from radioresistant S phase. Hence, a large radiation dose will preferentially kill radiosensitive cells, leaving a high number of hypoxic, radioresistant cells. Therefore, the computer program will overestimate the tumor effect of a single large dose per fraction (unless a resensitization factor is introduced).

The LQ equation does not take into account the proliferation of tumor cells. This factor is small if the treatments are performed over a short duration. However, if the treatments are highly protracted (e.g., there is a long time interval between EBRT and HDR), or in cases of tumors with high proliferation rates, the LQ model will overestimate the actual tumor effect. It also must be noted that individual α/β values are very variable. The α/β values for early reactions vary from 6 to 13 (the default in the program is set at 10); the α/β values for late reactions vary from 1 to 7 (the default being set at 3), while α/β values for tumors vary from 0.4 to 13 (the default being set at 10). However, α/β values for a particular patient are not known and may vary even within the same tissue. The isoeffective doses obtained will therefore depend on the α/β values used for that particular calculation. The LQ model assumes complete repair between fractions. If the time interval between fractions is too short (<6 hours) or the half-time of repair is very long, the repair of normal tissues will be incomplete, and the LQ formula will underestimate the biologic effect. Hence, it is important to have a sufficient time interval (at least 6 hours) between treatment fractions.

The infinite variation of the dwell times that is possible with HDR (or pulsed-dose rate) allows better optimization of the doses than can be achieved with LDR. Better packing or retraction of normal tissues is possible with HDR, due to the short treatment duration. This factor is not usually taken into account in the LQ model (unless the DMF is altered). Another difference not accounted for in the LQ model is that the dose stated in brachytherapy is generally the minimum tumor dose. The doses within the tumor are much higher. Hence, the effective dose (for tumor control probability) is much higher for brachytherapy than for EBRT.

In view of the many limitations of the LQ model, it must be stressed that, as with any mathematical model, the LQ model should be used judiciously only as a guide and should always be correlated with clinical judgment and outcome results. Due to the reasons mentioned earlier, caution is especially warranted whenever large fraction sizes, a short time interval between fractions, or highly protracted treatments are used.

Common Uses of High–Dose-Rate Brachytherapy

Although HDR brachytherapy has been used in almost every site in the body, it is now most commonly used to treat cancers of the cervix, endometrium, prostate, and breast. Less commonly treated sites for HDR include the lung, esophagus, bile duct, rectum, head and neck, skin, soft tissues, and blood vessels (coronary and peripheral arteries). HDR is generally used as a component of multimodality treatment that includes EBRT and/or chemotherapy and surgery. A summary of the clinical uses of HDR is included in this chapter, while the details of the physics and radiobiology of HDR are provided in other chapters.

Carcinoma of the Cervix

Brachytherapy is a necessary component in the curative treatment of cervical cancers.[8] HDR brachytherapy has been utilized more frequently compared to LDR brachytherapy over the past two decades due to the ability to deliver therapy on an outpatient basis, avoidance of long-term bed rest, and avoidance of cervical dilation. Additionally, greater sparing of the rectum and bladder by temporary retraction, dose optimization, and integration with EBRT to the pelvis is possible.[14] These advantages must be counterbalanced with the greater number of treatments required (typically four to six treatments, lasting approximately 10 to 15 minutes each). A recent international survey revealed that 85% of centers now utilize HDR brachytherapy.[15]

The ABS recommends keeping the total duration of treatment (EBRT and HDR) to <8 weeks because prolongation adversely affects local control and survival.[8] To maintain this treatment duration, the HDR is interdigitated during the course of EBRT. However, it should be noted that neither EBRT nor chemotherapy is given on the day of an HDR treatment. Typically, if the tumor is small and the vaginal geometry is optimal, HDR brachytherapy begins approximately 2 weeks after starting EBRT. HDR is then continued one time per week with the EBRT given on the other 4 days of the week. If large tumor volume requires delaying the start of HDR brachytherapy, it may be necessary to perform two implants per week after the EBRT has been completed to keep the total treatment duration to <8 weeks.

The insertion of the applicator is usually performed under intravenous sedation. However, if the cervix needs to be dilated, general or spinal anesthesia will likely be required. It should be emphasized that rectal and bladder retraction (by the use of packing or retractors) is essential in HDR as it is for LDR. The use of an external immobilization device (EID) to fix the position of the applicator is controversial; some centers prefer to use an EID to fix the position of the applicators, while others feel that the use of the EID is detrimental. Various types of applicators (tandem and ovoid being the most common) have been used and depend on the preference of the radiation oncologist.

Treatment Planning

Traditionally the HDR dose was prescribed to an arbitrary applicator-based definition of point A.[4,8] Unfortunately, point A does not necessarily reflect the dose to the tumor. Given this fact and in conjunction with the proliferation of improved imaging modalities, there has been a shift toward image-based treatment planning in brachytherapy for carcinoma of the cervix. It is well established that magnetic resonance imaging (MRI) is superior to other current imaging modalities in delineating gross tumor involving the cervix and adjacent normal tissues.[16] The use of MRI can lead to better delineation of the target volume, which then could translate to dose escalation for better tumor control while simultaneously limiting dose to normal tissues.

TABLE 25.2 GEC-ESTRO IMAGE-BASED PLANNING VOLUME DEFINITIONS FOR CERVICAL CANCER

Volume		*Description*
GTV_D	GTV at diagnosis	Macroscopic tumor extension at diagnosis as detected by clinical examination and visualized on MRI
$GTV_{B1,B2,B3...}$	GTV at each BT procedure	Macroscopic tumor extension at time of BT as detected by clinical examination and as visualized on MRI
HR $CTV_{B1,B2,B3...}$	HR CTV at each BT procedure	Includes $GTV_{B1,B2...}$, the whole cervix, and presumed extracervical tumor extension at time of BT by means of clinical examination and by MRI
IR $CTV_{B1,B2,B3...}$	IR CTV at each BT procedure	Encompasses HR CTV with a safety margin of 5 to 15 mm (safety margin is chosen according to tumor size and location, potential tumor spread, tumor regression, and treatment strategy). The IR CTV is never less than GTV_D.

GEC-ESTRO, Groupe European de Curietherapie and European Society for Therapeutic Radiology and Oncology; GTV, gross tumor volume; MRI, magnetic resonance imaging; BT, brachytherapy; HR, high risk; CTV, clinical target volume; IR, intermediate risk.

A gynecologic working group was formed by the Groupe European de Curietherapie and European Society for Therapeutic Radiology and Oncology (GEC-ESTRO) in 2000 to formulate and describe new terminology regarding three-dimensional (3D) image-based treatment planning in cervical cancer brachytherapy. Their recommendations are summarized in Table 25.2.[17] This working group recognized that most patients with cervical cancer are treated with combined-modality therapy including external radiotherapy, chemotherapy, and brachytherapy and that there is significant change of gross tumor during such treatment. Because of this, a fluid description of treatment volumes during the course of treatment is required to have a better understanding of dose-to-volume relationships throughout treatment and to more accurately compare treatments between institutions and patients. They devised definitions of gross tumor volume (GTV) at diagnosis and at each brachytherapy procedure as well as high-risk and intermediate-risk clinical target volumes (CTVs). Each of these volumes would be determined via clinical examination and MRI (preferably T2 weighted) at their respective times during the course of treatment. The CTVs are based on tumor load and represent risk of recurrence. Thus, "high risk" (HR-CTV) is that which includes macroscopic tumor, "intermediate risk" (IR-CTV) is that which includes significant microscopic disease, and "low risk" (LR-CTV) is that which includes potential microscopic tumor spread. It is assumed that the low-risk region is successfully treated with surgery and/or external-beam radiotherapy. Their recommendations were expanded in 2006 to include descriptions of dose–volume parameters for organs at risk and a stepwise procedure for transition from the traditional dose prescription (i.e., point A) to the 3D image-based volume prescription.[18] The group recommended for organs at risk that the minimum dose in the most irradiated tissue volumes of 0.1 cm^3, 1 cm^3, and 2 cm^3 be reported.

The recommended combined EBRT and HDR dose to at least 90% (D_{90}) of the HR-CTV is an isoeffective dose of 75 to

90 Gy.[17,18] The lower dose range can be utilized for early-stage disease (defined as nonbulky stage I or II <4 cm in diameter) and the higher dose range is used for advanced stage disease (defined as stage I or IIA >4 cm in diameter or stage IIIB). The total pelvic sidewall dose recommendations are 50 to 55 Gy for smaller lesions and 55 to 60 Gy for larger ones. The ratio of EBRT to brachytherapy is dependent on the stage, with a larger EBRT dose used for the more advanced stages. Most centers use a schedule of about 6 to 8 Gy per fraction in four to six fractions (a smaller number of fractions is used by those using larger doses per fraction).[8,14,19–24] The HDR dose is also dependent on the stage of the disease and the dose of pelvic EBRT.

The University of Vienna has extensive experience with image-based dosimetry for intracavitary brachytherapy for cervical cancer. Their evaluations have resulted in suggestions to keep the $D_{2\ mL}$ dose to the rectum <75 Gy and the $D_{2\ mL}$ to the bladder to <100 Gy.[25,26] The optimal dose constraint for the sigmoid is less clear, but applying the same constraint as used for the rectum is reasonable. As an example, in a patient who has received 45 Gy of EBRT and is planned to undergo five intracavitary brachytherapy treatments, the fractional HDR $D_{2\ mL}$ dose to the rectum and bladder should be kept to approximately <4.2 Gy and <6.1 Gy, respectively. These doses would need to be altered based on the total EBRT dose and number of planned intracavitary brachytherapy treatments.

In certain clinical situations (e.g., a narrow fibrotic vagina, bulky tumors, the inability to enter the cervical os, extension to the lateral parametria or pelvic sidewall, lower vaginal extension, and suboptimal applicator placement), the normal tissue tolerance may be exceeded if the aforementioned doses are used. In these situations, either repacking or reoptimization may be attempted. If this fails to reduce the normal tissue doses, the HDR fraction size can be decreased (which requires an increase in the fraction number), or the EBRT dose increased while decreasing the HDR total dose. At our centers, we prefer to use an interstitial implant (either LDR or HDR) in these situations. In the event of reduced vaginal capacity and if an interstitial technique is not available, Sharma et al.[27] have described an intracavitary technique that utilizes a central tandem with a single ovoid alternating with the contralateral ovoid with subsequent insertions.

Results of 3D Image-Based Treatment Planning

The ABS distributed a survey to its members in 2007 focusing on the utilization of 3D treatment planning for intracavitary brachytherapy of cervical cancer that was subsequently published in 2010.[28] Fifty-five percent of respondents utilized computed tomography (CT), while 43% used plain film and only 2% used MRI for treatment-planning purposes. Point A was still utilized as the primary prescription point in just over 75% of respondents, while 14% used a 3D clinical target volume only. A survey distributed to the international community and published in 2011 showed similar results.[15]

Over the last few years there has been accumulating clinical evidence supporting image-guided brachytherapy for cervical cancer. Potter et al.[29] reported their results of 145 patients with stages IB to IVA cervical cancer treated with EBRT and four image-guided brachytherapy treatments with or without cisplatin chemotherapy. MRI was used at each brachytherapy treatment and target volumes and organs at risk were contoured as per the GEC-ESTRO guidelines. Three-year local control and overall survival was 85% and 58%, respectively, with an overall mean HR-CTV D_{90} of 86 Gy. They further divided their experience into an early period (1998–2000) and late period (2001–2003) to better reflect the treatment-planning changes employed with the release of the GEC-ESTRO guidelines. At 3 years, complete remission was 96% for tumors 2 to 5 cm in both time periods but increased from 71% to 90% for tumors >5 cm between the two time periods. Additionally, overall survival for patients with tumors >5 cm increased from 28% to 58% between the two time periods. Grade 3 and 4 gastrointestinal and genitourinary complications decreased from 10% to 2% between the two time periods. Dimopoulos et al.[30] performed a further analysis of 141 of the original 145 patients and found that an HR CTV D_{90} >87 Gy resulted in a local recurrence rate of 4% versus 20% if the D_{90} was <87 Gy.

Additional studies have compared 3D image-guided brachytherapy to previous cohorts treated with traditional two-dimensional (2D) planning and have shown improvements in local control[31,32] and reductions in toxicity[31,33] with 3D planning. Appropriate concerns to the feasibility of MRI-based treatment planning for brachytherapy include the increased cost of obtaining serial MRIs during a course of treatment (on average at least four to six during a normal course of treatment) and the limited availability and high cost of MRI-compatible applicator instrumentation for brachytherapy procedures. While early results are encouraging, further studies are needed to show that the increase in cost will be offset by improvements in local control and quality of life for patients with cervical carcinoma.

Results of HDR Versus LDR Brachytherapy

LDR brachytherapy has been used with good results in carcinoma of the cervix for almost 100 years. Hence, it is important to critically analyze how the results obtained with HDR brachytherapy, which has a much shorter history, compare with those obtained with LDR. Unfortunately, most of the published reports have been nonrandomized studies. The earlier studies showed good local control and survival rates that compared well to those obtained with LDR; however, initially some increased late complications were noted. Subsequent studies using improved techniques demonstrated good control comparable to LDR without increased morbidity.[20,21,23,24,34–35,37,38] Table 25.3 summarizes the HDR fractionation and results of the most recently published retrospective literature.

Meta-analyses and published literature reviews have compared HDR with LDR brachytherapy. Orton et al.[14] published the classic meta-analysis comparing HDR and LDR obtained from a survey of 56 institutions treating 17,068 patients with HDR and 5,666 patients with LDR. Five-year survival data were available for 6,939 HDR patients and 3,365 LDR patients and was 82.7% versus 82.4% for stage I, 66.6% versus 66.8% for stage II, and 47.2% versus 42.6% for stage III, respectively. In 1999, Petereit and Peracey[22] published a literature review that included 5,619 patients treated with HDR brachytherapy and demonstrated 5-year pelvic control rates of 91%, 82%, and 71% in stage I, II, and III patients, respectively. Five-year overall survival by stage and complication rates was similar to previous meta-analyses. Statistically quantifiable conclusions cannot be drawn from comparisons of the results of uncontrolled studies using different methodologies from various centers; however, this anecdotal evidence suggests that the results of HDR are at least as good as those achieved by LDR brachytherapy. Table 25.4 summarizes the HDR fractionation and results by stage of the meta-analyses and review literature.

Four randomized studies have compared the use of HDR with the use of LDR brachytherapy in carcinoma of the cervix.[39–42,43] Shigematsu et al.[42] reported on 143 patients treated with HDR brachytherapy compared to 106 patients treated with LDR for stage IIB and III disease. Although the randomization technique was suboptimal (i.e., some patients who were randomized to LDR were actually treated with HDR because of limited LDR availability), the HDR arm achieved superior local control with no difference in survival as compared to the LDR arm. In a randomized study of LDR versus HDR brachytherapy reported from India, there was no difference in local control, survival, or severe complications between the two treatment modalities in 482 patients.[41] However, there was

TABLE 25.3 SUMMARY OF RETROSPECTIVE ANALYSIS OF HIGH-DOSE-RATE BRACHYTHERAPY IN THE TREATMENT OF CERVICAL CANCER

Author (Reference)	Stage	Number of Patients	EBRT (Gy)	HDR (Gy × Fractions)	Local Control	Survival	Late Complications
Lorvidhaya et al.[35]	I–III	1,992	30–50	7–7.5 × 4 5.5–6 × 6	75.2%	68.2% (5 year)	4.8% Gr 3, 4 Bowel 3.5% Gr 3, 4 Bladder
Potter et al.[37]	I–IV	189	48.6–50	7 × 3–6	77.6% (3 year)	58.2% (3 year)	6% Gr 3, 4 Rectal 4% Gr 3, 4 Bowel 2.9% Gr 3, 4 Bladder
Toita et al.[38]	I–III	88	50	6 × 3	82% (3 year)	77% (3 year)	12% Proctitis 11% Cystitis 14% Enterocolitis
Sood et al.[23]	I–III	49	45 9-Gy boost	9–9.4 × 2	77% w/o chemo 88% w/chemo (3 year)	78% (5 year)	4.1% ≥Gr 2
Patel et al.[21]	II–III	121	Gr 1: 40 Gy (CS) Gr 2: 46 Gy	9 × 5 9 × 2	87.5% (5 year) 71.1% (5 year)	–	None ≥Gr 3 Rectal 1.7% ≥Gr 3 Bladder
Ferrigno et al.[34]	I–III	118	40–50	6 × 4	65% (5 year)	55% (5 year)	6% Rectal 6% Small bowel 1.7% Urinary tract
Souhami et al.[24]	I–IVA	282	45	8 × 3	75% (15 year)	57% (5 year)	6.3% Gr 3, 4 Bowel 3.5% Gr 3, 4 Bladder
Patel et al.[20]	II–III	52	46	9 × 2	81% (3 year)	64% (3 year)	4.5% Gr 3, 4 Rectal 0% Gr 3, 4 Bladder

EBRT, external-beam radiation therapy; HDR, high-dose-rate; Gr, grade; CS, central shielding.

a statistical difference in rectal complications, with a 20% rate in the LDR group and only a 6% rate in the HDR group. In 2002, Hareyama et al.[39] reported their results of 132 patients with stage II and IIIB cervical carcinoma. The 5-year disease-specific survival of LDR versus HDR for stage II was 87% versus 69%, respectively, and for stage IIIB 60% versus 51%, respectively. The difference between survival rates was not statistically significant. The most recent randomized study was reported from Thailand in 2004.[40] In this trial, 237 patients were evaluated and there was no difference in overall survival, relapse-free survival, or pelvic control between LDR and HDR brachytherapy. In addition, there was no statistical difference in complication rates for the rectum, bladder, or small bowel. A recent meta-analysis of these randomized studies demonstrated that there was no significant difference between HDR and LDR brachytherapy regarding overall survival, local control, and treatment-related complications.[44] Tables 25.5 and 25.6 summarize the results and complications, respectively, of the available randomized studies.

In summary, the available data from randomized trials, retrospective analyses, and meta-analyses suggest that survival and local control of HDR treatments are probably equivalent to that of LDR, with similar or lower morbidity.

CARCINOMA OF THE ENDOMETRIUM

HDR brachytherapy is commonly used for adjuvant treatment of the vaginal cuff after hysterectomy in patients with an intermediate or high risk for vaginal recurrence (high-grade, deep myometrial invasion or advanced stage). Additionally, brachytherapy may be used for primary treatment in inoperable endometrial carcinoma and for treatment of recurrences after hysterectomy.

Vaginal Cuff Irradiation

The standard management for operable carcinoma of the endometrium is total abdominal hysterectomy with bilateral salpingo-oophorectomy (TAH-BSO). Patients at high risk for vaginal recurrences (deep myometrial invasion, high histologic grade and stage, lymphovascular invasion, cervical or extra-uterine spread, squamous cell or papillary histology) should receive radiation therapy. Two previous published randomized trials, Post Operative Radiation Therapy in Endometrial Carcinoma (PORTEC-1)[45,46] and Gynecologic Oncology Group (GOG)-99,[47] demonstrated general benefit of postoperative pelvic radiation therapy compared to observation in regards to local control with early-stage endometrial carcinoma and intermediate- to high-risk features for recurrence. Neither trial demonstrated improvement in survival. Following these two studies PORTEC-2[48] was undertaken to better answer how best to deliver adjuvant radiotherapy. As the majority of the recurrences in PORTEC-1 and GOG-99 occurred at the vaginal cuff in the observation arms, PORTEC-2 compared whole-pelvic radiation therapy to vaginal cuff brachytherapy. Eligible patients for PORTEC-2 included patients 60 years or older with inner half myometrial invasion and histologic grade 3, or outer half myometrial invasion and histologic grade 1 or 2. Those with cervical glandular involvement and grade 1 or 2 histology, or cervical glandular involvement and grade 3 histology, and <50% myometrial invasion of any age were also eligible. The results of PORTEC-2 were published in 2010 and demonstrated that vaginal cuff recurrence was equal (1.8% vs.

TABLE 25.4 SUMMARY OF META-ANALYSIS AND REVIEW LITERATURE OF HIGH-DOSE-RATE VS. LOW-DOSE-RATE BRACHYTHERAPY IN CERVICAL CANCER

Author (Reference)	Stage	Number of HDR Patients	Number of LDR Patients	HDR (Gy × Fractions)	5-Year Control (HDR Only)	5-Year Survival		Late Complications
						HDR	LDR	
Orton et al.[14]	I	1,327	630	7.5 × 5	–	82.7%	82.4%	9.05%
	II	2,891	1,271			66.6%	66.8%	(Moderate + Severe)
	III	2,721	1,464			47.2%	42.6%	
Petereit and Peracey[22]	I	1,048	–	7 × 4	91%	85%	–	5% Overall
	II	1,995	–		82%	68%	–	
	III	2,576	–		71%	47%	–	

HDR, high-dose-rate; LDR, low-dose-rate.

TABLE 25.5 SUMMARY OF RESULTS OF RANDOMIZED TRIALS OF HIGH-DOSE-RATE VS. LOW-DOSE-RATE BRACHYTHERAPY IN CERVICAL CANCER

			Number of Patients		*Local Control*		*5-Year Survival*	
Author (Reference)	*Stage*	*EBRT (Gy)*	*LDR*	*HDR*	*LDR (%)*	*HDR (%)*	*LDR (%)*	*HDR (%)*
Shigematsu et al.[42]	IIB–III	40	106	143	77	90	55	55
Teshima et al.[43,a]	I	40	171	259	73	76	89	66
	II						73	61
	III						45	47
Patel et al.[41]	I–III	35–45	246	236	80	76	58	58
Hareyama et al.[39]	II	50	71	61	–	–	87[b]	69[b]
	III						60[b]	51[b]
Lertsanguansinchai et al.[40]	I–III	40–54	109	112	89	86	71[c]	68[c]

EBRT, external-beam radiation therapy; LDR, low-dose-rate; HDR, high-dose-rate.
[a]Update of Shigematsu et al. [b]Disease-specific survival. [c]Three-year survival.

1.6% at 5 years) in both arms. Additionally, it demonstrated that there were fewer acute grade 1 and 2 gastrointestinal toxicities with vaginal cuff brachytherapy (12.6% vs. 53.8%). This has led to an increase in the utilization of vaginal cuff brachytherapy alone in patients with a high intermediate risk of recurrence. There still remains some controversy of which patients fall into the high intermediate-risk group as the three mentioned studies had subtle differences in patient eligibility. Thus, clinical judgement is needed when evaluating patients potentially eligible for vaginal cuff brachytherapy alone.

Technique

A vaginal cylinder is commonly used to deliver HDR brachytherapy. The largest-diameter cylinder that comfortably fits the vagina should be used to increase the depth dose. The length of vaginal vault treated varies. Some treat the superior 3 or 5 cm, while others treat the superior half or two-thirds of the vagina.[5,48,49–51] For serous and clear cell histologies, treatment of the entire vaginal canal should be considered. The use of a single-line iridium 192 (^{192}Ir) source creates a dose inhomogeneity at the vaginal apex due to source anisotropy. However, the clinical significance of source anisotropy is debatable. The use of ovoids, circular rings, or an angled source may reduce the dose inhomogeneity at the apex created by the ^{192}Ir source anisotropy.[5] The applicator should be placed in the midline, as horizontal as possible and parallel to the longitudinal axis of the body for appropriate dose distribution. Placement of a radio-opaque seed or clip at the vaginal apex helps to verify that the applicator is in contact with the vaginal apex on fluoroscopy or radiographs. However, these clips or seeds can sometimes fall off or migrate deep to the mucosa and, therefore, may not always indicate the position of the apex. Some centers prefer to use an external immobilization device to minimize movement; however, this is not mandatory. The use of a multichannel vaginal applicator such as the Miami applicator or the inflatable Capri balloon applicator may allow the radiation oncologist to better sculpt the desired radiation dose distribution for the individual patient compared to a single-channel device.

The dose distribution should be optimized to deliver the prescribed dose either at the vaginal surface or at a 0.5-cm depth, depending on the institutional policy. It is important to place dose optimization points not only along the lateral aspect of the vaginal wall but also at specified points about the dome of the vaginal cylinder to avoid higher vaginal apex doses, which can lead to vaginal vault necrosis.[2] Regardless of the prescription method, doses at both the vaginal surface and the 0.5-cm depth should be reported.[5]

The dose per fraction used has varied from 4.5 to 16 Gy, and the number of fractions has varied from two to seven, with the interval between fractions of 1 to 2 weeks.[49–53] The lower doses per fraction are usually given using either a larger number of fractions or in combination with EBRT to the pelvis. Sorbe et al.[54] evaluated two fractionation schemes (2.5 Gy × 6 vs. 5 Gy × 6) in a randomized trial and found no difference in locoregional recurrence rates but an increase in vaginal shortening, mucosal atrophy, and bleeding in the 5-Gy-per-fraction arm. The ABS dose suggestions[5] for HDR alone or in combination with 45 Gy EBRT are given in Table 25.7. Because some institutions specify the dose to the vaginal surface and others specify the dose at 0.5-cm depth, suggested HDR doses have been given for both specification methods.

From retrospective analysis, the 5-year survival rates of HDR therapy vary from 72% to 97%, depending on the stage, grade, and depth of myometrial invasion.[49–53,55,56] The severe (grade III or IV) late complication rate is usually <2% and depends on the dose per fraction.[49,50,52,57,58] The incidence of vaginal shortening is also very much dose dependent, reportedly ranging from as high as 70% when 9 Gy per fraction was prescribed at 1-cm depth to 31% when the dose was reduced to 4.5 Gy per fraction.[59] Other factors that increase morbidity include the use of a small (2-cm) diameter vaginal cylinder, the addition of pelvic external-beam radiation, and a dose specification point beyond 0.5 cm.[60]

Petereit and Peracey[22] published a literature review analyzing 1,800 cases of postoperative HDR brachytherapy alone in patients with low- to intermediate-risk endometrial cancer.

TABLE 25.6 SUMMARY OF COMPLICATIONS OF RANDOMIZED TRIALS OF HIGH-DOSE-RATE VS. LOW DOSE-RATE BRACHYTHERAPY IN CERVICAL CANCER

	Bladder				*Rectum*			
	Grade 1 + 2		*Grade 3 + 4*		*Grade 1 + 2*		*Grade 3 + 4*	
Author (Reference)	*LDR (%)*	*HDR (%)*	*LDR (%)*	*HDR (%)*	*LDR (%)*	*HDR (%)*	*LDR (%)*	*HDR (%)*
Shigematsu et al.[42]	–	–	–	–	–	–	–	–
Teshima et al.[43]	–	3[a]	–	–	3[a]	4[a]	–	–
Patel et al.[41]	3.7	3.8	–	–	17.5	5.9	2.4	0.4
Hareyama et al.[39]	–	–	7.5	4	–	–	8.7	3.5
Lertsanguansinchai et al.[40]	21	14	2.7	0.9	31	15	0.9	4.5

LDR, low-dose-rate; HDR, high-dose-rate.
[a]Includes grade 2 and 3.

TABLE 25.7 AMERICAN BRACHYTHERAPY SOCIETY–SUGGESTED DOSES OF HIGH-DOSE-RATE BRACHYTHERAPY ALONE OR IN COMBINATION WITH PELVIC EXTERNAL-BEAM RADIATION THERAPY TO BE USED FOR ADJUVANT TREATMENT OF POSTOPERATIVE ENDOMETRIAL CANCER

EBRT (Gy) at 1.8 Gy/Fraction	Number of HDR Fractions	HDR per Fraction (Gy)	Dose Specification Point
0	3	7.0	0.5-cm depth
0	4	5.5	0.5-cm depth
0	5	4.7	0.5-cm depth
0	3	10.5	Vaginal surface
0	4	8.8	Vaginal surface
0	5	7.5	Vaginal surface
45	2	5.5	0.5-cm depth
45	3	4.0	0.5-cm depth
45	2	8.0	Vaginal surface
45	3	6.0	Vaginal surface

EBRT, external-beam radiation therapy; HDR, high-dose-rate.

They found an overall vaginal control rate of 99.3%. Late morbidity was significantly higher with isoeffective doses for late-responding tissues exceeding 100 Gy. Patient education regarding the use of frequent vaginal dilation following HDR brachytherapy is important to minimize vaginal stenosis and sexual dysfunction.[61,62] The National Forum of Gynecological Oncology Nurses (NFGON) has published best practice guidelines for the use of vaginal dilators following radiation therapy treatments.[63]

Treatment of Recurrences at the Vaginal Cuff

A combination of pelvic EBRT and brachytherapy is generally used to treat recurrences at the vaginal cuff. With distal vaginal recurrences, the entire vagina and medial inguinal nodes are included in the EBRT field. Intracavitary vaginal brachytherapy should be used only for nonbulky recurrences (thickness <5 mm after the completion of EBRT).[5] Interstitial brachytherapy is to be used for bulky recurrences (thickness >5 mm after the completion of EBRT) and for previously irradiated patients. Apical recurrences are often more extensive superiorly than can be judged on physical examination, thus favoring the use of interstitial brachytherapy. These patients are best treated at centers with considerable experience in interstitial brachytherapy. Radio-opaque marker seeds or surgical clips should be placed at the margins of gross disease to delineate disease extent. If the relapse is limited to one wall of the vagina, consideration should be given to limiting the dose to the opposite wall. The ABS-suggested doses for HDR brachytherapy (in combination with 45 Gy EBRT) are provided in Table 25.8.[5]

Inoperable Endometrial Carcinoma

Patients with adenocarcinoma of the endometrium who are not candidates for surgery because of severe medical problems are treated with radiation therapy. A combination of pelvic EBRT and brachytherapy is preferred whenever possible. However, many of the conditions that do not allow surgery in these cases are also relative contraindications for EBRT and for LDR brachytherapy. In such cases, these patients may be treated with HDR alone.

TABLE 25.8 AMERICAN BRACHYTHERAPY SOCIETY–SUGGESTED DOSES OF HIGH-DOSE-RATE BRACHYTHERAPY TO BE USED IN COMBINATION WITH PELVIC EXTERNAL-BEAM RADIATION THERAPY FOR TREATING VAGINAL CUFF RECURRENCES FROM ENDOMETRIAL CANCER

EBRT (Gy) at 1.8 Gy/Fraction	Number of HDR Fractions	HDR per Fraction (Gy)	Dose Specification
45	3	7.0	0.5-cm depth
45	4	6.0	0.5-cm depth
45	5	6.0	Vaginal surface
45	4	7.0	Vaginal surface

EBRT, external-beam radiation therapy; HDR, high-dose-rate.

TABLE 25.9 AMERICAN BRACHYTHERAPY SOCIETY–SUGGESTED DOSES OF HIGH-DOSE-RATE BRACHYTHERAPY ALONE OR IN COMBINATION WITH EXTERNAL-BEAM RADIATION THERAPY FOR TREATMENT OF INOPERABLE PRIMARY ENDOMETRIAL CANCER

EBRT (Gy) at 1.8 Gy/Fraction	Number of HDR Fractions	HDR per Fraction (Gy)[a]
45	2	8.5
45	3	6.3
45	4	5.2
0	4	8.5
0	5	7.3
0	6	6.4
0	7	5.7

EBRT, external-beam radiation therapy; HDR, high-dose-rate.
[a]HDR doses are specified at 2 cm from the midpoint of the intrauterine sources.

Numerous applicators can be used for treatment of primary endometrial cancer. The tandem and ovoid applicator, while often used, does not irradiate the uterine fundus homogeneously. Others have therefore used a curved tandem, turning it to the left and right in alternate insertions. A Y-shaped applicator irradiates the fundus more evenly. Other possibilities include modified Heyman capsules or multiple tandems. The dose is commonly specified at 2 cm from the source, although CT- or MRI-based treatment planning to ensure a more homogeneous dose to the entire myometrium is preferred. The dose per fraction has ranged from 5 to 12 Gy, and three to six fractions are commonly employed.[64,65–68] The dose and/or the dose per fraction are reduced if EBRT can be added. The ABS-suggested doses for HDR brachytherapy alone or in combination with 45 Gy EBRT are given in Table 25.9.[5] The survival at 5 years for stage I is about 70% to 80%, which is slightly lower than that obtained by surgery. Coon et al.[69] reported a 5-year cause-specific survival of 87% for patients treated with 35 Gy HDR (treated twice a day) in five fractions without EBRT or with 20 Gy HDR in five fractions along with EBRT. The toxicity is higher (about 7%) when patients are treated with high doses per fraction.[59]

Carcinoma of the Prostate

Currently, permanent implantation of iodine 125 (^{125}I) or palladium 103 (^{103}Pd) seeds is the most common type of prostate brachytherapy. However, several centers have used HDR brachytherapy as a boost to EBRT[70–85] for the treatment of prostate cancer with encouraging results (Table 25.10). Galalae et al.[76] reported the results of 611 patients (some of which are included in Table 25.10) treated at three institutions (Kiel, Germany; William Beaumont Hospital; Seattle Prostate Institute) with EBRT and HDR brachytherapy for localized prostate cancer. Different fractionation schemes were used as seen in Table 25.11. Five-year biochemical control for low-risk, intermediate-risk, and high-risk patients was 96%, 88%, and 69%, respectively. One of the major advantages of HDR is that the dose distribution can be intraoperatively optimized by varying the dwell times at various dwell positions, potentially allowing reliable and reproducible delivery of the prescribed dose to the target volume while keeping the doses to normal structures (i.e., rectum, bladder, and urethra) within acceptable limits.[86] Another potential advantage of HDR brachytherapy in prostate cancer is the theoretical consideration that prostate cancer cells behave more like late-reacting tissue with a low α/β ratio and they should, therefore, respond more favorably to higher-dose fractions rather than to the lower-dose rate delivered in LDR brachytherapy.[87,88,89]

Patients with stages T1b to T3b prostate cancers without evidence of distant metastases are candidates for HDR brachytherapy as a boost to EBRT. Patients with distant metastases,

TABLE 25.10 RESULTS OF TREATMENT WITH INTERSTITIAL HIGH-DOSE-RATE BRACHYTHERAPY AS A BOOST TO EXTERNAL-BEAM RADIATION THERAPY FOR PROSTATE CANCER

Author (Reference)	*Number of Patients*	*EBRT Dose (Gy)*	*HDR (Gy × Fractions)*	*5-Year % bNED*	*% Complications Grade 3 (GU/GI)*
Neviani et al.[82]	403	45	5.5-6 × 3	94.3 (low risk)	2/1.3 (early)
			6-6.5 × 3	86.9 (int risk)	[illegible] (late)
			6.5-7 × 3	86.6 (high risk)	
Kaprelian et al.[79]	64	45	6 × 3	93.5[a]	3.1/0
	101	45	9.5 × 2	87.3[a]	1/0
Zwahlen et al.[84]	196	44–50.6	5 × 4	82.5	17.3/3 (early)
			6 × 3		7.1/0 (late)
Deutsch et al.[74]	160	45–50.4	5.5–7 × 3	98	NS
Bachand et al.[71]	153	40–44	6–6.5 × 3	96	NS
			9–10 × 2		
Hoskin et al.[77]	109	35.75	8.5 × 2	80	NS
Martinez et al.[80]	305	46	9.5–11.5 × 2	81.1[b]	2.0/0.5
	167	46	5.5–6.5 × 3	56.9[b]	3/0.5
			8.75 × 2		
Astrom et al.[70]	214	50	10 × 2	92 (low risk)	10/0
				87 (int. risk)	
				56 (high risk)	
Demanes et al.[73]	209	36	5.5–6 × 4	90 (low risk)[b]	6.7/0
				87 (int. risk)[b]	
				69 (high risk)[b]	
Deger et al.[72]	442	40–50.4	9–10 × 2	81 (low risk)	11
				65 (int. risk)	
				59 (high risk)	
Jo et al.[78]	98	36.8–45	5.5–6 × 3–4	92.9	8.1/0
Stevens et al.[83]	82	45	5.5 × 3	91[c]	6/1
Galalae et al.[75]	144	40–50	15 × 2	72.9[d]	2.3/4.1
Eulau[85]	104	50.4	3–4 × 4	91 (PSA <10)[b]	8.7/2
Mate et al.[81]				65 (PSA 10–20)[b]	
				59 (PSA ≥20)[b]	

EBRT, external-beam radiation therapy; HDR, high-dose-rate; bNED, biologically without evidence of recurrence; GU/GI, genitourinary/gastrointestinal; int, intermediate; NS, not stated; PSA, prostate-specific antigen.

[a]Median follow-up of 105 months for 6 × 3 group and 43 months for 9.5 × 2 group. [b]Ten-year bNED. [c]Three-year bNED. [d]Eight-year bNED.

with a life expectancy of <5 years, or who are medically unfit for anesthesia or in whom it is technically not feasible to implant the entire prostate should be excluded. Relative contraindications include large gland size (>60 mL), significant urinary obstructive symptoms, recent transurethral resection of the prostate (TURP) within the last 6 months, large TURP defects, infiltration of the external sphincter of the bladder neck, pubic arch interference, and a rectum–prostate distance on transrectal ultrasound of <5 mm.[86] These patients have, however, been implanted by experienced brachytherapists by using modified techniques.

Various implant techniques and treatment-planning methods have been used. As in permanent seed implantation, the procedure is performed under general or spinal anesthesia. Transrectal ultrasound is utilized for catheter placement and cystoscopy may be performed to exclude the urethra and bladder. At some institutions real-time transrectal ultrasound-guided treatment planning is performed. Other institutions use CT-based treatment planning. Fiducial markers are placed in the prostate so that radiographic comparison of the markers to catheter location can be confirmed prior to each delivery of each treatment.[90] Typically, 15 to 17 catheters are placed (although some institutions have used fewer) with fraction doses ranging from 3 to 15 Gy prescribed to the prostate (CTV 1) depending on the clinical situation. Additionally, it is recommended to identify the peripheral zone (CTV 2) and any areas of macroscopic tumor (CTV 3) so that these areas can potentially receive a higher fractional dose. As in permanent seed implantation, the D_{90}, D_{100}, V_{100}, V_{150}, and V_{200} should be reported. Simultaneously, the organs at risk should be contoured and the D^3_{2cm} of the rectum and bladder and $D^3_{0.1cm}$ of the urethra should be reported.[86] The interested reader should review the GEC/ESTRO guidelines for more specific information.[86]

Standard fractionation EBRT of 39.6 to 50.4 Gy or hypofractionated EBRT of 40 Gy in 16 fractions is given before,

TABLE 25.11 DOSE FRACTIONATION AND ISOEFFECTIVE DOSES (AS IF GIVEN AT 2 GY/FRACTION) OF COMBINED EXTERNAL-BEAM RADIATION THERAPY AND HIGH-DOSE-RATE BRACHYTHERAPY DOSES USED FOR PROSTATE CANCER

EBRT Dose (Gy)	*Number of EBRT Fractions*	*Total HDR (Gy)*	*HDR per Fraction (Gy)*	*Number of HDR Fractions*	*Isoeffective Dose (Gy) (α/β = 1.5)*	*Isoeffective Dose (Gy) (α/β = 5)*	*Isoeffective Dose (Gy) (α/β = 10)*
35.75	13	17	8.5	2	92	72	64
36	20	22–24	5.5–6	4	80–87	69–74	64–68
45	25	18	6	3	81	72	68
45	25	19	9.5	2	102	83	75
46	23	17.5–23	8.75–11.5	2	97–131	80–100	73–87
50	25	20	10	2	116	93	83
50.4	28	19.5	6.5	3	92	81	76

EBRT, external-beam radiation therapy; HDR, high-dose-rate.

TABLE 25.12 RESULTS OF TREATMENT WITH INTERSTITIAL HIGH-DOSE-RATE BRACHYTHERAPY AS MONOTHERAPY FOR PROSTATE CANCER

Author (Reference)	*Number of Patients*	*T Stage*	*HDR (Gy × Fractions)*	*Total HDR (Gy)*	*3 Year % bNED*	*% Late Complications Grade 3 (GU/GI)*
Demanes et al.[90]	157	1–2	7 × 6	42	97[a]	3/<1
	141		9.5 × 4	38		
Yoshioka et al.[93]	15	Low Risk	6 × 9	54	85[b]	1/1.8
	29	Int Risk			93[b]	
	68	High Risk			79[b]	
Corner et al.[91]	110	1–3	8.5 × 4	34	100[c]	1.8/0
			9 × 4	36		
			10.5 × 3	31.5		
Martin et al.[92]	52	1–2	9.5 × 4	38	NS	3.8/0 (acute)

HDR, high-dose-rate; bNED, biologically without evidence of recurrence; GU/GI, genitourinary/gastrointestinal; Int, Intermediate; NS, not stated.
[a]8-year biochemical control.
[b]5-year prostate-specific antigen failure free.
[c]No prostate-specific antigen failures with median follow-up of 30, 18, and 11.8 months, respectively, of the three dose groups.

concurrently with, or after HDR brachytherapy. The minimum volume treated should include the entire prostate and seminal vesicles with a margin, with or without pelvic lymph nodes. The HDR dose is given in multiple fractions in one or two implant procedures. A variety of dose and fractionation schemes may be appropriate for same-stage disease as shown in Table 25.11.[70,72,73,75,77,79–80,81] The HDR fractions are generally given twice a day with a minimum of 6 hours between fractions. The most commonly encountered acute genitourinary (GU) morbidities include urinary irritative symptoms, hematuria, hematospermia, and/or urinary retention, similar to LDR permanent implants.

HDR brachytherapy is also being used as monotherapy in a few centers, but long-term results are still forthcoming (Table 25.12).[90,91–92,93] HDR doses of 38 Gy delivered in four fractions (two times daily over 2 days), 54 Gy in nine fractions given twice a day over 5 days, and 42 Gy in six fractions over two separate implants have all been reported.[90,91,93] Demanes et al.[90] reported the combined results of 298 patients with low- to intermediate-risk prostate cancer treated at California Endocurietherapy (CET) or William Beaumont Hospital (WBH) between 1996 and 2005. HDR brachytherapy was delivered in either four fractions to a total dose of 38 Gy over 2 days in one implant (WBH) or a total dose of 42 Gy over six fractions with two implants 1 week apart (CET). With a median follow-up of 5.2 years, the 8-year biochemical control was 97%. Grade 3 genitourinary toxicity was 3% (urinary retention), while gastrointestinal toxicity was <1%. These results compare favorably to traditional permanent seed implant.[90]

Treatment of recurrent prostate cancer as well as treatment of de novo prostate cancer in patients who have previously received pelvic radiation is challenging. HDR brachytherapy has been used as salvage therapy after prostatectomy, EBRT, and permanent seed implant.[94–97] Overall patient numbers are low, so firm conclusions of its effectiveness are difficult; however, it does appear feasible in various clinical situations. Niehoff et al.[96] have reported their results of using HDR brachytherapy along with EBRT as salvage treatment for local recurrences after radical prostatectomy. Thirty-five patients were treated with either 30 or 40 Gy EBRT plus an HDR brachytherapy dose of 15 Gy in two fractions. Thirty-four patients had a decrease in prostate-specific antigen (PSA), and at a mean follow-up of 27 months 91% were alive. Mean duration of biochemical nonevidence of disease was 12 months, and there were no reported Radiation Therapy Oncology Group (RTOG) grade III or IV side effects.

HDR brachytherapy as a boost to EBRT for localized prostate cancer is being used more commonly and its role has been well defined. Its use as monotherapy is increasing and the early results are promising. Further studies are needed to more clearly define the role of HDR brachytherapy for recurrent disease after radical prostatectomy, previous EBRT, or permanent seed implant.

Breast

EBRT is the standard radiation modality used after lumpectomy in the conservative management of breast cancer. Over the past decade there has been an increase in use of brachytherapy as the sole modality of treatment[98–100,101,102–103] to decrease the 6-week treatment duration required for a course of EBRT to about 5 days. Table 25.13 lists the patients in whom an accelerated (4 to 5 days) brachytherapy treatment course can be an attractive alternative to 6 weeks of EBRT.[104] The ABS recommends a total dose of 34 Gy in 10 fractions to the CTV (lumpectomy site with 1- to 2-cm margin) when HDR brachytherapy is used as the sole modality.[104] The HDR treatments of 3.4 Gy are generally given at two fractions per day separated by at least 6 hours. This was also the dose used in a phase II RTOG trial.[98] as well as in the phase III National Surgical Adjuvant Breast and Bowel Project (NSABP) B-39 trial. Other prescriptive dosimetric parameters to be met recommended by the ABS include (a) ≥90% of the CTV should receive ≥90% of the dose; (b) V_{150} and V_{200} should be <50 cm^3 and <10 cm^3, respectively, for balloon catheters; and (c) maximum skin isodose should be <145% for balloon catheters.[104]

The results of HDR brachytherapy as the sole modality are included in Table 25.14.[98–100,102,103,105–110] Depending on the selection criteria, final pathologic assessment is necessary to completely evaluate a patient for partial breast brachytherapy, and, therefore, the ABS does not advocate intraoperative treatment delivery at this time.[3] The use of a single-channel

TABLE 25.13 BRACHYTHERAPY IN THE CONSERVATIVE MANAGEMENT OF BREAST CANCER

Indications for Brachytherapy as the Sole Modality	*Indications for Brachytherapy as a Boost to EBRT*
1. The patient lives a long distance from radiation oncology treatment facilities.	1. For patients with close, positive, or unknown margins
2. The patient lacks transportation.	2. For patients with EIC
3. The patient is a professional whose schedule will not accommodate a 6-week course of therapy.	3. For younger patients
4. The patient is elderly, frail, or in poor health and therefore unable to travel for a prolonged course of daily treatment.	4. For deep tumor location in a large breast
5. The patient's breasts are sufficiently large that they may have unacceptable toxicity with EBRT.	5. For CTV of irregular thickness

EBRT, external-beam radiation therapy; EIC, extensive intraductal component; CTV, clinical target volume.

TABLE 25.14 RESULTS OF BREAST-CONSERVING THERAPY WITH LUMPECTOMY PLUS HIGH-DOSE-RATE BRACHYTHERAPY OR AS A BOOST TO EXTERNAL-BEAM RADIATION THERAPY

Author (Reference)	Number of Patients	Technique	HDR (Gy × Fractions)	Total Dose (Gy)	Median Follow-Up (Months)	Local Recurrence (%)	Good/Excellent Cosmetic Results (%)
HDR Alone							
Perera et al.[110]	39	Interstitial	3.72 × 10	37.2	91	16.2	90
King et al.[109]	26	Interstitial	4 × 8	32	75	2[a]	67[b]
Polgar et al.[99]	88	Interstitial	5.2 × 7	36.4	66	4.7[c]	81.2
Polgar et al.[100]	37	Interstitial	5.2 × 7	36.4	133	9.3	77.8
	8		4.33 × 7	30.3			
Kaufman et al.[108]	32	Interstitial	3.4 × 10	34	83.9	6.1	88.9
Chen et al.[106]	79	Interstitial	4 × 8	32	76.8	1.5[d]	95–99[e]
			3.4 × 10	34			
Strnad et al.[102]	274	Interstitial	4 × 8	32	63	2.9	90
			PDR 0.6 Gy	49.8			
Arthur et al.[98]	66	Interstitial	3.4 × 10	34	78.6	3	Not stated
Benitez et al.[105]	43	MammoSite	3.4 × 10	34	65.2[f] (mean)	0	83.3[f]
Vicini et al.[103,d]	1,449	MammoSite	3.4 × 10	34	53.7	2.6	90.6
Harper et al.[107]	111	Mammosite	3.4 × 10	34	46	6.3	Not stated
HDR Boost							
Hennequin et al.[119]	106		5 × 2	10	45	5.1	63
Manning et al.[114]	18		2.5 × 6	15	50	0	68
Polgar et al.[123]	19		4 × 3	12	63.6	7.7	88.5
	33		4.75 × 3	14.25			
Resch et al.[125]	274		7–12 × 1	7–12	104 (mean)	1.5	38
Henriquez et al.[120]	294		2–2.5 × 8–11		69.6	9	96
Neumanova et al.[122]	215		8–12 × 1	8-12	69.6	1.5	73
Budrukkar et al.[117]	153		10 × 1	10	36	8	83
Guinot et al.[118]	125		4.4 × 3	13.2	84	4.2	77
Polgar et al.[124]	88		4–4.75 × 3	12–14.25	75	4.5	57
	10		8–10.35 × 1	8–10.35			
Knauerhase et al.[121]	75		8–12 × 1	8–12	93.6	5.9	Not stated

HDR, high-dose-rate; PDR, pulsed-dose-rate; LDR, low-dose-rate.
[a]Percentage of local recurrence of 51 patients treated either by LDR or HDR. [b]Twenty months' follow-up.
[c]Includes patients treated via partial breast irradiation with 50 Gy in 25 fractions with electrons, $n = 128$. [d]Reported at median follow-up of 45.6 months.
[e]Includes patients treated with LDR. [f]Includes 36 patients only.

MammoSite applicator has simplified the brachytherapy procedure.[101] Benitez et al.[105] reported a good to excellent cosmetic result of 83% and no local recurrences at a median follow-up of 65.2 months in 43 patients treated with the MammoSite applicator (Cytyc Corporation, Marlborough, MA). In addition, a multi-institutional registry trial performed by the American Society of Breast Surgeons to evaluate the clinical use of the MammoSite applicator reported a good to excellent cosmetic result of 90.6% of the 371 patients with 60-month follow-up. Of the total 1,449 cases with a median follow-up of 53.7 months, the ipsilateral local recurrence rate was 2.6%.[103] Newer devices such as the SAVI applicator (Cianna Medical, Aliso Viejo, CA) and the Contura applicator (SenoRx Inc., Irvine, CA) are multichanneled and can allow improved dose shaping.

In March 2005, the RTOG, in conjunction with the NSABP, opened a phase III randomized study (NSABP B-39) investigating standard whole-breast radiotherapy versus partial-breast radiotherapy after lumpectomy for women with early-stage breast cancer. The partial-breast treatment arm consists of three therapeutic options: intensity-modulated radiation therapy; HDR brachytherapy via MammoSite, Contura, or SAVI; and HDR brachytherapy via a multicatheter interstitial implant. The required dose for the brachytherapy treatment is 34 Gy given in 10 fractions over 5 days. Target accrual is 4,300 patients, and as of June 2011, 3,980 patients have been enrolled. It is hoped that over time the data will shed some light on the usefulness of partial-breast irradiation and brachytherapy as a sole modality of treatment. Various medical societies have published consensus statement guidelines for the selection of appropriate patients for breast brachytherapy as a sole modality treatment with slight variations.[104,111] According to the American Society of Therapeutic Radiology and Oncology (ASTRO) consensus statement, "suitable" patients for accelerated partial-breast irradiation include women 60 years of age and older, with unifocal tumors 2 cm in size or less, negative margins, positive estrogen receptor status, invasive ductal histology in the absence of ductal carcinoma in situ, and absence of nodal involvement. The consensus statement also outlined criteria for "cautionary" and "unsuitable" candidates. The reader is encouraged to review the original consensus statement for full details.[111] Thus far local control and cosmesis are similar to whole-breast EBRT with one group quoting 12-year follow-up.[100] However, further clinical studies are required to define the most appropriate candidates for breast brachytherapy as a sole modality treatment and to determine the best delivery method of brachytherapy (multicatheter interstitial implant vs. balloon brachytherapy) in such patients.

A newer device, the Axxent (Xoft Inc., Sunnyvale, CA), uses a miniaturized x-ray source to deliver low-energy x-rays within a needle or catheter, thereby mimicking HDR brachytherapy. The reduced radiation protection required for these devices due to limited penetration is a great advantage because it allows brachytherapy to be delivered in a nonshielded procedure room or a regular (unshielded) hospital operating suite. Although longer follow-up is needed to assess the risk of recurrence, early results with the use of this device for accelerated partial-breast irradiation reveal that the procedure is tolerated well and grade 3 adverse events are minimal, with 100% excellent or good cosmetic results at 1 year in one study evaluating 69 patients.[112,113] Brachytherapy has been used to boost the EBRT dose in select high-risk patients.[114,115–116]

Data on the use of HDR as a boost are limited (see Table 25.14).[114,117–125] Polgar et al.[123] reported the results of a randomized trial involving 207 women with stage I or II breast cancer treated with breast-conserving surgery and whole-breast radiotherapy and subsequently randomized to either no further therapy or radiation boost to the tumor bed. The radiation boost consisted of either 16 Gy of electron irradiation or 12 to 14.5 Gy fractionated HDR brachytherapy. Fifty-two patients were treated with HDR brachytherapy and the 5-year local tumor control rate was 91.4%. Excellent to good cosmesis was reported in 88.5% of patients. Similar results were noted in the group of patients receiving an electron irradiation boost. Because brachytherapy is an invasive procedure, it should be used selectively as a boosting technique. Situations in which brachytherapy may be advantageous as a boost are listed in Table 25.13. The brachytherapy boost can be given before or after EBRT, usually with a 1- to 2-week gap between EBRT and brachytherapy. The ABS recommends a dose fractionation scheme that yields early and late effects approximately equivalent to those of 10 to 20 Gy LDR following 45 to 50 Gy EBRT.[7] Biomathematic models are often used to estimate equivalent HDR regimens.[12,13] For example, an HDR regimen of five fractions of 310 cGy per fraction should approximate the early and late effects of 20 Gy LDR delivered at 0.5 Gy/hour. Although biomathematic models can be used to estimate the appropriate dose, there is no standardized HDR fractionation schedule that can be recommended for the use of HDR as a boost. Controlled clinical studies are required to further define the most appropriate doses to be used for boost treatment.

Use of interstitial HDR brachytherapy as neoadjuvant treatment in select patients not amenable to breast-conserving surgery at presentation has been reported by Roddiger et al.[126] Fifty-three patients who were unable to undergo breast-conserving surgery either because of initial tumor size or an unfavorable breast–tumor ratio were treated with systemic chemotherapy and HDR brachytherapy with 5 Gy twice per day for 3 days (total dose 30 Gy). Of these patients 56.6% went on to receive breast-conserving surgery, and with a median follow-up of 56 months the local recurrence rate was 2%. Further studies are needed to fully define the role of interstitial HDR brachytherapy as neoadjuvant treatment, but these results are encouraging.

Another clinical situation in which HDR brachytherapy has been evaluated is in the setting of salvage therapy to continue maintaining the breast in previously irradiated patients.[127,128] Current standard of care of recurrent disease following breast conservation is total mastectomy. Guix et al.[127] reported their series of 36 patients who had previously been treated with lumpectomy, external-beam radiation, and HDR brachytherapy boost who subsequently developed an ipsilateral breast recurrence and underwent excision only of the recurrence. Following excision, all patients underwent an HDR brachytherapy implant delivering 30 Gy in 12 fractions over 5 days. With a median follow-up of 89 months, 10-year local control was 89.4% and 10-year disease-free survival was 64.4%. They reported a 90.4% satisfactory cosmetic result. Again, while numbers are small, the possibility of continuing to provide breast conservation in the setting of recurrent disease is encouraging.

Endobronchial Radiation

The use of HDR brachytherapy is well established for palliation of cough, dyspnea, pain, and hemoptysis in patients with advanced or metastatic lung cancer. The use of brachytherapy as a boost to EBRT in curative cases should be restricted to a select group of patients who have predominantly endobronchial disease, are medically inoperable, or have small/occult carcinomas of the lung.

An initial bronchoscopy is performed to evaluate the airway and locate the site of obstruction. Either a 5- or 6-French (Fr) catheter (inserted through the brush channel of the bronchoscope) can be used to deliver the brachytherapy. Use of a 6-Fr catheter allows the HDR source to negotiate tight curves, which is not possible with the 5-Fr catheter. If a 6-Fr catheter is used, a large bronchoscope (with brush channel diameter of at least 2.2 mm) is required. The bronchoscope can be connected to a teaching head or a video monitor so that the radiation oncologist can also visualize the lesion and the catheter. It is extremely important to note the distances between the proximal extent of the tumor and fixed structures such as the carina. The catheter is inserted through the brush channel of the bronchoscope, passed through the tumor, and lodged in one of the smaller bronchi. Fluoroscopic confirmation of the catheter's position is desirable. The radiation oncologist then pushes the afterloading catheter in while the pulmonologist slowly withdraws the bronchoscope. The use of fluoroscopy assists in keeping the catheter in place during this push–pull technique of bronchoscope removal. The catheter is then secured with tape at the nose, and its position is marked in ink to alert the radiation oncologist in case of displacement. As an additional precautionary measure, the external length of the catheter from the tip of the nostril is noted. If multiple catheters are to be used, the procedure is repeated, taking care to clearly label each catheter. Localization x-rays with radio-opaque dummy wires in the catheter are then obtained. The location of the obstruction and the target length are marked on the x-rays to determine the length to be irradiated and the initial dwell position.

The dose has been prescribed at various points from 0.5 to 2 cm, although 1 cm from the source is commonly used.[6] The length to be irradiated usually includes the endobronchial tumor and 1.0- to 2.0-cm proximal and distal margins. If a single catheter is used and there is minimal curvature of the catheter in the area to be irradiated, it is possible to minimize the treatment-planning time by using preplanned dosimetry. For example, Ohio State University has precalculated treatment plans for 3-, 5-, 7-, and 10-cm lengths to be irradiated to 5 or 7.5 Gy at 1 cm from the source using equal dwell times. This allows the treatment to be performed without any delay if standard lengths and doses are used. Individualized image-based treatment planning must be performed if multiple catheters are used.

Palliative Endobronchial Brachytherapy

Candidates for palliative endobronchial brachytherapy include:[6,129–131]

1. Patients with a significant endobronchial tumor component that causes symptoms such as shortness of breath, hemoptysis, persistent cough, and other signs of postobstructive pneumonitis. Tumors with a predominantly endobronchial component are considered suitable, as opposed to extrinsic tumors that compress the bronchus or the trachea. Endobronchial brachytherapy can generally give quicker palliation of obstruction than EBRT. Furthermore, brachytherapy can be more convenient than 2 to 3 weeks of daily EBRT.
2. Patients who are unable to tolerate any EBRT because of poor lung function.
3. Patients with previous EBRT of sufficient total dose to preclude further EBRT.

A variety of doses have been successfully used by various centers. Total doses ranging from 15 Gy to 30 Gy HDR in one to five fractions calculated at 1 cm have been reported.[129,130] The ABS suggests using three weekly fractions of 7.5 Gy each or two fractions of 10 Gy each or four fractions of 6 Gy each prescribed at 1 cm when HDR is used as the sole modality for palliation.[6] These fractionation regimens have similar radiobiologic equivalence using the linear-quadratic model,[13] and there is no evidence of superiority for one regimen over the other. The benefits of fewer bronchoscopic applications should be weighed against the risks of higher dose per fraction. Additional treatments or doses higher than those suggested can be considered for nonirradiated patients or those who have received limited radiation. When HDR is used as a planned boost to supplement palliative EBRT of 30 Gy in 10 to 12 fractions, the ABS suggests using two

TABLE 25.15 SUMMARY OF HIGH-DOSE-RATE ENDOBRONCHIAL BRACHYTHERAPY FOR PALLIATION

Author (Reference)	*Number of Patients*	*HDR per Fraction (Gy)*^{a}	*Number of Fractions*	*Percentage Improved*	
				Symptoms	*Bronchoscopy*
Stout et al.[144]	100	15–20	1	50–86	NA
Speiser and Spratling[143]	144	10	3	85–99	80
	151	7.5	3		
Macha et al.[161]	365	5	3–4	66	NA
Kelly et al.[138]	175	15	1–2	66	78
Celebioglu et al.[132]	95	7.5–10	2–3	100	100
Escobar-Sacristan et al.[134]	81	5^b	4	85	97
Taulelle et al.[145]	189	8–10	3–4	54–74	79
Gejerman et al.[135]	41	5	3	72	54
Kubaszewska et al.[139]	270	8–10		76-92	80
Ozkok et al.[141]	74^c	7.5	2	57–94	77
	41	7.5	3	55–78	72
Skowronek et al.[142]	303	7.5	3		88.4
	345	10	1		
Guarnashcelli et al.[136]	52	5–7.5	1–3	92	87
Dagnault et al.[133]	81	5	4	77–100	95
Hauswald et al.[137]	41	5	3	58	73
Totals	2,548		1–4	55%–100%	72%–100%

HDR, high–dose-rate; NA, not available.

^{a}Dose prescribed at 1 cm. ^{b}Dose prescribed at 0.5 to 1 cm. ^{c}Received external-beam radiation therapy of 30 Gy in 10 fractions.

fractions of 7.5 Gy each or three fractions of 5 Gy each or four fractions of 4 Gy each (prescribed at 1 cm) in patients with no previous history of thoracic irradiation.[6] The interval between fractions is generally 1 to 2 weeks. The brachytherapy dose should be reduced when aggressive chemotherapy is given. Concomitant chemotherapy should be avoided during brachytherapy, unless it is in the context of a clinical trial.

The results from various centers (summarized in Table 25.15) show clinical improvement from 50% to 100% and bronchoscopy response from 59% to 100%.[132–145] Comparison of these results is difficult because of the differences in patient population and the variability in dose and fractionation employed. Complications include radiation bronchitis and stenosis, which may occur after endobronchial brachytherapy,[146] necessitating close follow-up. Another more serious complication is fatal hemoptysis. The hemoptysis could be a radiation therapy complication resulting from the high dose delivered to the area of the pulmonary artery, or it could represent the failure of treatment due to the progression of disease.[147] Multiple courses of brachytherapy, a high previous external-beam radiation dose, a left upper lobe location, or long irradiated segments increase the rate of hemoptysis.[148,149] Incidence of fatal hemoptysis varies from 0% to 50% with a median value of 8%.[130]

Curative Endobronchial Brachytherapy

The standard, definitive therapy for unresectable lung cancer is a combination of chemotherapy and EBRT. Select patients (i.e., those with predominantly endobronchial tumor) may benefit from endobronchial brachytherapy, either alone or as a boost to EBRT.

The ideal patients for curative endobronchial radiation alone are those with occult carcinomas of the lung confined to the bronchus or trachea. Additionally, these patients tend to have early-stage disease and are medically inoperable because of decreased pulmonary function, advanced age, or refusal of surgery. Results of a few reported series are encouraging[150–153] (Table 25.16). The largest series to date with 226 patients reported an 81% survival rate at 2 years utilizing four to six fractions of 5 to 7 Gy each.[150] Late complications did include a 5% fatal hemoptysis rate.

Endobronchial brachytherapy can be used in combination with EBRT for selected patients with inoperable non–small cell lung carcinoma (Table 25.17).[140,154–160] In cases of postobstructive pneumonia or lung collapse, brachytherapy can be used to open the bronchus and aerate the lung such that the tumor volume is better defined. This allows some sparing of normal lung from the EBRT field. Muto et al.[159] performed a nonrandomized prospective study evaluating three endobronchial brachytherapy schemes concomitantly with EBRT on 320 patients with advanced inoperable non–small cell lung cancer. Endobronchial brachytherapy consisted of either 10 Gy in one fraction, 14 Gy in two fractions, or 15 Gy in three fractions. Median survival for all patients was 11.1 months with a symptomatic response rate ranging from 82% to 94%. Complications were the least in the group of patients receiving 15 Gy in three fractions.

Endobronchial brachytherapy can be used as adjuvant treatment in cases with minimal residual disease after surgical resection. Macha et al.[161] reported tumor-free survival up to 4 years in 19 patients with doses of 20 Gy delivered in four fractions at 1 cm from the source axis.

The ABS suggests an HDR dose of three 5-Gy fractions or two 7.5-Gy fractions as a boost to EBRT (either 60 Gy in 30 fractions or 45 Gy in 15 fractions).[6] The HDR dose should be prescribed at a distance of 1 cm from the central axis of the catheter and given weekly. If endobronchial brachytherapy is used alone (in previously nonirradiated patients), HDR doses of five 5-Gy fractions or three 7.5-Gy fractions prescribed to 1 cm may be used.

New Approaches with Combination Therapy

HDR brachytherapy in combination with either sublobar resection, metallic stent placement, photodynamic therapy (PDT), or yttrium-aluminum-garnet (YAG) laser have been described. McKenna et al.[162] reported their series of 48 patients who had poor pulmonary function not amenable to lobectomy

TABLE 25.16 SUMMARY OF ENDOBRONCHIAL BRACHYTHERAPY WITHOUT EXTERNAL-BEAM RADIATION THERAPY FOR OCCULT CARCINOMAS OF THE LUNG

Author (Reference)	*Number of Patients*	*HDR per Fraction (Gy)*	*Prescription Depth (cm)*	*Number of Fractions*	*Total HDR (Gy)*	*Cause-Specific Survival (%)*	*Mean Follow-Up (Months)*	*Complications*
Perol et al.[153]	19	7	1	3–5	35	78	28	NA
Marsiglia et al.[152]	34	5	0.5–1	6	30	78	24	1 PNX
Hennequin et al.[151]	106	5–7	0.5–1.5	6	30–42	67.9 (2 year) 48.5 (5 year)	NA	2 FH, 3 BN, 13 RB
Aumont-Le Guilcher et al.[150]	226	5–7	1	4–6	24–35	81 (2 year) 56 (5 year)	30.4	44 RB, 21 S, 7 BN, 10 FH

HDR, high–dose-rate; NA, not available; PNX, pneumothorax; FH, fatal hemoptysis; BN, bronchial necrosis; RB, radiation bronchitis; S, stenosis.

TABLE 25.17 SUMMARY OF ENDOBRONCHIAL HIGH-DOSE-RATE BRACHYTHERAPY WITH SUPPLEMENTARY EXTERNAL-BEAM RADIATION THERAPY FOR CURATIVE THERAPY IN LOCALLY ADVANCED LUNG CANCER

Author (Reference)	*Number of Patients*	*EBRT (Gy)*	*Dose per Fraction/ Depth (Gy/cm)*	*Number of Fractions*	*Total HDR (Gy)*	*Median Survival (Months)*	*Complications*
Reddi and Marbach[160]	32	60	7.5/1	3	22.5	8	NA
Aygun et al.[155]	62	50–60	5.0/1	3–5	15.0–25.0	13	9 FH, S
Mehta et al.[140]	22	60	4.0/2	2	16.0	8.5	NA
Chang et al.[156]	54	20–70	7.0/1	3	21.0	NA	2 FH
Cotter et al.[157]	65	55–66	2.7–10.0/1	2–4	6.0–35.0	8	9 N, 4 S, 1 FH, 3 TEF
Huber et al.[158]	56	60	4.8/1	2	9.6	10	11 FH
Muto et al.[159]	84		10.0/1	1	10		
	47	60	7.0/1	2	14	11.1	10 FH, 3 BEF, 51 S
	50		5.0/1	3	15		
	139		5.0/0.5	3	15		
Anacak et al.[154]	30	60	5/1	3	15	11	6 S, 2 FH

EBRT, external-beam radiation therapy; HDR, high–dose-rate; NA, not available; FH, fatal hemoptysis; S, stenosis; N, necrosis; TEF, tracheoesophageal fistula; BEF, bronchoesophageal fistula.

who underwent wedge resection, lymph node dissection, and brachytherapy. Brachytherapy consisted of seven fractions of 350 cGy each prescribed to a depth of 1 cm delivered twice daily. Four recurrences were recorded with follow-up ranging from 1 to 27 months. Allison et al.[163] noted a significant improvement in Karnofsky performance status and pulmonary palliation with the use of a metallic stent placed in the endobronchial lumen followed by HDR brachytherapy of three 6-Gy fractions prescribed to a depth of 0.5 cm over a 2-week period. Finally, the use of HDR brachytherapy in combination with photodynamic therapy (PDT) or YAG laser has been described. Freitag et al.[164] reported their results of 32 patients with bulky endobronchial non–small cell lung cancer treated initially with PDT followed 6 weeks later with five fractions (one per week) of 4 Gy each prescribed at a distance of 1 cm. Eighty-one percent of patients were free of endobronchial tumor at a mean follow-up of 24 months. Chella et al.[165] performed a small randomized trial comparing YAG laser alone versus YAG laser plus HDR brachytherapy in 29 patients. HDR brachytherapy consisted of three fractions (one per week) of 5 Gy each prescribed at a distance of 0.5 cm. Combination therapy resulted in a statistical improvement in symptom-free period from 2.8 months to 8.5 months. Disease progression–free period improved from 2.2 months to 7.5 months as well.

Cancer of the Esophagus

Nonoperable definitive treatment of esophageal cancer has evolved over the last two decades to now frequently include concurrent EBRT and chemotherapy. HDR brachytherapy for palliative purposes has been evaluated in a few randomized trials and is well established, but its role in conjunction with concurrent EBRT and chemotherapy is less defined. HDR brachytherapy can be used either alone or in combination with EBRT.[166–167,168–169,170,171–172]

Brachytherapy is relatively simple to perform, because a single catheter is used for the treatment. A nasogastric tube or a specially designed esophageal applicator is used to deliver the treatments. The largest-diameter applicator that can be inserted easily (either intraorally or intranasally) should be used to minimize the mucosal dose relative to the dose at depth. The site to be irradiated, which includes the tumor and a distal and proximal margin of 2 to 5 cm, can be confirmed by fluoroscopy or endoscopy. The ABS recommends an HDR dose of 10 Gy in two fractions, prescribed at 1 cm from the source, to boost 50 Gy EBRT.[166] HDR brachytherapy can be given before, concurrently with, or after EBRT. The advantage of giving brachytherapy after EBRT is that a more uniform dose can be delivered to the residual tumor after it has been reduced by EBRT. Brachytherapy given initially provides rapid relief of dysphagia. HDR brachytherapy at doses of 16 Gy in two fractions or 18 Gy in three fractions delivered weekly or every other day has been used without additional EBRT to palliate esophageal cancers.[170,171]

A few randomized studies have evaluated esophageal HDR brachytherapy and are summarized in Table 25.18. Historically, primary treatment of esophageal cancer included definitive radiotherapy. Results with external-beam radiation alone in general were poor. In 1992, Sur et al.[172] reported a randomized trial of 50 patients with squamous cell carcinoma of the esophagus and compared EBRT alone with the combination of EBRT and HDR brachytherapy (12 Gy in two fractions) as a primary treatment. While perhaps not clinically relevant today given the advent and utilization of concurrent chemotherapy, this study did show an improvement in 12-month survival (78% vs. 44%) as well as relief of dysphagia at 6 months (90.5% vs. 53.5%) with the addition of HDR brachytherapy. For medically inoperable patients with submucosal esophageal cancer, external-beam radiation with the addition of intraluminal brachytherapy is an attractive approach. Ishikawa et al.[173] demonstrated a 5-year cause-specific survival of 86% with intraluminal brachytherapy compared to 62% with EBRT alone in a cohort of 56 patients.

In the palliative setting to relieve dysphagia, HDR brachytherapy is more defined. As was seen in definitive therapy, the combination of EBRT and HDR brachytherapy as compared to EBRT alone has resulted in an improvement in relief of dysphagia as well as survival. Sur et al.[169] reported a randomized trial of 50 patients with squamous cell carcinoma of the esophagus, with all patients receiving EBRT of 35 Gy in 15 fractions. The group treated additionally with HDR brachytherapy (12 Gy in two fractions) demonstrated a 6-month rate of relief of dysphagia of 84% compared to 13%. One-year survival was also improved (69% vs. 16%).

More recent studies have evaluated various HDR fractionation schemes as well as comparing HDR brachytherapy alone to combination EBRT and HDR brachytherapy. Sur et al.[171] evaluated three fractionation schemes given weekly (12 Gy in two fractions, 16 Gy in two fractions, and 18 Gy in three fractions) among 172 patients with advanced esophageal cancer. The higher dose fractionation schemes had a trend toward improved dysphagia-free survival (25% to 38% at 12 months). Subsequently, a multicenter, prospective randomized study conducted under the auspices of the International Atomic Energy Agency (IAEA) evaluated two HDR regimens in 232 patients.[170] Patients were randomized to receive 18 Gy in three fractions over 5 days or 16 Gy in two fractions over 3 days. The authors concluded that dose fractions of 6 Gy × 3 and 8 Gy × 2 within 1 week gave similar results for dysphagia-free survival (approximately 30% at 12 months), overall survival, and incidence of strictures and fistulas.

The addition of EBRT to HDR brachytherapy has yielded mixed results. Sur et al.[168] reported on a prospective pilot-randomized trial of 60 patients comparing HDR brachytherapy alone versus HDR brachytherapy plus EBRT for palliative treatment of advanced esophageal cancer. All patients

TABLE 25.18 SUMMARY OF ESOPHAGEAL HIGH-DOSE-RATE BRACHYTHERAPY

Author (Reference)	*Number of Patients*	*EBRT Dose (Gy)*	*Number of HDR Fractions*	*HDR per Fraction (Gy)*	*Relief of Dysphagia at 6 Months (%)*	*Relief of Dysphagia at 1 Year (%)*	*Survival at 1 Year*
Definitive							
Sur et al.[172]	25	55	–	–	53.5	37.5	44%
	25	35	2	6	90.5	70.6	78%
Palliation							
Sur et al.[169]	25	35	–	–	12.5	–	16%
	25	35	2	6	84.2	58.3	69%
Sur et al.[171]	36	–	2	6	40[a]	10[a]	9%
	68	–	2	8	52[a]	30[a]	22%
	68	–	3	6	50[a]	40[a]	35%
Sur et al.[170]	112	–	3	6	~75	~75	~25%
	120	–	2	8	~75	~60	~25%
Sur et al.[168]	30	–	2	8	>50	–	7.2 months[b]
	30	30	2	8	>50%	–	7.5 months[b]
Rosenblatt et al.[167]	109	–	2	8	~50%	~37%	~10%
	110	30	2	8	~70%	~45%	~18%

EBRT, external-beam radiation therapy; HDR, high-dose-rate.
[a]Approximate disease-free survival based on graph. [b]Median survival.

received 16 Gy in two fractions over a 3-day period and were then randomized to observation (Group A) versus EBRT (Group B) of 30 Gy in 10 fractions. At 12 months, there was no difference in dysphagia-free survival, overall survival, or incidence of strictures and fistulas for the two groups. However, the follow-up prospective multicenter randomized study in a larger patient group as reported by Rosenblatt et al.[167] utilizing the same regimen did show a sustained improvement in dysphagia-free survival at 12 months with the combined HDR brachytherapy and EBRT. There was no difference between the complication rates or overall survival between the two treatments.

In summary, retrospective studies as well as prospective, randomized clinical trials show that there is improved local control and survival when HDR brachytherapy is added to EBRT and that HDR brachytherapy alone can be used for palliation of advanced esophageal cancers. Because a high dose is delivered to the esophageal mucosa, side effects may include ulcerations, fistulas, and esophageal strictures. Additionally, the use of HDR brachytherapy as a boost to concurrent chemotherapy and EBRT has been evaluated.[174–177] Results have varied and thus caution should be exercised with this approach.

Biliary Cancers

Cholangiocarcinomas are rare malignancies and optimal adjuvant therapy remains unclear. A Surveillance, Epidemiology and End Results (SEER) database analysis suggested that brachytherapy may improve overall survival.[178] Tumors of the bile duct are often unresectable and are treated palliatively by biliary drainage and EBRT. The biliary drainage tube can be accessed to provide brachytherapy to the area of obstruction either by LDR, ^{192}Ir brachytherapy[179] or by HDR brachytherapy[179–183] alone or in combination with EBRT. Although brachytherapy is commonly delivered through a transhepatic cholangiogram catheter,[179] it has also been delivered using an endoscopic retrograde technique.[183] A size 12-Fr biliary drainage catheter is required to accommodate a 6-Fr HDR brachytherapy catheter. Therefore, the in-dwelling biliary drainage catheter is upsized to a size 12-Fr biliary drainage catheter, if required. Under fluoroscopy, the brachytherapy catheter is inserted into the biliary drainage catheter and advanced past the area of obstruction. A Tuohy-Borst (Y-shaped) adapter attached to the end of the biliary catheter allows concurrent external biliary drainage while holding the HDR catheter in place. The area of the obstruction is irradiated along with 1- to 2-cm proximal and distal margins. The dose per fraction delivered is variable, but about 5 Gy per fraction at a distance of 1 cm from the source is commonly used for three or four fractions (15 to 20 Gy total) to boost 45 Gy EBRT.[179] If EBRT is not delivered, a palliative dose of 30 Gy in six fractions can be used.[179] Concurrent chemotherapy (5-FU) is often added. It is important to leave the biliary drainage catheter in place after therapy to minimize biliary stricture.

Head and Neck Cancers

Brachytherapy, especially using manually afterloaded ^{192}Ir, has been widely used to treat head and neck cancers. HDR brachytherapy has been used in selected cases to reduce radiation exposure and permit optimization as summarized in Table 25.19.[184–199] However, these advantages are offset by the need for multiple fractions because the head and neck area does not tolerate high doses per fraction. Both the ABS and GEC-ESTRO have separately published general recommendations of utilizing HDR brachytherapy in the various sites of head and neck cancer.[10,200]

The nasopharynx is a site within the head and neck area that is easily accessed by an intracavitary HDR applicator.[201–203] Levendag et al.[201] have extensive experience in treating nasopharyngeal lesions with HDR brachytherapy. They have shown that patients most suitable for an HDR brachytherapy boost are those with T1 and T2 lesions following 60 (T1, T2a) to 70 Gy (T2b) of EBRT. HDR doses of 18 Gy in six fractions are delivered by a special nasopharynx applicator. T3 and T4 lesions are better suited to be boosted with intensity-modulated radiation therapy or stereotactic external-beam techniques.

The use of HDR brachytherapy catheters incorporated in removable dental molds allows repeated, highly reproducible, fractionated outpatient brachytherapy of superficial (<0.5-cm thick) tumors without requiring repeated catheter insertion into the tumor.[204] Suitable sites for mold therapy include the scalp, face, pinna, lip, buccal mucosa, maxillary antrum, hard palate, oral cavity, external auditory canal, and orbital cavity after exenteration. HDR can be used as the sole modality or in conjunction with EBRT. A total HDR dose equivalent to about 60 Gy LDR (prescribed at 0.5-cm depth) is recommended when used as the sole modality.[10] The HDR can also be used as a boost to 45 to 50 Gy EBRT, in which case the HDR doses are appropriately reduced to LDR equivalent doses of 15 to 30 Gy. The actual HDR dose per fraction and number of fractions can be varied to suit individual situations (including site and treatment volume). Biomathematic (LQ) modeling can be used to assist in the conversion of LDR to HDR.[13]

Local regional recurrence remains the primary pattern of failure in head and neck cancers despite advancements in surgery and concurrent chemotherapy and EBRT. Surgical salvage is generally the preferred treatment; however, it is not

TABLE 25.19 HIGH-DOSE-RATE BRACHYTHERAPY FOR HEAD AND NECK CANCERS

Author (Reference)	*Site*	*EBRT Dose (Gy)*	*HDR per Fraction (Gy)*	*Number of Fractions*	*Isoeffective Dose (Gy)*[a]	*Number of Patients*	*5-Year Local Control (%)*
Lau et al.[188]	Tongue	0	6.5	7	63	27	53
Inoue et al.[187]	Tongue	0	6	10	80	25	87
Leung et al.[189]	Tongue	0	4.5–6.3	10	54–86	19	95[b]
Guinot et al.[185]	Lip	0	4.5–5.5	8–10	54–57	39[c]	88[d]
Levendag et al.[191]	Nasal vestibule	0	3–4	14	48.3	64	92[e]
Yu et al.[199]	Various	50	2.7	6	67	12	79[f]
Dixit et al.[184]	Various	40–48	3	7	63–71	18	80[g]
Nag et al.[195]	Sinus	45–50	10–12.5	1	66–68	27	65
		45–63	15–20	1	94–95	7	
Lu et al.[192]	Nasopharynx	66	5	2	79	33	94[d]
Nose et al.[197]	Oropharynx	0	6	8–9	64–72	14	82
		14.4–66.6	6	3–6	62–90	68	
Ng et al.[195]	Nasopharynx	43.2–70.4	2.5–3	2–7	65–79	38	96
Nag et al.[194]	Various	45–50	7.5–20	1	61–95	65	59
Leung et al.[190]	Nasopharynx	66	10–12	2	99–110	145	95.8[h]
Yeo et al.[198]	Nasopharynx	66	10	2	99	178	91.6
Martinez-Monge et al.[193]	Oral cavity	45	4	4	63	8	86[i]
	Oropharynx		4	6	72	31	
Guinot et al.[186]	Tongue	0	4	11	51	17	79
		55	3	6	63	33	

EBRT, external-beam radiation therapy; HDR, high-dose-rate.
[a]Isoeffective dose for tumor effects as if given at 2 Gy/day using the linear-quadratic model with an α/β ratio of 10. [b]Four-year local control.
[c]One patient received 50 Gy EBRT with 3.5 Gy × 6 HDR. [d]Three-year local control. [e]Five-year relapse-free survival. [f]Two-year local control.
[g]Median follow-up of 14 months. [h]Five-year local failure free survival. [i]Seven-year local control.

possible in all cases. EBRT is effective as salvage treatment but comes with high toxicity. HDR brachytherapy has been used in a few limited series for recurrent disease of previously irradiated patients. Various fractionation schemes with or without EBRT or surgical resection have been utilized. Initial results appear comparable to other modalities.[205–209]

Another innovative approach is the use of intraoperative HDR brachytherapy, which permits normal tissues to be retracted or shielded during brachytherapy. Intraoperative HDR brachytherapy can reach many sites in the head and neck area that are difficult to treat or are inaccessible by either LDR brachytherapy or intraoperative electron beam radiation. The catheters are removed immediately after the single dose of radiation, hence minimizing inconvenience and permitting the use of brachytherapy in areas such as the base of the skull.[194,195] Doses of 7.5 to 15 Gy are given when EBRT of 45 to 50 Gy can be added. In recurrent tumors where no further EBRT can be given, a single intraoperative dose of 15 to 20 Gy can be given.[194,195]

Soft-Tissue Sarcomas

Excellent results are obtained with a combination of wide excision of the tumor and adjuvant EBRT. However, irradiation of large volumes after surgery gives rise to morbidity, especially normal-tissue fibrosis. To minimize morbidity, a few centers historically have used LDR brachytherapy.[210,211] The major problem with LDR brachytherapy of large volumes is the radiation exposure involved. Hence, a few centers have investigated the use of HDR brachytherapy for soft-tissue sarcomas.[212–225] HDR brachytherapy catheters are implanted along the tumor bed and radio-opaque clips indicate the margins. A 2- to 5-cm margin proximally and distally is used after gross excision of tumor. Optimized treatment planning can be used to deliver a more homogeneous dose. Doses of 40 to 50 Gy are given in 12 to 15 fractions if the HDR is given alone.[9] If EBRT (45 to 50 Gy) is added, the brachytherapy dose is limited to 18 to 25 Gy in four to seven fractions.[9] It is important to delay the start of brachytherapy for about 4 to 7 days after surgery to allow for wound healing.[9] An alternative technique not widely available is intraoperative HDR brachytherapy.[213,226] An intraoperative HDR brachytherapy dose of 12 to 15 Gy is given to the tumor bed in a single fraction intraoperatively to boost EBRT doses of 45 to 50 Gy. Nerve tolerance to a high dose per fraction is poor, and HDR should be used with caution when catheters have to be placed in contact with neurovascular structures. The ABS suggests the following interventions to minimize morbidity in soft-tissue sarcomas[9]:

1. When brachytherapy is used as adjuvant monotherapy, the source loading should start no sooner than 5 to 6 days after wound closure. However, the radioactive sources may be loaded earlier (as soon as 2 to 3 days after surgery) if doses of <20 Gy are given with brachytherapy as a supplement to EBRT.
2. Minimize dose to normal tissues (e.g., gonads, breasts, thyroid, skin) whenever possible, especially in children and patients of childbearing age.
3. Limit the allowable skin dose—the 40-Gy isodose line (LDR) to <25 cm^2 and the 25-Gy isodose line to <100 cm^2.

Outcomes of nonrandomized studies using HDR doses in the range of 2 to 9 Gy per fraction given once or twice daily or single-fraction intraoperative HDR brachytherapy are outlined in Table 25.20.[212–226]

A recent nonrandomized study has demonstrated that intensity-modulated radiation therapy achieved better local control over brachytherapy in patients with high-grade soft-tissue sarcomas of the extremity and thus has questioned the use of brachytherapy in this patient population.[227] Despite this, HDR brachytherapy still has a role to play in the management of soft-tissue sarcomas.

Pediatric Tumors

LDR brachytherapy has been used in children to reduce the deleterious effects of EBRT.[228,229] However, LDR brachytherapy is difficult to perform in young children and infants because they require prolonged sedation and immobilization with close monitoring, which increases the risk of radiation exposure to nursing staff and parents. HDR is therefore very appealing in infants and younger children and has undergone various trials.[230–232,233–234] The recommended dose for HDR as monotherapy is 36 Gy in 12 fractions given at 3 Gy per fraction (prescribed at 0.5 cm) twice a day.[9,230,234] The interval between fractions is at least 6 hours. There are no good published dose recommendations for HDR when used as a boost to EBRT. The linear-quadratic model[13] can be used to calculate a fractionation scheme equivalent to that of an LDR implant boost dose of 15 to 25 Gy (prescribed

TABLE 25.20 OUTCOME OF NONRANDOMIZED STUDIES OF HIGH-DOSE-RATE BRACHYTHERAPY USED FOR PRIMARY SOFT-TISSUE SARCOMAS

Author (Reference)	*Number of Patients*	*Median Follow-Up (Months)*	*Local Control (%)*	*Complications (%)*
Donath et al.[216]	19	12	70	16
Alekhteyar et al.[212]	13	16	77	NS
Ryan et al.[223]	32	50	82	48
Yoshida et al.[225]	13	24	72	8
Crownover et al.[215]	10	12	100	0
Koizumi et al.[218]	16	30	50	6
Chun et al.[214]	11	31	100	9
Rachbauer et al.[226,a]	39	26	100	28
Kretzler et al.[219,a]	11	51[b]	91	–
Alektiar et al.[213]	12[c]	33	74	34
	20[d]		54	
Mierzwa et al.[220]	43	39	88	7
Pohar et al.[222]	17	17	94	18
Petera et al.[221]	45	38.4	74	20
Itami et al.[217]	26	49.2	78	15
San Miguel et al.[224]	60	49.2	76	30 (Grade 3)
				10 (Grade 4)

HDR, high-dose-rate; NS, not stated

[a]Intraoperative single-fraction HDR. [b]Mean follow-up. [c]Primary disease.

[d]Recurrent disease.

at 0.5 cm). The recommended dose for intraoperative HDR brachytherapy as a boost to EBRT is 10 to 15 Gy (prescribed at 0.5 cm), depending on the extent of residual disease.[235–239] According to the Inter-group Rhabdomyosarcoma Study (IRS), the standard EBRT dose for pediatric soft-tissue sarcomas is 40 Gy for microscopic disease and 50 Gy for gross disease. Intraoperative HDR allows reduction in the dose of EBRT to 27 to 30 Gy so that concerns for impaired growth and organ function is greatly reduced.[230,236,240] The results of HDR brachytherapy in the treatment of pediatric tumors are summarized in Table 25.21.[233,236,238,241–246] Although the long-term morbidity of HDR brachytherapy in young children is not fully known, one may expect preservation of organ functions similar to that seen with LDR brachytherapy.[228,247] Due to the complexities involved in pediatric HDR brachytherapy, it is recommended that the use of HDR brachytherapy in pediatric tumors be limited to centers that have experience with pediatric implants.[9]

Skin Cancer

The widespread availability of HDR remote afterloading brachytherapy units allows the use of surface molds as an alternative to electron beam and for cases where surface irregularity, proximity to bone, or poor intrinsic tolerance of tissues does not allow for satisfactory treatment by electron beam. For most cases, a satisfactory mold can be made from 5-mm-thick sheets of wax with the HDR catheters spaced 1 cm apart. A simpler alternative is to use commercially available surface template applicators (e.g., Freiburg flab from Nucletron Corp., Columbia, MD, and HAM applicator from Mick Radionuclear Instruments Inc., Bronx, NY) that are used for intraoperative HDR brachytherapy.[248–250]

In addition to melanoma and nonmelanoma skin cancers, Merkel cell lesions as well as benign keloids have been treated with HDR brachytherapy. There is a wide range of recommended doses and fractionation schemes for treating skin cancer. Doses in the range of 3,500 cGy in five fractions to 5,000 cGy in 10 fractions have been used with success in HDR molds. Standard, more prolonged fractionation schemes with 180 to 200 cGy daily or twice-daily fractions can also be used. The linear-quadratic radiobiologic model can be used to determine the total dose for a given fractionation scheme.[12,13] Kuribayashi et al.[251] recently reported a 90% control rate postkeloidectomy utilizing 20 Gy in four fractions or 15 Gy in three fractions based on the site of the keloid.

Intraoperative High–Dose-Rate Brachytherapy

Intraoperative high–dose-rate (IOHDR) brachytherapy is an extreme example of reduced fractionation in that only a single HDR brachytherapy dose is applied.[249,252–254] This results in an inherent radiobiologic disadvantage, because the advantages of fractionation (repair of normal tissue damage, reoxygenation of hypoxic tumor cells, and movement of tumor cells from the radioresistant S phase to the more radiosensitive mitotic phase of the cell cycle) are lost. LQ model calculations show that there has to be a dose reduction of 20% to 25% to the late-reacting normal tissues for isoeffect. However, the dose reduction achieved by 1- to 4-cm displacement of normal tissue is much more (closer to 60% to 90% reduction).[254] Hence, HDR in these situations becomes advantageous. However, if such a dose reduction cannot be achieved in normal tissues, HDR brachytherapy becomes disadvantageous. Intraoperative HDR brachytherapy also has the advantage that normal tissues can be temporarily displaced and/or partially shielded during irradiation.

In IOHDR brachytherapy, the surgery is performed in a shielded operating room with remote anesthesia and a video monitoring system. Maximum surgical debulking is attempted whenever possible. Then the tumor bed is irradiated using special intraoperative applicators containing HDR catheters that are 1 cm apart and parallel to each other. The use of a fixed geometry applicator allows the patient to be treated without delay using preplanned dosimetry for the selected applicator. Normal tissues are either retracted from the high-dose area or shielded. Doses of 10 to 20 Gy are usually given as a single fraction over 10 to 30 minutes.[253] The advantages of

TABLE 25.21 RESULTS OF HIGH-DOSE-RATE BRACHYTHERAPY USED FOR TREATMENT OF PEDIATRIC TUMORS

Author (Reference)	*Number of Patients*	*Brachytherapy*	*HDR (Gy)*	*EBRT Dose (Gy)*	*Median Follow-Up (Months)*	*Local Control (%)*	*Late Toxicity (%)*
Nag et al.[233]	15	F-HDR	36 (3 Gy ×12)	0	120	80	20
Martınez-Monge et al.[243]	5	F-HDR	24 (4 Gy × 6)	27–45	27	100	0
Nakamura et al.[245]	16	F-HDR	10 (5 Gy × 2)	45–55	54	94	–
Viani et al.[246]	18	F-HDR	18–24	30.6–50	79.5[a]	90	16.5[a]
			21–40	0		100	
Laskar et al.[242]	21	F-HDR	36 (4 Gy × 9)	0	51	92	
			21 (3 Gy × 7)	30.6–45		100	
Schuck et al.[238]	20	IOHDR	10	45–55	24	65	40 (postop)
Nag et al.[236]	13	IOHDR	10–15	27–30	47	95	23
Goodman et al.[241]	66	IOHDR	4–15	0–56	12	56	12
Nag et al.[244]	13	IOERT	10–15	0–50.4	42	72	31

HDR, high–dose-rate; EBRT, external-beam radiation therapy; F-HDR, fractionated high–dose-rate (given twice a day); IOHDR, intraoperative high–dose-rate; IOERT, intraoperative electron beam radiation therapy.

[a]Whole group.

TABLE 25.22 ADVANTAGES OF SURGICAL DEBULKING WITH INTRAOPERATIVE HIGH-DOSE-RATE BRACHYTHERAPY OVER PERIOPERATIVE BRACHYTHERAPY OR ELECTRON BEAM INTRAOPERATIVE RADIATION THERAPY

Advantages Over Perioperative Brachytherapy	*Advantages Over Electron Beam IORT*
1. It is possible to use retraction or shielding to reduce the dose to normal tissues. 2. Normal structures can be temporarily moved while the radiation is given and then replaced in their normal position. For example, to access the base of the skull, the maxilla can be removed and later regrafted. Ureters can be severed and then reimplanted into the bladder. During liver transplantation procedures, the liver hilum can be irradiated during the interval between the removal of the host liver and reimplantation of the donor liver. 3. The process is rapid. Using a surface applicator eliminates the need to individually suture the catheters to the tumor bed. 4. HDR brachytherapy allows the treatment to be delivered at sites into which catheters cannot be sutured. 5. Because catheters are not left in the patient, there is no risk of catheter displacement, extrusion, or infection.	1. Electron beam IORT can only be delivered to areas accessible to the electron cone and, therefore, cannot treat steeply sloping surfaces, narrow cavities, or areas such as the diaphragm, pubis, and anterior abdominal wall. Intraoperative HDR brachytherapy has fewer anatomic constraints than electron beam IORT. 2. The HDR machine costs less than an electron beam linear accelerator. 3. Because the HDR afterloader can be transported between the radiation department and the operating room, dedicated equipment is not required.

IORT, intraoperative radiation therapy; HDR, high-dose-rate.

IOHDR brachytherapy over perioperative brachytherapy or electron beam intraoperative radiation therapy (IORT) are listed in Table 25.22. Unfortunately, the relative scarcity of shielded operating rooms has currently limited its availability to just a few centers.[235,239,249,252,253,255]

Reduction of Brachytherapy Errors

The International Commission on Radiological Protection (ICRP)[256] released Publication 97 in November 2005, which outlines quality assurance (QA) procedures necessary to prevent accidents with HDR brachytherapy. The ICRP gave general and specific recommendations for HDR brachytherapy programs, which are summarized in Tables 25.23 and 25.24. The general recommendations include the establishment of a written comprehensive QA program, formation of a hospital radiation safety committee, external auditing of procedures, peer reviewing of each case, and reporting of every incident or accident. The specific recommendations cover a broad range of topics. Training in HDR brachytherapy should commence prior to acquisition of machines, follow a team approach, and be sequential in the introduction of techniques, with simpler techniques first, followed by more complex treatments. For example, multiple-plane flexible implants should not be attempted first. Transport regulations of sources should be adhered to and performed by a factory-trained and -certified operator. In addition, new sources should be measured in a calibrated well chamber to verify reported activity, at which time it is advisable to do a full commissioning including physics and mechanical QA checks. It is recommended that all systems of delivery (i.e., catheters) be closed ended, that the step size at a particular center be constant (i.e., 5 mm) for all treatments, and that a dedicated self-contained brachytherapy suite exist to house all equipment. Prior to initiating treatment with the HDR machine, a few standard procedures should be employed. These include manually inserting a test wire to verify programmed treatment length and identify any kinks or obstructions, verifying applicator position with an appropriate imaging modality (i.e., fluoroscopy), and ensuring that all tubes outside the patient's body are as far away as possible to minimize unintended doses. Following treatment, a survey of the patient by a portable radiation monitor is essential. Finally, emergency plans and security procedures should be in place and strictly adhered to. "False alarms" and "interlock failures" should be thoroughly investigated, and persons responsible for emergency procedures should remain in the vicinity of the brachytherapy suite during the entire treatment. In some countries it is a requirement that both the clinician and physicist remain in the vicinity of the HDR suite. The possibility of theft of an

TABLE 25.23 INTERNATIONAL COMMISSION ON RADIOLOGICAL PROTECTION PUBLICATION 97: PREVENTION OF HIGH-DOSE-RATE BRACHYTHERAPY ACCIDENTS—GENERAL RECOMMENDATIONS

1. Written comprehensive QA program.
2. Compliance to QA procedures will contribute to minimizing the occurrence of errors, both in number and magnitude.
3. Hospital Radiation Safety committee (QA committee) needs to exist and interact with regulatory and health authorities.
4. Maintenance is an indispensable component of QA.
5. External audits of procedures reinforce good and safe practice and identify potential causes of errors.
6. Peer review of each case improves quality.
7. Every incident or accident should be reported as required to the appropriate authority.

QA, quality assurance.

TABLE 25.24 INTERNATIONAL COMMISSION ON RADIOLOGICAL PROTECTION PUBLICATION 97: PREVENTION OF HIGH-DOSE-RATE BRACHYTHERAPY ACCIDENTS—SPECIFIC RECOMMENDATIONS

1. Training in an HDR center should commence prior to machine acquisition and should include the specific techniques to be used.
2. Training should be directed toward ensuring a team approach involving clinician, physicist, technician, and nurse.
3. Training and introduction of techniques should be sequential, commencing with simpler techniques before attempting more complex activities. Fixed geometry applicators and implants are less likely to result in errors.
4. Transport regulations should be adhered to and performed by a factory-trained and certified operator. This includes on-site container inspection for damage, removal of the old source and its transfer to the container, and installation of the new one into the safe.
5. New sources should be measured in a calibrated well chamber to verify the manufacturer's reported activity and the results entered immediately into the software. At this time it is advisable to do a full commissioning (physics and mechanical QA checks).
6. All systems of delivery must be closed ended (catheters, needles, and fine tubes).
7. Manual insertion of a test wire (check cable) clearly marked at the programmed treatment length before each treatment should be done to ensure that the total length of the transfer tube plus applicator equals the programmed treatment length. A manual check cable also helps to identify any kinks or obstruction in the catheter or transfer tube.
8. The step size in a particular center should be kept constant (e.g., 5 mm) for all treatments to avoid errors of using incorrect step size.
9. Keeping all tubes outside of the body as far distant as possible from the patient's skin will help to minimize unintended doses.
10. Dedicated self-contained brachytherapy suite with adequate shielding housing all requirements is highly advisable.
11. Applicator positioning should be verified before each treatment.
12. So-called false alarms and interlock failures should be thoroughly investigated and appropriated action taken to repair them.
13. Survey of patient by portable radiation monitor should be done after each treatment.
14. An emergency plan should be prepared and practiced with commencement of operations.
15. The person responsible for performing an emergency procedure should remain in the brachytherapy suite during the entire treatment.
16. The HDR machine and source should be kept secure at all times.

HDR, high-dose-rate; QA, quality assurance.

TABLE 25.25 COMPARISON OF DIFFERENT BRACHYTHERAPY TECHNIQUES

	LDR ^{192}*Ir*	*LDR Remote*	*MDR*	*PDR*	*HDR*	*IOHDR*
Dose rate	Low	Low	Medium	High	High	High
Duration of each treatment	2–6 days	2–4 days	1 day	Minutes	Minutes	Minutes
Overall duration of treatment	2–6 days	2–4 days	1 day	2–4 days	4–6 weeks	Minutes
Radiation hazards	High	Small	Small	Small	Small	Small
Availability (worldwide)	High	Low	Low	Low	High	Low
Ease of optimization	Low	Low	Low	High	High	High
Dose as sole modality (Gy)	60	60	40	60	30–40	15–20
Dose as boost to EBRT (Gy)	20–40	20–40	20–30	20–40	20–30	10–15

LDR, low–dose-rate; MDR, medium–dose-rate; PDR, pulsed–dose-rate; HDR, high–dose-rate; IOHDR, intraoperative high–dose-rate; EBRT, external-beam radiation therapy.

HDR source for use as a weapon for nuclear terrorism is real, and the machine and source should be kept secure at all times. Particular attention should be paid if the facility or machine is decommissioned. It is believed that if a HDR brachytherapy center follows these general and specific recommendations, errors and accidents will be minimized.

HIGH-DOSE-RATE BRACHYTHERAPY IN DEVELOPING COUNTRIES

HDR brachytherapy has special relevance for developing countries where resources may be scarce. In this regard, the IAEA has issued recommendations for the use of HDR brachytherapy in developing countries.[257] A brief summary is given here; however, readers interested in the details are referred to the original article. An HDR treatment system should be purchased as a complete unit that includes the ^{192}Ir radioactive source, source-loading unit, applicators, treatment-planning system, and control console. Infrastructure support may require additional or improved buildings and procurement of or access to new imaging facilities. A supportive budget is needed for quarterly source replacement and the annual maintenance necessary to keep the system operational. The radiation oncologist, medical physicist, and technologist should be specially trained before HDR can be introduced. Training for the oncologist and medical physicist is an ongoing process as new techniques or sites of treatment are introduced. Procedures for QA of patient treatment and the planning system must be introduced. Emergency procedures with adequate training of all associated personnel must be in place. The decision to select HDR in preference to alternate methods of brachytherapy is influenced by the ability of the machine to treat a wide variety of clinical sites. In departments with personnel and budgetary resources to support this equipment appropriately, economic advantage becomes evident only if large numbers of patients are treated. With HDR it is possible to treat a large number of patients in institutions that have a high volume of brachytherapy patients but insufficient in-patient facilities for LDR brachytherapy or insufficient finances for the purchase of ^{125}I or ^{103}Pd seeds for permanent implants. Intangible benefits of source safety, personnel safety, and easy adaptation to fluctuating demand for treatments also require consideration when evaluating the need to introduce this treatment system.

SUMMARY

Although brachytherapy is a very effective modality, case selection and proper patient evaluation are essential. If the tumor is very large or widely metastatic, one is doomed to fail due to the physics of dose distribution in the former case and due to the biology of the tumor in the latter case. There are some differences between various brachytherapy modalities (Table 25.25). These differences should be kept in mind when selecting the brachytherapy modality in a particular situation. When HDR brachytherapy is used, the treatments must be executed carefully because the short treatment times do not allow any time for correction of errors, and mistakes can result in harm to patients. Hence, it is very important that all personnel involved in HDR brachytherapy be well trained and constantly alert. However, with proper case selection and delivery technique, HDR brachytherapy has great promise and convenience because of avoidance of radiation exposure, short treatment times, and outpatient therapy.

One of the disadvantages of HDR brachytherapy is that it requires a shielded room. A newer device, the Axxent (Xoft Inc., Sunnyvale, CA), uses a miniaturized x-ray source to deliver low-energy x-rays within a needle or catheter, thereby mimicking HDR brachytherapy. The reduced radiation protection required for these devices due to limited penetration is a great advantage because it allows brachytherapy to be delivered in a nonshielded procedure room or a regular (unshielded) hospital operating suite. Currently, the Xoft Axxent system has only a single channel and therefore has the limitation of being able to treat only small-volume tumor beds. It is being used at a few centers in the United States to treat breast cancer via a balloon device similar to the Mammosite balloon, the vaginal cuff with a single-channel cylinder applicator, and skin cancers with a surface applicator.[112,113,258,259]

It is expected that the use of HDR brachytherapy will continue to expand over the coming years and that refinements in the integration of imaging (computed tomography, magnetic resonance imaging, intraoperative ultrasonography) and optimization of dose distribution will foster this expansion.[17,260] The development of well-controlled randomized trials addressing issues of efficacy, toxicity, quality of life, and costs versus benefits will ultimately define the role of HDR brachytherapy in the therapeutic armamentarium.

SELECTED REFERENCES

A full list of references for this chapter is available online.

1. International Commission on Radiation Units and Measurements. *ICRU report 38: dose and volume specification for reporting intracavitary therapy in gynecology.* Bethesda, MD: International Commission on Radiation Units and Measurements, 1985.
2. Nag S, Samsami N. Pitfalls of inappropriate optimization. *J Brachyther Int* 2000; 16:187–198.
3. Arthur DW, Vicini FA, Kuske RR, et al. Accelerated partial breast irradiation: an updated report from the American Brachytherapy Society. *Brachytherapy* 2003;2:124–130.
4. Nag S, Chao C, Erickson B, et al. The American Brachytherapy Society recommendations for low-dose-rate brachytherapy for carcinoma of the cervix. *Int J Radiat Oncol Biol Phys* 2002;52:33–48.
5. Nag S, Erickson B, Parikh S, et al. The American Brachytherapy Society recommendations for HDR brachytherapy for carcinoma of the endometrium. *Int J Radiat Oncol Biol Phys* 2000;48:779–790.
6. Nag S, Kelly J, Horton J, et al. The American Brachytherapy Society recommendations for HDR brachytherapy for carcinoma of the lung. *Oncology* 2001;15:371–381.
7. Nag S, Kuske R, Vicini F, et al. The American Brachytherapy Society recommendations for brachytherapy for carcinoma of the breast. *Oncology* 2001;15:195–207.
8. Nag S, Orton C, Petereit D, et al. The American Brachytherapy Society recommendations for HDR brachytherapy of the cervix. *Int J Radiat Oncol Biol Phys* 2000;48:201–211.
9. Nag S, Shasha D, Janjan N, et al. The American Brachytherapy Society recommendations for brachytherapy of soft tissue sarcomas. *Int J Radiat Oncol Biol Phys* 2001;49:1033–1043.
10. Nag S, Vikram B, Demanes J, et al. The American Brachytherapy Society recommendations for HDR brachytherapy for head and neck carcinoma. *Int J Radiat Oncol Biol Phys* 2001;50:1190–1198.
11. Nag S, Dobelbower R, Glasgow G, et al. Inter-society standards for brachytherapy: a joint report from AAPM, ABS, ACMP, and ACRO. *Crit Rev Oncol Hematol* 2003;48:1–17.
13. Nag S, Gupta N. A simple method of obtaining equivalent doses for use in HDR brachytherapy. *Int J Radiat Oncol Biol Phys* 2000;46:507–513.
14. Orton CG, Seyedsadr M, Somnay A. Comparison of high and low dose rate remote afterloading for cervix cancer and the importance of fractionation. *Int J Radiat Oncol Biol Phys* 1991;21:1425–1434.
15. Viswanathan A, Creutzberg C, Craighead P, et al. International brachytherapy practice patterns: a survey of the Gynecologic Cancer Intergroup (GCIG). *Int J Radiat Oncol Biol Phys* 2012;82(1):250–255.
17. Haie-Meder C, Potter R, Van Limbergen E, et al. Recommendations from Gynaecological (GYN) GEC-ESTRO Working Group (I): concepts and terms in 3D image based 3D treatment planning in cervix cancer brachytherapy with emphasis on MRI assessment of GTV and CTV. *Radiother Oncol* 2005;74:235–245.

18. Potter R, Haie-Meder C, Van Limbergen E, et al. Recommendations from Gynaecological (GYN) GEC ESTRO working group (II): concepts and terms in 3D image-based treatment planning in cervix cancer brachytherapy-3D dose volume parameters and aspects of 3D image-based anatomy, radiation physics, radiobiology. *Radiother Oncol* 2006;78:67–77.
21. Patel FD, Rai B, Mallick I, et al. High-dose-rate brachytherapy in uterine cervical carcinoma. *Int J Radiat Oncol Biol Phys* 2005;62:125–130.
22. Petereit D, Peracey R. Literature analysis of high dose rate brachytherapy fractionation schedules in the treatment of cervical cancer: is there an optimal fractionation schedule? *Int J Radiat Oncol Biol Phys* 1999;43:359–366.
25. Georg P, Kirisits C, Goldner G, et al. Correlation of dose-volume parameters, endoscopic and clinical rectal side effects in cervix cancer patients treated with definitive radiotherapy including MRI-based brachytherapy. *Radiother Oncol* 2009;91:173–180.
26. Georg P, Lang S, Dimopoulos JC, et al. Dose-volume histogram parameters and late side effects in magnetic resonance image-guided adaptive cervical cancer brachytherapy. *Int J Radiat Oncol Biol Phys* 2011;79:356–362.
28. Viswanathan AN, Erickson BA. Three-dimensional imaging in gynecologic brachytherapy: a survey of the American Brachytherapy Society. *Int J Radiat Oncol Biol Phys* 2010;76:104–109.
29. Potter R, Dimopoulos J, Georg P, et al. Clinical impact of MRI assisted dose volume adaptation and dose escalation in brachytherapy of locally advanced cervix cancer. *Radiother Oncol* 2007;83:148–155.
30. Dimopoulos JC, Lang S, Kirisits C, et al. Dose-volume histogram parameters and local tumor control in magnetic resonance image-guided cervical cancer brachytherapy. *Int J Radiat Oncol Biol Phys* 2009;75:56–63.
33. Narayan K, van Dyk S, Bernshaw D, et al. Comparative study of LDR (Manchester system) and HDR image-guided conformal brachytherapy of cervical cancer: patterns of failure, late complications, and survival. *Int J Radiat Oncol Biol Phys* 2009;74:1529–1535.
34. Ferrigno R, Nishimoto IN, Novaes PE, et al. Comparison of low and high dose rate brachytherapy in the treatment of uterine cervix cancer. Retrospective analysis of two sequential series. *Int J Radiat Oncol Biol Phys* 2005;62:1108–1116.
35. Lorvidhaya V, Tonusin A, Changwiwit W, et al. High-dose-rate afterloading brachytherapy in carcinoma of the cervix: an experience of 1992 patients. *Int J Radiat Oncol Biol Phys* 2000;46:1185–1191.
38. Toita T, Kakinohana Y, Ogawa K, et al. Combination external beam radiotherapy and high-dose-rate intracavitary brachytherapy for uterine cervical cancer: analysis of doses and fractionation schedule. *Int J Radiat Oncol Biol Phys* 2003;56:1344–1353.
39. Hareyama M, Sakata K, Oouchi A, et al. High-dose-rate versus low-dose-rate intracavitary therapy for carcinoma of the uterine cervix: a randomized trial. *Cancer* 2002;94:117–124.
40. Lertsanguansinchai P, Lertbutsayanukul C, Shotelersuk K, et al. Phase III randomized trial comparing LDR and HDR brachytherapy in treatment of cervical carcinoma. *Int J Radiat Oncol Biol Phys* 2004;59:1424–1431.
41. Patel F, Sharma S, Pritam S, et al. Low dose rate versus high dose rate brachytherapy in the treatment of carcinoma of the uterine cervix: a clinical trial. *Int J Radiat Oncol Biol Phys* 1994;28:335–341.
42. Shigematsu Y, Nishiyama K, Masaki N, et al. Treatment of carcinoma of the uterine cervix y remotely controlled afterloading intracavitary radiotherapy with high-does rate: a comparative study with a low-dose rate system. *Int J Radiat Oncol Biol Phys* 1983;9:351–356.
45. Creutzberg CL, van Putten WL, Koper PC, et al. Surgery and postoperative radiotherapy versus surgery alone for patients with stage-1 endometrial carcinoma: multicentre randomised trial. PORTEC Study Group. Post Operative Radiation Therapy in Endometrial Carcinoma. *Lancet* 2000;355:1404–1411.
46. Scholten AN, van Putten WL, Beerman H, et al. Postoperative radiotherapy for stage 1 endometrial carcinoma: long-term outcome of the randomized PORTEC trial with central pathology review. *Int J Radiat Oncol Biol Phys* 2005;63:834–838.
47. Keys H, Roberts J, Brunetto V, et al. A phase III trial of surgery with or without adjunctive external pelvic radiation therapy in intermediate risk endometrial adenocarcinoma: a Gynecologic Oncology Group study. *Gynecol Oncol* 2004;92:744–751.
48. Nout RA, Smit VT, Putter H, et al. Vaginal brachytherapy versus pelvic external beam radiotherapy for patients with endometrial cancer of high-intermediate risk (PORTEC-2): an open-label, non-inferiority, randomised trial. *Lancet* 2010;375:816–823.
54. Sorbe B, Straumits A, Karlsson L. Intravaginal high-dose-rate brachytherapy for stage I endometrial cancer: a randomized study of two dose-per-fraction levels. *Int J Radiat Oncol Biol Phys* 2005;62:1385–1389.
58. Sorbe BG, Smeds AC. Postoperative vaginal irradiation with high dose rate afterloading technique in endometrial carcinoma stage I. *Int J Radiat Oncol Biol Phys* 1990;18:305–314.
59. Sorbe B, Kjellgren O, Stenson S. Prognosis of endometrial carcinoma stage I in two Swedish regions. A stúdy with special regard to the effects of intracavitary irradiation with high dose rate afterloading technique or with low dose-rate radium. *Acta Oncol* 1990;29:29–37.
64. Knocke TH, Kucera H, Weidinger B, et al. Primary treatment of endometrial carcinoma with high-dose-rate brachytherapy: results of 12 years of experience with 280 patients. *Int J Radiat Oncol Biol Phys* 1997;37:359–365.
69. Coon D, Beriwal S, Heron DE, et al. High-dose-rate Rotte "Y" applicator brachytherapy for definitive treatment of medically inoperable endometrial cancer: 10-year results. *Int J Radiat Oncol Biol Phys* 2008;71:779–783.
74. Deutsch I, Zelefsky MJ, Zhang Z, et al. Comparison of PSA relapse-free survival in patients treated with ultra-high-dose IMRT versus combination HDR brachytherapy and IMRT. *Brachytherapy* 2010;9:313–318.
77. Hoskin PJ, Motohashi K, Bownes P, et al. High dose rate brachytherapy in combination with external beam radiotherapy in the radical treatment of prostate cancer: initial results of a randomised phase three trial. *Radiother Oncol* 2007;84:114–120.
79. Kaprealian T, Weinberg V, Speight JL, et al. High-dose-rate brachytherapy boost for prostate cancer: comparison of two different fractionation schemes. *Int J Radiat Oncol Biol Phys* 2012;82(1):222–227.
80. Martinez AA, Gonzalez J, Ye H, et al. Dose escalation improves cancer-related events at 10 years for intermediate- and high-risk prostate cancer patients treated with hypofractionated high-dose-rate boost and external beam radiotherapy. *Int J Radiat Oncol Biol Phys* 2011;79:363–370.
86. Kovacs G, Potter R, Loch T, et al. GEC/ESTRO-EAU recommendations on temporary brachytherapy using stepping sources for localised prostate cancer. *Radiother Oncol* 2005;74:137–148.
87. Duchesne G, Peters L. What is the α/β ratio for prostate cancer? Rationale for hypofractionated high-dose-rate brachytherapy. *Int J Radiat Oncol Biol Phys* 1999;44:747–748.
89. Williams SG, Taylor JM, Liu N, et al. Use of individual fraction size data from 3756 patients to directly determine the alpha/beta ratio of prostate cancer. *Int J Radiat Oncol Biol Phys* 2007;68:24–33.
90. Demanes DJ, Martinez AA, Ghilezan M, et al. High-dose-rate monotherapy: safe and effective brachytherapy for patients with localized prostate cancer. *Int J Radiat Oncol Biol Phys* 2011;81(5)1286–1292.
93. Yoshioka Y, Konishi K, Sumida I, et al. Monotherapeutic high-dose-rate brachytherapy for prostate cancer: five-year results of an extreme hypofractionation regimen with 54 Gy in nine fractions. *Int J Radiat Oncol Biol Phys* 2011;80:469–475.
98. Arthur DW, Winter K, Kuske RR, et al. A phase II trial of brachytherapy alone after lumpectomy for select breast cancer: tumor control and survival outcomes of RTOG 95-17. *Int J Radiat Oncol Biol Phys* 2008;72:467–473.
99. Polgar C, Fodor J, Major T, et al. Breast-conserving treatment with partial or whole breast irradiation for low-risk invasive breast carcinoma–5-year results of a randomized trial. *Int J Radiat Oncol Biol Phys* 2007;69:694–702.
100. Polgar C, Major T, Fodor J, et al. Accelerated partial-breast irradiation using high-dose-rate interstitial brachytherapy: 12-year update of a prospective clinical study. *Radiother Oncol* 2010;94:274–279.
102. Strnad V, Hildebrandt G, Potter R, et al. Accelerated partial breast irradiation: 5-year results of the German-Austrian multicenter phase II trial using interstitial multicatheter brachytherapy alone after breast-conserving surgery. *Int J Radiat Oncol Biol Phys* 2011;80:17–24.
103. Vicini F, Beitsch P, Quiet C, et al. Five-year analysis of treatment efficacy and cosmesis by the American Society of Breast Surgeons MammoSite Breast Brachytherapy Registry Trial in patients treated with accelerated partial breast irradiation. *Int J Radiat Oncol Biol Phys* 2011;79:808–817.
104. Keisch M, Arthur D, Patel R, et al. American Brachytherapy Society—Breast Brachytherapy Task Group—guidelines. Available at: http://www.americanbrachytherapy.org/guidelines/abs_breast_brachytherapy_taskgroup.pdf 2007
111. Smith BD, Arthur DW, Buchholz TA, et al. Accelerated partial breast irradiation consensus statement from the American Society for Radiation Oncology (ASTRO). *Int J Radiat Oncol Biol Phys* 2009;74:987–1001.
115. Poortmans P, Bartelink H, Horiot J, et al. The influence of the boost technique on local control in breast conserving treatment in the EORTC 'boost versus no boost' randomised trial. *Radiother Oncol* 2004;72:25–33.
116. Romestaing P, Lehingue Y, Carrie C, et al. Role of a 10-Gy boost in the conservative treatment of early breast cancer: results of a randomized clinical trial in Lyon, France. *J Clin Oncol* 1997;15:963–968.
158. Huber R, Fischer R, Haútmann H, et al. Does additional brachytherapy improve the effect of external irradiation? A prospective, randomized study in central lung tumors. *Int J Radiat Oncol Biol Phys* 1997;38:533–540.
166. Gaspar LE, Nag S, Herskovic A, et al. American Brachytherapy Society (ABS) consensus guidelines for brachytherapy of esophageal cancer. Clinical Research Committee, American Brachytherapy Society, Philadelphia, PA. *Int J Radiat Oncol Biol Phys* 1997;38:127–132.
167. Rosenblatt E, Jones G, Sur RK, et al. Adding external beam to intra-luminal brachytherapy improves palliation in obstructive squamous cell oesophageal cancer: a prospective multi-centre randomized trial of the International Atomic Energy Agency. *Radiother Oncol* 2010;97:488–494.
170. Sur R, Levin C, Donde B, et al. Prospective randomized trial of HDR brachytherapy as a sole modality in palliation of advanced esophageal carcinoma: an International Atomic Energy Agency study. *Int J Radiat Oncol Biol Phys* 2002;53:127–133.
175. Gaspar LE, Winter K, Kocha WI, et al. A phase I/II study of external beam radiation, brachytherapy, and concurrent chemotherapy for patients with localized carcinoma of the esophagus (Radiation Therapy Oncology Group Study 9207): final report. *Cancer* 2000;88:988–995.
194. Nag S, Koc M, Schuller DE, et al. Intraoperative single fraction high-dose-rate brachytherapy for head and neck cancers. *Brachytherapy* 2005;4:217–223.
195. Nag S, Tippin D, Grecula J, et al. Intraoperative high-dose-rate brachytherapy for paranasal sinus tumors. *Int J Radiat Oncol Biol Phys* 2004;58:155–160.
200. Mazeron JJ, Ardiet JM, Haie-Meder C, et al. GEC-ESTRO recommendations for brachytherapy for head and neck squamous cell carcinomas. *Radiother Oncol* 2009;91:150–156.
211. Harrison L, Franzese F, Gaynor J, et al. Long-term results of a prospective randomized trial of adjuvant brachytherapy in the management of completely resected soft tissue sarcomas of the extremity and superficial trunk. *Int J Radiat Oncol Biol Phys* 1992;27:259–265.
227. Alektiar KM, Brennan MF, Singer S. Local control comparison of adjuvant brachytherapy to intensity-modulated radiotherapy in primary high-grade sarcoma of the extremity. *Cancer* 2011;117:3229–3234.
228. Gerbaulet A, Panis X, Flamant F, et al. Iridium afterloading curietherapy in the treatment of pediatric malignancies. The Institut Gustave Roussy experience. *Cancer* 1985;56:1274–1279.
229. Merchant TE, Parsh N, del Valle PL, et al. Brachytherapy for pediatric soft-tissue sarcoma. *Int J Radiat Oncol Biol Phys* 2000;46:427–432.
233. Nag S, Tippin D, Ruymann FB. Long-term morbidity in children treated with fractionated high-dose-rate brachytherapy for soft tissue sarcomas. *J Pediatr Hematol Oncol* 2003;25:448–452.
234. Nag S, Tippin DB. Brachytherapy for pediatric tumors. *Brachytherapy* 2003, 2:131–138.
236. Nag S, Tippin D, Ruymann F. Intraoperative high-dose-rate brachytherapy for the treatment of pediatric soft tissue sarcomas. *Int J Radiat Oncol Biol Phys* 2001; 51:729–735.
242. Laskar S, Bahl G, Ann Muckaden M, et al. Interstitial brachytherapy for childhood soft tissue sarcoma. *Pediatr Blood Cancer* 2007;49:649–655.
249. Nag S, Gunderson L, Harrison L. Techniques of intraoperative radiation therapy vs. intraoperative high dose rate brachytherapy. In: Gunderson L, et al., ed. *Intraoperative irradiation: techniques and results.* Totowa, NJ: Humana Press, 1999:111–130.
255. Nag S, Hu KS. Intraoperative high-dose-rate brachytherapy. *Surg Oncol Clin N Am* 2003;12:1079–1097.
256. International Commission on Radiological Protection 2001-2005. ICRP publication 97: Prevention of high-dose-rate brachytherapy accidents. *Ann ICRP* 2005;351–51.
257. Nag S, Dally M, De la Torre M, et al. Recommendations for implementation of high dose rate 192-Ir brachytherapy in developing countries by the Advisory Group of International Atomic Energy Agency. *Radiother Oncol* 2002;64:297–308.

Chapter 26
Radioimmunotherapy and Unsealed Radionuclide Therapy

Tod W. Speer

IMMUNOLOGY AND TARGETING CONSTRUCTS

Immunity refers to protection from disease or infectious agents.[1] Our immune system is composed of the cells and molecules responsible for the immune response, which can be divided into an early (1- to 12-hour) reaction, termed *innate immunity,* and a late (1- to >7-day) reaction, termed *adaptive immunity.* The innate immune system comprises biochemical and cellular mechanisms that exist prior to the introduction of a "foreign" or infectious agent and results in a rapid response. The innate immune system consists of epithelial barriers, phagocytic cells (neutrophils, macrophages), natural killer cells, the complement system, and cytokines. The adaptive immune system develops over time, becoming more effective with subsequent exposures of antigen. It exhibits the ability to "remember" and to respond more quickly with continued exposures to the same antigen. The adaptive immune system consists of lymphocytes and secreted antibodies. The adaptive immune system can be divided into humoral immunity and cell-mediated immunity. Concerning humoral immunity, B lymphocytes secrete antibodies for protection. Concerning cell-mediated immunity, helper T lymphocytes either activate macrophages or cytotoxic T lymphocytes, which then directly destroy pathologic (infectious or malignant) cells.

It is well known that the host's immune system is important for preventing the growth and development of cancer.[2] A large body of literature exists supporting the concept that the host immune system interacts with tumorigenesis and tumor progression. It has been shown in animal models and in the clinic that cancer immune surveillance is exceedingly important. For example, mice with an impaired innate or adaptive immune system will be more susceptible to develop chemically induced or spontaneous cancers. Additionally, the malignant transformation of cells in animals and humans, caused by the accumulation of somatic mutations and/or the deregulation of oncogenes or tumor suppressor genes, results in the expression of tumor antigens (TAs). These TAs are often recognized by the immune system as documented by TA-specific T-cell precursors and natural killer cells, found in the peripheral blood of cancer patients, capable of killing tumor cells. Further evidence of cancer immune surveillance exists in patients with genetic or drug-induced immunosuppression. Transplant patients exhibit a predisposition for certain malignancies (squamous cell carcinoma, basal cell carcinoma, Kaposi's sarcoma, melanoma, and lymphoma). Patients with Chediak-Higashi and Wiskott-Aldrich syndrome demonstrate an increased rate of lymphoproliferative malignancies. Discontinuing immunosuppressive drugs in solid organ allograph patients with occult malignant melanoma has resulted in tumor regression.

Despite the evidence of cancer genesis and progression in immune-compromised hosts, the majority of cancers develop in seemingly immune-competent individuals. The last decade of research has revealed that cancer cells have developed means to avoid immune detection and surveillance, either through the selection of nonimmunogenic tumor cells and/or the active suppression of the immune response. It has therefore been rightfully suggested that "tumor immune escape" be added to Hanahan and Weinberg's six hallmarks of cancer (self-sufficiency in growth signals, insensitivity to antigrowth signals, tissue invasion and metastasis, limitless replicative potential, sustained angiogenesis, and evasion of apoptosis).

The targets for radioimmunotherapy (RIT) typically consist of tumor-associated antigens (TAAs). The reason for this is because the cytotoxic radionuclide must be delivered preferentially to malignant tissue and should avoid normal tissue. To date, >2,000 TAAs have been identified (http://www2.licr.org/CancerImmunomeDB). One of the main methodologies used to identify TAAs is termed *SEREX* (serologic analysis of recombinant cDNA libraries). SEREX involves a bacteriophage recombinant cDNA expression library, prepared from various malignancies (isolated tumors or malignant cell lines) or testis tissue.[3] This cDNA expression library is transduced in *Escherichia coli* to produce a recombinant protein library. These various proteins (clones) are then tested against the serum from autologous cancer patients. Clones that react to IgG antibodies are identified and are then further characterized as TAAs. Many of these SEREX-identified TAAs have been elucidated by other processes and laboratories. This has led to the concept of a finite number of TAAs that are produced in cancer patients and are potentially identified by the immune system. These finite TAAs are collectively referred to as the cancer immunome. SEREX-defined antigens, representing broad categories, may be organized as follows: mutational antigens, amplified or overexpressed antigens, differentiation antigens, and cancer/testis antigens. Within these categories, only a limited number of TAAs have been used as targets for RIT (Table 26.1).

TABLE 26.1 SELECT MONOCLONAL ANTIBODIES EVALUATED FOR RADIOIMMUNOTHERAPY

Malignancy	*Antigen*	*Antibody*
Colorectal cancer	CEA	cT84.66, hMN-14, A5B7
	TAG-72	B72.3, CC49
	A33	anti-A33
	EpCAM	NR-LU-10, NR-LU-13
	DNA histone H1	chTNT-1/B
Breast cancer	MUC1	huBrE-3, m170
	L6	chL6
	TAG-72	CC49
	CEA	cT84.66
Ovarian cancer	MUC1	HMFG1
	Folate receptor	cMov18
	TAG-72	B72.3, CC49
Prostate cancer	PSMA	huJ591
	TAG-72	CC49
Lung cancer	DNA histone H1	chTNT-1/B
	TAG-72	CC49
Head and neck cancer	CD44v6	U36, BIWA4
Glioma	EGFR	425
	Tenascin	816 C, BC4
Melanoma	p97	96.5
Renal cancer	G250 glycoprotein	cG250
Medullary thyroid cancer	CEA	cT84.66, hMN-14, NP-4
Neuroblastoma	Ganglioside GD2	3F8
	NCAM	UJ13 A, ERIC-1

CEA, carcinoembryonic antigen; PSMA, prostate-specific membrane antigen; EGFR, epidermal growth factor receptor; NCAM, neural cell adhesion molecule.

From Wong YC, Williams LE, Yazaki PJ. Radioimmunotherapy of colorectal cancer. In: Speer TW, ed. *Targeted radionuclide therapy.* Philadelphia: Lippincott Williams & Wilkins, 2011:325.

The ideal target for RIT targeting constructs would be one that is overexpressed on cancer cells, is uniformly expressed, is not found to any significant level in normal tissue, is not shed into the circulation, and exhibits an important role in tumor growth and progression.[4] TAAs, as the name implies, are antigens "associated" with tumors but are also present in normal tissue. True tumor-specific antigens have not yet been identified and utilized. Overexpression is necessary because typical targeting constructs require antigen densities $\geq 10^5$ receptors on each cell for adequate targeting. A homogenous antigen expression is desired so that a uniform activity distribution of the radionuclide will result. Nonuniform activity distributions (heterogeneity of antigen in target tissue being one potential cause) will significantly lower the effectiveness of RIT by subsequently resulting in nonuniform or heterogeneous dose distributions.[5] This is particularly important for radionuclides with short path lengths of the emitted particles (i.e., Auger and α-particle emitters). Radionuclides with longer path lengths, such as high-energy β-emitters, can partly overcome the problem of nonuniform dose distributions through the crossfire effect. If the target antigen is significantly shed into the circulation, the targeting construct may bind and "complex" with the antigen. This will result in a more rapid clearance of the RIT agent and a much less effective treatment. If the TAA has an important signaling role, then subsequent binding of the targeting construct will most likely add to the cytotoxicity of the radionuclide because of the blockade or promotion of intracellular signaling, potentially resulting in disruption of growth pathways important for tumor growth. Some TAAs (receptors) will internalize when bound by the targeting construct. In truth, most receptors internalize, although they do so at different rates. A rapid internalization process will have an impact on the type of radionuclide that is selected and potentially on the delivery strategy of the RIT agent.

A multitude of agents have been used as carriers (targeting constructs) for the targeted delivery of radiation to cancer. These consist of antibodies, antibody fragments, peptides, affibodies, aptamers, and nanostructures (i.e., liposomes, nanoparticles, microparticles, nanoshells, and minicells). By an exceedingly large margin, intact monoclonal antibodies (mAbs) have dominated the field of RIT as targeting constructs[6] (Fig. 26.1). In humans, there are five classes or isotypes of antibodies (IgA, IgD, IgE, IgG, and IgM). IgG is the most commonly used mAb for RIT because it is the most prevalent antibody in serum and has the longest serum half-life, typically measured in weeks (approximately 23 days). IgG is further divided into four subtypes, IgG_{1-4}. IgG antibodies are large glycoprotein macromolecules, with an atomic mass of approximately 150,000 dalton (Da) or 150 kDa. The "y-shaped structure" (Fig. 26.1A) consists of two Fab fragments (fragment antigen binding; approximately 50,000 Da each) and an Fc fragment (crystallizable fragment; approximately 50,000 Da).

The "tip" of each Fab fragment has a variable amino acid sequence, from one mAb to another. Accordingly, each tip is an antigen binding site (ABS) and is responsible for antigen recognition. Each ABS forms a noncovalent bond (electrostatic forces, van der Waals forces, hydrophobic interactions, and hydrogen bonds) with the target or antigen. The specific region of an antigen, which binds to the ABS, is referred to as an epitope. It has been proposed that a million or more different antibodies exist in various individuals. Theoretically, $>10^9$ different antibodies can be produced. The outer core of the mAb consists of two identical light chains (outer portion of the Fab fragment) designated with an "L." The inner core, consisting of the Fc region

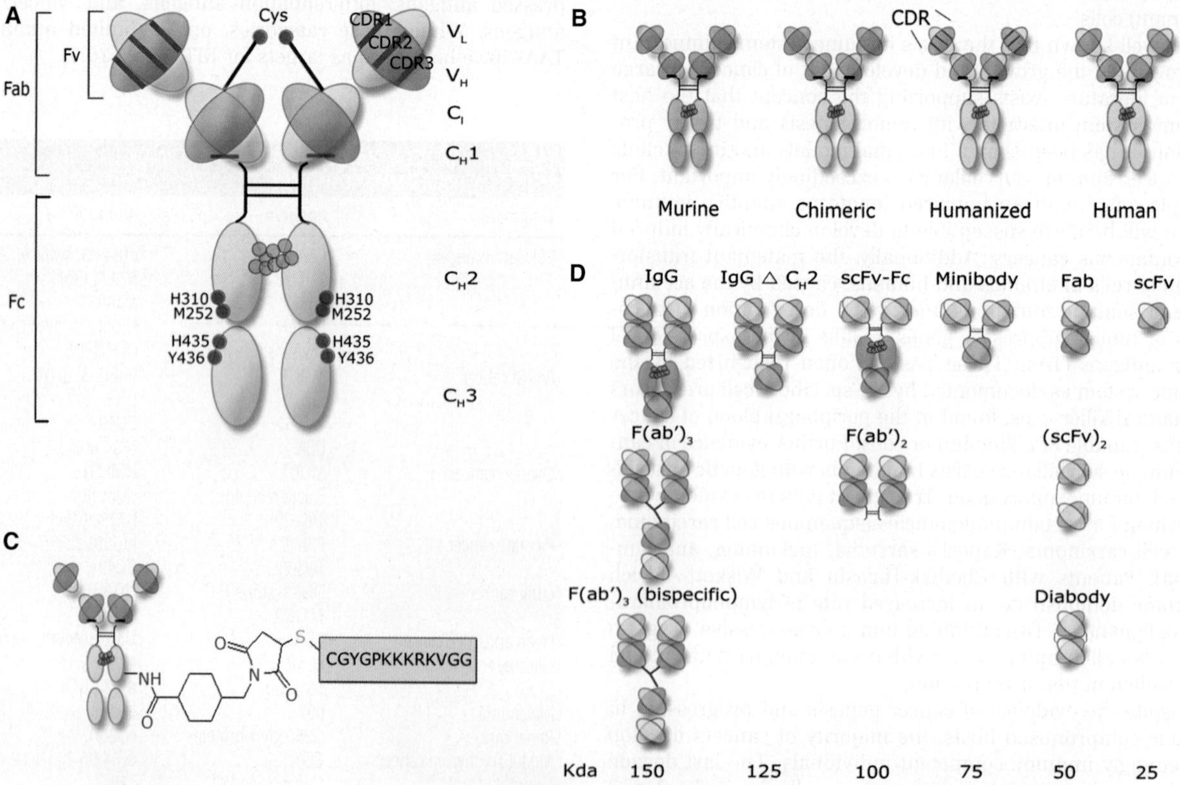

FIGURE 26.1. Antibody engineering: strategies to improve the therapeutic index in radioimmunotherapy. **A:** Typical structure of a humanized IgG antibody. The following engineering strategies are presented: *Red dots,* mutations in amino acids involved in FcRn binding that influence the pharmacokinetics of the IgG; *CDR1-3,* murine CDRs grafted into a human IgG backbone to humanize the antibody; *Cys,* engineered cysteine residues for site-specific conjugation. **B:** Humanization strategies: *purple,* indicating the murine portion of the IgG, and *blue,* indicating the human portion of the IgG **(C)** introducing a nuclear localizing signal **(D)** monospecific and bispecific fragments used in radioimmunotherapeutic strategies. CDR, complementarity-determining regions; CH, constant domain heavy chain; CL, constant domain light chain; Fc, crystallizable fragment; Fv, variable fragment. (From Burvenich IJG, Scott AM. The delivery construct: maximizing the therapeutic ratio of targeted radionuclide therapy. In: Speer TW, ed. *Targeted radionuclide therapy.* Philadelphia: Lippincott Williams & Wilkins, 2011:238.)

and the inner Fab region, is designated as heavy or "H." Both the light and heavy chains contain homologous, 110 amino acid sequences that fold on one another and are connected by a disulfide bridge, resulting in "globular" motif or loop, called an Ig domain. There are three constant heavy domains (C_H1-3) and only one constant light (C_L), one variable heavy (V_H), and one variable light (V_L) domain. The ABS consists of a V_L and a V_H region. Within each variable domain, there are three hypervariable regions (about 10 amino acid residues per hypervariable region) that form a three-dimensional surface that is "complementary" to the shape of the antigen surface; they are called complementarity-determining regions (CDRs). A total of six CDRs come together to form the ABS. There are two ABS for each IgG mAb; hence, each IgG mAb is considered bivalent.

Affinity refers to the strength of the bond between the ABS and the antigen. The strength of this bond is represented by the dissociation constant (K_d). Avidity refers to the overall strength of the ABS-antigen interaction, depending on both the affinity and the valency of the interaction. It should be noted that a high-affinity interaction can improve specific delivery of the RIT agent and reduce overall dosing requirements. Increasing the affinity indefinitely, however, may decrease tumor penetration. It has been demonstrated that an affinity of 10^{-7} to 10^{-8} M is needed for tumor retention, whereas affinities in the range of $\geq 10^{-10}$ to 10^{-11} M will result in retention in normal tissue and asymmetric binding in tumor tissue, termed the *binding site barrier*.[7] The binding site barrier phenomenon may be at least partially overcome by increasing the antibody mass, or the overall delivered quantity of antibody.

Unconjugated antibodies—those not attached to a radionuclide or cytotoxic agent—will also mediate biologic activities. These activities may be mediated by the Fc region of the mAb or may be Fc independent. Fc-mediated interactions are termed *effector functions* and consist of antibody-dependent cell-mediated cytotoxicity (ADCC) and complement-dependent cytotoxicity (CDC).[7] Concerning ADCC, interaction of the Fc region of the antibody with Fc receptors (located on immune effector cells) results in the subsequent phagocytosis or lysis of the antibody-bound cancer cell. CDC is initiated by the interaction of soluble blood proteins and the Fc region. Epitope-dependent (Fc-independent) functions of the mAb may result in the inhibition of ligand binding, inhibition of ligand-induced dimerization, and inhibition of receptor shedding. These epitope-dependent functions are characteristic of modern-day biologics that target growth factor receptors, such as cetuximab and trastuzumab.

The original technology used to produce mAbs was first published by Kohler and Milstein[8] in 1975 and is referred to as the hybridoma technique. The technique has propagated the use of murine mAbs for research and for therapy in the clinic. In fact, the two U.S. Food and Drug Administration (FDA) RIT agents used to treat non-Hodgkin lymphoma (NHL; ibritumomab tiuxetan and tositumomab) are murine mAbs. Although these agents are delivered as single instillations in patients typically with decreased immune recognition capabilities, there is a concern that human antiglobulin antibodies (HAGAs) will develop. If this phenomenon occurs in response to murine antibodies, then the resulting HAGAs will be called human antimouse antibodies (HAMAs). The formation of HAMAs will expedite blood clearance of the antibody and decrease targeting capabilities as well as potentially cause various adverse symptoms. Two main strategies, through the use of genetic engineering, have emerged[6] that reduce the immunogenicity of mAbs: (a) the production of antibody chimeras derived from both murine and human DNA and (b) the production of humanized or fully human antibodies (Fig. 26.1B). Chimeric antibodies retain murine V_H and V_L domains, whereas humanized antibodies retain murine CDRs. Fully human antibodies retain no murine components. Although the development of HAGA may not be important after a single dose of mAb in lymphoma patients, its induction will have a greater detrimental impact for patients with solid tumors when treated with RIT.[4] As can be seen in Table 26.2, as the targeting construct moves from a murine to humanized forms, the immunogenicity is lessened. This concept is important to employ multiple doses or fractions of RIT agents. Figure 26.1C illustrates the concept of adding a nuclear localizing signal to bring the mAb from the cell surface or cytoplasm into the cell nucleus.

Another factor that is critical and influences antibody targeting and pharmacokinetics is antibody molecular size (Fig. 26.1D). As stated previously, RIT has been less successful for treating solid tumors than hematologic malignancies. This is largely because of the lack of radiosensitivity of epithelial tumors (compared to hematologic malignancies) and the poor penetration of mAbs into large tumors. The decreased penetration of 150 kDa antibodies into large tumors is a direct result of increased tumor interstitial pressure, an aberrant tumor vasculature, and an abnormal tumor extracellular matrix.[9,10–12] Additionally, 150 kDa antibodies need longer periods of time to accrete into tumors and have long serum half-lives. When radiolabeled, a long serum half-life of the targeting construct will increase exposure of the bone marrow to radiation, which causes hematologic toxicity and limits the amount of antibody and radionuclide that can be given. To overcome some of these issues, methods have been used to generate antibody fragments of varying size and valency. These smaller fragments

TABLE 26.2 ANTIBODY IMMUNOGENICITY FOLLOWING A SINGLE ADMINISTRATION (SELECT SOLID TUMOR RADIOIMMUNOTHERAPY TRIALS)

First Author of Study (Year)	*Antibody*	*Type*	*Number of Patients*	*Percent Antibody Response (%)*
Breitz (1992)	^{186}Re-NR-LU-10	Murine	15	100
Meredith (1994)	^{131}I-CC49	Murine	15	100
Welt (1994)	^{131}I-mAb A33	Murine	23	100
Mulligan (1995)	^{177}Lu-CC49	Murine	9	100
Yu (1996)	^{131}I-COL-1	Murine	18	83 (prevented additional RIT in 2 patients)
Behr (1997)	^{131}I-NP-4	Murine	32	94
Juweid (1997)	^{131}I-MN-14	Murine	14	100
Meredith (1992)	^{131}I-cB72.3	Chimeric	12	58
Weiden (1993)	^{186}Re-NR-LU-13	Chimeric	8	75
Meredith (1995)	^{125}I-17-1 A	Chimeric	15	13
Wong (2000)	^{90}Y-cT84.66	Chimeric	21	52 (prevented additional RIT in 8 patients)
Kramer (1998)	^{111}In-huBrE3	Humanized	7	14
Hajjar (2002)	^{131}I-hMN-14	Humanized	15	47
Goldsmith (2002)	^{90}Y-huJ591	Humanized	19	0
Borjesson (2003)	^{186}Re-BIWA 4	Humanized	20	10

RIT, radioimmunotherapy.

Modified from Wong YC, Williams LE, Yazaki PJ. Radioimmunotherapy of colorectal cancer. In: Speer TW, ed. *Targeted radionuclide therapy*. Philadelphia: Lippincott Williams & Wilkins, 2011:321–351.

TABLE 26.3 TARGETING AND PHARMACOKINETICS OF INTACT IgG AND VARIOUS ANTIBODY FRAGMENTS

	IgG	F(ab')2	CH2-Deletion	Minibody	Fab	Diabody	scFv
MW	150	100	120	80	50	40–50	20–25
Serum half-life	2–3 d[a]	1 d	Hours	Hours	Hours	Hours	1 hr
Metabolism	Liver	Liver	Liver	Liver	Kidney	Kidney	Kidney
Tumor uptake[b]	*****	****	***	***	**	**	*
Time to accretion	Days	1 d	Hours	Hours	Hours	Hours	1 hr

MW, molecular weight (kDa).
[a]Serum half-life for fully human IgG is approximately 23 days.
[b]Tumor uptake values range from large (*****) to small (*).

exhibit superior tumor penetration and clear more rapidly from the circulation. However, if clearance from the circulation is too rapid, this can further limit tumor penetration. Table 26.3 summarizes these general concepts for targeting constructs of various molecular weights.

Although mAbs and their fragments represent the most commonly used targeting constructs for the delivery of a radionuclide to malignant tissue, other agents are either in use or are being investigated, consisting of peptides,[13,14,15,16] affibody molecules,[17,18–19] and aptamers.[20,21–23] Nanostructures are also being investigated as carriers of radionuclides.[24,25–26,27] In their unmodified form, the targeting capabilities of nanostructures are rather nonspecific.[24,28]

Peptides are small amino acid sequences (typically 7 to 14 amino acids) that serve as opioids, hormones, sweeteners, protein substrate inhibitors, releasing factors, antibiotics, and cytoprotectors.[29] The overexpression of receptors that are specific for various peptides has led to the development of peptide-based radiopharmaceuticals.[30] Somatostatin is one of the most common peptides and is overexpressed in a multitude of malignancies, including breast cancer, small cell lung cancer, medullary thyroid cancer, and neuroendocrine tumors (NETs). Somatostatin is rapidly degraded; however, its derivative, octreotide, is very stable. Octreoscan (indium-111 diethylenetriamine pentaacetic acid [^{111}In-DTPA]) has been shown to be highly diagnostic for NETs. Affibody molecules[17] are classified as affinity ligands or scaffold proteins that are approximately 7 to 9 kDa. These proteins are based on a 58 amino acid residue derived from staphylococcus protein A, which binds immunoglobulin. Various applications have been applied to affibody use, including radiolabeled targeting for therapy. Aptamers are small (8 to 12 kDa; 10 to 100 bases) single- or double-stranded oligonucleotides that are selected in vitro from a random library termed *SELEX* (systemic evolution of ligands by exponential enrichment). Aptamers are an attractive alternative to larger mAbs because they are easy to produce, have a low cost of production, exhibit high affinities, have a small size, are rapidly cleared from the circulation, have an unlimited shelf life, and are of low immunogenicity. Their major detriment is a short serum half-life (measured in minutes to hours) in their unmodified form. Aptamers are amazingly versatile and can recognize nearly any type of target, from metal ions to whole cells and even entire organisms. A complete database of known aptamers can be found at the Ellington Lab Web site (http://aptamer.icmb.utexas.edu). The current lack of radiolabeled aptamers is simply a portrayal of a very promising technology in its infancy.

THE PHYSICS AND RADIOBIOLOGY OF RADIOIMMUNOTHERAPY

RIT delivers radiation to the target tissue in a continuous, although declining, low dose rate (LDR) fashion. Typical dose rates for RIT are in the range of 10 to 20 cGy per hour. The total dose delivered by RIT is low, in the range of 1,500 to 2,000 cGy,[31] with an effective half-life of 24 to 72 hours. This can be compared to the high dose rate (HDR) delivery of radiation by external-beam radiation therapy (EBRT). EBRT typically will deliver radiation at a dose rate of 100 to 500 cGy per minute. It should be noted that these total dose ranges for RIT occur despite overall very low percent injected doses (0.1% to 10.0%) that ultimately localize in target tissue.[32] Regardless, radiation-induced apoptosis is still induced.

The most radiosensitive component of a cell is the DNA.[33] Irradiation of tissue results in DNA damage. This damage may be either repaired or result in permanent damage. Permanent damage will cause cell death. By using a target-hit model, the tissue response end point of cell death may be used to relate absorbed dose of ionizing radiation to cell death. When the log surviving fraction of irradiated cells is plotted on the ordinate and the dose (Gy) is plotted on the abscissa, a cell survival curve is generated (Fig. 26.2). The "hit" that results in most lethal events is a double-strand break (DSB) of DNA. The mathematical term, α, represents the initial slope of the cell survival curve. It is a constant for a given tumor (or tissue) and can be thought of as the probability, per unit of absorbed dose, of creating a lethal DSB.[34] The target is the resulting DSB, and the cell survival versus absorbed dose is a pure exponential function:

$$S = e^{-\alpha D}, \quad (1)$$

where S is the surviving cell fraction and D is the mean absorbed dose. Ionizing irradiation may also cause nonlethal single-strand breaks (SSBs). If these events accumulate, they may become lethal. The constant, β, is used to describe this phenomenon and represents the more distant, "linear" portion of the cell survival curve. The linear-quadratic (LQ) model combines the two processes into a continuously bending curve:

$$S = e^{-\alpha D - \beta D^2} \quad (2)$$

The shoulder on the cell survival curve is typically observed when HDRs of radiation are employed (green line in Fig. 26.2). In RIT, the dose rate is 1,000-fold lower; therefore, the quadratic portion of the curve will have a much lower impact on survival because many SSBs, considered sublethal damage, will

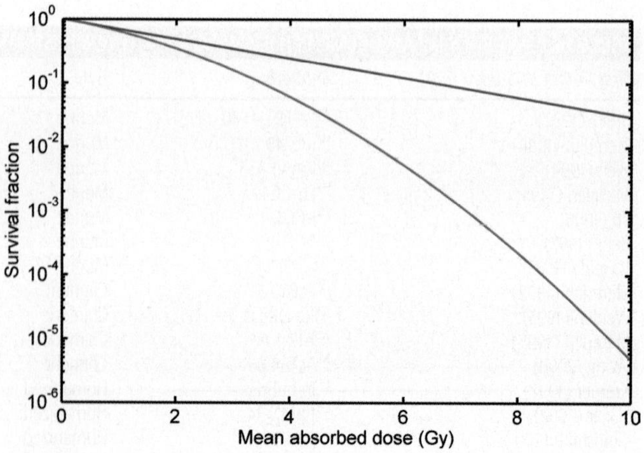

FIGURE 26.2. Cell survival curves following treatment with radiotherapy. The *blue curve* represents low dose rate radiotherapy; the *green curve* represents high dose rate radiotherapy. (From Bernhardt P, Speer TW. Modeling the systemic cure with targeted radionuclide therapy. In: Speer TW, ed. *Targeted radionuclide therapy.* Philadelphia: Lippincott Williams & Wilkins, 2011:265.)

TABLE 26.4 COMMONLY USED RADIONUCLIDES FOR RADIOIMMUNOTHERAPY

Radionuclide	*Physical Half-Life*	*E_{max} (MeV)*	*Maximum Range in Tissue*	*LET (keV/μm)*	*Approximate Cell Diameters*
β-Emitters		*β-Particle*		**0.2**	
Yttrium-90	2.7 d	2.30	12.0 mm		400–1,100
Iodine-131	8.0 d	0.81	2.0 mm		10–230
Lutetium-177	6.7 d	0.50	1.5 mm		4–180
Rhenium-186	3.8 d	1.10	3.6 mm		15–360
Rhenium-188	17.0 hr	2.10	11.0 mm		200–1,000
Copper-67	2.6 d	0.60	2.8 mm		5–210
α-Emitters		*α- Particle*		**80**	
Bismuth-213	45.7 min	5.87	70–100 μm		7–10
Astatine-211	7.2 hr	5.87	55–60 μm		5–6
Low-Energy Electron Emitters		*Low-Energy Electron*		**4–26**	
Iodine-125	60.1 d	0.35	2–500 nm		<1
Gallium-67	3.3 d	0.18	2–500 nm		<1
Indium-111	2.83 d	0.04–0.2	2–500 nm		<1

LET, linear energy transfer; E_{max}, maximum energy.

be repaired during the more lengthy delivery of LDR radiation. This will result in a "small" or absent observable shoulder. Thus, when estimating cell survival for RIT, α alone will define the radiosensitivity of the tumor (blue line in Fig. 26.2). Considering dose rate, RIT is approximately 20% less effective than HDR EBRT.[31] RIT, however, does appear to be relatively effective. This phenomenon can be attributed to many radiobiologic processes that appear to cause greater than predicted rates of apoptosis. These processes include low-dose/dose rate apoptosis, low-dose hyperradiosensitivity-increased radioresistance, inverse dose rate effect (G_2 synchronization), radiation-induced biologic bystander effect, and the crossfire effect.[32]

Various radionuclides have been used for RIT (Table 26.4), and their physical properties have been extensively reviewed in the nuclear medicine literature. They can be grouped into three basic categories depending on the type of emitted particulate radiation. Radionuclides that emit high-energy electrons are referred to as β-emitters. These electrons have maximum path lengths in tissue from 1.5 to 12.0 mm. This translates into a range of approximately 130 to 1,100 cell diameters. The most commonly used β-emitters for RIT are yttrium-90 [^{90}Y] and iodine-131 [^{131}I]. The maximum range of electrons in tissue for ^{90}Y and ^{131}I is 12 mm and 2 mm, respectively. It should be noted however, that 90% of the electron energy is deposited over 5.2 mm for ^{90}Y and 0.7 mm for ^{131}I. This range of 90% energy deposition is referred to as the R_{90}. The most commonly used α-emitter for RIT is ^{211}At. An α-particle is a helium nucleus that has a maximum range in tissue of 55 to 100 μm (5 to 10 cell diameters). Although it has a short range, the α-particle is very destructive and has a high linear energy transfer (LET). Low-energy electron emitters also emit radiation that is high LET and have path lengths between 2 and 500 nm (width of a double strand helix). Auger emitters, such as ^{111}In or iodine-125 [^{125}I], are most effective if delivered to the nucleus of a cell or incorporated into the DNA.

Because radionuclides have different energy spectra for their emitted particulate radiation, they will each interact with tissue and deposit their energy over varying distances. There is therefore a relation between type of radionuclide, tumor size, absorbed dose, and ultimately tumor cure probability (TCP). If it is assumed that a tumor has a spherical volume and contains a uniform and identical activity concentration of a radionuclide, then the TCP can be calculated for different radionuclides and tumor size.[35] Figure 26.3 illustrates the relation between tumor mass and TCP for astatine-211 [^{211}At], lutetium-177 [^{177}Lu], ^{131}I, and ^{90}Y. As can be seen, there is an optimum tumor size for the different energy spectra for each radionuclide such that the TCP is maximized. If the tumor is small relative to the emission range, then much of the energy will be lost to the surrounding tissue and the absorbed dose will be low. As the tumor size increases, more energy is absorbed until the maximum TCP is reached. As the tumor further increases in size, the absorbed energy remains high, although fewer cells are affected by the radiation and TCP begins to decrease.[35]

Labeling the targeting construct with the appropriate radionuclide (radiochemistry) is exceedingly important and equally complex. Radionuclides are attached to targeting constructs by either using a "linker" molecule, termed a *bifunctional chelating agent* (BCA) or by a chemical reaction that forms a covalent bond between the radionuclide and the targeting construct. Three basic scientific fields converged to make radiochemistry a reality: coordination chemistry, directed biologic targeting, and the medical application of radiopharmaceuticals.[36] In general, metallic radionuclides will require a BCA for labeling, and radiohalogens will require a chemical reaction (halogenation). The most prevalent therapeutic radionuclides used in RIT are ^{90}Y (metallic radionuclide) and ^{131}I (radiohalogen). One of the most commonly used BCAs is DTPA—a polyaminopolycarboxylate straight chain ligand. Tiuxetan, a modified DTPA molecule, is used as a linker molecule to chelate ^{90}Y to ibritumomab (^{90}Y ibritumomab tiuxetan; Zevalin, Spectrum Pharmaceuticals, Inc., Irvine, CA). Tiuxetan forms a urea-type bond[37] to the antibody (ibritumomab), and its five carboxyl groups interact with and chelate ^{90}Y to form a stable coordination sphere. The halogenation reaction that bonds ^{131}I to the targeting construct (^{131}I tositumomab; Bexxar, GlaxoSmithKline, Philadelphia, PA) is called

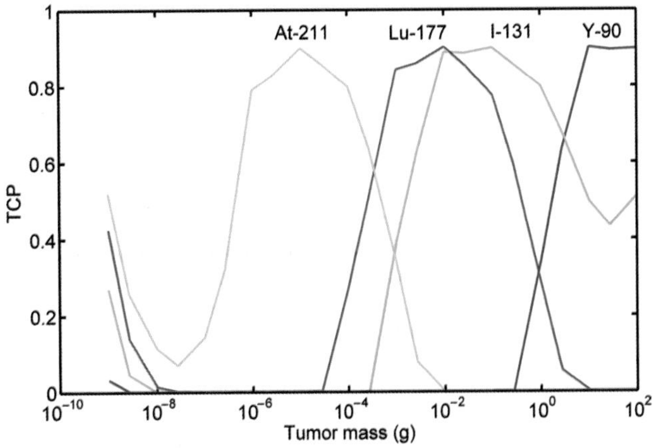

FIGURE 26.3. Tumor control probability (TCP) for various radionuclides. TCP = 0.9 versus tumor mass. The optimal TCP for various tumor masses when treated with ^{211}At, ^{177}Lu, ^{131}I, and ^{90}Y. This corresponds to approximately 10^{-5}, 10^{-2}, 0.1, and 10 g, respectively. (From Bernhardt P, Speer TW. Modeling the systemic cure with targeted radionuclide therapy. In: Speer TW, ed. *Targeted radionuclide therapy.* Philadelphia: Lippincott Williams & Wilkins, 2011:266.)

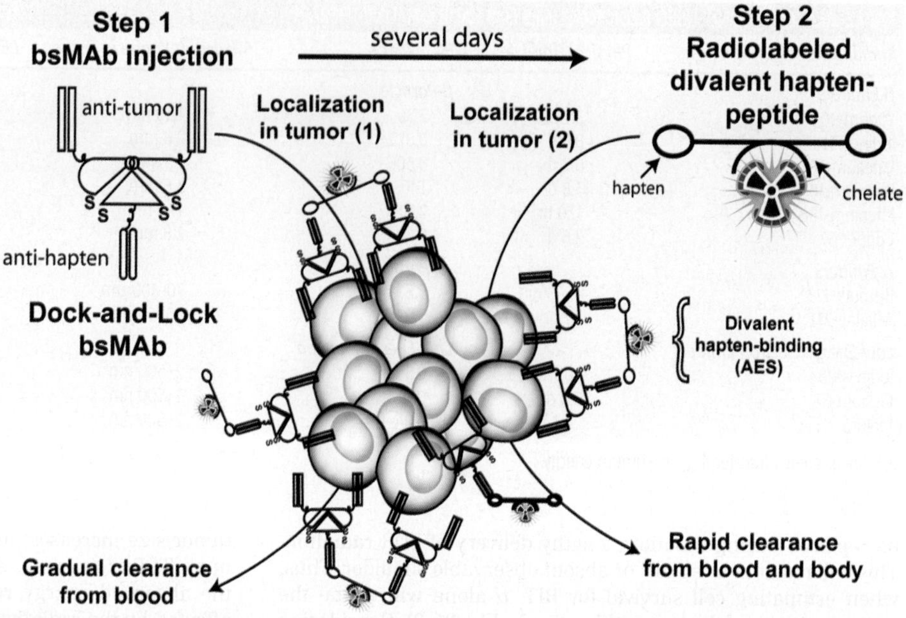

FIGURE 26.4. Bispecific pretargeting procedure. The bsMAb is injected, and over several days it will localize in the tumor and clear from the blood. The bsMAb shown in this example is based on the dock-and-lock method for preparing recombinant bsMAb that has two binding arms for the tumor and one for the hapten. Once the molar concentration of the bsMAb is low enough, the radiolabeled hapten-peptide is given. The hapten-peptide has two haptens for more stable binding within the tumor, perhaps by cross-linking two adjacent bsMAb through a process known as the affinity-enhancement system (AES). The peptide portion usually contains four to five D-amino acids with a single chelator bound to one of the amino acids that is used to capture the radionuclide. (From Sharkey RM, Goldenberg DM. Pretargeted radioimmunotherapy. In: Speer TW, ed. *Targeted radionuclide therapy.* Philadelphia: Lippincott Williams & Wilkins, 2011:194.)

iodination. Although there are many permutations of the iodination reaction, it basically inserts ^{131}I into a tyrosine group on the mAb without the need for a chelation molecule. Regardless of the required labeling technique, it is incumbent that a reasonably high labeling yield, unaltered biodistribution, stability of the radionuclide, and immunoreactivity are preserved.

To date, a single instillation or fraction of the RIT agent is delivered systemically (i.e., Zevalin and Bexxar). It is well known that although relatively effective for hematologic malignancies, RIT is much less effective for treating solid tumors. Therefore, a number of strategies are being developed that will potentially increase the effectiveness of RIT. These strategies include modulating the tumor microenvironment, using pretargeting techniques, extracorporeal delivery, combined modality therapy (CMT), fractionation, multiple radionuclides (radionuclide cocktail), increasing antibody mass (the amount of antibody delivered systemically), alteration of the physical properties (size and affinity) of the targeting construct, and employing different types of LET radiation (i.e., β-emitter vs. α-emitter). All in all, these strategies are designed to—either alone or in combination—deliver more radiation to the tumor, make the radiation more cytotoxic, or decrease the exposure of radiation to bone marrow. As a result, the tumor to blood ratio will increase, and ultimately the therapeutic ratio will increase. The pretargeting strategy warrants further discussion.[38–40,41]

Because radiolabeled mAbs take 2 to 3 days to localize or accrete into tumors, antibody-based RIT results in a prolonged exposure of the bone marrow to radiation, causing hematologic toxicity and rendering the bone marrow as the dose-limiting normal tissue. Accordingly, the tumor/blood ratios of mAb will only slightly favor the tumor. This situation can seriously limit the successful prospects of antibody-based RIT, especially for treating solid tumors. Truly, smaller targeting constructs (antibody fragments) can be used for RIT, and they will exhibit pharmacokinetics that result in a more rapid blood clearance, allowing for the administration of higher activities. Unfortunately, because of the lower overall tumor accretion and retention of antibody fragments, the advantage of a more rapid blood clearance is usually offset. Therefore, the ideal delivery construct would manifest the targeting properties of an intact mAb but exhibit the blood clearance pattern of a small molecular weight construct. Because no known such construct exists, pretargeting strategies have been developed. The basic premise of pretargeting is to separate the delivery of a large, macromolecule-targeting construct (prolonged circulation time) from the delivery of a much smaller cytotoxic radioconjugate (more rapid circulation time). Two main approaches have been employed: a bispecific monoclonal antibody (bsmAb) system and a streptavidin-biotin system. In the bsmAb system (Fig. 26.4), a portion of the antibody has affinity for the tumor (antitumor), and another portion has affinity for the radionuclide carrier ligand or hapten-peptide (antihapten). Initially (step 1), a large "saturation" dose of the unlabeled bsmAb is administered, and the antibody localizes in the tumor over several days. Occasionally, a clearing step is used to facilitate the clearance of the bsmAb from the circulation. Subsequently (step 2), a radionuclide conjugated to a hapten-peptide is administered that has high affinity for the antihapten portion of the bsmAb. This step results in a rapid distribution of the radionuclide in the tumor owing to the high affinity of the hapten-peptide for the bsmAb. Because the hapten-peptide has a small molecular weight, it will clear rapidly from the body and result in a low bone marrow exposure to radiation.[42] In the streptavidin-biotin system, streptavidin is conjugated to the initial pretargeting macromolecule, and biotin is conjugated to the radionuclide. Streptavidin and biotin have a very high affinity for each other (10^{15} M^{-1}). When either system is used, the tumor/blood ratios of the targeting agent are significantly increased.[43,44]

CONJUGATED THERAPY

To date, considerable progress has been made in the field of RIT for many different malignancies including NHL, Hodgkin lymphoma, leukemia, multiple myeloma, colorectal carcinoma, hepatocellular carcinoma (HCC), central nervous system (CNS) malignancies, medullary thyroid cancer, ovarian cancer, head and neck cancer, prostate cancer, renal cell carcinoma, osteosarcoma, NETs, melanoma, and pediatric malignancies. Although promising data is emerging for most disease sites, the hematologic malignancies appear to be the most radioresponsive. Progress has been less sanguine for solid tumor malignancies, and phase III trials are lacking.[45,46–47,48–49] For the sake of clarity and brevity, this section will focus only on clinically relevant phase II/III trials and U.S. FDA (or its international equivalent)-approved RIT therapeutics.

Hematologic Trials and Approved Therapeutic Agents

Currently, there are two U.S. FDA-approved RIT agents in the United States: ^{90}Y ibritumomab tiuxetan (Zevalin; 2002) and ^{131}I tositumomab (Bexxar; 2003). Zevalin has U.S. FDA approval for relapsed or refractory follicular NHL and as a frontline adjuvant agent for follicular NHL achieving a complete response (CR) or partial response (PR) to induction chemotherapy. Bexxar has U.S. FDA approval for the relapse or refractory setting as well as transformed NHL. Both are murine IgG mAbs that target the CD20 surface antigen on follicular NHL.[50] ^{90}Y ibritumomab tiuxetan utilizes ^{90}Y, a pure β-particle emitter with a physical half-life of 2.7 days. The β-particle has an energy of 2.3 MeV and a maximum tissue penetration of approximately 12.0 mm (R_{90} = 5.2 mm). Tiuxetan is a DTPA-type chelate that attaches ^{90}Y to the mAb, ibritumomab. Because there is no gamma emission in the spectrum of this isotope, it is not visualized by gamma camera scans. As a result, a biodistribution assessment cannot be performed. Therefore, a surrogate imaging radionuclide that emits gamma radiation (^{111}In) is required. In contrast, ^{131}I tositumomab is a mixed β/gamma emitter. The gamma spikes at 364 keV, and the beta emission has energy of 0.6 MeV. The maximum range in tissue of the β-particle is 2.3 mm (R_{90} = 0.7 mm). This agent can be imaged on gamma camera to calculate total body clearance. Although theoretical arguments can be rendered as to why one or the other therapeutic agent may have an advantage based on physical characteristics of the emission spectra, there is no convincing evidence that either Zevalin or Bexxar provides a clinical benefit for treating follicular NHL over each other, and they both appear to be mutually supportive.

For both agents, the treatment is delivered over 1 to 2 weeks. On day 1, both protocols deliver an infusion of nonradioactive (cold) anti-CD20 antibody (Zevalin employs rituximab; Bexxar employs tositumomab) designed to saturate the CD20 antigen sink (depletion of peripheral B-cells and the binding of nonspecific sites in the liver and spleen) and provide antibody mass, which improves biodistribution and tumor targeting.[51,52] The administered activity for Zevalin is based on weight (0.4 mCi/kg for a platelet count ≥150,000; 0.3 mCi/kg for a platelet count of 100,000 to 149,000; maximum of 32 mCi). A single gamma scan (^{111}In ibritumomab tiuxetan) is used to confirm a normal biodistribution on days 3 to 4. A review of the Zevalin imaging registry reveals that only 0.6% of scans exhibited an altered biodistribution. The administered activity for Bexxar is based on a calculated total body clearance (three scans over 1 week) that delivers a total body (red bone marrow) dose of 75 cGy. This calculation is reduced to a total body dose of 65 cGy for a platelet count <150,000. Eligible patients for both Zevalin and Bexxar are also required to have an absolute neutrophil count (ANC) ≥1,500 and a bone marrow biopsy that reveals <25% involvement with lymphoma.

Relapse Setting

Table 26.5 summarizes significant prospective phase II/III clinical trials providing evidence for the use of RIT for treating relapsed or refractory follicular NHL. Together they represent >200 patients treated with either Zevalin or Bexxar. Both agents appear to suggest an overall response rate (ORR) of 60% to 80% and a CR rate of 20% to 50%.

A phase III study comparing Zevalin versus rituximab for patients with relapsed or refractory low-grade follicular B-cell NHL or transformed NHL was performed.[53] Patients were randomized to either a single intravenous (IV) dose of Zevalin 0.4 mCi/kg (n = 73) or IV rituximab 375 mg/m^2 weekly for four doses (n = 70). The RIT group was pretreated with two rituximab doses (250 mg/m^2) to improve biodistribution and tumor targeting. After the first rituximab dose on day 1, ^{111}In ibritumomab tiuxetan was administered to assess biodistribution and to aide in dosimetry. No patients received the therapeutic dose of ^{90}Y ibritumomab tiuxetan (Zevalin) if >20 Gy or 3 Gy was calculated to any nontumor organ or the red marrow, respectively. Zevalin was administered after the second rituximab dose approximately 1 week (days 7 to 9) after the first dose of rituximab and ^{111}In ibritumomab tiuxetan. The administered activity of Zevalin was capped at 32 mCi. Patients in both arms of the study received two prior chemotherapy regimens. The ORR was 80% for Zevalin and 56% for rituximab ($p = 0.002$). The CR rates were 30% and 16% ($p = 0.04$), respectively, in the Zevalin and rituximab group. Durable responses ≥6 months were 64% versus 47% ($p = 0.030$) for Zevalin versus rituximab. The conclusion of the study was that RIT with Zevalin was well tolerated and resulted in statistically significant and clinically significant higher ORRs and CRs than rituximab alone.

In a pivotal, nonrandomized, phase III multicenter trial, patients with relapsed, refractory, or transformed follicular B-cell NHL were treated with Bexxar (n = 60), and the outcome was compared to patients' last qualifying chemotherapy (LQC) regimen (n = 28).[54] Eligible patients were required to have been treated with at least two prior protocol0specific chemotherapy regimens (median of four regimens in the study) and to either have not responded or progressed within 6 months of therapy. A PR or CR was observed in 39 patients (65%) after Bexxar compared to 17 patients (28%) after LQC (p <0.001). The median duration of response was 6.5 months for Bexxar and 3.5 months for the LQC group (p <0.001). The CR rate was 20% for Bexxar and 3% for the LQC group (p <0.001). The conclusion of the study was that a single dose of Bexxar was significantly more efficacious than the LQC received by heavily pretreated patients with relapse or refractory follicular B-cell NHL.

Techniques, Modalities, and Modifiers in Radiation Oncology

TABLE 26.5 SUMMARY OF MAJOR PUBLISHED TRIALS OF RADIOIMMUNOTHERAPY FOR RELAPSED OR REFRACTORY LOW-GRADE NON-HODGKIN LYMPHOMA

RIT (Author & Year)	*Study Design*	*OR (%)*	*CR (%)*	*PFS (TTP) [MDR]*
^{90}Y-IT (Witzig 1990)	Treatment failure to an anthracycline or 2 prior regimens or intermediate grade or mantle cell NHL in relapse	67	26	(12.9 in responders) [11.7 mo]
^{90}Y-IT (Witzig 2002)	No prior RTX; phase III study comparing RTX to ^{90}Y-IT	80	30	(11.2) [14.2 mo]
^{90}Y-IT (Witzig 2002)	Prior treatment with RTX and either no response to RTX or time to progression after RTX of <6 months	74	15	(6.8) [6.4 mo]
^{90}Y-IT (Wiseman 2002)	RTX naïve; platelet counts 100,000–150,000/ml	83	37	(9.4) [11.7 mo]
^{90}Y-IT (Tobinai 2009)	Prior RTX eligible	83	68	(9.6)
^{131}I-Tos (Kaminski 2000)	Original report; prior stem cell transplant allowed	71	34	(12 for all responders)
^{131}I-Tos (Vose 2000)	No prior RTX	57	32	(5.3) [9.9 mo]
^{131}I-Tos (Kaminski 2001)	At least 2 prior chemotherapy regimens with either no response or relapse within 6 months of completing the last regimen; no prior RTX	65	20	(8.4 for all responders) [6.5 mo]
^{131}I-Tos (Davies 2004)	No prior RTX	76	49	(0.8 y) [1.3 years]
^{131}I-Tos (Davis 2004)	Trial comparing ^{131}I-Tos to unlabeled tositumomab	55	33	(6.3) [not reached]
^{131}I-Tos (Horning 2005)	At least 1 prior course of RTX	65	38	(10.4) [24.5 mo]

RIT, radioimmunotherapy; OR, overall response; CR, complete response; PFS, progression-free survival; TTP, median time to progression for all patients in study; MDR, median duration of response in responders; ^{90}Y-IT, yttrium-90 ibritumomab tiuxetan; NHL, non-Hodgkin lymphoma; RTX, rituximab; ^{131}I-Tos, ^{131}I tositumomab.

Modified from Burdick M, Macklis RM. Radioimmunotherapy for non-Hodgkin lymphoma: a clinical update. In: Speer TW, ed. *Targeted radionuclide therapy.* Philadelphia: Lippincott Williams & Wilkins, 2011:435.

Frontline Therapy

Considering the concerns about RIT for treating large bulky tumors (tumor penetration, overall required dose, nonuniform dose distributions owing to antigen tissue heterogeneity), it would appear that bringing RIT into a frontline therapeutic setting after induction chemotherapy and maximum cytoreduction would be the next logical direction. A phase III first-line indolent trial (FIT) of consolidation with Zevalin compared to no additional therapy after first remission was reported for follicular B-cell NHL.[55] Patients with CD20+ stage III/IV follicular B-cell NHL who achieved a PR or CR to induction chemotherapy were randomized to Zevalin (n = 208) or to the control arm, representing no further treatment (n = 206). Prior to chemotherapy, patients had documented <25% bone marrow involvement. After induction chemotherapy, blood counts had to recover such that the ANC was ≥1.5, platelets were ≥150,000, and hemoglobin was ≥9. Patients in the Zevalin arm were treated with an activity of 0.4 mCi/kg; a maximum activity of 32 mCi was allowed. Although two doses of rituximab (250 mg/m^2) were used, an ^{111}In biodistribution scan was not required. The data was analyzed with a median follow-up of 3.5 years. Zevalin consolidation resulted in a median progression-free survival (PFS) advantage of 36.5 versus 13.3 months in the control arm (p <0.0001). The PFS benefit was maintained in the Zevalin arm regardless if patients achieved a PR (29.3 vs. 6.2 months; p <0.0001) or CR (53.9 vs. 29.5 months; p = 0.0154). The benefit of Zevalin consolidation was maintained across all Follicular Lymphoma International Prognostic Index (FLIPI) subgroups. In patients with a PR after induction chemotherapy, 77% were further converted to a CR when treated with Zevalin. This resulted in a final CR rate of 87% in the treatment arm, and this result compares well with established data. In the treatment arm, 90% of patients who were Bcl-2 positive converted to a negative status (90% molecular CR). Toxicity was well managed and primarily hematologic. A total of 8% of patients experienced a grade 3 to grade 4 infection. There were no treatment-related deaths. Data from the FIT trial have been updated.[56] With a median follow-up of 66.2 months, the PFS advantage of Zevalin was maintained in patients undergoing a PR/CR. The overall survival was 93% and 89% for Zevalin versus the control arm, respectively (p = 0.561).

Results of a phase III randomized trial (S0016) was recently reported in abstract form.[57] This study randomized 532 patients with bulky stage II through stage IV follicular NHL to cyclophosphamide, doxorubicin, vincristine, and prednisone (CHOP) regimens, specifically CHOP-R (n = 267) or CHOP-RIT (n = 265). The RIT consisted of a single consolidation dose of ^{131}I-tositumomab, calculated to deliver 75 cGy to the total body; the chemotherapy consisted of six cycles of CHOP. In the CHOP-R arm, Rituximab was given on days 1, 6, 48, 90, 134, and 141. With a median follow-up of 4.9 years, the 2-year estimated PFS was 76% and 80% in the CHOP-R and the CHOP-RIT arms, respectively (p = 0.11). The overall survival was similar in both arms (p = 0.08).

SOLID TUMOR TRIALS AND APPROVED THERAPEUTICS

Lung cancer remains the leading cause of cancer mortality in the world. Clearly, new strategies are required to help improve local and systemic control. To date, most RIT-targeting constructs will bind to cell surface or extracellular matrix antigens, on or in surrounding viable malignant cells. Each antigenic target (disease site) requires a specific targeting construct (typically an mAb or antibody fragment). There is, however, emerging data to support the concept of targeting necrotic and hypoxic regions of tumors.[58] The selective targeting of dead or dying cells will allow a cytotoxic event of nearby malignant cells by the bystander and crossfire effect. Additionally, only one type of targeting construct needs to be manufactured to target many different types of malignancies. If the cell surface antigen does not internalize to any significant degree, then a typical targeting construct will remain on the cell surface. Because dead and dying cells (undergoing apoptosis) exhibit disruption of their cell membrane, constructs that target intracellular products of apoptosis will then be able to gain access the cells' cytoplasm and nucleus. Although several "dead cancer cell antigens" are under investigation, tumor necrosis therapy or treatment (TNT) has been investigated in human trials. TNT is an IgG_{2a} mAb that targets nuclear histones.[59–61]

A pivotal trial of iodine-131-chimeric tumor necrosis treatment (^{131}I-chTNT) in advanced lung cancer patients was performed.[62] A total of 107 patients (n = 97, non–small cell; n = 10, small cell) were enrolled from 1999 to 2002. All patients had failed at least one prior therapeutic regimen (mean = 3; range = 1 to 5), and 86.9% of the patients had stage III to stage IV disease at study entry. In all cases, the patients received two instillations of ^{131}I-chTNT administered over 2 to 4 weeks. Sixty-two patients received IV administrations, and 45 patients received intratumoral injections of ^{131}I-chTNT. IV administrations were delivered at an activity 0.8 mCi/kg and intratumoral injections were delivered at an activity of 0.8 mCi/cm^3 of tumor size. In all patients (n = 107), the ORR was 34.6% (3.7% CR; 30.8% PR; 55.1% no change or stable disease; 10.3% progressive disease). Of the 62 patients receiving a systemic administration of ^{131}I-chTNT, the ORR was 35.5% (3.2% CR; 32.2% PR). Of the 45 patients receiving intratumoral injection of ^{131}I-chTNT, the ORR was 33.3% (5% CR; 20.9% PR). In 58 evaluable patients, the median survival was 11.7 months, and the 1-year survival rate was 41.4%. The average absorbed doses for tumor and normal lung were 8.45 Gy and 2.35 Gy for patients receiving systemic ^{131}I-chTNT and 30.0 Gy and 2.65 Gy for patients receiving intratumoral ^{131}I-chTNT. The major toxicity was hematologic and reversible. As expected, the hematologic toxicity was lower in the intratumoral injection group. In 2003, ^{131}I-chTNT was approved by the Chinese State Food and Drug Administration to treat refractory bronchogenic carcinoma. As a result, ^{131}I-chTNT became the first solid tumor TRIT agent in the world approved for therapy. Recently, two studies using ^{131}I-chTNT-1/B were completed for the treatment of CNS malignancies. The first trial was a phase I study using ^{131}I-chTNT-1/B to treat progressive and recurrent glioblastoma multiforme (NCT00128635). The second trial was a phase II study using ^{131}I-chTNT-1/B to treat patients with glioblastoma or anaplastic astrocytoma after conventional surgery.

HCC, or liver carcinoma, represents a significant worldwide malignancy and has several potential etiologies: viral, metabolic (hemochromatosis, alcoholic cirrhosis), toxins (aflatoxin), hormonal, or chemical (oil industry). In addition to resection, orthotopic liver transplantation (OLT) represents the only other potential curative option. In 1989, the Radiation Therapy Oncology Group (RTOG) reported a phase III study comparing EBRT and chemotherapy to the same treatment plus ^{131}I antiferritin antibody. None of the patients receiving EBRT and chemotherapy only were converted to a resectable state. In a separate analysis, 11 patients crossing over from the EBRT and chemotherapy arm to further therapy with ^{131}I antiferritin antibody were converted to resection. There was, however, no significant difference in the initial "intent to treat" treatment arms based on response rate and survival.[63–64,65,66] Of course, the most promising role of radiolabeled antibody therapy is in the treatment of minimal residual microscopic disease.

Licartin is an antibody fragment, F(ab')$_2$, that targets HAb18G/CD147, a HCC TAA. More recently, the safety and pharmacokinetics of Licartin (^{131}I metuximab) were investigated in phase I/II trials. The initial phase I trial evaluated 28 patients with HCC. They were treated with 0.25 to 1.0 mCi/kg of Licartin via hepatic artery infusion. In a subsequent phase II trial,

106 patients with HCC received 0.75 mCi/kg of Licartin on day 1 of a 28-day cycle. Life-threatening toxicities did not occur. In 73 patients (completing two cycles), 6 patients (8.22%) exhibited a PR, 14 patients (19.18%) had a minor response, and 43 patients (58.9%) maintained stable disease. The cohort had a 21-month survival of 44.54%. It was concluded that Licartin was safe and active in patients with HCC.[67]

Realizing that TRIT is most suited for treating microscopic disease, Licartin was tested in the adjuvant setting for patients with HCC undergoing OLT.[64,68] A total of 60 patients with HCC who were undergoing OLT were randomized to Licartin (0.42 mCi/kg) for three fractions at 28-day intervals versus placebo. Analysis at 1 year post-therapy revealed that the recurrence rate was significantly decreased by 30.4% ($p = 0.0174$) and the survival rate was significantly increased by 20.6% ($p = 0.0289$) in the Licartin group. No significant toxicities were observed. The Chinese State Food and Drug Administration has approved Licartin as adjuvant therapy after OLT for HCC in 2005. There are two trials using Licartin that are ongoing but not recruiting patients. The first trial (NCT00819650) randomizes patients with HCC undergoing an R0 resection to postoperative Licartin or no further treatment. Licartin is delivered in three doses (fractions) at 28-day intervals beginning at week 4 after liver resection. In the second trial (NCT00829465), patients with unresectable HCC are randomized to transcatheter arterial chemoembolization (TACE) or Licartin combined with TACE.

Currently, the most common antigen targets for CNS malignancies consist of the epidermal growth factor receptor (EGFR), tenascin, neural cell adhesion molecule (NCAM), placental alkaline phosphatase (PLAP), and phosphatidyl inositide. The EGFR is variably amplified in malignant tissue and is also present, to some extent, in benign tissue. Tenascin is an extracellular glycoprotein that is uniformly expressed in glioma, and NCAM is present on both benign and malignant glioma cells. Clinical trials using RIT to treat CNS malignancies have been extensively reviewed.[69] A phase III trial was reported in 2002.[70] A total of 12 patients with malignant glioma were randomized to surgical resection and radiotherapy (60 Gy) (n = 5) versus surgical resection, radiotherapy, and RIT (n = 7). The RIT agent was a ^{125}I-anti-EGFR antibody 425 that was administered intravenously in three weekly doses (50 mCi) beginning during week 4 of the EBRT. All patients in the treatment arm had a recurrence at the time of publication. Considering that the EGFR was not tested in submitted tissue, the trial had a small number of patients, and the 150-kDa antibody was administered intravenously, significant conclusions could not be drawn.

Most of the CNS RIT trials to date are of "dose searching pilot" or phase I design. The evolution of the trials has seen the delivery route move from systemic (intra-arterial or IV) to local instillation of the RIT agent into a surgically created resection cavity (SCRC). Even though the blood–brain barrier (BBB) is often disrupted by a rapidly growing CNS malignancy, this phenomenon is not well defined and 150 kDa antibodies would still not likely cross to a significant degree, although there does appear to be an element of nonspecific uptake from a systemic delivery.[71] As a result, studies using the systemic approach often deliver EBRT in conjunction with TRT. It has been well documented that EBRT will cause an increase in the permeability of the BBB and increase vascular leakage.[72–73,74] Regardless, it has been disappointingly estimated that only 0.001% to 0.01% of the systemically delivered antibody will penetrate each gram of solid tumor. Furthermore, biopsy data has revealed that a single systemic injection of radiolabeled anti-EGFR antibody will deliver only 0.02% of the injected activity per gram of tumor, resulting in a dose of only 100 to 200 cGy.[71]

Direct instillation of the TRT agent into the SCRC is an attractive alternative to the systemic approach. Unlike other malignant sites where the potential for systemic spread mandates a systemic approach, this is not the case for malignant gliomas. The local approach is accomplished by injecting or instilling the RIT agent directly into the SCRC via an Ommaya or Rickham catheter. Preliminary dosimetry is performed to ensure localization within the surgical bed and that no direct communication with the ventricular system has occurred. Institutions using this technique have utilized murine, chimeric, or humanized mAbs attached to ^{131}I, ^{90}Y, ^{188}Re, and ^{211}At. Other important treatment variances include fractionation, pretargeting, and a combined modality approach using EBRT and chemotherapy. The success of this approach will depend on meaningful penetration of the RIT agent into the local brain parenchyma such that the mAbs (or targeting construct) can bind to areas of microscopic extension of malignant cells at some distance from the SCRC margin. It is still unknown as to what impact the healing process/inflammation at the surgical margin has on the success of antibody penetration. As well, it is well known that binding site barrier phenomena, interstitial tumor pressure, aberrant tumor vasculature, and a recusant extracellular tumor matrix will significantly impede antibody penetration.[75]

Hopkins et al.[76] obtained biopsy data from three patients with glioma who received two to three cycles of either ^{131}I or ^{90}Y-ERIC-1 (anti-NCAM antibody) directly instilled into a SCRC. Relevant assumptions were that the SCRCs were spherical, the radionuclide was spread evenly around the resection margin, 100% of the RIT agent was bound to its target, and diffusion into the resection margin was uniform. It was shown that "modest" diffusion occurred and the process was exponential. The peak dose occurred between 0.16 and 0.18 cm beyond the resection margin, and 4.4% to 5.8% of the peak dose was delivered to a depth of 2 cm. Of note, NCAM is expressed on benign and malignant cells and perhaps a more tumor-specific antigen would allow for greater depth of penetration. Certainly, smaller targeting constructs have been shown to penetrate to a greater depth in brain parenchyma compared to intact antibodies.[77] Using the same antibody, radiolabeled with ^{131}I and instilled into a SCRC, Papanatassiou[73] showed that diffusion occurred from 0.5 to 1.0 cm (single-photon emission computed tomography [SPECT]). The range of antibody binding to the target was 8% to 80% of total injected activity. Because the R_{95} (thickness of tissue where 95% of the β energy is deposited) for ^{131}I is only 0.992 mm, it was concluded that a more optimal radionuclide would potentially be ^{90}Y with an R_{95} of 5.94 mm.[78] Assuming a 2-cm SCRC and 100% binding, as much as 351 Gy could be delivered to the tumor with a single instillation of 18.2 mCi of ^{90}Y-ERIC-1. This calculation resulted in an impressive minimum tumor/whole brain dose ratio of 140:1.

Using ^{131}I-81C6 (antitenascin mAB), dose-limiting toxicity was reached with a single injection of 80 mCi for leptomeningeal disease (intrathecal delivery), 100 mCi for heavily pretreated and recurrent glioma (into SCRC), and 120 mCi for de novo glioma (into SCRC) also receiving EBRT and chemotherapy.[79] Using a standard, fixed, mCi dose, a wide range of absorbed doses (18 to 186 Gy) will be delivered to a depth of 2 cm beyond the SCRC margin.[80] On further analysis, an optimal dose of 44 Gy to 2 cm beyond SCRC was identified. Doses <44 Gy resulted in increased recurrence rates, and doses >44 Gy resulted in a higher rate of necrosis. A trend toward significant improvement in median survival was shown for patients receiving 40 to 48 Gy versus <40 Gy.[78] Refining the technique further, it was shown that 20 of the 21 patients could be successfully dosed to 44 Gy by varying the initial injection activity and considering the volume of the SCRC.[81] Zalutsky et al.[82] showed that a high LET, α-emitting radioconjugate (^{211}At-ch81C6) could be safely delivered in a small cohort of glioma patients. Interestingly, histopathology appears to correlate with prognosis. Biopsy data from patients with a suspected recurrence, after receiving ^{131}I-labeled antitenascin 81C6 antibody, were analyzed. Three types of histologic patterns were evident: proliferative glioma, quiescent glioma, and negative for neoplasm. The median survival for each histopathologic pattern was 3.5, 15.0, and 27.5 months, respectively (p <0.0001). Considering total dose (EBRT plus radiolabeled antibody), patients receiving <86 Gy or >86 Gy had median survivals of 7 and 19 months, respectively (p <0.002).[83]

A review of the major RIT CNS trials[69] indicates that the range of maximum tolerated activity is between 10 and 120 mCi. There are many variables that could potentially account for the noted range. In general, by performing dosimetry for a given radionuclide delivery construct, a specific absorbed dose can be calculated to a predetermined depth from the SCRC margin. It has been shown that ^{131}I-antitenascin 81C6 can deliver 2,000 Gy, 90 Gy, and 34 Gy to the cavity interface at 1 cm and at 2 cm depth, respectively.[78,83] The median survival for TRT in treating glioma appears extremely favorable when compared to other treatment approaches. For de novo lesions, the median survival range is 50.9 to 57.6 months (three studies not reaching median survival at the time of the report) for anaplastic astrocytoma and 13.4 to 35.5 months for glioblastoma. For recurrent lesions, the median survival range is 13.0 to 52.0 months (one study not reaching median survival at the time of the report) for anaplastic astrocytoma and 14.0 to 25.0 months for glioblastoma.[69] Further improvements can be expected as this field matures and phase II and III data is generated. Unlike sealed source brachytherapy, there appears to be a very low rate of CNS toxicity and a reduced subsequent need for surgical intervention to remove necrotic regions.

Building on the data generated by Duke University, Bradmer Pharmaceuticals has developed two clinical trials using the ^{131}I-antitenascin antibody (Neuradiab) for treating glioblastoma (World Health Organization [WHO] grade IV astrocytoma). The first trial (Glass-Art) is a phase III study that randomizes patients with untreated glioblastoma to standard therapy (surgery, radiotherapy, and temozolomide) versus standard therapy plus Neuradiab. In the experimental arm, dosimetry is performed and a calculated dose of radiolabeled antibody is delivered via a Rickham catheter. The Neuradiab therapeutic dose is given after surgery and prior to the initiation of radiotherapy and temozolomide. The second trial is a phase II study designed to treat patients with recurrent glioblastoma with surgery, Neuradiab, and bevacizumab. This trial is not yet open for patient recruitment. The Glass-Art trial began enrolling patients in 2008. Although "ongoing," the trial is not recruiting participants at this time. Bradmer Pharmaceuticals continues to seek development partners and has submitted multiple grants for potential funding. On March 3, 2010, the company submitted a proposal for private placement. Funding continues to be problematic.

Initial promising investigations evaluated the long-term survival of patients with advanced ovarian cancer treated with RIT following cytoreductive surgery and platinum-based chemotherapy.[84] Eligibility criteria included patients with histologic evidence of ovarian cancer from stage IC to stage IV. Fifty-two patients entered the study: 31 patients had residual disease following standard chemotherapy, and 21 patients had achieved CR. The treatment consisted of a single intraperitoneal (IP) administration of 25 mg HMFG1 labeled with 666 MBq (18 mCi)/m^2 of ^{90}Y, with survival being the primary end point. In the group of 21 patients who had achieved CR following surgery, conventional chemotherapy, and IP RIT, the median survival had not been reached with a maximum follow-up of 12 years. Survival at >10 years was 78%. The conclusion of this study was that a substantial proportion of patients who achieve a CR with conventional therapy can achieve a long-term survival benefit if treated with IP ^{90}Y-HMFG1.

A phase III study was subsequently performed.[85] This multinational (74 centers, 17 countries, recruiting patients between 1998 and 2003), open-label, randomized phase III study compared ^{90}Y-HMFG1 (against the MUC 1 antigen) plus standard treatment versus standard treatment alone in patients with epithelial ovarian cancer (EOC) who had attained a complete clinical remission after cytoreductive surgery and platinum-based chemotherapy. Stage IC to stage IV patients were screened (n = 844), of whom 447 with a negative second-look laparoscopy (SLL) were randomly assigned to receive either a single dose of ^{90}Y-HMFG1 plus standard treatment (224 patients) or standard treatment alone (223 patients). Patients in the active treatment (RIT) arm received an IP dose of 25 mg ^{90}Y-HMFG1 to provide 666 MBq (18 mCi)/m^2. After a median follow-up of 3.5 years, 70 patients had died in the active treatment arm compared with 61 patients in the control arm. Cox proportional hazards analysis of survival demonstrated no difference between treatment arms. In the RIT arm, 104 patients experienced relapse compared with 98 patients in the standard treatment arm. No difference in time to relapse was observed between the two study arms. The conclusion was that a single IP administration of ^{90}Y-HMFG1 to patients with EOC, who had a negative SLL after primary therapy, did not extend survival or time to relapse. The reason for failure of the treatment could perhaps be explained by the choice of radionuclide. When treating microscopic disease with high-energy β-particles emitted from ^{90}Y, the electron will have too long of a range to deliver high enough energy to the tumor cell nuclei. It has been extensively modeled that high-energy β-particle emissions will not deposit large amounts of energy (absorbed energy) into tumor spheroids below a certain size. However, there are other concerns about this study that warrant comment:

1. Entry was allowed onto the study even if dispersal of the TRT agent (^{90}Y-HMFG1) could not occur in an entire quadrant of the abdomen because of adhesions. The adhesions were assessed by laparoscopy, computed tomography (CT) scan, or isotope diffusion scan. Although it is rather intuitive that a diffusion scan will allow a reasonable assessment of adhesions, it is less obvious that laparoscopy or a CT scan will discern between one or two quadrants of adhesions. This allowance could potentially result in a significant underdosing ≤25% of the abdominal cavity. Importantly, there was no mention of how these patients (no adhesions vs. one quadrant with adhesions) were stratified between each treatment arm.
2. The RIT arm contained 3% more stage III/IV patients.
3. The RIT arm had a higher mean CA-125 level after laparoscopy (never explained).
4. The RIT arm had 8% more patients with residual disease after initial surgery (44.2% vs. 35.9%).
5. In the standard arm, 7% (19.7% vs. 12.5%) more patients received consolidation chemotherapy.
6. The overall antibody mass (25 mg) may have been insufficient to help provide a concentration gradient to help "push" the radiolabeled antibody into the tumors.[52] This can be contrasted to the 250 mg/m^2 of cold antibody used with Zevalin or the 450-mg total antibody dose used with Bexxar.
7. With regard to the injected dose, 20% can enter the systemic circulation.
8. The radiolabeling process was performed by each institution and not centralized. Although a radiolabeling efficiency of 95% was confirmed with thin-layer chromatography, there was no mention of immunoreactivity quality assurance (potential loss of affinity of the antibody for the antigen as a result of the radiolabeling process).
9. During the accrual time period, single-institution experiences tended to report higher conversion rates to an open laparotomy (from an SLL) than was reported in the current study (59% vs. 5%).[85]
10. In the RIT arm, 18% of patients had ≤60% MUC1 staining (unknown impact).
11. There was no pattern of failure analysis (IP vs. distant).

The patterns-of-failure analysis eventually came to fruition.[86] Case report forms of all patients with disease recurrence were reviewed to determine site and date of recurrent disease. The 447 patients were included with a median follow-up of

3.5 years. Relapse was seen in 104 of 224 patients in the RIT arm and 98 of 223 patients in the control arm. Significantly fewer IP ($p < 0.05$) and more extraperitoneal ($p < 0.05$) relapses occurred in the RIT arm. Time to IP recurrence was significantly longer ($p = 0.0019$) and time to extraperitoneal recurrence was significantly shorter for the RIT arm ($p < 0.001$). In a subset analysis, the impact of IP RIT on IP relapse-free survival was even greater and could only be seen in a subgroup of patients with residual disease after primary surgery. Although there was no survival benefit for ^{90}Y-HMFG1 IP instillation as consolidation treatment for EOC, an improved control of IP disease was found, which appeared to be offset by increased extraperitoneal recurrences. It was proposed that the transient myelosuppression (alteration of the immune system) induced by therapy with ^{90}Y-HMFG1 indirectly caused the greater number of extraperitoneal metastases. Most likely, this observation is simply the result of an alteration in the failure pattern owing to a greater number of patients in the treatment arm benefiting from a greater IP control, as distant metastases will not be observed because of overwhelming local symptoms. In addition, for reasons mentioned previously, it is possible that the treatment arm was skewed with more advanced disease. Future trials should focus on both the IP and systemic delivery of RIT.

UNSEALED RADIONUCLIDE THERAPY

Unsealed radionuclide therapy (URT) refers to the medical application of radiopharmaceuticals that are not conjugated to a targeting agent and thereby localize in diseased tissue by virtue of biologic, chemical, or physical avidity.[87] These radionuclides are considered "unsealed" because they are not confined within a container that could be inserted or implanted into a tumor, as is performed with conventional brachytherapy techniques. Because they are not conjugated to a traditional targeting construct, this class of therapeutics has also been referred to as "naked" radiopharmaceuticals.[88] Oversight for the utilization of URT is governed by the U.S. FDA.[89] Safety issues, radioactive material shipping, and licensing are regulated by the U.S. Nuclear Regulatory Commission (NRC). A state may enter into an agreement with the NRC to perform its own regulation and to monitor of the use of radioactive material (agreement state), with the exception of fuel facilities and nuclear reactors. States that continue to allow monitoring by the NRC are referred to as nonagreement states.[90] The NRC receives advice regarding radiopharmaceuticals from the Advisory Committee on the Medical Use of Isotopes (ACMUI). Regulations for the practice of nuclear medicine reside in U.S. NRC Title 10 of the Code of Federal Regulations, Parts 20 and 35. Part 20 largely governs the standards for radiation protection, and Part 35 governs the medical use of radioactive material.[91,92]

Bone-seeking radiopharmaceuticals, used for palliation of painful bone metastases, represent one of the more common uses of URT. A few of the earlier radionuclides used for this purpose include phosphorus-32 [^{32}P], samarium-153 [^{153}Sm], and strontium-89 [^{89}Sr];[93] however, newer agents are being investigated and are in various stages of development.[94–95,96–101] As with RIT, the radionuclides used in the application of URT can be classified as β-, α-, and Auger emitters. The radionuclides used in URT target bone by either an intrinsic affinity (i.e., ^{89}Sr, radium-223 [^{223}Ra]) or by using bone-seeking phosphonate ligands attached to the radionuclide (i.e., samarium-153 ethylenediaminetetramethylenephosphonate [^{153}Sm-EDTMP] or rhenium-188 hydroxyethylidine diphosphate [^{188}Re-HEDP]).[95,102] Localization properties of individual agents and the clinical circumstances involved will determine routes of administration. These agents have been delivered by IV, intra-arterial, intracavitary, intra-articular (radiosynovectomy), and direct intralesional approaches. This variability of administration has been especially true for ^{32}P, which has been uniquely studied using IV, oral, IP, and intrathoracic routes.[103]

The initial use of a β-emitting radioisotope for the management of intractable malignant bone pain was reported in 1942.[104] Because URT demonstrates a chemical affinity for bone, the predominant thrust of clinical investigation has been for primary and secondary malignancies of bone and bone marrow. Other target sites, however, have been considered. In some instances, these alternative uses have remained a part of the therapeutic armamentarium; however, for many indications, the use of URT has yielded to nonradioactive approaches (corticosteroids, systemic chemotherapy, hormone therapy, analgesia, and surgery) and to EBRT. The lack of access to innovative candidate radionuclides, diminished trial participation, and absence of utilization and teaching from many training programs have further exacerbated the problem.[87] Regardless, a review of 15 randomized controlled trials (1,146 analyzed patients) comparing URT to placebo or another radionuclide for the treatment of metastatic bone pain confirms the efficacy of URT for pain management. This review also provides evidence that URT resulted in significant and complete pain relief during a 1- to 6-month period.[105] Practice guidelines have been established for URT,[106] and evidence-based guidelines for palliation of bone metastases include URT as a reasonable therapeutic option.[107]

The most common malignant sites that develop bone metastases are prostate, breast, and lung cancer.[93] URT exhibits increased targeting of bone in areas of osteoblastic activity and exerts this propensity because of a chemical similarity to calcium, which is classified as an alkaline earth metal in the periodic table (as are ^{89}Sr and ^{223}Ra). These therapeutic agents may either directly substitute for stable analogues in hydroxyapatite or may be chemisorbed on the hydroxyapatite surface of the phosphate moiety of phosphonate chelates.[102] Radionuclide decay profiles that include gamma emissions may be utilized for imaging and for documentation of therapeutic uptake in regions of bone pathology. Bone scans (technetium-99 m [^{99m}Tc]) are typically performed to verify disseminated osseous disease. The intensity of uptake on pretherapeutic scanning does not necessarily coincide with therapeutic efficacy, and widely disseminated disease may actually produce "dilution" of dose and potentially reduced effectiveness.[102]

Regardless of the precise method of chemical or physical affinity, all agents studied for palliation of osseous metastatic bone pain have fared better than placebos in randomized trials.[107] There is, however, limited evidence that the response or morbidity profile of the different radiopharmaceuticals vary significantly among themselves. Additionally, there is little evidence that dose escalation either in individual or cumulative doses will improve effectiveness. Sequenced administration has been investigated; however, if an initial intervention has not produced a significant level or duration of response, there is little evidence that additional administrations will increase effectiveness but they may potentially increase morbidity.[102]

Rapid and significant localization in bone by all agents will generally limit potential morbidity to myelosuppression, which in patients with adequate marrow reserve will usually be mild and be manifest initially within 1 week post-administration with evidence of thrombocytopenia. Leukopenia may develop somewhat later; however, all side effects typically reverse without intervention within 8 to 10 weeks. Circulating isotope not immediately incorporated into bone is typically excreted in urine; therefore, patients with reduced renal function may not be ideal candidates for the agents and, if used, should have blood counts monitored carefully. Administration is routinely on an outpatient basis, thus radiation protection measures for low-level radiation in urine should be practiced.[90]

Palliative effects may be observed within 3 to 5 days but usually peak at approximately 7 to 10 days, and the beneficial effects may last for months. At this point in time, subsequent administrations may be considered. When used for management of bone pain, all bone-seeking radiopharmaceuticals can exhibit a flare in pain within 24 to 72 hours post-injection that may last for 5 to 7 days. Appropriate analgesic management must be provided during this period. In the treatment of metastatic prostate cancer, prostate-specific antigen (PSA) levels may begin to decline within several days; however, the rapidity of decline, nadir of the PSA level, and duration of PSA response are not satisfactory predictors of improved outcomes.[102]

The bone-seeking agents have been and continue to be used primarily in metastatic prostate cancer, and evidence of effectiveness in breast and lung cancer is limited with responses noted primarily in osteoblastic metastases. Plain radiographs of symptomatic metastatic sites should be obtained prior to the use of systemic agents for palliation of bone pain. If there is evidence of possible impending fracture, stabilization and/or EBRT should be initiated prior to systemic radionuclide therapy. If painful vertebral metastasis is apparent clinically, CT or magnetic resonance imaging (MRI) of the painful vertebral segments should be obtained prior to administration of isotope to ensure that no epidural disease is present. If this pathology is discovered, EBRT or surgery should be carried out prior to systemic isotope therapy. IV administration of all agents should be carried out slowly over 1 to 5 minutes, through indwelling catheters with clear and unobstructed flow clearly validated, adequate hydration, and careful radiation precautions for patients and staff.

Radiopharmaceuticals

Iodine-131

Physical Properties: $t_{½}$ = 8.0 days; radiation decay: β (606 keV maximum and 190 keV mean); γ (364 keV).

Clinical Utility: Radioiodine (^{131}I) was first used to treat benign thyroid disease in the late 1920s and early 1930s.[108,109] The first reports of using ^{131}I to treat well-differentiated thyroid cancer (WDTC) were published in the 1940s.[110,111] To date, ^{131}I has become the standard of care, in conjunction with surgery, for the management of WDTC; its use and indications have been extensively reviewed.[110,112,113] Benign thyroid tissue (follicular cells) and certain thyroid carcinomas (follicular, papillary, and Hürthle cell carcinoma) will actively transport iodine into the cell via the sodium iodide symporter to initiate the synthesis thyroid hormone.[114,115] As a result, this innate targeting system has been exploited for many decades to treat locally persistent, recurrent, or metastatic thyroid carcinoma. The majority of data concerning the treatment of WDTC with ^{131}I has been generated by large retrospective series of patients, with the resulting clinical data often spanning several decades. Frequently, these institutions used unchanged protocols and fixed activities for therapy. Regardless, considerable evidence exists concerning local control, decreased metastases, and a survival benefit when ^{131}I is used as part of the treatment regimen.[116,117–118,119]

In general, ^{131}I therapy for WDTC is considered either ablation or treatment. Ablation is the use of ^{131}I to sterilize normal remnant thyroid tissue or microscopic disease that remains after thyroidectomy. Treatment refers to the therapeutic application of ^{131}I against cancer persistence, local recurrence, or distant metastatic disease. Whereas the treatment aspect of ^{131}I is well accepted, ablation is more controversial.[120,121] Recent decades have revealed a decrease in mortality for WDTC, owing to the early diagnosis and aggressive treatment of WDTC with near-total thyroidectomy and ^{131}I ablation in selected patients at high risk for recurrence and mortality, followed by thyroid-stimulating hormone (TSH) suppression.[122] If it is determined that ablation will be performed, patients are placed on a low-iodine diet and TSH stimulation is performed by withholding thyroid hormone.[113] Standard fixed activities of 30 to 100 mCi are used for ablation, whereas higher activities in the range of 100 to 300 mCi are used for known residual disease, recurrence, or metastatic disease. If possible, patient-specific dosimetry should be used to determine the activity in the metastatic setting.[122] Using this approach, a dose <200 cGy is calculated to the blood (bone marrow) and ≤120 mCi of ^{131}I being retained after 48 hours. This can result in administered activities between 75 and 659 mCi without the development of leukemia, permanent bone marrow suppression, or pulmonary fibrosis.[123] Diagnostic ^{131}I scanning and thyroglobulin measurement are required for follow-up.

Phosphorus-32

Physical Properties: $t_{½}$ = 14.3 days; radiation decay: β (1.71 MeV maximum and 1.69 MeV mean); γ (none).

Clinical Utility: Phosphorus-32 (^{32}P) represents one of the earliest agents in this class and perhaps is the most frequently studied for a wide variety of indications and routes of administration. In its aqueous form (Na2PO3), the agent was employed for the systemic therapy of chronic myelogenous leukemia and polycythemia vera. Orthopedic surgeons and rheumatologists have evaluated the agent for intra-articular management of persistent synovial effusions and hemarthroses secondary to hemophilia and leukemias.[124,125] The agent has been placed in indwelling catheters to treat CNS lesions.

The colloidal form of the agent (as chromic phosphate) became a standard modality for management of malignant pleural and peritoneal effusions in the 1960s and 1970s, driving numerous clinical investigations. Anecdotal reports suggesting significant activity were infrequently corroborated in randomized clinical trials. Following drainage of abdominal ascites or pleural effusions, up to 5 mCi of the agent was instilled and patients were placed in various positions to enhance distribution. The nature of the disease processes and prior therapy often predisposed patients to preinstillation adhesions with bowel or lung immobility, and distribution of the agent proved difficult. This indication has largely been replaced by instillations of various antibiotic or chemotherapeutic compounds.[126,127–128]

Following identification of a subset of early-stage, high-risk ovarian cancer patients (FIGO stage Ia or Ib [grade 3], or stage 1c or II [any grade], or any stage I/II patient with clear-cell histology), the Gynecologic Oncology Group (GOG), North Central Cancer Treatment Group (NCCTG), and Southwest Oncology Group (SWOG) undertook a randomized trial assigning patients to either a single dose of 15 mCi of IP ^{32}P versus cyclophosphamide 1 g/m^2 and cisplatin 100 mg/m^2 every 21 days for three cycles. Prior to instillation of the radioactive material through multiperforated indwelling peritoneal dialysis catheters, ^{99m}Tc was instilled to ensure free-flow and even distribution of the therapeutic agent. IP ^{32}P was administered within 10 days but not >6 weeks following laparotomy. Ten-year follow-up of the study population suggested a modest reduction in intra-abdominal recurrence rate for the chemotherapy population but only a small and nonsignificant improvement in survival. These findings were corroborated by other reports.[129]

In the 1990s, Order et al.[130] reported a series of patients treated with direct intralesional infusions of ^{32}P colloidal chromic phosphate for unresectable tumors of the liver, CNS, pancreas, and head and neck. The observation of extralesional extravasation of isotope was apparently overcome by preinstillation of macroaggregated albumin to induce capillary and arteriole blockade prior to isotope infusion. Intense activity and doses were documented; however, improvements in local control and survival were inconclusive.[131]

^{32}P localization in bone created interest in use of the orthophosphate form of the isotope for painful skeletal metastases with 85% of the administered dose ultimately incorporated into bone. However, priming regimens including androgenic agents prior to isotope administration were prolonged, beneficial results modest, and myelotoxicity significant; use of the agent for this indication has largely been abandoned.

Strontium-89 Chloride (Metastron, GE Healthcare, Chalfont St. Giles, UK)

Physical Properties: $t_{1/2}$ = 50.5 days; radiation decay: β (1.463 MeV maximum and 0.583 MeV mean); γ (none).

^{89}Sr, a calcium analogue, is administered as an IV injection at doses of 4 mCi, given slowly.

Clinical Utility: Porter et al.,[132] in a Trans-Canada study, compared ^{89}Sr to bisphosphonates in the prophylactic setting in an attempt to reduce subsequent development of additional osseous metastasis. Results were comparable in both arms, with a reduced cost of therapy in the ^{89}Sr arm. Low-grade hematologic toxicity in the radiation arm did not require intervention. In an attempt to build on currently established palliative results, a randomized phase III trial is under way to investigate the use of weekly doxorubicin (20 mg/m^2) with ^{89}Sr after response to induction chemotherapy.[133]

Samarium-153 Lexidronam (Quadramet, Cytogen, Princeton, NJ)

Physical Properties: $t_{1/2}$ = 46.3 hours; radiation decay: β (0.81 MeV maximum and 0.23 MeV mean); γ (maximum energy 103 keV).

Clinical Utility: Samarium-153 EDTMP (^{153}Sm) is a bone-seeking agent consisting of radioactive samarium and a telephosphonate chelator, EDTMP. The recommended therapeutic dose is 1.0 mCi/kg, administered intravenously over a period of 1 minute through a secure indwelling catheter and followed by a saline flush. Extensive preclinical and clinical investigations have demonstrated the safety and effectiveness profile of ^{153}Sm-EDTMP.[134] Although primarily used alone, there is increasing interest in consideration of combination therapy with the bisphosphonates and taxane-based chemotherapeutics.

The use of ^{153}Sm-EDTMP has been evaluated in osseous metastases for primary osteosarcomas. Anderson et al.[135] investigated the use of gemcitabine as a radiosensitizer to increase ^{153}Sm-EDTMP effectiveness. Using 30 mCi/kg (average of 1,640 mCi), they found acceptable toxicity and objective response in 8 of 14 patients investigated.

Radium-223 Chloride

Physical Properties: $t_{1/2}$ = 11.4 days; radiation decay: α (6 MeV maximum); γ (270 keV maximum).

Clinical Utility: Although not available for commercial distribution in the United States, there has been interest in ^{223}Ra in the treatment of metastatic hormone-refractory prostate cancer involving multiple bones. Nilsson et al.[136] at the Karolinska University Hospital and Institute in Stockholm reported initial findings in 2005, evaluating the safety and effectiveness of ^{223}Ra. The group had carried out preclinical studies prior to this phase I investigation. They concluded that at relevant dose levels, the agent was well tolerated and justified extension into phase II and III studies. Following focal EBRT to selected sites, patients were randomly assigned to treatment with ^{223}Ra or placebo in a double-blinded manner. One primary end point—bone-alkaline phosphatase levels—was significantly decreased in the treatment arm, and the time to PSA increase was significantly lengthened. Hematologic toxicity in both groups was equivalent. The time to first skeletal-related event (SRE) was significantly increased in the ^{223}Ra cohort and can be considered as a measure of quality of life, taking into account increase in pain or analgesic requirements; new neurologic symptoms or fractures; or additional surgical, radiologic, or systemic therapy. In this limited report, survival in the treated group was significantly extended. Subsequent reports have confirmed these findings, and a commercially prepared formulation of the agent (Alpharadin, Algeta ASA, Oslo, Norway) was granted approval by the U.S. FDA in February 2008 for phase I/II trials in the United States.[137] Currently, U.S. patients are eligible for ALSYMPCA (Alpharadin in Symptomatic Prostate Cancer), an international phase III trial randomizing patients with hormone-refractory prostate cancer to Alpharadin plus best standard of care versus placebo plus best standard of care.

Rhenium-186 HEDP (Etidronate)

Physical Properties: $t_{1/2}$ = 3.8 days; radiation decay: β (1.07 MeV maximum and 0.336 mean); γ (0.137 MeV maximum).

Clinical Utility: Although not commercially available in the United States, ^{186}Rh-HEDP has been studied in phase I trials in Europe in association with autologous peripheral blood stem cell rescue in the management of hormone-refractory prostate cancer metastatic to bone.[138] Promising results have led to initiation of phase II trials.

Rhenium-188 HEDP (Etidronate)

Physical Properties: $t_{1/2}$ = 16.9 hours; radiation decay: β (2.1 MeV maximum and 0.779 mean); γ (0.155 MeV maximum and 0.061 mean).

Clinical Utility: Although not commercially available in the United States, ^{188}Re-HEDP has been studied in Europe for some time. The agent is produced by a generator similar to that used to produce ^{99}mTc, enabling wide availability at relatively low cost. Liepe et al.[139] reported treatment of 46 patients with multiple bone metastases from breast and prostate cancer with pain. Thirty-one patients received ^{188}Re-HEDP (3,300 MBq) and 25 patients received ^{153}Sm-EDTMP (37 MBq/kg of body weight). All patients had a single injection of isotope. Patients with prostate cancer received hormone therapy for 6 months before isotope therapy and during the post-isotope observation period. Thirty-nine patients received bisphosphonates for 6 months prior to study treatment with discontinuance of the agents 1 month prior to isotope administration. In post-therapy evaluation, only the ^{188}Re-HEDP group had a statistically significant improvement in the Karnofsky Performance score. Pain relief within 2 weeks of treatment was noted in 77% of the ^{188}Re-HEDP group and in 73% of the ^{153}Sm-EDTMP group. These results were not statistically significant, and there was no significant difference between responses in the patients with prostate or breast cancer. A brief flare reaction was noted in 17% of patients in both groups within 14 days of therapy, and the majority of patients demonstrated a maximum of grade I anemia within 12 weeks of therapy based on the 1979 WHO criteria. Grade I thrombocytopenia was noted in 2 patients with each isotope, and 1 patient in the ^{188}Re-HEDP group experienced grade II thrombocytopenia. Grade I leukopenia was noted in 1 patient in each group. All cases of thrombocytopenia and leukopenia reversed within 12 weeks after therapy. Similar findings have been reported by other investigators.[140,141]

SELECTED REFERENCES

A full list of references for this chapter is available online.

1. Abbas AK, Lichtman AH, Pillais S, eds. *Cellular and molecular immunology.* Philadelphia: Saunders Elsevier, 2007.
2. Campoli M, Ferrone S. Cancer immune surveillance and tumor escape mechanisms. In: Speer TW, ed. *Targeted radionuclide therapy.* Philadelphia: Lippincott Williams & Wilkins, 2011:3–21.
3. Jeoung DI. Employing SEREX for identification of targets for anticancer targeted therapy. In: Speer TW, ed. *Targeted radionuclide therapy.* Philadelphia: Lippincott Williams & Wilkins, 2011:159–167.
4. Wong JYC, Williams LE, Yazaki PJ. Radioimmunotherapy of colorectal cancer. In: Speer TW, ed. *Targeted radionuclide therapy.* Philadelphia: Lippincott Williams & Wilkins, 2011:321–351.
5. O'Donoghue JA. Dosimetric principles of targeted radiotherapy. In: Abrams PG, Fritzberg AR, eds. *Radioimmunotherapy of cancer.* New York: Marcel Dekker, 2000:1–20.
6. Burvenich IJG, Scott AM. The delivery construct: maximizing the therapeutic ratio of targeted radionuclide therapy. In: Speer TW, ed. *Targeted radionuclide therapy.* Philadelphia: Lippincott Williams & Wilkins, 2011:236–248.
7. DiCara D, Nissim A. Methods for development of monoclonal antibody therapeutics. In: Speer TW, ed. *Targeted radionuclide therapy.* Philadelphia: Lippincott Williams & Wilkins, 2011:22–31.
8. Kohler G, Milstein C. Continuous cultures of fused cells secreting antibody of predefined specificity. *Nature* 1975;256(5517):495–497.
9. Jain M, Kaur S, Batra SK. Modulation of biologic impediments for radioimmunotherapy of solid tumors. In: Speer TW, ed. *Targeted radionuclide therapy.* Philadelphia: Lippincott Williams & Wilkins, 2011:182–190.

13. Zwanziger D, Beck-Sickinger AG. Malignancies treated with peptides. In: Speer TW, ed. *Targeted radionuclide therapy.* Philadelphia: Lippincott Williams & Wilkins, 2011:483–497.
15. Imhof A, Brunner P, Marincek N, et al. Response, survival, and long-term toxicity after therapy with the radiolabeled somatostatin analogue [90Y-DOTA]-TOC in metastasized neuroendocrine cancers. *J Clin Oncol* 2011;29:2416–2423.
17. Stahl S, Friedman M, Carlsson J, et al. Affibody molecules for targeted radionuclide therapy. In: Speer TW, ed. *Targeted radionuclide therapy.* Philadelphia: Lippincott Williams & Wilkins, 2011:49–58.
20. Missailidis S, Perkins A. Radiolabeled aptamers for imaging and therapy. In: Speer TW, ed. *Targeted radionuclide therapy.* Philadelphia: Lippincott Williams & Wilkins, 2011:59–70.
24. Burvenich IJG, Scott AM. The delivery construct: maximizing the therapeutic ratio of targeted radionuclide therapy. In: Speer TW, ed. *Targeted radionuclide therapy.* Philadelphia: Lippincott Williams & Wilkins, 2011:236–248.
27. Chithrani BD, Stewart J, Allen C, et al. Intracellular uptake, transport, and processing of nanostructures in cancer cells. *Nanomedicine* 2009;5:118–127.
28. Maeda H, Sawa T, Konno T. Mechanism of tumor-targeted delivery of macromolecules drugs, including the EPR effect in solid tumor and clinical overview of the prototype polymeric drug SMANCS. *J Control Release* 2001;74:47–61.
29. Tesauro D, Morelli G, Pedone C, et al. Radiolabeled peptides, structure and analysis. In: Speer TW, ed. *Targeted radionuclide therapy.* Philadelphia: Lippincott Williams & Wilkins, 2011:32–48.
30. Pedone C, Morelli G, Tesauro D, et al. Peptide structure and analysis. In: Chinol M, Paganelli G, eds. *Radionuclide peptide cancer therapy.* New York: Taylor & Francis Group, 2006:1–30.
31. Fowler JF. Radiobiological aspects of low dose rate in radioimmunotherapy. *Int J Radiat Oncol Biol Phys* 1990;18:1261–1269.
32. Murry D, McEwan AJ. Radiobiology of systemic radiation therapy. *Cancer Biother Radiopharm* 2007;22:1–23.
33. Speer TW, Khuntia D. Introduction to radiation therapy. In: Mehta MP, ed. *Principles and practice of neuro-oncology: a multidisciplinary approach.* New York: Demos Medical Publishing, 2011:719–743.
34. Speer TW, Limmer JP, Henrich D, et al. Evolution of radiotherapy toward a more targeted approach for CNS malignancies. In: Speer TW, ed. *Targeted radionuclide therapy.* Philadelphia: Lippincott Williams & Wilkins, 2011:356–376.
35. Bernhardt P, Speer TW. Modeling the systemic cure with targeted radionuclide therapy. In: Speer TW, ed. *Targeted radionuclide therapy.* Philadelphia: Lippincott Williams & Wilkins, 2011:263–280.
36. Wilson AD, Brechbiel MW. Chelation chemistry. In: Speer TW, ed. *Targeted radionuclide therapy.* Philadelphia: Lippincott Williams & Wilkins, 2011:88–107.
37. Witzig TE. Radioimmunotherapy for B-cell non-Hodgkin lymphoma. In: Reilly RM, ed. Monoclonal antibody and peptide-targeted radiotherapy of cancer. Hoboken, NJ: John Wiley & Sons, 2010:169–218.
41. Rossi EA, Sharkey RM, McBride W, et al. Development of new multivalent-bispecific agents for pretargeting tumor localization and therapy. *Clin Cancer Res* 2003;9:3886S–3896S.
42. Sharkey RM, Goldenberg DM. Pretargeted radioimmunotherapy. In: Speer TW, ed. *Targeted radionuclide therapy.* Philadelphia: Lippincott Williams & Wilkins, 2011:191–208.
43. Axworthy DB, Reno JM, Hylarides MD, et al. Cure of human carcinoma xenographs by a single dose of pretargeted yttrium-90 with negligible toxicity. *Proc Natl Acad Sci* 2000;97:1802–1807.
45. Sharkey RM, Goldenberg DM. Cancer radioimmunotherapy. *Immunotherapy* 2011;3:349–370.
48. Chatal JF, Davodeau F, Cherel M, et al. Different ways to improve the clinical effectiveness of radioimmunotherapy in solid tumors. *J Cancer Res Ther* 2009;5:S36–S40.
49. Boerman OC, Koppe MJ, Postema EJ, et al. Radionuclide therapy of cancer with radiolabeled antibodies. *Anticancer Agents Med Chem* 2007;7:335–343.
50. Burdick M, Macklis RM. Radioimmunotherapy for non-Hodgkin lymphoma: a clinical update. In: Speer TW, ed. *Targeted radionuclide therapy.* Philadelphia: Lippincott Williams & Wilkins, 2011:426–440.
52. Pandit-Taskar N, O'Donoghue JA, Morris MJ, et al. Antibody mass escalation study in patients with castration-resistant prostate cancer using 111In-J591:lesion delectability and dosimetric projections for 90Y radioimmunotherapy. *J Nucl Med* 2008;49:1066–1074.
53. Witzig TE, Gordon LI, Cabanillas F, et al. Randomized, controlled trial of yttrium-90-labeled ibritumomab tiuxetan radioimmunotherapy versus rituximab immunotherapy for patients with relapsed refractory low-grade, follicular, or transformed B-cell non-Hodgkin's lymphoma. *J Clin Oncol* 2002;20:2453–2463.
54. Kaminski MS, Zelenetz AD, Press OW, et al. Pivotal study of iodine I-131-tositumomab for chemotherapy-refractory, low-grade, or transformed low-grade B-cell non-Hodgkin's lymphomas. *J Clin Oncol* 2001;19:3918–3928.
55. Morschhauser F, Radford J, Van Hoof A, et al. Phase III trial of consolidation therapy with yttrium-90-ibritumomab tiuxetan compared with no additional therapy after first remission in advanced follicular lymphoma. *J Clin Oncol* 2008;26:5156–5164.
56. Hagenbeek A, Radford J, Hoof AV, et al. 90Y-ibritumomab tiuxetan (Zevalin) consolidation of first remission in advanced-stage follicular non-Hodgkin's lymphoma: updated results after a median follow-up of 66.2 months from the international, randomized, phase III first-line indolent trial (FIT) in 414 patients [abstract 594]. 52nd ASH Annual Meeting and Exposition, December 6, 2010, Orlando, FL. Available at: http://ash.confex.com/ash/2010/webprogram/Paper28386.html. Accessed January 1, 2012.
57. Press OW, Unger JM, Rimsza LM, et al. A phase III randomized intergroup trial (SWOG S0016) of CHOP chemotherapy plus rituximab Vs. CHOP plus iodine-131-tositumomab for the treatment of newly diagnosed follicular non-Hodgkin's lymphoma [abstract 98]. 53rd ASH Annual Meeting and Exposition, December 11, 2011, San Diego, CA. Available at: http://ash.confex.com/ash/2011/webprogram/Paper39037.html. Accessed January 1, 2012.
58. Al-Ejeh F, Brown MP. Combined modality therapy: relevance for targeted radionuclide therapy. In: Speer TW, ed. *Targeted radionuclide therapy.* Philadelphia: Lippincott Williams & Wilkins, 2011:220–235.
62. Chen S, Yu L, Jiang C, et al. Pivotal study of iodine-131-labeled chimeric tumor necrosis treatment radioimmunotherapy in patients with advanced lung cancer. *J Clin Oncol* 2005;23:1538–1547.
63. Order SE, Stillwagon GB, Klein JL, et al. Iodine 131 antiferritin, a new treatment modality in hepatoma: a Radiation Therapy Oncology Group study. *J Clin Oncol* 1985;3:1573–1582.
64. Order S. Radioimmunotherapy of unresectable hepatocellular carcinoma. In: Speer TW, ed. *Targeted radionuclide therapy.* Philadelphia: Lippincott Williams & Wilkins, 2011:352–355.
66. Order SE, Pajak T, Leibel S, et al. A randomized prospective trial comparing full dose chemotherapy to 131I antiferritin: an RTOG study. *Int J Rad Oncol Biol Phys* 1989;20:953–963.
68. Xu J, Shen Z-Y, Chen X-G, et al. A randomized controlled trial of Licartin for preventing hepatoma recurrence after liver transplantation. *Hepatology* 2007;45:269–276.
69. Speer TW, Limmer JP, Henrich D, et al. Evolution of radiotherapy toward a more targeted approach for CNS malignancies. In: Speer TW, ed. *Targeted radionuclide therapy.* Philadelphia: Lippincott Williams & Wilkins, 2011:356–376.
70. Wygoda Z, Kula D, Bierzynska-Macyszyn G, et al. Use of monoclonal anti-EGFR antibody in the radioimmunotherapy of malignant gliomas in the context of EGFR expression in grade III and IV tumors. *Hybridoma* 2006;26(3):125–132.
74. Hopkins K, Chandler C, Bullimore J, et al. A pilot study of the treatment of patients with recurrent malignant gliomas with intratumoral yttrium-90 radioimmunoconjugates. *Radiother Oncol* 1995;34(2):121–131.
75. Thurber GM. Kinetics of antibody penetration into tumors. In: Speer TW, ed. *Targeted radionuclide therapy.* Philadelphia: Lippincott Williams & Wilkins, 2011:168–181.
76. Hopkins K, Chandler C, Eatough J, et al. Direct injection of 90Y MoAbs into glioma tumor resection cavities leads to limited diffusion of the radioimmunoconjugates into normal brain parenchyma: a model to estimate absorbed radiation dose. *Int J Radiation Oncol Biol Phys* 1998;40:835–844.
78. Akabani G, Reardon DA, Coleman RE, et al. Dosimetry and radiographic analysis of 131I-labeled anti-tenascin 81C6 murine monoclonal antibody in newly diagnosed patients with malignant gliomas: a phase II study. *J Nucl Med* 2005;46:1042–1051.
79. Reardon DA, Akabani G, Coleman RE, et al. Phase II trial of murine 131I-labeled antitenascin monoclonal antibody 81C6 administered into surgically created resection cavities of patients with newly diagnosed malignant gliomas. *J Clin Oncol* 2002;20:1389–1397.
80. Reardon DA, Akabani G, Coleman RE, et al. Salvage radioimmunotherapy with murine iodine-131-labeled antitenascin monoclonal antibody 81C6 for patients with recurrent primary and metastatic malignant brain tumors: phase II study results. *J Clin Oncol* 2006;24:115–122.
81. Reardon DA, Zalutsky MR, Akabani G, et al. A pilot study: 131I-antitenascin monoclonal antibody 81C6 to deliver a 44-Gy resection cavity boost. *Neuro Oncol* 2008;10(2):182–189.
82. Zalutsky MR, Reardon DA, Akabani G, et al. Clinical experience with α-particle-emitting 211At: treatment of recurrent brain tumor patients with 211At-labeled chimeric antitenascin monoclonal antibody 81C6. *J Nucl Med* 2008;49(1):30–38.
83. McLendon RE, Akabani G, Friedman HS, et al. Tumor resection cavity administered iodine-131-labeled antitenascin 81C6 radioimmunotherapy in patients with malignant glioma: neuropathology aspects. *Nucl Med Biol* 2007;34:405–413.
85. Verheijen RH, Massuger LF, Benigno BB, et al. Phase III trial of intraperitoneal therapy with yttrium-90-labeled HMFG1 murine monoclonal antibody in patients with epithelial ovarian cancer after a surgically defined complete remission. *J Clin Oncol* 2006;24:571–578.
86. Oei AL, Verheijen RH, Seiden MV, et al. Decreased intraperitoneal disease recurrence in epithelial ovarian cancer patients receiving intraperitoneal consolidation treatment with yttrium-90-labeled murine HMFG1 without improvement in overall survival. *Int J Cancer* 2007;120:2710–2714.
87. Wallner PE. Unconjugated radiopharmaceuticals. In: Speer TW, ed. *Targeted radionuclide therapy.* Philadelphia: Lippincott Williams & Wilkins, 2011:294–297.
93. Reisfield GM, Silberstein EB, Wilson GR. Radiopharmaceuticals for the palliation of painful bone metastases. *Am J Hosp Palliat Care* 2005;22:41–46.
96. Liepe K. Alpharadin, a 223Ra-based alpha-particle-emitting pharmaceutical for the treatment of bone metastases in patients with cancer. *Curr Opin Investig Drugs* 2009;10:1346–1358.
97. Zafeirakis A, Zissimopoulos A, Baziotis N, et al. Introduction of a new semi-quantitative index with predictive implications in patients with painful osseous metastases after (186)Re-HEDP therapy. *Q J Nucl Med Mol Imaging* 2011;55:91–102.
98. Biersack HJ, Palmedo H, Andris A, et al. Palliation and survival after repeated (188)Re-HEDP therapy of hormone-refractory bone metastases of prostate cancer: a retrospective analysis. *J Nucl Med* 2011;52:1721–1726.
99. Liu C, Brasic JR, Liu X, et al. Timing and optimized acquisition parameters for the whole-body imaging of 177Lu-EDTMP toward performing bone pain palliation treatment. *Nucl Med Commun* 2012;33:90–96.
100. Ogawa K, Kawashima H, Shiba K, et al. Development of [(90)Y]DOTA-conjugated bisphosphonate for treatment of painful bone metastases. *Nucl Med Biol* 2009;36:129–135.
101. Das T, Chakraborty S, Sarma HD, et al. (170)Tm-EDTMP: a potential cost-effective alternative to (89)SrCl(2) for bone pain palliation. *Nucl Med Biol* 2009;36:561–568.
102. Silberstein EB. Teletherapy and radiopharmaceutical therapy of painful bone metastases. *Sem Nuc Med* 2005;35:152–158.
105. Roque I, Figuls M, Martinez-Zapata MJ, et al. Radioisotopes for metastatic bone pain. *Cochrane Database Syst Rev* 2011;(6):CD003347.
106. Dillehay GL, Ellerbroek NA, Balon H, et al. Practice guideline for the performance of therapy with unsealed radiopharmaceutical sources. *Int J Radiat Oncol Biol Phys* 2006;64:1299–1307.
107. Lutz S, Berk L, Chang E, et al. Palliative radiotherapy for bone metastases: an ASTRO evidence-based guideline. *Int J Radiat Oncol Biol Phys* 2011;79:965–976.
110. International Atomic Energy Agency. *Nuclear medicine in thyroid cancer management: a practical approach.* Vienna, Austria: International Atomic Energy Agency, 2009.
112. Kulkarni K, Van Nostrand D, Atkins F. 131-I ablation and treatment of well-differentiated thyroid cancer. In: Speer TW, ed. *Targeted radionuclide therapy.* Philadelphia: Lippincott Williams & Wilkins, 2011:281–293.
113. Reiners C, Dietlein M, Luster. Radio-iodine therapy in differentiated thyroid cancer: indication and procedure. *Best Pract Res Clin Endocrinol Metab* 2008;22:989–1007.
116. Mazzaferri EL, Jhiang SM. Long-term impact of initial surgical and medical therapy on papillary and follicular thyroid cancer. *Am J Med* 1994;97:418–428.

119. Hay ID, McConahey WM, Goellner JR. Managing patients with papillary thyroid carcinoma: insights gained from the Mayo Clinic's experience of treating 2,512 consecutive patients during 1940 through 2000. *Trans Am Clin Climatol Assoc* 2002;113:241–260.
122. Mazzaferri EL, Kloos RT. Using recombinant human TSH in the management of well-differentiated thyroid cancer: current strategies and future directions. *Thyroid* 2000;10:767–778.
123. Dorn R, Kopp J, Vogt H, et al. Dosimetry-guided radioactive iodine treatment in patients with metastatic differentiated thyroid cancer: largest safe dose using a risk-adapted approach. *J Nucl Med* 2003;44:451–456.
126. Potter ME, Partridge EE, Shingleton HM, et al. Intraperitoneal chromic phosphate in ovarian cancer: risks and benefits. *Gynecol Oncol* 1989;32:314–318.
129. Young RC, Brody MF, Nieberg RK, et al. Adjuvant treatment for early ovarian cancer: a randomized phase III trial of intraperitoneal 32P or intravenous cyclophosphamide and cisplatin—a Gynecologic Oncology Group study. *J Clin Oncol* 2003;21:4350–4355.
132. Porter AT, McEwan AJ, Powe JE, et al. Results of a randomized phase-III trial to evaluate the efficacy of strontium-89 adjuvant to local field external beam irradiation in the management of endocrine resistant metastatic prostate cancer. *Int J Radiat Oncol Biol Phys* 1993;25:805–813.
134. Sartor O. Overview of samarium Sm 153 lexidronam in the treatment of painful metastatic disease of bone. *Rev Urol* 2004;6(Suppl 10):S3–S12.
135. Anderson PM, Wiseman GA, Erlandson L, et al. Gemcitabine radiosensitization after high-dose samarium for osteoblastic osteosarcoma. *Clin Cancer Res* 2005; 11:6895–6900.
137. Nilsson S, Franzen L, Parker C, et al. Bone-targeted radium-223 in symptomatic, hormone-refractory prostate cancer: a randomised, multicentre, placebo-controlled phase II study. *Lancet Oncol* 2007;8:587–594.
138. O'Sullivan JM, McCready VR, Flux G, et al. High activity rhenium-186 HEDP with autologous peripheral blood stem cell rescue: a phase I study in progressive hormone refractory prostate cancer metastatic to bone. *Br J Cancer* 2002;86: 1715–1720.
139. Liepe K, Runge R, Kotzerke J. The benefit of bone-seeking radiopharmaceuticals in the treatment of metastatic bone disease. *J Cancer Res Clin Oncol* 2005; 131:60–66.
140. Li S, Liu J, Zhang H, et al. Rhenium-188 HEDP to treat painful bone metastases. *Clin Nuc Med* 2001;26:919–922.
141. Zhang H, Tian M, Li S, et al. Rhenium-188-HEDP therapy for the palliation of pain due to osseous metastases in lung cancer patients. *Cancer Biother Radiopharm* 2003;18:719–726.

Chapter 27 Photodynamic Therapy

Harry Quon, Charles B. Simone, II, Keith A. Cengel, Jarod C. Finlay, Timothy C. Zhu, and Theresa M. Busch

The first report of cytotoxicity (in paramecium) observed by combining a drug (acridine) and visible light can be traced to the medical student Oscar Raab working in the laboratory of Herman von Tappeiner in 1900.[1] This observation laid the foundation for the 1903 descriptions by von Tappeiner and Jesioneck who combined topical eosin and visible light for the treatment of a skin tumor.[2] Modern investigations of photodynamic therapy (PDT) have since been attributed to Lipson et al.[3] in 1960, with the discovery of hematoporphyrin derivative (HPD) by Samuel Schwartz,[4] a water-soluble mixture of porphyrins and a series of preclinical and clinical investigations led by Dougherty et al.[5]

Despite its deep historical origins and modern research investigations dating back 40 years, the clinical application of PDT remains limited to specific clinical situations. In part, this has been due to the superficial depth of cytotoxicity achievable with past photosensitizers and light delivery techniques. It is also due to the complexity of its application, requiring familiarity with safe photosensitizer administration coupled with the technical requirements for effective light delivery and the optical expertise to prescribe and deliver an activating light energy in a selective manner.

Despite these disadvantages, there are several compelling reasons to evaluate PDT as a major therapeutic approach in the management of cancer. Central to this is its unique mechanism of action allowing for nonoverlapping toxicities with traditional cancer therapeutics. As such, PDT does not exclude the subsequent administration of these treatment modalities. Technical advances with interstitial light delivery techniques (and advancements in modeling its dosimetry[6]) along with the clinical development of photosensitizers capable of absorbing and being activated at longer wavelengths now offer the potential for more penetrating cytotoxicity.[7] Unlike traditional chemotherapeutics and ionizing radiation therapy, there has also been a paucity of any long-term genotoxic effects with the use of PDT, an observation consistent with several *in vitro* studies.[8–10] The explosion in our understanding of tumor biology and the influence of the microenvironment has also provided tremendous insights into the development of novel strategies to optimize the clinical efficacy of PDT, including its combination with biologic therapeutics. This also includes the potential for PDT to enhance the effects of traditional cancer therapeutics and its promising role to more effectively induce adaptive cell-mediated immunity.

PRINCIPLES OF PHOTODYNAMIC THERAPY

Photosensitizers

PDT represents a treatment modality that combines the selective photochemical activation of photosensitizers with electromagnetic radiation in the visible energy range (i.e., light). Photosensitizers (PS) may be introduced into the cancer patient either systemically, topically, or injected locally, but it is its chemical structure that can significantly influence the effectiveness of a PDT treatment. These include influencing its biodistribution and subcellular localization along with how efficiently it absorbs light (referred to as its *molar extinction coefficient*) to generate reactive oxidative species (ROS), including singlet oxygen (referred to as its *quantum yield*) (Table 27.1). A PS with a low molar extinction coefficient will require large concentrations of the PS and light energy to be effectively delivered for photoactivation.

There are now a multitude of PS that have been generated with many under preclinical evaluation and several receiving regulatory approval for clinical application in the United States, European Union, and other countries. The first PS to receive regulatory approval was a semipurified preparation of HPD known as Photofrin (porfimer sodium). Porfimer sodium represents a complex mixture of hematoporphyrin oligomers whose chemical composition has been difficult to fully characterize and reproduce consistently. It has an absorption peak at 630 nm with a relatively low molar extinction coefficient, thus requiring large concentrations of drug and light energy (fluence) to be delivered. It has also been shown to have a prolonged risk of skin photosensitivity reflecting its relative lack of tumor selectivity; and while used routinely in clinical practice, these disadvantages have spurred ongoing PS development.

TABLE 27.1 FACTORS AFFECTING THE EFFICACY OF PHOTODYNAMIC THERAPY

Photosensitizer (PS)	Effectiveness of the tumor vasculature to deliver PS, extracellular and intracellular location of PS, PS extinction coefficient, singlet oxygen quantum yield, PS photobleaching
Light	Drug-light interval, fluence, fluence rate
Microenvironment	Oxygenation, status of immune system
Tumor response	Complex interaction between pro-apoptotic and pro-survival signals, angiogenic response

Several ideal characteristics have been well articulated in the area of PS development. These include a PS that has a well-established structure, ideally a pure compound with a constant composition and a stable shelf-life. Without light activation, it should have little toxicity and tumor specificity when administered. With light, a PS with spectral absorption peaks that demonstrate a high extinction coefficient will be more efficiently activated. However, it is not entirely clear if this is always desired. Strong PS absorption at a specific wavelength can further contribute to reduced light penetration, a phenomenon referred to as *self-shielding*. Moreover, potent PS such as temoporfin/m-THPC (Foscan) that thus require little drug and light for its efficient activation have been associated with significant complications necessitating even more vigilance to the light dosimetry (see below).[11] The wavelengths of a photosensitizer's absorption peaks also influences how the PS will be used clinically, with absorption at longer wavelengths (i.e., 700 nm range) offering deeper light penetration in human tissues. Lastly, some PS may undergo a process of *photobleaching,* whereby the PS in turn reacts with the singlet oxygen or other ROS created in the photoactivation process altering its ability to act as a PS. Typically, photobleaching decreases a photosensitizer's reactivity, which may or may not be desirable depending on the context of its clinical application.

Structurally, photosensitizers are generally classified as porphyrin-based or nonporphyrins with the former sharing a common backbone that consists of the tetrapyrrole ring. Other structural backbones that have demonstrated photosensitizing capabilities include the presence of four phenol rings and polycyclic ring compounds based on the pyrrole ring especially the tetrapyrrollic PS. Extensive reviews are available regarding the specific physicochemical properties (i.e., primary structures, the presence of complexed heavy metals, and specific side chain substitutions) and the impact on its systemic biodistribution, cellular uptake, and photosensitizing properties.[7] In general, the ability for hydrophobic compounds with two or less negative charges can still cross the plasma membrane. Otherwise, intracellular uptake is through active endocytosis. The charge of the hydrophobic PS can also influence where a PS localizes with cationic charges (positive), tending to localize to the mitochondria and anionic PS with a net charge of negative two or greater tending to localize in the lysosomes.[12] Cationic PS localizing to the mitochondria have been suggested to be more effective in mediating direct cytotoxicity.[13]

Although tumor specificity is in part mediated by selective light administration and its natural energy attenuation, specific extracellular and intracellular PS delivery is felt to further contribute to this process. Human tissue studies in patients receiving porfimer sodium-mediated intraperitoneal PDT have confirmed PS selectivity, even if narrow.[14] Systemically administered photosensitizers, especially those with the tetrapyrrole backbone, will associate with serum proteins, including albumin and low-density lipoproteins (LDL). The association with LDL proteins has been suggested to be a potential mechanism that may contribute to specific tumor localization.[15] In this model, it has been proposed that tumor selectivity occurs due to a preferential up-regulation of LDL receptors in tumor cells due to the rapid plasma membrane turnover rate and the need for constituents in its biosynthesis. Alternatively, the functionally altered tumor vasculature resulting from overexpression of vascular endothelial growth factor[16] and its impaired lymphatic clearance of the extravasated PS have also been advanced as a working model.[17] Although this may lead to increased PS retention, the extracellular distribution of the PS can be inhomogeneous and can impact the effectiveness of a PDT treatment. Korbelik and Grosl[18] demonstrated that direct tumor cell killing was a function of the distance from a tumor's vascular supply. In turn, photosensitizers that tend to be located in the intravascular space can increase the effectiveness of PDT through mediating vascular damage and tumor infarction.[19]

The subcellular localization of a PS can similarly influence the mechanism of cellular injury and has been well studied and recently summarized.[20] In general, photosensitizers that localize to the plasma membrane and lysosomes are likely to cause injury by necrosis. Those localizing to the mitochondria and endoplasmic reticulum are likely to initiate cell death by way of apoptosis.[5,20,21] However, mitochondrial injury can also mediate a necrotic cell death with severe inner mitochondrial membrane damage.[20]

Most photosensitizers tend not to accumulate in the nucleus, possibly explaining the paucity of genotoxicity and observed carcinogenesis.[8,22] Although DNA damage has been reported in cell culture experiments for various photosensitizers,[8–10,23] especially for 5-aminolevulinic acid,[23,24] efficient DNA repair has also been observed, suggesting that the damage may not be sufficient to overwhelm a cell's repair capacity.[10,25] As PDT can mediate cell death through non-DNA targets, the potential mutagenic effects of any DNA injury is likely to be further limited by its cell death.

Photosensitizer Activation

Following photosensitizer administration, the drug–light interval (DLI) that is prescribed warrants consideration. Preclinical studies have demonstrated that varying the DLI can influence both the PS extracellular and intracellular localization.[19,26] In general, longer DLI will promote PS extravasation and intracellular uptake, provided it has a sufficient long pharmacokinetic lifetime. However, this passive targeting of either the vascular (short DLI) or tumor compartment can be compounded by the lipophilicity of the PS and which proteins it associates with within the vasculature. It would also appear that targeting both the vascular and tumor compartment with repeat PS administration, combining both a short DLI and a long DLI, can further improve the effectively of PDT. However, the order of the repeat PS administration and activation may be particularly important. Prescribing an initial short DLI that targets the vasculature can create subsequent hypoxia that limits the efficacy of the repeat PS with a long DLI.[19]

PS activation involves the absorption of wavelength specific energy, causing specific changes in the electron energy states of the PS. Energy absorption can cause a PS electron to move from its ground state to a higher energy level or what is referred to as an excited energy state. While in the excited energy state, transition back to the ground state may occur, with energy released in the form of fluorescence or heat dissipation. Thus, some of the light absorbed by a PS may be re-emitted at a different wavelength, allowing for fluorescence detection of the PS or *photodynamic diagnosis* (PDD). Figure 27.1 demonstrates the Jablonski energy diagram that depicts the energy transitions that may occur with PDT. Two possible excited energy states may be possible: a singlet state (S1) or the triplet state (T1), which has a longer half-life. The distinction depends on the spin direction of the excited electron relative to its paired electron in the ground state. The triplet state has both electrons parallel to each other,

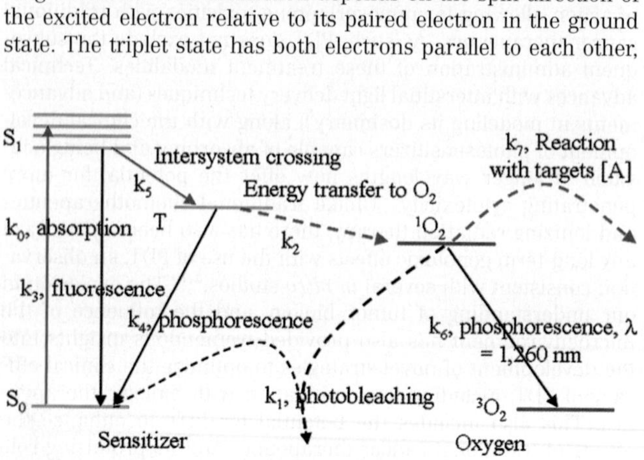

FIGURE 27.1. Jablonski energy diagram following type II photosensitizer activation.

and its ability to return to a ground state emitting fluorescence is impeded due to this spin direction.

Transition to the triplet state through a process referred to as *intersystem crossing* is critical to the generation of cytotoxic ROS. This is largely due to the longer half-life of the triplet state that increases the probability of interacting with a nearby organic molecule (i.e., in the plasma membrane), generating reactive anions or cations that in turn may react with molecular oxygen generating ROS (referred to as a type I reaction). Alternatively, a PS in its triplet state may directly transfer its energy to molecular oxygen to form an excited state singlet oxygen ($^1O_2$) (type II reaction). Both types of reactions may occur simultaneously, though direct singlet oxygen production is felt to be the dominant mechanism of cytotoxicity.[27,28]

Singlet oxygen within the cell has a limited half-life (estimated to be <0.04 μs) and thus a limited range of diffusion and activity (<0.02 μm).[22,29] As such, PS cytotoxicity is limited to its extracellular and intracellular (commonly referred to as subcellular) localization and adjacent potential targets for reactivity.[22] For example, photosensitizers that tend to biodistribute or favor being localized in the vasculature will favor an antivascular necrotic mechanism of injury. The specific subcellular localization offers an added degree of specificity to its cytotoxicity, as already described.

Physics of Light Dosimetry

Photodynamic therapy is inherently a dynamic process. All three principal components—photosensitizer, light, and oxygen—interact dynamically over the time period of a PDT prescription.[5] As light interacts with human tissue, its energy distribution is influenced by surface reflection and with absorption and scatter at depth. Light scatter in human tissues can be affected by many factors. Tissue architecture, its geometry, and its heterogeneity at the histologic and cellular levels can contribute to photon scattering, limiting the energy deposited at depth. Thus, it is important to recognize that light scatter is likely to be different from one tissue type to another. Although this factor remains to be fully characterized such that it can be accounted for in the prescription of PDT, selecting longer wavelengths for photoactivation can help to reduce photon scatter, thus increasing light penetration.

The deposition of light, or its *dosimetry,* is determined by the light source characteristics and the tissue optical properties, both on the surface and at depth, in contrast to ionizing radiation. In turn, the tissue optical properties are influenced by the spatiotemporal distribution and concentration of both the photosensitizer and oxygen in the illuminated tissues. During illumination, the light dosimetry also dynamically changes as the photodynamic process consumes oxygen and can also alter the blood flow.[30] For some photosensitizers, self-shielding can influence the light dosimetry at depth. Finally, the distribution of a photosensitizer may change as a result of photobleaching, a process whereby the photodynamic modification of the photosensitizer itself typically reduces its ability to further be photoactivated.

Quantifying the distribution of the light that is used in photoactivation is important oncologically and for quality assurance reasons, as in the practice of ionizing radiation. The ability to relate the treatment outcome to the effective light fluence and its rate of delivery (*fluence rate*) facilitates not only an understanding of its relationship to the treatment outcome but also to any potential toxicities, as areas of high fluence and fluence rates have been associated with treatment toxicities. Several approaches to quantifying light dosimetry may be outlined.

Explicit dosimetry refers to the prediction of a singlet oxygen dose on the basis of measurable quantities that contribute to the photodynamic effect.[31] In clinical practice, the quantity most amenable to measurement is the PDT dose, defined as the light energy deposited to a photosensitizer. This quantity is proportional to the product of the absorption coefficient of the photosensitizer and light fluence. The absorption coefficient of the photosensitizer is, in turn, proportional to the photosensitizer concentration. PDT dose calculated in this way is a good predictor of outcome if one is operating in a drug- or light-limited situation when there is ample oxygen supply. To generally account for the oxygen effect, the concentration of reacted singlet oxygen (i.e., the concentration of reactions between singlet oxygen and molecular targets within the tumor cells) needs to be modeled as a function of PDT dose and tissue oxygenation. It has been shown that the reacted singlet oxygen concentration can be expressed as the integration of the product of the PDT dose rate and the photosensitizer's singlet oxygen quantum yield.[32]

Implicit dosimetry refers to the use of photobleaching of the sensitizer as a measure of the light dose. For sensitizers where the photobleaching is mediated by singlet oxygen, it can be shown that on the microscopic scale, the fractional photobleaching is indicative of the concentration of singlet oxygen reactions induced by PDT.[33] Although the relationship to tissue response is more complex, photobleaching has been shown to be predictive of response in animal models[34] and used to design protocols for pain reduction during the treatment of patients.[35]

Accurate light dosimetry presents significant challenges in the clinic. Although it is relatively straightforward to measure the irradiance of light delivered to the surface of a tissue, the light absorbed by the sensitizer also includes the light scattered by tissue not too dissimilar from ionizing radiation. Unlike ionizing radiation, this scattered light contribution may also occur on a surface and is an important concept to consider in the practice of PDT. In hollow organs or any concave surface with surface secretions that further increase the reflective index, light can be reflected from one surface onto another surface, increasing the effective surface light fluence rate. This effect is often referred to as the *integrating sphere effect.* In the extreme case, multiple reflections can significantly magnify the fluence rate within a hollow organ. This integrating sphere effect has been extensively modeled in the case of bladder treatment.[36] In complex concave mucosal surfaces such as in the head and neck, scattered light photons have been demonstrated to increase the effective fluence rate by factors of three- to fourfold.[37,38]

Light scattering can also occur within tissues, leading to a significant difference between the incident fluence rate that is delivered and the fluence rate within the tissue. In practice, the integrating sphere effect and multiple scattering within the tissue occur simultaneously. Accurate dosimetry requires accounting for both of these effects, ideally through real-time measurements using an isotropic light photon detector capable of capturing both directly incident and scattered light.[39] A comparison of measurements using fiber-based isotropic detectors and photodiode detectors that capture only incident light indicated significant difference in the measured light dose with significant variation in the contribution from scattered light.[40] Through measurements with a series of light sources and detectors, tissue optical properties can be assessed. However, PDT treatment can significantly change the optical properties. This requires the ability to assess the optical properties in real time for there to be effective feedback to compensate for the influence of varying light transmission on the deposited light dose within the target tissue.[41,42] Recently, the first clinical experiences using an automated 18-channel system accommodating optical fibers for light delivery and monitoring was described in patients treated with temoporfin interstitial PDT.[6]

Biology of Photodynamic Therapy

Mechanisms of Tumor Cytotoxicity

Photodynamic therapy can induce cytotoxicity through all three death morphologies: apoptosis, autophagy, and necrosis. The multitude of signaling pathways (apoptotic and nonapoptotic) and the molecular interplay between various cell death pathways (balanced with the induction of pro-survival signals) that are activated with exposure of the cell to photodynamic oxidative stress have been the focus of intense investigations and the subject of a recent extensive review.[43] Of these modes of cell death, apoptosis is a major pathway of PDT-mediated cytotoxicity and reflects the near ubiquitous ability of PDT to induce mitochondrial injury.[44,45]

Photodynamic therapy can also induce tumor cell injury through direct damage of the endothelial cells of the tumor vasculature. In turn, thrombus formation and the release of various vasoactive molecules, with an increase in the vascular permeability and deterioration of vascular status, ensue. Leukocyte infiltration further compounds this response, all contributing to secondary hypoxia[46] with ischemic tumor death and tumor control.[47] Preclinical studies also suggest that beyond direct tumor and vascular cytotoxicity, long-term tumor control can only occur in immunocompetent animals.[48]

Influence of the Tumor Microenvironment on the Photodynamic Therapy Response

As PDT is dependent on the presence and distribution of a photosensitizer, light, and oxygen, the normal tissue microenvironment within which a tumor is located can significantly determine the treatment response of the tumor to PDT. All three key PDT components are subject to effects from the tissue microenvironment. For example, tumor vascular density, permeability, or perfusion can affect photosensitizer delivery,[49] which could undoubtedly contribute to the heterogeneities detected in photosensitizer levels among tumors within and among patients.[50–52,53–54] Tumor-associated hypoxia can limit PDT-created damage.[55,56–58] Even the distribution of the treatment light is affected by the microenvironment due to differences in the penetration of red light as a function of the oxygenation status of hemoglobin. Compared to deoxyhemoglobin, oxygenated hemoglobin is less absorptive of red light (630 or 650 nm), thereby allowing deeper light penetration in tissues with a higher proportion of oxygenated hemoglobin.[59]

Much research has been performed on the dependence, as well as the effects of, PDT on tumor oxygenation. With conventional photosensitizers, the photochemical process can consume tissue oxygen faster than its delivery, leading to a hypoxic state that limits PDT-mediated cytotoxicity.[60,61–62] Even intratumor heterogeneities in tumor oxygenation can have consequences to PDT-mediated cytotoxicity. This has been shown in murine studies that identify the presence of more severe PDT-created hypoxia in the base of subcutaneous tumors accompanied by a relative protection of this area from clonogenic cell death.[58]

PDT-mediated vascular effects are another cause of hypoxia during PDT. These effects can take the form of PDT-triggered vasoconstriction.[63] Additionally or alternatively, PDT can cause endothelial cell rounding, leading to intracellular gaps[64] and activation of the coagulation cascade. Ischemia then results, as leukocyte and platelet aggregation with secondary thrombosis within the vessels can further alter the blood flow.[63,65] Dynamic changes in tumor blood flow, including treatment-initiated decreases in the blood flow, have been observed for several photosensitizers including porfimer sodium, 5-aminolevulinic acid (5-ALA; Levulan), motexafin lutetium (Lutrin), verteporfin (Visudyne), palladium bacteriopherophorbide (Tookad), and 2-(1-hexyloxyethyl)-2-devinyl pyropheophorbide-a (HPPH; Photochlor).[63,66–72] In fact, PDT-triggered reductions in tumor blood flow during light delivery are not only therapy limiting, but also directly correlate with outcome measures. Yu et al.[68] showed that the duration (long) and the slope (shallow) of the Photofrin-PDT–induced decrease in tumor blood flow correlated with the time-to-tumor regrowth (prolonged) in an animal. Similarly, Standish et al.[73] and Pham et al.[74] reported PDT-induced decreases in tumor blood flow and $\%StO_2$ (tissue hemoglobin oxygen saturation), respectively, correlated with necrosis development. These findings show the value in the development and application of noninvasive approaches to measure tumor blood flow during clinical applications of PDT.[69,75,76] Thus, although PDT-induced ischemia can limit the effectiveness of PDT, in the setting of sufficient light and drug doses, the persistent ischemia that is induced can provide incremental cytotoxicity that can improve the effectiveness.[47,77]

Experimental strategies directed at modulating the vascular response to PDT are also consistent with the importance of its contribution to the PDT effect. For example, inhibitors of nitric oxide have been effective in increasing tumor and vascular damage to porfimer sodium or ALA-PDT in a protocol-dependent manner.[78–80] Also, the vascular disrupting agent, vadimezan (5,6-dimethylxanthenone-4-acetic acid; DMXAA) has been successful in improving PDT responses when administered in such a way as to decrease tumor perfusion after illumination.[70,81] It is even possible to deliver PDT in two fractions so that a vascular-damaging protocol follows one in which oxidative damage to tumor cells is the major cytotoxic mechanism.[19] This approach has been studied in preclinical models using verteporfin as photosensitizer by first employing a longer interval between drug administration and light delivery to allow drug accumulation in the tumor cells, leading to direct light-induced cytotoxicity, followed by a second round of drug administration and light delivery that utilizes a short drug-light interval, which causes more extensive vascular damage due to drug localization in the blood vessels at the time of light delivery.[19] Similar observations have been reported with the photosensitizer MV6401.[26]

Tumor Stress Response to Photodynamic Therapy

The oxidative stress initiated with PDT can induce the expression of genes that can mediate various modes of cell death as well as survival signals. Using c-DNA microarrays, the cellular effects of hypericin-mediated PDT was studied on the expression of a panel of genes involved in apoptosis, metabolism, and proliferation, among other cellular processes.[82] Twenty-five genes were significantly up-regulated by PDT, including dual specificity phosphatase-1 (DUSP1), which can induce apoptosis; the stress response proto-oncogenes, *FOSB* and *JUN*, whose protein products dimerize to contribute to the transcription factor AP-1, another effector (both positive and negative) of apoptotic response; and *MYC*, which codes for the pro-apoptotic transcription factor c-myc. Among the genes down-regulated by PDT were *THBS1*, whose protein product thrombospondin-1 is an effector of cell interaction with the extracellular matrix, angiogenesis, apoptosis, and cell migration; *ADAM10*, which codes for a family of cell surface proteins with roles in epithelial cell–cell adhesion, migration, and proliferation; and several genes in the integrin family that mediate cell-to-cell and cell-to-matrix attachments, thereby facilitating signal transduction along pathways controlling apoptosis and metastasis, among other functions.[82]

In other studies, PDT-induced apoptosis was associated with activation of p38 in the mitogen-activated protein kinase (MAPK) family,[83–85] which along with its other family members (including ERK and JNK) regulate cell proliferation, differentiation, and survival. Furthermore, expression of pro-apoptotic and anti-apoptotic proteins of the Bcl-2 family can also be modulated by PDT in a context-dependent matter, which depends on factors such as cell type and subcellular localization of photosensitizer.[83,86,87] Similarly, PDT-induced expression and phosphorylation of survivin, capable of inhibiting apoptosis through inhibiting caspase-9, has also been an active area of investigation to therapeutically improve PDT cytotoxicity.[88] Signal transduction in PDT-induced apoptosis, autophagy, and necrosis is an area of much and expanding interest, and for the interested reader, several comprehensive reviews[43,89,90] are available on the current state of knowledge on this topic.

Immunologic Response to Photodynamic Therapy

The altered microenvironment generated by PDT can also serve to stimulate the host immune responses. Both the activation of an innate (nonspecific) and an adaptive antigen-specific immune response may be seen following PDT. These findings have raised considerable hopes that a localized treatment with PDT may lead to broader and possibly systemic oncologic benefits. For example, PDT-induced damage is associated with the local influx of neutrophils and other cell types, such as macrophages, natural killer cells, and dendritic cells, which contribute to local damage and inflammation while also initiating a broader systemic immune response.[91] Both preclinical and clinical studies show this to be accompanied by the release of immune-modulating factors, such as interleukin (IL) 1-β, tumor necrosis factor (TNF)-α, IL-6, IL-10 and granulocyte colony-stimulating factor (G-CSF).[92,93–94]

The resulting activation of the innate immune response plays a major role in tumor control after PDT, and neutrophils are key to this process. *In vitro* studies demonstrate neutrophil adhesion to an extracellular matrix exposed by PDT-mediated endothelial cell damage.[95] *In vivo* studies find neutrophils to attach to PDT-treated blood vessels,[96] while various approaches toward depleting neutrophil influx into the PDT-treated tissues have been to the detriment of therapeutic outcome.[97,98] In fact, a systemic neutrophilia is known to accompany PDT of various tumor types, sites, and photosensitization protocols.[99–101] PDT can also activate the complement system with opsonization and fixation of the complement C3 protein to tumor cells, which also promotes a strong neutrophilia. This serves to not only target cells for destruction by the innate immune system but can induce the release of pro-inflammatory mediators further contributing to the migration of neutrophils.[102]

In addition to the induction of an innate immune response, PDT can also stimulate an adaptive cell-mediated immunity. In fact, these types of immune responses are intricately connected processes. It has been proposed that a critical aspect of PDT-induced adaptive immunity is the generation of a high antigen load with tumor cell death that is presented for adaptive immunity. Tumor cell death is further promoted by the strong neutrophilia through its release of lysosomal enzymes, including myeloperoxidase and the generation of further ROS. This strong neutrophilia also appears to be a critical factor for the development of PDT-induced adaptive immunity,[103] as neutrophils degranulate and release a family of mediators referred to as alarmins. *Alarmins* are a critical link between the innate inflammatory response and adaptive immunity as they are capable of recruiting and activating the maturation of antigen-presenting dendritic cells.[104] With a strong innate immune response, this antigen presentation can be more effectively recognized, inducing an adaptive cell-mediated immunologic response and memory.[105]

Dendritic cells (DCs) typically exist in the immature state within the tissue microenvironment actively surveying and capturing antigens then migrating and presenting these to T cells in adjacent draining lymph nodes. For dendritic cells to mature and affect adaptive immunity, the expression of costimulatory molecules that are involved in antigen-presentation to T cells is important. Several aspects of this innate response, including the strong neutrophilia[103] and the release of damage-associated molecular patterns (DAMPs), consist of various markers of normal tissue injury. Among these, the extracellular release of heat shock protein-70 (HSP-70) and its association with tumor antigens by PDT-treated cells appears to be particularly effective in being recognized by DCs through surface receptors leading to their activation and maturation.[106]

HSPs, in particular HSP-70, have been a DAMP of particular interest in PDT for some time.[107] HSPs are molecular chaperones crucial for proper protein folding. HSPs can facilitate cell survival during intracellular functioning, but become immunostimulatory when extracellular or membrane bound.[108] In studies of PDT, HSP-70 is rapidly exposed on the surface of tumor cells treated *in vitro*,[109] and its antibody-based blockage served to inhibit maturation of dendritic cells.[110] Moreover, surface or extracellular expression of HSP-70 after PDT has been shown to correlate with curative outcome in temoporfin-treated murine tumors.[111] Research in these and other aspects of PDT-generated antitumor immunity has spawned interest in the use of PDT to develop cancer vaccines, the history and progress of which have been recently reviewed.[112]

Vascular Response to Photodynamic Therapy

Despite the therapeutic benefits to be gained from PDT-created vascular damage and inflammation, it comes at a cost. In a post-PDT tumor microenvironment characterized by inflammatory infiltrates, cytokine overexpression, eicosanoid production, and hypoxia, there is a strong pro-angiogenic stimulus to support the growth of new tumor blood vessels.[113] Such angiogenesis can counteract the intended effects of treatment by providing a means for delivery of oxygen and nutrients to tumor cells that escaped direct (oxidative) or secondary (vascular or immune-mediated) damage by PDT. Vascular endothelial growth factor (VEGF) is one of the most common angiogenic molecules whose expression is stimulated by PDT, and its increase has been measured following PDT with a variety of photosensitizers and tumor models.[114–116] Moreover, studies of human tumors grown as murine xenografts find PDT to induce modest increases in host-derived (mouse) VEGF in addition to the increases in human VEGF that originate from the treated tumor.[117,118] The molecular mechanisms of PDT-initiated increases in VEGF can include increases in hypoxia-inducible factor (HIF)-1α, a transcription factor that promotes the activation of many hypoxia-responsive genes such as VEGF,[119,120] as well as activation of the p38 MAPK pathway.[121] In the case of the latter, an inhibitor of p38 MAPK significantly attenuated the PDT-induced increase in VEGF.[121]

Cyclo-oxygenase (COX) 2 is another pro-angiogenic molecule that is up-regulated by PDT under a variety of treatment conditions.[122,123–124] The COX-2 enzyme serves to catalyze the production of prostaglandin (PG) H_2, a substrate for multiple eicosanoid mediators (including additional prostaglandins and thromboxane) known to contribute to PDT-created ischemia.[125,126] The pro-angiogenic activity of COX-2 can be mediated through the enzyme's role in production of PGE_2, which in turn can promote increases in VEGF.[113] Moreover, PDT-stimulated pro-inflammatory cytokines such as IL-1β and TNF-α may also stimulate angiogenesis through a COX-2 dependent pathway. This is supported by findings that decrease in PGE_2 after COX-2 inhibition is accompanied by a reduction in protein levels of IL-1β and TNF-α.[127]

Biologic Strategies to Improve Photodynamic Therapy Cytotoxicity

With a growing understanding of the biological and molecular mechanisms that underlie PDT-derived cytotoxicity has come the development of alternative, more effective approaches toward PDT delivery. These include the development of new targeted PS that exploit specific signatures or functions in diseased tissue in order to deliver, or even to activate, the PS.[128] These are commonly referred to as *PDT molecular beacons*, where the PS and a singlet oxygen-quenching or -scavenging molecule are both coupled to a linker that can interact with a cancer-specific target.[129] In this way, the PS photoactivity is silenced due to the proximity of the singlet oxygen-quenching molecule. The PS is only capable of being photoactivated when the linker interacts with the cancer-specific target, which results in physical separation of the singlet oxygen-scavenging molecule from the PS. Examples of novel targeted linker constructs include an antisense oligonucleotide complementary to a target messenger RNA that is conformationally restricted until the oligonucleotide interacts with its target.

Modulation of light delivery has also proven successful in mitigating the microenvironment limitations imposed by PDT. For example, lowering the fluence rate of light delivery can conserve tumor oxygenation during PDT, increasing direct tumor cell cytotoxicity as well as vascular and immune effects.[56,58,97,130,131–132] Similarly, fractionation of the light with or without repeat administration of the PS before each light fraction has improved treatment response in various preclinical protocols[46,133–134,135–138] and in early clinical studies.[139] Without repeat PS administration, preclinical studies suggest that the light fractionation is improving oxygenation[46] with more effective vascular injury[138] and necrosis.[134] The duration of the light that is first administered[133] and the duration of time between each light fraction[134] may be particularly important in improving the oxygen delivery between light fractions. When the PS has been readministered before the second light fraction, a short DLI has demonstrated improved tumor control in preclinical models through vascular targeting with various photosensitizers such as verteporfin,[19] MV6401,[26] and m-tetrahydroxyphenylchlorin (mTHPC).[140]

As described above, PDT causes cytotoxic oxidative stress and induces the expression of pleiotropic pro-survival molecules such as COX-2.[84] Understanding the mechanisms leading to pro-survival molecule induction is relevant to the design of more effective treatments. PDT in combination with various targeted agents designed to reduce the effect of the tumor stress response has demonstrated improved tumor responses in various preclinical models. Antiangiogenic agents lead to decreases in VEGF expression after PDT,[115,141–143] along with improvements in tumor response.[114,115,117,119,141–144] Inhibition of HSP increases the curative potential of PDT through decreased expression of angiogenic and pro-survival proteins in the treated tumors,[145] while disruption of HSP-90 function *in vitro* leads to increases in PDT-induced apoptosis.[88] The COX-2 pathway has also been targeted in combination with PDT and can improve therapeutic outcome through inhibition of post-PDT angiogenesis, as well as, under some circumstances, through increases in direct PDT cytotoxicity.[127,146–148]

PRACTICE OF PHOTODYNAMIC THERAPY

Light Delivery and Dosimetry

The ability to achieve PS activation is dependent on effective administration of light not only with a wavelength that matches the spectral absorption of the PS, but also on depositing a sufficient amount of energy to the target tissue (total fluence). Wavelengths >800 nm are unable to deposit sufficient energy to activate a PS. Delivering sufficient fluence is influenced not only by the technique of its administration (i.e., surface vs. interstitial), but also by the ability of the light energy to penetrate sufficiently at depth to treat the intended target volume. As light photons interact with human tissues, photons scatter and are absorbed by endogenous chromophores such as hemoglobin, myoglobin, melanin, and cytochromes. Hemoglobin is especially important to consider. Hemoglobin has spectral absorption peaks <600 nm (i.e., hemoglobin absorbs all colors except red), and its ability to absorb light energy is affected by its oxygenation status. Oxygenated hemoglobin is less likely to absorb between 600 and 800 nm compared to deoxygenated hemoglobin. Thus, most activating light that has been used for PDT has typically been between 600 and 800 nm, depending on the spectral absorption characteristics of the PS.

The rate at which the light energy is delivered (fluence rate) is also an important treatment factor that can affect the efficacy of PDT. It primarily affects the tissue microenvironment such as the vascular flow and oxygenation. In general, it is important to recognize that high fluence rates can rapidly consume and reduce the local oxygen levels such that it limits the efficacy of the remaining light fluence.[149] Although the prescribed fluence rate is typically based on the power output of the light source, surface and internal scattering of light photons may result in areas of higher fluence rates. Strategies to reduce at least the surface scatter effect or to modify the prescribed power output of the light source should be considered (see below).

At present, the prescription of PDT typically used clinically remains limited to rudimentary power output calculations for surface illumination:

$$\text{Incident irradiance (mW/cm}^2\text{)} = \text{power (mW)/area (cm}^2\text{)},$$

$$\text{Time (t) required} = \text{prescription dose (J/cm}^2\text{)/irradiance (mW/cm}^2\text{)*1,000},$$

where the prescription dose is given in terms of the energy per unit area incident on the surface.

Various light delivery devices have been developed to perform PDT treatment. Most of them are fiber based. These include linear source, endotracheal-tube–modified point source, collimated light source, and flat-cut fiber (Fig. 27.2). The flat-cut and linear sources are suitable for inserting into the tissue for interstitial PDT application for the treatment of bulky tumors. The collimated light source is suitable for superficial treatment.

It is therefore helpful to recognize that various illumination techniques may be employed depending on the geometry of the target lesion that is to be treated. The most common clinical situation requires surface illumination, where several technical approaches may be considered. Where the geometry of the target lesion is flat or may be modified to be a near flat surface, the use of a light fiber with a diffusing lens at the tip of the fiber (i.e., microlens) offers the ability to achieve homogeneous light distribution across the surface target. Inhomogeneities due to different distances between points on the surface of the target and the light source can result in different fluence rates and the total light dose (fluence) that is effectively delivered. Unlike ionizing radiation, the surface scattering of photons due to surface concavities or reflective surfaces (i.e., any adjacent metal surfaces) can further increase the risk of high surface dose inhomogeneities. In a similar manner, surface convexities may create regions of shadowing that can create regions of low fluence and fluence rate. Areas of high light fluence (and its fluence rate) may also contribute to an increased risk of normal tissue complications.

When the target lesion is cylindrical, a cylindrical diffusing fiber with the light dose prescribed along its length has commonly been used. However, it is important to note that where the target surface is not rigid (i.e., esophagus), mucosal folds that are not in apposition to the light fiber may become underdosed. To reduce this risk, the cylindrical diffusing fiber can be placed within a balloon diffuser that can be expanded to increase its surface apposition with the mucosal surface. Similar considerations can be applied to spherical surface targets such as the mucosa of the bladder.

The use of a balloon diffuser may be helpful for certain complex three-dimensional surfaces, such as the lateral oral tongue and its adjacent floor of mouth where the surface to be treated can be molded in apposition to the balloon diffuser. In such situations, it is important to verify that the mucosal surface is in direct contact with the balloon's surface before the light is delivered. Other strategies for such complex three-dimensional surfaces may include dividing the target volume into separate targets and individually treating each area with a microlens (patching technique). With this approach, it is important to bear in mind that areas of potential overlap, when illuminated, may increase the risk of normal tissue complications. Other surface illumination techniques under development include a light blanket that attempts to mold the light source to such complex three-dimensional surfaces.

Interstitial light fibers can also be placed when volume illumination is required. As with interstitial brachytherapy techniques, the geometry of the light fibers can significantly affect the overall distribution and amount of light that is delivered. Thus, the use of rigid templates guiding the insertion of the trocar needles (Fig. 27.3) can be very helpful in ensuring accurate interfiber spacing. These templates may be used to facilitate the advancement of rigid trocar needles whose track can

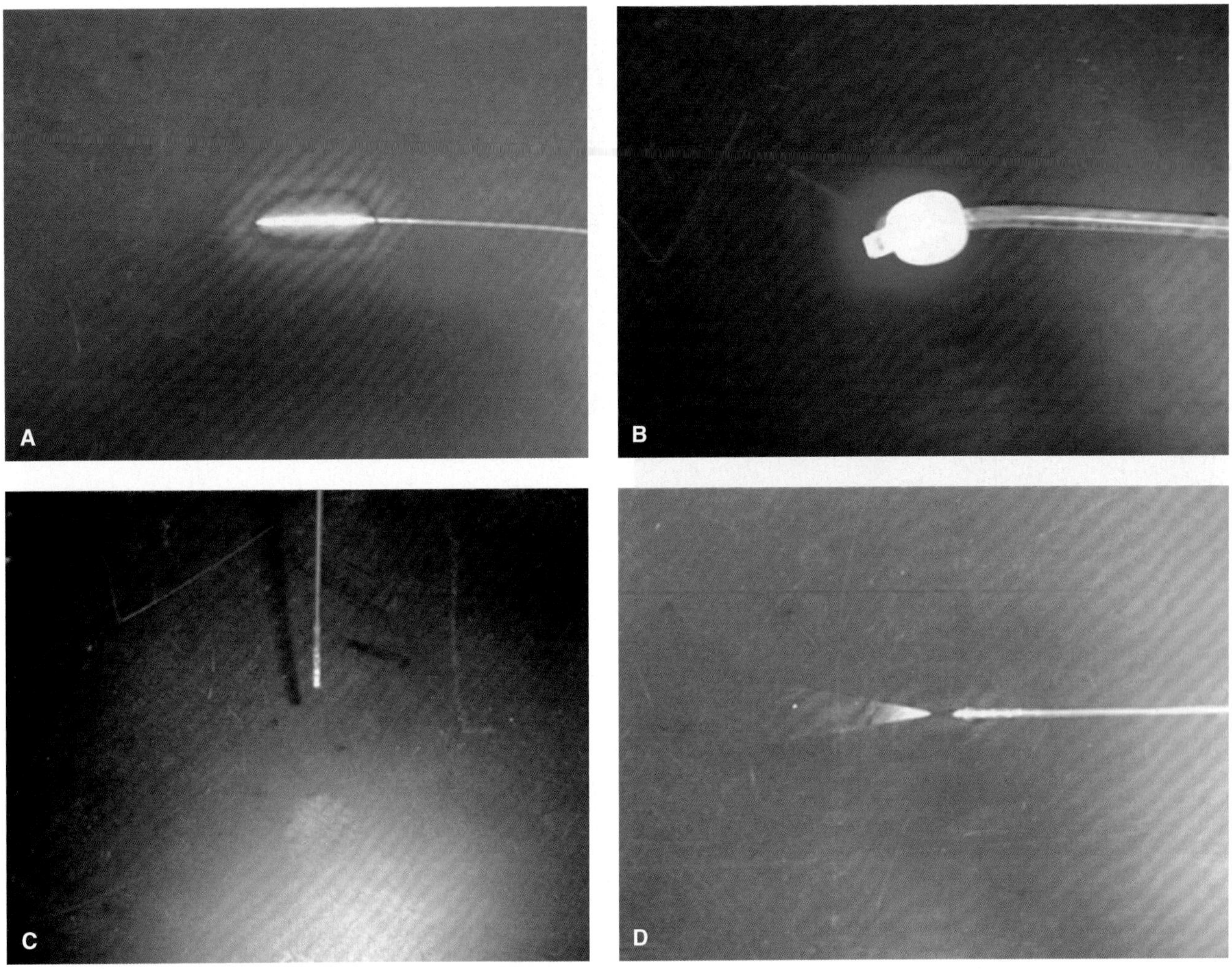

FIGURE 27.2. Various fiber-based light sources. These include a linear source **(A)**, an endotracheal-tube modified point source **(B)**, collimated light fiber **(C)**, and a flat cut fiber **(D)**.

then be replaced with light fibers. Alternatively, traditional low-dose rate after-loading plastic catheters may be used instead to allow the use of the needle track for both light detection fibers or treatment fibers where prescription is based on light dosimetry. The placement of the catheters can also facilitate several quality assurance measures. This can include verifying the geometry of the implant, allowing additional catheters to be placed or removed to optimize the geometry. It may also include verification or modification of the location of the light fiber in its catheter relative to the tumor volume.

Whether the optical properties of the tissue being treated are different by staging the placement of the implant and its illumination is not clear. However, where significant tissue trauma occurs with the placement of the implant, staging the illumination may offer some potential advantages especially where significant tissue bleeding with the introduction of the trocar needles has occurred. Other theoretical advantages may also include improved oxygenation of the implanted tissue, both improving the photosensitization process and reducing hemoglobin absorption of the activating light energy.

Although the optimal interstitial PDT prescription parameters remain to be defined, it is heartening to see successful interstitial light implants having been reported in patients. For such results to become generalizable, the development of a robust and easy-to-use dosimetry system will be needed that will facilitate characterizing the impact of different prescription factors (i.e., intercatheter distance, fluence rate) on normal tissue complications and oncologic results.

Additional Technical Considerations

A significant property of the visible light energy used for photoactivation is its ability to reflect on a surface when light is delivered with a microlens technique. This can in turn increase the fluence and fluence rate delivered especially when the surface is concave and is often referred to as the *integrating sphere effect*. Strategies to minimize this may include manipulating the surface geometry to reduce concavities and convexities (which can reduce the fluence delivered), removing surface mucosal secretions, including the use of anticholinergics such as glycopyrrolate, and considering alternative illumination techniques, as already discussed. Where the target lesion lies adjacent to reflective metal surfaces that may be used in exposing and possibly flattening the target lesion, surface reflection may be reduced by placing dyed surgical towels over these surfaces. Alternatively, these metal surfaces may be coated with a dark pigment. Similarly, surface scatter may increase the light that is delivered to the adjacent normal skin or mucosa adjacent but outside of the target lesion. These areas may be protected by covering the surface with a dark pigmented towel or dye.

For small surface target lesions treated with a microlens technique, movement of the light fiber due to hand tremor can have a significant impact on the light dosimetry across a small surface area. For example, this is especially a concern when the glottic laryngeal mucosa is being illuminated while working down a laryngoscope. For these reasons, adding rigidity to the flexible light fiber by fixing it to a rigid stylet and immobilizing

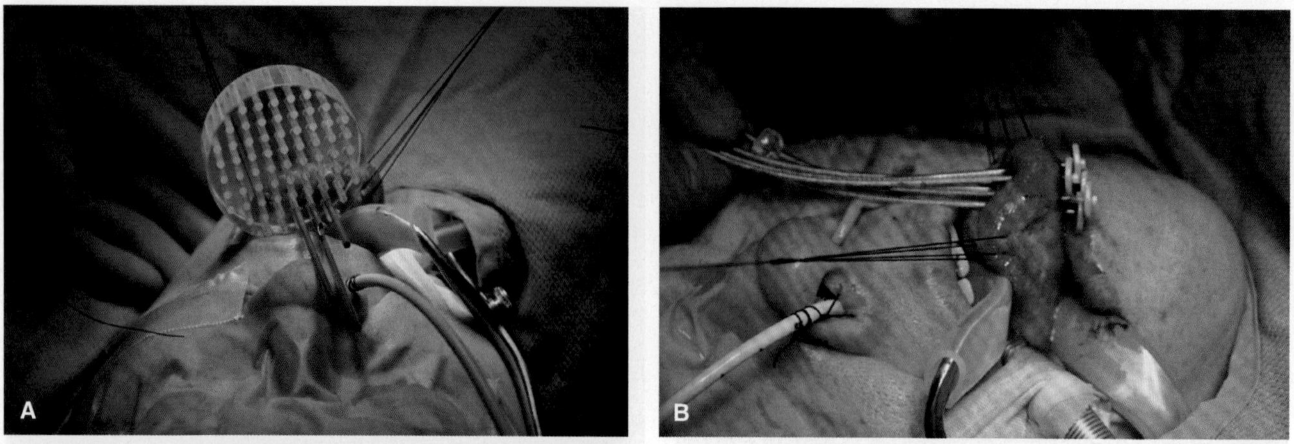

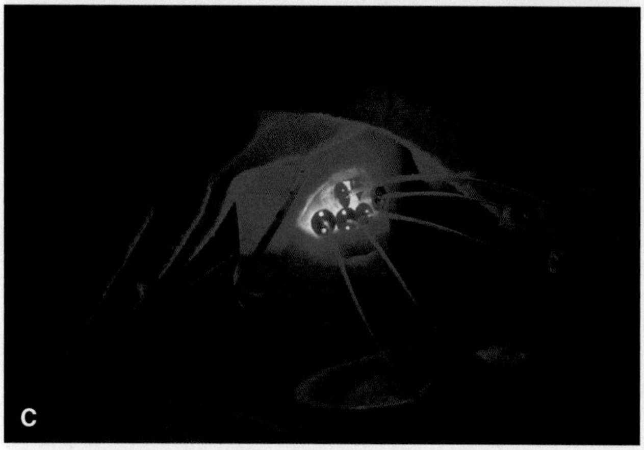

FIGURE 27.3. Example of an interstitial tongue photodynamic therapy implant. A traditional interstitial brachytherapy implant using a template **(A)** to facilitate the placement of trocars guiding the insertion of hollow plastic catheters **(B)** that are modified for linear light sources **(C)**.

it with various commercially available fixation devices should be considered.

As discussed above, the mechanism of action for PDT is dependent on various microenvironment factors, such as blood flow and the effective tissue oxygenation. Practically, these principles require attention to the handling of the tissues to be treated and to not compromise its vascular supply, especially when exposing the surface for treatment. Surface cautery and vasoconstrictive agents used to control bleeding should be judiciously used if at all. This is particularly important when using strategies of tumor debulking to improve the depth of penetration with superficial illumination. For interstitial techniques, precise placement of the light fibers minimizing the use of multiple passages of the needle trocar should be considered. Whether the use of steroids to manage the potential adverse effects of PDT-induced edema (i.e., for airway management) adversely affects the immune response is not clear, but judicious use is recommended at this time.

CLINICAL PHOTODYNAMIC THERAPY

The clinical study of PDT has been an active area of investigation, despite only three PS being approved for clinical use in cancer management. These include porfimer sodium for the treatment of esophageal and lung cancers and superficial papillary bladder carcinomas, temoporfin for head and neck carcinomas, and ALA for skin actinic keratosis and basal cell carcinoma. These trials have generally established clinical activity and the potential for cure in the appropriate cancer application. Despite these efforts, rigorous clinical development of PDT is generally lacking and has not evaluated important comparative questions of its activity to established treatment modalities or, where more appropriate, its value as an adjunctive modality. In general, clinical investigations have also not established the optimal PDT treatment parameters. A systematic evaluation of the quality of evidence supporting PDT in clinical practice is outside the scope of this chapter, and the reader is referred to the recent systematic review by Fayter et al.[150]

Skin

The dermatologic applications of PDT are perhaps the most established and scientifically robust of all the anatomic sites for which PDT has been evaluated, with established consensus statements regarding its use.[151] The success of PDT for skin malignancies is a testament to both its strengths and its weakness, with a multitude of randomized trials having been completed for various nonmelanomatous skin malignancies leading to its U.S. Food and Drug Administration (FDA) approval for the management of basal cell carcinomas and the premalignant nonhyperkeratotic actinic keratosis (AK).

PDT has been used extensively in the treatment of both premalignant and malignant skin tumors, typically with surface illumination.[151,152] PDT of nonhyperkeratotic actinic keratosis, squamous cell carcinoma *in situ* (Bowen's disease), and basal cell carcinoma (BCC) can be performed using systemically administered porfimer sodium or topically applied aminolevulinic acid (ALA) and ALA derivatives such as methyl-ALA (MAL). For example, in a placebo-controlled trial of PDT for AK, ALA-PDT showed a significantly superior complete response rate as compared to sham PDT using vehicle plus light of 89% versus 13% ($p < .001$).[153] PDT for AK shows similar efficacy with less toxicity as compared to cryotherapy, topical 5-fluorouracil cream, or curettage. For example, a study in which 119 subjects with 1,501 AK lesions of the scalp and face were randomly assigned to receive MAL-PDT to either the left- or right-sided lesions, with cryotherapy used to treat the contralateral side.[154] Twenty-four weeks after therapy, both treatment groups showed a high response rate (89% for MAL-PDT vs. 86% for cryotherapy; $p = .2$), but MAL-PDT showed superior cosmesis and patient preference. In contrast, the results for PDT of squamous cell carcinomas (SCC) of the skin using topical photosensitizers have been disappointing, with recurrence rates of >50%.[151,152] Perhaps the most significant potential value of ALA-PDT may be its ability to prevent the development of nonmelanoma skin cancers in patients with AK, as recently demonstrated in a randomized trial of prophylactic ALA-PDT.[155]

Other indications for ALA-PDT include superficial and nodular BCC.[156–158] In a large single institution series, high rates of local control (>90% complete response rate, <10% local failure at 3 to 5 years) can be achieved with PDT for superficial BCC. However, the response rate and local control rate for nodular BCC drops to 70% and 40%, respectively. In a multicenter randomized trial of MAL-PDT versus cryotherapy for superficial BCC, complete response rates at 3 months were 97% and 95%, with 22% and 20% 5-year recurrence rates for MAL-PDT and cryotherapy, respectively.[159] In this study, the excellent to good cosmetic outcome was 89% for MAL-PDT and 50% for cryotherapy. However, when topical PDT is compared to surgery for BCC, topical ALA or MAL-PDT consistently shows a small increase in recurrence rate as compared to surgery for both superficial and nodular BCC. However, the cosmetic outcomes for PDT are typically superior to surgery with good to excellent cosmetic outcome in >90% of PDT patients with PDT and 60% to 70% with surgery. In summary, PDT can be an appropriate and effective treatment alternative to cryosurgery or surgical excision for selected BCC. PDT is currently approved in the United States, Canada, and the European Union for the treatment of AK and approved in the European Union and Canada for treatment of BCC.

Brain

Photodynamic therapy has primarily been evaluated as adjunctive therapy treating the surgical bed often combined with its use for PDD as a fluorescent guide to (surgical) resection (FGR). Yang et al.[160] demonstrated that porfimer sodium fluorescence at 640 nm could be clearly visualized in the resection bed in patients with supratentorial gliomas not seen under white light. Biopsy of these areas of fluorescence confirmed the presence of residual tumor, demonstrating the concept of FGR. Similar high tumor specificity was also observed with hypericin-mediated FGR for glioblastoma multiforme (GBM)[161] and protoporphyrin-IX (PpIX) fluorescence (that was produced following administration of the photosensitizer ALA) of the surgical bed in GBM patients.[162] All biopsies of fluorescent tissue contained GBM.[161,162] The oncologic benefits of FGF could not be clearly evaluated in a phase III study (n = 27) as all patients receiving ALA also had received porfimer sodium and received PDT to the surgical cavity. Eljamel et al.[162] demonstrated that the mean survival significant increased with ALA-mediated FGR and porfimer sodium PDT ($p < .01$). However, in a phase III study of 322 patients with suspected malignant gliomas randomized to ALA-FGF or conventional surgery, Stummer et al.[163] reported an improved progression-free survival (41% vs. 21%, respectively; $p = .0003$) following a median survival of 35.5 months. No significant increased complications have been observed with photosensitizer-based PDD and FGR.[163]

Further evidence in support of PDT activity for GBM particularly comes from several institutional experiences where PDT was used to treat the resection cavity for various histologies, including newly diagnosed[164–165,166] and recurrent[165] GBM and anaplastic astrocytoma (AA).[164] Other histologies evaluated have also included malignant ependymomas[167] and meningiomas.[168] Muller and Wilson[166] reported the results of a retrospective institutional review of adjuvant porfimer sodium PDT (mean fluence of 58 J/cm^2 with only 18 patients receiving >100 J/cm^2) in 96 patients with supratentorial gliomas. Of these 96 patients, 49 patients presented with either newly diagnosed (n = 12) or recurrent (n = 37) GBM; a median survival of 8.25 and 7.25 months was reported, respectively. In contrast, Stylli et al.[165] reported a median survival of 14.3 and 14.9 months, respectively, with hematoporphyrin derivative (HpD)-mediated PDT. Though Muller and Wilson indicate that such differences may have been due to selection factors, they also suggest that this may be consistent with a dose–response effect, as Stylli et al. treated the majority of patients with 220 J/cm^2 (60–260 J/cm^2). Stylli et al. also observed a light-dose effect on overall survival for both GBM and AA. This has formed the basis for an ongoing randomized trial of low versus high light dose porfimer sodium–mediated PDT as adjuvant therapy following surgical resection for supratentorial gliomas.[169]

Head and Neck

The evaluation of PDT for head and neck malignancies has typically been for head and neck squamous cell carcinomas (HNSCC). Case reports or series have also demonstrated that PDT may have activity for other histologies such as Kaposi's sarcoma and salivary gland malignancies such as adenoid cystic carcinomas.[170] Although there have been significant numbers of clinical evaluations of PDT in the management of HNSCC, the vast majority represent single institutional experiences demonstrating activity either for definitive management or for palliation. Definitive management has typically evaluated surface illumination for premalignant dysplastic lesions or early primary invasive mucosa malignancies where the risk of nodal metastases was regarded as low. Common sites have included the oral cavity and the larynx with novel illumination techniques for the nasopharynx[37] and base of tongue[171] having been reported.

Superficial premalignant mucosal lesions are attractive for PDT due to the ability to achieve wide-field mucosal ablation given the uncertainties that are commonly encountered in defining the peripheral extent of the lesion. For these reasons, treatment of the larynx is particularly attractive due to the defined nature of this anatomic site, where tissue-preserving therapies such as PDT can offer further function-preserving advantages. To date, clinical experience suggests that this treatment approach can be effective in obtaining a complete response for the treated lesion, but long-term follow-up is limited and has recently been extensively reviewed.[172] However, this limitation is not dissimilar from other treatment modalities that have been used for mucosal dysplasia. To date, clinical experience has also included large retrospective reviews[173] and several prospective studies of porfimer sodium,[174] temoporfin,[175,176] and topical[177] and systemic[139] ALA that have demonstrated high complete response rates typically >80%. Further research efforts are needed to define both the long-term in-field and out-of-field relapses risks along with the risk of malignant transformation following PDT treatment.

PDT for the treatment of superficial invasive carcinomas has also been evaluated, typically with porfimer sodium and temoporfin, especially with the EU regulatory approval of temoporfin for the palliative management of HNSCC. Prospective studies of porfimer sodium[174,178] and temoporfin[179] have demonstrated complete response rates typically >80%, with both surface and interstitial illumination techniques used. Long-term in-field control rates have also been reported in approximately 70% to 90% of treated patients.[178,179]

The head and neck site has also been the main focus for the development of interstitial illumination techniques, offering an array of potential treatment possibilities. These include the ability to treat deeper invasive carcinomas where the risk of nodal metastases remains low, such as early tongue carcinomas (see Fig. 27.2) or the promise of less toxic salvage therapy,[180] palliation of local–regional relapses that require tumor responses,[181,182] and the treatment of benign tumors such as vascular malformations,[183] which would otherwise require potentially debilitating surgery or the administration of radiotherapy. Lastly, a potential role for intraoperative PDT using porfimer sodium as adjuvant therapy following surgical resection for local–regionally recurrent HNSCC has been reported. With a minimum follow-up of 24 months, four of five treated patients were without local–regional recurrence with no wound complications noted.[184]

Thoracic

Since 1998, PDT has been FDA approved for the treatment of microinvasive endobronchial and advanced partially obstructing non–small cell lung cancer (NSCLC).[185] Endobronchial light delivery has typically been used limiting treatment to central lesions with techniques under development to extend PDT to treat peripheral lesions.[186] It has been used as definitive therapy in treating endobronchial, roentgenographically occult, or synchronous primary carcinomas where the bronchoscopically visible lesions are ≤1 cm in surface dimension with no extracartilaginous invasion. Less effective results have been observed when PDT is used to treat larger tumors without prior surgical debulking and has largely been used for palliative indications. PDT has also been investigated for malignant mesothelioma and pleural involvement by NSCLC with promising findings suggestive of activity and benefit.

Roentgenographically Occult Bronchogenic Non–Small Cell Lung Cancer

Fewer than 1% of patients with roentgenographically occult bronchogenic carcinoma that are endoscopically visible but lack cartilaginous invasion have metastatic lymph node involvement, indicating a potential for a less invasive focal therapy to be curative.[187] With demonstrated efficacy of PDT in this setting, it has emerged as a first-line therapy for roentgenographically occult lesions, particularly for tumors ≤1 cm that have no extracartilaginous invasion or lymph node involvement. Investigators from the National Kinki Central Hospital for Chest Diseases used PDT to treat roentgenographically occult bronchogenic carcinoma in 25 patients with 29 lesions.[188] A complete remission was achieved in 72% of lesions, including 89% (17/19) of lesions ≤1 cm and 86% (18/21) of visible peripheral area lesions. In another series of 33 patients, with 40 roentgenographically occult carcinomas treated with PDT, a complete response was achieved in all lesions ≤1 cm (n = 32), but in only three of eight larger tumors.[189] Among the 39 roentgenologically occult lesions treated at Osaka Prefectural Habikino Hospital with PDT, a complete response was achieved in 64% of lesions, more likely in superficially infiltrating than for nodular lesions (76% vs. 43%).[190] Tohoku University Hospital investigators treated 48 medically operable patients with roentgenographically occult bronchogenic squamous cell carcinomas with tumor lengths of ≤1 cm with PDT, observing a complete response in 94% of patients and a 10-year overall survival rate of 71%.[191]

Radiographically Visible Early-Stage and Endobronchial Non–Small Cell Lung Cancer

Similar to roentgenologically occult bronchogenic carcinomas, early-stage and endobronchial NSCLC can be effectively treated with PDT. Although often used for patients unsuitable for surgical resection, PDT has became an established alternative treatment modality to surgery for patients with early-stage, small central NSCLC lesions.

At Tokyo Medical University Hospital, 240 patients with 283 central lung cancer lesions were treated from 1980 to 1995 with PDT. The overall response rate was 99%, with a complete response in 40%. A complete response was achieved in 83% (79/95) of early-stage lesions, with a 94% (65/69) complete response rate for lesions <1 cm. Several institutional experiences also made similar observations of durable complete responses in over 75% of patients treated at a minimum of 12 months' follow-up.[192,193] However, the complete response rate fell to 54% (14/26) for lesions ≥1 cm and 38% (6/16) for lesions ≥2 cm ($p = .00001$).[194] A more recent report from Tokyo Medical University Hospital demonstrated that among 93 patients treated with PDT for 114 central early-stage lung cancers, the complete response rate was higher for lesions <1 cm (77/83) than ≥1 cm (18/31; 93% vs. 58%; $p < .001$). The recurrence rate was 12% for lesions <1 cm with an initial complete response to PDT, and many recurrences could successfully be salvaged with additional PDT.[195] In a review of 15 trials of 626 patients with 715 central early-stage bronchogenic cancers treated typically for surgery ineligibility patients, PDT-related toxicity was limited, with one PDT-related death (0.15%), photosensitivity skin reactions in 5% to 28%, respiratory complications in 0% to 18%, and nonfatal hemoptysis in 0% to 8%. A complete response was achieved in 30% to 100% of patients for a 2- to 120-month duration, and the 5-year overall survival was 61%.[196]

Synchronous multiple primary lung cancers occur in 1% to 15% of patients with lung malignancies and have been increasing in incidence due to improvements in imaging. These cases may warrant considerations for aggressive management. Incorporating PDT in the management of central lesions, especially when small in size, can significantly reduce the pulmonary morbidity. In a study of 22 patients with synchronous early lung cancers treated with PDT alone for each lesion (n = 11) or surgery for the more peripheral lesions and PDT for the more central lesions (n = 11), PDT achieved a complete response in all 39 central tumors at 2 months following therapy.[197] All patients were alive with variable follow-up of up to 5 years.

Advanced-Stage Non–Small Cell Lung Cancer

For patients with locally advanced or metastatic NSCLC, PDT has most commonly been used for palliation. In a randomized trial comparing PDT to neodymium:yttrium-aluminum-garnet (Nd:YAG) laser therapy in the NSCLC patients with an obstructed airway, both PDT and Nd:YAG laser therapy were comparable with regard to symptom relief and response rates. The time to failure ($p = .03$) and the median survival ($p = .007$) were significantly longer in the cohort receiving PDT.[198] In combination with radiotherapy, prolonged response of the luminal tumor mass may be observed and warrants further investigation.[199,200]

Preoperative PDT has been reported in several small institutional series of patients with NSCLC. Although small in numbers, these series have independently observed that preoperative PDT may help reduce the extent of definitive resection needed for locally advanced NSCLC by down-staging patients who would otherwise require a pneumonectomy to undergo lobectomy instead or to convert patients originally deemed inoperable to be surgical candidates.[201–203] Okunaka et al.[201] reported on the results of 26 patients with NSCLC treated with preoperative PDT alone for the purposes of reducing the extent of resection or converting inoperable disease to an operable status. These surgical goals were achieved in 85% of patients, with four of five originally inoperable patients converted to resectable, and 18 of 21 patients originally candidates only for pneumonectomy were able to undergo lobectomy. Ross et al.[202] reported on 41 patients with locally advanced NSCLC treated with induction PDT and chemotherapy or radiation therapy. PDT induction allowed 57% of initially unresectable patients to undergo definitive surgical resection and 27% of those initially deemed in need of pneumonectomy to undergo lobectomy. Pathological down-staging occurred in 64%, and 46% of patients were alive at 3 years' following therapy.

PDT may also be used as part of multimodality management for patients with NSCLC with pleural spread. A phase II trial of 22 such patients at the University of Pennsylvania assessed the oncologic outcome of patients treated with surgery, achieving either a complete resection (n = 17) or partial tumor debulking (n = 3) followed by hemithoracic pleural PDT (porfimer sodium) (n = 20) or PDT alone (n = 2).[204] The 6-month local control rate for the cohort was 73.3% and the median overall survival was 21.7 months, suggesting promising activity.

Malignant Pleural Mesothelioma

The use of PDT to treat malignant pleural mesothelioma was pioneered at the National Cancer Institute in 1980s and has since become increasingly more integrated into multimodality therapy for mesothelioma.[205] In a National Cancer Institute phase I trial, 54 patients with pleural malignancies isolated to one hemithorax were evaluated, including 40 patients with mesothelioma. Among the 42 patients who underwent optimal tumor debulking to $\leq$5 mm of residual tumor thickness followed by PDT, PDT was relatively well tolerated; toxicities included a patient with an empyema and a late hemorrhage, bronchopleural fistulas in two patients, and esophageal perforations in two patients. The median survival among mesothelioma patients was 10 months.[206] In the perioperative period, however, intraoperative PDT for mesothelioma can be associated with acute bleeding, severe generalized vascular atherosclerosis, generalized edema, intrathoracic fluid accumulation, respiratory distress, and death.[207]

In a phase II study at Roswell Park Cancer Institute, 40 patients underwent extrapleural pneumonectomy or pleurectomy followed by intracavitary PDT.[208] The median survival was significantly better for stages I and II patients (n = 13) than stages III and IV patients (n = 24; 36 months vs. 10 months; $p < .0001$). PDT dose was found to be an independent prognostic indicators for survival ($p < .009$).[208] Dutch investigators treated 28 predominantly advanced-stage mesothelioma patients with pleuropneumonectomy followed by intraoperative PDT. Half of the patients in the cohort had persistent local tumor control for at least 9 months following PDT, and the median overall survival of the cohort was 10 months.[207] At the University of Pennsylvania, 28 patients with malignant pleural mesothelioma, including 86% with stages III and IV disease, were treated from 2004 to 2008 with macroscopic complete resection and intraoperative PDT. Patients who underwent radical pleurectomy (n = 14) had a significantly improved median survival (not reached at a median follow-up of 2.1 years vs. 8.4 months; $p = .009$) compared with those who underwent modified extrapleural pneumonectomy.[209]

The only randomized phase III trial assessing the role of PDT in the management of malignant pleural mesothelioma involved 63 patients at the National Cancer Institute undergoing maximum debulking surgery, postoperative cisplatin, interferon α-2b, and tamoxifen with or without first-generation intraoperative intrapleural PDT (630 nm, porfimer sodium, 30 J/cm^2 using intraoperative real-time light dosimetry).[210] Most patients (79%) had stage III disease. The median survival for the 15 nonoptimally cytoreduced patients with >5 mm residual disease was 7.2 months, compared to 14.4 months for the remaining 48 patients. PDT did not influence the pattern of recurrence, median survival (14.1 vs. 14.4 months), or median progression-free time (8.5 vs. 7.7 months).[210] Whether survival may have been improved with optimal debulking and PDT is not clear at this time.

Gastrointestinal Malignancies

Photodynamic Therapy for Malignancies of the Gastrointestinal Tract

Of the gastrointestinal (GI) tract tumors that can be treated with PDT, Barrett's esophagus (BE) with dysplasia and early-stage esophageal cancer are the best studied.[211,212] Overholt et al.[213] demonstrated in a multicenter randomized trial that PDT for premalignant BE can eliminate dysplastic cells and is associated with a lower incidence of development of invasive carcinoma. In this trial, 208 patients were randomly assigned to receive either PDT with proton pump inhibitor (PPI) or PPI alone in a two-to-one randomization schema. PDT-treated patients received porfimer sodium (2 mg/kg) 40 to 50 hours prior to the first light delivery. Areas of BE were exposed to 130 J/cm with 630 nm light using a cylindrical fiberoptic diffuser encased in an inflated esophageal balloon so that the fiber would be centered and the esophageal folds flattened. Ninety-six to 120 hours later, a repeat endoscopy was performed to assess response and an additional 50 J/cm could be given to areas of insufficient mucosal damage. If BE was found to persist on follow-up endoscopy, additional PDT treatments could be performed as described above to a maximum of three total treatments given at least 3 months apart. All patients (in both arms) received omeprazole therapy at a dose of 20 mg given twice daily. The results of this trial showed that PDT plus PPI was superior to PPI alone, both in terms of ablation of high-grade dysplasia (HGD) and progression to adenocarcinoma.

Updated 5-year results confirm the long-term benefits with a 50% relative risk reduction in the incidence of invasive carcinoma.[214] At 5 years of follow-up, Overholt et al.[213] demonstrated that 77% of patients treated with PDT-PPI showed ablation of HGD versus 39% of patients treated with PPI alone ($p < .0001$). More significantly, 15% of the patients in the PDT-PPI arm showed progression to cancer versus 29% of patients on the PPI arm ($p < .006$). The most serious toxicity of the PDT-PPI treatment was esophageal stricture, with the majority of cases successfully managed with esophageal dilatation. Mucosal injury prior to PDT and repeat PDT treatments appear to increase this risk.[213,215] Cost-effectiveness analysis proposes suggest that PDT even when repeated is a relatively safe and effective management option of patients with BE-HGD.

PDT has also been studied in a variety of tumor types in the GI tract beyond the esophagus. Significant clinical efficacy has been observed in early studies of PDT for gastric,[216] early duodenal, and ampullary cancers.[217–219] Promising results have been achieved in the treatment of cholangiocarcinomas (CC). Early case reports and pilot studies of PDT for CC demonstrated significant promise.[220,221] In a randomized, controlled trial of stenting with or without PDT, the median survival of patients treated with PDT plus stenting was a remarkable 493 days compared with only 98 days in the stenting alone group.[222] Other studies have shown similar results.[223–225] Consequently, a multicenter clinical trial has been recently initiated to obtain regulatory approval in the United States and Canada.[226]

Other clinical applications of PDT in the GI tract have included unresectable pancreatic cancers[227] and numerous reports using PDT to eliminate colon polyps as well as to palliate bulky colon and rectal cancers.[219,228–230] In addition, PDT may have efficacy in treating hepatocellular carcinoma. Early results have been promising, and a phase III study is currently under way to evaluate the efficacy of Talaporfin-mediated PDT using interstitial LEDs compared with institution-specific standard treatment.[231]

Photodynamic Therapy for Intraperitoneal Malignancies

Peritoneal carcinomatosis presents a very difficult problem for standard cancer treatment modalities. The superficial nature of PDT combined with its ability to treat large surface areas lends itself to this particular problem. However, adequate and homogeneous light distribution to all peritoneal surfaces remains an ongoing technical challenge to date. In a phase I trial of 70 subjects with predominantly recurrent ovarian carcinomatosis, intraoperative PDT following maximal surgical debulking resulted in a 76% complete cytologic response rate with tolerable toxicity.[232] In the follow-up phase II study, patients were enrolled and stratified according to cancer type (ovarian, gastrointestinal, or sarcoma) and given doses of porfimer sodium and light at the phase I defined maximally tolerated dose.[233] Other than capillary leak syndrome and skin photosensitivity, the complication rates were similar to the complication rates typically observed after similarly extensive surgery in the absence of PDT.[234] With a median follow-up of 51 months, the median failure-free survival and overall survival rates for the patients who received PDT were 3 months and 22 months in ovarian cancer patients and 3.3 months and 13.2 months in gastrointestinal cancer patients, respectively. Six months after therapy, the pathologic complete response rate was 3 of 33 (9.1%) and 2 of 37 (5.4%) for the patients with ovarian cancer and gastrointestinal cancer, respectively. These results in heavily pretreated patients suggest that PDT for peritoneal carcinomatosis may have clinical benefit, warranting further study.

Genitourinary Malignancies

Photodynamic Therapy for Prostate Carcinomas

The role of interstitial PDT for prostate adenocarcinoma has been investigated by several groups studying various PS including temoporfin,[6,235] motexafin lutetium,[52,233,236] and padoporfin.[237] The majority of these phase I and II trials have been in patients with locally recurrent adenocarcinoma, where the standard management option has not been well defined, typically following failure of radiotherapy. Several important observations can be generalized. Of these, it is clear that traditional brachytherapy techniques can be adopted to administer diffusing light fibers with potentially effective light delivery and oncologic efficacy. Oncologically, the results would suggest that a dose–response relationship may exist with higher light doses delivered, increasing the probability of acute tissue injury with an increase in PSA in the first 24 hours posttreatment,[52] pathologic complete response,[238] and possibly a more durable PSA response.[52] The early rise in PSA has been suggested to be a possible surrogate for treatment efficacy.[52]

At this time, the optimal light dose and other PDT prescription parameters remain to be determined for durable oncologic benefits to be realized. However, delivering a minimum and sufficient light fluence to 90% of the prostate may be important.[238] This is further complicated by the significant inter- and intra-patient heterogeneity[239,240] in the optical properties of the prostate that changes dynamically during the administration of the light.[6] However, analysis of the heterogeneity in the tissue injury as assessed by magnetic resonance imaging demonstrates that light dosimetry may not be sufficient to completely predict for prostate and surrounding normal tissue injury, such as the risk of urorectal fistulas.[241] That is, other factors such as the PS and oxygen concentrations and the effectiveness of the singlet oxygen generation along with unknown patient factors may be important and remain subjects of ongoing investigation.[242] In the interim, careful attention to minimize trauma to the rectal wall[235] and the light dosimetry for interstitial PDT remains important, and it may be prudent to establish a lower light fluence to the rectal wall as this tissue may have a lower intrinsic threshold for interstitial PDT injury.[241]

Photodynamic Therapy for Bladder Carcinomas

Bladder carcinomas are typically superficial and diffuse across the mucosa, lending to the application of intracavitary PDT. In fact, the first-generation photosensitizer hematoporphyrin and its derivative (HpD) was used as early as 1975, leading to the regulatory approval of the purified active component (porfimer sodium) for the treatment of recurrent superficial papillary carcinoma typically failing intravesical therapy such as bacille Calmette-Guérin (BCG). Several institutional experiences have demonstrated activity with HpD or porfimer sodium PDT to the whole bladder with high initial response rates of ≥70% with long-term (>2 years) control rates between 30% and 60%.[243,244–245,246] These response rates are not too dissimilar to those observed with many intravesical agents, suggesting comparable activity that was recently supported in a recent multicenter randomized study comparing BCG to porfimer sodium PDT in patients with superficial (nonmuscle invasive) carcinoma.[247] Bladder contracture due to fibrosis was observed to be a significant complication in the early experience of porfimer sodium PDT that was subsequently demonstrated could be reduced by measuring the light fluence on the surface accounting for both the incident and scattered light.[248] Other strategies that reduced the risk of late bladder injury included porfimer sodium PDT with less penetrating light (514 nm),[249] reducing the porfimer sodium and light dose administered,[243] and the use of topical ALA, which is a more superficial photosensitizer with comparable outcomes suggested.[250,251]

CONCLUSION

A significant body of preclinical and clinical evidence supports the conclusion that PDT can have significant cancer cytotoxicity with cure possible in several clinical applications. There has been a tremendous body of advancement in the physics of light dosimetry, sophisticated PS development for photodiagnosis and photoactivation, and our understanding of the cellular and microenvironment effects of PDT. These offer an array of potential translational opportunities to advance both the indications and the efficacy of PDT both alone and in combination with traditional therapeutics.

ACKNOWLEDGMENTS

Harry Quon is a consultant with Pinnacle Biologics, and Theresa M. Busch is a consultant with Pharmacyclics, Inc. Support for the authors during the writing of this contribution was provided through grants R01-CA-129554, R01-CA-085831, and P01-CA-087971.

SELECTED REFERENCES

A full list of references for this chapter is available online.

5. Dougherty TJ, Gomer CJ, Henderson BW, et al. Photodynamic therapy. *J Natl Cancer Inst* 1998;90:889–905.
6. Swartling J, Axelsson J, Ahlgren G, et al. System for interstitial photodynamic therapy with online dosimetry: first clinical experiences of prostate cancer. *J Biomed Opt* 2010;15:058003.
7. O'Connor AE, Gallagher WM, Byrne AT. Porphyrin and nonporphyrin photosensitizers in oncology: preclinical and clinical advances in photodynamic therapy. *Photochem Photobiol* 2009;85:1053–1074.
14. Hahn SM, Putt ME, Metz J, et al. Photofrin uptake in the tumor and normal tissues of patients receiving intraperitoneal photodynamic therapy. *Clin Cancer Res* 2006;12:5464–5470.
18. Korbelik M, Krosl G. Cellular levels of photosensitisers in tumours: the role of proximity to the blood supply. *Br J Cancer* 1994;70:604–610.
19. Chen B, Pogue BW, Hoopes PJ, et al. Combining vascular and cellular targeting regimens enhances the efficacy of photodynamic therapy. *Int J Radiat Oncol Biol Phys* 2005;61:1216–1226.
20. Buytaert E, Dewaele M, Agostinis P. Molecular effectors of multiple cell death pathways initiated by photodynamic therapy. *Biochim Biophys Acta* 2007;1776:86–107.
22. Moan J, Berg K. The photodegradation of porphyrins in cells can be used to estimate the lifetime of singlet oxygen. *Photochem Photobiol* 1991;53:549–553.
31. Wilson BC, Patterson MS, Lilge L. Implicit and explicit dosimetry in photodynamic therapy: a new paradigm. *Lasers Med Sci* 1997;12:182–199.
36. van Staveren HJ, Keijzer M, Keesmaat T, et al. Integrating sphere effect in whole-bladder-wall photodynamic therapy: III. Fluence multiplication, optical penetration and light distribution with an eccentric source for human bladder optical properties. *Phys Med Biol* 1996;41:579–590.
38. Tan IB, Oppelaar H, Ruevekamp MC, et al. The importance of in situ light dosimetry for photodynamic therapy of oral cavity tumors. *Head Neck* 1999;21:434–441.
41. Johansson A, Axelsson J, Andersson-Engels S, et al. Realtime light dosimetry software tools for interstitial photodynamic therapy of the human prostate. *Med Phys* 2007;34:4309–4321.
43. Buytaert E, Dewaele M, Agostinis P. Molecular effectors of multiple cell death pathways initiated by photodynamic therapy. *Biochim Biophys Acta* 2007;1776:86–107.
46. Curnow A, Haller JC, Bown SG. Oxygen monitoring during 5-aminolaevulinic acid induced photodynamic therapy in normal rat colon. Comparison of continuous and fractionated light regimes. *J Photochem Photobiol B* 2000;58:149–155.
47. Henderson BW, Fingar VH. Relationship of tumor hypoxia and response to photodynamic treatment in an experimental mouse tumor. *Cancer Res* 1987;47:3110–3114.
48. Korbelik M, Krosl G, Krosl J, et al. The role of host lymphoid populations in the response of mouse EMT6 tumor to photodynamic therapy. *Cancer Res* 1996;56:5647–5652.
50. Busch TM, Hahn SM, Wileyto EP, et al. Hypoxia and Photofrin uptake in the intraperitoneal carcinomatosis and sarcomatosis of photodynamic therapy patients. *Clin Cancer Res* 2004;10:4630–4638.
51. Hahn SM, Putt ME, Metz J, et al. Photofrin uptake in the tumor and normal tissues of patients receiving intraperitoneal photodynamic therapy. *Clin Cancer Res* 2006;12:5464–5470.
52. Patel H, Mick R, Finlay J, et al. Motexafin lutetium-photodynamic therapy of prostate cancer: short- and long-term effects on prostate-specific antigen. *Clin Cancer Res* 2008;14:4869–4876.

56. Henderson BW, Busch TM, Snyder JW. Fluence rate as a modulator of PDT mechanisms. *Lasers Surg Med* 2006;38:489–493.
57. Foster TH, Hartley DF, Nichols MG, et al. Fluence rate effects in photodynamic therapy of multicell tumor spheroids. *Cancer Res* 1993;53:1249–1254.
58. Busch TM, Xing X, Yu G, et al. Fluence rate-dependent intratumor heterogeneity in physiologic and cytotoxic responses to Photofrin photodynamic therapy. *Photochem Photobiol Sci* 2009;8:1683–1693.
60. Busch TM. Local physiological changes during photodynamic therapy. *Lasers Surg Med* 2006;38:494–499.
63. Fingar VH, Taber SW, Haydon PS, et al. Vascular damage after photodynamic therapy of solid tumors: a view and comparison of effect in pre-clinical and clinical models at the University of Louisville. *In Vivo* 2000;14:93–100.
64. Chen B, Pogue BW, Hoopes PJ, et al. Vascular and cellular targeting for photodynamic therapy. *Crit Rev Eukaryot Gene Expr* 2006;16:279–305.
67. Busch TM, Wang HW, Wileyto EP, et al. Increasing damage to tumor blood vessels during motexafin lutetium-PDT through use of low fluence rate. *Radiat Res* 2010;174:331–340.
68. Yu G, Durduran T, Zhou C, et al. Noninvasive monitoring of murine tumor blood flow during and after photodynamic therapy provides early assessment of therapeutic efficacy. *Clin Cancer Res* 2005;11:3543–3552.
71. Gross S, Gilead A, Scherz A, et al. Monitoring photodynamic therapy of solid tumors online by BOLD-contrast MRI. *Nature Med* 2003;9:1327–1331.
73. Standish BA, Lee KK, Jin X, et al. Interstitial Doppler optical coherence tomography as a local tumor necrosis predictor in photodynamic therapy of prostatic carcinoma: an in vivo study. *Cancer Res* 2008;68:9987–9995.
74. Pham TH, Hornung R, Berns MW, et al. Monitoring tumor response during photodynamic therapy using near-infrared photon-migration spectroscopy. *Photochem Photobiol* 2001;73:669–677.
86. Kessel D, Oleinick NL. Initiation of autophagy by photodynamic therapy. *Methods Enzymol* 2009;453:1–16.
89. Reiners JJ Jr, Agostinis P, Berg K, et al. Assessing autophagy in the context of photodynamic therapy. *Autophagy* 2010;6:7–18.
90. Ortel B, Shea CR, Calzavara-Pinton P. Molecular mechanisms of photodynamic therapy. *Frontiers Biosci* 2009;14:4157–4172.
91. Mroz P, Hashmi JT, Huang YY, et al. Stimulation of anti-tumor immunity by photodynamic therapy. *Expert Rev Clin Immunol* 2011;7:75–91.
92. Gollnick SO, Evans SS, Baumann H, et al. Role of cytokines in photodynamic therapy-induced local and systemic inflammation. *Br J Cancer* 2003;88:1772–1779.
97. Henderson BW, Gollnick SO, Snyder JW, et al. Choice of oxygen-conserving treatment regimen determines the inflammatory response and outcome of photodynamic therapy of tumors. *Cancer Res* 2004;64:2120–2126.
98. Sun J, Cecic I, Parkins CS, et al. Neutrophils as inflammatory and immune effectors in photodynamic therapy-treated mouse SCCVII tumours. *Photochem Photobiol Sci* 2002;1:690–695.
102. Korbelik M, Cecic I. Complement activation cascade and its regulation: relevance for the response of solid tumors to photodynamic therapy. *J Photochem Photobiol* 2008;93:53–59.
103. Kousis PC, Henderson BW, Maier PG, et al. Photodynamic therapy enhancement of antitumor immunity is regulated by neutrophils. *Cancer Res* 2007;67:10501–10510.
104. Yang D, de la Rosa G, Tewary P, et al. Alarmins link neutrophils and dendritic cells. *Trends Immunol* 2009;30:531–537.
105. Korbelik M. PDT-associated host response and its role in the therapy outcome. *Lasers Surg Med* 2006;38:500–508.
106. Todryk S, Melcher AA, Hardwick N, et al. Heat shock protein 70 induced during tumor cell killing induces Th1 cytokines and targets immature dendritic cell precursors to enhance antigen uptake. *J Immunol* 1999;163:1398–1408.
107. Gomer CJ, Ryter SW, Ferrario A, et al. Photodynamic therapy-mediated oxidative stress can induce expression of heat shock proteins. *Cancer Res* 1996;56:2355–2360.
108. Garg AD, Nowis D, Golab J, et al. Photodynamic therapy: illuminating the road from cell death towards anti-tumour immunity. *Apoptosis* 2010;15:1050–1071.
111. Mitra S, Giesselman BR, De Jesus-Andino FJ, et al. Tumor response to mTHPC-mediated photodynamic therapy exhibits strong correlation with extracellular release of HSP70. *Lasers Surg Med* 2011;43:632–643.
113. Gomer CJ, Ferrario A, Luna M, et al. Photodynamic therapy: combined modality approaches targeting the tumor microenvironment. *Lasers Surg Med* 2006;38:516–521.
119. Ferrario A, von Tiehl KF, Rucker N, et al. Antiangiogenic treatment enhances photodynamic therapy responsiveness in a mouse mammary carcinoma. *Cancer Res* 2000;60:4066–4069.
122. Bhuvaneswari R, Gan YY, Soo KC, et al. The effect of photodynamic therapy on tumor angiogenesis. *Cell Mol Life Sci* 2009;66:2275–2283.
128. Verma S, Watt GM, Mai Z, et al. Strategies for enhanced photodynamic therapy effects. *Photochem Photobiol* 2007;83:996–1005.
129. Zheng G, Chen J, Stefflova K, et al. Photodynamic molecular beacon as an activatable photosensitizer based on protease-controlled singlet oxygen quenching and activation. *Proc Natl Acad Sci USA* 2007;104:8989–8994.
130. Busch TM, Wileyto EP, Emanuele MJ, et al. Photodynamic therapy creates fluence rate-dependent gradients in the intratumoral spatial distribution of oxygen. *Cancer Res* 2002;62:7273–7379.
133. Curnow A, McIlroy BW, Postle-Hacon MJ, et al. Light dose fractionation to enhance photodynamic therapy using 5-aminolevulinic acid in the normal rat colon. *Photochem Photobiol* 1999;69:71–76.
134. Messmann H, Mlkvy P, Buonaccorsi G, et al. Enhancement of photodynamic therapy with 5-aminolaevulinic acid-induced porphyrin photosensitisation in normal rat colon by threshold and light fractionation studies. *Br J Cancer* 1995;72:589–594.
149. Henderson BW, Busch TM, Vaughan LA, et al. Photofrin photodynamic therapy can significantly deplete or preserve oxygenation in human basal cell carcinomas during treatment, depending on fluence rate. *Cancer Res* 2000;60:525–529.
150. Fayter D, Corbett M, Heirs M, et al. A systematic review of photodynamic therapy in the treatment of pre-cancerous skin conditions, Barrett's oesophagus and cancers of the biliary tract, brain, head and neck, lung, oesophagus and skin. *Health Technol Assess* 2010;14:1–288.
151. Nestor MS, Gold MH, Kauvar AN, et al. The use of photodynamic therapy in dermatology: results of a consensus conference. *J Drugs Dermatol* 2006;5:140–154.
152. Braathen LR, Szeimies RM, Basset-Seguin N, et al. Guidelines on the use of photodynamic therapy for nonmelanoma skin cancer: an international consensus. International Society for Photodynamic Therapy in Dermatology, 2005. *J Am Acad Dermatol* 2007;56:125–143.
153. Piacquadio DJ, Chen DM, Farber HF, et al. Photodynamic therapy with aminolevulinic acid topical solution and visible blue light in the treatment of multiple actinic keratoses of the face and scalp: investigator-blinded, phase 3, multicenter trials. *Arch Dermatol* 2004;140:41–46.
155. Apalla Z, Sotiriou E, Chovarda E, et al. Skin cancer: preventive photodynamic therapy in patients with face and scalp cancerization. A randomized placebo-controlled study. *Br J Dermatol* 2010;162:171–175.
160. Yang VXD, Muller PJ, Herman P, et al. A multispectral fluorescence imaging system: design and initial clinical tests in intra-operative Photofrin-photodynamic therapy of brain tumors. *Lasers Surg Med* 2003;32:224–232.
162. Eljamel MS, Goodman C, Moseley H. ALA and Photofrin fluorescence-guided resection and repetitive PDT in glioblastoma multiforme: a single centre phase III randomised controlled trial. *Lasers Med Sci* 2008;23:361–367.
163. Stummer W, Pichlmeier U, Meinel T, et al. Fluorescence-guided surgery with 5-aminolevulinic acid for resection of malignant glioma: a randomised controlled multicentre phase III trial. *Lancet Oncol* 2006;7:392–401.
166. Muller PJ, Wilson BC. Photodynamic therapy of brain tumors—a work in progress. *Lasers Surg Med* 2006;38:384–389.
172. Quon H, Grossman CE, Finlay JC, et al. Photodynamic therapy in the management of pre-malignant head and neck mucosal dysplasia and microinvasive carcinoma. *Photodiagnosis Photodyn Ther* 2011;8:75–85.
174. Rigual NR, Thankappan K, Cooper M, et al. Photodynamic therapy for head and neck dysplasia and cancer. *Arch Otolaryngol Head Neck Surg* 2009;135:784–788.
178. Biel MA. Photodynamic therapy treatment of early oral and laryngeal cancers. *Photochem Photobiol* 2007;83:1063–1068.
184. Biel MA. Photodynamic therapy as an adjuvant intraoperative treatment of recurrent head and neck carcinomas. *Arch Otolaryngol Head Neck Surg* 1996;122:1261–1265.
191. Endo C, Miyamoto A, Sakurada A, et al. Results of long-term follow-up of photodynamic therapy for roentgenographically occult bronchogenic squamous cell carcinoma. *Chest* 2009;136:369–375.
193. Furuse K, Fukuoka M, Kato H, et al. A prospective phase II study on photodynamic therapy with photofrin II for centrally located early-stage lung cancer. The Japan Lung Cancer Photodynamic Therapy Study Group. *J Clin Oncol* 1993;11:1852–1857.
196. Moghissi K, Dixon K. Update on the current indications, practice and results of photodynamic therapy (PDT) in early central lung cancer (ECLC). *Photodiagnosis Photodyn Ther* 2008;5:10–18.
202. Ross P Jr, Grecula J, Bekaii-Saab T, et al. Incorporation of photodynamic therapy as an induction modality in non-small cell lung cancer. *Lasers Surg Med* 2006;38:881–889.
204. Friedberg JS, Mick R, Stevenson JP, et al. Phase II trial of pleural photodynamic therapy and surgery for patients with non-small-cell lung cancer with pleural spread. *J Clin Oncol* 2004;22:2192–2201.
206. Pass HI, DeLaney TF, Tochner Z, et al. Intrapleural photodynamic therapy: results of a phase I trial. *Ann Surg Oncol* 1994;1:28–37.
207. Schouwink H, Rutgers ET, van der Sijp J, et al. Intraoperative photodynamic therapy after pleuropneumonectomy in patients with malignant pleural mesothelioma: dose finding and toxicity results. *Chest* 2001;120:1167–1174.
208. Moskal TL, Dougherty TJ, Urschel JD, et al. Operation and photodynamic therapy for pleural mesothelioma: 6-year follow-up. *Ann Thorac Surg* 1998;66:1128–1133.
209. Friedberg JS, Mick R, Culligan M, et al. Photodynamic therapy and the evolution of a lung-sparing surgical treatment for mesothelioma. *Ann Thorac Surg* 2011;91:1738–1745.
210. Pass HI, Temeck BK, Kranda K, et al. Phase III randomized trial of surgery with or without intraoperative photodynamic therapy and postoperative immunochemotherapy for malignant pleural mesothelioma. *Ann Surg Oncol* 1997;4:628–633.
213. Overholt BF, Lightdale CJ, Wang KK, et al. Photodynamic therapy with porfimer sodium for ablation of high-grade dysplasia in Barrett's esophagus: international, partially blinded, randomized phase III trial. *Gastrointest Endosc* 2005;62:488–498.
214. Overholt BF, Wang KK, Burdick JS, et al. Five-year efficacy and safety of photodynamic therapy with Photofrin in Barrett's high-grade dysplasia. *Gastrointest Endosc* 2007;66:460–468.
222. Ortner ME, Caca K, Berr F, et al. Successful photodynamic therapy for nonresectable cholangiocarcinoma: a randomized prospective study. *Gastroenterology* 2003;125:1355–1363.
235. Nathan TR, Whitelaw DE, Chang SC, et al. Photodynamic therapy for prostate cancer recurrence after radiotherapy: a phase I study. *J Urol* 2002;168:1427–1432.
236. Verigos K, Stripp DCH, Mick R, et al. Updated results of a phase I trial of motexafin lutetium-mediated interstitial photodynamic therapy in patients with locally recurrent prostate cancer. *J Environ Pathol Toxicol Oncol* 2006;25:373–388.
237. Trachtenberg J, Bogaards A, Weersink RA, et al. Vascular targeted photodynamic therapy with palladium-bacteriopheophorbide photosensitizer for recurrent prostate cancer following definitive radiation therapy: assessment of safety and treatment response. *J Urol* 2007;178:1974–1979.
238. Trachtenberg J, Weersink RA, Davidson SR, et al. Vascular-targeted photodynamic therapy (padoporfin, WST09) for recurrent prostate cancer after failure of external beam radiotherapy: a study of escalating light doses. *BJU Int* 2008;102:556–562.
240. Svensson T, Andersson-Engels S, Einarsdottir M, et al. In vivo optical characterization of human prostate tissue using near-infrared time-resolved spectroscopy. *J Biomed Opt* 2007;12:014022.
241. Davidson SR, Weersink RA, Haider MA, et al. Treatment planning and dose analysis for interstitial photodynamic therapy of prostate cancer. *Phys Med Biol* 2009;54:2293–2313.
243. Nseyo UO, DeHaven J, Dougherty TJ, et al. Photodynamic therapy (PDT) in the treatment of patients with resistant superficial bladder cancer: a long-term experience. *J Clin Laser Med Surg* 1998;16:61–68.
246. Nseyo UO, Shumaker B, Klein EA, et al. Photodynamic therapy using porfimer sodium as an alternative to cystectomy in patients with refractory transitional cell carcinoma in situ of the bladder. Bladder Photofrin Study Group. *J Urol* 1998;160:39–44.
248. D'Hallewin MA, Baert L. Long-term results of whole bladder wall photodynamic therapy for carcinoma in situ of the bladder. *Urology* 1995;45:763–767.

Techniques, Modalities, and Modifiers in Radiation Oncology

Chapter 28
Radiation Oncology in the Developing World

Timothy P. Hanna

One of the greatest challenges facing the international radiation oncology community and all other domains of cancer control is the burden of cancer in low- and middle-income countries. Low-income countries had a 2010 per capita gross national income of US $1,005 or less, and for middle-income countries the range was US $1,006 to $12,275.[1] Nations falling into these income groups are often described as developing countries. This chapter will describe the unique characteristics of cancer in this setting and the challenges to health service provision. It will also provide reasons for hope that the global challenge of cancer can be met.

GLOBAL BURDEN OF DISEASE

Based on projections for 2008, an estimated 14% of all deaths worldwide are due to cancer.[2] In comparison to the worldwide burden of cancer, cardiovascular disease and other chronic conditions are responsible for, respectively, 30% and 19% of deaths globally. In total, 63% of mortality worldwide is the result of noncommunicable disease. Eighty percent of these deaths occur in low- and middle-income countries (LMCs).[2] In low-income countries, where deaths from communicable disease and other related causes are common, chronic disease was the cause of almost as many deaths in 2008 and is expected to surpass them by 2015 or earlier.[2]

In 2008, 56% of cancers worldwide occurred in less developed countries, as did 64% of all cancer deaths.[3] The burden of cancer in developing countries relates to increasing life expectancy in developing countries, population growth patterns, and rising incidence of risk factors for chronic diseases in developing countries.[4,5] For example, an estimated 65% of people ≥60 years of age lived in less developed countries in 2010, and this is expected to rise to 79% by 2050.[4] The growing burden of cancer and other noncommunicable diseases in LMCs represents a significant epidemiologic transition and a dual challenge for disease control efforts.

EPIDEMIOLOGY OF CANCER WORLDWIDE

Worldwide, there were 12.7 million new cases of cancer and 7.6 million cancer deaths in 2008.[3] Lung cancer is the most common cause of cancer worldwide (1.61 million new cases in 2008), followed by breast cancer (1.38 million) and colorectal cancer (1.24 million) (Fig. 28.1).[3] Lung cancer is also the most common cause of cancer death, with 1.38 million deaths in 2008.[3] Gastric cancer (0.74 million) and liver cancer (0.70 million) are the second and third most common causes of cancer death, respectively. Age-standardized incidence rates of cancer in developed countries are nearly double the rates in developing countries, though mortality rates are far more similar. These findings reflect variation in prevalence and distribution of major risk factors and limitations in early detection and treatment resources in developing countries.[6]

Although cervix cancer is the 10th most commonly diagnosed cancer among women in developed countries, it is second only to breast cancer in developing nations.[3] This reflects a lack of sufficient prevention of cervical cancer in many LMCs. Cervix cancer is an extremely common cancer in Latin America, Sub-Saharan Africa, and parts of Asia such as India (Fig. 28.2).[3] Gastric cancer and hepatocellular carcinoma are also common in many LMCs, with 47% of all cases of gastric cancer in the world occurring in China alone (Fig. 28.2).[3] Kaposi's sarcoma is a common cancer in Sub-Saharan Africa because of the AIDS epidemic,[7] and esophageal cancer has the highest incidence rates worldwide in regions of Asia and Africa.[3] Oral cancer has a high incidence in South Asia, particularly among men.[3]

Among nine common modifiable risk factors for cancer, tobacco smoking is associated with the largest proportion of attributable risk.[8] In the developing world, an estimated 49% of men and 8% of women were current smokers in 1995.[9] With large populations and high tobacco use in China and India, tobacco is an extremely important risk factor for cancer in Asia.[10] In general, many LMCs have demonstrated increased tobacco use during the past three decades. National consumption continues to rise in many countries, and in others, a peak occurred in the 1980s and 1990s.[11] History has shown a 30- to

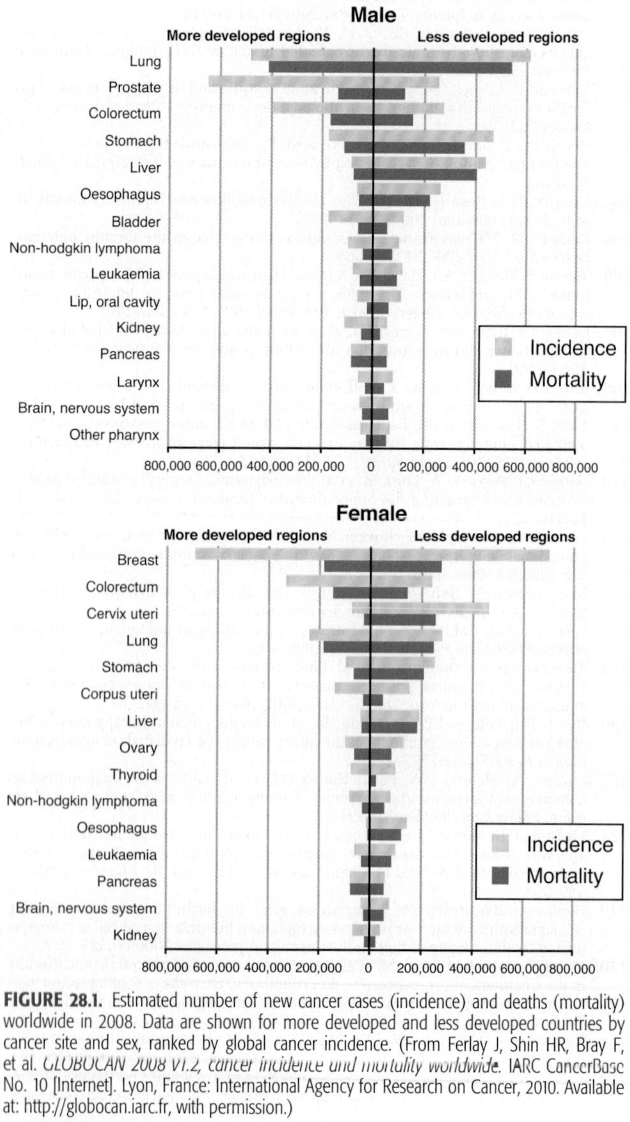

FIGURE 28.1. Estimated number of new cancer cases (incidence) and deaths (mortality) worldwide in 2008. Data are shown for more developed and less developed countries by cancer site and sex, ranked by global cancer incidence. (From Ferlay J, Shin HR, Bray F, et al. *GLOBOCAN 2008 V1.2, cancer incidence and mortality worldwide.* IARC CancerBase No. 10 [Internet]. Lyon, France: International Agency for Research on Cancer, 2010. Available at: http://globocan.iarc.fr, with permission.)

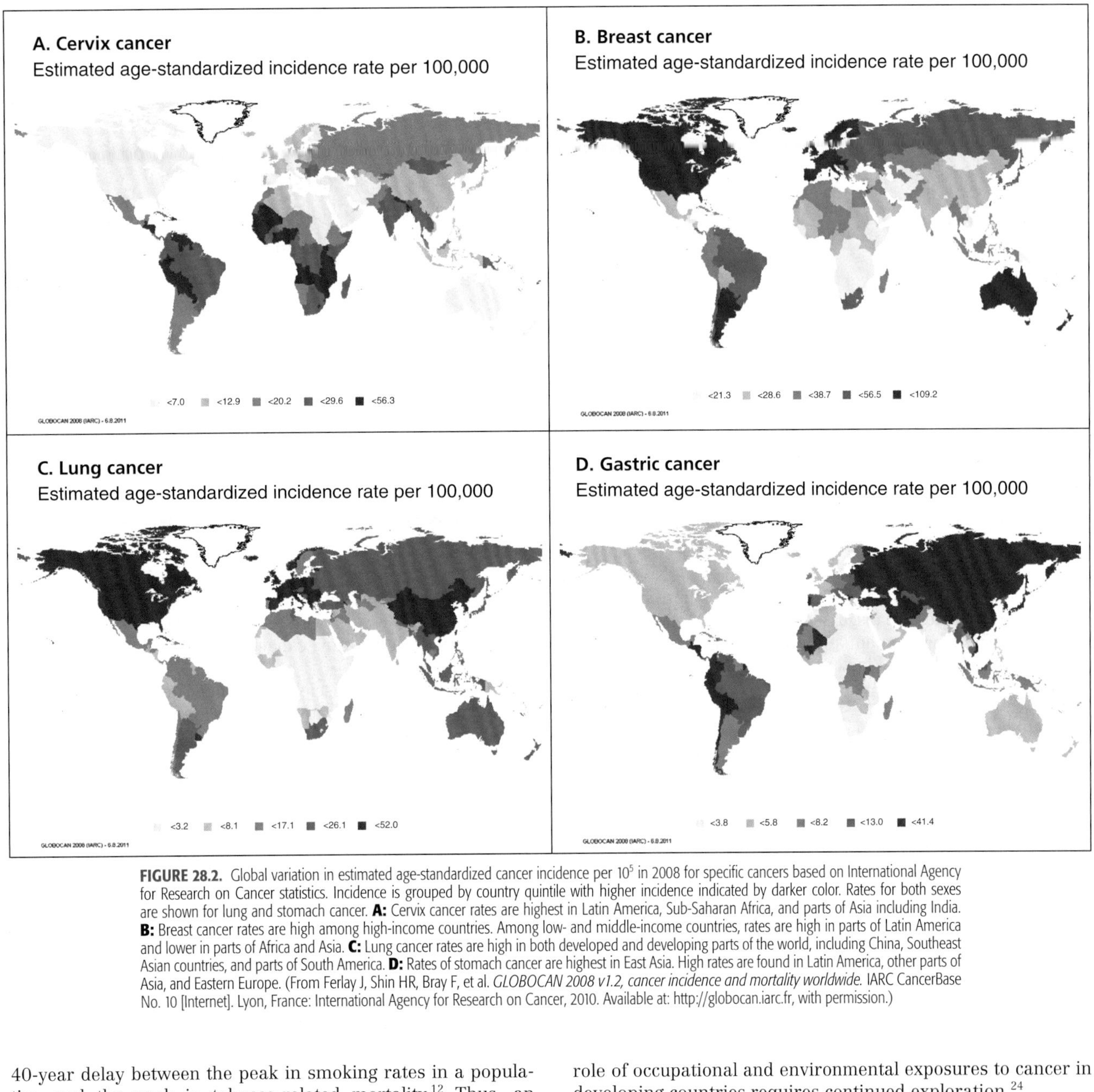

FIGURE 28.2. Global variation in estimated age-standardized cancer incidence per 10^5 in 2008 for specific cancers based on International Agency for Research on Cancer statistics. Incidence is grouped by country quintile with higher incidence indicated by darker color. Rates for both sexes are shown for lung and stomach cancer. **A:** Cervix cancer rates are highest in Latin America, Sub-Saharan Africa, and parts of Asia including India. **B:** Breast cancer rates are high among high-income countries. Among low- and middle-income countries, rates are high in parts of Latin America and lower in parts of Africa and Asia. **C:** Lung cancer rates are high in both developed and developing parts of the world, including China, Southeast Asian countries, and parts of South America. **D:** Rates of stomach cancer are highest in East Asia. High rates are found in Latin America, other parts of Asia, and Eastern Europe. (From Ferlay J, Shin HR, Bray F, et al. *GLOBOCAN 2008 v1.2, cancer incidence and mortality worldwide.* IARC CancerBase No. 10 [Internet]. Lyon, France: International Agency for Research on Cancer, 2010. Available at: http://globocan.iarc.fr, with permission.)

40-year delay between the peak in smoking rates in a population and the peak in tobacco-related mortality.[12] Thus, an increasing rate of tobacco-related malignancies is expected in LMCs during the next half century.[13,14]

Over 26% of cancers in developing countries are attributed to infectious causes.[15] Hepatitis B is a major risk factor for hepatocellular carcinoma in developing countries. Other factors are hepatitis C[16] and aflatoxin produced from *Aspergillus* in certain poorly preserved foods.[17] Human papillomavirus (HPV) and *Helicobacter pylori* are important etiologic agents, and there are numerous other infectious agents relevant to cancer in the developing world. These include Epstein-Barr virus, HIV, schistosomiasis, human T-cell leukemia virus type 1 (HTLV-1), and human herpesvirus 8 (HHV-8).[15,18] The prevalence of infectious causes is notable given the preventability of many of these causes through public health measures (e.g., hepatitis B, HPV vaccines).

There are a number of other factors that are relevant to patterns of global cancer incidence. Diet[19] and obesity are risk factors for some cancers.[20] This is notable given increasing trends in unhealthy diet and sedentary lifestyle among developing countries.[21] The impact of genetic polymorphisms on patterns of global cancer incidence has not been fully elucidated, but there is some suggestion of their relevance.[22,23] Similarly, the role of occupational and environmental exposures to cancer in developing countries requires continued exploration.[24]

In many developing countries, cancer often presents in advanced stages, due to factors such as lack of comprehensive screening and poor access to effective treatments.[25] As a result, case fatality rates are much higher in developing countries, with rates for breast and cervical cancer in low-income countries being more than double rates in high-income countries.[26] With cervical cancer being so common in developing countries and the high frequency of advanced cancer presentations requiring local therapy, radiation therapy has an extremely important role in developing countries. The following sections will describe radiation oncology in developing countries in terms of access, quality, and economics.

GLOBAL STATUS OF ACCESS TO RADIATION THERAPY

Access to radiation therapy is a multifactorial issue. Availability of machines and personnel for treatment is a key part of access to care. Other considerations include spatial accessibility, acceptability, affordability, accommodation, and awareness.[27,28]

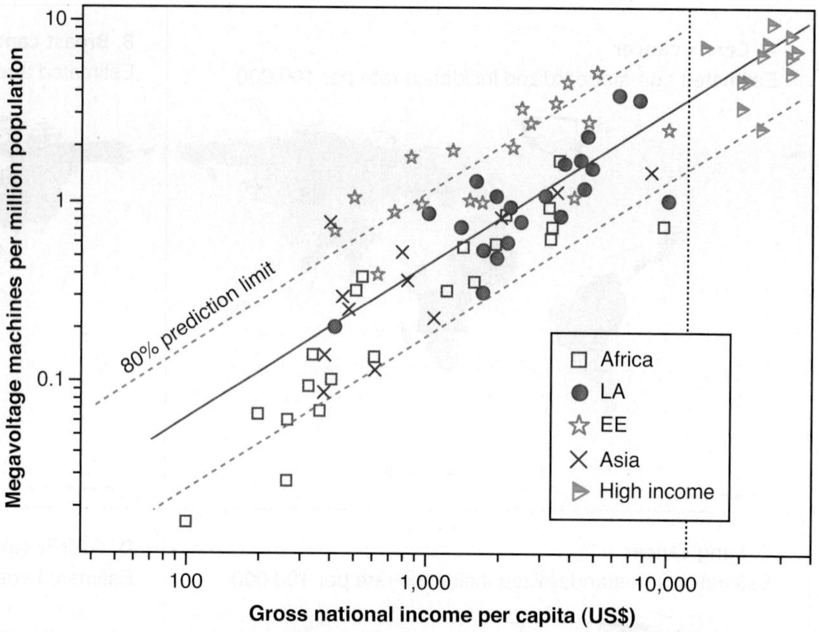

FIGURE 28.3. Megavoltage machines per million population versus gross national income per capita on a log-log scale. Countries are divided by income more than US $12,000 (high income) and then by region: Africa, Latin America (LA), Eastern Europe (EE), and Asia. The *solid line* is a linear regression line and *dotted lines* are the 80% confidence limit. The *vertical dotted line* represents the cutoff for high income. (From Levin V, Tatsuzaki H. Radiotherapy services in countries in transition: gross national income per capita as a significant factor. *Radiother Oncol* 2002;63:147–150, with permission from Elsevier.)

The most pertinent elements of access to radiation therapy in developing countries are discussed here.

Availability of equipment and personnel for radiation therapy are common limiting factors in developing countries. Less than 5% of global medical spending on cancer is in developing countries.[29] This is despite developing countries containing over 80% of the world's population[4] and almost 80% of the world's premature death, disability, and ill health from cancer.[2] Insufficient medical training programs make it difficult to address the lack of key personnel for radiation oncology.[30–33,34] International Atomic Energy Agency (IAEA) data suggest that developing countries only have about a third of the world's 12,206 megavoltage radiation therapy units despite an estimated need for between double and triple the current number.[35] There are currently 23 countries with populations over 1 million with no known machines, mostly in Africa.[35]

The greatest limitations in machine supply are strongly associated with low national economic status (Fig. 28.3).[36] Given the expected rise in cancer incidence in LMCs, these large mismatches between need and availability will only increase if current machine supply is not improved. In addition to machine availability, one must also consider the need for other physical resources. These include clinical space, bunkers, other equipment (brachytherapy, simulation, immobilization, treatment planning, beam modification, dosimetry, quality assurance), a reliable power supply for linear accelerators, and the availability of parts (and technical support) for machine maintenance and repair.[37]

The state of radiation therapy resources varies between developing countries and regions.[31,32,36,38] Some selected examples are provided for illustration. In 1999, Levin et al.[38] documented the availability and distribution of radiation therapy equipment in Africa. Only 22 of 56 countries in Africa were confidently known to have megavoltage radiation therapy facilities. In total, more than 400 million Africans had effectively no access to radiation therapy. Although machine supply has since modestly increased, there are still dramatic shortfalls in machine supply in Sub-Saharan Africa.[35]

In the Asia and Pacific Region, Tatsuzaki and Levin[31] found an 82-fold variation in the number of megavoltage machines per million population for 1999. China's and India's machine supply has increased in recent years, though capacity is still well below what is needed to treat all patients (Table 28.1).[3,35,39] Workforce resources vary considerably between countries, and most countries have less than two radiation oncologists per 1,000 incident cancers annually.[3,33,35] More physicists are required if radiotherapy capacity is to expand in the Asia Pacific region.[33]

In the era of multidisciplinary cancer therapy, for instance, for head and neck squamous cell carcinoma, availability of other elements of diagnosis and therapy such as surgical oncology, medical oncology, oncology nursing, pathology, radiology, rehabilitation, supportive care, and palliative care are all important to effective cancer management.[40] Without adequate pathology and radiology, it is not possible to effectively diagnose cancer and distinguish curative from palliative cases. The need for surgical capacity is especially noted, given its central role in curative treatment of the most common cancers globally, especially in their early stages. Access to palliative care, including pain control for moderate to severe pain, is also a major issue. The World Health Organization (WHO) estimates 5 billion people live in countries with limited or no access to narcotic analgesics and other controlled substances, with an estimated 5.5 million patients with terminal cancer dying each year without adequate treatment.[41]

Spatial accessibility refers to the geographic accessibility of medical treatments. Available information suggests spatial accessibility is a major issue in LMCs.[35,42] With radiation therapy centers often in large cities, rural populations may face substantial financial challenges when traveling into cities for the duration of radiation treatment.

Acceptability of available options can impact an individual's willingness to take advantage of services and adhere to recommended therapies. For example, a small study from Cameroon found beliefs, fears, cultural factors, and awareness were among explanations for delay in seeking medical attention for cancer.[43] Values surrounding effects of pelvic radiation treatment on fertility, loss of hair with some chemotherapy, and anatomic changes associated with surgery such as mastectomy are some potential factors in need of further description and quantification in developing countries. Culturally appropriate cancer control plans sensitive to a region's social and political concerns are needed, including initiatives to overcome stigma and improve awareness.[44]

Affordability of radiation therapy and other forms of cancer therapy are a major concern in LMCs.[45] Households often have limited or no health insurance coverage, especially in low-income and lower middle-income countries and more often

TABLE 28.1 MEGAVOLTAGE MACHINE SUPPLY AND CANCER BURDEN IN 17 ASIA PACIFIC COUNTRIES

Country	*2010 Per Capita Gross National Income ($US)*	*Population (Millions) 2010*	*Incident Cancers 2010*	*Megavoltage (MV) Machines 2011*	*Incident Cancers per MV Machine*
Myanmar	n.a.	48.0	69,952	6	11,659
Bangladesh	640	148.7	150,271	15	10,018
Pakistan	1,050	173.6	147,738	44	3,358
Vietnam	1,100	87.9	119,374	32	3,730
India	1,340	1,224.6	1,001,749	477	2,100
Mongolia	1,890	2.8	4,603	2	2,302
Philippines	2,050	93.3	82,468	30	2,749
Sri Lanka	2,290	20.9	25,802	12	2,150
Indonesia	2,580	239.9	309,582	34	9,105
Thailand	4,210	69.1	118,601	66	1,797
China	4,260	1,348.9	2,978,386	1,521	1,958
Malaysia	7,900	28.4	34,386	22	1,563
Korea, Rep	19,890	48.2	179,187	108	1,659
New Zealand	29,050[a]	4.4	21,080	25	843
Singapore	40,920	5.1	14,495	12	1,208
Japan	42,150	126.5	637,963	905	705
Australia	43,740[a]	22.3	112,023	131	855
Total		**3,692.6**	**6,007,660**	**3,442**	

n.a., not available.

[a]2009 data. As a simple estimate, countries with more than 1,000 new cancers annually per radiation machine most likely have a shortfall of radiation machines. 2010 gross national income per capita information provided by the World Bank Group (Atlas method), http://data.worldbank.org/about/country-classifications. 2010 population data from the World Population Prospects 2010 revision, http://esa.un.org/unpd/wpp/index.htm. Projected cancer incidence in 2010 from GLOBOCAN 2008, http://globocan.iarc.fr/. Reported number of megavoltage radiation machines from Directory of Radiotherapy Centers (DIRAC) August 2011, http://www-naweb.iaea.org/nahu/dirac/default.shtm.

among the poor in LMCs.[46,47] This is notable as cancer-related public health care may be inadequate or nonexistent. The cost of travel to the nearest cancer center can itself be another major financial obstacle, and costs of staying for the length of radiation treatment in another location can mean lost income and more cost to the patient and family.[45] A family may lose additional income due to caregiver absence from work.[45,48]

Awareness of the basic cancer principles and the value of cancer screening and early detection may limit timely access to cancer services for the public in LMCs. A large Union for International Cancer Control (UICC) survey of multiple LMCs found substantial lack of awareness of common preventable causes of cancer and found that a quarter or more of respondents in Asia and Africa did not think cancer could be cured.[49] Limited awareness of principles of cancer diagnosis and appropriate referral among nonspecialist health care workers may be further limiting factors for access to cancer treatment. Health care worker training in oncologic principles may be extremely basic or insufficient in some cases.[50]

QUALITY OF RADIATION ONCOLOGY IN DEVELOPING COUNTRIES

Key dimensions of quality are described by the Institute of Medicine as safety, effectiveness, patient-centeredness, timeliness, efficiency, and equity.[51] Quality can be assessed through consideration of a health system's structure, process, and outcomes.[52] Elements of structure are physical resources, human resources, and organizational structure. Limitations in physical and human resources in LMCs have already been described. The access issues that relate to late presentation and failure to receive indicated treatment arguably have the greatest impact on outcomes and quality of radiation therapy in developing countries. Quality may be further degraded by the inequitable access of the few available resources between country and city, rich and poor.

The organizational structure of health care in developing countries has historically revolved around communicable disease, nutritional deficiencies, and child and maternal health. The additional burden of noncommunicable disease in developing countries, commonly cancer, cardiovascular disease, chronic lung disease, and mental illness, impose a major strain on current resources and health care models. Challenges to the structure of cancer control and radiation therapy in limited-resource settings may also include insufficient priority of cancer control among some governments and donor agencies with many competing priorities. Other issues may include political or social instability, conflict, corruption, and fragmented service provision.

The process of health care refers to what occurs while care is provided. For radiation oncology, this includes technical elements of quality assurance, treatment prescription, treatment planning, and treatment delivery. It also includes the integration of multidisciplinary services needed alongside radiation oncology for effective cancer management. A major process issue in some countries is system-related delay in diagnosis.[53,54] This probably contributes to high rates of advanced disease at presentation. System-related diagnostic delay can relate to weak or nonexistent referral systems or limited resources for diagnosis. It is compounded by patient-related delay in seeking medical attention due to previously described access issues.[55] The additional impact on delay due to waiting times for radiation following radiation oncology consultation requires further characterization in LMCs.

The technical process of radiotherapy is a vital element of quality. For this reason, the IAEA and WHO have maintained a postal dose audit program using thermoluminescent devices (TLDs). A report focusing on measurements from developing countries found acceptable results, with most machines calibrated within the ± 5% dose acceptance limit. Sixteen percent of machines registered measurements outside this range in the first round of testing, with 93% measuring dose within 5% of the standard after the second round.[56] Notably, a dosimetric audit in Latin America and the Caribbean suggested an association between on-duty medical physics support and acceptable TLD results.[57] This emphasizes the importance of adequate staffing to a radiation department's quality assurance process.

Current reports are too limited to comment on the quality of general patterns of the radiation oncology clinical process in regions of the developing world. There are most certainly specific opportunities for gains. Taking advantage of hypofractionation to increase throughput where there is supportive evidence has not always occurred, as one survey on patterns of palliative radiation for bone metastasis in Africa suggests.[58] Implementation of multidisciplinary decision making among oncologists in LMCs is important but not always present.[59,60] Treatment refusal or nonadherence by patients can be a major problem in some cases and is an important area for quality improvement where it exists.[42,48,61] Audits of the clinical decision-making and the treatment-planning process may provide a useful means of ensuring patient safety, improving processes, and creating opportunities for continuing education.[62,63] This is particularly important with the introduction of technology at new locations. For example, initial experience with this approach in a new radiation therapy center in an Asian developing country found suboptimal management in 52% of cases.[62]

Adverse event rates in developing countries treating with radiation are largely unknown. A report examining the risk profile of radiation therapy for the WHO could not identify any detailed reports of adverse events from Africa or Asia.[64] It is important to highlight the need for adverse event recording and reporting for the purpose of patient safety and quality improvement for all countries utilizing radiation therapy.

Finally, quality of radiation oncology in developing countries relates to outcomes. Of all cancer outcomes, there is the most information on survival. Generally, overall survival for cancer patients is lower, and sometimes dramatically so, for populations in developing countries. In a large multinational series from the International Agency for Research on Cancer (IARC), 5-year age-standardized relative survival for cervix cancer was 79% in Seoul, South Korea, but 46% in Mumbai, India; 22% in The Gambia; and only 13% in Kampala, Uganda.[65] Similarly, for breast cancer, survival rates ranged from 90% in Hong Kong SAR to 13% in The Gambia. When absolute survival was stratified by extent of disease, in many cases, treatment outcomes were still inferior in regions with less developed health services compared to regions with more developed services (e.g., local and regional extent breast cancer and larynx cancer). This may reflect access and quality issues in diagnosis, treatment, and follow-up and/or limitations of the available data.

ECONOMICS OF RADIATION THERAPY IN DEVELOPING COUNTRIES

Radiation therapy has been shown to be cost-effective in numerous developed world settings.[66,67–68] A study by the Breast Health Global Initiative (BHGI) suggests that a comprehensive breast cancer program involving early detection and treatment, including radiotherapy, can be cost-effective in developing world settings.[69] Notably, the BHGI study found that it was more cost-effective to invest in early detection in addition to comprehensive cancer therapy resources for breast cancer than in cancer therapy resources alone. This finding reflects the ability of early detection to increase the chances of cure due to earlier stage presentation and to some degree the lower cost of treating earlier stage versus locally advanced disease. In other situations, preventing cancer reduces the number of patients needing treatment, which can also impact on overall cost of therapy for a population.

In addition to cost-effectiveness, the actual cost of delivering interventions must be taken into account when planning. Though per-patient costs of radiation can be quite low compared to other modalities given the long usage cycle of megavoltage radiotherapy units, large up-front costs can serve as a major deterrent to establishing services. Unfortunately, there is little context-specific information on the economics of cancer therapies in developing countries. One exception is an IAEA-supported study demonstrating wide variation in the cost of delivering a fraction of radiation between a sample of units in developing and developed countries.[70] For the costs considered, the median cost per fraction delivered by a cobalt machine was less than half that for linear accelerators. Cost variation was most associated with radiation machine cost and machine usage for linear accelerators, and for cobalt machines, machine cost, usage, and personnel cost.

Undoubtedly, applications of various radiation therapy techniques and modern equipment will yield opportunities to maximize the cost–benefit ratio of radiation treatment in developing countries. Hypofractionation yields opportunities to treat more patients with the same supply of equipment.[71] Hypofractionation for cervical cancer and lung cancer are examples of identified areas for research.[72–74] Investigation of brachytherapy or intraoperative radiation therapy (IORT) may provide means of delivering adjuvant treatments rapidly. High-dose-rate (HDR) brachytherapy markedly increases patient throughput (e.g., for cervical cancer) compared to low-dose-rate (LDR) brachytherapy per machine.[75] An IAEA study of accelerated radiation therapy for head and neck cancer in developing countries suggests an opportunity for increasing effectiveness of treatment without increasing departmental resources, though with increased, but tolerable, acute toxicity.[76]

There has been some debate about the relative merits of cobalt-60 versus linear accelerator technology for limited resource settings. The ideal mix of machines will change depending on site-specific considerations and future market dynamics. Regarding the latter, development of lower-cost entry-level linear accelerators and, on the other hand, increases in costs of new and more sophisticated cobalt equipment would affect decision making.[77] It is useful to remember that quality assurance costs, maintenance costs, and associated personnel requirements of cobalt machines are estimated to be substantially less than for linear accelerators and reliability is generally higher.[70,77]

TRANSLATING KNOWLEDGE INTO ACTION

Recognized priorities for action fall into six categories: (a) advocacy, (b) investment, (c) planning, (d) capacity building, (e) quality, and (f) research.[47,77–82] The varying resources, priorities, and disease burden seen in countries at different stages of development mean that there is no single solution that will apply in all cases.[81] In low-income countries with extreme resource limitations, a strategy focusing on cost-effective prevention, raising awareness of cancer within the population, monitoring of process and outcomes, good palliative care, and focused early detection and treatment goals would be a reasonable starting point.[83]

Advocacy. An international coalition to support cancer control and cancer care in developing countries is emerging. The UICC plays an important role as an umbrella organization for advocacy. Other groups range from international agencies (e.g., IAEA, WHO, IARC), to national organizations (e.g., U.S. National Cancer Institute), to professional groups (e.g., American Society for Radiation Oncology [ASTRO], European Society for Radiotherapy and Oncology [ESTRO], American Society of Clinical Oncology [ASCO], International Organization for Medical Physics [IOMP]), to nongovernmental organizations (NGOs) (e.g., Lance Armstrong Foundation, International Network for Cancer Treatment and Research [INCTR], Axios International, AfrOx, American Cancer Society), to academic institutions and hospitals (e.g., the Global Task Force on Expanded Access to Cancer Care and Control in Developing Countries [GTF.CCC] convened by Harvard, St. Jude Children's Research Hospital). Through the advocacy of the UICC and many other partners (e.g., NCD Alliance), the Political Declaration[84] of the United Nations High-Level Meeting on the Prevention and Control of Non-communicable Diseases (September 19–20, 2011) was an important acknowledgment by governments of the global problem of cancer and other non-communicable diseases. It was also a substantial step toward specific and concerted action by the international community.

Investment. The advocacy and work of the many cancer control groups range from local to global, and from grassroots to high-level agencies. All approaches are extremely important for generating the political will to invest in cancer control. Particularly in middle-income countries, incorporation of cancer care into public health insurance for those living in poverty is an important, and challenging, goal to meet.[47,85] Given the shortage of national funding for cancer care in poorer countries, international private and public donor support and advocacy for tiered pricing will be notably important in improving access to cancer therapy.

Planning. Development of radiation therapy capacity can not occur in isolation. Radiation therapy resources must be integrated into a broader context of multidisciplinary cancer care and cancer control and into a functional health system capable of tackling the double burden of communicable and noncommunicable diseases afflicting developing countries.[86] A national cancer control plan and collection of cancer registry and health data are central in organizing resources in an equitable and appropriate fashion.[87] Notably, the GTF.CCC has published an important resource for planning, advocacy, and priority setting entitled *Closing the Cancer Divide: A Blueprint to Expand Access in Low and Middle Income Countries.*[88]

Prevention (e.g., tobacco control, hepatitis B and HPV vaccination) and early detection are crucial in reducing the burden of advanced cancers in developing countries. When early detection and prevention are combined with timely access to effective cancer therapy, there is great potential for dramatically reducing deaths from cancer in developing countries as well as minimizing national costs of cancer therapy.[47] Numerous relevant resources on cancer control and other noncommunicable diseases have been published online by the WHO, including a series of modules on cancer control planning,[89] and the Framework Convention on Tobacco Control.

The IAEA plays a prominent role in quality assurance, safety standards, and dose calibration of radiation therapy equipment internationally. It has also been involved in numerous technical cooperation projects and radiation therapy clinical trials in developing countries. In 2004, the IAEA launched the Program of Action for Cancer Treatment (PACT) to widen the scope of its work in radiation therapy planning and capacity building. Its wide-ranging plan started with the development of sustainable demonstration radiation treatment sites in six countries throughout the developing world (Albania, Nicaragua, Sri Lanka, Tanzania, Vietnam, and Yemen). The PACT program situates the delivery of radiation therapy within a comprehensive framework including prevention, early detection, treatment, and palliation. Plans sensitive to the target country's social and political situation are developed through local and international partnerships. Other IAEA initiatives for developing countries include strengthening pediatric radiation oncology and quality audits.

At a global level, breast cancer guidelines stratified by availability of resources have been developed through the Breast Health Global Initiative.[90] This is a useful paradigm for developing resource-appropriate and stepwise, scalable goals and guidelines for cancer care that is being adopted for other cancers.[91] A related approach has been used by the IAEA to describe additional resource requirements, benefits, and risks for specific approaches in lung cancer treatment, including curative and palliative radiation.[92]

Developing innovative means of organizing and funding cancer services is needed. The IAEA's PACT program offers opportunities to identify successful models of service delivery and planning. A model of radiotherapy service provision utilizing geographically dispersed telemedicine-linked sites with varying levels of capacity has also been proposed by an Indian group to maximize available resources.[93] Another concept that is being explored is utilizing community health workers and primary care to expand cancer-related service provision. Proposed activities are cancer prevention, early detection, some treatment (e.g., systemic therapy), palliation, and follow-up.[47] A social business model is one potential solution to financing radiation therapy services.[94] This is being explored as part of a Bangladesh initiative.

Capacity Building. The importance of improving human resources for radiation oncology and oncology in general cannot be overstated given the global workforce shortage of trained health care professionals. Some initial efforts have been made in developing curricula and educational approaches specific to the discipline of radiation medicine.[95,96] The IAEA has been notably involved in these efforts. The issue of loss of trained staff from developing to developed countries is especially important to consider in developing educational programs. Urban regions in LMCs may have high-level expertise that can be utilized in developing national training programs. A complementary approach is online training. This is the approach of the Virtual University for Cancer Control and Regional Training Network (VUCCnet) initiative in Africa. A growing number cancer centers, regional groups, and specific nations have been involved in twinning projects building capacity for cancer therapy in limited-resource countries. These initiatives have been particularly strong in pediatric oncology, with demonstrated success.[97,98] They provide an appealing means for broad participation in improving cancer control in developing countries.

Numerous oncology societies in developed and developing countries support initiatives to build capacity in developing countries. The African Organization for Research and Training in Cancer (AORTIC) is an Africa-based collaboration with an advocacy, research, and training focus in cancer control for Africa. ESTRO, ASTRO, and a number of other radiation oncology societies support initiatives for education and capacity building in developing countries. ASCO has developed a number of ongoing initiatives in training, mentoring, and continuing education of oncologists in developing countries, including translation by local editors of their flagship journal into 12 languages.[99] The U.S. National Cancer Institute Radiation Research Program is partnering with other oncology groups to develop a capacity-building Cancer Expert Corps.

Regional and national initiatives are very important for improving the capacity to treat cancer in developing countries. For example, the Forum for Nuclear Cooperation in Asia (FNCA) organizes radiation therapy protocols in the Asian region for the common problems of cervical cancer and nasopharyngeal cancer.[100] The FNCA involves Asian countries at a wide range of economic levels. At a national level, the Association of Radiation Oncologists of India (AROI) publishes a scientific journal and supports various educational and professional activities.[101]

Quality. Embedded within the themes of investment, planning, and capacity building is the implicit theme of structure-related quality improvement. Process-related initiatives in quality are another very important part of ensuring optimal outcomes. These are often referred to indirectly (e.g., safety, effectiveness, patient-centeredness, timeliness, efficiency, equity).[51] Quality improvement relating to process and organizational structure is important as it holds the potential for improving some outcomes more rapidly than other drivers of health, such as economic growth.[102] One important element of quality for radiation oncology in developing countries is safety, given the potential for unsafe treatment to negate any benefit of available treatment.[103] Safety includes the clinical process, the various elements of technical quality assurance, maintenance, worker safety, public safety, and source security.[104,105] Safety requires investment in appropriate dosimetry equipment, sufficiently trained human resources, and time for quality assurance activities.[105] Internal and external audits, peer review, regulation, accreditation, certification, checklists, adverse event reporting, common protocols, quality improvement, and independent checking are examples of interventions ensuring safety and quality assurance in radiation oncology.[64,106,107]

Research. There are many fundamental questions that remain unanswered specific to cancer in developing countries. For instance, it cannot be assumed that approaches to treating cancer from developed settings will produce the same results when applied in other countries. Considerations include potential differences in disease bulk, malnutrition, rates of chronic infections such as HIV/tuberculosis/hepatitis B, and genetic polymorphisms affecting disease biology and treatment response.[108–112] Resources for supportive care and quality assurance are also considerations. There are many unknowns in cancer epidemiology and basic science, and, as mentioned, more health services research is emphatically needed into areas such as access, quality, and economics.[87]

Supporting research on cancer by investigators in the developing world is important as it can build local research capacity and provide a means of adapting scientific knowledge to local circumstances to meet national health priorities.[113] The U.S. National Cancer Institute has also been involved with numerous international collaborations. Protocol-driven clinical research can also strengthen local treatment capacity. The INCTR has been involved in designing clinical trials relevant to developing world situations, as has the IAEA.

International research partnerships are essential in the interconnected and interdependent world we live in.[113] Many developing countries have quite advanced resources to sustain research activities; for instance, a number of clinical trials for cervical cancer radiotherapy have occurred in India (e.g., HDR vs. LDR brachytherapy, radiation vs. chemoradiation).[114,115] India is also home of the Advanced Center for Treatment, Research and Education in Cancer (ACTREC), part of the Tata Memorial Center. Regional research collaborations are developing, for example, the FNCA. In addition, of note, a number of research/teaching twinning partnerships between developed and developing countries have been formed.[97,98,116]

Undoubtedly, industry and development will play an important role in improving access to quality radiation therapy equipment. Equipment that is affordable, safe, and technically suitable for developing country conditions is needed.[77] The IAEA has taken leadership in advocacy for such equipment, and there is hope that new solutions will proliferate. Creative public–private partnerships will be important, as will be innovative equipment design. This last point has been exemplified by a group in Canada that has pioneered cobalt-60 tomotherapy.[117]

CONCLUSION

Cancer in the developing world is an urgent problem, reaching critical proportions. Almost 60% of all cancer cases occur in the developing world. Vast numbers of people in developing countries have either limited access or no access to radiation therapy. At a time when new gains in oncology outcomes in the developed world are incremental, oncologists have the chance to help make some of the largest survival gains in history in the developing world. In addition, the potential for health care gains through cancer prevention and early detection, and the relief of suffering through palliative care are enormous. The poor deserve fair access to quality cancer care. The challenge will now be to deliver this in a thoughtful and contextually appropriate way.

SELECTED REFERENCES

A full list of references for this chapter is available online.

1. World Bank. *World Bank country classifications.* 2010. Available at: http://data.worldbank.org/about/country-classifications. Accessed August 13, 2011.
2. World Health Organization. *Projections of mortality and burden of disease, 2004-2030.* 2008. Available at: http://www.who.int/healthinfo/global_burden_disease/projections/en/index.html. Accessed August 13, 2011.
3. Ferlay J, Shin HR, Bray F, et al. *GLOBOCAN 2008 v.1.2, Cancer incidence and mortality worldwide.* IARC CancerBase No. 10 [Internet]. 2010. Available at: http://www-dep.iarc.fr. Accessed August 14, 2011.
6. Jemal A, Bray F, Center MM, et al. Global cancer statistics. *CA Cancer J Clin* 2011;61(2):69–90.
8. Danaei G, Vander Hoorn S, Lopez AD, et al. Causes of cancer in the world: comparative risk assessment of nine behavioural and environmental risk factors. *Lancet* 2005;366(9499):1784–1793.
15. Parkin DM. The global health burden of infection-associated cancers in the year 2002. *Int J Cancer* 2006;118(12):3030–3044.
26. Beaulieu N, Bloom DE, Reddy Bloom L, et al. *Breakaway: the global burden of cancer- challenges and opportunities.* New York: Economist Intelligence Unit: The Economist, 2009.
27. Penchansky R, Thomas JW. The concept of access: definition and relationship to consumer satisfaction. *Med Care* 1981;19(2):127–140.
28. Mackillop WJ. Health services research in radiation oncology: towards achieving the achievable for patients with cancer. In: Gunderson LL, Tepper JE, eds. *Clinical radiation oncology,* 2nd ed. New York: Churchill Livingstone, 2006.
30. Frenk J, Chen L, Bhutta ZA, et al. Health professionals for a new century: transforming education to strengthen health systems in an interdependent world. *Lancet* 2010;376(9756):1923–1958.
31. Tatsuzaki H, Levin CV. Quantitative status of resources for radiation therapy in Asia and Pacific region. *Radiother Oncol.* 2001;60(1):81–89.
32. Zubizarreta EH, Poitevin A, Levin CV. Overview of radiotherapy resources in Latin America: a survey by the International Atomic Energy Agency (IAEA). *Radiother Oncol* 2004;73(1):97–100.
33. Kron T, Cheung K, Dai J, et al. Medical physics aspects of cancer care in the Asia Pacific region. *Biomed Imaging Interv J* 2008;4(3):e33.
35. International Atomic Energy Agency. *Directory of radiotherapy centers (DIRAC).* Available at: http://www-naweb.iaea.org/nahu/dirac/default.shtm. Accessed August 7, 2011.
36. Levin V, Tatsuzaki H. Radiotherapy services in countries in transition: gross national income per capita as a significant factor. *Radiother Oncol* 2002;63(2): 147–150.
38. Levin CV, El Gueddari B, Meghzifene A. Radiation therapy in Africa: distribution and equipment. *Radiother Oncol* 1999;52(1):79–84.
39. Barton MB, Frommer M, Shafiq J. Role of radiotherapy in cancer control in low-income and middle-income countries. *Lancet Oncol* 2006;7(7):584–595.
47. Farmer P, Frenk J, Knaul FM, et al. Expansion of cancer care and control in countries of low and middle income: a call to action. *Lancet* 2010;376(9747):1186–1193.
51. Institute of Medicine Committee on Quality of Health Care in America. *Crossing the quality chasm: a new health system for the 21st century.* Washington, DC: National Academy Press, 2001.
56. Izewska J, Andreo P, Vatnitsky S, et al. The IAEA/WHO TLD postal dose quality audits for radiotherapy: a perspective of dosimetry practices at hospitals in developing countries. *Radiother Oncol* 2003;69(1):91–97.
58. Sharma V, Gaye PM, Wahab SA, et al. Patterns of practice of palliative radiotherapy in Africa, part 1: bone and brain metastases. *Int J Radiat Oncol Biol Phys* 2008;70(4):1195–1201.
59. Cazap E, Buzaid AC, Garbino C, et al. Breast cancer in Latin America: results of the Latin American and Caribbean Society of Medical Oncology/Breast Cancer Research Foundation expert survey. *Cancer* 2008;113(8 Suppl):2359–2365.
60. El Saghir NS, El-Asmar N, Hajj C, et al. Survey of utilization of multidisciplinary management tumor boards in Arab countries. *Breast* 2011;20(Suppl 2):S70–S74.
62. Shakespeare TP, Back MF, Lu JJ, et al. External audit of clinical practice and medical decision making in a new Asian oncology center: results and implications for both developing and developed nations. *Int J Radiat Oncol Biol Phys* 2006;64(3):941–947.
64. Barton M, Shafiq J, eds. *Radiotherapy risk profile: technical manual.* Geneva: World Health Organization, Radiotherapy Safety Team within the World Alliance for Patient Safety, 2008.
65. Sankaranarayanan R, Swaminathan R, eds. *Cancer survival in Africa, Asia, the Caribbean and Central America. IARC Scientific Publications No. 162.* Lyon, France: International Agency for Research on Cancer, 2011.
66. Barton MB, Gebski V, Manderson C, et al. Radiation therapy: are we getting value for money? *Clin Oncol (R Coll Radiol)* 1995;7(5):287–292.
69. Groot MT, Baltussen R, Uyl-de Groot CA, et al. Costs and health effects of breast cancer interventions in epidemiologically different regions of Africa, North America, and Asia. *Breast J* 2006;12(Suppl 1):S81–S90.
70. Van Der Giessen PH, Alert J, Badri C, et al. Multinational assessment of some operational costs of teletherapy. *Radiother Oncol* 2004;71(3):347–355.
72. Kitchener HC, Hoskins W, Small W, Jr, et al. The development of priority cervical cancer trials: a Gynecologic Cancer InterGroup report. *Int J Gynecol Cancer* 2010;20(6):1092–1100.
73. van Lonkhuijzen L, Thomas G. Palliative radiotherapy for cervical carcinoma, a systematic review. *Radiother Oncol* 2011;98(3):287–291.
74. Kepka L, Casas F, Perin B, et al. Radiochemotherapy for lung cancer in developing countries. *Clin Oncol (R Coll Radiol)* 2009;21(7):536–542.
76. Overgaard J, Mohanti BK, Begum N, et al. Five versus six fractions of radiotherapy per week for squamous-cell carcinoma of the head and neck (IAEA-ACC study): a randomised, multicentre trial. *Lancet Oncol* 2010;11(6):553–560.
77. Salminen EK, Kiel K, Ibbott GS, et al. International Conference on Advances in Radiation Oncology (ICARO): outcomes of an IAEA meeting. *Radiat Oncol* 2011;6:11.
79. Anderson BO, Cazap E, El Saghir NS, et al. Optimisation of breast cancer management in low-resource and middle-resource countries: executive summary of the Breast Health Global Initiative consensus, 2010. *Lancet Oncol* 2011;12(4): 387–398.
80. Anderson BO, Ballieu M, Bradley C, et al. *Access to cancer treatment in low- and middle-income countries-an essential part of global cancer control.* A CanTreat Position Paper. 2010. Available at: http://axios-group.com/index.php/download_file/view/85/151/. Accessed July 6, 2011.
81. Sloan FA, Gelband H, eds. *Cancer control opportunities in low- and middle-income countries.* Washington, DC: National Academy Press, 2007.
82. Union for International Cancer Control. *The world cancer declaration 2008.* 2011. Available at: http://www.uicc.org/declaration/download-declaration. Accessed July 31, 2011.
83. World Health Organization. *National cancer control programmes: policies and managerial guidelines.* Geneva: World Health Organization, 2002.
84. United Nations General Assembly 66th Session. *Political declaration of the high-level meeting of the General Assembly on the Prevention and Control of Non-communicable Diseases. A/66/L.1. Sept. 16, 2011.* New York: United Nations, 2011.

87. Hanna TP, Kangolle AC. Cancer control in developing countries: using health data and health services research to measure and improve access, quality and efficiency. *BMC Int Health Hum Rights* 2010;10:24.
88. Knaul FM, Frenk J, Shulman LN, for the Global Task Force on Expanded Access to Cancer Care and Control in Developing Countries. *Closing the cancer divide: a blueprint to expand access in low and middle income countries.* Boston, MA: Harvard Global Equity Initiative, 2011.
89. World Health Organization. *Cancer control: knowledge into action: WHO guide for effective programs: module 4. Diagnosis and treatment.* Geneva: World Health Organization, 2008.
90. Anderson BO, Shyyan R, Eniu A, et al. Breast cancer in limited-resource countries: an overview of the Breast Health Global Initiative 2005 guidelines. *Breast J* 2006;12(Suppl 1):S3–S15.
92. Macbeth FR, Abratt RP, Cho KH, et al. Lung cancer management in limited resource settings: guidelines for appropriate good care. *Radiother Oncol* 2007; 82:123–131.
93. Datta NR, Rajasekar D. Improvement of radiotherapy facilities in developing countries: a three-tier system with a teleradiotherapy network. *Lancet Oncol* 2004;5(11):695–698.
95. Coffey M, Engel-Hills P, El-Gantiry M, et al. A core curriculum for RTTs (radiation therapists/radiotherapy radiographers) designed for developing countries under the auspices of the international atomic energy agency (IAEA). *Radiother Oncol* 2006;81:324–325.
96. Podgorsak EB. *Radiation oncology physics: a handbook for teachers and students.* Vienna: IAEA, 2005.
97. Ribeiro RC, Pui CH. Saving the children–improving childhood cancer treatment in developing countries. *N Engl J Med* 2005;352(21):2158–2160.
98. Masera G, Baez F, Biondi A, et al. North-South twinning in paediatric haemato-oncology: the La Mascota programme, Nicaragua. *Lancet* 1998;352(9144):1923–1926.
102. Peabody JW, Taguiwalo MM, Robalino DA, et al. Improving the quality of care in developing countries. In: Jamison DT, Breman JG, Measham AR, et al., eds. *Disease control priorities in developing countries.* Washington, DC: World Bank and Oxford University Press, 2006.
103. Borras C. Overexposure of radiation therapy patients in Panama: problem recognition and follow-up measures. *Rev Panam Salud Publica* 2006;20(2–3):173–187.
106. Mytton OT, Velazquez A, Banken R, et al. Introducing new technology safely. *Qual Saf Health Care* 2010;19(Suppl 2):i9–i14.
107. Newton RC, Mytton OT, Aggarwal R, et al. Making existing technology safer in healthcare. *Qual Saf Health Care* 2010;19(Suppl 2):i15–i24.
109. McArdle O, Kigula-Mugambe JB. Contraindications to cisplatin based chemoradiotherapy in the treatment of cervical cancer in Sub-Saharan Africa. *Radiother Oncol* 2007;83(1):94–96.
113. Frenk J, Chen L. Overcoming gaps to advance global health equity: a symposium on new directions for research. *Health Res Policy Syst* 2011;9(1):11.
117. Schreiner LJ, Kerr A, Salomons G, et al. The potential for image guided radiation therapy with cobalt-60 tomotherapy. In: Ellis RE, Peters TM, eds. *Lecture notes in computer science: Proc. 6th Annual International Conference on Medical Image Computing and Computer Assisted Intervention (MICCAI).* Vol 8. Heidelberg: Springer-Verlag, 2003:449–456.

Chapter 29
Chemical Modifiers of Radiation Response

David S. Yoo and David M. Brizel

Chemical agents have been administered in conjunction with radiotherapy (RT) for both the enhancement of antitumor therapeutic efficacy and the amelioration of treatment-induced toxicity. Two concepts are fundamental to understanding the rationale for chemical modification of radiation response and to interpreting the studies that have addressed this issue. The first is the therapeutic ratio (TR), which is defined as the TCP/NTCP where TCP is the tumor control probability and NTCP is the normal tissue complication probability. Both of these parameters have sigmoid dose–response curves (Fig. 29.1). The horizontal separation between these two curves for any given treatment will often determine its overall utility. As the separation between these curves increases, the likelihood increases the odds that the treatment will be effective without causing an unacceptable level of morbidity. Conversely, when the two curves are closer together, the treatment may be less effective while causing an unacceptable level of morbidity.

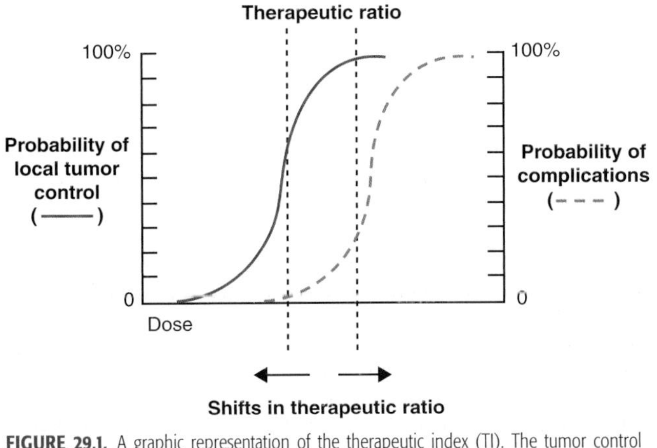

FIGURE 29.1. A graphic representation of the therapeutic index (TI). The tumor control probability (TCP) is to the left of the normal tissue complication probability (NTCP) and both are displayed as sigmoid dose–response curves. Larger separations are indicative of higher TIs. Ideally, normal tissue protection strategies would move the NTCP curve to the right without compromising TCP (moving the TCP curve to the right). Ideal therapeutic intensification strategies would move the TCP curve to the left without worsening NTCP (moving the NTCP curve to the left).

The second concept is the efficacy/toxicity profile of the putative chemical modifier, which can directly affect the TR. A radiosensitizing agent that exacerbates toxicity to the same extent that it improves efficacy (shifting both NTCP and TCP curves to the left) may leave the TR unchanged or worsened and not be clinically practical. Conversely, a radioprotective agent that also reduces RT efficacy against the tumor (shifting both NTCP and TCP curves to the right) also may not affect or even reduce the TR. The intrinsic toxicity of a radioprotector must also be considered when reduction of NTCP is the primary goal of a given chemical modification strategy. A compound that causes significant side effects of its own may render it unsuitable even if it can reduce the treatment-induced toxicity in question. This chapter will explore chemical radiosensitization and radioprotective strategies. The primary focus will be on treatments that have been clinically tested in head and neck cancer in order to amplify these concepts.

CHEMICAL RADIOSENSITIZATION

The Oxygen Effect

Tumor cell killing is produced by direct ionizations within critical cellular targets as well as by the indirect effect of energy deposited in other cellular molecules including water. Ionizing radiation generates free radicals, which can lead to cellular death via the creation of single strand and double strand breaks in DNA. This damage can be fixed or repaired by the chemical processes of oxidation and reduction, respectively.[1] The addition of molecular oxygen to target free radicals produces altered chemical structures that are potentially lethal. Tumor hypoxia reduces radiosensitivity *in vitro* and *in vivo*.[2,3] Well-oxygenated cells (partial pressure of oxygen or Po_2 >10 mm Hg) are approximately 2.5 times more sensitive to a given dose of ionizing radiation than their hypoxic counterparts.

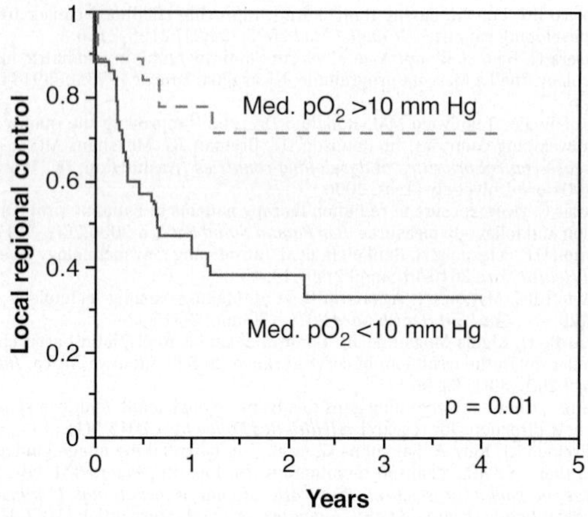

FIGURE 29.2. The correlation between pretreatment head and neck tumor oxygenation and local-regional disease control after radiotherapy with or without concurrent chemotherapy. Dashed line represents tumor median partial pressure of oxygen (Po_2) >10 mm Hg. Solid line represents tumor median Po_2 <10 mm Hg.

Clinical data clearly demonstrate the existence of tumor hypoxia in head and neck cancer[4,5] and extremely strong correlations between hypoxia and both in-field treatment failure and overall survival (Figs. 29.2 and 29.3).[6] This effect is independent of presenting stage of disease.[7] Tumor hypoxia has also been correlated with local and distant recurrence in carcinoma of the cervix treated with surgery[8,9] or RT[10] and with distant failure in soft tissue sarcomas treated with surgery and adjuvant RT.[11]

Augmentation of Tumor Oxygenation

Therapeutic attempts to overcome the deleterious effect of tumor hypoxia have followed three general lines of investigation: increased delivery of oxygen to tumor, preferential sensitization of hypoxic cells with oxygen mimetic agents, or cytotoxic agents that selectively target hypoxic tumor cells. Hemoglobin concentration is the major determinant of the oxygen delivery capability of blood to tissue. Hemoglobin oxygen saturation exceeds 90% when the arterial Po_2 is >70 mm Hg. Still, oxygen is relatively insoluble in plasma under normobaric conditions. Under hyperbaric conditions, considerable quantities of oxygen can be dissolved into plasma and thus be potentially available for delivery to hypoxic tissues.

Clinical trials of hyperbaric oxygen (HBO) and RT were conducted from the 1950s to the 1970s. Trials conducted in patients with cancers of the central nervous system,[12] lung,[13] bladder,[14] and skin[15] showed no benefit from the addition of HBO. Randomized trials conducted in carcinoma of the cervix[16] and head and neck[17,18] did, however, show improvements in locoregional control and overall survival. The cumbersome logistics associated with HBO delivery in conjunction with RT necessitated the utilization of nonconventional hypofractionated treatment regimens. This reality has prevented HBO from being incorporated into routine clinical use.

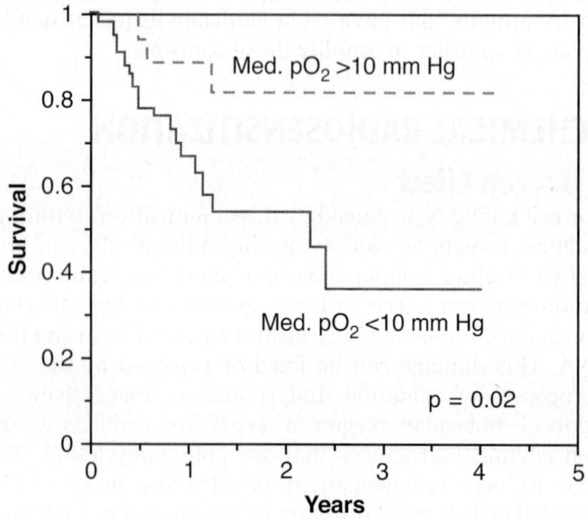

FIGURE 29.3. The correlation between pretreatment head and neck tumor oxygenation and local-regional disease control after radiotherapy with or without concurrent chemotherapy. Dashed line represents tumor median partial pressure of oxygen >10 mm Hg.

Carbogen (95% oxygen [O_2]/5% carbon dioxide [CO_2]) breathing, with or without concurrent nicotinamide administration, has also been utilized in attempts to improve tumor oxygenation and enhance RT response. The rationale for CO_2 addition in the gas breathing mixture is the generation of a mild acidosis that right shifts the oxyhemoglobin association curve, facilitating more unloading of oxygen into the most hypoxic tissues. The rationale for adding nicotinamide, a vitamin B derivative, is based on preclinical studies showing enhancement of tumor blood flow.[19,20] Polarographic electrode assessments in cervix and head and neck cancer have demonstrated that carbogen breathing and nicotinamide administration improve tumor oxygenation in some patients.[21–23]

A randomized trial of hyperfractionated RT with or without carbogen was conducted at the University of Florida from 1996 to 2002.[24] The study included patients with T2 to T4 squamous cell carcinoma of the oropharynx, larynx, and hypopharynx and was designed to detect a 20% improvement in 2-year local control in the carbogen arm relative to the RT alone arm, with a 15% improvement in 4-year cause-specific survival. Virtually all enrolled patients in both arms completed their prescribed courses of treatment. The addition of carbogen to RT did not appear to improve any of the planned end points of this trial. Most important, however, was the fact that while the design of this trial called for the enrollment of 675 patients, only 101 were entered over a 5-year period. The trial was therefore significantly underpowered in terms of its ability to detect the desired treatment effects. The inability to accrue patients, however, also called into question the overall viability of strategies utilizing carbogen.

The use of accelerated RT with carbogen and nicotinamide was tested in a phase II trial of 215 head and neck cancer patients.[25] Ninety-seven percent had stage III or IV disease, and the primary tumor site was laryngeal in 46%, hypopharyngeal in 23%, and oropharyngeal in 23%. Full compliance with carbogen breathing during RT was obtained in 88% of patients. Nicotinamide was administered 1 to 1.5 hours prior to RT at 60 to 80 mg/kg. Nicotinamide-induced nausea and vomiting necessitated discontinuation of the drug in 10% of patients receiving the lower dose and 31% of patients receiving the higher dose. Five-year locoregional control rates were 48% for hypopharynx primaries, 77% for larynx and 72% for oropharynx primaries.[26]

Allosteric modifiers of hemoglobin structure have been identified that can shift the oxyhemoglobin dissociation curve to the right and increase O_2 delivery to hypoxic tissues.[27] One such compound, RSR-13 (efaproxiral) has been tested in animal models and shown to improve tumor oxygenation[28] and enhance the effectiveness of RT.[29] A phase III open label trial of whole-brain RT and oxygen breathing with or without daily infusion of efaproxiral was conducted in 538 patients with brain metastases.[30] Fifty-four percent of the patients had metastatic non–small cell lung cancer and 20% had metastatic breast cancer. Overall, no improvement in survival was detected. A planned subset analysis suggested significant improvement in median survival time in breast cancer patients with sufficient levels of efaproxiral in their erythrocytes.[31] However, the phase III ENRICH trial, which examined efaproxiral and supplemental oxygen with whole-brain radiotherapy in breast cancer patients with brain metastases, showed no significant difference in overall survival.[32]

Anemia is a very powerful adverse prognostic factor in various malignancies, including carcinomas of the lung,[33] cervix,[34] and head and neck.[35–37] Polarographic electrode oxygen measurements in head and neck cancer have demonstrated that anemic patients are significantly more likely to have poorly oxygenated tumors than nonanemic patients, but significant tumor hypoxia has also been detected in patients who are not anemic.[6,38] Whether correction or prevention of anemia with blood transfusions or erythropoiesis-stimulating agents can improve treatment outcomes has been investigated in multiple studies.

The use of blood transfusions in cervical cancer patients gained traction after an initial publication from Princess Margaret Hospital showing an improvement in pelvic control and cure rates associated with correction of anemia.[39] However, subsequent publications from the same group showed no survival benefit to transfusion when the data were critically reexamined and analyzed on an intent-to-treat basis.[40] In head and neck cancer patients, studies suggest that blood transfusions may have a negative effect on survival.[41,42] Correction of anemia via erythropoietin (EPO) administration was evaluated in a double-blind, placebo-controlled randomized trial in 351 head and neck patients treated with RT.[43] The primary end point was local-regional progression-free survival. Eighty-two percent of patients (54) who received EPO maintained >14 g/dL (women) or 15 g/dL (men), while only 15% of the patients in the placebo arm attained this benchmark. The relative risk of locoregional progression, however, was 1.62 in the EPO arm, compared to placebo ($P = .0008$) with a similar, detriment seen for survival in those patients who received EPO (relative risk 1.39; $P = .02$). A systematic review pooling data from five randomized studies with a total of 1,397 patients showed significantly worse overall survival in head and neck cancer patients with the addition of EPO to radiotherapy (odds ratio 0.73; $P = .005$).[44] These poorer outcomes may have been the result of overcorrection of hemoglobin levels with increased thromboembolic events.[45] Tumor cells have also been found to express EPO receptors, with stimulation of downstream signaling pathways that may promote a more invasive phenotype.[46,47]

Sensitization of Hypoxic Cells

Electron-affinic compounds can oxidize radiation-induced free radical damage in the cell to produce increased kill.[48] The use of these agents would be particularly attractive in the hypoxic tumor microenvironment, where low oxygen concentrations impair the effectiveness of RT. The 2-nitroimidazoles are one such class of compounds that are metabolized into their active form under hypoxic conditions. Misonidazole, the prototype 2-nitroimidazole, was tested in two randomized trials. The Danish Head and Neck Cancer Study-2 (DAHANCA-2) performed a double-blind randomized trial evaluating the effect of misonidazole given in two drug schedules with split-course irradiation in the treatment of carcinoma of the larynx and pharynx.[49] Patients were stratified according to tumor site (larynx vs. pharynx), nodal status, and institution. The total misonidazole dose was 11 g/m^2. The study assessed 626 patients. Overall, the misonidazole group did not have significantly better local tumor control than the placebo group. Serious peripheral neuropathy, the dose-limiting toxicity of all nitroimidazole compounds, occurred in 26% of misonidazole-treated patients. The European Organisation for Research and Treatment of Cancer conducted a randomized study of conventional fractionation RT versus modified fractionation RT (three fractions per day) with or without misonidazole in 523 advanced head and neck cancer patients. No differences were seen in treatment outcome.[50]

Etanidazole (SR2508) is an analog of misonidazole with lower lipid solubility and less neurotoxicity in phase II studies in head and neck cancer.[51] A Radiation Therapy Oncology Group (RTOG) phase III study with etanidazole in head and neck tumors entered 521 patients who received conventionally fractionated irradiation with or without etanidazole 2 mg/m^2 3 times per week.[52] Of those on the etanidazole arm, 77% received at least 14 doses of the drug. No grade III or IV central nervous system or peripheral neuropathy was observed. The 2-year actuarial local tumor control was 40% in each arm, and the survival was 41% and 43%, respectively, in the irradiation alone and the irradiation plus etanidazole arms. A similar study of 374 patients performed in Europe did not show any overall benefit to treatment with etanidazole but did demonstrate increased neurotoxicity in the patients who received the drug.[53]

Nimorazole is a 5-nitroimidazole of the same structural class as metronidazole.[54] Its dose-limiting toxicity is nausea and vomiting; however, the drug can be administered with each radiation treatment. DAHANCA conducted a phase III trial of nimorazole (1.2 g/m^2 vs. placebo) for squamous cell cancer of the supraglottic larynx and pharynx.[55] There was a statistically significant improvement in locoregional tumor control (49% vs. 33% at 5 years; $P = .002$) but not for survival, which is consistent with the DAHANCA misonidazole trial. The use of nimorazole has become the standard of care in Denmark but has not been adopted in other countries.

Pharmacologic Targeting of Hypoxic Cells

Mitomycin C (MMC) is an alkylating agent metabolized in regions of low oxygen concentration and preferentially cytotoxic to hypoxic cells. MMC plays an integral role in conjunction with RT and 5-FU (fluorouracil) in the definitive nonsurgical management of squamous cell carcinomas of the anus.[56] Yale University investigators examined the concurrent use of MMC in 195 head and neck cancer patients treated on two randomized trials.[57] Their treatment program consisted of 68 Gy with or without MMC on days 1 and 43 of RT. Local regional recurrence-free survival was improved with the addition of MMC from 54% to 76% ($P = .003$). Overall survival improved from 42% to 48%, but this was not statistically significant. The majority of patients in these trials received adjuvant postoperative or preoperative irradiation. Only 74 (38%) received definitive primary RT, and the benefit from the addition of MMC in this subset is unclear.

A three-armed randomized trial conducted by the University of Vienna compared conventionally fractionated (CF) RT (2 Gy daily to 70 Gy) against variation of continuous hyperfractionated accelerated RT with or without MMC (V-CHART + MMC and V-CHART, respectively).[58] RT was given as an initial 2.5-Gy fraction followed by 1.65 Gy twice a day to a total dose of 55.3 Gy in 17 days. MMC was given as a 20 mg/m^2 bolus on day 5 of RT. Of the 239 patients enrolled, 85% had T3 or T4 primaries and 79% had nodal involvement. Three-year actuarial locoregional control was 48% for V-CHART plus MMC versus 32% for V-CHART and 31% for CF ($P = .05$ and $.03$, respectively). Survival including death from all causes was also improved to 41% in the V-CHART plus MMC arm as compared with 31% for V-CHART and 24% for CF ($P = .03$). The incidence of confluent mucositis was 90% in both experimental arms as compared with 33% in the CF arm. The median time to complete resolution of mucositis was 6 to 7 weeks in all three arms. Grade 3 or 4 hematologic toxicity, primarily thrombocytopenia, developed in 18% of the V-CHART plus MMC patients.

Porfiromycin, a derivative of MMC, provides greater differential cytotoxicity between hypoxic and oxygenated cells *in vitro*.[59] The Yale investigators also conducted a phase III study that compared patients treated with conventionally fractionated radiation plus MMC versus radiation plus porfiromycin.[60] Hematologic and nonhematologic toxicity was equivalent in the two treatment arms. With a median follow-up >6 years, MMC was superior to porfiromycin with respect to 5-year local relapse-free survival (91.6% vs. 72.7%; $P = .01$), local-regional relapse-free survival (82% vs. 65.3%; $P = .05$), and disease-free survival (72.8% vs. 52.9%; $P = .03$). There were no significant differences between the two arms with respect to overall survival (49% vs. 54%) or distant metastasis-free rate (80% vs. 76%). Their data supported the continued use of MMC as an adjunct to radiation therapy in advanced head and neck cancer and will become the control arm for future studies.

Tirapazamine (also known as SR-4233; WIN 59075; 3-amino-1,2,4-benzotriazine 1,4-dioxide) is a bioreductive agent preferentially cytotoxic to hypoxic cells *in vitro*. Twenty-five to 200 times more drug is required to produce the same level of cell killing in aerobic compared to anaerobic conditions.[61,62] Under hypoxic conditions, a free radical one-electron reduction product rapidly forms and is believed to be the toxic species, causing oxidative damage to pyrimidines and inducing DNA strand breaks.[63] Analysis of DNA and chromosomal breaks following hypoxic exposure to tirapazamine suggests that DNA double-strand breaks are the primary lesions involved in cell death.

This bioreductive agent differs from oxygen-mimetic sensitizers, such as the nitroimidazoles, in that it is itself cytotoxic to hypoxic tissues. Therefore, unlike the oxygen-mimetic sensitizers, tirapazamine-mediated therapeutic enhancement occurs whether the drug is given before or after irradiation.[64,65] In fractionated radiation therapy of murine tumors, tirapazamine is as effective as, if not superior to, etanidazole.[66] The efficacy of this radiation modifier depends on the number of "effective doses" that can be administered during a course of radiation therapy and the presence of hypoxic tumor cells.[67] Tirapazamine can also enhance the cytotoxicity of cisplatin.[68]

Rischin et al.[69] investigated the use of concurrent tirapazamine, cisplatin, and RT in advanced head and neck cancer in a series of trials. A phase I trial established the dosing schedule for tirapazamine given with RT and cisplatin. A randomized phase II study compared RT with cisplatin/tirapazamine versus RT with cisplatin/5-FU and suggested a benefit in the tirapazamine treatment arm (3-year local regional failure-free survival 84% vs. 66%; $P = .07$).[70] Tumor hypoxia imaging was performed with 18-fluorodeoxyglucose-misonidazole positron emission tomography (PET) scanning in 45 of the patients on these studies.[71] Hypoxia was identified in primary or nodal sites in 71% of the patients. Eight of 13 (62%) patients with hypoxic tumors who received cisplatin/5-FU experienced subsequent local-regional failure compared to only 1 of 19 (5%) patients with hypoxic tumors who received tirapazamine (hazard ratio [HR] = 15; $P = .001$). Only 1 of 10 patients with nonhypoxic tumors who received cisplatin/5-FU had a local-regional failure. These findings strongly suggested that the benefit of tirapazamine resulted from improved treatment efficacy against tumor hypoxia.

Two phase III trials were initiated to validate the use of tirapazamine in head and neck cancer. The HeadSTART study enrolled 861 patients and compared standard fractionation RT (70 Gy) with concurrent cisplatin/tirapazamine versus concurrent cisplatin alone.[72] The primary end point was overall survival, with 2-year rates of 65.7% in the cisplatin alone arm and 66.2% in the cisplatin/tirapazamine cohort. No differences were seen in failure-free survival, time to locoregional failure, or quality of life. Of note, the patients in this study were not selected based on the presence of tumor hypoxia. Moreover, 12% had major RT planning deficiencies, with those patients having significantly worse locoregional control and overall survival compared to those in protocol compliance.[73] A second trial with a planned enrollment of 550 patients was closed early due to excess number of deaths in the cisplatin/tirapazamine arm.[74]

Biologic Modifiers of Radiation Response

Overexpression of the epidermal growth factor receptor-1 (EGFR-1) is associated with an adverse outcome in squamous head and neck cancer.[75] Cetuximab (C225) is a chimeric monoclonal antibody to EGFR. Preclinical studies have demonstrated that cetuximab sensitizes cells to the cytotoxic effects of ionizing irradiation.[76,77] Preliminary studies demonstrated that this drug could be safely administered in conjunction with a course of RT for head and neck cancer.[78] An open-label phase III trial tested the impact of weekly injections of cetuximab added to a course of RT alone.[79] Most patients received accelerated fractionation with concomitant boost, although hyperfractionation and standard fractionation schemes were also permitted. Oral cavity primary tumors were ineligible for enrollment. Two-year local regional increased from 48% with RT to 56% with RT and cetuximab ($P = .02$). The initial survival advantage seen with the addition of cetuximab to RT has persisted, with updated 5-year overall survival rates of 45.6% versus 36.4% ($P = .018$).[80]

This trial provided an important proof of principle that adding a biologically targeted agent to a physically targeted modality improved therapeutic outcome. One-third of the patients enrolled had stage III disease, however, and thus had less advanced disease with more favorable prognoses than a significant proportion of patients who typically undergo chemoradiotherapy (CRT). A more favorable prognosis and improved treatment response has also been seen in patients with oropharyngeal squamous cell cancers associated with the human papillomavirus (HPV).[81] Whether RT with cetuximab is as effective or less toxic than RT with cisplatin in this select population is being examined by the phase III RTOG-1016 study.

A separate phase III study, RTOG-0522, randomized patients with locally advanced head and neck cancer to receive RT and concurrent cisplatin with or without cetuximab. Results of the study were presented at the American Society of Clinical Oncology annual meeting in 2011.[82] Treatment intensification with the addition of cetuximab to CRT did not improve 2-year progression-free or overall survival. Subset analyses of HPV-positive and HPV-negative patients are currently being performed. Still, EGFR inhibition remains a very active area of investigation in head and neck cancer. Agents currently in clinical trial include fully humanized monoclonal antibodies and orally administered small molecule inhibitors of the tyrosine kinase domains of the EGFR family of receptors.

CHEMICAL RADIOPROTECTION

The protection of normal tissues from the deleterious effects of radiation is a critical component in the development of a comprehensive treatment plan. Strategies for the accomplishment of this aim include the physical manipulation of the beam, modification of the fractionation schedule, and pharmacologic manipulation of the radiation response. Physical radiation protection rests on the principle of exclusion of normal tissue from the high-dose region and may be accomplished by contouring the shape of the radiation beam, the use of multiple treatment fields, the use of different beam energies, and modulation of the dose delivery from each beam (intensity-modulated radiation therapy [IMRT]). Modified fractionation typically uses multiple fractions of treatment per day as opposed to the conventional once daily paradigm in order to exploit the differing radiation repair capabilities of normal tissues as opposed to tumors. Physical modification of the treatment beam and altered fractionation are discussed elsewhere.

Protection

Pharmacologic radioprotection itself can be classified into three categories: protection, mitigation, and treatment. The direct cytotoxicity of ionizing irradiation results from the generation of free radicals that cause DNA strand breaks and lead to mitotic cell death. Amifostine (WR2721; Ethyol, Medimmune Inc, Gaithersburg, MD) is the prototype pharmacologic radioprotector that functions via free radical scavenging. Amifostine is a thiol containing pro drug that preferentially accumulates in the kidneys and salivary glands where it is metabolized to its active moiety, WR1065.[83]

An open-label phase III randomized trial was conducted from 1995 to 1997 to assess the ability of this drug to reduce the incidence of grade 2 or higher acute and late xerostomia and grade 3 or higher acute mucositis.[84] Patients enrolled in this trial received curative intent or adjuvant postoperative irradiation without concurrent chemotherapy. All treatment was delivered with conventional once daily fractionation of 1.8

to 2.0 Gy. Curative intent delivery consisted of 66 to 70 Gy total dose, and postoperative irradiation was delivered at 50 to 60 Gy total dose depending on the patient's assessed risk for recurrence. IMRT was not utilized, and inclusion of >75% of both parotid glands was required for inclusion in the study. Those patients who were randomized to receive amifostine were given a daily dose of 200 mg/m^2 intravenously for 15 to 30 minutes every day prior to each fraction of radiotherapy.

Three hundred three patients were enrolled in this trial, and minimum follow-up was 2 years. Amifostine did not reduce the incidence of grade 3 mucositis but did significantly reduce the incidence of acute and long-term grade >2 xerostomia. One-year post-RT, the incidence was 34% versus 56% for patients who had received amifostine versus those who had not (P = .002). Unstimulated saliva production >0.1 g was also more common in patients who had received amifostine (72% vs. 49%; P = .003). Two years post-RT, amifostine use was still associated with a significantly lower incidence of xerostomia, although the magnitude of benefit was lower (19% vs. 36%; P = .05). The lower incidences in both groups of patients also suggest some late recovery of salivary function. Reinforcing this idea of late recovery of salivary function is the fact that the percentage of patients who did not receive amifostine but who could exceed the >0.1 g of unstimulated saliva threshold had increased to 57%.[85]

Severe toxicity (CTC grade >3) attributable to amifostine occurred in <10% of patients in this trial and consisted of nausea and vomiting and transient hypotension. Nearly two-thirds of the patients had less severe grades of these side effects. Drug-related toxicity did cause approximately 20% of patients to discontinue amifostine prior to completing radiotherapy. Subcutaneous administration of the drug causes less nausea, vomiting, and hypotension than intravenous dosing but is associated with an increased risk of cutaneous toxicity, which again causes 15% to 20% of patients to not complete a full course of amifostine in conjunction with their radiation.[86] The incidence of severe cutaneous toxicity, including erythema multiforme, Stevens-Johnson syndrome, and toxic epidermal necrolysis, is 6 to 9 in 100,000.[87]

Some have argued that the size of this trial made it underpowered to detect a very small compromise in survival caused by amifostine (tumor protection).[88] This argument is technically correct but overlooks the reality that absolute refutation of a small compromise of antitumor efficacy attributable to amifostine would have required an equivalence trial. Demonstration that amifostine reduced survival from a hypothetical 45% to 40% (P = .05; 80% power) would have necessitated >1,200 patients per study arm.[89] Such a large study cannot be performed in head and neck cancer, because patient resources are too scarce. The largest randomized head and neck trial ever conducted, RTOG-9003, required 8 years to enroll 1,113 patients into four treatment arms.[90] A meta-analysis with individual patient data from 12 trials and 1,119 patients examined the impact of amifostine on survival in patients treated with RT or CRT. The majority of patients (65%) had head and neck cancers, with 33% lung cancers and 2% pelvic carcinomas. The hazard ratio of death was 0.98 (95% confidence interval, 0.84 to 1.14; P = .78).[91]

The potential of amifostine as a protector against radiation-induced esophagitis during the treatment of non–small cell lung cancer was studied in a randomized trial conducted by the RTOG.[92,93] No reduction in the incidence of grade 3 esophagitis was observed, although less swallowing dysfunction was observed in the patients who received amifostine. Part of the explanation for this absence may be attributable to the study design, which utilized a hyperfractionated radiation schedule 5 days per week (69.6 Gy total dose) and concurrent carboplatin/paclitaxel. Amifostine 500 mg intravenous was delivered 4 days per week prior to the afternoon fraction only. Moreover, 28% of the patients did not complete the full course of the drug either because of toxicity or refusal. Consequently, approximately 50% of the RT was delivered in the absence of the radioprotective drug in those patients who were randomized to receive it. Preclinical study of amifostine delivered daily in conjunction with fractionated lung and esophageal irradiation has demonstrated morphologic and immunohistochemical evidence of radioprotection.[94–96]

Amifostine is approved by the U.S. Food and Drug Administration for xerostomia in the setting of RT alone. The majority of both curative intent and adjuvant postoperative RT for head and neck cancer, with large target volumes that put the parotid glands at risk, is now delivered in conjunction with concurrent chemotherapy. Small phase II and III trials suggest that amifostine has a cytoprotective benefit in the chemoradiation setting, but level 1 evidence is lacking.[97,98] Moreover, the widespread adoption of IMRT with its ability to spare one or both parotid glands and reduce the incidence of xerostomia compared to conventional, non-IMRT techniques has further reduced the role for this drug.[99] The utility of amifostine in conjunction with IMRT has been investigated in small settings with inconclusive results.[100]

Mitigation

Administration of compounds that mitigate damage caused by previous radiation exposure constitutes a different approach to the management of radiation-induced toxicity. This strategy contrasts to the classical free radical scavenging radioprotective mechanism of drugs such as amifostine. The leading drug under development in this category is palifermin. Palifermin is a recombinant human keratinocyte growth factor that belongs to the fibroblast growth factor (FGF-7) family of cytokines. It stimulates cellular proliferation and differentiation in a variety of epithelial tissues including mucosa throughout the alimentary tract, salivary glands, and type II pneumocytes. Palifermin also regulates intrinsic glutathione-mediated cytoprotective mechanisms. Administration of palifermin in preclinical rodent models leads to a significant thickening of oral tongue mucosa.[101] Preclinical studies of fractionated RT have revealed that the administration of palifermin leads to increases in the dose of RT necessary to induce ulcerative mucositis and to reductions in the duration of this ulceration when it does occur.[102,103] Parotid gland production of saliva is also preserved when palifermin is administered in the setting of RT in preclinical systems. Preclinical evaluation of palifermin in a rodent model has also demonstrated that administration of a single dose of this drug after completion of a course of fractionated thoracic irradiation significantly reduces the severity and duration of pneumonitis and the severity of pulmonary fibrosis (Fig. 29.4).[104]

The ability of palifermin to reduce mucositis in a clinical setting has been tested in a pivotal phase III double-blind placebo-controlled trial of patients with non-Hodgkin lymphoma undergoing bone marrow transplantation.[105] The bone marrow ablative regimen consisted of 12 Gy of total-body irradiation (TBI) given at 1.5 Gy twice a day. Thereafter, etoposide (VP-16) and cyclophosphamide were administered. Palifermin was delivered prior to the initiation of TBI and again after the completion of chemotherapy, which also corresponded to 5 days after the completion of TBI. The dose schedule of palifermin was 60 mcg/kg/d 3 times for both administrations. This trial enrolled 212 patients who were equally divided between the placebo and palifermin arms. The World Health Organization (WHO) scoring system was used. The incidence of grade 3 or 4 mucositis approached 90% in the placebo arm as opposed to approximately 60% in the palifermin arm. For those patients who developed this level of toxicity, the duration was significantly reduced from 10.4 days in the placebo arm to 3.7 days in the palifermin arm (P <.001). Grade IV mucositis developed in 62% of the placebo arm patients and only 20% of the palifermin arm patients (P >.001). Mean duration of grade IV mucositis was reduced from 6.2 days to 3.3 days with the use of this drug (P <.001).

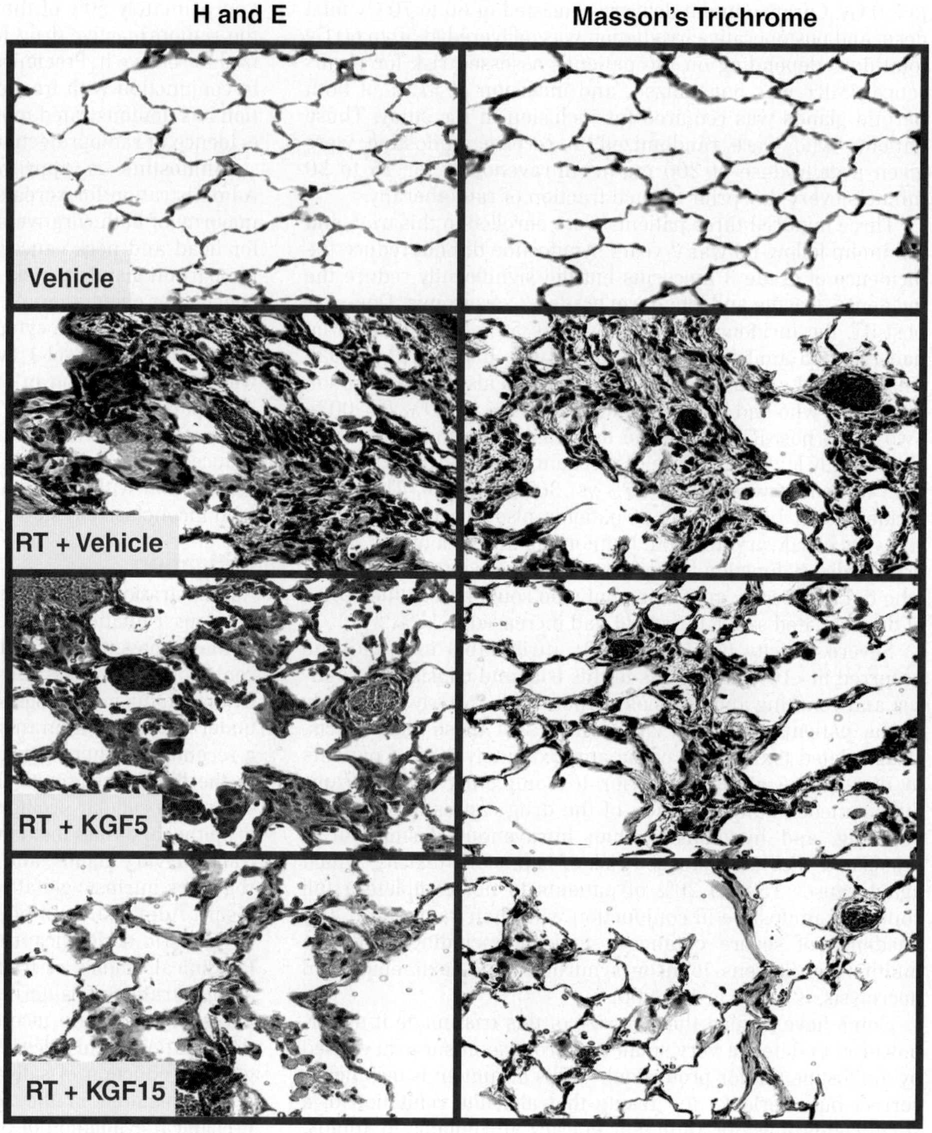

FIGURE 29.4. Mitigation of radiation-induced fibrosis attributable to single dose of recombinant human keratinocyte growth factor (KGF) administered after a course of fractionated hemithorax irradiation. The hematoxylin and eosin slides show the morphologic changes in the alveoli induced by irradiation including the inflammatory infiltrate and alveolar wall thickening. The Masson's trichrome panels show the collagen deposition that is characteristic of fibrosis. KGF was given either at 5 mg/kg or 15 mg/kg. Less injury is seen with the higher dose of KGF, suggesting that a dose–response effect exists.

A phase II study examined the safety and efficacy of palifermin in locally advanced head and neck cancer patients.[106] Patients were randomized 2 to 1 between palifermin and placebo. Palifermin was delivered at a dose of 60 mcg/kg. Institutions had the discretion to deliver RT via conventional once-daily 2-Gy fractions or with an accelerated hyperfractionated regimen of 1.25 Gy twice daily. One hundred patients were enrolled, of whom 34 received accelerated hyperfractionation and the remainder received standard fractionation. The first dose was delivered prior to the initiation of CRT and then every Friday afternoon after the last fraction of radiation. Two additional doses of palifermin were given 1 and 2 weeks after the completion of RT for a total of 10 doses of the drug. Palifermin did not reduce the incidence or duration of mucosal or salivary gland toxicity. The subset of patients receiving hyperfractionated radiation, however, showed significant improvements in the duration and severity of mucositis (Fig. 29.5). They also had improved swallowing function and less salivary gland toxicity relative to patients who received placebo.

A subsequent randomized phase III study examined a higher dose of palifermin at 180 mcg/kg to reduce oral mucositis in 188 patients with locally advanced head and neck cancer treated with CRT.[107] Palifermin was administered prior to starting CRT and once weekly for 7 weeks. The incidence of severe oral mucositis, the primary end point, was significantly lower in the palifermin arm compared to placebo (54% vs. 69%; $P = .041$). Both overall survival and progression-free survival were similar as well. However, no statistically significant differences emerged in secondary efficacy end points such as narcotic doses and duration of treatment breaks. A similar randomized phase III study examined palifermin at 120 mcg/kg in 186 head and neck cancer patients treated with postoperative CRT.[108] Palifermin again reduced the time to development and duration of WHO grade 3 or 4 oral mucositis without differences in patient-reported pain scores, treatment breaks, or efficacy. The precise role for palifermin in the management of head and neck cancer remains to be established.

Treatment

Radioprotectors and radiation mitigators are both designed to minimize the risk of clonogenic death of normal cells and subsequent disruption of the protective mucosal barrier. Head and neck RT also initiates a local cytokine cascade, which includes interleukin-1 and -6 and tumor necrosis factor-α (TNF-α). An inflammatory response results, which contributes to the ultimate anatomic disruption of the mucosa. Secondary bacterial

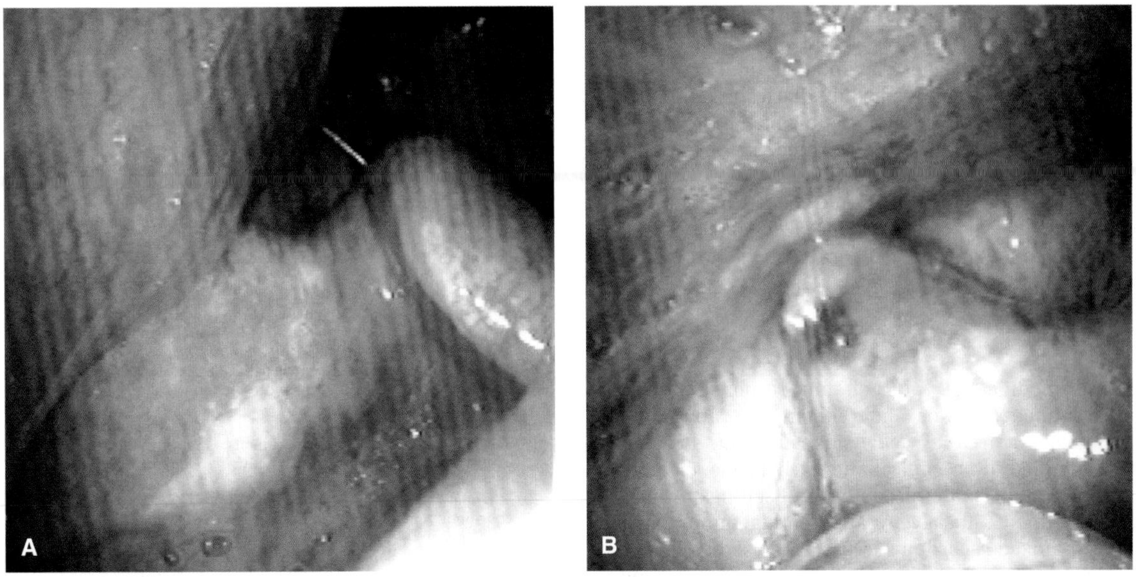

FIGURE 29.5. Confluent mucositis induced by concurrent chemoradiation in the base of tongue and supraglottic larynx regions. **A:** Demonstrates normal mucosa prior to the initiation of treatment. **B:** Demonstrates the pseudomembranous exudate, hemorrhage, and edema that are characteristic of this condition.

and fungal overgrowth are thought to exacerbate the local pathophysiology.

Sucralfate, a basic aluminum salt of sucrose, is used in the treatment of peptic ulcer disease. It provides a protective coating to ulcerated tissue by means of binding to exposed proteins in damaged cells.[109] It also stimulates mucus production, mitosis, and surface migration of cells. Sucralfate has been tested in several double-blind placebo-controlled randomized trials. Despite the attractive conceptual nature of using it to ameliorate mucositis, the clinical data do not show any benefit from sucralfate.[1,110–112]

Benzydamine hydrochloride is a nonsteroidal anti-inflammatory drug that also possesses antimicrobial activity.[113] It is a potent inhibitor of TNF-α.[114] Expression of this proinflammatory cytokine is up-regulated in mucosal tissue of the head and neck regions, with peak levels typically at approximately 20 Gy (conventionally fractionated) just prior to the first signs of mucosal ulceration. The ability of benzydamine to reduce mucositis during head and neck RT was tested in a randomized double-blind placebo-controlled trial.[115] The primary end point of this trial was the area under the curve for the mean mucositis score over a cumulative RT dose up to a total dose of 50 Gy. Secondary end points included use of concomitant pain medication, oral pain at rest and with eating, body weight, and the use of enteral nutritional support.

Benzydamine therapy resulted in a 30% reduction in mucosal erythema and ulceration. Most of this benefit was observed once doses >25 Gy had been delivered. One-third of the benzydamine patients did not develop any mucosal ulceration, compared with only 18% of the placebo-treated patients (P = .04). There was a nonsignificant trend toward reduction in mouth pain at rest for the patients who received benzydamine. Importantly, benzydamine was no more effective than placebo with respect to the reduction of pain during meals. Cumulative weight loss during RT was equivalent in the two treatment groups. There was no difference in the proportion of patients who required enteral nutritional support between the two treatment arms.

The data from the benzydamine trials suggest that this agent is active against mucositis but are inconclusive regarding whether it has any clinical role in treating this condition. There was no significant benefit regarding the functional sequelae of mucositis. Mucosal assessment was not performed beyond 50 Gy, and most patients received radiotherapy doses of 64 to 74 Gy. The study design may thus explain the discordance between the improvement in the anatomic assessment of mucosal integrity associated with benzydamine and the lack of any functional benefit, as the latter parameters were assessed throughout a patient's entire course of RT. The most severe mucositis during a course of head and neck RT occurs beyond the 50 Gy level. Fewer than 10% of the patients enrolled in this trial received concurrent chemotherapy, even though most of them had stage III or IV disease. Concurrent CRT has become the standard of care for most patients with this extent of disease. Consequently, the clinical value of benzydamine has not been proven for patients receiving high-dose RT with or without concurrent chemotherapy.

Endogenous oral flora may exacerbate the mucosal inflammatory process once the mucosal integrity is disrupted. Secondary infections may prolong the course of mucositis and compromise overall patient well-being. Protegrins are naturally occurring peptides that have broad-spectrum antimicrobial activity.[116] Iseganan is a synthetic analog of this class of compounds. A placebo-controlled trial in patients receiving chemotherapy suggested that iseganan reduced the incidence of ulcerative stomatitis and decreased both mouth pain and swallowing difficulty.[117]

A phase III double-blind, placebo-controlled trial was subsequently conducted to test this concept in patients receiving head and neck RT.[118] This trial mandated that a minimum dose of 60 Gy be delivered but allowed different fractionation schemes. Forty percent of the patients enrolled received concurrent chemotherapy. The study contained three treatment arms: standard-of-care (SOC) oral hygiene only, placebo plus SOC, and iseganan plus SOC. Iseganan and placebo were equivalent to one another with respect to all end points in the trial. Interestingly, both iseganan and placebo arms were superior to SOC oral hygiene alone. Two-thirds of the patients in both arms had confluent mucositis compared with 79% in the SOC alone arm (P = .02). Only 2% of the SOC patients had no mucosal ulceration versus 9% in both the iseganan and placebo arms (P = .04). Peak mouth pain and difficulty swallowing were also significantly worse for the patients assigned to SOC alone. RT dose reductions were also significantly more common in the SOC patients.

The iseganan trial showed no benefit from the administration of the study drug. It did, however, reveal the importance of adherence to a strict regimen of oral hygiene during head and neck RT. Patients on both the drug and placebo arms were instructed to swish and gargle prior to each administration of study drug. They also maintained study diaries to help ensure adequate compliance with administration of the study drug. These interventions were not performed in the patients assigned to SOC alone. This trial provides an important foundation in the evaluation of new therapies for mucositis through its demonstration of the value of organized and systematic attention to the maintenance of good oral hygiene throughout a course of head and neck CRT.

SUMMARY

The chemical modification of radiation response both for enhancing treatment efficacy and reducing therapy-induced toxicity remains an area of active investigation. Promising candidates identified in preclinical and early phase trials have been less successful in randomized phase III settings. Attempts to improve treatment efficacy by augmenting tumor oxygen delivery have a mixed record of success. The use of drugs that are preferentially cytotoxic to hypoxic cells holds promise, although improved tools to identify those patients most likely to benefit from targeted therapy are needed. Proof of principle for chemical radioprotection has been established in salivary glands but not elsewhere and is associated with significant toxicity in its own right. Growth factor utilization appears to protect against treatment-induced mucositis but not to an extent to change clinical practice. As radiotherapy regimens evolve and new technological advances continue to improve treatment delivery, investigators will continue to seek agents that optimize the therapeutic ratio.

REFERENCES

1. Chapman JD, Reuvers AP, Borsa J, et al. Chemical radioprotection and radiosensitization of mammalian cells growing in vitro. *Radiat Res* 1973;56(2):291–306.
2. Gray LH, Conger AD, Ebert M, et al. The concentration of oxygen dissolved in tissues at the time of irradiation as a factor in radiotherapy. *Br J Radiol* 1953;26(312):638–648.
3. Thomlinson RH, Gray LH. The histological structure of some human lung cancers and the possible implications for radiotherapy. *Br J Cancer* 1955;9(4):539–549.
4. Becker A, Hansgen G, Bloching M, et al. Oxygenation of squamous cell carcinoma of the head and neck: comparison of primary tumors, neck node metastases, and normal tissue. *Int J Radiat Oncol Biol Phys* 1998;42(1):35–41.
5. Brizel DM, Sibley GS, Prosnitz LR, et al. Tumor hypoxia adversely affects the prognosis of carcinoma of the head and neck. *Int J Radiat Oncol Biol Phys* 1997;38(2):285–289.
6. Brizel DM, Dodge RK, Clough RW, et al. Oxygenation of head and neck cancer: changes during radiotherapy and impact on treatment outcome. *Radiother Oncol* 1999;53(2):113–117.
7. Nordsmark M, Bentzen SM, Rudat V, et al. Prognostic value of tumor oxygenation in 397 head and neck tumors after primary radiation therapy. An international multi-center study. *Radiother Oncol* 2005;77(1):18–24.
8. Hockel M, Knoop C, Schlenger K, et al. Intratumoral pO2 predicts survival in advanced cancer of the uterine cervix. *Radiother Oncol* 1993;26(1):45–50.
9. Hockel M, Schlenger K, Aral B, et al. Association between tumor hypoxia and malignant progression in advanced cancer of the uterine cervix. *Cancer Res* 1996;56(19):4509–4515.
10. Fyles AW, Milosevic M, Wong R, et al. Oxygenation predicts radiation response and survival in patients with cervix cancer. *Radiother Oncol* 1998;48(2):149–156.
11. Brizel DM, Scully SP, Harrelson JM, et al. Tumor oxygenation predicts for the likelihood of distant metastases in human soft tissue sarcoma. *Cancer Res* 1996;56(5):941–943.
12. Chang CH. Hyperbaric oxygen and radiation therapy in the management of glioblastoma. *Natl Cancer Inst Monogr* 1977;46:163–169.
13. Cade IS, McEwen JB. Clinical trials of radiotherapy in hyperbaric oxygen at Portsmouth, 1964–1976. *Clin Radiol* 1978;29(3):333–338.
14. Cade IS, McEwen JB, Dische S, et al. Hyperbaric oxygen and radiotherapy: a Medical Research Council trial in carcinoma of the bladder. *Br J Radiol* 1978;51(611):876–878.
15. Sealy A, Hockly J, Shepstone B. The treatment of malignant melanoma with cobalt and hyperbaric oxygen. *Clin Radiol* 1974;25(2):211–215.
16. Watson ER, Halnan KE, Dische S, et al. Hyperbaric oxygen and radiotherapy: a Medical Research Council trial in carcinoma of the cervix. *Br J Radiol* 1978;51(611):879–887.
17. Henk JM. Late results of a trial of hyperbaric oxygen and radiotherapy in head and neck cancer: a rationale for hypoxic cell sensitizers? *Int J Radiat Oncol Biol Phys* 1986;12(8):1339–1341.
18. Henk JM, Kunkler PB, Smith CW. Radiotherapy and hyperbaric oxygen in head and neck cancer. Final report of first controlled clinical trial. *Lancet* 1977;2(8029):101–103.
19. Horsman MR, Brown JM, Hirst VK, et al. Mechanism of action of the selective tumor radiosensitizer nicotinamide. *Int J Radiat Oncol Biol Phys* 1988;15(3):685–690.
20. Horsman MR, Overgaard J, Christensen KL, et al. Mechanism for the reduction of tumour hypoxia by nicotinamide and the clinical relevance for radiotherapy. *Biomed Biochim Acta* 1989;48(2–3):S251–S254.
21. Aquino-Parsons C, Lim P, Green A, et al. Carbogen inhalation in cervical cancer: assessment of oxygenation change. *Gynecol Oncol* 1999;74(2):259–264.
22. Falk SJ, Ward R, Bleehen NM. The influence of carbogen breathing on tumour tissue oxygenation in man evaluated by computerised p02 histography. *Br J Cancer* 1992;66(5):919–924.
23. Laurence VM, Ward R, Dennis IF, et al. Carbogen breathing with nicotinamide improves the oxygen status of tumours in patients. *Br J Cancer* 1995;72(1):198–205.
24. Mendenhall WM, Morris CG, Amdur RJ, et al. Radiotherapy alone or combined with carbogen breathing for squamous cell carcinoma of the head and neck: a prospective, randomized trial. *Cancer* 2005;104(2):332–337.
25. Kaanders JH, Pop LA, Marres HA, et al. ARCON: experience in 215 patients with advanced head-and-neck cancer. *Int J Radiat Oncol Biol Phys* 2002;52(3):769–778.
26. Hoogsteen IJ, Pop LA, Marres HA, et al. Oxygen-modifying treatment with ARCON reduces the prognostic significance of hemoglobin in squamous cell carcinoma of the head and neck. *Int J Radiat Oncol Biol Phys* 2006;64(1):83–89.
27. Teicher BA, Wong JS, Takeuchi H, et al. Allosteric effectors of hemoglobin as modulators of chemotherapy and radiation therapy in vitro and in vivo. *Cancer Chemother Pharmacol* 1998;42(1):24–30.
28. Hou H, Khan N, O'Hara JA, et al. Effect of RSR13, an allosteric hemoglobin modifier, on oxygenation in murine tumors: an in vivo electron paramagnetic resonance oximetry and bold MRI study. *Int J Radiat Oncol Biol Phys* 2004;59(3):834–843.
29. Khandelwal SR, Kavanagh BD, Lin PS, et al. RSR13, an allosteric effector of haemoglobin, and carbogen radiosensitize FSAII and SCCVII tumours in C3H mice. *Br J Cancer* 1999;79(5–6):814–820.
30. Suh JH, Stea B, Nabid A, et al. Phase III study of efaproxiral as an adjunct to whole-brain radiation therapy for brain metastases. *J Clin Oncol* 2006;24(1):106–114.
31. Stea B, Shaw E, Pinter T, et al. Efaproxiral red blood cell concentration predicts efficacy in patients with brain metastases. *Br J Cancer* 2006;94(12):1777–1784.
32. Suh J. Results of the phase III ENRICH (RT-016) study of efaproxiral administered concurrent with whole brain radiation therapy (WBRT) in women with brain metastases from breast cancer. *Int J Radiat Oncol Biol Phys* 2008;72(1 Suppl):(abstr 110).
33. Robnett TJ, Machtay M, Hahn SM, et al. Pathological response to preoperative chemoradiation worsens with anemia in non-small cell lung cancer patients. *Cancer J* 2002;8(3):263–267.
34. Dunst J, Kuhnt T, Strauss HG, et al. Anemia in cervical cancers: impact on survival, patterns of relapse, and association with hypoxia and angiogenesis. *Int J Radiation Oncol Biol Phys* 2003;56(3):778–787.
35. Frommhold H, Guttenberger R, Henke M. The impact of blood hemoglobin content on the outcome of radiotherapy. The Freiburg experience. *Strahlenther Onkol* 1998;174(Suppl 4):31–34.
36. Lee WR, Berkey B, Marcial V, et al. Anemia is associated with decreased survival and increased locoregional failure in patients with locally advanced head and neck carcinoma: a secondary analysis of RTOG 85-27. *Int J Radiat Oncol Biol Phys* 1998;42(5):1069–1075.
37. Prosnitz RG, Yao B, Farrell CL, et al. Pretreatment anemia is correlated with the reduced effectiveness of radiation and concurrent chemotherapy in advanced head and neck cancer. *Int J Radiat Oncol Biol Phys* 2005;61(4):1087–1095.
38. Becker A, Stadler P, Lavey RS, et al. Severe anemia is associated with poor tumor oxygenation in head and neck squamous cell carcinomas. *Int J Radiat Oncol Biol Phys* 2000;46(2):459–466.
39. Bush RS, Jenkin RD, Allt WE, et al. Definitive evidence for hypoxic cells influencing cure in cancer therapy. *Br J Cancer Suppl* 1978;3:302–306.
40. Fyles AW, Milosevic M, Pintilie M, et al. Anemia, hypoxia and transfusion in patients with cervix cancer: a review. *Radiother Oncol* 2000;57(1):13–19.
41. Bhide SA, Ahmed M, Rengarajan V, et al. Anemia during sequential induction chemotherapy and chemoradiation for head and neck cancer: the impact of blood transfusion on treatment outcome. *Int J Radiat Oncol Biol Phys* 2009;73(2):391–398.
42. Hoff CM, Lassen P, Eriksen JG, et al. Does transfusion improve the outcome for HNSCC patients treated with radiotherapy? Results from the randomized DAHANCA 5 and 7 trials. *Acta Oncol* 2011;50(7):1006–1014.
43. Henke M, Laszig R, Rube C, et al. Erythropoietin to treat head and neck cancer patients with anaemia undergoing radiotherapy: randomised, double-blind, placebo-controlled trial. *Lancet* 2003;362(9392):1255–1260.
44. Lambin P, Ramaekers BL, van Mastrigt GA, et al. Erythropoietin as an adjuvant treatment with (chemo) radiation therapy for head and neck cancer. *Cochrane Database Syst Rev* 2009;3:CD006158.
45. Bennett CL, Silver SM, Djulbegovic B, et al. Venous thromboembolism and mortality associated with recombinant erythropoietin and darbepoetin administration for the treatment of cancer-associated anemia. *JAMA* 2008;299(8):914–924.
46. Arcasoy MO, Amin K, Chou SC, et al. Erythropoietin and erythropoietin receptor expression in head and neck cancer: relationship to tumor hypoxia. *Clin Cancer Res* 2005;11(1):20–27.
47. Mohyeldin A, Lu H, Dalgard C, et al. Erythropoietin signaling promotes invasiveness of human head and neck squamous cell carcinoma. *Neoplasia* 2005;7(5):537–543.
48. Adams GE. Hypoxia-mediated drugs for radiation and chemotherapy. *Cancer* 1981;48(3):696–707.
49. Overgaard J, Hansen HS, Andersen AP, et al. Misonidazole combined with split-course radiotherapy in the treatment of invasive carcinoma of larynx and pharynx: report from the DAHANCA 2 study. *Int J Radiat Oncol Biol Phys* 1989;16(4):1065–1068.
50. Van den Bogaert W, van der Schueren E, Horiot JC, et al. The EORTC randomized trial on three fractions per day and misonidazole (trial no. 22811) in advanced head and neck cancer: long-term results and side effects. *Radiother Oncol* 1995;35(2):91–99.
51. Wasserman TH, Lee DJ, Cosmatos D, et al. Clinical trials with etanidazole (SR-2508) by the Radiation Therapy Oncology Group (RTOG). *Radiother Oncol* 1991;20(Suppl 1):129–135.
52. Lee DJ, Cosmatos D, Marcial VA, et al. Results of an RTOG phase III trial (RTOG 85-27) comparing radiotherapy plus etanidazole with radiotherapy alone for locally advanced head and neck carcinomas. *Int J Radiat Oncol Biol Phys* 1995;32(3):567–576.
53. Eschwege F, Sancho-Garnier H, Chassagne D, et al. Results of a European randomized trial of etanidazole combined with radiotherapy in head and neck carcinomas. *Int J Radiat Oncol Biol Phys* 1997;39(2):275–281.

54. Overgaard J, Overgaard M, Nielsen OS, et al. A comparative investigation of nimorazole and misonidazole as hypoxic radiosensitizers in a C3H mammary carcinoma in vivo. *Br J Cancer* 1982;46(6):904–911.
55. Overgaard J, Hansen HS, Overgaard M, et al. A randomized double-blind phase III study of nimorazole as a hypoxic radiosensitizer of primary radiotherapy in supraglottic larynx and pharynx carcinoma. Results of the Danish Head and Neck Cancer Study (DAHANCA) Protocol 5-85. *Radiother Oncol* 1998;46(2):135–146.
56. Flam M, John M, Pajak TF, et al. Role of mitomycin in combination with fluorouracil and radiotherapy, and of salvage chemoradiation in the definitive nonsurgical treatment of epidermoid carcinoma of the anal canal: results of a phase III randomized intergroup study. *J Clin Oncol* 1996;14(9):2527–2539.
57. Haffty BG, Son YH, Papac R, et al. Chemotherapy as an adjunct to radiation in the treatment of squamous cell carcinoma of the head and neck: results of the Yale mitomycin randomized trials. *J Clin Oncol* 1997;15(1):268–276.
58. Dobrowsky W, Naude J. Continuous hyperfractionated accelerated radiotherapy with/without mitomycin C in head and neck cancers. *Radiother Oncol* 2000;57(2): 119–124.
59. Rockwell S, Hughes CS. Effects of mitomycin C and porfiromycin on exponentially growing and plateau phase cultures. *Cell Prolif* 1994;27(3):153–163.
60. Haffty BG, Wilson LD, Son YH, et al. Concurrent chemo-radiotherapy with mitomycin C compared with porfiromycin in squamous cell cancer of the head and neck: final results of a randomized clinical trial. *Int J Radiat Oncol Biol Phys* 2005;61(1): 119–128.
61. Zeman EM, Brown JM, Lemmon MJ, et al. SR-4233: a new bioreductive agent with high selective toxicity for hypoxic mammalian cells. *Int J Radiat Oncol Biol Phys* 1986;12(7):1239–1242.
62. Zeman EM, Hirst VK, Lemmon MJ, et al. Enhancement of radiation-induced tumor cell killing by the hypoxic cell toxin SR 4233. *Radiother Oncol* 1988;12(3): 209–218.
63. Zeman EM, Brown JM. Pre- and post-irradiation radiosensitization by SR 4233. *Int J Radiat Oncol Biol Phys* 1989;16(4):967–971.
64. Brown JM, Lemmon MJ. Potentiation by the hypoxic cytotoxin SR 4233 of cell killing produced by fractionated irradiation of mouse tumors. *Cancer Res* 1990;50(24):7745–7749.
65. Brown JM, Lemmon MJ. SR 4233: a tumor specific radiosensitizer active in fractionated radiation regimes. *Radiother Oncol* 1991;20(Suppl 1):151–156.
66. Brown JM, Lemmon MJ. Tumor hypoxia can be exploited to preferentially sensitize tumors to fractionated irradiation. *Int J Radiat Oncol Biol Phys* 1991;20(3): 457–461.
67. Brown JM. Therapeutic targets in radiotherapy. *Int J Radiat Oncol Biol Phys* 2001; 49(2):319–326.
68. Goldberg Z, Evans J, Birrell G, et al. An investigation of the molecular basis for the synergistic interaction of tirapazamine and cisplatin. *Int J Radiat Oncol Biol Phys* 2001;49(1):175–182.
69. Rischin D, Peters L, Hicks R, et al. Phase I trial of concurrent tirapazamine, cisplatin, and radiotherapy in patients with advanced head and neck cancer. *J Clin Oncol* 2001;19(2):535–542.
70. Rischin D, Peters L, Fisher R, et al. Tirapazamine, cisplatin, and radiation versus fluorouracil, cisplatin, and radiation in patients with locally advanced head and neck cancer: a randomized phase II trial of the Trans-Tasman Radiation Oncology Group (TROG 98.02). *J Clin Oncol* 2005;23(1):79–87.
71. Rischin D, Hicks RJ, Fisher R, et al. Prognostic significance of [18F]-misonidazole positron emission tomography-detected tumor hypoxia in patients with advanced head and neck cancer randomly assigned to chemoradiation with or without tirapazamine: a substudy of Trans-Tasman Radiation Oncology Group Study 98.02. *J Clin Oncol* 2006;24(13):2098–2104.
72. Rischin D, Peters LJ, O'Sullivan B, et al. Tirapazamine, cisplatin, and radiation versus cisplatin and radiation for advanced squamous cell carcinoma of the head and neck (TROG 02.02, HeadSTART): a phase III trial of the Trans-Tasman Radiation Oncology Group. *J Clin Oncol* 2010;28(18):2989–2995.
73. Peters LJ, O'Sullivan B, Giralt J, et al. Critical impact of radiotherapy protocol compliance and quality in the treatment of advanced head and neck cancer: results from TROG 02.02. *J Clin Oncol* 2010;28(18):2996–3001.
74. Seiwert TY, Salama JK, Vokes EE. The chemoradiation paradigm in head and neck cancer. *Nat Clin Pract Oncol* 2007;4(3):156–171.
75. Ang KK, Berkey BA, Tu X, et al. Impact of epidermal growth factor receptor expression on survival and pattern of relapse in patients with advanced head and neck carcinoma. *Cancer Res* 2002;62(24):7350–7356.
76. Huang SM, Harari PM. Modulation of radiation response after epidermal growth factor receptor blockade in squamous cell carcinomas: inhibition of damage repair, cell cycle kinetics, and tumor angiogenesis. *Clin Cancer Res* 2000;6(6): 2166–2174.
77. Huang SM, Bock JM, Harari PM. Epidermal growth factor receptor blockade with C225 modulates proliferation, apoptosis, and radiosensitivity in squamous cell carcinomas of the head and neck. *Cancer Res* 1999;59(8):1935–1940.
78. Robert F, Ezekiel MP, Spencer SA, et al. Phase I study of anti-epidermal growth factor receptor antibody cetuximab in combination with radiation therapy in patients with advanced head and neck cancer. *J Clin Oncol* 2001;19(13):3234–3243.
79. Bonner JA, Harari PM, Giralt J, et al. Radiotherapy plus cetuximab for squamous-cell carcinoma of the head and neck. *N Engl J Med* 2006;354(6):567–578.
80. Bonner JA, Harari PM, Giralt J, et al. Radiotherapy plus cetuximab for locoregionally advanced head and neck cancer: 5-year survival data from a phase 3 randomised trial, and relation between cetuximab-induced rash and survival. *Lancet Oncol* 2010;11(1):21–28.
81. Fakhry C, Westra WH, Li S, et al. Improved survival of patients with human papillomavirus-positive head and neck squamous cell carcinoma in a prospective clinical trial. *J Natl Cancer Inst* 2008;100(4):261–269.
82. Ang KK, Zhang QE, Rosenthal DI, et al. A randomized phase III trial (RTOG 0522) of concurrent accelerated radiation plus cisplatin with or without cetuximab for stage III–IV head and neck squamous cell carcinomas (HNC). *ASCO Meet Abstr* 2011; 29(15 Suppl):5500.
83. Yuhas JM, Spellman JM, Culo F. The role of WR-2721 in radiotherapy and/or chemotherapy. *Cancer Clin Trial* 1980;3(3):211–216.
84. Brizel DM, Wasserman TH, Henke M, et al. Phase III randomized trial of amifostine as a radioprotector in head and neck cancer. *J Clin Oncol* 2000;18(19):3339–3345.
85. Wasserman TH, Brizel DM, Henke M, et al. Influence of intravenous amifostine on xerostomia, tumor control, and survival after radiotherapy for head-and-neck cancer: 2-year follow-up of a prospective, randomized, phase III trial. *Int J Radiat Oncol Biol Phys* 2005;63(4):985–990.
86. Koukourakis MI, Kyrias G, Kakolyris S, et al. Subcutaneous administration of amifostine during fractionated radiotherapy: a randomized phase II study. *J Clin Oncol* 2000;18(11):2226–2233.
87. Boccia R, Anne PR, Bourhis J, et al. Assessment and management of cutaneous reactions with amifostine administration: findings of the ethyol (amifostine) cutaneous treatment advisory panel (ECTAP). *Int J Radiat Oncol Biol Phys* 2004; 60(1):302–309.
88. Lindegaard JC, Grau C. Has the outlook improved for amifostine as a clinical radioprotector? *Radiother Oncol* 2000;57(2):113–118.
89. Simon R. Design and analysis of clinical trials. In: DeVita V, Lawrence T, Rosenberg S, eds. *Cancer: principles and practice of oncology.* 8th ed. Philadelphia: Lippincott-Raven, 2008:571–590.
90. Fu KK, Pajak TF, Trotti A, et al. A Radiation Therapy Oncology Group (RTOG) phase III randomized study to compare hyperfractionation and two variants of accelerated fractionation to standard fractionation radiotherapy for head and neck squamous cell carcinomas: first report of RTOG 9003. *Int J Radiat Oncol Biol Phys* 2000;48(1):7–16.
91. Bourhis J, Blanchard P, Maillard E, et al. Effect of amifostine on survival among patients treated with radiotherapy: a meta-analysis of individual patient data. *J Clin Oncol* 2011;29(18):2590–2597.
92. Movsas B, Scott C, Langer C, et al. Randomized trial of amifostine in locally advanced non-small-cell lung cancer patients receiving chemotherapy and hyperfractionated radiation: Radiation Therapy Oncology Group trial 98-01. *J Clin Oncol* 2005;23(10):2145–2154.
93. Movsas B. Exploring the role of the radioprotector amifostine in locally advanced non-small cell lung cancer: Radiation Therapy Oncology Group trial 98-01. *Semin Radiat Oncol* 2002;12(1 Suppl 1):40–45.
94. Vujaskovic Z, Feng QF, Rabbani ZN, et al. Assessment of the protective effect of amifostine on radiation-induced pulmonary toxicity. *Exp Lung Res* 2002; 28(7):577–590.
95. Vujaskovic Z, Feng QF, Rabbani ZN, et al. Radioprotection of lungs by amifostine is associated with reduction in profibrogenic cytokine activity. *Radiat Res* 2002; 157(6):656–660.
96. Vujaskovic Z, Thrasher BA, Jackson IL, et al. Radioprotective effects of amifostine on acute and chronic esophageal injury in rodents. *Int J Radiat Oncol Biol Phys* 2007;69(2):534–540.
97. Antonadou D, Pepelassi M, Synodinou M, et al. Prophylactic use of amifostine to prevent radiochemotherapy-induced mucositis and xerostomia in head-and-neck cancer. *Int J Radiat Oncol Biol Phys* 2002;52(3):739–747.
98. Buntzel J, Glatzel M, Kuttner K, et al. Amifostine in simultaneous radiochemotherapy of advanced head and neck cancer. *Semin Radiat Oncol* 2002;12(1 Suppl 1): 4–13.
99. Nutting CM, Morden JP, Harrington KJ, et al. Parotid-sparing intensity modulated versus conventional radiotherapy in head and neck cancer (PARSPORT): a phase 3 multicentre randomised controlled trial. *Lancet Oncol* 2011;12(2):127–136.
100. Thorstad WL, Chao KS, Haughey B. Toxicity and compliance of subcutaneous amifostine in patients undergoing postoperative intensity-modulated radiation therapy for head and neck cancer. *Semin Oncol* 2004;31(6 Suppl 18):8–12.
101. Potten CS, O'Shea JA, Farrell CL, et al. The effects of repeated doses of keratinocyte growth factor on cell proliferation in the cellular hierarchy of the crypts of the murine small intestine. *Cell Growth Differ* 2001;12(5):265–275.
102. Dorr W, Spekl K, Farrell CL. Amelioration of acute oral mucositis by keratinocyte growth factor: fractionated irradiation. *Int J Radiat Oncol Biol Phys* 2002; 54(1):245–251.
103. Dorr W, Spekl K, Farrell CL. The effect of keratinocyte growth factor on healing of manifest radiation ulcers in mouse tongue epithelium. *Cell Prolif* 2002;35(Suppl 1): 86–92.
104. Chen L, Brizel DM, Rabbani ZN, et al. The protective effect of recombinant human keratinocyte growth factor on radiation-induced pulmonary toxicity in rats. *Int J Radiat Oncol Biol Phys* 2004;60(5):1520–1529.
105. Spielberger R, Stiff P, Bensinger W, et al. Palifermin for oral mucositis after intensive therapy for hematologic cancers. *N Engl J Med* 2004;351(25):2590–2598.
106. Brizel DM, Murphy BA, Rosenthal DI, et al. Phase II study of palifermin and concurrent chemoradiation in head and neck squamous cell carcinoma. *J Clin Oncol* 2008;26(15):2489–2496.
107. Le QT, Kim HE, Schneider CJ, et al. Palifermin reduces severe mucositis in definitive chemoradiotherapy of locally advanced head and neck cancer: a randomized, placebo-controlled study. *J Clin Oncol* 2011;29(20):2808–2814.
108. Henke M, Alfonsi M, Foa P, et al. Palifermin decreases severe oral mucositis of patients undergoing postoperative radiochemotherapy for head and neck cancer: a randomized, placebo-controlled trial. *J Clin Oncol* 2011;29(20):2815–2820.
109. Martin F, Farley A, Gagnon M, et al. Comparison of the healing capacities of sucralfate and cimetidine in the short-term treatment of duodenal ulcer: a double-blind randomized trial. *Gastroenterology* 1982;82(3):401–405.
110. Makkonen TA, Bostrom P, Vilja P, et al. Sucralfate mouth washing in the prevention of radiation-induced mucositis: a placebo-controlled double-blind randomized study. *Int J Radiat Oncol Biol Phys* 1994;30(1):177–182.
111. Meredith R, Salter M, Kim R, et al. Sucralfate for radiation mucositis: results of a double-blind randomized trial. *Int J Radiat Oncol Biol Phys* 1997;37(2):275–279.
112. Pfeiffer P, Madsen EL, Hansen O, et al. Effect of prophylactic sucralfate suspension on stomatitis induced by cancer chemotherapy. A randomized, double-blind cross-over study. *Acta Oncol* 1990;29(2):171–173.
113. Segre G, Hammarstrom S. Aspects of the mechanisms of action of benzydamine. *Int J Tissue React* 1985;7(3):187–193.
114. Sironi M, Pozzi P, Polentarutti N, et al. Inhibition of inflammatory cytokine production and protection against endotoxin toxicity by benzydamine. *Cytokine* 1996; 8(9):710–716.
115. Epstein JB, Silverman S Jr, Paggiarino DA, et al. Benzydamine HCl for prophylaxis of radiation-induced oral mucositis: results from a multicenter, randomized, double-blind, placebo-controlled clinical trial. *Cancer* 2001;92(4):875–885.
116. Bellm L, Lehrer RI, Ganz T. Protegrins: new antibiotics of mammalian origin. *Expert Opin Investig Drugs* 2000;9(8):1731–1742.
117. Giles FJ, Miller CB, Hurd DD, et al. A phase III, randomized, double-blind, placebo-controlled, multinational trial of iseganan for the prevention of oral mucositis in patients receiving stomatotoxic chemotherapy (PROMPT-CT trial). *Leuk Lymphoma* 2003;44(7):1165–1172.
118. Trotti A, Garden A, Warde P, et al. A multinational, randomized phase III trial of iseganan HCl oral solution for reducing the severity of oral mucositis in patients receiving radiotherapy for head-and-neck malignancy. *Int J Radiat Oncol Biol Phys* 2004;58(3):674–681.

Chapter 30
Oncologic Imaging/Oncologic Anatomy

Christopher R. Kelsey, Junzo P. Chino, Jared D. Christensen, and Lawrence B. Marks

This chapter addresses two topics central to the management of patients with cancer: oncologic anatomy and oncologic imaging. Although these topics are relevant for all specialties involved in the treatment of cancer, they are particularly germane for radiation oncologists. A sound understanding of anatomy, especially pertaining to malignant processes, facilitates interpretation of imaging studies. Likewise, understanding the advantages and limitations of individual imaging modalities assists in defining rational clinical target volumes (CTVs) that maximize the therapeutic ratio.

Advances in diagnostic imaging have increased our ability to visualize macroscopic disease, referred to as gross tumor volume (GTV). Imaging is currently unable to identify microscopic tumor extension around a primary tumor or occult nodal involvement. A CTV is created to account for both of these uncertainties (Table 30.1). A rational definition of the CTV should reflect the clinician's knowledge regarding the patterns of spread for each particular cancer. This involves both local spread around the primary site and patterns of lymphatic drainage. Appropriate expansion of a GTV to a CTV minimizes the risk of local failure (i.e., marginal miss), while reducing the risk of complications by avoiding regions at low risk of involvement (Fig. 30.1).

Radiation treatment planning has undergone considerable evolution during the past 20 years. With conventional planning, the physician conceives of beam orientations and aperture shapes based on the interpretation of available clinical and diagnostic information, including three-dimensional (3D) imaging data such as computed tomography (CT) or magnetic resonance imaging (MRI). The beam is then applied to the patient using a fluoroscopy-based conventional simulator, relying on an understanding of tumor and normal tissue anatomy and its association with fluoroscopic bony anatomy and surface anatomy. Relatively generous margins are used to account for inherent uncertainties of the process.

With 3D treatment planning, anatomic information from a planning CT scan is transferred to a computer where the images are segmented to define the tumor and normal tissues. Software allows this 3D information to be displayed and viewed from any orientation. Beam orientation and shape are chosen to encompass the target, yet minimize, as much as possible, normal tissue exposure. Thus, 3D planning tools allow the 3D anatomy to be more accurately incorporated into the planning process than with conventional techniques. The computer allows the planner to use beam orientations that are nonstandard (e.g., nonaxial beams). Beam apertures are typically smaller than with conventional simulation due to reduced uncertainty in the entire process. Current technology also allows data from other imaging modalities (MRI, positron emission tomography [PET], etc.) to be fused with the planning CT dataset and hence considered in the planning process. It is advantageous to position the patient similarly during the imaging and treatment planning scans to facilitate accurate image correlation.

Intensity modulated radiation therapy (IMRT) requires the clinician to explicitly delineate target volumes, including elective nodal basins and avoidance structures. The introduction of IMRT has revolutionized radiation treatment planning, and in the process, has required clinicians to become more proficient in 3D anatomy and malignant patterns of spread. Several groups have published guidelines demarcating elective nodal stations on axial CT images, including head and neck cancer,[1,2] lung cancer,[3] anorectal cancer,[4] and others. These stations are somewhat artificial but facilitate rational demarcation of nodal stations at risk, reporting of patterns of spread and failure, and communication with surgical colleagues.

One of the risks of 3D and IMRT is a false sense of security in the accuracy of imaging to portray the *in vivo* extent of disease. Further, imaging obtained at the time of initial treatment planning may not be representative of the *in vivo* anatomy throughout a multiweek course of therapy. Indeed, there have been several published examples of inferior outcomes with highly conformal treatment planning.[5,6] Modern imaging tools are clearly not perfect. The rapid embrace of newer technologies to visualize gross tumor and to address uncertainties related to organ motion and setup errors may be counterproductive if relied on too heavily in the treatment planning process. It is likely that we have, in the past, been able to sterilize microscopic tumor at the edge of radiotherapy fields that were expanded to account for setup errors and organ motion (i.e., not expanded with the intent of covering the microscopic disease). Furthermore, the clinical history or examination and imaging can be discordant, and one needs to be careful not to be overly reliant on imaging when defining target volumes. For example, in a patient with cancer of the nasopharynx with cranial nerve deficits, the target volume should include the

TABLE 30.1 VOLUME DEFINITIONS FOR RADIATION THERAPY PLANNING

Structure	Defined	Method of Assessment
Gross tumor volume (GTV)	Palpable or visible disease	Physical examination, imaging studies
Clinical target volume (CTV)	GTV + expansion for microscopic spread	Knowledge of patterns of spread (oncologic anatomy)
Planning target volume (PTV)	CTV + expansion for setup error and organ motion	Imaging studies (fluoroscopy or 4D CT to define degree of motion) and reproducibility/stability of mobilization/localization systems

4D, four dimensional; CT, computed tomography.

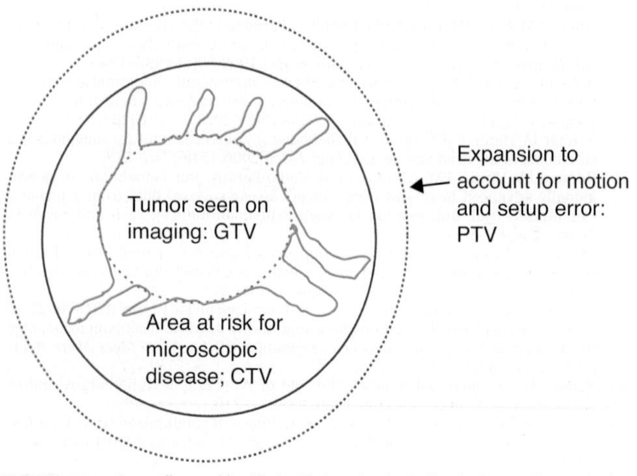

FIGURE 30.1. Gross disease identified with imaging is depicted, along with appropriate expansions to encompass surrounding microscopic disease (CTV) and setup/motion uncertainties (PTV).

corresponding anatomic site of likely extension, even in the absence of an abnormality on imaging. Thus, a sound understanding of oncologic anatomy and imaging modalities is vital in the treatment planning process.

IMAGING MODALITIES

Radiologic imaging is an integral component in the management of cancer patients. Imaging is utilized in the diagnosis and initial staging of disease, treatment planning, and posttreatment surveillance. Radiation oncologists must be familiar with the available imaging modalities and understand the appropriate utilization and limitations of each, which often varies based on the tumor site and study indication. In particular, a general sense of the sensitivity, specificity, and positive and negative predictive values of an imaging study helps the clinician assimilate and interpret imaging information that can be misleading or even contradictory. A detailed review of each imaging modality and its associated physics is beyond the scope of this chapter. However a general overview of the imaging modalities most frequently utilized in clinical practice is provided, with disease-specific applications addressed in the systems-based anatomy sections.

Radiography

Conventional radiography creates a two-dimensional grayscale image produced by the differential attenuation of x-rays that pass through soft tissues of varying density. Tissues that are very dense, such as bone, will absorb more x-rays than tissues that are less dense, such as lung. Radiographs are therefore best suited to detect pathology when a lesion differs greatly in density from adjacent structures, such as a soft tissue mass surrounded by aerated lung or a lytic lesion surrounded by dense bone. Radiographs have excellent spatial resolution: the ability to detect a small object within a given volume. However, they are suboptimal when there are only subtle differences in tissue density. Therefore, even large lesions can be missed if they are of similar density to surrounding structures. Given this and other limitations, additional imaging modalities are often obtained to supplement plain radiographs. In addition, although conventional radiography has limited utility in oncologic imaging, the basic principles underlie more advanced imaging modalities such as CT.

Cross-Sectional Imaging

CT, MRI, and ultrasound (US) generate two-dimensional cross-sectional images. The benefits of cross-sectional imaging include visualization of superimposed structures obscured on planar images, improved anatomic detail of individual organs and their precise relationship to adjacent structures, and the ability to perform multiplanar reconstructions. Furthermore, some applications provide functional in addition to morphologic information and can be acquired in real time, permitting image guidance for procedures. For these reasons, cross-sectional modalities are the mainstay of oncologic imaging.

Computed Tomography

CT generates cross-sectional images from the transmission of radiation through tissue. A patient lies on the scanner table within a gantry that houses an x-ray generator opposite multiple rows of detectors, hence the term *multidetector CT* (MDCT). Current generation scanners (e.g., 64 or 128 MDCT) are able to acquire high-resolution image data much faster due to improvements in the number of detectors and computer processing. As the gantry rotates, the detectors measure x-ray transmission through the rotation, or slice. The patient is moved through the scanner as the gantry rotates, resulting in a helical or spiral course at a very thin slice thickness, typically 0.625 mm. The spatial and temporal data from multiple projections are then processed by a Fourier transform mechanism generating two-dimensional axial images. The thin-slice volume dataset is isotropic, meaning that images can be reconstructed in orthogonal and oblique planes without a loss in image quality. Furthermore, thin-slice acquisition improves contrast resolution and decreases partial volume artifacts, thereby improving imaging quality and accuracy.

Images are displayed within a matrix composed of voxels, each representing a volume of radiodensity that is quantified by a linear attenuation value called a Hounsfield unit (HU). Each voxel is assigned a HU in the range of –1,000 to 1,000 corresponding to a shade of gray to represent the attenuation difference between a given material and water. By convention, air is the least dense material with a HU value of –1,000, while water has a HU value of 0. Soft tissues have a range of attenuation with typical HU values as follows: fat (–120), blood (30), muscle (40), bone (>300). HU analysis is more accurate than visual assessment of tissue composition and is particularly useful in characterizing enhancement postcontrast administration, a feature critical in the assessment of many solid organ lesions.

Both intravenous (IV) and oral contrast agents may be utilized to improve spatial resolution. Oral contrast agents are routinely used for abdominal and pelvic imaging to distinguish bowel from adjacent organs, lymph nodes, and tumors. The use of an intravascular contrast agent during CT depends on the study indication, target organ, and patient status. IV contrast agents contain variable concentrations of iodine compounds that attenuate, or absorb, x-rays, which allows for enhanced detection of vascular structures. Administration of IV contrast media is required for thorough assessment of vessels (e.g., aorta, pulmonary arteries), solid organs (e.g., liver, kidneys), and characterization of lesion vascularity. Contrast-enhanced CT is often necessary to detect solid organ metastases (e.g., liver, adrenal gland, brain). Contrast is usually not necessary for routine pulmonary imaging due to the inherent contrast of solid lesions within a background of aerated lung, although it does improve the characterization of hilar lymph nodes.

Given that the administration of contrast media can alter tissue attenuation, the HU value of a lesion or tissue may differ depending on whether the study was performed with or without contrast and based on the timing of image acquisition (e.g., arterial vs. portal venous phase). HUs are used during radiation treatment planning dose calculations; therefore, contrast can affect these calculations. If indicated, the HU within a structure enhanced by contrast (e.g., the bladder when planning for prostate cancer treatment) can be set to an alternate value prior to dose calculations. A similar phenomenon often occurs when materials with a high atomic number are within the scanned volume. These materials (e.g., dental fillings, hip prostheses) can cause artifacts that can make it challenging to accurately segment the image or affect dose calculations. The latter can also be corrected by setting the HU within the affected area to the desired value.

IV contrast agents are excreted through the kidneys, are nephrotoxic, and are not typically administered to patients with impaired renal function (glomerular filtration rate [GFR] <60, creatine [Cr] <1.8) unless on dialysis or out of emergent medical necessity. IV contrast media should also not be given to patients with a known contrast allergy resulting in anaphylaxis or laryngeal edema. More minor reactions, such as pruritus, are not an absolute contraindications and contrast may be administered following a proper steroid pretreatment protocol. Alternative imaging modalities should be considered if a contrast-enhanced study is required in the setting of a severe contrast allergy. An allergy to shellfish is no longer considered a contraindication to iodinated contrast administration.[7]

In part due to its availability, rapid acquisition, and high-yield anatomic data, CT has become one of the most widely used medical imaging modalities in the United States, with over 70 million scans performed annually, and it serves as the core modality for oncologic imaging.[8] Although CT is noninvasive, it is not entirely benign. CT utilizes radiation to generate images, and although dose modulation and optimal scanning parameters can significantly reduce patient radiation exposure, the cumulative effects of CT radiation are of clinical concern. Alternative imaging modalities should always be considered and performed in lieu of CT when appropriate.

Magnetic Resonance Imaging

MRI generates cross-sectional images without ionizing radiation. MRI utilizes strong magnets, typically 1.5 or 3.0 T for clinical applications. A 3.0 T magnet is 60,000 times greater than the earth's magnetic field. The magnetic field uniformly aligns the nuclei of hydrogen protons within tissue. Applying a radiofrequency (RF) pulse sequence and gradient to the magnetic field disrupts this alignment and equilibrium. When the RF pulse is removed, the protons realign, or relax, within the field and emit a measurable resonance radio signal. The detected radio signals, referred to as *echoes* or *spin echoes,* are then used to generate an image. The most important tissue properties for image generation are the proton density, the spin-lattice relaxation time (T1) and the spin-spin relaxation time (T2). Different tissues have different proton density and relaxation times, absorbing and releasing radio wave energy at different rates, which in part accounts for the high tissue contrast obtained by MRI.

Different RF pulse sequences can accentuate different tissue characteristics by varying parameters such as the repetition time (TR)—the time between RF pulses in the sequence, which determines how much time protons have to realign within the magnetic field—and the echo time (TE)—the time between the RF pulse and the peak returning signal. TR and TE dramatically affect image contrast and determine which tissue properties are selected. T1-weighted images, in which fluid is dark and fat is bright, are generally good at depicting anatomy; T1-weighted images are generated by selecting short TR (typically ≤800 ms) and short TE values (≤30 ms). T2-weighted images, in which fluid is bright and fat is dark, are fluid-sensitive and can depict areas of pathology; T2-weighted images are generated by selecting long TR (≥2,000 ms) and long TE values (≥60 ms) (Table 30.2). Scan sequences are composed of variations in RF pulses and TR and TE settings. Although these vary by MRI scanner manufacturer using proprietary names, the underlying principles are similar. Common sequence techniques include:

Spin-echo (SE) sequences produce standard T1- and T2-weighted images.

Multiple spin-echo (MSE) sequences allow for faster image acquisition and are also referred to as turbo spin echo, fast spin echo, or rapid-acquisition relaxation-enhanced imaging. The signal intensity and image quality is less than that of conventional SE sequences. Furthermore, fat is bright on MSE T2-weighted images, which can limit sensitivity for detecting pathology. Fat-suppression techniques can be used to offset this limitation. Fast low-angle acquisition with relaxation enhancement and half-Fourier acquisition single-shot turbo spin-echo sequences are MSE variations.

TABLE 30.2 MAGNETIC RESONANCE IMAGING SIGNAL INTENSITIES (SPIN-ECHO IMAGING)

	T1WI	T2WI	FLAIR
Cerebrospinal fluid	Dark	Bright	Dark
Fat[a]	Bright	Dark	Bright
Solid mass (tumor)	Dark	Bright	Bright
Edema	Dark	Bright	Bright
Cyst	Dark	Bright	Dark

T1WI, T1-weighted image; T2WI, T2-weighted image; FLAIR, fluid-attenuation inversion recovery; bright, hyperintense; dark, hypointense.

[a]Fat is bright on T2 fast spin echo (FSE) or gradient echo sequences.

Inversion recovery (IR) pulse sequences emphasize differences in T1 properties of tissues. A time of inversion (TI) is added to the sequence that can be set to target specific tissues. Short time of inversion recovery sequences suppress tissues with short T1 relaxation times, such as fat, and enhance tissues with high T2 properties, such as fluid, resulting in added tissue contrast. The opposite effect may be achieved with fluid-attenuation inversion recovery sequences. In addition to IR, tissue suppression may be achieved with fat or fluid saturation and opposed-imaging techniques.

Gradient-recalled echo (GRE) pulse sequences are used for rapid image acquisition, which minimizes motion artifact associated with breathing, the cardiac cycle, vessel pulsation, and bowel peristalsis. GRE sequences have low tissue contrast, with the exception of flowing blood, which is bright in signal, and are therefore ideal for cardiac and vascular applications. Fast low-angle shot (FLASH) and true fast imaging with steady-state precession (FISP) are examples of this technique.

Although the inherent tissue contrast with MRI is excellent, the administration of contrast media can further improve the detection of pathology and subtle differences in tissue properties. Gadolinium chelates are the most commonly used MRI contrast agents, which, like the iodinated CT equivalents, are confined to the vasculature and do not cross an intact blood–brain barrier. Gadolinium is a heavy metal ion with paramagnetic effects that shorten T1 and T2 relaxation times. Although there are flow-related techniques for vascular imaging that do not require contrast media (e.g., time of flight imaging), the use of a contrast agent is essential for characterizing tissue perfusion. Once considered safe for patients with impaired renal function, the use of gadolinium-based contrast agents have now been associated with nephrogenic systemic fibrosis (NSF), a debilitating and potentially fatal condition of fibrin deposition within the skin and other organs.[9] Although the precise mechanism is not understood, patients with severe renal dysfunction (GFR <30) who receive gadolinium-based contrast media are at increased risk of developing NSF.

One of the advantages of MRI over CT is that it can provide functional in addition to anatomic information. This is particularly beneficial in oncologic imaging. MRI techniques allow for tissue diffusion and perfusion imaging, quantification of blood flow by velocity phase encoding, and magnetic resonance proton spectroscopy, which provides biochemical quantification of tissues.

As with other imaging techniques, MRI has modality-specific artifacts that can limit image quality. Motion artifact can be problematic with MRI due to long scan times. Chemical shift artifact results in a loss of signal at the interface of tissues with highly variable contrast properties. MRI is also highly sensitive to magnetic field distortions that can produce artifacts. Susceptibility artifact is one of the most common problems with MRI and is frequently attributable to objects that alter the magnetic field, resulting in signal voids or distortion of MRI images, such as metallic hardware or devices. The magnetization of such objects also presents a safety hazard as items can overheat or become displaced, resulting in serious harm or injury. Patients must be carefully screened to ensure that any medical devices or surgical hardware are MRI compliant.

Ultrasonography

US is an imaging modality utilizing pulse-echo techniques rather than radiation to produce an image. The US transducer coverts electrical energy into a high-frequency pulse that is transmitted through tissues. The pulse interacts at tissue interfaces, generating a reflected echo signal that is detected by the transducer. The returning sound waves are transformed into a gray scale image in real time. Image quality is, in large part, determined by the pulse frequency. High-frequency transducers

(5–12 MHz) produce high-resolution images but have limited ability to penetrate. Therefore, they are best suited to imaging superficial structures such as the breast or thyroid. Low-frequency transducers (1–3.5 MHz) generate lower quality images but have better tissue penetration and are most often used for imaging abdominal and pelvic organs. The degree to which tissues are visualized by US is called *echogenicity*. Fat is highly echogenic (bright), whereas fluid-containing structures, such as simple cysts, are anechoic (dark).

The quality of US images is highly dependent on the sonographer. Variability in user experience can be problematic in the performance, reproducibility, and interpretation of US exams. Furthermore, US is prone to artifacts. Bone almost completely absorbs sound waves, resulting in acoustic shadowing that completely obscures tissues located beyond the bone. Air is also problematic as it almost completely reflects sound waves, leaving little pulse energy to penetrate tissues deep to the air. The application of a water-soluble gel between the transducer and the patient's skin eliminates air at the skin surface and ensures transmission of the US beam. Artifacts secondary to air markedly limit evaluation of lesions near the lung or bowel. In contrast to air, fluid readily transmits sound and makes an excellent "acoustic window" for imaging. This is the reason that patients are encouraged to drink plenty of fluids prior to a pelvic US examination—so that the bladder is fully distended.

Color Doppler US is an important adjunct to conventional gray-scale sonography. The Doppler effect is a change in frequency of returning sound waves reflected by a moving object, such as flowing blood. If blood flows away from the transducer, the echo frequency decreases; whereas if blood flows toward the transducer, the echo frequency increases. The change in frequency is directly proportional to the flow velocity and produces a color overlay in areas of flow on the standard gray-scale US image. Color Doppler US is useful in characterizing blood flow within lesions and assisting in image-guided procedures.

Endoscopic ultrasound (EUS) was introduced in the early 1980 s and has become a tool important in oncologic staging. It allows for high-resolution images of internal structures not typically accessible by high-frequency transducers by passing the probe through bowel or airways. It is most widely applied in the setting of gastrointestinal (GI) malignancies, especially esophageal and rectal carcinomas. A 5 to 12 MHz transducer can readily identify five of the layers of the gastrointestinal tract (Table 30.3 and Fig. 30.2).[10] Higher frequency transducers can identify additional layers, such as the muscularis mucosa and lamina propria of the esophagus, which has important staging implications. EUS is also utilized for characterization and image-guided sampling of regional lymph nodes in GI or bronchopulmonary disease. The ability of EUS to predict the tumor (T) stage is generally superior to its ability to predict the node (N) stage, although some imaging patterns of nodal involvement are recognized. Normal lymph nodes are usually ovoid, <10 mm in short axis, and have a homogeneous but variable echogenic appearance that may be isoechoic, hyperechoic, or hypoechoic to surrounding tissues. An echogenic (bright) center is common and represents the normal fatty hilum. Suspicious lymph nodes are typically round, >10 mm in short axis, have distinct margins, and are typically hypoechoic. If all four features are present, the likelihood of malignancy is 80% to 100%.[11] There is, however, considerable overlap between benign and malignant features of lymph nodes on EUS in addition to wide interobserver variability. Tissue sampling is therefore recommended for accurate staging. When describing clinical T and N staging by EUS, the prefix *u* should be utilized (e.g., uT3N1).

TABLE 30.3 ENDOSCOPIC ULTRASOUND WALL LAYERS OF THE ESOPHAGUS

Layer	EUS Characteristic	Histologic Layer	AJCC T Stage
1	Hyperechoic	Superficial mucosa	T1 *m*
2	Hypoechoic	Deep mucosa	T1 *m*
3	Hyperechoic	Submucosa	T1 *sm*
4	Hypoechoic	Muscularis propria	T2
5	Hyperechoic	Subserosa, serosa, adventitia	T3

EUS, endoscopic ultrasound; AJCC, American Joint Committee on Cancer; *m*, mucosa; *sm*, submucosa.

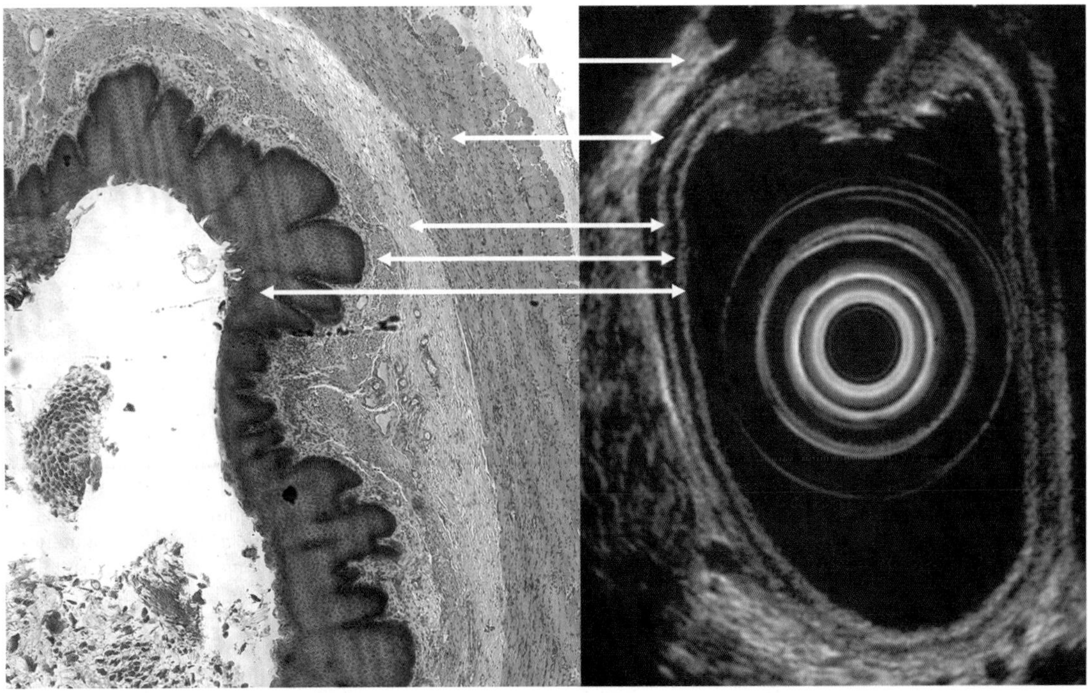

FIGURE 30.2. Axial endoscopic ultrasound image (*right*) and histologic specimen (*left*) from a normal esophagus. The endoscopic ultrasound layers and histologic layers of the esophagus are correlated (see Table 30.3). (Endoscopic ultrasound image courtesy of Dr. Frank Gress. Histologic image courtesy of Dr. Daniel Goodenough.)

Nuclear Imaging

Although radiographic and cross-sectional studies provide important anatomic information regarding pathologic processes, nuclear radiology provides physiologic information based on the distribution of an injected or ingested radiopharmaceutical. Radiopharmaceuticals consist of a radioactive substrate (radionuclide, radioisotope, or radiotracer) that is coupled with a physiologically active compound or analog. For example, technetium-99 m is a radioisotope that is coupled to pertechnetate, an iodine analog, which can enter thyroid follicular cells. The timing of imaging depends on the kinetics of absorption, metabolism, and half-life of the radionuclide. Gamma rays emitted by nuclear decay of the radionuclide are then detected using a γ-camera corresponding to radiotracer activity that is described in terms of uptake.

There are numerous available nuclear imaging studies that take advantage of differing radiopharmaceuticals for oncologic imaging. Many of these play a primary role in the management of oncology patients with specific malignancies. For example, indium-111 capromab pendetide (ProstaScint) can be utilized for prostate cancer and gallium-67 can be used for lymphomas—both of which will be discussed in greater detail later in the chapter. However, the primary nuclear imaging studies relevant to general oncologic imaging are PET and bone scintigraphy. These studies have broad application for many malignant processes in the diagnosis, staging, and surveillance of disease.

Positron Emission Tomography

Although several radionuclides for PET are available, the most common is 18-fluorodeoxyglucose (FDG). FDG is a glucose analog that concentrates in areas of high metabolic activity. Tumor cells are often highly metabolic, with rapid cell division and an increased number of glucose transporters. However, FDG uptake is not specific for malignancy and accumulates in any cell with increased metabolic activity, including myocardium, gastric mucosa, brain tissue, thyroid, and salivary glands, which limits evaluation of these organs. Furthermore, FDG tracer is excreted within the urinary system; therefore, activity within the kidneys, collecting system, and bladder can obscure malignancy of these structures. Notwithstanding these limitations, PET-CT has become the preferred imaging modality for clinical staging, facilitating the characterization of benign versus malignant pathology, detecting sites of unsuspected disease, identifying optimal sites for tissue sampling, assessing treatment response, and monitoring for recurrence for multiple malignancies.

Initially performed in isolation, PET is now routinely obtained in conjunction with CT. PET-CT combines the physiologic assessment of PET with the anatomic assessment of CT, resulting in improved diagnostic accuracy.[12] PET and CT may be obtained independently on the same day but is more commonly performed on a combined PET-CT scanner, which more precisely aligns the two imaging datasets for fusion as the patient does not have to move between examinations. Patients must fast for 4 to 6 hours prior to scanning in order to limit metabolic activity within the GI tract. Blood glucose levels should be well controlled (<150 mg/dL) to limit glucose receptor competition with FDG, as high glucose levels can result in a false-negative scan. Speech and motion should be restricted to minimize muscle uptake, which could obscure pathology. Approximately 1 hour following FDG administration, a CT scan is performed immediately followed by PET imaging, which can take up to 60 minutes. CT and PET datasets are then reconstructed in separate axial, coronal, and sagittal series as well as fused PET-CT images.

FDG uptake is nonspecific, localizing to any tissue with increased metabolic activity. Although most malignant tumors are hypermetabolic relative to normal tissues, nonmalignant processes also concentrate FDG, including foci of infection, inflammation, and benign neoplasms. FDG uptake is quantified by the standard uptake value (SUV). Most malignant tumors have a maximum SUV >2.5, while physiologic uptake is typically <2.5. SUVs are not absolute and can be affected by the timing of imaging, improper attenuation correction, partial volume affects, patient weight, FDG dose, and factors affecting FDG uptake, as previously described. It is therefore difficult to accurately compare SUVs between scans. However, if care is taken to ensure that variables between studies are similar, such as performing the examination on the same scanner with similar patient preparation, FDG dosing, and image timing, comparing SUVs between studies may be reliable. Clinical studies to date have documented that under such uniform conditions, changes in SUV have prognostic value, indicating that most tumors responding to therapy show a 20% to 40% decrease in SUV early in course of treatment.[13–15]

Bone Scintigraphy

Normal bone undergoes continuous remodeling, maintaining a delicate balance between osteoblastic and osteoclastic activity. Most bone metastases originate as intramedullary lesions, having gained access to the bone through the vasculature. As the lesions enlarge, reactive osteoblastic and osteoclastic changes result in characteristic radiographic changes indicative of bone metastases (sclerotic, lytic, or mixed lesions). Rapidly growing metastases tend to produce lytic lesions, while more slowly growing metastases typically produce sclerotic (or blastic) lesions. Metastases from multiple myeloma, thyroid cancer, and renal cell carcinoma are predominantly lytic, while blastic lesions are associated with breast and prostate cancers. The primary utility of bone scintigraphy in oncologic imaging is the detection of osseous metastatic disease.

Bone scintigraphy or bone scan imaging utilizes radiopharmaceuticals composed of bisphosphonates; the most common of which is the radionuclide technetium-99 m methylene diphosphonate (^{99m}Tc-MDP). ^{99m}Tc-MDP localizes to areas of new bone mineralization, which occurs in a wide array of bone pathology and is therefore highly sensitive to osseous disease, but is not very specific. Although a 30% to 50% reduction in bone density must occur before bone metastases are detected on radiographs, as little as 5% to 10% change is required to detect such on a bone scan.[16,17] Furthermore, bone scans are relatively inexpensive, convenient, and visualize the entire skeleton, including sites that are difficult to assess on plain films (e.g., ribs, sternum, scapula, sacrum). Reported sensitivities range from 62% to 100% with similar specificity rates (78% to 100%).[18]

Two primary patterns of radiotracer activity can be associated with malignancy: increased or decreased activity. Increased uptake occurs in areas of increased blood flow and osteoblastic activity; this is a common finding in metabolically active tumors and small sclerotic metastatic foci. Decreased radiotracer activity occurs as a "cold" area on bone scan and is associated with lytic bone disease and aggressive tumors that outgrow their blood supply. Rapidly progressing and purely lytic disease are the main causes of false-negative findings on bone scintigraphy, while false-positive findings can be related to trauma, healing, benign bone tumors, or arthritic changes.

Bone metastases are considered "nonmeasurable" using the Response Evaluation Criteria in Solid Tumors.[19] Although a decrease in the intensity of radionuclide uptake is often ascribed to a response to treatment and an increase is attributed to progressive disease, several points must be considered. First, tumor response may cause a "flare phenomenon," resulting from increased activity secondary to new osteoblastic activity concomitant with new bone formation. This may be falsely attributed to progressive disease. Similarly, lytic lesions that were previously "cold" on bone scan can transform into "hot" spots (areas of uptake) after treatment. Second, rapidly progressive disease with overwhelming bone destruction without new bone formation can be misinterpreted as stable or responding disease on bone scan.

Many patients are at low risk of harboring occult osseous metastatic disease and, in the absence of symptoms, a bone scan can be omitted from the staging workup. In prostate cancer, only approximately 1% of patients with a prostate-specific antigen (PSA) <10 will have a positive bone scan.[20,21] Patients with a Gleason score ≤7 and a PSA of 10 to 20 have a similar low risk of bone metastases.[22] In these patients, a bone scan should be omitted in the absence of symptoms. Similarly, a bone scan may be omitted in asymptomatic patients with node-negative breast cancer and lung cancer. Although studies have shown that MRI may be more sensitive than bone scans, especially for vertebral metastases, whole-body MRI is impractical and bone scintigraphy is considered sufficiently sensitive that MRI should be reserved for equivocal bone scans in the context of high clinical suspicion or for patients with positive bone scans but low clinical suspicion. Like MRI, PET has been shown to be more sensitive than scintigraphy for the diagnosis of osseous metastatic disease with sensitivity of 91% and 75%, and specificity values of 96% and 95%, respectively.[23] FDG-PET also provides earlier detection of metastases than bone scans, attributable to the fact that increased glucose metabolism in neoplastic cells occurs prior to increased osteogenesis (required for bone scintigraphy uptake). PET also has the advantage of providing more comprehensive imaging in that it can detect soft tissue metastases in addition to bone disease, whereas scintigraphy only evaluates osseous structures. As a general rule, patients with isolated osteoblastic metastases may be monitored by serial bone scans, while other clinical scenarios are likely best suited for PET.

BRAIN AND SPINE

Oncologic Anatomy

The Brain

The central nervous system consists of the brain and spinal cord. Both are covered with three meningeal layers—the dura mater, arachnoid mater, and pia mater. Meningiomas are the most common tumors arising from the meninges. They arise from arachnoid cells but are typically affixed to the underside of the dura mater. They are well-circumscribed tumors that do not typically invade the underlying brain parenchyma. Thus, when planning a course of radiation therapy, only minimal margins are required to account for surrounding microscopic disease extent in the direction of the brain parenchyma. Many meningiomas will have a linear area of enhancement on MRI, extending from the tumor along the dura. This so-called dural tail is generally not felt to represent direct extension of tumor but rather vascular congestion within the dura, leading to the characteristic enhancement.[24,25] Thus, enlarging the target volumes to include this linear area of enhancement is probably unnecessary unless other imaging abnormalities are apparent (e.g., nodularity).

The arachnoid mater and pia mater are considered the leptomeninges with the intervening space (subarachnoid space) filled with cerebrospinal fluid (CSF). Cancer can breach the CSF space through several routes, including hematogenous spread (via the Batson venous plexus or the arterial system) or by direct extension. Once cancer breaches the subarachnoid space, the entire craniospinal axis is at risk, and tumor deposits can lead to increased intracranial pressure, cranial nerve deficits, radiculopathies, and seizures. Leptomeningeal involvement occurs most frequently with pediatric brain tumors (e.g., medulloblastoma), acute lymphoblastic leukemia, and some solid cancers (e.g., breast cancer, melanoma, and lung cancer in particular).[26]

The major units of the brain include the cerebral hemispheres, diencephalon, cerebellum, and brainstem. The cerebral hemispheres consist of the frontal, parietal, temporal, and occipital lobes, basal ganglia, and lateral ventricles. The diencephalon includes the thalamus, hypothalamus, and third ventricle. The brainstem consists of the midbrain, the pons, and the medulla oblongata. The fourth ventricle lies between the pons and the cerebellum. Although more than half of pediatric brain tumors arise in the posterior fossa (cerebellum and brainstem), the vast majority of primary brain tumors in adults arise in the cerebral hemispheres or diencephalon.

Cranial Nerves

The cranial nerves consist of 12 paired nerves whose nuclei (with the exception of CN I) are located in the brainstem and upper spinal cord. They are termed cranial nerves because they exit the cranium through foramina in the base of skull and are encased by sheaths formed from the meninges. Nerve pathways connecting the cerebral cortex with the cranial nerves are complex. Although spinal motor neurons are innervated by the corticospinal tracts, many of the lower motor neurons in the brainstem are innervated by the corticobulbar tracts. These upper motor neurons innervate the cranial motor nuclei bilaterally (with some exceptions), in contrast to the nerves within the corticospinal tracts, which largely cross in the medulla leading to contralateral innervation.

Multiple tumors, both benign and malignant, commonly involve the cranial nerves, leading to serious neurologic deficits. Some of the more common include meningiomas involving the optic nerves (CN II), vestibular schwannomas (CN VIII), parotid gland tumors (CN VII), nasopharyngeal carcinoma (multiple), and brainstem gliomas (multiple).

The classic presenting symptoms of diffuse pontine gliomas illustrate the intricate anatomy of the pons. A unilateral lesion in the ventral pons with involvement of the pyramidal tracts (upper motor neurons) might cause contralateral motor weakness in the arms or legs. In addition, cranial nerves within the pons might also be affected, unilaterally, without complete paralysis because of bilateral innervation of the cranial nerves by fibers in the corticobulbar tracts. Ataxia, denoting impairment of coordination without weakness, can be caused by involvement of fibers projecting from the pons to the cerebellum within the middle cerebellar peduncle. Through this pathway, the cerebellum receives a copy of the information for muscle movement that the corticospinal tracts relay to lower motor neurons, facilitating the complicated act of coordination.

The cranial nerves should also be carefully examined when evaluating a patient with nasopharyngeal carcinoma (NPC). One-fifth of patients with NPC present with symptoms of cranial nerve involvement (Table 30.4). The most commonly involved cranial nerves are the abducent nerve (CN VI) and the trigeminal nerve (CN V). CN VI originates in the ventral aspect of the brainstem, ascends on the clivus, and crosses the internal carotid artery near the superior aspect of foramen lacerum before entering the cavernous sinus. It then exits the skull through the superior orbital fissure. The motor and sensory nerve roots of CN V exit the pons, pass underneath the free edge of the tentorium cerebelli into Meckel's cave, forming the trigeminal (Gasserian) ganglion. From the ganglion, V_1 and V_2 enter the cavernous sinus and subsequently exit the skull through the superior orbital fissure and foramen rotundum, respectively. V_3 exits the skull through foramen ovale.

The nasopharynx is in close proximity to foramen lacerum, rotundum, and ovale, explaining the frequent tumor involvement of CN V and VI. Invasion superiorly to the foramen lacerum and involvement of the trigeminal ganglion could lead to dysfunction in all three branches of CN V. In fact, most patients with NPC and CN V involvement have isolated deficits of V_2 or V_3. This occurs due to extension into foramen rotundum and ovale, respectively (Fig. 30.3). After gaining access to the middle cranial fossa, NPC may extend superiorly into the cavernous sinus. Four cranial nerves, including two branches of CN V, pass through the cavernous sinus. Within the sinus, the oculomotor nerve (CN III) is located most superiorly, while the maxillary nerve (CN V_2) is located most inferiorly. One would

TABLE 30.4 MAJOR FORAMINA AND OTHER APERTURES IN THE CRANIAL FOSSAE AND THEIR PRIMARY CONTENTS AND CLINICAL ASSOCIATION WITH NASOPHARYNGEAL CANCER

Foramina/Opening	*Contents*	*Frequency of Involvement by NPC (152) (%)*
Anterior Cranial Fossa		
Foramina in cribriform plate	Axons of olfactory cells (CN I)	0
Middle Cranial Fossa		
Optic canal	Optic nerve (CN II)	6
	Ophthalmic artery	
Superior orbital fissure	Oculomotor nerve (CN III)	9
	Trochlear nerve (CN IV)	17
	Abducent nerve (CN VI)	44
	Ophthalmic nerve (CN V_1)	45
Foramen rotundum	Maxillary nerve (CN V_2)	67
Foramen ovale	Mandibular nerve (CN V_3)	48
Foramen spinosum	Meningeal branch of CN V_3	14
	Middle meningeal artery/vein	
Foramen lacerum	Internal carotid artery[a]	
Petrous Portion of the Temporal Bone		
Internal acoustic meatus	Facial nerve (CN VII)[b]	
	Vestibulocochlear nerve (CN VIII)	9
	Labyrinthine artery	0
Posterior Cranial Fossa		
Jugular foramen	Glossopharyngeal nerve (CN IX)	20
	Vagus nerve (CN X)	20
	Spinal accessory nerve (CN XI)	14
	Internal jugular vein (superior bulb)	
Foramen magnum	Spinal roots of spinal accessory nerve (CN XI)	14
	Medulla	
	Vertebral artery	
	Anterior/posterior spinal artery	
Hypoglossal canal	Hypoglossal nerve (CN XII)	24

NPC, nasopharyngeal carcinoma.
[a]After entering the skull through the carotid canal.
[b]The facial nerve exits the skull through the stylomastoid foramen.

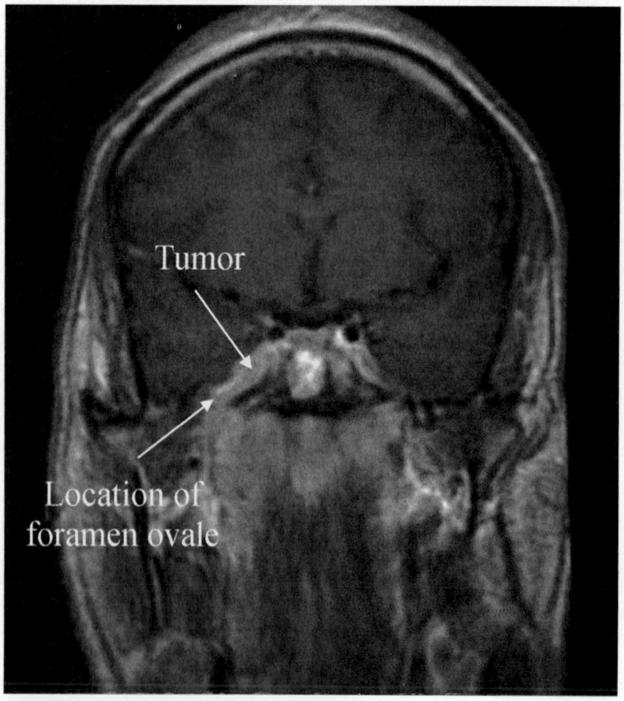

FIGURE 30.3. Coronal T1 magnetic resonance image with contrast demonstrating nasopharyngeal carcinoma extending through foramen ovale into Meckel's cave.

suspect that cranial nerves located more superiorly in the cavernous sinus would be involved less frequently than those located closer to the base of skull. This is consistent with what is observed clinically (see Table 30.4).

Lower cranial nerve involvement can occur without intracranial extension. The fossa of Rosenmüller is the most common site of origin of NPC. The lateral border of the fossa of Rosenmüller is the pharyngeal space. Direct tumor extension laterally into the parapharyngeal space or lymphatic metastases to high parapharyngeal lymph nodes can affect the cranial nerves exiting the jugular foramen (CN IX, X, and XI), and hypoglossal canal (CN XII). This may result in loss of the gag reflex (CN IX), hoarseness or dysphagia (CN X), atrophy or paralysis of trapezius and sternocleidomastoid (CN XI), as well as tongue deviation (CN XII).

Spine

The vertebral column typically consists of 33 bones (7 cervical, 12 thoracic, 5 lumbar, 5 sacral, and 4 coccygeal). The sacral and coccygeal vertebral bodies are fused. Although all individuals have seven cervical vertebral bodies, variations in the number of the other vertebral levels are occasionally observed. The spinal cord is housed within the spinal canal and encased by the meninges. Spinal cord levels do not correspond with levels of the vertebral column. In adults, the spinal cord typically ends at the L1-2 interspace (termed the *conus medullaris*). In an infant, the spinal cord terminates at L2 or L3. However, the spinal nerves continue to descend within the spinal canal (termed the cauda equina). The subarachnoid space, containing CSF, typically extends to the second sacral vertebral body. At this level the meninges fuse together and extend caudally as the filum terminale, which anchors the spinal cord to the coccyx. These anatomical issues have implications when evaluating a patient with spinal cord compression, designing craniospinal fields, and when setting up palliative spine fields.

Oncologic Imaging

Intracranial Metastases

Approximately 50% of adult intracranial neoplasms are metastatic, with lung, breast, melanoma, renal, and colon cancers being the most common, in order of decreasing frequency. Among individual primaries, melanoma is associated with the highest frequency of brain metastases.[27] Most metastases gain access to the brain through the vasculature and typically arise at the junction of the gray and white matter,[28] presumably because the caliber of blood vessels decreases at this point, acting as a trap for tumor emboli. Approximately 80% of brain metastases are found in the cerebral hemispheres, with less frequent involvement of the cerebellum (15%) and brainstem (5%), reflecting their smaller volume and blood flow.

The detection of brain metastases is an important part of initial staging. Furthermore, due to improved treatment strategies and overall cancer survival, the overall incidence of brain metastases is increasing. The preferred imaging modality for the diagnosis of intracranial metastasis is contrast-enhanced MRI. Brain metastases are typically well circumscribed and avidly enhance (Fig. 30.4). They are also typically associated with a disproportionate amount of surrounding edema best depicted on T2-weighted sequences. MRI is more sensitive than CT in detecting intracranial metastases, and approximately 20% of patients with solitary metastatic lesions by CT show multiple lesions on MRI.[29] Furthermore, for patients with a single brain metastasis detected with a conventional single-dose MRI-contrasted study, triple-dose studies will depict additional metastases in up to 25% of patients.[30] The detection of multiple lesions aids in directing appropriate treatment and helps to distinguish metastases from primary brain tumors, which are more commonly solitary.

Conventional PET-CT has limited utility in the assessment of brain metastases due to the high metabolic rate of normal

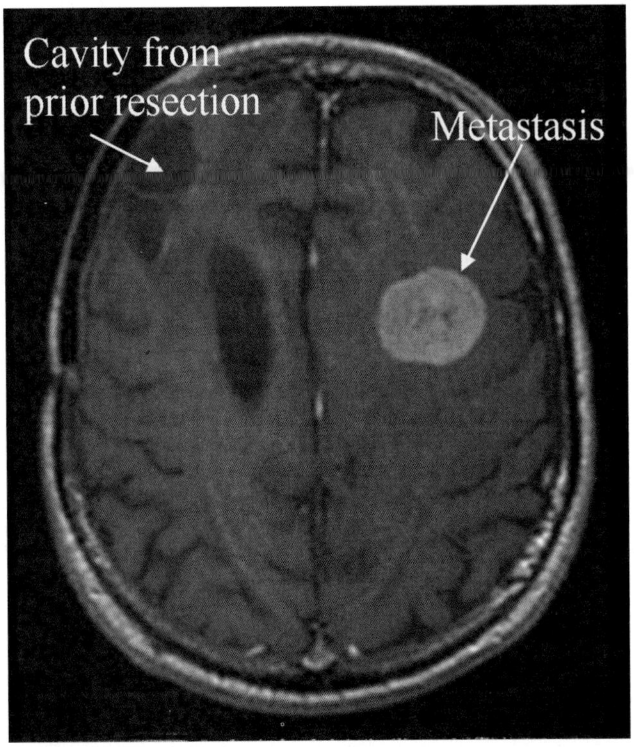

FIGURE 30.4. Axial T1 magnetic resonance image with contrast demonstrating a 2.5-cm melanoma brain metastasis in the left frontal lobe. Note the prior resection cavity in the right frontal lobe.

brain tissue. However, delayed phase PET, performed approximately 3.5 hours following FDG injection, allows for washout of FDG from normal brain cells, while abnormal tissue retains FDG. Delayed phase PET has been shown to be beneficial in detecting both primary and metastatic brain lesions as well as differentiating between residual or recurrent tumor and radiation necrosis following treatment.[31,32] The utility of delayed phase PET may be further enhanced through fusion with MRI.

Primary Brain Malignancy

Primary brain tumors account for approximately 50% of adult intracranial masses, of which half are malignant. The most common malignant primary brain tumor in adults is glioblastoma multiforme (GBM), which usually arises in the cerebral hemispheres. Compared with CT, MRI is more accurate in delineating the local gross extent of disease. In a series of 52 patients with primary brain tumors, the MRI signal abnormality was larger than that identified by CT in 62% of patients. Furthermore, 10 patients with equivocal CT scans had clear abnormalities on MRI.[33] GBMs are characterized by an expansile mass that is iso- to hypointense to surrounding tissue on T1-weighted images, with central necrosis and peripheral ring enhancement postcontrast administration. T2-weighted imaging shows a heterogeneous mass with high signal of the tumor nidus and surrounding T2-signal abnormality corresponding to vasogenic edema, in which malignant cells are known to frequently reside.[34] Central areas of low signal reflect a combination of blood products, necrosis, and vascular flow voids.

GBM most commonly grows along white matter tracts and does not typically involve the dura or skull. GBM is one of two entities that may spread into the contralateral cerebral hemisphere via tracts of the corpus callosum; central nervous system lymphoma is the other. Other potential routes of spread, including subependymal extension with CSF contamination or hematogenous dissemination, are possible but unusual.

Advanced imaging techniques are also beneficial in characterizing intracranial malignancy. Magnetic resonance spectroscopy (MRS) provides metabolic and biochemical information about tumors in relation to normal brain tissue by quantifying five metabolite peaks: choline (Cho)-containing compounds, Cr, *N*-acetylaspartate (NAA), lactate, and lipid: the Cho peak reflects cell membrane turnover, Cr is a surrogate for energy synthesis, and NAA is a marker exclusive to neuronal cells. Lactate is detected in necrotic tumors and infarcted tissue and results from anaerobic metabolism. Lipid peaks are produced by cellular and myelin breakdown products. The hallmark spectroscopic pattern of brain tumors is an increase in Cho-containing compounds and a decrease in NAA relative to normal brain tissue. MRS can also aid in the evaluation of tumor type and grade. High-grade gliomas tend to exhibit higher Cho:Cr and Cho:NAA ratios. High-grade gliomas also typically have higher lipid and lactate peaks as the result of necrosis.[35] MRS can also distinguish metastatic disease from high-grade gliomas, particularly when combined with perfusion MRI.[36] Differentiating radiation necrosis from tumor is also possible using MRS; however, newer techniques, such as dynamic susceptibility-weighted contrast-enhanced perfusion MRI, may be even more accurate and are currently being studied.[37]

Spinal Metastases

Osseous metastases are common in many malignancies, and the vertebral bodies are frequently involved due to the vascular distribution to the spine. MRI is more sensitive at detecting early vertebral body metastases than both radiographs and CT as it can image changes within the marrow space before cortical destruction occurs. Given that PET has similar sensitivity as MRI for osseous metastatic disease, is performed as part of routine staging, and can image the entire body, MRI is reserved for troubleshooting, such as determining extent of invasion into adjacent tissues. One notable exception is the use of urgent MRI for identification of cord compression in the setting of acute neurologic compromise. In this situation, it is often the T2-weighted sequences that are most useful: the high-signal CSF provides contrast to identify disease encroaching into the spinal canal. Spinal cord edema can also be identified. One should consider screening the entire spine when evaluating for cord compression.

Spinal cord compression is often considered an oncologic emergency, because the longer the duration of symptoms, the less likely the patient will regain function. Thus, therapy is often instituted emergently in these cases (e.g., with radiation, steroids, surgery, or sometimes chemotherapy in sensitive tumors). There is often discordance between the imaging and clinical examination findings. It is the *clinical* findings that determine the acuity of the situation rather than the imaging findings. A radiologic finding of cord compression certainly warrants an evaluation but does not necessarily warrant emergent intervention.

HEAD AND NECK

Oncologic Anatomy

The anatomy of the head and neck is complex, and it is important that oncologists have an intimate understanding of the location, function, and radiographic appearance of the various subsites. The potential for significant morbidity associated with local tumor progression and recurrence in the head and neck region, as well as the associated late effects of curative treatment, necessitates attention to detail. The impact of anatomy is such that the Accreditation Council for Graduate Medical Education mandates cadaver lab experience for otolaryngology residency.

Lymphatic Drainage of the Head and Neck

The lymphatics in the head and neck region largely proceed in an orderly fashion from sites in the upper aerodigestive tract into the common jugular chains, which eventually empty into systemic circulation near the junction of the internal jugular and subclavian veins. There are notable exceptions to this orderly drainage that can influence radiation treatment planning. In order to discuss this in a systematic fashion, the lymphatic basins of the neck are divided into six distinct levels, with surgical and radiographic boundaries.[38]

Level I is defined as both the submental basins (level IA) and the submandibular basins (level IB) and receive drainage from the oral cavity, although this basin may also be at risk from other sites in the setting of advanced nodal disease (N2b or greater). Level II contains the upper jugular nodes, extending from the C1 vertebral body to the hyoid bone, including the contents of the carotid sheath and the space deep to the sternocleidomastoid muscle (SCM). Level II is subdivided into anterior (level IIA) and posterior (level IIB) regions, as defined by the posterior border of the jugular vein. Level II contains the jugulodigastric node at the level of the jugular vein as it crosses the posterior belly of the digastric muscle, and is a common lymphatic pathway for the majority of the upper aerodigestive tract. Level III follows the carotid sheath and space posterior to the SCM from the hyoid bone to the cricoid and receives efferent lymph drainage from level II. Level IV continues to follow the same jugular chain to the level of the clavicle. Level V contains the posterior triangle of the neck, boarded by the trapezius posteriorly, the SCM anteriorly, and the clavicle inferiorly and is at particular risk for nasopharyngeal primaries. Level VI are the prelaryngeal lymph nodes (Delphian nodes), which extend from the inferior edge of the thyroid cartilage to the sternal notch, bounded laterally by the sternal heads of the SCM. Level VI is at risk in laryngeal cancers with subglottic or transglottic extension and for hypopharyngeal cancers with esophageal extension.[39]

In addition, there are two other regions not included in this level classification that are worthy of consideration. Just superior to level II, following the carotid sheath to the skull base are the junctional or retrostyloid nodes, which may be at risk when there is ipsilateral nodal disease. Medial to these nodes and to level II lie the retropharygeal nodes (or nodes of Rouviere), which lie in the regions anterior to the prevertebral fascia, which in turn surrounds the longus capitis and the longus colli muscles. The retropharyngeal nodes extend superiorly to the skull base and inferiorly to the hyoid bone and are at risk of cancers arising from the nasopharynx, posterior pharyngeal wall, and the pyriform sinus.[40]

The Oral Cavity

The oral cavity encompasses three major subsites: the oral tongue, the floor of mouth, and the buccal mucosa. Carcinomas originating from the oral tongue have potential to spread locally through the intrinsic and extrinsic muscles of the tongue, inferiorly to the floor of mouth, and posteriorly to the anterior tonsillar pillar. For the floor of mouth, the genioglossus, geniohyoid, and root muscles of the tongue are at risk for local disease spread, as well as levels IA and IB of the neck, laterally to the alveolar ridge and mandible. Tumors of the buccal mucosa may extend superiorly to the infratemporal fossa, inferiorly to the submandibular region, anteriorly to the lip commissure, and posteriorly to the retromolar trigone.[40]

The Oropharynx

The oropharynx anteriorly is bounded by the base of tongue, laterally by the tonsils, superiorly by the soft palate, and posteriorly by the posterior pharynx. Tumors arising from the base of tongue are often difficult to assess for extent of disease; therefore, the entire base of tongue, proximal oral tongue, and vallecula are at risk for subclinical disease. MRI may aid in delineation of the gross tumor volume for this site.[41] Tonsillar cancers may involve the base of tongue, palate, and buccal mucosa, although in locally advanced cases, they may also involve the nasopharynx, parapharyngeal space, and pterygoid muscles. Soft palate tumors may extend laterally to the tonsillar pillars and superiorly to the pterygopalatine fossa.

Nasopharynx, Oropharynx, and Hypopharynx

The nasopharynx is bounded superiorly and posteriorly by the sphenoid sinus, clivus, and the prevertebral fascia of C1 and C2. The parapharyngeal space lies laterally to the nasopharynx, which in turn is bounded laterally by the medial pterygoid muscle. The parapharyngeal space offers few anatomic barriers for the direct invasion of tumors superiorly and laterally to the base of skull, resulting in cranial nerve deficits as noted above. The eustachian tube empties into the nasopharynx at the torus tubarius; just posterior to the torus is the pharyngeal recess (or fossa of Rosenmüller), a fold of mucosa that is a frequent site for primary malignancies of this region.

Carcinoma arising from the posterior and lateral pharyngeal walls may spread superiorly to the nasopharynx and inferiorly to the hypopharynx. Similarly, primaries of the hypopharynx may spread superiorly through the oropharynx and nasopharynx. Malignancies of the pyriform sinus may also place the ipsilateral larynx at risk.

Larynx

The larynx is subdivided into three anatomic regions: the supraglottis (containing the epiglottis, the arytenoid and aryepiglottic folds, and the ventricular bands or false cords), the glottis (a 1-cm plane extending inferiorly from the lateral margin of the ventricle, including the true vocal cords and commissures), and the subglottis (from the inferior border of the glottis to the inferior aspect of the cricoid). The true cords have essentially no lymphatic drainage, allowing for focal treatment of a limited primary tumor without elective nodal treatment. In contrast, the supraglottic larynx has a rich and bilateral lymphatic system, requiring either dissection or elective nodal radiotherapy for even early primary tumors. The subglottis is a rare site of primary tumors and may invade locally into soft tissue as well as metastasize to laryngeal and tracheal lymphatics.[42]

Oncologic Imaging

For cancer of the head and neck, staging relies on careful physical examination, fiberoptic and direct laryngoscopy, directed biopsies, and integration of imaging modalities. Contrast-enhanced CT is the standard imaging modality for carcinomas of the head and neck region (Fig. 30.5). MRI may be a superior imaging modality for evaluating the extent of primary tumors of the oral cavity, oropharynx, and nasopharynx.[43] Novel approaches with MRI have shown promise in evaluating tumor responses to treatment by measuring physiologic changes within the tumor. Dynamic contrast-enhanced MRI may give insight into the vascular permeability (k-trans) in the tumor microenvironment; k-trans was found to be significantly higher in complete responders to concurrent chemoradiation therapy in one series.[44] Diffusion-weighted MRI may also provide information about the cellularity of a tumor mass or involved lymph node; an increase in the apparent diffusion coefficient (corresponding to a decrease in cellularity) during chemoradiation has been correlated with improved 2-year local control in another series.[45]

FDG-PET imaging for head and neck cancer has been useful as an adjunct to MRI and CT, particularly in clarifying the significance of intermediate lesions on MRI or CT. In one series, the addition of FDG-PET imaging improved the accuracy of tumor delineation from 40% to 70% with MRI or CT alone to 97% to 100%, altering the management of 23% of the patient under study.[46] Another series found FDG-PET to have a sensitivity of 88% in determining the primary tumor and a sensitivity of 82% and specificity of 100% for lymph node metastases.[47] However, in initial staging, no noninvasive imaging modality has a high enough negative predictive value to forgo appropriate

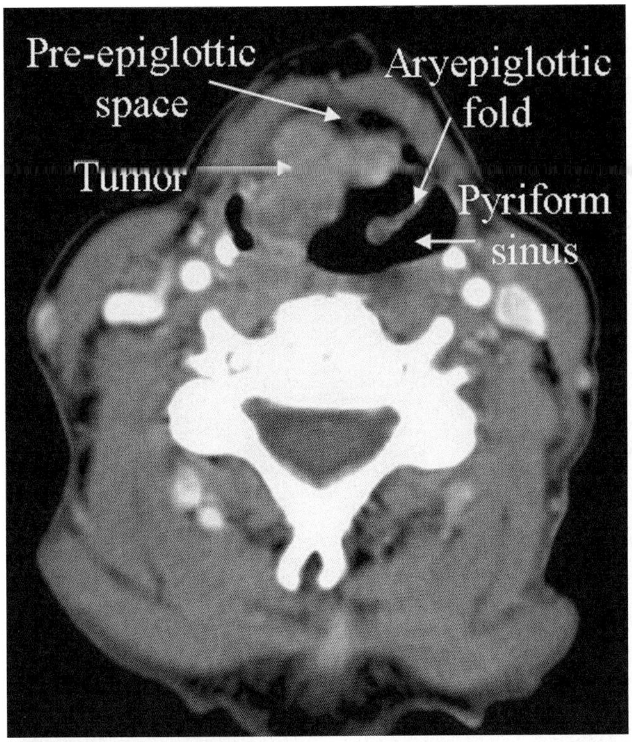

FIGURE 30.5. Axial computed tomography image demonstrating a squamous cell carcinoma involving the right aryepiglottic fold with anterior extension into the pre-epiglottic space.

dissection or elective nodal irradiation when the characteristics of the primary tumor suggest a significant risk of spread. That is in contrast to the value of FDG-PET after chemoradiation for the detection of residual nodal disease. The sensitivity for detection of persistent disease was 96% with a specificity of 72% in a posttreatment series, with a negative predictive value in some series as high as 99%, allowing for the abandonment of routine posttreatment neck dissections in patients with a complete clinical and PET response.[48,49] Novel PET tracers such as Cu64-ATSM and F18-misonidasole, designed to evaluate hypoxia within the tumor, may also prove to be clinically useful.[50]

THE BRACHIAL PLEXUS

Oncologic Anatomy

The brachial plexus originates from the primary rami of the C5 through the T1 vertebral levels and joins to form three nerve trunks (upper, middle, and lower) in the neck. These trunks divide as they course beneath the clavicle, forming three cords (lateral, medial, and posterior) in close approximation to the axillary artery, posterior to the pectoralis minor. The cords then form the three primary terminal nerves for the arm (the median, ulnar, and radial nerves) as well as the musculocutaneous nerve. These peripheral nerves are of particular importance due to the significant morbidity associated with injury, either from tumor invasion or from treatment-related toxicity. As the plexus traverses the neck and axilla, it is of particular relevance when treating tumors of the head and neck, upper thorax, and breast.

Oncologic Imaging

Identifying the brachial plexus is difficult on CT imaging and may be most directly visualized on MRI.[51] However, one may accurately contour the position of the trunks, divisions, and cords on noncontrast CT imaging based on bony, muscular, and vascular landmarks.[52] The method put forward by Hall et al.[52] begins contouring at the origination of the vertebral foramina of C5 through T1. The anterior and middle scalene muscles are then identified, with the trunks lying in the space between these muscles. The middle scalene will end at the superior aspect of the first rib just as the divisions of the plexus will be joining with the axillary artery as a neurovascular bundle. The artery then can be followed laterally as a surrogate for the remainder of the cords into the upper arm. Of interest to breast treatment, the course of the plexus will be brought superior and lateral with the upper arm with abduction, though still constrained by its course underneath the clavicle (Fig. 30.6).

THE THORAX

Oncologic Anatomy

The thorax consists of the superior part of the trunk and contains several important structures, including the heart, lungs, esophagus, and pleura. Primary tumors of the heart are extremely rare. On the other hand, lung cancer is the leading cause of cancer mortality in the United States, and the incidence of esophageal carcinoma is rising. Other common malignancies that arise in the thorax include malignant pleural mesothelioma, thymic malignancies, and malignant lymphomas.

There are many clinically relevant anatomical issues when evaluating patients with cancers of the thorax. These include (a) lobe-specific patterns of lymphatic spread, (b) the complex anatomy surrounding the lung apex, (c) the extent of the pleural space, (d) esophageal landmarks, and (e) thymic architecture.

Patterns of Lymphatic Spread

Lung malignancies frequently metastasize to regional lymph nodes. A basic understanding of mediastinal lymph node stations and lobe-specific lymphatic spread is helpful when evaluating and planning treatment for patients with lung cancer. The mediastinal nodes are a complex system, and it is challenging to predict where lymph node metastases will develop. However, these basic patterns provide a framework for customizing local treatment approaches (surgery and radiation therapy).

Both anatomical and clinical studies have shown that bronchogenic tumors frequently spread directly into mediastinal lymph nodes, bypassing intrapulmonary and hilar lymph nodes. This phenomenon appears to occur more frequently for upper lobe tumors.[53] For right-sided tumors, these pathways most frequently lead to ipsilateral paratracheal and subcarinal lymph node stations. For left-sided tumors, direct spread to anterior mediastinal lymph node stations (prevascular, para-aortic, and anterior-posterior window) is more common than to other mediastinal nodal stations. Second, right lung segments drain predominantly into the ipsilateral mediastinum. Conversely, left lung tumors commonly spread to both sides of the mediastinum,[54,55] especially left lower lobe tumors. Third, direct passageways to the supraclavicular fossa exist but are rare. Clinically, supraclavicular failures are uncommon and are usually associated with failure in upper paratracheal lymph node stations.[56] Fourth, most clinical studies have shown that subcarinal lymph nodes are frequently involved by both upper and lower lobe tumors.

The Superior Sulcus

The superior sulcus of the lung is surrounded by multiple critical structures. The subclavian artery and vein pass anterior to the lung apex, the brachial plexus and its branches cross over the apex of the lung toward the arm, and the stellate ganglia lie posteriorly alongside the exiting nerve roots of the lower cervical and upper thoracic spine. Other structures that can be involved by superior sulcus tumors are the vertebral bodies, trachea, and esophagus. Patients with superior sulcus tumors present with a variety of presentations (arm edema, arm

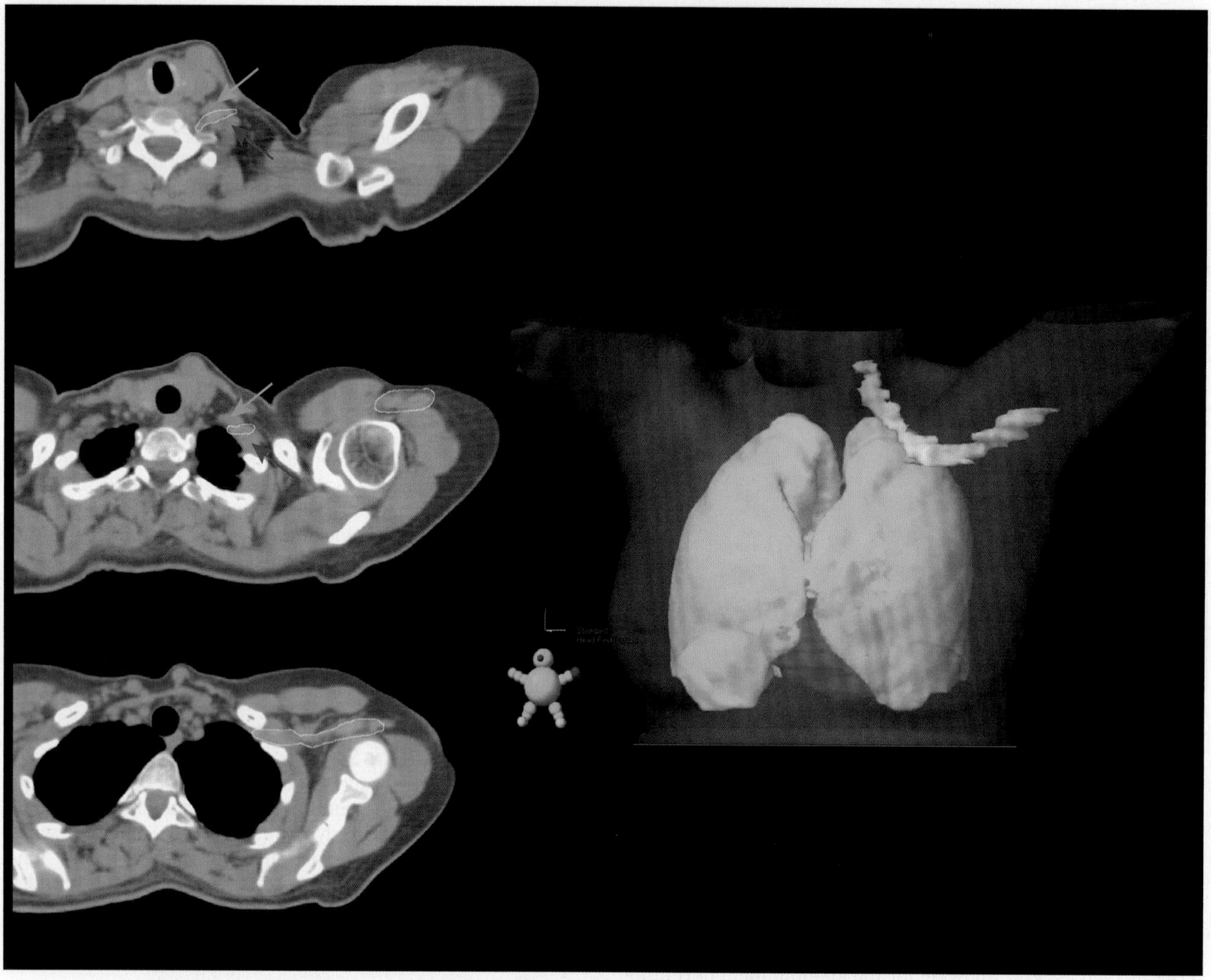

FIGURE 30.6. The brachial plexus (*yellow contour*) is delineated on axial computed tomography images on a woman undergoing treatment to the left breast. The anterior scalene (*green arrow*) and middle scalene (*red arrow*) are identified. The brachial plexus is delineated in the space between these muscles, originating at the C5-T1 roots and continuing to the axillary neurovascular bundle. The course of the plexus is contoured more distally than clinically necessary to emphasize the course and location when the arm is abducted.

weakness, and sensory deficits or Horner syndrome) related to the local extent of their disease.

The Pleura

The lungs are enclosed within a pleural sac. The visceral pleura is adherent to all of the surfaces of the lung, including the individual lobes where the pleura extends into the fissures. The parietal pleura is adherent to the thoracic wall, mediastinum, and diaphragm. The pleural recesses are potential spaces where portions of opposed parietal pleura are in contact during quiet respiration (Fig. 30.7). The inferior extension of the costodiaphragmatic recess can be easily underestimated, as can the medial extent of the costomediastinal recess (see Fig. 30.7). The inferior aspect of the costodiaphragmatic recess often extends to the level of the midkidney. The posteromedial extent of the pleura often wraps anteriorly over the descending aorta.

Malignant mesothelioma is a rare pleural neoplasm associated with prior asbestos exposure. Pathologically, it can be categorized into epithelial, sarcomatoid, and mixed histologic subtypes. Mesothelioma initially involves the pleura and grows by contiguous spread from the pleural space into the lung, chest wall, mediastinum, pericardium, and diaphragm. The extent of the pleural spaces has implications for postoperative radiation target volumes (Fig. 30.8).

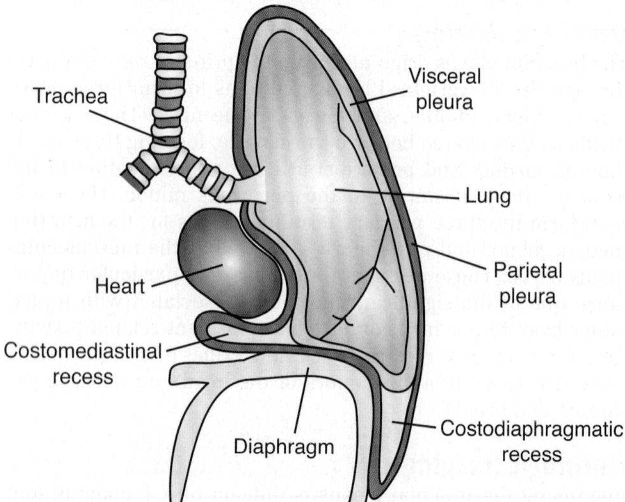

FIGURE 30.7. The extent of the pleura is illustrated. Note the inferior extension of the costodiaphragmatic recess and the medial extension of the costomediastinal recesses. (Courtesy of the University of Bristol, Department of Anatomy.)

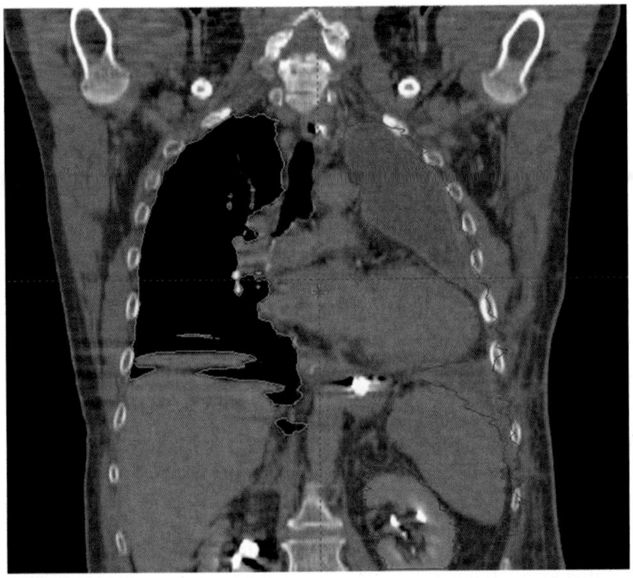

FIGURE 30.8. Digitally reconstructed coronal image from a treatment planning computed tomography scan illustrating the inferior extent of the costodiaphragmatic recess, which extends to the level of the midkidney. The patient had previously undergone an extrapleural pneumonectomy at which time metallic clips were placed, demarcating the inferior extent of the recess. The clinical target volume is illustrated in *red*.

TABLE 30.5 "ACCURACY" OF COMPUTED TOMOGRAPHY AND POSITRON EMISSION TOMOGRAPHY FOR MEDIASTINAL STAGING OF NON–SMALL CELL LUNG CANCER

End Point	*Toloza et al. (153)*	*Gould et al. (154)*	*Dwamena et al. (155)*	*Darling et al. (156) (%)*	*Bille et al. (157) (%)*
Computed Tomography (CT)					
Sensitivity	0.57	0.61	0.60		
Specificity	0.82	0.79	0.77		
Positive predictive value	0.56		0.50		
Negative predictive value	0.83		0.85		
Positron Emission Tomography (PET)					
Sensitivity	0.84	0.85	0.79		
Specificity	0.89	0.90	0.91		
Positive predictive value	0.79		0.90		
Negative predictive value	0.93		0.93		
Positron Emission Tomography/Computed Tomography (PET/CT)					
Sensitivity				70	54
Specificity				94	92
Positive predictive value				64	74
Negative predictive value				95	82

Esophageal Anatomy

The esophagus extends from the cricopharyngeus muscle at the level of the cricoid cartilage to the gastroesophageal junction in the abdomen. The cervical esophagus extends from the cricopharyngeus muscle (approximately15 cm from the incisors) to the level of the thoracic inlet (approximately 18 cm from the incisors). The thoracic esophagus extends from the thoracic inlet to the diaphragm and is sometimes divided into upper, middle, and lower sections. The carina is located at approximately 25 cm from the incisors and the gastroesophageal junction is located at approximately 40 cm. These general numbers are helpful when planning radiation fields based on staging studies that include endoscopy, EUS, and PET.

Thymus Architecture

The thymus is an encapsulated, bilobed gland situated in the superior anterior mediastinum and is involved in adaptive immunity. Although prominent in size during infancy and early childhood, it begins to involute during adolescence. The thymus decreases significantly in size in most patients after administration of chemotherapy, but typically regrows during the recovery phase, sometimes to a larger size than at baseline.[57]

The thymus gland is composed of both lymphocytes and epithelial cells. Thymic neoplasms are a common cause of anterior mediastinal masses and include both benign and malignant pathologies, including thymomas from epithelial cells and leukemias or lymphomas from lymphocytes.

Thymomas are the second most common primary mediastinal neoplasm in adults following lymphoma and are classified on a histologic spectrum from benign encapsulated thymoma to malignant thymic carcinoma. Once thymomas extend through the capsule, they can invade other regional structures, including the lungs and great vessels, sometimes rendering them inoperable. The thymus gland lies within the pleural envelope. The most common pattern of spread is within the pleural and pericardial spaces. Lymphatic and hematogenous metastases are rare.

Oncologic Imaging

Non–Small Cell Lung Cancer

Treatment decisions are often predicated on the status of the mediastinum in patients with operable non–small cell lung cancer (NSCLC). Patients without mediastinal disease generally proceed directly to resection, while those with mediastinal spread often receive induction therapy or definitive chemoradiotherapy. The standard noninvasive staging tool has been CT. In general, the sensitivity and specificity of CT is less than optimal[58–60] (Table 30.5). Thus, mediastinoscopy is often utilized to pathologically stage the mediastinum. Mediastinoscopy is associated with a low rate of morbidity. Nevertheless, if noninvasive studies proved highly accurate, this procedure might be avoided in some patients.

Numerous studies and meta-analyses[58–62] have assessed the ability of CT, PET, and integrated PET-CT to accurately stage the mediastinum in patients with NSCLC (see Table 30.5). Although significant heterogeneity exists among the individual studies, several conclusions can be drawn. First, the positive predictive value of CT is poor (around 50%). PET and PET-CT is somewhat better (80% to 90%). Still, 10% to 20% of patients with PET abnormalities in the mediastinum will have no evidence of disease at mediastinoscopy, although insufficient sampling may be explanatory in some cases. Therefore, many still advocate mediastinoscopy in the setting of a positive PET. The negative predictive value of PET and PET-CT appears to be better, especially when there are no enlarged lymph nodes visible on CT.[63] Nonetheless, most guidelines recommend mediastinoscopy prior to resection given the inherent limitations of PET.

Presently, pathology is considered the gold standard in studies that assess the accuracy of imaging. In a recent analysis in patients who had surgery for NSCLC with negative mediastinal nodes by pathology, patients with abnormalities in the mediastinal nodes on preoperative PET had worse disease outcomes than those with a negative PET in the mediastinum.[64] Thus, PET may have predictive value beyond the information provided by histology.

Localization of the esophagus is important during treatment planning of lung cancer. The esophagus is often well visualized on CT. However, its course can be tortuous and its exact location is often uncertain. Having the patient swallow dilute contrast during the planning CT can assist in localization of the esophagus. The heart and spinal canal (as a surrogate for the spinal cord) are also well seen on CT. The substructures of

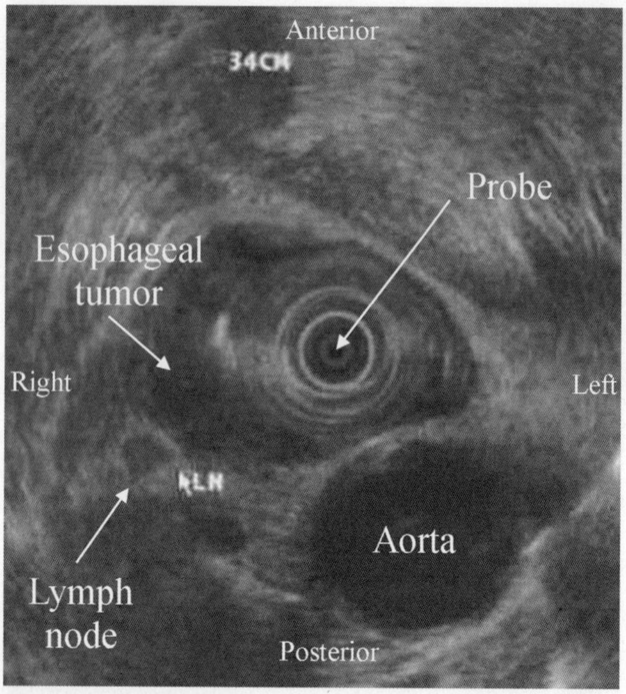

FIGURE 30.9. Endoscopic ultrasound image demonstrating a T3 esophageal tumor with an abnormal peritumoral lymph node. (Image courtesy of Dr. Frank Gress.)

the heart, however, are often challenging to define on CT. If one were to try to preferentially spare or consider the dose to cardiac substructures, an MRI or nuclear medicine cardiac image might provide additional information.

Esophageal Carcinoma

The most commonly used staging tools for esophageal carcinoma are barium swallow, EUS, CT, and PET. EUS, as previously discussed, is the most accurate modality to assess depth of invasion (T stage) but is less accurate in assessing nodal involvement (N stage) (Fig. 30.9). The ability to perform fine-needle aspiration biopsies of suspicious nodes, primarily disease in the celiac axis, has increased the ability of EUS to stage regional nodes. The reported accuracy of EUS for T and N stage is approximately 85% to 90% and 75%, respectively.[65,66] CT is primarily used to assess for metastatic disease. It is fairly unreliable in predicting T or N stage. The optimal role of PET in esophageal cancer staging is undefined, but it is generally used to evaluate for local or regional nodal disease and distant metastases. However, the sensitivity of PET for local or regional nodal disease does not appear to be superior to EUS.[67] PET may be most helpful in detecting distant metastases and differentiating patients who have residual disease after neoadjuvant chemoradiotherapy, requiring surgical resection, from those who are complete responders and may be spared the morbidity of surgery.[68]

Mesothelioma

CT best evaluates suspected mesothelioma for initial diagnosis and surgical planning. The characteristic CT appearance is focal or diffuse nodular pleural thickening, which demonstrates enhancement postcontrast administration.[69] CT is better than MRI at depicting the extent of disease; however, neither modality is particularly sensitive at detecting diaphragmatic or pericardial invasion unless it is extensive. PET is often performed for staging to detect distant and nodal metastases. However, it can also be helpful in establishing the initial diagnosis when CT findings are subtle, as even small foci of disease are typically highly FDG avid.

Superior Sulcus

Imaging plays a crucial role in the diagnosis and staging of superior sulcus tumors. Although radiographs are commonly the initial study to identify an abnormality at the lung apex, the precise location, extent of invasion, and assessment of resectability are best performed by a combination of CT, MRI, and PET. CT is best to define the primary tumor and detect rib or vertebral body invasion. CT may also identify suspicious pulmonary nodules that may be below the threshold for PET detection. Contrast-enhanced MRI using T1-weighted sequences is best for determining resectability by assessing the brachial plexus.[70] The primary role of PET is to identify distant and nodal metastases.

Superior sulcus tumors are staged according to the American Joint Commission on Cancer (AJCC) guidelines for staging of NSCLC and are classified as at least stage IIB disease due to direct invasion of the chest wall.[71] It is important to note that involvement of the brachial plexus or subclavian vessels is not part of the AJCC staging classification. Superior sulcus tumors, by definition, invade the chest wall; rib destruction and involvement of the lower brachial plexus roots (C8, T1) is considered T3 disease, whereas invasion of brachial plexus roots C5-7, the esophagus, vertebral body, or subclavian vessels constitutes T4 disease. Contraindications to surgery include invasion of brachial plexus roots or trunks above T1, invasion of >50% of a vertebral body, invasion of the esophagus or trachea and mediastinal (N2) or contralateral supraclavicular (N3) nodes; therefore, some T4-designated tumors may still be resectable, again highlighting the importance of accurate imaging.

Thymic Malignancy

Thymic neoplasms often go undetected until they are quite large and become symptomatic, at which time they may be depicted as a mediastinal mass on chest radiography. Contrast-enhanced CT is best for characterizing thymomas and detecting local invasion. High-grade tumors tend to be larger in size, have irregular margins, enhance heterogeneously, and have regions of necrosis; mediastinal lymphadenopathy may also be present. Direct invasion into the pleura, pericardium, and vessels is often difficult to detect by CT unless extensive. A preserved fat plane between tumor and adjacent structures is a negative predictor of invasion; however, this finding has poor positive predictive value.[72] Therefore, mere contiguity of tumor with a structure or loss of normal anatomic planes is not sufficient to preclude surgical resection.

THE BREAST

Oncologic Anatomy

Breasts are present in both males and females, although they are only well developed in the latter with the onset of puberty. In the male, generally only a few ducts are present, which nonetheless can rarely develop into malignancy, particularly in the context of *BRCA2* mutations.[73] In the female, the breast originates from a roughly circular base or bed extending from the lateral border of the sternum to the midaxillary line from medial to lateral, and from the second through sixth ribs superior to inferior. The upper outer quadrant extends along the pectoralis major toward the axilla, forming the axillary tail of Spence. This is also the most frequent quadrant for primary breast cancer (approximately 40%), which may be simply due the additional breast tissue associated with the tail.[74] Just posterior to the breast is the retromammary space, consisting of loose connective tissue, allowing for movement on the breast on the chest wall. Two-thirds of the breast rests on the deep pectoral fascia, which lies over the pectoralis major; the remainder rests on the fascia of the serratus anterior.

The breast tissue consists of lactiferous ducts that each drain 15 to 20 mammary gland lobules, and it is these ducts

TABLE 30.6 RISK OF INTERNAL MAMMARY LYMPH NODE INVOLVEMENT BASED ON STATUS OF AXILLA AND LOCATION WITHIN THE BREAST

Scenario	*Livingston and Arlen (158) (%)*	*Urban and Marjani (159) (%)*	*Noguchi et al. (160) (%)*
Negative Axilla	*8*	*8*	*5*
Outer quadrant primary	5	10	ns
Medial/central primary	14	16	ns
Positive Axilla	*33*	*52*	*35*
Outer quadrant primary	23	43	ns
Medial/central primary	48	55	ns
1–3 + axillary nodes	ns	ns	20
≥4 + axillary nodes	ns	ns	52

ns, not stated.

that are the origin of the majority of both noninvasive (ductal carcinoma *in situ*) and invasive disease (invasive ductal carcinoma). The breast is then anchored to the skin by suspensory ligaments (or Cooper's ligaments) and interspersed with fat lobules. These ligamentous attachments to the skin become more prominent with breast edema or congestion due to tumor involving the dermal lymphatics, resulting in the characteristic appearance of peau d'orange.

The lymphatic drainage of the breast is primarily to the axilla, although the upper outer quadrant may drain to the intermediary intrapectoral nodes (or Rotter's nodes) lying between the pectoralis major and pectoralis minor muscles, and the inner quadrants may drain to the internal mammary nodes (IMN). The axilla is divided into three sections with relation to the pectoralis minor muscle; the nodes found inferolateral to the muscle are termed level I, those beneath the muscle are termed level II, and those medial to the muscle are level III. Level I and II are generally removed in a standard axillary dissection, while the level III and the subsequent infraclavicular and supraclavicular basins are generally not considered resectable and are the target of radiotherapy if the more proximal basins have disease.

In a study of the location of sentinel nodes from various breast quadrants, the majority of drainage in all breast quadrants was to the axilla, and isolated drainage to the IMN was very rare (<6% in any quadrant).[75] However, identification of an additional IMN sentinel was found in 10% to 50% of cases dependent on quadrant (the upper outer quadrant was lowest at 10%, and the lower inner quadrant was most frequent at 52%). In surgical series in which the IMNs were routinely dissected, the incidence of isolated IMN disease was limited to 5% to 15%.[76–78] The risk of involvement increased when the axilla was also involved (20% to 55%), dependent on the axillary disease burden and location of the involved quadrant of the breast (Table 30.6). When IMNs were involved, the majority were located in the first three intercostal interspaces (first interspace 80%, second 75%, third 40%, and fourth 5%).[77] That stated, irradiation of the IMN nodes is controversial, and randomized data have not confirmed a survival benefit to routine treatment, although the treatment is well tolerated with modern techniques.[79–81]

Oncologic Imaging

Mammography remains the preferred imaging modality for the diagnosis and follow-up of both invasive and noninvasive disease. Multiple randomized trials have shown that screening mammography reduces the risk of breast cancer mortality by 20% to 35% in women aged 50 to 69.[82–86] The efficacy of screening in younger women (aged 40 to 49) and elderly women (aged 70 or older) is less certain. Most published guidelines suggest initiating screening at age 40. Screening mammography includes two standard views of each breast: a craniocaudal (CC) view and a mediolateral oblique (MLO) view. These images are taken at approximately 45-degree angulation to each other (i.e., they are not orthogonal). Although the CC view is oriented in the long axis of the patient (i.e., superior/inferior), the MLO is oriented in the medial-superior/lateral-inferior direction. The MLO view increases visualization of the upper outer quadrant and tail of the breast, while the CC view ensures adequate visualization of the inferior and medial aspects of the breast. Additional views, such as spot compression, can be utilized to further evaluate suspicious lesions.

The majority of women (approximately 95%) with abnormalities on a screening mammogram do not have breast cancer; thus, the positive predictive value is low. Overall, the sensitivity of screening mammography is approximately 75% (i.e., 25% of women diagnosed with breast cancer have a history of a normal mammogram 12 to 24 months prior to diagnosis). Sensitivity and specificity vary widely depending on breast density; for fatty versus dense fibroglandular breasts, reported sensitivities are 87% versus 63%, while specificities are 92% versus 68%, respectively.[87–89] Furthermore, sensitivity and specificity differ between screen-film versus digital mammography, with digital systems generally having higher diagnostic accuracy in women with dense breast tissue compared to film mammography.[90]

Systematic interpretation and unambiguous reporting is important for any screening study. Given the prevalence of breast malignancy and its clinical implications, the Breast Imaging Reporting and Data System (BI-RADS) was developed and constitutes guidelines for standardized reporting and quality assurance of screening mammography within the United States (Table 30.7). Mammographers are ahead of their radiology colleagues in this regard as the BI-RADS system affords a clear unambiguous means of quantifying the "suspiciousness" of mammographic findings. Systems similar to BI-RADS would be helpful for other imaging modalities as a means to reduce the risks of misunderstanding and miscommunication between radiologists and other care providers.

Features of concern for malignancy at mammography include a focal mass, irregular borders, and microcalcifications. Spiculation can be due to invasion into, or reactive changes within, the surrounding breast parenchyma. However, spiculated masses can also be secondary to fat necrosis, postoperative scarring, or other nonmalignant processes. Calcifications

TABLE 30.7 BREAST IMAGING REPORTING AND DATA SYSTEM (BIRADS) CATEGORIES USED FOR MAMMOGRAPHY EXAMINATIONS AND RISK OF MALIGNANCY

Assessment Category	*Assessment*	*Definition*	*Risk of Malignancy*
0	Need additional imaging evaluation	A lesion is noted for which additional imaging is needed	n/a
1	Negative	Breasts appear normal	<0.1%
2	Benign finding	A negative mammogram result but the radiologist wishes to describe a finding	<0.1%
3	Probably benign finding; short-interval follow-up suggested	Lesion with a high probability of being benign	<2%
4	Suspicious abnormality–biopsy should be considered	A lesion is noted for which the radiologist has sufficient concern to recommend a biopsy	25%–50%
5	Highly suggestive of malignancy	A lesion is noted that has a high probability of being cancer	75%–99%

n/a, not available.

Adapted from Elmore JG, Armstrong K, Lehman CD, et al. Screening for breast cancer. *JAMA* 2005;293:1245–1256.

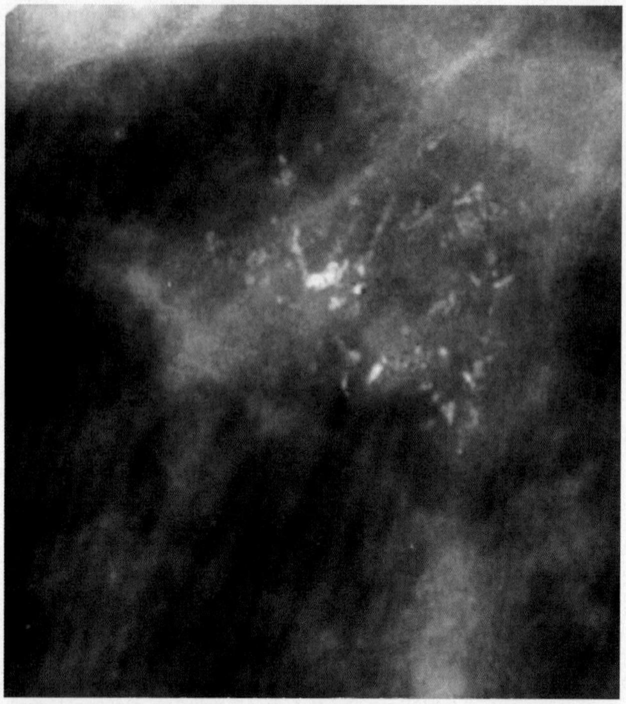

FIGURE 30.10. Clustered, pleomorphic calcifications visualized on mammography. The patient was found to have ductal carcinoma *in situ.*

associated with ductal carcinoma *in situ* or invasive carcinoma are typically pleomorphic (heterogeneous) in appearance and clustered in a localized area (Fig. 30.10). Linear, branching calcifications are suggestive of intraductal carcinoma. Round, well-circumscribed lesions, with or without coarse calcifications, are often benign.

Abnormalities on screening mammogram are generally followed with a diagnostic mammogram, in which supplemental and magnified views may be obtained to detect and characterize microcalcifications. Breast US is often performed to further characterize suspicious lesions, guide core biopsy, and assess regional lymph nodes. It is most helpful in differentiating fluid-filled cysts from solid tumors. MRI is not routinely recommended for upfront screening, except in patients with dense breast tissue and those at very high risk for primary breast malignancy, including those with *BRCA* mutations or women who received chest radiation therapy at a young age (typically <30 years old).[91] In addition to T1 and T2 lesion characteristics, patterns of MRI enhancement and washout kinetics are beneficial in evaluating concerning lesions. MRI can also be used for biopsy image guidance. After biopsy confirmation of disease, MRI has been examined in an attempt to better diagnose multifocal or contralateral disease preoperatively. One trial found contralateral cancers on MRI in 3% of their cohort, at the cost of performing a biopsy in 12%.[92] Preoperative MRI, however, did not improve the requirement for reoperation in a randomized UK trial.[93] The only clinically relevant outcome that routine use of preoperative MRI appears to have changed is that more women are having mastectomies as opposed to breast conservation.[94]

THE ABDOMEN

Oncologic Anatomy

Many diverse malignancies arise from abdominal structures. The most common are epithelial cancers of the stomach, pancreas, colon, liver, kidney, and biliary tract, including the gallbladder. Cancers of the kidney and colon are not often managed with radiation therapy and are not discussed further. Several relevant anatomical issues include (a) site-specific patterns of lymphatic spread for gastric cancer, (b) local disease extension of pancreatic cancer rendering a tumor inoperable, and (c) anatomy of the biliary tree.

Gastric Cancer: Patterns of Lymphatic Spread

The stomach is a distensible organ located in the left upper abdomen. It is classically divided into four parts: the gastroesophageal junction (cardia), fundus, body, and pylorus (antrum). Although the incidence of epithelial malignancies of the distal stomach has declined in Western countries over the past century, the incidence of malignancies of the gastroesophageal junction is increasing. Lymph node involvement is common in gastric cancer, likely due to the extensive submucosal and subserosal lymphatic networks. This rich lymphatic network places all lymph node regions within the abdomen at risk of harboring regional metastases, irrespective of the part of the stomach involved. However, some general patterns have been observed, which can facilitate rational radiation treatment planning for gastric cancer.

For tumors within the stomach, the perigastric region located along the greater and lesser curvatures of the stomach are typically the initial draining lymph node basin. The other primary lymph node regions are those along the three arterial branches of the celiac axis (common hepatic, left gastric, splenic). Secondary and tertiary drainage sites include lymph nodes in the hepatoduodenal, peripancreatic, para-aortic, mesenteric, and middle colic region.

A large surgical series from Japan demonstrated that the most common site of lymph node involvement was along the lesser and greater curvature (perigastrics), regardless of the part of the stomach involved (11% to 40%).[95] As expected, lymph node involvement around the cardia was unusual for distal stomach tumors (0% to 7%) but common for proximal tumors (13% to 31%). Similarly, infrapyloric lymph nodes were commonly involved for distant gastric cancers (49%) but rare for proximal tumors (3%). Other common sites of lymph node involvement included those along the left gastric artery (19% to 23%), common hepatic artery (7% to 25%, greatest for distal tumors), and celiac axis (8% to 13%). The risk of splenic hilar involvement has varied among surgical series but is generally highest for proximal tumors.[95–97] Based on these and other data, guidelines have been published outlining proposed radiation fields for gastric cancer based on site of involvement within the stomach.[98,99]

Pancreas

The pancreas is an elongated digestive gland posterior to the stomach. It is classically divided into four parts: the head, neck, body, and tail. The pancreatic head is nestled within the curve of the duodenum and this is where most pancreatic carcinomas arise. The pancreas has a rich lymphatic network and is in close proximity to multiple other abdominal organs and structures, making surgical resection difficult and negatively affecting long-term cure rates (resectability is the most important prognostic factor).

Biliary Tree

Hepatocytes within the liver secrete bile (an important agent for digestion) into bile canaliculi, the initial branches of the intrahepatic duct system. These canaliculi drain bile into larger and larger channels that eventually become the left and right hepatic ducts, draining bile from the left and right lobes of the liver, respectively. These exit the liver from the porta hepatis and join to form the common hepatic duct (approximately 4 cm in length). The cystic duct joins the common hepatic duct to form the common bile duct (approximately 10 cm in length). The common bile duct extends to, and empties into, the duodenum. It lies alongside the hepatic artery and portal vein.

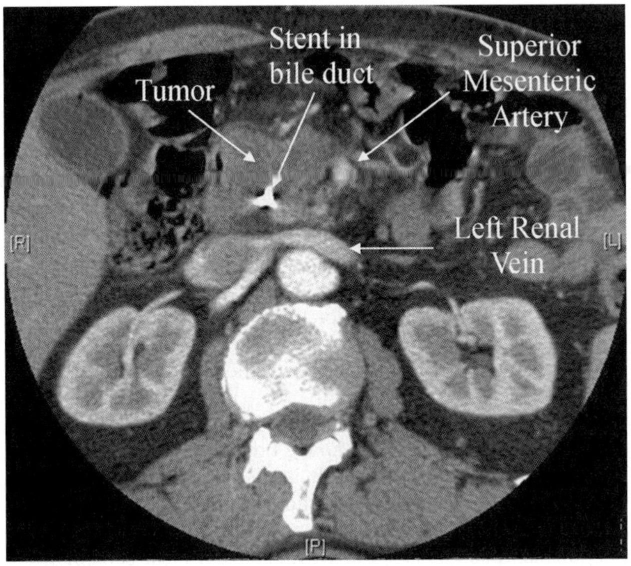

FIGURE 30.11. Axial computed tomography image demonstrating an adenocarcinoma of the pancreatic head with tumor abutting the superior mesenteric artery.

Biliary tract cancers include adenocarcinomas of the gallbladder and bile ducts, the latter referred to as cholangiocarcinomas. Cholangiocarcinomas include intrahepatic, perihilar, and distant extrahepatic biliary malignancies. Klatskin tumors are perihilar tumors that involve the bifurcation of the common hepatic duct. Both resectability and prognosis increase for more distally located biliary tumors.

Oncologic Imaging

Pancreatic Cancer

The pancreas can be imaged with US, CT, and MRI. MDCT with IV contrast and thin-section reconstructions optimize pancreatic tissue characterization and allow for detection of small tumors as well as vascular and ductal invasion. CT also defines the surgical anatomy to determine resectability and can detect regional and distant metastases (Fig. 30.11).

Adenocarcinoma of the pancreas most frequently arises in the head of the gland, to the right of the superior mesenteric or portal vein. It usually appears as a hypodense mass relative to the normally enhancing pancreas. Surgical resection typically provides the only chance of cure, and CT with thin-section reconstructions and IV contrast enhancement is an important technique to assess resectability. Encasement of the superior mesenteric artery (SMA) or celiac trunk defines an unresectable T4 tumor. On the other hand, the presence of a fat plane around the celiac trunk and SMA, along with a patent superior mesenteric or portal vein, defines potentially resectable disease. Borderline cases include those with tumor abutment on the SMA, severe unilateral SMV or portal vein impingement, or adjacent organ invasion. CT does not, however, detect small volume peritoneal or surface liver metastases that can be identified with laparoscopy. Oral contrast during radiation planning scans can be helpful to define the stomach and duodenum.

Hepatic Imaging

MDCT with IV contrast allows for morphologic characterization of the liver and biliary system. The administration of IV contrast is essential as many hepatic tumors are of similar attenuation as normal liver parenchyma and are not identifiable until central necrosis is present. MDCT with contrast is performed in both arterial and portal-venous phases of enhancement. This allows for detection of both early- and late-enhancing lesions, as well as characterization of enhancement patterns that can differentiate between benign and malignant disease. For example, hemangiomas are classically low attenuating on noncontrast images, have peripheral enhancement on the arterial phase, and demonstrate central filling on portal-venous phase imaging. Hepatocellular carcinoma is the most common primary hepatic malignancy and is characteristically hypervascular with pronounced enhancement throughout the solid tumor components on arterial phase images and diminished enhancement on the portal-venous phase. Contrast-enhanced CT can also identify invasion of tumor into the portal and hepatic veins and is frequently associated with portal vein thrombosis. As with other malignancies, PET is recommended for staging and identification of extrahepatic disease.

The liver is one of the most common sites of metastatic disease for many cancers. In patients with a known extrahepatic primary malignancy, evaluation of the liver is an important part of staging. Contrast-enhanced CT has a high sensitivity (73%) and specificity (96%) for detecting hepatic metastases.[100] MDCT of the liver for metastatic disease is typically performed with biphasic technique. Although most metastases are identified on the portal-venous phase, some hypervascular tumors (e.g., melanoma, renal cell carcinoma) may only be identified on arterial phase imaging. MRI has similar accuracy for the diagnosis of hepatic metastases as CT and may be performed in patients with an allergy to iodinated contrast media. However, CT outperforms MRI in detecting extrahepatic lesions, particularly within the lungs.

Biliary Imaging

US is typically the initial imaging study for patients with suspected biliary or pancreatic disease. The primary goals of evaluation include assessment for biliary and pancreatic ductal dilatation (abnormal is >3 mm), identify the presence of stones, characterize the gallbladder wall, and exclude a pancreatic head mass. US does not, however, image the entire pancreatic and biliary ductal system. In the presence of an US abnormality, further imaging is required.

Endoscopic retrograde cholangiopancreatography (ERCP) is a minimally invasive procedure that involves passing an endoscope into the duodenum and cannulating the main bile duct at the ampulla of Vater. Contrast is then infused to image both the biliary and pancreatic ductal system. In addition to being minimally invasive, ERCP carries risks associated with conscious sedation and can induce pancreatitis in 1.3% to 8.6% of patients.[101] Any evidence of biliary obstruction in the absence of calculi typically prompts further evaluation with cross-sectional imaging to exclude malignancy. ERCP can directly visualize ampullary carcinomas and permits tissue diagnosis achieved using needle aspiration, brush cytology, or forceps biopsy. ERCP may also provide palliation via stent placement in the setting of known obstructive biliary malignancy.

Magnetic resonance cholangiopancreatography (MRCP) is a noninvasive method of imaging the intra- and extrahepatic biliary and pancreatic ducts. MRCP does not require IV contrast; imaging relies heavily on T2-weighted sequences and high-resolution techniques resulting in the pancreatic and biliary ducts appearing very bright while surrounding tissues are dark in signal.[102] MRCP and ERCP have similar sensitivities and specificities in detecting ductal obstruction in the setting of malignancy, although MRCP is better at defining the anatomical extent and type of tumor involved (pancreatic vs. cholangiocarcinoma).[103,104]

Normal Tissue

During RT planning for cancers of the upper abdomen, consideration of the dose to the kidneys may be important. The kidneys are well visualized on CT. However, regional differences in kidney function cannot be readily assessed on CT. Nuclear medicine renal scans provide quantitative information regarding delivery of fluid into the kidneys from the bloodstream, concentration of wastes in the kidney, and excretion from the kidneys into the ureters and filling of the bladder. This information is useful when significant portions of one or both kidneys will be exposed to doses of RT expected to cause regional dysfunction. The liver, stomach, and small bowel are other organs whose location is often important to consider during RT planning. These are usually well seen on CT, although the use of oral contrast can be helpful.

THE PELVIC LYMPH NODES

Oncologic Anatomy

The lymphatic drainage of pelvic organs follows the iliac vessels throughout their branching within the pelvis. Most superiorly within the pelvis, the common iliac chains receive the majority of lymph drainage from intrapelvic organs, which then empty to the para-aortic chains superiorly in the region of the bifurcation of the abdominal aorta. The gonadal veins and arteries are notable exceptions to this orderly flow of lymph from the pelvis and are discussed separately below. Also of note, the rectum, sigmoid, and distal colon have a separate path for lymphatic metastasis via the inferior mesenteric chain to the preaortic basin.

The common iliac pathway receives lymphatic drainage from three primary routes: the external iliac chain, the internal iliac chain, and the presacral chain. The external iliac pathway begins at the point where the femoral vessels cross the inguinal ligament to become the external iliac chains, which courses more proximally to the common bifurcation. The internal iliac chain (also termed the hypogastric chain) is a more complex plexus, flowing back from the distal elaborations of the same artery. Just as these branches of the internal iliac vessels provide blood supply for the pelvic organs, the corresponding lymph node chains provide the majority of lymph drainage. The obturator nodes are part of the internal iliac system and may be found at the point in which the obturator vessels perforate the obturator internus muscle. Radiographically these nodes lay medial to the femoral head, just superior to the bony obturator foramen. The presacral chain is located just anterior to the sacrum and receives lymphatic drainage from the rectum, the cervix, and posterior vagina in the female and the prostate in the male.[4,94,105]

The testicles have an interesting lymphatic drainage that differs with laterality, essentially mirroring the differences in venous drainage of the two testicles. On the right, the testicle drains into the para-aortic nodes along the lower portion of the inferior vena cava at about the level of L3-L4 following the left testicular vein. On the left, the testicle drains to the renal hilar nodes following the left testicular vein.

Oncologic Imaging

CT is the current preferred means of identifying vessels within the pelvis and is an acceptable method of delineating the pelvic lymph node basins for elective radiotherapy. A 7-mm margin may be applied to the internal and external iliac vessels to arrive at a nodal CTV, with uninvolved bone, muscle (such as the psoas), and bowel excluded from the volume. The 7-mm margin was developed by investigators in London, who determined the minimum margin on CT visible vessels needed to cover 95% of all nodes identified using ultrasmall iron oxide particles (USPIO) as an MRI contrast agent.[106,107] Special care, however, should be taken to include visualized lymph nodes, even if they lie outside of this margin. One centimeter of soft tissue anterior to the sacrum, bridging between the common and internal nodal CTVs, should be added when presacral coverage is desired. The Radiation Therapy Oncology Group has release several atlases to aid the clinician in the contouring of pelvic CTVs that are available at its website. With 3D CT imaging, bony landmarks may not be the ideal determinant of block or multileaf collimator shapes when treating the pelvis.[108,109]

THE RECTUM

Oncologic Anatomy

The rectum is the final, straight portion of the large bowel, measuring approximately 12 cm in length, beginning at the transition from the sigmoid colon with the fusion of the tenia into the circumferential longitudinal muscle. It terminates with the ampulla, leading to the anal canal and dentate (or pectinate) line. Posteriorly, the entire rectum is extraperitoneal, whereas anteriorly, the peritoneal reflection occurs at approximately 7 to 9 cm from the anal verge in males at the posterior aspect of the bladder (superior to the prostate), and 5 to 8 cm from the verge in females, forming the rectouterine pouch (or pouch of Douglas). Below this point, the distal third of the rectum is entirely extraperitoneal.

The mesorectum is the supportive mesentery of the rectum, lying in the extraperitoneal space between the rectum anteriorly and sacrum posteriorly. It is of critical importance as a potential area of both direct and lymphatic spread of rectal cancers. High-quality total mesorectal excision with sharp dissection has been associated with excellent local control when compared to blunt dissections. However, this has not obviated the need for perioperative radiation therapy, as demonstrated by an increase in local failures if this is omitted.[110–112]

Oncologic Imaging

Endorectal US is the preferred nonsurgical staging tool for determining the T stage of rectal malignancy, with an overall accuracy of approximately 85% to 90%.[113] US is probably not needed in cases where there is a large mass with clear extension into the deep portions of the wall (or surrounding tissues) based on CT or examination. There is some tendency to overstage T2 lesions as T3 (beyond the muscularis propria); however, the accuracy remains superior to other imaging modalities.[114] The nodal staging accuracy is somewhat less at approximately 80%, which is comparable to results with either MRI or CT.[113] Accurate staging is critical when determining treatment for rectal cancer. Although surgery alone is sufficient for patients with stage I disease, surgery and chemoradiotherapy are indicated for patients with stage II or III tumors. The German Rectal Cancer Study Group showed that preoperative chemoradiotherapy is associated with improved local control with less acute and late toxicity than postoperative chemoradiotherapy.[115] In this study, 18% of patients in the immediate surgery group, believed to have stage II or III disease by EUS, were found to have stage I disease after surgical resection. Thus, further improvements in preoperative staging are needed to appropriately select patients for neoadjuvant therapy.

THE BLADDER AND URETHRA

Oncologic Anatomy

The bladder is a distensible muscular organ, which may be contained completely within the pelvis when empty or may extend far into the abdominal cavity with distention. The trigone is the posterior and inferior portion of the bladder, defined by the two ureteral orifices posteriorly and the urethral orifice inferiorly. The trigone remains fixed at the base with distension, while the superior most surface expands to accommodate urine. Due to this distensibility, this bladder is surrounded by loose connective tissue and fat. Anterior to the bladder this loose connective tissue is termed the space of Retzius, or retropubic space.

The urethra inferiorly has a short course to the introitus in the female, measuring approximately 4 to 5 cm in length. In the male, it is approximately 20 cm in length and traverses the prostate and penis to the meatus.

The lymphatic drainage of the base and posterior wall of the bladder may preferentially drain to the obturator and internal iliac basins via anterior pathways. In contrast, the external iliac chain may receive primary drainage from the lateral and superior bladder wall, and tumors arising from the bladder neck may also spread to the presacral nodal basins.[105]

Oncologic Imaging

Bladder tumors are often inadequately evaluated with conventional imaging techniques such as radiographic intravenous urograms and US. CT urography is useful for the diagnosis of superficial tumors but provides limited visualization of the depth of tumor invasion within the bladder wall. PET has limited utility in the primary diagnosis due to urinary excretion of FDG that can obscure bladder disease. Notwithstanding, PET is still performed as part of staging in order to identify distant metastases. Given the imaging limitations, cystoscopy with biopsy is the preferred method of confirming diagnosis and characterizing the primary tumor stage. Regional nodal involvement is best initially characterized by contrast-enhanced CT; however, the role of MRI is evolving, particularly for evaluation of lymph nodes utilizing novel contrast agents including USPIO.[116]

CERVIX, UTERUS, AND OVARIES

Oncologic Anatomy

The uterus lies between the bladder anteriorly and the rectum posteriorly, covered by a layer of peritoneum. Laterally lie the fallopian tubes and ovaries, which are anchored medially by the ovarian ligament (or utero-ovarian ligament) and laterally by the suspensory ligament of the ovary (or infundibulopelvic [IP] ligament). The ovarian arteries originate from the abdominal aorta, just inferior to the renal vessels, following a course anterior to the psoas on the left and crossing anterior to the inferior vena cava to the psoas on the right, both sides crossing anterior to the ureter and then crossing medially with the IP ligament to the ovaries. The fold of the peritoneum over the uterus continues laterally over these structures, forming the broad ligament. Similar to the testes, the right ovarian vein drains to the inferior vena cava, while the left ovary drains to the left renal vein.

The uterine corpus or body is the cephalad two-thirds of the organ and is lined internally by the endometrium, which varies in thickness by the menstrual cycle and by menopausal status. The middle muscular layer, the myometrium, is primarily smooth muscle. The final outer layer is the serosa or perimetrium and is continuous with the peritoneum. The caudal one-third of the organ is the uterine cervix, which consists of firm connective tissue, approximately one-half of which extends into the vagina. The intravaginal portion is lined by nonkeratinized squamous epithelium (the ectocervix), whereas the cervical canal is lined by columnar epithelium (the endocervix).

Lateral to the uterine cervix and corpus is the parametrium that caudally consists of the paracervical tissue, including the cardinal ligament, uterine artery and vein, and the ureter as it courses anteriorly to the bladder. This caudal portion of the parametrium is of importance for evaluation of lateral spread of cervical cancer and can be staged on physical examination by the bimanual examination and, perhaps more importantly, with the rectovaginal examination, where the examining rectal finger can palpate these structures. Cephalad to this, the parametrium continues as the broad ligament, terminating at the suspensory ligament of the ovary. Posteriorly the cervix is anchored to the sacrum via the uterosacral ligament, which classically attaches at the third sacral foramen, although recent MRI studies would suggest a fair amount of individual variation.[117]

Oncologic Imaging

MRI of the pelvis is the most useful modality outside of the physical examination to determine the extent of disease within the uterus and cervix with an accuracy of approximately 85%.[118–120] For endometrial carcinoma, T2- and postcontrast T1-weighted sequences are beneficial in staging, such as identifying the primary tumor, extent of invasion, and involvement of regional pelvic lymph nodes. In the setting of cervical cancer, T2-weighted sequences are often the most useful in determining the extent of disease and are preferred for MRI-guided brachytherapy.[121] US can be useful during intracavitary brachytherapy to ensure the proper placement of a uterine tandem.

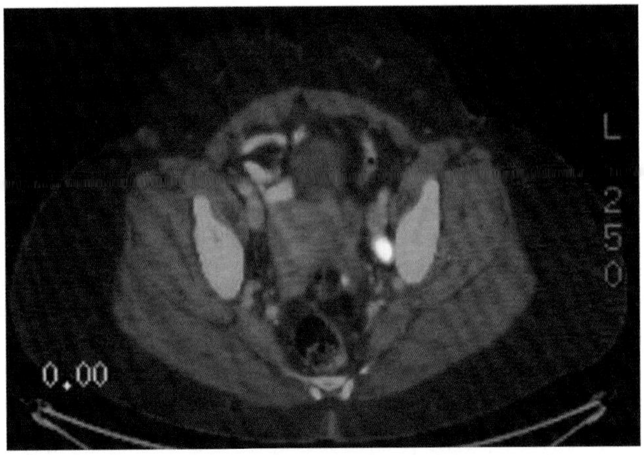

FIGURE 30.12. Positron emission tomography imaging of a patient with cervical cancer showing an 18-fluorodeoxyglucose-avid left external iliac lymph node.

PET-CT has been proven to be sensitive and specific in the evaluation of lymph nodes within the pelvic and para-aortic chains with squamous cell carcinoma of the cervix (sensitivity approximately 85%, and specificity 95% for para-aortic nodes), although it is less well studied in endometrial and other primary gynecologic sites[122] (Fig. 30.12). Investigators from Washington University have extensively studied FDG-PET in cervical cancer, showing that the initial maximum SUV of the primary tumor is predictive of response to treatment.[123] Additionally, they found that a complete metabolic response to treatment was highly predictive of progression free survival (PFS); at 3 years, with complete response, PFS was 78% versus 33% in partial responders and 0% with PET progression.[124] The prognostic significance of PET response to treatment has been confirmed by investigators in Melbourne.[125]

PROSTATE

Oncologic Anatomy

The prostate lies in the center of the male pelvis, with its widest portion, the base, in close approximation to the bladder neck superiorly, narrowing to the apex inferiorly, supported by the urogenital diaphragm (UGD). Posteriorly, the gland is closely related to the ampulla of the rectum. The seminal vesicles are located superior to the prostate and extend somewhat laterally and posteriorly and are immediately posterior to the posterior wall of the bladder. Anteriorly lies the retropubic space filled with fat.

Within the prostate five distinct zones exist: the peripheral zone, the central zone, the transitional zone, the periurethral glandular tissue, and the anterior fibromuscular stroma.[126] The peripheral zone accounts for the majority of the gland (70% of glandular tissue) as well as the majority of cancers (60% to 70%). The peripheral zone is located posteriorly and laterally within the gland. This zone is hyperintense on T2 MRI and care should be taken to include it when treatment planning with MRI. The central zone accounts for an additional 25% of glandular tissue and lies near the origin of the seminal vesicles, accounting for 10% of cancers. The transitional zone surrounds the urethra cephalad to the insertion of the ejaculatory duct, may hypertrophy with age, and is the origin of 10% to 20% of cancer within the prostate.

The Batson venous plexus is a series of valveless veins anterior to the vertebral bodies, which received drainage from the deep pelvic veins and prostate gland.[127,128] It has been postulated that due to the lack of valves, this may represent a pathway of spread for metastases and provide an anatomic basis for the propensity of prostate cancer to involve the lumbosacral vertebral bodies.

The T staging of prostate cancer remains based primarily on the physical examination, where the examining rectal finger may palpate the size and extent of discrete ridges and nodules within the gland. It is important to palpate and document the presence of the lateral sulci of the gland, as evidence of effacement is highly suggestive of extracapsular extension (ECE) of disease. The examiner should also attempt to palpate the base of the seminal vesicles, although this is not always possible given body habitus and individual anatomy.

Oncologic Imaging

Transrectal US is invaluable for guiding biopsies for diagnosis of disease; however, it has limited specificity and sensitivity (approximately 40% to 50%) for determination of seminal vesicle involvement and ECE. CT has similar limitations, as the prostate gland has similar attenuation characteristics as the anterior and lateral venous plexus, the inferior UGD, and the bladder wall superiorly. CT can determine suspicious pelvic nodes and is currently the standard for defining pelvic radiation target volumes, if indicated. If CT alone is used for definition of the prostate for treatment planning, the penile bulb may provide a useful reference point for ascertaining the apex of the gland, which lies approximately 15 to 18 mm superior to the bulb, although there is significant interpatient variation.[129] A retrograde urethrogram can be useful to identify the inferior aspect of the UGD and aid in the delineation of the apex approximately 12 to 15 mm superiorly.

MRI may be the optimal imaging modality for evaluation of the prostate itself and is an invaluable aid in treatment planning. As noted previously, the zonal anatomy of the prostate is only visible on T2-weighted imaging, and the apex can be clearly distinguished from the UGD and other neighboring structures (Fig. 30.13). The joint maximum sensitivity and specificity of determining extraprostatic disease on MRI is approximately 70%, although this may be improved with endorectal coils.[130,131] Due to the increased tissue contrast, planning based on MRI results in a reduction of interobserver variability and a reduction in the volume of the prostate contours.[132] In general, the prostate identified on CT is larger than that identified on MRI. Therefore, with MRI-based treatment planning, the accurate delineation of the GTV is more important (compared to CT where the GTV tends be slightly overestimated).

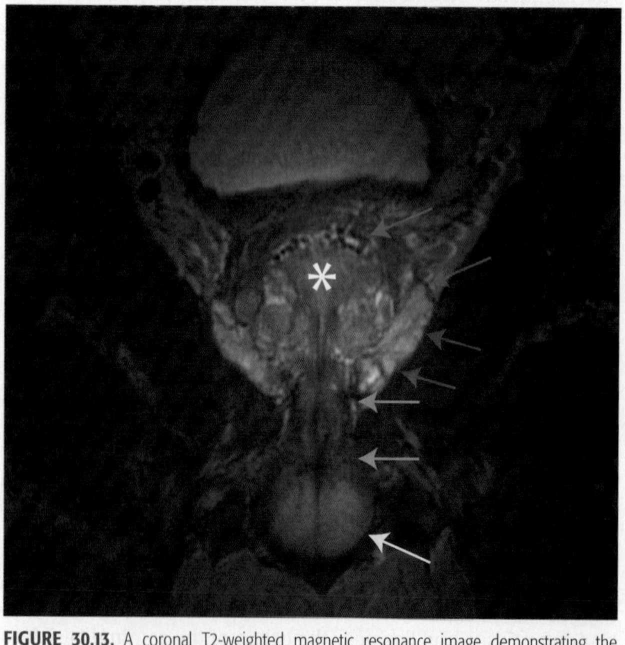

FIGURE 30.13. A coronal T2-weighted magnetic resonance image demonstrating the anatomy of the prostate. The regional anatomy is labeled as follows: the asterisk (*) is the central gland–a combination of the central zone and transitional zone; *red arrows* indicate the peripheral zone (PZ); *blue arrows* indicate the seminal vesicles (SV) and their insertion in the base; *green arrows* indicate the urogenital diaphragm (UGD); *yellow arrows* indicate the penile bulb (PB).

Many novel imaging modalities have been developed for prostate cancer but remain of uncertain utility in current practice. MRS has been explored to further define sites of disease within the prostate. However, the spatial resolution remains too low to accurately define regions for partial prostatic treatment.[133] Similarly, radiolabeled antibodies to the prostate specific membrane antigen are commercially available and may aid in the detection of recurrent disease, but specificity and the impact on clinical outcomes again remain unclear.[134] The use of lymphotrophic nanoparticle–enhanced MRI has also been explored for improved detection of involved lymph nodes with encouraging initial results.[135]

Radiolabeled antibodies to the prostate-specific membrane antigen may aid in initial staging of prostate cancer and the detection of recurrent disease. ProstaScint (Cytogen Corp, Princeton, NJ) imaging utilizes the radiolabeled monoclonal antibody indium-111 capromab pendetide, which is the most widely commercially available of the PSA-specific radiopharmaceuticals, to identify sites of local or metastatic disease. The use of ^{111}In-ProstaScint scans is generally indicated for newly diagnosed patients with intermediate or high Gleason score at risk of advanced disease and patients with suspected residual or recurrent disease following definitive treatment, typically in the setting of a rising PSA. One of the earliest multicenter trials with ProstaScint validated the imaging study for diagnosing lymph node involvement with specificity, sensitivity, accuracy, and positive predictive values of 86%, 75%, 81%, and 79%, respectively.[136] However, there is little consistency in available reported data, which has been attributed to high interobserver variability as the scans are difficult to interpret. ProstaScint single-photon emission computed tomography in conjunction with conventional CT or MRI has therefore been advocated to facilitate improved specificity by distinguishing sites of active disease from physiologic bone and vascular uptake.[137] ProstaScint is most commonly utilized to help distinguish patients with a localized recurrence after surgery from those with systemic progression, the former being appropriate candidates for salvage radiotherapy.[134] However, despite its potential utility, the precise role of ProstaScint and its impact on clinical outcomes remain unclear.

Prostate imaging and pathologic analyses can be somewhat discordant. The lesions seen on imaging can often appear focal. However, prostatectomy specimens usually demonstrate the microscopic presence of cancer in multiple regions of the gland. Thus, attempts to severely restrict the therapeutic radiation dose distribution to focal areas of the prostate need to be done with care.

The normal rectum and bladder are commonly avoided structures during pelvic RT, and their location relative to surrounding tissues can be readily determined on planning CT. The interface between the bladder and prostate can be challenging and may be improved with placement of contrast agents within the bladder.

THE LYMPHATIC SYSTEM

Oncologic Anatomy

The lymphatic system is a component of the circulatory system, and wherever arteries and veins pass, lymphatic vessels are also present (with the notable exceptions of the placenta and central nervous system). In the central nervous system, lymph is carried within perivascular lymph sheaths, as opposed to actual lymphatic vessels. The lymphatic system includes lymphatic vessels, lymph nodes, lymphatic organs such as the spleen, and the lymphocytes themselves. The lymphatic system is a loosely organized system but generally follows somewhat predictable paths. Small lymphatic vessels form within the tissues of the body, drain into one or more lymph nodes, and eventually drain into larger lymph trunks. These unite to form either the thoracic duct or right lymphatic duct, which empties into the venous system at the subclavian vein–internal jugular vein junction. The lymphatics are primarily involved in returning plasma from the interstitial space to the venous system, although they are also involved in absorption and transport of fat and in defense mechanisms. Radiation oncologists must become versed in an understanding of site-specific lymphatic spread, which is discussed at length within this chapter and elsewhere.

The primary tumors arising from the lymphatic system are leukemias and lymphomas. Leukemias are primarily managed with chemotherapy, although radiation therapy is often utilized in the setting of stem cell transplant (total body irradiation), central nervous system involvement (cranial or craniospinal irradiation), or in palliative settings. Lymphomas consist of multiple distinct entities that are often managed with radiation therapy.

Oncologic Imaging

Nodal Metastases

The accurate identification and characterization of lymph nodes have important diagnostic and prognostic implications in patients with both primary and secondary nodal disease. Prior to the advent of cross-sectional imaging, bipedal lymphangiography was the standard test for evaluating and staging nodal disease in the abdomen and pelvis. CT and MRI have supplanted lymphangiography in the morphologic assessment of nodal disease, which is further supplemented by the physiologic assessment offered by PET imaging. The utility of CT, MRI, and PET in the diagnosis of secondary nodal disease for various malignancies has been detailed earlier in this chapter.

Lymphoma

FDG PET-CT imaging plays an integral role in the management of both Hodgkin lymphoma (HL) and many non-Hodgkin lymphomas (NHL). Prior to PET, two nuclear medicine radionuclides—gallium-67 (Ga-67) and thallium-201 (Tl-201)—were routinely used in the staging of lymphoma. Activity on Ga-67 correlates with histopathologic grade, with high-grade lesions having more uptake. Tl-201, conversely, has avidity for low-grade but not high-grade lymphomas; therefore Tl-201 and Ga-67 scans were deemed complementary. However, the detection of abdominal disease is limited as both gallium and thallium are excreted into the bowel. Compared to Ga-67 scintigraphy, PET appears to have higher patient and site sensitivity.[138] However Ga-67 may be better at detecting certain indolent NHLs, specifically splenic marginal zone and small lymphocytic lymphomas, which are routinely not FDG avid.[139]

Numerous studies have demonstrated the value of PET for initial staging of lymphoma and assessment of response to treatment. A recent meta-analysis showed a median sensitivity of 90.3% and a median specificity of 91.1% for lymphoma staging with dedicated PET with a maximum accuracy of 87.8%.[140] In a review assessing combined PET-CT systems, the overall sensitivity and specificity for initial staging of NHL and HL was even higher.[141] Compared with CT alone, PET-CT staging often leads to up-staging or down-staging, with the former occurring in 15% to 30% of patients and the latter in 1% to 15% of patients.[142,143]

In addition to diagnosis and staging, PET is useful in monitoring initial treatment response. Several studies have shown that residual PET abnormalities after chemotherapy strongly predict for subsequent relapse, either with chemotherapy alone[144–146] or with combined modality therapy[147,148] (Fig. 30.14). Mikhaeel et al.[145] showed that posttreatment PET scans predicted outcome far better than posttreatment CT scans. Of 45 patients with aggressive NHL treated with chemotherapy, the relapse rate was 100% (9/9) for patients with residual FDG-avid disease versus 17% (4/36) for patients with negative posttreatment PET scans. Of these 45 patients, 33 also had posttreatment CT imaging. Only 41% of patients with abnormal CT imaging failed, while 25% of patients with negative CT scans eventually relapsed.

However, a negative PET after chemotherapy does not necessarily mean that all disease has been eradicated, simply that an excellent response to chemotherapy was achieved. This point was confirmed in a randomized trial in which patients with HL were randomized to observation or consolidation RT after achieving a PET compete response after chemotherapy.

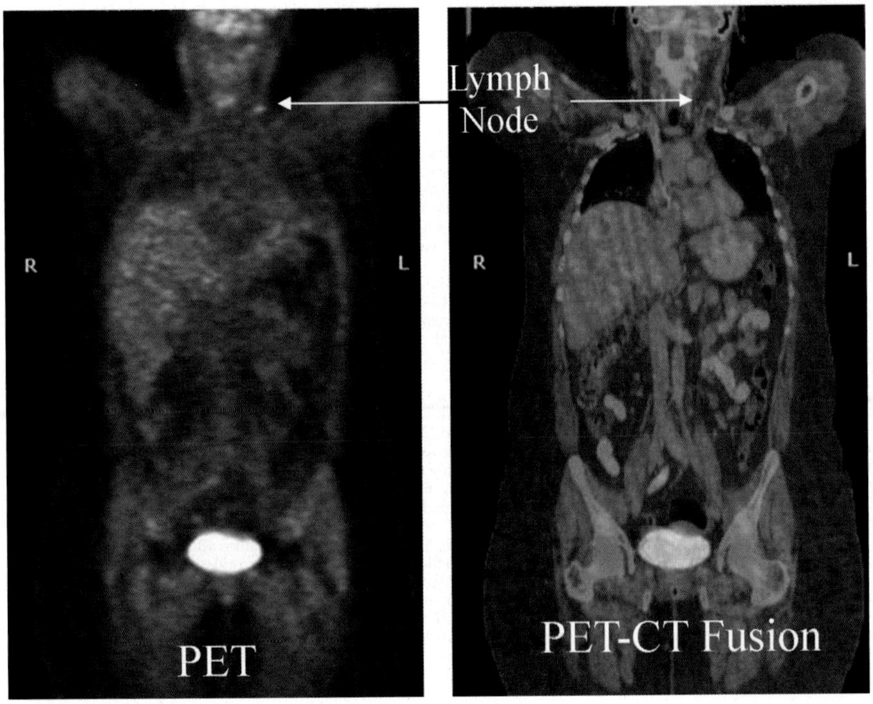

FIGURE 30.14. Postchemotherapy coronal positron emission tomography (PET) scan images of a patient with stage IVa Hodgkin's disease demonstrating a hypermetabolic left supraclavicular lymph node. The lymph node was <1 cm on computed tomography (CT) and would not be considered suspicious. Biopsy confirmed persistent disease. *Left:* PET image. *Right:* PET-CT fusion image. (Image courtesy of Dr. Edward Coleman.)

Even in the setting of a negative PET, consolidation RT still decreased the risk of recurrence.[149]

SUMMARY

The term *oncoanatomy* describes the fusion of clinical oncology and anatomy, for the betterment of both. The successful practice of radiation oncology requires a thorough understanding of anatomy. Likewise, the study of malignancy and observations regarding spread of malignant tumors aids in the understanding and instruction of anatomy. Radiation oncologists have a unique opportunity to assist in the instruction of anatomy. For most medical students, gross anatomy is an early first-year course before significant clinical experience is obtained. Over the ensuing years of medical school and residency, much of this knowledge is lost as it is not routinely applied during clinical practice. It is incumbent on those who seek advanced training in fields such as surgery, radiology, and radiation oncology to again become students of anatomy, as the successful practice of such disciplines requires an in-depth understanding of anatomical principles.

An oncoanatomy course has been described.[150,151] It consists of a monthly conference where the anatomy of a particular disease site is reviewed along with pertinent clinical implications. Following this didactic session, the presentation continues in the gross anatomy suite where anatomy faculty demonstrate on prosections. This course is attended by medical students, residents, and faculty members from multiple disciplines. The expertise of all involved contributes to a valuable educational environment.

REFERENCES

1. Gregoire V, et al. CT-based delineation of lymph node levels and related CTVs in the node-negative neck: DAHANCA, EORTC, GORTEC, NCIC,RTOG consensus guidelines. *Radiother Oncol* 2003;69:227–236.
2. Wijers OB, et al. A simplified CT-based definition of the lymph node levels in the node negative neck. *Radiother Oncol* 1999;52:35–42.
3. Chapet O, et al. CT-based definition of thoracic lymph node stations: an atlas from the University of Michigan. *Int J Radiat Oncol Biol Phys* 2005;63:170–178.
4. Myerson RJ, et al. Elective clinical target volumes for conformal therapy in anorectal cancer: a radiation therapy oncology group consensus panel contouring atlas. *Int J Radiat Oncol Biol Phys* 2009;74:824–830.
5. Pfeffer MR, et al. Orbital lymphoma: is it necessary to treat the entire orbit? *Int J Radiat Oncol Biol Phys* 2004;60:527–530.
6. Engels B, et al. Conformal arc radiotherapy for prostate cancer: increased biochemical failure in patients with distended rectum on the planning computed tomogram despite image guidance by implanted markers. *Int J Radiat Oncol Biol Phys* 2009;74:388–391.
7. Bettmann MA. Frequently asked questions: iodinated contrast agents. *Radiographics* 2004;24(Suppl 1):S3–S10.
8. Brenner DJ. Slowing the increase in the population dose resulting from CT scans. *Radiat Res* 2010;174:809–815.
9. Kuo PH, et al. Gadolinium-based MR contrast agents and nephrogenic systemic fibrosis. *Radiology* 2007;242:647–649.
10. Ingram M, Arregui ME. Endoscopic ultrasonography. *Surg Clin North Am* 2004;84:1035–1059.
11. Catalano MF, et al. Endosonographic features predictive of lymph node metastasis. *Gastrointest Endosc* 1994;40:442–446.
12. Lardinois D, et al. Staging of non-small-cell lung cancer with integrated positron-emission tomography and computed tomography. *N Engl J Med* 2003;348:2500–2507.
13. Wahl RL, et al. From RECIST to PERCIST: evolving considerations for PET response criteria in solid tumors. *J Nucl Med* 2009;50(Suppl 1):122S–150S.
14. Francis RJ, et al. Early prediction of response to chemotherapy and survival in malignant pleural mesothelioma using a novel semiautomated 3-dimensional volume-based analysis of serial 18F-FDG PET scans. *J Nucl Med* 2007;48:1449–1458.
15. Adams MC, et al. A systematic review of the factors affecting accuracy of SUV measurements. *AJR Am J Roentgenol* 2010;195:310–320.
16. Blake GM, et al. Quantitative studies of bone with the use of 18F-fluoride and 99mTc-methylene diphosphonate. *Semin Nucl Med* 2001;31:28–49.
17. Even-Sapir E. Imaging of malignant bone involvement by morphologic, scintigraphic, and hybrid modalities. *J Nucl Med* 2005;46:1356–1367.
18. Hamaoka T, et al. Bone imaging in metastatic breast cancer. *J Clin Oncol* 2004;22:2942–2953.
19. Therasse P, et al. New guidelines to evaluate the response to treatment in solid tumors. European Organization for Research and Treatment of Cancer, National Cancer Institute of the United States, National Cancer Institute of Canada. *J Natl Cancer Inst* 2000;92:205–216.
20. Gleave ME, et al. Ability of serum prostate-specific antigen levels to predict normal bone scans in patients with newly diagnosed prostate cancer. *Urology* 1996;47:708–712.
21. Kosuda S, et al. Can initial prostate specific antigen determinations eliminate the need for bone scans in patients with newly diagnosed prostate carcinoma? A multicenter retrospective study in Japan. *Cancer* 2002;94:964–972.
22. O'Sullivan JM, et al. Broadening the criteria for avoiding staging bone scans in prostate cancer: a retrospective study of patients at the Royal Marsden Hospital. *BJU Int* 2003;92:685–689.
23. Cheran SK, Herndon JE 2nd, Patz EF Jr. Comparison of whole-body FDG-PET to bone scan for detection of bone metastases in patients with a new diagnosis of lung cancer. *Lung Cancer* 2004;44:317–325.
24. Kawahara Y, et al. Dural congestion accompanying meningioma invasion into vessels: the dural tail sign. *Neuroradiology* 2001;43:462–465.
25. Nagele T, et al. The "dural tail" adjacent to meningiomas studied by dynamic contrast-enhanced MRI: a comparison with histopathology. *Neuroradiology* 1994;36:303–307.
26. Chamberlain MC. Neoplastic meningitis. *J Clin Oncol* 2005;23:3605–3613.
27. Johnson JD, Young B. Demographics of brain metastasis. *Neurosurg Clin North Am* 1996;7:337–344.
28. Delattre JY, et al. Distribution of brain metastases. *Arch Neurol* 1988;45:741–744.
29. Sze G, et al. Detection of brain metastases: comparison of contrast-enhanced MR with unenhanced MR and enhanced CT. *AJNR Am J Neuroradiol* 1990;11:785–791.
30. Sze G, et al. Comparison of single- and triple-dose contrast material in the MR screening of brain metastases. *AJNR Am J Neuroradiol* 1998;19:821–828.
31. Spence AM, et al. 18F-FDG PET of gliomas at delayed intervals: improved distinction between tumor and normal gray matter. *J Nucl Med* 2004;45:1653–1659.
32. Horky LL, et al. Dual phase FDG-PET imaging of brain metastases provides superior assessment of recurrence versus post-treatment necrosis. *J Neurooncol* 2011;103:137–146.
33. Lee BC, et al. MR recognition of supratentorial tumors. *AJNR Am J Neuroradiol* 1985;6:871–878.
34. Kelly PJ, et al. Imaging-based stereotaxic serial biopsies in untreated intracranial glial neoplasms. *J Neurosurg* 1987;66:865–874.
35. Howe FA, et al. Metabolic profiles of human brain tumors using quantitative in vivo 1H magnetic resonance spectroscopy. *Magn Reson Med* 2003;49:223–232.
36. Law M, et al. High-grade gliomas and solitary metastases: differentiation by using perfusion and proton spectroscopic MR imaging. *Radiology* 2002;222:715–721.
37. Barajas RF Jr, et al. Differentiation of recurrent glioblastoma multiforme from radiation necrosis after external beam radiation therapy with dynamic susceptibility-weighted contrast-enhanced perfusion MR imaging. *Radiology* 2009;253:486–496.
38. Som PM. Detection of metastasis in cervical lymph nodes: CT and MR criteria and differential diagnosis. *AJR Am J Roentgenol* 1992;158:961–969.
39. Harrison LB, Sessions RB, Hong WK. *Head and neck cancer: a multidisciplinary approach*, 3rd ed. Philadelphia: Lippincott Williams & Wilkins, 2009.
40. Eisbruch A, et al. Intensity-modulated radiation therapy for head and neck cancer: emphasis on the selection and delineation of the targets. *Semin Radiat Oncol* 2002;12:238–249.
41. Ahmed M, et al. The value of magnetic resonance imaging in target volume delineation of base of tongue tumours—a study using flexible surface coils. *Radiother Oncol* 2010;94:161–167.
42. Edge SB, et al. *AJCC cancer staging manual*, 7th ed. New York: Springer-Verlag, 2010.
43. Dammann F, et al. Rational diagnosis of squamous cell carcinoma of the head and neck region: comparative evaluation of CT, MRI, and 18FDG PET. *AJR Am J Roentgenol* 2005;184:1326–1331.
44. Kim S, et al. Prediction of response to chemoradiation therapy in squamous cell carcinomas of the head and neck using dynamic contrast-enhanced MR imaging. *AJNR Am J Neuroradiol* 2010;31:262–268.
45. Vandecaveye V, et al. Predictive value of diffusion-weighted magnetic resonance imaging during chemoradiotherapy for head and neck squamous cell carcinoma. *Eur Radiol* 2010;20:1703–1714.
46. Wong WL, et al. Validation and clinical application of computer-combined computed tomography and positron emission tomography with 2-[18F]fluoro-2-deoxy-D-glucose head and neck images. *Am J Surg* 1996;172:628–632.
47. Hannah A, et al. Evaluation of 18F-fluorodeoxyglucose positron emission tomography and computed tomography with histopathologic correlation in the initial staging of head and neck cancer. *Ann Surg* 2002;236:208–217.
48. Wong RJ, et al. Diagnostic and prognostic value of [(18)F]fluorodeoxyglucose positron emission tomography for recurrent head and neck squamous cell carcinoma. *J Clin Oncol* 2002;20:4199–4208.
49. Yao M, et al. Clinical significance of postradiotherapy [18F]-fluorodeoxyglucose positron emission tomography imaging in management of head-and-neck cancer-a long-term outcome report. *Int J Radiat Oncol Biol Phys* 2009;74:9–14.
50. Rischin D, et al. Prognostic significance of [18F]-misonidazole positron emission tomography-detected tumor hypoxia in patients with advanced head and neck cancer randomly assigned to chemoradiation with or without tirapazamine: a substudy of Trans-Tasman Radiation Oncology Group Study 98.02. *J Clin Oncol* 2006;24:2098–2104.
51. Todd M, Shah GV, Mukherji SK. MR imaging of brachial plexus. *Top Magn Reson Imaging* 2004;15:113–125.
52. Hall WH, et al. Development and validation of a standardized method for contouring the brachial plexus: preliminary dosimetric analysis among patients treated with IMRT for head-and-neck cancer. *Int J Radiat Oncol Biol Phys* 2008;72:1362–1367.
53. Riquet M, Hidden G, Debesse B. Direct lymphatic drainage of lung segments to the mediastinal nodes. An anatomic study on 260 adults. *J Thorac Cardiovasc Surg* 1989;97:623–632.
54. Nohl-Oser HC. An investigation of the anatomy of the lymphatic drainage of the lungs as shown by the lymphatic spread of bronchial carcinoma. *Ann R Coll Surg Engl* 1972;51:157–176.
55. Hata E, et al. Rationale for extended lymphadenectomy for lung cancer. *Theor Surg* 1990;5:19–25.
56. Kelsey CR, Light KL, Marks LB. Patterns of failure after resection of non-small-cell lung cancer: implications for postoperative radiation therapy volumes. *Int J Radiat Oncol Biol Phys* 2006;65:1097–1105.
57. Choyke PL, et al. Thymic atrophy and regrowth in response to chemotherapy: CT evaluation. *AJR Am J Roentgenol* 1987;149:269–272.
58. Dwamena BA, et al. Metastases from non-small cell lung cancer: mediastinal staging in the 1990s—meta-analytic comparison of PET and CT. *Radiology* 1999;213:530–536.

59. Gould MK, et al. Test performance of positron emission tomography and computed tomography for mediastinal staging in patients with non-small-cell lung cancer: a meta-analysis. *Ann Intern Med* 2003;139:879–892.
60. Toloza EM, Harpole L, McCrory DC. Noninvasive staging of non-small cell lung cancer: a review of the current evidence. *Chest* 2003;123(1 Suppl):137S–146S.
61. Bille A, et al. Preoperative intrathoracic lymph node staging in patients with non-small-cell lung cancer: accuracy of integrated positron emission tomography and computed tomography. *Eur J Cardiothorac Surg* 2009;36:440–445.
62. Darling GE, et al. Positron emission tomography-computed tomography compared with invasive mediastinal staging in non-small cell lung cancer: results of mediastinal staging in the early lung positron emission tomography trial. *J Thorac Oncol* 2011;6:1367–1372.
63. Pozo-Rodriguez F, et al. Accuracy of helical computed tomography and [18F] fluorodeoxyglucose positron emission tomography for identifying lymph node mediastinal metastases in potentially resectable non-small-cell lung cancer. *J Clin Oncol* 2005;23:8348–8356.
64. Xie L, et al. FDG-PET vs. histologic staging of the mediastinum in patients with pathologic N0-1 non-small cell lung cancer (NSCLC): what should be the gold standard? *J Thorac Oncol* 2010;5:S511–S512.
65. Lightdale CJ, Kulkarni KG. Role of endoscopic ultrasonography in the staging and follow-up of esophageal cancer. *J Clin Oncol* 2005;23:4483–4489.
66. Rosch T. Endosonographic staging of esophageal cancer: a review of literature results. *Gastrointest Endosc Clin North Am* 1995;5:537–547.
67. van Westreenen HL, et al. Systematic review of the staging performance of 18F-fluorodeoxyglucose positron emission tomography in esophageal cancer. *J Clin Oncol* 2004;22:3805–3812.
68. Westerterp M, et al. Esophageal cancer: CT, endoscopic US, and FDG PET for assessment of response to neoadjuvant therapy—systematic review. *Radiology* 2005;236:841–851.
69. Wang ZJ, et al. Malignant pleural mesothelioma: evaluation with CT, MR imaging, and PET. *Radiographics* 2004;24:105–119.
70. Bruzzi JF, et al. Imaging of non-small cell lung cancer of the superior sulcus: part 2: initial staging and assessment of resectability and therapeutic response. *Radiographics* 2008;28:561–572.
71. Kligerman S, Abbott G. A radiologic review of the new TNM classification for lung cancer. *AJR Am J Roentgenol* 2010;194:562–573.
72. Tomiyama N, et al. Using the World Health Organization classification of thymic epithelial neoplasms to describe CT findings. *AJR Am J Roentgenol* 2002;179:881–886.
73. Fentiman IS, Fourquet A, Hortobagyi GN. Male breast cancer. *Lancet* 2006;367:595–604.
74. Lee AH. Why is carcinoma of the breast more frequent in the upper outer quadrant? A case series based on needle core biopsy diagnoses. *Breast* 2005;14:151–152.
75. Estourgie SH, et al. Lymphatic drainage patterns from the breast. *Ann Surg* 2004;239:232–237.
76. Livingston SF, Arlen M. The extended extrapleural radical mastectomy: its role in the treatment of carcinoma of the breast. *Ann Surg* 1974;179:260–265.
77. Noguchi M, et al. A multivariate analysis of en bloc extended radical mastectomy versus conventional radical mastectomy in operable breast cancer. *Int Surg* 1992;77:48–54.
78. Urban JA, Marjani MA. Significance of internal mammary lymph node metastases in breast cancer. *Am J Roentgenol Radium Ther Nucl Med* 1971;111:130–136.
79. Kaija H, Maunu P. Tangential breast irradiation with or without internal mammary chain irradiation: results of a randomized trial. *Radiother Oncol* 1995;36:172–176.
80. Matzinger O, et al. Toxicity at three years with and without irradiation of the internal mammary and medial supraclavicular lymph node chain in stage I to III breast cancer (EORTC trial 22922/10925). *Acta Oncol* 2010;49:24–34.
81. Romestaing P, et al. Ten-year results of a randomized trail of internal mammary chain irradiation after mastectomy. *Int J Radiat Oncol Biol Phys* 2009;75:S1.
82. Alexander FE, et al. 14 years of follow-up from the Edinburgh randomised trial of breast-cancer screening. *Lancet* 1999;353:1903–1908.
83. Andersson I, Janzon L. Reduced breast cancer mortality in women under age 50: updated results from the Malmo Mammographic Screening Program. *J Natl Cancer Inst Monogr* 1997;22:63–67.
84. Miller AB, et al. Canadian National Breast Screening Study-2: 13-year results of a randomized trial in women aged 50–59 years. *J Natl Cancer Inst* 2000;92:1490–1499.
85. Nystrom L, et al. Long-term effects of mammography screening: updated overview of the Swedish randomised trials. *Lancet* 2002;359:909–919.
86. Tabar L, et al. Efficacy of breast cancer screening by age. New results from the Swedish two-county trial. *Cancer* 1995;75:2507–2517.
87. Rosenberg RD, et al. Effects of age, breast density, ethnicity, and estrogen replacement therapy on screening mammographic sensitivity and cancer stage at diagnosis: review of 183,134 screening mammograms in Albuquerque, New Mexico. *Radiology* 1998;209:511–518.
88. Carney PA, et al. Individual and combined effects of age, breast density, and hormone replacement therapy use on the accuracy of screening mammography. *Ann Intern Med* 2003;138:168–175.
89. Boyd NF, et al. Mammographic density and the risk and detection of breast cancer. *N Engl J Med* 2007;356:227–236.
90. Pisano ED, et al. Diagnostic performance of digital versus film mammography for breast-cancer screening. *N Engl J Med* 2005;353:1773–1783.
91. Saslow D, et al. American Cancer Society guidelines for breast screening with MRI as an adjunct to mammography. *CA Cancer J Clin* 2007;57:75–89.
92. Lehman CD, et al. MRI evaluation of the contralateral breast in women with recently diagnosed breast cancer. *N Engl J Med* 2007;356:1295–1303.
93. Turnbull L, et al. Comparative effectiveness of MRI in breast cancer (COMICE) trial: a randomised controlled trial. *Lancet* 2010;375:563–571.
94. Katipamula R, et al. Trends in mastectomy rates at the Mayo Clinic Rochester: effect of surgical year and preoperative magnetic resonance imaging. *J Clin Oncol* 2009;27:4082–4088.
95. Maruyama K, et al. Lymph node metastases of gastric cancer. General pattern in 1931 patients. *Ann Surg* 1989;210:596–602.
96. Fly OA Jr, Waugh JM, Dockerty MB. Splenic hilar nodal involvement in carcinoma of the distal part of the stomach. *Cancer* 1956;9:459–462.
97. Gunderson LL, Sosin H. Adenocarcinoma of the stomach: areas of failure in a re-operation series (second or symptomatic look) clinicopathologic correlation and implications for adjuvant therapy. *Int J Radiat Oncol Biol Phys* 1982;8:1–11.
98. Smalley SR, et al. Gastric surgical adjuvant radiotherapy consensus report: rationale and treatment implementation. *Int J Radiat Oncol Biol Phys* 2002;52:283–293.
99. Tepper JE, Gunderson LL. Radiation treatment parameters in the adjuvant postoperative therapy of gastric cancer. *Semin Radiat Oncol* 2002;12:187–195.
100. Kinkel K, et al. Detection of hepatic metastases from cancers of the gastrointestinal tract by using noninvasive imaging methods (US, CT, MR imaging, PET): a meta-analysis. *Radiology* 2002;224:748–756.
101. Cheng CL, et al. Risk factors for post-ERCP pancreatitis: a prospective multicenter study. *Am J Gastroenterol* 2006;101:139–147.
102. Mortele KJ, Ros PR. Anatomic variants of the biliary tree: MR cholangiographic findings and clinical applications. *AJR Am J Roentgenol* 2001;177:389–394.
103. Yeh TS, et al. Malignant perihilar biliary obstruction: magnetic resonance cholangiopancreatographic findings. *Am J Gastroenterol* 2000;95:432–440.
104. Lopera JE, Soto JA, Munera F. Malignant hilar and perihilar biliary obstruction: use of MR cholangiography to define the extent of biliary ductal involvement and plan percutaneous interventions. *Radiology* 2001;220:90–96.
105. Pano B, et al. Pathways of lymphatic spread in male urogenital pelvic malignancies. *Radiographics* 2011;31:135–160.
106. Taylor A, et al. Mapping pelvic lymph nodes: guidelines for delineation in intensity-modulated radiotherapy. *Int J Radiat Oncol Biol Phys* 2005;63:1604–1612.
107. Vilarino-Varela MJ, et al. A verification study of proposed pelvic lymph node localisation guidelines using nanoparticle-enhanced magnetic resonance imaging. *Radiother Oncol* 2008;89:192–196.
108. Kim RY, et al. Conventional four-field pelvic radiotherapy technique without computed tomography-treatment planning in cancer of the cervix: potential geographic miss and its impact on pelvic control. *Int J Radiat Oncol Biol Phys* 1995;31:109–112.
109. Chun M, et al. Radiation therapy of external iliac lymph nodes with lateral pelvic portals: identification of patients at risk for inadequate regional coverage. *Radiology* 1995;194:147–150.
110. Kapiteijn E, Putter H, van de Velde CJ. Impact of the introduction and training of total mesorectal excision on recurrence and survival in rectal cancer in the Netherlands. *Br J Surg* 2002;89:1142–1149.
111. Kapiteijn E, et al. Preoperative radiotherapy combined with total mesorectal excision for resectable rectal cancer. *N Engl J Med* 2001;345:638–646.
112. Quirke P, et al. Effect of the plane of surgery achieved on local recurrence in patients with operable rectal cancer: a prospective study using data from the MRC CR07 and NCIC-CTG CO16 randomised clinical trial. *Lancet* 2009;373:821–828.
113. Harewood GC, et al. A prospective, blinded assessment of the impact of preoperative staging on the management of rectal cancer. *Gastroenterology* 2002;123:24–32.
114. Puli SR, et al. How good is endoscopic ultrasound in differentiating various T stages of rectal cancer? Meta-analysis and systematic review. *Ann Surg Oncol* 2009;16:254–265.
115. Sauer R, et al. Preoperative versus postoperative chemoradiotherapy for rectal cancer. *N Engl J Med* 2004;351:1731–1740.
116. Deserno WM, et al. Urinary bladder cancer: preoperative nodal staging with ferumoxtran-10-enhanced MR imaging. *Radiology* 2004;233:449–456.
117. Umek WH, et al. Quantitative analysis of uterosacral ligament origin and insertion points by magnetic resonance imaging. *Obstet Gynecol* 2004;103:447–451.
118. Van Vierzen PB, et al. Fast dynamic contrast enhanced MR imaging of cervical carcinoma. *Clin Radiol* 1998;53:183–192.
119. Chung HH, et al. Accuracy of MR imaging for the prediction of myometrial invasion of endometrial carcinoma. *Gynecol Oncol* 2007;104:654–659.
120. Sheu MH, et al. Preoperative staging of cervical carcinoma with MR imaging: a reappraisal of diagnostic accuracy and pitfalls. *Eur Radiol*, 2001;11(9):1828–1833.
121. Dimopoulos JC, et al. Systematic evaluation of MRI findings in different stages of treatment of cervical cancer: potential of MRI on delineation of target, pathoanatomic structures, and organs at risk. *Int J Radiat Oncol Biol Phys* 2006;64:1380–1388.
122. Havrilesky LJ, et al. FDG-PET for management of cervical and ovarian cancer. *Gynecol Oncol* 2005;97:183–191.
123. Kidd EA, et al. The standardized uptake value for F-18 fluorodeoxyglucose is a sensitive predictive biomarker for cervical cancer treatment response and survival. *Cancer* 2007;110:1738–1744.
124. Schwarz JK, et al. Association of posttherapy positron emission tomography with tumor response and survival in cervical carcinoma. *JAMA* 2007;298:2289–2295.
125. Siva S, et al. Impact of post-therapy positron emission tomography on prognostic stratification and surveillance after chemoradiotherapy for cervical cancer. *Cancer* 2011;117:3891–3898.
126. Villeirs GM, et al. Magnetic resonance imaging anatomy of the prostate and periprostatic area: a guide for radiotherapists. *Radiother Oncol* 2005;76:99–106.
127. Batson OV. The function of the vertebral veins and their role in the spread of metastases. *Ann Surg* 1940;112:138–149.
128. Geldof AA. Models for cancer skeletal metastasis: a reappraisal of Batson's plexus. *Anticancer Res* 1997;17:1535–1539.
129. Plants BA, et al. Bulb of penis as a marker for prostatic apex in external beam radiotherapy of prostate cancer. *Int J Radiat Oncol Biol Phys* 2003;56:1079–1084.
130. Engelbrecht MR, et al. Local staging of prostate cancer using magnetic resonance imaging: a meta-analysis. *Eur Radiol* 2002;12:2294–2302.
131. Futterer JJ, et al. Standardized threshold approach using three-dimensional proton magnetic resonance spectroscopic imaging in prostate cancer localization of the entire prostate. *Invest Radiol* 2007;42:116–122.
132. Villeirs GM, et al. Magnetic resonance assessment of prostate localization variability in intensity-modulated radiotherapy for prostate cancer. *Int J Radiat Oncol Biol Phys* 2004;60:1611–1621.
133. Chabanova E, et al. Prostate cancer: 1.5 T endo-coil dynamic contrast-enhanced MRI and MR spectroscopy-correlation with prostate biopsy and prostatectomy histopathological data. *Eur J Radiol*, 2010;80:292–296.
134. Liauw SL, et al. Salvage radiotherapy after postprostatectomy biochemical failure: does pretreatment radioimmunoscintigraphy help select patients with locally confined disease? *Int J Radiat Oncol Biol Phys* 2008;71:1316–1321.
135. Harisinghani MG, et al. Noninvasive detection of clinically occult lymph-node metastases in prostate cancer. *N Engl J Med* 2003;348:2491–2499.
136. Hinkle GH, et al. Multicenter radioimmunoscintigraphic evaluation of patients with prostate carcinoma using indium-111 capromab pendetide. *Cancer* 1998;83:739–747.
137. Ellis RJ, et al. Single photon emission computerized tomography with capromab pendetide plus computerized tomography image set co-registration independently predicts biochemical failure. *J Urol* 2008;179:1768–1774.

Techniques, Modalities, and Modifiers in Radiation Oncology

138. Kostakoglu L, et al. Comparison of fluorine-18 fluorodeoxyglucose positron emission tomography and Ga-67 scintigraphy in evaluation of lymphoma. *Cancer* 2002; 94:879–888.
139. Tsukamoto N, et al. The usefulness of (18)F-fluorodeoxyglucose positron emission tomography ((18)F-FDG-PET) and a comparison of (18)F-FDG-pet with (67)gallium scintigraphy in the evaluation of lymphoma: relation to histologic subtypes based on the World Health Organization classification. *Cancer* 2007;110:652–659.
140. Isasi CR, Lu P, Blaufox MD. A metaanalysis of 18F-2-deoxy-2-fluoro-D-glucose positron emission tomography in the staging and restaging of patients with lymphoma. *Cancer* 2005;104:1066–1074.
141. Kwee TC, Kwee RM, Nievelstein RA. Imaging in staging of malignant lymphoma: a systematic review. *Blood* 2008;111:504–516.
142. Raanani P, et al. Is CT scan still necessary for staging in Hodgkin and non-Hodgkin lymphoma patients in the PET/CT era? *Ann Oncol* 2006;17:117–122.
143. Schaefer NG, et al. Non-Hodgkin lymphoma and Hodgkin disease: coregistered FDG PET and CT at staging and restaging—do we need contrast-enhanced CT? *Radiology* 2004;232:823–829.
144. Jerusalem G, et al. Whole-body positron emission tomography using 18F-fluorodeoxyglucose for posttreatment evaluation in Hodgkin's disease and non-Hodgkin's lymphoma has higher diagnostic and prognostic value than classical computed tomography scan imaging. *Blood* 1999;94:429–433.
145. Mikhaeel NG, et al. 18-FDG-PET as a prognostic indicator in the treatment of aggressive non-Hodgkin's lymphoma-comparison with CT. *Leuk Lymphoma* 2000; 39:543–553.
146. Spaepen K, et al. Prognostic value of positron emission tomography (PET) with fluorine-18 fluorodeoxyglucose ([18 F]FDG) after first-line chemotherapy in non-Hodgkin's lymphoma: is [18F]FDG-PET a valid alternative to conventional diagnostic methods? *J Clin Oncol* 2001;19:414–419.
147. Sher DJ, et al. Prognostic significance of mid- and post-ABVD PET imaging in Hodgkin's lymphoma: the importance of involved-field radiotherapy. *Ann Oncol* 2009;20:1848–1853.
148. Dorth JA, et al. The impact of radiation therapy in patients with diffuse large B-cell lymphoma with positive post-chemotherapy FDG-PET or gallium-67 scans. *Ann Oncol* 2011;22:405–410.
149. Picardi M, et al. Randomized comparison of consolidation radiation versus observation in bulky Hodgkin's lymphoma with post-chemotherapy negative positron emission tomography scans. *Leuk Lymphoma* 2007;48:1721–1727.
150. Cabrera AR, et al. Incorporating gross anatomy education into radiation oncology residency: a 2-year curriculum with evaluation of resident satisfaction. *J Am Coll Radiol* 2011;8:335–340.
151. Chino JP, et al. Teaching the anatomy of oncology: evaluating the impact of a dedicated oncoanatomy course. *Int J Radiat Oncol Biol Phys* 2011;79:853–839.
152. Leung SF, et al. Cranial nerve involvement by nasopharyngeal carcinoma: response to treatment and clinical significance. *Clin Oncol (R Coll Radiol)* 1990; 2:138–141.
153. Toloza EM, Harpole L, McCrory DC. Noninvasive staging of non-small cell lung cancer: a review of the current evidence. *Chest* 2003;123:137S–146S.
154. Gould MK, et al. Test performance of positron emission tomography and computed tomography for mediastinal staging in patients with non-small-cell lung cancer: a meta-analysis. *Ann Intern Med* 2003;139:879–892.
155. Dwamena BA, et al. Metastases from non-small cell lung cancer: mediastinal staging in the 1990s—meta-analytic comparison of PET and CT. *Radiology* 1999;213:530–536.
156. Darling GE, et al. Positron emission tomography-computed tomography compared with invasive mediastinal staging in non-small cell lung cancer: results of mediastinal staging in the early lung positron emission tomography trial. *J Thorac Oncol* 2011;6:1367–1372.
157. Bille A, et al. Preoperative intrathoracic lymph node staging in patients with non-small-cell lung cancer: accuracy of integrated positron emission tomography and computed tomography. *Eur J Cardiothorac Surg* 2009;36:440–445.
158. Livingston SF, Arlen M. The extended extrapleural radical mastectomy: Its role in the treatment of carcinoma of the breast. *Ann Surg* 1974;179:260–265.
159. Urban JA, Marjani MA. Significance of internal mammary lymph node metastases in breast cancer. *Am J Roentgenol Radium Ther Nucl Med* 1971;111:130–136.
160. Noguchi M, et al. Reappraisal of internal mammary node metastases as a prognostic factor in patients with breast cancer. *Cancer* 1991;68:1918–1925.

Chapter 31
Hyperthermia as a Treatment Modality

Mark W. Dewhirst, Paul Stauffer, Zeljko Vujaskovic, Chelsea D. Landon, and Leonard R. Prosnitz

The rationale for combining hyperthermia (HT) with radiation (RT) rests on several mechanisms. HT is known to cause direct cytotoxicity and also acts as a radiosensitizer. Studies performed *in vitro* yield a pattern of survival curves similar to RT survival curves. The mechanisms of action of HT appear to be complementary to the effects of RT with regard to inhibition of potentially lethal damage and sublethal damage repair, cell cycle sensitivity, and effects of hypoxia and nutrient deprivation. In addition, HT has effects on blood flow and tumor physiology, which may be of particular interest with regard to tumor oxygenation and combination therapy with drug-carrying nanoparticles.

Implementation of HT in the clinic presents significant challenges. It is difficult to heat tumor tissue volumes with uniformity and precision. There is no standardized equipment to effect locoregional HT. Techniques for measuring temperature and the actual definition and calculation of thermal dose remain significant problems.

The biologic rationale for HT is compelling and is founded on principles of classic radiobiology, molecular biology, and tumor physiology. Further improvements in technologies to deliver HT and measure thermal dose remain crucial. Nonetheless, there are now 17 randomized trials of HT in human cancer patients, the majority of which demonstrate a local control and/or survival advantage with the addition of HT to standard therapy, providing strong impetus for continuing work in this field.

THE BIOLOGY OF HYPERTHERMIA

Definition of Hyperthermia

HT means elevation of temperature to a supraphysiologic level. When cells or tumor tissues are subjected to elevated temperatures, a number of events follow that have important biologic consequences for cancer therapy. HT can kill cells in its own right, but perhaps more important, it can sensitize tumor cells to other forms of therapy, including RT and chemotherapy (CT). Some of the physiologic consequences of HT have implications for radiotherapy as well, such as thermally induced reoxygenation. Changes induced in microvessel pore size can lead to increased delivery of nanoparticle drugs[1,2,3,4] as well as macromolecular therapeutic agents, such as monoclonal antibodies[5] or drug-carrying polymers.[6] The adaptive response to hyperthermic exposure (thermotolerance) may augment host immune responses against tumor cells.[7] This chapter will not deal directly with the use of whole-body HT and will discuss the emerging field of thermal ablation only briefly[8] since neither has been combined with RT in the clinic.

Effects of Hyperthermia Alone on Cell Survival

HT kills cells in a log-linear fashion, depending on the time at a defined temperature (Fig. 31.1). Resulting survival curves typically have an initial shoulder region, followed by an exponential portion. The initial shoulder region indicates that damage has to accumulate to a certain level before cells begin to die, analogous to the sublethal damage that is seen with ionizing radiation. At lower temperatures, a resistant tail may appear at the end of the heating period. This resistant tail is not a resistant subpopulation, as might be seen for RT when there is a hypoxic subfraction, but rather is due to the induction of thermotolerance, which develops during the heating period. At temperatures >43°C the tail does not develop because thermotolerance is not observed at temperatures greater than this. More details on the mechanism of thermotolerance and its potential clinical significance are discussed later.

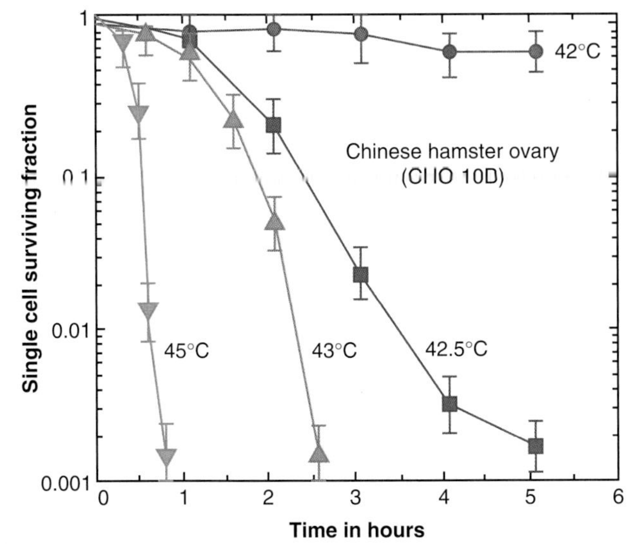

FIGURE 31.1. Cell survival curves for the Chinese hamster ovary cell line, plotted as a log of surviving fraction as a function of time of heating at a defined temperature. Note that the rate of cell killing is highly temperature dependent. For example, 5 hours of heating at 42°C kills very few cells, whereas 5 hours of heating at 0.5°C higher (42.5°C) results in nearly three logs of cell killing. (From Roizin-Towle L, Pirro JP. The response of human and rodent cells to hyperthermia. *Int J Radiat Oncol Biol Phys* 1991;20:751–756; with permission from Elsevier.)

Thermal Isoeffect Dose: The Arrhenius Relationship

The temperature dependence of the rate of cell killing by heat is referred to as the *Arrhenius relationship*. Typically, one plots the log of the slope ($1/D_0$) of cell survival curves as a function of temperature (Fig. 31.2). Characteristically, Arrhenius plots have a biphasic curve; the point at which the slope changes is referred to as a *breakpoint*. Above the breakpoint for nearly all cell types, a change in temperature of 1°C will double the rate of cell killing. Below the breakpoint, the rate of cell killing drops by a factor of 4 to 8 for every drop in temperature of 1°C. The change in slope below the breakpoint is due to the development of thermotolerance during heating.

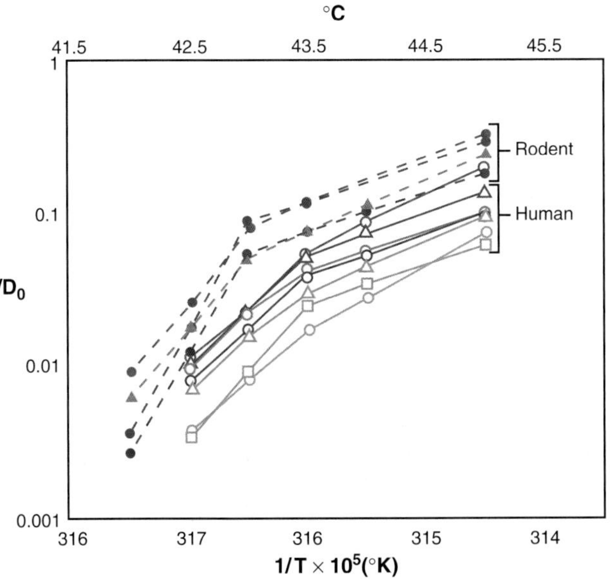

FIGURE 31.2. Arrhenius plots for a variety of rodent and human tumor cell lines, as assessed *in vitro*. Note that all human cells are below and to the right of the rodent cell lines. This means that for a given temperature, the slope of the cell-killing curve is less steep for human than for rodent cells. In addition, the breakpoint of the Arrhenius plot appears to be about 0.5°C higher for human than for rodent cells. These observations mean that human cells are more thermally resistant than rodent cells.[198] (From Roizin-Towle L, Pirro JP. The response of human and rodent cells to hyperthermia. *Int J Radiat Oncol Biol Phys* 1991;20:751–756; with permission from Elsevier.)

The recognition that there is a definable relationship between the rate of cell killing and temperature led Sapareto and Dewey[9] to propose using this relationship to normalize thermal data from HT. HT results in temperatures within tumors that are almost always nonuniform, with variable time–temperature history. The formulation for this relationship is as follows:

$$\text{CEM } 43°\text{C} = tR^{(43 - T)} \qquad (1)$$

where CEM 43°C is the cumulative equivalent minutes at 43°C (the temperature suggested for normalization), t is the time of treatment, T is the average temperature during the interval of heating, and R is a constant. When above the breakpoint, which is usually assumed to be 43°C, $R = 0.5$. When below the breakpoint, $R = 0.25$.

For a complex time–temperature history, the heating profile is broken into intervals of time (t) where the temperature remains relatively constant. CEM 43°C is calculated using the average T (T_{avg}) for each interval, and the resultant data are summed to give a final CEM 43°C for the entire heating regimen:

$$\text{CEM } 43°\text{C} = \sum tR^{(43 - T_{avg})} \qquad (2)$$

The CEM 43°C (thermal isoeffect dose) formulation has been used extensively and successfully in clinical trials to describe thermal dose despite its derivation from rodent studies.

Mechanisms of Hyperthermic Cytotoxicity

Cellular and Tissue Responses to Hyperthermia: Targets for Hyperthermic Cytotoxicity

The predominant molecular target for hyperthermic cell killing appears to be protein.[10] For many cells and tissues (both tumor and normal), the heat of inactivation for cell killing is in the range of that necessary for protein denaturation (130 to 170 kcal/mole). Additional evidence for proteins being the primary target is the importance of heat shock proteins in protecting cells from thermal damage. When cells are exposed to heat, the synthesis of nearly all proteins is stopped, with the exception of heat shock proteins, the synthesis of which is upregulated.[11] One of the primary functions of heat shock proteins is to refold other proteins that have been denatured or damaged.[12]

Some cellular organelles are especially important in controlling the thermal response. For example, modification of cellular membrane lipid content or use of membrane-active agents such as alcohols can sensitize cells to heat killing, but the sensitization is probably related to destabilization of the membrane as it relates to lipid–protein interactions.[10] The cytoskeleton of cells is particularly heat sensitive.[13] Cytoskeletal collapse also disrupts cytoskeletal-dependent signal transduction pathways.[14,15] Enzymes in the respiratory chain are more heat sensitive than enzymes in the glycolytic pathway.[16] The heat sensitivity of the centriole leads to chromosomal aberrations following thermal injury.[17] Finally, many DNA-repair proteins are heat sensitive. This may be one of the mechanisms that lead to heat-induced radiosensitization and chemosensitization.[18,19]

Little information is available from human tumors to know what proportion of cells is killed with heat alone or what the underlying mechanisms of cell death might be. Such information may be important with respect to reoxygenation, which has been seen in rodent, canine, and human tumors[20] after HT. Induction of apoptosis could lead to reoxygenation following heating as a result of reduced oxygen consumption, which could in turn increase RT sensitivity. Alternatively, induction of necrosis is not likely to affect hypoxia since both vessels and tumor cells would be killed in the process.

Thermotolerance

Thermotolerance is defined as a transient adaptation to thermal stress that renders surviving heated cells more resistant to additional heat stress. Whether or not a cell dies as a result of thermal insult is dependent on the net balance between how much protein is damaged and how much is protected and repaired via thermotolerance. Thermotolerance can develop either during or after heat stress and can persist for several days. If cells are not exposed to thermal stress again, thermotolerance will decay. The time of peak thermal resistance and the time of decay are related to the severity of the heat shock.

Concerns over the persistence of thermotolerance after HT has affected the design of many clinical trials of thermoradiotherapy. In most trials, a minimum of 48 hours has been suggested between HT fractions in order to avoid re-treatment during thermotolerance. This concern has proscribed the use of daily HT in conjunction with daily radiotherapy in most clinical trials or alternatively led to the use of hypofractionated RT, for example, large fractions twice weekly with concurrent heat.

Some investigators have suggested that one should take advantage of heat radiosensitization rather than hyperthermic cytotoxicity and ignore the issue of thermotolerance. The degree of HT-mediated cytotoxicity may be low with HT as it is currently practiced because temperatures achieved are largely below that needed for direct cell killing. Furthermore, heat radiosensitization is relatively unaffected by thermotolerance.[21]

Does thermotolerance occur in humans after heating? Heat shock protein synthesis was evaluated in a small group of human patients (n = 23) with chest wall recurrences of breast cancer who underwent RT with or without HT. Elevated levels of heat shock proteins in biopsy specimens after treatment correlated with lower probability of attaining a complete response.[22] In another study of patients treated with fluorouracil (5-FU) plus thermoradiotherapy for colorectal cancer, no correlation between HSP27 or HSP70 levels, either before or after treatment, and outcome was seen.[23] Interpretation of clinical studies is complicated by the fact that heat shock protein expression is frequently upregulated in tumors in the absence of heat stress.[11] Stresses other than HT, such as hypoxia and hypoxia–reoxygenation injury, can cause elevations in heat shock protein levels. Thus the question of the relevance of thermotolerance to the clinic and the best HT/RT fractionation scheme remains unsettled.

Immunologic Implications of the Heat Shock Response

There is emerging evidence that HT can augment the immunologic response toward tumors. Examples of effects that are known to occur after heating include (a) increased immunogenicity,[24–27] (b) increased T-cell, NK-cell, and dendritic cell maturation and activity,[28–34] and (c) enhanced trafficking of immune effector cells into tumors and lymphatic organs.[35,36] The trafficking is likely mediated by cytokines such as interleukin 6.[37,38]

Hyperthermia and Physiology

In this section, we discuss what is known about the physiologic consequences of HT and then discuss how physiology can be manipulated to enhance the efficacy of HT.

As temperatures are elevated, tissue perfusion increases. In muscle, cyclic variations in temperature have been observed when delivered power is kept constant, demonstrating that thermoregulation is controlled by a threshold temperature.[39] The temperature threshold for this change is 41°C to 41.5°C in skin.[40] Changes in vascular permeability also occur, leading to edema formation in the heated volume. As temperature or time-at-temperature is increased, vascular stasis and hemorrhage develop.

The change in normal tissue perfusion upon heating is typically much greater than what one sees in tumors. Muscle and skin perfusion increase by about 10-fold, whereas tumor perfusion may increase by 1.5- to 2-fold.[41] The mechanism of vascular stasis in tumors is not fully determined, but potential sources include arteriovenous shunting, thrombus formation, and leukocyte plugging.[42] Hemorrhage probably occurs as a result of enlarged endothelial cell gaps or loss of endothelial cell and basement membrane integrity along the vessel wall.

These vascular effects may be exploited clinically. HT causes extravasation of nanoparticles into tumor parenchyma. Heating to 40°C to 42°C results in a marked increase in extravasation of liposomes in tumor but not in normal tissue vasculature. Above 42°C vascular stasis and hemorrhage occur with reduced liposomal extravasation. These results are consistent with the hypothesis that the increase in extravasation is due to cytoskeletal collapse in the vessel wall (endothelial cell). The increase in liposomal extravasation can be exploited as a drug delivery vehicle, particularly since the effect appears to be preferential to tumors. Many investigators have shown that HT increases liposomal drug accumulation in tumors, leading to enhanced antitumor efficacy of a variety of drugs compared with liposome administration alone or free drug administered with HT.[4] When temperature-sensitive liposomes are used, even better antitumor effects can be achieved, particularly using low-temperature–sensitive liposomes that have entered into human clinical trials.[1,43,44] The improved effectiveness of these drugs when combined with HT is directly related to the increase in drug delivery.[1,45,46]

Although the changes in perfusion in tumors are relatively small in comparison with normal tissues, there have been a number of efforts to exploit them as a means to augment drug delivery to tumors. For relatively small agents, such as most chemotherapeutic drugs, there is no real advantage to using heat to augment delivery, although increased cellular uptake has been seen with a number of drugs.[47] For drugs with molecular weight <1,000, the primary mechanism that governs drug transport is diffusion, which is controlled by the concentration gradient across the vascular wall.[48] The temperature dependence of diffusion is not large, so HT has relatively little effect.

However, convection is the primary driving force for transvascular transport for molecules >1,000 molecular weight. This is controlled by the pressure gradient across the blood vessel wall. HT increases transvascular delivery of monoclonal antibodies[5] and polymeric peptides that can carry drugs or radioisotopes.[6]

Effects of Hyperthermia on Tumor Metabolism and Oxygenation

Enzymes for aerobic metabolism are more heat sensitive than those involved in anaerobic metabolism.[16] The net result of this difference in heat sensitivity is that nutrient stores are more rapidly depleted during heat shock, leading to a reduction in adenosine triphosphate (ATP) and buildup of lactic acid. A number of rodent studies have demonstrated changes in energy balance and pH after heating. Kelleher et al.[49] reported decreases in ATP and increases in lactate concentration occurring concomitantly with reduction in tumor blood flow after heating. In a series of human patients with soft tissue sarcomas who were treated preoperatively with HT and RT, a reduction in magnetic resonance spectroscopy ATP/inorganic phosphate was significantly correlated with a higher probability for tumor response.[50] HT reduces oxygen consumption rates in murine and human tumor lines.[51] These results are consistent with the theory that a reduction in tumor respiration occurs after HT.

A shift toward anaerobic metabolism would decrease oxygen consumption rates, which could improve tumor oxygenation. Oleson[52] suggested that some of the benefits of HT in the clinical setting may result from improvements in oxygenation. Results from several studies in rodent tumors and human tumor xenografts support the notion that an overall improvement in tumor oxygenation can result from time–temperature

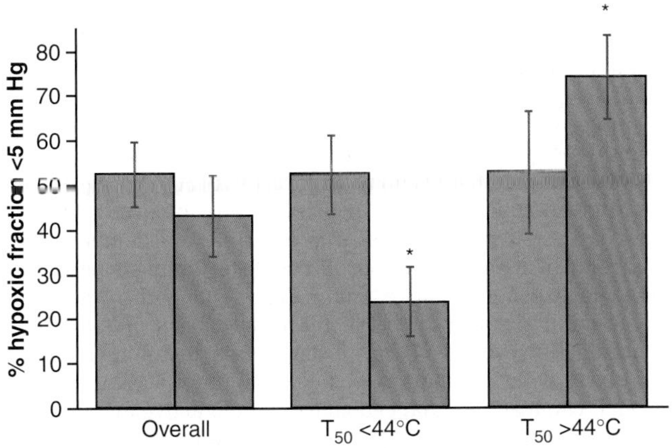

FIGURE 31.3. Effects of median temperature during hyperthermia treatment on oxygenation of canine tumors, as measured 24 hours postheating. When the median temperature is less than 44°C, there is significant reduction in hypoxic fraction. When median temperature exceeds 44°C, hypoxic fraction increases. Closed bar indicates measurements taken before hyperthermia, and open bar indicates measurements taken 24 hours after hyperthermia treatment. (Data replotted from Vujaskovic Z, Poulson J, Gaskin A, et al. Temperature-dependent changes in physiologic parameters of spontaneous canine soft tissue sarcomas after combined radiotherapy and hyperthermia. *Int J Radiat Oncol Biol Phys* 2000;46(1):179–185; with permission from Elsevier.)

combinations below those that cause vascular damage (e.g., 41°C to 41.5°C for 60 minutes). Higher thermal doses that cause vascular damage (e.g., >43°C, 60 minutes) may lead to decreases in tumor oxygenation.[20]

HT improves tumor oxygenation in canine and human tumors.[53–55] In a human study of soft tissue sarcomas, failure to reoxygenate after the first HT fraction led to a significantly lower probability of achieving pathologic complete response at the time of surgery.[54] In women with locally advanced breast cancer treated with neoadjuvant thermochemoradiotherapy, reoxygenation after the first heat treatment was associated with higher likelihood for achieving a clinical response.[56] In a canine soft tissue sarcoma study involving thermoradiotherapy treatment, there was an overall improvement in partial pressure of oxygen at 24 hours after the first heat treatment, but for those tumors in which the median temperature was greater than 44°C, perfusion and tumor oxygenation decreased (Fig. 31.3). This threshold temperature for vascular damage is about 44°C for human and canine tumors. It is difficult, however, to attain this temperature in nonanesthetized human patients.

Zywietz et al.[57] reported that twice-weekly heating to 43°C for 60 minutes in combination with 60 Gy delivered in 20 fractions over 4 weeks resulted in a steady decline in partial pressure of oxygen of a rat rhabdomyosarcoma. However, Thrall et al. reported that there were long-term improvements in oxygenation of canine tumors treated with fractionated thermoradiotherapy.[53] Thus, it is not known with certainty whether reoxygenation or deoxygenation predominates after fractionated thermoradiotherapy and how this relates to treatment outcome. The sarcoma and breast clinical studies cited previously argue in favor of a positive effect on oxygen status, but only a few HT treatments may be necessary to achieve this.

It has been reported that fractionated HT (42.5°C for 60-minute conditioning dose followed by 44.5°C for up to 90 minutes) can lead to vascular thermotolerance.[58] This means that the likelihood of vascular damage decreases if a second HT treatment is given within 1 to 2 days after the first treatment, at a time when thermotolerance may still be present. It was reported that vascular thermotolerance is associated with vessel normalization.[59] Normalization is a phenomenon popularized by Jain to explain the beneficial effects of antiangiogenic treatments to improve transport properties of tumors.[60] It is associated with a decrease in microvessel density and an increase in pericyte coverage, conditions reflective of a more mature vasculature.

The process of vascular normalization after heating may be mediated in part by upregulation of the transcription factor hypoxia-inducible factor-1 (HIF-1). This transcription factor is known to regulate angiogenesis by controlling levels of vascular endothelial growth factor in tissue. Moon et al. reported that HT increases HIF-1 in tumors by activating the enzyme NADPH oxidase.[51] The reactive oxygen species produced by this enzyme inhibited degradation of the labile subunit of HIF-1, HIF-1α.[51] The upregulation of HIF-1 levels was accompanied by increases in levels of vascular endothelial growth factor and perfused vascular density in heated tumors.

Physiologic Approaches to Enhance Thermal Cytotoxicity: pH Modification

It is well established that an acute reduction in extracellular pH can greatly enhance sensitivity to HT. Cells adapted to grow at low pH, as occurs in tumors, have little reserve to further increase proton pumping. It is the reduction in intracellular pH that is actually responsible for the increase in cytotoxicity.[61] The potential degree of enhancement in killing is substantial, and, as a result, considerable effort has been made to accomplish this feat *in vivo*. The most widely studied method has been induction of hyperglycemia. The rationale is that excess glucose load to the tumor will push it toward glycolysis and lactic acid production because most tumors have a limited oxygen supply and also have defects in respiratory pathways. Induction of a hyperglycemic state may also reduce blood flow by increasing blood viscosity. Reduced perfusion compromises heat exchange capacity, thereby increasing temperatures in tumor during heating. When glucose has been administered intravenously, there has been little effect on perfusion, but reduction in extracellular pH has been observed.[62,63]

In humans, the induction of hyperglycemia has been accomplished by either oral or intravenous glucose administration. Results using this approach have been mixed. On average, the drop in extracellular pH is about 0.17 pH unit, which is near the goal of 0.2 pH unit.[62] However, there is considerable variation from one patient to another in terms of how effective this approach is. Furthermore, in prediabetic patients, the trend is toward an increase in pH rather than a decrease. In canines with soft tissue sarcomas, induction of hyperglycemia via intravenous administration did not result in any significant change in either intracellular or extracellular pH.[64]

The use of hyperglycemia resulted in improved response to thermochemotherapy and thermoradiotherapy in rodents.[65,66] Data in human tumors are sparse. One study in a limited number of patients suggested improvement in response with the use of hyperglycemia combined with thermoradiotherapy.[67] However, pH was not measured, and the study was not randomized.

The addition of agents that can selectively drive down tumor intracellular pH, such as glucose combined with the respiratory inhibitor metaiodobenzylguanidine, has the potential to further enhance hyperthermic cytotoxicity selectively in tumor tissues.[68,69] Some groups have also focused on the use of pharmacologic agents that block the extrusion of hydrogen ions from cells, which is normally accomplished via membrane-bound pumps. Use of such agents, in combination with acidification of the extracellular space, can lead to enhanced hyperthermic cell killing both *in vitro* and *in vivo*.[70]

Blood Flow Manipulation

Blood perfusion is a major impediment to effective heating. This is because perfusion is the primary mechanism for conducting heat and maintaining homeostasis. Thus, if tumor blood flow can be effectively reduced, temperatures in the tumor will increase. A number of vasoactive agents have been shown to reduce tumor blood flow, including some that are normally considered to be vasodilators. Agents investigated include hydralazine, nitroprusside, and angiotensin II; the first two drugs are vasodilators and the last is a vasoconstrictor. Clinically, changes in blood pressure have limited doses that can be safely used, minimizing effects on tumor blood flow. New agents are needed. It also makes sense to consider combinations of approaches that might reduce both tumor blood flow and pH and lead to improved temperature distributions, as well as to heat sensitization.

Radiation and Hyperthermia

Rationale for Combining Hyperthermia with Radiotherapy

When RT is combined with HT, complementary effects occur. Cells in the S phase of the cell cycle are relatively radioresistant, but when heated, these cells are most sensitive. Hypoxic cells are known to be three times more resistant to RT as compared with aerobic cells. With HT, there is no difference in sensitivity between aerobic and hypoxic cells. As discussed in detail earlier, there is good evidence that HT can lead to reoxygenation, which will further improve RT response.[20,54,55] Finally, HT inhibits the repair of both sublethal and potentially lethal damage via its effects in inactivating crucial DNA repair pathways.[71–73]

Factors to Consider When Combining Hyperthermia with Radiotherapy

The interaction between RT and HT is described by the "thermal enhancement ratio" (TER), defined as the ratio of doses of RT to achieve an isoeffect for RT/RT + HT. TERs for local control have been estimated for a number of human tumors using historical control data for RT alone.[74] In most tumor types examined, these ratios were greater than 1. Assessment of normal tissue TER has not been attempted, except in a few cases. For those examples, TER values for normal-tissue damage have been less than those for tumor in the same patient population, suggesting potential for therapeutic gain for RT+ HT compared with RT alone.[74] Prospective, randomized trials in dogs with spontaneous tumors have also shown evidence for improved local tumor control with RT + HT compared with RT alone,[75–76,77–78] with no observable increase in the frequency of clinically relevant late normal-tissue complications. In one canine trial, enhancement of late RT damage (as assessed histologically) was reported and the duration of acute RT complications was prolonged.[78] There is evidence, however, that excessively high intratumoral temperatures (i.e., >45°C for 60 minutes) can lead to damage to surrounding normal tissues, an effect that is often caused by rapid tumor regression.[76,79] Such damage is not easily repaired and can lead to chronic tissue consequences, such as fibrosis, fistula formation, and bone necrosis.

In summary, most available data from preclinical and clinical studies indicate that therapeutic gain is achievable for the combination of HT with RT. There is little evidence to suggest that HT enhances the incidence or severity of late normal-tissue complications from RT, particularly when excessively high intratumoral temperatures are avoided.

Hyperthermia and Chemotherapy

Rationale for Using Hyperthermia with Chemotherapy

Many chemotherapeutic agents have demonstrated synergism with HT, including cisplatin and related compounds, melphalan, cyclophosphamide, nitrogen mustards, anthracyclines, nitrosoureas, bleomycin, mitomycin C, and hypoxic cell sensitizers.[80] The mechanisms may include (a) increased cellular uptake of drug, (b) increased oxygen free radical production, and (c) increased DNA damage and inhibition of repair.[47] Hypoxia and pH appear to be important in the thermochemotherapeutic response.

An important factor in the potential use of HT with many drugs is its ability to reverse, at least partially, drug resistance. Examples of drugs for which this has been shown include cisplatin,[81,82] melphalan,[83] nitrosoureas,[84] and doxorubicin, when combined with the MDR inhibitor verapamil.[85]

In vitro and *in vivo* results may not correlate. Paclitaxel, for example, shows little *in vitro* activity, but clinical results in combination with HT and RT have been encouraging.[56]

Most antimetabolites do not interact with HT synergistically when given concomitantly.[47] However, it is important to consider issues such as time of drug exposure and temperature, both of which may be important in determining where and when to expect a positive interaction. When 5-FU has been given simultaneously with HT, there have been only additive effects.[86] However, 5-FU has been shown to interact supra-additively with HT under specific conditions. Heating to 39°C to 41°C can lead to enhanced conversion to active metabolites, thereby increasing drug cytotoxicity. In addition, continuous-infusion protocols with this drug may lead to cell cycle block in S phase, a relatively sensitive part of the cell cycle to HT.[87]

For most drugs (excluding 5-FU and perhaps other antimetabolites), the optimal sequence between heat and drug is to administer them simultaneously or to give the drug immediately before the onset of heating. For platinum-containing drugs, the tissue extraction rate of drug may be increased with HT, further substantiating the rationale for use of this sequence.[88] The degree of interaction between drugs and HT is temperature and cell line dependent.[47]

There are also some classes of drugs for which there has been no demonstrated synergistic interaction. Interactions with etoposide have been unpredictable, and current recommendations are that one cannot expect synergistic interactions with it.[47] There is also no evidence for synergistic interaction between vinca alkaloids and HT.

The term *trimodality therapy* has been used to describe combination therapy of HT, drugs, and RT. It has been studied in both preclinical and clinical models and will be discussed at length in the clinical section of this chapter.

Hyperthermia and Thermosensitive Liposomally Encapsulated Drugs

In a classic paper, Yatvin et al.[89] suggested that a temperature-sensitive liposome could be used to selectively deliver drug to tumors. Several papers have been published using formulations similar to that of Yatvin et al. The combination of HT with such drug carriers increased drug delivery and efficacy as compared with using drug carrier alone or free drug with HT.[4] However, the thermal properties of the original Yatvin formulation were not amenable to clinical application. The release temperature was too high, and the rate of drug release was relatively slow.[90] A breakthrough occurred when Needham et al.[91] reported the formulation for a low-temperature-sensitive liposome that rapidly released drug at 41.4°C. A second formulation with similar drug release properties was reported by Lindner et al.[92] This type of liposome is referred to as a low-temperature-sensitive liposome (LTSL).

Direct comparison of the relative efficacy of a doxorubicin-containing LTSL, the Yatvin formulation, a traditional non–thermally sensitive liposome formulation similar to Doxil, and free drug has been made. The LTSL was clearly more effective than any other formulation, as assessed using tumor growth delay as an endpoint. The difference in effectiveness was demonstrated to be related to a significant improvement in drug delivery to tumor, as well as to increased drug binding to DNA.[1] Further preclinical work with this formulation demonstrated that it has broad activity when combined with local HT across a range of different tumor types.[93] The formulation was tested in a phase I trial of canine tumors, where the maximum tolerated dose was associated with bone marrow toxicity.[94] This has been the dose-limiting feature of the toxicity in phase I trials in humans as well.[43,44] The drug was tested in a double-blind, phase III trial in combination with thermal ablation for hepatocellular carcinoma

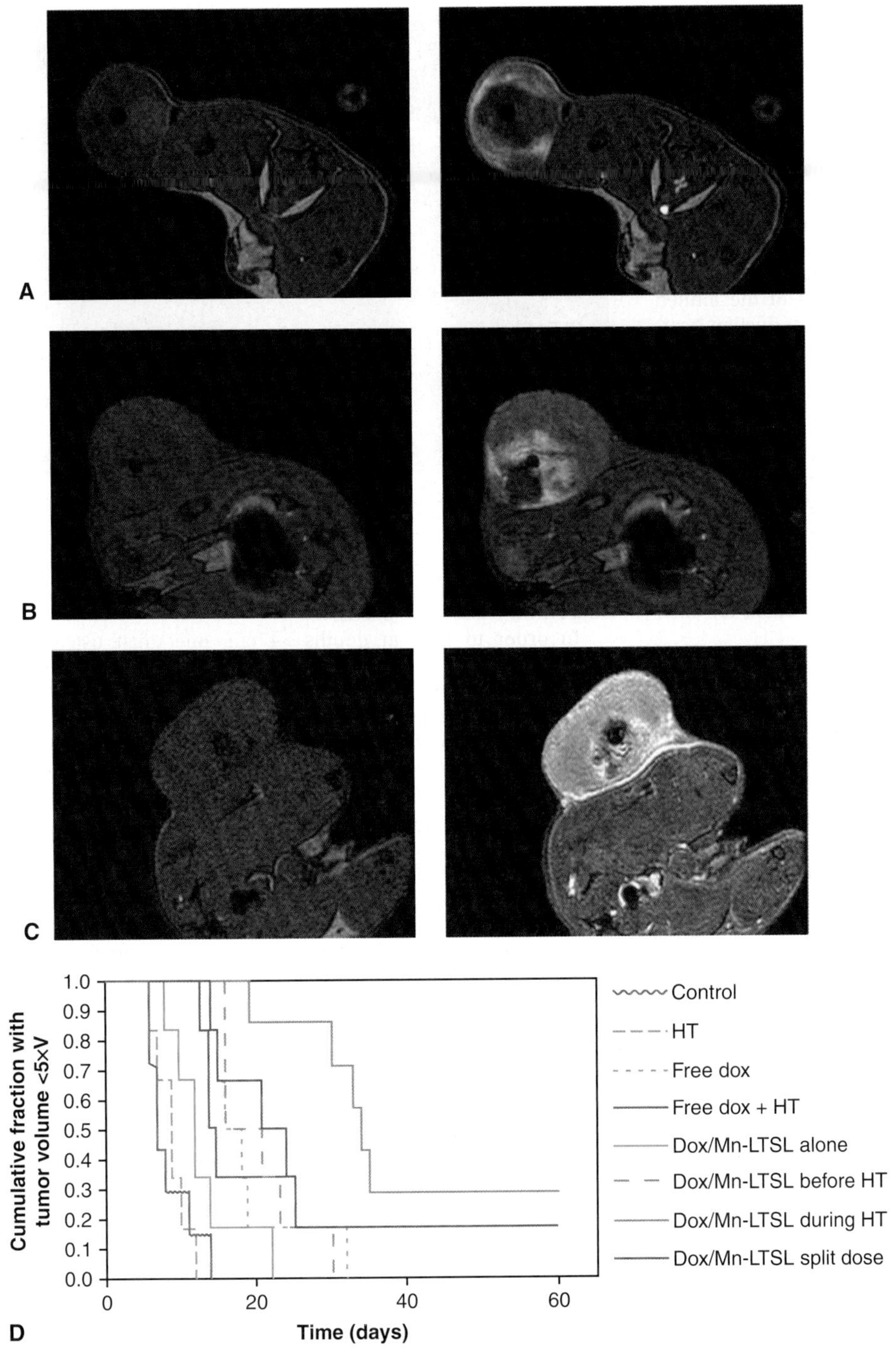

FIGURE 31.4. Tumor drug distributions and antitumor effect following various low-temperature-sensitive liposome (LTSL) and hyperthermia treatment protocols. Rats bearing fibrosarcomas were treated with doxorubicin- and manganese-containing LTSLs during hyperthermia **(A)**, prior to hyperthermia **(B)**, or in two equal doses, one prior to hyperthermia and the other after steady-state hyperthermia had been reached **(C)**. Tumors are shown prior to treatment (Before) and after LTSL and hyperthermia treatment (After). Liposome content release corresponds to the white regions. The corresponding antitumor effect is also depicted **(D)**. Treatment A resulted in peripheral enhancement at the edge of the tumor, whereas the split-dose treatment (C) led to uniform enhancement. Treatment B resulted in central enhancement, as well as delayed tumor growth. (A to C, unpublished data; D, from Ponce AM, Viglianti BL, Yu D, et al. Magnetic resonance imaging of temperature-sensitive liposome release: drug dose painting and antitumor effects. *J Natl Cancer Inst* 2007;99(1):53–63; Oxford University Press, with permission.)

(104-06-301, NCT00617981). The trial is now completed, and the sponsor is waiting for follow-up before reporting the results. The formulation has also been used as a magnetic resonance (MR) imaging agent, where drug and contents have been loaded in the same liposome.[45,46] Changes in MR signal intensity were used to determine drug concentration in preclinical models. Concentrations measured with MRI were associated with antitumor activity in individual animals[45] (Fig. 13.4).

HYPERTHERMIA PHYSICS

The objective of local or regional hyperthermia therapy is to achieve tumor temperatures in the range of 40°C to 45°C and to maintain that temperature for a time period on the order of 1 hour. Attaining this thermal dose goal throughout a tumor volume requires the delivery of power with sufficient spatial and temporal variation to balance the heterogeneous and time-varying heat transfer processes within the target volume. Heat transfer from thermal conduction and blood perfusion redistribution of energy within living tissue are complex, and achieving the desired thermal uniformity across large tissue regions is difficult. Thermal conduction is a well-understood process, but in practical delivery of clinical hyperthermia the thermal conductivity is complicated by the irregularities of patient anatomy and tissue interfaces and varies by more than factor of two between high-water-content tissues and fat or bone. An even larger uncertainty in heat transfer is caused by blood perfusion, which varies dramatically among tissue types, and as a function of time and local temperature. Even with excellent control of the power deposition, knowledge of tissue thermal properties is needed in order to preplan temperature uniformity within a given target volume. In addition, since blood flow changes rapidly, temperature should be measured continuously during treatment in order to readjust the heating pattern for uniform temperature.

Clinical hyperthermia can be accomplished using one of three modalities: *thermal conduction* (e.g., circulating hot water in a needle, a catheter, or a surface pad), nonionizing *electromagnetic radiation* (EM), or *ultrasound* (US). In each case, heating is sensitive to tissue geometry, heterogeneity of tissue properties (especially blood perfusion), and issues with coupling energy into tissue from practical-sized applicators. Because of the limited penetration of heat from a hot source, thermal conduction heating is largely restricted to interstitial applications with closely spaced implant arrays. Energy can be delivered deeper into tissue using EM or US fields that deposit energy directly in tissue, with effective penetration dependent on frequency and applicator type. For either source, the absorbed power distribution is commonly normalized by the respective tissue density and referred to as the *specific absorption rate* (SAR) distribution, with units of watts per kilogram. The underlying physical principles are described in several excellent review articles[95–96,97–99,100] and in books that cover the field of hyperthermia.[101–102,103] Representative examples of typical heating equipment for each modality are given in the following subsections.

Electromagnetic Heating

When a radiofrequency electric field (*E* field) is applied to tissue, heating occurs from resistive losses as a result of electric current in a resistive media (tissue). At higher microwave frequencies, heat is generated from mechanical interactions between adjacent polar water molecules aligning to the alternating EM field. In either case, energy deposition is proportional to the electrical conductivity and square of the time-averaged *E* field. Electrical conductivity varies 50-fold depending on tissue type and frequency, with higher conductivity for high-water-content tissues like muscle and internal organs and much lower conductivity for fat and bone. The electrical properties of most tissues have been characterized over a large range of frequencies and published previously.[104] Power deposition has better penetration with lower-frequency, longer-wavelength fields, but the longer the wavelength, the broader is the focus of heating. To obtain deep penetration in the body, multiple-antenna arrays are required to diffuse surface heating, and in combination with the longer wavelengths this produces regional energy deposition that involves substantial volumes of tissue.

EM heating devices can be separated into two categories: superficial HT applicators, with effective penetration into tissue in the range of 1 to 4 cm; and deep HT devices, which have effective penetration >4 cm. Superficial HT devices include waveguides, modified horns,[105] capacitive and inductively coupled sheet antennas,[106,107] and microstrip[108,109] or patch antennas[110] that typically operate at 433, 915, or 2,450 MHz. In recent years, multiple-antenna planar and conformal array applicators have become more common to increase the size of tumor that can be heated, as well as to provide lateral adjustment of power deposition to accommodate heterogeneous tissue. These devices provide lateral adjustment of the power deposition pattern to equilibrate hot and cold regions across a tumor. Superficial microwave applicators are usually coupled into tissue through a deionized water bolus to accommodate surface irregularity. In addition, the bolus is usually temperature controlled to help maintain skin temperature below 44°C. Although current developmental multiantenna array applicators should be available commercially in the near future, the majority of superficial clinical HT is performed with BSD Medical (Salt Lake City, UT) waveguide applicators in the United States and Lucite cone applicators[105] or contact flexible microwave applicators[111] in Europe. Figure 31.5 shows typical

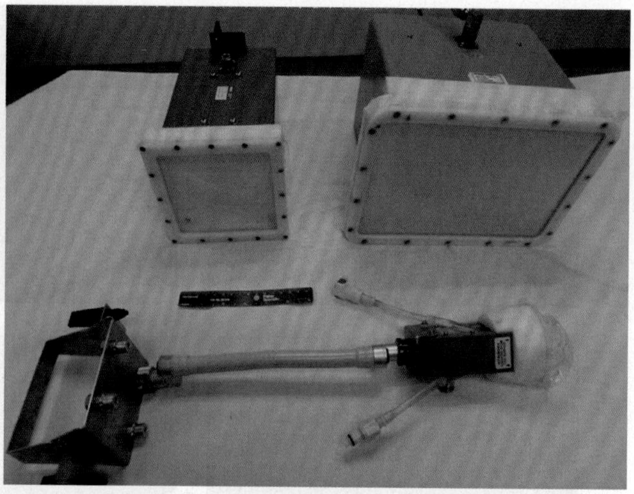

FIGURE 31.5. Photograph of three different-size microwave waveguide applicators used with the BSD 500 Hyperthermia system from BSD Medical (Salt Lake City, UT).

waveguide applicators used for heating up to 20 × 15 cm superficial chest-wall disease.

In order to heat at depths >4 cm, one must use lower frequencies in the radiofrequency (RF) band from 50 kHz to 150 MHz. There are three basic techniques for EM power deposition deep in tissue: magnetic induction heating, capacitively coupled RF current heating, and RF phased-array heating. Magnetic fields penetrate to the body axis but induce local eddy current loops that are governed by paths of least resistance and cause power deposition peaks and nulls that cannot be controlled externally. Although regional heating with magnetic induction failed to show sufficient control clinically,[112] there is interest in using magnetic fields to couple energy into implanted ferromagnetic seeds[113] and nanoparticles.[114]

The capacitive coupling technique uses RF fields from 5 to 30 MHz to drive currents between two or more saline pad electrodes. Heat is concentrated under the electrodes in tissues with high resistance (e.g., fat). The electrodes are generally aggressively cooled to prevent hot spots on the skin surface and superficial fat.[115] Although there is lack of real-time adjustment of heat distribution during treatment, energy can be concentrated on one side using a smaller electrode. The technique has been used effectively in the clinic for superficial and moderate depth tumors, predominantly in Asian patients with thin fat layers that can be cooled sufficiently with surface cooling.[116–117,118,119] Another possible approach is to drive RF current between an interstitial needle and a large-surface-area return electrode to focus heating at depth around the implanted electrode. Similarly, this can be done with an implanted balloon electrode for intracavitary applications (e.g., esophagus).[120]

The third option for noninvasive deep heating is the RF phased-array technique, which uses a body-concentric array of dipole antennas[121,122] or large waveguides.[123] Driving multiple antennas with equal phase produces a heat focus centrally in a concentric array, providing much deeper penetration than is possible operating the antennas noncoherently. By applying a phase delay to some of the antennas, one can steer the central focus laterally. Systems in the 1990s included four separate phase- and amplitude-controlled antennas in a single concentric array around the body. Since then, both dipole and waveguide array systems have been expanded to include two or three rings of antennas to provide axial as well as lateral adjustment of heating at depth.[123,124–125] In general, RF phased arrays have more flexibility in adjusting the SAR pattern than magnetic induction and capacitive heating techniques. The capacitive approach, such as Yamamoto Thermotron RF-8 (Yamamoto Vinita, Osaka, Japan), and RF phased-array applicators like the BSD Medical Sigma Ellipse and Sigma Eye are

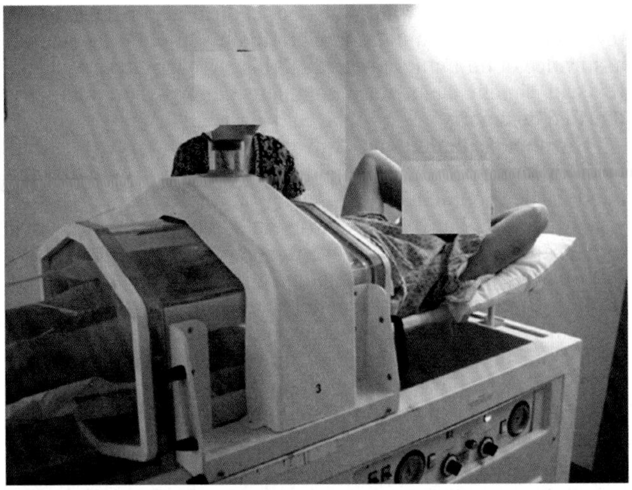

FIGURE 31.6. Photograph of non–muscle-invasive bladder cancer patient during deep regional hyperthermia treatment in BSD 2000 Sigma Ellipse applicator (BSD Medical, Salt Lake City, UT).

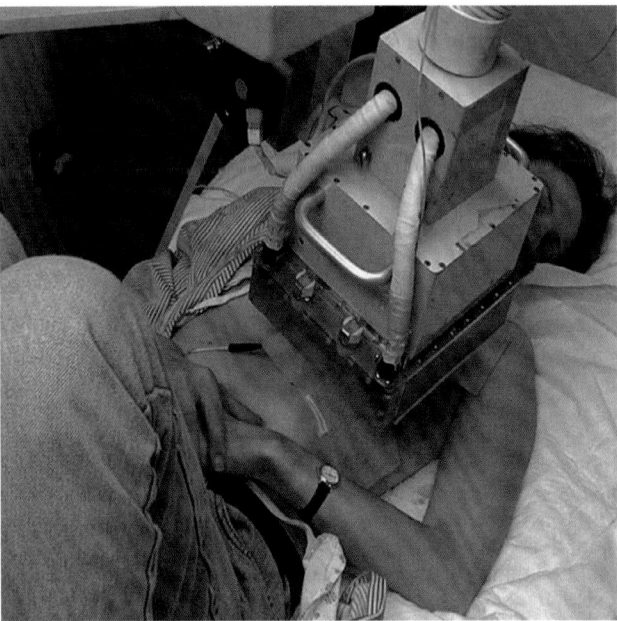

FIGURE 31.7. Sonotherm 1000 (Labthermics Technologies, Urbana, IL) 4 × 4 planar array ultrasound applicator treatment of chest-wall disease.

the most frequently used deep heat systems. Figure 31.6 shows a patient setup in the Sigma Ellipse applicator for treatment of non–muscle-invasive bladder cancer.

Ultrasound Heating

Energy transfer from an acoustic field results from the mechanical losses of viscous friction. The penetration of a US field decreases with increasing frequency, just as for EM energy. However, the wavelength of US is orders of magnitude smaller than that of an EM field of similar penetration capabilities, so that US energy can be focused into small tissue volumes. The use of small US applicators is an advantage for producing controllable sizes and shapes of focal regions at depth. However, anatomic geometry and tissue heterogeneity limit the use of US in many regions of the body because air reflects and bone preferentially absorbs US energy. The availability of an adequate "acoustic window" (path for US beam unobstructed by bone or air proximal or distal to the target) is the primary consideration for clinical applications.

Superficial tissue disease may be heated with a single unfocused US transducer, but array applicators are preferred for larger volumes typical of human disease. One popular clinical system involves a 4 × 4 transducer planar array applicator that treats up to 15-cm-square area.[126] Effective penetration of this lightly focused array is 2 to 6 cm using frequencies in the 1- to 3.5-MHz range. Transducers are coupled with a temperature-regulated conformal water bolus to control skin temperature, and good contact is ensured with US coupling gel. With all 16 transducers at the same frequency, the power deposition pattern can be adjusted laterally by varying power to the transducers, but only minor adjustment of penetration depth is possible by changing the water cooling temperature. The Sonotherm 1000 device (Labthermics Technologies, Champaign IL) shown in Figure 31.7 has been used successfully since the early 1980s for superficial tumors up to 6 cm deep.[127]

Deep heating with US may be obtained using stationary arrays of focused transducers, electronically phase focused arrays, or mechanically scanned focused arrays in the 0.5- to 2-MHz range. At these frequencies, penetration in soft tissue is substantial, and care must be taken to avoid problems with bony structures both in front of and behind the target volume. In addition, careful consideration of the beam path both entering and exiting the body is required to avoid potential surface burns from reflections at body/air interfaces. Ultrasound arrays have been used successfully for treating relatively small tissue regions at depth in the body, which is particularly appropriate for image-guided thermal ablation. Extension of ultrasound arrays for treating large tumors deep in the body has been attempted[128,129] but has not proven practical for clinical use.

Interstitial Hyperthermia

Interstitial heating shares many of the characteristics of interstitial brachytherapy—highly localized and inhomogeneous dose distributions, invasiveness, and sensitivity to specific site and approach. Heat treatments are usually combined close in time with brachytherapy, making dual use of implants for both hyperthermia and radiation. Some techniques permit simultaneous delivery, but most clinical experience has been with heat and radiation delivered sequentially.[130] As reviewed previously, there are numerous technologies for interstitial hyperthermia.[99,131]

The simplest approach involves heating the implants themselves with resistive heating elements, circulating hot water, or coupling energy into ferromagnetic implants from an external magnetic field.[132] Dense implant spacing (~1.0 cm between sources) is required because heat transfer is by thermal conduction only. More commonly, interstitial heating is accomplished within closely spaced arrays of 0.5- to 30-MHz radiofrequency electrodes[133,134] or 433- to 2,450-MHz microwave antennas.[135] With RF electrodes, heating occurs from currents between the exposed metal, and there is no mechanism to adjust heating along the electrode length during treatment. High current density in tissue near the electrode surface requires close electrode spacing (1 to 1.5 cm). Heterogeneous tissue conductivity or nonparallel RF electrodes compromise temperature uniformity. By raising the frequency from about 500 kHz to 10 to 30 MHz, current is coupled capacitively through the catheter wall, and electrodes may be segmented to enable adjustment of heating along the implant length.[136]

Interstitial microwave antennas have been designed for operation at frequencies of 433, 915, and 2,450 MHz, which produce different heating lengths in tissue (approximately 9, 4, and 2 cm, respectively). Although the antenna radiation pattern cannot be adjusted during treatment to accommodate different tumor dimensions, some designs offer the ability to select antennas of different heating lengths.[99] Although heating is generally not uniform along the length of interstitial microwave antennas, the radial penetration is higher than with RF or thermal conduction sources, permitting slightly larger spacing (e.g., 1.5 to 2 cm). In addition, EM fields from adjacent coherently phased antennas can interact constructively, resulting in maximum temperature rise centrally in an array rather than adjacent to the antenna surface.

In recent years, interstitial US has emerged as the most controllable interstitial heating approach, demonstrating the potential to adjust power deposition in tissue axially along the implant length, radially into tissue, and directionally around the implant.[137,138] Small tubular piezoelectric transducers with lengths on the order of millimeters may be aligned in a linear array to match any tumor length. The cylindrical elements radiate US pressure waves in the frequency range of 3 to 10 MHz. Penetration at these frequencies permits implant array spacing of ≥2 cm with better temperature uniformity than with other interstitial power sources, due to improved penetration, directional control of ultrasound radiation, and independent power control of each segment of tumor-length arrays.

Although considerable effort has gone into the development of interstitial heating technology, interstitial hyperthermia has lost its popularity due to decline in brachytherapy use and nonuniform distributions. Because of the excellent localization, the same technologies are seeing rapidly expanding use for thermal ablation procedures, which have a larger range of therapeutic temperature.[139]

Determination of Thermal Dose

Accurate real-time thermal dosimetry has been the limiting factor in the delivery of quality hyperthermia treatments. Temperature distributions are highly nonuniform and cannot be predicted accurately with present bioheat transfer modeling because the parameters used as input do not accurately model the spatial and temporal variation of actual properties. Clinical measurements of complete three-dimensional (3D) temperature distributions have not been technically feasible because most treatments have been monitored with only a limited number of invasive temperature measurements.

Numerous publications report correlation of various temperature-related parameters to clinical response based on sparse sampling with invasive probes. This effort has not been definitive in identifying quantitative parameters for prospective delivery of quality hyperthermia treatments. Minimum tumor temperature is one of the most-quoted prognostic temperature descriptors.[80,140,141] Biologically, it is reasonable to expect that treatment outcome will be associated with minimum temperature attained by all tumor cells. However, the true minimum of a distribution is never recorded with typical sparse sampling. Recognizing this limitation, investigators have looked at surrogates for biologically significant minimum temperature, such as the 90th-percentile temperature (T_{90}) or the temperature exceeded by 90% of measured points. Although they are less sensitive to clinical outcome than actual minimum tumor temperature, some investigators have found these surrogates to be reliable predictors for prescribing effective hyperthermia prospectively.[141,142,143] Going forward, it is expected that as our knowledge of minimum tumor temperature improves, parameters like fraction of tumor achieving temperatures greater than various indices (e.g., T40°C, T41°C, T42°C, etc.) will be increasingly predictive for response.

Typical clinical treatments are characterized with *invasive thermometry*, which samples 8 to 16 points continuously during heating. In some cases, 30 or more points are sampled using multisensor probes or by mechanically translating sensors through implanted catheters. Thermal mapping to achieve a higher density of measured points is now a quality assurance requirement for multi-institutional clinical trials.[144] Even so, the number of measurement points is extremely low and placement within the tumor ill defined. Strategies for choosing the spatial sampling of measurement points are highly variable, ranging from uniform spacing, to centrally or peripherally enhanced spacing, to just randomly placed sensors. Invasive thermometry has been firmly established as a basic requirement for monitoring and control of clinical hyperthermia, but there are serious limitations of random sampling as regards assurance of minimum prescribed dose. Clearly, future clinical HT will benefit from more complete noninvasive volumetric thermal dosimetry.

The obvious limitations of invasive thermometry for characterizing complex *in vivo* temperature distributions have stimulated the development of *noninvasive thermometry* approaches, which include backscatter ultrasound, electrical impedance tomography, active microwave imaging, passive microwave radiometry, and magnetic resonance thermal imaging (MRTI). Of these approaches, the volumetric average readings possible with microwave radiometry show most promise for control of superficial heat applicator distributions,[145] and the complete 3D characterization of tissue temperature distributions possible with multiple-slice MR thermal imaging shows most promise for monitoring and control of deep hyperthermia. Although several MR parameters are sensitive to temperature, proton resonance frequency shift–based MRTI has been shown to provide excellent temperature sensitivity and stability, with approximately 0.3°C to 0.5°C resolution in 1-cm^3 volumes in phantom studies[146] and 0.5°C to 1°C per 1 cm^3 in clinical monitoring of deep-tissue hyperthermia.[147–148,149] Although research is ongoing to correct image distortion and motion artifacts caused by breathing, organ movement, or circulating cooling water,[150–152] MR thermal imaging has clearly demonstrated its usefulness for monitoring clinical HT.

Numerical modeling of SAR and thermal distributions has experienced a dramatic improvement in accuracy in recent years due to advances in EM and thermal modeling software, tissue segmentation programs, and available computing power. Because the electrical properties of tissue are known with more certainty than thermal properties, current numerical modeling approaches are more accurate in calculating SAR patterns than steady-state temperature distributions. Investigators are reporting increasingly accurate results of patient treatment planning from SAR optimization[146,153] based on high-resolution, patient-specific anatomy derived from computed tomography or MRI scans. Current software can complete 3D SAR distribution calculations in a matter of hours. Until recently, validation of calculated SAR patterns has been performed primarily in simplified phantom models, using infrared thermography, Schottky diode sheet array,[154] or fiberoptic thermal monitoring sheet array[155] measurements of 2D cross-sectional planes in split phantom layered tissue models or 3D scanning of electric field probes through liquid muscle tissue–equivalent materials.[156] With the increasing availability of MR thermal imaging to provide complete noninvasive 3D characterization of thermal distributions, it is now possible to characterize heating patterns *in vivo* with high resolution during heating. This dynamic vision allows validation of preplanned SAR distributions or real-time adjustment of heating parameters to rectify errors in preplanned heating from unexpected tissue properties or misalignment of patient position in the applicator.

Along with the advent of more controllable heat applicators like the Academic Medical Center (Amsterdam, The Netherlands) three-ring waveguide array[123] and the BSD Sigma Eye three-ring dipole array,[157] pretreatment optimization of phase and amplitude drive parameters has become increasingly complex.[158] Even with high-resolution thermal feedback, rapid manual adjustment of multiple power sources for correction for unintended hot spots is challenging. Thus, new approaches are under investigation that use MR thermal feedback to correct errors in preplanned power excitation parameters via real-time adjustments to the power control algorithm.[159,160] The path is now clear for increasing use of noninvasive thermometry to provide high-resolution volumetric thermal feedback for real-time power adjustments, as well as adaptive correction of preplanned control algorithms. This includes increasing use of microwave radiometry for monitoring/control of superficial HT and MRTI for monitoring/control of deep HT. This new vision, combined with improving theoretical models, should lead to significantly enhanced uniformity of thermal dose, which should in turn produce large gains in efficacy of thermal therapy for cancer in the coming years.

CLINICAL HYPERTHERMIA

General Considerations

As mentioned in the biology section, HT is defined as elevation of temperatures to a supraphysiologic range. Typically this is in the range of 40°C to 45°C with heating durations of 1 hour. Much higher temperatures, in the range of 50°C to 100°C for a few minutes, have been used in single-treatment thermal ablative procedures for a variety of clinical sites, most often for the treatment of metastatic disease. Excellent recent reviews are available[161,162] Thermal ablation will not be discussed further in this chapter.

HT as defined is almost always used as an adjunctive treatment in conjunction with RT, CT, and more often today with the combination of CT and RT. There have been a number of investigations of the use of HT alone as cancer treatment. For superficial tumors a very transient response may be observed, but no long-term tumor control has been reported. HT alone is widely practiced in certain alternative and complementary medicine clinics, most often in Europe, but occasionally in the United States as well. The data offer no support for this practice. HT when used alone should not be confused with thermal ablative therapy, in which heat is used alone but to much higher temperatures and for which there is considerable supporting scientific evidence.

Radiotherapy Trials

Historically, HT was developed as an adjunctive treatment to RT because of the biological considerations cited earlier. A large number of reports, mostly phase II trials, involving patients with superficial malignant disease have suggested the efficacy of adjunctive HT.[163–164,165] There are, in addition, a moderately large number of phase III trials that attest to the efficacy of adjunctive HT combined with RT. These trials will be discussed in detail subsequently. In general, clinical response rates with the addition of HT to RT have approximately doubled from 25% to 35% with RT alone to 50% to 70% with the combination of RT and HT. Many of the phase III trials demonstrated improvements in disease-free survival, as well as overall survival.

Chemotherapy Trials

Local regional HT has also been combined with CT in a variety of clinical situations, including intraperitoneal carcinomatosis from ovarian carcinoma, colorectal carcinoma, appendiceal carcinoma, and primary peritoneal carcinomatosis, limb perfusion primarily for malignant melanoma, the treatment of locally advanced soft tissue sarcomas, the treatment of chest wall recurrences, primarily from breast carcinoma, the treatment of recurrent bladder carcinoma with intravesical CT, the treatment of locally advanced esophageal carcinoma, and finally as a part of trimodality therapy (RT, CT and HT) for locally advanced rectal carcinoma, cervical carcinoma, esophageal carcinoma, and head and neck carcinomas.

Most of the studies reported are phase II trials. The Rotterdam group treated 19 patients with locally recurrent cervix carcinoma after RT with a combination of HT and cisplatin. An overall response rate of 53% was observed, with one complete response, and that patient remaining free of disease 4 years later.[166] The use of CT and HT in locally advanced rectal carcinoma has also been explored. Nine patients were treated by Hildebrandt and colleagues with this combination, all patients having failed RT with or without surgery. The CT (oxaliplatin, folinic acid, and 5-FU) in combination with HT was moderately well tolerated and proved quite feasible in this phase I/II trial.[167] Another area of very active investigation has been the use of CT and RT for soft tissue sarcomas. Numerous phase II reports have been published, but more significantly, a large multi-institutional phase III trial has just been published and will be described subsequently in the section on phase III trials.

Intraperitoneal Chemotherapy and Hyperthermia

Two other areas of active interest involving the use of CT with HT are (a) the use of intraperitoneal CT at the time of cytoreductive surgery in conjunction with HT and (b) the combination of HT and infusion CT for limb perfusion in the management of extremity malignancies (hyperthermic isolated limb perfusion). Hyperthermic intraperitoneal chemotherapy was introduced approximately 20 years ago for the treatment of peritoneal carcinomatosis, primarily by the group at Washington Hospital Center (Washington, DC).[168] This procedure is an aggressive attempt to treat a situation generally considered incurable, that is, widespread peritoneal carcinomatosis. It is a complex, technically demanding procedure involving extensive cytoreductive surgery and a variety of chemotherapeutic agents subsequently installed into the peritoneal cavity with the perfusate heated to a temperature of 40°C to 43°C. Typically, the CT is infused over an approximately 5-day period. In highly selected patients this procedure has been associated with a significant cohort of long-term survivors but also significant morbidity and mortality. Survival rates ranging between 27% and 50% have now been reported from a number of studies, with the mortality of the treatment being reduced to less than 10% and the morbidity in the range of 30%. One randomized trial has been performed suggesting that this treatment is superior to palliative surgery and systemic CT,[169] but almost all other reports are phase I/II trials. The primary lesions most often treated have been colorectal cancer and ovarian cancer. Success and patient selection are very much dependent on the ability to achieve surgical resection of visible abdominal disease, leaving only microscopic intraperitoneal disease to be treated by the hyperthermic CT perfusate.

Results of these phase II trials have been reviewed extensively.[170,171,172] Although the phase II data and the one phase III trial look quite promising in comparison with standard CT and palliative surgery, it is unclear which components of the treatment are essential to its success. For example, would cytoreductive surgery combined with intraperitoneal CT without the HT component achieve results as good as cytoreductive surgery and hyperthermic intraperitoneal chemotherapy? Definitive phase III trials are necessary to answer this question.

Limb Perfusion Chemotherapy and Hyperthermia

Another application of HT has been in conjunction with limb perfusion with CT, primarily for the treatment of in-transit malignant melanoma and locally advanced soft tissue sarcomas that might otherwise require amputation. This procedure is commonly referred to as hyperthermic isolated limb perfusion (HILP). It was initiated almost 50 years ago. The rationale was that much higher doses of chemotherapeutic agents could be used by isolating the extremity circulation. The initial agent employed was melphalan; this has remained the standard of care. HT was added in an attempt to achieve chemosensitization. The current procedure calls for the use of a membrane oxygenator to maintain acid–base balance, as well as oxygenation of the isolated limb in the physiologic range. HT is achieved by heating the perfusate, as well as using external warming blankets. Temperatures are generally in the range of 38°C to 40°C. Isolation from the systemic circulation is achieved by the placing of a tourniquet proximal to the cannulated blood vessels.

The data have been reviewed by several authors.[173,174–175] For melanoma, complete response rates in the range of 50% to 70% are achieved, with overall 5-year survival in the range of 30% for this generally poor prognostic clinical scenario. For extremity sarcomas, complete response rates have ranged from 10% to 50% and partial response rates from 17% to 64%, with most reports toward the higher end of the range. Limb salvage has generally been achieved in about 60% to 85% of patients. The use of HILP for extremity sarcoma is a more recent procedure than that for melanoma. It was introduced in Europe with experience gained at many European centers but has not been approved by the U.S. Food and Drug Administration for use in the United States.

Few randomized trials are available comparing HILP with systemic CT, nor has the use of HT as a component of the procedure been compared with the use of infused CT alone. Phase II data, however, suggest a very poor response for systemic CT alone in the circumstances in which isolated limb perfusion is employed. The extensive experience with external applicator HT combined with CT for the treatment of locally advanced soft tissue sarcomas suggests that HT is an important component of the limb perfusion therapeutic package.

Trimodality Therapy Trials

The combination of CT, RT, and HT was explored in an international collaborative study for locally advanced cervix carcinoma.[176] Sixty-eight patients were treated in Europe and the United States with this program. Whole-pelvic RT to a dose of 45 to 50 Gy was delivered, followed by a brachytherapy boost, with the total dose to point A being approximately 86 Gy. All patients received weekly concurrent cisplatin. External microwave HT was delivered once weekly with different equipment, depending on the institution. The 2-year survival was 78% and the disease-free survival was 71%—encouraging data compared with historic controls, but needing to be confirmed in a phase III trial.

Rau and colleagues from Berlin also explored the use of preoperative trimodality therapy for locally advanced, untreated rectal carcinoma (RT, HT, and 5-FU/leucovorin).[177] RT was given to 45 Gy. External microwave HT was administered once weekly with the BSD 2000. Thirty-six patients were treated with this program, which was generally well tolerated. Thirty-two of 36 patients subsequently were surgically resectable. In 5 patients pathologic complete response (CR) was observed, with a partial response in an additional 17 patients. After surgery, overall survival was 86% at 38 months with no local recurrences. Again, these were quite encouraging results compared with historic controls, but phase III validation remains necessary.

Kang et al. from Korea reported on the treatment of 235 patients with locally advanced rectal cancer with concurrent preoperative radiochemotherapy with or without heat, although the patients were not randomized.[178] The CT consisted of 5-FU, leucovorin, and mitomycin C in most patients. HT was delivered twice weekly with a radiofrequency capacitive heating device. Intrarectal temperature was recorded, with the highest temperatures in the range of 40°C. One hundred thirty-seven patients were treated without HT and 108 with HT. Fifty-eight percent of the patients treated with trimodality therapy were downstaged, compared with 38% in the group receiving CT and RT without heat. The radiation dose was 40 to 45 Gy. Survival also seemed somewhat increased in the group of patients receiving HT. Again, confirmatory phase III data are necessary.

The use of trimodality therapy has also been reported for locally recurrent breast cancer.[179,180] Twenty-seven patients were treated, 23 of whom had been previously irradiated and 22 of whom had received prior CT. Patients were treated with superficial HT and RT to a dose of 45 Gy and capecitabine CT in 21 patients, vinorelbine in 2 patients, and paclitaxel in 4. Eighty percent of patients achieved a CR, with 76% locally controlled at 1 year. The treatment was quite well tolerated.

Investigators at Duke University also tested a novel approach of liposomal CT combined with HT for locally advanced breast cancer.[181] This approach is based on preclinical studies demonstrating that HT augments liposomal CT delivery to tumors and consequently will deposit a higher dose of CT at the heated tumor compared with surrounding normal tissue. A phase I/II trial enrolled 43 patients with stage IIB-III locally advanced breast cancer. Fourteen of these 43 patients had inflammatory cancer. The overall clinical response rate was 72%, with a 10% pathologic CR rate. The 4-year disease-free survival in these patients was 63%, and overall survival was 75%, again results that are quite promising but in need of confirmation.

A number of studies, principally from Japan, reported on the use of trimodality therapy for patients with esophageal carcinoma. Kuwano et al.[182] reported on 136 patients receiving preoperative trimodality therapy, with the CT consisting of cisplatin and bleomycin and 30 Gy of RT combined with heat from an endocavitary radiofrequency heating device. Approximately two-thirds of patients with locally advanced esophageal carcinoma achieved pathologic CR. The program was well tolerated. Five-year survival rates of 22% were obtained, compared with 13% in a matched group of patients receiving only preoperative CT and RT without HT. Phase III confirmatory trials are lacking.

Normal-Tissue Damage from Hyperthermia

With the use of HT—either superficial or deep heating—the most commonly encountered toxicities are superficial tissue burns. They are generally first or second degree in nature, occurring in approximately 5% to 10% of patients in the Duke experience and characteristically being relatively small in volume, generally less than 4 cm in maximum diameter. Careful monitoring of surface temperatures is necessary to keep this problem at a low incidence, but hot spots do occur. Third-degree burns are fortunately very unusual—<1% of patients in our experience. With deep regional heating, subcutaneous fat necrosis may be encountered with a frequency of about 10%. Usually this presents as firm small (1 to 2 cm) subcutaneous nodules. They are rarely painful and gradually resolve with time. They may be confused with local recurrence of cancer. Monitoring of intratumoral temperatures is frequently done in our institution, and catheter complications may occur if they are left in place throughout the course of HT (e.g., for several weeks). The most frequently reported complication in this instance is infection at the catheter site. If intratumoral temperature measurement catheters are removed and replaced with each treatment, catheter complications then become infrequent—less than 5%.[183]

There are potential medical contraindications to deep regional HT related to the potential physiologic stress of the procedure. Both the Radiation Therapy Oncology Group and the European Society of Hyperthermic Oncology have guidelines for the use of regional HT.[184,185–186]

Thermal Dosimetry and Clinical Outcome

The description, prescription, and delivery of a thermal dose is a complex problem. Although many advances have been made, the issue is far from solved and remains a work in progress. Thermal dose delivery is very different from conventional RT, where a dose may be precisely prescribed and delivered. Biologic tissue effects from heat are related to both the amount of temperature rise and the time of exposure. The rise in temperature depends not only on the energy deposited, but also on how much is carried away by thermal conduction and tissue blood perfusion. These factors almost always result in nonuniformity of tumor/tissue heating. Time–temperature relationships vary from patient to patient and may vary from treatment to treatment within the same patient. Accordingly, a method is necessary to normalize time–temperature measurements and convert them into a standard dosimetry unit so that different heat treatments may be compared. This is the basis for the concept of the cumulative equivalent minutes at 43°C described

TABLE 31.1 SELECTED PHASE III TRIALS OF CHEMOTHERAPY WITH OR WITHOUT RADIATION AND WITHOUT HYPERTHERMIA VERSUS CHEMOTHERAPY PLUS HYPERTHERMIA OR TRIMODALITY THERAPY

Author, Year	*Site*	*Treatment*	*Number of Patients*	*Outcome (%)*		
				CR	*LC*	*OS*
Kitamura, 1995	Esophagus	CRT	32	6	–	24.2
		CRT + HT	34	25[a]	–	50.4[a]
Columbo, 2003	Bladder	CT	41	–	35	–
		CT + HT	42	–	80[a]	–
Issels, 2010	Sarcomas	CT	172	1	55	57
		CT + HT	169	2.5	66[a]	59

CR, complete remission; CRT, combined radiotherapy; CT, chemotherapy; HT, hyperthermia; LC, local control; OS, overall survival.
[a]Statistically significant.

earlier (CEM 43°C). Typically during a heat treatment, temperature measurements are made at multiple points throughout the tumor, and minimal, average, and maximum temperatures are recorded. It has been found useful to describe temperature distribution in terms of percentile ranking. The T_{90}, for example, indicates that 90% of measured points exceed that temperature value. The T_{50} would indicate that 50% of measured points exceed the value in question. Taking into account the time of heating leads to the calculation of parameters such as the CEM 43°C T_{90}, which converts the temperature–time profile of any given heating session into the equivalent number of minutes for which 90% of the tumor exceeds 43°C.

Retrospective evaluation of many phase II and III trial results has often (but not always) shown a positive relationship between the thermal dose delivered and the treatment outcome, with higher doses producing a better outcome. Retrospective studies by our group suggested that a minimum thermal dose of 10 CEM 43°C T_{90} is necessary for clinical effectiveness.

We then attempted to confirm this in prospective trials with soft tissue sarcomas,[141] as well as in a randomized trial involving superficial chest-wall recurrences of breast carcinoma.[187] The sarcoma trial was unsuccessful, in that despite delivery of appropriate thermal doses, the obtained pathologic response rate was not as predicted. The phase III trial with superficial chest-wall recurrences, however, with the thermal dose prescribed prospectively showed a clear relationship of thermal dose administered to outcome. A third trial in pet dogs with soft tissue sarcomas also demonstrated a clear correlation between thermal dose and clinical outcome.[188] It thus appears that prospective control of thermal dose will lead to improved clinical outcomes, but the issue is by no means settled. Work continues on delineating the appropriate descriptors of thermal dose and how to integrate and normalize different patient and institutional data.

Phase III Clinical Trials

A surprising number of phase III trials have been conducted involving the use of HT and RT, HT and CT, or trimodality therapy. These trials have involved both superficial and the deep malignancies in various sites throughout the body and in patients in whom the treatment attempt was either curative or palliative. For the most part, the reported trials have shown benefit to the addition of HT. The more significant trials are summarized in Tables 31.1 and 31.2.

Breast Cancer Hyperthermia Trials

Locally recurrent breast cancer on the chest wall is probably the primary clinical situation in which the use of HT has been investigated because of the frequency of this clinical scenario, as well as its superficial nature, which facilitates heating. Many phase II trials have been published, generally showing positive effect for the addition of HT to RT. Five separate phase III trials were combined for analysis in an international collaborative study by Vernon.[189] Patients were randomized to either RT alone or RT combined with HT. Heating techniques differed somewhat among institutions. Nonetheless, significant improvement in the complete response rate of patients receiving HT + RT was demonstrated, with 59% complete response in the combined treatment group and 41% of those receiving RT alone. No survival differences were apparent, which is not unexpected, given that most patients had widespread disease. The differences were most pronounced in those patients who had been previously irradiated and were being re-treated.

A second important trial was carried out by Jones et al.,[187] in which superficial heatable tumors were randomly allocated to RT alone or RT + HT. This trial is unique, in that the HT dose was prospectively prescribed and administered. One hundred eight patients were entered into the trial, approximately evenly divided between the two arms, with significant improvements

TABLE 31.2 SELECTED PHASE III TRIALS OF RADIOTHERAPY ALONE VERSUS COMBINED RADIOTHERAPY AND HYPERTHERMIA

Author, Year	*Site*	*Treatment*	*Number of Patients*	*Outcome (%)*		
				CR	*LC*	*OS*
Datta, 1990	Head and neck	RT	32	31	19	–
		RT + HT	33	55	33	–
Valdagni, 1993	Head and neck (nodes)	RT	22	41	24	0
		RT + HT	18	83[a]	69	53[a]
Overgaard, 1995	Melanoma	RT	65+	35	28	–
		RT + HT	63	62[a]	46[a]	–
Vernon, 1996	Breast	RT	135	41	–	40
		RT + HT	171	59[a]	–	40
Sneed, 1998	Brain	RT	33	–	–	15
		RT + HT	36	–	–	31[a]
van der Zee, 2000	Cervix	RT	56	57	41	27
		RT + HT	58	83[a]	61[a]	51[a]
	Rectal	RT	71	15	8	22
		RT + HT	72	21	16	13
	Bladder	RT	49	51	33	22
		RT + HT	52	3[a]	742	28
Jones, 2005	Chest wall (breast)	RT	52	42	25	23
		RT + HT	56	66[a]	48[a]	21
Hua, 2011	Nasopharynx	RT + CT	90	81	79	63
		RT + HT + CT	90	96[a]	91[a]	73[a]

CR, complete remission; CT, chemotherapy; HT, hyperthermia; LC, local control; OS, overall survival; RT, radiotherapy.
[a]Statistically significant.

in CR rate, as well as in duration of local control for the HT-treated patients, although no survival differences were seen.

These two reports, as well as the numerous phase II trials in the literature for locally recurrent breast cancer, have led some to conclude HT should be a standard component of therapy for this clinical situation, particularly when local recurrence has developed following prior RT and consequently the dose of reirradiation is limited. Although there are no phase III trials comparing trimodality therapy for locally recurrent breast cancer, it is our usual practice to treat with a combination of superficial HT, RT, and CT, most often oral capecitabine. This combination is effective and quite well tolerated.

Head and Neck Carcinoma

Three randomized trials investigating the efficacy of HT in head and neck carcinoma have been published over the last 20 years. The first, by Datta et al.,[190] randomized 65 patients to receive RT alone or RT + HT for stage I-IV head and neck carcinoma of various primary sites. Fifty-two of the 65 patients had stage III/IV disease. Although a benefit was seen for the addition of HT to RT, it was significant only in the stage III/IV patients, where the 2-year disease-free survival was 25% in the RT/HT group, compared with 8% in the RT-alone group. No CT was used in this trial. The RT doses were approximately 65 Gy, and the heat was delivered via a diathermy machine.

Valdagni et al.[191] evaluated the treatment of cervical lymph nodes in patients with locally advanced head and neck cancer, randomizing 41 patients to treatment with either RT alone or RT + HT. Eighty-five percent of patients in the RT/HT arm achieved CR. Local control was 69% in the combined group at 5 years, and survival was 53%, compared with 24% and 0% in the RT-alone group. All differences were statistically significant. There was no enhancement of normal-tissue toxicity in the RT/HT group and no clear relationship between thermal dose received and outcome. Heat was delivered with an external microwave applicator.

The third trial was an investigation of nasopharynx carcinoma by Hua et al.[192] These investigators randomized 180 patients with advanced nasopharynx cancer to receive HT + RT or RT alone. HT treatment was carried out with an intracavitary microwave applicator. The CR rate was 95.6% in the RT/HT group, compared with 81% in the RT-alone group; local control was 91% versus 79%, and survival was 72.7% versus 63.1%, all differences statistically significant. The RT dose was 70 Gy in 2-Gy fractions. HT treatments were once weekly for 30 minutes following RT. All patients received concurrent cisplatin/5-FU CT as well.

Malignant Melanoma Trials

Overgaard and colleagues randomized 129 melanoma superficial/skin lesions in 70 patients between RT alone and RT + HT.[193] CR rate was 35% for those treated with RT alone, compared with 62% for those treated with the combination. Two-year local control rate was 46% in the RT/HT group, compared with 28% in the RT-alone group. All differences were statistically significant. Only 14% of the treatments in this study achieved the recommended thermal parameters of 43°C for 60 minutes. The heating was carried out with microwave applicators. Nonetheless, the observed benefits were seen with no apparent relationship to thermal dose.

Glioblastoma Multiforme Trials

At the University of California, San Francisco, Sneed and coworkers evaluated the use of interstitial HT combined with a brachytherapy boost for selected patients with glioblastoma multiforme.[135] Eligible patients were those whose tumor was implantable with interstitial seeds following external beam RT to 59.4 Gy. Such patients were randomized to brachytherapy alone or the same plus interstitial HT. Of the 79 randomized patients, 69 were evaluable; 33 were randomized to RT alone and 36 to RT + HT. Time to treatment failure and 2-year overall survival were significantly prolonged in the HT arm, with 31% vs. 15% survival for RT alone. CEM 43°C T_{90} ranged from 0 to 771, with a median of 14.1. Adequate thermal dose was achieved for most patients, but there was no clear correlation between thermal dose and outcome.

Dutch Deep Hyperthermia Trials

Among the more significant deep HT trials are those carried out by the Dutch group involving patients with cervical, rectal, and bladder cancer.[194] In these trials, 258 patients with previously untreated, locally advanced pelvic carcinomas were randomized to receive RT alone or RT + HT. HT treatments were generally given once weekly for a total of five treatments. Generally, thermal goals were not achieved, and again there was no clear relationship between thermal dose and outcome. For the entire group of patients, the CR rates were 39% and 55%, respectively, for the RT-alone group or RT+ HT (p >.001). The observed benefits, however, were largely confined to patients with cervical carcinoma. The CR rate for this group was 83% with RT + HT compared with 57% for RT alone; the overall survival at 3 years was 51% for the RT + HT group, compared with 27% for the RT-alone group. Local control was 61% at 3 years for the combined group versus 41% for the RT-alone patients.

This trial was criticized for the apparent suboptimal outcome in the control group. In addition, the demonstration of the efficacy of CT combined with RT in cervix cancer in several recent phase III trials has resulted in a new standard therapy—namely HT and CT combined for locally advanced cervix carcinoma—and raised the question of whether the addition of HT to RT and CT would be beneficial. Nonetheless, the Dutch trial is an important demonstration of the worth of HT combined with RT for deep-seated malignancies.

Phase III Trials of Hyperthermia Plus Chemotherapy

Selected phase III trials involving the use of HT and CT are shown in Table 31.1. Kitamura et al.[195] investigated the use of RT and CT for esophageal carcinoma compared with trimodality therapy (CT, RT, HT). Sixty-six patients were randomized. Intraluminal heating was delivered by a microwave applicator. Six HT treatments were delivered with a thermal goal of 42°C to 44°C at the tumor surface for 30 minutes. The treatment was given preoperatively and consisted of 30-Gy RT combined with either bleomycin or cisplatin. Subsequently, esophagectomy was performed. The pathologic CR rate was 25% for the trimodality group versus 6% in the CT/RT group. Three-year survival was 50.4% in the trimodality group and 24.2% in the CT/RT group, and the difference was statistically significant.

Columbo et al.[196] investigated the use of intravesical CT alone compared with the same plus HT for bladder carcinoma. Eighty-three patients were randomized to receive either mitomycin CT alone intravesically or the same plus HT. Each patient group, following complete transurethral resection of any bladder tumors, received eight weekly sessions of intravesical therapy, followed by a maintenance regimen of four monthly sessions. The duration of each treatment was 60 minutes. HT was delivered via an intravesical applicator. The temperature goal was a median temperature of 42°C ± 2°C for at least 40 minutes per session. The primary endpoint was recurrence-free survival, which was 35% at 2 years in the CT-alone patients and 80% in the CT + HT patients, a highly statistically significant result.

A third very important trial investigating the use of CT and HT for soft tissue sarcomas was published by Issels et al.[197] These investigators, in a multi-institutional European and North American study, randomized 241 patients with high-risk soft tissue sarcomas to receive neoadjuvant CT alone (etoposide, ifosfamide, doxorubicin) or the same CT with deep HT. The primary endpoint was local progression-free survival. Treatment was given on days 1 and 4 of each CT cycle with a goal of achieving tumor temperatures of 42°C for 60 minutes. Four cycles of CT were planned, followed by definitive surgical resection when possible and typically followed by postoperative RT as well. Neither the surgery nor the RT was randomized but was given to all suitable patients. At 4 years, local progression-free survival was 66% in the CT/HT group, compared with 55% in those receiving CT alone. This difference was highly statistically significant. Overall survival was comparable in the two groups as were distant metastasis. Nonetheless, this study provides high-quality evidence for the chemosensitization apparently achieved by locoregional HT. The failure to achieve a survival benefit emphasizes the need for better systemic therapy in this disease.

Summary of Phase III Clinical Trials

Results of the published phase III trials cited previously are intriguing and encouraging, despite significant problems in study design, with small numbers of patients in most trials and difficulties with HT administration, with failure to achieve thermal goals in many instances. The pattern of a beneficial effect from the addition of HT is striking and strongly suggests the worth of future trials and more widespread clinical application of HT.

Future Directions

Technical Challenges

The use of HT for the treatment of deep-seated tumors remains mostly experimental, with only one device, the BSD 2000, approved by the Food and Drug Administration for limited use in the United States. Deep heating often requires the use of invasive thermometry catheters; thus, particularly for deep heating, a team of skilled physicists, engineers, physicians, and nurses is required. Advances in noninvasive, MRI-based thermometry will assist greatly in helping to accurately determine and control thermal dose, but much work remains to be done in this area. The encouraging clinical data cited here for bladder tumors and soft tissue sarcomas will, it is hoped, stimulate further efforts along these lines. Small phase II investigations of other deep sites, such as locally advanced breast cancer, prostate, and rectal cancer, suggest a role for HT if technological advances proceed. Partnerships between academia and industry to facilitate equipment development are vitally necessary.

Multimodality Therapy

For the great majority of malignancies, single-modality therapy is a thing of the past. Successful treatment approaches often involve combinations of RT, CT, and surgery. HT must be considered in this context. The old model of investigating the combination of RT and HT without the use of CT is, for the most part, no longer applicable. Future trials addressing the value of HT need to ensure that best current treatment practice represents the control arm.

The combination of HT and CT without RT is an exciting new area. Drug delivery to tumors remains a major challenge due to a number of physiologic barriers, as discussed earlier. HT offers much potential in this area. The clinical evidence from the sarcoma and bladder trials cited earlier is impressive, as is the phase II evidence from intraperitoneal CT and limb perfusion studies. In addition, HT may serve as a trigger for temperature-sensitive drug delivery systems such as liposomes, polymers, and hydrogels.

Finally, a word about cost. Most new oncologic therapies are associated with significant cost profiles. Consider, for example, monoclonal antibodies, drugs that target angiogenesis, tyrosine kinase inhibitors, new RT technologies such as IMRT, proton beams, and the like. In this regard HT is relatively inexpensive. Given the results already achieved, further implementation and investigation seem clearly warranted.

SELECTED REFERENCES

A full list of references for this chapter is available online.

2. Kong G, Braun RD, Dewhirst MW. Hyperthermia enables tumor-specific nanoparticle delivery: effect of particle size. *Cancer Res* 2000;60(16):4440–4445.
4. Kong G, Dewhirst MW. Hyperthermia and liposomes. *Int J Hyperthermia* 1999; 15(5):345–470.
9. Sapareto SA, Dewey WC. Thermal dose determination in cancer therapy. *Int J Radiat Oncol Biol Phys* 1984;10(6):787–800.
16. Streffer C. Metabolic changes during and after hyperthermia. *Int J Hyperthermia* 1985;1(4):305–319.
19. Kampinga HH, Dikomey E. Hyperthermic radiosensitization: mode of action and clinical relevance. *Int J Radiat Biol* 2001;77(4):399–408.
20. Song CW, Park H, Griffin RJ. Improvement of tumor oxygenation by mild hyperthermia. *Radiat Res* 2001;155(4):515–528.
22. Liu FF, Miller N, Levin W, et al. The potential role of HSP70 as an indicator of response to radiation and hyperthermia treatments for recurrent breast cancer. *Int J Hyperthermia* 1996;12(2):197–208; discussion 9–10.
23. Rau B, Gaestel M, Wust P, et al. Preoperative treatment of rectal cancer with radiation, chemotherapy and hyperthermia: analysis of treatment efficacy and heat-shock response. *Radiat Res* 1999;151(4):479–488.
40. Dewhirst MW, Sim D, Gross J. Effects of heating rate on normal and tumor microcirculatory function. In: Diller K, Roemer RB, eds. *Heat and mass transfer in the microcirculation of thermally significant vessels*. Anaheim, CA: ASME, 1986: 75–80.
41. Song CW. Effect of local hyperthermia on blood flow and microenvironment: a review. *Cancer Res* 1984;44(10 Suppl):4721s–4730s.
42. Reinhold HS. Physiological effects of hyperthermia. *Recent Results Cancer Res* 1988;107:32–43.
43. Poon RT, Borys N. Lyso-thermosensitive liposomal doxorubicin: an adjuvant to increase the cure rate of radiofrequency ablation in liver cancer. *Future Oncol* 2011;7(8):937–945.
45. Ponce AM, Viglianti BL, Yu D, et al. Magnetic resonance imaging of temperature-sensitive liposome release: drug dose painting and antitumor effects. *J Natl Cancer Inst* 2007;99(1):53–63.
47. Dahl O. Interaction of heat and drugs *in vitro* and *in vivo*. In: Seegenschmiedt M, Fessenden P, Vernon C, eds. *Thermoradiotherapy and thermochemotherapy*. Berlin: Springer-Verlag, 1995:103–155.
49. Kelleher DK, Engel T, Vaupel PW. Changes in microregional perfusion, oxygenation, ATP and lactate distribution in subcutaneous rat tumours upon water-filtered IR-A hyperthermia. *Int J Hyperthermia* 1995;11(2):241–255.
50. Prescott DM, Charles HC, Sostman HD, et al. Therapy monitoring in human and canine soft tissue sarcomas using magnetic resonance imaging and spectroscopy. *Int J Radiat Oncol Biol Phys* 1994;28(2):415–423.
52. Oleson JR. Eugene Robertson Special Lecture. Hyperthermia from the clinic to the laboratory: a hypothesis. *Int J Hyperthermia* 1995;11(3):315–322.
53. Thrall DE, Larue SM, Pruitt AF, et al. Changes in tumour oxygenation during fractionated hyperthermia and radiation therapy in spontaneous canine sarcomas. *Int J Hyperthermia* 2006;22(5):365–373.
54. Brizel DM, Scully SP, Harrelson JM, et al. Radiation therapy and hyperthermia improve the oxygenation of human soft tissue sarcomas. *Cancer Res* 1996;56 (23):5347–5350.
55. Vujaskovic Z, Poulson JM, Gaskin AA, Thrall DE, Page RL, Charles HC, et al. Temperature-dependent changes in physiologic parameters of spontaneous canine soft tissue sarcomas after combined radiotherapy and hyperthermia treatment. *Int J Radiat Oncol Biol Phys* 2000;46(1):179–185.
56. Jones EL, Prosnitz LR, Dewhirst MW, et al. Thermochemoradiotherapy improves oxygenation in locally advanced breast cancer. *Clin Cancer Res* 2004;10(13): 4287–4293.
57. Zywietz F, Reeker W, Kochs E. Changes in tumor oxygenation during a combined treatment with fractionated irradiation and hyperthermia: an experimental study. *Int J Radiat Oncol Biol Phys* 1997;37(1):155–162.
59. Dings RP, Loren ML, Zhang Y, et al. Tumour thermotolerance, a physiological phenomenon involving vessel normalisation. *Int J Hyperthermia* 2011;27(1):42–52.
60. Jain RK. Normalization of tumor vasculature: an emerging concept in antiangiogenic therapy. *Science* 2005;307(5706):58–62.
62. Leeper DB, Engin K, Thistlethwaite AJ, et al. Human tumor extracellular pH as a function of blood glucose concentration. *Int J Radiat Oncol Biol Phys* 1994;28(4):935–943.
64. Prescott DM, Charles HC, Sostman HD, et al. Manipulation of intra- and extracellular pH in spontaneous canine tumours by use of hyperglycaemia. *Int J Hyperthermia* 1993;9(5):745–754.
67. Nagata K, Murata T, Shiga T, et al. Enhancement of thermoradiotherapy by glucose administration for superficial malignant tumours. *Int J Hyperthermia* 1998;14(2):157–167.
74. Overgaard J. The current and potential role of hyperthermia in radiotherapy. *Int J Radiat Oncol Biol Phys* 1989;16(3):535–549.
75. Gillette SM, Dewhirst MW, Gillette EL, et al. Response of canine soft tissue sarcomas to radiation or radiation plus hyperthermia: a randomized phase II study. *Int J Hyperthermia* 1992;8(3):309–320.
76. Dewhirst MW, Sim DA. The utility of thermal dose as a predictor of tumor and normal tissue responses to combined radiation and hyperthermia. *Cancer Res* 1984;44(10 Suppl):4772s–4780s.
80. Hand JW, Machin D, Vernon CC, et al. Analysis of thermal parameters obtained during phase III trials of hyperthermia as an adjunct to radiotherapy in the treatment of breast carcinoma. *Int J Hyperthermia* 1997;13(4):343–364.
82. Hettinga JV, Konings AW, Kampinga HH. Reduction of cellular cisplatin resistance by hyperthermia—a review. *Int J Hyperthermia* 1997;13(5):439–457.
90. Landon CD, Park JY, Needham D, et al. Nanoscale drug delivery and hyperthermia: the materials design and preclinical and clinical testing of low temperature-sensitive liposomes used in combination with mild hyperthermia in the treatment of local cancer. *Open Nanomed J* 2011;3:38–64.

91. Needham D, Anyarambhatla G, Kong G, et al. A new temperature-sensitive liposome for use with mild hyperthermia: characterization and testing in a human tumor xenograft model. *Cancer Res* 2000;60(5):1197–1201.
93. Yarmolenko PS, Zhao Y, Landon C, et al. Comparative effects of thermosensitive doxorubicin-containing liposomes and hyperthermia in human and murine tumours. *Int J Hyperthermia* 2010;26(5):485–498.
97. Hynynen K. Ultrasound heating technology. In: Seegenschmiedt MH, Fessenden P, Vernon CC, eds. *Thermoradiotherapy and thermochemotherapy*. Berlin: Springer-Verlag, 1995:253–277.
98. Lee ER. Electromagnetic superficial heating technology. In: Seegenschmiedt MH, Fessenden P, Vernon CC, eds. *Thermoradiotherapy and thermochemotherapy*. Berlin: Springer-Verlag, 1995:193–217.
99. Stauffer PR, Diederich CJ, Seegenschmiedt MH. Interstitial heating technologies. In: Seegenschmiedt MH, Fessenden P, Vernon CC, eds. *Thermoradiotherapy and thermochemotherapy. Vol. 1, Biology, physiology and physics*. Berlin: Springer-Verlag, 1995:279–320.
103. Seegenschmiedt MH, Fessenden P, Vernon CC, eds. *Thermoradiotherapy and thermochemotherapy. Vol. 1, Biology, physiology and physics*. Berlin: Springer-Verlag, 1995.
109. Lee ER, Wilsey TR, Tarczy-Hornoch P, et al. Body conformable 915 MHz microstrip array applicators for large surface area hyperthermia. *IEEE Trans Biomed Eng* 1992;39(5):470–483.
110. Stauffer P, Maccarini P, Arunachalam K, et al. Conformal microwave array (CMA) applicators for hyperthermia of diffuse chestwall recurrence. *Int J Hyperthermia* 2010;26(7):686–698.
111. van Wieringen N, Wiersma J, Zum Vorde Sive Vording P, O et al. Characteristics and performance evaluation of the capacitive contact flexible microstrip applicator operating at 70 MHz for external hyperthermia. *Int J Hyperthermia* 2009; 25(7):542–553.
118. Ohguri T, Imada H, Yahara K, et al. Radiotherapy with 8-MHz radiofrequency-capacitive regional hyperthermia for stage III non-small-cell lung cancer: the radiofrequency-output power correlates with the intraesophageal temperature and clinical outcomes. *Int J Radiat Oncol Biol Phys* 2009;73(1):128–135.
121. Franckena M, Fatehi D, de Bruijne M, et al. Hyperthermia dose-effect relationship in 420 patients with cervical cancer treated with combined radiotherapy and hyperthermia. *Eur J Cancer* 2009;45(11):1969–1978.
123. Kok HP, de Greef M, Borsboom PP, et al. Improved power steering with double and triple ring waveguide systems: the impact of the operating frequency. *Int J Hyperthermia* 2011;27(3):224–239.
127. Samulski TV, Grant WJ, Oleson JR, et al. Clinical experience with a multi-element ultrasonic hyperthermia system: analysis of treatment temperatures. *Int J Hyperthermia* 1990;6(5):909–922.
135. Sneed PK, Stauffer PR, McDermott MW, et al. Survival benefit of hyperthermia in a prospective randomized trial of brachytherapy boost +/– hyperthermia for glioblastoma multiforme. *Int J Radiat Oncol Biol Phys* 1998;40(2):287–295.
137. Diederich CJ. Thermal ablation and high-temperature thermal therapy: overview of technology and clinical implementation. *Int J Hyperthermia* 2005;21(8): 745–753.
142. Leopold KA, Dewhirst MW, Samulski TV, et al. Cumulative minutes with T90 greater than Tempindex is predictive of response of superficial malignancies to hyperthermia and radiation. *Int J Radiat Oncol Biol Phys* 1993;25(5):841–887.
145. Jacobsen S, Stauffer PR. Can we settle with single-band radiometric temperature monitoring during hyperthermia treatment of chestwall recurrence of breast cancer using a dual-mode transceiving applicator? *Phys Med Biol* 2007;52(4):911–928.
147. Craciunescu O, Stauffer P, Soher B, et al. Accuracy of real time noninvasive temperature measurements using magnetic resonance thermal imaging in patients treated for high grade extremity soft tissue sarcomas. *Med Phys* 2009;36(11):4848–4858.
148. Gellermann J, Hildebrandt B, Issels R, et al. Noninvasive magnetic resonance thermography of soft tissue sarcomas during regional hyperthermia: correlation with response and direct thermometry. *Cancer* 2006;107(6):1373–1382.
153. Paulides MM, Bakker JF, Linthorst M, et al. The clinical feasibility of deep hyperthermia treatment in the head and neck: new challenges for positioning and temperature measurement. *Phys Med Biol* 2010;55(9):2465–2480.
157. Gellermann J, Weihrauch M, Cho CH, et al. Comparison of MR-thermography and planning calculations in phantoms. *Med Phys* 2006;33(10):3912–3920.
162. Webb H, Lubner MG, Hinshaw JL. Thermal ablation. *Semin Roentgenol* 2011; 46(2):133–141.
163. Wust P, Hildebrandt B, Sreenivasa G, et al. Hyperthermia in combined treatment of cancer. *Lancet Oncol* 2002;3(8):487–497.
164. Horsman MR, Overgaard J. Hyperthermia: a potent enhancer of radiotherapy. *Clin Oncol* 2007;19(6):418–426.
169. Verwaal VJ, van Ruth S, de Bree E, et al. Randomized trial of cytoreduction and hyperthermic intraperitoneal chemotherapy versus systemic chemotherapy and palliative surgery in patients with peritoneal carcinomatosis of colorectal cancer. *J Clin Oncol* 2003;21(20):3737–3743.
170. Roviello F, Caruso S, Marrelli D, et al. Treatment of peritoneal carcinomatosis with cytoreductive surgery and hyperthermic intraperitoneal chemotherapy: state of the art and future developments. *Surg Oncol* 2011;20(1):e38–e54.
172. Chua TC, Robertson G, Liauw W, et al. Intraoperative hyperthermic intraperitoneal chemotherapy after cytoreductive surgery in ovarian cancer peritoneal carcinomatosis: systematic review of current results. *J Cancer Res Clin Oncol* 2009;135(12):1637–1645.
174. Turley RS, Raymond AK, Tyler DS. Regional treatment strategies for in-transit melanoma metastasis. *Surg Oncol Clin North Am* 2011;20(1):79–103.
175. Deroose JP, Eggermont AM, van Geel AN, et al. Long-term results of tumor necrosis factor alpha- and melphalan-based isolated limb perfusion in locally advanced extremity soft tissue sarcomas. *J Clin Oncol* 2011;29(30):4036–4044.
176. Westermann AM, Jones EL, Schem BC, et al. First results of triple-modality treatment combining radiotherapy, chemotherapy, and hyperthermia for the treatment of patients with stage IIB, III, and IVA cervical carcinoma. *Cancer* 2005;104 (4):763–770.
178. Kang MK, Kim MS, Kim JH. Clinical outcomes of mild hyperthermia for locally advanced rectal cancer treated with preoperative radiochemotherapy. *Int J Hyperthermia* 2011;27(5):482–490.
179. Zagar TM, Oleson JR, Vujaskovic Z, et al. Hyperthermia for locally advanced breast cancer. *Int J Hyperthermia* 2010;26(7):618–624.
180. Zagar TM, Higgins KA, Miles EF, et al. Durable palliation of breast cancer chest wall recurrence with radiation therapy, hyperthermia, and chemotherapy. *Radiother Oncol* 2010;97(3):535–440.
181. Vujaskovic Z, Kim DW, Jones E, et al. A phase I/II study of neoadjuvant liposomal doxorubicin, paclitaxel, and hyperthermia in locally advanced breast cancer. *Int J Hyperthermia* 2010;26(5):514–521.
185. Waterman FM, Dewhirst MW, Fessenden P, et al. RTOG quality assurance guidelines for clinical trials using hyperthermia administered by ultrasound. *Int J Radiat Oncol Biol Phys* 1991;20(5):1099–1107.
186. Lagendijk JJ, Van Rhoon GC, Hornsleth SN, et al. ESHO quality assurance guidelines for regional hyperthermia. *Int J Hyperthermia* 1998;14(2):125–133.
187. Jones EL, Oleson JR, Prosnitz LR, et al. Randomized trial of hyperthermia and radiation for superficial tumors. *J Clin Oncol* 2005;23(13):3079–3085.
189. Vernon CC. Radiotherapy with or without hyperthermia in the treatment of superficial localized breast cancer: results from randomized controlled trials. *Int J Radiat Oncol Biol Phys* 1996;35(4):731–744.
192. Hua Y, Ma S, Fu Z, et al. Intracavitary hyperthermia in nasopharyngeal cancer: a phase III clincal stuudy. *Int J Hyperthermia* 2011;27(2):180–186.
194. van der Zee J. Comparison of radiotherapy alone with radiotherapy plus hyperthermia in locally advanced pelvic tumors: a prospective randomised multicentre trial. *Lancet* 2000;355:1119–1125.
196. Colombo R, Da Pozzo LF, Salonia A, et al. Multicentric study comparing intravesical chemotherapy alone and with local microwave hyperthermia for prophylaxis of recurrence of superficial transitional cell carcinoma. *J Clin Oncol* 2003; 21(23):4270–4276.
197. Issels RD, Lindner LH, Verweij J, et al. Neo-adjuvant chemotherapy alone or with regional hyperthermia for localised high-risk soft-tissue sarcoma: a randomised phase 3 multicentre study. *Lancet Oncol* 2010;11(6):561–570.
198. Roizin-Towle L, Pirro JP. The response of human and rodent cells to hyperthermia. *Int J Radiat Oncol Biol Phys* 1991;20(4):751–756.

Chapter 32
Basic Concepts of Chemotherapy and Irradiation Interaction

D. Nathan Kim, Michael Story, and Hak Choy

For decades, radiation therapy has been a major treatment modality for locally or regionally confined cancers. The rate of treatment failure is still high, particularly for large tumors or advanced disease. Technologic improvements in radiation therapy have continuously been made that allow delivery of higher radiation doses to the tumor or lower doses to normal tissues, and in the implementation of strategies that modulate the biologic response of tumors or normal tissues to radiation. These strategies include altered fractionation scheduling including extreme hypofractionation (e.g., stereotactic body radiotherapy, stereotactic radiosurgery), combined-modality treatments using chemical or biologic agents, and, more recently, targeting molecular processes and signaling pathways that have become dysregulated in cancer cells.

The combination of chemotherapeutic drugs with radiation has perhaps had one of the strongest impacts on current cancer radiation therapy practice. This is particularly true for concurrent chemoradiation therapy, which has been shown in many recent clinical trials to be superior to radiation therapy alone in controlling locoregional disease and in improving patient survival. Combining chemotherapeutic drugs with radiation therapy has a strong biologic rationale. Such agents reduce the number of cells in tumors undergoing radiation therapy by their independent cytotoxic action and by rendering tumor cells more susceptible to killing by ionizing radiation. An additional benefit of combined treatment is that chemotherapeutic drugs, by virtue of their systemic activity, may also act on metastatic disease. Most drugs have been chosen for combination with radiation therapy based on their known clinical activity in particular disease sites. Alternatively, agents that are effective in overcoming resistance mechanisms associated with radiation therapy could be chosen. There have been clinical successes with concurrent chemoradiation therapy using traditional drugs, such as cisplatin and 5-fluorouracil (5-FU), and these studies have led to extensive research on exploring newer chemotherapeutic agents for their interactions with radiation. A number of potent chemotherapeutic agents, subsequently, have entered clinical trials or practice. These agents were selected after strong preclinical studies demonstrated that they are potent enhancers of the radiation response and thus might further improve the therapeutic outcome of chemoradiation therapy. Also, there are rapidly emerging molecular targeting strategies aimed at improving the efficacy of radiation therapy.

This chapter reviews the biologic rationale and principles fundamental to the use of chemotherapy and molecular targeted agents in conjunction with radiation treatments and discusses mechanistic interactions between drugs and radiation, the knowledge of which is essential in developing the optimal treatment strategies and designing appropriate clinical trials. It also provides a brief overview of current treatment applications and advances in the clinic. Owing to limited space, this review is far from comprehensive; additional information can be found in other reviews on this subject.[1,2,3–4,5]

THERAPEUTIC INDEX

Both radiation and chemotherapeutic drugs are cytotoxic to tumor and normal tissue cells. This lack of specificity is a major limitation in their use when applied either as individual treatments or in combination. Radiation inflicts damage to tumor and normal tissues in the radiation treatment field, whereas drugs, because of their systemic action, can affect any tissue in the body. Damage is often accentuated when the two agents are combined and when they affect the same tissue. In general, both the antitumor effectiveness and the severity of normal-tissue damage produced by either radiation or drugs are increased as their dose is increased. This dose–effect relationship is sigmoidal and enables estimation of the therapeutic index (ratio), which is defined as the ratio between the doses (radiation, drug) that produce the same level (probability) of antitumor efficacy and normal-tissue damage. To be therapeutically beneficial, the therapeutic ratio must be positive (>1); that is, individual agents or their combination must be more effective against tumors than normal tissues. To define therapeutic benefit in clinical settings, many factors must be taken into account, such as whether the treatment is curative or palliative, which tissues are dose limiting (critical tissues), what degree of tissue damage is acceptable, and so forth. The balance between a given level of antitumor efficacy and acceptable normal-tissue complications gives a measure of the therapeutic ratio of a treatment.

EXPLOITABLE STRATEGIES IN CHEMORADIATION THERAPY

The goals of combining chemotherapeutic drugs with radiation therapy are to increase patient survival by improving locoregional tumor control, decrease or eliminate distant metastases, or both, while preserving organ and tissue integrity and function. Combined-modality treatment can further improve positive therapeutic outcome of individual treatments through a number of specific strategies, which Steel and Peckham[6] classified into four groups: "spatial cooperation," independent toxicity, enhancement of tumor response, and protection of normal tissues.

Spatial cooperation was the initial rationale for combining chemotherapy with radiation therapy, in which the action of radiation and chemotherapeutic drugs is directed toward different anatomic sites. Localized tumors would be the domain of radiation therapy because large doses of radiation can be given. On the other hand, chemotherapeutic drugs are likely to be more effective in eliminating disseminated micrometastases than in eradicating larger primary tumors. Thus, the cooperation between radiation and chemotherapy is achieved through the independent action of two agents. Spatial cooperation is the basis for adjuvant chemoradiation therapy, in which radiation is given first to control the primary tumor and chemotherapy is given later to cope with micrometastases. The concept of spatial cooperation is also applied in the treatment of hematologic malignancies that have spread to "sanctuary" sites, such as the brain. These sites are poorly accessible to chemotherapeutic agents, and thus they are more appropriately treated with radiation therapy.

Independent toxicity is another important strategy for increasing the therapeutic ratio of chemoradiation therapy. Normal-tissue toxicity is the main dose-limiting factor for both chemotherapy and radiation therapy. Therefore, combinations of radiation and drugs would be better tolerated if drugs were selected such that toxicities to specific cell types and tissues do not overlap with, or minimally add to, radiation-induced toxicities. This strategy requires a thorough knowledge of drug toxicity, underlying mechanisms, and drug pharmacokinetics. Another strategy in chemoradiation therapy is to exploit the ability of chemotherapeutic agents to *enhance tumor radioresponse*. The enhancement denotes the existence of some type of interaction between drugs and radiation at the molecular, cellular, or pathophysiologic (microenvironmental, metabolic) level, resulting in an antitumor effect greater than would be expected on the basis of additive actions. Many mechanisms may be involved in drug–radiation interactions leading to tumor radio enhancement, and some of them are elaborated on further in the text. The enhancement must be selective or preferential to tumors compared with critical normal tissues to achieve therapeutic gain. The ability of chemotherapeutic agents to enhance tumor radioresponse by counteracting determinants associated with tumor radioresistance is a major rationale for concurrent radiation therapy.

An additional strategy is to *protect normal tissues* so that higher doses of radiation can be delivered to the tumor. This can be achieved through technical improvements in radiation delivery or administration of chemical or biologic agents that selectively or preferentially protect normal tissues against the damage by radiation or drugs. A separate section in this chapter discusses radioprotectors in more detail.

ASSESSMENT OF DRUG–RADIATION INTERACTION

Any drug considered for use in combination with radiation therapy needs to undergo preclinical evaluation for its interaction with radiation both in *in vitro* cell culture systems and *in vivo,* with the aim of assessing antitumor activity and normal-tissue toxicity. The interaction between two agents is more easily defined and quantified *in vitro* because complete cell survival curves are readily obtained. The *in vitro* cell survival assay measures the ability of cells to produce colonies of a defined minimum size. Cell survival is determined after treatment with a drug or radiation alone, given at different doses, or after treatment with both agents, in which case the cells are exposed to the drug before, during, or after irradiation. Survival curves are usually plots of the surviving fraction of cells on a logarithmic scale and the dose of radiation or drugs on a linear scale.

The cell survival curve after irradiation characteristically has a "shoulder" of varying width that denotes the capacity of cells to repair radiation damage. The curves that describe survival after chemotherapeutic agents show much more variation both in absolute sensitivity to drugs and their shape than those after radiation, all depending on the drug tested. Some curves possess shoulders, some lack them, and some show resistant "tails" at higher drug doses. The tails denote the existence of cell subpopulations resistant to chemotherapeutic agents.

To assess the effect of the drug on cell radiosensitivity, the combined drug–radiation curve is commonly plotted after the cytotoxicity produced by the drug alone is excluded ("normalized"). The radiation cell survival curve is not changed if the drug does not influence cell radiosensitivity regardless of whether the drug is cytotoxic on its own. In this case, the cytotoxicity of the drug contributes only to the overall cell killing by the combined treatment (*additive effect*) of both agents. Chemotherapeutic agents may interact with radiation by altering cell radiosensitivity such that the combination results in a *supra-additive* or *subadditive effect*, depending on whether the cell killing is greater or smaller than the sum of cell killings produced by individual agents. Drugs may eliminate the shoulder on the radiation survival curve, implying that drugs can inhibit cell repair from radiation damage, or they may change the slope of the exponential portion of the survival curve. A steeper slope indicates increased sensitization to radiation, whereas a shallower slope indicates protection.

Because of nonlinear dose-related characteristics in cell killing by both chemotherapeutic agents and radiation, the effects of the combined treatment are best assessed using the "isobologram," an isoeffect plot for the dose response to the combination of two agents[6] (Fig. 32.1). Dose–response curves are determined for each agent to generate the isobologram, an envelope of additivity, which denotes expected additive response over a range of doses of the agents used. If the interaction between drugs and radiation is supra-additive or synergistic (i.e., the effect is caused by lower doses of the two agents than the envelope of additivity would predict), the effect is shown at the left side of the envelope. In contrast, the effect of the subadditive or antagonistic interaction is shown to the right of the envelope: the effect required higher doses of the two agents than predicted. The width of the envelope of additivity depends on the degree of the nonlinearity in the dose response to individual agents. The envelope is wider as the degree of nonlinearity increases. In the case of a linear dose–response relationship for each agent, which is rare, the isobologram is also linear, represented by a single straight line.

In vitro testing is often followed by *in vivo* exploration of drug–radiation interactions, which allows assessment of the combined treatment on both tumors and normal tissues. This

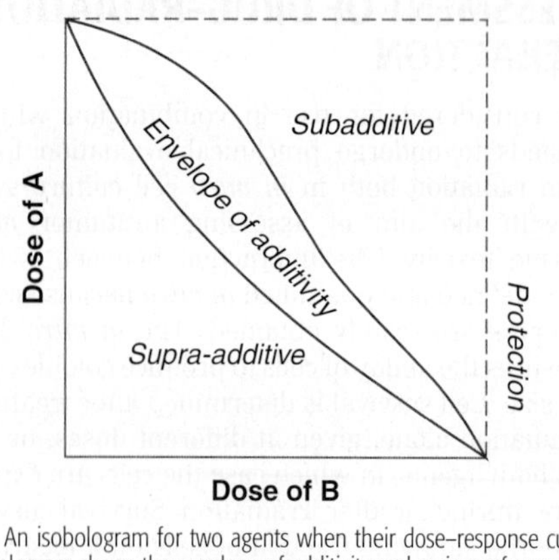

FIGURE 32.1. An isobologram for two agents when their dose–response curves are nonlinear. The isobologram shows the envelope of additivity and regions of supra-additivity and subadditivity. (Modified from Steel GG, Peckham MJ. Exploitable mechanisms in combined radiotherapy-chemotherapy: the concept of additivity. *Int J Radiat Oncol Biol Phys* 1979;5: 85–91, with permission. Copyright 1979 by Elsevier Science, Inc.)

is essential for determination of therapeutic gain, as discussed earlier in this chapter. Syngeneic animal tumors or human tumor xenografts in nude mice are most often used for this purpose. The efficacy of the treatment is determined by the extent of tumor growth delay or the rate of tumor cure. In normal tissues, the effect of chemotherapeutic drugs on radiation response of acutely and late-responding tissues can be assessed using a variety of available assays. Some of these assays are clonogenic, such as the jejunal crypt assay, where the end point depends directly on the reproductive integrity of individual cells. More frequently, however, dose–response relationships for normal tissues are based on functional end points (such as breathing rate in lung damage and paralysis in spinal cord damage). These end points tend to reflect the minimum number of functional cells remaining in tissues or organs and not the proportion of cells retaining reproductive integrity.

MECHANISTIC CONSIDERATIONS IN DRUG–RADIATION INTERACTIONS

Increasing Initial Radiation Damage

Radiation induces many different lesions in the DNA molecule, which is the critical target for radiation damage. The lesions consist of single-strand breaks (SSBs), double-strand breaks (DSBs), base damage, DNA–DNA and DNA–protein cross-links, and so forth. DSBs and chromosome aberrations that occur in association with or as a consequence of DSBs are usually considered to be the principal damage that results in cell death.[7] Any agent that makes DNA more susceptible to radiation damage may enhance cell killing. Certain drugs, such as halogenated pyrimidines, incorporate into DNA and make it more susceptible to radiation damage.[8]

Inhibition of Cellular Repair

Both sublethal[9] and potentially lethal[10,11] damage inflicted by radiation can be repaired. Although sublethal damage repair (SLDR) denotes the increase in cell survival when the radiation dose is split into two fractions of radiation separated by a time interval, potentially lethal damage repair (PLDR) designates the increase in cell survival as the result of postirradiation environmental conditions. SLDR is rapid, with a half-time of approximately 1 hour, and is complete within 4 to 6 hours after irradiation. This time between two radiation fractions allows radiation-induced DSBs in DNA to rejoin and repair. SLDR is expressed as the restitution of the shoulder on the cell survival curve for the second dose. PLDR occurs when environmental conditions prevent cells from dividing for several hours, such as keeping *in vitro* growing cells in plateau phase after irradiation. Preventing cells from division allows the completion of repair of DNA lesions that would have been lethal had DNA undergone replication within several hours after irradiation. PLDR is considered to be a major determinant responsible for radioresistance in some tumor types, such as melanomas. The repair can be achieved through restoration of damaged molecules by reducing species that donate electrons to oxidized substrates or through involvement of enzymes mediating homologous and nonhomologous recombination repair of DNA DSBs, base excision repair of base damage, and nucleotide excision repair of DNA–protein cross-links.

Many chemotherapeutic agents used in chemoradiation therapy interact with cellular repair mechanisms and inhibit repair, and hence may enhance cell or tissue response to radiation. The aforementioned halogenated pyrimidines enhance cell radiosensitivity not only through increasing initial radiation damage but also by inhibiting cellular repair.[8,12] Nucleoside analogs, such as gemcitabine, are a class of chemotherapeutic agents potent in inhibiting the repair of radiation-induced DNA and chromosome damage.[13,14] They have been shown strongly to enhance tumor radioresponse in preclinical studies and have been, and are continuing to be, extensively investigated for such activity in patients with cancer.[15,16]

Cell Cycle Redistribution

Both chemotherapeutic agents and radiation are more effective against proliferating than nonproliferating cells. Their cytotoxic action further depends on the position of cells in the cell cycle. Cell cycle dependency in response to radiation was first described almost 40 years ago.[17] Terasima and Tolmach.[17] reported that the sensitivity of the cell response to radiation varied widely depending on which phase of the cell cycle the cells were in at the time of irradiation, and that cells in the G_2 and M cell cycle phases were approximately three times more sensitive than cells in the S phase. The exact reason for this variability is still unknown.

The influence of the cell cycle on cell response to cytotoxic agents can be therapeutically exploited in chemoradiation therapy using cell cycle redistribution strategies. For example, some chemotherapeutic drugs, such as taxanes, can block transition of cells through mitosis, with the result that cells accumulate in the radiosensitive G_2 and M phases of the cell cycle. Radiation delivered at the time of significant accumulation of cells in both the G_2 and M phases results in enhanced radioresponse of cells *in vitro*[18,19] and of tumors *in vivo*.[20,21] However, this cell cycle mechanism of taxane-induced enhancement of tumor radioresponse is dominant only in tumors that are resistant to paclitaxel or docetaxel as a single treatment. Although tumor growth in taxane-resistant tumors is not substantially affected by the drug, tumors do exhibit significant transient accumulation of cells in mitosis 6 to 12 hours after the treatment.[21] Taxanes also enhance the radioresponse of tumors that respond by significant tumor growth delay to taxanes given as a single treatment modality, but a major mechanism for radio enhancement in such tumors is reoxygenation of radioresistant hypoxic cells, as discussed later.[20]

Elimination of the radioresistant S-phase cells by the chemotherapeutic agents may be another cell cycle redistribution strategy in chemoradiation therapy. Nucleoside analogs, such as fludarabine or gemcitabine, are good examples of the agents that become incorporated into S-phase cells and eliminate them by inducing apoptosis.[13,15] In addition to purging S-phase cells, the analogs induce the surviving cells to undergo parasynchronous movement to accumulate in the G_2 and M phases of the cell cycle between 1 and 2 days after drug administration, a time when the highest enhancement of tumor radioresponse was observed.[15] Tumors with a high cell growth fraction are likely to respond better to the cell cycle redistribution strategy in chemoradiation therapy than tumors with a low cell growth fraction.

Counteracting Hypoxia-Associated Tumor Radioresistance

Solid malignant tumors usually are characterized by defective vascularization, both in the number of blood vessels and vessel function. Because of this, blood supply to tumor cells is inadequate, cells lack oxygen and nutrients, and multiple tumor microregions become hypoxic, acidic, and eventually necrotic. Hypoxia occurs at distances from blood vessels larger than 100 to 150 μm. The hypoxic cell content in tumors varies widely and can be more than 50%. The presence of hypoxia makes tumors more aggressive (hypoxia is conducive to the emergence of more virulent tumor cell variants and stimulates metastatic spread[22,23]) and more resistant to radiation as well as most chemotherapeutic agents. Hypoxic cells are 2.5 to 3 times more resistant to radiation than well-oxygenated cells. The fact that hypoxia may be a cure-limiting factor in radiation therapy, at least in some clinical situations, is suggested by the findings that reduced hemoglobin levels[24] and low tumor pO_2[25,26] are associated with higher treatment failure rates. Also, there are reports showing that local tumor control by radiation therapy can be improved by the use of hypoxic cell radiosensitizers[27] or hyperbaric oxygen.[28,29] With respect to the effects of chemotherapy, hypoxic regions are less accessible to chemotherapeutic drugs; in addition, hypoxic tumor cells are either nonproliferating or they proliferate poorly, and as such do not respond well to drugs.

Combining chemotherapeutic agents with radiation therapy can reduce or eliminate hypoxia or its negative influence on tumor radioresponse. Most chemotherapeutic drugs preferentially kill proliferating cells, primarily found in well-oxygenated regions of the tumor. Because these regions are located close to blood vessels, they are easily accessible to chemotherapeutic agents. Destruction of tumor cells in these areas leads to an increased oxygen supply to hypoxic regions, and hence reoxygenates hypoxic tumor cells. Massive loss of cells after chemotherapy lowers the interstitial pressure, which then allows the reopening of previously closed capillaries and the re-establishment of blood supply. It also causes tumor shrinkage so that previously hypoxic areas are closer to capillaries and thus accessible to oxygen. Finally, by eliminating oxygenated cells, more oxygen becomes available to cells that survived chemotherapy. It was recently shown that tumor reoxygenation is a major mechanism underlying the enhancement of tumor radioresponse induced by taxanes in tumors sensitive to these drugs.[20]

Another approach to counteract the negative impact of hypoxia is selective killing of hypoxic cells through bioreductive drugs, such as tirapazamine,[22] which undergo reductive activation in a hypoxic milieu, rendering them cytotoxic. A related possibility is to exploit the acidic state (low pH) of tumors, which develops as a result of hypoxia-driven anaerobic metabolism that produces lactic acid,[30] through the use of drugs that selectively accumulate in acidic environments or become activated by a low pH.[31]

The use of agents that selectively radiosensitize hypoxic cells to reduce their negative impact has been considered and tested in clinical trials for some time. These drugs increase radiation damage by mimicking the effect of oxygen. Many clinical trials have tested these drugs, particularly misonidazole, in combination with radiation therapy, but few of them have shown an improved treatment outcome. The exception is nimorazole, which also does not elicit the neurotoxicity commonly associated with hypoxic cell sensitizers that prevented the delivery of clinically effective doses of these agents.[32]

Inhibition of Tumor Cell Repopulation

The constant balance between cell production and cell loss maintains the integrity of normal tissues. When this balance is perturbed by cytotoxic action of chemotherapeutic drugs or radiation, the integrity of tissues is re-established by an increased rate of cell production. The cell loss after each fraction of radiation during radiation therapy induces compensatory cell regeneration (repopulation), the extent of which determines tissue tolerance to radiation therapy. In contrast to normal tissues, malignant tumors are characterized by an imbalance between cell production and cell loss in favor of cell production. As with normal tissues, tumors also respond to radiation or drug-induced cell loss with a compensatory regenerative response. Preclinical studies provided ample evidence demonstrating that the rate of cell proliferation in tumors treated by radiation or chemotherapeutic drugs is higher than that in untreated tumors.[33–35] This increased rate of treatment-induced cell proliferation is commonly termed *accelerated repopulation*. Accelerated repopulation of tumor clonogens has been shown to occur during clinical radiation therapy as well. Withers et al.[36] showed that the total dose of radiation needed to control 50% of head and neck carcinomas progressively increased with time whenever radiation therapy treatment was prolonged beyond 1 month. This increase in radiation dose required to achieve tumor control was greater than what would be anticipated based on the pretreatment tumor volume doubling time of approximately 60 days for head and neck tumors. The increase was attributed to accelerated repopulation, and it was estimated to average approximately 0.6 Gy/day,[36] but may be as high as 1 Gy/day.[37]

Although accelerated cell proliferation is beneficial for normal tissues because it spares them from radiation damage, it has an adverse impact on tumor control by radiation therapy or chemotherapy. Chemotherapeutic drugs, because of their cytotoxic or cytostatic activity, can reduce the rate of proliferation when given concurrently with radiation therapy, and hence increase the effectiveness of the treatment. Caution must be taken to select drugs that preferentially affect rapidly proliferating cells and preferentially localize in malignant tumors. However, the main limitation of concurrent chemoradiation therapy is the enhanced toxicity of rapidly dividing normal tissues because most available chemotherapeutic agents show poor tumor selectivity. Moreover, accelerated repopulation induced by chemotherapeutic drugs may have a negative influence on the outcome of tumor response to radiation when drugs are used in induction or neoadjuvant chemotherapy protocols. In this strategy, chemotherapy precedes radiation therapy. Treatment outcomes after induction chemotherapy followed by radiation therapy have not been overly encouraging in terms of both local tumor control and patient survival, even if a large proportion of tumors initially responded with total or partial clinical regression by the time of radiation therapy implementation. Some experimental evidence suggests that the drug-induced accelerated cell repopulation can actually make the tumor more difficult to control with radiation.[33,34]

Other Potential Interactions

Molecular Signaling Pathways That May Be Responsible for Radioresistance. Significant strides have been made in elucidating molecular pathways that may be involved in resistance to cytotoxic therapy including radiation treatments. These molecular determinants are being scrutinized in preclinical and clinical settings as potential targets for cancer therapy, of which some agents are being studied for the potential for enhancing radiation effects.[38] For example, the efficacy of combining the epidermal growth factor receptor (EGFR) inhibitor cetuximab with radiation therapy has been demonstrated in randomized clinical studies in head and neck cancer patients.[39] Molecular targeting has become an immensely important topic, and effective integration of these strategies with radiation therapy to foster improved efficacy of therapy is an active area of investigation. This topic is further discussed in significant detail in the section to follow.

Targeting the Tumor Microenvironment. Tumor microenvironment has been postulated as being a potential therapeutic target for cancer therapy. Tumor microenvironment is a complex system of many cell types including endothelial cells, smooth muscle cells, fibroblasts, and cells involved with the immune system (lymphocytes, macrophages, etc.).[40] Among these different cells that make up the different components of the tumor microenvironment, the most studied preclinically and clinically are the cells that make up the tumor microvasculature. Preclinical studies have suggested the potential role for radiosensitization of the tumor microvasculature using compounds directed at targeting angiogenesis.[41] Clinical studies have been performed with efforts to combine antiangiogenic agents with radiation therapy, with mixed results.[41] Studies are ongoing, as many antiangiogenic agents are approved for cancer therapy, and are detailed in the section on antiangiogenesis agents.

Cancer Stem Cells. Cancer stem cells are defined as being cells within a tumor that possess the capacity to self-renew and generate the heterogeneous lineages of cancer cells that make up the tumor.[42] Cancer stem cells as a source of radiation resistance for solid tumors is an area of active investigation. Potential for the need to eradicate cancer stem cells for effective cure by radiotherapy has been postulated, and while radioresistance of cancer stem cells has been noted in *in vitro* studies,[43] this notion has been challenged as some have demonstrated radiosensitivity of cancer stem cells.[44] But, if in fact cancer stem cells are radioresistant, one possible strategy may be to identify molecular pathways that could influence cancer stem cell radiosensitivity and investigate the use of such agents in combination with radiotherapy at different stages during the course of therapy.[45]

TIMING OF DRUG ADMINISTRATION IN RELATION TO RADIATION THERAPY

Most clinical chemoradiation therapy regimens evolved empirically: increasingly, information from preclinical studies is being considered in planning the optimal timing of drug administration in relation to radiation therapy. Depending on the principal aim of the therapy, drugs are administered before (*induction* or *neoadjuvant chemotherapy*), during (*concurrent* or *concomitant chemotherapy*), or after (*adjuvant chemotherapy*) the course of radiation therapy. The advantages and disadvantages of each approach are summarized in Table 32.1.

In regard to the primary tumor, induction chemotherapy may reduce the number of clonogenic cells and cause the reoxygenation of the surviving hypoxic cells, both of which render tumors more controllable by radiation. In addition, chemotherapy-induced tumor shrinkage may allow the use of smaller radiation fields, in which case less normal tissue is exposed and damaged by radiation. This treatment approach is often used in the therapy of solid tumors in children and of lymphomas. Induction chemotherapy precedes radiation therapy for a few weeks to a few months, which improves tolerability of the combined treatment.

TABLE 32.1 ADVANTAGES AND DISADVANTAGES OF DIFFERENT CHEMORADIATION SEQUENCING STRATEGIES

Strategy	*Advantages*	*Disadvantages*
Sequential chemoradiation	• Least toxic • Maximizes systemic therapy • Smaller radiation fields if induction shrinks tumor	• Increased treatment time • Lack of local synergy
Concurrent chemoradiation	• Shorter treatment time • Radiation enhancement	• Compromised systemic therapy • Increased toxicity • No cytoreduction of tumor
Concurrent chemoradiation and adjuvant chemotherapy	• Maximizes systemic therapy • Radiation enhancement • Both local and distant therapy delivered up front	• Increased toxicity • Increased treatment time • Difficult to complete chemotherapy after chemoradiation
Induction chemotherapy and concurrent chemoradiation	• Maximizes systemic therapy • Radiation enhancement	• Increased toxicity • Increased treatment time • Difficult to complete chemoradiation after induction therapy

Induction chemotherapy has resulted in therapeutic improvement in a number of clinical trials compared with radiation therapy, but in general the therapeutic benefits are below expectations. A number of factors could account for this, including accelerated proliferation of tumor cell clonogens and selection or induction of drug-resistant cells that are cross-resistant to radiation. The preclinical findings provide solid evidence for the existence of accelerated repopulation in tumors treated with chemotherapeutic agents. On the other hand, although development of drug resistance is a significant problem in chemotherapy, the evidence that cells that acquire drug resistance are also resistant to radiation is not convincing.

When chemotherapy is given during a course of radiation therapy, it is referred to as *concurrent chemotherapy*. This form of treatment is intended to cope with both disseminated lesions and the primary tumor, but it takes advantage of drug–radiation interactions to maximize tumor radioresponse. The drug scheduling in relation to individual radiation fractions is highly important, and the selection of optimal timing of drug administration must be based on mechanisms of tumor radio enhancement by a given drug, the drug's normal tissue toxicity, and the conditions under which the highest enhancement is achieved. The data from preclinical studies can greatly contribute to the selection of the most optimal schedules. For example, it has been demonstrated that murine tumors sensitive to taxanes show enhanced radioresponse, but the best effect is achieved if drug treatment precedes radiation by 1 to 3 days.[20] A major mechanism for tumor radio enhancement was reoxygenation of hypoxic cells. Based on this preclinical information, one would anticipate that in clinical protocols such tumors would best respond to a bolus of a taxane given once or twice weekly during radiation therapy. In contrast, tumors resistant to taxanes on their own would call for daily administration of a taxane because they show accumulation of radiosensitive G_2- and M-phase cells 6 to 12 hours after drug administration. If the objective is to counteract rapid repopulation of tumor cell clonogens induced by radiation, then administration of cell cycle–specific chemotherapeutic agents during the second half of radiation therapy, when accelerated repopulation is more expressed, might be more effective. At present, the enhancement in normal-tissue complications remains the major limitation of concurrently combining chemotherapy with radiation therapy. Nevertheless, as is made evident later in the text, concurrent chemoradiation therapy has provided better clinical results both in terms of local tumor control and patient survival than have other modes of chemoradiation therapy combinations.[46,47]

Adjuvant chemotherapy designates a treatment modality in which chemotherapeutic drugs are given some time after completion of radiation therapy. The primary objective is to eradicate disseminated disease; however, the control of the primary tumor may also be improved by the ability of drugs to deal with tumor cells that survived radiation.

INTERACTION OF SPECIFIC CHEMOTHERAPIES AND RADIATION IN THE TREATMENT OF CANCER

This section provides an overview of the evidence that exists for combining particular chemotherapies with radiation. In many cases, the level of support that exists for combined therapy mirrors the age of the drug. However, as would be expected, newer drugs have generally been subject to more rigorous preclinical assessment of their efficacy before their introduction into the clinical setting (Table 32.2).

Platinum-Based Drugs

This group of compounds, distinguished from most others by its metallic element base, has come to be recognized as one of the most potent chemotherapies available to date. Cisplatin (*cis*-diamminedichloroplatinum II), which is the prototype drug, has been acknowledged to be a potent radiosensitizer for many years and has a significant role in clinical practice to date. Preclinical work done using murine models by Rosenberg et al.[64] in the late 1960s showed that cisplatin is an effective antitumor chemotherapy. Subsequent efforts have shown that its primary mechanism of inhibition of tumor growth appears to involve the inhibition of DNA synthesis.[65,66] Another secondary mechanism includes the inhibition of transcription elongation by DNA interstrand cross-links.[67]

TABLE 32.2 MECHANISMS OF CHEMOTHERAPY-INDUCED RADIATION SENSITIZATION

Class of Compound	*Mechanism of Radiosensitization*	*References*
Platinum-based compounds	Inhibition of DNA synthesis Inhibition of transcription elongation by DNA interstrand cross links Inhibition of repair of radiation-induced DNA damage	48–51
Taxanes	Cellular arrest in the G_2M phase of the cell cycle Induction of apoptosis Reoxygenation of tumor cells	20,21,52,53
Topoisomerase I inhibitors	Inhibition of repair of radiation-induced DNA strand breaks Redistribution into G_2 phase of the cell cycle Conversion of radiation-induced single-strand breaks into double-strand breaks	54–56
Hypoxic cell cytotoxins	Complementary cytotoxicity with radiation on euoxic and hypoxic tumor cells	58,59
Antimetabolites	Nucleotide pool perturbation Lowering apoptotic threshold Cell cycle redistribution Tumor cell reoxygenation	13,14,60,61
Temozolomide	DNA repair inhibition (radiosensitization effect may be subject to MGMT status)	62,63

Work on nonmammalian systems first demonstrated the radiosensitizing abilities of platinum-based compounds.[68–70] This was confirmed in several mammalian systems as well.[48,71,72] This makes inherent sense because these platinum compounds have a high electron affinity and react preferentially with hydrated electrons. The exact mechanism for the increased cell death seen with combinations of ionizing radiation and platinum drugs is not known for certain; however, the evidence would seem to point to the inhibition of PLDR[49] and to the radiosensitization of hypoxic tumor cells.[73] Cisplatin free radical–mediated sensitization may involve the ability to scavenge free electrons formed by the interaction between radiation and DNA. The reduction of the platinum moiety may serve to stabilize DNA damage that would otherwise be repairable.[74] Greater than additive effects of cisplatin and radiation are seen in tumor models most reliably when the drug is administered with fractionated radiation,[74] explained by its inhibition of SLDR.

Carboplatin, a second-generation platinum compound with a different toxicity profile, has also been studied as a radiosensitizer.[50,51] Its potential efficacy as a radiosensitizer has allowed for its incorporation into regimens used in several randomized trials. Interest exists in the combination of radiation with other platinum analogs, including oxaliplatin[75] as well as orally administered compounds like satraplatin.[76–78]

Oxaliplatin, although sharing a similar mode of action as other platinum compounds, has been shown to have activity in cisplatin-resistant systems *in vitro*.[4] One potential explanation for this is that oxaliplatin is not affected by loss of mismatch repair, which leads to cisplatin resistance *in vitro*,[79] and there are those who postulate that adducts formed by oxaliplatin are less well recognized by DNA repair systems.[80] Whether oxaliplatin is truly active against cisplatin-resistant cancer clinically is an area of active investigation,[81] and after encouraging findings in phase I to II rectal cancer studies, it entered into phase III studies, some of which have closed to accrual.[80]

Antimicrotubules

Taxanes

The radiosensitizing properties of plant-derived chemotherapeutic agents, the taxanes, have been studied extensively in both preclinical models and in clinical trials. Paclitaxel (Taxol) and docetaxel (Taxotere) act as mitotic spindle inhibitors through their promotion of microtubule assembly and inhibition of disaggregation.[82] Both taxanes bind to the *N*-terminal 31–amino-acid sequence of the β-tubulin subunit of cellular tubulin polymers, stabilizing the polymers by shifting the dynamic equilibrium that exists between tubulin dimers and microtubules in favor of the polymerized state.[83,84] Although there is preclinical evidence that docetaxel has both a higher affinity for the tubulin-binding site and greater *in vitro* cytotoxicity than paclitaxel, this has not necessarily translated into greater clinical efficacy because the toxicity profiles of the two drugs also differ.[85,86]

The administration of a taxane leads to cellular arrest in the G_2/M phase of the cell cycle, which is the precise point associated with increased sensitivity to the lethal effects of ionizing radiation.[87] Early laboratory studies with a human lung cancer cell line[19] and human astrocytoma cells[18] bore out the prospect of significant radiosensitization, with relative enhancement ratios in the 1.48 to 1.8 range when paclitaxel was administered before irradiation.

The exact conditions used in various studies appear to determine the strength of the interaction between radiation and paclitaxel because subadditive effects have been seen in addition to the more widely reported additive and supra-additive effects.[21] In general, enhancement of radiation effects is seen when proliferating cells have been incubated with moderate concentrations of paclitaxel for 24 hours before irradiation. Conditions leading to a less-than-optimal response include paclitaxel-mediated G_1 arrest, wherein a more resistant cell subpopulation counteracts the effects of a G_2/M block; paclitaxel-induced cell cycle effects such as the G_2/M block in cells destined to die before irradiation; and incubation conditions insufficient to exert cellular effects. The fact that nonproliferating cells are also sensitized to the effects of radiation by the use of paclitaxel suggests that mechanisms other than the cell cycle arrest in the G_2/M phase underlie paclitaxel's sensitizing abilities.

Paclitaxel also acts to induce programmed cell death; work from the M.D. Anderson Cancer Center[21] has examined the relationship between mitotic arrest, apoptosis, and the antineoplastic activity of paclitaxel in 16 murine tumors. Single-dose paclitaxel (40 mg/kg) induced mitotic arrest to varying degrees in all tumors; however, apoptosis was induced in only 50% of tumors. This study also revealed that pretreatment levels of apoptosis correlated with both paclitaxel-induced apoptosis and tumor growth delay. Therefore, both the pretreatment apoptotic rate and paclitaxel-induced apoptotic rate could potentially act as predictors of the response to paclitaxel.

Milas et al.[21] summarized observations that showed that (a) there was massive loss of tumor cells though the apoptotic pathway was restricted to the perivascular region, and (b) radio enhancement occurring during this period of cell loss became even more impressive when apoptotic cells were removed from the tumor. Experiments in which tumor xenografts were treated with paclitaxel and exposed to radiation under hypoxic or air-ambient conditions were pursued.[20] It was found that the creation of hypoxic conditions greatly reduced the efficacy of paclitaxel in its enhancement of radioresponse. It appears that a combination of cell cycle effects, drug-induced reoxygenation, and drug-induced apoptosis underlies paclitaxel's radiosensitizing abilities.

Docetaxel has also been found to be a respectable radiosensitizer in both *in vitro*[52] and *in vivo* models.[53] Radiation response in the presence of docetaxel was examined in three different cell lines that have widely different responses to radiation alone.[88] Their findings suggest that the p53 status of tumor cells may have a profound effect on the radiosensitizing effects of a taxane. Other novel taxanes and analogs that continue to attract the interest of investigators for their potential to enhance radiation effects include Abraxane, paclitaxel poliglumex, larotaxel, cabazitaxel,[89,90] and orally available taxanes.[91]

Epothilones

Epothilones are a novel class of antimicrotubule agents, originally derived from the myxobacterium *Sorangium cellulosum.* These agents bind to the site near the taxane binding site, and mechanism of action is similar to taxanes[89,92,93]; however, their chemical structures are unrelated, and their binding is specific and independent of the taxanes. Several epothilones are undergoing investigation in clinical trials: patupilone, ixabepilone, BMS-310705, ZK-EPO, and epothilone D.[94] Epothilones enhance microtubule stability, formation of abnormal mitotic spindles inducing G_2 and M arrest, and apoptosis. Interestingly, patupilone has been shown to cross the blood–brain barrier, and studies with concurrent radiation therapy for central nervous system (CNS) malignancies have been performed at the phase I level.[95] The potential for patupilone to work as a radiosensitizer for multidrug-resistant cancer cells *in vitro* has been reported,[96] as well as for medulloblastoma cells,[97] lung cancer, and prostate cancer cells.[98,99]

Antimetabolites

5-Fluorouracil (5-FU)

The radiosensitizing properties of 5-FU have been known for years.[100] Several mechanisms have been proposed for the cytotoxicity of this drug:

a. Its incorporation into RNA, which leads to a disruption of RNA function;
b. Inhibition of thymidylate synthetase function and subsequently of DNA synthesis; and
c. Direct incorporation of the drug into DNA.

It is believed that a combination of these effects underlies its radiosensitizing properties.[101] Optimization of its schedule of delivery is crucial to obtaining an effect with this combination, and it is accepted that cytotoxic doses of 5-FU are needed to obtain a radiosensitizing effect. In general, it is thought that a continuous infusion of the drug is needed to obtain the desired drug levels after irradiation.[102] Long-standing clinical experience with this drug bears out much of the laboratory studies of its effectiveness as a radiation sensitizer.

Capecitabine

Capecitabine is an oral prodrug of 5-FU. It is converted to its cytotoxic form in three enzymatic steps, the last of which is mediated by thymidine phosphorylase. One of the potential advantages of this mechanism for increasing tumor cytotoxicity is that thymidine phosphorylase is overexpressed in tumor tissues. Interestingly, radiation has been shown to stimulate expression of thymidine phosphorylase, which provides a further rationale for considering combined therapy with radiation treatments.[103] Several phase I/II studies of radiation therapy and capecitabine primarily in rectal cancer have been completed,[104,105] and a large phase III study from the National Surgical Adjuvant Breast and Bowel Project (NSABP) is under way.[105]

Gemcitabine

Gemcitabine is another nucleoside analog that acts as a very potent radiosensitizer. The biologic action of gemcitabine is due almost completely to its effects on DNA metabolism. Early studies of this drug in leukemic cell lines found that notable decreases in cellular deoxynucleotide triphosphates occurred with the use of the drug.[106]

Direct incorporation of the drug into DNA and drug-induced apoptosis are also thought to underlie its cytotoxicity.[106] The metabolism of gemcitabine in the cell is complex, and it is able to potentiate its cytotoxicity as a sole therapy.[106] Depending on the conditions, relative enhancement ratios in the range of 1.1 to 2.5 have been reported.

Gemcitabine is S-phase specific and as such should be selectively toxic to proliferating cells,[107] decreasing the amount of proliferation that can occur during fractionated radiation therapy. In addition, cell cycle redistribution induced by these agents may improve cell kill by allowing more cells to be treated in the more sensitive parts of the cell cycle.[108] As DNA synthesis inhibitors, these drugs may act to inhibit the repair of radiation-induced DNA damage.[13] Finally, as DNA chain terminators, they may serve to trigger the apoptotic response.[14]

There is strong preclinical evidence to suggest that the radiosensitizing abilities of gemcitabine are intimately linked to cellular deoxyadenosine triphosphate levels.[14] Interesting results from Latz et al.[60] show quite clearly that cells that are pretreated with gemcitabine no longer show a progressive increase in radioresistance as they progress toward DNA replication, and sensitization, therefore, appears to be greatest in the S phase.

Milas et al.[15] found the largest enhancement of growth delay when gemcitabine was delivered 24 to 60 hours before irradiation in a murine sarcoma tumor model. The use of gemcitabine with radiation also decreased the risk for development of lung metastases in those mice that attained durable local control (73% in the radiation-alone group vs. 40% in the combined-modality group), which was confirmed in a second study with a larger number of mice.[61] This preclinical work is supportive of the principles of combined-modality therapy in that better local control translated into decreased systemic spread of tumor cells. The same authors also report a dose-dependent increase in the apoptotic rate after the administration of gemcitabine,[15] which they believe correlates with the elimination of the more radioresistant S-phase population of cells and a redistribution of the remaining cells into more radiosensitive parts of the cell cycle. They also report that reoxygenation of the resistant hypoxic fraction of tumor cells is a mechanism for the radiosensitizing action of gemcitabine.[61]

In summary, the preclinical evidence suggests that gemcitabine acts through several mechanisms (nucleotide pool perturbation, lowering of the apoptotic threshold, cell cycle redistribution, and tumor cell reoxygenation) to enhance the effect of ionizing radiation on tumors. Clinical experience has shown that this drug is indeed a potent sensitizer with the potential for significant toxicity as well as improvement in tumor control when combined with radiation.[109,110,111–115]

Pemetrexed

Pemetrexed is a novel multitargeted agent, exerting its effect via simultaneous inhibition of multiple folate-requiring enzymes, including thymidylate synthase, dihydrofolate reductase, and glycinamide ribonucleotide formyl-transferase.[116] Pemetrexed has shown synergistic activity with radiation treatments, likely due to interference with DNA synthesis.[117] There are indications that radiosensitization by pemetrexed is not cell cycle phase specific[118] *in vitro*. Others have suggested that a combination of radiation therapy and pemetrexed results in supra-additive effects, which may be in part due to apoptosis induction.[119] Phase I/II studies in non–small cell lung cancer (NSCLC) and esophageal cancer combining pemetrexed-based chemotherapy with radiation therapy have been completed demonstrating tolerability and encouraging results.[120,121,122,123–126]

Topoisomerase I Inhibitors

Camptothecin is a plant alkaloid obtained from the *Camptotheca acuminata* tree. Its initial clinical evaluation in the 1960s and 1970s was abandoned because of severe and unpredictable hemorrhagic cystitis.[127,128] Camptothecin and its derivatives (e.g., irinotecan, topotecan, 9-aminocamptothecin, SN-38) target DNA topoisomerase I.[129–130,131] This enzyme relaxes both positively and negatively supercoiled DNA and allows for diverse essential cellular processes, including replication and transcription, to proceed. In the presence of camptothecin, a camptothecin–topoisomerase I–DNA complex becomes stabilized with the 5′-phosphoryl terminus of the enzyme-catalyzed DNA SSB bound covalently to a tyrosine residue of topoisomerase I. These stabilized cleavable complexes interact with the advancing replication fork during the S phase or during unscheduled DNA replication after genomic stress and cause the conversion of SSBs into irreversible DNA DSBs, resulting in cell death.[130]

Several investigators have reported that camptothecin enhances the cytotoxic effect of radiation *in vitro* and *in vivo*.[54–55,56] Chen et al.[55] showed that cells exposed to 20(S)-10,11 methylenedioxycamptothecin before or during radiation had sensitization ratios of 1.6, whereas those treated with the drug after radiation had substantially less enhancement of radiation-induced DNA damage. There are several hypotheses regarding the mechanism of interaction between radiation and irinotecan: (a) inhibition of topoisomerase I by irinotecan leads to inhibition of repair of radiation-induced DNA strand breaks; (b) irinotecan causes a redistribution of the cells into the more radiosensitive G_2 phase of the cell cycle; (c) topoisomerase I–DNA adducts are trapped by irinotecan at the sites of radiation-induced SSBs, leading to their conversion into DSBs.[57] While there is currently insufficient evidence to identify the underlying mechanism with certainty, the primary mechanism involved with radiosensitization may depend on which camptothecin derivative is being used.

Data from *in vivo* experiments demonstrate that combination 9-aminocamptothecin and irradiation is more effective when fractionated, compared with single doses.[132] There is also evidence for circadian-dependent cytotoxicity and radiation sensitization when camptothecin derivatives like 9-aminocamptothecin are used as radiation sensitizers.[132] The integration of this group of drugs into clinical treatments with radiation therapy have been explored in NSCLC and brain tumors.[133–135,136]

Alkylating Agents

Temozolomide

Temozolomide, a relatively new drug, is a second-generation alkylating agent, which is orally administered, is readily bioavailable, and demonstrates broad-spectrum activity in a variety of difficult-to-treat malignancies including glioma and melanoma.[137] It is unique in its ability to cross the blood–brain barrier (about 30% to 40% of plasma concentration found in CSF). *In vitro* studies demonstrate increased inhibition of cell growth in combination with radiotherapy.[138] Radiosensitization appears to occur via inhibition of DNA repair, leading to an increase in mitotic catastrophe.[62] It has proven efficacy as a first-line therapy for glioblastoma multiforme (GBM) patients in conjunction with radiotherapy based on a randomized phase III clinical study demonstrating survival benefit.[139] Temozolomide spontaneously converts to the reactive methylating agent MTIC and transfers methyl groups to DNA, the most important one being at the O6 position of guanine, an important site for DNA alkylation.[140] The MGMT gene encodes a DNA repair protein that removes the alkyl group from the O6 position of guanine, and high MGMT activity levels abrogate the effectiveness of alkylating agents. *In vitro*, temozolomide enhances the radiation response most effectively in MGMT-negative glioblastomas, and likely due to decreased double-strand DNA repair capacity and increased DNA double-strand break damage, which occurs when the combination of temozolomide and radiation therapy was administered.[63] Analysis of a randomized study by the European Organization for Research and Treatment of Cancer (EORTC) and National Cancer Institute of Canada (NCIC) demonstrated that loss of MGMT expression by promoter methylation is correlated with a better outcome after treatment with radiation and temozolomide.[141]

Other Agents

Mitomycin-C

Mitomycin-C is a quinone, whose mechanisms of action include inhibition of DNA and RNA synthesis.[142] When combined with radiation, the rationale for the use of mitomycin-C is based on its ability to target hypoxic cells that are known to be relatively radiation resistant.[143] There is preclinical evidence to suggest that mitomycin-C administered before irradiation leads to a supra-additive interaction.[58,144] The postulated mechanisms of action for supra-additivity include prevention of repopulation and hypoxic cell sensitization, although the definitive action is not fully elucidated. Given that normal tissues are not hypoxic, the selective targeting of this cell population with mitomycin-C has the potential to improve cures without compromising normal-tissue complication rates. The use of mitomycin-C is limited by its hematologic toxicities. Mitomycin-C combined with radiation therapy remains the standard-of-care therapy for anal carcinoma based on multiple clinical studies.[145]

Tirapazamine

Investigators have pursued a similar strategy as outlined previously with the development of tirapazamine, a hypoxic cell cytotoxin.[22,59] Brown[59] has discovered that tirapazamine, which is a benzotriazine di-*N*-oxide, is toxic to hypoxic cells at concentrations much lower than what is needed to radiosensitize cells. It has the greatest differential toxicity known between hypoxic and well-oxygenated cells. Essentially, this drug functions through its intracellular reduction to form a highly reactive radical capable of causing both SSBs and DSBs.[146] In the presence of oxygen, a free electron is absorbed, and the compound is back-oxidized to the parent compound with the concomitant release of a superoxide radical, which is much less cytotoxic than the tirapazamine radical. Clinical trials are ongoing or have been completed in multiple tumor sites including cervix, head and neck, glioblastoma multiforme, and lung malignancies (small cell lung cancer).[147–159] A phase III study by the TransTasman group (TROG 02.02) suggested no significant improvement in survival outcome in locally advanced head and neck cancer patients, unselected for hypoxia, with the addition of tirapazamine to a standard platinum-based chemoradiation regimen.[157] A subset analysis of the phase II study from the TransTasman Group suggested that tumors with a hypoxic component as assessed by 18F fluoromisonidazole positron emission tomography (FMISO-PET) imaging had a higher likelihood of locoregional failure, while an improvement in local control was identified for those treated with the addition of tirapazamine, suggesting that it specifically targets hypoxic tumor cells.[153] While most studies have demonstrated a reasonable toxicity profile, several studies have suggested caution in the appropriate selection of a dose and delivery regimen when combining tirapazamine to a standard chemoradiation regimen.[151,154]

EMERGING STRATEGIES FOR IMPROVEMENT OF CHEMORADIATION THERAPY

In spite of increasing therapeutic achievements of chemoradiation therapy, the use of this form of therapy is still very much restricted by its narrow therapeutic index. The available agents are either insufficiently effective on their own or in combination with radiation against tumors, or normal-tissue toxicity prevents the use of effective doses of drugs or radiation. Significant research efforts, both preclinical and clinical, have been undertaken to improve chemoradiation therapy. They include developing more selective and more effective chemotherapeutic agents, incorporating additional agents into chemoradiation therapy that protect normal tissues from injury by drugs or radiation, and improving the technique of radiation therapy delivery to minimize treatment of adjacent normal tissue while maximizing tumor dose delivery.

Increasing Antitumor Efficacy of Chemotherapeutic Drugs

A number of newer chemotherapeutic agents are being developed with the goal of enhancing antitumor effects by improving on the selective targeting of tumor cells via strategies such as chemical modification of known compounds including agents currently in use with radiation therapy due to their radiosensitizing properties.

Approaches for improvement of drug safety, convenience, or efficacy could include chemical modifications, or modifications of the formulation of a known drug. One example is that of Abraxane (nab-paclitaxel, ABI-007). Abraxane is a 130-nM particle form of paclitaxel that is bound to albumin and is solvent free. This avoids the need for Cremophor-based vehicles and lowers the risk of hypersensitivity reactions.[89] Such vehicles have the potential for altered pharmacokinetics by drug entrapment, leading to decreased drug clearance, decreased volume of distribution, and ultimately nonlinear pharmacokinetics. Interestingly, Abraxane has been demonstrated to have higher antitumor activity compared to Taxol in preclinical studies. This is in part mediated via utilization of albumin receptor–mediated endothelial transport, which leads to higher intracellular accumulation compared to standard paclitaxel.[160] Clinically, Abraxane has shown demonstrated efficacy in metastatic breast cancer in a phase III study.[161] Phase I/II studies in advanced NSCLC, melanoma, bladder cancer, high-risk prostate cancer, and gynecologic malignancy have been reported.[161,162,163–172] Preclinical studies have demonstrated Abraxane to have radiosensitizing properties.[173] Therefore, there is significant interest in determining the potential efficacy of Abraxane in disease sites where combined therapy with taxanes and radiation has demonstrated therapeutic advantage, and clinical trials are under way.

Another approach to make current chemotherapeutic drugs more effective against tumors and at the same time less toxic to normal tissues is compound modification via conjugation with water-soluble polymeric drugs, such as polyglutamic acid. These conjugates accumulate in tumors and release the active drug into the tumor in high concentrations and for a longer time. The enhancement in uptake by and prolongation of drug release in tumors are thought to be due to the enhanced permeability and retention effect of macromolecular compounds in solid tumors.[174,175] The abnormal vasculature in tumors is porous to macromolecules, but high concentrations of drug can build up in tumors owing to inadequate lymphatic drainage, whereas polymer–drug conjugates are confined to the bloodstream in normal tissue.[174] This leads to improved spatial localization of the cytotoxic drug within tumor. A highly promising polyglutamic acid–paclitaxel conjugate was recently developed. It is less toxic, more effective against tumors, and more enhancing of tumor radioresponse in preclinical studies than unconjugated paclitaxel.[175,176] Furthermore, there are *in vivo* laboratory data suggesting that radiation adds to the accumulation of drug within tumors by modification of tumor vasculature.[177] Therefore, multiple mechanisms for spatial localization and cooperation, including inherent drug properties, radiation modification of vasculature, and radiation-based targeting of sites within the body, could make this an attractive strategy for combining this agent with radiation treatments. Clinical trials in esophageal cancer (phase II) and gastric cancer (phase I) have been reported in combination with radiation treatments.[178,179]

Normal-Tissue Protection

Because normal-tissue toxicity represents a major limitation of concurrent chemoradiation therapy, every effort must be taken to prevent or minimize complications. This could be achieved through the incorporation into the treatment of radioprotective or chemoprotective agents or through improvements of radiation delivery. A number of chemical and biologic compounds are available that exhibited either selective or preferential protection of normal tissues in preclinical *in vivo* testing.[180–183,184] In addition, there are many candidate compounds, particularly extracts from plants used in traditional medicine settings, that are undergoing *in vitro* evaluation.[185–186,187] The most commonly tested radioprotectors are thiol compounds, such as WR-2721 (amifostine), a prodrug that must be converted *in vivo* to its active metabolite WR-1065. Amifostine is currently the only Food and Drug Administration (FDA)-approved radioprotector. The principal mechanisms of protection by these agents include scavenging of free radicals generated by ionizing radiation and some chemotherapy agents, such as alkylating agents, and donating hydrogen atoms to facilitate direct chemical repair of DNA damage. However, amifostine modulates transcriptional regulation of genes involved in apoptosis, cell cycle regulation, and DNA repair as well.[188] The protector is taken up preferentially by normal tissues, where the entry into cells is accomplished by active transport. In contrast, the drug diffuses passively into tumors, where its availability is also reduced by deficient tumor vasculature. Amifostine has been shown to reduce normal-tissue toxicity in a number of clinical settings, including protection of salivary glands in head and neck radiation therapy,[189,190] prevention of acute and late normal-tissue toxicities from chemoradiation in cancers of the head and neck[191] and the esophagus in chemoradiation therapy of lung cancer,[192,193] without adversely affecting tumor response to treatment. The drug significantly protects against cisplatin-induced nephrotoxicity, ototoxicity, and neuropathy.

Emerging Strategies to Improve Radiation Therapy

Technology-Based Strategies

Several technologic strategies to improve the efficacy and decrease the toxicity of radiation therapy have been developed. These advances include improvements in radiation therapy delivery, such as three-dimensional treatment planning, conformational radiation therapy, intensity-modulated radiation therapy (IMRT), and image-guided radiation therapy (IGRT). Use of heavy particles, such as protons or carbons, which have a more favorable beam profile, is another approach likely to minimize the toxicity, and combining such treatments with chemotherapy may lead to enhancement of the effectiveness of not only radiation therapy but also chemoradiation treatments. The principle primarily exploited with this would be that of maximizing spatial localization, with technologic advances and/or heavy particles being used to maximize radiation therapy's spatial localization. Further advances in imaging, with the advent of molecular-based imaging applications in oncology, will lead to further refinement of IGRT techniques. Because there are significant discussions of three-dimensional conformational radiation therapy (3DCRT), IMRT, IGRT, and heavy particles detailed in other chapters, we refer readers to those chapters for more in-depth discussion.

Altering Fractionation Schemes to Improve Therapeutic Ratio for Chemoradiation Treatments

Accelerated fractionation regimens are designed to counteract tumor repopulation, and accelerated fractionation with concomitant boost technique has shown superiority in terms of local control over the standard fractionation regimen in a large randomized study for head and neck cancer patients.[194] Head and neck cancer remains one of the best paradigms for effectiveness of accelerated fractionation methods in clinical use. However, when combined with chemotherapy, a benefit to accelerated fractionation over standard fractionation was not demonstrated.[195]

Hyperfractionation is another strategy aimed at increasing the tumoricidal dose by delivering smaller doses/fractions, which allows a higher total dose to be administered as smaller doses/fractions lead to improved tolerance of late-responding normal tissues.[87] The efficacy of hyperfractionation over standard fractionation has been demonstrated in several disease sites, including lung and head and neck cancer.[194,196,197] In head and neck cancer, hyperfractionated radiation therapy with chemotherapy has yielded superior outcomes compared to hyperfractionated radiation therapy (RT) alone[198]; however, there has been no trial to demonstrate superiority of hyperfractionated RT and chemotherapy compared to conventional RT and chemotherapy. Perhaps, given the limited success of concurrent therapy, methods of combining systemic agents sequentially either before or after radiation treatments with altered fractionation can be considered.

MOLECULAR-TARGETED THERAPIES: NEW AGENTS AND NOVEL PARADIGMS FOR OPTIMIZING COMBINED MODALITY THERAPY

Recent discoveries in molecular biology have identified a number of molecular pathways involving receptors, enzymes, or growth factors that may be responsible for resistance of cancer cells to radiation or other cytotoxic agents and as such may serve as targets for augmentation of radiation response or chemotherapy response. It is becoming more evident that with advances in the understanding of the molecular processes that are associated with various malignancies, a molecular profile of a tumor may prove to be as important as its pathologic profile. Further classification of a patient's tumor molecular profile should, among other things, aid in selection of the appropriate targeted agents. The challenge for radiation oncologists in this molecular era is determining what would be the best method of integrating cytotoxic radiation treatments with a molecular-based therapeutic plan.

Among this expanding list of molecular targets are epidermal growth factor (EGF) and its receptor (EGFR); vascular endothelial growth factor (VEGF) and its receptor (VEGFR); mammalian target of rapamycin (mTOR); anaplastic lymphoma kinase (ALK) fusion proteins; heat shock protein 90 (hsp90); poly(adenosine diphosphate [ADP]-ribose) polymerase (PARP); mutated *ras;* histone deacetylase (HDAC) inhibitors; cell cycle checkpoint control proteins such as checkpoint kinase 1 (CHK1); a number of the DNA repair enzymes, including DNA-dependent protein kinase (DNA-PK), ataxia telangiectasia mutated (ATM), and RAD51; the proteosome; angiogenic molecules; and various other molecules that regulate different steps in their signal transduction pathways.[199] A handful of agents have now gained FDA approval for cancer therapy in patients, and many are undergoing clinical trials to determine their efficacy when used in combination with radiation therapy. Some agents are potentially single-pathway targets, and others are able to target multiple molecular signaling pathways. Some newly emerging molecular strategies to improve chemoradiation therapy are shown in Table 32.3. The most clinically advanced of these strategies include agents targeting EGFR, VEGF and VEGFR, and ALK1 pathways. The scope of this section will be a discussion of relevant molecularly targeted agents that have been FDA approved for use, and which hold promise for use in conjunction with radiation treatments.

TABLE 32.3 MOLECULAR TARGETING POSSIBILITIES IN COMBINATION WITH CHEMORADIATION OR RADIATION

Class	*Agents*	*Status in Combination with RT*
Epidermal growth factor receptor inhibitors	Cetuximab	Head and neck cancer–phase III, approved for use Other sites–phase I, phase II
	Gefitinib	Phase I/II reported
	Erlotinib	Phase I/II reported
Antiangiogenics	Bevacizumab	Phase I/II reported
	Thalidomide	Brain metastases–phase III, negative study Other sites–phase I/II reported
Multitargeted tyrosine kinase inhibitors (TKIs)	Sunitinib (inhibits PDGFR, VEGFR, KIT, RET, CSF-1R, FLT3)	Phase I reported
	Sorafenib (inhibits Raf kinase, PDGF, VEGFR2/3, cKit)	None reported
	Pazopanib (inhibits VEGFR1–3, PDFR-α, PDFR-β, c-Kit, FGFR-1, FGFR-3, Lck, c-Fms)	None reported
MTOR inhibitors	Temsirolimus	Phase I reported
	Everolimus	Phase I reported
ALK inhibitor	Crizotinib	None reported
HDAC inhibitors	Vorinostat	Phase I reported
	Romidepsin	None reported

RT, radiation therapy; PDGFR, platelet-derived growth factor receptor; VEGFR, vascular endothelial growth factor; CSF-1R, colony stimulating factor 1 receptor; FLT3, fms-related tyrosine kinase 3; FGFR, fibroblast growth factor receptor.

EGFR

Targeting EGFR is one of the current model paradigms for the combination of molecular-based therapy and radiation. EGFR is also known as ErbB1, a member of the ErbB family of receptor tyrosine kinases, which also includes ErbB2 (HER2/neu). EGFR is a 170-kD transmembrane glycoprotein with an intracellular domain possessing intrinsic tyrosine kinase activity. On binding to a ligand, such as EGF or transforming growth factor-α, EGFR undergoes autophosphorylation and initiates transduction signals regulating cell division, metastases, angiogenesis, proliferation, and differentiation (Fig. 32.2). EGFR plays an important role in tumor growth and response to cytotoxic agents, including ionizing radiation. The receptor is frequently expressed in high levels in many types of cancer, which

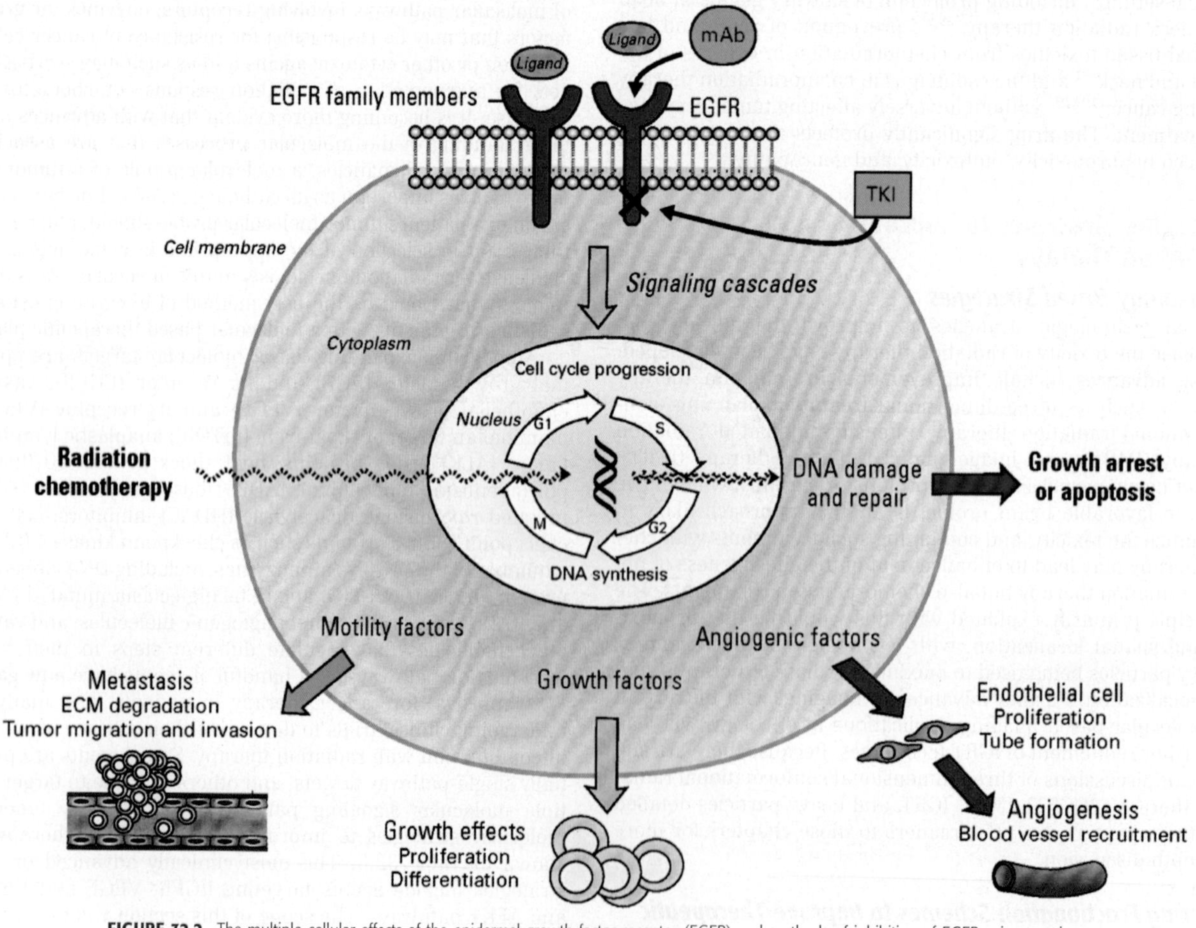

FIGURE 32.2. The multiple cellular effects of the epidermal growth factor receptor (EGFR) and methods of inhibition of EGFR using tyrosine kinase inhibitors (TKIs) or monoclonal antibody (mAB). The potential interactions of EGFR pathways with radiation and chemotherapy are shown. (From Harari PM, Allen GW, Bonner JA. Biology of interactions: antiepidermal growth factor receptor agents. *J Clin Oncol* 2007;25:4057–4065. Adapted with permission from American Society of Clinical Oncology, Inc.)

is often associated with more aggressive tumors, poor patient prognosis, and tumor resistance to treatment with cytotoxic agents including radiation.[200–204] *In vitro* experimental studies have provided solid evidence linking EGFR with resistance to cytotoxic drugs. Although transfection of EGFR into tumor cells increases their resistance to drugs[205] and radiation,[206] the blockade of the EGFR-mediated signaling pathway with antibodies to EGFR enhances the sensitivity of tumor cells to drugs[203] and ionizing radiation.[207] *In vivo* studies have shown that blockade of EGFR, such as with cetuximab, anti-EGFR monoclonal antibody, or interference with its downstream signaling processes, can improve tumor treatment with both chemotherapeutic agents and radiation.[208,209] Furthermore, overexpression of constitutively active EGFR vIII has been correlated with enhanced radioresistance.[210]

Broadly speaking, the two most developed strategies for inhibiting EGFR include the use of monoclonal antibodies (mABs) against EGFR and small molecule tyrosine kinase inhibitors (TKIs) (Fig. 32.2). Cetuximab and panitumumab are examples of mABs, and their mechanism includes blocking the extracellular binding domain, thus inhibiting dimer formation. TKIs such as gefitinib or erlotinib target the intracellular tyrosine kinase domain. However, the activity of EGFR is complicated by the signal diversity due to the formation of homo- and heterodimers with other members of the ErbB family and by the specific autophosphorylation patterns within each ErbB family member. This is further compounded by the identification of specific mutations within EGFR that confer sensitivity to certain EGFR inhibitors. The approach of combining an anti-EGFR therapy with cytotoxic agents including radiation in the treatment of patients with cancer remains an area of active investigation,[39,211–214,215] and some of these key agents warrant further discussion.

Cetuximab (Erbitux). Cetuximab is a chimeric mouse anti-EGFR mAB and is perhaps the most widely studied and developed mAB in this class. It has been studied in a large randomized phase III trial for locally advanced head and neck squamous cell carcinoma patients. This study included 424 patients treated with either radiation therapy alone or radiation therapy with concurrent cetuximab. Medial survival was nearly doubled (49 vs. 29 months, $p = .03$), and progression-free survival (PFS) and locoregional control were both improved with the addition of cetuximab.[39] This resulted in FDA approval in 2006 for use of cetuximab in combination with radiation treatments for locoregionally advanced head and neck cancer. One of the issues that remains is how this compares to concurrent chemoradiation therapy with platinum-based agents for the same population of patients. Radiation Therapy Oncology Group (RTOG) 0522 is a randomized study comparing the addition of cetuximab to standard concurrent cisplatinum and radiation treatments in head and neck cancer patients. Although publication is pending, initial reports suggest no additional survival benefit with the use of cetuximab.[216]

Interestingly, recent phase II studies for stage III NSCLC were reported by the RTOG 0324 and Cancer and Leukemia Group B (CALGB) groups.[114,217] In the randomized phase II CALGB study, two novel chemotherapy regimens in combination with concurrent radiation therapy were investigated in stage III NSCLC patients. The first group received carboplatin (area under the curve [AUC] = 5) and pemetrexed (500 mg/m^2) every 21 days for four cycles with 70 Gy of RT. The second group received the same with the addition of cetuximab. Both groups received four cycles of pemetrexed as consolidation therapy. The primary end point was 18-month survival with a goal of ≥55%, at which point the regimens would be deemed worthy of further study. The carboplatin/pemetrexed/RT arm demonstrated 18-month overall survival (OS) of 58%, and the group with cetuximab, 54%. The combination of thoracic radiation, pemetrexed, and carboplatin, with or without cetuximab, was demonstrated to be feasible and fairly well tolerated.[114]

In the RTOG study, patients were treated with a combination of Taxol, carboplatin, and cetuximab (225 mg/m^2) for six weekly cycles, with 63 Gy of daily radiation therapy. All patients received a loading dose (400 mg/m^2) of cetuximab 1 week prior to RT, and patients received carboplatin/Taxol/cetuximab for two additional cycles after completion of radiation treatments. This study demonstrated median survival of 22.7 months, and 2-year OS of 49.3%.[217] Due to these very promising results, cetuximab was included in the RTOG 0617 trial, which was initially designed to compare two different radiation doses (60 vs. 74 Gy) with concurrent chemotherapy. Current randomization includes chemotherapy + cetuximab + RT versus chemotherapy + RT, followed by adjuvant chemotherapy versus chemotherapy + cetuximab; results are pending.

Gefitinib (Iressa). Gefitinib is approved for use as a single agent in the treatment of chemotherapy-refractory NSCLC.[206] It is known to inhibit primarily the EGFR tyrosine kinase but also has shown some activity for HER-2 kinase, albeit at a much lower level.[206] This agent demonstrated promise in phase II studies ('Iressa' dose evaluation in advanced lung cancer [IDEAL-1] and IDEAL-2)[218,219] but had disappointing results in phase III trials (Iressa NSCLC trial assessing combination treatment [INTACT-1] and INTACT-2), where it failed to demonstrate additional benefit to standard chemotherapy for advanced lung cancer patients.[220,221] However, a subset of patients were noted to have a significant response to gefitinib, and subsequently this led to the discovery that mutations in the EGFR tyrosine kinase domain may predict for a positive response to gefitinib.[222,223] Since then, studies involving gefitinib and combined-modality therapy have also been reported.

The Southwest Oncology Group performed a large phase III trial where stage III NSCLC patients were treated with standard chemoradiation therapy, and after consolidation with docetaxel for three cycles, patients were randomized to maintenance therapy with a placebo or gefitinib 250 mg/day. This was an unselected patient population. At interim analysis, patients on the gefitinib maintenance arm had a worse overall survival, and therefore the study was closed.[215] CALEB 30106[224] was a phase II study designed to evaluate the addition of gefitinib to sequential or concurrent chemoradiotherapy in patients with unresectable NSCLC. Patients were categorized into poor-risk (performance status [PS] ≥2, weight loss ≥5%) and good-risk stratum (PS 0 to 1, weight loss <5%). All patients received induction chemotherapy with two cycles of carboplatin (AUC = 6) and paclitaxel (200 mg/m^2), plus gefitinib 250 mg from days 1 to 21. Gefitinib was removed from induction in May 2004 when a randomized phase III trial did not demonstrate benefit to adding gefitinib with chemotherapy. The poor-risk group received 66 Gy of RT delivered in 33 fractions, with gefitinib 250 mg/day. Good-risk-stratum patients received the same RT and gefitinib but also received weekly carboplatin (AUC = 2) and paclitaxel (50 mg/m^2). Consolidation gefitinib was given until progression. For the poor-risk stratum, PFS was 13.4 months, and median OS was 19 months. For the good-risk stratum, PFS was 9.2 months, and median OS was 13 months. Thirteen of 45 tumors had activating EGFR mutations, and two of 13 had T790M mutations. Seven of 45 tumors had KRAS mutations. When analyzed by these molecular phenotypes, no significant difference in outcome was noted. Interestingly, the poor-risk stratum who received radiation + gefitinib after induction chemotherapy demonstrated promising survival and PFS outcomes. This will lead to further studies designed to elucidate the role of gefitinib and radiation therapy in poor-performance-status patients with stage III NSCLC. Meanwhile, the good-risk-stratum patients did not demonstrate a very good outcome, suggesting that the addition of gefitinib to the chemoradiation therapy regimen may not be beneficial. This is consistent with studies of erlotinib and chemoradiation therapy.[225]

Erlotinib (Tarceva). Erlotinib is also an EGFR TKI that has been approved for use by the FDA. Erlotinib is a potent inhibitor of EGFR autophosphorylation and, like gefitinib, also has some activity against HER-2. It also seems to be a fairly potent inhibitor of signaling mediated by the mutant EGFR vIII.[206] Findings from two large phase III studies, the Tarceva Lung Cancer Investigation (TALENT)[226] and Tarceva Responses in Conjunction with Paclitaxel and Carboplatin (TRIBUTE)[227] trials, demonstrated no significant benefit of the addition of erlotinib to chemotherapy to overall survival in patients with advanced lung cancer.[226,227] Similar to the gefitinib studies, the lack of a demonstrable global benefit to erlotinib pointed to the need for stringent patient selection criteria. In the TRIBUTE study, addition of erlotinib to carboplatin and Taxol improved PFS and OS only in a subset of never smokers. NCIC conducted a phase III study of patients with stage IIIB or IV NSCLC who had failed one to two prior chemotherapy regimens. Overall survival was improved with erlotinib over placebo (6.7 vs. 4.7 months), and response rate, time to symptomatic progression, and PFS were also improved.[228] Meanwhile, erlotinib has been studied in combination with gemcitabine for advanced pancreatic cancer patients demonstrating an OS benefit (median 6.24 vs. 5.91 months) compared to gemcitabine alone[229] by NCIC.

Because EGFR TKIs appear to be most effective in never smokers and those with EGFR mutations, these issues were studied in a phase II study (CALGB 30406), which to date has only been reported in abstract form. This study evaluated patients who were never/light smokers. Patients were randomized to erlotinib alone or erlotinib with carboplatin and paclitaxel. At a median follow-up of 30 months, there was no statistically significant difference in PFS with the addition of erlotinib. However, patients with EGFR mutations had significantly improved PFS and OS in both treatment groups compared to patients who did not harbor the EGFR mutation.[230] There have been a few phase I and II studies that examine the combination of erlotinib and radiation therapy. For instance, adding erlotinib to radiation therapy and temozolomide has been studied for glioblastoma multiforme in a phase I/II setting. The North Central Cancer Treatment Group (NCCTG) demonstrated no significant benefit for the addition of erlotinib,[231] and Cleveland Clinic's phase II study demonstrated detrimental effects.[232] Interestingly, a phase II study by Prados et al.[233] demonstrated superior median survival compared to historical controls treated without erlotinib (19.3 months), with good tolerance to therapy. Erlotinib with chemoradiation (gemcitabine, paclitaxel, and radiation) demonstrated tolerability in a phase I study for locally advanced inoperable pancreatic cancer patients,[234,235] and another study demonstrated tolerability of IMRT-based radiation therapy with erlotinib and capecitabine for pancreatic cancer patients in the postoperative setting.[236] A phase I study of the combination of chemoradiation therapy with erlotinib has been completed in cervical squamous cell carcinoma and a phase II study in locally advanced esophageal cancer, both demonstrating the feasibility of such approaches.[237,238]

In head and neck cancer patients, the addition of erlotinib has been studied with chemoradiation both in newly diagnosed patients and in early phase trials for reirradiation of patients with recurrent head and neck cancer.[239–241] The group from the Sarah Cannon consortium has recently reported on a phase II study of erlotinib, bevacizumab, and radiation therapy and the feasibility of such an approach in a community-based setting with a high level of efficacy and tolerability.[242]

Choong et al.[225] reported on a ping-pong–design phase I study of erlotinib with chemoradiotherapy in patients with NSCLC. One group received induction carboplatin and paclitaxel followed by carboplatin/paclitaxel/radiation + erlotinib, while a second group received cisplatin/etoposide/radiation + erlotinib followed by Taxotere. The erlotinib dose was escalated from 50 mg to 150 mg in three levels in each arm. Median survival in each group was 13.7 months and 10.2 months respectively, with patients who developed rash having an improvement in OS and PFS. This study demonstrated tolerability for such a regimen but with fairly disappointing survival data, once again pointing to the need for improved patient selection when using EGFR-based treatments.

Summary. Several studies have demonstrated the feasibility and tolerability of combining EGFR inhibitors with chemoradiation therapy in different tumor types. Of note, the importance of molecular profiling and patient selection, such as EGFR mutation status, and smoking status in predicting the efficacy of an anti-EGFR-based regimen has become apparent. Future studies involving anti-EGFR treatments in combination with radiation treatments should also incorporate such stringent patient selection criteria to maximize the chance of providing a benefit for the appropriate patients. Finally, when combining EGFR inhibitors with radiation, the efficacy may vary by tumor type, molecular profile, and the sequencing of the EGFR inhibitor therapy with respect to radiation treatments.

Antiangiogenesis

The formation of tumor vasculature, a prerequisite for progressive tumor growth, is initiated and sustained by angiogenic mediators secreted by tumor cells and cells from the surrounding stroma. Many different angiogenic factors have been identified, including vascular endothelial growth factor/vascular permeability factor (VEGF), members of the fibroblast growth factor (FGF) family, platelet-derived growth factor (PDGF), interleukin-8, and prostaglandins. In addition to angiogenic factors, tumors secrete substances that inhibit angiogenesis, such as angiostatin, endostatin, thrombospondin-1, and interferons, so that the final outcome of angiogenesis (and hence tumor growth) depends on the balance between proangiogenic and antiangiogenic activities.

Inhibitors of angiogenesis have undergone extensive preclinical testing, with some agents moving into clinical trials. However, as monotherapeutic agents, the early agents have not been as promising as their preclinical evaluations had suggested.[243] Even though it was assumed that an antiangiogenic agent would impair the efficacy of radiation therapy via the enhancement of hypoxia, early evidence for radiation therapy in combination with angiostatin showed both improved oxygenation and reduced oxygenation.[244–246] However, the first clinical trial with a specific inhibitor of angiogenesis, angiostatin, showed a synergistic effect.[247] Since then, the role of specific factors in vascular growth and maintenance has become clearer. VEGF receptors, in particular, play a critical role in vascular integrity, including angiogenesis and endothelial cell survival, via their tyrosine kinase activities.[248] VEGF expression induces endothelial cell proliferation by creating a vascular sprout that subsequently organizes into a capillary tube.[249,250] VEGF also promotes angiogenesis through the formation of a hyperpermeable immature vascular network.[251] VEGF expression is enhanced following radiation, which is likely a survival response for vascular endothelial cells, ultimately in support of tumor survival. Receptor tyrosine kinases, EGFR in particular, up-regulate VEGF, and cyclo-oxygenase-2 (COX-2) inhibitors limit the up-regulation of VEGF by prostaglandins. One proposed mechanism for resistance to a specific targeted antiangiogenic agent such as VEGF or VEGF receptor inhibitors is that tumor cells may be able to up-regulate alternate angiogenic factors such as PDGF and FGF.[252] Therefore, multitargeted agents that can inhibit multiple pathways have been developed and are also under investigation.

A model of normalization of tumor vasculature has been described by Jain.[253] In this model, proangiogenic factors from tumors can cause abnormal neovascularization, and inhibition of tumor angiogenesis transiently normalizes the tumor vasculature. This, therefore, has the counterintuitive effect of decreasing tumor hypoxia and improving effectiveness of radiation therapy. Preclinical studies and a phase I study of bevacizumab, 5-FU, and radiation therapy preoperatively in locally advanced rectal cancer patients also supported this notion.[254]

There are other biologic mechanisms associated with angiogenesis that suggest combining radiation treatments with antiangiogenic agents, including induction of expression of DNA repair enzymes and targeting of the tumor microenvironment with combined-modality therapy. Data from a number of preclinical studies suggest that at higher doses of radiation, tumor radiosensitivity is directly linked to efficacy of endothelial cell death,[255] and that the conventional fractionation dose (~2 Gy) may not be effective at targeting endothelial cells.[41] However, in preclinical studies, endothelial cell apoptosis may be induced at lower radiation doses by the addition of antiangiogenic drugs or by blocking targets such as PI3K/AKT pathways, which are activated by ionizing radiation on endothelial cells.[256] Finally, radioresistance of some tumors is thought to be mediated in part by the presence of cancer stem cells, which secrete significant amounts of VEGF,[257] and raises the question of whether these tumor cells can become a more sensitive target to radiation treatments when combined with antiangiogenic agents.[258]

Antiangiogenic compounds can also be broadly classified as monoclonal antibodies or tyrosine kinase inhibitors. The most clinically developed agents that have been FDA approved include the mAB bevacizumab and the TKIs sorafenib, sunitinib, and pazopanib.

Bevacizumab. Bevacizumab is a recombinant humanized monoclonal antibody that targets VEGF to inhibit its interaction with the VEGF receptor.[259] It has a long circulating half-life after intravenous infusion of up to 21 days. Bevacizumab was the first drug to receive approval by FDA when used as first-line therapy with 5-FU in patients with advanced colorectal cancer. It has since demonstrated efficacy and activity in NSCLC, renal cell carcinoma, glioblastoma multiforme (GBM), and ovarian cancer.[41] A number of studies have also been performed in different disease sites with bevacizumab in conjunction with radiation therapy. Phase I and II studies with rectal cancer have demonstrated feasibility, and recommendations for appropriate doses to be used with radiation and 5-FU or capecitabine have been established.[260–263] A phase II study of bevacizumab, capecitabine, and radiotherapy for locally advanced rectal cancer in the preoperative setting was reported. Twenty-five patients with clinically staged T3N1 or T3N0 rectal cancer received 50.4 Gy with bevacizumab every 2 weeks (5 mg/kg) and capecitabine 900 mg/m^2 orally bid followed by surgery. Thirty-two percent of patients had pathologic complete response, and 24% of patients had <10% viable tumor cells in the specimen. Three wound complications required surgical interventions.[264] Thirty-two patients were enrolled in a phase I/II study of neoadjuvant bevacizumab, radiation therapy, and fluorouracil in advanced rectal cancer.[261] This treatment yielded 5-year OS and local control of 100% and 5-year disease-free survival of 75%. Toxicity was acceptable, and bevacizumab was shown to decrease tumor interstitial fluid pressure. Biomarkers showed significant correlation to outcome.

Phase I and II studies by Crane et al.[266] have been performed of bevacizumab with capecitabine-based chemotherapy and radiation treatments for pancreatic cancer.[265,266] In the phase II study RTOG 0411, overall median survival was not compromised, but there was a 35.4% rate of grade 3 or greater gastrointestinal-related toxicity (22% during chemoradiation therapy and 13.4% during maintenance chemotherapy). However, there was a significant correlation with grade 3 toxicity during the chemoradiation therapy phase and protocol deviation in terms of generous treatment volumes. A need for prospective quality assurance in future trials was recommended.[266]

Efforts to improve the therapeutic ratio by addition of bevacizumab to chemoradiation therapy have been attempted in multiple studies for both small cell lung cancer and NSCLC patients. Unfortunately, these studies have demonstrated that this regimen was associated with an incidence of tracheoesophageal fistula in both small cell and non–small cell lung cancer settings.[267] A number of studies using bevacizumab have been reported for CNS malignancies. A phase II study by Gruber et al.[268] was reported at the American Society of Clinical Oncology (ASCO) 2009 meeting. Postoperative radiation therapy with temozolomide was given with or without bevacizumab, and bevacizumab maintenance therapy was delivered. Median PFS was reported to be higher in the bevacizumab group at 17 months versus 7 months in their initial reports. Out of 20 patients treated with bevacizumab, two cases of grade 3 to 4 toxicity was related to bevacizumab (pulmonary embolism with thrombocytopenia and leg ulcer with cellulitis). A multicenter phase II study[269] consisting of 70 patients with newly diagnosed GBM examined the response of patients who received postoperative therapy with standard RT, daily temozolomide, and biweekly bevacizumab. Maintenance temozolomide and bevacizumab was given after the completion of therapy. Patients demonstrated improved PFS of 13.6 months (vs. 7.6 months) compared to the University of California Los Angeles/Kaiser Permanente Los Angeles control group, but not an improvement of overall survival. Another study examined patients with recurrent GBM and anaplastic gliomas. Patients in this cohort were treated with bevacizumab (10 mg/kg) every 2 weeks until tumor progression. They also were treated with 30 Gy of hypofractionated radiotherapy in five fractions after the first cycle of bevacizumab. Twenty-five patients were treated (20 with GBM and five with anaplastic gliomas). For the GBM cohort, a response rate of 50% and 6-month PFS of 65% were reported. Median OS was 12.5 months and 1-year survival was 54%. Three patients had to discontinue therapy due to grade 3 effects (CNS intratumor hemorrhage, wound dehiscence, and bowel perforation). No radiation necrosis was seen in these previously irradiated patients.[270]

The University of Chicago group has published phase I and phase II studies combining bevacizumab with 5-FU and hydroxyurea-based radiation therapy in advanced head and neck cancer patients.[271,272] In the phase I study, bevacizumab at 10 mg/m^2 was reported to be integrateable in this chemoradiotherapy regimen, but five patients with fistula formation and four with ulceration/tissue necrosis were reported. It was felt that the fistula and tissue necrosis could have been bevacizumab related. The randomized phase II study enrolled 26 patients with newly diagnosed T4N0/1 head and neck cancers. Patients received hydroxyurea, 5-FU, and bid radiotherapy with or without bevacizumab (10 mg/kg every 14 days). Unexpectedly, there was significant locoregional progression seen in the bevacizumab arm. Two patients died during therapy, and one died shortly after therapy. This led to study termination, and it was felt that addition of bevacizumab to chemoradiotherapy should be limited to clinical trials for head and neck squamous cell carcinoma.

Thalidomide. Thalidomide is an agent that was originally marketed as a sedative and was initially taken off the market due to concerns of teratogenicity. There has been a resurgence in use and interest in this agent, as it has since been found to have potent immunomodulatory effects as well as antiangiogenic properties.[273] Although its effects are not limited to angiogenesis, there are suggestions that thalidomide stimulates vessel maturation with implications for vascular normalization, which may be an important strategy for antineoplastic therapy.[274] Therefore, use of thalidomide with or without radiation therapy has been investigated in both preclinical and clinical settings.[275]

A phase III study (RTOG 0118) was performed to study the efficacy of WBRT (37.5 Gy in 15 fractions) when combined with thalidomide, in patients with 4 or more, or large (>4 cm) tumor, or midbrain brain metastases. Median survival was 3.4 months for both arms (with or without thalidomide), and thalidomide was not well tolerated in this population (48% of patients discontinued thalidomide due to side effects).[276] The efficacy of thalidomide, temozolomide, and 30 Gy in 10 fractions of whole-brain radiation therapy was studied in patients with brain metastases from melanoma. The efficacy was found to be low, and further therapy with this approach was not recommended.[277] A phase II study of thalidomide and radiation in children with newly diagnosed brainstem gliomas and GBM also yielded negative results.[278] A phase II study of temozolomide and thalidomide in patients with newly diagnosed GBM did not demonstrate significant improvement compared to temozolomide alone.[279] Similarly, concurrent thalidomide during radiotherapy of hepatocellular carcinoma did not demonstrate additional benefits in a phase II setting.[280] Eastern Cooperative Oncology Group (ECOG) 3598 was a randomized study comparing chemoradiation therapy ± thalidomide in patients with stage III NSCLC. There was no difference in PFS or OS with the addition of thalidomide.[281]

Summary Antiangiogenesis Agents. It is clear from these studies that the efficacy and safety of antiangiogenic agents in combination with radiation and chemoradiation therapy, while promising in many regards, need to be approached with great caution. It also appears that the location of the tumor and agents used in combination with radiation and antiangiogenic agents such as bevacizumab may factor into determining the feasibility and tolerability of such regimens. The potential for improved efficacy over chemoradiation therapy has been raised in particular for gastrointestinal and CNS malignancies, and further larger studies to help clarify the potential role for antiangiogenic agents in chemoradiation therapy are warranted.

Multitargeted Tyrosine Kinase Inhibitors

Several tyrosine kinase inhibitor agents have been developed that have demonstrable antitumor and antiangiogenesis activities. These include sorafenib (Nexavar), sunitinib (Sutent), and pazopanib (Votrient). All three agents are approved for use in treatment of patients with advanced renal cell carcinoma. Preclinical studies have demonstrated promising findings when combining multitargeted receptor tyrosine kinase inhibitors with radiation therapy.[256,282–288]

Sunitinib is an oral, multitargeted receptor tyrosine kinase inhibitor, which was approved by the FDA for treatment of advanced renal cell carcinoma and imatinib-resistant gastrointestinal stromal tumor (GIST) in January of 2006. Its targets include platelet-derived growth factor receptor (PDGFR), VEGFR, KIT, RET, CSF-1R, and flt3. Several preclinical studies have suggested that sunitinib may be an appropriate agent to consider for use in combination with radiation therapy for a number of solid tumors.[256,285–288] In the clinical setting, a few studies have been reported to date. Wuthrick et al.[289] have completed a phase I trial of 37.5 mg of sunitinib daily with radiation therapy (doses ranged from 14 to 70 Gy [1.8 to 3.5 Gy per fraction]) in 15 patients with primary ($n = 3$) and metastatic ($n = 12$) CNS malignancies.[289] Six patients developed grade 2 or less toxicities, and grade 3 toxicities occurred in seven patients. No grade 3 to 5 intracerebral hemorrhagic events or hypertensive events were reported. Two grade 5 adverse events attributed to disease progression were reported. With a median follow-up of 34.2 months, 13% achieved partial response, 60% had stable disease, and 13% had progressive disease. Six-month PFS for patients with brain metastasis was 58%. The authors recommended consideration for further phase II studies. Kao et al.[290] reported on a phase I study designed to determine the safety and maximum-tolerated dose of concurrent sunitinib and radiation therapy using image-guided technologies for patients with oligometastases (one to five sites) from renal cell carcinoma. The most common treatment sites were bone, liver, and lung. Sunitinib was given at 25 to 37.5 mg/day with either 40 or 50 Gy of radiation therapy delivered in 10 fractions in a ping-pong design of either sunitinib or radiotherapy dose escalation. Twenty-one patients with 36 metastatic lesions were enrolled. No dose-limiting toxicity (DLT) was noted for sunitinib at 37.5 mg plus 40 Gy. At 37.5 mg sunitinib with 50 Gy, and 50 mg sunitinib with 50 Gy, one out of 10 patients, and two out of five patients, respectively, experienced DLTs (grade 4 myelosuppression and grade 3 nausea). The 1-year overall survival rate was 75%, and progression-free survival rate was 44%. They have proceeded to a phase II trial for sunitinib at 37.5 mg/day and a 50-Gy dose regimen.

Sorafenib is a small-molecule TKI that has been approved for treatment of advanced renal cell carcinoma and more recently has received a "fast track" designation for treatment of advanced hepatocellular carcinoma. It is also a multikinase inhibitor of Raf kinase, PDGF, VEGFR2 and R3, and cKit.[291] Pazopanib is also a multitargeted TKI that was approved by the FDA in October 2009 and inhibits the intracellular tyrosine kinase portion of VEGFR1–3, PDGFR-α and -β, c-Kit, FGF receptor-1 (FGFR-1), FGFR-3, Lck, and c-Fms.[292] Phase I and II studies combining these agents with radiation therapy are ongoing.

Mammalian Target of Rapamycin (mTOR)

The mTOR pathway has been shown to be dysregulated in a number of solid tumors.[293] A number of rapamycin analogs exist and have been approved by the FDA, such as temsirolimus (Torisel) or everolimus (Afinitor). Temsirolimus is approved for treating patients with advanced renal cell carcinoma. Everolimus is approved for treatment of patients with advanced renal cell carcinoma that has progressed after other therapies, or patients with pancreatic neuroendocrine tumors who are not surgical candidates. The potential for radiosensitization effects of these agents has been studied in a preclinical setting in a number of different cancer types.[294–302] Temsirolimus was studied in combination with chemoradiation therapy in newly diagnosed GBM patients in a dose-escalation phase I study.[303] Unfortunately, concomitant and adjuvant use of temsirolimus was associated with a high rate (three of 12 patients) of grade 4/5 infections. This was reduced with antibiotic prophylaxis and by limiting the duration of temsirolimus therapy. Therefore, based on this study, a dose of 50 mg/week of temsirolimus combined with radiation and temozolomide is the recommended phase II dose and schedule. The North Central Cancer Treatment Group has also reported a phase I trial of everolimus and temozolomide in combination with radiation therapy in newly diagnosed GBM patients.[304] Eighteen patients were enrolled, and everolimus was well tolerated. The recommended dose for the phase II study is 70 mg/week in combination with standard temozolomide/radiation therapy. Further studies involving the use of agents inhibiting the signaling pathway downstream of mTOR are in development.

Anaplastic Lymphoma Kinase (ALK) Inhibitors

ALK fusion protein results in constitutive activation of ALK tyrosine kinase. Although studies specifically addressing ALK inhibitors with radiation therapy have not yet been reported, because of the impact this molecular has made in the NSCLC therapy paradigm, this topic will be briefly discussed. Soda et al.[305] discovered the fusion of the ALK gene with echinoderm microtubule-associated proteinlike 4 (ELM4-ALK). This *ELM4-ALK* fusion oncogene has become a very important potential biomarker for patients with NSCLC. The frequency of *ALK* rearrangement ranges from 3% to 7% in unselected NSCLC patients. Furthermore, similar to EGFR mutations, this rearrangement is seen more frequently in adenocarcinomas and patients with never or light smoking history. *ALK* rearrangements appear to be mutually exclusive with *EGFR* and *KRAS* mutations.[306] Several ALK inhibitors have been identified, and the furthest developed is crizotinib. Crizotinib was initially designed as an MET inhibitor but has been found to be clinically effective as an ALK inhibitor in NSCLC patients harboring *ALK* rearrangements.[306] In a phase I trial of 82 patients selected for ALK rearrangement (out of over 1,500 patients), an impressive response rate of 57% was noted.[307] Based on a very promising phase I study, this agent has entered phase III studies directly. There are no significant data to suggest a radiosensitizing or synergistic effect when combined with radiation therapy concurrently, but sequential use of this agent with a chemoradiation regimen is being considered.

Histone Deacetylase (HDAC) Inhibitors

HDACs contribute to oncogenic transformation, and involvement of acetylation and HDAC activity in cancer development provides a mechanistic rationale for considering HDAC inhibitors as an anticancer therapy. Inhibitors of histone deacetylase relax chromatin structure. This can lead to increased radiosensitivity through enhanced DNA damage.[308,309] However, some histone deacetylase inhibitors have also been shown to down-regulate the expression of both EGFR and ErbB2 and to inhibit PI3K and AKT signaling,[310–312] all strong potentiators of tumor cell survival and modulators of DNA DSB repair.[313] This combination of DNA damage enhancement, inhibition of DNA repair, and down-regulation of strong survival highlights the utility of agents that attack multiple signaling pathways.

The most clinically developed HDAC inhibitors include vorinostat and romidepsin, both of which have FDA approval for use in cutaneous T-cell lymphoma. While their indications are supported by data suggesting activity in hematologic malignancies, studies in solid tumors have also been reported. Preclinical studies of radiation therapy and HDAC inhibitors have been reported in squamous cells, medulloblastoma cells, breast cancer brain metastatic cells, colorectal models, GBM cells, pancreatic cells, neuroblastoma cells, osteosarcoma, and rhabdomyosarcoma cells.[310,314–325] Of note, 18 HDAC enzymes have been identified and classified into four groups (classes I through IV).

Vorinostat is a hydroxamic acid multi-HDAC inhibitor that blocks the enzymatic activity of both class I and II HDACs at low nanomolar concentrations.[321] Vorinostat is active in inducing differentiation, cell growth arrest, or apoptosis in a wide variety of transformed cells in preclinical studies.[321] Vorinostat is FDA approved for treatment of cutaneous T-cell lymphoma (CTCL) that has persisted, progressed, or recurred after treatment with other first-line agents. Therefore, primary efficacy of vorinostat has been demonstrated in hematologic malignancies. However, it is also being studied in a number of different solid tumor types with mixed success (NSCLC, colorectal cancer, breast cancer, prostate cancer, GBM) in phase I and II clinical settings in combination with other standard cytotoxic agents, including radiation therapy.[326–330] Ree et al.[320] reported on combining vorinostat with pelvic palliative radiotherapy for gastrointestinal carcinoma patients. Sixteen patients were evaluable. Patients received palliative radiotherapy (30 Gy in 10 fractions) with escalating vorinostat dose, administered orally daily 3 hours before each radiotherapy fraction. Maximum tolerated dose was determined to be 300 mg/day. Histone hyperacetylation was detected, indicating biologic activity of vorinostat.

Romidepsin is a novel HDAC inhibitor with recent FDA approval for treatment of CTCL, approved as second-line therapy.[331] Studies in small cell lung cancer, recurrent glioma, and castrate-resistant prostate cancer have been performed with mixed success.[332–334] As yet there are no reported studies demonstrating efficacy of romidepsin in combination with radiation treatments.

Miscellaneous Molecular Targets

K-Ras

Activating mutations in the ras oncogene are found in many tumors including lung, colon, head and neck, glioblastoma, pancreas, and others. The overall rate of ras mutations in human cancers is 25% to 30%, but for some cancers the mutation rate can be quite high. These activating mutations drive key intracellular signaling pathways that confer proliferative and survival advantages to tumor cells, including radioresistance, through the chronic activation of the PI3K and the Ras/MAP kinase pathways.[335,336–337] Ras must be prenylated in order to be membrane bound, where it becomes active. Prenylation can occur by two enzymatic processes, farnesylation and geranylgeranylation. Inhibitors of farnesylation, specifically farnesyltransferase inhibitors (FTIs), have had some success in limiting the negative impact of ras activation, particularly in inhibiting tumor cell radioresistance *in vitro* and *in vivo*.[23,335,338–340] FTIs selectively affect tumors because the *ras* genes in normal tissues are not mutated. The activity of FTIs has had limited success, partly because of the activity against a given ras species, H-ras versus n-Ras or K-ras, and partly because of the FTI resistance of geranylgeranylated K-ras.[335,338,341,342,343] However, new compounds that target both farnesylation and geranylgeranylation have been shown to be effective in preclinical studies, and new molecular targets for radiosensitization by FTIs have been identified,[337,344] which may enhance their clinical utility.

Targeting DNA

Many therapy agents target the DNA of cells, preferably tumor cells. This can be through DNA damage induction, inhibition of cell cycle traversal, or inhibition of DNA replication, for example, and targeting the enzymes that manage the integrity of the DNA of cells represents a sound therapeutic strategy. Furthermore, differences between tumor and normal cells in cell cycle checkpoint controls, DNA repair capabilities, and even chromatin architecture have been identified that could be taken advantage of by combined therapies.

There are multiple strategies to targeting DNA repair pathways with drugs or small molecules. First, DNA damage must be sensed, and there are several key enzymes that are considered damage sensors. The most established sensors are telomeric repeat-binding factor 2 (TRF2), the Mre11-Rad50-Nbs1 (MRN) complex, and ATM.[345,346] These proteins set off the cascade of events that alter chromatin, recruit repair enzymes to the break site, and initiate cell cycle checkpoint control following DNA damage. Key regulatory proteins within each of these areas are being successfully targeted in preclinical studies. Examples include a specific inhibitor of ATM, Ku55933, which has shown enhanced radiosensitivity in *in vitro* experiments[347]; small molecules that reconstitute the wild-type p53 protein structure in mutant p53 molecules[348]; and radiotherapy combined with adenoviral wild-type p53 delivered *in vivo* by liposomal carriers in clinical trials for lung cancer.[349] Preclinical evaluations of compounds that target DNA repair components directly, particularly when combined with radiation and radiosensitizing compounds such as cisplatin or gemcitabine, are ongoing. Inhibitors of DNA-PKcs, a critical enzyme in nonhomologous end joining (NHEJ), have been successful in preclinical studies on tumor cell lines; however, a treatment advantage for normal tissue may provide a challenge.[350–355]

There are novel therapeutic targets within the DNA repair pathway known as *homologous recombination* (HR). For instance, RAD51 and BRCA1/2 defective cell lines are radiosensitive, and antisense strategies against RAD51 have been used against a number of cancer cell lines. Interestingly, targeting HR may have a distinct advantage over the NHEJ pathway. NHEJ occurs throughout the cell cycle, whereas HR is considered to be a dominant repair pathway during the S and G_2 phases of the cell cycle because of the need for a template strand of DNA. This implies that for most normal tissues, where there is little to no cellular turnover and where NHEJ is the dominant DNA repair pathway, there would be a survival advantage compared to tumors where cells are traversing the cell cycle and are more likely to be found in the S or G_2 phase. Finally, specific inhibitors such as small interfering RNA (siRNA), antisense, small molecules, and antibodies that target DNA repair are still relatively new, and while the *in vitro* data are encouraging, clinical efficacy remains to be seen.

PARP is an enzyme whose specific function is to repair SSBs, and with recent advances in agents that block this pathway, a discussion of such agents is warranted. PARP catalyzes the transfer of ADP-ribose units from intracellular NAD^+ to nuclear receptor proteins, leading to the formation of ADP-ribose polymers. Nicotinamide was the first PARP inhibitor identified, and since then second-generation PARP inhibitors have been developed. While significant current interest is in the role of PARP inhibitors in BRCA-deficient tumors, they have also been studied as chemosensitizers. Therefore, initial studies primarily were based on nonselected tumor types to determine the efficacy of PARP inhibition in combination with chemotherapy agents. However, because radiotherapy damages cells by causing DNA breaks, and PARP inhibitors impair DNA repair mechanisms, studies in combination with radiation therapy have been performed *in vitro* and *in vivo* demonstrating effectiveness in cancer cell lines, including glioma cells.[356–358,359] Furthermore, with exciting preclinical data suggesting that PARP inhibitors may have a significantly and selectively high impact in BRCA-deficient cells,[360,361] a new paradigm for a clinical trial was born in which patients with BRCA mutations or BRCA-ness were selected for treatment with PARP inhibitors.[362,363] BRCA-ness refers to abnormal function of BRCA1/2 genes, or other genes implicated in similar DNA repair pathways to BRCA1 and BRCA2, which is seen in triple-negative breast cancer patients, for example, without necessarily having the hereditary mutations.[363] After encouraging preclinical data in solid tumors with chemotherapy, and particularly in selected tumor cells with BRCA deficiency, multiple PARP inhibitors have been studied or are being studied in solid tumors in phase I/II settings. In combination with chemotherapy agents, multiple agents including AG014699, INO-1001, KU-0059436/AZD2281, ABT-888, and BSI-201 have completed phase I studies, which have been reported primarily for solid tumors. BSI-201 has been studied in a phase II setting in triple-negative breast cancers.[363] Ongoing studies with these and other agents together with chemotherapy in solid tumors, and also interestingly in selected tumors with BRCA mutation or possible BRCA-ness, are in progress. Of note, ABT-888 is a PARP inhibitor that appears to cross the blood–brain barrier, and its efficacy in combination with whole-brain radiation for brain metastases and with temozolomide and radiation for patients with primary brain tumors is being studied in phase I and phase I/II studies, respectively.[363] FDA approval for these agents remains pending.

Future Directions: Era of Personalized Medicine Using Molecularly Tailored Therapeutics

While high-impact molecular discoveries and effective combined-modality treatment realizations have been of significant importance in the field of oncology, another area that has made significant strides and impact on cancer therapeutics is the concept of molecular selection of patients for appropriate therapy. One of the first such examples is in the field of breast cancer where hormonal therapy and Herceptin treatments are selectively given to patients whose tumors demonstrate appropriate molecular criteria (estrogen receptor positivity and HER2/neu positivity).[364] Other examples include imatinib for treatment of patients with c-kit harboring GIST tumors,[365] anti-EGFR therapy for lung cancer patients with EGFR tyrosine kinase mutations, crizotinib for lung cancer patients with ALK fusion gene translocation, and the predictive value of KRAS mutation status for anti-EGFR therapy for patients with metastatic colorectal cancer.[366]

Meanwhile, abundant studies are in progress and/or have been performed to attempt to determine biomarkers that may provide prognostic or therapeutic information. Multigene assays (Oncotype DX),[367] for example, are already in use in clinical practice for patients with breast cancer. Genomic signatures or biomarkers of response to chemotherapy of tumor, to survival, or to metastatic potential of tumor have been studied.[368] Similarly, efforts to study and identify biomarkers for radiation response, sensitivity, resistance, or toxicity are being investigated, but mature data for use in a clinical setting have not yet been elucidated.

Therefore, clinical trial design for combined-modality therapy in the next decade will require a level of complexity beyond formulaic addition of two cytotoxic agents to elucidate a synergistic response. It will require an in-depth understanding of molecular pathways of the individual cytotoxic agents, including chemotherapy, targeted agents, and ionizing radiation. Appropriate incorporation of validated biomarkers and studies designed to elucidate other important biomarkers for prediction of treatment response will be essential. Incorporation of molecular selection strategies using appropriate biomarkers, to design tailored studies, and incorporation of appropriate molecular agents into our combined-modality regimens will be essential as we enter this era of personalized medicine.

TABLE 32.4 CHEMORADIATION THERAPY AS STANDARD OF CARE BY SELECTED DISEASE SITES

Disease Site	*Commonly Used Chemotherapeutic Agents*	*Sequencing and Intent of Therapy*	*Benefit of Combined-Modality Approach*
Locally advanced head and neck cancer	Cisplatin, 5-FU, hydroxyurea, carboplatin, cetuximab	• Definitive concurrent • Postoperative concurrent	Definitive: Organ preservation/survival benefit Postoperative: DFS/LRC benefit; overall survival benefit in subset of patients
Glioblastoma multiforme	Temozolomide	• Postoperative concurrent • Definitive concurrent in unresectable cases	Overall survival
Locally advanced/unresectable non–small cell lung cancer	Cisplatin, carboplatin, paclitaxel, cisplatin, etoposide, vinblastine	• Definitive concurrent • Sequential	Overall survival
Limited-stage small cell lung cancer	Cisplatin/etoposide	• Definitive concurrent	Overall survival
Esophageal cancer	Cisplatin/5-FU	• Preoperative concurrent • Definitive concurrent	Local control, overall survival
Gastric cancer	5-FU, leucovorin	• Postoperative concurrent	Overall survival
Pancreatic cancer	5-FU, gemcitabine	• Postoperative concurrent • Definitive concurrent in unresectable patients	Locoregional control, possibly survival
Locally advanced rectal cancer	5-FU, Xeloda	• Preoperative concurrent	Improved sphincter preservation, improved DFS
Anal cancer	5-FU, mitomycin-C	• Definitive concurrent	Improved colostomy-free survival
Cervical cancer	Cisplatin, 5-FU, hydroxyurea	• Definitive concurrent	Overall survival benefit
Bladder cancer	Cisplatin, 5-FU, mitomycin-C	• Definitive concurrent	Bladder preservation

5-FU, 5-fluorouracil; DFS, disease-free survival; LRC, locoregional control.

TABLE 32.5 THE LONG-TERM TOXICITY OF COMBINED CHEMORADIATION THERAPY

Agent	Toxicity	Mechanism	References
Bleomycin	Pneumonitis/pulmonary fibrosis	Undefined but related to total drug dose and effects on pulmonary macrophages, type I and II alveolar cells; effects/lethality exacerbated by the administration of radiation.	369–371
Actinomycin D	Hepatopathy	Altered liver function postradiation leads to decreased metabolism of agents, including actinomycin, which in turn worsens the hepatopathy.	372,373
Doxorubicin	Cardiomyopathy	There is an additive interaction between doxorubicin and radiation with recall of radiation effects occurring. Primary radiation effect is on the endothelial cell, whereas doxorubicin affects the connective tissue stroma of the myocardium.	374–377
Methotrexate	Leukoencephalopathy	Methotrexate may cause this syndrome on its own. Radiation effects on the blood–brain barrier and the choroid plexus can alter methotrexate clearance, leading to higher levels in the brain. Effects are increased when both modalities are used.	378–380
Cisplatin	Sensorineural hearing loss	While cisplatinum alone can cause this, reports suggests radiation therapy concurrently with cisplatin may contribute to sensorineural hearing loss.	381–384

THE CLINICAL EXPERIENCE WITH CHEMORADIATION IN CANCER THERAPY

The level of clinical experience with the combination of radiation and chemotherapy has increased dramatically during the years. In many tumor types, the sequencing and method of administration of the combination have been very important in attaining improved outcomes seen in randomized trials. Improved local control and better overall survival rates have resulted from combination therapy in a number of diseases, including rectal cancer, limited-stage small cell lung cancer, locally advanced NSCLC, esophageal cancer, gastric cancer, cervical cancer, glioblastoma, and rhabdomyosarcomas. Equally important are the successes seen in the realm of organ preservation in sarcomas of the extremity, bladder cancers, carcinomas of the anal canal, head and neck cancers, and breast cancer.

As the role for combined-modality therapy and studies leading to such for each of the tumor types are well represented in individual chapters addressing the disease site, readers will be referred to individual disease site chapters in the text for details. Briefly summarized in Table 32.4, however, are some representative disease sites in adult malignancies, where combined-modality therapy with chemotherapy and/or targeted biologic agents and radiation therapy is accepted as the standard of care. The table also summarizes the commonly used systemic agent for these different disease sites. As one can see, the list, while not comprehensive, is certainly extensive and impressive, and the clinical impact that combined-modality therapy has had in each of these disease sites cannot be understated.

As outcomes in each of the solid tumors improve with concurrent therapy, we need to become cognizant of the potential for significant long-term toxicity from combination chemoradiation and do our best to minimize the risks that these side effects pose to patient survival and quality of life. Several well-documented chemoradiation-imposed late effects are summarized in Table 32.5.

CONCLUDING REMARKS

The combination of chemotherapy and radiation therapy has become a common strategic practice in the therapy of locally advanced cancers, with emphasis on the concurrent delivery of both modalities. Improvements in treatment outcome in terms of both local control and patient survival have been achieved with traditional chemotherapeutic agents such as cisplatin and 5-FU. However, there is considerable room for improvement of the combined treatment strategies. Selection of the most effective drug or the optimal treatment approach remains a significant challenge.

Newer chemotherapies, and novel molecularly based targeted therapeutic agents, are becoming available at an increasing rate. These agents have high potential for increasing the therapeutic effectiveness of radiation therapy, and therefore their evaluation—both in the laboratory and in the clinic, in combination with radiation therapy—is essential for improvement of cancer treatment. Preclinical studies not only provide a biologic rationale for the use of a given drug with radiation but also are able to generate information that is critical to the design of effective treatment schedules in clinical settings. Studies of the mechanisms of molecular agents/chemotherapy–radiation therapy interaction at the genetic–molecular, cellular, and tumor (or normal tissue) microenvironmental levels are essential for obtaining clear insight into the radiomodulating potential of these agents and their ability to increase radiotherapeutic effects.

Biomarkers, molecular therapeutics, advanced imaging technology, and advances in understanding of effective chemotherapy and radiation treatment integration have led to an era where personalized medicine for cancer therapy is becoming a reality. Many studies have pointed toward the need for careful patient selection when designing clinical trials incorporating molecular-targeted agents. Effective biomarker development and integration of such into clinical trial design are essential as it becomes more and more clear that cancer is truly a heterogeneous entity. There are certainly challenges that we can anticipate along the way toward an era of personalized medicine. For example, once numerous biomarkers have been elucidated, how will we decide which biomarkers are most important to test for further clinical trials? Furthermore, how will these studies be financed? In the era of tenuous health care finances, will we have the funds to implement the needed studies and be able to support payment for all the novel drugs coming out of the pipeline?

Finally, despite significant improvements rendered to cancer therapy in the past decades, it is sobering to realize that cancer, particularly when advanced, remains a deadly disease for many. As we embark on this era of abundant molecular therapeutics, novel chemotherapeutic agents, better-established chemoradiation regimens, and more sophisticated imaging technology and radiation delivery methods, it will be essential to design well-thought-out and effective combined-modality-therapy clinical trials to further improve the odds in the battle against cancer.

SELECTED REFERENCES

A full list of references for this chapter is available online.

1. Herscher LL. Principles of chemoradiation: theoretical and practical considerations. *Oncology (Williston Park)* 1999;13(10 Suppl 5):11–22.
3. Phillips T. Radiation-chemotherapy interactions. In: Pass HI, Johnson DH, eds. *Lung cancer: principles and practice*. Philadelphia: Lippincott-Raven, 1996.
4. Seiwert TY, Salama JK, Vokes EE. The concurrent chemoradiation paradigm–general principles. *Nat Clin Pract Oncol* 2007;4(2):86–100.
6. Steel GG, Peckham MJ. Exploitable mechanisms in combined radiotherapy-chemotherapy: the concept of additivity. *Int J Radiat Oncol Biol Phys* 1979;5(1):85–91.
7. Radford IR. Evidence for a general relationship between the induced level of DNA double-strand breakage and cell-killing after X-irradiation of mammalian cells. *Int J Radiat Biol Relat Stud Phys Chem Med* 1986;49(4):611–620.

8. Kinsella TJ, et al. Enhancement of X ray induced DNA damage by pre-treatment with halogenated pyrimidine analogs. *Int J Radiat Oncol Biol Phys* 1987; 13(5):733–739.
9. Elkind MM, Sutton H. X-ray damage and recovery in mammalian cells in culture. *Nature* 1959;184:1293–1295.
10. Iliakis G. Radiation-induced potentially lethal damage: DNA lesions susceptible to fixation. *Int J Radiat Biol Relat Stud Phys Chem Med* 1988;53(4):541–584.
11. Little JB, et al. Repair of potentially lethal radiation damage in vitro and in vivo. *Radiology* 1973;106(3):689–694.
12. Wang Y, Pantelias GE, Iliakis G. Mechanism of radiosensitization by halogenated pyrimidines: the contribution of excess DNA and chromosome damage in BrdU radiosensitization may be minimal in plateau-phase cells. *Int J Radiat Biol* 1994; 66(2):133–142.
13. Gregoire V, et al. Radiosensitization of mouse sarcoma cells by fludarabine (F-ara-A) or gemcitabine (dFdC), two nucleoside analogues, is not mediated by an increased induction or a repair inhibition of DNA double-strand breaks as measured by pulsed-field gel electrophoresis. *Int J Radiat Biol* 1998;73(5):511–520.
14. Lawrence TS, et al. Radiosensitization of pancreatic cancer cells by 2',2'-difluoro-2'-deoxycytidine. *Int J Radiat Oncol Biol Phys* 1996;34(4):867–872.
19. Choy H, et al. Investigation of taxol as a potential radiation sensitizer. *Cancer* 1993;71(11):3774–3778.
22. Brown JM, Giaccia AJ. The unique physiology of solid tumors: opportunities (and problems) for cancer therapy. *Cancer Res* 1998;58(7):1408–1416.
23. Brunner TB, et al. Farnesyltransferase inhibitors as radiation sensitizers. *Int J Radiat Biol* 2003;79(7):569–576.
24. Bush RS, et al. Definitive evidence for hypoxic cells influencing cure in cancer therapy. *Br J Cancer Suppl* 1978;3:302–306.
25. Hockel M, et al. Intratumoral pO2 predicts survival in advanced cancer of the uterine cervix. *Radiother Oncol* 1993;26(1):45–50.
26. Nordsmark M, Overgaard M, Overgaard J. Pretreatment oxygenation predicts radiation response in advanced squamous cell carcinoma of the head and neck. *Radiother Oncol* 1996;41(1):31–39.
27. Dische S. A review of hypoxic cell radiosensitization. *Int J Radiat Oncol Biol Phys* 1991;20(1):147–152.
29. Henk JM, Kunkler PB, Smith CW. Radiotherapy and hyperbaric oxygen in head and neck cancer. Final report of first controlled clinical trial. *Lancet* 1977;2 (8029):101–103.
31. Tannock IF, Rotin D. Acid pH in tumors and its potential for therapeutic exploitation. *Cancer Res* 1989;49(16):4373–4384.
32. Overgaard J, et al. A randomized double-blind phase III study of nimorazole as a hypoxic radiosensitizer of primary radiotherapy in supraglottic larynx and pharynx carcinoma. Results of the Danish Head and Neck Cancer Study (DAHANCA) Protocol 5–85. *Radiother Oncol* 1998;46(2):135–146.
33. Stephens TJ. Regeneration of tumors after cytotoxic treatment. In: Meyn RE, Withers HR, eds. *Radiation biology in cancer research.* New York: Raven Press, 1980.
34. Milas L, et al. Dynamics of tumor cell clonogen repopulation in a murine sarcoma treated with cyclophosphamide. *Radiother Oncol* 1994;30(3):247–253.
35. Hermens AF, Barendsen GW. The proliferative status and clonogenic capacity of tumour cells in a transplantable rhabdomyosarcoma of the rat before and after irradiation with 800 rad of X-rays. *Cell Tissue Kinet* 1978;11(1):83–100.
36. Withers HR, Taylor JM, Maciejewski B. The hazard of accelerated tumor clonogen repopulation during radiotherapy. *Acta Oncol* 1988;27(2):131–146.
39. Bonner JA, et al. Radiotherapy plus cetuximab for squamous-cell carcinoma of the head and neck. *N Engl J Med* 2006;354(6):567–578.
40. Albini A, Sporn MB. The tumour microenvironment as a target for chemoprevention. *Nat Rev Cancer* 2007;7(2):139–147.
43. Koch U, Krause M, Baumann M. Cancer stem cells at the crossroads of current cancer therapy failures–radiation oncology perspective. *Semin Cancer Biol* 2010; 20(2):116–124.
45. Hittelman WN, et al. Are cancer stem cells radioresistant? *Future Oncol* 2010;6 (10):1563–1576.
48. Douple EB, Lognan ME. Therapeutic potentiation in a mouse mammary tumour and an intracerebral rat brain tumour by combined treatment with cis-dichlorodiammineplatinum (II) and radiation. *J Clin Hematol Oncol* 1977;30:585–603.
49. Carde P, Laval F. Effect of cis-dichlorodiammine platinum II and X rays on mammalian cell survival. *Int J Radiat Oncol Biol Phys* 1981;7(7):929–933.
50. Begg AC, et al. Radiosensitization in vitro by cis-diammine (1,1-cyclobu tanedicarboxylato) platinum(II) (carboplatin, JM8) and ethylenediamminemalonatoplatinum(II) (JM40). *Radiother Oncol* 1987;9(2):157–165.
51. O'Hara JA, Douple EB, Richmond RC. Enhancement of radiation-induced cell kill by platinum complexes (carboplatin and iproplatin) in V79 cells. *Int J Radiat Oncol Biol Phys* 1986;12(8):1419–1422.
52. Amorino GP, Hamilton VM, Choy H. Enhancement of radiation effects by combined docetaxel and carboplatin treatment in vitro. *Radiat Oncol Investig* 1999;7(6):343–352.
56. Kim JS, et al. Radiation enhancement by the combined use of topoisomerase I inhibitors, RFS-2000 or CPT-11, and topoisomerase II inhibitor etoposide in human lung cancer cells. *Radiother Oncol* 2002;62(1):61–67.
57. Amorino GP, et al. Preclinical evaluation of the orally active camptothecin analog, RFS-2000 (9-nitro-20(S)-camptothecin) as a radiation enhancer. *Int J Radiat Oncol Biol Phys* 2000;47(2):503–509.
59. Brown JM. The hypoxic cell: A target for selective cancer therapy - eighteenth Bruce F. Cain Memorial Award Lecture. *Cancer Res* 1998;59:5863–5870.
60. Latz D, et al. Radiosensitizing potential of gemcitabine (2',2'-difluoro-2'-deoxycytidine) within the cell cycle in vitro. *Int J Radiat Oncol Biol Phys* 1998; 41(4):875–882.
61. Mason KA, et al. Maximizing therapeutic gain with gemcitabine and fractionated radiation. *Int J Radiat Oncol Biol Phys* 1999;44(5):1125–1135.
64. Rosenberg B, et al. Platinum compounds: a new class of potent antitumour agents. *Nature* 1969;222(5191):385–386.
71. Wodinsky I, et al. Combination radiotherapy and chemotherapy for P388 lymphocytic leukemia in vivo. *Cancer Chemother Rep [2]* 1974;4(1):73–97.
72. Szumiel I, Nias AH. The effect of combined treatment with a platinum complex and ionizing radiation on Chinese hamster ovary cells in vitro. *Br J Cancer* 1976; 33(4):450–458.
73. Stratford IJ, Williamson C, Adams GE. Combination studies with misonidazole and a cis-platinum complex: cytotoxicity and radiosensitization in vitro. *Br J Cancer* 1980;41(4):517–522.
74. Dewit L. Combined treatment of radiation and cisdiamminedichloroplatinum (II): a review of experimental and clinical data. *Int J Radiat Oncol Biol Phys* 1987;13(3):403–426.
76. Amorino GP, et al. Radiopotentiation by the oral platinum agent, JM216: role of repair inhibition. *Int J Radiat Oncol Biol Phys* 1999;44(2):399–405.
77. Choy H. Satraplatin: an orally available platinum analog for the treatment of cancer. *Expert Rev Anticancer Ther* 2006;6(7):973–982.
78. Choy H, Park C, Yao M. Current status and future prospects for satraplatin, an oral platinum analogue. *Clin Cancer Res* 2008;14(6):1633–1638.
84. Manfredi JJ, Horwitz SB. Taxol: an antimitotic agent with a new mechanism of action. *Pharmacol Ther* 1984;25(1):83–125.
86. Ringel I, Horwitz SB. Studies with RP 56976 (taxotere): a semisynthetic analogue of Taxol. *J Natl Cancer Inst* 1991;83(4):288–291.
87. Hall EJ. *Radiobiology for the radiologist.* 4th ed. Philadelphia: Lippincott, 1994.
93. Altmann KH, Wartmann M, O'Reilly T. Epothilones and related structures–a new class of microtubule inhibitors with potent in vivo antitumor activity. *Biochim Biophys Acta* 2000;1470(3):M79–M91.
96. Hofstetter B, et al. Patupilone acts as radiosensitizing agent in multidrug-resistant cancer cells in vitro and in vivo. *Clin Cancer Res* 2005;11(4):1588–1596.
102. McGinn CJ, Kinsella TJ. The experimental and clinical rationale for the use of S-phase-specific radiosensitizers to overcome tumor cell repopulation. *Semin Oncol* 1992;19(4 Suppl 11):21–28.
106. Plunkett W, et al. Gemcitabine: metabolism, mechanisms of action, and self-potentiation. *Semin Oncol* 1995;22(4 Suppl 11):3–10.
110. Choy H, et al. RTOG 0017: a phase I trial of concurrent gemcitabine/carboplatin or gemcitabine/paclitaxel and radiation therapy ("ping-pong trial") followed by adjuvant chemotherapy for patients with favorable prognosis inoperable stage IIIA/B non-small cell lung cancer. *J Thorac Oncol* 2009;4(1):80–86.
116. Norman P. Pemetrexed disodium (Eli Lilly). *Curr Opin Investig Drugs* 2001;2 (11):1611–1622.
117. Bischof M, et al. Interaction of pemetrexed disodium (ALIMTA, multitargeted antifolate) and irradiation in vitro. *Int J Radiat Oncol Biol Phys* 2002;52(5): 1381–1388.
122. Govindan R, et al. Randomized phase II study of pemetrexed, carboplatin, and thoracic radiation with or without cetuximab in patients with locally advanced unresectable non-small-cell lung cancer: Cancer and Leukemia Group B trial 30407. *J Clin Oncol* 2011;29(23):3120–3125.
131. Hsiang YH, Liu LF. Identification of mammalian DNA topoisomerase I as an intracellular target of the anticancer drug camptothecin. *Cancer Res* 1988;48 (7):1722–1726.
136. Chakravarthy A, Choy H. A phase I trial of outpatient weekly irinotecan/carboplatin and concurrent radiation for stage III unresectable non small-cell lung cancer: a Vanderbilt-Ingram Cancer Center Affiliate Network Trial. *Clin Lung Cancer* 2000;1(4):310–311.
139. Stupp R, et al. Radiotherapy plus concomitant and adjuvant temozolomide for glioblastoma. *N Engl J Med* 2005;352(10):987–996.
140. Hegi ME, et al. MGMT gene silencing and benefit from temozolomide in glioblastoma. *N Engl J Med* 2005;352(10):997–1003.
142. Sartorelli AC, et al. Mitomycin C: a prototype bioreductive agent. *Oncol Res* 1994;6(10–11):501–508.
143. Bristow RG. Molecular and cellular basis of radiotherapy. In: Tannock IF, Hill R, eds. *The basic science of oncology.* Montreal: McGraw-Hill, 1998.
162. Green MR, et al. Abraxane, a novel Cremophor-free, albumin-bound particle form of paclitaxel for the treatment of advanced non-small-cell lung cancer. *Ann Oncol* 2006;17(8):1263–1268.
173. Wiedenmann N, et al. 130-nm albumin-bound paclitaxel enhances tumor radiocurability and therapeutic gain. *Clin Cancer Res* 2007;13(6):1868–1874.
184. Yuhas JM, Storer JB. Differential chemoprotection of normal and malignant tissues. *J Natl Cancer Inst* 1969;42(2):331–335.
187. Arora R, et al. Radioprotection by plant products: present status and future prospects. *Phytother Res* 2005;19(1):1–22.
190. Brizel DM, et al. Phase III randomized trial of amifostine as a radioprotector in head and neck cancer. *J Clin Oncol* 2000;18(19):3339–3345.
194. Fu KK, et al. A Radiation Therapy Oncology Group (RTOG) phase III randomized study to compare hyperfractionation and two variants of accelerated fractionation to standard fractionation radiotherapy for head and neck squamous cell carcinomas: first report of RTOG 9003. *Int J Radiat Oncol Biol Phys* 2000; 48(1):7–16.
195. Ang K, Zhang Q, Wheeler RH, et al. A phase III trial (RTOG 0129) of two radiation-cisplatin regimens for head and neck carcinomas (HNC): impact of radiation and cisplatin intensity on outcome. *J Clin Oncol* 2010;28(15s, 2010 [suppl; abstr 5507]).
196. Belani CP, et al. Phase III study of the Eastern Cooperative Oncology Group (ECOG 2597): induction chemotherapy followed by either standard thoracic radiotherapy or hyperfractionated accelerated radiotherapy for patients with unresectable stage IIIA and B non-small-cell lung cancer. *J Clin Oncol* 2005;23(16): 3760–3767.
197. Saunders M, et al. Continuous hyperfractionated accelerated radiotherapy (CHART) versus conventional radiotherapy in non-small-cell lung cancer: a randomised multicentre trial. CHART Steering Committee. *Lancet* 1997;350 (9072):161–165.
198. Brizel DM, et al. Hyperfractionated irradiation with or without concurrent chemotherapy for locally advanced head and neck cancer. *N Engl J Med* 1998;338(25): 1798–1804.
206. Harari PM, Allen GW, Bonner JA. Biology of interactions: antiepidermal growth factor receptor agents. *J Clin Oncol* 2007;25(26):4057–4065.
207. Huang SM, Bock JM, Harari PM. Epidermal growth factor receptor blockade with C225 modulates proliferation, apoptosis, and radiosensitivity in squamous cell carcinomas of the head and neck. *Cancer Res* 1999;59(8):1935–1940.
215. Kelly K, et al. Phase III trial of maintenance gefitinib or placebo after concurrent chemoradiotherapy and docetaxel consolidation in inoperable stage III non-small-cell lung cancer: SWOG S0023. *J Clin Oncol* 2008;26(15):2450–2456.
216. Ang KK, Zhang QE, Rosenthal DI, et al. A randomized phase III trial (RTOG 0522) of concurrent accelerated radiation plus cisplatin with or without cetuximab for stage III-IV head and neck squamous cell carcinomas (HNC). *J Clin Oncol* 2011; 29(suppl; abstr 5500).
220. Giaccone G, et al. Gefitinib in combination with gemcitabine and cisplatin in advanced non-small-cell lung cancer: a phase III trial–INTACT 1. *J Clin Oncol* 2004;22(5):777–784.

221. Herbst RS, et al. Gefitinib in combination with paclitaxel and carboplatin in advanced non-small-cell lung cancer: a phase III trial–INTACT 2. *J Clin Oncol* 2004;22(5):785–794.
222. Lynch TJ, et al. Activating mutations in the epidermal growth factor receptor underlying responsiveness of non-small-cell lung cancer to gefitinib. *N Engl J Med* 2004;350(21):2129–2139.
253. Jain RK. Normalization of tumor vasculature: an emerging concept in antiangiogenic therapy. *Science* 2005;307(5706):58–62.
254. Willett CG, et al. Direct evidence that the VEGF-specific antibody bevacizumab has antivascular effects in human rectal cancer. *Nat Med* 2004;10(2):145–147.
255. Garcia-Barros M, et al. Tumor response to radiotherapy regulated by endothelial cell apoptosis. *Science* 2003;300(5622):1155–1159.
256. Kim DW, et al. Molecular strategies targeting the host component of cancer to enhance tumor response to radiation therapy. *Int J Radiat Oncol Biol Phys* 2006;64(1):38–46.
267. Spigel DR, et al. Tracheoesophageal fistula formation in patients with lung cancer treated with chemoradiation and bevacizumab. *J Clin Oncol* 2010;28(1):43–48.
274. Lebrin F, et al. Thalidomide stimulates vessel maturation and reduces epistaxis in individuals with hereditary hemorrhagic telangiectasia. *Nat Med* 2010;16(4):420–428.
305. Soda M, et al. Identification of the transforming EML4-ALK fusion gene in non-small-cell lung cancer. *Nature* 2007;448(7153):561–566.
307. Kwak EL, et al. Anaplastic lymphoma kinase inhibition in non-small-cell lung cancer. *N Engl J Med* 2010;363(18):1693–1703.
335. Bernhard EJ, et al. Direct evidence for the contribution of activated N-ras and K-ras oncogenes to increased intrinsic radiation resistance in human tumor cell lines. *Cancer Res* 2000;60(23):6597–6600.
342. McKenna WG, et al. The role of the H-ras oncogene in radiation resistance and metastasis. *Int J Radiat Oncol Biol Phys* 1990;18(4):849–859.
359. Chalmers A, et al. PARP-1, PARP-2, and the cellular response to low doses of ionizing radiation. *Int J Radiat Oncol Biol Phys* 2004;58(2):410–419.
360. Bryant HE, et al. Specific killing of BRCA2-deficient tumours with inhibitors of poly(ADP-ribose) polymerase. *Nature* 2005;434(7035):913–917.
361. Farmer H, et al. Targeting the DNA repair defect in BRCA mutant cells as a therapeutic strategy. *Nature* 2005;434(7035):917–921.
367. Paik S, et al. A multigene assay to predict recurrence of tamoxifen-treated, node-negative breast cancer. *N Engl J Med* 2004;351(27):2817–2826.
369. Coppin CM, et al. Improved local control of invasive bladder cancer by concurrent cisplatin and preoperative or definitive radiation. The National Cancer Institute of Canada Clinical Trials Group. *J Clin Oncol* 1996;14(11):2901–2907.
371. Samuels ML, et al. Large-dose bleomycin therapy and pulmonary toxicity. A possible role of prior radiotherapy. *JAMA* 1976;235(11):1117–1120.
374. Billingham ME, et al. Adriamycin cardiotoxicity: endomyocardial biopsy evidence of enhancement by irradiation. *Am J Surg Pathol* 1977;1(1):17–23.
378. Allen JC, et al. Leukoencephalopathy following high-dose intravenous methotrexate chemotherapy: quantitative assessment of white matter attenuation using computed tomography. *Neuroradiology* 1978;16:44–47.
379. Keime-Guibert F, Napolitano M, Delattre JY. Neurological complications of radiotherapy and chemotherapy. *J Neurol* 1998;245(11):695–708.

SECTION III CLINICAL RADIATION ONCOLOGY

Part A Skin

Chapter 33
Skin

William M. Mendenhall, Anthony A. Mancuso, Jessica M. Kirwan, John W. Werning, and Franklin P. Flowers

The purpose of this chapter is to discuss cutaneous carcinoma and melanoma. Uncommon cutaneous malignancies, such as angiosarcoma and dermatofibrosarcoma protuberans, will be addressed elsewhere. Most skin cancers are managed surgically. Because of the functional cosmetic deficits that may occur after surgery for skin cancers of the head and neck, the discussion will occasionally focus on lesions in this area.

Skin cancer is the most common of all malignancies. The American Cancer Society estimates that approximately two million basal cell carcinomas (BCCs) and squamous cell carcinomas (SCCs) are diagnosed annually in the United States, although the precise number is unknown because they are not reported.[1] The risk for carcinoma of the skin increases with sun exposure. A low incidence occurs in dark-skinned people; a corresponding increase occurs in those with a fair, ruddy, Scotch-Irish complexion. The mortality rate is about 1,800 per year, or 0.45%.

Several conditions are associated with carcinoma of the skin, including the following:

- Actinic exposure
- Ionizing radiation
- Scar (e.g., burn scar)
- Chronic draining of sinus or fistulous tract (e.g., pilonidal sinus)
- Immune disorders
  - Chronic lymphocytic leukemia
  - Solid organ transplant patients
  - Discoid lupus erythematosus
- Chemicals
  - Arsenicals (herbicides, pesticides)
  - Psoralens and ultraviolet light (PUVA) treatment for psoriasis[54]
  - Nitrates
  - Tars, oils, and paraffins
- Hereditary disorders
  - Xeroderma pigmentosum
  - Basal cell nevus syndrome
  - Albinism
  - Congenital epidermolysis bullosa

Melanoma is less common than BCCs and SCCs. Jemal et al.[2] estimated that approximately 68,130 melanomas will be diagnosed in the United States in 2010 and that about 8,700 deaths owing to the disease will occur.

ANATOMY

The epidermis is thinner in the face than in most portions of the body, measuring approximately 0.04 mm. No consistent change in the thickness of the epidermis occurs with increasing age, and no difference in skin thickness exists between men and women.

The dermis, which contains the blood and lymphatic vessels, adnexa, hair follicles, sweat glands, and sebaceous glands, is 1 to 2 mm thick; the dermis of the eyelid is thinner, ≤0.6 mm. Beneath the dermis lies the subcutaneous tissue containing the fat and the superficial fascia. No distinct transition occurs from the dermis to the subcutaneous layer.

Lymphatics

No lymphatics exist in the epidermis. A superficial capillary lymphatic plexus lies in the dermis and is without valves.[3] The deep lymphatic trunks in the dermis and subcutaneous tissues have valves. The density of the capillary lymphatics has been noted to be about the same in all areas, except the sole of the foot and palm of the hand, where it is denser. Observation suggests that SCCs and melanomas occurring on the skin of the temple are particularly prone to develop lymphatic metastasis.[4] During the healing of wounds, such as incisions or burns, a regeneration of lymphatic capillaries across the scar occurs, similar to the regrowth of small blood vessels.[3]

The first-echelon lymph nodes for carcinomas of the face and scalp are the superficial network of lymph nodes that form a ring around the top of the neck: submental (level IA), submandibular (level IB), parotid area, postauricular (mastoid), and occipital lymph nodes as well as inconstant facial lymph nodes.

PATHOLOGY

The most common carcinomas of the skin are BCC (65%), SCC (30%), or one of their variants and the adnexal carcinomas. Merkel cell carcinoma (MCC) is a rare neuroendocrine malignancy arising in the skin that was first described by Toker[5] in 1972. Verrucous carcinoma, a variant of SCC, occurs most often on the foot and is rare in the head and neck area. Carcinoma in situ (CIS) occurs frequently in the head and neck. Perineural invasion (PNI) is observed in 2% to 3% of patients with BCCs and SCCs.[6]

Noncutaneous carcinomas (e.g., renal cell carcinoma) may metastasize to the skin and subcutaneous tissues.

Basal Cell Carcinoma

The common BCC, which arises from the basal layer of the epithelium, may have a variety of growth patterns merge into one another in the same tumor, and the different names applied to the gross and microscopic appearances have clinical implications. The morphea type (sclerosing BCC) shows little surface disease and a marked infiltrating pattern; it is an important subtype because of the higher risk for recurrence. Microcystic BCC is a histologic variant of BCC that exhibits the same natural history as the more common variety. Some lesions will have mixed BCC and SCC (basosquamous cell carcinoma or metatypical BCC).

Melanin pigment may be seen on both gross and microscopic examination of BCC.

Squamous Cell Carcinoma

SCC and its variants (i.e., verrucous carcinoma, spindle cell SCC) are similar histologically to SCC occurring in other sites. Most are well differentiated. Evans and Smith[7] identified two categories of spindle cell tumors of skin: one was composed of SCC mixed with a spindle cell component; the other was predominantly spindle cells. The spindle cell component is similar in both groups; mitoses, giant cells, and epithelioid cells may be seen.

Keratoacanthoma

Keratoacanthoma is a benign tumor of the skin that grossly resembles a cystic BCC and microscopically resembles SCC or squamous papilloma. Part of the difficulty in histologic diagnosis is owing to an inadequate biopsy specimen. Ackerman[8] concluded that "the diagnosis of keratoacanthoma can only be made with absolute certainty by biologic behavior in the form of eventual involution."

Adnexal Carcinoma

Carcinomas may arise from the epithelium of the sweat glands, sebaceous glands, or hair follicles and microscopically resemble the tissue of origin. Carcinoma of the sweat gland can arise from either the eccrine or apocrine glands; however, no reliable histologic criteria exist to differentiate the origin. It is difficult to distinguish between benign tumors and malignant carcinomas of the sweat gland in the absence of metastases. The differential diagnosis includes adenocarcinoma metastatic to skin and BCCs and SCCs with an adenoid cystic growth pattern. They are frequently misdiagnosed at the time of the first biopsy. Malignant trichilemmoma arising from hair follicles is extremely rare.

Microcystic adnexal carcinoma (sclerosing sweat duct carcinoma) is a rare variant of adnexal carcinoma first described in 1982. The lesion usually presents on the upper lip or skin of the periorbital area as an indurated plaque without direct invasion of the overlying epidermis. It tends to be slow growing and locally invasive.[9–11] Microcystic adnexal carcinoma exhibits a propensity for local recurrence after excision and is associated with PNI; lymph node metastases are rare. The role of radiation therapy (RT) in the treatment of this rare malignancy is undefined.

Merkel Cell Carcinoma

MCC is a small cell neuroendocrine carcinoma arising in the skin. As in neuroendocrine carcinomas arising in other primary sites, MCC produces a neuron-specific enolase and has been found to contain membrane-bound neurosecretory granules within the tumor cell. In the past, the correct diagnosis often was not obtained until an extensive recurrence was noted. MCC was often misdiagnosed as BCC, lymphoma, adnexal carcinoma, or carcinoma metastatic to the skin from another primary site (i.e., small cell carcinoma of the lung or medullary carcinoma of the thyroid).[12]

Melanoma

Melanoma arises from melanocytes, which are present in the epidermis as well as in other parts of the body including the eye and respiratory, gastrointestinal, and genitourinary tracts.

PATTERNS OF SPREAD

The patterns of spread for individual anatomic sites are outlined in the Selection of Treatment Modality section. Some lesions remain confined to the epidermis (CIS) and may involve a large area of skin. Large in situ lesions occur more often on the trunk; however, small areas of CIS are common on the head and neck.

Basal Cell and Squamous Cell Carcinomas

Both BCC and SCC usually are well differentiated, and most have an indolent growth with distinct margins; a small proportion are poorly differentiated and grow rapidly. BCC occurs more frequently around the central portion of the face, whereas SCC occurs more often on the ears, preauricular and temporal area, scalp, and skin of the neck.

Most lesions remain superficial and invade the adjacent epidermis in a circumferential growth pattern. Invasion of the dermis usually is confined to the superficial (papillary) dermis. Eventually, penetration of the reticular dermis, subcutaneous tissues, and other underlying structures occurs. A few skin carcinomas tend to grow beneath the skin, and the surface lesion gives little indication of their extensive growth; this is more often seen in recurrent tumors. Most early BCCs and SCCs show an orderly invasion of the superficial dermis, which allows successful local therapy. Both BCCs and SCCs invade cartilage and bone, develop PNI spread, and eventually enter the lymphatics, although the latter is not common. BCC, in particular, has a low incidence of lymphatic involvement unless it is recurrent, whereas the incidence of lymph node spread for SCC is estimated to be 10% to 15%.

SCCs may develop distant metastases, whereas BCCs rarely produce metastases.

Metatypical BCC is intermediate between BCC and SCC as far as recurrence rates and the risk of metastases.[13]

Spindle cell tumors of the skin have a gross appearance and growth pattern similar to SCCs.

Carcinoma of the Sweat Gland

Carcinoma of the sweat gland occurs with equal frequency in males and females. It predominantly affects elderly people, although it may occur even in early adulthood. The lesion is generally a subcutaneous nodular mass, which may be solitary or multiple, and the larger lesions may be ulcerated. Carcinoma of the sweat gland most often occurs on the eyelid, face, and scalp. The growth rate varies from indolent to rapid. The tumor may be present for several years with little change and then suddenly begin to enlarge. PNI is frequent. Regional and distant metastases may develop. Scalp lesions are the ones most likely to develop metastases to regional lymph nodes.

Recurrence after excision is frequent, and often multiple recurrences are reported.[14,15] Little information exists on the response to RT.[15] In our limited experience, carcinoma of the sweat gland is sufficiently radioresponsive to justify RT, particularly in association with excision.

The mucin-producing sweat gland adenocarcinoma is a rare tumor. The eyelid is the primary site in about one-half of cases and the face and scalp in another one-fourth of cases. The tumor presents most often in middle-aged men. Wright and Font[16] reported 21 cases that originated on the eyelid. Eight patients (38%) developed one or more local recurrences, one patient died with extensive persistent disease in the face after a 15-year interval, and only one patient had metastasis to the submandibular lymph nodes successfully treated by radical neck dissection.[16] Regional or distant metastasis is a relatively infrequent event for lesions arising in the head and neck area.

Sebaceous Gland Carcinoma

Sebaceous gland carcinoma is rare. It occurs most often on the eyelids, predominantly on the upper lid in elderly women, although the lower lid and caruncle are also sites of origin; it may occur on other parts of the head and neck skin as well. It is often indolent in its growth; however, it may be locally aggressive and develop regional and distant metastases. Local recurrence is common after excision because the lesions often have significant deep and lateral spread beyond the obvious lesion. Metastasis to regional lymph nodes is reported in about 20% of cases, and a small percentage of patients develop distant metastases.[17] Inadequate treatment often occurs because of incorrect histologic diagnosis.

Keratoacanthoma

Keratoacanthoma benign lesions start as a firm, round skin nodule and grow to 1 to 2 cm in a short time, usually a few weeks. As the lesion matures, the center becomes separate and can be removed, revealing a small crater. The lesion occurs most often in the exposed area of the head and neck. Keratoacanthoma is an unlikely diagnosis for a lesion of the lip vermillion. Typically, keratoacanthoma is twice as common in men as women. It occurs most often in patients older than 40 years of age, although it may be seen as early as the second decade of life.

Basal Cell Nevus Syndrome

The basal cell nevus syndrome is an autosomal-dominant disorder with a high level of penetrance but a variable clinical picture. The clinical syndrome may be composed of any or all of the following:

- Multiple BCCs (differing only in their tendency to develop at an early age and on unexposed skin areas)
- Jaw cysts (common)
- Palmar or plantar pits
- Skeletal abnormalities (short fingers, hypertelorism)
- Ectopic calcification
- Eye muscle palsies
- Hamartomas
- Epidermal cysts

The age at onset is frequently in the second or third decade of life, and a family history is often positive for the disorder.[18]

Merkel Cell Carcinoma

MCC occurs primarily in white men between 60 and 80 years of age.[19] The lesion often presents as a painless, raised skin nodule or mass that is red, pink, or blue and may have diffuse margins, and is covered with an intact epidermis. Most lesions are ≤2 cm in size at diagnosis.[19] Human polyomavirus is thought to be etiologic in a significant proportion of patients; human polyomavirus DNA in the MCC cells may be associated with an improved prognosis.[19]

MCC displays an aggressive growth pattern. Mojica et al.[20] reported on 1,665 patients from the National Cancer Institute's Surveillance Epidemiology and End Results (SEER) database and observed the following extent of disease at diagnosis: localized, 55%; positive regional nodes, 31%; distant metastases, 6%; and no data, 8%.

Melanoma

Melanoma is more aggressive and prone to metastasize to regional lymph nodes and exhibit hematogenous dissemination compared with BCC and SCC. The likelihood of regional and/or distant metastases is related to the depth of invasion of the primary tumor. The incidence of positive sentinel lymph node biopsies (SLNBs) versus depth of penetration is depicted in Table 33.1.

Lymphatics

The overall risk of lymphatic metastases is estimated to be 10% to 15% for cutaneous SCC of the skin. The risk increases with the size of the lesion, depth of the penetration, histologic grade, and recurrence.

The risk of lymph node metastases from previously untreated BCCs is <1% and is not related to size, depth of penetration, or histologic subtype; the risk increases for recurrent BCCs, especially those with multiple recurrences over several years. Lymph node metastases, however, are seen on rare occasions without a history of recurrence, and an interval of several years may occur between the treatment of the primary lesion and the appearance of involvement in lymph nodes. When they do occur, lymph node metastases often are solitary.

CLINICAL PICTURE

Presenting Symptoms

The common history for BCC or SCC is a slowly enlarging growth on or just beneath the skin surface. Often a history exists of a sore that will not completely heal. Other symptoms such as bleeding or pain are unusual until the lesion becomes large, and even then symptoms are relatively mild and infrequent. Patients with PNI may complain of paresthesia, especially the sensation of worms crawling under skin (formication). PNI is usually observed with midface lesions and most often involves cranial nerves V2 and/or VII.[6] Advanced, neglected lesions with bone and cartilage destruction, orbit invasion, and regional metastases may be seen; these advanced lesions often produce few, if any, symptoms, and patients simply delay consulting a physician.

Melanomas usually present as a pigmented skin lesion associated with a change in color, shape, and/or size. Although most probably arise de novo, some may arise in a previously benign nevus. Occasionally, patients present with regional or distant metastases without an apparent primary tumor.

Physical Examination

The site, size, and mobility of the primary lesion is documented. Depending on location, evidence of PNI is assessed as well as any findings that might suggest involvement of underlying bone on cartilage. The regional lymph nodes must be carefully examined, even though they are not often involved. Because of the infrequent appearance of regional lymphatic metastases, and because cases of skin cancer often are not followed diligently, lymph node metastases frequently are missed. Although lymphatic metastases may appear within a few months of the management of the primary lesion, in some cases many years intervene before the regional lymph nodes become apparent. It is not at all unusual for ≥5 years

TABLE 33.1 PRIMARY DEPTH OF INVASION VERSUS SENTINEL LYMPH NODE BIOPSY POSITIVITY

		Depth of Invasion (Number of Patients)			
Series	*Primary Site*	*≤1 mm*	*1.01–2.00 mm*	*2.01–4.00 mm*	*>4.00 mm*
Rousseau et al., 2003[21] University of Texas MD Anderson Cancer Center	Various	4% (388)	12% (522)	28% (314)	44% (151)
Emery et al., 2007[22] University of Oregon	Various	2% (41)	13% (85)	20% (35)	27% (11)
Paek et al., 2007[23] University of Michigan	Various	–	19% (490)	32% (301)	45% (119)
Kruper et al., 2006[24] University of Pennsylvania	Various	5% (251)	10% (228)	20% (140)	38% (63)
Leong et al., 2006[25] Multicenter study	Head and neck	3% (134)	7% (230)	21% (160)	13% (63)
Berk et al., 2005[26] Stanford University	Various	0% (45)	18% (115)	19% (64)	16% (32)

From Mendenhall WM, Amdur RJ, Grobmyer SR, et al. Adjuvant radiotherapy for cutaneous melanoma. *Cancer* 2008;112(6):1189–1196, with permission.

to intervene between the primary lesion and the appearance of metastases. Patients with chronic lymphocytic leukemia and concomitant skin cancer often have enlarged lymph nodes from both processes and may have elements of SCC and leukemia in the same lymph nodes.

METHODS OF DIAGNOSIS AND STAGING

Biopsy should be performed on the majority of lesions before deciding on treatment. We do not always insist on biopsy for elderly patients who have a typical skin carcinoma and are to be treated by RT.

Small lesions occurring on the free skin areas (i.e., not involving the eyelid, ear, or periorbital areas) usually can undergo biopsy and be treated simultaneously with surgical excision. Larger lesions, or those involving areas where functional or cosmetic deficit might occur from excision, first undergo biopsy with a small excisional biopsy or with a skin punch. Biopsy with a skin punch should include the subcutaneous fat; punch biopsy is contraindicated when differentiating between keratoacanthoma and SCC because of the small sample size.

The following is a partial list of conditions to be considered in the differential diagnosis of BCC and SCC:

- Senile keratosis
- Keratoacanthoma
- Nonpigmented nevi
- Melanoma
- Cutaneous horn
- Psoriasis
- Lymphoma (mycosis fungoides)
- Soft tissue sarcomas (dermatofibrosarcoma protuberans)
- Hemangiosarcoma
- Metastatic carcinoma
- Adnexal carcinoma of skin
- MCC

Staging

The 2010 American Joint Committee on Cancer (AJCC) systems for BCC/SCC and melanoma are depicted in Tables 33.2 and 33.3, respectively. Although there is an AJCC staging system for MCC, we prefer the Yiengpruksawan system for this rare entity because of its simplicity: stage I, localized; stage II, regional lymph node metastases; and stage III, distant metastases.[27]

TABLE 33.2 2010 AJCC STAGING SYSTEM FOR BASAL CELL AND SQUAMOUS CELL CARCINOMAS

Primary Tumor (T)[a]			
TX	Primary tumor cannot be assessed		
T0	No evidence of primary tumor		
Tis	Carcinoma in situ		
T1	Tumor ≤2 cm in greatest dimension with <2 high-risk features		
T2	Tumor >2 cm in greatest dimension or tumor any size with ≥2 high-risk features		
T3	Tumor with invasion of maxilla, mandible, orbit, or temporal bone		
T4	Tumor with invasion of skeleton (axial and appendicular) or perineural invasion of skull base		
Depth/Invasion	>2 mm thickness		
	Clark level ≥IV		
	Perineural invasion		
Anatomic location	Primary site ear		
	Primary site non–hair-bearing lip		
Differentiation	Poorly differentiated or undifferentiated		
Regional Lymph Nodes (N)			
NX	Regional lymph nodes cannot be assessed		
N0	No regional lymph node metastases		
N1	Metastasis in a single ipsilateral lymph node, ≤3 cm in greatest dimension		
N2	Metastasis in a single ipsilateral lymph node, >3 cm but ≤6 cm in greatest dimension; or in multiple ipsilateral lymph nodes, none >6 cm in greatest dimension; or in bilateral or contralateral lymph nodes, none >6 cm in greatest dimension		
N2a	Metastasis in a single ipsilateral lymph node, >3 cm but ≤6 cm in greatest dimension		
N2b	Metastasis in multiple ipsilateral lymph nodes, none >6 cm in greatest dimension		
N2c	Metastasis in bilateral or contralateral lymph nodes, none >6 cm in greatest dimension		
N3	Metastasis in a lymph node, >6 cm in greatest dimension		
Distant Metastasis (M)			
M0	No distant metastases		
M1	Distant metastases		
Stage	***T***	***N***	***M***
Stage 0	Tis	N0	M0
Stage I	T1	N0	M0
Stage II	T2	N0	M0
Stage III	T3	N0	M0
	T1	N1	M0
	T2	N1	M0
	T3	N1	M0
Stage IV	T1	N2	M0
	T2	N2	M0
	T3	N2	M0
	T Any	N3	M0
	T4	N Any	M0
	T Any	N Any	M1

[a]High-risk features for the primary tumor (T) staging.

From American Joint Committee on Cancer. Cutaneous squamous cell carcinomas and other cutaneous carcinomas. In: *Cancer staging handbook*, 7th ed. Chicago, IL: Springer, 2010:359–376, with permission.

Diagnostic Imaging

Computed tomography (CT) and magnetic resonance imaging (MRI) are only necessary in a carefully chosen group of patients being treated for skin cancer. CT is the primary modality for showing bone invasion and nodal metastases. High-resolution MRI is better than CT for demonstrating PNI.[28] Positron emission tomography (PET) is useful to detect regional and distant metastases in patients with MCC and melanoma.

SELECTION OF TREATMENT MODALITY

Basal Cell and Squamous Cell Carcinomas

The likelihood of cure is similar after surgery or RT for early-stage BCCs and SCCs.[29] Therefore, selection of one modality over another is based on other parameters such as function, cosmesis, age of the patient, convenience, cost, availability of appropriate RT equipment, and the wishes of the patient. Patients with advanced cancers are often best treated with surgery and adjuvant RT if the cancer is resectable and the functional and cosmetic outcomes are acceptable.

Radiotherapy Alone

Small skin cancers located on "free skin," such as the cheek or forehead, may be easily excised with a good cosmetic result and minimal inconvenience; therefore, surgery is usually the treatment of choice for such lesions. It is also desirable to avoid RT in young patients because the late effects of irradiation progress gradually with time and, with very long-term follow-up, may be associated with a suboptimal cosmetic result compared with resection and reconstruction. In contrast, resection of an early-stage skin cancer of the eyelid, external ear, or nose may result in a significant cosmetic deformity and necessitate complex reconstruction that compares unfavorably with RT. This is particularly relevant in the case of older patients who have a limited life expectancy and who are at higher risk for a perioperative complication.

TABLE 33.3 2010 AJCC STAGING SYSTEM FOR MELANOMA

Definitions of TNM

Primary Tumor (T)

TX	Primary tumor cannot be assessed (e.g., curettage or severely regressed melanoma)
T0	No evidence of primary tumor
Tis	Melanoma in situ
T1	Melanomas ≤1.0 mm in thickness
T2	Melanomas 1.01–2.0 mm
T3	Melanomas 2.01–4.0 mm
T4	Melanomas >4.0 mm

Note: The "a" and "b" subcategories of T are assigned based on ulceration and number of mitoses per mm^2 as shown below:

T Classification	*Thickness (mm)*	*Ulceration Status/Mitoses*
T1	≤1.0	a: without ulceration and mitosis <1/mm^2
		b: with ulceration or mitoses ≥1/mm^2
T2	1.01–2.0	a: without ulceration
		b: with ulceration
T3	2.01–4.0	a: without ulceration
		b: with ulceration
T4	>4.0	a: without ulceration
		b: with ulceration

Regional Lymph Nodes (N)

NX	Patients in whom the regional nodes cannot be assessed (e.g., previously removed for another reason)
N0	No regional metastases detected
N1–3	Regional metastases based on the number of metastatic nodes and presence or absence of intralymphatic metastases (in-transit or satellite metastases)

Note: N1–3 and a–c subcategories assigned as show below:

N Classification	*Number of Metastatic Nodes*	*Nodal Metastatic Mass*
N1	1 node	a: micrometastasis[a]
		b: macrometastasis[b]
N2	2–3 nodes	a: micrometastasis[a]
		b: macrometastasis[b]
		c: in-transit metastasis(es)/satellite(s) without metastatic nodes
N3	≥4 metastatic nodes, or matted nodes, or in-transit metastasis(es)/satellite(s) with metastatic nodes	

Distant Metastasis (M)

M0	No detectable evidence of distant metastases
M1a	Metastases to skin, subcutaneous, or distant lymph nodes
M1b	Metastases to lung
M1c	Metastases to all other visceral sites or distant metastases to any site combined with an elevated serum LDH

Note: Serum LDH is incorporated into the M category as shown below:

M Classification	*Site*	*Serum LDH*
M1a	Distant skin, subcutaneous, or nodal metastases	Normal
M1b	Lung metastases	Normal
M1c	All other visceral metastases	Normal
	Any distant metastasis	Elevated

Anatomic Stage/Prognostic Groups

Clinical Staging[c]				*Pathologic Staging*[d]			
Stage 0	Tis	N0	M0	0	Tis	N0	M0
Stage IA	T1a	N0	M0	IA	T1a	N0	M0
Stage IB	T1b	N0	M0	IB	T1b	N0	M0
	T2a	N0	M0		T2a	N0	M0
Stage IIA	T2b	N0	M0	IIA	T2b	N0	M0
	T3a	N0	M0		T3b	N0	M0
Stage IIB	T3b	N0	M0	IIB	T3b	N0	M0
	T4a	N0	M0		T4a	N0	M0
Stage IIC	T4b	N0	M0	IIC	T4b	N0	M0
Stage III	Any T	≥N1	M0	IIIA	T1–4a	N1a	M0
				IIIB	T1–4a	N2a	M0
				IIIC	T1–4b	N1a	M0
					T1–4b	N2a	M0
					T1–4a	N1b	M0
					T1–4a	N2b	M0
					T1–4a	N2c	M0
					T1–4b	N1b	M0
					T1–4b	N2b	M0
					T1–4b	N2c	M0
					Any T	N3	M0
Stage IV	Any T	Any N	M1	IV	Any T	Any N	M1

[a]Micrometastases are diagnosed after sentinel lymph node biopsy and completion of lymphadenectomy (if performed).

[b]Macrometastases are defined as clinically detectable nodal metastases confirmed by therapeutic lymphadenectomy or when nodal metastasis exhibits gross extracapsular extension.

[c]Clinical staging includes microstaging of the primary melanoma and clinical/radiologic evaluation for metastases. By convention, it should be used after complete excision of the primary melanoma with clinical assessment for regional and distant metastases.

[d]Pathologic staging includes microstaging of the primary melanoma and pathologic information about the regional lymph nodes after partial or complete lymphadenectomy. Pathologic Stage 0 or Stage IA patients are the exception; they do not require pathologic evaluation of their lymph nodes.

AJCC, American Joint Committee on Cancer; LDH, lactate dehydrogenase.

From American Joint Committee on Cancer. Melanoma of the skin. In: *Cancer staging handbook*, 7th ed. Chicago, IL: Springer, 2010:387–415, with permission.

Patients with locally advanced skin cancers present a difficult problem because, although the likelihood of cure may be better with combined RT and surgery in some situations, the cosmetic result is sometimes unacceptable. Patients receive postoperative RT if surgery is indicated and feasible. If surgery is not feasible, the patient is managed with RT alone. Although it might seem that the risk of bone and/or cartilage necrosis would be high after RT for a skin cancer invading these structures, the observed risk of complications is relatively low.[30,31] Exceptions are advanced cancers of the scalp and those overlying the anterior aspect of the tibia where there is little tissue between the skin surface and the bone. Following definitive RT, bone exposure is likely and may progress to an osteoradionecrosis (ORN) requiring surgical intervention.

Patients with lesions associated with clinical PNI with gross tumor extending to sites that render complete resection unlikely or unfeasible, such as the cavernous sinus, are treated with RT alone. Subtotal resection does not enhance the likelihood of cure and only increases the morbidity of treatment.

Adjuvant Radiotherapy

Postoperative RT is added after surgery if pathologic examination of the surgical specimen reveals findings indicative of a high risk for local recurrence, such as close or positive margins and/or invasion of nerve, cartilage, or bone. A significant proportion of patients with positive margins after resection of an early-stage skin cancer may never develop a local recurrence. Postoperative RT may be withheld if the lesion is a BCC, the primary site is located on the free skin, the patient is reliable and will return for close follow-up, and if salvage treatment would have a high likelihood of eradicating recurrent tumor with a good cosmetic result. BCCs of the nose, eyelid, or ear and lesions that would have immediate access to major nerve trunks are usually retreated immediately when resection margins are positive. The risk of recurrence is probably greater than for lesions of the free skin, and the consequences of recurrence may be significant. Observation is particularly attractive for the elderly patient in poor medical condition who may not live to experience a local recurrence. Metatypical BCCs behave more aggressively than BCCs, and those with positive margins after surgery should be re-excised and/or treated with postoperative RT.

Patients with BCC and focal incidental PNI involving a small nerve trunk and widely negative margins may be safely observed. Otherwise, patients with incidental PNI should be considered for postoperative RT, particularly if the lesion is SCC.

The usual policy for patients with positive margins from SCC is immediate retreatment by either re-excision, RT, or both, depending on the situation. There is evidence that this approach leads to a reduced risk of metastasis and reduced likelihood of death from cancer.

Management of Regional Lymph Node Metastases

Carcinoma of the skin metastatic to the parotid lymph nodes is managed as a high-grade parotid neoplasm, usually with superficial or total parotidectomy followed by postoperative RT.[29,32–34] If only one node is involved and there is no extracapsular extension, it may be safe to withhold RT. However, if the tumor recurs in the parotid area after parotidectomy, the likelihood of salvage is remote.[32] Therefore, it has been our practice to use combined treatment in all patients. If the parotid lymph node metastasis is fixed and thought to be incompletely resectable, the patient is treated with high-dose preoperative RT (6,000 to 7,000 cGy) followed by parotidectomy. RT alone is used only in patients who are inoperable because of tumor extent or poor medical condition.

Cervical lymph node metastases are managed just as they would be for other carcinomas of the head and neck. Neck dissection alone is adequate treatment if only one node is involved and there is no extracapsular extension. If two or more nodes contain tumor or if extracapsular extension is noted, neck dissection is followed by postoperative RT.

Merkel Cell Carcinoma

The preferred treatment for MCC is resection of the primary tumor and any clinically positive regional nodes. Our bias is to treat both the primary site and regional lymphatics with postoperative RT. The dose-fractionation schedule is the same as that employed for SCC. The role of adjuvant chemotherapy is ill defined. Patients who should be considered for adjuvant chemotherapy are those with positive nodes and/or satellite lesions. Drugs employed are often those used for small cell carcinomas and include etoposide and cisplatin.

Melanoma

The preferred treatment for melanoma is resection of the primary lesion and any grossly positive regional nodes. Patients with desmoplastic melanoma are usually suitable for surgery alone unless there is extensive PNI associated with a lesion near a named nerve, in which case postoperative RT is considered. Postoperative RT is also employed to treat the primary site when there are in-transit metastases and the margins are equivocal. Patients who have lesions with a depth of invasion exceeding 1 mm and clinically negative nodes should be considered for SLNB. We also perform SLNB for lesions with depth of invasion ≤1 mm if there is also ulceration or invasion into Clark's level IV or V. Adjuvant postoperative RT is often employed for positive regional nodes. Patients who are at high risk for regional lymph node metastases and are unable to undergo SLNB and/or elective node dissection should be considered for elective nodal irradiation of the first-echelon lymphatics. The dose-fractionation schedule is usually the MD Anderson hypofractionation technique consisting of 3,000 cGy in five fractions over 2.5 weeks with a reduction off of the spinal cord and/or central nervous system (CNS) at 2,400 cGy.[35] Alternatively, conventional fractionation may be employed if late effects and suboptimal cosmesis are a concern.[36]

Definitive RT using orthovoltage RT or electrons may be employed for elderly patients with lentigo maligna or lentigo malignant melanoma where excision is not feasible because of cosmesis function and/or medial comorbidities.[37–39] The dose-fractionation schedules are the same as those described for postoperative RT.

TREATMENT TECHNIQUES

Treatment techniques vary for primary lesions and for regional lymph node metastases.

Primary Lesion

RT of the primary lesion is usually accomplished using one of three basic external-beam techniques (orthovoltage RT, electron beam, and high-energy x-rays or photons) or with an interstitial implant either alone or in combination with external-beam techniques. Most early skin cancers are managed with orthovoltage RT with beam energies of 100 to 250 Kvp. The advantages of this technique, compared with electron beam, are that the maximum dose is at the skin surface; bolus is not required; there is less beam constriction both at the surface and at depth so that smaller fields can be used (Fig. 33.1); shielding of the eye is easier and more effectively accomplished, particularly if electron energies ≥10 MeV are used (Table 33.4)[40]; it is less expensive; and the likelihood of tumor control may be higher, possibly as a result of increased radiobiologic effectiveness (RBE) but more likely because of technical problems that are difficult to overcome when using electrons alone. The disadvantages of orthovoltage x-rays, compared with electron beam, are that there is a higher dose to deeper tissues and to underlying bone and cartilage.

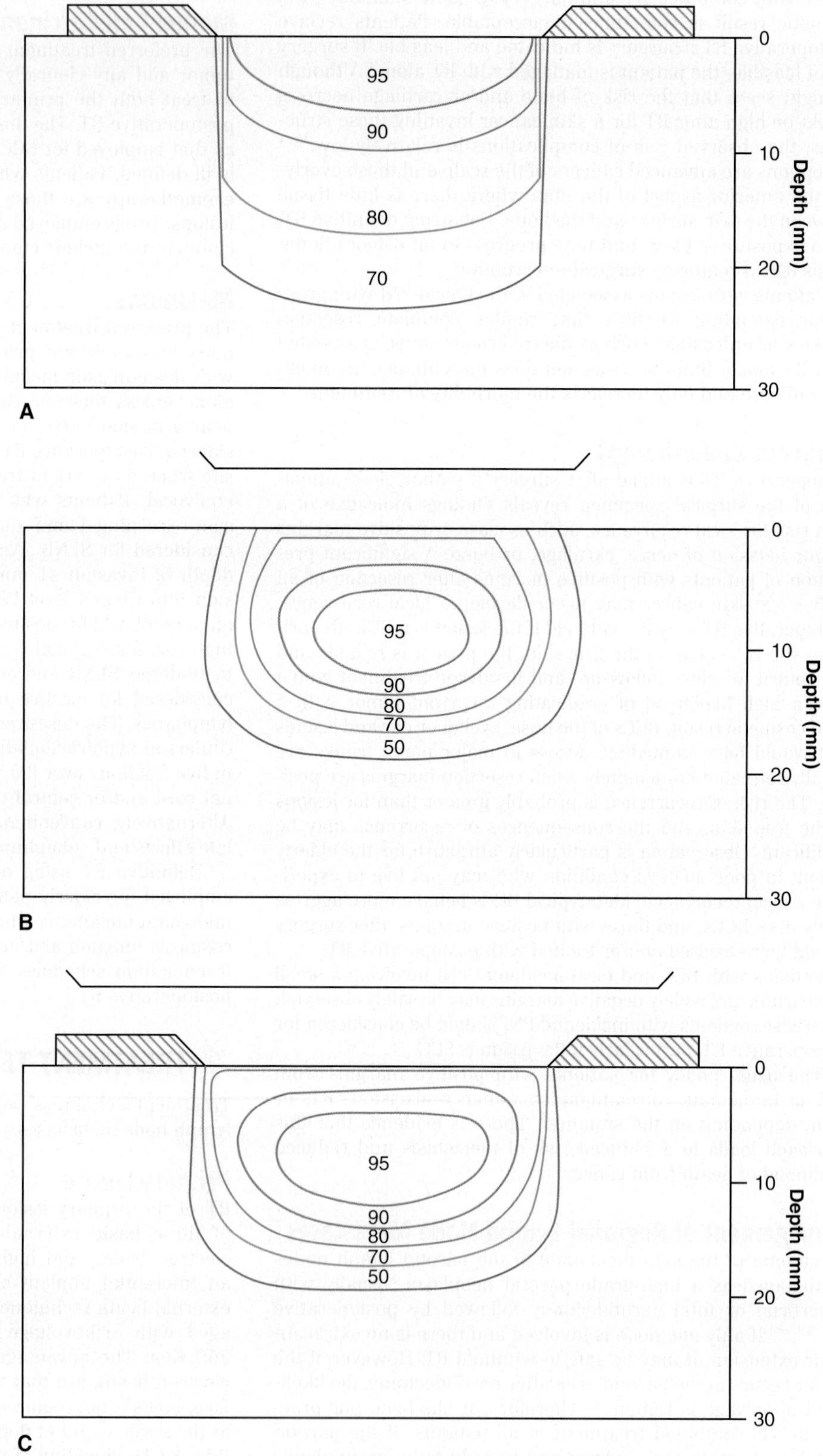

FIGURE 33.1. A: 250-kVp x-rays (HVL 1.4 mm Cu) with secondary collimation on the phantom surface. Source-to-surface distance (SSD) = 50 cm; isodose %: 95, 90, 80, 70. **B:** 6-MeV electron beam with secondary collimation 5 cm above the phantom surface (at the level of the electron cone). Source of collimator distance (SCD) = 95 cm; SSD = 100 cm; isodose %: 95, 90, 80, 70, 50. **C:** 6-MeV electron beam with tertiary collimation on the phantom surface. SSD = 100 cm; SCD = 100 cm; isodose %: 95, 90, 80, 70, 50.

The latter problem can be largely eliminated by using heavily filtered orthovoltage beams for tumors involving or overlying cartilage or bone. Another significant problem associated with orthovoltage RT is that most radiation oncology departments do not have an orthovoltage machine, and thus it is unavailable. Electron beam is usually used for lesions of the scalp to reduce the dose to the underlying brain; orthovoltage x-rays are used to treat most other skin cancers. Orthovoltage RT is particularly useful for lesions of the head and neck.

Before treatment with either electron-beam or orthovoltage x-rays, a customized lead mask is constructed to collimate the beam directly on the skin surface. A 1.0- to 1.5-cm margin is

TABLE 33.4 OCULAR PROTECTION: DOSE BENEATH THE EYE SHIELD

Structure (Depth)	250 kVp X-ray (HVL 1.4 mm Cu)	Electron-Beam Energy (MeV)						
		6	8	10	12	14	17	20
Cornea (1 mm)	10%	18%	37%	64%	75%	93%	98%	102%
Lens (8 mm)	9%	9%	19%	36%	46%	61%	70%	87%
Retina (23 mm)	10%	19%	22%	22%	21%	23%	25%	29%

HVL, half-value layer.

Dose is expressed as a percentage of the dose to D_{max} (depth of maximum dose deposition).

From Amdur RJ, Kalbaugh KJ, Ewald LM, et al. Radiation therapy for skin cancer near the eye: kilovoltage x-rays versus electrons. *Int J Radiat Oncol Biol Phys* 1992;23: 769–779, with permission from Elsevier.

TABLE 33.5 GUIDELINES FOR SELECTION OF EXTERNAL-BEAM DOSE

Orthovoltage Dose (cGy)[a]	Examples
6,500 over 7 wk	Large untreated lesion with bone/cartilage invasion or large recurrent tumor.[b]
6,000 over 7 wk	Large untreated lesion with minimal or suspected bone/cartilage invasion.[b]
5,500 over 6 wk	Moderate to large inner canthus, eyelid, nasal, or pinna lesions (20–30 cm^2 area).
5,000 over 4 wk	Small, thin lesion (<1.5 cm) around eye, nose, or ear (10 cm^2 area).
4,500 over 3 wk	Moderate-sized lesion on free[c] skin or postoperative treatment of moderate-sized cancer on free skin with positive margins.
4,000 over 2 wk or 3,000 over 1 wk	Small lesions (1 cm) on free skin.
The following schemes are used when the late cosmetic result is not important and travel for the patient is difficult:	
4,000 in 10 fractions or 3,000 in 5 fractions or 2,000 in 1 fraction	Rapid fractionation schemes produce a high cure rate for small lesions, although the cosmetic result may be less than optimal after 5 years.

[a]Add 10% to dose for supervoltage therapy.

[b]All or a portion of the therapy given with supervoltage photons and/or electrons.

[c]"Free" refers to not involving the ear, nose, eye, or eyelid.

From Mendenhall WM, Million RR, Mancuso AA, et al. Carcinoma of the skin. In: Million RR, Cassisi NJ, eds. *Management of head and neck cancer: a multidisciplinary approach*, 2nd ed. Philadelphia, PA: JB Lippincott, 1994:643–691.

adequate for a well-defined T1 lesion treated with orthovoltage RT. An additional 1 cm is added to the margin when the electron beam is used to account for beam constriction. For larger and/or ill-defined tumors, a 2-cm margin is usually necessary. If the tumor is located near the eye, a gold-plated lead eye shield is placed directly on the anesthetized cornea to minimize the irradiation dose to underlying structures (Fig. 33.2). The dose beneath the eye shield is depicted for orthovoltage x-rays and electron beams of various energies in Table 33.4. Isodose distributions for the two techniques are shown in Figure 33.1; note that the dose distribution is better for orthovoltage RT than for electron beam, particularly if a lead mask is not used with the electron beam.

Advanced skin cancers that are deeply invasive are often treated with high-energy photons to adequately cover the deep extent of the tumor. Bolus is used to ensure an adequate surface dose. Field arrangement varies with primary site. For example, a wedge-pair technique may be used for lesions involving the external ear, whereas a three-field technique (similar to that used for paranasal sinus cancer) is frequently used for skin cancers with extension proximally along the second division of the fifth cranial nerve. The target volume includes the entire course of the involved nerve, which would include the gasserian ganglion in this case, to the brain stem. Intensity-modulated radiotherapy (IMRT) may be used in some patients to produce a more conformal dose distribution to reduce the dose to surrounding normal structures. Proton-beam radiotherapy may also be used to produce a very conformal dose distribution with steep dose gradients to limit the dose to the visual apparatus and the CNS.[41,42]

The extent of RT fields for patients with PNI varies with histology and the extent of PNI. Patients with BCC or SCC and focal incidental PNI are treated with a wide local field. Those with extensive incidental PNI are treated with fields that include the at-risk nerves to the skull base, particularly if margins are positive or equivocal. The at-risk nerves receive 50 to 70 Gy depending on the extent of PNI and margin status. Patients with clinical PNI receive definitive RT to fields that include the primary site and involved nerves to the skull base.

The regional lymph nodes are electively irradiated if the suspected risk of subclinical disease exceeds 10% to 15%.[43] Patients with SCC and PNI should be considered for elective nodal RT, particularly if the lesion is located on the head or neck.

Dose-fractionation schedules used for irradiation of skin cancers are outlined in Table 33.5. We have recently used twice-daily RT with megavoltage photons or protons at 1.2 Gy per fraction to doses of 74.4 Gy in a continuous course with a minimum 6-hour interfraction interval for advanced lesions near radiosensitive structures. The suggested maximum doses for short-course orthovoltage RT are listed in Table 33.6.

Parotid-Area Lymph Node Metastases

The parotid gland and upper neck are treated with an en face mixed beam of 6-MV x-rays and high-energy electrons (usually

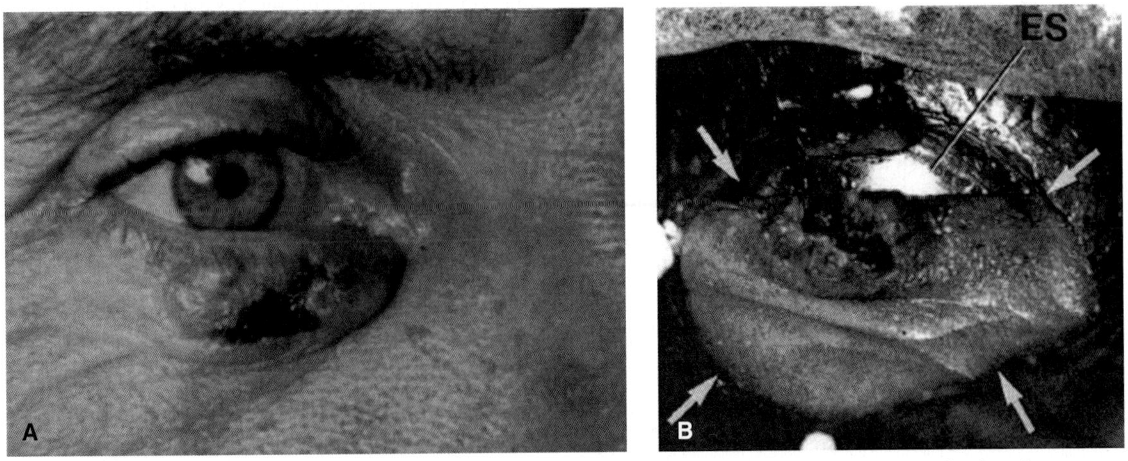

FIGURE 33.2. **A:** 1-cm × 1-cm basal cell carcinoma of the midportion of the lower lid. **B:** Treatment setup that was used to irradiate the patient. *Arrows* indicate the field edge. ES, eye shield.

TABLE 33.6 SUGGESTED MAXIMUM SKIN DOSES[a] FOR PALLIATION WITH 250 KVP X-RAYS (BELOW MOIST DESQUAMATION LEVEL FOR THE AVERAGE PATIENT)

	Total Dose (cGy)						
Field Size (Area in cm²)	1 Day (1 Exposure)	2 Days (2 Exposures)	4 Days (4 Exposures)	5 Days (5 Exposures)	2 Weeks (10 Exposures)	3 Weeks (15 Exposures)	5 Weeks (25 Exposures)
Small fields							
10	2,000	2,750	3,500	3,750	5,000	5,500	6,000
50	1,750	2,500	3,250	3,500	4,500	5,000	5,500
Medium fields							
100	1,500	2,000	2,500	2,750	3,750	4,250	5,000
150	1,250	1,750	2,250	2,500	3,250	3,750	4,500
Large fields							
200	1,000	1,500	2,000	2,250	3,000	3,500	4,250
300	Not recommended	Not recommended	Not recommended	2,000	2,750	3,250	4,000

[a]The total doses listed are administered over a treatment course of the indicated length, divided into the indicated number of fractional treatments.

From Mendenhall WM, Million RR, Mancuso AA, et al. Carcinoma of the skin. In: Million RR, Cassisi NJ, eds. *Management of head and neck cancer: a multidisciplinary approach*, 2nd ed. Philadelphia, PA: JB Lippincott, 1994:643–691.

20 MeV), weighted 1.0:0.67 in favor of the electron beam. The electron-beam field is 1 cm larger than the x-ray field to account for the beam constriction of the electrons, except where the field abuts the low-neck field (Fig. 33.3). This field arrangement is treated to 4,600 cGy in 23 fractions, specified at a depth of 4 to 5 cm from the skin surface. An anterior field is matched to the lateral mixed-beam field to treat the ipsilateral low neck and is irradiated to 5,000 cGy in 25 fractions, specified at D_{max}.

At 4,600 cGy tumor dose, the primary field is reduced off of the spinal cord, and the dose to the tumor bed is boosted with an anteriorly angled 20-MeV electron-beam field or an appositional mixed-beam field with an abutting posterior electron strip. The final dose for patients treated at 200 cGy per fraction with negative margins is 6,000 cGy; with positive margins, 6,600 cGy; and with gross residual disease, 7,000 cGy. If the dose per fraction is reduced to 180 cGy, the total dose is increased by 500 cGy. An alternative to the mixed electron–photon beam is a wedge-pair technique using 4 to 6 MV photon beams. IMRT may also be considered to reduce the dose to the temporal lobe and cerebellum, particularly if the margins are positive and/or tumor involves the deep lobe of the parotid.

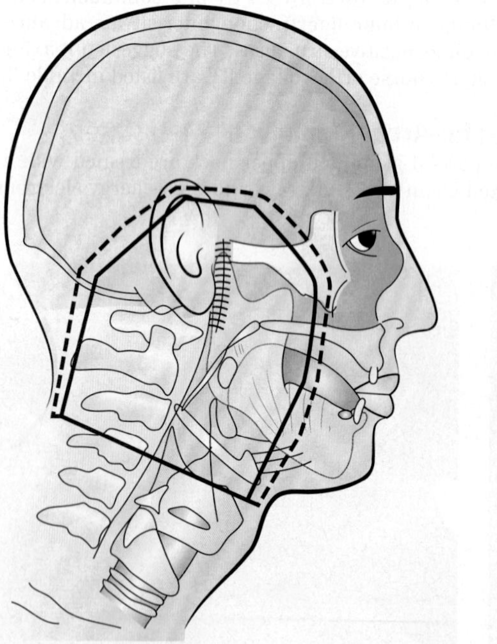

FIGURE 33.3. Typical en face mixed-beam field used in the treatment of parotid node metastases to encompass the entire parotid bed and surgical scar. Patients are treated supine with a face mask made of low-temperature thermal plastic (polycaprolactone) for immobilization and a lead lollipop to decrease the dose to the contralateral salivary gland. A bolus of petrolatum-coated gauze is applied to all scars.

Axillary Metastases

Axillary lymph node metastases are irradiated with opposed anterior and posterior portals that include the supraclavicular fossa. The dose-fractionation schedule is 4,500 cGy in 25 fractions with a reduction and boost depending on margin status.

Ilioinguinal Lymph Node Metastases

Ilioinguinal lymph nodes are usually irradiated with IMRT to reduce the volume of tissue irradiated, particularly small bowel. The femoral and external iliac vessels are contoured on the treatment planning CT and a 1.5- to 2-cm margin is added to obtain the clinical target volume (CTV).

FOLLOW-UP AND MANAGEMENT OF RECURRENCE

After RT, patients are evaluated every 2 to 3 months for the first and second years, every 4 months for the third year, every 6 months for the fourth and fifth years, and annually thereafter. Chest roentgenograms are obtained annually, and a follow-up CT, MRI, and/or PET is obtained as needed for patients irradiated for advanced lesions.

Treatment of local-regional recurrences after RT alone or combined with surgery is usually resection. If a local recurrence is amenable to en bloc surgical resection with frozen section control of the margins, this may be preferable for selected cases. Local recurrences after RT may be significantly more extensive than is clinically apparent; thus, wide margins are preferred. Retreatment with RT is rarely indicated because of the high likelihood of complications. The most common scenario for recurrence in the neck nodes is failure in a solitary submandibular location; the success rate of salvage neck dissection is high in this circumstance.

RESULTS

Basal Cell and Squamous Cell Carcinomas

Most series reporting the results of treatment for skin cancer contain a preponderance of early lesions and do not employ a staging system, making it difficult to compare various series and the relative efficacy of different treatment modalities.

Primary Lesion

The likelihood of local control after irradiation for skin carcinomas of various sizes managed at the Mallinckrodt Institute of Radiology is outlined in Table 33.7.[44] The probability of local control is higher for smaller lesions, for BCC compared with SCC, and for previously untreated lesions compared with recurrent cancers. The results of RT using various beam energies are listed in Table 33.8; treatment with orthovoltage irradiation

TABLE 33.7 LOCAL TUMOR CONTROL WITH RADIOTHERAPY ACCORDING TO SIZE, CELL TYPE, AND PRESENTATION (FROM MALLINCKRODT INSTITUTE OF RADIOLOGY–339 PATIENTS)

Size	*Basal Cell, Previously Untreated*	*Basal Cell, Recurrent*	*Squamous Cell, Previously Untreated*	*Squamous Cell, Recurrent*
≤1 cm	64/66 (97%)	22/23 (96%)	11/11 (100%)	10/12 (83%)
1.1–3 cm	71/75 (95%)	27/36 (75%)	19/21 (90%)	7/13 (54%)
3.1–5 cm	11/13 (85%)	7/9 (78%)	7/8 (88%)	6/9 (67%)
>5 cm	12/13 (92%)	1/2 (50%)	3/5 (60%)	6/11 (55%)
Size not specified	4/4 (100%)	1/1 (100%)	0/1 (0%)	4/6 (67%)
Total	**162/171 (95%)**	**58/71 (82%)**	**40/46 (87%)**	**33/51 (65%)**

From Lovett RD, Perez CA, Shapiro DL, et al. External irradiation of epithelial skin cancer. *Int J Radiat Oncol Biol Phys* 1990;19:235–242, with permission from Elsevier.

yields local control rates that are as good as, or better than, local control rates yielded by other treatment modalities.[44]

Schulte et al.[45] reported on 1,113 patients treated with orthovoltage RT for 1,267 skin cancers and followed for a median of 82 months (Table 33.9). Patients were usually treated at 5 Gy per fraction. The incidence of soft tissue necrosis was 6.3%; 83% healed with conservative treatment.[45]

Al-Othman et al.[46] reported on 85 patients with 88 clinical T4 SCCs (37), BCCs (41), and metatypical BCCs (10) treated with definitive RT at the University of Florida (Gainesville, FL) between 1964 and 1997. Forty-three lesions were previously untreated, and 45 cancers were recurrent after prior surgery. The 5-year outcomes were as follows: local control, 53%; ultimate local control, 90%; regional control, 93%; ultimate regional control, 100%; distant metastasis-free survival, 95%; cause-specific survival, 76%; and overall survival, 56%. Thirteen (15%) of 85 patients developed a severe treatment-related complication.

Balamucki et al.[47] reported on 216 patients treated at the University of Florida for skin carcinomas with incidental (107 patients) or clinical (109 patients) PNI; median follow-up for living patients was 6 years (range, 0.6 to 2.3 years). One hundred eighty-five patients (86%) had SCCs, and the remainder had BCCs or metatypical BCCs. Patients with incidental PNI were treated with surgery and postoperative RT (99 patients), preoperative RT and surgery (4 patients), and RT alone (4 patients). Eight patients received adjuvant chemotherapy. Twenty six of 107 patients (24%) presented with clinically positive nodes. The outcomes for patients treated with incidental PNI are depicted in Table 33.10. Seventeen of 107 patients (16%) developed treatment complications. Patients with clinical PNI were treated with surgery and postoperative RT (58 patients), preoperative RT and surgery (2 patients), or RT alone (49 patients). Fifteen of 109 patients (14%) presented with clinically positive nodes. The outcomes for patients treated for clinical PNI are depicted in Table 33.11. Fourteen of 62 patients (23%) who had achieved continuous local control experienced symptomatic improvement in clinical neuropathic symptoms after treatment. Thirty nine of 109 patients (36%) developed treatment complications.

Galloway et al.[48] reported on a subset of these patients and compared their outcomes with radiographic extent of PNI and found that the extent of PNI was inversely related to the likelihood of local control and survival (Table 33.12).

TABLE 33.8 LOCAL CONTROL RATES ACCORDING TO EXTERNAL-BEAM TECHNIQUE (FROM MALLINCKRODT INSTITUTE OF RADIOLOGY–339 PATIENTS)

	Size			
Modality	*≤1 cm (%)*	*1.1–5 cm (%)*	*>5 cm (%)*	*Not Specified (%)*
Basal Cell Carcinoma				
Superficial x-ray	69/71 (97%)	84/90 (93%)	4/4 (100%)	3/3 (100%)
Electron beam	11/12 (92%)	16/22 (73%)	4/5 (80%)	1/1 (100%)
Combination	5/5 (100%)	13/16 (81%)	5/6 (83%)	0/0
Photons (1.2–4 MV)	1/1 (100%)	3/5 (60%)	0/0	1/1 (100%)
Squamous Cell Carcinoma				
Superficial x-ray	12/12 (100%)	10/11 (91%)	1/1 (100%)	0/0
Electron beam	3/4 (75%)	7/10 (70%)	3/4 (75%)	0/1 (0%)
Combination	4/5 (80%)	19/26 (73%)	4/8 (50%)	2/4 (50%)
Photons (1.2–4 MV)	2/2 (100%)	3/4 (75%)	1/3 (33%)	2/2 (100%)

Significance levels: basal cell carcinoma 1.1–5 cm, superficial x-ray (84/90) versus electron beam/combination (29/38), $p = .013$; squamous cell carcinoma ≤1 cm, superficial x-ray (12/12) versus electron beam/combination (7/9), $p = .17$; squamous cell carcinoma 1.1–5 cm, superficial x-ray (10/11) versus electron beam/combination (26/36), $p = .41$.

From Lovett RD, Perez CA, Shapiro DL, et al. External irradiation of epithelial skin cancer. *Int J Radiat Oncol Biol Phys* 1990;19:235–242, with permission from Elsevier.

TABLE 33.9 RAW AND CUMULATIVE RECURRENCE RATES OF BASAL CELL AND SQUAMOUS CELL CARCINOMAS AFTER SOFT X-RAY THERAPY

		Recurrence Rates (%)			
			Cumulative After:		
Tumor	*Number*	*Raw*	*5 Years*	*10 Years*	*15 Years*
BCCs and SCCs, total[a]	1,267	5.1	4.7	6.9	7.4
BCCs, total	1,019	4.5	4.2	6.1	6.1
T1[b]	615	2.4[c]	3.9	4.7	4.7
T2[b]	366	5.2[c]	4.2	8.6	8.6
T3[b]	22	9.1[c]	11.4	11.4	
Previously untreated (primary)	964	4.4	4.2	5.7	5.7
Previously treated and recurrent	55	7.3	4.3	13.2	13.2
SCCs, total	245	6.9	6.0	10.5	12.8
Tis[b]	13	7.7[d]	11.1		
T1[b]	79	1.3[d]	1.7	1.7	1.7
T2[b]	138	8.7[d]	7.4	14.2	19.0
T3[b]	14	21.4[d]	25.9	25.9	
Previously untreated (primary)	233	6.4	5.8	9.6	12.0
Previously untreated and recurrent	12	16.7	30.0	30.0	

BCC, basal cell carcinoma; SCC, squamous cell carcinoma.

[a]Including three patients with combinations of BCCs and SCCs.

[b]Multiple (>1) tumors in same irradiated field were excluded.

[c]Difference of the raw recurrence rate of BCCs Tis–T3 were statistically significant (X^2, 6.99; $p < 0.05$).

[d]Differences of the raw recurrence rate of SCCs Tis–T3 were statistically significant (X^2, 9.13; $p < 0.05$).

From Schulte KW, Lippold A, Auras C, et al. Soft x-ray therapy for cutaneous basal cell and squamous cell carcinomas. *J Am Acad Dermatol* 2005;53:993–1001, with permission from Elsevier.

TABLE 33.10 OUTCOMES AFTER TREATMENT FOR SKIN CARCINOMA WITH INCIDENTAL PERINEURAL INVASION (107 PATIENTS)

Parameter	*5-Year Outcome*
Local control	80%
Ultimate local control	82%
Local-regional control	70%
Ultimate local-regional control	74%
Cause-specific survival	73%
Overall survival	55%

From Balamucki CJ, Mancuso AA, Amdur RJ, et al. Skin carcinoma of the head and neck with perineural invasion. *Am J Otolaryngol* 2012;33(4):447–454, with permission.

TABLE 33.11 OUTCOMES AFTER TREATMENT FOR SKIN CARCINOMA WITH CLINICAL PERINEURAL INVASION (109 PATIENTS)

Parameter	5-Year Outcome
Local control	54%
Ultimate local control	57%
Local-regional control	51%
Ultimate local-regional control	56%
Cause-specific survival	64%
Overall survival	54%

From Balamucki CJ, Mancuso AA, Amdur RJ, et al. Skin carcinoma of the head and neck with perineural invasion. *Am J Otolaryngol* 2012;33(4):447–454, with permission.

TABLE 33.12 CLINICAL PERINEURAL INVASION: 5-YEAR OUTCOME VERSUS PRETREATMENT RADIOGRAPHIC FINDINGS (45 PATIENTS)

	Radiographic Findings			
5-Year Outcome	Imaging Negative (n = 10)	Minimal or Moderate Peripheral PNI (n = 14)	Central and/or Macroscopic PNI (n = 21)	P
Local control	76%	57%	25%	0.2027
Cause-specific survival	100%	56%	61%	0.0206
Overall survival	90%	50%	58%	0.0817

PNI, perineural invasion.

From Galloway TJ, Morris CG, Mancuso AA, et al. Impact of radiographic findings on prognosis for skin carcinoma with clinical perineural invasion. *Cancer* 2005;103: 1254–1257, with permission.

TABLE 33.13 MERKEL CELL CARCINOMA 5-YEAR OUTCOMES VERSUS STAGE

Outcomes	Stage I (n = 24)	Stage II (n = 16)	All Patients	P-value
Local control	96%	87%	92%	.3240
Regional control	87%	65%	78%	.1587
Local-regional control	87%	67%	79%	.1607
Distant metastasis-free survival	71%	37%	57%	.0073
Cause-specific survival	58%	27%	45%	.0090
Overall survival	48%	18%	36%	.0037

Mendenhall WM, Kirwan JM, Morris CG, et al. Cutaneous Merkel cell carcinoma. *Am J Otolaryngol* 2012;33(1):88–92.

Regional Nodes

Veness et al.[32] reported on 167 patients treated at Westmead Hospital (Sydney, Australia) between 1980 and 2000 for cutaneous SCCs metastatic to the parotid and/or cervical nodes. Twenty-one patients (13%) were treated with surgery alone, and the remainder received surgery and adjuvant RT. The median time to recurrence after treatment was 8 months. The 5-year local-regional recurrence and disease-free survival rates were as follows: surgery and RT, 20% and 73%, and surgery alone, 43% and 54%, respectively. Multivariate analysis revealed that multiple positive nodes and treatment with surgery alone were significantly associated with decreased survival.

Hinerman et al.[33] reported on 117 patients with 121 clinically positive parotids treated at the University of Florida between 1969 and 2005. Patients were treated with preoperative RT and surgery (17 parotids), surgery and postoperative RT (87 parotids), and RT alone (17 parotids). The 5-year outcomes were as follows: local (parotid) control, 78%; local-regional control, 74%; distant metastasis-free survival, 92%; disease-free survival, 70%; and overall survival, 54%. The 5-year local-regional control rate was 83% after surgery and postoperative RT versus 47% after preoperative RT and surgery or RT alone. Three (3%) patients developed severe complications.

Merkel Cell Carcinoma

Mendenhall et al.[19] reported on 40 patients treated with RT alone (3 patients) or combined with surgery (37 patients) at the University of Florida between 1984 and 2009. Eleven patients received adjuvant chemotherapy. Twenty-four patients had stage I disease, and 16 patients had stage II MCC. Median follow-up on survivors was 4.2 years (range, 2.2 to 14.2 years). No patient was lost to follow-up. The 5-year outcomes are depicted in Table 33.13. No severe late complications were observed.

Melanoma

One of the largest experiences with adjuvant RT for melanoma has been reported by investigators from the MD Anderson Cancer Center (Houston, TX; Table 33.14). Although RT may be used to treat gross disease, this would only occur by default and in mostly palliative situations.

Tsang et al.[37] reported on 36 patients treated between 1968 and 1988 with definitive RT for lentigo maligna at the Princess Margaret Hospital (Toronto, Canada) and followed for a median 6 years. The 5-year local control rate was 86%. Farshad et al.[39] reported an 150 patients treated at the University of Zurich with definitive RT for lentigo maligna (93 patients), lentigo maligna melanoma (54 patients), or both (3 patients). One hundred one patients were followed for at least 2 years (mean, 8 years); the local control rate was 93%.

TABLE 33.14 OUTCOMES AFTER SURGERY AND POSTOPERATIVE RADIOTHERAPY AT THE UNIVERSITY OF TEXAS MD ANDERSON CANCER CENTER FOR LYMPH NODE–POSITIVE MELANOMA PATIENTS

Series	Number of Patients	Site	Follow-Up[a]	RC[b]	DMFS[b]	Survival[b]
Ballo, 2002[50]	89	Axilla	Median, 58 mo (range, 7–159 mo)	87% (5 y)	49% (5 y)	OS, 50% (5 y)
Ballo, 2003[49]	160	Cervical	Median, 78 mo (range, 6–224 mo)	94% (10 y)	43% (10 y)	CSS, 48% (10 y)
Ballo, 2004[51]	40	Ilioinguinal	Median, 23 mo (range, 4–107 mo)	74% (3 y)	35% (3 y)	OS, 38% (3 y)

RC, regional control; DMFS, distant metastasis-free survival; CSS, cause-specific survival; OS, overall survival.

[a]Follow-up for surviving patients.

[b]Outcome (interval).

From Mendenhall WM, Amdur RJ, Grobmyer SR, et al. Adjuvant radiotherapy for cutaneous melanoma. *Cancer* 2008;112:1189–1196, with permission.

CONCLUSIONS

RT is an effective modality for the primary treatment of skin cancer as well as in the adjuvant setting. It is used to treat the primary skin lesion when resection would result in an unacceptable functional and/or cosmetic outcome as well as in the patient who is medically unsuitable for, or who declines, surgery. Adjuvant RT is usually indicated after surgery for close or positive margins, PNI, bone and/or cartilage involvement, metastatic parotid-area lymph nodes, multiple lymph node metastases, and extracapsular extension.

REFERENCES

1. American Cancer Society. Skin cancer: basal and squamous cell overview. Available at: http://www.cancer.org/Cancer/SkinCancer-BasalandSquamousCell/OverviewGuide/index. Accessed March 29, 2011.
2. Jemal A, Siegel R, Xu J, et al. Cancer statistics, 2010. *CA Cancer J Clin* 2010;60:277–300.
3. Yoffey JM, Courtice FC. *Lymphatics, lymph and lymphoid tissue*. Cambridge, MA: Edward Arnold, 1956.
4. Taylor BW Jr, Brant TA, Mendenhall NP, et al. Carcinoma of the skin metastatic to parotid area lymph nodes. *Head Neck* 1991;13:427–433.
5. Toker C. Trabecular carcinoma of the skin. *Arch Dermatol* 1972;105:107–110.
6. Mendenhall WM, Amdur RJ, Hinerman RW, et al. Skin cancer of the head and neck with perineural invasion. *Am J Clin Oncol* 2007;30:93–96.
7. Evans HL, Smith JL. Spindle cell squamous carcinomas and sarcoma-like tumors of the skin: a comparative study of 38 cases. *Cancer* 1980;45:2687–2697.
8. Ackerman AB. Histopathology of keratoacanthoma. In: Andrade R, Gumport SL, Popkin GL, et al., eds. *Cancer of the skin: biology, diagnosis, management*. Philadelphia, PA: WB Saunders, 1976:781–796.
9. Chow WC, Cockerell CJ, Geronemus RG. Microcystic adnexal carcinoma of the scalp. *J Dermatol Surg Oncol* 1989;15:768–771.
10. Mayer MH, Winton GB, Smith AC, et al. Microcystic adnexal carcinoma (sclerosing sweat duct carcinoma). *Plast Reconstr Surg* 1989;84:970–975.
11. Requena L, Marquina A, Alegre V, et al. Sclerosing-sweat-duct (microcystic adnexal) carcinoma—a tumor from a single eccrine origin. *Clin Exp Dermatol* 1990;15:222–224.
12. Goepfert H, Remmler D, Silva E, et al. Merkel cell carcinoma (endocrine carcinoma of the skin) of the head and neck. *Arch Otolaryngol* 1984;110:707–712.
13. Schuller DE, Berg JW, Sherman G, et al. Cutaneous basosquamous carcinoma of the head and neck: a comparative analysis. *Otolaryngol Head Neck Surg* 1979;87:420–427.
14. Fierstein JT, Thawley SE, Druck NS, et al. Metastatic sweat gland carcinoma. *Laryngoscope* 1978;88:1691–1696.
15. Harari PM, Shimm DS, Bangert JL, et al. The role of radiotherapy in the treatment of malignant sweat gland neoplasms. *Cancer* 1990;65:1737–1740.
16. Wright JD, Font RL. Mucinous sweat gland adenocarcinoma of eyelid: a clinicopathologic study of 21 cases with histochemical and electron microscopic observations. *Cancer* 1979;44:1757–1768.
17. Mellette JR, Amonette RA, Gardner JH, et al. Carcinoma of sebaceous glands on the head and neck. A report of four cases. *J Dermatol Surg Oncol* 1981;7:404–407.
18. Southwick GJ, Schwartz RA. The basal cell nevus syndrome: disasters occurring among a series of 36 patients. *Cancer* 1979;44:2294–2305.
19. Mendenhall WM, Kirwan JM, Morris CG, et al. Cutaneous Merkel cell carcinoma. *Am J Otolaryngol* 2012;33(1):88–92.
20. Mojica P, Smith D, Ellenhorn JD. Adjuvant radiation therapy is associated with improved survival in Merkel cell carcinoma of the skin. *J Clin Oncol* 2007;25:1043–1047.
21. Rousseau DL Jr, Ross MI, Johnson MM, et al. Revised American Joint Committee on Cancer staging criteria accurately predict sentinel lymph node positivity in clinically node-negative melanoma patients. *Ann Surg Oncol* 2003;10:569–574.
22. Emery RE, Stevens JS, Nance RW, et al. Sentinel node staging of primary melanoma by the "10% rule": pathology and clinical outcomes. *Am J Surg* 2007;193:618–622.
23. Paek SC, Griffith KA, Johnson TM, et al. The impact of factors beyond Breslow depth on predicting sentinel lymph node positivity in melanoma. *Cancer* 2007;109:100–108.
24. Kruper LL, Spitz FR, Czerniecki BJ, et al. Predicting sentinel node status in AJCC stage I/II primary cutaneous melanoma. *Cancer* 2006;107:2436–2445.
25. Leong SP, Accortt NA, Essner R, et al. Impact of sentinel node status and other risk factors on the clinical outcome of head and neck melanoma patients. *Arch Otolaryngol Head Neck Surg* 2006;132:370–373.
26. Berk DR, Johnson DL, Uzieblo A, et al. Sentinel lymph node biopsy for cutaneous melanoma: the Stanford experience, 1997–2004. *Arch Dermatol* 2005;141:1016–1022.
27. Yiengpruksawan A, Coit DG, Thaler HT, et al. Merkel cell carcinoma. Prognosis and management. *Arch Surg* 1991;126:1514–1519.
28. Mancuso AA, Hanafee WN. *Head and neck radiology*, 2nd ed. Philadelphia, PA: Lippincott Williams & Wilkins, 2011.
29. Mendenhall WM, Million RR, Mancuso AA, et al. Carcinoma of the skin. In: Million RR, Cassisi NJ, eds. *Management of head and neck cancer: a multidisciplinary approach*, 2nd ed. Philadelphia, PA: JB Lippincott, 1994:643–691.
30. Million RR. The myth regarding bone or cartilage involvement by cancer and the likelihood of cure by radiotherapy. *Head Neck* 1989;11:30–40.
31. Mendenhall WM, Amdur RJ, Hinerman RW, et al. Radiotherapy for cutaneous squamous and basal cell carcinomas of the head and neck. *Laryngoscope* 2009;119:1994–1999.
32. Veness MJ, Morgan GJ, Palme CE, et al. Surgery and adjuvant radiotherapy in patients with cutaneous head and neck squamous cell carcinoma metastatic to lymph nodes: combined treatment should be considered best practice. *Laryngoscope* 2005;115:870–875.
33. Hinerman RW, Amdur RJ, Morris CG, et al. Cutaneous squamous cell carcinoma metastatic to parotid-area lymph nodes. *Laryngoscope* 2008;118:1989–1996.
34. Andruchow JL, Veness MJ, Morgan GJ, et al. Implications for clinical staging of metastatic cutaneous squamous carcinoma of the head and neck based on a multicenter study of treatment outcomes. *Cancer* 2006;106:1078–1083.
35. Mendenhall WM, Amdur RJ, Grobmyer SR, et al. Adjuvant radiotherapy for cutaneous melanoma. *Cancer* 2008;112:1189–1196.
36. Chang DT, Amdur RJ, Morris CG, et al. Adjuvant radiotherapy for cutaneous melanoma: comparing hypofractionation to conventional fractionation. *Int J Radiat Oncol Biol Phys* 2006;66:1051–1055.
37. Tsang RW, Liu FF, Wells W, et al. Lentigo maligna of the head and neck. Results of treatment by radiotherapy. *Arch Dermatol* 1994;130:1008–1012.
38. Khan N, Khan MK, Almasan A, et al. The evolving role of radiation therapy in the management of malignant melanoma. *Int J Radiat Oncol Biol Phys* 2011;80:645–654.
39. Farshad A, Burg G, Panizzon R, et al. A retrospective study of 150 patients with lentigo maligna and lentigo maligna melanoma and the efficacy of radiotherapy using Grenz or soft X-rays. *Br J Dermatol* 2002;146:1042–1046.
40. Amdur RJ, Kalbaugh KJ, Ewald LM, et al. Radiation therapy for skin cancer near the eye: kilovoltage x-rays versus electrons. *Int J Radiat Oncol Biol Phys* 1992;23:769–779.
41. Bhandare N, Monroe AT, Morris CG, et al. Does altered fractionation influence the risk of radiation-induced optic neuropathy? *Int J Radiat Oncol Biol Phys* 2005;62:1070–1077.
42. Monroe AT, Bhandare N, Morris CG, et al. Preventing radiation retinopathy with hyperfractionation. *Int J Radiat Oncol Biol Phys* 2005;61:856–864.
43. Garcia-Serra A, Hinerman RW, Mendenhall WM, et al. Carcinoma of the skin with perineural invasion. *Head Neck* 2003;25:1027–1033.
44. Lovett RD, Perez CA, Shapiro DL, et al. External irradiation of epithelial skin cancer. *Int J Radiat Oncol Biol Phys* 1990;19:235–242.
45. Schulte KW, Lippold A, Auras C, et al. Soft x-ray therapy for cutaneous basal cell and squamous cell carcinomas. *J Am Acad Dermatol* 2005;53:993–1001.
46. Al-Othman MOF, Mendenhall WM, Amdur RJ. Radiotherapy alone for clinical T4 skin carcinoma of the head and neck with surgery reserved for salvage. *Am J Otolaryngol* 2001;22:387–390.
47. Balamucki CJ, Mancuso AA, Amdur RJ, et al. Skin carcinoma of the head and neck with perineural invasion. *Amer J Otolaryngol* 2012;33(4):447–454.
48. Galloway TJ, Morris CG, Mancuso AA, et al. Impact of radiographic findings on prognosis for skin carcinoma with clinical perineural invasion. *Cancer* 2005;103:1254–1257.
49. Ballo MT, Bonnen MD, Garden AS, et al. Adjuvant irradiation for cervical lymph node metastases from melanoma. *Cancer* 2003;97:1789–1796.
50. Ballo MT, Strom EA, Zagars GK, et al. Adjuvant irradiation for axillary metastases from malignant melanoma. *Int J Radiat Oncol Biol Phys* 2002;52:964–972.
51. Ballo MT, Zagars GK, Gershenwald JE, et al. A critical assessment of adjuvant radiotherapy for inguinal lymph node metastases from melanoma. *Ann Surg Oncol* 2004;11:1079–1084.

Part B AIDS-Related Malignancies

Chapter 34
Neoplasms Associated with Acquired Immunodeficiency Syndrome

Bernadine R. Donahue and Jay S. Cooper

> We cannot deal with AIDS by making moral judgments or refusing to face unpleasant facts, and still less by stigmatizing those who are infected.
>
> —Kofi Annan, former U.N. secretary general

HUMAN IMMUNODEFICIENCY VIRUS

One of the greatest public health challenges of the latter half of the 20th century has been emergence of human immunodeficiency virus (HIV). Although the biology of the virus has been elucidated, diagnostic tests have been created, and effective drugs and care systems have been established, HIV remains an epidemic in the 21st century, particularly in the developing world. HIV infection, immunosuppression, and enhanced tumor growth characterize the acquired immunodeficiency syndrome (AIDS).

Nearly 30 million people have died of AIDS in the past 30 years,[1] and despite gains that have been made, AIDS remains a health catastrophe in those parts of the world with little or no access to life-sustaining drugs. In 2009, the most recent year for which worldwide statistics are available, over 33 million people were living with AIDS (including 2.5 million children under the age of 15 years), 2.6 million people became infected, and 1.8 million people died of AIDS. Nearly 70% of these events occurred in Sub-Saharan Africa.[1] Although the toll of HIV infection in North America can be viewed as relatively small in comparison to other parts of the world, the statistics remain concerning. In 2009, 1.5 million persons in North America were living with HIV and there were 25,000 deaths attributable to AIDS.[1] Many HIV-infected persons in the United States do not receive optimal care: for some, the monetary cost of highly active antiretroviral therapy (HAART) is prohibitive, while for others, the toxicity associated with HAART is unbearable. Despite funded programs aimed at reducing the incidence of AIDS, 70,000 persons became infected with HIV in North America during 2009.[1] Thus, even in such resource-rich areas as North America, AIDS is likely to remain a serious problem in the foreseeable future.

Human Immunodeficiency Virus and Malignancy

AIDS-associated malignancies are a well-recognized, not-infrequent, and potentially lethal consequence of the disease. Early in the epidemic, three types of malignancies showed a sufficiently increased incidence that they qualified as AIDS-defining conditions when they occurred in conjunction with HIV infection: Kaposi's sarcoma (KS), non-Hodgkin lymphoma (NHL), and carcinoma of the cervix. In 1981, the appearance of KS in young homosexual men heralded the association of tumors and HIV infection.[2] Intermediate- or high-grade B-cell lymphomas in HIV-infected individuals were classified as AIDS-defining events in 1985.[3] Cervical carcinoma was recognized in 1993 as an AIDS-defining illness for HIV-infected women.[4] Data reported from the AIDS Cancer Match Registry Study (including more than 300,000 adult persons with HIV/AIDS) demonstrated the expected increased relative risks of developing the three AIDS-defining tumors,[5] however, in addition, this study as well as others suggested an increase in some other tumors, such as Hodgkin lymphoma, anal carcinomas, skin cancers, and prostate cancer, as well as unusual pediatric age malignancies in HIV-infected children.[6,7,8,9–10]

By 1993, the Centers for Disease Control (CDC) dropped the requirement of an AIDS-defining malignancy or other overt illnesses for a diagnosis of AIDS[4]; however, the burden of cancer in the HIV-infected population remains a substantial and potentially growing problem. The raw numbers from the HIV/AIDS Cancer Match Study and the CDC reflect the overall decrease in AIDS-defining neoplasms over the past decades: from 1991–1995 to 2001–2005, the estimated number of AIDS-defining cancers decreased from 34,587 to 10,325, whereas non-AIDS-defining cancers increased from 3,193 to 10,059,[11] and this finding is corroborated by multiple other datasets.[8,12] It is likely that this trend will continue as the HIV-infected population ages,[13–14,15–17,18,19] and given that the AIDS population in the United States expanded fourfold from 1991 to 2005 primarily because of an increase in the number of people aged 40 years or older,[11] cancer in the setting of HIV infection will continue to require our attention.

This chapter subsequently is organized by histologic type of HIV-associated malignancy. Epidemiology, patterns of disease, pathology, diagnostic evaluation, treatment, and prognosis are included. The use of radiation as it relates specifically to each malignancy in the setting of HIV is discussed. For additional details regarding the *delivery* of radiation, the chapters in this text addressing each specific neoplasm should be consulted.

It is of historical interest to note that in June 2001, the International Atomic Energy Agency issued a monograph, "The Role of Radiotherapy in the Management of Cancer Patients Infected by Human Immunodeficiency Virus (HIV)," which, given the paucity of data and the immense scope of the problem, attempted to provide some guidance for the treatment of HIV-associated malignancies.[20] At the time, AIDS was an almost uniformly fatal disease, and it was against this background that the authors stated that for HIV-associated malignancies:

> [T]he usual oncological rules of practice do not apply: cure at any cost is not a sensible option. Very often the best decision is simply to treat with the simplest, most effective, palliative

regimen available. Any decision to treat radically has to be tempered by the realisation that the patient's life span will be limited, regardless of the success or failure of the treatment for the malignant disease. Nowhere in oncology is an individualised approach to decision-making more important than in HIV oncology...for a patient with asymptomatic malignancy and HIV infection, active observation is a perfectly reasonable policy.[20]

Fortunately, a decade later, the outlook for HIV-infected persons is much improved, and the era of therapeutic nihilism has past. There is now solid rationale for including patients with HIV and cancer in clinical trials. The Cancer Therapy Evaluation Program has advised researchers that individuals known to be HIV positive should not be arbitrarily excluded from participation in clinical cancer treatment trials, and the National Cancer Institute has advocated that persons with HIV and cancer should only be excluded from cancer trials if there is a scientific reason for doing so.[21] In general, for persons with HIV, the procedure is to attempt to utilize "standard" stage-directed treatments for each malignancy discussed. However, the authors do so with the major caveat that the "standard" treatment may need to be modified based on the immunologic status, the viral load, coexisting opportunistic infections, and comorbidities in any given individual.

Treatment-related toxicity will continue to be a concern as HIV infection yields to better therapies and the incidence of unrelated tumors increases. Laboratory data suggest that certain protease inhibitors may increase radiosensitivity; however, this has not been borne out in the clinic. See et al.[22] compared the toxicity rates of radiation therapy in patients who were taking or not taking a second-generation protease inhibitor and observed no difference. Baeyens et al.[23] demonstrated heightened sensitivity of HIV-infected T lymphocytes to damage from radiation, but the *in vivo* data are not uniformly supportive. Kaminuma et al.[24] concluded that radiotherapy is safe, but HIV infection was associated with earlier onset (i.e., with lower dose) and more severe acute skin and mucosal toxicity. Mallik et al.,[25] in a review of the literature, concluded that local control and disease-specific survival are not affected by HIV infection if the CD4 count exceeds 200 cells per cubic millimeter. This appears to be true even for tumors that are treated with relatively aggressive combinations of chemotherapy and radiation, such as carcinomas of the anal canal or of the head and neck region.[26,27] Thus, in general, it appears that curative radiation therapy (with or without chemotherapy as the extent of disease dictates) provides disease control without imparting a degree of toxicity substantially beyond that traditionally seen in HIV-uninfected individuals. Nevertheless, the myelosuppressive nature of some of the agents incorporated into HAART regimens and the neurotoxicity of others raise concern when radiation therapy is being delivered to large volumes of bone marrow or over the central nervous system (CNS).[28] If we are to continue to improve the outcome of HIV-infected persons with malignancies, close monitoring for toxicity, attention to immunologic parameters, and a strong emphasis on supportive care are essential when treating such patients with standard treatments.

LYMPHOMA

The incidence of lymphoma in association with HIV infection was reported as approximately 60 to 100 times greater than expected in the general population during the early years of the epidemic.[29,30] Although primary central nervous system lymphoma (PCNSL) was one of the initial CDC-approved criteria for a diagnosis of AIDS,[31] the inclusion of systemic high-grade B-cell NHL did not occur until 1985.[3] Its incidence was shown to correlate with the duration of immunosuppression, CD4 count 1 year prior to the diagnosis of NHL, and B-cell stimulation.[32] Epstein-Barr virus (EBV) was implicated in its etiology by the finding of anti-EBV immunoglobulins and circulating EBV-infected B cells in the setting of HIV.[33] Where available, HAART appears to have decreased the incidence of both PCNSL and NHL, most likely secondary to an overall decrease in the proportion of patients with low CD4 counts.[12]

Primary Central Nervous System Lymphoma

Epidemiology and Risk Factors

At its height, the incidence of NHL originating in the brain without evidence of systemic involvement in persons with AIDS was 3,600-fold higher than in the general population.[34] HAART has decreased the high risk of developing this disorder in persons who are infected with HIV.[35]

Patterns of Disease

In most patients who have HIV-associated PCNSL, the diagnosis is suggested by the onset of headaches or a change in mental status.[36,37] Unfortunately, PCNSL can be clinically and radiographically indistinguishable from other pathologic processes in HIV-infected patients. Neurocognitive dysfunction in HIV-infected patients is associated with a long differential diagnosis, including PCNSL, toxoplasmosis, herpetic infections, cryptococcus, progressive multifocal leukoencephalopathy, neuroimmune reconstitution inflammatory syndrome (IRIS), and HIV-associated dementia, leukoencephalopathy, and demyelination. In general, the typical radiographic findings of PCNSL are that of multiple contrast-enhancing lesions, often, but not exclusively, in a periventricular location (Fig. 34.1).

Diagnostic Workup

Prior to HAART, it was common for an HIV-infected patient to present with a clinical and radiographic picture that could be consistent with either toxoplasmosis or PCNSL (Fig. 34.2). A negative toxoplasmosis titer did not eliminate the diagnosis of toxoplasmosis, and similarly a positive toxoplasmosis titer did not preclude the presence of PCNSL.[38,39] Because there was a high incidence of toxoplasmosis in the HIV-infected population, the standard first-line treatment for an HIV-infected patient who developed a neurologic abnormality and had a radiographically visible brain lesion consistent with either toxoplasmosis or CNS lymphoma was the institution of antitoxoplasmosis antibiotics. During the first decade of the epidemic, it was common to administer *empiric* cranial radiation therapy in patients who

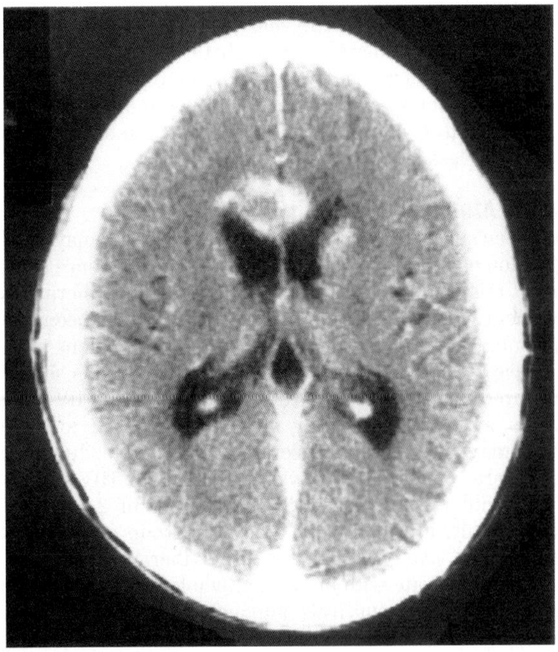

FIGURE 34.1. Example of periventricular location of human immunodeficiency virus–associated primary central nervous system lymphoma.

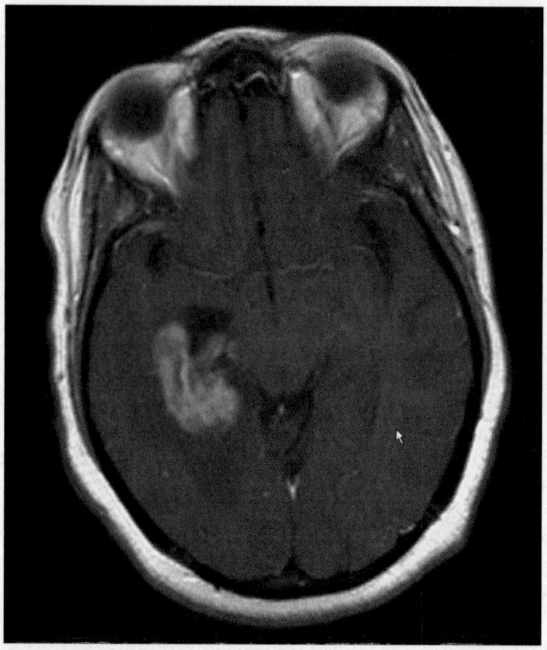

FIGURE 34.2. Magnetic resonance image findings in a patient who presented with a change in mental status and was found to be human immunodeficiency virus positive. Differential diagnosis included primary central nervous system lymphoma; biopsy proved toxoplasmosis.

did not manifest clinical or radiographic improvement by the second or third week of antitoxoplasmosis treatment. However, as our knowledge of the myriad HIV-related opportunistic infections expanded and the poor outcome with this empiric approach was recognized, the emphasis shifted to recommending biopsy for definitive diagnosis.[40]

Pathology and Prognostic Factors

The majority of PCNSL are B-cell large immunoblastic types, and EBV DNA is identifiable in nearly all cases.[41] Polymerase chain reaction amplification of EBV DNA in the cerebrospinal fluid is usually positive in these patients and may become negative following treatment.[42] In general, PCNSL is seen later in the course of HIV infection than is systemic NHL. Patients usually have CD4 counts <50 cells per cubic millimeter before PCNSL becomes evident.[43] Although the overall median survival of these patients is poor, patients no older than 35 years who have Karnofsky performance scores of at least 80% tended to survive 5 to 6 months, rather than the 2 months typically observed in less favorable subgroups.[44]

General Management

It has been suggested that the institution of HAART may result in regression of existing PCNSL, but to date scant evidence exists to support this claim.[45–47] Methotrexate-based chemotherapy with or without whole-brain radiation therapy (RT) has been shown to prolong the median survival in immunocompetent patients who have PCNSL,[48] and when possible, this approach should be considered for patients with HIV. However, many HIV-infected patients who are sufficiently immunosuppressed to develop PCNSL may be unable to tolerate methotrexate. In the pre-HAART era, chemotherapy was evaluated for HIV-associated PCNSL, with median survival on the order of 2 months.[49,50] More recently, in the HAART era, a subgroup of HIV-positive patients who can tolerate aggressive therapy consisting of either methotrexate with or without whole-brain radiotherapy, may achieve longer survivals, although their outcome remains worse than the median survival of 41 months reported in immunocompetent patients treated with methotrexate-based chemotherapy.[48,51]

Radiation

Cranial irradiation alone in the treatment of PCNSL was essentially palliative, produced short-lived clinical and radiographic evidence of tumor response, and resulted in mean overall survival of 2 months.[36,44,49,52–54,55,56–57,58] Recent intriguing data from Japan showed a survival rate of 64% at 3 years in a cohort of irradiated patients who were receiving HAART.[59] Patients who received (or who were able to receive) doses 30 Gy or more fared better than those receiving lower doses. Unfortunately, one-third of persons who lived more than 12 months manifested leukoencephalopathy.

Although HAART appears to have decreased the incidence of HIV-associated PCNSL, it remains to be determined what the precise influence of aggressive antiretroviral treatment will be on the outcome of HIV-infected patients with PCNSL. However, it appears that survival is prolonged by HAART.[60,61] There are anecdotal reports of regression of PCNSL with the institution of HAART and case reports of survival 2 years or more.[45–47,62] Cohort data from Australia showed that in a subset analysis of 47 patients with biopsy-proven PCNSL, antiretroviral therapy with at least two agents along with RT was associated with better survival.[63] In addition to immunomodulation by targeting HIV, attempts have been made to target EBV, which is nearly uniformly found in HIV PCNSL. Combinations of zidovudine, ganciclovir, and interleukin-2 were piloted by the AIDS Malignancy Consortium.[64] The incidence of myelosuppression with this was high, and this remains an experimental approach.

Systemic Non-Hodgkin Lymphoma

Epidemiology and Risk Factor

The incidence of NHL decreased with introduction of HAART, and this reflected the decreased number of HIV-infected persons with low CD4 counts.[65] Although it appears that non-nucleoside transcriptase inhibitor–based HAART is as protective as protease inhibitor–based HAART and more protective than nucleoside analogs alone,[66] cases of NHL among patients with multiclass antiretroviral resistance have been described as developing soon after newer-class antiretrovirals were initiated; this has raised the potential of IRIS-mediated NHL.[67,68]

Diagnosis

Rapidly developing adenopathy or constitutional B symptoms (fevers, unexplained weight loss, night sweats) are the most common presentations of HIV-associated systemic NHL. Nearly 75% of all patients will present with advanced-stage disease (stage III or IV), will manifest B symptomatology, and frequently have extranodal involvement.[69] The most common histologic subtypes are high-grade B-cell lymphoma or Burkitt's lymphoma; however, intermediate-grade (diffuse large cell type) lymphomas are not uncommon. As patients who have AIDS-NHL frequently have extranodal involvement, staging evaluation should include chest, abdomen, and pelvic computerized tomograms, bone marrow biopsy, and cerebrospinal fluid analysis.

Treatment

Treatment for AIDS-NHL lymphoma initially was based on high-dose chemotherapy regimens that proved to be toxic. Subsequently, therapy relied on attenuated doses of cytotoxic chemotherapy or standard-dose chemotherapy plus cytokine support; however, outcomes were still poor.[70–74] Further study helped to define a regimen with high efficacy with acceptable toxicity using infusional cyclophosphamide, doxorubicin, and etoposide (CDE), and a multicenter trial employing this regimen showed that the median 1-year survival of 48% achieved with CDE was approximately twice as high as was achievable with previously standard regimens such as methotrexate with leucovorin rescue, bleomycin, doxorubicin, cyclophosphamide, vincristine, and dexamethasone.[75] The advent of rituximab, an anti-CD20 antibody that has improved survival for patients with non-HIV-associated NHL, may improve the outcome in HIV-associated NHL. An AIDS Malignancies Consortium phase III trial that randomized patients to cyclophosphamide, doxorubicin, vincristine, and prednisone (CHOP) versus CHOP plus rituximab (R-CHOP) showed a higher complete response rate (57%) in the R-CHOP arm as compared with CHOP alone (47%); this, however, was not statistically significant and there was an increased risk of death from infection in the R-CHOP arm.[76] A French trial also evaluated the safety and efficacy of R-CHOP for the treatment of AIDS-related NHL.[77] This trial included 61 patients, two-thirds of whom achieved a complete response. The overall survival at 2 years was 75%, and although infections were seen, only one patient died from infection. The AIDS Malignancies Consortium (AMC034) trial randomized patients to EPOCH (etoposide, prednisone, vincristine, cyclophosphamide, and doxorubicin) with concurrent rituximab versus EPOCH followed sequentially by rituximab.[78,79] The patients who received concurrent rituximab achieved a complete response of 73%.

CNS prophylaxis with intrathecal chemotherapy has been controversial in the setting of high-grade NHL and HIV infection, but frequently was used, especially in patients with extranodal disease. However, it appears that patients who do not have EBV-infected tumors may not require such prophylaxis. The risk of CNS involvement was 10 times higher in patients who were EBV positive, as compared with those who were EBV negative.[80] It may be that prophylaxis can be reserved for a selected subset of patients. The sustained-release formulation of intrathecal cytarabine may have an important role to play in both the prophylaxis and treatment of CNS meningeal involvement.[81]

A previously unrecognized form of lymphoma, called primary effusion or body cavity lymphoma, was identified in HIV-infected patients during the second decade of the epidemic.[82] It appeared to be associated with human herpesvirus-8,[83] and it accounted for approximately 4% of AIDS-related NHL.[84] Typically, such patients present with an effusion in a body cavity, in the absence of widespread lymphadenopathy. The effusion contains numerous atypical lymphoid cells with a plasmacytoid appearance and an indeterminate (non-B or T cell) immunophenotype and clonal immunoglobulin heavy- and light-chain gene rearrangements. Multiple myeloma-1/interferon regulatory factor-4 protein expression can be used to differentiate primary effusion lymphoma from other lymphomas.[85] Survival of patients who have primary effusion lymphoma remains very short, on the order of 2 to 5 months, even with aggressive therapy.

It is clear that with the availability of HAART, it became feasible to employ standard chemotherapy regimens, and a major question now is whether HAART should be administered in conjunction with, or after, chemotherapy. In general, it is recommended that zidovudine be avoided because of its myelosuppressive effects. The current thinking is that HIV-infected persons should be treated in the same aggressive fashion as noninfected persons, however, patients much be chosen carefully and monitored closely for toxicity.[86,87]

Radiation Therapy

The role of consolidative radiation therapy following systemic treatment in AIDS patients who have NHL has not been evaluated methodically. It had been suggested that radiation should be used as a consolidative boost in patients with bulky disease who have demonstrated slow or partial response to chemotherapy.[88,89] More obviously, it also was indicated for palliation of bulky lesions and was used to provide palliative therapy for patients who develop lymphomatous meningitis. In lymphomatous meningitis, this approach was shown to result in a 60% to 70% clinical or cytological response, however, median time to progression was on the order of only 2 to 2.5 months.[90,91]

Results and Prognosis

Despite our best current therapies, patients who have AIDS-NHL generally have a poor overall survival. Early in the epidemic prognostic factors were identified that correlated with the length of survival.[92–94] Patients who had bone marrow involvement, low Karnofsky performance status at diagnosis (<70%), low CD4 counts, or a prior diagnosis of AIDS had a median survival on the order of 4 months; those without these adverse features had a median survival of 11 months. Rossi et al.[95] reported that the International Prognostic Index (IPI), a model designed to predict the outcome of NHL in general, is a reliable prognostic indicator of outcomes for patients who have AIDS-related NHL. Both the likelihood of complete response and median survival after treatment correlated appropriately with IPI score. Moreover, the IPI score correlated with the CD4 cell count, suggesting that the degree of immunodeficiency imparted by HIV infection influenced the aggressiveness of NHL. Ultimately, a prognostic model for systemic AIDS-related NHL treated in the era of highly active antiretroviral therapy was established based solely on the IPI and the CD4 count.[96]

NHL remains an important cause of morbidity and mortality in AIDS patients. Registry data from San Diego suggest an improvement in median survival for these patients from approximately 4 months to 9 months after the introduction of HAART,[35] however, data from Kaiser Permanente in California demonstrate that HIV-infected patients with NHL in the HAART era continue to endure substantially higher mortality compared with HIV-uninfected patients with NHL, with 59% of HIV-infected patients dying within 2 years after NHL diagnosis as compared with 30% of HIV-uninfected patients.[97] There is hope that newer targeted agents, such as rituximab, which has shown an improvement in survival for patients with non-HIV-associated NHL, will improve the outcome in HIV-associated NHL. It is of interest that in developing countries challenged by the lack of HAART, efficacious regimens employing dose-modified oral chemotherapy have been developed, which result in outcomes comparable to the pre-HAART experience in the United States.[98]

Hodgkin Lymphoma

The relative risk of developing Hodgkin lymphoma in the setting of HIV infection (HIV-HL) is increased as compared with the general population as demonstrated by a joint Danish and U.S study of 302,824 HIV-infected patients that showed a relative risk of 11.5.[99] Although data from the Multicenter AIDS Cohort Study showed a stable incidence of this disease before and after the introduction of HAART,[12] there is recent evidence that the incidence of this disease in the HIV-infected population increased after the introduction of HAART. Data from a large European cohort showed a rising standardized incidence ratio from 1983 through 2007, with multivariate analysis showing that HAART was associated with an increased risk of disease.[18]

The explanation for the rise in HIV-HL after combined antiretroviral therapy became widely available is unclear, however, one intriguing explanation involves the relationship between Reed-Sternberg cells and CD4 cells.[100] The risk of Hodgkin lymphoma appears to peak when HAART reconstitutes the immune system and CD4 cells reach levels of 150 to 190 cells per cubic millimeter. It is postulated that Reed-Sternberg cells produce growth factors that increase the influx of CD4 cells, which in turn provide signals that cause the proliferation of Reed-Sternberg cells. If CD4 cells stimulate the growth of Reed-Sternberg cells, it would stand to reason that as HAART improves the CD4 cell count, more of these cells are available to stimulate growth of the cell associated with Hodgkin lymphoma.

Hodgkin lymphoma in HIV-infected individuals tends to be advanced, associated with B symptoms, and can present with unusual manifestations, such as presentation with a gastric or intracranial mass.[101,102] In addition to the usual prognostic factors for Hodgkin lymphoma, low CD4 count and preexisting AIDS confer a worse prognosis.

In the past, only 50% of patients had a complete response following combination chemotherapy, and 2-year survival was on the order of 45%.[103,104] How to integrate RT into the management of HIV-HL was also problematic. A report from M.D. Anderson Cancer Center suggested that radiation therapy was "appropriate" for approximately 50% of patients who had HIV-HL, usually in combination with chemotherapy; nevertheless, even in that series (with a median follow-up of 64 months), 5-year overall survival was only 54%.[105]

However, the outcome may be improving in the setting of HAART and combination chemotherapy.[106] A phase II study in 59 patients with HIV-HL (52 of whom also received concurrent HAART) resulted in a complete response rate of 81% with the Stanford V regimen, although 3-year overall survival was only 51%.[107] A more recent series from Germany reported a risk-adapted approach in 93 patients with HIV-HL.[108] Patients with early-stage favorable Hodgkin lymphoma were treated with 2 cycles of adriamycin, bleomycin, vinblastine, dacarbazine (ABVD) and 30 Gy involved field RT, those with unfavorable early-stage disease received 4 cycles of BEACOPP (bleomycin, etoposide, doxorubicin, cyclophosphamide, vincristine, procarbazine, prednisone) and 30 Gy involved field, and those with advanced stage disease were treated with 6 to 8 cycles of BEACOPP. Importantly, BEACOPP was replaced with ABVD for patients with "far-advanced" HIV infection, and HAART was given concomitantly with chemotherapy. Early results are encouraging with a 1-year overall survival of 88%, although the outcome was worse for those patients with advanced stage disease. Additionally, of concern, even with careful attention to the risks of toxicity, four patients died of neutropenic sepsis.

In general, radiation therapy should be considered for HIV-HL for the same indications it is considered in non-HIV-associated Hodgkin lymphoma; however, there continues to be a paucity of data on its use and tolerance in this setting.

KAPOSI'S SARCOMA

Epidemiology and Risk Factors

At the start of the epidemic, AIDS often was identified by the diagnosis of KS, and KS in this setting became known as epidemic Kaposi's sarcoma (EKS). People infected with HIV had at least a 20,000 times greater risk of developing KS than uninfected individuals.[109] The discovery that HIV-infected gay or bisexual men were more likely than HIV-infected heterosexual men to develop KS was one of the first clues that KS or its etiologic agent might somehow be sexually transmitted.

With the introduction of progressively more effective antiretroviral therapies, the incidence of KS in the United States, as a component of AIDS, has diminished over time. A report from the International Collaboration on HIV and Cancer evaluating the cancer incidence from 23 prospective studies that included 47,936 HIV-seropositive individuals from North America, Europe, and Australia showed that the adjusted incidence rate for KS declined from 15.2 in the period of time from 1992 through 1996 to 4.9 between 1997 and 1999.[110] A report from the Swiss HIV Cohort Study showed that the risk of developing KS declined by 66% during the 15 months after HAART was initiated ($p = .001$), as compared to the pre-HAART era.[111]

In December 1994, a herpes virus that appeared to be associated with the etiology of Kaposi's sarcoma was identified.[112] This was called human herpesvirus-8 (HHV-8) as well as KS-associated herpesvirus (KSHV). The virus was detected in both the epidemic (AIDS-related) and endemic (previously typical African) forms of KS, as well as classic (elderly men of Eastern European or Mediterranean ancestry) KS. In a 1996 report from the Multicenter AIDS Cohort Study, antibodies to HHV-8 were detected in 80% of HIV-infected men who subsequently went on to develop KS.[113] This suggested that KS resulted from infection with HHV-8, rather than being a direct result of HIV itself, or to cytokines induced by the HIV virus; HIV produced the immunosuppression that facilitated HHV-8 expression as KS. HHV-8 has a large number of genes that can encode homologues of host genes, many of which are involved in angiogenesis and the cell cycle. At present, six major subtypes (called A, B, C, D, E, and F) of HHV-8 are recognized based on the specific amino acid sequences of the gene *K1* (*ORF-K1*) of the virus and further divided into subgroups known as clades (e.g., A1, A2, A3). Additionally, increased levels of interleukin-6, which is thought to be an important growth factor in HHV-8 associated neoplasms, have been found in tissues affected by HHV-8.[114]

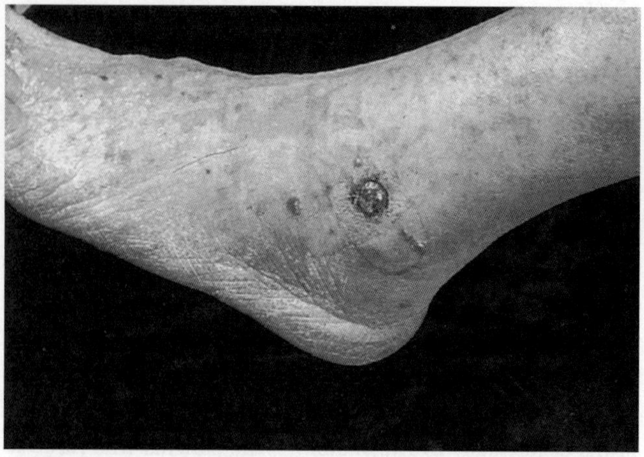

FIGURE 34.3. Purple, 1.5-cm nodular classic Kaposi's sarcoma on the ankle of an elderly man. (From Krigel RL, Friedman-Kien AE. Kaposi's sarcoma of AIDS: diagnosis and treatment. In: DeVita VT Jr, Hellman S, Rosenberg SA, eds. *AIDS: etiology, diagnosis, treatment, and prevention,* 2nd ed. Philadelphia: JB Lippincott, 1988, with permission.)

Patterns of Disease

KS is characterized by purplish lesions on the skin or mucosal surfaces. The lesions can be macular, plaque-like, or nodular, with or without associated lymphadenopathy or lymphedema (Figs. 34.3–34.5). At presentation, skin lesions can be either single or multiple and may cause pain, bleeding, or disfigurement. As involvement of lymph nodes and lymphatic spaces occurs, progressive edema can result. This is seen most commonly in lesions involving the lower extremity, the inguinal regions, the genitalia, and the face. Visceral KS typically involves the aerodigestive tracts. Oropharyngeal lesions can result in life-threatening airway obstruction. Pulmonary involvement can result in life-threatening respiratory failure.

Diagnostic Workup

In addition to inspection of all visible skin and mucosal surfaces, the likelihood of visceral KS is sufficiently high that endoscopic evaluation of the gastrointestinal (GI) tract is appropriate for any patient with GI symptoms. In any patient who develops KS as the first sign of AIDS, a more comprehensive workup for HIV should be undertaken: complete physical examination, blood count and chemistries including CD4 lymphocyte count and viral load, chest x-ray, tuberculin test, anergy screen, and screen for sexually transmitted diseases.

Pathology

It is generally agreed that KS is a neoplasm of mesenchymal origin, and the histologic diagnosis of KS requires the identification of both spindle cell and vascular elements within the lesion. The spindle-shaped cells look much like fibroblasts and are generally considered the neoplastic element. Overall, the appearance often is suggestive of slitlike embryonic vascular channels filled with red blood cells; however, red cells characteristically are also found mixed within the spindle cell framework of the tumor.

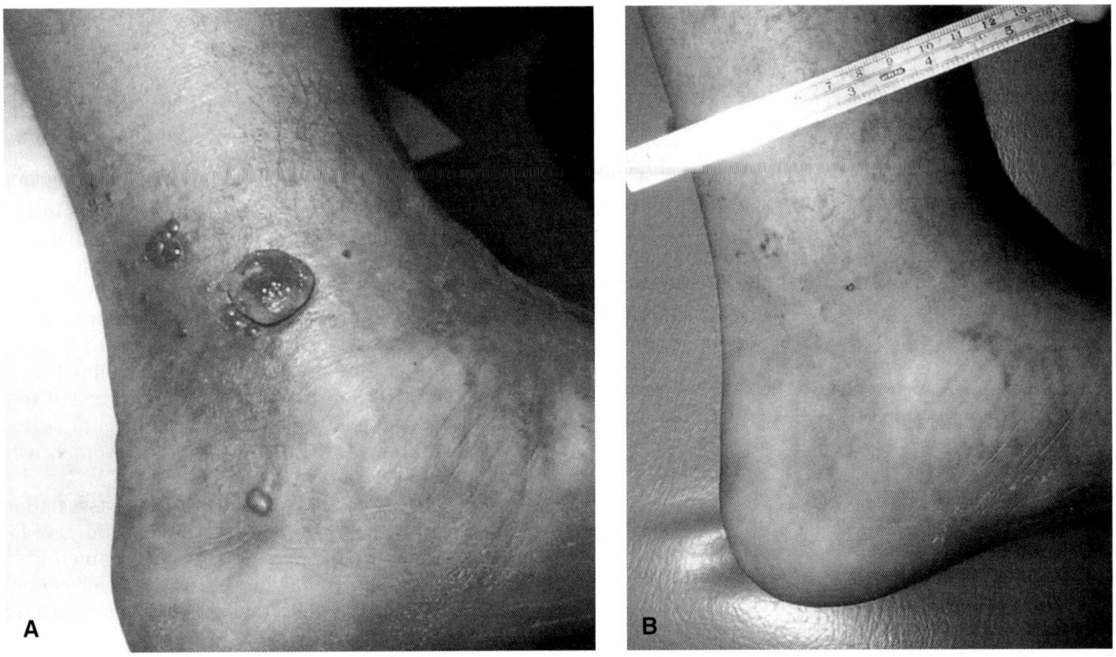

FIGURE 34.4. A: Epidemic Kaposi's sarcoma of the foot before treatment. B: Same patient approximately 1.5 years after 30 Gy was delivered in 10 fractions over 2 weeks by 6-MeV electron beam therapy (with bolus).

Treatment

Alternatives to or in Association with Radiation Therapy

EKS typically exhibits multifocal distribution at the time of presentation, and radiation therapy has played a smaller and smaller role in its management over time as better alternatives have been discovered. The role of HAART is now well established and appears to result in durable clinical response rates of over 60% of patients.[115] In one prospective cohort study of good risk (confined to skin or nodes or minimal oral disease) KS, treatment with HAART alone allowed 74% of patients to survive systemic-treatment free for 5 years.[116] It is important to recognize, however, that a small subset of patients may experience a worsening of symptoms when HAART is instituted. Bower et al.[117] have reported that after commencing HAART, 6.6% of patients with HIV-associated KS developed progressive immune reconstitution inflammatory syndrome KS (i.e., a worsening in their clinical status), despite control of virologic and immunologic parameters, felt to be secondary to an immune response against a preexisting pathogen.[117]

Systemic chemotherapy has been used for patients with advanced disease. A concern had been that cytotoxic chemotherapy potentially could further compromise the immune system and accelerate the effects of HIV infection. Also, the standard doses of chemotherapy used for solid tumors often resulted in unacceptable morbidity for these patients.[118,119] Consequently, treatment protocols were developed with low-dose chemotherapy to which epidemic KS was responsive.[120] The regimen of ABV became the gold standard in the 1990s.

Liposomal daunorubicin and doxorubicin were approved subsequently by the U.S. Food and Drug Administration (FDA) for the treatment of EKS. Randomized studies comparing these drugs with the standard ABV showed at least comparable

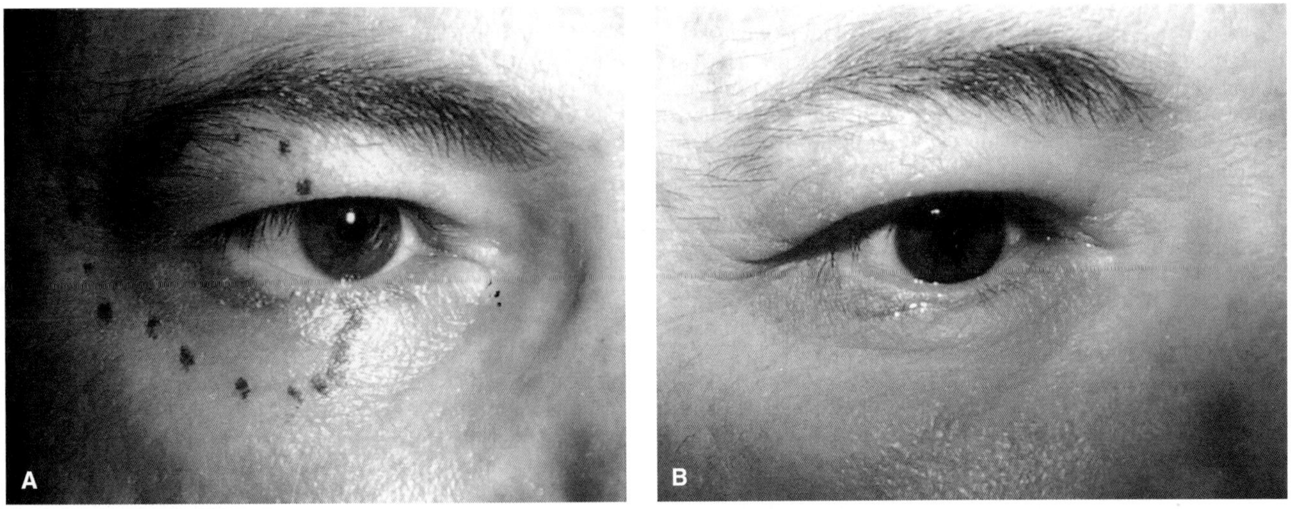

FIGURE 34.5. A: Epidemic Kaposi's sarcoma of the upper and lower lateral eyelids before treatment. B: Same patient approximately 1 month after 30 Gy was delivered in 10 fractions over 2 weeks by kilovoltage x-rays. An eye shield was used to protect the lens of the eye. Residual pigmentation is visible.

activity with a more favorable toxicity profile,[121,122] and the liposomal drugs are generally now used as first-line therapy. Response rates of 25% with a median duration of 4 months can be expected.[121,122]

Paclitaxel is also approved for treatment. Toxicity is mild except for myelosuppression, which can be dealt with by growth factors when necessary.[123,124] Gill et al.[123] reported a 60% response rate (nearly all partial responses) with a 10-month median duration of response in one phase II trial. Although there are other active drugs available, such as VP-16, paclitaxel has become a common second- or third-line drug following the liposomal agents, due to its activity and acceptable toxicity.

Without HAART, patients often require ongoing therapy to control symptomatic KS. However, when HAART is available and decreases HIV RNA to undetectable levels, chronic chemotherapy frequently can be discontinued.[125]

Radiation Therapy

Radiation therapy can also be useful for palliation of pain, bleeding, or edema. Typically, small fields that include only the distressing lesion and a small margin are treated, either with superficial quality x-rays or low-energy electrons (and bolus). One of the more commonly used dose-fractionation schemes is 30 Gy in 10 fractions delivered over 2 weeks, which has resulted in substantial benefit without substantial toxicity for the typical patient.[126] More than 90% of lesions respond to therapy and approximately 70% respond completely.[127] Stelzer and Griffin's[128] prospective randomized trial demonstrated a correlation between dose and response within the tested range of 8 Gy in 1 fraction to 40 Gy in 20 fractions over 4 weeks. Greater dose was associated with a higher response rate, a lower incidence of residual pigmentation, and a longer duration of tumor control. However, these data should not be interpreted as a blanket recommendation for higher dose; rather, this suggests that doses should be tailored to individual patients' needs. For patients who have far-advanced AIDS (where a briefer duration of palliation will suffice and the appearance of the lesion is not as important), a dose of 8 Gy in 1 fraction often is preferable.[129] In contrast, relatively healthy patients, who are treated to improve their cosmetic appearance, should receive relatively higher doses. Even then, it is prudent to remember that some residual purple pigmentation remains in approximately 55% of treated patients.[128]

Gratifying short-term palliation of painful swollen extremities secondary to far advanced KS can be achieved by covering the limb in bolus (or placing it in a water bath) and delivering a single fraction of 8 Gy by parallel opposed photon portals.

Despite the relative sensitivity of KS to radiation, toxicity of treatment needs to be considered in every situation. Treatment of symptomatic oropharyngeal lesions with radiation has been problematic because of the high degree of radiation-induced mucositis that these patients develop even following low-dose radiation therapy.[130] Palliation of symptomatic visceral or mucosal disease should nearly always be attempted first with chemotherapy and HAART. However, there are rare instances in which patients' lesions have failed to respond to systemic chemotherapy or in which patients are unable to tolerate systemic chemotherapy. These patients may benefit from attenuated doses of local radiation to palliate bleeding or obstructive lesions. Piedbois et al.[131] have reported 88% objective response and "good palliation of symptoms" following 10 to 20 Gy (2.5 Gy per fraction, 4 fractions per week) for delicate anatomic sites, such as the penis, the palms, oral mucosa, or the conjunctivae. In one report of 25 patients who had pulmonary lesions treated with radiation therapy (10.5–15 Gy at 1.5 Gy per fraction), subjective improvement was observed in nearly 90% of patients, although only one-third of patients survived for 3 months.[132]

CERVICAL CANCER

Epidemiology

Cervical carcinoma in the presence of HIV infection was accepted by the CDC as an AIDS-defining illness in 1993.[4] The association between HIV and cervical cancer is complex and, although it has been clearly demonstrated that there is an increased incidence of preinvasive lesions in HIV-infected women, it is not clear that there is a substantially higher incidence of invasive disease.[133] Some authors argued that since the introduction of HAART, there was little evidence to support the continued status of cervical cancer as an AIDS-defining illness, because cervical cancer did not appear to have a strong relationship to immune function as determined by CD4 count or responsiveness to HAART.[134] However, recent reports from Africa, where the AIDS epidemic continues to rage, suggest a doubling of the risk of cervical cancer in women with AIDS as compared to African women without AIDS.[135]

Not surprisingly, there appears to be an association between human papilloma virus (HPV) infection and risk for cervical epithelial abnormalities in HIV-infected women.[136,137–139] Data suggest that the introduction of HAART reduces the burden of HPV infection and intraepithelial neoplasia, which may in turn explain why rates of cervical cancer do not appear to have increased during the HAART era.[140,141] A report on a prospective cohort of 286 HIV infected women who initiated HAART and were assessed semiannually for HPV infection and intraepithelial lesions showed that HAART initiation among adherent women was associated with a significant reduction in prevalence and incident detection of oncogenic HPV infection as well as a decreased prevalence and more rapid clearance of oncogenic HPV-positive intraepithelial lesions.[142]

Diagnosis

Routine gynecologic evaluation, including Papanicolaou (PAP) smears (and colposcopy when warranted), is the most successful means of detecting the dysplastic and *in situ* lesions (cervical intraepithelial neoplasia [CIN]) that give rise to invasive lesions. Unfortunately, HIV-infected women often presented with advanced-stage disease, and, thus, in addition to vaginal bleeding and dyspareunia, the disease frequently manifested with abdominal or back pain, weight loss, or palpable cervical adenopathy. During the early years of the AIDS epidemic, up to 50% of HIV-infected women were diagnosed as having stage III or IV disease when they first sought care, as compared to approximately 20% of noninfected women.[143,144]

Treatment

Treatment should be dictated by the extent of disease, taking into account the patient's history of opportunistic infections and overall medical status. HIV-infected women treated with CIN should be approached in a fashion similar to non-HIV infected women, albeit with attention to the possible increased risk of complications.[145] Patients who have early-stage, nonbulky disease are usually treated with a radical hysterectomy and pelvic lymph node dissection. Patients who have more advanced local-regional disease should be treated in the same fashion as their non-HIV-infected counterparts. Although previously this would have been radiation therapy alone, in one series of patients treated by radiation alone for advanced disease, 50% had no or minimal response to treatment, and at a median follow-up of 3 months all had progression of disease.[146] In a series of 42 HIV-positive patients treated with definitive radiotherapy at Tata Memorial Hospital in India, only 22 patients completed the full course of RT; 50% achieved a complete response.[147] It should be noted that when RT alone was used to treat cervical cancer, the rates of acute toxicity in HIV-infected women, particularly genitourinary, GI, and cutaneous toxicity, were observed to be higher than expected.[148]

The current standard of care for advanced cervical cancer is a combination of radiation therapy and cisplatin-based chemotherapy. At present there are insufficient data to demonstrate the routine feasibility or efficacy of this approach in the setting of AIDS; however, based on the tolerability of combined modality approaches in other AIDS-related malignancies and the evidence of improved outcome in advanced cervical cancer in the general population, it is believed that advanced cervical cancers in women who do not have a specific contraindication for chemotherapy should receive concurrent chemotherapy, external-beam radiotherapy, and an intracavitary boost. Patients who have hematogenously borne metastatic disease may benefit from palliative chemotherapy or radiation therapy in an effort to reduce symptoms such as pain and bleeding.

Results and Prognosis

Although there initially was concern over the ability to deliver standard treatment to HIV-infected patients with cervical carcinoma, available data suggest treatment can be delivered, albeit with a higher risk of complications and perhaps a worse outcome. In a study from the early years of the epidemic, 9 of 16 HIV-infected women who had cervical carcinoma died at a mean interval of only 9.2 months from diagnosis.[146] Data on the outcomes with chemoradiation in the HAART era are lacking.

Prevention and early diagnosis of cervical abnormalities prior to the development of invasive cancer appear to be critical if the outcomes for patients are to improve. Prospective data from the Women's Interagency HIV Study have confirmed that with close monitoring (i.e., PAP smears every 6 months) and appropriate intervention, the incidence of invasive cervical cancer among women with HIV is not higher than in HIV-negative women.[149] The widespread use of the FDA-approved recombinant vaccine targeting HPV-16 and HPV-18 may further decrease the incidence of cervical cancer in the setting of HIV.

ANAL CANCER

Anal carcinomas, like cervical carcinomas, appear to be related to sexually transmitted HPV (primarily HPV-16), with anal intercourse being a risk factor.[150] HIV-infected homosexual men have increased serum HPV DNA as compared with HIV-seronegative homosexual men.[151] In one study, more than 60% of HIV-infected men with abnormal anogenital examinations were found to have squamous intraepithelial lesions on biopsy.[152] How HAART has impacted the development of anal intraepithelial neoplasia and the subsequent development of invasive anal cancer is still being defined. Some authors reported that antiretroviral treatment did not protect against the development of premalignant or malignant lesions,[153] while others reported that HAART decreased the prevalence of anal intraepithelial neoplasia in men with persistent HPV but did not affect the HPV.[154] However, recent data from a large European cohort of people with HIV evaluating the incidence of non-AIDS defining cancers showed an elevated incidence of anal cancer during the pre-HAART era (1983–1995), the early HAART era (1996–2001), and the established HAART era (2002–2007) with similar standardized incidence ratios in all three periods.[18] Thus, at present, it appears that HAART does not diminish the excess risk of anal cancer in the HIV-positive population.

Early-stage lesions may present as an incidental finding during excision of condylomata or hemorrhoids or may be identified when patients present with anal fissures. However, many patients with HIV anal carcinoma present with more advanced disease, and signs and symptoms may include perianal or rectal pain, tenesmus, bleeding, mucous drainage, or palpable groin nodes. Evaluation and workup should include digital rectal examination, inguinal node evaluation with biopsy or fine-needle aspiration of suspicious nodes, anoscopy, gynecologic examination in women, body computed tomography, and consideration of positron emission tomography scan.

Carcinoma *in situ* frequently can be approached with measures employed for the treatment of genital warts (i.e., topical podophyllin, topical 5-fluorouacil [5-FU], and laser therapy). In patients with low-grade, early-stage lesions (T1) without any evidence of nodal involvement, local excision with wide margins may be acceptable if the sphincter function is preserved. However, for the patients with HIV anal carcinoma who present with more advanced T stages or nodal involvement, if treatment is to be definitive, chemoradiation (with 5-FU/mitomycin-C and radiation therapy as the standard of care in immunocompetent persons) is the treatment of choice when possible. Unfortunately, the administration of mitomycin-C to patients with advanced HIV may be associated with the potential for severe myelosuppression and hemolytic uremic syndrome, thus limiting its use in some patients. In early series, there was evidence that patients with HIV infection required longer breaks from chemoradiation because of severe skin reactions and almost uniformly required chemotherapy dose reductions because of neutropenia.[155,156–157] These toxicities led to various attempts to render treatment more tolerable in the setting of HIV.

In the early years of the AIDS epidemic, HIV-infected patients who had anal carcinoma appeared to have a shorter survival and a higher incidence of local failure as compared with non-HIV infected persons.[155,158] It appears that after the introduction of HAART, the outcome for persons with HIV-anal cancer improved.[159] Recent series have shown that with modern management, including intensity-modulated radiation therapy and growth factor support, hematologic toxicity in HIV patient was similar to immunocompetent patients.[160,161] Additionally, in selected patients, local control and survival rates may now approach those of the non-HIV population when 5-FU/mitomycin–based chemotherapy and full-dose RT is delivered.

Seo et al.[162] showed that at a median follow-up of 3 years, 14 HIV-infected patients had no differences in overall survival (91%) as compared with immunocompetent patients; disease-specific survival and colostomy-free survival were also similar. There were no differences in acute and late toxicity profiles between the two groups. In a multicentric cohort study comparing 40 HIV-positive patients with 81 HIV-negative patients treated for anal cancer, the 5-year overall survival was 61% and 65%, respectively; however, the local control was only 38% in the HIV-positive patients as compared with 87% in the HIV-negative patients.[163] In a series of 34 HIV-infected patients with anal carcinoma treated with various combinations of chemotherapy and irradiation, actuarial local control and overall survival at 3 years were 63% and 69%, respectively.[26] A series reported by Fraunholz et al.[160] from Germany described 21 HIV-positive patients who were receiving highly active antiretroviral therapy and who were treated with standard chemoradiation. Five patients required chemotherapy dose reduction and five patients required an interruption of RT. At a median follow-up of more than 4 years, the 5-year local control, cancer-specific, and overall survival rates were 59%, 75%, and 67%, respectively. There was one treatment-related death. The authors also noted that in the 3 to 7 weeks following completion of treatment, CD4 counts decreased, and one-third of patients experienced an increase in viral load. Thus, although standard chemoradiation should be considered in HIV-anal cancer, careful attention must be paid to immunologic parameters and risks of toxicity.

Newer strategies employing targeted agents, such as in an AIDS Malignancy Consortium phase II study employing cetuximab in addition to 5-FU, cisplatin, and radiation (1.8 Gy per fraction to a total of 45 Gy without a planned break), may improve the outcome of HIV-associated anal carcinoma.[164] This trial has accrued 45 patients and results are pending. However, it may be that, given an etiology similar to cervical carcinoma, a key to improving outcome in anal cancer would be to employ similar strategies as are used for cervical cancer with prevention and early diagnosis of mucosal abnormalities.[165] Rigorous surveillance for anal intraepithelial neoplasia with cytology and anoscopy in the population at risk should be considered,[166] and there is hope that widespread vaccination for HPV would be a major public health advance against anal cancer.

LUNG CANCER

The higher incidence of smoking in the HIV population has been a confounding variable in studies reporting an increased incidence of lung cancer in persons with HIV infection (HIV-LC),[167,168] however, after controlling for smoking, it appears that the rates of lung cancer are higher in HIV-infected than uninfected patients with large cohort studies and meta-analysis showing standardized incidence ratios of 2 to 4 for HIV-LC.[15,169,170]

The presentation of lung cancer in the HIV population is marked by young age at presentation (38–50 years) and advanced disease at diagnosis (75% of patients).[171] The most common subtype of non–small cell lung cancer in this group has been reported to be adenocarcinoma.[172]

In the pre-HAART the median survival of HIV-LC was only 4 to 5 months.[172,173–174] Case reports documented increased toxicity (particularly esophageal) in patients with HIV irradiated for lung cancer,[175] however, larger series do not necessarily report increased toxicity,[171] although doses of >60 Gy usually were not employed.

It is unclear as to whether combined antiretroviral therapy improves the outcome in these patients.[176] The largest cohort study in the HAART era included 30 patients, 27 of whom presented with stage IIB to IV disease. Although patients diagnosed with very early-stage disease could undergo surgery, the median survival was only 5 months for those with advanced disease.[177] How to incorporate antiretroviral drug regimens into lung cancer treatment regimens remains undefined. In general, an attempt should be made to deliver standard treatment based on the stage of the disease with the caveat that the treatment approach may need to be modified based on the patient's immunological status, viral load, and coexisting opportunistic infections.

HEAD AND NECK TUMORS

Given the increased smoking rate and HPV infection rate in persons with HIV, it would not be surprising to see an increased incidence of both squamous cell and HPV-related head and neck tumors in HIV-infected persons. Persons with HIV-AIDS have a threefold higher prevalence of oral HPV infection than the non-HIV population, and thus we may anticipate an increased incidence of HPV-associated oropharyngeal cancers in this population.[178] North American data provide some evidence that since the beginning of the HAART era, there has been an increased incidence of head and neck cancers in persons with HIV infection.[16] A recent report of a large European cohort of HIV-infected persons documented a trend in increasing incidence from the pre-HAART era through the present, but this did not reach statistical incidence.[18]

A recent review of carcinomas arising in the head and neck region in HIV-positive patients indicates that patients with HIV-AIDS are at an increased risk of developing mucosal squamous cell carcinoma, nasopharyngeal carcinoma, lymphoepithelial carcinoma of the salivary gland, and Merkel cell carcinoma.[179] This review also suggested that HIV-positive patients with these cancers present at a younger age, with more aggressive disease and worse prognosis compared to HIV-negative patients.

Case reports describing the treatment of head and neck malignancies in patients with HIV do not suggest the same increased mucosal sensitivity as is seen in patients with HIV-KS.[180,181] Larger series appear to corroborate this. Sanfilippo et al.[182] reported a series of 12 HIV-positive patients with squamous cell carcinoma of the head and neck who underwent irradiation. Median radiation dose was 66.4 Gy and median duration of treatment was 51 days. Nearly two-thirds of patients developed grade 3 toxicity, but only one patient developed grade 4 confluent moist desquamation. Similar results were reported by Klein et al.[27] Twelve HIV-infected patients received a median dose of 68 Gy for squamous cell carcinomas of the head and neck; half also received chemotherapy. Local-regional control at 3 years was estimated to be 92% and survival was estimated at 78%. Nearly half the patients required treatment breaks of more than 10 days, however, no hospitalizations or treatment-related fatalities occurred. Toxicity appeared comparable to historical controls as did tumor control. However, it must be remembered that these patients were a relatively "healthy" group of HIV-infected persons, with all having Karnofsky performance status of 80 or higher and a median CD4 count of 460.

There is a paucity of data examining the tolerance and outcome in HIV-infected persons treated with combined chemoradiation; however, there is some hope that biologic agents such as cetuximab, a monoclonal antibody already approved for use in combination with radiation therapy for the treatment of locally or regionally advanced squamous cell carcinoma of the head and neck, may offer a viable option for HIV-infected patients with locally advanced disease.[183]

LIVER CANCER

Increased levels of hepatitis B and C coinfections in the HIV population may explain the higher standardized incidence ratios of hepatocellular carcinoma reported in both North American and European datasets,[13,18] although the data are conflicting as to whether the incidence is higher for persons receiving combined antiretroviral therapy. The French have published on the feasibility of liver transplant for cirrhosis in persons with hepatitis and HIV,[184] but data on the treatment of hepatocellular carcinoma in the setting of HIV are lacking. A recent report detailing serious adverse effects in an HIV-positive patient who was also coinfected with HBV and treated with sorafenib reminds us that we have much to learn about potential interactions between the newer targeted agents for this disease and HAART.[185]

PROSTATE CANCER

Recent data have shown an increase in the number of cases of prostate cancer in HIV-infected persons.[11] From 1991–1995 to 2001–2005, estimated counts increased from 87 to 759 cancers, seemingly driven by growth and aging of the AIDS population. There are no data to support approaching prostate cancer any differently in an otherwise healthy HIV-infected man than in a non-HIV infected one.[186–188] Pantanowitz et al.[189] reported on 17 HIV-positive patients from multiple institutions treated for prostate cancer with various standard treatments, including surgery, hormonal therapy, and radiotherapy. No serious treatment-related side effects were reported. Ng et al.[190] reported a series of 14 HIV-positive patients with prostate cancer treated with external beam radiation therapy with or without brachytherapy at St. Vincent's Hospital in New York City. Following treatment, only one patient's prostate-specific antigen (PSA) level remained above 1.1 ng/mL, the average CD4 count remained stable, and the viral load increased in only 2 of 14 patients. There were no unusual complications, and no infections related to treatment. Silberstein et al.[191] reported on eight HIV-positive men who underwent robotic-assisted laparoscopic prostatectomy for treatment of prostate cancer. Preoperatively, all eight were on HAART and had undetectable viral loads.

HIV-positive men required more perioperative transfusions and had a higher incidence of perioperative ileus as compared with HIV-negative men. The PSA level in all eight HIV-positive patients remained undetectable at the short median follow-up time of 2.6 months. Thus, although long-term treatment outcomes in HIV-positive patients remain uncertain, early results suggest acceptable response rates and toxicities in HIV-negative patients treated with standard treatments.

PEDIATRIC MALIGNANCIES

A major triumph in the war against AIDS has been the virtual elimination of the vertical transmission of HIV in the developed world. However, in Africa, 1,000 babies still acquire the virus every day,[192] an appalling figure given that it has been more than 15 years since the first study that demonstrated the efficacy of zidovudine in reducing mother-to-child transmission of the virus.[193] Children who go on to develop AIDS appear to be at increased risk of developing tumors,[6] particularly NHL (Burkitt's lymphomas accounted for the most common histologic subtype), but also including leiomyosarcomas, primary CNS lymphomas, and KS.[194–195,196] The Pediatric Oncology Group reported 28 NHL, 4 B-cell acute lymphoblastic leukemias, 1 Hodgkin lymphoma, 8 leiomyosarcomas, 1 hepatoblastoma, and 1 schwannoma in a cohort of HIV-infected children.[197] Hopefully, the prevention of pediatric HIV ultimately will lead to a further decline in these cancers.

It appears that HAART has decreased the incidence of pediatric HIV malignancies.[198,199] In a study of more than 5,000 children who were under 15 years of at the time they were diagnosed as having AIDS, cancer was 40 times more frequent in children with HIV than in the general population in the pre-HAART era, as compared with 17 times more frequent in the HAART era.[200]

SUMMARY

HIV infection fosters immunosuppression, and immunosuppression fosters the appearance of malignancies. Progress requires therapies that counteract the immunosuppression associated with HIV infection. HAART appears to have decreased the incidence of KS and PCNSL; however, there appears to be an increase in many non-AIDS-defining malignancies in HIV-infected persons in the era of HAART. Data regarding the influence of HAART on prognosis of malignancies remain difficult to interpret, with some studies claiming improved survival and others claim no influence. Furthermore, even in areas where HAART is widely available, individual patients may not access or comply with treatment, and, if general adherence to or effectiveness of therapy is poor, the overall immune status of the population will remain low, and, consequently, there will be no decline in the incidence of HIV-associated malignancies. Although HAART has dramatically changed the face of AIDS, major challenges, not the least of which is the emergence of viral resistance, unfortunately ensure that improvements in the treatment of AIDS-associated malignancies will continue to be needed. Ultimately, the key to eradicating AIDS-associated malignancies will lie in the prevention of HIV transmission.

SELECTED REFERENCES

A full list of references for this chapter is available online.

2. Centers for Disease Control. Kaposi's sarcoma and pneumocystis pneumonia among homosexual men—New York City and California. *Morb Mortal Wkly Rep* 1981;30:305–308.
3. Centers for Disease Control. Revision of the case definition of acquired immunodeficiency syndrome for national reported: United States. *Ann Intern Med* 1985; 103:402–403.
4. Centers for Disease Control. 1993 revised classification system for HIV infection and expanded surveillance case definition for AIDS among adolescents and adults. *JAMA* 1993;269:729–730.
5. Frisch M, Biggar RJ, Engels EA, et al. For the AIDS-Cancer Match Registry Study Group. Association of cancer with AIDS-related immunosuppression in adults. *JAMA* 2001;85:1736–1745.
6. Biggar RJ, Frisch M, Goedert JJ. For the AIDS-Cancer Match Registry Group. Risk of cancer in children with AIDS. *JAMA* 2000;284:205–209.
8. Engels EA, Biggar RJ, Hall HI, et al. Cancer risk in people infected with human immunodeficiency virus in the United States. *Int J Cancer* 2008;123:187–194.
11. Shiels MS, Pfeiffer RM, MH Gail, et al. Cancer burden in the HIV-infected population in the United States. *J Natl Cancer Inst* 2011;103:753–762.
12. Seaberg EC, Wiley D, Martínez-Maza O, et al. Cancer incidence in the multicenter AIDS cohort study before and during the HAART era: 1984 to 2007. *Cancer* 2010; 116:5507–5516.
13. Bedimo RJ, McGinnis KA, Dunlap M, et al. Incidence of non-AIDS-defining malignancies in HIV-infected versus noninfected patients in the HAART era: impact of immunosuppression. *J Acquir Immune Defic Syndr* 2009;52:203–208.
14. Clifford GM, Polesol J, Rickenbach M, et al. Cancer in the Swiss HIV cohort study: association with immunodeficiency, smoking, and highly active antiretroviral therapy. *J Natl Cancer Inst* 2005;97:425–432.
18. Powles T, Robinson D, Stebbing J, et al. Highly active antiretroviral therapy and the incidence of non-AIDS-defining cancers in people with HIV infection. *J Clin Oncol* 2008;27:884–890.
22. See AP, Zeng J, Tran PT, et al. Acute toxicity of second generation HIV protease-inhibitors in combination with radiotherapy: a retrospective case series. *Radiat Oncol* 2011;6:25.
23. Baeyens A, Slabbert JP, Willem P, et al. Chromosomal radiosensitivity of HIV positive individuals. *Int J Radiat Biol* 2010;86:584–592.
24. Kaminuma T, Karasawa K, Hanyu N, et al. Acute adverse effects of radiation therapy on HIV-positive patients in Japan: study of 31 cases at Tokyo Metropolitan Komagome Hospital. *J Radiat Res* 2010;51:749–753.
25. Mallik S, Talapatra K, Goswami J. AIDS: a radiation oncologist's perspective. *J Cancer Res Ther* 2010;6:432–441.
26. Hauerstock D, Ennis RD, Grossbard M, et al. Efficacy and toxicity of chemoradiation in the treatment of HIV-associated anal cancer. *Clin Colorectal Cancer* 2010;9:238–242.
27. Klein EA, Guiou M, Farwell G, et al. Primary radiation therapy for head-and-neck cancer in the setting of human immunodeficiency virus. *Int J Radiat Oncol Biol Phys* 2011;79:60–64.
28. Housri N, Yarchoan R, Kaushal A. Radiotherapy for patients with the human immunodeficiency virus: are special precautions necessary? *Cancer* 2010;116: 273–283.
29. Beral V, Peterman T, Berkleman R, et al. AIDS-associated non-Hodgkin's lymphoma. *Lancet* 1991;337:805–809.
31. Centers for Disease Control. Update on acquired immune deficiency syndrome (AIDS)—United States. *Morb Mortal Wkly Rep* 1981;31:507–514.
35. Diamond C, Taylor TH, Aboumrad T, et al. Changes in acquired immunodeficiency syndrome-related non-Hodgkin lymphoma in the era of highly active antiretroviral therapy. *Cancer* 2006;106:128–135.
36. Donahue B, Cooper J, Rush S, et al. Results of empiric radiotherapy for HIV associated primary CNS lymphomas. *Int J Rad Oncol Biol Phys* 1989;17(Suppl abstr 1028):223.
37. Donahue BR, Sullivan JW, Cooper JS. Additional experience with empiric radiotherapy for HIV-associated primary CNS lymphoma. *Cancer* 1995;76:328–332.
40. Corn BW, Trock BJ, Curran WJ. Management of primary central nervous system lymphoma for the patient with acquired immunodeficiency syndrome. *Cancer* 1995;76:163–166.
49. Ambinder RF, Lee S, Curran WJ, et al. Phase II intergroup trial of sequential chemotherapy and radiotherapy for AIDS-Related primary central nervous system lymphoma. *Cancer Ther* 2003;1:215–221.
50. Jacomet C, Girard PM, Lebrette MG, et al. Intravenous methotrexate for primary central nervous system non-Hodgkin's lymphoma in AIDS. *AIDS* 1997;11: 1725–1730.
51. Diamond C, Taylor TH, Im T, et al. Highly active antiretroviral therapy is associated with improved survival among patients with AIDS-related primary central nervous system non-Hodgkin's lymphoma. *Curr HIV Res* 2006;4:375–378.
52. Baumgartner JE, Rachlin JR, Beckstead JH, et al. Primary central nervous system lymphomas: natural history: response to radiation therapy in 55 patients with acquired immunodeficiency syndrome. *J Neurosurg* 1990;73:206–211.
53. Corn BW, Donahue BR, Rosenstock JG, et al. Palliation of AIDS-related primary lymphoma of the brain: observations from a multi-institutional database. *Int J Rad Oncol Biol Phys* 1997;38:601–605.
54. Formenti SC, Gill PS, Lean E, et al. Primary central nervous system lymphoma in AIDS—results of radiation therapy. *Cancer* 1989;63:1101–1107.
56. Kasamon YL, Ambinder RF. AIDS-related primary central nervous system lymphoma. *Hematol Oncol Clin North Am* 2005;19:665–687.
57. Ling SM, Roach M, Larson DA, et al. Radiotherapy of primary central nervous system lymphoma in patients with and without human immunodeficiency virus—ten years of treatment experience at the University of California San Francisco. *Cancer* 1994;73:2570–2582.
59. Nagai H, Odawara T, Ajisawa A, et al. Whole brain radiation alone produces favourable outcomes for AIDS-related primary central nervous system lymphoma in the HAART era. *Eur J Haematol* 2010;84:499–505.
60. Kreisl TN, Panageas KS, Elkin EB, et al. Treatment patterns and prognosis in patients with human immunodeficiency virus and primary central system lymphoma. *Leuk Lymphoma* 2008;49:1710–1716.
61. Skiest DJ, Crosby C. Survival is prolonged by highly active antiretroviral therapy in AIDS patients with primary central nervous system lymphoma. *AIDS* 2003; 17:1787–1793.
63. Newell E, Hoy JF, Cooper SG, et al. Human immunodeficiency virus-related primary central nervous system lymphoma: factors influencing survival in 111 patients. *Cancer* 2004;100:2627–2636.
64. Aboulafia DM, Ratner L, Miles SA, et al., and AIDS Associated Malignancies Clinical Trials Consortium. Antiviral and immunomodulatory treatment for AIDS-related primary central nervous system lymphoma: AIDS Malignancies Consortium pilot study 019. *Clin Lymphoma Myeloma* 2006;6:399–402.
67. Huhn GD, Badri S, Vibhakar S, et al. Early development of non-Hodgkin lymphoma following initiation of newer class antiretroviral therapy among HIV-infected patients—implications for immune reconstitution. *AIDS Res Ther* 2010; 7:44.

68. Jaffe HW, De Stavola BL, Carpenter LM, et al. Immune reconstitution and risk of Kaposi sarcoma and non-Hodgkin lymphoma in HIV-infected adults. *AIDS* 2011;25:1395–1403.
76. Kaplan LD, Lee JY, Ambinder RF, et al. Rituximab does not improve clinical outcome in a randomized phase 3 trial of CHOP with or without rituximab in patients with HIV-associated non-Hodgkin lymphoma: AIDS-Malignancies Consortium Trial 010. *Blood* 2005;106:1538–1543.
77. Boue F, Gabarre J, Gisselbrecht C, et al. Phase II trial of CHOP plus rituximab in patients with HIV-associated non-Hodgkin's lymphoma. *J Clin Oncol* 2006;24: 4123–4128.
79. Sparano JA, Lee JY, Kaplan LD, et al. Rituximab plus concurrent infusional EPOCH is highly effective in HIV-associated B-cell non-Hodgkin lymphoma. *Blood* 2010;115:3008–3016.
81. Mazhar D, Stebbing J, Bower M. Non-Hodgkin's lymphoma and the CNS: prophylaxis and therapy in immunocompetent and HIV-positive individuals. *Expert Rev Anticancer Ther* 2006;6:335–341.
83. Jaffe ES. Primary body cavity-based AIDS-related lymphomas. Evolution of a new disease entity. *Am J Clin Pathol* 1996;105:141–143.
84. Simonelli C, Spina M, Cinella R, et al. Clinical features and outcome of primary effusion lymphoma in HIV-infected patients: a single-institution study. *J Clin Oncol* 2003;21:3948–3954.
86. Spano JP, Costagliola D, Katlama C, et al. AIDS-related malignancies: state of the art and therapeutic challenges. *J Clin Oncol* 2008;26:4834–4842.
87. Sparano, JA. HIV-associated lymphoma: the evidence for treating aggressively but with caution. *Curr Opin Oncol* 2007;19:458–463.
89. Swift PS. Radiation therapy for malignancies in the setting of HIV disease. *Oncology* 1997;11:683–694.
90. Chamberlain MC, Dirr L. Involved-field radiotherapy and intra-ommaya methotrexate/cytarabine in patients with AIDS-related lymphomatous meningitis. *J Clin Oncol* 1993;11:1978–1984.
96. Bower M, Gazzard B, Mandalia S, et al. A prognostic index for systemic AIDS-related non-Hodgkin lymphoma treated in the era of highly active antiretroviral therapy. *Ann Intern Med* 2005;143:265–273.
97. Chao C, Xu L, Abrams D, et al. Survival of non-Hodgkin lymphoma patients with and without HIV infection in the era of combined antiretroviral therapy. *AIDS* 2010;24:1765–1770.
105. Tsimberidou AM, Sarris AH, Medeiros LJ, et al. Hodgkin's disease in patients infected with human immunodeficiency virus: frequency, presentation and clinical outcome. *Leuk Lymphoma* 2001;41:535–544.
106. Biggar RJ, Jaffe ES, Goedert JJ, et al. Hodgkin lymphoma and immunodeficiency in persons with HIV/AIDS. *Blood* 2006;108:3786–3791.
107. Spina M, Gabarre J, Rossi G, et al. Stanford V regimen and concomitant HAART in 59 patients with Hodgkin disease and HIV infection. *Blood* 2002;100:1984–1988.
108. Hentrich M, Berger M, Hoffman C, et al. HIV-associated Hodgkin's lymphoma (HIV-HL): results of a prospective multicenter trial. *J Clin Oncol* 2010;28(15 Suppl): 8035.
112. Chang Y, Cesarman E, Pessin MS, et al. Identification of herpesvirus-like DNA sequences in AIDS-associated Kaposi's sarcoma. *Science* 1994;266:1865–1869.
115. Aversa SM, Cattelan AM, Salvango L, et al. Treatments of AIDS-related Kaposi's sarcoma. *Crit Rev Oncol Hematol* 2005;53:253–265.
116. Bower M, Weir J, Francis N, et al. The effect of HAART in 254 consecutive patients with AIDS-related Kaposi's sarcoma. *AIDS* 2009;23:1701–1706.
117. Bower M, Nelson M, Young AM, et al. Immune reconstitution inflammatory syndrome associated with Kaposi's sarcoma. *J Clin Oncol* 2005;23:5224–5228.
121. Gill PS, Wernz J, Scadden D, et al. Randomized phase III trial of liposomal daunorubicin versus doxorubicin, bleomycin, and vincristine in AIDS-related Kaposi's sarcoma. *J Clin Oncol* 1996;14:2353–2364.
123. Gill PS, Tulpule A, Espina BM, et al. Paclitaxel is safe and effective in the treatment of advanced AIDS-related Kaposi's sarcoma. *J Clin Oncol* 1999;17:1876–1883.
126. Cooper JS, Steinfeld AS, Lerch IA. The prognostic significance of residual pigmentation following radiotherapy of epidemic Kaposi's sarcoma. *J Clin Oncol* 1989; 7:619–621.
127. Cooper J, Steinfeld A, Lerch, I. Intentions and outcomes in the radiotherapeutic management of epidemic Kaposi's sarcoma. *Int J Radiation Oncology Biol Phys* 1991;20:419–422.
128. Stelzer KJ, Griffin TW. A randomized prospective trial of radiation therapy for AIDS-associated Kaposi's sarcoma. *Int J Radiat Oncol Biol Phys* 1993;27: 1057–1061.
129. Berson AM, Quivey JM, Harris JW, et al. Radiation therapy for AIDS-related Kaposi's sarcoma. *Int J Radiat Oncol Biol Phys* 1990;19:569–575.
130. Cooper JS, Fried PR. Toxicity of oral radiotherapy in patients having AIDS. *Arch Otolaryngol* 1987;113:327–328.
131. Piedbois P, Frikha H, Martin L, et al. Radiotherapy in the management of epidemic Kaposi's sarcoma. *Int J Radiat Oncol Biol Phys* 1994;30:1207–1211.
133. Chirenje ZM. HIV and cancer of the cervix. *Best Pract Res Clin Obstet Gynaecol* 2005;19:269–276.
136. Chaturvedi AK, Madeleine MM, Biggar RJ, et al. Risk of human papillomavirus-associated cancers among persons with AIDS. *J Natl Cancer Inst* 2009;101: 1120–1130.
142. Minkoff H, Zhong Y, Burk RD, et al. Influence of adherent and effective antiretroviral therapy use on human papillomavirus infection and squamous intraepithelial lesions in human immunodeficiency virus-positive women. *J Infect Dis* 2010; 201:681–690.
146. Chadha M, Sood B, Stanson R. Patients with human immunodeficiency virus (HIV): infections and cervical neoplasia. *Int J Rad Oncol Biol Phys* 1984;30(S1): 284.
147. Shrivastava SK, Engineer R, Rajadhyaksha S, et al. HIV infection and invasive cervical cancers, treatment with radiation therapy: toxicity and outcome. *Radiother Oncol* 2005;74:31–35.
148. Gichangi P, Bwayo J, Estimable B, et al. HIV impact on acute morbidity and pelvic tumor control following radiotherapy for cervical cancer. *Gynecol Oncol* 2006;100:405–411.
149. Massad LS, Seaberg EC, Watts DH, et al. Long-term incidence of cervical cancer in women with human immunodeficiency virus. *Cancer* 2009;115:524–530.
153. Berry JM, Palefsky JM, Welton ML. Anal cancer and its precursors in HIV-positive patients: perspectives and management. *Surg Oncol Clin North Am* 2004;13: 355–373.
156. Holland JM, Swift PS. Tolerance of patients with human immunodeficiency virus and anal carcinoma to treatment with combined chemotherapy and radiation therapy. *Radiology* 1994;193:251–254.
157. Kim JH, Sarani B, Orkin BA, et al. HIV-positive patients with anal carcinoma have poorer treatment tolerance and outcome than HIV-negative patients. *Dis Colon Rectum* 2001;44:1496–1502.
159. Barriger RB, Calley C, Cárdenes HR. Treatment of anal carcinoma in immune-compromised patients. *Clin Transl Oncol* 2009;11:609–614.
160. Fraunholz I, Weiss C, Eberlein K, et al. Concurrent chemoradiotherapy with 5-fluorouracil and mitomycin c for invasive anal carcinoma in human immunodeficiency virus-positive patients receiving highly active antiretroviral therapy. *Int J Radiat Oncol Biol Phys* 2010;76:1425–1432.
161. Salama JK, Mell LK, Schomas DA, et al. Concurrent chemotherapy and intensity-modulated radiation therapy for anal canal cancer patients: a multicenter experience. *J Clin Oncol* 2007;25:4581–4586.
162. Seo Y, Kinsella MT, Reynolds HL, et al. Outcomes of chemoradiotherapy with 5-fluorouracil and mitomycin C for anal cancer in immunocompetent versus immunodeficient patients. *Int J Radiat Oncol Biol Phys* 2009;75:143–149.
163. Oehler-Jänne C, Huguet F, Provencher S, et al. HIV-specific differences in outcome of squamous cell carcinoma of the anal canal: a multicentric cohort study of HIV-positive patients receiving highly active antiretroviral therapy. *J Clin Oncol* 2008;26:2550–2557.
165. Chiao EY, Giordano TP, Palefsky JM, et al. Screening HIV-infected individuals for anal cancer precursor lesions: a systematic review. *Clin Infect Dis* 2006;43: 223–233.
167. Cadranel J, Garfield D, Lavole A, et al. Lung cancer in HIV infected patients: facts, questions and challenges. *Thorax* 2006;61:1000–1008.
169. Grulich AE, van Leeuwen MT, Falster MO, et al. Incidence of cancers in people with HIV/AIDS compared with immunosuppressed transplant recipients: a meta-analysis. *Lancet* 2007;370:59–67.
171. Spano JP, Massiani MA, Bentata M, et al. Lung cancer in patients with HIV Infection and review of the literature. *Med Oncol* 2004;21:109–115.
172. Tirelli U, Spina M, Sandri S, et al. Lung carcinoma in 36 patients with human immunodeficiency virus infection. The Italian Cooperative Group on AIDS and tumors. *Cancer* 2000;88:563–569.
175. Leigh BR, Lau DH. Severe esophageal toxicity after thoracic radiation therapy for lung cancer associated with the human immunodeficiency virus: a case report and review of the literature. *Am J Clin Oncol* 1998;21:479–481.
177. Hakimian R, Fang H, Thomas L, et al. Lung cancer in HIV-infected patients in the era of highly active antiretroviral therapy. *J Thorac Oncol* 2007;2:268–272.
179. Purgina B, Pantanowitz L, Seethala RR. A review of carcinomas arising in the head and neck region in HIV-positive patients. *Patholog Res Int* 2011;2011: 469150.
182. Sanfilippo NJ, Mitchell J, Grew D, et al. Toxicity of head-and-neck radiation therapy in human immunodeficiency virus-positive patients. *Int J Radiat Oncol Biol Phys* 2010;77:1375–1379.
186. Levinson A, Nagler EA, Lowe FC. Approach to management of clinically localized prostate cancer in patients with human immunodeficiency virus. *Urology* 2005;65:91–94.
187. O'Connor JK, Nedzi LA, Zakris EL. Prostate adenocarcinoma and human immunodeficiency virus: report of 3 cases and review of the literature. *Clin Genitourin Cancer* 2006;5:85–88.
188. Wosnitzer MS, Lowe FC. Management of prostate cancer in HIV-positive patients. *Nat Rev Urol* 2010;7:348–357.
189. Pantanowitz L, Bohac G, Cooley TP, et al. Human immunodeficiency virus-associated prostate cancer: clinicopathological findings and outcome in a multi-institutional study. *BJU Int* 2008;101:1519–1523.
190. Ng T, Stein NF, Kaminetsky J, et al. Preliminary results of radiation therapy for prostate cancer in human immunodeficiency virus-positive patients. *Urology* 2008;72:1135–1138.
196. Granovsky MO, Mueller BU, Nicholson HS, et al. Cancer in human immunodeficiency virus infected children: a case series from the Children's Cancer Group and the National Cancer Institute. *J Clin Oncol* 1988;16:1729–1735.
199. Nachman SA, Chernoff M, Gona P, et al. Incidence of noninfectious conditions in perinatally HIV-infected children and adolescents in the HAART era. *Arch Pediatr Adolesc Med* 2009;163:164–171.

Part C Central Nervous System

Chapter 35
Primary Intracranial Neoplasms

Vinai Gondi, Michael A. Vogelbaum, Sean Grimm, and Minesh P. Mehta

ANATOMY

The central nervous system (CNS) is enveloped by three meningeal layers: the *dura mater* (also known as the pachymeninges), the *arachnoid mater*, and the *pia mater*. The pia and arachnoid layers are also referred to as the leptomeninges, and within them is the subarachnoid space, which is filled with cerebrospinal fluid (CSF). Dural folds separate the two hemispheres of the cerebrum (falx cerebri) and the cerebrum from the cerebellum and brainstem (tentorium or falx cerebelli). The frontal and parietal lobes are separated by a well-defined sulcus ("central sulcus"). The frontal and temporal lobes are separated by the Sylvian fissure, and the parietal and occipital lobes are separated by the calcarine sulcus (Fig. 35.1).

The diencephalon consists of the thalamus and the pineal region and is situated between the cerebrum and the mesencephalon, adjacent to the third ventricle. Lateral to the thalamus is the internal capsule, which carries the motor fibers (upper motor neurons) from the cortex en route to the brainstem and spinal cord.

At the tentorial notch, the mesencephalon rides on the upper part of the clivus. Its interior, the tectum, is partially occupied by cranial nerve nuclei (for the oculomotor, trochlear, and proprioceptive portions of the trigeminal nerves). The dorsal plate houses the superior and inferior colliculi, which regulate eye movements and hearing impulses, respectively. The trochlear nerve is the only cranial nerve that exits from this dorsal location.

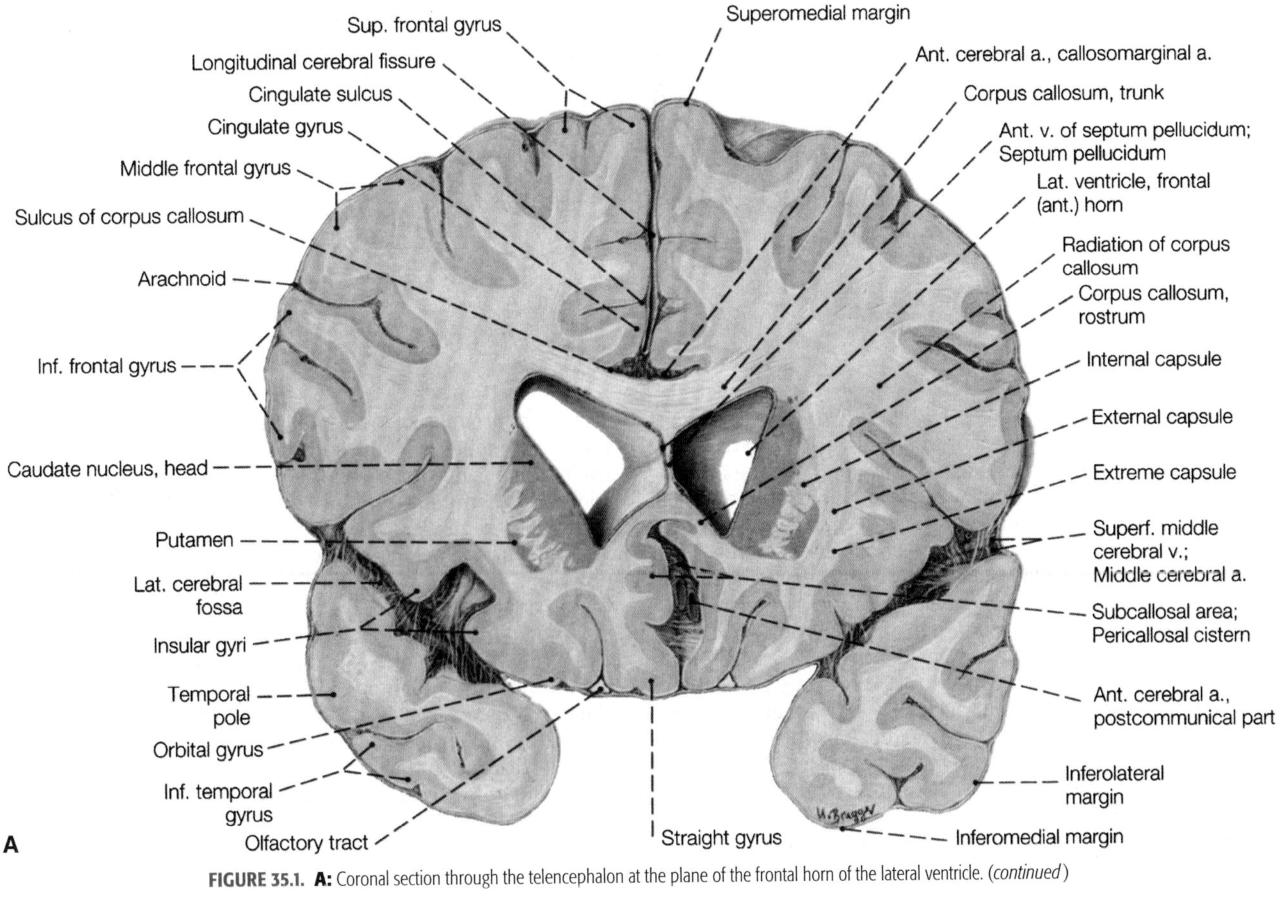

FIGURE 35.1. A: Coronal section through the telencephalon at the plane of the frontal horn of the lateral ventricle. (*continued*)

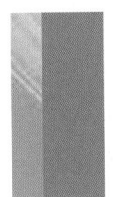

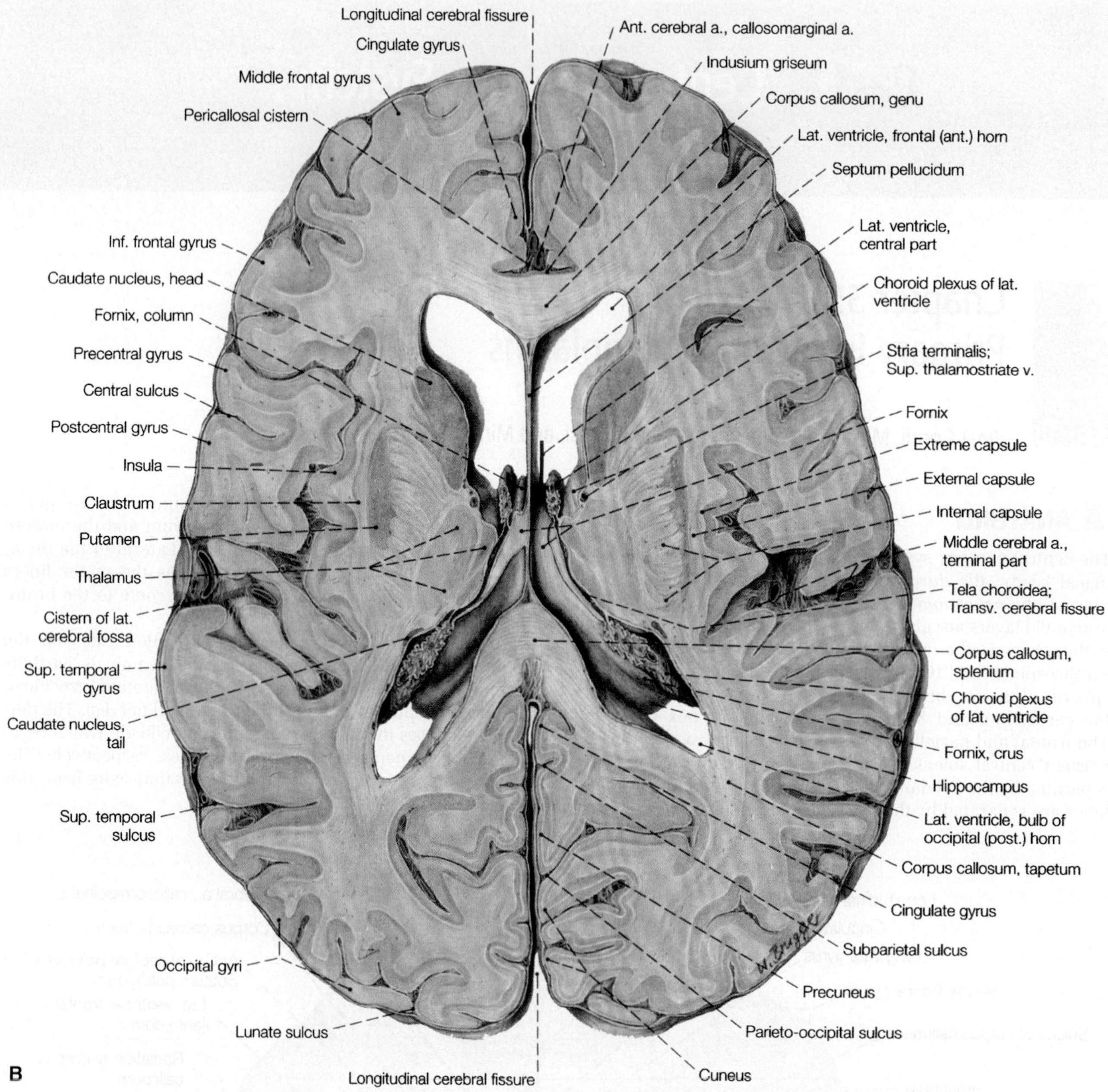

FIGURE 35.1. *(continued)* **B:** Transverse section at the level of the floor of the central part of the lateral ventricle. View of the superior surface of the plane of sectioning.

The pons relays information between the two cerebellar hemispheres and from the spinal cord to the cerebellum, carries the major ascending and descending pathways between the mesencephalon and the medulla oblongata, and contains the major motor and tactile sensory nuclei for the trigeminal nerve, which emerges from its lateral surface. The border between the pons and the medulla oblongata is noteworthy for the emergence of the abducens, facial, and vestibulocochlear (acoustic) cranial nerves.

The cerebellum develops laterally and posteriorly from the pons and differentiates into the median vermis cerebelli and the bilateral hemispheres, which are flattened by the sloping tentorium on both sides. Anteriorly, the cerebellum faces the dorsal aspects of the pons and the medulla oblongata (the floor of the fourth ventricle).

The medulla oblongata forms the link between the pons, the spinal cord, and the cerebellum. It houses the majority of the cranial nerve nuclei (abducens, facial, vestibulocochlear, glossopharyngeal, vagal, accessory, and hypoglossal).

CSF is produced by the choroid plexus, which lies in the roofs of the fourth and third ventricles, as well as in the medial walls of the central body and inferior horns of the lateral ventricles. The foramina of Munro transmit CSF between the third and lateral ventricles at the superolateral corners of the third ventricle. The aqueduct of Sylvius in the midbrain transmits CSF from the third to the fourth ventricles. It is the narrowest canal of the intracranial nervous system and is therefore the most common location of obstruction of flow by compression or tumor deposits, resulting in noncommunicating (obstructive) hydrocephalus. CSF in the fourth ventricle flows out of the ventricular system through the midline foramen of Magendie and the two lateral foramina of Luschka to the subarachnoid space.

CSF resorption back into the venous system occurs at arachnoid (or Pacconian) granulations—special outpouching structures from the arachnoid membrane that enhance fluid movement from the CSF space into the venous sinus system. Scarring from infection or inflammation or clogging of the

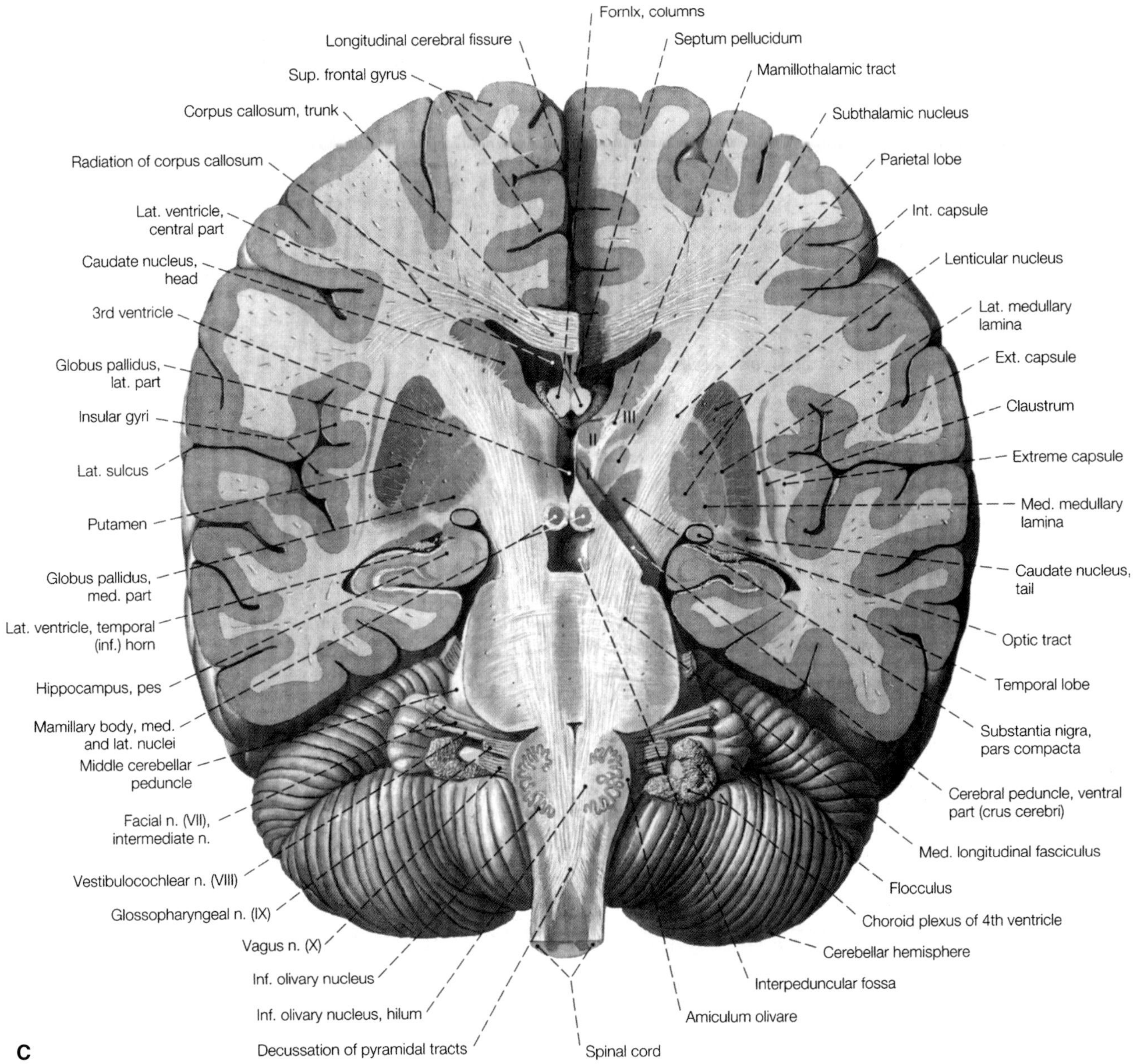

C

FIGURE 35.1. *(continued)* **C:** Section through telencephalon and brainstem parallel with the cerebral peduncles. View of the posterior surface of the plane of sectioning. On the right side of the figure, the section reaches back to approximately the middle of the cerebral peduncle (oblique section). I to III indicate thalamic nuclei: I, medial nucleus; II, anterior nucleus; III, lateral nucleus. (A to C, from Sobotta J, Figge FHJ. *Atlas of human anatomy,* Vol. 2, 9th ed. Munich, Germany: Urban & Schwarzenberg, 1977. © Urban & Schwarzenberg, with permission.)

arachnoid granulations causes increased pressure in the CSF space and communication hydrocephalus.

EPIDEMIOLOGY

In 2010, there were an estimated 22,020 new cases of primary CNS tumors in the United States and 13,140 deaths,[1] for an incidence of approximately 6.5 per 100,000 persons. The incidence of brain tumors increases with age to reach 50 per 100,000 at age >75 years.[1]

Occupational and environmental exposures have been associated with the development of CNS tumors. Farmers and petrochemical workers have been shown to have a higher incidence of primary brain tumors. A variety of chemical exposures have been linked, as reviewed by Ohgaki and Kleihues.[2] The use of cellular phones has been questioned as a contributing factor to the development of brain tumors. The World Health Organization (WHO) recently classified radiofrequency electromagnetic fields, such as those emitted by wireless phones, as "possibly carcinogenic to humans" (group 2B) based on limited clinical evidence.[3] Although prior cohort, case–control, and time–trend analyses showed no association between cell phone use and brain tumor risk,[4–6] more recent case–control studies suggested a potential increased risk of glioma among individuals with the greatest cumulative lifetime cell phone use (≥ more hours in one study, >2,000 hours in another).[7,8] However, significant concerns with respect to recall and selection biases in both studies prevent a causal association from being concluded.

Prior exposure to ionizing radiation is a known risk factor for development of primary CNS tumors, particularly meningiomas, but also gliomas, sarcomas, and other tumor types.[9] There is a 2.3% incidence of primary brain tumors in children treated with prophylactic cranial irradiation for acute leukemia, a 22-fold increase over expected.[10,11]

Development of intracranial malignancy is also associated with several hereditary diseases, such as neurofibromatosis types 1 and 2, von Hippel-Lindau disease, and tuberous sclerosis. Other hereditary associations are with retinoblastoma and Li-Fraumeni syndrome.

NATURAL HISTORY

The natural history of a primary brain neoplasm is determined by its histology, grade, and location. The majority of adult gliomas spread invasively without forming a natural capsule. They frequently cause edema in surrounding tissue. This edema is usually vasogenic but may be ischemic or cytotoxic. It is seen best on T2-weighted magnetic resonance imaging (MRI) and is responsible for at least some of the clinical symptoms and signs. The edema is a consequence of altered blood–brain barrier (BBB) permeability. Different tumors cause varying amounts of edema (in descending order: metastases, astrocytomas, meningiomas, and oligodendrogliomas).

Some high-grade neoplasms metastasize by "seeding" the subarachnoid and ventricular spaces. Because of gravity or flow, these metastatic deposits are often present in the caudal portion of the spinal canal. Tumors that have a propensity for CSF spread include medulloblastomas, primitive neuroectodermal tumors (PNETs), and CNS lymphoma. The exact frequency of CSF spread among other histologies (e.g., germ cell tumors, ependymomas) is debated in the literature. Extracranial metastases from primary brain tumors are rare but can occur with medulloblastomas, germinomas, and high-grade astrocytomas.

CLINICAL PRESENTATION

The presenting symptoms of a primary brain tumor are classified as generalized or focal. Headache is more prevalent in patients with fast-growing, high-grade tumors. Seizures are a more common presenting feature in low-grade tumors. Focal neurologic deficits such as weakness, language dysfunction, or sensory loss are more frequent presentations of high-grade tumors. Acute events such as hemorrhage markedly alter the tempo of symptom onset regardless of tumor grade. Table 35.1 summarizes common clinical presentations of the more common CNS tumors.

Because brain parenchyma is anesthetic, headaches associated with brain tumors are due to increased intracranial pressure or to local pressure on sensitive intracranial structures (mainly dura and vessels). Headaches associated with increased intracranial pressure classically occur in the morning. Associated findings may include focal neurologic deficits, behavioral changes, and papilledema. Cushing's triad is classically associated with increased intracranial pressure, but the full triad (hypertension, bradycardia, respiratory irregularity) is seen in only one-third of the cases of increased intracranial pressure. Long-standing increases in intracranial pressure may lead to optic atrophy and blindness because of transmission of the pressure to the optic nerves.

DIAGNOSTIC WORKUP

The initial workup of patients with brain tumors must include a complete history and physical examination. Information obtained from relatives and friends is helpful because many tumors cause changes in mentation not appreciated by the patient. In patients with symptoms, signs, or imaging suggestive of systemic dissemination, biopsy confirmation of the primary tumor or at least one of the extracranial metastatic sites is recommended. Solitary brain lesions in adult patients with certain types of known systemic cancer (e.g., lung, breast, or colon cancers or melanoma) are far more likely to be a cerebral metastasis than a primary CNS tumor, although this is not always the case.

Imaging Studies

MRI with a gadolinium-containing contrast agent is the imaging modality of choice for most CNS tumors. Computed tomography (CT) is generally reserved for those situations in which

TABLE 35.1 SYMPTOMS, SIGNS, AND DIAGNOSTIC CHARACTERISTICS OF VARIOUS INTRACRANIAL TUMORS

Tumor	*Common Symptoms*	*Common Signs*	*Imaging Characteristics*
Glioblastoma multiforme	Headache, seizure, unilateral weakness, mental changes	Focal presentation related to tumor location	Enhancing MRI or CT lesion, hypodense interior, often with associated edema
Meningioma	Localized headache	Focal presentation related to tumor location	Enhancing MRI or CT lesion associated with dura
Astrocytoma	Headache, seizure, unilateral weakness, mental changes	Focal presentation related to tumor location	May not enhance on CT or MRI
Cerebral	Headache, seizure, unilateral weakness, mental changes	Focal presentation related to tumor location	
Cerebellar	Occipital headache	Increased intracranial pressure (i.e., papilledema), abducens and oculomotor nerve deficits; coordination	
Brainstem or thalamus	Nausea, vomiting, ataxia	Increased intracranial pressure (i.e., papilledema), abducens and oculomotor nerve deficits; ataxia	May be seen only on MRI
Optic nerve	Ocular changes	Ocular changes	Uniform enhancement on MRI or CT scan
Medulloblastoma	Morning headaches, nausea, vomiting	Coordination, increased intracranial pressure (i.e., papilledema), abducens and oculomotor nerve deficits	Heterogeneously enhancing on MRI or CT, typical lateral location in adults
Ependymoma	Morning headaches, nausea, vomiting	Coordination, increased intracranial pressure (i.e., papilledema), abducens and oculomotor nerve deficits	Heterogeneous enhancement on MRI or CT with or without calcification
Neurilemoma, schwannoma, neurinomas	Unilateral deafness, vertigo	Ipsilateral acoustic and facial or trigeminal nerve deficits	Homogeneous enhancing mass on MRI or CT, arising from cranial nerve
Oligodendroglioma	Insidious headache, mental changes	Focal presentation related to tumor location	Heterogeneous lesion that may or may not enhance on MRI or CT, frequently with calcification, cystic regions, or hemorrhage
Lymphoma	Focal presentation related to tumor location	Focal presentation related to tumor location	Homogeneous, intense enhancement on MRI, may have a diffuse or "cotton wool" appearance
Craniopharyngioma	Headache, mental changes, hemiplegia, seizure, vomiting, visual impairment	Cranial nerve deficits (II–VII)	Mixed cystic, calcified lesion on MRI and CT, arising from suprasellar region

CT, computed tomography; MRI, magnetic resonance imaging.

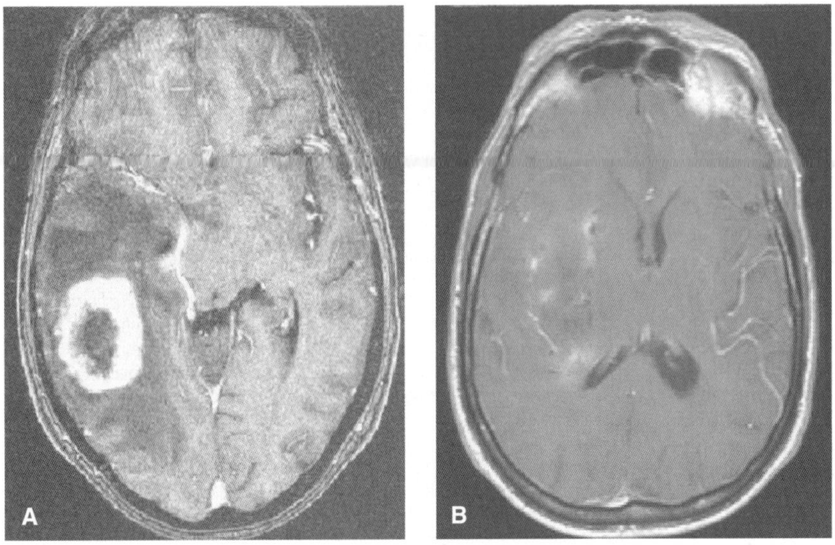

FIGURE 35.2. Magnetic resonance image of brain showing **(A)** glioblastoma, demonstrating a contrast-enhancing lesion with central necrosis and vasogenic edema, and **(B)** low-grade glioma, illustrating a nonenhancing lesion difficult to delineate from normal parenchyma.

MRI is contraindicated, such as implanted pacemaker, metal fragment, or paramagnetic surgical clips, or where there is a need to image the extent of calcification or hemorrhage.

Magnetic Resonance Imaging

The most useful imaging studies are T1-weighted sagittal images, gadolinium (Gd)-enhanced (usually obtained in high-resolution modes such as spoiled gradient echo or magnetization-prepared rapid gradient echo) and unenhanced T1 axial images, T2-weighted axial images, and fluid-attenuated inversion recovery (FLAIR) sequences. As is the case with CT contrast agents, gadolinium-based contrast leaks into parenchyma in areas with BBB breakdown, and the paramagnetic properties of gadolinium generate hyperintense signal on T1 scans. T1 images usually are better at demonstrating anatomy and areas of contrast enhancement. T2 and FLAIR images are more sensitive for detecting edema and infiltrative tumor. Tumor appearance on T1-weighted MRI is similar to that on CT, although tumor volumes are better delineated on MRI, particularly with low-grade neoplasms that do not demonstrate contrast enhancement (Fig. 35.2). With the increasing incidence of posttreatment "pseudoprogression," additional specialized diffusion, perfusion, and spectroscopic sequences are being increasingly used to distinguish tumor from necrosis or pseudoprogression, and positron emission tomography (PET) imaging may also have some role in this; in the United States, only fluorodeoxyglucose-PET is approved, but amino acid, fluorothymidine, and F-DOPA PET imaging is being evaluated (Fig. 35.3). Diffusion-weighted and functional MR also has utility in guiding resection, and in this context, magnetoencephalography is also being studied.

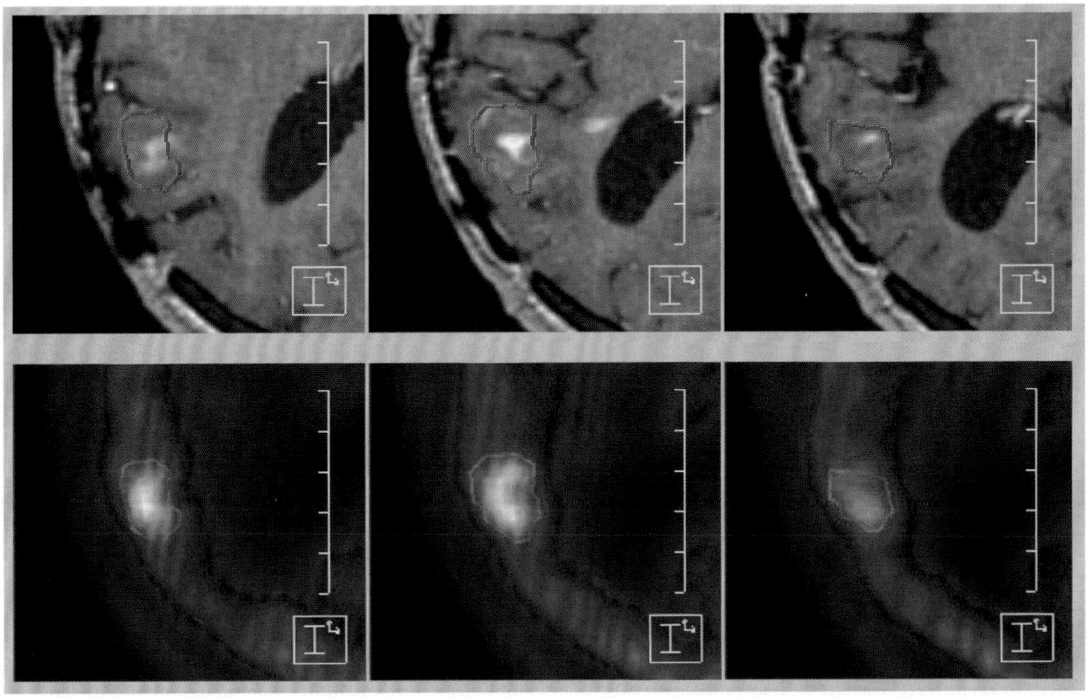

FIGURE 35.3. Oligodendroglioma imaged using an anatomic imaging technique, contrast-enhanced three-dimensional, spoiled gradient echo, T1-weighted magnetic resonance imaging (*top*) and a functional imaging technique, fluorodeoxyglucose positron emission tomography (*bottom*). The red contour delineates the extent of increased metabolic activity seen using functional imaging. Looking at the top panel, one can appreciate the fact that if the anatomic image set alone were to be used for target definition, it would yield a gross underestimation of the target volume as compared with the functional imaging technique.

Neuraxis Imaging

For neoplasms with high risk of CSF spread, staging of the neuraxis is essential. Gd-enhanced MRI of the spine is the imaging modality of choice. Ideally, neuraxis imaging should be performed before surgery. In the immediate postoperative period, spinal MRI scans may be difficult to interpret because arachnoiditis and blood products in the CSF can mimic leptomeningeal metastasis. Delayed spinal MRI (>3 weeks after surgery), combined with an increased dose of intravenous gadolinium, is a sensitive imaging study to detect leptomeningeal disease.

Histologic Confirmation of Diagnosis

The morbidity of biopsy has decreased significantly with improvements in operative technique and anesthesia, as well as with the availability of stereotactic biopsy techniques. Exception might be made in selected patients, such as those patients with known active systemic cancer and multiple lesions that are radiographically consistent with brain metastases, patients with typical clinical and MRI findings of a brainstem glioma or optic nerve meningioma, HIV-positive patients with CT or MRI findings consistent with primary CNS lymphoma and positive Epstein-Barr virus polymerase chain reaction in the CSF, or patients with secretory germ-cell tumors.

Cerebrospinal Fluid Cytology

CSF cytology is essential for staging tumors with a propensity for CSF spread (e.g., medulloblastoma, PNET, germ cell tumors, CNS lymphoma). Sampling of the CSF in the immediate postoperative period may lead to false-positive results, however, and is best done before surgery or more than 3 weeks after surgery, as long as intracranial pressure is not elevated. CSF spread of tumor may be associated with several abnormal CSF findings. These include CSF pressure >150 mm H_2O at the lumbar level in a laterally positioned patient, elevated protein level (>40 mg/dL in the lumbar cistern), a reduced glucose level (<50 mg/mL), and the finding of tumor cells by cytologic examination. Tumor markers in the CSF may help in making the diagnosis.

Differential Diagnosis

Most adults with new or persistent neurologic findings (focal deficit, increased intracranial pressure, seizures, altered mentation) are investigated using CT or MRI. There are a number of classical imaging features that help to refine the differential diagnosis (Table 35.2).

TABLE 35.2 DIFFERENTIAL DIAGNOSIS OF SPACE-OCCUPYING LESIONS ON COMPUTED TOMOGRAPHY OR MAGNETIC RESONANCE IMAGING

Pathology	*Features on CT or MRI*
Neoplasm	
Primary	Solitary, no prior cancer, thick nodular CE
Metastatic	Multiple, prior cancer, + edema, located at gray/white junction
Infectious	
Abscess	Fever, acutely ill, ± systemic infection, cyst cavity with smooth, thin walls, CE, and restricted diffusion within cavity
Cerebritis	Fever, acutely ill, ± systemic infection, diffuse T2 change, no CE mass
Meningitis	Diffuse enhancement of meninges on T1-weighted imaging (may simulate leptomeningeal metastases)
Vascular	
Infarct	Gray and white matter involvement, wedge-like vascular distribution associated with restricted diffusion and low ADC signal
Bleeding	Homogeneous, clears quickly, residual hemosiderin ring
Treatment-related necrosis	Central hypodensity, ring CE, edema, >6 mo after radiation therapy or chemotherapy, metabolic scan shows low activity

ADC, apparent diffusion coefficient; CE, contrast enhancement; CT, computed tomography; MRI, magnetic resonance imaging.

TABLE 35.3 HISTOLOGIC CLASSIFICATION OF TUMORS OF THE CENTRAL NERVOUS SYSTEM

Neuroepithelial tumors	Tumors of the meninges
Astrocytic tumors	Meningioma
Astrocytoma	Benign meningioma
Anaplastic astrocytoma	Atypical meningioma
Glioblastoma multiforme	Malignant meningioma
Oligodendroglial tumors	Mesenchymal tumors, benign
Oligodendroglioma	Mesenchymal tumors, malignant
Anaplastic oligodendroglioma	Hemangiopericytoma
Ependymal tumors	Chondrosarcoma
Ependymoma	Malignant fibrous histiocytoma
Anaplastic ependymoma	Rhabdomyosarcoma
Mixed gliomas	Uncertain histogenesis
Oligoastrocytoma	Hemangioblastoma
Anaplastic oligoastrocytoma	Hematopoietic neoplasms
Choroid plexus tumors	Malignant lymphomas
Neuronal tumors	Plasmacytoma
Ganglioglioma	Cysts/tumor-like lesions
Anaplastic ganglioglioma	Rathke cleft cyst
Neurocytoma	Epidermoid cyst
Pineal parenchymal tumors	Dermoid cyst
Pineocytoma	Germ cell tumors
Pineoblastoma	Germinoma
Embryonal tumors	Yolk-sac tumor
Medulloblastoma	Choriocarcinoma
Ependymoblastoma	Teratoma
Primitive neuroectodermal tumors	Mixed-germ cell tumors
Tumors of cranial/spinal nerves	Sellar tumors
Schwannoma (neurilemoma)	Pituitary adenoma
Neurofibroma	Craniopharyngioma

PATHOLOGY

Primary intracranial tumors are of ectodermal and mesodermal origin and arise from the brain, cranial nerves, meninges, pituitary, pineal, and vascular elements. The WHO classification system is the mostly widely used and lists approximately 100 distinct pathologic subtypes of CNS malignancies in broad categories (Table 35.3).[12] Guidelines for assigning grade of malignancy are provided, where applicable.

GENERAL MANAGEMENT

The medical management of patients with brain tumors includes management of increased intracranial pressure, seizures, and venous thromboembolic disease.

Cerebral Edema

Glucocorticoids are used to control neurologic signs and symptoms caused by cerebral edema. Lower doses of steroids (e.g., 2 to 4 mg dexamethasone) twice daily have been shown to be as effective as higher doses. Prolonged steroid use is associated with multiple medical problems, and therefore steroids should be discontinued or tapered to the lowest dose necessary, as soon as possible. Dexamethasone is the most common corticosteroid used for historical reasons and because of minimal mineral-corticoid effects. As with all corticosteroids, a slow taper is necessary to prevent a rebound in cerebral edema and also to allow the pituitary–adrenal axis to recover.

Seizures

Patients with seizures require anticonvulsants. Because anticonvulsants such as carbamazepine, phenobarbital, and phenytoin induce hepatic cytochrome P450 isozymes, which increase the metabolism and clearance of several cancer chemotherapy agents such as paclitaxel and irinotecan,[13,14] non–enzyme-inducing anticonvulsants, such as levetiracetam, lacosamide, lamotrigine, and pregabalin are preferred.

Prophylactic anticonvulsant use (in patients who have never experienced a seizure) remains controversial, although practice guidelines from the American Academy of Neurology recommended against their use because of lack of data.[15]

SURGERY

Surgical procedures can be summarized as biopsy for diagnosis only, resection for cure, surgical debulking for management of mass effect–related symptoms, CSF diversion procedures to relieve acute symptoms caused by increased intracranial pressure or hydrocephalus, and, increasingly, re-resection to distinguish and manage the effects of progressive tumor from symptomatic necrosis or pseudoprogression. Other roles of surgery include the placement of chemotherapy wafers, brachytherapy devices, and catheters for interstitial drug delivery and for monitoring tumor drug concentrations. Complete resection of tumor is associated with a survival advantage for some tumor types.[16,17] However, for some radiosensitive and/or chemosensitive malignancies such as primary CNS lymphoma, aggressive resection is unnecessary, and the surgeon's role is limited to providing diagnostic material.

Operative Technique

Ultrasound-, CT-, and MRI-guidance systems provide surgeons with intraoperative navigation based upon preoperative and/or intraoperative data. In general, these consist of a workstation into which the relevant imaging studies have been loaded, together with infrared or ultrasound detectors that recognize the three-dimensional (3D) orientation and position in space of various tools. Once the patient is registered, the tumor's margins are "visualized" below the scalp so that the surgeon can plan the smallest and safest approach. Resection is assisted by use of the intraoperative microscope and guided by the appearance and consistency of tumor tissue compared with surrounding normal brain. Intraoperative CT, MRI, or ultrasonography can be used to evaluate the completeness of tumor resection. In the case of lesions that are in or near suspected functional cortex, cortical mapping can be performed to localize areas that are critical for motor or speech function. Endoscopy can be used to minimize access for resection of intraventricular lesions or pituitary tumors, as well as for re-establishing pathways of CSF flow, for example, in cases of tumors that have obstructed the cerebral aqueduct, thereby avoiding the need for a CSF shunt. In addition to intraoperative image guidance, the use of ultraviolet-fluorescent tumor-localizing dyes such as 5-aminolevulinec acid has gained acceptance in Europe to enhance the completeness of resection and is being investigated in the United States.

Stereotactic biopsy is performed with either a stereotactic frame or scalp fiducials; a CT or MRI is performed and the data loaded into an image guidance system. Target and entry points are selected, and the trajectory is visualized on a workstation. The entry point is located on the patient's scalp, and a small burr hole or twist drill hole is made. The biopsy needle is oriented using the image guidance system and passed to the appropriate depth, and tissue samples are obtained. Multiple tissue samples may be obtained along the needle tract, until the pathologist can provide an intraoperative diagnosis. The volume of tissue removed is insufficient to relieve mass effect, and patients who are symptomatic are better treated by open resection.

RADIOTHERAPY

Radiobiologic Considerations Underlying Tissue Injury

The process of radiation injury in the brain is highly complex and dependent on a variety of technical factors, including dose, volume, fraction size, and the specific target cell population, as well as secondary mechanisms of expression of injury such as vascular leak causing edema, vascular endothelial loss resulting in hypoxic injury, reactive gliosis, and to-date inadequately studied host factors. Some structures (e.g., optic chiasm, hypothalamus, lacrimal gland, lenses, etc.) appear to be substantially more sensitive to radiation than others. Even focal lesions may result in widespread radiographic and/or functional perturbations. The time course for the manifestation of injury can be highly variable and the clinical picture easily confounded with tumor progression. The effect on endothelial cells often becomes manifest as an early T2 signal abnormality on MRI, possibly due to disruption of the BBB and edema formation. Metabolic perturbations observed with PET may reflect oligodendroglial demyelination. Further vascular perturbation and regeneration in response to injury results in an enhancing lesion on imaging. Delayed effects include white matter necrosis and vascular obliteration. The time course can be shortened from several months to a few weeks by increasing the volume of brain irradiated or increasing the fraction size or total dose.

Historically, late injury from radiotherapy has been reported as the "tolerance" dose at either the 5% or 50% risk level at 5 years (TD 5/5 or TD 50/5, respectively). The values for whole-brain fractionated radiotherapy at 2 Gy per fraction are 60 and 70 Gy, respectively. With partial-brain irradiation, the corresponding values are 70 and 80 Gy, respectively. In the setting of fractionated radiotherapy with a fraction size <2.5 Gy, recent Quantitative Analysis of Normal Tissue Effects in the Clinic estimates are 5% and 10% rates of symptomatic necrosis at 72- and 90-Gy maximum equivalent doses in 2-Gy fractions, respectively.[18] For larger fraction sizes (≥2.5 Gy), incidence and severity of toxicity are unpredictable. In children, cognitive dysfunction has largely been seen after whole-brain doses.

General Concepts

Pertinent Anatomic Landmarks

With conventional simulation, radiographic and surface topographic reference points for appreciation of beam-to-head projection geometry are necessary. The external auditory meatii define anatomic reference planes such as Reid's baseline and the Frankfort horizontal plane, connecting points in the two external auditory meatii and one anterior infraorbital edge. Unless marked at simulation, the external auditory meatii may be difficult to see on lateral projections because of the overlying temporal bone. The two lateral parts of the anterior cranial fossa, the two anterior parts of the middle cranial fossa floors, and the two mandibular angle points, with their lateral locations, represent appropriate reference points. With CT-based planning, the need for identifying these is obviated.

In a lateral radiograph, the sella turcica is centrally located and marks the lower border of the medial telencephalon and diencephalon. The hypothalamic structures are located an additional 1 cm superior to the sellar floor, and the optic canal runs at most 1 cm superior and 1 cm anterior to that point. The pineal body (or the tentorial notch) usually sits approximately 1 cm posterior and 3 cm superior to the external auditory meatus. The cribriform plate is the most inferior part of the anterior cranial fossa; it is an important reference point for the inferior border of whole-brain irradiation fields. In most patients, little distance is found between the lateral projections of the lens and the most inferior part of the cribriform plate. The temporal lobes are situated in the middle cranial fossae, the floor of which is easily identified on lateral radiographs. Individualized blocks should always be used to delineate the field inferior border for whole-brain radiotherapy.

On an anteroposterior radiograph with a Frankfort horizontal plane (ear markers and one inferior orbital edge in a horizontal plane), the temporal bones (pyramids) project in the orbits. This implies that the ethmoid sinuses and the sphenoid sinus will project between the orbits, the sella just above these air cavities, and the foramen magnum just below the connection line between the inferior orbital edges. The frontal and occipital lobes therefore project above the orbits, and the temporal lobes and cerebellum in and somewhat below the orbits.

Treatment Setup

The head should be positioned so that its major axes are parallel with and perpendicular to the central axis incident beam and the treatment table. It may be preferable to fully flex or extend the neck in some patients, depending on tumor location and choice of beams, although the use of noncoplanar fields and intensity-modulated radiotherapy (IMRT) techniques makes this less necessary.

Reproducibility of head positioning is achieved by using a fixation device. Many devices are available for this, with reproducibility precision ranging from 1 to 5 mm. With the advent of image-guided radiation therapy and intrafraction motion detection, unprecedented accuracy can be achieved in delivering radiotherapy. This permits substantial reduction in margins for setup variability.[19]

Target Volume Definition

Two major factors drive margin selection: the inaccuracy of estimating the clinical target volume (CTV) and the specific dosimetric and setup variability components that are institution specific and determine the planning target volume (PTV).

Common sense and practice dictate that these CTV expansion margins should not traverse anatomically discontiguous structures or include areas unlikely to be infiltrated by tumor. Inclusion of the bony skull is unnecessary unless direct tumor extension is suspected. With some exceptions, "compartmental crossing" to the contralateral hemisphere or, for example, into the posterior fossa or the brainstem for a supratentorial cortical tumor is not necessary, but because many infiltrating gliomas "cross" through the anterior and/or posterior corpus callosal tracts, these should be adequately included in CTV margin selection.

Radiotherapy Techniques

The most commonly employed radiotherapy techniques in the management of CNS tumors are partial-brain irradiation, whole-brain radiotherapy (WBRT), craniospinal irradiation (CSI), stereotactic radiosurgery (SRS), fractionated stereotactic radiotherapy (FSRT), and, less commonly, brachytherapy. The indications for each of these techniques are discussed under the sections on the individual tumor types. CSI is more frequently used in management of pediatric CNS tumors and is discussed in detail in Chapter 82.

Whole-Brain Radiotherapy

WBRT is used most often for patients with brain metastases but also for patients with primary CNS lymphomas and glioblastomatosis cerebrii and as a component of CSI.

Whole-brain irradiation is administered through parallel-opposed lateral portals. The inferior field border should be inferior to the cribriform plate, the middle cranial fossa, and the foramen magnum, all of which should be distinguishable on simulation or portal localization radiographs (Fig. 35.4). The safety margin depends on penumbra width, head fixation, and anatomic factors but should be at least 1 cm, even under optimal conditions. A special problem arises anteriorly because sparing of the ocular lenses and lacrimal glands may require blocking with margins <5 mm at the cribriform plate.

The anterior border of the field should be approximately 3 cm posterior to the ipsilateral eyelid for the diverging beam to exclude the contralateral lens. However, this results in only approximately 40% of the prescribed dose to the posterior eye. A better alternative is to angle the beam approximately 3 degrees or more (100- or 80-cm source-to-axis distance midline, but also field size dependent) against the frontal plane so that the anterior beam border traverses posterior to the lenses (approximately 2 cm posterior to eyelid markers). Placing a radiopaque marker on both lateral canthi and aligning the markers permits individualization in terms of the couch angle. This arrangement provides full dose to the posterior eyes. However, the eyelid-to-lens and eyelid-to-retina topography is individually more constant than the canthus, and lateral beam eye shielding is better individualized with the aid of CT or MRI scans.[20] When in doubt about tumor coverage or lens sparing for tumors in a subfrontal or middle cranial fossa location, one should consider CT-based contouring and planning.

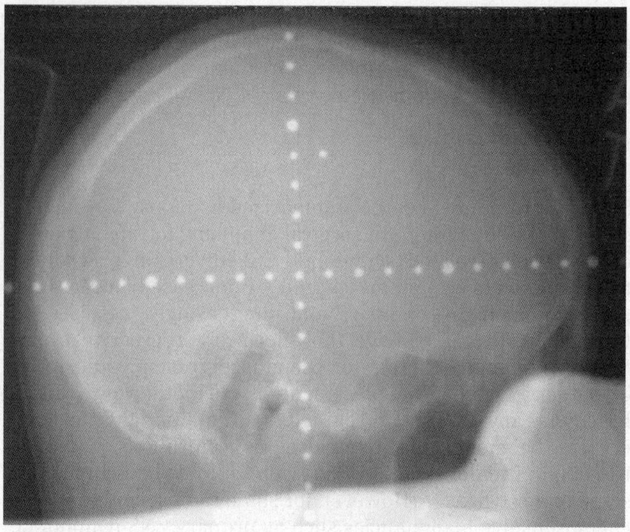

FIGURE 35.4. Lateral portal localization film of whole brain, illustrating adequate inclusion of the cribriform plate and the anterior and middle cranial fossae.

Craniospinal Irradiation

Traditional CSI techniques use opposed lateral cranial fields and one or more posterior spinal fields, depending on patient size. The junctioning of noncoplanar fields in the cervical region is potentially hazardous because of the risk of overlap resulting in radiation myelitis. Consequently, great attention needs to be paid to precise immobilization, and a variety of immobilization devices are available for this purpose. Image guidance during radiotherapy can help in ensuring day-to-day reproducibility. The prone position permits direct visualization of the light field from the linear accelerator on the patient, thereby allowing daily adjustments of the junctions. However, if anesthesia or sedation is required, as may be the case with young children, a supine setup may be considered safer.[21] To avoid the risk of dose overlap, at least two techniques (with numerous variations) are commonly used, and several variations of these have also been reported. In the first, a gap is used between abutting fields such that the beam edges intersect deep to the spinal cord. This gap could result in a cold spot in a small segment of the spinal cord. If the beam intersection point were raised dorsally, a hot spot would result.

The second technique attempts to avoid this problem by using a half-beam technique in which the caudal edge of the brain is matched precisely with the cephalad edge of the abutting spine field without cold or hot spots. This requires collimator angulation and sometimes a couch rotation as well. For both techniques, the use of moving junctions (known as "feathering") smoothes out any dose inhomogeneity.[22] Several studies have demonstrated that adequate coverage of the subfrontal region, posterior fossa, and depth assessment of the cord requires CT-based planning. Given the complexity of CSI, we recommend that it be delivered at centers with adequate staff, experience, and expertise.

With sophisticated techniques such as helical intensity modulated, image-guided tomotherapy and volumetric arc-modulated radiotherapy, it is possible to treat the entire neuraxis in a single setup.[23] In recent years, protons, as well as other techniques, have been used for CSI.

Stereotactic Radiosurgery

Stereotactic radiosurgery requires a team comprised at a minimum of a neurosurgeon, radiation oncologist, and radiation oncology physicist, in addition to appropriate support staff. SRS can be delivered using a conventional or modified linear accelerator (LINAC) system, a Gamma Knife (Elekta Corp., Stockholm), or a robotically controlled miniaturized linear accelerator (CyberKnife; Accuray, Sunnyvale, CA). In LINAC radiosurgery circular or oval collimators ranging from 4 to 40 mm are used to collimate the treatment beam into a circular pencil beam, and treatment is delivered using multiple noncoplanar arcs that intersect at a single point to treat an approximately spherical target of <4 cm in diameter. Newer miniaturized multileaf collimators allow beam shaping. The Gamma Knife is a fixed-beam, multisource radiation unit containing 201 cobalt-60 (^{60}Co) sources that are collimated using a helmet with circular apertures ranging from 4 to 18 mm that are focused onto a single target point. The newer Gamma Knife technology obviates the need for "helmet changes" and can effectively allow IMRT-like dose distributions to be created. For irregularly shaped lesions, treatments delivered using either noncoplanar arcs delivered through a single circular collimator or a single collimator helmet lead to the inclusion of a large amount of normal brain and yield inferior conformality. In these cases it is advantageous to use multiple circular collimators or collimator helmets placed on different target points (and in the newest version of the Gamma Knife [Perfexion], different segments can be treated with different collimator diameters, and differential weighting is also possible), or to consider the use of multileaf collimated beams.

Radiation Therapy Oncology Group (RTOG) study 90-05 established the maximum tolerated dose of single faction SRS to be 24, 18, and 15 Gy for tumors ≤20 mm, 21 to 30 mm, and 31 to 40 mm in maximum diameter, respectively, and these and other parameters are frequently used to guide prescription doses.[24]

Fractionated Stereotactic Radiotherapy

For lesions larger than 4 cm and/or located in critical regions, the delivery of a single large-fraction treatment as in SRS is not desirable because of a high risk of CNS toxicity. Fractionated stereotactic radiotherapy (FRST) is a hybrid between conventionally fractionated radiotherapy and SRS that combines fractionation with stereotactic localization and targeting techniques. Various systems for FSRT have been developed, with a reported accuracy of 1 to 3 mm.[25–27] As for SRS, the use of multiple arcs and circular collimators for irregularly shaped lesions leads to the inclusion of a large amount of normal tissue. The use of multiple noncoplanar fixed fields each having a unique entrance and exit pathway is preferable because of better conformality because multileaf collimators are almost always used.[19,28] With the Perfexion device, the use of the "Extend" frame permits FSRT, as well as targeting of lower cranial lesions.

Heavy Charged Particles

Heavy-charged-particle beams deposit their dose at a depth that depends on their energy over a distance of few millimeters when the heavy charged particles come to rest, the so-called Bragg peak. To cover a larger volume, the particle beam can be modulated, in effect adding up multiple Bragg peaks. The very sharp dose gradient at the distal edge permits the use of high-dose radiotherapy for tumors in critical locations, such as at the clivus and base of skull, and provides better normal-tissue sparing in other situations, especially, for example, in craniospinal irradiation.[29] A small number of European and Japanese centers are treating CNS tumors with carbon ions, which putatively have higher linear energy of transfer and presumed superior biologic effect, but no substantial clinical data are available to back these claims. There are no U.S. centers using these technologies, although neutron-beam irradiation, with or without coadministration of boronated agents to increase the cross-sectional area of interaction, continues to be used in some U.S. centers.

Brachytherapy and Radiocolloid Solutions

Selection criteria for brachytherapy include tumor confined to one hemisphere, no transcallosal or subependymal spread, small size (<5 to 6 cm), well circumscribed on CT or MRI, and accessible location for the implant. A balloon-based system, GliaSite (IsoRay Medical, Richland, WA), placed into the cavity at the time of surgery has been employed in the treatment of recurrent malignant gliomas whose largest spatial dimension is <4 cm and are roughly spherical.[30] After treatment planning the balloon is filled with a liquid that contains organically bound iodine-125 (^{125}I), and treatment is completed within 3 to 7 days. Direct infusion of radioimmunoglobulins has been used in primary and recurrent brain gliomas.[31]

CHEMOTHERAPY AND TARGETED AGENTS

Conventional Chemotherapy

Many conventional chemotherapy agents do not adequately penetrate normal or nonenhancing tumor-infiltrated brain, whereas some drugs, despite having a molecular weight and chemical structure that make them appear capable of crossing the BBB, are *p*-glycoprotein and other active transporter substrates that are actively effluxed out of the brain parenchyma. Even when drug delivery is adequate, most CNS tumors are resistant to most chemotherapeutic agents. Alkylating agents such as carmustine (BCNU) and lomustine (CCNU) have been the most widely studied drugs in CNS tumors. These agents cross the BBB, but prolonged use is difficult because of cumulative myelotoxicity and the dose-related risk of pulmonary fibrosis. Despite radiographic responses in 15% to 40% of patients, the impact on survival has been modest at best. Procarbazine has similar efficacy but is better tolerated. Cisplatin and carboplatin have been used as either single agents or in combination regimens. Response rates have been modest and their impact on survival is unclear. Topoisomerase I (CPT-11, irinotecan) and topoisomerase II inhibitors (etoposide) have shown only modest activity. Taxanes, such as paclitaxel, have not demonstrated activity as single agents. Temozolomide, an oral agent with excellent bioavailability, has a good toxicity profile and is the only agent to demonstrate a survival benefit for glioblastoma patients in randomized clinical trials.

Combination regimens, such as BCNU and temozolomide, are not more efficacious,[32] because of the need to reduce the dose of each agent due to overlapping myelotoxicity.

Direct Delivery of Therapeutic Agents

Methods for circumventing the BBB include implantation of slow-release chemotherapy wafers into a tumor resection cavity,[33,34] pharmacologic or osmotic BBB disruption,[35,36] and convection enhanced drug delivery (CED). CED involves the use of intracerebrally implanted catheters to deliver a drug into the brain parenchyma or tumor at a slow but continuous rate of flow. Unlike diffusion, in which a drug distributes along an exponentially decaying concentration gradient depending on the size of the molecule, drug distribution by CED is less size dependent, occurs over a larger volume of brain tissue, and results in a more uniform drug concentration within the volume of distribution.[37] Large and/or hydrophilic agents that do not cross the BBB are ideal candidates for delivery via CED. Examples of agents used in CED studies include viruses,[38] paclitaxel,[39] topotecan,[40] and a variety of engineered, targeted protein toxins. These toxins are engineered to include a targeting ligand (e.g., interleukin-4, interleukin-13, tumor growth factor-α, and transferrin) and a genetically altered bacterial toxin that is effective only when internalized by a cell that expresses the target of the ligand.[41–44] Two phase III clinical trials have evaluated the use of CED. The PRECISE trial[45] studied CED of interleukin-13 linked to *Pseudomonas* exotoxin (cintredekin besudotox) as compared to Gliadel (Eisai, Woodcliff Lake, NJ) wafers in glioblastoma patients at first recurrence. No difference in overall survival was observed, but cintredekin besudotox was associated a higher pulmonary embolism rate. The TransMID trial evaluated the efficacy of transferrin-CRM107 delivered by CED to patients with inoperable recurrent or progressive glioblastoma. The trial was terminated early in 2007 because it was deemed unlikely to meet the prespecified criteria for efficacy.

BCNU impregnated in a polymer and made into a wafer has been used for local delivery, placed on the walls of the resection cavity at the time of surgery. The wafer slowly undergoes biodegradation, releasing the active drug. This local delivery system has the advantages of minimal systemic toxicity, no limitation posed by the BBB, and delivery of very high local concentrations of chemotherapy. Studies in glioblastoma multiforme (GBM) have shown only marginal benefit.[34,46]

Targeted Agents

The molecular changes in gliomas offer opportunities for targeted therapies. Signal transduction pathways, for example, are often markedly enhanced and may contribute to the cancer phenotypic and biologic changes. Molecules that block signal transduction pathways are undergoing extensive investigation.[47] These include agents that block angiogenesis (vascular endothelial growth factor receptor); proliferation, tumor cell invasion, and survival (EGFR); and cell survival (platelet-derived growth factor receptor); as well as inhibitors of downstream signaling molecules such as Akt, Ras, Raf kinase, and mTOR. Because single-agent strategies have shown minimal efficacy, clinical trials are now focusing on combination regimens.[47]

FOLLOW-UP

The follow-up schedule for a brain tumor patient must be frequent enough to check on side effects and to taper steroids shortly after completion of treatment. Periodic MRIs are used to detect tumor recurrence at a stage when further therapy may be contemplated. Assessment of intellectual functioning and quality of life is important, and patients must be monitored for neuroendocrine and ophthalmologic side effects.

SEQUELAE OF TREATMENT

Surgery

With appropriate patient selection, diligent surgical technique, and use of surgical adjuncts such as speech and/or motor mapping, the rate of complications can be minimized. Even in the best of hands new temporary neurologic deficits can be seen in 15% or more of patients, although the rate of permanent new deficits is typically now <5%.[48] The incidence and types of deficits seen following surgery depend upon the location of the tumor and the deficits present preoperatively. The most common complications associated with surgery are bleeding and infection, particular in the case of reoperation in a patient who has received prior radiotherapy and/or chemotherapy or when chemotherapy wafers are placed into a resection cavity.[49] It has been suggested that the use of linear incisions (as opposed to U-shaped flaps) can help reduce the incidence of incision-related complications, such as infection.[50] Posterior fossa resections, particularly in children with medulloblastoma, may be associated with posterior fossa syndrome (mutism plus bulbar symptoms). Transient perioperative edema, within about 48 hours of surgery, may be responsible for early postoperative neurologic worsening and can often be mitigated with the use of a short course of high-dose steroid therapy.

Patients with postoperative neurologic deterioration require careful clinical assessment, and in most cases a CT or MRI is required to determine the cause of the deterioration. MRI diffusion-weighted sequences can be used to detect the presence of a new infarct. A high index of suspicion should be maintained for postoperative infection because symptoms may be masked by perioperative steroid use, and the headache and fever associated with craniotomy may obscure the classic signs of meningitis.

Radiotherapy

The response of intracranial tissues to radiation has been classically divided into three phases based on the timing of onset of symptoms: acute, subacute, and late.

Acute Toxicity

Transient worsening of pretreatment deficits may develop during the course of treatment, and further acute toxicities may manifest up to 6 weeks following completion of irradiation. These symptoms are believed to be the consequence of a transient peritumoral edema and usually respond to a short-term increase or the institution of corticosteroids. Persistent or refractory symptoms may be caused by tumor progression, and repeat imaging while under treatment may be indicated if the clinical condition worsens despite steroids.

General symptoms such as fatigue, headache, and drowsiness may be seen, especially in individuals treated with large brain fields or with CSI. A mild dermatitis that develops in irradiated areas may be treated with topical agents if necessary. Alopecia within the irradiated areas is common and may be permanent with higher total doses. Nausea and vomiting independent of changes in intracranial pressure may occur, particularly with posterior fossa or brainstem irradiation. Otitis externa can be seen if the ear is included in the irradiation fields, and serous otitis media also may occur. Patients treated with CSI with photons are at risk for mucositis and esophagitis because of the exit dose from the spinal fields through the oropharynx and mediastinum. Hematologic toxicity may also be seen in these patients due to irradiation of the vertebral bodies, a major depot of bone marrow in adults.

Subacute Toxicity

Subacute or "early-delayed" toxicity that develops during the 6-week to 6-month period following irradiation is attributed to changes in capillary permeability, as well as to transient demyelination due to damage to oligodendroglial cells. Symptoms, which include headache, somnolence, fatigability, and deterioration of pre-existing deficits, usually respond to steroids. The main challenge is to distinguish the clinical and imaging findings from tumor recurrence. The phenomenon of pseudoprogression temporally fits within the subacute toxicity time frame.

Late Sequelae

Late sequelae of radiotherapy appear from 6 months to many years following treatment and are usually irreversible and progressive. They are believed to be due to white matter damage from vascular injury, demyelination, and necrosis. The pathophysiology of radiation-induced neurocognitive damage is complex and involves intercellular and intracellular interactions between vasculature and parenchymal cells, particularly oligodendrocytes, which are important for myelination. Oligodendrocyte death occurs either due to direct p53-dependent radiation apoptosis or due to exposure to radiation-induced tumor necrosis factor-α.[51,52] Postradiation injury to the vasculature involves damage to the endothelium leading to platelet aggregation and thrombus formation, followed by abnormal endothelial proliferation and intraluminal collagen deposition.[53]

The most serious late reaction to radiotherapy is radiation necrosis, which has a peak incidence at 3 years. Radiation necrosis can mimic recurrent tumor clinically by the reappearance and worsening of initial symptoms and neurologic deficits and radiographically with the development of a progressive, irreversible, enhancing mass with associated edema on imaging. PET, MR spectroscopy, and nuclear and dynamic CT scanning procedures may aid in the differentiation of radiation necrosis from recurrent tumor. The best treatment for symptomatic necrosis is control of symptoms with steroids, followed by surgical debulking, although even after resection necrosis may progress. Given the central role of capillary leakage to radiation necrosis, bevacizumab, an antibody against vascular endothelial growth factor (VEGF), has been tested clinically as treatment for radiation necrosis and has shown encouraging results.[54] Other measures include use of corticosteroids with anticoagulation or hyperbaric oxygen, although randomized trials have not shown these to be useful. Although focal necrosis is usually due to radiotherapy alone, diffuse leukoencephalopathy is more commonly associated with the combination of radiotherapy and chemotherapy, particularly methotrexate.

Inclusion of the middle ear may result in high-tone hearing loss and vestibular damage, especially in patients who receive cisplatin. Retinopathy or cataract formation may be seen if the eye is in the radiation field. Optic chiasm and nerve injury may manifest as a decrease in visual acuity, visual field changes, or blindness at doses >54 to 60 Gy. Onset of hormone insufficiency from irradiation of the hypothalamic–pituitary axis is variable but may be seen with doses as low as 20 Gy.

Cranial irradiation can produce neuropsychologic changes and neurocognitive impairment; other factors, such as tumor-related morbidity, as well as the effects of surgery and chemotherapy, may also contribute.[53,55] Decline in list-learning recall has been observed in prospective clinical trials of therapeutic and prophylactic cranial irradiation.[56,57] These changes are believed to be due to interactions between the vasculature and parenchymal cells. Hippocampal-dependent functions of new learning, memory, and spatial information processing appear to be most affected.[58] Doses as low as 2 Gy can induce apoptosis in the proliferating cells in the hippocampus.[59] Agents such as methylphenidate and memantine or radiotherapeutic strategies such as hippocampal avoidance may improve neurocognitive function.[60–62]

MANAGEMENT OF INDIVIDUAL TUMORS

Malignant Glioma

Malignant or high-grade gliomas account for approximately half of all primary brain tumors in adults. They are rapidly growing tumors that directly invade the brain parenchyma but almost never metastasize outside the CNS. They present in any age group, although most occur in late adulthood. Malignant gliomas correspond to anaplastic gliomas (WHO grade III) and GBM (WHO grade IV). Molecular genetics and results from clinical series have shown these to be two distinct diseases with unique behavior, response to treatment, and prognosis. Historical trials that included grade III and IV gliomas are described in the section on GBM because patients with GBM comprised the majority of subjects, and anaplastic gliomas are discussed in further detail in the following section.

Glioblastoma

GBM accounts for approximately 75% of all high-grade gliomas. The histopathologic features of GBM include nuclear atypia, mitotic activity, vascular proliferation, and necrosis; any three of these suffice to make the diagnosis. GBM is diffusely infiltrative, involving large portions of the brain. MRI characteristically shows vasogenic edema and ring enhancement around central necrotic regions.

The prognosis for patients with GBM is poor, with median survival time of approximately 14 months in highly selected patients receiving contemporary treatment. Pretreatment patient and tumor characteristics such as age at diagnosis, tumor histology, and Karnofsky performance status (KPS) are the best predictors of outcome. Extent of resection, duration of neurologic symptoms, and radiographic response to treatment have also been suggested as predictors of survival.

Curran et al.[63] used nonparametric recursive partitioning analysis (RPA; a statistical tool that allows for the identification of significant prognostic factors and subsequent classification of patients into groups with similar outcomes) to analyze data from three RTOG trials that included 1,578 patients with malignant gliomas. Age was the most important predictor of survival, with patients younger than 50 years faring best; KPS ≥70 was the next-most-significant prognostic factor. Taking into account these and other variables, it is possible to divide patients into groups with similar outcomes, with 2-year overall survival ranging from 4% to 76% and median survival ranging from 2.7 to 58.6 months (Table 35.4). Although developed in patients receiving radiotherapy alone, the RPA classification retains prognostic significance in patients treated with radiotherapy plus temozolomide.[64] More recent studies integrated molecular data from O^6–methylguanine-DNA methyltransferase (MGMT) promoter methylation status and other novel biomarkers to develop novel risk-stratification models.[65,66]

Molecular Genetics

Glioblastoma may arise *de novo* (primary) or from a low-grade glioma that has transformed into a higher-grade tumor (secondary). Some series report that up to 40% of GBM are

TABLE 35.4 RADIATION THERAPY ONCOLOGY GROUP RECURSIVE PARTITIONING ANALYSIS OF MALIGNANT GLIOMA

Class	Patient Characteristics	Median Survival (Months)
I, II	Anaplastic astrocytoma	40–60
	Age ≤50 yr, normal mental status or age >50 yr, KPS >70, symptoms >3 mo	
III, IV	Anaplastic astrocytoma	11–18
	Age ≤50 yr, abnormal mental status	
	Age >50 yr, symptoms <3 mo	
	Glioblastoma	
	Age <50 yr	
	Age >50 yr, KPS ≥70	
V, VI	Glioblastoma	5–9
	Age >50 yr, KPS <70 or abnormal mental status	

KPS, Karnofsky performance status.

Clinical Radiation Oncology

secondary. Secondary GBMs arise in younger patients and are associated with a more favorable prognosis than for those with primary GBM. The more favorable prognosis may be related to the impact of younger age and better performance status of this group. Emerging data suggest that promoter methylation of the PTEN gene in low-grade gliomas may be causally linked to secondary malignant transformation to GBM. Secondary GBMs usually have a mutation in the isocitrate dehydrogenase gene and often have p53 mutations.

Treatment

Standard treatment consists of maximal safe surgical resection followed by radiotherapy with concurrent temozolomide chemotherapy and subsequent adjuvant temozolomide chemotherapy. Other approaches including alterations in the delivery of radiotherapy, newer chemotherapeutic agents, and radiosensitizers, and other agents are the subject of ongoing research.

Radiotherapy Target Volume

Randomized trials have demonstrated a clear survival benefit to the use of radiotherapy after surgery.[67] Localized irradiation volumes are recommended despite the fact that GBM is usually more widely disseminated. Dandy,[68] for example, identified recurrences in the contralateral hemisphere even after hemispherectomy, showing the phenomenal capability of malignant gliomas to spread along white matter tracts. Such findings, as well as autopsy studies,[69–71] led to recommendations that the entire intracranial contents should be irradiated. However, Hochberg and Pruitt[72] reported that in 35 patients who had a CT scan within 2 months prior to autopsy, 78% of recurrences of GBM were within 2 cm of the margin of the initial tumor bed and 56% were within ≤1 cm of the volume outlined by the CT scan. These findings were confirmed by Wallner et al.,[73] who showed that 78% of unifocal tumors (25 of 32) recurred within 2 cm of the initial tumor volume, defined as the enhancing edge of the tumor on CT scan, and 56% of tumors (18 of 32) recurred within 1 cm of the initial tumor margin. No unifocal tumor recurred as a multifocal lesion, and large tumors were not more likely to recur farther from the initial tumor margin than were smaller tumors.

In a correlative study, Halperin et al.[74] reviewed CT scans and pathologic sections of 15 brains of patients with GBM who received minimal or no radiotherapy. If radiation treatment portals had been designed to cover the contrast-enhancing volume and peritumoral edema with a 1-cm margin, the portals would have covered histologically identified tumor in only 6 of 11 cases. However, treatment of the contrast-enhancing area and all surrounding edema with a 3-cm margin around the edema would have covered histologically identified tumor in all cases.

Kelly et al.[75] reported on 40 patients with intracranial glial neoplasms who underwent CT- and MRI-guided stereotactic serial biopsies. Histologic analysis of 195 biopsy specimens showed that contrast enhancement most often corresponded to tumor tissue without intervening parenchyma, and hypodensity most often corresponded to parenchyma infiltrated by isolated tumor cells, tumor in low-grade gliomas, or edema. Isolated tumor cell infiltration extended at least as far as T2 changes on MRI. T2-weighted MRI revealed much larger volumes of infiltrated parenchyma than shown by low attenuation on CT scans.

Therefore, inclusion of all radiographic evidence of tumor and associated edema with generous margins is the rule in the design of treatment portals. With advances in MRI technology, the definition of tumor margins may change. For example, Pirzkall et al.[76] showed metabolically active tumor extending outside the region defined on T2-weighted MRI in 88% of patients. PET imaging with methionine and/or thymidine may also prove useful.

Radiotherapy Dose

Standard therapy is a total dose of 60 Gy in 30 to 33 fractions. Walker et al.[77] reported a dose–response analysis using data from 420 patients treated on Brain Tumor Cooperative Group protocols. Doses ranged from <45 to 60 Gy, using daily fractions of 1.7 to 2 Gy; only one-third of the patients received <60 Gy. A significant improvement in median survival from 28 to 42 weeks in the groups treated with doses of 50 to 60 Gy was found. A Medical Research Council study of 443 patients also showed a significant survival advantage in patients who received 60 Gy compared to those who received 45 Gy (12 vs. 9 months; $p = .007$).[78]

For patients with poor pretreatment prognostic factors and a limited expected survival who are not able to tolerate conventional treatment, a shorter course of treatment may provide good palliation. Older patients (>65 years), especially those with poor performance status, have been shown to experience limited posttreatment improvement or rapid neurologic deterioration following conventional radiotherapy. Short-course radiotherapy has been tested in older patients, and results are described later.

Dose Escalation and Altered Fractionation

With the vast majority of tumor recurrences occurring within the previous irradiation field and the poor outcomes associated with standard therapy, regimens designed to deliver a larger dose have been attempted to improve local control and enhance survival.

A benefit for doses >60 Gy using conventional treatment has not been demonstrated. The RTOG and Eastern Cooperative Oncology Group (ECOG) randomized 253 patients to either whole-brain irradiation to 60 Gy given in 6 to 7 weeks or 60 Gy plus a 10-Gy boost to a limited volume given in 7 to 8 weeks.[79] There was no benefit for the higher irradiation dose. Median survival was 9.3 months for patients receiving 60 Gy and 8.2 months for those receiving 70 Gy.

Dose intensification using 3D conformal radiotherapy or IMRT also has not consistently shown to improve clinical outcome. Chan et al.[80] published the results of 34 patients with high-grade gliomas treated using 3D conformal IMRT to a dose of 90 Gy. At median follow-up of 11.7 months, median survival was found to be 11.7 months, and 1- and 2-year survivals were 47.1% and 12.9%, respectively, comparable to historical controls. In contrast, a retrospective study by Tanaka et al.[81] suggested a survival advantage for patients treated with high-dose conformal radiotherapy.

Several groups have used hyperfractionated or accelerated regimens as a means to escalate dose, using twice-daily, three-times-daily, and even four-times-daily fractionation.[82–84] Only the study of Shin et al.[84] showed an improvement in survival using daily fractionation. In this study, 81 patients were randomized to 61.4 Gy in 69 fractions of 0.89 Gy given three times daily over 4.5 weeks or conventional fractionation to 58 Gy in 30 fractions given once daily over 6 weeks. Median survival in the two groups was 39 and 27 weeks, respectively, and the 1-year survival rates were 41% and 20%, respectively ($p < .001$).

Others have failed to confirm these results. In a prospective, randomized, phase I/II trial, RTOG 83-02 examined dose escalation using twice-daily fractionation in patients with malignant gliomas. Hyperfractionated regimens studied were 64.8, 72.0, 76.8, and 81.6 Gy given in 1.2-Gy fractions twice daily, and accelerated hyperfractionated regimens were 48 and 54.4 Gy given in 1.6-Gy twice-daily fractions. Patients also received chemotherapy with BCNU. In the final report on all 747 patients, there were no significant differences between the treatment arms with regard to median survival time.[85] Late toxicities were slightly increased with higher doses. A phase III trial compared conventional radiotherapy to 60 Gy in 30 daily fractions to hyperfractionated radiotherapy to 72 Gy in 60 fractions of 1.2 Gy given twice daily.[86] No difference in survival was found. Several other accelerated hyperfractionation regimens to doses over 70 Gy have been investigated, also without significant improvement in survival.[87,88]

Dose Escalation Using Radiosurgery and FSRT

A radiosurgical boost was reported as effective in patients with newly diagnosed malignant glioma in a retrospective analysis of 115 patients treated at three institutions with a combination of surgery, external-beam radiotherapy, and LINAC-based radiosurgery on similar institutional protocols.[89] The actuarial 2-year and median survival for all patients was 45% and 96 weeks, respectively. In comparison to results for 1,578 patients treated on three RTOG external-beam radiotherapy protocols from 1974 to 1989, patients treated with radiosurgery had significantly improved 2-year and median survival ($p = .01$). This improvement in survival was seen predominantly for the worse prognostic classes (RPA classes 3 to 6). Patient selection may in part account for these results: it has been estimated that selection criteria limit the application of radiosurgery to approximately only 20% to 30% of patients with GBM.

In a prospective randomized trial, Souhami et al.[90] compared conventional radiotherapy (60 Gy) plus adjuvant BCNU with and without radiosurgery in 203 patients with GBM. At a median follow-up of 61 months, no significant improvement in median survival was observed (13.5 vs. 13.6 months). There was no difference in failure pattern between the two groups, and measurements of quality of life and cognitive decline were found to be comparable as well.

The use of a boost using FSRT was tested prospectively in RTOG 0023.[91] 76 patients with GBM with postoperative residual tumor plus tumor cavity diameter <60 mm were treated with 50-Gy standard radiotherapy in daily 2-Gy fractions plus four FSRT treatments given once weekly during weeks 3 to 6 of radiotherapy. The FSRT dose was either 5 or 7 Gy per fraction for a cumulative dose of 70 or 78 Gy in 29 treatments over 6 weeks. Significant toxicity included three patients with acute grade 4 toxicity (neurologic, constitutional, metabolic) and one with grade 3 late necrosis. The median survival time was 12.5 months. Overall, no survival advantage was seen when compared to the RTOG historical database.

Dose Escalation Using Brachytherapy

Laperriere et al.[92] used brachytherapy as a boost to conventional radiotherapy in patients with malignant gliomas. Patients were randomized to external-beam radiotherapy (50 Gy in 25 fractions) alone ($n = 69$) or external-beam radiotherapy plus a temporary stereotactic ^{125}I implant delivering a minimum peripheral tumor dose of 60 Gy ($n = 71$). Median survival was not significantly different between the two arms (13.8 vs. 13.2 months; $p = .49$).

The results of the Brain Tumor Cooperative Group National Institutes of Health Trial 8701 reported by Selker et al.[93] support these findings. In this randomized, prospective trial, 299 patients with newly diagnosed malignant glioma received surgery, external-beam radiotherapy, and BCNU with or without an interstitial radiotherapy boost with ^{125}I. Treatment with an interstitial boost did not prolong survival as compared to conventional treatment.

Radiotherapy delivered by an inflatable balloon catheter is a newer approach to brachytherapy. Tatter et al.[30] evaluated the safety and performance of one such device (GliaSite Radiation Therapy System; Cytyc, Marlborough, MA). Twenty-one patients with recurrent malignant gliomas underwent surgical resection and implantation of a subcutaneous port. At 1 to 2 weeks following implantation, the catheter was filled with an aqueous solution of organically bound ^{125}I for delivering a minimum of 40 to 60 Gy over 3 to 6 days, with subsequent removal of the device. This treatment was well tolerated with no serious adverse effects. Median survival was 12.7 months. Prospective, randomized trials are needed for further evaluation.

Dose Escalation Using Proton Therapy

Dose escalation up to ^{60}Co gray equivalent (CGE) with mixed photon and proton beam irradiation has been tested in two prospective trials.

Fitzek et al.[94] reported on a phase II study of 23 patients with newly diagnosed GBM. The 2-year overall survival was 34%, and median overall survival was 20 months, which compared favorably to historical data. Recurrence was observed in regions treated to 60 to 70 CGE, but only 1 recurrence was observed in regions treated to 90 CGE. More recently, Mizumoto et al.[95] reported on a phase I/II study of 20 patients with supratentorial GBM treated with mixed photon and proton beam irradiation to 96.6 Gy in 56 twice-daily fractions with concomitant nimustine chemotherapy. MRI-defined T2-enhancing region was treated to 50.4 CGE in 28 daily morning fractions. In daily evening fractions, patients were treated to 23.1 CGE for the first 14 fractions to the T1-enhancing region plus 1 cm and then 23.1 CGE for the subsequent 14 fractions to the T1-enhancing region only. Median survival was 22 months, and 2-year overall survival was 45%. Late radiation necrosis was noted in 1 patient, and late leukoencephalopathy was observed in a second patient. Given its high cost, proton therapy requires further prospective, randomized trials to validate these single-institution findings.

Radiosensitizers

Studies using radiation modifiers in conjunction with radiotherapy to overcome the hypoxia present in malignant gliomas have shown disappointing results. Chang[96] reported on 38 patients treated with hyperbaric oxygen and irradiation using fractionation schedules ranging from 36 Gy given in 3 weeks to 60 Gy given in 6 to 7 weeks and compared them with 42 patients treated with radiotherapy alone. An improvement in 18-month survival rate from 10% to 28% and an increase of median survival from 31 to 38 weeks was noted. The increased cost and difficulty of the widespread application of this treatment make this approach impractical. Perfluorocarbon emulsions, such as Fluosol, which have enormous oxygen-carrying capacity, have been tested as hypoxic sensitizers without significant benefit.[97] Randomized studies failed to show significant improvement with the addition of the hypoxic cell sensitizer misonidazole.[82,98]

Miralbell et al.[99] reported the results of a European Organisation for Research and Treatment of Cancer (EORTC) trial examining the addition of carbogen and nicotinamide to overcome the effects of proliferation and hypoxia presumed responsible for radioresistance in GBM. In this prospective phase I and II trial, 107 eligible patients received radiotherapy (60 Gy) with carbogen breathing during each treatment session ($n = 23$), a daily oral dose of nicotinamide ($n = 28$), or both ($n = 56$). Patients receiving nicotinamide had higher rates of acute toxicity. Overall survival was similar in all three groups (median survival 10.1 vs. 9.7 vs. 11.1 months) and did not differ from results of series using radiotherapy alone.

The redox-modulating radiosensitizer motexafin gadolinium (MGd) showed encouraging results in a phase I clinical trial[74]; however, results from a single-arm phase II trial, RTOG 0513, of MGd and conventional therapy in newly diagnosed GBM showed no survival improvement.

Chemotherapy

The use of cytotoxic chemotherapeutic agents for glioblastoma dates back to the 1960s when the Brain Tumor Study

Group conducted a controlled study using carmustine.[100] After surgery, patients were assigned to one of four treatment groups: (a) no further therapy, (b) carmustine alone, (c) radiation therapy, and (d) radiation therapy followed by carmustine. At 18 months 23% of patients who received radiation therapy plus carmustine were still alive as compared to 5% with carmustine or radiotherapy alone. The U.S. Food and Drug Administration (FDA) approved carmustine and lomustine for the treatment of brain tumors (including glioblastoma) in the 1970s. Subsequent prospective studies failed to demonstrate a survival advantage to carmustine or other cytotoxic chemotherapy for glioblastoma, although two meta-analyses demonstrated a small survival benefit from chemotherapy.[101,102]

The only chemotherapeutic agent that has demonstrated efficacy in a randomized, controlled clinical trials is temozolomide, an oral imidazotetrazine derivative of dacarbazine that is metabolized *in vivo* to an active agent. Like the nitrosureas, it alkylates the O^6 position on guanine, producing single-strand DNA breaks. It is well tolerated by patients; fatigue, constipation, and nausea are the most common toxicities. The drug is myelosuppressive in a minority of patients. Approval for the treatment of recurrent anaplastic astrocytoma was obtained from the FDA in 1999 based on the work of Yung et al.[103] Its approval for use as adjuvant therapy for glioblastoma was based on a large phase III clinical trial conducted by the EORTC and the National Cancer Institute of Canada (NCIC).[104,105] This phase III trial randomized 573 patients with newly diagnosed glioblastoma (between the ages of 18 and 70 years and KPS > 70) to either radiation therapy alone (total 60 Gy in 30 fractions; control arm) or temozolomide chemotherapy in combination with radiation therapy (total 60 Gy in 30 fractions; experimental arm). Patients on the experimental arm received temozolomide daily during radiation therapy (because of its radiosensitization effect in preclinical studies) at a dose of 75 mg/m^2, followed by monthly temozolomide at a dose of 150 to 200 mg/m^2 on a 5 of every 28 days schedule for six cycles.

Patients randomized to the experimental arm had a median survival of 14.6 months as compared to 12.1 months for the control arm. The 2-year survival of patients treated with radiation therapy plus chemotherapy was 26% as compared to 6% for radiation alone. This impressive increase in 2-year survival with minor improvement in overall survival suggested that there was an unspecified subpopulation of patients that responded to chemotherapy. Toxicity with chemoradiotherapy was acceptable with 7% grade 3 or 4 hematologic toxicities, compared to none in the group treated with radiotherapy alone.

The survival benefit from the addition of temozolomide has now been demonstrated for at least 5 years out from initial treatment and in all clinical prognostic subgroups, including patients aged 60 to 70 years and in RPA classes III through V.[105] Five-year overall survival was 9.8% for patients who received combined temozolomide and radiotherapy as compared to 1.9% for those who received radiotherapy alone.

The RTOG recently completed a 1,100-patient, randomized, phase III trial comparing standard adjuvant temozolomide with a dose-dense schedule in newly diagnosed glioblastoma.[66] A total of 833 patients were randomized to receive either standard therapy (temozolomide plus radiotherapy followed by 6 to 12 cycles of temozolomide at a dose of 150 to 200 mg/ m^2 on a 5/28 day schedule) or dose-intense temozolomide (temozolomide plus radiotherapy followed by 6 to 12 cycles of temozolomide at a dose of 150 mg/ m^2 on a 21/28 day schedule). There was no statistical difference between the experimental and standard arms for overall survival (16.6 vs.14.9 months, p = .63) or progression-free survival (5.5 vs. 6.7 months, p = .06), indicating no additional benefit from dose-intense temozolomide. The trial prospectively stratified for MGMT methylation status, and no survival benefit with dose-intense therapy was identified in any subgroup. As expected, the dose-intense arm resulted in increased toxicity. Thus, at the present time, there is no role for dose-intense temozolomide for newly diagnosed glioblastoma patients.

Because only a subgroup of patients benefit from temozolomide, their identification is desirable to avoid exposing them to the toxicity of a potentially ineffective therapy. Recent work has focused on identifying potential predictive laboratory markers. Epigenetic silencing of the MGMT DNA repair gene by promoter methylation has been associated with longer survival for malignant glioma patients treated with alkylating agents.[106] A retrospective analysis of assessable cases from the EORTC/NCIC temozolomide study demonstrated a survival benefit for patients treated with temozolomide and radiotherapy if their tumor contained a methylated MGMT promoter (median, 21.7 months) as compared to patients with nonmethylated MGMT promoters (median, 12.7 months).[107] Prospective data supporting the prognostic value of MGMT promoter methylation were obtained in the RTOG dose-intense temozolomide study (RTOG 0525).[66] MGMT methylation was associated with improved median overall survival (21.2 vs. 14 months, p <.0001), median progression-free survival (8.7 vs. 5.7 months, p <.001), and response (p = .012).

Other chemotherapeutic regimens, such as the combination of CPT-11 and temozolomide, have shown promising results in a phase II trial with an objective response rate of 25% and 6-month progression-free rate of 38%.[108] When tested prospectively in a single-arm RTOG trial, the regimen did not show improved survival. Buckner et al.[109] reported on a phase III trial of carmustine with or without cisplatin before and concurrently with radiotherapy and observed increased toxicity but no survival benefit with the addition of cisplatin.

Conventional cytotoxic chemotherapeutic agents have also been combined with agents designed to modulate tumor biology. Two large phase III, randomized clinical trials investigating the addition of bevacizumab to the EORTC/NCIC regimen have completed accrual, and results are pending.

Investigational Approaches

Radioimmunotherapy

Radioimmunotherapy using monoclonal antibodies against EGFR tagged with ^{125}I has been evaluated in the treatment of high-grade gliomas. In a phase II trial by Brady et al.,[110] 25 patients with malignant gliomas (10 with anaplastic astrocytoma and 15 with GBM) were treated with surgical resection or biopsy, followed by definitive external-beam radiotherapy and one or multiple doses (35 to 90 mCi per intravenous or intra-arterial infusion) of ^{125}I-labeled monoclonal antibody. The total cumulative dose ranged from 40 to 224 mCi. At 1 year, 60% of patients were alive, and the median survival was 15.6 months. In an updated report of this study that included a total of 180 patients with a minimum follow-up of 5 years, median survival was 13.4 months for those with GBM.[111]

Another potential target is tenascin, an extracellular protein overexpressed in malignant gliomas but not found in normal tissue. Radiolabeled monoclonal antibodies to tenascin have been evaluated in phase I or II trials showing activity against newly diagnosed and recurrent malignant gliomas.[112,113] In a phase II trial by Reardon et al.,[112] ^{131}I-labeled murine antitenascin monoclonal antibody was injected directly into the surgical resection cavity in 33 patients with untreated malignant glioma. Patients were subsequently treated with external-beam radiotherapy and 1 year of alkylator-based chemotherapy. Even after accounting for prognostic factors, median survival

(86.7 weeks) was longer than that of historical controls. Treatment-related toxicities were mild; only 1 patient required reoperation for radionecrosis.

Targeted Therapies

EGFR gene amplification is seen in approximately 40% to 50% of patients with GBM. EGFR is associated with control of cell growth through autocrine and paracrine effects of growth factors. Inhibitors of EGFR tyrosine kinase such as gefitinib and erlotinib and EGFR antibodies have shown activity against GBM in early clinical trials.[114,115] However, in a study by Chakravarti et al.,[116] EGFR levels as measured by quantitative immunohistochemistry were not of prognostic value for patients with newly diagnosed GBM. Response to gefitinib did not correlate with tumor EGFR status in a study by Uhm et al.[117] The presence of an EGFR deletion mutant variant III (EGFRvIII), leading to a constitutively active variant of a key cell survival pathway, and the presence of intact PTEN, a downstream inhibitor of this signaling pathway, have been found to be significantly associated with clinical response to EGFR kinase inhibitors in patients with GBM.[118]

More recently, immunotherapeutic approaches involving peptide vaccines targeting EGFRvIII have been tested in multicenter phase II trials of newly diagnosed EGFRvIII-expressing GBM following gross total resection and conventional radiotherapy with concurrent temozolomide. Both peptide vaccines rindopepimut (CDX-110) and PEPvIII consist of 13 amino acids unique to EGFRvIII and conjugated to keyhole limpet hemocyanin. In a phase II study of rindopepimut,[119] the primary endpoint of progression-free rate at 5.5 months was 66%. At a median follow-up of 29.5 months, overall survival was 21.3 months. In a phase II trial of PEPvIII,[120] median progression-free survival and overall survival were 14.2 and 26 months, respectively. In both trials, results compared favorably to historical controls, although such comparisons are troublesome because patients enrolled in these studies were required to have good performance status and gross total resection, both of which are positive prognostic factors. Of interest, 82% of cases in the PEPvIII trial lost EGFRvIII expression at recurrence, suggesting the capacity of the EGFRvIII-targeted vaccine to potentially eliminate EGFRvIII-expression tumor cells in most patients. Similar results have been observed in preclinical models.[121] Efforts to test these EGFRvIII vaccination strategies in the phase III setting are ongoing. Further data are needed to define the significance of EGFR mutations and downstream regulators of associated pathways.

Mutations and loss of the PTEN gene are encountered in approximately 70% of patients with GBM. PTEN inhibits signaling through the phosphoinositide 3-kinase and Akt signaling pathway. Loss of PTEN results in loss of effectiveness of EGFR inhibitors, probably due to constitutive signaling through phosphoinositide 3-kinase, which bypasses any upstream EGFR inhibitor effect. Specific inhibitors such as CCI-779 and everolimus are ineffective as single agents. Preclinical experiments suggest that these agents are potential radiosensitizers.[122]

Neovascularization is a major feature of GBM, and many studies demonstrate that GBMs secrete VEGF in abundance. The supporting endothelium strongly expresses receptors for VEGF. Bevacizumab, an anti-VEGF antibody, is FDA approved for the treatment of recurrent glioblastoma (see later discussion). Multiple phase II studies have demonstrated an impressive radiographic response rate and reduction in peritumoral edema. Other agents, such as enzastaurin, which inhibits VEGF signaling by inhibiting protein kinase cβ2, have been tested with approximately 40% response rates.[123]

Treatment of Elderly Patients

Approximately one-third of patients with GBM are 65 years or older. Older age has been demonstrated to be an important adverse prognostic factor in GBM. In a population-based survey of 3,298 patients with GBM in Ontario,[124] each decade increase in age was associated with a reduction in overall survival, with patients older than 70 years having a median survival of 4 to 5 months. In the updated results from the EORTC/NCIC trial, Stupp et al.[105] observed a survival advantage to radiotherapy with concomitant and adjuvant temozolomide compared to radiotherapy alone in all age subgroups, including patients older than 60 years of age.

However, due to concerns over the tolerance of conventional chemoradiotherapy for older patients, particularly those with poor performance status, nonconventional approaches to adjuvant therapy have been tested. A phase III Association des Neuro-Oncologue d'Expression Française (ANOCEF) group trial[125] observed improved median survival (6.7 vs. 3.9 months) and progression-free survival but equivalent toxicity with adjuvant radiotherapy to 50 Gy compared to best supportive care in patients 70 years and older with KPS ≥70.

Short-course radiotherapy and single-agent temozolomide have also been investigated. As described previously, Roa et al.[126] observed no difference between standard radiotherapy of 60 Gy in 30 fractions or a shorter course of 40 Gy in 15 fractions in GBM patients older than 50 years. A more recent European trial compared overall survival between standard radiotherapy (60 Gy in 30 fractions), short-course radiotherapy (34 Gy in 10 fractions), and single-agent temozolomide in patients 60 years or older.[127] Preliminary results have demonstrated inferior median survival with 60-Gy radiotherapy versus temozolomide with subgroup analysis limiting this survival difference only to patients older than age 70. No other survival differences were observed. Toxicities have not yet been reported. Preliminary results from the NOA-08 phase III trial[128] demonstrated inferior survival but higher toxicity with 1-week-on/1-week-off temozolomide compared to radiotherapy to 54 to 60 Gy in patients 65 years or older with anaplastic astrocytoma or GBM.

Treatment at Recurrence

Although several therapeutic options have been considered for patients with recurrent GBM, none are curative, and therefore the management goals should be palliative. Hospice referral for palliative care is reasonable for many patients. Palliative debulking may help selected patients by relieving mass effect and probably extends survival by about 4 to 6 months on average. Based on an impressive radiographic response rate in two nonrandomized, phase II clinical trials,[129,130] single-agent bevacizumab was approved by the FDA in 2009 for the treatment of recurrent glioblastoma. In a study of 49 glioblastoma patients, Kreisl et al.[130] reported objective response rate of 35%, 6-month progression-free survival of 29%, 3.7-month median progression-free survival, and 7.2-month median overall survival. Similarly, Friedman et al.[129] reported an objective response rate of 28%, 6-month progression-free survival of 43%, median progression-free survival of 4.2 months, and median overall survival of 9.2 months in a total of 85 patients. Although approved as a single agent, controversy remains on whether bevacizumab should be combined with a cytotoxic agent as with other solid tumors.

Polymer-based local chemotherapy (carmustine wafers) has been tested in a randomized trial that included 222 patients with recurrent glioma (mostly GBM); survival increased from 44% to 64% at 6 months (p = .02) for patients with GBM, and median survival increased from 23 to 31 weeks.[46] Systemic chemotherapeutic agents have been tested mostly in the context of clinical trials and have been uniformly disappointing,[131] as have targeted agents, with the notable exception of EGFR tyrosine kinase inhibitors in patients with recurrent GBM expressing wild-type PTEN and mutant EGFR.[118] Of 37 patients with recurrent GBM treated with EGFR tyrosine kinase inhibitors at UCLA there were 7 responders, whereas 19 had early progression. Coexpression of mutant EGFR and wild-type PTEN had 86% sensitivity, 89% specificity, and a positive predictive value of 75% for response.

Repeat radiotherapy using one of several different methods (including radiosurgery, brachytherapy, GliaSite balloon brachytherapy, and even repeat external-beam radiotherapy) may be considered for carefully selected patients.[132] Hypofractionated reirradiation with bevacizumab has shown promising results in small single-institutional reports, with surprisingly limited toxicity, attributed to "vascular stabilization and protection" resulting from bevacizumab, and more investigations of this approach are being considered.[133] The hypofractionated approach with temozolomide and bevacizumab has been extended to the newly diagnosed setting, and at the Society of Neuro-oncology 2011 meeting, investigators from the Memorial Sloan-Kettering Cancer Center reported median survival of >21 months in a small cohort of unmethylated MGMT GBM patients.[134]

Evidence-Based Treatment Summary

1. Maximal surgical resection, although not tested in a prospective trial, is generally fit.
2. Postoperative radiotherapy has been shown to provide a survival advantage in several clinical trials. The typical radiotherapy dose is 60 Gy in 6 weeks; dose escalation strategies have generally failed. Although there is much interest in incorporating advanced imaging in treatment planning and in using newer treatment modalities, their benefits in GBM remain to be demonstrated.
3. Temozolomide, given during and after radiotherapy, provides a significant survival advantage that is greatest in patients with methylation of the promoter region of the MGMT gene.

Anaplastic Glioma

Anaplastic gliomas (WHO grade III gliomas: anaplastic astrocytoma, anaplastic oligoastrocytoma, and anaplastic oligodendroglioma) constitute approximately 25% of high-grade gliomas in adults, generally occurring during young to middle adulthood. Histologically, these tumors have increased cellularity, nuclear atypia, and marked mitotic activity, without necrosis or neovascularization. On imaging, anaplastic gliomas may show enhancement and necrosis similar to GBM, although up to one-third of tumors may not enhance.[135]

The prognosis for patients with anaplastic glioma is heavily influenced by a number of molecular genetic factors. Based upon traditional histology alone, patients with anaplastic astrocytoma have a median survival of approximately 3 years following diagnosis, although there is clinical and biologic heterogeneity. Prognostic factors include age at diagnosis, mental status, and performance status (see Table 35.4). Patients with histologically defined anaplastic oligodendroglioma, in general, have a better prognosis. However, the prognosis of these patients is better defined by whether or not chromosome changes characterized by loss of heterozygosity of 1p and 19q are present (see later discussion). The prognosis for patients with a mixed tumor, anaplastic oligoastrocytoma, varies depending on the dominant histologic cell type.[136]

Molecular Genetics

Allelic loss of 1p and 19q is believed to be an early genetic alteration in the transformation and progression of oligodendrogliomas. Combined 1p and 19q deletions have been found in 63% of patients with anaplastic oligodendroglioma and 52% of patients with mixed anaplastic oligoastrocytoma, whereas astrocytic tumors have a low incidence (8% to 11%) of combined 1p and 19q deletions.[137] Deletions in 1p and 19p have been associated with longer progression-free survival and chemosensitivity and radiosensitivity.[137–138,139]

The impact of 1p19q codeletion status on outcome has been confirmed in two recent phase III trials. RTOG 94-02 retrospectively assessed 1p and 19q status in 206 of 289 enrolled patients (71%) with anaplastic oligodendroglioma/oligoastrocytoma randomized to receive chemotherapy with procarbazine, CCNU, and vincristine (PCV) followed by radiotherapy or radiotherapy alone.[27] Combined loss of 1p and 19q was present in 43% of patients in the PCV plus radiotherapy arm and 50% in the radiotherapy-alone arm. Combined loss of 1p and 19q resulted in a longer median survival time of >7 years versus 2.8 years (p <.001). There was no effect of tumor genotype on overall survival by treatment. At first analysis, PCV did not appear to improve survival for any patient subgroup. In EORTC 26951, 368 patients with anaplastic oligodendroglioma/oligoastrocytoma were randomized to receive radiotherapy followed by PCV or radiotherapy alone.[140] Patients with codeletions of 1p and 19q had significantly longer overall survival irrespective of treatment, and similar to the RTOG trial, the addition of PCV did not result in a better outcome compared to radiotherapy alone. Presence of 1p or 19q loss was found to be the most important predictor of outcome, with a hazard ratio of 0.27, confirming that patients with loss of 1p or 19q represent a unique biologic subset.

In a recent updated analysis of RTOG 9402, the RTOG reported survival benefit from the addition of PCV chemotherapy in the 1p19q codeleted subset.[141] The analysis was performed with median follow-up of >11 years. For the entire study population, the median overall survival for patients receiving radiotherapy alone or radiotherapy plus PCV chemotherapy was similar. However, the 126 patients with 1p19q codeleted tumors had much longer median survival times than the 135 patients whose tumors did not carry the 1p19q codeletion: 8.7 versus 2.7 years. Even more impressive, however, was the finding that 1p19q codeletion predicted the benefit from adding chemotherapy to radiotherapy. Patients with 1p19q codeleted tumors who received PCV chemotherapy plus radiotherapy (59 patients) had a median overall survival time of 14.7 years, compared with only 7.3 years for patients with codeleted tumors who received radiotherapy alone (67 patients), therefore establishing 1p19q codeletion as both a prognostic and predictive marker.

Others molecular factors with clinical implications include MGMT promoter methylation and somatic mutations in the isocitrate dehydrogenase 1 (IDH1) gene. MGMT promoter methylation has demonstrated prognostic significance for anaplastic oligodendroglial tumors. However, unlike grade IV astrocytoma tumors, in which MGMT promoter methylation predicts survival benefit from temozolomide added to radiotherapy, MGMT promoter methylation has not shown similar predictive significance for outcome to PCV chemotherapy in anaplastic oligodendroglial tumors.[142] Identified through genome-wide mutational analysis of grade IV glioma, IDH1 mutations have been observed in 55% to 80% of grade II and III gliomas.[143,144] Although rarely present in primary grade IV gliomas, IDH1 mutations are frequently present in secondary grade IV gliomas that develop from lower-grade tumors, providing a biologic explanation for this clinical categorization.[145] Prospective trials of anaplastic gliomas demonstrated IDH1 mutations to be a strong prognostic factor. EORTC 26951 observed IDH1 mutations in 46% of patients and demonstrated prognostic significance, independent of 1p/19q codeletion, in both arms of the trial for both progression-free survival and overall survival.[146] A German multicenter phase III trial of up-front radiotherapy versus up-front chemotherapy for newly diagnosed anaplastic gliomas observed IDH1 mutations to be a stronger prognostic factor than 1p19q codeletion or MGMT promoter hypermethylation.[145] Of note, however, is that both MGMT promoter hypermethylation and IDH1 mutations are correlated with 1p19q chromosomal loss.

Treatment

The current standard of care for patients with anaplastic gliomas is maximal surgical resection followed by postoperative radiotherapy.[147] The radiotherapy target volume and dose are the same as for GBM.

Chemotherapy

Adjuvant chemotherapy added to radiotherapy has been justified on the basis of prospective trials, and a meta-analysis showing a small long-term survival benefit in patients with anaplastic glioma treated with alkylating agents plus radiotherapy.[102,147] However, because treatment is associated with significant toxicity and because of the marginal survival benefit, the use of chemotherapy has not been universally adopted. Phase 3 studies are currently enrolling patients to more clearly define the role of chemotherapy for patients with anaplastic astrocytoma, or non-codeleted anaplastic gliomas, whereas for the codeleted subset of anaplastic gliomas, chemotherapy is now considered "standard of care."

Anaplastic Astrocytoma

Levin et al.[148] randomized patients with anaplastic gliomas or GBM to receive radiotherapy with adjuvant BCNU or PCV. The use of PCV was found to be associated with an improved outcome in patients with anaplastic glioma. In contrast, a retrospective review of 432 patients with newly diagnosed anaplastic astrocytoma treated with BCNU or PCV in RTOG studies showed no improvement in survival with chemotherapy.[149]

A prospective phase III trial by the United Kingdom Medical Research Council randomized 674 patients, of whom 117 (17%) had anaplastic astrocytoma after surgery, to radiotherapy alone or radiotherapy followed by PCV.[150] There was no advantage for adjuvant PCV in any subgroup. The median survival of patients with anaplastic astrocytoma, 13 to 15 months, was substantially lower than the median survival of 2 to 3 years reported in previous trials, which has led to debate over the applicability of these results.

Temozolomide has shown activity in patients with recurrent anaplastic astrocytoma. In a phase II trial by Yung et al.,[103] 162 patients with anaplastic astrocytoma were treated with temozolomide (150 to 200 mg/m^2 per day on days 1–5 every 28 days) at first relapse. The 6-month progression-free survival was 46%, and overall survival was 13.6 months. The objective response rate was 35% (complete response 8%, partial response 27%). The agent was well tolerated, with mild to moderate hematologic toxicity in <10% of patients. The results of this trial suggest that temozolomide has antitumor activity with an acceptable safety profile for anaplastic astrocytoma. Although it is controversial, many neuro-oncologists treat anaplastic astrocytoma patients with concurrent temozolomide chemotherapy and radiation therapy followed by adjuvant temozolomide chemotherapy based on the EORTC/NCIC clinical trial in glioblastoma. This practice is being investigated in an ongoing phase III clinical trial of non–1p19q-codeleted anaplastic glioma patients (the CATNON Intergroup trial).

Anaplastic Oligodendroglioma/Oligoastrocytoma

Anaplastic oligodendroglioma and oligoastrocytoma are generally thought of as chemosensitive primarily based on high response rates to PCV in several studies. Two large randomized trials, described earlier, investigated the use of sequential chemoradiotherapy compared to radiotherapy alone with chemotherapy reserved for salvage in patients with anaplastic oligodendroglioma and oligoastrocytoma.[27,140] With 11-year follow-up, no difference in survival was found for the entire cohort, but for the codeleted patients, there was a near-doubling of survival, establishing chemoradiotherapy as a standard for this subset.

Because of the significant toxicity associated with PCV, many clinicians now use temozolomide, which is much better tolerated. The optimal number of chemotherapy cycles has not been established. Temozolomide has produced high response rates in patients with anaplastic oligodendroglioma. Chinot et al.[151] administered temozolomide to 48 patients with anaplastic oligodendroglioma/oligoastrocytoma who had previously failed PCV chemotherapy. The objective response rate was 43.8% (complete response 16.7%, partial response 27.1%). Grade 3 thrombocytopenia occurred in 6.3% patients. Vogelbaum et al.[152] reported the results of RTOG 01-31, a phase II trial in which temozolomide was given preradiotherapy to newly diagnosed patients with anaplastic oligodendroglioma/oligoastrocytoma. In the 27 patients available for review, the objective response rate was 33.3% (complete response 3.7%, partial response 29.6%). The 6-month-progression rate was 10.3%. Toxicity was acceptable. In a retrospective series from Ducray et al.,[153] up-front temozolomide for patients older than 70 years with anaplastic oligodendroglioma or anaplastic oligoastrocytoma demonstrated median progression-free survival of 6.9 months and median survival of 12.1 months, with improved outcomes in patients with MGMT methylation. Response to temozolomide has also been shown to be significantly associated with loss of 1p in a small retrospective study.[35]

In addition, a recent international retrospective study of more than 1,000 adults with anaplastic oligodendroglial tumors observed that combination chemotherapy and radiotherapy was associated with longer time to progression and overall survival than either modality alone.[127] In cases without 1p19q codeletion, Lassman et al.[154] observed that combination chemotherapy and radiotherapy was associated with longer time to progression and overall survival than either modality alone. In cases with 1p19q codeletion, combination chemotherapy and radiotherapy was associated with longer median time to progression compared to either modality alone, but this difference was not associated with a survival advantage. In addition, longer time to progression was observed with PCV compared to temozolomide in codeleted cases. Therefore, although temozolomide is widely used in lieu of PCV, the data supporting this practice are weak at best and, based on Lassman's retrospective review, is possibly deleterious.

Radiosensitizers

Prados et al.[155] randomized patients with anaplastic astrocytomas to receive conventional radiotherapy with or without bromodeoxyuridine (BrdU) given as an infusion during each week of radiotherapy plus adjuvant PCV. The study was closed before full accrual, based on an interim analysis that predicted no survival advantage for the BrdU arm. In the 190 patients who were eligible for analysis, there was no survival benefit found with the addition of BrdU.

Evidence-Based Treatment Summary

1. Maximal resection, although not tested in a prospective trial, is generally associated with more favorable outcome and is recommended whenever feasible.
2. Postoperative radiotherapy has been shown to provide a survival advantage in several clinical trials. These trials included patients with WHO grade III and IV tumors; no trial for only grade III tumors has been conducted. The standard of care is as for GBM in terms of radiotherapy target volume and dose, typically 60 Gy in 6 weeks.
3. The role of chemotherapy remains undefined for the non-codeleted anaplastic gliomas. The most widely tested agent, BCNU, and combination, with PCV, have no definite survival benefit. Temozolomide is active in recurrent anaplastic astrocytoma and is currently being tested in the up-front setting.

4. Patients with codeletions of 1p and 19q have a more favorable prognosis and respond better to both chemotherapy and radiotherapy, and in this subset, PCV chemoradiotherapy has a proven survival advantage over radiotherapy alone. The exact role of temozolomide has not been defined.

Low-Grade Glioma

Low-grade gliomas are slow-growing tumors that are divided into pilocytic and nonpilocyitc subtypes. They account for 20% and 10% of gliomas and primary intracranial tumors in adults, respectively.

Pilocytic Astrocytoma

Pilocytic astrocytoma, also known as juvenile pilocytic astrocytoma, corresponds to WHO grade I. They are more common in children. On imaging, they are well circumscribed enhancing lesions, often with a cystic component.

Treatment

Pilocytic astrocytomas are more amenable to total resection than other low-grade gliomas. Fenestration of the cyst and resection of the mural nodule are usually curative. In tumors in which the wall of the cyst enhances, cystic degeneration of a larger tumor is more likely, and resection of the entire cyst is necessary. Complete resection of pilocytic astrocytomas is associated with excellent survival, with the majority (>90%) of patients cured of the tumor; no adjuvant therapy is necessary.

Incomplete resection is associated with long-term survival rates of 70% to 80% at 10 years. The benefit of postoperative radiotherapy is unclear. Although the usual recommendation is for close follow-up, there is evidence of improved progression-free survival in this situation,[156] and immediate postoperative irradiation may be appropriate in some relatively uncommon cases, depending on the location of the tumor, the extent of residual disease, the feasibility of repeated surgical excision, and availability for follow-up. If radiotherapy is indicated, the dose is typically 50 to 55 Gy (1.8- to 2-Gy fractions).

Evidence-Based Treatment Summary

1. Maximal surgical resection, although not tested in a prospective trial, is associated with more favorable outcome and is recommended whenever feasible.
2. Postoperative radiotherapy may be considered in patients with incompletely resected tumors, based on risk factors for progression and consequences of progression.
3. Chemotherapy does not have an established role in pilocytic astrocytoma in adults.

Nonpilocytic/Diffusely Infiltrating Gliomas

Nonpilocytic or diffusely infiltrating low-grade gliomas are classified as WHO grade II tumors. They may arise from astrocytic, oligodendrocytic, or mixed lineage. Presentation usually occurs in the third or fourth decade of life, and only a small percentage of patients are younger than 19 years or older than 65 years. CT typically demonstrates an ill-defined, diffuse, nonenhancing low-density region, often in the frontal or temporal lobes. Calcifications are commonly seen with oligodendrogliomas. MRI is more sensitive in detecting and defining these lesions, which are hypointense and nonenhancing on T1-weighted images and hyperintense on T2-weighted images. Because these tumors are highly infiltrative, tumor always extends beyond the abnormality observed on imaging.

Histologically, there is increased cellularity compared to normal brain tissue, with mild to moderate nuclear pleomorphism and no evidence of mitotic activity, vascular proliferative changes, or necrosis. Differentiation from reactive gliosis can be difficult. Histologic subtypes are often identified in low-grade astrocytomas. Fibrillary and protoplasmic subtypes convey no specific prognostic information. Gemistocytic subtypes behave in a fashion more consistent with a malignant glioma.

Factors associated with improved outcome include young age, good neurologic status, oligodendroglial subtype, and low proliferation indices. Median survival is approximately 5 years for patients with astrocytoma and approximately 10 years for patients with oligodendroglioma.[157] The 5-year survival rate is 37% for patients with astrocytoma, 56% for mixed oligoastrocytoma, and 70% for oligodendroglioma.[34] A Ki-67 (MIB-I) index >3% has been shown to correlate with a worse prognosis.[158] Malignant transformation portends a poor outcome.

Molecular Diagnosis and Prognosis

Smith et al.[137] found loss of 1p and 19q in 44% of 52 patients with oligodendrogliomas, of which 34 (65%) were low grade. Combined loss of 1p and 19q was associated with an improved probability of survival, independent of other factors, such as age. Fallon et al.[159] examined 139 tumor samples from 80 patients with primary and recurrent oligodendrogliomas, of which 74% were grade II at initial diagnosis. Combined loss of 1p and 19q occurred in 71% of patients, more commonly in pure oligodendrogliomas (75%) than in mixed oligoastrocytomas (39%). Patients with combined loss of 1p and 19q had an overall median survival of 14.9 years, compared to 4.7 years for those without 1p and 19q deletions.

Okamota et al.[160] found a similar frequency of loss of 1p and 19q of 70% in patients with low-grade oligodendrogliomas in a population-based study. In a review of 44 cases of low-grade oligodendrocytic tumors, Sasaki et al.[161] considered half of the cases classical oligodendroglioma and the remainder nonclassical oligodendroglioma with more astrocytic features on histopathology. Deletion of 1p was detected in 86% and 27% of these groups, respectively. Response to chemotherapy was assessed at time of recurrence in 13 patients. Of the 11 who responded to chemotherapy, 10 had loss of 1p. Both of the nonresponders were found not to have loss of 1p. A small prospective trial by Hoang-Xuan et al.[162] found a similar trend. Loss of 1p with or without loss of 19q, which was detected in 12 of 26 patients with low-grade oligodendrocytic tumors treated with temozolomide, was found to have a significant association with response to chemotherapy ($p < .004$).

IDH1 mutations may be predictive of a better prognosis in patients with low-grade gliomas, but this marker does not appear to predict response to chemotherapy.[163] Promoter methylation of the PTEN gene has been associated with poorer prognosis and a higher likelihood of malignant transformation.[164] Other small studies have not shown an association between other molecular findings and chemosensitivity.[165,166]

Clinical Prognostic Variables

In addition to histology and molecular characteristics, several clinical variables have been found to be of prognostic importance. Pignatti et al.[167] performed the most comprehensive of these analyses and constructed a scoring system to identify patients at low and high risk. This trial was based on data from two large European phase III trials for low-grade glioma designed to examine the dose and timing of postoperative radiotherapy, EORTC 22844 and 22845. Cox regression analysis was used to identify prognostic variables from 322 patients from EORTC 22844 and then validated on 288 patients from EORTC 22845. Multivariate analysis showed that age 40 years or older, astrocytoma histology, maximum diameter ≥6 cm, tumor crossing the midline, and presence of neurologic deficits negatively affected survival. A prognostic scoring system was derived: patients with up to two of these factors were considered low risk (median survival, 7.7 years), and patients with three or more were considered high risk (median survival, 3.2 years).

Treatment

Treatment—in particular the timing of intervention for patients with diffusely infiltrative low-grade tumors remains controversial. The clinical course is variable, with some patients having long survival even without treatment and others suffering from progressive deterioration despite treatment. In general, early intervention is indicated for patients with increasing symptoms, radiographic progression, and high-risk features suggestive of transformation to a higher-grade tumor. Adequate tissue sampling is critical to ensure accurate diagnosis, and maximal surgical resection in this context may be advisable in appropriately selected patients. In younger patients (<40 years) who have undergone complete resection, observation with serial imaging are options. In those who have undergone a subtotal resection or those with high-risk features, postoperative radiotherapy may be recommended, typically 50 Gy in 1.8-Gy fractions. Recent evidence suggests that chemotherapy may have a role, particularly in patients with loss of 1p and 19q. Accrual of patients into well-designed clinical trials is imperative to define optimal treatment, and newer trials are also focusing on the effect of treatment or tumor progression on neurocognitive functioning.

Surgery

Although surgery is considered an integral part of treatment, the goal of surgery and its timing are still debated. In practice, most patients undergo surgery at presentation in order to establish the diagnosis and to determine histology, grade, and molecular characteristics that affect treatment. However, even under the best circumstances, total resection with an adequate margin is rarely achieved due to the diffusely infiltrative nature of these tumors and involvement of eloquent regions.[168] Although it is controversial, most studies have found total or subtotal (>90%) resection to be associated with improved outcome.[168–170] Moreover, with the advent of imaging to assist in identifying critical areas of the brain, resection may be achieved with less morbidity and mortality than in the past. Proponents of aggressive resection are also supported by studies that suggest that radical surgery results in more accurate histopathologic diagnosis.[171] However, surgical resection is unlikely to be curative. In RTOG 98-02, 5-year progression-free survival in 111 good-risk patients, defined as patient age younger than 40 years and gross total tumor resection, was 48%.[172] Review of postoperative MR imaging demonstrated crude recurrence rates of 26%, 68%, and 89% for residual disease <1 cm, 1 to 2 cm, and >2 cm, respectively.

Radiotherapy

Three recent phase III trials provide the best evidence with respect to the indications for radiotherapy, as well as the dose (Table 35.5).

Patients considered favorable by the scoring system introduced by Pignatti et al.[167] are typically observed postoperatively and given radiotherapy at disease progression or recurrence. This practice is based on the results of a phase III trial by van den Bent et al.[173] in EORTC 22845. In this multi-institutional trial, 314 patients with low-grade gliomas were randomized to receive postoperative radiotherapy to 54 Gy in fractions of 1.8 Gy (n = 157) or radiotherapy at progression (n = 157). A significant improvement in median progression-free survival was found with early radiotherapy (5.3 vs. 3.4 years; p <.0001), but there was no difference in median survival (7.4 vs. 7.2 years; p = .872). It is of note that only 65% the patients in the

TABLE 35.5 PHASE III TRIALS OF PATIENTS WITH LOW-GRADE GLIOMA TREATED WITH RADIOTHERAPY

Study	*Treatment Arm*	*Number of Patients*	*Five-Year Survival (%)*
EORTC 22845	Observation[a]	157	66
	54 Gy (30 fractions)	157	68
EORTC 22844	45 Gy (25 fractions)	171	58
	59.4 Gy (33 fractions)	172	59
NCCTG	50.4 (28 fractions)	101	72
	64.8 (36 fractions)	102	64

EORTC, European Organization for Research and Treatment of Cancer; NCCTG, North Central Cancer Treatment Group.

[a]Treatment with radiotherapy at progression.

delayed-radiotherapy group received radiotherapy at progression. Malignant transformation occurred in 65% to 72% of patients, with no difference between the two groups. Although seizure control was superior in the early radiotherapy group, adequate data on quality of life were not obtained. The authors concluded that although early radiotherapy may be appropriate in some situations—for example, patients with symptomatic lesions—withholding radiotherapy until tumor progression does not jeopardize survival.

For patients given radiotherapy postoperatively, the dose has been established by two phase III trials. In EORTC 22844, 379 patients were randomized to receive 45 Gy in 5 weeks or 59.4 Gy in 6.6 weeks postoperatively.[174] With a median follow-up of 74 months, overall survival (58% vs. 59%) and progression-free survival (47% vs. 50%) were similar in both arms.

In a joint North Central Cancer Treatment Group, RTOG, and ECOG study, 203 patients were randomized to low-dose radiotherapy to 50.4 Gy in 28 fractions (n = 101) or high-dose radiotherapy to 64.8 Gy in 36 fractions.[175] There was no significant difference in progression-free survival or overall survival. Survival at 2 and 5 years was 94% and 72%, respectively, with low-dose radiotherapy and 85% and 64%, respectively, with high-dose radiotherapy. Grade 3 to 5 neurotoxicity occurred in 5% of patients in the high-dose cohort and 2.5% of patients in the low-dose cohort.

Consequently, low-dose radiotherapy—50 Gy in 1.8-Gy fractions—is the standard of care for patients with low-grade gliomas. The target volume is local, with a margin of 2 cm beyond changes demonstrated on traditional MRI sequences. Using FLAIR images, which usually show abnormality beyond any enhancing or nonenhancing tumor, a smaller margin of 0.8 to 1 cm may be used.

Chemotherapy

There is no categorically established role for chemotherapy in adult patients with low-grade gliomas. A Southwest Oncology Group (SWOG) study by Eyre et al.[176] randomly assigned 60 patients with incompletely excised low-grade gliomas to receive radiotherapy alone (55 Gy in 6.5 to 7 weeks) or radiotherapy plus CCNU. Median survival was 4.5 years for radiotherapy alone and 7.4 years for radiotherapy plus CCNU (p = .7). This trial was closed early due to slow accrual. It has been argued that continued enrollment may have led to a significant difference in survival considering the large difference between the two arms.[177]

Multiagent chemotherapy, in particular PCV, appeared promising, with response rates ranging from 50% to 80% in recurrent and newly diagnosed tumors,[165,166] but proved no better than radiotherapy alone in RTOG 98-02.[172] In this phase III trial, 251 unfavorable patients (age 40 years or older with subtotal resection or biopsy) were randomized to receive radiotherapy alone to 54 Gy in 30 fractions or radiotherapy followed by six cycles of standard dose PCV. With a median follow-up of 6 years, 5-year overall survival was not different between arms (63% for radiotherapy alone; 72% for radiotherapy plus PCV), but a trend to improved 5-year progression-free survival was observed with the addition of PCV chemotherapy (46% for radiotherapy alone; 63% for radiotherapy plus PCV; $p = .06$). In addition, an overall survival advantage to PCV chemotherapy was detected in patients who survived beyond 2 years. However, acute grade 3 or 4 toxicity occurred in 67% of patients who received radiotherapy plus PCV, as compared with 9% of patients who received radiotherapy alone.

Temozolomide has been shown to have activity in phase II trials in newly diagnosed and recurrent low-grade gliomas.[162,177–179] The EORTC has completed accrual to a phase III trial (EORTC 22041) comparing radiotherapy to 50.4 Gy and temozolomide with stratification of 1p and 19q allele status. A North American Intergroup trial is comparing radiotherapy versus chemoradiotherapy (based on temozolomide).

Evidence-Based Treatment Summary

1. Maximal surgical resection, although not tested in a prospective trial, is generally associated with more favorable outcome and is recommended whenever feasible.
2. Postoperative radiotherapy has not been shown to provide a survival advantage in the only clinical trial testing this question, although progression-free survival and seizure control were superior. The typical radiotherapy dose is 45 to 54 Gy; randomized trials do not show a survival advantage with higher doses.
3. CCNU and PCV do not provide a survival advantage over radiotherapy alone. In RTOG 9802, survival advantage from chemoradiotherapy was detected in patients surviving beyond 2 years. Temozolomide is being tested in phase III trials.

Gliomatosis Cerebri

Gliomatosis cerebri is a rare condition with diffuse involvement of multiple parts of the brain (greater than two lobes), sparing neurons and normal structures. On MRI, there is typically diffuse increased signal on T2-weighted and FLAIR images and low or absent signal in the affected areas on T1-weighted images. Treatment remains undefined. Perkins et al.[180] reviewed the treatment outcomes of 30 patients with gliomatosis cerebri treated with radiotherapy at MD Anderson Cancer Center. Transient radiographic improvement or disease stabilization was achieved in 87% of patients, with clinical improvement observed in 70%. Patients younger than 40 years and those with nonglioblastoma histology had significantly improved overall survival.

In a French study, 63 patients with gliomatosis cerebri were treated initially with PCV or temozolomide.[181] Objective responses were observed in 33% of patients and radiologic responses in 26%, with no significant difference between the two regimens. Median progression-free survival and overall survival were 16 and 29 months, respectively. Regardless of regimen, patients with an oligodendroglial component had significantly better outcomes in terms of progression-free and overall survival.

A recent German phase II trial[182] treated 35 gliomatosis cerebri patients with procarbazine and lomustine. Median progression-free survival was 14 months, and median overall survival was 30 months. Twelve patients received salvage radiotherapy at progression. IDH1 mutation was a strong independent prognostic factor.

A retrospective review of 296 patients with gliomatosis cerebri from the literature ($n = 206$) and the ANOCEF network ($n = 90$) demonstrated median survival of 14.5 months.[183] Patients younger than 42 years and with better KPS, low-grade histology, or oligodendroglial subtype had better outcomes. The impact on survival of radiotherapy remained unclear.

Evidence-Based Treatment Summary

1. Maximal surgical resection is not an achievable goal.
2. Radiotherapy is considered the standard, but no trials have validated its role.
3. The role of chemotherapy remains ill defined.

Adult Brainstem Glioma

Brainstem gliomas account for 15% of all pediatric brain tumors[184] but are rare in adults. They can be divided into several distinct types. The diffuse intrinsic pontine tumors are generally high-grade astrocytomas, either anaplastic astrocytomas or GBM, whereas focal, dorsally exophytic, or cervicomedullary are usually low grade and have a much better prognosis. Although rare, other aggressive tumors such as PNETs and atypical teratoid-rhabdoid tumors can occur in the brainstem.[185,186] Nonneoplastic processes that may be confused with a primary brainstem tumor include neurofibromatosis, demyelinating diseases, arteriovenous malformations, abscess, and encephalitis.

Diffuse intrinsic pontine glioma remains one of the most challenging brain tumors. Even biopsy is rarely performed because of the substantial risk of morbidity and mortality. The diagnosis is usually based on a clinical presentation of rapidly developing neurologic findings of multiple cranial nerve palsies (most commonly VI and VII), hemiparesis, and ataxia, in combination with MRI finding of diffuse enlargement and poorly marginated T2 signal involving >50% of the pons.[187] Most diffuse intrinsic pontine gliomas are nonenhancing. Enhancement, particularly in a focal lesion, may suggest a juvenile pilocytic astrocytoma rather than a high-grade glioma; these lesions should be biopsied.

Treatment

Corticosteroids may be necessary to manage neurologic symptoms until treatment is instituted. Patients with hydrocephalus may require placement of a ventriculoperitoneal shunt. The approach to treatment should be based on the type of brainstem glioma as determined by both the clinical presentation and radiographic findings. Surgery is the treatment of choice for operable lesions (i.e., accessible focal tumors, dorsally exophytic and cervicomedullary tumors). For low-grade tumors amenable to surgical resection, as in other low-grade gliomas, the role of postoperative radiotherapy is controversial, and many would advocate close observation. For unresectable low-grade tumors radiotherapy should be delivered using volumes and doses as for low-grade gliomas in other locations.

Involved field radiotherapy is the primary treatment for infiltrating pontine gliomas. The GTV is usually best defined using T2-weighted or FLAIR MRI. A margin of 1 to 1.5 cm is added to create a CTV and further expanded by 0.3 to 0.5 cm to create a PTV. Margins may not need to be uniform in all directions, particularly where bone limits tumor extension. These lesions should be treated with doses on the order of 55.8 to 60 Gy using daily fractions of 1.8 to 2.0 Gy per day. Although radiotherapy provides short-term benefits, long-term results have remained dismal. There is no advantage to the use of higher doses given using hyperfractionation. Chemotherapy has no established role. Chapter 82 provides more details as most data on intrinsic pontine gliomas come from pediatric trials.

Fewer data exist with respect to brainstem glioma in adults, but there is some evidence that these tumors may be less aggressive in adults, with overall survival that ranges from

45% to 66% at 2 to 5 years, perhaps because of a greater frequency of more favorable tumor types.[188] Kesari et al.[189] published a series of 101 adults with brainstem gliomas and observed 5- and 10-year overall survival rates of 58% and 41%, respectively. Of 24 candidate factors, they observed prognostic significance associated with ethnicity, tumor location, age of diagnosis, and tumor grade. In the series from ANOCEF, 48 adult patients with brainstem gliomas were grouped on the basis of their clinical, radiologic, and histologic features.[190] Nearly half had nonenhancing, diffusely infiltrative tumors and had symptoms that were present for more than 3 months. Eleven of these 22 patients underwent biopsy, and 9 had low-grade histology. Nearly all underwent radiotherapy and had a median survival of 7.3 years. A second group of 15 patients who had presented with rapid progression of symptoms and had contrast enhancement on MRI were described. Fourteen of these patients underwent biopsy, and anaplasia was identified in all 14 specimens. Despite radiotherapy, the median survival in this group was 11.2 months, which approximates the survival in pediatric series.

Evidence-Based Treatment Summary

1. Surgical resection is indicated for patients with favorable tumor types but is not an achievable goal in patients with intrinsic pontine gliomas.
2. For intrinsic pontine tumors, radiotherapy is considered the standard. Dose-escalation strategies have been ineffective.

Ependymoma

Ependymoma accounts for only 1.8% of all adult brain tumors.[1] Rosette formation is a hallmark of ependymoma on pathologic specimens. The presence of increased cellularity, cytologic atypia, and microvascular proliferation suggests a diagnosis of anaplastic ependymoma. Unlike pediatric ependymomas, which largely arise intracranially, 75% of ependymomas in the adult population arise in the spinal canal. Spinal ependymomas typically present with sensory deficits. Ependymomas may expand locally, extend along ependymal spaces, and occasionally disseminate through the CSF. However, the predominant pattern of relapse is local, even when anaplasia is present.[191–193,194,195]

Treatment

Maximal surgical resection, including second surgery if necessary, is the initial treatment for ependymoma. Surgery alone may be sufficient in selected patients based on the results of pediatric series described in Chapter 82. However, the standard of care for most adults is postoperative irradiation. There appears to be a radiation dose response, with improved tumor control with doses >50 Gy, and doses of 54 to 59.4 Gy are typically prescribed. Radiation dose for spinal ependymomas can be limited by spinal cord tolerance. At 1.8 to 2 Gy/fraction, the estimated risk of radiation myelopathy is <1% at 54 Gy and <10% at 61 Gy.[196]

Historically, for posterior fossa tumors, the entire posterior fossa has been irradiated. However, Paulino[197] showed the pattern of failure to be "local," that is, within the tumor bed itself. In nine patients who received radiation therapy to the tumor bed plus a 2-cm margin, the two failures in this group were within the tumor bed (i.e., there were no failures within the posterior fossa outside the tumor bed). For most patients, a more usual volume now consists of the tumor bed and any residual disease (GTV) plus an anatomically defined margin of 1 to 1.5 cm to create a CTV. Larger margins may be required in areas of infiltration, and special attention must be paid to areas of spread along the cervical spine because 10% to 30% of fourth ventricular tumors extend down through the foramen magnum to the upper cervical spine.[195,198] Radiotherapy field size for spinal ependymomas commonly includes two cranial and two caudal vertebral bodies. Sacral ependymomas should include coverage of nerve roots, with the caudal border extending to S4/S5 and lateral borders extending to the sacroiliac joints.

In the past, craniospinal irradiation was recommended for patients with high-grade and infratentorial tumors who were believed to be at an increased risk of CSF spread.[193] Modern series document that local recurrence is the primary pattern of failure and that the incidence of isolated spinal relapses is low even among the highest-risk patients, with the majority of spinal failures associated with local recurrences.[191,194] As a result, the current recommendation for patients with ependymomas is limited-field radiation if the spinal MRI scan and CSF cytology are negative. Patients with neuraxis spread (positive MRI or positive CSF cytology) should receive craniospinal irradiation (40 to 45 Gy), with boosts to the areas of gross disease and to the primary tumor to total doses of 50 to 54 Gy.

Chemotherapy has not been proven useful in ependymoma. However, a regimen consisting of preirradiation cyclophosphamide, vincristine, cisplatin, and etoposide used in a recent Children's Cancer Group study (CCG-9942) for patients with residual ependymoma appears more promising than agents and regimens used in the past. In addition, cisplatin-based chemotherapy has shown some activity in recurrent ependymoma in adults.[199]

Results of Treatment

In modern series that used mostly local fields for patients with nondisseminated disease, 5-year survival is on the order of 70%.[193,198,200–203]

Several authors have attempted to identify variables associated with improved outcome in adults. Ferrante et al.[201] analyzed 20 patients with fourth ventricle ependymomas. The 5-year survival rate in patients older than 16 years was 60%. The use of postoperative irradiation was associated with a markedly improved 5-year survival of 68% versus 18% without radiotherapy ($p = .011$).

Reni et al.[204] reported on a series of 70 adult intracranial ependymomas and observed 5-year overall and progression-free survival rates of 67% and 43%, respectively. Older age and supratentorial location were poor prognostic factors, and the use of postoperative radiotherapy was associated with improved progression-free survival and a trend toward improved overall survival.

Metellus et al.[205] evaluated 114 adult patients with intracranial ependymoma and observed incomplete resection and supratentorial location to be significant predictors of recurrence and poor survival. For incompletely resected tumors, postoperative radiotherapy improved both overall and progression-free survival. In a study of spinal myxopapillary ependymomas from the Rare Cancer Network,[206] use of postoperative radiotherapy was an independent predictor of progression-free survival.

A retrospective study of 23 adult patients with supratentorial ependymomas treated at Columbia-Presbyterian Medical Center with a variety of radiotherapy field sizes and doses (including stereotactic radiosurgery) showed a 5-year survival rate of 100% for hemispheric tumors and 73% for third ventricular tumors.[197] Of interest, six patients with low-grade tumors did not receive postoperative irradiation. Five remained free of recurrence during a mean follow-up period of 69 months.

Five-year survival was 62% for a French series of 34 adult patients with ependymoma, 17 of whom had anaplastic histology.[207] Gross total resection was performed in 27 patients. Half of the 34 patients were irradiated; 13 of these received local fields to a mean dose of 56 Gy. Univariate analysis showed that anaplasia and location in the brain parenchyma predicted poor outcome.

Evidence-Based Treatment Summary

1. Maximal surgical resection should be performed when feasible.
2. Postoperative radiotherapy is considered the standard, but no prospective trials have validated its role. Craniospinal irradiation is used only in patients with disseminated disease.
3. The role of chemotherapy remains to be defined.

Medulloblastoma

Medulloblastoma is a relatively rare tumor in adults, with an incidence of 0.5 per 100,000.[1,208] The majority arise in the 20- to 40-year age group. Adult medulloblastomas are more frequently located laterally than those in childhood (50% vs. 10%), and are more frequently desmoplastic.[209] In addition, the incidence of severe anaplasia is lower than in the pediatric population.[210] Medulloblastoma is a densely cellular tumor with small, darkly staining ovoid cells with hyperchromatic nuclei and frequent mitoses. Homer Wright rosettes (clustered cells surrounding a central eosinophilic core) are characteristic. CSF dissemination may manifest as positive cytology or macroscopic seeding of the subarachnoid space and is not uncommon. Systemic spread is seen in approximately 5% of patients, mostly to bone and bone marrow. Shunt procedures have been suggested as a cause, although modern series dispute this.[211]

In children, adverse prognostic factors include male gender and age younger than 3 years.[212] Patients with total or near-total resections fare better than those with subtotal resection or biopsy only, and residual tumor >1.5 cm^2 on postoperative scans is an adverse prognostic factor. Patients with CSF spread have a worse prognosis. Patients are classified as "average risk" if there is <1.5 cm^2 of residual tumor and no dissemination; patients with >1.5 cm^2 of residual tumor and/or dissemination are considered "high risk."

Treatment

All patients with nondisseminated medulloblastoma should undergo complete resection if feasible. In some cases, extension into the brainstem precludes complete resection without significant morbidity.

Although it is not clear whether the biology of adult medulloblastoma is different from that of pediatric medulloblastoma, long-term survival seems comparable, and in general the treatment guidelines for pediatric medulloblastoma detailed in Chapter 82 should probably be followed. Postoperative radiotherapy should begin within 28 to 30 days following surgical resection whenever possible. Radiotherapy is delivered to the entire craniospinal axis. This is followed by a boost to the entire posterior fossa using parallel-opposed portals or, more commonly, posterior oblique fields or other multifield techniques to spare the cochlea. Although there may be less concern over long-term toxicity of full-dose CSI in adults as compared with children, adults treated for medulloblastoma with a mean dose to the whole brain of 35 Gy have been shown to have long-term cognitive deficits.[213] It may be reasonable to extrapolate from the pediatric experience and to treat healthy young adults with average risk disease with reduced-dose CSI (23.4 Gy) as long as appropriate chemotherapy is administered. The total dose to the posterior fossa should be 54 to 55.8 Gy. However, many adult patients, particularly those who are "older" or who have comorbidities, may not tolerate the postradiation chemotherapy as well as their pediatric counterparts, and the long-term outcome in adults treated with reduced-dose craniospinal irradiation and chemotherapy is not known. Full-dose CSI (36 Gy) should be delivered in the setting of high-risk disease. This is then followed by a boost to the posterior fossa as for average-risk disease. Intracranial and spinal metastases should be boosted as well, to total doses on the order of 45 to 50 Gy for spinal metastases and 50 to 54 Gy for intracranial metastases. Treatment is usually delivered at 1.8 Gy per day.

The role of adjuvant chemotherapy in children with medulloblastoma is well established but remains unclear in adults. A series of 32 adults with medulloblastoma from Germany has shown a nonsignificant trend to prolonged survival with adjuvant chemotherapy.[214] In general treatment in adults should probably parallel that in children, even though, as noted, treatment may be compromised by poorer tolerance to chemotherapy.

Results of Treatment

Brandes et al.[215] reported on long-term results from a prospective phase II trial of adult medulloblastoma, with average-risk patients treated with radiotherapy alone and high-risk patients treated with two cycles of up-front chemotherapy followed by radiotherapy and adjuvant chemotherapy. At a median follow-up of 7.6 years, 5-year overall and progression-free survival rates were 75% (average risk, 80%; high risk, 73%) and 72% (average risk, 80%; high risk, 69%), respectively.

The largest series to date of adult medulloblastoma is a retrospective review of 253 patients older than the age of 18 years treated at 13 different French institutions between 1975 and 2004.[216] The median follow-up in this series was 7 years. On multivariate analysis, brainstem involvement, fourth ventricular floor involvement, and posterior fossa radiation dose <50 Gy were negative prognostic factors. Overall survival was 72% at 5 years and 55% at 10 years. One hundred twenty-four patients were classified as having average-risk disease, and 67 of these received chemotherapy along with CSI. Overall survival was not different between patients treated with full-dose CSI alone and patients treated with CSI doses <34 Gy in combination with chemotherapy. However, it should be noted that this was a heterogeneous group of patients, and only 12 of these patients received a spinal dose ≤29 Gy. Thus, long-term outcome of adults treated with reduced-dose CSI to 23.4 Gy and chemotherapy is still unknown.

Evidence-Based Treatment Summary

1. There are no prospective, randomized trials evaluating major therapeutic issues in this disease in adults.
2. Maximal surgical resection should be performed, where feasible.
3. Standard treatment consists of postoperative radiotherapy to the craniospinal axis followed by a boost to the posterior fossa.
4. The use of chemotherapy generally follows the pediatric indications and guidelines.

Primary Central Nervous System Lymphoma

Primary central nervous system lymphoma (PCNSL) is a non-Hodgkin lymphoma that is restricted to the central nervous system (brain, spinal cord, meninges, and eye) and accounts for <3% of primary intracranial malignancies. It occurs in two distinct patient populations: immunocompromised (HIV, post-transplant, etc.) and immunocompetent. Immunodeficiency is the only known risk factor. Immunocompetent patients present typically in the sixth and seventh decades of life, whereas immunosuppressed individuals more commonly present in the third and fourth decades of life.

The majority of primary CNS lymphomas are B-cell lymphomas of intermediate or high grade that are indistinguishable from high-grade non-Hodgkin lymphomas occurring elsewhere in the body. In immunocompetent patients, PCNSL typically presents with one or multifocal (in 30%) mass lesions primarily located in the frontal lobes, corpus callosum, and deep periventricular brain structures. Although the lesions appear focal, diffuse involvement of the parenchyma is invariably present. As a consequence of this deep localization, patients usually present with cognitive dysfunction or personality change. Other symptoms include headache or focal neurologic dysfunction such as hemiparesis or hemisensory loss; seizures are rare. Symptoms often progress over weeks to months before a diagnosis is made.

On MRI, PCNSL is hypointense on T1 and hypointense to isointense on T2/FLAIR sequences with variable surrounding edema. There is usually homogeneous enhancement with intravenous contrast. Ring enhancement is uncommon, except in immunocompromised patients. The appearance on T2 sequences and lack of central necrosis help to differentiate PCNSL from glioma.

Even with the "classic" imaging appearance, histology is essential for diagnosis. If PCNSL is suspected, sterotactic biopsy is the best approach; extensive resection does not improve survival. Corticosteroids should be held at presentation unless absolutely necessary (e.g., pending brain herniation) because their "lytic" effect on lymphoma may lead to a false-negative biopsy. Once a diagnosis of PCNSL is established, an extent of disease workup is required. At diagnosis of PCNSL, ocular disease is present in 20% (often misdiagnosed as idiopathic uveitis) and demonstrable leptomeningeal disease is present in 25% (usually asymptomatic until late). A complete staging workup consists of contrast-enhanced brain MR, lumbar puncture (for CSF cytology, flow cytometry, and Epstein-Barr virus polymerase chain reaction), slit-lamp ocular exam (to look for intraocular lymphoma), HIV serology, and contrast-enhanced spine MRI. Systemic staging (body CT, bone marrow biopsy) is rarely positive in patients with typical findings of CNS lymphoma but should be performed if systemic symptoms are present (weight loss, night sweats, fever).

Age and performance status are the most important prognostic factors. An RPA analysis of 338 patients at Memorial Sloan-Kettering Cancer Center led to the identification of three RPA classes: class I (age, <50 years) was associated with median survival of 8.5 years; class II (age, >50 years, and KPS ≥ 70) with that of 3.2 years; and class III (age, >50 years, and KPS < 70) with that of 1.1 years.[217] The International Extranodal Lymphoma Study Group evaluated 378 patients and observed age older than 60 years, ECOG >1, elevated lactate dehydrogenase, high CSF protein, and deep regions of the brain as prognostic.[218]

Treatment

The role of surgery is limited to establishing the tissue diagnosis. This is best achieved by stereotactic biopsy; extensive tumor resection offers no survival benefit. Because primary CNS lymphoma often responds dramatically to corticosteroid therapy, corticosteroids should be avoided unless absolutely necessary until after tissue is obtained.

PCNSL is exquisitely sensitive to radiotherapy and chemotherapy. Although never studied in a prospective fashion, WBRT is believed to be more effective that focal radiotherapy due to the extensive infiltration of lymphoma throughout the brain. The optimal dose is 45 to 50 Gy, and there is no benefit of adding a boost to the tumor site. With WBRT alone, median survival is 12 to 18 months, and the 5-year survival rate is only 4%.

The standard systemic lymphoma chemotherapy regimens are ineffective for PCNSL, as demonstrated in prospective clinical trials.[219–221] High-dose systemic methotrexate, administered at a high dose (1 to 8 g/m^2) and at a rapid rate of infusion to overcome the BBB, is the only agent that has demonstrated improved survival over WBRT alone. A recent randomized, phase II study suggests that combination chemotherapy with methotrexate results in superior disease control and survival as compared to single-agent methotrexate.[222] High-dose methotrexate regimens produce adequate levels of drug in the CSF so that direct instillation of chemotherapy (e.g., using an Ommaya reservoir) into the CSF is not necessary, unless CSF cytology is positive.[223]

Whole-brain radiotherapy is typically used as postchemotherapy consolidation in patients younger than 60 years, as a salvage strategy for recurrence, or as up-front therapy alone for patients with poor performance status (KPS < 40) or renal failure. Patients 60 years of age or older are at high risk of developing treatment-related neurotoxicity following treatment with methotrexate and WBRT; WBRT is often deferred in this subgroup except for recurrence.

Neurotoxicity after PCNSL treatment is characterized by dementia, ataxia, and urinary incontinence, occurring a mean of 7 months from treatment. Both methotrexate and radiotherapy can cause this syndrome, and the combination is synergistic. The risk is greatest in patients 60 years of age or older at diagnosis and when methotrexate is administered concurrently or following radiotherapy. In one phase II trial, patients 60 years old or older had a 100% incidence of neurotoxicity at 24 months, whereas those younger than 60 years had a 30% incidence at 96 months.[224]

The commonly used radiotherapy schedule for primary CNS lymphoma in immunocompetent patients is 40 to 45 Gy to the whole brain. The posterior orbits should be included in the whole-brain fields. In patients with ocular involvement, the whole eye can be treated to 30 to 40 Gy, with shielding of the anterior chamber and lacrimal apparatus after this dose. However, most treating physicians reserve the use of ocular radiotherapy for failure of intravitreal methotrexate and rituximab. CSI has been advocated for patients with documented CSF involvement. However, intrathecal chemotherapy is preferred because it may be equally efficacious but less toxic, with less impact on bone marrow reserve.

For immunosuppressed patients with primary CNS lymphoma, modification of the irradiation dose and schedule may be necessary. Patients with poor prognostic features (low KPS, CD4 counts of <200, advanced AIDS) may be treated with an abbreviated course of radiotherapy (e.g., 36 to 40 Gy).

Results of Treatment

Unlike non-CNS lymphoma, there appears to be a radiotherapy dose response with a threshold between 30 and 50 Gy, with a median of 40 Gy. A study by Bessell et al.[225] showed a higher relapse rate and reduced survival rate in patients who received WBRT 30.6 Gy as compared to 45 Gy in patients who had complete response to chemotherapy. This was significant for patients younger than 60 years of age. However, radiation doses beyond 45 to 50 Gy are associated with a plateau in radiation response. The RTOG conducted a phase II study (RTOG 83-15) to evaluate WBRT as first-line treatment. Median survival was 12 months, and recurrence in the brain occurred in 61% of patients, with more relapses in the 60-Gy region, suggesting no clear dose response at >40 Gy.

The most widely used treatment regimen is based on a phase II study (RTOG 93-10)[226] that treated 102 newly diagnosed PCNSL patients with five cycles of high-dose methotrexate (2.5 g/m^2), vincristine, and procarbazine followed by 45 Gy WBRT and high-dose cytarabine (3.0 g/m^2) postradiotherapy. Approximately halfway through the study, the dose of WBRT was decreased to 36 Gy delivered by hyperfractionation to those that achieved a complete response after preradiotherapy chemotherapy. Fifty-eight percent of patients achieved a complete response, and 36% had a partial response after preradiotherapy chemotherapy. Median progression-free and overall survival were 24 and 37 months, respectively.

Long-term results with various combination chemotherapy regimens that include intravenous and intrathecal methotrexate, cranial radiotherapy, and intravenous cytarabine have been encouraging, especially in patients younger than 50 years of age (5-year survival rate of 60%). In older patients (>50 years of age), results are poor (5-year survival of rate of <10%), and toxicity is greater with dementia and ataxia in a substantial proportion of patients.[227]

Chemotherapy has also been used without radiotherapy or as a means of delaying radiotherapy particularly in patients older than age 60 years because of their substantial risk of developing treatment-related neurotoxicity.[228] Complete responses occur in >50% of patients. Single-agent methotrexate using a dose of 8 g/m^2 had a high response rate, but responses were of a relatively short duration, with a median progression-free survival of approximately 1 year.[229]

Eliminating WBRT from treatment regimens results in higher recurrence incidence. Current work is focusing on methods to eliminate or reduce the risk of neurotoxicity without compromising long-term disease control. Shah et al.[230] reported a phase II study that evaluated the effectiveness and toxicity of reduced-dose WBRT (23.4 Gy) in patients who achieved a complete response following methotrexate-based chemotherapy. The estimated 2-year overall survival and progression-free survival in these 19 patients were 89% and 79%, respectively. At a follow-up of 12 months, none of the patients treated with reduced-dose radiotherapy developed treatment-related dementia on neurocognitive studies.

The use of high-dose chemotherapy with autologous stem transplant (HDC/ASCT) in newly diagnosed PCNSL patients is another strategy that has been explored as an alternative to WBRT. Because available data are limited to a few small, nonrandomized, phase 2 studies[231] and these studies differ in induction and condition regimens, defining the efficacy of this strategy is difficult. Cumulative results suggest that there may be a curative effect in young patients. High-dose methotrexate–based polychemotherapy induction is more active than monochemotherapy, and conditioning regimens containing thiotepa seem to be more effective and more toxic. The BEAM regimen (carmustine, etoposide, cytarabine, and melphalan) was ineffective, with median event-free survival of only 9.3 months. Two ongoing clinical trials (NCT01011920; NCT00863460) randomizing patients to consolidative WBRT versus HDC/ASCT will help to establish the highest tolerated and most effective consolidation strategy. Until more data are available, HDC/ASCT consolidation to primary chemotherapy can only be recommended as an experimental approach.

In patients with immunosuppression and primary CNS lymphoma, results are discouraging, although selected patients (non-HIV immunosuppression, favorable-prognosis patients with AIDS) may have survival comparable with that of nonimmunosuppressed populations when treated in a standard fashion.[232]

Evidence-Based Treatment Summary

1. Surgical resection is not necessary.
2. Avoiding or deferring WBRT results in inferior progression-free survival but without significantly affecting overall survival. Because of the toxicities associated with WBRT, its role is being evaluated in a risk-adapted approach by the RTOG.
3. High-dose systemic methotrexate is the only agent that has demonstrated improved survival over WBRT alone. High-dose methotrexate–based chemotherapy followed by whole-brain radiotherapy is the standard treatment for patients younger than 60 years of age with a good performance status.
4. High-dose methotrexate–based chemotherapy alone with deferred radiotherapy may be preferred in elderly patients because of substantial risk of neurotoxicity associated with combined chemotherapy–radiotherapy regimens.

Meningioma

Meningiomas account for approximately 30% of primary intracranial neoplasms and are the most common benign intracranial tumor in adults.[1] The peak age of incidence is in the sixth and seventh decades, although they may occur at any age. They are more common in women. Typical locations for meningiomas include the cerebral convexities, falx cerebri, tentorium cerebelli, cerebellopontine angle, and sphenoid ridge. Malignant varieties with invasive growth and aggressive behavior occasionally occur.

Grossly, meningiomas are well-circumscribed, firm, tan, or grayish lesions arising from the meninges. Hyperostosis of adjacent bone may be present. Microscopically benign meningiomas usually have a bland, whorled appearance, with little anaplasia or mitotic activity. Psammoma bodies may be present. Histologic variants (e.g., fibrous, transitional, angiomatous) can be identified but are of little prognostic significance. Malignant varieties are identified on the basis of clinical behavior (rapid growth or recurrence, invasiveness), pathologic features such as microscopic features of malignancy (cellular or nuclear anaplasia, mitotic figures), or specific histologic type (rhabdoid, papillary, anaplastic). The 2007 updated WHO grading criteria incorporate mitotic activity, nuclear-to-cytoplasmic ratio, spontaneous necrosis, brain invasion, and certain mengingioma variants to assign a grade I through III (Table 35.6).[233] Benign meningiomas (~78% to 80%) are classified as WHO grade I and associated with slower growth and lower risk of recurrence, atypical meningiomas (20%) are WHO grade II with an increased likelihood of aggressive behavior, and anaplastic or malignant gliomas (3% to 5%) are WHO grade III and associated with high invasiveness and the worst prognosis.

Meningiomas are known to be induced by ionizing radiation, with an average interval to diagnosis of 19 to 35 years, depending on the dose of radiation. They may be multiple, particularly in patients with neurofibromatosis type 2 (NF2) and in non-NF2 families with a hereditary predisposition to meningioma.

The most common cytogenetic alteration in meningiomas involves a deletion of chromosome 22. Molecular genetics findings indicate that approximately 50% of

TABLE 35.6 WORLD HEALTH ORGANIZATION 2007 TUMOR GRADE

Grade I (Benign)	Grade II (Atypical)	Grade III (Anaplastic/Malignant)
Any major variant other than clear cell, chordoid, papillary or rhabdoid OR Does not fulfill criteria for grades II or III	Frequent mitoses (>4 per 10 hpf) OR Three or more of the following: Sheeting architecture Hypercellularity (focal or diffuse) Prominent nucleoli Small cells with high nuclear-to-cytoplasmic ratio Foci of spontaneous necrosis OR Additional subtypes/features Chordoid meningioma Clear cell meningioma Brain invasion	Excessive mitotic index (>20 per 10 hpf) OR Frank anaplasia defined as focal or diffuse loss of meningothelial differentiation resembling sarcoma, carcinoma, or melanoma OR Additional subtypes/features Papillary meningioma Rhabdoid meningioma

hpf, high-power fields.

meningiomas have allelic losses that involve band q12 on chromosome 22. Allelic losses of chromosomal arms 6q, 9p, 10q, and 14q are seen in both atypical and anaplastic meningiomas. Genetic and cytogenetic alterations accumulate with progression from WHO grade I to WHO grade III in 60% of sporadic meningiomas.

The incidental finding of a meningioma on CT or MRI is not uncommon, particularly in the elderly. Many meningioma patients are asymptomatic and may remain so for a long time.[234,235] Lesions in the cerebellopontine angle commonly present with symptoms of cranial neuropathy. Cerebral convexity meningioma may present with symptoms of headache or a seizure. Meningiomas of the sphenoid wing or optic nerve may be associated with visual loss. The differential diagnosis of meningioma in the base of the skull or spine includes bone metastasis or primary bone tumors (chondrosarcoma, chordoma, osteosarcoma). In the cerebellopontine angle, acoustic neuromas may resemble meningiomas on imaging.

Meningiomas typically grow slowly. In 47 asymptomatic patients with meningioma diagnosed incidentally by MRI, Nakamura et al.[236] reported a mean annual growth measured using serial MRI of 14.6% and a mean tumor doubling time of 21.6 years. Higher annual growth rates were seen in young patients and lower annual growth rates in patients with calcification and hypointense or isointense T2 signals on MRI. The location of the lesion, extent of surgical resection, and histopathologic features of the tumor (benign or malignant) are the most important determinants of prognosis.[237]

After surgery, the average time to recurrence is approximately 4 years. In a review of 38 patients who underwent subtotal resection, the mean diameter increase was 0.37 cm/year and mean tumor doubling time was 8 years.[238]

Treatment

Grade I Meningioma

Patients with asymptomatic lesions may be observed and followed with serial imaging. The treatment of choice for symptomatic or progressive benign meningiomas is complete surgical resection if it can be accomplished with acceptable morbidity. Resection of these typically vascular tumors may be facilitated by preoperative angiography with or without embolization. Even after complete resection, 7% to 12% of these tumors recur at 5 years, and 20% to 25% recur at 10 years,[239,240] so that follow-up with serial imaging is necessary.

Complete resection of skull-based, cerebellopontine angle, or cavernous sinus meningiomas may be difficult without significant morbidity. Subtotal resections are associated with higher relapse rates of 39% to 47% at 5 years and 60% to 61% at 10 years without adjuvant therapy.[239,240] For these patients, conservative subtotal resection followed by postoperative irradiation may give good local control with less morbidity than an aggressive base-of-skull resection. An alternative approach for patients who have undergone subtotal resection is follow-up with further surgery, if feasible, and radiotherapy delayed to time of recurrence.

In patients with subtotally excised unresectable or recurrent meningiomas the typical radiotherapy dose is 50 to 54 Gy in 25 to 30 fractions over 5 to 6 weeks. The target volume for radiotherapy is defined by CT or MRI scan and modified according to the neurosurgeon's description of the location of residual tumor. The margin expansion for meningiomas is based on the knowledge of direction of spread, especially through neural foramina, bony invasion, dural tails, and so forth. The GTV is the enhancing abnormality on contrast-enhanced MRI. Margin expansions then incorporate setup errors and block margins; these can vary from 0.5 to 1 cm in total, depending on the precision of the immobilization and delivery systems. Multiple fields with wedges or rotational fields and 3D conformal techniques are used for maximal sparing of normal brain tissue. IMRT or proton therapy may be helpful in avoiding adjacent surrounding structures.

Postoperative irradiation after less-than-complete resection improves local control, prolongs the interval to recurrence, and improves survival. In series by Condra et al.,[239] subtotal resection with postoperative irradiation had a local control rate of 87% at 15 years, compared to 76% following total excision and 30% after subtotal excision (p = .0001). In modern series using MRI and CT localization, 5-year local control is reported to be >90%.[241]

Radiosurgery as the sole modality or as postoperative adjuvant therapy may be of interest for selected patients, generally those with smaller tumors. In recent series, 5-year progression-free survival rates are >80%.[242–246]

Chemotherapy has not been useful in the treatment of benign meningiomas. Given the high estrogen and progesterone receptor expression on meningiomas, progesterone receptor antagonists have been tested but have not been found beneficial.

Grade II and III Meningioma

For atypical or malignant meningiomas, the recurrence rate after surgery alone is high (41% to 100% at 5 years), even after complete surgical resection,[247] and postoperative irradiation after maximal resection is recommended for all patients. The target volume is more generous than that used for benign meningiomas. The GTV is typically expanded by 1.5 to 2 cm around the contrast-enhancing visible tumor to account for microscopic invasion of brain parenchyma. The recommended dose is on the order of 54 Gy in 30 fractions for atypical meningioma and 60 Gy in 33 fractions for malignant meningioma, although some have reported improved local control with higher doses.[248]

In a review of 38 patients with malignant meningiomas by Dziuk et al.,[241] use of postoperative radiotherapy resulted in superior local control. At 5 years, irradiation following initial resection improved 5-year disease-free survival from 15% to 80% (p = .002). Progression-free survival was 57% in patients treated with total resection and radiotherapy, compared to 28% in patients treated with total resection alone.

Systemic therapy has no defined role. Combined chemotherapy with vincristine, Adriamycin, and cyclophosphamide has shown some efficacy in patients with malignant meningiomas.[249]

Unresectable or Recurrent Meningioma

In patients in whom aggressive surgery is not an option, radiotherapy may relieve symptoms and decrease the rate of tumor progression.

Radiotherapy may be useful in the treatment of recurrent meningioma. In a review by Miralbell et al.,[250] progression-free survival at 8 years for patients treated with subtotal resection and radiotherapy at first recurrence was 78%, compared to 11% in patients treated with resection alone (p = .001).

Various chemotherapy treatments that have been used in patients with recurrent meningiomas include combined doxorubicin and dacarbazine or ifosfamide and mesna.[251] Long-term, low-dose daily hydroxyurea may have some activity.[252]

Hormonal manipulation, including tamoxifen and the antiprogesterone drug RU486, showed some activity in a SWOG phase II evaluation of tamoxifen in unresectable or refractory meningiomas.[253] However, a subsequent SWOG phase III study of mifepristone for unresectable meningioma was negative.[254]

Evidence-Based Treatment Summary

1. Small asymptomatic meningiomas in noncritical locations, especially in the elderly or in patients with other comorbidities, can be observed.

2. The goal of surgery is to completely resect the meningioma with negative margins, as patients with WHO grade I completely resected meningiomas have low rates of relapse and can be observed postoperatively.
3. For subtotally resected or unresectable progressive meningioma radiotherapy is frequently used but has not been tested in a prospective clinical trial. Local control appears to be improved with postoperative radiotherapy. Both radiosurgery and radiotherapy have been used in this context but have not been directly compared.
4. For grades II and III meningioma, postoperative radiotherapy is routinely recommended.
5. Primary radiotherapy or radiosurgery could be used for unresectable, progressive meningiomas.
6. Systemic therapy does not have a defined role in meningioma.

Craniopharyngioma

Craniopharyngiomas arise from epithelial remnants of the Rathke pouch and are typically found in the suprasellar region in children or adolescents. They account for <5% of all CNS neoplasms in adults. They are slowly growing tumors that often have solid and cystic components, the latter filled with lipoid, cholesterol-laden ("crankcase oil") fluid. Although appearing well encapsulated, craniopharyngiomas typically demonstrate invaginations into adjacent brain and may provoke a vigorous glial reaction.

The cystic nature of craniopharyngiomas is usually evident on CT and MRI and helps to distinguish these tumors from other base-of-skull lesions and pituitary adenomas. The solid portion is often calcified and enhancing, whereas the cystic portion typically demonstrates a thin rim of enhancement. The finding of multiple cysts of varying intensity on T1- and T2-weighted MRI is characteristic of craniopharyngioma.

Intrasellar lesions may compress the pituitary gland and hypothalamus, producing hormonal abnormalities, especially antidiuretic and growth hormone deficits. Prechiasmal lesions may compress the optic pathway, leading to visual field cuts or decreased central visual acuity. Retrochiasmal lesions may grow into the third ventricle and cause hydrocephalus or compress the optic tracts. Craniopharyngiomas can occasionally reach enormous size and produce neurologic impairment by direct impingement on brain parenchyma. Surgical decompression is the optimal treatment for rapid symptom relief. However, the location, proximity, and adhesiveness of the tumor to adjacent structures often preclude complete resection.

Treatment

A discussion of craniopharyngioma in the pediatric context is provided in Chapter 82. Management options include complete resection, subtotal resection alone, or subtotal resection or biopsy followed by postoperative radiotherapy.

Complete surgical resection, which is applicable only to a minority of patients, is associated with local control and long-term survival in 70% to 90% of patients.[255] However, aggressive resection may be associated with significant morbidity, with up to 10% incidence of perioperative mortality and up to 30% severe morbidity, especially diabetes insipidus or other endocrine deficits, visual impairment, obesity, and memory impairment.

Partial resection or cyst aspiration and biopsy rapidly relieve local compressive symptoms and have less operative morbidity but are associated with eventual tumor progression in most cases. Long-term survival and local control are achieved only in approximately 30% of patients. In contrast to aggressive resections, subtotal resections carry a mortality of about 1%.

With a limited surgical procedure (partial resection or cyst aspiration plus biopsy) followed by radiotherapy, local control and survival rates are nearly equivalent to those achieved with complete resection, with survival rates of 89% and 77% at 5 and 10 years, respectively, as compared with 53% to 37% for patients who have had subtotal resection alone. Typically, doses of 50 to 54 Gy in 25 to 30 fractions (1.8 Gy) over 6 weeks are delivered to the preoperative tumor volume with a 1- to 1.5-cm margin, depending on the accuracy of the imaging used for planning and the reproducibility of the treatment setup. In patients with compressive symptoms, surgical decompression before irradiation is essential because the tumor typically responds slowly to radiotherapy, and radiation-induced edema may worsen compressive symptoms.

With these dose recommendations (i.e., 1.8-Gy fractions to 50 to 54 Gy), the risk of visual impairment is very low (1% and 1.5%). In a retrospective analysis of patients treated with 51.3 to 70 Gy, a higher incidence of radiation-related complications was seen in those who received more than 60 Gy (with an actuarial incidence of optic neuropathy of 30% and brain necrosis of 12.5%), without any concomitant improvement in tumor control.[256]

Radiotherapy may be given as salvage rather than immediately after subtotal resection. In a series of 76 patients treated at the University of Pennsylvania, long-term survival rates were equivalent.[257] In another series radiotherapy given at recurrence yielded a 10-year progression-free survival rate of >70%.[258] Recurrences occur from 3 to 192 months (median, 12 months) after subtotal resection, so that close surveillance is necessary during the first years following incomplete resection.

Other modalities used in the treatment of craniopharyngioma have included intralesional bleomycin and radioactive colloid instillations for cystic tumors. Radiosurgery may be useful in ablating small residual or recurrent tumors.[259] With radiosurgery, dose to the optic chiasm and nerves must be kept below 8 Gy, estimated to be radiobiologic tolerance for optic neuropathy with single-fraction radiosurgical doses. As a result, radiosurgery use should be restricted to tumors <3 cm in size and located >3 to 5 mm from the optic apparatus.

Evidence-Based Treatment Summary

1. Surgical resection is recommended, when feasible.
2. The use of postoperative radiotherapy has not been tested in prospective trials but reduces the risk of recurrence and improves survival in incompletely resected tumors. Cyst decompression and biopsy followed by radiotherapy may be an acceptable treatment for patients for whom resection is not considered feasible.
3. Intracavitary bleomycin or radiocolloids may be useful in cystic tumors.

Vestibular Schwannoma and Neurofibroma

Neurilemomas, also known as schwannomas and neurinomas, arise from the Schwann cells of the myelin sheath of the peripheral nerves. When occurring close to the eighth cranial nerve, they are also called vestibular schwannomas or acoustic neuromas. These tumors account for approximately 6% of CNS neoplasms in adults. They may be sporadic or associated with NF2, with bilateral vestibular schwannomas being pathognomonic of this disease. Most sporadic vestibular schwannomas are unilateral and occur in the fourth and fifth decades of life. Those arising in patients with NF2 tend to occur in the second or third decades. These tumors grow slowly in a well-circumscribed, expansile fashion, displacing adjacent nerves rather than invading them. Most arise from cranial nerve VIII in the medial internal auditory canal. Less commonly, they may arise from other cranial nerves, the trigeminal nerve being the most common alternate site.

Growth in the internal auditory canal gives rise to vestibular and hearing abnormalities in up to 95% of patients. A progressive unilateral sensorineural hearing loss is characteristic. Expansion into the cerebellopontine angle may lead to trigeminal symptoms, and a unilateral absent corneal reflex is an early sign of trigeminal involvement. Large tumors may impinge on the cerebellum and brainstem, leading to ataxia and long tract signs, as well as involvement of cranial nerves IX, X, XI, and XII.

Pure tone and speech audiometry are the most useful screening tests. Selective loss of speech discrimination in excess of pure tone loss is particularly suggestive of vestibular schwannoma. Brainstem auditory–evoked responses typically demonstrate a slowing of conduction, and electronystagmography may detect a decrease in caloric response on the ipsilateral side. Thin-slice, Gd-enhanced MRI through the cerebellopontine angle is the imaging modality of choice for suspected vestibular schwannoma. Thin-slice, contrast-enhanced, high-resolution CT scan is an acceptable alternative when MRI is not obtainable. An intensely enhancing lesion close to the internal auditory canal is highly suggestive of this diagnosis. Patients with suspected neurofibromatosis should have complete imaging of the craniospinal axis to document other neurilemomas, neurofibromas, and meningiomas that may be present.

Neurofibromas differ from neurilemomas in their cellular composition and growth pattern. Although neurofibromas also arise from peripheral nerves, they are most commonly multiple and associated with NF1. Neurofibromas expand rather than displace the nerve of origin. Histologically, neurofibromas are composed of a hypertrophied mass of fibroblasts and Schwann cells through which run normal neurons. Symptoms are caused primarily through compression of the involved or adjacent nerves.

Treatment

Treatment should offer a high chance of local control, as well as preservation of cranial nerve function. Observation alone may be appropriate in patients willing to undergo regular clinical and imaging follow-up and may allow treatment to be deferred for some time. The mainstay of treatment has been microsurgical resection. Retrosigmoid (suboccipital) middle fossa and translabyrinthine approaches offer the possibility of hearing preservation but are associated with higher incidences of seventh nerve damage and postoperative complications. The translabyrinthine approach is associated with low operative morbidity and mortality but sacrifices hearing. At centers with expertise in microsurgical resection, total or near-total resection rates of 90% are routinely obtained with a surgical mortality rate of <2%. Anatomic preservation of the facial nerve may be achieved in 90% of patients and functional preservation in more than two-thirds. Preservation of useful hearing is reported in 30% to 50%. In patients in whom a near-total or total resection is achieved, the tumor recurrence rate is <10%. In patients in whom a subtotal resection is achieved, tumor recurrence may occur in one-third to one-half. Adjuvant radiotherapy may reduce the rate of recurrence to that of complete resection.

In patients with a medical contraindication to surgery, treatment with external-beam irradiation alone is an option. A dose of 50 to 55 Gy in 25 to 30 fractions over 5 to 6 weeks is recommended. Maire et al.[140] evaluated 24 patients with stage III and IV cerebellopontine angle schwannomas treated with external irradiation. With median follow-up of 60 months, there was an 88% tumor control rate with no injuries to the cranial nerve V or VIII.

Radiosurgery may be an alternative to microsurgical resection. The well-circumscribed nature of these tumors, coupled with their typical intense enhancement on MRI, facilitates their localization and treatment using stereotactic techniques. The progression-free survival rate with radiosurgery is nearly 90% at 20 years. Radiosurgical treatment with higher doses yielded high rates of tumor growth arrest (>80%) and tumor shrinkage in up to two-thirds of patients, although facial or trigeminal neuropathy develops in nearly one-third of patients as long as 2 years after therapy. The volume of the lesion is a significant risk factor for complications involving cranial nerve V, VII, or VIII. Temporary enlargement may occur up to 2 years following radiosurgery.[260]

Noren[261] reviewed the results of 669 patients with vestibular schwannoma treated with Gamma Knife radiosurgery between 1969 and 1997. Long-term growth control was achieved in 95%. Facial weakness and/or numbness occurred in approximately one-third of patients during the 1970s but in <2% in the 1990s. Hearing was preserved in 65% to 70% of patients, although tinnitus was rarely changed by treatment. With dose reduction to 12 to 13 Gy, high rates of tumor control and cranial nerve preservation may be achieved. Flickinger et al.[262] reported the results of 313 patients treated with radiosurgery to median dose of 13 Gy. The actuarial 6-year tumor control rate was 98.6%. The actuarial 6-year rates for preservation of seventh nerve function, normal fifth nerve function, unchanged hearing level, and useful hearing were 100%, 95.6%, 70.3%, and 78.6%, respectively. Hayhurst et al.[263] reported on their clinical series of 200 patients treated with radiosurgery to 12 Gy and observed 5 cm^3 to be the target volume threshold above which adverse treatment effects were more likely. In addition, they observed a maximum dose threshold of 9 Gy to cranial nerve V as significantly associated with trigeminal neuropathy.

Radiosurgery provides similar local control with less morbidity than surgery for small (<3 cm) unilateral tumors. In a series from the University of Pittsburgh, radiosurgery was found to have improved preservation of facial function (p <.05) and hearing (p <.03) with decreased associated morbidity (p <.01) when compared to surgical resection.[264]

FSRT has been shown to give local control rates of 91% to 97% with similar effects on cranial nerves V and VII.[265–268] However, in one series FSRT resulted in 2.5-fold greater preservation of hearing compared to radiosurgery.[265] FSRT may be an option for tumors too large to receive radiosurgery.

Bevacizumab has been used in patients with progressive bilateral vestibular schwannomas associated with NF2, usually in the context of bilateral hearing loss, producing both tumor regression and restoration of hearing in some patients. This has led to this approach being actively investigated at present. Sporadic and NF2-related vestibular schwannomas express VEGF, and bevacizumab binds VEGF with high affinity. In the initial experience reported by Plotkin et al.,[269] 10 NF2 patients at risk for complete hearing loss or brainstem compression were treated with bevacizumab on a compassionate-care basis and demonstrated promising results, with 6 of 10 patients experiencing ≥20% tumor volume reduction and 4 of 7 patients experiencing significantly improved hearing.

Evidence-Based Treatment Summary

1. Small nonprogressive tumors can be observed.
2. Surgical resection is generally considered the standard of care for symptomatic lesions.
3. Radiosurgery produces outcomes equivalent to surgery, although these modalities have not been prospectively compared.
4. Fractionated stereotactic radiotherapy is being increasingly employed, with institutional reports suggesting a lower incidence of cranial neuropathies than radiosurgery, but this has not been prospectively validated.
5. The role of bevacizumab in NF-2-associated progressive bilateral vestibular schwannomas is being explored.

Hemangioblastoma and Hemangiopericytoma

Hemangioblastomas are benign vascular tumors that present during the third and fourth decades of life. They account for 1% to 2% of primary CNS tumors in adults. Most arise in the cerebellum, constituting the most common primary cerebellar tumors in adults. An association with von Hippel-Lindau disease is noted in 10% of patients. Histologically, the tumor consists of closely packed, thin-walled blood vessels in a stroma of large, oval foamy cells. The lesions are intensely enhancing on CT and MRI, and angiography confirms the vascular nature of the lesion. Imaging of the craniospinal axis often documents multiple lesions in patients with von Hippel-Lindau disease. Treatment is surgical, and complete resection is curative. Radiosurgery has also been shown to be useful in patients with unresectable disease but is associated with higher rates of recurrence.[270–272]

Hemangiopericytoma is a sarcomatous lesion developing from smooth muscle in blood vessels usually along the base of the skull, although intraparenchymal lesions may be seen. In contrast to other primary CNS tumors, hemangiopericytomas commonly develop systemic metastases. There is a 90% 9-year actuarial risk for local failure following surgical resection only. Postoperative radiotherapy to total doses of 50 to 60 Gy reduces the risk of recurrence rate and improves overall survival. Tumor control is dose dependent, with doses >50 Gy associated with superior outcomes. Radiographic response is slow. Radiosurgery has been used for recurrent hemangiopericytomas, with reported local control rates of approximately 80% following treatment.[273]

Evidence-Based Treatment Summary

1. Surgical resection is recommended, when feasible, for both of these diseases.
2. Radiotherapy is generally reserved for subtotally resected progressive hemangioblastoma, but there are no prospective data.
3. Postoperative radiotherapy is recommended for subtotally resected hemangiopericytoma, but there are no prospective data.
4. Radiotherapy or radiosurgery may be considered for unresectable tumors.

SELECTED REFERENCES

A full list of references for this chapter is available online.

3. Baan R, Grosse Y, Lauby-Secretan B, et al. Carcinogenicity of radiofrequency electromagnetic fields. *Lancet Oncol* 2011;12:624–626.
12. Kleihues P, Scheithauer BW. *Histologic typing of tumors of the central nervous system*. 2nd ed. Berlin: Springer-Verlag, 1993.
16. Lacroix M, Abi-Said D, Fourney DR, et al. A multivariate analysis of 416 patients with glioblastoma multiforme: prognosis, extent of resection, and survival. *J Neurosurg* 2001;95:190–198.
18. Lawrence YR, Li XA, el Naqa I, et al. Radiation dose-volume effects in the brain. *Int J Radiat Oncol Biol Phys* 2010;76:S20–S27.
24. Shaw E, Scott C, Souhami L, et al. Single dose radiosurgical treatment of recurrent previously irradiated primary brain tumors and brain metastases: final report of RTOG protocol 90-05. *Int J Radiat Oncol Biol Phys* 2000;47:291–298.
53. Crossen JR, Garwood D, Glatstein E, et al. Neurobehavioral sequelae of cranial irradiation in adults: a review of radiation-induced encephalopathy. *J Clin Oncol* 1994;12:627–642.
56. Chang EL, Wefel JS, Hess KR, et al. Neurocognition in patients with brain metastases treated with radiosurgery or radiosurgery plus whole-brain irradiation: a randomised controlled trial. *Lancet Oncol* 2009;10:1037–1044.
58. Monje ML, Palmer T. Radiation injury and neurogenesis. *Curr Opin Neurol* 2003;16:129–134.
63. Curran WJ Jr, Scott CB, Horton J, et al. Recursive partitioning analysis of prognostic factors in three Radiation Therapy Oncology Group malignant glioma trials. *J Natl Cancer Inst* 1993;85:704–710.
64. Mirimanoff RO, Gorlia T, Mason W, et al. Radiotherapy and temozolomide for newly diagnosed glioblastoma: recursive partitioning analysis of the EORTC 26981/22981-NCIC CE3 phase III randomized trial. *J Clin Oncol* 2006;24:2563–2569.
66. Gilbert MR, Wang M, Aldape KD, et al. RTOG 0525: A randomized phase III trial comparing standard adjuvant temozolomide with a dose-dense schedule in newly diagnosed glioblastoma. *J Clin Oncol* 2011;29:abstr 2006.
67. Walker MD, Green SB, Byar DP, et al. Randomized comparisons of radiotherapy and nitrosoureas for the treatment of malignant glioma after surgery. *N Engl J Med* 1980;303:1323–1329.
91. Cardinale R, Won M, Choucair A, et al. A phase II trial of accelerated radiotherapy using weekly stereotactic conformal boost for supratentorial glioblastoma multiforme: RTOG 0023. *Int J Radiat Oncol Biol Phys* 2006;65:1422–1428.
102. Stewart LA. Chemotherapy in adult high-grade glioma: a systematic review and meta-analysis of individual patient data from 12 randomised trials. *Lancet* 2002;359:1011–1018.
104. Stupp R, Mason WP, van den Bent MJ, et al. Radiotherapy plus concomitant and adjuvant temozolomide for glioblastoma. *N Engl J Med* 2005;352:987–996.
105. Stupp R, Hegi ME, Mason WP, et al. Effects of radiotherapy with concomitant and adjuvant temozolomide versus radiotherapy alone on survival in glioblastoma in a randomised phase III study: 5-year analysis of the EORTC-NCIC trial. *Lancet Oncol* 2009;10:459–466.
107. Hegi ME, Diserens AC, Gorlia T, et al. MGMT gene silencing and benefit from temozolomide in glioblastoma. *N Engl J Med* 2005;352:997–1003.
119. Lai RK, Recht LD, Reardon DA, et al. Long-term follow-up of ACT III: A phase II trial of rindopepimut (CDX-110) in newly diagnosed glioblastoma. *Neuro-oncology* 2011;13(Suppl 3):iii34–iii40.
120. Sampson JH, Heimberger AB, Archer GE, et al. Immunologic escape after prolonged progression-free survival with epidermal growth factor receptor variant III peptide vaccination in patients with newly diagnosed glioblastoma. *J Clin Oncol* 2010;28:4722–4729.
125. Gallego Perez-Larraya J, Ducray F, Chinot O, et al. Temozolomide in elderly patients with newly diagnosed glioblastoma and poor performance status: an ANOCEF phase II trial. *J Clin Oncol* 2011;29:3050–3055.
126. Roa W, Brasher PM, Bauman G, et al. Abbreviated course of radiation therapy in older patients with glioblastoma multiforme: a prospective randomized clinical trial. *J Clin Oncol* 2004;22:1583–1588.
127. Malmstrom A, Gronberg BH, Stupp R, et al. Glioblastoma in elderly patients: A randomized phase III trial comparing survival in patients treated with 6-week radiotherapy versus hypofractionated radiotherapy over 2 weeks versus temozolomide single-agent chemotherapy. *J Clin Oncol* 2010;28(18s):LBA2002.
136. Donahue B, Scott CB, Nelson JS, et al. Influence of an oligodendroglial component on the survival of patients with anaplastic astrocytomas: a report of Radiation Therapy Oncology Group 83-02. *Int J Radiat Oncol Biol Phys* 1997;38:911–914.
139. Cairncross JG, Ueki K, Zlatescu MC, et al. Specific genetic predictors of chemotherapeutic response and survival in patients with anaplastic oligodendrogliomas. *J Natl Cancer Inst* 1998;90:1473–1479.
142. van den Bent MJ, Dubbink HJ, Sanson M, et al. MGMT promoter methylation is prognostic but not predictive for outcome to adjuvant PCV chemotherapy in anaplastic oligodendroglial tumors: a report from EORTC Brain Tumor Group Study 26951. *J Clin Oncol* 2009;27:5881–5886.
145. Yan H, Parsons DW, Jin G, et al. IDH1 and IDH2 mutations in gliomas. *N Engl J Med* 2009;360:765–773.
146. van den Bent MJ, Dubbink HJ, Marie Y, et al. IDH1 and IDH2 mutations are prognostic but not predictive for outcome in anaplastic oligodendroglial tumors: a report of the European Organization for Research and Treatment of Cancer Brain Tumor Group. *Clin Cancer Res* 2010;16:1597–1604.
167. Pignatti F, van den Bent M, Curran D, et al. Prognostic factors for survival in adult patients with cerebral low-grade glioma. *J Clin Oncol* 2002;20:2076–2084.
172. Shaw EG, Berkey BA, Coons SW, et al. Initial report of Radiation Therapy Oncology Group (RTOG) 9802: Prospective studies in adult low-grade glioma. *Proc Am Soc Clin Oncol* 2006;24(18s):1500.
173. van den Bent MJ, Afra D, de Witte O, et al. Long-term efficacy of early versus delayed radiotherapy for low-grade astrocytoma and oligodendroglioma in adults: the EORTC 22845 randomised trial. *Lancet* 2005;366:985–990.
174. Karim AB, Maat B, Hatlevoll R, et al. A randomized trial on dose-response in radiation therapy of low-grade cerebral glioma: European Organization for Research and Treatment of Cancer (EORTC) Study 22844. *Int J Radiat Oncol Biol Phys* 1996;36:549–556.
175. Shaw E, Arusell R, Scheithauer B, et al. Prospective randomized trial of low- versus high-dose radiation therapy in adults with supratentorial low-grade glioma: initial report of a North Central Cancer Treatment Group/Radiation Therapy Oncology Group/Eastern Cooperative Oncology Group study. *J Clin Oncol* 2002;20:2267–2276.
194. Timmermann B, Kortmann RD, Kuhl J, et al. Combined postoperative irradiation and chemotherapy for anaplastic ependymomas in childhood: results of the German prospective trials HIT 88/89 and HIT 91. *Int J Radiat Oncol Biol Phys* 2000;46:287–295.
217. Abrey LE, Ben-Porat L, Panageas KS, et al. Primary central nervous system lymphoma: the Memorial Sloan-Kettering Cancer Center prognostic model. *J Clin Oncol* 2006;24:5711–5715.
218. Ferreri AJ, Blay JY, Reni M, et al. Prognostic scoring system for primary CNS lymphomas: the International Extranodal Lymphoma Study Group experience. *J Clin Oncol* 2003;21:266–272.
226. DeAngelis LM, Seiferheld W, Schold SC, et al. Combination chemotherapy and radiotherapy for primary central nervous system lymphoma: Radiation Therapy Oncology Group Study 93-10. *J Clin Oncol* 2002;20:4643–4648.
229. Batchelor T, Carson K, O'Neill A, et al. Treatment of primary CNS lymphoma with methotrexate and deferred radiotherapy: a report of NABTT 96-07. *J Clin Oncol* 2003;21:1044–1049.
230. Shah GD, Yahalom J, Correa DD, et al. Combined immunochemotherapy with reduced whole-brain radiotherapy for newly diagnosed primary CNS lymphoma. *J Clin Oncol* 2007;25:4730–4735.
233. Perry A, Louis DN, Scheithauer BW, et al. In: Louis DN, Ohgaki H, Wieslter OD, et al., eds. *WHO classification of tumours of the central nervous system*. Lyon, France: IARC, 2007.
262. Flickinger JC, Kondziolka D, Niranjan A, et al. Acoustic neuroma radiosurgery with marginal tumor doses of 12 to 13 Gy. *Int J Radiat Oncol Biol Phys* 2004;60:225–230.
263. Hayhurst C, Monsalves E, Bernstein M, et al. Predicting nonauditory adverse radiation effects following radiosurgery for vestibular schwannoma: a volume and dosimetric analysis. *Int J Radiat Oncol Biol Phys* 2012;82:2041–2046.
264. Pollock BE, Lunsford LD, Kondziolka D, et al. Outcome analysis of acoustic neuroma management: a comparison of microsurgery and stereotactic radiosurgery. *Neurosurgery* 1995;36:215–224; discussion 224–229.
269. Plotkin SR, Stemmer-Rachamimov AO, Barker FG 2nd, et al. Hearing improvement after bevacizumab in patients with neurofibromatosis type 2. *N Engl J Med* 2009;361:358–367.

Chapter 36
Pituitary Gland Cancer

Theodore E. Yaeger

ANATOMIC CONSIDERATIONS

The pituitary gland, also known as the hypophysis cerebri, is an important endocrine organ. It is an ovoid body, the main portion of which is situated in the hypophysial fossa of the sphenoid bone (Fig. 36.1). The main portion is connected to the brain by the infundibulum. The diaphragma sellae forms a dural roof for the greater part of the hypophysis and is pierced by the infundibulum. In front of the infundibulum, the superior aspect of the gland is related directly to the arachnoid and pia[1] and the subarachnoid space then extends below the diaphragma.[2] The gland is surrounded in the fossa by a fibrous capsule that fuses with the endosteum.[3]

The hypophysis is related above to the optic chiasma and below to the intercavernous venous sinus and the sphenoid air sinus, allowing an endonasal approach for surgical purposes[4] and laterally to the cavernous sinuses. By causing pressure on the chiasma, hypophysial tumors commonly result in visual defects such as superior temporal anopsia or bilateral temporal hemianopsia.

The hypophysis is best divided on embryological bases into two main parts[5]: the adenohypophysis and the neurohypophysis. The former comprises the pars infundibularis (or pars tuberalis), the pars intermedia, and the pars distalis. The latter comprises the median eminence, the infundibular stem, and the infundibular process or neural lobe. The median eminence is frequently also classified as part of the tuber cinereum. The term infundibulum or neural stalk is used for the median eminence and the infundibular stem. The term hypophysial stalk usually refers to the pars infundibularis and the infundibulum.

The adenohypophysis constitutes about 80% of the total volume of the pituitary gland[6] and is a diverticulum of the buccopharyngeal region. The pars distalis area secretes a number of hormones. The neurohypophysis develops as a diverticulum from the floor of the third ventricle. Specifically, it is not an actual endocrine-producing gland but more appropriately should be considered a storage gland for neurosecretions produced by the hypothalamus, which are then carried down via the axona of the supraopticohypophysial tracts.

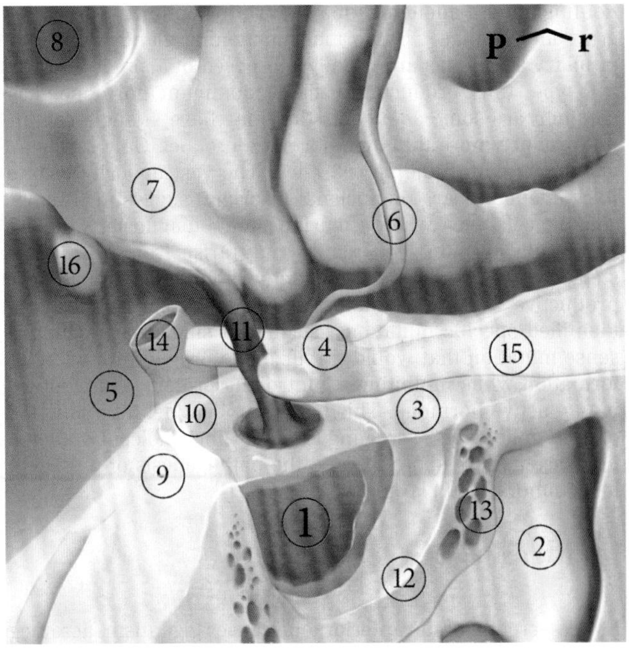

FIGURE 36.1. Posterolateral view of the pituitary gland. P, posterior; r, right. 1, pituitary gland; 2, sphenoid sinus; 3, diaphragm sellae; 4, optic chiasm; 5, chiasmatic cistern; 6, anterior cerebral artery; 7, hypothalamus; 8, third ventricle; 9, dorsum sellae; 10, posterior clinoid; 11, pituitary stalk; 12, sella turcica; 13, cavernous sinus; 14, internal carotid artery; 15, right optic nerve; 16, mamillary body.

Blood Supply and Innervations

The hypophysis is supplied by a series of hypophysial arteries from the internal carotids. The maintenance and regulation of the activity of the adenohypophysis are dependent on the blood supply by way of the hypophysial portal system.[7–11] Nerve fibers from the hypothalamus liberate releasing factors into the capillary beds in the infundibulum, and these substances are then carried by the portal vessels to the distal parts of the gland, causing the effects relevant to the specific secretions. The neurohypophysis receives its main nerve supply from the hypothalamus by way of fibers known collectively as the hypothalamohypophysial tract. This tract contains two sets of fibers: the supraopticohypophysial tract and the tuberohypophysial tract.

Gross Appearance

Upon gross examination, the pituitary gland is a small, gray, rounded gland that developed from ingrown oral epithelium known as Rathke's pouch as an extension of the developing oral cavity. Developmentally it is eventually cut off from its origins by the growth of the sphenoid bone and settles into a saddle-shaped, base-of-brain, bone depression called the sella turcica. The anterior pituitary has a portal vascular system that is the conduit for the transport of hypothalamic-releasing hormones from the hypothalamus to the anterior pituitary. Hypothalamic neurons have terminals in the median eminence where the hormones are released into the portal systems. This vascular supply traverses the pituitary stalk and then enters the anterior pituitary lobe. Most pituitary hormones are controlled predominately by releasing factors from the hypothalamus, with the exception of prolactin, which is controlled by the dopamine system via an inhibitory mechanism. It is attached to the lower surface of the hypothalamus by the infundibular stalk. The Rathke's pouch portion forms the anterior lobe and the intermediate area. The posterior pituitary is embryologically derived from an out-pouching from the floor of the third ventricle and grows inferiorly along the stalk of the anterior lobe. In contrast to the anterior lobe, this posterior lobe is supplied by the inferior hypophyseal artery, which will drain into the venous sinus system to directly release into the systemic circulation. As such, the pituitary gland has a dual circulation; one is composed of arteries and veins, the other a portal venous system that links the hypothalamus and the anterior lobe. The neural tissue of the infundibular stalk forms the posterior lobe. In general, the pituitary gland averages $1.3 \times 1.0 \times 0.5$ cm in size and weighs

0.55 to 0.6 g but enlarges during pregnancy.[12] Overall, it is about the smallest functioning gland in the human body, having an important role in physiologic regulation.[6]

Physiology

There are five cell types that are revealed using specific antibody staining:

1. *Somatotrophs.* Growth hormone–producing acidophilic cells constituting about 50% of the anterior lobe.
2. *Lactotrophs.* Prolactin producing acidophic cells (also known as mammotrophs).
3. *Corticotrophs.* Basophilic-appearing cells that produce adrenocortitrophic hormone, pro-opiomelanocortin, melanocytic-stimulating hormone, endorphins, and lipotropin.
4. *Thyrotrophs.* Very pale appearing cells that produce thyroid-stimulating hormone.
5. *Gonadotrophs.* Basophilic cells that produce follicle-stimulating hormone and luteinizing hormone.

MORPHOLOGY

The most common pituitary adenoma is a soft, well-circumscribed lesion that may be confined to the sella turcica. Larger lesions typically extend superiorly through the diaphragm sella into the suprasellar region. This can cause compression of the optic chiasm and adjacent structures, including cranial nerves. Continued expansion eventually erodes the sella turcica, the anterior clinoid process, and even into the cavernous and sphenoid sinuses. As many as 30% of cases adenomas can be nonencapsulated and infiltrate adjacent bones, dura, and the brain proper, although rarely.[13] Foci of hemorrhage and necrosis are hallmarks of these invasive larger adenomas. Pituitary apoplexy occurs when an acute hemorrhage causes a rapidly enlarging mass, resulting in sudden onset of mass effect symptoms.

CLINICAL COURSE

The signs and symptoms of pituitary adenomas include endocrine abnormalities and mass effects. Abnormalities associated with excessive secretions of anterior pituitary hormones are specific to the particular aberrant cell line, as described below. Local mass effect can be associated with any type of pituitary tumor, including a rare metastatic tumor from another site. The earliest changes in local anatomy result in radiographic changes with local deformation of the sella, the diaphragm, and bone erosions. Ultimately, compression of surrounding normal soft tissues results in visual field abnormalities with headache, nausea, and vomiting; eventually compressing the nonneoplastic pituitary and resulting in hypopituitarism. This can occur rapidly if there is hemorrhage resulting in pituitary apoplexy with excruciating headache, diplopia from pressure on the oculomotor nerves, and hypopituitarism.

The posterior pituitary or neurohypophysis consists of pituicytes—modified glial cells—and axonal processes extending from nerve cell bodies in the supraoptic and paraventricular nuclei of the hypothalamus. These cells transit through the pituitary stalk to the posterior lobe where the two posterior lobe hormones, oxytocin and vasopressin, are stored.

Hormones are secreted in the following lobes:

- *Intermediate lobe:* no effects are known in warm-blooded mammals.
- *Anterior lobe:* Growth hormone–regulating cell division and protein synthesis; adrenocorticotrophic hormone, which regulates the functional activity of the adrenal cortex; thyroid-stimulating hormone, which regulates the functional activity of the thyroid gland; follicle-stimulating hormone, which regulates ovarian follicles and spermatogenesis; luteinizing hormone (in women), which stimulates ovulation, formation of the corpus luteum, and secretion of estrogen and progesterone. In men, it can be called interstitial cell–stimulating hormone, which stimulates testosterone secretion. Also in women there is prolactin, which induces secretion of breast milk.
- *Posterior lobe:* Hormones are secreted by the neurosecretory cells of the hypothalamus and pass through the fibers of the supraopticohypophyseal tracts in the infundibular stalk to the neurohypophysis where they are stored. These stored secretions are oxytocin, which acts on smooth muscles of the female uterus to increase contractility. There is also antidiuretic hormone, which increases water reabsorption of the renal system via the kidney tubules, and a derivative known as vasopressin to regulate blood pressure.

DISORDERS

Diseases of the pituitary are divided into those that affect the anterior lobe and those that affect the posterior lobe. The former are either hypersecretory or hyposecretory in nature. In most cases, hypersecretion is caused by a functioning adenoma within the anterior lobe. Hypopituitarism may be caused by a variety of destructive processes, including ischemic injury, radiation exposure (including therapeutic radiation), inflammatory responses, and nonfunctioning tumors such as a squamous "pearl" from cell rests that occurs during embryo development. Other than endocrine abnormalities, diseases of the anterior pituitary may manifest by a local mass effect. Radiographically this can usually be seen by enlargement of the sella turcica, clinically by visual field defects or visual cuts, and evidence of increased intracranial pressure by optic examination or a patient's complaint of headache and nausea. The posterior pituitary may provide clinical evidence of antidiuretic hormone abnormalities.

Hyperpituitarism and Pituitary Anterior Adenomas

Excess production of hormones related to the anterior pituitary is often caused by a benign adenoma arising from the anterior lobe. Less commonly, there can be hyperplasia or, rarely, actual carcinoma of glandular elements. Interestingly nonfunctioning adenomas may cause hypopituitarism as they grow and displace the normal functioning gland. Functional pituitary adenomas are usually composed of a single aberrant cell type, thus producing a single dominant hormone. Less common are some adenomas that may have a single cell line but produce more than one hormone product. Only rarely are adenomas with multiple cell lines. The vast majority of pituitary adenomas are monoclonal in origin, suggesting a single somatic cell, even when a plurihormonal diagnosis is made.[14] Some plurihormonal adenomas may arise from a primitive stem cell, which may subsequently differentiate to different productive cell lines simultaneously. Molecular studies have identified specific mutations, such as a single base-pair missense mutation that would stabilize one protein into an active formation while inhibiting a controlling protein, thus mimicking an active hormone. This has been identified in about 40% of growth hormone–secreting tumors. Other molecular aberrations seem more sporadic, and the pathogenesis of most pituitary tumors is still largely unknown.

PHYSIOLOGY

Hyperpituitarism of the Pituitary Lobes

Hypersecretion of the anterior lobe causes gigantism, acromegaly, and Cushing disease (pituitary basophilism). Hyposecretion of the anterior lobe causes dwarfism, Simond disease (pituitary cachexia), postpartum pituitary necrosis of Sheehan syndrome, acromicria, eunuchoidism, and hypogonadism. A posterior lobe deficiency is a hypothalamic lesion that causes diabetes insipidus. Anterior and posterior lobe deficiencies plus a hypothalamic lesion causes Frohlich syndrome (adiposogenital dystrophy) and pituitary obesity.

Anterior Lobe

In the anterior lobe, the most common tumor, accounting for about 30% of all adenomas, is a prolactinoma (lactotroph adenoma).[15] These range from small or microadenomas (Fig. 36.2) to very large and expanded tumors associated with clinical mass effects. Microscopically, they are chromophobic or weakly acidophilic.

Immunohistochemistry can identify prolactin within the cells as secretory granules. Prolactin is a very efficient hormone, and even microadenomas can produce enough excess prolactin to cause hyperprolactin syndrome. Serum concentrations of prolactin tend to be proportional with the size of the tumor. Patients between 20 and 40 years of age presenting with amenorrhea, galactorrhea, loss of libido, and infertility should be checked for serum prolactin.[16] Almost 25% of cases of female amenorrhea are related to increased prolactin. At an older age, the clinical manifestations could be very subtle, leading to patients presenting with mass effects as the primary symptoms. Hyperprolactinemia also occurs normally during pregnancy and reaches a peak at delivery. It can continue postpartum by suckling in lactating women. Interference with a dopamine feedback mechanism by damage to the dopaminergic neurons within the pituitary stalk (via head trauma) in the hypothalamic region or the use of drugs (reserpine, haloperidol, phenothiazines, estrogens) that block the lactotroph cell receptors can result in lactotroph hyperplasia. Moreover, any mass within the stalk can disturb this inhibition influence, causing a mild elevation in serum prolactin. As such, a mild elevation does not necessarily indicate a prolactin-secreting adenoma. Finally, renal failure and hypothyroidism can elevate prolactin.

Prolactinomas are typically treated with bromocriptine (Box 36.1), a dopamine receptor agonist that causes the lesions to diminish in size and function. Growth hormone (somatotroph cell) –secreting tumors are the second most common functional tumors. Approximately 40% of somatotroph tumors express an oncogene (*GSP*), which is a mutant GTPase deficient alpha subunit of the G protein designated Gs.[17] Histologically these tumors are composed of acidophilic to chromophobic granulated cells. Immunohistochemistry can demonstrate growth hormone associated with small amounts of prolactin.[18] Children who develop hypersecretion adenomas before the epiphyses are closed develop gigantism. If the epiphyseal plates have fused, such as in young adults, then acromegaly can occur. This is usually manifested clinically with enlarged hands and feet, increased bone density, enlarged thyroid, heart, liver, adrenal, and broadening of the lower face with jaw protrusion, developing into prognathism. Patients often have associated prolactinemia, with gonadal dysfunction, hypertension, congestive heart failure, and a risk of gastrointestinal cancer. The goals of treatment are to control serum growth hormone and decrease mass effects of the primary adenoma while preventing deficiencies. Most commonly, the tumors are removed surgically via a transsphenoid approach in younger patients, treatment with external-beam radiotherapy (see the Radiation Techniques section), or drug therapy. Eventually, good growth hormone control over a long period allows the characteristic tissue overgrowth and related symptoms to recede, with improvement in metabolic abnormalities. It is important to remember that because clinical manifestations of growth hormone is subtle, these adenomas usually present with mass effects from large tumor sizes. Corticotrophin cell adenomas usually present as microadenomas. Histologically, these tumors are basophilic, but they can be chromophobic and stain for the periodic acid stain (Schiff stain) due to presence of carbohydrate in the precursor adrenocorticotrophic hormone (ACTH). Excess ACTH eventually leads to Cushing syndrome, with a chronic hypersecretion of cortisol from adrenal stimulation. However, when the hypercortisolism comes directly from the pituitary adenoma, the process is Cushing disease. Nelson syndrome occurs in most cases by a loss of inhibitory feedback of adrenal cortisol of the pituitary when hyperfunctioning adrenals are surgically excised and a subclinical pituitary corticotroph microadenoma exists. The microadenoma is stimulated, but hypercortisolism does not occur due to the absence of the adrenals. However, mass effects can occur, and ACTH precursor molecules can also affect melanocytes, thus producing hyperpigmentation.

Mixed adenomas, gonadotroph, and thyrotroph adenomas can occur, but these are less frequent than nonsecreting or null-cell adenomas (Table 36.1). Mostly gonadotroph adenomas are luteinizing or follicle-stimulating producing tumors of middle-age men and women with complaints of chronic fatigue or menorrhea.[19] Like null-cell adenomas, these tumors can

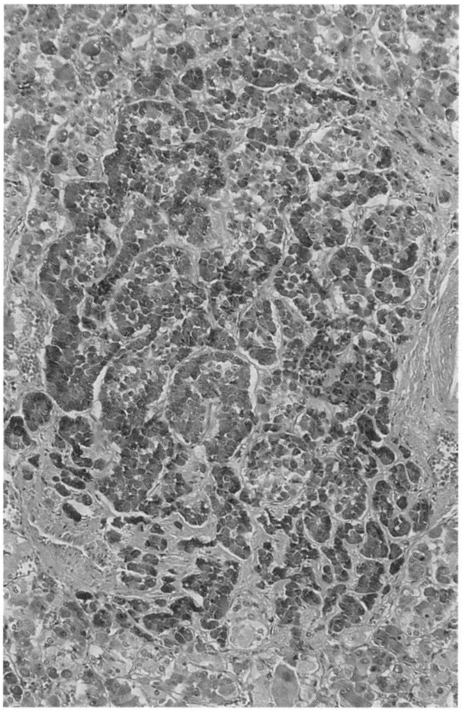

FIGURE 36.2. Photomicrograph of microadenoma. (From Damjanov I. *Histopathology: a color atlas and textbook*. Baltimore: Williams & Wilkins, 1996, with permission.)

Box 36.1

Pituitary Adenoma Management Overview

Symptomatic adenomas present for medical attention as a result of hormone secretions, compression of nearby normal structures with neurologic symptoms, or compression of the pituitary stalk causing hypopituitarism. An initial therapy for most prolactinomas is with a dopamine agonist such as bromocriptine, lysuride, or pergolide. Medical intervention usually decreases adenoma function and size. Initial therapy for other pituitary adenomas is transsphenoidal surgical resection. Surgery is generally safe and reverses neurologic symptoms, with most patients normalizing hormone levels. It is mostly useful to cure microadenomas. Radiation therapy is often reserved for patients with residual disease after surgery, such as after a debulking surgery. It is also considered for recurrence after definitive surgery or for medically inoperable patients. Typically, conventional radiation delivers a dose of 45 Gy at 1.8 Gy daily fractions. At this dose, good control can usually be achieved with a very low risk of optic neuropathy. Normalization of hormone levels, however, can take months to years to achieve.

TABLE 36.1 PITUITARY ADENOMA DISTRIBUTIONS

Type	Frequency (%)
Prolactinoma	20–30
Growth hormone adenoma	5
Mixed growth/prolactin adenoma	5
Adrenocorticotrophic hormone adenoma	10–15
Gonadotroph adenoma	10–15
Null cell adenoma	20
Thyroid-stimulating hormone adenoma	1
Plurihormonal adenoma	15

From Pituitary neoplasia. In: Berger PC, Scheithauer BW, Vogel FS, eds. *Surgical pathology of the nervous system and its coverings,* 3rd ed. New York: Churchill Livingstone, 1991; with permission from Elsevier.

become substantial in size with mass effects (Table 36.2). Thyrotrophs are rare, found in about 1% of patients, and are a rare source of hyperthyroidism.[20] Primary pituitary carcinomas are quite rare, typically not functional, and have variable polymorphisms. A clinical diagnosis of an actual carcinoma requires the demonstration of metastases, usually to lymph nodes, brain, bone, or liver, and rarely elsewhere. Radiation therapy to the primary pituitary site can be palliative.

Hypopituitarism

Decreased secretions of pituitary hormones can result from diseases of the hypothalamus or the pituitary proper, which cause syndromes of hypopituitarism. Most cases of a hypofunctioning pituitary result from the destruction of more than 75% of the anterior gland. Metastatic tumors, involuted primary tumors, ischemic necrosis, or surgical or radio-ablated pituitary can produce empty sella syndrome. A Rathke's cleft cyst can accumulate proteinaceous fluids, expanding and destroying the normal pituitary. Primary necrosis can be caused by Sheehan syndrome[21] or by disseminated intravascular coagulopathy and, more rarely, sickle cell crisis. Also causative is elevated intracranial pressure from hydrocephalus, head trauma, or severe shock. Destroying all or part of the functioning pituitary can result in a clinical diagnosis of empty sella syndrome.[22]

Histologically there is a small fibrotic nidus of tissue in a radiographically expanded sella turcica. Two distinct types are identified: primary empty syndrome, which occurs in obese women with multiple pregnancies, and a defect of the diaphragma sella, which allows arachnoid matter and cerebrospinal fluid to herniate into an expanded sella, thus compressing the pituitary gland. Hyperprolactinemia can occur to due to the loss of dopamine inhibition. Only rarely does actual hypopituitarism occur because enough functioning residual tissue usually remains. Secondary syndromes usually occur from surgical removal, radiation ablation, or spontaneous infarction. These patients express hypopituitarism syndromes. Rare congenital defects are known,[23] such as a gene that encodes Pit-1, a transcription factor related to important pituitary-specific genes such as growth hormone, prolactin, and thyroid-stimulating hormones. The genetically altered protein will bind to the appropriate cell receptors but can activate the expression of the gene, thus causing the patient to fail to produce the hormone(s). Less frequently, diseases of the hypothalamus or hypothalamic stalk can cause the pituitary to become dysfunctional. These can include craniopharyngiomas (Box 36.2),[24] metastases, sarcoidosis, or tuberculous meningitis and infiltrative diseases such as opportunistic infections. Radiotherapy to nearby structures such as the brain, base of brain, optic chiasm, and nasopharynx can also cause hypothalamic disorders. Dysfunction of the adrenal cortex, thyroid, and gonads, the loss of melanocyte-stimulating hormone, atrophy of the genitalia, amenorrhea, impotency, loss of libido, and pubic and axillary hair are changes related to the cause and type(s) of deficiencies in pituitary hypofunction.

Box 36.2

Craniopharyngiomas

Craniopharyngiomas are frequently calcified and can be visualized radiographically. They are usually about 3.5 cm in diameter, encapsulated, and solid but can be cystic or multilobulated. They can displace cranial nerves and the optic chiasm and protrude into the floor of the third ventricle. They are thought to be vestigial remnants of the Rathke's pouch, representing about 2% of intracranial tumors, occurring about half the time in children and young adults. In children, they can cause growth retardation. Adults usually present with visual disturbances. Both can demonstrate hormonal disturbances and diabetes insipidus. Histologically there can be two forms. The adamantinomatous form has nests or cords of squamous to columnar epithelium in a background of spongy-like reticulum. Because keratin formation occurs, these tumors are frequently calcified. A brisk glial reaction can occur if in direct contact with brain tissue. The second type is a papillary craniopharyngioma. These are usually solid sections of squamous cells typically lacking a cystic component and calcification.

Posterior Lobe

The posterior pituitary is composed of pituicytes—modified glial cells—with associated axonal processes extending from nerve origins in the supraoptic and paraventricular nuclei within the hypothalamus. Two proteins are produced: antidiuretic hormone and oxytocin. These hormones are stored in the posterior pituitary and released with the appropriate stimuli. Oxytocin functions to stimulate the smooth muscle contractions of the uterus during delivery as well as stimulating smooth muscle of the lactiferous mammary gland ducts within the gravid breasts. No known clinical abnormalities are known for inappropriate secretions. Antidiuretic hormone (ADH) is a nonpeptide produced primarily in the supraoptic nucleus. ADH is released from axon terminals from the neurohypophysis directly into the general circulation secondary to appropriate stimulation(s). ADH is causative for two distinct clinical syndromes: diabetes insipidus and the syndrome of inappropriate secretion (SIADH). Diabetes insipidus can result from head trauma, surgical or radiation damage, tumors, and inflammatory conditions. It causes the inappropriate oversecretion of urine and can lead to life-threatening dehydration. SIADH is causative in the absorption of excessive water, thus causing hematologic dilution and hyponatremia. The most frequent cause is from ectopic ADH produced by malignant neoplasms such as lung carcinoma

TABLE 36.2 ENDOCRINE SECRETIONS AND CLINICAL PRESENTATIONS

Type of Secretion	Frequency (%)	Symptoms	Size at Diagnosis
Prolactinoma	43	Women: amenorrhea, galactorrhea	Microadenoma
		Men: impotence, hypopituitarism	Microadenoma
Nonsecreting	30	Hypopituitarism	Microadenoma
Gonadotrophin	17	Children: Gigantism	Microadenoma
Growth hormone		Adults: Acromegaly	Microadenoma
Adrenocorticotrophic hormone	7	Cushing's disease	Microadenoma
		Nelson's disease	
Thyroid-stimulating hormone	1	Hyperthyroidism	Microadenoma or microadenoma

From Oruckaptan HH, Senmevsim O, Ozcan OE, et al. Pituitary adenomas: results of 684 surgically treated patients and review of the literature. *Surg Neurol Int* 2000;53:211–219, with permission.

and nonneoplastic lung disease as a paraneoplastic syndrome. However, direct or compression injury to the hypothalamus or posterior pituitary is known. Glial tumors such as primary central nervous system (CNS) neoplasms or craniopharyngiomas can have direct mechanical or stimulatory effects. SIADH causes hyponatremia, cerebral edema, and neurologic dysfunction; patients are typically initially evaluated because of changes in cognition.[25] Peripheral edema does not usually develop because blood is diluted but normal in volume.

RADIATION THERAPY

Radiation therapy can be a highly effective form of intervention to control pituitary adenomas. In current practice, it is rarely the sole means of treatment and is usually reserved for patients with residual surgical disease or the medically inoperable patient. The overall 10-year control rates are consistently reported in the range of 85% or higher,[26–29] including two recent reports from the University of Florida[28,30] reporting a 93% control rate at 9.2 years and the absences of "late-recurrences" with long-term follow-up using doses of 45 Gy or higher. In the former report,[27] patients were analyzed as to whether they experienced surgery followed by radiation versus radiotherapy alone. Combined approaches achieved a 95% control rate, whereas radiotherapy alone achieved 90% at 10 years of follow-up. Importantly, an 80% control rate was achieved for patients treated by initial surgery who then developed a recurrence after application of delayed radiotherapy. This result is consistent with a report from Princess Margaret Hospital analyzing 166 patients with similar treatment and results.[26]

Pediatric pituitary adenomas have similar results when comparing surgery and radiation with radiotherapy alone. In the study by Grigsby et al.,[31] 19 patients were treated who were younger than 19 years of age, and at 15 years' of follow-up only two had failed. A sentinel paper that was published in 1971 arguably solidified the use of about 45 Gy as the threshold dose for acceptable local control and tolerance.[32] It has been confirmed many times by both American and European authors.[33]

Although there is a lack of tumor progression, clinically and radiographically, many patients who have elevated hormone level at the outset of definitive therapy do not achieve complete normalization following radiotherapy alone. The University of Heidelberg reported on 68 patients with hormone active adenomas. The complete response rate for normalization occurred in only 38%.[28] Again, Princess Margaret Hospital reported on 145 patients receiving radiation alone for hormonally active pituitary adenomas. Although the progress-free rate was 96%, the long-term biochemical remission rate was 40%.[34] Therefore, radiation is proven to be highly effective for controlling pituitary adenoma growth and progression. However, radiotherapy alone is less effective in normalizing hormone activity when patients present with a hormone active tumor.

A newer technique is rapidly becoming available for using radiotherapy intervention for pituitary adenomas: stereotactic radiosurgery (SRS). A number of institutions have reports using SRS either as a single fraction or with a fractionated schedule, called fractionated stereotactic radiotherapy (FSRT).[35] In FSRT, conventional doses of 45 to 50 Gy are delivered using a relocatable head-frame technique. With SRS, a single fraction is delivered in doses from 10 to 27 Gy using cranial hard-fixation techniques.[35–37] The local control rates using these advanced techniques have been reported as >90%, and the yet-to-be-proven hypothesis is that the hormone response rates would be higher than with conventional doses. In an encouraging article, Yoon et al.[37] reported that 11 of 13 patients had normalization of prolactin-secreting adenomas within 1 year. Unfortunately, Mitsumori et al.[36] reported that the 3-year actuarial rate for an adverse CNS event was 38% for a single fraction versus 0% for

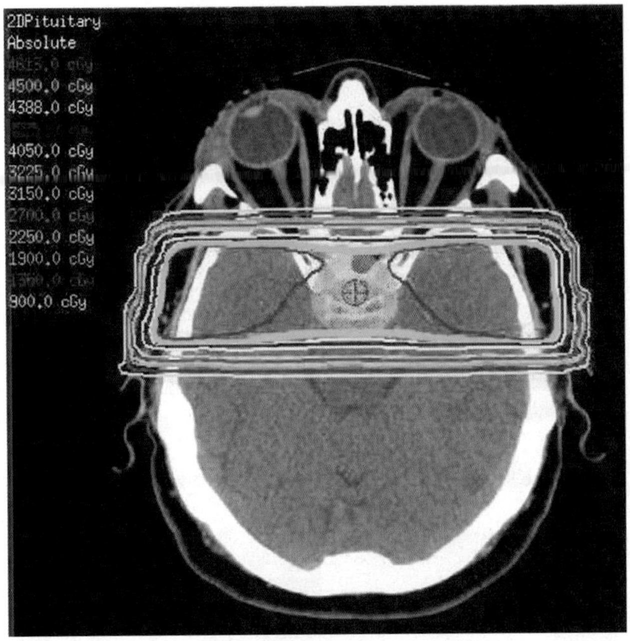

FIGURE 36.3. Two-dimensional parallel opposed pair radiotherapy planning.

the FSRT technique. Presently, many radiation oncologists are using modified fraction schemes via various technologies, acutely aware of the nearby critical anatomic structures and the likely potential that patients will live long enough to develop late sequelae.

Radiation Techniques

Radiation therapy planning and delivery has evolved from a two-dimensional calculated, parallel-opposed small open or minimally blocked bitemporal fields (Fig. 36.3) to three-dimensional, computer tomographic–assisted planning (Fig. 36.4) that uses a multiple field approach with custom blocks or multileaf collimation (MLC) blocked portals designed to concentrate therapeutic doses and minimize risks to surrounding normal

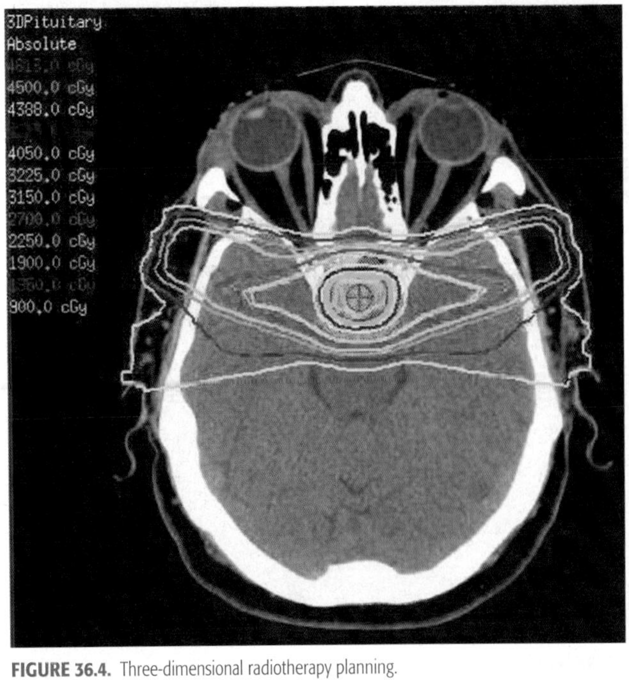

FIGURE 36.4. Three-dimensional radiotherapy planning.

Clinical Radiation Oncology

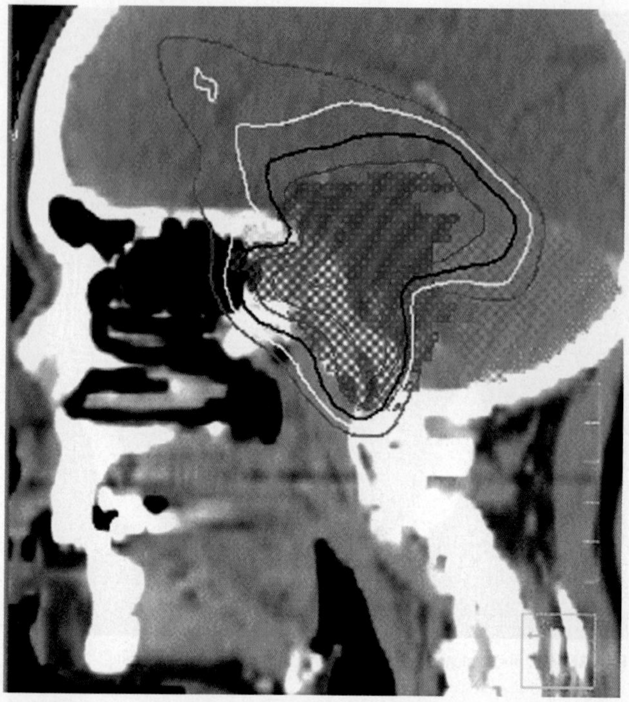

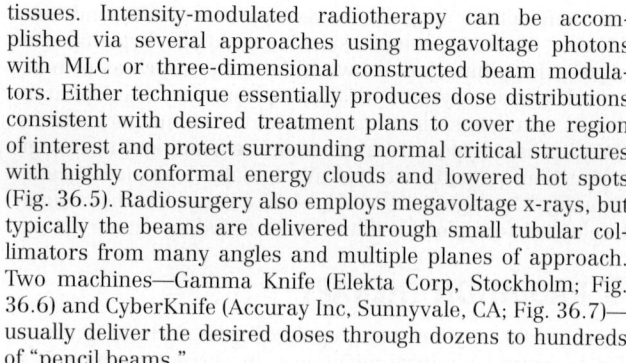

FIGURE 36.5. Intensity-modulated radiotherapy.

tissues. Intensity-modulated radiotherapy can be accomplished via several approaches using megavoltage photons with MLC or three-dimensional constructed beam modulators. Either technique essentially produces dose distributions consistent with desired treatment plans to cover the region of interest and protect surrounding normal critical structures with highly conformal energy clouds and lowered hot spots (Fig. 36.5). Radiosurgery also employs megavoltage x-rays, but typically the beams are delivered through small tubular collimators from many angles and multiple planes of approach. Two machines—Gamma Knife (Elekta Corp, Stockholm; Fig. 36.6) and CyberKnife (Accuray Inc, Sunnyvale, CA; Fig. 36.7)—usually deliver the desired doses through dozens to hundreds of "pencil beams."

At present there are an increasing number of facilities that are investigating treatments with protons.[38] Proton therapy, while still exceedingly expensive, utilizes the unique advantage of the Bragg-Peak phenomenon to deliver doses mostly confined to the region of interest (Fig. 36.8).

Late Effects

A worrisome potential in using higher doses to a pituitary adenoma is the possibility of developing late radiation-induced optic neuropathies. Although it has been reported that the incidence of optic nerve damage is low, ranging from 0.7% to 2%, the risk of optic nerve or chiasm injury is dependent on both the total dose and dose per fraction.[27,28,34] Even with conventional doses

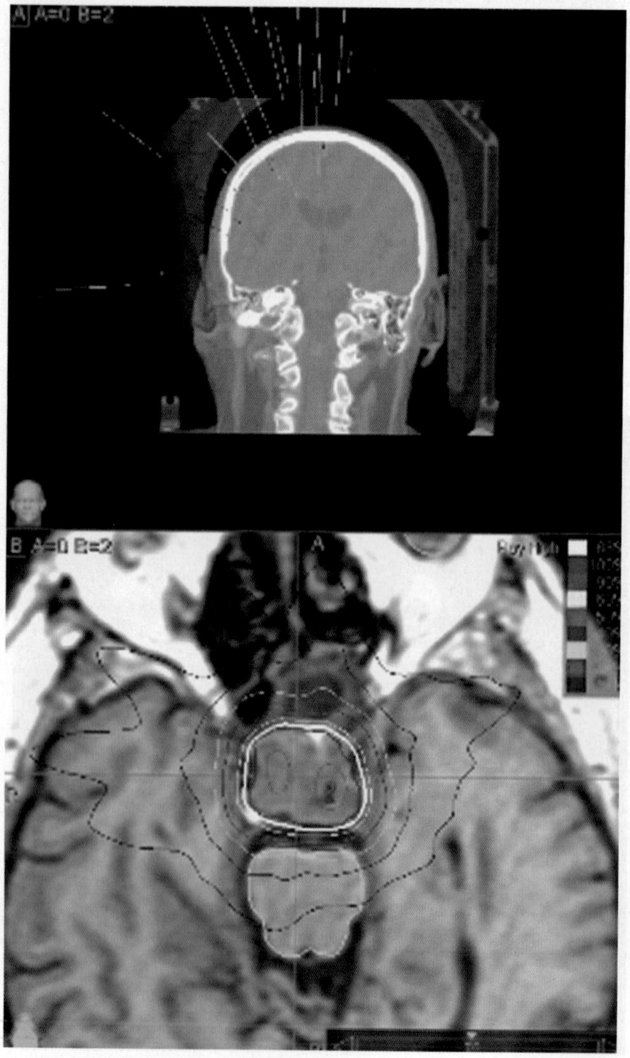

FIGURE 36.6. Gamma Knife.

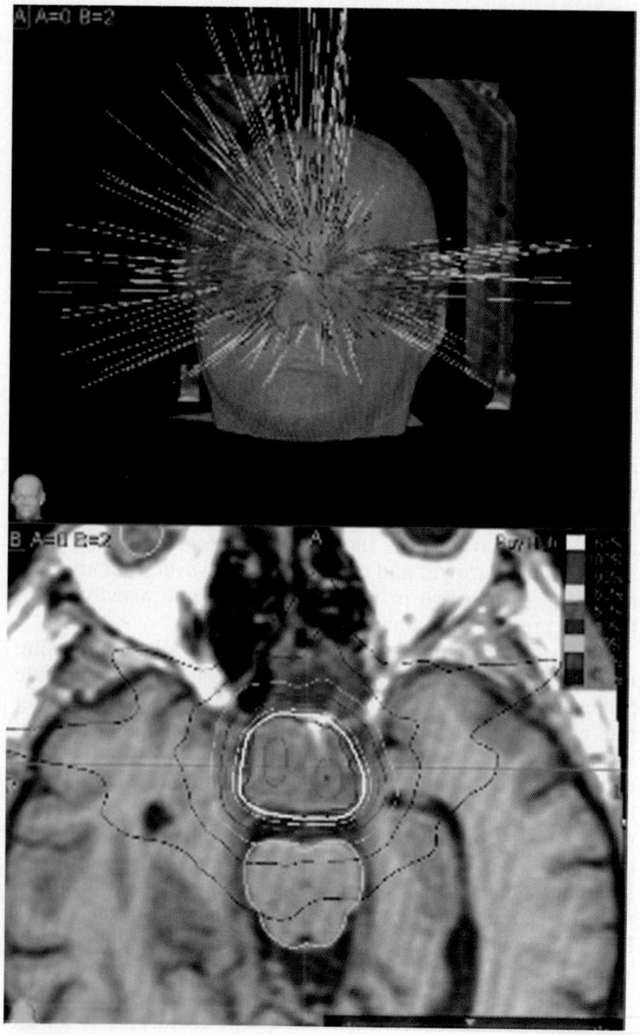

FIGURE 36.7. CyberKnife.

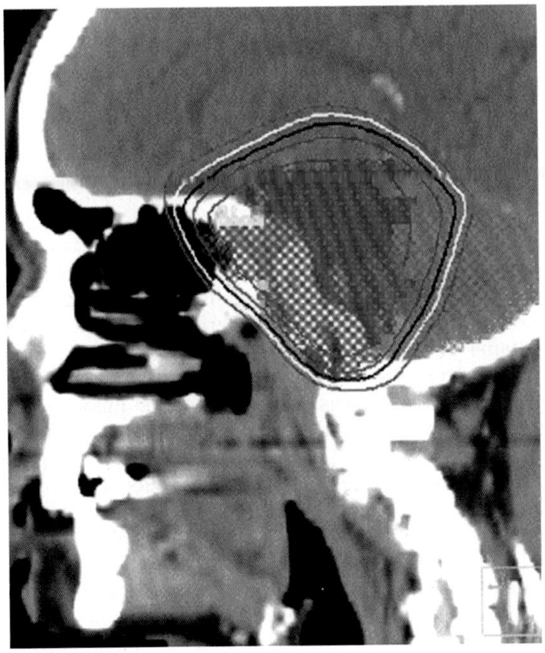

FIGURE 36.8. Proton therapy.

of 45 to 50 Gy, the risk is very low but it is not zero. Additionally, doses ranging from 45 to 50 Gy to the whole pituitary gland carry substantial risk of causing hypopituitarism. This is reported in the range of 10% to 30% in some series,[26–29,35] and potentially half of all patients treated to 45 Gy will develop a deficiency of at least one pituitary hormone within 5 years after definitive radiotherapy. Therefore, the patient must be followed indefinitely for this complication risk. Second malignant neoplasms are always a concern in long-term survivors who have received therapeutic doses of radiation. The Royal Marsden Hospital looked at 334 patients irradiated for pituitary adenomas to a media dose of 45 Gy. Five patients developed a secondary brain tumor, for an actuarial risk of 1.3% at 10 years and 1.9% at 20 years.[39] Thus, the relative risk of developing a second tumor compared with the normal, unexposed, population was 9.3%. Princess Margaret Hospital reported similarly with four gliomas from 306 treated patients over a latency period of 8 to 15 years. The actuarial risk was 1.7% at 10 years and 2.7% at 15 years for a relative risk of 16%.[40]

CONCLUSION

The Hypophysis Cerebri or pituitary gland may be the smallest functioning gland in humans, but it represents one of the most critical functioning endocrine glands for normal development, growth, organ regulation, reproductive regulation, and birthing functions as well as regulation of other hormone glands in the total body system(s). The physical gland may be small but its capabilities are great. Dysfunction of any part of this hormone gland has wide-reaching implications for endocrine abnormalities and for local mass effects. The latter especially affects the optic nerves and proliferates a cascade of additional and potentially devastating hormonal dysfunctions. The former influences cellular division, protein synthesis, regulation of the adrenal cortex and the thyroid, follicle and sperm production, formation and function of the gravid uterus, testosterone secretion, and milk production. Lasting effects from chronic hypopituitarism also increased mortality from cardiac and cardiovascular events.[41,42] To summarize, adequate medical knowledge and understanding of the pituitary gland include understanding multiple feedback mechanisms required for the hormone normal-regulatory processes of the human body. Knowledge of therapy mechanisms for abnormalities plays an essential role for medical intervention, especially for the appropriate use of radiotherapy.

REFERENCES

1. Sutherland S. The meningeal relations of the human hypophysis cerebri. *J Anatomy London* 1945;79:33.
2. Ferner H. The hypophyseal cistern of man and its relation to the pathogenesis mechanisms of secondary sella dilation. *Anatomy Entw Gesch* 121:407, 1960.
3. Boyd WH. Pituitary. *Anatomy Rec* 1960;137:437.
4. Radojevic S, Jovanovic S, Lotric N. Anatomic notes on trans-sphenoidal approach to the pituitary gland. *Arch Anatomy Path* 1969;17:274.
5. McK Ricoh D, Wislocki GB, O'Leary JL. Visual effects of hypophyseal tumors. *Res Publ Assoc Nerve Mental Dis* 1940;20:3.
6. Ramzi S, Vinay K, Collins T. *Robbins pathologic basis of disease,* 6th ed. Philadelphia: WB Saunders, 1999.
7. Morin F. Pituitary blood supply. *Arch Ital Anatomy Embriol* 1940;45:94.
8. Xuereb GP, Pritchard ML, Daniel PM. The hypophyseal portal system of vessels in man. *Q J Exp Physiol* 1954;39:219–230.
9. Stanfield JP. The blood supply of the human pituitary gland. *J Anatomy London* 1960; 94:257.
10. Harris GW. *Neural control of the pituitary gland.* London: Arnold, 1955.
11. O'Rahilly R. Anatomy. In: *A regional study of the human structure,* 4th ed. Philadelphia: WB Saunders, 1975.
12. Craven RH Jr. *Taber's encyclopedic medical dictionary.* Philadelphia: FA Davis, 1997.
13. Yeh PJ, Chen JW. Pituitary tumors: surgical and medical management. *Surg Oncol* 1997;6:67.
14. Alexander JM. Clinically nonfunctioning pituitary tumors are monoclonal in origin. *J Clin Invest* 1990;86:336.
15. Schlechte J, Dolan K, Sherman B, et al. The natural history of untreated hyperprolactinemia. *J Clin Endrocrinol Metab* 1989;68:412.
16. Mindermann T, Wilson CB. Age-related and gender-related occurrences of pituitary adenomas. *Clin Endocrinol* 1994;41:359.
17. Lyons J, Landis CA, Harsh G, et al. Two G protein oncogenes in human endocrine tumors. *Science* 1990;249:655.
18. Melmed S, Ho K, Kalbinski A, et al. Recent advances in pathogenesis, diagnosis and management of acromegaly. *J Clin Endocrinol Metab* 1995;80:3395.
19. Ho DM, Hsu CY, Ting LT, et al. The clinicopathological characteristics of gonadotroph cell adenomas: a study of 118 cases. *Hum Pathol* 1997;28:905–911.
20. Beck-Peccoz P. Thyrotropin secreting pituitary tumors. *Endoc Rev* 1997;17:610.
21. Sheehan H. Postpartum necrosis of the anterior pituitary. *J Pathol Bacteriol* 1987; 45:189.
22. Barkin A. Pituitary atrophy in patients with Sheehan's syndrome. *Am J Med Sci* 1989;298:39.
23. Pfaffle RW, DeMattia GE, Parks JS, et al. Mutation of POU specific domain of Pit-1 and hypopituitarism without pituitary hypoplasia. *Science* 257:1118–1121.
24. DeVile CJ, Grant DB, Hayward RD, et al. Growth and endocrine sequelae of craniopharyngioma. *Arch Dis Child* 1996;75:108–114.
25. Maesaka JK. An expanded view of SIADH. *Clin Nephrol* 1996;46:79.
26. Tsang RW, Brierley JD, Panzarella T, et al. Radiation therapy for pituitary adenoma: treatment outcome and prognosis factors. *Int J Radiat Oncol Biol Phys* 1994;30: 557–565.
27. McCord MW, Buatti JM, Fennell EM, et al. Radiotherapy for pituitary adenoma: long term outcome and sequelae. *Int J Radiat Oncol Biol Phys* 1997;39:437–444.
28. Zierhut D, Flentje M, Adolph J, et al. External radiotherapy of pituitary adenomas. *Int J Radiat Oncol Biol Phys* 1995;33:307–314.
29. Breen P, Flickinger JC, Kondziolka D, et al. Radiotherapy for non-functional pituitary adenoma: analysis of long term tumor control. *J Neurosurg* 1998;89: 933–938.
30. McCollugh WM, Marcus R, Rhoton AL, et al. Long-term follow up of radiotherapy for pituitary adenomas: the absence of late recurrence after >4500 cGy. *Int J Radiat Oncol Biol Phys* 1991;21:607.
31. Grigsby PW, Thomas PR, Simpson JR, et al. Long term results of radiotherapy in the treatment of pituitary adenomas in children and adolescents. *Am J Clin Oncol* 1998;11:607.
32. Hayes TP, Davis RA, Raventos A. The treatment of pituitary chromophobe adenomas. *Radiology* 1971;98:149.
33. Zierhut D, Flentje M, Adolph J, et al. External radiotherapy of pituitary adenomas. *Int J Radiat Oncol Biol Phys* 1995;33:307.
34. Tsang RW, Brierley JD, Panzarella T, et al. Role of radiation therapy in clinical hormonally active pituitary adenomas. *Radiother Oncol* 1996;41:45.
35. Milker-Zabel S, Debus J, Thilmann C, et al. Fractionated stereotactically guided radiotherapy and radiosurgery in the treatment of functional and non-functional adenomas of the pituitary gland. *Int J Radiat Oncol Biol Phys* 2001;50:1279.
36. Mitsumori M, Shrieve DC, Alexander E 3rd, et al. Initial clinical results of LINAC-based stereotactic radiosurgery and stereotactic radiotherapy for pituitary adenomas. *Int J Radiat Oncol Biol Phys* 1998;42:573–580.
37. Yoon SC, Suh TS, Jang HS, et al. Clinical results of 24 pituitary adenomas with LINAC-based radiosurgery. *Int J Radiat Oncol Biol Phys* 1998;42:849.
38. Malyapa R. Clinical outcomes study of proton therapy for pituitary adenoma. University of Florida Proton Therapy Institute. Protocol 0701-P101.
39. Brada M, Ford D, Ashley S, et al. Risk of second brain tumor after conservation surgery and radiotherapy for pituitary adenoma. *BMJ* 1992;304:1343.
40. Tsang RW, Laperriere NJ, Simpson WJ. Glioma arising after radiation therapy for pituitary adenoma. A report of four patients and estimation of risk. *Cancer* 1993; 72:2227.
41. Bates T, Bengtsson A-G. Premature mortality due to cardiovascular disease in hypopituitarism. *Lancet* 1990;336:285.
42. Bulow B, Hagman I, Mikczy Z, et al. Increased cerebrovascular mortality in patients with hypopituitarism. *Clin Endocrinol* 1997;46:75.

Chapter 37
Spinal Canal

Jiayi Huang*, Cliff Robinson*, and Jeff M. Michalski

Tumors of the spinal cord and cauda equina account for 3% to 4% of central nervous system (CNS) tumors overall and 6% of CNS tumors in children.[1] Spinal canal tumors are classified by the World Health Organization (WHO) according to histological types. Clinically, they are also characterized by their location relative to the protective layers of the spinal cord as either extradural, intradural–extramedullary, or intramedullary (Fig. 37.1). Intramedullary lesions arise from the intrinsic substance of the spinal cord. Histologically, intramedullary spinal cord neoplasms include gliomas such as astrocytoma, ependymoma, and oligodendroglioma. Intradural–extramedullary tumors arise from the connective tissues, blood vessels, or coverings adjacent to the cord or cauda equina. Common histologies include nerve sheath tumor, meningioma, and ependymoma. Extradural tumors are most commonly metastatic, although primary tumors in this compartment may occur as well. Primary extradural tumors arising from the vertebral bodies may include benign tumors such as osteoid osteoma, osteoblastoma, or aneurysmal bone cysts, or as malignant tumors such as plasmocytoma or myeloma, chordoma or chondrosarcoma, osteosarcoma, and Ewing's sarcoma. Other primary extradural tumors arising outside of the vertebral body include epidural hemangiomas, lipomas, extradural meningiomas, nerve sheath tumors, and lymphomas.

Radiation therapy is an important modality in the management of both primary and metastatic tumors involving the spinal canal. This chapter focuses primarily on the management of primary spinal cord tumors. Primary extradural tumors are usually managed in a manner similar to histopathologically identical tumors arising at other locations and will not be discussed here in detail. The management of metastatic tumors involving the spinal canal is discussed in Chapter 93.

ANATOMY

Spinal Cord

The spinal cord is a slender cylinder composed of functional segments corresponding to 31 pairs of spinal nerves: 8 cervical, 12 thoracic, 5 lumbar, 5 sacral, and 1 coccygeal. In contrast to the brain, the white matter of the spinal cord is located in the periphery and surrounds the central gray matter. The gray matter contains the cell bodies of sensory, motor, and autonomic neurons. On cross-section, the gray matter is a butterfly-shaped region with anterior horns controlling motor function, lateral horns (in the thoracic and upper lumbar region) controlling autonomic functions, and posterior horns involved in sensation. The white matter contains the axonal elements of neurons that transmit impulses to and from the brain. As in the brain, the axons of the spinal cord white matter possess a myelin sheath formed by the cytoplasmic extension of glial cells. Schwann cells sheath the spinal nerves that enter and exit the spinal cord. The spinal cord is organized into somatotopically distinct regions (Fig. 37.2). The lateral and anterior spinal cord white matter contains the nerve tracts that are involved with fine motor control and tone, including the corticospinal tracts. The spinocerebellar tracts transmit muscle stretch and tone sensation from the extremities to the cerebellum. The lateral spinal thalamic tract is located laterally near the spinal cord surface and carries ascending crossed pain fibers to the thalamus. The dorsal columns transmit fine touch and positional sensation from the extremities to the brain. Because of its serial organization, injury to the spinal cord results in characteristic neurologic findings that depend on the location of the insult.

The spinal cord is surrounded by the meninges, which is composed (from outer to inner) of the dura mater, arachnoid, and pia mater. The pia mater covers the spinal cord and its blood vessels. This layer condenses laterally into approximately 20 pair of dentate ligaments, which suspend the cord to the dura mater. The dura mater forms a dense, fibrous barrier between the bony spinal canal and the spinal cord. The dural sac ends inferiorly at S2-3 but the dura continues with the filum terminale down to the coccyx. The arachnoid mater resides between the dura mater and the pia mater. The arachnoid encloses the subarachnoid space filled with cerebrospinal fluid (CSF). The subarachnoid space follows the arachnoid down to the end of the dural sac.

The growth of the vertebral column during childhood takes place at a rate and extent greater than that of the spinal cord

*Both authors contributed equally to this work.

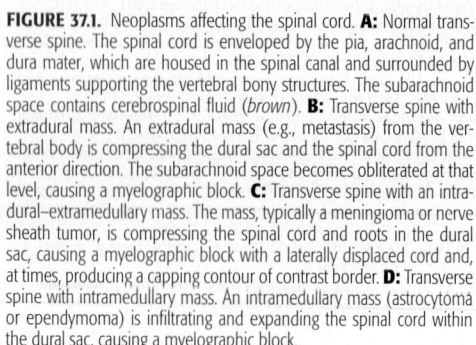

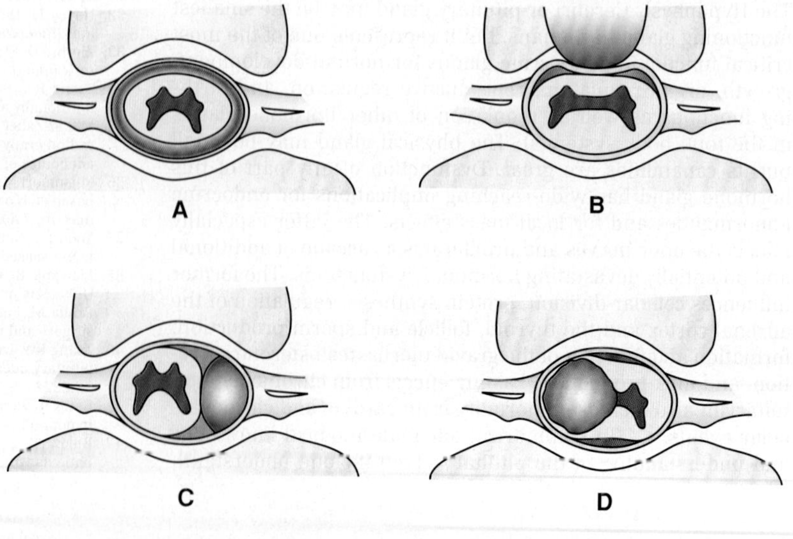

FIGURE 37.1. Neoplasms affecting the spinal cord. **A:** Normal transverse spine. The spinal cord is enveloped by the pia, arachnoid, and dura mater, which are housed in the spinal canal and surrounded by ligaments supporting the vertebral bony structures. The subarachnoid space contains cerebrospinal fluid (*brown*). **B:** Transverse spine with extradural mass. An extradural mass (e.g., metastasis) from the vertebral body is compressing the dural sac and the spinal cord from the anterior direction. The subarachnoid space becomes obliterated at that level, causing a myelographic block. **C:** Transverse spine with an intradural–extramedullary mass. The mass, typically a meningioma or nerve sheath tumor, is compressing the spinal cord and roots in the dural sac, causing a myelographic block with a laterally displaced cord and, at times, producing a capping contour of contrast border. **D:** Transverse spine with intramedullary mass. An intramedullary mass (astrocytoma or ependymoma) is infiltrating and expanding the spinal cord within the dural sac, causing a myelographic block.

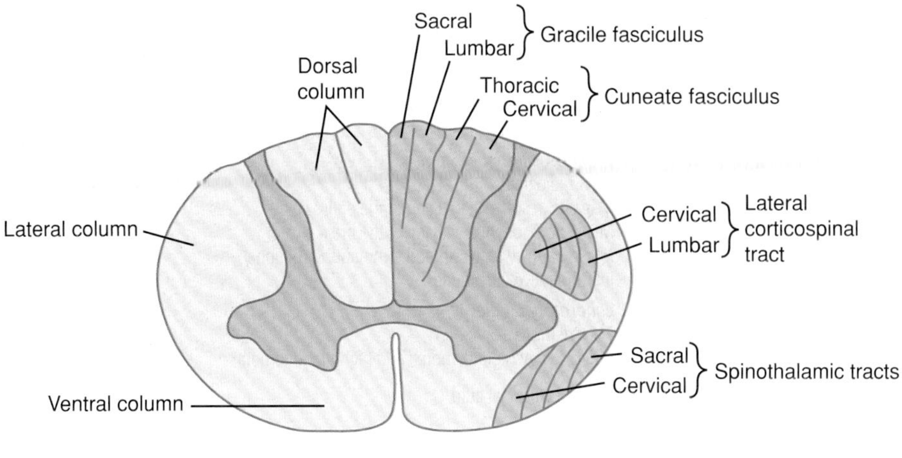

FIGURE 37.2. Somatotopic organization of the cervical spinal cord in transection. (From Waxman S, *Clinical neuroanatomy*. New York: McGraw-Hill, 2010, with permission.)

itself. By adulthood, the spinal cord is nearly 25 cm shorter than the vertebral column and ends near the level of the L1 vertebral body. Because of this differential growth, the exit level of each pair of spinal nerves in the spinal cord is usually higher than the corresponding vertebral body level. For example, in adults the C8 nerve root leaves the cord at the C6 vertebral body, the T6 nerve at the T3 vertebral level, and the T12 nerve at the T9 vertebral level. All of the lumbar nerves exit the spinal cord from vertebral levels T10 through T12, and all of the sacral nerves exit the spinal cord near the L1 vertebral level. The lower lumbar, sacral, and coccygeal nerves form the cauda equina, the collection of nerves that fills the thecal sac below L1. At its most caudal extent, the cord tapers to a thin segment, the conus medullaris. It is tethered to the coccyx by the filum terminale, a dense thread of pia mater.

Spinal Canal

The posterior body surfaces and neural arches of the vertebrae form the vertebral foramina, which in continuity form the spinal canal. Vertebral foramina are triangular in the lumbar and cervical regions, where the cord is mostly mobile, and round in the thoracic region. The spinal canal is lined with ligaments, including the posterior longitudinal ligament on its anterior wall, the flaval ligaments between adjacent arches, and the interspinous ligaments between the spinous processes. At each vertebral level, a spinous process protrudes from the posterior aspect of the neural arch, and transverse processes extend from the lateral edges of each arch. The laminae are those portions of the neural arch between the spinous and transverse processes, and the pedicles lie between the transverse processes and the body. At the intersection between the laminae and pedicles are superior and inferior paired articular facets. The superior articular facets are synovial joints that articulate with the inferior articular facets of the vertebra immediately above. The paired pedicles of each vertebra are notched at their superior and inferior edges such that the notches from two contiguous vertebra form an intervertebral foramen, through which the spinal nerve courses.

EPIDEMIOLOGY

Primary spinal canal tumors comprise 3% to 4% of all primary CNS tumors.[1] Their incidences vary by location and age. Primary spinal canal tumors appear to be more common in non-Hispanic whites than Hispanics or non-Hispanic blacks.[2] Although the incidence of spinal cord ependymoma has increased significantly over the past 30 years, the incidence of other glioma subtypes has remained stable.[3]

In adults, nearly two-thirds of all intradural tumors are extramedullary and are typically nerve sheath tumors, meningiomas, or ependymomas. The other third of intradural tumors are intramedullary, with the most common histologies being astrocytoma and ependymoma, followed by hemangioblastoma and other tumor types (Table 37.1). Overall, extramedullary nerve sheath tumors and meningiomas represent the most common spinal canal neoplasms, followed by intramedullary ependymomas and astrocytomas.

Primary tumors of the spinal canal are relatively more frequent in children, accounting for 6% of pediatric CNS tumors.[1] More than 50% of pediatric patients are younger than 10 years of age.[4,5] In a review of 872 children with intraspinal tumors, 36% had intramedullary tumors, 27% had intradural extramedullary tumors, and 24% had extradural tumors (13% were unclassified).[5] Nearly 75% of pediatric intramedullary tumors were astrocytomas or gangliogliomas and a few were ependymomas. Approximately 25% of the intradural–extramedullary tumors were ependymomas, followed in incidence by dermoids

TABLE 37.1 PRIMARY SPINAL CANAL TUMORS: LOCATIONS, TYPES, AND FREQUENCIES

Location	*Frequency (%)*	*Type*	*Comments*
Extradural	Few	Meningioma	~10% of spinal meningiomas
Intradural–extramedullary	70	Nerve sheath tumor	45% of primary tumors in this location, thoracic preference
		Meningioma	<40% of primary tumors at this location, thoracic preference
		Ependymoma in cauda	60% of all spinal ependymomas
		Vascular tumor	<10% of primary tumors at this location
		Teratoma, dermoid, squamous cell neoplasia	10% of primary tumors at this location, sacrococcygeal preference
		Lipoma	Few, subpial
Intradural–intramedullary	30	Ependymoma in cord	<40% of all spinal canal ependymomas
		Astrocytoma	<45% of primary tumors at this location
		Hemangioblastoma	Rare
		Oligodendroglioma	~15% of primary tumors at this location
		Teratoma	Rare

(23%), teratomas (16%), nerve sheath tumors (14%), lipomas (13%), and meningiomas (9%).[6]

NATURAL HISTORY

Most primary tumors of the spinal canal are histologically benign. Despite this, they are often the cause of significant disability because they compress or invade the spinal cord and interfere with neurologic function. Intramedullary tumors produce neurologic damage by local invasion or cystic compression of the cord, whereas extramedullary lesions compress, stretch, or distort the cord or the spinal nerves. Primary spinal cord tumors may be focal or relatively localized in some patients but may involve nearly the entire length of the cord in others. In one report, 73% of affected children presented with widening of the entire spinal cord from the medulla or cervical medullary junction to the conus medullaris.[7] These "holocord" tumors typically consist of a discrete solid mass and an associated cystic component or syrinx that extends over a significant length of the spinal cord. Local tumor progression is the dominant form of treatment failure of spinal cord tumors. CSF seeding is possible but uncommon.[8–10,11] Because the CNS has no lymphatics, spread to lymph nodes is not seen with spinal canal tumors. Extraneural spread is rare, occurring with an overall incidence of 0.96% in a cohort of 28,441 CNS cancers identified in a Surveillance, Epidemiology, and End Results (SEER) analysis. Interestingly, cancers of the spinal cord had a higher risk of extraneural spread relative to cerebral tumors.[12] The major causes of death in patients with spinal canal tumors are complications of paraplegia or quadriplegia such as infection or respiratory compromise.

CLINICAL PRESENTATION

Pain is the most common presenting symptom, affecting approximately 72% of patients.[13] Often the pain is localized to the region of involvement and may be present for a long time before the patient manifests localizing neurologic signs. Radicular pain, a result of pressure on nerve roots, reflects the distribution of the involved root and indicates that conduction is intact. Numbness replacing pain is a more advanced sign that indicates compromise of spinal nerve or nerve tract conduction. Extramedullary tumors can cause distention of the dura with severe pain in the region of the tumor that is characteristically aggravated by recumbency because of venous congestion. Thus, pain is often worse at night.[7] Movement or the Valsalva maneuver also may worsen pain. Less commonly, pain is characterized as a burning sensation in one or more extremities.

Other symptoms of CNS involvement include weakness (55% of patients), sensory deficits (39%), and sphincter dysfunction (15%).[13] Low-grade tumors generally have a more prolonged duration of symptoms than high-grade tumors. Bladder and bowel dysfunction as presenting symptoms are relatively uncommon except for tumors that involve the conus medullaris and filum terminale.

Tumors involving the lumbosacral spine present with a cauda equina nerve root compression syndrome. Patients may have radicular pain in the anterior (L4), lateral (L5), or posterior (S1) thigh with corresponding paresthesias followed by muscle wasting of the glutei, hamstrings, or tibialis anterior muscles. Saddle anesthesia, absent ankle reflexes (S1), or plantar (S2) responses may be present. Impotence and loss of anal or bulbar cavernous reflexes also may occur.

DIAGNOSTIC WORKUP

History and Physical Findings

Table 37.2 shows the diagnostic workup for primary tumors of the spinal cord. A meticulous and accurate patient history and physical examination are critical aspects of the initial assessment and can often localize suspected spinal tumors. The neurologic examination should concentrate on testing motor and sensory functions and reflexes. The differential diagnosis of a patient with a spinal cord tumor may include syringomyelia, multiple sclerosis, amyotrophic lateral sclerosis, diabetic neuropathy, viral myelitis, or paraneoplastic syndromes.

TABLE 37.2 DIAGNOSTIC WORKUP FOR PRIMARY SPINAL CORD TUMORS
General
History
Physical examination
Complete neurologic examination
Diagnostic Imaging Studies
Plain radiography
Magnetic resonance imaging of the entire spine
Magnetic resonance imaging of the brain
Myelography with computed tomography (optional)
Intraoperative ultrasound
Laboratory Studies
CSF chemistry (optional)
CSF cytology (ependymoma and high-grade tumors)

CSF, cerebrospinal fluid.

A cutaneous sensory level may be definable, although the level of cord compression is a few segments higher than the superior level of sensory loss because of pathway crossing characteristics. Loss of pain and heat and cold sensation below a specific dermatomal level indicates compromise of the spinothalamic pathway in the lateral columns. Impaired posture, gait, and coordination and loss of vibration sense indicate compromise of the posterior spinocerebellar pathways or the posterior columns.

At the level of the lesion, flaccid weakness and loss of tendon reflexes may occur. Below the lesion, the same signs are noticed in acute stages, but spastic paralysis and hyperactive tendon reflexes plus an upward Babinski toe sign ensue in subacute and chronic stages. These findings are consistent with lower and upper motor neuron involvement, respectively. The signs and symptoms of neurologic dysfunction may be asymmetric. In some cases, a classic Brown-Séquard syndrome may be present with ipsilateral loss of motor function and fine touch sensation and contralateral loss of pain and temperature sensation below the level of the lesion.

Autonomic reflexes (e.g., sweating) frequently are increased below the level of the lesion and may encompass the whole body if the lesion is cervical.[14] Sweating disappears at the level of the compressed cord. Disruption of urinary and bowel function usually occurs later than sensory and motor dysfunction. Early loss of bladder function, saddle anesthesia, and later pain characterize neoplasms of the conus medullaris and filum terminale.

Radiographic Studies

Although plain films are not typically used as the principal imaging modality for the evaluation of suspected spinal canal tumors, abnormalities can be detected from increased intracanal pressure including erosion of vertebral pedicles, enlargement of the anteroposterior diameter of the bony canal, or scalloping of the posterior wall of the vertebral bodies. Calcification may be seen in extramedullary tumors, especially meningiomas, and less frequently in nerve sheath tumors. Overall, plain radiographs of the spine show abnormalities in approximately 50% of patients with primary spinal canal neoplasms.[15–18] Changes are more likely to be detected on plain radiographs in children than in adults, such as kyphoscoliosis or scalloping of the vertebral bodies.[4,5,19,20]

Myelography, once considered the standard examination in evaluation of the spinal cord and canal, is now used principally

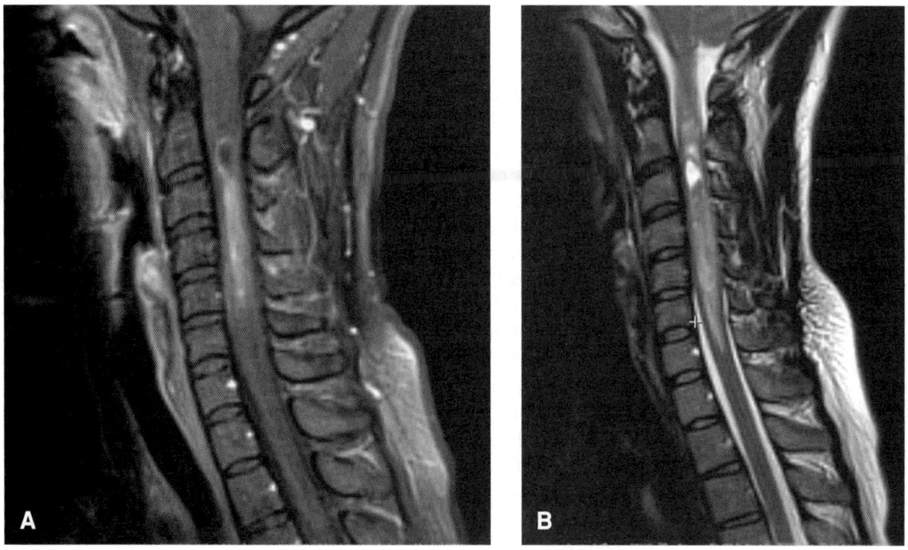

FIGURE 37.3. Sagittal magnetic resonance imaging scans of a 30-year-old female with a low-grade astrocytoma involving the cervical spine. **A:** T1-weighted image demonstrates an intramedullary lesion that expands the cord from the level of the craniocervical junction to the level of C7. The enhancing component extends from mid C2 to C5, and there is an associated cystic component at the cranial aspect of the lesion. **B:** T2-weighted image demonstrates T2 hyperintensity within the lesion suggestive of edema and hypointensity suggestive of blood products.

in patients who are unable to undergo magnetic resonance imaging (MRI) because of the presence of implanted ferromagnetic materials or for whom images at the level of concern are distorted by the presence of surgical hardware. In this situation, computed tomography (CT) scanning combined with myelography will give better spatial resolution. CT myelography may be particularly beneficial as part of radiotherapy treatment planning in the postoperative setting, where the spinal cord may be obscured by artifact on the MRI.[21]

Computed Tomography

CT is most helpful in evaluating the spine for extradural pathologic processes. Bone tumors or paraspinal soft tissue masses that secondarily involve the spinal cord (e.g., dumbbell tumors) can be imaged with contrast-enhanced CT scans. Nerve sheath tumors can enlarge the intervertebral foramina or spinal canal and cause smooth erosion of bone. Meningiomas are occasionally calcified. Both of these neoplasms are partially outlined by

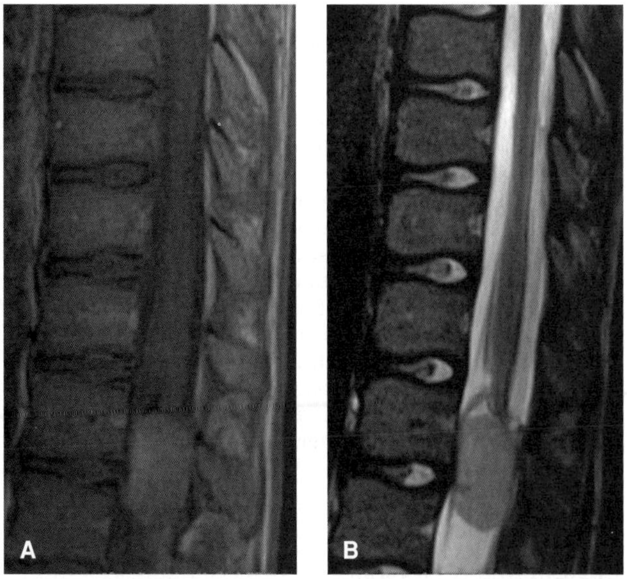

FIGURE 37.4. Sagittal magnetic resonance imaging scans of a 12-year-old male with a myxopapillary ependymoma involving the lumbar spine. **A:** T1-weighed image demonstrates a homogenously enhancing intradural extramedullary mass at the level of L1. **B:** T2-weighted image demonstrates hyperintensity of the mass. (Courtesy Aseem Sharma, MD, Mallinckrodt Institute of Radiology.)

CSF and produce extramedullary deformity by displacement of the spinal cord.[22]

Magnetic Resonance Imaging

MRI has replaced myelography and CT as the imaging study of choice in evaluation of tumors of the spinal canal. Sagittal and axial images give a three-dimensional appreciation of the patient's anatomy and help plan therapy. The various signal characteristics of the CSF—white and gray matter, bone and bone marrow, fat, and flowing blood—all facilitate the interpretation of the study. Some cystic tumors, vascular lesions, or lipomas can be diagnosed based on their characteristic signals on T1- and T2-weighted images without contrast injection. Intravenous gadolinium-diethylenetriamine pentaacetic acid (Gd-DTPA) administration improves the sensitivity of MRI by enhancing the solid component of intramedullary tumors and differentiating them from surrounding edema or syrinx cavities (Figs. 37.3 and 37.4). Unlike low-grade gliomas in the brain, nearly all spinal cord gliomas, regardless of grade, enhance with Gd-DTPA.[23] Sagittal T1-weighted images usually localize intramedullary mass neoplasms along with adjacent cysts. Intradural–extramedullary lesions also show enhancement on T1-weighted images after administration of Gd-DTPA. The use of Gd-DTPA also increases the sensitivity of detecting leptomeningeal metastases.[23]

MRI of the brain should be performed in patients with ependymomas or high-grade astrocytomas to exclude the possibility of neuraxis seeding or the presence of an intracranial primary tumor.

Cerebrospinal Fluid

A patient suspected of having a spinal canal neoplasm should not be subjected to a lumbar puncture before MRI. Symptoms may be exacerbated after a spinal tap because of shifting of the spinal cord and incarceration before the tumor can be localized adequately.[20] The CSF usually has increased protein levels and may exhibit xanthochromia, especially with extradural compression conditions, but lower values can be found in cases of intramedullary disease and with compression in the cervical region.[14] The incidence of leptomeningeal spread in patients with primary spinal cord glioma is low overall but is substantially more common with malignant tumors. Leptomeningeal dissemination has been reported to be as high as 60% for intramedullary glioblastoma.[24,25] Cytological examination of the cerebrospinal fluid should be done in patients with ependymomas (especially anaplastic and myxopapillary types) and high-grade astrocytomas.

Tissue Diagnosis

Suspected primary tumors of the spinal cord and spinal canal must be pathologically confirmed in all circumstances. Strong consideration should also be given to biopsy of any presumed metastatic tumors if they are the first site of disease recurrence after successful management of a previous malignant primary tumor. In rare circumstances in which emergency radiation therapy is indicated to relieve spinal cord compression in the absence of a confirmed cancer diagnosis, a patient should be made aware of the consequences of treatment in the absence of a definitive diagnosis, including the inability to tailor therapy based on histology and possible delay of appropriate treatment for nonmalignant etiologies.

PATHOLOGIC CLASSIFICATION

The current comprehensive classification system of spinal tumors was published by the WHO in 2007. It groups the CNS neoplasms by the tumor type and provides a grading system to predict prognosis and guide therapy. Tumor types include neuroepithelial (i.e., astrocytoma, ependymoma, ganglioglioma), nerve sheath (i.e., schwannoma, neurofibroma), meningioma, lymphoma, germ cell, and metastatic tumors.[26] Clinically, they are also characterized by their location as either extradural, intradural–extramedullary, or intramedullary.

Intramedullary Tumors

Most intramedullary tumors of the spinal cord are glial in origin, with astrocytomas and ependymomas accounting for the majority.

Astrocytomas are the most common intramedullary spinal cord tumors, comprising approximately 45% of reported cases in adults. In contrast to intracranial astrocytoma, the majority of intramedullary astrocytomas are low grade (WHO grade I or II), including 75% in adults and 85% to 90% in children.[27,28,29] Juvenile pilocytic astrocytomas (grade I) in particular, as in other locations in the CNS, are not infiltrative in nature. Recognition of this feature, along with advances in surgical techniques and intraoperative monitoring, has led neurosurgeons to manage these tumors with more radical resections.[19,30,31–32] However, many fibrillary astrocytomas (grade II) as well as anaplastic astrocytomas (grade III) and glioblastoma multiforme (grade IV) are infiltrative, and complete resection carries a significant risk of neurologic disability. In these cases, a subtotal resection or biopsy may be the only safe surgical option.

Astrocytomas are more likely to occur in the cervical and thoracic regions than ependymomas. Low-grade astrocytomas are typically confined to a focal segment of the spinal cord. Rarely, astrocytomas may involve a large part of the spinal cord, at which point they are designated a holocord tumor. These holocord tumors may result entirely from tumor involvement or from a large syrinx in addition to the original tumor. The term "holocord" must be used with caution, however, as many of the previously reported cases were made by myelography, and recent series using MRI suggest a significantly decreased frequency of these tumors.[33]

A discriminating feature of intramedullary spinal cord tumors is the presence or absence of a syrinx. Syringes associated with spinal cord astrocytoma occur in 20% to 40% of patients.[34] Syringes can span the entire length of the cord, although they tend to favor more rostrally located tumors, as well as favoring the more rostral portion of the tumor itself.[34] In certain instances, a syrinx may even extend into the medulla, producing an obstructive hydrocephalus.[35] The syrinx itself can be responsible for significant neurologic deficit.

Approximately 40% of intramedullary tumors are ependymomas. Ependymomas are derived from glial cells similar to those lining the ventricular system. Several histologic types have been reported and include cellular, epithelial, tanycytic, subependymoma, myxopapillary, or mixed types. Cellular (classic) ependymomas (WHO grade II or III) typically develop in the cervical and thoracic spinal cord. Myxopapillary ependymomas (grade I) often arise from within the filum terminale and typically occur in the lumbosacral region.[36–38,39–40] Myxopapillary ependymomas frequently can be completely excised. In many circumstances, however, these tumors tightly envelope the nerve roots of the cauda equina, making *en bloc* excision difficult. Gross total resection of these tumors often requires piecemeal removal. The myxopapillary variant may be biologically less aggressive than the cellular variant, but late recurrences can occur even after complete gross excision; therefore, long-term follow-up of these patients is required.[40–44]

A variety of vascular neoplasms can arise from within the spinal cord, including arteriovenous malformations, hemangiomas, and hemangioblastomas. Approximately one-third of hemangioblastomas are associated with von Hippel-Lindau disease. These are benign neoplasms that are usually well circumscribed and amenable to surgery.[45] Unresectable or recurrent hemangioblastomas may be treated with stereotactic radiosurgery.[46]

Intradural–Extramedullary Tumors

Most intradural–extramedullary neoplasms are meningiomas, nerve sheath tumors, or myxopapillary ependymomas. They usually are amenable to complete surgical excision.

Meningiomas are usually benign, well-encapsulated neoplasms that are easily separated from the spinal cord; most can be completely excised, and they rarely recur. They may arise anywhere within the intradural space but are found in the thoracic region in approximately 80% of patients.[47–49] Meningiomas are uncommon in the lumbar region and rare in the sacrum. At least 80% of meningiomas occur in women 40 years of age or older.[47,48]

Nerve sheath tumors arise from the Schwann cell, the cell responsible for insulating peripheral nerves and contributing to impulse conduction. Nerve sheath tumors have been called, neurofibroma, schwannoma, neuroma, and neurilemoma in the past. More recently, a distinction between neurofibroma and schwannoma has been made. Although both tumors arise from Schwann cells, certain gross, microscopic, and clinical features help distinguish the two.[29] Neurofibromas typically encase involved nerve roots, while schwannomas commonly displace the nerve roots due to their asymmetric growth. The plexiform neurofibroma is associated with type 1 neurofibromatosis, and the presence of multiple tumors helps establish the diagnosis of this genetic condition. In contrast, schwannoma is associated with type 2 neurofibromatosis. Patients with type 1 neurofibromatosis may be at risk for malignant tumor transformation following radiotherapy.[50] Nerve sheath tumors usually are solitary and may occur in any section of the spinal canal. They are evenly distributed in the cervical, thoracic, and lumbar regions; they are least common in the sacrum. They occur in men and women with equal frequency and are most commonly diagnosed in the fourth through sixth decades of life. Most of these tumors are completely intradural, although 10% to 15% may have an extradural component as well (so-called dumbbell tumors). Most nerve sheath tumors are benign, well-encapsulated lesions that are amenable to total surgical excision. The rare malignant nerve sheath tumors have a natural history similar to soft tissue sarcomas, and they should be treated as such.[51–53]

Miscellaneous Neoplasms

Unusual intradural–extramedullary tumors include lipomas, dermoids, and epidermoid tumors. They are typically benign and amenable to complete resection. Even if incompletely excised, recurrences are usually slow.

Extradural Tumors

Most extradural tumors are metastatic, and the presentation and management of these is discussed in Chapter 94. A variety of primary bone and soft tissue tumors may arise from an extradural location and involve the spinal canal. Bone tumors include osteosarcoma, chordomas, chondrosarcoma, and Ewing's sarcoma. Soft tissue tumors include soft tissue sarcomas, including malignant nerve sheath tumors, lymphomas, and neuroblastomas. These tumors and their management are discussed in Chapters 78 (lymphoma), 82 (osteosarcoma/chordoma), 83 (soft tissue sarcoma), 86 (neuroblastoma), and 88 (Ewing's tumor), respectively.

PROGNOSTIC FACTORS

The major prognostic factors in patients with primary spinal canal tumors are tumor type and grade, tumor extent and location, patient age, and presenting neurologic function. Treatment-related factors that influence the outcome include tumor resectability and the use of radiation therapy for certain tumor types. Many of these factors are interdependent. For example, ependymomas occur most frequently in the distal spinal canal and are more often resectable than astrocytic tumors.

Recently, Milano et al.[54] analyzed 664 patients with spinal cord astrocytomas and 1,057 patients with spinal cord ependymomas using the SEER database. In this largest study to date on prognostic factors for long-term outcome, lower grade, younger age, and surgical resection were associated with significantly better overall survival and cause-specific survival for both astrocytomas and ependymomas. Radiotherapy was associated with worse cause-specific survival, but this is likely due to adverse selection bias. The 5-year overall survival of grades 1, 2, 3, and 4 astrocytomas was 82%, 70%, 28%, 14% and the 5-year cause-specific survival was 89%, 77%, 36%, 20%, respectively. The 5-year overall survival of grades 1, 2, and 3 ependymomas was 92%, 97%, and 58% and the 5-year cause-specific survival was 100%, 98%, and 64%, respectively.

Several investigators have reported that patients with rostral tumors have a worse survival and neurologic outcome than patients with more caudal tumors.[8,55–57] Guidetti et al.[56] stated that patients with cervical lesions had a higher surgical risk and complication rate, which made thorough resection of tumors in this location difficult and sometimes inadvisable. In a series of 62 patients with exclusively intramedullary ependymomas, patients with high cervical presentations (above C5) accounted for 4 of 6 postoperative deaths because of apneic respiratory complications.[57] In the Mallinckrodt Institute of Radiology experience, Garcia[8] reported that the primary tumor location was the most important prognostic feature. It was suggested that a greater concentration of function per unit volume of the upper spinal cord compared with that of the cauda equina accounted for the worst neurologic outcome and survival in patients with rostral tumors. Chun et al.,[55] from the Medical College of Virginia, also reported that patients with cervical lesions had significantly worse outcomes than patients with tumors in other sites. In both the Mallinckrodt Institute of Radiology and the Medical College of Virginia experiences, tumors affecting the rostral or cervical spinal cord were more likely to be astrocytomas, and tumors in the caudal spinal cord, filum terminale, or cauda equina were more likely to be ependymomas. The anatomic dependence of various tumor types may also contribute to the better prognosis seen in patients with tumors of the lower spinal canal.

Extensive involvement of the spinal cord with an ependymoma is associated with a worse outcome. Linstadt et al.[10] reported a 93% 10-year disease-specific survival rate with localized ependymoma compared with 50% for patients with diffuse tumors. Extensive tumors have a 50% local failure rate after surgery and radiation therapy, compared with only 20% for limited disease (one to three vertebral body segments).[39] However, extent of disease has not been a prognostic factor in other series.[58] Myxopapillary ependymomas that most commonly involve the cauda equina are felt to be less aggressive than other ependymomas,[40–42] but they have been reported to seed the CSF.[59,60] Encapsulated myxopapillary tumors of the cauda equina are frequently amenable to complete *en bloc* excision, and the recurrence rate is very low. Unencapsulated or adherent tumors often are removed piecemeal and are associated with a high local recurrence rate after surgery alone.[39,40,43,61,62]

Neurologic function at diagnosis is an important clinical prognostic factor. In general, the fewer the symptoms and the better the neurologic function at presentation, the greater the likelihood the tumor will be controlled with fewer long-term adverse neurologic sequelae.[8,31,56,57,63] Poor neurologic function in patients with spinal cord tumors is often attributable to the disease process and a prolonged delay in diagnosis rather than the effect of surgery or radiation therapy.[4,27,28,61,64,65]

SURGICAL MANAGEMENT

Intramedullary Tumors

Intramedullary tumors, most of which are astrocytomas and ependymomas, present a surgical challenge. Complete surgical excision is the treatment of choice if it can be achieved without compromising neurologic function. Ependymomas are more frequently amenable to gross total excision than are astrocytomas.[30,56,66] Complete resection of intramedullary tumors with preservation of neurologic function was not possible until 1940, when Greenwood[20] introduced the bipolar coagulation forceps. Since then, other technological advancements have emerged, including the dissecting microscope, intraoperative ultrasound, ultrasonic aspirator, contact laser scalpel, and intraoperative neurophysiologic monitoring.[67] These modern surgical techniques have increased the complete resectability of intramedullary tumors while minimizing neurologic injury.[68–70]

Intraoperative ultrasonography is used to localize the lesion, define its extent, and assess the progress of tumor resection.[71] The ultrasonic aspirator allows removal of tissue fragments from within 1 mm of the vibrating tip, permitting dissection immediately adjacent to vital neural tissue.[72] The contact laser scalpel only delivers thermal energy to tissue upon direct contact, and the laser beam resides entirely within a coated sapphire crystal probe tip. It provides precise dissection of tumor with little mechanical or thermal injury to normal spinal cord parenchyma.[73]

Intraoperative neurophysiologic monitoring is considered standard of care for resection of intramedullary tumors. It is dependent on two key components: somatosensory-evoked potentials (SEPs) and motor-evoked potentials (MEPs). SEPs are monitored continuously during the incision of the dorsal midline of the spinal cord to avoid injuring the dorsal column, as the cord anatomy is often distorted by the tumor. MEPs are monitored once the surgeon starts to dissect the tumor to avoid irreversible damage to the corticospinal tract. MEPs should be monitored using a combination of epidural electrodes (D waves) and signals from limb muscle (mMEPs). Typically, a decrement of 50% or more of D-wave amplitude is considered a major indication to stop surgery.[74] Sala et al.[75] reported that the use of intraoperative neurophysiologic monitoring during resection of intramedullary tumors significantly improved long-term ambulatory status as compared to historical controls.

The risk of paralysis after surgery is less than 1% of patients with minimal or no preoperative neurologic deficits, but may be much higher for those who present with more substantial deficits. Approximately one-third of patients will develop temporary motor deficits after surgery and most will have at least some postoperative deterioration in neurologic status.[76,77] If complete excision of low-grade spinal cord tumors is achieved, the local recurrence rate is low and prognosis is excellent without additional adjuvant therapy. In patients who recur, tumor regrowth is often slow and second resection may be possible.[78–80]

Intradural–Extramedullary Tumors

The treatment of choice for most tumors in this location is maximal surgical excision with preservation of neurologic function. Most benign nerve sheath tumors and meningiomas can be completely resected using a posterior approach with a standard posterior laminectomy.[29] Nerve sheath tumors rarely recur after satisfactory surgical removal. In contrast, as much as 15% of spinal meningiomas recur as late as 10 years after gross total or near total removal.[81] Piecemeal resection of ependymomas of the filum terminale can be accomplished with little neurologic disability; however, the risk of recurrence in these patients is significant, and adjuvant radiation therapy is warranted.[39,40,62,82,83]

In young children, posterior laminectomy is being abandoned and replaced with posterior osteoplastic laminotomy. Replacing the posterior bony elements of the spinal canal is less likely to cause significant kyphotic deformity and affords better protection of the spinal cord.[69,84,85]

CHEMOTHERAPY

The reported use of chemotherapy for primary spinal canal tumors is limited. Outside of a clinical trial, chemotherapy is often reserved for patients with progression of disease following surgery and radiotherapy with no other treatment options. Combined with the low incidence of the disease, most studies are retrospective with very few patients, which limits any definitive conclusion regarding their efficacy. The use of chemotherapy for spinal canal tumors is often extrapolated based on the experience for intracranial tumors. However, such assumption requires further validation as the underlying oncogenesis and biological pathways may be different between the two entities.[86]

Platinum and etoposide are generally considered the most active agents for ependymomas. In the setting of recurrent ependymoma, platinum-based chemotherapy has been shown to produce higher response rates than nitrosourea-based chemotherapy, but most patients in the studies had intracranial ependymomas.[87,88] In a prospective phase II study, 10 consecutive patients with recurrent cellular spinal cord ependymomas were treated with oral etoposide. Two patients had partial responses, and five patients had stable disease. The median overall survival was 17.5 months.[89]

Temozolomide is an attractive agent for primary spinal cord glioma given its success in treating intracranial astrocytoma.[90] Kim et al.[91] reported their experience of treating two patients with primary spinal cord glioblastoma multiforme with concurrent radiotherapy and temozolomide followed by adjuvant temozolomide. The two patients survived 12 and 16 months, respectively, in contrast with a median survival time of 9 months in other reports. Chamberlain[92] reported a series of 22 patients with recurrent WHO grade II glioma treated with temozolomide. Overall, there were 18% partial response and 55% with stable disease. The median survival was 23 months and progression-free survival at 2 years was 27%.

For young children, especially those less than 3 years of age, there is an even greater interest in identifying effective and minimally toxic chemotherapy to delay or eliminate radiation therapy. There are two prospective cooperative group trials that have included children with primary spinal cord astrocytomas. In one clinical trial conducted by the French Society of Pediatric Oncology, eight children with unresectable or recurrent intramedullary low-grade gliomas were treated with a planned 16-month course of carboplatin, procarbazine, vincristine, cyclophosphamide, etoposide, and cisplatin. Seven of the patients had a clinical or radiographic response to the chemotherapy. Five of the patients remained progression free, with follow-up ranging from 16 to 59 months.[93] In the Children's Cancer Group 945 trial, 13 children with high-grade astrocytic spinal cord neoplasms were assigned to receive two cycles of "8-drugs-in-1-day" chemotherapy before radiation therapy, then eight additional cycles thereafter. At 5 years, 46% of the children had no progression and 54% were alive. The authors argued that more intensive therapy was necessary.[94] Mora et al.[95] recently reported a small but thought-provoking study of three infants with spinal cord astrocytomas (WHO grade II or III) treated with irinotecan and cisplatin. All three infants had subtotal resection and progressed on conventional carboplatin-based chemotherapy. After switching to irinotecan and cisplatin, all three patients had remarkable radiologic and clinical response. At the time of the last follow-up, they had remained in remission at 12, 20, and 48 months after diagnosis. The authors hypothesized that irinotecan and cisplatin may provide synergistic effect without overlapping toxicities. Currently, children with high-grade astrocytomas of the spinal cord are eligible to enroll in a phase II Children's Oncology Group clinical trial of adjuvant radiation and concurrent temozolomide followed by additional temozolomide and lomustine chemotherapy for high-grade gliomas (COG-ACNS0423).

RADIATION THERAPY

There are currently no randomized controlled trials to guide the role of radiation therapy for primary spinal canal tumors. Clinical use of postoperative radiation therapy is generally guided by patterns of failure and the prevailing attitude of many radiation centers.[96] Patients with completely resected low-grade astrocytomas[19,29,31,32,97] and ependymomas[78,80,98–100] typically have an excellent prognosis, with local failure rates of less than 10% without additional therapy. Most centers do not advocate routine use of adjuvant radiation therapy in this setting, but long-term follow-up is indicated as late failures can occur.

In contrast, adjuvant radiation therapy after incomplete resection or piecemeal excision of low-grade ependymomas and astrocytomas is supported by retrospective analyses. Guidetti et al.[56] first reported a beneficial outcome in patients receiving radiation therapy after an incomplete excision of an ependymoma. Patients who have undergone complete excision of a cauda equina ependymoma by piecemeal removal have a local failure rate that ranges from 20% to 43%.[39,40,62] The addition of radiation therapy in patients who have undergone piecemeal excision of a cauda equina ependymoma produces a local recurrence rate equal to that of patients undergoing gross total resection.[39,62,83] In a multi-institutional series, adjuvant radiation therapy significantly improved progression-free survival in the 40 patients with low- and intermediate-grade astrocytomas.[30] After adjuvant radiotherapy, the cumulative incidence of local failure ranges from approximately 20% for low-grade ependymoma to 40% for low-grade astrocytoma.[96]

Nonetheless, there are clinical circumstances in which careful follow-up after incomplete resection is appropriate, with a second surgery or radiation therapy considered at the time of progression or recurrence. Radiation therapy of the spine in a child may produce a spinal deformity (i.e., scoliosis or kyphosis) because of retardation of bone growth from damage to epiphyseal plates of the vertebral bodies as well as soft tissue fibrosis and contracture.[101] Most spinal cord tumors in young children are either low-grade astrocytomas or well-differentiated ependymomas that have a very low growth rate. Delaying radiation therapy until recurrence or tumor progression may allow the child to grow at a normal rate for several years before receiving radiation therapy. Constantini et al.[102] reported a series of 164 patients younger than 21 years of age treated with radical surgery alone without adjuvant radiotherapy. Gross total resection or subtotal resection was achieved in 77%

and 20% of patients, respectively. The 3-month neurologic function was 60% stable, 16% improved, and 24% deteriorated compared with preoperative function. The 5-year progression-free survival rate for low-grade and high-grade tumors was 78% and 30%, respectively.

The prognosis of high-grade astrocytomas and ependymomas is dismal, and multimodality treatment is recommended, ideally on a clinical trial. Adjuvant radiation therapy is routinely recommended regardless of the extent of resection. The role of concurrent and adjuvant chemotherapy for high-grade intramedullary astrocytoma remains inconclusive as discussed earlier. Despite aggressive treatments, few patients with high-grade astrocytomas survive beyond 2 years.[96,103] As with intracranial high-grade glioma, novel therapies beyond traditional radiotherapy and cytotoxic chemotherapy are desperately needed.

Relapse can occur years after treatment and is predominantly local. In a series of 37 spinal ependymomas treated with adjuvant radiotherapy, more than 50% of failures developed 5 years after diagnosis, and the extent of surgical resection correlated with time to progression.[104] These findings were confirmed in another series of patients with spinal myxopapillary ependymoma, where Chao et al.[105] reported a median time to recurrence of 7.7 years.

The prognosis is excellent for most patients with intradural–extramedullary tumors, which rarely recur after total excision. However, subtotally resected meningiomas may recur late after surgery.[81] Some investigators have advocated postoperative radiation therapy using either conventional fractionated external-beam radiotherapy or stereotactic radiosurgery.[106,107] Radiation therapy is beneficial to patients undergoing subtotal resection or piecemeal excision of intradural–extramedullary ependymomas.[10,39,40,62] Data supporting the routine use of radiation therapy in the management of patients with nerve sheath tumors, vascular malformations, lipomas, hemangiomas, teratomas, and dermoids are limited.

RADIATION THERAPY TECHNIQUES

Target Volume

Historically, it had been recommended that superior and inferior field borders encompass two vertebral bodies above and below a tumor defined by myelography, with the width of the field approximated between the tips of the lateral processes of the vertebral bodies. With the advancement of CT simulation and MRI fusion, the gross tumor volume (GTV) can be more accurately defined and smaller margins may be used. For low-grade astrocytomas or ependymomas, a clinical target volume (CTV) margin of 0.5 to 1 cm is appropriate. The CTV should encompass the preoperative GTV plus any associated intratumoral cysts. It is not necessary to include an intramedullary syrinx that extends above or below the primary tumor unless there is radiographic or surgical evidence of tumor extension to these regions. Planning treatment volume (PTV) margins of 0.5 cm or less may be used to account for setup error, with smaller PTV margins necessitating adequate patient immobilization and optimal daily localization techniques (orthogonal kilovoltage imaging, cone-beam CT, etc.).

High-grade astrocytomas and ependymomas can be more infiltrative, and a larger CTV margin of at least 1.5 cm craniocaudally should be used. Merchant et al.[108] described a diffuse failure pattern in children with high-grade gliomas shortly after completing radiation therapy, suggesting that the tumor was not adequately covered in the irradiated volume and the need for larger CTV margins of 1.5 cm. The intervertebral foramina should be included within the CTV if tumor extension is suspected.

For myxopapillary ependymomas involving the conus, a 1.5-cm CTV margin cephalad and caudad to the GTV is used, but not beyond the thecal sac, which is typically at the level of S2-3. If the cauda equina is involved, the CTV should extend inferiorly to encompass the entire thecal sac, with the volume widened at the sacroiliac joints to ensure adequate coverage of the meningeal sleeves in the intervertebral foramina. Failure to adequately encompass the thecal sac has been associated with an increased rate of treatment failure.[62]

Craniospinal or spinal axis irradiation usually is not indicated in the treatment of most spinal cord tumors; local failure accounts for most tumor recurrences.[8,10,30,39,97,109] However, neuraxis dissemination may be seen in patients with anaplastic ependymomas,[110] malignant astrocytomas,[24,111] and myxopapillary ependymomas.[59,60] Craniospinal irradiation may be considered in these situations.

Radiation Technique

For conventional external-beam field arrangements, cervical cord tumors are typically treated with parallel opposed lateral fields to reduce dose to the oral cavity, larynx, and pharynx. Thoracic cord tumors are commonly treated with direct posterior or posterior wedge fields to limit dose to the anterior structures such as the lungs, esophagus, and heart. Lumbar and cauda equina tumors are mostly treated with opposed anteroposterior–posteroanterior portals because of the lumbar lordosis and the deep location of the vertebral canal. Conformal or intensity-modulated radiation therapy (IMRT) methods may reduce normal tissue toxicity[60] and should be considered when exit dose to the anterior midline structures of the trunk would otherwise be excessive (Fig. 37.5). However, IMRT may increase the volume of normal tissue receiving low doses and is theoretically associated with a higher risk of secondary malignancy.[112]

In female patients requiring treatment to the lumbosacral spine for cauda equina tumors, a lateral technique may be used to avoid exit irradiation to the ovaries and uterus. This technique prevents the anterior pelvic structures from receiving significant irradiation dose, which is desirable in young women and girls to minimize incidental irradiation of the ovaries. The superior aspect of this field can be matched to the divergence of a superior posteroanterior field in a fashion similar to the junction of a cranial portal to a spinal portal in craniospinal irradiation. Beam modifiers such as wedges or tissue compensators may be required with this lateral beam arrangement. Care should be taken to avoid irradiating the kidneys at the L1 through L3 levels with this technique. Arms should be positioned appropriately to avoid entrance or exit irradiation from the lateral beams.

The depth of the vertebral surface of the cord beneath the skin surface is determined from CT or MRI, and for short field lengths this depth is used for dose prescription. The treatment plan should provide a homogeneous dose distribution. For small lesions of the cervical spinal cord, where lateral fields will be used, radiation beam energies of 4 to 6 MV photons achieve a homogeneous dose distribution. Lesions involving the thoracic and lumbar spine often require combinations of low-energy (4 to 6 MV) and high-energy (18 to 25 MV) photons to achieve a homogeneous dose distribution when posterior fields are used. Attention to the exit dose delivered to anterior anatomical structures needs to be considered against dose heterogeneity in the target volume. Parallel-opposed posterior and anterior fields or paired oblique wedge fields can give homogeneous dose distributions with x-ray energies as low as 4 or 6 MV.

Radiation Dose

Low-grade astrocytomas and ependymomas should be irradiated to a total dose of 50.4 Gy, given in 1.8 Gy daily fractions. High-grade astrocytomas can be treated to a dose of 54 Gy with 1.8 Gy daily fractions. High-grade ependymomas and multifocal low-grade astrocytoma should be treated to a dose

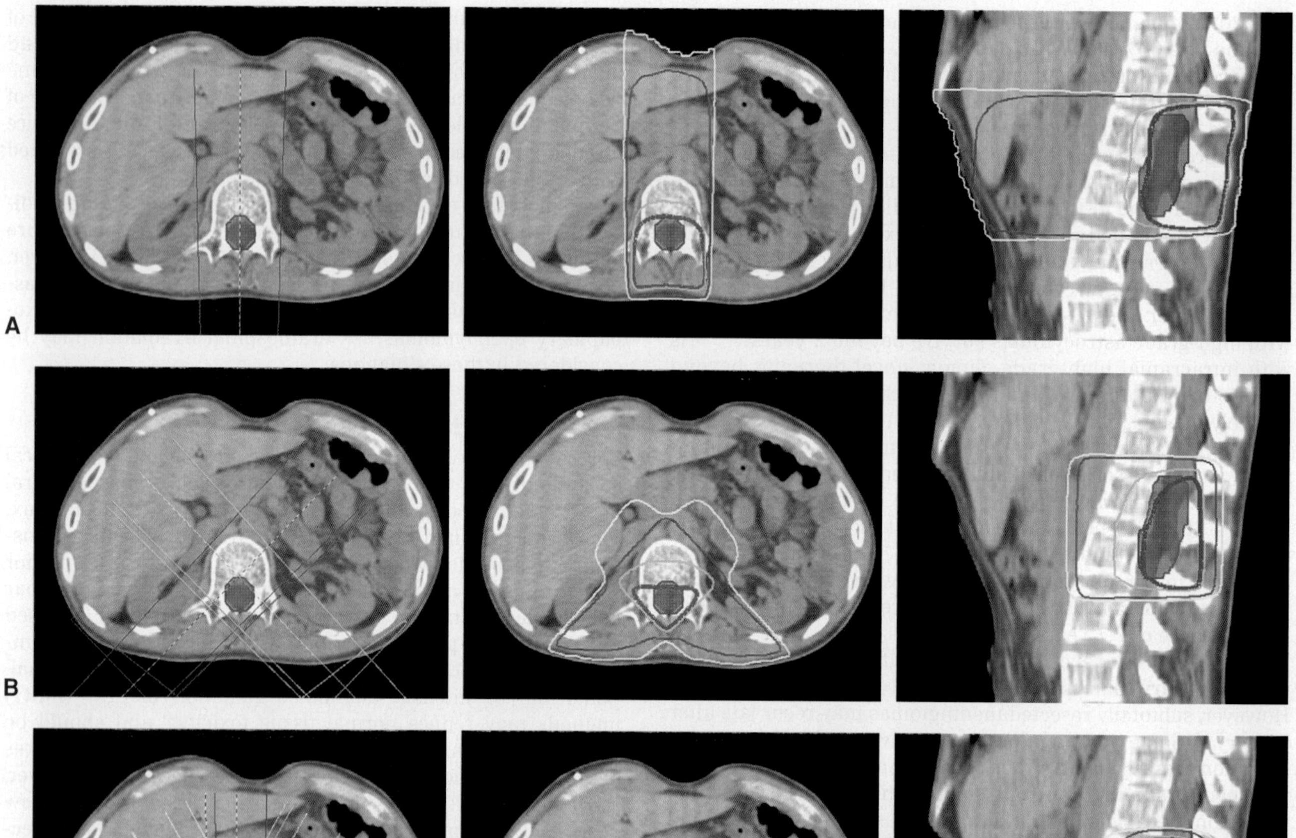

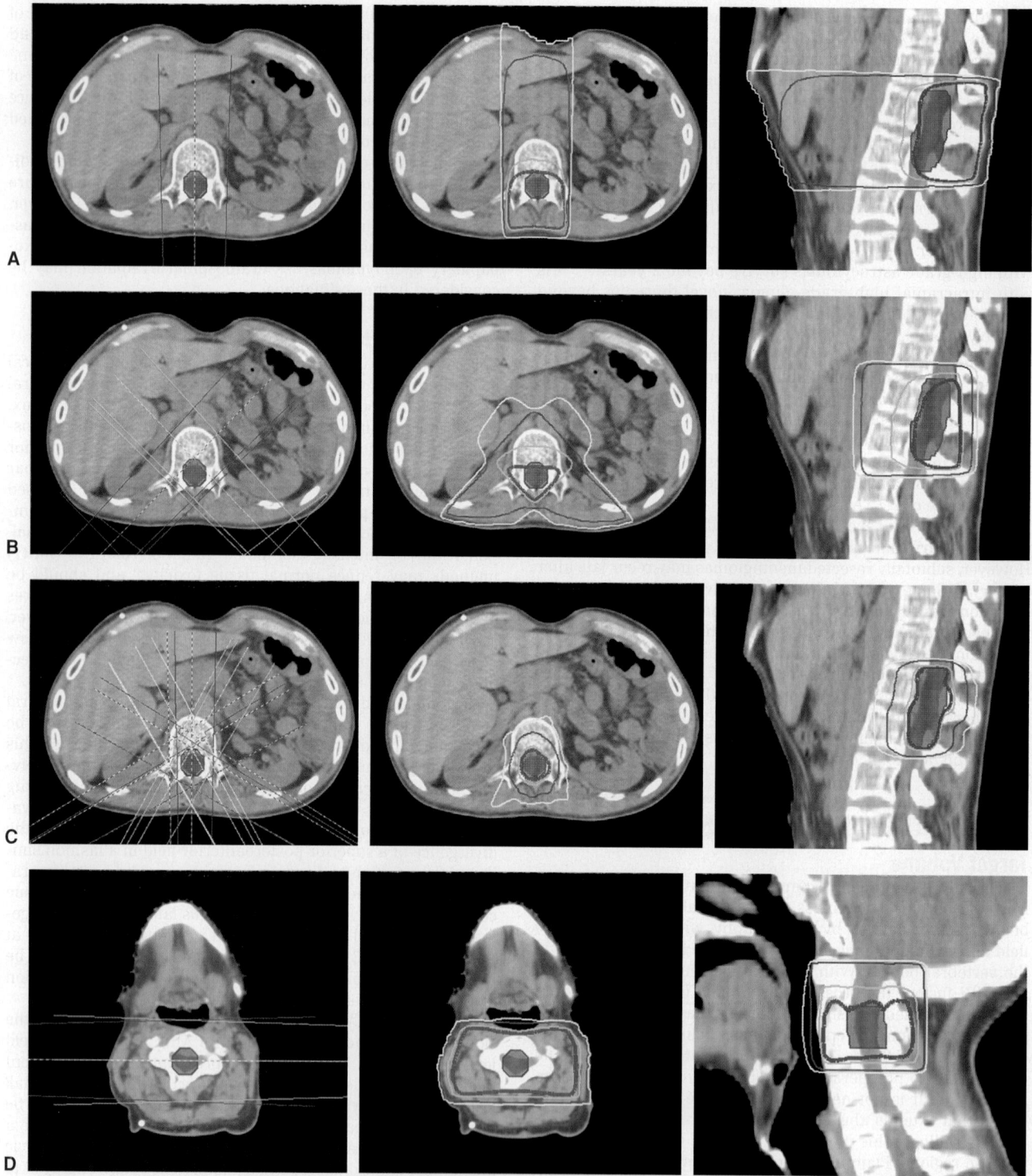

FIGURE 37.5. Treatment planning for spinal cord tumors. Planning treatment volume (PTV) in *solid blue*. *Red line,* prescription dose of 50.4 Gy; *Green line,* 95% of prescription dose of 47.88 Gy; *Blue line,* 30 Gy; *Yellow line,* 20 Gy. **A:** A single posteroanterior field. The advantages of this beam arrangement include simplicity and near-universal applicability in most spinal cord radiation therapy treatments. One disadvantage of this field arrangement is the large volume of tissue that receives a significant exit dose. The axial and sagittal isodose displays reflect a 6-MV x-ray beam treated to a point just anterior to the PTV. **B:** Paired posterior oblique wedge fields. The advantage of this technique is a decrease in high exit-dose irradiation to anterior tissues with a more conformal irradiation dose distribution near the target volume. Disadvantages include more complicated treatment setup and verification. The axial and sagittal isodose displays reflect a 45-degree wedged pair of 6-MV x-ray beams treated to the same point with a 90-degree hinge angle. **C:** Intensity-modulation radiation therapy (IMRT). An advantage is a highly conformal dose distribution with excellent sparing of adjacent critical structures. Disadvantage are complexity and high integral dose. The axial and sagittal isodose displays reflect a five-field static IMRT plan with 6-MV x-rays. **D:** Opposed lateral fields. An advantage is a homogeneous dose distribution in the target volume with sparing of anterior structures from significant irradiation dose. A disadvantage is limited applicability in cervical and lower lumbosacral sites. Exclusive use of this field arrangement in the thorax and upper abdomen is inappropriate because of limited lung and kidney tolerance. The axial isodose display reflects a pair of laterally directed 6-MV x-ray fields treated to the midplane of the cervical spine. (C, Courtesy Andrew Lindsey, Washington University in St. Louis Department of Radiation Oncology.)

of 50.4 to 54 Gy.[96] Limited dose response data exist for spinal cord tumors. In the Mallinckrodt series of 37 patients with primary spinal cord tumors, local control and survival were significantly better for those received 40 Gy or higher.[8] Shaw et al.[39] reported that the local failure rate of ependymomas was 35% in patients receiving 50 Gy or less compared with only 20% in patients receiving more than 50 Gy. However, doses beyond 50.4 Gy have not been shown to improve local control or survival.[10,66,113] In patients with high-grade ependymomas or other spinal cord gliomas with evidence of CSF dissemination, craniospinal irradiation should be considered. Typical doses to the craniospinal axis range from 36 to 45 Gy, with a boost to sites of gross tumor to 50.4 to 54 Gy.

Stereotactic Radiosurgery

Stereotactic radiosurgery (SRS) provides the ability to deliver highly conformal, high-dose radiation in such a manner as to mitigate normal tissue injury while escalating dose to the target volume. Most spine SRS reports to date have focused on its use in the management of metastatic disease to the spine. In a recent review, Hsu et al.[114] found local control rates in excess of 80% in most series, with significant pain improvement in 43% to 97%.

A few reports have also detailed spine SRS in the management of patients with intradural tumors. In the largest series reported to date, Gerszten et al.[107] treated 73 patients with benign intradural spinal tumors (meningioma, schwannoma, neurofibroma) using CyberKnife (Accuray Inc, Sunnyvale, CA) spine SRS to doses ranging from 16 to 30 Gy in 1 to 5 fractions. At a median of 37 months follow-up, the local control rate was 98% and pain improved in 70% of meningiomas, 50% of schwannomas, and 0% of neurofibromas. Three patients developed radiotherapy-related spinal cord toxicity 5 to 13 months after treatment. Overall radiographic response rates for benign intradural tumors in the series reported to date range from 28% to 39%.[114]

Investigators from Stanford University have reported their experience treating spinal cord ependymomas and hemangioblastomas using spine SRS delivered with the CyberKnife system (Fig. 37.6). In the earliest report, 7 patients with 10 intramedullary spinal tumors (7 hemangioblastomas, 3 ependymomas) received spine SRS to a dose of 18 to 25 Gy in 1 to 3 fractions.[46]

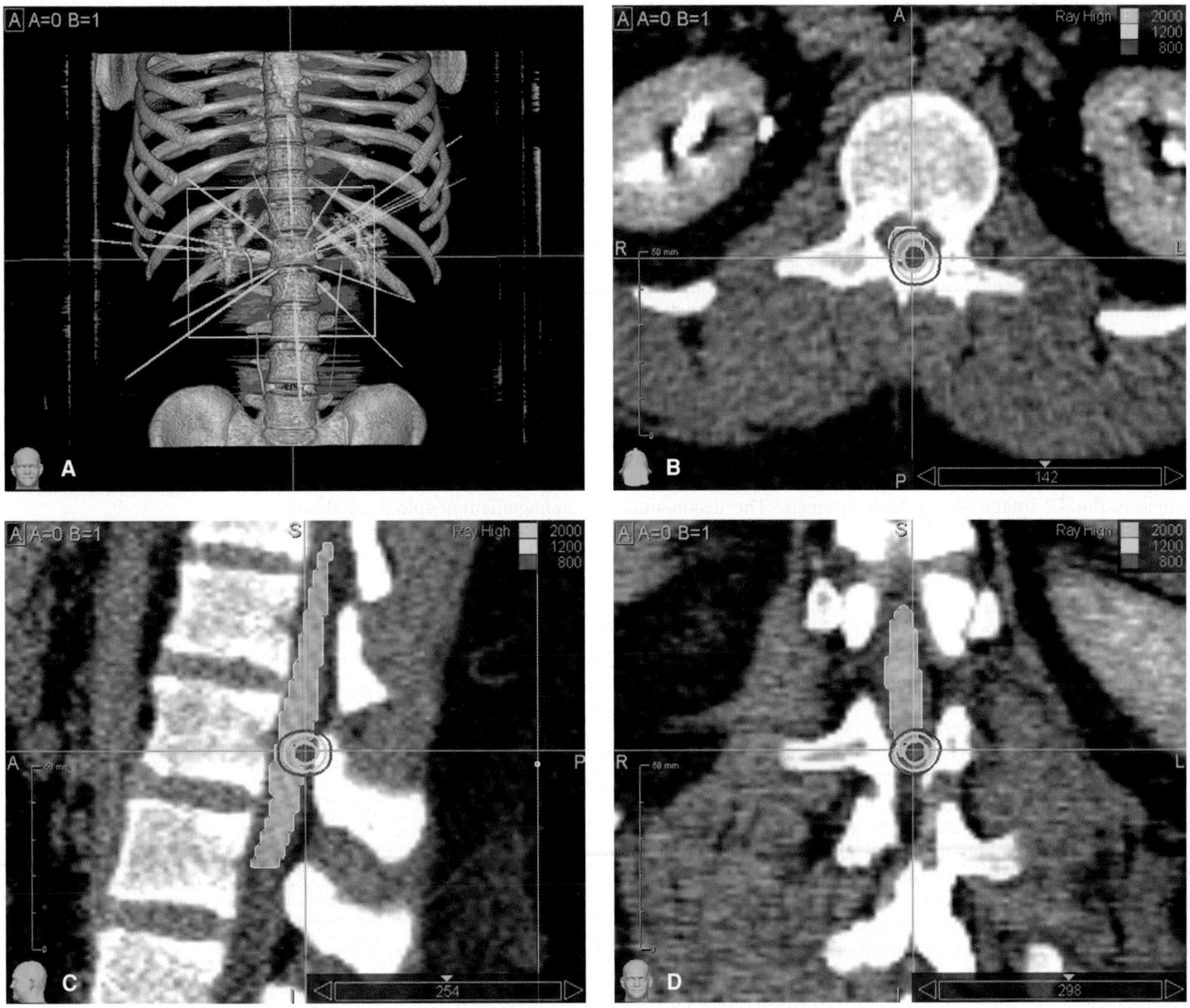

FIGURE 37.6. Stereotactic radiosurgery for an L1 hemangioblastoma. A single dose of 20 Gy was delivered with CyberKnife using 87 noncoplanar beams as shown in *blue*. As is typical of treatment delivery with this unit, the plan is nonisocentric. Gross tumor volume is shown in *solid red*, spinal cord in *solid yellow. Green line,* prescription dose of 20 Gy; *Light blue line,* 12 Gy; *Dark blue line,* 8 Gy. **A:** Three-dimensional representation of select noncoplanar beam paths. **B:** Axial isodose display reveals a sharp dose gradient between the prescription dose and the 12 and 8 Gy isodose lines. **C:** Sagittal isodose display. **D:** Coronal isodose display. (Courtesy Scott Soltys, MD, and Megan Daly, MD, Stanford University Department of Radiation Oncology.)

At a mean follow-up of 12 months, one ependymoma and two hemangioblastomas were smaller on follow-up imaging, with the remainder stable. No significant treatment-related complications were reported. In a follow-up study, Daly et al.[115] reported a 3-year actuarial control rate for 27 spinal hemangioblastomas treated with spine SRS to 18 to 25 Gy in 2 to 3 sessions. One patient developed a grade 2 foot drop 4 months after SRS, and two patients developed grade 1 sensory deficits.

Early results of spine SRS for intradural–extramedullary or intramedullary lesions are promising, and with the rapidly increasing availability of extracranial radiosurgery devices, SRS for these patients will no doubt increase in utilization. However, with such few reports and limited follow-up to date, caution certainly seems warranted given the potential for late toxicity in these patients with high rates of long-term survival. Issues related to spinal cord tolerance after spine SRS are discussed below.

SPINAL CORD TOLERANCE

A reversible myelopathy can occur within 2 to 6 months after radiation therapy. L'Hermitte's sign, characterized by shocklike sensations radiating to the hands and feet when the neck is flexed, is the classic finding. It is believed that this phenomenon is related to transient demyelination of the treated length of the spinal cord.[116,117] This syndrome usually lasts a few weeks, and no therapy is required. It is not associated with chronic progressive myelitis.

Chronic, progressive, or delayed myelopathy can occur months to years after radiation therapy. The latency period of chronic myelopathy has been reported to be bimodal with peaks of incidence occurring at 13 and 29 months.[118] The early peak may correspond to white matter injury with subsequent demyelination, and the latter peak may correspond to microvascular injury.[118] Permanent myelopathy is characterized by progressive motor weakness, paresthesias, and loss of pain or temperature sensation. Patients ultimately lose bowel and bladder control and experience complete sensory and motor function loss. Diagnosis of radiation myelopathy requires that the dominant neurologic abnormality be localized to a segment irradiated and other causes have been ruled out. MRI may assist in the diagnosis, with cord edema frequently being present in the early delayed phase. Within 8 months of the onset of symptoms, the T1-weighted image may show low intensity, whereas the T2 image shows high intensity. The lesion may enhance with Gd-DTPA. Late changes in patients with permanent delayed myelopathy may include atrophy.[119] Even with modern imaging, it may be difficult to determine whether neurologic deficits after radiotherapy are related to tumor progression or treatment-induced myelopathy.

The occurrence of chronic progressive myelopathy depends on total dose, fraction size, volume, and region irradiated.[120,121] Historically, the spinal cord has been limited to maximum doses of 45 to 50 Gy with fractionation schedules of 1.8 to 2 Gy per day. These estimates came from an era of inexact dose estimation with a bias toward reporting injury in highly selected populations. More recently, data have been published from institutions that have treated large groups of patients in systematic and reliable fashion. The Quantitative Analysis of Normal Tissue Effects in the Clinic (QUANTEC) initiative comprehensively reviewed modern radiotherapy toxicity data and published new guidelines on spinal cord tolerance.[122] For conventional external-beam radiation therapy at 1.8 to 2 Gy per day, a dose of 50 Gy, 60 Gy, and 69 Gy is associated with a 0.2%, 6%, and 50% rates of myelopathy, respectively. However, pediatric patients and patients receiving potentially neurotoxic chemotherapy may have decreased spinal cord tolerance, with reports of myelopathy at doses 50 Gy or less.[123–125]

Dose–volume data for myelopathy after spine SRS is evolving. In a multi-institutional review of 1,075 patients treated with spine SRS principally for metastatic disease, the rate of spinal cord toxicity was 0.6%.[126] Data from the QUANTEC initiative indicate that the rate of myelopathy will be less than 1% with the maximum dose to the spinal cord limited to the equivalent of 13 Gy in a single fraction or 20 Gy in 3 fractions.[122] The most commonly employed dose constraint for SRS is to keep less than 10% of the spinal cord (defined as 3 to 6 mm above and below the target volume) to less than 10 Gy.[114] Intriguing data from investigators at Stanford University utilizing SRS for spinal hemangioblastoma suggest that spinal cord tolerance may be higher than predicted by conventional modeling.[115,127] Maximum cord dose delivered in 2 to 3 sessions in their series was an average of 22.7 Gy (range, 17.8 to 30.9 Gy) to small volumes, with only 1 of 24 treatments resulting in myelopathy. Such a phenomenon may at least in part be explained by preclinical experiments suggesting a dramatic length and partial volume effect to spinal cord tolerance after radiation. For example, in one animal study, the ED_{50} (dose at which 50% of animals developed limb paralysis) for single fraction full thickness radiation to the spinal cord was 20.4 Gy for a 20 mm cord length, compared with 53.7 Gy for 4 mm and 87.8 Gy for 2 mm cord lengths.[128]

Both animal and human studies have demonstrated that irradiated spinal cord may recover at least partially over time. Animal experiments of reirradiation using Rhesus monkeys estimated cord recovery of 76%, 85%, and 100% at 1, 2, and 3 years, respectively.[129,130] In human studies, where reirradiation is at least 6 months after the initial radiation course, essentially no cases of myelopathy were observed when the cumulative 2-Gy equivalent doses are 60 Gy or less.[122,131]

CONCLUSIONS

Spinal canal tumors are relatively rare and consist of diverse histological entities. Surgery remains the primary treatment modality, aided by gradual advances in neurosurgical techniques. Adjuvant radiotherapy is generally considered for incomplete resection, recurrent tumors, or high-grade tumors. New radiotherapy techniques such as intensity modulated radiotherapy or stereotactic radiosurgery have shown promising potential to improve the therapeutic ratio. The role of chemotherapy is not clearly defined and is often extrapolated from intracranial counterparts. Continued long-term follow-up of clinical outcomes and innovation of novel approaches are essential for improving the management of spinal canal tumors.

SELECTED REFERENCES

A full list of references for this chapter is available online.

1. Central Brain Tumor Registry of the United States. *CBTRUS statistical report: primary brain and central nervous system tumors diagnosed in the United States in 2004–2007. 2011.* Available at: http://www.cbtrus.org/2011-NPCR-SEER/WEB-0407-Report-3-3-2011.pdf.
2. Schellinger KA, et al. Descriptive epidemiology of primary spinal cord tumors. *J Neurooncol* 2008;87(2):173–179.
3. Hsu S, et al. Incidence patterns for primary malignant spinal cord gliomas: a Surveillance, Epidemiology, and End Results study. *J Neurosurg Spine* 2011;14(6): 742–747.
4. DeSousa AL, et al. Intraspinal tumors in children. A review of 81 cases. *J Neurosurg* 1979;51(4):437–445.
5. Constantini S, Epstein F. Intraspinal tumors in infants and children. In: Youman J, ed. *Neurological surgery.* Philadelphia: WB Saunders, 1996.
8. Garcia DM. Primary spinal cord tumors treated with surgery and postoperative irradiation. *Int J Radiat Oncol Biol Phys* 1985;11(11):1933–1939.
9. Hely M, Fryer J, Selby G. Intramedullary spinal cord glioma with intracranial seeding. *J Neurol Neurosurg Psychiatry* 1985;48(4):302–309.
10. Linstadt DE, et al. Postoperative radiotherapy of primary spinal cord tumors. *Int J Radiat Oncol Biol Phys* 1989;16(6):1397–1403.
12. Smoll NR, Villanueva EV. The epidemiology of extraneural metastases from primary brain, spinal cord, and meningeal tumors. *Neurosurgery* 2010;67(5): E1470–E1471.
13. Raco A, et al. Long-term follow-up of intramedullary spinal cord tumors: a series of 202 cases. *Neurosurgery* 2005;56(5):972–981.
20. Greenwood J. Spinal cord tumors. In: Youman J, ed. *Neurological surgery.* Philadelphia: W.B. Saunders, 1982.
21. Uhl M, et al. CT-myelography for high-dose irradiation of spinal and paraspinal tumors with helical tomotherapy: revival of an old tool. *Strahlenther Onkol* 2011;187(7):416–420.

23. Sze G. Neoplastic disease of the spine and spinal cord. In: Atlas SW, ed. *Magnetic resonance imaging of the brain and spine*. Philadelphia: Lippincott-Raven, 1996.
24. Cohen AR, et al. Malignant astrocytomas of the spinal cord. *J Neurosurg* 1989; 70(1):50–54.
25. Bell WO, et al. Leptomeningeal spread of intramedullary spinal cord tumors. Report of three cases. *J Neurosurg* 1988;69(2):295–300.
26. Louis DN, et al. The 2007 WHO classification of tumours of the central nervous system. *Acta Neuropathol* 2007;114(2):97–9109.
28. McCormick PC, Stein BM. Intramedullary tumors in adults. *Neurosurg Clin North Am* 1990;1(3):609–630.
30. Abdel-Wahab M, et al. Spinal cord gliomas: a multi-institutional retrospective analysis. *Int J Radiat Oncol Biol Phys* 2006;64(4):1060–1071.
33. Bouffet E, et al. Prognostic factors in pediatric spinal cord astrocytoma. *Cancer* 1998;83(11):2391–2399.
34. Samii M, Klekamp J. Surgical results of 100 intramedullary tumors in relation to accompanying syringomyelia. *Neurosurgery* 1994;35(5):865–873; discussion 873.
39. Shaw EG, et al. Radiotherapeutic management of adult intraspinal ependymomas. *Int J Radiat Oncol Biol Phys* 1986;12(3):323–327.
40. Sonneland PR, Scheithauer BW, Onofrio BM. Myxopapillary ependymoma. A clinicopathologic and immunocytochemical study of 77 cases. *Cancer* 1985;56(4): 883–893.
41. Chan HS, et al. Myxopapillary ependymoma of the filum terminale and cauda equina in childhood: report of seven cases and review of the literature. *Neurosurgery* 1984;14(2):204–210.
42. Mork SJ, Loken AC. Ependymoma: a follow-up study of 101 cases. *Cancer* 1977;40(2): 907–915.
43. Ross DA, et al. Myxopapillary ependymoma. Results of nucleolar organizing region staining. *Cancer* 1993;71(10):3114–3118.
44. Schweitzer JS, Batzdorf U. Ependymoma of the cauda equina region: diagnosis, treatment, and outcome in 15 patients. *Neurosurgery* 1992;30(2):202–207.
46. Ryu SI, Kim DH, Chang SD. Stereotactic radiosurgery for hemangiomas and ependymomas of the spinal cord. *Neurosurg Focus* 2003;15(5):E10.
50. Evans DGR, et al. Malignant transformation and new primary tumours after therapeutic radiation for benign disease: substantial risks in certain tumour prone syndromes. *J Med Genet* 2006;43(4):289–294.
51. Grobmyer SR, et al. Malignant peripheral nerve sheath tumor: molecular pathogenesis and current management considerations. *J Surg Oncol* 2008;97(4): 340–349.
52. Wanebo JE, et al. Malignant peripheral nerve sheath tumors. A clinicopathologic study of 28 cases. *Cancer* 1993;71(4):1247–1253.
53. Wong WW, et al. Malignant peripheral nerve sheath tumor: analysis of treatment outcome. *Int J Radiat Oncol Biol Phys* 1998;42(2):351–360.
54. Milano MT, et al. Primary spinal cord glioma: a Surveillance, Epidemiology, and end results database study. *J Neurooncol* 2010;98(1):83–92.
55. Chun HC, et al. External beam radiotherapy for primary spinal cord tumors. *J Neurooncol* 1990;9(3):211–217.
56. Guidetti B, Mercuri S, Vagnozzi R. Long-term results of the surgical treatment of 129 intramedullary spinal gliomas. *J Neurosurg* 1981;54(3):323–330.
57. Ferrante L, et al. Intramedullary spinal cord ependymomas—a study of 45 cases with long-term follow-up. *Acta Neurochir (Wien)* 1992;119(1-4):74–79.
58. Goh KY, Velasquez L, Epstein FJ. Pediatric intramedullary spinal cord tumors: is surgery alone enough? *Pediatr Neurosurg* 1997;27(1):34–39.
59. Fassett DR, Pingree J, Kestle JRW. The high incidence of tumor dissemination in myxopapillary ependymoma in pediatric patients. Report of five cases and review of the literature. *J Neurosurg* 2005;102(1 Suppl):59–64.
60. Merchant TE, et al. Pediatric low-grade and ependymal spinal cord tumors. *Pediatr Neurosurg* 2000;32(1):30–36.
61. Malis LI. Intramedullary spinal cord tumors. *Clin Neurosurg* 1978;25:512–539.
62. Wen BC, et al. The role of radiation therapy in the management of ependymomas of the spinal cord. *Int J Radiat Oncol Biol Phys* 1991;20(4):781–786.
66. Kopelson G, et al. Management of intramedullary spinal cord tumors. *Radiology* 1980;135(2):473–479.
67. Sciubba DM, et al. The evolution of intramedullary spinal cord tumor surgery. *Neurosurgery* 2009;65(6 Suppl):84–91; discussion 91–92.
68. Matsuyama Y, et al. Surgical results of intramedullary spinal cord tumor with spinal cord monitoring to guide extent of resection. *J Neurosurg Spine* 2009;10(5): 404–413.
69. McGirt MJ, et al. Resection of intramedullary spinal cord tumors in children: assessment of long-term motor and sensory deficits. *J Neurosurg Pediatr* 2008; 1(1):63–67.
70. Garces-Ambrossi GL, et al. Factors associated with progression-free survival and long-term neurological outcome after resection of intramedullary spinal cord tumors: analysis of 101 consecutive cases. *J Neurosurg Spine* 2009;11(5): 591–599.
74. Sala F, et al. Surgery for intramedullary spinal cord tumors: the role of intraoperative (neurophysiological) monitoring. *Eur Spine J* 2007;16(Suppl 2):130–139.
75. Sala F, et al. Motor evoked potential monitoring improves outcome after surgery for intramedullary spinal cord tumors: a historical control study. *Neurosurgery* 2006;58(6):1129–1143.
81. Mirimanoff RO, et al. Meningioma: analysis of recurrence and progression following neurosurgical resection. *J Neurosurg* 1985;62(1):18–24.
82. Miller DC. Surgical pathology of intramedullary spinal cord neoplasms. *J Neurooncol* 2000;47(3):189–194.
83. Shirato H, et al. The role of radiotherapy in the management of spinal cord glioma. *Int J Radiat Oncol Biol Phys* 1995;33(2):323–328.
84. Abbott R, et al. Osteoplastic laminotomy in children. *Pediatr Neurosurg* 1992; 18(3):153–156.
85. Inoue A, Ikata T, Katoh S. Spinal deformity following surgery for spinal cord tumors and tumorous lesions: analysis based on an assessment of the spinal functional curve. *Spinal Cord* 1996;34(9):536–542.
86. Chamberlain MC, Tredway TL. Adult primary intradural spinal cord tumors: a review. *Curr Neurol Neurosci Rep* 2011;11(3):320–328.
87. Brandes AA, et al. A multicenter retrospective study of chemotherapy for recurrent intracranial ependymal tumors in adults by the Gruppo Italiano Cooperativo di Neuro-Oncologia. *Cancer* 2005;104(1):143–148.
88. Gornet MK, et al. Chemotherapy for advanced CNS ependymoma. *J Neurooncol* 1999;45(1):61–67.
89. Chamberlain MC. Etoposide for recurrent spinal cord ependymoma. *Neurology* 2002;58(8):1310–1311.
90. Stupp R, et al. Effects of radiotherapy with concomitant and adjuvant temozolomide versus radiotherapy alone on survival in glioblastoma in a randomised phase III study: 5-year analysis of the EORTC-NCIC trial. *Lancet Oncol* 2009; 10(5):459–466.
91. Kim WH, et al. Temozolomide for malignant primary spinal cord glioma: an experience of six cases and a literature review. *J Neurooncol* 2011;101(2): 247–254.
92. Chamberlain MC. Temozolomide for recurrent low-grade spinal cord gliomas in adults. *Cancer* 2008;113(5):1019–1024.
93. Doireau V, et al. Chemotherapy for unresectable and recurrent intramedullary glial tumours in children. Brain Tumours Subcommittee of the French Society of Paediatric Oncology (SFOP). *Br J Cancer* 1999;81(5):835–840.
94. Allen JC, et al. Treatment of high-grade spinal cord astrocytoma of childhood with "8-in-1" chemotherapy and radiotherapy: a pilot study of CCG-945. Children's Cancer Group. *J Neurosurg* 1998;88(2):215–220.
95. Mora J, et al. Successful treatment of childhood intramedullary spinal cord astrocytomas with irinotecan and cisplatin. *Neuro Oncol* 2007;9(1):39–46.
96. Isaacson SR. Radiation therapy and the management of intramedullary spinal cord tumors. *J Neurooncol* 2000;47(3):231–238.
102. Constantini S, et al. Radical excision of intramedullary spinal cord tumors: surgical morbidity and long-term follow-up evaluation in 164 children and young adults. *J Neurosurg* 2000;93(2 Suppl):183–193.
103. Kim MS, et al. Intramedullary spinal cord astrocytoma in adults: postoperative outcome. *J Neurooncol* 2001;52(1):85–94.
104. Gomez DR, et al. High failure rate in spinal ependymomas with long-term follow-up. *Neuro Oncol* 2005;7(3):254–259.
105. Chao ST, et al. The role of adjuvant radiation therapy in the treatment of spinal myxopapillary ependymomas. *J Neurosurg Spine* 2011;14(1):59–64.
106. Gezen F, et al. Review of 36 cases of spinal cord meningioma. *Spine (Phila Pa 1976)* 2000;25(6):727–731.
107. Gerszten PC, et al. Radiosurgery for benign intradural spinal tumors. *Neurosurgery* 2008;62(4):887–895.
108. Merchant TE, et al. High-grade pediatric spinal cord tumors. *Pediatr Neurosurg* 1999;30(1):1–5.
110. Whitaker SJ, et al. Postoperative radiotherapy in the management of spinal cord ependymoma. *J Neurosurg* 1991;74(5):720–728.
111. Kopelson G, Linggood RM. Intramedullary spinal cord astrocytoma versus glioblastoma: the prognostic importance of histologic grade. *Cancer* 1982;50(4): 732–735.
112. Hall EJ, Wuu C-S. Radiation-induced second cancers: the impact of 3D-CRT and IMRT. *Int J Radiat Oncol Biol Phys* 2003;56(1):83–88.
113. Abdel-Wahab M, et al. Prognostic factors and survival in patients with spinal cord gliomas after radiation therapy. *Am J Clin Oncol* 1999;22(4):344–351.
114. Hsu W, et al. Stereotactic radiosurgery for spine tumors: review of current literature. *Stereotact Funct Neurosurg* 2010;88(5):315–321.
115. Daly ME, et al. Tolerance of the spinal cord to stereotactic radiosurgery: insights from hemangioblastomas. *Int J Radiat Oncol Biol Phys* 2011;80(1):213–220.
120. Phillips TL, Buschke F. Radiation tolerance of the thoracic spinal cord. *Am J Roentgenol Radium Ther Nucl Med* 1969;105(3):659–664.
121. Wara WM, et al. Radiation tolerance of the spinal cord. *Cancer* 1975;35(6):1558–1562.
122. Kirkpatrick JP, van der Kogel AJ, Schultheiss TE. Radiation dose-volume effects in the spinal cord. *Int J Radiat Oncol Biol Phys* 2010;76(3 Suppl):S42–S49.
123. Townsend N, et al. Intramedullary spinal cord astrocytomas in children. *Pediatr Blood Cancer* 2004;43(6):629–632.
124. Chao MW, et al. Radiation myelopathy following transplantation and radiotherapy for non-Hodgkin's lymphoma. *Int J Radiat Oncol Biol Phys* 1998;41(5):1057–1061.
125. Seddon BM, et al. Fatal radiation myelopathy after high-dose busulfan and melphalan chemotherapy and radiotherapy for Ewing's sarcoma: a review of the literature and implications for practice. *Clin Oncol (R Coll Radiol)* 2005;17(5): 385–390.
127. Daly ME, et al. Normal tissue complication probability estimation by the Lyman-Kutcher-Burman method does not accurately predict spinal cord tolerance to stereotactic radiosurgery. *Int J Radiat Oncol Biol Phys* 2012;82(5): 2025–2032.
128. Bijl HP, et al. Regional differences in radiosensitivity across the rat cervical spinal cord. *Int J Radiat Oncol Biol Phys* 2005;61(2):543–551.
129. Ang KK, et al. Extent and kinetics of recovery of occult spinal cord injury. *Int J Radiat Oncol Biol Phys* 2001;50(4):1013–1020.
130. Ang KK, et al. The tolerance of primate spinal cord to re-irradiation. *Int J Radiat Oncol Biol Phys* 1993;25(3):459–464.
131. Milano MT, et al. Stereotactic radiosurgery and hypofractionated stereotactic radiotherapy: normal tissue dose constraints of the central nervous system. *Cancer Treat Rev* 2011;37(7):567–578.

Part D Head and Neck

Chapter 38
Eye and Orbit

Nicholas J. Sanfilippo and Silvia C. Formenti

Tumors of the eye and orbit are rare. The American Cancer Society estimates that in 2011 there will be 2,570 new cases with 240 deaths.[1] Male to female incidence is similar, with 1,270 cases occurring in men and 1,300 in women. In adults, melanoma is the most common primary intraocular cancer, followed by lymphoma, while in children retinoblastoma is the most common tumor, followed by medulloepithelioma. Metastases, or secondary intraocular tumors, are more common than primary tumors and typically come from breast or lung cancers.[2] Numerous other tumors such as rhabdomyosarcoma, optic nerve glioma, conjunctival tumors, and eyelid carcinomas also occur in the orbit. Radiation therapy has been effective in the treatment of many of these tumors and can be delivered externally or by brachytherapy, depending on the clinical situation, and can be used exclusively or in concert with other treatments such as surgery or chemotherapy. Technological advances such as intensity modulated radiation therapy (IMRT), proton beam therapy, and stereotactic radiotherapy have a key role in management of these tumors given the anatomy proximity of structures in this location. This chapter will outline the most relevant malignant and benign conditions of the eye and orbit with emphasis on radiotherapeutic management.

ANATOMY

The eye is not an exact sphere, but rather a fused two-piece unit. The smaller, more curved frontal unit is the cornea and is linked to the larger unit called the sclera. The corneal segment is typically about 8 mm in radius. The sclera constitutes the remainder of the eyeball, with a radius of approximately 12 mm. The cornea and sclera are connected by the limbus. The iris and the pupil are seen instead of the cornea due to the cornea's transparency. The area opposite the pupil, the fundus, shows the characteristic pale optic disc or papilla, where vessels enter the eye and optic nerve fibers depart the globe. Dimensions of the globe differ among adults by only 1 or 2 mm. The vertical measure, generally less than the horizontal distance, is about 24 mm in adults. The eye is made up of three coats or tunics, enclosing three transparent structures (Fig. 38.1). The outermost layer is composed of the cornea and sclera. The middle layer consists of the choroid, ciliary body, and iris. The innermost is the retina, where the blood supply is from the vessels of the choroid as well as the retinal vessels. The lens is suspended to the ciliary body by the suspensory ligament, made up of fine transparent fibers.

RADIATION TOLERANCE OF OCULAR STRUCTURES

Eyelid

Acute radiosensitivity of eyelid skin is comparable to skin at other sites, and loss of eyelashes may occur at doses as low as 20 Gy using standard fractionation.[3] Late effects can include telangiectasia and atrophy. Xerophthalmia can result from doses as low as 24 to 26 Gy and may be the result of dysfunction of the Meibomian glands, lacrimal acinar cells, or both.[4] Significant xerophthalmia can cause corneal desiccation and pain. It is generally believed that smaller fraction sizes, longer treatment schedules, and smaller volumes will reduce late effects, but this must be weighed against the potential for ocular trauma when using shielding on a daily basis.[5] Optimum management of eyelid toxicity includes cleanliness, dressings for moist desquamation, healing time, and artificial tears for Meibomian gland dysfunction.

Conjunctiva

Acute conjunctivitis is common with doses ≥30 Gy and secondary bacterial or rarely viral infections may occur.[6] Conjunctivitis can be reduced by treating with an open eye with megavoltage equipment if the clinical situation permits. Treatment of acute conjunctivitis involves artificial tears to relieve symptoms and treatment of an underlying infection when indicated.

Lacrimal System

The lacrimal gland system includes the main lacrimal glands, accessory lacrimal glands, and lacrimal duct system, and symptoms of dryness can occur if any of these structures receive radiation. The most concerning late effect is dry-eye syndrome, where patients can experience tearing, redness, discharge, foreign body sensation, blurred vision, and photophobia. Moderate-dose orbital radiation therapy (RT) (30–45 Gy) can cause dry-eye syndrome 4 to 11 years after treatment, while higher doses (>57 Gy) can produce it in 9 to 10 months.[7] Lacrimal shielding should be used if tumor control will not be compromised, and shielding the accessory lacrimal glands may reduce toxicity if the main gland is irradiated. IMRT can help minimize the risks of RT-induced xerophthalmia, and prophylactic nasolacrimal duct intubation with silicon tubing may be considered in high-risk patients.[8,9] Treatments available for RT-induced xerophthalmia include topical lubricants, moist chamber goggles, punctual occlusion with plugs, or tarsorrhaphy.

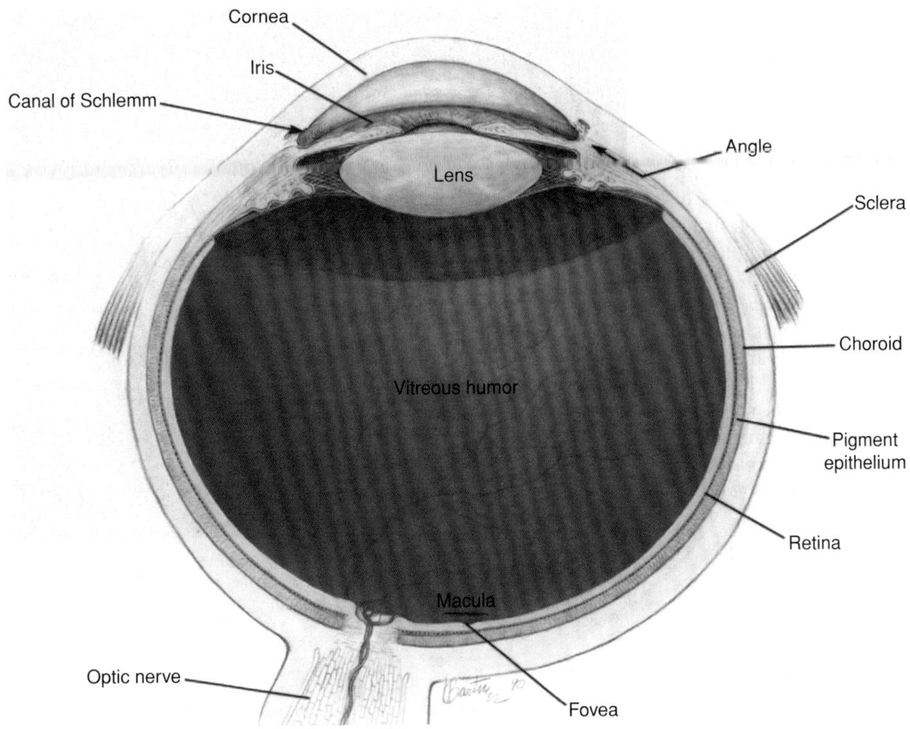

FIGURE 38.1. Normal eye anatomy. (Courtesy of National Eye Institute, National Institutes of Health.)

Cornea

Although RT can directly injure the cornea, most acute corneal toxicity results from loss of the tear film with secondary keratitis sicca. Punctate epithelial erosions are common after conventionally fractionated RT doses of 30 to 50 Gy.[10] They typically subside within several weeks but can persist for years. At higher doses, corneal edema (40–50 Gy) or perforation (60 Gy) may occur, causing pain, tearing, foreign body sensation, or reduced vision. Corneal toxicity can be reduced by using megavoltage equipment and reducing the surface dose or by using careful RT planning to minimize corneal irradiation so long as the tumor dose is not compromised. Commercially available eye shields may also be used, particularly for electron beam RT.[11] There are few published data on management of corneal toxicity from RT. Close ophthalmologic follow-up is recommended so topical treatment with steroids or antibiotics can be administered when indicated.

Iris

The iris is relatively radioresistant and thus, acute iritis is rare. However, persistent iritis, with symptoms such as pain, red eye, and blurred vision, has been observed after hypofractionated RT doses of 30 to 40 Gy and after doses ≥70 Gy given with conventional fractionation.[12] A problematic late effect of the iris is neovascular glaucoma, where patients may present with ocular pain, headache, photophobia, decreased vision, and redness.[13] Risk factors include higher radiation dose, diabetes, vitreous hemorrhage, and retinal detachment. Where possible, techniques that spare the anterior chamber should be used. The primary treatments for iritis and neovascular glaucoma are topical steroids and cycloplegic drops, respectively. Laser panretinal photocoagulation or peripheral cryotherapy may prevent or slow the progression of glaucoma if performed early. However, in many cases more aggressive intervention such as trabeculectomy may be required. Occasionally progression to a blind, painful eye may necessitate enucleation. Novel therapies such as intravitreal bevacizumab as an adjunctive treatment to retinal ablative procedure appear to be promising for the management of iris neovascularization associated with neovascular glaucoma.[14]

Lens

Age at time of treatment, total dose, and fractionation contribute to cataract formation.[15,16] Hall et al.[15] estimated an increased risk of approximately 50% for 1-Gy exposure to the lens during childhood. In adults, higher doses are associated with cataract: after 2.5 to 6.5 Gy, the latent period is 8 years with a 33% of progressive cataract, while after 6.51 to 11.5 Gy, the latent period is 4 years, with a 66% risk.[16] Cataract risk can be reduced by using customized lens shields and lens-sparing techniques or by using fully fractionated RT schedules. IMRT may be used to reduce cataract risk by reducing overall lens dose and relative fraction size. The definitive treatment for RT-induced cataract is surgery, which yields excellent results.

Retina

Radiation retinopathy is a late effect of RT that typically presents 6 months to 3 years after treatment, although cases have been reported as long as 15 years after therapy.[17] Patients may be asymptomatic or may complain of floaters or reduced visual acuity, and clinical signs include microaneurysms, telangiectasia, hard exudates, cotton wool spots, and neovascularization. The threshold dose for retinal damage is usually considered to be 30 to 35 Gy. In a Cochrane database review of RT for macular degeneration, no retinopathy or optic nerve damage was reported in 1,154 patients treated with doses up to 24 Gy.[18] The risk of retinopathy increases dramatically when doses exceed 50 Gy using standard fractionation.[19] Incidence as well as severity are also increased by coexistent diabetic retinopathy, hypertension, collagen vascular disease, simultaneous chemotherapy, and pregnancy.[20] No proven therapy exists for radiation retinopathy, although local treatments such as photocoagulation may improve symptoms and there is interest in intravitreal bevacizumab.[21]

Optic Nerve

Like the retina, the optic nerve manifests toxicity months or years after RT, with a peak incidence at 18 months.[22] Radiation-induced optic neuropathy (RION) has a variable presentation and is related to the nerve fibers most affected, usually causing visual field defects. In a recent review by the Mayo Clinic, risk of RION was almost zero with conventionally fractionated doses ≤50 Gy and the occurrence of RION is still rare with a maximum dose <55 Gy. The risk of RION increases from 3% to 7% at 55 to 60 Gy and is substantial (>7% to 20%) at doses >60 Gy.[23] Parsons et al.,[24] in a series of 131 patients (215 optic nerves) treated with RT for extracranial head and neck tumors, found no RION in nerves that received <59 Gy. Fraction size was of primary importance; in cases where >60 Gy was received, fraction size was more important than total dose in producing RION. The 15-year actuarial risk was 11% when fraction size was <1.9 Gy compared with 47% when fraction size was >1.9 Gy. A significant exception in development of RION appears to exist for patients treated for pituitary tumors, where toxicity has been reported at doses as low as 46 Gy in 1.8-Gy fractions.[23] Because there is no known effective therapy for RION, efforts must be made to minimize optic nerve dose through sophisticated treatment planning and delivery with an effort to minimize treatment volume, total dose, and especially dose per fraction received.

MANAGEMENT OF BENIGN OCULAR DISEASES

Pterygium

Pterygium is a benign growth of fibrovascular tissue on the conjunctiva that can cause irritation, erythema of the cornea, and obstructed vision in advanced cases. The exact cause of pterygium is unknown, but it is associated with excessive exposure to wind, sunlight, or sand. It has also been postulated that ultraviolet light exposure may increase the risk of pterygium development.[25] At present, no reliable medical treatment exists to reduce or even prevent pterygium progression. If symptoms are severe, the only definitive treatment is surgical removal, which requires removal of the head, neck, and body of the pterygium. Without adjuvant treatment, surgical resection alone, commonly referred to as bare sclera excision, carries recurrence rates of 20% to 80%.[25–27] Therefore, adjunctive measures are recommended, which can be broadly classified as medical methods, beta-irradiation, and surgical methods. Intraoperative and postoperative mitomycin-C are the most commonly used medical adjuncts, and recurrence rates of 3% to 37% have been reported.[28] However, topical chemotherapy is not commonly used out of concern for late complications, including scleral sclerosis, infectious scleritis, perforation, or endophthalmitis, all of which can impair vision.[29] Beta-irradiation has a historical role in management of pterygium. In a prospective randomized study, 96 eyes with primary pterygium received beta-irradiation with a strontium-90 after resection or sham radiation[27] Local control was 93.2% for the irradiated group versus 33.3% for the sham radiation group. Like topical chemotherapy, however, beta-irradiation has generally been abandoned due to the risk of sight-threatening complications such as scleral necrosis, infectious scleritis, corneal perforation, and endophthalmitis.[30] Surgical adjuvant therapy is thus the mainstay of management for primary and recurrent pterygium. Conjunctival autografting is generally regarded as the procedure of choice because of its efficacy and long-term safety, with recurrence rates of 2% to 39% without the attendant sight-threatening complications of topical chemotherapy or beta-irradiation.[31] Other surgical techniques include amniotic membrane transplantation, limbal conjunctival transplantation, and cultivated conjunctival translation, but none appear to be more effective than conjunctival autografting.[32–34]

Choroidal Hemangiomas

Choroidal hemangiomas are benign vascular tumors of the choroid. Although probably congenital in all cases, they are frequently undetected until after the second decade of life and can have a wide range of clinical features and treatment options.[35]

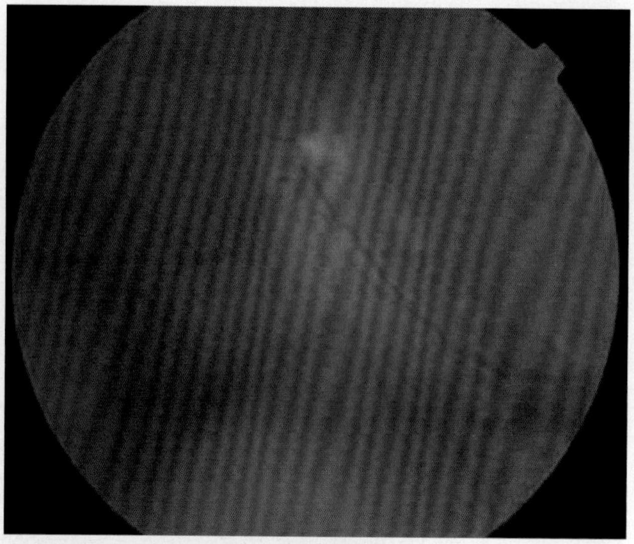

FIGURE 38.2. Diffuse choroidal hemangioma with exudative retinal detachment. (From Kubicka-Trząska A, Kobylarz J, Romanowska-Dixon B. Ruthenium-106 plaque therapy for diffuse choroidal hemangioma in Sturge-Weber syndrome. *Case Rep Ophthalmol Med* 2011, art. 785686.)

These tumors are characterized as either circumscribed or diffuse type. Most circumscribed choroidal hemangiomas are first noted when they produce visual symptoms caused by accumulation of serous subretinal fluid, degenerative changes in the macular retina, or both. In contrast to circumscribed choroidal hemangiomas, the diffuse variety is large and is associated with manifestations of the Sturge-Weber syndrome.[35] Diffuse tumors are usually diagnosed in young patients either due to examination of the fundus prompted by a facial hemangioma or due to visual impairment secondary to serous retinal detachment or hyperopic amblyopia (Fig. 38.2). The clinical course of either form of choroidal hemangioma is highly variable, with visual impairment ranging from none to total blindness. Neither variety of choroidal hemangioma metastasizes or transforms to malignancy. Therefore, the primary indication for treatment is loss of visual acuity.

Treatment alternatives include laser photocoagulation, thermotherapy, photodynamic therapy, and radiotherapy. Photocoagulation is beneficial for circumscribed lesions, but diffuse lesions have high recurrence rate and retinal damage is possible.[34] Low to moderate dose radiation using lens-sparing external beam photon irradiation, episcleral plaque therapy, proton beam therapy, and stereotactic radiotherapy have been used in the treatment of choroidal hemangioma.[35,36] Total doses of 18 to 30 Gy delivered in 10 to 18 fractions of external beam photon radiation therapy can result in partial flattening of the hemangioma, resorption of subretinal fluid, and reattachment of the retina within 6 to 12 months.[36,37] Heimann et al.[37] reported no recurrence of subretinal fluid with at a mean follow-up of 3.6 years. In another series, Kivela et al.[38] found subretinal fluid had reaccumulated in only 1 of 12 patients treated with follow-up of 66 months, thus illustrating response durability. In very advanced cases with retinal detachment, a higher dose of 36 Gy in fractions of 1.8 Gy has been described and appears to be efficacious, but clearly larger series with longer follow-up are needed to describe response durability and delayed side effects, including retinopathy and cataract formation.[37,38] Lens-sparing techniques, including three-dimensional conformal radiation therapy with computed tomography (CT) planning, should be considered to reduce the incidence of cataract formation[39,40] Brachytherapy has also been used for choroidal hemangioma treatment and particularly for circumscribed lesions, given the focused dose distribution of brachytherapy. This treatment usually achieves resolution of subretinal fluid and reattachment of the retina with preservation of pretreatment visual acuity.[41] Radiation dose varies with the isotope, but in one study using iodine-125, a target dose of 48 Gy to the apex was prescribed and tumor regression was noted in eight of eight cases.[41] More recently results of proton beam therapy have been reported from investigators at the Institut Curie. In a series of 71 cases with circumscribed choroidal hemangioma treated with 20 cobalt gray equivalent (CGE), retinal reattachment occurred in all cases and a completely flat scar was obtained in 91.5%.[42] The main complications during the surveillance period were cataract (28%) and radiation-induced maculopathy (8%). No cases of eyelid complications or neurovascular glaucoma were observed.

Capillary Hemangioma

Capillary hemangiomas are benign endothelial cell neoplasms that rarely occur on the eyelids or skin of the orbit. Retinal capillary hemangiomas may represent a component of the von Hippel-Lindau syndrome, and lesions of the face that occupy the distribution of the trigeminal nerve can be a component of Sturge-Weber syndrome. The natural history of these lesions is usually spontaneous regression over 3 to 4 years, therefore, conservative management is the treatment of choice.[43] Occasionally, however, lesions may be large enough to obstruct vision and amblyopia may occur. Treatment options then include corticosteroids, interferon alfa-2a, laser therapy, embolization, immunomodulators, surgery, and systemic propranolol.[44] Radiation therapy in the management of capillary hemangiomas is primarily of historical interest, with historical studies showing that doses in the 16 to 20 Gy range provide effective local control.[45]

Orbital Pseudotumor

Orbital pseudotumor is a rare inflammatory process that affects the soft tissue components of the orbit. Clinically, it presents in the fourth and fifth decades with signs and symptoms including proptosis, swelling, increased orbital pressure, and restricted ocular motion.[46] The diagnosis is based on history, imaging of the orbit, and pathologic examination of tissue in accessible lesions. Characteristic imaging features include extraocular muscle enlargement, optic nerve thickening, and inflammation of retrobulbar adipose tissue. Treatment options for orbital pseudotumor include corticosteroids, external beam radiation therapy (EBRT), immunotherapy, chemotherapy, and surgery; corticosteroids are typically used as primary treatment.[47] EBRT is usually reserved for cases that are refractory to corticosteroid treatment, with local control rates of 67% to 83%.[48,49] Matthiesen et al.[50] recently described 20 orbits treated with EBRT to a median dose of 20 Gy with follow-up of 16.5 months and found 87.5% had improved symptoms or reduction of corticosteroid dose and 56% were able to discontinue steroid treatment completely. Based on these observations, EBRT appears to achieve durable control in orbital pseudotumor and is an effective strategy in patients who respond poorly to medical treatment.

Thyroid-Associated Orbitopathy

Thyroid-associated orbitopathy (TAO), frequently termed Graves' ophthalmopathy, is part of an autoimmune process that can affect the orbital and periorbital tissue, the thyroid gland, and, rarely, the pretibial skin or digits (thyroid acropathy).[51–52,53] Although the use of the term thyroid ophthalmopathy is pervasive, the disease process is actually an orbitopathy in which the orbital and periocular soft tissues are primarily affected with secondary effects on the eye. TAO may compromise a patient's vision by causing diplopia, decreased ocular motion, exposure keratitis, or optic neuropathy. A variety of treatments exist including thyroid hormone regulation, corticosteroids, external beam radiotherapy, or surgical decompression.[54] Radiation therapy historically has been used in cases refractory to medical therapy. Doses of 20 Gy using standard fractionation have been effective in ameliorating symptoms and providing durable control, with one series reporting 87% of patients having improvement in symptoms.[55] However, prospective studies examining the use to radiation therapy for TAO suggest that its role is unclear. Nine randomized controlled trials have tested orbital RT in 465 patients with TAO, although studies differed with respect to severity of TAO on trial entry, radiation dose and fractionation, and inconsistency in the use of concurrent corticosteroids.[56–64] Three of these studies, which compared orbital RT with sham control, reported only minor improvement in outcome. Mourits et al.[60] randomized 59 patients to either 20 Gy in 10 fractions to both orbits or sham RT and found improved globe motility and elevation, but no difference in change in lid fissure, soft tissue swelling, proptosis, or clinical activity score (a measure of disease activity and propensity to progress). The authors concluded that RT should be used only for motility impairment. Gorman et al.[64] randomized 42 subjects to orbit RT to one orbit and sham RT to the other followed by the reverse therapy 6 months later. No clinically or statistically significant differences were observed at 6 months. At 12 months, muscle volume and proptosis were slightly more improved in the orbit that was first treated. Prummel et al.[63] conducted a trial where 88 patients with mild TAO were randomly assigned to bilateral RT or sham RT. Irradiation was effective in improving motility and decreasing severe diplopia, but no differences in health-related quality of life were detected, although lack of complete quality-of-life data on 58% of subjects resulted in low power to detect a difference. Complications of orbital RT are rare but not insignificant. Even in the absence of known diabetes mellitus, the risk of definite retinopathy is 1% to 2% in the first 10 years after treatment.[65,66] Based on these randomized data, the role of RT for TAO is thus controversial. In a 2008 report on orbital RT for TAO by the American Academy of Ophthalmology, the investigators concluded that while extraocular motility may improve with RT, the evidence of treatment effect is mixed in clinical trials, and future studies are needed to determine if improved motility translates into improved quality of life.[67] Radiation technique for TAO usually involves treatment of both orbits with parallel opposed lateral portals with low energy (6 MV) photons. A downward 5-degree tilt or use of half-beam block should be used to avoid direct radiation of the contralateral lens.

OCULAR AND ORBITAL MALIGNANT TUMORS

Metastatic Carcinoma to the Uvea

Tumor metastases to the eye are more common than primary ocular cancers, with the uvea representing the most common site affected.[68] Shields et al.[2] described a comprehensive series of usual metastases and found that within the uvea, 88% of metastases are to the choroid (Fig. 38.3), followed by metastases to the iris (9%) and ciliary body (2%). This large difference is thought to be due to the distribution of blood supply, which heavily favors the choroid as compared to the iris or ciliary body. The most common primary cancer sites for uveal metastasis in males were lung (40%), gastrointestinal (9%), and kidney (8%). The primary site was unknown at the time of presentation in 29% of males. In females, the most common sites included breast (68%), lung (12%), and other (4%). Metastases can be either unilateral or bilateral. In a study of 264 patients with uveal metastases from breast cancer reported by Demirci et al.,[69] 62% of patients had unilateral metastasis at presentation. Patients with breast cancer metastatic to the uvea show survival rates of 65% at 1 year, 35% at 3 years, and 24% at 5 years.

Numerous treatment options exist for choroidal metastases, including systemic chemotherapy, hormonal therapy, EBRT,

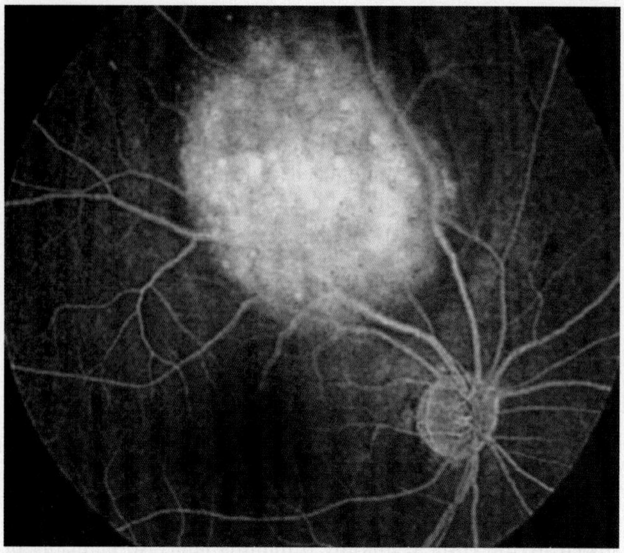

FIGURE 38.3. Fundus fluorescein angiography of choroidal metastasis from non–small cell lung cancer showing hyperfluorescence from the surface of the choroidal tumor in its late phase with the accumulation of subretinal fluid. (From Singh A, Singh P, Sahni K, et al. Non-small cell lung cancer presenting with choroidal metastasis as first sign and showing good response to chemotherapy alone: a case report. *J Med Case Rep* 2010;4:185.)

brachytherapy, or photodynamic therapy. Individualized treatment should be considered, taking into account disease extent and life-expectancy with the primary goal of maintaining visual acuity. As systemic treatments for metastatic cancers improve, clinicians may be faced with treatment of symptomatic choroidal metastases. For cases with multifocal or diffuse presentations, EBRT has been effective with doses in the range of 20 to 40 Gy. Rosset et al.[70] described 58 patients (88 eyes) treated with external radiation with a median dose of 35.5 Gy (range 20–53 Gy) in 10 to 30 fractions. Various techniques were used and lens sparing was used when possible. Visual acuity improved in 62% of patients, with significantly better results when doses >35.5 Gy were used. Five complications were noted, including three cataracts, retinopathy in a single patient who underwent biopsy, and one case of glaucoma from subretinal hemorrhage. In cases of unilateral disease, the authors noted no cases of new contralateral lesions when bilateral radiation was performed, but did describe new contralateral lesions in 3 of 26 patients when unilateral technique was used. They have thus recommended bilateral irradiation even in cases of unilateral disease (Fig. 38.4).

Plaque brachytherapy is usually reserved for solitary metastases. This modality offers precise, controlled radiation delivery to the eye and requires only 3 to 4 days of treatment, which is an important consideration in uveal metastases because many patients have limited survival expectancy. Key clinical factors to consider for plaque therapy include the size and thickness of the lesion, the distance of the lesion from the optic nerve, and the distance of the lesion from the foveola. Investigators from the Wills Eye Hospital studied 36 patients who received plaque radiotherapy either as primary or salvage treatment (after external radiation) for uveal metastases.[71] The mean duration of treatment was 86 hours and mean dose to the apex and base of the tumor was 68.8 Gy and 235.6 Gy, respectively. Tumor regression was documented in 94% of cases with mean follow-up of 11 months. In six cases where plaque therapy was used after suboptimal response to external irradiation, five eyes were successfully salvaged. Complications from plaque radiotherapy are similar to those of EBRT, including dryness, radiation retinopathy, papillopathy, and cataract, but these side effects are uncommon, especially given the short life-expectancy of many patients. The investigators concluded that plaque radiation is an effective, time-efficient method for treatment of selected solitary uveal metastases. Thus, both EBRT and plaque therapy are effective therapies for uveal metastases, with the optimal treatment depending on the extent of intraocular disease, symptoms, and overall condition and prognosis of the patient. Close collaboration of ophthalmologists, radiation oncologists, and medical oncologists is imperative to develop an appropriate treatment strategy.

Malignant Melanoma of the Uvea

Uveal melanomas represent <5% of all malignant melanomas with approximately 1,400 new cases per year in the United States.[72] These tumors may arise from any of the three parts of the uvea and are sometimes referred to by their location, such as iris melanoma (Fig. 38.5A), ciliary body melanoma, or choroidal melanoma (Fig. 38.5B). True iris melanomas, originating from within the iris as opposed to originating elsewhere and invading the iris, are distinct in their etiology and prognosis, such that the other tumors are often referred to collectively as posterior uveal melanomas. Although uveal melanoma is rare among nonwhites, the role of sunlight and other environmental factors is unknown.[73] Detection of uveal melanoma is often by routine examination with or without symptoms; a study from

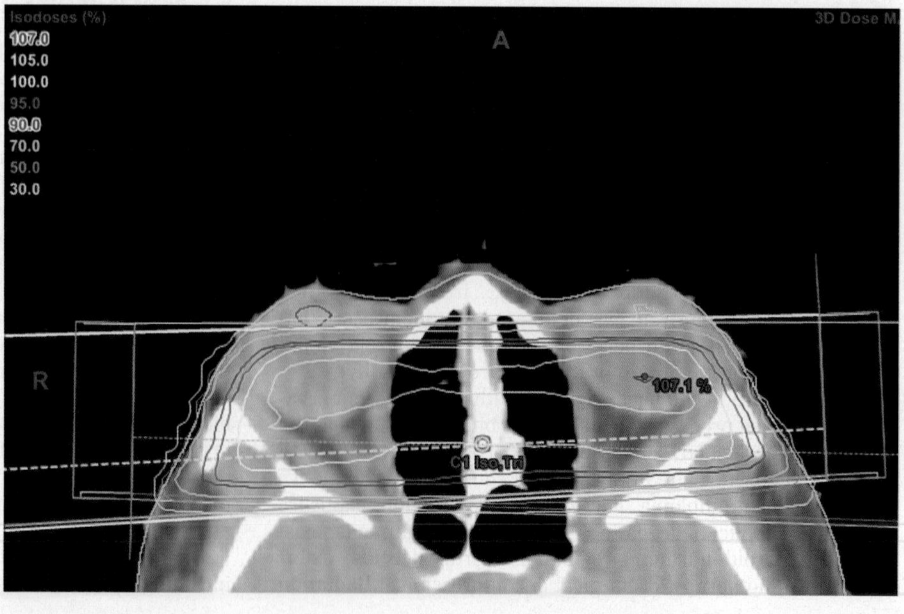

FIGURE 38.4. Bilateral radiation therapy for uveal metastases in a patient with widely metastatic lung cancer.

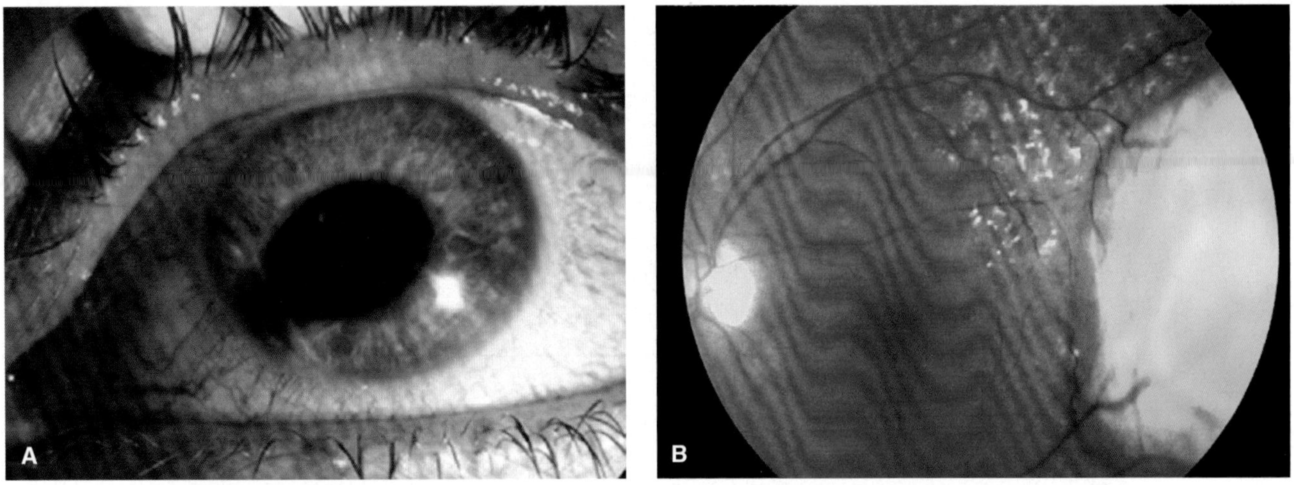

FIGURE 38.5. A: Iris melanoma located at the inferonasal aspect of the eye. B: Typical choroidal melanoma with associated nonrhegmatogenous retinal detachment. (From Papastefanou VP, Cohen VML. Uveal melanoma. *J Skin Cancer* 2011, art. 573974.)

the United Kingdom showed that 45% of patients were asymptomatic when their tumor was detected.[74] Advances in diagnostic techniques such as binocular indirect ophthalmoscopy, angiography, and B-scan ultrasonography have aided ocular oncologists in the evaluation and management of patients with uveal melanoma.[75,76] Staging of iris differs from ciliary body and choroidal lesion, with thickness being of primary importance in choroidal and ciliary body tumors (Table 38.1).

Several treatment options exist for uveal melanoma. Most patients are treated with the goal of eradication of disease and long-term survival. There is evidence that local tumor recurrence is associated with increased mortality.[77] Factors predictive of local recurrence include epithelioid cell type, large tumor size, and posterior tumor extension.[78] When possible, curative treatment should be sought with the goal of preserving vision with acceptable cosmesis. In patients with known metastatic disease, the main objective is to preserve vision and remove any threat of the eye becoming painful within the patient's life-expectancy. Many factors influence treatment selection, including tumor size, location, and extent; secondary effects, such as cataract; concurrent ocular disease, such as diabetic retinopathy; the patient's general health and life-expectancy; and the cost and duration of the treatment.[79] In cases where maintaining useful vision is feasible, organ-preservation therapy should be considered, and thus radiation therapy, delivered either externally or by brachytherapy, has been instrumental in the primary management of uveal melanoma.

Observation

It is not uncommon for indeterminate pigmented uveal tumors to be observed without treatment until growth is documented. The probability of malignancy can be estimated according to tumor thickness, serous retinal detachment, orange pigment, and symptoms.[80] Patients and clinicians can then make a combined decision on when to commence therapy after discussion of risks and benefits.

Enucleation

Enucleation was traditionally the standard of care for choroidal melanoma since the late 19th century, but its effectiveness in improving survival has never been clearly demonstrated.[81] A study from the Helsinki University Hospital looked at the long-term prognosis of patients treated by enucleation between 1962 and 1981 and found death was attributable to melanoma in 61% of cases.[82] They also reported that cause-specific mortality (CSM) increased with longer follow-up. The 5-, 15-, 25-, and 35-year CSMs were 31%, 45%, 49%, and 52%, respectively, thus illustrating that a substantial number of patients die of metastatic disease more than 5 years after enucleation. The desire to improve survival and preserve vision stimulated the development of alternative, organ-preserving therapies for uveal melanoma. Still, enucleation is required in a subset of patients, either because tumor is too extensive at presentation or because complications of conservative therapy, namely vision loss, would be too high. General guidelines for enucleation include tumor diameter >17 mm, thickness >6 to 7 mm, involvement of the optic disc, invasion of more than 30% of the iris, ciliary body, or angle, retinal perforation, or poor general health of the patient.[79] It was once postulated that surgical manipulation during enucleation could disseminate tumor cells into blood vessels and thereby increase the possibility of metastatic spread.[81] This spawned an interest in preoperative radiotherapy in an effort to prevent dissemination, but a more recent study showed no improvement in survival when preenucleation radiation was used.[83]

Endoresection

Transretinal endoresection is controversial, mainly because of fears of seeding tumor cells, but has been advocated for juxtopapillary tumors up to 10 mm in diameter.[79] The operation involves vitrectomy; tumor removal with a vitrector either via a retinotomy or after lifting a retinal flap; fluid–air exchange to drain any subretinal fluid; endolaser photocoagulation to destroy any residual tumor in the sclera and to achieve retinopexy; air–silicone exchange; and, if possible, adjunctive brachytherapy.[84] Given the seemingly heightened risk of tumor seeding with endoresection, some investigators have recommended preoperative stereotactic radiation, but this practice is similarly controversial.[85] Endoresection carries approximately 10% risk of local recurrence, which can arise from microscopic disease in the scleral bed or at the margins of resection.[84]

Transscleral Resection

Transscleral local resection has been promoted for tumors >6-mm thick in patients highly motivated to retain vision and in patients with severe exudative retinal detachment after radiotherapy.[79] The procedure carries substantial operative risk. Choroidectomy and cyclochoroidectomy, for example, require hypotensive anesthesia with systolic blood pressure lowered to approximately 40 mm Hg.[86] The operation involves the preparation of a lamellar scleral flap, ocular decompression by limited pars plana vitrectomy, resection of the tumor together with the deep scleral lamella, suturing of the scleral flap, intraocular injection of balanced salt solution, and adjunctive brachytherapy either at the end of the operation or a several weeks later. This procedure has approximately 30%

TABLE 38.1 UVEAL MELANOMA STAGING

Thickness (mm)							
>15					4	4	4
12.1–15				3	3	4	4
9.1–12		3	3	3	3	3	4
6.1–9	2	2	2	2	3	3	4
3.1–6	1	1	1	2	2	3	4
<3.0	1	1	1	1	2	2	4
	<3.0	3.1–6	6.1–9	9.1–12	12.1–15	15.1–18	>18
Largest basal diameter (mm)							

NOTES: Categories for ciliary body and choroid uveal melanoma based on thickness and diameter: T size noted as category 1–4.

Thickness (mm); Largest basal diameter (mm)

Primary Tumor (T)

All Uveal Melanomas	
Tx	Primary tumor cannot be assessed.
T0	No evidence of primary tumor.
Iris	
T1	Tumor limited to the iris.
T1a	Tumor limited to the iris not more than 3 clock hours in size.
T1b	Tumor limited to the iris more than 3 clock hours in size.
T1c	Tumor limited to the iris with secondary glaucoma.
T2	Tumor confluent with or extending to the ciliary body, choroid, or both.
T2a	Tumor confluent with or extending to the ciliary body, choroid, or both, with secondary glaucoma.
T3	Tumor confluent with or extending into the ciliary body, choroid, or both, with scleral extension.
T3a	Tumor confluent with or extending into the ciliary body, choroid, or both, with scleral extension and secondary glaucoma
T4	Tumor with extrascleral extension.
T4a	Tumor with extrascleral extension <5 mm in diameter.
T4b	Tumor with extrascleral extension >5 mm in diameter.
Ciliary Body and Choroid: Classified According to Categories 1–4.	
T1	Tumor size category 1.
T1a	Tumor size category 1 without ciliary body involvement and extraocular extension.
T1b	Tumor size category 1 with ciliary body involvement.
T1c	Tumor size category 1 without ciliary body involvement, but with extraocular extension ≤5 mm in diameter.
T1d	Tumor size category 1 with ciliary body involvement and extraocular extension ≤ 5 mm in diameter.
T2	Tumor size category 2.
T2a	Tumor size category 2 without ciliary body involvement and extraocular extension.
T2b	Tumor size category 2 with ciliary body involvement.
T2c	Tumor size category 2 without ciliary body involvement, but with extraocular extension ≤5 mm in diameter.
T2d	Tumor size category 2 with ciliary body involvement and extraocular extension ≤5 mm in diameter.
T3	Tumor size category 3.
T3a	Tumor size category 3 without ciliary body involvement and extraocular extension.
T3b	Tumor size category 3 with ciliary body involvement.
T3c	Tumor size category 3 without ciliary body involvement, but with extraocular extension ≤5 mm in diameter.
T3d	Tumor size category 3 with ciliary body involvement and extraocular extension ≤5 mm in diameter.
T4	Tumor size category 4.
T4a	Tumor size category 4 without ciliary body involvement and extraocular extension.
T4b	Tumor size category 4 with ciliary body involvement.
T4c	Tumor size category 4 without ciliary body involvement, but with extraocular extension ≤5 mm in diameter.
T4d	Tumor size category 4 with ciliary body involvement and extraocular extension ≤5 mm in diameter.
T4e	Any tumor size category with extraocular extension >5 mm in diameter.
Regional Lymph Nodes (N)	
Nx	Regional lymph nodes cannot be assessed.
N0	No regional lymph node metastases.
N1	Regional lymph node metastases.
Distant Metastases (M)	
M0	No distant metastases
M1	Distant metastases
M1a	Largest diameter of largest metastasis ≤3 cm.
M1b	Largest diameter of largest metastasis 3.1–8.0 cm.
M1c	Largest diameter of largest metastasis ≥8 cm.
Anatomic Stage/Prognostic Groups	
I	T1aN0M0
IIA	T1b-dN0M0
	T2aN0M0
IIB	T2bN0M0
	T3aN0M0
IIIA	T2c-dN0M0
	T3b-cN0M0
	T4aN0M0
IIIB	T3dN0M0
	T4b-cN0M0
IIIC	T4d-eN0M0
IV	Any TN1M0
	Any T Any N M1a-c

incidence of local relapse when performed exclusively, but this probability declines to approximately 10% when perioperative brachytherapy is delivered.[87]

Transpupillary Thermotherapy

Photocoagulation of choroidal melanoma using brief flashes of light has also been investigated, but was superseded by low-energy, long-duration krypton laser photocoagulation, which has greater penetration.[88] This modality was surpassed by transpupillary thermotherapy, in which 1-minute applications of 3-mm spots of low-energy diode laser are administered to the tumor and the surrounding choroid.[89] The objective is not immediate thermoablation, but rather heating the tumor by only a few degrees so that following treatment, tumor regression occurs slowly, often resulting in a white scar. This technique may be used for indeterminate choroidal tumors. Some advocates of transpupillary thermotherapy recommend adjunctive brachytherapy, while others have attempted phototherapy without radiotherapy.[90]

Plaque Brachytherapy

Plaque brachytherapy is the mainstay of treatment in many centers, with iodine-125 and ruthenium-106 being the most common isotopes, although palladium-103 has also been used effectively.[91] Iodine emits γ-rays, which have a range sufficient for tumors up to 8- to 10-mm thick, while ruthenium delivers beta-particles that have a more limited range, which is suitable for tumors up to approximately 5 mm. The general objective with all plaques is to deliver approximately 80 Gy to the tumor apex by fixing the plaque in the exact location of the tumor (Fig. 38.6). Computer modeling has been developed, as seen in general radiotherapy planning, to create a three-dimensional model of the eye and determine the appropriate treatment time and estimated dose to the optic nerve, macula, and lens.[92] The largest prospective experience of patients treated by plaque brachytherapy was conducted by the Collaborative Ocular Melanoma Study (COMS) group. From 1986 to 2003, COMS conducted two multicenter trials of brachytherapy with iodine-125 versus enucleation in selected patients with choroidal melanoma. Long-term results were subsequently published in COMS report 28 in 2006, which evaluated 1,317 patients.[93] Eligible patients had unilateral choroidal melanoma with an apical height of 2.5 to 10 mm and a maximum basal tumor diameter (MBTD) of 16 mm. Patients whose tumors were contiguous with the optic disc were ineligible, as were patients with metastases from melanoma or another malignancy. Patients were followed for 5 to 15 years, and within 12 years after enrollment, 471 of 1,317 (36%) had died. Overall cause-specific mortality at 5 and 10 years for both treatment arms were 19% and 35%, respectively. Cumulative all-cause mortality was 43% in the iodine-125 arm and 41% in the enucleation arm, indicating that with long-term follow-up no survival difference existed between plaque brachytherapy and enucleation. Age older than 60 years and MBTD >11 mm were the primary predictors of time to death from all causes and death with melanoma metastases. Local control was excellent in the COMS series, with only 12.5% of patients requiring salvage enucleation.[94] Visual acuity after plaque brachytherapy depends on a number of features. Shields et al.[95] examined 1,106 patients with visual acuity of 20/100 or better who underwent brachytherapy for uveal melanoma. They found 34% of patients had poor visual acuity at 5 years and 68% at 10 years, defined as 20/200 to no light perception. Factors adversely affecting visual acuity were age over 60 years, poor vision at baseline, increasing tumor thickness (>8 mm), proximity to the foveola of <5 mm, recurrent tumor, subretinal fluid, and history of diabetes or hypertension. Best results were obtained in eyes with small tumors outside a radius of 5 mm from the optic disc and foveola. Whether improvements in tumor imaging and localization and radiation planning will improve functional results will be determined with further investigation.

Proton Beam Therapy

Proton beam therapy may be used to treat uveal melanoma and is usually indicated for tumors that extend close to or are contiguous with the optic disc, referred to as parapapillary and peripapillary tumors, respectively.[96] Large tumors and lesions of the iris and ciliary body may also be candidates for this modality as are patients who are not fit for operative therapy.[79] Because a proton beam delivers a homogeneous dose to tumor and has a sharp edge, a high tumor dose can be delivered with relative sparing of the optic nerve. The decision to use proton therapy over other forms of external therapy, such as helium ions or stereotactic radiotherapy, often depends on the availability of treatment facilities in addition to clinical factors. One of the largest experiences in proton beam therapy for uveal melanoma is from the Harvard Medical School.[97] Treatment planning involves intraoperative examination by transillumination or indirect ophthalmoscopy, and the edges of the tumor are delineated by four tantalum rings sutured to the sclera.

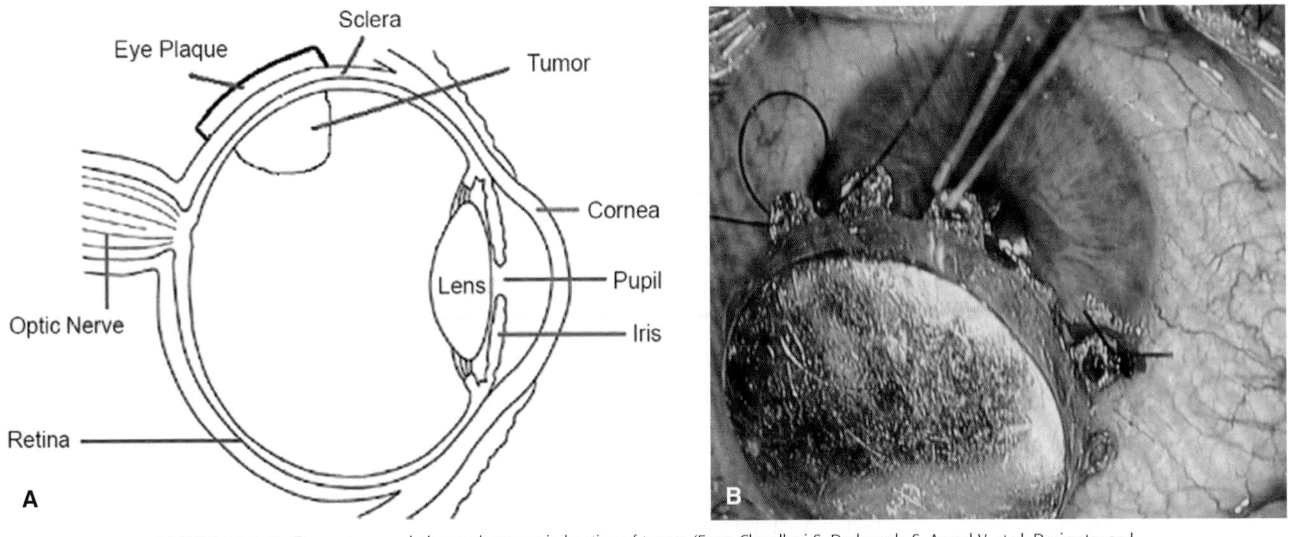

FIGURE 38.6. A: Eye anatomy and plaque placement in location of tumor. (From Chaudhari S, Deshpande S, Anand V, et al. Dosimetry and treatment planning of Occu-Prosta I-125 seeds for intraocular lesions. *J Med Phys* 2008;33:14–18.) **B:** Plaque brachytherapy for melanoma of the iris. (From Khan MK, Khan N, Almasan A, et al. Future of radiation therapy for malignant melanoma in an era of newer, more effective biological agents. *Onco Targets Ther* 2011;4:137–148.)

For tumors of the ciliary body and peripheral choroid, surgery is not performed; transillumination is instead used to define tumor margins in relation to the iris and cornea. Radiation planning is done with an interactive three-dimensional computer system to define the beam aperture and range modulation needed to adequately encompass the tumor and a 1.5-mm margin is included to allow for motion during treatment, setup error, and possible microscopic extension.[98] Patients receive a total dose of 70 CGE, which is delivered in 5 equal fractions over 7 to 10 days (63.6 proton Gy × 1.1 relative biological effectiveness = 70 CGE).[97] The Harvard group recently reported long-term follow-up in a series of 573 patients with peripapillary and parapapillary melanomas with median surveillance of 96.3 months.[96] Local recurrence was rare, with 5- and 10-year local recurrence of 3.3% and 6%, respectively, and similarly high rates of local control have been observed in a larger series from the same institution.[99] Enucleation rates were 13.3% and 17.1% at 5 and 10 years after treatment, respectively. Of 450 patients with baseline visual acuity of 20/200 or better, two-thirds had visual acuity <20/200 years after treatment, although 56% could count fingers. The most common complications were radiation maculopathy and papillopathy. By 3 years the cumulative rate of both complications was 49%, and by 10 years, this increased to 61% for papillopathy and 68% for maculopathy. The visual outcome after proton therapy depends on the height of the tumor and its location relative to the fovea and optic nerve.[99] Anterior segment complications, such as rubeosis iridis and neovascular glaucoma, are the most serious, but occur less frequently, with each occurring in approximately 15% of cases at 5 years postradiation.[100] These results indicate that although visual acuity is compromised with proton beam therapy, particularly in patients with juxtapapillary lesions, some preservation is possible and eye conservation is likely with extremely low rates of local recurrence.

Stereotactic Radiotherapy

Stereotactic radiation can be delivered by linear accelerator (LINAC) or by specialized devices for focused radiation such as the Leksell Gamma Knife (Elekta, Norcross, GA), which provides focused radiation with a multitude of sources. Because gamma knife treatment is usually done in a single fraction, the term radiosurgery is applied, whereas for LINAC-based treatment, single fraction or multifraction treatment is possible. Gamma knife radiosurgery (GKR) for uveal melanoma was first introduced in 1998 by investigators at the Indiana University School of Medicine.[101] Nineteen patients with uveal melanoma were treated to a dose of 40 Gy prescribed to the 50% isodose line. With median follow-up was 40 months, 3- and 5-year overall survival rates were 86 and 55%, respectively. The 3- and 5-year tumor control rates were both 94%. Six of the 19 treated patients (32%) developed distant metastasis 31 to 75 months after GKR. Of the 19 patients treated, 2 had improved, 4 had stable, and 13 had worse vision in the treated eye. Similar results were reported in a larger series of 78 patients from investigators in Milan.[102] The dose was adjusted over the treatment period: 7 patients received 50 Gy at the 50% isodose line (1994–1995), 21 patients received 40 Gy to the 50% isodose line (1995–1999), and 47 patients received 35 Gy to the 50% isodose line (2000–2006). Local tumor control was achieved in 91.0% of patients and the eye retention rate was 89.7%. A significant relative reduction of visual acuity was observed during follow-up. The most frequently encountered complications were exudative retinopathy (33.3%), neovascular glaucoma (18.7%), radiogenic retinopathy (13.5%) and vitreous hemorrhage (10.4%).

One theoretical disadvantage of single-dose stereotactic radiosurgery is the potential for complications, which has prompted investigators to explore fractionated stereotactic radiotherapy (SRT) treatment of uveal melanoma.[103] In particular, severe radiation retinopathy is dose dependent with respect to both total dose (>25 Gy) and dose per fraction (>2 Gy).[104,105] Muller et al.[103] conducted a prospective study on 102 patients with uveal melanoma treated with fractionated SRT between 1999 and 2007. Patients had uveal melanoma of the choroid or ciliary body with a tumor thickness <12 mm and diameter <16 mm with no metastases. The technique, like GKR, utilized a fixed immobilization system, and a dose of 50 Gy was delivered in 5 equal fractions on 5 consecutive days using 6 MV photons with stereotactic arcs. With median follow-up of 32 months, local control was achieved in 96% of patients. Fifteen enucleations were performed 2 to 85 months after radiation, and best corrected visual acuity (defined as 20/x while using glasses if needed) decreased from a mean of 0.26 at diagnosis to 0.16, 3 months after radiation and then declined to 0.03, 4 years after therapy. Deterioration of visual acuity was in part related to complications of treatment. Grade 3 or 4 neurovascular glaucoma occurred in 9 patients, 8 of which required enucleation. In these 9 patients, tumors were not anteriorly located nor did they receive a high dose to the ciliary body, as one might expect, but were associated with grade 3 retinopathy, which was seen in 19 patients. The authors hypothesized that the physical reaction of ischemic retinopathy might also affect vessels in the ciliary body. Thirteen patients (13%) developed grade 3 or 4 optic neuropathy, which was associated with posterior tumors and optic nerve dose, which was limited to 4 Gy per fraction. Grade 3 cataracts occurred in 10 patients (10%), which were managed by extraction and lens implantation. Cataract formation was dose related, with a median dose of 5 Gy per fraction to the lens, causing cataract in 50% of cases. The authors concluded that while local control was excellent, the number of secondary enucleations was substantial, particularly from neurovascular glaucoma. These data suggest that further follow-up is needed to determine response durability and late side effects of this treatment program.

Retinoblastoma

Retinoblastoma (Rb), the most common ocular malignancy in childhood, affects approximately 300 children per year in the United States.[104] The incidence is higher in developing countries, and while the reason for this is not clear, lower socioeconomic status and the presence of certain human papilloma virus sequences have been implicated.[105] Rb has a heritable form and a nonheritable form, with approximately 55% of children having the nonheritable form. If there is no family history, the disease is labeled sporadic, but this does not necessarily indicate that it is the nonheritable form, because bilateral cases, most of which are heritable, often have no family history of Rb. It can present with unilateral disease (two-thirds of cases), bilateral disease, or rarely with tumor in both eyes and the pineal gland, which is called trilateral disease.[106] Approximately 80% of children in Rb are diagnosed before the age of 3, with unilateral cases diagnosed at an earlier age (14–16 months) than those with bilateral presentations (29–30 months).[107–110] Histologically, Rb develops from immature retinal cells and replaces the retina and other intraocular tissues. Macroscopically, viable tumor cells are found near blood vessels, while zones of necrosis are found in relatively avascular areas. Microscopically, both undifferentiated and differentiated elements may be present. Undifferentiated elements appear as collections of small, round cells with hyperchromatic nuclei; differentiated elements include Flexner-Wintersteiner rosettes, Homer-Wright rosettes, and fluerettes from photoreceptor differentiation.[111]

The study of Rb has provided insights into the genetic basis of cancer. The Rb gene (*RB1*) is located on the long arm of chromosome 13 (13q14). In order for Rb to develop, both copies of the gene at the 13q14 locus must be lost, deleted, mutated, or inactivated. If either the maternal or paternal copy of the gene that is inherited by an individual is defective, then that individual is heterozygous for the mutant allele. Tumor formation requires both alleles of the gene to be mutant or inactive. These two mutations correlate to the two "hits" theorized by Knudson[112]

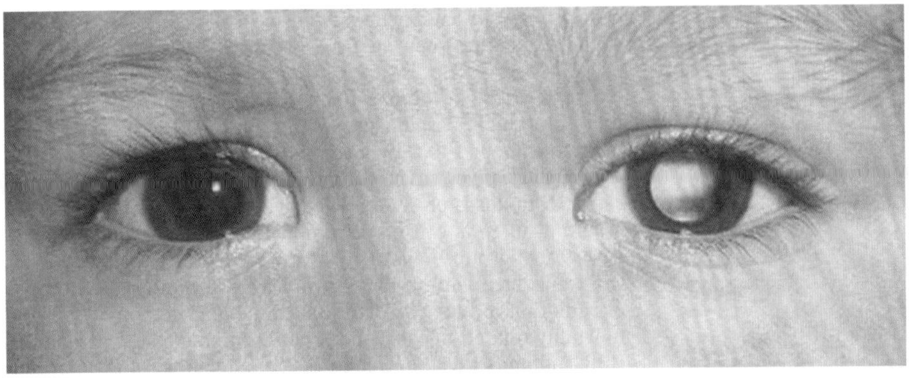

FIGURE 38.7. Leukokoria from retinoblastoma. (From Aerts I, Lumbroso-Le Rouic L, Gauthier-Villars M, et al. Retinoblastoma. *Orphanet J Rare Dis* 2006;1:31.)

and Hethcote and Knudson,[113] which was based on the finding that children with bilateral Rb developed multifocal, bilateral tumors at an earlier age than those with unifocal, unilateral tumors. The first "hit" can be inherited and would be present in all cells in the body, and the second "hit" results in loss of the remaining normal allele and occurs within a particular retinal cell or cells with dysregulation of the cell cycle.[114] In sporadic, nonheritable Rb, both hits occur within a single retinal cell after fertilization (somatic events), thus resulting in unilateral Rb. Identifying the *RB1* mutation can have management implications both in the affected child as well as siblings and future offspring. For example, if *RB1* mutation is detected, then siblings, children, and other relatives can be tested for the mutation. If they do not carry the mutation, they need not undergo rigorous examinations under anesthesia.[115]

The most common and obvious sign of Rb is leukokoria, a discoloration of the pupil (Fig. 38.7). Other less common and less specific signs and symptoms are deterioration of vision, a red or irritated eye, faltering growth, or developmental delay.[116] Some children with retinoblastoma can develop a squint, commonly referred to as cross-eyed or wall-eyed, indicating strabismus.[117] In advanced disease in developing countries, eye enlargement is a common finding. Funduscopy typically reveals a white-colored main tumor (Fig. 38.8), frequently with satellite lesions in the retina, subretinal space, or vitreous referred to as "seeds." Secondary serous retinal detachment may be associated with large lesions. To confirm these findings, a detailed examination under anesthesia through dilated pupils is performed.

Ultrasonography of the eyes is often performed to evaluate the intraocular mass with attention to heterogeneity and calcifications, which support a diagnosis of Rb. Ultrasonography is not as sensitive as CT, which is the ideal imaging format to detect intraocular calcifications. CT, however, raises the concern of exposure to radiation in children younger than 1 year of age with germline mutations,[118] but it is still frequently used to confirm the diagnosis. Magnetic resonance imaging (MRI) of the brain and orbits is the most sensitive means of evaluating for extraocular extension and also provides better delineation of the optic nerve and the pineal area.[119] MRI of the brain and spinal cord and cerebral spinal fluid examination are indicated when there is gross invasion of the optic nerve by imaging studies or microscopic involvement beyond the lamina cribrosa on histopathologic examination of the enucleated eye. A bone marrow examination and a bone scan are indicated only in cases of an abnormal blood count or clinical symptoms suggesting osseous metastases. The diagnosis of retinoblastoma is based on examination by an ophthalmologist and imaging studies. Biopsy is generally not performed due to the theoretical risk for extraocular dissemination, which could convert an intraocular, curable tumor into extraocular, metastatic disease. Therefore, in the absence of a tissue diagnosis, benign conditions that can resemble retinoblastoma must be carefully excluded.

Rb can spread in a variety of ways, including direct invasion of the optic nerve into the chiasm or dissemination through the subarachnoid space to the brain and spinal cord. Tumors can also invade the choroid and the vascular layer and spread via blood to the bone and bone marrow.[120,121] Anterior spread can occur and involve the aqueous venous channels, conjunctiva, and lymphatics or invade the sclera into the orbit with eventual spread to regional lymph nodes.

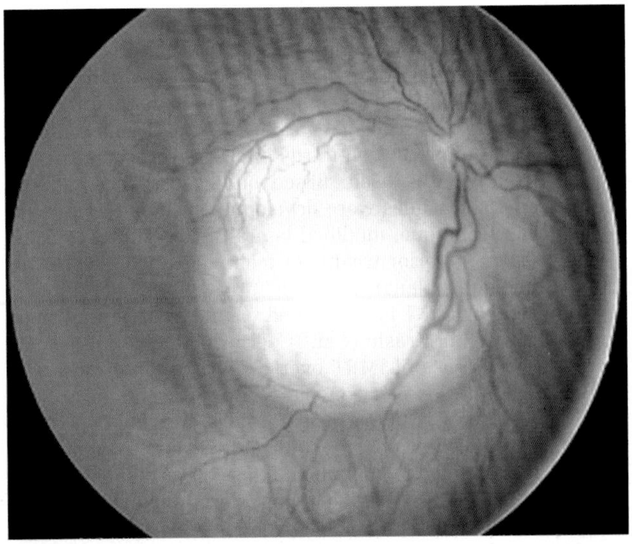

FIGURE 38.8. Retinoblastoma on fundoscopic exam. (From Aerts I, Lumbroso-Le Rouic L, Gauthier-Villars M, et al. Retinoblastoma. *Orphanet J Rare Dis* 2006;1:31.)

Treatment

Management of Rb requires close cooperation of a multidisciplinary team of ophthalmologists, pediatric oncologists, pediatric radiation oncologists, pathologists, genetic counselors, social workers, nurses, and others. Most unilateral cases present with advanced intraocular disease and require enucleation, which is also indicated for eyes with recurrent disease and no useful vision. Children with bilateral presentations typically require multimodality therapy with chemotherapy and local therapy. Staging and classification schemes have been developed to assess outcomes, particularly for intraocular Rb. The Reese-Ellsworth (R-E) classification, developed in the 1960s, was the first of these (Table 38.2).[122] Specifically, the R-E classification, which has five groups, was devised to predict prognosis in eyes that were treated with EBRT. Eyes with disease consistent with the lower groups have a lower risk for enucleation following EBRT, while group V eyes have the highest risk for enucleation. In recent years, chemotherapy has diminished the role EBRT for intraocular disease, and thus the R-E scheme is less useful and alternative schemes have been proposed by Shields et at.[123] and Murphree,[124] among others. The International Retinoblastoma Classification was developed by a group of experts in 2003 in Paris, which is used by many

TABLE 38.2 REESE-ELLSWORTH CLASSIFICATION OF RETINOBLASTOMA

Group 1: Very Favorable for Maintenance of Sight
A. Solitary tumor, smaller than 4 disc diameters (DD), at or behind the equator.
B. Multiple tumors, none larger than 4 DD, all at or behind the equator.

Group 2: Favorable for Maintenance of Sight
A. Solitary tumor, 4 to 10 DD at or behind the equator.
B. Multiple tumors, 4 to 10 DD behind the equator.

Group 3: Possible Maintenance of Sight
A. Any lesion anterior to the equator.
B. Solitary tumour, larger than 10 DD behind the equator.

Group 4: Unfavorable for Maintenance of Sight
A. Multiple tumors, some larger than 10 DD.
B. Any lesion extending anteriorly to the ora serrata.

Group 5: Very Unfavorable for Maintenance of Sight
A. Massive tumors involving more than one half of the retina.
B. Vitreous seeding.

cooperative study groups (Table 38.3). An additional system has been proposed by Chantada et al.,[125] which was designed to address extraocular disease and microscopic disease following enucleation.

Enucleation

Most children with unilateral Rb present with advanced disease and require enucleation. Other indications for enucleation are cases of bilateral disease where the eye with more advanced disease does not respond to chemotherapy or other treatments, when active tumor is present in an eye with no vision, when glaucoma is present as a result of neovascularization of the iris or tumor invasion into the anterior chamber, and when direct visualization of an active tumor is obstructed by conditions including hemorrhage, corneal opacity, or cataract.[126] Enucleation is curative in >95% of patients with unilateral disease. Orbital implants are used at most treatment centers, and by connecting them to orbital muscles, excellent cosmesis can be achieved.

TABLE 38.3 INTERNATIONAL CLASSIFICATION OF RETINOBLASTOMA

Group	Subgroup	Quick Reference	Features
A	A	Small tumor	Retinoblastoma ≤ 3 mm in size[a]
B	B	Larger tumor	Retinoblastoma > 3 mm in size[a] or
		Macula	Macular retinoblastoma location (<3 mm to foveola)
		Juxtapapillary	Juxtapapillary retinoblastoma location (≤1.5 mm to disc)
		Subretinal fluid	Clear subretinal fluid ≤3 mm from margin
C		Focal seeds	Retinoblastoma with
	C1		Subretinal seeds ≤3 mm from retinoblastoma
	C2		Vitreous seeds ≤3 mm from retinoblastoma
	C3		Both subretinal and vitreous seeds ≤3 mm from retinoblastoma
D		Diffuse seeds	Retinoblastoma with
	D1		Subretinal seeds >3 mm from retinoblastoma
	D2		Vitreous seeds >3 mm from retinoblastoma
	D3		Both retinal and vitreous seeds >3 mm from retinoblastoma
E		Extensive	Extensive retinoblastoma occupying >50% globe or Neovascular glaucoma Opaque media from hemorrhage in anterior chamber, vitreous, or subretinal space Invasion of postlaminar optic nerve, choroid (>2 mm), sclera, orbit, anterior chamber

[a]Refers to 3 mm in basal dimension or thickness.

External Beam Radiation Therapy

Rb is a highly radiosensitive tumor as first shown by Hilgartner[127] in 1903. By virtue of its radiosensitive nature, Rb was historically treated with first-line EBRT in a majority of cases, with doses of 42 to 50 Gy given in 1.5- to 2-Gy fractions, resulting in 87% eye preservation in R-E groups I to IV versus 29% in group V eyes.[128] However during the past 15 years, the trend has been to move away from radiotherapy because of radiation-induced growth deformities of the bony orbit and mortality related to osteosarcoma development.[129–131] However, EBRT still has a viable role in the management of Rb, particularly as salvage, or perhaps more accurately termed, consolidative treatment in tumors that are refractory to chemotherapy and other local therapies. Other indications include lesions that are too large, numerous, or close to the optic disc or fovea for focal therapy out of concern for preserving central vision. EBRT also has a special role in treating eyes with vitreous seeds.[132] Chan et al.[133] reported on 36 eyes that received EBRT after incomplete response to primary chemotherapy and focal therapies in 22 patients with bilateral Rb. Thirty-two received lens-sparing EBRT and the remainder received whole-eye EBRT to a dose of 40 to 44 Gy in 20 to 22 fractions. The rate of eye preservation was 83%, and 67% required no further treatment after EBRT. Visual acuity was recorded for 19 eyes, of which 10 read 6/9-6/5, 3 read 6-18-6/36, and 6 read 6/60 or worse. Side effects were limited to cataracts and dry eyes, although follow-up (median 40 months) was insufficient to assess second malignancies. The investigators concluded that EBRT was highly effective in preserving eyes with useful vision in bilateral Rb in cases refractory to chemotherapy and focal therapies. In a more advanced population, Kingston et al.[134] evaluated consolidative EBRT (40–44 Gy) in 14 patients with R-E group V eyes after induction chemotherapy with carboplatin, etoposide, and vincristine. Four eyes were enucleated primarily for severe disease at presentation and of the remaining 20, 6 required enucleation (4 for recurrence, 2 for neovascular glaucoma). Of the 12 surviving children, 5 have visual acuity of better than 1/60 in at least one eye. Thus, while most group V eyes could be salvaged, the resultant visual acuity was often poor.

Radiation techniques in Rb should provide uniform coverage of the entire retina approaching the ora serrata and coverage of up to 10 mm of the optic nerve while sparing the lens and bony anatomy to the extent possible.[132] In practice, the dual goals of including the entire retina in the beam and protecting the lens have represented a challenge. Historically, a single lateral field was used in the radiotherapeutic management of one eye and parallel-opposed fields for the management of both eyes. The traditional border for these "D-shaped" fields was the lateral rim of the bony orbit, which could result in underdosing of the anterior retina with associated local failure. McCormick et al.[135] reported local failure in two-thirds of cases when lens-sparing lateral technique was used. Based on these concerns, more sophisticated techniques were developed, such as the anterior lens-sparing technique, modified lateral field techniques using oblique angles, anterior treatment techniques using electrons, and multiple noncoplanar arcs.[136–139]

Conformal or IMRT is well suited for the treatment of small tumors such as Rb. Krasin et al.[140] performed a planning study that favored the use of IMRT over conformal, anterior-lateral photon and anterior electron plans for the treatment of the entire globe. IMRT resulted in the greatest sparing of the surrounding bony orbit and other normal tissues. As acute and late toxicity is related to volume and dose of normal tissue irradiated, proton therapy has been considered for the treatment of Rb, with the added advantage of reducing low-dose irradiation of normal tissue. Lee et al.[141] compared protons with three-dimensional conformal radiation therapy, IMRT, and electron therapy when treating the entire retina and vitreous cavity. Protons provided superior coverage with greater sparing of normal tissue, which in theory may result in a superior therapeutic ratio. Krengli et al.[142] came to a similar conclusion looking at target coverage and lens sparing using protons for various intraocular tumor locations and beam arrangements. Focused techniques such as proton beam irradiation should be strongly considered in the management of Rb due to the high risk of second malignancy. Patients with hereditary disease who received EBRT have a cumulative incidence of second cancers of 35%, compared with 6% for those who did not receive EBRT, and the risk is even higher if treatment takes place before 1 year of age.[143,144] Cataracts, optic nerve damage, total retinal vascular occlusion, vitreous hemorrhage, and facial and temporal bone hypoplasia are other complications associated with EBRT therapy.[145]

Brachytherapy

Brachytherapy with either iodine-125, gold, and more recently ruthenium have been used in selected cases of Rb.[146] The intention is to deliver a dose of 40 to 45 Gy transclerally to the apex of the tumor over a period of 2 to 4 days. This treatment is limited to tumors that are <16 mm in base and 8 mm in thickness, and can be used as the primary treatment or, more frequently, in patients who had failed initial therapy, including previous EBRT.[147–150] Shields et al.[151] described 79% local control at 5 years using this method. Side effects are generally less common than with EBRT and include optic neuropathy, radiation retinopathy, and cataract formation. Second malignancies do not appear to be associated with this type of local therapy. Relative contraindications include larger tumors and those that involve the macula.

Thermotherapy

Thermotherapy involves the application of heat directly to the tumor with infrared radiation. A temperature between 45°C and 60°C is reached, which is below the coagulative threshold and therefore spares the retinal vessels from coagulation.[151,152] Thermotherapy alone can be used for small lesions that are ≤3 mm in diameter without vitreous or subretinal seeds. In a study of 91 tumors, 92% of the tumors that were <1.5 mm in diameter were controlled with thermotherapy alone.[153]

Chemothermotherapy and Laser Photocoagulation

Larger tumors or tumors with subretinal seeds are usually treated with a combination of thermotherapy and chemotherapy (chemothermotherapy), usually delivered within hours of each other. In one study of 188 retinoblastomas, tumor control was achieved in 86% of cases.[154] Complications included focal iris atrophy, paraxial lens opacity, sector optic disk atrophy, retinal traction, optic disk edema, retinal vascular occlusion, retinal detachment, and corneal edema. Chemothermotherapy may be especially useful for patients with small tumors adjacent to the fovea and optic nerve, where radiation therapy or laser photocoagulation may result in significant visual loss. Laser photocoagulation is recommended only for small posterior tumors with the goal of coagulating the tumor's blood supply.[155] Effective therapy usually requires two or three sessions at monthly intervals. Complications of this treatment include retinal detachment, retinal vascular occlusion, retinal traction, and preretinal fibrosis.

Cryotherapy

Cryotherapy induces tumor tissue to freeze rapidly, resulting in damage to the vascular endothelium with secondary thrombosis and infarction of the tumor tissue. It may be used as primary therapy for small peripheral tumors or for small recurrent tumors previously treated with other modalities. Tumors are typically treated three times per session, with one or two sessions at monthly intervals. Ninety percent of tumors <3 mm in diameter are cured permanently, and complications are few and rarely serious.[156] Transient conjunctival edema and transient localized serous retinal detachments can occur. Vitreous hemorrhage can be observed in large or previously irradiated tumors.

Chemotherapy

Chemotherapy has been used to treat intraocular retinoblastoma since the early 1990s. Chemotherapy is used to reduce the size of the tumor to allow local ophthalmological therapies, including cryotherapy and laser photocoagulation, or thermotherapy, to eradicate the remaining disease. This combination of therapies has been promoted to avoid EBRT or enucleation and thereby decreases the potential for long-term side effects while salvaging useful vision. The common indications for chemotherapy for intraocular Rb include tumors that cannot be effectively treated with local therapies alone, usually due to size. Chemotherapy may be indicated in children with unilateral or bilateral disease, but many patients with unilateral disease are diagnosed with advanced disease and require enucleation. Numerous studies have been published that show that chemotherapy is very effective in eliminating the need for EBRT or enucleation in R-E group I to III eyes, while proving to be significantly less successful in eyes with group IV or V disease.[157–161,162,163–165] Carboplatin, vincristine, and etoposide are generally used, and cyclosporine has been added to the regimen in some institutions in order to reduce drug resistance.[166] Chemotherapy regimens from different investigators vary in the number and frequency of cycles, but they are generally well tolerated, with the expected side effects of myelosuppression and associated risk of infection. There is still the potential risk for second malignancies, especially when using etoposide.[167] Chemotherapy alone is not very effective in avoiding EBRT or enucleation in patients with R-E group V eyes, especially those with vitreous seeds. Friedman et al.[165] showed that only 53% of 30 group V eyes could be controlled with chemotherapy alone. Based on these data, newer regimens incorporate carboplatin, vincristine, and etoposide along with subtenon carboplatin for more advanced eyes.[168,169] Eyes with diffuse vitreous seeding rarely respond to chemotherapy alone, and while EBRT is modestly successful, new approaches are needed. Novel therapies for patient with vitreous or subretinal seeding include intra-arterial chemotherapy (IAC) with selective catheterization of the ophthalmic artery.[170] Gobin et al.[170] described 78 patients (95 eyes) treated with IAC with melphalan with or without topotecan and evaluated procedure success, event-free (RT or enucleation) ocular survival, and ocular and extraocular complications. The procedure succeeded in 98.5% of cases and the ocular event-free survival rates at 2 years were 70% for all eyes, 82% for eyes that received IAC as primary treatment, and 58% for eyes that had prior treatment with chemotherapy or EBRT, and there were no permanent complications. Abramson et al.[171] reported similarly encouraging results in 67 patients (76 eyes) treated with IAC. Among treatment-naïve eyes, the ocular salvage rate was 83% for eyes with subretinal seeding only, 64% for eyes with vitreous seeding only, and 80% for eyes with both. Other strategies have also been investigated. A recent phase I study using adenoviral vectors to deliver the herpes simplex thymidine kinase gene followed by ganciclovir demonstrated durable clinical and histopathologic responses in patients heavily pretreated with vitreous seeds.[172] Clinical trials using these novel therapies should be encouraged in this population.

Management of Extraocular Disease

Patients with extraocular disease historically have had a poor prognosis, but recent studies using combinations of chemotherapy and EBRT have been encouraging. Chantada et al.[173] reported a 5-year event-free survival rate of 84% in 15 patients with orbital or preauricular disease treated with chemotherapy that included vincristine, doxorubicin, and cyclophosphamide or vincristine, idarubicin, cyclophosphamide, carboplatin, and etoposide. These patients also received EBRT of 45 Gy administered to the optic chiasm for patients with orbital disease and to the involved nodes for those with preauricular lymphadenopathy. There are several reports suggesting that high-dose chemotherapy with stem cell rescue combined with EBRT for areas of bulky disease at diagnosis is beneficial, with some long-term survivors among patients with metastatic disease not involving the central nervous system.[174–176,177]

Primary Intraocular Lymphoma

Primary intraocular lymphoma (PIOL), formally known as ocular reticulum cell sarcoma, is an uncommon clinical manifestation of non-Hodgkin lymphoma, which arises in the retina or the vitreous humor.[178] It usually develops in patients in the fifth and sixth decades of life as a chronic, relapsing, and steroid-resistant uveitis and vitritis. Patients often complain of blurred vision, a painless loss of vision, and floaters. Intraocular lymphoma may occur independently, prior or subsequent to a primary central nervous system lymphoma. PIOL progresses to intracranial involvement in 60% to 85% of cases.[179,180] Historically PIOL has been difficult to diagnose, often taking several years from the onset of symptoms to establishing a diagnosis, which likely contributed to suboptimal outcome in many cases.[181] Given the tumor's rarity, the optimal treatment of PIOL is unclear. Radiation therapy has been used with durable control after 35 to 45 Gy given exclusively to both eyes in the absence of central nervous system disease.[179,182] However, concerns of central nervous system relapse have led investigators to use chemotherapy as initial treatment and radiation as a consolidative therapy.[183,184] Methotrexate and cytosine arabinoside are most commonly used, given their ability to cross the blood–ocular barrier.

Optic Pathway Glioma

Optic pathway gliomas, with or without contiguous involvement of the hypothalamus, have an incidence of approximately 1 in 100,000, with 90% presenting in the first two decades of life[185] Most of these neoplasms are pilocytic or low-grade astrocytomas.[186] Untreated, the clinical course is that of deterioration of visual acuity, progressive visual field deficits, endocrine or intellectual impairment, and death in up to 30% due to local tumor progression.[187,188] Multiple treatment strategies exist, including surveillance, chemotherapy, radiation therapy, surgery, or some combination of therapies. Advances in management have resulted in cause-specific survival rates of 90% to 100% except in cases associated with neurofibromatosis, which carry a worse prognosis.[189,190] Therefore, multidisciplinary management of optic pathway gliomas is critical with an emphasis on reducing treatment-related sequelae. The role of surgery is limited but may be a reasonable treatment option in patients where tumor is confined to a single optic nerve with no useful vision. Local failure rates of approximately 5% can be achieved after complete resection.[185] Radiation therapy has resulted in 10-year survival rates ranging from 40% to 93%, but with potentially severe long-term sequelae, including endocrine problems, neurodevelopmental disorders, and second malignancy.[191] Concerns of these toxicities are significant enough such that at most centers, children of any age are initially treated with chemotherapy in order to delay irradiation until progression. Investigators have found that a 2.5- to 3-year delay in RT can be achieved with this approach.[189]

The main indication of RT is for progressive disease, and radiation doses in the range from 45 to 60 Gy in 1.8- to 2.0-Gy fractions have been effective.[190,192] Erkal et al.[190] reported on 33 cases of optic pathway gliomas (OPG) treated between 1973 and 1994. Twenty-four children had OPGs and nine had chiasmatic-hypothalamic gliomas. Evidence of neurofibromatosis was present in six children. Subtotal resection was performed in 22 and biopsy in 7. Median total dose was 50 Gy in 25 fractions and mean follow-up was 13.6 years. Ten-year overall, progression-free, and cause-specific survival rates were 79%, 77%, and 88%, respectively. Differences in any of the survival endpoints between optic pathway and chiasmatic-hypothalamic gliomas were not statistically significant, but absence of neurofibromatosis correlated with significantly better progression-free and cause-specific survival. Grabenbauer et al.[192] also reported a series of OPG but also assessed visual outcomes. Twenty-five patients received radiation therapy following surgery or biopsy. Treatment volume included a 0.5- to 1-cm margin around the tumor as depicted on CT or MRI. Age-adjusted radiation doses ranged from 45 to 60 Gy with a fraction size of 1.6 to 2 Gy. Overall survival and progression-free survival rates were 94% and 69% at 10 years, respectively. Age older than 10 years at time of treatment and total radiation dose >45 Gy significantly improved progression-free survival. Hypothalamic deficiency also correlated with age, with 69% patients aged below 10 years compared with 25% above 10 years experiencing this condition. As for visual acuity, 36% had an improvement, 52% remained stable, and 12% had measurable deterioration. The authors concluded that postoperative RT with a total dose above 45 Gy should be considered for patients with progressive OPG. Lifelong yearly evaluation for growth hormone, thyroid, and adrenal function is also crucial because the need for replacement therapy is high, particularly in children under 10 years of age.

As in other pediatric malignancies, radiation technique should be approached with an emphasis on normal tissue sparing. Combs et al.[193] reported on 15 patients treated with fractionated stereotactic RT (FSRT) to a median total dose of 50.2 Gy at 1.8 Gy per fraction. The progression-free survival rate at 3 and 5 years was 92% and 72%, respectively. Functional results were encouraging, with only two patients having worsening of vision after RT. Seven had preexisting endocrinopathy, but only one additional patient had endocrine dysfunction after treatment, suggesting FSRT is an effective option for OPG. Still, conformal RT, IMRT, and FSRT carry concerns of second malignancy due the large volume of intracranial tissue receiving a low, potentially mutagenic dose of radiation. For this reason, proton beam therapy has been advocated.[194] Fuss et al.[194] evaluated dosimetry plans for proton versus conformal plans in seven cases of OPG and found proton therapy offered substantial normal tissue sparing both at high- and low-dose areas. The difference was more apparent in tumors >80 cm^3, but even in tumors <20 cm^3, conformity of conformal RT came at the expense of a larger amount of normal tissue receiving low to moderate doses of radiation.

Orbital Tumors

Primary Orbital Lymphoma

Orbital non-Hodgkin lymphomas (NHL) account for only 0.01% of NHL and are typically B-cell lymphomas.[195] Depending on the stage and grade of disease, observation, first-line chemotherapy, or chemotherapy followed by RT are all treatment options, but RT is generally the treatment of choice for NHL localized to the orbital cavity.[196,197] Local control at the rate of 90% to 100% can be achieved using doses of 30 to 36 Gy.[197] Historically, radiation was delivered with an anterior portal prescribed to the orbital apex or by wedged anterior and later fields. Late effects from these techniques include cataract formation, lens ulceration, glaucoma, and lacrimal complications.[197] More recently, investigators have described the use of IMRT in orbital lymphoma and were able to reduce dose to the contralateral orbit, lacrimal gland, and lens (Fig. 38.9).[198]

Conjunctival Tumors

Conjunctival tumors comprise a variety of conditions, from benign papilloma to malignant lesions such as squamous cell carcinoma (SCC). Radiotherapeutic management of these

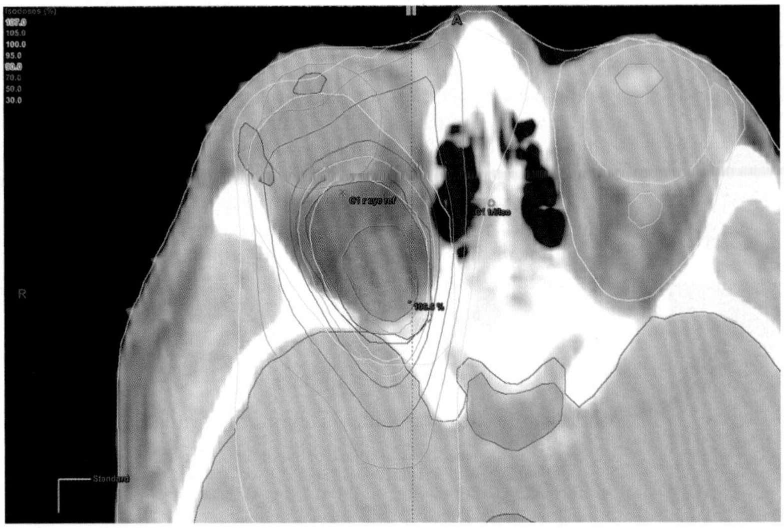

FIGURE 38.9. Primary orbital lymphoma treated with intensity modulated radiation therapy illustrating sparing of lens, lacrimal gland, and contralateral orbit.

tumors is related to the histologic type, as is the case in tumors found elsewhere. Mucosa-associated lymphoid tissue (MALT) lymphoma, for example, has been effectively managed with exclusive RT with local control rates approaching 100%.[199] In a series of patients with MALT lymphoma of the ocular adnexa that included 37 patients with conjunctival disease, Hashimoto et al.[200] reported local control rates of 100% with a median dose of 30.6 Gy. Electron beam therapy was frequently used with eye lens shielding when possible depending on the extent of disease (Fig. 38.10). Treatment options for SCC include excision with or without adjuvant cryotherapy or topical chemotherapy, while advanced cases may require orbital exenteration.[201,202] RT has been used in the primary, adjuvant, and salvage settings with a variety of methods, including photon, proton, and electron beam therapy.[203,204] Most frequently, however, radiation is used in patients with relapsed disease. The treatment volume typically includes gross tumor with margins of approximately 1 cm and doses of approximately 60 Gy, as in cases of SCC from other sites.[205]

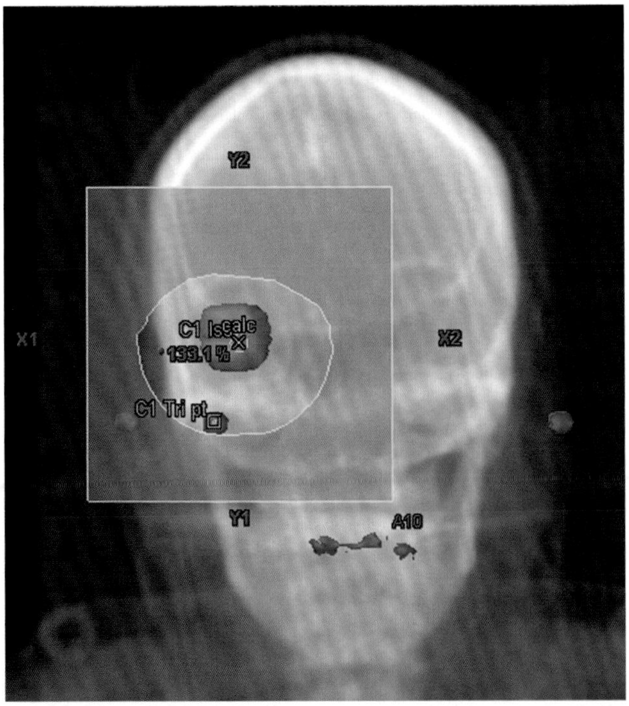

FIGURE 38.10. Electron beam therapy for mucosa-associated lymphoid tissue lymphoma of the conjunctiva. The patient received 30.6 Gy using 9 MeV electrons. Lens shielding was not used due to the extent of disease at presentation.

Sebaceous Carcinoma of the Eyelid

Sebaceous gland adenocarcinoma occurs in the periorbital area, usually in the eyelid.[206] It can exhibit aggressive local behavior and can metastasize to regional lymph nodes and distant organs. Older individuals tend to be affected, but it occurs with greater frequency and at an earlier age in patients with hereditary retinoblastoma with treated with radiation.[207–209] The main systemic association is Muir-Torre syndrome, an autosomal dominant condition characterized by greater frequency of sebaceous adenoma, sebaceous carcinoma, keratoacanthoma, and gastrointestinal malignancies.[210] The most common method of metastasis of eyelid sebaceous carcinoma is through the lymphatic channels to regional lymph nodes. Historically, regional node metastasis occurred in about 30% of cases, but metastases have become less frequent in recent years.[211,212] Tumors that originate in the upper eyelid tend to metastasize to preauricular and parotid nodes, which represent the most common sites of metastasis. Tumors of the lower eyelid region can metastasize to submandibular and cervical nodes, which warrant consideration in RT planning. Until recently, orbital exenteration was widely believed to be the only reasonable option in the management of sebaceous carcinoma that involved most of the conjunctiva and invaded the orbit. However, local excision with adjuvant therapies, such as topical chemotherapy or cryotherapy, have become more accepted.[213,214] EBRT, with doses of approximately 60 Gy, is rarely used for primary treatment, but should be considered for adverse features such as regional lymph node involvement or for recurrent disease.[215]

Orbital Rhabdomyosarcoma

Rhabdomyosarcoma (RMS) affects 250 to 300 children per year in the United States. In 1950, Stobbe and Dargeon[216] demonstrated improvement in the outcome in head and neck sites when radiation therapy was added after incompletely resected RMS. In 1961, Pinkel and Pinkren[217] advocated adjuvant chemotherapy after complete surgical excision and postoperative radiation therapy, which was the beginning of the multimodal approach to solid tumors. Recognizing the value of this multimodal approach as well as the relative rarity of these tumors, the leadership of the three U.S. cooperative pediatric cancer research groups formed the Intergroup Rhabdomyosarcoma Study (IRS) group in 1972 to investigate the biology and treatment of RMS. Since then, five successive clinical protocols involving almost 5,000 patients have been completed: IRS-I (1972–1978); IRS-II (1978–1984); IRS-III (1984–1991); IRS-IV Pilot (for patients with advanced disease

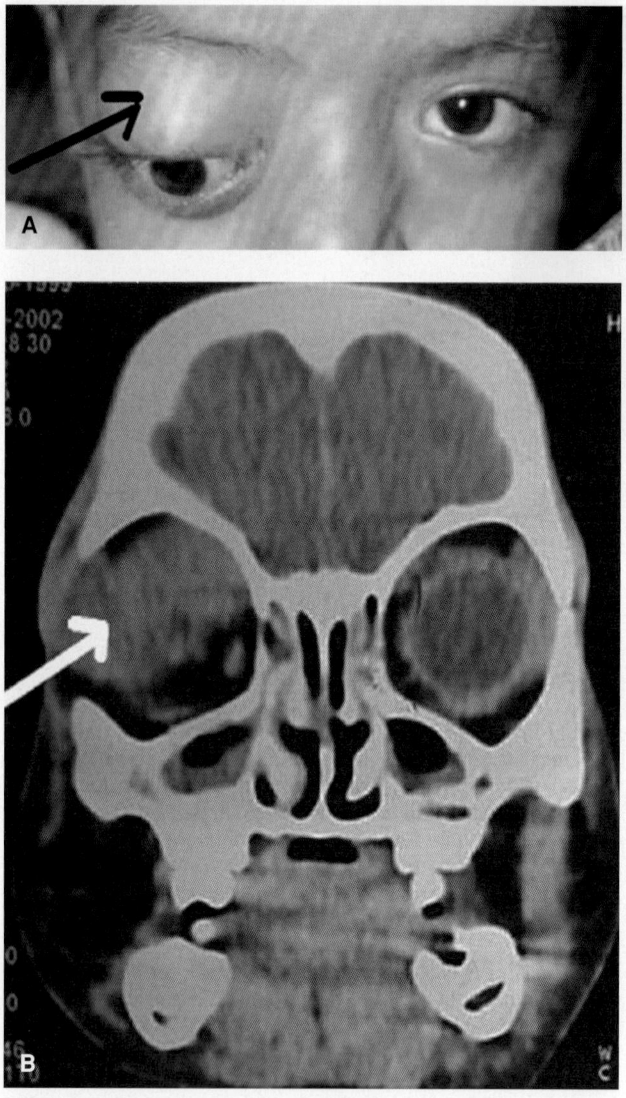

FIGURE 38.11. A: Orbital rhabdomyosarcoma with proptosis. **B:** Coronal computed tomography scan of patient with orbital rhabdomyosarcoma. (From Das JK, Tiwary BK, Paul SB, et al. Primary orbital rhabdomyosarcoma with skeletal muscle metastasis. *Oman J Ophthalmol* 2010;3:91–93.)

only; 1987–1991); and IRS-IV (1991–1997).[218,219–223] The head and neck region is the most common site of presentation and accounts for about 35% of the patients in the IRS studies.[224] These tumors are most commonly of the embryonal subtype and rarely spread to regional lymph nodes. Orbital tumors produce proptosis and, occasionally, ophthalmoplegia (Fig. 38.11). Modern management of RMS comprises multiagent chemotherapy followed by RT. Prechemotherapy as well as postchemotherapy tumor volume must be considered when planning RT. McDonald et al.[225] reported on 20 patients with head and neck RMS (two orbit) treated with IMRT to a total dose of 50 Gy, in accordance with cooperative group protocols. The initial targeting of the prechemotherapy tumor volume with 1- to 2-cm margin to 30.6 to 36 Gy followed by a cone-down boost to the postchemotherapy tumor volume with a 0.5- to 1-cm margin allowed for significant sparing of normal tissues and only one patient developed an in-field recurrence after 50 months. The 3-year event-free survival, overall survival, and risk of central nervous system failure were 74%, 76%, and 7%, respectively.

Periorbital Skin Cancers

Skin cancers of the eyelid and periorbital skin include, most frequently, basal cell carcinoma (BCC), SCC, but also rare histologies such as Merkel cell carcinoma (MCC).[203,226] For small BCC and SCC, single-modality treatment with surgery or RT results in good local control, but RT is frequently used due to cosmetic concerns. For more advanced tumors or more aggressive histologies, such as MCC, combined surgery and RT is typically recommended. Low energy electron beam therapy is useful in this setting and can be delivered with an eye shield. RT for skin tumors requires doses of 60 Gy or more for definitive treatment using standard fractionation, but altered fraction can be employed to shorten treatment duration and minimize ocular trauma of shield placement.

SELECTED REFERENCES

A full list of references for this chapter is available online.

2. Shields CL, Shields JA, Gross N, et al. Survey of 520 eyes with uveal metastases. *Ophthalmology* 1997;104:1265–1276.
4. Stephens LC, Schultheiss TE, Peters LJ, et al. Acute radiation injury of ocular adnexa. *Arch Ophthalmol* 1988;106:389–391.
6. Stafford SL, Kozelsky TF, Garrity JA, et al. Orbital lymphoma: radiotherapy outcome and complications. *Radiother Oncol* 2001;59:139–144.
8. Goyal S, Cohler A, Camporeale J, et al. Intensity-modulated radiation therapy for orbital lymphoma. *Radiat Med* 2008;26:573–581.
12. Merriam GRSA, Focht EF. The effects of ionizing radiations on the eye. *Radiat Ther Oncol* 1972;6:346–385.
15. Hall P, Granath F, Lundell M, et al. Lenticular opacities in individuals exposed to ionizing radiation in infancy. *Radiat Res* 1999;152:190–195.
19. Parsons JT, Bova FJ, Fitzgerald CR, et al. Radiation retinopathy after external-beam irradiation: analysis of timedose factors. *Int J Radiat Oncol Biol Phys* 1994;30:765–773.
35. Singh A D, Kaiser P K. Uveal vascular tumors. In: Singh AD, Damato BE, Pe'er J, et al., eds. *Clinical ophthalmic oncology*. Philadelphia: Saunders-Elsevier, 2007:289–299.
39. Freire JE, DePotter P, Brady LW, et al. Brachytherapy in primary ocular tumors. *Semin Surg Oncol* 1997;13:167–176.
50. Matthiesen C, Bogardus C Jr, Thompson JS, et al. The efficacy of radiotherapy in the treatment of orbital pseudotumor. *Int J Radiat Oncol Biol Phys* 2011;79:1496–1502.
53. Bartalena L, Baldeschi L, Dickinson A, et al. Consensus statement of the European Group on Graves' orbitopathy (EUGOGO) on management of GO. *Eur J Endocrinol* 2008;158:273–285.
67. Bradley EA, Gower EW, Bradley DJ, et al. Orbital radiation for graves ophthalmopathy: a report by the American Academy of Ophthalmology. *Ophthalmology* 2008;115:398–409.
68. Shields JA, Shields CL. *Metastatic tumors to the intraocular structures. Intraocular tumors: a text and atlas.* Philadelphia: WB Saunders, 1992:207–238.
69. Demirci H, Shields CL, Chao AN, et al. Uveal metastasis from breast cancer in 264 patients. *Am J Ophthalmol* 2003;136:264–271.
70. Rosset A, Zografos L, Coucke P, et al. Radiotherapy of choroidal metastases. *Radiother Oncol* 1998;46: 263–268.
71. Shields CL, Shields JA, De Potter P, et al. Plaque radiotherapy for the management of uveal metastasis. *Arch Ophthalmol* 1997;115:203–209.
80. Shields CL, Shields JA, Kiratli H, et al. Risk factors for growth and metastasis of small choroidal melanocytic lesions. *Ophthalmology* 1995;102:1351–1361.
83. Earle JD. Results from the Collaborative Ocular Melanoma Study (COMS) of enucleation versus preoperative radiation therapy in the management of large ocular melanomas [letter]. *Int J Radiat Oncol Biol Phys* 1999;43:1168–1169.
91. Finger PT, Chin KJ, Duvall G. Palladium-103 for Choroidal Melanoma Study Group. Palladium-103 ophthalmic plaque radiation therapy for choroidal melanoma: 400 treated patients. *Ophthalmology* 2009;116:790–796.
95. Shields CL, Shields JA, Cater J, et al. Plague radiotherapy for uveal melanoma: long term visual outcome in 1106 consecutive patients treated between 1976 and 1992. *Arch Ophthalmol* 2000;118:1219–1228.
96. Lane AM, Kim IK, Gragoudas ES. Proton irradiation for peripapillary and parapapillary melanomas. *Arch Ophthalmol* 2011;129:1127–1130.
97. Gragoudas ES, Lane AM. Uveal melanoma: proton beam irradiation. *Ophthalmol Clin North Am* 2005;18:111–118.
99. Gragoudas E, Li W, Goitein M, et al. Evidence-based estimates of outcome in patients irradiated for intraocular melanoma. *Arch Ophthalmol* 2002;120:1665–1671.
102. Modorati G, Miserocchi E, Galli L, et al. Gamma knife radiosurgery for uveal melanoma: 12 years of experience. *Br J Ophthalmol* 2009;93:40–44.
112. Knudson AG Jr. Mutation and cancer: statistical study of retinoblastoma. *Proc Natl Acad Sci USA* 1971;68:820–823.
123. Shields CL, Mashayekhi A, Demirci H, et al. Practical approach to management of retinoblastoma. *Arch Ophthalmol* 2004;122:729–735.
124. Murphree AL. Intraocular retinoblastoma: the case for a new group classification. *Ophthalmol Clin North Am* 2005;18:41–53.
125. Chantada G, Doz F, Antoneli CB, et al. A proposal for an international retinoblastoma staging system. *Pediatr Blood Cancer* 2006;47:801–805.
135. McCormick B, Ellsworth R, Abramson D, et al. Radiation therapy for retinoblastoma: comparison of results with lens-sparing versus lateral beam techniques. *Int J Radiat Oncol Biol Phys* 1988;15:567.
140. Krasin MJ, Crawford BT, Zhu Y, et al. Intensity-modulated radiation therapy for children with intraocular retinoblastoma: potential sparing of the bony orbit. *Clin Oncol (R Coll Radiol)* 2004;16:215–222.
141. Lee CT, Bilton SD, Famiglietti RM, et al. Treatment planning with protons for pediatric retinoblastoma, medulloblastoma, and pelvic sarcoma: how do protons compare with other conformal techniques? *Int J Radiat Oncol Biol Phys* 2005;63:362–372.

151. Shields CL, Shields JA, Cater J, et al. Plaque radiotherapy for retinoblastoma: Long-term tumor control and treatment complications in 208 tumors. *Ophthalmology* 2001;108:2116–2121.
162. Kingston JE, Hungerford JL, Madreperla SA, et al. Results of combined chemotherapy and radiotherapy for advanced intraocular retinoblastoma. *Arch Ophthalmol* 1996;114:1339–1343.
168. Abramson DH, Frank CM, Dunkel IJ. A phase I/II study of subconjunctival carboplatin for intraocular retinoblastoma. *Ophthalmology* 1999;106:1947–1950.
170. Gobin YP, Dunkel IJ, Marr BP, et al. Intra-arterial chemotherapy for the management of retinoblastoma: four-year experience. *Arch Ophthalmol* 2011;129:732–737.
171. Abramson DH, Marr BP, Dunkel IJ, et al. Intra-arterial chemotherapy for retinoblastoma in eyes with vitreous and/or subretinal seeding: 2-year results. *Br J Ophthalmol* 2012;96:499–502.
177. Kremens B, Wieland R, Reinhard H, et al. High-dose chemotherapy with autologous stem cell rescue in children with retinoblastoma. *Bone Marrow Transplant* 2003;31:281–284.
184. Isobe K, Ejima Y, Tokumaru S, et al. Treatment of primary intraocular lymphoma with radiation therapy: a multi-institutional survey in Japan. *Leuk Lymphoma* 2006;47:1800–1805.
192. Grabenbauer GG, Schuchardt U, Buchfelder M, et al. Radiation therapy of optico-hypothalamic gliomas (OHG)-radiographic response, vision and late toxicity. *Radiother Oncol* 2000;54:239–245
193. Combs SE, Schulz-Ertner D, Moschos D, et al. Fractionated stereotactic radiotherapy of optic pathway gliomas: tolerance and long-term outcome. *Int J Radiat Oncol Biol Phys* 2005;62:814–819.
197. Bolek TW, Moyses HM, Marcus RB Jr, et al. Radiotherapy in the management of orbital lymphoma. *Int J Radiat Oncol Biol Phys* 1999;44:31–36.
200. Hashimoto N, Sasaki R, Nishimura H, et al. Long-term outcome and patterns of failure in primary ocular adnexal mucosa-associated lymphoid tissue lymphoma treated with radiotherapy. *Int J Radiat Oncol Biol Phys* 2012;82:1509–1514.
211. Shields JA, Demirci H, Marr BP, et al. Sebaceous carcinoma of the eyelids. Personal experience with 60 cases. *Ophthalmology* 2004;111:2151–2157.
218. Anderson GJ, Tom LW, Womer RB, et al. Rhabdomyosarcoma of the head and neck in children. *Arch Otolaryngol Head Neck Surg* 1990;116:428.
225. McDonald MW, Esiashvili N, George BA, et al. Intensity-modulated radiotherapy with use of cone-down boost for pediatric head-and-neck rhabdomyosarcoma. *Int J Radiat Oncol Biol Phys* 2008;72:884–891.

Chapter 39
Ear

Tony J.C. Wang and K.S. Clifford Chao

ANATOMY

The external, middle, and inner components of the ear develop from the three embryonic layers: ectoderm, mesoderm, and endoderm.

The external ear consists of the auricle or pinna, the external auditory meatus (canal), and the tympanic membrane (Fig. 39.1). The auricle is composed of elastic cartilage covered with skin. The external auditory meatus connects the tympanic membrane to the exterior and is approximately 2.4 cm long. The outer third is cartilaginous, and the inner two-thirds is bony and slightly narrower. The external auditory canal is anterior to the mastoid process and posterior to the parotid gland at the temporomandibular joint. The inferior border of the canal lies near the jugular bulb and the facial nerve as it descends through the stylomastoid foramen. The skin lining the auditory canal is continuous with that of the auricle, and in the outer one-third of the canal, it contains hair follicles and sebaceous and ceruminous glands. The tympanic membrane, which is made of multiple layers of squamous epithelium, separates the auditory canal from the middle ear.

The middle ear houses the auditory ossicles, the tympanic cavity, and opens into the eustachian tube to communicate with the pharynx. The middle ear cavity is lined with a mucoperiosteal membrane, and the eustachian tube is lined with stratified columnar epithelium and has numerous mucous glands in the two-thirds of the tube closer to the pharynx. The overall length of the eustachian tube is 3.5 cm.[1]

The inner or internal ear lies in the petrous portion of the temporal bone and consists of the bony labyrinth and the membranous labyrinth. The membranous labyrinth, which holds the organ of hearing, is housed within the bony labyrinth. The

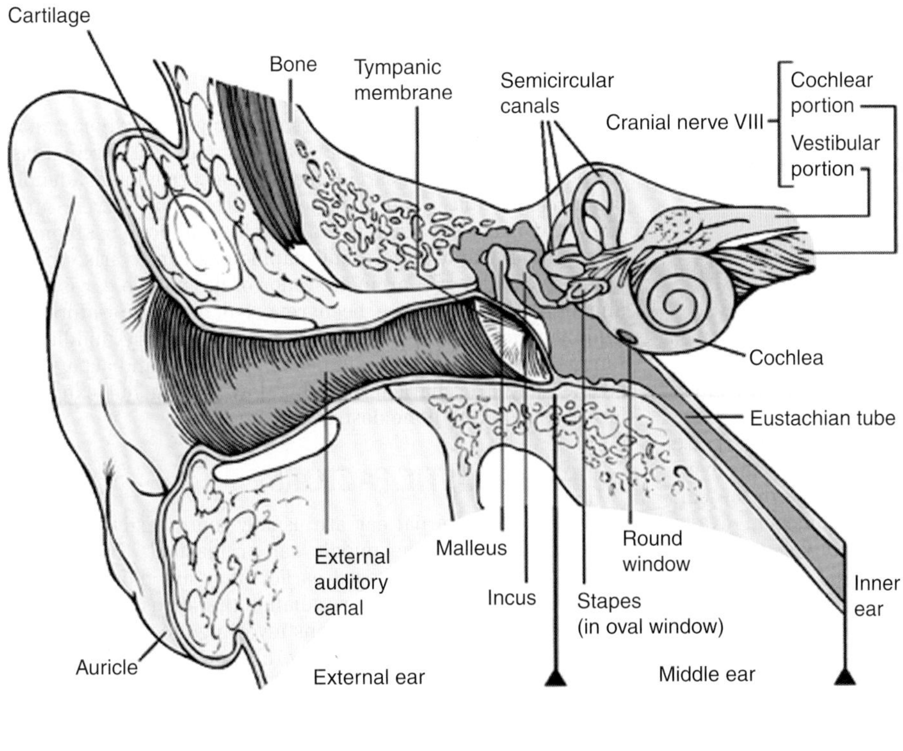

FIGURE 39.1. Ear anatomy.

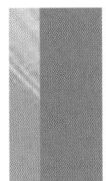

cochlea, which is responsible for hearing, and the vestibule, which is responsible for balance, are part of the inner ear.

Blood supply to the auricle and the external auditory canal come from branches of the posterior auricular artery and the superficial temporal artery, which arise from the external carotid artery. Blood is supplied to the middle ear region from branches of ascending pharyngeal and middle meningeal arteries and from the artery of the pterygoid canal. The inner ear is supplied by the internal auditory artery, which is a branch of the basilar artery, and from the anterior inferior cerebellar artery.

The nerves innervating the ear include cranial nerves V, VIII, IX, and X. The eighth cranial nerve or vestibulocochlear nerve is responsible for auditory and vestibular function. It exits from the brainstem between the pons and the medulla and follows the internal acoustic meatus.

For the external ear, lymphatic vessels of the tragus and anterior external portion of the auricle drain into the superficial parotid lymph nodes. The posterior and superior aspects of the auricle drain into the retroauricular lymph nodes, and the lobule drains into the superficial cervical group of lymph nodes. Lymphatics from the middle ear and the mastoid antrum pass into the parotid nodes and into the upper deep cervical lymph nodes. The lymphatics in the middle ear and eustachian tube are rather sparse, and the inner ear has no lymphatics.

EPIDEMIOLOGY

Malignant disease of the auricle is common, but cancers of the middle ear and external auditory canal are rare, with an incidence of approximately 1 per million people.[2,3] Tumors of the external ear are most often cutaneous malignancies and may be related to sun exposure.[4,5] Other predisposing factors described, although their significance is in question, are otorrhea, chronic eczema, chronic dermatologic conditions, and chronic ulcerations from trauma.[6]

Tumors of the external ear most commonly occur in patients 60 to 70 years of age; tumors of the middle ear and the mastoid are more common in patients 40 to 60 years of age.[7,8] More women than men have middle ear tumors, but more men have tumors of the external ear.[9,10]

CLINICAL PRESENTATION

External Ear

Basal cell carcinomas are more common than squamous cell carcinomas in the external ear, with a ratio of 1.3 to 1.[7] They present as small ulcerations, mostly on the helix.[11,12] For squamous cell carcinomas, lymph node metastases occur in approximately 10% to 15%.[13] The common sites of lymph node metastases in order of frequency are the parotid gland, the upper deep cervical chain, and the postauricular nodes.[8,13] The rate of regional metastasis is higher in advanced disease and may involve the level 5 cervical lymph node group.[14]

External Auditory Canal

Most patients present with symptomatic lesions of the external auditory canal. Pruritus and pain are common. Swelling behind the ear, decreased hearing, and facial paralysis are seen in advanced cases. Spread of the tumor into the lymphatic areas is more common than to other areas of the ear. Tumors arising in the cartilaginous portion of the canal invade the cartilaginous walls and spread into the bony canal areas. However, those arising in the bony canal have a more effective barrier (preventing spread), and therefore progress predominantly along the main axis of the canal, eventually invading the middle ear or the cartilaginous part of the canal. Distant metastases are rare.

TABLE 39.1 DIAGNOSTIC EVALUATION FOR CARCINOMA OF THE EAR

History
Physical examination
Otoscopy
Neurologic exam for cranial nerve function
Careful assessment of regional lymph nodes
Laboratory tests
Complete blood count
Blood chemistry
Radiographic studies
High-resolution computed tomography (standard)
Magnetic resonance imaging (selected patients)
Arteriography (optional)
Biopsy
Other studies
Audiology testing

DIAGNOSTIC WORKUP

Table 39.1 summarizes workup and diagnostic procedures. A history and physical including otoscopy and careful lymph node exam should be performed. Neurologic exam finding of cranial nerve deficits may be an indication of advanced disease. A baseline audiology testing should be performed prior to any treatment.

Both multidetector computed tomography (CT) and magnetic resonance imaging (MRI) play an important role in visualizing tumors of the ear.[15] CT can show abnormal soft tissue, soft tissue enhancement, distortion of the normal tissue planes, and bone destruction (Fig. 39.2). Recent advances in CT allows evaluation not only of temporal bone, infratemporal fossa, and base of skull, but also of the anatomic structures of the middle and inner ear in greater detail.[16] CT scans can help to determine the extension and the operability of tumors.[17,18] Sometimes magnetic resonance imaging can provide excellent delineation of soft tissue tumor margins, muscle infiltration, intracranial extension, and vessel encasement.[19,20] Except in selected cases, angiography and jugular venography have also been abandoned in favor of CT.

Diagnosis is always established by biopsy and occasionally by aspiration of the exudative material or by surgical exploration. A bone scan may be done to determine the changes in the temporal bone around the tumor, but it provides very nonspecific information and is not a recommended method of evaluation.

PATHOLOGIC CLASSIFICATION

Approximately 85% of the tumors involving the auditory canal, middle ear, and mastoid area are squamous cell carcinomas. Infrequently, basal cell carcinomas, adenocarcinomas, adenoid cystic carcinomas, and melanomas are seen.[21] Even rarer are sarcomas, specifically embryonic rhabdomyosarcomas. Ceruminous gland tumors and papillomas rarely arise in the auditory canal.[6,21,22] Carcinoid tumor of the middle ear is rare, and only 50 cases have been reported in the literature.[23,24] Endolymphatic sac tumor, or aggressive papillary middle ear tumors, are distinct from middle ear adenomas and act aggressively. They are characterized by slow growth but extensive local invasion and bone destruction.[25,26]

PROGNOSTIC FACTORS

Lesions of the external ear are usually more easily controlled than are lesions of the middle ear or mastoid. External ear lesions are usually diagnosed earlier; they are mostly cutaneous, and adequate surgery or radiation therapy is usually effective.[8,27,28] Presence of large lesions involving the middle ear and those with extension into the temporal bone is a poor prognostic sign and more difficult to treat.[2,29,30] There does not appear to be

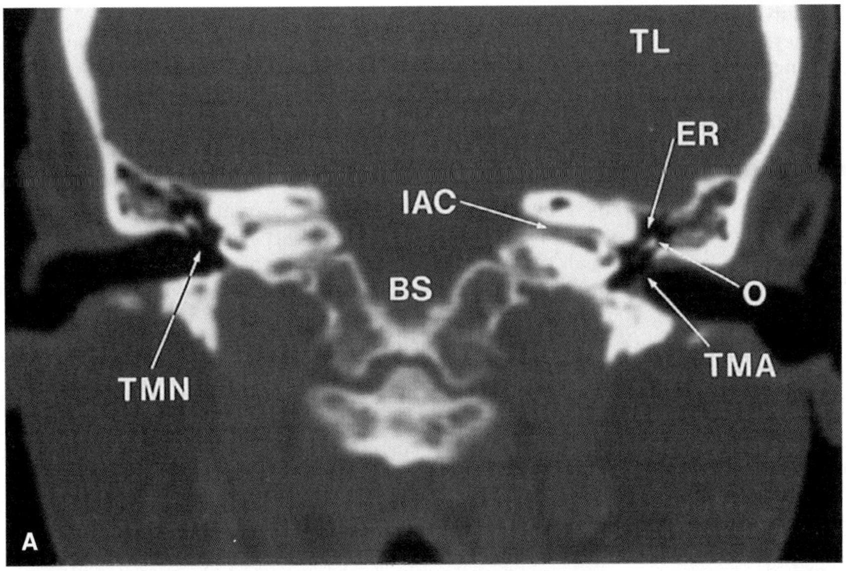

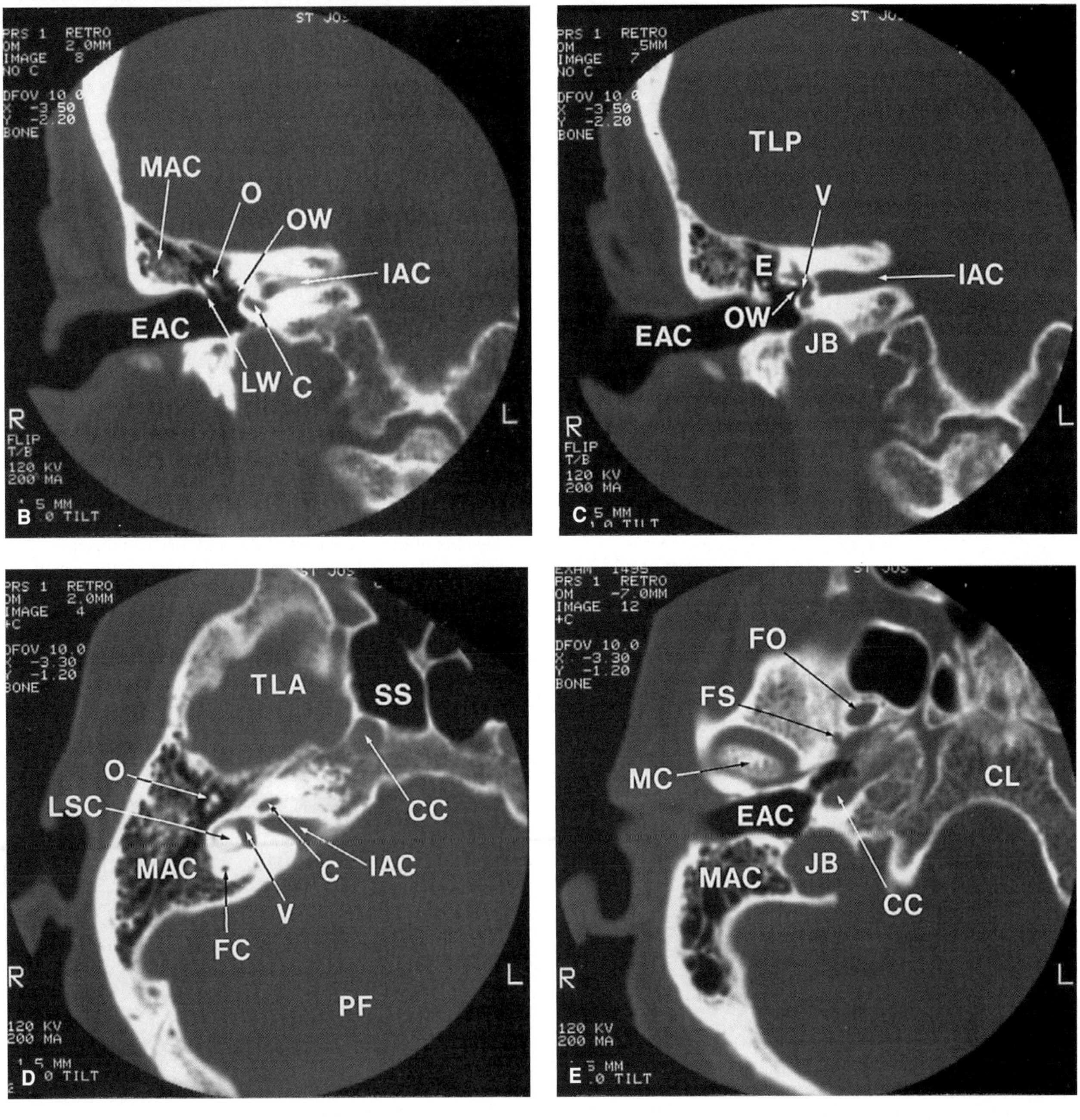

FIGURE 39.2. Normal anatomy of the ear. **A–C:** Coronal sections. **D, E:** Transverse sections. BS, brainstem; C, cochlea; CC, carotid canal; CL, clivus; E, epitympanum; EAC, external auditory canal; ER, epitympanic recess; FC, facial canal; FO, foramen ovale; FS, foramen spinosum; IAC, internal auditory canal; JB, jugular bulb; LSC, lateral semicircular canal; LW, lateral wall, epitympanic recess (scutum); MAC, mastoid air cells; MC, mandibular condyle; OS, ossicles; OW, oval window; PF, posterior fossa; TLA, temporal lobe, anterior portion; TLP, temporal lobe, posterior portion; TMN, tympanic membrane, normal appearance; TMA, tympanic membrane, abnormally thickened; SS, sphenoid sinus; V, vestibule. (Courtesy of Robert Gresick, MD, DePaul Health Center, St. Louis, MO.)

a correlation between tumor differentiation, positive margins, or perineural disease and survival, although they may serve as a predictor for local control in tumors involving the temporal bone.[29,31,32] Seventh nerve palsy associated with middle ear tumors indicates poor local control.[32,33] Spread of tumors to the lymph nodes usually indicates a poor prognosis because this is often a late event in the natural history of the disease.[34]

STAGING

The seventh edition of the American Joint Committee on Cancer (AJCC) staging manual[35] includes the external ear in its staging system under Cutaneous Squamous Cell Carcinoma and Other Cutaneous Carcinomas (Table 39.2). A group from the University of Pittsburgh proposed a staging system for squamous cell carcinoma of the external auditory canal and temporal bone, which was updated in 2002.[36–38] The primary tumor stage is determined by the level of bony erosion, size, and involvement of the middle ear. Lymph node disease is considered advanced stage with poor prognosis. This staging system has often been cited in the literature.[2,39–48]

TABLE 39.2 THE AMERICAN JOINT COMMITTEE ON CANCER AND INTERNATIONAL UNION AGAINST CANCER STAGING SYSTEM FOR EAR CANCER

Stage	*Staging Criteria*		
T Category			
Tx	Primary tumor cannot be assessed		
T0	No evidence of primary tumor		
Tis	Carcinoma *in situ*		
T1	Tumor 2 cm or less in greatest dimension with fewer than two high-risk features[a]		
T2	Tumor >2 cm in greatest dimension or tumor any size with two or more high-risk features[a]		
T3	Tumor with invasion of maxilla, mandible, orbit, or temporal bone		
T4	Tumor with invasion of skeleton (axial or appendicular) or perineural invasion of skull base		
N Category			
Nx	Regional lymph nodes cannot be assessed		
N0	No regional lymph node metastases		
N1	Metastasis in a singly ipsilateral lymph node, 3 cm or less in greatest dimension		
N2a	Metastasis in a single ipsilateral lymph node, >3 cm but not >6 cm in greatest dimension		
N2b	Metastasis in multiple ipsilateral lymph nodes, none >6 cm in greatest dimension		
N3c	Metastasis in bilateral or contralateral lymph nodes, none >6 cm in greatest dimension		
N3	Metastasis in a lymph node, >6 cm in greatest dimension		
M Category			
M0	No distant metastases		
M1	Distant metastases		
Stage Grouping			
0	Tis	N0	M0
I	T1	N0	M0
II	T2	N0	M0
III	T3	N0	M0
	T1	N1	M0
	T2	N1	M0
	T3	N1	M0
IV	T1	N2	M0
	T2	N2	M0
	T3	N2	M0
	T any	N3	M0
	T4	N any	M0
	T any	N any	M1

[a]High-risk features for the primary tumor (T) staging include depth of invasion >2-mm thickness, Clark level ≥ IV, and perineural invasion; anatomic location primary site on ear or hair-bearing lip; poorly differentiated or undifferentiated.

Used with the permission of the American Joint Committee on Cancer (AJCC), Chicago, Illinois. The original source for this material is American Joint Committee on Cancer. *AJCC cancer staging handbook,* 7th ed. New York: Springer, 2010.

GENERAL MANAGEMENT

External Ear

Tumors of the external ear are most often treated with limited surgery or external radiation therapy. Treatment in early stages with irradiation is usually in the form of megavoltage electron beam therapy or orthovoltage.[49,50] Most radiation techniques have been fairly successful in the treatment of lesions in this area, with local control rates of 80% to 97%.[27,51–53] Caccialanza et al.[27] reported a 5-year cure rate of 78% with a mean follow-up of 2.4 years for 115 carcinomas of the pinna treated with definitive kilovoltage radiation to a total dose of 45 to 70 Gy in 2.5- to 5-Gy fractions given two to three times per week. Surgery is beneficial if the lesion has invaded the cartilage of the ear or extends medially into the auditory canal. If squamous cell carcinoma of the external ear is treated with surgery alone, there is a recurrence rate of 14% to 19%.[8,54] Mohs surgery is another option, with reported local recurrence rates of 5% to 7%.[28,55] Advanced lesions involving a significant portion of the ear canal are managed with a combination of irradiation and surgery. Palmer and Snell[56] describe the use of radical soft tissue and subtotal temporal bone excision with deltopectoral flap coverage for extensive tumors of the auricular area.

Treatment of draining lymphatics is normally not required for early stages of external ear tumors.[12] Afzelius et al.[11] indicate that lesions >4 cm and those with cartilage invasion have an increased risk of nodal spread; they recommend prophylactic neck dissection.[57] Most investigators do not agree with this approach because the overall chance of lymph node involvement in tumors of the external ear is only 16%. Osborne et al.[58] reported that parotidectomy may be unnecessary in management of advanced auricular carcinoma without clinically positive parotid disease.

Interstitial irradiation using afterloading ^{192}Ir, particularly for tumors smaller than 4 cm, is also an effective method of treatment, affording excellent local control with good cosmesis[31,53] (Table 39.3).

Radical surgery followed by postoperative radiation therapy is an acceptable method of treatment for more advanced lesions of the external auditory canal and lesions in the middle ear and mastoid.[30,46,59] Pfreundner et al.[30] recommended a postoperative radiotherapy dose of 54 to 60 Gy for patients with negative margins. Positive margins warrant higher doses of 66 Gy because of higher recurrence rates. Except in tumors that are detected early, neither modality alone is considered optimal, and a combination of the two produces the best results.

Lesions of the outer part of the auditory canal require local excision with at least a 1-cm margin between the lesion and the tympanic membrane if there is no radiographic evidence of invasion of the mastoid. Surgery for tumors of the auditory canal is performed through a U-shaped incision with elevation of the flap from below. A split-thickness skin graft is usually required to cover the deficit along the auditory canal.

When the tumor involves the bony auditory canal and impinges on the tympanic membrane but does not involve the middle ear or the mastoid, a partial temporal bone resection

TABLE 39.3 TREATMENT OF CARCINOMA OF THE EXTERNAL EAR

	Modality	
Result	*Surgery*	*Irradiation*
Cure at 3 yr (34)	330/358 (92%)[a]	141/174 (81%)
Cure at 5 yr (27)		(78%)
Local control at 2 yr (28,52)	82/87 (94%)[b]	60/62 (97%)
Local control at 2 yr (50)		(86%)[c]
Local control at 4 yr (53)		60/61 (99%)
Local control at 5 yr (51)		128/138 (93%)
Local control at 5 yr (50)		(79%)[c]

[a]Results given as number of successful outcomes/patient population.
[b]Treatment by Mohs micrographic surgery.
[c]Included advanced primary tumors.

may be necessary; in this procedure, the auditory canal, tympanic membrane, malleus, and incus are removed along with the temporomandibular joint, and the defect is grafted with a split-thickness skin graft. Postoperative radiation may be indicated, depending on margin status.

Middle Ear and Temporal Bone

In management of temporal bone tumors originating from the middle ear and mastoid area, surgical options include subtotal temporal bone resection, total temporal resection, lateral temporal resection, or mastoidectomy. Complete resection with clear margins may be difficult to achieve, given that important structures reside around the temporal bone.[40,57,60–63] Postoperative radiation therapy is recommended and increases local tumor control.[30,40,64,65] In studies that suggest limited benefit of postoperative irradiation, the results may be related to the extent of the tumor.[66] Given that total and subtotal temporal bone resection can result in significant morbidity, some investigators favor limited surgery with postoperative or perioperative radiation.[67,68] Chemotherapy has not been beneficial in tumors of the ear. A study on preoperative chemoradiotherapy suggested improvement in estimated survival of advanced disease, but additional trials are necessary to determine efficacy.[69]

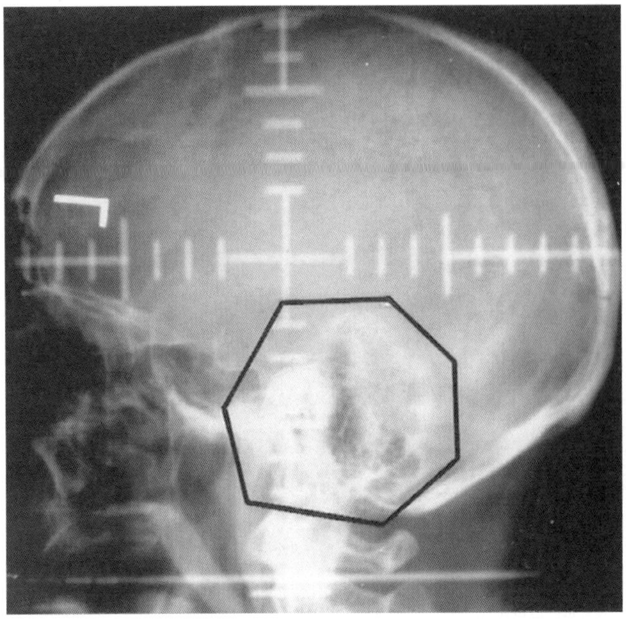

FIGURE 39.3. Example of treatment portal for tumor of the middle ear involving the petrous bone. The mastoid is included in irradiated volume.

RADIATION THERAPY TECHNIQUES

Tumors involving the pinna can be treated with megavoltage electrons or with superficial or orthovoltage irradiation. The fields can be round or polygonal, drawn around the tumor to spare surrounding normal tissues. For small, superficial tumors, margins of 1 cm are adequate. However, more extensive lesions require large portals, which may encompass the entire pinna or external canal and require 2- to 3-cm margins around the clinically apparent tumor (Fig. 39.3). Lesions involving the pinna must be treated with slow fractionation (1.8 to 2 Gy daily) to prevent cartilage necrosis. Doses of 66 Gy over a period of 6.5 weeks are required to achieve adequate tumor control.

Large lesions of the external auditory canal are treated with radiation or combined with surgery; the portals should encompass the entire ear and temporal bone with an adequate margin (3 cm). The volume treated should include the ipsilateral preauricular, postauricular, and subdigastric lymph nodes. Treating lymphatics beyond the jugulodigastric area is usually not necessary.

The use of intensity-modulated radiotherapy (IMRT) can help improve target coverage and spare normal critical structures. Careful understanding of lymphatic drainage and tumor extension is crucial for target delineation and to avoid geographic miss. Pretreatment CT or MRI scans should be reviewed along with any operative or pathology reports.

In the definitive treatment of advanced external auditory canal or middle ear cancers, gross target volume (GTV) should include the clinical and radiographic gross disease (Fig. 39.4). Clinical target volume 1 (CTV1) should encompass the GTV with a 0.3- to 0.5-cm margin to a dose of 66 to 70 Gy at 2 Gy per fraction. CTV2 should include CTV1 with a 0.5- to 0.7-cm

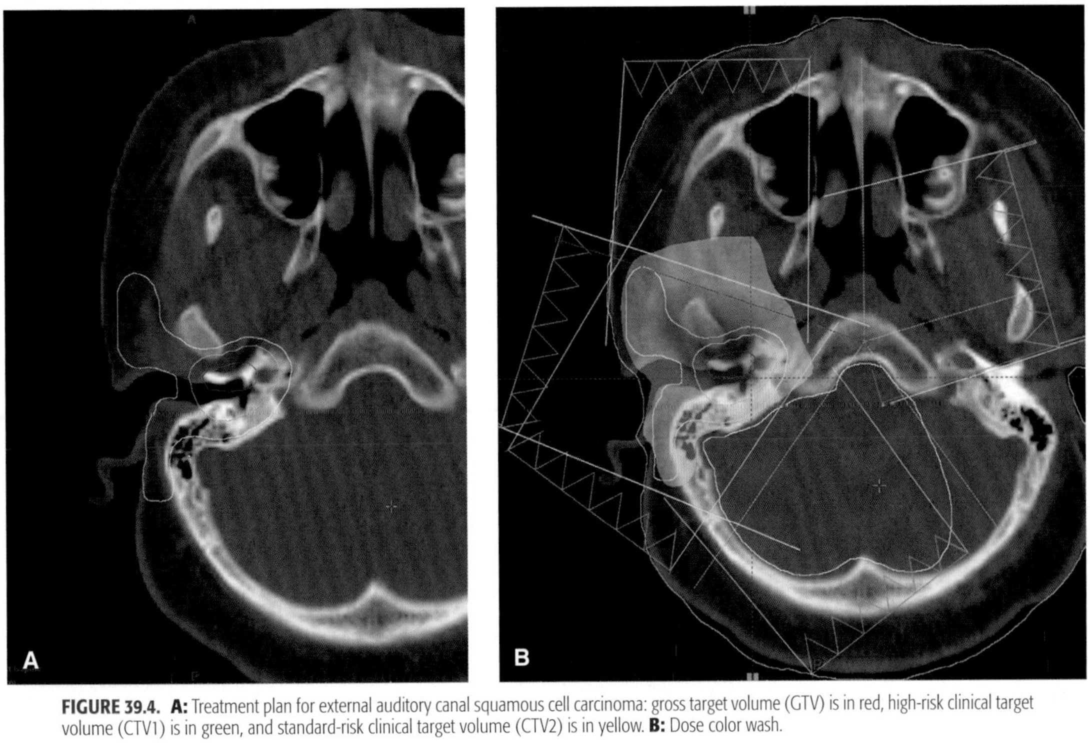

FIGURE 39.4. A: Treatment plan for external auditory canal squamous cell carcinoma: gross target volume (GTV) is in red, high-risk clinical target volume (CTV1) is in green, and standard-risk clinical target volume (CTV2) is in yellow. **B:** Dose color wash.

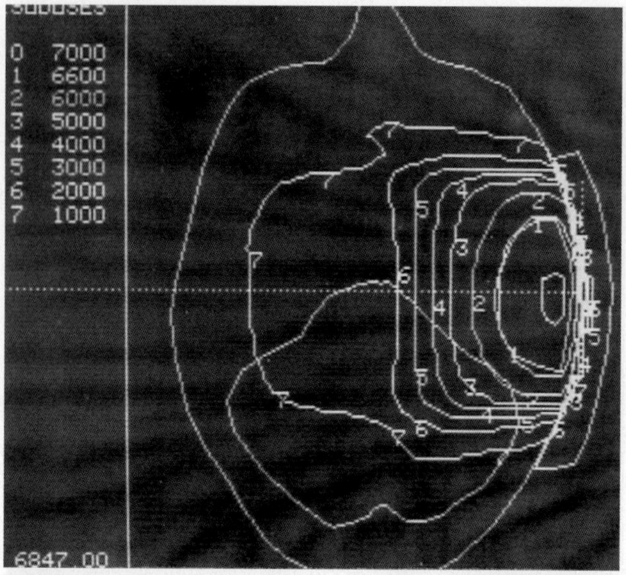

FIGURE 39.5. Computerized isodose distribution for treatment of a middle ear tumor using a combination of 4-MV photons (20%) and 16-MeV electrons (80%).

margin, as well as the preauricular nodes, postauricular nodes, ipsilateral upper cervical neck (level II), and parotid gland to a dose of 63 Gy at 1.8 Gy per fraction. A CTV3 can be considered for some patients with more advanced and aggressive tumors for treatment of the ipsilateral middle and lower neck (level III and IV) and contralateral upper neck (level II) to a dose of 56 Gy at 1.6 Gy per fraction. Planning target volumes are created with a 3- to 5-mm margin around the CTVs.

Chen et al.[64] described the target volumes for postoperative IMRT of the external auditory canal and middle ear. In the postoperative setting, CTV1 includes the original tumor region, surgical bed, soft tissue invasion, areas with positive residual disease, or positive margins to a dose of 60 to 66 Gy at 2 Gy per fraction. CTV2 includes CTV1 with a 0.5- to 0.7-cm margin, depending on the anatomy, and the ipsilateral upper neck (level II), including the parotid region, to a dose of 54 to 60 Gy at 1.8 Gy per fraction. In some patients, CTV3 is included to cover the ipsilateral middle to low neck (level III and IV) with or without the contralateral upper neck (level II) to a dose of 50 to 54 Gy at 1.6 Gy per fraction. Plans should be optimized to cover 95% of the planning target volume with 100% of the prescribed dose.

Extremely advanced tumors that are unresectable should be treated with high-energy ipsilateral electron beam therapy (16 to 20 MeV) alone or mixed with photons (4 to 6 MV), wedge pair (superior inferiorly angled beams) techniques using low-energy photons, or IMRT. IMRT is a reasonable option if nodal coverage is indicated. Doses of 60 to 70 Gy over 6 to 7 weeks are required. Doses higher than this may produce osteoradionecrosis of the temporal bone. If various types of radiation therapy beams are available, individualized treatment plans should be devised (Fig. 39.5). Most patients receiving radiation therapy to the middle ear and temporal bone regions benefit from immobilization devices such as the Aquaplast system. When electron beam radiation therapy is used, use of water bolus in the external auditory canal and concha may reduce the auricular complications.

Palliative Radiation Therapy

Radiation therapy offers significant palliation in recurrent or advanced disease. Pain relief is reported in 61% of patients with tumors of the auditory canal and middle ear.[70] Recurrences developing after previous irradiation may be re-treated with low-dose radiation therapy and hope for control of tumor in approximately 20% of patients.[71] When a small-volume local recurrence occurs after previous radiation therapy, fractionated high–dose-rate treatment may be considered.

TABLE 39.4 TREATMENT OF CARCINOMA OF THE EXTERNAL AUDITORY CANAL AND MIDDLE EAR

		Modality		
Investigators	*Published*	*Surgery*	*Radiation Therapy*	*Surgery and Radiation Therapy*
Madsen et al.[2]	2008	11/18 (61%)[a]	7/26 (27%)	12/24 (50%)
Pemberton et al.[72]	2006		49/123 (40%)	
Moody et al.[38]	2000	4/4 (100%) early[b] 0/5 (0%) advanced		7/8 (88%) early 4/15 (27%) advanced
Pfreundner et al.[30]	1999			13/21 (62%)
Zhang et al.[68]	1999		3/11 (27%)	12/20 (60%)
Testa et al.[47]	1997	29/44 (66%)	3/9 (33%)	9/15 (60%)
Gabriele et al.[71]	1994		9/15 (60%)	9/11 (82%)
Liu et al.[32]	1993		3/13 (23%)	8/15 (54%)
Birzgalis et al.[33]	1992		8/10 (80%) early 10/39 (26%) advanced	
Tiwari et al.[73]	1992			10/23 (41%)[c]
Spector[76]	1991			26/34 (76%)[d]
Korzeniowski and Pszon[74]	1990			18/29 (53%)[e]

[a]Results given as patients surviving 5 yr/patient population.
[b]Two-year overall survival. [c]Three-year overall survival.
[d]Three-year disease-free survival. [e]Some patients had biopsy only.

RESULTS OF THERAPY

The series of patients reported from several institutions are small. Results of treatment with various modalities are shown in Table 39.4. In more extensive lesions, combinations of surgery and irradiation have yielded satisfactory results. Overall 5-year survival rates with combination therapy for tumors involving the middle ear and external auditory canal range from 40% to 60%, whereas patients with early-stage tumors achieve a 70% 5-year survival rate with no evidence of disease.

Data from a multi-institutional series (Fig. 39.6) indicate that there is a negative association between disease-free survival and extent of disease using the University of Pittsburgh staging system.[46] These data also provide evidence of the

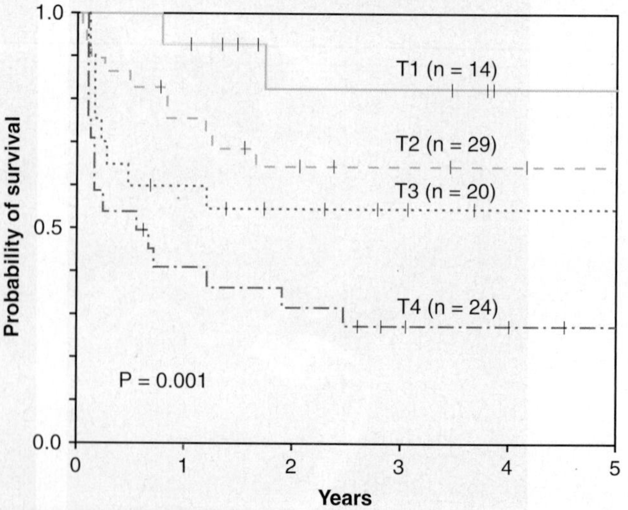

FIGURE 39.6. Data from patients with tumors of middle ear and external auditory canal from a multi-institutional series demonstrate the association between disease-free survival and extent of disease using the University of Pittsburgh staging system. (From Ogawa K, Nakamura K, Hatano K, et al. Treatment and prognosis of squamous cell carcinoma of the external auditory canal and middle ear: a multi-institutional retrospective review of 87 patients. *Int J Radiat Oncol Biol Phys* 2007;68:1326–1324; with permission from Elsevier.)

TABLE 39.5 NORMAL TISSUE DOSE CONSTRAINTS	
Structure	Constraints
Brainstem	Maximum <60 Gy
Spinal cord	Maximum <45 Gy
Cochlea	Mean dose <45 Gy
Optic nerve	Maximum <55 Gy
Optic chiasm	Maximum <55 Gy
Lens	Maximum <45 Gy
Larynx	Mean dose <44 Gy; maximum <66 Gy
Oral Cavity	Mean dose <35 Gy
Parotid gland	Combined parotid glands mean dose <25 Gy or spare one parotid gland mean dose <20 Gy
Temporal bone	Limit to <70 Gy to reduce osteoradionecrosis chance

success of combined surgery and postoperative irradiation for malignancies of the temporal bone.[31,75,76]

NORMAL-TISSUE COMPLICATIONS

Organs at risk should include the brainstem, spinal cord, cochlea, eye, optic nerve, chiasm, lens, larynx, oral cavity, parotid glands, and temporal bone. Normal-tissue constraints are given in Table 39.5.

For conventionally fractionated radiation therapy, the mean dose to the cochlea should be limited to less or equal to 45 Gy, or more conservatively 35 Gy, to reduce sensorineural hearing loss.[77] Modeling of some of the sensorineural hearing loss data from the Quantitative Analysis of Normal Tissue Effects in the Clinic studies are presented in (Fig. 39.7). The phenomenological binomial equation of Zaider and Amols was used.[78] Chen et al.[79] noted that hearing loss at a given radiation dose increased as frequency of the sound increased. The data are reasonably covered by theoretical curves having a characteristic dose (parameter α_2) of about 10 Gy.

SEQUELAE OF TREATMENT

Possible sequelae with surgery are hemorrhage, infection, loss of facial nerve function, and, rarely, carotid artery thrombosis. Occasionally, vertigo is reported after temporal bone resection. Vertigo may last for 2 weeks, and a period of unsteadiness may last for a few months. Permanent deafness usually occurs on the operated side.

Radiation therapy sequelae include cartilage necrosis of the external auditory canal and osteoradionecrosis of temporal bone.[12,80] Very rarely, secondary infection and meningitis are reported.[10] Because of the proximity of the brainstem and medulla oblongata, it is extremely difficult to deliver a high dose of irradiation to the temporal bone without a significant risk of injury to these structures. An overall 10% incidence of bone necrosis can be expected after administration of 60 to 65 Gy. After external ear lesions are treated with interstitial irradiation, there is a 4% incidence of late cutaneous and cartilage necrosis. Risk of necrosis increases for lesions >4 cm.[53] A majority of patients can experience acute grade 2 and 3 skin toxicities with postoperative IMRT.[64] Following definitive or postoperative radiation, there is a 30% incidence of xerostomia.[59]

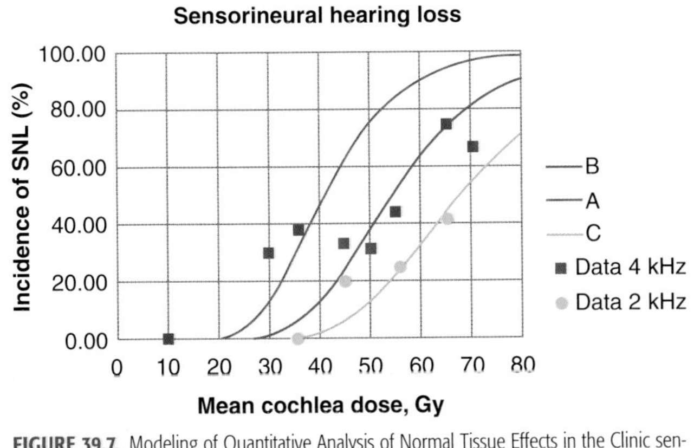

FIGURE 39.7. Modeling of Quantitative Analysis of Normal Tissue Effects in the Clinic sensorineural hearing loss data using the phenomenological binomial equation of Zaider and Amols.[77,78] Data for 2 kHz are shown as circles and those for 4 kHz as squares. All points are taken from Figure 1a, b of Bhandare et al.[77] Theoretical curves use a simple two-parameter variant of the nested exponential equation (10) of Zaider and Amols[78]: $P(D) = 100\ \exp[-\alpha_1 \exp(-\alpha_2 D)]$. The three curves are drawn with $\alpha_1 = 40$; the central curve has $1/\alpha_2 = 13.3$ Gy **(B)**, and outer curves are for $1/\alpha_2 =$ **(A)** green, 10 Gy and **(C)** blue, 16 Gy. SNHL, sensorineural hearing loss. (From Burri RJ. Ear. In: Chao C, Perez CA, Brady LW, eds. *Radiation oncology: management decisions.* Philadelphia: Lippincott Williams & Wilkins, 2011:203–209.)

SELECTED REFERENCES

A full list of references for this chapter is available online.

2. Madsen AR, Gundgaard MG, Hoff CM, et al. Cancer of the external auditory canal and middle ear in Denmark from 1992 to 2001. *Head Neck* 2008;30:1332–1338.
7. Ahmad I, Das Gupta AR. Epidemiology of basal cell carcinoma and squamous cell carcinoma of the pinna. *J Laryngol Otol* 2001;115:85–86.
11. Afzelius LE, Gunnarsson M, Nordgren H. Guidelines for prophylactic radical lymph node dissection in cases of carcinoma of the external ear. *Head Neck Surg* 1980;2:361–365.
13. Clark RR, Soutar DS. Lymph node metastases from auricular squamous cell carcinoma. A systematic review and meta-analysis. *J Plast Reconstr Aesthet Surg* 2008;61:1140–1147.
14. Peiffer N, Kutz JW Jr, Myers LL, et al. Patterns of regional metastasis in advanced stage cutaneous squamous cell carcinoma of the auricle. *Otolaryngol Head Neck Surg* 2011;144:36–42.
17. Arriaga M, Curtin HD, Takahashi H, et al. The role of preoperative CT scans in staging external auditory meatus carcinoma: radiologic-pathologic correlation study. *Otolaryngol Head Neck Surg* 1991;105:6–11.
27. Caccialanza M, Piccinno R, Kolesnikova L, et al. Radiotherapy of skin carcinomas of the pinna: a study of 115 lesions in 108 patients. *Int J Dermatol* 2005;44:513–517.
28. Silapunt S, Peterson SR, Goldberg LH. Squamous cell carcinoma of the auricle and Mohs micrographic surgery. *Dermatol Surg* 2005;31:1423–1427.
30. Pfreundner L, Schwager K, Willner J, et al. Carcinoma of the external auditory canal and middle ear. *Int J Radiat Oncol Biol Phys* 1999;44:777–788.
32. Liu FF, Keane TJ, Davidson J. Primary carcinoma involving the petrous temporal bone. *Head Neck* 1993;15:39–43.
36. Arriaga M, Curtin H, Takahashi H, et al. Staging proposal for external auditory meatus carcinoma based on preoperative clinical examination and computed tomography findings. *Ann Otol Rhinol Laryngol* 1990;99:714–721.
37. Hirsch BE. Staging system revision. *Arch Otolaryngol Head Neck Surg* 2002;128:93–94.
38. Moody SA, Hirsch BE, Myers EN. Squamous cell carcinoma of the external auditory canal: an evaluation of a staging system.*Am J Otol* 2000;21:582–588.
40. Cristalli G, Manciocco V, Pichi B, et al. Treatment and outcome of advanced external auditory canal and middle ear squamous cell carcinoma. *J Craniofac Surg* 2009;20: 816–821.
46. Ogawa K, Nakamura K, Hatano K, et al. Treatment and prognosis of squamous cell carcinoma of the external auditory canal and middle ear: a multi-institutional retrospective review of 87 patients. *Int J Radiat Oncol Biol Phys* 2007;68:1326–1334.
47. Testa JR, Fukuda Y, Kowalski LP. Prognostic factors in carcinoma of the external auditory canal. *Arch Otolaryngol Head Neck Surg* 1997;123:720–724.
50. Silva JJ, Tsang RW, Panzarella T, et al. Results of radiotherapy for epithelial skin cancer of the pinna: the Princess Margaret Hospital experience, 1982-1993. *Int J Radiat Oncol Biol Phys* 2000;47:451–459.
51. Hayter CR, Lee KH, Groome PA, et al. Necrosis following radiotherapy for carcinoma of the pinna. *Int J Radiat Oncol Biol Phys* 1996;36:1033–1037.
52. Lim JT. Irradiation of the pinna with superficial kilovoltage radiotherapy. *Clin Oncol (R Coll Radiol)* 1992;4:236–239.
53. Mazeron JJ, Ghalie R, Zeller J, et al. Radiation therapy for carcinoma of the pinna using iridium 192 wires: a series of 70 patients. *Int J Radiat Oncol Biol Phys* 1986; 12:1757–1763.
59. Prabhu R, Hinerman RW, Indelicato DJ, et al. Squamous cell carcinoma of the external auditory canal: long-term clinical outcomes using surgery and external-beam radiotherapy. *Am J Clin Oncol* 2009;32:401–404.
64. Chen WY, Kuo SH, Chen YH, et al. Postoperative intensity-modulated radiotherapy for squamous cell carcinoma of the external auditory canal and middle ear: treatment outcomes, marginal misses, and perspective on target delineation. *Int J Radiat Oncol Biol Phys* 2012;82:1485–1493.
68. Zhang B, Tu G, Xu G, et al. Squamous cell carcinoma of temporal bone: reported on 33 patients. *Head Neck* 1999;21:461–466.
71. Gabriele P, Magnano M, Albera R, et al. Carcinoma of the external auditory meatus and middle ear. Results of the treatment of 28 cases. *Tumori* 1994;80:40–43.
72. Pemberton LS, Swindell R, Sykes AJ. Primary radical radiotherapy for squamous cell carcinoma of the middle ear and external auditory canal—an historical series. *Clin Oncol (R Coll Radiol)* 2006;18:390–394.
74. Korzeniowski S, Pszon J. The results of radiotherapy of cancer of the middle ear. *Int J Radiat Oncol Biol Phys* 1990;18:631–633.
76. Spector JG. Management of temporal bone carcinomas: a therapeutic analysis of two groups of patients and long-term followup. *Otolaryngol Head Neck Surg* 1991;104:58–66.

Chapter 40
Locally Advanced Squamous Carcinoma of the Head and Neck

David M. Brizel and David J. Adelstein

Approximately 50,000 patients are diagnosed annually with squamous cell head and neck cancer (HNC) in the United States. Worldwide, approximately 600,000 patients are afflicted. Nearly 60% of this population presents with locally advanced but nonmetastatic disease. Locoregional failure constitutes the predominant recurrence pattern, and most fatalities result from uncontrolled local and/or regional disease.

Radiotherapy (RT) alone was long the standard nonsurgical therapy for locally advanced disease. The state of the art regarding radiation dose fractionation has evolved from once-daily treatment to hyperfractionation and accelerated fractionation.[1,2,3–4] These newer strategies lead to a 7% to 10% improvement in locoregional control relative to once-daily treatment schemes. A recent meta-analysis of randomized trials testing modified fractionation schemes against conventional once-daily fractionation demonstrated that hyperfractionation was the most effective strategy, leading to an 8% absolute improvement in 5-year survival.[5] Nonetheless, even the most effective RT regimens result in local control rates of 50% to 70% and disease-free survivals (DFSs) of 30% to 40%.

This circumstance has stimulated the investigation of treatments combining RT and chemotherapy. Review articles describe in detail the different chemotherapeutic agents and RT schemes of these treatment programs.[6,7] Most trials have used sequential or neoadjuvant (induction) chemotherapy followed by RT. Randomized trials of induction cisplatin and 5-fluorouracil (5-FU) chemotherapy followed by standard fractionation versus laryngectomy and postoperative RT in advanced larynx and hypopharynx cancer performed by the Veterans Administration Cooperative Group[8] and the European Organization for the Research and Treatment of Cancer (EORTC), respectively, initially showed that larynx preservation could be achieved without compromising overall survival.

Most randomized clinical trials show the superiority of combined RT and chemotherapy to RT alone for the treatment of locally advanced, nonmetastatic HNC. A meta-analysis of individual patient data from >17,346 participants in 93 trials conducted from 1965 to 2000 (Meta-Analysis of Chemotherapy on Head and Neck Cancer [MACH-NC]) demonstrated that the use of radiotherapy and concurrent chemotherapy (CRT) resulted in a 19% reduction in the risk of death and an overall 6.5% improvement in 5-year survival compared to treatment with RT alone ($p < .0001$).[9] This benefit was predominantly attributable to a 13.5% improvement in local regional control. The 2.9% reduction in the risk of distant metastases was not statistically significant (Fig. 40.1).

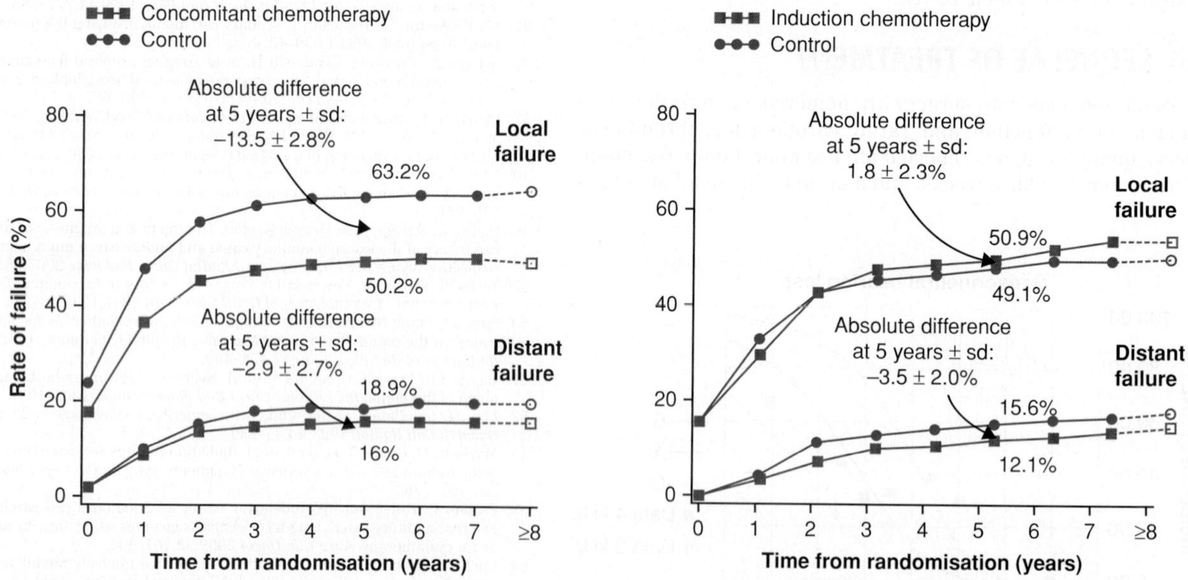

Local failure and distant failure/person-years by period

	Years 0–2	Years 3–5	Years ≥6	Years 0–2	Years 3–5	Years ≥6
Local failure						
Control	493/1648	22/406	2/165	497/2627	38/1073	10/684
Chemotherapy	373/1837	20/603	1/240	519/2749	58/1142	22/751
Distant failure						
Control	82/1756	8/416	1/166	90/2788	18/1116	8/711
Chemotherapy	83/1915	6/616	0/241	62/2929	23/1204	9/773

FIGURE 40.1. Data from the Meta-Analysis of Chemotherapy In Head and Neck Cancer (MACH-NC) illustrating that the major therapeutic benefit of platinum-based chemotherapy results from an improvement in local-regional disease control when the drugs are given concurrently with radiotherapy. No significant improvement occurs with induction chemotherapy followed by radiotherapy.

The MACH-NC also demonstrated a 2% improvement in 5-year survival from the use of induction chemotherapy followed by RT, which was not significant. A subset analysis of trials that used cisplatin and 5-FU as the induction regimen did show a 4% improvement in overall survival.[10]

Randomized comparisons of concurrent chemoradiation versus induction chemotherapy followed by radiotherapy alone are few but confirm that the former strategy is superior.[11,12] The Radiation Therapy Oncology Group (RTOG) conducted a three-arm trial of radiation alone versus radiation and concurrent cisplatin versus induction cisplatin followed by irradiation in larynx carcinoma. Concurrent therapy constituted the most effective means of larynx preservation and provided the best disease control, albeit without a statistically significant survival benefit.[12] Neoadjuvant chemotherapy followed by RT was no more efficacious than RT alone. Despite the lack of evidence supporting sequential chemoradiation strategies, this strategy was the most common method of integrating the two modalities in the community practice setting until recently.[13] A more contemporary survey has demonstrated that concurrent RT and chemotherapy is now used more frequently.[14]

RT and concurrent chemotherapy represents the most commonly used strategy and is a more attractive approach because some chemotherapeutic agents may both radiosensitize cells and provide additive cytotoxicity. The superiority of concurrent CRT relative to RT alone has been demonstrated in randomized trials in squamous cell carcinoma of other anatomic sites including the esophagus and uterine cervix.[15–17]

Certain issues must be considered when evaluating randomized trials of CRT for advanced head and neck cancer. The first consideration relates to the effectiveness of the RT-alone control arm. Specifically, does it represent optimal single-modality treatment? If the CRT regimen is more effective than RT alone but the radiation is suboptimal, then it is difficult to accurately gauge whether or not the combined-modality regimen represents a true improvement in therapy. The second consideration concerns the toxicity of CRT itself. Typically, both acute and late toxicity from CRT are greater than from RT alone.[18–20]

Acute mucositis constitutes the most significant impediment to the timely delivery of concurrent therapy. Because prolongation of total treatment time adversely affects the success of RT in HNC,[21,22–23] a major challenge has been the development of treatment schedules that integrate RT and chemotherapy and yet do not excessively increase total treatment time. A thorough understanding of toxicity is mandatory as avoidance of the functional morbidity associated with surgery in advanced head and neck cancer is one of the main reasons for the utilization of concurrent therapy in the first place.

HISTORICAL DEVELOPMENT OF RADIATION AND CONCURRENT CHEMOTHERAPY

CRT may be administered in synchronous or alternating schemes. Synchronous administration results in the delivery of RT and chemotherapy (CT) on the same days. Typically, chemotherapy will be given for 1 or more days at the initiation of RT and then repeated in the same fashion several weeks later. Alternating regimens usually sandwich RT and CT around one another. Radiation and drugs are therefore not necessarily given on the same days. In such a scheme, CT would be given during the first week of treatment with RT following in subsequent week(s) before CT is given again.

Synchronous Radiation and Single-Agent Chemotherapy

Synchronous treatment is completed more quickly than alternating treatment. It is therefore preferable from a theoretical standpoint in terms of addressing the issue of accelerated repopulation, albeit at the expense of increased acute side effects. Early randomized trials of conventionally fractionated RT and CT used single-agent chemotherapy. These studies are summarized in Table 40.1. The experimental arms of RTOG 90-03,[1] EORTC 22791,[3] and DAHANCA 6-7[4] are included to provide a basis for comparison with optimal regimens of RT alone.

Both the Northern California Oncology Group (NCOG) and the EORTC tested radiation and synchronous bleomycin against radiation therapy alone.[24,25] Acute toxicity was worse in the combined-modality arm in both trials, but the outcomes were quite different with respect to efficacy. The EORTC trial showed no improvement in DFS or survival and the RT/bleomycin combination in the NCOG program led to a statistically significant doubling of locoregional control and DFS, as well as a near-significant improvement in overall survival from 24% to 43%.

Differences in study design and execution may explain the discrepancy between outcomes in the EORTC and NCOG trials. Fractionation was similar in the two studies, but patients in the EORTC trial received 15 mg of bleomycin twice weekly during the first 5 weeks of RT for a total dose of 150 mg, whereas the NCOG patients received 5 mg twice weekly for a total dose of 70 mg. Acute mucosal and skin toxicity was worse in the RT/bleomycin arm in both trials. Toxicity significantly prolonged the RT delivery time in 30% of the combined-modality patients in the EORTC trial but not in any of the RT-alone patients. This prolongation of treatment time and associated tumor repopulation in such a large proportion of patients may have negated any benefit accrued from the use of concurrent therapy. There were no differences in overall treatment time between the two treatment arms in the NCOG trial. An important lesson from these two studies is that the dose administration schedules of concurrent chemotherapy must be carefully designed so that toxicity does not adversely affect overall treatment compliance.

The Christie Hospital in Great Britain evaluated RT and 100 mg/m^2 of single-agent methotrexate (MTX) given at the commencement of and after 2 weeks of a 3-week course of treatment.[26] Most of the 313 patients in this protocol received 50 to 55 Gy in 15 or 16 fractions. Mucositis was significantly greater in the patients receiving MTX, but there was no difference in long-term toxicity. The addition of MTX increased local control from 50% to 70% (p = .02) and survival from 37% to 47% (p = .07). The greatest benefit was seen in patients with oropharyngeal primary tumors who constituted one-third of the study population. Local control with RT/MTX was 78% versus 38% with RT alone (p = .002) in this patient subset. Survival was 25% with RT alone and 50% with RT/MTX (p = .009). Unfortunately, the data from this trial are not generally applicable to current clinical practice because of the large radiation fraction sizes that were used.

5-FU has been used in conjunction with RT more frequently than any other chemotherapeutic agent. Lo et al.[27] reported the first study to show a significant improvement in local control and survival with the addition of bolus 5-FU to RT in squamous carcinoma of the oral cavity. Browman et al.[28] compared RT and continuous infusion 5-FU against RT alone in a placebo-controlled randomized trial sponsored by the National Cancer Institute of Canada. All 175 patients received 66 Gy in 2-Gy fractions. 5-FU was given at 1,200 mg/m^2/day for the first 3 days of the first and third weeks of irradiation. Confluent mucositis was more frequent in the 5-FU arm than in the placebo arm (32% vs. 11%; p = .001), as was weight loss >15% from pretreatment baseline (41% vs. 11%; p < .0001). This increased acute toxicity did not prolong the delivery of RT in the RT/5-FU arm relative to the RT/placebo arm. Two-year DFS and survival were 30% and 50% for RT/placebo patients and 50% and 63% for RT/5-FU patients (p = .06 and .08), respectively.

The relative radioresistance of hypoxic cells *in vitro* is well understood.[29] Clinically, the existence of hypoxia both in head and neck primary tumors and metastatic lymph nodes has been described, and its adverse impact on the prognosis of patients treated with RT has been demonstrated.[30,31] Investigators from

TABLE 40.1 RANDOMIZED TRIALS OF ONCE-DAILY IRRADIATION AND CONCURRENT CHEMOTHERAPY IN ADVANCED HEAD AND NECK CANCER

Institution	*N*	*Radiotherapy*	*Chemotherapy*	*Outcome RT vs. RT/CCT; p Value*	*Comments*
RTOG 90-03 Accelerated fractionation	268	72 Gy/42 days	None	LC: 54% DFS: 39% S: 51%	
Hyperfractionation	263	81 Gy/49 days	None	LC: 54% DFS: 38% S: 54%	
DAHANCA 6-7	1,476	70 Gy/39 days	None	LC: 76% DFS: 73%	
EORTC 22791	356	80.5 Gy/47 days	None	LC: 59%	
NCOG	104	70 Gy (1.8 Gy/day)	Bleo 5 mg/m²/week weeks 1–7; synchronous	LC: 35% vs. 70%; .001 DFS: 15% vs. 31%; .04 S: 24% vs. 43%; .11	RT/CCT → ↑ acute toxicity, but RT not delayed
EORTC	224	64 Gy (1.8–2.0 Gy/day)	Bleo 15 mg/m²/week weeks 1–5; synchronous	DFS: 22% vs. 23%; NS S: 23% vs. 22%; NS	RT/CCT → ↑ acute toxicity with RT delayed in 30%
Christie Hospital	313	50–55 Gy (3.3 Gy/day)	MTX 100 mg/m² days 0, 14; synchronous	LC: 50% vs. 70%; .02 S: 37% vs. 47%; .07	Statistically significant benefit in LC and S for oropharynx
NCI Canada	175	66 Gy (2.0 Gy/day)	5-FU 1,200 mg/m² days 1–3 and 15–17; synchronous	DFS: 30% vs. 50%; .06 S: 50% vs. 63%; .08	Placebo-controlled trial
Yale University	195	68 Gy (1.8–2.0 Gy/day)	MMC 15 mg/m² days 5, 43; synchronous	LC: 54% vs. 76%; .003 S: 42% vs. 48%; NS	Predominantly postop series 1° RT in 74 patients Benefit unclear in this patient group
Cleveland Clinic	100	66–72 Gy (1.8–2.0 Gy/day)	5-FU 1,000 mg/m² CI CDDP 20 mg/m² CI Days 1–4 and 22–25; synchronous	LC: 35% vs. 55%; .02 DFS: 52% vs. 67%; .03 S: 58% vs. 58%; NS	RT/CCT ↑ toxicity but RT not delayed LC means survival with 1° site organ preservation
Princess Margaret Hospital	209	50 Gy (2.5 Gy/day)	MMC 10 mg/m² 5-FU 1,000 mg/m² CI; synchronous	LC: ~40% vs. ~40% S: ~40% vs. ~40%	RT only: continuous course RT/CTT: 4-week break after 25 Gy
NICR Italy	157	RT/CCT: 60 Gy RT: 66 Gy	5-FU 200 mg/m² bolus CDDP 20 mg/m² bolus Days 1–5, 22–26, 43–47, and 64–68; alternating	LC: 32% vs. 64%; .04 DFS: 9% vs. 21%; .008 S: 10% vs. 24%; .01	Unresectable disease RT/CCT: RT on weeks 2, 3, 5, 6, 8, and 9 RT only: ≥2 week delay in >30%
GORTEC 94-01	226	70 Gy (2 Gy/day)	Carboplatin (CBDCA) 70 mg/m² 5-FU 600 mg/m²/day CI	LC: 25% vs. 48%; .002 DFS: 15% vs. 27%; .01 S: 16% vs. 23%; .05	Significantly increased acute and late toxicity with RT/CCT
Intergroup Nasopharynx	193	70 Gy (2 Gy/day)	CDDP 100 mg/m² Days 1, 22, and 43 Post-RT CDDP/5-FU	DFS: 24% vs. 69%; <.001 S: 47% vs. 78%; .005	Early trial closure

RT/CCT, radiotherapy and concurrent chemotherapy; RTOG, Radiation Therapy Oncology Group; LC, local control; DFS, disease-free survival; S, survival; b.i.d, twice daily; EORTC, European Organization for the Research and Treatment of Cancer; NCOG, Northern California Oncology Group; Bleo, bleomycin; NS, not significant; MTX, methotrexate; 5-FU, 5-fluorouracil; NCI, National Cancer Institute; MMC, mitomycin-C; CDDP, cisplatin; CI, continuous infusion; NICR, National Institute for Cancer Research.

Yale University designed their treatment strategy around this principle. They treated 195 patients in two randomized trials with mitomycin-C (MMC). This agent is predominantly metabolized in and preferentially cytotoxic to hypoxic cells. The Yale treatment program consisted of 68 Gy ± MMC on days 1 and 43 of RT. Local control was improved with the addition of MMC from 54% to 76% (p = .003). Survival improved from 42% to 48%, but this was not statistically significant. The majority of patients in these trials received adjuvant postoperative or preoperative irradiation, however. Only 74 (38%) received definitive, primary RT, and the benefit from the addition of MMC in this subset is unclear.[32]

Synchronous Radiation and Multiagent Chemotherapy

Cisplatin (CDDP) is a radiosensitizer, too.[33] The combination of CCDP and 5-FU is also one of the most active cytotoxic drug combinations against squamous cell HNC. Consequently, investigators have incorporated both of these drugs into a variety of concurrent treatment strategies. A randomized trial from the Cleveland Clinic assigned patients to receive 66 to 72 Gy ± two cycles of synchronous CDDP (20 mg/m²/day × 4) and infusional 5-FU (1,000 mg/m²/d × 4) during weeks 1 and 4 of RT.[34] The main objective of this study was primary site organ preservation. Surgical salvage was allowed for patients with persistent disease. Acute toxicity was significantly greater in the combined-modality treatment arm, especially with respect to weight loss. Mucosal recovery usually required 8 to 12 weeks after completion of RT and chemotherapy. There were no differences in the total time required for RT delivery, however. Three-year DFS was significantly better for the patients receiving chemoradiotherapy (67% vs. 52%; p = 0.03). Three-year survival with primary site preservation was also higher in the combined-modality group (57% vs. 35%, p = .02), although there was no significant difference in overall survival.

MMC and 5-FU were used together in a trial of 209 patients conducted at the Princess Margaret Hospital.[35] Patients were treated with continuous course RT alone at 2.5 Gy/day to 50 Gy in 28 days. Patients randomized to receive RT/chemotherapy received the same dose fractionation scheme as those receiving RT alone but over a total time of 56 days due to a planned 4-week treatment interruption after 25 Gy. Bolus MMC (10 mg/m²) was given on days 1 and 43. Two cycles of continuous infusion 5-FU (1,000 mg/m²/day) were given on days 1 to 4 and 43 to 46. The intent of the treatment break was to maintain comparable levels of acute toxicity in the two treatment arms. Acute toxicity was, in fact, equivalent in the two groups. Unfortunately, however, there was no difference in 4-year local control (~40%) or survival (~40%).

The Princess Margaret trial raises an important question: can one quantify the contribution provided by concurrent chemotherapy in terms of the delivery of an equivalent dose of irradiation? Approximately 0.6 Gy/day is necessary to compensate for the tumor repopulation that transpires with each day of prolongation of standard course RT.[23] Thus, the total dose in the

Princess Margaret Hospital RT/chemotherapy arm would have to have been about 67 Gy [(2.5 Gy × 20) + (0.6 Gy/day × 28 days)] in order to have been isoeffective with the 50-Gy regimen in the RT-alone arm. The equivalent efficacy of the two treatments in this trial therefore suggests that the chemotherapy compensated for the tumor repopulation that occurred during the treatment break. Thus, one could argue that the chemotherapy was equivalent to approximately 17 Gy of additional irradiation. There can be no doubt as to the inferiority of the split-course fractionation scheme in this trial had it been delivered without chemotherapy and compared head to head against the continuous course RT regimen. Conversely, if the combined-modality treatment had been given with continuous course RT, it would quite probably have been more efficacious than the RT-only regimen.

A Spanish three-arm randomized trial (N = 859) provides additional information that is pertinent to the estimation of the radiotherapeutic dose equivalent provided by the delivery of concurrent chemotherapy.[36] Patients were assigned to receive one of the following regimens:

A. 2 Gy/day to 60 Gy/42 days,
B. 1.1 Gy twice daily to 70.4 Gy/44 days, or
C. 2 Gy/day to 60 Gy/42 days with concurrent bolus 5-FU 250 mg/m^2 given every other day.

Progression-free survival and overall survival were significantly worse in arm A as compared with arms B and C, as one would expect. Arms B and C were equally efficacious. Not accounting for the different fractionation in arms B and C and the unconventional administration of chemotherapy, it is still clear that the addition of 5-FU was comparable to dose escalation of approximately 10 Gy. A recent modeling analysis of phase III trials comparing CRT with RT only suggests that concurrent chemotherapy provides the equivalent of a 10- to 12-Gy dose escalation.[37]

Neither the Princess Margaret nor the Spanish trial delivered maximally intensive radiotherapy in their respective control arms. The rationale for treatment intensification with the addition of concurrent chemotherapy as opposed to simple RT dose escalation is weak in such a context. The situation may be dramatically different, however, when the RT-alone arm is maximally intensive such as in RTOG 90-03 or EORTC 22791. Dose escalations of 10 to 12 Gy are not possible with accelerated regimens that already deliver 72 Gy during 6 weeks or with hyperfractionated regimens delivering 79 Gy in 7 weeks (see Radiation Fractionation Scheme section). Concurrent chemotherapy, however, can be added to modified fractionation regimens ≥70 Gy.

Alternating Radiotherapy and Chemotherapy

Alternating therapy produces less acute mucosal toxicity than synchronous therapy but may prolong the overall treatment time by several weeks. Although longer treatment times adversely affect efficacy in programs of standard RT alone due to tumor repopulation, the significance of overall treatment time (for RT) in a continuous course of alternating RT and chemotherapy is controversial. Some investigators have suggested that the usual time–dose relationships do not apply.[38]

The National Institute for Cancer Research in Italy conducted a phase III trial comparing RT with alternating RT and chemotherapy in 157 patients with unresectable head and neck cancer.[39,40] The RT arm was designed to give 70 Gy/7 weeks via standard fractionation. The combined-therapy arm scheduled chemotherapy on weeks 1, 4, 7, and 10 and radiation (60 Gy) on weeks 2 to 3, 5 to 6, and 8 to 9. Each 2-week cycle of radiation consisted of 20 Gy/10 fractions. Each cycle of chemotherapy included 5 days of bolus CDDP (20 mg/m^2/day) and bolus 5-FU (200 mg/m^2/day). The incidence of grade 3/4 mucositis (18% to 19%) was the same in both treatment groups. However, RT treatment delays occurred more often in the RT-alone patients: 32% with a 1-week prolongation and 25% with a ≥2-week prolongation. Corresponding delays in the combined-modality treatment group were 11% and 15%, respectively. The median dose of RT delivered in the combined-modality-treatment group matched the planned dose of 60 Gy, but it was only 62 Gy in the RT-alone group. Five-year actuarial survival was significantly better in the combined-modality-treatment patients (24% vs. 10%; p = .01), as were DFS (21% vs. 9%, p = .008) and local control (64% vs. 32%; p = .04).

Given the similar levels of acute toxicity, it is unclear why treatment times were prolonged and total doses reduced so extensively in the RT-only patients. Better protocol compliance in the control arm might well have changed the outcome of this trial. There are no other randomized trials of RT and alternating chemotherapy. Further randomized trials of alternating therapy will be necessary to determine its true value because the deficiencies of the National Institute for Cancer Research study prevent definitive conclusions.

Despite its drawbacks, the Italian study, like the Princess Margaret Hospital trial, strongly reinforces the idea that in some settings, chemotherapy counteracts tumor repopulation during treatment. The total RT treatment time was prolonged in the combined-modality arms in both studies. The fundamental difference between these two trials is that patients received no treatment during the RT break in the Princess Margaret Hospital trial and the patients in the Italian trial received chemotherapy during each interruption of RT.

CONTEMPORARY RANDOMIZED TRIALS OF RADIOTHERAPY AND CONCURRENT CHEMOTHERAPY

Curative Intent Treatment

The French cooperative group trial, GORTEC 94-01, was performed in patients who had stage III/IV oropharyngeal carcinoma.[19,41] Radiotherapy consisted of conventional 2 Gy, once-daily fractionation to 70 Gy. Patients on the CRT arm also received three cycles of concurrent carboplatin (70 mg/m^2) and continuous infusion 5-FU (600 mg/m^2/day × 4 days). Two hundred twenty-six patients were enrolled in the trial. CRT resulted in significant improvement in 5-year locoregional control (48% vs. 25%; p = .002), DFS (27% vs. 15%; p = .01), and survival (23% vs. 16%; p = .05). This improvement in efficacy was accompanied by a significant increase in acute mucositis (grade ≥2) from 39% to 71% (p = .005). Severe acute cutaneous and hematologic toxicity and worse nutritional status were also significantly more prevalent in the patients who received combined-modality therapy. Severe late toxicity, primarily cervical fibrosis, occurred in 27% of the combined-modality patients and in 12% of those treated with RT alone (p = .04). Severe dental complications were twice as frequent in the combined-modality patients (37% vs. 18%; p = .01).

Wendt et al.[42] conducted a multi-institutional trial of CRT versus RT for patients with unresectable stage III/IV head and neck cancer. CRT patients received three cycles of cisplatin, 5-FU, and leucovorin during a 7-week period. Cisplatin was given as a 60 mg/m^2 bolus. 5-FU was given as an initial 350 mg/m^2 bolus followed by a 4-day continuous infusion of 350 mg/m^2/day. Leucovorin was also given for 4 days at 100 mg/m^2/day. Radiotherapy was given as three cycles of 23.4 Gy at 1.8 Gy bid in both treatment arms. It coincided with the chemotherapy on the CRT arms. Planned treatment breaks were given between the cycles of treatment to ameliorate treatment-induced mucositis. The cumulative dose of radiation therapy in both treatment arms was 70.2 Gy in 7 weeks.

One-third of the 270 patients enrolled had oropharynx primary tumors. CRT doubled both 3-year local control (35% vs. 17%; $p < .004$) and survival (49% vs. 24%; $p < .003$) (Fig. 40.2). As in the GORTEC 94-01 oropharyngeal trial, confluent mucositis was significantly higher (38% vs. 16%; $p < .001$) with the use of CRT.

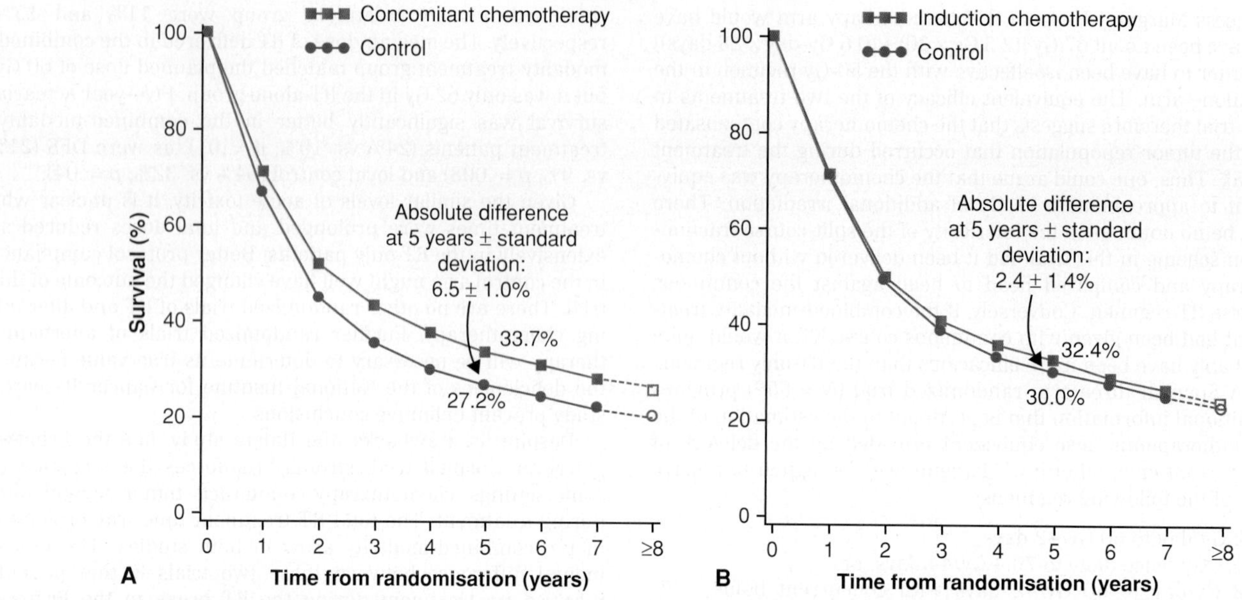

A Death/person-years by period

	Years 0–2	Years 3–5	Years ≥6
Control	2500/6298	672/3658	217/2487
Chemotherapy	2187/6647	706/4576	278/3194

B Death/person-years by period

	Years 0–2	Years 3–5	Years ≥6
Control	1283/3535	393/2276	137/1417
Chemotherapy	1318/3820	392/2608	167/1530

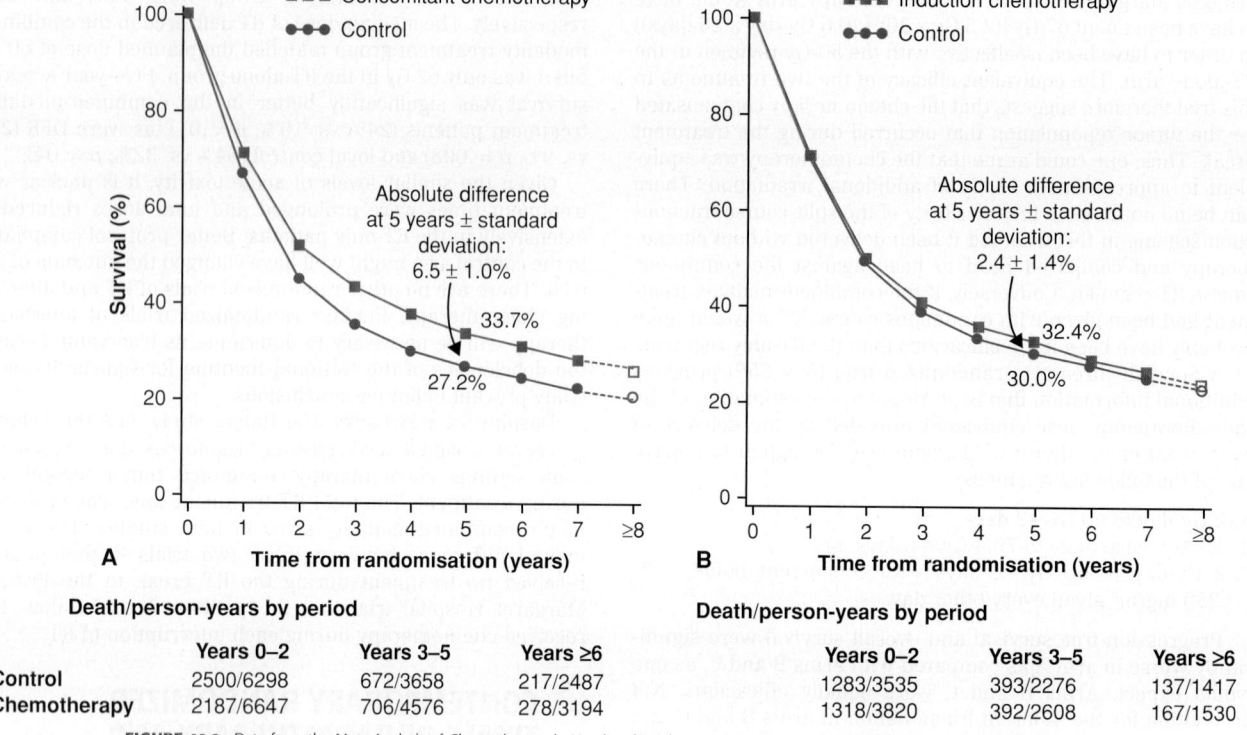

FIGURE 40.2. Data from the Meta-Analysis of Chemotherapy in Head and Neck Cancer (MACH-NC), which demonstrates that adding concurrent chemotherapy to radiotherapy provides a significant improvement in survival but that induction chemotherapy does not. **A:** Concomitant chemotherapy. **B:** Induction chemotherapy.

Treatment of advanced nasopharynx carcinoma with radiation and concurrent chemotherapy was the subject of an intergroup study in which patients in both arms received conventionally fractionated RT (1.8 to 2.0 Gy/day) to a total dose of 70 Gy.[43] Those patients who were randomized to concurrent chemotherapy also received three cycles of cisplatin during RT at a dose of 100 mg/m^2. After the completion of RT, they received an additional three cycles of cisplatin at 80 mg/m^2 as well as 4-day continuous infusions of 5-FU at 1,000 mg/m^2/day. All patients had stage III/IV, M0 disease. In spite of the initial plan of enrolling 270 patients, the trial was terminated early when an interim analysis demonstrated the superiority of the combined-modality regimen. One hundred ninety-three patients were enrolled, and the median follow-up is 2.7 years. Three-year progression-free survival favored the combined-modality patients (69% vs. 24%; $p < .001$). Similarly, 3-year survival was 78% versus 47% ($p = .005$) in favor of the patients who received concurrent chemotherapy (Fig. 40.3). Table 40.1 summarizes the data from the trials of conventionally fractionated irradiation and concurrent chemotherapy.

One must ask not only whether CRT is more effective than conventionally fractionated RT, but also whether it is superior

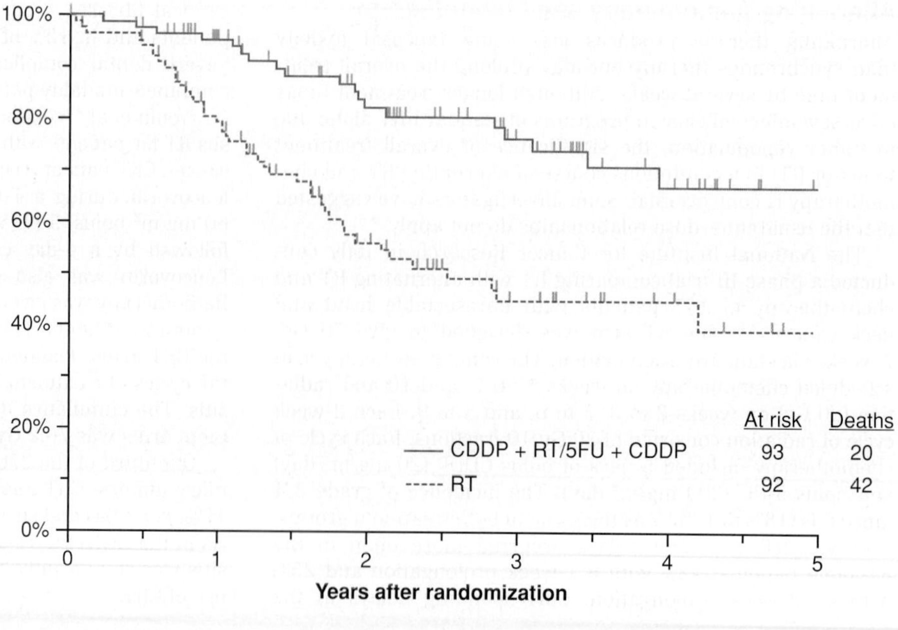

FIGURE 40.3. Three-year survival in the Intergroup Nasopharynx Carcinoma Trial was significantly better ($p = .005$) for those patients who received concurrent cisplatin and postirradiation adjuvant cisplatin/5-fluorouracil (78%) than for those who received radiotherapy alone (47%). These results led to early trial closure.

to hyperfractionated or accelerated fractionation irradiation as these strategies represent the most efficacious single-modality treatment strategies. A prospective randomized trial from Duke University provides some insight into this issue.[44] Patients with locally advanced head and neck cancer were randomized to hyperfractionated irradiation alone versus split-course hyperfractionation with concurrent CDDP/5-FU chemotherapy. Patients in the RT-alone arm received 1.25 Gy bid continuous course to 75 Gy in 6 weeks, whereas those patients on the CRT arm received 1.25 Gy bid split course to 70 Gy in 7 weeks. Chemotherapy was given during weeks 1 and 6 of irradiation (CDDP 12 mg/m^2/day × 5 days; 5-FU continuous infusion was 600 mg/m^2/day × 5 days).

The time–dose aspects of the RT in the combined-modality arm are similar to those of the previously discussed trials. The time–dose characteristics of the RT in the control arm were similar to certain aspects of both the concurrent boost arm (decreased treatment time) and the hyperfractionation arm (increased total dose) of RTOG 90-03. Most importantly, these characteristics made the RT more intensive in the control arm than in the experimental CRT arm. This study design was intentional because a primary objective of the trial was to determine whether a lower dose of RT with concurrent chemotherapy would be superior to maximally intensive/effective RT alone.

Fifty-four percent of the patients presented with unresectable disease, and approximately 40% of the primaries were located in the oropharynx. One hundred sixteen patients were enrolled, and the updated median follow-up now exceeds 5 years. Locoregional control was 70% versus 44% (p = .006), favoring the combined-modality patients. An unpublished update of the 5-year survival revealed superiority in the combined-modality patients (42% vs. 27%; p = .04) (Fig. 40.4). Confluent (grade 3) mucositis was seen in approximately 75% of the patients in both arms, the main difference being that the mean time to resolution of mucositis was 50% longer in the patients receiving radiation and concurrent chemotherapy (6 vs. 4 weeks).

Jeremic et al.[45] evaluated hyperfractionated irradiation (1.1 Gy bid to 77 Gy) with or without concurrent low-dose daily cisplatin (6 mg/m^2) in stage III/IV patients. One hundred thirty patients were enrolled; primary tumors originated in the oropharynx in approximately one-third of the population. Fifty-nine percent presented with T3 or T4 primaries, and 80% had nodal involvement. Five-year locoregional control (50% vs. 36%; p = .04), progression-free survival (46% vs. 25%; p = .007), and overall survival (46% vs. 25%; p = .007) (Fig. 40.5) were all significantly improved with the addition of concurrent chemotherapy. Of note, the distant metastasis-free survival was also improved in the concurrent therapy patients (86% vs. 57%; p = .01).

A German multicenter trial also confirmed that CRT is superior to maximally intensive single-modality irradiation.[18]

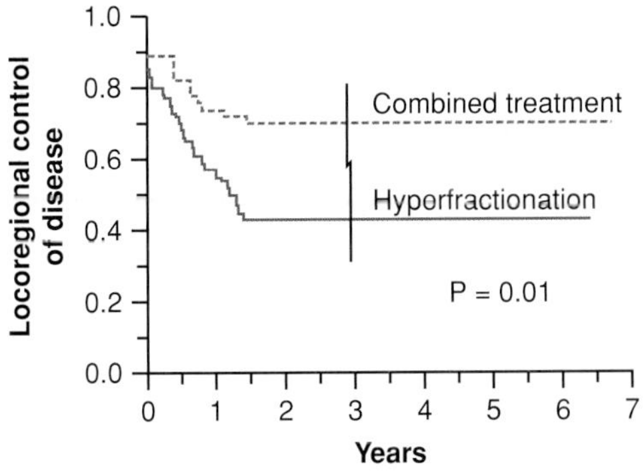

FIGURE 40.4. Five-year locoregional control in the Duke University randomized trial of continuous course accelerated hyperfractionation (44%) versus split-course accelerated hyperfractionation and concurrent cisplatin/5-fluorouracil (p = .01). Extended follow-up has demonstrated that the survival benefit of combined-modality treatment is also statistically significant.

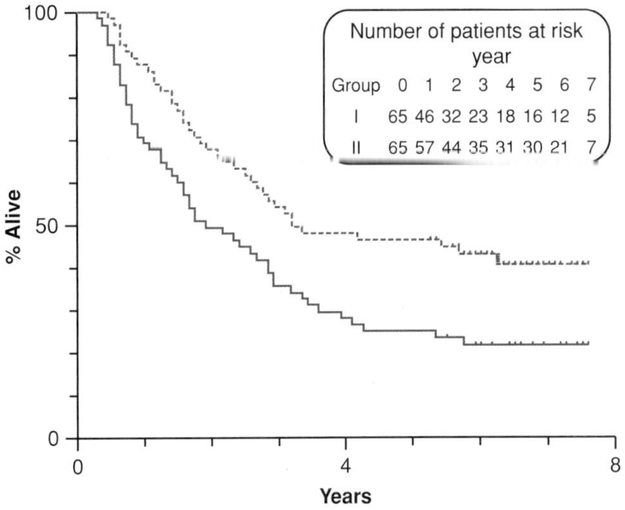

FIGURE 40.5. Five-year survival in the Yugoslavian trial of hyperfractionated irradiation alone (25%) or with daily low-dose concurrent cisplatin (46%) (p = .007).

Three hundred eighty-four patients, 93% of whom had either stage III or IV oropharyngeal or hypopharyngeal primaries, were enrolled. As in the Duke trial, the total dose of RT delivered in the CRT arm was lower than that in the RT control arm. RT patients received 77.6 Gy in 6 weeks (14 Gy at 2 Gy once daily followed by 63.6 Gy at 1.4 Gy twice daily), and CRT patients received 70.6 Gy during 6 weeks (30 Gy at 2 Gy per day followed by 40.6 Gy at 1.4 Gy twice daily). Chemotherapy consisted of mitomycin-C (10 mg/m^2) on days 5 and 35 and 5-FU given as a single bolus of 350 mg/m^2 and a 5-day continuous infusion of 600 mg/m^2/day. Two-year survival was significantly better in the combined-modality arm (54% vs. 45%; p = .05), as was locoregional control (61% vs. 45%; p = .001). Acute and chronic toxicity were equivalent in the two treatment populations.

A French cooperative group (FNLCC-GORTEC) tested a related concept in 163 patients with technically unresectable carcinomas of the oropharynx and hypopharynx.[46] RT was administered at 1.2 Gy twice daily to a total dose of 80.4 Gy/46 days to oropharyngeal primary tumors and 75.6 Gy/44 days to hypopharyngeal primary tumors. The experimental arm received the same RT and concurrent CDDP (100 mg/m^2) on days 1, 22, and 43 of RT. Three 5-day cycles of continuous infusion 5-FU were also administered. The first cycle was 750 mg/m^2/day and the second and third cycles were 430 mg/m^2/day. Three-year DFS favored the concurrent chemoradiation arm (48% vs. 25%; p = .002), as did overall survival (38% vs. 20%; p = .04). Post hoc subset analyses demonstrated that the larger (and statistically significant) benefit was confined to the patients with oropharyngeal carcinomas. However, the trial was not designed to compare treatment efficacy in these two different primary sites of origin.

A three-armed randomized trial from the University of Vienna compared conventionally fractionated RT (2 Gy daily to 70 Gy) against continuous hyperfractionated accelerated RT with and without mitomycin C (V-CHART + MMC and V CHART, respectively).[47] Radiotherapy was given as an initial 2.5-Gy fraction followed by 1.65 Gy twice daily to a total dose of 55.3 Gy in 17 days. MMC was given as a 20 mg/m^2 bolus on day 5 of RT. Of the 239 patients enrolled, 85% had T3/4 primary tumors, and 79% had nodal involvement.

Three-year actuarial locoregional control was 48% for V-CHART + MMC versus 32% for V-CHART and 31% for conventional fractionation (CF) (p = .05 and.03, respectively). Survival including death from all causes was also improved to 41% in the V-CHART + MMC arm as compared with 31% for V-CHART and 24% for CF (p = .03).

TABLE 40.2 RANDOMIZED TRIALS OF ACCELERATED OR HYPERFRACTIONATED RADIOTHERAPY AND CONCURRENT CHEMOTHERAPY IN ADVANCED HEAD AND NECK CANCER

Institution	*N*	*Radiotherapy*	*Chemotherapy*	*Outcome RT RT/CCT p Value*	*Comments*
RTOG 90-03 Accelerated fractionation and conc. boost	268	72 Gy/42 days 1.8 Gy q day and 1.5 Gy concurrent boost	None	LC: 54% DFS: 39% S: 51%	
RTOG 90-03 Hyperfractionation	263	81 Gy/49 days 1.2 Gy bid	None	LC: 54% DFS: 38% S: 54%	
University of Munich	308	70.2 Gy/51 days 1.8 Gy bid in both arms 23.4 Gy × 3 cycles 10-day split between cycles	5-FU 350 mg/m² bolus on day 2 5-FU 350 mg/m²/day × 4 CI Leucovorin 50 mg/m²/day × 4 CDDP 60 mg/m² × 1 Days 1–4, 22–25, 42–45	LC: 17% 34%; .01 S: 24% 48%; <.0003	Unresectable disease Toxicity not reported
University of Vienna	239	55 Gy/2.5 weeks for V-CHART ± MMC 70 Gy/7 weeks CF control	MMC 20 mg/m² on day 5	LC: 32% 48%; .05 S: 31% 49%; .03	V-CHART vs. V-CHART/MMC
Yugoslavian Cooperative	130	77 Gy/49 days in both arms 1.1 Gy bid	CDDP 6 mg/m²/day	LC: 36% 50%; .04 DFS: 25% 46%; .007 S: 25% 46%; .007	Daily chemotherapy
Charite' University, Berlin	384	RT/CT: 70.6 Gy/6 weeks RT: 77.6 Gy/6 weeks	MMC 10 mg/m² day 5,36 5-FU 350 mg/m² bolus 5-FU 600 mg/m² 5 days CI	LC: 45% 61%; .001 S: 24% 29%; .009	
Duke University	116	RT/CCT: 70 Gy/48 days (1-week break @ 40 Gy) RT: 74 Gy/42 days (continuous course) 1.25 Gy bid both arms	5-FU 600 mg/m²/day CI CDDP 12 mg/m²/day bolus Days 1–5 and 36–40	LC: 44% 70%; .007 DFS: 41% 61%; .06 S: 34% 55%; .04	Acute and chronic toxicity comparable between RT and RT/CCT
FNLCC-GORTEC	163	80 Gy/47 days (oropharynx) 76 Gy/44 days (hypopharynx)	80 Gy/47 days CDDP 100 mg/m² on days 1, 22, and 43 5-FU 750 mg/m² × 5 days cycle 1 and 430 mg/m² × 5 days cycles 2 and 3	LC: DFS: 25% 48%; .002 S: 20% 38%; .04	All patients with unresectable disease
Swiss Cooperative Group	224	74.4 Gy/44 days 1.2 Gy bid	74 Gy/40 days 1.2 Gy bid CDDP 20 mg/m²/day Two 5-day cycles	LC: 33% 51%; .04 DFS: 24% 27%; >.10 S: 32% 46%; .15	

RT/CCT, radiotherapy and concurrent chemotherapy; RTOG, Radiation Therapy Oncology Group; LC, local controls; DFS, disease-free survival; S, survival; bid, twice daily; 5-FU, 5-fluorouacil; CI, continuous infusion; CDDP, cisplatin; V-CHART, Vienna-Continuous Hyperfractionated Accelerated Radiation Therapy; MMC, mitomycin-C; CF, conventional fractionation.

The incidence of confluent mucositis was 90% in both experimental arms as compared with 33% in the CF arm. The median time to complete resolution of mucositis was 6 to 7 weeks in all three arms. Grade 3/4 hematologic toxicity, primarily thrombocytopenia, developed in 18% of the V-CHART + MMC patients. Table 40.2 summarizes the data from the trials that used modified fractionation and concurrent chemotherapy and includes the RTOG 90-03 and EORTC 22791 data as a point of reference for optimally delivered RT alone.

Adjuvant Postoperative Irradiation

The role of chemotherapy for patients receiving primary resection and postoperative irradiation has been studied less extensively than in the definitive irradiation setting. The National Cancer Institute Head and Neck Contracts Program[48] conducted a three-arm trial that evaluated the addition of one cycle of preoperative cisplatin and bleomycin with or without six cycles of sequential cisplatin (80 mg/m²) maintenance chemotherapy after surgery and postoperative irradiation. The control arm consisted of surgery and postoperative irradiation alone. This trial enrolled 443 patients and demonstrated no benefit with respect to locoregional control or survival from the addition of chemotherapy. Nearly half of the patients who were randomized to receive maintenance chemotherapy never received it. Despite this flaw in study execution, the incidence of distant metastases as the site of first relapse was 9% in the patients assigned to maintenance chemotherapy as opposed to 19% in those who were not ($p = .02$).

Intergroup Study 0034 readdressed the issue of postoperative chemotherapy in a trial that randomized patients after surgery to three 21-day cycles of sequential cisplatin (100 mg/m²) and infusion 5-FU (1,000 mg/m²/day for 5 days) followed by 50 to 60 Gy versus 50 to 60 Gy alone with no chemotherapy.[49] Again, there was no significant improvement in locoregional control or overall survival associated with the use of chemotherapy, but the incidence of distant metastases was reduced from 30% to 20% ($p = .02$).

In contrast to the use of sequential postoperative RT and chemotherapy, the EORTC conducted a randomized trial in which patients were given either postoperative RT alone (2 Gy daily to 66 Gy) or the same RT with three cycles of cisplatin (100 mg/m²) on days 1, 22, and 43 of irradiation.[50] Three hundred thirty-four patients were enrolled. Two-thirds of patients in the combined-modality arm received all three cycles of chemotherapy. The median follow-up is 5 years. Three-year DFS was increased from 41% to 59% ($p = .001$), and 3-year survival was increased from 49% to 65% ($p = .006$) in favor of the group of patients receiving concurrent therapy. Acute mucosal toxicity greater than grade 3 was significantly higher in the concurrent treatment arm (41% vs. 21%; $p = .001$). An analysis of 10-year outcomes is in progress.

The RTOG led an intergroup trial that randomized 459 high-risk postoperative patients to receive 60 to 66 Gy with or without concurrent CDDP in the same dose and schedule as in the EORTC study.[51] Sixty-one percent of patients in the concurrent therapy arm received all three cycles of CDDP. The median follow-up for this study is 4 years; 2-year actuarial local regional control favored the combined-modality arm by 82% versus 72% (hazard ratio [HR], 0.61; $p = .61$), with only eight local or regional recurrences occurring beyond the 2-year point. DFS also favor concurrent therapy (HR, 0.78; $p = .04$). There was no statistically significant difference in survival (HR, 0.84; $p = .19$). Acute toxicity grade 3 or higher was higher in the concurrent therapy patients (77% vs. 34%; $p < .001$), but late toxicity was similar (21% vs. 17%).

PRINCIPLES FOR THE CHOICE OF CONCURRENT TREATMENT REGIMENS

Three general statements can summarize the previously reviewed randomized trials:

a. RT with concurrent chemotherapy is more efficacious than conventionally fractionated RT alone in advanced head and neck cancer;
b. Concurrent therapy appears to be more effective than maximally intensive single-modality RT administered via a modified fractionation regimen; and
c. Acute and late toxicity are increased with the use of concurrent chemotherapy.

No consensus exists, however, regarding either the optimal radiation dose fractionation scheme or the optimal scheduling of chemotherapy in these concurrent regimens. These controversies pose a decision-making dilemma to the physician when it is time to devise a treatment plan. The application of certain principles may serve as a guide in this selection process, though. The radiochemotherapy regimen should be more effective than maximally effective single-modality radiation. The use of an RT/chemotherapy regimen, which is superior to a suboptimal RT-alone regimen, does not offer the potential for a therapeutic gain to the patient.[36]

Radiation Fractionation Scheme

One rational approach to the choice of radiation dose fractionation within the context of concurrent chemotherapy would start with the selection of an optimal single-modality therapy and a definition of both its clinical efficacy and toxicity. Different dose-fractionation schemes in concurrent treatment programs could then be normalized to one another using the biologically equivalent dose (BED) concept.[52] The BED = $nd[1 + d/(\alpha/\beta)]$, where n = the number of fractions delivered, d = the dose per fraction, and $\alpha/\beta = 10$ for tumors and acute responding normal tissues and 2 for late-responding tissues. The intent of this normalization process is to allow a comparison of these different treatment programs in order to identify those having a favorable profile in terms of maximizing the probability of tumor control while minimizing the risk of late toxicity. Kasibhatla et al.[37] evaluated prospective trials of CRT in order to estimate the radiotherapeutic dose equivalence of the concurrent chemotherapy. They concluded that, with respect to the tumor, the administration of concurrent chemotherapy was equivalent to the delivery of an additional 10 to 12 Gy. Subsequently, Lee and Eisbruch[53] estimated that concurrent chemotherapy was equivalent to the delivery of an additional 8 Gy when the development of acute mucositis was used as the end point.

Whether modified fractionation irradiation and concurrent chemotherapy is superior to conventionally fractionated irradiation and concurrent chemotherapy has been addressed in the RTOG 0129 clinical trial. Both RT and chemotherapy constituted experimental variables in this trial. Patients ($N = 720$) were randomized to receive accelerated fractionation/concomitant boost to 72 Gy/6 weeks as per RTOG 90-03 and two cycles of concurrent bolus cisplatin (100 mg/m^2) or conventionally fractionated RT 70 Gy/7 weeks and three cycles of concurrent bolus cisplatin (100 mg/m^2). A preliminary report has revealed no differences in outcome between the two arms, suggesting that one could compensate for the elimination of the third dose of cisplatin by the more intensive radiation schedule. It should also be pointed out that on the conventionally fractionated arm only 69% of patients could tolerate all three doses of CDDP, a common occurrence with the use of high-dose CDDP regimens.[54] Outcome was also the same in the conventionally fractionated arm patients who only received two cycles of CDDP versus all three cycles.

Chemotherapy Scheduling Considerations

Many investigators consider 100 mg/m^2 bolus dosing of CDDP on days 1, 22, and 43 of RT to be standard. This schedule was originally developed for use in clinical trials of induction chemotherapy and later incorporated into CRT regimens. This traditional cyclical approach to delivery of concurrent CDDP has not been compared directly with schedules that use smaller, more frequent doses. In fact, randomized clinical trials comparing so-called nonstandard schedules of platinum-based CRT against RT alone[42,43,55,56] have treated large numbers of patients with efficacy that compares favorably with bolus CDDP CRT regimens.[12,43,57]

Schedules that deliver smaller and more frequent doses of chemotherapy are also quite effective in improving outcome.[45] Given the efficacy of these nonstandard platinum schedules, they may be preferable to cyclical bolus administration on two counts. More frequent administration could provide radiosensitizing chemotherapy during a larger proportion of the course of RT. Smaller individual doses of drug may lead to less chemotherapy-induced morbidity without compromise of efficacy.[58,59] Concurrent CRT using such schedules has proven very effective and become the standard of care in squamous carcinoma of the uterine cervix.[16,60–62]

Compliance is a significant problem with the standard three-cycle concurrent CDDP paradigm. Nearly one-third of patients do not receive all cycles, and subset analyses suggest that two cycles are as effective as three.[12,46,50,51] RTOG 0129 and other studies have suggested that there may be a minimum cumulative threshold dose of approximately 200 mg/m^2 of cisplatin that is required to achieve maximal benefit when used concomitantly with radiation.[63–64,65] Schedules that administer chemotherapy more frequently throughout the course of RT deliver approximately the same cumulative dose as would result from two cycles of bolus CDDP, with treatment-related morbidity being the outcome that is most affected by drug administration schedule and cumulative dose >200 mg/m^2.[63]

Weekly cisplatin regimens have been increasingly used, in large part because of their relative ease of administration and the clinical impression of reduced toxicity. It is important to stress the limitations of this experience. No direct comparison has been made between the weekly and the every-three-week regimens. The randomized data justifying weekly drug administration are equivocal. The North American Head and Neck Intergroup, in an older trial, compared radiation alone with radiation and weekly cisplatin (20 mg/m^2/week) in patients with unresectable disease. This study was recently updated and reported by Quon et al.[66] No survival difference was observed between the two treatment arms, but it is very important to recognize that the total cisplatin dose was only 140 mg/m^2.

In nasopharyngeal cancer, Chan et al.[67] reported a comparison of radiation with radiation and concurrent cisplatin (40 mg/m^2/week). Progression-free survival was not different between the two treatment arms and a marginal overall survival difference was only appreciated after adjustment for stage and age. This survival difference was restricted to those patients with T3 or T4 tumors, and no difference was observed in the likelihood of distant metastatic disease. Thus, despite the enthusiasm for weekly cisplatin dosing regimens, there is little objective evidence supporting their use, and the every-three-week regimen must still be considered standard.

Recently, a Chinese trial compared 70 Gy of conventionally fractionated irradiation against the same regimen given with weekly concurrent cisplatin (30 mg/m^2) in 230 patients with World Health Organization stage II nasopharynx cancer.[68] No adjuvant chemotherapy was given. Five-year overall survival was significantly better in the combined-modality arm (95% vs. 86%; $p = .007$). The benefit was due to an improvement in distant metastases–free survival (95% vs. 84%; $p = .007$). Interestingly, concurrent chemotherapy did not improve local-regional control most likely because of the excellent results in the control arm (93% vs. 91%).

Phase III comparisons of platin- and non-platin-based concurrent treatment regimens are almost nonexistent, and the relative benefit of concurrent platin versus fluorouracil or taxane therapy is unknown. Meta-analysis data have suggested that fluorouracil or cisplatin regimens are more successful than carboplatin- or mitomycin-based treatments[69] and that concurrent platin monotherapy is better than non-platin monotherapy.[9] In a single small phase III trial, a weekly paclitaxel concurrent regimen appeared equivalent to a weekly cisplatin concurrent schedule.[70] Overall, however, the data must be considered limited.

Most concurrent chemotherapy regimens use a single agent, an approach that, in general, suboptimally exploits the potential systemic adjuvant benefits of this modality. In most other diseases multiagent chemotherapy has been considered a better approach in controlling distant disease. In head and neck cancer multiagent induction chemotherapy regimens have clearly demonstrated an impact on distant metastases, a benefit observed both from single trials and in large meta-analyses.[9] This same meta-analysis demonstrated a significant but less pronounced impact on distant metastases from concurrent treatment schedules. No clear survival difference has been identified when comparing concurrent single-agent platin regimens and concurrent multiagent schedules.

Radiation has also been administered in conjunction with concurrent high-dose intra-arterial cisplatin. This approach has the hypothetical advantage of allowing selective delivery of chemotherapy to the tumor while sparing uninvolved organs and allowing for the administration of intravenous sodium thiosulfate, a systemic cisplatin neutralizing agent designed to protect the kidneys. Although the procedure proved technically challenging, a phase II multi-institutional trial proved feasible.[71] A phase III trial comparing concurrent radiation and intra-arterial versus intravenous cisplatin revealed no benefit, however, and enthusiasm for this regimen has waned.[72]

The most frequently utilized regimen for concurrent chemoradiotherapy remains single-agent high-dose cisplatin given every 3 weeks, despite strong feelings and considerable rhetoric. Limited evidence suggests that cisplatin may be more effective than carboplatin.[73] Taxanes are also active agents against squamous head and neck cancer but have not been studied extensively as components of CRT regimens.

Radiotherapy and Molecularly Targeted Agents

Recent efforts to integrate radiation and systemic therapy have focused on molecularly targeted agents. The epidermal growth factor receptor (EGFR) is the target most often addressed and best studied in head and neck cancer. The EGFR is upregulated in approximately 90% of patients with squamous cell head and neck cancer and has been associated with a poor prognosis.[74,75–76] In patients with recurrent or metastatic disease, a modest response rate has been observed with the anti-EGFR monoclonal antibody cetuximab, both with and without systemic chemotherapy, as well as with the oral tyrosine kinase inhibitors gefitinib and erlotinib.[77,78–79,80,81] Even more impressive is the disease stability that has been identified after treatment with these agents. This experience has prompted further exploration of these agents in definitive management.

Bonner et al.[82] reported the results of the first phase III randomized trial exploring the role anti-EGFR therapy in the definitive management of a solid tumor. This trial compared the use of radiation therapy alone with radiation and concurrent cetuximab in the treatment of patients with stage III or IV nonmetastatic squamous cell carcinoma of the oropharynx, hypopharynx, or larynx. Cetuximab therapy consisted of a loading dose of 400 mg/m^2 followed by a weekly dose of 250 mg/m^2 for the duration of the radiation therapy. An updated analysis reported in 2010 confirmed the initial results.[83] The addition of cetuximab to radiation therapy improved the median overall survival from 29 months to 49 months ($p = .018$), and the 5-year overall survival from 36% to 46%. The incidence of grade 3 or greater toxicity including mucositis did not differ between the two groups, except for a greater incidence of acneiform rash and infusion reactions in those patients treated with cetuximab. An interesting but unplanned subgroup analysis suggested that the benefit was greater in the cetuximab-treated patients with oropharynx cancers, smaller primary tumors, and more advanced nodal involvement. Males, patients with a better performance status, and patients who were younger also seemed to do better. This demographic distribution suggested the possibility that the drug was more effective in those patients with human papillomavirus (HPV)-associated disease, although HPV testing of the tumor specimens was not performed. It was also notable that survival was better in the cetuximab-treated patients who developed a cetuximab-induced rash.

It is important to recognize that the control arm of this trial, radiation therapy alone, is no longer considered a treatment standard for most patients with stage III and IV locoregionally advanced squamous cell head and neck cancer. Consequently, the relative benefit of cetuximab and radiation compared to a more standard radiation and concurrent chemotherapy combination is unknown. RTOG attempted to define this better in its 0522 trial reported preliminarily at the 2011 meeting of the American Society of Clinical Oncology.[84] This study compared concurrent radiation, cetuximab, and cisplatin with radiation and cisplatin alone. As expected, the skin reactions were worse in those patients given cetuximab. No differences were observed in any survival outcome including progression-free survival, overall survival, or patterns of disease failure. Approximately 50% of the patients were p16 positive (and by inference HPV positive), but somewhat unexpectedly, no outcome differences were observed as a function of p16 status either. Given the results of this study, there is currently no justification for adding cetuximab to the standard radiation and cisplatin regimens used in definitive management outside of a clinical trial.

The findings in RTOG 0522 conflict with the observation made in the metastatic disease setting. There, a phase III randomized trial compared cisplatin and fluorouracil with cisplatin, fluorouracil, and cetuximab.[80] This study demonstrated an improvement in survival from the addition of cetuximab to standard chemotherapy, and it remains unclear why the RTOG 0522 trial did not demonstrate a similar outcome improvement.

The question also remains unanswered as to whether concurrent radiation and cetuximab is equivalent or even superior to radiation and cisplatin. This issue is currently being addressed by the RTOG 1016 study, which compares these two regimens in a more selected patient population with HPV-positive oropharynx cancer. It is anticipated that the survival outcomes on the two treatment arms will be equivalent but that a difference may emerge in terms of late toxicity, function, or quality of life. It is of note that a retrospective study reported from Memorial Sloan-Kettering Cancer Center suggested the possibility that locoregional control and survival were better in patients treated with radiation and cisplatin when compared to patients given radiation and cetuximab.[85] Although these results were upheld on multivariate analysis, prospective validation is required given the very significant differences in patients selected for these treatments. The randomized phase II TREMPLIN study prospectively compared the two regimens administered after three-drug induction chemotherapy. Given the nature and size of this trial, however, it is difficult to interpret any outcome comparisons.[86]

DEVELOPMENTAL ASPECTS OF COMBINED-MODALITY THERAPY

Induction Chemotherapy and Sequential Chemoradiation

The use of induction chemotherapy for locoregionally advanced squamous cell head and neck cancer continues to be an attractive treatment option. The dramatic tumor shrinkage seen in previously untreated patients after cisplatin-based chemotherapy regimens would intuitively suggest that an improvement in locoregional control and even survival should also result. Multiple phase III clinical trials, however, have failed to demonstrate any reproducible impact from induction treatment schedules on overall outcome.[87,88] A marginal survival benefit was identified by the large Meta-Analysis of Chemotherapy on Head and Neck Cancer (MACH-NC) using fluorouracil and platin induction chemotherapy, but this survival improvement was dwarfed by that obtained with the use of concurrent treatment regimens (Fig. 40.2).[9,89]

A frequent observation from these induction trials, however, has been a reduction in distant metastases.[8,90,91] The fact that this did not impact on overall survival likely reflects the historically limited importance of distant metastases in the natural history of this disease. Recently, however, with the increasing locoregional control achieved by concurrent treatment regimens, distant metastases have emerged as a more frequent cause of treatment failure.[92,93] This observation has led to the suggestion that there may be a role for the reintroduction of chemotherapy into current multimodality treatment schedules.[94]

Coincident with this resurgent interest in induction schedules has been the recognition that the widely used and very successful cisplatin and fluorouracil combination may not be the optimal induction regimen. Considerable phase III experience now exists demonstrating the superiority of three-drug fluorouracil, cisplatin, and taxane–containing regimens when compared to fluorouracil and cisplatin alone[95–98] (Table 40.3). In these studies, successful induction was followed by definitive radiation therapy with or without concurrent chemotherapy.

It is important to note that three of these studies demonstrated a survival benefit favoring the three-drug induction regimen. This should not be interpreted as evidence that three-drug induction chemotherapy is a new standard of care. Induction chemotherapy followed by definitive radiation or chemoradiation is not a generally established sequence of treatment modalities, and the superiority of one induction regimen over another does not define induction chemotherapy as a standard of care.

Nonetheless, there are several situations where induction chemotherapy may have a role. In the larynx preservation setting, induction fluorouracil and cisplatin followed by definitive radiation in responders has been compared directly with concurrent chemoradiation with single-agent cisplatin and with radiation therapy alone.[12] Although the laryngeal preservation and locoregional control were superior in the concurrent chemoradiotherapy arm, laryngectomy-free survival and distant metastatic control were equivalent between the two chemotherapy regimens.[99] It is of note that overall survival was unchanged by the addition of chemotherapy. Thus, induction chemotherapy can be considered an acceptable larynx preservation strategy. The superiority of the three-drug docetaxel, cisplatin, and fluorouracil regimen when compared to fluorouracil and cisplatin in the larynx preservation setting has been established,[98] although the subsequent use of concurrent treatment regimens after three-drug induction has proven difficult.[86]

TABLE 40.3 TAXANE, CISPLATIN, AND FLUOROURACIL (TPF) VERSUS CISPLATIN AND FLUOROURACIL (PF) INDUCTION CHEMOTHERAPY: RANDOMIZED TRIALS

	Hitt 2005[95]	*Vermorken 2007*[96]	*Posner 2007*[97]	*Pointreau 2009*[98]
Taxane	Paclitaxel	Docetaxel	Docetaxel	Docetaxel
Definitive treatment	Variable	Radiation	Radiation/weekly carboplatin	Variable
Response rate				
PF	68%	54%	64%	59%
TPF	80%	68%	72%	80%
p value	<.001	.006	.07	.002
Survival	2 years	3 years	3 years	3 years
PF	54%	26%	48%	60%
TPF	67%	37%	62%	60%
p value	.06	.02	.002	.57

Of greater interest has been the use of induction chemotherapy in what has been termed *sequential treatment* regimens, that is, induction chemotherapy followed by concurrent chemoradiotherapy.[100] The rationale for this approach is that the addition of induction chemotherapy can, by improving the distant metastatic control, improve upon the overall survival achieved after concurrent chemoradiotherapy alone. These treatment schedules are intensive and require considerable commitment from both patient and physician. Toxicity, when compared to concurrent chemoradiotherapy alone, will be increased, and the administration of multiple doses of both induction and concurrent cisplatin is challenging.[86]

A preliminary report by Hitt and Lopez-Pousa[101] from their study of three-drug induction chemotherapy followed by chemoradiotherapy compared with chemoradiotherapy alone suggested a benefit for the induction arm. Significant methodologic flaws existed in this initial report, and the results may ultimately prove to be uninterpretable. A successful phase II randomized experience has been reported by Paccagnella et al.[102] comparing induction docetaxel, cisplatin, and fluorouracil before chemoradiotherapy with chemoradiotherapy alone. This experience has now been expanded to a phase III trial, which also includes an assessment of the role of concurrent cetuximab. Similarly, a phase III trial comparing induction followed by concurrent chemoradiotherapy with concurrent treatment alone has been completed by the University of Chicago consortium, and the results are eagerly anticipated.

A third rationale for induction chemotherapy has been explored by University of Michigan investigators. Their premise is that induction chemotherapy can serve as a predictive tool and allow for the appropriate selection of the subsequent definitive head and neck cancer management strategy. Patients responding to induction chemotherapy can be approached nonoperatively, while those in whom induction is unsuccessful should proceed to surgical resection. This strategy is based on the long-standing recognition that patients responding to induction chemotherapy are also those who respond best to radiation therapy.[103]

This approach has been used successfully in patients with advanced larynx cancer.[104] The treatment schedule began with a single cycle of induction cisplatin and fluorouracil, followed by concurrent chemoradiotherapy with high-dose single-agent cisplatin in responders. At least a partial response to single-cycle induction was achieved in 75% of patients, and larynx preservation ultimately proved possible in 70% of the entire patient cohort. It was of particular import that those patients requiring laryngectomy because of a failure to respond to induction chemotherapy achieved an overall survival equivalent to the chemotherapy responders.

This experience proved less successful in their patients with oropharynx and oral cavity cancer, however.[105,106] Furthermore, the relegation of induction chemotherapy to a purely predictive tool is disquieting to both medical and radiation oncologists. Induction adds significant cost and toxicity, and one would hope that it might provide an additional survival benefit or an improvement in distant metastatic disease control. Perhaps other less toxic predictive "biomarkers" than responsiveness to induction chemotherapy might emerge in the future.

Thus, induction chemotherapy, particularly using the three-drug cisplatin, fluorouracil, and taxane combination, remains a very active but incompletely developed tool. Its ultimate impact on survival, distant metastases, and our treatment paradigms remains to be seen. The results of current phase III trials must be awaited before sequential treatment schedules can be considered standard treatment approaches. Toxicity considerations will play an important role in the choice of therapeutic strategies. Overall, more treatment means more toxicity as treatment is escalated along the continuum from conventional once-daily RT only to the most intensive combined-modality regimens. The total toxicity burden imposed upon a patient may increase as much as fivefold.[107] These considerations are particularly relevant to sequential therapy programs. Compliance rates with an entire course of treatment with these regimens is only 65% to 70% in the most experienced hands.[95,97,108]

Other Targeted Agents

Other EGFR monoclonal antibodies are also being explored in the head and neck cancer patient population, both in the metastatic setting and in conjunction with radiation, including panitumumab and zalutumumab.[109,110] The oral tyrosine kinase inhibitors including gefitinib, erlotinib, and others have undergone limited phase II testing as part of definitive treatment schedules. Results from these studies have been mixed and enthusiasm restrained.[71,111–114]

Treatments directed against other molecular targets, most notably the vascular endothelial growth factor receptor (VEGFR), are also now being integrated with definitive radiation therapy schedules.[115,116] Overexpression of VEGF in head and neck cancer is associated with a twofold increase in the risk of death from disease.[117] Yoo et al.[118] performed a pilot study in 29 patients that integrated dual targeting of EGFR with erlotinib and VEGFR with the antibody bevacizumab into a regimen of platinum-based chemoradiation for newly diagnosed, locally advanced, nonmetastatic disease. Three-year progression-free survival was 82%. One of the most important facets of this trial was that it utilized functional metabolic imaging with the performance of serial dynamic contrast-enhanced magnetic resonance imaging (DCE-MRI) scans to assess response to treatment. DCE-MRI quantitatively measures tumor perfusion and vascular permeability, which is expressed by the parameter K^{trans}. Patients whose disease recurred after treatment had lower baseline pretreatment median K^{trans} values, which rose during the earliest phases of therapy. Patients who did not fail, however, had higher baseline median K^{trans} values that decreased during therapy. These data suggest that K^{trans} could potentially serve as an imaging biomarker to guide initial treatment selection based on pretreatment prognosis or to guide treatment modification based on a favorable or unfavorable response to the early phases of treatment.[119]

Hypoxia is one of the most important characteristics of the aggressive malignant phenotype.[120–123] Poorly oxygenated tumors are less likely to respond to surgery,[124] radiotherapy,[120,125–127] and chemotherapy. Hypoxic primary tumors are more likely to develop distant metastases after treatment.[128] A recent review of nearly 400 HNC patients who underwent tumor oxygenation measurement demonstrated that hypoxia was strongly associated with treatment failure independently of stage and therapeutic modality.[31]

Tirapazamine, a bioreductively activated compound, is one to two orders of magnitude more cytotoxic to hypoxic cells than well-oxygenated cells and also potentiates the activity of cisplatin.[129–131] Phase I/II studies in advanced squamous HNC demonstrated efficacy with acceptable toxicity when this drug was incorporated into cisplatin-containing CRT regimens and suggested that the benefit of the drug was restricted to those patients who had hypoxic tumors as assessed by ^{18}F-misonidazole positron emission tomography (PET) scanning.[132,133]

Two phase III trials were conducted to determine whether targeting of hypoxic cells with tirapazamine/cisplatin CRT was superior to cisplatin CRT. The first trial (HeadSTART) enrolled 880 patients. No benefit was observed from the addition of tirapazamine.[134] A large number of patients had significant protocol deviations with respect to the delivery of radiotherapy, however. A subset analysis of patients who correctly received all of their treatment according to the protocol guidelines did demonstrate an advantage in patients who received tirapazamine.[135] Another important consideration is that patients enrolled into this trial were not selected according to whether or not they had hypoxic tumors, which would have increased the power to detect a benefit from the drug if in fact one existed. A second trial with the same treatment schema was launched with a planned enrollment of 550 patients but was prematurely closed because of an unexplainable excess of deaths during treatment in the tirapazamine arm.

SUMMARY

The use of modified daily fractionation as opposed to conventional once-daily fractionation improves the prognosis of patients who receive curative intent RT for advanced head and neck cancer. Radiation therapy and concurrent chemotherapy in turn are superior to both single-modality conventional and modified fractionation radiation therapy in the nonsurgical management of advanced head and neck cancer. Anti-EGFR-targeted therapy also enhances the effectiveness of RT. The role of EGFR inhibition in a chemoradiation setting is under investigation. Likewise, the benefit of adding induction chemotherapy to a platform of chemoradiation is being tested. Hypoxia-targeted therapy remains investigational.

The increased acute and late toxicity that results from combining these multiple modalities poses immediate challenges. These include the need to develop criteria for *a priori* selection of those patients with advanced-stage disease who can still be adequately treated with radiotherapy alone and the need to create effective strategies for toxicity prophylaxis and management. These efforts will allow for the optimal integration of radiotherapy, chemotherapy, and biologically targeted therapy for those patients requiring combined modality therapy.

SELECTED REFERENCES

A full list of references for this chapter is available online.

1. Fu KK, Pajak TF, Trotti A, et al. A Radiation Therapy Oncology Group (RTOG) phase III randomized study to compare hyperfractionation and two variants of accelerated fractionation to standard fractionation radiotherapy for head and neck squamous cell carcinomas: first report of RTOG 9003. *Int J Radiat Oncol Biol Phys* 2000;48:7–16.
3. Horiot JC, Le Fur R, N'Guyen T, et al. Hyperfractionation versus conventional fractionation in oropharyngeal carcinoma: final analysis of a randomized trial of the EORTC cooperative group of radiotherapy. *Radiother Oncol* 1992;25:231–241.
4. Overgaard J, Hansen HS, Specht L, et al. Five compared with six fractions per week of conventional radiotherapy of squamous-cell carcinoma of head and neck: DAHANCA 6 and 7 randomised controlled trial. *Lancet* 2003;362:933–940.
5. Bourhis J, Overgaard J, Audry H, et al. Hyperfractionated or accelerated radiotherapy in head and neck cancer: a meta-analysis. *Lancet* 2006;368:843–854.
8. Induction chemotherapy plus radiation compared with surgery plus radiation in patients with advanced laryngeal cancer. The Department of Veterans Affairs Laryngeal Cancer Study Group. *N Engl J Med* 1991;324:1685–1690.
9. Pignon JP, le Maitre A, Maillard E, et al. Meta-analysis of chemotherapy in head and neck cancer (MACH-NC): an update on 93 randomised trials and 17,346 patients. *Radiother Oncol* 2009;92:4–14.
12. Forastiere AA, Goepfert H, Maor M, et al. Concurrent chemotherapy and radiotherapy for organ preservation in advanced laryngeal cancer. *N Engl J Med* 2003;349:2091–2098.
18. Budach V, Stuschke M, Budach W, et al. Hyperfractionated accelerated chemoradiation with concurrent fluorouracil-mitomycin is more effective than dose-escalated hyperfractionated accelerated radiation therapy alone in locally advanced head and neck cancer: final results of the radiotherapy cooperative clinical trials group of the German Cancer Society 95-06 Prospective Randomized Trial. *J Clin Oncol* 2005;23:1125–1135.
19. Denis F, Garaud P, Bardet E, et al. Final results of the 94-01 French Head and Neck Oncology and Radiotherapy Group randomized trial comparing radiotherapy alone with concomitant radiochemotherapy in advanced-stage oropharynx carcinoma. *J Clin Oncol* 2004;22:69–76.
20. Denis F, Garaud P, Bardet E, et al. Late toxicity results of the GORTEC 94-01 randomized trial comparing radiotherapy with concomitant radiochemotherapy for advanced-stage oropharynx carcinoma: comparison of LENT/SOMA, RTOG/EORTC, and NCI-CTC scoring systems. *Int J Radiat Oncol Biol Phys* 2003;55:93–98.
22. Overgaard J, Hjelm-Hansen M, Johansen LV, et al. Comparison of conventional and split-course radiotherapy as primary treatment in carcinoma of the larynx. *Acta Oncol* 1988;27:147–152.
23. Withers HR, Taylor JM, Maciejewski B. The hazard of accelerated tumor clonogen repopulation during radiotherapy. *Acta Oncol* 1988;27:131–146.
27. Lo TC, Wiley AL Jr, Ansfield FJ, et al. Combined radiation therapy and 5-fluorouracil for advanced squamous cell carcinoma of the oral cavity and oropharynx: a randomized study. *AJR Am J Roentgenol* 1976;126:229–235.
29. Gray LH, Conger AD, Ebert M, et al. The concentration of oxygen dissolved in tissues at the time of irradiation as a factor in radiotherapy. *Br J Radiol* 1953;26:638–648.

30. Brizel DM, Dodge RK, Clough RW, et al. Oxygenation of head and neck cancer: changes during radiotherapy and impact on treatment outcome. *Radiother Oncol* 1999;53:113–117.
31. Nordsmark M, Bentzen SM, Rudat V, et al. Prognostic value of tumor oxygenation in 397 head and neck tumors after primary radiation therapy. An international multi-center study. *Radiother Oncol* 2005;77:18–24.
32. Haffty BG, Son YH, Papac R, et al. Chemotherapy as an adjunct to radiation in the treatment of squamous cell carcinoma of the head and neck: results of the Yale Mitomycin Randomized Trials. *J Clin Oncol* 1997;15:268–276.
33. Bartelink H, Kallman RF, Rapacchietta D, et al. Therapeutic enhancement in mice by clinically relevant dose and fractionation schedules of cis-diamminedichloroplatinum (II) and irradiation. *Radiother Oncol* 1986;6:61–74.
34. Adelstein DJ, Lavertu P, Saxton JP, et al. Mature results of a phase III randomized trial comparing concurrent chemoradiotherapy with radiation therapy alone in patients with stage III and IV squamous cell carcinoma of the head and neck. *Cancer* 2000;88:876–883.
35. Keane TJ, Cummings BJ, O'Sullivan B, et al. A randomized trial of radiation therapy compared to split course radiation therapy combined with mitomycin C and 5 fluorouracil as initial treatment for advanced laryngeal and hypopharyngeal squamous carcinoma. *Int J Radiat Oncol Biol Phys* 1993;25:613–618.
36. Sanchiz F, Milla A, Torner J, et al. Single fraction per day versus two fractions per day versus radiochemotherapy in the treatment of head and neck cancer. *Int J Radiat Oncol Biol Phys* 1990;19:1347–1350.
37. Kasibhatla M, Kirkpatrick JP, Brizel DM. How much radiation is the chemotherapy worth in advanced head and neck cancer? *Int J Radiat Oncol Biol Phys* 2007; 68:1491–1495.
39. Merlano M, Benasso M, Corvo R, et al. Five-year update of a randomized trial of alternating radiotherapy and chemotherapy compared with radiotherapy alone in treatment of unresectable squamous cell carcinoma of the head and neck. *J Natl Cancer Inst* 1996;88:583–589.
42. Wendt TG, Grabenbauer GG, Rodel CM, et al. Simultaneous radiochemotherapy versus radiotherapy alone in advanced head and neck cancer: a randomized multicenter study. *J Clin Oncol* 1998;16:1318–1324.
43. Al-Sarraf M, LeBlanc M, Giri PG, et al. Chemoradiotherapy versus radiotherapy in patients with advanced nasopharyngeal cancer: phase III randomized Intergroup study 0099. *J Clin Oncol* 1998;16:1310–1317.
44. Brizel DM, Albers ME, Fisher SR, et al. Hyperfractionated irradiation with or without concurrent chemotherapy for locally advanced head and neck cancer. *N Engl J Med* 1998;338:1798–1804.
45. Jeremic B, Shibamoto Y, Milicic B, et al. Hyperfractionated radiation therapy with or without concurrent low-dose daily cisplatin in locally advanced squamous cell carcinoma of the head and neck: a prospective randomized trial. *J Clin Oncol* 2000;18:1458–1464.
46. Bensadoun RJ, Benezery K, Dassonville O, et al. French multicenter phase III randomized study testing concurrent twice-a-day radiotherapy and cisplatin/5-fluorouracil chemotherapy (BiRCF) in unresectable pharyngeal carcinoma: results at 2 years (FNCLCC-GORTEC). *Int J Radiat Oncol Biol Phys* 2006;64:983–994.
47. Dobrowsky W, Naude J. Continuous hyperfractionated accelerated radiotherapy with/without mitomycin C in head and neck cancers. *Radiother Oncol* 2000;57: 119–124.
50. Bernier J, Domenge C, Ozsahin M, et al. Postoperative irradiation with or without concomitant chemotherapy for locally advanced head and neck cancer. *N Engl J Med* 2004;350:1945–1952.
51. Cooper JS, Pajak TF, Forastiere AA, et al. Postoperative concurrent radiotherapy and chemotherapy for high-risk squamous-cell carcinoma of the head and neck. *N Engl J Med* 2004;350:1937–1944.
53. Lee IH, Eisbruch A. Mucositis versus tumor control: the therapeutic index of adding chemotherapy to irradiation of head and neck cancer. *Int J Radiat Oncol Biol Phys* 2009;75:1060–1063.
54. Ang KK, Harris J, Wheeler R, et al. Human papillomavirus and survival of patients with oropharyngeal cancer. *N Engl J Med* 2010;363:24–35.
56. Huguenin P, Beer KT, Allal A, et al. Concomitant cisplatin significantly improves locoregional control in advanced head and neck cancers treated with hyperfractionated radiotherapy. *J Clin Oncol* 2004;22:4665–4673.
57. Adelstein DJ, Li Y, Adams GL, et al. An intergroup phase III comparison of standard radiation therapy and two schedules of concurrent chemoradiotherapy in patients with unresectable squamous cell head and neck cancer. *J Clin Oncol* 2003;21:92–98.
63. Ang KK. Concurrent radiation chemotherapy for locally advanced head and neck carcinoma: are we addressing burning subjects? *J Clin Oncol* 2004;22:4657–4659.
64. Loong HH, Ma B, Mo F, et al. The effect of cisplatin dose administered during concurrent chemoradiotherapy in patients with locoregionally advanced nasopharyngeal carcinoma. *J Clin Oncol* 2011;29:abstr 5532.
66. Quon H, Leong T, Haselow R, et al. Phase III study of radiation therapy with or without cis-platinum in patients with unresectable squamous or undifferentiated carcinoma of the head and neck: an intergroup trial of the Eastern Cooperative Oncology Group (E2382). *Int J Radiat Oncol Biol Phys* 2011;81:719–725.
67. Chan AT, Leung SF, Ngan RK, et al. Overall survival after concurrent cisplatin-radiotherapy compared with radiotherapy alone in locoregionally advanced nasopharyngeal carcinoma. *J Natl Cancer Inst* 2005;97:536–539.
68. Chen QY, Wen YF, Guo L, et al. Concurrent chemoradiotherapy vs radiotherapy alone in stage II nasopharyngeal carcinoma: phase III randomized trial. *J Natl Cancer Inst* 2011;103:1761–1770.
69. Budach W, Hohr T, Budach V, et al. A meta-analysis of hyperfractionated and accelerated radiotherapy and combined chemotherapy and radiotherapy regimens in unresected locally advanced squamous cell carcinoma of the head and neck. *BMC Cancer* 2006;6:28.
72. Rasch CR, Hauptmann M, Schornagel J, et al. Intra-arterial versus intravenous chemoradiation for advanced head and neck cancer: results of a randomized phase 3 trial. *Cancer* 2010;116:2159–2165.
73. Fountzilas G, Ciuleanu E, Dafni U, et al. Concomitant radiochemotherapy vs radiotherapy alone in patients with head and neck cancer: a Hellenic Cooperative Oncology Group Phase III Study. *Med Oncol* 2004;21:95–107.
75. Ang KK, Berkey BA, Tu X, et al. Impact of epidermal growth factor receptor expression on survival and pattern of relapse in patients with advanced head and neck carcinoma. *Cancer Res* 2002;62:7350–7356.
76. Chung CH, Ely K, McGavran L, et al. Increased epidermal growth factor receptor gene copy number is associated with poor prognosis in head and neck squamous cell carcinomas. *J Clin Oncol* 2006;24:4170–4176.
77. Burtness B, Goldwasser MA, Flood W, et al. Phase III randomized trial of cisplatin plus placebo compared with cisplatin plus cetuximab in metastatic/recurrent head and neck cancer: an Eastern Cooperative Oncology Group study. *J Clin Oncol* 2005;23:8646–8654.
80. Vermorken JB, Mesia R, Rivera F, et al. Platinum-based chemotherapy plus cetuximab in head and neck cancer. *N Engl J Med* 2008;359:1116–1127.
82. Bonner JA, Harari PM, Giralt J, et al. Radiotherapy plus cetuximab for squamous-cell carcinoma of the head and neck. *N Engl J Med* 2006;354:567–578.
83. Bonner JA, Harari PM, Giralt J, et al. Radiotherapy plus cetuximab for locoregionally advanced head and neck cancer: 5-year survival data from a phase 3 randomised trial, and relation between cetuximab-induced rash and survival. *Lancet Oncol* 2010;11:21–28.
84. Ang KK, Zhang QE, Rosenthal DI, et al. A randomized phase III trial (RTOG 0522) of concurrent accelerated radiation plus cisplatin with or without cetuximab for stage III-IV head and neck squamous cell carcinomas (HNC). *J Clin Oncol* 2011;29:360s.
86. Lefebvre J, Pointreau Y, Rolland F. Sequential chemoradiotherapy (SCRT) for larynx preservation (LP): results of the randomized phase II TREMPLIN study. *J Clin Oncol* 2011;29:360s.
89. Pignon JP, Bourhis J, Domenge C, et al. Chemotherapy added to locoregional treatment for head and neck squamous-cell carcinoma: three meta-analyses of updated individual data. MACH-NC Collaborative Group. Meta-Analysis of Chemotherapy on Head and Neck Cancer. *Lancet* 2000;355:949–955.
91. Paccagnella A, Orlando A, Marchiori C, et al. Phase III trial of initial chemotherapy in stage III or IV head and neck cancers: a study by the Gruppo di Studio sui Tumori della Testa e del Collo. *J Natl Cancer Inst* 1994;86:265–272.
94. Brockstein B, Haraf DJ, Rademaker AW, et al. Patterns of failure, prognostic factors and survival in locoregionally advanced head and neck cancer treated with concomitant chemoradiotherapy: a 9-year, 337-patient, multi-institutional experience. *Ann Oncol* 2004;15:1179–1186.
95. Hitt R, Lopez-Pousa A, Martinez-Trufero J, et al. Phase III study comparing cisplatin plus fluorouracil to paclitaxel, cisplatin, and fluorouracil induction chemotherapy followed by chemoradiotherapy in locally advanced head and neck cancer. *J Clin Oncol* 2005;23:8636–8645.
96. Vermorken JB, Remenar E, van Herpen C, et al. Cisplatin, fluorouracil, and docetaxel in unresectable head and neck cancer. *N Engl J Med* 2007;357:1695–1704.
97. Posner MR, Hershock DM, Blajman CR, et al. Cisplatin and fluorouracil alone or with docetaxel in head and neck cancer. *N Engl J Med* 2007;357:1705–1715.
98. Pointreau Y, Garaud P, Chapet S, et al. Randomized trial of induction chemotherapy with cisplatin and 5-fluorouracil with or without docetaxel for larynx preservation. *J Natl Cancer Inst* 2009;101:498–506.
102. Paccagnella A, Ghi MG, Loreggian L, et al. Concomitant chemoradiotherapy versus induction docetaxel, cisplatin and 5 fluorouracil (TPF) followed by concomitant chemoradiotherapy in locally advanced head and neck cancer: a phase II randomized study. *Ann Oncol* 2010;21:1515–1522.
104. Urba S, Wolf G, Eisbruch A, et al. Single-cycle induction chemotherapy selects patients with advanced laryngeal cancer for combined chemoradiation: a new treatment paradigm. *J Clin Oncol* 2006;24:593–598.
105. Worden FP, Kumar B, Lee JS, et al. Chemoselection as a strategy for organ preservation in advanced oropharynx cancer: response and survival positively associated with HPV16 copy number. *J Clin Oncol* 2008;26:3138–146.
107. Bentzen SM, Trotti A. Evaluation of early and late toxicities in chemoradiation trials. *J Clin Oncol* 2007;25:4096–4103.
108. Adelstein DJ, Moon J, Hanna E, et al. Docetaxel, cisplatin, and fluorouracil induction chemotherapy followed by accelerated fractionation/concomitant boost radiation and concurrent cisplatin in patients with advanced squamous cell head and neck cancer: a Southwest Oncology Group phase II trial (S0216). *Head Neck* 2010;32:221–228.
115. Lee NY, Zhang Q, Pfister DG, et al. Addition of bevacizumab to standard chemoradiation for locoregionally advanced nasopharyngeal carcinoma (RTOG 0615): a phase 2 multi-institutional trial. *Lancet Oncol* 2012;13:172–180.
116. Seiwert TY, Haraf DJ, Cohen EE, et al. Phase I study of bevacizumab added to fluorouracil- and hydroxyurea-based concomitant chemoradiotherapy for poor-prognosis head and neck cancer. *J Clin Oncol* 2008;26:1732–1741.
117. Kyzas PA, Cunha IW, Ioannidis JP. Prognostic significance of vascular endothelial growth factor immunohistochemical expression in head and neck squamous cell carcinoma: a meta-analysis. *Clin Cancer Res* 2005;11:1434–1440.
118. Yoo D, Kirkpatrick J, Craciunescu O, et al. Prospective trial of synchronous bevacizumab, erlotinib, and concurrent chemoradiation in locally advanced head and neck cancer. *Clin Cancer Res* 2012;18:1404–1414.
119. Brizel DM. Head and neck cancer as a model for advances in imaging prognosis, early assessment, and posttherapy evaluation. *Cancer J* 2011;17:159–165.
120. Koukourakis MI, Giatromanolaki A, Sivridis E, et al. Hypoxia-inducible factor (HIF1A and HIF2A), angiogenesis, and chemoradiotherapy outcome of squamous cell head-and-neck cancer. *Int J Radiat Oncol Biol Phys* 2002;53:1192–1202.
121. Graeber TG, Osmanian C, Jacks T, et al. Hypoxia-mediated selection of cells with diminished apoptotic potential in solid tumours. *Nature* 1996;379:88–91.
122. Koukourakis MI, Giatromanolaki A, Sivridis E, et al. Hypoxia-regulated carbonic anhydrase-9 (CA9) relates to poor vascularization and resistance of squamous cell head and neck cancer to chemoradiotherapy. *Clin Cancer Res* 2001;7:3399–3403.
123. Moeller BJ, Cao Y, Li CY, et al. Radiation activates HIF-1 to regulate vascular radiosensitivity in tumors: role of reoxygenation, free radicals, and stress granules. *Cancer Cell* 2004;5:429–441.
124. Hockel M, Schlenger K, Aral B, et al. Association between tumor hypoxia and malignant progression in advanced cancer of the uterine cervix. *Cancer Res* 1996;56: 4509–4515.
126. Brizel DM, Dodge RK, Clough RW, et al. Oxygenation of head and neck cancer: changes during radiotherapy and impact on treatment outcome. *Radiother Oncol* 1999;53:113–117.
128. Brizel DM, Scully SP, Harrelson JM, et al. Tumor oxygenation predicts for the likelihood of distant metastases in human soft tissue sarcoma. *Cancer Res* 1996;56: 941–943.
132. Rischin D, Peters L, Fisher R, et al. Tirapazamine, Cisplatin, and Radiation versus Fluorouracil, Cisplatin, and Radiation in patients with locally advanced head and neck cancer: a randomized phase II trial of the Trans-Tasman Radiation Oncology Group (TROG 98.02). *J Clin Oncol* 2005;23:79–87.
134. Rischin D, Peters LJ, O'Sullivan B, et al. Tirapazamine, cisplatin, and radiation versus cisplatin and radiation for advanced squamous cell carcinoma of the head and neck (TROG 02.02, HeadSTART): a phase III trial of the Trans-Tasman Radiation Oncology Group. *J Clin Oncol* 2010;28:2989–2995.
135. Peters LJ, O'Sullivan B, Giralt J, et al. Critical impact of radiotherapy protocol compliance and quality in the treatment of advanced head and neck cancer: results from TROG 02.02. *J Clin Oncol* 2010;28:2996–3001.

Chapter 41
Nasopharynx

Benjamin H. Lok, Jeremy Setton, Felix Ho, Nadeem Riaz, Shyam S. Rao, and Nancy Y. Lee

ANATOMY

The nasopharynx is a cuboidal chamber that is slightly broader in the transverse dimension than in the anterior–posterior dimension (Fig. 41.1). Anteriorly it is continuous with the nasal cavity via the posterior choanae, while inferiorly it communicates with the oropharynx. The roof of the nasopharynx is formed by the basilar portion of the sphenoid and occipital bones and the floor by the superior surface of the soft palate and nasopharyngeal isthmus. The lateral walls of the nasopharynx contain the pharyngotympanic tube (*Eustachian tube*) openings, which are bounded by a prominence known as the *torus tubarius*. The *torus* is formed by the cartilage of the pharyngotympanic tube elevating the mucous membrane of the lateral nasopharynx. Posterior to the torus is the pharyngeal recess otherwise known as the *fossa of Rosenmüller*. The lateral walls, including the pharyngeal recess (*fossa of Rosenmüller*), are the most common origin of nasopharyngeal malignancies. The posterior wall of the nasopharynx contains the superior pharyngeal constrictor muscle, pharyngobasilar fascia, and buccopharyngeal fascia.

The superior pharyngeal constrictor only extends superiorly to the skull base in the midline, and laterally the pharyngobasilar fascia serves to attach the constrictor muscle to the base of the skull at the basiocciput and petrous portion of the temporal bone. This lateral area of muscular deficiency is otherwise known as the *sinus of Morgagni*, through which the pharyngotympanic tube and levator veli palatini pass. The pharyngobasilar fascia is continuous with the foramen lacerum and is in close proximity to the foramen ovale, foramen spinosum, jugular foramen, hypoglossal canal, and carotid space. The proximity of these foramina to the sinus of Morgagni assumes importance in the consideration of intracranial extension (Fig. 41.2). A summary of the various foramina located in the base of skull is presented in Table 41.1.

The afferent innervation of the nasopharynx anterior to the pharyngotympanic tube orifice is provided by the maxillary division of the trigeminal nerve (V_2), and posterior to the tubal orifice by the glossopharyngeal nerve. Motor supply is via the pharyngeal branches of the glossopharyngeal nerve, vagus nerve, and sympathetic fibers from the superior cervical ganglion. The arterial supply of the nasopharynx is provided by the ascending pharyngeal artery, sphenopalatine artery, and the artery of the pterygoid canal. Venous drainage is provided by the pharyngeal plexus, which drains into the internal jugular veins directly or via communication with the pterygoid plexus.

EPIDEMIOLOGY AND ETIOLOGY

Nasopharyngeal carcinoma is an uncommon cancer in most parts of the world. The age-adjusted incidence rate (per 100,000 people per year) among men ranges from 0.6 in the United States and Japan to 5.4 in Algeria, 5.8 in the Philippines, 11.0 in Singapore, 17.2 among Eskimos, Indians, and Aleuts in Alaska to 17.8 and 26.9 in Hong Kong and Guangdong Province in Southern China, respectively.[1–2,3]

A bimodal age distribution is observed in low-risk populations. The first peak incidence arises between 15 to 25 years of age, with the second peak at 50 to 59 years of age.[4,5–6] In high-risk populations, the peak incidence occurs in the fourth and fifth decades of life.[4] Both genders have a similar age distribution; however, the male-to-female incidence ratio is 2:1 to 3:1.[7]

This distinct racial and geographic distribution of nasopharyngeal carcinoma suggests a multifactorial cause. Current epidemiologic and experimental data identify at least three important etiologic factors: (i) genetic, (ii) environmental, and (iii) viral.

The high incidence of nasopharyngeal carcinoma among Southern Chinese and populations of Southern Chinese descent suggests a component of genetic susceptibility. A genome-wide

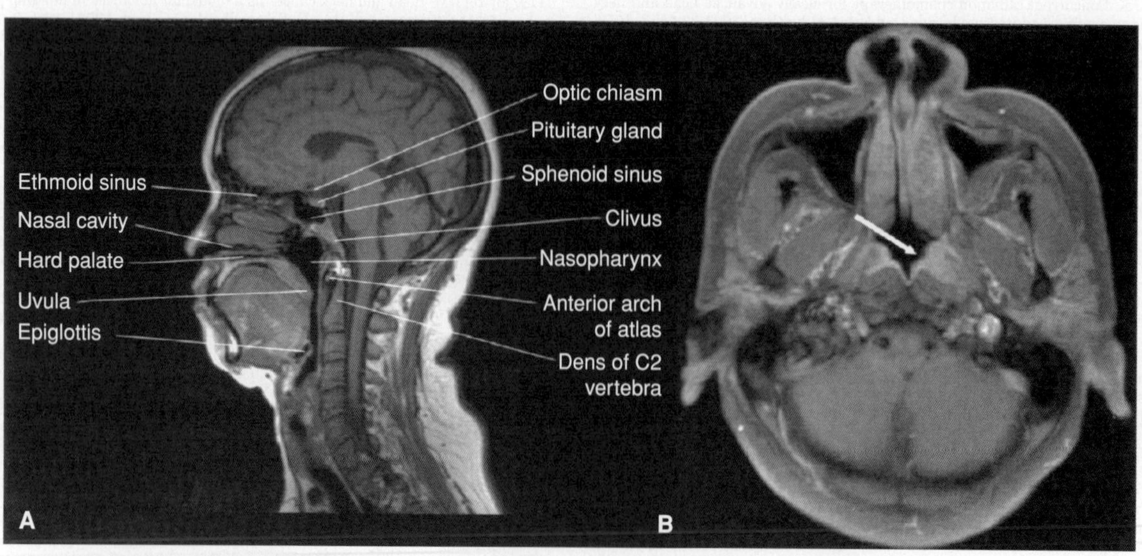

FIGURE 41.1. **A:** Midsagittal magnetic resonance image (MRI) of the head, showing the nasopharynx and related structures. **B:** Axial contrast-enhanced MRI showing a small tumor in the left *fossa of Rosenmüller* (*arrow*) and normal structures in the rest of the nasopharynx.

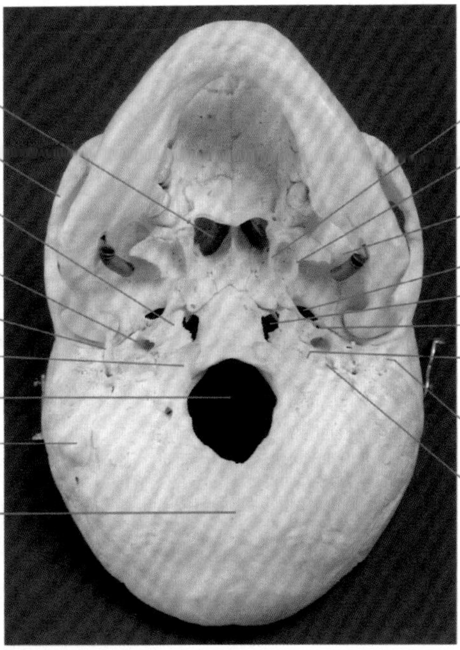

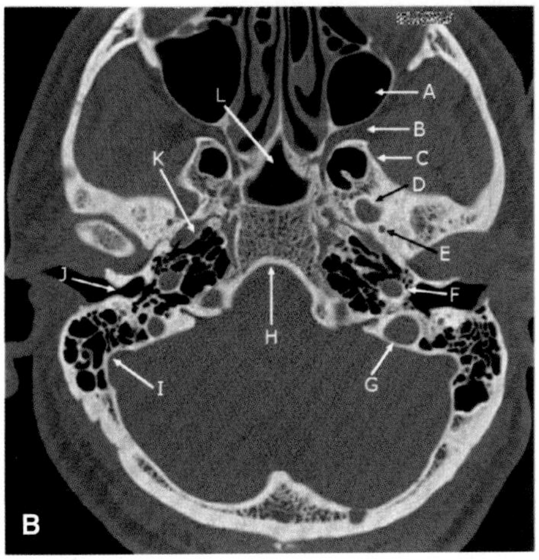

FIGURE 41.2. A: Basal view of skull illustrating the foramina of the base of the skull and the occupying structures. **B:** Axial computed tomography scan illustrating the bony anatomy.

TABLE 41.1 FORAMINA OF THE BASE OF THE SKULL AND ASSOCIATED ANATOMIC STRUCTURES

Foramen/Fissure	*Cranial Nerve*	*Other Structures*
Cribriform plate	Olfactory nerve (I)	Anterior ethmoidal nerve
Optic foramen	Optic nerve (II)	Ophthalmic artery
Superior orbital fissure	Oculomotor (III), trochlear (IV), ophthalmic division of trigeminal (V_1) nerve, abducent (VI) nerves	Ophthalmic vein, orbital branch of middle meningeal and recurrent branch of lacrimal arteries, sympathetic plexus, filaments from carotid plexus
Foramen rotundum	Maxillary division of trigeminal (V_2) nerve	
Foramen ovale	Mandibular division of trigeminal (V_3) nerve	Accessory meningeal artery, lesser superficial petrosal nerve
Foramen lacerum		Internal carotid, sympathetic carotid plexus; vidian nerve, meningeal branch of ascending pharyngeal artery, emissary vein
Foramen spinosum	Recurrent branch of V_3 nerve	Middle meningeal artery and vein
Stylomastoid foramen	Facial (VII) nerve	
Internal acoustic meatus	Auditory (VIII) nerve	Internal auditory artery
Jugular foramen	Glossopharyngeal (IX), vagus (X), spinal accessory (XI) nerves	Inferior petrosal sinus, transverse sinus, meningeal branches from occipital and ascending pharyngeal arteries
Hypoglossal canal	Hypoglossal (XII) nerve	Meningeal branch of ascending pharyngeal artery
Foramen magnum		Spinal cord, spinal accessory nerve, vertebral vessels, anterior and posterior spinal vessels

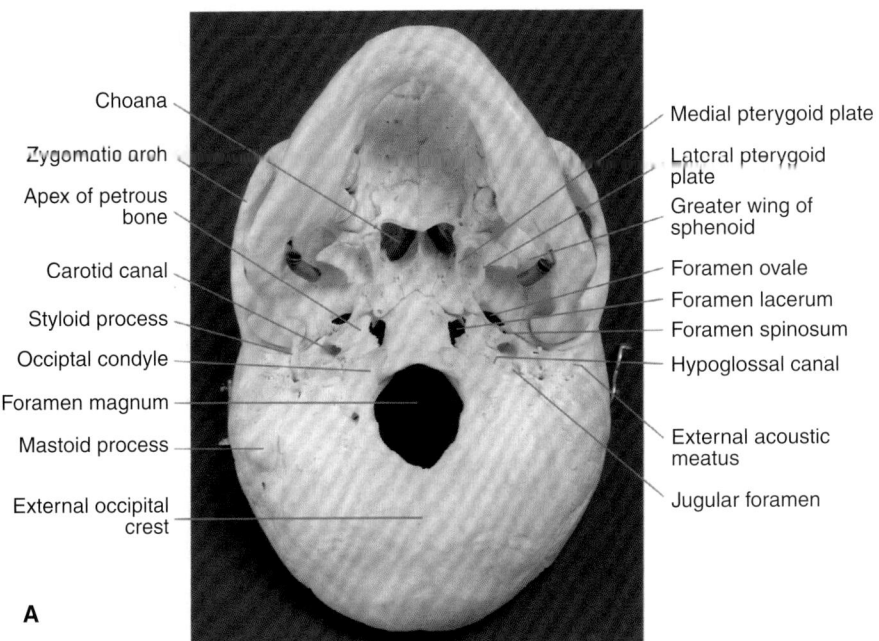

association study of nasopharyngeal cancer found three susceptibility loci[8] and confirmed a linkage study that found a gene closely linked to the HLA locus conferred a greatly increased risk of this disease.[9] In addition, several HLA haplotypes, including A2, B46, and B17, are associated with an increased risk of developing nasopharyngeal carcinoma.[10,11]

The high consumption of salted fish in Southern China has been implicated as an important environmental factor.[12–13,14–15] Dimethylnitrosamine, a carcinogen found in salted fish, has been shown to induce carcinoma in the upper respiratory tract in rats.[13] Other potential environmental etiologic factors that have been associated with nasopharyngeal carcinoma include alcohol consumption and exposure to dust, fumes, formaldehyde, and cigarette smoke,[16,17] although definitive conclusion has been elusive. Descendents from Chinese who have migrated from endemic areas to Western countries show progressively lower risk, but their incidence remains higher than that of the indigenous populations.[18–20] Buell[18] observed that American-born second-generation Chinese had a lower risk than the Asian-born first generation, while whites born in Southeast Asia had an increased risk compared to American-born whites. Dickson and Flores[20] reported that the incidence rate in Chinese who were natively born in China was 20.5, compared with 1.3 for Chinese and 0.2 for whites born in Canada. Taken together, environmental factors appear to play a role in the etiology of nasopharyngeal cancer.

Epstein-Barr virus (EBV) has been associated with nasopharyngeal carcinoma, especially the nonkeratinizing type, irrespectively of ethnic or geographic origin.[21] Premalignant lesions of nasopharyngeal epithelium show increased levels of EBV, suggesting that EBV infection may influence the early stages of tumorigenesis in nasopharyngeal carcinoma (NPC).[22] Detection of a single form of EBV DNA in tumors suggests that clonal expansion from an initial EBV infected and ultimately transformed cell is likely. EBV's tumorigenic potential is due to a set of latent genes: latent membrane proteins (LMP1, LMP2A, and LMP2B) and EBV-determined nuclear antigens (EBNA1 and EBNA2), which are the proteins predominantly expressed in NPC.[23] LMP1 is the principal oncogene, with evidence that the C-terminal activating regions of the protein activate a variety of signaling pathways, including mitogen-activated protein kinases, phosphoionositol-3-kinase, nuclear factor κ-B, and epidermal growth factor receptor (EGFR).[24,25] LMP1 is also required for cell immortalization and is present in 80% to 90% of NPC tumors.[26] This mounting evidence highlights the likely etiologic role for EBV in NPC.

NATURAL HISTORY

Local Extension

A summary of structures locally infiltrated by nasopharyngeal carcinoma at diagnosis is provided in Table 41.2.

Anterior

Anteriorly, it is common for the extension and infiltration of tumor to occur into the nasal fossa. Invasion of the lateral wall of the nasal fossa can lead to involvement and destruction of the pterygoid plates. Beyond these structures, albeit less common, is invasion of the posterior ethmoid and maxillary sinuses. In advanced disease, infiltration of the orbital apex (typically through the inferior orbital fissure) can occur.

Superior and Posterior

Superiorly, tumors can directly invade the base of skull, sphenoid sinus, and the clivus. The foramen lacerum, positioned directly above the pharyngeal recess (*fossa of Rosenmüller*), is a vulnerable spot through which tumor may enter the cavernous sinus and the middle cranial fossa to invade cranial nerves II to VI (Fig. 41.3). Figure 41.4 demonstrates involvement of the trigeminal cave (*Meckel's cave*) and the maxillary branch of the trigeminal nerve (V_2). The foramen ovale also allows access for tumor to invade the middle cranial fossa, in addition to the petrous portion of the temporal bone, and the cavernous sinus. Posteriorly, invasion of the prevertebral (longus capitus) muscles is commonly seen.

Inferior

Extension inferiorly to the oropharynx is not unlikely, with potential involvement of the tonsillar pillars, the tonsillar fossa, and the lateral and posterior oropharyngeal walls. In advanced disease, invasion of the C1 vertebra posteriorly and inferiorly can occur. Direct invasion of the soft palate is uncommon.

Lateral

Lateral extension occurs early, with involvement of the lateral parapharyngeal space along with invasion of the levator and tensor veli palatini muscles (Fig. 41.5). In advanced disease,

TABLE 41.2 STRUCTURES LOCALLY INFILTRATED BY NASOPHARYNGEAL CARCINOMA AT DIAGNOSIS[a]

Structures Involved	*Frequency (%)*
Adjacent soft tissue	
Nasal cavity	87
Parapharyngeal space, carotid space	68
Pterygoid muscle (medial, lateral)	48
Oropharyngeal wall, soft palate	21
Prevertebral muscle	19
Bony erosion/paranasal sinus	
Clivus	41
Sphenoid bone, foramina lacerum, ovale, rotundum	38
Pterygoid plate(s), pterygomaxillary fissure, pterygopalatine fossa	27
Petrous bone, petro-occipital fissure	19
Ethmoid sinus	6
Maxillary antrum	4
Jugular foramen, hypoglossal canal	4
Pituitary fossa/gland	3
Extensive/intracranial extension	
Cavernous sinus	16
Infratemporal fossa	9
Orbit, orbital fissure(s)	4
Cerebrum, meninges, cisterns	4
Hypopharynx	2

[a]Based on magnetic resonance imaging of 308 patients from Pamela Youde Nethersole Eastern Hospital, Hong Kong.

Modified from Chan J, Bray F, McCarron P, et al. Nasopharyngeal carcinoma. In: Barnes L, Eveson JW, Reichart P, et al., eds. *Pathology and genetics of head and neck tumours.* Lyon, France: IARC Press; 2005:85–97.

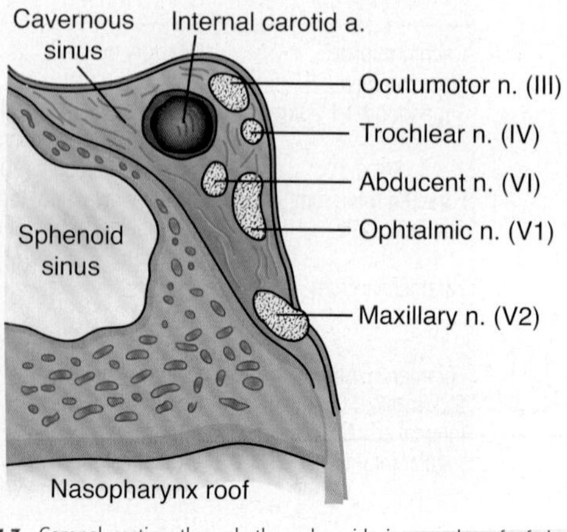

FIGURE 41.3. Coronal section through the sphenoid sinus and roof of the nasopharynx showing the relative positions of the cranial nerves III to VI. (Modified from Chao KSC. *Practical essentials of intensity-modulated radiation therapy.* Philadelphia: Lippincott Williams & Wilkins; 2005:138.)

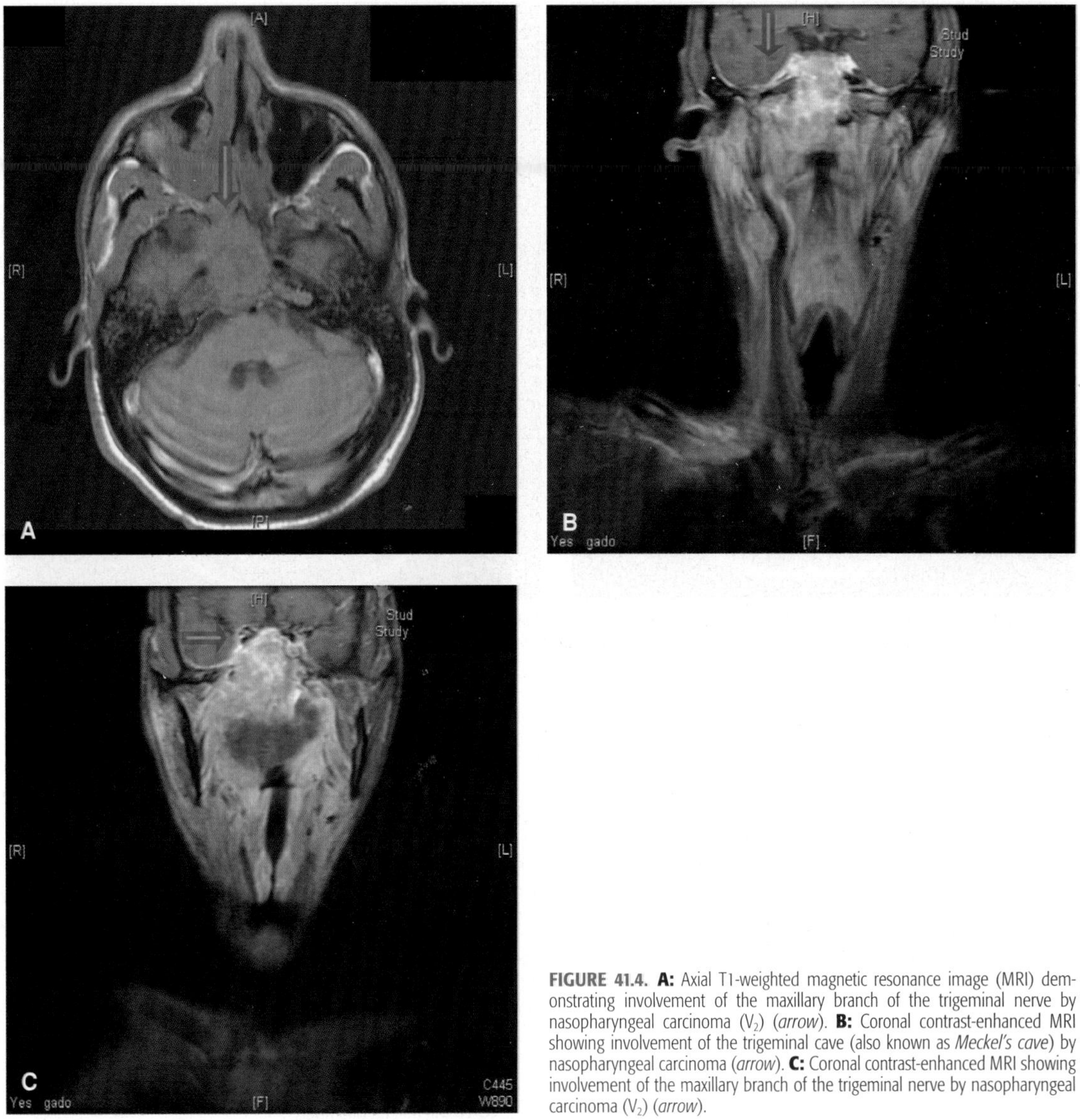

FIGURE 41.4. **A:** Axial T1-weighted magnetic resonance image (MRI) demonstrating involvement of the maxillary branch of the trigeminal nerve by nasopharyngeal carcinoma (V_2) (*arrow*). **B:** Coronal contrast-enhanced MRI showing involvement of the trigeminal cave (also known as *Meckel's cave*) by nasopharyngeal carcinoma (*arrow*). **C:** Coronal contrast-enhanced MRI showing involvement of the maxillary branch of the trigeminal nerve by nasopharyngeal carcinoma (V_2) (*arrow*).

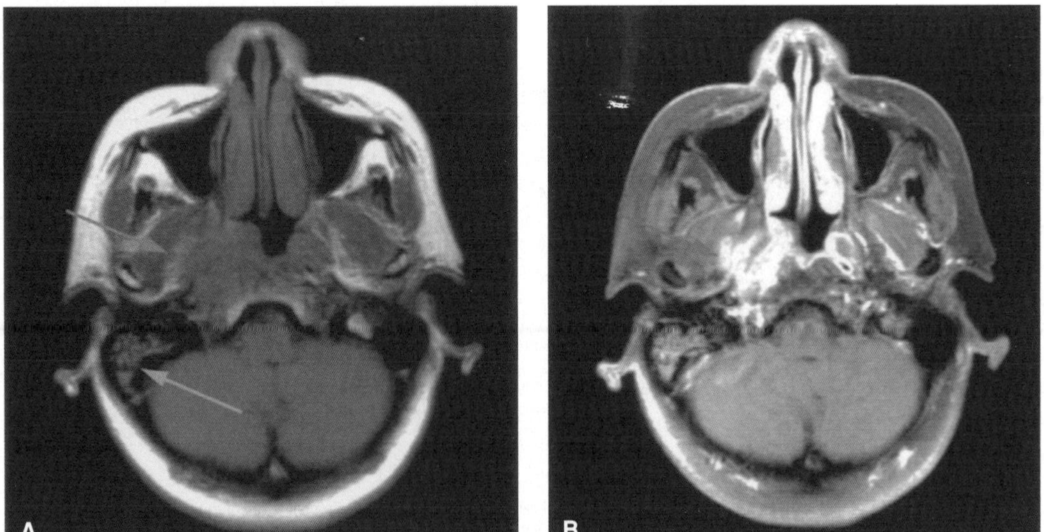

FIGURE 41.5. **A:** Axial T1-weighted magnetic resonance image (MRI) showing tumor infiltration of the right parapharyngeal space (*left arrow*). Note the resultant serous otitis media (*right arrow*). **B:** Axial contrast-enhanced MRI showing enhanced tumor involving the parapharyngeal space and medial pterygoid muscles (*arrow*).

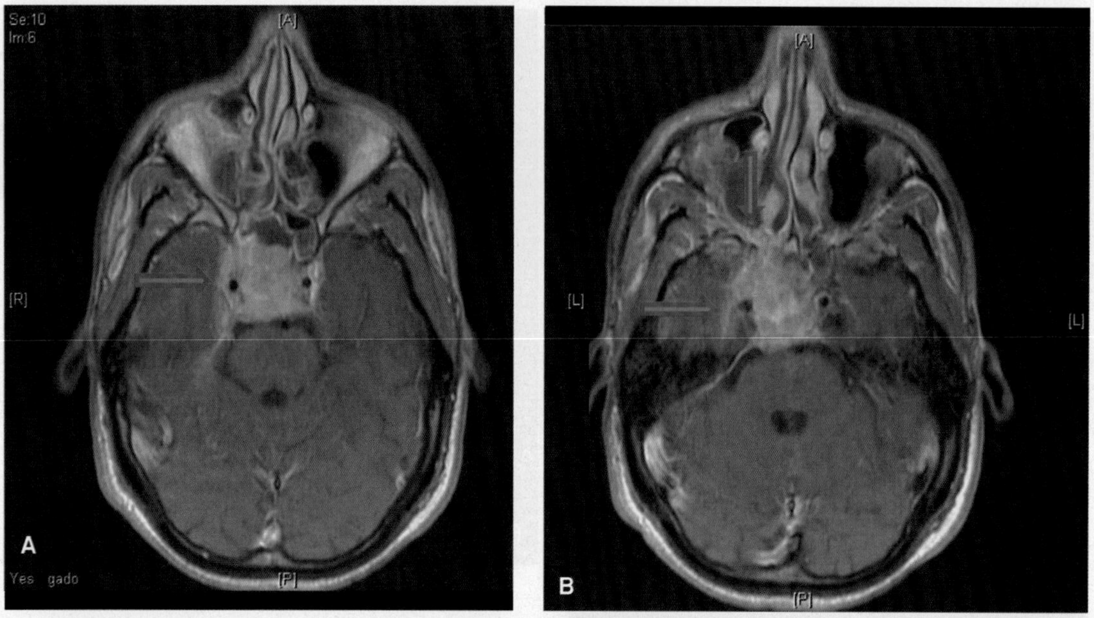

FIGURE 41.6. A: Axial contrast-enhanced magnetic resonance image (MRI) demonstrating involvement of the cavernous sinus by nasopharyngeal carcinoma. **B:** Axial contrast-enhanced MRI showing invasion of pterygopalatine fossa (*vertical arrow*) with spread to cavernous sinus (*horizontal arrow*).

invasion of the pterygoid muscles can occur. Direct extension of the tumor or lateral retropharyngeal lymph node metastasis in the parapharyngeal space may lead to invasion or compression of cranial nerves IX to XI as they transpire the jugular foramen, cranial nerve XII as it emerges from the hypoglossal canal, and the cervical sympathetic nerves. Direct invasion or compression of the internal carotid artery can occur in advanced disease (Fig. 41.6). Tumor can directly invade the middle ear through the pharyngotympanic tube (Eustachian tube).

Lymphatic Spread

The nasopharynx is comprised of a vast avalvular lymph capillary network that exists in the mucous membrane, leading to frequent involvement of regional neck nodes (Fig. 41.7). As

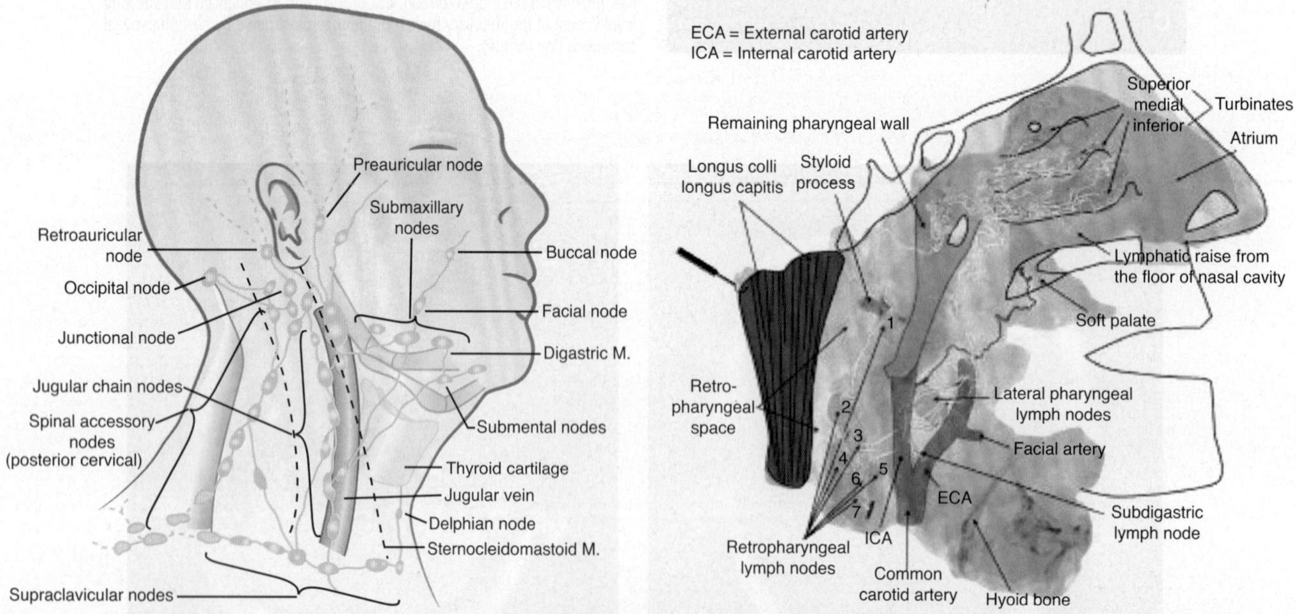

FIGURE 41.7. A: Pathways for lymphatic spread of nasopharyngeal carcinoma. **B:** Two major lymph collectors of the nasopharynx: (i) lateral lymph collector and (ii) posterior lymph collector. Yellow, lymphatic vessels from nasal cavity. Blue, lymphatic vessels from soft palate. Green, lymph nodes. Retropharyngeal nodes are numbered. Red, carotid artery. Dark brown, longus muscles. Light brown, remaining pharyngeal and nasal wall. (A, Redrawn from Rouviere H. *Anatomy of the human lymphatic system.* Ann Arbor, MI: Edward Brothers; 1938:27. B, From Pan WR, Suami H, Corlett RJ, et al. Lymphatic drainage of the nasal fossae and nasopharynx: Preliminary anatomical and radiological study with clinical implications. *Head Neck* 2009;31:52–57, with permission.)

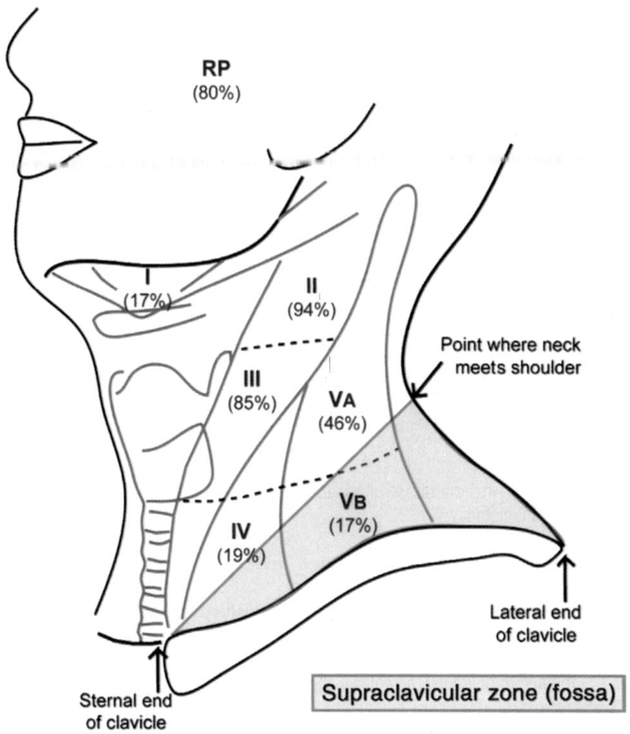

FIGURE 41.8. Distribution of positive nodes at different radiologic levels based on magnetic resonance imaging of 202 patients with nasopharyngeal carcinoma treated at Pamela Youde Nethersole Eastern Hospital (Hong Kong). Note the anatomic boundaries of the supraclavicular fossa as defined by the American Joint Committee on Cancer/International Union Against Cancer staging system.

many as 85% to 90% of cases present with lymphatic spread to the ipsilateral nodes.[27–29] Bilateral spread is present in approximately 50% of cases. The distribution of NPC involved nodes at diagnosis is shown in Figure 41.8. An anatomic and radiographic study that directly examined lymphatic vasculature concluded that there are two major lymph collectors of the nasopharynx (Fig. 41.7B).[30] One lymph collector runs along the lateral side of the pharyngeal wall, while the second runs more posteriorly. The lateral lymph collector empties into multiple first-tier nodes, which include the lateral pharyngeal node, the jugulodigastric/subdigastric node, and the third, fourth, and fifth nodes of the retropharyngeal group.[30] The posterior lymph collector empties into the first node (*node of Rouviere*) of the retropharyngeal group (Fig. 41.9). This direct study is corroborated clinically by frequent observation of lateral and retropharyngeal lymph node involvement by magnetic resonance imaging (MRI) or computed tomography (CT) scans, even though they remain impalpable. Metastasis to the jugulodigastric and superior posterior cervical nodes is also common. From these first-tier nodes, further metastatic spread to the midjugular, lower jugular, and posterior cervical and supraclavicular nodes can develop. Seldom, submental and occipital nodes can be involved secondary to lymphatic obstruction caused by widespread cervical lymphadenopathy. Mediastinal lymph nodes and, occasionally, axillary nodes may be involved with the presence of supraclavicular lymphadenopathy.

Hematogenous Dissemination

Distant metastasis is present in 3% to 6% of the cases at presentation and may occur in 18% to 50% of cases during the disease course.[31,32,33–34,35] The rate of distant metastasis is highest in patients with advanced neck node metastasis,[27,36,37] especially with low-neck involvement.[38,39] Bone is the most common distant metastatic site, followed by the lungs and liver,[40] with lung metastasis being associated with better prognosis than other sites. Brain and skin metastases rarely occur.[41,42]

CLINICAL PRESENTATION

Nasopharyngeal carcinoma presents in patients with symptoms in one or more of the following three categories: (i) neck masses, usually appearing in the upper neck; (ii) presence of tumor mass in the nasopharynx (epistaxis, nasal obstruction and discharge); (iii) skull-base erosion and palsy of cranial nerves V and VI due to tumor extension superiorly (headache, diplopia, facial pain and numbness).

The frequency of various presenting symptoms and signs is summarized in Table 41.3. A neck mass is the most common presenting symptom, followed by nasal and aural symptoms. The physical signs commonly present at diagnosis are enlarged

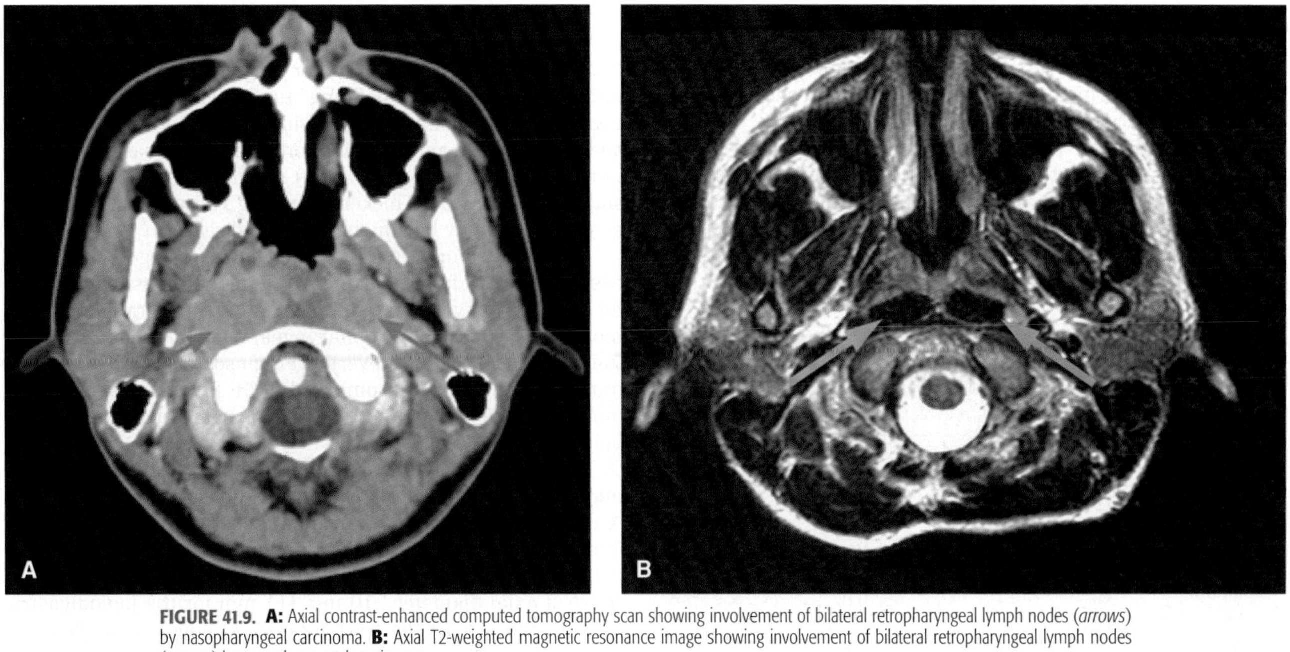

FIGURE 41.9. A: Axial contrast-enhanced computed tomography scan showing involvement of bilateral retropharyngeal lymph nodes (*arrows*) by nasopharyngeal carcinoma. **B:** Axial T2-weighted magnetic resonance image showing involvement of bilateral retropharyngeal lymph nodes (*arrows*) by nasopharyngeal carcinoma.

TABLE 41.3 SYMPTOMS AND PHYSICAL SIGNS OF NASOPHARYNGEAL CARCINOMA AT PRESENTATION

Symptom/Sign	*Chao and Perez*[355] *(n = 164) (%)*	*Lee et al.*[29] *(n = 4768) (%)*
Neck mass	66	76
Enlarged neck node(s)		75
Nasal (discharge, bleeding, obstruction)	>37	73
Aural (tinnitus, hearing impairment)	41	62
Headache	40	35
Cranial nerve palsy	23	20
Neurologic symptoms		
Ophthalmic (diplopia, squint)		11
Facial numbness		8
Slurring of speech		2
Sore throat	16	
Weight loss		7
Trismus		3
Distant metastases		3
Dermatomyositis		1

neck node(s) and, less often, cranial nerve palsy. The cranial nerves V and VI are frequently involved, while I, VII, and VIII are rarely involved (Table 41.4).[29,43]

Cervical lymphadenopathy is present in up to 87% of patients.[44] Typically, a mass is observable in the upper posterior neck and palpable beneath the superior portion of the sternocleidomastoid muscle close to the mastoid process. This is caused by metastasis to the parapharyngeal nodes or superior posterior cervical nodes of the spinal accessory chain.

DIAGNOSTIC AND STAGING WORKUP

Diagnosis of nasopharyngeal carcinoma is made by biopsy of the primary tumor. This can typically be performed with local anesthesia in an outpatient setting. Biopsy by direct visualization with general anesthesia may be necessary for diagnosis when the tumor is not visible or when the patient cannot cooperate. Not uncommonly the tumor is submucosal and not visible. For suspicious cases of a nasopharyngeal primary tumor with lack of visible tumor, random biopsies of the most commonly involved sites are warranted: pharyngeal recess (*fossa of Rosenmüller*) on each of the lateral walls and superior posterior wall of the nasopharynx. Fine-needle aspiration of a suspicious neck mass may establish the presence of metastatic nasopharyngeal carcinoma in the regional lymphatics. This may be performed prior to the biopsy of the nasopharynx when the primary tumor is not clinically detectable.

Table 41.5 lists the pretreatment diagnostic evaluations and staging evaluations that are generally recommended for NPC.

Complete physical examination should include thorough palpation of the neck, cranial nerve examination, percussion and auscultation of the chest, palpation of the abdomen for possible liver involvement, and percussion of the spine and bones for possible bone metastasis. CT and MRI of the head and neck are useful in the evaluation of tumor erosion into the bony structures of the base of skull along with retropharyngeal and cervical lymphadenopathy. However, MRI is the preferred imaging technique in the staging evaluation of nasopharyngeal carcinoma.[45–47] The current American Joint Committee on Cancer (AJCC) T-classification requires a search for tumor invasion into the soft tissue (e.g., parapharyngeal space) and bony structures. MRI may be necessary for proper staging because CT has limitations in accurately defining tumor extension into these regions.[48] MRI is superior to CT in delineating muscle, soft tissue involvement, and examination of the skull base.[48–50] When utilizing MRI, thin slices (3 mm) should be used for accurate staging (Fig. 41.10). Thicker slices (e.g., ≥5 mm) risk misdiagnosis of what may be a higher-T-stage disease.

Ng et al.[51] compared MRI and CT in assessing extent of disease. The study found a significantly higher sensitivity of MRI for skull base involvement (60% vs. 40%), intracranial involvement (57% vs. 36%), retropharyngeal node (58% vs. 21%), and tumor infiltration of prevertebral muscles (i.e., longus colli muscles) (51% vs. 22%) compared to CT. By MRI, T-staging was modified in 27% of patients, with 22% being upstaged and 4% being downstaged.

MRI and CT scans can detect lymph node metastasis that may not be clinically evident on physical examination.[52] According to a study by Van den Brekel et al.,[53] lymph node metastases are commonly recommended to be radiologically defined by presence of central necrosis, extracapsular spread, shortest axial diameter ≥10 mm (11 mm for the juglodigastric node and 5 mm for the retropharyngeal node), or a cluster of three or more lymph nodes that are borderline in size.

TABLE 41.4 INCIDENCE OF CRANIAL NERVE INVOLVEMENT BY NASOPHARYNGEAL CARCINOMA AT DIAGNOSIS

Cranial Nerve	*Chao and Perez*[355] *(n = 164) (%)*	*Chan et al.*[82] *(n = 722) (%)*
I	–	–
II	1.3	0.8
III	3.5	1.3
IV	2.4	0.6
V	7.8	V_1, 3.5; V_2, 5.8; V_3, 3.9
VI	13.3	5.1
VII	3.6	0.1
VIII	4.8	–
IX–XII	IX, 2; X, 5.4; XI, 1.3; XII, 4.8	2.4

TABLE 41.5 RECOMMENDED PRETREATMENT DIAGNOSTIC EVALUATIONS FOR NASOPHARYNGEAL CARCINOMA

- General
  - Medical history
  - Physical examination:
    - Palpation of neck node (record size, laterality, and lowest extent of enlarged nodes)
    - Testing of cranial nerve (including assessment of vision and hearing functions)
    - Exclusion of gross signs of distant metastases
- Fiberoptic endoscopy examination
  - Nasopharyngoscopy and biopsies
  - ± Panendoscopy
- Otologic assessment
  - Inspection of tympanic membranes (as clinically indicated)
  - Baseline audiologic testing (preferable)
- Laboratory studies
  - Complete blood count
  - Liver function tests
  - Urinalysis
  - Epstein-Barr virus–specific serologic tests
    - Immunoglobulin A
    - Antiviral capsule antigen titers
    - Serum Epstein-Barr virus DNA levels
- Radiographic studies
- Assessment of locoregional extent (imaging of nasopharynx, paranasal sinuses, base of skull, nasal cavity, and the neck)
  - Magnetic resonance imaging (study of choice)
  - Computed tomography (acceptable alternative)
- Chest radiograph (posterior–anterior and lateral)
- Additional metastatic workup if clinically indicated or N3 disease
  - Positron emission tomography (study of choice)
  - Computed tomography of chest and abdomen
    - In patients with abnormal liver function tests or clinical suspicion of lung or liver metastasis
  - Bone scan
    - In patients with advanced locoregional disease, symptoms suggestive of bone metastasis or an elevated serum alkaline phosphatase

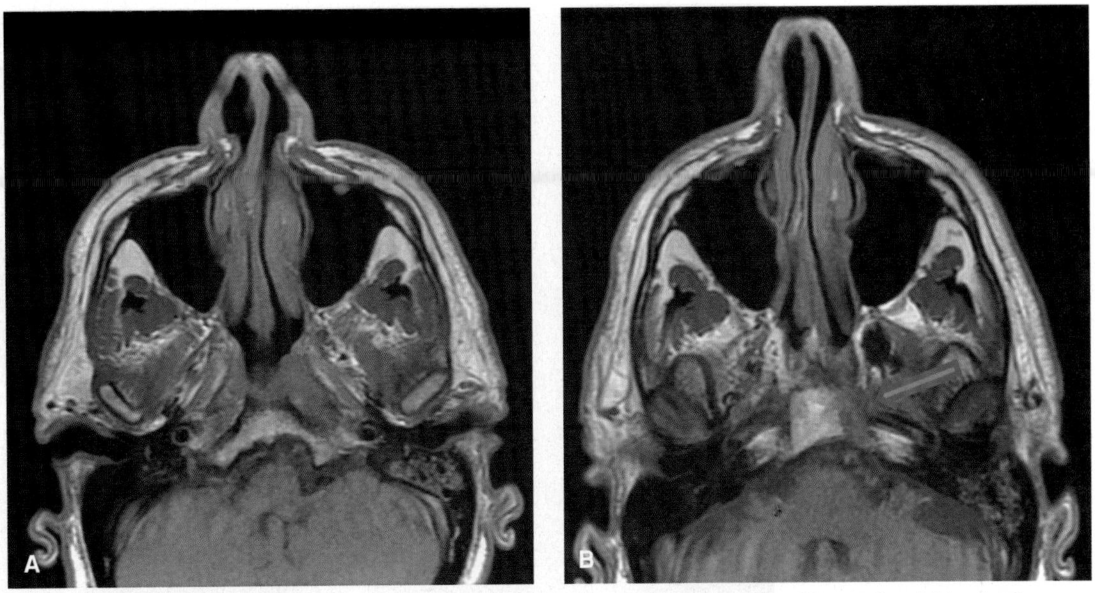

FIGURE 41.10. A: Axial T1-weighted magnetic resonance image (MRI) with 5-mm slices. **B:** Axial T1 MRI with 3-mm slices; skull-base invasion (*arrow*) upstaged this tumor from T1 to T3.

Detailed evaluation of nodal enlargement by palpation and imaging should consist of the size and location of the node, unilateral/bilateral involvement, and assessment of supraclavicular fossa involvement. Figure 41.8 defines the anatomical boundaries of the supraclavicular fossa, and Figure 41.11 demonstrates an example of bilateral cervical lymph node involvement seen by radiologic studies.

A complete search for distant metastasis is recommended for patients with advanced logoregional disease (e.g., N3 disease) or patients with suspicious clinical or laboratory findings. Positron emission tomography (PET) CT scanning (Fig. 41.12) is now commonly utilized in place of conventional staging by CT, bone, scans and ultrasound and appears to be at least as sensitive. Chang et al.[54] demonstrated that [^{18}F] fluorodeoxyglucose (FDG)-PET was superior to conventional work-up (i.e., chest x-ray, isotope bone scan, and abdominal ultrasound) in detection of distant metastases, where 12% of patients were upstaged to stage IVC. PET, in the study, offered sensitivity and specificity of 100% and 90.1%, respectively. However, large comparative studies of these various staging modalities have yet to be reported.[54,55–56]

The intimate association of EBV with nasopharyngeal carcinoma, independent of geographic and ethnic background, has provided clinicians with a tumor marker for disease diagnosis. Immunoglobulin (Ig) A anti-viral capsid antigen (VCA) and IgG anti–early antigen (EA) antibodies are both sensitive for diagnosing nasopharyngeal carcinoma; however, IgA anti-VCA has better specificity.[57] More than 90% of untreated nasopharyngeal carcinoma patients from California, East Africa, and Hong Kong have elevated IgA antibody titers.[58–60] Elevated IgA anti-VCA and IgG anti-EA antibody titers are typically associated with nonkeratinizing carcinoma (both the differentiated and undifferentiated histologic subtypes). Neel et al.[61] reported 82% and 86% of patients with nonkeratinizing carcinoma had elevated IgA anti-VCA and IgG anti-EA antibody titers, respectively, contrasted with only 16% and 35%, respectively, in

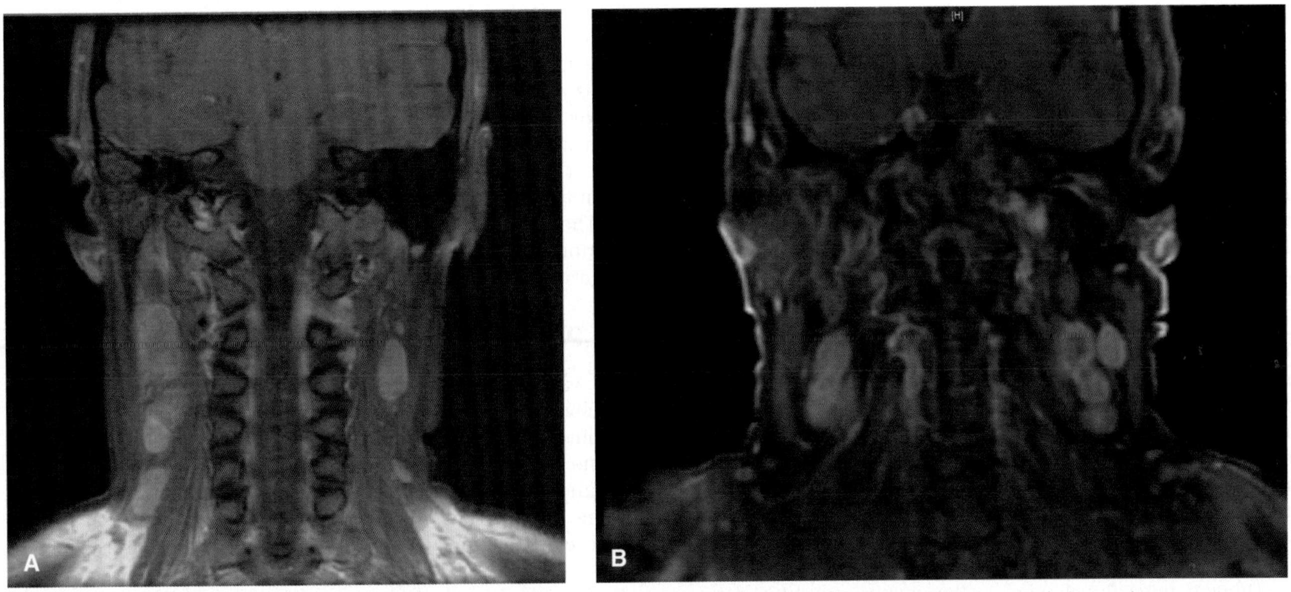

FIGURE 41.11. Two examples of coronal magnetic resonance images showing bilateral cervical lymphadenopathy. There is orderly downward lymphatic spread toward the supraclavicular fossa.

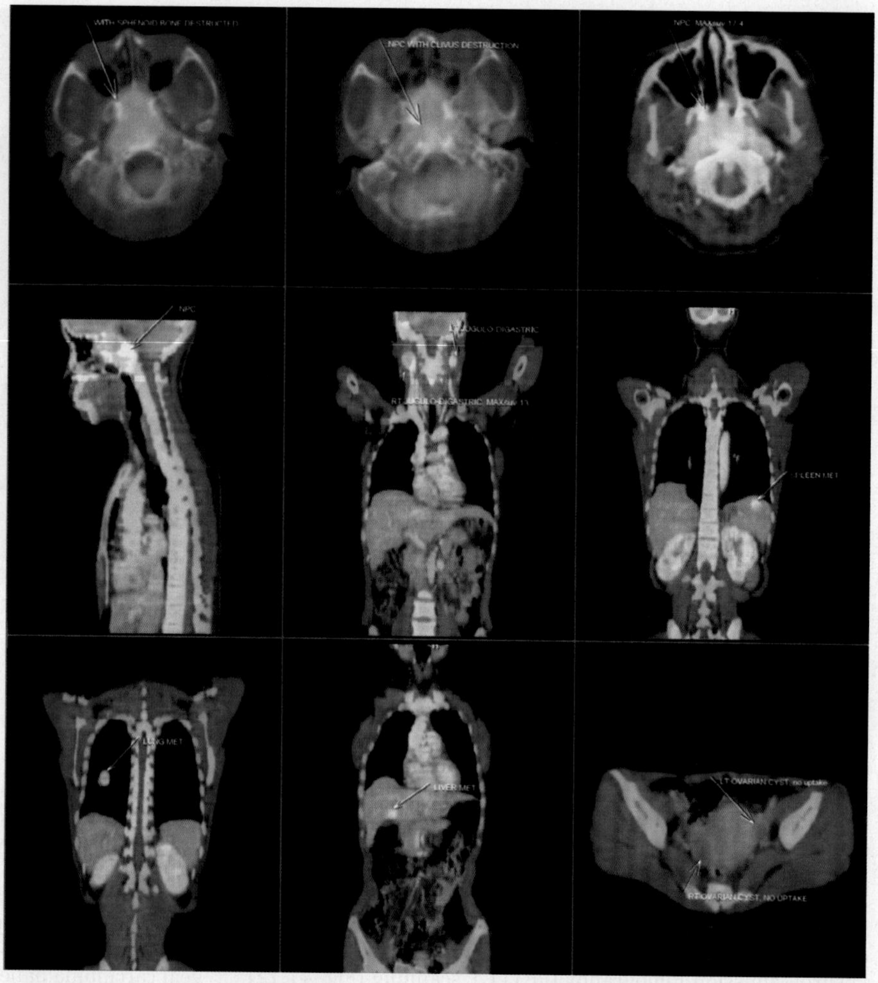

FIGURE 41.12. Positron emission tomography coupled with computed tomography (PET-CT) for a patient with nasopharyngeal carcinoma. Physical examination and biochemistry did not show any sign suggestive of distant metastases. X-ray of chest was normal. PET-CT revealed multiple distant metastases in lung, liver, and spleen, in addition to extensive local infiltration and bilateral cervical lymph nodes. (From Chan J, Bray F, McCarron P, et al. Nasopharyngeal carcinoma. In: *Pathology and genetics of head and neck tumours.* Lyon, France: IARC Press; 2005:85–97, with permission.)

patients with the keratinizing histologic type. IgA anti-VCA antibodies may serve as a screening test in high-risk patients, as they can be found elevated in patients months before the onset of symptoms.[62,63] A baseline test of plasma EBV DNA may be useful for prognosis, and levels over time can be utilized as surveillance in a posttreatment setting.[64,65]

STAGING SYSTEM

Various staging systems have been devised to predict prognosis and guide treatment strategy for patients with nasopharyngeal carcinoma.[66–69,70] The AJCC, International Union Against Cancer (UICC), and Ho staging systems are the most commonly used systems in the English-language literature. The AJCC and UICC systems are virtually identical in their 2002 version, and this continues in the 2010 update. Each system has particular limitations; however, they continually evolve and build upon each other's experience. Table 41.6, left, displays the AJCC staging system currently in use. One advantage of the Ho system is its approach to N-stage classification, which uses level or location of nodal involvement. This N-staging appears superior to that of the AJCC/UICC system, which is primarily based upon the laterality, size, and number of lymph node involvements.[14,38,71] However, for the first time, the 2010 AJCC system includes spread of disease to retropharyngeal lymph nodes as N1 classification. These nodal sites are considered the first echelon of nodal metastasis and were involved in 83% of nasopharyngeal carcinoma patients, compared with 74% with involvement of level II to IV neck nodes.[72]

Other noteworthy changes in the most recent AJCC system are in regard to the T-stage classification. In the 2002 AJCC system (Table 41.6, right), invasion of the nasopharynx soft tissue was used to separate T1 and T2 tumors, however, studies have shown that this distinction has no prognostic significance.[71,73,74] Parapharyngeal extension had been found to have prognostic value[75–76,77] and had been used to segregate T2a and T2b. The new 2010 AJCC system now separates tumors with parapharyngeal involvement into the T2 subgroup, while all tumors confined to the nasopharynx or with extension into oropharynx or nasal cavity without parapharyngeal involvement are classified as T1 (i.e., former 2002 AJCC T1 and T2a is now 2010 AJCC T1). Base-of-skull involvement has a significantly better prognosis than cranial nerve involvement,[27,38,78–80] but both were included in the T4 subgroup in the 2002 AJCC system. The 2010 AJCC system downstages base-of-skull involvement to T3.

These modifications to the staging classifications will require continued examination to determine if they improve prognostic accuracy.

PATHOLOGIC CLASSIFICATION

The vast majority of malignant nasopharyngeal tumors are carcinoma (80% to 99%), with the remainder of these lesions (about 5%) being lymphomas.[81] Other rare malignant tumors of the nasopharynx include adenocarcinoma, plasmacytoma, melanoma, and sarcomas. Regarding nasopharyngeal carcinoma, the current World Health Organization (WHO) pathologic classification,[82] released in 2005, includes three major types (Fig. 41.13). Keratinizing squamous cell carcinoma is distinguished by the presence of keratin pearls or intracellular keratin. Nonkeratinizing carcinoma is characterized by the

TABLE 41.6 AMERICAN JOINT COMMITTEE ON CANCER STAGING OF NASOPHARYNGEAL CANCER, 2010 AND 2002

Stage	Staging Criteria		
2010 Staging			
T category			
TX	Primary tumor cannot be assessed		
T0	No evidence of primary tumor		
Tis	Carcinoma *in situ*		
T1	Tumor confined to the nasopharynx, or tumor extends to nasal cavity[a] and/or oropharynx[b] without parapharyngeal extension[c]		
T2	Tumor with parapharyngeal extension[c]		
T3	Tumor involves bony structures of skull base and/or paranasal sinuses		
T4	Tumor with intracranial extension and/or involvement of cranial nerves, hypopharynx, orbit, or with extension to the infratemporal fossa/masticator space[d]		
N category			
NX	Regional lymph nodes cannot be assessed		
N0	No regional lymph node metastasis		
N1	Unilateral metastasis in cervical lymph node(s), ≤6 cm in greatest dimension, above the supraclavicular fossa, and/or unilateral or bilateral retropharyngeal lymph node(s), ≤6 cm in greatest dimension		
N2	Bilateral metastasis in cervical lymph node(s), ≤6 cm in greatest dimension, above the supraclavicular fossa[e,f]		
N3	Metastasis in lymph node(s)[e] >6 cm and/or to supraclavicular fossa[f]		
	N3a. >6 cm in dimension		
	N3b. Extension to the supraclavicular fossa[f]		
M category			
M0	No distant metastasis		
M1	Distant metastasis		
Stage grouping			
0	Tis	N0	M0
I	T1	N0	M0
II	T1	N1	M0
	T2	N0	M0
	T2	N1	M0
III	T1	N2	M0
	T2	N2	M0
	T3	N0	M0
	T3	N1	M0
	T3	N2	M0
IVA	T4	N0	M0
	T4	N1	M0
	T4	N2	M0
IVB	Any T	N3	M0
IVC	Any T	Any N	M1

Stage	Staging Criteria		
2002 Staging			
T category			
TX	Primary tumor cannot be assessed		
T0	No evidence of primary tumor		
Tis	Carcinoma *in situ*		
T1	Tumor confined to the nasopharynx		
T2	Tumor extends to adjacent soft tissues: nasal cavity,[a] oropharynx[b]		
	T2a. Tumor without parapharyngeal extension[c]		
	T2b. Tumor with parapharyngeal extension		
T3	Tumor involves bony structures and/or paranasal sinuses		
T4	Tumor with intracranial extension, involvement of cranial nerves, hypopharynx, orbit, infratemporal fossa,[d] or masticator space[d]		
N category			
NX	Regional lymph nodes cannot be assessed		
N0	No regional lymph node metastasis		
N1	Unilateral metastasis in lymph node(s), ≤6 cm in greatest dimension, above the supraclavicular fossa		
N2	Bilateral metastasis in lymph node(s), ≤6 cm in greatest dimension, above the supraclavicular fossa		
N3	Metastasis in lymph node(s)		
	N3a. >6 cm in dimension		
	N3b. Extension to the supraclavicular fossa[f]		
M category			
MX	Distant metastasis cannot be assessed		
M0	No distant metastasis		
M1	Distant metastasis		
Stage grouping			
0	Tis	N0	M0
I	T1	N0	M0
IIA	T2a	N0	M0
IIB	T1	N1	M0
	T2a	N1	M0
	T2b	N0	M0
	T2b	N1	M0
III	T1	N2	M0
	T2a	N2	M0
	T2b	N2	M0
	T3	N0	M0
	T3	N1	M0
	T3	N2	M0
Stage IVA	T4	N0	M0
	T4	N1	M0
	T4	N2	M0
Stage IVB	Any T	N3	M0
Stage IVC	Any T	Any N	M1

[a]Nasal cavity: anterior extension beyond the posterior margins of the choanal orifices.

[b]Oropharynx: inferior extension beyond the level of the free border of the soft palate. The junction at C1/C2 level is recommended as a more consistent radiologic landmark.[344]

[c]Parapharyngeal extension: posterolateral infiltration beyond the pharyngobasilar fascia.

[d]Masticator space and infratemporal fossa: extension beyond the anterior surface of the lateral pterygoid muscle, or lateral extension beyond the posterolateral wall of the maxillary antrum, and the pterygomaxillary fissure.

[e]Midline nodes are considered ipsilateral nodes.

[f]Supraclavicular fossa: triangular region defined by the superior margin of the sternal end of the clavicle, the superior margin of the lateral end of the clavicle, and the point where the neck meets the shoulder.

Used with the permission of the American Joint Committee on Cancer (Chicago, IL). The original source for this material is the *AJCC Cancer Staging Handbook,* 7th ed. New York: Springer; 2010 and *AJCC Cancer Staging Handbook,* 6th ed. New York: Springer; 2002.

complete absence of keratin formation and is further subdivided into differentiated and undifferentiated subtypes. The third type is known as basaloid squamous cell carcinoma[83] and is composed of closely packed small tumor cells that form a lobular and, at times, pallisading pattern along with focal squamous carcinoma elements. Basaloid squamous cell carcinoma is quite rare, with a frequency of <0.2%[82] (Fig. 41.13). The nonkeratinizing type has a strong association with EBV positivity.[84] The keratinizing type may have a correlation with HPV; however, the small sample size of these studies necessitates continued investigation.[85]

The histologic differences between these three types are by no means distinct. Lesions can share intermediate features, and some may be histologic hybrids. Lymphoepithelioma or lymphoepithelial carcinoma is considered a morphologic variant of undifferentiated carcinoma in which many lymphocytes are found among the tumor cells. Geography, race, and national origin affect the distribution of the WHO histologic types (Table 41.7). The frequency of nonkeratinizing carcinoma varies from 99% in Hong Kong to 75% in the United States.[82]

Of note, the former WHO classification remains quite commonly used and classifies the three histologic types as follows: (I) squamous cell carcinoma, (II) nonkeratinizing carcinoma, and (III) undifferentiated carcinoma.[66] This leads to unnecessary confusion with the new WHO classification, as the former classification was used in the majority of older studies.

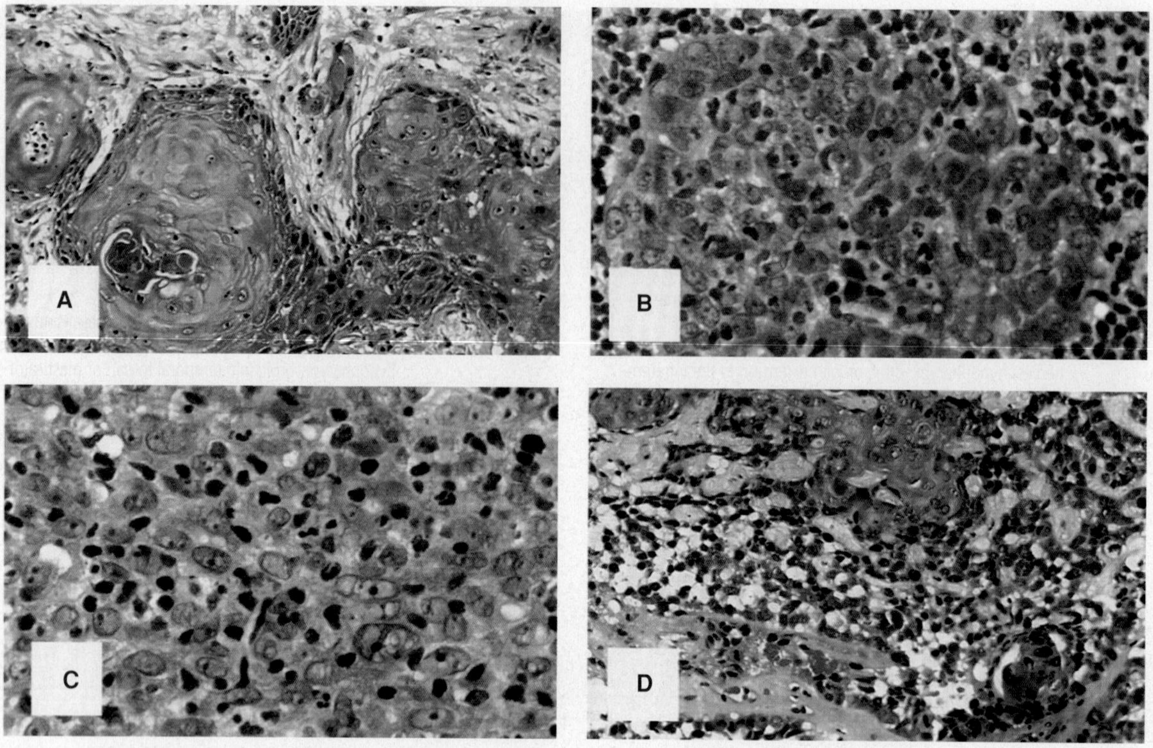

FIGURE 41.13. Photomicrographs of nasopharyngeal carcinoma. **A:** Keratinizing squamous cell carcinoma. **B:** Nonkeratinizing carcinoma, differentiated subtype. **C:** Nonkeratinizing carcinoma, undifferentiated subtype. **D:** Basaloid squamous cell carcinoma. (From Chan J, Bray F, McCarron P, et al. Nasopharyngeal carcinoma. In: *Pathology and genetics of head and neck tumours.* Lyon, France: IARC Press; 2005:85–97, with permission.)

PROGNOSTIC FACTORS

The extent of local invasion, regional lymphatic spread, and distant metastasis, as reflected by the TNM staging, is the most important prognostic factor. In general, advanced T-category is associated with worse local control and overall survival; advanced N-category predicts increased risk of distant metastasis and worse survival. Presence of distant metastasis (M1) upon presentation usually indicates poor prognosis, and treatment has conventionally been palliative in nature. A summary of the patterns of failure and survival rate for the different stages can be found in the Results of Treatment section.

The association of bone erosion, cranial nerve palsy, and lower nodal level with poorer survival is largely undisputed.[86–87,88–89] However, the prognostic significance of parapharyngeal extension has been a topic of controversy. In a study of 364 patients, Chua et al.[90] showed that greater tumor extension as defined by extension to the prestyloid space or extension to the anterior part of the masticator space was associated with a worse local failure-free rate (L-FFR; 72% vs. 86%) and lower distant failure-free survival rate (D-FFR; 68% vs. 87%) compared to tumors with no extension or extension only to the retrostyloid space. Other investigators reported similarly significant findings.[75,76,88,91,92] Cheng et al.[93] found parapharyngeal space extension to be the key factor in distant metastasis, even in N1 and N2 NPC.

However, Teo et al.[87] did not find parapharyngeal space involvement to be an independent significant prognosticator in a study of 903 patients. Au et al.,[94] using the AJCC/UICC definition of extension beyond the pharyngobasilar fascia in a study of 1,294 patients, also found that parapharyngeal extension was not a significant factor upon multivariate analysis.

These contradictory findings may be attributed to varying definitions of parapharyngeal space and incidence in the different series,[75,87,88,91] prompting some to advocate for consideration of the degree of parapharyngeal space extension in future staging systems.[76] In addition, suboptimal imaging by CT and conflation with retropharyngeal node enlargement likely contribute to the debate.[95,96]

Nevertheless, the most recent 2010 AJCC staging system (Table 41.6) downgraded involvement of oropharynx and/or nasal cavity without parapharyngeal extension from T2a to T1 while designating the presence of parapharyngeal extension to be the sole determinant of T2 classification. This was in light of recent multiple large retrospective studies that found no significant difference in disease failure hazard ratios between former AJCC 2002 T2a and T1.[73,77,93,97]

One recent topic of interest has been the prognostic significance of prevertebral space involvement (PSI). Recent MRI-based studies reported PSI to be an independent prognostic factor in cases of NPC treated with two-dimensional (2D) radiation therapy.[98,99] In a study of 506 patients treated with intensity-modulated radiotherapy (IMRT), Zhou et al.[100] found PSI to

TABLE 41.7 FREQUENCY OF DIFFERENT HISTOLOGIC SUBTYPES OF NASOPHARYNGEAL CARCINOMA

	High-Incidence Population: Hong Kong (%)	*Intermediate-Incidence Population: Tunisia (%)*	*Low-Incidence Population: United States (%)*
Keratinizing squamous cell carcinoma	1	8	25
Nonkeratinizing carcinoma	99	92	75
Undifferentiated	92	76	NA
Differentiated	7	16	NA
Basaloid-squamous carcinoma	<0.2	NA	NA

NA, not available.

Modified from Chan J, Bray F, McCarron P, et al. Nasopharyngeal carcinoma. In: *Pathology and genetics of head and neck tumours.* Lyon, France: IARC Press; 2005:85–97.

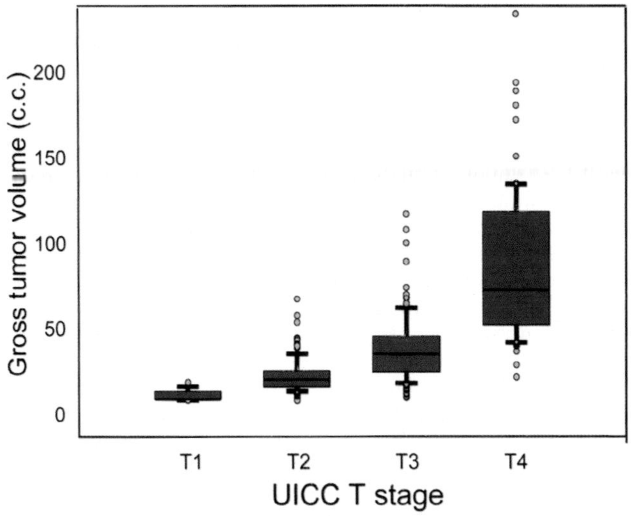

GTV_P				
Median	2.7cc	13.2cc	28.1cc	65.5cc
Range	2-12	2-60	3-110	15-219

FIGURE 41.14. The correlation between T-category and gross volume of primary tumor (GTV-P). UICC, International Union Against Cancer. (Modified from Sze W, Lee A, Yau T, et al. Primary tumor volume of nasopharyngeal carcinoma: Prognostic significance for local control. *Int J Radiat Oncol Biol Phys* 2004;59:21–27.)

independently predict overall survival (OS) and distant metastasis-free survival (DMFS) rates similar to those of T4 disease and advocated for its inclusion as a T4 parameter in future AJCC staging systems.

Another prognostic factor to consider is the gross volume of the primary tumor (GTV-P). Although it is highly correlated to T-stage, considerable variability in tumor volume exists within the same T-stage, and evidence increasingly suggests that tumor volume as an independent significant factor can better predict prognosis than T-category as specified by both AJCC/UICC and Ho systems[101,102–103,104,105] (Fig. 41.14).

In a study of 308 patients staged with MRI, Sze et al.[103] showed that those with GTV-P of <15 cm^3 had significantly higher L-FFR than those with a value of ≥15 cm^3 (97% vs. 82% at 3 years; $p < 0.01$). Multivariate analysis confirmed GTV-P to be a strongly significant factor independent of T-category by the 1997 fifth edition of the AJCC/UICC; the risk of local failure increased by 1% for every 1-cm^3 increase in volume. A similar observation between GTV and clinical outcomes was observed in other head and neck tumors, including oropharyngeal cancers.[106] Further study is required to determine how tumor volume may be optimally incorporated into future staging systems.

Most series found significantly better prognosis for females and younger patients.[86,94,107] In 759 patients, Sham and Choy[86] showed a higher 5-year survival rate in females compared with males (45% vs. 28%) and in patients younger than 40 vs. older than 40 years of age (50% vs. 40%, $p = .002$). However, they did not find age to significantly affect the 10-year survival rate. Multivariate analysis of 1,294 patients by Au et al.[94] also showed worse cancer specific death rates in males (hazard ratio [HR] = 1.28, $p = .02$) and patients older than 50 years (HR = 1.79, $p < 0.001$).

Although not all studies found histology to be an independent prognostic factor,[27,108] many found nonkeratinizing and undifferentiated carcinomas (formerly known as lymphoepitheliomas) to be more radiosensitive and offer better prognosis than keratinizing squamous cell carcinoma.[31,109,110] Of note, regarding ethnicity as a prognostic factor, a study by Corry et al.[111] showed no prognostic difference between ethnic Asian and non-Asian patients with nonkeratinizing carcinoma.

EBV and Other Biomarkers

Because of the association of EBV with NPC, various anti-EBV antibodies have long been studied for their potential as biomarkers. While some studies showed that elevated level of serum anti-EBV antibodies could indicate presence[60,112,113] of disease, others showed anti EBV antibody titers to have little value for posttreatment surveillance.[61,114,115] The prognostic value of such titers prior to treatment has also been controversial. While Xu et al.[116] found that high EBV DNase-specific neutralizing antibody at diagnosis predicted significantly worse event-free and overall survival, others found that a number of antibodies (VCA-IgG, VCA-IgA, EA-IgG, EA-IgA, EBNA-IgG, EBNA-IgA) could not predict prognosis.[113,117,118]

Circulating cell-free DNA of EBV in the plasma of NPC patients is a significant prognostic marker and has been found to be superior to serum anti-EBV antibodies.[118] Lo et al.[119] showed that plasma EBV DNA had high sensitivity (96%) and specificity (93%) for detecting NPC, while Ma et al.[120] showed that circulating EBV DNA levels correlated significantly with tumor burden. Studies by Lo et al.[121] and Lin et al.[64] found that high pretreatment levels were associated with advanced stages and poor prognosis. Meanwhile, Leung et al.[65] showed that pretreatment plasma EBV DNA load was an independent prognostic factor for OS in 376 patients and could be used to segregate early-stage patients into poor-risk and high-risk subgroups. Thus, pretreatment EBV DNA assays have the potential to complement TNM staging in guiding treatment.

Although Le et al.[122] found no correlation between pretreatment EBV DNA levels and survival, they did find posttreatment levels to be a strongly significant predictor of outcome; patients with no detectable EBV DNA had a 2-year OS rate of 94% versus 55% for patients with detectable posttreatment levels ($p < 0.002$).

Other studies also consistently reported that patients with elevated posttreatment EBV DNA load had higher risk of tumor recurrence.[64,121,123–125] Using multivariate analysis to compare various prognostic factors for NPC, Lin et al.[126] found that the combined EBV DNA load (pretreatment and 1-week posttreatment) was the most significant factor.

More recently, both Wang et al.[127] and An et al.[128] demonstrated that the clearance rate of plasma EBV DNA during the first month of salvage chemotherapy could predict tumor response and overall survival in patients with metastatic/recurrent NPC; undetectable levels after the first cycle indicated significantly better survival. These data suggest that early evaluation of plasma EBV DNA can offer oncologists timely insight for potential alterations in the therapeutic regimen for patients with a slow clearance rate. In addition, Wang et al.[129] prospectively monitored the plasma EBV DNA of 245 NPC patients in clinical remission with assays every 3 to 6 months and found the plasma EBV DNA assay to have much greater sensitivity, specificity, and accuracy than FDG-PET in predicting relapse, suggesting its utility for posttreatment surveillance.

As with other head and neck squamous cell carcinomas, EGFR is commonly expressed in patients with NPC. Chua et al.[130] found expression of EFGR in 89% of patients, in which overexpression was associated with significantly poorer disease-specific survival. Others reported similar findings of prognostic significance.[24,131,132] Ma et al.[131] performed multivariate analysis on several biomarkers in 78 patients, including microvessel density, Ki67 antigen, p53 oncoprotein, HER2, and EGFR, and found EGFR to be the only independent prognostic factor.

The study by Hui et al.[133] showed that 58% of NPC patients had expression of hypoxia-inducible factor 1α (HIF-1α), 57% had carbonic anhydrase IX (CA IX), and 60% had vascular endothelial growth factor (VEGF). Those with positive hypoxic profile (high expression of HIF-1α and CA IX) had a worse progression-free survival ($p = .04$); those with both positive hypoxic and angiogenic profile (high VEGF) were strongly associated with worse progression-free survival ($p = .0095$). Multiple other studies have also showed that overexpression of these markers, particularly VEGF, is associated with poorer survival.[134–136]

Other biologic factors that might have prognostic significance include E-cadherin and β-catenin,[137] c-erbB2,[138] p53,[139] NM23-HI,[140,141] and interleukin-10.[142] Further validation of these potential biomarkers is needed.

TREATMENT STRATEGY

Because of the anatomic location—proximity to critical structures—surgical exposure and tumor resection with sufficient margins have been very challenging.[143] Primary surgical intervention was rare after the 1950s for these reasons, with surgical interventions employed mainly for biopsy to gain histologic confirmation and salvage therapy for persistent or recurrent cancer. Primary treatment since has typically employed radiotherapy (RT) alone and, more recently, in combination with chemotherapy.

Radiation Therapy

To achieve the best therapeutic ratio, every single step in the RT procedures (localization of gross tumor and target volumes, immobilization, optimization of dose fractionation, determination of treatment techniques, and precision in RT delivery) is important.

For planning, the patient should be set up in a supine position with head extended for adequate separation between the primary tumor/retropharyngeal nodes and the upper neck nodes. The tip of the uvula and the base of the occiput should be on a parallel plane to the beam axis. The patient is immobilized with a thermoplastic mask covering the head-to-shoulder region (Fig. 41.15). For patients to be treated by conventional 2D technique, a mouth bite is useful to minimize the dose to the oral cavity, with enlarged neck nodes to be marked with wire before imaging.

Dose, Time, and Fractionation

A significant dose–response relation was observed in the majority of retrospective studies, based on patients irradiated with 2D techniques. Marks et al.[144] and Vikram et al.[145] showed that local control was significantly improved in patients who received >67 Gy to the tumor target. Perez et al.[27] observed that patients with T1-2 tumors had a local tumor control rate of 100% for those given >70 Gy, compared with 80% for those treated with 66 to 70 Gy. However, local control for patients with T3-4 tumors remained <55%, even with total dose >70 Gy. Similar findings were reported by Mesic et al.,[146] where ≥70 Gy achieved better local control for T1-2 tumors than 60 Gy (94% vs. 76%), but higher doses or larger fields did not significantly improve outcomes in T3-4 tumors. These observations suggest that, besides consideration of the prescribed dose, the problem of sufficient coverage has to be overcome for advanced tumors.

Lee et al.[147] reported a study of 1,008 patients with T1 tumors irradiated by four different fractionation schedules and demonstrated that total dose was the most important radiation factor ($p = .01$). Dose fraction did not affect local control; however, it was a significant risk factor for temporal lobe necrosis.[148,149] Therefore, a fractional dose of >2 Gy should be avoided[150] (see section Sequelae of Treatment).

The impact of the time factor is more contentious. A randomized study by Marcial et al.[151] in which 62 patients were treated with split-course irradiation (30 Gy in 10 fractions over 2 weeks, then a 3-week rest period, followed by an additional 30 Gy in 10 fractions) and compared with 59 patients with 66 Gy in 33 fractions in 6.5 to 7 weeks demonstrated no significant difference in 5-year local control (86% vs. 80%), nodal control (86% vs. 78%), or disease-free survival (40% vs. 30%).

However, Vikram et al.[145] observed that patients with interruption of RT for ≥21 days had significantly poorer local tumor control than patients without interruptions (34% vs. 67%). Similar findings have been subsequently reported,[152,153] with the general consensus that prolongation is likely to be detrimental, even for nonkeratinizing NPC.

In general, the prescription recommended for NPC is to a total dose of about 70 Gy over 7 weeks to the gross tumor along with 50 to 60 Gy for elective treatment of potential risk sites.

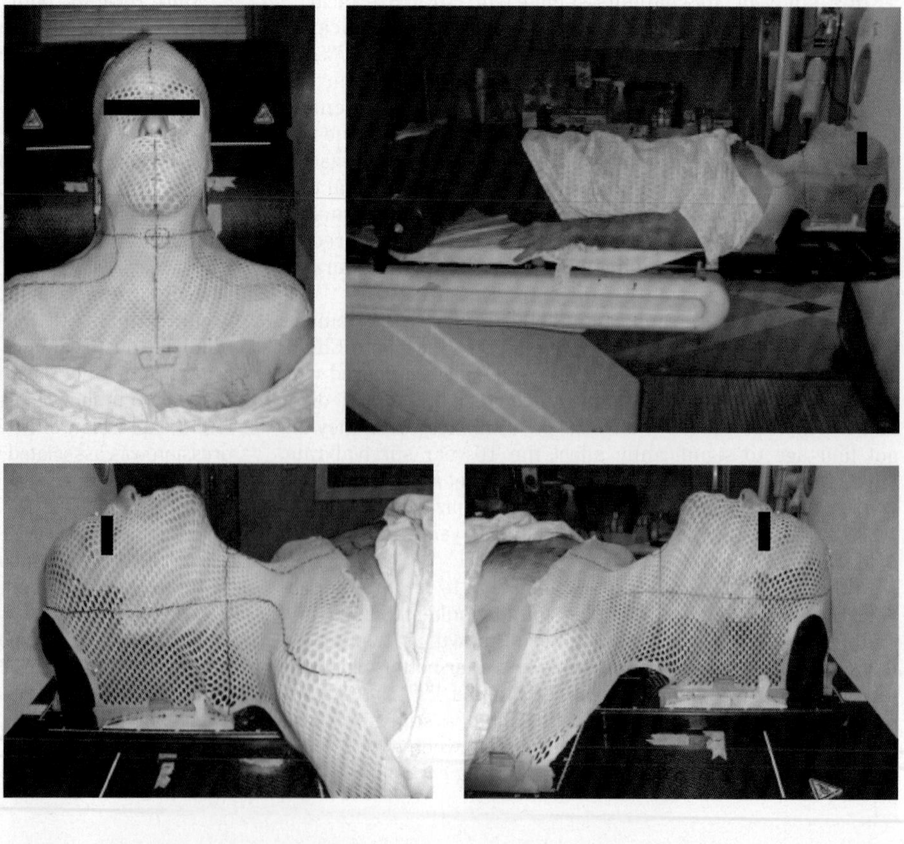

FIGURE 41.15. Immobilization of patient in a customized thermoplastic mask covering the whole head-to-shoulder region.

Tumor Target Volumes

The GTV should encompass the primary nasopharyngeal tumor, gross retropharyngeal lymphadenopathy, and gross nodal disease as determined by clinical, endoscopic, and radiologic examinations. Presence of lymph nodes of ≥1 cm or with evidence of central necrosis is considered gross nodal disease. For patients given induction chemotherapy, it is recommended that the targets be determined by the prechemotherapy extent.

Prophylactic neck radiation is usually recommended in N0 patients because of the high incidence of occult neck node involvement. Lee et al.[35] found that patients with a clinically negative neck who underwent elective neck irradiation had a significantly lower nodal recurrence rate than those who were untreated (11% vs. 40%). In addition, even with successful salvage by subsequent treatment, patients with nodal recurrence had a significantly greater incidence of distant metastases than those without recurrence (21% vs. 6%).

The clinical target volume (CTV) includes the GTV, regions of microscopic disease, and potential infiltrative spread. Different centers may have different philosophies in defining the margins and dose level. For example, Table 41.8 shows the delineation criteria for the various CTVs currently employed at Memorial Sloan-Kettering Cancer Center. A gross disease CTV (CTV_{70}) is defined as the GTV plus an additional margin of 5 mm to 1 cm surrounding all gross disease. The margin may be decreased to as small as 1 mm in critical regions near the brainstem or spinal cord. The high-risk subclinical CTV ($CTV_{59.4}$) encompasses the GTV including all potential areas of microscopic spread of disease. This volume should include at a minimum the entire nasopharynx; retropharyngeal lymph nodal regions; clivus; skull base; pterygoid fossae; parapharyngeal space; sphenoid sinus; posterior one-fourth to one-third of the nasal cavity; and posterior one-fourth to one-third of the maxillary sinuses. This $CTV_{59.4}$ should also include lymph nodal groups that are at risk of potential microscopic disease spread: bilateral upper deep jugular (junctional, parapharyngeal), submandibular, subdigastric (jugulodigastric), midjugular, posterior cervical, and retropharyngeal lymph nodes. In patients with clinically N0 neck, it is not necessary to include level I nodal regions.

The planning target volume (PTV) is defined as the CTV including a circumferential margin of typically 3 to 5 mm to all the CTVs to account for setup errors and potential patient motion. The PTV margin may be decreased to as small as 1 mm in regions near critical normal structures such as the brainstem or spinal cord.

Conventional Two-Dimensional Treatment Techniques

One of the most common RT approaches employed is comprised of two phases.[154] Phase I consists of large lateral opposing faciocervical fields that encompass the primary tumor and the upper neck nodes in one volume, with a matching lower anterior cervical field for the lower cervical lymphatics. Phase II is used after 40 Gy to limit the dose to the spinal cord. This three-field technique includes lateral opposing facial fields coupled with anterior facial field for the primary tumor. Typical treatment fields and radiologic landmarks are shown in Figure 41.16. Shrinking treatment fields by cone-down after 50 to 60 Gy should be done, when possible, to increase protection of critical structures.

The three-field technique in phase II allows the dose to be minimized to the temporomandibular joints and the bilateral temporal lobes. However, coverage may not be sufficient for tumors with extensive posterolateral extension to the parapharyngeal spaces or caudal extension to the oropharynx. To

TABLE 41.8 EXAMPLE OF GUIDELINE ON ANATOMIC STRUCTURES/BOUNDARIES FOR DELINEATING CLINICAL TARGET VOLUMES FOR INTENSITY-MODULATED RADIATION THERAPY[a]

	Delineation of CTV	
CTV	Structure	Anatomic Boundaries
CTV_{70}	GTV + ≥5-mm margin (can be reduced to as low as 1 mm for tumors in close proximity to critical structures/neurologic structures)[b]	
$CTV_{59.4}$	CTV_{70} + ≥5-mm margin (as low as 1 mm when close to critical structures)[b]	
	Entire nasopharynx	From 5 to 10 mm from mucosal surface of nasopharynx Anterior: junction with nasal choana Lateral: medial border of parapharyngeal space Caudal: caudal border of C1 vertebra
	Base of skull	Posterior: anterior 1/2 to 2/3 of clivus (entire clivus, if involved) Lateral: lateral border of foramen ovale
	Parapharyngeal spaces	Lateral: lateral border of styloid processes
	Inferior sphenoid sinus	Cranial: lower half of sphenoid sinus (in T3-T4 disease, include entire sphenoid sinus)
	Posterior nasal cavity	Anterior: posterior 1/4 to 1/3 of nasal cavity
	Posterior maxillary sinuses	Anterior: posterior 1/4 to 1/3 of maxillary sinuses (to ensure pterygopalatine fossae coverage)
	Cavernous sinus, include in high-risk patients (T3, T4 bulky disease involving roof of nasopharynx)	
	High-risk nodal levels (include all bilaterally)	a. Upper deep jugular (junctional, parapharyngeal) b. Submandibular (level I)[c] c. Subdigastric (jugulodigastric) (level II) d. Midjugular (level III) e. Low jugular and supraclavicular (level IV) f. Posterior cervical (level V) g. Retropharyngeal

CTV, clinical target volume; GTV, gross tumor volume: all gross primary tumor and involved lymph nodes; PTV, planning target volume: CTV + 3- to 5-mm margin. Total dose prescription at PTV_{70}, 70 Gy in 33 fractions (2.12 Gy per fraction); at $PTV_{59.4}$, 59.4 Gy in 33 fractions (1.8 Gy per fraction).

[a]Based on guideline currently used at Memorial Sloan-Kettering Cancer Center and detailed in RTOG 0615 (http://www.rtog.org/ClinicalTrials/ProtocolTable/StudyDetails.aspx?study=0615).

[b]CTV margins may also be limited to exclude bone NOT at risk for subclinical disease or air.

[c]Bilateral IB lymph nodes can be spared if patient is node negative. The treatment of level IB may result in the delivery of clinically significant radiation doses to normal structures such as the floor of mouth, mandible, and upper pharyngeal mucosa above the hyoid. At the discretion of the treating radiation oncologist, level IB may also be spared or limited to the anterior border of the submandibular gland in low-risk, node-positive patients. Patients presenting with isolated retropharyngeal nodes or isolated level IV nodes are considered low risk for level IB involvement. Treatment of level IB should be considered in node-negative patients with extensive involvement of the hard palate, nasal cavity, or maxillary antrum.

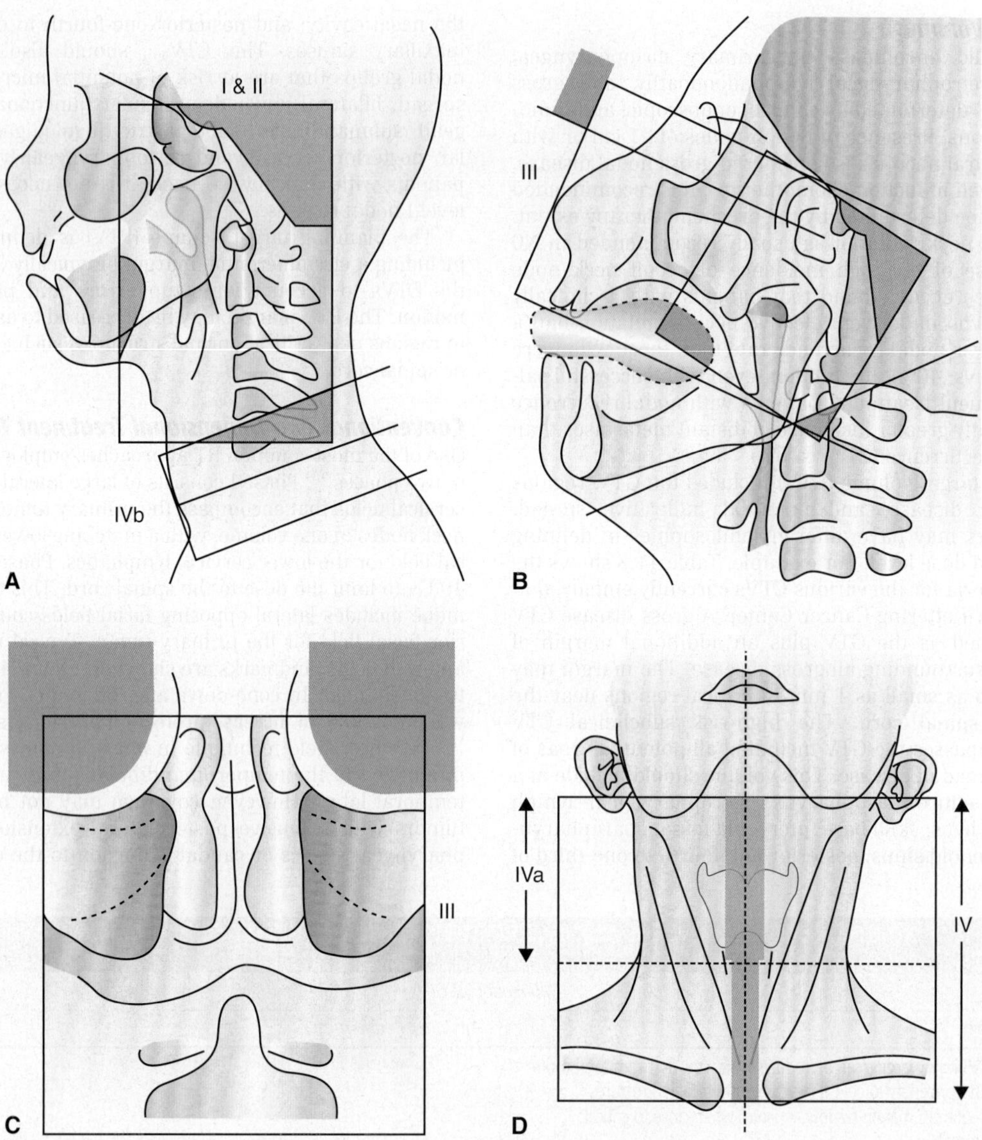

FIGURE 41.16. Conventional two-dimensional radiotherapy using Ho's technique. **A:** Phase I, lateral-opposed faciocervical fields (I–II) and lower anterior cervical field (IVb). **B:** Phase II, sagittal view showing lateral-opposed facial fields and noncoplanar anterior facial field (III). **C:** Coronal view of anterior facial field (III). **D:** Anterior cervical field for whole neck (IV).

remedy this deficit, an additional dose is delivered by a posterolateral field with avoidance of neurologic structures.[155]

Three-Dimensional Conformal Treatment Techniques

Nasopharyngeal carcinoma presents most typically as a concave tumor, allowing for computerized three-dimensional (3D) treatment plans to be an important technical advance for improved radiation delivery. Several investigators designed multifield conformal plans, including the seven-field technique used at Memorial Sloan-Kettering Cancer Center (MSKCC) (New York, NY)[156] and the "Boomerang" technique used at Peter MacCallum Cancer Institute (East Melbourne, Australia).[157] When compared to conventional 2D plans, 3D planning demonstrated better tumor dose coverage while decreasing normal tissue dose in several studies.[87,158,159]

Leibel et al.[160] from MSKCC demonstrated that the target volume underdosed at the 95% isodose level was lowered with 3D plans when compared with 2D plans (7% vs. 22%). On average, the mean tumor dose increased 13%, leading to an estimation that tumor control would increase by 15%. However, a subsequent study in which 68 patients received this technique for a boost of 19.8 to 25.2 Gy following phase I conventional 2D treatment for 50.4 Gy to a total dose of 70.2 to 75.6 Gy did not show significant improvement; the 5-year L-FFR was 77% and late toxicity grade ≥3 was 25%.[156]

More encouraging results were obtained by Jen et al.,[161] who compared 72 patients treated with 3D conformal technique with 108 patients treated with 2D technique. A significant improvement in 3-year L-FFR for T4 (86% vs. 47%) and event-free survival for both stage III (80% vs. 56%) and stage IV (82% vs. 33%) was observed. Furthermore, the incidence of xerostomia at 3 years was significantly less with 3D conformal treatment (69.2% vs. 98.0%), although for most other late toxicities little difference was seen.

IMRT Techniques

IMRT has supplanted conventional radiotherapy in the treatment of NPC in an increasing number of institutions throughout the world. The intensity of the radiation beams can be modulated to deliver a high dose to the tumor with a superior target volume coverage while significantly limiting the dose to surrounding normal tissues.[162–165,166,167] Following the initial publication[168] and the subsequent update on IMRT for NPC from the University of California, San Francisco (UCSF),[166] several other institutions have utilized IMRT with similar excellent treatment outcomes.[169–170,171–175]

TABLE 41.9 INTENSITY-MODULATED RADIATION THERAPY FOR NASOPHARYNGEAL CARCINOMA: METHODS AND RESULTS BY DIFFERENT CENTERS

	UCSF[166,177]	MSKCC[169]	PWH[171]	SYS[345]	QMH[170]	QMH[178]	CUHK[346]	NCCS[307]	PYNEH[311]
No. of patients	118	74	63	104	50	50	865	195	193
Patient characteristics									
Treatment period	1995–2003	1998–2004	2000–2002	2001–2001	2000–2002	2000–2004	2001–2008	2002–2005	2005–2007
T-category	All	All	All	All	T1-T2	T3-T4	All	All	All
Intensity-modulated RT									
PTV-G									
Margin around GTV (mm)	–	5–10	2	–	–	–	–	3–5	5–8
Total dose (Gy)	70	70.2	66	64–70	68–70	76	68	66–70	70
Dose per fraction (Gy)	2.12	2.34	2	2.33–2.56	2–2.06	2.17	2	2–2.12	2.12
Additional treatment									
Accelerated fractionation (%)	–	80	–	–	–	–	–	–	62
Boost	22% ICB		32% ICB 24% 3D	–	–	–	–	10% ICB	–
Chemotherapy (%)	90	93	30	23	0	68	65	>57	84
Median follow-up (mo)	30	35	29	19	14	25	40	36.5	30
Tumor control									
Time point (y)	4	3	3	3	2	2	5	3	2
Local-FFR (%)	96	91	92	99	100	96	90.4	89.6	95
Nodal-FFR (%)	98	93	98	99	94	–	–	–	96
Distant-FFR (%)	72	78	79	88	94	94	84	89.2	90
Overall survival (%)	74	83	90	86	NR	92	83	94.3	92
Late toxicities									
Xerostomia (grade ≥2) (%)	2[a] (2 years)	32 (1 year)	23 (2 year)	–	–	–	–	–	–
Deafness (grade >2) (%)	7[a]	>15	15	–	–	42	–	–	–
Fibrosis (grade >2) (%)	–	–	11	–	–	14	–	–	–
Dysphagia (grade >2) (%)	1[a]	–	5	–	–	–	–	–	–
Hypopituitarism (%)	–	0	23	–	–	–	–	–	–
Osteonecrosis (%)	0.8	0	2	–	–	–	–	–	–
Temporal lobe necrosis (%)	0.8	0	3	–	–	4	–	–	–
Carotid pseudoaneurysm/ epistaxis (%)	0.8[a]	–	–	–	–	4	–	–	–

MSKCC, Memorial Sloan Kettering Cancer Center (New York, NY); PWH, Prince of Wales Hospital (Hong Kong); QMH, Queen Mary Hospital (Hong Kong); SYS, Sun Yat-sen Cancer Center (Guangzhou, China); UCSF, University of California, San Francisco (San Francisco, CA).

3D, three-dimensional conformal boost; FFR, failure-free rate; GTV, gross tumor volume; ICB, intracavitary brachytherapy; NR, not reported; PTV-G, planning target volume for gross tumor; RT, radiation therapy.

[a]Based on data reported by Lee et al.[166]

Another point of interest is the possibility of biologic enhancement by simultaneous modulated accelerated-radiation therapy (SMART), also known as dose painting, as a new way of delivering an accelerated fractionation (AF) schedule, a concept that was first reported by Butler et al.[176] for the treatment of other head and neck cancers with IMRT.

These differing methods and dose fractionation regimens for IMRT are being investigated by different groups. Table 41.9 summarizes the key features along with reported results. The majority of the patients in these series received additional chemotherapy and/or enhanced RT with boosts or AF. All reported encouraging early results, with local control in >90% at 2 to 4 years.

At UCSF patients were typically prescribed 70 Gy to the $PTV_{gross\ disease}$ and involved lymph nodes in 2.12- to 2.25-Gy fractions, while $PTV_{high\text{-}risk\ subclinical}$ patients were prescribed 59.4 Gy in 1.8 fractions, and a clinically negative neck ($PTV_{low\text{-}risk\ subclinical}$) patient received 54 Gy at 1.64-Gy fractions, all in conventional once-daily fractions.[166,177] Bucci et al.[177] reported the updated results of 118 patients and confirmed excellent locoregional control of 96%. Nonetheless, distant failure remained high (28%) despite broad use of concurrent-adjuvant CRT. OS was 74% at 4 years.

At MSKCC, Wolden et al.[169] reported their experience with 74 patients: 59 were treated with AF using the concomitant boost method and 15 by the SMART method/dose painting. For the SMART cohort, a total dose of 70.2 Gy at 2.34 Gy/fraction was given to the gross disease, and the "microscopic" PTV received 54 Gy at 1.8 Gy/fraction. There was a trend, but no statistically significant improvement, in 3-year L-FFR than for patients treated by 3D conformal boost (91% vs. 79%, $p = .11$) Additional dose escalation by SMART boost in 50 patients with T3 to T4 tumors was reported by Kwong et al.[178] from Queen Mary Hospital (Hong Kong). They sought to deliver a total dose of 76 Gy at 2.17 Gy/fraction to the gross tumor. The early result for locoregional control was excellent (96% at 2 years); however, serious late toxicities were observed, including 4% of patients having a life-threatening hemorrhage from carotid artery pseudoaneurysm, and another 4% developing temporal lobe necrosis with a median follow-up of 2.1 years.

Two different IMRT approaches are being utilized by different centers: (i) an extended-whole field (EWF) IMRT technique, in which the total target volume is encompassed in the IMRT plan, or (ii) a split-field (SF) IMRT technique, in which the target volumes superior to the vocal cords are treated with an IMRT plan and the lower neck nodes are treated with a conventional low anterior neck field.[179–181] Discussions among practitioners on which IMRT technique is best have been persistent. Concerns of potential failures at the SF matchline due to potential underdosing, or even complications resulting from overdosing, have caused many centers to implement EWF IMRT even when no clinically involved neck nodes are evident in the matchline region. These concerns may be caused by the treatment delivery system that is used at centers where a perfect match between the IMRT fields and the low anterior neck field is not possible. However, with a EWF technique, an unnecessary dose of radiation is delivered to the normal glottic larynx,[182] whereas with the SF IMRT technique, the dose to the vocal cords is minimal due to shielding by a midline Cerrobend block or the multileaf collimator (MLC). No IMRT matchline failures or complications have been reported with the SF IMRT technique.[168]

Figures 41.17 and 41.18 show examples of MSKCC IMRT plans delivered with the dynamic MLC system using a sliding-window technique to patients with early and advanced disease,

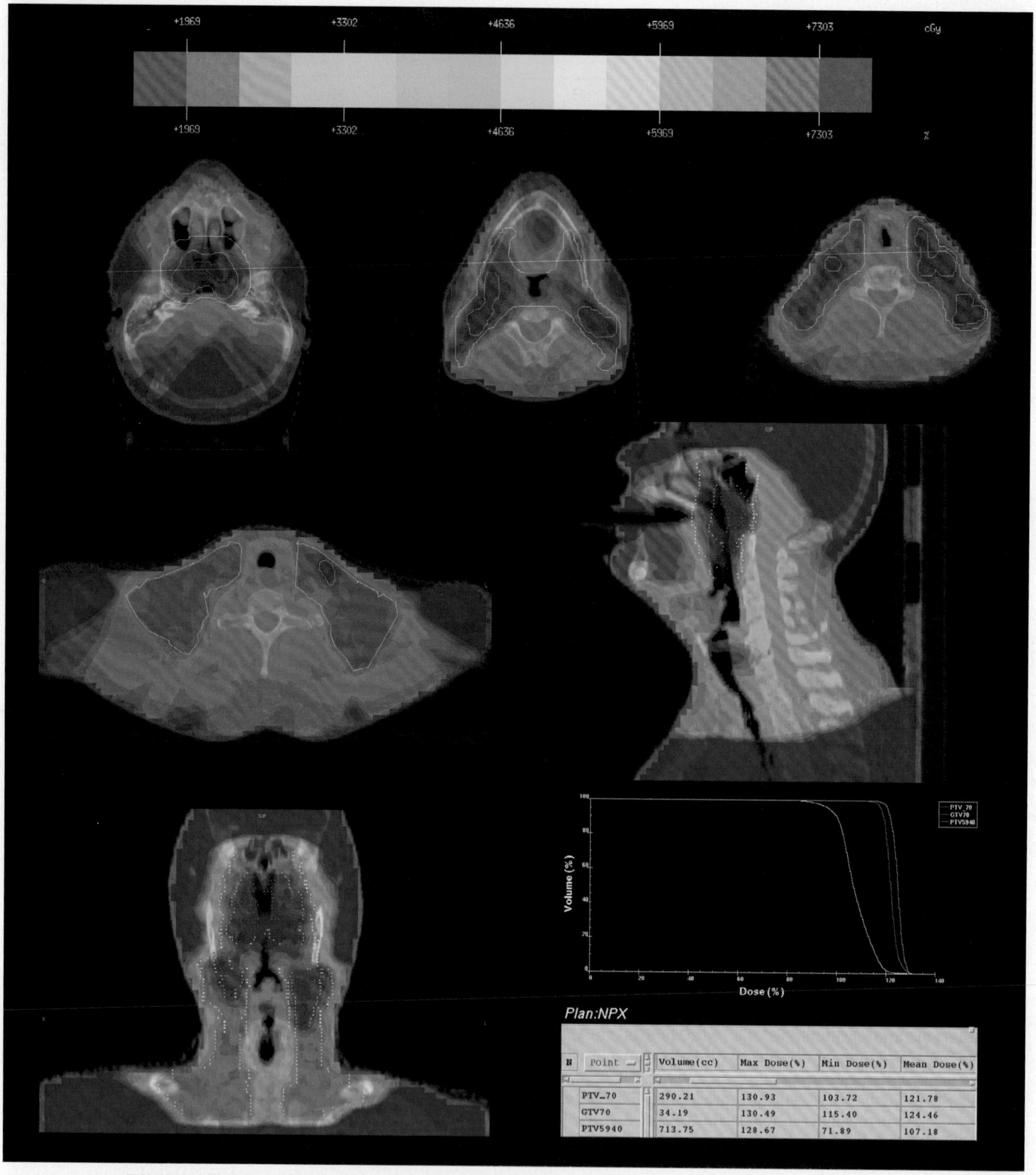

FIGURE 41.17. Intensity-modulated radiation therapy for a patient with T2N2M0 nasopharyngeal carcinoma treated at Memorial Sloan-Kettering Cancer Center, showing delineation of gross tumor target (GTV) and planning target volume (PTV) for 70 and 54 Gy, the dose distribution, and the dose volume histogram (DVH) for GTV, PTV_{70}, and $PTV_{59.4}$.

respectively. A total dose of 70 Gy at 2.12 Gy/fraction to the $PTV_{gross\ disease}$ and 59.4 Gy to the $PTV_{high\text{-}risk\ subclinical}$ patients is given over 33 once-daily fractions (Table 41.8). For the low neck, if split-field IMRT is used, a dose of 50.4 Gy at 1.8 Gy/fraction/day is generally prescribed. However, if the low neck is included in the IMRT fields and is considered at low risk for nodal involvement, the $PTV_{low\text{-}risk\ subclinical}$ patient typically receives 54 Gy at 1.64 Gy/fraction per day.

Inverse planning involves the appropriate specification of normal tissue dose constraints. It is important to note that overstringent use of normal tissue constraints might result in inadequate cover of tumor targets, and therefore optimal balance is essential. Different dose constraint guidelines have been suggested.[183,184] An example of dose-constraint guidelines is provided in Table 41.10, which displays the guidelines used at Memorial Sloan-Kettering Cancer Center.

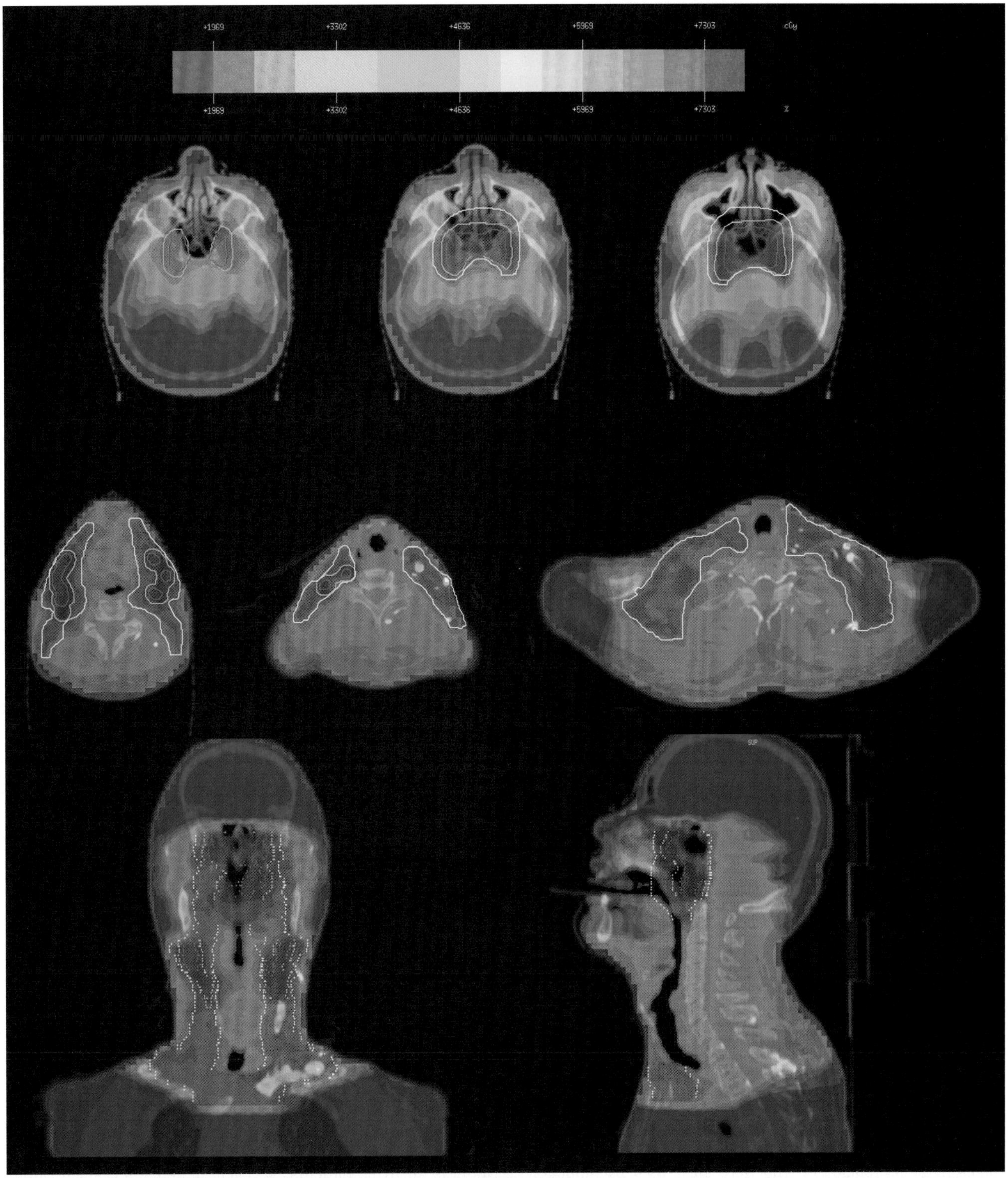

FIGURE 41.18. Intensity-modulated radiation therapy for a patient with T4, N2, M0 nasopharyngeal carcinoma treated at Memorial Sloan-Kettering Cancer Center, showing delineation of gross tumor volume (GTV) and planning target volume (PTV) for 70 and 54 Gy and the dose distribution.

Dose Escalation

Excellent local tumor control has been reported by delivering an additional boost to patients with early disease treated by conventional 2D technique.

Brachytherapy

The most commonly used method is brachytherapy. Intracavitary insertions[185–193] or interstitial implants[194–197] have been used in T1 to T3 nasopharyngeal carcinomas as a boost treatment following external beam irradiation (EBRT) or in the treatment of recurrent disease, either alone or in combination with EBRT. Brachytherapy is not suitable for treatment of tumors with intracranial extension because of the rapid reduction of dose as distance from the radioactive source increases. Since the advent of IMRT as primary radiotherapy for nasopharyngeal carcinoma and with its demonstration of excellent local control, the use of brachytherapy as a boost treatment following definitive IMRT has dramatically declined.

TABLE 41.10 INTENSITY-MODULATED RADIATION THERAPY FOR NASOPHARYNGEAL CARCINOMA: AN EXAMPLE OF NORMAL TISSUE DOSE CONSTRAINTS[a]

Structure	Constraint
Critical Structures	
Brainstem	Maximum <5 Gy or 1% of PTV cannot exceed 60 Gy
Optic nerves	Maximum <54 Gy or 1% of PTV cannot exceed 60 Gy
Optic chiasm	Maximum <54 Gy or 1% of PTV cannot exceed 60 Gy
Spinal cord	Maximum <45 Gy or 1 cc of the PTV cannot exceed 50 Gy
Mandible and temporomandibular joint	Maximum <70 Gy or 1 cc of the PTV cannot exceed 75 Gy
Brachial plexus	Maximum <66 Gy
Temporal lobes	Maximum <60 Gy or 1% of PTV cannot exceed 65 Gy
Other Normal Structures	
Oral cavity	Mean <40 Gy
Parotid gland	Mean ≤26 Gy (should be achieved in at least one gland) or at least 20 cc of the combined volume of both parotid glands will receive <20 Gy or at least 50% of the gland will receive <30 Gy (should be achieved in at least one gland)
Cochlea	V_{55} <5%
Eyes	Mean <35 Gy, Max <50 Gy
Lens	Max <25 Gy
Glottic larynx	Mean <45 Gy
Esophagus, postcricoid pharynx	Mean <45 Gy

[a]Based on guidelines currently used at Memorial Sloan-Kettering Cancer Center (New York, NY).

PTV, planning target volume.

Multiple applicators and techniques have been developed for the delivery of intracavitary brachytherapy.[187,188,189,191,193,198] In the past, intracavitary brachytherapy was delivered using low–dose rate (LDR) techniques. However, at present, remote afterloading, fractionated high–dose rate (HDR) techniques are more commonly used (Fig. 41.19).[198]

Table 41.11 summarizes reports on the use of brachytherapy as a boost for dose escalation. Most studies demonstrated that local control of up to 90% to 95% could be achieved for T1-2 tumors without excessive late damages. A retrospective comparison by Wang[188] from Massachusetts General Hospital (Boston, MA) reported that T1 to T2 patients who received a 10- to 15-Gy LDR brachytherapy boost after 60 to 64 Gy by EBRT had a 5-year L-FFR of 90% versus 54%, respectively, with $p = .001$ for patients receiving EBRT alone to 65 to 70 Gy. A similar study by Teo et al.[199] in which delivery of 18 to 24 Gy in three fractions by HDR brachytherapy showed significant improvement of the 5-year L-FFR of 95% compared with 90% 5-year L-FFR for EBRT-only patients ($p = .016$).

However, a report by Ozyar et al.[200] of patients with T1 to T4 tumors treated with HDR brachytherapy boost of 12 Gy in three fractions did not show improvement over EBRT alone (3-year L-FFR,86% vs. 94%; $p = .23$). More recently, a prospective trial by the International Atomic Energy Agency studied 275 patients with locoregionally advanced NPC disease (TNM stages III or M0 stage IV) who were all treated by induction chemotherapy followed by concurrent chemoradiotherapy to 70 Gy; one randomized arm then received a brachytherapy boost of 11-Gy LDR or three fractions of 3-Gy HDR. With a median follow-up of 29 months, the authors reported no additional benefit of brachytherapy boost compared with chemoradiotherapy alone toward 3-year OS (63.3% vs. 62.9%, $p = .742$, respectively), locoregional-FFR (54.4% vs. 60.5%, $p = .647$), or distant-metastasis–free survival (52.6% vs. 59.8%, $p = .496$).[201]

One major limitation of brachytherapy is that the dose delivered is adequate only for superficial nonbulky tumors. Furthermore, optimal positioning of the applicators depends both on the individual clinician's skill and the patient's anatomic features.

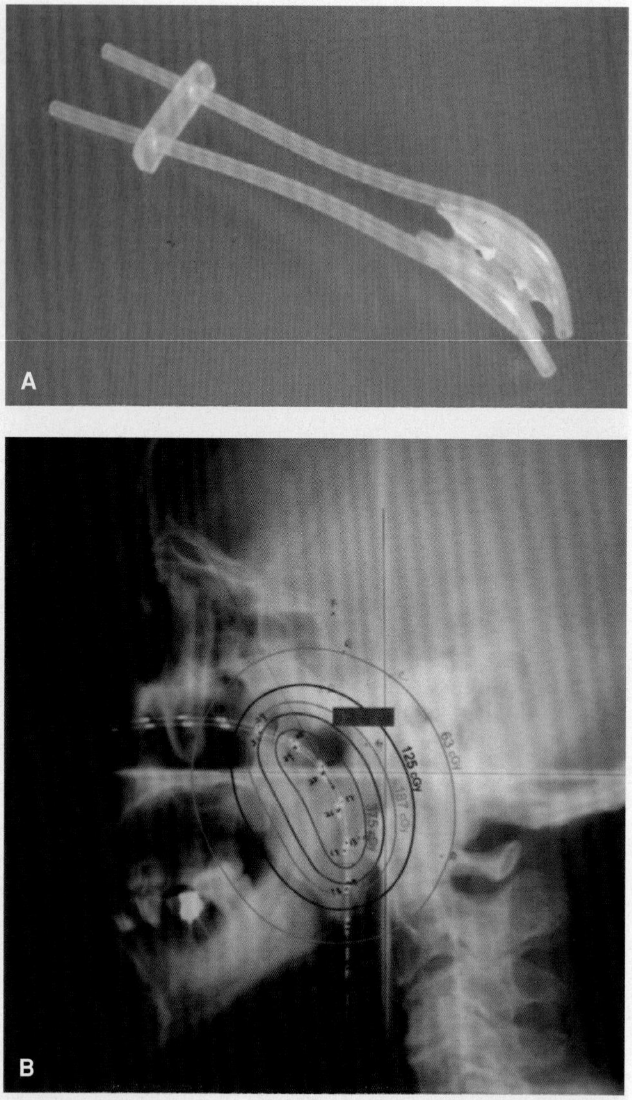

FIGURE 41.19. Endocavitary brachytherapy for nasopharyngeal carcinoma. **A:** The Rotterdam nasopharyngeal applicator. **B:** The simulator check-film showing the position of the radioactive sources and the dose distribution.

Stereotactic Radiosurgery

Stereotactic radiosurgery (SRT) or fractionated radiotherapy allows for precise delivery of highly conformal RT with a rapid dose falloff and provides an alternative for dose escalation. Hara et al.[202] reported a study of 82 patients with T1 to T4 tumors showing excellent 5-year L-FFR of 98% after receiving a median SRT boost of 12 Gy (range, 7 to 15 Gy) following EBRT to 66 Gy. However, despite the addition of concurrent chemotherapy in 76% of the patients, the distant failure rate was 32% and OS was 69%. With a median follow-up of 40.7 months for living patients, 12.1% of patients developed radiographic temporal lobe necrosis (only 2.4% were symptomatic with seizures), and 3.6% developed retinopathy. The risk was especially high in patients with T4 tumors.

Altered Fractionation

Over the last few decades, studies have been conducted to explore the role of altered fractionation regimens in head and neck cancers, along with nasopharyngeal cancers. Hyperfractionation, accelerated fractionation, and a combination were explored in conjunction with concurrent chemotherapy.

Sanchiz et al.[203] conducted a large randomized trial examining twice-daily (BID) versus once-daily (QD) irradiation for head and neck cancer, including tumors of the nasopharynx. A total

TABLE 41.11 ADJUVANT BRACHYTHERAPY BOOST FOR PRIMARY TREATMENT OF NASOPHARYNGEAL CARCINOMA

			Brachytherapy			Local Control		
Author	T-Category[a]	External Radiotherapy Dose (Gy)	Modality	Dose (Gy)	Fraction	Day	Year	Rate (%)
Chang et al.[347]	T1	65–68	HDR-ICB	5–11	1–2	1–8	5	94
		65–68	HDR-ICB	15–16.5	3	15		80 vs. 74
		60–72	Control					(p = .01)
Lee et al.[190]	T1-3	54–72	HDR-ICB or LDR-ICB	5–7 10–54	2	1	5	89
Levendag et al.[186]	T1-2a	60	HDR-ICB	15	5	3	5	92
	T2b	70	HDR-ICB	11	2			
Lu et al.[348]	T1-2	66	HDR-ICB	10	2	8	2	94
Ng et al.[349]	T1-4	43–70	HDR-ICB	6–15	2–5	2–5	5	96
Ozyar et al.[200]	T1-4	59–71	HDR-ICB	12	3	3	5	86 vs. 94
		59–74	Control	–				(p = .23)
Ren et al.[350]	T2b	60	HDR-ICB	12–20	1	1	5	98 vs. 80
		68	Control	–				(p =.012)
Syed et al.[197]	T1-4	50–60	ICB + interstitial	33–37	1	3	5	93
Teo et al.[199]	T1-2a	60–71	HDR-ICB	18–24	3	15	5	95 vs. 90
		60–71	Control	–				(p = .17)
Vikram[351]	T1-4	60–66	Interstitial	160 in 1 yr			5	96
Wang[188]	T1-2	60–64	LDR-ICB	7–10	1	1	5	91 vs. 60
		65–70	Control	–				(p <.01)

HDR, high-dose-rate; ICB, intracavitary brachytherapy; LDR, low-dose-rate; NR, not reported.

[a]Based on *AJCC Cancer Staging Handbook,* 6th ed. New York: Springer; 2002 or *AJCC Cancer Staging Handbook,* 5th ed. New York: Springer; 1997.

of 859 patients with advanced head and neck cancers (T3-T4, N0-3, M0 by UICC staging), which included 92 patients with nasopharyngeal carcinoma, was randomly assigned to QD irradiation (group A), BID irradiation (group B), or QD irradiation with concurrent 5-fluorouracil (5-FU) chemotherapy (group C). Groups B and C showed a significant improvement in median duration of response and OS when compared to group A. No significant differences were seen between groups B and C.

The first randomized trial on accelerated fractionation (AF) for NPC by Teo et al.[204] used an uncommon schedule of 2.5 Gy/fraction QD for 8 fractions before randomization to an experimental arm using 1.6 Gy BID for an additional 32 fractions versus a control arm treated with 2.5 Gy QD for another 16 fractions. The trial was terminated early because of excessive neurologic toxicities in the AF arm (49% vs. 23%). For this series of 159 patients (62% with T1-2 tumors), the AF arm did not achieve significant improvement in tumor control (5-year L-FFR, 89% vs. 85%). Jen et al.[205] reported on a study of 222 patients in which 76 patients received hyperfractionated RT at 1.2 Gy/fraction BID and 12 patients received accelerated-hyperfractionated RT at 1.6 Gy BID, to a median dose of 80 Gy for these twice-daily RT groups. The remaining 134 patients treated by conventional QD fractionation to a median dose of 70 Gy. The patients treated by BID fractionation did not demonstrate a statistically significant difference in 5-year L-FFR when compared to QD fractionation (T1-3, 93% vs. 86%; T4, 44% vs. 37%, respectively). The 1.2-Gy/fraction regimen did not cause excessive toxicity; however, patients treated with 1.6 Gy/fraction had a 27% incidence of temporal lobe necrosis.[206] See section Sequelae of Treatment for more details regarding the influence of dose fractionation on brain necrosis.

To minimize the risk of late damage, the more moderate AF schedule of the Danish Head and Neck Cancer Study Group 6–7 Trials using 2 Gy/fraction, six fractions per week[207] of 1,476 patients with head and neck cancer, of which 435 had pharyngeal tumors, including nasopharynx, demonstrated that accelerated fractionation resulted in significantly improved 5-year L-FFR (76% vs. 64% for six and five fractions, respectively, p = .0001) and disease-specific survival (73% vs. 66%, for six fractions and five fractions, respectively, p = .01) but not OS. This same fractionation schedule was tested retrospectively for NPC by Lee et al.[208] They reported that patients irradiated to a total dose of 66 Gy with 2D technique when on an AF schedule had significantly higher L-FFR than those treated with conventional five fractions per week. The benefit was significant particularly for T3-4 tumors (87% vs. 62%; p <0.01), and multivariate analyses confirmed that fractionation was an independent prognostic factor for overall progression (AF group: HR = 0.63, 95% confidence interval [CI], 0.41 to 0.98, p = .04). In addition, no significant increase in late toxicity was observed at 3 years (20% vs. 15%).

This schedule was then used in the subsequent NPC-9902 trial initiated by the Hong Kong Nasopharyngeal Carcinoma Study Group,[209] which aimed to assess the therapeutic benefit of AF and/or concurrent-adjuvant chemoradiotherapy (CRT). It randomized 189 patients with locally advanced NPC (T3-T4, N0-1, M0) to four arms: (i) conventional fractionation (CF) alone, (ii) AF (six fractions/week) alone, (iii) CF with concurrent chemotherapy, and (iv) AF with concurrent chemotherapy. Preliminary results with a median follow-up of 2.9 years showed that AF per se did not demonstrate a significant improvement in event-free survival (EFS) when compared with CF (AF vs. CF: HR 0.68, 95% CI 0.37 to 1.25, p = .22). However, AF combined with CRT (arm 4) achieved a strongly significant improvement when compared with CF alone (EFS: 94% vs. 70%, p = .008) but without an improvement in OS. A significant increase in acute and late toxicity in the AF plus CRT arm was also noted.

From these and other experiences with altered fractionation schedules in the treatment of nasopharyngeal carcinoma, in addition to other head and neck cancers, it has been concluded that both total dose and overall treatment time are important factors in determining outcomes.[210] With the increasing use of IMRT, dose escalation—to allow ample dose delivery to gross and subclinical disease—has become achievable without associated changes in rates of toxicity, considerably improving the therapeutic ratio of concurrent chemoradiation and causing the aforementioned fractionation schemes to fall out of favor.

Chemotherapy

Nasopharyngeal carcinoma is generally regarded to be a highly chemosensitive disease. While radiotherapy alone is the standard treatment for stage I NPC, concurrent CRT with or without adjuvant chemotherapy is the current standard for locally advanced disease (stage III–VB) based on multiple randomized, controlled trials and meta-analysis (Table 41.12). Although

TABLE 41.12 RANDOMIZED PROSPECTIVE TRIALS WITH CONCURRENT CHEMORADIOTHERAPY

Author	Year	Patients (n)	Control Arm	Radiotherapy Dose (Gy)	Experimental Arm (Chemotherapy)			Time Point (year)	Tumor Control (%)[a]		
					Induction	Concurrent	Adjuvant		LRC	DMFS	OS
Concurrent ± Adjuvant Chemoradiotherapy (Phase III Trials)											
Al-Sarraf[214]	1998	193	RT	70	–	P	PF	5	NR	NR	63 vs. 37
Lin[222]	2003	284	RT	70–74	–	PF	–	5	89 vs. 73	79 vs. 70	72 vs. 54
Kwong[352]	2004	222	RT	52.5–68		U	PF/VBM	3	80 vs. 72	85 vs. 71	87 vs. 77
Chan[228]	2005	350	RT	66	–	P	–	5	NR	NR	70 vs. 59
Wee[215]	2005	221	RT	70	–	P	PF	5	NR	83 vs. 63	67 vs. 49
Zhang[229]	2005	115	RT	70–74	–	O	–	2	NR	92 vs. 80	100 vs. 77
Chen[317]	2008	316	RT	70	–	P	PF	2	98 vs. 92	87 vs. 79	90 vs. 80
Lee[318]	2010	348	RT	70	–	P	PF	5	88 vs. 78	74 vs. 68	68 vs. 64
Lee[353]	2011	189	RT	70	–	P	PF	5	81 (C)–90 (A) vs. 85 (C)–75 (A)	75 (C)–95 (A) vs. 75 (C)–74 (A)	78 (C)–85 (A) vs. 66 (C, A)
Chen[b,213]	2011	230	RT	68–70	–	P	–	5	93 vs. 91	95 vs. 84	95 vs. 86
Induction-Concurrent Chemoradiotherapy (Phase II Trials)											
Hui[238]	2009	65	CCRT	66	DP	P	–	2	NR	NR	94 vs. 68
Fountzilas[354]	2012	141	CCRT	66–70	PET	P	–	3	NR	NR	72 vs. 67

A, accelerated fractionation; C, conventional fractionation; CCRT, concurrent chemoradiation; D, docetaxel; DMFS, distant metastasis–free survival; E, epirubicin; F, fluorouracil; LRC, locoregional control rate; M, methotrexate; NR, not reported; O, oxaliplatin; OS, overall survival; P, cisplatin; RT, radiotherapy alone; T, paclitaxel; U, uracil and tegafur; V, vincristine.

[a]Experimental arm vs. control arm.

[b]Stage II by Chinese 1992 staging system (equivalent to stage II-III by *AJCC Cancer Staging Handbook*, 7th ed. New York: Springer; 2010); 13% of patients were AJCC stage III.

there is less evidence for CRT in intermediate stage (2010 AJCC stage II) disease, it is recommended that such patients be treated with CRT in light of pooled data from two phase III trials[211,212] and a more recent phase III trial from Chen et al.[213] In more detail, Chen et al.[213] demonstrated that Chinese stage II NPC patients (equivalent to AJCC II-III; only 13% of the study's patients are AJCC 2010 stage III) that received concurrent chemoradiotherapy resulted in a 5-year OS benefit compared to radiation alone (94.5% vs. 85.8%, $p = .007$), with improved distant control (94.8% vs. 83.9%, $p = .007$). Multivariate analyses found that number of chemotherapy cycles was the only independent factor associated with improved OS, progression-free survival, and distant control. With the addition of chemotherapy, an increase in acute side effects was observed, but no significant increase in late effects was reported.

Concurrent Chemoradiotherapy

The landmark Intergroup 0099 trial was the first to document a significant survival benefit for CRT versus RT alone.[214] This trial randomized 147 patients with locally advanced NPC to either RT alone or CRT at centers located in the United States. Chemotherapy consisted of concurrent cisplatin (CDDP; 100 mg/m^2 on days 1, 22, and 43), followed by three cycles of adjuvant CDDP (80 mg/m^2 on day 1) and 5-FU (1000 mg/m^2/d on days 1 to 4) every 4 weeks. Radiotherapy was delivered in 1.8- to 2-Gy fractions to a total dose of 70 Gy. The trial was closed early due to a significant overall survival benefit in favor of CRT (78% vs. 47% at 3 years). A 5-year update confirmed progression-free survival (58% vs. 29%) and overall survival (67% vs. 37%) in favor of CRT. Reactions to these findings were initially tempered by several limitations of the trial. Results achieved in the RT arm were much poorer than those generally obtained at centers treating endemic NPC. Outcomes in the CRT arm were in fact more consistent with outcomes obtained in endemic areas using RT alone. Another concern was that 24% of the enrolled patients had disease of keratinizing histology, and it was unknown whether the same benefit would be seen in endemic areas with predominantly undifferentiated disease.

Subsequent trials confirmed the benefit of concurrent CDDP-based chemotherapy in endemic populations. Wee et al.[215] reported the results of 221 stage III-IVB patients from Singapore randomized to receive either RT alone or CRT. Chemotherapy consisted of a slightly modified version of the Intergroup regimen: CDDP (25 mg/m^2 on days 1 to 4) for three cycles every 3 weeks, followed by adjuvant CDDP (20 mg/m^2 on days 1 to 4) and 5-FU (1000 mg/m^2 per day on days 1 to 4) for three cycles. Radiotherapy was delivered to a dose of 70 Gy in 2-Gy fractions. Three-year overall survival for the CRT and RT arms was 85% and 65%, respectively ($p = .006$). CRT reduced the incidence of distant metastasis by 17% at 2 years ($p = .003$).

Langendijk et al.[216] performed a meta-analysis of 10 trials that randomized NPC patients to conventional RT or CRT. The 10 studies included 4 neoadjuvant trials,[217–220] 3 concurrent (with/without adjuvant) trials,[214,221,222] 2 adjuvant trials,[223,224] and 1 neoadjuvant plus adjuvant trial.[225] The authors found a pooled hazard ratio for death of 0.82, with an absolute survival benefit of 4% at 5 years. Subgroup analysis revealed that the overall survival benefit was only significant for those patients receiving concurrent chemotherapy, with a hazard ratio for death of 0.48 and absolute survival benefit of 20% at 5 years. Analysis of the neoadjuvant chemotherapy trials found a significant reduction in locoregional recurrence and distant metastasis but no overall survival benefit.

These results, in combination with results from a second meta-analysis[226] and the Singapore trial reported by Wee et al.,[215] confirmed CRT as the standard approach in stage III, IVA, and IVB NPC. At many centers, the standard course of chemotherapy has been based on the U.S. Intergroup regimen, which consisted of concurrent high-dose CDDP (100 mg/m^2 for three cycles) and adjuvant CDDP/5-FU for three cycles. This regimen is associated with significant acute and late toxicities, and patient compliance is frequently difficult to achieve. In the Intergroup 0099 trial, for example, only 63% completed all three cycles of concurrent chemotherapy, and only 55% were able to receive all three courses of adjuvant therapy.[214] As a result, weekly CDDP has been adopted by many institutions, especially for patients with poor nutritional status.[227] In a phase III trial comparing CRT versus RT alone in 350 patients with locally advanced disease, Chan et al.[228] demonstrated good efficacy and tolerability for a regimen consisting of weekly CDDP (40 mg/m^2). Seventy-eight percent of patients in the CRT arm received at least four cycles of CDDP, and CRT was associated with a statistically significant survival benefit after adjusting for age and disease stage.

Other Chemotherapy Agents

Weekly oxaliplatin (70 mg/m^2) has been demonstrated to have good tolerability and efficacy, albeit in the setting of a small phase III trial of 115 patients randomized to CRT or RT alone.[229] Carboplatin has also been employed as a substitute to high-dose CDDP, with comparable efficacy, in a noninferiority trial reported by Chitapanarux et al.[230] Two hundred and six patients were randomized to either concurrent high-dose CDDP and adjuvant CDDP/5-FU or concurrent weekly carboplatin and adjuvant carboplatin/5-FU. The trial had 80% power to detect a hazard ratio for death of 1.25 at 3 years. No significant difference in disease-free survival or overall survival was seen at median follow-up of 26 months. Disease-free survival was 59.6% and 64.7% ($p = 0.522$) for the carboplatin and CDDP arms, respectively.

Cetuximab to target epidermal growth factor receptor (EGFR; EGFR overexpression is observed in >80% of NPC patients) was examined in a phase II trial, with optimistic findings.[231] The 2-year rates of OS, locoregional progression–free survival, distant metastasis–free survival, and progression-free survival were 89.9%, 93.0%, 82.8%, and 86.5%, respectively. Bevacizumab, to exploit the angiogenesis pathway (VEGF is overexpressed in about two-thirds of NPC patients), was studied in a phase II trial in which the agent was added to the standard chemoradiotherapy schedule and demonstrated promising results.[232] Lee et al. reported, with a median follow-up of 2.5 years, 2-year OS, locoregional progression–free survival, distant metastasis–free survival, and progression-free survival of 90.9%, 83.7%, 90.8%, and 74.7%, respectively.

Adjuvant Chemotherapy

While good efficacy and tolerability have been shown for select alternative regimens, the greatest body of evidence for concurrent CRT has been with the CDDP-based U.S. Intergroup regimen of concurrent plus adjuvant chemotherapy. Nevertheless, it is unknown whether the adjuvant chemotherapy component of the U.S. Intergroup regimen contributed to its survival benefit.

Compliance with adjuvant chemotherapy can be especially difficult, as patients are recovering from the acute effects of CRT. Randomized trials comparing RT alone to RT plus adjuvant chemotherapy have all been negative.[224,225] Moreover, there are data to suggest a survival benefit for concurrent CRT without adjuvant chemotherapy.[222,228]

In 2011, Chen et al.[233] reported a randomized trial that compared concurrent CRT to concurrent CRT plus adjuvant chemotherapy (CDDP/5-FU) in 508 patients. With a median follow-up of 38 months, there were fewer failures at any site in the concurrent chemoradiotherapy plus adjuvant chemotherapy group versus the chemoradiotherapy-only group (14% vs. 16%); however, this difference was not statistically significant ($p = .13$). It is important to note that this trial was not designed as a noninferiority trial against the standard. In addition, compliance was an issue in this study, in which about 18% of patients randomized to the adjuvant arm did not receive adjuvant chemotherapy.[233] Until further data emerge, adjuvant chemotherapy is considered by many to be optional in the setting of concurrent CRT, although it may have a role in patients with residual EBV DNA after CRT.

Neoadjuvant Chemotherapy

The effect of adding neoadjuvant chemotherapy to concurrent CRT is a topic of much current interest and the subject of two ongoing phase III randomized trials. Multiple phase II trials have shown excellent outcomes and tolerability with a variety of regimens.[234–237] Figure 41.20 demonstrates the potential value of induction chemotherapy in tumor control. One recent randomized phase II trial demonstrated an overall survival benefit for docetaxel/CDDP followed by CDDP-RT when compared to concurrent CDDP-RT alone.[238] Although the difference in 3-year progression-free survival did not reach statistical significance

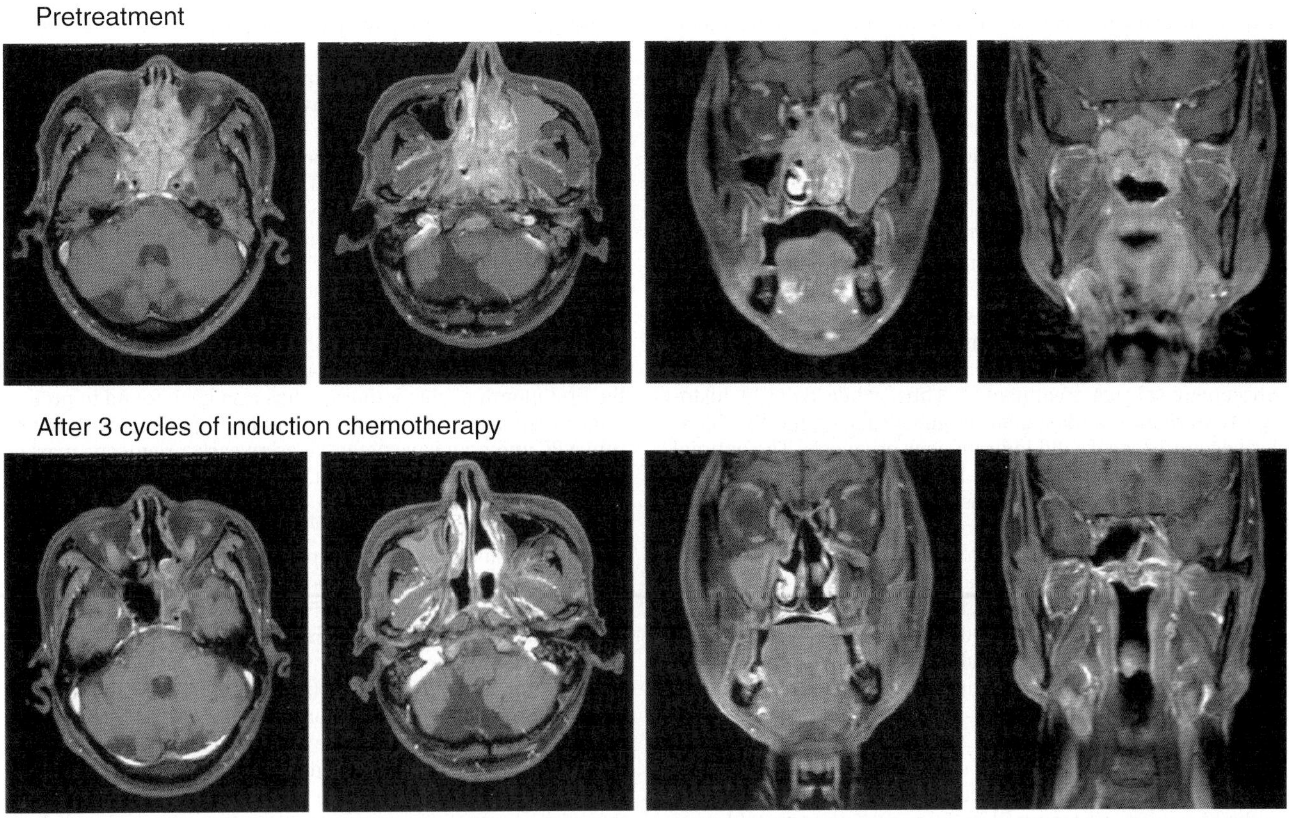

FIGURE 41.20. Magnetic resonance imaging showing shrinkage of primary tumor by induction chemotherapy using cisplatin and 5-fluorouracil before proceeding to concurrent cisplatin and radiotherapy. (From Lee AW, Lau KY, Hung WM, et al. Potential improvement of tumor control probability by induction chemotherapy for advanced nasopharyngeal carcinoma. *Radiother Oncol.* 2008;87(2):204–210, with permission from Elsevier.)

(88.2% vs. 59.2%, p = .12), 3-year overall survival was significantly improved in the neoadjuvant arm (94.1% v 67.7%, p = .012).

An ongoing phase III trial opened by the National Health Research Institute, Taiwan (http://clinicaltrials.gov/ct2/show/NCT00201396), is randomizing patients to concurrent CRT versus induction chemotherapy (CDDP, mitomycin, epirubicin, and leucovorin) plus concurrent CRT. The enrollment goal is 480 patients with an estimated completion date of December 2013. Another ongoing phase III trial, organized by the Hong Kong Nasopharyngeal Cancer Study Group Limited (http://clinicaltrials.gov/ct2/show/NCT00379262), is enrolling patients to one of three arms: (i) CDDP/5-FU induction chemotherapy plus concurrent CDDP-RT, (ii) concurrent CDDP-RT plus adjuvant CDDP/5-FU, or (iii) CDDP/capecitabine induction chemotherapy plus concurrent CDDP-RT. In addition, patients in each of these three arms will be randomized to either conventional or accelerated RT. The enrollment goal is 798 patients, with an estimated study completion date of April 2017.

PERSISTENT/RECURRENT NPC

Because long-term survival can be achieved for a substantial proportion of patients with early locoregional recurrence and useful palliation for those with extensive disease, aggressive salvage treatment is usually advocated. Several approaches can be used successfully, including surgery, brachytherapy, and EBRT. Chemotherapy is generally used in conjunction with local treatment in patients with advanced disease.

Early Detection and Diagnosis

While progress in surgical and reconstructive techniques and radiotherapy delivery methods has led to improvements in the control rate for primary treatment of NPC, local failure remains a problem for patients with advanced T-category disease. Distinction should be made between persistent disease (tumors that do not completely regress following primary treatment) and recurrent disease (tumors that reemerge after initial complete regression) because the prognoses and therapeutic considerations are different, with better survival and control rates for persistent disease.[239]

As tumors regress at different rates following RT, one difficult decision is when to consider residual tumors as genuine persistence and proceed with salvage treatment. In one prospective study by Kwong et al.,[240] serial biopsies of the nasopharynx were performed on 803 patients after RT treatment to observe the time course of histologic remission for NPC and determine its prognostic significance. The 5-year L-FFR was 82% for patients who achieved early histologic remission (<5 weeks), 77% for those with delayed remission (5 to <12 weeks), but only 40% for those with persistent disease at 12 weeks, despite subsequent salvage treatment.[240] Thus, while delayed histologic remission was not a poor prognostic factor, positive biopsies beyond 12 weeks did indicate poor prognosis. The optimal time for intervention remains uncertain, but because it is important to avoid both unnecessary overtreatment and excessive delay in treatment, the authors recommended an observation period of 10 weeks before additional treatment.[240]

Early detection of locoregional failure is crucial for a better chance of salvage, and regular follow-up after completion of primary treatment is recommended. Frequently used methods include manual palpation, rigid nasopharyngeal endoscopy and nasopharyngeal biopsies, imaging techniques (e.g., CT and MRI), and serologic tests (e.g., anti-EBV titers, plasma EBV DNA levels).

Nasopharyngoscopy is more sensitive than CT and MRI in detecting tumor persistence/recurrence and is the preferred method for initial screening.[241,242] If a patient presents with suspicious endoscopic findings or elevated anti-EBV titers, a nasopharyngeal biopsy is performed to confirm diagnosis. CT or MRI is performed upon a confirmed diagnosis to delineate the tumor extent.[243] Although MRI has limitations in separating tumor recurrence from radiation fibrosis,[244] it is superior to CT in demonstrating extent of soft tissue tumors, as well as in identifying submucosal infiltration, marrow infiltration in the skull base, perineural invasion, and intracranial spread.[241,245,246]

Technetium-99m methoxyisobutylisonitrile single-photon emission computed tomography may be a useful tool for differentiating persistent or recurrent tumor from radiation fibrosis[247] and was shown by Kostakoglu et al.[248] to be superior to MRI performed at 3 to 6 months post-RT in diagnosing complete response. The advent of FDG-PET is another valuable development. FDG-PET and MRI were compared in 67 NPC patients 4 to 70 months after completion of RT, and FDG-PET was found to be superior to MRI in all aspects in detection of local recurrence, with increased sensitivity (100% vs. 62%) and specificity (93% vs. 44%).[249] It may also contribute useful information to questionable findings on MRI.[250,251]

Paraneoplastic syndrome (PNS) can signal a silent neoplasm and may precede the clinical manifestation itself of persistent or recurrent NPC. PNS can follow the course of the tumor and can sometimes be used to diagnose recurrence and monitor its evolution, with the most common dermatologic manifestation being dermatomyositis and the syndrome of inappropriate secretion of antidiuretic hormone being a common endocrinologic presentation.[252]

Circulating cell-free DNA of EBV may be another useful tool for early detection of treatment failure. A longitudinal study by Lo et al.[121] showed that elevation of EBV DNA levels was noted in patients with relapse up to 6 months before detectable clinical disease. In addition, EBV DNA copy number has been shown to predict margin status post salvage nasopharyngectomy. Wei et al.[253] reported that in early recurrent NPC patients with elevated EBV DNA copies, surgical resection reduced the EBV DNA copy number postoperatively and that negative surgical margins are associated with zero EBV DNA copies postoperatively.

The incorporation plasma EBV DNA measurements as screening prior to PET in detecting posttreatment failures of NPC has been investigated. In a prospective study by Wang et al.,[129] 245 NPC patients in remission were monitored prospectively via plasma EBV DNA assay every 3 to 6 months, in which 36 patients with abnormal EBV DNA tests and 5 patients with clinically suggestion signs of recurrence but undetectable EBV DNA levels underwent FDG-PET scans. Elevated EBV DNA levels correctly predicted all 36 recurrences, while the 5 patients who presented with clinical signs suggestive of recurrent disease but with undetectable EBV DNA levels did not have recurrent disease. The authors concluded that plasma EBV DNA appears to be a useful biomarker for posttreatment surveillance in NPC.

In addition, the clearance rate of plasma EBV DNA during the first month of chemotherapy has also been found to predict tumor response and patient survival in 30 patients with recurrent NPC and may have potential as an early prognostic marker to help guide salvage treatment.[127]

Additional Radiation for Persistent Disease

Excellent results have been reported when using brachytherapy for locally persistent disease after a full course of EBRT (Table 41.13), with 5-year L-FFR in the range of 87% to 95% for patients with initial T1 tumors (AJCC 2002 T1-2a).[199,239,254–256] Preliminary evidence suggests that patients with disease persisting from initial T2 tumors (AJCC 2002 T2b) could also be effectively treated by brachytherapy.[257]

Stereotactic RT is a valuable alternative for delivering additional EBRT. Yau et al.[258] studied 755 patients with T1-4 tumors and found that 7% had positive biopsies 8 weeks after completion of primary RT. Twenty-one patients were treated with fractionated stereotactic RT to a median dose of 15 Gy and achieved a 3-year L-FFR of 82%, which was similar to the corresponding

TABLE 41.13 RESULTS OF LOCALLY PERSISTENT/RECURRENT NASOPHARYNGEAL CARCINOMA TREATED WITH BRACHYTHERAPY

			Brachytherapy			Local Control	
Author	T-Category	Modality	Dose (Gy)	Fraction	Day	Time (Years)	Rate (%)
Local Persistence							
Kwong et al.[239]	T1	Interstitial gold grain	60			5	87
Law et al.[255]	T1-2a	Iridium mold	40			5	90
Leung et al.[254]	T1-2	HDR-ICB	22.5–24	3	15	5	95
Leung et al.[257]	T2b	HDR-ICB	22.5–24	3	15	5	97
Zheng et al.[256]	T1	HDR-ICB	15–30	5–6	15–18	5	100
	T2	HDR-ICB	15–30	5–6	15–18		90
Local Recurrence							
Kwong et al.[239]	rT1	Interstitial gold grain	60			5	63
Law et al.[255]	rT1-2a	Iridium mold	50–55[a]			5	89
Leung et al.[267]	rT1-2	EBRT + HDR-ICB	50 + 14.8[a]	3	15	3	72

EBRT, external beam radiotherapy; HDR-ICB, high-dose-rate intracavitary brachytherapy.
[a]Median dose.

L-FFR of 86% in the complete responders and was significantly better than the corresponding L-FFR of 71% in 24 patients treated with high dose-rate brachytherapy to a median dose of 20 Gy.

Reirradiation for Recurrent Disease

Various radiation therapy modalities are used to treat recurrent NPC, including intracavitary brachytherapy, external beam irradiation, interstitial implantation, particle beam radiotherapy, and stereotactic radiosurgery (Table 41.14).[187,192,193,195,196,259] IMRT has also been used with excellent preliminary results, with control rates of up to 100% for rT1-3.[260]

The most important prognostic factors are the TNM stage of the tumor at the time of recurrence and reirradiation dose. Thorough restaging, including metastatic workup, is necessary. A study of 891 patients with local recurrence from 1976 to 1985 by Lee et al.[261] showed that only 32% of reirradiated patients achieved local salvage, with 54% developing regional and/or distant failure. Most series using conventional 2D technique showed that doses ≥60 Gy were associated with better outcome.[187,193,262,263] For IMRT, 60 to 70 Gy is recommended, taking into account factors such as previous radiation amount, overlap between previously treated area and target for reirradiation, interval between RT courses, tumor bulk, and whether concurrent chemotherapy will be given.[264]

Lee et al.[265] retrospectively compared the symptomatic late toxicity rate in 487 patients with two courses of EBRT versus 3,635 patients with one course. They found that the major determinant of late complications was severity of damage during the initial course and that the sum of total biologic dose tolerated (BED-Σ) was higher than expected with a single-course treatment (BED-1). This suggested partial recovery of normal

TABLE 41.14 RESULTS ON REIRRADIATION FOR LOCAL RECURRENCE OF NASOPHARYNGEAL CARCINOMA

					Treatment Outcome (Actuarial Rate)		Major Late Toxicity (Cumulative Incidence)	
Author	Year	Number	Reirradiation Technique	Time (Years)	Local Control (%)	Survival (%)	Overall (%)	Brain Necrosis (%)
Fu et al.[266]	1975	39	All 2D	5	26	41	23	NR
Yan et al.[356]	1983	219[a]	All 2D	5	NR	18	>29	>12
Wang[187]	1987	51	All 2D	5	NR	33	6	2
Pryzant et al.[193]	1992	53	All 2D	5	35	18	NR	NR
Lee et al.[262]	1997	654	All 2D	5	rT1: 35 rT2: 28 rT3-4: 11	16	26	3
Teo et al.[263]	1998	123	All 2D	5	rT1: 43 rT2: 31 rT3-4: 16	rT1: 63 rT2: 48 rT3-4: 31	NR	
Chua et al.[357]	1998	97	All 2D	5	NR	rT1-2: 57 rT3: 42 rT4: 17	NR	16
Leung et al.[267]	2000	91	All 2D	5	38	30	57	27
Chang et al.[273]	2000	186	81% 2D, 19% 3D	3	NR	rT1: 39 rT2: 24 rT3: 28 rT4: 4	2D: 23 3D: 9	2D: 14 3D: 0
Zheng et al.[278]	2005	86	All 3D	5	rT1: 92 rT2: 81 rT3: 68 rT4: 41	rT1: 70 rT2: 52 rT3: 32 rT4: 10	49	16
Lu et al.[279]	2004	49	IMRT	3/4	100	NR	NR	NR
Chua et al.[260]	2005	31	IMRT	1	rT1-3: 10% rT4: 35	63	19	7
Koutcher et al.[268]	2010	29	83% IMRT, 4% 2D, 13% 3D	5	52	60	31	17
Ozyigit et al.[275]	2011	51	47% SBRT, 53% 3D	2	rT1-2: 75 rT3-4: 54	rT1-2: 85 rT3-4: 46	3D: 48 SBRT: 21	3D: 19 SBRT: 4
Qiu et al.[280]	2011	70	IMRT	2	66	67	36	NR

2D, conventional two-dimensional external radiotherapy and/or brachytherapy; 3D, three-dimensional conformal radiotherapy; IMRT, intensity-modulated radiotherapy; NR, not reported; SBRT, stereotactic body radiation therapy.
[a]Patients with regional relapse included.

tissue (especially in patients reirradiated after 2 or more years) and higher tolerance for reirradiation when primary treatment was given, with better sparing of normal tissues. Assuming α/β ratio of 3 Gy, it was found that the BED-Σ that incurred 20% toxicity at 5 years was 129% that of BED-1.

Brachytherapy has been widely used for treatment of recurrent NPC (Table 41.13) and can be used effectively on its own for early-stage recurrent NPC.[239,255] Using interstitial implants with radioactive gold grains, Kwong et al.[239] reported a 5-year L-FFR of 63%; complications included headache (28%), palatal fistula (19%), and mucosal necrosis (16%). Law et al.[255] achieved excellent local salvage up to 89% using iridium mold, but the complication rate was 53%.

The combination of brachytherapy and EBRT is useful, particularly when conventional 2D technique is used. Lee et al.[262] showed that patients reirradiated by combined modalities had an improved 5-year L-FFR of 45% compared with 32% by EBRT alone and 29% by brachytherapy alone. The superiority of the combined method has been supported by other studies.[187,193,266,267] A recent study from MSKCC found that combined-modality treatment (CMT), consisting of EBRT followed by brachytherapy, achieved similar L-FFR with previous historical series. CMT also demonstrated fewer late grade 3 or higher events compared with patients receiving EBRT alone (8% vs. 73%, respectively).[268]

Stereotactic radiosurgery or fractionated stereotactic radiotherapy is another useful tool for retreatment of local recurrence, as it allows for rapid fall-off of radiation dose outside tumor volume and near surrounding critical structures and can be used either alone for smaller lesions or in combination with EBRT for larger ones. Control rates ranging from 53% to 86% have been reported.[269–272] For advanced recurrence with extension beyond the nasopharynx, this method offers better dose coverage than brachytherapy. A higher salvage rate from adding stereotactic radiation as a boost after EBRT has been reported.[270,273,274] Although most series reported a low risk of complications, massive hemorrhage with potential fatal outcome has been described.[270] Radiosurgery should thus be avoided when there is direct tumor encasement of the carotid artery or when a high cumulative dose has already been delivered. Fractionated stereotactic radiotherapy has shown improved late toxicity profile compared to 3D conformal RT[275] and single-dose radiosurgery[276] and may also give better local control rates compared with single-fraction radiosurgery.[277]

Advances in imaging technology and radiotherapy techniques have made it possible to reduce target volume without jeopardizing local control, reducing complication rates. Table 41.15 summarizes the treatment outcome and severe late complications by external beam reirradiation. Past series using 2D technique achieved 5-year survival rates in the range of 16% to 63%, and the incidence of temporal lobe necrosis ranged from 2% to 27%. The use of 3D conformal radiotherapy showed improving results. In a study by Chang et al.,[273] none of the patients reirradiated by 3D technique developed temporal lobe necrosis, compared with 14% of those reirradiated by 2D technique. Zheng et al.[278] reported a 5-year local salvage rate of 71% from 3D technique, but the actuarial rate of late toxicities (grade 4) was still as high as 49%.

The use of IMRT for reirradiation has shown very encouraging short-term results. Using IMRT to deliver 68 to 70 Gy, Lu et al.[279] reported 100% salvage rate without any severe late complications in a series of 49 patients with a median follow-up of 9 months. Using IMRT to a median dose of 54 Gy in 31 patients (with or without induction chemotherapy and stereotactic boost), Chua et al.[260] reported a 1-year control rate of 100% for rT1-T3 and 35% for rT4, with late complications (greater than grade 3) of 25% (at 1 year). Using a median dose of 70 Gy in 70 patients, Qiu et al.[280] reported a locoregional salvage rate of 66% with similar toxicity rate at 2 years. While rT staging did not predict control rate, original T classification remained a significant adverse prognostic factor and may serve as a strong marker for the underlying locally aggressive biology of the original disease. Longer follow-up is needed to better evaluate treatment results and sequelae resulting from IMRT.

Chemoradiotherapy may also improve treatment outcome for recurrent NPC in certain patients, and most recent salvage radiation series have included cisplatin-based chemotherapy for advanced-stage disease.[260,268,280,281] Using gemcitabine and cisplatin as induction chemotherapy followed by reirradiation with IMRT in 20 patients (95% rT3-4), Chua et al.[260] reported a 1-year local salvage rate of 75%. In a study of 35 patients (66% rT3-4), Poon et al.[281]

TABLE 41.15 INCIDENCE OF LATE TOXICITY FOLLOWING RADIATION WITH CONVENTIONAL TECHNIQUE (WITHOUT CONCURRENT CHEMOTHERAPY) FOR NASOPHARYNGEAL CARCINOMA

Severe Late Complication	*Sanguineti et al.*[28] *(n = 378)*	*Chao and Perez*[355] *(n = 164)*	*Lee et al.*[39] *(n = 4527)*	*Yeh et al.*[356] *(n = 849)*	*Leung et al.*[320] *(n = 880)*[a]
Period	1954–1992	1956–1991	1976–1985	1983–1998	1990–1998
Radiotherapy					
Total dose (Gy)	61–70	56–69	65[b]	68–76	62.5–66[b]
Dose per fraction (Gy)	NR	1.8–2	2.5–4.2	1.8	2–2.5
Altered fractionation (%)	8	Nil	Nil	Nil	Nil
Sequential chemotherapy (%)	Nil	Nil	8	Nil	20
Overall incidence (%)					
Grading of toxicity	≥3	≥3	≥2	≥1	?
Crude rate	30.4	14	30.8	NR	16.5
Actuarial rate	19 (10-year)	NR	60 (10-year)	NR	14 (5-year)
Treatment mortality (%)	3.2	3	1.4	NR	0.9
Types of complications (%)					
Temporal-lobe necrosis	1.1	1.2	3	6[c]	1.1
Brainstem encephalopathy/myelopathy	2.4		1		
Cranial neuropathy	4.5		5.3	3.3	6.8
Endocrine dysfunction	7.9		3.5		8.6
Severe epistaxis		1.2	0.6		0.3
Carotid rupture		0.6			
Hearing loss	2.6		8.2	54[c]	
Persistent otitis			2.5	32[c]	
Trismus	2.9	0.6	5.1	12[c]	0.7
Bone damage[d]	2.6	2.4	0.4		
Eyeball damage[e]			0.2		
Soft-tissue necrosis/fistula	1.1	1.8	0.4		0.5
Pharynx stricture/dysphagia		4.2		6[c]	
Soft-tissue fibrosis	4.2		15.9	25[c]	1.4
Persistent lymphedema	0.5	0.6	0.1		
Radiation-induced malignancy			<0.1		

NR, not reported.
[a]Patients with one course of radiotherapy. [b]Median dose equivalent to 2 Gy/fraction. [c]Five-year actuarial rate.
[d]Bone necrosis, fracture, or osteomyelitis. [e]Cataract, retinitis, corneal ulcer.

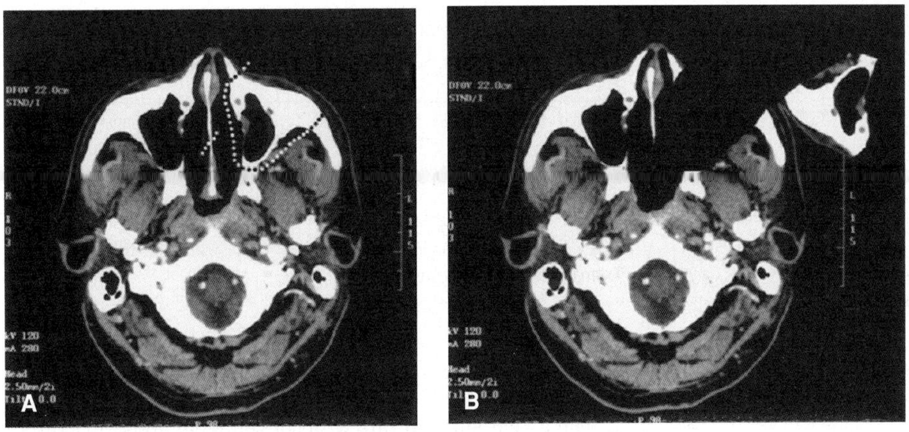

FIGURE 41.21. A: Computed tomography shows planned osteotomies of the maxilla and the posterior part of the nasal septum (*broken line*). **B:** The maxilla is swung laterally while still attached to the anterior cheek flap.

reported a 1-year EFS of 42% by concurrent cisplatin followed by adjuvant chemotherapy with cisplatin and 5-fluorouracil. However, while concomitant chemoirradiation is increasingly used to treat primary NPC, it remains uncertain whether concomitant chemoirradiation is appropriate for retreatment of purely local recurrences (rT1-2), due to high rates of toxicity and potential complications.

Surgical Treatment

For patients with persistent nodal disease, radical neck dissection is the preferred treatment for persistent or recurrent lymph node involvement in the neck when there is no distant metastasis[282] and may achieve a 5-year nodal control rate of 66% and disease-free survival rate of 37%.[283] In cases with extension of disease beyond lymph nodes into nearby structures, additional afterloading brachytherapy to tumor bed may improve local control.[284]

Surgical management at the primary site is hampered by difficulties in obtaining adequate exposure and obtaining adequate surgical margins.[143,285–287] Various approaches have been employed, including an infratemporal approach from the lateral aspect,[288] transpalatal, transmaxillary, and transcervical approaches from the inferior aspect,[287,289] and an anterolateral approach.[290] More recently, minimally invasive techniques, such as a transnasal approach and an endoscopic approach, have also been employed successfully.[291] Although controversial, salvage surgery by nasopharyngectomy can be a viable option in certain patients in whom disease is localized in the nasopharynx, with acceptable results reported for rT1-3 tumors.[247] Wei et al.[292] reported a 5-year control rate of 62% and 5-year disease-free survival rate of 49% in 60 patients who received curative resections. Typically, all patients with recurrence have undergone prior radical RT, with associated complications of trismus and palatal fistula being common; however, the mortalities associated with these surgical procedures are low.

Recurrent NPC is frequently located in the pharyngeal recess on the lateral wall. Access to this region is crucial for complete tumor extirpation. Wei and Sham[293] advocated the anterolateral approach or maxillary swing approach for localized recurrence in the nasopharynx. After facial incisions and the necessary osteotomies, the maxilla bone is swung laterally while remaining attached to the anterior cheek flap as one osteocutaneous entity (Figs. 41.21 and 41.22). The nasopharynx with the tumor and its surrounding area, including the paranasopharyngeal region, are then widely exposed for resection. Upon completion of nasopharyngectomy, the maxilla is replaced and attached to the remainder of the facial skeleton with miniplates.

Wei et al.[290] reported 161 patients with salvage nasopharyngectomy employing this approach performed at Queen Mary Hospital (Hong Kong) for recurrent NPC following primary treatment by radical RT. Twelve patients had prior brachytherapy as a salvage procedure. All patients were recurrent stage T1, with 78% of these patients achieving negative tumor resection margins, confirmed by frozen section, with the remaining patients demonstrating microscopic tumor at the internal carotid artery or the skull base during surgery, making further complete resection unattainable. All patients recovered from this anterolateral approach and were discharged. Regarding treatment-associated morbidities, trismus of varying grades was present in 60% and palatal fistula in 25% of patients. Recent modification of the palatal incision has eliminated the problem of palatal fistula.[294]

Satisfactory long-term results can be achieved when persistent/recurrent tumor are completely resected. Several recent surgical series reported locoregional control and OS rates of

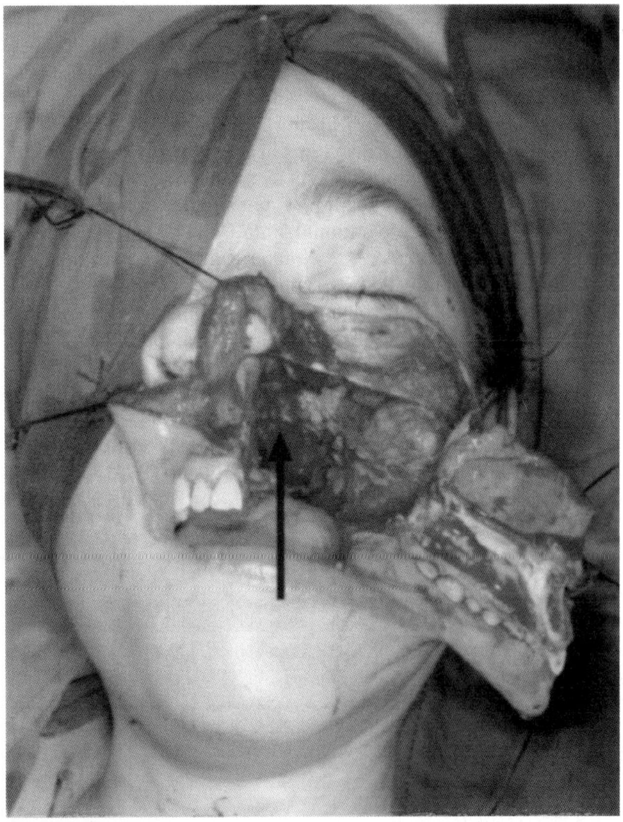

FIGURE 41.22. The left maxilla is swung laterally, exposing the nasopharynx (*arrow*).

TABLE 41.16 LOCAL TUMOR CONTROL AFTER CONVENTIONAL RADIOTHERAPY

Author	Year	5-Year Local Control Rate by T-Stage[a] (%)			
		T1	T2	T3	T4
Hoppe[32]	1976	87	94	68	44
Mesic[146]	1981	97	84	73	71
Chu[31]	1984	76	79	37	55
Vikram[145]	1985		74	100[b]	63
Wang[302]	1990	76	54	34	42
		67[c]	84[c]	78[c]	52[c]
Perez[27]	1992	85[d]	75[d]	67[d]	40[d]
Bailet[301]	1992	64	61		

T, primary tumor stage.
[a]By 1992 AJCC T-stage. [b]With only 3 patients in this group.
[c]Treated by twice-daily accelerated fractionation. [d]The 10-year actuarial rate.

40% to 72% and 30% to 54% respectively.[291,295–297] Postoperative reirradiation is recommended for patients with positive surgical margins and/or advanced disease[292,298,299] and may be beneficial even when surgical margins are negative.[247]

For recurrent tumors, margin status, adjuvant treatment type, and parapharyngeal space involvement were significant prognostic factors for local control, whereas dura or brain involvement, local recurrence, and adjuvant treatment type predicted survival.[291] Preoperative EBV DNA levels and PET-CT can assist in predicting the outcome of salvage nasopharyngectomy, and PET-CT may predict presence of extracapsular spread of metastatic lymph nodes.[300]

RESULTS OF TREATMENT

Specific results of various treatments are mentioned in the previous respective sections. This section focuses on summarizing these results.

The local and regional control rates in select conventional radiotherapy series are listed in Tables 41.16 and 41.17. Control of the primary lesion using conventional radiotherapy varied with the T classification (Table 41.16), ranging from 64% to 97% for T1 lesions, 54% to 94% for T2 lesions, 34% to 100% for T3 lesions, and 40% to 71% for T4 lesions.[27,31,32,145,146,301,302] Dose escalation with intracavitary brachytherapy if using non-IMRT treatment techniques[188] has been shown to improve local control. Stereotactic radiosurgery boost after external beam radiotherapy (both conventional and IMRT) has also shown improved local control.[202,303] Nonkeratinizing squamous cell carcinoma (both differentiated and undifferentiated subtypes) had improved local control rates when compared to keratinizing squamous cell carcinoma in T2 to T3 lesions but not in T1 or T4 lesions.[27,214,216]

Excellent nodal control rates in the neck have been demonstrated by conventional radiotherapy even after involvement of extensive cervical lymph node metastasis (Table 41.17). The neck nodal control rates ranged from 82% to 100% for N0, 86% to 92% for N1, and 78% to 89% for N2 to N3 disease.[27,32,146] Five-year survival rates ranged from 36% to 58% (Table 41.18).[27,31,32,146,301,302,304]

TABLE 41.17 NODAL CONTROL AFTER CONVENTIONAL RADIOTHERAPY

Author	Year	5-Year Nodal Control Rate by N-Stage[a] (%)			
		N0	N1	N2	N3
Hoppe[32]	1976	96	92	87	89
Mesic[146]	1981	100	90	88	82
Perez[27]	1992	82[b]	86[b]	78[b]	

N, regional lymph node stage.
[a]By 1992 AJCC N-stage. [b]The 10-year actuarial rate.

TABLE 41.18 OVERALL SURVIVAL AFTER CONVENTIONAL RADIOTHERAPY

Author	Year	Patients (n)	5-Year Survival Rate (%)	Analysis
Hoppe[32]	1976	82	57	Actuarial
Mesic[146]	1981	251	52	Actuarial disease-free
Chu[31]	1984	80	36	Actuarial
Vikram[145]	1985	107	56	Actuarial[a]
Wang[302]	1990	185	43	Absolute
Bailet[301]	1992	103	58	Actuarial

[a]Estimated from survival curve.

The 5-year survival rate with conventional non-IMRT radiotherapy correlated with the T-stage, as well as with the N-stage (Table 41.19), being 60% to 76% for T1, 48% to 68% for T2, 27% to 55% for T3, and 0% to 29% for T4 lesions[32,302] and 42% to 78% for N0, 27% to 70% for N1, and 32% to 52% for N2 to N3 disease. When nodes in the lower neck and/or the supraclavicular fossa are involved prognosis is poor.

Contemporary series with IMRT demonstrated excellent local and regional control achieved in 97% and 98% of the patients treated at UCSF, respectively.[166] An update of the UCSF experience continued to show excellent local control of approximately 96%.[177] Subsequently, several other institutions also recently published their results, which further demonstrate excellent local control rates ranging from 91% to 100% and regional control rates ranging from 91% to 98% (Table 41.20).[150,169–170,171,178,231,232,305,306–310,311,312–313]

The Radiation Therapy Oncology Group conducted a phase II trial using IMRT with/without chemotherapy in the treatment of nasopharyngeal carcinoma in which patients with ≥T2 (i.e., ≥T2b by AJCC 2002) and/or node-positive disease also received concurrent CDDP followed by adjuvant CDDP and 5-FU chemotherapies. The results showed that a multi-institutional setting can reproduce the excellent results (local control rate of 92.3%) observed from single-institution studies.[305] This reproducibility of excellent locoregional control rates in a multi-institutional trial, along with several single-institution studies, with IMRT is encouraging; however, distant metastases remains a therapeutic challenge despite extensive use of chemotherapy. The distant recurrence rate ranges from 10% to 15% at 2 years,[305,311] with 4-year rates as high as 34% (Table 41.20).[166] Novel systemic therapies or regimens are needed for improved distant control and overall survival of this disease.

SEQUELAE OF TREATMENT

Overall Incidence and Types

Due to the anatomic proximity of the nasopharynx to critical structures and the need for high radiation doses and adequate

TABLE 41.19 OVERALL SURVIVAL BY T- AND N-STAGE AFTER CONVENTIONAL RADIOTHERAPY

Author	Year	5-Year Local Control Rate by T-Stage (%)				5-Year Survival Rate by N-Stage (%)			
		T1	T2	T3	T4	N0	N1	N2	N3
Hoppe[32]	1976	76[a]	68[a]	55[a]	0[a]	78[a]	70[a]	42[a]	39[a]
Chu[31]	1984					42[b]	27[b]	52[b]	27[b]
Wang[302]	1990	60[c]	48[c]	27[c]	29[c]	60[c]	42[c]		32[c]

N, regional lymph node stage; T, primary tumor stage. By *AJCC Cancer Staging Handbook*, 4th ed. New York: Springer; 1992 T-stage and N-stage.
[a]Actuarial disease-free survival.
[b]Actuarial survival. [c]Absolute survival.

TABLE 41.20 RESULTS FROM CONTEMPORARY IMRT SERIES WITH OR WITHOUT CHEMOTHERAPY

Study	*Year*	*Stage*	*Number*	*Median Follow-up (Months)*	*Time Point (Years)*	*Local Control Rate (%)*	*Regional Control Rate (%)*	*Distant-Metastasis–Free Rate (%)*	*OS (%)*
Lee et al.[166] (UCSF)	2002	All	67	31	4	97	98	66	88
Kwong et al.[170] (Hong Kong)	2004	T1 N0-1[a]	33	24	3	100	92	100	100
Kam[171] (Hong Kong)	2004	All	63	29	3	92	98	79	90
Wolden et al.[169] (MSKCC)	2006	All	74	35	3	91	93	78	83
Kwong et al.[178] (Hong Kong)	2006	III-IVB[a]	50	25	2	96	NA	94	92
Lee et al.[305] (MSKCC)	2009	All	68	31	2	93	91	85	80
Tham et al.[307] (Singapore)	2009	All	195	37	3	90	NA	89	94
Lin et al.[306] (China)	2009	II-IV[a]	323	30	3	95	98	90	90
Wong et al.[357] (China)	2010	All	175	34	3	94	93	87	87
Lin et al.[309] (China)	2010	IIB-IVB[a]	370	31	3	95	97	86	89
Kam et al.[308] (Hong Kong)	2010	All	231	59	6	82	91	75	66
Ng et al.[311] (Hong Kong)	2011	All	193	30	2	95	96	90	92
Xiao et al.[310] (China)	2011	III-IVA[a]	81	54	5	95	NA	NA	75
Bakst et al[150] (MSKCC)	2011	II-IVB[a]	25	33	3	91	91	91	89
Xiayun et al.[313] (China)	2011	IIB-IVB[b]	54	30	3	95	98	86	88
Ma et al.[231] (Hong Kong)	2011	III-IVB[b]	30	32	2	93	93	93	90
Lee et al.[232] (MSKCC)	2011	IIB-IVB[c]	42	30	2	NA	NA	91	91
Su et al.[312] (China)	2012	I-IIB[b]	198	51	5	97	98	98	NA

NPC, nasopharyngeal carcinoma; IMRT, intensity-modulated radiation therapy; MSKCC, Memorial Sloan-Kettering Cancer Center; NA, not available; UCSF, University of California, San Francisco.

T, primary tumor stage; N, regional lymph node stage; M, distant metastasis stage.

[a]By *AJCC Cancer Staging Handbook,* 5th ed. New York: Springer; 1997 stage.

[b]By *AJCC Cancer Staging Handbook,* 6th ed. New York: Springer; 2002 stage.

[c]By *AJCC Cancer Staging Handbook,* 7th ed. New York: Springer; 2010 stage.

field coverage, the risks of radiation-induced toxicities are substantial. The overall complication rate from conventional treatment ranged from 31% to 66%, with severe sequelae including temporal lobe necrosis, hearing loss, xerostomia, neck fibrosis, cranial nerve dysfunction, endocrine dysfunction, soft tissue necrosis, osteonecrosis, and transverse radiation myelitis.[28,32,39] The diagnosis of irradiation injury can be difficult, as other possible causes (tumor recurrence in particular) must be excluded.

The toxicity results of five major series using conventional irradiation for NPC are summarized in Table 41.21.

The series of 378 patients treated at MDACC during 1954–1992 showed an actuarial frequency rate in grade ≥4 toxicity of 16%, 19%, and 29% at 5, 10, and 20 years, respectively.[28] Despite the use of higher radiation doses, Sanguineti et al.[28] showed a reduction in the 10-year actuarial rate of severe toxicity from 14% in 1954–1971 to 5% in 1983–1992. Other investigators reported similar findings.

The decreased rates of complications over time were likely due to the use of newer oblique and opposed lateral field techniques instead of single central field, custom blocking, and image-guided (CT) treatment planning.[28]

Due to the extremely narrow therapeutic treatment margin of NPC, maximum conformity and precision in RT delivery are crucial for minimizing the risk of late damage. The emergence of IMRT is a major advance for improving physical dose distribution and has increased the potential for protecting normal tissues. Studies on patients treated with IMRT thus far have shown substantial sparing of salivary function,[166,170,171] while other benefits will require longer follow-up to confirm.

The improved conformity offered by IMRT has led to attempts at dose escalation in order to achieve better tumor coverage for patients with extensive locoregional infiltration. However, studies have shown that dose escalation together with concurrent chemotherapy may lead to severe toxicities.[178,314] Furthermore, extensive use of concurrent CRT independent of incorporation of dose escalation has been shown to significantly increase toxicities (grade ≥3) compared to RT alone.[209,214,215,315–318]

Temporal Lobe Necrosis

Temporal lobe necrosis (TLN) is perhaps the most troublesome complication. Studies on NPC patients treated with conventional 2D RT found that TLN accounted for up to 65% of all irradiation-induced deaths; large fractions (>2 Gy) and overacceleration of treatment schedule greatly increased risk, with incidence as high as 33%.[39,148,149]

Diagnosis of TLN was often difficult and thus delayed. In Lee et al.'s examination of 102 patients with late TLN following conventional 2D RT,[319] only 31% presented with classic symptoms of TLN (hallucinations, absence attacks, déjà vu), while 14% had headaches, confusion, convulsions, or hemiparesis. Thirty-nine percent had vague symptoms of dizziness, poor memory, or sudden changes in behavior, while 16% were asymptomatic.

TLN remains a serious concern in patients treated with IMRT, with incidence of 3% to 4% being reported for schedules of 70 Gy at 2.12 Gy/fraction,[177] 66 to 74 Gy at 2 Gy/fraction,[171] and 76 Gy at 2.17 Gy/fraction.[178] Series using larger fractions (70.2 Gy at 2.34 Gy/fraction and 68 Gy at 2.27 Gy/fraction) had incidence rates as high as 12% to 14%.[150,310] Bakst et al.,[150] in a prospective trial of hypofractionated dose-painting IMRT using 2.34-Gy fractions to deliver a total dose of 70.2 Gy, had favorable disease control and survival outcomes; however, 12% of treated patients developed temporal lobe necrosis, and the conclusion was that large fractional doses should be avoided to prevent in-field brain radiation necrosis.

Cranial Neuropathy

Cranial nerves IX through XII, particularly XII, are the most frequently impaired by radiation.[39,320,321] This is related to marked radiation fibrosis, especially in patients who receive an additional boost dose to parapharyngeal space. Common symptoms include slurring of speech, twitching of neck muscles, and/or dysphagia. In a study of 31 NPC patients with post-RT dysphagia, Wu et al.[322] found that 77% aspirated after the act of swallowing, raising concerns of fatal aspiration pneumonia.

Cranial nerve VI is also frequently affected, particularly in patients with TLN, while isolated palsy of branches of cranial nerve V is less common.[39] Optic neuropathy is rare with careful

TABLE 41.21 INCIDENCE OF LATE TOXICITY FOLLOWING RADIATION WITH CONVENTIONAL TECHNIQUE (WITHOUT CONCURRENT CHEMOTHERAPY) FOR NASOPHARYNGEAL CARCINOMA

Severe Late Complication	*Sanguineti et al.[28] (n = 378)*	*Chao and Perez[355] (n = 164)*	*Lee et al.[39] (n = 4527)*	*Yeh et al.[356] (n = 849)*	*Leung et al.[320] (n = 880)[a]*
Period	1954–1992	1956–1991	1976–1985	1983–1998	1990–1998
Radiotherapy					
Total dose (Gy)	61–70	56–69	65[b]	68–76	62.5–66[b]
Dose per fraction (Gy)	NR	1.8–2	2.5–4.2	1.8	2–2.5
Altered fractionation (%)	8	Nil	Nil	Nil	Nil
Sequential chemotherapy (%)	Nil	Nil	8	Nil	20
Overall incidence (%)					
Grading of toxicity	≥3	≥3	≥2	≥1	?
Crude rate	30.4	14	30.8	NR	16.5
Actuarial rate	19 (10-year)	NR	60 (10-year)	NR	14 (5-year)
Treatment mortality (%)	3.2	3	1.4	NR	0.9
Types of complications (%)					
Temporal-lobe necrosis	1.1	1.2	3	6[c]	1.1
Brainstem encephalopathy/myelopathy	2.4		1		
Cranial neuropathy	4.5		5.3	3.3	6.8
Endocrine dysfunction	7.9		3.5		8.6
Severe epistaxis		1.2	0.6		0.3
Carotid rupture		0.6			
Hearing loss	2.6		8.2	54[c]	
Persistent otitis			2.5	32[c]	
Trismus	2.9	0.6	5.1	12[c]	0.7
Bone damage[d]	2.6	2.4	0.4		
Eyeball damage[e]			0.2		
Soft-tissue necrosis/fistula	1.1	1.8	0.4		0.5
Pharynx stricture/dysphagia		4.2		6[c]	
Soft-tissue fibrosis	4.2		15.9	25[c]	1.4
Persistent lymphedema	0.5	0.6	0.1		
Radiation-induced malignancy			<0.1		

NR, not reported.
[a]Patients with one course of radiotherapy. [b]Median dose equivalent to 2 Gy/fraction.
[c]Five-year actuarial rate. [d]Bone necrosis, fracture, or osteomyelitis. [e]Cataract, retinitis, corneal ulcer.

attention to the RT technique and should be considered when treating lesions with base-of-skull involvement.[323] The possibility of intracranial recurrence may confound the diagnosis of radiation injury, and exclusion of recurrence is necessary.

Oral Complications

Xerostomia is an almost universal complication from treatment with conventional RT and may lead to dental caries. Jen et al.[324] showed that the salivary flow dropped by half with a dose of 7.2 Gy, reached the nadir after 36 Gy, and then further dropped after completion of RT without recovery during the following 2 years.

However, Lee at al.[166] reported marked recovery of salivary function in patients treated with parotid-sparing IMRT (mean parotid dose, 34 Gy); the rate of grade 2 xerostomia decreased from 64% at 3 months to 2.4% at 2 years. Randomized trials comparing 2D RT and IMRT in patients with T1-2 tumors confirmed IMRT's advantage in this regard.[325,326] Nevertheless, it is important to rule out tumor invasion of the parotid gland prior to parotid-sparing IMRT, as recurrences have been reported. Cannon and Lee[327] concluded that PET alone may be insufficient for detection of intraparotid lymph node involvement in patients with multilevel nodal disease, including disease in level II nodes. Even with negative PET findings, these patients may require additional evaluation of any benign-appearing parotid nodules before parotid-sparing IMRT by fine-needle aspiration or CT-guided biopsy.

Dental sequelae frequently accompany xerostomia. In a series of 1,758 patients, 2.7% developed osteoradionecrosis at the maxilla and 1.7% at the mandible. Tong et al.[328] reported a 29% complication rate in patients who had post-RT extraction of posterior maxillary teeth, with 10.5% developing osteonecrosis. Prophylactic fluoride treatment should be employed to prevent dental decay, and decayed teeth should be extracted prior to RT to reduce this risk.[328,329]

Aural Toxicity

Hearing loss has always been a common radiation sequela, and the increasing use of cisplatin-based concurrent CRT has resulted in deafness rates as high as 42%.[330]

Sensorineural hearing loss (SNHL), particularly in the high-frequency range, was found in at least 30% of patients assessed with audiograms following RT, with higher rates in patients treated by concurrent CRT.[39,331,332,333] The primary determinant of high-frequency SNHL is mean cochlea dose, which should be kept below 48 Gy to minimize damage.[39,331,332,333] Due to the location of the primary tumor in the nasopharynx, pharyngotympanic tube (Eustachian tube) damage resulting in otitis media is difficult to avoid. However, lowering the dose to the external auditory canal and mastoid air cells can reduce the incidence and severity of acute external otitis and chronic serous otitis media, respectively.

Carotid Artery Injury

Carotid stenosis is a potentially fatal complication reported in patients who undergo irradiation of the head and neck region. Interval from radiotherapy was a significant independent predictor for severe carotid stenosis. Some have advocated for routine duplex ultrasound screening for high-risk patients (age >60 years, smoking, hypertension, hypercholesterolemia, cerebrovascular symptoms).[334,335] Severe cases may require carotid endarterectomy or endoplasty.

Massive bleeding from ruptured pseudoaneurysms at the petrous portion of the internal carotid has been reported following IMRT with dose escalation.[178,336] Urgent diagnosis and intervention with endovascular occlusion or stenting may be needed to prevent fatal consequences. Other concerns include severe telangiectasia and hypervascularization in the internal maxillary artery territory, for which emergency embolization may be considered.

Endocrine Dysfunction

The most common endocrine sequelae are amenorrhea and/or galactorrhea from hyperprolactinemia in female patients, followed by hypothyroidism and hypoadrenalism.

Lee et al.[39] observed symptomatic hypothalamic–pituitary dysfunction in 5% of patients, with a median latency of 5 years, while a longitudinal study by Lam et al.[337] with detailed endocrine assessment found a 5-year incidence of 62%, with dysfunction detected as early as 1 year following RT.[338] The deficiency of releasing or inhibitory factors indicated that the hypothalamus is the primary location of damage.[339,340] As many of these dysfunctions may be corrected pharmacologically, routine evaluation of hypothalamic, pituitary, and thyroid function should be considered in the follow-up examination of long-term survivors.

Shielding may help lessen endocrine dysfunction when using 2D technique.[341] The need for maximum conformity to protect normal tissues during radiotherapy is paramount.

Second Malignancies

Radiation-induced malignancy is rare, with an incidence of 0.04% and latency period of >10 years. The most common histologic types are maxillary osteosarcoma[342] and soft tissue sarcoma.[72] Surgery presents the only chance of cure, but the prognosis is often poor. While second primary head and neck cancer is relatively uncommon for NPC patients, Teo et al.[343] reported an excessive incidence rate of tongue cancer at 0.13% per patient-year. The possibility of radiation carcinogenesis cannot be excluded.

SELECTED REFERENCES

A full list of references for this chapter is available online.

3. Curado M, Edwards B, Shin H, et al. *Cancer incidence in five continents.* IARC Scientific Publications, 2007. IX(160).
4. Ferlay J, Shin H, Bray F, et al. *GLOBOCAN 2008, Cancer incidence and mortality worldwide: IARC CancerBase No. 10.* [Internet]. Lyon, France: International Agency for Research on Cancer, 2010.
9. Lu SJ, Day NE, Degos L, et al. Linkage of a nasopharyngeal carcinoma susceptibility locus to the HLA region. *Nature* 1990;346(6283):470–471.
14. Teo PM, Leung SF, Yu P, et al. A comparison of Ho's, International Union Against Cancer, and American Joint Committee stage classifications for nasopharyngeal carcinoma. *Cancer* 1991;67(2):434–439.
15. Yu MC, Ho JH, Lai SH, et al. Cantonese-style salted fish as a cause of nasopharyngeal carcinoma: report of a case-control study in Hong Kong. *Cancer Res* 1986; 46(2):956–961.
27. Perez CA, Devineni VR, Marcial-Vega V, et al. Carcinoma of the nasopharynx: factors affecting prognosis. *Int J Radiat Oncol Biol Phys* 1992;23(2):271–280.
28. Sanguineti G, Geara FB, Garden AS, et al. Carcinoma of the nasopharynx treated by radiotherapy alone: determinants of local and regional control. *Int J Radiat Oncol Biol Phys* 1997;37(5):985–996.
29. Lee AW, Foo W, Law SC, et al. Nasopharyngeal carcinoma: presenting symptoms and duration before diagnosis. *Hong Kong Med J* 1997;3(4):355–361.
30. Pan WR, Suami H, Corlett RJ, et al. Lymphatic drainage of the nasal fossae and nasopharynx: preliminary anatomical and radiological study with clinical implications. *Head Neck* 2009;31(1):52–57.
32. Hoppe RT, Goffinet DR, Bagshaw MA. Carcinoma of the nasopharynx. Eighteen years' experience with megavoltage radiation therapy. *Cancer* 1976;37(6):2605–2612.
35. Lee AW, Poon YF, Foo W, et al. Retrospective analysis of 5037 patients with nasopharyngeal carcinoma treated during 1976–1985: overall survival and patterns of failure. *Int J Radiat Oncol Biol Phys* 1992;23(2):261–270.
38. Teo P, Shiu W, Leung SF, et al. Prognostic factors in nasopharyngeal carcinoma investigated by computer tomography–an analysis of 659 patients. *Radiother Oncol* 1992;23(2):79–93.
39. Lee AW, Law SC, Ng SH, et al. Retrospective analysis of nasopharyngeal carcinoma treated during 1976–1985: late complications following megavoltage irradiation. *Br J Radiol* 1992;65(778):918–928.
48. Sievers KW, Greess H, Baum U, et al. Paranasal sinuses and nasopharynx CT and MRI. *Eur J Radiol* 2000;33(3):185–202.
51. Ng SH, Chang TC, Ko SF, et al. Nasopharyngeal carcinoma: MRI and CT assessment. *Neuroradiology* 1997;39(10):741–746.
53. van den Brekel MW, Stel HV, Castelijns JA, et al. Cervical lymph node metastasis: assessment of radiologic criteria. *Radiology* 1990;177(2):379–384.
54. Chang JT, Chan SC, Yen TC, et al. Nasopharyngeal carcinoma staging by (18) F-fluorodeoxyglucose positron emission tomography. *Int J Radiat Oncol Biol Phys* 2005;62(2):501–507.
61. Neel HB 3rd, Taylor WF. Epstein-Barr virus-related antibody. Changes in titers after therapy for nasopharyngeal carcinoma. *Arch Otolaryngol Head Neck Surg* 1990;116(11):1287–1290.
63. Zong YS, Sham JS, Ng MH, et al. Immunoglobulin A against viral capsid antigen of Epstein-Barr virus and indirect mirror examination of the nasopharynx in the detection of asymptomatic nasopharyngeal carcinoma. *Cancer* 1992;69(1):3–7.
64. Lin JC, Wang WY, Chen KY, et al. Quantification of plasma Epstein-Barr virus DNA in patients with advanced nasopharyngeal carcinoma. *N Engl J Med* 2004; 350(24):2461–2470.
65. Leung SF, Zee B, Ma BB, et al. Plasma Epstein-Barr viral deoxyribonucleic acid quantitation complements tumor-node-metastasis staging prognostication in nasopharyngeal carcinoma. *J Clin Oncol* 2006;24(34):5414–5418.
70. Edge SB, American Joint Committee on Cancer. *AJCC cancer staging manual,* 7th ed. New York: Springer, 2010:xiv, 648.
72. King AD, Ahuja AT, Leung SF, et al. Neck node metastases from nasopharyngeal carcinoma: MR imaging of patterns of disease. *Head Neck* 2000;22(3):275–281.
73. Liu MZ, Tang LL, Zong JF, et al. Evaluation of sixth edition of AJCC staging system for nasopharyngeal carcinoma and proposed improvement. *Int J Radiat Oncol Biol Phys* 2008;70(4):1115–1123.
77. Mao YP, Xie FY, Liu LZ, et al. Re-evaluation of 6th edition of AJCC staging system for nasopharyngeal carcinoma and proposed improvement based on magnetic resonance imaging. *Int J Radiat Oncol Biol Phys* 2009;73(5):1326–1334.
82. Chan J, Bray F, McCarron P, et al. Nasopharyngeal carcinoma. In: *Pathology and genetics of head and neck tumours. World Health Organization classification of tumours.* Lyon, France: IARC Press, 2005:85–97.
86. Sham JS, Choy D. Prognostic factors of nasopharyngeal carcinoma: a review of 759 patients. *Br J Radiol* 1990;63(745):51–58.
87. Teo P, Yu P, Lee WY, et al. Significant prognosticators after primary radiotherapy in 903 nondisseminated nasopharyngeal carcinoma evaluated by computer tomography. *Int J Radiat Oncol Biol Phys* 1996;36(2):291–304.
90. Chua DT, Sham JS, Kwong DL, et al. Prognostic value of paranasopharyngeal extension of nasopharyngeal carcinoma. A significant factor in local control and distant metastasis. *Cancer* 1996;78(2):202–210.
100. Zhou GQ, Mao YP, Chen L, et al. Prognostic value of prevertebral space involvement in nasopharyngeal carcinoma based on intensity-modulated radiotherapy. *Int J Radiat Oncol Biol Phys* 2012;82(3):1090–1097.
102. Chen MK, Chen TH, Liu JP, et al. Better prediction of prognosis for patients with nasopharyngeal carcinoma using primary tumor volume. *Cancer* 2004;100 (10):2160–2166.
103. Sze WM, Lee AW, Yau TK, et al. Primary tumor volume of nasopharyngeal carcinoma: prognostic significance for local control. *Int J Radiat Oncol Biol Phys* 2004;59(1):21–27.
106. Lok BH, Setton J, Caria N, et al. Intensity-modulated radiation therapy in oropharyngeal carcinoma: effect of tumor volume on clinical outcomes. *Int J Radiat Oncol Biol Phys* 2011.
107. Perez CA, Ackerman LV, Mill WB, et al. Cancer of the nasopharynx. Factors influencing prognosis. *Cancer* 1969;24(1):1–17.
110. Marks JE, Phillips JL, Menck HR. The National Cancer Data Base report on the relationship of race and national origin to the histology of nasopharyngeal carcinoma. *Cancer* 1998;83(3):582–588.
116. Xu J, Wan XB, Huang XF, et al. Serologic antienzyme rate of Epstein-Barr virus DNase-specific neutralizing antibody segregates TNM classification in nasopharyngeal carcinoma. *J Clin Oncol* 2010;28(35):5202–5209.
119. Lo YM, Chan LY, Lo KW, et al. Quantitative analysis of cell-free Epstein-Barr virus DNA in plasma of patients with nasopharyngeal carcinoma. *Cancer Res* 1999;59(6):1188–1191.
120. Ma BB, King A, Lo YM, et al. Relationship between pretreatment level of plasma Epstein-Barr virus DNA, tumor burden, and metabolic activity in advanced nasopharyngeal carcinoma. *Int J Radiat Oncol Biol Phys* 2006;66(3):714–720.
121. Lo YM, Chan LY, Chan AT, et al. Quantitative and temporal correlation between circulating cell-free Epstein-Barr virus DNA and tumor recurrence in nasopharyngeal carcinoma. *Cancer Res* 1999;59(21):5452–5455.
122. Le QT, Jones CD, Yau TK, et al. A comparison study of different PCR assays in measuring circulating plasma epstein-barr virus DNA levels in patients with nasopharyngeal carcinoma. *Clin Cancer Res* 2005;11(16):5700–5707.
127. Wang WY, Twu CW, Chen HH, et al. Plasma EBV DNA clearance rate as a novel prognostic marker for metastatic/recurrent nasopharyngeal carcinoma. *Clin Cancer Res* 2010;16(3):1016–1024.
129. Wang WY, Twu CW, Lin WY, et al. Plasma Epstein-Barr virus DNA screening followed by (1)F-fluoro-2-deoxy-D-glucose positron emission tomography in detecting posttreatment failures of nasopharyngeal carcinoma. *Cancer* 2011; 117(19):4452–4459.
130. Chua DT, Nicholls JM, Sham JS, et al. Prognostic value of epidermal growth factor receptor expression in patients with advanced stage nasopharyngeal carcinoma treated with induction chemotherapy and radiotherapy. *Int J Radiat Oncol Biol Phys* 2004;59(1):11–20.
133. Hui EP, Chan AT, Pezzella F, et al. Coexpression of hypoxia-inducible factors 1alpha and 2alpha, carbonic anhydrase IX, and vascular endothelial growth factor in nasopharyngeal carcinoma and relationship to survival. *Clin Cancer Res* 2002;8(8):2595–2604.
143. Wilson CP. The approach to the nasopharynx. *Proc R Soc Med* 1951;44(5): 353–358.
144. Marks JE, Bedwinek JM, Lee F, et al. Dose-response analysis for nasopharyngeal carcinoma: an historical perspective. *Cancer* 1982;50(6):1042–1050.
149. Lee AW, Kwong DL, Leung SF, et al. Factors affecting risk of symptomatic temporal lobe necrosis: significance of fractional dose and treatment time. *Int J Radiat Oncol Biol Phys* 2002;53(1):75–85.
150. Bakst RL, Lee N, Pfister DG, et al. Hypofractionated dose-painting intensity modulated radiation therapy with chemotherapy for nasopharyngeal carcinoma: a prospective trial. *Int J Radiat Oncol Biol Phys* 2011;80(1):148–153.

151. Marcial VA, Hanley JA, Chang C, et al. Split-course radiation therapy of carcinoma of the nasopharynx: results of a national collaborative clinical trial of the Radiation Therapy Oncology Group. *Int J Radiat Oncol Biol Phys* 1980;6(4):409–414.
154. Ho JHC. Nasopharynx. In: Halnan KE, ed. *Treatment of cancer.* New York: Igaku-Shoin, 1982:249–268.
156. Wolden SL, Zelefsky MJ, Hunt MA, et al. Failure of a 3D conformal boost to improve radiotherapy for nasopharyngeal carcinoma. *Int J Radiat Oncol Biol Phys* 2001;49(5):1229–1234.
160. Leibel SA, Kutcher GJ, Harrison LB, et al. Improved dose distributions for 3D conformal boost treatments in carcinoma of the nasopharynx. *Int J Radiat Oncol Biol Phys* 1991;20(4):823–833.
166. Lee N, Xia P, Quivey JM, et al. Intensity-modulated radiotherapy in the treatment of nasopharyngeal carcinoma: an update of the UCSF experience. *Int J Radiat Oncol Biol Phys* 2002;53(1):12–22.
168. Sultanem K, Shu HK, Xia P, et al. Three-dimensional intensity-modulated radiotherapy in the treatment of nasopharyngeal carcinoma: the University of California-San Francisco experience. *Int J Radiat Oncol Biol Phys* 2000;48(3):711–722.
169. Wolden SL, Chen WC, Pfister DG, et al. Intensity-modulated radiation therapy (IMRT) for nasopharynx cancer: update of the Memorial Sloan-Kettering experience. *Int J Radiat Oncol Biol Phys* 2006;64(1):57–62.
170. Kwong DL, Pow EH, Sham JS, et al. Intensity-modulated radiotherapy for early-stage nasopharyngeal carcinoma: a prospective study on disease control and preservation of salivary function. *Cancer* 2004;101(7):1584–1593.
176. Butler EB, Teh BS, Grant WH 3rd, et al. Smart (simultaneous modulated accelerated radiation therapy) boost: a new accelerated fractionation schedule for the treatment of head and neck cancer with intensity modulated radiotherapy. *Int J Radiat Oncol Biol Phys* 1999;45(1):21–32.
178. Kwong DL, Sham JS, Leung LH, et al. Preliminary results of radiation dose escalation for locally advanced nasopharyngeal carcinoma. *Int J Radiat Oncol Biol Phys* 2006;64(2):374–381.
182. Amdur RJ, Li JG, Liu C, et al. Unnecessary laryngeal irradiation in the IMRT era. *Head Neck* 2004;26(3):257–263; discussion 263–264.
188. Wang CC. Improved local control of nasopharyngeal carcinoma after intracavitary brachytherapy boost. *Am J Clin Oncol* 1991;14(1):5–8.
198. Levendag PC, Peters R, Meeuwis CA, et al. A new applicator design for endocavitary brachytherapy of cancer in the nasopharynx. *Radiother Oncol* 1997;45(1):95–98.
201. Rosenblatt E, El-Gantiry M, Elattar I, et al. Brachytherapy Boost In Locoregionally Advanced Nasopharyngeal Carcinoma: A Prospective Randomized Trial Of The International Atomic Energy Agency [abstract]. 2011.
204. Teo PM, Leung SF, Chan AT, et al. Final report of a randomized trial on altered-fractionated radiotherapy in nasopharyngeal carcinoma prematurely terminated by significant increase in neurologic complications. *Int J Radiat Oncol Biol Phys* 2000;48(5):1311–1322.
209. Lee AW, Tung SY, Chan AT, et al. Preliminary results of a randomized study (NPC-9902 Trial) on therapeutic gain by concurrent chemotherapy and/or accelerated fractionation for locally advanced nasopharyngeal carcinoma. *Int J Radiat Oncol Biol Phys* 2006;66(1):142–151.
210. Fu KK, Pajak TF, Trotti A, et al. A Radiation Therapy Oncology Group (RTOG) phase III randomized study to compare hyperfractionation and two variants of accelerated fractionation to standard fractionation radiotherapy for head and neck squamous cell carcinomas: first report of RTOG 9003. *Int J Radiat Oncol Biol Phys* 2000;48(1):7–16.
213. Chen QY, Wen YF, Guo L, et al. Concurrent chemoradiotherapy vs radiotherapy alone in stage II nasopharyngeal carcinoma: phase III randomized trial. *J Natl Cancer Inst* 2011;103(23):1761–1770.
214. Al-Sarraf M, LeBlanc M, Giri PG, et al. Chemoradiotherapy versus radiotherapy in patients with advanced nasopharyngeal cancer: phase III randomized Intergroup study 0099. *J Clin Oncol* 1998;16(4):1310–1317.
215. Wee J, Tan EH, Tai BC, et al. Randomized trial of radiotherapy versus concurrent chemoradiotherapy followed by adjuvant chemotherapy in patients with American Joint Committee on Cancer/International Union against cancer stage III and IV nasopharyngeal cancer of the endemic variety. *J Clin Oncol* 2005;23(27):6730–6738.
216. Langendijk JA, Leemans CR, Buter J, et al. The additional value of chemotherapy to radiotherapy in locally advanced nasopharyngeal carcinoma: a meta-analysis of the published literature. *J Clin Oncol* 2004;22(22):4604–4612.
226. Baujat B, Audry H, Bourhis J, et al. Chemotherapy in locally advanced nasopharyngeal carcinoma: an individual patient data meta-analysis of eight randomized trials and 1753 patients. *Int J Radiat Oncol Biol Phys* 2006;64(1):47–56.
227. Chan AT. Nasopharyngeal carcinoma. *Ann Oncol* 2010;21(Suppl 7):vii308–vii312.
231. Ma BB, Kam MK, Leung SF, et al. A phase II study of concurrent cetuximab-cisplatin and intensity-modulated radiotherapy in locoregionally advanced nasopharyngeal carcinoma. *Ann Oncol* 2011.
232. Lee NY, Zhang Q, Pfister DG, et al. Addition of bevacizumab to standard chemoradiation for locoregionally advanced nasopharyngeal carcinoma (RTOG 0615): a phase 2 multi-institutional trial. *Lancet Oncol* 2011.
233. Chen L, Hu CS, Chen XZ, et al. Concurrent chemoradiotherapy plus adjuvant chemotherapy versus concurrent chemoradiotherapy alone in patients with locoregionally advanced nasopharyngeal carcinoma: a phase 3 multicentre randomised controlled trial. *Lancet Oncol* 2011.
235. Chan AT, Ma BB, Lo YM, et al. Phase II study of neoadjuvant carboplatin and paclitaxel followed by radiotherapy and concurrent cisplatin in patients with locoregionally advanced nasopharyngeal carcinoma: therapeutic monitoring with plasma Epstein-Barr virus DNA. *J Clin Oncol* 2004;22(15):3053–3060.
238. Hui EP, Ma BB, Leung SF, et al. Randomized phase II trial of concurrent cisplatin-radiotherapy with or without neoadjuvant docetaxel and cisplatin in advanced nasopharyngeal carcinoma. *J Clin Oncol* 2009;27(2):242–249.
239. Kwong DL, Wei WI, Cheng AC, et al. Long term results of radioactive gold grain implantation for the treatment of persistent and recurrent nasopharyngeal carcinoma. *Cancer* 2001;91(6):1105–1113.
240. Kwong DL, Nicholls J, Wei WI, et al. The time course of histologic remission after treatment of patients with nasopharyngeal carcinoma. *Cancer* 1999;85(7):1446–1453.
242. Ragab SM, Erfan FA, Khalifa MA, et al. Detection of local failures after management of nasopharyngeal carcinoma: a prospective, controlled trial. *J Laryngol Otol* 2008;122(11):1230–1234.
247. King WW, Ku PK, Mok CO, et al. Nasopharyngectomy in the treatment of recurrent nasopharyngeal carcinoma: a twelve-year experience. *Head Neck* 2000;22(3):215–222.
253. Wei WI, Yuen AP, Ng RW, et al. Quantitative analysis of plasma cell-free Epstein-Barr virus DNA in nasopharyngeal carcinoma after salvage nasopharyngectomy: a prospective study. *Head Neck* 2004;26(10):878–883.
257. Leung TW, Tung SY, Wong VY, et al. Nasopharyngeal intracavitary brachytherapy: the controversy of T2b disease. *Cancer* 2005;104(8):1648–1655.
260. Chua DT, Sham JS, Leung LH, et al. Re-irradiation of nasopharyngeal carcinoma with intensity-modulated radiotherapy. *Radiother Oncol* 2005;77(3):290–294.
262. Lee AW, Foo W, Law SC, et al. Reirradiation for recurrent nasopharyngeal carcinoma: factors affecting the therapeutic ratio and ways for improvement. *Int J Radiat Oncol Biol Phys* 1997;38(1):43–52.
264. Chen AM, Phillips TL, Lee NY. Practical considerations in the re-irradiation of recurrent and second primary head-and-neck cancer: who, why, how, and how much? *Int J Radiat Oncol Biol Phys* 2011;81(5):1211–1219.
265. Lee AW, Foo W, Law SC, et al. Total biological effect on late reactive tissues following reirradiation for recurrent nasopharyngeal carcinoma. *Int J Radiat Oncol Biol Phys* 2000;46(4):865–872.
268. Koutcher L, Lee N, Zelefsky M, et al. Reirradiation of locally recurrent nasopharynx cancer with external beam radiotherapy with or without brachytherapy. *Int J Radiat Oncol Biol Phys* 2010;76(1):130–137.
280. Qiu S, Lin S, Tham IW, et al. Intensity-modulated radiation therapy in the salvage of locally recurrent nasopharyngeal carcinoma. *Int J Radiat Oncol Biol Phys* 2011.
290. Wei WI, Lam KH, Sham JS. New approach to the nasopharynx: the maxillary swing approach. *Head Neck* 1991;13(3):200–207.
293. Wei WI, Sham JS. Nasopharyngeal carcinoma. *Lancet* 2005;365(9476):2041–2054.
300. Chan JY, Chow VL, Mok VW, et al. Prediction of surgical outcome using plasma epstein-barr virus dna and (18) F-FDG PET-CT scan in recurrent nasopharyngeal carcinoma. *Head Neck* 2011.
305. Lee N, Harris J, Garden AS, et al. Intensity-modulated radiation therapy with or without chemotherapy for nasopharyngeal carcinoma: radiation therapy oncology group phase II trial 0225. *J Clin Oncol* 2009;27(22):3684–3690.
311. Ng WT, Lee MC, Hung WM, et al. Clinical outcomes and patterns of failure after intensity-modulated radiotherapy for nasopharyngeal carcinoma. *Int J Radiat Oncol Biol Phys* 2011;79(2):420–428.
324. Jen YM, Lin YC, Wang YB, et al. Dramatic and prolonged decrease of whole salivary secretion in nasopharyngeal carcinoma patients treated with radiotherapy. *Oral Surg Oral Med Oral Pathol Oral Radiol Endod* 2006;101(3):322–327.
327. Cannon DM, Lee NY. Recurrence in region of spared parotid gland after definitive intensity-modulated radiotherapy for head and neck cancer. *Int J Radiat Oncol Biol Phys* 2008;70(3):660–665.
328. Tong AC, Leung AC, Cheng JC, et al. Incidence of complicated healing and osteoradionecrosis following tooth extraction in patients receiving radiotherapy for treatment of nasopharyngeal carcinoma. *Aust Dent J* 1999;44(3):187–194.
330. Lee AW, Ng WT, Hung WM, et al. Major late toxicities after conformal radiotherapy for nasopharyngeal carcinoma-patient- and treatment-related risk factors. *Int J Radiat Oncol Biol Phys* 2009;73(4):1121–1128.
332. Chen WC, Jackson A, Budnick AS, et al. Sensorineural hearing loss in combined modality treatment of nasopharyngeal carcinoma. *Cancer* 2006;106(4):820–829.
335. Lam WW, Leung SF, So NM, et al. Incidence of carotid stenosis in nasopharyngeal carcinoma patients after radiotherapy. *Cancer* 2001;92(9):2357–2363.
342. Dickens P, Wei WI, Sham JS. Osteosarcoma of the maxilla in Hong Kong Chinese postirradiation for nasopharyngeal carcinoma. A report of four cases. *Cancer* 1990;66(9):1924–1926.

Chapter 42
Cancer of the Nasal Cavity and Paranasal Sinuses

Steven J. Frank, Anesa Ahamad, and K. Kian Ang

ANATOMY

Nasal Cavity

The nasal cavity extends from the hard palate inferiorly to the base of the skull superiorly. It is above and behind the vestibule and is defined anteriorly by the transition from skin to mucous membrane and posteriorly by the choanae, which open directly into the nasopharynx.[1] The nasal cavity consists of four subsites: the nasal vestibule, the lateral walls, the floor, and the septum.

The *nasal vestibule* is the triangular space located inside the aperture of the nostril as a slight dilatation that extends as a small recess toward the apex of the nose. It is defined laterally by the alae; medially by the membranous septum, the distal end of the cartilaginous septum, and columella; and inferiorly by the adjacent floor of the nasal cavity. It is lined by skin containing hairs and sebaceous glands; therefore, tumors at this location are often those that arise from the skin, usually squamous cell cancers[2] but may occasionally be basal cell carcinoma[3] sebaceous carcinoma,[4] melanoma,[5] or non-Hodgkin lymphoma.[6]

The *lateral walls* correspond with the medial walls of the maxillary sinuses and consist of thin bony structures that have three shell-shaped projections (superior, middle, and inferior conchae or turbinates) into the nasal cavity. The *floor* extends from the vestibule to the nasopharynx above the hard palate of the maxilla. The *septum* divides the nasal cavity into right and left halves.

Paranasal Sinuses

The paranasal sinuses are named according to the bones in which they are located: the ethmoid, maxilla, sphenoid, and frontal.

Ethmoid Sinuses

The ethmoid sinuses are composed of several small cavities, the ethmoid air cells, within the ethmoid labyrinth located below the anterior cranial fossa and between the nasal cavity and the orbit. They are separated from the orbital cavity by a thin, porous bone, the *lamina papyracea*, and from the anterior cranial fossa by a portion of the frontal bone, the *fovea ethmoidalis*. They are in close proximity to the optic nerves laterally and the optic chiasm posteriorly. The ethmoid sinuses are divided into anterior, middle, and posterior groups of air cells. The middle ethmoid cells open directly into the middle meatus. The anterior cells may drain indirectly into the middle meatus via the infundibulum. The posterior cells open directly into the superior meatus.

Maxillary Sinuses

The maxillary sinuses, the largest of the paranasal sinuses, are pyramid-shaped cavities located in the maxillae. The lateral walls of the nasal cavity form the base and the roofs correspond to the orbital floors, which contain the infraorbital canals. The floors of the maxillary sinuses are composed of the alveolar processes. The apices extend toward and frequently into the zygomatic bones. Secretions drain by mucociliary action into the middle meatus via the hiatus semilunaris through an aperture near the roof of the maxillary sinus. Ohngren's line is a theoretical plane dividing each maxillary sinus into the suprastructure and infrastructure; it is defined by connecting the medial canthus with the angle of the mandible.

Sphenoid Sinus and Frontal Sinuses

The sphenoid bone forms a midline inner cavity that communicates with the nasal cavity through an aperture in its anterior wall. It is directly apposed superiorly to the pituitary gland and optic chiasm, laterally to the cavernous sinuses, anteriorly to the ethmoid sinuses and nasal cavity, and inferiorly to the nasopharynx. The paired, typically asymmetric frontal sinuses are located between the inner and outer tables of the frontal bone. They are anterior to the anterior cranial fossa, superior to the sphenoid and ethmoid sinuses, and superomedial to the orbits. They usually communicate with the middle meatus of the nasal cavity.

EPIDEMIOLOGY

Cancers of the nasal cavity and paranasal sinuses are relatively uncommon. Fewer than 4,500 cases are diagnosed each year in the United States, an incidence of 0.75 per 100,000.[7] Cancers of the maxillary sinus are twice as common as those of the nasal cavity; cancers of the ethmoid, frontal, and sphenoid sinuses are extremely rare. They generally develop after the age of 40 years, except for esthesioneuroblastoma, which has a unique bimodal age distribution[8] and occurs twice as often in men than in women.[9] These tumors are most common in Japan and South Africa.

The etiologic factors vary by tumor type and location. Adenocarcinomas of the nasal cavity and ethmoid sinus have been reported to occur more frequently in carpenters and sawmill workers who are exposed to wood dust,[10,11,12] Synthetic wood, binding agents, and glues may also be involved as cocarcinogens.[13] Squamous cell carcinomas of the nasal cavity have been seen more often in nickel workers.[14] Maxillary sinus carcinomas have been associated with radioactive thorium-containing contrast material (Thorotrast) used for radiographic visualization of the maxillary sinuses in the past. Occupational exposure in the production of chromium, mustard gas, isopropyl alcohol, and radium also may increase the risk of sinonasal carcinomas.

Cigarette smoking is reported to increase the risk of nasal cancer, with a doubling of risk among heavy or long-term smokers and a reduction in risk after long-term cessation. After adjustment for smoking, a significant dose–response relationship has also been noted between alcohol consumption and risk of nasal cancer.[15]

NATURAL HISTORY

Nasal Vestibule

Nasal vestibule carcinomas can spread by direct invasion of the upper lip, gingivolabial sulcus, premaxilla (early events), or nasal cavity (late events), as shown in Figure 42.1. Vertical invasion may result in septal (membranous or cartilaginous) perforation or alar cartilage destruction. Lymphatic spread from nasal vestibule carcinomas is usually to the ipsilateral facial (buccinator and mandibular) and submandibular nodes. Large lesions extending across the midline may spread to the contralateral facial or submandibular nodes. The incidence of nodal

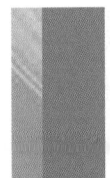

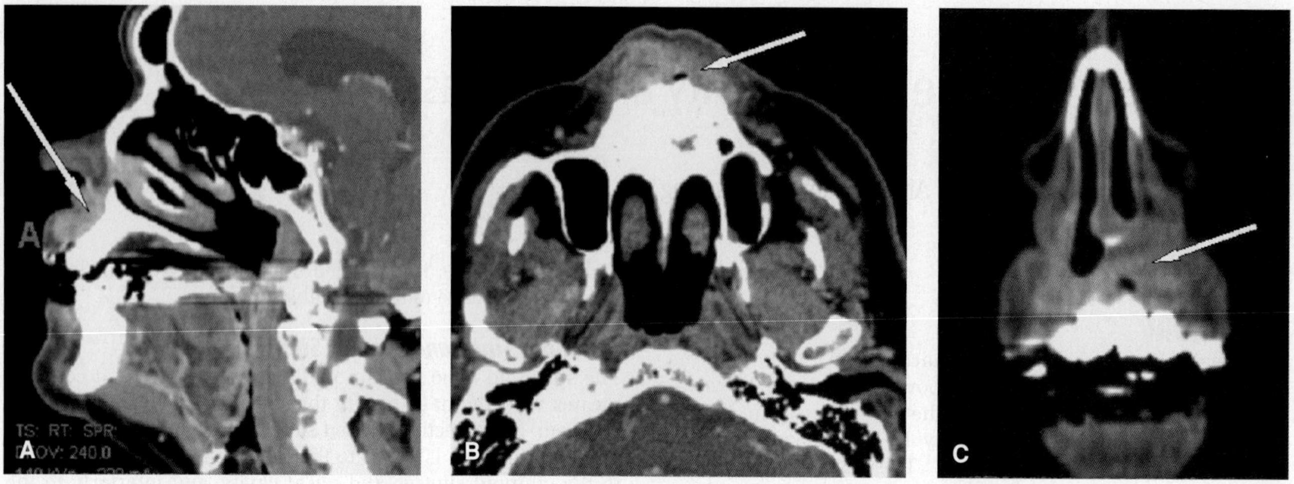

FIGURE 42.1. Computed tomography scans of a nasal vestibule squamous cell carcinoma that has spread by direct invasion of the upper lip (*arrow* in **A**) and gingivolabial sulcus and premaxilla (*arrow* in **B** and **C**).

metastasis at diagnosis is approximately 5%.[16,17] Without elective nodal treatment, approximately 15% of patients develop nodal relapse. Hematogenous metastases are rare.

Nasal Cavity and Ethmoid Sinuses

The pattern of contiguous spread of carcinomas varies with the location of the primary lesion. Tumors arising in the upper nasal cavity and ethmoid cells can extend to the orbit through the thin lamina papyracea and to the anterior cranial fossa via the cribriform plate, or they may grow through the nasal bone to the subcutaneous tissue and skin. Lateral wall primaries invade the maxillary antrum, ethmoid cells, orbit, pterygopalatine fossa, and nasopharynx. Primaries of the floor and lower septum may invade the palate and maxillary antrum. Perineural extension (typically involving branches of the trigeminal nerve) is seen most often with adenoid cystic carcinomas.

Lymphatic spread of nasal cavity primaries is uncommon, although spread to retropharyngeal and cervical lymph nodes is possible. In a series of 51 patients reported by the University of Texas MD Anderson Cancer Center,[18] only 1 patient had palpable subdigastric nodes at diagnosis. Of the 36 patients who did not receive elective lymphatic irradiation, 2 (6%) experienced subdigastric nodal relapse. Hematogenous dissemination is rare. In the MD Anderson Cancer Center series, for example, distant metastasis to bone, brain, or liver occurred in only 4 of 51 patients.[18]

The olfactory region is the site of origin of esthesioneuroblastoma and, occasionally, adenocarcinomas. Esthesioneuroblastoma is a tumor of neural crest origin first reported by Berger and Luc in 1924 as esthesioneuroepithelioma olfactif[19]; other names include olfactory neuroblastoma and esthesioneurocytoma. Esthesioneuroblastoma constitutes approximately only 3% of all intranasal neoplasms. About 250 cases have been reported between 1924 and 1990.[20] The tumor typically is composed of round, oval, or fusiform cells containing neurofibrils with pseudorosette formation and diffusely increased microvascularity.[21]

Esthesioneuroblastoma may be mistaken for any other "small round-cell tumor," that is, a group of aggressive malignant tumors composed of small and monotonous undifferentiated cells that includes Ewing's sarcoma, peripheral primitive neuroectodermal tumor (also known as extraskeletal Ewing's), rhabdomyosarcoma, lymphoma, small cell carcinoma (undifferentiated or neuroendocrine), and mesenchymal chondrosarcoma. The clinical presentations of these entities often overlap, but clinicopathologic features and immunohistochemical staining may help in distinguishing among them.

The route of contiguous spread of esthesioneuroblastomas is similar to that of ethmoid carcinomas. Lymph node involvement and distant metastasis are uncommon at diagnosis.[22,23]

Maxillary Sinuses

The pattern of spread of maxillary sinus cancers varies with the site of origin. Suprastructure tumors extend into the nasal cavity, ethmoid cells, orbit, pterygopalatine fossa, infratemporal fossa, and base of skull (Fig. 42.2A–C). Invasion of these structures gives lesions of the suprastructure a poorer prognosis. Their treatment is also associated with greater morbidity as a consequence of craniofacial resection or radiation of intracranial and ocular structures. Infrastructure tumors often infiltrate the palate, alveolar process, gingivobuccal sulcus, soft tissue of the cheek, nasal cavity, masseter muscle, pterygopalatine space, and pterygoid fossa (Fig. 42.2D–J).

The maxillary sinuses are believed to have a limited lymphatic supply[24] and a correspondingly low incidence of lymphadenopathy at diagnosis.[25,26] Only 6 of the 73 patients (8%) in the MD Anderson Cancer Center series had palpable lymphadenopathy at diagnosis. The incidence of nodal spread, however, varies with the histologic type (17%, or 5 of 29 patients with squamous cell or poorly differentiated carcinomas vs. 4%, or 1 of 27 for patients with adenocarcinoma, adenoid cystic carcinoma, or mucoepidermoid carcinoma). The incidence of subclinical disease, as reflected in the rate of nodal relapse in patients who did not receive elective neck treatment, also varies with histologic type (38%, or 9 of 24 patients with squamous cell or poorly differentiated carcinomas vs. 8%, or 2 of 26 patients with adenocarcinoma, adenoid cystic carcinoma, or mucoepidermoid carcinoma). The cumulative incidence of nodal involvement (gross and microscopic) for patients with squamous cell and poorly differentiated carcinomas is about 30%. The risk of regional recurrence after treatment is 20% to 30% or higher, depending on the extent of disease and elective neck treatment.[27] Ipsilateral subdigastric and submandibular nodes are most often involved. Hematogenous spread is uncommon.

CLINICAL PRESENTATION

Nasal Vestibule

Carcinomas of the nasal vestibule usually present as asymptomatic plaques or nodules, often with crusting and scabbing. Advanced lesions may extend beyond the vestibule and may cause pain, bleeding, or ulceration. Large ulcerated lesions may

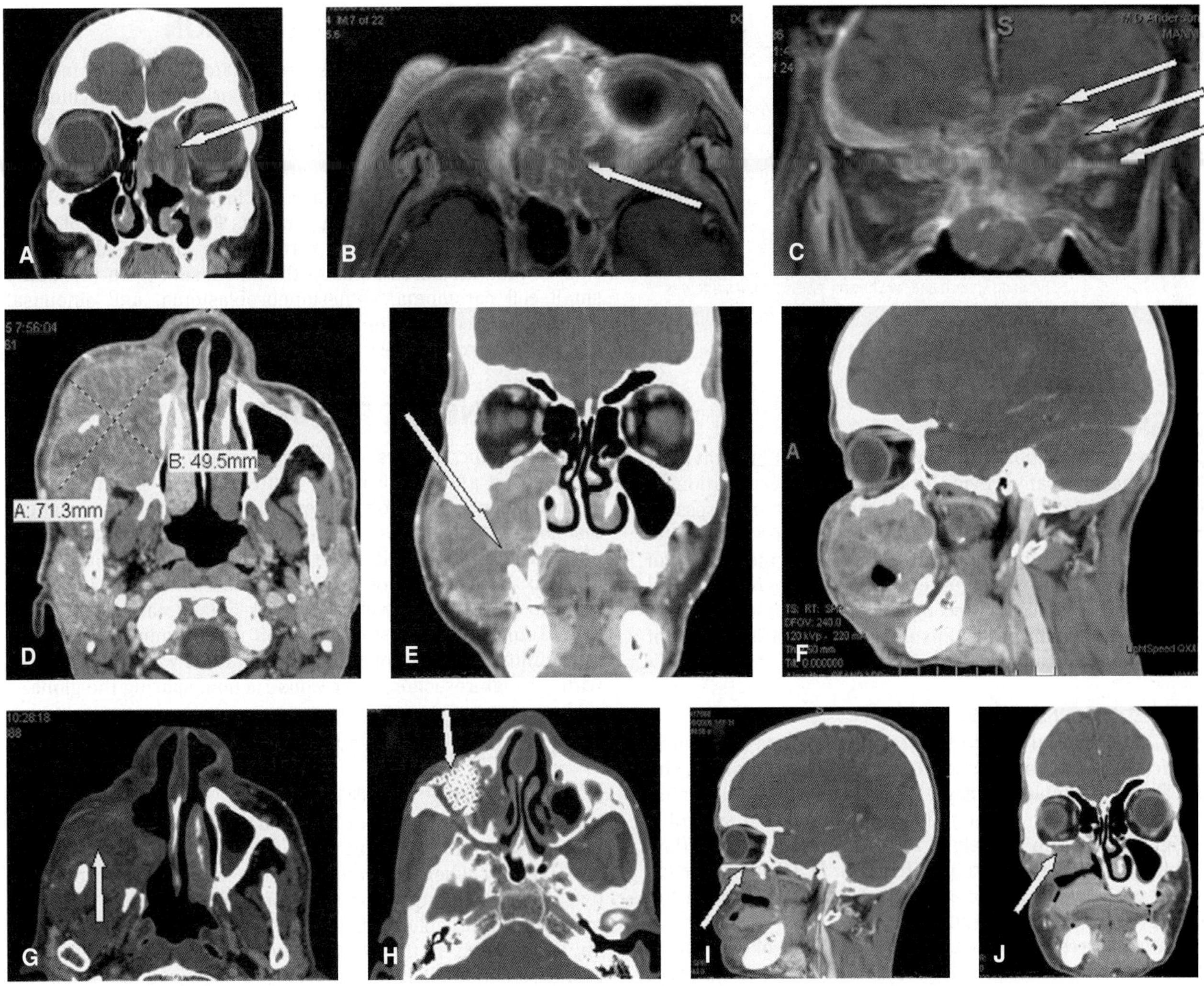

FIGURE 42.2. The pattern of spread of maxillary sinus cancers. **A–C:** Suprastructure tumors are shown, with arrows indicating the involvement of the nasal cavity and ethmoid cells **(A)**, the orbit **(B)**, and the base of skull **(C)**. **D–J:** Advanced tumor is shown, with arrows indicating alveolar process destruction with loosening of a tooth **(E)** and abutment of the orbital floor without frank intraorbital invasion **(F)**. The patient had a maxillectomy and orbital floor resection with an anterolateral thigh (ALT) flap (*arrow* in **G**), and titanium mesh reconstruction of the orbital floor (**H, I,** and **J**).

become infected, leading to severe tenderness that requires anesthesia for complete clinical assessment.

Nasal Cavity

Nasal cavity tumors present with symptoms and signs of nasal polyps (e.g., chronic unilateral discharge, ulcer, obstruction, anterior headache, and intermittent epistaxis), hence delaying the diagnosis. Additional symptoms and signs develop as the lesion enlarges: medial orbital mass, proptosis, expansion of the nasal bridge, diplopia resulting from invasion of the orbit, epiphora due to obstruction of the nasolacrimal duct, anomaly of smell or anosmia from involvement of the olfactory region, or frontal headache due to extension through the cribriform plate.

The common presenting symptoms of esthesioneuroblastomas are nasal obstruction and epistaxis. Spaulding et al.[28] found that anosmia could precede diagnosis by many years. Other symptoms are related to contiguous disease extension into the orbit (proptosis, visual-field defects, orbital pain, epiphora), paranasal sinuses (medial canthus mass, facial swelling), or anterior cranial fossa (headache) or are due to inappropriate antidiuretic hormone secretion.[28]

Ethmoid Sinuses

The presenting symptoms and signs of ethmoid sinus tumors are central or facial headaches and referred pain to the nasal or retrobulbar region, a subcutaneous mass at the inner canthus, nasal obstruction and discharge, diplopia, and proptosis. In one study of 34 patients with ethmoid sinus cancers treated at MD Anderson Cancer Center between 1969 and 1993,[29] nasal cavity symptoms (nasal obstruction, epistaxis, discharge) were reported in 25 patients (74%), orbital symptoms (diplopia, orbital pain, vision loss, proptosis, inner canthus mass, tearing) in 12 (35%), headache in 6 (18%), and hyposmia or anosmia in 5 (15%).

Maxillary Sinuses

Maxillary sinus cancers usually are diagnosed at advanced stages. Symptoms and signs are facial swelling, pain, or paresthesia of the cheek induced by disease extension to the premaxillary region, epistaxis, nasal discharge and obstruction related to tumor spread to the nasal cavity, ill-fitting dentures, alveolar or palatal mass, unhealed tooth socket after extraction from spread to the oral cavity, and proptosis, diplopia, impaired vision, or orbital pain due to orbital invasion.[30]

DIAGNOSTIC WORKUP

The recommended pretreatment physical, diagnostic, and staging evaluations are listed in Table 42.1.

TABLE 42.1 PRETREATMENT EVALUATION FOR TUMORS OF THE NASAL CAVITY AND PARANASAL SINUSES

General	Complete history and physical examination
	Fiberoptic endoscopic examination with biopsies
Radiographic	Computed tomography/magnetic resonance imaging of the primary site and neck
	Chest x-ray; computed tomography of thorax if adenoid cystic or neuroendocrine carcinoma
Laboratory	Complete blood count
Other	Dental evaluation with extractions/restorations as needed
	Baseline ophthalmologic examination
	Baseline speech and swallowing assessment if surgery is planned

Physical Examination

Inspection and palpation of the orbits, nasal and oral cavities, and nasopharynx can provide preliminary determination of tumor extent. Bimanual palpation is important in assessing contiguous extension of nasal vestibule lesions and in identifying buccinator and submandibular nodal involvement. Careful examination of cranial nerves is required. Fiberoptic nasal endoscopy after mucosal decongestion and topical analgesia allows assessment of local extent and facilitates biopsy of tumor involving the nasal cavity or nasopharynx.

Radiographic Evaluation

Imaging has a crucial role in the staging of sinonasal tumors. Magnetic resonance imaging (MRI) and computed tomography (CT) scans are complementary.[31] MRI is superior at detecting direct intracranial or perineural or leptomeningeal spread.[32] T2-weighted MRI can be helpful in distinguishing tumor (low signal) from obstructed secretions (bright).[33] CT is superior for detecting early cortical bone erosion or extension through the cribriform plate or orbital walls.

Certain features provide clues as to the nature of the tumors in this region. Slowly progressive lesions tend to deform instead of destroy bony structures. Intermediate-grade tumors can cause sclerosis of adjacent bone. Lymphomas tend to permeate bone without frank destruction, and carcinomas and sarcomas infiltrate and destroy adjacent bone.

Biopsy

Transnasal biopsy is preferred for tumors arising from or extending into the nasal cavity or nasopharynx. Some paranasal sinus tumors may be more easily sampled using transoral procedures or an open Caldwell-Luc approach.

Laboratory Studies

Complete blood counts and serum chemistries can be used to screen for the presence of distant metastases. Abnormalities of these tests can be further investigated as necessary.

STAGING

The seventh edition of the American Joint Committee on Cancer's (AJCC) *AJCC Cancer Staging Manual* tumor-node-metastasis (TNM) classification includes staging for cancers of the maxillary sinus, ethmoid sinus, and the nasal cavity.[34] Significant updates from the sixth edition affect classifications of T4 lesions and hence stage IV disease. Specifically, T4 lesions are now considered either T4a (moderately advanced local disease) or T4b (very advanced local disease), which leads to stratification of stage IV disease as either IVA (moderately advanced local or regional disease, IVB (very advanced local or regional disease), or IVC (distant metastatic disease). Definitions of anatomic stage prognostic groupings and TNM classifications are given in Table 42.2.

PATHOLOGIC CLASSIFICATION

Most nasal vestibule cancers are squamous cell carcinomas; the remaining tumors are basal cell or adnexal carcinomas. Most cancers of the nasal cavity and paranasal sinuses are also squamous cell carcinomas, although minor salivary gland neoplasms (adenocarcinoma, adenoid cystic carcinoma, and mucoepidermoid carcinoma) account for 10% to 15% of lesions in these locations. Melanoma accounts for 5% to 10% of nasal cavity malignancies but is rare in the paranasal sinuses. Neuroendocrine carcinomas of the sinonasal region (including small cell carcinoma, esthesioneuroblastoma, and sinonasal undifferentiated carcinomas), lymphomas, sarcomas, and plasmacytomas are even less common.

PROGNOSTIC FACTORS

Patient-specific factors (primarily prognostic for survival) include age and performance status. Disease-specific factors (primarily prognostic for locoregional control) include location, histology, and locoregional extent (reflected in TNM stage), and perineural invasion. Extensive local disease involving the nasopharynx, base of skull, or cavernous sinuses markedly increases surgical morbidity as well as the risk of subtotal surgical excision. Tumor extension into the orbit may require enucleation, but minimal invasion of the floor or medial wall may be dealt with through resection and reconstruction, sparing the globe.

GENERAL MANAGEMENT

Nasal Vestibule Tumors

Nasal vestibule tumors can be treated definitively with surgery, primary radiation therapy, or postoperative (adjuvant) radiation therapy when indicated because of tumor size or positive surgical findings. For small superficial tumors, standard treatment approaches are surgery or primary radiation therapy. Depending on the location and size of the primary tumor, radiation can be delivered as external beam radiation therapy, brachytherapy, or a combination of the two. Primary radiation therapy may be preferable for nasal vestibule carcinoma for better cosmetic outcome, although surgery can yield high control rates with excellent cosmetic results for selected small superficial tumors. Adjuvant radiation is indicated for cases involving positive surgical margins, positive lymph nodes, or perineural invasion. Cartilaginous invasion is not a contraindication for radiation therapy because fractionated treatment carries a low risk of necrosis.[35] For large invasive tumors with extensive tissue destruction and distortion, the combination of surgery and radiation therapy, with the radiation given either before or after surgery, is the mainstay of treatment. However, some clinicians favor primary radiation with salvage surgery for this situation.[36] Cosmesis can be enhanced by having experienced prosthodontists design aesthetically satisfactory custom-made nasal prostheses after radical surgery. Patients who are older or who have poor performance status can be treated with radiation therapy alone. No role for systemic chemotherapy has been established for tumors of this type.

Nasal Fossa Tumors

Either surgery or primary radiation therapy can produce similarly high control rates for early-stage nasal fossa lesions. The choice of treatment modality is generally guided by the size and location of the tumor as well as the anticipated cosmetic outcome. Posterior nasal septum lesions or locally advanced lesions are generally treated surgically, but small anterior-inferior septal lesions (≤1.5 cm) can be treated effectively with interstitial brachytherapy (iridium-192 [^{192}Ir] implant). For lateral wall lesions extending to the nasal ala, primary external beam radiation therapy may produce the best cosmetic results.

TABLE 42.2 2010 AMERICAN JOINT COMMITTEE ON CANCER STAGING SYSTEM FOR CANCER OF THE NASAL CAVITY AND PARANASAL SINUSES

Definitions of TNM

Primary Tumor (T)	
TX	Primary tumor cannot be assessed
T0	No evidence of primary tumor
Tis	Carcinoma in situ
Maxillary Sinus	
T1	Tumor limited to maxillary sinus mucosa with no erosion or destruction of bone
T2	Tumor causing bone erosion or destruction including extension into the hard palate and/or middle nasal meatus, except extension to posterior wall of maxillary sinus and pterygoid plates
T3	Tumor invades any of the following: bone of the posterior wall of maxillary sinus, subcutaneous tissues, floor or medial wall of orbit, pterygoid fossa, ethmoid sinuses
T4 a	Moderately advanced local disease Tumor invades anterior orbital contents, skin of cheek, pterygoid plates, infratemporal fossa, cribriform plate, sphenoid or frontal sinuses
T4b	Very advanced local disease Tumor invades any of the following: orbital apex, dura, brain, middle cranial fossa, cranial nerves other than maxillary division of trigeminal nerve (V2), nasopharynx, or clivus
Nasal Cavity and Ethmoid Sinus	
T1	Tumor restricted to any one subsite, with or without bony invasion
T2	Tumor invading two subsites in a single region or extending to involve an adjacent region within the nasoethmoidal complex, with or without bony invasion
T3	Tumor extends to invade the medial wall or floor of the orbit, maxillary sinus, palate, or cribriform plate
T4a	Moderately advanced local disease Tumor invades any of the following: anterior orbital contents, skin of nose or cheeks, minimal extension to anterior cranial fossa, pterygoid plates, sphenoid or frontal sinuses
T4b	Very advanced local disease Tumor invades any of the following: orbital apex, dura, brain, middle cranial fossa, cranial nerves other than (V2), nasopharynx, or clivus
Regional Lymph Nodes (N)	
NX	Regional lymph nodes cannot be assessed
N0	No regional lymph node metastasis
N1	Metastasis in a single ipsilateral lymph node. 3 cm or less in greatest dimension
N2	Metastasis in a single ipsilateral lymph node, more than 3 cm but not more than 6 cm in greatest dimension, or in multiple ipsilateral lymph nodes or contralateral lymph nodes, none more than 6 cm in greatest dimension
N2a	Metastasis in a single ipsilateral lymph node, more than 3 cm but not more than 6 cm in greatest dimension
N2b	Metastasis in multiple ipsilateral lymph nodes, none more than 6 cm in greatest dimension
N2c	Metastasis in bilateral or contralateral lymph nodes, none more than 6 cm in greatest dimension
N3	Metastasis in a lymph node, more than 6 cm in greatest dimension
Distant Metastasis (M)	
M0	No distant metastasis
M1	Distant metastasis

Anatomic Stage/Prognostic Groups

Stage 0	Tis	N0	M0
Stage I	T1	N0	M0
Stage II	T2	N0	M0
Stage III	T3	N0	M0
	T1	N1	M0
	T2	N1	M0
	T3	N1	M0
Stage IVA	T4a	N0	M0
	T4a	N2	M0
	T1	N2	M0
	T2	N2	M0
	T3	N2	M0
	T4a	N2	M0
Stage IVB	T4b	Any N	M0
	Any T	N3	M0
	Any T	Any N	M1

Used with the permission of the American Joint Committee on Cancer, Chicago, Illinois. The original source for this material is the *AJCC Cancer Staging Manual,* 7th ed. (2010) published by Springer Science and Business Media LLC, www.springerlink.com.

Paranasal Sinus Tumors

Surgery can produce excellent control rates for T1 and T2 tumors and is generally the mainstay of treatment. The combination of surgery and postoperative radiation therapy is the treatment of choice for patients with more advanced but resectable disease who are medically fit to undergo surgery. Maxillary sinus and ethmoid sinus tumors often present as locally advanced disease (large T3 or T4) and are commonly managed with surgery and postoperative radiation therapy. Ethmoid sinus carcinomas can be treated with radiation alone or with concurrent chemotherapy to avoid structural or functional deficits.[37] Surgery generally involves medial maxillectomy and *en bloc* ethmoidectomy; a craniofacial approach is required if tumor extends superiorly to the ethmoid roof or olfactory region.[38,39] Primary radiation therapy, with or without concurrent chemotherapy, can be considered for patients who are not fit to undergo surgery owing to significant comorbid conditions or poor performance status, or for patients who decline radical surgery.

For patients presenting with Kadish stage A esthesioneuroblastoma, either surgery or radiation therapy ultimately yields locoregional control rates exceeding 90%.[8] Single-modality therapy has also been used for lesions involving the nasal cavity and one or more paranasal sinuses (stage B), as has surgery followed by adjuvant radiation therapy. However, the optimal therapy for stage B lesions is not clear because of the heterogeneity of these tumors. Surgery with adjuvant radiation is generally used for disease that extends beyond the nasal cavity and paranasal sinuses (stage C). Overall, local therapy with surgery and postoperative radiation therapy yields excellent results at 5 years with regard to both overall survival (93.1%) and local control (96.2%).[36] Elective nodal irradiation is not generally recommended because the incidence of nodal relapse is <15%. Distant metastasis is uncommon (10%) even among patients presenting with locally advanced disease.

CHEMOTHERAPY: NEOADJUVANT AND CONCOMITANT

Neoadjuvant chemotherapy (i.e., chemotherapy given before surgery) can reduce tumor volumes, which may allow a less extensive surgical resection than would be possible otherwise. Similarly, chemotherapy given before primary radiation therapy can also reduce tumor volumes and facilitate radiotherapy planning by increasing the distance between tumor borders and critical organ structures such as brain, chiasm, optic nerve, or spinal cord. Investigations are ongoing to determine whether the response (or lack of same) to neoadjuvant chemotherapy can help in the choice of definitive treatment. For example, if neoadjuvant chemotherapy produces a complete response, then primary radiation therapy, with or without chemotherapy, can be considered; a less-than-complete response would prompt surgical excision of the lesion followed by adjuvant radiation therapy.

Concurrent chemoradiation therapy can also be used for patients with medical conditions that preclude surgery if those patients have good performance status. Depending on the patient's performance status and renal function, single-agent cisplatin or carboplatin can be used concurrently with external beam radiation for locally advanced, unresectable squamous cell carcinoma. Neoadjuvant chemotherapy or concurrent chemoradiation with etoposide and cisplatin or carboplatin can be used to treat sinonasal undifferentiated carcinoma, neuroendocrine carcinoma, or small cell carcinoma. Chemotherapy is not used routinely for esthesioneuroblastoma, and its role in the management of this disease is under investigation. Chemotherapy may have a role in the management of Kadish stage C disease, and although responses to chemotherapy have been reported, they are usually of limited duration.[40] Concurrent chemotherapy during radiation may be considered for inoperable cases.

PALLIATION

Symptoms of incurable sinonasal cancer are particularly distressing. Multidisciplinary input is required even for very advanced cases, as palliation may involve limited surgery, radiation therapy, chemotherapy, investigational studies, or best supportive care. The morbidity of each modality must be balanced with the potential benefits in symptom control and improved quality of life. Particular attention is required to address the control of pain and discomfort as a first priority, and the impact of disfigurement and dysfunction, which is often present.

Chemotherapy can be given as single-agent therapy in investigational settings. If radiation therapy is given, large doses per fraction are usually given to reduce the duration of treatment. However, if concurrent chemotherapy is added, treatment with 2-Gy fractions should be considered to avoid severe acute effects. Radiation or chemotherapy is often effective in reducing tumor bulk and relieving symptoms associated with disfiguring masses, proptosis, discomfort or neuropathic pain, headache, epistaxis or other bleeding, nasal obstruction or discharge, and trismus.

RADIATION THERAPY TECHNIQUES

Tumors of the Nasal Cavity

Nasal Vestibule Tumors

Target Volumes

For small, well-differentiated lesions that are ≤1.5 cm in diameter, small fields with a 1- to 2-cm margin are appropriate. The initial target volume for all poorly differentiated tumors and well-differentiated primary tumors larger than 1.5 cm without palpable lymphadenopathy should include both nasal vestibules with at least 2- to 3-cm margins around the primary tumor (wider margins for infiltrative tumor) as well as bilateral facial, submandibular, and subdigastric nodes. When lymph node involvement is present at diagnosis, the lower neck is also irradiated. For larger nasal vestibule lesions, the lower half of the nose and the upper lip are treated as well as the regional lymphatics, including the facial lymphatics and upper neck nodes. For postoperative radiation therapy, the initial target volume includes the operative bed plus a 1- to 1.5-cm margin and the elective nodal regions.

Treatment Techniques

External Beam Radiation. Thin superficial nasal vestibule lesions can be treated with orthovoltage x-rays or electrons with skin bolus, whereas thicker lesions are generally treated with electrons. In definitive therapy, the target volume is treated to a dose of 66 to 70 Gy, with a small reduction in the treatment fields after 50 Gy to boost the dose to the gross disease. For patients presenting with palpable neck adenopathy, the entire neck is treated with at least a subclinical dose of 50 Gy, and the gross disease plus a 1- to 2-cm margin is then treated with an additional 16 to 20 Gy. A technique for external beam irradiation using electrons is illustrated in Figure 42.3. The patient lies supine, immobilized with the neck slightly flexed by using a custom mask to align the anterior surface of the maxilla parallel with the top of the couch. For larger nasal vestibule lesions, the lower half of the nose and the upper lip are treated with an anterior appositional field using 20-MeV electrons and 6-MV photons weighted 4 to 1. Skin collimation is used to minimize scatter irradiation to the eye and reduce the penumbra of the beam and reduce the field size required. Custom beeswax bolus material is prepared to allow a relatively flat surface contour onto which the electron beam is incident, avoiding inhomogeneity due to oblique incidence and surface irregularity. A bolus is also used to fill the nares to avoid the dose perturbation from the air cavity with electron beams. In photon treatments, the bolus is removed to spare the skin unless the overlying skin is involved. An intraoral Cerrobend-containing stent is used to displace the tongue posteriorly and partially shield the upper alveolar ridge.

When indicated, the right and left facial lymphatics are irradiated with appositional fields; these require an approximately 15-degree gantry rotation to the respective side with 6-MeV electron fields, each abutting the appositional primary lesion portal and the upper neck fields. The medial border is matched to the lateral border of the anterior primary field. The anterior border extends down from the oral commissure to the middle of the horizontal ramus of the mandible, whereas the posterior border extends from the upper edge of the anterior field to just above the angle of the mandible. The inferior border splits the horizontal ramus of the mandible and is matched to the upper neck field. The junctions are moved twice during the course of treatment to reduce dose heterogeneity. The submandibular and subdigastric nodes are treated with lateral parallel-opposed photon fields. For patients with involved nodes, these upper neck fields are matched inferiorly to an anterior portal treating the middle and lower neck nodes.

For definitive treatment, the external beam radiation schedule for lesions up to 1.5 cm in diameter for which a combination

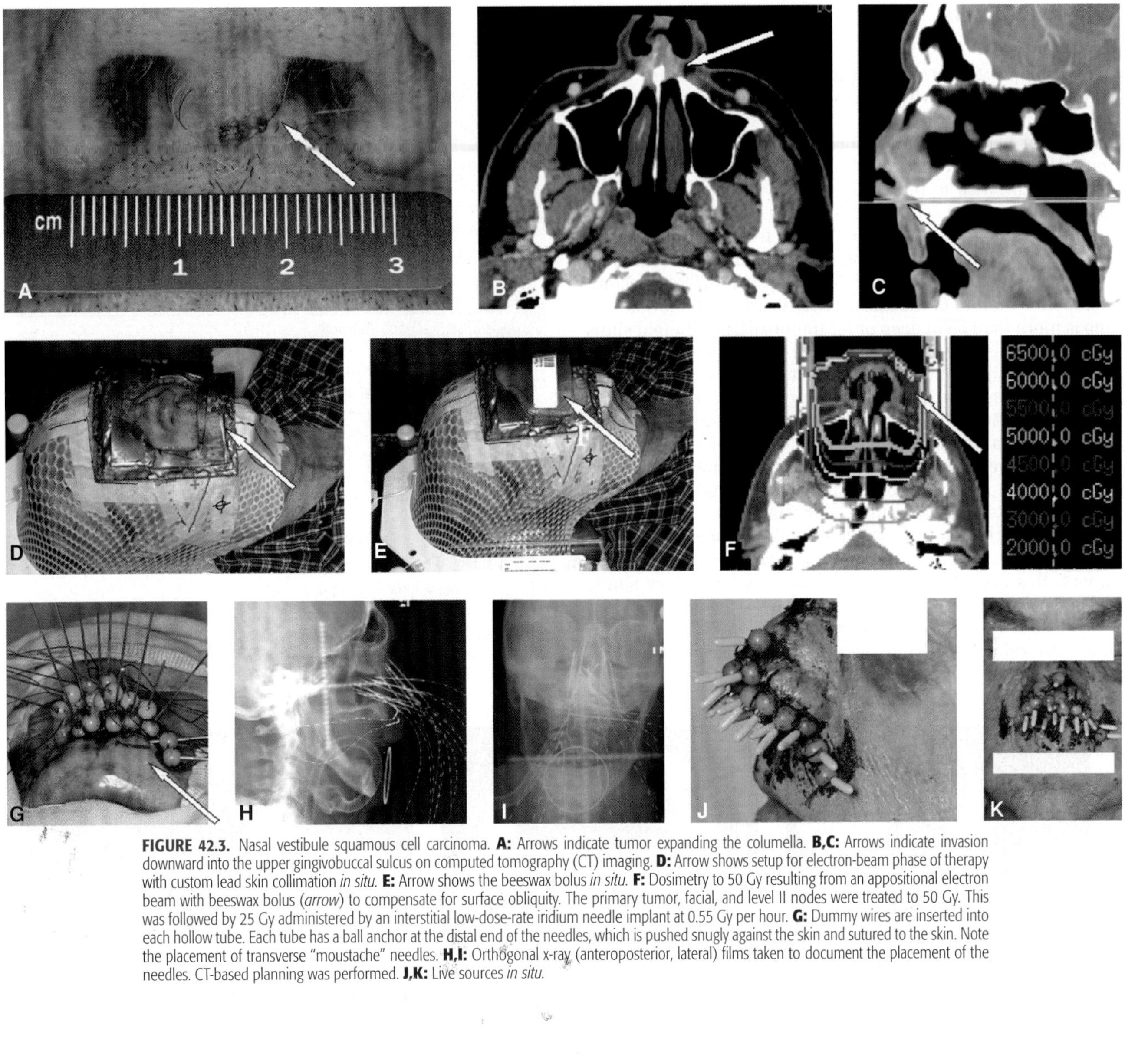

FIGURE 42.3. Nasal vestibule squamous cell carcinoma. **A:** Arrows indicate tumor expanding the columella. **B,C:** Arrows indicate invasion downward into the upper gingivobuccal sulcus on computed tomography (CT) imaging. **D:** Arrow shows setup for electron-beam phase of therapy with custom lead skin collimation *in situ.* **E:** Arrow shows the beeswax bolus *in situ.* **F:** Dosimetry to 50 Gy resulting from an appositional electron beam with beeswax bolus (*arrow*) to compensate for surface obliquity. The primary tumor, facial, and level II nodes were treated to 50 Gy. This was followed by 25 Gy administered by an interstitial low-dose-rate iridium needle implant at 0.55 Gy per hour. **G:** Dummy wires are inserted into each hollow tube. Each tube has a ball anchor at the distal end of the needles, which is pushed snugly against the skin and sutured to the skin. Note the placement of transverse "moustache" needles. **H,I:** Orthogonal x-ray (anteroposterior, lateral) films taken to document the placement of the needles. CT-based planning was performed. **J,K:** Live sources *in situ.*

of electrons and photons is used is typically 50 Gy in 25 fractions followed by a boost of 10 to 16 Gy in 5 to 8 fractions (prescribed at the 90% isodose line). Larger lesions to be treated by external beam radiation alone receive 50 Gy in 25 fractions plus a boost of 16 to 20 Gy in 8 to 10 fractions. The schedule for elective nodal irradiation is 50 Gy in 25 fractions. Palpable nodes are given a boost to a total dose of 66 to 70 Gy in 33 to 35 fractions, depending on the size. For postoperative treatment, the volume is reduced off the undissected nodal regions after 50 Gy (25 fractions) to deliver an additional 6 Gy to the surgical bed. At 56 Gy, a final "cone down" is done to include a 4-Gy dose to the preoperative tumor bed, for a total dose of 60 Gy. If the excision was limited or positive margins are present, the final cone-down dose is 10 Gy for a total dose of 66 Gy.

Brachytherapy. Brachytherapy for small lesions is accomplished by using a ^{192}Ir wire implant or, in selected cases, by using an intracavitary ^{192}Ir mold. Hollow needles for after loading are inserted under general anesthesia, which allows good exposure of the tumor and protects the airway in the event of bleeding from the vascular Kiesselbach plexus on the anterior nasal septum or from posterior hemorrhages originating from larger vessels near the sphenopalatine artery, behind the middle turbinate. Implantation of a T2 squamous cell carcinoma of the columella is shown in Figure 42.3. The recommended doses for low-dose–rate brachytherapy have evolved empirically and range from 60 to 65 Gy delivered during 5 to 7 days.

Brachytherapy can be used instead of an external beam boost for patients with T1 or T2 nasal vestibule tumors after initial larger-field radiation therapy. After delivery of 50 Gy, the patient is assessed and if the tumor volume has been substantially reduced, a boost of 20 to 25 Gy may be administered in about 2 days by using low-dose–rate brachytherapy.

High-dose–rate brachytherapy has also been used to deliver the boost. A custom mold of the nasal vestibule is fabricated and tumor is marked in the mold. Two to four plastic tubes are inserted in the mold alongside the tumor at 1-cm intervals. For tumors of the lateral part of the vestibule, two catheters are placed on the inner aspect of the nasal vestibule. For medially localized tumors, catheters are placed on both sides of the vestibule. After external beam radiation to 50 Gy in 5 weeks, high-dose–rate brachytherapy is delivered in week 6. The dose is typically 3 Gy per fraction, given twice a day, to a total dose of 18 Gy specified at the center of the tumor. With a median overall treatment time (external beam radiation plus brachytherapy) of 36 days, this technique has been reported to yield 2-year local control rates of 86% and ultimate locoregional control rates of 100%.[41]

Nasal Fossa Tumors

Target Volume

The technique for primary or postoperative external beam irradiation of nasal cavity tumors depends on the depth of the neoplasm. For tumors located <3.5 or 4.0 cm from the skin of the apex of the nose, electrons can be used, as 20 MeV electrons will provide coverage up to 5 cm in depth. A margin of at least 1 cm deep to the posterior edge must be included in the full-dose volume. The technique is as previously described for nasal vestibule carcinoma. CT-based treatment planning is necessary for accurate target localization and dose calculation.

Intensity-modulated radiation therapy (IMRT) is recommended for tumors of the nasal cavity in which the target volume is more than 5 cm deep or for tumors of the ethmoid sinus (Fig. 42.4). This technique delivers the desired dose to the target volume while minimizing the dose to critical organs such as cornea, lens, lacrimal glands, retina, optic nerve, optic chiasm, brain, and brainstem. For postoperative radiation therapy, the primary clinical target volume (CTV) descriptions are given in Table 42.3. The CTV_1 consists of the primary tumor bed with a 1.0- to 1.5-cm margin. A boost subvolume consisting of high-risk regions (sites of positive margins, gross macroscopic residual tumor) to be treated to higher doses may be outlined. The CTV_2 includes the entire operative bed. For ethmoid sinus tumors, this might include the frontal sinus, maxillary sinus, and sphenoid sinus. The bony orbit is part of the operative bed when orbital exenteration is performed because of tumor invasion. For lesions involving the ethmoid sinuses or olfactory

TABLE 42.3 TARGET VOLUMES FOR INTENSITY MODULATED RADIATION THERAPY OF SINONASAL CANCERS

Target	*Description*	*Dose (33–35 Fractions) (Gy)*
Primary Radiation Therapy		
GTV	GTV (= prechemotherapy volume)	66–70
CTV_1 (primary CTV)	GTV + 1.0–1.5 cm	66–70
CTV_2 (intermediate-dose CTV)	Primary CTV + 1.0–1.5 cm	59–63
CTV_3 (elective CTV)	Nodal volumes, nerve tract, and base of skull margin	54–57
Target	*Description*	*Dose (30 Fractions) (Gy)*
Postoperative Radiation Therapy		
CTV_{HR} (high-risk CTV)	Sites of suspected positive margins, gross macroscopic residual tumor, extracapsular nodal disease	66–70[a]
CTV_1 (primary CTV)	Primary tumor bed with 1.0–1.5 cm margin	60
CTV_2 (intermediate dose CTV)	Surgical bed	57
CTV_3 (low-dose CTV)	Trigeminal nerve perineural invasion is present, additional skull base margin, elective nodal volume if indicated	54

GTV, gross tumor volume; CTV, clinical target volume.

[a]70 Gy may be given by adding a second boost plan or increasing the number of fractions to 35.

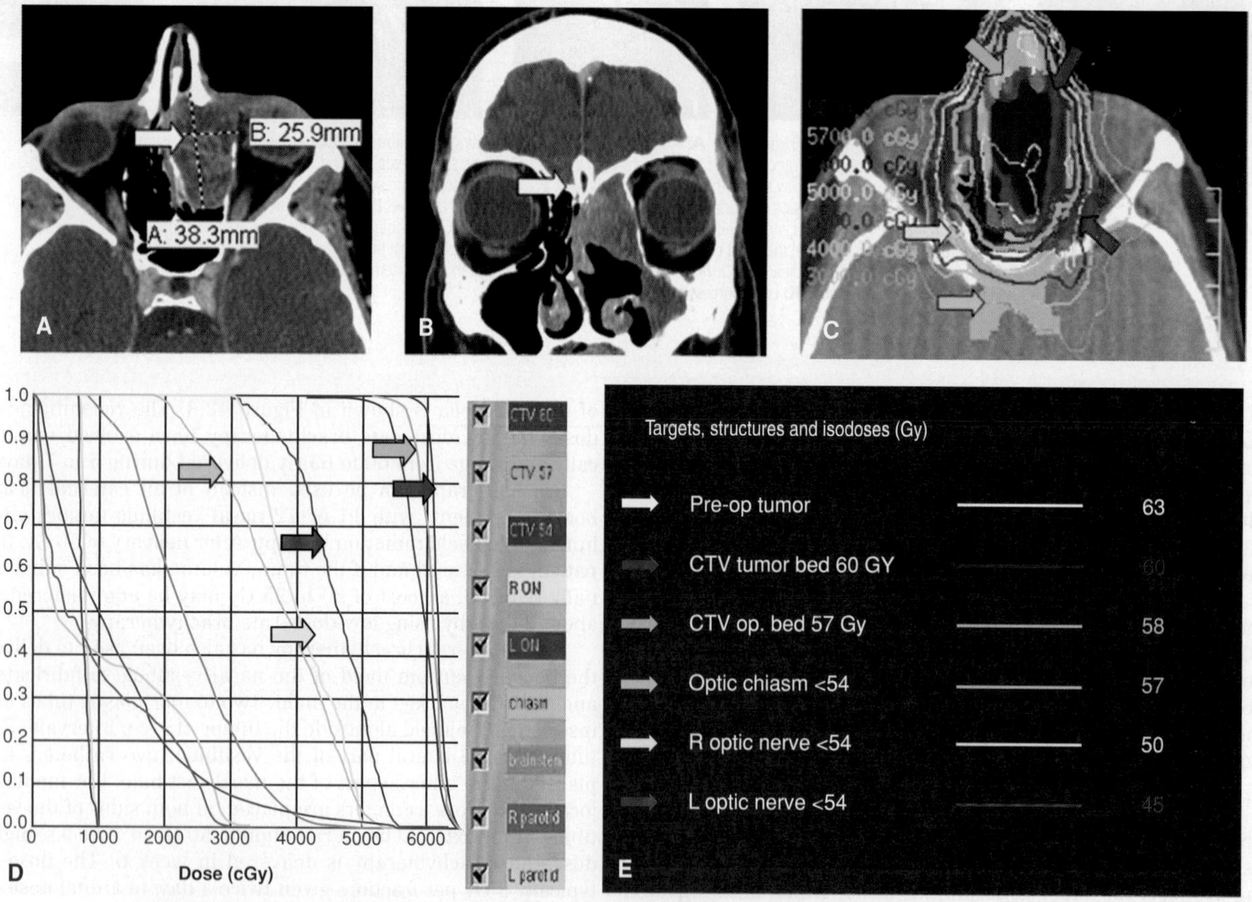

FIGURE 42.4. Intensity-modulated radiotherapy for adjuvant radiotherapy for an adenoid cystic carcinoma of the ethmoid sinus, anterior skull base, nasal cavity, and medial orbit following endoscopic anteroposterior ethmoidectomy with resection of tumor, left maxillary antrostomy with disease removal, bilateral sphenoidotomy, and frontal sinusotomy with anterior approach to the anterior skull base including a left lateral rhinotomy and medial maxillectomy and extradural resection of anterior cranial base. **A,B:** Preoperative computed tomography scans with tumor indicated by white arrow. **C:** Transverse section at the level of the orbit that show sharp dose gradient at the interface of the clinical target volume and the optic nerves and chiasm. **D,E:** Cumulative dose volume (*y*-axis) histogram.

region, the CTV should also include the cribriform plate. A third CTV may be delineated to encompass the tract of cranial nerve V2 to the foramen rotundum if perineural invasion is present. For primary radiation therapy given as IMRT, the CTV_1, consisting of the gross tumor volume plus a margin of 1 to 2 cm, receives the full dose of 66 to 70 Gy. For patients receiving neoadjuvant chemotherapy, target volume definition is based on the extent of disease before chemotherapy.

For three-dimensional (3D) conformal radiation therapy, the initial target volume for postoperative radiation consists of the surgical bed with 1- or 2-cm margins, depending on the surgical pathology findings and the proximity of critical structures. The boost volume consists of areas at greatest risk of recurrence, such as close or positive resection margins or regions of perineural invasion, with 1- to 2-cm margins.

For small anteroinferior septal lesions, brachytherapy can be accomplished by using a single-plane implant of the lesion with 2-cm margins. Elective neck irradiation is not given routinely even for patients with large tumors or esthesioneuroblastoma.

Setup and Field Arrangement

For target volumes <5 cm deep, an electron technique similar to that described for nasal vestibule carcinomas is used. Treatment devices include lead skin collimation to obtain a sharp penumbra as well as bolus material in the nasal cavity, in postoperative defects, and on skin scars. An intraoral stent is used to depress the tongue, provide a patent airway, and aid in immobilization. Tungsten internal eye shields may be used if the target volume approaches the orbits (see Fig. 42.3).

For 3D-conformal therapy or IMRT, the patient is immobilized in a supine position with the head positioned such that the hard palate is perpendicular to the treatment couch. Scars are marked with thin radio-opaque wires, bolus and other devices are positioned, and transverse CT images are obtained from the vertex to the upper mediastinum. For IMRT, rigid immobilization is necessary, including use of special head and shoulder thermoplastic masks that extend down to the upper thorax. The shoulders can be additionally depressed and fixed by using wrist straps tethered to a footboard. Target volumes are delineated as previously described.

For IMRT, multiple gantry angles are used based on beam-optimization algorithms. An example of a 10-field noncoplanar arrangement with two vertex beams is shown in Figure 42.4. The beam angle selections are based on the same principles as for 3D-conformal therapy:

1. Preference for the shortest path to the target;
2. Avoidance of direct irradiation of the critical structures (e.g., avoid beam entry through the contralateral eye after ipsilateral exenteration); and
3. Use of as large a beam separation as possible.

Inverse planning is usually done and multiple iterations may be necessary to ensure that the following are accomplished:

1. Targets are covered;
2. Normal tissue constraints are respected; and
3. Dose is relatively homogenous.

Dose calculations should include heterogeneity corrections because of the significant amounts of air and bone in the sinuses. Radiation oncologists must work closely with physicists and dosimetrists. It is important to realize that the criteria for accepting or rejecting the plan may not be evident from the dose–volume histogram.

For 3D-conformal radiation therapy, anterior oblique wedge-pair photon fields are appropriate for lesions located in the anterior lower half of the nasal cavity. Opposed-lateral fields can be used to treat tumors at the posterior part of the nasal fossa, provided the ethmoid cells are not involved. The optic pathway can be excluded from the radiation fields with this setup. For primaries of the upper nasal cavity and ethmoidal air cells, a three-field setup allows coverage of the ethmoid cells while sparing the optic apparatus. CT-based treatment planning is necessary to select beam and wedge angles (usually 45 to 60 degrees) and the relative loading of the fields, as well as to evaluate the dose to critical structures such as brain, brainstem, and optic structures.

Proton beam therapy techniques for treating nasal fossa tumors are rapidly evolving and include both passive scattering and discrete spot scanning beams. Theoretically, the advantage of proton therapy derives from the unique physical properties of protons that allow deposition of most of the particle's energy at the end of its range. Descriptions of the various techniques by which proton therapy can be delivered are beyond the scope of this chapter. Nevertheless, with optimization of dosimetry, the conformality and heterogeneity within the target volumes provided by proton therapy should be equivalent to what can be achieved with either electron or photon therapy, with the added advantage of minimizing the unnecessary dose or "dose bath" from IMRT to the surrounding normal tissue structures.

Dose Fractionation Schedule

The dose schedule for low-dose–rate brachytherapy is 60 to 65 Gy during 5 to 7 days. The external beam regimen for primary radiation therapy is 50 Gy in 25 fractions followed by a boost of 16 to 20 Gy in 8 to 10 fractions, depending on the size of the lesion. Postoperative radiation therapy consists of 50 Gy to elective tissue, 56 Gy to the operative bed, and 60 Gy to the tumor bed, with an optional boost to close or positive surgical margins, all given at 2 Gy per fraction. Dose regimens for intensity-modulated therapy, whether with photons or protons, are summarized in Table 42.3.

Tumors of the Paranasal Sinuses

Target Volume

Because maxillary cancers are usually diagnosed at a locally advanced stage and surgery is the primary therapy, most patients receive postoperative radiation therapy. Delineation of target volumes is based on physical examination, pretreatment imaging, intraoperative findings (tumor extension relative to critical structures such as orbital wall, cribriform plate, cranial nerve foramina, and ease of resection), and pathologic findings (such as positive margin or perineural invasion).

IMRT is the preferred treatment method as it generally yields better dose distribution in terms of both tumor coverage and sparing of normal tissues than can be achieved with 3D-conformal radiation therapy. IMRT is rapidly becoming the standard of care technique for external beam therapy for sinonasal malignancies.[42,43] Proton therapy may offer additional advantages over IMRT in terms of further reducing the dose to normal tissues while achieving equivalent doses to the target volume. The CTV_1 consists of the primary tumor bed with 1.0- to 1.5-cm margin of normal tissue. The CTV_2 encompasses the operative bed, including the bony orbit after orbital exenteration and the ethmoid, frontal, or sphenoid sinuses if explored during surgery. A third CTV may be delineated to encompass the tract of cranial nerve V2 to the foramen rotundum if perineural invasion is present. A CTV for high-risk areas (CTV_{HR}; see Table 42.3) may also be outlined to cover, for example, gross macroscopic residual tumor or positive margins to which a higher dose may be delivered.

For primary radiation therapy using IMRT, the prescription doses are 66 to 70 Gy to the gross tumor volume (the prechemotherapy volume for those receiving systemic treatment), plus a 1- to 1.5-cm margin of normal-appearing tissue (CTV_1), 59 to 63 Gy to other secondary clinical target volumes such as the rest of the involved sinus and wider region around the primary target, and 54 to 57 Gy to the tracts of nerves (if perineural invasion is present) and to elective nodal regions. An example

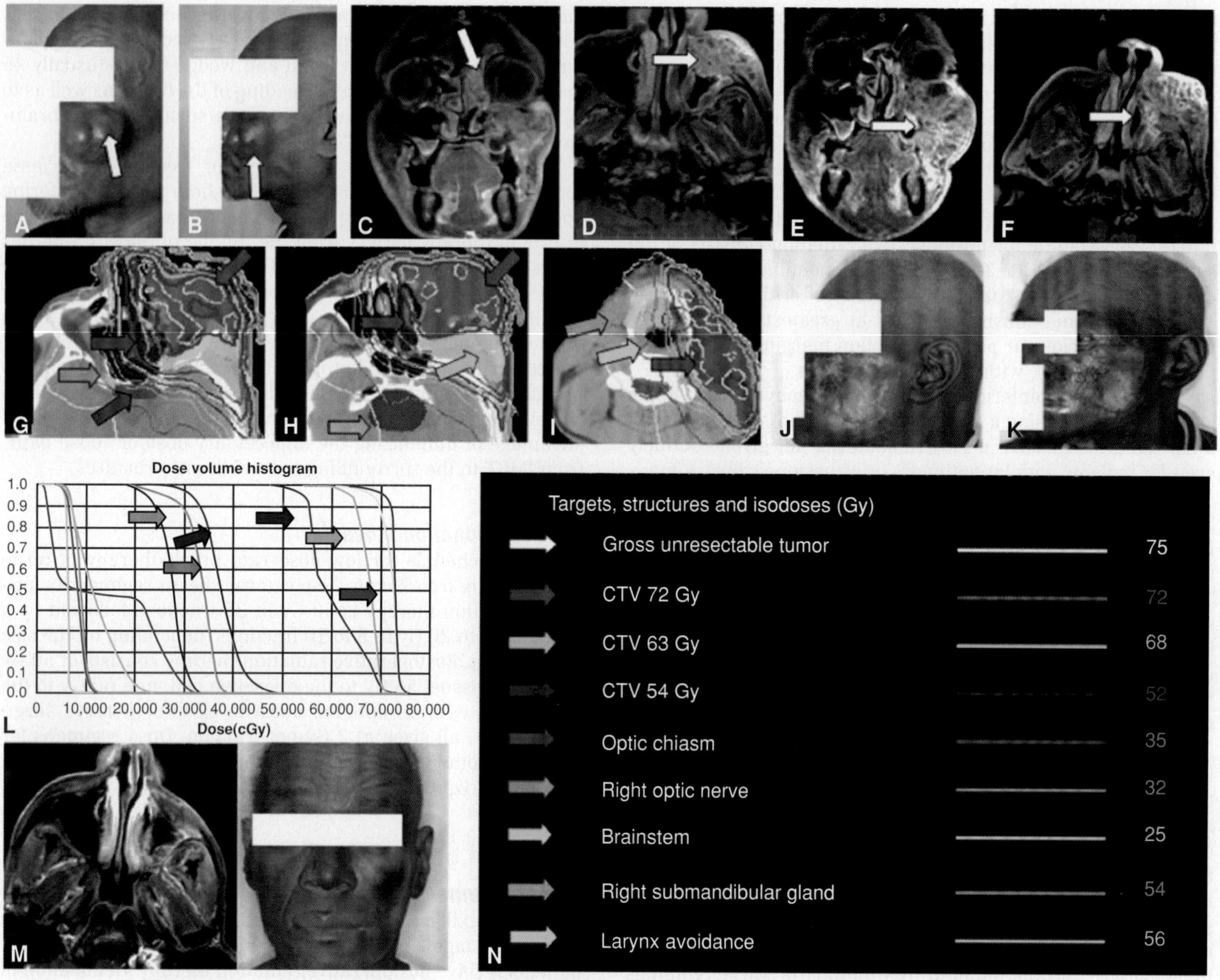

FIGURE 42.5. Intensity-modulated radiotherapy (IMRT) for definitive radiotherapy for T4N0 squamous cell carcinoma of the maxillary sinus. **A,B:** Pretreatment photographs showing skin of cheek involvement. **C,D:** Magnetic resonance image (MRI) scans with tumor indicated by *white arrow*. **E,F:** MRIs following induction chemotherapy showed progressive disease involving left maxilla, left nasoethmoid region, extending inferiorly into the premaxillary soft tissues. **G–I:** IMRT plan with sections showing coverage of the target volumes. The patient was treated using concomitant boost fractionation. The primary plan delivered 57 Gy and a concomitant boost plan administered an additional 15 Gy. **G** and **H** also show avoidance of the normal tissues, as listed in the key and illustrated further in the cumulative dose–volume histogram in **L**. **J,K:** The skin reaction during final week of radiotherapy. **M,N:** MRI and patient photo at follow-up, showing healed skin with hyperpigmentation. The tumor was in complete remission at the last visit 7 months after therapy.

of an IMRT plan for primary definitive radiation therapy of a T4N0 squamous cell carcinoma is shown in Figure 42.5.

For postoperative radiation therapy using a 3D-conformal technique, the initial target volume consists of the operative bed with 1- to 2-cm margins. The boost field consists of the primary tumor bed and areas at higher risk of recurrence, such as positive resection margins or perineural invasion. Radiation is administered to the neck after node dissection if multiple nodes are involved or extracapsular extension is present. Elective radiation of ipsilateral submandibular and subdigastric nodes is given for patients with squamous cell or poorly differentiated carcinoma. An example of an intensity-modulated proton plan for postoperative radiation therapy is shown in Figure 42.6.

Setup and Field Arrangement

Patients undergoing treatment of paranasal tumors are immobilized in a supine position with the head slightly hyperextended to bring the floor of the orbit parallel to the axis of the anterior field. An intraoral stent is used to open the mouth and depress the tongue out of the radiation field. After palatectomy, the stent can be designed to hold a water-filled balloon to obliterate the large air cavity in the surgical defect to improve dose homogeneity. An orbital exenteration defect can also be filled directly with a water-filled balloon to decrease the dose delivered to the temporal lobe. Marking of the lateral canthi, oral commissures, external auditory canals, and external scars facilitates target volume delineation. The planning CT scan should include the entire head to allow the use of vertex beams. The principles of target delineation and plan evaluation for IMRT of maxillary sinus cancer are the same as those described for nasal cavity and ethmoid tumors.

For 3D-conformal radiation, a three-field technique consisting of an anterior and right and left lateral fields is used for tumors involving the suprastructure or extending to the roof of the nasal cavity and ethmoid cells. The lateral fields may have a 5-degree posterior tilt and 60-degree wedges. The relative loading varies from 1:0.15:0.15 to 1:0.07:0.07 depending on the tumor location and photon energy. For the initial target volume, the superior border of the anterior portal is above the crista galli to encompass the ethmoids and, in the absence of orbital invasion, at the lower edge of the cornea to cover the orbital floor. The inferior border is 1 cm below the floor of the sinus and the medial border is 1 to 2 cm (or more if necessary) across the midline to cover contralateral ethmoidal extension. The lateral border is 1 cm beyond the apex of the sinus or falling off the skin.

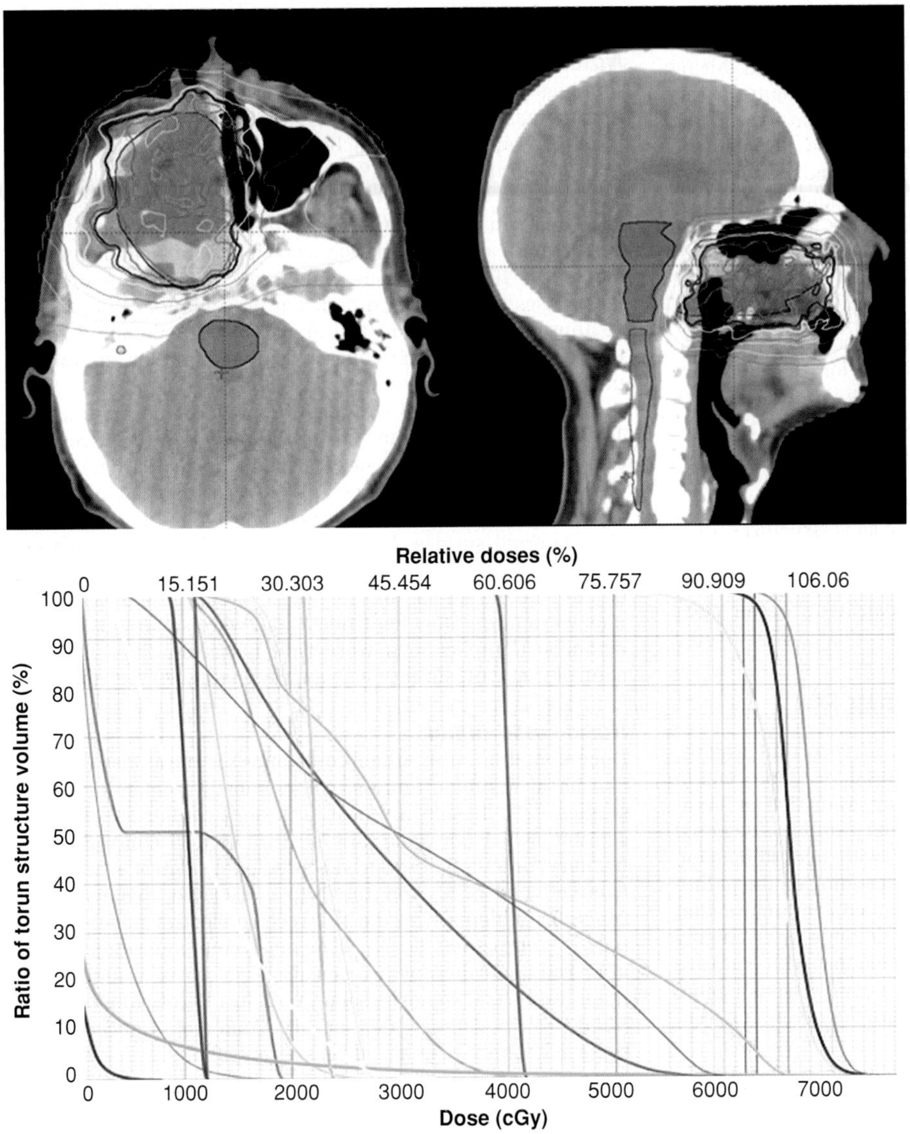

FIGURE 42.6. Proton therapy for recurrent adenoid cystic carcinoma (ACC) of the right hard palate. The patient had a palatectomy with radial forearm free flap reconstruction followed by postoperative external beam radiation therapy with IMRT to 60 Gy in 30 fractions. One year later, the ACC recurred with enhancement in right V1 and V2, involvement of the right cavernous sinus, and an enhancing mass in the infratemporal fossa and pterygopalatine fossa. Salvage surgery involved a right total maxillectomy with orbital preservation, pterygomaxillary space dissection and resection, and an extracranial dissection of vidian nerve and cranial nerve 5, V2. With evidence of skull base and cavernous sinus involvement after surgery he was treated with postoperative chemoradiation with IMPT and cisplatin to a dose of 66 Gy(RBE) in 33 fractions. No evidence of disease was present at 6 months after salvage therapy. The figure represents the axial, sagittal, and dose–volume histogram (DVH) of the IMPT plan. (DVH for the IMPT plan, from *left* to *right* on the graph: *red*, spinal cord; *green*, whole brain; *black*, brainstem; *pink*, left parotid; *white*, left eye; *brown*, right cochlea; *dark green*, left lens; *sky blue*, right parotid; *brown*, oral cavity; *violet*, optic chiasm; *red*, right eye; *green*, mandible; *light green*, left optic nerve; *soft pink*, right lens; *dark green*, right optic nerve; *yellow*, CTV or CTV_3; *blue*, CTV_2; *orange*, CTV_1.)

The superior border of the lateral portals follows the floor of the anterior cranial fossa, the anterior border is behind the lateral bony canthus parallel to the slope of the face, the posterior border covers the pterygoid plates, and the inferior border corresponds to that of the anterior portal. The boost volume encompasses the tumor bed while sparing the optic pathway.

Anterior and ipsilateral wedge-pair (usually 45-degree wedges) photon fields are used for tumors of the infrastructure with no extension into the orbit or ethmoids. If necessary, the lateral portal can have a 5-degree inferior tilt to avoid beam divergence into the contralateral eye. Lateral-opposed photon fields are preferred for tumors of the infrastructure spreading across midline through the hard palate. If necessary, the fields can be slightly angled (5-degree inferior tilt from the ipsilateral side and 5-degree superior tilt from the contralateral side) to avoid irradiating the contralateral eye. The use of a half beam with the isocenter placed at the level of the orbital floor and the upper half of the fields shielded further reduces exposure of the eyes by beam divergence.

The eyes and the optic pathway are of particular concern. With 3D-conformal techniques, the cornea can generally be shielded (to avoid keratitis) in patients with limited involvement of the medial or inferior orbital wall. If the tumor invades the orbital cavity without necessitating orbital exenteration, care should be taken to avoid irradiating the lacrimal gland to prevent xerophthalmia. It is important to keep the dose to the contralateral optic nerve as well as the optic chiasm below 54 Gy in 27 fractions to prevent bilateral blindness.

Treatment of the Neck

For squamous and undifferentiated carcinoma, elective neck irradiation is recommended.[47] Ipsilateral upper neck treatment is delivered by using a lateral appositional electron field (usually 12 MeV). With conventional radiation techniques, careful matching is required to prevent hot or cold spots. The superior border of the field slopes up from the horizontal ramus of the mandible anteriorly to match the inferior border of the primary portal posteriorly, leaving a small triangle over the cheek untreated. The anterior border is just behind the oral commissure, the posterior border is at the mastoid process, and the inferior border is at the thyroid notch (above the arytenoids). The nodal volume can also be covered by using IMRT with sparing of the parotid gland. Alternatively, the primary tumor bed and the upper neck can be treated with IMRT with the isocenter above the arytenoids and matched to a separate unmodulated lower neck field. This allows the laryngeal structures to be spared by using a larynx block.

If the maxillary sinus is being treated with conventional non-IMRT techniques, the central axes of the primary (sinus) fields and the opposed-lateral upper neck fields all are placed in the plane of the inferior border of the maxillary fields (i.e., usually 1 cm below the floor of the maxillary sinus). An independent collimator jaw is used to shield the caudal half of the maxillary fields and the cephalad half of the neck field. The junction between the primary and the neck fields can be moved during the course of treatment to reduce dose heterogeneity in this region. Portals are reduced after 42 Gy, and treatment to the posterior neck continues with abutting electron fields to the desired dose. The middle and lower neck is irradiated with an anterior appositional photon field matched to the inferior border of the opposed-lateral upper neck fields.

Dose Fractionation Schedule

Table 42.3 summarizes the dose regimens for IMRT. With 3D-conformal techniques, the dose for postoperative radiation therapy at 2 Gy per fraction is 50 Gy for elective nodal treatment, 56 Gy to the operative bed, 60 Gy to the tumor bed if resection margins are negative, and 66 Gy if margins are positive. For primary radiation therapy, the total dose to the primary tumor at 2 Gy per fraction is 66 to 70 Gy. The contralateral optic nerve and chiasm are excluded from the field after a dose of 50 to 54 Gy. When the tumor invades structures adjacent to the optic chiasm, a dose of up to 60 Gy to the chiasm may be acceptable because of the higher probability of control and the relatively low risk of visual impairment,[36] after clear discussion with the patient.

FOLLOW-UP AND RECURRENCES

Salvage is possible for some persistent or recurrent lesions. In particular, recurrent cancers of the nasal vestibule remain curable with salvage surgery after primary radiation or occasionally with salvage radiation after primary surgery. Regional recurrences can be treated successfully with neck dissection with or without postoperative radiation depending on the pathologic features. Treatment options are limited for tumors that recur after combined-modality therapy, although a few highly selected patients may qualify for reirradiation with curative intent. Cumulative doses of radiation to neural tissues (spinal cord, brainstem, brain, optic structures) are the main limitation to reirradiation.

Most oncologists recommend a second baseline physical examination together with CT, MRI, or positron emission tomography with CT for patients with nasal cavity or paranasal sinus tumors at 3 months after treatment. Common practice is to repeat clinical examination and imaging when indicated every 4 months for the first 3 years after treatment, every 6 months for the fourth and fifth years after treatment, and annually thereafter. In addition to monitoring possible tumor recurrence, these follow-up visits are critical for identifying and managing side effects of treatment.

RESULTS OF TREATMENT

The results of treatment have improved from the 1960s through the 1990s, with overall survival rates increasing progressively from 33% ± 18% in the 1960s to 42% ± 15% in the 1970s, 54% ± 15% in the 1980s, and 56% ± 13% in the 1990s (P <.001).[48] In a systematic review of published series spanning 40 years, Dulguerov et al.[48] demonstrated progressive improvements in outcome for all treatment modalities (surgery, surgery with radiation, and radiation). However, a more recent review of the experience at the University of California, San Francisco showed no significance differences in 5-year overall survival rates or local control rates by decade of treatment (1960s through 2000s; overall survival, 46% to 56%; local control 55% to 62%) or by radiation technique (conventional, 3D conformal, or IMRT; overall survival 47% to 57%; local control 59% to 65%). However, the incidence of severe (grade 3 or 4) side effects declined significantly over time from 50% in the 1960s to 16% in the 2000s.[49]

Tumors of the Nasal Cavity

Nasal Vestibule Tumors

Findings from several retrospective studies of radiation therapy for nasal vestibule tumors[3,17,36,41,50–58] suggest that either brachytherapy or external beam radiation therapy can produce cure rates of up to 90% for small (<2-cm) lesions (Table 42.4).[3,17,41,50–53,55–57] For 2- to 4-cm lesions, external beam radiation can control 70% to 80% of tumors. Although nodal spread of disease is relatively rare for lesions smaller than 2 cm, up to 40% of patients with larger primary tumors have metastases to the cervical nodes at presentation. With the use of appropriate radiation techniques and fractionation schedules, severe and late complications after radiation therapy are uncommon (see Table 42.4).

An analysis by the Groupe Europeen de Curietherapie of 1,676 carcinomas of the skin of the nose and nasal vestibule treated by brachytherapy or external beam irradiation revealed an overall local control rate of 93%.[3] Local control depended on tumor size (<2 cm, 96%; 2–3.9 cm, 88%; ≥4 cm, 81%), tumor site (external surface, 94%; vestibule, 75%), and status (new, 95%; recurrent, 88%). Local control was independent of histology for tumors <4 cm, but for those >4 cm, basal cell carcinomas were more often controlled than were squamous cell carcinomas. Complications were rare (necrosis, 2%). The local control rate with surgery was approximately 90%.

Nasal Fossa Tumors

Documentation of treatment outcomes for nasal fossa tumors, like nasal vestibule tumors, comes mostly from retrospective studies.[18,59–61] Results are best for lesions confined to the nasal septum, which are generally small and well controlled with primary radiation therapy. Locoregional control rates range from 60% to 85%, and the rate of isolated regional recurrence for patients who did not receive elective nodal irradiation is approximately 5%. The most common complications after radiation therapy are soft tissue necrosis, visual impairment, and nasal stenosis, seen in 5% to 11% of patients (Table 42.5).[18,59,60,61] Ang et al.[18] at MD Anderson Cancer Center reported better primary disease control and survival rates for patients with tumors located in the septum (86%) versus patients with tumors on the lateral wall or floor of the nasal fossa (68%). In that study no patients with nasal septum carcinomas who underwent elective nodal irradiation had nodal relapses, whereas two of eight patients who did not undergo nodal irradiation experienced recurrence in the ipsilateral subdigastric nodes. Distant metastasis was more common among patients with lateral wall and floor disease, and ultimately survival rates were best among patients with nasal septum tumors. However, other groups[59,61] found no differences in results for tumors at various sites within the nasal cavity. Results of treatment for early-stage tumors are equally good after radiation therapy or surgery. Indeed, T1 lesions in particular can be well controlled with either modality, and in one study were associated with a 5-year overall survival rate of 91%.[62]

An analysis of 783 patients with nasal cavity cancer included in the Surveillance, Epidemiology, and End Results (SEER) database from 1988 through 1998[63] revealed squamous cell carcinoma to be the most common tumor type (49.3%), followed by esthesioneuroblastoma (13.2%). More than half of the cases presented with a small primary tumor (T1), and only 5% had positive nodes at diagnosis. Overall mean survival time was 57 months and the 5-year survival rate was 40.3%. On multivariate analysis, male sex, increasing age, T status, N status, and poorer tumor grade all adversely affected survival (P <.05). Radiation therapy, given to 50.5% of patients, also independently predicted poorer survival (P = .03), probably because those patients had had poor prognostic features such as perineural invasion, positive margins, or poor performance status (medically unfit for surgery). Five-year survival rates by tumor

TABLE 42.4 LOCAL AND REGIONAL CONTROL RATES OF NASAL VESTIBULE CARCINOMAS TREATED BY DEFINITIVE RADIOTHERAPY

Series (Reference)	*Patients*	*Local Control*	*Regional Control*	*Comments/Complications*
MD Anderson 1967–1984 (51)	32	BT: 11/11 controlled EB: 20/21 (95%) controlled	Small lesions, no ENI: 11/11 Large lesions, no ENI: 5/9 (56%) Large lesions, ENI: 12/12 (100%)	Osteonecrosis, epistaxis: 1 patient each
Princess Margaret Hospital 1958–1983 (17)	54	<2 cm (n = 34): 97% ≥2 cm (n = 16) + size not reported (n = 6): 57%	No ENI: 51/54 (94%)	Osteonecrosis: 2 patients; nasal stenosis: 2 patients; massive epistaxis: 1 patient
Daniel den Hoed Cancer Center, Rotterdam 1968–1978 (55)	32	EB: <1.5 cm: 72% (5-yr); >1.5 cm: 50% (5-yr) Dose <54 Gy: 37%; >54 Gy: 82%	Data not available	External beam radiotherapy was hypofractionated (2.5–3 Gy/fraction)
VU University, Amsterdam (41)	56	Overall at 2 years: 79% (ultimate at 5 years after salvage: 95%) <1.5 cm (n = 32): 83% (ultimate: 94%) ≥1.5 cm (n = 24): 74% (ultimate: 96%)	Routine ENI to the mustache region 2-yr control rate: 87% (6 of 7 neck relapses were salvaged). 5-yr Ultimate control rate: 97%	Rhinorrhea: 45%; nasal dryness 39%; epistaxis 15%; adhesions 4%. Skin necrosis: 3 patients (all in IDR BT group) Sarcoma in the nasal vestibule: 1 patient.
U. of Florida 1970–1995 (56)	56 4	Overall at 5 years: 87% EB: 60/71 (86%) Surgery and EB: 8/8 (100%) (Ultimate LC: 94%)	T1-T2: 39/43 (91%) T4: 30/36 (83%) N0 LC: 87% (Ultimate: 97%) N0/no ENI: 47/54 (87%) (Ultimate neck control: 97%)	Soft tissue necrosis: 15 patients Severe complications: 3 patients
Queens Medical Centre, Nottingham, UK (52)	23	EB only: 8/13 Surgery only: 8/10	Not reported	Radionecrosis: 1 patient
DAHANCA, Denmark (50)	174	5-yr locoregional control: 67% T1: 79% T2:54% T3: 35%	No ENI: 89%	Not reported
Queensland Radium Institute, Australia (57)	28	Surgery and EB: 4/6 (66%) EB: 13/22 (59%)	Surgery and EB: 57% EB: 86%	Septal necrosis: 2 patients; nasobuccoalveolar fistula and fistula: 1 patient each
French Groupe Europeen de Curietherapie (3)	1676	Skin of nose and nasal vestibule carcinoma treated by BT or EB (ortho- or megavoltage). Overall LC = 93% (FU ≥2 yr); <2 cm: 96%; 2–3.9 cm: 88%; ≥4 cm: 81% LC of nose skin: 94% LC of vestibule: 75%. LC for previously untreated tumors: 95% vs. 88% for recurrent tumors		
Daniel den Hoed Cancer Center, Rotterdam (53)	64	Local relapse-free survival: 92% at 5 years T1: 89% T2: 100%		Not reported

RT, radiotherapy; ENI, elective nodal irradiation; BT, brachytherapy; EB, external beam; LC, local control; IDR, intermediate dose rate; FU, follow-up.

TABLE 42.5 TREATMENT OUTCOMES FOR NASAL FOSSA TUMORS

Series (Reference)	*Patients*	*Treatments*	*Survival Rates at 5 Years*	*Late Complications*
MD Anderson 1969–1985 (18)	45	RT alone: 18 patients RT+ surgery: 2 patients Surgery + RT: 25 patients Median time to relapse: 9 months	Overall: 75% Disease-specific: 83%	Radiation-induced blindness: 2 patients Surgical blindness: 2 patients Maxilla necrosis: 3 patients Nasal stenosis: 2 patients Septal perforation: 1 patient Severe dental decay: 1 patient
Roswell Memorial Park Institute 1942–1964 (59)	57	RT alone: 30 patients Surgery alone: 13 patients Surgery + RT: 14 patients	Crude overall: 56% Disease-free: 56%	Not reported
University of Puerto Rico 1976 (60)	40	RT alone: 34 patients Surgery alone: 6 patients	Overall: 56%	Not reported
Mallinckrodt Institute of Radiology 1969–1984 (61)	56	RT alone: 28 patients RT + surgery: 18 patients Surgery + RT: 10 patients	Overall: 52%	Soft tissue necrosis: 2 patients Cataract: 1 patient Nasal synechiae: 1 patient Severe otitis media: 2 patients Hemorrhage (fatal): 2 patients Optic neuropathy: 1 patient Brain necrosis: 1 patient

RT, radiation therapy.

Clinical Radiation Oncology

TABLE 42.6 TREATMENT RESULTS FOR NASAL CAVITY CANCER FROM THE SURVEILLANCE, EPIDEMIOLOGY AND END RESULTS DATABASE FOR 1988 THROUGH 1998[a]

Tumor Type	5-Year Survival Rate (%)	T or N Classification	5-Year Survival Rate (%)
Adenocarcinoma	49.0	T1	66.4
Adenoid cystic carcinoma	59.1	T2	51.8
Melanoma	22.1	T3	45.6
Other tumors	59.5	T4	40.2
Sarcoma	78.0	Overall	56.7
Squamous cell carcinoma	61.6		
Esthesioneuroblastoma	63.6	N0	62.3
SNUC	49.5	N+	28.4

SNUC, sinonasal undifferentiated carcinoma.

[a]Results are shown by tumor type and by T and N stage. Because of rounding, percentages may not total 100.

From Bhattacharyya N. Cancer of the nasal cavity: survival and factors influencing prognosis. *Arch Otolaryngol Head Neck Surg* 2002;128:1079–1083, with permission.

type, T status, and N status are shown in Table 42.6.[63] Five-year survival rates also correlated with extent of tumor dedifferentiation, being 75.3%, 61.9%, 47.6%, and 36.8% for well-, moderately, poorly, and undifferentiated cancers, respectively.

Esthesioneuroblastoma

Either surgery or primary radiation therapy as single-modality therapy can produce locoregional control rates exceeding 90% for tumors are confined to the nasal cavity (Kadish stage A).[8] Single-modality therapy has also been used for lesions involving the nasal cavity and one or more paranasal sinuses (stage B), as has surgery followed by adjuvant radiation therapy. However, the optimal therapy for stage B lesions is not clear because of the heterogeneity of these tumors. Disease that extends beyond the nasal cavity and paranasal sinuses (stage C) seems to be best treated with a combination of surgery and radiation, and the role of chemotherapy, if any, is being investigated. Elective nodal irradiation is not generally recommended because the incidence of nodal relapse is <15%. Distant metastasis is uncommon (10%) even among patients presenting with locally advanced disease.

Among 783 nasal cavity cancers identified from the SEER database, 103 (13.2%) were esthesioneuroblastomas; the median survival time for patients with these tumors was 88 months and the overall 5-year survival rate was 63.6%.[63] Tables 42.7[48,64–68] and 42.8[8] summarize the results of treatment. The prognosis for patients with stage A disease is excellent. Overall, 30% of patients with stage B tumor died of the disease. About 60% of patients with stage C tumors died of the disease, primarily because of failure to control the primary tumor. As noted above, distant metastasis is uncommon (10%) even in locoregionally advanced disease.

Spaulding et al.[28] reported results for 25 patients treated at the University of Virginia Medical Center from 1959 through 1986 who were followed for 2 years after therapy. Treatment approaches had gradually evolved during that period, with progressive introduction of craniofacial resections, complex field megavoltage radiation, and, for stage C disease, the addition of chemotherapy. Therefore, patients were assigned to two groups, based on treatment era, for comparative analysis. Although this series is relatively small, it revealed two interesting findings on this rare disease: first, that extensive craniofacial resection does not seem to confer a major advantage over wide local excision for patients with stage B lesions, and second, that the addition of chemotherapy to craniofacial resection and radiation therapy for patients with stage C tumors may yield higher disease-specific survival rates.

A larger series of 72 patients with sinonasal neuroendocrine tumors treated at MD Anderson Cancer Center between 1982 and 2002[64] included a spectrum of histologies: esthesioneuroblastoma (31 patients), sinonasal undifferentiated carcinoma (SNUC, 16 patients), neuroendocrine carcinoma (18 patients), and small cell carcinoma (7 patients). The overall survival rates at 5 years were 93.1% for patients with esthesioneuroblastoma, 62.5% for those with SNUC, 64.2% for neuroendocrine carcinoma, and 28.6% for small cell carcinoma (P = .0029; log-rank test). The local control rates at 5 years also were superior for patients with esthesioneuroblastoma (96.2%) compared with patients who had SNUC (78.6%), neuroendocrine carcinoma (72.6%), or small cell carcinoma (66.7%) (P = .04). The corresponding regional failure rate at 5 years were 8.7% for patients with esthesioneuroblastoma, 15.6% for SNUC, 12.9% for neuroendocrine carcinoma, and 44.4% for small cell carcinoma, and distant metastasis rates were 0%

TABLE 42.7 OVERALL TREATMENT RESULTS OF ESTHESIONEUROBLASTOMA

Series (Reference)	Patients	Local Control	Regional Control and Survival	Comments/Complications
MD Anderson 1982–2002 (64)	31	5-yr: 96.2%	5-yr: 91.3% 5-yr OS: 93.1%; DM: 0%	
UCLA 1970–1990 (48)	26	Overall: 18/26 (69%) S alone: 1/7 (14%) RT alone: 2/5 (40%) S + RT: 10/12 (83%)	4/26 (15%) patients had nodal disease (at presentation or after initial therapy) 5-yr CSS: 74%. 5-yr RFS: 58%	Postoperative cerebrospinal fluid leak, epiphora, radiation retinopathy (3/17 patients)
Mayo Clinic 1951–1990 (65)	49	5-yr: 65% (all patients) S alone: 73% S + RT: 86%	3/49 (6%) had N1 at presentation and 8/46 (17%) had regional relapse (7/8 with concurrent local failure). 5-yr DFS and OS: 55% and 69% (all patients)	Osteonecrosis of trephine bone plate (4 patients)
U. of Virginia 1959–1991 (66)	40	Overall: 30/40 (75%) controlled	4/40 (10%) clinically N1 at presentation and 4/36 (11%) developed regional relapse. 5-yr OS: 78%	–
U. of Virginia Health System, 1976–2004 treated with a standardized protocol (67)[a]	50	17 patients (34%) developed recurrent disease, which was locoregional in 12 patients	5-yr DFS: 86.5% Possibility for surgical salvage.	–
Hospital do Cancer Instituto Nacional de Cancer, Rio de Janeiro, Brazil 1983–2000 (68)	36	S + RT: 18; RT only: 14; S only: 1 RT and chemotherapy: 2	5- and 10-yr DFS: 46% and 24% 5- and 10-yr OS: 55% and 46% N+ and DM adversely affected prognosis (P <.001 and P = .01, respectively).	Kadish classification best predicted disease-free survival

OS, absolute overall survival; DM, distant metastases; S, surgery; RT, radiation therapy; CSS, cause-specific survival; RFS, relapse-free survival; DFS, disease-free survival.

[a]Kadish A or B received preoperative RT followed by craniofacial resection; Kadish stage C disease was treated with preoperative chemotherapy and RT followed by a craniofacial resection.

TABLE 42.8 PATTERN OF FAILURE AND RESULTS OF SALVAGE TREATMENT OF ESTHESIONEUROBLASTOMA BY STAGE AND TREATMENT

Kadish Stage	*Therapy*	*Local Control*	*Nodal Relapse*	*Salvage by Subsequent RT or S*	*Distant Metastasis*	*Died of Disease*
A (n = 24)	RT	3/5	1/5	3/3	0/5	0/5
	S	5/9	1/9	1/1	0/9	0/9
	S + RT	9/10	2/10	2/2	1/10	1/10
	All	17/24 (71%)	4/24 (17%)	9/9	1/24 (4%)	1/24 (4%)
B (n = 33)	RT	6/7	2/7	0/1	0/7	3/7
	S	3/6	0/6	1/2	0/6	2/6
	S + RT	15/20	1/20	3/4	3/20	5/20
	All	24/33 (73%)	3/33 (9%)	4/7	3/33 (9%)	10/33 (30%)
C (n = 21)	RT	2/5	2/7	0/0	1/5	4/5
	S	1/1	0/6	0/0	0/1	0/1
	S + RT	9/15	1/20	1/1	1/15	8/15
	All	12/21 (57%)	3/33 (9%)	1/1	2/21 (10%)	12/21 (57%)

RT, radiotherapy; S, surgery.

Modified from Elkon D, Hightower SI, Lim ML, et al. Esthesioneuroblastoma. *Cancer* 1979;44:1087–1094.

for esthesioneuroblastoma, 25.4% for SNUC, 14.1% for neuroendocrine carcinoma, and 75.0% for small cell carcinoma. Moreover, local therapy alone produced excellent local and distant control rates for esthesioneuroblastoma. Among 8 patients treated for esthesioneuroblastoma since 2000 with surgery and adjuvant IMRT to 60 Gy (1 with stage B disease and 7 with stage C [5 of whom had intracranial extension]), there were no local recurrences and one nodal recurrence was salvaged surgically. All eight patients were alive with no evidence of disease at the last follow-up.

Tumors of the Paranasal Sinuses

Five-year outcomes from studies reported since 1998 continue to illustrate that local control after treatment of paranasal sinus tumors remains problematic[30,42,46,47,67–78] (Table 42.9). For patients with carcinoma of the maxillary sinuses, the combination of surgery and radiation yields 5-year local control and survival rates ranging from 44% to 80%. These rates are better than those achieved with either surgery or radiation therapy alone. For radiation therapy alone, the 5-year local control rates range from 22% to 39% and the 5-year overall survival rates from 22% to 40%. Findings from a large multicenter retrospective analysis of 418 patients with ethmoid sinus adenocarcinoma indicated that the size of the lesion (T4) the extent of nodal involvement (N+), and the presence of brain extension were the most significant prognostic factors for overall survival.[79] Although the authors concluded that surgery followed by postoperative radiation therapy remains the treatment of choice, they did note that 51% of the patients developed recurrences, 74% of which were local.

A 1991 review of outcomes after treatment of 73 patients with maxillary sinus carcinomas at MD Anderson Cancer Center reported 5-year local and regional control rates according to pathologic T category as follows: for T1 and T2 tumors, 91% local and 71% regional control; for T3, 77% local and 80% regional; and for T4, 65% local and 93% regional.[30] Five-year regional control rates according to N category were 84% for N0 disease and 82% for N1 or N2 disease. The most common histologic subtypes were squamous cell carcinoma (48%) and adenoid cystic carcinoma (27%); 5-year local and regional control rates were 62% (local) and 86% (regional) for squamous cell tumors and 82% (local) and 94% (regional) for adenoid tumors. Perineural invasion and nodal disease at presentation were poor prognostic factors. An update of this report published in 2007[47] showed that increasing the radiation portals to cover the skull base for patients with perineural invasion reduced the risk of local recurrence and that adding elective nodal irradiation for patients with squamous or undifferentiated tumors improved the rates of nodal control, distant metastasis, and recurrence-free survival.

IMRT has emerged as the standard of care for tumors of the paranasal sinuses with low toxicity and high local control rates.[42,62,73,78] Madani et al.[73] reported the largest series to date, in which 105 patients (most of whom [56%] had ethmoid sinus tumors) were treated with IMRT. At a median follow-up time of 40 months, the 5-year actuarial local control and overall survival rates were 70.7% and 58.5%. In multivariate analysis, invasion of the cribiform plate was found to predict worse local control ($P < .001$) and lower overall survival ($P < .001$).

The extent of neuroendocrine differentiation of sinonasal carcinomas also influences the patterns of failure. In one study, the 5-year actuarial rates of local, regional, and distant failure according to tumor histology were as follows: esthesioneuroblastoma 4% local failure, 9% regional failure, and 0% distant failure; neuroendocrine carcinoma 27% local, 13% regional, and 12% distant; sinonasal undifferentiated carcinoma 21% local, 16% regional, and 25% distant; and small cell carcinoma 33% local failure, 44% regional failure, and 75% distant failure.[64]

Future Directions in Radiation Therapy

IMRT has rapidly become the standard of care in external beam therapy for sinonasal malignancies.[42,43,62,73] Nevertheless, proton beam therapy may confer further benefits for nasal and paranasal sinus tumors, and investigators at MD Anderson Cancer Center have demonstrated the clinical feasibility of intensity-modulated proton therapy for this purpose (see Fig. 42.6). The additional advantages of this technique over photon-based IMRT are its ability to limit the radiation "dose bath" to normal critical tissue structures and allow escalation of dose to the target. Well-designed clinical trials in a cooperative group setting will be necessary to provide the evidence required for widespread adoption of proton therapy over IMRT for these rare malignancies. Finally, further improvements in the local control of sinonasal malignancies will require incorporating systemic agents as neoadjuvant or concurrent therapy. Again, the rarity of sinonasal cancer will most likely require international cooperative group trials to facilitate timely analyses of outcomes and design of future trials.

SEQUELAE OF TREATMENT

Soft Tissue and Bone

The formation of nasal cavity synechiae (fibrous mucosal bands causing airway stenosis) can be prevented by intermittent dilation of the nasal passages with a petroleum-coated cotton swab until mucositis has resolved. Dry mucous membranes can be managed symptomatically with saline nasal spray. Soft-tissue or cartilage necrosis is uncommon after therapy, at an estimated incidence of 5% to 10%.[26,66,71,80]

Eyes and Optic Pathway

Chronic keratitis and iritis (dry-eye syndrome) can develop after radiation therapy if tumor extension to the orbital cavity mandates irradiation of the lacrimal gland to doses of more

TABLE 42.9 OUTCOME OF PATIENTS WITH LOCALLY ADVANCED CANCER OF THE PARANASAL SINUSES TREATED WITH COMBINED SURGERY AND RADIATION THERAPY

Study (Reference)	*Year*	*Patients*	*5-Year Survival (%)*	*Local Recurrence (%)*	*Distant Metastasis (%)*
A. Results from Surgery and Conventional Radiation Therapy					
Lavertu et al. (71)	1989	54	38	52	–
Spiro et al. (75)	1989	105	38	49	15
Zaharia et al. (76)	1989	149	36	43	–
Paulino et al. (46)	1998	48	47	46	17
Le et al. (72)	1999	97	34	54	34
Myers et al. (74)	2002	141	52	56	33
Jiang et al. (30)	1991	67[a]	53[b]	24	27
Katz et al. (70)	2002	31		21	
Blanco et al. (69)	2004	106	27	42	29
Dirix et al. (42)	2007	127	54	47	20
Bristol et al. (47)	2007	90 G1 (1969–1991) 56 G2 (>1991–2002)			
Study (Reference)	*Year*	*Patients*	*Survival (%)*	*Local Recurrence (%)*	*Distant Metastasis (%)*
B. Results from Surgery and Intensity-Modulated Radiation Therapy					
Duthoy et al. (77)	2005	39	2-yr OS 68 4-yr OS 59	2-yr 27 4-yr 32	–
Ahamad et al. (unpublished)[c]	2005	53	Crude: 88.6	Crude: 15.1 2-yr 20 4-yr 25	20.7
Daly et al. (62)	2007	36	45	2-yr 38	
Hoppe et al. (78)	2008	37	80	2-yr 25	
Madani et al. (73)	2009	84	58.5	41.5	18
Dirix et al. (42)	2010	40	89	2-yr 24	

C. Side Effects of Combined Surgery and Radiation Therapy in Patients with Paranasal Sinus Cancer

Vestibulo-cochlear	Vestibular dysfunction, persistent otitis, tinnitus, hearing impairment
Ophthalmologic (lacrimal gland, eyes, lens, optic nerves and chiasm)	Retinopathy, xerophthalmia, keratopathy, cataracts, visual impairment
Neurologic (brain, brainstem, spinal cord, temporal lobe)	Neurocognitive impairment, cranial neuropathy, myelopathy, brain necrosis
Endocrine (pituitary gland, hypothalamus, thyroid gland if neck irradiated)	Multiple endocrine dysfunction: hyperprolactinemia, syndromes associated with decreased GH, FSH, LH, T4, TSH, ACTH, and their downstream hormones
Oral (major salivary glands, oral mucosa, mandible and temporomandibular joint)	Xerostomia, dental caries, dysgeusia, mandible exposure, and necrosis, trismus
Connective tissue complications (oral cavity, soft palate musculature, pharynx, larynx, skin and subcutaneous tissues, skull bones)	Soft tissue necrosis, skin changes, persistent lymphedema, subcutaneous fibrosis, cartilage necrosis, nasal dryness, choanal stenosis, swallowing and voice dysfunction, bone necrosis

OS, overall survival; GH, growth hormone; FSH, follicle-stimulating hormone; LH, luteinizing hormone; TSH, thyroid-stimulating hormone; ACTH, adrenocorticotropic hormone.

[a]Patients with node-negative disease. [b]Five-year relapse-free survival.

[c]Patients treated at MD Anderson Cancer Center with intensity-modulated radiation therapy.

than 30 to 40 Gy.[26,80] Without lacrimal irradiation, fewer than 20% of patients treated with up to 55 Gy to the cornea develop chronic corneal injury.[81] The risk of cataract formation at 5 years is approximately 5% after doses of up to 10 Gy to the lenses using conventional fractionation; this risk increases to 50% at 5 years after 18 Gy.[82]

Radiation retinopathy generally occurs within 18 months to 5 years after treatment.[83] It is rare after doses of <45 Gy, but the incidence increases to about 50% after doses of 45 to 55 Gy.[84] Optic neuropathy tends to develop between 2 and 4 years after radiation therapy, but it has been reported as late as 14 years after treatment.[84] The reported incidence of optic neuropathy is <5% after 50 to 60 Gy but increases to around 30% for doses of 61 to 78 Gy. Factors that influence the risk of radiation-induced optic neuropathy were reported in 2006 for 273 patients treated between 1964 and 2000 in whom the radiation fields included the optic nerves or chiasm.[85] The likelihood of developing optic neuropathy was primarily influenced by the total dose, but fraction size was marginally significant. The 5-year rates of freedom from optic neuropathy were 95% for doses ≤63 Gy treated once daily, 98% for doses ≤63 Gy treated twice daily, 78% for doses >63 Gy treated once daily, and 91% for doses >63 Gy treated twice daily. On multivariate analysis, the risk of optic neuropathy was found to correlate with increasing total dose ($P = .0047$) and possibly with increasing patient age ($P = .091$), once daily versus twice-daily fractionation ($P = .068$), and overall treatment time ($P = .097$). When the target volumes include the optic pathway, special attention must be paid to hot spots and dose per fraction to avoid optic neuropathies.

Optimizing the technique for paranasal sinus tumors is crucial so that the radiation dose to the optic apparatus is limited to the greatest extent possible to minimize the risk of complications. Investigators at the University of Florida, reviewing 464 patients treated from 1964 through 2001,[44] reported a 20% incidence of ipsilateral radiation retinopathy at 5 and 10 years after conventional or 3D radiation therapy. In that study, patients were deemed functionally blind when visual acuity dropped to 20/100 on the Snellen chart, and neovascularization (rubeosis iridis or neovascular glaucoma) was coincident with radiation retinopathy. Use of IMRT has been shown to limit the doses to the optic apparatus without compromising local control. Indeed, Chen et al.[49] reported findings for 127 patients treated between 1960 and 2005 with a variety of radiation therapy techniques that had evolved over that period, namely conventional, 3D conformal, and IMRT. They concluded that the incidence of severe (grade ≥3) complications depended on the radiation treatment technique used: 54% for conventional therapy, 22% for 3D-conformal therapy, and 13% for IMRT. Specifically, the incidence of grade 3 or 4 late ocular toxicity decreased from 20% with conventional techniques to 0% with IMRT, whereas grade 3 or 4 late auditory toxicity decreased from 15% with conventional to 4% with IMRT ($P < .001$). Moreover, to date no radiation-induced blindness has been reported among the collective experience, with 308 patients treated with IMRT as either definitive or postoperative therapy for nasal and paranasal malignancies.[42,49,61,62,73,77,84]

REFERENCES

1. Bridger MW, van Nostrand AW. The nose and paranasal sinuses—applied surgical anatomy. A histologic study of whole organ sections in three planes. *J Otolaryngol* 1978;7:1–33.
2. Goepfert H, Guillamondegui OM, Jesse RH, et al. Squamous cell carcinoma of nasal vestibule. *Arch Otolaryngol* 1974;100:8–10.

3. Mazeron JJ, Chassagne D, Crook J, et al. Radiation therapy of carcinomas of the skin of nose and nasal vestibule: a report of 1676 cases by the Groupe Europeen de Curietherapie. *Radiother Oncol* 1988;13:165–173.
4. Murphy J, Bleach NR, Thyveetil M. Sebaceous carcinoma of the nose: multi-focal presentation? *J Laryngol Otol* 2004;118:374–376.
5. Prasad ML, Patel SG, Busam KJ. Primary mucosal desmoplastic melanoma of the head and neck. *Head Neck* 2004;26:373–377.
6. Su K, Xu J, Qiao M, et al. CT characteristics of primary nasal non-Hodgkin lymphoma. *J Clin Otorhinolaryngol* 2003;17:261–263.
7. Roush G. Epidemiology of cancer of the nose and paranasal sinuses: current concepts. *Head Neck Surg* 1979;2:3–11.
8. Elkon D, Hightower SI, Lim ML, et al. Esthesioneuroblastoma. *Cancer* 1979;44:1087–1094.
9. Lewis JS, Castro EB. Cancer of the nasal cavity and paranasal sinuses. *J Laryngol Otol* 1972;86:255–262.
10. Acheson ED, Cowdell RH, Hadfield E, et al. Nasal cancer in woodworkers furniture industry. *Br Med J* 1968;2:587–596.
11. Acheson ED, Hadfield EH, Macbeth RG. Carcinoma of the nasal cavity and accessory sinuses in woodworkers. *Lancet* 1967;1:311–312.
12. Klintenberg C, Olofsson J, Hellquist H, et al. Adenocarcinoma of the ethmoid sinuses. A review of 28 cases with special reference to wood dust exposure. *Cancer* 1984;54:482–488.
13. Schwaab G, Julieron M, Janot F. Epidemiology of cancers of the nasal cavities and paranasal sinuses. *Neurochirurgie* 1997;43:61–63.
14. Torjussen W, Solberg LA, Hogetveit AC. Histopathological changes of the nasal mucosa in active and retired nickel workers. *Br J Cancer* 1979;40:568–580.
15. Zheng W, McLaughlin JK, Chow WH, et al. Risk factors for cancers of the nasal cavity and paranasal sinuses among white men in the United States. *Am J Epidemiol* 1993;43:61–63.
16. Bars G, Visser AG, Van Andel JG. The treatment of squamous cell carcinoma of the nasal vestibule with interstitial iridium implantation. *Radiother Oncol* 1985;4:121–125.
17. Wong CS, Cummings BJ, Elhakim T, et al. External irradiation for squamous cell carcinoma of the nasal vestibule. *Int J Radiat Oncol Biol Phys* 1986;12:1943–1946.
18. Ang KK, Jiang G-L, Frankenthaler RA, et al. Carcinomas of the nasal cavity. *Radiother Oncol* 1992;24:163–168.
19. Beitler JJ, Fass DE, Brenner HA, et al. Esthesioneuroblastoma: is there a role for elective neck treatment? *Head Neck* 1991;13:321–326.
20. Goldsweig HG, Sundaresan N. Chemotherapy of recurrent esthesioneuroblastoma. Case report and review of the literature. *Am J Clin Oncol* 1990;13:139–143.
21. Kadish S, Goodman M, Wang CC. Olfactory neuroblastoma. A clinical analysis of 17 cases. *Cancer* 1976;37:1571–1576.
22. Howell MC, Branstetter BF 4th, Snyderman CH. Patterns of regional spread for esthesioneuroblastoma. *AJNR Am J Neuroradiol* 2011;32:929–933.
23. Ozsahin M, Gruber G, Olszyk O, et al. Outcome and prognostic factors in olfactory neuroblastoma: a rare cancer network study. *Int J Radiat Oncol Biol Phys* 2010; 78:992–997.
24. Rouviere H, Tobias MJ. *Anatomy of the human lymphatic system.* Ann Arbor, MI: Edwards, 1938.
25. Le Q-T, Fu KK, Kaplan MJ, et al. Lymph node metastasis in maxillary sinus carcinoma. *Int J Radiat Oncol Biol Phys* 2000;46:541–549.
26. Paulino AC, Fisher SG, Marks JE. Is prophylactic neck irradiation indicated patients with squamous cell carcinoma of the maxillary sinus? *Int J Radiat Oncol Biol Phys* 1997;39:283–289.
27. Mendenhall WM, Mendenhall CM, Riggs CEJ, et al. Sinonasal undifferentiated carcinoma. *Am J Clin Oncol* 2006;29:27–31.
28. Spaulding CA, Kranyak MS, Constable WC, et al. Esthesioneuroblastoma: a comparison of two treatment eras. *Int J Radiat Oncol Biol Phys* 1988;15:581–590.
29. Jiang GL, Morrison WH, Garden AS, et al. Ethmoid sinus carcinomas: natural history and treatment results. *Radiother Oncol* 1998;49:21–27.
30. Jiang GL, Ang KK, Peters LJ, et al. Maxillary sinus carcinomas: natural history and results of postoperative radiotherapy. *Radiother Oncol* 1991;21:193–200.
31. Kondo M, Horiuchi M, Inuyama Y, et al. Value of computed tomography for radiation therapy of tumors of the nasal cavity and paranasal sinuses. *Acta Radiol Oncol Radiat Phys Biol* 1983;22:3–7.
32. Shapiro MD, Som PM. MRI of the paranasal sinuses and nasal cavity. *Radiol Clin North Am* 1989;27:447–475.
33. Som PM, Shapiro MD, Biller HF, et al. Sinonasal tumors and inflammatory tissues: differentiation with MR imaging. *Radiology* 1988;167:803–808.
34. Edge SB, Byrd DR, Compton CC, et al., eds. Nasal cavities and paranasal sinuses. In: *AJCC cancer staging manual,* 7th ed. New York: Springer, 2010:69–78.
35. Million RR. The myth regarding bone or cartilage involvement by cancer and the likelihood of cure by radiotherapy. *Head Neck* 1989;11:30–40.
36. McCollough WM, Mendenhall NP, Parsons JT, et al. Radiotherapy alone for squamous cell carcinoma of the nasal vestibule: management of the primary site and regional lymphatics. *Int J Radiat Oncol Biol Phys* 1993;26:73–79.
37. Waldron JN, O'Sullivan B, Warde P, et al. Ethmoid sinus cancer: twenty-nine cases managed with primary radiation therapy. *Int J Radiat Oncol Biol Phys* 1998;41: 361–369.
38. Bridger GP, Kwok B, Baldwin M. Craniofacial resection for paranasal sinus cancers. *Head Neck* 2000;22:772–780.
39. Lund VJ, Howard DJ, Wei WI, et al. Craniofacial resection for tumors of the nasal cavity and paranasal sinuses. A 17-year experience. *Head Neck* 1998;20:97–105.
40. Wade PMJ, Smith RE, Johns ME. Response of esthesioneuroblastoma to chemotherapy. Report of five cases and review of the literature. *Cancer Bull* 1984;53: 1036–1041.
41. Langendijk JA, Poorter R, Leemans CR, et al. Radiotherapy of squamous cell carcinoma of the nasal vestibule. *Int J Radiat Oncol Biol Phys* 2004;59:1319–1325.
42. Dirix P, Vanstraelen B, Jorissen M, et al. Intensity-modulated radiotherapy for sinonasal cancer: improved outcome compared to conventional radiotherapy. *Int J Radiat Oncol Biol Phys* 2010;78:998–1004.
43. Hoppe BS, Stegman LD, Zelefsky MJ, et al. Treatment of nasal cavity and paranasal sinus cancer with modern radiotherapy techniques in the postoperative setting—the MSKCC experienced. *Int J Radiat Oncol Biol Phys* 2007;67:691–702.
44. Monroe AT, Bhandare N, Morris CG, et al. Preventing radiation retinopathy with hyperfractionation. *Int J Radiat Oncol Biol Phys* 2005;61:856–864.
45. Parsons JT, Bova FJ, Fitzgerald CR, et al. Radiation retinopathy after external-beam irradiation: analysis of time-dose factors. *Int J Radiat Oncol Biol Phys* 1994;30: 765–773.
46. Paulino AC, Marks JE, Bricker P, et al. Results of treatment of patients with maxillary sinus carcinoma. *Cancer* 1998;83:457–465.
47. Bristol IJ, Ahamad A, Garden AS, et al. Postoperative radiotherapy for maxillary sinus cancer: long-term outcomes and toxicities of treatment. *Int J Radiat Oncol Biol Phys* 2007;68:719–730.
48. Dulguerov P, Jacobsen MS, Allal AS. Nasal and paranasal sinus carcinoma: are we making progress? *Cancer* 2001;92:3012–3029.
49. Chen AM, Daly ME, Bucci MK, et al., Carcinomas of the paranasal sinuses and nasal cavity treated with radiotherapy at a single institution over five decades: are we making improvement? *Int J Radiat Oncol Biol Phys* 2007;69:141–147.
50. Agger A, von Buchwald C, Madsen AR, et al. Squamous cell carcinoma of the nasal vestibule 1993–2002: a nationwide retrospective study from DAHANCA. *Head Neck* 2009;31:1593–1599.
51. Chobe R, McNeese M, Weber R, et al. Radiation therapy for carcinoma of the nasal vestibule. *Otolaryngol Head Neck Surg* 1988;98:67–71.
52. Dowley A, Hoskison E, Allibone R, et al. Squamous cell carcinoma of the nasal vestibule: a 20-year case series and literature review. *J Laryngol Otol* 2008;122: 1019–1023.
53. Levendag PC, Nijdam WM, van Moolenbourgh SE, et al., Interstitial radiation therapy for early stage nasal vestibulae cancer: a continuing quest for optimal tumor control and cosmesis. *Int J Radiat Oncol Biol Phys* 2006;66:160–169.
54. Levendag PC, Pomp J. Radiation therapy of squamous cell carcinoma of the nasal vestibule. *Int J Radiat Oncol Biol Phys* 1990;19:1363–1367.
55. Mak AC, Van Andel JG, van Woerkom-Eijkenboom WM. Radiation therapy of carcinoma of the nasal vestibule. *Eur J Cancer* 1980;16:81–85.
56. Mendenhall WM, Stringer SP, Cassisi NJ, et al. Squamous cell carcinoma of the nasal vestibule. *Head Neck* 1999;21:385–393.
57. Poulsen M, Turner S. Radiation therapy for squamous cell carcinoma of the nasal vestibule. *Int J Radiat Oncol Biol Phys* 1993;27:267–272.
58. Wallace A, Morris CG, Kirwan J, et al. Radiotherapy for squamous cell carcinoma of the nasal vestibule. *Am J Clin Oncol* 2007;30:612–616.
59. Badib AO, Kurohara SS, Webster JH, et al. Treatment of cancer of the nasal cavity. *Am J Roentgenol Radium Ther Nucl Med* 1969;106:824–830.
60. Bosch A, Vallecillo L, Frias Z. Cancer of the nasal cavity. *Cancer* 1976;37:1458–1463.
61. Hawkins RB, Wynstra JH, Pilepich MV, et al. Carcinoma of the nasal cavity–results of primary and adjuvant radiotherapy. *Int J Radiat Oncol Biol Phys* 1988;15: 1129–1133.
62. Daly ME, Chen AM, Bucci MK, et al. Intensity-modulated radiation therapy for malignancies of the nasal cavity and paranasal sinuses. *Int J Radiat Oncol Biol Phys* 2007;67:151–157
63. Bhattacharyya N. Cancer of the nasal cavity: survival and factors influencing prognosis. *Arch Otolaryngol Head Neck Surg* 2002;128:1079–1083.
64. Rosenthal DI, Barker JLJ, El-Naggar AK, et al. Sinonasal malignancies with neuroendocrine differentiation. *Cancer* 2004;101:2567–2573.
65. Foote RL, Morita A, Ebersold MJ, et al. Esthesioneuroblastoma: the role of adjuvant radiation therapy. *Int J Radiat Oncol Biol Phys* 1993;27:835–842.
66. Eden BV, Debo RF, Larner JM, et al. Esthesioneuroblastoma. Long-term outcome and patterns of failure—the University of Virginia experience. *Cancer* 1994;73: 255–2562.
67. Loy AH, Reibel JF, Read PW, et al. Esthesioneuroblastoma: continued follow-up of a single institution's experience. *Arch Otolaryngol* 2006;132:134–138.
68. Dias FL, Sa GM, Lima RA, et al. Patterns of failure and outcome in esthesioneuroblastoma. *Arch Otolaryngol* 2003;129:1186–1192.
69. Blanco AI, Chao KSC, Ozyigit G, et al. Carcinoma of paranasal sinuses: long-term outcomes with radiotherapy. *Int J Radiat Oncol Biol Phys* 2004;59:51–58.
70. Katz TS, Mendenhall WM, Morris GC, et al. Malignant tumors of the nasal cavity and paranasal sinuses. *Head Neck* 2002;24:821–829.
71. Lavertu P, Roberts JK, Kraus DH, et al. Squamous cell carcinoma of the paranasal sinuses: the Cleveland Clinic experience 1977–1986. *Laryngoscope* 1989;99: 1130–1136.
72. Le QT, Fu KK, Kaplan M, et al. Treatment of maxillary sinus carcinoma: a comparison of the 1997 and 1977 American Joint Committee on cancer staging systems. *Cancer* 1999;86:1700–1711.
73. Madani I, Bonte K, Vakaet L, et al. Intensity-modulated radiotherapy for sinonasal tumors: Ghent University Hospital update. *Int J Radiat Oncol Biol Phys* 2009;73: 424–432.
74. Myers LL, Nussenbaum B, Bradford CR, et al. Paranasal sinus malignancies: an 18-year single institution experience. *Laryngoscope* 2002;112:1964–1969.
75. Spiro JD, Soo KC, Spiro RH. Squamous carcinoma of the nasal cavity and paranasal sinuses. *Am J Surg* 1989;158:328–332.
76. Zaharia M, Salem LE, Travezan R, et al. Postoperative radiotherapy in the management of cancer of the maxillary sinus. *Int J Radiat Oncol Biol Phys* 1989;17: 967–971.
77. Duthoy W, Boterberg T, Claus F, et al. Postoperative intensity-modulated radiotherapy in sinonasal carcinoma. *Cancer* 2005;104:71–82.
78. Hoppe BS, Wolden SL, Zelefsky MJ, et al. Postoperative intensity-modulated radiation therapy for cancers of the paranasal sinuses, nasal cavity, and lacrimal glands: technique, early outcomes, and toxicity. *Head Neck* 2008;30:925–932.
79. Choussy O, Ferron C, Vedrine P, et al. Adenocarcinoma of ethmoid: A GETTEC retrospective multicenter of 418 cases. *Laryngoscope* 2008;118:437–443.
80. Parsons JT, Bova FJ, Fitzgerald CR, et al. Severe dry-eye syndrome following external beam irradiation. *Int J Radiat Oncol Biol Phys* 1994;30:775–780.
81. Jiang GL, Tucker SL, Guttenberger R, et al. Radiation-induced injury to the visual pathway. *Radiother Oncol* 1994;30:17–25.
82. Emami B, Lyman J, Brown A, et al. Tolerance of normal tissue to therapeutic irradiation. *Int J Radiat Oncol Biol Phys* 1991;21:109–122.
83. Takeda A, Shigematsu N, Suzuki S, et al. Late retinal complications of radiation therapy for nasal and paranasal malignancies: relationship between irradiated-dose area and severity. *Int J Radiat Oncol Biol Phys* 1999;44:599–605.
84. Combs SE, Konkel S, Schultz-Ertner D, et al. Intensity-modulated radiotherapy (IMRT) in patients with carcinomas of the paranasal sinuses: clinical benefit for complex shaped target volumes. *Radiat Oncol* 2006;1:23.
85. Bhandare N, Monroe AT, Morris CG, et al. Does altered fractionation influence the risk of radiation-induced optic neuropathy? *Int J Radiat Oncol Biol Phys* 2005;62: 1070–1077.

Chapter 43
Salivary Gland Cancer

Chris H.J. Terhaard

The salivary glands consist of the three large, paired major glands—parotid, submandibular, and sublingual (Fig. 43.1)—and many smaller, minor glands located throughout the upper aerodigestive tract. Salivary gland malignancies make up only approximately 0.4% of all cancers and account for <5% of the annual incidence of head and neck malignancies in the United States. The international variation in the incidence is between 0.4 and 2.6/100,000 per year, with a mean of approximately 1.2/100,000.[1,2] No significant change in incidence has been shown in recent decades.[1–3]

ANATOMY

Major Salivary Glands

Parotid Gland

The parotid gland is located superficial to and partly behind the ramus of the mandible and covers the masseter muscle. Superficially, it overlaps the posterior part of the muscle and largely fills the space between the ramus of the mandible and the anterior border of the sternocleidomastoid muscle. One or more isthmi that wrap around the branches of the facial nerve connect the superficial and deep lobes of the gland. The nerve enters the deep surface of the gland as a single trunk, passing posterolateral to the styloid process. It usually leaves the gland as five or more branches, emerging at the anterior, upper, and lower borders of the gland. The facial nerve runs superficial to the main blood vessels that traverse the gland but is interwoven within the glandular tissue and its ducts. Thus, removal of all or part of the parotid gland demands meticulous dissection if the nerve is to be spared.

The parotid gland contains an extensive lymphatic capillary plexus, many aggregates of lymphocytic cells, and numerous intraglandular lymph nodes in the superficial lobe. Lymphatics drain from more lateral areas on the face, including parts of the eyelids, diagonally downward and posterior toward the parotid gland, as do the lymphatics from the frontal region of the scalp. Associated with the gland, both superficially and more deeply, are parotid nodes. These drain downward along the retromandibular vein to empty in part into the superficial lymphatics and nodes along the outer surface of the sternocleidomastoid muscle and in part into upper nodes of the deep cervical chain. Lymphatics from the parietal region of the scalp drain partly to the parotid nodes in front of the ear and partly to the retroauricular nodes in back of the ear, which, in turn, drain into upper deep cervical nodes.[4]

Submandibular Gland

The submandibular gland largely fills the triangle between the two bellies of the digastric and the lower border of the mandible and extends upward deep to the mandible. It lies partly on the lower surface of the mylohyoid and partly behind the muscle against the lateral surface of the muscle of the tongue, the hypoglossus. The submandibular gland has a larger superficial part, or body, and a smaller deep process. The inferior surface is adjacent to the submandibular lymph nodes, and the deep process of the submandibular gland lies between the mylohyoid laterally and the hyoglossus medially and between the lingual nerve above and the hypoglossal nerve below.[5] Bimanual palpation with one finger in the floor of the mouth and one under the edge of the mandible facilitates clinical detection of masses in this gland.

A rich lymphatic capillary network lies in the interstitial spaces of the gland (Fig. 43.2). From the lateral and superior portions of the gland, lymph flows to the prevascular or preglandular submandibular lymph nodes. The posterior portion of

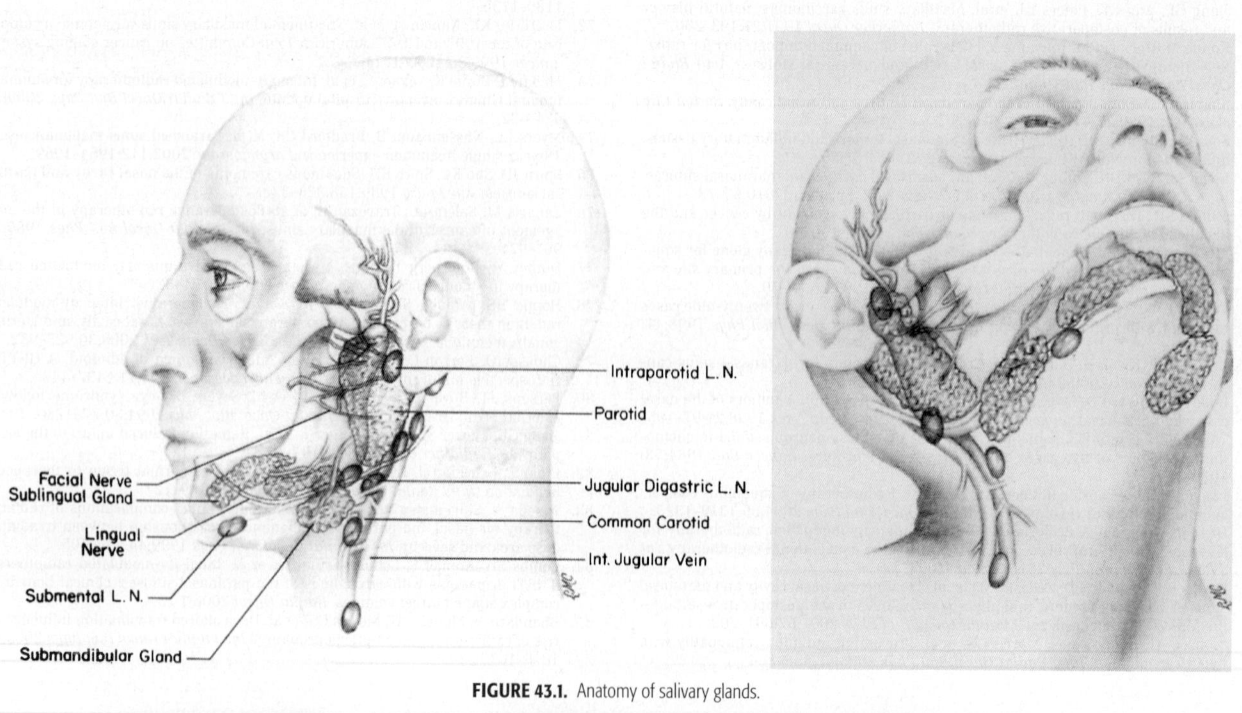

FIGURE 43.1. Anatomy of salivary glands.

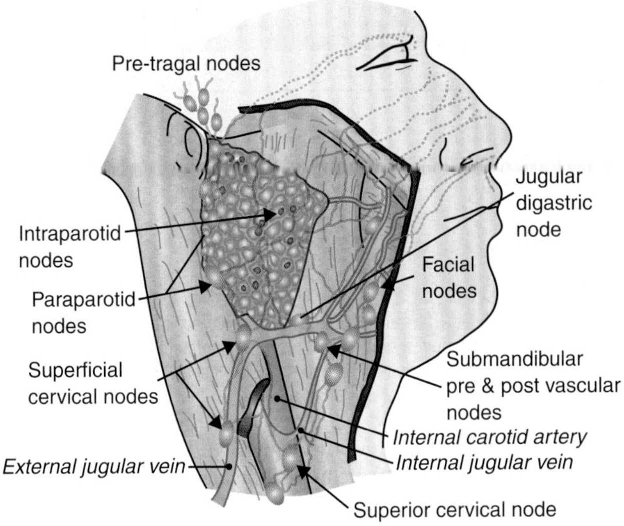

FIGURE 43.2. Lymph node distribution in and around the parotid gland.

the gland gives rise to one or two lymphatic trunks, which follow the facial artery and go directly to the anterior subdigastric nodes of the internal jugular chain.[6] The nodes overlying the submandibular gland, followed by the subdigastric and high midjugular lymph nodes, are those involved in nodal metastases.

Sublingual Gland

This smallest of the three major salivary glands, along with many minor salivary glands, lies between the mucous membrane of the floor of the mouth above and the mylohyoid muscle below, the mandible laterally, and the genioglossus muscles of the tongue medially. This is a rare site for malignant neoplasms; they are difficult to distinguish from cancer of the floor of the mouth, accounting for <2% of all reported cases of salivary gland tumors.[1,7] The sublingual gland drains either to the submandibular lymph nodes or more posterior into the deep internal jugular chain between the digastric and omohyoid muscles. Rarely, the lymphatics of the sublingual gland drain into a submental node or supraomohyoid jugular node.

Minor Salivary Glands

Minor salivary glands are widely distributed in the upper aerodigestive tract, palate, buccal mucosa, base of tongue, pharynx, trachea, cheek, lip, gingiva, floor of mouth, tonsil, paranasal sinuses, nasal cavity, and nasopharynx.

EPIDEMIOLOGY

Seventy percent of all salivary tumors arise in the parotid gland, 8% in the submandibular gland, and 22% in the minor salivary glands.[7] The proportion of malignant tumors increases from parotid (25%) to submandibular (43%) to minor salivary glands (65%).[7,8] There is a preponderance of benign tumors in women; malignant tumors exhibit an equal sex distribution.[2] Patients with benign tumors are younger (mean age, 46 years) compared with those with malignant tumors (mean age, 54 years), with a trend to an older age for submandibular and minor salivary gland locations.[7] From 2% to 3% of salivary neoplasms occur in children, in whom half of the tumors are malignant.[9] The majority of cancers are located in the parotid gland, with mucoepidermoid cancers predominating. The tumors in children are mostly less advanced, and a 95% 5-year survival is reached.[9]

Etiologic factors are not clearly defined. Nutrition may be a factor because Eskimos in the Arctic, who have low intake of vitamins A and C, have a high incidence. Cigarette smoking and alcohol consumption are in general not related to salivary gland cancer,[10] although cigarette consumption of >80 pack-years may contribute to salivary gland cancer.[11] Irradiation can also be a cause, as evidenced by the increased incidence in survivors of the atomic bombs dropped on Hiroshima and Nagasaki and in those irradiated to the head and neck for benign conditions during childhood.[12–15] Saku et al.[13] studied salivary gland tumors in atomic bomb survivors of Hiroshima and Nagasaki. Two-thirds of all cases were parotid, and the remainder were equally distributed between submandibular and minor salivary glands. Mucoepidermoid cancer and Warthin's tumor (benign) were particularly elevated compared with nonexposed persons and disproportionately high at high radiation doses. Modan et al.[12] found a clear dose–response effect in a matched control study of patients who had low-dose head–neck irradiation in childhood; there was a 2.6-fold increase of benign tumors and a 4.5-fold increase of cancer. The majority of these tumors are mucoepidermoid cancers[14,15]; however, <1% of salivary gland tumors may be caused by former irradiation.[16]

Workers in various occupations experience an increased risk of salivary gland cancer.[17] For women employed as hairdressers or working in beauty shops, a significant elevated risk was observed in a study by Swanson and Burns.[11]

Women with salivary gland cancer may have a 2.5-fold elevated breast cancer risk.[18] After treatment for salivary gland cancer, there is an increased risk for subsequent cancer of the oral cavity (hazard ratio [HR] = 3.5) and thyroid (HR = 2.7), lung and kidney cancer (HR = 1.7), and second salivary gland cancer (HR = 10), especially after acinic cell cancer (HR = 31). For adenoid cystic cancer the risk of developing nasopharyngeal is increased by a factor 17.[19]

NATURAL HISTORY

Local invasion is the initial route of spread of malignant tumors of the salivary glands, depending on location and histologic type. For parotid tumors, this may result in fixation to structures in around 20% of cases.[20] Skin invasion is more often seen in parotid tumors (8%–10%) compared with submandibular tumors (3%).[21,22]

Approximately 25% of patients with a malignant parotid salivary gland tumor present with facial palsy from cranial nerve invasion.[7,20,22,23,24]

A detailed study by the Dutch Head and Neck Oncology Group (NWHHT) concerning patients with a salivary gland malignancy found an overall incidence of clinically positive nodes of 14% and clinically occult, pathologically positive nodes in an additional 11% of patients.[21] This percentage depends on the number of neck dissections performed, the tumor location, histology, and T stage. The number of elective neck dissections performed varies among the tumor locations. Stennert et al.[25] performed a neck dissection in all malignant *parotid* tumors and found 53% unilateral positive nodes and 0% contralateral nodes. In selected patients in other studies, the percentage positive nodes varied between 20%[26] and 38%.[24] Three of four involved lymph nodes in early parotid malignancies (21% occult nodes) were localized in intraparotideal nodes by Stenner et al.[27] Resection of *submandibular* tumors is combined with a (partial) neck dissection in most cases. Pathologic neck nodes may be seen in up to 42% of cases.[24] The risk of positive lymph nodes in *minor salivary gland* cancer depended on four prognostic factors; male sex, T3-T4, pharyngeal site, and histology (high-grade mucoepidermoid and high-grade adenocarcinoma). Based on these factors, a scoring system from 0 to 4 was developed by Lloyd et al.[28] The risk of positive nodes in minor salivary gland cancer is <10% for score 0 to 1, 17% for score 2, 41% for score 3, and 70% for score 4. Salivary gland tumors arising in the oral cavity produce an incidence of

TABLE 43.1 RISK ESTIMATION (%) FOR POSITIVE NECK NODES

Summation: T Score + Histologic Type Score	Parotid Gland	Submandibular Gland	Oral Cavity	Other Locations
2	4	0	4	0
3	12	33	13	29
4	25	57	19	56
5	33	60	–	–
6	38	50	–	–

T1 = 1, T2 = 2, T3–4 = 3; acinic/adenoid cystic/carcinoma ex pleomorphic adenoma = 1, mucoepidermoid = 2, squamous/undifferentiated = 3.

From Terhaard CHJ, Lubsen H, Rasch CRN, et al. The role of radiotherapy in the treatment of malignant salivary gland tumors. *Int J Radiat Oncol Biol Phys* 2005;61:103–111.

TABLE 43.2 DISTRIBUTION OF PRESENTING SITES OF INTRAORAL MINOR SALVARY GLAND TUMORS

Site	Number of Patients (%)	Percentage Malignant
Palate	206 (54)	43
Upper lip	64 (17)	9
Buccal mucosa	54 (14)	37
Retromolar region	20 (5)	95
Lower lip	18 (5)	56
Floor of mouth	13 (3)	69
Tongue	5 (1)	60
Total	**380**	**41**

Adapted from Buchner A, Merrell PW, Carpenter WM. Relative frequency of intra-oral minor salivary gland tumors: a study of 380 cases from northern California and comparison to reports from other parts of the world. *J Oral Pathol Med* 2007;36:207–214.

cervical node metastases of <10%.[8,24,29,30] Nasopharyngeal salivary gland tumors have a high risk of occult metastases (50%).[30] In general, the risk of positive findings in the neck, including *all salivary gland malignancies,* may be based on a combination of T stage, tumor localization, and histology. The highest risk is seen for squamous cell, undifferentiated, and salivary duct cancers.[24,31] There is an intermediate risk for mucoepidermoid cancer and a low risk for acinic cell, adenoid cystic carcinoma, and carcinoma ex pleomorphic adenoma.[24] A 15% risk is found for T1 tumors, 26% for T2, and 33% for T3–4.[24] An example of a rating scale to estimate the risk of positive neck nodes based on tumor location, T stage, and histologic type is shown in Table 43.1.

Distant metastases overall are encountered in 3% of patients at presentation and in 33% after 10 years.[21] They are fairly common with adenoid cystic, salivary duct, squamous cell, and undifferentiated carcinomas; in the case of adenoid cystic carcinomas, they may occur quite late in the course of the disease, without recurrence of the primary tumor.[21,32,33] Distant metastases are primarily to lung, bone, and occasionally liver.[21] Reported incidence of distant metastases in patients with adenoid cystic carcinoma after 10 years of follow-up is approximately 40%.[21,33,34] Five years after diagnosis of distant metastases of adenoid cystic carcinoma and acinic cell cancer, more than one-third of the patients are still alive; 10% are alive

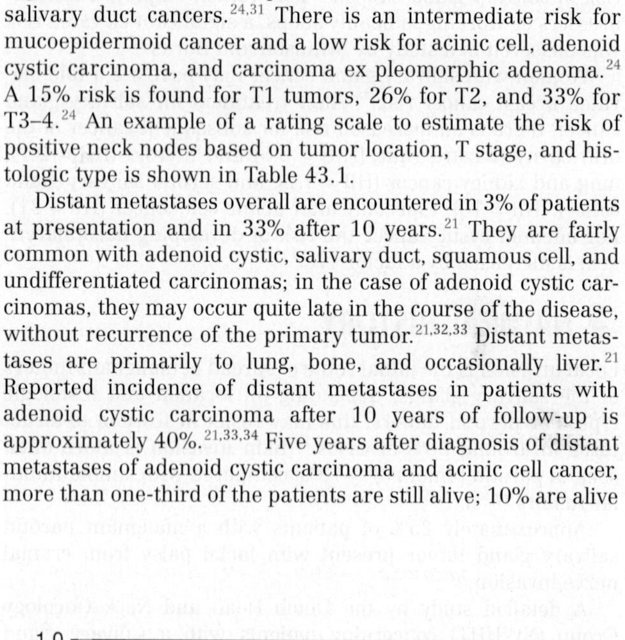

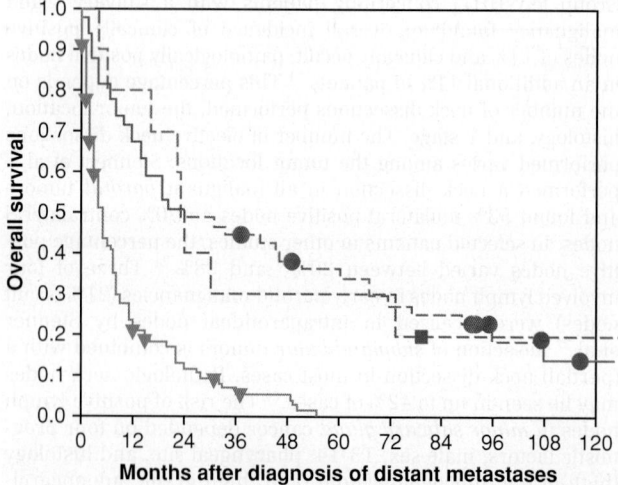

FIGURE 43.3. Survival after diagnosis of distant metastases, depending on histology; update of the nationwide Dutch study. (●) Adenoid cystic carcinoma[49]; (■) acinic cell carcinoma[11]; (▲) others[99]; $p < .001$. (From Terhaard CHJ, Lubsen H, Van der Tweel, et al. Salivary gland carcinoma: independent prognostic factors for locoregional control, distant metastases, and overall survival: Results of the Dutch Head and Neck Oncology Cooperative Group. *Head Neck* 2004;26(8):681–693.)

after 10 years. An update of the survival data of the NWHHT study after diagnosis of distant metastases of salivary gland cancer is shown in Figure 43.3.

CLINICAL PRESENTATION

Three of four parotid masses are benign.[7] Patients most often have a painless, rapidly enlarging mass, often present for years before a sudden change in its indolent growth pattern prompts the patient to seek medical attention. Duration of clinical symptoms before diagnosis may last >10 years.[7,21] For malignant tumors, the median duration of clinical symptoms generally is shorter (3 to 6 months)[21,35] than that of benign tumors, although for some minor salivary gland tumors, median periods of 2 years have been reported.[29,36]

Pain is more frequently associated with malignant disease.[7] Although as many as one-third of parotid cancers may have facial nerve involvement, only 10% to 20% of patients complain of pain.[7,20,21] Pain may appear with involvement of deeper structures (masseter, temporal, and pterygoid muscles). Rarely, tumors of the parotid may involve the base of the skull and cause intractable pain and paralysis of various cranial nerves. Asymptomatic swelling of the floor of the mouth is the primary presentation in sublingual salivary gland cancer, with pain and tongue numbness as symptoms of advanced disease.[37]

The signs and symptoms associated with tumors of the minor salivary glands vary because of their diverse locations. The distribution of presenting sites and risk of malignancy for 380 cases of intraoral minor salivary gland tumors are shown in Table 43.2.[38] A painless lump is the most common presenting symptom. Almost all extraoral minor salivary gland tumors are malignant.[7] Extraoral minor salivary gland tumors are most frequently seen in the nasal cavity (52%), followed by the larynx (18%), the oropharynx (14%, mostly localized in the tonsil), nasopharynx (8%), and ethmoid (8%).[7] For tumors arising in the nasal cavity or sinuses, facial pain is the most common presenting symptom, followed by nasal obstruction. Laryngeal primary tumors most frequently cause hoarseness or voice change.

Clinical features suggesting a malignant salivary gland tumor are rapid growth rate, pain, facial nerve palsy, childhood occurrence, skin involvement, and cervical adenopathy.

DIAGNOSTIC WORKUP AND STAGING

Major Salivary Glands

The diagnostic workup of major salivary gland tumors includes a careful history and physical examination, with particular attention to signs of local fixation or regional adenopathy.

For superficial lesions of the parotid gland, the submandibular gland, and the sublingual gland and evaluation of the cervical lymph nodes, ultrasound (US) is the first diagnostic step, combined with fine-needle aspiration cytology (FNAC). In US,

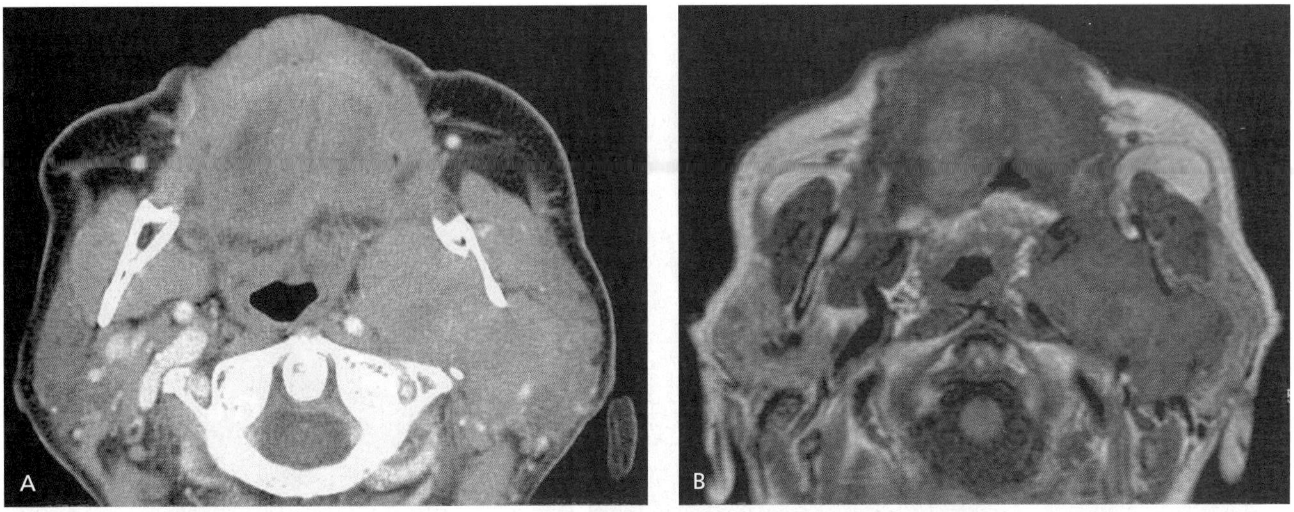

FIGURE 43.4. A patient with acinic cell cancer of the left parotid gland. **A:** Axial contrast-enhanced computed tomography image. **B:** T1-weighted magnetic resonance image. Both images show an infiltrating soft tissue mass involving the deep and superficial lobe. The tumor has widened the left stylomandibular tunnel, with infiltration in the pterygoid musculature. The left internal carotid artery is displaced medially. (Courtesy of Dr. F. A. Pameijer, radiologist, University Medical Center, Utrecht, Netherlands.)

signs of malignancy are ill-defined borders with heterogonous architecture, internal necrosis, and cystic changes.[39] Benign salivary tumors are well defined and hypoechoic. FNAC is very useful for differentiating between yes and no neoplastic lesions, with a specificity of >95%. The sensitivity for malignancy may vary according to country, with a mean of around 80%.[40] In a systematic review Colella et al.[41] found concordant cytology in 80%, 96%, and 94%, respectively, for patients with a histologic diagnosis of a malignant tumor, a benign tumor, or a nonneoplastic lesion. False-negative findings may be seen as result of lack of representative material or a cyst. The relative low negative predictive value of fine-needle aspiration will be improved if magnetic resonance imaging (MRI) and fine-needle aspiration are combined.

The next imaging tool in salivary gland tumors suspected for malignancy is MRI. MRI is superior to computed tomography (CT), especially when malignancy is suspected, based on the excellent soft-tissue contrast (Fig. 43.4). T1-weighted (W) images are excellent to assess the margins, extension into the deep tissues, and patterns of infiltration because the (fatty) background of the gland is hyperintensive. With T1-W gadolinium series, tumor infiltration and heterogeneous enhancement may be visualized, as seen in high-grade tumors.[39] With fat-suppressed T2-W images the fluid content of a tumor is visualized. In general, benign tumors are hyperintensive, and malignant tumors show intermediate or low intensity at T2-W MR images. Early contrast enhancement and slow washout are signs of malignancy on dynamic MRI.[42] A low apparent diffusion coefficient (ADC), derived from diffusion-weighted MRI using high *b* values, is associated with malignancy.[43] However, Warthin's tumors (benign) may also show low ADC values.[44] Perineural invasion of adenoid cystic carcinoma may be evaluated with both CT (foraminal enlargement) and MRI (thickened nerve with enhancement on the fat-suppressed T1-weighted images).[39] The tumor extension along the facial nerve (VII; foramen styloideum), the cranial nerve V-3 (foramen ovale), or nerve V-2 (foramen rotundum), as seen in tumors of the deep parotid lobe, may be visualized by T1-weighted images.[43] This is of special importance for the delineation of these nerves in case of postoperative radiotherapy for extensive perineural invasion; see Figure 43.5 for the trigeminal and facial nerves. Cortical involvement is best evaluated by CT.

Fluorodeoxyglucose (FDG) uptake in salivary glands is quite unpredictable, resulting in a low sensitivity of FDG-positron emission tomography (PET) for the diagnosis of malignancy in salivary glands. However, the combination of FDG-PET with CT imaging was a deciding image modality in 15% of cases in a study of Razfar et al.[45] The recently developed combined FDG-PET/MRI scans could be a valuable extension of the diagnostic imaging modalities in salivary gland cancer.

The seventh edition of the manual of the American Joint Committee on Cancer and the seventh edition of the classification system of the International Union Against Cancer are identical for major salivary glands (Table 43.3).[46] They are based on size, extension, and nodal involvement. Relative

TABLE 43.3 INTERNATIONAL UNION AGAINST CANCER STAGING SYSTEM FOR MAJOR SALIVARY GLAND CANCER (PAROTID, SUBMANDIBULAR, SUBLINGUAL)

Primary Tumor (T)			
T1	≤2 cm without extraparenchymal extension		
T3	>4 cm and/or extraparenchymal extension		
T4a	Invasion skin, and/or mandible, and/or ear canal, and/or facial nerve		
T4b	Invasion skull base and/or pterygoid plates and/or carotid artery		
Regional Lymph Nodes (N)			
N0	No regional lymph node metastasis		
N1	Ipsilateral single lymph node, ≤3 cm		
N2a	Single ipsilateral lymph node >3 cm but <6 cm		
N2b	Multiple ipsilateral lymph nodes, none >6 cm		
N2c	Bilateral or contralateral lymph nodes, none >6 cm		
N3	Lymph node >6 cm		
Distant Metastases (M)			
MX	Presence of distant metastasis cannot be assessed		
M0	No distant metastasis		
M1	Distant metastasis		
Stage Grouping			
I	T1	N0	M0
II	T2	N0	M0
III	T3	N0	M0
	T1, T2, T3	N1	M0
IVA	T1, T2, T3, T4	N2	M0
	T4a, T4b	N0, N1	M0
IVB	T4b	Any N	M0
	Any T	N3	M0
IVC	Any T	Any N	M1

From Sobin LH, Gospodarowicz MK, Wittekind Ch. *TNM classification of malignant tumors,* 7th ed. Hoboken, NJ: Wiley-Blackwell, 2009.

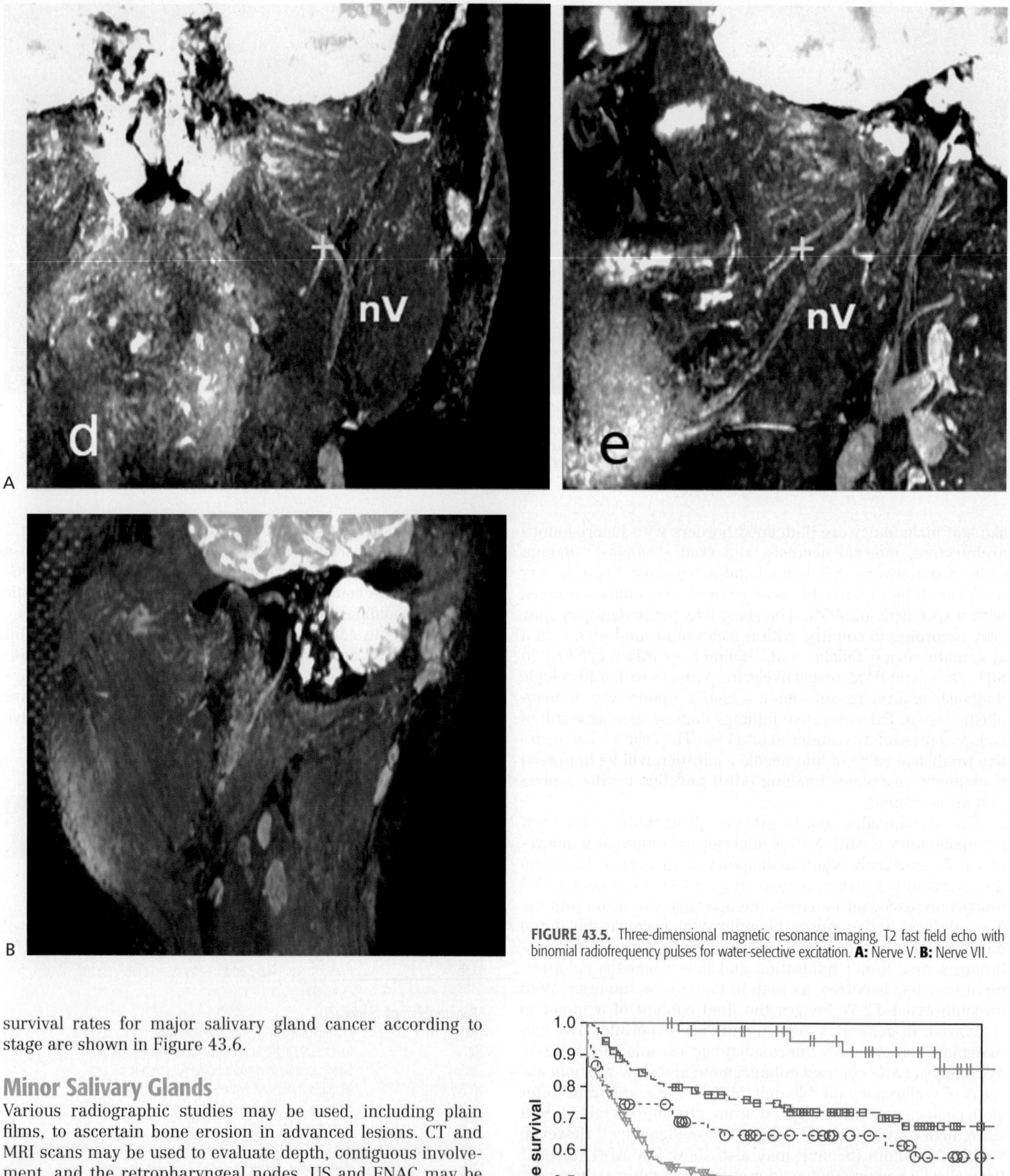

FIGURE 43.5. Three-dimensional magnetic resonance imaging, T2 fast field echo with binomial radiofrequency pulses for water-selective excitation. **A:** Nerve V. **B:** Nerve VII.

survival rates for major salivary gland cancer according to stage are shown in Figure 43.6.

Minor Salivary Glands

Various radiographic studies may be used, including plain films, to ascertain bone erosion in advanced lesions. CT and MRI scans may be used to evaluate depth, contiguous involvement, and the retropharyngeal nodes. US and FNAC may be used to examine the neck nodes. The definitive diagnostic procedure is an excisional biopsy, particularly if malignancy is clinically expected. Unplanned incisional biopsies should be avoided, and fine-needle biopsies are impractical because of the polymorphism of most malignant salivary gland tumors.

A formal staging system has not been developed for minor gland tumors. The same staging system for minor salivary glands as for squamous cell carcinoma in sites other than the parotid or submandibular glands may be used. The American Joint Committee on Cancer and International Union Against Cancer classification and stage regrouping system has been reported to be a major long-term outcome predictor in minor salivary gland carcinoma.[47]

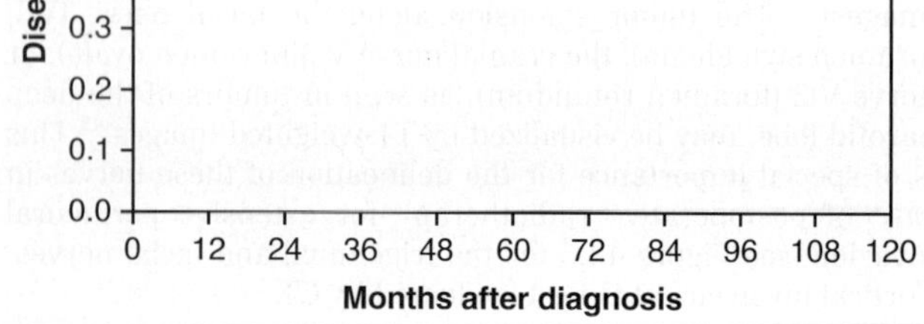

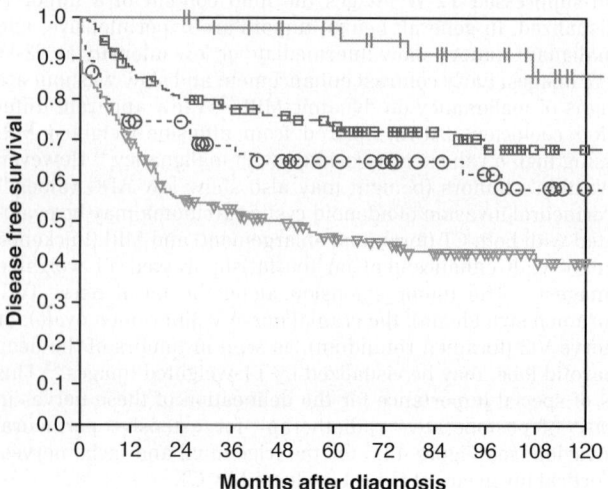

FIGURE 43.6. Disease-free survival for major salivary glands according to the 2002 classification of the American Joint Committee on Cancer. Results of the nationwide Dutch study: +, stage I; □, stage II; ○, stage III; ∇, stage IV.

PATHOLOGIC CLASSIFICATION

Salivary glands are composed of acinar–ductal units, with acinar cells on the inside of the acinic, and ductal epithelial cells on the inside of the striated and excretory ducts. Myoepithelial cells are located in the outside of acini and intercalated and striated ducts. Basal (reserve) cells are found on the outside of the excretory ducts.[48] Carcinomas may arise from all these cell types, separately or combined. The histologic classification of these salivary gland tumors is very demanding for the head and neck pathologist. In 1991 the World Health Organization classification for salivary gland tumors of 1972 was expanded from 7 to 20 subtypes. Various types of carcinomas were distinguished based on precise histologic definitions, prognosis, and treatment (discussed more in detail by Seifert and Sobin[49]). In 2005 the WHO classification of malignant salivary gland tumors was extended again; 24 subtypes were specified (Table 43.4).[48] Classification may be difficult, as shown in a re-evaluation of 101 intraoral salivary gland tumors by experienced pathologists; major disagreement was seen in 8, and there was minor disagreement in 33.[50]

Most salivary gland subtypes are very rare. The percentage of the histologic subtypes varies from series to series and according to the localization of the tumor (Fig. 43.7). In 666 patients with a salivary gland carcinoma in a study performed in the Netherlands, for which the pathology was revised, adenoid cystic carcinoma was most frequently diagnosed (27%), followed by mucoepidermoid carcinoma (16%), acinic cell carcinoma (14%), carcinoma ex pleomorphic adenoma (8%), undifferentiated carcinoma (7%), salivary duct carcinoma and adenocarcinoma not otherwise specified (both 6%), polymorph low-grade adenocarcinoma (PLGA) and squamous cell carcinoma (both 5%), and epithelial–myoepithelial carcinoma in 2%. In this large study, all other subtypes were rarely or not at all diagnosed.

Salivary gland carcinomas may be graded as of low and high malignancy, particularly for mucoepidermoid tumors. However, there is a disparity in grading, even among experienced pathologists.[51] Low-grade mucoepidermoid, PLGA, epithelial–myoepithelial, and acinic cell carcinomas comprise a group of low to moderate malignancy; high-grade mucoepidermoid, malignant mixed, adenoid cystic, squamous, undifferentiated, and salivary duct carcinomas represent higher-grade malignancies.[52]

Adenoid cystic carcinoma is most common in minor salivary glands,[8,21,30,47] followed by the submandibular gland.[21,53,54,55] Perineural invasion is common in adenoid cystic carcinoma.[56]

TABLE 43.4 WORLD HEALTH ORGANIZATION 2005 CLASSIFICATION OF TUMORS OF THE SALIVARY

Malignant Epithelial Tumors	***Benign Epithelial Tumors***
Acinic cell carcinoma	Pleomorphic adenoma
Mucoepidermoid carcinoma	Myoepithelioma
Adenoid cystic carcinoma	Basal cell adenoma
Polymorphous low-grade adenocarcinoma	Warthin's tumor
Epithelial–myoepithelial carcinoma	Oncocytoma
Clear cell carcinoma NOS	Canalicular adenoma
Basal cell adenocarcinoma	Sebacceous adenoma
Sebaceous carcinoma	Lymphadenoma
Sebaceous lymphadenocarcinoma	Sebaceous
Cystadenocarcinoma	Nonsebaceous
Low-grade cribriform cystadenocarcinoma	Ductal papilloma
Mucinous adenocarcinoma	Inverted ductal papilloma
Oncocytic carcinoma	Intraductal papilloma
Salivary duct carcinoma	Sialadenoma papilliferum
Adenocarcinoma NOS	Cystadenoma
Myoepithelial carcinoma	***Soft-Tissue Tumors***
Carcinoma ex pleomorphic adenoma	Hemangioma
Carcinosarcoma	***Hematolymphoid Tumors***
Metastasizing pleomorphic adenoma	Hodgkin lymphoma
Squamous cell carcinoma	Diffuse large B-cell lymphoma
Small cell carcinoma	Extranodal marginal zone B-cell lymphoma
Large cell carcinoma	
Lymphoepithelial carcinoma	
Sialoblastoma	

NOS, not otherwise specified.

From Seifert G, Sobin LH. The World Health Organization's histological classification of salivary gland tumors. *Cancer* 1992;70:379–385.

The adenoid cystic variety has a tubular pattern that has been associated with the best prognosis, a cribriform pattern with an intermediate prognosis, and a solid pattern with the worst prognosis.[57]

In parotid tumors in children and adults, the most common malignant subtype is *mucoepidermoid carcinoma* (MEC).[9,55,58–60] MEC contains squamous cells, mucus-producing cells, and cells of intermediate type. Several grading criteria and a cell cycle–based Ki-67 proliferation index for MEC have been published.[48] *Acinic cell* cancer derives from cells of the terminal ducts and intercalated ducts. Grading for acinic cell cancer is controversial.[61] Most tumors (86%) are located in the parotid gland.[61] As in MEC, the Ki-67 proliferation index is a

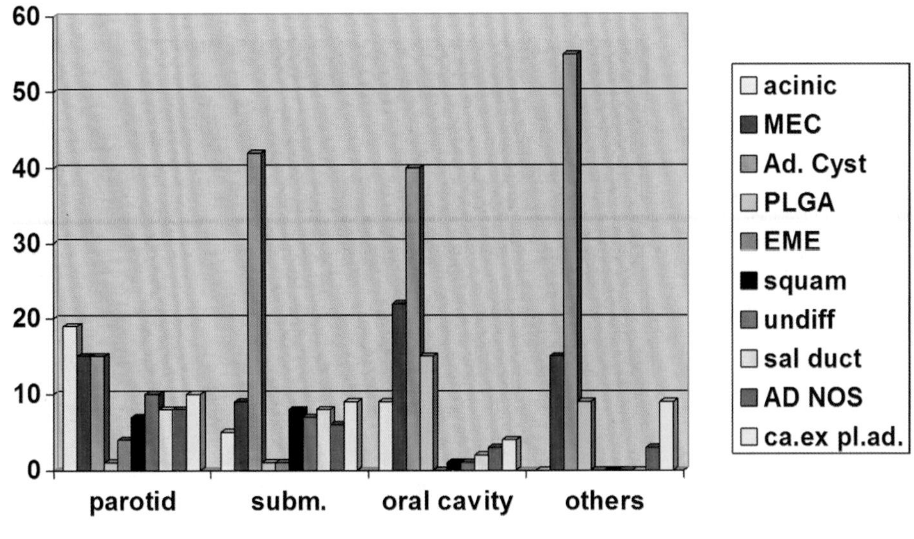

FIGURE 43.7. Distribution of cell types (%) in various series from the Dutch study, depending on site, AD NOS, not otherwise specified. Ad. Cyst, adenoid cystic; ca.ex pl. ad., carcinoma ex pleomorphic adenoma; subm, submandibular; EME, epithelial–myoepithelial carcinoma; MEC, mucoepidermoid cancer; PLGA, polymorphous low-grade adenocarcinoma; sal duct, salivary duct carcinoma; squam, squamous cell carcinoma; undiff, undifferentiated.

prognostic factor for disease-free survival.[48] *Carcinoma ex pleomorphic adenoma* may be localized in all salivary glands, although the majority is found in the parotid gland. In the development of carcinoma ex pleomorphic adenoma a progressive loss of heterozygosity of chromosome 8q, 12 G, and 17P is seen.[62] The prognosis is poor, with a high risk of distant metastases.[21] *Undifferentiated and squamous cell carcinomas* are mainly localized in the parotid gland. The prevalence of comorbidity for patients with squamous cell carcinoma of the salivary gland is comparable to that of other head and neck cancers, whereas the prevalence of comorbidity in all other malignant salivary gland cancer subtypes is significantly less.[63] In addition, patients with squamous cell carcinoma of the salivary glands are mostly older.[2] Thus, squamous cell carcinoma of the salivary gland may be a different entity among salivary gland cancers. PLGA, salivary duct, and epithelial–myoepithelial carcinoma are the most common new subtypes of the World Health Organization 1991 classification. *PLGA* is a solid, ovoid, noncapsulated mass with a highly variable growth pattern (Fig. 43.8A). Most are located in the palate, and the prognosis generally is good, with a tendency to local and sometimes regional recurrences.[64,65] No distant metastases were seen in 34 patients with PLGA in the retrospective Dutch study. *Salivary duct carcinoma* resembles ductal breast cancer morphologically (Fig. 43.8B). They derive from excretory duct cells. They are usually located in the parotid gland and are highly aggressive.[32,66] They are frequently positive for androgen receptors and positive for HER-2/neu protein. However, gene amplification is seen in <50% of cases.[48] There is also a low-grade subtype, resembling breast atypical ductal hyperplasia and low-grade ductal carcinoma in situ. The prognosis is excellent.[67] *Epithelial–myoepithelial carcinoma* is mainly localized in the parotid gland. The tumors are composed of myoepithelial cells surrounded by epithelial-lined ducts resembling intercalated ducts. It is a low-grade tumor; all 14 patients of the Dutch study remained disease free. However, local recurrences may be encountered.[68] *Myoepithelial carcinomas* have exclusive myoepithelial differentiation. They are commonly seen in the parotid gland and the palate. Differentiation with other salivary glands cancers may be difficult. The prognosis is poor, with a 40% 5-year disease-free survival.[69] *Basal cell adenocarcinoma* is a low-grade tumor, predominantly seen in the parotid gland, with a high risk of local recurrence but a low risk of regional recurrences or distant metastases.[70] *Malignant oncocytoma* is a high-grade malignant tumor, characterized by oncocytes, with necrosis, perineural spread, vascular invasion, and a high risk of cervical lymph nodes.[71] Most tumors are found in the parotid or submandibular gland. Salivary gland cystadenocarcinoma is a low-grade tumor; two of three are localized in the parotid gland, with others in the oral cavity.[72] *Mucinous adenocarcinoma* is a high-grade malignancy of the palate and floor of the mouth, with a high risk for neck node and distant metastases.[73] Sebaceous carcinoma is mainly localized in the parotid gland and is a slow-growing, low-grade tumor.[74]

PROGNOSTIC FACTORS

A number of prognostic variables have been studied in the management of salivary gland cancer. In these studies, multivariate analyses have been performed considering locoregional control, distant metastases, and survival. Results of studies with a sufficient number of patients and follow-up are summarized in Table 43.5. Local control and overall survival are influenced by site, favoring tumors of the oral cavity.[21,75] T and N stages are independent variables for locoregional control, distant metastases, and survival, regardless of site.[8,21,34,52,58,59,75–77,78–79] As can be concluded from Table 43.5, in almost all studies histologic subtype is not an independent prognostic factor for locoregional control, but it plays a role in risk for distant metastases and overall survival.[21,75] The added prognostic value of cytologic and/or histologic factors in salivary carcinoma is limited, largely due to the combined prognostic value of other prognostic factors such as tumor size, N and M classification, and comorbidity.[80] Comorbidity is associated with overall survival, but not with disease-free survival.[63]

Oncogene expression has been evaluated in the search for additional prognostic factors. Expression of the oncoprotein p53 was found in an Italian study to be higher in malignant tumors than in benign tumors.[81] Furthermore, tumors with moderate-to-high expression of p53 were more frequently associated with regional and distant metastasis and a lower disease-free and overall actuarial survival rate compared with patients with no p53 expression. Univariate and multivariate analyses confirmed the independent prognostic value of p53 expression. Vascular endothelial growth factor significantly correlates with p53 expression and is an independent prognostic factor for survival for salivary gland cancer.[82] Overexpression of HER-2/neu was seen in approximately one-third of mucoepidermoid carcinomas in a series of 50 parotid gland cancers[83] and in approximately 20% of salivary duct carcinomas.[66,84] Overexpression was seen and appeared to be an independent marker of poor prognosis. It also has been associated with poor prognosis in carcinomas of the breast, ovary, and endometrium. Another molecular feature studied in relationship to prognosis is the DNA content in adenoid cystic carcinomas. DNA aneuploidy is correlated with the solid type and thus with poor prognosis.[57]

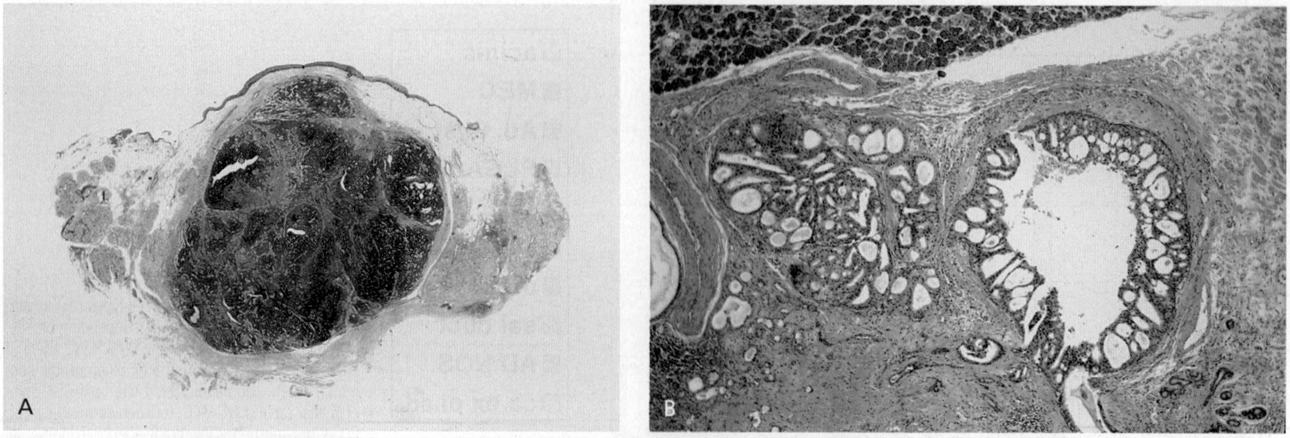

FIGURE 43.8. Examples of polymorphous low-grade adenocarcinoma **(A)** and salivary duct carcinoma **(B)**. (Courtesy of Prof. Dr. P. Slootweg, pathologist, Radboud University Medical Center, Nijmegen, Netherlands.)

TABLE 43.5 PROGNOSTIC FACTORS FOR SALIVARY GLAND CANCER–SELECTION OF MULTIVARIATE ANALYZED STUDIES

Study (by Name of First Author)	Number	Locoregional Control	Distant Metastases	Survival
General				
Terhaard[21,63]	565	L: T, site, bone+ R: N VII dysfunction, N L + R: Margin, therapy[a]	Sex, T, N, skin, histology, Perineural+	OS: Sex, age, T, skin+, bone invasion, comorbidity
Therskilden[75]	251	L: Histology, site, N, margin, therapy		DFS: Histology, stage, margin
Mendenhall[78]	224	L: T	Stage	DFS: Stage
Bjorndal[79]	871	L+R: Stage, margin, vascular invasion, grade		OS: Age, latency, stage, margin,vascular invasion
Chen, adenoid cystic[88]	140	L+R: T4, perineural invasion, no PORT, major nerve involvement		
Chen, surgery alone[91]	207	L+R: pN+, grade, margin, T3-T4		
Parotid				
Spiro[60]	470			OS: Stage, age, histology, site
Bhattacharryya[58]	903			OS: Age, T, N, extraglandular extension
Van der Poorten[22]	237			DFS: Age, pain, T, N, skin invasion, N VII dysfunction, perineural, margin
Poulsen[90]	209	L: Age, N, margin, grade		DFS: >4 nodes, sex, named nerve+, extraglandular extension
Garden[116]	166	L: N VII dysfunction, N		
Submandibular				
Bhattachatyya[53]	370			OS: Age, grade,
Storey[54]	83	Grade, histology, margin, early years		DS: Early years
Minor				
Jones[8]	103	L: T, N R: Stage		OS: T, general condition
Lopes[29]	103	N, histology, bone invasion		DFS: Stage, therapy[b]
Beckhardt[35]	116	Histology		DFS: Grade, T, margin
Parsons[30]	95	L: Stage, therapy[a]		DFS: Stage, therapy[a]

DFS, disease-free survival; L, local; OS, overall survival; R, regional; SG, salivary glands.
[a]Surgery + Radiotherapy > Surgery. [b]Surgery + Radiotherapy > Radiotherapy.

Major Salivary Glands

The survival of patients with submandibular cancers is inferior to that of patients with parotid cancers according to a study by Spiro et al.[60] Extraglandular extension[58,59] and skin invasion[22,52,85] in parotid cancers result in decreased disease-free survival. More-advanced age was found to be a negative prognostic factor for locoregional control in some studies[20,31,76] and for disease-free and overall survival in most studies.[22,52,58,60,77] Impairment of function of the facial nerve is a known prognostic factor, influencing not only locoregional control,[21,59,85] but also disease-free survival.[52,77,85,86] Pain at presentation may be associated with reduced disease-free survival.[52] Perineural invasion and pain are closely related: in some studies, not pain but perineural growth is an independent prognostic factor for distant metastases[21] or disease-free survival.[59,87,88]

The importance of histologic subtype for major salivary gland cancer varies in published studies. In most studies, histologic types are subdivided into low and high grade. The main prognostic significance of grading relates to disease-free survival,[58,79,82] although grade was not a prognostic factor in most studies. The best prognosis is seen for acinic cell and (low-grade) mucoepidermoid cancer,[21,60] the worst for undifferentiated[21,85] and squamous cell cancer.[21,60] At the Netherlands Cancer Institute, a prognostic score for patients with parotid carcinoma was developed and validated.[22,52] The preoperative prognostic score is based on a weighted combination of prognostic factors (age, pain, clinical T and N stages, skin invasion, and facial nerve dysfunction); histology and grading are not incorporated. Four subgroups were formed, with markedly different prognoses. In the postoperative score, perineural invasion and positive surgical margins were also included. In adenoid cystic carcinoma, named major nerve involvement is a prognostic factor; however, this may not be true for microscopic invasion only.[89] Positive or close surgical margins result in an increase in local recurrence rate.[21,54,75,79,90,91] Radiation therapy in addition to surgery improves locoregional control in patients with adverse prognostic factors.[20,24,75,85,88,92,93] Improvement of survival has only been shown in two studies[53,85] and for stage III and IV major salivary glands in a matched-pair analysis.[94]

Minor Salivary Glands

The poorest prognosis is associated with adenoid cystic carcinoma.[29,35] Stage, base-of-skull involvement, and bone invasion are risk factors for locoregional recurrence and survival in minor salivary gland cancers.[8,29,35,90,95] Locoregional control may be improved by adding postoperative radiotherapy.[30]

GENERAL MANAGEMENT

The general management of salivary gland malignancies in most patients includes surgical excision, followed by radiation therapy for unfavorable prognostic factors (Table 43.5). Postoperative radiotherapy to enhance local control is recommended for T3–4 tumors, close or incomplete resection, bone involvement, perineural invasion, high-grade cancer, and recurrent cancer.[21,35,54,59,76,85] Postoperative radiotherapy is indicated for patients with neck node lymph metastases.[21,91] Elective neck radiotherapy prevents nodal relapses in a selected group of patients, but in general is not indicated for acinic cell or adenoid cystic carcinoma.[96] According to Chen et al.,[88,93] for carcinoma ex pleomorphic adenoma of the parotid gland and adenoid cystic carcinoma, surgery and postoperative local radiotherapy is the standard. Concurrent postoperative platinum- and/or paclitaxel-based chemoradiotherapy for high-risk patients (nodal involvement, microscopic positive margins, T3/T4, perineural involvement) may result in 3-year locoregional control of >90%, although in the published data the number of patients is small, the follow-up is short, and the acute toxicity is more severe.[97,98] In a small (n = 24) matched control study, postoperative platinum-based chemoradiation for locally advanced major salivary gland cancer improved overall survival significantly compared to postoperative radiation alone; of interest, progression-free survival was only 55% for both groups.[99] In general, there is little proof that for salivary gland cancer concurrent postoperative chemoradiotherapy is superior to postoperative radiation alone. For advanced, inoperable, and recurrent salivary gland cancers, primary neutron therapy may lead to superior local control rates compared with primary photon therapy, without evidence of improved survival rates.[95,100,101] The use of conventional radiation therapy along with hyperthermia has been reported to have similar efficacy in this patient population.[102]

Major Salivary Glands

Surgical technique depends on location and extent of primary disease and regional adenopathy. Preservation of the facial nerve, at least partially, followed by postoperative radiotherapy is the preferable treatment unless the facial nerve is involved by tumor.[103] Aggressive surgery does not improve disease-free survival. A decrease in extended surgery, resulting in a decrease of sacrifice of the facial nerve, has been shown in the course of years.[60] Cable facial nerve grafting with the greater auricular or sural nerve graft decreases the incidence of facial palsy postoperatively, especially if branches and not the main trunk are involved.[104] Adjuvant postoperative radiotherapy has no negative effect on facial nerve function.[104]

Surgical treatment includes neck dissection in cases of clinically positive nodes, followed by postoperative radiotherapy.[24] The risk of occult nodal disease depends on T stage and histologic type.[24,96] As shown in the scoring system in Table 43.1, the decision to treat the neck for parotid tumors is indicated by a score of at least 4.[24] When local prognostic factors indicate postoperative radiotherapy, no elective neck dissection has to be performed; the neck nodes will also be irradiated.[25,105] Parotid tumors with facial nerve weakness are associated with frequent occult neck nodes; elective treatment is also indicated.[105] The first echelon neck nodes in parotid salivary gland cancer are the intraparotideal,[27,106] followed by level II, III, and IV nodes.[96,107] Involvement of level I nodes is an independent risk factor for disease-free survival.[106] Level I and V nodes are only involved if other levels are positive.[107] Contralateral nodes are not at risk. Thus, in case of prophylactic treatment of the clinical N0 neck, at least levels II and III should be incorporated, followed by postoperative radiotherapy in case of pathologic positive nodes of levels I to V. In most cases, elective neck dissection of levels I to III combined with a local resection is performed for submandibular tumors. There is no indication for neck dissection for T1 acinic or T1 adenoid cystic tumors (Table 43.1).[24,54,96]

Minor Salivary Glands

The treatment of minor salivary gland tumors varies with location but usually involves an attempt at adequate surgical excision first. Irradiation has been used in surgically inaccessible sites or combined with surgery because of locally aggressive tumor behavior and the occurrence of incomplete resection.[21,30,35,108] For tumors arising in the palate, tongue, floor of the mouth, oral cavity, or oropharynx, surgical exposure is readily available, and resection usually can be accomplished with acceptable morbidity. Tumors arising in the posterior nasal cavity, nasopharynx, or sphenoid region, however, are relatively inaccessible and are mostly treated with radiation therapy.[108] The indication of elective neck treatment may depend on a prognostic index (sore 0 to 4) using four clinicopathologic factors associated with increased risk on positive nodes: male sex, stage T3/T4, pharyngeal location, and high grade.[28] For a score of ≥2, elective treatment of the neck nodes is indicated. Surgery alone may be used to treat early-stage hard-palate lesions without evidence of positive margins, perineural spread, or bone invasion; simple excision must be avoided.[35] Patients with adenoid cystic carcinoma can have a long natural history with late recurrences,[108] and consideration should be given to careful surgical reconstruction and rehabilitation because even patients who are not cured can live many years before dying of disease (see Fig. 43.3).[21] Occasionally, a patient may present after simple excision (shelling out) of a lesion, and the pathologic examination shows adenoid cystic carcinoma. If re-excision would cause significant functional or cosmetic sequelae, irradiation alone may be used.[30] However, simple excision is not recommended as the initial management of these tumors because of the potential for a significant volume of residual disease.

RADIATION THERAPY TECHNIQUES

Pleomorphic Adenoma

Pleomorphic adenoma (benign mixed tumor) is histologically benign, occurs frequently in a relatively young population, and comprises 65% to 75% of all parotid epithelial tumors.[60] Standard therapy has been conservative (superficial) parotidectomy, with recurrence rates of about 0% to 5%.[109] Simple excision results in a high recurrence rate of around 25%, as focal capsular exposure occurs in virtually all cases.[109] In the past at some institutions, local excision and radiation therapy were used to lower the frequency of facial nerve injury and Frey's syndrome.[110] Dawson and Orr[110] reported results for 311 patients. They found a 2.5% recurrence rate at 10 years and an additional 5.5% by 20 years. None of the patients had malignant recurrences at 10 years, 0.5% had such recurrences at 15 years, and 3% had recurrences at 20 years. The later recurrences were more likely to show malignant transformation. The authors concluded that the primary treatment should be surgery because of the patient's young age, the benign histology, and the remote possibility of subsequent radiation-induced malignancy. However, certain patients may be referred for radiation therapy.[111] In a study by Riad et al.[112] tumor size of >4 cm, adherence to the facial nerve, and close safety margins, were confounding factors for recurrence, however, because were they correlated with tumor puncture and spillage. Indications for postoperative irradiation may include recurrent disease; microscopically positive margins after surgical resection; and large, deep-seated lesions that may not allow complete surgical excision with adequate margins or would require sacrificing the facial nerve.[110,111,113,114] Radiotherapy may decrease the risk of a second recurrence in case of multinodular recurrence only but not for uninodular disease.[114] The entire parotid area should be irradiated with a dose of 50 to 60 Gy in 5 to 6 weeks. Figure 43.9 shows an example of a large, multicystic pleomorphic adenoma with a close safety margin and spillage during parotidectomy; postoperative radiotherapy was indicated.

Parotid Gland

The volume of irradiation is determined by pathologic findings, such as perineural invasion of a major nerve. Typically, the entire ipsilateral parotid gland is delineated on the postoperative CT scan performed in a custom-made head and neck mold.[59,115] The delineation of the clinical target volume is individualized based on the extent of the disease and surgery.[59] In case of a tumor of the deep lobe, the parapharyngeal space and the infratemporal fossa have to be covered adequately.[115] In general it is not necessary to treat the scar to full skin dose because only 1% of the patients have a scar failure.[76] For very superficial localized tumors and in case of skin invasion, a bolus over the scar is required. In tumors with named perineural invasion (e.g., adenoid cystic carcinoma) the nerve provides a route to the base of skull. Thus, it is important to cover the cranial nerve pathways from the parotid up to the base of the

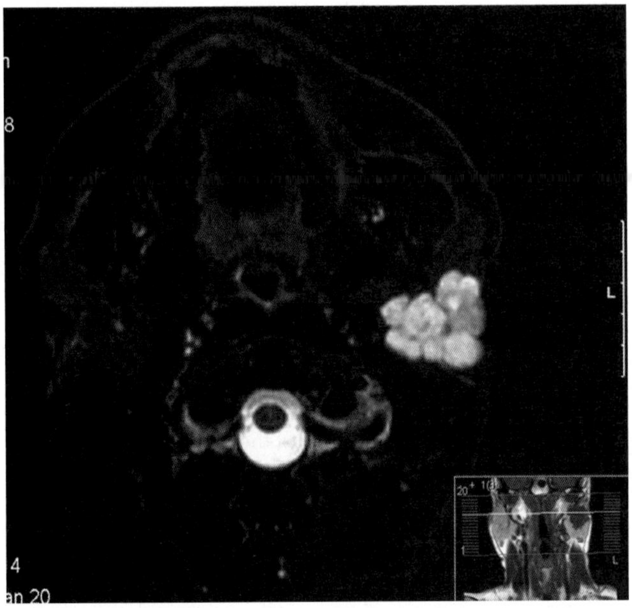

FIGURE 43.9. Multicystic pleomorphic adenoma, T2 short tau inversion recovery, transverse slice.

skull.[89,116] In perineural invasion, postoperative radiotherapy with a dose of 50 Gy, including the base of the skull, decreased local recurrence rate from 15% with surgery alone to 5% with combined surgery and radiotherapy in a study by Chen et al.[117] Focal perineural invasion only is not an indication for routine inclusion of the nerve pathways.[116] A clear relationship between dose and local control was only found by Chen et al.,[88] a dose of ≥60 Gy resulted in significant higher local control rates. In general, a dose of at least 60 Gy postexcision is recommended[24,88,115,116] and at least 66 Gy (33 fractions) for high-risk patients with positive margins (<1 mm).[59,116]

The ipsilateral neck is treated after a neck dissection has been performed for positive nodes; levels I to V should be included.[24] There is no indication for bilateral elective neck treatment.[25,27,96] The recommended postoperative dose for positive nodes is at least 60 Gy (30 fractions) and is 66 Gy for extranodal disease.[24] Elective irradiation of the neck should be considered for advanced T stage, certain histologic subtypes (Table 43.1), facial nerve dysfunction at presentation, and recurrent disease. The intraparotideal nodes should be included.[27,106] At least in early high-risk parotid cancer, levels II and III should be included.[27] Levels I and V are seldom positive if only one positive node is diagnosed. However, because in elective treatment the number of possible positive nodes is unknown, most authors advise treatment of levels Ib to IV prophylactically.[24,105,118] A dose of approximately 46 to 50 Gy is recommended.[24,59]

Three basic radiation therapy approaches are used, depending on available equipment: conventional, three-dimensional conformal radiation therapy (3DCRT), and intensity-modulated radiation therapy (IMRT). The first involves unilateral anterior and posterior wedged pair fields using ^{60}Co or 4- to 6-MV photons (Fig. 43.10A). Typical field boundaries are the zygomatic arch superiorly, the masseter muscle anteriorly, the pterygoid muscle and ramus mandibulae laterally, the mastoid process posteriorly, and the posterior belly of the digastric muscle inferiorly.[93] A slight inferior angulation of the beams avoids an exit dose through the contralateral eye. A simpler technique uses

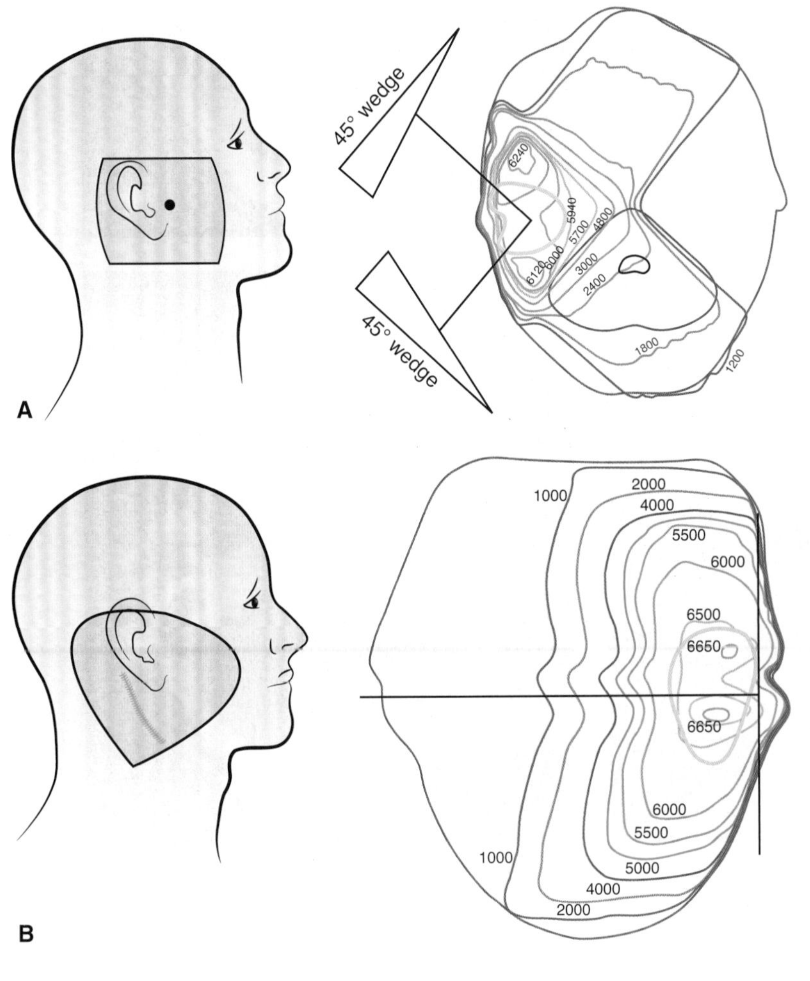

FIGURE 43.10. Conventional radiotherapy for parotid cancer. **A:** Unilateral wedge arrangement and isodose distribution using wedged pair. **B:** Ipsilateral 16-MeV electrons plus ^{60}Co (4:1) electron beam field.

homolateral fields with 12- to 16-MeV electrons in combination with photons.[69,119] Usually, 80% of the dose is delivered with electrons and 20% with ^{60}Co or 4- to 6-MV photons to spare the opposite salivary gland, reduce mucositis, and decrease the skin reaction produced by electrons (Fig. 43.10B). Yaparpalvi et al.[119] compared nine conventional treatment techniques. Ipsilateral wedge pair technique with 6-MV photons, wedged anteroposterior and posteroanterior and lateral technique with 6-MV photons, and mixed beam using 6-MV photons and 16-MeV electrons (1:4 weighted) were most optimal, considering dose homogeneity within the target and dose to normal tissues. Electron beam (9 to 12 MeV) and tangential photon fields are effective conventional techniques for sparing the underlying spinal cord (from doses >45 Gy) and the opposite parotid gland in elective neck irradiation. Conventional techniques do not allow for tissue heterogeneity (air cavity, dense bones, and tissues); underdose and overdose may be seen. Thus, conformal techniques should be the treatment of choice.

After outlining of the target volumes and critical normal tissues on the planning CT scan, a more conformal 3DCRT plan may be reached by the use of geometrically shaped beams of uniform intensity.[115] More normal tissue may be spared with this technique.[115,120] In case of named perineural invasion a 3D maximum-intensity projection T2 MRI technique performed in treatment position may be used to delineate the cranial nerves (see Fig. 43.5). Probably the most conformal radiation technique is IMRT. It can produce convex dose distributions and steep dose gradients. Five- to seven-field inverse IMRT allows excellent coverage of the tumor with sparing of mandible, cochlea, spinal cord, brain, and oropharynx[121,122–123] compared with conformal 3DCRT. In particular, the dose to the cochlea and Eustachian tube should be <45 to 50 Gy.[124,125] IMRT may spare the inner ear if the distance of the planning target volume is >6 mm.[122] Figure 43.11 shows a comparison of 3DCRT and IMRT planning for a postoperative radiotherapy plan for a parotid cancer, without named nerve involvement, treated with a dose of 66 Gy. The mean dose to the mastoid, meatus acusticus externus, and contralateral parotid gland was 53 and 43 Gy, 57 and 51 Gy, 1 and 9 Gy for 3DCRT and IMRT, respectively. The maximum dose to the cochlea was 39 and 32 Gy,

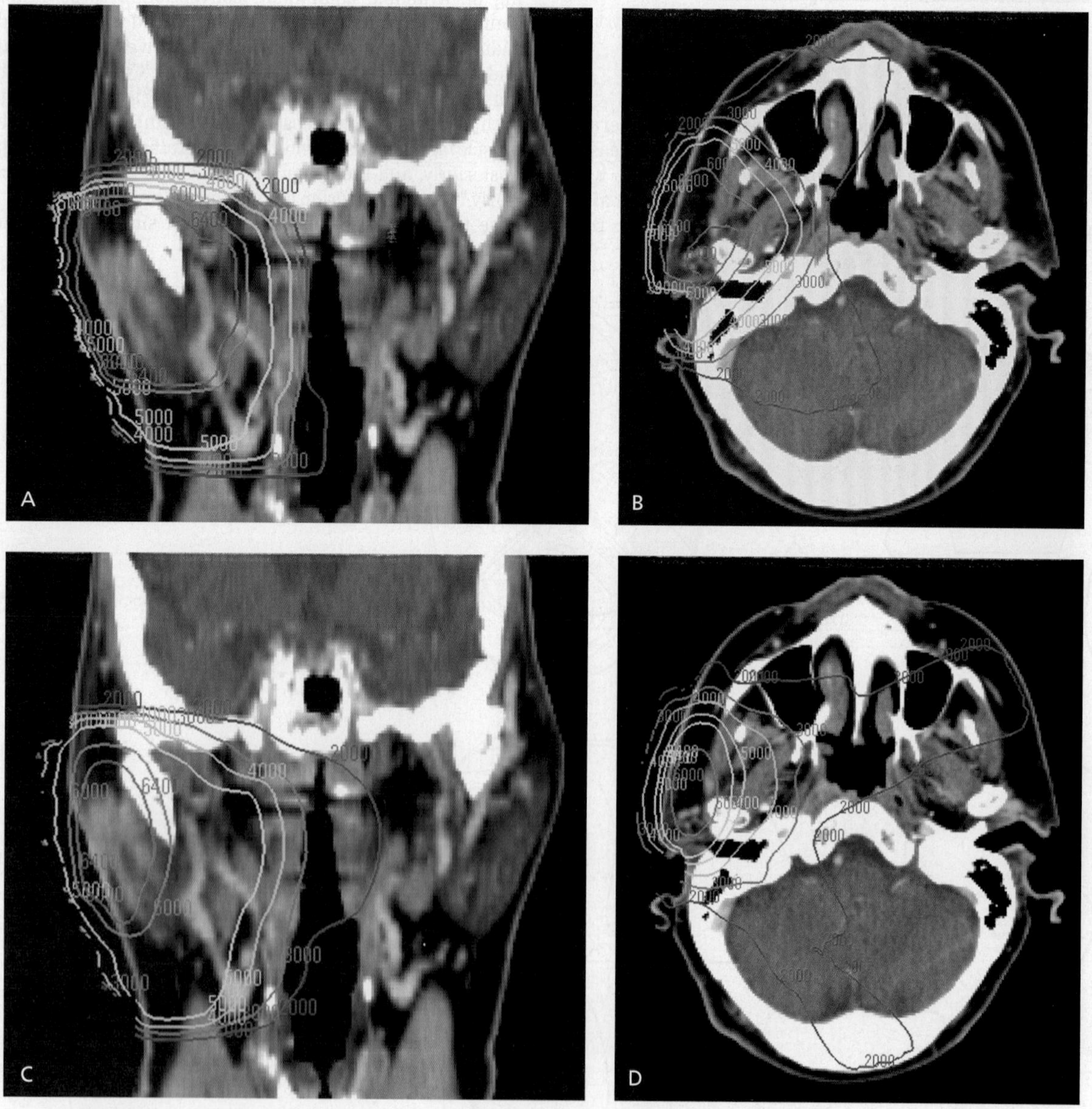

FIGURE 43.11. Postoperative radiation therapy of a parotid cancer, microscopically incompletely resected. Coronal **(A,C)** and transverse **(B,D)** dose distribution for three-dimensional conformal radiation therapy (25 × 2 Gy primary field, 8 × 2 Gy boost) **(A,B)** and intensity-modulated radiation therapy (inverse, seven fields and 39 segments; simultaneously moderated accelerated radiotherapy: 33 × 1.6 Gy primary field, 33 × 2 Gy boost) **(C,D)**.

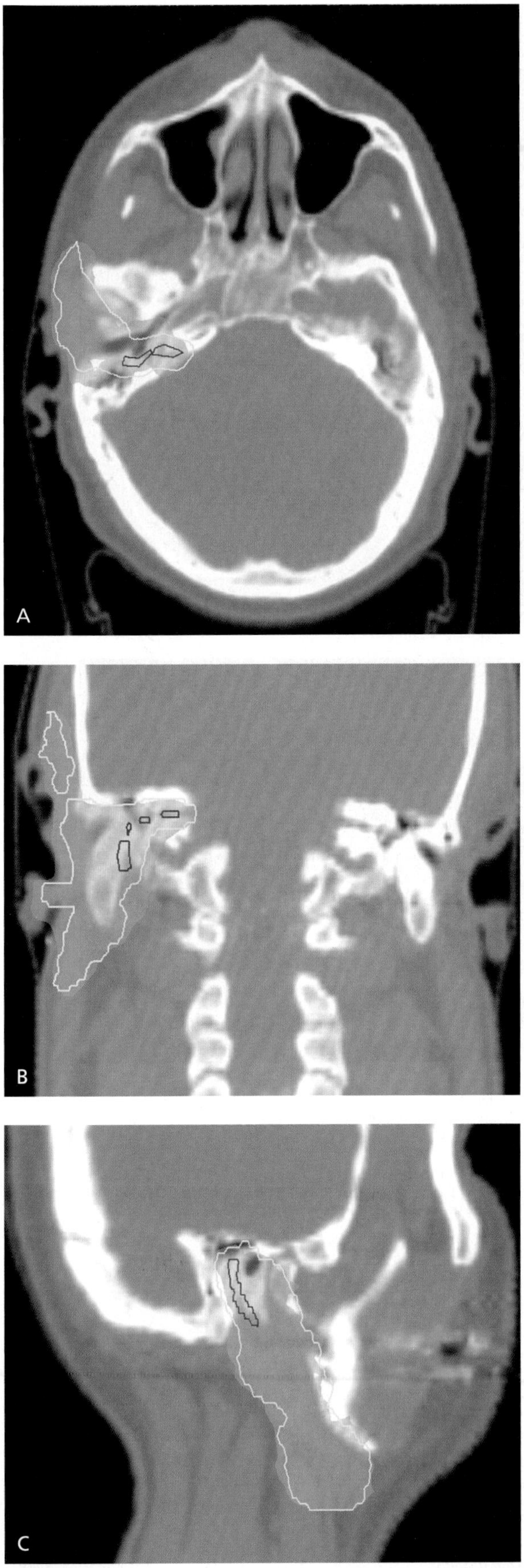

FIGURE 43.12. Recurrent adenocarcinoma of the parotid gland with named nerve involvement (nerve VII, in blue) delineated on base of magnetic resonance image (Fig. 43.5B). A unilateral intensity-modulated radiation therapy technique was used (yellow, 50 Gy isodose; boost not shown). Transverse **(A)**, coronal **(B)**, and sagittal **(C)** planes.

respectively. Figure 43.12 shows a patient with a recurrent adenocarcinoma of the parotid gland with named perineural involvement, for whom a total parotidectomy was performed. The resection was incomplete. The facial nerve was delineated based on MRI (see Fig. 43.5B). A unilateral IMRT technique was used.

Submandibular Gland

Except for small acinic cell and adenoid cystic cancers (Table 43.1), the neck node levels I to IV[118] should be irradiated electively, following the indications outlined for parotid tumors; technical considerations are similar. Bilateral fields may be required for tumor extension toward the midline. Five-year locoregional control was significant higher for a dose of >56 Gy in a study by Mallik et al.[126] If there is named perineural invasion of a major nerve, a tumor dose of 60 to 66 Gy in 6 to 6.5 weeks is recommended, and the nerve path to the base of skull should be treated, preferably by 3DCRT or IMRT. For an adenoid cystic carcinoma of the submandibular gland with only focal perineural invasion, an attempt to encompass the base of the skull would require a significant change in the treatment volume and may not be warranted because of potential morbidity and the low rate of relapse at that site.[108] An example of 3DCRT for a T2 adenoid cystic carcinoma of the submandibular gland is shown in Figure 43.13.

Sublingual Gland

These tumors are mostly malignant, mostly adenoid cystic carcinoma, mostly advanced disease, and high grade, although with a low risk of positive neck nodes. Aggressive surgery is required, with postoperative local radiotherapy in almost all cases.[37] In case of named nerve involvement the lingual and/or hypoglossic nerve should be included in the radiation portals.

Minor Salivary Glands

The radiation therapy technique for treating minor salivary gland tumors depends on the area involved and is similar to the treatment for squamous cell carcinomas in these areas, with two significant exceptions. First, when a named branch of a cranial nerve is involved by adenoid cystic carcinoma, the nerve pathways to the base of the skull should be electively treated. When only focal perineural invasion of small, unnamed nerves is present, treatment of the base of the skull depends on the site. Second, for tumors of the palate or paranasal sinuses, the base of the skull is included because of its proximity to the tumor bed. In case of an adenoid cystic carcinoma with perineural invasion, IMRT may reduce the high-dose volume compared to conventional bilateral opposed fields. Figure 43.14 shows an example for a patient with a minor salivary gland cancer of the palate. IMRT is a useful strategy for irradiating minor salivary gland sites such as the ethmoid sinuses while sparing the optic pathways.[127]

In addition, because the incidence of lymph node metastases is usually lower than that for squamous cell carcinomas of similar size, the radiation therapy fields are rarely extended to cover such areas if there are no palpable lymph node metastases. Indications for elective treatment of the neck nodes may depend on a scoring system.[28] Typically, for male patients with a T3/T4 N0 pharyngeal-site tumor neck nodes should be treated prophylactically. In minor salivary gland cancers of the oral cavity elective radiation of the neck nodes is seldom indicated. Postoperative radiotherapy is indicated after resection of metastatic neck lymphadenopathy.

For patients receiving postoperative irradiation after surgical resection, a dose of 60 Gy is given for negative margins and 66 Gy for microscopically positive margins. For gross residual disease after surgery or for lesions treated with irradiation alone, a total dose of 70 Gy is recommended at 2 Gy per fraction.

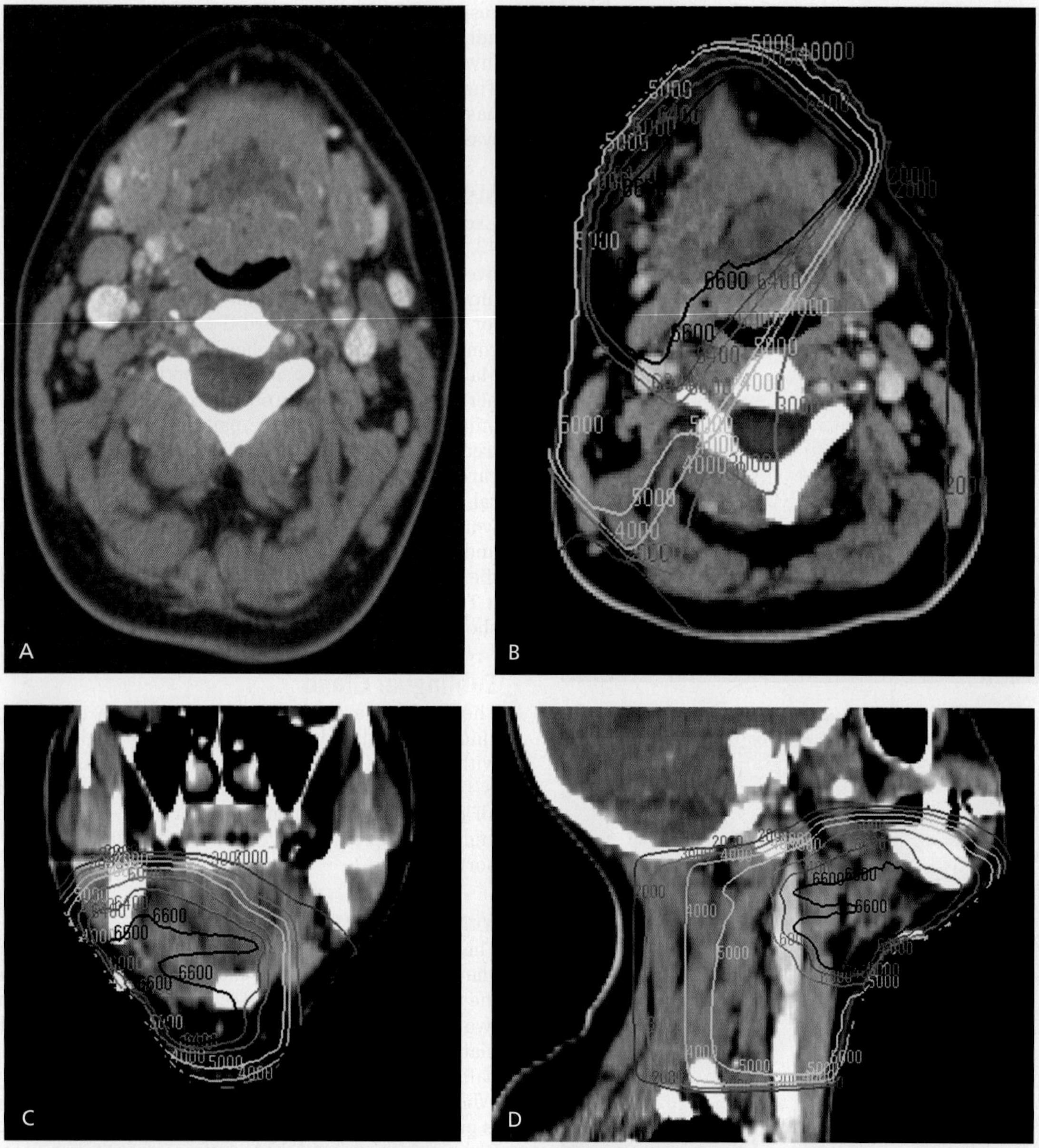

FIGURE 43.13. Dose distribution for a T2 N0 adenoid cystic cancer of the right submandibular gland. Computed tomography performed before microscopically incomplete local excision **(A)**. Three-dimensional conformal radiation therapy, three fields (one right and two left oblique): 25 × 2 Gy, 5 × weekly primary tumor and level I to III nodes, 8 × 2 Gy boost; transverse **(B)**, coronal **(C)**, and sagittal **(D)** planes. Mean dose to contralateral submandibular gland is 27 Gy.

RESULTS OF THERAPY

Surgery With or Without Postoperative Radiotherapy

Tables 43.6 through 43.8 list local control rates and 5- and 10-year survival rates for several series reporting the surgical, irradiation, and combination treatment of carcinomas of the major and minor salivary glands. Little adverse effect of delay between surgery and radiotherapy may be predicted for what are, in general, slow-growing salivary gland cancers. In three studies—one concerning submandibular cancer,[54] one for minor salivary gland,[108] and another for adenoid cystic cancer[88]—impaired locoregional control rates were seen for a delay of >6 weeks, which was not confirmed in the Dutch study.[24] The prognosis for children with a malignant salivary gland cancer (mostly mucoepidermoid cancer of the parotid gland) is excellent, with a 5-year overall survival of >90%.[9] Most are treated with surgery alone because of the possible risk of radiation-induced malignancies.

TABLE 43.6 RESULTS OF STANDARD THERAPY FOR CANCER OF THE PAROTID

Study (by Name of First Author)	*Number of Patients*	*Treatment*	*Five-Year Survival (%)*	*Ten-Year Survival (%)*	*Local Control (%)*
Bhattacharyya[58]	903	S ± R	67	50	NA
Spiro[7]	623	S	55	47	61
Terhaard[21]	37	S	67	61	51 (10 yr)
	254	S + R	65	51	88 (10 yr)
Garden[59]	166	S + R	78	60	90 (10 yr)
North[85]	19	S	59	NA	74
	50	S + R	75	NA	98
Poulsen[90]	209	S + R	71	65	76
Renehan[92]	37	S	77	63	57 (locoreg)
	66	S + R	78	67	85 (locoreg)
Pohar[20]	56	S	65	50	63 (locoreg)
	91	S + R	55	40	89 (locoreg)
Chen[93] (CexPA)	23	S	44	NA	49 (5 yr)
	40	S + R	59	NA	75 (5 yr)

CexPA, carcinoma ex pleomorphic adenoma; locoreg, locoregional; NA, not available; R, irradiation; S, surgery.

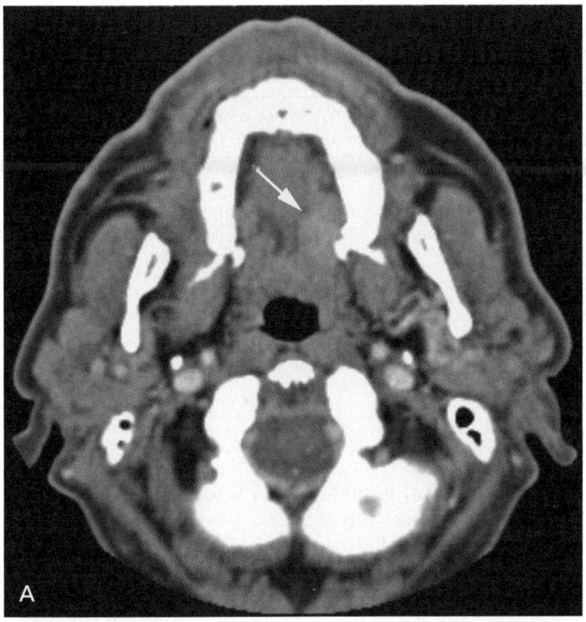

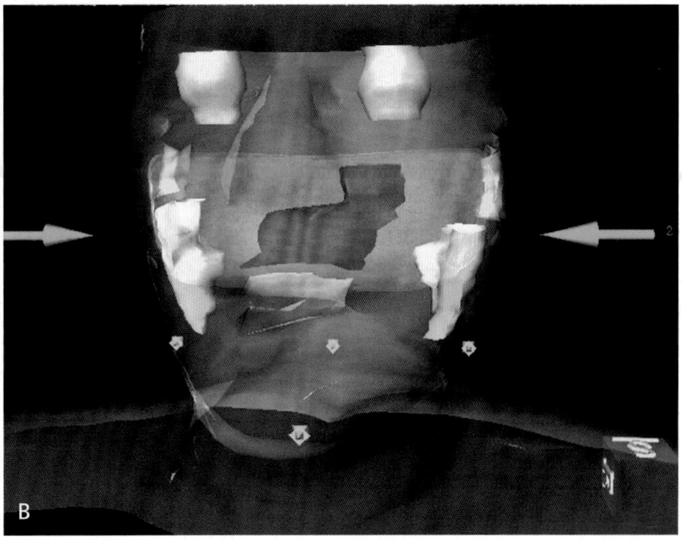

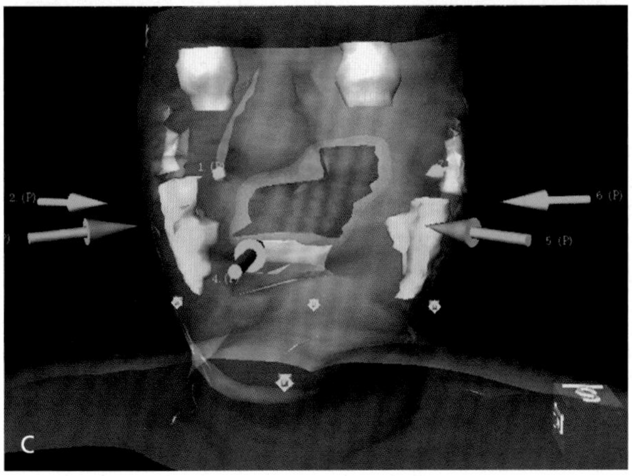

FIGURE 43.14. T2 N0 adenoid cystic cancer of the palate with major perineural invasion. Computed tomography performed before local excision (**A**, arrow: tumor); target includes right palatinus major nerve until the base of the skull. Dose distribution (25 × 2 Gy primary field) in transverse planes; conventional bilateral opposed fields **(B)**; intensity-modulated radiation therapy (seven fields, 40 segments) **(C)**; 95% isodose of 50 Gy in red.

Long-term follow-up is recommended because failures may appear after 5 years, especially for minor salivary gland tumors and adenoid cystic cancer.[8,21,64,65,88] Recurrent tumors in general are more difficult to control than are primary ones, so high initial locoregional control rates should be the goal. Because of high rates of local failure of approximately 40% for parotid, 60% for submandibular, and 65% for minor salivary glands with surgery alone in the past,[7] many institutions have advocated postoperative irradiation especially to reduce the incidence of local failure. Local tumor control appears to be improved by the combination of surgery and irradiation,

TABLE 43.7 RESULTS OF STANDARD THERAPY FOR CANCER OF THE SUBMANDIBULAR GLANDS

Study (by Name of First Author)	Number of Patients	Treatment	Five-Year Survival (%)	Ten-Year Survival (%)	Local Control (%)
Spiro[7]	129	S	31	22	40 (locoreg)
Terhaard[21]	68	S + R	57	45	91 (10 yr)
Storey[54]	83	S + R	60 (DFS)	53 (DFS)	88 (locoreg)
Bhattacharyya[53]	370	S ± R	60	NA	NA

DFS, disease-free survival; locoreg, locoregional; NA, not available; R, irradiation; S, surgery.

although randomized, controlled trials have not been performed. Evidence of a positive role of postoperative radiotherapy is based on retrospective studies and a matched-pair analysis. In the study by Armstrong et al.,[94] postoperative radiotherapy significantly improved locoregional control from 17% to 51% for stage III and IV, but not for stage I and II, major salivary gland cancer. Locoregional control for patients with positive nodes increased from 40% to 69%. In most studies, an imbalance in prognostic factors is seen when comparing surgery alone with combined therapy, favoring surgery alone. Despite this imbalance, locoregional control with combined surgery and postoperative radiotherapy is superior to surgery alone for patients with negative prognostic factors, irrespective of site.[21,24,54,75,78,88,93] In the nationwide Dutch study, the relative risk for surgery alone compared with combined treatment was 9.7 for local recurrence and 2.3 for regional recurrence.[24] In a study from Denmark, the relative risk of no radiotherapy versus radiotherapy was 4.7 for locoregional control.[75] Postoperative radiotherapy is particularly effective if there are close and microscopic positive resection margins, enhancing local control from around 50% to 80% to 95%.[24,75,88,90] Comparable results are noted for T3-T4 tumors and pathologically confirmed bone and perineural invasion.[24,78] For adenoid cystic carcinoma with perineural invasion, postoperative radiotherapy increased 10-year local control rates from 30% to 80% in a study by Chen et al.[88]

TABLE 43.8 RESULTS OF STANDARD THERAPY FOR MINOR SALIVARY GLANDS

Study (by Name of First Author)/Site	Number of Patients	Treatment	Five-Year Survival (%)	Ten-Year Survival (%)	Local Control (%)
Spiro[93]	526	S	48	37	35 (locoreg)
Garden[108]	160	S + R	81	65	88 (15 yr)
Terhaard[21]/oral cavity	67	S	87	76	91
	54	S + R	85	72	98
Lopes[29]/oral cavity	59	S	86	83	90 (locoreg)
	32	S + R	88	56	78 (locoreg)
	15	R	46	–	13 (locoreg)
Beckhardt[35]/palate	79	S	90 (DSS)	80 (DSS)	NA
	35	S + R	87 (DSS)	83 (DSS)	NA
Vander Poorten[47]	55	S ± R	66	57	76 (locoreg)
Schramm[31]/nasopharynx	23	S + R	67 (DSS)	48 (DSS)	77 (5 yr)

DSS, disease-specific survival; locoreg, locoregional; NA, not available; R, irradiation; S, surgery.

However, for a T1 or T2 tumor that was completely resected with no bone or perineural invasion, surgery alone will result in >90% 10-year local control rate, and radiotherapy is not indicated.[24]

Treatment results also may depend on histopathologic status. However, after review, histologic type may change, even among experienced pathologists. In general, the best prognosis is shown for acinic cell and mucoepidermoid cancers, with a 15% risk of distant metastases after 10 years and a 10-year locoregional control rate of approximately 85%. Ten-year overall survival is around 80% and 65%, respectively.[7,21,53,61] In one of three patients, postoperative radiotherapy is indicated.[21,61] Squamous cell and undifferentiated tumors have been associated with a 10-year overall survival of 35% or less, caused by a high risk of distant metastases (35% and 50%, respectively) and locoregional recurrence.[7,21,90] Postoperative radiotherapy is indicated in all cases to improve locoregional control. The intermediate-risk group consists of adenoid cystic cancer and cancer ex pleomorphic adenoma. Distant failure after 10 years is approximately 35%.[21,34,116] Although the risk of nodal recurrence is low (5% to 10%), local recurrence is diagnosed more often (20% to 30%). A precipitous decrease in relapse-free survival is noted at 5 (~70%), 10 (~50%), and 15 years (~45%) for patients with adenoid cystic carcinomas, which are well known for late recurrences.[21,88,116] Significant improvement was reported in local control for adenoid cystic cancer with combined surgery and irradiation in several studies,[54,88,92,116] regardless of site. Local tumor control rates with combined modality therapy for these tumors approach 85% to 90% at 10 years. Postoperative radiotherapy is also able to improve locoregional control rates, with a rate of approximately 20% for high-grade tumors.[54,77,92]

In the World Health Organization classification of 1991, among others, three new subtypes were described that are diagnosed relatively frequently. PLGA is situated almost solely in the palate. Treatment consists of wide local excision. In a report by Castle et al.,[64] treatment results on 164 tumors were analyzed, with 90% treated with surgery alone. Local control was 90%, with only few patients dying from PLGA. However, local failures may be seen even after long follow-up. In a series from Evans and Luna[65] of 40 patients with PLGA, local recurrence was seen in 43% of patients treated with surgery alone, mainly because of close and microscopic positive resection margins. No recurrence was seen in the 9 patients treated with postoperative radiotherapy.

Salivary duct carcinoma is a very aggressive disease, and postoperative locoregional radiotherapy is indicated in all cases. Most patients die of the disease, despite often successful locoregional combined therapy. Because of the high percentage of distant metastases, 5-year survival is only approximately 10% to 15%. The prognosis correlates with HER-2/*neu* receptor status; 3-year survival is 56% and 17% for (+)HER-2/*neu* and (+++)HER-2/*neu*, respectively.[66]

Epithelial–myoepithelial cancers have a very favorite outcome, with a risk of distant metastases <5% and a disease-free survival of >80% after 10 years. However, local recurrences may be seen in one out of three, and postoperative local radiotherapy is indicated in case of incomplete margin, tumor necrosis, lymphatic invasion, and myoepithelial anaplasie.[68]

Minor salivary gland tumors of the oral cavity have a more favorable prognosis than paranasal sinus tumors (maxillary and ethmoid sinus and nasal cavity).[108] Patients with hard-palate lesions tend to be diagnosed when they have small asymptomatic lumps, which are easily detected on physical examination. On the other hand, paranasal sinus tumors usually do not cause symptoms until they are locally advanced. The surgical approach for these tumors is more difficult, with a greater chance for leaving behind residual disease, leading to high recurrence rates. A combined approach with surgery and postoperative irradiation is recommended.

Primary Radiotherapy

The poor results for salivary gland cancer with irradiation alone in several series have been attributed to the use of primary radiotherapy for patients with locally advanced lesions or distant metastases at presentation, who were essentially treated for palliation. Locoregional control rates after conventional photon or electron therapy are approximately 25%.[78,100,101] For treatment with photons with curative intent, a clear dose–response relationship has been described.[24,128] A dose of at least 66 to 70 Gy should be adopted, resulting in a 5-year local control of 50& to 70%. Wang and Goodman[129] reported local control as high as 85% with accelerated hyperfractionated photon therapy. The follow-up was rather short, and the results have not been updated. The generally slow rate of regression of advanced salivary gland tumors has made them a logical target for alternative radiation therapy approaches, such as fast neutrons.

Neutron Therapy

Patients with inoperable primary or recurrent major or minor salivary glands were included in the Radiation Therapy Oncology Group–Medical Research Council randomized phase III clinical trial. Patients were randomized between 70 Gy for 7.5 weeks or 55 Gy for 4 weeks of photon therapy and neutron therapy. The study had to be stopped because of a statistically significant difference in 2-year locoregional control after inclusion of only 32 patients. The 10-year locoregional control probability was 17% after photon therapy and 56% after neutron therapy.[101] However, survival was identical. Late morbidity was somewhat higher for neutron therapy. Douglas et al.[95]

published results on 279 patients treated with neutrons. Almost all patients had evidence of gross residual disease. Major and minor salivary gland sites were equally distributed. Total dose, administered with neutrons, varied from 17.4 to 20.7 Gy. The 6-year locoregional control and cause-specific survival were 59% and 49%, respectively, conforming to the results of most studies. Locoregional control was only 19% for base of skull involvement and 67% for no involvement. Locoregional control was 72% for minor sites and 61% for major sites. The 6-year actuarial grade 3 and 4 toxicity was 10%. Less severe late morbidity may occur if neutron therapy is combined with photons. A study from Heidelberg for advanced, inoperable, recurrent, or incompletely resected adenoid cystic carcinoma compared results of treatment with neutrons, photons, or mixed beams.[100] Severe late grade 3 and 4 toxicity was 19% with neutrons, compared to 10% with mixed-beam and 4% with photon therapy. The 5-year local control was 75% for neutrons and 32% for mixed beams and photons; survival was identical.

In an effort to improve poor results for tumors invading the base of skull, several new techniques have been developed. A combination of neutron therapy with, after a 4-week split, a Gamma Knife stereotactic radiosurgical boost has been used for tumors invading the base of the skull.[130] Compared to a historical control group treated with neutrons only, in 34 patients treated with combined neutrons and Gamma Knife the actuarial local control rate at 40 months was 82% versus 39% for the control group. Complications grades were equal.[130] Another option is a combination of photon (54 Gy) and carbon-ion (18 Gy) radiotherapy.[131] In a series of 16 patients with adenoid cystic cancer invading the base of skull, the 3-year local control was 65%, without late effects exceeding grade 2. Longer follow-up results of these new techniques are awaited.

In conclusion, neutron beam therapy seems to be the treatment of choice for unresectable, residual, or recurrent salivary gland tumors. Despite high locoregional control, survival is not improved, and late toxicity is of concern.

SYSTEMIC THERAPY

The rarity of these neoplasms and their localized nature provide limited opportunities for trials with chemotherapy. Most published studies concern small series with different histological subtypes, using a large variety of chemotherapy regimens. In a series of 17 cases from Katori and Tsukuda,[132] *combined* chemotherapy (cyclophosphamide, pirabucin, cisplatin) with radiotherapy (mean 64 to 72 Gy) for high-risk, stage III/IV untreated salivary gland cancer showed a pathologic complete response in only 24% of cases. Better results were shown for *concurrent* postoperative chemotherapy (paclitaxel, 5-fluorouracil, hydroxyurea) and radiotherapy (twice a day, 1.5 Gy; mean dose, 65 Gy) in high-risk salivary gland cancer by Pederson et al.[97] In 24 patients, a 5-year locoregional progression-free survival of 96% and a 5-year overall survival of 59% were reached. In a small case–control study of 24 patients comparing postoperative platinum-based chemoradiotherapy with postoperative chemoradiotherapy alone, 3-year overall survival was significant higher for the combined group (83% vs. 44%, respectively).[99] However, 3-year local progression-free survival was poor in both groups (61% vs. 44%, respectively). Thus, in general there is no proof of superiority for concurrent chemoradiotherapy in the curative setting.

In a phase II study *chemotherapy alone* (platinum and gemcitabine) for advanced, metastatic, or locoregionally recurrent salivary gland cancer showed an objective, modest response of 8 of 30 patients with a mean duration of 6 months.[133]

In the *palliative* setting cisplatin as monotherapy showed a 20% response rate for locoregional disease and only 7% for distant failures, with duration of 6 to 9 months. A combination of 5-fluorouacil, cyclophosphamide, cisplatin, and doxorubicin gave a response rate of 50%.[134] Palliative chemotherapy may be beneficial in patients who have progressive, symptomatic disease with no other treatment options. In adenoid cystic carcinoma (ACC) single-agent vinorelbine, epirubicin, and mitoxantrone are first-line options, and for combined regimens cisplatin and antracyclines are recommended.[135]

Molecular targeting therapy is a promising cancer treatment option. A variety of drugs targeting specific pathways are used in the palliative treatment of salivary gland cancer. The molecular pathology of salivary gland cancer was reviewed by Stenner and Klussman.[136] Locati et al.[137] performed treatment-relevant target immunophenotyping in a large series of 139 patients with primary, recurrent, and metastatic salivary gland cancer. Tyrosine kinase receptors and epidermal growth factor receptor (EGFR) were positive in 70% for all histologic subtypes. C-KIT was positive in 78% of the ACC. HER-2/NEU was positive in 44% of salivary duct carcinomas (SDCs) and in 21% of adenocarcinomas not otherwise specified (NOS). Hormonal receptor status was also determined. In SDC and adenocarcinoma NOS, androgen receptor was positive in 43% and 21%, respectively.[137] Her-2/NEU and EGFR were positive in 26% and 70%, respectively, in a study with 66 SDCs.[84] These findings could be exploited for selection of patients for molecular targeting treatment. However, the response rate of the investigated targeted therapy is limited. A promising role for antiandrogen deprivation has been shown in 10 patients with recurrent/metastatic SDC. Clinical benefit (palliation of symptoms, even for brain metastases) was seen in 50%, with a mean duration of 1 year.[138]

In the future, the role of molecular-targeted therapy for these salivary gland cancers has to be further established.

SEQUELAE OF TREATMENT

The most notable complication of treatment of parotid malignancies is facial nerve paralysis, which is often caused by the initial or a repeated surgical procedure. However, various series have shown that facial nerve sacrifice is rarely necessary unless the nerve is directly involved by tumor, particularly when postoperative irradiation is given.[60,90] When facial nerve sacrifice is required, facial nerve grafting and postoperative radiation therapy achieve comparable facial nerve function compared with unirradiated graft despite more negative prognostic factors.[104] Other postoperative sequelae, such as salivary fistulae and neuromas of the greater auricular nerve, are sometimes seen. Frey's syndrome (i.e., gustatory sweating) may occur in a few patients after parotid surgery, but it is rarely bothersome.[76]

Partial xerostomia after irradiation of the parotid gland is frequently observed and may be permanent. Trismus may result from radiation-induced fibrosis of the temporomandibular joint or the masseter muscles. It usually occurs when there is extensive tumor infiltration of the masseter muscle and high doses are given.

Radiotherapy to the parotid gland may result in complications along the auditory system. As late toxicity, external canalis stenosis, dryness, skin atrophy, and chronic otitis externa, resulting in conductive hearing loss, although rare, may be seen. Chronic otitis media has been documented in 35% to 40% of cases due to damage to the muscles of the Eustachian tube. This may lead to conductive hearing loss, and repeated myringotomies may be indicated.[123] Radiation-induced hearing loss mostly is caused by progressive endothelial damage to the vascularization of the inner ear. This will cause sensorineurinal hearing loss, cognitive impairment, and at the end decrease quality of life. However, most hearing loss is seen at >4,000 Hz; for daily use normal frequency ranges from 1,000 to 3,000 Hz. In a prospective study of patients treated for head and neck cancer a hearing loss of ≥10 dB at 2 years after radiotherapy was seen in 40% for 8,000 Hz and in 50% for 3,000 Hz.[125] A threshold of 45 Gy was seen at ≥2,000 Hz, also depending on age and baseline hearing loss.[125] In published results, the mean threshold dose for the cochlea and Eustachian tube for sensorineural hearing loss varies between 40 and 50 Gy.[123–125] The latency is around 1.5 to 2 years; after this time hearing loss stabilizes. The risk of sensorineural hearing loss depends on radiation technique. From 2D conventional to 3D conformal radiotherapy the mean dose to the cochlea may decrease from >50 Gy to approximately 40 Gy,[115,120] and further improvement is noted with the use of IMRT.[115,122] No dose–response relationship has been published for vestibular damage.[123]

Garden et al.[108] reported complications of irradiation in 51 of 160 patients receiving postoperative conventional 2D irradiation for minor salivary gland tumors. The most common complication was decreased hearing in 26 patients, 20 of whom had myringotomies or myringotomy tubes placed for serous otitis media. Bone necrosis or exposure was observed in several patients; however, this complication has been seen infrequently during the last decade with improved radiation therapy techniques and treatment of multiple, as opposed to single, fields per day. Complications to the eyes or optic pathways were most common in patients with paranasal sinus primary tumors. At least six cases of contralateral optic atrophy occurred. Other eye complications included dry eye syndrome, nasolacrimal duct obstruction, cataract, retinopathy, and perforated globe.[108] To reduce the incidence of bilateral blindness, the dose to the optic chiasm and contralateral optic nerve is limited to 54 Gy. In patients with extensive tumor involvement of the orbit, it may be preferable to remove the eye surgically rather than to subject the entire orbit to high doses. Radiation-induced injury to the visual pathway is dose dependent. None of the patients receiving a dose of <50 Gy developed optic neuropathy or chiasm injury, whereas the 10-year actuarial incidences of optic nerve chiasm injury is 5% and 30% for patients receiving 50 to 60 Gy and 61 to 78 Gy, respectively.[139]

Radiotherapy of tumors of the pharynx, and less frequently the oral cavity, may result in permanent complaints of xerostomia. In the largest published series the mean dose to the parotid glands that relates to 1-year xerostomia was 39 Gy; no threshold was seen.[140] A dose of <25 Gy is preferable to reach a low risk on xerostomia.[140] This serious late complication may be significantly reduced by the use of IMRT.[141,142] For patients with a dose to both parotid glands that exceeds at least 39 Gy, amifostine administration during head and neck radiotherapy may reduce the severity and duration of xerostomia 2 years after radiotherapy[143] without compromising locoregional control.

TREATMENT OF RECURRENCE

Re-treatment usually involves additional surgery, if feasible, and postoperative irradiation in previously unirradiated patients (Fig. 43.15). In the re-treatment of parotid neoplasms, preserving facial nerve function and obtaining local control are more difficult than for the initial tumor. Therapy consisting of surgery with postoperative irradiation has demonstrated enhanced local control, and facial nerve sacrifice may be necessary less often if this combination is used. In certain histologic subtypes (e.g., adenoid cystic carcinoma), re-treatment of locally recurrent disease yields prolonged survival. Aggressive local therapy for recurrent disease is indicated if the probability of long-term survival is high. Multimodality treatment may be beneficial for recurrence disease of minor salivary gland if initial tumor classification was T1/2.[144]

Chemotherapy also has been used for recurrent disease. Polychemotherapy for recurrent high-grade disease may result in around 45% response rate, with a median duration of 7.5

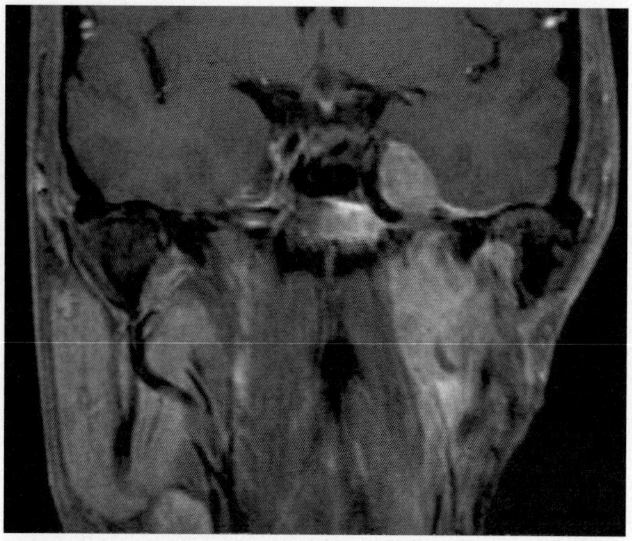

FIGURE 43.15. Coronal fat-suppressed, contrast-enhanced magnetic resonance image shows a recurrence of squamous cell cancer of the parotid gland after total parotidectomy. The tumor is centered in the left masticator space with perineural spread along the nV3. Retrograde perineural spread of the tumor through the foramen ovale on the left side. (Courtesy of Dr. F. A. Pameijer, radiologist, University Medical Center, Utrecht, Netherlands.)

months.[145] However, in view of its significant toxicity and modest response rates in a population that may have recurrent yet indolent progressive disease, trials of aggressive cytotoxic therapy are recommended only on carefully drafted protocols. In the future, molecular-targeted agents may be tested in selected recurrent salivary gland cancers.

SELECTED REFERENCES

A full list of references for this chapter is available online.

7. Spiro RH. Salivary neoplasms: Overview of a 35-year experience with 2,807 patients. *Head Neck Surg* 1986;8:177–184.
9. Sultan L, Rodriguez-Galindo C, Al-Sharabati S, et al. Salivary gland carcinomas in children and adolescents: a population-based study, with comparison to adult cases. *Head Neck* 2011;1476–1481.
21. Terhaard CHJ, Lubsen H, Van Der Tweel, et al. Salivary gland carcinoma: independent prognostic factors for locoregional control, distant metastases, and overall survival: results of the Dutch Head and Neck Oncology Cooperative Group. *Head Neck* 2004;26:681–693.
22. Van de Poorten V, Hart A, Vauterin T, et al. Prognostic index for patients with parotid carcinoma. *Cancer* 2009;115:540–550.
24. Terhaard CHJ, Lubsen H, Rasch CRN, et al. The role of radiotherapy in the treatment of malignant salivary gland tumors. *Int J Radiat Oncol Biol Phys* 2005;61:103–111.
26. Zbären P, Schüpbach J, Nuyens M, et al. Elective neck dissection versus observation in primary parotid carcinoma. *Otolaryngol Head Neck Surg* 2005;132: 387–391.
31. Régis de Brito Santos I, Kowalski LP, Cavalcante de Araujo V, et al. Multivariate analysis of risk factors for neck metastases in surgically treated parotid carcinoma. *Arch Otolaryngol Head Neck Surg* 2001;127:46–60.
38. Buchner A, Merrell PW, Carpenter WM. Relative frequency of intra-oral minor salivary gland tumors: a study of 380 cases from northern California and comparison to reports from other parts of the world. *J Oral Pathol Med* 2007;36: 207–214.
39. Lee YYP, Wong KT, King AD, et al. Imaging of salivary gland tumours. *Eur J Radiol* 2008;66:419–436.
41. Colella G, Cannavale R, Flamminio F, et al. Fine-needle aspiration cytology of salivary gland lesions: a systematic review. *J Oral Maxillofac Surg* 2010;68:2146–2153.
43. Thoeny HC. Imaging of salivary gland tumours. *Cancer Imaging* 2007;7:52–62.
46. Sobin LH, Gospodarowicz MK, Wittekind C. *TNM classification of malignant tumors*, 7th ed. Hoboken, NJ: Wiley-Blackwell, 2009.
48. Leivo I. Insights into a complex group of neoplastic disease: advances in histopathologic classification and molecular pathology of salivary gland cancer. *Acta Oncol* 2006;45:662–668.
49. Seifert G, Sobin LH. The World Health Organization's histological classification of salivary gland tumors. *Cancer* 1992;70:379–385.
52. Vander Poorten VLM, Balm AJM, Hilgers FJM, et al. The development of a prognostic score for patients with parotid carcinoma. *Cancer* 1999;85:2057–2067.
54. Storey MR, Garden AS, Morrison WH, et al. Postoperative radiotherapy for malignant tumors of the submandibular gland. *Int J Radiat Oncol Biol Phys* 2001; 51:952–958.
59. Garden AS, el-Naggar AK, Morrison WH, et al. Postoperative radiotherapy for malignant tumors of the parotid gland. *Int J Radiat Oncol Biol Phys* 1997; 79–85.

63. Terhaard CHJ, Schroeff MP, Schie K. The prognostic role of comorbidity in salivary gland carcinoma. *Cancer* 2008;113(7)1572–1579.
66. Jaehne M, Roeser K, Jaekel T, et al. Clinical and immunohistologic typing of salivary duct carcinoma. A report of 50 cases. *Cancer* 2005;103:2526–2533.
78. Mendenhall WM, Morris CG, Amdur RJ, et al. Radiotherapy alone or combined with surgery for salivary gland carcinoma. *Cancer* 2005;103:2544–2550.
79. Bjørndal K, Krogdahl A, Therkildsen MH, et al. Salivary gland carcinoma in Denmark 1990–2005: outcome and prognostic factors. Results of the Danish Head and Neck Cancer Group (DAHANCA). *Oral Oncol* 2012;48:179–185.
91. Chen AM, Granchi PJ, Garcia J, et al. Local regional recurrence after surgery without postoperative irradiation for carcinomas of the major salivary glands: implications for adjuvant therapy. *Int J Radiat Oncol Biol Phys* 2007;67:982–987.
94. Armstrong JG, Harrison LB, Spiro RH, et al. Malignant tumors of major salivary gland origin. *Arch Otolaryngol Head Neck Surg* 1990;116:290–293.
96. Chen AM, Garcia J, Lee NY, et al. Patterns of nodal relapse after surgery and postoperative radiation therapy for carcinomas of the major and minor salivary glands: what is the role of elective neck irradiation? *Int J Radiat Oncol Biol Phys* 2007;67:988–994.
101. Laramore GE, Krall JM, Griffin TW, et al. Neutron versus photon irradiation for unresectable salivary gland tumors: final report of an RTOG-MRC randomized clinical trial. *Int J Radiat Oncol Biol Phys* 1993;27:235–240.
105. Ferlito A, Pellitteri PK, Robbins T, et al. Management of the neck in cancer of the major salivary glands, thyroid and parathyroid glands. *Acta Otolaryngol* 2002;122:673–678.
110. Dawson AK, Orr JA. Long-term results of local excision and radiotherapy in pleomorphic adenoma of the parotid. *Int J Radiat Oncol Biol Phys* 1985;11:451–455.
115. Nutting CM, Rowbottom CG, Cosgrove VP, et al. Optimisation of radiotherapy for carcinoma of the parotid gland: a comparison of conventional, three-dimensional conformal, and intensity-modulated techniques. *Radiother Oncol* 2001;60:163–172.
120. Jereczek-Fossa BA, Rondi E, Zarowski A, et al. Prospective study on the dose distribution to the acoustic structures during postoperative 3D conformal radiotherapy for parotid tumors. *Strahlenther Onkol* 2011;187:350–356.
121. Bragg CM, Conway J, Robinson MH. The role of intensity-modulated radiotherapy in the treatment of parotid tumors. *Int J Radiat Oncol Biol Phys* 2002;52:729–738.
125. Pan CC, Eisbruch A, Lee JS, et al. Prospective study of inner ear radiation dose and hearing loss in head-and-neck cancer patients. *Int J Radiat Oncol Biol Phys* 2005;61:1393–1402.
128. Chen AM, Bucci MK, Quivey JM, et al. Long-term outcome of patients treated by radiation therapy alone for salivary gland carcinomas. *Int J Radiat Oncol Biol Phys* 2006;66:1044–1050.
130. Douglas JG, Goodkind R, Laramore GE. Gamma knife stereotactic radiosurgery for salivary gland neoplasms with base of skull invasion following neutron radiotherapy. *Head Neck* 2008;30:492–496.
133. Laurie SA, Ho AL, Fury MG, et al., Systemic therapy in the management of metastatic or locally recurrent adenoid cystic carcinoma of the salivary glands: a systematic review. *Lancet Oncol* 2011;12:815–824.
136. Stenner M, Klussmann JP. Current update on established and novel biomarkers in salivary gland carcinoma pathology and the molecular pathways involved. *Eur Arch Otorhinolaryngol* 2009;266:333–341.
138. Jaspers HCJ, Verbist BM, Schoffelen R, et al. Androgen receptor-positive salivary duct carcinoma: a disease entity with promising new treatment options. *J Clin Oncol* 2011;16:473–476.

Chapter 44
Oral Cavity

Rafael R. Mañon, Jeffrey N. Myers, Heath D. Skinner, and Paul M. Harari

The oral cavity consists of the lips, oral tongue, floor of the mouth, retromolar trigone, alveolar ridge, buccal mucosa, and hard palate (Figs. 44.1 to 44.3). Classification of tumors by subsite is useful because patterns of spread and clinical outcomes vary by specific subsite, partly reflecting the variable risk of nodal spread by anatomic site of presentation. Cancer of the oral cavity makes up approximately 30% of head and neck region tumors and 3% of all cancers in the United States.[1] Surveillance Epidemiology and End Results (SEER) program data estimate 23,880 cases of cancer of the oral tongue, mouth, and oral cavity for 2010 in the United States.[2] The incidence rate of oral cancer is more than twice as high in men as in women.[3–5] For all stages, the estimated 1-year survival rate after diagnosis is 84%, while the 5-year and 10-year survival rates are 61% and 51%, respectively.[3,6] The incidence has been declining by more than 1.4% per year in men and by 1.1% in women since 1992.[6] According to American Cancer Society statistics, mortality rates from carcinoma of the oral cavity and pharynx have decreased by 2% per year over the past three decades.[4]

Worldwide, the incidence of oral cancer parallels the tobacco epidemic. Global estimates suggest 263,900 new cases of oral cancer and 128,000 deaths related to oral cancer in 2008.[7] International Agency for Research on Cancer data indicate that the highest rates of oral cancer are found in Melanesia, South-Central Asia, and Eastern Europe. Over the past two decades, oral cancer mortality rates appear to be decreasing in most countries. However, mortality rates in several Eastern European countries, including Hungary and Slovakia, continue to increase.[2,8] This unfavorable trend may be associated with the increase of tobacco consumption in women in several countries.[8]

ANATOMY

The anterior boundary of the oral cavity is the skin–vermilion junction. The superior portion of the oral cavity extends posteriorly to the junction between the hard and soft palate, while the inferior portion extends to the circumvallate papillae. The specific anatomic subsites of this region are listed in the following sections.

Lip

The lips begin at the junction of the vermilion border with the skin and form the anterior aspect of the oral vestibule. The lips are composed of the vermilion surface, which is the portion of the lip that comes in contact with the opposing lip. The lips are well defined into an upper and lower. The primary motor control of the lips is provided by the buccal and mandibular branches of the facial nerve.

Oral Tongue

The anterior two-thirds of the tongue is mobile and considered part of the oral cavity. The oral tongue extends anteriorly from the circumvallate papillae to the undersurface of the tongue at the junction of the floor of the mouth. The fibrous septum divides the tongue into right and left halves. The oral tongue can be demarcated into four anatomic areas: the tip, lateral borders, dorsal surface, and undersurface (ventral surface). There are six pairs of muscles that form the oral tongue. Three of these muscles are extrinsic, while the other three are intrinsic. The extrinsic muscles include the genioglossus, hyoglossus, and styloglossus. The intrinsic muscles include the lingual, vertical, and transverse muscles. The for-

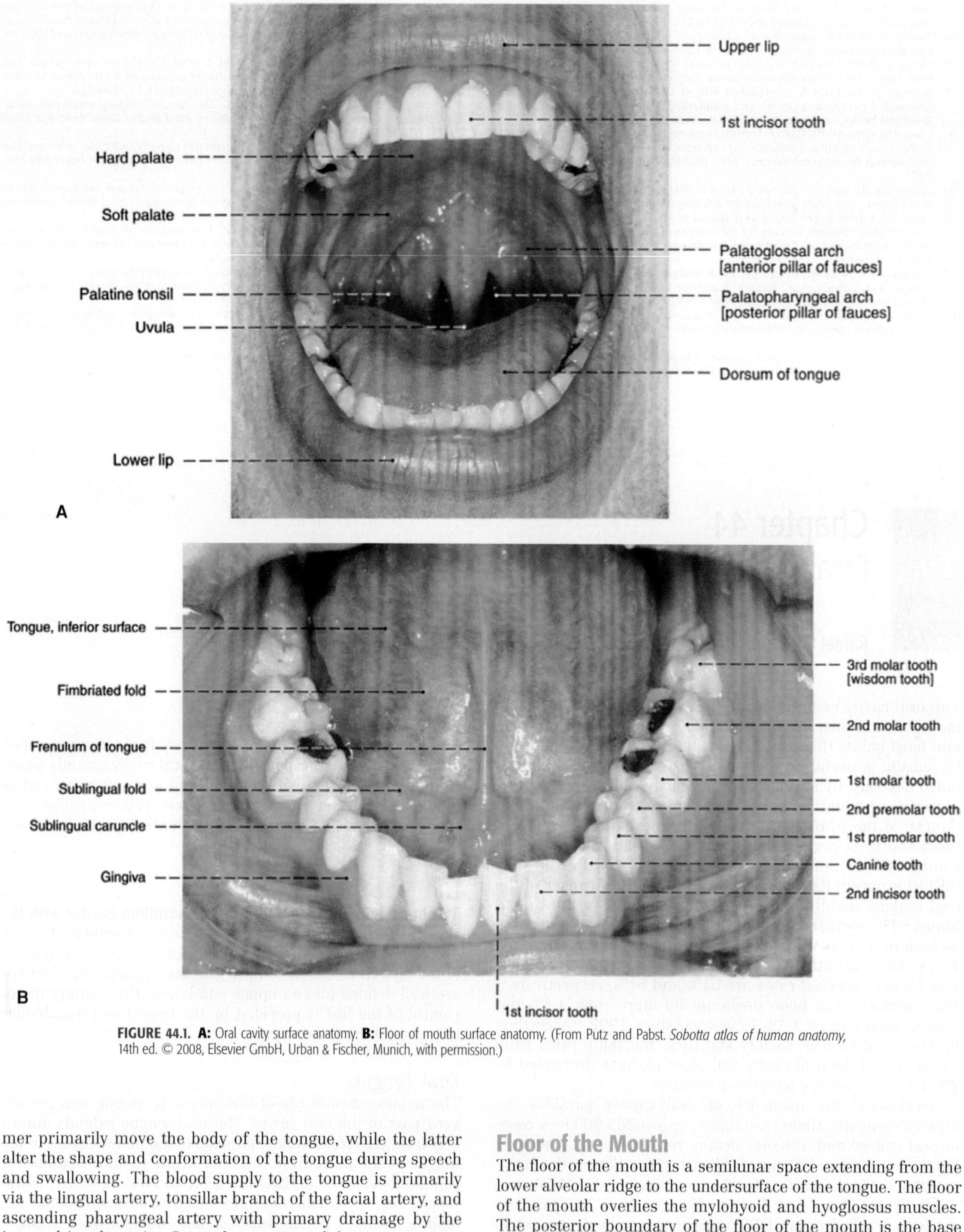

FIGURE 44.1. A: Oral cavity surface anatomy. **B:** Floor of mouth surface anatomy. (From Putz and Pabst. *Sobotta atlas of human anatomy,* 14th ed. © 2008, Elsevier GmbH, Urban & Fischer, Munich, with permission.)

mer primarily move the body of the tongue, while the latter alter the shape and conformation of the tongue during speech and swallowing. The blood supply to the tongue is primarily via the lingual artery, tonsillar branch of the facial artery, and ascending pharyngeal artery with primary drainage by the internal jugular vein. General sensation of the anterior two-thirds of the tongue is supplied by the lingual nerve. Excluding the circumvallate papillae, taste fibers from the anterior two-thirds of the tongue run in the chorda tympani branch of the facial nerve; the glossopharyngeal nerve provides sensation and taste to the posterior third of the tongue and circumvallate papillae.

Floor of the Mouth

The floor of the mouth is a semilunar space extending from the lower alveolar ridge to the undersurface of the tongue. The floor of the mouth overlies the mylohyoid and hyoglossus muscles. The posterior boundary of the floor of the mouth is the base of the anterior tonsillar pillar. This region is divided into right and left by the frenulum of the tongue and contains the ostia of the submandibular and sublingual salivary glands. A sling formed by the mylohyoid muscles medially supports the anterior floor of the mouth, and the hyoglossus supports the posterior floor of the mouth. The lingual and hypoglossal nerves are lateral to the hyoglossus, while the lingual artery is medial

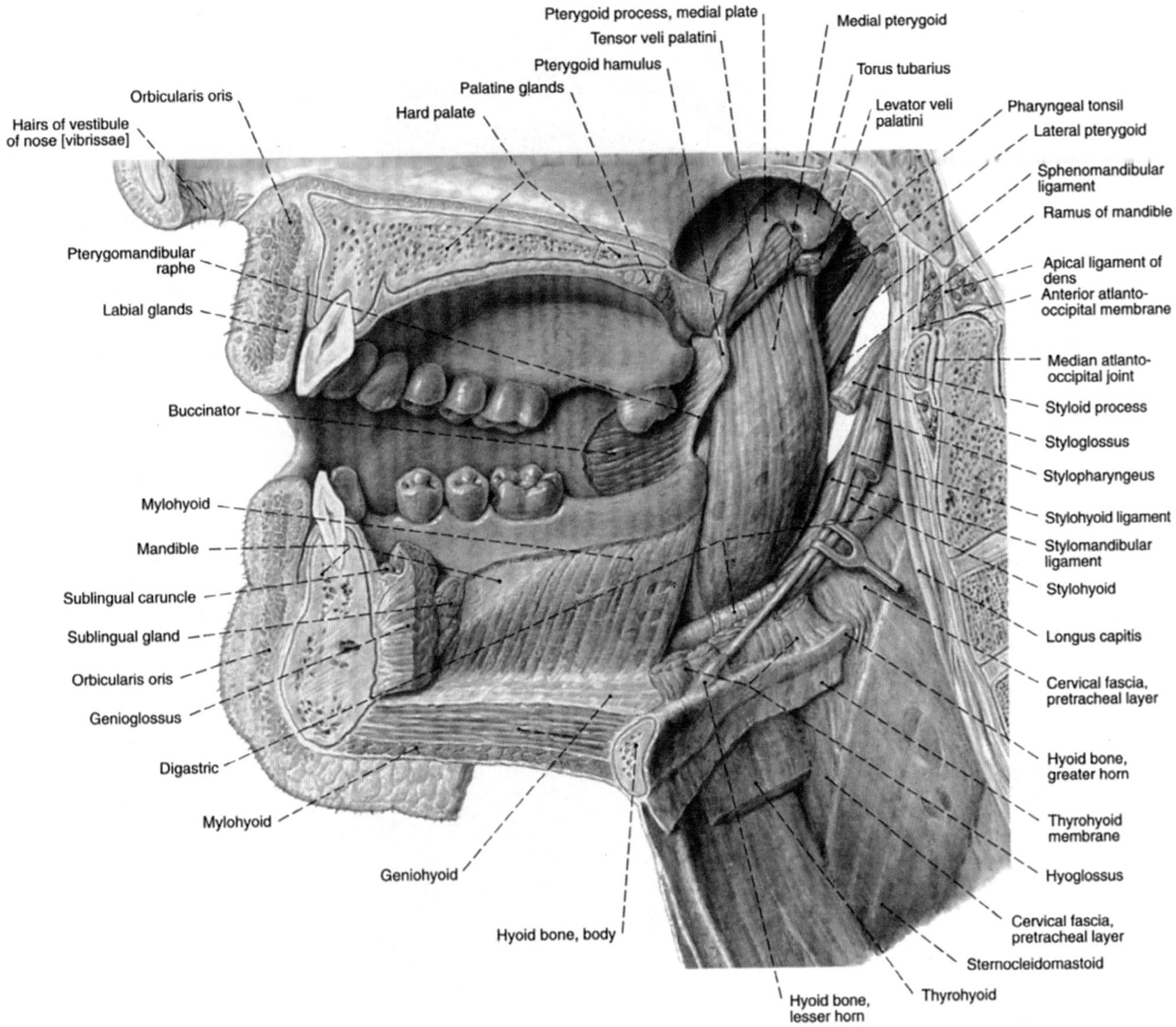

FIGURE 44.2. Oral cavity; paramedian section depicting regional anatomy. (From Putz and Pabst. *Sobotta atlas of human anatomy,* 14th ed. © 2008, Elsevier GmbH, Urban & Fischer, Munich, with permission.)

to the hyoglossus. Innervation of the floor of the mouth is provided by the lingual nerve.

Hard Palate

The hard palate extends from the inner surface of the superior alveolar ridge to the posterior edge of the palatine bone. This is a semilunar area between the superior alveolar ridge and the mucous membrane covering the palatine process of the maxillary palatine bones.

Alveolar Ridge

The alveolar ridges include the alveolar processes of the maxilla and mandible and the overlying mucosa. The mucosal covering of the lower alveolar ridge extends from the line of attachment of mucosa in the buccal gutter to the line of free mucosa of the floor of the mouth. The lower alveolar ridge extends to the ascending ramus of the mandible posteriorly. The superior alveolar ridge mucosa extends from the line of attachment of mucosa in the upper gingival buccal gutter to the junction of the hard palate. The posterior margin is the upper end of the pterygopalatine arch.

Retromolar Trigone

The retromolar trigone is the triangular area overlying the ascending ramus of the mandible. The base of the triangle is formed by the posteriormost molar, and the apex lies at the maxillary tuberosity.

Buccal Mucosa

The buccal mucosa includes the mucosal surfaces of the cheek and lips from the line of contact of the opposing lips to the pterygomandibular raphe posteriorly. This extends to the line of attachment of the mucosa of the upper and lower alveolar ridge superiorly and inferiorly. Innervation is supplied by the buccal nerve, a branch of the mandibular nerve.

EPIDEMIOLOGY

The epidemiology of oral cancer strongly reflects exposure to certain environmental agents, particularly tobacco and alcohol. Worldwide, the incidence of oral cancer varies considerably. The International Agency for Research on Cancer notes that the age-standardized incidence rate of oral cavity cancer in

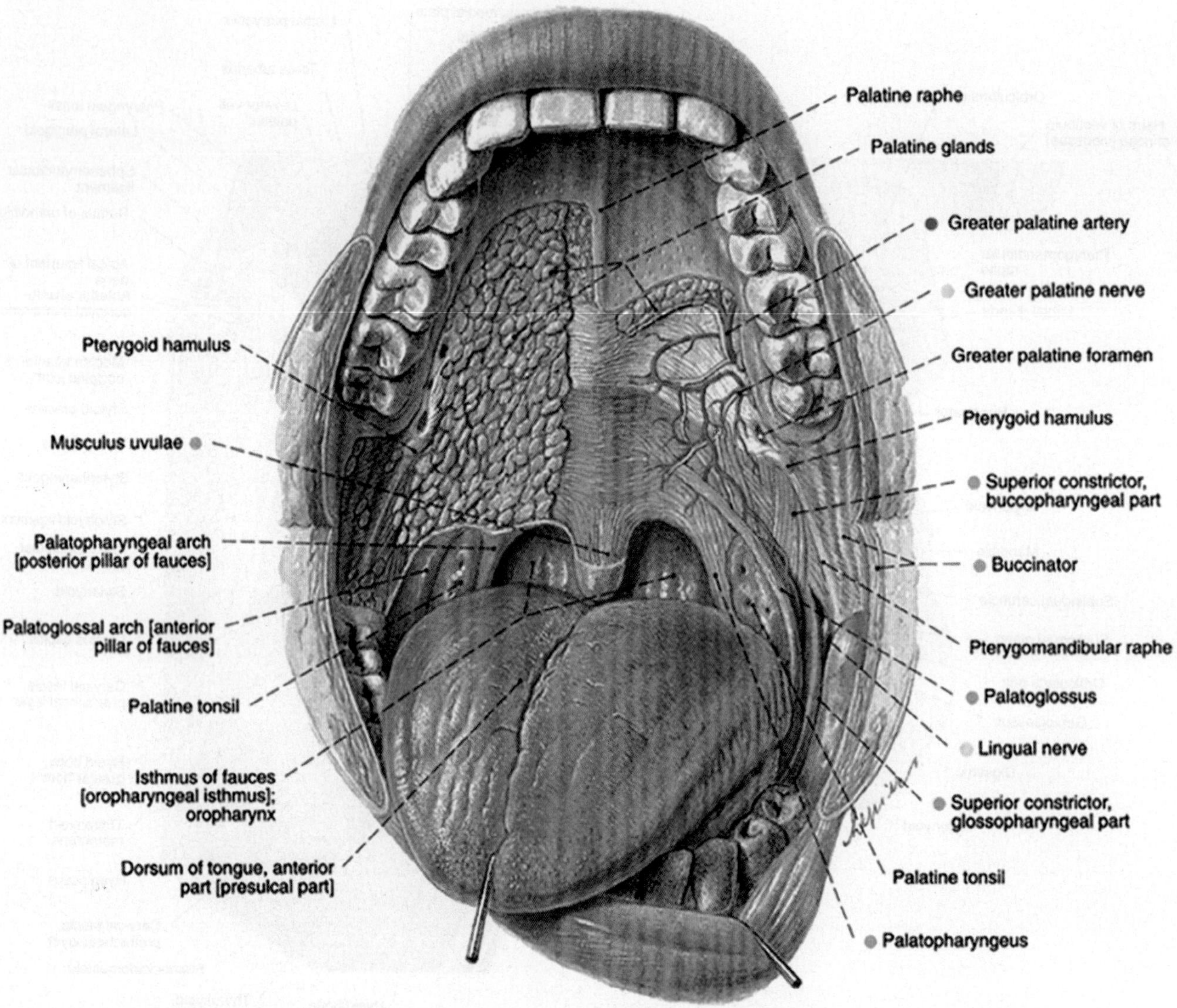

FIGURE 44.3. Oral cavity illustration depicting regional anatomy. (From Putz and Pabst. *Sobotta atlas of human anatomy,* 14th ed. © 2008, Elsevier GmbH, Urban & Fischer, Munich, with permission.)

economically developed areas in 2008 was 6.9 per 100,000; the age-adjusted rate in economically developing areas was 4.6 per 100,000.[7] In Western Europe and the United States the age-adjusted incidence of oral cavity cancer is approximately 7.0 per 100,000 in men, and about half that number in women.[7] The incidence of oral cancer in both men and women is highest in Melanesia where the rate is 24.0 per 100,000 in men and 12.0 per 100,000 in women.[7] In Central Asia and Eastern Europe the incidence of oral cancer in men is also among the highest in the world: 9.4 and 9.1 per 100,000, respectively. The lowest incidence of oral cancer is found in Middle Africa and Eastern Asia.[7]

There is a strong causal relationship between smoking and cancer of the oral cavity. Smoking is identified as an independent risk factor in 80% to 90% of patients.[9–11] Tobacco users have a fivefold to 25-fold higher risk of oral cavity and oropharyngeal cancer.[12] Cessation of smoking is associated with a decline in the risk of cancer of the oral cavity. Abstaining from the use of cigarettes results in a 30% reduction in the risk of cancer in those who quit after 1 to 9 years; the risk is reduced by 50% in those who quit for more than 9 years.[11] In India the habit of chewing betel nut leaves rolled with lime and tobacco (mixture known as "pan"), which results in prolonged carcinogen exposure to the oral mucosa, is thought to be the leading cause of oral cancer.[13,14] The practice of "reverse smoking" (smoking with the lighted end of the cigar in the mouth, also known as Chutta), peculiar to certain parts of India, is associated with an increase in cancer of the hard palate.[15] The combined use of alcohol and tobacco may have a synergistic effect on carcinogenesis.[12] International Head and Neck Epidemiology Consortium (INHANCE) pooled analysis data demonstrate a greater than multiplicative joint effect between tobacco and alcohol on head and neck cancer risk, which is most pronounced in pharyngeal and oral cavity cancer.[16] Data from a large Japanese cohort study suggest that male smokers have a 2.6 relative risk of death from oral and pharyngeal cancer compared to nonsmokers; the relative risk of death for smoking and drinking combined is 3.3.[17]

The oral cavity is the most common site for head and neck cancer in the United States.[18] Carcinoma of the oral cavity commonly afflicts patients in the sixth to seventh decades of life.[5,18,19] Recent SEER data indicate that the age-standardized incidence rate (ASR per 100,000 persons) of oral cavity and pharyngeal cancer in the United States is 15.7 in men and 6.2 in women.[3] Although the incidence rates of oral and pharyngeal cancer between Caucasians and African Americans are similar, the mortality rate for African American males is 6.3/100,000, nearly double that of Caucasian males (3.1/100,000).[3]

Although there has been a declining trend in the overall incidence of oral cavity squamous cell carcinoma over the past 30 years, recent studies suggest the incidence of this disease in young adults may be on the rise worldwide.[5,19] SEER data suggest that 11.3% of oral cancer cases occur in patients under the age of 45.[19] Institutional series suggest that 4% to 6% of oral cancers now occur at ages younger than 45 years.[19,20] A recent study by Patel et al.[5] suggests that this increasing trend is most pronounced in young white women.[5] Reports examining risk factors for oral cancer in the young provide evidence that many younger patients have never smoked or consumed alcohol; predisposition to genetic instability has been hypothesized as a causative factor. Early published series suggest that young patients with oral cancer have a worse prognosis.[19] However, recent matched-control studies and national database reviews suggest that outcomes in this population of patients are probably similar to that of older patients.[5,19]

Ultraviolet radiation has been associated with carcinoma of the lip. In geographic regions where there are long daily periods of sun exposure, cancer of the lip may represent up to 60% of all cancers of the oral cavity.[21] Herpes simplex virus (HSV) and human papilloma virus (HPV) have also been implicated in the etiology of oral cavity cancer. The former has been shown to act as a cocarcinogen with tobacco and ultraviolet light in animal models.[22,23] The relationship between HPV and oropharyngeal cancer has been well established,[24,25] but the association with oral cavity cancer is less clear. Approximately 50% of patients with oropharyngeal cancer and 0% to 20% with oral cavity cancer are positive for HPV 16 DNA.[5] A meta-analysis of 17 studies demonstrated a weak association between HPV and oral cancer.[26]

Certain syndromes such as Plummer-Vinson (characterized by iron-deficiency anemia, hypopharyngeal webs, weight loss, and dysphagia) have been associated with oral cavity cancer. However, Plummer-Vinson syndrome is rare and accounts for a small number of cancers of the oral cavity. Disorders such as xeroderma pigmentosum, ataxia telangiectasia, Bloom syndrome, and Fanconi's anemia are a result of defective "caretaker" genes. Because such defects result in genetic instability, an increased incidence of second primary malignancies has been reported in this population.[27] For instance, an aggressive form of early adulthood head and neck carcinomas, including oral cancer, is seen in patients with Fanconi's anemia.[19] By contrast, with the exception of Li Fraumeni syndrome, abnormalities in "gatekeeper" genes, which inhibit cell proliferation and/or promote cell death, do not appear to predispose to oral cancer. However, despite such reports, the genetics of oral cavity cancer have not been well delineated.[28]

In patients with cancer of the oral cavity the risk of developing a second primary cancer is well recognized. The concept of field cancerization described by Slaughter and Smejkal[29] in 1953 and Day et al.[30] may explain the significantly higher rate of second malignancy in patients with head and neck cancers compared to the general population. In an analysis of 851 patients with squamous cell carcinoma of the head and neck, 19% of the study population developed a secondary head and neck carcinoma 5 years after undergoing initial therapy.[31] The probability of developing a second metachronous malignancy at 5 years was 22% (18% for the subset of patients with oral cavity cancer).[31] Day and Blot[32] evaluated the risks of subsequent malignancies in 21,371 patients with oral and pharyngeal cancers between 1973 and 1987. The rate of development of second tumors was 3.7% per year. The risk of second primary cancer was 2.8 times greater than expected, with a 20-fold increase of oral or esophageal cancers and a fourfold to sevenfold increase of respiratory cancers. In a meta-analysis patients with carcinoma of the oral cavity had the highest rate of second primary cancers, most of which occurred in the upper aerodigestive tract.[33] An analysis of results from a large intergroup randomized chemoprevention study demonstrated that the incidence of second primary cancers is highly influenced by smoking.[34] Second primary cancers have an adverse effect on prognosis and are the major cause of treatment failure in patients with early-stage disease.[31,35]

MOLECULAR BIOLOGY

In parallel to the Fearon and Vogelstein model describing the genetic basis of colon cancer,[36] there are a series of specific genetic events that precede the development of oral squamous cell carcinoma.[37,38] Cancer progression models describe several steps that occur during tumor development: oncogenes become activated and tumor-suppressor genes become deactivated and a series of these alterations are required for carcinogenesis. In the oral mucosa this genetic progression is reflected histologically by the transformation from normal mucosa to dysplastic epithelium and ultimately to frankly invasive squamous cell carcinoma. Data to support this model come from studies that reveal genetic alterations in histologically normal tissues and in premalignant lesions, including loss of heterozygosity at chromosomes 3p14 and 9p21. Furthermore, mutations in the region of chromosome 17p13, which encompasses the tumor-suppressor gene *TP53*, are among early events that contribute to malignant transformation. Indeed, biopsies of normal mucosa from patients with upper aerodigestive tract carcinomas frequently harbor *TP53* mutations.

Additional mutations have been observed in known cancer-related genes encoding proteins such as p16, H-ras, phosphatidylinositol-3-kinase (PI3 K), and F-box/WD repeat-containing protein 7 isoform 1 (FBXW7). Recent whole exome sequencing studies indicate that inactivating mutations in Notch1 are found in close to 15% of tumors evaluated.[39] This gene is primarily associated with cellular development and differentiation and encodes a transmembrane receptor with an extracellular domain containing numerous EGF-like repeats. Upon ligand activation, Notch1's intracellular portion is cleaved and translocated to the nucleus where it can induce genes that are both prosurvival and differentiation as well as antiproliferative. This duality appears to be cell type specific, leading to the observation of Notch1 being either tumorigenic or a tumor suppressor depending on the cancer type. The precise role of Notch1 inactivation in oral squamous carcinoma is currently under investigation; but structural abnormalities in the Notch1 gene found in oral squamous carcinoma specimens suggest that Notch1 functions more like a tumor suppressor in this tumor type.

The aforementioned mutations contribute to changes in critical cellular processes that regulate growth, survival, immortality, tissue invasion, and new blood vessel formation that subsequently lead to changes in the biology of epithelial cells whereby they acquire distinct histologic characteristics. How the same environmental exposures lead to tumor development in some individuals and not others may be explained in part by genetic susceptibility to tobacco carcinogens.[40] This susceptibility has been linked to the ability to repair DNA damage and/or metabolize tobacco-related carcinogens. Adding to the complexity of carcinogenesis in this setting is the possibility that alterations in multiple enzymes participating in carcinogen metabolism may be required to exert a sensitizing effect, thus confounding efforts to establish a relationship to any one specific alteration.[41]

NATURAL HISTORY AND PATTERNS OF SPREAD

Premalignant Lesions

Leukoplakia

Leukoplakia and erythroplakia are gross clinical descriptors that do not always correspond directly to specific pathologic entities.[28,42] The World Health Organization defines leukoplakia

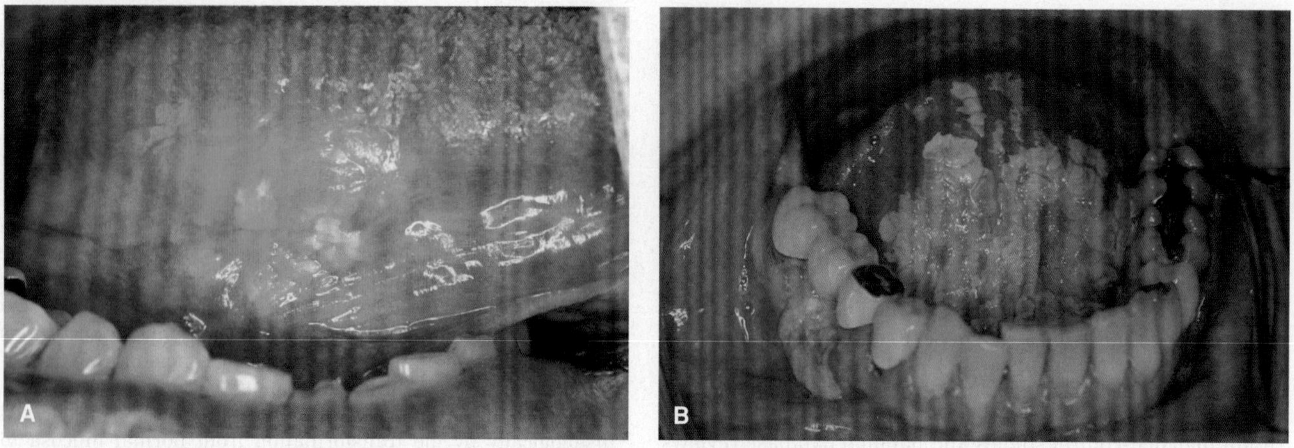

FIGURE 44.4. A: Superficial patches of leukoplakia involving the lateral and ventral surfaces of the oral tongue. **B:** Extensive leukoplakia involving the ventral oral tongue, floor of the mouth, and mandibular alveolus.

as a white patch or plaque that cannot be rubbed off or characterized clinically or pathologically as any other disease[42] (Fig. 44.4). Leukoplakia is not related to the presence or absence of dysplasia; however, it is the most common precursor of cancer of the oral cavity. Leukoplakia has a varied clinical appearance, and its appearance frequently changes over time. This is primarily a clinical entity, with certain key pathologic features. These features include hyperkeratosis and acanthosis. Leukoplakias begin as thin gray or gray/white plaques that may appear somewhat translucent, are sometimes fissured or wrinkled, and are typically soft and flat. They frequently have sharply demarcated borders but occasionally blend gradually into normal surrounding mucosa.

Homogenous leukoplakia is a uniform white lesion that is prevalent in the buccal mucosa. These lesions represent the most common variety of leukoplakia and have a low malignant potential. Conversely, high-risk oral leukoplakia demonstrates abnormal orientation of cells, nuclear hyperchromatism, increased mitosis, and a nuclear cytoplasmic ratio.[28] Clinically these lesions are nonhomogenous, nodular, speckled, or verrucous, with central ulceration or erosion.[42,43] Follow-up studies demonstrate that between <1% and 18% of oral leukoplakias develop into oral cancer, with the latter clinical subtype conferring a higher risk of malignant transformation.[44,45]

The natural history of leukoplakia is variable. Leukoplakia may regress spontaneously without therapy. A baseline biopsy can be performed to establish diagnosis and rule out malignant transformation. Leukoplakia with clinically or histologically aggressive features, demonstrating dysplasia, should be excised.

Erythroplakia

The term *erythroplakia* describes a chronic, red, generally asymptomatic lesion or patch on the mucosal surface that cannot be attributed to a traumatic, vascular, or inflammatory cause. Erythroplakia, like leukoplakia, is a clinical diagnosis of exclusion that requires the clinician to rule out all other erythematous oral lesions.[46] However, erythroplakia is associated with a higher risk of malignant transformation than leukoplakia. Transformation rates are considered to be the highest among all precancerous oral lesions and conditions.[47] Histopathologically it has been documented that in homogenous oral erythroplakia, 51% showed invasive carcinoma, 40% carcinoma *in situ,* and 9% mild or moderate dysplasia.[47] The treatment of choice for erythroplakia is surgical excision.

Oral Submucous Fibrosis

The term describes a generalized fibrosis of the oral cavity tissues resulting in marked rigidity and trismus. At early stages these premalignant lesions are characterized by blanching of the mucosa with a marble-like appearance. At more advanced stages, palpable fibrous bands become evident around the buccal mucosa and the mouth opening. Once oral submucous fibrosis reaches advanced stages, approximately 25% of cases biopsied demonstrate epithelial dysplasia in addition to subepithelial alterations.[12] Oral submucous fibrosis is associated with the use of betel quid (with or without tobacco) or pan masala.[12] In India, it is estimated that as many as 5 million individuals are afflicted with oral submucous fibrosis.[12]

Oral Cavity Cancer

Relative Distribution

The most common subsite for squamous cell carcinoma of the oral cavity (excluding the lip) is the oral tongue (Fig. 44.5). In a review of 3,308 cases of oral cavity cancer treated at the University of Texas M.D. Anderson Cancer Center between 1970 and 1999, 32% involved the oral tongue.[28] The floor of the mouth is the second most common subsite where oral cavity carcinomas may arise. Carcinoma of the alveolar ridge accounts for approximately 10% of oral cavity carcinomas. Squamous cell carcinoma of the retromolar trigone and hard palate is rare. Similarly, carcinoma of the buccal mucosa is rare in the United States but is the most common carcinoma of the oral cavity in Southeast Asia because of the widespread use of betel nut.[28]

Patterns of Spread

Local Spread

Carcinoma from distinct anatomic subsites may exhibit different tendencies for spread based on natural anatomic barriers and location. For instance, the majority of lip cancers are local

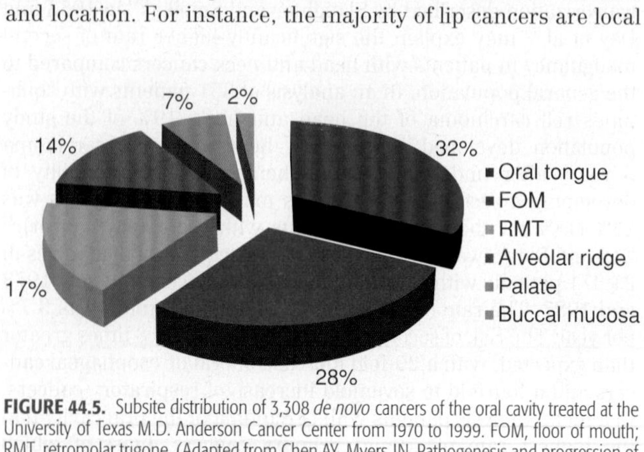

FIGURE 44.5. Subsite distribution of 3,308 *de novo* cancers of the oral cavity treated at the University of Texas M.D. Anderson Cancer Center from 1970 to 1999. FOM, floor of mouth; RMT, retromolar trigone. (Adapted from Chen AY, Myers JN. Pathogenesis and progression of squamous cell carcinoma of the oral cavity. *Dis Mon* 2001;47:275–361.)

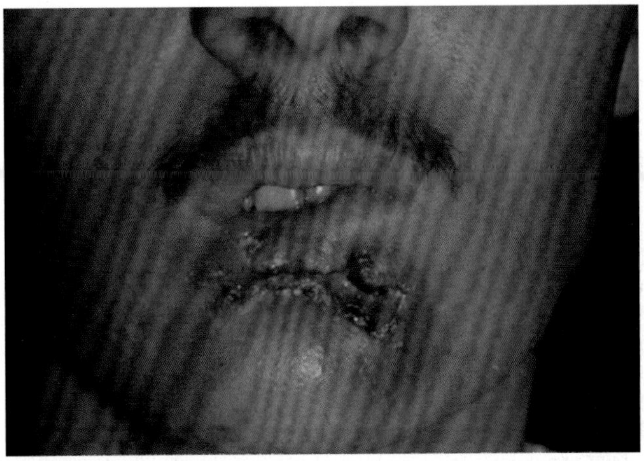

FIGURE 44.6. Advanced, destructive, ulcerative squamous cell carcinoma involving the lower lip, buccogingival soft tissues, and skin in a patient with long-term habit of tobacco chewing.

growths that do not invade deeply into the tissues of the oral cavity or mandible.[48] However, a select few lip carcinomas may be deeply invasive with perineural involvement, posterior spread to involve cortical bone, extension to the inferior alveolar nerve, or spread to the skin of the face (Fig. 44.6). Squamous cell carcinoma of the floor of the mouth can secondarily involve the ventral tongue, extend along the lingual nerve or submandibular duct, or invade the cortex of the mandible. Tumors in this location can invade deeply, involving the muscles of the floor of the mouth. There is an anatomic gap between the mylohyoid and hyoglossus muscles through which a carcinoma can gain access to submandibular and sublingual areas. Carcinomas of the alveolar ridge and retromolar trigone tend to invade bone early. Tumors of the inferior alveolar ridge may access the mandibular canal and the inferior alveolar nerve, while tumors of the superior alveolar ridge may pass into the maxillary antrum or floor of the nose. Infiltrating lesions of the buccal mucosa can invade the buccinator muscle, extend to the buccal fat pad, and invade the subcutaneous tissue. The hard palate has a relatively dense mucoperiosteum that is relatively resistant to tumor invasion. However, the primary and secondary palates are fused at the incisive fossa, where tumors can gain access into the nasal cavity. The greater palatine foramina can allow tumors to spread posteriorly and enter the pterygopalatine fossa and skull base.

Lymphatic Metastases

For the purpose of staging and treatment planning, the neck is generally divided into five primary levels. Level I includes the submental (Ia) and submandibular (Ib) triangles. Level II includes the upper jugular chain lymph nodes from the base of the skull to the carotid bifurcation and from the sternohyoid muscle anteriorly to the posterior border of the sternocleidomastoid posteriorly. Level III includes the midjugular nodes, which extend from the carotid bifurcation to the omohyoid muscle inferiorly, the sternohyoid medially, and the posterior aspect of the sternocloidomastoid posteriorly. Level IV includes the inferior jugular nodes, bounded by the omohyoid muscle superiorly, the clavicle inferiorly, and the posterior aspect of the sternocleidomastoid posteriorly. Level V includes nodes in the posterior triangle, bordered by the base of the skull superiorly, clavicle inferiorly, and posterior aspect of the sternocleidomastoid anteriorly.

The oral cavity has an extensive group of lymphatics that manifest a fairly predictable lymph node drainage pattern based on location (subsite) within the oral cavity[49] (Table 44.1). The upper and lower lip demonstrates distinct patterns of lymphatic drainage. The principal lymphatic drainage of the upper

TABLE 44.1 RELATIVE INVOLVEMENT OF LYMPH NODE REGIONS BY ORAL CAVITY SUBSITE

	Percentage Involved			
	Submaxillary	Submental	Upper Jugular	Midjugular
Oral tongue	18	9	73	18
FOM	64	7	43	0
RMT	25	0	63	12.5

FOM, floor of mouth; RMT, retromolar trigone.

From Byers RM, Wolf PF, Ballantyne AJ. Rationale for elective modified neck dissection. *Head Neck Surg* 1988;10:160–167.

lip is to preauricular, periparotid, submental, and submandibular lymph nodes, which secondarily drain to deep jugular lymph nodes. The medial portion of the lower lip drains primarily to the submental lymph nodes, while the lateral portion drains to the submandibular triangle.

A classical study by Lindberg[50] demonstrated that the superior deep jugular nodes are most frequently involved by cancers of the oral cavity. The oral tongue has an extensive lymphatic drainage. The anterior portion of the tongue drains to the submental nodes (level Ia), and the lateral portion drains to the submandibular (level Ib) and deep jugular nodes (level II). The posterior oral tongue drains into the upper jugulodigastric group of lymph nodes (level II). The lymphatics of the oral tongue also have extensive communication across the midline; thus, carcinomas of the oral tongue can metastasize bilaterally. Studies suggest that some carcinomas of the lateral oral tongue may metastasize to level IV lymph nodes without involving levels I, II, or III.[51] This implies that there may be separate lymphatic channels draining from the oral tongue directly to level IV nodes, allowing for apparent "skip metastases."

Dye injection studies have shown that the floor of the mouth has superficial and deep lymphatic drainage systems.[51] The superficial system crosses randomly in the midline and drains into both the ipsilateral and contralateral submandibular lymph nodes. The deep lymphatic system is thought to penetrate the periosteum and drains into the submandibular and upper jugular lymph nodes. Lymphatics from the buccal mucosa drain into the periparotid, submental, and submandibular nodes. Tumors of the alveolar ridge may drain into the submental and submandibular triangles, upper deep jugular, and retropharyngeal lymph nodes. Tumors of the inferior alveolus are more likely to metastasize to the neck than tumors of the superior alveolus. The main lymphatic drainage from the retromolar trigone is into the superior-deep jugular lymph nodes; however, there may be some drainage into periparotid and retropharyngeal lymph nodes. Lymphatics in the hard palate are few, but drainage is into submandibular, superior deep jugular, and retropharyngeal nodes.

The risk of neck metastases depends on several factors including site and size of the primary tumor. Overall, for patients with squamous cell carcinoma of the oral cavity, cervical metastases occur in approximately 30% of cases.[43] The rate of neck metastases for carcinoma of the lip is approximately 10%.[43] Squamous cell cancer of the oral tongue carries the highest risk of nodal metastases. The frequency of neck metastases can range from 15% to 75%, depending on the size of the primary lesion.[50,52] Approximately 25% of patients with carcinoma of the oral cavity will have occult nodal metastases, and 3% of patients will have contralateral metastases.[50,52] Contralateral metastases are more common in tumors that approach or cross the midline. Early tumors of the floor of the mouth have approximately a 12% to 30% incidence of occult nodal metastases depending on the thickness of the lesion, while larger lesions can have an incidence of nearly 50%.[53] Approximately 15% to 20% of upper alveolar ridge tumors will involve the neck at presentation; the risk of occult metastases in

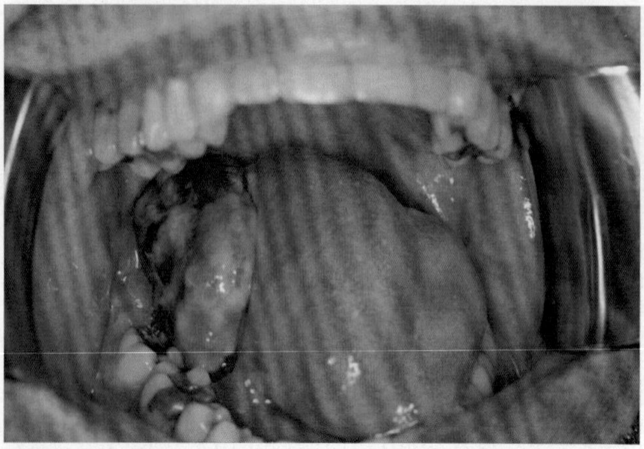

FIGURE 44.7. Unusual oral cavity metastasis in a patient with known renal cell carcinoma. This advanced, hemorrhagic metastasis showed identical pathology to the patient's known renal cell carcinoma.

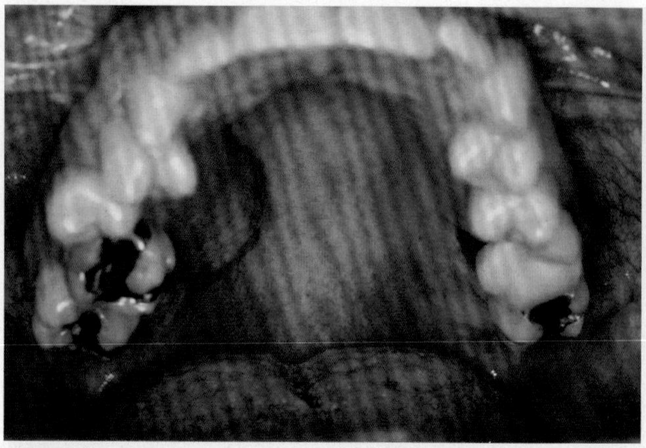

FIGURE 44.8. Kaposi's sarcoma involving the hard palate and maxillary alveolus in a patient with human immunodeficiency virus.

a clinically negative neck is approximately 15% to 20%.[50] The incidence of neck metastases in lower alveolar ridge tumors is higher than for tumors of the upper alveolar ridge.[50] For cancers of the buccal mucosa, the incidence of positive cervical lymph nodes at diagnosis is 10% to 30%; the incidence of pathologically positive nodes in a clinically negative neck is about 15%. Similar rates of occult metastases occur for squamous cell carcinoma of the retromolar trigone; however, patients tend to present with more advanced disease, resulting in a somewhat higher rate of regional metastases.[43] The incidence of lymph node involvement from carcinoma of the hard palate is low, approximately 15%.[48,54]

Distant Metastases

The majority of oral cavity cancers present as localized disease and remain localized until late in the course of their development. Distant metastasis occurs in approximately 15% to 20% of patients who eventually die of their disease.[43] The risk of distant metastasis increases with the degree of lymph node involvement. Patients with recurrent disease are also at higher risk for distant metastases.[55] Patients without clinically appreciable neck disease rarely fail distantly after treatment. In general terms with respect to head and neck cancer, 66% of distant metastases are to the lungs, 22% to the bones, and 9.5% to the liver.[56] On rare occasion, the oral cavity will serve as a site for distant metastasis from another anatomic primary tumor site (Fig. 44.7).

PATHOLOGIC CLASSIFICATION

The predominant histopathologic type of cancer in the oral cavity is squamous cell carcinoma. There are several variants of squamous cell carcinoma, including basaloid and verrucous carcinoma. Basaloid squamous cell carcinoma is believed to have a worse prognosis than traditional squamous cell carcinoma. In a retrospective comparison between basaloid squamous cell carcinoma and traditional poorly differentiated squamous cell carcinoma, the former had a higher incidence of advanced disease at presentation, distant metastases, and poorer overall survival rate.[57] Verrucous carcinoma is a less common variant of squamous cell carcinoma. It is generally considered a low-grade malignancy with low metastatic potential and good overall prognosis, although often with challenges for local control in elderly patients.[28] For most cases, adjuvant radiation and elective neck dissection are not indicated. Sarcomatoid carcinomas can be found in the oral cavity and larynx. This variant of squamous cell carcinoma carries a poor prognosis with a mean survival of approximately 2 years.[58]

Less than 10% of neoplasms of the oral cavity have non-squamous histology. Most of these are minor salivary gland tumors, which tend to arise in the hard palate. Adenoid cystic carcinoma accounts for approximately 30% to 40% of minor salivary gland cancers of the oral cavity.[59] Other histologies that can occur in the oral cavity include adenocarcinomas, melanoma, ameloblastoma, lymphoma, and Kaposi's sarcoma (Fig. 44.8). Approximately 50% of acquired immunodeficiency syndrome–related cases of Kaposi's sarcoma have oral cavity involvement.[43] Most lymphomas in the head and neck arise in Waldeyer's ring (tonsil, base of tongue, and nasopharynx). Only 2% of all lymphomas are found in the oral cavity.[60] Fortunately, melanoma of the oral cavity is very rare and represents only 0.2% to 8% of all melanomas.[61] Mucosal melanomas generally have a worse prognosis than cutaneous melanomas.

CLINICAL PRESENTATION

The oral cavity is an anatomic region that is readily accessible to visual inspection and palpation. Despite this fact, many patients with oral cavity tumors present with advanced-stage disease as initial symptoms may be vague and painless. Tumors of the oral tongue often present as small ulcers and gradually invade the musculature of the tongue. Advanced lesions may be either ulcerative or exophytic and are usually quite evident. Some cancers of the oral tongue are painful even in their early stages. Cervical metastases occur early in the natural history of the disease, with 30% to 40% of patients harboring cervical lymph node metastases at diagnosis. Squamous cell carcinomas of the oral tongue most often arise along the lateral borders of the tongue[28] (Fig. 44.9).

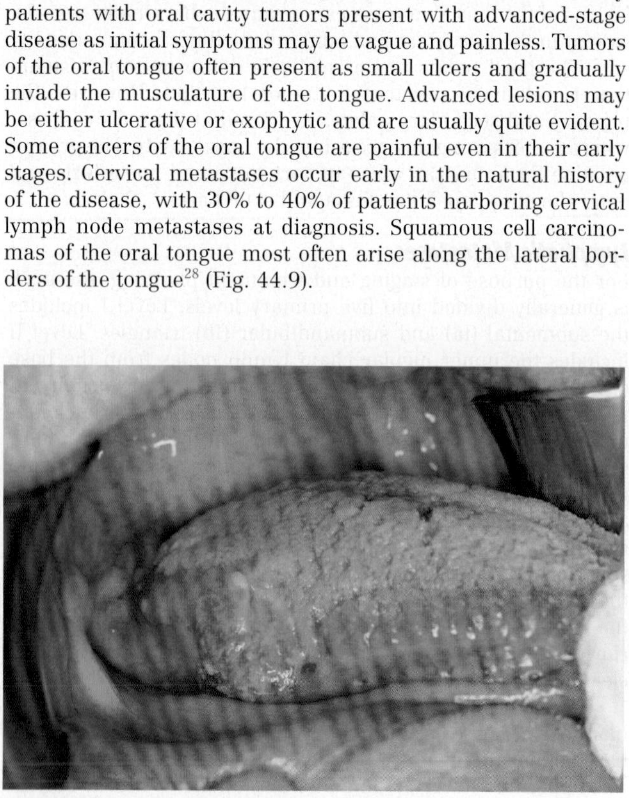

FIGURE 44.9. T2N0M0 squamous cell carcinoma involving the right lateral oral tongue.

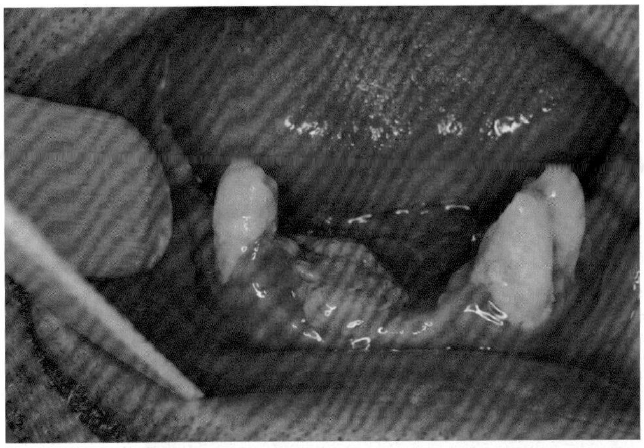

FIGURE 44.10. T1N0M0 squamous cell carcinoma of the mandibular alveolus. No evidence of bone invasion identified on Panorex or computed tomography imaging.

Lesions of the floor of the mouth are often infiltrative and may invade bone, the muscles of the floor of the mouth, and the tongue. The frenulum is frequently a site of involvement. Clinical fixation of the tumor to the mandible suggests periosteal involvement, which may occur early.

Tumors of the alveolar ridge may present with pain while chewing, loose teeth, or ill-fitting dentures in edentulous patients. These cancers often arise in edentulous areas or along the free margin of the mandibular alveolus (Figs. 44.10 and 44.11). Anesthesia of the lower lip and teeth may indicate involvement of the mandibular canal and inferior alveolar nerve.

Tumors involving the retromolar trigone region may present with an exophytic growth pattern and limited involvement of underlying bone (Fig. 44.12), or they may infiltrate cortical bone and spread along regional tissue planes to involve the pterygoid complex and parapharyngeal space. These latter lesions often induce trismus early in the clinical course.

Carcinoma of the buccal mucosa is rarely symptomatic early in its course. Lesions may be papillary or erosive and located near the dental occlusal line. These tumors are often relatively asymptotic and therefore seldom come to medical attention as T1 lesions. Often, these tumors manifest associated leukoplakia. Multiple primary sites and local recurrence are also common. These tumors most frequently arise adjacent to the lower molars along the occlusal line of the teeth.

Carcinoma of the hard palate is often painless, and the sole presenting symptom may be an irregularity in the mucosa or ill-fitting dentures. Other presenting symptoms include nonhealing ulcers of the hard palate, intermittent bleeding, and pain.

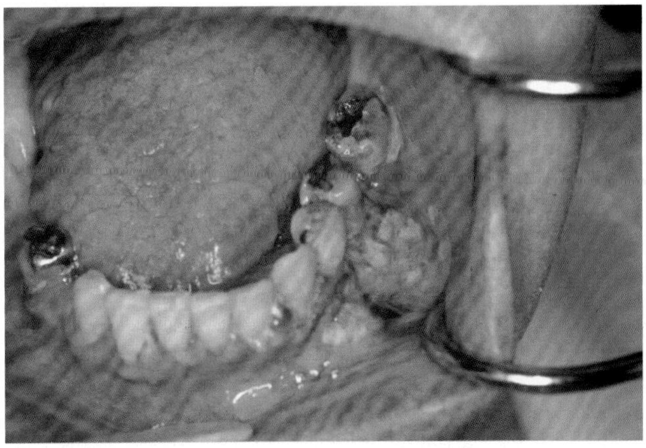

FIGURE 44.11. Squamous cell carcinoma involving the mandibular alveolus and buccogingival space.

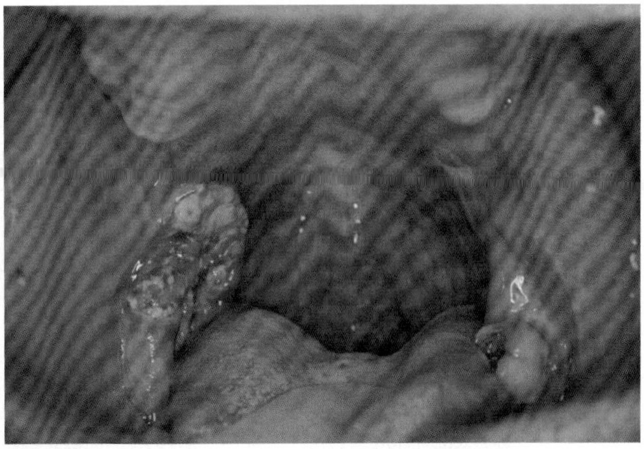

FIGURE 44.12. Exophytic T3 carcinoma involving the right retromolar trigone, anterior tonsillar pillar, and proximal soft palate with minimal infiltration into the right base of the tongue.

DIAGNOSTIC EVALUATION

Patients with oral cavity cancer should undergo a comprehensive history and physical examination. Detailed examination is particularly important for oral cavity tumors in that much can be learned about cancers that afford opportunity for direct visual inspection and digital palpation. A biopsy of lesions in question should be obtained as well as a thorough dental assessment. Computed tomography (CT) scans, panoramic radiographs, magnetic resonance imaging (MRI), and other imaging studies may also be important for accurate staging of the tumor and in treatment planning.

The history of present illness should address the following issues: tobacco and alcohol use; dysphagia; odynophagia; pain; trismus; difficulties with speech; hoarseness; loose teeth; ill-fitting dentures; hypoesthesia of the face, lips, or mandible; weight loss; and malnutrition. Otalgia suggests involvement of the ninth or 10th cranial nerve; facial numbness may suggest involvement of the fifth cranial nerve. Hypoesthesia usually results from perineural invasion, often from penetration of the mandible and perineural spread along the inferior alveolar nerve. The presence of trismus may indicate extension into the pterygoid musculature, signifying locally advanced disease. Other symptoms include a persistent ulcer, bleeding, drooling, or respiratory distress. A patient's comorbid illnesses must also be taken into account in the treatment plan.

A detailed examination of the head and neck should be performed, with particular focus on the oral cavity and oropharynx. This usually begins with a full inspection of the oral cavity, including a thorough inspection of the teeth. Palpation of the oral cavity can help assess bony involvement, tongue fixation, and depth of involvement. Deviation or fixation of the tongue suggests involvement of extrinsic muscles of the tongue. Bimanual palpation can help assess the depth of tumor invasion into musculature of the tongue and floor of the mouth. A thorough palpation of the neck is important to assess regional nodal disease.

Imaging can complement the physical examination in determining the extent of disease. A chest x-ray should be performed to exclude lung metastases or a second primary cancer. CT is the modality most commonly used to determine the extent of soft-tissue and bony involvement and occult disease in the neck (Fig. 44.13). CT may be used to determine the extent of invasion into the deep musculature of the tongue and adjacent structures. Moreover, CT is a valuable modality for visualizing invasion of the mandible, palate, and pterygopalatine fossa. If CT scanning is not available, then panoramic radiographs can be used to demonstrate mandibular invasion. MRI may be used in case of contrast allergy or a lesion that is not well visualized on CT. For instance, MRI may be used if a patient has significant dental artifact that obscures visualization

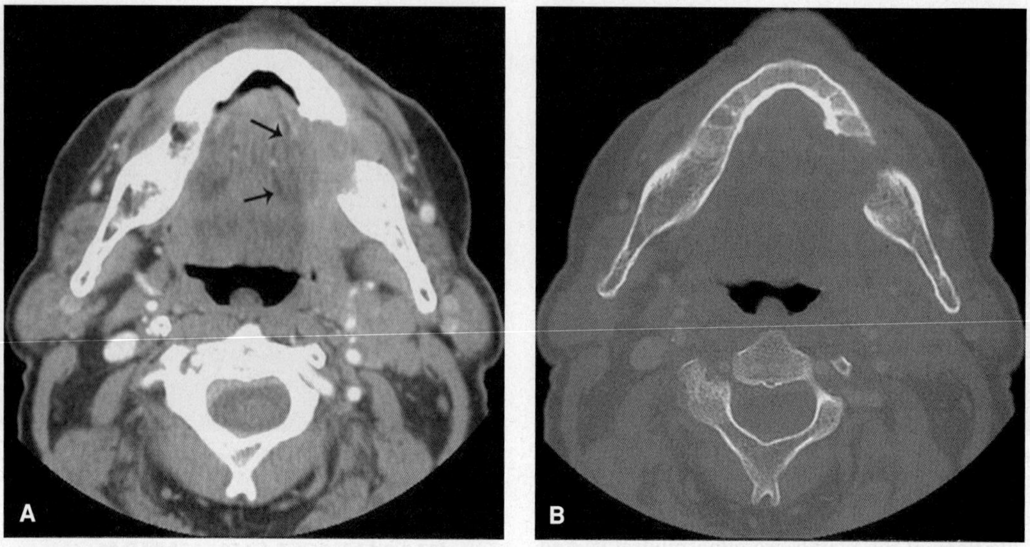

FIGURE 44.13. A: Transverse computed tomography image with contrast depicting infiltrative squamous cell carcinoma of the left lateral oral tongue and floor of the mouth with associated bone destruction. There is posterior tumor extension to involve the retromolar trigone and tonsillar complex. **B:** Corresponding computed tomography bone window views demonstrating destruction of the mandibular body.

of the primary tumor on CT. MRI provides excellent definition of tumor involving the tongue and is a good modality for evaluating the possibility of perineural spread. Ultrasound may be used to screen for enlarged lymph nodes that are not clinically detectable. In experienced hands, the accuracy of ultrasound when combined with fine needle aspiration may be superior to CT or MRI for staging the neck.[62]

Positron emission tomography (PET) and PET/CT have been used increasingly in head and neck cancer evaluation for staging disease in the neck, evaluation of perineural and skull base involvement, identification of distant metastases, and detection of recurrence. Several studies suggest that PET is more sensitive and specific in evaluating lymphatic metastases compared to CT and MRI.[63,64] PET/CT may improve the anatomic localization of abnormalities identified on PET and decrease the number of equivocal PET findings.[65] Liao et al.[66] prospectively evaluated 473 patients with oral cavity squamous cell carcinoma and reported a sensitivity of 77.7% and a specificity of 58% for PET/CT after histopathologic correlation of nodal metastases to the neck. Maddipatla et al.,[67] in a prospective study evaluating 552 lymph nodes dissected after oral cancer surgery, reported a 97% negative predictive value (NPV) for PET/CT. Pentenero et al.[68] reported an accuracy of 66.7%, a specificity of 76.9%, and an NPV of 83.3% for staging of the neck with PET/CT. Despite the improved overall accuracy, clinical application of PET/CT is limited by the suboptimal detection of small metastases. Therefore, the decision to pursue a neck dissection should not be based solely on PET/CT findings.

Reports have indicated that the overall sensitivity and specificity of PET may be superior to CT and MRI for evaluating persistent or recurrent disease, particularly in patients who have received previous radiotherapy.[69,70] The accuracy of PET in detecting disease recurrence or persistence may be influenced by the time posttreatment when images are acquired. It is recommended that a PET scan not be performed until 8 to 12 weeks posttreatment to minimize the risk of both false-negative and false-positive interpretations.[71–74]

CLINICAL STAGING

The American Joint Committee on Cancer has established a staging system for all cancers of the oral cavity (Table 44.2).[75] Nonepithelial malignancies and melanoma of the lip and oral cavity are not included.

TABLE 44.2 STAGING OF ORAL CAVITY CARCINOMA

A	
Tis	Carcinoma *in situ*
T1	Tumor ≤2 cm in greatest dimension
T2	Tumor >2 cm in greatest dimension, but ≤4 cm
T3	Tumor >4 cm in greatest dimension
T4 (lip)	Tumor invades through cortical bone, inferior alveolar nerve, floor of mouth, or skin of face (i.e., chin or nose)
T4a (oral cavity)	Tumor invades adjacent structures (e.g., through cortical bone, into deep [extrinsic] muscles of the tongue, maxillary sinus, skin of face)
T4b	Tumor invades masticator space, pterygoid plates, or skull base and/or encases carotid artery
B	
Nx	Regional lymph nodes cannot be assessed
N0	No regional lymph nodes
N1	Metastases in a single ipsilateral lymph node ≤3 cm in greatest dimension
N2	Metastases in a single ipsilateral lymph node >3 cm, but <6 cm in greatest dimension; or in multiple lymph nodes none >6 cm in greatest dimension; or in bilateral or contralateral lymph nodes
N2a	Metastases in a single ipsilateral lymph node >3 cm, but ≤6 cm in greatest dimension
N2b	Metastases in multiple lymph nodes none ≤6 cm in greatest dimension
N2c	Metastases in bilateral or contralateral lymph nodes, none 6 cm in greatest dimension
N3	Metastases in a lymph node >6 cm in greatest dimension

C			
Stage 0	Tis	N0	M0
Stage I	T1	N0	M0
Stage II	T2	N0	M0
Stage III	T3	N0	M0
	T1–3	N1	M0
Stage IVA	T4a	N0	M0
	T4a	N1	M0
	T1–4a	N2	M0
Stage IVB	Any T	N3	M0
	T4a	Any N	M0
Stage IVC	Any T	Any N	M1

Used with the permission of the American Joint Committee on Cancer (AJCC), Chicago, Illinois. The original source for this material is the *AJCC Cancer Staging Handbook,* Seventh Edition (2010) published by Springer Science and Business Media LLC, www.springerlink.com.

GENERAL MANAGEMENT

The choice of treatment modality, either singly or in combination, depends on the stage and size of the tumor and relevant patient factors such as toxicity, performance status, comorbid disease, and convenience. The overall health and functional status of the patient are important determinants in choosing between surgical and nonsurgical approaches. A multidisciplinary approach is paramount in the management of oral cancer patients. It is important and valuable for patients to undergo evaluation by relevant members of the multidisciplinary team, including head and neck surgery, radiation and medical oncology, nursing, dentistry, dietary, speech pathology, and social work, before treatment is delivered. Multidisciplinary evaluation prior to treatment disposition helps to ensure that broad consensus treatment recommendations are made and interdisciplinary coordination of care is facilitated.

Surgery is most commonly the treatment of choice. Surgical resection is expeditious, effective, and often associated with modest morbidity and good functional outcome particularly for patients with small to moderate-size lesions. Radiation therapy can be considered for patients with early-stage disease who either are not surgical candidates or refuse surgical management. For patients with advanced lesions of the oral cavity, a combined-modality approach is generally recommended. In patients with high-risk pathologic features, the addition of concurrent chemotherapy during the postoperative radiation treatment course may further augment tumor control rates provided the chemotherapy can be tolerated.[76–78] High-risk features commonly include extracapsular tumor spread and positive resection margins.[77,79–81]

SURGICAL MANAGEMENT

Cancer of the oral cavity is most commonly treated surgically when the disease is in its early stages.[28] Because successful treatment of oral cavity carcinoma relies on effective management of the regional lymphatics as well as the primary cancer, the neck should be addressed in treatment planning. Elective neck surgical treatment is often used for management of the clinically node-negative patient with oral cancer, and therapeutic neck dissections are performed for patients with clinically apparent nodal disease. Postoperative radiation or chemoradiation is administered to those patients with pathologic evidence of extensive nodal disease and/or extracapsular spread. Because of the high occult metastatic rate for many cancers, elective neck treatment is encouraged in all but the earliest stages of primary site disease.

Management of the Oral Cavity

Surgical approaches to cancers of the oral cavity may either be transoral, transcervical (pull-through), or, alternatively, via mandibulectomy, which is sometimes necessary to obtain the exposure required to achieve adequate margins. In cases where the mental or alveolar nerve is involved with tumor, the nerve should be proximally resected and analyzed microscopically. A tracheotomy is often necessary to maintain a patent airway because of the large amount of oral edema resulting from extensive resection and placement of myocutaneous flaps in the oral cavity.

Tumors that approximate the gingiva should be resected with the gingiva and periosteum as an additional deep margin, while those that appear to involve the periosteum should be resected with an additional deep margin of bone. This last procedure is termed a *marginal mandibulectomy*. Depending on the extent of tumor involvement, this may involve resection of a bicortical rim of bone at the upper aspect of the alveolus (rim mandibulectomy) or, alternatively, selective removal of the inner cortex using a vertical or oblique resection (sagittal mandibulectomy). It is commonly recommended to leave at least a 1-cm-thick segment of bone inferiorly following a rim mandibulectomy to reduce the risk of pathologic fracture. Those lesions that directly invade bone should be resected with a segment of bone. This often requires soft-tissue or osseous reconstruction of the resected bone segment.

Regarding reconstruction after tumor resection, small surgical defects may not require reconstruction and therefore are often allowed to heal by secondary intention. Larger defects may be reconstructed by primary closure, skin graft, regional flap, or free-tissue transfer from different sites. Goals of reconstruction are to replicate the function and appearance of the resected tissue. Urken et al.[82] have developed a systematic approach to functional reconstruction of the oral cavity. Their approach to reconstruction is based on the extent and functional status of the residual tongue and the presence or absence of an associated mandibulectomy.

Split-thickness skin grafts are often used for reconstruction and are usually most expedient and efficacious for small defects. Larger defects may require a local or regional flap. Small intraoral defects can be reconstructed effectively with palatal, tongue, and buccal mucosa flaps but usually at the cost of decreased function. Regional flaps that are used in the reconstruction of the oral cavity include the pectoralis major flap, trapezius flap, and latissimus dorsi flap. Continuing developments in microvascular surgery have allowed for head and neck reconstructive surgeons to perform free-tissue transfer to reconstruct oral cavity defects. The free flaps most commonly utilized in the oral cavity are the radial forearm flap, the anterolateral thigh flap, the rectus abdominis flap, and the fibula flap.

Total glossectomy defects are well suited for free flap reconstruction. Reconstruction of the mandible often requires free flaps that contain bone and soft tissue such as the fibula flap, the iliac crest flap, and the scapular flap. Compared to reconstruction plates, free flaps also allow the potential for a sensate flap through neural anastomosis. A sensate flap may result in improved swallowing and speech function, but few studies have unequivocally demonstrated an improvement in these functional outcomes.[76,83–87]

Management of the Neck

Lymphadenectomy in the presence of known neck disease can be therapeutic as well as provide prognostic information (i.e., presence of extracapsular extension). For midline tumors, regardless of the type of dissection, bilateral surgical management is recommended. However, for well-lateralized tumors, unilateral dissection, followed by bilateral postoperative radiation, is reasonable. Generally, in patients with nodal disease ≥6 cm (N3), extracapsular extension, or clinically evident disease in levels IV or V, the most common approach is a modified radical nodal dissection (MRND). This includes the removal of nodal levels I through V (including the submental nodes), with sparing of the sternocleidomastoid muscle, internal jugular vein, and accessory nerve, if they are uninvolved with disease. However, as MRND can lead to significant morbidity, the use of selective neck dissection has gained favor in patients with more limited nodal disease.[88] This procedure involves the removal of at least levels I through III, with the possible addition of level IV depending on the interpretation of the surgeon. Outcomes for selective neck dissection in this patient population compare favorably to those observed with MRND; however, the possibility of skip metastases is always a concern.[89]

Heretofore, we have discussed the role of nodal dissection in patients with clinically evident nodal disease. However, further neck management questions arise in the patient with a clinically negative neck. The decision to proceed with a selective neck dissection in this context is usually guided by the invasion of the primary oral tumor, with a depth >2 to 4 mm thought to require surgical intervention. Further guidance on this topic is provided by two recent trials investigating the role of sentinel lymph node biopsy (SLNB) in patients with small volume (T1–2) oral squamous cell carcinoma.[90,91] Similar to other cancer types, SLNB provides excellent sensitivity (~90% to 100%) and negative predictive value (~95%) with no compromise of local control in the neck. Although a promising approach, SLNB in oral cavity squamous cell carcinoma has yet to become a standard practice in North America.

RADIATION THERAPY

General Principles

Evidence-based practice guidelines in oncology published by the National Comprehensive Cancer Network (NCCN) recommend single-modality treatment (i.e., surgery or radiation) for early-stage T1 or T2 lesions[92]; however, a primary surgical approach is generally preferred. For more advanced lesions, NCCN guidelines recommend a combined-modality approach involving surgery followed by adjuvant radiation or chemoradiation.[92] In considering primary radiation as a treatment option, it must be borne in mind that the keratinizing, well-differentiated histology of many oral cancers may portend radioresistance. It is also important to consider that the bony structures of the mandible and maxilla may impact the transmission of ionizing radiation. A combined approach including both external-beam radiation and interstitial brachytherapy is often recommended for optimal outcome. Thus, a course of radiation can require several weeks of daily therapy followed by an interstitial implant. The normal-tissue toxicity risks of xerostomia, dental and gum injury, and occasional osteoradionecrosis may render radiation therapy a less attractive option for single-modality treatment of patients who are candidates for surgery.

Historically, sites commonly treated with single-modality radiation include the lip, floor of the mouth, and oral tongue.[93,94] Early work indicates that the success rate of radiotherapy is higher if some or all of the treatment is administered with brachytherapy.[95,96] Decroix and Ghossein[97] reported outcomes in 602 patients with cancer of the oral tongue treated with radium implantation or implantation plus external-beam radiation. In this series, recurrence at the primary site or at the primary site and neck was 14% and 22% for T1 and T2 lesions, respectively. The Royal Marsden Hospital reported local control rates of 90% at 5 years for T1 and T2 tumors treated with interstitial radiation with or without external-beam radiation.[98] Pernot et al.[99] reported local control rates of 96% for T1, 85% for T2, and 64% for T3 lesions of the oral cavity treated with brachytherapy and neck dissection. In this series, locoregional control rates were 83%, 70%, and 44%, respectively. Retrospective studies suggest that control rates at the primary site of early oral cavity lesions treated with brachytherapy alone or a combination of brachytherapy plus external-beam radiation range from approximately 70% to >95%.[97–100] For tumors that either involve the mandible or are immediately adjacent to it, definitive radiotherapy is contraindicated because it compromises control and increases the risk of osteoradionecrosis.

Intraoral cone, like interstitial brachytherapy, is a localized radiation therapy technique that has been used to boost the dose to the primary tumor in the oral cavity. Institutions with significant experience with this technique have reported results that rival those obtained by interstitial brachytherapy.[101,102] Either technique for boosting the primary tumor has resulted in improved outcomes compared to high-dose radiation therapy alone.[103,104] In general, external-beam radiation therapy followed by either technique is preferable over radiation therapy alone. As with all specialized procedures, the skill and experience of the radiation oncologist is of critical importance to the successful delivery and outcome of interstitial radiation or intraoral cone therapy.

The outcomes for advanced lesions of the oral cavity (T3 and T4) are less than satisfactory with either surgery or radiation alone. In most advanced-stage cancers single-modality therapy is inferior to combined-modality therapy.[96,105,106] Adjuvant radiation therapy can be delivered preoperatively or postoperatively.[101,105] Although each strategy has potential advantages and disadvantages, postoperative radiation therapy is generally preferred. Notable disadvantages of preoperative radiation therapy include a delay in definitive surgical treatment and limitations on the dose of radiation that can be delivered due to the risk of wound complications after surgery. Postoperative radiation treatment carries the advantage of no delay in the implementation of surgical resection and complete pathologic staging of the tumor. However, it must be borne in mind that postoperative wound complications may delay the implementation of postoperative radiation, and the regional hypoxia that can accompany the postoperative state may diminish the effectiveness of radiation compared to that achievable under conditions of full oxygenation.

Adjuvant Radiation

Although surgery is the preferred initial treatment approach for the majority of patients with tumors of the oral cavity, adjuvant radiation is commonly recommended to enhance the likelihood of locoregional tumor control. Robertson et al.[107] conducted a phase III study in the United Kingdom of 350 patients with T2–4/N0–2 oral cavity or oropharyngeal cancers comparing surgery and postoperative radiation versus radiation alone. Because a difference in survival was identified, the study was closed early. The authors found that after 23 months, overall survival, cause-specific survival, and local control were all improved in the surgery plus radiation arm. Traditionally, indications for postoperative radiation therapy include multiple cervical metastases, positive or close margins, extracapsular extension, perineural invasion, advanced T stage, and mandibular bone involvement. A phase III study conducted at the University of Texas M.D. Anderson Cancer Center established the relative prognostic significance of clusters of two or more clinicopathologic features.[108] The adverse clinicopathologic features in this study included (a) close or positive margins, (b) nerve involvement, (c) two or more positive lymph nodes, (d) largest node >3 cm, (e) treatment delay >6 weeks, and (f) Zubrod performance status ≥2. The presence of extracapsular extension was the only factor independently predictive of locoregional recurrence. Moreover, the authors concluded that escalation of dose beyond 63 Gy (in 1.8 Gy per fraction) to sites of increased risk did not yield improved locoregional control.

It is well appreciated that head and neck tumors are rapidly proliferating. Several retrospective series have demonstrated an association between diminished outcomes and a delay beyond 6 weeks in initiating postoperative radiation.[109–111] A multi-institutional prospective study by Ang et al.[112] demonstrated that the total treatment time from the completion of surgery to the completion of radiation may affect the likelihood of ultimate disease control. This study illustrated the impact of overall treatment time on 5-year locoregional control: patients with overall treatment times <11 weeks demonstrated a locoregional control rate of 76%, compared to 62% for 11 to 13 weeks, and 38% for times beyond 13 weeks. Hence, it is recommended that adjuvant radiation proceed as soon as surgical wounds are well healed, optimally 4 to 6 weeks after completion of surgery.

There has been significant interest in the use of intensified radiation fractionation schedules to counter rapid tumor cell repopulation as a means of improving outcomes in head and neck cancer patients treated with radiation. Altered fractionation regimens such as hyperfractionation or accelerated fractionation have been considered for patients being treated with radiation alone, as this approach has been demonstrated to improve the likelihood of locoregional tumor control in the definitive setting.[113] However, the use of altered fractionation in the postoperative setting has not been resolved. Ang et al.[112]

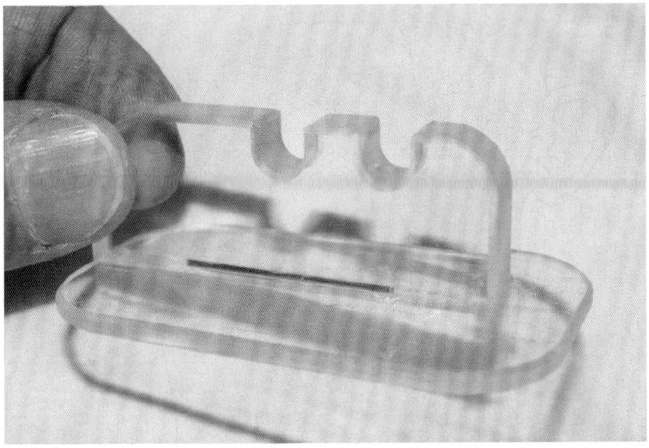

FIGURE 44.14. Lucite oral cavity mouthpiece fabricated at the University of Wisconsin for patients with oral cavity carcinomas. Upper dentition or maxillary alveolus links to U-shaped notch and tongue rests beneath smooth undersurface of mouthpiece. Note embedded solder wire in mouthpiece floor to facilitate visualization of tongue positioning at the time of simulation and beam design.

reported a trend toward higher locoregional control and survival with a concomitant boost schedule compared to a standard fractionation schedule. However, in a subsequent study, Sanguineti et al.[114] demonstrated no benefit for accelerated fractionation, except in patients for whom postoperative radiation was delayed.

There has been recent interest in postoperative chemoradiation for patients with high-risk pathologic features. The results of two randomized trials suggest that postoperative chemoradiation may be beneficial for improving local-regional control and disease-free survival among selected patients with specific high-risk features.[77,80] The impact of chemoradiotherapy appears to be most pronounced in patients with extracapsular extension and/or microscopically involved surgical margins.[79,80]

Neoadjuvant Therapy

At the current time, neoadjuvant radiation and chemotherapy remain largely experimental for cancer of the oral cavity. The use of preoperative chemotherapy has been studied in at least two randomized trials. Licitra et al.[115] conducted a phase III study of 195 patients with T2–4 (>3 cm)/N0–2 squamous cell carcinoma of the oral cavity and randomized patients to surgery alone versus three cycles of cisplatin and 5-fluorouacil (5-FU) followed by surgery. The authors found no difference in overall survival but did comment on the possibility of neoadjuvant chemotherapy as potentially improving resectability and reducing the need for adjuvant radiation therapy. In a similarly designed trial, Volling et al.[116] also reported no difference in overall survival with the use of neoadjuvant chemotherapy, although there was an improvement in disease-free survival.

Preoperative chemoradiation has been studied prospectively by Mohr et al.[117] The authors randomized 268 patients with T2–4/N0–3 oral cavity and oropharyngeal cancers to either preoperative chemoradiation with cisplatin or surgery alone. Results of this study revealed an improvement in overall survival and local control with the use of preoperative therapy. This regimen, however, has not shown common adoption in other centers around the world.

Radiation Techniques

Carcinoma of the oral cavity has traditionally been treated with opposed lateral fields, using either two-dimensional or three-dimensional (CT-based) techniques. During simulation and treatment, patients are commonly immobilized with a thermoplastic mask. Patients are placed in the supine position with a bite block (for oral tongue and floor of mouth cases) to depress the tongue away from the hard palate (Fig. 44.14); some institutions use a cork and tongue blade or a custom intraoral stent[92] for this purpose. For patients with a short neck, the shoulders are depressed by having the patient pull on a tensioning device looped beneath the feet. Custom masking of the head and neck and shoulders can also help accomplish optimal positioning. Generally, the oral cavity tumor bed and upper echelon lymph nodes are included within the initial lateral fields (Fig. 44.15). The upper border of the field is positioned to provide a 1.5- to 2.0-cm border on the tumor bed in an attempt to partially spare parotid glands and the hard palate if possible without compromising coverage of the tumor bed and regional lymphatics. The inferior border of the field resides at approximately the thyroid notch, just above the true vocal cords. The posterior border is set at the midvertebral body level if level V nodal coverage is not required. The nodal volume should include level Ia–b, II, and III. For patients with more advanced neck disease or positive level V lymph nodes, where the posterior chain requires radiation, the initial fields should be set behind the C1 vertebral body spinous process. The portals are then reduced at approximately 45 Gy to spare high dose to the spinal cord. If patients harbor cervical lymph node metastases, or high-risk disease, then the lower neck will also be treated.

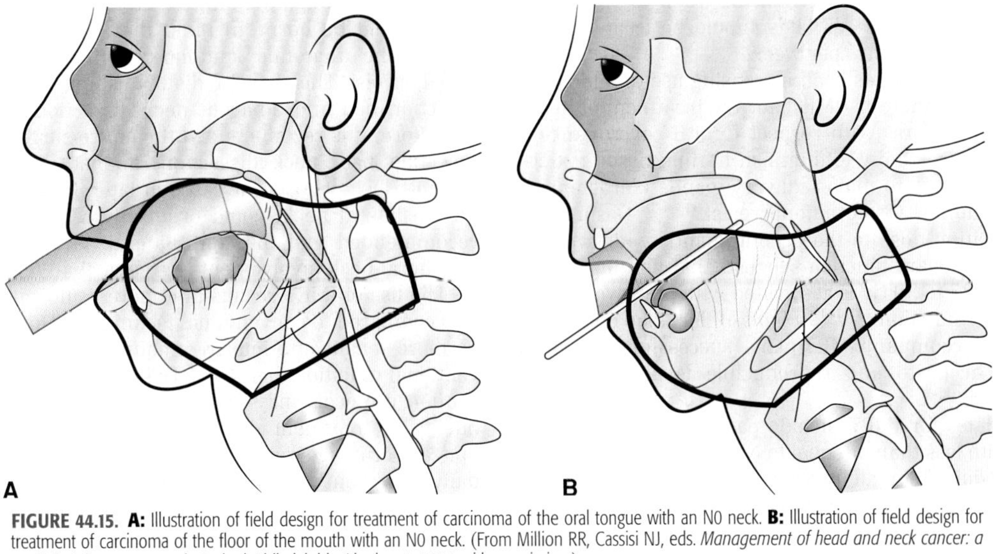

FIGURE 44.15. **A:** Illustration of field design for treatment of carcinoma of the oral tongue with an N0 neck. **B:** Illustration of field design for treatment of carcinoma of the floor of the mouth with an N0 neck. (From Million RR, Cassisi NJ, eds. *Management of head and neck cancer: a multidisciplinary approach,* 2nd ed. Philadelphia: Lippincott, 1994, with permission.)

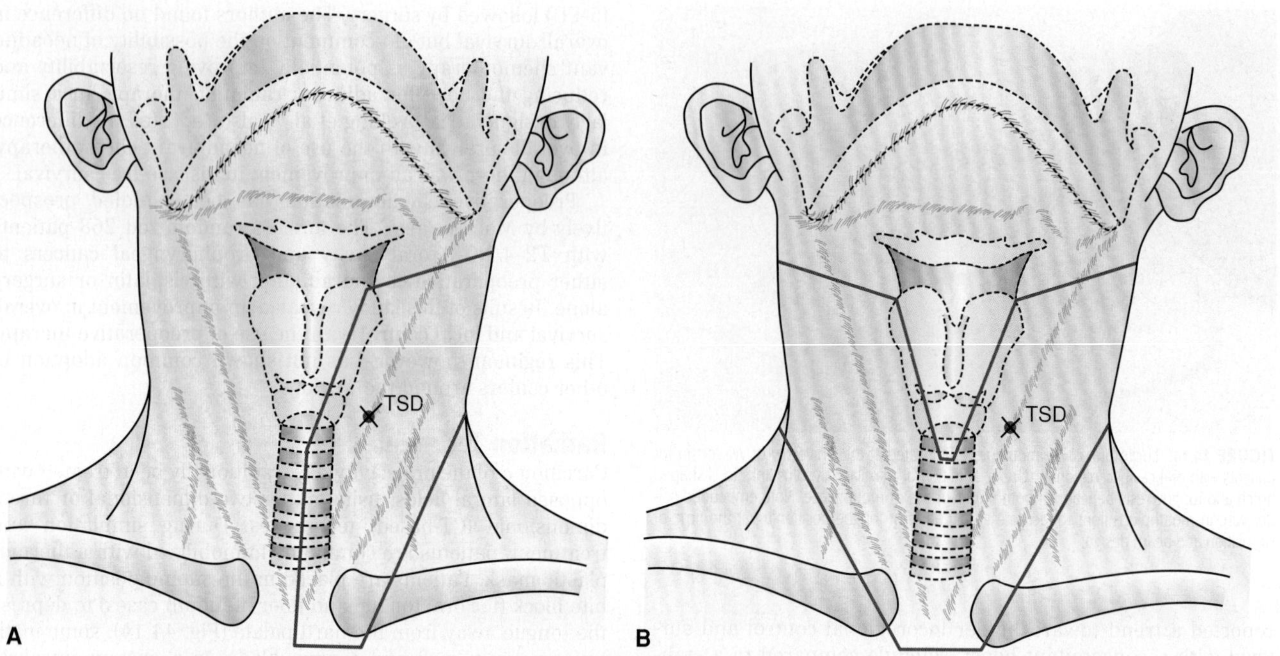

FIGURE 44.16. Illustration of field design for treatment of the neck. **A:** Well-lateralized lesion with clinically negative neck. **B:** Elective bilateral neck irradiation. (From Million RR, Cassisi NJ, eds. *Management of head and neck cancer: a multidisciplinary approach*, 2nd ed. Philadelphia: Lippincott, 1994, with permission.)

In this case, a single half-beam-blocked anteroposterior field is matched to the inferior border of the opposed lateral fields at the level of the thyroid notch (Fig. 44.16). An anterior larynx block is used, which not only protects the central larynx from unnecessary radiation dose but also protects against spinal cord overdose due to three-field overlap.

Megavoltage beams with an energy range between 4 and 6 MV are most suitable for treatment of cancers involving the oral cavity. Cobalt-60 (similar average energy to that from 4-MV linear accelerators) remains a very acceptable radiation delivery unit for cancers in this anatomic region owing to the small lateral separation distances in the head and neck area. When higher-energy beams are used, bolus material may be necessary to bring the dose to the surface as required for tumors that extend to the skin. This is particularly important in patients with large-volume nodal disease or extracapsular extension where particular attention should be paid to adequate dosing of superficial tissues. Tissue-compensating filters should be used with opposed lateral fields when the variation of the separation is >3 cm. All fields should be treated daily with at least 5 treatment days per week.

In recent years, there has been increasing use of intensity-modulated radiation therapy (IMRT) for the treatment of head and neck region tumors. With respect to oral cavity cancer, IMRT offers the opportunity to diminish normal-tissue toxicities, including damage to major salivary glands (xerostomia) and to the mandible (osteoradionecrosis).[118–120] Dosimetric analysis of radiation dose to the parotid glands with evaluation of resultant salivary function suggests that limiting mean parotid dose to <25 to 30 Gy is associated with improved post-radiation salivary function.[121–123] In light of the steep dose gradients that often accompany IMRT plans, successful delivery is dependent on accurate and reproducible localization and immobilization.[124,125]

Ideal candidates for IMRT include patients with T1–4 primary lesions with less than or equal to N2b neck disease. IMRT may not be required in all patients with T1–2/N0 disease because the bulk of both parotid glands can be excluded from opposed lateral portals. In patients who have ipsilateral positive neck nodes IMRT may allow dose limitation to the contralateral parotid gland without compromising treatment results.[126] In patients with bilateral (N2c) neck disease it may be difficult to effectively spare the parotid glands, particularly when superior level II cervical lymph nodes are involved.

A comprehensive discussion regarding target volume delineation and treatment planning for IMRT is outside the scope of this chapter. However, in the following discussion we will provide some broad principles and illustrations (Fig. 44.17). Generally, most cases of oral cavity cancer will be treated postoperatively. In this setting, the high-risk clinical target volume (CTV1) should include the primary tumor bed (based on preoperative imaging, physical examination, and operative findings) plus regions of grossly involved adenopathy. The intermediate-risk clinical target volume (CTV2) should include the pathologically positive hemineck; this frequently requires coverage of nodal levels I, IIa–b, III, and IV for most cases. The low-risk clinical target volume (CTV3) usually includes the prophylactically treated neck felt to have a low risk of harboring microscopic disease (e.g., the uninvolved low or contralateral neck).

It should be borne in mind that neck dissection tends to disrupt the anatomic landmarks defining borders between nodal levels. The task of distinguishing the primary tumor resection bed and adjacent neck dissection may be difficult. Therefore, it is recommended the entire surgical bed (primary resection bed, neck dissection, and scar) be encompassed within CTV1.[127] Also, for cases of lateralized disease in which the ipsilateral neck would ordinarily require treatment, it is recommended that the contralateral neck be included when ipsilateral neck involvement is greater than N1.[127]

The use of IMRT results in a more conformal dose distribution compared to conventional techniques. However, IMRT may be more sensitive to intertreatment setup variations than conventional radiation therapy.[125] Daily imaging and strict immobilization protocols may decrease setup error and improve the fidelity of treatment delivery.[125,128,129] At several centers, an optically or image-guided localization system is used to enhance daily treatment precision for IMRT delivery.[125] Tomotherapy, which involves the helical delivery of intensity-modulated radiation, enables a high degree of target conformality coupled with the capacity for diagnostic CT scanning, thereby allowing image

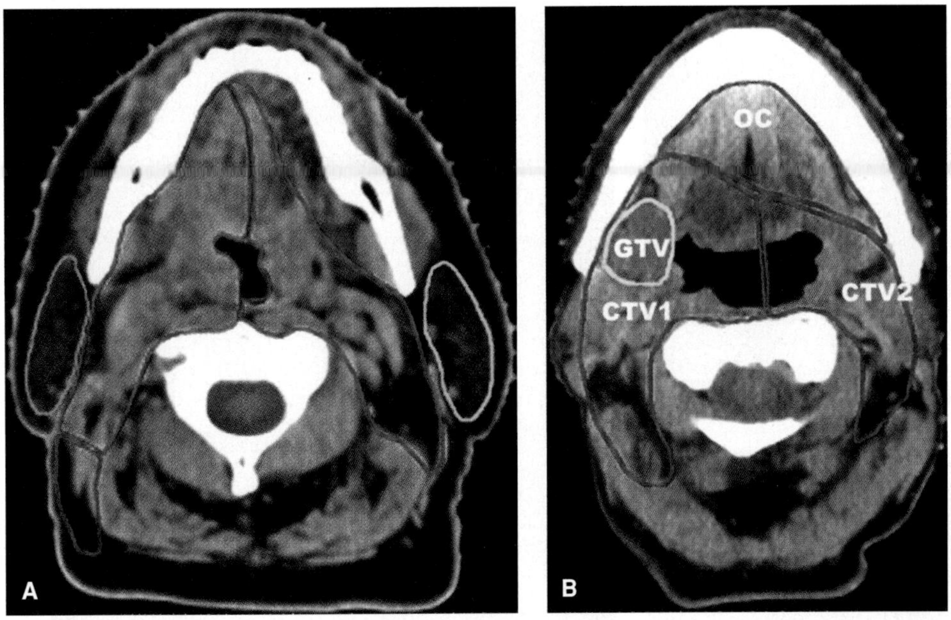

FIGURE 44.17. A: Clinical target volume (CTV) delineation for patient with T2/N2b oral tongue carcinoma receiving postoperative intensity-modulated radiation therapy (IMRT). CTV1 (*red line*), CTV2 (*dark blue line*), and parotid glands also noted. **B:** CTV delineation for patient with T3N2b retromolar trigone carcinoma receiving definitive IMRT. Gross tumor volume (GTV) (*yellow line*), CTV1 (*red line*), CTV2 (*dark blue line*), and oral cavity (*magenta line*) are shown. (From Chao KS, Ozyigit, G, eds. *Intensity modulated radiation therapy for H&N cancer.* Philadelphia: Lippincott Williams & Wilkins, 2003, with permission.)

guidance for adaptive radiotherapy and daily setup verification.[130,131] Cone-beam CT and daily orthogonal digital portal images are also strategies that have been implemented to enhance daily setup reproducibility for head and neck IMRT treatment.[124,125] With the use of these techniques, planning treatment volume (PTV) expansions on the CTV may be limited to 2 to 5 mm. However, larger margins may be necessary if daily imaging and immobilization protocols that address the shoulders as well as the head and neck[132] are not used. Shoulder immobilization is particularly important if the low neck is included in an extended IMRT plan (i.e., rather than treated with a single anteroposterior field matched to upper neck IMRT fields).[127,132–134]

The delivery of a single IMRT plan throughout the course of treatment provides better dose conformality compared to the delivery of several consecutive (sequential) plans.[135] The high-risk PTV (PTV1) should be treated to doses in the range of 60 to 66 Gy in 2.0 Gy per fraction. If microscopically positive margins or extracapsular spread is noted, this region should receive 64 to 66 Gy.[120,126] Intermediate-risk regions (i.e., without extracapsular extension [ECE] or microscopically positive margins) may receive 60 Gy. It is recommended that the intermediate-risk PTV (PTV2) and the low-risk PTV (PTV3) receive 60 Gy and 50 to 54 Gy, respectively. Optimally, treatment to low- and intermediate-risk regions should be given in fractions of 1.6 to 2.0 Gy.

External-Beam Dose and Fractionation

When postoperative radiation is used for oral cavity cancer, the most common dose fractionation in the United States is 1.8 to 2.0 Gy per day. Dissected tissues that harbored the original tumor should generally receive on the order of 60 Gy. However, for close or positive microscopic margins or extracapsular nodal extension, a 4- to 6-Gy localized boost should be considered. If there is gross residual disease, either further surgical resection or focal boosting up to 70 Gy is advisable. Regions of somewhat lesser risk (i.e., clinically or pathologically uninvolved necks) should receive on the order of 50 to 54 Gy.

When definitive radiation is used for oral cavity cancer, boosting the primary tumor with either interstitial implantation, submental, or intraoral cone therapy can result in increased tumor control and decreased complications, particularly osteoradionecrosis.[103] When external-beam radiation therapy is used as the sole treatment modality, even small lesions that cannot be excised or treated with brachytherapy require doses in the range of 66 Gy in 2-Gy fractions for reliable control. For larger tumors, improved local control rates are likely to be achieved with doses ≥70 Gy, but there is an increasingly significant price to pay in terms of normal-tissue toxicity for doses in this range.

Brachytherapy

Historically, brachytherapy has played an important role in the treatment of oral cavity carcinoma. Brachytherapy has been used to boost the primary site in the oral cavity before or following external-beam radiation (Fig. 44.18). This technique has also been used as a sole modality in the treatment of selected (early-stage) tumors of the oral cavity with good results.[99,100,136] When brachytherapy is used as a sole treatment modality, doses of 65 to 75 Gy are commonly prescribed over 6 to 7 days. Traditionally, radiation has been delivered using low-dose rates of 0.4 to 0.6 Gy per hour to the target volume.[137,138] However, there has been recent interest in high–dose-rate (HDR) (Fig. 44.19) and pulsed–dose-rate techniques (PLDR),[139,140] although there is no compelling evidence that these techniques are superior to traditional low–dose-rate radiation in the treatment of head and neck cancer. There have been several dose and fractionation schedules published for HDR brachytherapy in the treatment of oral cavity cancer.[141–144] Although the American Brachytherapy Society has not provided a consensus as to optimal dose and fractionation,[145] there is concern regarding the potential morbidity with fraction sizes ≥6.0 Gy in this setting.[145]

Many techniques for brachytherapy in the oral cavity have been described.[146,147] Brachytherapy can be accomplished with either rigid cesium needles or with iridium-192 (^{192}Ir) sources afterloaded into Angiocaths. The most common technique is afterloading with ^{192}Ir.[148] Guide needles can be inserted either freehand or with the aid of a custom template to help maintain optimal source spacing.

Depending on the size of the lesion, a single-plane, double-plane, or volume implant can be used to cover the tumor with a 1-cm margin. For tumors <1 cm in thickness, single-plane implants are adequate. Surface mold radiation can also be considered for small tumors with <1-cm depth or superficial lesions of the lip, hard palate, lower gingiva, and floor of the mouth. However, when lesions exceed 2.5 cm, it is difficult to avoid significant cold spots in the implant volume. For this reason, it is recommended that for lesions >2.5 cm, part of the treatment

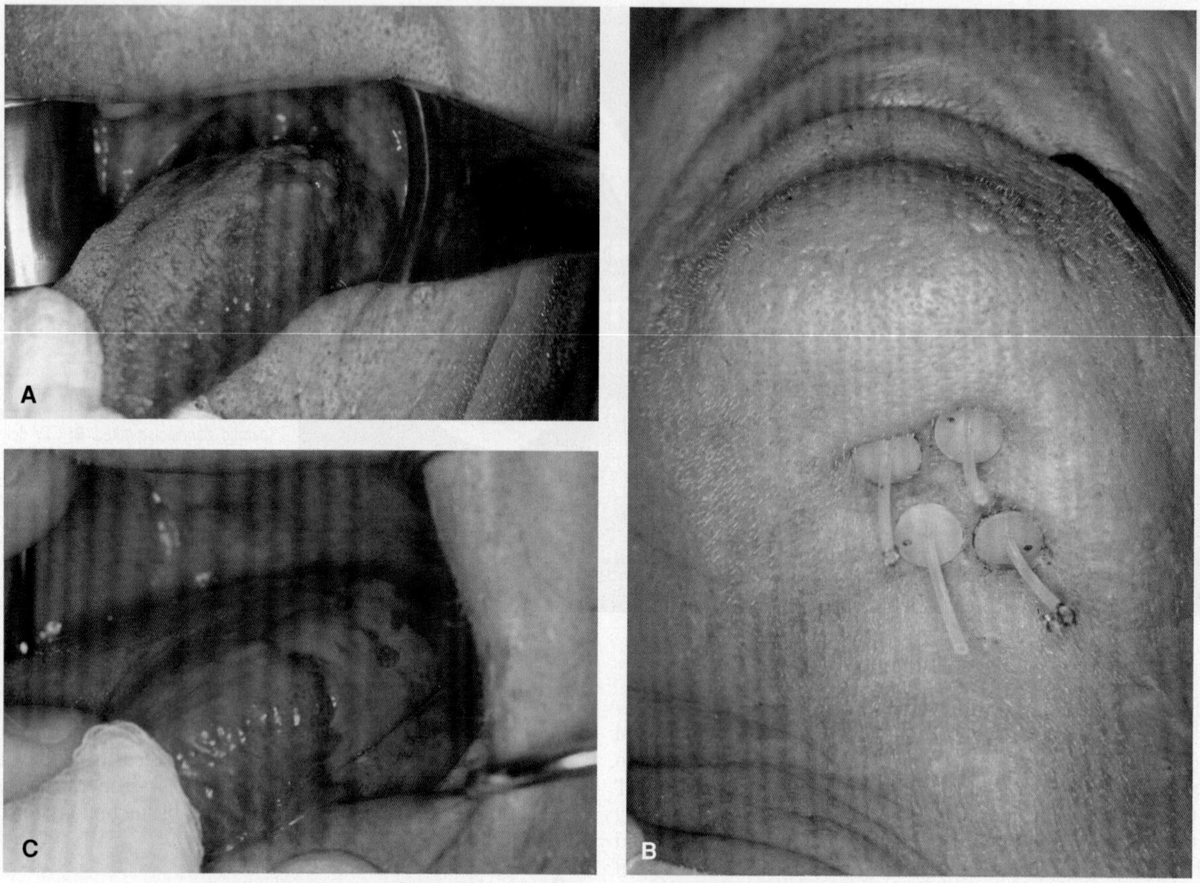

FIGURE 44.18. A: T2N0M0 squamous cell carcinoma involving the left lateral oral tongue. **B:** Submental view of interstitial implantation catheters housing ^{192}Ir seeds for delivery of 25-Gy tumor boost following external-beam radiation of 50 Gy. **C:** Implantation bed mucositis conforming to the tumor distribution 7 days following 25-Gy implant boost.

should be given with external-beam radiation to supplement the dose to the cold spots. In this setting, a combined treatment plan typically gives 50 Gy over 5 weeks with external-beam radiation followed by 30 Gy with a brachytherapy implant. What must be borne in mind is that as tumors get too close to the mandible or become large in volume, the risk of osteoradionecrosis increases.[149]

Over the past decade or more, stepwise improvements in reconstructive surgery techniques have diminished the practice frequency of brachytherapy in the treatment of oral cavity carcinoma. In addition, a diminishing percentage of radiation oncologists remain highly skilled and experienced with the requisite implant techniques. Finally, the steady advancement of highly conformal external-beam techniques (IMRT, tomotherapy) has contributed to less frequent practice of brachytherapy in head and neck cancer overall. The identical comments parallel the use of the intraoral cone radiation treatment described further in the next section.

Intraoral Cone

The intraoral cone is another delivery tool to enable boosting of radiation dose to sites within the oral cavity while avoiding

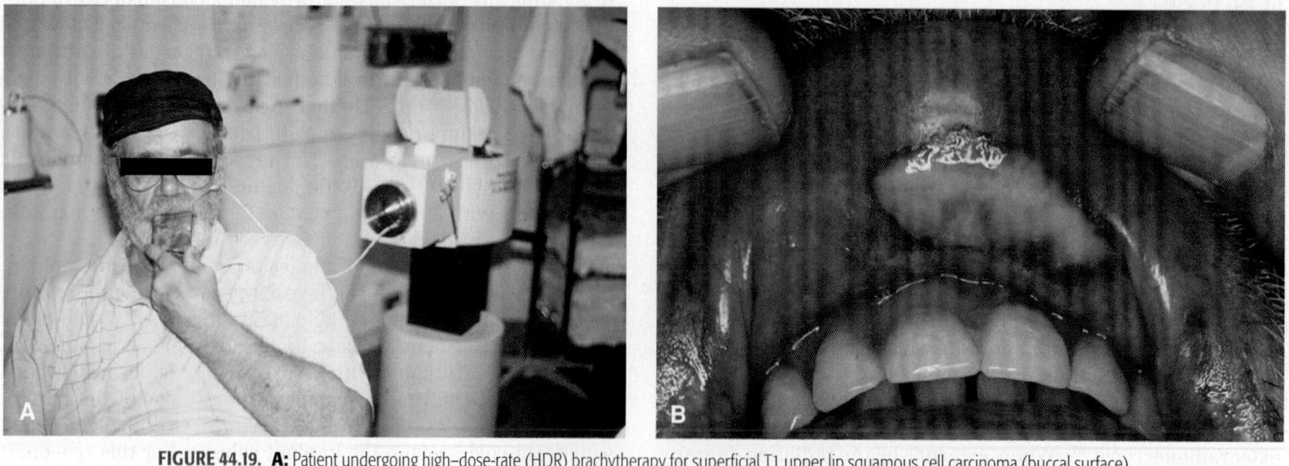

FIGURE 44.19. A: Patient undergoing high–dose-rate (HDR) brachytherapy for superficial T1 upper lip squamous cell carcinoma (buccal surface) using a single interstitial catheter for source delivery. **B:** Focal mucositis 1 week following completion of HDR brachytherapy treatment course.

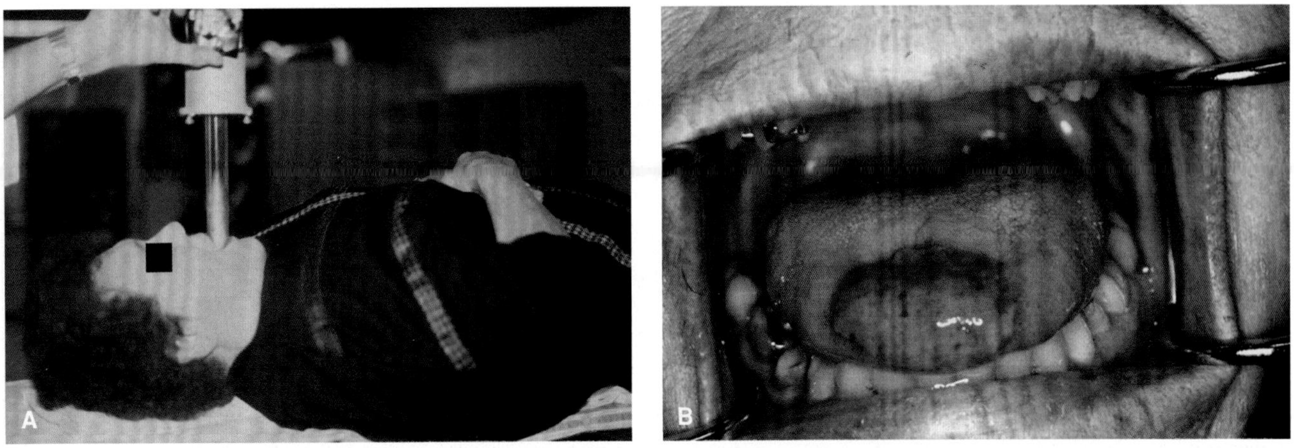

FIGURE 44.20. A: Intraoral cone boost technique at the University of Wisconsin for focal delivery of electron beam radiation. The electron cone is mounted directly to the accelerator gantry with a side view periscope enabling direct vision and positioning for daily treatment. **B:** Focal mucositis involving the distal oral tongue following treatment of a 1-cm tumor in this location with intraoral cone technique.

direct dose to the mandible (Fig. 44.20). This technique is generally best suited for anterior oral cavity lesions in edentulous patients. However, palatal arch sites can be targeted with the intraoral cone as well. Treatment with intraoral cone involves either 100- to 250-kilovolt (peak) (kvp) x-rays or electron beams in the 6- to 12-MeV range.[101,102,146] Lesions up to 3 cm are amenable to treatment with intraoral cone as long as they are accessible. Intraoral cone therapy requires careful daily positioning and verification by the physician. For this purpose the device is equipped with a periscope to visualize the lesion. The cone abuts the mucosa and is centered directly over the lesion. Intraoral cone treatment should take place prior to external-beam radiation so that the lesion can be adequately visualized. A major advantage of cone therapy is that it is highly focal to the tumor bed but noninvasive. Hence, when available, for suitable lesions, it may be preferred over brachytherapy. However, as noted for brachytherapy delivery, operator experience and dedication are essential to optimize outcome.

Chemotherapy and Radiation

The application of chemotherapy to the treatment of head and neck cancer dates back to the 1960s. Over the decades the role of chemotherapy has advanced from initial use only in the recurrent or metastatic setting to active current use in the definitive treatment setting. There are a number of studies that demonstrate a benefit of concurrent chemotherapy administration in the definitive treatment of head and neck cancer with radiation.[150–156] Although these trials vary with respect to radiation dose, fractionation schedule, and chemotherapy regimen, they have in common a randomized comparison between radiotherapy and radiotherapy plus chemotherapy. The advantage of concurrent chemotherapy with radiation has been further examined in the context of several meta-analyses.[157–160] These meta-analyses generally identify a small overall survival benefit for the use of chemotherapy on the order of 1% to 8%.[161] Summary analyses suggest no significant survival benefit for the use of neoadjuvant and adjuvant chemotherapy but do suggest a clear benefit for the use of concurrent chemoradiation. However, in many of the randomized studies comparing radiation alone to chemoradiation, oral cavity cancer patients are either excluded or make up only a small proportion of the study population.

Several studies have focused on the use of chemoradiation in patients with high-risk pathologic features following initial surgery. Cooper et al.[77] reported the results of a randomized study comparing radiation alone (60 to 66 Gy) to chemoradiation (same radiation dose plus three cycles of 100 mg/m^2 cisplatin) in patients with head and neck carcinoma demonstrating high-risk features after gross total resection. High-risk disease was defined as any or all of the following: two or more involved lymph nodes, extracapsular extension of nodal disease, and microscopically involved resection margins. This study demonstrated a benefit in local-regional control and disease-free survival for the chemoradiation arm, but no overall survival benefit was appreciated. Bernier et al.[80] randomized patients to essentially equivalent treatment arms following head and neck cancer surgery. Eligibility criteria included patients with pathologic T3 or T4 disease (except T3N0), or patients with any T-stage disease with two or more involved lymph nodes, or patients with T1–2 and N0–1 disease with unfavorable pathologic findings (extranodal spread, positive margins, perineural involvement, or vascular embolism). Local control, progression-free survival, and overall survival were superior for patients in the chemoradiation arm. In a subsequent comparative analysis using pooled data from these two studies, ECE and/or microscopically involved surgical margins were the risk factors for which the impact of concurrent chemoradiation was significant.[79] However, there was a trend favoring concurrent chemoradiation in the subset of patients with stage III to IV disease, vascular embolism, perineural infiltration, and/or positive lymph nodes at level IV and V with oral cavity or oropharyngeal primary cancers.[79] The subset of patients with two or more involved lymph nodes, without evidence of ECE, did not appear to benefit from chemotherapy in this analysis. These studies suggest that the addition of chemoradiation following surgery may be beneficial in selected patients with high-risk head and neck cancer, although with increased toxicity profiles.

Dental Care

Prior to the initiation of head and neck radiation, a careful oral and dental evaluation, including a panoramic radiograph, should be performed. Dentition in poor condition should be identified and considered for extraction to minimize the subsequent risk of osteoradionecrosis. Specifically, those teeth that will reside within the high-dose radiation volume that demonstrate significant periodontal disease, advanced caries, or abscess formation or are otherwise in a state of disrepair should be extracted. In addition, impacted teeth, unopposed teeth, and teeth that could potentially oppose a segment of a resected jawbone should be considered for extraction if they are anticipated to reside within the high-dose radiation treatment volume. Extraction of marginal teeth should also be considered in patients who are deemed unable to maintain adequate oral hygiene.

Radiation can induce several chronic effects in the oral cavity that warrant routine surveillance. Radiation can impair

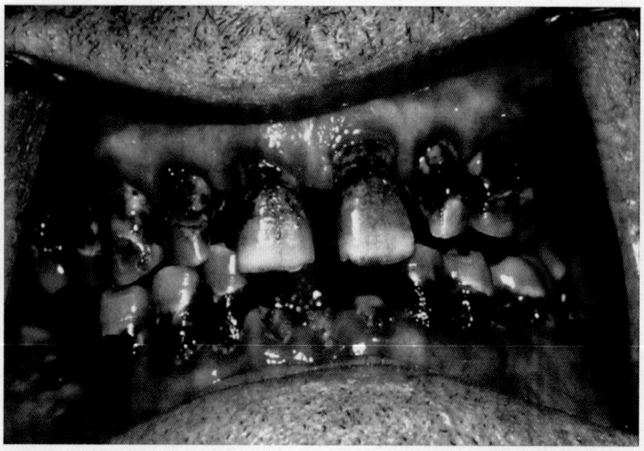

FIGURE 44.21. Advanced dental caries in a patient with profound radiation xerostomia and lack of attention to dental hygiene over many years following treatment.

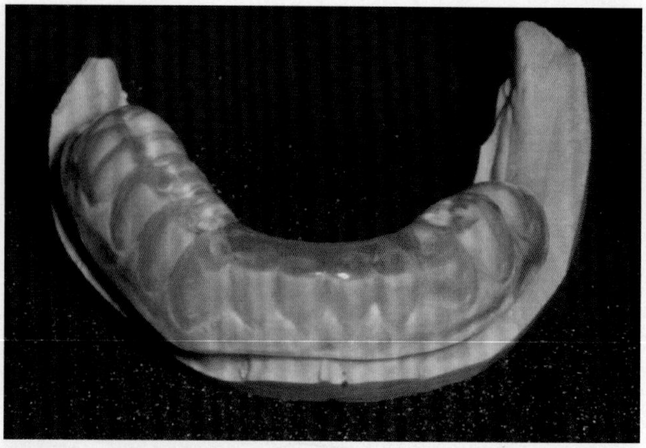

FIGURE 44.23. Custom-designed fluoride carrier trays to facilitate daily fluoride application to existing dentition.

bone healing and diminish the capacity for successful recovery following trauma or oral surgery. For this reason, elective oral surgical procedures including extractions must be very carefully considered after radiation. Escalation of dental caries deriving from xerostomia following radiation is well recognized (Fig. 44.21). Radiation of the major salivary glands changes the nature of salivary secretions,[48] which can increase the accumulation of plaque and debris, reduce salivary pH, and reduce the buffering ability of saliva.[162] This creates an environment in the oral cavity, which predisposes patients to caries. During a course of radiation to the oral cavity, simple techniques such as the use of custom molds to absorb electron backscatter can diminish hot-spot mucositis from dental fillings and improve treatment tolerance (Fig. 44.22). Attention to oral hygiene with frequent dental follow-up examinations and cleanings, daily fluoride therapy (Fig. 44.23), flossing, and brushing should be an integral component of the education and postradiation care of patients who undergo radiation to the oral cavity.

PROGNOSTIC AND PREDICTIVE FACTORS

The most significant prognostic factor for outcome in oral cavity carcinoma is the presence of cervical metastases.[163] In patients with positive cervical metastases the 5-year survival is reduced by approximately 50% compared to those without cervical metastases.[164] The prognosis diminishes further when patients harbor multiple levels of nodal involvement or ECE. In a retrospective review, Myers et al.[163] found that 5-year

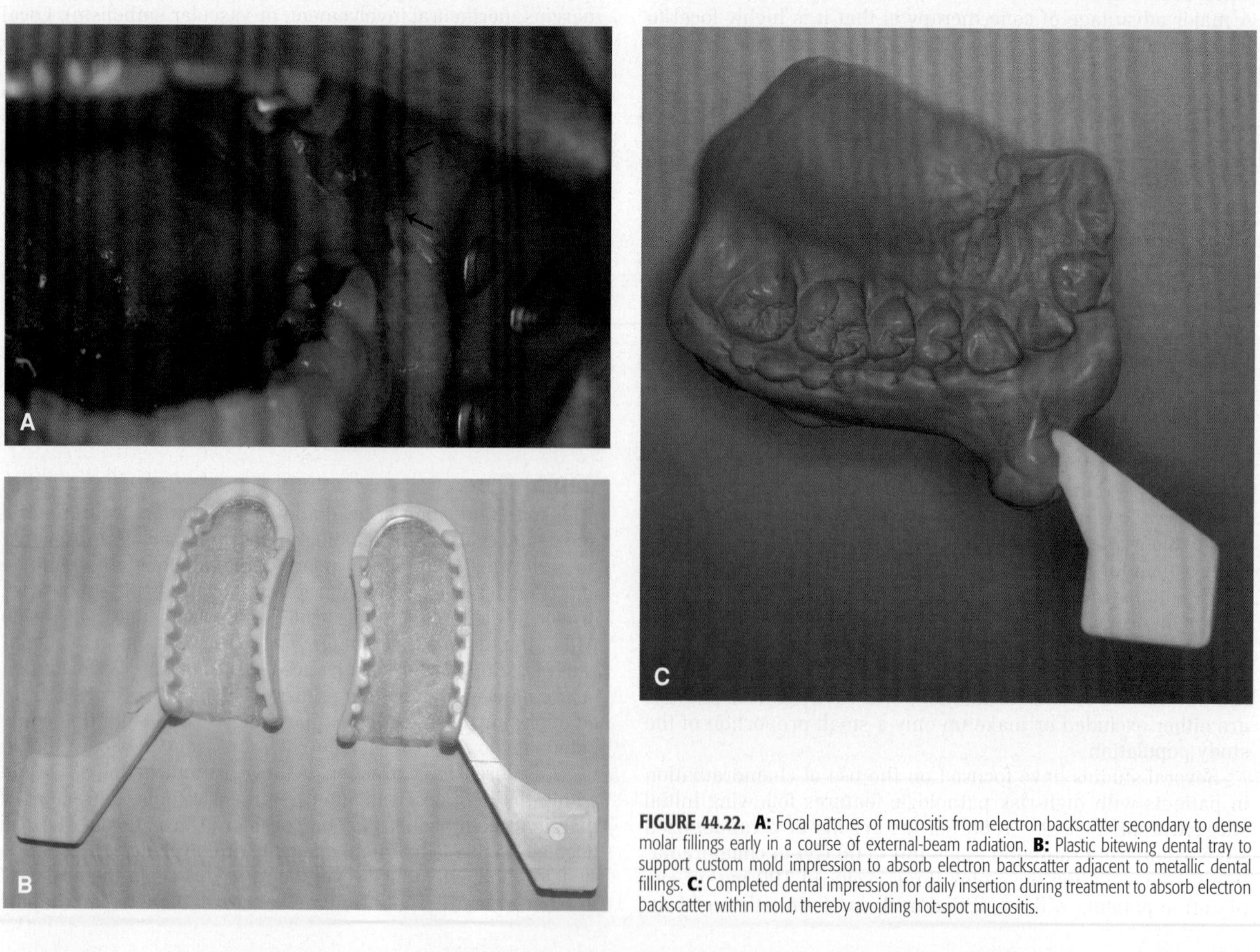

FIGURE 44.22. **A:** Focal patches of mucositis from electron backscatter secondary to dense molar fillings early in a course of external-beam radiation. **B:** Plastic bitewing dental tray to support custom mold impression to absorb electron backscatter adjacent to metallic dental fillings. **C:** Completed dental impression for daily insertion during treatment to absorb electron backscatter within mold, thereby avoiding hot-spot mucositis.

disease-specific and overall survival rates for pathologically N0 patients were 88% and 75%, respectively; these decreased to 65% and 50%, respectively, if patients were node positive but without evidence of ECE. Patients who were node positive with evidence of ECE had 5-year disease-specific and overall survival rates of 48% and 30%, respectively.

Several histopathologic factors in the primary lesion are associated with adverse prognosis. Tumor thickness and depth of invasion have been shown to confer a higher risk of regional metastases.[28] Perineural invasion has been correlated with cervical lymph node metastases, extracapsular extension, and diminished survival.[165–167] Microvascular invasion has also been correlated significantly with cervical lymph node metastases.[168,169] However, lymphatic invasion has not been correlated significantly with cervical lymph node invasion.[28] The prognostic significance of grade has also been evaluated.[170] Because of the wide variation in pathologic interpretation, it is difficult to discern the independent value of histologic grading as a prognostic or predictive value.[28]

SUBSITE-SPECIFIC TREATMENT AND RESULTS

Lip

Early-stage carcinoma of the lip can be managed with surgery or radiation therapy. However, surgery is generally preferred for tumors <2 cm. Although the local control of T1 and T2 squamous cancers of the lip is excellent with surgical resection, disruption of the oral sphincter provided by the orbicularis muscle can lead to oral incompetence if not properly reconstructed. Therefore, a number of reconstructive methods have been developed to help preserve oral sphincteric function even following large excisions for T3 and T4 lesions. For these larger lesions, surgery followed by radiotherapy remains a standard therapy.

When primary radiotherapy is used to treat lip cancer, the target volume should include the primary tumor plus a 1.5- to 2.0-cm margin. For early-stage lesions, orthovoltage photons (100 to 200 keV) or electrons may be used. The electron energy should be chosen based on the thickness of the lesion (commonly 6 to 9 MeV). Effort should be made to shield the underlying gum, dentition, and mandible as appropriate. This can be accomplished with the use of oral shields or Cerrobend stents. The recommended dose is 50 Gy in 4.5 to 5 weeks for smaller lesions and 60 Gy in 5 to 6 weeks for larger lesions. Some institutions have used an approach where external-beam radiation is given to approximately 40 to 50 Gy followed by a brachytherapy boost, or smaller lesions are treated by primary brachytherapy alone (Fig. 44.24).

An important consideration in managing lip cancer is the risk of regional metastatic disease. Generally, the risk of regional lymph node metastatic disease for T1 and T2 cancers of the lip is lower than for stage-matched tumors of other oral cavity sites. Thus, elective neck dissection is recommended for patients with T3 and T4 carcinomas of the lip; however, it may not be warranted for all T1 and T2 lesions. Some institutions have used a "moustache field" for elective irradiation of the perifacial lymphatics (approximately 50 Gy) for more advanced upper lip lesions.[171] Sentinel lymph node biopsy may prove to be useful in the management of patients of node-negative lip cancers, but further clinical investigation in this area is needed.

Oral Tongue

Although primary radiation therapy and surgery are potential treatment options for early-stage carcinoma of the oral tongue, most oral tongue cancers in the United States are treated surgically.[28] Surgical resection and reconstruction as appropriate is generally preferred for medically operable patients. Postoperative radiation therapy is recommended for patients with large primary tumors (T3, T4), close or positive surgical margins, evidence of perineural spread, multiple positive nodes, or extracapsular extension.[171] Postoperative chemoradiation should be considered for patients with adverse risk factors who are able to tolerate combined-modality treatment.[77,79–81] Primary radiotherapy techniques can be used for patients who refuse or are unable to tolerate surgery.

Superficial T1 lesions can be treated with brachytherapy or intraoral cone therapy alone. ^{192}Ir temporary implants are used to deliver 50 to 60 Gy with dose rates of 40 to 60 cGy per hour. For infiltrating T1 or T2 lesions, a combined approach using external beam and a brachytherapy or intraoral cone boost should be considered. More advanced lesions should be treated with an approach combining surgery and radiation therapy. Postoperative treatment should include the site of primary tumor, dissected neck, and draining lymphatics. Opposing lateral fields are used to encompass the tongue and upper neck bilaterally, and this volume should be treated to 50 to 54 Gy (see Fig. 44.15A and Table 44.1). High-risk areas (primary surgical bed, positive/close margins, extracapsular extension, perineural spread) should receive additional boost treatment up to 60 to 66 Gy. In patients treated with IMRT, the high-risk CTV should include the intrinsic and extrinsic muscles of the tongue, floor of the mouth, base of the tongue, glossotonsillar sulcus, and anterior tonsillar pillar.[127] The adjacent dissected neck should also be included in this volume. The appropriate draining lymphatics should be included in the low- to intermediate-risk

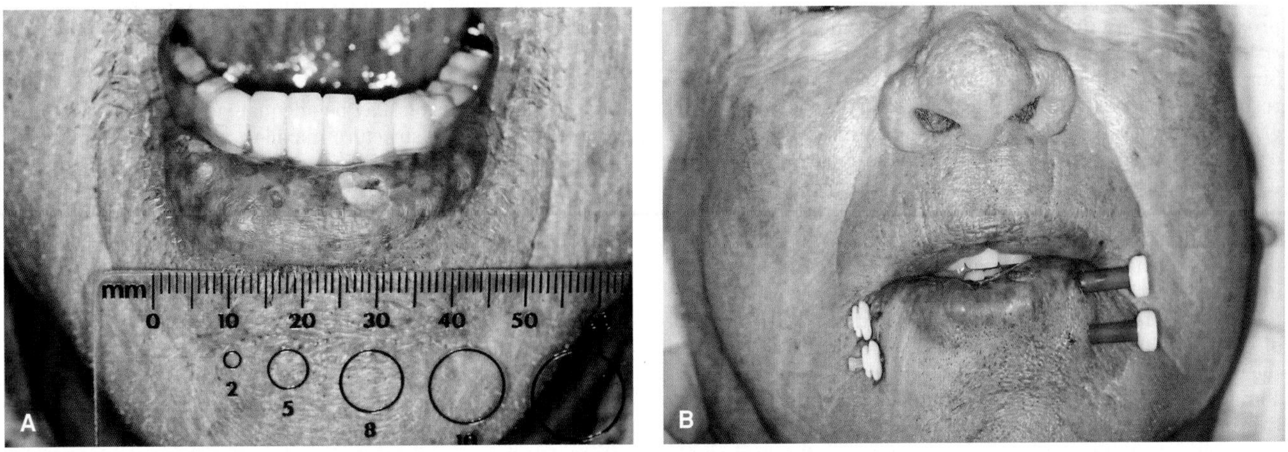

FIGURE 44.24. A: Infiltrative T2N0 squamous cell carcinoma of the lower lip measuring 3.5 × 1.2 × 1.2 cm. **B:** Interstitial iridium-192 implant performed (two catheters) for high-dose-rate (HDR) brachytherapy delivery over 11 elapsed days as sole treatment: the patient remains with no evidence of disease at 1 year with excellent cosmetic and functional status.

CTV (see Table 44.1 and Intensity-Modulated Radiation Therapy section).

Surgical approaches to oral tongue cancers can either be transoral, transcervical, or alternatively via mandibulectomy to obtain the exposure necessary to achieve adequate margins. Partial glossectomy is the most common procedure performed for oral tongue cancers, and the extent of resection depends on the size and growth pattern of the tumor, as some lesions are relatively infiltrative while others may be more exophytic. Because the tongue is essentially composed of skeletal muscle covered by mucosa, the tissue is extremely elastic, and wide margins are encouraged at the onset of resection to avoid retraction of muscle fibers with microscopic tumor cells that could serve as a source of local recurrence.

Total glossectomy may be indicated for extensive tumors or those that involve the intrinsic tongue musculature. Total glossectomy, even with reconstruction, can result in difficulty with deglutition and maintenance of an adequate airway. Aspiration may be a chronic problem, and thus, laryngectomy may be necessary in some cases. However, properly selected patients with adequate postoperative rehabilitation can be treated with total glossectomy without laryngectomy. If the larynx is preserved, laryngeal suspension and palatal augmentation may help with the rehabilitative efforts.

Tumor size and depth of invasion are currently the most reliable indicators for predicting cervical metastases in patients with oral tongue squamous cell carcinoma. Because of the high risk of nodal metastases, the neck should be addressed with either surgery or radiation in all but the earliest tumors of the oral tongue. Patients with small oral tongue cancers should be considered for neck therapy, particularly if the primary tumor exhibits extension onto the floor of the mouth or there is increased tumor thickness. Treatment of the clinically negative neck is most often accomplished by supraomohyoid neck dissection. Elective neck dissection appears to result in better overall cancer outcome than observation. Potential pitfalls of observation include a salvage rate of only one-third for patients who do not undergo elective neck dissection along with resection of the oral cavity primary cancer. For patients with a clinically and radiographically N0 neck, with well-lateralized disease, or those who do not undergo neck dissection, 50 to 54 Gy should be considered to the ipsilateral neck as elective nodal irradiation (Fig. 44.16). Patients with advanced lesions and high-risk disease (particularly with multiple positive nodes) should receive radiation treatment to the bilateral necks.

Floor of the Mouth

Early-stage floor of the mouth cancer can be treated effectively by radiation therapy or surgery. Surgery is usually preferred in patients who are medically operable because proximity of the tumor to the mandible confers a significant risk of radiation-induced ulceration and osteoradionecrosis. Small lesions of the floor of the mouth are most commonly resected transorally. The surgical defect can be left to heal by granulation or reconstructed with a split-thickness skin graft or local flap. Advanced-stage floor of the mouth cancers are usually managed by a combination of surgery and radiation or chemoradiation.

Small (T1 and T2) lesions may be treated with a combination of external-beam radiation and boost with interstitial implant or intraoral cone. For lesions that are very close to the mandible, brachytherapy is contraindicated because of the risk of osteoradionecrosis. Infiltrative lesions that are tethered to the mandible and advanced lesions following surgical resection should receive postoperative radiation. Portals for postoperative treatment are similar to that for oral tongue carcinoma. Opposing lateral fields are used to encompass the oral cavity tumor bed and upper neck bilaterally, and this volume is commonly treated to 50 to 54 Gy. High-risk areas (primary surgical bed, positive/close margins, extracapsular extension, perineural spread) may receive additional boost treatment up to 60 to 66 Gy. In cases where IMRT is used, the high-risk CTV should include genioglossus and geniohyoid muscles bilaterally, the sublingual and submandibular glands ipsilaterally (bilaterally if the tumor is midline), the adjoining alveolar ridge and mandible, the muscles at the root of the tongue, and the dissected necks.[127] The low- to intermediate-risk CTV should include the appropriate electively treated necks (Table 44.1).

In the surgical management of floor of the mouth cancer, special attention should be paid to mandibular invasion. A cancer that appears to involve only the periosteum or that only superficially invades the mandible can be removed via a transoral or transcervical approach in which a marginal mandibulectomy is performed. However, segmental mandibulectomy may be necessary for patients with a limited mandibular height when there is no direct bone invasion, because marginal mandibulectomy may leave these patients with insufficient bone, placing them at high risk for radionecrosis or pathologic fracture. A full-thickness segmental resection may be necessary if there is frank bone invasion. For advanced cancers, resection of the anterior arch of the mandible may be necessary. Defects of the anterior segment of the mandible require reconstruction with bone, usually with a free fibular or iliac crest graft.

Management of the neck is similar to that for other tumors of the oral cavity. Patients with lesions <2 mm thick with no adverse pathologic factors and a clinically and radiographically negative neck may be observed after primary resection and observation. Otherwise, most N0 patients should receive either selective neck dissection or radiation therapy. Patients with advanced lesions and high-risk disease (particularly with multiple positive nodes) should receive radiation treatment to bilateral necks.

Hard Palate and Upper Alveolar Ridge

Tumors of the hard palate are quite rare, accounting for only 0.5% of all oral cancers in the United States. Most carcinomas manifest as a granular superficial ulceration of the hard palate. Initial growth tends to be superficial, although these tumors can extend through the periosteum of bone into regions adjacent to the oral cavity, such as the paranasal sinuses and floor of the nose. Although radiation can be used to treat carcinomas of this site, surgery is preferred. Postoperative radiation therapy should be delivered when there are adverse features, that is, close/positive margins, perineural extension, vascular invasion, high-grade histology, multiple positive nodes, or extracapsular extension. The radiation field should encompass the entire surgical bed. In most cases it is necessary to treat with opposed lateral fields to cover the volume at risk. However, for well-lateralized lesions of the upper alveolar ridge, ipsilateral radiation with a wedge pair may be adequate. Conformal treatment techniques, including IMRT, can also be used to tailor the radiation coverage to the high-risk tissue bed and draining lymphatics as appropriate.

Wide local excision may be adequate to obtain surgical margins. However, infrastructure maxillectomy may in some cases be necessary. For tumors that extensively involve the adjacent bony and soft-tissue structures, a total maxillectomy, with or without orbital exenteration, may be required. A defect in the maxilla results in lack of oral/nasal separation that can impair the ability to speak and swallow effectively. An obturator with or without a skin graft is the most common method used to restore oral/nasal separation. The obturator is commonly fabricated from a synthetic polymer and provides oronasal separation that can yield improved speech and swallowing function. Regional pedicled flaps and free-tissue transfers may provide alternatives to obturation. However, their use is somewhat controversial for reconstruction of palatal defects because these nonremovable flaps may mask local recurrences that can be more readily identified in patients whose defects are obturated.

Elective treatment of the neck is controversial for hard palate region tumors. Although some series have shown lower rates of occult metastases for palatal tumors when compared to other oral cavity sites, preoperative imaging should be performed to evaluate for the presence of metastases to the retropharyngeal nodes because these are difficult to evaluate on clinical examination and are at some risk for spread from primary palatal tumors. Elective treatment of the clinically negative neck should be considered in high-grade tumors or lesions that present with advanced T stage.

Retromolar Trigone

Squamous cell carcinoma of the retromolar trigone is uncommon, and the true incidence is difficult to determine because these cancers often involve both the retromolar trigone and adjacent sites, thereby making it difficult in some cases to identify the original tumor epicenter. Cancers of the retromolar trigone may be advanced at presentation because only a thin layer of soft tissue overlies the bone in this region and invasion of the underlying bone may occur early. In addition, there are multiple pathways for spread from this site including the buccal mucosa, tonsillar fossa, glossopharyngeal sulcus, floor of the mouth, base of the tongue, hard and soft palate, masticator space, and maxillary tuberosity. Because patients tend to present with advanced disease of the retromolar trigone, many have regional metastases at the time of presentation.

The treatment of carcinoma of the retromolar trigone has been controversial.[172] Traditionally, surgery and radiation have been felt to be comparable modalities of treatment. However, recent reports suggest that surgery with adjuvant or neoadjuvant radiotherapy may be associated with better outcomes compared to radiation alone.[173,174] Although early-stage T1 and T2 cancers may be treated equally effectively with surgery or radiation, the probability of osteoradionecrosis is likely higher with definitive radiation.[172] Stage III and IV lesions commonly require combined surgery and radiation. The resection of advanced cancer of the retromolar trigone usually requires a composite resection of soft tissue and bone. A limiting factor for the achievement of adequate surgical resection margins for tumors in this area includes extension of tumor posterosuperiorly into the pterygopalatine fossa and into the base of the skull. Well-lateralized lesions of the retromolar trigone can be treated by ipsilateral mixed-beam techniques or angled-wedge techniques.

Buccal Mucosa

Verrucous carcinoma accounts for <5% of all oral cavity carcinomas, occurs most often in the buccal mucosa, has a more favorable prognosis, and is considered a low-grade malignancy. Surgical resection remains the preferred mode of treatment for primary lesions of the buccal mucosa. Adjuvant radiation treatment is usually not indicated. Because verrucous carcinomas rarely metastasize, elective neck dissection is often not indicated for patients with this disease. Careful pathology review with clinical correlation is important in the categorization of verrucous carcinomas, as this diagnosis can influence subsequent treatment recommendations.

Squamous cell carcinoma of the buccal mucosa can be an especially aggressive cancer of the oral cavity, as buccal cancers have multiple potential routes of spread to adjacent areas in the head and neck. Posteriorly, they can extend to involve the pterygoid muscles, and superiorly, they can grow to involve the alveolar ridge, palate, or maxillary sinus. The majority of patients have cancer that extends beyond the buccal mucosa. Metastasis to the cervical lymph nodes most commonly affects the submandibular nodes.

T1 and T2 tumors of the buccal mucosa can be managed with equal effectiveness by either surgery or radiation. Transoral resection is preferred and is most convenient for small lesions. Tumors approximating the gingiva should be resected with the gingiva and periosteum as an additional deep margin, while those that involve the periosteum should be resected with an additional deep margin of bone. When radiation therapy is used for small lesions, brachytherapy or external beam may be employed. Cancers that directly invade bone should be resected with a segment of bone. Larger tumors (T3 or T4) may require surgery combined with radiation therapy.

Management of Recurrent Disease

The appropriate management of recurrent oral cavity cancer depends largely on the extent of disease, the prior therapy administered, and whether the recurrences are local, regional, or both. Obviously, if there is distant disease recurrence, systemic therapy approaches will likely assume primary importance. In the case of small recurrences at the primary site for patients treated with primary excision only, further excision with or without postoperative radiotherapy is often recommended. For larger recurrences in patients who received radiation as part of their initial management, the rate of surgical salvage is quite low. In some cases, further resection may be considered for palliation or curative treatment attempt, particularly in the setting of a clinical trial. Systemic therapy, reirradiation, and palliative care are other options for this group of patients, and the risks and benefits of each should be discussed with the individual patient.

SELECTED REFERENCES

A full list of references for this chapter is available online.

1. Greenlee RT, et al. Cancer statistics, 2000. *CA Cancer J Clin* 2000;50(1):7–33.
2. Jemal A, et al. Cancer statistics, 2010. *CA Cancer J Clin* 2010;60(5):277–300.
3. Surveillance, Epidemiology, and End Results (SEER) Program. Research data (1973–2008), National Cancer Institute, DCCPS, Surveillance Research Program, Cancer Statistics Branch, released April 2011, based on the November 2010 submission. http://www.seer.cancer.gov.
4. American Cancer Society. *Cancer facts and figures 2010.* Atlanta: American Cancer Society. http://www.cancer.org/Research/CancerFactsFigures/cancer-facts-figures-2010
5. Patel SC, et al. Increasing incidence of oral tongue squamous cell carcinoma in young white women, age 18 to 44 years. *J Clin Oncol* 2011;29(11):1488–1494.
6. American Cancer Society. *Cancer Facts and Figures 2011.* Atlanta: American Cancer Society. http://www.cancer.org/Research/Cancer FactsFigures/cancer-facts-figures-2011
7. Jemal A, et al. Global cancer statistics. *CA Cancer J Clin* 2011;61(2):69–90.
8. Garavello W, et al. The oral cancer epidemic in central and eastern Europe. *Int J Cancer* 2010;127(1):160–171.
9. Boyle P, Macfarlane GJ, Scully C. Oral cancer: necessity for prevention strategies. *Lancet* 1993;342(8880):1129.
10. Kurumatani N, et al. Time trends in the mortality rates for tobacco- and alcohol-related cancers within the oral cavity and pharynx in Japan, 1950–94. *J Epidemiol* 1999;9(1):46–52.
11. Macfarlane GJ, et al. Alcohol, tobacco, diet and the risk of oral cancer: a pooled analysis of three case-control studies. *Eur J Cancer B Oral Oncol* 1995;31B(3):181–187.
12. Lambert R, et al. Epidemiology of cancer from the oral cavity and oropharynx. *Eur J Gastroenterol Hepatol* 2011;23(8):633–641.
13. Pande P, et al. Prognostic impact of Ets-1 overexpression in betel and tobacco related oral cancer. *Cancer Detect Prev* 2001;25(5):496–501.
14. Sharma DC. Betel quid and areca nut are carcinogenic without tobacco. *Lancet Oncol* 2003;4(10):587.
15. Reddy CR, Kumari KR. Microinvasive carcinoma of hard palate in reverse smoking females. *Indian J Cancer* 1974;11(4):386–393.
16. Hashibe M, et al. Interaction between tobacco and alcohol use and the risk of head and neck cancer: pooled analysis in the International Head and Neck Cancer Epidemiology Consortium. *Cancer Epidemiol Biomarkers Prev* 2009;18(2):541–550.
17. Ide R, et al. Cigarette smoking, alcohol drinking, and oral and pharyngeal cancer mortality in Japan. *Oral Dis* 2008;14(4):314–319.
18. Salom A. Dismissing links between HPV and aggressive tongue cancer in young patients. *Ann Oncol* 2010;21(1):13–17.
19. Goldstein DP, Irish JC. Head and neck squamous cell carcinoma in the young patient. *Curr Opin Otolaryngol Head Neck Surg* 2005;13(4):207–211.
20. Llewellyn CD, Johnson NW, Warnakulasuriya KA. Risk factors for squamous cell carcinoma of the oral cavity in young people–a comprehensive literature review. *Oral Oncol* 2001;37(5):401–418.
21. Antoniades DZ, et al. Squamous cell carcinoma of the lips in a northern Greek population. Evaluation of prognostic factors on 5-year survival rate–I. *Eur J Cancer B Oral Oncol* 1995;31B(5):333–339.
22. Burns JC, Murray BK. Conversion of herpetic lesions to malignancy by ultraviolet exposure and promoter application. *J Gen Virol* 1981;55(Pt 2):305–313.
23. Larsson PA, et al. Snuff tumorigenesis: effects of long-term snuff administration after initiation with 4-nitroquinoline-N-oxide and herpes simplex virus type 1. *J Oral Pathol Med* 1989;18(4):187–192.
24. D'Souza G, et al. Case-control study of human papillomavirus and oropharyngeal cancer. *N Engl J Med* 2007;356(19):1944–1956.

25. Fakhry C, Gillison ML. Clinical implications of human papillomavirus in head and neck cancers. *J Clin Oncol* 2006;24(17):2606–2611.
26. Hobbs CG, et al. Human papillomavirus and head and neck cancer: a systematic review and meta-analysis. *Clin Otolaryngol* 2006;31(4):259–266.
27. Prime SS, et al. A review of inherited cancer syndromes and their relevance to oral squamous cell carcinoma. *Oral Oncol* 2001;37(1):1–16.
28. Chen AY, Myers JN. Cancer of the oral cavity. *Dis Mon* 2001;47(7):275–361.
29. Slaughter DP, et al. Field cancerization in oral cavity stratified squamous epithelium: Clinical implications and multicentric origin. *Cancer* 1953;6:963–968.
30. Day GL, et al. Second cancers following oral and pharyngeal cancers: role of tobacco and alcohol. *J Natl Cancer Inst* 1994;86(2):131–137.
31. Schwartz LH, et al. Synchronous and metachronous head and neck carcinomas. *Cancer* 1994;74(7):1933–1938.
32. Day GL, Blot WJ. Second primary tumors in patients with oral cancer. *Cancer* 1992;70(1):14–19.
33. Haughey BH, et al. Meta-analysis of second malignant tumors in head and neck cancer: the case for an endoscopic screening protocol. *Ann Otol Rhinol Laryngol* 1992;101(2 Pt 1):105–112.
34. Khuri FR, et al. The impact of smoking status, disease stage, and index tumor site on second primary tumor incidence and tumor recurrence in the head and neck retinoid chemoprevention trial. *Cancer Epidemiol Biomarkers Prev* 2001; 10(8):823–829.
35. Lippman SM, Hong WK. Second malignant tumors in head and neck squamous cell carcinoma: the overshadowing threat for patients with early-stage disease. *Int J Radiat Oncol Biol Phys* 1989;17(3):691–694.
36. Fearon ER, Vogelstein B. A genetic model for colorectal tumorigenesis. *Cell* 1990;61(5):759–767.
37. Califano J, et al. Genetic progression model for head and neck cancer: implications for field cancerization. *Cancer Res* 1996;56(11):2488–2492.
38. Shavers VL, et al. Racial/ethnic patterns of care for cancers of the oral cavity, pharynx, larynx, sinuses, and salivary glands. *Cancer Metastasis Rev* 2003;22(1): 25–38.
39. Agrawal N, Frederick FM, Pickering CR, et al. Exome sequencing of head and neck squamous cell carcinomas reveals inactivating mutations in *NOTCH1*. *Science* 2011;333(6046)1154–1157.
40. Lentsch EJ, Myers JN. *Cancer of the head and neck*, 4th ed. Philadelphia: WB Saunders and Company, 2004.
41. Ho T, Wei Q, Sturgis EM. Epidemiology of carcinogen metabolism genes and risk of squamous cell carcinoma of the head and neck. *Head Neck* 2007;29(7):682–699.
42. Monteil RA. [Oral leukoplakia: clinical or histologic entity?]. *Ann Pathol* 1983;3 (3):257–261.
43. Myers E. *Cancer of the head and neck*, 4th ed. Philadelphia: Saunders, 2003.
44. Kannan S, et al. Ultrastructural variations and assessment of malignant transformation risk in oral leukoplakia. *Pathol Res Pract* 1993;189(10):1169–1180.
45. Reibel J. Prognosis of oral pre-malignant lesions: significance of clinical, histopathological, and molecular biological characteristics. *Crit Rev Oral Biol Med* 2003; 14(1):47–62.
46. Shafer WG, Waldron CA. Erythroplakia of the oral cavity. *Cancer* 1975;36(3): 1021–1028.
47. Reichart PA, Philipsen HP. Oral erythroplakia–a review. *Oral Oncol* 2005;41 (6):551–561.
48. Wang C. *Radiation therapy for head and neck neoplasms*, 3rd ed. New York: Wiley-Liss, 1997.
49. Byers RM, Wolf PF, Ballantyne AJ. Rationale for elective modified neck dissection. *Head Neck Surg* 1988;10(3):160–167.
50. Lindberg R. Distribution of cervical lymph node metastases from squamous cell carcinoma of the upper respiratory and digestive tracts. *Cancer* 1972;29(6): 1446–1449.
51. Byers RM, et al. Frequency and therapeutic implications of "skip metastases" in the neck from squamous carcinoma of the oral tongue. *Head Neck* 1997; 19(1):14–19.
52. Strong EW. Carcinoma of the tongue. *Otolaryngol Clin North Am* 1979;12(1): 107–114.
53. Spiro RH, et al. Predictive value of tumor thickness in squamous carcinoma confined to the tongue and floor of the mouth. *Am J Surg* 1986;152(4):345–350.
54. Shear M, Hawkins DM, Farr HW. The prediction of lymph node metastases from oral squamous carcinoma. *Cancer* 1976;37(4):1901–1907.
55. Merino OR, Lindberg RD, Fletcher GH. An analysis of distant metastases from squamous cell carcinoma of the upper respiratory and digestive tracts. *Cancer* 1977;40(1):145–151.
56. Ferlito A, et al. Incidence and sites of distant metastases from head and neck cancer. *ORL J Otorhinolaryngol Relat Spec* 2001;63(4):202–207.
57. Winzenburg SM, et al. Basaloid squamous carcinoma: a clinical comparison of two histologic types with poorly differentiated squamous cell carcinoma. *Otolaryngol Head Neck Surg* 1998;119(5):471–475.
58. Ellis GL, Corio RL. Spindle cell carcinoma of the oral cavity. A clinicopathologic assessment of fifty-nine cases. *Oral Surg Oral Med Oral Pathol* 1980;50(6): 523–533.
59. Weber RS, et al. Minor salivary gland tumors of the lip and buccal mucosa. *Laryngoscope* 1989;99(1):6–9.
60. Freeman C, Berg JW, Cutler SJ. Occurrence and prognosis of extranodal lymphomas. *Cancer* 1972;29(1):252–260.
61. Smyth AG, et al. Malignant melanoma of the oral cavity–an increasing clinical diagnosis? *Br J Oral Maxillofac Surg* 1993;31(4):230–235.
62. van den Brekel MW, et al. Modern imaging techniques and ultrasound-guided aspiration cytology for the assessment of neck node metastases: a prospective comparative study. *Eur Arch Otorhinolaryngol* 1993;250(1):11–17.
63. Adams S, et al. Prospective comparison of 18F-FDG PET with conventional imaging modalities (CT, MRI, US) in lymph node staging of head and neck cancer. *Eur J Nucl Med* 1998;25(9):1255–1260.
64. Kim SY, et al. Utility of FDG PET in patients with squamous cell carcinomas of the oral cavity. *Eur J Surg Oncol* 2008;34(2):208–215.
65. Schoder H, et al. Head and neck cancer: clinical usefulness and accuracy of PET/CT image fusion. *Radiology* 2004;231(1):65–72.
66. Liao CT, et al. PET and PET/CT of the neck lymph nodes improves risk prediction in patients with squamous cell carcinoma of the oral cavity. *J Nucl Med* 2011;52(2):180–187.
67. Maddipatla S, Madero-Visbal RA, Graves T, et al. Preoperative staging of oral cavity carcinoma with FDG-PET/CT. *J Clin Oncol* 2008;26(suppl):abstr 6044.
68. Pentenero M, et al. Accuracy of 18F-FDG-PET/CT for staging of oral squamous cell carcinoma. *Head Neck* 2008;30(11):1488–1496.
69. Anzai Y, et al. Recurrence of head and neck cancer after surgery or irradiation: prospective comparison of 2-deoxy-2-[F-18]fluoro-D-glucose PET and MR imaging diagnoses. *Radiology* 1996;200(1):135–141.
70. Farber LA, et al. Detection of recurrent head and neck squamous cell carcinomas after radiation therapy with 2-18F-fluoro-2-deoxy-D-glucose positron emission tomography. *Laryngoscope* 1999;109(6):970–975.
71. Andrade RS, et al. Posttreatment assessment of response using FDG-PET/CT for patients treated with definitive radiation therapy for head and neck cancers. *Int J Radiat Oncol Biol Phys* 2006;65(5):1315–1322.
72. Greven KM, et al. Serial positron emission tomography scans following radiation therapy of patients with head and neck cancer. *Head Neck* 2001;23(11):942–946.
73. Isles MG, McConkey C, Mehanna HM. A systematic review and meta-analysis of the role of positron emission tomography in the follow up of head and neck squamous cell carcinoma following radiotherapy or chemoradiotherapy. *Clin Otolaryngol* 2008;33(3):210–222.
74. Lowe VJ, et al. Surveillance for recurrent head and neck cancer using positron emission tomography. *J Clin Oncol* 2000;18(3):651–658.
75. Edge SB, Byrd DR, Compton CC, et al. American joint committee on cancer staging. Lip and oral cavity. In *AJCC cancer staging manual*. Springer: New York, 2010.
76. Aviv JE, et al. Surface sensibility of the floor of the mouth and tongue in healthy controls and in radiated patients. *Otolaryngol Head Neck Surg* 1992;107(3): 418–423.
77. Cooper JS, et al. Postoperative concurrent radiotherapy and chemotherapy for high-risk squamous-cell carcinoma of the head and neck. *N Engl J Med* 2004; 350(19):1937–1944.
78. Day TA, et al. Oral cancer treatment. *Curr Treat Options Oncol* 2003;4(1):27–41.
79. Bernier J, et al. Defining risk levels in locally advanced head and neck cancers: a comparative analysis of concurrent postoperative radiation plus chemotherapy trials of the EORTC (#22931) and RTOG (# 9501). *Head Neck* 2005;27(10):843–850.
80. Bernier J, et al. Postoperative irradiation with or without concomitant chemotherapy for locally advanced head and neck cancer. *N Engl J Med* 2004;350(19): 1945–1952.
81. Bernier J, Vermorken JB, Koch WM. Adjuvant therapy in patients with resected poor-risk head and neck cancer. *J Clin Oncol* 2006;24(17):2629–2635.
82. Urken ML, et al. A systematic approach to functional reconstruction of the oral cavity following partial and total glossectomy. *Arch Otolaryngol Head Neck Surg* 1994;120(6):589–601.
83. Urken ML. Composite free flaps in oromandibular reconstruction. Review of the literature. *Arch Otolaryngol Head Neck Surg* 1991;117(7):724–732.
84. Urken ML. Advances in head and neck reconstruction. *Laryngoscope* 2003;113 (9):1473–1476.
85. Urken ML, et al. The scapular osteofasciocutaneous flap: a 12-year experience. *Arch Otolaryngol Head Neck Surg* 2001;127(7):862–869.
86. Urken ML, et al. Microvascular free flaps in head and neck reconstruction. Report of 200 cases and review of complications. *Arch Otolaryngol Head Neck Surg* 1994;120(6):633–640.
87. Urken ML, et al. Oromandibular reconstruction using microvascular composite free flaps. Report of 71 cases and a new classification scheme for bony, soft-tissue, and neurologic defects. *Arch Otolaryngol Head Neck Surg* 1991;117(7):733–744.
88. Ow TJ, Myers JN. Current management of advanced resectable oral cavity squamous cell carcinoma. *Clin Exp Otorhinolaryngol* 2011;4(1):1–10.
89. Byers RM. A word of caution: the skip metastases. *Head Neck* 1995;17(4): 359–360.
90. Civantos FJ, et al. Sentinel lymph node biopsy accurately stages the regional lymph nodes for T1-T2 oral squamous cell carcinomas: results of a prospective multi-institutional trial. *J Clin Oncol* 2010;28(8):1395–1400.
91. Ross GL, et al. Sentinel node biopsy in head and neck cancer: preliminary results of a multicenter trial. *Ann Surg Oncol* 2004;11(7):690–696.
92. Kaanders JH, et al. Devices valuable in head and neck radiotherapy. *Int J Radiat Oncol Biol Phys* 1992;23(3):639–645.
93. Harrison LB, Fass DE. Radiation therapy for oral cavity cancer. *Dent Clin North Am* 1990;34(2):205–222.
94. Nag S, et al. The American Brachytherapy Society recommendations for brachytherapy of soft tissue sarcomas. *Int J Radiat Oncol Biol Phys* 2001;49(4):1033–1043.
95. Fu KK, et al. Time, dose and volume factors in interstitial radium implants of carcinoma of the oral tongue. *Radiology* 1976;119(1):209–213.
96. Fu KK, et al. External and interstitial radiation therapy of carcinoma of the oral tongue. A review of 32 years' experience. *AJR Am J Roentgenol* 1976;126(1): 107–115.
97. Decroix Y, Ghossein NA. Experience of the Curie Institute in treatment of cancer of the mobile tongue: I. Treatment policies and result. *Cancer* 1981;47(3):496–502.
98. Dearnaley DP, et al. Interstitial irradiation for carcinoma of the tongue and floor of mouth: Royal Marsden Hospital Experience 1970–1986. *Radiother Oncol* 1991;21(3):183–192.
99. Pernot M, et al. [Evaluation of the importance of systematic neck dissection in carcinoma of the oral cavity treated by brachytherapy alone for the primary lesion (apropos of a series of 346 patients)]. *Bull Cancer Radiother* 1995;82(3):311–317.
100. Pernot M, et al. Epidermoid carcinomas of the floor of mouth treated by exclusive irradiation: statistical study of a series of 207 cases. *Radiother Oncol* 1995; 35(3):177–185.

Chapter 45
Oropharynx

Joseph K. Salama, Maura L. Gillison, and David M. Brizel

The incidence of oropharyngeal carcinoma is increasing. This is in contrast to the decreasing incidence of head and neck cancer arising in other anatomic sites. The classic etiologic factors of tobacco abuse and alcohol use continue to play a significant role. However, a significant increase in rates of oropharyngeal cancers in nonsmokers and nondrinkers caused by oncogenic human papillomaviruses (HPVs) is occurring, predominantly among men. Although both HPV–associated and HPV-unassociated malignancies are classified as squamous cell carcinomas, the behavior of these cancers markedly differs as HPV-associated cancers have a significantly more favorable prognosis after the delivery of standard treatments. The recognition that HPV-associated oropharyngeal cancer is a distinct clinical entity, as well as the impact of standard therapies on speech, swallowing, degustation, and psychological well-being, has led to significant multidisciplinary interest in defining different treatment paradigms for HPV-associated and HPV-unassociated oropharyngeal cancers. Treatment recommendations for these two clinical entities remain the same, however, until ongoing investigations are completed.

Based on the critical function of the oropharynx in speech and swallowing, the treatment of oropharyngeal carcinomas can significantly impact patient quality of life. Appropriate treatment strategies should focus on maintaining high cure rates while minimizing long-term, treatment-induced functional morbidity. Early-stage oropharyngeal cancers are managed with single modality therapy (radiation or surgery), with the choice based on anticipated posttherapy consequences. Treatment of locoregionally advanced tumors involves multiple modalities with the use of either concomitant chemotherapy and radiotherapy or surgery followed by adjuvant radiotherapy with or without chemotherapy based on pathologic risk factors.

Novel surgical and radiation delivery modalities, as well as molecularly targeted chemotherapeutics, are the current focus of clinical investigation, with an intent to maximize the therapeutic index for HPV-associated oropharyngeal cancers. Transoral surgical advances including laser and robotic interventions have the potential to reduce morbidity. Advances in radiotherapy allow for improved dosing to the primary tumor and involved nodes while reducing radiation exposure of normal tissues, particularly the parotids and pharyngeal constrictors. Further studies are needed to more completely integrate molecularly targeted agents into the treatment of oropharyngeal cancers.

EPIDEMIOLOGY

Oropharyngeal cancers account for approximately 10% of the annual worldwide incidence of head and neck squamous cell carcinomas. The incidence of oropharyngeal cancer differs significantly by geography.[1] In the United States, the annual incidence of oropharyngeal squamous cell carcinoma is 4.8 in 100,000,[2] which is similar to other developed countries. This rate increased by 28% from 1988 to 2004, largely because of the 225% increase in HPV-associated oropharyngeal cancer, whereas HPV-unassociated oropharyngeal cancer declined by 50% over the same time period.[3] The incidence of oropharyngeal cancer in developing countries is lower at approximately 3 in 100,000.[1] This rise in developed countries is unique because other mucosal head and neck cancer incidences have decreased over this same time period. The putative cause is the increasing incidence of HPV-associated cancers, which is discussed in detail later. Worldwide, the majority of oropharyngeal cancers remain attributable to tobacco smoking and/or the ingestion of excessive amounts of alcoholic beverages. For these cases, incidence rates are generally higher for men than women (4:1), who are diagnosed more commonly in the sixth and seventh decades of life.

HUMAN PAPILLOMAVIRUS–ASSOCIATED OROPHARYNGEAL CANCER

Human Papillomavirus

HPV is a circular, double-stranded DNA virus, first determined to be oncogenic when it was found to be the associated with cervical cancer in 1983[4] and subsequently established as a significant human carcinogen in 1996.[5] To date, approximately 150 HPV types have been identified. HPV subtypes are classified as high or low risk based on epidemiologic associations with cervical cancer in case-control studies.[6] HPV 16 is the most common HPV type identified in human tumors and is associated with more than 90% of all HPV-associated related oropharyngeal cancers.[7] Infection with HPV 16 confers an approximate 14-fold increase in risk for oropharyngeal cancer.[8]

The HPV genome encodes three oncoproteins (E5, E6, and E7), in addition to regulatory genes (E1 and E2) as well as capsid protein genes (L1 and L2). Oncogenesis is primarily mediated via the E6 and E7 proteins. HPV E6 complexes with E3 ubiquitin ligase and E6-associated protein, promoting ubiquitin-mediated destruction of p53. Loss of cellular p53 function results in dysregulation of the G1/S and G2/M checkpoints. An E7/cullin 2 complex ubiquitinates the Rb protein, resulting in loss of G1/S checkpoint control.[9] E7 is believed to be the major transforming oncogene during early carcinogenesis, with E6 functioning later.[10] A diagram of the pathways affecting the malignant transformation of keratinocytes by HPV is shown in Figure 45.1. Although E6 and E7 oncoprotein function is necessary for development of an HPV-associated malignancy, it is not sufficient. It is believed that as yet undefined genetic events are required for HPV malignant transformation.[11]

Several different techniques are used to detect HPV in oropharyngeal cancer biopsy specimens. The gold standard is demonstration of HPV E6/E7 in clinical specimens. However, this approach is clinically impractical because it is very difficult to detect viral RNA from cytologic fluid and paraffin embedded tissues. Polymerase chain reaction (PCR) of HPV DNA is a technique with high sensitivity but low specificity, as cross contamination or transcriptionally inactive DNA can be detected. In situ hybridization (ISH) uses oligonucleotide probes designed to anneal to complementary HPV DNA in the tumor specimen. Advantages of this technique include localization of DNA within the tumor specimen and allow for identification of a single viral copy.[12] A consequence of HPV E7-mediated Rb inhibition is induction of demethylases resulting in expression of $p16^{INK4A}$, an upstream tumor suppressor cyclin-dependent kinase inhibitor.[13] Immunohistochemistry staining for $p16^{INK4A}$ is frequently used as a surrogate for HPV status. There is a small (7%) discordance between HPV ISH and $p16^{INK4A}$ IHC (approximately 7%), which is likely related to a combination of infection with non-HPV-16 subtypes or low viral copy numbers not detectable by IHC and true p16-positive/HPV-negative cases.

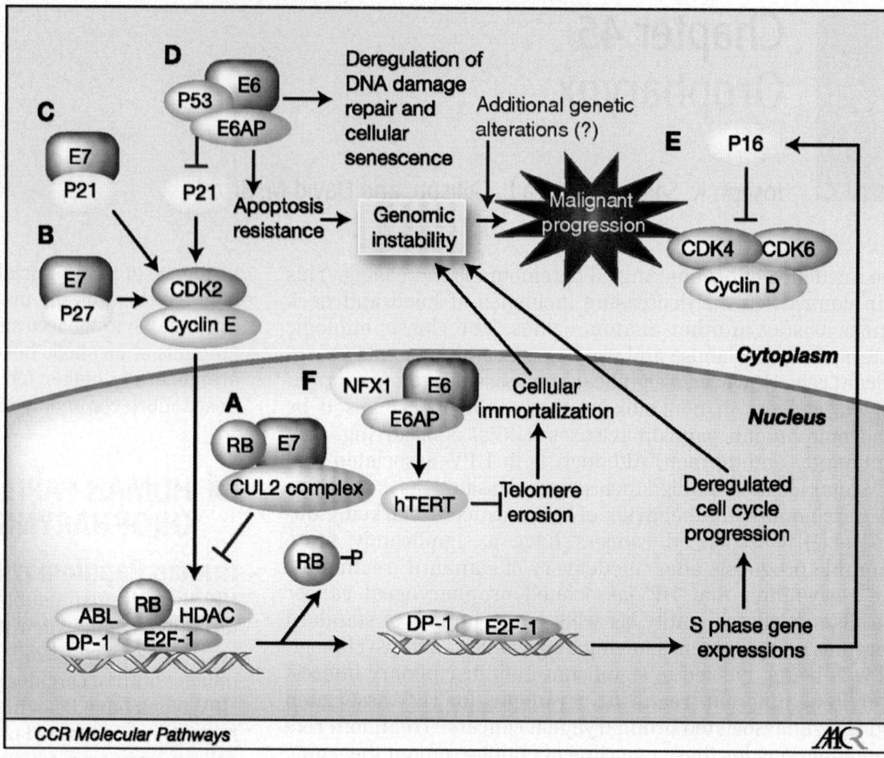

FIGURE 45.1. Diagram of malignant transformation in keratinocytes caused by the HPV oncoproteins E6 and E7. Clockwise from *A*, ubiquitination by E7 and the cullin 2 ubiquitin ligase complex leading to pRb degradation (23, 25, 56, 57); *B*, interaction between E7 and $p27^{Kip1}$ resulting in inhibition of cell cycle arrest contributing to carcinogenesis (58); *C*, interaction between E7 and $p21^{Cip1}$ resulting in inhibition of cell cycle arrest contributing to carcinogenesis (31, 59); *D*, ubiquitination by E6 and ubiquitin ligase E6AP leading to p53 degradation (19–21); *E*, increased expression of $p16^{INK4A}$ by a consequent of feedback loops from the absence of pRb function (42); and *F*, degradation of NFX1, a transcriptional repressor of hTERT, by association with E6/E6AP resulting in hTERT activation and cellular immortalization (60). (From Chung CH, Gillison ML. Human papillomavirus in head and neck cancer: its role in pathogenesis and clinical implications. *Clin Cancer Res* 2009;15(22):6758–6762, with permission.)

Clinical Characteristics of Human Papillomavirus–Associated Oropharyngeal Cancer

HPV-associated oropharyngeal cancers are more likely to occur among men and than women (3:1), most of whom (80%) will not have a smoking history. These cancers are more common among white individuals than other races, are diagnosed in individuals who are 5 to 10 years younger than HPV-unassociated oropharyngeal cancers, and are associated with higher socioeconomic status. Furthermore, when compared to patients with HPV-unassociated cancers, these patients are more likely to be married, college educated, and have a median income of more than $55,000. The use of marijuana also elevates odds of HPV-associated oropharyngeal cancer.[14] Analogous to cervical cancers, patients with HPV-associated oropharyngeal cancer have been associated with certain sexual behaviors. These include high number of vaginal or oral sex partners, infrequent condom use, engagement in casual sex, and early age of first intercourse.[15] Whether or not HPV acts in a synergistic manner with tobacco or alcohol exposure in patients to increase the risk of HPV-associated oropharyngeal cancer is a matter of ongoing controversy.

HPV-associated oropharyngeal cancers are characterized frequently as poorly differentiated, nonkeratinizing, or basaloid in histopathology.[16] HPV-associated and HPV-unassociated carcinomas are also different with regard to molecular alterations. HPV-associated oropharyngeal cancers demonstrate wild-type p53, p16 expression, and infrequent amplification of cyclin D, whereas the converse is true for HPV-unassociated cancers. A subset of HPV-associated oropharyngeal cancer patients with more extensive smoking histories will have tumors exhibiting *TP53* mutations, higher epidermal growth factor receptor (EGFR), and Bcl-xL expression and have outcomes similar to those of HPV-unassociated patients.[9]

Response of Human Papillomavirus–Associated Oropharyngeal Cancer to Standard Therapy

Patients with HPV-associated oropharyngeal cancers have significantly better outcomes compared to HPV-unassociated oropharyngeal tumors.[17,18] In a reanalysis of Radiation Therapy Oncology Group (RTOG) 0129, a randomized study comparing cisplatin administered with either accelerated concomitant boost radiotherapy or conventionally fractionated radiotherapy, HPV status was independently associated with improved outcomes. Three-year overall survival was 82% in HPV-positive patients compared with 54% in HPV-negative patients. Even after adjustment for age, tumor stage, nodal stage, treatment assignment, and tobacco use, HPV status independently predicted for improved survival (hazard ratio [HR] 0.42, 95% confidence interval [CI] 0.27 to 0.66). Additionally, locoregional progression (13.6% vs. 24.8%) and progression-free survival

TABLE 45.1 HUMAN PAPILLOMAVIRUS STATUS AND SURVIVAL OUTCOMES IN PROSPECTIVE TRIALS

Cooperative Group	Number of Patients	RT	Induction	Concurrent	HPV+	Survival HPV+	Survival HPV–	p-Value
ECOG	96	70 Gy	Paclitaxel 175 mg/m^2 Carboplatin AUC = 6 2 cycles	Weekly paclitaxel 30 mg/m^2	40%	95%	62%	0.005
TROG	195	70 Gy	None	CDDP +/– tirapazamine	28%	94%	77%	0.007
RTOG	323	70 Gy	None	CDDP 100 mg/m^2	64%	79%	46%	0.002
DAHANCA	156	62–68 Gy	None	Nimorazole 1,200 mg/m^2/d	22%	62%	26%	0.003

RT, radiotherapy; HPV+, human papillomavirus positive; HPV–, human papillomavirus negative; ECOG, Eastern Cooperative Oncology Group; AUC, area under the curve; TROG, Trans-Tasman Radiation Oncology Group; CDDP, cisplatin; RTOG, Radiation Therapy Oncology Group; DAHANCA, Danish Head and Neck Cancer Group.

(71.8% vs. 50.4%) were significantly improved in HPV-positive cases. Other large cooperative group studies have demonstrated similar findings.[18,19] It is important to realize that the prognostic significance of HPV was independent of the chemoradiotherapy platform and applies to treatment with radiotherapy alone,[20] as shown in Table 45.1. In fact HPV-related tumors have a better prognosis regardless of the treatment modality (surgery, radiotherapy, or chemoradiotherapy) used.

ANATOMY

The oropharynx is contiguous with the oral cavity anteriorly, the larynx and hypopharynx posterior-inferiorly, and superiorly with the nasopharynx. Three main subregions compose the oropharynx including the tonsil, base of tongue, and soft palate. Normal function of the oropharynx is critical for speech and swallowing.

The tonsillar region contains the anterior and posterior tonsillar pillars as well as the palatine tonsil. The palatine tonsils are lymphoid aggregates incompletely encapsulated with a keratinized stratified squamous epithelial mucosal lining positioned in the tonsillar bed, which is a part of the tonsillar cleft between the anterior (palatoglossal) and posterior (palatopharyngeal) tonsillar pillars.

The base of tongue comprises the posterior third of the tongue and is bounded anteriorly by the circumvallate papillae, sitting in front of the sulcus terminalis. The base of tongue is bounded posterior-inferiorly by the hyoid and epiglottis and laterally by the glossopharyngeal sulci. Underlying the mucosa of the base of tongue are lymphatic nodules collectively known as the lingual tonsil. The vallecula is a 1-cm mucosal strip that serves as a transition between the base of tongue and epiglottis and is considered a part of the base of tongue. The sensory innervation of the base of tongue is via the glossopharyngeal nerve (cranial nerve [CN] IX) with a small aspect of the base of tongue supplied by the internal laryngeal nerve (CN X).

The soft palate is a fibromuscular structure bounded anteriorly by the hard palate, laterally coursing into the anterior tonsillar pillars and posterior-inferiorly forming a free edge, and the midline uvula. The soft palate is composed of five muscles (levator veli palatini, tensor veli palatini, palatoglossus, palatopharyngeus, and musculus uvulae) posteriorly and the palatine aponeurosis an expanded tendon of the tensor veli palatini anteriorly. The muscles of the soft palate are supplied through the pharyngeal plexus (which is composed of the pharyngeal branches of CNs IX and X, as well as sympathetic branches from the superior cervical ganglion, except for the tensor veli palatini, which is supplied by CN V2). The sensory supply is from CN IX.

The oropharynx serves many functions, including that of degustation, respiration, and speech. Advanced tumors arising in the oropharynx can infiltrate muscles and nerves, thus significantly impeding these functions. A major goal of successful therapy is to limit the impact of the treatment on long-term function.

TABLE 45.2 ANATOMIC BOUNDARIES OF NECK NODE LEVELS

I	Bounded by posterior belly of digastric, hyoid bone inferiorly, and body of mandible superiorly
II	Bounded by skull base superiorly to level of hyoid bone inferiorly
III	Bounded by hyoid bone superiorly to cricothyroid membrane inferiorly
IV	Bounded by cricothyroid membrane superiorly to clavicle inferiorly
V	Bounded by anterior border of trapezius posteriorly, posterior border of sternocleidomastoid anteriorly, and clavicle inferiorly
VI	Bounded by level of hyoid bone superiorly to suprasternal notch inferiorly, lateral border formed by medial border of carotid sheath

ROUTES OF SPREAD

Primary routes of spread for oropharyngeal cancers include direct extension and lymphatic spread, with hematogenous metastases being less common. Oropharyngeal cancers have a predilection for submucosal extension, often visualized as raised erythematous regions without distinct borders or ulceration. This can best be appreciated by direct visualization rather than on radiographic imaging.

Lymphatic Spread of Oropharyngeal Cancer

The lymphatic drainage of the oropharynx and the neck was first described by Rouviere[21] in 1938 and has since been refined by others.[22] Originally grouped by lymph node chains located in particular anatomic regions, nodal groups are now classified by the level system[23] with the location of lymph nodes in the neck being defined by surgical-anatomic landmarks (Table 45.2). Recently, this system (levels I to VI) was refined with the addition of sublevels (Ia/Ib, IIa/IIb, and Va/Vb) (as shown in Table 45.2), also incorporating radiologically defined landmarks[24] (as shown in Table 45.3 and Fig. 45.2).

TABLE 45.3 RADIOGRAPHIC BOUNDARIES OF NECK NODE LEVELS

Level	Cranial	Caudal	Anterior	Posterior	Lateral	Medial
Ia	Geniohyoid m., plane tangent to basilar edge of mandible	Plane tangent to body of hyoid bone	Symphysis menti, platysma m.	Body of hyoid bone	Medial edge of ant. belly of digastric m.	NA
Ib	Mylohyoid m., cranial edge of submandibular gland	Plane through central part of hyoid bone	Symphysis menti, platysma m.	Post. edge of submandibular gland	Inner side of mandible, platysma m., skin	Lateral edge of ant. belly of digastric m.
II	Caudal edge of lateral process of C1	Caudal edge of body of hyoid bone	Post. edge of submandibular gland; ICA; post. edge of post. belly of digastric m.	Post. edge of SCM m.	Medial edge of SCM m.	Int. edge of ICA, paraspinal m.
III	Caudal edge of body of hyoid bone	Caudal edge of cricoid cartilage	Posterolateral edge of sternohyoid m.; ant. edge of SCM m.	Post. edge of SCM m.	Medial edge of SCM m.	Int. edge of ICA, paraspinal m.
IV	Caudal edge of cricoid cartilage	2 cm cranial to sternoclavicular joint	Anteromedial edge of SCM m.	Post. edge of SCM m.	Medial edge of SCM m.	Medial edge of ICA, paraspinal m.
V	Cranial edge of body of hyoid bone	CT slice including transverse cervical vessels	Post. edge of SCM m.	Ant. border of trapezius m.	Platysma m., skin	Paraspinal m.
VI	Caudal edge of body of thyroid cartilage	Sternal manubrium	Skin, platysma m.	Separation between trachea & esophagus	Medial edge of SCM, thyroid gland, skin	NA
RP	Base of skull	Cranial edge of body of hyoid bone	Fascia under pharyngeal mucosa	Prevertebral m.	Medial edge of ICA	Midline

m., muscle; ant., anterior; NA, not applicable; post., posterior; ICA, internal carotid artery; SCM, sternocleidomastoid; Int., interior; CT, computed tomography.

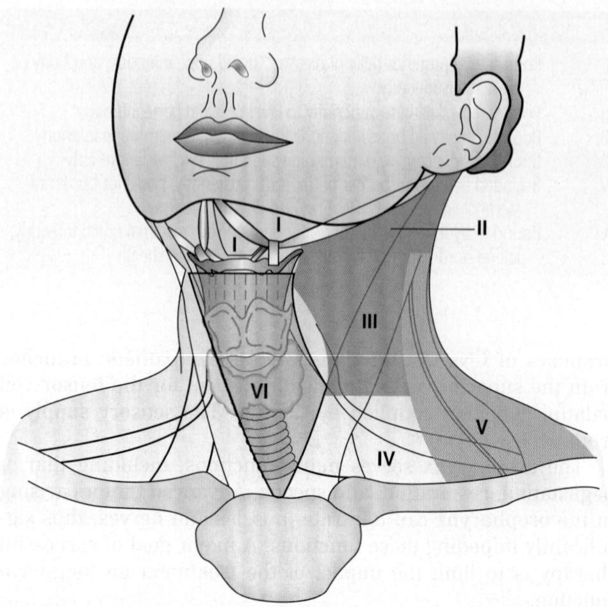

FIGURE 45.2. Schematic diagram indicating the location of the lymph node levels in the neck based on anatomic boundaries. (Used with the permission of the American Joint Committee on Cancer (AJCC), Chicago, Illinois. The original source for this material is the AJCC *Cancer Staging Handbook*, Seventh Edition [2010] published by Springer Science and Business Media LLC, www.springerlink.com.)

The most common location for lymph node metastases from oropharyngeal cancers is the ipsilateral level II. The probability of lymphatic (regional) metastasis is related to the size and location of the primary tumor within the oropharynx. The typical order of metastatic progression is systematic, from the upper jugular chain nodes superiorly (level I/II; first echelon), to midcervical (level III), and to lower cervical nodes (level IV), inferiorly. In large series of oropharyngeal cancer patients, isolated skip metastases are rare (0.3%), and level I or V involvement is usually associated with the involvement of other levels. Additionally, tumors encroaching or crossing midline or involving the posterior pharyngeal wall exhibited a higher propensity for bilateral lymphadenopathy.

Knowledge of the probability of occult pathologic lymphadenopathy for each involved oropharynx anatomic subsite and extent of disease is critical to modern radiotherapy and surgery planning, as selective neck dissections and limited radiotherapy volumes are the norm. Standardized contouring atlases have been published to aid clinicians in development of appropriate radiotherapy volumes to cover potential occult microscopic lymphatic spread in the N0 neck.[25–27] Additionally, information about probabilities of occult pathologic lymphatic involvement has been compounded from series of patients undergoing elective neck dissection.[28] The use of this knowledge to develop appropriate radiotherapy volumes will be discussed in more detail in the radiotherapy volumes section. The rate of pathologic lymphadenopathy for the pathologically involved neck is outlined in Table 45.4.

Distant Metastatic Spread of Oropharyngeal Cancer

Distant metastatic spread in oropharyngeal cancer is relatively uncommon, affecting approximately 15% of all patients during the course of their disease.[29] The most common locations for distant metastatic spread of oropharyngeal cancers are the lung parenchyma,[29] followed by osseous and hepatic metastases. Metastases are more common in patients presenting with locoregionally advanced or recurrent tumors, with the risk increasing with primary tumor stage as well as the burden of pathologic lymphadenopathy (N2-N3 disease).[29,30] Extranodal extension, lower cervical pathologic lymphadenopathy (level IV), and lymphovascular invasion have also been associated with increased rates of distant metastases.[31]

Metastatic deposits within the lung parenchyma typically appear radiographically as well-circumscribed, peripherally located nodules. Care should be taken to differentiate between pulmonary metastases and primary pulmonary malignancies, characterized as spiculated irregularly shaped masses commonly associated with hilar and mediastinal lymphadenopathy, given their differing prognostic implications. This distinction often is impossible, even after biopsy, as both can be of squamous cell histology. In such instances, physically fit patients should be given the benefit of the doubt and treated as if they have two separate primary tumors. In patients with limited pulmonary metastases, who are technically resectable and fit for surgery, resection of pulmonary oropharyngeal cancer metastases may improve survival.[32–34] For nonsurgical candidates, hypofractionated image-guided radiotherapy to all known metastatic sites can result in long-term disease control and should be considered for patients with limited metastatic disease.[35]

CLINICAL PRESENTATION

Oropharyngeal cancers present with a constellation of symptoms that depend on the location of the primary tumor, invasion of nearby organs, and extent of nodal disease. Often, patients will present with a painless neck mass, which is usually mobile, firm, and nontender but can be fixed, indicating extranodal extension and invasion into surrounding structures. Such masses are frequently treated with an initial course of antibiotics; however, persistence or growth in this context mandates further evaluation. Some patients complain of a deep-seated otalgia located within the auditory canal. This is mediated via irritation of the glossopharyngeal nerve (CN IX) with referral via the petrosal ganglion to the tympanic nerve of Jacobson. Regurgitation of foods can occur with invasion of the soft palate, inhibiting its ability to elevate during swallowing.

TABLE 45.4 DISTRIBUTION OF CLINICAL METASTATIC NECK NODES FROM HEAD AND NECK SQUAMOUS CELL CARCINOMAS

		Distribution of Metastatic Lymph Nodes Per Level (Percentage of the N+ Patients Ipsilateral/Contralateral)					
Tumor Site	*N+ Patients (%)*	*I*	*II*	*III*	*IV*	*V*	*Other*
Oral cavity (n = 787)	36	42/3.5	79/8	18/3	5/1	1/0	1.4/0.3
Oropharynx (n = 1,479)	64	13/2	81/24	23/5	9/2.5	13/3	2/1
Hypopharynx (n = 847)	70	2/0	80/13	51/4	20/3	24/2	3/1
Supraglottic larynx (n = 428)	55	2/0	71/21	48/10	18/7	15/4	2/0
Nasopharynx (n = 440)	80	9/5	71/56	36/32	22/15	32/26	15/10

N+, node positive.

From Grégoire V, Coche E, Cosnard G, et al. Selection and delineation of lymph node target volumes in head and neck conformal radiotherapy: proposal for standardizing terminology and procedure based on the surgical experience. *Radiother Oncol* 2000;56:135–150, with permission.

Trismus is seen with more advanced tumors and reflects invasion of the pterygoid fossa and/or musculature. Odynophagia and dysphagia are other common presenting symptoms that occur with invasion into the pharyngeal musculature or obstruction by pathologic lymphadenopathy.

DIAGNOSTIC EVALUATION

Physical Examination

A complete examination of all mucosal head and neck sites should be performed in any patient with a known or suspected diagnosis of oropharyngeal cancer. This process not only characterizes the primary tumor but also evaluates for other malignancies given the high propensity for second primary upper aerodigestive tract tumors. A thorough physical examination is essential for diagnosis and understanding of the complete extent of disease, and it helps to guide the surgeon on the choice of optimal biopsy site. Inspection of the oropharynx should be performed under adequate illumination and be well practiced, systematic, and reproducible. Following examination of the oral cavity, where attention should be directed to the number and health of the patient's teeth and to the mucosal sites, one should closely examine the anterior tonsillar pillars, the tonsillar fossae, and posterior tonsillar pillars followed by the soft palate. Proper exposure can be achieved either with gloved index fingers or with two disposable tongue depressors used in unison. Palpation of the tonsillar fossa and the base of tongue should be performed because these locations can harbor occult primary tumors, with the base of tongue performed at the completion of the examination owing to its propensity to trigger the gag reflex. Direct visualization should be followed by fiberoptic examination whenever possible, because this allows optimal inspection of the base of tongue, posterior-inferior tonsil vallecula, as well as documenting spread to laryngeal and pharyngeal subsites. Fiberoptic examinations should be recorded and compared to assess response during the course of therapy. Indirect mirror examination is less informative than fiberoptic evaluation; however, it should be performed if fiberoptic capabilities are not available.

Oropharyngeal tumors often appear as ulcerated masses, with surrounding erythema, neovascularization, and mucositis. Tenderness, evidence of recent bleeding, obstruction of the airway, skin invasion, alteration of gag reflex, and extent of trismus (measured from upper to lower incisors) should be documented. Bulging of the parapharyngeal space should also be noted because this could represent retropharyngeal lymphadenopathy.

Careful examination of the neck is also important for staging and management. Palpation of the neck should focus on neck levels defined by standard anatomic relationships. The neck should gently be turned to the side while being examined to relax the sternocleidomastoid muscle, which facilitates the detection of smaller involved lymph nodes. Care should be taken not to palpate too firmly in older patients or those with known vascular disease, as aggressive carotid massage can be associated with syncope. Lymph nodes should be recorded in terms of the level in which they arise, their size, and the character of their firmness, as well if they are fixed and whether or not they penetrate and involve the skin.

Confirmatory biopsy of the primary site should be performed. Adequate exposure is usually possible for in-office biopsies of the proximal oropharynx. Posterior oropharyngeal tumors are often biopsied under general anesthesia in the operating room, often as part of a comprehensive examination under anesthesia as well as comprehensive endoscopic evaluation (laryngoscopy, bronchoscopy, and esophagoscopy).

Computed Tomography

Computed tomography (CT) imaging of the head and neck with intravenous contrast should be performed for all newly diagnosed oropharyngeal cancer patients to assess the extent of primary tumors and to determine the presence or absence of cervical lymph node metastases. Scan slice thickness <5 mm is desirable to optimize the detection of smaller pathologically involved lymph nodes and to provide the best anatomic delineation of both primary and nodal disease. Pathologically involved lymph nodes are characterized on CT imaging as those that are enlarged, enhance with contrast, and have a necrotic center. Primary tumors appear as contrast-enhancing masses, distorting normal anatomic relationships. Whereas ulceration and invasion into surrounding organs are readily assessed, submucosal spread is often difficult to characterize with CT. As multiplanar image reconstruction is routinely available, lymph node and primary tumor size should be measured in both longitudinal and cross-sectional dimensions to more accurately stage patients. Unfortunately, dental artifact on CT imaging may often obscure complete visualization with neutral head position, requiring further scanning with an adjusted head position. Thoracic CT should be performed routinely to assess for pulmonary spread of oropharyngeal cancer patients with N2 or greater nodal disease, as well as those with advanced primary tumors, given the risks of pulmonary metastases described previously. A diagnostic CT image of a patient with locoregionally advanced head and neck cancer is shown in Figure 45.3.

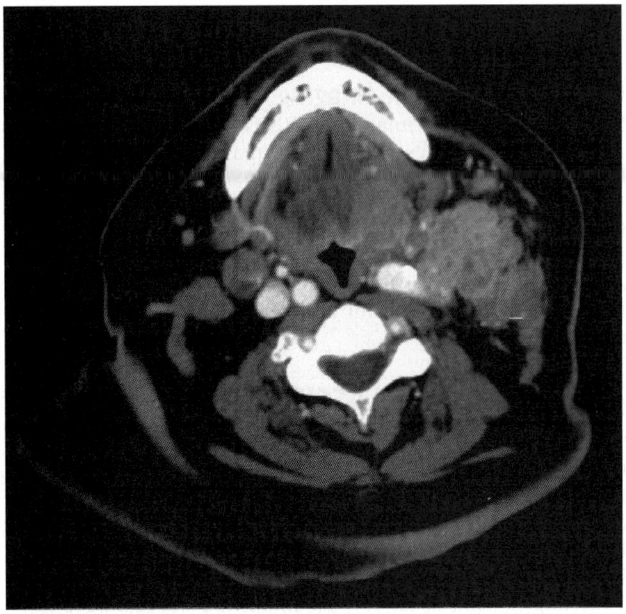

FIGURE 45.3. Diagnostic computed tomography image demonstrating locoregionally advanced oropharyngeal cancer with extensive ipsilateral cervical lymphadenopathy.

Positron Emission Tomography

Positron emission tomography (PET) and/or PET/CT imaging incorporating tumor physiology in conjunction with anatomic information are now routinely recommended for the initial staging of oropharyngeal cancer patients. From a practical standpoint, PET-based imaging can assess not only the locoregional burden of disease but also detect and quantify distant metastases. For oropharyngeal cancer patients specifically, the ability to detect clinically and radiographically occult pathologic cervical lymphadenopathy renders PET a powerful clinical tool, as ipsilateral radiotherapy volumes are used in specific circumstances.[36] Although commonly reported as the maximum standard uptake value (SUV_{max}), alternative measurements such as SUV_{mean} may have greater prognostic value.[37] The utility of PET/CT for oropharyngeal cancer patients demonstrates high sensitivity approaching 100%, although only about 60% specificity for pathologically proven tumor. Clinical status and knowledge of prior procedures is critical to PET interpretation, because recent biopsies and infections can cause artificially elevated metabolic activity.

Magnetic Resonance Imaging

Magnetic resonance imaging (MRI) can be a useful imaging tool for oropharyngeal tumors. Squamous cell carcinoma appears as low signal in T1 MRI and corresponding high signal in T2 sequences. The ability of MRI to differentiate tumor from soft tissues is particularly useful when determination of the extent of base of tongue or oral tongue invasion is needed. Additionally, MRI is useful in patients with compromised renal function who are not able to receive iodine-based CT contrast agents.

PATHOLOGIC CLASSIFICATION

Squamous cell carcinomas are the most common histologic subtype comprising more than 95% of all oropharyngeal cancers. Uncommonly, minor salivary gland and mesenchymal tumors can affect this region. Given the proportionally high content of lymphoid tissue in the region within Waldeyer's ring, malignant Hodgkin and non-Hodgkin lymphomas also arise in this region. This chapter will discuss only squamous cell and related (poorly differentiated and lymphoepithelioma) histologic subtypes. Malignant lymphomas are discussed in Chapters 77–78. Minor salivary gland tumors are discussed in Chapter 43, and sarcomas are discussed in Chapters 48 & 83.

STAGING

Staging for oropharyngeal cancer is based on the American Joint Committee on Cancer (AJCC)/Union for International Cancer Control (UICC) system, shown in Table 45.5. Clinical staging is based on all available history, physical examination, endoscopic, radiographic, metabolic, and scintigraphic data. For all subsites, the size of the primary tumor contributes to the T-stage, with T1 being <2 cm, T2 >2 cm but <4 cm, and T3 >4 cm. T4a describes tumors invading the larynx, extrinsic muscles of the tongue, medial pterygoid, hard palate, or mandible. T4b disease describes oropharyngeal tumors invading the lateral pterygoid, pterygoid plates, lateral nasopharynx, skull base, or surrounding the carotid artery. Nodal staging for each of the subsites is the same: N0 indicates no clinical or radiographic evidence of pathologic lymphadenopathy; N1 indicates a single lymph node <3 cm in the ipsilateral cervical chains; N2a indicates a single lymph node >3 cm and <6 cm in the ipsilateral cervical chain; N2b indicates multiple ipsilateral cervical lymph nodes all <6 cm in size; N2c indicates bilateral pathologically involved cervical lymph nodes with the largest node <6 cm; and N3 indicates the presence of at least one lymph node >6 cm. Distant metastatic disease is classified as M1.

Stage grouping is shown in Table 45.6. Stage I comprises T1N0 tumors, and stage II is made up of T2N0 tumors. Stage III includes patients with T3N0–1 or T1-T2N1. Stage IV is divided into three subgroups: stage IVa is made up of patients with T4aN0–2a-c, T1–3N2a-c tumors; stage IVb disease basically describes patients who are technically unresectable, including patients with an extensive primary tumor (T4b) or those with any primary stage who have extensive lymphadenopathy (T any N3); stage IVc disease is reserved for patients with distant metastases.

TABLE 45.5 TNM STAGING SYSTEM FOR OROPHARYNGEAL CANCER

Primary Tumor (T)	
T1	Tumor ≤2 cm in greatest dimension
T2	Tumor >2 cm but not >4 cm in greatest dimension
T3	Tumor >4 cm in greatest dimension
T4a	Tumor invades the larynx, deep/extrinsic muscle of the tongue, medial pterygoid, hard palate, or mandible
T4b	Tumor invades lateral pterygoid muscle, pterygoid plates, lateral nasopharynx, or skull base or encases carotid artery
Regional Lymph Nodes (N)	
N0	No regional lymph node metastasis
N1	Metastasis in a single ipsilateral node, ≤3 cm
N2a	Metastasis in a single ipsilateral node, >3 cm but <6 cm
N2b	Metastasis in multiple ipsilateral nodes, >3 cm but <6 cm
N2c	Metastasis in bilateral or contralateral lymph nodes, none >6 cm
N3	Metastasis in a lymph node >6 cm
Distant Metastasis (M)	
M0	No distant metastasis present
M1	Distant metastasis present

Used with the permission of the American Joint Committee on Cancer (AJCC), Chicago, Illinois. The original source for this material is the AJCC *Cancer Staging Handbook*, Seventh Edition (2010) published by Springer Science and Business Media LLC, www.springerlink.com.

TABLE 45.6 STAGE GROUPING FOR OROPHARYNGEAL CANCER

	T1	*T2*	*T3*	*T4a*	*T4b*
N0	I	II	III	IVa	IVb
N1	III	III	III	IVa	IVb
N2a-c	IVa	IVa	IVa	IVa	IVb
N3	IVb	IVb	IVb	IVb	IVb
M1	IVc	IVc	IVc	IVc	IVc

MANAGEMENT STRATEGIES

Functional organ preservation with minimal toxicity is the management goal for all oropharyngeal cancer patients. Based on AJCC stage, patients are usually grouped into two different treatment groups to help guide therapy decisions. Those with locally confined disease (stage I and stage II tumors) are considered as early stage, whereas those with stages III and IV (nonmetastatic) disease are considered as having locoregionally advanced disease. For all subsites, early-stage tumors are usually well controlled with a single local modality, either radiotherapy or surgery. Selection of local modality should be based on the primary tumor size, extent of local spread, and subsite involved. Small tumors of the tonsil and small exophytic tumors of the base of tongue can be well managed surgically, whereas the morbidity of surgery on the soft palate favors radiotherapy. For locoregionally advanced disease, two appropriate treatment strategies are used: (a) either surgery followed by radiation therapy with or without chemotherapy based on pathologic risk factors or (b) radiotherapy usually given with chemotherapy.

SURGICAL TECHNIQUES, APPROACHES, AND RESULTS

Base of Tongue

Surgery plays a limited role in the management of base of tongue tumors given the inherent morbidity of a near-total or total glossectomy, which is required for large and/or midline tumors. For select, well-lateralized base of tongue tumors with minimal cervical lymphadenopathy, a partial glossectomy can be performed. Given the high propensity for occult microscopic nodal involvement, bilateral cervical lymph node dissection is often performed. Base of tongue tumors in close proximity to the laryngeal apparatus, such as those arising in the vallecula, often require a supraglottic or total laryngectomy to achieve adequate margins of resection.

Traditional surgical approaches for base of tongue tumors include the midline mandibulotomy (splitting the lip, mandible, and oral tongue midline), the lateral mandibulotomy (dividing the mandible near the angle and approaching the base of tongue from the side), and the floor drop procedure (elevating the inner periosteum from the mandible from angle to angle, which releases the entire floor of mouth and oral tongue into the neck, exposing the base of tongue).

Tonsil Cancers

For small (<1 cm) early-stage tonsil cancers confined to the anterior pillar, a wide local excision can achieve adequate tumor-free margins, whereas tumors involving the palatine tonsil often require a radical tonsillectomy. For both of these situations, the tonsil is approached transorally, with primary closure. Larger tumors with extension onto the tongue, onto the mandible or into surrounding tissue often require a composite resection, usually including resection of the tonsil, tonsillar fossa, pillars, a portion of the soft palate, tongue, and mandible. For tumors not adjacent or adherent to the mandible, a midline mandibulotomy approach is used. For tumors adherent to the mandible, a partial mandibulectomy is used. Defects are often closed with a myocutaneous flap. Complications from surgery depend on the extent of resection, with impairment in swallowing possible by removal of part of the tongue or soft palate.

Soft Palate Cancers

Surgical resection is rarely recommended as initial therapy for soft palate tumors. Resection of the soft palate is often associated with significant reflux into the nasopharynx during swallowing, even with the use of custom prostheses. Additionally, because of the midline location, primary disease spreads bilaterally to the neck with frequency high enough to require elective treatment. However, when surgery is performed, the tumors are approached transorally and a full-thickness wide local resection is performed for tumors limited to the soft palate. A more extensive composite resection is required if disease extends to surrounding structures. Flaps or prostheses are used to preserve velopharyngeal competence. Nasal speech is also often a consequence.

Transoral Surgical Approaches

Transoral surgical approaches, routinely used for limited tonsillar resections, are increasingly being used for other oropharyngeal cancer operations as an alternative to open surgical procedures. By limiting the need for open surgical exposure, these operations can have a quicker recovery time and less morbidity. More recently, endoscopic approaches have been adopted to enhance the utility of transoral surgery. However, limited prospective data support the benefit of transoral operations over traditional approaches. Prospective data are needed to further elucidate the benefits of these surgical advances and better integrate them with the other standard oncologic therapies.

Transoral Laser Surgery

Small series report favorable outcomes for selected patients with stage I through stage IV oropharyngeal tumors treated with transoral laser microsurgery with or without neck dissection, followed by adjuvant radiotherapy or chemoradiotherapy.[38–40] Positive margin rates are variable (3% to 24%) and appear to vary based on primary site, being more common in base of tongue tumors. Complications include postoperative hemorrhage (5% to 10%). Temporary tracheostomy placement is relatively common (17% to 30%) and needed for exposure, airway control, or aspiration following extensive resection. High rates of locoregional control following this procedure have been reported, primarily for stage I/II patients (87% to 100%), although for stage III/IV patients, local recurrence is more common (20% to 30%). Swallowing outcomes are favorable with series reporting most patients tolerating a normal diet.[40]

Transoral Robotic Surgery

The use of a computer-aided interaction between the surgeon and the patient is commonly referred to as robotic surgery. The most common robotic surgical system, the da Vinci Surgical System, is comprised of three surgical instruments and a binocular endoscope controlled by robotic arms and inserted under direct or endoscopic guidance by the surgeon from a patient-side apparatus. The surgeon controls the instruments from a console separated from the patient. The operative environment is visualized virtually, in a three-dimensional (3D) environment created via a computer that links the environment provided by the binocular endoscope to the position of the instruments. The surgeon's movements are translated into the micromovements of the instruments. The advantages of this system include motion scaling, which can increase precision as well as reduce hand tremor and fatigue. When the system is used for transoral surgeries, an assistant is often positioned by the patient's head.

There are no prospective randomized studies supporting the use of transoral robotic surgery (TORS) for oropharyngeal tumor resection over conventional surgery. All studies to date are small single-institution series. Proponents of TORS highlight an enhanced visualization of the surgical field over traditional transoral techniques. Some have hypothesized that perhaps local control could be enhanced via TORS debulking with minimal acute sequelae. However, this claim has yet to be tested prospectively. Prospective studies have shown that TORS can be used safely with a low risk of laceration or fracture to a patient.[41] In a series of 27 patients with tonsillar cancer who underwent TORS tonsillectomy, morbidity was "acceptable," including one case of musical bleeding and two cases of moderate trismus; one patient required a tracheostomy, and negative margins were obtained in 25 of 27 patients.[42]

Until mature prospective multi-institutional series and randomized data are available, the true utility of transoral laser microsurgery and TORS remains unknown. Although early results are favorable and associated with shorter hospital stays, long-term data are needed. Additionally, standard oncologic principles limiting the number of modalities used to minimize treatment related side effects should be carefully considered prior to widespread adoption of the surgical techniques.

ADJUVANT THERAPY FOLLOWING DEFINITIVE SURGICAL RESECTION

Following surgical resection of oropharyngeal cancers, pathologic features including advanced primary T-stage (T3 or T4), lymphovascular space invasion, perineural invasion, positive margins, multiple pathologically involved cervical lymph nodes, and extranodal extension place patients at high risk for locoregional recurrence.[43] In these cases, postoperative radiotherapy (PORT), often in conjunction with chemotherapy, has been shown to reduce the risk of locoregional relapse.[44,45,46] PORT was shown in RTOG 73–03 to results in superior locoregional control (70% vs. 58%) when compared to preoperative radiotherapy but did not affect survival.[47]

Adjuvant Chemoradiotherapy for Oropharyngeal Cancer

The addition of cisplatin-based chemotherapy to PORT has been compared to PORT alone for medically fit head and neck cancer patients of any site in several randomized studies.[48–51] All of these studies have demonstrated statistically significant[48–50] or strong statistical trends[51] for improved locoregional control and disease-free survival with the addition of chemotherapy to PORT. Additionally, two of these studies have demonstrated statistically significant improvements in overall survival,[48,49] whereas the other two have shown numerically improved but not statistically significant survival improvements.[50,51] A significant portion of patients in these studies had oropharyngeal cancer (European Organisation for Research and Treatment of Cancer [EORTC] 30% and RTOG 43%) generalizing these results to oropharyngeal patients with high-risk pathologic features.

Concurrent Chemotherapy Regimens for Adjuvant Chemoradiotherapy

The optimal chemotherapy regimen delivered with PORT is currently unknown. Schedules of bolus cisplatin 100 mg/m² were tested in two[48,51] randomized studies mentioned earlier, one tested 50-mg weekly cisplatin[49] and the other tested cisplatin 20 mg/m² and 5-fluorouracil (5-FU) 600 mg/m² days 1 through 5 and days 29 through 33.[50] There have been no randomized comparisons of these cisplatin-based schedules. Randomized studies have been attempted to identify the role of carboplatin-based chemotherapy concurrently with PORT compared to PORT alone.[52] Unfortunately, these studies closed before accrual goals were met, and no significant benefit was found with the addition of carboplatin to PORT. RTOG 0234 randomized high-risk postoperative patients (positive margin, extranodal extension, and/or ≥2 pathologically involved cervical nodes) to PORT in combination with cetuximab (400 mg/m² loading dose followed by 250 mg/m² weekly) and weekly docetaxel 15 mg/m² or to PORT with cetuximab (400 mg/m² loading dose followed by 250 mg/m² weekly) and 30 mg/m² cisplatin weekly. Results of this randomized phase II study are maturing. Currently, no randomized data support the use of taxanes or cetuximab in the postoperative setting.[53] Based on the available data, many consider cisplatin 100 mg/m² every 3 weeks as the standard.

Adjuvant Radiotherapy Dose

The optimal radiation therapy dose for PORT is also not well defined. Most of the randomized studies demonstrating the benefit of concurrent chemotherapy with PORT used radiotherapy doses of 60 to 66 Gy in 2-Gy daily fractions to high-risk areas (primary tumor bed with positive margin or nodal regions with extracapsular spread). Doses of 50 to 54 Gy in 2-Gy fractions were usually given to areas at risk for microscopic involvement. There is little evidence supporting the higher PORT doses used in these randomized trials over those recommended from the PORT-alone dose-finding studies of 63 Gy for extranodal extension and 57.6 Gy for all others. In three of four randomized studies testing the utility of chemotherapy concurrently with PORT, doses of more than 65 Gy were delivered to high-risk areas.[48–51] The fourth study, RTOG 95-01, allowed a dose of 60 Gy with or without an optional 6-Gy boost. As these studies were associated with significant benefits for patients with extracapsular extension and positive margins, we recommend similar dosing schedules.

Postoperative Radiotherapy Treatment Volume

The typical treatment volume used in PORT for head and neck cancer includes the bilateral neck and the primary tumor site. However, it is unclear whether both the neck and primary always need to be within the PORT volume. In those with completely resected primary tumors with negative margins whose sole indication for PORT is pathologic cervical adenopathy, some would direct therapy only to the neck. Additionally, for patients with a positive margin as the sole indication for treatment in the setting of a comprehensive neck surgery without pathologically involved cervical lymph nodes, some would direct treatment to the primary resection bed only. For well-lateralized primary tumors, patterns of progression would suggest that PORT to the ipsilateral neck only may be appropriate.[53]

DEFINITIVE RADIOTHERAPY

For early-stage oropharyngeal cancers, the use of radiation therapy as a single modality is associated with good outcomes and functional preservation.[54] Although there is not consensus on the optimal dose fractionation schedule for oropharyngeal cancer patients receiving radiotherapy alone, randomized data[55–57] and meta-analyses[58,59] support an overall survival benefit with the use of accelerated fractionation or hyperfractionated radiotherapy. Therefore, for oropharyngeal cancer treated with radiotherapy alone, strong consideration should be given to altered fractionation of some sort.

Hyperfractionated Radiotherapy

The benefit of hyperfractionated radiotherapy for oropharyngeal cancer was clearly demonstrated in EORTC 22791, in which patients with T2-3N0-1 non–base of tongue oropharyngeal cancers were randomized to conventionally fractionated radiotherapy at 70 Gy (2 Gy per day) or to 80.5 Gy hyperfractionated at 1.15 Gy twice daily. Hyperfractionated radiotherapy was associated with statistically significant improvements in locoregional control (5-year, 59% vs. 40%). Additionally, there was a trend toward improved overall survival ($p = 0.08$) particularly in stage III patients.[57]

Accelerated Radiotherapy

Accelerated radiotherapy has also been shown to benefit oropharyngeal cancer patients; however, this may depend on the exact regimen used. For example, a randomized study comparing an accelerated regimen of 66 to 70 Gy delivered in 2-Gy daily fractions 6 days a week to the same dose delivered 5 days a week with oropharyngeal cancer affecting the majority of patients demonstrated improved locoregional control (42% vs. 30%, $p = 0.004$), disease-free survival (50% vs. 40%, $p = 0.03$), and a trend toward improved overall survival (35% vs. 28%, $p = 0.07$).[60] When analyzed as a separate subgroup, pharyngeal primary sites had improved locoregional control (HR 0.6, 95% CI 0.41–0.86).[56] Of note, accelerated fractionation improved local control for both p16-positive (HR 0.56, CI 0.33–0.96) as well as p16-negative tumors (HR 0.77, CI 0.60–0.99).[61] However, when a more intensive accelerated regimen of 1.8 Gy twice daily to 59.4 Gy was compared to 70 Gy in 2-Gy fractions in stage III/IV head and neck cancer patients, no statistical benefits were seen in terms of locoregional control or overall survival.[62] It is unknown if the lack of benefit seen was due to the regimen used or to inclusion criteria because the benefit for acceleration in some randomized studies was less significant for those with stage IV disease as well as those with a larger nodal disease burden.[60]

Accelerated Versus Hyperfractionated Radiotherapy

For oropharyngeal cancer patients in particular, and head and neck cancer patients in general, it is not known if hyperfractionated or accelerated radiotherapy is superior. The meta-analysis of radiotherapy in carcinoma of the head and neck collaborative group pooled 15 randomized studies (including 6,515 patients) comparing conventionally fractionated radiotherapy to either accelerated radiotherapy or hyperfractionated radiotherapy. Oropharyngeal cancer patients were the largest subsite, representing 44% of all patients (1,585 patients). Altered fractionation radiotherapy regimens were associated with a 3.4% absolute improvement in 5-year overall survival. Heterogeneity in patients included on accelerated and hyperfractionated trials obscure direct comparison, although hyperfractionated patients had an absolute 8.2% improvement in overall survival at 5 years compared to a 2% absolute benefit with accelerated radiotherapy.[59]

One of the studies included in the meta-analysis, RTOG 90-03, compared conventional fractionation (70 Gy in 2-Gy daily fractions) to hyperfractionation (81.6 Gy in 1.2 Gy twice daily) to accelerated fractionation with a split course (67.2 Gy in 1.6 Gy twice daily with a 2-week rest after 38.4 Gy) to accelerated fractionation with concomitant boost regimen (72 Gy in 1.8-Gy fractions for 14 fractions followed by a 1.8-Gy morning and a 1.5-Gy afternoon boost to gross disease). Although all primary sites other than the nasopharynx were included, 60% of patients included had oropharyngeal primary tumors.

Improved locoregional control was seen in both the hyperfractionated and accelerated concomitant boost arms.[63] These improvements resulted in trend toward improved disease-free survival for patients treated with hyperfractionation (37.6% vs. 31.7%, p = 0.067) and accelerated concomitant boost (39.3% vs. 31.7%, p = 0.054), which almost reached statistical significance at the p = 0.05 level. These improvements were associated with an increase in both acute and late toxicity in all three accelerated treatment arms. No significant difference in overall survival was seen.

Simultaneous Integrated Boost Radiotherapy

With the increasing use of intensity-modulated radiotherapy (IMRT), simultaneous integrated boost radiotherapy has been investigated for oropharyngeal cancer patients. The RTOG completed a study (00-22) in early-stage (T1-2, N0-2) oropharyngeal cancer patients treated with bilateral neck radiotherapy[54] using doses of 2.2 Gy, 2 Gy, and 1.8 Gy to gross tumor, intermediate-risk, and low-risk planning target volumes (PTVs), respectively. The 2-year risk of local progression was 9% and was higher in patients who had significant underdosing of known tumor. Additionally, no local recurrences, distant metastases, or second cancers were seen in never smokers, possibly representing a surrogate for HPV-related disease, compared to seven locoregional recurrences, five second cancers, and one case of distant metastases in smokers. Two-year overall survival was 95%, and disease-free survival was 82%. Therefore, it appears that for patients with early-stage oropharyngeal cancer treated with radiotherapy alone, simultaneous integrated boost radiotherapy is a viable treatment option.

CONCURRENT CHEMORADIOTHERAPY FOR LOCOREGIONALLY ADVANCED OROPHARYNGEAL CANCER

For patients with locoregionally advanced oropharyngeal cancer, concurrent chemoradiotherapy is the standard treatment. Resection is generally not recommended given the associated surgical morbidity. Additionally, adjuvant chemoradiotherapy is frequently necessary and has similar morbidity to definitive intent chemoradiotherapy. Comparisons of outcomes with radiotherapy with or without neck dissection or surgery with or without adjuvant radiotherapy resulted in similar outcomes with higher complication rates with surgery.[64]

Evidence for Concurrent Chemoradiotherapy

The use of concurrent chemoradiotherapy for most stage III and IV (nonmetastatic) oropharyngeal cancer patients is based on the results of the meta-analysis of chemotherapy in head and neck cancer (MACH-NC), which demonstrated a 6.2% absolute improvement in overall survival at 5 years from the use of concurrent chemoradiotherapy compared to radiotherapy alone. This benefit was also observed in the oropharyngeal cancer subgroup.[65] Additionally, level I evidence from multiple randomized studies restricted to oropharyngeal cancer patients supports the use of concurrent chemoradiotherapy for stage III/IV oropharyngeal cancer.[66,67] The Groupe d'Oncologie Radiothérapie Tête Et Cou (GORTEC) compared 2-Gy daily conventional radiotherapy to 70 Gy concomitantly administered with daily bolus carboplatin and continuous infusion 5-fluorouracil 600 mg/m^2/day on days 1 through 4 every 3 weeks for three cycles. A total of 222 patients (113 assigned to radiotherapy alone and 109 assigned to combined treatment) were eligible for analysis. With a median follow-up of 5.5 years, absolute 5-year overall survival was significantly higher in the combined modality arm (15.8% with radiotherapy alone to 22.4% with chemoradiotherapy), as shown in Figure 45.4. Five-year locoregional control was also significantly improved with concomitant therapy (from 24.7% vs. 47.6% for the combined-treatment group, p = 0.002).[68] Combined modality therapy was associated with increased hematologic toxicity, increased mucositis, and weight loss. Severe late toxicity was also increased with combined modality therapy (14% vs. 9% radiotherapy alone), including increased mandibular toxicity and cervical fibrosis. These patients were treated with two-dimensional (2D) treatment planning, typically including parallel-opposed fields with dosimetric hotspots located in the mandible and neck soft tissues. The extent to which concurrent chemotherapy contributes to these specific late toxicities in the setting of IMRT is not clearly understood.

Outcomes of locoregionally advanced oropharyngeal cancer have improved in the era of concurrent chemoradiotherapy and modern radiotherapy planning and delivery techniques. This improvement is likely influenced by newer imaging techniques leading to more informed patient selection and radiotherapy planning and the influence of a rise in HPV-related oropharyngeal cancer cases. A recent analysis of more than 300 locoregionally advanced oropharyngeal cancer patients treated with primary chemoradiotherapy with a median follow-up of 34 months reported low 2-year rates of local progression (6.1%),

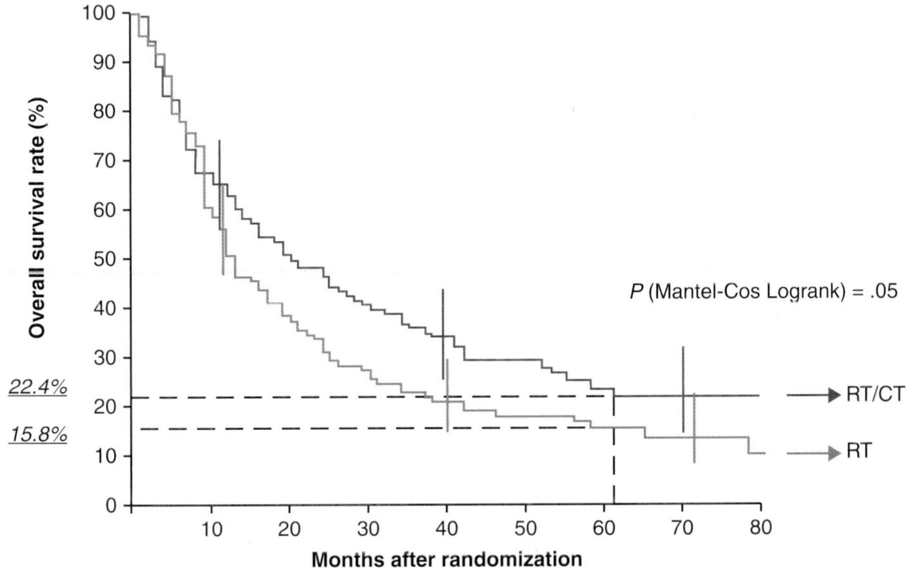

FIGURE 45.4. Overall survival among patients with oropharyngeal cancer treated with radiotherapy alone (RT) or with radiotherapy with concomitant chemotherapy (RT/CT) as analyzed by the Kaplan-Meier method on GORTEC 94-01. (From Denis F, Garaud P, Bardet E, et al. Final results of the 94-01 French Head and Neck Oncology and Radiotherapy Group randomized trial comparing radiotherapy alone with concomitant radiochemotherapy in advanced-stage oropharynx carcinoma. *J Clin Oncol* 2004;22[1]:69–76. Reprinted with permission. © 2004 American Society of Clinical Oncology.)

regional progression (5.2%), and distant progression (12.2%).[69] Base of tongue cancers have historically been associated with poor outcomes when treated with surgery or radiotherapy alone or in combination (5-year disease-specific and overall survival of 27.8% and 40.3%, respectively).[70] However, recent single-institution series using chemoradiotherapy highlight high rates of locoregional control for BOT cancers with the use of either 3D conformal radiotherapy (5-year, 82%) or IMRT (5-year, 97.4%),[71] which could represent the influence of HPV-related oropharyngeal cancer.

Acute Toxicity of Chemoradiotherapy

For oropharyngeal cancer patients, a course of concurrent chemoradiotherapy is a life-changing event given the associated toxicities, including fatigue, nausea, emesis, thickened secretions, xerostomia, mucositis, dysphagia, odynophagia, alopecia, dermatitis, anemia, neutropenia, hoarseness, Lhermitte's syndrome, and infection. Dysphagia is perhaps the most difficult acute complication of chemoradiotherapy for oropharyngeal cancer. Oropharyngeal patients are less likely to be affected than those with laryngeal or hypopharyngeal tumors.[72] Older patients and those with worse performance status are more likely to have worsening of their swallowing following chemoradiotherapy. Those with more advanced tumors are more likely to have swallowing improvement likely owing to reduction of tumor bulk.[73] Given the adverse effect of dysphagia on nutritional status, management recommendations include early therapeutic intervention with swallowing exercises designed to strengthen the pharyngeal musculature. Patients should be instructed to swallow as large a volume as possible during and after treatment and to perform exercises shown to improve swallowing ability.[74] Dysphagia has been associated retrospectively, with the exceeding of specific dosimetric thresholds to the pharyngeal constrictors or laryngeal apparatus, which should be incorporated into radiotherapy planning as discussed later.

Late Toxicity of Chemoradiotherapy

Late toxicities of chemoradiotherapy for oropharyngeal cancer patients can be quite significant and may include fibrosis, osteoradionecrosis, trismus, xerostomia, dental caries, feeding tube dependence, and neuritis. Late toxicities of chemoradiotherapy have been catalogued by the RTOG in a pooled analysis of 230 patients treated on three prospective chemoradiotherapy trials with a median follow-up of 3 years. Oropharyngeal primaries affected 34% of all patients. Older patients and those with larger (T3, T4) tumors were more likely to experience late toxicity, as were those who underwent a posttreatment neck dissection.[75] When late toxicity was analyzed by primary tumor site, patients with oropharyngeal and oral cavity primary tumors were statistically less likely to experience late toxicity. Long-term analysis of the aforementioned GORTEC randomized trial demonstrated that 56% of patients treated with chemoradiotherapy had at least one grade 3 to 4 late toxicity compared to 30% treated with radiotherapy alone ($p = 0.12$). The small number of long-term survivors probably reduced the power to detect statistically significantly differences between these groups.[68]

Alternative Concurrent Chemoradiotherapy Regimens

The toxicities of concurrent chemoradiotherapy have stimulated the search for improvements in this platform. Some questions still remain unanswered, including what constitutes the optimal chemotherapy regimen. Cisplatin at 100 mg/m^2 every 3 weeks for 2–3 cycles is often cited as a standard regimen. The aforementioned GORTEC randomized study demonstrated an overall survival advantage using a carboplatin/5-FU regimen specifically chosen to avoid cisplatin-related tinnitus, renal dysfunction, and emesis. There are no randomized studies comparing alternative cisplatin dosing schedules (such as 30 to 40 mg/m^2 weekly, 20 mg/m^2/day, days 1 through 5 and days 22 through 26) to bolus cisplatin or to other chemoradiotherapy platforms. However, multiple randomized studies that compared radiotherapy alone to concurrent chemoradiotherapy using nonbolus cisplatin schedules including daily cisplatin (6 mg/m^2/day),[76] weekly cisplatin 40 mg/m^2 weekly,[77] or cisplatin 20 mg/m^2/day, days 1 through 5 repeated every 3 weeks,[78] had comparable outcomes to bolus cisplatin. The relative merits of various chemoradiotherapy platforms will be discussed in more detail in Chapter 40.

Induction Chemotherapy Prior to Definitive Local Therapy

The use of neoadjuvant chemotherapy prior to surgical resection or radiotherapy for oropharyngeal cancer patients has been tested in randomized studies. In particular, a phase III study restricted to oropharyngeal cancer patients compared cisplatin 100 mg/m^2 on day 1 and 5-fluorouracil 1,000 mg/m^2/day, days 1 through 5, repeated every 3 weeks for three cycles followed by definitive local therapy to definitive local therapy alone. At the time of the study, standard local therapies included either radiotherapy alone (70 Gy to the primary, 50 Gy to the neck) or composite surgery with PORT (50 to 65 Gy based on pathologic findings). Although only 318 of a planned 760 patients were enrolled, a statistically significant improvement in overall survival was seen in the induction chemotherapy arm at 5 years (5.1 years vs. 3.3 years) with a median follow-up of 5 years.[79] This study suggests a benefit to neoadjuvant chemotherapy. The applicability of this trial in the chemoradiotherapy era is questionable, however, because the patients in the control arm of the study received surgery or 70 Gy of daily radiotherapy, which is known to be inferior to accelerated or hyperfractionated radiotherapy. The value of this treatment compared to concurrent chemoradiation is also unknown.

Whether or not induction chemotherapy prior to concurrent chemoradiotherapy improves survival when compared to chemoradiotherapy is currently unknown and waiting maturation of data from completed randomized studies. Induction chemotherapy has been advocated by some given that distant metastases is frequently a site of first failure for patients with locoregionally advanced head and neck cancer in general.[80] This is particularly true for patients with oropharyngeal cancer because local regional therapy (chemoradiotherapy) has become so much more effective.[69] Induction chemotherapy has resulted in low rates of distant metastases in single-arm phase II studies,[81,82] suggesting a role for some oropharyngeal patients at increased risk for distant metastases. Randomized studies assessing the role of induction chemotherapy were initiated prior to robust knowledge of the behavior of HPV-associated oropharyngeal cancers. Therefore, inclusion of these patients with their favorable outcomes were not accounted for in the study design and may complicate interpretation of these studies.

Targeted Agents and Radiotherapy

A randomized study compared radiotherapy, 70 to 76.8 Gy with or without weekly cetuximab, (loading dose of 400 mg/m^2 followed by 250 mg/m^2) for locoregionally advanced head and neck cancer patients. The combination therapy was found to improve locoregional control, disease-free survival, and overall survival.[83] The majority of patients had oropharyngeal primary tumors (60%). When analyzed alone, patients with oropharyngeal cancer treated with cetuximab had demonstrated improved 2-year locoregional control (50% vs. 41%) and median locoregional disease-free duration: 49 months versus 23 months (HR 0.61) with the use of cetuximab. Furthermore, the median overall survival for oropharyngeal cancer patients treated with cetuximab and radiotherapy was >66 months compared to 30.3 months in those treated with radiotherapy alone (HR 0.62), a larger difference than those with laryngeal

(32.8 months vs. 31.6 months) or hypopharyngeal (13.7 months vs. 13.5 months) primary sites. Therefore, for oropharyngeal cancer patients meeting the inclusion criteria for this study, stage III/IV, nonmetastatic, Karnofsky performance status score >60, and normal hematopoietic, hepatic, and renal function, cetuximab and radiotherapy is an alternative treatment platform. Consideration should be given to the use of altered radiation fractionation with cetuximab because improved overall survival was seen in patients who were treated with accelerated concomitant boost and hyperfractionated radiotherapy.

Cetuximab should be avoided in specific regions (particularly the southeastern United States) where severe anaphylactic reactions mediated by an immunoglobulin E response to the galactose-alpha-1,3-galactose oligosaccharide found on the Fab portion of the cetuximab heavy chain are seen.[84] A fully humanized monoclonal antibody to the EGFR, panitumumab, has a much lower rate of severe allergic reactions; however, there is no level-1 evidence to support its equivalent efficacy in this clinical setting. Aside from these geographic limitations, it is unclear which patient populations should receive concurrent chemotherapy and which should receive cetuximab plus radiotherapy. Some physicians use cetuximab plus radiotherapy preferentially over cisplatin plus radiotherapy in patients with renal dysfunction or overall poor functional status, although there is no level-1 evidence to support this indication. In fact, these same medical conditions constituted exclusion criteria for the randomized trial proving its benefit.

Given the improved outcomes of HPV-associated oropharyngeal cancer with standard treatments, deintensification of therapy is being considered in this patient population. Randomized studies comparing standard chemoradiotherapy to combined EGFR inhibition and radiotherapy are ongoing in the cooperative group setting. RTOG 1016 is comparing bolus cisplatin 100 mg/m^2 days 1 and 23 with accelerated radiotherapy (70 Gy, 2 Gy/day, 6 days per week) to the same radiotherapy and cetuximab 400 mg/m^2 loading dose and 250 mg/m^2 weekly with radiotherapy. This noninferiority study has a primary end point of comparable 5-year survival. The National Cancer Institute of Canada (NCIC) is conducting a similar study, although with the use of panitumumab with radiotherapy given the lower rates of dermatologic and anaphylactic reactions. Other investigations are attempting radiation dose reduction by aiming to keep locoregional control high while reducing acute toxicity, with some using induction chemotherapy before chemoradiotherapy. Mature reports from these studies will help to determine how to optimally treat this unique patient population.

Targeted Agents in Combination with Cytotoxins and Radiotherapy

To date, there are no comparisons of cytotoxic agents and radiation with and without cetuximab for oropharyngeal cancer patients. Oropharyngeal cancer patients comprised 70% of RTOG 0522, which compared two concurrent cycles of 100 mg/m^2 cisplatin and accelerated concomitant boost to 72-Gy radiotherapy with or without the addition of a loading dose of 400 mg/m^2 followed by weekly 250 mg/m^2 cetuximab. The combination of cisplatin, cetuximab, and radiotherapy did not improve locoregional control, disease-free survival, or overall survival. However, this triplet therapy was associated with increased grade 3/4 mucositis (45% vs. 35%, P = 0.003) and skin reactions (40% vs. 17%, P <0.0001) without increasing grade 3/4 dysphagia rates (62% vs. 66%, P = 0.27).[85] Fifty-one percent of oropharyngeal tumor specimens were evaluated for p16 expression, and 73% of these specimens were positive. No differences in outcome were seen as a function of differences in HPV status.

Oropharyngeal cancer patients have also been included in studies evaluating the addition of bevacizumab to chemoradiotherapy. The addition of bevacizumab to 5-fluorouracil, hydroxyurea, and twice-daily radiotherapy (FHX) did not confer any benefit in a study of locoregionally advanced head and neck cancer patients. The study was terminated early because of toxicity and because only 5 of 26 participants had oropharyngeal primary tumors.[86] Bevacizumab has also been integrated with erlotinib (synchronous dual inhibition of vascular endothelial growth factor [VEGF] and EGFR) and cisplatin (33 mg/m^2 cisplatin days 1 through 3, weeks 1 and 5) together with 1.25-Gy twice-daily radiotherapy to 70 Gy. Seventy-one percent of patients had oropharyngeal primary tumors. At a median follow-up of 46 months, 3-year locoregional control and overall survival were promising at 86% and 85%, respectively, compared to historical series.[87] Soft tissue and osteoradionecrosis occurred in both series, and careful attention should be paid to the results of ongoing studies integrating bevacizumab to multiple chemoradiotherapy platforms for locoregionally advanced head and neck cancer patients, including those with oropharyngeal tumors.

EXTERNAL-BEAM RADIOTHERAPY SIMULATION AND TREATMENT PLANNING

Radiotherapy Simulation

Prior to a course of radiotherapy or chemoradiotherapy, patients should undergo simulation, preferably CT based, to allow for optimal radiotherapy planning. A peripheral IV should be placed prior to simulation for the delivery of low osmolar iodinated contrast to optimize the distinction between vascular structures and lymph nodes. Patients are positioned supine, with a rigid head holder cradling the posterior calvarium. Generally, an extended head position is preferable. The shoulders should be positioned as caudally as possible to allow adequate exposure of the neck. This can be achieved either with shoulder pulls or with commercially available devices. Tongue immobilization can be useful for oropharyngeal cancer patients with oral tongue involvement. Bite blocks are also useful because they often elevate the hard palate with its minor salivary glands. The head should be immobilized with a thermoplastic mask. Care should be taken to ensure that the mask is tight and should not allow movement of the nose, chin or, forehead. Images should be taken from above the calvarium to the carina to ensure that appropriate volumes can be drawn. The addition of metabolic imaging and MRI has been found to be complementary for gross tumor volume (GTV) delineation.[88]

Radiotherapy Volumes

Radiotherapy volumes for oropharyngeal cancer patients are based on the International Commission on Radiation Units and Measurements (ICRU) 50. The GTV includes all known primary and cervical lymph node tumor extension based on clinical, endoscopic, and imaging findings. Care should be taken to look for fat stranding, which could be indicative of extranodal extension. This is usually expanded to include a margin for microscopic extension forming the high-dose clinical target volume (CTV). The true CTV indicating the margin needed to cover microscopic extension not visible on clinical and imaging modalities is not known. Current RTOG guidelines specify an extension of 0.5 to 1 cm from the GTV to form the high-dose CTV. Nodal regions at risk for occult microscopic spread are usually included in a low-risk CTV. Many studies using clinical presentation data as well as elective surgical series have attempted to define the risk based on primary tumor site and extent of involvement as shown in Table 45.7. In general, this includes at least bilateral level II to IV. Typically, one nodal region beyond those pathologically involved is included—that is, for a patient with level II pathologic lymphadenopathy, level IB should be included. The inclusion of the retropharyngeal nodes routinely in the low-risk PTV is controversial as it often increases radiation dose to the pharyngeal constrictors, which

TABLE 45.7 INCIDENCE (%) OF PATHOLOGIC LYMPH NODE METASTASIS IN SQUAMOUS CELL CARCINOMAS OF THE OROPHARYNX

	Distribution of Metastatic Lymph Nodes Per Level (Percentage of the Neck Dissection Procedures)											
	Prophylactic RND						Therapeutic RND					
Tumor Site	Number of RNDs	I	II	III	IV	V	Number of RNDs	I	II	III	IV	V
Base of tongue & vallecula	21	0	19	14	9	5	58	10	72	41	21	9
Tonsillar fossa	27	4	30	22	7	0	107	17	70	42	31	9
Total	48	2	25	19	8	2	165	15	71	42	27	9

RND, regional node dissection.

From Grégoire V, Coche E, Cosnard G, et al. Selection and delineation of lymph node target volumes in head and neck conformal radiotherapy: proposal for standardizing terminology and procedure based on the surgical experience. *Radiother Oncol* 2000;56:135–150, with permission.

has been associated with dysphagia[89] and should depend on the extent of the primary tumor and cervical lymphadenopathy. The incidence of retropharyngeal lymphadenopathy is demonstrated in Tables 45.8 and 45.9. Coverage of the retropharyngeal nodes up to the base of skull is associated with a low risk of progression;[90] however, absence of coverage is not necessarily associated with an increased risk of recurrence. Certainly, retropharyngeal coverage (i.e., extending the superior border of level II to include the retrostyloid space) should be considered for oropharyngeal tumors extending into the nasopharynx or pterygoid region, those with gross retropharyngeal nodal involvement, and those with high level II lymphadenopathy.[26]

Consensus guidelines for contouring the clinically node-negative neck have been published and endorsed by international head and neck cancer cooperative groups, including the RTOG, EORTC, Danish Head and Neck Cancer Group (DAHANCA), GORTEC, and NCIC.[27] These guidelines are clinically useful aids for delineating specific nodal treatment volumes. Similar guidelines have been proposed for the node-positive neck and postoperative patients.[26] Specific recommendations for node-positive patients include coverage of the supraclavicular fossa for patients with level IV or Vb lymphadenopathy and inclusion of the entire thickness of muscles invaded by pathologic lymphadenopathy in the CTV. Additionally, pathologic lymphadenopathy spanning adjacent levels should trigger inclusion of the full extent of both levels in the CTV. For postoperative patients, coverage of the entire operative bed in the neck is recommended to account for potential tumor spillage. Coverage of the retrostyloid space was recommended for all patients with pathologic level II lymphadenopathy. Similar to the nondissected node-positive neck, inclusion of muscles invaded by tumor is recommended, as is coverage of all levels spanned by pathologic lymphadenopathy.

TABLE 45.8 INCIDENCE OF RETROPHARYNGEAL LYMPH NODES IN HEAD AND NECK PRIMARY TUMORS

	Incidence of Retropharyngeal Lymph Nodes (Percentage of the Total Number of Patients)		
Primary Site	Overall	N0 Neck	N+ Neck
Oropharynx			
Pharyngeal wall	18/93 (19)	6/37 (16)	12/56 (21)
Soft palate	7/53 (13)	1/21 (5)	6/32 (19)
Tonsillar fossa	16/176 (9)	2/56 (4)	14/120 (12)
Base of tongue	5/121 (4)	0/31 (0)	5/90 (6)

N+, node positive.

From Grégoire V, Coche E, Cosnard G, et al. Selection and delineation of lymph node target volumes in head and neck conformal radiotherapy: proposal for standardizing terminology and procedure based on the surgical experience. *Radiother Oncol* 2000;56:135–150, with permission.

CTVs are expanded to account for organ motion and setup uncertainty ideally based on institution-specific data to form the PTV. For oropharyngeal cancer patients, movement of the base of tongue should be considered (particularly with swallowing) when designing an appropriate PTV margin. The expansion from CTV to PTV should account for imaging methods used to assess daily setup. In general, if more frequent image guidance is performed, the margin needed for setup uncertainty should be less. The RTOG currently recommends 5 to 10 mm for patients treated with standard weekly megavoltage port films and 0.25 to 5 mm if more frequent kV image or cone-beam CT guidance is used. Representative contours for a patient with locoregionally advanced oropharyngeal cancer are shown in Figures 45.5, 45.6, and 45.7.

Indications for Ipsilateral Radiotherapy

For well-lateralized tonsillar cancer cases not involving the base of tongue and with minimal involvement of the soft palate (>1-cm margin between medial extent of tumor and midline), the CTV can be limited to the ipsilateral neck, which will significantly limit the exposure of the contralateral parotid, submandibular gland, and pharyngeal musculature.[91] The ability to forgo treatment to the contralateral neck is based on the extremely low risk of occult contralateral neck lymph node involvement. Surgical series demonstrate that the risk of contralateral cervical lymph node involvement is owing to primary tumor size (more common in T3 and T4 tumors).[92,93] Additionally, an analysis of tonsillar cancer patients, mostly

TABLE 45.9 INCIDENCE OF PATHOLOGIC RETROPHARYNGEAL LYMPH NODE METASTASES IN HEAD AND NECK PRIMARY TUMORS

		Incidence of Retropharyngeal Lymph Nodes (Percentage of the Total Number of Patients)		
Authors	Primary Site	Overall	pN0 Neck[a]	pN+ Neck[b]
Ballantyne[137]	Oropharynx (pharyngeal wall)	15/34 (44[c])	NA	NA
Hasegawa & Matsuura[138]	Oropharynx	4/11 (36%)	1/2 (50%)	3/9 (33%)
	Hypopharynx	8/13 (62%)	0/3 (0%)	9/10 (90%)
Okumura et al.[139]	Oropharynx & hypopharynx	6/42 (14%)	Not stated	Not stated
Byers et al.[140]	Oropharynx (pharyngeal wall)	2/45 (4%)	Not stated	Not stated

NA, not applicable.

[a]Pathologically negative nodes in levels I through V.

[b]Pathologically positive nodes in levels I through V.

[c]Numbers in parentheses are in percentages.

From Grégoire V, Coche E, Cosnard G, et al. Selection and delineation of lymph node target volumes in head and neck conformal radiotherapy: proposal for standardizing terminology and procedure based on the surgical experience. *Radiother Oncol* 2000; 56:135–150, with permission.

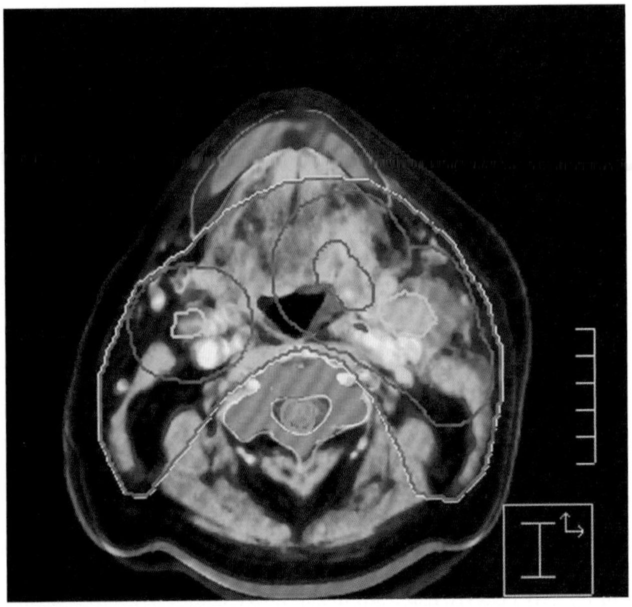

FIGURE 45.5. Axial image of a patient with locoregionally advanced oropharyngeal cancer with gross tumor volume and planning treatment volumes.

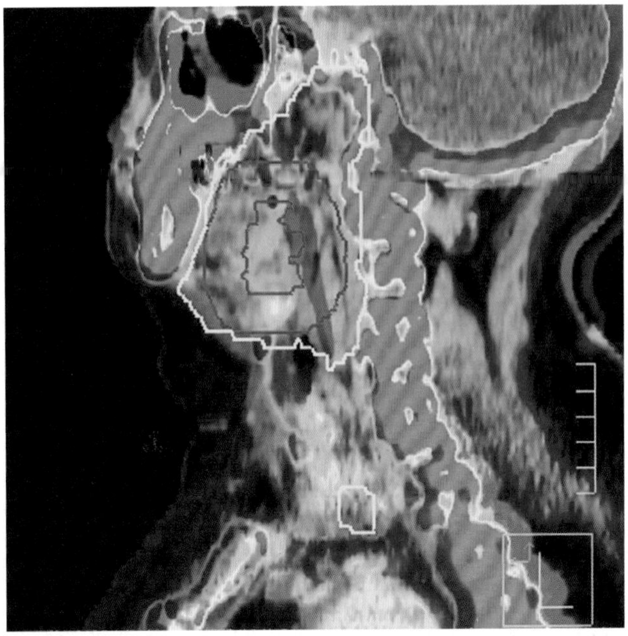

FIGURE 45.7. Sagittal image of a patient with locoregionally advanced oropharyngeal cancer with gross tumor volume and planning treatment volumes.

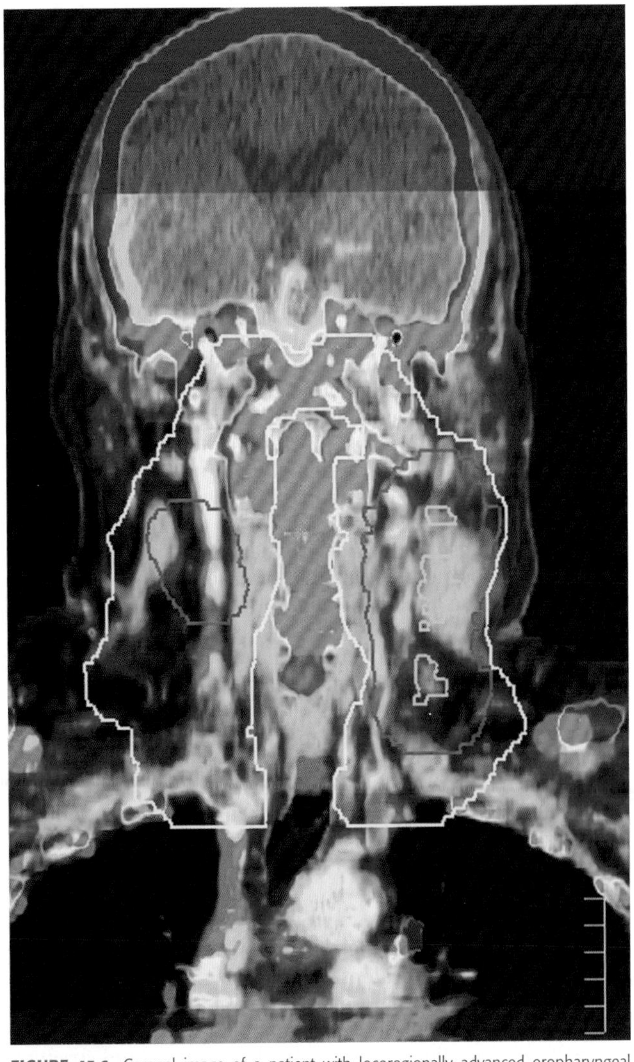

FIGURE 45.6. Coronal image of a patient with locoregionally advanced oropharyngeal cancer with gross tumor volume and planning treatment volumes.

T1-2 (79%) and N0-1 (88%), who underwent resection of the primary tumor often with ipsilateral lymph node dissection showed that only 5% of patients progressed in the contralateral neck.[94] The low incidence of progression seen in early-stage tonsil cancers is likely owing to a lack of invasion of the soft palate and base of tongue, which have a richer lymphatic network and access to the contralateral nodes. Patients with contralateral cervical lymph node involvement usually have extensive involvement of ipsilateral cervical lymph nodes[95] or tumors approaching or crossing the midline.

In properly selected tonsil cancer patients, ipsilateral-only radiotherapy results in low rates of contralateral neck progression. Large series of patients undergoing ipsilateral radiotherapy only demonstrated no contralateral neck progression in patients with T1 tumors and only 1% to 2% in those with T2 tumors. In the few patients with T3 tumors, contralateral nodal progression was 3% to 10%.[96,97] Further analysis of these series shows that contralateral nodal progression was associated with both base of tongue and soft palate involvement (13%), T3 stage (10%), and involvement of the midline of the soft palate (16.5%). No contralateral nodal progression was seen in patients with N2b or higher neck disease, although there were not many patients with this presentation.

Studies evaluating the role of ipsilateral treatment in the context of concurrent chemoradiation are sparse. An analysis of tonsil cancer patients treated at MD Anderson Cancer Center from 1970 to 2007 included only three patients who received concurrent systemic therapy for N2b disease. In these patients, there was no contralateral neck progression.[98] An analysis of 20 locoregionally advanced tonsillar cancer patients with N2b nodal disease, 18 of whom received concurrent chemoradiotherapy, demonstrated high rates of primary and nodal disease control along with a low risk of contralateral nodal progression. A caveat to this study is that all of these patients were staged with a PET scan, and most of these patients underwent surgery at the primary (80%) and/or at the neck (70%).[99] There appears to be little progression in properly selected patients treated with ipsilateral-only radiotherapy; however, care should be taken to ensure that patients with more advanced tumors are not treated in this fashion.

Ipsilateral External-Beam Radiotherapy Planning Techniques

Techniques for ipsilateral radiotherapy traditionally include a wedge pair or mixed photon electron field arrangement. The wedge pair technique includes ipsilateral anterior and posterior oblique fields with the head hyperextended to move the orbits out of the treatment field. Adequate sparing of normal tissue with this technique is achieved as the anterior beam spares the oral cavity and the contralateral parotid gland, although this usually contributes dose to the spinal cord. The posterior field aperture also spares the contralateral parotid, although this contributes dose to the spinal cord and oral cavity. With the wedge pair technique, hot spots are typically located peripherally near the surface and are between 110% and 115%. These hot spots can be reduced or eliminated if necessary with the addition of a lightly weighted (10%) third lateral field. The contralateral parotid dose is usually negligible at zero to 10%.

Alternatively, a combination of photons and electrons can be delivered through two ipsilateral fields. Traditional energies used 14 to 16 MeV electrons and 4 to 6 MV photons but should now be based on optimal 3D planning dosimetry. Bolus is often used to reduce dose to the temporal lobe. Often an off-cord reduction is used to limit the spinal cord to 45 Gy with low-energy electrons supplementing the region over the spinal cord. Recently, the use of IMRT for ipsilateral-only treatment has been increasing.

Bilateral External-Beam Radiotherapy Planning Techniques

Radiotherapy planning should be performed with 3D conformal radiotherapy or IMRT as available. Standard beam arrangements for 3D conformal radiotherapy are opposed lateral upper fields that are exactly matched to a low neck/supraclavicular field treated with either a single anterior or anterior-posterior–posterior-anterior (AP-PA) fields. Once spinal cord tolerance is reached, electron fields can be used to increase dose to gross disease as needed. Caution must be exercised to ensure that AP-PA and lateral fields do not overlap, causing an overdose to the spinal cord. Multiple techniques can be employed to prevent this complication.

Intensity-Modulated Radiotherapy

IMRT has been widely adopted for the treatment of head and neck cancers.[100] Although hypothetical consideration of second cancers exists with IMRT,[101] this technology has the ability to minimize normal organ exposure to radiation. This is particularly important for oropharyngeal cancer patients because pharyngeal constrictor dose and parotid dose are associated with dysphagia and xerostomia, respectively.[102] In addition, IMRT has the potential to decrease acute dermatitis.[103]

Care should be taken during IMRT to minimize dose to the uninvolved larynx to limit radiation-related speech disorders. Different techniques are available to achieve this objective. The two most commonly used techniques are (a) using IMRT to cover the entire head and neck volume or (b) using an upper IMRT field matched to a low anterior neck field. Comparisons of these two techniques have demonstrated significantly reduced mean dose to the larynx and inferior pharyngeal constrictor with the use of a low anterior neck field matched to the IMRT field.[104] Whole-field IMRT is preferable when gross disease is present, close to, or below the level of the larynx because coverage is better with this technique.[105]

Impact of Intensity-Modulated Radiotherapy on Xerostomia

The impact of IMRT on reduction of xerostomia in pharyngeal cancer patients (oropharynx or hypopharynx) was prospectively tested in a randomized trial.[103] Patients with pharyngeal squamous cell carcinoma (either oropharynx or hypopharynx) not involving the parotid glands, with good performance status and without distant metastatic spread (T1-4 N0-3), were recommended to receive either definitive or adjuvant radiotherapy without concurrent chemotherapy and were randomized 1:1 to either conventional radiotherapy or IMRT. The primary end point was the proportion of patients with grade 2 or worse xerostomia at 12 months, assessed via the late effects of normal tissues (LENT SOMA) scale.[103] Additionally, salivary flow was assessed prior to radiotherapy, during week 4 of radiotherapy, then 2, 3, 6, 12, 18, and 24 weeks after radiotherapy. Unstimulated and sodium citrate–stimulated parotid saliva from each parotid orifice and floor of mouth were also collected. Patient-reported quality of life was collected via the EORTC QLQC30 instrument and with the head and neck–specific instrument HN35. Patients could not receive prophylactic pilocarpine or amifostine. Radiotherapy dose was 65 Gy in 30 fractions for definitively treated patients or postoperative patients with macroscopic residual disease (2.17/fraction) or 60 Gy in 30 fractions (2 Gy/fraction) for postoperatively treated patients without macroscopic residual disease. Uninvolved nodal regions at risk for microscopic spread were treated to 50 Gy (2 Gy/fraction) in the conventional arm and 54 Gy (1.8 Gy/fraction) in the IMRT arm.

Six centers in the United Kingdom participated and recruited 94 patients (47 to each arm). Eighty-five percent of participants had oropharyngeal primary tumors. Eighty-one percent of patients in the IMRT arm were N0–1 compared to 53% in the conventional arm. This correlated with the statistical difference in stage with 83% of the conventional arm being stage 3 to 4 compared to 68% of the IMRT group. In addition, there were numerically more patients who received PORT in the conventional group (32% vs. 17%).

IMRT significantly reduced mean radiotherapy dose to the ipsilateral (47.6 Gy vs. 61 Gy) and contralateral (25.4 Gy vs. 61 Gy) parotid glands ($p < 0.0001$). Median follow-up was 44 months. At each planned observation time point, a smaller proportion of IMRT patients reported grade 2 or worse LENT SOMA subjective xerostomia compared to conventional radiotherapy. At 12 months, only 38% of patients treated with IMRT had grade 2 or higher xerostomia compared to 74% in the conventional arm. These were independent of tumor site, radiotherapy indication, stage, and use of neoadjuvant chemotherapy. Additionally, both unstimulated (47% vs. 0%) and stimulated contralateral parotid saliva flow were increased in the IMRT group. Interestingly, grade 2 and higher fatigue was increased in the IMRT group (74% vs. 41%). Locoregional progression (IMRT 78%, conventional 80%, $p = 0.34$) and overall survival (IMRT 78%, conventional 76%) were similar between the two arms.

These findings in primarily oropharyngeal patients are consistent with those found in studies of nasopharyngeal patients. It is unclear if the benefit of salivary reduction seen with IMRT continues when pharmacologic agents to reduce xerostomia such as pilocarpine and amifostine are employed. Ongoing cooperative group trials recommend limiting the mean dose to the parotids as low as possible and be at least <26 Gy. Furthermore, the mean dose to the submandibular gland is recommended to be limited to 36 Gy (RTOG 1016).

Impact of Intensity-Modulated Radiation Therapy on Dysphagia

IMRT planning should take into consideration the risk of dysphagia. Many studies have attempted to correlate dosimetric parameters with functional swallowing consequences following radiotherapy or chemoradiotherapy. As highlighted in the studies that follow, radiation dose to the larynx and pharyngeal constrictors should be limited as reasonably as possible to reduce the risks of aspiration, feeding tube dependence, and stricture. Consensus on dosimetric parameters does not exist because the studies to date have all been retrospective, and their findings are not completely concordant.

Careful correlation of videofluoroscopic findings to radiotherapy dose to normal tissues has been performed in oropharyngeal cancer patients treated with chemoradiotherapy. Based on this analysis, the dose with a 25% or 50% risk (TD_{25} or TD_{50}) of dysphagia to the pharyngeal constrictors was 56 and 63 Gy, respectively. Similarly, TD_{25} and TD_{50} were 39 Gy and 56 Gy for the glottis and supraglottic larynx.[106] Mean dose to the esophagus was associated with the development of strictures. There were no threshold doses found in this analysis, thus it is reasonable to use the TD_{25} as a planning goal, and if not achieved, then trying to keep the dose to these structures as low as possible.

Others have analyzed radiotherapy doses to normal tissues and correlated to clinical outcomes the persistent use of percutaneous endoscopic gastrostomy (PEG) tubes, aspiration rates, and stricture rates.[107] In this analysis, mean dose to the larynx and mean dose to the inferior pharyngeal constrictor predicted for persistent use of PEG tubes and aspiration. Additionally, the volume of larynx receiving 35 to 70 Gy (V_{35} to V_{70}) and inferior pharyngeal constrictor V_{40} through V_{65} was associated with PEG tube dependence, and larynx V_{55} through V_{70} and inferior pharyngeal constrictor V_{60} and V_{65} were significantly associated with aspiration. Patients with a mean dose of approximately 50 Gy to the larynx and inferior constrictor all had PEG tubes removed by 12 months.

Concurrent Chemotherapy and Accelerated Radiotherapy

Two recently reported randomized studies showed that there was no benefit to accelerated radiotherapy over conventionally fractionated radiotherapy when delivered with concurrent platinum based chemotherapy.[108] GORTEC 99–02 randomized locoregionally advanced head and neck cancer patients to either very accelerated radiotherapy at 64.8 Gy (1.8 Gy twice daily), 70 Gy (2 Gy daily over 7 weeks) with concurrent carboplatin 70 mg/m^2 and 5-FU 600 mg/m^2/day on days 1 through 4, days 22 through 25, and days 43 through 46, or 70 Gy (2 Gy daily to 40 Gy, then 1.5 Gy twice daily) with carboplatin 70 mg/m^2 and 5-FU 600 mg/m^2/day on days 1 through 4 and days 29 through 33. Outcome in both chemoradiotherapy arms was similar, and both were superior to very accelerated radiotherapy with lower rates of acute toxicity and percutaneous gastrostomy tube placement during therapy and at 5 years. Similarly, RTOG 0129 randomized patients to 72-Gy accelerated concomitant boost radiotherapy with two cycles of cisplatin 100 mg/m^2 or to 70 Gy daily radiotherapy with three cycles of cisplatin 100 mg/m^2. Again, there was no benefit to accelerated chemoradiotherapy seen in 3-year overall survival (accelerated 59% vs. conventional 56%), locoregional progression (31% vs. 29%), or worst grade 3 to 4 toxicity (26% vs. 21%). The value of acceleration via the use of a simultaneous integrated boost, a commonly used approach for IMRT delivery, must therefore be questioned when concurrent chemotherapy is being used as part of the treatment program.

Brachytherapy

Brachytherapy, the application of radioactive materials in close proximity to tumors, was developed in the pre-IMRT, preconcurrent chemoradiotherapy era as a means to deliver a tumoricidal dose to gross tumors while minimizing dose to the mandible. The advent of improved radiotherapy planning and delivery techniques, in addition to a recognition that osteoradionecrosis secondary to brachytherapy is significantly underreported, has corresponded to a major decrease in the utilization of brachytherapy for oropharyngeal tumors.

For oropharyngeal tumors, brachytherapy has historically played a role in boosting gross disease following external-beam therapy, as oropharyngeal tumors have a high propensity for occult nodal spread. Typically, catheters are implanted under general anesthesia in the operating room, with two capable physicians present to handle unexpected events, highlighting the fact that brachytherapy is an operator-dependent procedure. Although low dose rate brachytherapy has previously been the most common type of brachytherapy used, high dose rate (HDR) and pulsed dose rate (PDR) techniques are becoming much more common and sometimes preferred given the ability to control dwell times and develop more customized dose distributions. Given the historically poor locoregional control rates for tumors of the base of tongue, intensifying the treatment with brachytherapy makes logical sense. High rates of locoregional control have been achieved using an integrated treatment approach of external-beam radiotherapy directed at the primary and bilateral neck, followed by a brachytherapy boost.[109] Complications of brachytherapy for base of tongue tumors include osteoradionecrosis of the mandible. The risk of complication appears to be related to the technique of implantation but may approach 30%. There is limited information regarding the use of brachytherapy and chemotherapy concurrently, which should be avoided.

When brachytherapy is planned following external-beam radiotherapy, care should be taken to delineate the pretreatment tumor extent because regression is not always uniform. Tattoos and gold seeds have been used to accomplish this. The CTV used is recommended by the European Society for Radiotherapy and Oncology (ESTRO) to be 5 mm at minimum and more commonly 1 to 1.5 cm for base of tongue tumors. The PTV is usually equal to the CTV as the implanted catheters move with the tumor. Catheters are typically positioned parallel and equidistant at 1 to 1.5 cm apart. Whereas traditional methods of calculating dose have been used in the past based on the Paris, Manchester, or New York systems, computer-derived brachytherapy plans are now routine.

Brachytherapy Guidelines

The American Brachytherapy Society (ABS) has published guidelines for the use of HDR brachytherapy for head and neck tumors and oropharyngeal tumors in particular. Prophylactic tracheostomy is recommended because posterior and large tumors are at risk to cause airway obstruction. Expert panel evidence, as well as single-institution series, recommend external-beam radiotherapy doses of 45 to 60 Gy followed by an HDR brachytherapy boost of 3 to 4 Gy per fraction for 6 to 10 doses with locoregional control of implanted tumors reaching 82% to 94%.[110]

The European Brachytherapy Group (GEC) and ESTRO have also published joint guidelines for the use of brachytherapy for head and neck malignancies. Similar to the ABS, these were based on consensus recommendations reflecting limited data.[111] For oropharyngeal tumors, these guidelines recommend 45 to 50 Gy external-beam radiotherapy followed by 25 to 30 Gy boost for tonsillar tumors, and 30 to 35 Gy boost to base of tongue tumors. The total brachytherapy boost dose is fraction-size dependent: 21 to 30 Gy in 3-Gy fractions and 16 to 24 Gy in 4-Gy fractions. Quality of life analyses comparing a combined regimen of brachytherapy and external-beam radiotherapy to surgery and PORT favored a primary radiotherapy-only approach,[112] suggesting that in experienced hands, this is a reasonable treatment method.

Hypofractionated Image-Guided Radiotherapy for Oropharyngeal Cancer

Hypofractionated image-guided radiotherapy techniques, commonly referred to has stereotactic body radiotherapy (SBRT), have resulted in promising outcomes for the treatment of early-stage lung cancers[113] and limited metastases.[35] Consequently, investigators are attempting to incorporate these techniques into the treatment of oropharyngeal cancer. To date, data are limited,[114,115] and further investigations are needed to determine what role, if any, exists for this approach.

POSTTREATMENT MANAGEMENT AND SURVEILLANCE

Following definitive therapy for oropharyngeal cancer, patients should be seen regularly for clinical evaluation. Current guidelines suggest examination every 1 to 3 months for the first year posttherapy, every 2 to 4 months in the second year posttherapy, and every 4 to 6 months in the third through fifth years. The intensity of the examinations within the first 2 years coincides with the likelihood of recurrence in the interval. Given that radiation to the neck commonly causes hypothyroidism, thyroid-stimulating hormone levels should be evaluated every 6 months.

Following definitive radiotherapy or chemoradiotherapy, follow-up imaging should be performed within the first 3 months of treatment completion for patients with node-positive presentations. A radiographic complete response on CT imaging of the neck, defined as nonenhancing, nonnecrotic nodal tissue <1.5 cm, is associated with 100% long-term disease control in the neck, and no further therapy is needed.[116] Surveillance CT imaging of the primary site does not add additional information to physical/fiberoptic examination and should not be routinely performed.[117]

PET/CT is more widely available and is often used as the sole imaging modality following the completion of radiotherapy. An analysis of 121 node-positive predominately oropharyngeal (74%) head and neck cancer patients, prospectively followed with PET/CT at around 12 weeks posttherapy and again 4 weeks later if there was residual activity, helped to clarify the role of PET/CT scan following chemoradiotherapy. With or without residual CT abnormalities in the neck, a negative PET scan at 12 weeks, defined as the absence of metabolic activity, was associated with no isolated nodal progression.[118] Additionally, the negative predictive value of PET was 98.1% (95% CI 93.2% to 99.8%) compared to 96.8% in CT (95% CI 88.8% to 99.6%). However, more importantly, false-positive readings were seen in only 1.8% of PET scans compared to 38% of CT scans, resulting in a positive predictive value of 77.8% for PET/CT scan and 14% for CT. When the analysis was restricted to p16 positive patients, the results were similar with a negative predictive value of 98.2% (95% CI 90.4% to 100%) and 66.7% (95% CI 9.4% to 99.2%) for PET.

TREATMENT OF RECURRENT AND METASTATIC OROPHARYNGEAL CANCER

Systemic Therapy for Recurrent and Metastatic Oropharyngeal Cancer

The standard therapy for patients with recurrent or metastatic oropharyngeal cancer is systemic therapy with platinum-based chemotherapy. In phase II studies, many drugs in addition to platinum agents and methotrexate have shown single-agent activity, including paclitaxel,[119] docetaxel,[120] gemcitabine,[121] ifosphamide,[122] vinorelbine,[123] pemetrexed,[124] capecitabine,[125] and irinotecan.[126] Single-agent cisplatin (100 mg/m^2) has been shown to improve overall survival compared to best supportive care.[127] Cisplatin was also shown to be superior to single-agent methotrexate.[128] Multiple randomized studies have attempted to improve survival with combination cisplatin-based regimens. The combination of cisplatin (100 mg/m^2) with 5-FU (1,000 mg/m^2/day) demonstrated improved response rates (32% vs. 17%) but not improved median survival (5.7 months) over cisplatin alone.[129] Similar results were seen when the combination of cisplatin/5-FU, carboplatin/5-FU, and methotrexate alone were randomly compared. The combination of cisplatin and 5-FU was shown to have increased response rates compared to methotrexate (32% vs. 10%) as was carboplatin and 5-FU compared to methotrexate (21% vs. 10%); however, neither had improved median survival (6.6 and 5.6 months, respectively compared to 5.0 months) to methotrexate.[130] Response rates and survival are similar with cisplatin and paclitaxel versus cisplatin/5-FU, which provides a regimen that is easier to administer.[131] For oropharyngeal cancer specifically, a planned subset analysis of a phase III trial comparing cisplatin and pemetrexed to cisplatin and placebo demonstrated that oropharyngeal cancer patients receiving the combination regimen had improved survival (9.9 months vs. 6.1 months, p = 0.002) and improved progression-free survival (4 vs. 3.4 months, p = 0.047).[132]

The addition of agents targeted to the EGFR to platinum-based systemic therapy has been shown to improve overall survival compared to platinum agents alone in a phase III study with a large proportion of oropharyngeal cancer patients. The EXTREME study randomized recurrent and metastatic head and neck cancer patients to either cisplatin 100 mg/m^2 day 1 or carboplatin area under the curve (AUC) = 5 day 1 combined with 5-FU 1,000 mg/m^2/day 5-FU days 1 through 4 every 3 weeks, with or without cetuximab 250 mg/m^2 following a loading dose of 400 mg/m^2. Cetuximab was continued until disease progression or patient intolerance.[133] Median overall survival was improved from 7.4 months with chemotherapy alone to 10.1 months with the combination of systemic therapy and cetuximab, as was median progression-free survival (3.3 months to 5.6 months). No phase III data have suggested a benefit for the addition of tyrosine kinase inhibitors including gefitinib or erlotinib to platinum-based therapy. Ongoing investigations are determining the role of bevacizumab and other targeted agents.

Reirradiation for Locoregionally Confined Recurrent or Second Primary Disease

For the subgroup of recurrent oropharyngeal cancer patients with locoregionally confined disease, surgical resection is recommended, although this is possible only in a small proportion of patients.[134] Following surgery[135] in those with high-risk pathologic features or in those who are not surgical candidates,[136] a second course of full-dose radiotherapy with chemotherapy has been shown to result in long-term survival in approximately 20% of patients.[136] Patients who are able to undergo surgery prior to reirradiation as well as those who have not been exposed to prior chemotherapy and are treated to higher doses have improved outcomes. Because of the high risk of normal tissue toxicity including up to a 20% carotid rupture rate and 15% fatal toxicity, patients undergoing a second course of chemotherapy and radiation therapy should be managed at experienced centers. It is unknown if systemic therapy alone or chemotherapy and reirradiation is a better therapy for these patients, because a phase III comparison of these modalities failed to accrue. Therefore, treatment decisions will have to be individualized based on extent of disease, performance status, and preference.

SELECTED REFERENCES

A full list of references for this chapter is available online.

2. Ernster JA, Sciotto CG, O'Brien MM, et al. Rising incidence of oropharyngeal cancer and the role of oncogenic human papilloma virus. *Laryngoscope* 2007;117(12):2115–2128.
3. Chaturvedi AK, Engels EA, Pfeiffer RM, et al. Human papillomavirus and rising oropharyngeal cancer incidence in the United States. *J Clin Oncol* 2011;29(32):4294–4301.
4. Durst M, Gissmann L, Ikenberg H, et al. A papillomavirus DNA from a cervical carcinoma and its prevalence in cancer biopsy samples from different geographic regions. *Proc Natl Acad Sci U S A* 1983;80(12):3812–3815.
5. IARC. *Human papillomaviruses*. Lyon, France: IARC, 1995.
6. Munoz N, Bosch FX, de Sanjose S, et al. Epidemiologic classification of human papillomavirus types associated with cervical cancer. *N Engl J Med* 2003;348(6):518–527.
7. Kreimer AR, Clifford GM, Boyle P, et al. Human papillomavirus types in head and neck squamous cell carcinomas worldwide: a systematic review. *Cancer Epidemiol Biomark Prev* 2005;14(2):467–475.
8. Mork J, Lie AK, Glattre E, et al. Human papillomavirus infection as a risk factor for squamous-cell carcinoma of the head and neck. *N Engl J Med* 2001;344(15):1125–1131.
9. Chung CH, Gillison ML. Human papillomavirus in head and neck cancer: its role in pathogenesis and clinical implications. *Clin Cancer Res* 2009;15(22):6758–6762.

14. Gillison ML, D'Souza G, Westra W, et al. Distinct risk factor profiles for human papillomavirus type 16-positive and human papillomavirus type 16-negative head and neck cancers. *J Natl Cancer Inst* 2008;100(6):407–420.
15. D'Souza G, Kreimer AR, Viscidi R, et al. Case-control study of human papillomavirus and oropharyngeal cancer. *N Engl J Med* 2007;356(19):1944–1956.
17. Ang KK, Harris J, Wheeler R, et al. Human papillomavirus and survival of patients with oropharyngeal cancer. *N Engl J Med* 2010;363(1):24–35.
18. Fakhry C, Westra WH, Li S, et al. Improved survival of patients with human papillomavirus-positive head and neck squamous cell carcinoma in a prospective clinical trial. *J Natl Cancer Inst* 2008;100(4):261–269.
19. Rischin D, Young RJ, Fisher R, et al. Prognostic significance of p16INK4A and human papillomavirus in patients with oropharyngeal cancer treated on TROG 02.02 phase III trial. *J Clin Oncol* 2010;28(27):4142–4148.
20. Lassen P, Eriksen JG, Hamilton-Dutoit S, et al. Effect of HPV-associated p16INK4A expression on response to radiotherapy and survival in squamous cell carcinoma of the head and neck. *J Clin Oncol* 2009;27(12):1992–1998.
23. Robbins KT, Clayman G, Levine PA, et al. Neck dissection classification update: revisions proposed by the American Head and Neck Society and the American Academy of Otolaryngology-Head and Neck Surgery. *Arch Otolaryngol Head Neck Surg* 2002;128(7):751–758.
24. Som PM, Curtin HD, Mancuso AA. An imaging-based classification for the cervical nodes designed as an adjunct to recent clinically based nodal classifications. *Arch Otolaryngol Head Neck Surg* 1999;125(4):388–396.
25. Gregoire V, Coche E, Cosnard G, et al. Selection and delineation of lymph node target volumes in head and neck conformal radiotherapy. Proposal for standardizing terminology and procedure based on the surgical experience. *Radiother Oncol* 2000;56(2):135–150.
26. Gregoire V, Eisbruch A, Hamoir M, et al. Proposal for the delineation of the nodal CTV in the node-positive and the post-operative neck. *Radiother Oncol* 2006;79(1):15–20.
27. Gregoire V, Levendag P, Ang KK, et al. CT-based delineation of lymph node levels and related CTVs in the node-negative neck: DAHANCA, EORTC, GORTEC, NCIC,RTOG consensus guidelines. *Radiother Oncol* 2003;69(3):227–236.
28. Chao KS, Wippold FJ, Ozyigit G, et al. Determination and delineation of nodal target volumes for head-and-neck cancer based on patterns of failure in patients receiving definitive and postoperative IMRT. *Int J Radiat Oncol Biol Phys* 2002; 53(5):1174–1184.
29. Merino OR, Lindberg RD, Fletcher GH. An analysis of distant metastases from squamous cell carcinoma of the upper respiratory and digestive tracts. *Cancer* 1977;40(1):145–151.
30. McLeod NM, Jess A, Anand R, et al. Role of chest CT in staging of oropharyngeal cancer: a systematic review. *Head Neck* 2009;31(4):548–555.
31. Goodwin WJ. Distant metastases from oropharyngeal cancer. *ORL* 2001;63(4): 222–223.
38. Grant DG, Salassa JR, Hinni ML, et al. Carcinoma of the tongue base treated by transoral laser microsurgery, part one: untreated tumors, a prospective analysis of oncologic and functional outcomes. *Laryngoscope* 2006;116(12):2150–2155.
39. Steiner W, Fierek O, Ambrosch P, et al. Transoral laser microsurgery for squamous cell carcinoma of the base of the tongue. *Arch Otolaryngol Head Neck Surg* 2003;129(1):36–43.
40. Grant DG, Hinni ML, Salassa JR, et al. Oropharyngeal cancer: a case for single modality treatment with transoral laser microsurgery. *Arch Otolaryngol Head Neck Surg* 2009;135(12):1225–1230.
42. Weinstein GS, O'Malley BW Jr, Snyder W, et al. Transoral robotic surgery: radical tonsillectomy. *Arch Otolaryngol Head Neck Surg* 2007;133(12):1220–1226.
43. Cooper JS, Pajak TF, Forastiere A, et al. Precisely defining high-risk operable head and neck tumors based on RTOG #85–03 and #88–24: targets for postoperative radiochemotherapy? *Head Neck* 1998;20(7):588–594.
45. Lavaf A, Genden EM, Cesaretti JA, et al. Adjuvant radiotherapy improves overall survival for patients with lymph node-positive head and neck squamous cell carcinoma. *Cancer* 2008;112(3):535–543.
48. Bernier J, Domenge C, Ozsahin M, et al. Postoperative irradiation with or without concomitant chemotherapy for locally advanced head and neck cancer. *N Engl J Med* 2004;350(19):1945–1952.
49. Bachaud JM, Cohen-Jonathan E, Alzieu C, et al. Combined postoperative radiotherapy and weekly cisplatin infusion for locally advanced head and neck carcinoma: final report of a randomized trial. *Int J Radiat Oncol Biol Phys* 1996; 36(5):999–1004.
50. Fietkau R, Lautenschläger C, Sauer R, et al. Postoperative concurrent radiochemotherapy versus radiotherapy in high-risk SCCA of the head and neck: results of the German phase III trial ARO 96–3. *J Clin Oncol* 2006;24(18S):5507.
51. Cooper JS, Pajak TF, Forastiere AA, et al. Postoperative concurrent radiotherapy and chemotherapy for high-risk squamous-cell carcinoma of the head and neck. *N Engl J Med* 2004;350(19):1937–1944.
52. Racadot S, Mercier M, Dussart S, et al. Randomized clinical trial of post-operative radiotherapy versus concomitant carboplatin and radiotherapy for head and neck cancers with lymph node involvement. *Radiother Oncol* 2008;87(2):164–172.
53. Salama JK, Saba N, Quon H, et al. ACR Appropriateness Criteria® adjuvant therapy for resected squamous cell carcinoma of the head and neck. *Oral Oncol* 2011;47(7):554–559.
54. Eisbruch A, Harris J, Garden AS, et al. Multi-institutional trial of accelerated hypofractionated intensity-modulated radiation therapy for early-stage oropharyngeal cancer (RTOG 00–22). *Int J Radiat Oncol Biol Phys* 2010;76(5): 1333–1338.
55. Fu KK, Pajak TF, Trotti A, et al. A Radiation Therapy Oncology Group (RTOG) phase III randomized study to compare hyperfractionation and two variants of accelerated fractionation to standard fractionation radiotherapy for head and neck squamous cell carcinomas: first report of RTOG 9003. *Int J Radiat Oncol Biol Phys* 2000;48(1):7–16.
56. Overgaard J, Hansen HS, Specht L, et al. Five compared with six fractions per week of conventional radiotherapy of squamous-cell carcinoma of head and neck: DAHANCA 6 and 7 randomised controlled trial. *Lancet* 2003;362(9388):933–940.
57. Horiot JC, Le Fur R, N'Guyen T, et al. Hyperfractionation versus conventional fractionation in oropharyngeal carcinoma: final analysis of a randomized trial of the EORTC Cooperative Group of Radiotherapy. *Radiother Oncol* 1992;25(4): 231–241.
58. Budach W, Hehr T, Budach V, et al. A meta-analysis of hyperfractionated and accelerated radiotherapy and combined chemotherapy and radiotherapy regimens in unresected locally advanced squamous cell carcinoma of the head and neck. *BMC Cancer* 2006;6:28.
59. Bourhis J, Overgaard J, Audry H, et al. Hyperfractionated or accelerated radiotherapy in head and neck cancer: a meta-analysis. *Lancet* 2006;368(9538): 843–854.
60. Overgaard J, Mohanti BK, Begum N, et al. Five versus six fractions of radiotherapy per week for squamous-cell carcinoma of the head and neck (IAEA-ACC study): a randomised, multicentre trial. *Lancet Oncol* 2010;11(6):553–560.
61. Lassen P, Eriksen JG, Krogdahl A, et al. The influence of HPV-associated p16-expression on accelerated fractionated radiotherapy in head and neck cancer: evaluation of the randomised DAHANCA 6&7 trial. *Radiother Oncol* 2011;100 (1):49–55.
62. Poulsen MG, Denham JW, Peters LJ, et al. A randomised trial of accelerated and conventional radiotherapy for stage III and IV squamous carcinoma of the head and neck: a Trans-Tasman Radiation Oncology Group Study. *Radiother Oncol* 2001;60(2):113–122.
63. Fu KK, Pajak TF, Trotti A, et al. A Radiation Therapy Oncology Group (RTOG) phase III randomized study to compare hyperfractionation and two variants of accelerated fractionation to standard fractionation radiotherapy for head and neck squamous cell carcinomas: first report of RTOG 9003. *Int J Radiat Oncol Biol Phys* 2000;48(1):7–16.
64. Parsons JT, Mendenhall WM, Stringer SP, et al. Squamous cell carcinoma of the oropharynx: surgery, radiation therapy, or both. *Cancer* 2002;94(11):2967–2980.
65. Pignon JP, le Maitre A, Maillard E, et al. Meta-analysis of chemotherapy in head and neck cancer (MACH-NC): an update on 93 randomised trials and 17,346 patients. *Radiother Oncol* 2009;92(1):4–14.
66. Fallai C, Bolner A, Signor M, et al. Long-term results of conventional radiotherapy versus accelerated hyperfractionated radiotherapy versus concomitant radiotherapy and chemotherapy in locoregionally advanced carcinoma of the oropharynx. *Tumori* 2006;92(1):41–54.
67. Calais G, Alfonsi M, Bardet E, et al. Randomized trial of radiation therapy versus concomitant chemotherapy and radiation therapy for advanced-stage oropharynx carcinoma. *J Natl Cancer Inst* 1999;91(24):2081–2086.
68. Denis F, Garaud P, Bardet E, et al. Final results of the 94–01 French Head and Neck Oncology and Radiotherapy Group randomized trial comparing radiotherapy alone with concomitant radiochemotherapy in advanced-stage oropharynx carcinoma. *J Clin Oncol* 2004;22(1):69–76.
69. Lok BH, Setton J, Caria N, et al. Intensity-modulated radiation therapy in oropharyngeal carcinoma: effect of tumor volume on clinical outcomes. *Int J Radiat Oncol Biol Phys* 2012;82(5):1851–1857.
70. Zhen W, Karnell LH, Hoffman HT, et al. The National Cancer Data Base report on squamous cell carcinoma of the base of tongue. *Head Neck* 2004;26(8):660–674.
71. Pederson AW, Haraf DJ, Witt ME, et al. Chemoradiotherapy for locoregionally advanced squamous cell carcinoma of the base of tongue. *Head Neck* 2010; 32(11):1519–1527.
72. Stenson KM, MacCracken E, List M, et al. Swallowing function in patients with head and neck cancer prior to treatment. *Arch Otolaryngol Head Neck Surg* 2000;126(3):371–377.
73. Salama JK, Stenson KM, List MA, et al. Characteristics associated with swallowing changes after concurrent chemotherapy and radiotherapy in patients with head and neck cancer. *Arch Otolaryngol Head Neck Surg* 2008;134(10):1060–1065.
74. Rosenthal DI, Lewin JS, Eisbruch A. Prevention and treatment of dysphagia and aspiration after chemoradiation for head and neck cancer. *J Clin Oncol* 2006; 24(17):2636–2643.
75. Machtay M, Moughan J, Trotti A, et al. Factors associated with severe late toxicity after concurrent chemoradiation for locally advanced head and neck cancer: an RTOG analysis. *J Clin Oncol* 2008;26(21):3582–3589.
76. Jeremic B, Shibamoto Y, Milicic B, et al. Hyperfractionated radiation therapy with or without concurrent low-dose daily cisplatin in locally advanced squamous cell carcinoma of the head and neck: a prospective randomized trial. *J Clin Oncol* 2000;18(7):1458–1464.
77. Sharma A, Mohanti BK, Thakar A, et al. Concomitant chemoradiation versus radical radiotherapy in advanced squamous cell carcinoma of oropharynx and nasopharynx using weekly cisplatin: a phase II randomized trial. *Ann Oncol* 2010;21(11):2272–2277.
78. Huguenin P, Beer KT, Allal A, et al. Concomitant cisplatin significantly improves locoregional control in advanced head and neck cancers treated with hyperfractionated radiotherapy. *J Clin Oncol* 2004;22(23):4665–4673.
79. Domenge C, Hill C, Lefebvre JL, et al. Randomized trial of neoadjuvant chemotherapy in oropharyngeal carcinoma. French Groupe d'Etude des Tumeurs de la Tete et du Cou (GETTEC). *Br J Cancer* 2000;83(12):1594–1598.
80. Brockstein B, Haraf DJ, Rademaker AW, et al. Patterns of failure, prognostic factors and survival in locoregionally advanced head and neck cancer treated with concomitant chemoradiotherapy: a 9-year, 337-patient, multi-institutional experience. *Ann Oncol* 2004;15(8):1179–1186.
81. Salama JK, Stenson KM, Kistner EO, et al. Induction chemotherapy and concurrent chemoradiotherapy for locoregionally advanced head and neck cancer: a multi-institutional phase II trial investigating three radiotherapy dose levels. *Ann Oncol* 2008;19(10):1787–1794.
82. Machtay M, Rosenthal DI, Hershock D, et al. Organ preservation therapy using induction plus concurrent chemoradiation for advanced resectable oropharyngeal carcinoma: a University of Pennsylvania phase II trial. *J Clin Oncol* 2002; 20(19):3964–3971.
83. Bonner JA, Harari PM, Giralt J, et al. Radiotherapy plus cetuximab for squamous-cell carcinoma of the head and neck. *N Engl J Med* 2006;354(6):567–578.
84. Chung CH, Mirakhur B, Chan E, et al. Cetuximab-induced anaphylaxis and IgE specific for galactose-alpha-1,3-galactose. *N Engl J Med* 2008;358(11):1109–1117.
85. Ang KK, Zhang QE, Rosenthal DI, et al. A randomized phase III trial (RTOG 0522) of concurrent accelerated radiation plus cisplatin with or without cetuximab for stage III-IV head and neck squamous cell carcinomas (HNC). *J Clin Oncol* 2011;29(Suppl):5500.
86. Salama JK, Haraf DJ, Stenson KM, et al. A randomized phase II study of 5-fluorouracil, hydroxyurea, and twice-daily radiotherapy compared with bevacizumab plus 5-fluorouracil, hydroxyurea, and twice-daily radiotherapy for intermediate-stage and T4N0–1 head and neck cancers. *Ann Oncol* 2011;22(10):2304–2309.
87. Yoo DS, Kirkpatrick J, Craciunescu O, et al. Prospective trial of synchronous bevacizumab, erlotinib, and concurrent chemoradiation in locally advanced head and neck cancer. *Clin Cancer Res* 2012;18(5):1404–1414.
88. Thiagarajan A, Caria N, Schoder H, et al. Target volume delineation in oropharyngeal cancer: impact of PET, MRI, and physical examination. *Int J Radiat Oncol Biol Phys* 2012;83(1):220–227.

89. Eisbruch A, Schwartz M, Rasch C, et al. Dysphagia and aspiration after chemoradiotherapy for head-and-neck cancer: which anatomic structures are affected and can they be spared by IMRT? *Int J Radiat Oncol Biol Phys* 2004;60(5):1425–1439.
90. Eisbruch A, Marsh LH, Dawson LA, et al. Recurrences near base of skull after IMRT for head-and-neck cancer: implications for target delineation in high neck and for parotid gland sparing. *Int J Radiat Oncol Biol Phys* 2004;59(1):28–42.
91. Yeung AR, Garg MK, Lawson J, et al. ACR Appropriateness Criteria® ipsilateral radiation for squamous cell carcinoma of the tonsil. *Head Neck* 2012;34(5):613–616.
92. Lim YC, Lee SY, Lim JY, et al. Management of contralateral N0 neck in tonsillar squamous cell carcinoma. *Laryngoscope* 2005;115(9):1672–1675.
93. Olzowy B, Tsalemchuk Y, Schotten KJ, et al. Frequency of bilateral cervical metastases in oropharyngeal squamous cell carcinoma: a retrospective analysis of 352 cases after bilateral neck dissection. *Head Neck* 2011;33(2):239–243.
94. Foote RL, Schild SE, Thompson WM, et al. Tonsil cancer. Patterns of failure after surgery alone and surgery combined with postoperative radiation therapy. *Cancer* 1994;73(10):2638–2647.
96. O'Sullivan B, Warde P, Grice B, et al. The benefits and pitfalls of ipsilateral radiotherapy in carcinoma of the tonsillar region. *Int J Radiat Oncol Biol Phys* 2001; 51(2):332–343.
97. Jackson SM, Hay JH, Flores AD, et al. Cancer of the tonsil: the results of ipsilateral radiation treatment. *Radiother Oncol* 1999;51(2):123–128.
98. Chronowski GM, Garden AS, Morrison WH, et al. Unilateral radiotherapy for the treatment of tonsil cancer. *Int J Radiat Oncol Biol Phys* 2012;83(1):204–209.
99. Rusthoven KE, Raben D, Schneider C, et al. Freedom from local and regional failure of contralateral neck with ipsilateral neck radiotherapy for node-positive tonsil cancer: results of a prospective management approach. *Int J Radiat Oncol Biol Phys* 2009;74(5):1365–1370.
101. Hall EJ. Intensity-modulated radiation therapy, protons, and the risk of second cancers. *Int J Radiat Oncol Biol Phys* 2006;65(1):1–7.
102. Eisbruch A, Ship JA, Dawson LA, et al. Salivary gland sparing and improved target irradiation by conformal and intensity modulated irradiation of head and neck cancer. *World J Surg* 2003;27(7):832–837.
103. Nutting CM, Morden JP, Harrington KJ, et al. Parotid-sparing intensity modulated versus conventional radiotherapy in head and neck cancer (PARSPORT): a phase 3 multicentre randomised controlled trial. *Lancet Oncol* 2011;12(2):127–136.
104. Caudell JJ, Burnett OL III, Schaner PE, et al. Comparison of methods to reduce dose to swallowing-related structures in head and neck cancer. *Int J Radiat Oncol Biol Phys* 2010;77(2):462–467.
106. Eisbruch A, Kim HM, Feng FY, et al. Chemo-IMRT of oropharyngeal cancer aiming to reduce dysphagia: swallowing organs late complication probabilities and dosimetric correlates. *Int J Radiat Oncol Biol Phys* 2011;81(3):e93–e99.
107. Caudell JJ, Schaner PE, Desmond RA, et al. Dosimetric factors associated with long-term dysphagia after definitive radiotherapy for squamous cell carcinoma of the head and neck. *Int J Radiat Oncol Biol Phys* 2010;76(2):403–409.
108. Bourhis J, Sire C, Graff P, et al. Concomitant chemoradiotherapy versus acceleration of radiotherapy with or without concomitant chemotherapy in locally advanced head and neck carcinoma (GORTEC 99-02): an open-label phase 3 randomised trial. *Lancet Oncol* 2012;13(2):145–153.
110. Nag S, Cano ER, Demanes DJ, et al. The American Brachytherapy Society recommendations for high-dose-rate brachytherapy for head-and-neck carcinoma. *Int J Radiat Oncol Biol Phys* 2001;50(5):1190–1198.
111. Mazeron JJ, Ardiet JM, Haie-Meder C, et al. GEC-ESTRO recommendations for brachytherapy for head and neck squamous cell carcinomas. *Radiother Oncol* 2009;91(2):150–156.
114. Kodani N, Yamazaki H, Tsubokura T, et al. Stereotactic body radiation therapy for head and neck tumor: disease control and morbidity outcomes. *J Radiat Res* 2011;52(1):24–31.
115. Siddiqui F, Patel M, Khan M, et al. Stereotactic body radiation therapy for primary, recurrent, and metastatic tumors in the head-and-neck region. *Int J Radiat Oncol Biol Phys* 2009;74(4):1047–1053.
116. Liauw SL, Mancuso AA, Amdur RJ, et al. Postradiotherapy neck dissection for lymph node-positive head and neck cancer: the use of computed tomography to manage the neck. *J Clin Oncol* 2006;24(9):1421–1427.
117. Sullivan BP, Parks KA, Dean NR, et al. Utility of CT surveillance for primary site recurrence of squamous cell carcinoma of the head and neck. *Head Neck* 2011;33(11):1547–1550.
118. Porceddu SV, Pryor DI, Burmeister E, et al. Results of a prospective study of positron emission tomography-directed management of residual nodal abnormalities in node-positive head and neck cancer after definitive radiotherapy with or without systemic therapy. *Head Neck* 2011;33(12):1675–1682.
128. A phase III randomised trial of cisplatinum, methotrextate, cisplatinum +methotrexate and cisplatinum + 5-FU in end stage squamous carcinoma of the head and neck. Liverpool Head and Neck Oncology Group. *Br J Cancer* 1990;61(2):311–315.
129. Jacobs C, Lyman G, Velez-Garcia E, et al. A phase III randomized study comparing cisplatin and fluorouracil as single agents and in combination for advanced squamous cell carcinoma of the head and neck. *J Clin Oncol* 1992;10(2):257–263.
132. Urba S. Phase III study of pemetrexed in combination with cisplatin versus placebo plus cisplatin in patients with recurrent or metastatic squamous cell head and neck cancer. *Ann Oncol* 2010;21(Suppl 8):314.
133. Vermorken JB, Mesia R, Rivera F, et al. Platinum-based chemotherapy plus cetuximab in head and neck cancer. *N Engl J Med* 2008;359(11):1116–1127.
135. Janot F, de Raucourt D, Benhamou E, et al. Randomized trial of postoperative reirradiation combined with chemotherapy after salvage surgery compared with salvage surgery alone in head and neck carcinoma. *J Clin Oncol* 2008;26(34):5518–5523.
136. Choe KS, Haraf DJ, Solanki A, et al. Prior chemoradiotherapy adversely impacts outcomes of recurrent and second primary head and neck cancer treated with concurrent chemotherapy and reirradiation. *Cancer*. 2011 Jun 13. doi: 10.1002/cncr.26084. [Epub ahead of print]

Chapter 46
Hypopharynx

Timothy J. Kruser, Hiral K. Shah, Henry T. Hoffman, Nitin A. Pagedar, and Paul M. Harari

There is a strong association between tobacco use and the development of hypopharynx cancer.[1–3] Due to the rich lymphatic network in this anatomic region, patients commonly present with regional nodal metastases. Many hypopharynx cancer patients also carry significant medical comorbidities and social issues that present additional challenges to the successful delivery of aggressive cancer therapy. As for all complex tumors of the head and neck (H&N) region, multidisciplinary evaluation and management are critical and should involve the H&N surgeon, radiation oncologist, medical oncologist, nurse, nutritionist, speech or swallow therapist, and social worker. Although a selected cohort of early-stage tumors may be amenable to organ preservation surgery, more radical surgery such as laryngopharyngectomy is often required for patients who undergo a primary operative approach for hypopharynx cancer. This ablative procedure can induce significant cosmetic and functional changes, and postsurgical rehabilitation efforts guided by knowledgeable professionals are very important to assist in patient adaptation. Increasingly, hypopharynx cancer patients are being considered for nonoperative treatment approaches using definitive radiation or chemoradiation as a means of obtaining tumor control with preservation of organ function. Regardless of the specific treatment approach, all patients require active rehabilitation therapy in an effort to maximize their ultimate speech and swallow function. Despite stepwise advances in the diagnosis and treatment of hypopharynx cancer, the overall outcome for these patients is relatively poor compared with other H&N cancer sites.[4] As with most tumors of the H&N region, there is significant interest in combining molecular targeted therapies with traditional cytotoxic therapy in an effort to further improve outcomes.

ANATOMY

The hypopharynx, sometimes referred to as the laryngopharynx, is contiguous superiorly with the oropharynx and inferiorly with the cervical esophagus (Fig. 46.1). As general landmarks, the superior border of the hypopharynx is demarcated by the hyoid bone and the inferior border by the cricoid cartilage. With regard to cancer diagnosis and staging, there are three primary anatomic subsites within the hypopharynx: the bilateral pyriform sinuses, the postcricoid region, and the posterior pharyngeal wall.

The pyriform sinuses are essentially inverted pyramids with the medial, lateral, and anterior walls narrowing inferiorly to form the apices. Posteriorly, the pyriform sinuses are open and contiguous with the pharyngeal walls. Superiorly, the sinuses are surrounded by the thyrohyoid membrane through which passes the internal branch of the superior laryngeal nerve.

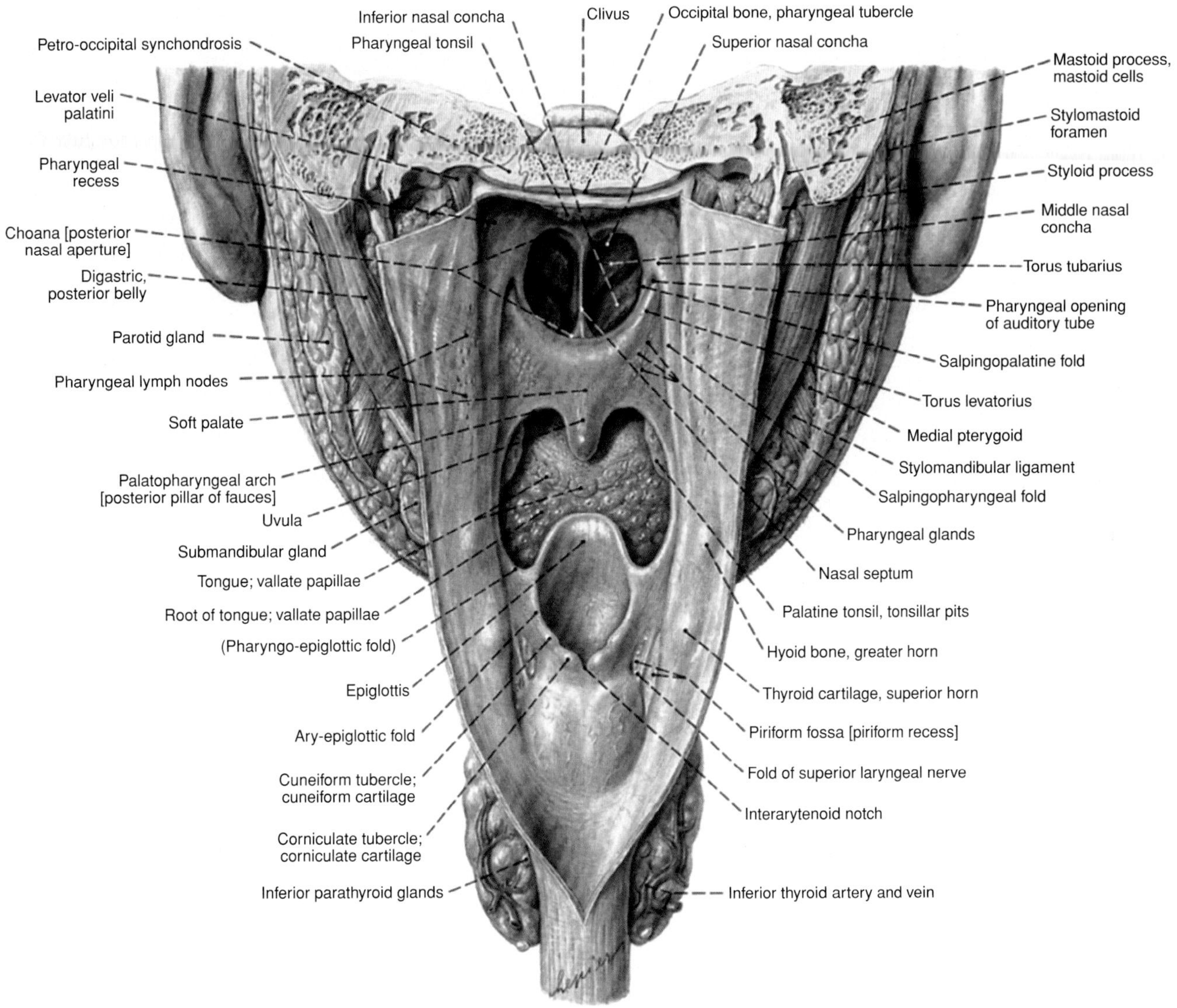

FIGURE 46.1. Posterior view of the hypopharynx shows the relationship of the pyriform sinus, pharyngeal wall, and postcricoid region within the head and neck. (From Putz R, Pabst R, *Sobotta: Atlas der Anatomie des Menschen,* 2001. © Elsevier GmbH, Urban & Fischer Verlag München, with permission.)

Tumor involvement of the sensory branches of this nerve can result in referred otalgia. The postcricoid region is comprised of the mucosa overlying the cricoid cartilage, with the arytenoid and esophageal mucosa forming the superior and inferior borders, respectively. The posterior pharyngeal wall predominantly comprises the squamous mucosa covering the middle and inferior pharyngeal constrictor muscles and is separated from the prevertebral fascia by the retropharyngeal space. Typically, the mucosa lining the pharyngeal wall is <1 cm in thickness and provides a minimal barrier to direct tumor infiltration. The posterior pharyngeal wall is contiguous with the lateral wall of the pyriform sinus (Fig. 46.2).

Sensory innervation of the hypopharynx is provided by the internal branch of the superior laryngeal nerve as well as fibers deriving from the glossopharyngeal nerve. The recurrent laryngeal nerve and the pharyngeal plexus provide the primary motor supply. The arterial supply of the hypopharynx is derived primarily from branches of the external carotid artery: superior thyroid arteries, ascending pharyngeal arteries, and lingual arteries.

There is a rich network of lymphatics within the hypopharynx that drain directly through the thyrohyoid membrane and into the jugulodigastric lymph nodes, most commonly involving the subdigastric node. Additionally, there may be direct drainage into the spinal accessory nodes. Tumors involving the posterior pharyngeal wall can also drain to the retropharyngeal nodes, including the most cephalad retropharyngeal nodes of Rouviere.

EPIDEMIOLOGY AND ETIOLOGY

Hypopharynx cancers are relatively uncommon. Approximately 1,800 cases per year were diagnosed annually in the United States from 1990 to 2004,[4] and the population-adjusted annual incidence rate in the United States was 0.7 per 100,000 from 2000 to 2008, according to the National Cancer Institute's Surveillance, Epidemiology, and End-Results (SEER) database.[5] Hypopharyngeal cancers accounted for 5.2% of upper aerodigestive tract cancers during that time. Approximately three-fourths of hypopharyngeal cancers occur in men, with a mean age of 65 years. Over 90% of patients with hypopharynx cancer report past cigarette use.[6] Alcohol appears to potentiate the carcinogenic effects of tobacco. Additionally, alcohol consumption at medium to high levels for a long period of time can increase the likelihood of hypopharynx cancer in nonsmoking patients.[7] The index hypopharynx cancer often occurs within

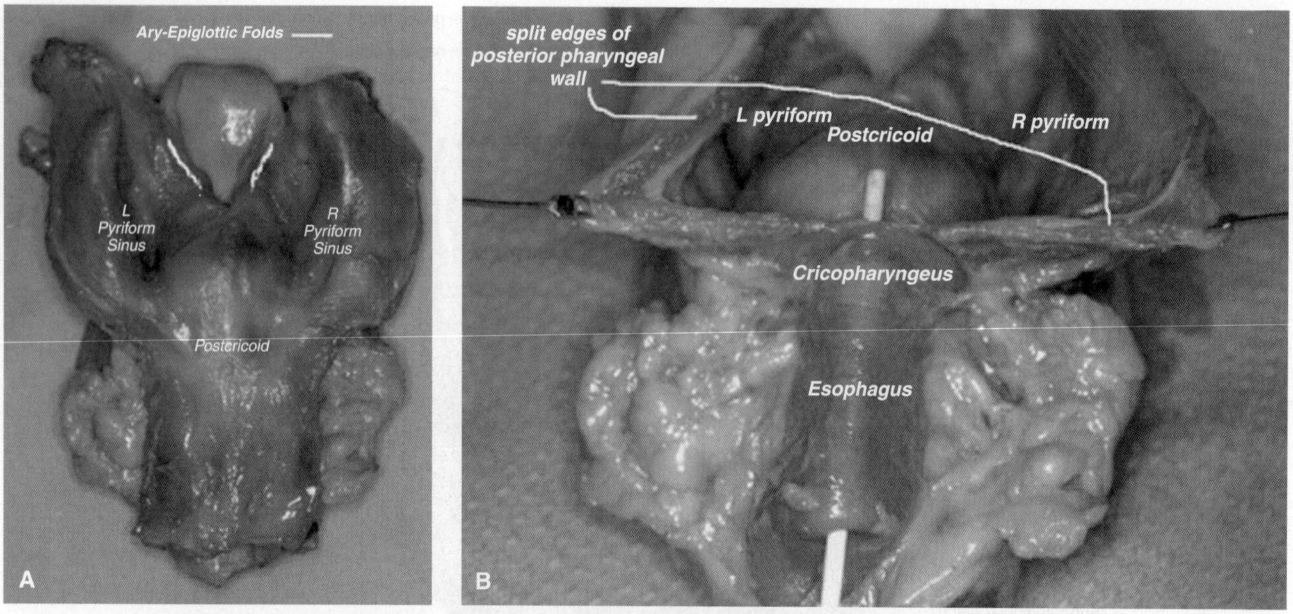

FIGURE 46.2. **A:** Posterior view of resected larynx and hypopharynx specimen afforded by incision through the posterior pharyngeal wall, cricopharyngeus, and cervical esophagus in the posterior midline. The aryepiglottic folds (*marked*) and arytenoids separate the pyriform sinuses (hypopharynx) from the larynx. **B:** The three primary anatomic subsites (posterior pharyngeal wall, postcricoid region, and pyriform sinuses) are revealed in this posterior view of the hypopharynx with the posterior pharyngeal wall incised.

a field of diseased mucosa characterized by high-grade dysplasia. This "field cancerization" reflects widespread mucosal exposure to carcinogens and is responsible for the high rate of synchronous and metachronous primary tumors identified in patients with hypopharynx cancer. Successful counseling with particular emphasis on smoking cessation can enhance treatment tolerance and diminish the risk of developing subsequent cancers of the upper aerodigestive tract. Patients with occupational exposure to coal dust, steel dust, iron compounds, and fumes have also shown an increased risk for developing hypopharynx cancer.[8,9] Overall, the incidence of hypopharynx cancer has shown some gradual decline in the United States. From 1975 to 2001, the incidence decreased by approximately 35%, perhaps as a result of smoking cessation efforts.[10]

Human papilloma virus (HPV) infection is well established as a risk factor for the development of squamous cell carcinoma of the gynecologic tract, particularly uterine cervix. The relation between HPV and H&N cancer is now becoming much better appreciated, particularly for cancers of the oropharynx, where it may approach 60% to 70% in some series. Studies have demonstrated that approximately 20% to 25% of patients with hypopharynx cancer test positive for HPV DNA,[11,12] and seropositivity for antibodies against the HPV-16 E6 and E7 antibodies has been associated with a significantly elevated risk of hypopharyngeal cancer.[13] The clinical implications of the presence of HPV in hypopharynx cancer are yet to be defined.

There is a recognized increased risk of developing cancers of the postcricoid region for patients with Plummer-Vinson syndrome, characterized by iron-deficiency anemia, hypopharyngeal webs, weight loss, and dysphagia.[7] Favorable changes in the epidemiology of hypopharynx cancer have resulted from

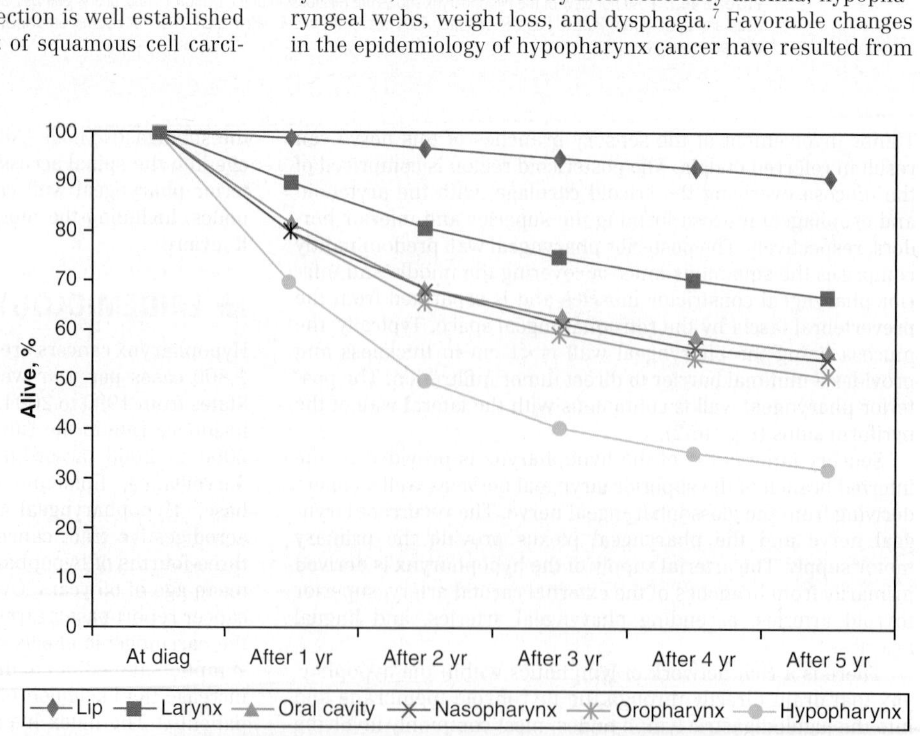

FIGURE 46.3. Five-year survival by mucosal site for head and neck cancers from 1990 to 1999 cases. (From Cooper JS, Porter K, Mallin K, et al. National Cancer Database report on cancer of the head and neck: 10-year update. *Head Neck* 2009;1:748–758, with permission.)

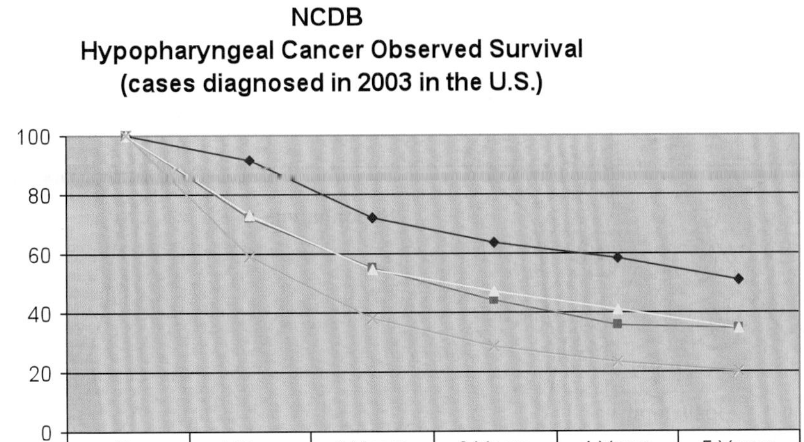

	Dx	1 Year	2 Years	3 Years	4 Years	5 Years
Stage I n=36	100	91.7	72.2	63.9	58.3	51.3
Stage II n=114	100	71.9	55.2	44.2	35.7	34.8
Stage III n=270	100	73.1	54.7	47.2	40.8	34.8
Stage IV n=790	100	59.1	37.7	28.5	23.3	19.8

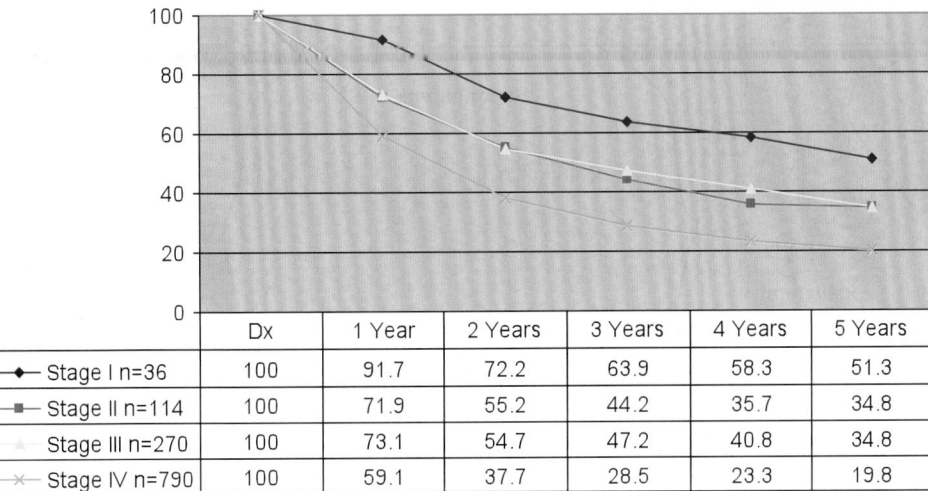

FIGURE 46.4. Observed survival for hypopharyngeal cancer in the United States is calculated for new cases identified in the NCDB in 2003 and includes all pathologic types and the selected anatomic sites: C129, C130, C131, C132, C138, C139. Staging according to sixth edition of the *AJCC Cancer Staging Handbook*. (From National Cancer Data Base. Commission on Cancer. American College of Surgeons. Benchmark Reports. Available at: http://cromwell.facs.org/BMarks/BMPub/Ver10/bm_reports.cfm, with permission.)

changes in nutrition. The addition of iron to flour has made Plummer-Vinson syndrome quite rare in the upper Midwestern United States and Scandinavian countries where it was formerly more common. An associated decrease in hypopharynx cancer involving the postcricoid region has followed.

PROGNOSTIC FACTORS

Several prognostic factors have been identified for patients with hypopharynx cancer. Age, particularly older than 70 years, has been identified as an unfavorable predictor of outcome.[7] This may simply reflect the diminished likelihood of elderly patients to successfully tolerate the aggressive therapy approaches required for locoregionally advanced cancers of the H&N. Women have been found to achieve somewhat improved outcomes compared to men, although this may in part be a manifestation of earlier-stage disease at diagnosis.[14,15] In addition, tumor location has an impact on outcome, with cancers of the pyriform sinus generally faring better than those arising in the postcricoid or posterior pharyngeal wall regions.[14,15] As a whole, hypopharynx cancer patients fare poorly in comparison with patients harboring tumors from other H&N sites (Figs. 46.3 and 46.4).[4,16] To a lesser extent, tobacco, alcohol, and dietary factors (carotenoids, vitamin C, vitamin E, and flavonoids) may also have an impact on outcome.[17]

Biologic factors have been investigated for their potential role in hypopharyngeal cancer. The presence of p53 gene mutations has been associated with bulkier tumors and younger patients along with higher expression of the epidermal growth factor receptor (EGFR). However, p53 has not shown correlation with multiple primary tumors, tumor grade, or DNA ploidy.[18,19] Further, there are conflicting data regarding the prognostic significance of EGFR expression for patients with hypopharyngeal cancer.[20] Some studies suggest EGFR overexpression portends a worse prognosis for patients undergoing (chemo)radiotherapy but not for patients treated with primary surgical resection.[21,22]

STAGING

The most commonly used staging system for hypopharynx cancer is the American Joint Committee on Cancer's (AJCC) 2009 seventh edition of the *AJCC Cancer Staging Handbook* and is based on a combination of clinical and radiographic data (Table 46.1).[23] No significant changes were made between the sixth and seventh editions other than to alter the classification of extension to the esophagus (previously T4a, from the tumor-node-metastasis [TNM] classification) toT3. The nodal and group staging is similar to other sites within the pharynx with the exception of nasopharynx. Although AJCC staging is a useful tool to broadly group similar cancer types, it should not be used as a blueprint for management. Patient factors, including age, comorbid medical conditions, and motivation for organ preservation, are beyond the scope of the staging system but nevertheless represent important factors for consideration with each individual patient.

PATTERNS OF SPREAD

Local Extension

It is sometimes difficult to definitively assign tumor origin to a specific subsite in the hypopharynx when the tumor overlaps more than one subsite. Of the hypopharynx cancer cases recorded in the National Cancer Institute's SEER database between 2000 and 2008, 83% of tumors with a known subsite arose in the pyriform sinus. An additional 9% arose from the posterior pharyngeal wall, and 4% originated in the postcricoid region.[5]

TABLE 46.1 AMERICAN JOINT COMMITTEE ON CANCER 2010 T STAGING FOR HYPOPHARYNX CANCER

T Stage	*Description*
T1	Limited to 1 subsite of the hypopharynx and ≤2 cm in greatest dimension
T2	Tumor invades more than 1 subsite of the hypopharynx or an adjacent site, or measures >2 cm but ≤4 cm in greatest diameter without fixation of hemilarynx
T3	Tumor measures >4 cm in greatest dimension or with fixation of hemilarynx or with extension to the esophagus
T4a	Invades thyroid/cricoid cartilage, hyoid bone, thyroid gland, or central compartment soft tissue, which includes prelaryngeal strap muscles and subcutaneous fat
T4b	Tumor invades prevertebral fascia, encases carotid artery, or involves mediastinal structures

Used with the permission of the American Joint Committee on Cancer, Chicago, Illinois. The original source for this material is the *AJCC Cancer Staging Handbook*, 7th Edition (2010) published by Springer Science and Business Media LLC, www.springerlink.com.

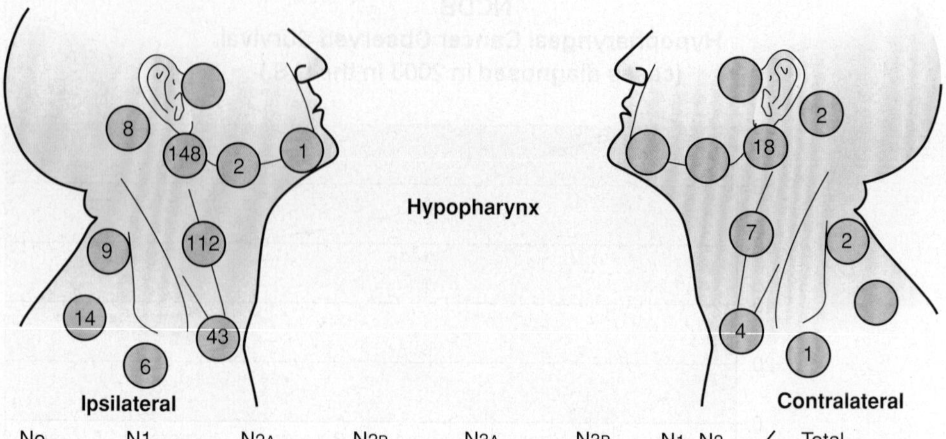

No	N1	N2A	N2B	N3A	N3B	N1–N3 / Total
65	51	27	45	51	28	202 / 267 = 75%

FIGURE 46.5. Nodal distribution patterns for a series of 267 patients with hypopharynx cancer as summarized by admission records at the M.D. Anderson Cancer Center. (From Lindberg R. Distribution of cervical lymph node metastases from squamous cell carcinoma of the upper respiratory and digestive tracts. *Cancer* 1972;29:1446–1449, with permission.)

Due to the high propensity for advanced primary disease as well as regional nodal involvement, the majority of hypopharynx cancer patients present with stages III and IV disease. In a retrospective study from Washington University, 87% of patients with cancers of the pyriform sinus and 82% of patients with posterior pharyngeal wall tumors presented with stage III or IV disease.[24]

Cancers arising from the pyriform sinus may spread superiorly to involve the aryepiglottic folds and arytenoids and invade the paraglottic and pre-epiglottic space. Lateral tumor extension can involve portions of the thyroid cartilage, allowing entry into the lateral compartment of the neck. High-resolution computed tomography (CT) or magnetic resonance imaging (MRI) is often useful for optimal assessment regarding the extent of tumor invasion. For tumors arising from the medial wall, the most common site of involvement for pyriform sinus tumors, there is a likelihood of tumor involvement of intrinsic muscles of the larynx resulting in vocal cord fixation. Inferior tumor extension beyond the apex can involve the thyroid gland.

Cancers arising within the postcricoid region can extend circumferentially to involve the cricoid cartilage or anteriorly to involve the larynx with resultant vocal cord fixation. Tumor involvement of the recurrent laryngeal nerve can also precipitate vocal cord fixation. Primary postcricoid tumors are often quite extensive and can involve the pyriform sinus, trachea, or esophagus. As a result, these tumors generally carry a worse prognosis in comparison to tumors from other subsites of the hypopharynx.[14] Nodal spread to the paratracheal nodes and inferior deep cervical nodes is not uncommon. Tumors arising from the posterior pharyngeal wall can extend to involve the oropharynx superiorly, the cervical esophagus inferiorly, and the prevertebral fascia and retropharyngeal space posteriorly.

Many cancers of the hypopharynx have a propensity for submucosal spread. It can therefore be difficult to accurately quantify the full microscopic extent of disease. This is particularly true for cancers of the posterior pharyngeal wall and postcricoid regions. Careful study through serial sectioning of surgical specimens has identified that 60% of hypopharynx cancers demonstrate subclinical spread with a range of 10 mm superiorly, 25 mm medially, 20 mm laterally, and 20 mm inferiorly.[25] This extensive pattern of tumor infiltration can present considerable challenge in the effort to achieve clear surgical margins or full dosimetric coverage with radiotherapy.

Regional Disease

Due to the rich lymphatic drainage of the hypopharynx, more than 50% of patients will manifest clinically positive cervical lymph nodes at the time of diagnosis, and ultimately 65% to 80% of patients will have nodal involvement, as 30% to 40% of N0 necks harbor micrometastatic disease when electively dissected.[26] Jugular chain nodes, levels II to IV, as well as retropharyngeal nodes are all at high risk of harboring regional metastases in patients with hypopharynx cancer. Postcricoid tumors may also spread directly to pre- and paratracheal nodal basins. In light of cross-draining lymphatics, there is a significant risk of bilateral cervical node metastasis (Fig. 46.5).[27,28]

Distant Metastases

The most common site for distant metastasis to develop in patients with cancer of the hypopharynx is the lung. Previously, approximately one-quarter of patients diagnosed with hypopharynx cancer presented with distant metastases, although this incidence in more recent reports is estimated at approximately 16%.[29] For those patients not rendered free of locoregional disease following initial therapy, the incidence of distant metastases increases notably with the length of time following initial treatment.[30]

Field Cancerization

Carcinogens can induce dysplastic changes throughout the mucosa of the upper aerodigestive tract, leading to an increased risk for field cancerization that enhances the likelihood of synchronous or metachronous secondary primary tumors. Approximately 7% of patients with hypopharynx cancer will manifest a second primary tumor at initial diagnosis and between 10% to 20% will develop a secondary primary tumor over time. In fact, this second tumor risk is a significant cause of mortality in patients who survive more than 2 years following initial treatment.[6]

CLINICAL PRESENTATION

In light of the nonspecific nature of early symptoms, the majority of patients with cancers of the hypopharynx present with advanced local or regional disease. Frequently, there is a delay between presentation and diagnosis as patients are often managed for presumed infectious or gastrointestinal etiology. The majority of symptoms are related to local tumor spread, including dysphagia and odynophagia. There may be frank pharyngeal obstruction, invasion of constrictor muscles, prevertebral space invasion, or strap muscle invasion. Common presenting signs and symptoms include dysphagia, sore throat, hoarseness, weight loss >10 pounds, and neck mass. The majority of patients present with more than one of these signs and symptoms.[31] Roughly 25% of patients will present with clinical stage III disease and 50% with clinical stage IV disease; however, reflux symptoms can be a common presentation leading to diagnosis

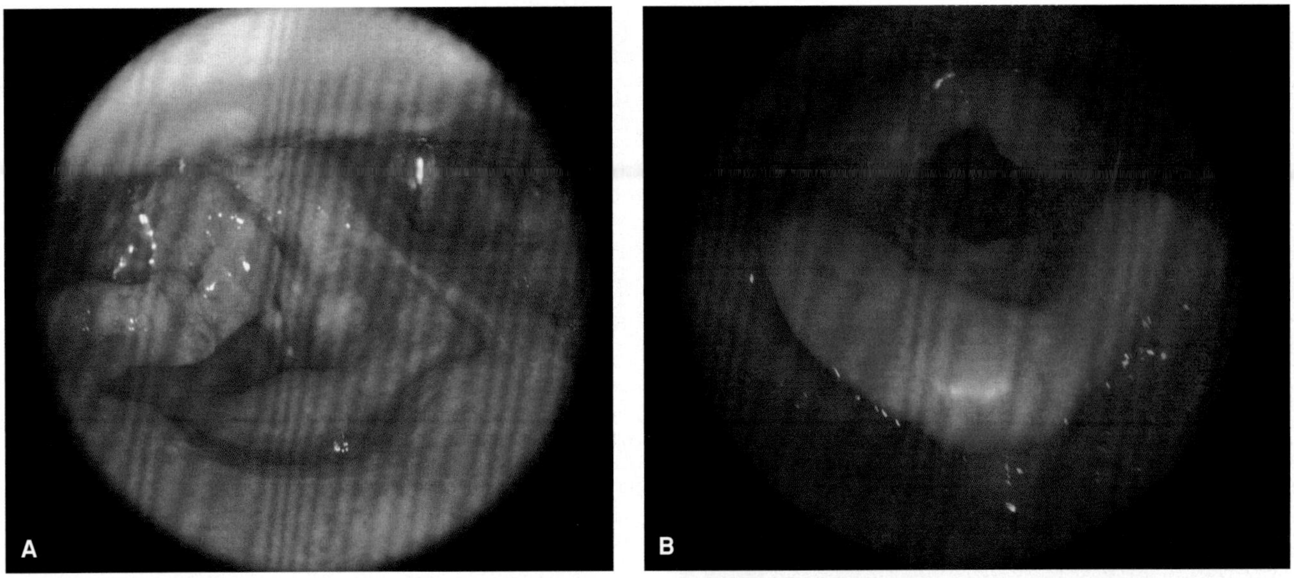

FIGURE 46.6. **A:** Outpatient clinic photograph taken through a rigid endoscope mounted with a 35-mm camera of a newly diagnosed exophytic T2 tumor arising from the right pyriform sinus with involvement of the adjacent aryepiglottic fold. There was no compromise of vocal cord mobility, and clinical staging of the primary lesion was T2. **B:** Photographic examination 1 year following 70-Gy radiation and concurrent cisplatin chemotherapy with complete tumor regression and excellent functional status of the laryngopharynx. Note mild to moderate mucosal edema of supraglottic structures following high-dose radiation.

of stage I or II hypopharyngeal tumors.[6] Selected patients may first come to medical attention with complaints of unilateral ear pain (referred otalgia) due to tumor involvement of the visceral sensory nerves of the pharynx.

PRETREATMENT EVALUATION AND STAGING WORKUP

A comprehensive workup for patients with cancers of the hypopharynx should include a detailed history focusing on the duration of symptoms, amount of weight loss, the presence of otalgia, changes in voice quality, and degree of dysphagia. A previous history of another upper aerodigestive tract malignancy and a history of tobacco smoking are commonly associated. The physical examination should include direct and indirect visualization of the full laryngopharyngeal axis with particular attention to the size, location, and anatomic positioning of the primary tumor as well as the mobility status of the true vocal cords. Dentition and oral health should be assessed. If the patient presents with cervical adenopathy, the size, number, location, texture, and mobility of these nodes should be documented.

Although cervical adenopathy associated with hypopharynx cancer may be analyzed with fine-needle aspiration (FNA) biopsy, there is little value in this approach, because most patients will receive advanced radiographic imaging to further define the nodal involvement. On rare occasions FNA may be useful to help distinguish other coexisting causes of lymphadenopathy such as lymphoma. Most patients will undergo a direct laryngoscopy under general anesthesia in conjunction with esophagoscopy. This panendoscopy allows not only biopsy confirmation of the primary tumor site, but also mapping of the extent of the tumor as well as the ability to survey for synchronous primary tumors (Fig. 46.6A). Use of transnasal fiberoptic techniques makes it possible for a panendoscopy to be done for selected patients without anesthesia in the clinic setting.

In addition to panendoscopy, patients should undergo either high-resolution CT with contrast (or MRI) extending from the skull base to below the clavicle to help assess the extent of the primary tumor and to quantitatively and qualitatively assess cervical adenopathy (Figs. 46.7 and 46.8).[27] Although a chest x-ray has traditionally been used to assess for the presence of pulmonary metastasis, 18-fluorodeoxyglucose positron emission tomography (^{18}FDG-PET) imaging (with accompanying CT for coregistration) is increasingly used to assess the extent of regional adenopathy and to survey for the presence of distant metastasis. FDG-PET is becoming an increasingly valuable adjunct to CT or MRI in the radiation treatment planning process, particularly for patients treated with conformal intensity modulated radiation therapy (IMRT) or tomotherapy techniques. Di Martino et al.[32] compared CT, PET, color-coded duplex sonography, palpation, and panendoscopy in assessment of tumor and nodal status. The results of this study are summarized in Table 46.2 and support the promising sensitivity and specificity of PET scanning in H&N cancers. Schwartz et al.[33] examined standardized uptake value (SUV) of primary and nodal metastasis in H&N cancer patients and their relationship to clinical outcome. A primary tumor SUV >9.0 was

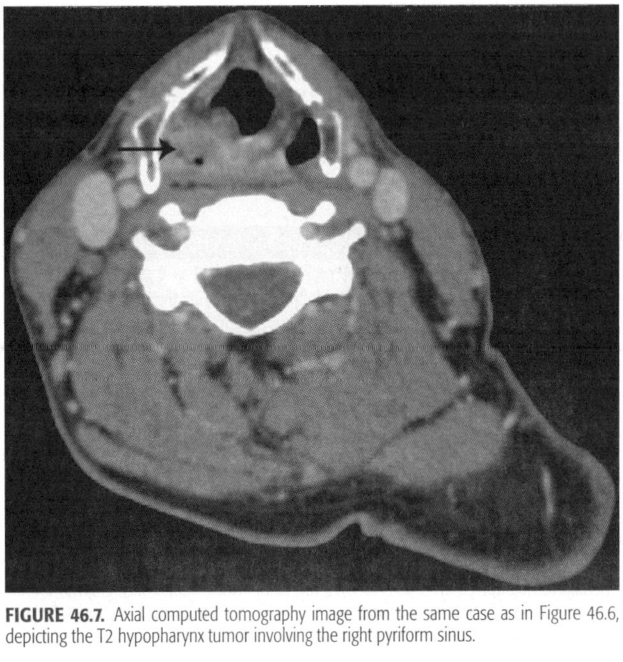

FIGURE 46.7. Axial computed tomography image from the same case as in Figure 46.6, depicting the T2 hypopharynx tumor involving the right pyriform sinus.

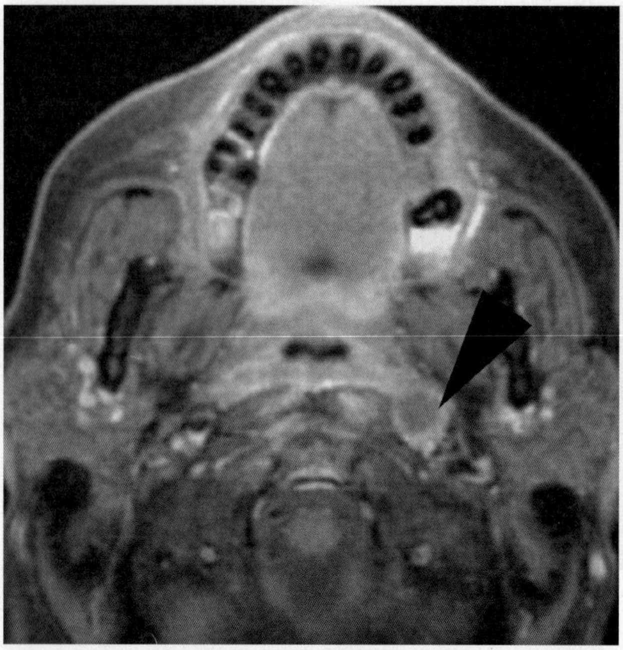

FIGURE 46.8. Axial gadolinium-enhanced T1-weighted magnetic resonance image scan with fat-saturation depicting metastatic lateral retropharyngeal node with evidence of central necrosis and peripheral enhancement.

associated with a significantly lower local recurrence-free survival and disease-free survival. However, there was no correlation between nodal SUV and clinical outcome.

A recent prospective multicenter study of 233 H&N squamous cell carcinoma (SCC) patients (including 46 hypopharyngeal cancer) highlighted the potential impact of PET imaging on H&N SCC management.[34] TNM staging and therapeutic decisions were first determined based on conventional workup, and then physicians were unblinded to FDG-PET data and asked to restage the patients and reanalyze their therapeutic decisions. PET and conventional workup revealed discordant TNM staging in 100 patients (43%). PET was deemed significantly more accurate than conventional staging and improved the staging in 20% of patients. Incorporation of PET data ultimately impacted management in 32 patients (13.7%) (Table 46.3), supporting the use of FDG-PET in H&N SCC staging.

Many patients with hypopharynx cancer present with concurrent medical and social comorbidities that require consideration before initiating cancer-directed therapy. Commonly, there is a progressive history of dysphagia and odynophagia with associated weight loss. Whether these patients are treated with surgical or nonsurgical approaches, a gastrostomy tube may need to be considered as a temporary measure. It is important to optimize or at least stabilize the patient's nutritional status prior to initiating definitive therapy.

TABLE 46.2 COMPARISON OF VARIOUS MODALITIES FOR STAGING

	Sensitivity (%)		Specificity (%)	
	T	N	T	N
Panendoscopy	95	–	85	–
PET	95	84	92	90
CDDS	74	84	75	96
CT	68	84	69	88
Palpation	–	63	–	96

PET, positron emission tomography; CDDS, color-coded duplex sonography; CT, computed tomography.

Adapted from Di Martino E, Nowak B, Hassan HA, et al. Diagnosis and staging of head and neck cancer: a comparison of modern imaging modalities (positron emission tomography, computed tomography, color-coded duplex sonography) with panendoscopic and histopathologic findings. *Arch Otolaryngol Head Neck Surg* 2000;126:1457–1461.

TABLE 46.3 IMPACT OF FDG-PET ON STAGING, MANAGEMENT FOLLOWING CONVENTIONAL WORKUP

Endpoint	Impact of FDG-PET on 233 Patients
Discordant TNM stage	100 (43%)
PET accurately upstaged	30 (13%)
PET accurately downstaged	17 (7.3%)
PET inaccurately changed stage	13 (5.6%)
No confirmed gold standard TNM	40 (17%)
Impact on Patient Management[a]	
Low	188 patients (80.7%)
Medium	12 patients (5.2%)
High	20 patients (8.6%)

FDG, fluorodeoxyglucose; PET, positron emission tomography; TNM, tumor-node-metastasis classification.

[a]Impact ratings: low, treatment modality and delivery unchanged; medium, change within the same treatment modality (planned procedure, dose, or mode of administration changed); high, change in treatment intent or treatment modality (e.g., curative to palliation, surgery to chemoradiation, and so on).

Adapted from Lonneux M, Hamoir M, Reychler H, et al. Positron emission tomography with [18F]fluorodeoxyglucose improves staging and patient management in patients with head and neck squamous cell carcinoma: a multicenter prospective study. *J Clin Oncol* 2010;28:1190–1195.

It is valuable for hypopharynx cancer patients to undergo evaluation by a speech and swallow therapist to determine the degree of dysfunction prior to therapy. This may be done as a bedside study of swallowing capacity, a fiberoptic endoscopic evaluation of swallowing, or (usually preferably) through the more definitive fluoroscopic barium swallow study. This modified barium swallow study is called a cookie swallow, video pharyngogram, or oropharyngeal motility study and is most commonly done with a speech pathologist in attendance. If objective swallowing dysfunction is present, patients may be taught adaptive techniques to improve the effectiveness and safety of their oral intake. Additionally, close follow-up with the same speech and swallow therapist is highly desirable during and after therapy to maximize the patient's long-term functional capabilities.

Because many hypopharynx patients have an active history of alcohol and tobacco use, it is important to counsel accordingly and encourage all patients to take advantage of methods and programs to facilitate smoking and alcohol cessation. All patients should undergo comprehensive dental evaluation and cleaning as well as basic education regarding oral hygiene. For patients treated with conventional radiation therapy techniques, there is a significant likelihood of long-term xerostomia that can promote dental decay. If existing dentition is in poor condition, dental extractions should be considered prior to therapy, particularly for teeth that will reside within the high-dose radiation region. Typically 10 to 14 days are required following dental extractions to allow for healing prior to the initiation of radiation therapy. Custom fluoride carrier trays should be fabricated and discussed for long-term use in an effort to diminish the rate of dental decay for patients with chronic xerostomia.

Finally, many patients with hypopharynx cancer will have social issues, including lack of family support, financial limitations, transportation issues, poor nutrition, and hygiene habits that may hamper their ability to successfully receive adequate care. Often, the involvement of a case manager or social worker is of central importance to assist patients who require support both during as well as following cancer therapy.

PATHOLOGICAL CLASSIFICATION

In SEER data from 2000 to 2008, 93.9% of hypopharynx cancers were squamous cell carcinoma, with lymphoma, sarcoma,

TABLE 46.4 GENERAL TREATMENT RECOMMENDATIONS BASED ON HYPOPHARYNX TUMOR STAGE

Stage I	Radiation alone or voice preservation surgery if feasible
Stage II	Radiation alone
Stage III and IV with functional laryngopharynx	Concurrent chemoradiation followed by selective neck dissection
Stage III and IV with dysfunctional laryngopharynx[a]	Laryngopharyngectomy with adjuvant RT or CRT

RT, radiation therapy; CRT, chemoradiation therapy.

[a]Patients with bulky, destructive tumors that severely compromise the airway or destroy cartilage, bone, and deep soft tissue are often best served with immediate laryngopharyngectomy and postoperative radiation or chemoradiation.

adenocarcinoma, and adenoid cystic carcinoma each accounting for approximately 0.5% of cases.[5] Similarly, the National Cancer Data Base (NCDB) Benchmark Reports evaluated 17,654 cases of hypopharyngeal cancer in the United States between the years of 2000 and 2008. Over 90% of cases were SCC.[16]

MANAGEMENT

For patients presenting with early-stage, resectable disease, voice-preserving surgery and definitive radiotherapy alone are viable and acceptable treatment options. The vast majority of patients, however, present with stage III or IV disease and warrant multimodality treatment. A key consideration in determining the favored approach for these patients is the likelihood and motivation to preserve laryngopharyngeal function (Table 46.4).

Primary Surgery

T1 and T2 Tumors

Contemporary indications for primary surgical management of patients with early cancers of the hypopharynx include those with a history of previous H&N radiation, those in whom organ conservation approaches are deemed possible, and those who refuse radiation. Even for hypopharynx cancer patients who will receive nonoperative treatment approaches, it remains critical for the H&N surgeon to remain actively involved. The role of the surgeon in these cases may include endoscopic biopsy with detailed assessment of tumor extent, methods to secure the airway (tracheotomy or laser debulking), and methods to ensure adequate nutrition (gastrostomy). The surgeon will also play a vital role in multidisciplinary oncologic follow-up after nonoperative treatment.

Selected T1 and T2 hypopharynx cancers may lend themselves to surgical excision. These favorable subsites include the upper pyriform sinus and the posterior pharyngeal wall. The standard supraglottic laryngectomy encompasses the aryepiglottic fold and may be extended to include part of the arytenoids, the base of the tongue, and the upper pyriform sinus. Small cancers isolated to the posterior pharyngeal wall may be removed by endoscopic laser resection or removal using an open approach. Dysphagia requiring nothing by mouth status is common from an open approach, especially if reconstruction of the posterior wall is effected with an adynamic and insensate free flap. Relative contraindications to organ conservation surgery for hypopharynx cancers include cartilage invasion, vocal fold fixation, postcricoid invasion, deep pyriform sinus invasion, and extension beyond the larynx.

Innovations with free flap reconstruction have allowed retention of speech, swallowing, and breathing functions of the larynx despite extensive resection by way of a hemilaryngopharyngectomy. The temporoparietal flap and radial forearm free flap coupled with rigid cartilaginous support have been employed to retain function in patients with hypopharynx cancers without extension to the postcricoid region or apex of the pyriform sinus.[35]

In recent years, advancements in organ preservation surgery have included the use of transoral laser microsurgery and transoral robotic surgery. For selected cases, these approaches can achieve oncologic tumor removal, while limiting normal tissue disruption, thereby potentially avoiding tracheostomy and the use of feeding tubes.[36–39] This approach may involve concurrent or delayed neck dissection following transoral resection of the primary lesion (to allow for final margin assessment). The necks in some T1N0 patients may be observed with close interval follow-up CT scans. Adjuvant (chemo)radiotherapy is utilized in the majority of patients using this approach (see "Postoperative Radiotherapy" below for indications) and should generally encompass the primary tumor site as well as bilateral necks and supraclavicular fossae. Recent results have demonstrated that appropriately selected T1 or T2 lesions can achieve negative margins by transoral laser microsurgery or transoral robotic surgery.[36] Oncologic outcomes appear similar to open surgical approaches using this technique and are likely accompanied by lower rates of permanent gastrostomy tube or tracheostomy placement (Table 46.5).

T3 or T4 Resectable Tumors

Favorable T3 hypopharynx cancers that present in the upper aspect of the pyriform sinus and allow full extirpation by either an extended supraglottic laryngectomy or extended vertical partial laryngopharyngectomy with free flap reconstruction are infrequent. Most T3 and T4 hypopharynx cancers that are treated surgically will require total laryngectomy with efforts to preserve a posterior strip of the hypopharynx spanning the oropharynx to the esophagus. This preserved posterior wall of the hypopharynx may be tubed and closed on itself in selected cases. In the past it was common practice to accept primary reconstruction of this segment as adequate for swallowing if closure over a nasogastric tube was possible. More recently primary closure has been discouraged for cases with less than a 3- to 3.5-cm width of posterior pharyngeal wall mucosa to tube on itself. Most commonly superior swallowing results when the anterior and lateral walls of the remaining hypopharynx are reconstructed with a pedicled or free flap.

For more bulky tumors of the hypopharynx, total laryngopharyngectomy, removal of the larynx and the entire hypopharynx, is required. This procedure creates a gap between the oropharynx and esophagus that must be reconstructed with a tubed fasciocutaneous flap such as the radial forearm free flap or anterolateral thigh flap, a free jejunum, or a tubed pedicled myocutaneous flap. The myocutaneous flaps are technically difficult to tube due to the bulk of the fat and muscle underlying the skin paddle.

Laryngopharyngectomy with esophagectomy may be performed if the hypopharynx cancer extends inferior to the cricopharyngeus to

TABLE 46.5 FIVE-YEAR ONCOLOGIC OUTCOMES FOR TRANSORAL MICROLASER SURGERY FOR T1 OR T2 HYPOPHARYNGEAL TUMORS

Study (Reference)	T Stage	N	Node (+)	LC	DSS	OS	Permanent Gastrostomies	Permanent Tracheostomies
Martin et al. (36)	pT1	20	62%	84%	NR	68% (stage I–II)	3.5%[a]	3.5%[a]
	pT2	48		70%	NR			
Karatzanis et al. (35)	pT1	45	56%	90%	78%	NR	0	0
	pT2	74	64%	83%	70%	NR	4%	2.5%

LC, local control; DSS, disease-specific survival; NR, not reported; OS, 5-year overall survival.

[a]Entire cohort, including T3 and T4 patients.

ensure the inferior margin. In this case, gastric pull-up or colon interposition are reconstructive options used to restore the conduit for food and saliva extending from the oropharynx to the stomach.

Palliative Surgery

For patients with incurable, metastatic disease at presentation, or with symptomatic local recurrence not amenable to curative salvage therapy attempts, surgery can play an important role in palliation. If aspiration of secretions (despite nothing by mouth status and enteral feedings) persists, laryngopharyngectomy may afford a reasonable option to discuss with the patient and family members. Similarly, complete stenosis of the pharynx or upper esophagus due to tumor (or following treatment) may leave a patient with the constant need for suctioning his or her own secretions. In selected patients, laryngopharyngectomy with gastric pull-up may be a reasonable palliative option. Finally, gastric feeding tube placement can be considered for patients who do not wish to pursue palliative radiation therapy or surgery.

Postoperative Radiation Therapy

Most advanced hypopharynx cancers that are treated with initial surgical resection have unfavorable features that warrant the addition of postoperative radiation therapy in an effort to enhance locoregional control rates. Classical indications for postoperative radiation include T4 primary tumors, close or positive microscopic margins, cartilage or bony invasion, more than one metastatic lymph node, or the presence of extracapsular extension (ECE). Conventional therapy involves the use of a shrinking-field technique to deliver 54 to 63 Gy to all areas at risk and a boost to 60 to 66 Gy to regions of ECE or positive margins. The entire cervical nodal chain from the skull base to the clavicle bilaterally should be included. IMRT techniques may be considered in an attempt to reduce radiation dose to normal tissue structures such as the contralateral parotid gland and thereby preserve better salivary function.

The Radiation Therapy Oncology Group (RTOG) and European Organisation for Research and Treatment of Cancer (EORTC) have evaluated the role of concurrent chemotherapy along with postoperative radiation in prospective randomized trials. Eligibility criteria in the RTOG trial included patients with two or more positive nodes, ECE, or microscopically positive margins. All patients received 60 Gy alone or with concurrent cisplatin 100 mg/m^2 every 3 weeks. This trial demonstrated an improvement in locoregional control and disease-free survival for patients who received concurrent chemoradiotherapy. However, no significant benefit in absolute survival was confirmed (Table 46.6).[40] The EORTC conducted a similar trial that included patients with stage III (except T3N0 larynx), stage IV, and patients with stage I or II with positive margins, lymphovascular invasion, and perineural invasion. All patients received 66 Gy alone or with cisplatin at 100 mg/m^2 every 3 weeks. This trial demonstrated a significant improvement in progression-free survival and overall survival with the addition of chemotherapy (Table 46.7).[41] A subsequently published *post hoc* analysis of the combined data from these trials suggested that patients with ECE and positive margins were most likely to benefit from the addition of chemotherapy, while those with two or more involved lymph nodes without ECE as their only risk factor did not appear to benefit from the addition of chemotherapy.[42]

Although the studies above identify that the addition of cisplatin chemotherapy to postoperative radiation can improve tumor control outcome for specific categories of high-risk patients, it is clear that this modest benefit comes at the expense of additional toxicity. Careful clinical judgment regarding the selection of patients most likely to tolerate and thereby benefit from this approach is warranted. A recently updated meta-analysis demonstrated similar modest benefit from the addition of concurrent chemotherapy in the postoperative setting as compared to the definitive setting. However, this analysis showed that patients older than 70 years of age derive little to no benefit from the addition of systemic chemotherapy to radiation in H&N cancer.[43] The inadvertent introduction of treatment breaks during the adjuvant radiation course can easily compromise the potential benefits of the combined modality therapy in this setting.

TABLE 46.6 RESULTS OF RTOG POSTOP CHEMORADIATION TRIAL

	Arm 1[a] (%)	Arm 2[b] (%)	P
2-yr LRC	72	82	.003
2-yr DM	23	20	NS

RTOG, Radiation Therapy Oncology Group; LRC, locoregional control; DM, distant metastasis; NS, not significant.

[a]Arm 1: 60 Gy in 6 weeks.

[b]Arm 2: 60 Gy in 6 weeks with concurrent cisplatin (100 mg/m^2) days 1, 22, and 43.

Adapted from Cooper JS, Pajak TF, Forastiere AA, et al. Postoperative concurrent radiotherapy and chemotherapy for high-risk squamous-cell carcinoma of the head and neck. *N Engl J Med* 2004;350:1937–1944.

TABLE 46.7 RESULTS OF EORTC POSTOPERATIVE CHEMORADIATION TRIAL

	Arm 1[a]		Arm 2[b]		
	Median	5 Year	Median	5 Year	p
PFS	23 months	36%	55 months	47%	0.04
OS	32 months	40%	72 months	53%	0.02

EORTIC, European Organisation for Research and Treatment of Cancer; PFS, progression-free survival; OS, overall survival.

[a]Arm 1: RT alone 66 Gy in 6 ½ weeks.

[b]Arm 2: 66Gy in 6½ weeks with concurrent cisplatin (100 mg/m^2) days 1, 22, and 43.

Adapted from Bernier J, Domenge C, Ozsahin M, et al. Postoperative irradiation with or without concomitant chemotherapy for locally advanced head and neck cancer. *N Engl J Med* 2004;350:1945–1952.

Definitive Radiation Therapy

T1 and T2 Tumors

Curative radiation therapy (RT) is generally the preferred treatment option for patients with T1 or T2 hypopharynx tumors (see Table 46.4). This approach affords good potential for organ preservation without compromise in clinical outcome. A classical course of radiation therapy for hypopharynx cancer lasts 6 to 7 weeks, with treatment delivered 5 days per week. Conventional treatment involves a shrinking-field technique that initiates with opposed lateral fields encompassing the primary tumor and upper neck lymphatics with a matched anterior field to complete treatment of the lower neck (Table 46.8). One of the most common worldwide fractionation regimens involves

TABLE 46.8 GENERAL ANATOMIC LANDMARKS FOR FIELD DESIGN USING CONVENTIONAL HEAD AND NECK RADIOTHERAPY FOR HYPOPHARYNX CANCER

Border	Description
Superior	Include base of skull
Posterior	Behind vertebral spinous processes (or further if required to cover metastatic cervical lymph nodes)
Inferior	Lower aspect of cricoid cartilage unless extensive caudal tumor extension
Anterior	Flash skin at level of thyroid cartilage

For T1 lesions, classical dose is 66–70 Gy in 2 Gy daily fractions. For T2–T4 lesions, consider altered fractionation regimens or concurrent cisplatin-based chemotherapy, particularly for patients over 70 years of age. Gross disease should generally receive 70 Gy with concurrent chemotherapy.

the delivery of 2 Gy daily fractions to 70 Gy over 7 weeks. Due to the high likelihood of subclinical nodal metastases even in the clinically N0 neck, patients traditionally receive comprehensive radiation to encompass nodal regions from the skull base to the clavicle. Due to the varying thicknesses of the head and neck, custom compensators or wedges should be used for the lateral fields to improve dose homogeneity. Shrinking field techniques to spare direct spinal cord dose after approximately 45 Gy, as well as final mucosal reductions after 54 to 60 Gy, are often appropriate with posterior neck boosting, with electrons to supplement posterior chain nodal dosing without excessive dose to the spinal cord.

SCC of the H&N are rapidly proliferating tumors. There has been significant interest over the past several decades in the use of intensified radiation fractionation schedules to counter rapid tumor cell repopulation as a means of improving outcomes in H&N cancer patients treated with radiation alone. Altered fractionation techniques, including hyperfractionation (e.g., 1.1–1.4 Gy twice daily) and accelerated fractionation (e.g., 6 fraction per week or concomitant boost regimens), have demonstrated improved locoregional control rates for H&N cancer patients.[44–46] A recent meta-analysis examined 15 trials that compared conventional fractionation to altered fractionation, either hyperfractionation or accelerated fractionation. This meta-analysis demonstrated a small but statistically significant survival benefit of 3.4% at 5 years with altered fractionation. The benefit was higher with hyperfractionation compared to accelerated fractionation and was more pronounced for patients younger than age 50.[47]

Early T-stage hypopharynx patients with N0 or N1 neck disease can be considered for treatment with radiation alone or concurrent radiation plus chemotherapy. In this setting, gross disease should receive 70 Gy and the contralateral neck (N0) should receive 50 to 54 Gy. With T1N0 lesions, patients may achieve 5-year disease-specific survival (DSS) on the order of 90%, while T2N0 lesions may achieve DSS above 70% (Tables 46.9 and 46.10).[48–52]

The use of three-dimensional CT-based planning has become routine in the management of H&N cancer patients (Fig. 46.9). CT-based planning allows precise delineation of target volume and visualization of dose distributions (Fig. 46.10). In the past several years, there has been significant interest in the use of IMRT in H&N cancer as a means of diminishing normal tissue toxicities, particularly xerostomia resulting from irradiation of major salivary glands. Excellent candidates for IMRT include patients with unilateral T1 to T3 primary lesions with N2b or less neck disease. In light of the high-dose gradients that can accompany highly conformal plans, a critical component of successful IMRT delivery is the use of an accurate and reproducible localization system. At several centers, the an optically guided localization system is used to enhance treatment precision for patients undergoing IMRT for H&N cancer.[53] The cephalad margin of the N0 contralateral neck may often be limited to the C1-2 interspace in an effort to further improve parotid gland sparing.[54,55] A recent randomized trial of conventional radiotherapy versus IMRT in patients with T1-4N0-3 oropharyngeal and hypopharyngeal tumors at high risk for xerostomia highlighted the benefits of IMRT for parotid sparing. Patients were treated either postoperatively or definitively, and the contralateral parotid was constrained to <24 Gy to the whole gland. Grade 2 or worse xerostomia was significantly reduced at both 12 months (74% conventional vs 38% IMRT) and at 24 months (83% conventional vs 29% IMRT).[56] These benefits translated to significantly better quality-of-life scores in the IMRT group and strongly support a role for IMRT in H&N SCC radiotherapy.

TABLE 46.9 LOCAL CONTROL FOR CARCINOMA OF THE POSTERIOR PHARYNGEAL WALL TREATED WITH RADIATION ALONE

	Local Control After RT		*Ultimate Local Control After Salvage*	
Stage	*2 Year (%)*	*5 Year (%)*	*2 Year (%)*	*5 Year (%)*
T1	100	100	100	100
T2	79	74	86	81
T3	59	49	66	66
T4	36	36	36	36

RT, radiation therapy.

Adapted from Amdur RJ, Mendenhall WM, Stringer SP, et al. Organ preservation with radiotherapy for T1-T2 carcinoma of the pyriform sinus. *Head Neck* 2001;23:353–362.

TABLE 46.10 CAUSE-SPECIFIC AND OVERALL SURVIVAL FOR CARCINOMA OF THE PYRIFORM SINUS TREATED WITH RADIATION ALONE

Stage	*5-Year Cause Specific Survival (%)*	*5-Year Overall Survival (%)*
I	96	57
II		61
III	02	41
IVa	49	29
IVb	33	25

Adapted from Amdur RJ, Mendenhall WM, Stringer SP, et al. Organ preservation with radiotherapy for T1-T2 carcinoma of the pyriform sinus. *Head Neck* 2001;23:353–362.

T3 and T4 Tumors

There are several reasons why hypopharynx cancer patients who are technically resectable may not undergo primary surgery. These include age (e.g., patients over 70 to 80 years old), the presence of significant medical comorbidities, or patient unwillingness to accept total laryngectomy. Curative-intent radiation or chemoradiation is often pursued in these settings. Conventional radiation therapy commonly involves a shrinking three-field technique to deliver approximately 70 Gy in 2-Gy daily fractions to areas of gross disease and 50 to 60 Gy to areas of microscopic disease. If patients are scheduled to undergo postradiotherapy neck dissection, then gross nodal disease can be limited to 60 to 63 Gy. If patients are not candidates for postradiotherapy neck dissection, then gross nodal disease should be carried to 70 Gy. Altered fractionation regimens such as hyperfractionation or accelerated fractionation should be considered for patients being treated with radiation alone given

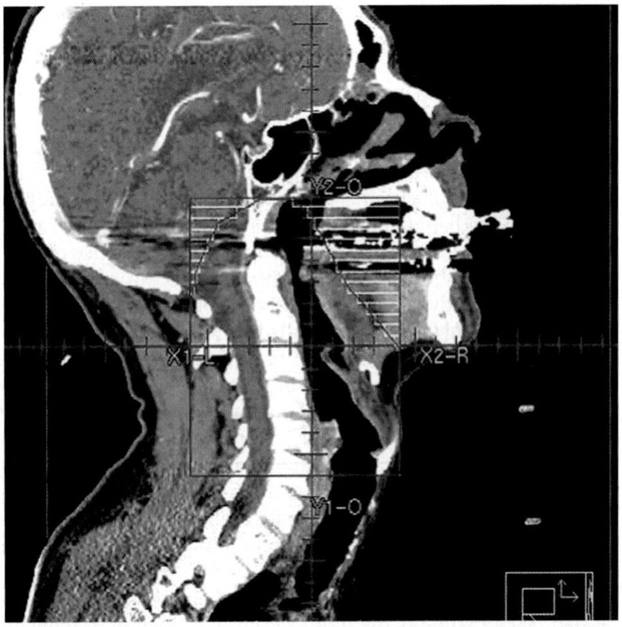

FIGURE 46.9. Digitally reconstructed radiograph depicting a classical lateral field designed to encompass the T2 pyriform sinus cancer from Figures 46.6 and 46.7 plus bilateral cervical lymphatics from skull base to cricoid, with a matching anterior low-neck field to extend the lymphatic coverage to the level of the clavicle.

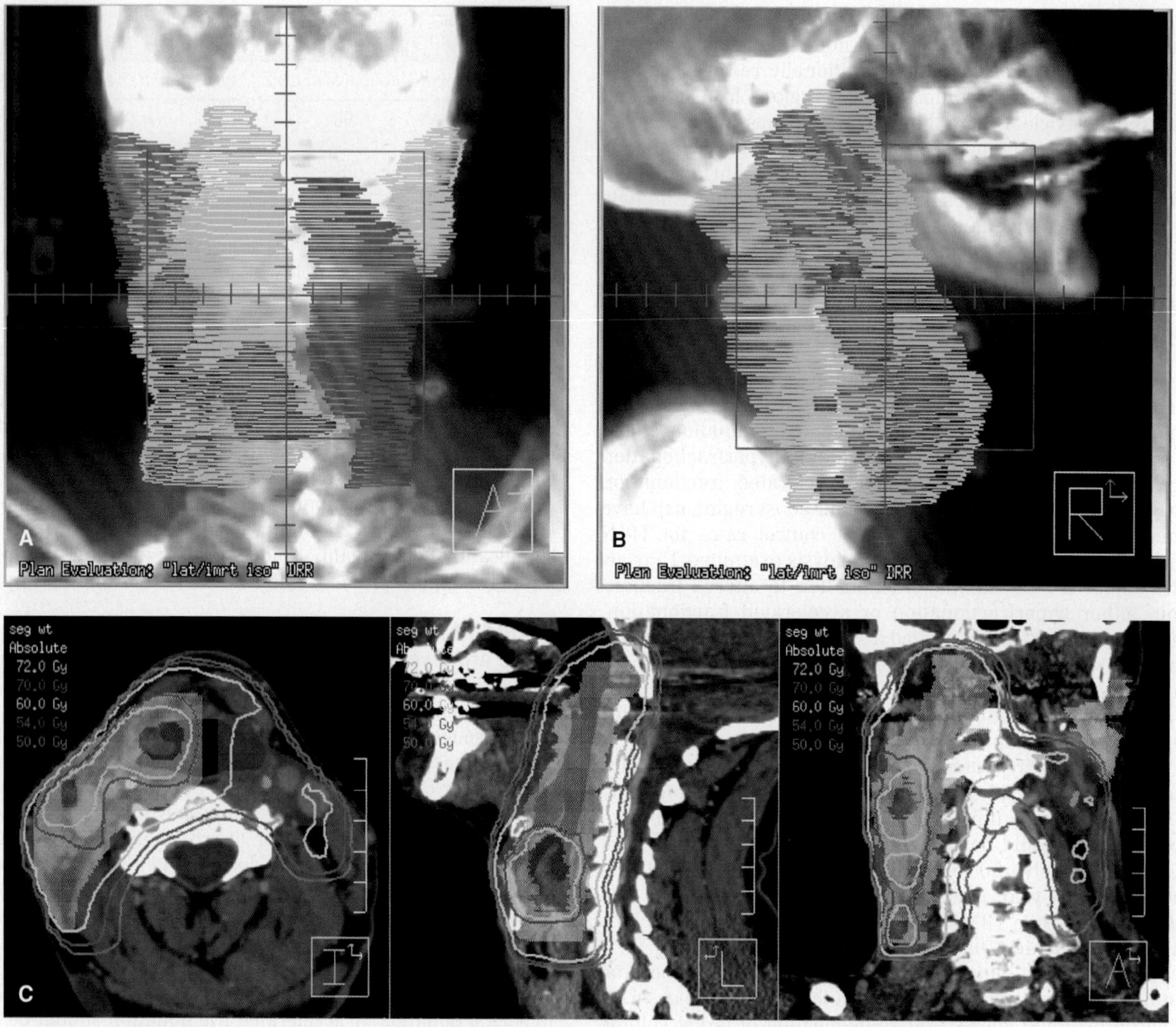

FIGURE 46.10. Beam's eye projections of intensity-modulated radiation therapy target contours for patient with T2N2bM0 tumor of the right pyriform sinus (same case as depicted in Figs. 46.6, 46.7 and 46.9). **A,B:** Depict anterior and lateral projections highlighting the GTV (*red,* 70 Gy), high-risk CTV1 (*green,* 60 Gy), low-risk CTV2 (*blue,* 54 Gy), and bilateral parotid glands. **C:** Demonstrates transverse, sagittal, and coronal treatment planning images depicting head and neck intensity-modulated radiation therapy isodose distributions for the same patient. The left parotid gland received a mean dose of 22 Gy.

the overall survival benefit observed with these approaches over standard fractionation in meta-analysis.[47]

In patients with adequate performance status, concurrent chemoradiation strategies using platinum-based chemotherapy should be considered. The recently updated meta-analysis to examine the benefit of chemotherapy in advanced H&N cancer confirms a significant survival advantage for the use of concomitant chemotherapy (6.5%), with the effect of single-agent platin significantly higher than other monochemotherapies.[43] However, this meta-analysis also confirms a steadily decreasing benefit for the use of chemotherapy with advancing patient age, such that no advantage is observed for patients over 70 years of age. This same loss of statistical benefit for patients over 70 years of age is also observed for the outcome gains derived from altered fractionation over conventional fractionation.[47] Therefore, once-daily radiation regimens without concurrent chemotherapy may be quite reasonable for hypopharynx patients over 70 years of age or for those patients with modest performance status.

Another alternative to concomitant chemotherapy or accelerated fractionation is the more recent introduction of molecular-targeted therapies in the treatment of H&N cancer patients. The most mature clinical dataset in H&N cancer involves the use of EGFR inhibitors such as cetuximab (monoclonal antibody against the EGFR). An international phase III trial comparing high-dose radiation alone versus radiation plus cetuximab in advanced H&N cancer patients confirmed a locoregional control improvement (10% at 5 years) and overall survival advantage (10% at 5 years) with the addition of cetuximab.[57,58] A relatively small subset of patients with hypopharynx cancer was enrolled in this study of 424 patients, and this subset did not demonstrate a clear advantage with use of the EGFR inhibitor treatment. Ongoing trials to examine the potential value of adding cetuximab to concurrent chemoradiation approaches in advanced H&N cancer are in progress in both the definitive and high-risk postoperative settings.

Management of hypopharynx cancer has gradually evolved over the past decades to reflect the steady advancement of nonsurgical therapy. Data from the NCDB Benchmark Reports addressing 16,136 cases diagnosed in 2000 to 2008 reveal the combination of radiation and chemotherapy to be the most common initial treatment overall for stage II (32.6%), stage III (47.8%), and stage IV (43.8%) disease.[16] Over 50% of stage III and stage IV cases received initial treatment with chemotherapy in some form—either alone or in combination with radiation or surgery. Radiation as a single-modality therapy was the most common initial treatment for stage I hypopharynx cancer (24.4%), followed by surgery alone (21.0%) as the next most

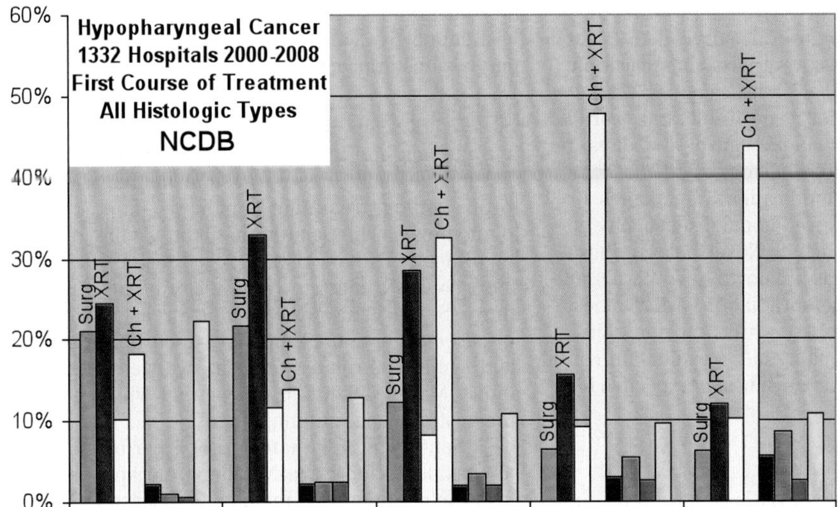

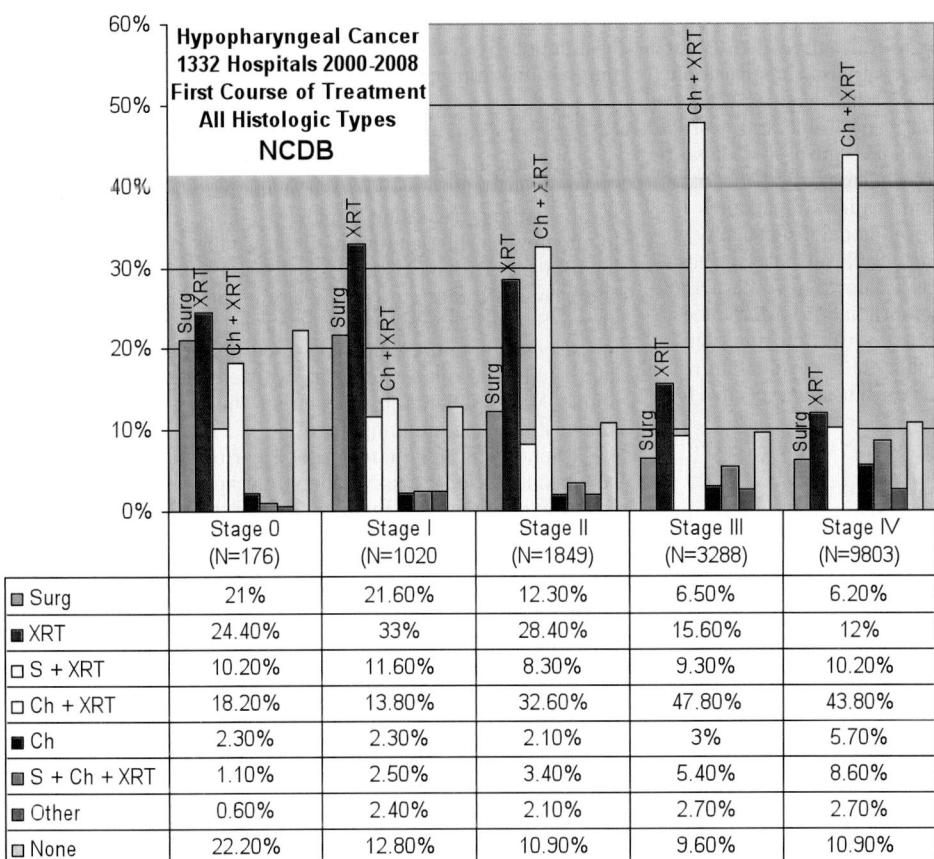

	Stage 0 (N=176)	Stage I (N=1020	Stage II (N=1849)	Stage III (N=3288)	Stage IV (N=9803)
Surg	21%	21.60%	12.30%	6.50%	6.20%
XRT	24.40%	33%	28.40%	15.60%	12%
S + XRT	10.20%	11.60%	8.30%	9.30%	10.20%
Ch + XRT	18.20%	13.80%	32.60%	47.80%	43.80%
Ch	2.30%	2.30%	2.10%	3%	5.70%
S + Ch + XRT	1.10%	2.50%	3.40%	5.40%	8.60%
Other	0.60%	2.40%	2.10%	2.70%	2.70%
None	22.20%	12.80%	10.90%	9.60%	10.90%

FIGURE 46.11. The stage-specific first course of treatment for hypopharyngeal cancer in the United States from 2000 to 2008 is presented with unknown stage excluded. S, surgery; XRT, radiotherapy; Ch, chemotherapy. (From National Cancer Data Base. Commission on Cancer. American College of Surgeons. Benchmark Reports. Available at: http://cromwell.facs.org/BMarks/BMPub/Ver10/bm_reports.cfm, with permission.)

common. It has been reported that approximately 35% to 45% of patients with advanced hypopharyngeal tumors treated with concurrent chemoradiotherapy utilizing IMRT can be expected to live 5 years, with laryngeal preservation in approximately two-thirds of survivors (Table 46.11).[59,60] These survival rates from single institutions utilizing IMRT should be interpreted cautiously in light of less favorable outcomes identified through a cross-sectional analysis of patients diagnosed with hypopharyngeal cancer in the United States in 2003. Review of the NCDB data identified 5-year observed survival for the majority of hypopharyngeal cancers (stage IV) to be only 19.8% (see Fig. 46.4).[16]

Induction Chemotherapy and Sequential (Chemo)radiation

Recently, there has been renewed interest in the concept of induction chemotherapy approaches for patients with locoregionally advanced H&N cancer. In an effort to examine the potential for organ preservation in patients with advanced cancers of the hypopharynx, the EORTC conducted a randomized trial for patients with tumors that would require total laryngectomy as the surgical approach. This trial randomly allocated patients to induction chemotherapy with cisplatin and 5-florouracil (5-FU) followed by definitive radiation versus primary surgical resection and postoperative radiation. With a median follow-up of 10 years, this trial demonstrated no significant difference in 5- or 10-year overall survival or progression-free survival. Of note, two-thirds of living patients in the chemoradiotherapy arm were able to retain their larynxes.[60]

More recently the introduction of taxane-containing regimens have been demonstrated to improve outcomes in patients receiving induction chemotherapy. Three randomized trials have been reported that compare induction 5-FU and cisplatin versus 5-FU, cisplatin, plus a taxane. The EORTC study (TAX-323) randomized patients with locoregionally advanced, unresectable disease to either induction cisplatin and fluorouracil (PF) versus induction docetaxel, cisplatin, and fluorouracil (TPF) followed by definitive radiation alone.[62] Treatment with TPF improved the median overall survival from 14.5 months to 18.8 months, with a 27% reduction in the risk of death. Similar results were noted in TAX-324, which utilized similar induction chemotherapy arms (TPF vs. PF), followed by concurrent chemoradiotherapy with carboplatin.[63] Five-year survival in the TPF arm was 52% versus 42% receiving PF, while no increased rates of gastric feeding tubes or tracheostomies were noted between groups. A subgroup analysis of larynx and hypopharynx patients demonstrated improved survival in these patients, as well as higher rates of laryngectomy-free survival.[64]

In addition to enhanced survival outcomes, a recent randomized French study demonstrated that TPF induction chemotherapy (compared to PF induction) results in superior tumor response rates (80% vs. 59%) as assessed by laryngoscopy and CT or MRI.[65] Those with response to induction chemotherapy were treated with organ-preserving (chemo)radiotherapy, while nonresponders received laryngectomy and postoperative (chemo)radiation. The higher response rates in the TPF arm

TABLE 46.11 ONCOLOGIC OUTCOMES FOR PATIENTS UNDERGOING CONCURRENT CHEMORADIOTHERAPY AND INTENSITY-MODULATED RADIATION THERAPY FOR ADVANCED HYPOPHARYNGEAL CANCERS

Study (Reference)	Total Patients in Study (n)	Stage	# of Patients per Stage (%)	Larynx Preservation Rate (%)	5-Year OS (%)
Huang et al. (58)	33	II	2 (6%)	67	44
		III	5 (15%)		
		IV	26 (79%)		
Liu et al. (59)	27	II	5 (19%)	63	35
		III	4 (15%)		
		IV	18 (66%)		

OS, overall survival.

allowed for higher rates of laryngeal preservation (70% vs. 57% at 3 years), without a detriment in overall survival (60% at 3 years in both arms). These aggressive approaches certainly appear worthy of consideration for H&N subsites such as hypopharynx where the organ preservation is desirable and overall outcomes are poor, with both locoregional control and distant metastases presenting a formidable challenge. Patients with good performance status, no contraindications to taxanes or platins, a high tumor burden or advanced nodal disease may be optimal candidates for this approach.[66] Nevertheless, these strategies are costly and toxic, and it is unknown how these outcomes compare to concurrent chemoradiation approaches. Careful assessment of tumor control, survival, and long-term functional outcome dovetailed with quality-of-life evaluation will be important to help place these regimens in best perspective for advanced H&N cancer patients.

Postradiotherapy Neck Dissection

Patients with hypopharynx cancer also require careful evaluation regarding regional nodal metastases. For N0 or N1 patients treated with primary radiation or chemoradiation approaches, adjuvant neck dissection is generally unnecessary. However, for patients presenting with N2 or N3 neck disease, careful evaluation of tumor response in the neck is important to help gauge the potential value of adjuvant neck dissection following radiation or chemoradiation. An increasing number of reports suggest that detailed imaging of the neck 12 weeks postradiation with FDG-PET can serve as a valuable guide to help select those patients warranting adjuvant neck dissection. One such study from the University of Iowa assessed the value of a postradiation FDG-PET to help select those patients who might benefit most from subsequent neck dissection. For complete clinical responders, the Iowa study concluded that FDG-PET in this setting has a very high negative predictive value. The authors suggest that FDG-PET may be a valuable tool to help determine which patients should undergo adjuvant neck dissection versus observation following the completion of H&N radiation or (chemo)radiotherapy.[67] Despite these emerging data, many institutions mandate adjuvant neck dissection for all patients presenting with N2 or N3 neck disease in an effort to maximize regional disease control.[68–70] Both approaches are readily defendable at present. If neck dissection is performed, this provides an opportunity for the surgeon to reassess the primary tumor site under anesthesia with directed biopsy if suspicious for residual disease. If residual disease at the primary site is highly suspected or confirmed by biopsy several months following completion of radiation or chemoradiation, this will prompt consideration regarding the feasibility and advisability of salvage surgery options.

Palliative Radiotherapy

The management of patients with unresectable locoregional disease without distant metastases is dependent on patient performance status. A patient with a good performance status may be offered definitive radiotherapy, concurrent chemoradiotherapy, or induction chemotherapy with sequential (chemo)radiotherapy, as discussed above. However, patients with poor performance status who are not considered candidates for aggressive radiation or chemoradiation approaches should be managed with palliative intent. This may include short course radiation regimens such as 4 to 5 Gy × 5 fractions over 1 to 2 weeks with repeat of the same 3 weeks hence if favorable initial tolerance and response is achieved. A recent study suggests using a 3.7 Gy fraction twice daily × 2 consecutive days for 3 cycles every 2 to 3 weeks, as described in RTOG-85-02, may have similar palliative efficacy with less toxicity as compared to other palliative regimens.[71] Other approaches described include 50 Gy in 16 fractions[72] and 30 Gy in 5 fractions, 2 fractions per week.[73] Systemic chemotherapy alone can be considered, although for poor performance status patients, best supportive care with medical therapy and airway control may also be appropriate.

Palliative Chemotherapy

As many as one-quarter of hypopharynx cancer patients will develop metastatic disease at some point in their clinical course. In this setting, treatment is palliative and should be delivered to maximize or help maintain quality of life. If patients are having difficulty with local pain, bleeding, or swallowing, palliative short-course radiation therapy can be delivered, as described above. Surgery may also provide a reasonable palliative option for selected patients who have incurable disease but significant symptoms related to their localized disease, as described above. Many patients in this setting will benefit from narcotic analgesics for pain management.

Patients with adequate or good performance status should be considered for palliative chemotherapy. Median overall survival for patients with metastatic disease is 6 to 10 months.[74] Single-agent cisplatin is usually the first regimen, as it has been shown to improve overall survival.[75] Combinations of cytotoxic chemotherapies have demonstrated improved response rates over cisplatin alone, but have not improved survival and are accompanied by increased toxicity[76] and therefore are uncommonly utilized. However, recent randomized studies have shown efficacy of the anti-EGFR monoclonal antibody cetuximab. In combination with cisplatin as first-line treatment, cetuximab improved overall survival from 7.4 months to 10.1 months over cisplatin alone.[77] As second-line therapy in patients who have progressed through platinum-based chemotherapy, cetuximab also has demonstrable activity as either monotherapy[78] or in combination with platinum-based chemotherapy.[79]

COMPLICATIONS

Surgery

The complications from surgery generally fall within the confines of bleeding, infection, reaction to the anesthesia, and damage to structures around or in the field of surgery. The damage to the laryngopharynx that occurs in the course of removing those tissues involved by cancer necessarily interferes with key laryngeal functions: breathing, swallowing, and speaking.

If an effort is made to preserve laryngeal function, some compromise may be required. A long-term tracheotomy, nothing by mouth status with the use of gastrostomy feedings, and significant dysphonia are not uncommon for patients with hypopharynx cancer treated with conservation laryngeal surgery. These same complications may attend the more comprehensive laryngopharyngectomy as well. Stenosis of the neopharynx, difficulty with alaryngeal speech, and stomal stenosis may compromise the same functions ordinarily ascribed to the larynx. For all open surgical approaches, the risk of a salivary fistula is greatest for those patients previously treated with radiation. Although salivary fistulas are rare with endoscopic approaches, they have occurred in cases requiring aggressive laser resection.

Radiation Therapy

During a course of H&N radiation therapy, there are predictable side effects that are experienced by the majority of patients: mucositis, fatigue, loss of taste acuity, radiation dermatitis, and xerostomia. Typically patients will begin to experience mucositis during the third week of radiotherapy. This initially manifests as mucosal blanching within the treatment field, but can progress to patchy or confluent mucositis. Initially patients can be treated with an over-the-counter pain reliever, but once patients develop grade II or III mucositis, they will commonly require narcotic analgesics for adequate pain control. The combination of dysphagia and mucositis can result in significant nutritional compromise necessitating intravenous hydration and parenteral nutritional supplementation. Nausea associated with treatment can also further complicate the nutritional status. These acute toxicities can become particularly pronounced in the setting of intensified radiation fractionation schedules or combined chemoradiotherapy. Patients may require prophylactic antiemetics. In patients receiving concurrent radiotherapy and platinum-based chemotherapy, there is clear potential for myelosuppression; therefore, blood counts should be monitored regularly. Signs or symptoms of infection should be addressed promptly. Finally, xerostomia can become problematic during the course of radiation. Ultimately, patients can be reassured that the majority of these side effects, with the exception of xerostomia, are temporary and will resolve several weeks to months following completion of therapy.

As noted, one of the acute side effects of radiotherapy that can become permanent is xerostomia. Chemical and physical modifiers of the radiation response have been utilized to reduce long-term xerostomia. The free radical scavenger amifostine has the potential to reduce radiation effects on normal tissues if administered just prior to each radiation fraction. A randomized phase III trial demonstrated a reduction in the severity of the acute and chronic grade 2 or higher xerostomia in patients who received amifostine during RT.[80] Dose-limiting toxicities commonly include hypotension and nausea. There has been concern over possible tumor-protective effects of amifostine, but a recent meta-analysis does not suggest this.[81] However, data supporting the use of amifostine to reduce xerostomia has been generated in the setting of conventional radiation, and the magnitude of benefit on xerostomia of parotid-sparing IMRT appears greater than that of amifostine.[55,56] Therefore, the ultimate value of amifostine in patients with advanced H&N cancer, especially in the setting of IMRT, has been called into question.[82] Currently there is no universal standard recommendation across treatment centers for the use of this radioprotector.

In some cases, hypopharynx cancer patients who complete a course of radiation therapy will be noted to have persistent laryngeal edema on subsequent follow-up visits. Although in the early posttreatment phase (in fact up to 24 months), significant or newfound edema should raise suspicion regarding the possibility of persistent or recurrent disease; the majority of patients who receive high-dose radiation across major segments of the larynx and hypopharynx will manifest some degree of edema, mucosal congestion, and eventual fibrosis (see Fig. 46.6B). Generally, this collateral damage is a tolerable chronic toxicity with modest impact on patient quality of life. However, in approximately 10% to 15% of patients, this edema is severe enough to cause significant airway and swallow function compromise requiring tracheostomy.

LONG-TERM FOLLOW-UP

Regardless of whether patients undergo primary surgery or radiation therapy, there is value in close posttreatment surveillance by H&N surgeon and radiation oncologist in a multidisciplinary fashion. Follow-up care is designed initially to survey for recurrence. As duration from time of intervention to clinic visits lengthen, the focus shifts to surveillance for second primaries (i.e., lung), to address morbidity from treatment, and to provide generalized support.

During the first 6 months after treatment, patients should be followed every 4 to 6 weeks with clinical examination, including fiberoptic nasopharyngoscopy. Recommended guidelines include a follow-up visit every 1 to 3 months during the first year, every 2 to 4 months for the second year, every 4 to 6 months for years 3 through 5, and every 6 to 12 months thereafter. Additionally, if the patient received comprehensive H&N radiation, the serum thyroid-stimulating hormone level should be measured every 6 to 12 months. Imaging evaluation of the neck, most commonly with CT or MRI scan, are obtained at 3- to 6-month intervals during the first 2 years or as indicated based on clinical findings. Functional imaging with ^{18}FDG-PET can sometimes prove valuable to help differentiate posttreatment fibrosis from persistent or recurrent disease.

A study by Hermans et al.[83] examined findings on CT scan of the neck 3 to 4 months following completion of radiation therapy for patients with larynx or hypopharynx cancer to examine correlation with long-term outcome. The authors suggest that in patients achieving complete radiographic resolution of all pretreatment disease, the likelihood of subsequent local failure is very small. These patients might therefore undergo routine clinical examination, with repeat imaging reserved for instances where the clinical examination becomes suspicious for recurrence. For patients who achieved <50% reduction in tumor volume or retained a mass 1 cm or larger on the posttreatment imaging study, the likelihood of local failure was 100% and 30%, respectively. In these patients, repeat CT at 3 to 4 months, FDG-PET, or biopsy is therefore recommended. Preliminary reports indicate that the results of the first post-RT FDG-PET scan may be a strong predictor of developing locoregional disease recurrence.[67]

In the posttreatment setting of hypopharynx cancer patients, the involvement of an experienced H&N radiologist is highly desirable for optimal interpretation of imaging results. Soft tissue changes following ablative surgery and reconstruction, or following high-dose radiation or chemoradiation with resultant edema and fibrosis, can be very difficult to differentiate from tumor, particularly for the inexperienced reader.

MANAGEMENT OF RECURRENCE

After completion of treatment, patients should be followed closely for signs of recurrent or persistent disease. If recurrence is suspected, this should be confirmed by biopsy. If biopsy is confirmatory, then the patient should undergo complete restaging to assess the extent of disease. In the setting of local or regional disease alone, patients treated with initial radiation or chemoradiation can be considered for surgical salvage therapy. Although salvage surgery following comprehensive H&N radiation and chemotherapy presents several resection and reconstructive healing challenges for the surgeon, selected patients may still derive long-term benefit from this approach. Select patients with low-volume localized disease may be candidates for transoral laser microsurgery for recurrent disease following radiation.[84] Recurrent patients who initially received comprehensive H&N radiation have traditionally not been considered good candidates for repeat high-dose radiation in light of normal tissue tolerances. However, two recent prospective RTOG studies have demonstrated that reirradiation to the H&N is feasible.[85,86] With the advent of highly conformal radiation delivery techniques, selected patients may benefit from reirradiation approaches in conjunction with systemic chemotherapy.[87] A retrospective study from Memorial Sloan-Kettering Cancer Center has suggested that IMRT is beneficial for local control in this setting,[88] and a recent prospective trial of reirradiation utilizing IMRT suggests long-term disease control can be achieved in select patients with tolerable toxicity.[89] Many patients with recurrent disease, however, are not good candidates for aggressive surgery or salvage radiation therapy and are best served with systemic chemotherapy or best supportive care approaches.

QUALITY OF LIFE

Assessment of parameters, including functional status, organ preservation, treatment cost, and patient-assessment of quality of life (QOL), play an increasingly important role in the evaluation of overall treatment efficacy. For larynx and hypopharynx cancer patients, a focus of contemporary clinical investigation has been the study of treatments designed to preserve laryngeal function for patients traditionally treated with total laryngectomy. A frequently cited but somewhat controversial study by McNeil et al.[90] employed a questionnaire administered to healthy individuals and concluded that some might forgo total laryngectomy in favor of alternative therapy, even if this choice diminished their ultimate chance for cure. A more recent report by El-Deiry et al.[91] evaluated long-term QOL in a matched pair analysis comparing the surgical and nonsurgical treatment of patients with advanced H&N cancer involving the oropharynx, hypopharynx and larynx. Although patients in the surgery arm demonstrated worse speech outcomes than those treated with chemoradiation, this difference did not carry over to the overall QOL score. These investigators concluded that, although it seems reasonable that organ preservation (nonsurgical) treatment will uniformly result in a higher QOL, the complexities of human adjustment and multitude of potential treatment effects render this assumption invalid for many patients. Alternatively, a study from the Medical University of South Carolina compared swallow-related QOL after surgery or radiotherapy for H&N cancer using a dysphagia symptom survey, the M.D. Anderson Dysphagia Inventory (MDADI). They found significantly better scores on the emotional and functional components of the MDADI for patients undergoing chemoradiation compared to those undergoing surgery followed by radiation.[92]

There have been relatively few prospective assessments of QOL following treatment for H&N cancer. In a subset of locally advanced patients requiring radical surgery, such as total laryngectomy and partial pharyngectomy, the functional deficits are predictable. However, for patients undergoing organ preservation with radiation alone or in combination with chemotherapy, it can be difficult to assess the true extent and quality of organ preservation. Regardless of the primary treatment approach, these patients often require long-term speech, swallow, and dental rehabilitation. A study from Meyer et al.[93] retrospectively assessed speech intelligibility and QOL in survivors of H&N cancer. A total of 64 patients were enrolled; 31 underwent RT alone, 5 surgery alone, and 28 received both. All patients underwent comprehensive subjective and objective testing of speech function and QOL. They found significant subjective and objective deficits in speech and QOL even 5 years after completion of therapy. Terrell et al.[94] reported the results of a self-administered health survey of 570 patients at a Veterans' Administration hospital that demonstrated that the single most notable event having a negative impact on QOL was placement of a feeding tube. This was followed by medical comorbid conditions, presence of a tracheotomy tube, chemotherapy, and neck dissection.

A prospective study on QOL utilizing the EORTC QLQ-C30 and QLQ-H&N35 questionnaires was conducted in Sweden on 357 patients. This study found that QOL issues were significantly associated with the site of origin, with stage at diagnosis being the most important predictor. Additionally, patients with hypopharynx cancer exhibited the poorest QOL.[95] Similarly, another study prospectively examining swallow function in H&N cancer patients demonstrated that worse swallowing was associated with hypopharyngeal tumor sites.[96] Although the use of IMRT can have a significant impact on xerostomia and QOL measures in H&N cancer patients,[97,98] the intimate approximation of hypopharyngeal tumors to pharyngeal constrictor musculature does not allow for sparing of these structures vital to long-term swallow function, likely contributing to the poorer QOL of hypopharynx patients in comparison to other H&N cancer patients.[99]

CONCLUSION

Patients with cancers of the hypopharynx commonly present with advanced disease associated with varying degrees of compromise in speech or swallow function. Many hypopharynx cancer patients also carry significant medical and social comorbidities. Typically, small T1 or T2 lesions can be managed with either primary radiation or surgery, with similar clinical outcome. For intermediate-stage disease that would require laryngopharyngectomy for the surgical approach, an increasingly preferred treatment option is combined chemoradiation that has demonstrated equivalence to immediate surgery in cancer survival, however, with improved organ preservation and functional outcome. For bulky hypopharynx tumors with significant airway compromise, laryngeal distortion, and cartilage destruction, it is generally best to proceed with definitive surgery with postoperative radiation or chemoradiation.

Despite an aggressive approach in the overall management of hypopharynx cancer patients, ultimate cure rates remain quite poor. There are relatively few early-stage patients; and for many advanced-stage patients, it is difficult to achieve long-term control. Even for those patients with excellent response to therapy, there exists a continuous risk for the development of second malignancies, particularly of the upper aerodigestive track with long-term follow-up. Posttreatment patients often require aggressive speech and swallow therapy to maximize their functional outcome. There is significant interest in the incorporation of molecular targeted therapies in combination with traditional cytotoxic therapy and radiation in an effort to improve outcomes.

REFERENCES

1. Brugere J, Guenel P, Leclerc A, et al. Differential effects of tobacco and alcohol in cancer of the larynx, pharynx, and mouth. *Cancer* 1986;57:391–395.
2. Schechter GL, Kalafsky JT. Cancer of the hypopharynx and cervical esophagus: management concepts. *Oncology (Williston Park)* 1988;2:17–24, 34–35.
3. Spitz MR. Epidemiology and risk factors for head and neck cancer. *Semin Oncol* 1994;21:281–288.
4. Cooper JS, Porter K, Mallin K, et al. National Cancer Database report on cancer of the head and neck: 10-year update. *Head Neck* 2009;31:748–758.
5. Surveillance E and End-Results (SEER) Program. SEER*Stat Database: Incidence—SEER 17 Regs Research Data, Nov. 2010 sub (2000–2008). National Cancer Institute, DCCPS, Surveillance Research Program, Cancer Statistics Branch. Released April 2011.
6. Hoffman HT, Karnell LH, Shah JP, et al. Hypopharyngeal cancer patient care evaluation. *Laryngoscope* 1997;107:1005–1017.
7. Popescu CR, Bertesteanu SV, Mirea D, et al. The epidemiology of hypopharynx and cervical esophagus cancer. *J Med Life* 2010;3:396–401.
8. Boffetta P, Richiardi L, Berrino F, et al. Occupation and larynx and hypopharynx cancer: an international case-control study in France, Italy, Spain, and Switzerland. *Cancer Causes Control* 2003;14:203–212.
9. Shangina O, Brennan P, Szeszenia-Dabrowska N, et al. Occupational exposure and laryngeal and hypopharyngeal cancer risk in central and eastern Europe. *Am J Epidemiol* 2006;164:367–375.
10. Davies L, Welch HG. Epidemiology of head and neck cancer in the United States. *Otolaryngol Head Neck Surg* 2006;135:451–457.
11. Klussmann JP, Weissenborn SJ, Wieland U, et al. Prevalence, distribution, and viral load of human papillomavirus 16 DNA in tonsillar carcinomas. *Cancer* 2001; 92:2875–2884.
12. Mineta H, Ogino T, Amano HM, et al. Human papilloma virus (HPV) type 16 and 18 detected in head and neck squamous cell carcinoma. *Anticancer Res* 1998; 18:4765–4768.
13. Ribeiro KB, Levi JE, Pawlita M, et al. Low human papillomavirus prevalence in head and neck cancer: results from two large case-control studies in high-incidence regions. *Int J Epidemiol* 2011;40:489–502.
14. Spector JG, Sessions DG, Emami B, et al. Squamous cell carcinoma of the pyriform sinus: a nonrandomized comparison of therapeutic modalities and long-term results. *Laryngoscope* 1995;105:397–406.
15. Spector JG, Sessions DG, Emami B, et al. Squamous cell carcinomas of the aryepiglottic fold: therapeutic results and long-term follow-up. *Laryngoscope* 1995; 105:734–746.
16. National Cancer Data Base. Commission on Cancer. American College of Surgeons Benchmark Reports. Available at: http://www.facs.org/cancer/ncdb/. Accessed August 24, 2011.
17. Dikshit RP, Boffetta P, Bouchardy C, et al. Lifestyle habits as prognostic factors in survival of laryngeal and hypopharyngeal cancer: a multicentric European study. *Int J Cancer* 2005;117:992–995.
18. Chang F, Syrjanen S, Syrjanen K. Implications of the p53 tumor-suppressor gene in clinical oncology. *J Clin Oncol* 1995;13:1009–1022.
19. Frank JL, Bur ME, Garb JL, et al. p53 tumor suppressor oncogene expression in squamous cell carcinoma of the hypopharynx. *Cancer* 1994;73:181–186.
20. Frank JL, Garb JL, Banson BB, et al. Epidermal growth factor receptor expression in squamous cell carcinoma of the hypopharynx. *Surg Oncol* 1993;2:161–167.
21. Pivot X, Magne N, Guardiola E, et al. Prognostic impact of the epidermal growth factor receptor levels for patients with larynx and hypopharynx cancer. *Oral Oncol* 2005;41:320–327.
22. Magne N, Pivot X, Bensadoun RJ, et al. The relationship of epidermal growth factor receptor levels to the prognosis of unresectable pharyngeal cancer patients treated by chemo-radiotherapy. *Eur J Cancer* 2001;37:2169–2177.
23. Edge SB, Byrd DR, Compton CC, et al. *AJCC cancer staging handbook,* 7th ed. New York: Springer, 2010.
24. Spector JG, Sessions DG, Haughey BH, et al. Delayed regional metastases, distant metastases, and second primary malignancies in squamous cell carcinomas of the larynx and hypopharynx. *Laryngoscope* 2001;111:1079–1087.

25. Ho CM, Lam KH, Wei WI, et al. Squamous cell carcinoma of the hypopharynx—analysis of treatment results. *Head Neck* 1993;15:405–412.
26. Koo BS, Lim YC, Lee JS, et al. Management of contralateral N0 neck in pyriform sinus carcinoma. *Laryngoscope* 2006;116:1268–1272.
27. Mukherji SK, Armao D, Joshi VM. Cervical nodal metastases in squamous cell carcinoma of the head and neck: what to expect. *Head Neck* 2001;23:995–1005.
28. Lindberg R. Distribution of cervical lymph node metastases from squamous cell carcinoma of the upper respiratory and digestive tracts. *Cancer* 1972;29:1446–1449.
29. Muir C, Weiland L. Upper aerodigestive tract cancers. *Cancer* 1995;75:147–153.
30. Marks JE, Kurnik B, Powers WE, et al. Carcinoma of the pyriform sinus. An analysis of treatment results and patterns of failure. *Cancer* 1978;41:1008–1015.
31. Thawley SE. *Comprehensive management of head and neck tumors.* Philadelphia: WB Saunders, 1999.
32. Di Martino E, Nowak B, Hassan HA, et al. Diagnosis and staging of head and neck cancer: a comparison of modern imaging modalities (positron emission tomography, computed tomography, color-coded duplex sonography) with panendoscopic and histopathologic findings. *Arch Otolaryngol Head Neck Surg* 2000; 126:1457–1461.
33. Schwartz DL, Rajendran J, Yueh B, et al. FDG-PET prediction of head and neck squamous cell cancer outcomes. *Arch Otolaryngol Head Neck Surg* 2004;130: 1361–1367.
34. Lonneux M, Hamoir M, Reychler H, et al. Positron emission tomography with [18F]fluorodeoxyglucose improves staging and patient management in patients with head and neck squamous cell carcinoma: a multicenter prospective study. *J Clin Oncol* 2010;28:1190–1195.
35. Gilbert RW, Neligan PC. Microsurgical laryngotracheal reconstruction. *Clin Plas Surg* 2005;32:293–301.
36. Karatzanis AD, Psychogios G, Waldfahrer F, et al. T1 and T2 hypopharyngeal cancer treatment with laser microsurgery. *J Surg Oncol* 2010;102:27–33.
37. Martin A, Jackel MC, Christiansen H, et al. Organ preserving transoral laser microsurgery for cancer of the hypopharynx. *Laryngoscope* 2008;118:398–402.
38. Steiner W, Ambrosch P, Hess CF, et al. Organ preservation by transoral laser microsurgery in piriform sinus carcinoma. *Otolaryngol Head Neck Surg* 2001; 124:58–67.
39. Boudreaux BA, Rosenthal EL, Magnuson JS, et al. Robot-assisted surgery for upper aerodigestive tract neoplasms. *Arch Otolaryngol Head Neck Surg* 2009; 135:397–401.
40. Cooper JS, Pajak TF, Forastiere AA, et al. Postoperative concurrent radiotherapy and chemotherapy for high-risk squamous-cell carcinoma of the head and neck. *N Engl J Med* 2004;350:1937–1944.
41. Bernier J, Domenge C, Ozsahin M, et al. Postoperative irradiation with or without concomitant chemotherapy for locally advanced head and neck cancer. *N Engl J Med* 2004;350:1945–1952.
42. Bernier J, Cooper JS, Pajak TF, et al. Defining risk levels in locally advanced head and neck cancers: a comparative analysis of concurrent postoperative radiation plus chemotherapy trials of the EORTC (#22931) and RTOG (#9501). *Head Neck* 2005;27:843–850.
43. Pignon JP, le Maitre A, Maillard E, et al. Meta-analysis of chemotherapy in head and neck cancer (MACH-NC): an update on 93 randomised trials and 17,346 patients. *Radiother Oncol* 2009;92:4–14.
44. Fu KK, Pajak TF, Trotti A, et al. A Radiation Therapy Oncology Group (RTOG) phase III randomized study to compare hyperfractionation and two variants of accelerated fractionation to standard fractionation radiotherapy for head and neck squamous cell carcinomas: first report of RTOG 9003. *Int J Radiat Oncol Biol Phys* 2000;48:7–16.
45. Overgaard J, Hansen HS, Specht L, et al. Five compared with six fractions per week of conventional radiotherapy of squamous-cell carcinoma of head and neck: DAHANCA 6 and 7 randomised controlled trial. *Lancet* 2003;362:933–940.
46. Skladowski K, Maciejewski B, Golen M, et al. Continuous accelerated 7-days-a-week radiotherapy for head-and-neck cancer: long-term results of phase III clinical trial. *Int J Radiat Oncol Biol Phys* 2006;66:706–713.
47. Bourhis J, Overgaard J, Audry H, et al. Hyperfractionated or accelerated radiotherapy in head and neck cancer: a meta-analysis. *Lancet* 2006;368:843–854.
48. Amdur RJ, Mendenhall WM, Stringer SP, et al. Organ preservation with radiotherapy for T1-T2 carcinoma of the pyriform sinus. *Head Neck* 2001;23:353–362.
49. Garden AS, Morrison WH, Clayman GL, et al. Early squamous cell carcinoma of the hypopharynx: outcomes of treatment with radiation alone to the primary disease. *Head Neck* 1996;18:317–322.
50. Nakamura K, Shioyama Y, Kawashima M, et al. Multi-institutional analysis of early squamous cell carcinoma of the hypopharynx treated with radical radiotherapy. *Int J Radiat Oncol Biol Phys* 2006;65:1045–1050.
51. Yoshimura R, Kagami Y, Ito Y, et al. Outcomes in patients with early-stage hypopharyngeal cancer treated with radiotherapy. *Int J Radiat Oncol Biol Phys* 2010;77:1017–1023.
52. Fein DA, Mendenhall WM, Parsons JT, et al. Pharyngeal wall carcinoma treated with radiotherapy: impact of treatment technique and fractionation. *Int J Radiat Oncol Biol Phys* 1993;26:751–757.
53. Hong TS, Tome WA, Chappell RJ, et al. The impact of daily setup variations on head-and-neck intensity-modulated radiation therapy. *Int J Radiat Oncol Biol Phys* 2005;61:779–788.
54. Eisbruch A, Ship JA, Dawson LA, et al. Salivary gland sparing and improved target irradiation by conformal and intensity modulated irradiation of head and neck cancer. *World J Surg* 2003;27:832–837.
55. Eisbruch A, Ten Haken RK, Kim HM, et al. Dose, volume, and function relationships in parotid salivary glands following conformal and intensity-modulated irradiation of head and neck cancer. *Int J Radiat Oncol Biol Phys* 1999;45: 577–587.
56. Nutting CM, Morden JP, Harrington KJ, et al. Parotid-sparing intensity modulated versus conventional radiotherapy in head and neck cancer (PARSPORT): a phase 3 multicentre randomised controlled trial. *Lancet Oncol* 2011;12:127–136.
57. Bonner JA, Harari PM, Giralt J, et al. Radiotherapy plus cetuximab for squamous-cell carcinoma of the head and neck. *N Engl J Med* 2006;354:567–578.
58. Bonner JA, Harari PM, Giralt J, et al. Radiotherapy plus cetuximab for locoregionally advanced head and neck cancer: 5-year survival data from a phase 3 randomised trial, and relation between cetuximab-induced rash and survival. *Lancet Oncol* 2010;11:21–28.
59. Huang WY, Jen YM, Chen CM, et al. Intensity modulated radiotherapy with concurrent chemotherapy for larynx preservation of advanced resectable hypopharyngeal cancer. *Radiat Oncol* 2010;5:37.
60. Liu WS, Hsin CH, Chou YH, et al. Long-term results of intensity-modulated radiotherapy concomitant with chemotherapy for hypopharyngeal carcinoma aimed at laryngeal preservation. *BMC Cancer* 2010;10:102.
61. Lefebvre JL, Chevalier D, Luboinski B, et al. Larynx preservation in pyriform sinus cancer: preliminary results of a European Organization for Research and Treatment of Cancer phase III trial. EORTC Head and Neck Cancer Cooperative Group. *J Natl Cancer Inst* 1996;88:890–899.
62. Vermorken JB, Remenar E, van Herpen C, et al. Cisplatin, fluorouracil, and docetaxel in unresectable head and neck cancer. *N Engl J Med* 2007;357:1695–1704.
63. Lorch JH, Goloubeva O, Haddad RI, et al. Induction chemotherapy with cisplatin and fluorouracil alone or in combination with docetaxel in locally advanced squamous-cell cancer of the head and neck: long-term results of the TAX 324 randomised phase 3 trial. *Lancet Oncol* 2011;12:153–159.
64. Posner MR, Norris CM, Wirth LJ, et al. Sequential therapy for the locally advanced larynx and hypopharynx cancer subgroup in TAX 324: survival, surgery, and organ preservation. *Ann Oncol* 2009;20:921–927.
65. Pointreau Y, Garaud P, Chapet S, et al. Randomized trial of induction chemotherapy with cisplatin and 5-fluorouracil with or without docetaxel for larynx preservation. *J Natl Cancer Inst* 2009;101:498–506.
66. Budach V. TPF sequential therapy: when and for whom? *Oncologist* 2010;15 (Suppl 3):13–18.
67. Yao M, Smith RB, Graham MM, et al. The role of FDG PET in management of neck metastasis from head-and-neck cancer after definitive radiation treatment. *Int J Radiat Oncol Biol Phys* 2005;63:991–999.
68. Boyd TS, Harari PM, Tannehill SP, et al. Planned postradiotherapy neck dissection in patients with advanced head and neck cancer. *Head Neck* 1998;20: 132–137.
69. Stenson KM, Haraf DJ, Pelzer H, et al. The role of cervical lymphadenectomy after aggressive concomitant chemoradiotherapy: the feasibility of selective neck dissection. *Arch Otolaryngol Head Neck Surg* 2000;126:950–956.
70. Wang SJ, Wang MB, Yip H, et al. Combined radiotherapy with planned neck dissection for small head and neck cancers with advanced cervical metastases. *Laryngoscope* 2000;110:1794–1797.
71. Chen AM, Vaughan A, Narayan S, et al. Palliative radiation therapy for head and neck cancer: toward an optimal fractionation scheme. *Head Neck* 2008;30: 1586–1591.
72. Al-mamgani A, Tans L, Van rooij PH, et al. Hypofractionated radiotherapy denoted as the "Christie scheme": an effective means of palliating patients with head and neck cancers not suitable for curative treatment. *Acta Oncol* 2009; 48:562–570.
73. Porceddu SV, Rosser B, Burmeister BH, et al. Hypofractionated radiotherapy for the palliation of advanced head and neck cancer in patients unsuitable for curative treatment—"Hypo Trial." *Radiother Oncol* 2007;85:456–462.
74. Argiris A, Karamouzis MV, Raben D, et al. Head and neck cancer. *Lancet* 2008; 371:1695–1709.
75. Morton RP, Rugman F, Dorman EB, et al. Cisplatinum and bleomycin for advanced or recurrent squamous cell carcinoma of the head and neck: a randomised factorial phase III controlled trial. *Cancer Chemother Pharmacol* 1985;15:283–289.
76. Clavel M, Vermorken JB, Cognetti F, et al. Randomized comparison of cisplatin, methotrexate, bleomycin and vincristine (CABO) versus cisplatin and 5-fluorouracil (CF) versus cisplatin (C) in recurrent or metastatic squamous cell carcinoma of the head and neck. A phase III study of the EORTC Head and Neck Cancer Cooperative Group. *Ann Oncol* 1994;5:521–526.
77. Vermorken JB, Mesia R, Rivera F, et al. Platinum-based chemotherapy plus cetuximab in head and neck cancer. *N Engl J Med* 2008;359:1116–1127.
78. Vermorken JB, Trigo J, Hitt R, et al. Open-label, uncontrolled, multicenter phase II study to evaluate the efficacy and toxicity of cetuximab as a single agent in patients with recurrent and/or metastatic squamous cell carcinoma of the head and neck who failed to respond to platinum-based therapy. *J Clin Oncol* 2007; 25:2171–2177.
79. Baselga J, Trigo JM, Bourhis J, et al. Phase II multicenter study of the antiepidermal growth factor receptor monoclonal antibody cetuximab in combination with platinum-based chemotherapy in patients with platinum-refractory metastatic and/or recurrent squamous cell carcinoma of the head and neck. *J Clin Oncol* 2005;23:5568–5577.
80. Brizel DM, Wasserman TH, Henke M, et al. Phase III randomized trial of amifostine as a radioprotector in head and neck cancer. *J Clin Oncol* 2000;18: 3339–3345.
81. Bourhis J, Blanchard P, Maillard E, et al. Effect of amifostine on survival among patients treated with radiotherapy: a meta-analysis of individual patient data. *J Clin Oncol* 2011;29:2590–2597.
82. Eisbruch A. Amifostine in the treatment of head and neck cancer: intravenous administration, subcutaneous administration, or none of the above. *J Clin Oncol* 2011;29:119–121.
83. Hermans R, Pameijer FA, Mancuso AA, et al. Laryngeal or hypopharyngeal squamous cell carcinoma: can follow-up CT after definitive radiation therapy be used to detect local failure earlier than clinical examination alone? *Radiology* 2000;214:683–687.
84. Grant DG, Salassa JR, Hinni ML, et al. Transoral laser microsurgery for recurrent laryngeal and pharyngeal cancer. *Otolaryngol Head Neck Surg* 2008;138: 606–613.
85. Langer CJ, Harris J, Horwitz EM, et al. Phase II study of low-dose paclitaxel and cisplatin in combination with split-course concomitant twice-daily reirradiation in recurrent squamous cell carcinoma of the head and neck: results of Radiation Therapy Oncology Group Protocol 9911. *J Clin Oncol* 2007;25:4800–4805.
86. Spencer SA, Harris J, Wheeler RH, et al. Final report of RTOG 9610, a multi-institutional trial of reirradiation and chemotherapy for unresectable recurrent squamous cell carcinoma of the head and neck. *Head Neck* 2008;30:281–288.
87. Wong SJ, Machtay M, Li Y. Locally recurrent, previously irradiated head and neck cancer: concurrent re-irradiation and chemotherapy, or chemotherapy alone? *J Clin Oncol* 2006;24:2653–2658.
88. Lee N, Chan K, Bekelman JE, et al. Salvage re-irradiation for recurrent head and neck cancer. *Int J Radiat Oncol Biol Phys* 2007;68:731–740.
89. Chen AM, Farwell DG, Luu Q, et al. Prospective trial of high-dose reirradiation using daily image guidance with intensity-modulated radiotherapy for recurrent and second primary head-and-neck cancer. *Int J Radiat Oncol Biol Phys* 2011;80:669–676.
90. McNeil BJ, Weichselbaum R, Pauker SG. Speech and survival: tradeoffs between quality and quantity of life in laryngeal cancer. *N Engl J Med* 1981;305:982–987.

91. El-Deiry M, Funk GF, Nalwa S, et al. Long-term quality of life for surgical and nonsurgical treatment of head and neck cancer. *Arch Otolaryngol Head Neck Surg* 2005;131:879–885.
92. Gillespie MB, Brodsky MB, Day TA, et al. Swallowing-related quality of life after head and neck cancer treatment. *Laryngoscope* 2004;114:1362–1367.
93. Meyer TK, Kuhn JC, Campbell BH, et al. Speech intelligibility and quality of life in head and neck cancer survivors. *Laryngoscope* 2004;114:1977–1981.
94. Terrell JE, Ronis DL, Fowler KE, et al. Clinical predictors of quality of life in patients with head and neck cancer. *Arch Otolaryngol Head Neck Surg* 2004;130:401–408.
95. Hammerlid E, Bjordal K, Ahlner-Elmqvist M, et al. A prospective study of quality of life in head and neck cancer patients. Part I: at diagnosis. *Laryngoscope* 2001;111:669–680.
96. Frowen J, Cotton S, Corry J, et al. Impact of demographics, tumor characteristics, and treatment factors on swallowing after (chemo)radiotherapy for head and neck cancer. *Head Neck* 2010;32:513–528.
97. Jabbari S, Kim HM, Feng M, et al. Matched case-control study of quality of life and xerostomia after intensity-modulated radiotherapy or standard radiotherapy for head-and-neck cancer: initial report. *Int J Radiat Oncol Biol Phys* 2005;63:725–731.
98. Vergeer MR, Doornaert PA, Rietveld DH, et al. Intensity-modulated radiotherapy reduces radiation-induced morbidity and improves health-related quality of life: results of a nonrandomized prospective study using a standardized follow-up program. *Int J Radiat Oncol Biol Phys* 2009;74:1–8.
99. Caudell JJ, Schaner PE, Desmond RA, et al. Dosimetric factors associated with long-term dysphagia after definitive radiotherapy for squamous cell carcinoma of the head and neck. *Int J Radiat Oncol Biol Phys* 2010;76:403–409.

Chapter 47
Laryngeal Cancer

William M. Mendenhall, Anthony A. Mancuso, Robert J. Amdur, and John W. Werning

ANATOMY

The larynx is divided into the supraglottis, glottis, and subglottis. The supraglottis consists of the epiglottis, false vocal cords, ventricles, aryepiglottic folds, and the arytenoids. The glottis includes the true vocal cords and the anterior commissure. The subglottis is located below the vocal cords (Figs. 47.1 and 47.2).[1]

The lateral line of demarcation between the glottis and supraglottic larynx is the apex of the ventricle. The demarcation between the glottis and subglottis is ill defined, but the subglottis is considered to extend from a point 5 mm below the free margin of the vocal cord to the inferior border of the cricoid cartilage or 10 mm below the apex of the ventricle.

The vocal cords vary from 3 to 5 mm in thickness and terminate posteriorly with their attachment to the vocal process. The posterior commissure is the mucosa between the arytenoids.

The shell of the larynx is formed by the hyoid bone, thyroid cartilage, and cricoid cartilage; the cricoid cartilage is the only complete ring. The more mobile interior framework is composed of the heart-shaped epiglottis and the arytenoid, corniculate, and cuneiform cartilages. The corniculate and cuneiform cartilages produce small, rounded bulges at the posterior end of each aryepiglottic fold.

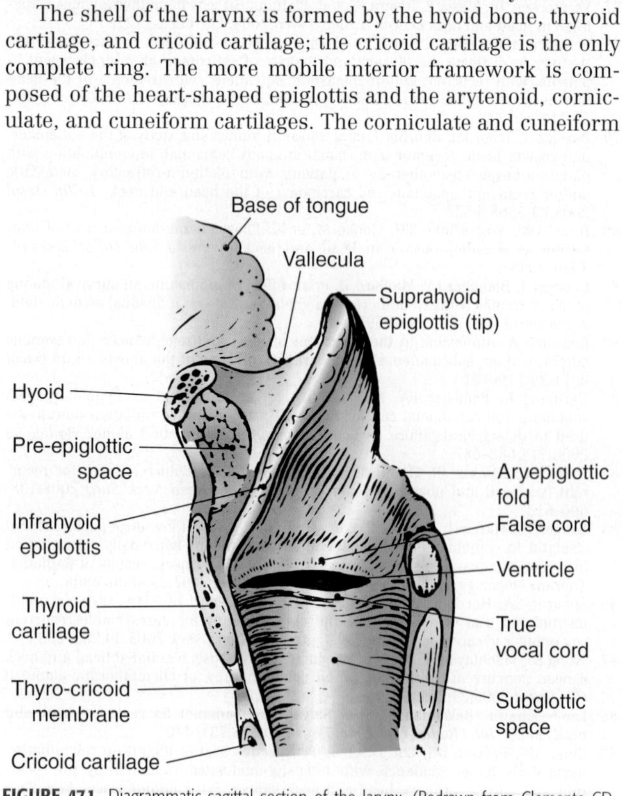

FIGURE 47.1. Diagrammatic sagittal section of the larynx. (Redrawn from Clemente CD. *Anatomy: a regional atlas of the human body.* Philadelphia: Lea & Febiger, 1975. Copyright Urban & Schwarzenberg, Munich, Germany, 1975.)

The thyroid and the cricoid cartilages and a portion of the arytenoid cartilage are hyaline cartilage and may partially ossify with age, particularly in men. The epiglottis is elastic cartilage; ossification does not occur, and even focal calcification is rare.[2]

The external laryngeal framework is linked together by the thyrohyoid, the cricothyroid, and the cricotracheal ligaments or membranes (Figs. 47.3 and 47.4).[1]

The epiglottis is joined superiorly to the hyoid bone by the hyoepiglottic ligament. The epiglottis is joined to the thyroid cartilage by the thyroepiglottic ligament at a point just below the thyroid notch and above the anterior commissure. The arrangement of the ligaments that connect the cricoid and arytenoid cartilages and form the vocal ligaments, which are part of the true vocal cords, is shown in Figure 47.2B.[1] The conus elasticus (cricovocal ligament) is the lower portion of the elastic membrane that connects the inferior framework. It connects the upper surface of the cricoid, the vocal process of the arytenoid, and the lower thyroid cartilage; its free border is thickened into the vocal ligament.

The vocal ligaments and muscles attach to the vocal process of the arytenoid posteriorly and the thyroid cartilage anteriorly. The intrinsic muscles of the larynx, which primarily control the movement of the cords, are presented in Figures 47.2 and 47.3.[1] The extrinsic muscles are concerned primarily with swallowing. The cricothyroid muscle produces tension and elongation of the vocal cords and is innervated by the superior laryngeal nerve (Fig. 47.4).[1]

The pre-epiglottic and paraglottic fat spaces are essentially one contiguous space lying between the external framework of the thyroid cartilage and hyoid bone and the inner framework of the epiglottis and intrinsic muscles. Lam and Wong[3] showed that there are thin membranous septa between the paraglottic and pre-epiglottic spaces that are capable of holding a tumor in check to a limited degree. The space is traversed by blood and lymphatic vessels and nerves. Because few capillary lymphatics arise in this area, invasion of the fat space should only indirectly be associated with lymph node metastases. The fat space is limited by the conus elasticus inferiorly, the thyroid ala, the thyrohyoid membrane, the hyoid bone anterolaterally, the hyoepiglottic ligament superiorly, and the fascia of the intrinsic muscles on the medial side. Posteriorly, it is adjacent to the anterior wall of the pyriform sinus.

The laryngeal surface of the epiglottis and the free margin of the vocal cords are squamous epithelium, and the remainder is usually pseudostratified ciliated columnar epithelium.

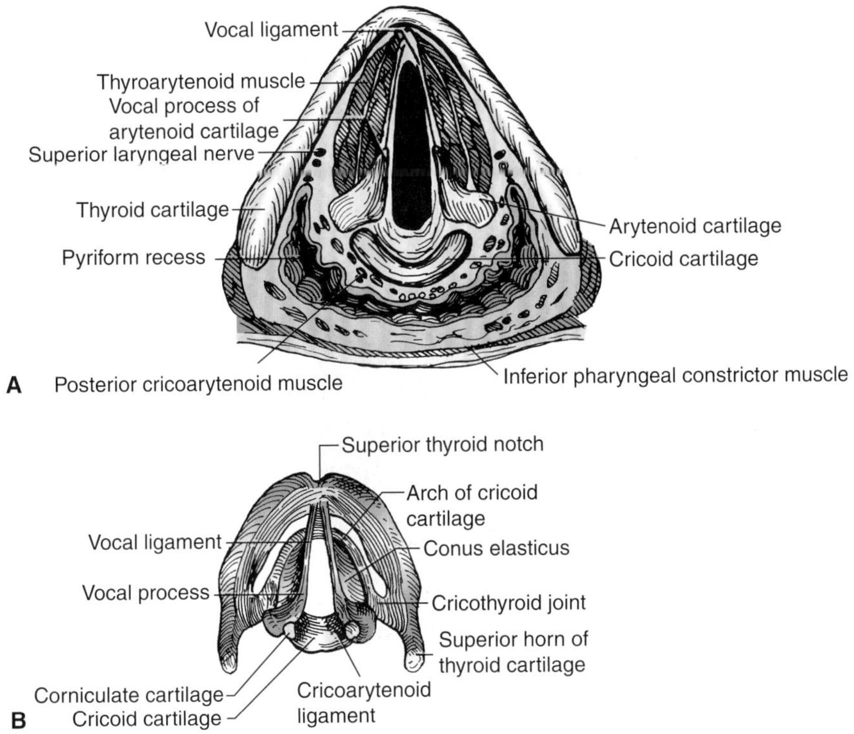

FIGURE 47.2. **A:** Cross section of the larynx at the level of the vocal cords. **B:** Framework of the larynx. (Redrawn from Clemente CD. *Anatomy: a regional atlas of the human body.* Philadelphia: Lea & Febiger, 1975. Copyright Urban & Schwarzenberg, Munich, Germany, 1975.)

Beneath the epithelium of the free edge of the vocal cord is the lamina propria, which can be divided into three layers. There is no true submucosal layer along the free margin of the vocal fold.[4] The laryngeal arteries are branches of the superior and inferior thyroid arteries.

The intrinsic muscles of the larynx are innervated by the recurrent laryngeal nerve. The cricothyroid muscle—an intrinsic muscle responsible for tensing the vocal cords—is supplied by a branch of the superior laryngeal nerve; isolated damage to this nerve causes a bowing of the true vocal cord, which continues to be mobile, but the voice may become hoarse.

The supraglottic structures have a rich capillary lymphatic plexus; the trunks pass through the pre-epiglottic space and the thyrohyoid membrane and terminate mainly in the subdigastric (level II) lymph nodes; a few drain to the middle internal jugular chain (level III) lymph nodes.

There are essentially no capillary lymphatics of the true vocal cords; as a result, lymphatic spread from glottic cancer occurs only if tumor extends to supraglottic or subglottic areas.

The subglottic area has relatively few capillary lymphatics. The lymphatic trunks pass through the cricothyroid membrane to the pretracheal (Delphian) lymph nodes in the region of the thyroid isthmus. The subglottic area also drains posteriorly through the cricotracheal membrane, with some trunks going to the paratracheal (level VI) lymph nodes and others continuing to the inferior jugular (level IV) chain.

EPIDEMIOLOGY AND RISK FACTORS

Cancer of the larynx represents about 2% of the total cancer risk and is the most common head and neck cancer (skin excluded). In 2010 in the United States, there were approximately 12,720

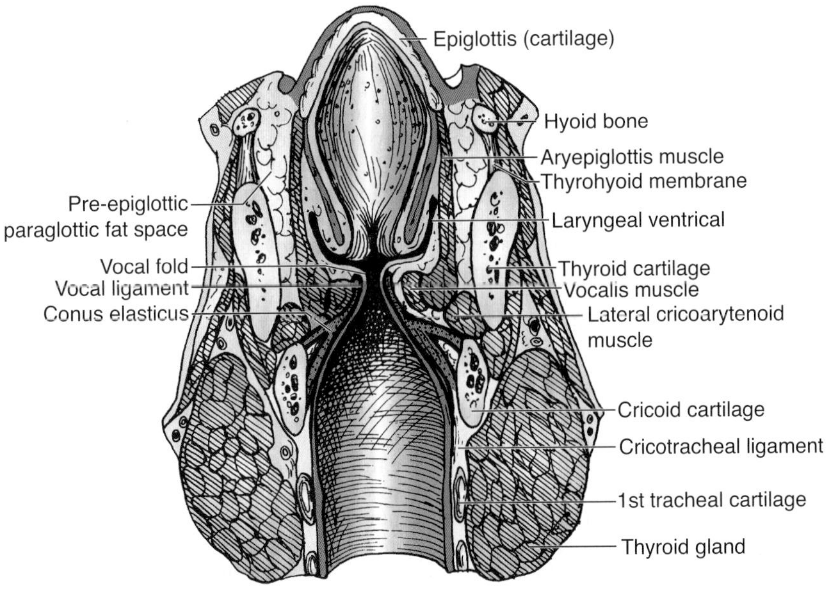

FIGURE 47.3. Diagram of the coronal view of the larynx. (Redrawn from Clemente CD. *Anatomy: a regional atlas of the human body.* Philadelphia: Lea & Febiger, 1975. Copyright Urban & Schwarzenberg, Munich, Germany, 1975.)

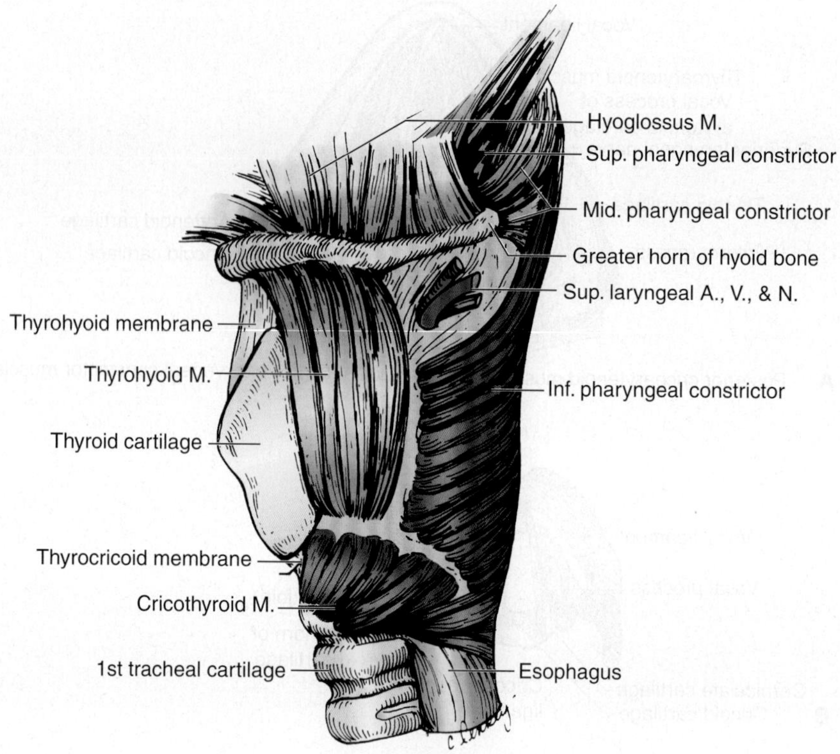

FIGURE 47.4. External view of the larynx. (Redrawn from Clemente CD. *Anatomy: a regional atlas of the human body.* Philadelphia: Lea & Febiger, 1975. Copyright Urban & Schwarzenberg, Munich, Germany, 1975.)

new cases of cancer of the larynx (10,110 men and 2,610 women) and about 3,600 deaths from laryngeal cancer.[5] Based on 1973–1998 U.S. data, at diagnosis, about 51% of the cases remain localized, 29% have regional spread, and 15% have distant metastases.[6] The ratio of glottic to supraglottic carcinoma is approximately 3:1.

Cancer of the larynx is strongly related to cigarette smoking. The risk of tobacco-related cancers of the upper alimentary and respiratory tracts declines among former smokers after 5 years and is said to approach the risk of nonsmokers after 10 years of abstention.[7] The role of alcohol in provoking laryngeal cancer remains unclear.[8] Some evidence exists that heavy marijuana smoking may be associated with laryngeal cancer in young patients.

PATTERNS OF SPREAD

Local Spread

Although supraglottic and glottic lesions tend to remain confined to their original compartments, there is no anatomic barrier to growth from one area to the next. Glottic lesions tend to be slow growing, but as they increase in size, they extend to the supraglottic and subglottic areas. Supraglottic lesions do not often start near the vocal cords. Involvement of the cords on their external epithelial surface is a late phenomenon, but submucosal extension by way of the paraglottic space occurs earlier.

The fat space is an important avenue of submucosal tumor spread for infrahyoid epiglottis, false cord, and true vocal cord lesions. As the false cord and the true vocal cord lesions penetrate anteriorly and laterally, they quickly encounter the tough perichondrium of the thyroid cartilage and may eventually be shunted by the conus elasticus (lateral cricothyroid membrane) out of the larynx via the cricothyroid space. Thyroid cartilage invasion usually occurs in the ossified section of the cartilage, commonly in the region of the anterior commissure tendon or the junction of the anterior one-fourth and the posterior three-fourths of the thyroid lamina.[9]

Fixation of the vocal cord from laryngeal cancer is usually caused by invasion or destruction of the vocal cord muscle, invasion of the cricoarytenoid muscle or joint, or, rarely, invasion of the recurrent laryngeal nerve. Perineural spread is uncommon.

Supraglottic Larynx

Suprahyoid Epiglottis

A lesion of the suprahyoid epiglottis may produce a huge exophytic mass with little tendency to destroy cartilage or spread to adjacent structures. Other lesions may infiltrate the tip and destroy cartilage. The destructive lesions tend to invade the vallecula and pre-epiglottic space, the lateral pharyngeal walls, and the remainder of the supraglottic larynx.

Infrahyoid Epiglottis

Lesions of the infrahyoid epiglottis tend to produce irregular tumor nodules and simultaneously invade the porous epiglottic cartilage and thyroepiglottic ligament into the pre-epiglottic fat space and extend toward the vallecula and base of the tongue. The thick hyoepiglottic ligament is an effective tumor barrier. However, the tumor may present in the vallecula and base of tongue without involving the suprahyoid epiglottis.

Lesions of the infrahyoid epiglottis grow circumferentially to involve the false cords, aryepiglottic folds, medial wall of the pyriform sinus, and the pharyngoepiglottic fold. Invasion of the anterior commissure and cords and anterior subglottic extension usually occur only in advanced lesions. Infrahyoid epiglottic lesions that extend onto or below the vocal cords are at a high risk for thyroid cartilage invasion, even if the cords are mobile.[10]

False Cord

Early false cord carcinomas, which are usually submucosal with little exophytic component, are difficult to delineate accurately. They involve the paraglottic fat space early in their development and may spread a considerable distance beneath the mucosa without producing physical signs. These carcinomas extend to the perichondrium of the thyroid cartilage quite early, but cartilage invasion is a late phenomenon. Extension to the lower portion of the infrahyoid epiglottis and invasion of the pre-epiglottic space are common. Submucosal extension involves the true vocal cord, which may appear normal. Vocal cord invasion is often associated with thyroid cartilage invasion. Submucosal extension to the medial wall of the pyriform sinus occurs early.

Aryepiglottic Fold/Arytenoid

Early lesions of the aryepiglottic fold/arytenoid are usually exophytic. It may be difficult to decide whether the lesion started on the medial wall of the pyriform sinus or on the aryepiglottic fold. As the lesions enlarge, they extend to adjacent sites and eventually cause fixation of the larynx, which is usually a result of involvement of the cricoarytenoid muscle or joint or, rarely, invasion of the recurrent laryngeal nerve. Computed tomography (CT) may distinguish the cause of fixation. Advanced lesions invade the thyroid, epiglottic, and cricoid cartilages and eventually invade the pyriform sinus and postcricoid area.

Glottic Larynx

Most lesions of the true vocal cord begin on the free margin and upper surface of the cord. When diagnosed, about two-thirds are confined to the cords, usually one cord. The anterior portion of the cord is the most common site. Anterior commissure involvement, which is common, is said to occur when no tumor-free cord can be seen anteriorly; if the lesion crosses to the opposite cord, anterior commissure invasion is certain. Small lesions isolated to the anterior commissure account for only 1% to 2% of cases. Extension to the posterior commissure is uncommon, occurring only in advanced lesions.

Tumors at the anterior commissure may extend anteriorly via the anterior commissure tendon (Broyles' ligament)[11] into the thyroid cartilage. Kirchner,[12] using whole-organ sections, showed that such extension is unusual unless the tumor extends off the vocal cord onto the base of the infrahyoid epiglottis and suggested that the tendon serves as more of a barrier than an avenue of tumor spread. Early subglottic extension is also associated with involvement of the anterior commissure, and tumor may grow through the cricothyroid membrane.

Lesions that arise on the posterior half of the vocal cord tend to extend along the submucosa toward the medial side of the vocal process and invade the cricoarytenoid joint and posterior commissure; this spread is difficult to appreciate by clinical examination.

Subglottic extension may occur by simple mucosal surface growth, but it more commonly occurs by submucosal penetration beneath the conus elasticus. One centimeter of subglottic extension anteriorly or 4 to 5 mm of subglottic extension posteriorly brings the border of the tumor to the upper margin of the cricoid, exceeding the anatomic limits for conventional hemilaryngectomy. Lesions may spread beneath the epithelium along the length of the vocal cord within Reinke's space.[13]

As vocal cord lesions enlarge, they extend to the false cord, vocal process of the arytenoid, and subglottis. Infiltrative lesions invade the vocal ligament and muscle and eventually reach the paraglottic space and the perichondrium of the thyroid cartilage. Advanced glottic lesions eventually penetrate through the thyroid cartilage or via the cricothyroid space to enter the neck, where they may invade the thyroid gland. Lesions involving the anterior commissure often exit the larynx via the cricothyroid space after they extend subglottically.[13]

A fixed cord that is associated with a lesion having <1 cm of subglottic extension and no false cord involvement does not ordinarily indicate invasion of the thyroid cartilage.[12] If the false cord is also involved, cartilage invasion is likely.

Subglottic Larynx

Subglottic cancers are rare. Most involve the inferior surface of the vocal cords by the time they are diagnosed, so it is difficult to know whether the tumor started on the undersurface of the vocal cord or in the true subglottic larynx. Because early diagnosis is uncommon, most lesions are bilateral or circumferential at discovery. They involve the cricoid cartilages in the early stage because there is no intervening muscle layer. Partial or complete fixation of one or both cords is common; misdiagnosis or diagnostic delay is frequent.

Lymphatic Spread

The location and stage of neck nodes detected on admission for previously untreated patients with squamous cell carcinoma of the supraglottic larynx are given in Figure 47.5.[14] The disease spreads mainly to the level II nodes. The level Ib nodes are rarely involved, and there is only a small risk of level V lymph node involvement. The incidence of clinically positive nodes is 55% at the time of diagnosis; 16% are bilateral.[14] Elective neck dissection shows pathologically positive nodes in 16% of cases; observation of initially node-negative necks eventually identifies the appearance of positive nodes in 33% of cases.[15,16] Spread to the pyriform sinus, vallecula, and base of the tongue increases the risk of lymph node metastases. The risk of late-appearing contralateral lymph node metastasis is 37% if the ipsilateral neck is pathologically positive, but the risk is unrelated to whether the nodes in the ipsilateral neck were palpable before neck dissection.

The incidence of clinically positive lymph nodes at diagnosis for vocal cord carcinoma approaches zero for T1 lesions and is

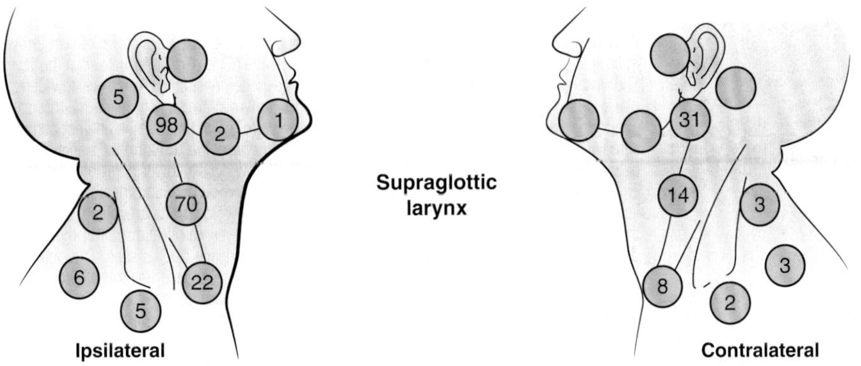

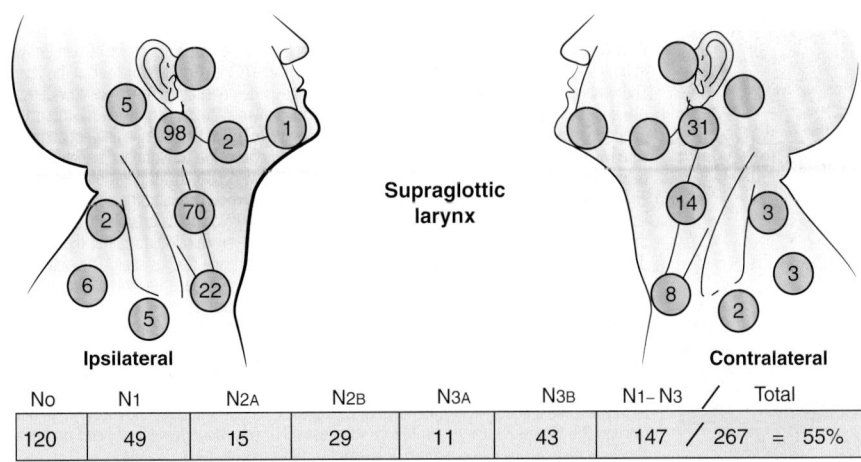

No	N1	N2A	N2B	N3A	N3B	N1–N3 / Total
120	49	15	29	11	43	147 / 267 = 55%

FIGURE 47.5. Nodal distribution on admission, MD Anderson Cancer Center, 1948–1965. (From Lindberg RD. Distribution of cervical lymph node metastases from squamous cell carcinoma of the upper respiratory and digestive tracts. *Cancer* 1972;29:1446–1449; with permission.)

<2% for T2 lesions.[17] The incidence of neck metastases increases to 20% to 30% for T3 and T4 lesions. Supraglottic spread is associated with metastasis to the level II nodes. Anterior commissure and anterior subglottic invasion are associated with involvement of the midline pretracheal lymph node (level VI).

Lederman[18] reported a 10% incidence of positive lymph nodes in 73 patients with subglottic carcinoma.

CLINICAL PRESENTATION

Carcinoma arising on the true vocal cords produces hoarseness at a very early stage. Sore throat, ear pain, pain localized to the thyroid cartilage, and airway obstruction are features of advanced lesions.

Hoarseness is not a prominent symptom of cancer of the supraglottis until the lesion becomes extensive. Pain on swallowing, usually mild, is the most frequent initial symptom, often described as a sore throat. Some patients report a sensation of a "lump in the throat." Pain is referred to the ear by way of the vagus nerve and auricular nerve of Arnold. A mass in the neck may be the first sign of a supraglottic cancer. Late symptoms include weight loss, foul breath, dysphagia, and aspiration.

DIAGNOSTIC WORKUP

Physical Examination

Flexible fiberoptic endoscopes are used routinely to complement the laryngeal mirror examination. The mirror often provides the best view of the posterior pharyngeal wall. The flexible fiberoptic laryngoscope is inserted through the nose and is useful in more difficult cases.

Determination of vocal cord mobility frequently requires multiple examinations because the subtle distinctions between mobile, partially fixed, and fixed cords are often challenging, apparently changing from examination to examination. A cord that appeared mobile before direct laryngoscopy may exhibit impaired motion or even fixation after biopsy.

Ulceration of the infrahyoid epiglottis or fullness of the vallecula is an indirect sign of pre-epiglottic space invasion. Palpation of diffuse, firm fullness above the thyroid notch with widening of the space between the hyoid and the thyroid cartilages signifies invasion of the pre-epiglottic space. The pre-epiglottic fat space is a low-density area on the CT scan, and changes resulting from tumor invasion are easily seen.

Postcricoid extension may be suspected when the laryngeal click disappears on physical examination. Postcricoid tumor may cause the thyroid cartilage to protrude anteriorly, producing a fullness of the neck.

Invasion of the thyroid cartilage remains a difficult clinical diagnosis. Localized pain or tenderness to palpation or a small bulge over one ala of the thyroid cartilage is suggestive.

Radiographic Studies

CT scan with contrast enhancement is the method of choice for studying the larynx (Fig. 47.6).[19] The CT scan should be performed before biopsy so that abnormalities that may be caused by the biopsy are not confused with tumor. CT is preferred to magnetic resonance (MR) imaging because the longer scanning time for MR results in motion artifact.[20] CT slices 1 to 2 mm thick are obtained at 1- to 2-mm intervals through the larynx and at 3-mm intervals for the remainder of the study. Thinner sections (1 to 2 mm through the larynx) facilitate high-quality multiplanar reformations. The gantry is angled so that the scan slices are parallel to the plane of the true vocal cords. It is also necessary to obtain a CT scan of the entire neck to detect positive, nonpalpable lymph nodes. Positive retropharyngeal nodes may be present at diagnosis in patients with laryngeal cancer who have advanced neck disease.[21] Retropharyngeal adenopathy is often

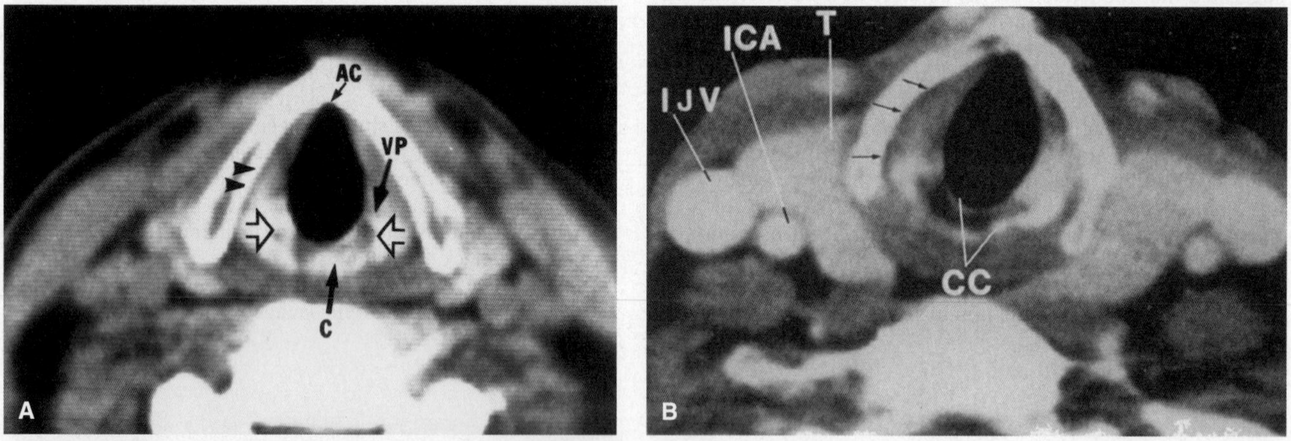

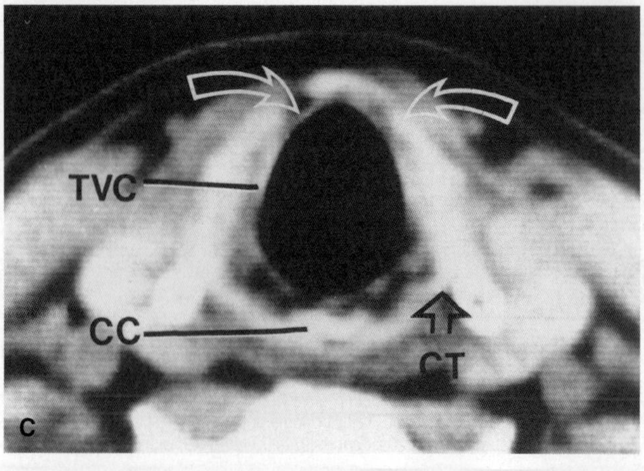

FIGURE 47.6. A: Normal CT anatomy of the midplane of the true vocal cords. Open arrows indicate arytenoid cartilages. The top of the cricoid cartilage (C) is partially visualized at this level. The vocal process (VP) of the left arytenoid cartilage is demonstrated. A narrow, low-density plane is seen between the right true vocal cord and the thyroid lamina (*arrowheads*); this is the inferior part of the paraglottic fat space. Notice the complete lack of tissue at the anterior commissure (AC). *Any tissue density here should be considered abnormal.* **B:** Normal CT anatomy just below the midplane of the vocal cords. Arrows indicate low-density lower paraglottic fat space. The fibrofatty tissue in this space facilitates separation of the vocal cord and the adjacent thyroid lamina. If this clear space is maintained in the face of the thyroid lamina irregularity adjacent to the tumor, the lamina abnormality can be attributed to uneven calcification rather than tumor destruction. The posterior portion (lamina) of the cricoid cartilage (*CC*) is seen. The outer and inner cortex of the cartilage is calcified; an intervening marrow space has lower density. The vertical height of the lamina is 2 to 3 cm. There is incomplete calcification of the thyroid cartilage anteriorly. ICA, internal carotid artery; IJV, internal jugular vein; T, thyroid gland. **C:** Normal CT anatomy 5 mm below the free margin of the true vocal cord (TVC). The vocal cord appears thin because of abduction during scanning. There is incomplete bilateral paramedian calcification and thinning of the thyroid lamina (*arrows*). Notice the normal lack of tissue density between the airway and the anterior arch of the thyroid cartilage. CC, cricoid cartilage; CT, cricothyroid joint. (Million RR, Cassisi NJ. Larynx. In Million RR, Cassisi NJ, eds. *Management of head and neck cancer: a multidisciplinary approach.* Philadelphia: JB Lippincott, 1984:315–364.)

not apparent on physical examination but is usually appreciated on CT scan.

Contrast enhancement helps to outline the blood vessels and thyroid gland. Tumor is often enhanced, probably because of reactive inflammatory changes. In addition to CT, MR may be obtained to define subtle exolaryngeal spread or early cartilage destruction. The value of MR for detecting early cartilage destruction is open to speculation. Sagittal MR may be useful in detecting early invasion of the base of the tongue.

Vocal Cord Carcinoma

Although the CT scan does not show minimal mucosal lesions and is generally not helpful for well-defined, easily visualized T1, or early T2 vocal cord carcinomas, it is almost always obtained. CT is excellent for determining subglottic extension and is often used in selected T1 and most T2 lesions for this reason alone. CT scanning is useful in the diagnosis of moderately advanced and advanced lesions; it is excellent for demonstrating extension outside the larynx into the soft tissues of the neck and has potential for determining thyroid or cricoid cartilage invasion, which tends to occur at the edges of the cartilage rather than on the faces. Early cartilage involvement is difficult to detect with axial scans, but it may be demonstrated by coronal or sagittal scanning techniques. If the low-density plane of the paraglottic space is intact, cartilage is probably not invaded by tumor.

Archer et al.[22] correlated CT findings with the incidence of cartilage or bone invasion on whole-organ sections. For 12 of 14 patients with pathologic evidence of cartilage invasion, the average diameter of the tumor in two dimensions was >16 mm, and the lesion was located below the top of the arytenoid. Lesions in which the maximum diameter lay above the top of the arytenoid had a low incidence of cartilage invasion.[22]

Supraglottic Carcinoma

The CT scan provides an excellent means for viewing the pre-epiglottic and paraglottic fat spaces. Soft-tissue extension into the neck or base of the tongue can also be seen. The CT scan is also useful for determining extension to the subglottis.[2]

Diagnostic procedures for laryngeal cancer at the University of Florida are summarized in Table 47.1.[23] A CT scan is usually performed for all patients; MR is obtained in a small subset of patients with questionable findings on CT. Positron emission tomography is not routinely obtained. Direct laryngoscopy and biopsy with frozen section are usually performed with the patient under general anesthesia. The ventricles, subglottis, apex of the pyriform sinus, and postcricoid area must be carefully examined because these areas are not consistently seen by indirect examinations. Fiberoptic telescopes (0 and 30 degrees) are introduced through the laryngoscope for inspection of these areas. A generous biopsy specimen is taken from the obvious lesion; additional biopsy specimens may be obtained from suspicious areas and from areas grossly involved. The mucosa of the margin of the cord may be stripped to provide adequate tissue if the lesion is distributed superficially along the cord and is not obviously a carcinoma.

TABLE 47.1 DIAGNOSTIC WORKUP FOR CARCINOMA OF THE LARYNX

General
History
Physical examination
Indirect laryngoscopy
Direct laryngoscopy
Biopsies
Radiographic studies
Chest x-ray films
Computed tomography with contrast enhancement (before biopsy)
Magnetic resonance imaging (selected cases)

From Mendenhall WM, Parsons JT, Mancuso AA, et al. Larynx. In Perez CA, Brady LW. *Principles and practice of radiation oncology,* 4th ed. Philadelphia: Lippincott-Raven, 1998:1094–1116.

TABLE 47.2 STAGING OF LARYNGEAL CANCER

Supraglottis	
T1	Tumor limited to one subsite of supraglottis with normal vocal cord mobility
T2	Tumor invades mucosa of more than one adjacent subsite of supraglottis or glottis or region outside the supraglottis (e.g., mucosa of base of tongue, vallecula, medial wall of pyriform sinus) without fixation of the larynx
T3	Tumor limited to larynx with vocal cord fixation and/or invades any of the following: postcricoid area, pre-epiglottic space, paraglottic space, and/or inner cortex of thyroid cartilage
T4a	Moderately advanced local disease; tumor invades through the thyroid cartilage and/or invades tissues beyond the larynx (e.g., trachea, soft tissues of neck including deep extrinsic muscle of the tongue, strap muscles, thyroid, or esophagus)
T4b	Very advanced local disease; tumor invades prevertebral space, encases carotid artery, or invades mediastinal structures
Glottis	
T1	Tumor limited to vocal cord(s) (may involve anterior or posterior commissure) with normal mobility
T1a	Tumor limited to one vocal cord
T1b	Tumor involves both vocal cords
T2	Tumor extends to supraglottis and/or subglottis, and/or with impaired vocal cord mobility
T3	Tumor limited to the larynx with vocal cord fixation and/or invades paraglottic space and/or inner cortex of the thyroid cartilage.
T4a	Moderately advanced local disease; tumor invades through the outer cortex of the thyroid cartilage and/or invades tissues beyond the larynx (e.g., trachea, soft tissues of neck including deep extrinsic muscle of the tongue, strap muscles, thyroid, or esophagus)
T4b	Very advanced local disease; tumor invades prevertebral space, encases carotid artery, or invades mediastinal structures

Used with the permission of the American Joint Committee on Cancer (AJCC), Chicago, Illinois. The original source for this material is American Joint Committee on Cancer. *AJCC Cancer Staging Handbook,* 7th ed. New York: Springer, 2010; published by Springer Science and Business Media LLC, www.springerlink.com.

STAGING

The 2010 American Joint Committee on Cancer (AJCC)[24] staging system for laryngeal primary cancer is listed in Table 47.2. T2 glottic cancers are stratified into those with normal (T2A) and impaired (T2B) vocal cord mobility. For lesions arising in the supraglottis, the sites of origin include false cords, aryepiglottic folds, suprahyoid epiglottis, infrahyoid epiglottis, pharyngoepiglottic folds, and arytenoids. Only in the early T stages can one identify the specific site of origin with certainty. As the lesion enlarges, the site of origin is an educated guess based on the location of the greatest bulk of tumor. The major difference between the 1998 and 2010 staging systems is that a glottic cancer that invades the paraglottic space is upstaged to T3 in the latter system, even with mobile vocal cords, resulting in significant stage migration.[25] In addition, T4 has been stratified into T4A and T4B, based on resectability.

PATHOLOGIC CLASSIFICATION

Nearly all malignant tumors of the larynx arise from the surface epithelium and therefore are squamous cell carcinoma or one of its variants.

Carcinoma in situ occurs frequently on the vocal cords. Differentiating among dysplasia, carcinoma in situ, squamous cell carcinoma with microinvasion, and true invasive carcinoma is a problem that the pathologist and the clinician frequently confront.

Most vocal cord carcinomas are well or moderately well differentiated. In a few cases, an apparent carcinoma and sarcoma occur together, but most of these are actually a spindle-cell carcinoma (i.e., squamous cell carcinoma with a spindle-cell stromal reaction).

Verrucous carcinoma occurs in 1% to 2% of patients with carcinoma of the vocal cord. The histologic diagnosis is difficult and must correlate with the gross appearance of the lesion.

Small-cell neuroendocrine carcinoma is rarely diagnosed in the supraglottic larynx, but it should be recognized because of its biologic potential for rapid growth, early dissemination, and responsiveness to chemotherapy.

Minor salivary gland tumors arise from the mucous glands in the supraglottic and subglottic larynx, but they are rare.[26] Even rarer are paragangliomas, carcinoids, soft-tissue sarcomas, malignant lymphomas, and plasmacytomas. Benign chondromas and osteochondromas are reported, but their malignant counterparts are rare.

PROGNOSTIC FACTORS

The extent of the primary lesion and neck disease are the major determinants of prognosis. The likelihood of local control is determined primarily by T stage; there are conflicting data pertaining to a possible inverse relationship between N stage and local control. The likelihood of local-regional control is affected primarily by the overall AJCC stage, which accounts for both T stage and N stage. AJCC stage and N stage are the major determinants of cause-specific survival. In addition, within each N stage, patients with positive nodes in the low neck below the level of the thyroid notch tend to have a lower cause-specific survival rate than those with disease confined to the upper neck. In general, women tend to have a better prognosis than men.

TREATMENT SELECTION AND TECHNIQUE: VOCAL CORD CARCINOMA

Selection of Treatment Modality

In treating vocal cord carcinoma, the goal is cure with the best functional result and the least risk of a serious complication. Patients may be considered to be in an early group if the chance of cure with larynx preservation is high, a moderately advanced group if the likelihood of local control is 60% to 70% but the chance of cure is still good, and an advanced group if the chance of cure is moderate and the likelihood of laryngeal preservation is relatively low. The early group may be treated initially by radiotherapy (RT) or, in selected cases, by partial laryngectomy. The moderately advanced group may be treated with either RT with laryngectomy reserved for relapse or by total laryngectomy with or without adjuvant postoperative RT. The obvious advantage of the former strategy, which we use at the University of Florida, is that there is a fairly good chance that the larynx will be preserved.[27] Although some patients may be rehabilitated with a tracheoesophageal puncture after laryngectomy, only about 20% of patients use this device long term, and the majority use an electric larynx.[28] The advanced group is treated with total laryngectomy and neck dissection with or without adjuvant RT or by RT and adjuvant chemotherapy.[29] Data suggest that if patients whose tumors show a partial or complete response to two to three cycles of neoadjuvant chemotherapy are then given high-dose RT, the cure rates are comparable with those obtained with initial total laryngectomy.[30] Another less expensive and less toxic method to select patients likely to be cured by RT alone is to calculate the primary tumor volume on pretreatment CT or MR. Data indicate that primary tumor volume is inversely related to the probability of local control after irradiation.[31,32] Recent data indicate that whereas induction chemotherapy probably does not improve the likelihood of local-regional control and survival, concomitant chemotherapy and RT results in an improved possibility of cure compared with RT alone.[33–35] There is a subset of patients with high-volume (>3.5 cc), unfavorable, advanced cancers who may be cured by chemoradiation but have a useless larynx and permanent tracheostomy and/or gastrostomy.[31] These patients are best treated with a total laryngectomy, neck dissection, and postoperative RT.

Carcinoma in Situ

Lesions diagnosed as carcinoma in situ may sometimes be controlled by stripping the cord. However, it is difficult to exclude the possibility of microinvasion on these specimens. Recurrence is frequent, and the cord may become thickened and the voice hoarse with repeated stripping. Localized carcinoma in situ can also be excised using the CO_2 laser.

Early RT for carcinoma in situ often means a better chance of preserving a good voice, especially since many patients with this diagnosis eventually receive this treatment.[36]

Many patients with a diagnosis of carcinoma in situ have obvious lesions that probably contain invasive carcinoma. We have often proceeded with RT rather than put the patient through a repeated biopsy procedure.

Early Vocal Cord Carcinoma

In most centers, RT is the initial treatment prescribed for T1 and T2 lesions, with surgery reserved for salvage after RT failure.[17,37,38] Although hemilaryngectomy or cordectomy produces comparable cure rates for selected T1 and T2 vocal cord lesions, RT is generally preferred.[37,39] Supracricoid laryngectomy, as reported by Laccourreye et al.,[40] is a procedure designed to remove moderate-sized cancers involving the supraglottic and glottic larynx. The larynx may be removed with preservation of the cricoid and the arytenoid with its neurovascular innervation; the defect is closed by approximating the base of the tongue to the remaining larynx. The oncologic and functional results of this procedure in selected patients are reported to be excellent. Transoral laser excision also may provide high cure rates for select patients with small, well-defined lesions limited to the mid one-third of one true cord.[41–45] A small subset of transoral laser surgeons successfully use this technique in moderately advanced cancers.[37] The major advantage of RT compared with partial laryngectomy is better quality of the voice. Partial laryngectomy finds its major use as salvage surgery in suitable cases after RT failure. Even if the patient has a local recurrence after salvage partial laryngectomy, there is a third chance with total laryngectomy, which may still be successful.

Verrucous lesions have the reputation of being unresponsive to RT and, in some instances, converting into invasive, often anaplastic, metastasizing lesions. Partial laryngectomy is recommended for early verrucous carcinoma of the glottis, but RT is recommended if the alternative is total laryngectomy. We have observed typical verrucous lesions that have disappeared with RT and not recurred. O'Sullivan et al.[46] also made this observation. In addition, a variety of tumors that recur after unsuccessful treatment (with surgery, RT, and/or chemotherapy) are more likely to exhibit more aggressive behavior.

Moderately Advanced Vocal Cord Cancer

Fixed-cord lesions (T3) may be subdivided into relatively favorable or unfavorable lesions. Patients with unfavorable lesions usually have extensive bilateral disease with a compromised airway and are considered to be in the advanced group. Patients with favorable T3 lesions have disease confined mostly to one side of the larynx, have a good airway, and are reliable for follow-up. Some degree of supraglottic and subglottic extension usually exists. The extent of disease and tumor volume, in particular, are related to the likelihood of control after RT.[31]

The patient with a favorable lesion is advised of the alternatives of RT with surgical salvage or immediate total laryngectomy. Recent data suggest that the likelihood of local-regional control is better after some altered fractionation schedules compared with conventional once-daily RT.[35,47] Follow-up examinations are recommended every 4 to 6 weeks for the first year, every 6 to 8 weeks for the second year, every 3 months for the third year, every 6 months for the fourth and fifth years, and annually thereafter. The patient must understand that total laryngectomy may be recommended purely on clinical grounds without biopsy-proven recurrence and that the risk of laryngeal osteochondronecrosis is about 5%.

Evaluation of cord mobility after 50.4 Gy or at the end of RT has not been helpful in predicting local control.[32] Some patients in whom the vocal cord remained fixed have had local tumor control of the disease for 2 years or longer after RT.

The major difficulty in using RT for the more advanced lesions is distinguishing radiation edema from local recurrence during follow-up examinations.[48] Progressive laryngeal edema, persistent throat pain, or fixation of a previously mobile vocal cord frequently signifies recurrent disease in the larynx, although a few patients with these findings remain disease-free with long-term follow-up.

Extended hemilaryngectomy has been used by a few surgeons in the treatment of well-lateralized fixed-cord lesions. A permanent tracheostomy is usually required because a portion of the cricoid is resected, but a useful voice may be retained.[49]

Advanced Vocal Cord Carcinoma

Advanced lesions usually show extensive subglottic and supraglottic extension, bilateral glottic involvement, and invasion of the thyroid, cricoid, and/or arytenoid cartilages.[9,22] The airway is compromised, necessitating a tracheostomy at the time of direct laryngoscopy in approximately 30% of patients. Clinically positive lymph nodes are found in about 25% to 30% of patients.

The mainstay of treatment is total laryngectomy, with or without adjuvant RT. The most frequent sites of local failure after total laryngectomy are the tracheal stoma, the base of the tongue, the neck lymph nodes, and/or or soft tissues of the neck. If the neck is clinically negative before surgery and if postoperative RT is planned, neck dissection may be withheld, and RT may be used to treat both sides of the neck. However, in practice, most surgeons prefer to perform elective bilateral selective (levels II to IV) neck dissections in conjunction with a total laryngectomy for T3 N0 or T4 N0 laryngeal cancer, even if postoperative RT is planned. If the lymph nodes are clinically positive, a therapeutic neck dissection is performed at the time of laryngectomy.

The indications for postoperative RT include close or positive margins, significant subglottic extension (1 cm or more), cartilage invasion, perineural invasion, endothelial-lined space invasion, extension of the primary tumor into the soft tissues of the neck, multiple positive neck nodes, extracapsular extension, and control of subclinical disease in the opposite neck.[50,51] Preoperative RT is indicated for patients who have fixed neck nodes, have had an emergency tracheotomy through tumor, or have direct extension of tumor involving the skin.

Definitive RT is prescribed for the patient who refuses total laryngectomy or is medically unsuitable for major surgery.

As previously stated, there is evidence that two to three cycles of induction chemotherapy followed by RT in patients obtaining at least a partial response may provide a moderate likelihood of larynx preservation without compromising cure.[30] Data suggest that concomitant chemotherapy and RT is more efficacious than RT alone or induction chemotherapy followed by RT.[33,34] The optimal combination of concomitant chemotherapy and irradiation is unclear.[35]

A randomized intergroup trial (RTOG 91-11) compared three treatment arms: arm A, three cycles of induction cisplatin and fluorouracil followed by RT in complete and partial responders; arm B, RT and concomitant cisplatin (100 mg/m^2 on days 1, 22, and 43 of RT); and arm C, once-daily RT (70 Gy in 35 fractions over 7 weeks) alone.[33] Five hundred forty-seven patients were randomized and followed for a median of 3.8 years; 518 patients were evaluable. The rates of larynx preservation were as follows: arm A, 72%; arm B, 84%; and arm C, 67%. The rates of larynx presentation were significantly improved for arm B; there was no significant difference between arms A and C. The 5-year survival rates were similar for the three treatment groups: arm A, 55%; arm B, 54%; and arm C, 56%. The likelihood of developing distant metastases was lower for the two groups of patients that received adjuvant chemotherapy.

Surgical Treatment

Cordectomy is an excision of the vocal cord and may be performed by the transoral approach usually with a laser or externally by a thyrotomy. Its use is usually confined to small lesions of the middle one-third of the cord. After cordectomy, a pseudocord is formed, and the patient has a useful, if somewhat harsh, voice.

Vertical partial laryngectomy (i.e., hemilaryngectomy) allows removal of limited cord lesions with preservation of voice. One entire cord with as much as one-third of the opposite cord with the adjacent thyroid cartilage is the maximum cordal involvement suitable for surgery in men; women have a smaller larynx, and usually only one vocal cord may be removed without compromising the airway. Partial fixation of one cord is not a contraindication to hemilaryngectomy; a few surgeons performed a hemilaryngectomy for selected fixed-cord lesions. The maximum subglottic extension suitable for hemilaryngectomy is 8 to 9 mm anteriorly and 5 mm posteriorly; this limit is necessary to preserve the integrity of the cricoid. Tumor extension to the epiglottis, false cord, or both arytenoids is a contraindication to hemilaryngectomy.

Supracricoid partial laryngectomy is used for selected T2 and T3 glottic carcinomas and entails removal of both true and false cords as well as the entire thyroid cartilage. The cricoid is sutured to the epiglottis and hyoid (cricohyoidoepiglottopexy).

Total laryngectomy with or without neck dissection is the operation of choice for advanced lesions and as a salvage procedure for RT failures in lesions that are not suited for conservation surgery. The entire larynx is removed, and the pharynx is reconstructed. A permanent tracheostomy is required. Speech may be reconstituted with a prosthesis or with an electrolarynx. One hundred four (63%) of 166 patients entered into the surgery and postoperative irradiation arm of the Veterans Affairs Laryngeal Cancer Study Group randomized trial were evaluable for communication status at 2 years after treatment.[52] Ninety-six patients had undergone a total laryngectomy and communicated as follows: tracheoesophageal, 27 (28%); esophageal, 5 (5%); artificial larynx, 47 (50%); nonvocal, 7 (7%); and no data, 10 (10%).[52] One hundred seventy-three patients underwent total laryngectomy and postoperative RT at the University of Florida, and 69 patients were evaluable for 5 years or longer.[28] Voice rehabilitation was accomplished as follows: tracheoesophageal, 19%; artificial larynx, 57%; esophageal, 3%; nonvocal, 14%; and no data, 7%.

Radiation Therapy Technique

RT for T1 or T2 vocal cord cancer is delivered by small portals covering only the primary lesion.[38] The cervical lymph node chain is not electively treated. For T1 lesions, RT portals extend from the thyroid notch superiorly to the inferior border of the cricoid and fall off anteriorly. The posterior border depends on the posterior extension of the tumor.[20] For T2 tumors, the field is extended depending on the anatomic distribution of the tumor. The field size ranges from 4 × 4 cm to 5 × 5 cm (plus an additional 1.0 cm of "flash" anteriorly) and is occasionally 6 × 6 cm for a large T2 lesion. Portals larger than this increase the risk of edema without improving the cure rate.

A commonly used dose-fractionation schedule at many institutions is 66 Gy for T1 lesions and 70 Gy for T2 cancers given in 2-Gy fractions. Evidence suggests that increasing the dose per fraction may improve the likelihood of local control.[53–57] Ample data suggest that 1.8 Gy once daily results in significantly lower local control rates compared with 2.0 Gy

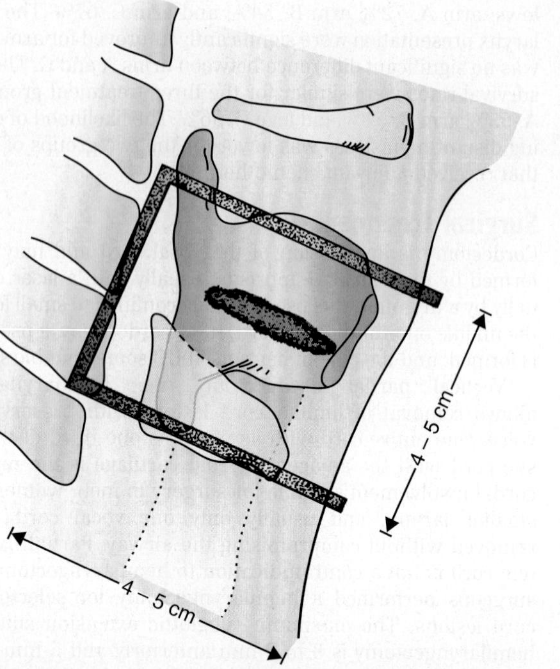

FIGURE 47.7. Treatment portal for early glottic carcinoma. The top border is adjusted according to the lesion. The middle of the thyroid notch is the landmark for very early lesions, and the top of the notch is the marker for larger lesions or those with minimal supraglottic extension. The posterior border is 1 cm posterior to the back edge of the thyroid cartilage if the lesion is confined to the anterior two-thirds of the vocal cord; if the posterior one-third of the vocal cord is involved, the posterior border is placed 1.0 to 1.5 cm behind the cartilage. The inferior border is placed at the bottom of the cricoid cartilage if there is no subglottic extension. (From Million RR, Cassisi NJ, Mancuso AA. Larynx. In: Million RR, Cassisi NJ, eds. *Management of head and neck cancer: a multidisciplinary approach,* 2nd ed. Philadelphia, JB Lippincott, 1994;431–497.)

once daily.[54] Yamakazi et al.[58] reported a prospective trial in which patients with T1 N0 squamous cell carcinoma of the glottic larynx were randomized to definitive RT at 2.0 Gy per fraction or 2.25 Gy per fraction. The 5-year local control rates were 77% after 2.0 Gy per fraction and 92% after Gy per fraction ($p = .004$); there was no difference in either acute or late toxicity. Patients with T1 or T2 vocal cord cancer treated with once-a-day fractionation at the University of Florida are irradiated with 2.25-Gy fractions; the dose-fractionation schemes used are as follows: Tis–T2 A, 63.0 Gy in 28 fractions, and T2B, 65.25 Gy in 29 fractions.

At the University of Florida, patients are treated in the supine position; the field borders for a patient with a T1 N0 cancer are depicted in Figure 47.7.[20] The field is checked by the physician at the treatment machine according to palpable anatomic landmarks. This allows the treatment volume to be kept at a minimum and reduces the risk of geographic miss. A three-field technique, using 4- or 6-MV x-rays, is used to deliver approximately 95% of the dose through opposed lateral wedged fields weighted to the side of the lesion; the remaining dose is delivered by an anterior field shifted 0.5 cm toward the side of the lesion (Fig. 47.8).[20] The tumor dose is usually specified at the 95% normalized isodose line.

RT of T3 and T4 lesions requires larger portals, which include the levels II and III lymph nodes (Fig. 47.9).[59,60] The level IV lymph nodes are included in a separate low-neck portal. Patients treated at the University of Florida are irradiated in a continuous course twice daily at 1.2 Gy per fraction to a total dose of 74.4 Gy. The portals are reduced after 45.6 Gy in 38 fractions; the reduced portals cover only the primary lesion.

Intensity-modulated RT (IMRT) is used if there is a clear advantage associated with this technique. Disadvantages associated with IMRT include increased dose inhomogeneity, increased total body dose, and increased labor and expense.[61] The most

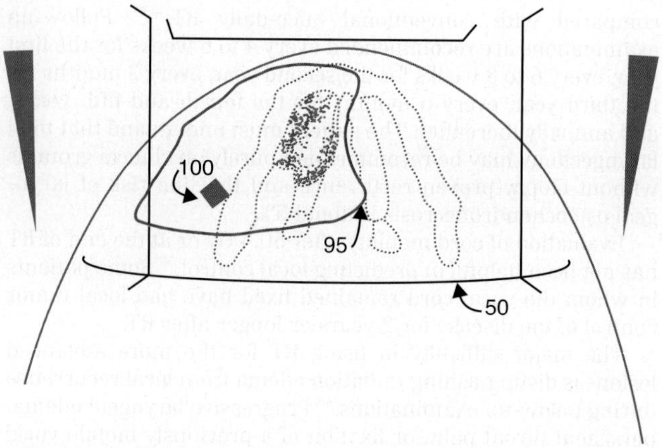

FIGURE 47.8. Normalized isodose distribution for three-field technique for treatment of a tumor involving the anterior two-thirds of one true vocal cord. The dose is specified at the 95% isodose line. (From Million RR, Cassisi NJ, Mancuso AA. Larynx. In: Million RR, Cassisi NJ, eds. *Management of head and neck cancer: a multidisciplinary approach,* 2nd ed. Philadelphia, JB Lippincott, 1994;431–497.)

common indications for IMRT for laryngeal cancers would be the occasional patients with a node-positive T3–T4 cancer, where the retropharyngeal nodes would be electively irradiated and the dose to the contralateral parotid gland reduced, and/or a difficult low match between the lateral fields used to treat the primary site and upper neck and the anterior low neck field in a patient with a short neck and large shoulders. In the latter instance, IMRT could be used to encompass the entire target volume and avoid the problem of field junctioning entirely. IMRT is especially useful for patients with extensive subglottic invasion, where achieving an adequate inferior margin with conventional lateral portals may not be possible.

Evidence from both retrospective and randomized trials points to improved therapeutic ratios with altered fractionation schedules.[35] Given that RT is effective treatment for head and neck primary squamous cell carcinoma, it should not be surprising that higher doses of RT given more intensively would be more effective at providing tumor control. Because most observers have noted no increase in late toxicity with the various regimens, it generally is concluded that these schedules yield an improved therapeutic ratio. A recently updated Radiation Therapy Oncology Group 90-03 trial reported on 1,073 patients who were randomly selected to receive one of four fractionation schedules[47,62]:

1. Standard fractionation: 2 Gy per fraction, once a day, 5 days a week, to a total dose of 70 Gy in 35 fractions over 7 weeks
2. Hyperfractionation: 1.2 Gy per fraction, twice daily (≥6 hours apart), 5 days a week, to a total dose of 81.6 Gy in 68 fractions over 7 weeks
3. Accelerated fractionation with split: 1.6 Gy per fraction, twice daily (≥6 hours apart), 5 days a week, to a total dose of 67.2 Gy in 42 fractions over 6 weeks, including a 2-week rest after 38.4 Gy
4. Accelerated fractionation with concomitant boost: 1.8 Gy per fraction, once a day, 5 days a week to a large field, plus 1.5 Gy per fraction once a day to a boost field given 6 or more hours after treatment of the large field for the last 12 treatments days, to a total dose of 72 Gy in 42 fractions over 6 weeks

The 5-year local-regional failure rates were as follows: standard fractionation, 59%; hyperfractionation, 51%; accelerated split course, 58%; and concomitant boost, 52%. Both the hyperfractionation and concomitant boost schedules yielded local-regional control rates that were significantly better than those with standard fractionation. There was a trend toward improved overall survival with hyperfractionation but no difference in cause-specific survival. Acute toxicity was increased

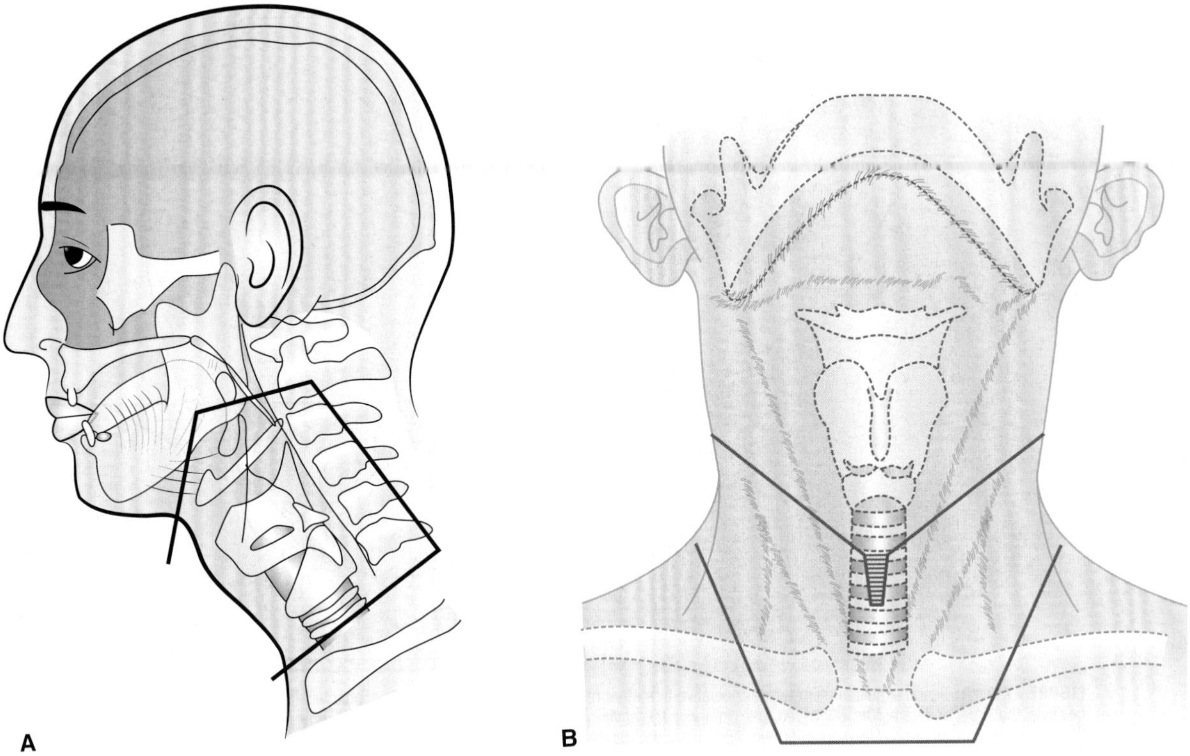

FIGURE 47.9. A: Radiation treatment technique for carcinoma of glottic larynx, stage T3-T4 N0. The patient is treated supine, and the field is shaped with Lipowitz's metal. Anteriorly, the field is allowed to fall off. The entire pre-epiglottic space is included by encompassing the hyoid bone and epiglottis. The superior border (just above the angle of the mandible) includes the jugulodigastric lymph nodes. Posteriorly, a portion of the spinal cord must be included within the field to ensure adequate coverage of the midjugular lymph nodes; spinal accessory lymph nodes themselves are at little risk of involvement. The lower border is slanted to facilitate matching with the low-neck field and to reduce the length of spinal cord in the high-dose field. The inferior border is placed at the bottom of the cricoid cartilage if the patient has no subglottic spread; in the presence of subglottic extension, the inferior border must be lowered according to the disease extent. **B:** Example of a low-neck portal for T3 N0 glottic carcinoma. The main nodes at risk are the low jugular and lateral paratracheal. The Delphian node would be in the primary portal. A very narrow and short midline shield is used. (A, from Parsons JT, Mendenhall WM, Mancuso AA, et al. Twice-a-day radiotherapy for squamous cell carcinoma of the glottic larynx. *Head Neck* 1989;11:123–128; with permission; B, from Million RR, Cassisi NJ, Mancuso AA, et al. Management of the neck for squamous cell carcinoma. In: Million RR, Cassisi NJ, eds. *Management of head and neck cancer: a multidisciplinary approach,* 2nd ed. Philadelphia: JB Lippincott Company, 1994:75–143.)

with all three altered fractionation schedules; there was a modest increase in late effects with the concomitant boost schedule.

The treatment technique used for postoperative RT after total laryngectomy is depicted in Figure 47.10.[50] The treatment technique for preoperative RT is essentially the same as that used for RT alone. Alternatively, IMRT may be employed for the indications discussed previously.

Treatment of Recurrence

Most recurrences appear within 18 months, but late recurrences may appear after 5 years. The latter are likely second primary malignancies. The risk of metastatic disease in lymph nodes increases with local recurrence.[17]

Recurrence After Radiation Therapy

With careful follow-up, recurrence is sometimes detected before the patient notices a return of hoarseness. There is often minimal lymphedema for 1 to 2 months after RT, which usually subsides or stabilizes. An increase in edema, particularly if associated with hoarseness or pain, suggests recurrence, even if there is no obvious tumor. Fixation of a previously mobile vocal cord usually implies local recurrence, but we have occasionally observed a patient who has experienced a fixed cord with an otherwise normal-appearing larynx and who has not shown evidence of recurrence.

It may be difficult to diagnose recurrence if the tumor is submucosal. Generous, deep biopsies are required. If recurrence is strongly suspected, laryngectomy may rarely be advised without biopsy-confirmed evidence of recurrence. Positron emission tomography may be useful to distinguish recurrent tumor from necrosis.

RT failures may be salvaged by cordectomy, hemilaryngectomy, supracricoid partial laryngectomy, or total laryngectomy. Biller et al.[63] reported a 78% salvage rate by hemilaryngectomy for 18 selected patients in whom RT failed; total laryngectomy was eventually required in 2 patients. Only 2 patients died of cancer. These investigators offered guidelines for using hemilaryngectomy: contralateral vocal cord is normal, arytenoid is not involved, subglottic extension does not exceed 5 mm, and vocal cord is not fixed. In our experience, 14 patients irradiated for T1 or T2 vocal cord cancers underwent a hemilaryngectomy after local recurrence, and 8 were successfully salvaged.[17]

Recurrence After Surgery

The rate of salvage by RT for recurrences or new tumors that appear after initial treatment by hemilaryngectomy is about 50%. Lee et al.[64] reported 7 successes among 12 patients; one lesion was later controlled by total laryngectomy. Total laryngectomy can be used successfully to treat hemilaryngectomy failures not suitable for RT. RT rarely cures patients with recurrence in the neck or stoma after total laryngectomy.

TREATMENT SELECTION AND TECHNIQUE: SUPRAGLOTTIC LARYNX CARCINOMA

Selection of Treatment Modality

Patients with supraglottic laryngeal carcinoma may be considered to be in an early or favorable group suitable for RT

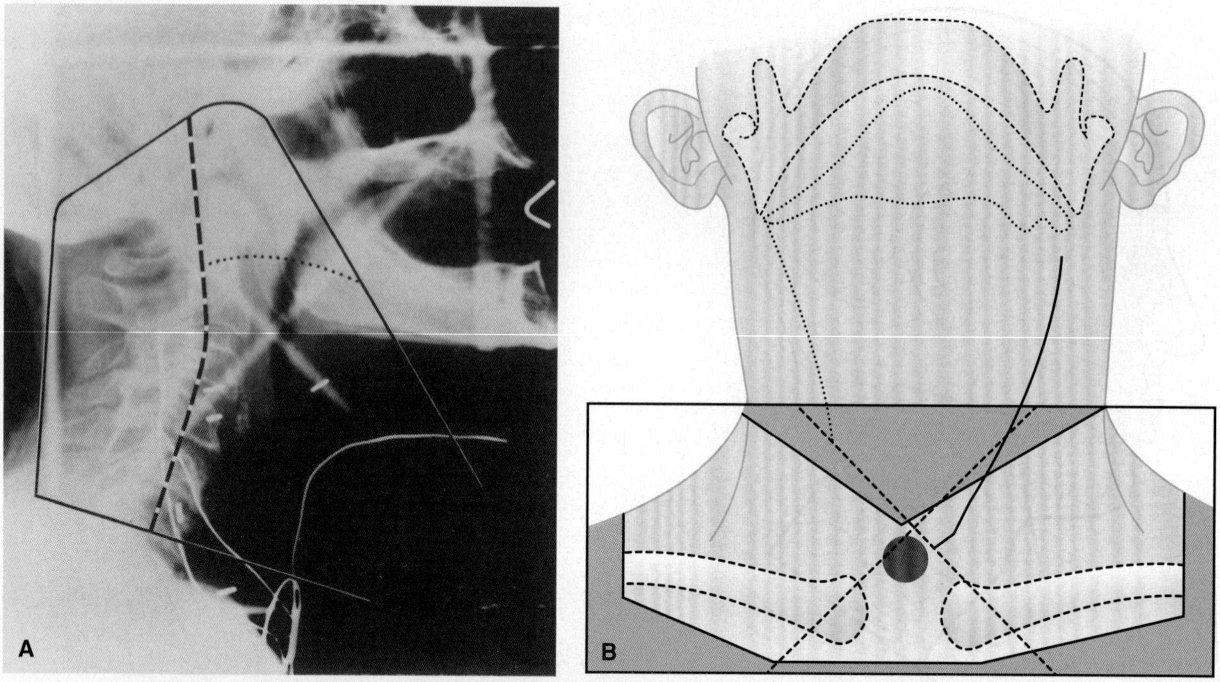

FIGURE 47.10. A: Typical simulation film for postoperative treatment of advanced cancer of the laryngopharynx. If the neck is pathologically negative, the superior field border is lowered to 2 cm above the angle of the mandible. The initial "off-cord" reduction (50 Gy) (*broken line*) and the final reduction (*dotted line*) are indicated. Wires mark the surgical scars and stoma. The slanting line used on the lower border reduces the length of spinal cord treated by the primary field, allows better caudal coverage of the mucosal surfaces while simultaneously bypassing the shoulders, and facilitates matching of the low-neck field. **B:** Schematic diagram of the low-neck field. The rectangle (*solid line*) represents the light field. The shaded areas represent the blocked portions of the field (stacked lead blocks). The superior border of the neck field is the inferior border of the primary field. The actual line is treated only in the primary field. The upper border of the low-neck field assumes a V shape. In the midline of the patient, the apex of the V generally is at or close to the central axis (*broken lines*), so that the portal that treats the spinal cord is not divergent in its upper portion and diverges away from the primary fields in its lower portion. At the junction of the three fields, a short (2 to 3 cm) segment of spinal cord remains untreated by any of the three fields. (From Amdur RJ, Parsons JT, Mendenhall WM, et al. Postoperative irradiation for squamous cell carcinoma of the head and neck: an analysis of treatment results and complications. *Int J Radiat Oncol Biol Phys* 1989;16:25–36; with permission from Elsevier.)

or conservation laryngectomy or an unfavorable group often requiring total laryngectomy.

Early and Moderately Advanced Supraglottic Lesions

Treatment of the primary lesion for the early group is by RT or supraglottic laryngectomy, with or without adjuvant RT.[65] Transoral laser excision is effective in experienced hands for small, selected lesions.[42] Total laryngectomy is rarely indicated as the initial treatment for this group of patients and is reserved for treatment failures.

RT and supraglottic laryngectomy are highly successful modes of therapy for early lesions.[65] Approximately 50% of supraglottic laryngectomies performed at the University of Florida have been followed by postoperative RT because of neck disease and, less often, positive margins.

The decision to use RT or supraglottic laryngectomy depends on several factors, including the anatomic extent of the tumor, medical condition of the patient, philosophy of the attending physician(s), and inclination of the patient and family. Overall, about 80% of patients are treated initially by RT. Approximately half of the patients seen in our clinic whose lesions are technically suitable for a supraglottic laryngectomy are not suitable for medical reasons (e.g., inadequate pulmonary status or other major medical problems); these patients are treated with RT.

Analysis of local control by anatomic site within the supraglottic larynx shows no obvious differences in local control by RT for similarly staged lesions. Invasion of the pre-epiglottic space is not a contraindication to supraglottic laryngectomy or RT. Primary tumor volume based on pretreatment CT is inversely related to local tumor control after RT.[31] A large, bulky (>6 cc) infiltrative lesion, especially one with extensive pre-epiglottic space invasion, is a common reason to select supraglottic laryngectomy.

The status of the neck often determines the selection of treatment of the primary lesion. Patients with clinically negative neck nodes have a high risk for occult neck disease and may be treated by RT or supraglottic laryngectomy and bilateral selective neck dissections (levels II to IV).

If a patient has an early-stage primary lesion but advanced neck disease (N2b or N3), combined treatment is frequently necessary to control the neck disease.[29] In these cases, the primary lesion is usually treated by definitive RT, with surgery added to the treatment of the involved neck site(s). If the same patient were treated with supraglottic laryngectomy, neck dissection, and postoperative RT, the portals would unnecessarily cover the primary site and the neck. If the patient has early, resectable neck disease (N1 or N2a) and surgery is elected for the primary site, postoperative RT is added only because of unexpected findings (e.g., positive margins, multiple positive nodes, or extracapsular extension). We prefer to avoid routine high-dose preoperative or postoperative RT in conjunction with a supraglottic laryngectomy because the lymphedema of the remaining larynx may be considerable, although it eventually subsides. However, Lee et al.[66] from the MD Anderson Cancer Center reported excellent results with combined supraglottic laryngectomy and postoperative RT for moderately advanced lesions.

Advanced Supraglottic Lesions

Although a subset of these patients may be suitable for a supraglottic or supracricoid laryngectomy, total laryngectomy is the main surgical option. Selected advanced lesions, especially those that are mainly exophytic, may be treated by RT and concomitant chemotherapy,[34] with total laryngectomy reserved for RT failures.

For patients whose primary lesion is to be treated by a total or partial laryngectomy and who have resectable neck disease, surgery is the initial treatment, and postoperative RT is added if needed. If the neck disease is unresectable, preoperative RT is used. The indications for preoperative and postoperative RT have been previously outlined.

Surgical Treatment

Supraglottic Laryngectomy

Supraglottic laryngectomy is voice-sparing surgery that can be used successfully for selected lesions involving the epiglottis, a single arytenoid, the aryepiglottic fold, or the false vocal cord. Extension of the tumor to the true vocal cord, the anterior commissure, or both arytenoids, fixation of the vocal cord, or thyroid or cricoid cartilage invasion precludes supraglottic laryngectomy. The supraglottic laryngectomy may be extended to include the base of the tongue if one lingual artery is preserved.

All patients have difficulty swallowing, with a tendency to aspirate immediately after surgery, but almost all learn to swallow again in a short time; motivation and the amount of tissue removed are key factors in learning to swallow again. Preoperatively, adequate pulmonary reserve is evaluated by blood gas determinations, function tests, chest roentgenography, and a work test involving walking the patient up two flights of stairs to determine tolerance to pulmonary stress. The voice quality is generally normal after supraglottic laryngectomy.

Supracricoid Laryngectomy

This procedure is an option for lesions extending from the supraglottis into one or both vocal cords. However, vocal cord fixation is a relative contraindication. At least one arytenoid must be preserved for successful decannulation and phonation. Extension to the cricoid and thyroid cartilage destruction also preclude its use. Phonation and respiratory function are reconstituted by approximating the cricoid to the hyoid (cricohyoidopexy).

Wide-Field Total Laryngectomy

Total laryngectomy is performed as previously described.

Radiation Therapy Technique

The primary lesion and both sides of the neck are treated with opposed lateral portals; wedges are used to compensate for the contour of the neck (Fig. 47.11).[20] The lower neck nodes are irradiated through a separate anterior portal. IMRT may be employed to spare one or both parotids and to avoid a low match line in the occasional patient with a short neck and large shoulders. We currently use either the concomitant boost fractionation schedule or hyperfractionation when employing IMRT.

In the case of clinically positive nodes, an electron beam portal may be used to increase the dose to the posterior cervical nodes after the fields are reduced to avoid the spinal cord at 45 Gy. CT is obtained 4 weeks after completing RT, and a neck dissection is added if the residual cancer in the nodes is believed to exceed 5%; otherwise the patient is observed and a CT is repeated in 3 months.[29]

Patients experience a sore throat, loss of taste, and moderate dryness during RT. Edema of the arytenoids may occur and give a sensation of a lump in the throat. Tracheostomy is rarely necessary, even for bulky lesions.

Edema of the larynx may persist for several months to a year. Patients who continue to smoke heighten the side effects of dryness, dysphagia, and hoarseness.

Preoperative and Postoperative Treatment Technique

If total laryngectomy is required and the lesion is resectable, postoperative RT is preferred because there is no evidence that

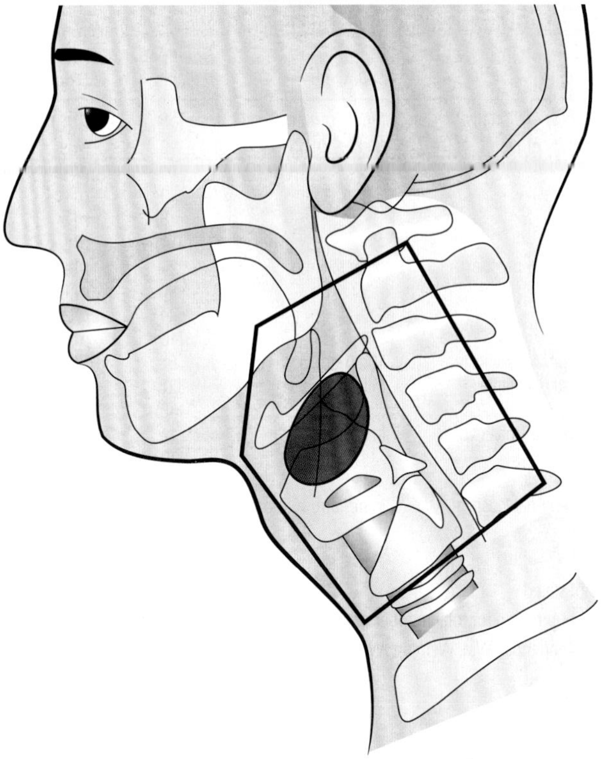

FIGURE 47.11. Example of the portal for a lesion of the lower epiglottis or false vocal cord and a clinically negative neck. The subdigastric nodes are included but not the junctional nodes. Depending on the anatomy and tumor extent, the anterior border may fall off (i.e., "flash") or a small strip of skin may be shielded. (From Million RR, Cassisi NJ, Mancuso AA, et al. Management of the neck for squamous cell carcinoma. In: Million RR, Cassisi NJ, ed. *Management of head and neck cancer: a multidisciplinary approach,* 2nd ed. Philadelphia: JB Lippincott, 1994:75–143.)

preoperative RT produces any better local-regional control or survival rates than surgery and postoperative RT. Irradiation is added for close or positive margins, invasion of soft tissues of the neck, significant subglottic extension (1 cm or more), thyroid cartilage invasion, multiple positive nodes, and extracapsular extension. The high-risk areas are usually the base of the tongue and the neck.

The dose for postoperative RT as a function of known residual disease is as follows: negative margins, 60 Gy in 30 fractions; microscopically positive margins, 66 Gy in 33 fractions; and gross residual disease, 70 Gy in 35 fractions. All patients are treated with a continuous course, one fraction per day, 5 days per week. The lower neck is treated with doses to 50 Gy in 25 fractions at D_{max}. If there is subglottic extension, the dose to the stoma is boosted with electrons (usually 10 to 14 MeV) for an additional 10 Gy in five fractions. The treatment technique is shown in Figure 47.10.[50] If postoperative RT is added after a supraglottic laryngectomy, the dose is lowered to 55.8 Gy given in 1.8-Gy fractions. This dose produces acceptable rates of local control and laryngeal edema.[66]

The treatment technique used for preoperative RT is essentially the same as that used for patients treated with RT alone, using doses of 50 to 60 Gy at 1.8 to 2.0 Gy per fraction. Thereafter, the dose is boosted to areas of unresectable disease (usually the neck) to total doses ranging from 65 to 70 Gy.

Treatment of Recurrence

Failures after supraglottic laryngectomy or RT can frequently be controlled by further treatment; therefore, recognition of recurrence should be vigorously pursued.[65] Salvage of patients with recurrence after combined total laryngectomy and RT is uncommon. Stomal recurrences are occasionally controlled by RT or surgery.

TABLE 47.3 LOCAL CONTROL AFTER TRANSORAL LASER EXCISION

Institution	*Follow-up[a]*	*Number of Patients*	*Stage*	*Local Control (%) (Interval)*	*Local Control with Larynx Preservation (%) (Interval)*	*Ultimate Local Control (%) (Interval)*
University of Göttingen[42]	Median, 78 mo	159	pTis-pT2	94 (NS)	99 (NS)	–
University of Kiel[76]	Mean, 40 mo	8	pTis	100 (NS)	–	–
		88	pT1a	92 (NS)	–	–
		10	pT1b	80 (NS)	–	–
		8	pT2	88 (NS)	–	–
		114	pTis-pT2	–	96 (NS)	–
University of Brescia[77]	Mean, 76 mo	21	pTis	81 (NS)	–	95^b (5 yr)
		96	pT1	82 (NS)	–	87^b (5 yr)
		23	pT2	74 (NS)	–	91^b (5 yr)
		140	pTis-pT2	80 (NS)	97 (NS)	–
Washington University[78]	Minimum, 3 yr	61	T1	77 (NS)	90 (NS)	98 (NS)
University of Naples[79]	Minimum, 5 yr	321	T1	82^b (NS)	89^c (NS)	–
		158	T2	60^b (NS)	~67^c (NS)	–
La Sapienza University[80]	Minimum, 3 yr	12	Tis	100 (NS)	100 (NS)	–
		120	T1a	94 (NS)	100 (NS)	–
		24	T1b	91 (NS)	100 (NS)	–
Tata Memorial Hospital[81]	Minimum, 18 mo	52	T1a	90 (NS)	94 (NS)	–
		17	T1b	65 (NS)	88 (NS)	–
		13	T2	77 (NS)	92 (NS)	–

NS, not stated.
[a]Follow-up period for total number of patients. [b]Ultimate local control with laser treatment alone. [c]Local-regional control rate.
From Mendenhall WM, Werning JW, Hinerman RW, et al. Management of T1–T2 glottic carcinomas. *Cancer* 2004;100:1786–1792.

RESULTS OF TREATMENT

Vocal Cord Cancer

The local control and survival rates after treatment of early-stage glottic carcinoma are depicted in Tables 47.3 to 47.6.[37] Sengupta et al.[36] recently reported on 37 patients treated at the University of Florida with definitive RT for carcinoma in situ and observed the following 5 year outcomes: local control, 91%; local control with larynx preservation, 91%; and ultimate local control, 91%. Chera et al.[38] reported on 585 patients at the University of Florida for T1-T2 N0 glottic carcinoma and observed the following 5-year local control rates: T1A1, 95%; T1B, 94%; T2 A, 81%; and T2B, 74%. Hinerman et al.[27] recently reported an update of the University of Florida experience treating fixed-cord T3 glottic cancers with definitive RT and reported a 5-year local control rate after RT of 63%. The local control and survival rates are similar for transoral laser excision, open partial laryngectomy, and RT. Larynx preservation rates are also comparable. Voice quality depends on the amount of tissue removed with partial laryngectomy and is probably similar for patients with limited lesions treated with laser to those undergoing RT and poorer for patients undergoing open partial laryngectomy.[37]

Foote et al.[67] reported on 81 patients who underwent laryngectomy for T3 cancers at the Mayo Clinic between 1970 and 1981. Seventy-five patients underwent a total laryngectomy and 6 underwent a near-total laryngectomy; 53 patients received a neck dissection. No patient underwent adjuvant irradiation or chemotherapy. The 5-year rates of local-regional control, cause-specific survival, and absolute survival were 74%, 74%, and 54%, respectively. The results of definitive RT patients with T3 glottic carcinoma are depicted in Table 47.7[59] and are similar to the surgical outcomes reported by Foote et al.[67]

The survival and control rates of patients with T3 fixed-cord lesions treated at the University of Florida are presented in Table 47.8.[68] There was no relationship between subsequent local control and whether the vocal cord remained fixed or became mobile during irradiation. The incidence of severe complications, including those after the initial treatment and any later salvage procedures, was 15% after RT alone and 15% after surgery alone or combined with adjuvant irradiation. The vocal quality varied from fair to nearly normal.

The results of treatment of T4 vocal cord carcinoma in four surgical series and two radiotherapy series are summarized in

TABLE 47.4 LOCAL CONTROL AFTER OPEN PARTIAL LARYNGECTOMY

Institution	*Follow-up*	*Number of Patients*	*Stage*	*Local Control (%) (Interval)*	*Local Control with Larynx Preservation (%) (Interval)*	*Ultimate Local Control (%) (Interval)*
Universitaire Timone[82]	NS	62	T1	100 (NS)	100 (NS)	–
		65	T2	92 (NS)	92 (NS)	–
Hôpital Saint Charles[83]	Minimum, 3 yr	18	T1a	100 (NS)	–	–
		40	T1b	95 (NS)	–	–
		23	T2a	83 (NS)	–	–
Mayo Clinic[84]	Median, 6.6 yr	159	Tis–T1	93 (5 yr)	94 (NS)	100 (NS)
Hôpital Laënnec[85]	Minimum, 3 yr	295	T1	89 (NS)	–	–
		90	T2a	74 (NS)	–	–
		31	T2b	68 (NS)	–	–
		416	T1–T2b	84 (NS)	–	97 (NS)
Washington University[78]	Minimum, 3 yr	404	T1	92 (NS)	93 (NS)	99 (NS)
Washington University[86]	Minimum, 5 yr	71	T2	93 (NS)	93 (NS)	99 (NS)

NS, not stated.
From Mendenhall WM, Werning JW, Hinerman RW, et al. Management of T1–T2 glottic carcinomas. *Cancer* 2004;100:1786–1792.

TABLE 47.5 LOCAL CONTROL AFTER RADIOTHERAPY

Institution	*Follow-up[a]*	*Number of Patients*	*Stage*	*Local Control (Interval) (%)*	*Local Control with Larynx Preservation (Interval)(%)*	*Ultimate Local Control (Interval) (%)*
University of Florida[17]	Minimum, 2 yr	230	T1a	94 (5 yr)	95 (5 yr)	98 (5 yr)
	Median, 9.9 yr	61	T1b	93 (5 yr)	95 (5 yr)	98 (5 yr)
		146	T2a	80 (5 yr)	82 (5 yr)	96 (5 yr)
		82	T2b	72 (5 yr)	76 (5 yr)	96 (5 yr)
Massachusetts General Hospital[87]	NS	665	T1	93 (5 yr)	–	–
		145	T2a	77 (5 yr)	–	–
		92	T2b	71 (5 yr)	–	–
University of California, San Francisco[88]	Median, 9.7 yr	315	T1	85 (5 yr)	–	96[b] (5 yr)
		83	T2	70 (5 yr)	–	91[b] (5 yr)
Princess Margaret Hospital[89]	Median, 6.8 yr	403	T1a	91 (5 yr)	–	–
		46	T1b	82 (5 yr)	–	–
		286	T2	69 (5 yr)	–	–
MD Anderson Hospital[90]	Median, 6.8 yr	114	T2a	74 (5 yr)	–	–
		116	T2b	70 (5 yr)	–	–
		230	T2	72 (5 yr)	–	91 (5 yr)

NS, not stated,

[a]Follow-up period for total number of patients. [b]Local-regional control rate.

From Mendenhall WM, Werning JW, Hinerman RW, et al. Management of T1–T2 glottic carcinomas. *Cancer* 2004;100:1786–1792.

TABLE 47.6 SURVIVAL DATA

Institution	*Treatment*	*Follow-up*	*Number of Patients*	*Stage*	*Cause-Specific Survival (Interval) (%)*	*Absolute Survival (Interval) (%)*
Washington University[78]	Laser	Minimum, 3 yr	61	T1	95 (5 yr)	84 (5 yr)
University of Göttingen[42]	Laser	Median, 6.5 yr	159	pTis–T2	100 (5 yr)	87 (5 yr)
University of Brescia[77]	Laser	Mean, 6.3 yr	140	pTis–T2	98 (5 yr)	93 (5 yr)
Washington University[78]	OPL	Minimum, 3 yr	404	T1	97 (5 yr)	84 (5 yr)
Mayo Clinic[84]	OPL	Median, 6.6 yr	159	Tis-T1	–	84 (5 yr)
Washington University[86]	OPL	Minimum, 5 yr	71	T2	–	~92 (5 yr)
University of Florida[17]	RT	Minimum, 2 yr	230	T1a	98 (5 yr)	82 (5 yr)
		Median, 9.9 yr	61	T1b	98 (5 yr)	79 (5 yr)
			146	T2a	95 (5 yr)	77 (5 yr)
			82	T2b	90 (5 yr)	77 (5 yr)
University of California San Francisco[88]	RT	Median, 9.7 yr	315	T1	96 (10 yr)	65 (10 yr)
			83	T2	91 (10 yr)	63 (10 yr)
Massachusetts General Hospital[87]	RT	NS	665	T1	98 (5 yr)	–
			145	T2a	92 (5 yr)	–
			92	T2b	84 (5 yr)	–
MD Anderson Hospital[90]	RT	Median, 6.8 yr	230	T2	92 (5 yr)	73 (5 yr)

NS, not stated; OPL, open partial laryngectomy; RT, radiotherapy.

From Mendenhall WM, Werning JW, Hinerman RW, et al. Management of T1–T2 glottic carcinomas. *Cancer* 2004;100:1786–1792.

TABLE 47.7 STAGE T3 GLOTTIC CARCINOMA TREATED WITH IRRADIATION ALONE (NO CHEMOTHERAPY)

Investigator	*Institution*	*Number of Patients*	*Minimum Follow-up (Year)*	*Local Control (%)*	*Ultimate Control After Salvage Surgery (%)*
Harwood et al.[91]	Princess Margaret (Toronto)	112	3	51	77
Wang[92]	Massachusetts General (Boston)	70	4	36	57
Fletcher et al.[93]	MD Anderson (Houston)	17	2	77	No data
Skolyszewski and Reinfuss[94]	15 European Centers	91	3	50	No data
Stewart et al.[95]	Manchester (England)	67	10	57	67
Mills[96]	Capetown, South Africa	18	2	44	78
Mendenhall et al.[32]	University of Florida (Gainesville)	75	2	63	86

Modified from Parsons JT, Mendenhall WM, Mancuso AA, et al. Twice-a-day radiotherapy for T3 squamous cell carcinoma of the glottic larynx. *Head Neck* 1989;11:123–128.

TABLE 47.8 T3 GLOTTIC CARCINOMA TREATED AT THE UNIVERSITY OF FLORIDA, 1965–1988: FIVE-YEAR RESULTS

Parameter	*Radiotherapy Alone (53 Patients)*	*Surgery With or Without Adjuvant Radiotherapy (65 Patients)*
Local-regional control (%)	62	75
Ultimate local-regional control (%)	84	82
Absolute survival (%)	55	45
Cause-specific survival (%)	75	71

Data from Mendenhall WM, Parsons JT, Stringer SP, et al. Stage T3 squamous cell carcinoma of the glottic larynx: a comparison of laryngectomy and irradiation. *Int J Radiat Oncol Biol Phys* 1992;23:725–732.

TABLE 47.9 TREATMENT OF STAGE T4 GLOTTIC CARCINOMAS

Investigator	Tumor Stage	Number of Patients	Method of Treatment	Results: No Evidence of Disease
Jesse[97]	T4 N0–N+	48	Laryngectomy	54% at 4 yr
Ogura et al.[98]	T4 N0	11	Laryngectomy	45% at 3 yr
Skolnick et al.[99]	T4 N0	7	Laryngectomy	30% at 5 yr
Vermund[100]	T4 N0	31	Laryngectomy	35% at 5 yr
Stewart and Jackson[101]	T4 N0	13	Radiotherapy with surgery for salvage	38% at 5 yr
Harwood et al.[53]	T4 N0	56	Radiotherapy with surgery for salvage	49% at 5 yr[a]

[a]Life-table method; uncorrected for deaths from intercurrent disease.

Modified from Harwood AR, Beal FA, Cummings BJ, et al. T4N0M0 glottic cancer: an analysis of dose-time-volume. *Int J Radiat Oncol Biol Phys* 1981;7:1507–1512.

Table 47.9.[53] Hinerman et al.[27] observed an 81% 5-year local control rate in 22 selected patients with favorable T4 cancers treated with definitive RT at the University of Florida.

Parsons et al.[69] reviewed the literature and reported a local control rate of 62% in a series of 87 patients treated with RT alone for T4 glottic carcinoma.

Supraglottic Cancer

The proportion of patients suitable for a supraglottic laryngectomy is depicted in Table 47.10.[65] Depending on the referral patterns, a modest subset of patients is suitable for this operation. The extent of neck disease for patients treated with either surgery or RT is shown in Table 47.11.[65] In general, patients treated with supraglottic laryngectomy appropriately have earlier-stage neck disease and would be anticipated to have a lower risk of distant failure and improved survival. The local control rates after transoral laser, RT, and supraglottic laryngectomy are summarized in Tables 47.12 to 47.14.[65] In general, the local control rates after transoral laser excision are fairly good for patients with T1–T2 tumors and tend to deteriorate for those with more advanced disease. The local control rate for patients selected for supraglottic laryngectomy is excellent. However, the incidence of severe complications tends to be higher after supraglottic laryngectomy compared with RT and transoral laser excision (Table 47.15).[65,70]

FOLLOW-UP POLICY

Follow-up of patients with early lesions is planned for every 4 to 8 weeks for 2 years, every 3 months for the third year, and every 6 months for years 4 and 5, and then annually for life.

Follow-up of patients with vocal cord or supraglottic larynx lesions treated by RT or conservative surgery is almost more important than the treatment itself because early detection of recurrence usually results in salvage that may include cure with voice preservation.

If recurrence is suspected but the biopsy is negative, patients are reexamined at 2- to 4-week intervals until the matter is settled. The value of follow-up CT scans for detecting early local recurrence is investigational.

Wagenfeld et al.[71] studied 740 cases of glottic larynx cancer treated from 1965 to 1974 to determine the incidence of second respiratory tract malignancies. There was a minimum follow-up of 5 years. There were 48 second respiratory tract malignancies, although only 14 were expected. Twenty-five were in the lung, and 23 were scattered among other head and neck sites. Only 7 of the 23 second head and neck primary lesions resulted in death; these second lesions were frequently diagnosed in an early stage during routine follow-up for the glottic lesion.

Because the risk of a lethal lung primary lesion is nearly as great as that of dying of an early glottic carcinoma, it makes sense to obtain annual chest roentgenograms. Approximately 50% of patients who receive moderate- to high-dose RT to the entire thyroid gland will develop hypothyroidism within 5 years, and so thyroid functions are checked every 6 to 12 months and thyroid replacement is initiated if the thyroid-stimulating hormone level begins to rise.[72]

SEQUELAE OF TREATMENT

Surgical Sequelae

Neel et al.[73] reported a 26% incidence of nonfatal complications for cordectomy. Immediate postoperative complications included atelectasis and pneumonia, severe subcutaneous emphysema in the neck, bleeding from the tracheotomy site or larynx, wound complications, and airway obstruction requiring tracheotomy. Late complications included granulation tissue that had to be removed by direct laryngoscopy to exclude recurrences, extrusion of cartilage, laryngeal stenosis, and obstructing laryngeal web.

TABLE 47.10 PROPORTION OF PATIENTS SUITABLE FOR SUPRAGLOTTIC LARYNGECTOMY

Series	Number of Patients	Number (Percentage) with Supraglottic Laryngectomy
Ogura et al., 1975[102]	263	177 (67%)
Lutz et al., 1990[103]	202	72 (36%)
Lee et al., 1990[66]	404	60 (15%)
Weems et al., 1987[104]	195	30 (15%)
Gregor et al., 1996[105]	89	26 (29%)
Spriano et al., 1997[106]	257	38 (14%)

Some values were estimated as closely as possible to fit the table format if the information was not specifically stated in the cited reference.

From Hinerman RW, Mendenhall WM, Amdur RJ, et al. Carcinoma of the supraglottic larynx: treatment results with radiotherapy alone or with planned neck dissection. *Head Neck* 2002;24:456–467.

TABLE 47.11 SUPRAGLOTTIC CARCINOMA: EXTENT OF NECK DISEASE VERSUS TREATMENT

Series	Treatment	Number of Patients	Extent of Neck Disease
Bocca, 1991[107]	SGL	537	94% N0–N1
Isaacs et al., 1998[108]	SGL	39	74% N0–N1
Ogura et al., 1975[102]	SGL	177	77% N0
Davis et al., 1991[109]	Laser	14	93% N0
Zeitels et al., 1994[110]	Laser	45	100% N0
Rudert et al., 1999[111]	Laser	34	82% N0–N1
Ghossein et al. 1974[112]	Radiation	203	53% N0
Hinerman et al., 2002[65]	Radiation	274	54% N0

SGL, supraglottic laryngectomy.

Some values were estimated as closely as possible to fit the table format if the information was not specifically stated in the cited reference.

From Hinerman RW, Mendenhall WM, Amdur RJ, et al. Carcinoma of the supraglottic larynx: treatment results with radiotherapy alone or with planned neck dissection. *Head Neck* 2002;24:456–467.

TABLE 47.12 SUPRAGLOTTIC CANCER: LOCAL CONTROL AFTER TRANSORAL LASER EXCISION

Series	Staging	Number of Patients	Percentage of Patients with T1 or T2 Tumors	Local Control (%)			
				T1	T2	T3	T4
Davis et al., 1991[109]	P	14 R	57	100	100	50	–
Steiner,[a] 1993[42]	P	81 R	72	–	76	77	100
Zeitels et al., 1994[110]	ND	22	100	100	100	–	–
Zeitels et al., 1994[110]	ND	23 R	65	100	92	63	–
Csanády et al., 1999[113]	ND	23	100	70[b]		–	–
Rudert et al., 1999[111]	P	34 R	50	100	75	78	38

Some values were estimated as closely as possible to fit the table format if the information was not specifically stated in the cited reference.

ND, type of staging not provided; P, pathologic staging; R, plus or minus radiotherapy.

[a]Fifty-one glottic and 30 supraglottic. [b]Overall local control rate for T1 and T2.

From Hinerman RW, Mendenhall WM, Amdur RJ, et al. Carcinoma of the supraglottic larynx: treatment results with radiotherapy alone or with planned neck dissection. *Head Neck* 2002;24:456–467.

TABLE 47.13 SUPRAGLOTTIC CANCER: LOCAL CONTROL AFTER RADIOTHERAPY

Series	Institution	Number of Patients	Local Control (%)			
			T1	T2	T3	T4
Fletcher and Hamberger, 1974[114]	MD Anderson Hospital	173	88	79	62	47
Ghossein et al., 1974[112]	Fondation Curie	203	94	73	46[a]	52
Wang and Montgomery, 1991[115]	Massachusetts General Hospital	229 q.d.	73	60	54	26
		209 b.i.d.	89	89	71	91
Nakfoor et al., 1998[116]	Massachusetts General Hospital	164	96	86	76	43
Sykes et al., 2000[117]	Christie Hospital	331[b]	92[c]	81[c]	67[c]	73[c]
Hinerman et al., 2002[65]	University of Florida[d]	274	100	86	62	62

Some values were estimated as closely as possible to fit the table format if the information was not specifically stated in the cited reference. b.i.d., twice a day; q.d., once a day.

[a]All had cord fixation. [b]All N0. [c]After 17 were salvaged by total laryngectomies.

[d]1998 American Joint Committee on Cancer staging.

From Hinerman RW, Mendenhall WM, Amdur RJ, et al. Carcinoma of the supraglottic larynx: treatment results with radiotherapy alone or with planned neck dissection. *Head Neck* 2002;24:456–467.

TABLE 47.14 LOCAL CONTROL AFTER SUPRAGLOTTIC LARYNGECTOMY

Series	Institution	Number of Patients	Patients with T1 and T2 Tumors (%)	Local Control (%)			
				T1	T2	T3	T4
Ogura et al., 1975[102]	Washington University	177	78		94[a]		
Bocca, 1991[107]	Milan University						
Stage I		47	100	94			
Stage II		252	100		82		
Stage III		205	53		80[b]		
Stage IV		33	70		67[c]		
Lee et al., 1990[66]	MD Anderson Cancer Center	60	58	100	100	100	100
DeSanto, 1990[118]	Mayo Clinic	70	100	100	100		
Steiniger et al., 1997[119]	Albany Medical College	29	83		97[a]		
Spriano et al., 1997[106]	Varese, Italy	54	100	96[d]			
Burstein and Calcattera, 1985[120]	University of California, Los Angeles	40	58	100[d]		85	94
Isaacs et al., 1998[108]	University of Florida	33	76	100[d]		78	71
Lutz et al., 1990[103]	University of Pittsburgh	72	No data			99[d]	

Some values were estimated as closely as possible to fit the table format if the information was not specifically stated in the cited reference. T stages were not specified.

[a]Overall local control rate for T1–T4. [b]Overall local control rate for T1–T3. [c]Overall local control rate for T2–T3.

[d]Overall local control rate for T1–T2.

From Hinerman RW, Mendenhall WM, Amdur RJ, et al. Carcinoma of the supraglottic larynx: treatment results with radiotherapy alone or with planned neck dissection. *Head Neck* 2002;24:456.

TABLE 47.15 SUPRAGLOTTIC CANCER: SEVERE COMPLICATIONS ACCORDING TO TREATMENT MODALITY

Series	Institution	Number (Percentage) of Severe Complications
Radiotherapy		
Fletcher and Hamberger, 1974[114]	MD Anderson Cancer Center	10/173 (6%)
Ghossein et al., 1974[112]	Fondation Curie	8/117 (7%)
Nakfoor et al., 1998[116]	Massachusetts General Hospital	12/169 (7%)
Sykes et al., 2000[117]	Christie Hospital	7/331 (2%)
Hinerman et al., 2002[65]	University of Florida	12/274 (4%)
Supraglottic Laryngectomy		
Lee et al., 1990[66]	MD Anderson Cancer Center	9/63 (14%)
Isaacs et al., 1998[108]	University of Florida	14/34 (41%)
Burstein and Calcaterra, 1985[120]	University of California, Los Angeles	14/41 (34%)
Steiniger et al., 1997[119]	Albany Medical College	12/29 (41%)
Spriano et al., 1997[106]	Varese, Italy	13/54 (24%)
Gall et al., 1977[74]	Washington University	20/133 (15%)
Weber et al., 1993[121]	University of Pittsburgh	12/69 (17%)
Beckhardt et al., 1994[122]	University of Wisconsin	15/50 (30%)
Transoral Laser Excision		
Rudert et al., 1999[111]	University of Kiel, Germany	3/34 (9%)
Zeitels et al., 1994[110]	Massachusetts Eye and Ear Infirmary	2/45 (4%)
Steiner,[a] 1993[42]	University of Göttingen, Germany	7/240 (3%)
Davis et al., 1991[109]	University of Utah, Salt Lake City	0/14 (0%)
Csanády et al., 1999[113]	Albert Szent Gyorgyi Medical University, Szeged, Hungary	0/23 (0%)

Some values were estimated as closely as possible to fit the table format if the information was not specifically stated in the cited reference.
[a]Includes patients with glottic cancer.
From Hinerman RW, Mendenhall WM, Amdur RJ, et al. Carcinoma of the supraglottic larynx: treatment results with radiotherapy alone or with planned neck dissection. *Head Neck* 2002;24:456–467.

The postoperative complications and sequelae of hemilaryngectomy include chondritis, wound slough, inadequate glottic closure, and anterior commissure webs.[74] The complications associated with supraglottic laryngectomy and total laryngectomy for supraglottic carcinomas include fistula (8%), carotid artery exposure or blowout (3% to 5%), infection or wound sloughing (3% to 7%), and fatal complications (3%).[74] The risk of complication increased if tumor margins were involved by tumor; there was no change in risk associated with age, sex, race, laryngeal site, stage of primary tumor, size of primary tumor, use of low-dose preoperative RT, or status of the positive nodes.

The incidence of complications after treatment of supraglottic carcinoma is given in Table 47.15.[65]

Radiation Therapy Sequelae

The acute reactions from the treatment of early vocal cord cancer using a tumor dose of 2.25 Gy per day to administer a total dose 63 Gy (4- or 6-MV photons, five fractions per week) are relatively mild. During the first 2 to 3 weeks, the voice may improve as the tumor regresses. The voice generally becomes hoarse again because of RT-induced changes, even though the tumor continues to regress. A mild sore throat develops beginning at the end of the second week, but medication is usually not required. The voice begins to improve approximately 3 weeks after completion of treatment, usually reaching a plateau in 2 to 3 months. Patients with extensive lesions often recover a normal voice, although not as frequently as those with small tumors.

Edema of the larynx is the most common sequela after RT for glottic or supraglottic lesions. The rate of clearance of the edema is related to the RT dose, volume of tissue irradiated, addition of a neck dissection, continued use of alcohol and tobacco, and size and extent of the original lesion. Edema may be accentuated by a radical neck dissection and may require 6 to 12 months to subside.

Soft-tissue necrosis leading to chondritis occurs in <1% of patients, usually in those who continue to smoke. Soft-tissue and cartilage necroses mimic recurrence, with hoarseness, pain, and edema; a laryngectomy may be recommended as a last resort for fear of recurrent cancer, even though biopsy specimens show only necrosis.

Corticosteroids such as dexamethasone (Decadron) have been used to reduce RT-induced edema after recurrence has been ruled out by biopsy. If ulceration and pain occur, administration of an antibiotic such as tetracycline may help. Of 519 patients with T1 N0 or T2 N0 vocal cord cancer treated at the University of Florida, 5 (1%) experienced severe complications,[17] including total laryngectomy for a suspected local recurrence (1 patient), permanent tracheostomy for edema (3 patients), and a pharyngocutaneous fistula after a salvage total laryngectomy (1 patient).

In patients irradiated for supraglottic carcinoma, sore throat persists 1 to 2 months after completion of treatment. There is an associated dry mouth from RT of the salivary and parotid glands, a loss of taste, and a sensation of a lump in the throat. It is unusual for patients to require a tracheotomy before RT unless severe lymphedema develops at the time of direct laryngoscopy and biopsy. However, in patients who have recovered from the direct laryngoscopy and biopsy without obstruction, a tracheotomy has rarely been required during a fractionated course of RT.

Patients treated twice a day with 1.2-Gy fractions (continuous-course technique) to a total dose of 74.4 Gy usually have more brisk acute reactions than those treated once a day with 2-Gy fractions. Approximately 30% treated with twice-a-day RT require temporary gastrostomy feeding tubes because they have difficulty in swallowing.[75]

Examples of acute chondritis requiring discontinuation of treatment have not been seen, although most epiglottic lesions exhibit cartilage invasion.

The epiglottis, both suprahyoid and infrahyoid portions, remains thicker than normal for long periods of time, but this is not often associated with difficulty in swallowing, respiratory obstruction, or aspiration. The patient is cautioned to eat and drink slowly until the edema resolves. The false cord and arytenoids may develop some edema.

Lesions of the suprahyoid epiglottis frequently destroy the tip of the epiglottis, and it may require some time for the exposed cartilage to heal. Successful RT of infrahyoid epiglottis tumors is not associated with a high rate of necrosis, even though most of these lesions penetrate the porous epiglottic cartilage.

The incidence of severe late complications in 274 patients treated with RT alone or combined with neck dissection at the University of Florida was 4%.[65]

ACKNOWLEDGMENT

We thank the research support staff of the Department of Radiation Oncology for their help with statistics, editing, and manuscript preparation.

REFERENCES

1. Clemente CD. *Anatomy: a regional atlas of the human body.* Philadelphia: Lea & Febiger, 1975.
2. Mancuso AA, Hanafee WN. *Head and neck radiology.* Philadelphia: Williams & Wilkins, 2011.
3. Lam KH, Wong J. The preepiglottic and paraglottic spaces in relation to spread of carcinoma of the larynx. *Am J Otolaryngol* 1983;4(2):81–91.
4. Hirano M. Structure and vibratory behavior of the vocal folds. In: Sawashima M, Cooper FS, editors. *Dynamic aspects of speech production: current results, emerging problems, and new instrumentation.* Tokyo: University of Tokyo Press, 1977:13–27.
5. Jemal A, Siegel R, Xu J, et al. Cancer statistics, 2010. *CA Cancer J Clin* 2010; 60(5): 277–300.
6. Ries LAG, Eisner MP, Kosary CL. *SEER cancer statistics review, 1973-1998.* Bethesda, MD: National Cancer Institute, 2001.
7. Wynder EL. The epidemiology of cancers of the upper alimentary and upper respiratory tracts. *Laryngoscope* 1978;88(1 Pt 2, Suppl 8): 50–51.
8. Vincent RG, Marchetta F. The relationship of the use of tobacco and alcohol to cancer of the oral cavity, pharynx or larynx. *Am J Surg* 1963;106:501–505.
9. Archer CR, Yeager VL, Herbold DR. Computed tomography vs. histology of laryngeal cancer: their value in predicting laryngeal cartilage invasion. *Laryngoscope* 1983;93(2):140–147.
10. Pillsbury HR, Kirchner JA. Clinical vs histopathologic staging in laryngeal cancer. *Arch Otolaryngol* 1979;105(3):157–159.
11. Broyles EN. The anterior commissure tendon. *Ann Otol Rhinol Laryngol* 1943; 52:342–345.
12. Kirchner JA. Staging as seen in serial sections. *Laryngoscope* 1975;85(11, Pt 1): 1816–1821.
13. Olofsson J, van Nostrand AW. Growth and spread of laryngeal and hypopharyngeal carcinoma with reflections on the effect of preoperative irradiation. 139 cases studied by whole organ serial sectioning. *Acta Otolaryngol Suppl* 1973;308: 1–84.
14. Lindberg R. Distribution of cervical lymph node metastases from squamous cell carcinoma of the upper respiratory and digestive tracts. *Cancer* 1972;29(6): 1446–1469.
15. Fletcher GH. Elective irradiation of subclinical disease in cancers of the head and neck. *Cancer* 1972;29(6):1450–1454.
16. Ogura JH, Biller HF, Wette R. Elective neck dissection for pharyngeal and laryngeal cancers. An evaluation. *Ann Otol Rhinol Laryngol* 1971;80(5):646–650.
17. Mendenhall WM, Amdur RJ, Morris CG, et al. T1-T2N0 squamous cell carcinoma of the glottic larynx treated with radiation therapy. *J Clin Oncol* 2001; 19(20):4029–4036.
18. Lederman M. The place of radiotherapy in the treatment of cancer of the larynx [in French]. *Ann Radiol (Paris)* 1961;4:433–454.
19. Million RR, Cassisi NJ. Larynx. In: Million RR, Cassisi NJ, ed. *Management of head and neck cancer: a multidisciplinary approach,* 1st ed. Phildelphia: JB Lippincott, 1984 315–364.
20. Million RR, Cassisi NJ, Mancuso AA. Larynx. In: Million RR, Cassisi NJ, ed. *Management of head and neck cancer: a multidisciplinary approach,* 2nd ed. Philadelphia: JB Lippincott, 1994:431–497.
21. McLaughlin MP, Mendenhall WM, Mancuso AA, et al. Retropharyngeal adenopathy as a predictor of outcome in squamous cell carcinoma of the head and neck. *Head Neck* 1995;17(3):190–198.
22. Archer CR, Yeager VL, Herbold DR. Improved diagnostic accuracy in laryngeal cancer using a new classification based on computed tomography. *Cancer* 1984;53(1):44–57.
23. Mendenhall WM, Parsons JT, Mancuso AA, et al. In: Carlos A, Perez LWB, eds. *Principles and practice of radiation oncology,* 3rd ed. Philadelphia: Lippincott-Raven, 1998:1069–1093.
24. American Joint Committee on Cancer, *AJCC cancer staging handbook,* 7th ed. New York: Springer, 2010.
25. Dagan R, Morris CG, Bennett JA, et al. Prognostic significance of paraglottic space invasion in T2N0 glottic carcinoma. *Am J Clin Oncol* 2007;30(2):186–190.
26. Gindhart TD, Johnston WH, Chism SE, et al. Carcinoma of the larynx in childhood. *Cancer* 1980;46(7):1683–1687.
27. Hinerman RW, Mendenhall WM, Morris CG, et al. T3 and T4 true vocal cord squamous carcinomas treated with external beam irradiation: a single institution's 35-year experience. *Am J Clin Oncol* 2007;30(2):181–185.
28. Mendenhall WM, Morris CG, Stringer SP, et al. Voice rehabilitation after total laryngectomy and postoperative radiation therapy. *J Clin Oncol* 2002;20(10):2500–2505.
29. Mendenhall WM, Villaret DB, Amdur RJ, et al. Planned neck dissection after definitive radiotherapy for squamous cell carcinoma of the head and neck. *Head Neck* 2002;24(11):1012–1018.
30. Induction chemotherapy plus radiation compared with surgery plus radiation in patients with advanced laryngeal cancer. The Department of Veterans Affairs Laryngeal Cancer Study Group. *N Engl J Med* 1991;324(24):1685–1690.
31. Mendenhall WM, Morris CG, Amdur RJ, et al. Parameters that predict local control after definitive radiotherapy for squamous cell carcinoma of the head and neck. *Head Neck* 2003;25(7):535–542.
32. Mendenhall WM, Parsons JT, Mancuso AA, et al. Definitive radiotherapy for T3 squamous cell carcinoma of the glottic larynx. *J Clin Oncol* 1997;15(6):2394–2402.
33. Forastiere AA, Goepfert H, Maor M, et al. Concurrent chemotherapy and radiotherapy for organ preservation in advanced laryngeal cancer. *N Engl J Med* 2003; 349(22):2091–2098.
34. Pignon JP, Bourhis J, Domenge C, et al. Chemotherapy added to locoregional treatment for head and neck squamous-cell carcinoma: three meta-analyses of updated individual data. MACH-NC Collaborative Group. Meta-Analysis of Chemotherapy on Head and Neck Cancer. *Lancet* 2000;355(9208):949–955.
35. Mendenhall WM, Riggs CE, Vaysberg M, et al. Altered fractionation and adjuvant chemotherapy for head and neck squamous cell carcinoma. *Head Neck* 2010; 32(7):939–945.
36. Sengupta N, Morris CG, Kirwan J, et al. Definitive radiotherapy for carcinoma in situ of the true vocal cords. *Am J Clin Oncol* 2010;33(1):94–95.
37. Mendenhall WM, Werning JW, Hinerman RW, et al. Management of T1-T2 glottic carcinomas. *Cancer* 2004;100(9):1786–1792.
38. Chera BS, Amdur RJ, Morris CG, et al. T1N0 to T2N0 squamous cell carcinoma of the glottic larynx treated with definitive radiotherapy. *Int J Radiat Oncol Biol Phys* 2010;78(2):461–466.
39. O'Sullivan B, Mackillop W, Gilbert R, et al. Controversies in the management of laryngeal cancer: results of an international survey of patterns of care. *Radiother Oncol* 1994;31(1):23–32.
40. Laccourreye H, Laccourreye O, Weinstein G, et al. Supracricoid laryngectomy with cricohyoidoepiglottopexy: a partial laryngeal procedure for glottic carcinoma. *Ann Otol Rhinol Laryngol* 1990;99(6, Pt 1): 421–426.
41. McGuirt WF, Blalock D, Koufman JA, et al. Comparative voice results after laser resection or irradiation of T1 vocal cord carcinoma. *Arch Otolaryngol Head Neck Surg* 1994;120(9):951–955.
42. Steiner W. Results of curative laser microsurgery of laryngeal carcinomas. *Am J Otolaryngol* 1993;14(2):116–121.
43. Rodrigo JP, Suarez C, Silver CE, et al. Transoral laser surgery for supraglottic cancer. *Head Neck* 2008;30(5):658–666.
44. Peretti G, Piazza C, Cocco D, et al. Transoral CO(2) laser treatment for T(is)-T(3) glottic cancer: the University of Brescia experience on 595 patients. *Head Neck* 2010;32(8):977–983.
45. Rodel RM, Steiner W, Muller RM, et al. Endoscopic laser surgery of early glottic cancer: involvement of the anterior commissure. *Head Neck* 2009;31(5):583–592.
46. O'Sullivan B, Warde P, Keane T, et al. Outcome following radiotherapy in verrucous carcinoma of the larynx. *Int J Radiat Oncol Biol Phys* 1995;32(3):611–617.
47. Fu KK, Pajak TF, Trotti A, et al. A Radiation Therapy Oncology Group (RTOG) phase III randomized study to compare hyperfractionation and two variants of accelerated fractionation to standard fractionation radiotherapy for head and neck squamous cell carcinomas: first report of RTOG 9003. *Int J Radiat Oncol Biol Phys* 2000;48(1):7–16.
48. Parsons JT, Mendenhall WM, Stringer SP, et al. Salvage surgery following radiation failure in squamous cell carcinoma of the supraglottic larynx. *Int J Radiat Oncol Biol Phys* 1995;32(3):605–609.
49. Pearson BW, Woods RD 2 nd, Hartman DE. Extended hemilaryngectomy for T3 glottic carcinoma with preservation of speech and swallowing. *Laryngoscope* 1980;90(12):1950–1961.
50. Amdur RJ, Parsons JT, Mendenhall WM, et al. Postoperative irradiation for squamous cell carcinoma of the head and neck: an analysis of treatment results and complications. *Int J Radiat Oncol Biol Phys* 1989;16(1):25–36.
51. Huang DT, Johnson CR, Schmidt-Ullrich R, et al. Postoperative radiotherapy in head and neck carcinoma with extracapsular lymph node extension and/or positive resection margins: a comparative study. *Int J Radiat Oncol Biol Phys* 1992;23(4):737–742.
52. Hillman RE, Walsh MJ, Wolf GT, et al. Functional outcomes following treatment for advanced laryngeal cancer. Part I—Voice preservation in advanced laryngeal cancer. Part II—Laryngectomy rehabilitation: the state of the art in the VA System. Research Speech-Language Pathologists. Department of Veterans Affairs Laryngeal Cancer Study Group. *Ann Otol Rhinol Laryngol Suppl* 1998;172:1–27.
53. Harwood AR, Beale FA, Cummings BJ, et al. T4NOMO glottic cancer: an analysis of dose-time volume factors. *Int J Radiat Oncol Biol Phys* 1981;7(11):1507–1512.
54. Kim RY, Marks ME, Salter MM. Early-stage glottic cancer: importance of dose fractionation in radiation therapy. *Radiology* 1992;182(1):273–275.
55. Schwaibold F, Scariato A, Nunno M, et al. The effect of fraction size on control of early glottic cancer. *Int J Radiat Oncol Biol Phys* 1988;14(3):451–454.
56. Woodhouse RJ, Quivey JM, Fu KK, et al. Treatment of carcinoma of the vocal cord. A review of 20 years experience. *Laryngoscope* 1981;91(7):1155–1162.
57. Mendenhall WM, Riggs CE, Cassisi NJ. Treatment of head and neck cancers. In: DeVita VT, Hellman S, Rosenberg SA, eds. *Cancer: principles and practice of oncology,* 8th ed. Philadelphia: Lippincott Williams & Wilkins, 2008:809–814.
58. Yamazaki H, Nishiyama K, Tanaka E, et al. Radiotherapy for early glottic carcinoma (T1N0M0): results of prospective randomized study of radiation fraction size and overall treatment time. *Int J Radiat Oncol Biol Phys* 2006;64(1):77–82.
59. Parsons JT, Mendenhall WM, Mancuso AA, et al. Twice-a-day radiotherapy for T3 squamous cell carcinoma of the glottic larynx. *Head Neck* 1989;11(2):123–128.
60. Million RR, Cassisi NJ, Mancuso AA, et al. Management of the neck for squamous cell carcinoma. In: Million RR, Cassisi NJ, eds. *Management of head and neck cancer: a multidisciplinary approach,* 2 nd ed. Philadelphia: JB Lippincott, 1994: 75–142.
61. Mendenhall WM, Mancuso AA. Radiotherapy for head and neck cancer—is the "next level" down? *Int J Radiat Oncol Biol Phys* 2009;73(3):645–646.
62. Trotti A, Fu KK, Pajak TF. Long term outcomes of RTOG 90-03: A comparison of hyperfractionation and two variants of accelerated fractionation to standard fractionation radiotherapy for head and neck squamous cell carcinoma. *Int J Radiat Oncol Biol Phys* 2005;63:S70–S71.
63. Biller HF, Barnhill FR Jr, Ogura JH, et al. Hemilaryngectomy following radiation failure for carcinoma of the vocal cords. *Laryngoscope* 1970;80(2):249–253.
64. Lee F, Perlmutter S, Ogura JH. Laryngeal radiation after hemilaryngectomy. *Laryngoscope* 1980;90(9):1534–1539.
65. Hinerman RW, Mendenhall WM, Amdur RJ, et al. Carcinoma of the supraglottic larynx: treatment results with radiotherapy alone or with planned neck dissection. *Head Neck* 2002;24(5):456–467.
66. Lee NK, Goepfert H, Wendt CD. Supraglottic laryngectomy for intermediate-stage cancer: U.T. M.D. Anderson Cancer Center experience with combined therapy. *Laryngoscope* 1990;100(8):831–836.
67. Foote RL, Olsen KD, Buskirk SJ, et al. Laryngectomy alone for T3 glottic cancer. *Head Neck* 1994;16(5):406–412.

68. Mendenhall WM, Parsons JT, Stringer SP, et al. Stage T3 squamous cell carcinoma of the glottic larynx: a comparison of laryngectomy and irradiation. *Int J Radiat Oncol Biol Phys* 1992;23(4):725–732.
69. Parsons JT, Mendenhall WM, Stringer SP, et al. T4 laryngeal carcinoma: radiotherapy alone with surgery reserved for salvage. *Int J Radiat Oncol Biol Phys* 1998;40(3):549–552.
70. Ganly I, Patel SG, Matsuo J, et al. Analysis of postoperative complications of open partial laryngectomy. *Head Neck* 2009;31(3):338–345.
71. Wagenfeld DJ, Harwood AR, Bryce DP, et al. Second primary respiratory tract malignancies in glottic carcinoma. *Cancer* 1980;46(8):1883–1886.
72. Garcia-Serra A, Amdur RJ, Morris CG, et al. Thyroid function should be monitored following radiotherapy to the low neck. *Am J Clin Oncol* 2005;28(3):255–258.
73. Neel HB 3rd, Devine KD, Desanto LW. Laryngofissure and cordectomy for early cordal carcinoma: outcome in 182 patients. *Otolaryngol Head Neck Surg* 1980; 88(1):79–84.
74. Gall AM, Sessions DG, Ogura JH. Complications following surgery for cancer of the larynx and hypopharynx. *Cancer* 1977;39(2):624–631.
75. Al-Othman MO, Amdur RJ, Morris CG, et al. Does feeding tube placement predict for long-term swallowing disability after radiotherapy for head and neck cancer? *Head Neck* 2003;25(9):741–747.
76. Rudert HH, Werner JA. Endoscopic resections of glottic and supraglottic carcinomas with the CO2 laser. *Eur Arch Otorhinolaryngol* 1995;252(3):146–148.
77. Peretti G, Nicolai P, Redaelli De Zinis LO, et al. Endoscopic CO2 laser excision for Tis, T1, and T2 glottic carcinomas: cure rate and prognostic factors. *Otolaryngol Head Neck Surg* 2000;123(1, Pt 1):124–131.
78. Spector JG, Sessions DG, Chao KS, et al. Stage I (T1 N0 M0) squamous cell carcinoma of the laryngeal glottis: therapeutic results and voice preservation. *Head Neck* 1999;21(8):707–717.
79. Motta G, Esposito E, Cassiano B, et al. T1-T2-T3 glottic tumors: fifteen years experience with CO2 laser. *Acta Otolaryngol Suppl* 1997;527:155–159.
80. Gallo A, de Vincentiis M, Manciocco V, et al. CO2 laser cordectomy for early-stage glottic carcinoma: a long-term follow-up of 156 cases. *Laryngoscope* 2002; 112(2):370–374.
81. Pradhan SA, Pai PS, Neeli SI, et al. Transoral laser surgery for early glottic cancers. *Arch Otolaryngol Head Neck Surg* 2003;129(6):623–625.
82. Giovanni A, Guelfucci B, Gras R, et al. Partial frontolateral laryngectomy with epiglottic reconstruction for management of early-stage glottic carcinoma. *Laryngoscope* 2001;111(4, Pt 1):663–668.
83. Crampette L, Garrel R, Gardiner Q, et al. Modified subtotal laryngectomy with cricohyoidoepiglottopexy—long term results in 81 patients. *Head Neck* 1999;21(2): 95–103.
84. Thomas JV, Olsen KD, Neel HB 3rd, et al. Early glottic carcinoma treated with open laryngeal procedures. *Arch Otolaryngol Head Neck Surg* 1994;120(3):264–268.
85. Laccourreye O, Weinstein G, Brasnu D, et al. A clinical trial of continuous cisplatin-fluorouracil induction chemotherapy and supracricoid partial laryngectomy for glottic carcinoma classified as T2. *Cancer* 1994;74(10):2781–2790.
86. Spector JG, Sessions DG, Chao KS, et al. Management of stage II (T2N0M0) glottic carcinoma by radiotherapy and conservation surgery. *Head Neck* 1999;21(2): 116–123.
87. Wang CC. Carcinoma of the larynx. In: Wang CC, ed. *Radiation therapy for head and neck neoplasms,* 3rd ed. New York: Wiley-Liss, 1997:221–255.
88. Le QT, Fu KK, Kroll S, et al. Influence of fraction size, total dose, and overall time on local control of T1-T2 glottic carcinoma. *Int J Radiat Oncol Biol Phys* 1997; 39(1):115–126.
89. Warde P, O'Sullivan B, Bristow RG, et al. T1/T2 glottic cancer managed by external beam radiotherapy: the influence of pretreatment hemoglobin on local control. *Int J Radiat Oncol Biol Phys* 1998;41(2):347–353.
90. Garden AS, Forster K, Wong PF, et al. Results of radiotherapy for T2N0 glottic carcinoma: does the "2" stand for twice-daily treatment? *Int J Radiat Oncol Biol Phys* 2003;55(2):322–328.
91. Harwood AR, Beale FA, Cummings BJ, et al. T3 glottic cancer: an analysis of dose time-volume factors. *Int J Radiat Oncol Biol Phys* 1980;6(6):675–680.
92. Wang CC. Radiation therapy of laryngeal tumors: curative radiation therapy. In: Thawley SE, Panje WR, eds. *Comprehensive management of head and neck tumors.* Philadelphia: WB Saunders, 1987:906–919.
93. Fletcher GH. Radiation therapy for cancer of the larynx and pyriform sinus. *Eye Ear Nose Throat Digest* 1969;31:58–67.
94. Skolyszewski J, Reinfuss M. The results of radiotherapy of cancer of the larynx in six European countries. *Radiobiol Radiother (Berl)* 1981;22(1):32–43.
95. Stewart JG, Brown JR, Palmer MK, et al. The management of glottic carcinoma by primary irradiation with surgery in reserve. *Laryngoscope* 1975;85(9):1477–1484.
96. Mills EE. Early glottic carcinoma: factors affecting radiation failure, results of treatment and sequelae. *Int J Radiat Oncol Biol Phys* 1979;5(6):811–817.
97. Jesse RH. The evaluation of treatment of patients with extensive squamous cancer of the vocal cords. *Laryngoscope* 1975;85(9):1424–1429.
98. Ogura JH, Sessions DG, Ciralsky RH. Supraglottic carcinoma with extension to the arytenoid. *Laryngoscope* 1975;85(8):1327–1331.
99. Skolnik EM, Yee KF, Wheatley MA, et al. Carcinoma of the laryngeal glottis therapy and end results. *Laryngoscope* 1975;85(9):1453–1466.
100. Vermund H. Role of radiotherapy in cancer of the larynx as related to the TNM system of staging. A review. *Cancer* 1970;25(3):485–504.
101. Stewart JG, Jackson AW. The steepness of the dose response curve both for tumor cure and normal tissue injury. *Laryngoscope* 1975;85(7):1107–1111.
102. Ogura JH, Sessions DG, Spector GJ. Conservation surgery for epidermoid carcinoma of the supraglottic larynx. *Laryngoscope* 1975;85(11, Pt 1):1808–1815.
103. Lutz CK, Johnson JT, Wagner RL, et al. Supraglottic carcinoma: patterns of recurrence. *Ann Otol Rhinol Laryngol* 1990;99(1):12–17.
104. Weems DH, Mendenhall WM, Parsons JT, et al. Squamous cell carcinoma of the supraglottic larynx treated with surgery and/or radiation therapy. *Int J Radiat Oncol Biol Phys* 1987;13(10):1483–1487.
105. Gregor RT, Oei SS, Baris G, et al. Supraglottic laryngectomy with postoperative radiation versus primary radiation in the management of supraglottic laryngeal cancer. *Am J Otolaryngol* 1996;17(5):316–321.
106. Spriano G, Antognoni P, Piantanida R, et al. Conservative management of T1-T2N0 supraglottic cancer: a retrospective study. *Am J Otolaryngol* 1997;18(5): 299–305.
107. Bocca E. Sixteenth Daniel C. Baker, Jr, memorial lecture. Surgical management of supraglottic cancer and its lymph node metastases in a conservative perspective. *Ann Otol Rhinol Laryngol* 1991;100(4, Pt 1):261–267.
108. Isaacs JH Jr, Slattery WH 3rd, Mendenhall WM, et al. Supraglottic laryngectomy. *Am J Otolaryngol* 1998;19(2):118–123.
109. Davis RK, Kelly SM, Hayes J. Endoscopic CO2 laser excisional biopsy of early supraglottic cancer. *Laryngoscope* 1991;101(6, Pt 1): 680–683.
110. Zeitels SM, Koufman JA, Davis RK, et al. Endoscopic treatment of supraglottic and hypopharynx cancer. *Laryngoscope* 1994;104(1, Pt 1):71–78.
111. Rudert HH, Werner JA, Hoft S. Transoral carbon dioxide laser resection of supraglottic carcinoma. *Ann Otol Rhinol Laryngol* 1999;108(9):819–827.
112. Ghossein NA, Bataini JP, Ennuyer A, et al. Local control and site of failure in radically irradiated supraglottic laryngeal cancer. *Radiology* 1974;112(1):187–192.
113. Csanady M, Ivan L, Czigner J. Endoscopic CO(2) laser therapy of selected cases of supraglottic marginal tumors. *Eur Arch Otorhinolaryngol* 1999;256(8):392–394.
114. Fletcher GH, Hamberger AD. Causes of failure in irradiation of squamous-cell carcinoma of the supraglottic larynx. *Radiology* 1974;111(3):697–700.
115. Wang CC, Montgomery WW. Deciding on optimal management of supraglottic carcinoma. *Oncology (Williston Park)* 1991;5(4):41–46; discussion 46, 49, 53.
116. Nakfoor BM, Spiro IJ, Wang CC, et al. Results of accelerated radiotherapy for supraglottic carcinoma: a Massachusetts General Hospital and Massachusetts Eye and Ear Infirmary experience. *Head Neck* 1998;20(5):379–384.
117. Sykes AJ, Slevin NJ, Gupta NK, et al. 331 cases of clinically node-negative supraglottic carcinoma of the larynx: a study of a modest size fixed field radiotherapy approach. *Int J Radiat Oncol Biol Phys* 2000;46(5):1109–1115.
118. DeSanto LW. Early supraglottic cancer. *Ann Otol Rhinol Laryngol* 1990;99(8): 593–597.
119. Steiniger JR, Parnes SM, Gardner GM. Morbidity of combined therapy for the treatment of supraglottic carcinoma: supraglottic laryngectomy and radiotherapy. *Ann Otol Rhinol Laryngol* 1997;106(2):151–158.
120. Burstein FD, Calcaterra TC. Supraglottic laryngectomy: series report and analysis of results. *Laryngoscope* 1985;95(7, Pt 1): 833–836.
121. Weber PC, Johnson JT, Myers EN. Impact of bilateral neck dissection on recovery following supraglottic laryngectomy. *Arch Otolaryngol Head Neck Surg* 1993; 119(1):61–64.
122. Beckhardt RN, Murray JG, Ford CN, et al. Factors influencing functional outcome in supraglottic laryngectomy. *Head Neck* 1994;16(3):232–239.

Chapter 48
Unusual Nonepithelial Tumors of the Head and Neck

Carlos A. Perez and Wade L. Thorstad

GLOMUS TUMORS

Anatomy

Glomus bodies are found in the jugular bulb and along the tympanic (Jacobson) and auricular (Arnold) branches of the tenth nerve in the middle ear or in other anatomic sites (Fig. 48.1). Depending on the location, glomus tumors (chemodectoma or paraganglioma) are classified as tympanic (middle ear), jugulare, or carotid vagal or designated as originating from other locations, such as the larynx, adventitia of thoracic aorta, abdominal aorta, or the surface of the lungs (Fig. 48.2).[1]

Glomus tumors (GT) or chemodectomas consist of large epithelioid (smooth muscle) cells with fine granular cytoplasm embedded in a rich capillary network and fibrous stroma with reticulin fibers, which derive from embryonic neural crest cells. Although histologically benign, they may extend along the lumen of the vein to regional lymph nodes, but rarely to distant sites. These tissues are responsive to changes in oxygen and carbon dioxide tensions and pH.

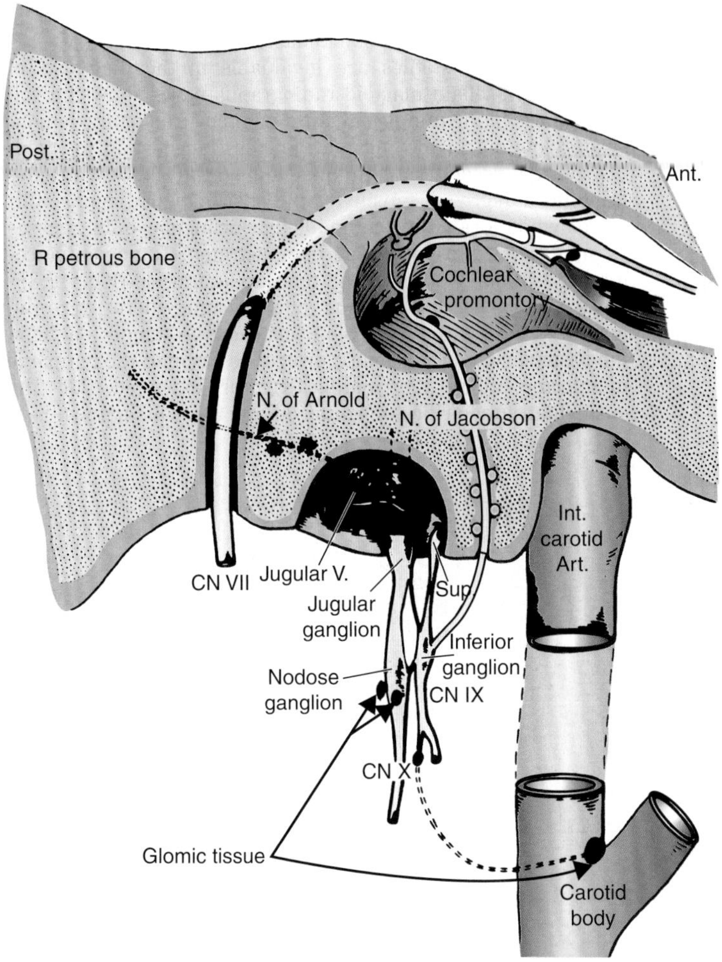

FIGURE 48.1. Anatomy of the region of the glomus jugulare. (From Hatfield PM, James AE, Schulz MN. Chemodectomas of the glomus jugulare. *Cancer* 1972; 30:1165–1168, with permission.)

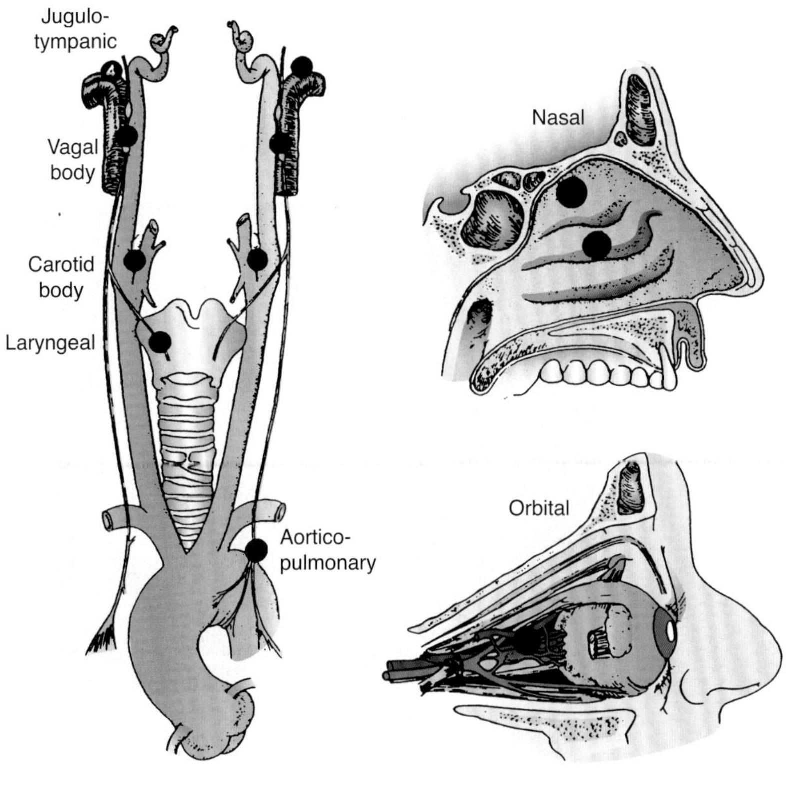

FIGURE 48.2. Distribution of paragangliomas of the head and neck region. Laterality was not specified in three patients with carotid body paragangliomas. The diagram does not include one left carotid body paraganglioma that was found incidentally at autopsy and a left vagal body paraganglioma that presented in a patient who had two other paragangliomas. (From Lack EE, Cubilla AL, Woodruff JM, et al. Paragangliomas of the head and neck region. *Cancer* 1977;39:3997–4009, with permission.)

Epidemiology

The mean age at diagnosis has been reported to be 44.7 years for carotid body tumors and 52 years for glomus tympanicum.[2] These tumors occur three or four times more frequently in women than in men, suggesting a possible estrogen influence.[2,3,4] Glomus tumors may be familial; they occur in multiple sites in 10% to 20% of patients.[5]

Recent advances in genetics identified three loci associated with hereditary paragangliomas, and genetic screening may detect affected patients.[6] Multiple paragangliomas of the head and neck are rare, with an incidence of 10% of all patients, but in familial cases it increases up to 35% to 50%.[5] In the head and neck region, the most common association is bilateral carotid body tumors or carotid body tumor associated with tympanic–jugular glomus.[7]

Clinical Presentation

Glomus tumors may arise along the nerve roots. In the middle ear they may initially cause earache or discomfort.[97] As they expand, eventually they produce pulsatile tinnitus, hearing loss, and, in later stages, cranial nerve paralysis resulting from invasion of the base of the skull in 10% to 15% of patients. If the tumor invades the middle cranial fossa, symptoms may include temporoparietal headache, retro-orbital pain, proptosis, and paresis of cranial nerves V and VI. If the posterior fossa is involved, symptoms may include occipital headache, ataxia, and paresis of cranial nerves V to VII, IX, and XII; invasion of the jugular foramen causes paralysis of nerves IX to XI. Chemodectoma of the carotid body usually presents as a painless, slowly growing mass in the upper neck. Occasionally the mass may be pulsatile and may have an associated thrill or bruit. As it enlarges, the mass may extend into the parapharyngeal space and be visible on examination of the oropharynx. Very rarely these tumors may be malignant.[8] Metastases occur in 2% to 5% of cases.[3]

Diagnostic Workup

Diagnostic evaluation for glomus tumors of the ear and base of skull is outlined in Table 48.1. In the majority of glomus tympanicum, physical examination demonstrates a red, vascular middle ear mass, although occasionally it may be bluish or white (the latter resembling a cholesteatoma).[2] Audiography may demonstrate conductive hearing loss in the ear involved by tumor as noted in 33 of 49 patients evaluated by Larson et al.;[2] 4 of 33 patients with conductive deficits also exhibited tympanic pulsations. Examination of the neck may occasionally demonstrate a mass in the neck that may be pulsatile or have a bruit or regional lymph node metastases.

Radiographic studies are invaluable in the diagnosis of these tumors. Plain mastoid radiographs never show the soft tissue mass in the middle ear, although they frequently demonstrate clouding of the mastoid air cells, suggesting mastoiditis.[157] High-resolution computed tomography (CT) with contrast has a degree of sensitivity and specificity to diagnose this tumor when located in the middle ear or jugular bulb; masses as small as 3 mm have been demonstrated. Tumor enhancement is similar to that of the temporalis muscle (Fig. 48.3).[2] In 46 patients with glomus tympanicum, there were no instances of local bony erosion; instead, the tumors engulfed the ossicular chain, bulged or protruded through the tympanic membrane, filled the middle ear, or extended into the eustachian tube orifice or aditus ad antrum. This pattern is in

TABLE 48.1 DIAGNOSTIC WORKUP FOR GLOMUS TUMORS OF THE EAR AND BASE OF SKULL, HEMANGIOPERICYTOMA, ESTHESIONEUROBLASTOMA, EXTRAMEDULLARY PLASMACYTOMA, AND SARCOMA OF THE HEAD AND NECK

General
Clinical history
General physical examination
Ear, nose, and throat examination
Radiographic studies
Computed tomography scan (with contrast) to define tumor extent and possible central nervous system involvement)
Magnetic resonance imaging with gadolinium
Arteriography to determine bilateral involvement and collateral cerebral blood flow (optional)
Jugular phlebography (optional)
Laboratory studies
Complete blood cell count
Blood chemistry profile
Urinalysis
Special tests
Audiograms to establish baseline hearing loss
Histologic staining to determine presence of catecholamines

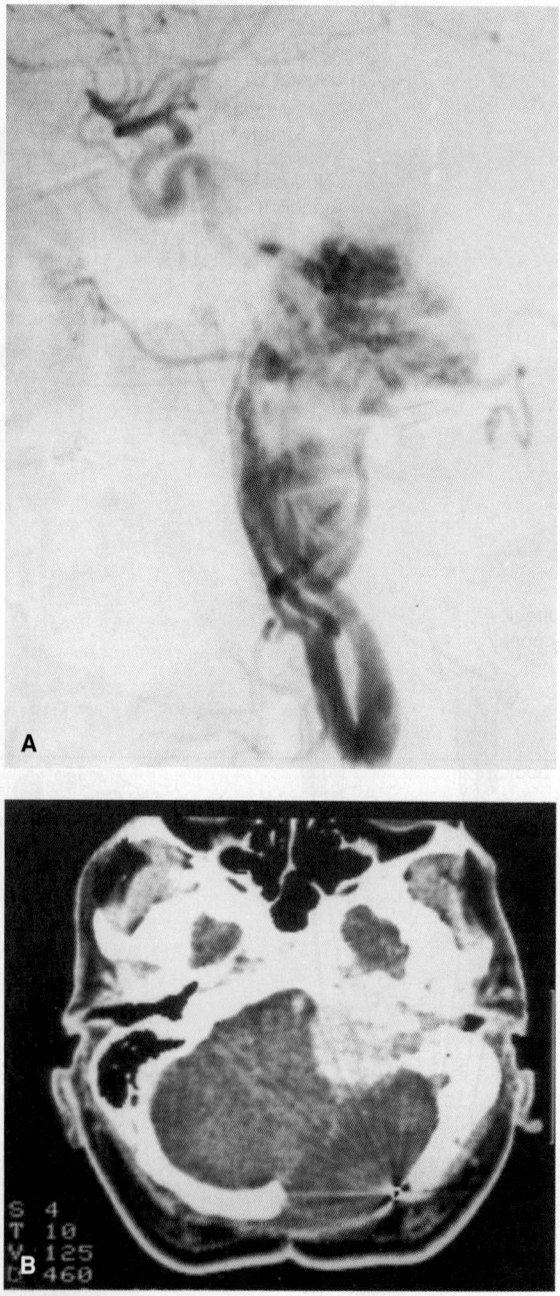

FIGURE 48.3. A: Late-phase arteriogram illustrating large glomus jugulare tumor with extension into the neck. **B:** Computed tomography scan with contrast enhancement showing intracranial component of lesion.

contrast to cholesteatomas, which typically destroy adjacent bony landmarks, including the ossicles, and progressively erode the petrous bones as they enlarge.[2]

Magnification angiography is a sensitive and specific means of detecting glomus tympanicum tumors. This procedure should be performed after high-resolution thin-section CT scan (with contrast material), only when there is a question regarding the nature of the lesion or the location of the carotid canal. Findings include a hypervascular middle ear mass that first appears in the middle to late arterial phase, persists through the capillary phase, and quickly disappears in the venous phase without demonstrably early draining veins. Biopsy of an aberrant internal carotid artery can result in major neurologic sequelae or death.

Vogl et al.[9] reported on 40 patients with glomus tumors of the skull; diagnostic interpretations were correlated with histologic examination, digital subtraction angiography, CT, and clinical follow-up. Sixteen of 18 proven tumors were detected with spin-echo images alone. Although four high-flying jugular bulbs were misinterpreted as tumors because of similar signal intensity, combined evaluation allowed differentiation between tumor and sinusal blood flow in all cases.

Drape et al.[10] described magnetic resonance imaging (MRI) findings in 31 patients with a clinical suspicion of glomus tumor; gadoterate meglumine was injected into 19 patients. Twenty-seven of 28 pathologically confirmed glomus tumors were detected with MRI; a peripheral capsule was present in most tumors. The investigators were able to differentiate three subtypes of glomus tumors (vascular, solid, and myxoid) on the basis of relaxation times and enhancement characteristics. Multidetector CT angiography was found to be more accurate in the diagnosis of six glomus tumors, with enhancement in the arterial phase, when compared with MRI.[11]

As GTs show high levels of somatostatin receptor (SSTR) subtypes 2 and 5, fluorine-(^{18}F)-octreotate positron emission tomography (PET) may be useful for diagnostic purposes in a semiquantitative manner and for improving target volume delineation in radiation therapy planning. Astner et al.[12] noted that preliminary findings with two different PET tracers for SSTR imaging have been reported: gallium-68 (^{68}Ga)-DOTATOC (DOTA-d-Phe(1)-Tyr(3)-octreotide [somatostatin analog]) PET was shown to detect SSTR-expressing tumors with high sensitivity and specificity. A second PET tracer, Gluc-Lys^{18}F-TOCA, allows fast, high-contrast imaging of SSTR-positive tumors with superior biokinetics and diagnostic performance as compared with indium-111 (^{111}In)-DTPA (diethylene triamine pentaacetic acid)-octreotide and—as far as can be determined from the literature—comparable to ^{68}Ga-DOTATOC.[13,14,15]

Cytochemical techniques demonstrate increased levels of serotonin, epinephrine, and norepinephrine in normal glomus tissue of the carotid body. Histologic staining techniques, including chromaffin and argentaffin reactions, identify patients with hormonally active tumors. This is important because the glomus tumor may coexist with a pheochromocytoma, which requires special preoperative preparation of the patient. Biopsy of glomus tumors may result in severe hemorrhage.

Staging

The prognosis of these tumors is closely related to the anatomic location and the volume of the lesion, which is reflected in the Glasscock-Jackson classification[16] shown in Table 48.2. An alternative classification proposed by McCabe and Fletcher[17] is presented in Table 48.3.

TABLE 48.2 GLASSCOCK-JACKSON CLASSIFICATION OF GLOMUS TUMORS

Glomus tympanicum	
I.	Small mass limited to promontory
II.	Tumor completely filling middle ear space
III.	Tumor filling middle ear and extending into the mastoid
IV.	Tumor filling middle ear, extending into the mastoid or through tympanic membrane to fill the external auditory canal; may extend anterior to carotid
Glomus jugulare	
I.	Small tumor involving jugular bulb, middle ear, and mastoid
II.	Tumor extending under internal auditory canal; may have intracranial canal extension
III.	Tumor extending into petrous apex; may have intracranial canal extension
IV.	Tumor extending beyond petrous apex into clivus or infratemporal fossa; may have intracranial canal extension

From Jackson CG, Glasscock ME III, Harris PF. Glomus tumors: diagnosis, classification, and management of large lesions. *Arch Otolaryngol* 1982;108:401–406, with permission.

General Management

Li et al.[18] published a historical perspective of various treatment modalities used to treat glomus tumors over the past 60 years.

Surgery

Surgery is generally selected for small tumors that can be completely excised. Glomus tympanicum tumors are particularly well managed with excision via tympanotomy or mastoidectomy. Percutaneous embolization of a low-viscosity silicone polymer has been used, frequently as preoperative preparation of the tumor embolization of feeding vessels allows meticulous microsurgery with virtually complete hemostasis.

Surgical treatment of a glomus tumor arising in the jugular bulb, however, often consists of piece-by-piece removal accompanied by significant intraoperative bleeding with damage to adjacent neurovascular structures and requires more complex surgical approaches involving the base of the skull. Preoperative embolization via a transarterial approach has proved beneficial but is often limited by vascular anatomy and unfavorable locations. Abud et al.[19] reported experience with preoperative devascularization using direct puncture and an intralesional injection of cyanoacrylate (acrylic glue) under fluoroscopic guidance in nine patients with head and neck paragangliomas. Ozyer et al.[20] performed devascularization with intralesional injection of *N*-butyl-cyanoacrylate (seven carotid and three jugular paragangliomas). The tumors were subsequently surgically removed.

The local tumor control rate with surgery alone is only about 60%, and there is significant morbidity, particularly cranial nerve injury and bleeding.

In a retrospective review of all skull-base surgery cases treated at Baylor University, 175 jugulotympanic glomus tumors

TABLE 48.3 MODIFICATION OF McCABE AND FLETCHER CLASSIFICATION OF CHEMODECTOMAS

Group I: Tympanic tumors
Absence of bone destruction on x-rays of the mastoid bone and jugular fossa
Absence of facial nerve weakness
Intact eighth nerve with conductive deafness only
Intact jugular foramen nerves (cranial nerves IX, X, and XI)
Group II: Tympanomastoid tumors
X-ray evidence of bone destruction confined to the mastoid bone and not involving the petrous bone
Normal or paretic seventh nerve
Intact jugular foramen nerves
No evidence of involvement of the superior bulb of the jugular vein on retrograde venogram
Group III: Petrosal and extrapetrosal tumors
Destruction of the petrous bone, jugular fossa, and/or occipital bone on x-rays
Positive findings on retrograde jugulography
Evidence of destruction of the petrous or occipital bones on carotid arteriogram
Jugular foramen syndrome (paresis of cranial nerves IX, X, or XI)
Presence of metastasis

From Wang M-L, Hussey DH, Doornbos JF, et al. Chemodectoma of the temporal bone: a comparison of surgical and radiotherapeutic results. *Int J Radiat Oncol Biol Phys* 1988;14:643–648, with permission.

and 9 malignant cases (5.1%) were identified.[8] The 5-year survival rate was 72%.

Radiation Therapy

Irradiation is frequently used in the treatment of glomus tumors, particularly for those in the tympanicum and jugulare bulb locations. Tumors with destruction of the petrous bone, jugular fossa, or occipital bone or patients with jugular foramen syndrome are more reliably managed with irradiation.[2,4,21,22] Some surgeons, such as Glasscock et al.[16] have questioned the effectiveness of radiation therapy in the treatment of chemodectomas because on histologic sections, obtained even many years after irradiation, it is possible to find chromophilic cells remaining in the tumor. However, there is also evidence of fibrosis and decreased vascularity.[23] Suit and Gallager[24] demonstrated in a murine mammary carcinoma model that morphologically intact cells may have lost their reproductive ability after irradiation, which is the ultimate end point of cell killing. Furthermore, it is extremely unusual to observe clinical regrowth of a glomus tumor after irradiation, even if they do not regress completely.

Some reports describe successful combinations of surgery with preoperative irradiation, in an attempt to make an unresectable tumor operable, or postoperatively when obvious tumor could not be resected.

Radiation Therapy Techniques

Radiation therapy techniques are determined by the location and extent of the tumor, which must be defined before treatment.[21,25,26] Limited, usually bilateral, portals were used for relatively localized glomus tumors, whether or not the treatment is combined with surgery (Fig. 48.4). Dickens et al.[27] used a three-field arrangement with a superior-inferior wedged and lateral open field, with a weighting of 1:1:0.33. A superior-inferior 60-degree and 45-degree wedged filtered field arrangement was also used. Electrons (15 to 18 MeV) with a lateral portal or combined with cobalt-60 (^{60}Co) or 4- to 6-MV photons (20% to 25% of total tumor dose) render a good dose distribution (Fig. 48.5). Several prosthetic materials have been used to enhance irradiation dose homogeneity.[28] In patients in whom tumor has spread into the posterior fossa, it may be necessary to use parallel opposed portals with 6- to 18-MV photons. Treatment is given at the rate of 1.8 to 2 Gy tumor dose per day with 5 treatments per week for a total tumor dose of 45 to 55 Gy in 5 weeks. Three-dimensional conformal radiation therapy (3D-CRT) or image-guided intensity-modulated radiation

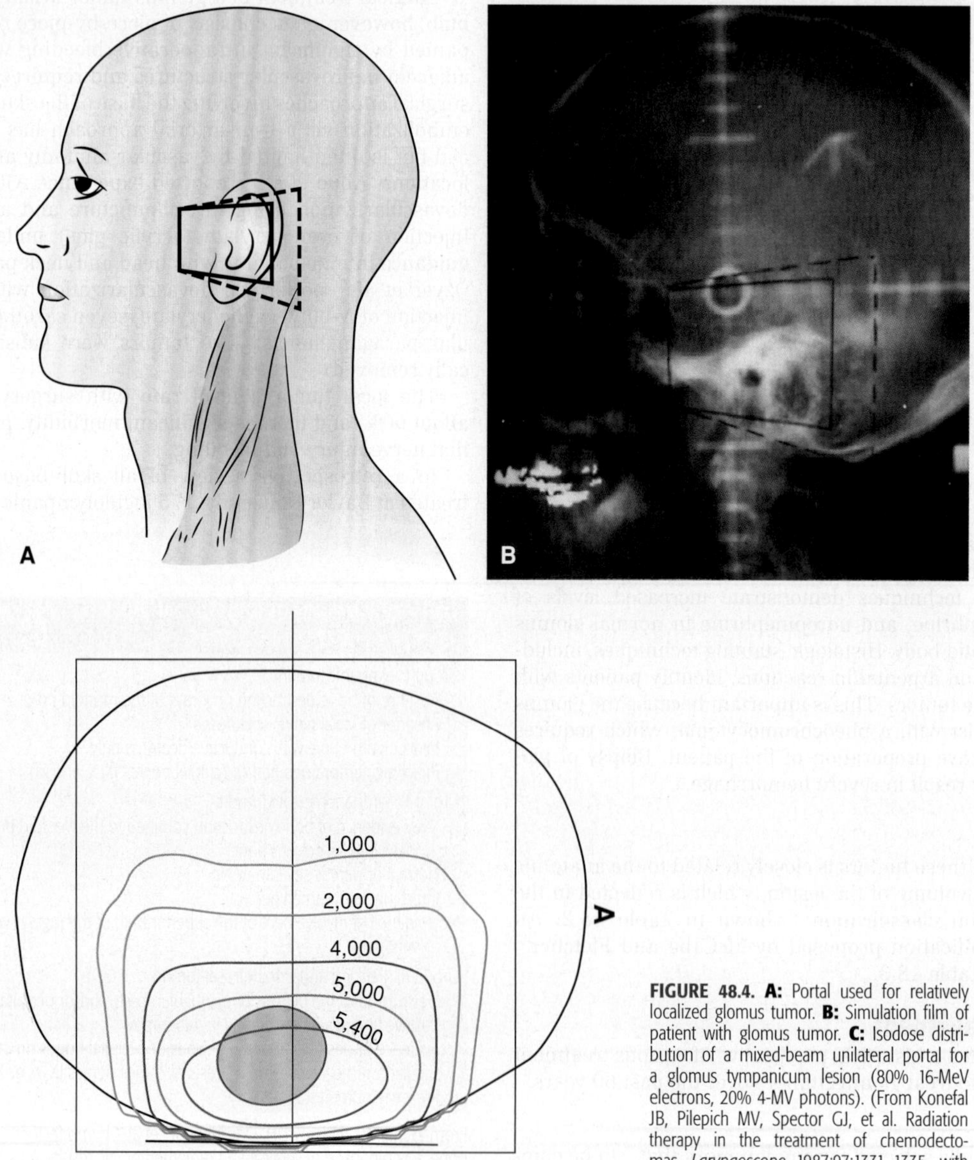

FIGURE 48.4. A: Portal used for relatively localized glomus tumor. **B:** Simulation film of patient with glomus tumor. **C:** Isodose distribution of a mixed-beam unilateral portal for a glomus tympanicum lesion (80% 16-MeV electrons, 20% 4-MV photons). (From Konefal JB, Pilepich MV, Spector GJ, et al. Radiation therapy in the treatment of chemodectomas. *Laryngoscope* 1987;97:1331–1335, with permission.)

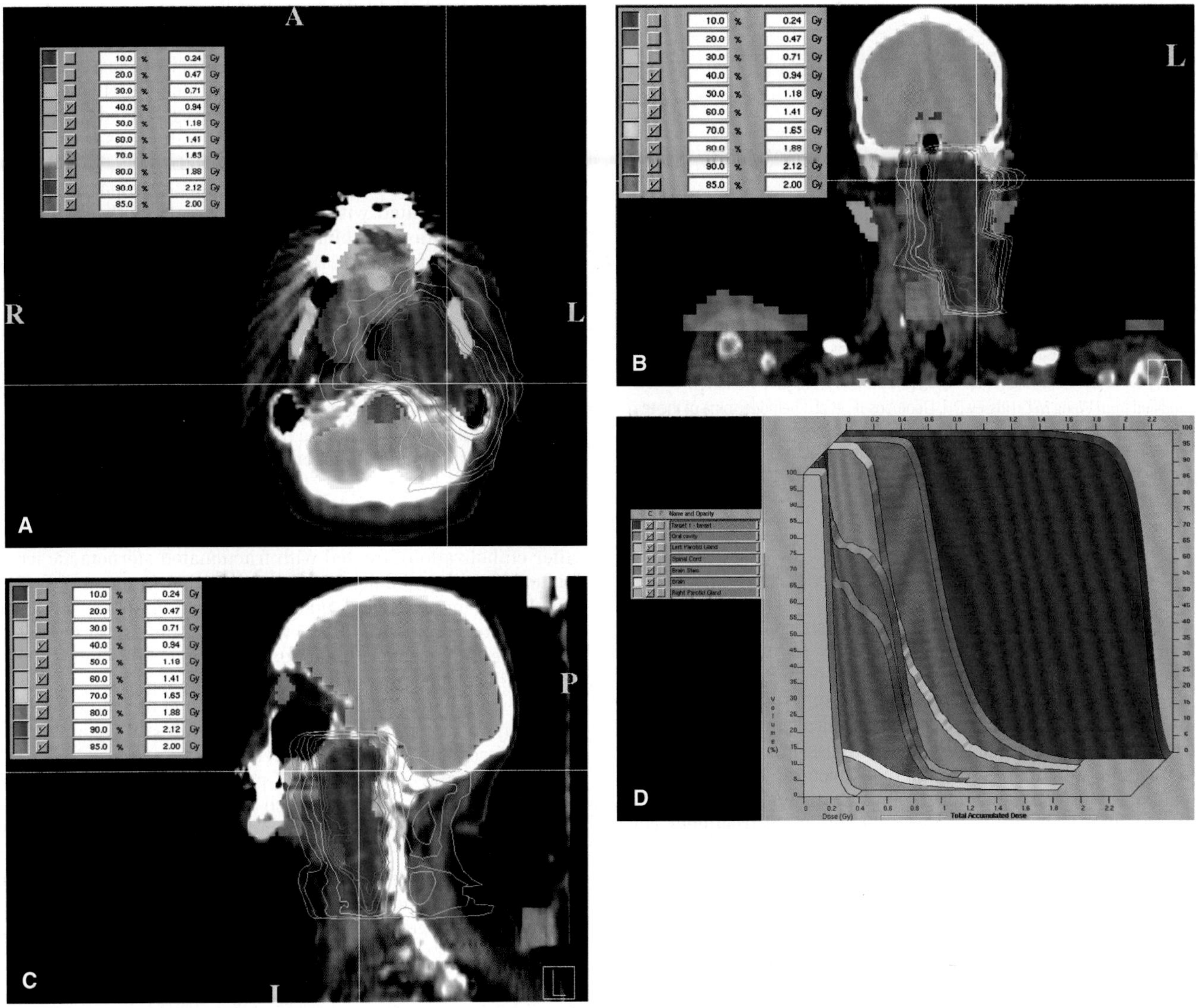

FIGURE 48.5. Fifty-nine-year-old woman with an unusual malignant left glomus jugulare, who had a metastatic left upper cervical lymph node. She was treated definitively with intensity-modulated radiation therapy (66 Gy in 2-Gy fractions). Cross **(A)**, coronal **(B)**, and sagittal **(C)** sections showing dose distributions at primary site and left neck, sparing normal structures **(D)** dose–volume histogram:

Structure	*Dose Range (Gy)*	*Mean Dose (Gy)*
Planning target volume (including left neck)	38–77	70
Brain	0–59	2
Brainstem	6–35	12
Spinal cord	0–32	13

therapy (IMRT) are highly desirable techniques to treat these tumors, with excellent dose distributions (Fig. 48.5). Table 48.4 summarizes the doses of irradiation recommended by several investigators and the probability of tumor control for each.[21,26,29]

Leber et al.[30] reported on 13 patients with glomus tumors treated with radiosurgery in 6, because of recurrences after surgical removal. Histology was not available in seven patients, diagnosis was made from neuroradiological features only. With mean follow-up of 42 months (range 14 to 72 months), there was no tumor progression and no clinical deterioration in any patient; 64% of the patients had improvement of symptoms, and in 36% the volume of the lesion decreased in size. There was no radiation-related morbidity. In recent years there has been an increasing number of reports in small series of patients with glomus tumors <2 or 3 cm treated with stereotactic radiation therapy, with tumor control over 80% and relatively minimal morbidity. The mean single dose is about 16 Gy (range 13 to 20 Gy).[31,32,33,34,35,36,37] A report on fractionated stereotactic irradiation (6 MV x-rays) of 17 patients has been published, with a dose of 57 Gy.[38] Pollock[39] reported on 42 glomus tumors (19 primary treatment and 23 recurrences after initial surgery) treated with Gamma Knife (Elekta Corp, Stockholm) stereotactic radiation (12 to 24 Gy single dose at 50% isodose, depending on tumor size). Twelve lesions (31%) decreased in size and 26 were unchanged. The most common complication was hearing loss (19%). Wegner et al.[40] treated 18 patients with carotid or jugular lesions with fractionated stereotactic CyberKnife (Accuray, Sunnyvale, CA) irradiation (21 Gy in 3 fractions or 25 Gy in 5 fractions) (Fig. 48.6). Tumor size was stable in 17 patients and decreased in 1 patient.

TABLE 48.4 LOCAL CONTROL WITH RADIATION THERAPY FOR CHEMODECTOMA OF THE TEMPORAL BONE (GLOMUS TYMPANICUM AND JUGULARE)

Institution (Reference)	Local Control	Nominal Dosage Schedule
Princess Margaret Hospital (41)	42/45[a]	35 Gy/3 wk
Queen Elizabeth Hospital, Birmingham (42)	19/20[b]	45–50 Gy/4–5 wk
University of Washington (43)	10/13	8–65 Gy/4–7 wk
Rotterdamsch Radio-Therapeutisch Instituut, Netherlands (44)	19/19	40–60 Gy/4–6 wk
University of Minnesota (8)	13/14	30–60 Gy/3.5–7.5 wk
University of Virginia (45)	14/17	40–50 Gy/4–5 wk
Total	**117/128 (91%)**	

[a]Two patients listed as failures were salvaged with further treatments.

[b]One patient listed as a failure was salvaged with further radiation therapy.

Modified from Wang M-L, Hussey DH, Doornbos JF, et al. Chemodectoma of the temporal bone: a comparison of surgical and radiotherapeutic results. *Int J Radiat Oncol Biol Phys* 1987;14:643–648; and Springate SC, Weichselbaum RR. Radiation or surgery for chemodectoma of the temporal bone: a review of local control and complications. *Head Neck* 1990;12:303–307.

Results of Therapy

The postirradiation change in tumor size is slow, with an increase in proliferative and perivascular fibrosis and minimal alterations in the chief epithelial cells. Histologic evaluation of tumor cell viability is not reliable.[24] Despite the persistence of tumor both clinically and angiographically, amelioration of symptoms, absence of disease progression, and occasional return of cranial nerve function have been reported. Seventeen patients were treated for glomus tympanicum tumors at Washington University.[3] In five patients, initial treatment consisted of irradiation alone, and all were tumor free at last follow-up (4.5 years in one patient) or at death. Seven of eight patients irradiated for surgical recurrence were free of disease 4.5 to 19 years after irradiation. The remaining four patients were treated preoperatively or postoperatively; only one had recurrence and was salvaged surgically and tumor free 10 years later. Of six patients with glomus jugulare lesions treated with irradiation, two with extensive lesions died of their disease, whereas the glomus tumor was controlled in four, including two patients with intracranial extension. Irradiation doses ranged from 46 to 52 Gy, with 86% to 100% tumor control with doses over 46 Gy and 50% (two of four) with doses below 46 Gy.

Wang et al.[46] reported on 32 patients with tympanic chemodectomas; 13 treated with surgery alone, 15 with irradiation alone, and 4 with a combination of both modalities. The initial tumor control rate was 46% with surgery alone; ultimately 84% of patients were tumor free after salvage with additional surgery. Although 78% survived 10 years, 31% developed complications. Of the patients treated with irradiation, 84% had initial local tumor control; 77% survived 10 years, and only 11% developed complications. The doses of irradiation used were slightly higher than those reported by others (mean 58.32 Gy). However, no improvement in tumor control was noted with higher doses. Complications occurred in two patients receiving 66 Gy.

Zabel et al.[47] described results in 22 patients with large chemodectomas of the skull base (8 after primary surgery and 4 after embolization), treated with fractionated stereotactic irradiation (median total dose 57 Gy with median fraction dose 1.8 Gy). With a median follow-up of 5.7 years, 5- and 10-year actuarial tumor control was 90%, with 7 patients (32%) having a partial response and 13 patients with (59%) stable tumors. No patient developed new neurological deficit.

In a compilation of several studies, Kim et al.[48] noted a 25% local failure rate in 83 patients treated with <40 Gy and 1.4% local failure in 142 patients receiving >40 Gy.

Powell et al.[22] reported on 84 patients with chemodectoma of the head and neck, 46 of which were in the glomus jugulare and tympanicum, treated with irradiation alone (45 to 50 Gy in 25 fractions). Local control of the lesion was 73% at 5 years. Thirty patients were treated with surgery after irradiation with no recurrences (median follow-up of 9 years). Four patients, treated with surgery alone, developed recurrences by 7 years. Four carotid body and glomus vagal tumors treated with

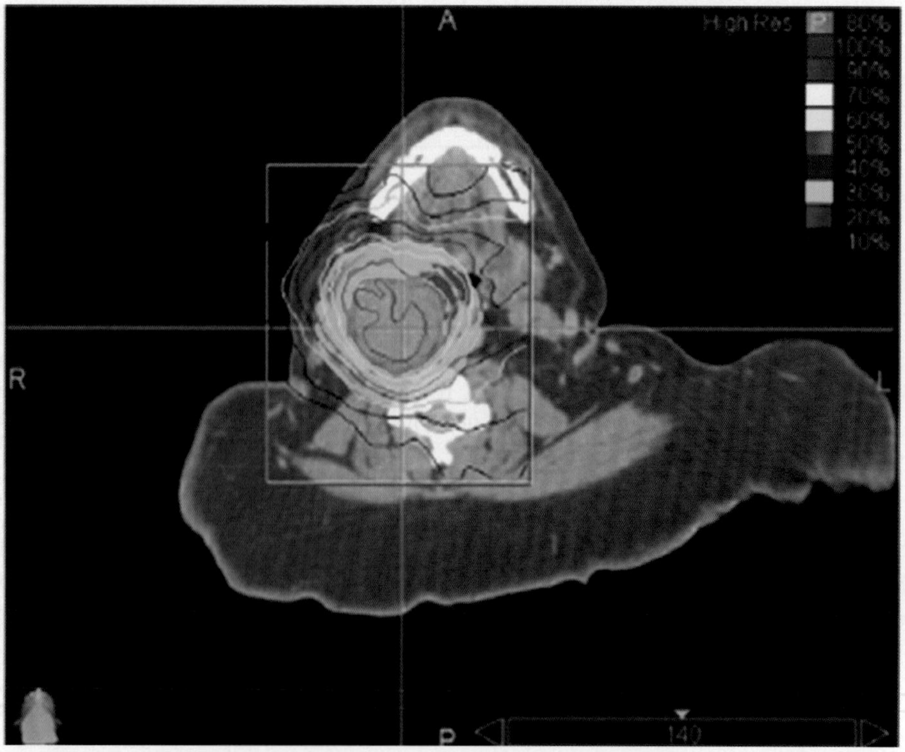

FIGURE 48.6. Dose distribution with stereotactic radiation therapy (radiosurgery) for glomus tumor. Patient was treated with 25 Gy in 5 fractions prescribed to the 80% isodose line; 98% of tumor received the prescribed dose. Thick *orange line* represents the 80% isodose. (From Wegner RE, Rodriguez KD, Heron DE, et al. Linac-based stereotactic body radiotherapy for treatment of glomus. *Radiother Oncol* 2010;97:395–398, with permission.)

irradiation were locally controlled at 1, 2, 8, and 11 years, respectively. In 13 patients treated with surgery alone, the 15-year local control rate was 54%.

Hinerman et al.[49,50] updated a previous report with 104 patients who had 121 chemodectomas of the temporal bone, carotid bone, or glomus vagal treated with radiation therapy alone in 104 patients or subtotal resection with or without radiation therapy (17 tumors). Seventeen patients had undergone a previous treatment (surgery 14, irradiation 1, or both 2). Eighty-nine patients were treated with megavoltage radiation therapy, 15 with stereotactic fractionated, 6 with stereotactic single dose, and 11 with IMRT. Median dose with fractionated irradiation was 45 Gy with daily fractions of 1.5 to 2 Gy delivered with ^{60}Co, 6-MV, or 8-MV x-rays, or a combination of different beam energies.[50] There were six tumor recurrences, with a local tumor control of 95%. No severe treatment complications were noted. In the initial report,[49] 18 patients had 25 chemodectomas of carotid body and/or glomus vagal; 15 tumors originated in the carotid body and 10 in the glomus vagal. Pathologic confirmation of chemodectoma was obtained in 10 patients, and diagnosis was based on physical and radiographic findings in the remaining 8 patients. Twenty-two lesions were treated with radiation therapy alone and two received postoperative radiation therapy after surgical resection for gross residual tumor with malignant changes and lymph node involvement. Patients with benign glomus tumors received 45 Gy in 25 fractions, in most instances, whereas patients with malignant carotid body tumors received 64.8 to 70 Gy in 1.8-Gy fractions. Local tumor control was obtained in 14 of 15 carotid body and 10 of 10 glomus vagal (overall 96% tumor control).[51]

Ivan et al.[52] published a meta-analysis based on 869 patients in 46 studies reported with glomus tumors, with follow-up ranging from 6 to 256 months. The tumor control rates were, for subtotal resection 69%, gross tumor resection (GTR) 86%, subtotal resection and radiosurgery 71%, and stereotactic radiosurgery (SRS) alone 95%. Posttreatment cranial nerve deficit was observed in 26% to 40% of patients treated with GTR and in about 10% of the SRS group. Guss et al.[53] reported on a meta-analysis of 19 studies (335 patients) with glomus tumors treated with stereotactic radiation therapy (radiosurgery), eight publications with a median follow-up of 36 months; tumor control (unchanged or reduced tumor volume) was 95% to 96%, with various stereotactic radiation therapy (RT) techniques.

In 29 patients with post surgical recurrent glomus tumors (16 jugular, 7 carotid, 5 tympanic and one thyroid) Elshaikh et al.[54] reported that the 5 year tumor conrol was 100% in 12 treated with radiation therapy and 62% in 17 treated surgically.

Cheesman and Kelly[55] emphasized the importance of evaluating preoperatively the swallowing function of patients with glomus jugulare undergoing surgery, as it is common for these patients to develop postsurgical dysphagia.

The results of primary treatment for temporal bone chemodectoma are summarized in Table 48.5.

The initial results of treatment for carotid body or glomus vagal are summarized in Table 48.6. Complications were rare in patients treated with chemodectoma of the head and neck.

TABLE 48.5 TEMPORAL BONE CHEMODECTOMAS: LOCAL CONTROL AFTER RADIATION THERAPY ALONE OR RADIATION THERAPY AND SURGERY

Author (Reference)	*Number of Patients*	*Local Control (%)*	*Follow-Up (Year)*
Larner et al. (56)	15	93 (RT alone)	Median, 16.2
Powell et al. (22)	46	90 (RT alone)	Median, 9
Wang et al. (46)	19	84 (RT ± surgery)	5–35
Koncfal et al. (3)	23	83 (RT ± surgery)	Mean, 10.5
Pryzant et al. (57)	19	95 (RT ± surgery)	Mean, 11
Cole and Beiler (58)	30	97 (RT alone)	3–27
Boyle et al. (59)	9	100 (RT alone)	1–12
Schild et al. (60)	8	100 (RT ± surgery)	Median, 7.5
deJong et al. (61)	38	89 (RT ± surgery)	Median, 11.5
Hinerman et al. (50)	53	93 (RT ± surgery)	Mean, 15

RT, radiation therapy.

From Hinerman RW, Mendenhall WM, Amdur RJ, et al. Definitive radiotherapy in the management of chemodectomas arising in the temporal bone, carotid body, and glomus vagale. *Head Neck* 2001;23:363–371, with permission.

TABLE 48.6 CHEMODECTOMAS OF CAROTID BODY/GLOMUS VAGALE: RADIATION THERAPY ALONE OR RADIATION THERAPY AFTER SURGERY

Author (Reference)	*Number of Patients*	*Local Control (%)*	*Follow-Up (Year)*
Valdagni and Amichetti (62)	7	100 (RT + subtotal resection)	1–19
Verniers et al. (51)	22	100 (RT ± subtotal resection	Mean, 10
Powell et al. (22)	4	100 (RT alone)	Median, 9
Schild et al. (60)	2	100 (Subtotal resection + RT)	Median, 7.5
Cole and Beiler (58)	30[a]	97 (RT alone)	3–27
Hinerman et al. (50)	18	96 (RT ± resection)	Mean, 9

RT, radiation therapy.

[a]Glomus jugulare and glomus vagale.

From Hinerman RW, Mendenhall WM, Amdur RJ, et al. Definitive radiotherapy in the management of chemodectomas arising in the temporal bone, carotid body, and glomus vagale. *Head Neck* 2001;23:363–371, with permission.

HEMANGIOPERICYTOMA

Hemangiopericytomas are rare soft tissue neoplasms that account for 3% to 5% of all soft tissue sarcomas and 1% of all vascular tumors. Some 15% to 30% of all hemangiopericytomas occur in the head and neck, and of these, approximately 5% occur in the sinonasal area. They may resemble meningiomas in the central nervous system (CNS), clinically and on imaging studies.[63] Vagal paragangliomas originate within the first 2 cm of the extracranial stretch of the vagus nerve and are associated with the inferior ganglion.[64] These tumors are believed to originate from the pericytes of Zimmerman extravascular cells, morphologically resembling smooth muscle, found around the capillaries or from primitive mesenchymal cells. The function of the pericyte is uncertain but is believed to provide mechanical support for the capillaries having contractile function.[65]

Epidemiology

Hemangiopericytomas is an unusual tumor; it represents approximately 1% of all vascular neoplasms; it occurs in both genders with equal frequency and is found primarily in adults. Only 45 cases of primary hemangiopericytomas of bone were described in the world literature in 1988.

In the head and neck, the most common sites are the nasal cavity and the paranasal sinuses, and, less frequently, the orbital region, the parotid gland, and the neck.[66,67,68,69] Hemangiopericytomas represent 3% to 4% of all meningeal and <1% of CNS tumors.

Pathology

Hemangiopericytomas are composed of a proliferation of tightly packed pericytes around thin-walled endothelial-lined vascular channels, ranging from capillary-sized vessels to large, gaping sinusoidal spaces.[66] The tumor has a tendency to grow slowly and invade locally into adjacent structures.[68,70] Although they are always well circumscribed and partially or completely surrounded by a pseudocapsule, benign tumors may be difficult to differentiate from malignant tumors. However, prominent mitoses (>4 per high-power field), foci of necrosis, and increased cellularity are suggestive of malignancy; the definitive sign is local recurrence or development of metastases. In general, tumors of the CNS, lower extremity, and mediastinum tend to be more malignant, with local recurrence occurring in up to 50% of cases.[66]

Kowalski and Paulino[71] reviewed 12 cases of hemangiopericytomas. Proliferation index was assessed using an immunoperoxidase stain for MIB-1 (Ki-67). The mitotic index per 10 high power fields varied from 0 or 1 to 15. Proliferation indices using MIB-1 ranged from 2.6% to 52.5%. Clinical follow-up revealed three cases with recurrence all possessing proliferation indices of approximately 10%, indicating a more aggressive subset of hemangiopericytomas. Vuorinen et al.[72] found the proliferation index to be a poor predictor of prognosis. In a review of 23 cases, Sundaram et al.[63] found that all hemangiopericytomas were negative for epithelial membrane antigen and S-100 and all were positive for vimentin.

Meningeal hemangiopericytomas almost always recur, despite seemingly complete removal, due to infiltrative properties of hemangiopericytoma cells and not just higher proliferation potential. They often metastasize.

Clinical Presentation

Soft tissue hemangiopericytoma is a firm, painless, slowly expanding mass that is often nodular and well localized. The skin overlying the mass does not have any discoloration or redness to indicate its vascular origin because the capillaries are emptied of the blood by compression of massive numbers of pericytes surrounding them.[64,66]

In the head and neck, the tumor may constitute a polypoid, soft gray or red mass that grows slowly and may cause nasal obstruction. Epistaxis and nasal obstruction are common symptoms. Orbital hemangiopericytomas account for 3% of orbital malignancies and most frequently occur with painless proptosis.[73] Hemangiopericytoma rarely originates in the lacrimal sac; it occurs in a younger age group than that of hemangiopericytoma of other locations. Charles et al.[74] reported on seven cases previously described and added one case.

Hemangiopericytoma may occur intracranially. When it arises in the brain, it is a solid mass attached to the meninges that grossly resembles a meningioma. These intracranial hemangiopericytomas carry a high risk of local failure (80%), as well as higher potential for dissemination. The mean time for local recurrence is 75 months.[75]

The incidence of metastasis, which depends on the site of origin, can be 50% to 80%. Late metastases occurring 10 years after diagnosis are not uncommon.

On plain radiographs, hemangiopericytoma appears as a soft tissue mass in the nasal cavity or other portions of the head and neck. A defect caused by pressure erosion of the surrounding bones may occur, and calcifications are rare. In the neck, the tumor appears as a well-circumscribed, homogeneously and intensely enhancing mass on CT. On MRI, the mass is iso- to slightly hyperintense to muscle on T1- and T2-weighted imaging. Multiple, branching flow voids are typically seen within the tumor on both T1- and T2-weighted images. On T2-weighted imaging, the punctate black flow voids in cross-section within the relatively bright tumor, creating a characteristic "salt and pepper" appearance in tumors >2 cm in diameter. Additionally, flow voids of large feeding arteries are seen at the periphery of the mass. Angiography demonstrates the characteristic appearance of a vascular tumor, with large feeding arteries, intense tumor stain, and early draining veins.[64] On arteriography, according to Yaghmai,[76] hemangiopericytoma is the only vascular tumor that has radially arranged or spiderlike branching vessels around and inside the tumor and a long-standing, well-demarcated tumor stain. Intracranial tumors typically have arterial blood supply from both meningeal and cerebral connections, with one to three main feeders supplying many small corkscrew-like vessels.[75] The most distinctive and constant feature of this tumor is its hypervascularity, which may be demonstrated with contrast-enhanced CT.[67] Intracranially, the diffusely enhancing tumor may closely resemble a meningioma on CT. However, some CT signs may suggest hemangiopericytoma rather than meningioma, such as a lack of calcification, scarce surrounding edema, and ringlike enhancement. Both CT and MRI scans are of special value in the delineation of the full extent of the tumor.

General Management

Complete surgical resection, if possible, combined with preoperative embolization of the tumor, is the treatment of choice. More extensive surgery is required in tumors that show features of malignancy. Many patients undergo surgical treatment after embolization of the feeding artery(ies).

For incompletely resected tumors, postoperative radiation therapy is used.[77,78] The role of chemotherapy in this tumor is not well determined; a few reports have described partial tumor regression in some lesions treated with cytotoxic agents. Doxorubicin, alone or in combination-drug regimens, is the most effective agent for metastatic hemangiopericytoma, producing complete and partial remissions in 50% of cases. Other drugs prescribed when metastasis occurs are cyclophosphamide, dacarbazine, vincristine, and actinomycin-D.[79] Park et al.[80] reported on 14 patients with soft tissue hemangiopericytoma treated with temozolomide 150 mg/m^2 orally on days 1 to 7 and days 15 to 21 and bevacizumab 5 mg/kg intravenously on days 8 and 22, repeated at 28-day intervals. Median follow-up period was 34 months. Eleven patients (79%) achieved a Choi partial response, with a median time to response of 2.5 months. The estimated median progression-free survival was 9.7 months, with a 6-month progression-free rate of 78.6%. The most frequently observed toxic effect was myelosuppression.

Radiation Therapy Techniques

The role of radiation therapy alone in the management of hemangiopericytoma is controversial. The main role of irradiation is as an adjuvant after complete excision of the lesion or postoperatively for minimal residual disease.[69,81,82] The tumor has been considered relatively radioresistant. Tumor doses of 60 to 65 Gy in 6 to 7 weeks are required to produce local tumor control in postoperative cases.[83] Orbital hemangiopericytoma has been cured by surgery and postoperative irradiation to 65 Gy.[73]

There appears to be a definite role for postoperative irradiation to the brain for primary hemangiopericytoma when radical surgery is performed because these tumors tend to recur after seemingly complete removal. Jha et al.[82] reported local tumor control in all patients treated with adjuvant external-beam irradiation postoperatively. Radiation therapy also has been used as a salvage procedure after local recurrence following initial surgery or chemotherapy.

The fields of irradiation should be wide to encompass the tumor bed with a margin of at least 5 cm to safely avoid marginal recurrence. Portal arrangement and beam selection are similar to those used in treatment of malignant brain tumors or soft tissue sarcomas.

Results of Therapy

Billings et al.[84] reported on 10 patients with hemangiopericytoma of the head and neck; seven tumors arose from soft tissue sites and three from the mucosa. All patients underwent wide excision of the primary lesion with a local recurrence rate of 40%. Three patients developed metastatic lung disease 0 to 8 years after initial diagnosis. Each patient who developed metastatic disease had abundant mitoses on pathological review compared with rare or absent mitoses in the lesions that took a more benign course.

Patrice et al.[85] reported on 18 primary hemangioblastoma tumors (16 had no prior surgical resection and 2 were subtotally resected lesions) and 20 lesions treated after surgical failure with stereotactic irradiation (radiosurgery). Minimum tumor doses ranged from 12 to 20 Gy (median 15.5 Gy). With a median follow-up of 24.5 months (range 6 to 77 months), the 2-year actuarial survival was 88%, and the 3-year freedom from progression was 86%. Four of 22 patients died. Thirty one of 36 evaluable tumors (86%) were controlled locally. None of the 18 primary tumors treated with definitive stereotactic irradiation failed. Of the 18 recurrent tumors, 13 (72%) were controlled. There were no significant permanent complications attributable to the stereotactic irradiation.

Spitz et al.[69] published a report on 36 patients with hemangiopericytoma. The median follow-up was 57 months. Twenty-eight patients (78%) underwent complete and potentially curative resection. Of the nine patients (32%) who had local recurrences, four (44%) had epidural tumors and three (33%) had retroperitoneal tumors, but none had extremity tumors. Ten patients had recurrences at distant sites. Of the 13 patients who experienced any form of disease recurrence, four had recurrences after a disease-free interval of more than 5 years. The 5-year actuarial survival rate for the entire group of 36 patients was 71%.

Carew et al.[86] reviewed the records of 12 patients with hemangiopericytomas of the head and neck: 5 had high or intermediate grade lesions and 7 had low-grade lesions. Nine patients were treated with curative intent; they underwent a variety of surgical resections dictated by tumor location and size. Four patients received postoperative radiation therapy, to a median dose of 60 Gy, for positive surgical margins (two patients), high-grade histology (one patient), or a recurrent lesion (one patient). The 5-year overall survival rate for patients treated surgically was 87.5%. A single mortality occurred in a patient with a recurrent high-grade lesion who failed at local, regional, and distant sites.

Staples et al.[87] reported on 12 patients with localized hemangiopericytoma, 7 treated with surgery alone (only 1 had long-term tumor control and 2 were salvaged with radiation therapy), 4 with resection and postoperative irradiation (all with long-term tumor control), and 1 with surgery and chemotherapy. Local tumor control was achieved at all sites treated with doses >55 Gy. Mitotic activity was not a reliable predictor of biologic behavior.

Kim et al.[48] evaluated 17 hemangiopericytomas in nine patients treated with Gamma Knife stereotactic radiation therapy. Mean and median marginal doses were 18.1 and 20 Gy (range 11 to 22 Gy), respectively, at the 50% isodose line. Mean clinical and radiological follow-up periods were 49 and 34 months, respectively. Successful tumor control was achieved in 14 of 17 lesions (82.4%). Actuarial local tumor control rates at 5 years was 67%. No adverse effects, such as radiation necrosis or marked peritumoral edema, were observed. Marginal dose (≥17 Gy) was the only statistically significant factor for local tumor control on univariate analysis.

Kano et al.[88] in a retrospective review of 20 patients who had undergone stereotactic radiation therapy for 29 hemangiopericytomas. All patients had undergone previous surgical resection. In addition, 12 patients underwent fractionated radiotherapy before stereotactic radiation therapy. Of the 20 patients, 16 patients had low-grade hemangiopericytomas (20 tumors) and 4 had high-grade anaplastic hemangiopericytomas (9 tumors). The median target volume was 4.5 cm^3 and the median marginal dose was 15 Gy (range 10 to 20 Gy). At an average of 48.2 months, the overall survival after radiosurgery was 85.9% and 13.8% at 5 and 10 years, respectively. Follow-up imaging studies demonstrated tumor control in 21 (72.4%) of 29 tumors. The progression-free survival rate after stereotactic radiation therapy at 3 and 5 years was 89.1% for low-grade hemangiopericytomas and 66.7% and 0%, respectively, for high-grade hemangiopericytomas. The factors associated with improved progression-free survival included lower grade and >14 Gy marginal radiation dose.

Olson et al.[89] published a review of 21 patients with 28 recurrent or residual hemangiopericytomas on whom radiosurgery was performed. Prior treatments included embolization (6 cases), transcranial resection (39 cases), transsphenoidal resection (2 cases), and fractionated radiotherapy (8 cases). The mean prescription and maximum radiosurgical doses to the tumors were 17.0 and 40.3 Gy, respectively. Repeat radiosurgery was used to treat 13 tumors. With median follow-up of 68 months (range 2 to 138 months), local tumor control was 47.6% (10 of 21 patients). Of the 28 tumors treated, 8 decreased in size on follow-up imaging (28.6%), 5 remained unchanged (17.9%), and 15 ultimately progressed. Progression-free survival at 5 years was 28.7%, and it improved to 71.5% after multiple radiosurgery treatments. Prior fractionated irradiation or radiosurgical prescription dose did not correlate with tumor control. In 4 of 21 (19%) patients, extracranial metastases developed. Redmond et al.[90] reported on 118 patients with hemangiopericytoma of the CNS, 9% of whom had distant metastases at the time of initial presentation; 112 patients underwent surgical resection (23% had GTR, 31% subtotal resection, and 46% had surgery not otherwise specified). Adjuvant RT was received by 31% of patients following GTR, 44% after subtotal tumor resection, and 50% of patients following surgery not otherwise specified. The 5- and 10-year overall survival for all patients was 76.7% and 50.1%, respectively. Patients receiving adjuvant RT (n = 42) had a significantly better overall survival than patients who did not (n = 67; 10-year overall survival was 66.2% vs. 40.7%; $P = .05$). There was no difference in 5- or 10-year overall survival for patients treated with subtotal resection plus RT (n = 16) compared with those treated with GTR alone (n = 14; 10-year overall survival 75% vs. 57.1%; $P = .53$).

CHORDOMAS

Anatomy

Chordomas are rare neoplasms of the axial skeleton that arise from the remnant of the primitive notochord (chorda dorsalis). About 50% arise in the sacrococcygeal area; 35% arise intracranially, where they typically involve the clivus, and the remaining 15% occur in the midline along the path of the notochord, primarily involving the cervical vertebrae.[91]

Epidemiology

Chordomas are more common in patients in their 50s and 60s but can occur in all age groups. In children and young adults, the prognosis and long-term survival appear to be better than in older patients. No risk factors have been identified. Male predominance is reported at a 2:1 to 3:1 ratio.

Natural History

Although slowly growing, chordomas are locally invasive, destroying bone and infiltrating soft tissues. Basisphenoidal chordomas tend to cause symptoms earlier and may be difficult to differentiate histologically from chondromas and chondrosarcomas and radiographically from craniopharyngiomas, pineal tumors, and hypophyseal and pontine gliomas. The lethality of these tumors rests on their critical location, aggressive local behavior, and extremely high local recurrence rate. The incidence of metastasis, which has been reported to be as high as 25%, is higher than previously believed and may be related to the long clinical history. The most common site of distant metastasis is the lungs, followed by liver and bone. Lymphatic spread is uncommon.

Pathology

Chordoma is a soft, lobulated tumor that may have areas of hemorrhage, cystic changes, or calcification. It is frequently encapsulated but may be nonencapsulated or pseudoencapsulated. Histologically, it is composed of cords or masses of large cells (physaliferous cells) with typical vacuoles and granules of glycogen in the cytoplasm and abundant intercellular mucoid material. Usually there are few mitotic cells.[92] A chondroid variant of chordoma may exist, being prevalent in the spheno-occipital area. Patients with this type of histologic variant have improved survival.

Aside from the previously mentioned histologic features, the prognostic factors that most influence the choice of treatment are location and local extent of tumor.

Clinical Presentation

Chordomas tend to originate from the clivus and chondrosarcomas from the temporal bone.[93] Clinical symptoms vary with the location and extent of the tumor. In the head, extension may be intracranial or extracranial, into the sphenoid sinus, nasopharynx, clivus, and sellar and parasellar areas, with a resultant mass effect. In chordomas of the spheno-occipital region, the most common presenting symptom is headache. Other presentations include symptoms of pituitary insufficiency, nasal stuffiness, bitemporal hemianopsia, diplopia, and other cranial nerve deficits. Volpe et al.[94] reviewed the clinical features of 48 patients with chordoma and 49 patients with low-grade chondrosarcoma of the skull base. Twenty-five patients (52%) with chordoma and 24 patients (49%) with chondrosarcoma had ocular symptoms (diplopia or visual impairment) as the initial manifestation of the disease. Of the 59 patients (both groups) with diplopia, the diplopia was initially intermittent in 25 (42%). Headache and diplopia from abducens nerve palsy occurred in 22 patients (46%) with chordoma and 23 (47%) with chondrosarcoma.

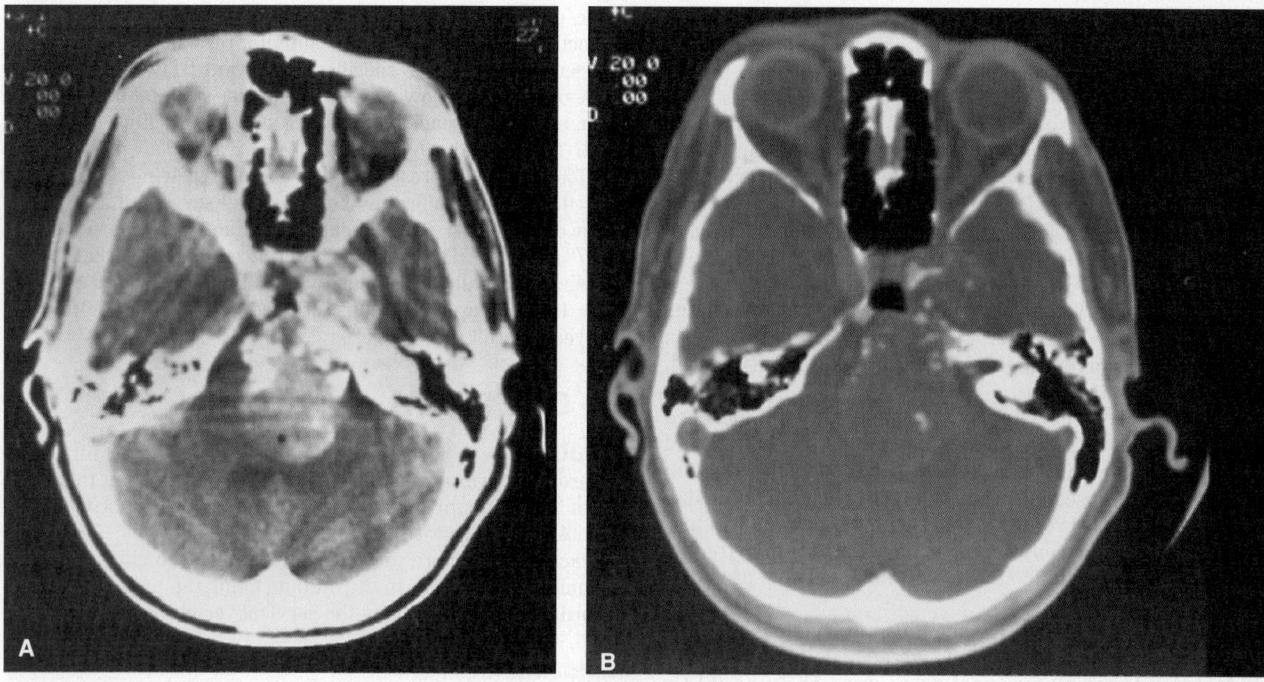

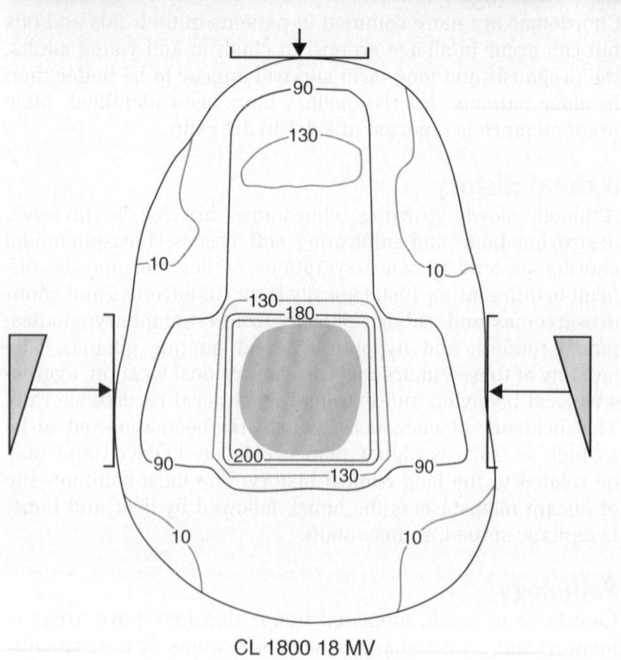

FIGURE 48.7. A: Contrast material-enhanced axial computed tomography scan demonstrates a large chordoma with extension into the posterior fossa and left parasellar region. **B:** Computed tomography scan photographed at bone windows shows the bony destruction and intratumoral calcifications. **C:** Treatment planning field arrangement for illustrated clivus chordoma using standard irradiation techniques with wedges on lateral ports.

TABLE 48.7 DIAGNOSTIC WORKUP FOR CHORDOMA

General
History
Physical examination
Radiologic studies
Plain radiographs
Computed tomography scan/magnetic resonance imaging
Laboratory studies
Complete blood cell count
Chemistry
Urinalysis
Special studies
Endocrinologic profile (clivus)
Visual evaluations (clivus)

Diagnostic Workup

The diagnostic workup varies with the primary location of disease. Most patients have significant bony destruction, and some may have calcifications in the tumor; hence, plain films and, specifically, CT scans or MRI are very useful (Table 48.7).[95] In most cases, the soft tissue component is much more extensive than initially appreciated, and a CT scan with contrast enhancement is required (Fig. 48.7A). CT and MRI are equivalent for demonstration of the presence and site of these tumors. MRI is inferior to CT in its ability to demonstrate bony destruction and intratumoral calcification (Fig. 48.7B).[96] MRI is superior to CT regarding the delineation of the exact extent of the tumor, which allows for better treatment planning.[95] Because of availability and lower cost, CT appears to be the technique of choice for routine follow-up of previously treated patients.[96]

Reliable signs of chordoma of the skull base are posterior extension to the pontine cistern; a lobulated, "honeycomb" appearance after gadolinium; the swollen appearance of the bone in the early stages; bone erosion on CT; and frequent extension to critical structures such as the circle of Willis, cavernous sinuses, and brainstem.[96]

General Management

Because of their surgical inaccessibility and relative resistance to radiation therapy, clivus chordomas represent a formidable therapeutic challenge. The general management of the patient is dictated by the anatomic location of the tumor and the direction and extent of spread. A surgical approach is recommended (when feasible), but complete surgical extirpation alone is unusual.[97] Regression of preoperative symptoms without additional postoperative morbidity could be achieved by radical transoral tumor extirpation documented by MRI. Intracranial spread usually requires steroid coverage and therapy directed to correction of neurologic deficits that may be present. Because of the high incidence of local recurrence, combined surgical excision and irradiation is frequently used. No effective chemotherapeutic agent or combination of drugs has been identified.

Radiation Therapy Techniques

Irradiation techniques vary considerably, depending on the location of the tumor along the craniospinal axis. Basisphenoidal tumors usually have been treated by a combination of parallel opposed lateral fields, anterior wedges, and photon and electron beam combinations, depending on the extent of the neoplasm. Precision radiation therapy planning, using CT and MRI, is required because high doses of external-beam radiation therapy are needed. Three-dimensional-CRT or IMRT provide optimal dose distributions.

The tumor usually surrounds the spinal cord and infiltrates vertebral bones. A combined technique using protons or electrons to boost the initial photon fields is generally applied. In the treatment of chordomas surrounding the spinal cord, IMRT can provide high-dose homogeneity and planning target volume (PTV) coverage (Fig. 48.8). Frequent digital portal image-based setup control reduces random positioning errors for head and neck cancer patients immobilized with conventional thermoplastic masks. Gabriele et al.[98] treated a patient with incomplete resection of a vertebral chordoma surrounding C2-3 with a total dose of 58 Gy in 2-Gy daily fractions. Beam arrangement consisted of seven 6 MV nonopposed coplanar IMRT fields using 120-leaf collimator in sliding window mode. To verify the daily setup, portal images at 0 degrees and 90 degrees were compared with the simulation images before treatment delivery (manual matching) and after treatment delivery (automatic anatomy matching). The mean dose to the PTV was 57.6 Gy covering 95% of the PTV with the 95% isodose. The minimum dose to the PTV (D99) was 53.6 Gy. The maximum dose to the spinal cord was 42.2 Gy and to the spinal cord planning risk volume (8 mm margin) 53.7 Gy. The mean dose to the parotids were 37.4 Gy (homolateral gland) and 19.5 Gy (contralateral gland). Because of the slow proliferative nature of chordomas, high linear energy transfer may prove useful in their management, as it will be discussed later. Brachytherapy can be used for recurrent tumors of the base of skull or adjacent to the spine when a more aggressive surgical exposure is offered.

Results of Therapy

Photons

Although survival in some patients with chordoma may be long term, the salient feature of this unusual neoplasm is local recurrence with eventual death. The course may be indolent, with multiple treatments for recurrences, but the overall 5-year disease-free survival rate is <10% to 20%. Catton et al.[99] analyzed the long-term results of treatment for patients with chordoma of the sacrum, base of skull, and mobile spine treated predominantly with postoperative photon irradiation. In 20 base of skull chordomas, most of them irradiated with conventionally fractionated radiation to a median dose of 50 Gy in 25 fractions for 5 weeks (range 25 to 50 Gy), median survival was 62 months (range 4 to 240 months) from diagnosis with no difference between clival and nonclival presentations. There was no survival advantage to patients receiving radiation doses >50 Gy (median 60 Gy) compared with lower doses <50 Gy (median 40 Gy). Hyperfractionation regimens did not influence the degree or duration of symptomatic response or progression-free survival. Median survival after retreatment was 18 months.

Forsyth et al.[100] reported on 51 patients with intracranial chordomas (19 classified as chondroid) treated surgically (biopsy in 11 patients and subtotal removal or greater in 40); 39 patients received postoperative irradiation. At the time of the analysis, 17 patients were alive. The 5- and 10-year survival rates were 51% and 35%, respectively; 5-year survival was 36% for biopsy patients and 55% for those who had resection. Patients who underwent postoperative irradiation tended to have longer disease-free survival times.

Gay et al.[101] analyzed the outcome of 46 patients with cranial base chordomas and 14 with chondrosarcomas after extensive surgical resection, 50% of them treated previously; 20% received postoperative irradiation. Nine patients with chordomas and two with chondrosarcomas died during the postoperative follow-up period. The 5-year recurrence-free survival for all patients was 76%. Chondrosarcomas had a better prognosis than chordomas (5-year recurrence-free survival of 90% and 65%, respectively; $P = .09$). Patients who had undergone previous surgery had a greater risk of recurrence than did those who had not undergone previous surgery (5-year recurrence-free survival rates of 64% and 93%, respectively; $P < .05$). Those with total or near-total resection had a better 5-year recurrence-free survival rate (84%) than did patients with partial or subtotal resection (64%; $P < .05$). Postoperative leakage of cerebrospinal fluid was the most frequent complication (30% of patients) and was found to increase the risk of permanent disability. Patients

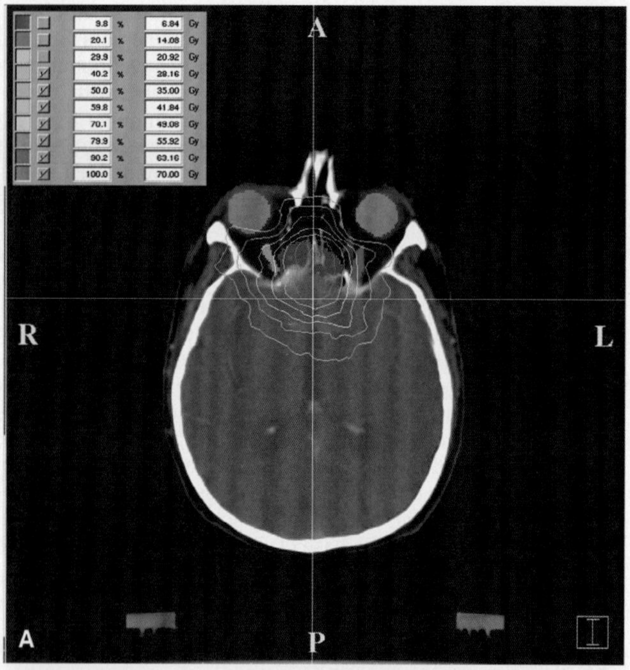

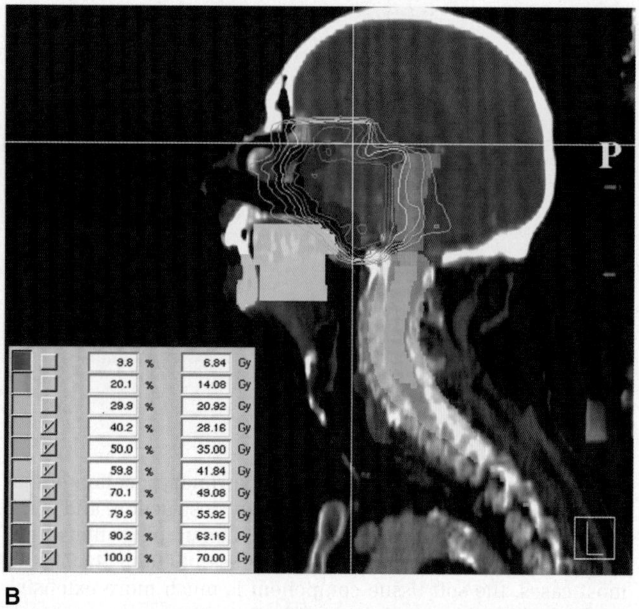

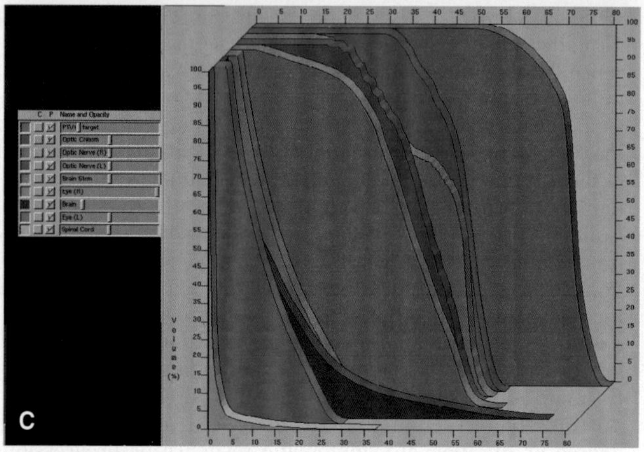

FIGURE 48.8. Chordoma of clivus in 81-year-old man treated with 70 Gy in 2-Gy fractions. Example of intensity-modulated radiation therapy plan: **A:** Cross-section in upper portion of planning target volume (PTV), demonstrating coverage of target volume with sparing of ocular structures. **B:** Sagittal plane dose distribution with excellent coverage of PTV. **C:** Dose–volume histogram:

Structure	*Dose Range (cGy)*	*Mean Dose (Gy)*
PTV (including left neck)	60–75	70
Optic nerves/chasm	25–50	41
Ocular globe	3–30	12

who had undergone previous irradiation had a greater risk of death in the postoperative period (within 3 months of operation) and during follow-up.

Tai et al.[91] reviewed the results of irradiation combined with surgery, irradiation alone, and surgery alone in 159 patients reported in the literature. An analysis of the optimal biologically equivalent dose was performed using the linear-quadratic formula on 47 patients. With conventional photon irradiation, no dose–response relationship was shown. Survival improved in patients undergoing surgery followed by irradiation.

Chetty et al.[102] reported on 18 chordomas, 61% of them occurred in the sphenoid region. Follow-up for 12 patients ranged from 3 to 170 months. Various combinations of surgery and radiation therapy were used. Mean survival was 73.4 months, with a survival rate of 50% (6 of 12 patients).

Keisch et al.[103] reported on 21 patients with chordoma treated at the authors' medical center: 5 had clival tumors, 2 had nasopharyngeal tumors, and 1 had a lumbar spine tumor. Nine patients were treated with surgery alone, eight had subtotal resection and postoperative irradiation, and four received irradiation alone after biopsy. The 5- and 10-year actuarial survivals were significantly better in patients treated with surgery alone or surgery and irradiation than in those treated with radiation therapy alone (52%, 32%, and 0%, respectively; $P = .02$). Disease-free survival of patients with base of skull tumors was not significantly different among the treatment groups.

Debus et al.[104] reported on 45 patients treated for chordoma or chondrosarcoma with postoperative fractionated 3D stereotactic radiation therapy. Median dose at isocenter was 66.6 Gy for chordomas and 64.9 Gy for chondrosarcomas. All chondrosarcomas achieved and maintained local tumor and recurrence-free status at 5-years follow-up. Local control rate of chordomas at 5 years was 50% and survival was 82%. Clinically significant late toxicity developed in only one patient.

Bugoci et al.[105] published results on 12 patients with skull-base chordoma treated with fractionated stereotactic RT and IMRT boost (total dose 74 Gy in 2-Gy fractions). With median follow-up of 34 months, local tumor control at 3 years was 65% and overall survival 92%.

Den et al.[106] described a multi-institutional study of 31 patients, 28 with clivus chordoma or chondrosarcoma, treated with various photon techniques (single-dose stereotactic, fractionated 3D-CRT, IMRT). Median fractionated total dose was 65 Gy. Actuarial 3-year local tumor control was 68% and overall survival 63%. Patients receiving 65 Gy or a higher dose had a 5-year tumor control of 78% and overall survival of 90%. No grade 2 or greater toxicity was observed.

Muthukumar et al.[107] published a report on 15 patients with skull-base chordoma and chondrosarcoma treated with stereotactic radiation therapy (13 had previous surgical resection). Median minimum marginal tumor single dose was 18 Gy (12 to 20 Gy) and the number of isocenters ranged from 1 to 10 (average, 4). Dose to optic nerve or chiasm was ≤9 Gy. With median follow-up of 40 months, eight patients had clinical improvement, three were stable, and four had died. No significant morbidity was noted.

Protons

The best results in the treatment of chordomas have been obtained with radical surgery followed by high-dose proton irradiation.[108] Berson et al.[109] described 45 patients with chordomas or chondrosarcomas at the base of the skull or cervical spine treated by subtotal resection and postoperative irradiation. Twenty-three patients were treated definitively by charged particles, 13 patients with photons and particles, and 9 were treated for recurrent disease. Doses ranged from 36 to 80 Gy equivalent (GyE). There appeared to be significant benefit for patients with smaller tumor volumes (80% vs. 33% actuarial survival rate at 5 years). Patients treated for primary disease had a 78% actuarial local tumor control at 2 years versus 33% for recurrent disease.

Austin et al.[110] evaluated 141 patients with chordoma and chondrosarcoma of the base of skull and cervical spine treated with proton and photon irradiation. The local disease was controlled in 111 patients. They reviewed 26 patients who had recurrent disease (21 nonchondroid chordomas, two chondroid chordomas, and three chondrosarcomas). The prescribed doses ranged from 67 to 72 cobalt Gray equivalent (CGE). Approximately 25% (6 of 26) of the cases failed in the prescribed dose region. More than half (15 of 26) failed in regions where tumor dose was limited by normal tissue constraints. Approximately 10% of the patients recurred in the surgical pathway and 10% were judged to be marginal misses. Overall, 75% of the patients failed in regions receiving less than the prescribed dose. All tumors that failed in the high-dose region had recurrences (10 of 26) and larger tumors (average volume of 102 cc) than those with base of skull disease (16 of 115) with an average volume of 63 cc.

O'Connell et al.[111] reported on 62 patients with base of skull chordomas treated with proton beam irradiation (65 to 73.5 GyE); 29 patients (19 women and 10 men) experienced local failure, and 14 women (48%) and 7 men (21%) died of disease. On histologic analysis, the presence of >10% necrosis, prominent nucleoli, and tumor >70 mm were significant predictors of short-term disease-specific survival. Chondroid chordoma and conventional chordomas had equivalent outcomes.

Fagundes et al.[112] updated the Massachusetts General Hospital experience with 204 patients treated for chordoma of the base of the skull or cervical spine. Sixty-three patients (31%) had treatment failures, which were local in 60 patients (29%) and the only site of failure in 49 patients. Two patients had regional lymph node relapse, and three developed surgical pathway recurrence. Thirteen patients relapsed in distant sites (especially lungs and bones). The 5-year actuarial survival rate after any relapse was 7%. There was no significant difference in survival for patients who had a local or distant failure. Two patients (1.4%) with local tumor control developed distant metastases in contrast with 10 of 60 patients (16%) who failed locally and distantly.

Terahara et al.[113] reported on 132 patients with skull-base chordoma treated with combined photon and proton irradiation; in 115 patients dose–volume data and follow-up were available. The prescribed doses ranged from 66.6 to 79.2 CGE (median 68.9 CGE). Dose to the optic structures (optic nerves and chiasm), the brainstem surface, and the brainstem center was limited to 60, 64, and 53 CGE, respectively. Local failure developed in 42 of 115 patients, with the actuarial local tumor control rates at 5 and 10 years being 59% and 44%, respectively. In a Cox multivariate analysis, the model's equivalent uniform dose suggests that the probability of recurrence of skull-base chordomas depends on gender, target volume, and target dose inhomogeneity; equivalent uniform dose was shown to be a useful parameter to evaluate dose distribution for the target volume.

Hug et al.[114] analyzed efficacy of fractionated proton radiation therapy for 33 skull-base chordomas and 25 chondrosarcomas. Following various surgical procedures, residual tumor was present in 91% of patients; 59% demonstrated brainstem involvement. Target doses ranged from 64.8 to 79.2 CGE (mean 70.7 CGE). The range of follow-up was 7 to 75 months (mean 33 months). In 10 patients (17%) the treatment failed locally, resulting in local control rates of 92% (23 of 25 patients) for chondrosarcomas and 76% (25 of 33 patients) for chordomas. All tumors with volumes of ≤25 mL remained locally controlled compared with 56% of tumors >25 mL (P = .02). Of patients without brainstem involvement, 94% did not experience recurrence; whereas with brainstem involvement (and dose reduction because of brainstem tolerance constraints), the tumor control rate was 53% (P = .04). Actuarial 5-year survival rates were 100% for patients with chondrosarcoma and 79% for patients with chordoma. Grade 3 and 4 late toxicities were observed in four patients (7%) and were symptomatic in three (5%).

Ares et al.[42] treated 42 patients with chordomas and 22 with chondrosarcomas of the skull base using spot-scanning protons (median doses 73.5 and 68.4 Gy, respectively, at 1.8 to 2.0 Gy relative biological effect). With median follow-up of 38 months, 5-year tumor control was 81% and 94% and overall survival 100% and 91%, respectively. Late toxicity consisted of one grade 3 and one grade 4 unilateral optic neuropathy and two patients with grade 3 CNS necrosis. No patient experienced brainstem toxicity.

Noel et al.[115] reported on 49 chordomas and 18 chondrosarcomas treated with high-energy photons (two-thirds of dose) and 201 MeV protons (one-third of dose). Median total dose was 67 CGE (60 to 70 CGE). With median follow-up of 32 months, 3-year local tumor control was 71% for chordomas and 85% for chondrosarcomas, and 4-year overall survival 88% and 75%, respectively. Fourteen tumors (21%) failed locally.

Recently, heavy particles have been used to treat some of these patients.[116, 210] Hasegawa et al.[79] reported on 54 patients with skull base or paracervical tumors (31 with chordomas) treated with carbon ions (escalating doses from 48 to 60.8 GyE in 16 fractions over 4 weeks). In the 31 chordoma patients, 5-year local tumor control and overall survival were 78% and 85%, respectively. Patients were divided into two groups; a low-dose group (n = 10) irradiated with doses ranging from 48 to 57.8 GyE, and a high-dose group (n = 21) irradiated with 60.8 GyE. The 5-year local tumor control was 60% for the low-dose group and 93% for the high-dose group and the overall survival was 90% and 84%, respectively. One late grade 2 brain sequela was noted in a patient treated with 60.8 GyE.

Likewise, Schulz-Ertner et al.[43] treated 24 chordomas and 13 chondrosarcomas with 3D planning carbon ions (median dose 60 GyE). With mean follow-up of 13 months, local tumor control at 2 years was 90%. Progression-free survival was 83% for chordomas and 100% for chondrosarcomas. No significant toxicity was observed.

Benk et al.[117] described results in 18 children 4 to 18 years of age with base of skull or cervical spine chordomas who received fractionated high-dose postoperative irradiation using mixed-photon and 160-MeV proton beams. Median tumor dose was 69 CGE with a 1.8-CGE daily fraction. With a median follow-up of 72 months, the 5-year survival was 68%, and the 5-year disease-free survival rate was 63%. Patients with cervical spine chordomas had a worse survival rate than did those with base of skull lesions (P = .008). The incidence of treatment-related morbidity was acceptable: two cases of growth hormone deficit corrected by hormone replacement, one temporal lobe necrosis, and one fibrosis of the temporalis muscle, improved after surgery.

A report on proton therapy for base of skull chordoma published by the Royal College of Radiologists[118] concluded that outcome after proton irradiation is superior to that reported for conventional photon irradiation. Radiation therapy schedules involving a mixed schedule of protons and photons have achieved an approximately 60% local tumor control rate at 5 years.

Sequelae of Treatment

In patients treated with high irradiation doses, as well as with charged particles, there is an increasing probability of sequelae, including brain damage, spinal cord injury, bone or soft tissue necrosis, and xerostomia. In a report by Berson et al.,[109] three patients experienced unilateral visual loss, and four patients had radiation injury to the brainstem.

Santoni et al.[119] reported on the temporal lobe damage rate in 96 patients (75 primary and 21 recurrent tumors) treated with postoperative high-dose proton and photon irradiation for chordomas and chondrosarcomas of the base of the skull. All the patients were randomized to receive 66.6 or 72 CGE with conventional fractionation (1.8 CGE per day, 5 fractions per week) using opposed lateral fields for the photon component and a noncoplanar isocentric technique for the proton component. Of the 96 patients, 10 developed temporal lobe damage (lateral in 2 and unilateral in 8). The cumulative temporal lobe damage incidence at 2 and 5 years was 7.6% and 13.2%, respectively. CT and MRI scans were evaluated for white matter changes; the MRI areas suggestive of temporal lobe damage in 10 patients were always separate from the tumor bed.

In patients receiving high-dose proton therapy for clivus tumors, Slater et al.[120] observed a 26% incidence of endocrine abnormalities at 3 years and 37% at 5 years, with hypothyroidism being the most frequent sequela. The dose to the pituitary in patients with abnormalities ranged from 63.1 to 67.7 GyE.

LETHAL MIDLINE GRANULOMA

Natural History and Pathology

Lethal midline granuloma (LMG) or midline malignant polymorphic reticulosis is a clinical entity characterized by progressive, unrelenting ulceration and necrosis of the midline facial tissues.[121,122] LMG is associated with Epstein-Barr virus, which has at least two subtypes with different biologic properties that can be identified by their genomic configuration. The occurrence of the rare subtype 2 in LMG may relate to a covert immune defect.[123] Considerable controversy exists regarding various disorders characterized by a necrotizing and granulomatous inflammation of the tissues of the upper respiratory tract and oral cavity. It is now clear that if infections and other known agents such as cocaine use, sarcoidosis, environmental toxins, and various neoplasms can be excluded, three clinicopathologic entities remain: Wegener's granulomatosis, LMG, and polymorphic reticulosis (PMR).[15] A review of the literature suggests that cases described as idiopathic midline destructive disease and PMR are a large evolutionary spectrum from almost benign to fatal malignant lymphoma.[124]

Wegener's granulomatosis is an epithelioid necrotizing granulomatosis with vasculitis of small vessels. Systemic involvement of the kidneys and lungs is common.

PMR is an unusual disorder with distinctive clinical and pathologic features. Histologically, PMR is characterized by an atypical mixed lymphoid infiltration of the submucosa with extensive areas of necrosis, sometimes extending to bone or cartilage. The lesion consists of variable zones of small lymphocytes with scattered immunoblastic forms, abundant plasma cells with occasional eosinophilia and histiocytosis.[125] PMR has been considered a lymphoproliferative disorder; most, if not all, cases are peripheral T-cell lymphomas. Several authorities believe that PMR and systemic lymphomatoid granulomatosis are the same disease, with the latter predominantly involving the lungs.[126]

Idiopathic LMG describes a localized disorder not characterized by visceral lesions but by destruction of the midfacial area, which, if left untreated, is uniformly fatal. The histopathologic findings are nonspecific, with a relatively nondescript inflammatory reaction with acute and chronic inflammation and necrosis. Despite specific clinicopathologic features, the distinction between LMG and PMR is often difficult; although controversial, they may represent two phases of the same disease, with LMG remaining histologically benign or evolving into PMR. LMG occurs more frequently in men.[98] Ages range from 21 to 64 years; almost half of the patients are in their 50s at presentation. Most patients have involvement of the nasal cavity (including destruction of the septum) and the paranasal sinuses (particularly maxillary antrum). The primary lesion may extend into the orbits, the oral cavity (palate, gingiva), and even the pharynx.

Characteristics of the three different diseases are outlined in Table 48.8.

Clinical Features and Diagnostic Workup

Clinical manifestations include progressive nasal discharge, obstruction, foul odor emanating from the nose, and, in later stages, pain in the nasal cavity, paranasal areas, and even in the orbits.

Examination discloses ulceration and necrosis in the nasal cavity, perforation or destruction of nasal septum and turbinates, and even ulceration of the nose. Edema of the face and eyelids may be noted, and the bridge of the nose may be sunken. Radiographic studies initially show soft tissue swelling, mucosal thickening, and findings consistent with chronic sinusitis.

CT is invaluable in demonstrating the full extent of the tumor, including bone or cartilage destruction. In 13 patients presenting with LMG, CT proved essential for determining the extent of the disease, guiding biopsy, and planning radiation therapy.[127] MRI was also helpful for the latter because it could

TABLE 48.8 DIFFERENTIAL FEATURES OF THREE CLINICOPATHOLOGIC ENTITIES

	Wegener's Granulomatosis	*Idiopathic Midline Granuloma*	*Polymorphic Reticulosis*
Disease features	Diffuse, inflammatory disease of upper airway, predominately sinuses and nose	Destructive extension to palate and facial soft tissues	Destructive lesion with destruction of bone and extension through soft tissues
Systemic involvement	Lungs, kidneys, small-vessel vasculitis may not have airway involvement	No	No
Associated with lymphoma	No	May remain benign or progress to lymphoma	Usually evolves to lymphoma
Histologic features	Necrotizing vasculitis with epithelioid granulomas, giant cells, and fibrinoid necrosis	Inflammatory reaction, nonspecific; granulomas and giant cells are infrequent	Characteristic atypical and polymorphic lymphoreticular cellular infiltrate; angiocentric growth patterns may simulate vasculitis, but fibrinoid necrosis is absent in vessel walls
Treatment	Chemotherapy	Radiation therapy	Chemotherapy; radiation therapy and chemotherapy

Modified from Bataskis JG. Wegener's granulomatosis and midline (non peeling) granuloma. *Head Neck Surg* 1979;1:213.

distinguish fluid retained within the paranasal sinuses from solid masses and tumor from granulation tissue; it was of little value for detecting bone lysis. Eight patients proved to have T-cell lymphoma, two had Crohn disease, in one the lesion was factitious, and two had granulomas without diagnostic histologic features.

General Management and Radiation Therapy Techniques

When treatment of these patients is planned, it is extremely important to exclude the diagnosis of Wegener's granulomatosis, a benign process that is commonly treated with antimicrobial agents, steroids, and systemic chemotherapy.[126] *Bona fide* LMG does not respond to steroids; the treatment of choice is radiation therapy.[128,129,130]

Target volume should encompass all areas of involvement, including adjacent areas at risk (i.e., for a lesion of the maxillary antrum, it will include the antrum as well as all of the paranasal sinuses) with a 2- to 3-cm margin.[131] Because marginal failures are a significant problem, wide margins are necessary for treatment of these patients.[125]

Irradiation techniques are similar to those described for tumors of the paranasal sinuses, nasal cavity, or nasopharynx. Several investigators have described complete responses with doses of 30 to 50 Gy; most patients are treated with 35 to 45 Gy in 3 to 4.5 weeks.[129,132] The authors recommend 45 to 50 Gy in 4.5 to 5.5 weeks in 1.8- to 2-Gy daily fractions.

Results of Therapy

Because of the rarity of this tumor, experience is limited. Fauci et al.[132] reported on 10 patients with extensive midline granuloma treated with irradiation. Three received 10 Gy, and all failed within 2 years (retreated with 40 to 46 Gy). The remaining seven patients received 40 to 50 Gy. Local control of disease was 77%; two patients had local recurrences, one outside the initially irradiated volume.

In a study of 34 patients with PMR treated with primary radiation therapy except for one patient, Smalley et al.[125] found that a minimum dose of 42 Gy or a time-dose factor of 70 was necessary to achieve long-term local control. The most frequent failure site was within the original irradiation field. Systemic failure occurred in 25% of their patients initially presenting with limited disease. The salvage of this subset of patients requires effective systemic chemotherapy. Multimodality treatment using intensive chemotherapy and radiation therapy might improve the prognosis of these patients.

Fauci et al.[132] published a prospective study of 15 patients with systemic lymphomatoid granulomatosis. Of 13 patients treated with cyclophosphamide and prednisone, seven sustained complete remission (mean duration of remission, 5.2 ± 0.6 years). Two patients receiving only prednisone and six receiving cyclophosphamide and prednisone died. Six deaths were associated with biopsy-proven lymphoma; one was caused by a lymphoma-like illness unproven by biopsy. The eighth death was caused by adenocarcinoma in a patient with lymphoma in remission. None of these patients received radiation therapy.

Chen et al.[133] reported their experience in 92 cases of LMG or centrofacial malignant lymphoma treated with radiation therapy. Twenty-five patients received combination chemotherapy, usually containing doxorubicin, cyclophosphamide, vincristine, and prednisone (CHOP) or other combinations, including CHOP or nitrogen mustard, vincristine, procarbazine, and prednisone (MOPP) in some patients. The nose was the most frequently involved site at initial presentation (85% of patients). Immunophenotyping in 36 patients showed T-cell lineage in 25 (69%) and B-cell lineage in 6 (17%). The irradiation technique consisted of treating all involved and adjacent areas with doses of 30 to 75 Gy. Sixteen patients received neck irradiation (30 to 60 Gy). Daily fractions were 2 to 3 Gy in 5 weekly fractions. Actuarial survival rates were 59.5% at 5 years, 56.2% at 10 years, and 40.5% at 20 years. There was no significant difference in survival in patients receiving <50 Gy. A relapse in the midfacial region was noted in seven patients. Other relapse sites were lung and skin in three patients, para-aortic or inguinal lymph nodes in two patients, and brain in one. Survival of patients with recurrences was poor; 73% died within 8 months.

Hatta et al.[134] reviewed 18 patients (15 males and 3 females) with LMG (polymorphic reticulosis), about 5.6% of patients with malignant head and neck tumors. Most of the 18 patients underwent both radiation therapy and chemotherapy (cyclophosphamide, vincristine, prednisone [COP], CHOP, methotrexate, leucovorin, doxorubicin, cyclophosphamide, vincristine, bleomycin, prednisone [MACOP-B]), but, because their disease had reached an advanced stage, three underwent radiation therapy only, three chemotherapy only, and one received no radical therapy. Of the 18 patients, 13 died of the disease; in 6 patients progress was confined to the local lesion. The 5-year cumulative survival rate was 15.7%. Fourteen autopsy studies revealed that tumor had invaded the liver (92.8%), lung (92.8%), and spleen (71.4%), and in all cases it was in leukemic patterns. Five cases were positive for ubiquitin carboxyl-terminal esterase L1 (ubiquitin thiolesterase) (CD45RO) and 10 cases were positive for lysozyme. All cases were positive for Ki-1 (CD30).

Sakata et al.[135] reported on 107 patients with stage I and II non-Hodgkin lymphoma of the head and neck treated with involved field radiation therapy for orbital, nasal, or paranasal lymphoma and extended field radiation for Waldeyer's ring or neck lymphoma (39 to 48 Gy). In the latter half of the study, adjuvant chemotherapy was administered. Of 107 patients, 95 achieved chemoradiation. Of the 12 patients who did not achieve chemoradiation, 9 had nasal T-cell lymphoma of the lethal midline granuloma (LMG-NTL) type. Only one patient who obtained chemoradiation relapsed in a previously irradiated area. LMG-NTL was the most significant prognostic factor on multivariate analysis (P <.001). Older patients also experienced a higher relative risk than patients aged ≤60 years (P = .0063). Dose of doxorubicin reached borderline significance (P = .0600). Radiotherapy is excellent for obtaining local control of head and neck non-Hodgkin lymphoma and LMG-NTL.

CHLOROMA

Natural History

Chloroma (granulocytic sarcoma, myeloblastoma) is a solid extramedullary tumor composed of early myeloid precursors usually associated with acute myelocytic or nonlymphocytic leukemia. These tumors have predilection for the skin, lymph nodes, and the spine; most common head and neck sites of presentation are in the orbit and other craniofacial bones. The name chloroma (from the Greek *chloros,* meaning green) derives from the green color of affected tissues resulting from the presence of myeloperoxidase. Because not all deposits exhibit the characteristic green tint, the term *granulocytic sarcoma* (GS) seems more appropriate.

GS, an extramedullary proliferation of malignant myeloid precursor cells, were identified in 3% of 478 patients with acute chronic granulocytic leukemia; they can be seen with other myeloproliferative disorders, including polycythemia vera, hypereosinophilia, and myeloid metaplasia. In the absence of acute leukemia, GS is usually an ominous sign, suggesting imminent conversion to acute myelocytic leukemia or blast crisis. As survival rates for myelogenous leukemias improve, the number of patients who relapse with chloromas is increasing.

Children are affected more often than adults. Of 33 patients with orbital chloromas reported by Zimmerman and Font,[136] 75% were in their first decade of life. Chloromas are found more frequently in children with the M4 and M5 acute myeloid leukemia subtypes of the French-American-British Cooperative Group Classification and are also associated with the 8:21 translocation. Chloromas may appear during bone marrow remission before an increase in blasts is detected in the bone marrow, so they may herald relapse.

Clinical Presentation and Diagnostic Workup

Intraorbital (retrobulbar) chloroma causes progressive exophthalmos or temporal swelling. CNS involvement causes both local pressure phenomena and generalized elevation of intracranial pressure with headaches, nausea, and vomiting. Intracerebral chloromas may manifest as the rare CNS (parenchymal) involvement of acute nonlymphocytic leukemia.[137,138]

Intracranial chloromas may exhibit intermediate or high attenuation in unenhanced CT scans, with intense, uniform enhancement with contrast material.[139,140] Confusion with meningioma, hematoma, solitary metastasis, and lymphoma may occur on CT scans.[125] MRI of GS is commonly used for a spinal or cranial location that demonstrates isointensity relative to gray matter on TI-weighted images and isointensity to white matter on T2-weighted images. GS demonstrate almost uniform enhancement with gadolinium, which further aids in delineating it.

General Management

Many of these patients are treated with anthracycline-based chemotherapy, although surgical excision or radiation therapy for masses are indicated.

Radiation Therapy Techniques

Chloromas are extremely radiosensitive; however, the optimal dose of irradiation has not been established. Response rates of leukemic infiltrates have been reported with doses as low as 4 Gy, yet the need for higher doses up to 30 Gy in certain locations of extramedullary leukemic infiltrates is well recognized. Although the literature is limited regarding the maximum dose needed for treatment of chloromas, Chak et al.,[141] in a study of 23 patients with GS, reported that 20 to 30 Gy yielded 85% to 89% local tumor control. In the authors' limited experience, there appears to be a relationship between the size of the chloroma and the total dose of irradiation required for control. The target volume is the tumor mass and an adequate margin (2 to 3 cm). Irradiation techniques depend on the location of the infiltrate. For superficial lesions, electron beam is recommended. Orbital chloroma may constitute a radiation therapy emergency because visual loss is possible if the patient is not treated promptly.

ESTHESIONEUROBLASTOMA

Esthesioneuroblastomas (ENB), first described by Berger and Luc,[142] are rare tumors thought to arise in the olfactory receptors in the nasal mucosa or the cribriform plate of the ethmoid bone. The olfactory nerves perforate grooves in the ethmoid bone in the cribriform plate and continue into the subarachnoid spaces, accounting for the high incidence of intracranial extension.[142]

Epidemiology

ENB constitutes 3% of all endonasal neoplasms. In the United States,[143] according to the data from the Surveillance, Epidemiology, and the End Results (SEER) program, 84 cases of ENB were registered from 1978 to 1990[144] and about 945 cases have been reported in the world literature.[145] The review authors' cases accounted for 198 and collaborative efforts accounted for 747 cases. Sex distribution was 53.6% male and 46.64% female. Kadish classification was applied to 563 cases; 103 (18.3%) class A, 182 (32.2%) class B, and 278 (49.4%) class C cases.

There appears to be a slight male predominance. The age incidence has a bimodal distribution, with peaks at 11 to 20 years and 40 to 60 years, the highest incidence at 51 to 60 years.

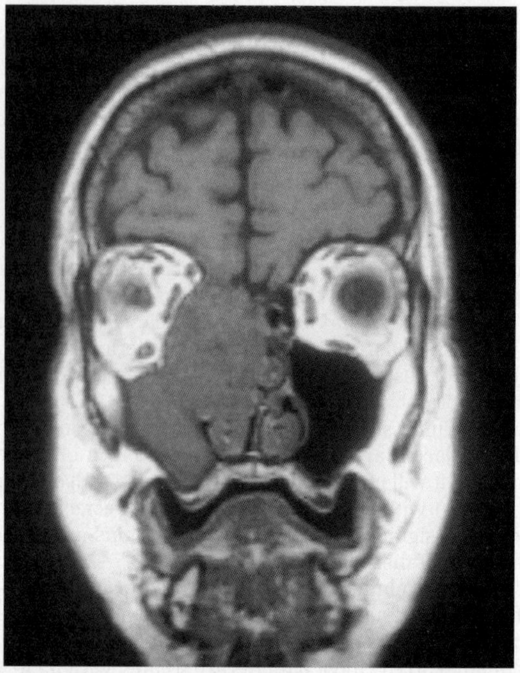

FIGURE 48.9. Coronal magnetic resonance imaging scan showing a large soft tissue mass and bone destruction in the right ethmoidal maxillary sinuses and nasal cavity secondary to extensive (Kadish stage C) esthesioneuroblastoma.

Natural History

Although others thought that ENB were of ectodermal origin, most observers believe the tumor to be of neuroectodermal origin in the olfactory epithelium.[14,146] Most of these tumors occur high in the nasal cavity or in the lateral wall adjacent to the ethmoid. The tumor may spread to the opposite ethmoid bone, superiorly to the frontal sinus and anterior cranial fossa, posteriorly to the sphenoid sinus, nasopharynx, and base of skull, laterally to the orbits, forward to the frontonasal angle, or inferiorly to the nasal cavity and antrum (Fig. 48.9). Lymphatic spread may be to the subdigastric, posterior cervical, submaxillary, or preauricular nodes, as well as to the nodes of Rouviere. The exact incidence of distant metastases is uncertain; it has been stated to be as high as 50%, but this rate is influenced by the use of chemotherapy in high-risk patients.

Clinical Presentation

These tumors tend to be friable and bleed easily. The most common clinical symptoms are epistaxis and nasal blockage. Patients also may have local pain or headache, visual disturbances, rhinorrhea, tearing, proptosis, or swelling in the cheek.[147] The symptoms may be associated with a mass in the neck.

Diagnostic Workup and Staging

Physical examination may show the inferior aspect of a polypoid friable mass in the nasal cavity. Ocular findings or a mass in the nasopharynx may be present. With early lesions, radiographs or CT or MRI may show only nonspecific opacification, soft tissue swelling, and occasionally bone destruction.[148] Octreotide is a somatostatin analog that, when coupled to a radioisotope, produces a scintigraphic image of neuroendocrine tumors (NETs) expressing somatostatin type-2 receptors. Octreotide scintigraphy may be useful in confirming the preoperative diagnosis of certain head and neck NETs, such as paragangliomas, Merkel cell carcinomas, medullary thyroid carcinomas, and esthesioneuroblastomas. Bustillo et al.[149]

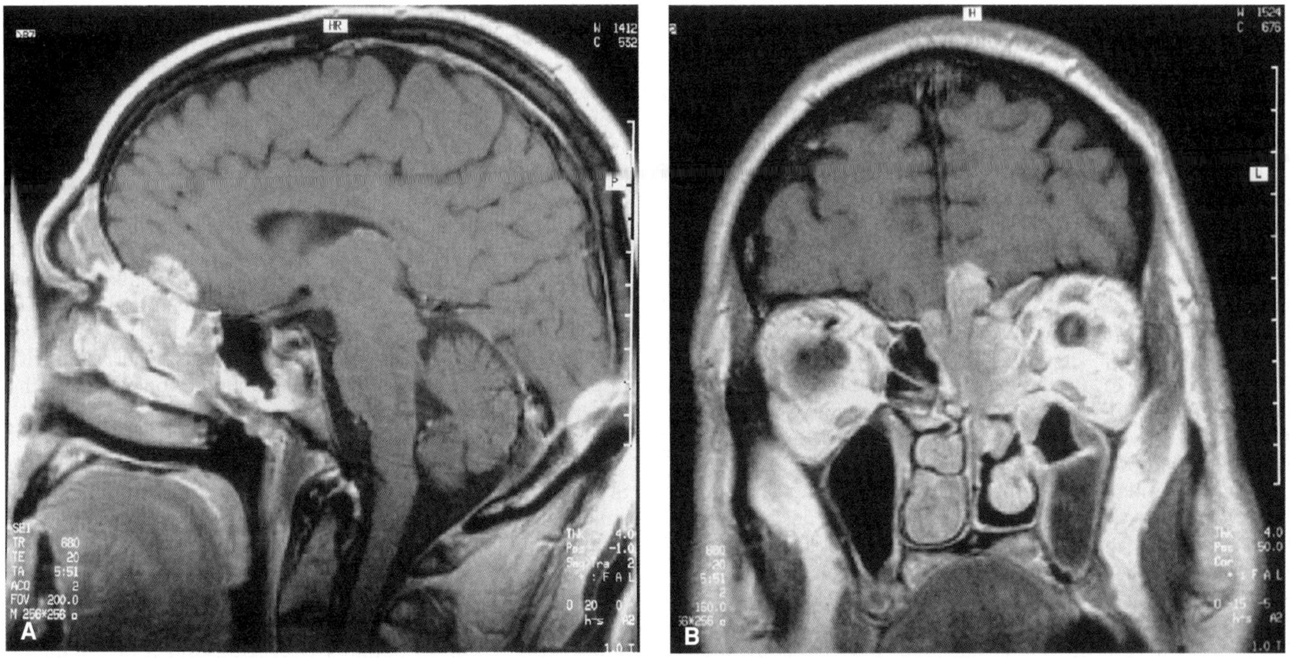

FIGURE 48.10. Sagittal **(A)** and coronal **(B)** views of a preoperative magnetic resonance imaging of a 56-year-old patient who was initially seen with a Kadish stage C tumor involving left nasal cavity and extending intracranially. (From Chao KSC, Kaplan C, Simpson JR, et al. Esthesioneuroblastoma: the impact of treatment modality. *Head Neck* 2001;23:749–757, with permission.)

carried out a retrospective study that compared the results of octreotide scintigraphy with the histopathologic diagnosis in 74 patients with head and neck NETs. Of the 60 patients undergoing evaluation for suspected paraganglioma, octreotide scintigraphy was correctly positive in 36 of 37 patients with paraganglioma and correctly negative in 19 of 23 patients who did not exhibit paraganglioma (sensitivity of 97% and a specificity of 82%). There were 14 patients in the nonparaganglioma group. Octreotide scintigraphy detected or diagnosed locoregional recurrences in two with esthesioneuroblastoma.

Table 48.1 outlines the suggested diagnostic workup. MRI, especially with gadolinium contrast, may be used as a supplement or alternative to CT scanning.[39] CT provides the best information about the tumor and its local invasion into surrounding bone structures. MRI allows an estimate of tumor spread into surrounding soft tissue areas, such as the anterior cranial fossa and the retromaxillary space. Bone scintigraphy scan is useful in detecting distant metastases.

The expansile tendency of olfactory neuroblastoma is characterized by bowing of the sinus walls. The destructive aspect is manifested as tumor replacing the turbinates, septum, and sinus walls with extension into contiguous areas (Figs. 48.9 and 48.10). The density or signal and enhancement characteristics are nonspecific of olfactory neuroblastoma.

Although dopamine β-hydroxylase and catecholamines are produced by these tumors, their measurements or vanillylmandelic acid excretion levels have not proven clinically useful.

A staging system has been proposed by Kadish et al.[147] (Table 48.9).

TABLE 48.9 KADISH SYSTEM FOR STAGING OF ESTHESIONEUROBLASTOMA

Stage	Characteristic
A	Disease confined to the nasal cavity
B	Disease confined to the nasal cavity and one or more paranasal sinuses
C	Disease extending beyond the nasal cavity or paranasal sinuses; includes involvement of the orbit, base of skull or intracranial cavity, cervical lymph nodes, or distant metastatic sites

From Kadish S, Goodman M, Wang CC. Olfactory neuroblastoma: a clinical analysis of 17 cases. *Cancer* 1976;37:1571–1576, with permission.

Pathologic Features and Prognostic Factors

ENBs are polypoid, frequently reddish, soft, and vascular tumors with neuroblasts and neurocytes. ENBs contain epithelial components serving as a supporting stroma and have a nerve component that corresponds to the olfactory cells. Rosettes are the main feature, consisting of several rows of cells arranged around the central area.[14] ENBs may be confused with lymphoma or anaplastic carcinoma and have diffuse, regular distribution. ENBs contain many fibrils, which fill the central space of the rosette (called a pseudorosette). It has been suggested that the presence of chromaffin granules indicates a derivative from primitive neural crest cells. ENB must be distinguished from other poorly differentiated neoplasms, including sinonasal undifferentiated carcinoma, which is derived from the Schneiderian epithelium. Sinonasal undifferentiated carcinoma lacks rosettes and intercellular fibrils.[14]

Extension of the primary tumor based on the Kadish staging system[147] has been identified as the most important determinant of treatment outcome, although this was not confirmed by Chao et al.[150] High-grade tumors had worse outcome in the reports from the Mayo Clinic and the University of California–Los Angeles (UCLA).[151]

Argiris et al.[152] found that in 16 patients with ENB, 11 of whom had Kadish stage C, 8 (50%) had brain involvement at presentation. Craniofacial resection was performed in 13 patients (81%); 14 received either preoperative or postoperative therapy (radiation therapy in 11 and chemotherapy in 4). The actuarial 5-year survival was 60%, disease-free survival 33%, with a median follow-up of 4.3 years. The first site of failure was locoregional alone in 10 of 12 patients who progressed, and in 6 patients involved the brain or the meninges. Two patients were successfully salvaged.

Hyams[83] proposed a histologic grading system for ENB in which grade I tumors have an excellent prognosis and grade IV tumors are uniformly fatal. The Hyams grading system predated advanced craniofacial techniques, extensive use of immunohistochemistry, and the recognition of sinonasal undifferentiated carcinoma (SNUC) as a distinct entity. Miyamoto et al.,[153] in a retrospective review of 12 patients with ENB and

14 with SNUC, used the Kadish clinical stage and Hyams histopathologic system. Kadish staging was available for 26 patients (2 patients with stage A tumors; 7 with stage B, and 17 with stage C). Of the eight evaluable patients with Kadish stage A or B tumors, six remained disease free for more than 2 years compared with only five of seven Kadish stage C tumors. Slides were available for Hyams grading in 21 patients (2 patients with grade I tumors, 4 with grade II, 4 with grade III, and 11 with grade IV). They concluded that both the Hyams grading and the Kadish staging system can be used as independent predictors of outcome; patients with either advanced clinical stage or pathologic grade of ENB or SNUC have poor prognosis, but long-term survival is possible in these patients if aggressive treatment is used.

Papadaki et al.[154] analyzed 18 formalin-fixed paraffin-embedded olfactory neuroblastoma specimens (12 primary tumors and 6 recurrences or metastases) from 14 patients and concluded that p53 point mutation does not play an important role in the initial development of olfactory neuroblastoma; however, p53 wild-type hyperexpression may occur in subsets, show local aggressive behavior, and have a tendency for recurrence.

General Management

Surgery alone appears to be adequate treatment for small, low-grade tumors confined to the ethmoids in which negative surgical margins can be obtained. An ethmoidomaxillary resection with or without orbital sparing is usually necessary. This procedure is combined with preoperative or postoperative irradiation.[151,155] A complete resection with preservation of vital structures is achievable by using a craniofacial approach.

Treatment, which could be classified in 898 reported cases in 1997, consisted of surgery alone in 24% (226 cases), radiation therapy alone in 18.4% (165 cases), combined surgery and radiation therapy in 43.2% (388 cases), chemotherapy in 13.2% (119 cases), and in 11 cases (1.2%) bone marrow transplant. In the reported cases follow-up could be evaluated in 477 cases, while in only 234 cases a 5-year follow-up was done; on these 20.5% had surgery only, 11.1% radiation therapy, and 68.4% combined surgery and radiation therapy. The best survival rates were obtained by combined therapy, 72.5% versus 62.5% with surgery alone and 53.8% with radiation therapy.[31]

Dias et al.[156] reported on 35 patients with ENB treated with gross tumor resection through a transfacial approach with postoperative RT in 11 patients, craniofacial resection and postoperative RT in 7, exclusive RT in 14, craniofacial resection alone in 1, and a combination of chemotherapy and RT in 2 patients. Radiation therapy median dose was 48 Gy. Craniofacial resection plus postoperative RT provided a better 5-year disease-free survival rate (86%) compared with the other therapies ($P = .05$). The 5-year disease-specific survival rate was 64% and 43% for the low- and high-grade tumors, respectively ($P = .20$). At 5 and 10 years disease-free survival was 46% and 24%, respectively and overall survival was 55% and 46%, respectively.

Early lesions involving the ethmoids with little or no bony destruction or nerve invasion can be treated adequately by high-energy (photon or electron) radiation therapy with good cosmetic and functional results.[81,103,157] Those with more extensive local disease benefit from surgery and adjuvant irradiation,[156,158] although some have advocated against combined surgery and radiation therapy because of complications. Patients with locally advanced disease or high-grade tumors should receive aggressive treatment with combined modalities, such as surgery, radiation therapy, and chemotherapy.

Monroe et al.[78] described treatment results in 22 patients who received RT for ENB (equal numbers of males and females, median age of 54 years). The modified Kadish stage was stage A in 1 patient, stage B in 4 patients, stage C in 15 patients, and stage D in 2 patients. Treatment modalities included primary RT in 6 patients, preoperative RT in 1 patient, postoperative RT after craniofacial resection in 12 patients, and salvage RT in 3 patients treated for recurrence after surgery. Elective neck RT was performed in 11 of 20 patients (2 patients had cervical metastases at presentation for RT). Rates of local tumor control, cause-specific survival, and absolute survival at 5 years were 59%, 54%, and 48%, respectively. The cause-specific survival rate at 5 years was lower after primary RT (17%) than after craniofacial resection and postoperative RT (56%). Cervical metastases occurred in 6 of 22 patients (27%). No neck recurrences occurred in 11 patients treated with elective neck RT compared with four neck recurrences in 9 patients (44%) not receiving elective neck RT ($P = .02$). Their data and review of the current literature suggest a higher cervical failure rate than previously recognized; elective neck RT seems to correlate with improved nodal tumor control and should be considered in the treatment of ENB.

Rosenthal et al.[155] treated 72 adults with nonmetastatic, primary sinonasal neuroendocrine tumors (31 with ENB, 16 with SNUC, 18 with neuroendocrine carcinoma [NEC], and 7 with small cell carcinoma [SmCC]). Patients with ENB usually were treated with surgery and/or radiotherapy; only 3 of 31 patients (9.7%) received radiation to regional lymphatics, and only 5 of 31 received chemotherapy. In contrast, patients with non-ENB histologies usually received chemotherapy (10 of 16 patients with SNUC, 12 of 18 patients with NEC, and 5 of 7 patients with SmCC). With a median follow-up for surviving patients of 81.5 months, overall survival at 5 years was 93.1% for patients with ENB, 62.5% for SNUC, 64.2% for NEC, and 28.6% for SmCC ($P = .0029$). The local control tumor rate at 5 years also was superior for patients who had ENB (96.2%) compared with patients who had SNUC (78.6%), NEC (72.6%), or SmCC (66.7%) ($P = .04$). The regional failure rate at 5 years was 8.7% for patients with ENB, 15.6% for patients with SNUC, 12.9% for patients with NEC, and 44.4% for patients with SmCC. Additional late events increased the regional failure rate for patients with ENB to 31.9% at 10 years. The distant metastasis rate at 5 years was 0.0% for patients with ENB, 25.4% for patients with SNUC, 14.1% for patients with NEC, and 75.0% for patients with SmCC.

Eich et al.[143] described 17 patients with ENB (4 Kadish stage B and 13 stage C), treated with incomplete surgery (2 patients), adjuvant radiation therapy (6 patients), definitive RT (7 patients), and for recurrent tumor (2 patients). Median postoperative dose was 56 Gy (40 to 60 Gy) and definitive 58 Gy (40 to 70 Gy). With a median follow-up of 7 years, 10 of 17 had no evidence of recurrence (5 of 6 treated with complete resection and postoperative RT and 3 of 7 treated with definitive RT).

Gruber et al.[159] described 28 patients with ENB treated with RT (median dose 60 Gy). In 13 patients total tumor resection (recommended by the authors) was performed. Chemotherapy (cisplatin, etoposide, cyclophosphamide, and vincristine) combined with RT were used in five patients. With median follow-up of 68 months, 54% of the patients were free of local tumor progression (51% at 10 years). Disease-free survival at 10 years was 25%.

Ozsahin et al.[160] described results of treatment in 13 European and North American centers for 77 patients with olfactory neuroblastoma, 11 with Kadish stage A, 29 with stage B, and 37 with stage C; 56 patients had surgery, 44 with total tumor excision. All but 5 patients received radiation therapy (50% with 3D-CRT) and 21 had chemotherapy. With median follow-up of 72 months locoregional tumor control was 62%, disease-free survival 57%, and overall survival 64%. Patients having total tumor resection or receiving ≥54 Gy had better overall survival than those treated with lower doses (Fig. 48.11). Six of the patients treated with RT (56 to 70 Gy) developed grade 3 or4 late complications (five osteonecrosis and one retinopathy).

Sperry et al.[161] treated 30 patients with ENB (70% with Kadish stage C) with surgery in 27 (52% craniofacial resection),

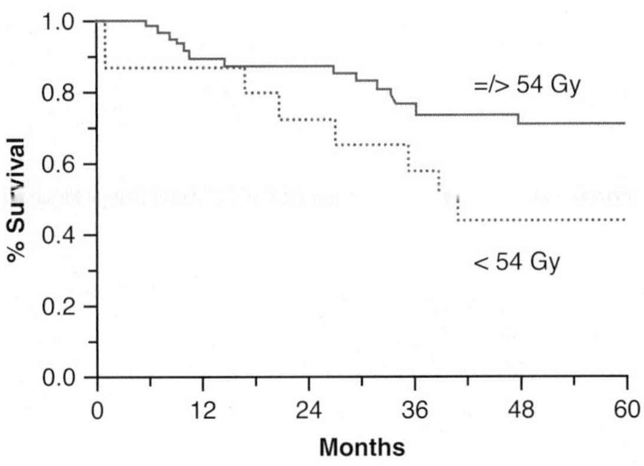

Patients at risk

RT ≥54 Gy	57	49	44	32	28	27
RT <54 Gy	15	13	11	9	7	6

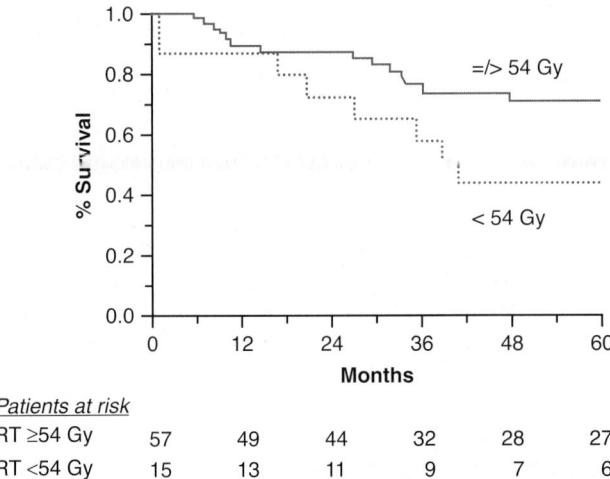

FIGURE 48.11. Overall survival correlated with radiation therapy dose in 72 patients with olfactory neuroblastoma. (From Ozsahin M, Gruber G, Olszik O, et al. Outcome and prognostic factors in olfactory neuroblastoma: a rare cancer network study. *Int J Radiat Oncol Biol Phys* 2010;78:993–997, with permission.)

combined with postoperative RT in 75.9% and chemoradiation in 23%. Local tumor failure at 5 years was 43.6% and regional failure 15.7%. The 5-year disease-free survival was 40.7% and overall survival 80%.

Madani et al.[162] published a report on 84 patients (73 with primary and 11 with local recurrent) sinonasal tumors, 9 of which were ENB, treated with IMRT (median dose 70 Gy in 35 fractions). Mean D50 to the optic chiasm was 37.2 Gy, to ipsilateral optic nerve 49.4 Gy, to contralateral optic nerve 47.1 Gy, and to the retina 37.7 and 28.4 Gy, respectively.

Protons have been used sparingly in the treatment of some of these patients. Nishimura et al.[163] reported on 14 patients with olfactory neuroblastoma treated with proton beam (65 CGE in 2.5-GyE fractions) in 6 patients combined with surgery, sometimes combined with chemotherapy.[164] With median follow-up of 40 months, 5-year local progression-free survival was 84%, disease-free survival 71%, and overall survival 93%.

For advanced lesions, in which disseminated disease is likely, chemotherapy may improve tumor control and decrease the incidence of distant metastases. A combination of thiotepa, cyclophosphamide, doxorubicin, vincristine, nitrogen mustard, and actinomycin-D has been used.[165,166] A retrospective review of 10 patients with recurrent esthesioneuroblastoma treated with chemotherapy at the Mayo Clinic suggested that cisplatin-based chemotherapy is active in advanced, high-grade tumors.[155] Survival from initial chemotherapy treatment was 44.5 months (range 3 to 130 months) in patients with low-grade tumors and 26.5 months (range 2 to 67 months) in patients with high-grade tumors (Table 48.10).

Elective Neck Treatment

ENB has been shown to metastasize to the neck and remote sites. Although the sites of metastases are widely variable and often atypical, Beitler et al.[167] found cervical node metastasis to be as frequent as local recurrence. Davis and Weissler[62] compiled a retrospective review of patients and found that the cumulative cervical metastasis rate reached 27% (55 of 207 patients). Noh et al.,[168] in a report of 19 patients with ENB treated with combinations of surgery, RT, and/or chemotherapy, noted that 4 patients with high risk factors received elective neck RT (45 to 70 Gy). There were no cervical node failures in 5 patients with Kadish stages A and B, 3 of 10 in patients with Kadish stage C treated surgically, and 0 in 9 receiving chemotherapy.

In general, because of the low incidence of cervical lymph node metastasis (≤10%) in early-stage disease, elective irradiation of the neck or a dissection is not indicated. However, in patients with Kadish stage C disease, the cervical metastatic rate climbed to 44% (25 of 57 patients). As noted previously, Monroe et al.[78] observed cervical node metastasis in 6 of 22 patients (27%). In 11 patients they treated with elective neck RT, no recurrences were noted, in contrast to 4 of 9 (44%) for patients not receiving elective neck RT. Thus, with advanced-stage disease, cervical nodes should be initially managed by irradiation, radical neck dissection, or a combination of both.[169]

Radiation Therapy Techniques

A combination of photons and electrons with conventional anterior fields provides good coverage for limited ethmoidal disease when the tumor is confined anteriorly. Beam arrangement can be modified for disease extending into the orbit or maxillary sinus. Obturator or bolus may be needed postoperatively to compensate for tissue deficit. When intracranial or posterior extension is present or tumor has spread into the maxillary sinus, a pair of perpendicular (anteroposterior and lateral) portals with wedges or two lateral wedge fields in conjunction with an open anterior photon field will give good coverage of the treatment volume, with the dose inhomogeneity around 10% to 20%. Incorporation of a vertex field eliminates the high inhomogeneous dose along the junction line of the conventional three-field technique. Treatment techniques are similar to those described for treatment of paranasal sinuses (see Chapter 42). The orbits can be spared or treated as the degree of extension dictates. Occasionally, an anterior electron beam field may be needed to supplement low-dose areas. When the electron beam is used over air cavities, some dosimetry problems result. Eye blocks must be positioned precisely to avoid undesirable side effects.

When combined therapy is used, preoperative doses of 45 Gy and postoperative doses of 50 to 60 Gy are indicated, depending on the status of the surgical margins. Doses of 65 to 70 Gy are delivered with irradiation alone in patients with inoperable tumors.[170] Usual fraction dose is 1.8 to 2.0 Gy. Contrast-enhanced CT or MRI scans before initiation of treatment are crucial to demarcate extension of the tumor. Treatment planning with CT for determination of tumor extension is extremely important.[171] Because of the proximity of esthesioneuroblastoma to the optic nerves, optic chasm, and the brainstem, the precision of treatment setup, target volume definition, and dose homogeneity dictate tumor control and the sequelae of treatment. Treatment techniques similar to those for paranasal sinuses may create "hot spots" along the optic

TABLE 48.10 RESULTS OF TREATMENT CORRELATED WITH MODALITY AND STAGE FOR ESTHESIONEUROBLASTOMA

	Stage A			*Stage B*			*Stage C*		
Modality[a]	*Initial Treatment*	*For Recurrence*	*Total Control Rate (%)*	*Initial Treatment*	*For Recurrence*	*Total Control Rate (%)*	*Initial Treatment*	*For Recurrence*	*Total Control Rate (%)*
Radiation therapy alone	2/5	5/5	70	4/7	3/4	64	1/5	1/1	33
Surgery alone	5/9	4/4	69	3/6	1/2	50	1/1	–	–
Radiation therapy and surgery	7/10	–	70	12/30	0/1	57	7/15	–	47

[a]All results reflect treatment of 78 patients, who were observed for 6 months to 32 years.

From Elkon D, Hightower SI, Lim ML, et al. Esthesioneuroblastoma. *Cancer* 1979;44:1087–1094, with permission.

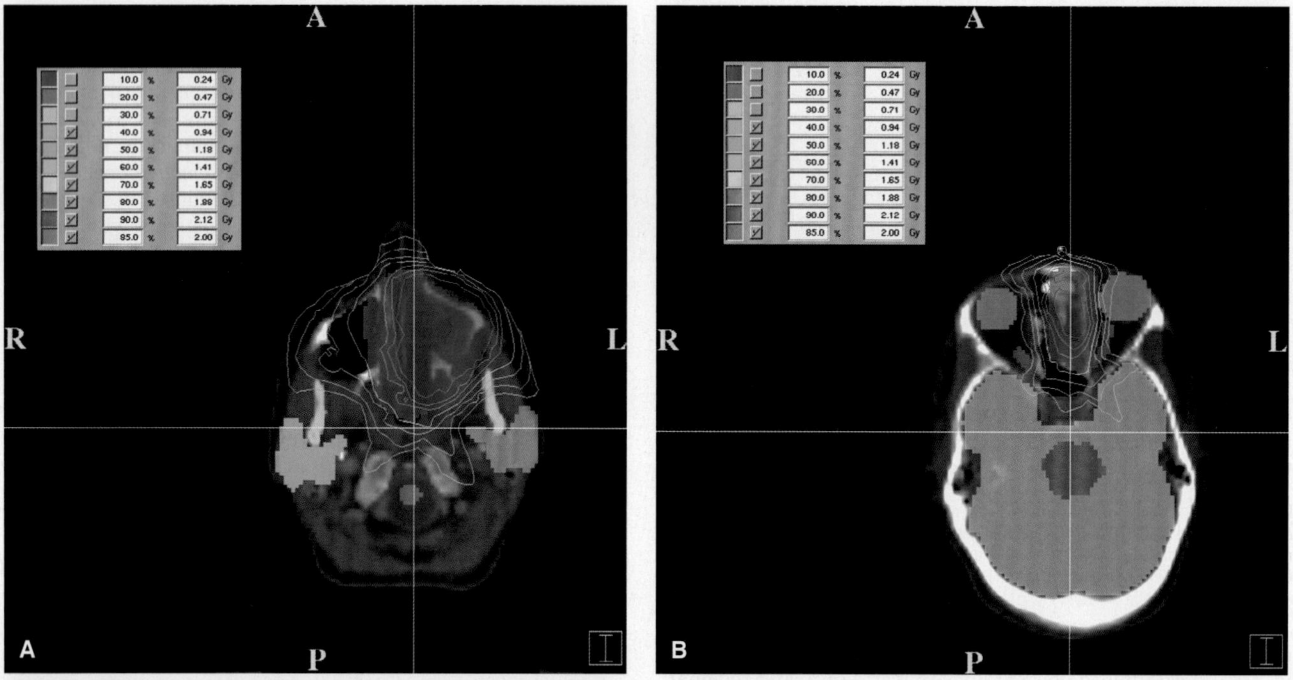

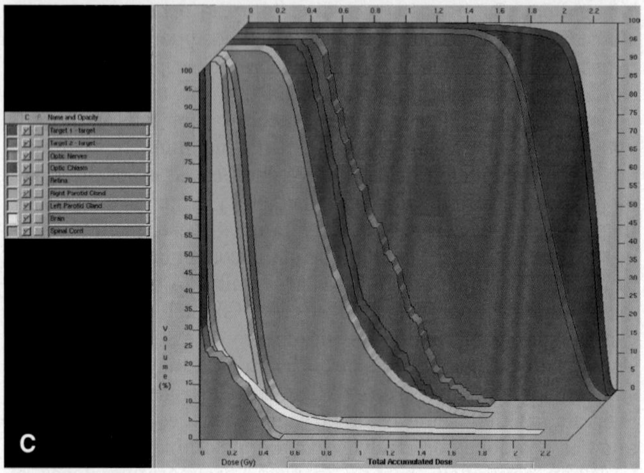

FIGURE 48.12. Esthesioneuroblastoma in a 35-year-old woman, initially treated with a craniofacial surgical resection. Patient received postoperative intensity-modulated radiation therapy (2-Gy fractions). **A:** Cross-section illustrating coverage of ethmoid nasal and left maxillary antrum volume. **B:** Cross-section showing dose distribution in target volume with excellent sparing of ocular structures. **C:** Dose–volume histogram:

Structure	*Dose Range (cGy)*	*Mean Dose (Gy)*
Planning target volume 1	30–70	65
Planning target volume 2	40–70	58
Optic chasm and nerves	13–42	24

tracks. High doses per fraction (exceeding 2 Gy) increase the possibility of late sequelae, such as blindness and bone and brain necrosis.

Three-dimension CRT or IMRT provides alternatives to the conventional three-field technique used to treat these tumors (Fig. 48.12). Special attention should be directed to reduce unnecessary irradiation to ocular structures, including optic nerve(s) and chiasma. When occasionally a patient presents with cervical node metastasis, IMRT is very helpful to optimally treat the primary tumor and the cervical lymphatics (Fig. 48.13).

Results of Therapy

Surgery and Irradiation

Platek et al.,[172] in an analysis of SEER data (1973–2005) of 135 cases of olfactory neuroblastoma, noted that 59% of the patients were treated with surgery and RT, 23% with surgery only, 12% with RT only, and 6% with neither. No data on chemotherapy administration were available. The 5-year survival with surgery plus RT was 66%, with surgery only 51%, with RT only 26%, and with other therapy 34% ($P = .003$).

Kased et al.[170] reported on 17 patients with ENB (15 undergoing a surgical procedure, 7 receiving concurrent chemotherapy, and 4 adjuvant chemotherapy) treated with IMRT (median dose 66 Gy in 2-Gy fractions). With median follow-up of 44.5 months, the 5-year freedom of locoregional tumor progression was 91%, progression-free survival 83%, and overall survival 81%. Four patients had acute complications (meningitis, sepsis, sinusitis requiring surgery, and brain abscess) and two patients developed late brain abscess, requiring surgical treatment.

Radiation therapy is an important component in the management of ENB, but the optimal sequence when integrated with surgery is unknown. Eden et al.[144] observed no significant difference in survival whether preoperative or postoperative irradiation was given, but suggested improved local tumor control with preoperative irradiation. Technical factors may have contributed to a higher incidence of postoperative radiation therapy failures because three of five postoperative cases received <50 Gy; all three patients were treated with a single anterior field, which gives less homogeneous dose distribution throughout the treatment volume.

Foote et al.[151] updated the experience of the Mayo Clinic. Seventeen patients had disease confined to nasal cavity or paranasal sinuses (Kadish stages A and B), and 32 patients had more advanced disease. Treatment included gross total resection alone or combined with radiation therapy. The 5-year actuarial survival, disease-free survival, and local tumor control rates were 69.1%, 54.8%, and 65.3%, respectively. Local tumor

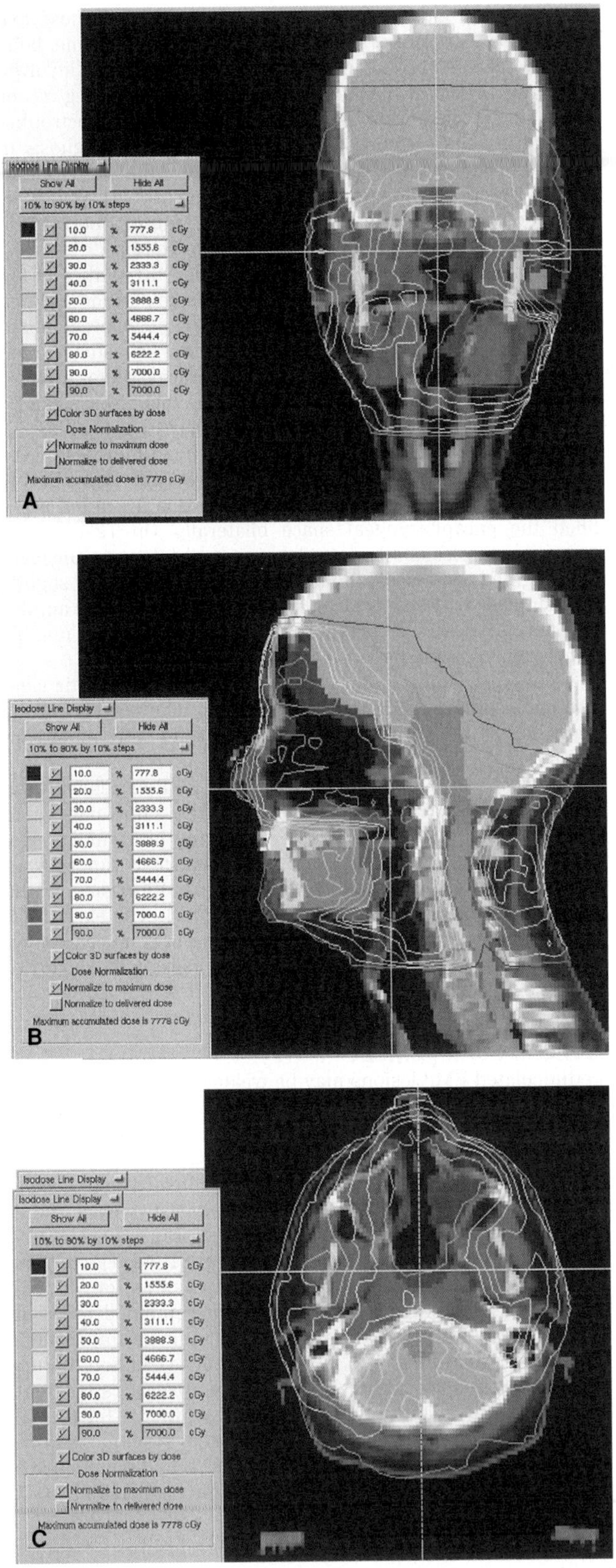

FIGURE 48.13. Patient with Kadish stage C esthesioneuroblastoma of ethmoid cells and nasal cavity who presented with a large left upper cervical lymph node metastasis. Intensity-modulated radiation therapy plans to deliver 70 Gy to primary tumor and cervical lymphadenopathy. **(A)** Coronal, **(B)**, sagittal, and **(C)** cross-section dose distributions illustrate excellent coverage of all target volumes.

control was improved in patients who received postoperative irradiation (55.5 Gy) even after complete tumor resection.

Levine et al.[173] conducted a retrospective review of 35 patients; 6% of them presented with cervical metastasis, and ultimately 25.7% developed cervical metastases. Fourteen percent of the patients had a local recurrence at an average of 6 years after diagnosis, and in 37% at least one episode of metastatic disease occurred. The disease-free survival was 80.4% at 8 years. CNS complications occurred in 25.7% of patients, orbital complications in 22.9%, systemic posttreatment problems in 20%, and chemotoxic sequelae in 18%.

Eriksen et al.[174] carried out a retrospective review of 13 patients with ENB (Kadish stage A 1 patient, stage B 5 patients, and stage C 7 patients). The 5-year disease-free survival was 51%. Forty-six percent of the patients experienced relapse, and despite intensive salvage therapy, median survival after recurrence was only 12 months.

Chao et al.[150] reported on 25 patients with ENB (Kadish stage A in 3 patients, stage B in 13 patients, C in 8 patients, and modified D in 1 cervical nodal metastasis patient); 17 patients were treated with surgery and radiation therapy, 6 with irradiation alone, and 2 with surgery only. Eight patients received neoadjuvant chemotherapy. Median follow-up was 8 years. The 5-year actuarial overall survival, disease-free survival, and local tumor control rates were 66.3%, 56.3%, and 73%, respectively. Kadish stage was not a significant prognosticator for local control or disease-free survival. Five-year local tumor control was 87.4% for combined surgery with RT and 51.2% for irradiation alone. Two patients with Kadish stages A and B disease underwent surgical resection alone; both failed locally. In contrast, only three of nine patients with Kadish stage A or B disease who received adjuvant radiation therapy had a local recurrence. With adjuvant radiation therapy, the surgical margin status did not influence local tumor control.

Simon et al.[171] reported on 13 patients with ENB or olfactory neuroblastoma (Kadish stage B 5 patients, and stage C 8 patients). The majority of the patients were treated with a craniofacial resection or tumor removal through a rhinotomy approach. Two patients received neoadjuvant chemotherapy before surgical resection (cisplatin, ifosfamide, and etoposide). Twelve of the 13 patients received RT either initially or for salvage. Median dose of postoperative irradiation was 59.4 Gy in 1.8-Gy fractions. The overall actuarial 5-year survival was 61% and 10-year survival 24%, and disease-free survival rates were 56% and 42%, respectively.

Chemotherapy and Irradiation

Eden et al.[144] described results in 16 patients with stage A or B disease and 24 patients with stage C disease treated with irradiation (median dose 50 Gy) and surgery for stages A and B disease, with the addition of chemotherapy (cyclophosphamide and vincristine) for stage C disease. Actuarial survival rates at 5 and 10 years were 78% and 71%, respectively. Locoregional failure developed in 15 of 40 patients; 68% of the failures were locoregional (including brain, neck, facial bone, and sinus). They had no recurrences at the primary tumor bed; all recurrences were either outside the irradiation field or at distant sites.

Preoperative neoadjuvant therapy may provide a valuable complement to radical craniofacial resection.[165]

Forty patients were treated for ENB at Institut Gustave Roussy, France.[146] Three patients had stage T1, 7 patients had T2, 15 patients had T3, and 15 patients had T4 lesions. At presentation the cervical metastatic rate was 18% and distant metastases were detected by bone marrow biopsy and bone scan in three patients. Treatment modalities included surgery alone in 8 patients, radiation therapy alone in 3 patients, surgery plus radiation therapy in 11 patients, chemotherapy alone in 2 patients, chemotherapy plus radiation therapy in 10 patients, and chemotherapy plus surgery and radiation therapy in 6 patients. The 5-year survival rate was 51%. Multimodality treatment offered better survival (63% at 5 years). Overall local, regional, and distant failure rates were 58%, 15%, and 40%, respectively. Distant metastases commonly occurred in bone (82%).

Noh et al.[168] summarized reports on patterns of failure of ENB treated with or without chemotherapy. Although the indications for high-dose chemotherapy and bone marrow transplantation must be better defined, it may be a promising alternative for patients with large tumors or those with recurrent tumor to whom no further local therapy (e.g., surgery or irradiation) can be safely given.[175]

Sequelae of Treatment

In a few patients, depending on the dose of irradiation, long-term sequelae include bone necrosis, brain necrosis or abscess, blindness, or painful eye reactions requiring enucleation.[176,177,178]

Simon et al.,[171] in 13 patients with olfactory ENB treated with surgery and radiation therapy, noted that one patient lost vision as a result of glaucoma and radiation retinopathy after 67.3 Gy in 34 fractions. One patient treated with 61.76 Gy in 34 fractions developed a visual field defect and optic atrophy; she also had a nasal cutaneous fistula. One patient sustained intraoperative rupture of the ocular globe and subconjunctival hemorrhage.

EXTRAMEDULLARY PLASMACYTOMAS

Solitary plasmacytomas are rare tumors of plasma cell origin, making up 4% of all plasma cell tumors. Multiple myeloma occurs about 40 times more frequently than solitary plasmacytoma. Monoclonal extramedullary plasmacytoma (EMP) is a rare, low-grade lymphoma found predominantly in the head and neck region. Only since the introduction of immunophenotyping techniques two decades ago has it been possible to differentiate EMP from benign polyclonal plasma cell proliferation. Hotz et al.[179] reviewed the records of 24 patients with morphologically diagnosed EMP treated at their institution; only 14 patients had true monoclonal plasmacytoma. No EMP-related deaths occurred. Two patients had local recurrence, and two patients developed multiple myeloma. Diagnostic procedures exclude a benign polyclonal plasmacytoma, multiple myeloma, and solitary bone plasmacytoma. The slow natural progression of the disease and the rarity of secondary multiple myeloma favor nonmutilating local surgery whenever possible to avoid the long-term sequelae of radiation.

Epidemiology

The annual incidence of EMP is 0.04 cases per 100,000 population.[180] They constitute only 0.5% of all upper respiratory tract malignancies. Male patients exceed female patients by a ratio of 4 to 1, and 75% of patients are 40 to 60 years of age.[181]

In a detailed literature search of more than 400 publications between 1905 and 1997, EMP mainly occurred between the fourth and seventh decades of life.[182] Seven hundred fourteen cases (82.2%) were found in the upper aerodigestive tract.

The most common sites in the head and neck are the nasopharynx, nasal cavity, paranasal sinuses, and tonsils.

Clinical Presentation and Diagnostic Workup

EMP of the head and neck area should be considered a separate entity because of its clinical behavior. The most common symptoms are nasal obstruction, local pain and swelling, and epistaxis.

Grossly, plasmacytomas tend to be sessile in the nasal cavity and paranasal sinuses and pedunculated in the nasopharynx and larynx. The masses are soft, pliable, and pale gray. The lesion may remain localized or may infiltrate and destroy the surrounding soft tissue and bone. The usual criteria for solitary plasmacytomas, either medullary or extramedullary, include a biopsy-proven plasma cell tumor with one or, at the most, two solitary foci, absence of Bence-Jones protein in the urine, bone marrow taken some distance from the primary site not involved by tumor (<10% of plasma cells), hemoglobin of 13 g/mL or more, and a normal serum protein level or serum electrophoresis at the time of the diagnosis. Basically, the diagnosis of solitary plasmacytoma is made by exclusion, that is, by eliminating the possibility of multiple myeloma.[183] Diagnosis is based on histology along with special immunoperoxidase staining for immunoglobulin -λ and -κ light chains.[29]

Strict staging criteria, including normal MRI studies of the axial skeleton and the long bones and absence of monoclonal plasma cells detected by flow cytometry or polymerase chain reaction, are required for diagnosis of solitary plasmacytoma. Careful microscopic and immunohistochemical studies are also required for the correct diagnosis, because this disease can be confused with other malignancies, particularly lymphomas.

Six patients with primary EMP in the head and neck were examined with MRI;[184] five lesions were oval and sharply demarcated without signs of infiltration, while the other lesion filled the parapharyngeal space bilaterally. On T2-weighted sequence, the lesions had moderate signal intensity. On plain T1-weighted sequences, the tumors were isointense or slightly hyperintense with respect to surrounding muscles; after administration of contrast medium, four lesions showed notable enhancement, with distinct central inhomogeneity.

Bone destruction is not a particularly bad prognostic sign, although some investigators report that it adversely affects prognosis.[184] Bony invasion is common in the more malignant types.[14]

Cervical lymph node metastasis from EMP varies with the site of the primary lesion and follows the same pattern of spread as squamous cell carcinoma arising in a similar site. The reported incidence of lymph node metastasis ranges from 12% to 26%. The diagnostic workup for EMP arising in the head and neck region is shown in Table 48.1. The exact relationship between EMP and multiple myeloma is unclear; however, approximately 20% to 30% of EMP cases will convert to multiple myeloma.[179,183]

General Management

Pedunculated EMP lesions may be treated by surgical excision because the chance of local recurrence is low. The treatment of choice for all other lesions is radiation therapy alone or combined with other modalities.[185,186] In a review of 714 cases in the literature, the following therapeutic strategies were used to treat patients with EMP of the upper aerodigestive tract: radiation therapy alone in 44.3%, combined therapy (surgery and irradiation) in 26.9%, and surgery alone in 21.9%. The median overall survival or recurrence-free survival was longer than 300 months for patients who underwent combined intervention (surgery and irradiation), for surgical intervention alone (median survival time, 156 months), and for radiation therapy alone (median survival time, 114 months). Overall, after treatment for EMP in the upper aerodigestive tract, 61.1% of all patients had no recurrence or conversion to systemic involvement (i.e., multiple myeloma); however, 22% had recurrence of EMP, and 16.1% had conversion to multiple myeloma.

Radiation Therapy Techniques

Irradiation techniques vary with the location of the primary tumor. The techniques are similar to those used for primary tumors in comparable locations (i.e., nasopharynx, tonsil, paranasal sinuses). Solitary plasmacytomas respond well to doses of 50 to 60 Gy in 2-Gy fractions. The local tumor control rate with radiation therapy alone is about 85%. Harwood et al.[186] summarized the literature but could not draw a dose–response curve from the data because of a lack of cases receiving low-dose radiation therapy. Nevertheless, there is a high

TABLE 48.11 FAILURE PATTERNS OF ESTHESIONEUROBLASTOMA: LITERATURE REVIEW

	Early Stages (Kadish A–B)						*Late Stages (Kadish C–D)*					
	Chemotherapy No			*Chemotherapy Yes*			*Chemotherapy No*			*Chemotherapy Yes*		
Author (Reference)	*Local*	*Regional*	*Distant*	*Local*	*Regional*	*Distant*	*Local*	*Regional*	*Distant*	*Local*	*Regional*	*Distant*
Kadish et al. (147)	2/5	0/5	0/5	–	–	–	3/4	1/4	0/4	–	–	–
Elkon et al. (187)	9/42	6/42	4/42	–	–	–	9/18	2/18	2/18	–	–	–
Dulquerov (188)	1/11	1/11	1/11	–	–	–	1/4	1/4	1/4	0/1	0/1	0/1
Zappia et al. (189)	1/6	1/6	0/6	–	–	–	1/6	1/6	0/6	1/2	0/2	0/2
Eich et al. (143)	0/4	0/4	0/4	–	–	–	0/12	2/12	3/12	0/1	0/1	0/1
Eich et al. (190)	NA	1/8	0/8	NA	0/3	0/3	NA	1/13	1/13	NA	1/16	1/16
Kim et al. (191)	–	–	–	–	–	–	1/6	2/6	0/6	0/8	1/8	2/8
Noh et al. (168)	–	–	–	0/2	0/2	0/2	0/3	3/3	0/3	1/7	0/7	2/7
Total	13/68	9/76	5/76	15/53	13/66	7/66	2/19	2/35	5/35			
Percent	19	12	6.6	28	19.7	10.6	10.5	6	14.3			

NA, not available.

Modified from Noh OK, Lee S-W, Yoon SM, et al. Radiotherapy for esthesioneuroblastoma: is elective nodal irradiation warranted in the multimodality treatment approach? *Int J Radiat Oncol Biol Phys* 2011;79:443–449.

risk of local recurrence with tumor doses below 30 Gy and a negligible risk for those treated at or above 40 Gy (Table 48.11).

Wax et al.[29] reported on seven patients, three treated with radiation therapy (31.75 to 60 Gy). All patients have maintained local tumor control and had been followed for a minimum of 1.5 years, with an average of 3 years. One patient, treated with surgical excision, experienced a relapse at a distant site 6 years later.

The response to therapy of 32 patients with localized plasmacytoma were described by Shih et al.;[192] 22 patients had solitary plasmacytoma of bone and 10 had EMP. Median age for EMP was 63 years. Most EMPs occurred in the oronasopharynx (six cases) and paranasal sinuses (two cases). Seven patients with EMP received radiation therapy (47 to 65 Gy), and all achieved initial local tumor control. There was one local recurrence and multiple myeloma conversion in the EMP group. Local recurrence or dissemination was associated with the appearance of or an increase in myeloma protein.

Holland et al.[193] reported on 14 cases of EMP, eight of which were in the head and neck. With doses of 46 to 62 Gy, the complete tumor response was 72%. No dose–response effect was observed.

Liebross et al.[194] described results in 22 patients with solitary EMP, in the head or neck in 19 patients, usually in the nasal cavity or maxillary sinuses, and bone destruction was found in 10 of 11 patients. Among all patients, serum myeloma protein was present in three patients (14%) and Bence-Jones protein alone in two (9%). Radiation therapy was the sole treatment in 18 of 22 patients (median dose 50 Gy; range 40 to 60 Gy); 5 of 7 patients with an EMP of oral cavity, oropharynx, nasopharynx, parotid, or larynx also received elective neck irradiation. Local tumor control was achieved in 21 of 22 patients (95%), and disease never recurred in regional nodes. Disappearance of myeloma protein occurred in three of five patients with an evaluable abnormality. Multiple myeloma developed in seven patients (32%), all within 5 years. The 5-year rate of freedom from progression to multiple myeloma was 56% and the median survival was 9.5 years. Chao et al.[150] reported on 16 patients with EMP and a median follow-up of 66 months. The head and neck region accounted for the majority of presentations (88%). A serum monoclonal paraprotein was found in three patients, and bone erosion was identified in seven patients. All patients received local RT, although two patients also received elective nodal irradiation. The median RT dose was 45 Gy (range 40 to 50.4 Gy). Local tumor control was achieved in all patients (100%), however, regional recurrence outside the RT fields occurred in 2 of 16. Multiple myeloma developed in five patients (31%) all within 5 years. The 10-year myeloma-free survival is 75% and 10-year overall survival is 54%.

Galieni et al.[195] reviewed 46 cases of EMP most frequently localized in the upper airways (37 of 46 patients, 80%), with the mass being limited to a single site in all but seven patients in whom two contiguous sites were involved. The most frequent form of treatment was local radiation therapy. Thirty-nine patients (85%) achieved complete remission, five (11%) a partial remission, and two (4%) did not respond to therapy. Local recurrence or recurrence at other sites occurred in 7.5% and 10%, respectively. Seven patients (15%) developed multiple myeloma. The 15-year survival rate was 78%.

Michalski et al.[180] described 10 patients with EMP treated with radiotherapy. One patient treated at relapse underwent surgical resection followed by postoperative RT. The disease was most frequently localized in the paranasal sinuses (50%). All nine patients who received definitive RT (40 to 50 Gy) achieved a complete response. Median follow-up period was 29 months. Four patients (40%) relapsed, three have died of their disease. Two patients with paranasal sinus disease subsequently relapsed with multiple myeloma at 10 months and 24 months, respectively. The relapse rate in neck nodes of 10% does not justify elective irradiation of the uninvolved neck.

Miller et al.[196] reported that tumor arose in the sinonasal or nasopharyngeal region in 11 of 20 patients (55%). The primary modality of treatment was radiation therapy (45 to 60 Gy). The mean follow-up was 60.2 months. In 15 to 20 cases, immunohistochemistry staining for immunoglobulin light chain production was conducted. One of the two cases (50%) classified as medullary plasmacytoma demonstrated conversion to multiple myeloma, whereas only 2 of 18 cases of EMP (11%) converted to multiple myeloma.

Ozsahin et al.[177] published a compilation of solitary plasmacytoma (42 cases) in the head and neck. There were 258 patients with bone (n = 206) or extramedullary (n = 52) plasmacytomas without evidence of multiple myeloma. Most (n = 214) of the patients received RT alone; 34 received chemotherapy and RT; and 8 had surgery alone. The median radiation dose was 40 Gy. Median follow-up was 56 months (range 7 to 245 months). The median time for multiple myeloma development was 21 moths (range 2 to 135 months), with a 5-year survival probability of 45% (Fig. 48.14A). The 5-year overall survival, disease-free survival, and local control rates were 74%, 50%, and 86% respectively (Fig. 48.14B). On multivariate analyses, favorable factors were younger age and tumor size <4 cm for survival; age, extramedullary localization, and RT for disease-free survival; and small tumor and RT for local control. Bone localization was the only predictor of multiple myeloma development. No dose–response relationship was found for doses >30 Gy, even for larger tumors.

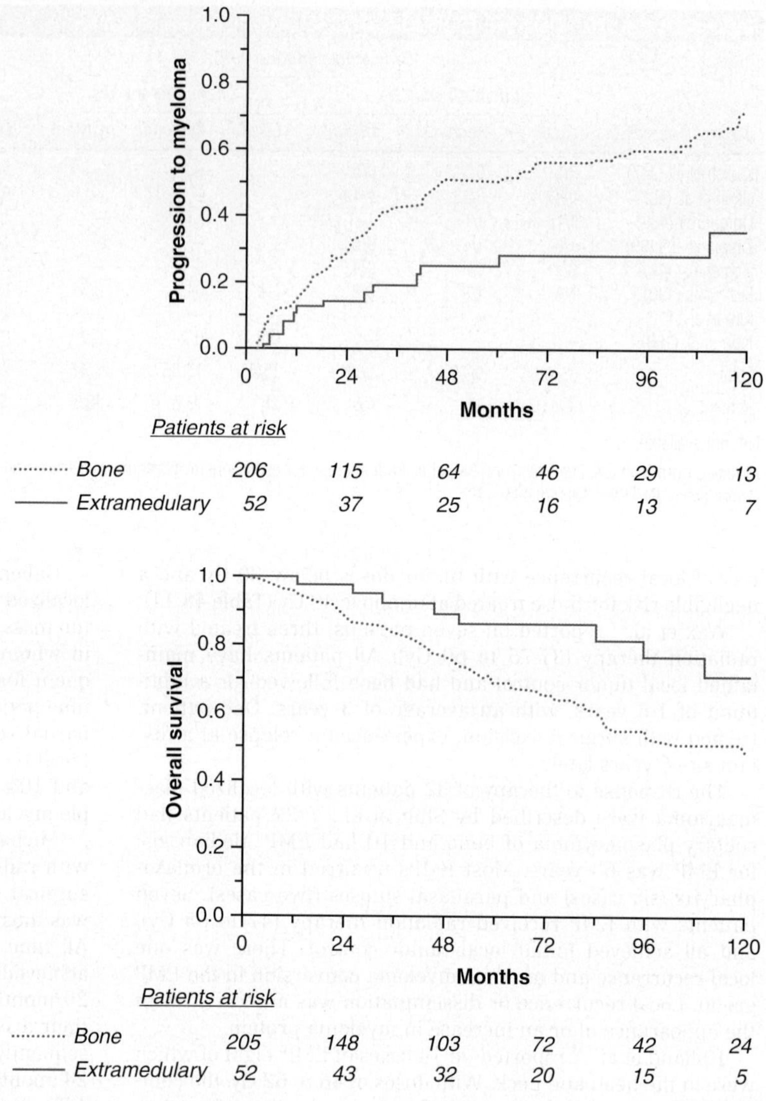

FIGURE 48.14. A: Probability of progression to multiple myeloma according to bone (*dotted line*) or extramedullary (*solid line*) solitary plasmacytoma (P = .0009). **B:** Overall survival correlated with bone (*dotted line*) or extramedullary (*solid line*) solitary plasmacytoma (P = .04). (From Ozsakin M, Tsang RW, Poortmans P, et al. Outcomes and patterns of failure in solitary plasmacytoma: a multicenter rare cancer: study of 258 patients. *Int J Radiat Oncol Biol Phys* 2006;64: 210–217, with permission.)

Tournier-Rangeard et al.,[197] in a review of 17 patients with solitary EMP in the head and neck, noted a local tumor control of 100% for patients who received ≥45 Gy dose to the CTV versus 50% with doses <45 Gy (P = .034). Prognostic factor for 5-year disease-specific survival (81.6%) was local tumor control (P = .058). Prognostic factors for disease-free survival (64.1%) were monoclonal immunoglobulin secretion (P = .008) and CTV dose >45 Gy (P = .056).

Bachard et al.[185] published outcomes of 68 patients with EMP of the head and neck, 39 treated with radiation (median dose 35 to 37 Gy in 15 fractions), 14 with surgery plus RT, 8 with surgery, and 3 with chemoradiation. With median follow-up of 8 years, 5-year local recurrence-free survival was 81% and survival 76%. Local recurrence was equivalent in patients treated with surgery or RT (12.5%). Multiple myeloma developed in 23% of the patients. Sasaki et al.[198] described results of radiation therapy in 67 patients with solitary plasmacytoma of the head and neck (in 44 combined with surgery) treated at 23 centers in Japan. Median RT dose was 50 Gy. With 63 months median follow up the 10 year local tumor control was 87% and overall survival 56%. The 10 year survival was 70% for patients treated with combined RT and surgery and 50% in those treared with RT alone (p = 0.004). Twelve patients (18%) developed distant metastasis and 8 (12%) converted to multiple myeloma.

Table 48.12 summarizes the doses of irradiation and probability of tumor control reported by various investigators. The

TABLE 48.12 EXTRAMEDULLARY PLASMACYTOMA OF HEAD AND NECK TREATED BY RADIATION THERAPY

Author (Reference)	*Number of Patients*	*Number of Males/ Number of Females*	*Number <50 Years of Age*	*Local Control*	*Number with Multiple Myeloma*	*Recommended Tumor Dose (Gy)[a]*
Kotner and Wang (199)	16	10/6	12	12/16	4	40–50
Wiltshaw (200)	14	10/4	10	11/14	N/A	–
Woodruff et al. (181)	15	8/7	11	14/15	1	40–50
Bush et al. (201)	10	5/5	5	8/10	2	50–55
Harwood et al. (186)	22	18/4	16	18/22	4	35 for 3 wk
Kapadia et al. (202)	12	9/3	10	11/12	3	–
MD Anderson Cancer Center[b]	15	12/3	12	13/15	4	50
Total	**104**	**72/32**	**76**	**87/104 (83.6)**	**18 (17.3)**	**40–50**

[a]10 Gy/wk unless otherwise stated. [b]Updated, unpublished data of Corwin J.

authors' limited experience confirms the efficacy of tumor doses of 45 to 50 Gy for local tumor control. In patients who had extensive disease, a higher dose (50 to 60 Gy) was used, as recommended by several investigators.[203]

NASOPHARYNGEAL ANGIOFIBROMA

Epidemiology

Juvenile nasopharyngeal angiofibroma (JNPAF) is found more frequently in young pubertal boys;[204] it has been shown to contain androgen receptors[205,206] and occasionally to regress with estrogen therapy. Hwang et al.,[207] in 24 nasopharyngeal angiofibromas, detected androgen receptors in 18 of 24 (75%) cases, whereas only two (8.3%) were positive to progesterone. None of the 24 cases was positive for antibodies to estrogen.

The tumor is believed to originate from the posterolateral wall of the nasal cavity where the sphenoidal process of the palatine bone meets the horizontal ala of the vomer and the roof of the pterygoid process because it is always involved.[208,209] Other investigators agree, because involution of tumor after irradiation usually occurs in this direction.[210]

JNPAF comprises <0.05% of head and neck tumors.[162] Patient age at presentation ranges from 9 to 30 years,[211,212] with a median of 15 years. Females comprise <4% of the total cases.[213] Some investigators have suggested chromosomal studies in affected women because this is mainly a male disease.[209]

Clinical Presentation and Pathology

Symptoms usually occur 2 to 48 months before diagnosis.[211] The most common complaints are nasal obstruction or epistaxis, followed by nasal voice or discharge, cheek swelling, proptosis, diplopia, hearing loss, and headaches.[211] Nasopharyngeal angiofibroma may initially extend into the nasal fossae and maxillary antrum and push the soft palate downward, then through the pterygopalatine fossa and superoanteriorly through the inferior orbital fissure or laterally through the pterygomaxillary fissure to the cheek and temporal regions.[27]

Beham et al.,[214] in a study of 32 cases of JNPAF, noted that most of the tumor vessels, which lacked elastic laminae, were characterized by vascular walls of irregular thickness and variable muscle content. In places, endothelial cells were separated from the stroma by only a single attenuated layer of contractile cells; in some more fibrotic hyaline areas, the stromal cells displayed reactivity for smooth muscle actin. The irregularity of the vascular walls, together with the lack of elastic laminae and stromal fibers, explains the pronounced tendency for hemorrhage in these lesions.

Differential diagnosis includes fibrosarcoma, rhabdomyosarcoma, chronic sinusitis, arteriovenous malformation, lymphangioma, neurofibroma, pleomorphic adenoma, lymphoma, pyogenic granuloma, polyps, and hemangioma.

Diagnostic Workup

After the history and physical examination, CT scans with and without contrast should be obtained. Characteristic findings are a mass in the posterior nasal or pterygopalatine fossa and bone erosion in the sphenopalatine foramen and extension to the pterygoid plate.[44] The pattern of enhancement in this highly vascular tumor is diagnostic,[215,216] and many investigators believe carotid angiograms are unnecessary[217] after CT diagnosis of the lesion, unless embolization, which is also controversial, is contemplated.

CT scans are especially helpful in regions involving thin bony structures (paranasal sinuses, orbits), where CT performs better than MRI. In the nasopharynx and parapharyngeal space, MRI is superior to CT. Obtaining tumor volumetric data with spiral CT or MRI facilitates 3D treatment planning.[218]

Seventy-two patients with JNPAF were evaluated with CT or MRI.[215] Origin of the tumor was in the pterygopalatine fossa at the aperture of the pterygoid (vidian) canal. The tumor extended posteriorly along the pterygoid canal with invasion of the cancellous bone of the pterygoid base and greater wing of the sphenoid in 60% of the patients. The inability to remove the tumor *in toto* was principally due to deep invasion of the sphenoid; 93% of recurrences occurred with this type of tumor extension.

If intracranial extension is noted and radiation therapy is contemplated, no further studies are indicated. If the lesion is extracranial and surgery is indicated, bilateral carotid angiograms will identify the feeding vessels and delineate the boundaries of the tumor.

Biopsies are not indicated in all patients because of the potential for severe hemorrhage. It is important to perform a biopsy of the lesion when the clinical picture (sex, age, location, and behavior of the lesion) is not consistent with JNPAF because some lesions have proven to be sarcomas or chronic sinusitis.[209] Two cases of fibrosarcoma have been reported in patients in their 40s.[219]

Staging and Prognostic Factors

Staging schemes have been proposed by Chandler et al.,[209] a radiographic staging system by Sessions et al.,[210] and a more detailed anatomical system by Radkowski et al.[220] (Tables 48.13 and 48.14). In a retrospective review of 44 cases of JNPAF, invasion of the skull affected two-thirds of the patients, and the rate of recurrence was 27.5%.[221] Extensions to the intratemporal fossa, sphenoid sinus, base of pterygoids and clivus, the cavernous sinus (medial), foramen lacerum, and anterior fossa were correlated with more frequent recurrence. In a review of 97 cases age at diagnosis, tumor size and Radkowski classification were significant prognostic factors for recurrence.[222]

General Management

Optimum management of these patients remains controversial[223] and the decision of whether surgery or radiation therapy should be used depends in part on the initial extent of the disease. In patients with extracranial tumors,[221] surgery is the treatment of choice and yields near-zero mortality or any long-term morbidity.[224] Tumor extension to the posterior infratemporal fossa or intracranially is associated with a higher risk of recurrence.[225]

TABLE 48.13 STUDIES REPORTING TREATMENT OUTCOME AND LATE GRADE 3 VISUAL IMPAIRMENT AFTER INTENSITY-MODULATED RADIATION THERAPY FOR SINONASAL TUMORS

Author (Reference)	Number of Patients	Treatment	Median Dose (Gy)	Follow-Up (Months)	Local Control (Year)	Overall Survival	Grade 3 Visual Morbidity
Claus et al. (226)	32	IMRT+/–S	70	15	NR	80% (1 yr)	0
Duthoy et al. (227)	39	IMRT+S	70	31	68% (4)	59% (4 yr)	2
Combs et al. (41)	46	IMRT+/–S	64	16	81% (2)	90% (2 yr)	0
Hoppe et al. (228)	30	IMRT+S	60	23	NR	NR	0
Daly et al. (229)	36	IMRT+/–S	70	39	58% (5)	45% (5 yr)	0
Dirix et al. (230)	25	IMRT+S	60	27	81% (2)	88% (2 yr)	0
Madani et al. (162)	84	IMRT+/–S	70	40	70% (5)	58.5% (5 yr)	1

IMRT, intensity-modulated radiation therapy; S, surgery; NR, no report.

Modified from Madani I, Bonte K, Vakaet L, et al. Intensity modulated radiotherapy for sinonasal tumors: Ghent University Hospital: Update. *Int J Radiat Oncol Biol Phys* 2009;73:424–432.

TABLE 48.14 STAGING OF NASOPHARYNGEAL ANGIOBROMA

IA	Limited to the nose or nasopharynx
IB	Extension into one or more paranasal sinuses
IIA	Minimal extension through sphenopalatine foramen medial pterygomaxillary fossa
IIB	Involvement of pterygomaxillary fossa displacing anteriorly posterior wall of maxillary antrum. Lateral or anterior displacement of maxillary artery branches or superior extension eroding orbital bones
IIC	Extension through pterygomaxillary fossa into the cheek and temporal fossa or posterior to pterygoid plates
IIIA	Erosion of skull base with minimal intracranial extension
IIIB	Erosion of skull base with extensive intracranial involvement with or without cavernous sines involvement

Modified from Radkowski D, McGill T, Healy GB, et al. Angiofibroma. Changes in staging and treatment. *Arch Otoraryngol Head Neck Surg* 1996;122:122–129.

Tumor remnants in symptom-free patients should be kept under surveillance by repeated CT scanning, because involution may occur. Recurrent symptoms may be treated by radiation therapy rather than by extended surgery or combined procedures.[209,231,221]

When there is intracranial tumor extension (seen in about 20% of patients), the risk of surgically related death increases. Some investigators recommend preoperative intra-arterial tumor vessel embolization at the time of diagnostic bilateral carotid angiography, claiming a decrease in operative bleeding.[232] Salvage with embolization of polyvinyl alcohol has been described.[233] Others have reported anecdotal evidence of partial regression with the use of estrogens, believed to be the result of feedback inhibition of the pituitary's production of gonadotropin-releasing hormone.

Although radiation therapy is equally effective in extracranial tumors, the low but existing risk of secondary malignancies should limit its use to the more advanced tumors only, such as those involving the orbital apex or the base of the skull.[225,234] In the experience of Cummings et al.[231] covering 20 years, only two radiation-related malignancies were noted (one skin, one thyroid).

Radiation Therapy Techniques

Photon irradiation should be used for these patients, and fields must be individualized to cover the tumor completely with a margin (1 to 2 cm). Treatment portals are similar to those used in carcinoma of the nasopharynx (without irradiating the cervical lymph nodes) or carcinoma of the paranasal sinuses when these structures or the nasal cavity is involved. Opposing lateral portals are suitable in most patients, with larger fields and compensators used for tumors extending into the nose (Fig. 48.15). More extensive disease requires three-field or wedge-pair arrangements of 3D-CRT or IMRT that can yield excellent dose distributions, particularly when there is nasopharyngeal or intracranial tumor extension. In all cases, the eyes are protected as much as possible.

The recommended tumor dose ranges from 30 Gy in 15 fractions in 3 weeks to 50 Gy in 24 to 28 fractions in 5 weeks.[235] A conventional setup uses 6- to 18-MV photons to treat the lesion with parallel-opposed fields to 50 Gy (2-Gy fractions).

The advantages of IMRT for the treatment of extensive or recurrent JNPAF were described in three patients on whom the tumor affected the base of skull, pterygopalatine, and intratemporal fossae, posterior orbit, and nasopharynx.[232] Tumor dose varied from 34 to 45 Gy. Chakraborty et al.[236] treated eight patients with IMRT for stage III tumors (median dose 39.6 Gy). Local control at 2 years was 87.5% and toxicity was minimal (persistent rhinitis in one patient).

Results of Therapy

In a surgical report, 18 patients were treated with gross tumor excision; 2 cases with intracranial involvement required a combined neurosurgical-otolaryngologic approach.[237] Recurrent intracranial disease was detected by MRI in three patients, who were treated with 35-, 36-, and 45-Gy external-beam irradiation. Extracranial tumor recurrences were re-excised in seven patients. All patients (followed up with serial MRI) are living without evidence of active disease.

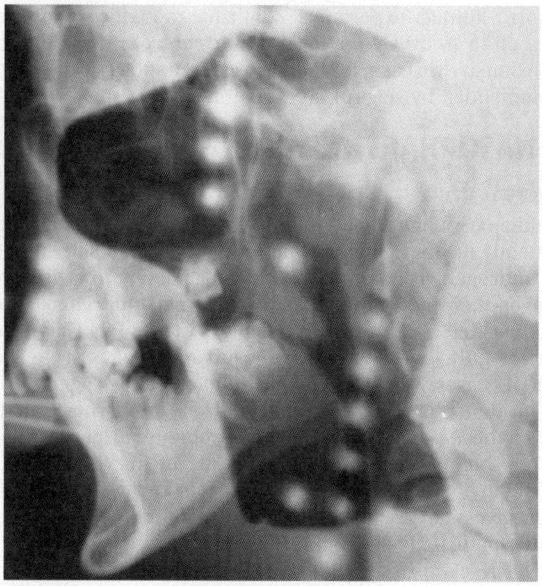

FIGURE 48.15. Example of conventional lateral portal used at the Mallinckrodt Institute of Radiology for nasopharyngeal angiofibroma.

Cummings et al.[231] treated 42 patients primarily with irradiation and 13 for postsurgical failures; all except 6 had biopsies. Nine had stage IV disease according to Chandler's staging system. Dose was 30 to 35 Gy in 14 to 16 fractions over a 3-week period. Follow-up ranged from 3 to 26 years. The control rate was 80% and was equivalent for all dose ranges. Local control was 89% and 74%, respectively, when three fields versus two fields were used. When the field size was more than 6-by-6 cm, the control rate was 83% versus 55% for smaller portals, indicating the importance of accurately determining the target volume, including any potential tumor extension. Of 11 recurrences, 8 were controlled by a second course of irradiation and 3 by surgery. These tumors regress slowly, with 50% still present at 12 months. At 24 months, 23% of tumors were still present, and half of those recurred. Of the complete responders, only 1 of 33 had a recurrence. Robinson et al.[238] also found that objective responses after irradiation were noted within 6 months in 60% of patients and within 6 to 20 months in the other 40%. Symptoms, however, resolved in all patients within 6 months of treatment.

At the Mallinckrodt Institute of Radiology, Fields et al.[239] reviewed the authors' experience with 13 patients: 11 surgical failures and 2 primarily treated with irradiation. Intracranial extension was noted in 38% of patients. Follow-up ranged from 40 to 173 months. Doses ranged from 36 to 52 Gy, with a median of 48 Gy (1.8 to 2 Gy per fraction, 5 days a week). The control rate was 85%; patients failing irradiation were salvaged with embolization. Late morbidity was mostly xerostomia and dental decay.

Ungkanont et al.[212] described results in 20 patients treated before 1974 and 23 treated between 1975 and 1993: 31 had surgery (18 with preoperative embolization), 3 had irradiation, 7 received chemotherapy (4 combined with surgery), and 2 were observed. Disease-free survival was 67%; 28% of patients survived with residual tumor, and 4.6% died of surgical complications. Roche et al.[240] treated 15 patients with JNPAF with various maxillofacial surgical resections, combined with Gamma Knife radiosurgery in 2 patients and external RT in 4 patients.

With median follow-up of 108 months, 12 patients were tumor-free and 2 had no progression. All patients had normal or nearly normal quality of life.

Tumor regression usually occurs slowly after either irradiation[231] or chemotherapy;[241] therefore, the presence of tumor up to 2 years after treatment is not an invariable sign of failure unless it is symptomatic or progressing. McAfee et al.[242] treated 22 patients with JNPAF with definitive RT (30 to 36 Gy); with median follow-up of 12.7 years, 20 patients (91%) had tumor control. The two patients failing were salvaged with surgery. No major treatment morbidity was noted. Kasper et al.,[243] in 9 patients treated with RT (30 to 35 Gy), observed 25% to 50% initial tumor regression within 1 year. Eventually seven of the patients had complete clinical tumor regression, but on CT or MRI only two of seven had no residual disease.

The management of large JNPAF with intracranial extension is complex. In 18 patients with JNPAF, preoperative MRI, embolization of feeding branches from the external carotid artery, and attempted complete resection were used in seven patients with intracranial disease;[237] serial MRI scans were used for follow-up. Intracranial disease that was persistent or recurrent and demonstrated subsequent growth was irradiated (35 to 45 Gy) or re-excised.

Wiatrak et al.[234] reported on three patients with extensive intracranial extension treated primarily with radiation therapy doses of 36.6, 40.0, and 50.4 Gy, respectively, without surgical tumor resection. Although there was no complete resolution of the tumors, significant improvement of symptoms was obtained without serious sequelae.

Ochoa-Carrillo et al.[216] reported on 31 patients treated with surgery or radiation therapy. Surgery was the treatment chosen in patients with stages II and III disease, while radiation therapy was the treatment in stage IV, but it had low effectiveness, indicating the need to carefully investigate the value of craniofacial approaches in these tumors. Radiation therapy (30 to 55 Gy) was administered to 16 patients; seven with stage III persistent or recurrent tumor, and eight patients as initial treatment for stage IV disease. The disease-free interval of patients with stages III and IV disease was 80.3% and 19%, respectively, after 36 months of follow-up.

Tranbahuy et al.[244] reported on seven patients with juvenile angiofibroma who underwent direct tumoral embolization. This technique induced marked devascularization and necrosis of the tumor. No neurologic sequelae were encountered.

Goepfert et al.[241] reported on five patients with aggressive nasopharyngeal angiofibromas recurrent after extracranial resection and irradiation who were treated with chemotherapy. Doxorubicin (60 mg/m^2 intravenous push for 1 day) and dacarbazine (250 mg/m^2 intravenous drip for 5 days) were given, with courses being repeated every 3 to 4 weeks. In a second regimen, vincristine, dactinomycin, and cyclophosphamide were administered at usual doses. Excellent tumor regression was noted in all patients. Patients were disease free at 2, 3, 6, and 10 years.

Sequelae of Therapy

Most investigators agree that surgical mortality increases with intracranial extension of the tumor. The most common radiation therapy sequelae include delayed growth secondary to hypopituitarism and decreased bone maturation.[158]

Malignant degeneration in JNPAF undergoing radiation therapy has been occasionally reported,[245,246] and there are several well-documented cases of radiation-induced sarcomas in these patients,[23,231] with doses ranging from 66 Gy to more than 90 Gy. Spagnolo et al.[23] reported on four patients treated with irradiation who later developed sarcoma. Cummings et al.[231] reported two neoplasms developing 13 and 14 years after irradiation; one was a basal cell carcinoma and one metastatic thyroid carcinoma. Both patients are alive without disease. Two patients developed cataracts.

NONLENTIGINOUS MELANOMA

Malignant melanoma accounts for 11% of primary head and neck malignancies.[110] Of all malignant melanomas, 20% to 35% are located in the head and neck area.[131]

Cutaneous Melanomas

In a review of the literature, Batsakis et al.[247] found that, of all head and neck malignant melanomas, 64% to 78% were cutaneous, 6% to 8% were mucosal, and 14% to 30% were ocular. The superficial spreading and nodular types of malignant melanoma have a metastatic potential of 10% to 30% and 50%, respectively.[248] Prognosis is correlated with location and stage of the tumor.[249] Neurotropic melanoma is an uncommon variant of cutaneous melanoma, with a higher propensity to invade peripheral nerves. A thorough evaluation with CT scans should determine if there is intracranial or base of the skull involvement.

Whole-body imaging with a CT or PET-CT scan is appropriate only for patients with regional nodal metastases. CT imaging detects occult disease in 0.5% to 3.7% of patients with microscopic nodal metastases on sentinel lymph node biopsy and in 4% to 16% of patients with clinically palpable nodal disease.[250] Only one metastatic lesion was identified in over 500 patients with invasive, node-negative melanoma evaluated in two large studies.[208]

Treatment of cutaneous melanomas has typically been wide excision of the lesion with a minimum 3-cm margin.[110] More recently, margins of at least 2 cm have been used in the head and neck for stage I melanomas, with equivalent success, with local failure rate of 3% to 6%.[208] In the absence of palpable regional lymphadenopathy, the decision to proceed with lymph node sampling after excision of a primary melanoma is frequently based on the probability of detecting nodal micrometastatic disease, which increases monotonically with the depth of the primary lesion. In several large clinical trials and meta-analyses, nodal metastases were uncommon in patients with melanoma primary lesions under 1-mm thick, with positive nodes seen in only 1% to 5.6% of patients. In contrast, thick lesions with Breslow depths >4 mm were associated with nodal metastases, with estimates ranging from 35% to 45%.[208]

Radiation therapy, combined with surgery is increasingly used in the treatment of patients with malignant melanoma (cutaneous or mucosal).[251] The Princess Margaret Hospital treated 16 patients with nodular melanomas with local excision and postoperative radiation therapy (50 Gy in 10 fractions over 2 weeks); 14 exhibited local tumor control, and 6 were alive and well 2 to 14 years after treatment. These results were comparable with those with wide local excision alone but with less morbidity and fewer cosmetic alterations. Later, at the same institution, Harwood and Cummings[110] treated five patients with definitive radiation therapy for superficial spreading melanoma of the head and neck area. All five lesions were locally controlled; one patient had a lymph node metastasis that was later controlled, and one died of distant metastases. They recommend treating these patients with 45 Gy in 10 fractions over 2 weeks to 50 Gy in 15 fractions in 3 weeks.[252,253]

Harwood and Cummings[248] also reported results in 74 patients treated with 3 fractions at 8 Gy given on days 0, 7, and 21 with shielding of the spinal cord, brain, and eye. Thirty patients were treated postoperatively after neck dissections if they had extracapsular tumor extension, multiple nodal involvement, a node >3 cm, or residual disease. Tumor control in the neck was achieved in 26 of 30 patients (86.6%) with follow-up of 1 to 4 years. In four patients with microscopic residual disease at the primary site, this postoperative regimen controlled three of four lesions with follow-up of 1 to 3.5 years. The other 40 patients were treated either for gross (13 patients) or recurrent (27 patients) cutaneous melanoma. Complete response was observed in 15 of 40 lesions (37.5%) and partial response in 12 lesions. An update of Harwood's data (personal communication, 1989) showed a neck tumor control rate of 94% in 41 adjuvantly treated patients versus 57% in 48 patients with gross residual or recurrent tumors. He concluded that irradiation alone should be considered for treatment of superficial spreading melanomas when surgery is contraindicated or after a simple excision in all cases of nodular melanoma in which a wide excision may be contraindicated because of age, location, or medical condition. For nodal disease, patients with poor prognostic pathologic factors should receive postoperative irradiation. Recurrent or unresectable tumors also should be irradiated. Harwood et al.[186] recommended high-dose fractions because the local control rate was 71% when the dose per fraction was >4 Gy and 25% with lower fractions.

Ang et al.[205] reported on 174 patients with head and neck cutaneous melanoma high-risk features (three or more positive nodes, extracapsular tumor extension) who after surgery were treated with elective postoperative RT (30 Gy in 5 fractions of 6 Gy in 2.5 weeks).With median follow-up of 35 months, locoregional tumor control was 88%. Lesion thickness strongly affected 5-year survival (100% for <1.5 mm, 72% for >1.5 to 4.0 mm, and 30% for >4 mm). Bibault et al.[254] treated 60 patients with cutaneous melanoma with node dissection (17 in the head and neck) and postoperative RT and 26 (4 in head and neck) with surgery alone. At 5 years, the regional tumor control was better in patients receiving >50 Gy (80% vs. 35% with lower doses), which was reflected on higher overall survival. Grade 2 toxicity was noted in 9% of the patients. In 49 patients with high-risk cutaneous melanoma in the head and neck, Chang et al.[158] used postoperative RT (30 Gy in 5 fractions or 60 Gy in 30 fractions). With median follow-up of 1.7 years and 4.4 years for living patients, the 5-year locoregional tumor control was 87% (no difference with either RT schedule), cause specific survival 57%, and overall survival 46%. Two patients in the hypofractionated group developed major complications (osteonecrosis of temporal bone and brachial plexopathy). Strojan et al.[255] reported on 83 patients with cutaneous melanoma in the head and neck, 40 treated with neck dissection only and 43 with dissection and postoperative RT (30 Gy in 5 fractions or 60 Gy in 30 fractions). In 20 patients, the primary site was included in the irradiated volume. With median follow-up of 2.1 years, the regional tumor control at 2 years was 56% with surgery alone and 78% with surgery plus RT, with survival 58% and 51%, respectively. Late toxicity was observed in 6 of 34 (17%) of surgery alone patients and in 10 of 36 (28%) of the surgery plus RT group. Chang et al.[158] summarized reports published on results of postoperative RT in head and neck cutaneous melanoma.

Another approach to the treatment of recurrent or unresectable cutaneous melanomas is combined hyperthermia and high-fraction radiation therapy, as reported by Emami et al.[255] and Engin et al.[257] These data support the use of high fractions for melanoma because Overgaard's complete response rate was 59% when fractions of more than 4 Gy were used and 33% for lower dose per fraction sizes. However, a randomized study by the Radiation Therapy Oncology Group comparing 4 fractions of 8 Gy given on days 0, 7, 14, and 21 and 20 fractions of 2.5 Gy in 5 weekly fractions showed no significant difference in tumor response (24.2% and 23.4% complete response and 35% partial response).[258]

Treatment with high doses of adjuvant interferon or interleukin-2 in high-risk stage II and III melanoma reduced the risk or disease recurrence and increased the median disease-free survival in several large trials.

Mucosal Melanomas

Primary mucosal melanomas of the head and neck area comprise 2% to 8% of the cases seen each year in the United States.[247] They occur more commonly in countries such as Japan, where mucosal melanoma is found in 22% to 32% of patients with malignant melanoma.[212] Most occur in the fifth to seventh decades of life; they are extremely rare in the first two decades (0.6% of mucosal melanomas).[259] The male-to-female ratio approaches 1 to 1.[259] A review by Batsakis[14] of 204 mucosal melanomas showed 56.4% to be from the upper respiratory tract and 44% from the oral cavity and pharynx. Nasal cavity or paranasal tumors comprise <1% of malignant melanomas and 2% to 9% of head and neck melanomas.[260] Pigmentation may precede the lesion in up to 28% of patients for more than 1 year.[261] In the oral cavity, the most common location is the hard palate (up to 80%), followed in order of decreasing frequency by the upper gingiva and lower gingiva.

Diagnostic Workup

An excisional biopsy should be performed when feasible because some reports have suggested possible local or metastatic spread secondary to a punch or incisional biopsy,[262] although this has not been noted in cutaneous melanomas.[45] Batsakis[14] found that one-third of these lesions were amelanotic, and Hoki et al.[260] noted that 25% were amelanotic.

Metastatic melanoma to the mucosa of the head and neck area is less common. It can be differentiated from primary tumors by the presence of normal tissue between subepidermal tumor and the basal layer of melanocytes.[14] The larynx, tongue, and tonsils are the most common locations for metastases.

Prognostic Factors

Batsakis et al.[247] found >0.5 mm invasion to be a poor prognostic factor. Trapp et al.[263] noted this to be true only in patients with >0.7-mm invasion. Lymph node involvement is not a prognostic factor. Mucosal melanomas fare worse than their cutaneous counterparts,[147] suggesting a lack of immunologic competence.[264]

Management and Results of Therapy

Surgical excision is usually recommended for these lesions. Because of the poor results obtained and because 37% of patients had associated adjacent pigmentation, some investigators recommend prophylactic excision of all melanocytic nevi. Because the results with irradiation are comparable with those of surgical series and because of the poor survival of these patients due to distant metastases and not locoregional failure, irradiation alone, with surgery for salvage, should be seriously considered as the primary treatment for mucosal melanomas of the head and neck.[253] Elective neck irradiation is not indicated in all patients, as only few develop nodal metastasis.[97]

Patients with nasal cavity or paranasal mucosal melanoma have a median survival of 24 months. Five-year disease-free survival rates of 25% have been reported.[259] Patients with laryngeal melanoma had a 13% 5-year disease-free survival rate.[147] In a review of the Japanese literature, Umeda et al.[265] found a local tumor control rate for stages I and II disease of 58% (7 of 12) in surgically treated patients with oral melanomas and a minimum follow-up of 3 years. Similar rates of failure have been reported, even with radical *en bloc* excisions (20% to 42%). Because the main cause of treatment failure is distant metastases and because almost no patient has clinically evident nodal metastases at presentation, an elective neck node dissection is not consistently recommended. This subject is still controversial, as 30% to 60% of patients may later develop nodal disease.[266]

Harwood and Cummings[248] treated 12 cases and added 12 cases from the literature for a total of 24 patients and 25 lesions. Local tumor control was achieved in 11 of 24 (9 to 54 months' follow-up). Six of seven tumors treated with 4-Gy fractions or larger were controlled, versus 5 of 18 treated with smaller fractions. Saigal et al.[97] treated 17 patients with mucosal melanomas (sinonasal tract in 11, oral cavity in 6) with surgery (16 combined with RT) and 1 with RT. Seven patients received adjuvant immunotherapy. With median follow-up of 35.2 months, local tumor control at 5 years was 81%, disease-free survival

44.5%, and overall survival 51.5%. Krengli et al.[267] reported on 74 patients with upper aerodigestive tract mucosal melanomas (31 nasal and 12 oral), 17 treated with surgery alone, 42 with surgery and RT (median dose 60 Gy, 2-Gy fractions), 11 with RT alone and 4 with chemoimmunotherapy. At 3 years, the local recurrence was 43% with surgery alone, 29% with surgery plus RT. Grade 3 mucositis was noted in nine patients.

Kingdom and Kaplan[268] described results in 13 patients with mucosal melanoma of the nasal cavity and paranasal sinuses treated with surgical resection. Eight had microscopically negative margins. Seven patients received postoperative irradiation (30 to 62 Gy). The neck was treated in three patients with doses of 30 to 50 Gy. The local tumor recurrence rate was 85% (11 of 13), with a mean interval from primary tumor treatment to recurrence of 16 months. Metastatic neck disease developed in two patients and distant metastases in four. Patients receiving postoperative irradiation had increased disease-free interval and prolonged survival. Negative surgical margins were not predictive of a more favorable outcome. The investigators recommend resection of tumor with negative margins and postoperative irradiation for the treatment of all patients with mucosal malignant melanoma.

Zenda et al.[250] treated 14 patients with head and neck mucosal melanomas using protons (60 Gy in 15 fractions, 3 fractions per week). With median follow-up of 36.7 months, the 3-year local tumor control was 85.7% and overall survival 58%. The most frequent failure site was the cervical nodes (six patients). Two patients developed late decreased visual acuity. Carbon ion therapy was used by Yanagi et al.[269] in the primary treatment of 72 patients with mucosal melanomas of the head and neck (dose ranging from 52.8 to 64 GyE in 16 fractions).With median follow-up of 49 months, local tumor control at 5 years was 84%, cause-specific survival 39.6%, and overall survival 27%. No grade 3 morbidity was observed. Jingu et al.[270] treated 37 patients with head and neck melanomas with carbon ions (57.6 GyE in 16 fractions) and chemotherapy. With median follow-up of 19 months, the local tumor control at 3 years was 65.3% and overall survival 81%. MRI minimum apparent diffusion coefficient was a prognostic factor for survival.

LENTIGO MALIGNA MELANOMA

Natural History

Lentigo maligna (Hutchinson's melanotic freckle[271] or circumscribed precancerous melanosis of Dubreuilh) and its invasive counterpart, lentigo maligna melanoma (LMM), are well-recognized clinicopathologic entities. LMM comprises about 10% of all melanomas in the head and neck, occurs predominantly on the face and ears of elderly persons, and generally has a very long natural history, frequently reaching a large size before diagnosis. Approximately one-third of lentigo maligna lesions, if left untreated, will eventually transform into invasive LMM.

Tannous et al.[272] hypothesized that lentigo maligna can be divided into two categories: one represents a pigmented lesion that is a precursor to melanoma, and the other melanoma *in situ*. Also, they hypothesized that in some patients there is a progression to malignant melanoma.

Clinical Presentation and Diagnostic Workup

These lesions appear as circumscribed and later as more diffuse areas of hyperpigmentation of the skin. They may develop some superficial nodularity and eventual ulceration as they become more invasive. In 10% of the latter patients, regional and distant metastases eventually develop. The 10% metastatic spread in LMM contrasts with the 25% metastatic tendency in nodular melanomas arising in superficial spreading melanomas and a 50% metastatic spread in nodular melanomas arising *de novo*.

The diagnostic workup of these patients is similar to that of patients suspected of having malignant melanoma. Biopsies of the lesion are required to obtain histopathologic confirmation of the diagnosis. Careful physical examination must rule out any areas of extension or regional or distant spread.

General Management

The usual treatment of lentigo maligna and LMM has been surgery, with approximately 5- to 10-mm margin of normal skin or Mohs surgery, although larger margins may be required for ill-defined lesions.[273] Radiation therapy is used for more extensive lesions or for postsurgical recurrences.[273] Hill and Gramp[274] reported on 66 cases of LMM; 38% of which required two excisions or more to clear the tumor and 32% of cases showed evidence of invasive melanoma. Only one case has recurred thus far, and none have developed metastatic disease. For larger lesions, wider surgical excision with skin grafting has been reported to give poor cosmetic results.

Cohen et al.[275] reported their experience with Mohs microsurgery, which was performed in 26 patients with lentigo maligna and 19 patients with LMM. After a median follow-up of 58 months (214.3 patient-years), there was one recurrence, in a patient with five prior recurrences before Mohs micrographic surgery. Kuflik and Gage[176] treated 30 patients with cryosurgery. Lesions ranged from 1.3 to 4.5 cm in diameter. Lesions recurred in two patients (recurrence rate of 6.6%) who were successfully retreated with cryosurgery. Eleven patients observed for more than 5 years showed no recurrences.

Because of the low incidence of regional lymph node metastases, elective lymph node dissection is not indicated.

Radiation therapy with various techniques has been frequently used in the treatment of these patients, particularly those with larger lesions, because of minimal morbidity and generally excellent cosmetic results (Fig. 48.16).

Radiation Therapy Techniques

As in other skin lesions, the portals should be carefully designed to include the entire tumor with adequate margin (1 cm for lesions <2 cm and 2 cm for larger tumors). Because Miescher's irradiation technique used very superficial x-rays, with 50% depth dose being at approximately 1 mm, there is the possibility of local recurrence if dermal extension is unrecognized. Therefore, Harwood and Lawson[253] recommend using minimum x-ray energies of 100 keVp and preferably 140 to 175 keVp to treat these patients. Superficial x-rays (100 to 200 keVp) with adequate filtration or electrons (6 to 9 MeV) with appropriate thickness of bolus (1 to 1.5 cm) are adequate for most patients. Doses of 45 to 50 Gy in 15 to 25 fractions delivered over 3 to 5 weeks will control the disease in most patients. The authors recommend delivering 3 to 3.5 Gy, 3 times weekly, every other day, to a total of 50 Gy, depending on the size and thickness of the lesion. Elective irradiation of the regional lymphatics is not necessary.

Careful follow-up with clinical examinations and photographs of the lesion is essential to ascertain the continuing regression of the tumor.

In patients on whom surgical excision is performed, postoperative irradiation is recommended if positive margins are found.[112] Doses are similar to those stated earlier.

Results of Therapy

Harwood and Lawson[253] described 13 patients with lentigo maligna treated with radiation therapy: 11 had local tumor control, 1 had an edge recurrence salvaged by irradiation, and 1 had residual tumor (alive and well 11 years after treatment for the recurrence). One patient alive at 2 years refused further treatment. Of 19 patients irradiated for LMM, 17 had tumor control with radiation therapy alone for periods ranging from 6 months to 6 years. One patient had a central recurrence that was salvaged by surgery (alive and well 5 years after treatment of recurrence). No patient has developed lymph node or distant metastases in either group.

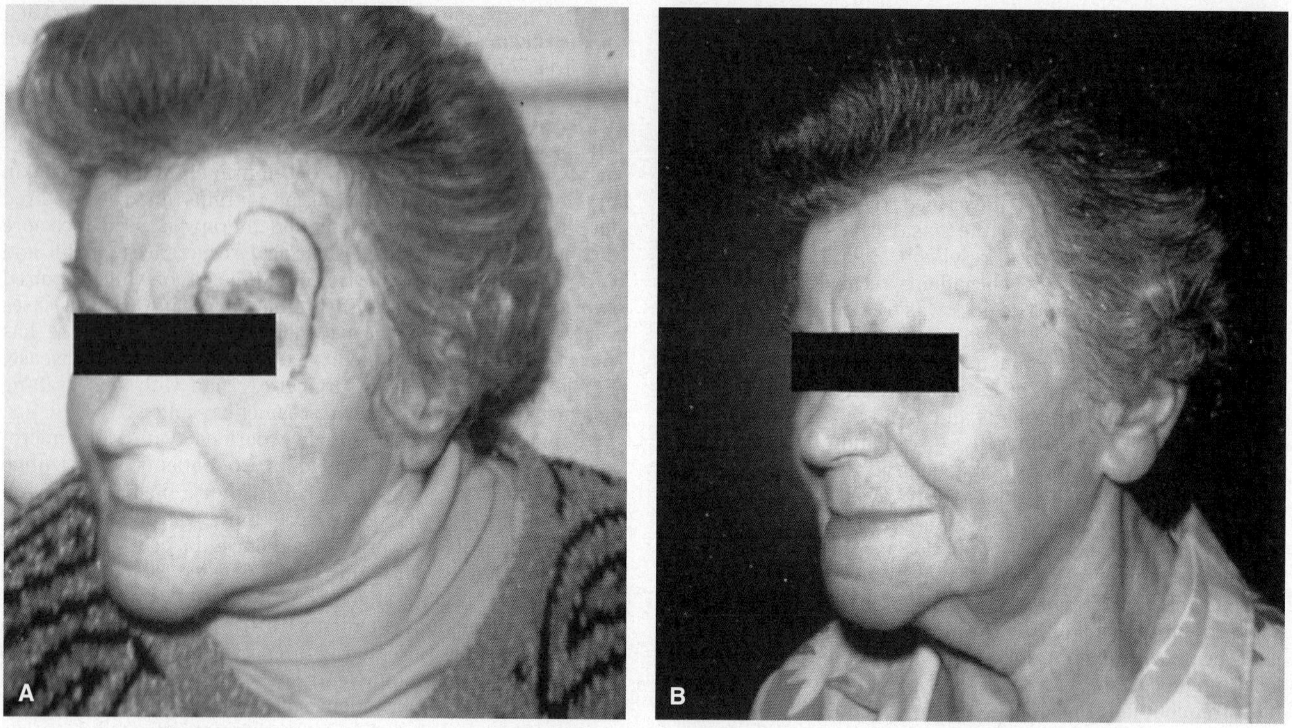

FIGURE 48.16. Lentigo maligna melanoma of face before **(A)** and 6 years after **(B)** 50 Gy in 25 fractions delivered with 9-MeV electrons and bolus.

Tsang et al.[259] described results in 54 patients treated with radiation therapy or surgery. Younger patients with smaller lesions were treated with surgical excision (18 patients) and achieved actuarial tumor control of 94% at 3 years. Older patients with larger lesions located in the head and neck area were treated by radiation therapy (36 patients), with an actuarial tumor control rate of 86% at 5 years. No patient developed metastatic melanoma. The late cosmetic appearance was acceptable in the majority of irradiated patients, with 11% showing poor cosmesis because of progressive skin pallor, atrophy, and telangiectasia in the treated area.

SARCOMAS OF THE HEAD AND NECK

Natural History

Sarcomas account for <1% of malignant neoplasms in the head and neck. The most frequent histological type is malignant fribohistiocytoma (29%), while the least common is liposarcoma (1%). The histology is complex and requires immunochemical analysis including angiosarcoma, chondrosarcoma, hemangiosarcoma, leiomyosarcoma, liposarcoma, malignant fibrous sarcoma, neurofibrosarcoma, osteosarcoma, rhabdomyosarcoma, malignant schwannoma, and synovial sarcoma. Fibrosarcoma, angiosarcoma, leiomyosarcoma, and rhabdomyosarcoma are the most common types, but this varies in published reports. Distribution of these sarcomas was 33% in the scalp or face, 26% in the orbit or paranasal sinuses, 14% arising from upper aerodigestive tract including larynx, and 27% in the neck. Synovial sarcomas are rare soft tissue malignancies in the head and neck region; they account for 3% to 5% of head and neck tumors. Histologic, immunohistochemical, and characteristic chromosomal translocation findings are necessary for diagnosis. The poor prognosis of this sarcoma justifies radical surgery with postoperative radiation.[277]

Radiation-induced sarcoma of the head and neck is a rare long-term complication of treatment. The rarity of this tumor is reflected in the very few series reported in the English language medical literature.[278,279] When they do occur, most appear at least 10 years following radiation therapy. There is a possibility of a postirradiation sarcoma whenever a suspicious lesion is seen, regardless of the amount of time that has passed since radiation therapy was administered. The original pathology should be re-examined to ensure that the original tumor was diagnosed correctly. Electron microscopy can be useful in differentiating sarcomatous-appearing epithelial lesions from true soft tissue sarcomas.

The incidence of radiation-induced sarcomas of the head and neck is, however, likely to increase due to progressive aging of the population combined with improved survival in head and neck cancer patients. This problem can be extremely challenging, and the overall outlook has been reported to be very bleak. Patel et al.[279] reviewed 69 cases reported in the English medical literature since 1966 and pooled this information with their experience in treatment of 10 patients. This group was compared for survival with 124 patients with a diagnosis of head and neck sarcoma registered on the Head and Neck Sarcoma database at the Royal Marsden Hospital. There was no site prediction for radiation-induced sarcoma of the head and neck, but malignant fibrous histiocytoma was the most common pathologic diagnosis. The period of latency between initial radiation therapy and diagnosis ranged from 9 to 45 years, with a median of 17 years. Surgery was the mainstay of treatment, and follow-up ranged from 6 months to 15 years with a median of 48 months. The actuarial 5-year disease-free survival rate in these patients was 60%.

Clinical Presentation and Diagnostic Workup

Clinical presentation varies with the primary site of disease. Tumors arising from the aerodigestive tract usually present with nasal bleeding, a palpable mass in the neck, or difficulty in swallowing or breathing. In tumors arising from the base of skull or the nerve sheath, cranial nerve deficit is the most common presentation. Diagnostic workup follows that of soft tissue sarcomas of other sites in the body. With early lesions, radiographs or CT may show only nonspecific opacification, soft tissue swelling, and occasionally bone destruction. Table 48.1 outlines the suggested diagnostic workup. MRI, especially with gadolinium contrast, may be used as a supplement or alternative to CT scanning.[280,281] A CT scan of the chest is also mandatory for staging workup.

The American Joint Committee on Cancer staging system for soft tissue sarcomas is based on histologic grade, the tumor size and depth, and the presence of distant or nodal metastases. The staging system is the same as for sarcomas of the extremities, although specific staging for head and neck sarcomas is not standardized.[213]

Prognostic Factors

Prognostic factors for predicting local recurrence or disease-free survival include anatomic site, treatment modality, tumor histology and grade, tumor size, extension of disease, lymph node metastasis, and surgical margins.[277,282,283,284]

A report from Royal Marsden Hospital showed anatomic location and treatment modality to be independent prognostic factors for local recurrence; tumors of the head had a better local recurrence-free survival than did those of the neck.[77] Patients treated with a combination of surgery and radiation therapy had a better recurrence-free survival than did those treated with surgery or irradiation alone. The only significant independent prognostic factor for overall survival was the implementation of definitive surgery versus biopsy. In the above report, the prognostic impact of tumor stage and grade did not reach statistical significance. In contrast, Tran et al.[285] reported that 90% of patients with low-grade tumors were free of disease versus only 16% with high-grade lesions.

Bentz et al.[157] reviewed 111 head and neck sarcoma patients; median duration of follow-up was 51 months; the actuarial 5-year relapse-free disease-specific, and overall survivals were 55%, 52%, and 44%, respectively. By multivariate analysis, size and grade significantly influenced all survivals, whereas margin status additionally influenced relapse-free survival.

In 109 soft tissue sarcomas of all sites, a French study demonstrated that quality of the surgery was one of the most important variables for predicting local recurrences. Tumor size, surgical margins, presence of tumor necrosis, and adequacy of the excision correlated with metastasis-free survival.[286]

General Management

Surgery is the preferred initial treatment modality for sarcomas.[235,287] Unfortunately, it is often difficult to achieve complete resection of the tumor, and a high recurrence rate has been observed with surgery alone.[288] Extracapsular enucleation of the tumor results in 90% local recurrence because of the presence of microscopic pseudopodia, which tend to grow through the pseudocapsule into the surrounding tissue, and the presence of skipped lesions some distance from the main tumor mass. Pathologic analysis of the surgical bed often discloses microscopic extension of tumor. Farhood et al.,[288] in a review of 176 cases of adult head and neck sarcomas, reported that the pathologic margins of surgical specimens obtained by wide local excision were positive in >50% of cases. This resulted in inferior overall survival for sarcomas of the head and neck when compared with extremity sarcomas.[238] Wide local excision, with a 5-cm margin around the pseudocapsule in extremity sarcomas, is associated with better outcome, although approximately 20% will have local recurrence. The criteria for surgical resection are impractical for head and neck sarcomas because of anatomic limitations;[213] wide local excision is rarely possible because the tumors extend beyond the confines of origin and in the proximity of vital neurovascular structures. Some retrospective studies have suggested improved local tumor control when combined surgery and external irradiation are used. In 130 patients with soft tissue sarcomas of the head and neck treated with surgery alone at Royal Marsden Hospital, the overall 5-year survival was 50%; local tumor control was only 47%, and local recurrence was the cause of death in 63% of cases. Patients treated with combined-modality treatment (surgery and irradiation) had less extensive surgery, yet local recurrence-free survival was longer.[283]

Synovial sarcoma in the head and neck is rare. In a report of 36 patients Al-Daraji et al.[289] noted there was a predilection for the parotid and the temporal regions, and nine involved skeletal muscle. Of 29 patients followed for a median 14 years after surgical treatment, 11 were alive and tumor free.

A multidisciplinary discussion before the initiation of treatment is required to formulate the best approach for radiation delivery, surgical technique, and mode of reconstruction.

Radiation Therapy

Radiation therapy, by external beam or brachytherapy, plays an important adjunctive role in disease management, especially for tumors where *en bloc* resection with negative margin is not possible.[284,290] Chemotherapy regimens are available for soft tissue neoplasms, primarily designed to improve local tumor control.[127] A systematic review of radiation therapy trials was performed by the Swedish Council of Technology Assessment in Health Care.[290] This synthesis of the literature on radiation therapy for soft tissue sarcomas is based on data from five randomized trials. Moreover, data from 6 prospective studies, 25 retrospective studies, and 3 other articles were used. In total, 39 scientific articles were included, involving 4,579 patients. The results were compared with those of a similar overview from 1996, which included 3,344 patients. There was evidence that adjuvant radiotherapy improves local tumor control in combination with conservation surgery with negative, marginal, or minimal microscopic positive surgical margins. There are still insufficient data to establish that preoperative radiotherapy is favorable compared to postoperative radiotherapy in patients presenting primarily with large tumors. The preoperative setting results in more wound complications. There is no randomized study comparing external-beam radiotherapy and brachytherapy. These data suggest that external-beam radiotherapy and low–dose-rate brachytherapy result in comparable local control for high-grade tumors. Some patients with low-grade soft tissue sarcomas benefit from external-beam radiotherapy in terms of local control. Brachytherapy with a low-dose rate for low-grade tumors seems to be of no benefit, but data are sparse. In two small studies investigating hyperfractionation schedules, there was no indication of improvements compared to daily fractions of 2 Gy.

Mesenchymal chondrosarcoma of the sinonasal tract is a rare, malignant tumor of extraskeletal origin.[93] Thirteen patients with sinonasal mesenchymal chondrosarcoma presented with nasal obstruction (n = 8), epistaxis (n = 7), mass effect (n = 4), or a combination of these. The maxillary sinus was the most common site of involvement (n = 9), followed by the ethmoid sinuses (n = 7) and the nasal cavity (n = 5). All cases were managed by surgery with adjuvant radiation therapy (n = 4) and/or chemotherapy (n = 3). The overall mean survival was 12.1 years, although five of six patients who developed local recurrences died of disease (mean survival, 6.5 years). Six patients were alive and disease free (mean survival, 17.3 years), and two patients were lost to follow-up.

Radiation Therapy Techniques

The general principles for radiation therapy of head and neck sarcomas are similar to those of soft tissue sarcomas. Complete coverage of the surgical bed and scar with adequate margins (3 to 5 cm) is required.[291] However, because of the proximity of critical and radiosensitive organs (eyes, spinal cord, brainstem), selecting optimal portal margins without seriously compromising the functioning of these organs is an art. Techniques similar to those used in epithelial tumors of the head and neck can be applied to sarcomas. In general, 55 to 60 Gy is needed for postoperative adjuvant irradiation, and an additional 10- to 15-Gy boost is recommended if the surgical margins are close (≤3 mm) or involved by tumor. Some institutions prefer preoperative irradiation of 45 to 50 Gy. Special attention should be directed to limiting the dose to critical structures. Use of a 3D or IMRT treatment technique can be considered as demonstrated in Fig. 48.8.

Protons or heavy ions have been used in selected patients.[292] Hug et al.[293] reported on 27 patients treated at Massachusetts General Hospital in Boston (18 primary and 9 recurrent sarcomas of the head and neck close or abutting critical structures with 160 MeV protons; mean dose 68.5 GyE in 2.1-GyE fractions). Local recurrence was seen in eight patients (29%) and regional recurrence in six patients (22%). Tumor grade had a significant impact on outcome. One patient developed Lhermitte sign and another hypothyroidism.

Jingu et al.[294] described results in 27 patients with head and neck unresectable bone and soft tissue sarcomas, treated with carbon ions (57.6, 64.0, or 70.4 GyE in 16 fractions). The 3-year local tumor control was 91.6% and survival 72%. Therapy was well tolerated.

TABLE 48.15 TREATMENT RESULTS OF ADULT SOFT TISSUE SARCOMAS OF THE HEAD AND NECK

Author (Reference)	Number of Patients	Modalities	5-Year Actuarial Rates: Local Control (%)	5-Year Actuarial Rates: Survival (%)
Weber et al. (299)	188	S, R, C	–	Overall: 49.4 (<5 cm) Overall: 30.4 (≥5 cm)
Greager et al. (300)	48	S, R, C	–	Disease free: 54
Farhood et al. (288)	176	S, R, C	–	Overall: 55
McKenna et al. (301)	16	S, R, C	75	Disease free: 63
Eeles et al. (283)	103[a]*	S, R, C	47	Overall: 50
LeVay et al. (280)	52	S, R, C	59	Cause specific: 63
Tran et al. (285)	164	S, R, C	41	Overall: 66
Willers et al. (284)	57	S, R, C	60	Overall: 66
Chao et al.[b]	33	S, R, C	49	Disease free: 40
Colville et al. (213)	60	S, R, C	50	60

C, chemotherapy; R, radiation therapy; S, surgery.
[a]Series based on adults and children, excluding angiosarcomas. [b]Unpublished data.

Results of Therapy

Because of the propensity for sarcomas to invade the surrounding tissues, complete surgical clearance may be difficult. In a series from UCLA, attempted *en bloc* resection left residual tumor at the surgical margins in 52 of 127 patients.[285] The incidence of local recurrence was high (60%) with surgery alone.

In a retrospective report of 73 patients with sarcomas of the head and neck treated at Princess Margaret Hospital, the 5-year cause-specific survival was 62%, with a local recurrence rate of 41% and a distant metastasis rate of 31%.[280] Extension to adjacent structures, high-grade tumor, and tumor >10 cm were associated with poor survival. Gross residual tumor after surgery was also associated with a high local recurrence rate (75%) despite the addition of radiation therapy. Patients with clear surgical margins or only microscopic involvement fared much more favorably and had a similar local tumor control rate (74% and 70%, respectively), provided adjuvant irradiation was given. Because of the difficulty in obtaining wide surgical margins, 68% of the patients died as a result of uncontrolled local disease. These data substantiate the importance of surgical margins as well as the contribution of adjuvant irradiation.[280]

Colville et al.[213] reported on 41 male and 19 female patients treated with head and neck soft tissue sarcomas, with an overall 5-year survival of 60%. Twenty-five patients had surgery alone, 20 had surgery and pre- or postoperative radiation therapy, and 15 received nonsurgical treatment. With mean follow-up of almost 4 years, the 5-year local tumor control was 56% in the surgical group and 40% in the nonsurgical group (more advanced and aggressive tumors). The 5-year survival was 70% and 40%, respectively.

Penel et al.[295] recorded their experience with 28 adult head and neck soft tissue sarcomas. The most common subtype was rhabdomyosarcoma (RMS) (seven cases). Twenty-two patients presented with previous inadequate resection performed elsewhere before admission. Nineteen patients had surgery (complete resection in 13 cases). Associated treatments were neoadjuvant chemotherapy, adjuvant chemotherapy, and postoperative radiotherapy in 4, 3, and 10 cases, respectively. The 2-year overall survival rate was 56%. Wolden et al.[296] treated 28 patients with head and neck RMS using IMRT (50–55 Gy in 1.8 Gy fractions) combined with chemotherapy. With median follow up of 24 months local tumor control was 95–100% and 3 year survival McDonald et al.[297] treated 20 children with RMS in the head and neck with IMRT (median dose 50.4 Gy, 1.8 per fraction). With 29 months median follow up the 3 year local tumor control was 100% and survival 76%.

Pandey et al.[298] reported on 22 cases of head and neck sarcomas (neck, lower jaw, tongue, cheek, scalp, and maxilla were the most common sites affected). None of the patients had palpable neck nodes or distant metastasis at presentation. All the patients were treated with primary surgical resection, followed by adjuvant treatment in 14 cases (63.6%). After a median follow-up of 14.5 months, two patients died, six developed local recurrence, four developed metastatic disease, and another patient developed a second primary sarcoma. The overall 5-year survival was 80%, while the 5-year disease-free survival rate was 24.1%.

Barker et al.[13] published a review of 44 patients with nonmetastatic soft tissue sarcoma in a head and neck. The most common tumor histologies included malignant fibrous histiocytoma (15 patients), angiosarcoma (9 patients), fibrosarcoma (6 patients), and leiomyosarcoma (6 patients). The median overall survival for all patients was 79 months. The actuarial 5-year local tumor control was 55% and was highly correlated with the extent of surgical excision: 25% for subtotal resection or debulking, 65% for wide local excision, and 100% for radical excision. Local tumor control at 5 years was 60% for patients treated with both surgery and radiotherapy, 54% surgery alone, and 43% for radiation alone. Adjuvant radiation therapy significantly improved the local control rates (from 25% to 54%) for patients with close (<2 mm) or positive surgical margins. Of 14 patients with locoregional failure in whom salvage was attempted, 9 (64%) were rendered disease free.

Rapidis et al.[302] reported on 25 patients with head and neck sarcomas with follow-up ranging from 8 to 144 months. Twenty-three patients were treated with surgery as the primary modality; 14 with surgery alone. Clear margins were obtained in all of them and local control was achieved in 12 of 13. The 5-year survival for the entire group was 40%. Reported results of treatment of soft tissue sarcomas is summarized in Table 48.15.

Tumor Characteristics

Several series have shown that tumor grade and size dictate the outcome of patients with head and neck sarcomas such as leiomyosarcoma, rhabdomyosarcoma, and malignant fibrous sarcoma.[275] Farhood et al.,[288] in a review of 176 adult head and neck sarcomas, found that only 20% of the patients with high-grade tumors were alive 10 years after treatment, compared with 88% of patients with low-grade tumors. Weber et al.[299] described a 45% 10-year survival rate for patients with tumors <5 cm versus 10% for those with tumors ≥5 cm.

Many series have reported that chondrosarcoma is not a radiosensitive tumor, and radiation therapy has no role in it treatment. However, some reports have demonstrated the contribution of radiation therapy in this histology. McNaney et al.[303] described a 65% survival rate at 2 years in 20 chondrosarcoma patients who received primary radiation therapy. Tumor grade was the most important prognostic factor.

Osteogenic sarcoma of the head and neck has a pattern of recurrence different from similar tumors elsewhere in the body. Head and neck osteosarcomas are usually high grade; they have a very high incidence of local recurrence but a lower risk of distant metastases. Several studies have used adjuvant irradiation and chemotherapy, which commonly results in improved locoregional tumor control and survival. Tran et al.[285] reported a 73% 5-year survival rate in patients with osteogenic sarcoma of the head and neck treated with high-dose preoperative irradiation followed by wide surgical excision.

Chemotherapy

Head and neck soft tissue sarcomas frequently metastasize; 25% of patients in a UCLA study had distant metastases.[265] The role of adjuvant chemotherapy to improve disease-free survival in sarcoma of the head and neck is controversial. Unlike with soft tissue sarcomas of the extremities, in which distant metastasis is the most common cause of death, the majority of deaths in sarcomas of the head and neck are associated with local failure. Approximately half of the distant metastases were detected after local recurrence occurred.[280] Chemotherapy did not appear to affect local tumor control.

In a series of 94 patients treated at UCLA,[244] local control was achieved in 52% of patients treated with surgery alone and 90% of those receiving adjuvant irradiation with or without chemotherapy.

For preoperative neoadjuvant chemotherapy, which supplements radiation therapy to downstage disease before surgery, satisfactory results are available only for sarcomas of extremities.[304] With the exception of rhabdomyosarcoma, postoperative adjuvant chemotherapy for head and neck sarcomas should be given only in a clinical trial setting.

SELECTED REFERENCES

A full list of references for this chapter is available online.

6. Semaan MT, Megerian CA. Current assessment and management of glomus tumors. *Curr Opin Otolaryngol Head Neck Surg* 2008;16:420–426.
14. Batsakis JG. In: *Tumors of the head and neck,* 2nd ed. Baltimore: Williams & Wilkins, 1979:474–475.
18. Li G, Chang S, Adler JR, et al. Irradiation of glomus jugulare tumors: a historical perspective. *Neurosurg Focus* 2007;23:E13.
22. Powell S, Peters N, Harmer C. Chemodectoma of the head and neck: results of treatment in 84 patients. *Int J Radiat Oncol Biol Phys* 1992;22:919–924.
25. Krych AJ, Foote RL, Brown PD, et al. Long-term results of irradiation for paraganglioma. *Int J Radiat Oncol Biol Phys* 2006;65:1063–1066.
32. Chen PG, Nguyen JH, Payne SC, et al. Treatment of glomus jugulare tumors with Gamma Knife radiosurgery. *Laryngoscope* 2010;120:1856–1862.
33. Genc A, Bicer A, Abacioglu U, et al. Gamma Knife radiosurgery for the treatment of glomus jugulare tumors. *J Neurooncol* 2010;97:101–108.
35. Lim M, Bower R, Nangiana JS, et al. Radiosurgery for glomus jugulare tumors. *Technol Cancer Res Treat* 2007;6:419–423.
37. Navarro MA, Maitz A, Grills IS, et al. Successful treatment of glomus jugulare tumors with Gamma Knife radiosurgery: clinical and physical aspects of management and review of the literature. *Clin Transl Oncol* 2010;12:55–62.
38. Henzel M, Hamm K, Gross MW, et al. Fractionated stereotactic radiotherapy of glomus tumors. Local control, toxicity, symptomatology and quality of life. *Strahlenther Onkol* 2007;183:557–562.
39. Pollock BE. Stereotactic radiosurgery in patients with glomus jugulare tumors. *Neurosurg Focus* 2004;17(2):E10.
41. Combs SE, Konkel S, Schulzertner D, et al. Intensity modulated radiotherapy (IMRT) in patients with carcinoma of the paranasal sinuses: clinical benefit for complex shaped target volumes. *Radiat Oncol* 2006;1:23.
43. Schulz-Ertner D, Haberer T, Jakel O, et al. Radiotherapy for chordomas and low grade chondrosarcomas of the skull base with carbon ions. *Int J Radiat Oncol Biol Phys* 2002;53;36–42.
44. Lloyd G, Howard D, Lund VJ, et al. Imaging for juvenile angiofibroma. *J Laryngol Otol* 2000;114:727–730.
47. Zabel A, Milker-Zabel S, Huber P. Fractionated sterotactic conformal radiotherapy in the management of large chemodectomas of the skull base. *Int J Radiat Oncol Biol Phys* 2004;58:1445–1450.
48. Kim JW, Kim DG, Chung HT, et al. Gamma Knife stereotactic radiosurgery for intracranial hemangiopericytomas. *J Neurooncol* 2010;99:115–122.
50. Hinerman RW, Morris CG, Mendenhall WM, et al. Paragangliomas of the head and neck treated with external-beam radiotherapy. *Int J Radiat Oncol Biol Phys* 2007;69(Suppl 3): S434 (abstr 2416).
51. Verniers DA, Keus RB, Schouwenburg PF, et al. Radiation therapy, an important mode of treatment for head and neck chemodectomas. *Eur J Cancer* 1992;27:1028–1033.
52. Ivan ME, Sughrue ME, Clark AJ, et al. A meta-analysis of tumor control rates and treatment related morbidity for patients with glomus jugulare tumors. *J Neurosurg* 2011;114:1299–1305.
53. Guss ZD, Batra S, Limb CJ, et al. Radiosurgery of glomus jugulare tumors: a meta-analysis. *Int J Radiat Oncol Biol Phys* 2011;81(4):e497–e502.
62. Valdagni R, Amichetti M. Radiation therapy of carotid body tumors. *Am J Clin Oncol* 1990;13:45–48.
68. Rutkoeski MJ, Sughrue ME, Kane AJ, et al. Predictors of mortality following treatment of intracranial hemangiopericytoma. *J Neurosurg* 2010;113:333–339.
69. Spitz FR, Bouvet M, Pisters PW, et al. Hemangiopericytoma: a 20-year single institution experience. *Ann Surg Oncol* 1998;5:350–355.
85. Patrice SJ, Sneed PK, Flickinger JC, et al. Radiosurgery for hemangioblastoma: results of a multi-institutional experience. *Int J Radiat Oncol Biol Phys* 1995; 32(Suppl 1):147(abstr).
87. Staples JJA, Robinson RAA, Wen B-CA, et al. Hemangiopericytoma—the role of radiotherapy. *Int J Radiat Oncol Bio Phys* 1990;19:445–451.
88. Kano H, Niranjan A, Kondziolka D, et al. Adjuvant stereotactic radiosurgery after resection of intracranial hemangiopericytomas. *Int J Radiat Oncol Biol Phys* 2008;72:1333–1339.
89. Olson C, Yen CP, Schlesinger D, et al. Radiosurgery for intracranial hemangiopericytomas: outcomes after initial and repeat Gamma Knife surgery. *J Neurosurg* 2010;112:133–139.
90. Redmond KJ, Gullett NP, Kleinberg L, et al. Hemangiopericytoma of the central nervous system: analysis of current national patterns of care. *Int J Radiat Oncol Bio Phys Proc* 2010:78(suppl 3):S615.
91. Tai PT, Craighead P, Bagdon F. Optimization of radiotherapy for patients with cranial chordoma: a review of dose-response ratios for photon techniques. *Cancer* 1995;75:749–756.
97. Saigal K, Palmer JD, Reis I, et al. Mucosal melanomas of the head and neck: a modern experience at the University of Miami. *Int J Radiat Oncol Bio Phys Proc* 2010:78(suppl 3):S479.
101. Gay E, Sckhar LN, Rubinstein E, et al. Chordomas and chondrosarcomas of the cranial base: results and follow-up of 60 patients. *Neurosurgery* 1995;36: 887–896.
107. Muthukumar N, Kondziolka D, Lundford LD, et al. Stereotactic radiosurgery for chordoma and chondrosarcoma: further experience. *Int J Radiat Oncol Biol Phys* 1998;41:387–392.
108. Suit HD, DeLaney T, Goldberg S, et al. Protons versus carbon ion beams in the definitive radiation treatment of cancer patients. *Radiother Oncol* 2010;95: 3–22.
112. Fagundes MA, Hug EB, Liebsch NJ, et al. Radiation therapy for chordomas of the base of skull and cervical spine: patterns of failure and outcome after relapse. *Int J Radiat Oncol Biol Phys* 1995;33:579–584.
115. Noel G, Jauffret E, de Crevoisier R, et al. Photon and proton therapy for chordoma and chondrosarcoma of the base of the skull and cervical spine: prognostic factors and patterns of failure. *Radiother Oncol* 2002;S81 (abstr 241).
116. Jakel O, Land B, Combs SE, et al. On the cost-effectiveness of carbon ion radiation therapy for skull base chordoma. *Radiother Oncol* 2007;83:133–138.
118. Royal College of Radiologists Proton Therapy Working Party. Proton therapy for base of skull chordoma: a report for the Royal College of Radiologists. *Clin Oncol (R Coll Radiol)* 2000;12:75–79.
121. Mendenhall WM, Olivier KR, Lynch JW Jr, et al. Lethal midline granuloma-nasal natural killer/T-cell lymphoma. *Am J Clin Oncol* 2006;29:202–206.
122. Rosignoli M, Pezzuto RW, Galli J, et al. Midline granuloma and Wegener's granulomatosis. *Acta Otorhinolaryngol Ital* 1992;38(Suppl 12):1–46.
135. Sakata K, Hareyama M, Oouchi A, et al. Treatment of localized non-Hodgkin's lymphomas of the head and neck: focusing on cases of non-lethal midline granuloma. *Radiat Oncol Invest* 1998;6:161–169.
146. Ganz JC, Abdelkarim K. Glomus jugulare tumors: certain clinical and radiologic aspects observed following Gamma Knife radiosurgery. *Acta Neurochir* 2009;151: 423–426.
147. Kadish S, Goodman M, Wang CC. Olfactory neuroblastoma: a clinical analysis of 17 cases. *Cancer* 1976;37:1571–1576.
151. Foote RL, Morita A, Ebersold MJ, et al. Esthesioneuroblastoma: the role of adjuvant radiation therapy. *Int J Radiat Oncol Biol Phys* 1993;27:835–842.
153. Miyamoto RC, Gleich LL, Biddinger PW, et al. Esthesioneuroblastoma and sinonasal undifferentiated carcinoma: impact of histological grading and clinical staging on survival and prognosis. *Laryngoscope* 2000;110:1262–1265.
156. Dias FL, Sa GM, Lima RA, et al. Patterns of failure and outcome in esthesioneuroblastoma. *Arch Otolaryngol Head Neck Surg* 2003;129:1186–1192.
157. Bentz BG, Singh B, Woodruff J, et al. Head and neck soft tissue sarcomas: a multivariate analysis of outcomes. *Ann Surg Oncol* 2004;11:619–628.
159. Gruber G, Laedrach K, Baumert B, et al. Esthesioneuroblastoma: irradiation alone and surgery alone are not enough. *Int J Radiat Oncol Biol Phys* 2002;54:486–491.
160. Ozsahin M, Gruber G, Olszik O, et al. Outcome and prognostic factors in olfactory neuroblastoma: a rare cancer network study. *Int J Radiat Oncol Biol Phys* 2010; 78:993–997.
161. Sperry JL, Reis I, Casiano RR, et al. Esthesioneuroblastoma: a modern experience at the University of Miami. *Int J Radiat Oncol Biol Phys* 2010;78(Suppl 3): S472 (abstr 2603).
162. Madani I, Bonte K, Vakaet L, et al. Intensity modulated radiotherapy for sinasal tumors: Ghent University Hospital update. *Int J Radiat Oncol Biol Phys* 2009;73: 424–432.
163. Nishimura H, Ogino T, Kawashima M, et al. Proton-beam therapy for olfactory neuroblastoma. *Int J Radiat Oncol Biol Phys* 2007;68:758–762.
166. Sohrabi S, Drabick JJ, Crist H, et al. Neoadjuvant concurrent chemoradiation for advanced esthesioneuroblastoma: a case series and review of the literature. *J Clin Oncol* 2011,29(13).e358–e361.
168. Noh OK, Lee S-w, Yoon SM, et al. Radiotherapy for esthesioneuroblastoma: is elective nodal irradiation warranted in the multimodality treatment approach? *Int J Radiat Oncol Biol Phys* 2011;79:443–449.
170. Kased N, El-sayed IH, Weinberg VK, et al. Intensity modulated radiation therapy for esthesioneuroblastoma: clinical outcomes and toxicity. Int J Radiat Oncol Biol Phys Proc 52th ASTRO Annual Meeting S447 (abstr 2545).
172. Platek ME, Mashtare TL, Popat SR, et al. Improved survival following surgery and radiation for olfactory neuroblastoma: analysis of the SEER database. *Int J Radiat Oncol Biol Phys* 2009;75(Suppl 3):S396 (abstr 2478).
175. Polin RS, Sheehan JP, Chenelle AG, et al. The role of preoperative adjuvant treatment in the management of esthesioneuroblastoma: the University of Virginia experience. *Neurosurgery* 1998;42:1029–1037.
178. Payne BR, Prasad D, Steiner M, et al. Gamma surgery for hemangiopericytomas. *Acta Neurochir (Wien)* 2000;142:527–536.
180. Michalski VJ, Hall J, Henk JM, et al. Definitive radiotherapy for extramedullary plasmacytomas of the head and neck. *Br J Radiol* 2003;76:738–741.

185. Bachard G, Goldstein D, Brown D, et al. Solitary extramedullary plasmacytoma of the head and neck-Long-term outcome analysis of 68 cases. *Head Neck* 2008;30:1012–1019.
193. Holland J, Trenkner DA, Wasserman TH, et al. Plasmacytoma: treatment results and conversion to myeloma. *Cancer* 1992;69:1513–1517.
197. Tournier-Rangeard L, Lapeyre M, Graff-Caillaud P, et al. Radiotherapy for solitary extramedullary plasmacytoma in the head-and-neck region: a dose greater than 45 Gy to the target volume improves the local control. *Int J Radiat Oncol Biol Phys* 2006;64:1013–1017.
198. Sasaki R, Yasuda K, Abe E, et al. Multi-institutional analysis of solitary extramedullary plasmacytoma of the head and neck treated with curative radiotherapy. *Int J Radiat Oncol Biol Phys* 2012;82(2):626–634.
203. Creach KM, Foote RL, Neben-Wittich MA, et al. Radiotherapy for extramedullary plasmacytoma of the head and neck. *Int J Radiat Oncol Biol Phys* 2009;73: 789–794.
204. Wu W, Shi JX, Cheng HL, et al. Hemangiopericytomas in the central nervous system. *J Clin Neurosci* 2009;16:519–523.
205. Ang KK, Peters LJ, Weber RS, et al. Postoperative radiotherapy for cutaneous melanoma of the head and neck region. *Int J Radiat Oncol Biol Phys* 1994;30: 795–798.
208. Algazi AP, Soon CW, Daud AI. Treatment of cutaneous melanoma: current approaches and future prospects. *Cancer Manag Res* 2010;2:197–211.
216. Ochoa-Carrillo FJ, Carrillo JF, Frias M. Staging and treatment of nasopharyngeal angiofibroma. *Eur Arch Otorhinolaryngol* 1997;254:200–204.
220. Radkowski D, McGill T, Healy GB, et al. Angiofibroma. Changes in staging and treatment. *Arch Otolaryngol Head Neck Surg* 1996;122:122–129.
222. Sun XC, Wang DH, Yu HP, et al. Analysis of reisk factors associated with recurrence of nasopharyngeal angiofibroma. *J Otoraryngol Head Neck Surg* 2010;39: 56–61.
224. Lee JT, Chen P, Safa A, et al. The role of radiation in the treatment of advanced juvenile angiofibroma. *Laryngoscope* 2002;112:1213–1220.
225. Carrillo JF, Maldonado F, Albores O, et al. Juvenile nasopharyngeal angiofibroma: clinical factors associated with recurrence and proposal for a staging system. *J Surg Oncol* 2008;98:75–80.
226. Claus F, Boterberg T, Ost P, et al. Short term toxicity profile for 32 sinonasal tumor patients treated with IMRT: Can we avoid dry eye syndrome? *Radiother Oncol* 2002;64:205–208.
227. Duthoy W, Boterberg T, Claus F, et al. Postoperative intensity modulated radiotherapy in sinonasal carcinoma: clinical results in 39 patients. *Cancer* 2005;104: 71–82.
228. Hoppe BS, Stegman LD, Zelefski MJ et al. Treatment of nasal cavity and paranasal sinus cancer with modern radiotherapy techniques in the postoperative setting: the MSKCC experience. *Int J Radiat Oncol Biol Phys* 2007;67: 691–702.
230. Dirix P, Nuyts S, Vanstraelen B, et al. Post-operative intensity modulated radiotherapy for malignancies of the nasal cavity and paranasal sinuses. *Radiother Oncol* 2007;69:1042–1050.
231. Cummings BJ, Blend R, Fitzpatrick P, et al. Primary radiation therapy for juvenile nasopharyngeal angiofibroma. *Laryngoscope* 1984;94:1599–1604.
240. Roche PH, Paris J, Regis J, et al. Management of invasive juvenile nasopharyngeal angiofibroma: the role of a multimodality approach. *Neurosurgery* 2007;61: 768–777.
242. McAfee WJ, Morris CG, Amdur RJ, et al. Definitive radiotherapy for juvenile nasopharyngeal angiofibroma. *Am J Clin Oncol* 2006;29:168–170.
243. Kasper ME, Parsons JT, Mancuso AA, et al. Radiation therapy for juvenile angiofibroma: evaluation by CT and MRI, analysis of tumor regression, and selection of patients. *Int J Radiat Oncol Biol Phys* 1993;25:689–694.
249. Tseng WH, Martinez SR. Tumor location predicts survival in cutaneous head and neck melanoma. *J Surg Res* 2011;167:192–198.
251. Khan N, Khan MK, Almasan A, et al. The evolving role of radiation therapy in the mangment of malignant melanoma. *Int J Radiat Oncol Biol Phys* 2011;80(3): 645–654.
254. Bibault J-E, Dewas S, Mirabel X, et al. Adjuvant radiation therapy in metastatic lymph nodes from melanoma. *Radiat Oncol* 2011;6:12–18.
262. Rapini RP, Golitz LE, Greer RO, et al. Primary malignant melanoma of the oral cavity: a review of 117 cases. *Cancer* 1985;55:1543–1551.
267. Krengli M, Masini L, Kaanders JHAM, et al. Radiotherapy in the treatment of mucosal melanoma of the upper aerodigestive tract: analysis of 74 cases. A rare cancer network study. *Int J Radiat Oncol Biol Phys* 2006;65:751–759.
269. Yanagi T, Mizoe J-E, Hasegawa A, et al. Mucosal malignant melanoma of the head and neck treated by carbon ion radiotherapy. *Int J Radiat Oncol Biol Phys* 2009;74:15–20.
273. Erickson C, Miller SJ. Treatment options in melanoma in situ: topcal and radiation therapy, excision and Mohs surgery. *Int J Dermatol* 2010;49:482–491.
277. VanDamme JP, Schmitz S, Machiels JP, et al. Prognostic factors and assessment of staging systems for head and neck soft tissue sarcomas in adults. *Eur J Surg Oncol* 2010;36:684–690.
280. LeVay J, O'Sullivan B, Catton C, et al. An assessment of prognostic factors in soft tissue sarcoma of the head and neck. *Arch Otolaryngol Head Neck Surg* 1994; 120:981–986.
284. Willers H, Hug E, Spiro I, et al. Adult soft tissue sarcomas of the head and neck treated by radiation and surgery or radiation alone: patterns of failure and prognostic factors. *Int J Radiat Oncol Biol Phys* 1995;33:585–593.
287. Ketabchi A, Kalavrezos N, Newman L. Sarcomas of the head and neck: a 10-year retrospective of 25 patients to evaluate treatment modalities, function and survival. *Br J Oral Maxillofac Surg* 2011;49:116–120.
290. Strander H, Turesson I, Cavallin-Stahl E. A systematic overview of radiation therapy effects in soft tissue sarcomas. *Acta Oncol* 2003;42:516–531.
292. Laramore GE. Role of particle radiotherapy in the management of head and neck cancer. *Curr Opin Oncol* 2009;21:224–231.
293. Hug EB, Hanssens PE, Liebsch NJ, et al. Soft tissue sarcomas of the head and neck: results of combined proton and photon radiation therapy using 3-D treatment planning. *Int J Radiat Oncol Biol Phys* YEAR;30(Suppl 1):222 (abstr 119).
294. Jingu K, Mizoe J-E, Hasegawa A, et al. Improvement in the prognosis of unresectable bone and soft tissue sarcomas in the adult head and neck by carbon ion radiation therapy: results of a phase I/I study. *Int J Radiat Oncol Biol Phys* 2009;75(Suppl 3):S524 (abstr 2760).
295. Penel N, Van Haverbeke C, Lartigau E, et al. Head and neck soft tissue sarcomas of adult: prognostic value of surgery in multimodal therapeutic approach. *Oral Oncol* 2004;40:890–897.
296. Wolden SL, Wexler LH, Kraus DH, et al. Intensity modulated radiation therapy for head and neck rhabdomyosarcoma. *Int J Radiat Oncol Biol Phys* 2005;61: 1432–1438.
297. McDonald MW, Esiashvili N, George BA, et al. Intensity modulated radiotherapy with cone-down boost for pediatric head and neck rhabdomyosarcoma. *Int J Radiat Oncol Biol Phys* 2008;72:884–891.
299. Weber DC, Rutz HP, Pedroni ES, et al. Results of spot-scanning proton radiation therapy of chordoma and chondrosarcoma of the skull base: the Paul Scherrer Institute experience. *Int J Radiat Oncol Bio Phys* 2005;83:401–409.

Chapter 49
Neck Cancer Including Unknown Primary Tumor

William M. Mendenhall, Anthony A. Mancuso, Robert J. Amdur, and John W. Werning

ANATOMY

The locations of the various lymph node groups in the head and neck are shown in Figure 49.1.[1] Under normal conditions, the right and left lymphatic networks do not shunt from one side to the other.[2]

The internal jugular chain (IJC) lymph nodes lie adjacent to the internal jugular vein and extend from the skull base to the clavicle. The most superior group of lymph nodes in this chain lies near the base of the skull in the posterior aspect of the lateral pharyngeal space and is often referred to as the parapharyngeal or junctional lymph nodes. These lymph nodes lie deep to the sternocleidomastoid muscle, the posterior belly of the digastric muscle, and the tail of the parotid gland. The remaining IJC lymph nodes are artificially divided into the subdigastric, middle jugular, and lower jugular groups.

The spinal accessory chain (SAC) lymph nodes are distributed along the course of cranial nerve XI. The superior nodes of the SAC blend with the upper IJC nodes. The supraclavicular lymph nodes merge laterally with the SAC lymph nodes and medially with the lower IJC lymph nodes.

There are three to six submandibular lymph nodes. They may be either preglandular or postglandular; there are no lymph nodes in the substance of the submandibular gland. The submental lymph nodes lie in the midline between the anterior bellies of the digastric muscles, anterior to the hyoid bone and external to the mylohyoid muscle. The lateral retropharyngeal lymph nodes lie within the retropharyngeal space, which is bounded anteriorly by the pharyngeal constrictor muscles, superiorly by the skull base, and posteriorly by the prevertebral fascia. They are usually at the level of the C1 and C2 vertebral bodies but may be found as inferiorly as C3. The medial retropharyngeal nodes are small, inconstant intercalated nodes that are located near midline and empty into the lateral retropharyngeal lymph nodes.

The neck nodes are divided into levels as follows: level I, submental (IA) and submandibular (IB) nodes; level II, upper internal jugular nodes, from the skull base to the level of the

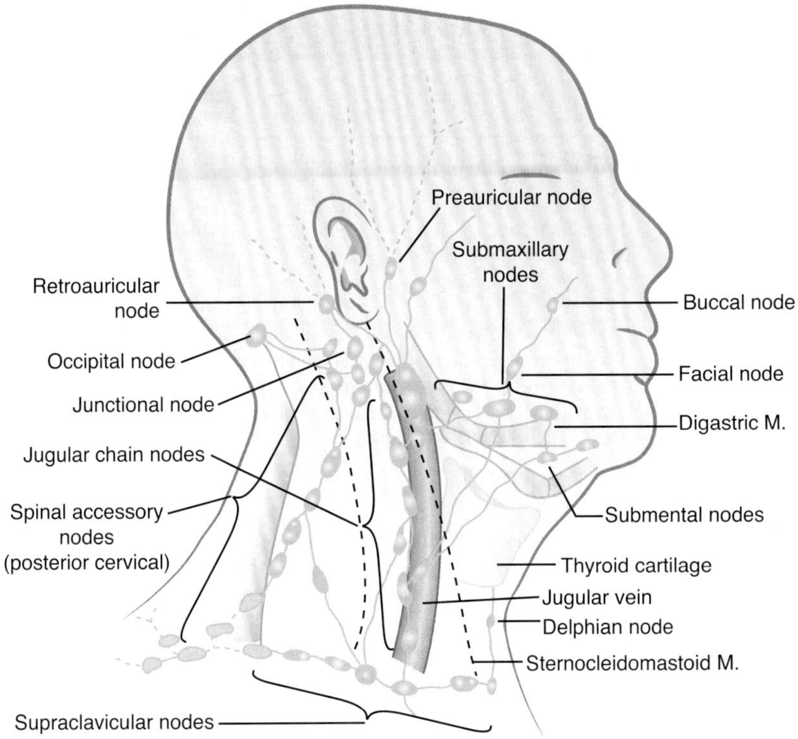

FIGURE 49.1. Arrangement of lymph nodes in the head and neck. (Redrawn from Rouviere H. *Anatomy of the human lymphatic system,* Tobias MJ [trans]: Ann Arbor, MI: Edwards Brothers, 1938:27.)

hyoid bone; level III, middle internal jugular nodes, from the level of the hyoid bone to the omohyoid muscle; level IV, inferior internal jugular nodes, from the level of the omohyoid muscle to the clavicle; level V, spinal accessory lymph nodes; and level VI, anterior neck nodes, bounded by the hyoid bone, the sternum, and the common carotid arteries. Included in level VI are the paratracheal, pretracheal, precricoid (Delphian), and tracheo-esophageal groove nodes.[3]

NATURAL HISTORY

The risk of lymph node metastases is influenced by the location of the primary tumor, histologic differentiation, size of the lesion, and the availability of capillary lymphatics.[4–7] The estimated risk of subclinical disease in the clinically negative neck

TABLE 49.1 DEFINITION OF RISK GROUPS

Group	*Estimated Risk of Subclinical Neck Disease*	*Stage*	*Site*
I: Low risk	<20%	T1	Floor of mouth, retromolar trigone, gingiva, hard palate, buccal mucosa
II: Intermediate risk	20% to 30%	T1	Oral tongue, soft palate, pharyngeal wall, supraglottic larynx, tonsil
		T2	Floor of mouth, oral tongue, retromolar trigone, gingiva, hard palate, buccal mucosa
III: High risk	>30%	T1–4	Nasopharynx, pyriform sinus, base of tongue
		T2–4	Soft palate, pharyngeal wall, supraglottic larynx, tonsil
		T3–4	Flour of mouth, oral tongue, retromolar trigone, gingiva, hard palate, buccal mucosa

From Mendenhall WM, Million RR. Elective neck irradiation for squamous cell carcinoma of the head and neck: analysis of time–dose factors and causes of failure. *Int J Radiat Oncol Biol Phys* 1986;12:741–746, with permission.

as a function of primary site and tumor (T) stage is shown in Table 49.1.[4] Recurrent lesions have a higher risk of lymphatic involvement than untreated lesions.

The relative incidence of clinically positive lymph nodes in the neck by anatomic site and T stage is shown in Table 49.2.[5] The most commonly involved lymph nodes in the head and neck are the level II lymph nodes, followed by the level III lymph nodes. Lesions that are well lateralized almost always spread first to the ipsilateral neck nodes. Lesions on or near the midline as well as lateralized base of tongue and nasopharyngeal lesions may spread to both sides of the neck.

Patients who have clinically positive lymph nodes on the ipsilateral side of the neck may be at risk for contralateral lymph node spread if the metastatic masses produce significant obstruction of the lymphatic trunks. In addition, patients who have undergone previous surgery on one side of the neck develop shunting of lymph across the submental region to the opposite side of the neck. When contralateral lymph node metastases occur, the level II lymph nodes are most frequently involved, followed by the level III and level IV lymph node groups.

As tumor grows within a lymph node, the node becomes indurated and more rounded, and enlarges. Tumor eventually extends through the capsule of the lymph node and invades surrounding structures. Extension to the neurovascular bundle is common and may produce a mass that is considered fixed to palpation. The incidence of tumor involvement and the likelihood of capsular penetration as a function of lymph node size are shown in Table 49.3.[6]

The risk of lateral retropharyngeal lymph node involvement is related to primary site and neck stage[7]; the medial retropharyngeal nodes are almost never the site of metastatic disease. The incidence of positive retropharyngeal nodes based on pretreatment computed tomography (CT) and, in selected cases, magnetic resonance imaging (MRI) is shown in Table 49.4.[7]

DIAGNOSTIC WORKUP

Physical Examination

The patient is examined in the sitting position, the examiner behind the patient with one hand on the occiput to flex the

TABLE 49.2 CLINICALLY DETECTED NODAL METASTASES ON ADMISSION CORRELATED WITH T STAGE

Primary Site	T Stage	N0 (%)	N1 (%)	N2–3 (%)
Oral tongue[a]	T1	86	10	4
	T2	70	19	11
	T3	52	16	31
	T4	24	10	66
Floor of mouth[a]	T1	89	9	2
	T2	71	18	10
	T3	56	20	24
	T4	46	10	43
Retromolar trigone/anterior tonsillar pillar[b]	T1	88	2	9
	T2	62	18	20
	T3	46	21	33
	T4	32	18	50
Soft palate[b]	T1	92	0	8
	T2	64	12	24
	T3	35	26	39
	T4	33	11	56
Tonsillar fossa[b]	T1	30	41	30
	T2	32	14	54
	T3	30	18	52
	T4	10	13	76
Base of tongue[b]	T1	30	15	55
	T2	29	14	56
	T3	26	23	52
	T4	16	8	76
Oropharyngeal walls[b]	T1	75	0	25
	T2	70	10	20
	T3	33	22	44
	T4	24	24	52
Supraglottic larynx[c]	T1	61	10	29
	T2	58	16	26
	T3	16	25	40
	T4	26	18	41
Hypopharynx[d]	T1	37	21	42
	T2	30	20	49
	T3	21	26	54
	T4	26	15	58
Nasopharynx[e]	T1	8	11	82
	T2	16	12	72
	T3	12	9	80
	T4	17	6	78

Data are those of 2,044 patients, M.D. Anderson Hospital, Houston, TX, 1948–1965.

[a]T stage defined by Lindberg.[5] [b]T stage defined by Fletcher et al.[78]

[c]T stage defined by Fletcher et al.[79] [d]T stage defined by MacComb et al.[80]

[e]T stage defined by Chen and Fletcher.[81]

Modified from Lindberg RD. Distribution of cervical lymph node metastases from squamous cell carcinoma of the upper respiratory and digestive tracts. *Cancer* 1972; 29:1446–1449.

patient's head forward and the other hand on the side of the neck to be examined. To examine the IJC lymph nodes, which lie deep to the sternocleidomastoid muscle along the internal jugular vein, place the thumb and index finger around the sternocleidomastoid muscle in the form of a "C" and then gently proceed from the sternal notch to the angle of the mandible. Both sides of the neck should not be examined simultaneously. The level Ib and level Ia nodes may be evaluated by direct palpation of these areas as well as by a bimanual examination with the index finger placed in the floor of the mouth.[8]

TABLE 49.3 RELATIONSHIP BETWEEN NODE SIZE, THE PRESENCE OF TUMOR IN THE NODE, AND CAPSULAR PENETRATION IN 519 NODES[a]

	Size of Node (cm)				
	1	2	3	4	≥5
Number of nodes	177	183	84	17	58
Percentage positive	33	62	81	88	100
Percentage positive with capsular penetration	14	26	49	71	76

[a]Institut Gustave-Roussy, Villejuif, France.

Modified from Richard JM, Sancho-Garnier H, Micheau C. Prognostic factors in cervical lymph node metastasis in upper respiratory and digestive tract carcinoma: study of 1713 cases during a 15-year period. *Laryngoscope* 1987;97:97–101.

TABLE 49.4 INCIDENCE OF POSITIVE RETROPHARYNGEAL NODES FOR VARIOUS PRIMARY SITES AND CLINICAL NECK STAGES (794 TUMORS)

	Clinical Neck Stage		
Primary Site	N0 Neck (%)	N+ Neck[a] (%)	Overall (%)
Nasopharynx	2/5 (40)	12/14 (86)	74
Pharyngeal wall	6/37 (16)	12/56 (21)	19
Soft palate	1/21 (5)	6/32 (19)	13
Tonsillar region	2/56 (4)	14/120 (12)	9
Pyriform sinus or postcricoid area	0/55 (0)	7/81 (9)	5
Base of tongue	0/31 (0)	5/90 (6)	4
Supraglottic larynx	0/87 (0)	4/109 (4)	2

[a]N+ are neck nodes clinically involved (stages N1–3B).

From McLaughlin MP, Mendenhall WM, Mancuso AA, et al. Retropharyngeal adenopathy as a predictor of outcome in squamous cell carcinoma of the head and neck. *Head Neck* 1995;17:190–198, with permission.

The following features of metastatic lymph nodes should be recorded: anatomic location, size, consistency, mobility, and clinical impression as to whether the node is involved with cancer.

Radiographic Evaluation

CT, MRI, fluorodeoxyglucose–positron emission tomography (FDG-PET), and ultrasound may be used to evaluate cervical metastatic disease.[9] At the University of Florida, CT remains the primary method of examination of most carcinomas arising in the upper aerodigestive tract and the regional lymphatic system. MRI is the primary study only in patients with nasopharyngeal malignancies. MRI also may be used in patients who are allergic to intravenous contrast medium. Ultrasound has been used mainly in Europe to evaluate the cervical nodes. FDG-PET may be used to evaluate equivocal suspicious lymph nodes if the results of the scan would alter the treatment plan. Positive nodes <1 cm will not be reliably detected on a PET scan. FDG-PET remains unproven with regard to improving accuracy rates over those available with properly performed and interpreted CT.

Small metastases may be seen as lucent foci in normal-sized nodes. Such metastases have been identified and surgically confirmed in nodes as small as 6 to 8 mm; however, most subclinical disease in normal-sized nodes remains undetected on CT. FDG-PET has a marginal capability to improve on CT in detecting the subclinical disease in small (<1 cm) nodes.

Lucent foci in normal-sized nodes must be differentiated from hilar fat or volume-averaging artifacts. As the metastasis grows, the node becomes more spherical than elliptical. Areas of necrosis are almost always present in nodal metastases larger than 2 cm. As the metastasis enlarges, the capsule of the node becomes hyperemic and is seen radiographically as a contrast-enhanced rim. When the capsule becomes indistinct and irregular along its outer margin, it is highly suggestive of early capsular penetration. Continued growth causes obliteration of the fat planes surrounding the nodes. Finally, no clear plane of normal tissue lies between the mass and the adjacent structures, at which point the clinician usually notes fixation (Fig. 49.2). Penetration of the prevertebral fascia and fixation to the scalene muscles are uncommon in untreated patients. Largely necrotic nodes may be negative on FDG-PET examinations.

If a node shows evidence of capsular penetration and envelops more than 50% of the circumference of the carotid artery, clinical evidence of fixation to the artery is likely. Ultrasound

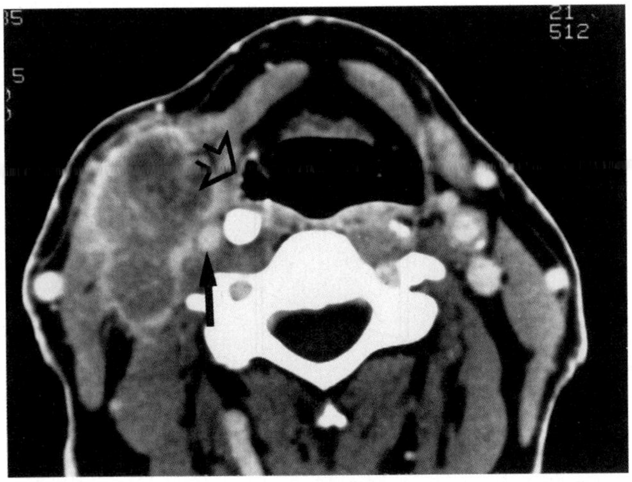

FIGURE 49.2. T1 squamous cell carcinoma of the lateral wall of the right pyriform sinus (*open arrow*) and a fixed N3B neck node that abuts but does not surround the carotid artery (*solid arrow*). Mendenhall WM, Parsons JT, Mancuso AA, et al. Head and neck: management of the neck. In: Perez CA, Brady LW, Halperin EC, et al., eds. *Principles and practice of radiation oncology.* Philadelphia: Lippincott Williams and Wilkins 2004:1158–1178.

and MRI may prove useful in evaluating tumor extension to the carotid, as suggested by CT. MRI tends to be better at excluding extension to the neurovascular bundle when it is suspected on CT, whereas ultrasound can help show invasion of the vessel wall, thus confirming focal extension to the artery.

STAGING

The staging systems shown in Table 49.5 are those of the American Joint Committee on Cancer (AJCC). Because all University of Florida data presented in this chapter were analyzed using the 1983 AJCC staging system,[10] both the 1983 and 2010 systems are outlined in Table 49.5. Stage N3C in the 1983 system is rare and should alert the clinician to search for another primary lesion. The 2010 AJCC staging system classifies bilateral or contralateral nodes not more than 6 cm in diameter as N2C; N3 is defined as a metastasis in a lymph node more than 6 cm in diameter.[11] The AJCC nodal staging system for head and neck cancer has not changed appreciably since the 1997 edition. The AJCC nodal staging for nasopharyngeal carcinoma differs from other head and neck primary sites and will be discussed in the chapter devoted to that topic.

SURGERY

Standard radical neck dissection involves removal of the superficial and deep cervical fascia with its lymph nodes in levels I to V in continuity with the sternocleidomastoid muscle, omohyoid muscle, internal and external jugular veins, spinal accessory nerve, and submandibular gland. Sacrifice of cranial nerve XI often, but not always, results in atrophy of the trapezius muscle, with shoulder drop and discomfort.

Modified radical neck dissection removes the superficial and deep cervical fascia with its enclosed lymph nodes and leaves one or more of the nonlymphatic structures such as the sternocleidomastoid and digastric muscles, internal jugular vein, and spinal accessory nerve. Currently, almost all of the patients treated with neck dissection at the authors' institution undergo this operation with at least preservation of cranial nerve XI. The advantages of the functional neck dissection are less cosmetic deformity and better function.

For a selective neck dissection, one or more of lymph node groups I to V are not removed. The advantage of the selective neck dissection is that it provides equivalent efficacy and less morbidity in appropriately selected cases. Supraomohyoid neck dissection removes the lymph nodes in levels I to III and is most commonly used for patients with small oral cavity cancers and

TABLE 49.5 1983 AND 2010 AMERICAN JOINT COMMITTEE ON CANCER STAGING FOR NECK LYMPH NODES

Stage	*Definition*
1983 Stage	
NX	Nodes cannot be assessed
N0	No clinically positive nodes
N1	Single clinically positive homolateral node 3 cm or less in diameter
N2	Single clinically positive homolateral node more than 3 cm but not >6 cm in diameter or multiple clinically positive homolateral nodes, none >6 cm in diameter
N2A	Single clinically positive homolateral node >3 cm but not >6 cm in diameter
N2B	Multiple clinically positive homolateral nodes, none >6 cm in diameter
N3A	Clinically positive homolateral node(s), one >6 cm in diameter
N3B	Bilateral clinically positive nodes (in this situation, each side of the neck should be staged separately (i.e., N3B, right; N2A, left, N1)
N3C	Contralateral clinically positive node(s) only
2010 Stage	
NX	Regional lymph nodes cannot be assessed
N0	No regional lymph node metastasis
N1	Metastasis in a single ipsilateral lymph node, 3 cm or less in greatest dimension
N2	Metastasis in a single ipsilateral lymph node, more than 3 cm but not more than 6 cm in greatest dimension; or in multiple ipsilateral lymph nodes, none more than 6 cm in greatest dimensions; or in bilateral or contralateral lymph nodes, none more than 6 cm in greatest dimension
N2A	Metastasis in single ipsilateral lymph node more than 3 cm but not more than 6 cm in greatest dimension
N2B	Metastasis in multiple ipsilateral lymph nodes, none more than 6 cm in greatest dimension
N2C	Metastasis in bilateral or contralateral lymph nodes, none more than 6 cm in greatest dimension
N3	Metastasis in a lymph node more than 6 cm in greatest dimension

Used with the permission of the American Joint Committee on Cancer (AJCC), Chicago, Illinois. The original source for this material is the *AJCC Cancer Staging Handbook,* 7th ed. (2010) published by Springer Science and Business Media LLC, www.springerlink.com

a clinically negative neck. The lateral neck dissection entails removal of level II to IV nodes and is most often used in the treatment of laryngeal, oropharyngeal, and hypopharyngeal cancers. If significant metastatic adenopathy is encountered during a selective neck dissection, it should be converted to a radical or modified radical dissection.

An extended radical neck dissection implies removal of additional lymph node groups or nonlymphatic structures in addition to the structures removed in a radical neck dissection. Bilateral neck dissections may be performed simultaneously or separately (staged) in patients with bilateral neck disease as long as one internal jugular vein can be preserved. At one time, simultaneous neck dissection appeared to be associated with a higher incidence of complications and operative mortality compared with staged neck dissections.[12,13] The authors' more recent experience suggests that this is no longer the case.

Complications of Neck Dissection

Complications of neck dissection include hematoma, seroma, lymphedema, wound infection, wound dehiscence, chyle fistula, damage to cranial nerves VII, X, XI, and XII, carotid exposure, and carotid rupture. The incidence of complications is higher when neck dissection is combined with resection of the primary lesion or when it follows a course of radiation therapy (RT). The postoperative mortality rate for unilateral neck dissection after RT was 3% for patients treated between 1964 and 1982.[14]

The incidence of postoperative complications in a series of patients treated with RT to the primary lesion and neck followed by unilateral or bilateral neck dissection(s) is shown in Tables 49.6[14] and 49.7.[15] Two of 10 patients undergoing a

TABLE 49.6 POSTOPERATIVE COMPLICATIONS OF UNILATERAL NECK DISSECTION AFTER IRRADIATION TO THE PRIMARY LESION AND NECK (143 PATIENTS)

Complications	Number Complications	Number Second Operations to Repair Complication	Death
Salivary fistula	1	0	0
Wound breakdown	23	15	0
Bleeding	2	1	1
Pneumonia	2	0	1
Orocutaneous fistula	1	1	0
Lymphatic fistula	2	0	0
Pulmonary embolus	1	0	0
Cardiovascular problem	2	0	1
Sepsis	1	0	1
Total complications	35[a]	17	4[b]
Incidence (%)	33/143 (23)	17/143 (12)	4/143 (3)

[a]Thirty-five complications in 33 patients.

[b]Deaths occurred 6, 7, 8, and 35 days after surgery.

From Mendenhall WM, Million RR, Cassisi NJ. Squamous cell carcinoma of the head and neck treated with radiation therapy: the role of neck dissection for clinically positive neck nodes. *Int J Radiat Oncol Biol Phys* 1986;12:733–740, with permission.

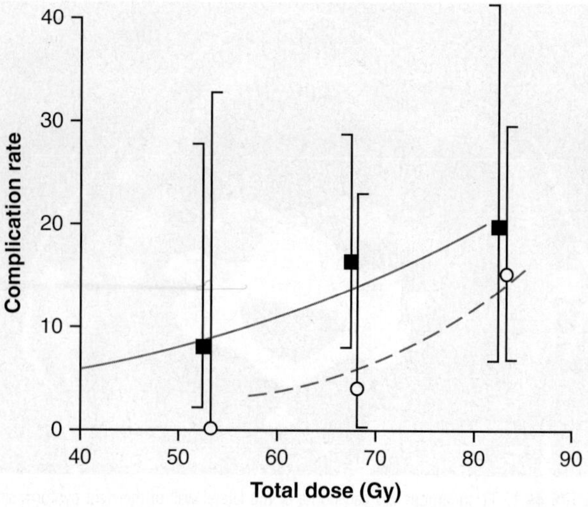

FIGURE 49.3. Complication rate (2+ or 3+) versus total dose. Separate analysis for once a day (filled square, *solid curve*) and twice a day (circle, *dashed curve*). Data are plotted at the midpoints of the range 45 to 60 Gy, 60 to 70 Gy, and 75 to 90 Gy. Error bars denote 95% confidence intervals. The curves are the results of separate logistic regression analysis. (From Taylor JMG, Mendenhall WM, Parsons JT, et al. The influence of dose and time on wound complications following post-radiation neck dissection. *Int J Radiat Oncol Biol Phys* 1992;23:41–46, with permission.)

staged bilateral neck dissection experienced a moderately severe complication compared with 4 of 40 patients undergoing a simultaneous bilateral neck dissection. None of the 10 patients who underwent a staged bilateral neck dissection experienced a severe complication, compared with 6 of 40 patients (15%) who underwent a simultaneous bilateral neck dissection ($P = .24$).[15]

Taylor et al.[16] analyzed the incidence of moderate (2+) and severe (3+) wound complications in a series of 205 patients who underwent a planned unilateral neck dissection after RT at the University of Florida. RT was given once daily in 123 patients, twice daily in 80 patients, and with both techniques in the remaining two patients. The incidence of wound complications increased with total dose and dose per fraction (Fig. 49.3).

RADIATION THERAPY

RT may be used in the treatment of cervical lymph node metastases as elective treatment when there are no palpable lymph nodes, as the only treatment for clinically positive lymph nodes,[17] or as preoperative or postoperative treatment in combination with neck dissection for clinically positive lymph nodes.[18]

The regional lymph nodes are considered in the treatment planning of the primary lesion. With clinically negative neck nodes, treatment planning depends on the estimated risk of subclinical disease in the nodes. With clinically positive lymph nodes, the plan is influenced by the number of lymph nodes, size, and location.

TABLE 49.7 COMPLICATIONS AFTER RADIATION THERAPY FOLLOWED BY A BILATERAL NECK DISSECTION (N = 50 PATIENTS)

Severity	Complication	Number of Patients
Moderate	Wound breakdown	2
	Bleeding	1
	Laryngeal edema	2
	Chyle fistula	1
Severe	Wound breakdown	4
	Fatal cardiac arrest	1
	Fatal acute laryngeal edema	1

From Somerset JD, Mendenhall WM, Amdur RJ, et al. Planned postradiotherapy bilateral neck dissection for head and neck cancer. *Am J Otolaryngol* 2001;22:383–386, with permission.

Elective Radiation Therapy of Cervical Lymph Nodes When the Primary Tumor Is Treated by Radiation Therapy

Factors that influence the decision to irradiate the neck electively are site and size of the primary lesion, histologic grade, difficulty in neck examination, relative morbidity for adding lymph node coverage, likelihood of the patient's returning for follow-up examinations, and suitability of the patient for a radical neck dissection if the tumor appears in the neck at a later date. Patients in whom the primary lesion is to be treated by RT, who have clinically negative nodes, and in whom the risk of subclinical disease is 20% or greater usually receive elective neck irradiation to a minimum dose equivalent to 45 to 50 Gy over 4.5 to 5 weeks (see Table 49.1). Patients with lesions arising in the lip, nasal vestibule, nasal cavity, or paranasal sinuses have a low risk of subclinical neck disease, and the neck is not treated electively unless the lesion is recurrent, advanced, or poorly differentiated. Similarly, the risk of occult neck disease is essentially 0% for T1 and 1.7% for T2 glottic carcinomas, and elective neck radiation therapy is not indicated.[19,20]

The lateral treatment portals used to encompass cancers in the oropharynx, supraglottic larynx, and hypopharynx include the upper jugular and often the midjugular chain lymph nodes. RT portals used for primary lesions of the oral cavity, nasopharynx, glottis, nasal cavity, and paranasal sinuses must be enlarged to include the lymph nodes. The treatment portals for irradiation of the cervical lymph nodes must be designed in such a way as to minimize additional mucosal irradiation. A common error in irradiating oropharyngeal and nasopharyngeal cancers is to enlarge the lateral (primary) portals inferiorly to unnecessarily include all of the larynx in the lateral portals (Fig. 49.4).[21] Because the midneck is smaller in circumference than the upper neck, the total dose and dose per fraction are higher in the larynx than along the central axis of the beam, leading to double trouble. Although a field junction through a positive node(s) may be avoided with intensity-modulated radiation therapy (IMRT), the larynx still receives a substantially higher dose compared with a separate anterior low neck portal with a midline laryngeal block junctioned at the thyroid notch (Figs. 49.5, 49.6, and 49.7).[22] Treating an unnecessarily large

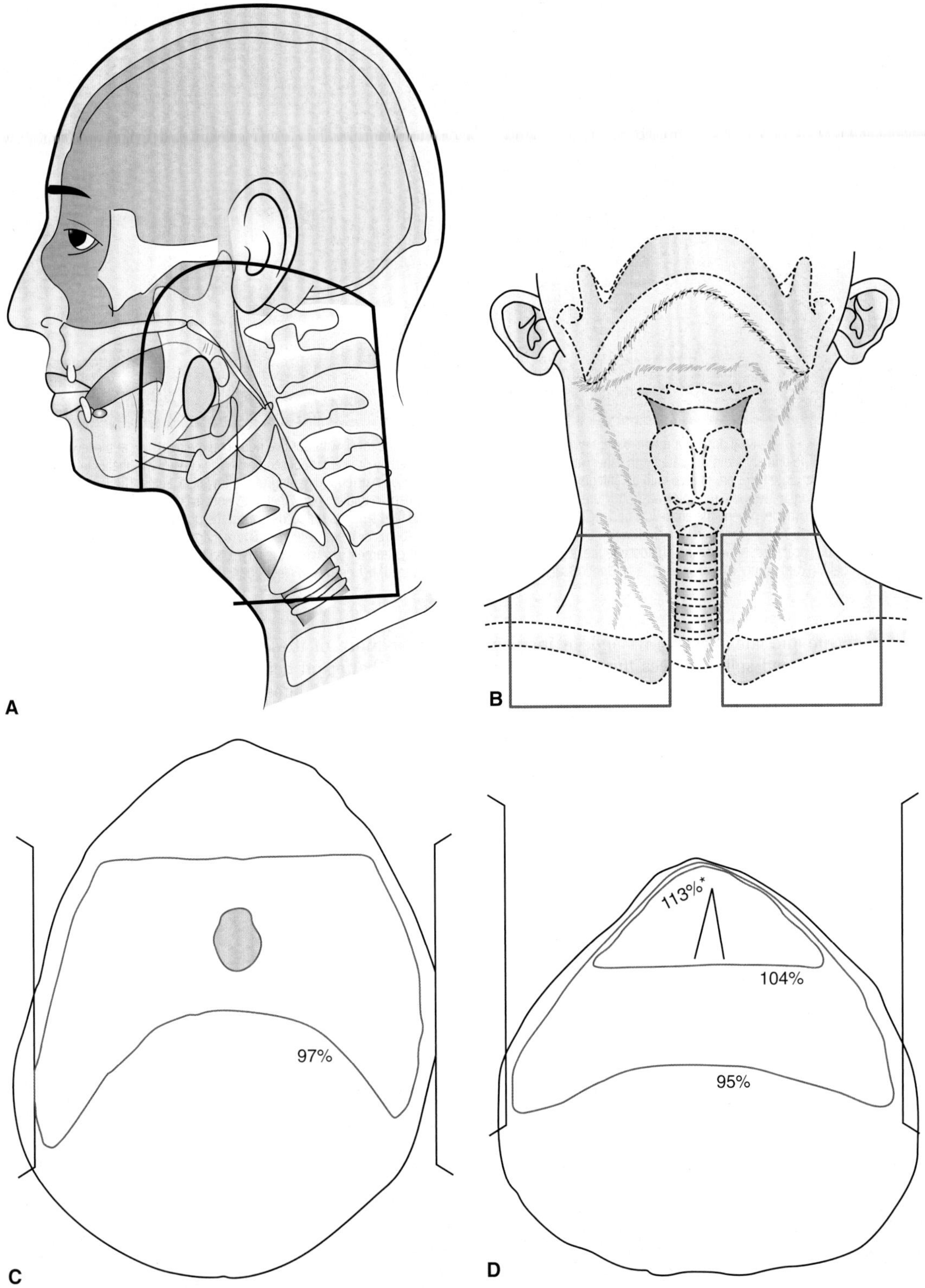

FIGURE 49.4. Carcinoma of the base of the tongue: large radiation portals. **A:** Parallel-opposed lateral portals include the primary lesion, larynx, hypopharynx, most of the cervical spinal cord, and the upper portion of the trachea and cervical esophagus. Treatment through this portal tangentially irradiates the skin of the anterior neck unnecessarily. If an anterior field is not used to irradiate the low neck, the inferior border of the lateral field may be placed near the clavicle (*dashed line*). **B:** Anterior low-neck portal. The wide midline tracheal block partially shields the low internal jugular lymph nodes, which are located adjacent to the trachea. The supraclavicular lymph nodes, which are less likely to be involved with tumor than the low jugular nodes, are adequately covered. **C:** Central axis dosimetry at the level of the base of tongue primary lesion. The contours were obtained from a RANDO phantom using parallel cobalt-60 fields weighted equally. The base of tongue tumor is outlined, and the tumor dose is specified at 97% of maximum dose. **D:** Off-axis contour through larynx. The minimum dose to the entire larynx is 104% of the maximum dose specified at the central axis, and the maximum dose on this off-axis contour is 113%. If the base of tongue tumor dose is specified as 50 Gy at 2 Gy per fraction, the minimum larynx dose is 53.61 Gy at 2.14 Gy per fraction, and the maximum larynx dose is 58.25 Gy at 2.33 Gy per fraction. If the tumor dose is specified as 60 Gy at 2 Gy per fraction, the minimum larynx dose is 64.33 Gy at 2.14 Gy per fraction, and the maximum larynx dose is 69.9 Gy at 2.33 Gy per fraction. (From Mendenhall WM, Parsons JT, Million RR. Unnecessary irradiation of the normal larynx [editorial]. *Int J Radiat Oncol Biol Phys* 1990;18:1531–1533, with permission.)

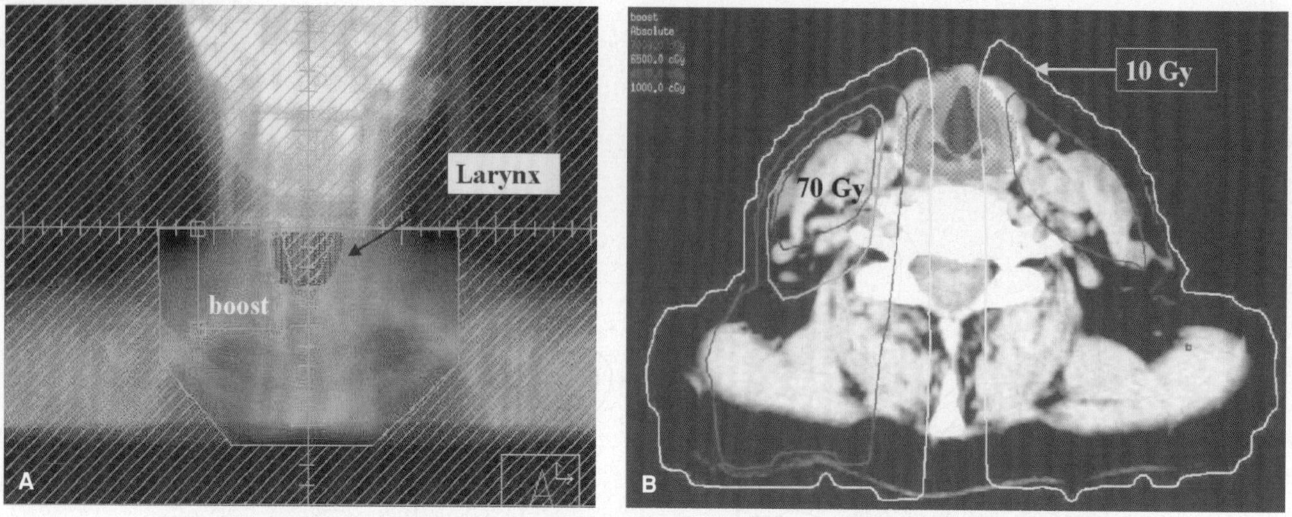

FIGURE 49.5. Laryngeal dose in a model patient with a stage T2N2b carcinoma of the tonsil with positive nodes on the right side at the level of the larynx. The primary site is irradiated with either intensity-modulated radiation therapy or lateral opposed fields. The cervical lymphatics inferior to the primary site fields are treated with an anterior low-neck field. **A:** Digitally reconstructed radiograph of the low-neck fields. The larynx was contoured and appears as a red color-wash structure. The larynx is shielded with a narrow midline block that does not cover the entire width of the larynx. In this model patient, the entire low-neck field received 50 Gy, and then the field size was reduced to boost the positive nodes on the right of the larynx to 70 Gy. Irradiation was given with a 6-MV photon beam with source to axis distance of 100 cm. **B:** Axial dose distribution at the level of the true vocal cords showing that the dose to the central portion of the larynx is extremely low when the larynx is shielded in the anterior low-neck field. (From Amdur RJ, Li JG, Liu C, et al. Unnecessary laryngeal irradiation in the IMRT era. *Head Neck* 2004;26:257–264, with permission.)

field increases the acute and late effects of RT and, by increasing the risk of an unplanned split, reduces the probability of disease control.[21,22]

IMRT may be used to treat patients if there is a goal that can be achieved to reduce the toxicity of irradiation. These goals are usually parotid sparing to reduce the risk of long-term xerostomia, avoiding a low neck match in patients with a low-lying larynx, and improved coverage of the poststyloid parapharyngeal space in patients with nasopharyngeal cancer.[23] If one or more of these goals cannot be achieved, the patients may be better off being treated with conventional RT because of the disadvantages of IMRT, which include increased risk of a marginal miss, less homogeneous dose distribution, and increased cost and complexity.[23]

Elective neck irradiation for early oral cavity lesions includes the level Ib and level II lymph nodes. The level III and level IV lymph nodes are treated as well by using a narrow anterior field. For primary lesions located in the oropharynx,

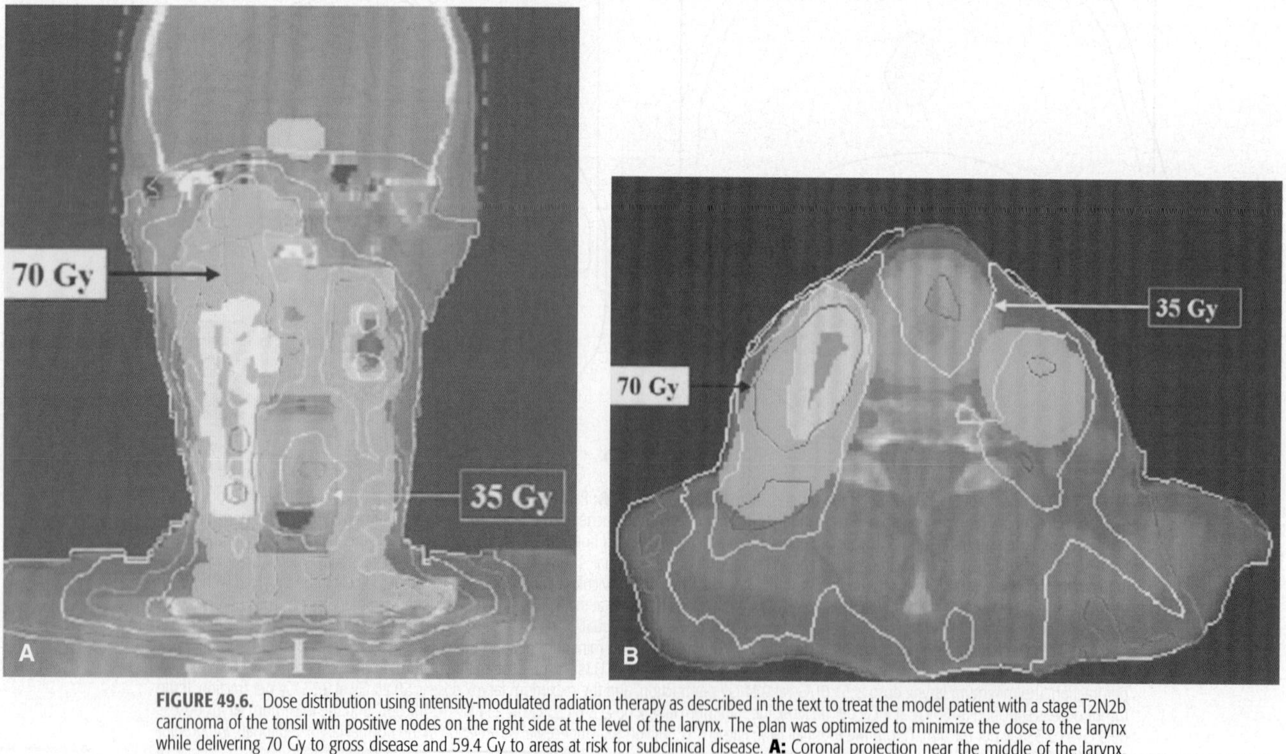

FIGURE 49.6. Dose distribution using intensity-modulated radiation therapy as described in the text to treat the model patient with a stage T2N2b carcinoma of the tonsil with positive nodes on the right side at the level of the larynx. The plan was optimized to minimize the dose to the larynx while delivering 70 Gy to gross disease and 59.4 Gy to areas at risk for subclinical disease. **A:** Coronal projection near the middle of the larynx. **B:** Axial projection at the level of the true vocal cords. A comparison of Figures 49.5B and 49.6B shows that sparing of the central portion of the larynx is shielded in an anterior low-neck field. (From Amdur RJ, Li JG, Liu C, et al. Unnecessary laryngeal irradiation in the IMRT era. *Head Neck* 2004;26:257–264, with permission.)

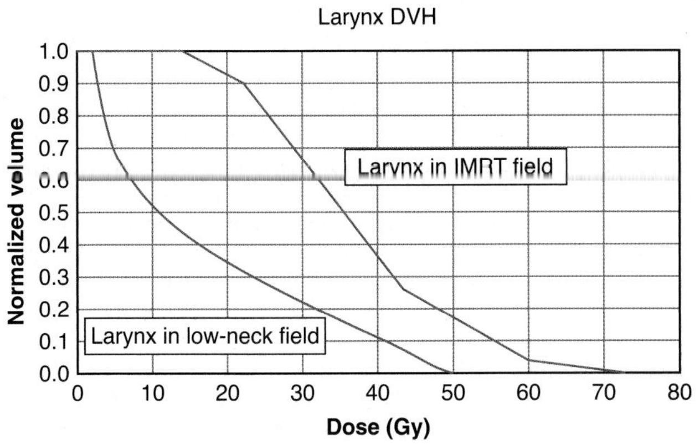

FIGURE 49.7. Dose–volume histogram of the larynx for the model patient described in Figures 49.5 and 49.6. The thicker line is the dose–volume histogram when the larynx is included in the intensity-modulated ration therapy (IMRT) fields shown in Figure 49.6. The thinner line is the dose–volume histogram when the larynx is shielded in the anterior low-neck field shown in Figure 49.5. There is a major difference in the portion of the larynx that receives an extremely low dose. For example, when the larynx is included in the IMRT fields, the entire larynx receives more than 10 Gy, whereas when the larynx is shielded in the low-neck field, approximately 45% of the larynx receives <10 Gy. (From Amdur RJ, Li JG, Liu C, et al. Unnecessary laryngeal irradiation in the IMRT era. *Head Neck* 2004;26:257–264, with permission.)

nasopharynx, supraglottic larynx, and hypopharynx, the lower neck nodes are also routinely included. The low neck is treated with a single anterior field (Fig. 49.8). A tapered midline larynx or trachea shield is added to protect the spinal cord, the larynx, and the pharynx. For primary lesions lying below the thyroid notch, a small midline tracheal block 5- to 10-mm wide is placed in the low-neck field, primarily to avoid field overlap at the spinal cord. A 1-cm wide midline block made of Lipowitz's metal may be used to shield the trachea, esophagus, and spinal cord below the level of the cricoid.

Treatment of Clinically Positive Cervical Lymph Nodes When the Primary Tumor Is Treated by Radiation Therapy

The dose required to control a clinically positive lymph node that is included within the RT portals depends on the size of the lymph node[17,24] and whether concomitant chemotherapy is administered. Relatively recent data suggest that advanced disease has a better chance of cure after altered fractionation or concomitant chemotherapy.[25] Patients treated at the authors' institution routinely receive hyperfractionation when using three-dimensional conformal RT and the concomitant boost technique when using IMRT, combined with weekly cisplatin 30 mg/m^2. Positive nodes receive approximately 70 to 74 Gy, regardless of size or rate of regression.

The decision to add a neck dissection after RT for multiple unilateral positive nodes or bilateral lymph node disease is individualized and is based on the diameter of the largest node, node fixation, and number of clinically positive nodes in the neck. If clinically positive lymph nodes disappear completely during RT, the likelihood of control by RT alone is improved and a neck dissection may be withheld.[26–29] Peters et al.[30] reported on 100 node-positive patients with squamous cell carcinoma of the oropharynx treated with concomitant boost RT between 1984 and 1993 at the MD Anderson Cancer Center (Houston, TX). Sixty-two patients had a complete response in the neck and received no further therapy. Three patients (5%) subsequently developed an isolated recurrence in the neck and four patients (6%) developed a recurrence in the neck in conjunction with other sites of relapse. The 2-year neck disease

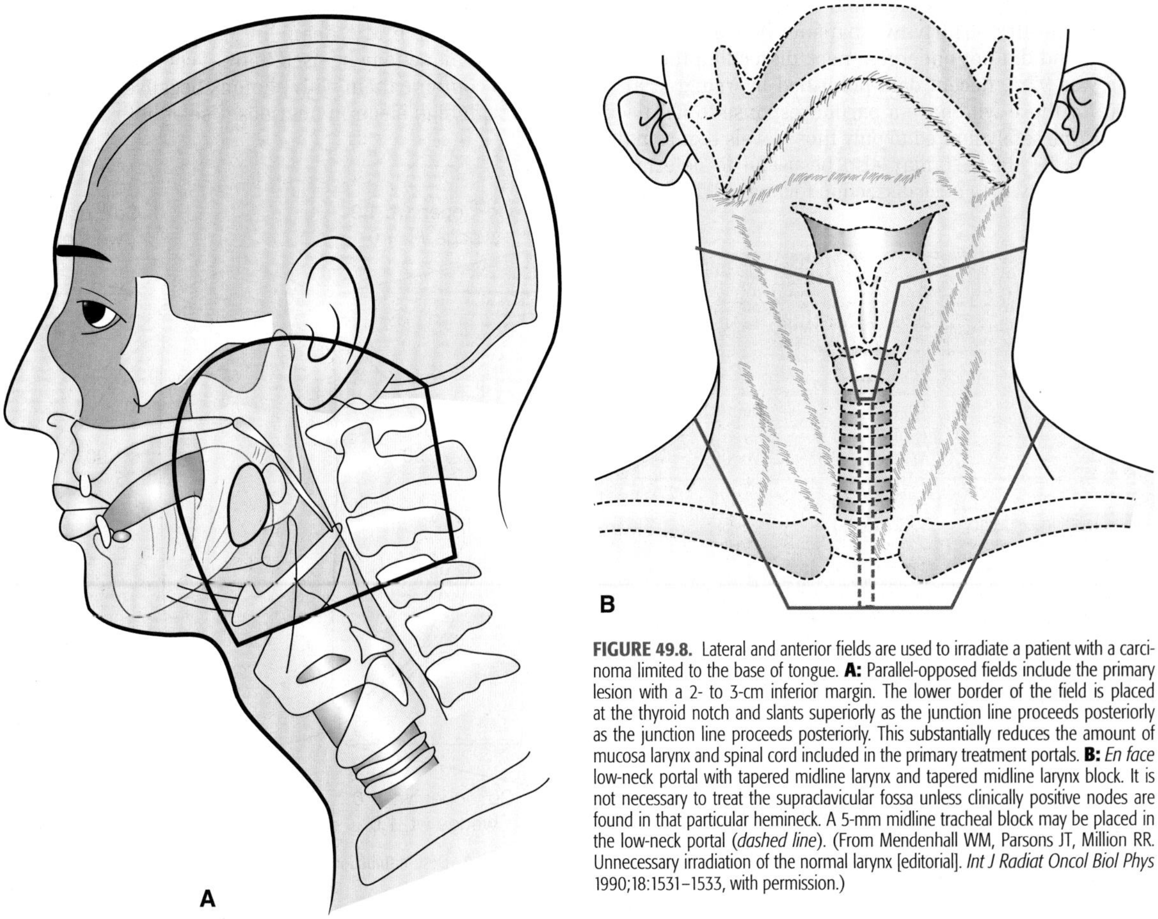

FIGURE 49.8. Lateral and anterior fields are used to irradiate a patient with a carcinoma limited to the base of tongue. **A:** Parallel-opposed fields include the primary lesion with a 2- to 3-cm inferior margin. The lower border of the field is placed at the thyroid notch and slants superiorly as the junction line proceeds posteriorly as the junction line proceeds posteriorly. This substantially reduces the amount of mucosa larynx and spinal cord included in the primary treatment portals. **B:** *En face* low-neck portal with tapered midline larynx and tapered midline larynx block. It is not necessary to treat the supraclavicular fossa unless clinically positive nodes are found in that particular hemineck. A 5-mm midline tracheal block may be placed in the low-neck portal (*dashed line*). (From Mendenhall WM, Parsons JT, Million RR. Unnecessary irradiation of the normal larynx [editorial]. *Int J Radiat Oncol Biol Phys* 1990;18:1531–1533, with permission.)

control rates did not vary significantly with pretreatment nodal size: ≤3 cm, 87%; and >3 cm, 85%. The incidence of subcutaneous fibrosis was similar following RT alone compared with another group of patients who underwent a neck dissection in addition to RT. Johnson et al.[31] reported on 81 patients with node-positive stages III and IV squamous cell carcinoma of the head and neck treated with concomitant boost accelerated hyperfractionated RT at the Medical College of Virginia (Richmond). Fifty-eight patients (72%) had a complete response in the neck and were followed; three patients (5%) subsequently developed an isolated recurrence in the neck and one additional patient developed recurrent cancer in the neck and in the primary site. The 3-year neck disease control rates were 94% for nodes ≤3 cm compared with 86% for those >3 cm.

Both of these series of patients received aggressive altered fractionated RT and it is unclear whether these data can be broadly extrapolated to patients with head and neck cancer from a variety of head and neck primary sites that are treated less aggressively. It is also unclear whether the addition of concomitant chemotherapy results in a lower likelihood of needing a neck dissection. However, multiple subsequent studies evaluating neck control rates after RT alone or combined with chemotherapy suggest that the likelihood of an isolated failure in the neck is low if there is a complete response after treatment.[18,32–36]

The authors' policy at the University of Florida has changed to the extent that we now evaluate patients with clinically positive nodes with CT 4 weeks after RT and withhold neck dissection in the subset of patients with a complete response thought to have ≤5% risk of residual disease.[37–41] Liauw et al.[40] evaluated a series of 550 patients treated with definitive RT at the University of Florida between 1990 and 2002; 341 patients (62%) underwent a post-RT planned neck dissection. CT images obtained at approximately 4 weeks post-RT were reviewed for 211 patients; radiographic complete response (rCR) was defined as no nodes >1.5 cm and no focal abnormalities such as focal lucency, enhancement, or calcification.[34] The outcomes are depicted in Table 49.8. Thirty-two patients had an rCR and were followed and did not undergo a neck dissection; the neck control rate was 97%. Recent data published by Yeung et al.[37] suggest that for those who have a partial response to RT, neck dissection may be safely limited to only those levels that remain suspicious after RT. PET-CT may also be useful to determine whether to proceed with a neck dissection following RT. Patients undergo PET-CT 3 months after completion of RT to minimize the risk of a false positive scan; those with a negative PET-CT are followed, the remainder undergo a neck dissection.

If a neck dissection is planned to follow RT in patients with clinically positive lymph nodes, the preoperative dose varies with the size and location of the lymph node, fixation, and response to RT. Preoperative doses of 50 Gy are sufficient for mobile lymph nodes 3 to 4 cm in size, but 60 Gy or more is recommended for 5- to 6-cm nodes and for fixed nodes. Lymph nodes measuring 7 to 8 cm are almost always fixed to adjacent structures and often require doses of 70 to 75 Gy for the surgeon to achieve a complete resection. If the lymph node lies behind the plane of the spinal cord, electrons may be used to boost the dose after the primary fields have been reduced off the spinal cord after 45 to 50 Gy.[14] Patients in whom the decision is made to add a neck dissection after completion of RT receive full-dose irradiation to the clinically positive neck nodes.

Another technique commonly used for boosting the dose to the neck mass after spinal cord tolerance has been reached and the treatment to the primary lesion has been completed is opposed anterior and posterior fields with wedges. The final dose to the neck node (not to the entire neck) may be 70 to 80 Gy without exceeding the spinal cord tolerance (Fig. 49.9). The anterior and posterior wedge-pair technique is preferable to an appositional electron boost field because high-energy electron beams increase the skin and mucosal dose.

When the cervical lymph nodes are located superficially, sometimes within 1 cm from the skin or fixed to it, treatment with high-energy photon beams (≥6 MV) may underdose these nodes. Treatment should be initiated with cobalt-60 or 4-MV x-rays for the initial 45 to 50 Gy, after which a higher energy photon beam can be used to continue RT of the primary tumor if the neck nodes are clinically negative or if a neck dissection is planned to follow RT (Fig. 49.10). Parallel-opposed 6-MV x-ray beams may adequately treat the upper neck nodes included in the primary treatment fields; however, the supraclavicular nodes in the *en face* low-neck field may be underdosed with a 6-MV beam in very thin patients. Although electrons alone may be used to treat cervical nodes, it is preferable to combine them with photons because of the high surface dose with high electron energies. Use of both 20-MeV electrons

TABLE 49.8 PREDICTIVE VALUE OF POSTRADIOTHERAPY COMPUTED TOMOGRAPHY FINDINGS AT 4 WEEKS IN THE HEMINECK CORRELATED TO NECK DISSECTION PATHOLOGY (N = 193 HEMINECKS)

	NPV		*PPV*	
Findings	*Number/Total Number*	*Percent*	*Number/Total Number*	*Percent*
Any lymph node >1.5 cm	85/118	72	24/75	32
Any lymph node with focal lucency	49/57	86	49/136	36
Any focally abnormal lymph node[a]	75/98	77	34/95	36
Any lymph node with enhancement	111/147	76	21/46	46
Any lymph node with calcification	102/144	71	15/49	31
Two or more focally abnormal lymph nodes[a]	90/113	80	34/80	43
Any lymph node >1.5 cm and any focally abnormal lymph node	32/34	94	55/159	35

NPV, negative predictive value; PPV, positive predictive value.

[a]Focally abnormal lymph nodes equal grade 3 or 4 focal lucency, focal enhancement, or focal calcification.

From Liauw SL, Mancuso AA, Amdur RJ, et al. Postradiotherapy neck dissection for lymph node-positive head and neck cancer: the use of computed tomography to manage the neck. *J Clin Oncol* 2006;24:1421–1427. Reprinted with permission. © 2008. American Society of Clinical Oncology. All rights reserved.

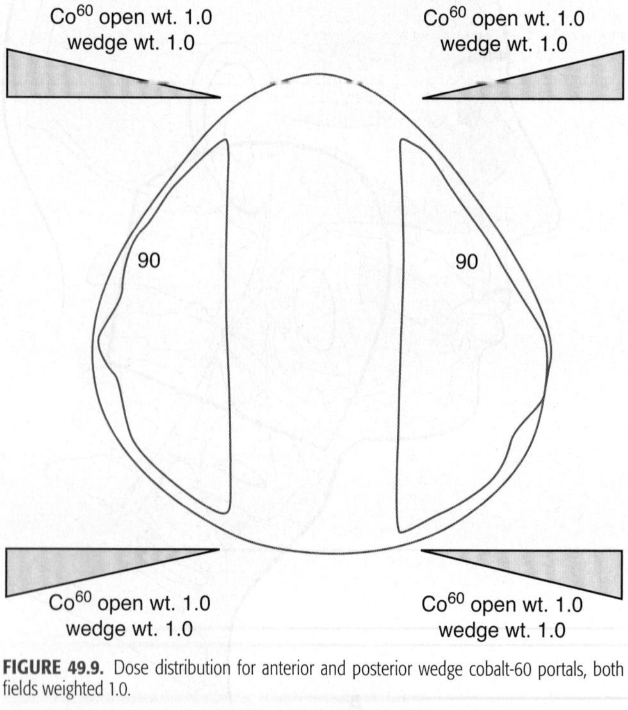

FIGURE 49.9. Dose distribution for anterior and posterior wedge cobalt-60 portals, both fields weighted 1.0.

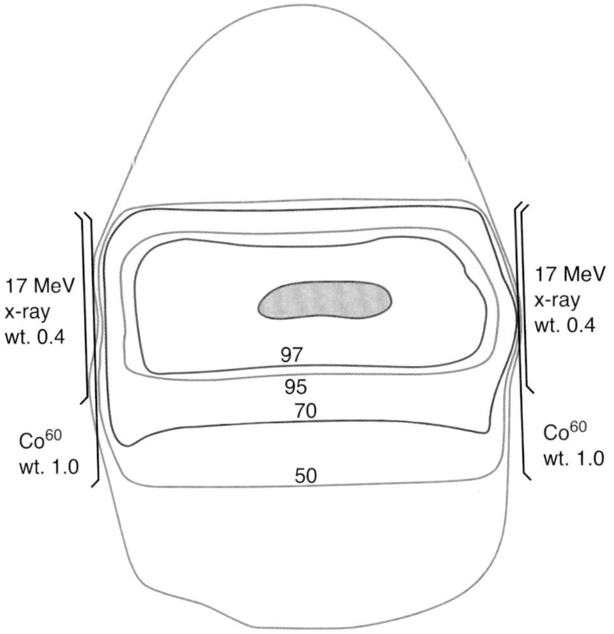

FIGURE 49.10. Dose distribution for parallel-opposed cobalt-60 portals, each weighted 1.0, with reduced 17-MV x-ray portals, each weighted 0.4.

and 17-MV x-rays is compared with treatment by 20-MeV electrons alone in a patient with a lateralized lesion of the oropharynx (Fig. 49.11).[42] The addition of the 17-MV x-rays to the 20-MeV electrons decreases the surface dose while still adequately irradiating the cervical nodes that are within the primary field. The addition of the x-ray beam also produces a dose distribution that is less affected by bone than that from the electron beam alone.

Large lymph nodes may not show much regression during the course of RT but often show significant regression from completion of treatment to the time the patient returns for neck dissection, usually after 4 to 6 weeks. The mass frequently has a thick capsule that facilitates its removal at the time of neck dissection.

Patients with bilateral neck disease require individualized treatment planning jointly by the radiation oncologist and the surgeon. If disease is minimal on one side, RT alone may be used to control the disease on that side of the neck, and a neck dissection may be used on the side with more disease. If major bilateral disease is present, bilateral neck dissection should follow RT.

Complications of Neck Irradiation

The complications of neck irradiation include subcutaneous fibrosis and lymphedema of the larynx and submentum. The latter complications may be minimized by sparing an anterior strip of skin when designing the parallel-opposed lateral portals used to encompass the primary lesion. The probability of complications is directly related to the radiation dose with little, if any, morbidity observed with the doses used for elective radiation therapy of the neck.

Complications of neck treatment in patients who receive RT in conjunction with resection of the primary lesion and a neck dissection are essentially the same as those occurring after neck dissection. However, they occur with an increased incidence depending on the RT dose and extent of surgery.

Treatment of the Neck After Incisional or Excisional Biopsy

Open biopsy of a clinically positive neck node before definitive treatment potentially spills tumor cells along tissue planes that may not be removed with a radical neck dissection. McGuirt and McCabe[13] reported that incisional or excisional biopsy of positive neck nodes before definitive surgery increased the risk of neck

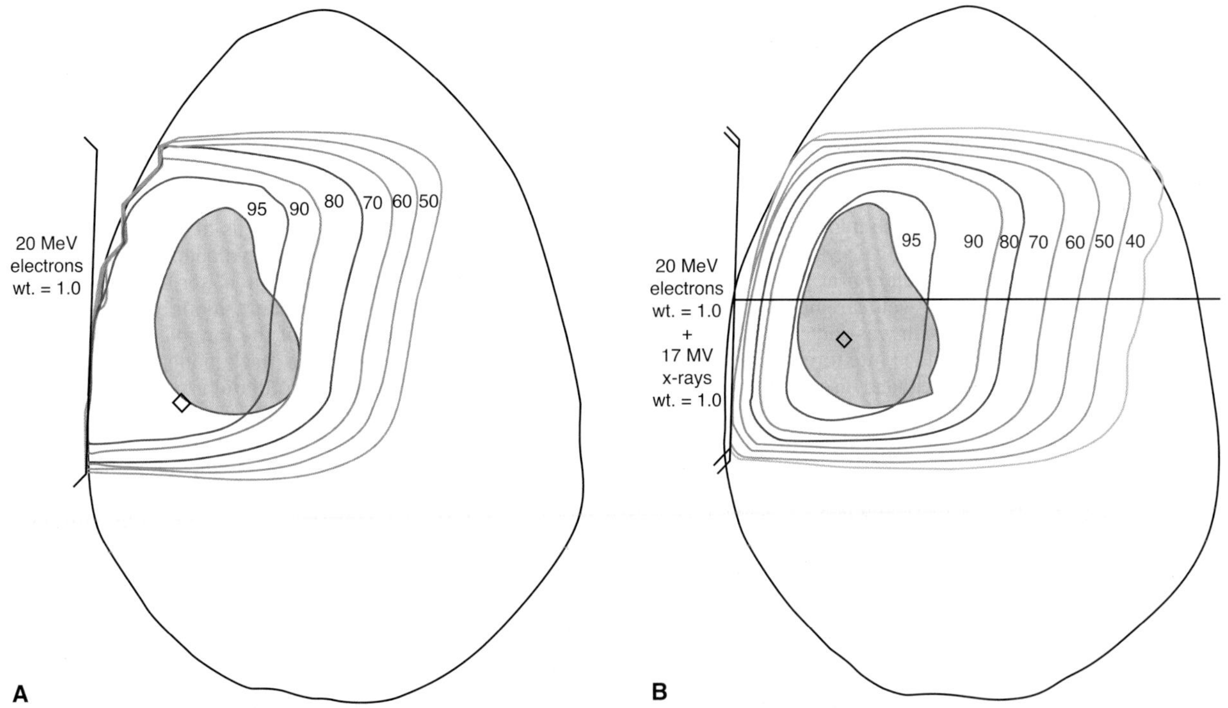

FIGURE 49.11. A: Dose distribution for 20-MeV electrons, field size 8.5 cm by 8.5 cm, SSD 100 cm. **B:** Dose distribution for 20-MeV electrons, field size 8.5 cm by 8.5 cm, and 17-MV x-rays, field size 7 cm by 7 cm, SSD 100 cm for both. The given doses are weighted 1 to 1. The addition of the 17-MV x-ray beam reduces the surface dose and gives a dose distribution that is affected less by bone. (From Bova FJ. Treatment planning for irradiation of head and neck cancer. In: Million RR, Cassisi NJ, eds. *Management of head and neck cancer: a multidisciplinary approach.* 2nd ed. Philadelphia: JB Lippincott, 1994: fig. 14–18:306, with permission.)

TABLE 49.9 CONTROL OF DISEASE IN THE CLINICALLY NEGATIVE NECK WITH ELECTIVE NECK IRRADIATION (NUMBER CONTROLLED/NUMBER TREATED)

Risk Group	No ENI (%)	Partial ENI (%)	Total ENI (%)
I (<20%)	13/15 (87)	16/17 (94)	1/1 (100)
II (20%–30%)	6/9 (67)	34/38 (89)	10/11 (91)
III (>30%)	3/4 (75)	32/33 (97)	61/62 (98)

ENI, elective neck irradiation.

From Mendenhall WM, Million RR. Elective neck irradiation for squamous cell carcinoma of the head and neck: analysis of time-dose factors and causes of failure. *Int J Radiat Oncol Biol Phys* 1986;12:741–746, with permission.

failure and worsened the prognosis for patients with squamous cell carcinoma of the head and neck. Parsons et al.[43] reported their experience with incisional or excisional biopsy of positive neck nodes followed by RT as the initial step in the treatment of the patient; these data were updated by Mack et al.[44] After excisional biopsy of a single lymph node, RT alone to the primary lesion and to the neck resulted in a 95% rate of neck control.[44] If residual disease remained in the neck after biopsy, RT followed by neck dissection was more successful than RT alone for controlling neck disease (see Table 49.17).

If the primary lesion is to be treated surgically, the patient's neck is also treated with preoperative RT to the primary lesion and neck, followed by resection. If the primary lesion is to be treated with RT, the patient is treated with RT. If there is no palpable disease remaining in the neck after excisional biopsy of a positive node, the neck may be treated with RT alone. If an incisional biopsy of the node has been performed (leaving gross disease) or if other positive nodes remain after an excisional neck node biopsy, RT is followed by a neck dissection. The dose of RT preceding a neck dissection depends on the amount of gross disease in the neck and the degree of fixation.[14]

RESULTS OF TREATMENT

Clinically Negative Nodes

Elective neck dissection and elective neck irradiation are equally effective in controlling subclinical disease. The decision whether to use surgery or RT for the purpose of electively treating the neck nodes depends on the method used to treat the primary lesion. Patients with a relatively early primary lesion and clinically negative nodes should be treated with one modality. Patients whose primary lesion is treated surgically may undergo an elective neck dissection, and those whose primary lesion is to be treated with RT should be considered for elective neck irradiation.

The results of elective neck irradiation at the University of Florida for patients with squamous cell carcinoma of the head and neck in whom the primary lesion was controlled are shown in Table 49.9.[4,45] Patients were divided into three risk categories based on the estimated risk of subclinical disease in the neck as follows: group I, low risk (<20% likelihood of occult disease); group II, moderate risk (20% to 30% risk of occult disease); and group III, high risk (more than 30% likelihood of occult disease). There were 6 neck failures (21%) in 28 patients who did not receive elective neck irradiation and 8 neck failures (5%) in 162 patients who received elective neck irradiation. Of the eight failures in patients receiving elective neck irradiation, two occurred within the irradiation fields, one at the field margin, and five in out-of-field areas. No correlation was found between the rate of tumor control in the first-echelon lymph nodes and the irradiation dose for doses ranging from 40 to 55 Gy or greater.[4] Only one failure occurred in the first-echelon lymph nodes, and this was after 48 Gy in 25 fractions using continuous-course irradiation.[4] The low neck, defined as that part of the neck located below the treatment portals used to treat the primary lesion, received either 50 Gy in 25 fractions or 40.5 Gy in 15 fractions, specified at D_{max} (0.5 cm depth). Both dose-fractionation protocols were equally effective in sterilizing subclinical disease in the low neck.[46] Elective neck irradiation is equally efficacious for squamous cell carcinoma arising from various head and neck primary sites.

If the primary lesion recurs, there is a renewed risk of lymphatic spread to the neck even after elective neck irradiation has been administered because of the possibility of reseeding the neck lymphatics. However, this risk is probably <10% in the first echelon lymph nodes because the prior elective neck irradiation likely fibrosed some of the lymphatic vessels.[47] In patients in whom primary failure occurs in addition to failure in the clinically negative nodes, the chances of surgical salvage are poor. In patients in whom the primary lesion is controlled and in whom failure develops in the initially negative neck, the chances of salvage with neck dissection are approximately 60%.

Although elective neck irradiation significantly reduces the risk of neck recurrence, there is no definite evidence that it improves survival. It would be necessary to conduct a large randomized trial to detect a survival difference, if one exists. Another problem is that the first-echelon lymph nodes are often included in the treatment portals used to treat the primary lesion so that it is often impossible to avoid at least partial elective neck irradiation. Therefore, such a trial would have to be restricted to primary sites where the portals would have to be enlarged to electively irradiate the neck or to patients treated with elective neck dissection rather than elective neck irradiation. Vandenbrouck et al.[48] and Fakih et al.[49] have conducted randomized trials comparing elective neck dissection with no elective neck treatment for patients with oral cavity carcinoma and oral tongue cancer, respectively. No survival advantage was noted for patients undergoing elective neck dissection in either study. However, because of the small number of patients in both trials, it is likely that even if a survival difference existed, it would have been missed.

Dearnaley et al.[50] reported on a series of 148 patients treated with an interstitial implant, alone or combined with external-beam RT, for cancer of the tongue or floor of mouth. Of 131 patients with negative neck nodes at diagnosis, 59 (45%) received elective neck irradiation to a dose of 40 Gy or greater. A multivariate analysis showed that elective neck irradiation significantly improved survival and reduced the risk of dying of cancer. Piedbois et al.[51] reported a series of 233 patients with T1-2N0 carcinoma of the oral cavity treated with interstitial iridium brachytherapy: 123 patients received no elective neck treatment, and 110 patients underwent an elective neck dissection. Patients who received an elective neck dissection tended to have more advanced primary

TABLE 49.10 FAILURE OF INITIAL IPSILATERAL NECK TREATMENT: 596 PATIENTS WITH CARCINOMA OF THE TONSILLAR FOSSA, BASE OF TONGUE, SUPRAGLOTTIC LARYNX, OR HYPOPHARYNX

	N0							
Treatment[a]	No Treatment	Partial Treatment	Complete Treatment	N1 (%)	N2A (%)	N2B (%)	N3A (%)	N3B (%)
Irradiation		15%	2%	15	27	27	38	34
Surgery	55% (16/29)	35%	7%	11	8	23	42	41
Combined		1/5	0/6	0	0	0	23	25

[a]MD Anderson Cancer Center data; patients treated 1948–1967.

Modified from Barkley HT Jr, Fletcher GH, Jesse RH, et al. Management of cervical lymph node metastases in squamous cell carcinoma of the tonsillar fossa, base of tongue, supraglottic larynx, and hypopharynx. *Am J Surg* 1972;124:462–467.

TABLE 49.11 FIVE-YEAR RATE OF NECK CONTROL BY 1983 AJCC STAGE AND TREATMENT (459 PATIENTS; 593 HEMINECKS)[a]

	Irradiation Alone		*Irradiation + Neck Dissection*		
Stage	*Number Heminecks*	*Control (%)*	*Number Heminecks*	*Control (%)*	*Significance*
N1	215	86	38	93	$P = .28$
N2A	29	79	24	68	$P = .6$
N2B	138	70	80	91	$P < .01$
N3A	29	33	40	69	$P < .01$

AJCC, American Joint Committee on Cancer.

[a]Excludes 67 heminecks on which incisional or excisional biopsy was done before treatment.

University of Florida data; patients treated October 1964 to October 1985; analysis December 1988 by Eric R. Ellis, MD.

TABLE 49.12 CERVICAL METASTASIS APPEARING IN THE CONTRALATERAL N0 NECK: 596 PATIENTS WITH CARCINOMA OF THE TONSILLAR FOSSA, BASE OF TONGUE, SUPRAGLOTTIC LARYNX, OR HYPOPHARYNX

	Stage				
Treatment[a]	*N0 (%)*	*N1 (%)*	*N2A (%)*	*N2B(%)*	*N3A (%)*
Irradiation	4	2	9	7	0
Surgery	25	17	23	43	33
Combined	0	0	0	11	0

[a]MD Anderson Hospital data; patients treated 1948–1967.

Adapted from Barkley HT Jr, Fletcher GH, Jesse RH, et al. Management of cervical lymph node metastases in squamous cell carcinoma of the tonsillar fossa, base of tongue, supraglottic larynx, and hypopharynx. *Am J Surg* 1972;124:462–467.

lesions. Although the ultimate rates of neck control were similar, a multivariate analysis showed that elective neck dissection was significantly associated with improved survival.

Clinically Positive Nodes

The incidence of treatment failure in the neck by N stage and treatment category has been reported by the MD Anderson Cancer Center (Table 49.10) and the University of Florida (Table 49.11 and Fig. 49.12).[52,53] In patients in whom the neck is treated with combined modalities, RT precedes surgery when the primary site is to be treated with irradiation or when the node is fixed. Surgery precedes RT when the primary site is to be treated operatively and the nodes are resectable.

When the initial treatment is surgery, a neck dissection is sufficient treatment for patients with a single positive lymph node <3 cm unless there is extracapsular spread of disease. RT may be added for control of subclinical disease in the contralateral side of the neck (Table 49.12).[52] The presence of multiple positive nodes in the surgical specimen is an indication for postoperative RT of the neck, especially when positive nodes are found at more than one level.[6,54,55]

Olsen et al.[56] reported a series of 284 patients who underwent neck dissection at the Mayo Clinic for pathologic stage N1 and N2 squamous cell carcinoma of the head and neck; no patient received adjuvant therapy. Neck recurrence-free survival rates at 5 years were as follows: N1, 76%; N2, 60%; and overall, 69%. A multivariate analysis showed that four or more positive nodes (P = .005), invasion of lymphatic or vascular spaces (P = .003), invasion of soft tissue (P = .0008), and a desmoplastic stromal pattern (P = .0001) were significantly associated with an increased risk of recurrence in the neck.[56]

The postoperative dose prescribed is usually 60 Gy in 30 fractions to 65 Gy in 35 fractions over 6 to 7 weeks for patients with negative margins; higher doses may be prescribed when residual disease is present in the neck.[54,57,58] If RT is to be added after surgery, it is usually initiated within 4 to 6 weeks after the operation, although it has been reported that a delay to 10 weeks is not associated with an increased risk of neck failure.[54]

The rate of control for neck nodes treated with RT alone as a function of node size, treatment scheme, and dose is shown in Table 49.13. RT alone is sufficient for patients with N1 (up to 2 cm) disease as long as the fraction size (2 Gy) and the total dose are sufficient.[38] RT followed by neck dissection has provided better rates of disease control than RT alone for patients with more advanced neck disease. The rate of neck disease control for patients treated with twice-daily RT, alone or followed by neck dissection, is shown in Figure 49.12 and shows a significant improvement in the control rates when neck dissection was added in selected cases.[59,60] As shown in a multivariate analysis by Ellis et al.[61] the addition of neck dissection after RT is independently related to a significantly decreased risk of dying from cancer. At least 50 Gy should be given preoperatively to the lymph nodes, although doses vary according to the size and degree of fixation of the lymph node. For example, large, fixed lymph nodes require 70 to 75 Gy of preoperative RT (Table 49.14). The likelihood of disease control in each side of the neck treated with irradiation and neck dissection is decreased when the node is fixed before treatment or when

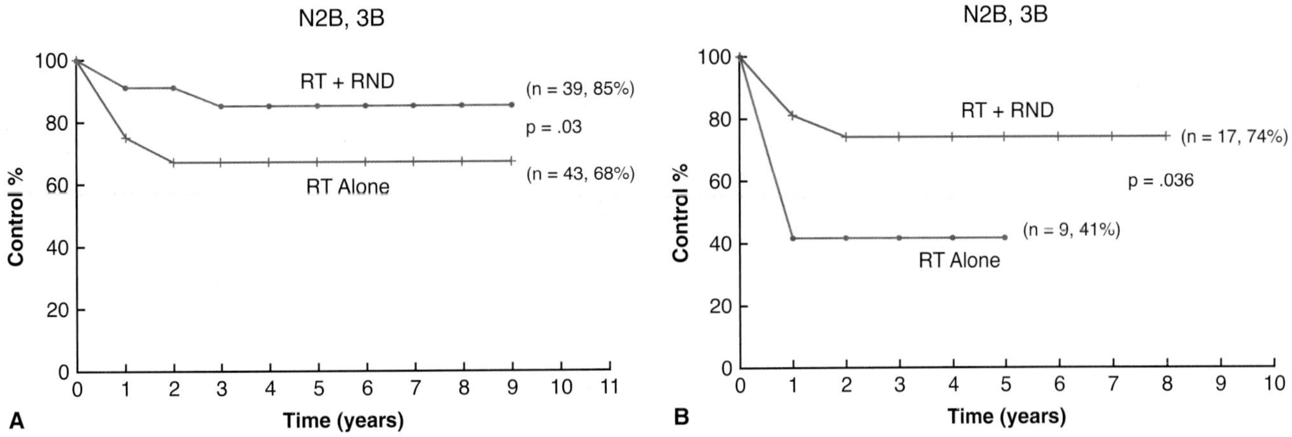

FIGURE 49.12. Rate of neck disease control (life table method[77]) for patients treated with twice-daily irradiation (RT) alone or combined with neck dissection (radiotherapy plus RND) for clinically positive neck nodes. **A:** N2B, N3B. **B:** N2 A, N3 A. (From Parsons JT, Mendenhall WM, Cassisi NJ, et al. Neck dissection after twice-a-day radiotherapy: morbidity and recurrence rates. *Head Neck* 1989;11:400–404, with permission.)

TABLE 49.13 LYMPH NODE DISEASE CONTROL BY RADIATION TREATMENT TECHNIQUE (NUMBER CONTROLLED/NUMBER TREATED)

Node Size (cm)	Continuous Course (%)	Split Course (%)	Excluded[a]	Total (%)
<1.0	5/5	2/2	1/1	8/8
1.0	29/35 (83)	19/23 (85)	3/4	51/62 (82)
1.5–2.0	43/49 (88)	20/24 (83)	5/9	68/82 (83)
2.5–3.0	14/19 (74)	10/18 (56)	0/3	24/40 (60)
3.5–6.0	14/20 (70)	10/17 (59)	0/1	24/38 (63)
≥7.0	0/2	0/5	0/1	0/8

[a]Less than 50 Gy for nodes equal to 1.0 cm and <55 Gy for nodes equal to 1.5 cm.

Modified from Mendenhall WM, Million RR, Bova FJ. Analysis of time-dose factors in clinically positive neck nodes treated with irradiation alone in squamous cell carcinoma of the head and neck. *Int J Radiat Oncol Biol Phys* 1984;10:639–643.

TABLE 49.15 CONTROL OF DISEASE IN THE NECK AS A FUNCTION OF NODE MOBILITY (109 PATIENTS; 121 HEMINECKS)

Size (cm)	Proportion of Fixed Nodes (%)	Number Heminecks Controlled/Number Treated: Mobile or Tethered (%)	Fixed (%)
<3	1/23 (4)	19/22 (86)	1/1 (100)
3–4	4/44 (9)	33/40 (83)	2/4 (50)
5–6	9/27 (33)	17/18 (94)	6/9 (67)
7–8	10/21 (48)	8/11 (73)	5/10 (50)
≥9	3/6 (50)	2/3 (67)	1/3 (33)

From Mendenhall WM, Million RR, Cassisi NJ. Squamous cell carcinoma of the head and neck treated with radiation therapy: the role of neck dissection for clinically positive neck nodes. *Int J Radiat Oncol Biol Phys* 1986;12:733–740, with permission.

residual tumor is found in the pathologic specimen (Tables 49.15 and 49.16).[14] No difference is seen in the rate of control as a function of the interval between RT and neck dissection when comparing patients who have surgery within 6 weeks with those who have neck dissection more than 6 weeks after RT.[14] If a local recurrence occurs, prior combined treatment of the neck does not diminish the chance of successful surgical salvage of the patient.[62] The likelihood of disease control at the primary site was not found to be related to neck stage at diagnosis in patients treated with RT alone or followed by neck dissection at the University of Florida;[63] this finding is different from what others have reported.[64]

Results After Incisional or Excisional Biopsy

Patients who have undergone an incisional or excisional biopsy of a metastatic lymph node before referral do not have an increased risk of neck failure or a decreased cure rate if RT is the next step in treatment.[43] The likelihood of control and the cure rate are probably diminished if an operation without prior RT follows incisional or excisional biopsy of a metastatic neck node because of the risk that the biopsy procedure disseminated tumor cells into tissues not removed by neck dissection.[13]

Ellis et al.[61] reported on 508 patients with 660 positive heminecks treated at the University of Florida with RT alone or followed by a planned neck dissection. Pretreatment node biopsy did not influence outcome when RT was the next step in treatment (Table 49.17).[61] The results of the forward stepwise log-rank tests of prognostic factors for predicting time to recurrence are shown in Table 49.18.[61]

CERVICAL LYMPH NODE METASTASIS WITH UNKNOWN PRIMARY TUMOR

In a small percentage of patients with enlarged cervical lymph nodes, the primary lesion cannot be found, even after extensive evaluation.[65–67] Patients with enlarged lymph nodes in the upper neck have a good prognosis when treated aggressively, compared with those with enlarged lymph nodes in the low internal jugular chain or supraclavicular fossa. The latter patients are more likely to have primary lesions located below the clavicles, which carry a much worse prognosis. The majority of patients have either squamous cell or poorly differentiated carcinoma. Those with adenocarcinoma almost always have a primary lesion below the clavicles, although if the nodes are located in the upper neck, one must exclude a salivary gland, thyroid, or parathyroid primary tumor. This section deals with patients presenting with squamous cell or poorly differentiated carcinoma in the upper or middle neck.

Patients should be evaluated with a thorough physical examination including careful evaluation of the head and neck. A needle biopsy of the lymph node should be performed. After chest roentgenography, a CT or MRI of the head and neck is obtained to detect an unknown primary lesion arising from the mucosa of the head and neck. It is unclear whether FDG-PET scans may identify primary lesions that would not otherwise be identifiable.[68] The available data suggest that some patients will benefit from these studies. Direct laryngoscopy and examination under anesthesia are performed with directed biopsies of the nasopharynx, tonsils, base of the tongue, and pyriform sinuses, and of any abnormalities noted on CT or MRI or suspicious mucosal lesions noted at laryngoscopy. Patients with adequate lymphoid tissue in their tonsillar fossae should undergo an ipsilateral tonsillectomy. The diagnostic evaluation

TABLE 49.14 CERVICAL LYMPH NODE DISEASE CONTROL WITH RADIATION THERAPY FOLLOWED BY NECK DISSECTION, WITH PRIMARY LESION TREATED INITIALLY BY RADIATION THERAPY (NUMBER CONTROLLED/NUMBER TREATED)

Minimum Node Diameter (cm)	Minimum Node Dose (Gy): <50	50–50.99	60–69.99	≥70
<3	5/5	1/2	5/5	3/3
3–4	6/8	10/14	9/9	5/7
5–6	4/7	5/5	7/8	4/4
7–8	2/3	2/4	4/6	3/4
≥9	No data	1/1	2/4	0/1

University of Florida data; patients treated 1964–1982; analysis 1984 by WM Mendenhall, MD. Ninety-one patients were treated with once-a-day fractionation, continuous- or split-course technique (100 heminecks).

From Mendenhall WM, Million RR, Cassisi NJ. Squamous cell carcinoma of the head and neck treated with radiation therapy: the role of neck dissection for clinically positive neck nodes. *Int J Radiat Oncol Biol Phys* 1986;12(5):733–740, with permission.

TABLE 49.16 NECK DISEASE CONTROL AS A FUNCTION OF PATHOLOGIC FINDINGS IN THE NECK DISSECTION SPECIMEN (108 PATIENTS; 120 EVALUABLE HEMINECKS)[a]

Size (cm)	Proportion with Positive Specimens (%)	Number Heminecks Controlled/Number Treated: Negative Specimen (%)	Positive Specimen (%)
<3	10/23 (43)	13/13 (100)	7/10 (70)
3–4	22/43 (51)	20/21 (95)	14/22 (64)
5–6	10/27 (37)	17/17 (100)	6/10 (60)
7–8	12/21 (57)	8/9 (89)	5/12 (42)
≥9	4/6 (67)	2/2 (100)	1/4 (25)

[a]One patient was excluded because data were unavailable.

From Mendenhall WM, Million RR, Cassisi NJ. Squamous cell carcinoma of the head and neck treated with radiation therapy: the role of neck dissection for clinically positive neck nodes. *Int J Radiat Oncol Biol Phys* 1986;12:733–740, with permission.

TABLE 49.17 EFFECT OF NECK NODE BIOPSY ON 5-YEAR RATE OF NECK CONTROL (660 HEMINECKS)

	No Neck Biopsy		Neck Biopsy		
Hemineck Stage	Number of Heminecks	Probability of Hemineck Control (%)	Number of Heminecks	Probability of Hemineck Control (%)	Significance of Difference Between Curves
N1	253	87 ± 3	12	100	P = .22
N2A	53	73 ± 8	15	93 ± 6	P = .18
N2B	218	78 ± 3	23	72 ± 11	P = .86
N3A	69	54 ± 7	17	81 ± 10	P = .30

From Ellis ER, Mendenhall WM, Rao PV et al. Incisional or excisional neck-node biopsy before definitive radiotherapy, alone or followed by neck dissection. *Head Neck* 1991;13:177–183, with permission.

for the patient with cervical metastasis from an unknown head and neck primary lesion is summarized in Table 49.19. The results of a diagnostic evaluation for an unknown primary site in 236 patients at the University of Florida are depicted in Table 49.20.[69] Overall, 132 primary sites were discovered in 126 patients (53%) and were most often located in the oropharynx: tonsillar fossa, 59 (45%); base of tongue, 58 (44%); pyriform sinus, 10 (8%); pharyngeal wall, 3 (2%); and supraglottic larynx, 1 (1%).[69]

Some patients may be cured with treatment directed only to the involved area of the neck[70]; however, the authors usually irradiate the nasopharynx and oropharynx as well as both sides of the neck. The hypopharynx and larynx were irradiated as well until 1997 when it was decided to eliminate them because they are rarely the site of the primary cancer and because irradiation of these sites significantly increases the morbidity of treatment. It is not necessary to irradiate the oral cavity unless the patient has submandibular adenopathy, in which case the authors either do a neck dissection and observe the patient or irradiate the oral cavity and oropharynx and not the nasopharynx. Patients are treated with parallel-opposed fields at 1.8 Gy per fraction to a midline dose of 64.8 Gy with reduction off the spinal cord at 45 Gy tumor dose (Fig. 49.13). An alternative is to use IMRT to spare the contralateral parotid gland in patients with ipsilateral neck nodes. The lower neck is treated through a separate *en face* anterior field. IMRT may be used if patients have unilateral neck disease to reduce the dose to the contralateral parotid.

TABLE 49.18 PROGNOSTIC FACTORS, IN ORDER OF THEIR IMPORTANCE, FOR PREDICTING THE TIME TO OCCURRENCE OF VARIOUS EVENTS

Event	Rank Order	Factor	Level of Significance
Recurrence in neck (n = 660 heminecks)	1	Increasing N stage	P = .0001
	2	Treatment of neck with RT alone	P = .0001
	3	Fixed nodes	P = .0001
	4	T stage[a]	P = .0350
Death with disease present (n = 508 patients)	1	Recurrence above clavicles	P = .0001
	2	Increasing N stage	P = .0003
	3	Fixed nodes	P = 0.0053
	4	Treatment of neck with RT alone	P = .0121
For occurrence of distant metastasis (n = 508 patients)	1	Recurrence above clavicles	P = .0001
	2	Increasing N stage	P = .0003
	3	Fixed nodes	P = .0704
	4	Nodes below thyroid notch	P = .1023

RT, radiation therapy.

[a]This factor is thought to be correlated with the censoring pattern.

From Ellis ER, Mendenhall WM, Rao PV, et al. Incisional or excisional neck-node biopsy before definitive radiotherapy, alone or followed by neck dissection. *Head Neck* 1991; 13:177–183, with permission.

Erkal et al.[66] reported on 126 patients treated with curative intent at the University of Florida between 1964 and 1997 with follow-up for at least 2 years. RT was delivered to head and neck mucosal sites and both sides of the neck in 119 patients and to the neck alone in 7 patients. Twelve patients (10%) developed squamous cell carcinoma in a head and neck mucosal site at 0.5 to 10.9 years (median, 1.8 years) after treatment. The 5-year results were as follows: head and neck mucosal failure, 13%; neck node control, 78%; distant metastases, 14%; absolute survival, 47%; and cause-specific survival, 67%. Wallace et al.[71] reported a combined series of 179 patients treated at the University of Florida (139 patients) and the University of Wisconsin (40 patients). The 5-year mucosal control rate was 92%; the head and neck mucosa was irradiated in 174 patients (97%). For the subset of 28 patients where the mucosal RT was limited to the nasopharynx and oropharynx, the 5-year mucosal control rate was 100%. Barker et al.[65] subsequently reported on 17 patients treated with the larynx-sparing technique described above between 1997 and 2002 at the authors' institution; none of these patients developed a head and neck mucosal squamous cell carcinoma after receiving RT.

Colletier et al.[72] reported on 136 patients treated with neck dissection followed by RT to head and neck mucosal sites and bilateral lymph nodes. Six percent of patients developed carcinomas in head and neck mucosal sites within RT portals, and 4% of patients developed carcinomas in head and neck mucosal sites outside the RT portals. The absolute survival rate at 5 years was 60%. The authors recommended RT to head and neck mucosal sites. Reddy and Marks[73] reported on 16 patients with RT to ipsilateral lymph nodes and 36 patients with RT to head and neck mucosal sites and bilateral lymph nodes. The authors concluded that RT reduced the rate of developing carcinomas in head and neck mucosal sites. For patients with

TABLE 49.19 DIAGNOSTIC WORKUP FOR CERVICAL LYMPH NODE METASTASES: UNKNOWN PRIMARY TUMOR

General
History
Physical examination
Careful examination of the neck and supraclavicular regions
Examination of oral cavity, pharynx, and larynx (indirect laryngectomy)

Radiographic Studies
Chest roentgenogram
Computed tomography or magnetic resonance imaging scans of head and neck (special attention to nasopharynx, pharynx, and larynx)

Laboratory Studies
Complete blood cell count
Blood chemistry profile

Direct Laryngoscopy and Directed Biopsies
Nasopharynx, both tonsils, base of tongue, both pyriform sinuses, and any suspicious or abnormal mucosal areas
Fine-needle aspirate or core needle biopsy of the cervical node
Tonsillectomy

TABLE 49.20 DETECTION OF PRIMARY SITE VERSUS PATIENT GROUP

Patient Group	Biopsy-Proven Primary Site/Number of Patients (%)
PE∅/RAD∅	21/72 (29.2)
PE∅/RAD+	51/82 (62.2)
PE+/RAD∅	15/25 (60.0)
PE+/RAD+	39/57 (68.4)
Total	126/236 (53.4)

PE∅, physical examination negative; PE+, physical examination suspicious, but not definitely positive; RAD∅, radiological examination negative; RAD+, radiological examination (computed tomography and/or magnetic resonance imaging) suspicious, not definitively positive.

From Cianchetti M, Mancuso AA, Amdur RJ, et al. Diagnostic evaluation of squamous cell carcinoma metastatic to cervical lymph nodes from an unknown head and neck primary site. *Laryngoscope* 2009;119:2348–2354, with permission.

no RT to head and neck mucosal sites, the rate of developing carcinomas in head and neck mucosal sites was 46% and the absolute survival rate at 5 years was 47%. For patients treated with RT to head and neck mucosal sites, the rates were 8% and 53%, respectively. Grau et al.[74] reported on 273 patients treated with curative intent at five cancer centers in Denmark between 1975 and 1995 with surgery alone (23 patients), RT to the ipsilateral neck alone or combined with surgery (26 patients), and RT to the neck and head and neck mucosa alone or combined with surgery (224 patients). The ipsilateral oropharynx unintentionally received some RT in patients treated to the ipsilateral neck alone, depending on the treatment technique. The 5-year rates of freedom from failure in the head and neck mucosa were as follows: surgery alone, 45%; RT with or without surgery to the ipsilateral neck, 77%; and RT to the head and neck mucosa with or without surgery, 87%. The oropharynx, particularly the base of tongue, was the most common location of mucosal site failure.

The incidence of subsequent mucosal primary lesions was compared by Erkal et al.[25] for 1,112 patients with a known primary site (oropharynx, hypopharynx, and supraglottis) and a series of 126 patients treated for an unknown primary site at the University of Florida. The incidence of a subsequent mucosal head and neck cancer was similar for both groups, suggesting either that mucosal irradiation significantly reduced the risk of primary site failure or that patients with unknown primary sites have a much lower risk of a second primary head and neck cancer developing subsequently (Fig. 49.14).[66]

A subset of patients presenting with squamous cell carcinoma metastatic to the neck nodes from an unknown head and neck primary site are treated with palliative intent because of poor medical condition, extensive nodal involvement, or distant metastases at presentation. Treatment of the neck depends on the extent and location of the adenopathy. Forty of 166 patients (24%) were treated palliatively at the University of Florida between 1964 and 1997.[75] Treatment was delivered to the neck alone to a dose of 30 Gy in 10 fractions over 2 weeks or 20 Gy in 2 fractions with a 1-week interfraction interval. The nodal response rate was 65% and the symptomatic response rate was 57% at 1 year. The 1-year absolute and cause-specific survival rates were 25%.

The main complication of RT for patients treated for an unknown head and neck primary tumor is xerostomia. The complications of treatment of the neck, which have been discussed previously, depend on whether a neck dissection is added.[76]

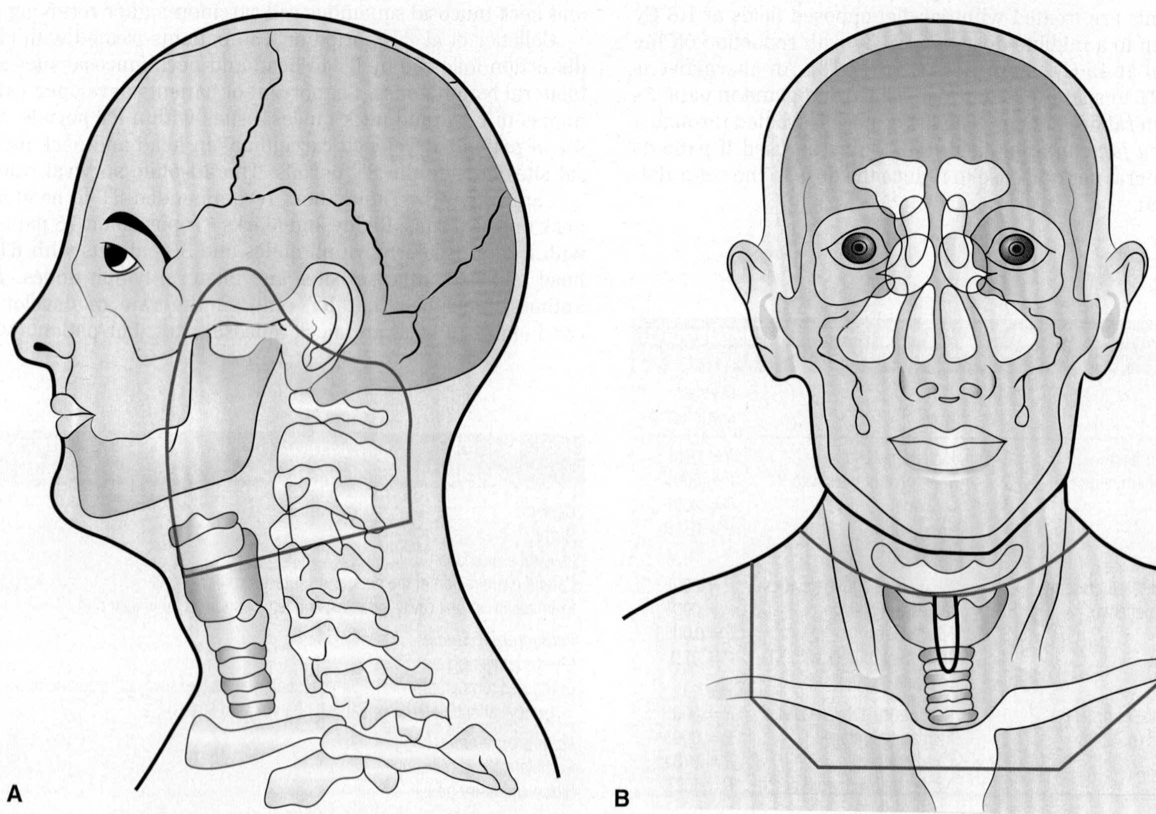

FIGURE 49.13. Radiation therapy portals used starting from 1997 to treat head and neck mucosal sites and upper cervical lymph nodes **(A)** and lower cervical and supraclavicular lymph nodes **(B)**. The inferior border for lateral portals is placed at the superior anterior border of the thyroid cartilage, shielding the hypopharynx and larynx. (From Erkal HS, Mendenhall WM, Amdur RJ, et al. Squamous cell carcinomas metastatic to cervical lymph nodes from an unknown head-and-neck mucosal site treated with radiation therapy alone or in combination with neck dissection. *Int J Radiat Oncol Biol Phys* 2001;50:55–63, with permission.)

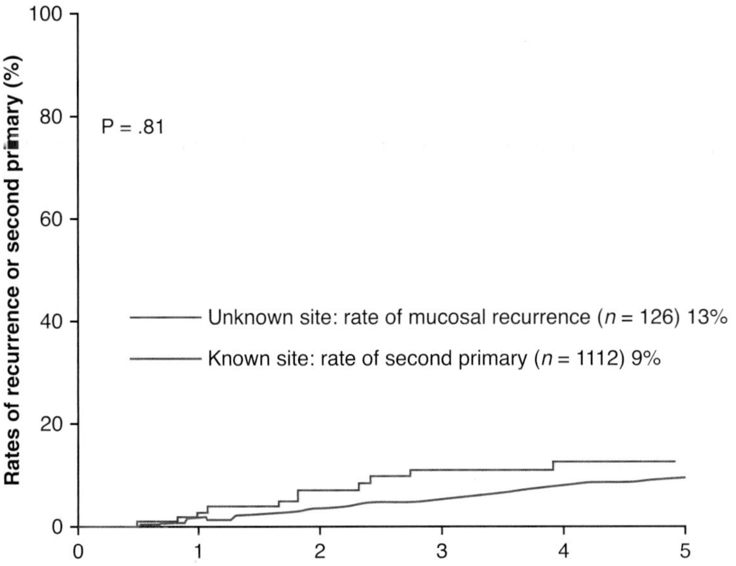

FIGURE 49.14. The rate of developing carcinomas in head and neck mucosal sites for patients treated for carcinomas with an unknown head and neck mucosal site compared to the rate of developing metachronous carcinomas in head and neck mucosal sites for patients treated for carcinomas with a known head and neck mucosal site. (From Erkal HS, Mendenhall WM, Amdur RJ, et al. Squamous cell carcinomas metastatic to cervical lymph nodes from an unknown head-and-neck mucosal site treated with radiation therapy alone or in combination with neck dissection. *Int J Radiat Oncol Biol Phys* 2001;50:55–63, with permission.)

ACKNOWLEDGMENT

We thank the research support staff of the Department of Radiation Oncology for their help with statistics, editing, and manuscript preparation.

REFERENCES

1. Rouviére H, Tobias MJ. *Anatomy of the human lymphatic system.* Ann Arbor, MI: Edwards Brothers, 1938.
2. Fisch U. [Lymphographic studies on the cervical lymphatic system]. *Fortschr Hals Nasen Ohrenheilkd* 1966;14.
3. Stringer SP. Current concepts in surgical management of neck metastases from head and neck cancer. *Oncology (Williston Park)* 1995;9(6):547–554.
4. Mendenhall WM, Million RR. Elective neck irradiation for squamous cell carcinoma of the head and neck: analysis of time-dose factors and causes of failure. *Int J Radiat Oncol Biol Phys* 1986;12(5):741–746.
5. Lindberg R. Distribution of cervical lymph node metastases from squamous cell carcinoma of the upper respiratory and digestive tracts. *Cancer* 1972;29(6): 1446–1449.
6. Richard JM, Sancho-Garnier H, Micheau C, et al. Prognostic factors in cervical lymph node metastasis in upper respiratory and digestive tract carcinomas: study of 1,713 cases during a 15-year period. *Laryngoscope* 1987;97(1):97–101.
7. McLaughlin MP, Mendenhall WM, Mancuso AA, et al. Retropharyngeal adenopathy as a predictor of outcome in squamous cell carcinoma of the head and neck. *Head Neck* 1995;17(3):190–198.
8. Million RR, Cassisi NJ, Mancuso AA, et al. Management of the neck for squamous cell carcinoma. In: Million RR, Cassisi NJ, eds. *Management of head and neck cancer: a multidisciplinary approach.* Philadelphia: JB Lippincott, 1994:75–142.
9. Mancuso AA, Hanafee WN. *Head and neck radiology.* Philadelphia: Williams & Wilkins, 2011.
10. American Joint Committee on Cancer. In: *Manual for staging of cancer.* 2nd ed. Philadelphia: JB Lippincott, 1983:37–42.
11. American Joint Committee on Cancer. Head and neck. In: *AJCC cancer staging manual.* 6th ed. New York: Springer, 2010:39–46,
12. Razack MS, Baffi R, Sako K. Bilateral radical neck dissection. *Cancer* 1981; 47(1):197–199.
13. McGuirt WF, McCabe BF. Significance of node biopsy before definitive treatment of cervical metastatic carcinoma. *Laryngoscope* 1978;88(4):594–597.
14. Mendenhall WM, Million RR, Cassisi NJ. Squamous cell carcinoma of the head and neck treated with radiation therapy: the role of neck dissection for clinically positive neck nodes. *Int J Radiat Oncol Biol Phys* 1986;12(5):733–740.
15. Somerset JD, Mendenhall WM, Amdur RJ, et al. Planned postradiotherapy bilateral neck dissection for head and neck cancer. *Am J Otolaryngol* 2001;22(6): 383–386.
16. Taylor JM, Mendenhall WM, Parsons JT, et al. The influence of dose and time on wound complications following post-radiation neck dissection. *Int J Radiat Oncol Biol Phys* 1992;23(1):41–46.
17. Dubray BM, Bataini JP, Bernier J, et al. Is reseeding from the primary a plausible cause of node failure? *Int J Radiat Oncol Biol Phys* 1993;25(1):9–15.
18. Mendenhall WM, Villaret DB, Amdur RJ, et al. Planned neck dissection after definitive radiotherapy for squamous cell carcinoma of the head and neck. *Head Neck* 2002;24(11):1012–1018.
19. Mendenhall WM, Parsons JT, Stringer SP, et al. T1-T2 vocal cord carcinoma: a basis for comparing the results of radiotherapy and surgery. *Head Neck Surg* 1988;10(6):373–377.
20. Mendenhall WM, Parsons JT, Brant TA, et al. Is elective neck treatment indicated for T2N0 squamous cell carcinoma of the glottic larynx? *Radiother Oncol* 1989;14(3):199–202.
21. Mendenhall WM, Parsons JT, Million RR. Unnecessary irradiation of the normal larynx. *Int J Radiat Oncol Biol Phys* 1990;18(6):1531–1533.
22. Amdur RJ, Li JG, Liu C, et al. Unnecessary laryngeal irradiation in the IMRT era. *Head Neck* 2004;26(3):257–263; discussion 63–64.
23. Mendenhall WM, Mancuso AA. Radiotherapy for head and neck cancer—is the "next level" down? *Int J Radiat Oncol Biol Phys* 2009;73(3):645–646.
24. Taylor JM, Mendenhall WM, Lavey RS. Time-dose factors in positive neck nodes treated with irradiation only. *Radiother Oncol* 1991;22(3):167–173.
25. Mendenhall WM, Riggs CE, Vaysberg M, et al. Altered fractionation and adjuvant chemotherapy for head and neck squamous cell carcinoma. *Head Neck* 2010; 32(7):939–945.
26. Bartelink H, Breur K, Hart G. Radiotherapy of lymph node metastases in patients with squamous cell carcinoma of the head and neck region. *Int J Radiat Oncol Biol Phys* 1982;8(6):983–989.
27. Bartelink H. Prognostic value of the regression rate of neck node metastases during radiotherapy. *Int J Radiat Oncol Biol Phys* 1983;9(7):993–996.
28. Bataini JP, Bernier J, Jaulerry C, et al. Impact of neck node radioresponsiveness on the regional control probability in patients with oropharynx and pharyngolarynx cancers managed by definitive radiotherapy. *Int J Radiat Oncol Biol Phys* 1987;13(6):817–824.
29. Maciejewski B. Regression rate of metastatic neck lymph nodes after radiation treatment as a prognostic factor for local control. *Radiother Oncol* 1987;8(4):301–308.
30. Peters LJ, Weber RS, Morrison WH, et al. Neck surgery in patients with primary oropharyngeal cancer treated by radiotherapy. *Head Neck* 1996;18(6):552–559.
31. Johnson CR, Silverman LN, Clay LB, et al. Radiotherapeutic management of bulky cervical lymphadenopathy in squamous cell carcinoma of the head and neck: is postradiotherapy neck dissection necessary? *Radiat Oncol Investig* 1998;6(1):52–57.
32. Ferlito A, Corry J, Silver CE, et al. Planned neck dissection for patients with complete response to chemoradiotherapy: a concept approaching obsolescence. *Head Neck* 2010;32(2):253–261.
33. Corry J, Peters L, Fisher R, et al. N2-N3 neck nodal control without planned neck dissection for clinical/radiologic complete responders-results of Trans Tasman Radiation Oncology Group Study 98.02. *Head Neck* 2008;30(6):737–742.
34. Rengan R, Pfister DG, Lee NY, et al. Long-term neck control rates after complete response to chemoradiation in patients with advanced head and neck cancer. *Am J Clin Oncol* 2008;31(5):465–469.
35. Yao M, Hoffman HT, Chang K, et al. Is planned neck dissection necessary for head and neck cancer after intensity-modulated radiotherapy? *Int J Radiat Oncol Biol Phys* 2007;68(3):707–713.
36. Yovino S, Settle K, Taylor R, et al. Patterns of failure among patients with squamous cell carcinoma of the head and neck who obtain a complete response to chemoradiotherapy. *Head Neck* 2010;32(1):46–52.
37. Yeung AR, Liauw SL, Amdur RJ, et al. Lymph node-positive head and neck cancer treated with definitive radiotherapy: can treatment response determine the extent of neck dissection? *Cancer* 2008;112(5):1076–1082.
38. Mendenhall WM, Million RR, Bova FJ. Analysis of time-dose factors in clinically positive neck nodes treated with irradiation alone in squamous cell carcinoma of the head and neck. *Int J Radiat Oncol Biol Phys* 1984;10(5):639–643.
39. Bernier J, Bataini JP. Regional outcome in oropharyngeal and pharyngolaryngeal cancer treated with high dose per fraction radiotherapy. Analysis of neck disease response in 1646 cases. *Radiother Oncol* 1986;6(2):87–103.
40. Liauw SL, Mancuso AA, Amdur RJ, et al. Postradiotherapy neck dissection for lymph node-positive head and neck cancer: the use of computed tomography to manage the neck. *J Clin Oncol* 2006;24(9):1421–1427.
41. Mabanta SR, Mendenhall WM, Stringer SP, et al. Salvage treatment for neck recurrence after irradiation alone for head and neck squamous cell carcinoma with clinically positive neck nodes. *Head Neck* 1999;21(7):591–594.
42. Bova FJ. Treatment planning for irradiation of head and neck cancer. In: Million RR, Cassisi NJ, eds. *Management of head and neck cancer: a multidisciplinary approach.* Philadelphia: JB Lippincott, 1984:209–230.
43. Parsons JT, Million RR, Cassisi NJ. The influence of excisional or incisional biopsy of metastatic neck nodes on the management of head and neck cancer. *Int J Radiat Oncol Biol Phys* 1985;11(8):1447–1454.
44. Mack Y, Parsons JT, Mendenhall WM, et al. Squamous cell carcinoma of the head and neck: management after excisional biopsy of a solitary metastatic neck node. *Int J Radiat Oncol Biol Phys* 1993;25(4):619–622.

45. Mendenhall WM, Million RR, Cassisi NJ. Elective neck irradiation in squamous-cell carcinoma of the head and neck. *Head Neck Surg* 1980;3(1):15–20.
46. Mendenhall WM, Parsons JT, Million RR. Elective lower neck irradiation: 5000 cGy/25 fractions versus 4050 cGy/15 fractions. *Int J Radiat Oncol Biol Phys* 1988; 15(2):439–440.
47. Dagan R, Morris CG, Kirwan JM, et al. Elective neck dissection during salvage surgery for locally recurrent head and neck squamous cell carcinoma after radiotherapy with elective nodal irradiation. *Laryngoscope* 2010;120(5):945–952.
48. Vandenbrouck C, Sancho-Garnier H, Chassagne D, et al. Elective versus therapeutic radical neck dissection in epidermoid carcinoma of the oral cavity: results of a randomized clinical trial. *Cancer* 1980;46(2):386–390.
49. Fakih AR, Rao RS, Borges AM, et al. Elective versus therapeutic neck dissection in early carcinoma of the oral tongue. *Am J Surg* 1989;158(4):309–313.
50. Dearnaley DP, Dardoufas C, A'Hearn RP, et al. Interstitial irradiation for carcinoma of the tongue and floor of mouth: Royal Marsden Hospital Experience 1970–1986. *Radiother Oncol* 1991;21(3):183–192.
51. Piedbois P, Mazeron JJ, Haddad E, et al. Stage I–II squamous cell carcinoma of the oral cavity treated by iridium-192: is elective neck dissection indicated? *Radiother Oncol* 1991;21(2):100–106.
52. Barkley HT Jr, Fletcher GH, Jesse RH, et al. Management of cervical lymph node metastases in squamous cell carcinoma of the tonsillar fossa, base of tongue, supraglottic larynx, and hypopharynx. *Am J Surg* 1972;124(4):462–467.
53. Mendenhall WM, Parsons JT, Stringer SP, et al. Squamous cell carcinoma of the head and neck treated with irradiation: management of the neck. *Semin Radiat Oncol* 1992;2(3):163–170.
54. Amdur RJ, Parsons JT, Mendenhall WM, et al. Postoperative irradiation for squamous cell carcinoma of the head and neck: an analysis of treatment results and complications. *Int J Radiat Oncol Biol Phys* 1989;16(1):25–36.
55. Lefebvre JL, Castelain B, De la Torre JC, et al. Lymph node invasion in hypopharynx and lateral epilarynx carcinoma: a prognostic factor. *Head Neck Surg* 1987;10(1):14–18.
56. Olsen KD, Caruso M, Foote RL, et al. Primary head and neck cancer. Histopathologic predictors of recurrence after neck dissection in patients with lymph node involvement. *Arch Otolaryngol Head Neck Surg* 1994;120(12):1370–1374.
57. Marcus RB Jr, Million RR, Cassissi NJ. Postoperative irradiation for squamous cell carcinomas of the head and neck: analysis of time-dose factors related to control above the clavicles. *Int J Radiat Oncol Biol Phys* 1979;5(11–12):1943–1949.
58. Million RR. Squamous cell carcinoma of the head and neck: combined therapy: surgery and postoperative irradiation. *Int J Radiat Oncol Biol Phys* 1979;5(11–12): 2161–2162.
59. Parsons JT, Mendenhall WM, Cassisi NJ, et al. Hyperfractionation for head and neck cancer. *Int J Radiat Oncol Biol Phys* 1988;14(4):649–658.
60. Parsons JT, Mendenhall WM, Cassisi NJ, et al. Neck dissection after twice-a-day radiotherapy: morbidity and recurrence rates. *Head Neck* 1989;11(5):400–404.
61. Ellis ER, Mendenhall WM, Rao PV, et al. Incisional or excisional neck-node biopsy before definitive radiotherapy, alone or followed by neck dissection. *Head Neck* 1991;13(3):177–183.
62. Mendenhall WM, Parsons JT, Amdur RJ, et al. Squamous cell carcinoma of the head and neck treated with radiotherapy: does planned neck dissection reduce the change for successful surgical management of subsequent local recurrence? *Head Neck Surg* 1988;10(5):302–304.
63. Mendenhall WM, Parsons JT, Amdur RJ, et al. Squamous cell carcinoma of the head and neck treated with radiation therapy: the impact of neck stage on local control. *Int J Radiat Oncol Biol Phys* 1988;14(2):249–252.
64. Wall TJ, Peters LJ, Brown BW, et al. Relationship between lymph nodal status and primary tumor control probability in tumors of the supraglottic larynx. *Int J Radiat Oncol Biol Phys* 1985;11(11):1895–1902.
65. Barker CA, Morris CG, Mendenhall WM. Larynx-sparing radiotherapy for squamous cell carcinoma from an unknown head and neck primary site. *Am J Clin Oncol* 2005;28(5):445–448.
66. Erkal HS, Mendenhall WM, Amdur RJ, et al. Squamous cell carcinomas metastatic to cervical lymph nodes from an unknown head-and-neck mucosal site treated with radiation therapy alone or in combination with neck dissection. *Int J Radiat Oncol Biol Phys* 2001;50(1):55–63.
67. Mendenhall WM. Unknown primary squamous cell carcinoma of the head and neck. *Curr Cancer Ther Rev* 2005;1:167–174.
68. Mukherji SK, Drane WE, Mancuso AA, et al. Occult primary tumors of the head and neck: detection with 2-[F-18] fluoro-2-deoxy-D-glucose SPECT. *Radiology* 1996;199(3):761–766.
69. Cianchetti M, Mancuso AA, Amdur RJ, et al. Diagnostic evaluation of squamous cell carcinoma metastatic to cervical lymph nodes from an unknown head and neck primary site. *Laryngoscope* 2009;119(12):2348–2354.
70. Coster JR, Foote RL, Olsen KD, et al. Cervical nodal metastasis of squamous cell carcinoma of unknown origin: indications for withholding radiation therapy. *Int J Radiat Oncol Biol Phys* 1992;23(4):743–749.
71. Wallace A, Richards GM, Harari PM, et al. Head and neck squamous cell carcinoma from an unknown primary site. *Am J Otolaryngol* 2011;32(4):286–290.
72. Colletier PJ, Garden AS, Morrison WH, et al. Postoperative radiation for squamous cell carcinoma metastatic to cervical lymph nodes from an unknown primary site: outcomes and patterns of failure. *Head Neck* 1998;20(8):674–681.
73. Reddy SP, Marks JE. Metastatic carcinoma in the cervical lymph nodes from an unknown primary site: results of bilateral neck plus mucosal irradiation vs. ipsilateral neck irradiation. *Int J Radiat Oncol Biol Phys* 1997;37(4):797–802.
74. Grau C, Johansen LV, Jakobsen J, et al. Cervical lymph node metastases from unknown primary tumours. Results from a national survey by the Danish Society for Head and Neck Oncology. *Radiother Oncol* 2000;55(2):121–129.
75. Erkal HS, Mendenhall WM, Amdur RJ, et al. Squamous cell carcinomas metastatic to cervical lymph nodes from an unknown head and neck mucosal site treated with radiation therapy with palliative intent. *Radiother Oncol* 2001;59(3):319–321.
76. Mendenhall WM, Amdur RJ, Hinerman RW, et al. Head and neck: management of the neck. In: Perez CA, Brady LW, Halperin EC, et al., eds. *Principles and practice of radiation oncology.* Philadelphia: Lippincott Williams & Wilkins, 2004:1158–1178.
77. Cutler SJ, Ederer F. Maximum utilization of the life table method in analyzing survival. *J Chronic Dis* 1958;8(6):699–712.
78. Fletcher GH, Jesse RH, Healey JE, et al. Oropharynx. In: MacComb WS, Fletcher GH, eds. *Cancer of the head and neck.* Baltimore: Williams & Wilkins, 1967:179–212.
79. Fletcher GH, Jesse RH, Lindberg RD, et al. The place of radiotherapy in the management of the squamous cell carcinoma of the supraglottic larynx. *Am J Roentgenol Radium Ther Nucl Med* 1970;108(1):19–26.
80. MacComb WS, Healey JE, McGraw JP, et al. Hypopharynx and cervical esophagus. In: MacComb WS, Fletcher GH, eds. *Cancer of the head and neck.* Baltimore: Williams & Wilkins, 1967:213–240.
81. Chen KY, Fletcher GH. Malignant tumors of the nasopharynx. *Radiology* 1971; 99(1):165–171.

Chapter 50
Thyroid Cancer

Roi Dagan and Robert J. Amdur

BASIC THYROID ANATOMY AND PHYSIOLOGY

Gross Anatomy

The thyroid gland is located in the central anterior neck at the cervical–thoracic junction. The bulk of the gland is located immediately anterior and inferior to the thyroid cartilage. It has two lateral lobes connected by a central isthmus. Approximately 50% of individuals have a pyramidal lobe that extends superiorly from the central aspect of the gland, which is a remnant of the gland's embryologic origin, the thyroglossal duct. The average adult thyroid gland measures approximately 5 × 5 cm and weighs 10 to 20 g.

The location of the gland in the central neck and its relation to critical structures explain the presenting symptoms of advanced neoplastic processes arising from the thyroid as well as potential complications of thyroid surgery and radiotherapy (Fig. 50.1). The lateral lobes extend superiorly to the level of the midthyroid cartilage overlying the larynx and inferiorly to the sixth tracheal ring. The gland wraps around 75% of the tracheal circumference, posteriorly encroaching on the esophagus. The lateral extent is just medial to the common carotid arteries. The recurrent laryngeal nerves, sympathetic trunks, vagus, and phrenic nerves are all found immediately posterior to the gland, and the gland is anteriorly bound by the strap muscles. Parathyroid glands are located posterior to the thyroid gland and vary in location and number.

Vasculature and Lymphatics

The arterial blood supply to the thyroid gland is provided by the paired superior thyroid arteries (branches of the external carotid arteries) and inferior thyroid arteries (branches of the thyrocervical trunk from the subclavian arteries). Venous blood drains via the paired superior and middle thyroid veins to the internal jugular veins and from the inferior thyroid veins to the subclavian and innominate veins. There is a dense lymphatic network

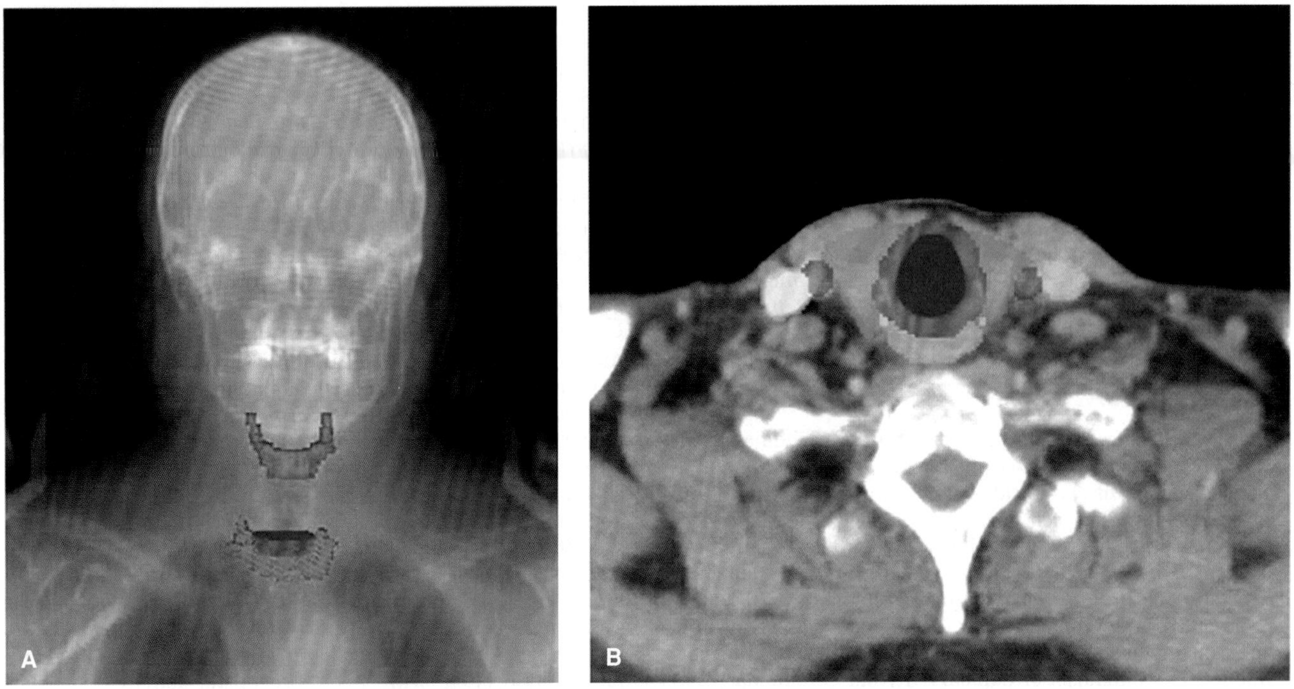

FIGURE 50.1. Anatomy of the thyroid gland. **A:** Digitally reconstructed radiograph of a patient's head and neck showing the relative position of the thyroid gland (*blue*) to the hyoid bone (*green*) and bottom of the cricoid cartilage (*purple*). **B:** Contrast-enhanced axial computed tomography slice at the level of the bottom of the cricoid cartilage (*purple*) showing the position of the thyroid gland (*blue*) relative to the esophagus (*orange*), carotid arteries (*red*), jugular vein (*lavender*) and the approximate position of the recurrent laryngeal nerves (*yellow-green*).

draining the gland in multiple directions, and bilateral involvement of lymph node metastases is common. According to the American Joint Committee on Cancer's (AJCC) seventh edition of the *AJCC Cancer Staging Handbook,* the first-echelon nodes for thyroid cancer metastases are located in level 6 (the central or "visceral" compartment) between the hyoid bone and the thoracic inlet.[1] Specifically, these are the paralaryngeal, paratracheal, and prelaryngeal (Delphian) nodes. Second-echelon nodal spread is to the mid- and lower cervical nodes (levels 3 and 4), supraclavicular nodes, upper mediastinal nodes (level 7), and to a lesser extent the upper cervical nodes (level 2). Retropharyngeal node involvement is unusual but can be encountered in the setting of advanced nodal disease. Level 1 (submental and submandibular) lymph nodes are rarely involved.

Microscopic Anatomy

Microscopically, the normal thyroid gland consists of numerous lobules comprising individual follicles forming the structural and functional unit of the gland. The supporting stoma and vasculature are intertwined around the follicles. Each follicle consists of a single layer of cuboidal surface epithelium comprising thyroid follicular cells surrounding a central lumen-containing colloid, a substance rich in thyroglobulin (Tg). Approximately 10% of the follicular epithelium contains parafollicular cells, or C cells, which are neural crest-derived cells containing granules of calcitonin. The gland is incompletely surrounded by a connective tissue capsule.

Physiology

The primary physiologic role of the thyroid gland is the production of thyroid hormone, which plays an important role in metabolic homeostasis. A secondary role is the production of calcitonin, a hormone involved in calcium homeostasis. The follicular cells of the thyroid gland synthesize and secrete Tg and thyroid hormone in two biologically active forms, thyroxine (3,5,3′,5′ iodothyronine or T_4) and triiodothyronine (3,5,3′ iodothyronine or T_3). It is useful to consider T_4 as the storage and transport form of thyroid hormone and T_3 as the metabolically active form. Most circulating thyroid hormone is bound to thyroxine-binding globulin. In peripheral tissues, where thyroid hormone executes its endocrine function, T_4 is rapidly converted to the more active form T_3 by the action of T_4 monodeiodinase. T_3 is transported to the nucleus where it binds to specific nuclear receptors and interacts with regulatory genes, influencing their expression. The gene products ultimately increase the cell's basal metabolic rate, protein synthesis, catecholamine effects, and growth of long bones and play an essential role in metabolism of proteins, fats, and carbohydrates. Thyroid hormone exerts it endocrine function on virtually all cells in the body.

Iodine is a critical component of thyroid hormone and is essential for thyroid function. The recommended daily intake is 150 μg, and at least 50 μg of daily intake is necessary to prevent deficiency, resulting in a goiter. The follicular cells of the thyroid gland possess a unique ability to actively uptake and concentrate iodine. The sodium iodine symporter (NaIS) actively transports sodium and iodine against an electrochemical gradient across the cell membrane in an energy-dependent fashion. This transmembrane protein is stimulated by thyroid-stimulating hormone (TSH or thyrotropin), which is synthesized in the anterior pituitary. Functional NaIS is present on malignant follicular cells seen in multiple variants of differentiated thyroid cancer. The unique ability to concentrate iodine within these malignant cells makes radioactive iodine (RAI) a potent targeted therapy. The central role of TSH in driving the internalization of iodine within follicular thyroid cells is exploited in preparation for RAI. To increase the efficacy of iodine-131 (I-131) therapy, T_4 deprivation, a low-iodine diet, and administration of recombinant human TSH (rhTSH) can be used to increases the effects of TSH on follicular thyroid cells (see the section on preparing patients for I-131). NaIS is also present in the parotid glands, breast tissues, gastric mucosa, and nasolacrimal ducts, placing them at risk for injury from RAI therapy.

Upon entering the follicular cells, iodine is transported across the apical membrane and oxidized to a form that binds to tyrosyl residues of Tg, a large (660 kDa) glycoprotein synthesized by the follicular cells. Iodinated Tg becomes the main component of the intraluminal colloid stores of the thyroid follicles. T_3 and T_4 are synthesized by the coupling of iodinated tyrosine. They remain attached to the Tg until leaving the gland. TSH stimulation results in endocytosis of colloid droplets from the lumen into the follicular cells where it is hydrolyzed and releases Tg, T_4, and, to lesser degree, T_3 into the circulation. Malignant differentiated follicular cells retain this function. Thus, serum Tg becomes a unique tumor marker after thyroidectomy and thyroid remnant ablation.[2]

A feedback loop between the thyroid, pituitary, and hypothalamus regulates thyroid hormone synthesis and secretion. Thyrotropin-releasing hormone (TRH) is synthesized in the hypothalamus, and its primary function is to increase the secretion of TSH in the pituitary. Both T_3 and T_4 in turn inhibit TRH release and TSH secretion.

CLASSIFICATIONS OF THYROID CANCER

Correct pathological classification of thyroid carcinoma is fundamental to the appropriate clinical management of the malignancy. A system of classification is shown in Table 50.1 and discussed below. The cell of origin, cytological features, and growth morphology determine the pathologic classification. All carcinomas of the thyroid gland are derived from the follicular epithelium, except medullary thyroid carcinoma (MTC), which is derived from the parafollicular C cells. Capsular invasion is important in the pathologic diagnosis of certain thyroid carcinomas. The diagnosis of papillary thyroid carcinoma (PTC) is entirely predicated on the presence of diagnostic nuclear features and does not require invasive growth, while follicular carcinoma (FC) requires the presence of capsular or vascular invasion.[3] Other rarely encountered malignant neoplasms of the thyroid gland include thyroid lymphoma and sarcomas. These two entities will not be discussed in this chapter and are better evaluated and managed under paradigms detailed in the chapters on lymphoma and sarcoma.

Differentiated (Follicular-Derived) Thyroid Carcinoma

The two major subgroups comprising differentiated thyroid carcinoma (DTC) are PTC and FC. They are distinguished by architectural and cytological features.

Papillary Thyroid Cancer

PTC is the most common histologic type, representing approximately 80% to 90% of all thyroid cancer diagnoses, and has the best prognosis of all thyroid malignancies.[4] Malignant nuclear cytological characteristics are the distinguishing feature of PTC and include nuclear enlargement, hypochromasia, intranuclear cytoplasmic inclusions (nuclear pseudoinclusions), nuclear grooves, and distinct nucleoli. After formalin fixation, nuclei may appear pale, optically clear, and resemble "Orphan Annie's eyes." PTC is strongly lymphotropic, and multicentric disease within the parenchyma of the gland is often present secondary to early lymphatic spread. All PTC stain strongly for Tg.[5–7]

In its classic variant, PTC has a tumor architecture comprising branching papillae with fibrovascular cores. Papillary microcarcinoma is used to describe incidentally identified papillary carcinoma measuring <1.0 cm in diameter. The encapsulated variant of PTC (approximately 10% of PTCs) is surrounded by a thick fibrous capsule, unlike most PTCs that are nonencapsulated and infiltrate the surrounding thyroid parenchyma. Although not as favorable as microcarcinoma, encapsulated PTC has a favorable prognosis compared with classic PTC. The follicular variant of PTC differs from the classic variant by its follicular growth pattern; however, it retains the nuclear features diagnostic of PTC. Its prognosis roughly mirrors that of classic PTC. Other variants include diffuse sclerosing, tall cell, and columnar cell PTC, which have a much poorer prognosis.

Diffuse sclerosing is a rare form of PTC, with histologic features of extensive sclerosis, lymphocytic infiltrate, and psammoma bodies. A greater percentage of patients with diffuse sclerosing PTC present with extrathyroidal extension or distant metastases. Likewise, tall cell and columnar variants are commonly associated with poor prognostic features such as advanced age, large tumor size, aggressive histologic features with early invasion, and distant metastases. The distinguishing feature of tall cell PTC is that at least 70% of the carcinoma is composed of cells that are at least twice as tall as they are wide because of abundant cellular cytoplasm. Columnar cell variant is extremely rare. These carcinomas histologically show striking nuclear stratification, usually with papillary architecture. However, the usual nuclear features of PTCs may be absent; therefore, some pathologists prefer to classify columnar cell as poorly differentiated carcinomas.

TABLE 50.1 PATHOLOGICAL CLASSIFICATION FOR THYROID CANCER

Cell of Origin
I. Follicular epithelial cell
A. Differentiated thyroid cancers
1. Papillary and mixed papillary variants
a. Classic
b. Papillary microcarcinoma
c. Encapsulated variant
d. Follicular variant
e. Aggressive variants
i. Diffuse sclerosing
ii. Tall cell variant
III. Columnar cell variant
2. Follicular cancer
a. Classic morphology–Follicular carcinoma
b. Hürthle cell variant
B. Poorly differentiated thyroid cancer
1. Insular carcinoma
C. Undifferentiated thyroid cancer (Anaplastic carcinoma)
II. Parafollicular cell (C cell)
A. Medullary carcinoma

Follicular Carcinoma

FC, like PTC, is a DTC of follicular cell origin. They comprise 15% to 30% of all thyroid carcinomas and share a similar prognosis to classic PTC. This malignant thyroid neoplasm lacks the cytological features of PTC. These carcinomas show evidence of thyroid follicle formation and are usually well circumscribed with a defined tumor capsule. They are grossly indistinguishable from follicular adenomas. The diagnosis of FC is dependent on the presence of one of two histologic features: (a) tumor invasion through the entire tumor capsule or (b) tumor invasion into a blood vessel located in the tumor capsule or immediately outside the tumor capsule. Minimally invasive forms of FC may present a pathologic challenge and often require serial sectioning to find evidence of capsular or vascular invasion, while widely invasive forms of FC are obviously invasive tumors both on gross and microscopic evaluation.

Hürthle Cell Carcinoma

This follicular epithelial-derived carcinoma, also known as oncocytic carcinoma, is characterized by large cells with abundant granular eosinophilic cytoplasms. Hürthle cells may be seen in both benign and other non-Hürthle cell malignant neoplastic lesions; however, at least 75% of the tumor must be comprised of Hürthle cells to designate it Hürthle cell carcinoma. Similar to FC, Hürthle cell carcinoma requires the presence of capsular or vascular invasion to classify it as a malignant neoplasm. Although Hürthle cell carcinoma is classically included under the subclassification FC, it is now apparent that there are both follicular and papillary types. Hürthle cell carcinoma has a less-favorable prognosis and usually presents with large tumor size, more invasive features, early regional and distant metastatic spread, and lower likelihood to concentrate RAI.

Poorly Differentiated Thyroid Carcinoma (Insular Carcinoma)

These follicular epithelial cell-derived tumors are intermediate between DTC and undifferentiated (anaplastic) thyroid cancers (ATC). Both their histologic appearance and biological behavior are more aggressive than DTC. They tend to be widely invasive and many will extend beyond the gland. Insular carcinoma is characterized by tumor cells that are arranged in discrete nests separated by a fibrous stroma. Microscopically, they are usually solid with some evidence of follicle formation. Mitoses and necrosis are often present. The presence of more differentiated areas of tumor admixed with insular carcinoma suggests that the latter represents "dedifferentiated" tumors.

Undifferentiated (Anaplastic) Thyroid Carcinoma

ATC comprise <5% of all malignant thyroid neoplasms. This is the most aggressive form of thyroid carcinoma, accounting for 14% to 50% of all thyroid cancer deaths. Most patients are diagnosed at the age of 65 years or older.[8] ATC originates from the thyroid follicular epithelium but shows little to no evidence of histologic differentiation. This tumor is defined as much by its clinical behavior as its histologic appearance. When diagnosed, most ATCs are widely invasive, replacing most if not all of the normal-appearing gland, and freely infiltrate the perithyroidal tissues. They are usually accompanied by bulky metastatic lymphadenopathy and distant metastatic spread. Gross pathologic evaluation is characterized by widely infiltrative disease with areas of necrosis and hemorrhage. Various microscopic patterns have been described, including small cell, spindle cell, giant cell, squamoid, or pleomorphic. They are hypothesized to be lesions that have dedifferentiated from more benign differentiated follicular neoplasms.

Medullary Thyroid Carcinoma

Medullary thyroid carcinoma (MTC) does not originate from the follicular epithelial cells, but from the parafollicular C cells, which are neural crest-derived cells whose function is to produce calcitonin. MTC comprises less that 5% to 10% of all thyroid cancers. Cases are seen sporadically (80%) or in association with familial multiple endocrine neoplasia (MEN IIa, MEN IIb, and pure familial MTC) syndromes. Multifocal and bilateral MTC are usually seen in patients with MEN, but, otherwise, familial and sporadic MTCs are indistinguishable. Grossly, these tumors are well circumscribed and nonencapsulated. Microscopically, tumors can have different appearances, including patterns that mimic other types of thyroid tumors. The most common pattern is of solid growth or nests similar to insular carcinoma. Amyloid, which is present in approximately 80% of cases, is a characteristic feature of MTC. Calcitonin stains are usually positive and specific for MTC, but up to 20% of cases may not stain for calcitonin; therefore, other neuroendocrine markers such as chromogrannin may be useful.

Classification Based on the Capacity to Concentrate Radioactive Iodine

Different pathologic classes of thyroid carcinoma concentrate RAI to various degrees. This characteristic is central to management decisions because the ability to concentrate RAI presents a useful therapeutic target. Table 50.2 presents a classification system that categorizes cancers based on whether they always concentrate RAI, infrequently concentrate RAI, or never concentrate RAI. Papillary and follicular carcinomas (with the exception of the more aggressive variants), usually concentrate RAI. The follicular variant of papillary cancer has the same avidity for RAI as papillary cancer with classic morphology. Therefore, from the treatment standpoint, the distinction between these types of DTCs is not important. The aggressive variants of papillary carcinoma and Hürthle cell carcinoma can

TABLE 50.2 A SYSTEM OF CLASSIFICATION FOR THYROID CANCER BASED ON THE ABILITY TO CONCENTRATE RADIOACTIVE IODINE

A. Usually concentrate RAI
I. Classic papillary carcinoma
II. Encapsulated papillary carcinoma
III. Follicular variant and mixed follicular-papillary carcinoma
IV. Follicular carcinoma
B. Frequently do not concentrate RAI
I. Tall cell and columnar cell variants of papillary carcinoma
II. Hürthle cell carcinoma
III. Poorly differentiated (insular) carcinoma
C. Never concentrate RAI
I. Anaplastic carcinoma
II. Medullary carcinoma

RAI, radioactive iodine.

concentrate RAI, but to a lesser degree than the classic morphologies. In fact, there is often no measurable iodine uptake in metastases of these tumors. Anaplastic and medullary cancers never concentrate RAI to a clinically useful degree.

EPIDEMIOLOGY OF THYROID CANCER

Thyroid cancer is the most commonly diagnosed endocrine cancer. There will be an estimated 48,000 new thyroid cancer diagnoses and 1,740 thyroid cancer deaths in the United States by the end of 2011.[9] The overall incidence is 7.7 per 100,000 persons per year.[10] There is a strong female prevalence with women being three times more likely than men to be diagnosed with thyroid cancer. Thyroid cancer is the fifth most common cancer diagnosis in women, accounting for approximately 5% of all new female cancer diagnoses.[9] DTC comprises the overwhelming majority (94%) of new thyroid cancer diagnoses. Approximately 5% are medullary thyroid carcinoma and 1% are anaplastic thyroid carcinoma.[11] Per the National Cancer Institute's Surveillance, Epidemiology, and End Results (SEER) database, the incidence of thyroid cancer has increased in the United States from 3.6 per 100,000 people in 1973 to 8.7 in 2002. The bulk of these cases result from an increase in detection of small primary cancer, with 49% and 87% of new cancers measuring <1 cm and 2 cm, respectively.[12] According to another SEER database analysis, the most commonly diagnosed PTC in 2006 was papillary microcarcinoma (<1 cm).[13] An even greater proportion of thyroid cancers remain clinically occult, and the prevalence of PTCs at autopsy has been reported as high as 35%.[14]

The incidence of thyroid cancer increases with age with a peak incidence at 40 to 44 years old for women and 65 to 69 years for men. The peak incidence for ATC is at 60 years for both sexes, and for MTC it can vary depending on whether it is familial or sporadic.[15] The incidence of PTC varies significantly across race, with Asian women having the highest incidence of PTC at 10.96 per 100,000 woman-years compared with the lowest incidence for African American women of 4.9 per 100,000 woman-years.[10]

The prevalence of thyroid cancer in the U.S. population is much higher than the incidence of new diagnoses, a phenomenon attributed to the indolent nature of most DTCs. In 2001, there were an estimated 300,000 individuals living in the United States with thyroid cancer, a number similar to much more commonly diagnosed fatal cancers such as primary carcinomas of the bronchus and lung.[15] Patients living with recurrent thyroid cancer comprise a substantial proportion of the prevalence of thyroid cancer. In a series of 1,355 patients with papillary and follicular thyroid cancers, the 30-year cumulative rate of recurrence was approximately 30%, while cancer-related mortality was <10% (Fig. 50.2).[16] Studies reporting the outcomes of patients treated for thyroid cancer must be interpreted with consideration of the length of follow-up. Roughly 25% of all

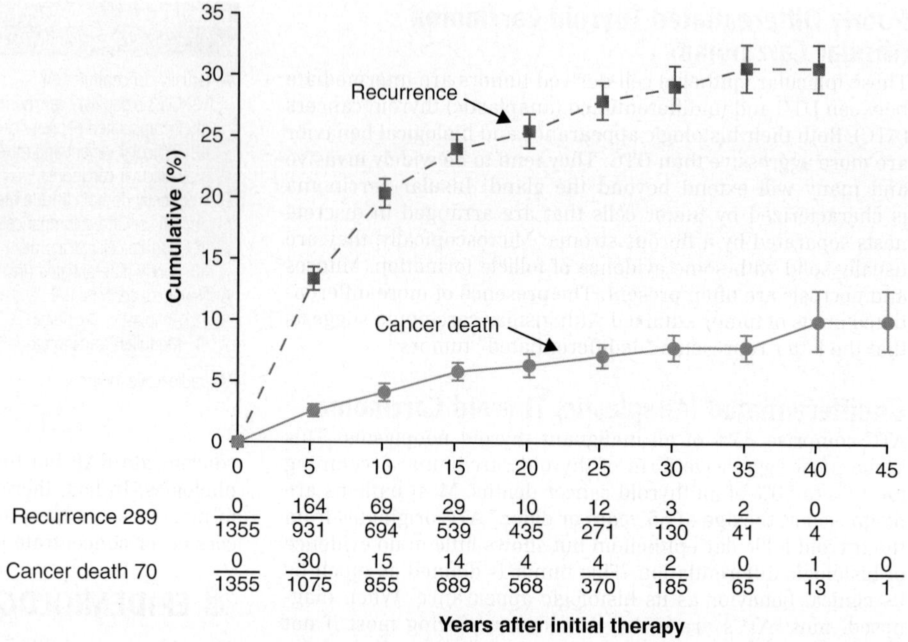

FIGURE 50.2. Tumor recurrence and cancer deaths in 1,355 patients treated for follicular and papillary thyroid carcinoma. (From Mazzaferri EL, Jhiang SM. Long-term impact of initial surgical and medical therapy on papillary and follicular thyroid cancer. *Am J Med* 1994;97:418–28, with permission from Elsevier.)

recurrences will present after 5 years of follow-up and as many as 16% will be detected after 15 years of follow-up.[15]

Radiation-Induced Thyroid Cancer

Exposure to ionizing radiation is an established risk factor for thyroid nodules and cancer. Well-recognized data come from survivors of atomic bombs in Hiroshima and Nagasaki and the nuclear reactor accident in Chernobyl.[17–18,19–20,21–23] A recent analysis of the 59,687 atomic bomb survivors in the Life Span Study demonstrated a total of 24.5% of cases of thyroid cancer in this cohort were attributed to radiation exposure with a strong dose response.[21] Women and young children appeared to be most susceptible. An estimated additional 1,000 cases of thyroid cancer throughout Europe have been attributed to the Chernobyl accident.[23] An increased risk of thyroid cancer has also been attributed to exposure to therapeutic radiation in children treated for Hodgkin lymphoma, tinea capitis, enlarged tonsils, and enlarged thymus.[24,25–26] Radiation-induced thyroid cancer is pathologically indistinguishable from spontaneous forms of the disease and is not associated with more aggressive biology or poorer prognosis.[27,28–30]

Familial Medullary Thyroid Carcinoma

Twenty-five percent of cases of MTCs are hereditary. All patients with MTC should be screened for familial disease, and genetic testing is considered the standard of care for all first-degree relatives of patients with newly diagnosed MTC. Heritable forms of MTC are associated with the familial MEN syndromes (MEN IIa, MEN IIb, and pure familial MTC) and have their own unique epidemiology. These disorders are inherited in an autosomal dominant fashion due to a germline-point mutation in the *RET* gene on chromosome 10q11.2. Men and women are affected equally given the pattern of inheritance. These patients typically present with bilateral and multifocal tumors compared to sporadic forms of MTC. The aggressiveness and age of onset of familial MTC differs depending on the specific genetic mutation. Prophylactic thyroidectomies are increasingly being performed on patients at risk for developing MTC.[31]

CLINICAL MANIFESTATIONS OF THYROID CANCER

The most common presentation of thyroid cancer is an asymptomatic thyroid nodule found incidentally by the patient, clinicians, or on an imaging study performed for other reasons. Palpable thyroid nodules occur in 3% to 4% of the normal population, and their incidence at autopsy has been reported as high as 50%.[32,33–34] However, <1% of thyroid nodules represent a cancer. The differential diagnosis of thyroid nodules includes adenomas (macrofollicular, microfollicular, Hürthle cell, and atypical), cystic lesions (simple cysts or hemorrhagic cysts), colloid nodules, thyroiditis, granulomatous disease, and cancer. Positive findings on history and physical examination that raise suspicion that a thyroid nodule is malignant include rapid growth, firmness, fixation, vocal cord paralysis, cervical adenopathy, stridor, dysphagia, or neurological compromise. In cases where two or more of these symptoms or signs are present, the incidence of thyroid cancer is over 70%, and surgery should be recommended even in the presence of a nondiagnostic fine-needle aspiration (FNA).[35]

Clinically occult thyroid cancer and benign thyroid nodules will often present on imaging studies performed for other diagnoses. Studies utilizing computed tomography (CT), magnetic resonance imaging (MRI), or ultrasound (US) have reported the incidence of clinically occult thyroid nodules to be 19% to 67%.[36] Fluorodeoxyglucose (FDG)-positron emission tomography (PET) studies have also reported the incidence of focal uptake within the thyroid gland at 2% to 3%, with only 25% to 50% ultimately representing cancer.[37,38] Many incidentally detected thyroid cancers will ultimately prove to be clinically significant lesions with pathologically identified extrathyroidal extension, lymph node metastases, or both.[39]

Alternatively, locally advanced thyroid cancer presents with symptoms from involvement of the critical structures intimately associated with the thyroid gland, massive cervical lymphadenopathy, or metastatic disease. These patients present with symptoms such as hoarseness from tumor compression of the recurrent laryngeal nerve, airway compromise, dysphagia or respiratory symptoms, and pain and weight loss resulting from metastatic dissemination.

DIAGNOSTIC EVALUATION OF THYROID CANCER

Laboratory Studies

All patients with thyroid nodules should undergo a serum TSH in addition to basic metabolic, renal, and liver function tests and a complete blood count. Other lab tests, such as Tg, T_3,

TABLE 50.3 ULTRASOUND FINDINGS USED TO SELECT THYROID NODULES FOR FINE-NEEDLE ASPIRATION

Ultrasound Characteristic	Tumor Size Requiring Biopsy
Size >1 cm in one dimension	All
Spherical shape	≤1 cm
Hypoechoic	≤1 cm
Microcalcification	≤1 cm
Irregular or indistinct margins	≤8 mm
Increased Doppler flow	≤8 mm
Invasion into surrounding tissue	≤8 mm
Suspicious cervical lymph node	≤8 mm

and T_4, are commonly obtained but are rarely useful in the initial management of thyroid cancer. Serum calcitonin can be measured during the initial evaluation of patients with MTC and is essential during follow-up for these patients.

Ultrasound and Ultrasound-Guided Fine-Needle Aspirate

Neck US with Doppler and US-FNA are the standard diagnostic approaches for evaluating thyroid nodules, both palpable and incidentally detected on imaging. The ultrasonographic features used to select thyroid nodules for FNA are shown in Table 50.3. For a more-detailed discussion on the use of US in the evaluation of thyroid nodules, please refer to a consensus statement by the Society of Radiologists in Ultrasound on the management of thyroid nodules detected by US[40] and the American Thyroid Association's recently updated management guidelines for patients with thyroid nodules and differentiated thyroid cancer.[41]

US-FNA has several benefits in the evaluation of thyroid nodules over other means of obtaining a tissue diagnosis: (a) the technique is minimally invasive and is usually performed as an outpatient procedure; (b) the operator can visually verify that the biopsy needle is in the nodule(s) of suspicion; and (c) it allows for evaluation of nonpalpable nodules and, in the setting of cystic lesions, lowers the rate of inadequate specimens.

US-FNA of thyroid nodules yields cytology that can be broadly classified into four categories: (a) insufficient for diagnosis, (b) benign, (c) positive for cancer, and (d) indeterminate for diagnosis. Approximately 5% to 10% of US-FNA specimens are insufficient for diagnosis, and the rate of insufficient biopsies can be reduced by 50% with repeated biopsies or evaluation by personnel trained in cytological evaluation of thyroid nodules at the time of the procedure. Sixty-five percent to 75% of US-FNA cytology will be benign. Approximately 5% of all US-FNAs of thyroid lesions yield specimens with the diagnostic cytological features of PTC, anaplastic carcinoma, medullary carcinoma, or other poorly differentiated carcinomas. Finally, 15% to 20% of US-FNA will be classified as "suspicious" or indeterminate for diagnosis. Other synonyms for this cytological classification are follicular neoplasm or follicular tumor. The diagnostic evaluation of these lesions is aided by the use of laboratory evaluation of thyroid function and nuclear imaging with RAI uptake studies if the TSH is suppressed. About 20% of these will ultimately show FC or Hürthle cell carcinoma on surgical specimens.[42]

The overall diagnostic accuracy of US-FNA will depend on the skill and experience of the operator and the cytologist in interpreting the specimen. In a large series of 1,135 cases, there were 1,127 satisfactory samples: 6% cancer (or suspicious for cancer), 10% follicular neoplasms, 82% benign, and 0.7% indeterminate; the false-negative rate was 0% and only 1.5% were false positives. Surgery was performed on 169 patients, and a review of final pathology yielded a sensitivity of 100% and specificity of 67%. The corresponding positive and negative predictive values of US-FNA were 87% and 100%, respectively.[43] Another study of 1,613 cases of FNA reported a sensitivity of 78%, specificity of 98%, and a predictive value of 100% for papillary carcinoma.[44] The major limitation of this diagnostic tool is the inability to distinguish benign follicular adenomas from FC and follicular PTC.

Cervical US is also an important staging tool because it is effective in identifying lymph node metastases. Cervical lymph node size, presence of calcification, and irregular diffuse intranodular blood flow are the most important US features suggestive of lymph node metastases.[45,46] Using criteria based on the ratio of largest to smallest lymph node diameter, nodule echogenicity, intranodal structure, and margin irregularity, the sensitivity and specificity of cervical US for identifying malignant cervical lesions were 90% and 82%, respectively, in a study of 112 patients followed for thyroid cancer by high-resolution US with Doppler.[47] Preoperative cervical US identified lymph node metastases that were occult on physical examination in 33% to 39% of patients in a large retrospective series.[48,49] Cervical US findings will alter the surgical approach in 14% to 24% of patients with PTC by identifying nonpalpable cervical lymph node metastases.[45,49]

Computed Tomography and Magnetic Resonance Imaging

CT and MRI commonly detect otherwise clinically occult thyroid nodules. Malignancy is likely with either imaging technique when there are findings of a mass with extrathyroidal extension, lymph node metastases, or both. In this setting, the studies are useful in presurgical planning by establishing the extent of extraglandular tumor and helping the surgeon determine the need for extended neck dissections (Fig. 50.3). MRI is superior to CT for establishing the local extent of a known cancer, because it will more clearly show esophageal or tracheal invasion (Fig. 50.4).[50] MRI is indicated in the presence of hoarseness, stridor, dysphagia, or other clinical signs of locally extensive thyroid cancer that cannot be adequately assessed by US.

A major downside to CT is that useful imaging of the neck requires contrast enhancement, which can interfere with subsequent RAI therapy. Because of their high concentration of iodine, CT contrast agents can seriously compromise the effectiveness of therapeutic RAI. When patients receiving iodinated contrast agents require RAI, therapy should be delayed in order to achieve adequate efficacy. Given this drawback as well as the effectiveness of US in defining the local-regional extent of tumor, the authors strongly discourage the use of CT in the staging evaluation of known thyroid cancer. In selected cases, a noncontrasted CT of the chest may be indicated to evaluate the presence of mediastinal and lung metastases, but, generally speaking, it is not necessary to perform a CT before primary therapy of most DTCs.

Nuclear Medicine Studies

The four major nuclear medicine studies related to thyroid cancer evaluation with iodine isotopes are radioactive iodine uptake (RAIU), thyroid scan, diagnostic whole-body scan (DxWBS), and posttreatment whole-body scan (RxWBS). Table 50.4 summarizes each of these studies.

RAIU tests are used to quantify the RAI-concentrating ability of remnant thyroid tissue after thyroidectomy. This value is required by federal regulation for outpatient I-131 therapy.

Thyroid scans produce images of the thyroid's ability to concentrate RAI and have a historical use in the evaluation of thyroid nodules, characterizing them as functional ("hot") or nonfunctional ("cold"). The authors do not use thyroid scans in the workup or management of patients with thyroid cancer.

The typical DxWBS involves a total body image several days after administering approximately 3 mCi of I-131. The current value of a DxWBS in thyroid cancer management is controversial. Some experts use a DxWBS to determine the

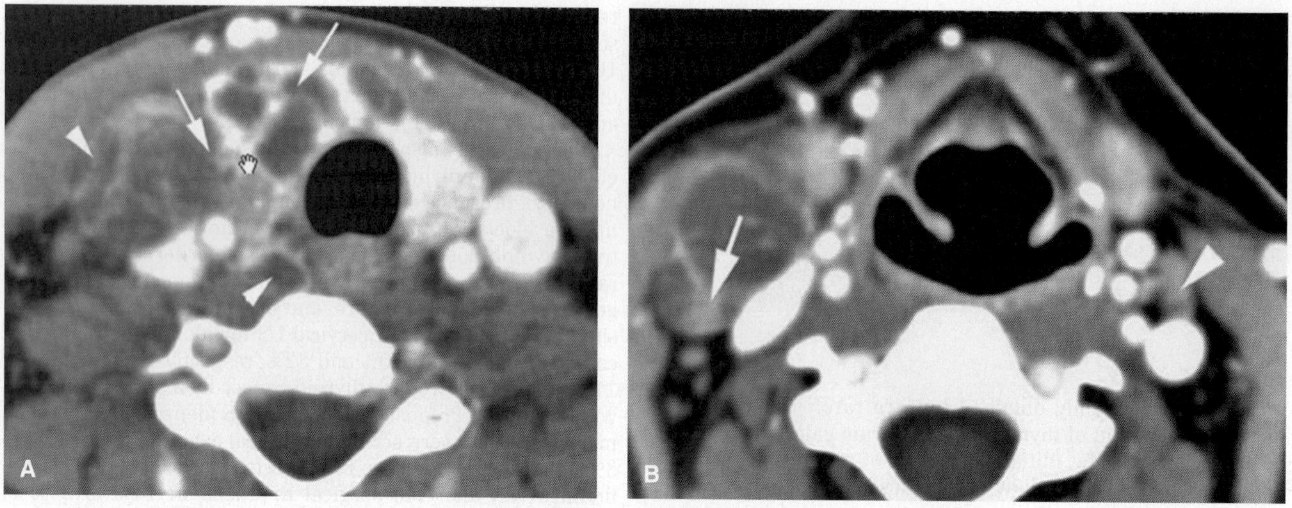

FIGURE 50.3. A patient presenting with a neck mass. **A:** Computed tomography study showing the mass to be due to a primary papillary thyroid carcinoma coming into contact with a related level 4 metastatic lymph node (*arrows*). The lymph node at level 4 and in the tracheoesophageal groove is shown by the *arrowheads*. **B:** A section more superiorly shows level 3 adenopathy that is multicystic in a pattern typical but not necessarily diagnostic of papillary thyroid carcinoma. There is upper level 4 cystic adenopathy with an enhancing mural nodule (*arrow*)—a morphology suggesting of thyroid carcinoma. A contralateral enhancing positive node with a focal low-density defect (*arrowhead*) is also present. (From Mancuso AA, Mendenhall WM, Vaysberg M. Thyroid: nodules and malignant tumors. In: Mancuso AA, ed. *Head and neck radiology*. Philadelphia: Lippincott Williams & Wilkins, 2010:1457–1481, with permission.)

dose of I-131 in a patient being treated for thyroid cancer. Some experts use a DxWBS as part of the surveillance program following initial treatment. A comprehensive discussion of the issues related to DxWBS is beyond the scope of this chapter. The main arguments against doing DxWBS are low sensitivity, stunning of residual cancer cells, and unnecessary radiation exposure. The bottom line is that reasonable people will disagree about the role of DxWBS in thyroid cancer management. The authors do not use DxWBS to stage or monitor thyroid cancer patients and have not ordered a DxWBS in over 5 years.

An RxWBS should be done in every patient who receives a therapeutic dose of RAI. The optimal interval between administration and scan in most patients is approximately 7 days. The primary purposes of an RxWBS is to detect gross residual disease in the regional lymphatics or in distant sites and to determine if known disease concentrates RAI.

FDG-PET is another nuclear medicine study that is commonly used to detect metastatic disease, but the predictive value of PET in thyroid cancer is not well defined. TSH stimulation increases the accuracy of FDG-PET in most types of DTC. A prospective trial comparing FDG-PET studies during thyroid

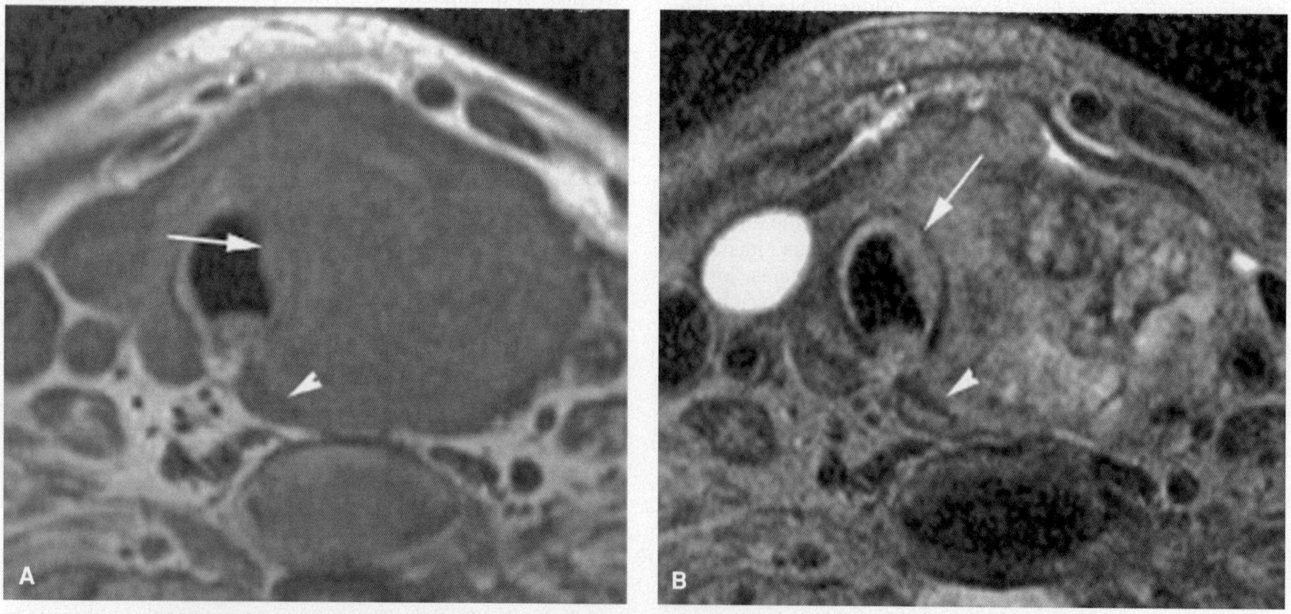

FIGURE 50.4. A patient demonstrating the value of magnetic resonance in the detection of invasion of the trachea and cervical esophagus, especially as it pertains to treatment planning. This patient has anaplastic carcinoma of the thyroid gland. In **A:** T1-weighted images show distortion of the trachea (*arrow*) and esophagus (*arrowhead*), but it is difficult to determine whether invasion is present. In **B:** the T2-weighted image shows obvious growth of tumor replacing the normal signal of cartilage of the trachea with growth on both sides of the cartilage (*arrow*) as well as replacement of the normal muscular wall signal of the cervical esophagus (*arrowhead*), indicating esophageal wall invasion. (From Mancuso AA, Mendenhall WM, Vaysberg M. Thyroid: nodules and malignant tumors. In: Mancuso AA, edr. *Head and neck radiology*. Philadelphia: Lippincott Williams & Wilkins, 2010:1457–1481, with permission.)

TABLE 50.4 NUCLEAR IMAGING STUDIES USED IN THE MANAGEMENT OF DIFFERENTIATED THYROID CARCINOMAS

Study	Isotope	Diagnostics	Results	Purpose	Comment
Radioactive uptake study (RAIU)	I-123 or I-131[a]	Counts are measured over the low neck 2 to 24 hr after administration	Not an image but a number. Normal findings after near total thyroidectomy are 0.5% to 5%	Quantifies the ability of thyroid tissue to concentrate iodine and estimate the amount of remaining thyroid tissue after thyroidectomy; required by federal regulation for outpatient therapy with I-131	Ideally should be done after restricting dietary iodine for 2 wk and elevating serum TSH to >30 U/mL with levothyroxine deprivation or rhTSH administration
Thyroid scan	I-123, I-131, or Tc-99	Same basic procedures as RAIU, but the thyroid is imaged with a gamma camera	Results are given as an image	Used in the evaluation of thyroid nodules to determine if the nodule is functional (i.e., "hot" or "cold")	Contributes little information to justify routine use in evaluating most thyroid nodules[160] In the setting of suppressed TSH, a "hot" nodule rarely harbors malignancy and cytology is not necessary[41]
Diagnostic whole-body scan (DxWBS)	Usually I-131 (2 to 5 mCi)	The entire body is imaged with a gamma camera ~3 days after RAI is administered (a delay allows washout of RAI from normal tissues)	Records images of the distribution of RAI throughout the entire body	To detect residual cancer	Patients are prepared with a low-iodine diet and TSH elevation. Some experts do not use this study in cancer management
Posttreatment whole-body scan (RxWBS)	I-131, 30 to 250 mCi (therapeutic dose range)	Same as DxWBS but performed ~7 days after RAI is administered	Same as DxWBS	Evaluates the quality of therapy for thyroid remnant ablation and identifies metastases	False positives are the only downside and their impact is mitigated when interpreted in the appropriate clinical context

RAI, radioactive iodine; TSH, thyroid-stimulating hormone; rhTSH, recombinant human TSH; yr, years; wk, weeks.
[a]The authors currently use I-123 at doses of 200 to 300 μCi.

hormone suppression to studies after administration of rhTSH showed increased detection of occult metastases in the stimulated studies.[51] Some insurers will not reimburse for FDG-PET for thyroid cancer without prior documentation of follicular-derived thyroid cancer with a suppressed or stimulated Tg over 10 ng/mL and a negative DxWBS.[41]

When FDG-PET is performed for reasons other than thyroid cancer and reveals a hypermetabolic thyroid nodule, a biopsy is warranted in most cases as these lesions carry a 15% risk of malignancy.[50] A recent study of 5,877 patients who received FDG-PET for cancer screening or staging or restaging purposes, 3.7% revealed hypermetabolic activity within the thyroid gland. Of the patients sent for US-FNA, 14% were diagnosed with thyroid malignancies.[52] A larger review of pooling data from over 55,000 FDG-PET studies reported a 1% prevalence of focal thyroid gland abnormalities, and the rate of confirmed thyroid malignancies in this group was as high as 33%.[53]

PROGNOSTIC FACTORS

The most important prognostic factor for disease recurrence and cancer mortality is the histologic classification. DTC, when diagnosed in an early stage, has a favorable prognosis. However, tall-cell variant can have a 10-year mortality of up to 25%.[54] Hürthle cell carcinoma carries a relatively poor prognosis, with a 25% rate of metastatic disease[55,56] and decreased survival at 10 years of 76%, compared with 93% and 85% for PTC and FC, respectively.[57] Columnar cell variant and diffuse-sclerosing variants likewise carry a poor prognosis relative to other forms of DTC. Contrarily, follicular-variant PTC and most FC share the same favorable prognosis as classic PTC relative to age and stage at diagnosis. ATC has an abysmal prognosis. All ATCs are considered stage IV under the current AJCC system and the overall 5-year survival is approximately 5%.[1]

Within the classification of DTC there are several important prognostic factors, including age, gender, family history, tumor size, extrathyroidal extension, vascular invasion, cervical and mediastinal lymph node metastases, degree of cytologic atypia and tumor necrosis, presence of distant metastases, and the degree to which the cancer can concentrate RAI. The prognostic variables are summarized in Table 50.5 and several of these factors are discussed in detail below.

Age

Age is a major prognostic variable that is accounted for in the current and previous AJCC staging systems (Fig. 50.5). The current AJCC system dichotomizes staging for DTC based on age under 45 years versus 45 years and older. In the current system, patients under 45 years of age with any T or N stage (based on tumor-node-metastasis [TNM] classification) are considered overall stage I, unless metastatic disease is present, which elevates the overall stage to stage II. Conversely, patients 45 years of age and older are given an overall stage I and II only if their T and N stages are T1N0 and T2N0, respectively. Thereby, this system considers age to be one of the most important prognostic variables. A limitation of this system is that it fails to account for the poor prognosis seen in patients diagnosed at a young age (<15 years old). Children present with more advanced tumors than young adults and have more recurrences and distant metastases.[58,59] In one series of 56 children (ages 4 to 20 years) with PTC or FC, the 10-year progression-free survival was only 61%, although survival remained favorable at 98%.[60] Another series of 21 children (ages 4 to 15 years) reported a 24% rate of distant metastases at presentation.[61]

Gender

Compared to women, men who develop DTC are diagnosed at an age approximately 20 years older, are twice as likely to develop distant metastases, and are 30% more likely to have regional metastases.[62,63] It is unclear why there is a gender bias toward increasing age at diagnosis for men, but it may be attributed to delayed access to the U.S. health care system for men. Delaying the diagnosis for more than 12 months is associated with a doubling in the chance of thyroid cancer mortality.[16]

Primary Tumor Size

A linear relationship exists between primary tumor size and cancer-specific mortality.[16,62,64,65–66] Very large tumors are

TABLE 50.5 PROGNOSTIC FACTORS IN DIFFERENTIATED THYROID CANCER

Variable	*Favorable*	*Unfavorable*	*Comment*
Age	15 to 44 yo	<15 yo or ≥45 yo	Older age is accounted for in the AJCC staging system, but children (<15 yo) have a 30% to 40% risk of recurrence
Gender	Female	Male	Twofold increase in distant metastases[62]
Family history	Absent	Present	Increased incidence of multifocalilty and aggressive tumors in patients with first-degree family members with DTC[161]
Tumor size	≤4 cm (<1 cm, very favorable)	>4 cm	A linear relation exists between primary tumor size and thyroid cancer mortality[16]
Focality/laterality	Unifocal or unilateral	Multifocal or bilateral	Twofold increase in the rate of nodal metastases and threefold increase in the distant metastases with multifocal tumors
Extrathyroid extension	Organ confined	Extrathyroidal extension	A 1.5-fold increase in 10-yr recurrence and fivefold increase in mortality
Histologic grade	Low grade	High grade	Tumors with increased necrosis, nuclear atypia, and vascular invasion have a worse prognosis
Lymph node metastases	Absent	Present	–
Distant metastases	Absent	Present	50% mortality with distant metastases
RAI concentration	Concentrate RAI	Inability/low capacity to concentrate RAI	–

AJCC, American Joint Committee on Cancer; DTC, differentiated thyroid cancer; RAI, radioactive iodine; yr, years; yo, years old.

associated with increased rates of extrathyroidal disease, lymph node and distant metastases, less-favorable histologies, and, in some cases, unresectable disease, all of which harbor a poor prognosis. Papillary microcarcinoma (<1 cm) have a disease course characterized by exceedingly favorable outcomes. These cancers, often found incidentally during surgery for benign thyroid conditions, are considered clinically insignificant malignancies and generally do not portend to decreased survival. Recurrences after total thyroidectomy in some series are nearly zero. Some small tumors, however, are associated with other poor prognostic factors that warrant more aggressive management. Lymph node metastases occur in as many as 20% to 60% of cases with small tumors; 30% to 40% can be multifocal, and 17% to 30% will have extrathyroidal extension.[67–68,69] These outcomes have led some investigators to argue that treatment for papillary microcarcinoma should be no different from that for PTC larger than 1 cm in size, advocating for the routine use of RAI.[70] The authors agree with other investigators that additional prognostic factors such as extrathyroidal extension, lymph node metastases,[71] age, and multifocality should drive the decision to treat with adjuvant RAI when managing papillary microcarcinoma.

Multifocality and Bilaterality

Anywhere from 20% to 80% of patients undergoing thyroidectomy for unifocal tumors are diagnosed with multifocal disease and 44% will have disease in the contralateral lobe.[6] This incidence of contralateral lobe disease is increased when multifocal disease is found in the incident lobe,[72] underscoring the need for completion thyroidectomy after a thyroid cancer is found at the hemithyroidectomy. Patients with multifocal disease have double the rate of nodal metastases and triple the rate in distant metastases.[73,74,75,76]

Extrathyroidal Extension

Extrathyroidal extension (ETE) is a key risk factor for lymph node and distant metastases.[77] The probability of primary tumor spread beyond the thyroid increases with tumor size,[65] but can be seen even in small tumors.[67–68,69] ETE predicts for

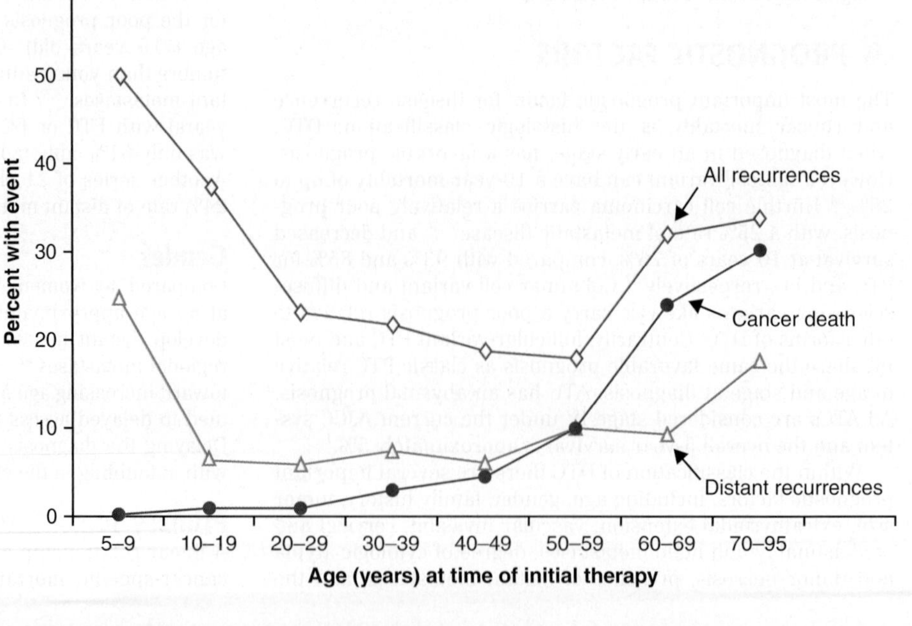

FIGURE 50.5. Effect of age on outcomes of patients with differentiated thyroid cancer. (From Mazzaferri EL, Kloos RT. Clinical review 128: current approaches to primary therapy for papillary and follicular thyroid cancer. *J Clin Endocrinol Metab* 2001;86:1447–1463. © 2001, The Endocrine Society.)

increased lymph node recurrences and distant metastases.[62,69] In its earliest form, ETE is clinically occult and seen only on pathologic evaluation. More advanced ETE presents with signs of local invasion of the muscles of the neck, blood vessels, recurrent laryngeal nerve, larynx, pharynx, esophagus, and even the spinal cord or brachial plexus. Gross ETE occurs in the majority (70%) of ATC.[78]

Lymph Node Metastases

Often a presenting symptom of a thyroid cancer, lymph node metastases are more common with PTC than FC (46% vs. 25%).[16] The prognostic importance of lymph node metastases has historically been somewhat controversial, but several studies have shown this to be predictive of recurrence and decreased survival; bilateral and mediastinal lymphadenopathy in particular portend to a poor prognosis.[16,79,80–81] Nevertheless, the absolute magnitude of negative impact on survival from lymph node metastases is marginal, decreasing 30-year survival from 94% to 90%.[16]

Distant Metastases

Although distant metastases are the leading cause of death in patients with DTC, they are not uniformly fatal. Roughly 10% of patients with PTC and 25% of those with FC develop distant metastases, with the lungs being the most common site of involvement. One-half of these metastases are present at diagnosis.[82] Patients with DTC who develop distant metastases have an increased thyroid cancer mortality of 40% to 50% compared with 10% to 15% for those with local recurrence.[62,74,82,83]

STAGING

The seventh edition (2010) of the AJCC staging system for thyroid cancer is shown in Table 50.6. Staging is based on the anatomic extent of disease as well as the patient's age and tumor histology. Both clinical and pathologic staging can be employed. Separate staging groups are recommended for differentiated, medullary, and anaplastic carcinomas.

SURGICAL MANAGEMENT OF THYROID CANCER

Surgery is the primary treatment of localized thyroid cancer of all histologies. A total thyroidectomy is the preferred oncologic procedure, because the gland is surgically accessible and its primary endocrine function can be replaced by exogenous therapy (levothyroxine). It is critical to understand that even a total thyroidectomy leaves residual thyroid tissue that will have major implications for subsequent therapy and disease monitoring. The clearest evidence of residual thyroid tissue after total thyroidectomy is seen on postoperative RAI thyroid studies, which nearly always show uptake in the region of the thyroid bed. The presence of residual thyroid tissue in this setting is not a sign of incomplete surgery, but a matter of practicality. The ligament connecting the posterior surface of the thyroid capsule to the trachea harbors microscopic nests of thyroid tissue and is rarely completely resected in order to reduce the risk of tracheal injury. Second, the recurrent laryngeal nerve is embedded in thyroid tissue at the point where the nerve enters the larynx, and it is not possible to remove all of this thyroid tissue without injuring the nerve and compromising voice quality and laryngeal function.

Several important complications can arise from thyroidectomy. The most common are recurrent laryngeal nerve injury (temporary 30% and permanent 2%) and hypoparathyroidism (temporary 5% and permanent 0.5%). These complications can be mitigated with the use of more conservative surgery.[84,85] Other structures at risk for operative injury include the vagus, spinal accessory and superior laryngeal nerves, trachea, esophagus, thoracic duct, and carotid arteries. The operative morbidity is reduced by increasing the surgical experience, intraoperative monitoring of the recurrent laryngeal nerves, and autotransplantation of parathyroid glands.[86]

There are several critical issues regarding the surgical management of thyroid cancer and nodules that warrant detailed discussion:

1. When is surgery indicated for the evaluation of a thyroid nodule with nondiagnostic cytology?
2. When is it safe to consider hemithyroidectomy for thyroid carcinoma?
3. What is the appropriate extent of neck dissection?

These issues are discussed in further detail below.

Surgical Evaluation of Thyroid Nodules

The 2009 revision of the American Thyroid Association (ATA) "Guidelines for Management of Patients with Thyroid Nodules and Differentiated Thyroid Cancer" contains several recommendations addressing the role of surgery in the evaluation of thyroid nodules.[41] Surgical evaluation of thyroid nodules is indicated for the following reasons: (a) cytology is suspicious for PTC; (b) cytology contains follicular cells with no concordant functioning nodule on an RAI scan, especially with a low- to normal-range serum TSH. (In these cases, lobectomy or total thyroidectomy should be considered.); (c) cytology contains Hürthle cell neoplasm, which does not warrant an RAI study and should be managed with either lobectomy or total thyroidectomy, depending on the lesion's size and other risk factors; and (d) growing nodules, even in the face of benign cytology, may be considered for surgical removal. In cases when a lobectomy reveals a thyroid cancer, completion thyroidectomy is recommended for all patients for whom the procedure would have been recommended had the diagnosis been available before surgery. The use of I-131 ablation as an alternative to completion surgery is not recommended.

Lobectomy in the Management of Thyroid Cancers

Although total thyroidectomy is considered the standard surgical approach for nearly all resectable thyroid carcinomas, there are published clinical guidelines that consider a more conservative surgery appropriate in some clinical scenarios. The 2011 National Comprehensive Cancer Network (NCCN) guidelines find lobectomy acceptable in patients between the ages of 15 and 45 years with PTC tumors <4 cm and without prior radiotherapy, distant metastasis, cervical lymph node metastasis, extrathyroidal extension, or aggressive histologic variants.[54] The 2009 ATA guidelines recommend considering lobectomy only in tumors with the above features that are <1 cm in size.[41] Advocates for lobectomy argue that operative morbidity is mitigated with the use of more conservative surgery.[84]

In a review of 52,173 patients from the National Cancer Database who underwent surgery for PTC, 82.9% underwent total thyroidectomy and 17.1% underwent lobectomy.[87] On multivariate analysis, when lobectomy was used, there was a 57% increase in recurrences and 21% increase in death compared with total thyroidectomy. For PTC <1 cm, the surgical approach did not impact recurrence or survival. The benefit of total thyroidectomy was seen across all tumors >1 cm, even when patients with tumors 1 to 2 cm were analyzed separately.[87] A previous SEER analysis of 4,402 patients with PTC failed to show a survival benefit to total thyroidectomy; however, patients undergoing total thyroidectomy in this analysis had larger tumors that were 10% more likely to have extrathyroidal extension and 20% more likely to have cervical lymph node metastases compared to patients who were not operated on.[88] The AMES (age, distant metastasis, extent, and size) and MACIS (metastases, age, completeness of resection, invasion, size [Mayo Clinic]) prognostic scoring system has been proposed for

TABLE 50.6 AMERICAN JOINT COMMITTEE ON CANCER (AJCC) 2010 TNM STAGING SYSTEM FOR THYROID CANCER

Primary Tumor (T)		
TX		Primary tumor cannot be assessed
T0		No evidence of primary tumor
T1		Tumor 2 cm or less in greatest dimension and limited to the thyroid gland
	T1a	Tumor 1 cm or less in greatest dimension and limited to the thyroid gland
	T1b	Tumor more than 1 cm but not more than 2 cm in greatest dimension and limited to the thyroid gland
T2		Tumor more than 2 cm but not more than 4 cm in greatest dimension and limited to the thyroid gland
T3		Tumor more than 4 cm in greatest dimension limited to the thyroid or any tumor with minimal extrathyroidal extension to the sternothyroid muscle or perithyroid soft tissues
T4		Advanced disease defined as more than minimal extrathyroidal extension
	T4a	Moderately advanced disease Tumor of any size extending beyond the thyroid capsule to invade subcutaneous soft tissues, larynx, trachea, esophagus, or recurrent laryngeal nerve
	T4b	Very advanced disease Tumor invades prevertebral fascia, encases carotid artery or mediastinal vessels
All anaplastic carcinomas are considered T4 tumors		
T4a		Intrathyroidal anaplastic carcinoma
T4b		Anaplastic carcinoma with gross extrathyroidal extension
Regional Lymph Nodes (N)		
NX		Regional lymph nodes cannot be assessed
N0		No evidence of regional lymph node metastasis
N1		Regional lymph node metastasis
	N1a	Metastasis to level VI (pretracheal, paratracheal, and prelaryngeal/Delphian lymph nodes)
	N1b	Metastasis to unilateral, bilateral, contralateral cervical (Levels I, II, III, IV, or V) or retropharyngeal or superior mediastinal lymph nodes (Level VII)
Distant Metastasis (M)		
M0		No distant metastasis
M1		Distant metastasis

Overall Staging Groups

(DTC) Papillary or Follicular Carcinoma			
Under 45 Years			
Stage I	Any T	Any N	M0
Stage II	Any T	Any N	M1
45 Years and Older			
Stage I	T1	N0	M0
Stage II	T2	N0	M0
Stage III	T3	N0	M0
	T1	N1a	M0
	T2	N1a	M0
	T3	N1a	M0
Stage IVA	T4a	N0	M0
	T4a	N1a	M0
	T1	N1b	M0
	T2	N1b	M0
	T3	N1b	M0
	T4a	N1b	M0
Stage IVB	T4b	Any N	M0
Stage IVC	Any T	Any N	M1
Medullary Carcinoma (All Age Groups)			
Stage I	T1	N0	M0
Stage II	T2	N0	M0
	T3	N0	M0
Stage III	T1	N1a	M0
	T2	N1a	M0
	T3	N1a	M0
Stage IVA	T4a	N0	M0
	T4a	N1a	M0
	T1	N1b	M0
	T2	N1b	M0
	T3	N1b	M0
	T4a	N1b	M0
Stage IVB	T4b	Any N	M0
Stage IVC	Any T	Any N	M1
Anaplastic Carcinoma (All Stage IV)			
Stage IVA	T4a	Any N	M0
Stage IVB	T4b	Any N	M0
Stage IVC	Any T	Any N	M1

Used with the permission of the American Joint Committee on Cancer (AJCC), Chicago, Illinois. The original source for this material is the *AJCC Cancer Staging Handbook*, 7th ed. (2010) published by Springer Science and Business Media LLC, www.springerlink.com.

selecting low-risk patients for more conservative initial resections[89–90,91]; however, most patients undergo total thyroidectomy even when classified as low risk,[92] and, overall, the use of total thyroidectomy is increasing.[93]

In general, total thyroidectomy is the appropriate initial surgical approach for most patients with differentiated thyroid cancer because it increases the effectiveness of adjuvant I 131, removes all intrathyroidal cancer, reduces recurrences, and facilitates the use of surveillance scans and Tg. The surgeon's experience with the operation is a large determinant of the ultimate outcome. In the hands of surgeons performing over 100 cases in a 5-year period, total thyroidectomy complication rates are comparable to less extensive surgeries and are two-thirds less likely than when performed by less experienced surgeons.[86]

Neck Dissection in Differentiated Thyroid Cancer

As with squamous cell carcinomas, a modified radical neck dissection is done for thyroid cancer when there is a visible or palpably positive node. However, elective neck dissection (removal of lymphatic regions at risk for subclinical disease) is generally not performed for DTC of follicular cell origin, unlike primary surgery for most other head and neck cancers. Despite a high incidence of subclinical lymph node involvement in even small PTCs, elective neck dissection is not included in the initial surgical approach because identifying microscopic regional metastases will not influence the recommendation for RAI nor will it affect prognosis.[63]

According to the 2009 ATA guidelines, central-compartment (level VI) dissection is recommended for all patients with clinically involved lymph nodes; however, for small T1 or T2 tumors without adverse clinical or pathologic features, a prophylactic central neck dissection can be omitted. In clinically N0 patients with other adverse features (T3 or T4), a prophylactic central neck dissection can be considered. A lateral level II to IV neck dissection should only be reserved for patients with biopsy-proven metastatic lateral cervical lymphadenopathy.[41] When a lateral neck dissection is indicated, levels II to IV should be resected *en bloc* in lieu of removing only abnormal lymph nodes.[94–95,96] Levels I, V, and VII should not be dissected unless clinically suspicious. Central and lateral neck dissections are part of the standard primary therapy for all patients with sporadic and hereditary forms of medullary thyroid carcinoma.[97,98]

Despite these ATA guidelines, there remains active controversy in the literature regarding the role of routine prophylactic central neck dissection in patients with DTC. Space limitation precludes a thorough discussion of this controversy, but details can be found in the articles referenced in the remainder of this paragraph. In general, the advocates for routine central neck dissection argue that it leads to more accurate staging, reduces central neck recurrences, avoids reoperations, and provides the optimal conditions for effective RAI therapy.[99–104,105] Detractors of this approach point to a lack of clear recurrence and survival benefits with prophylactic central neck dissection with an associated increase in the rate of surgical complications.[99,106,107–108] A recent meta-analysis with over 1,200 patients showed no improvement in recurrences with the addition of prophylactic central neck dissection.[109]

MANAGEMENT OF DIFFERENTIATED THYROID CANCER WITH RADIOACTIVE IODINE

Bioconcentration of Radioactive Iodine

RAI for DTC is arguably the most successful targeted therapy in all of oncology. The iodine-concentrating capacity of benign and neoplastic thyroid tissue makes an overwhelming majority of thyroid carcinomas amenable to RAI therapy. RAI is taken up by thyroid tissue, including DTC of follicular epithelial origin, at a rate 6.6 times more than most tissues in the body. The biological half-life in extrathyroidal tissue is merely 12 days compared to 80 days for thyroid tissue (Table 50.7).

TABLE 50.7 PHYSICAL, BIOLOGICAL, AND EFFECTIVE HALF-LIVES (T½) OF I-131

	Physical T½	Biological T½	Effective T½
Thyroid tissue	8 days	80 days	7.3 days
Extrathyroidal tissue	8 days	12 days	8 hours

Radioactive Decay of Iodine-131

I-131 is produced from the fission of uranium atoms during the operation of nuclear reactors or in the detonation of nuclear bombs. I-131 decays by negatron emission (beta-minus decay) to xenon-131 (Xe-131). A neutron from the I-131 nucleus converts to a proton and an electron (beta-particle) is emitted from the nucleus. This first transition results in a beta-particle with a range of energies from 250 to 800 keV. These beta-particles are core to I-131's ability to deliver targeted cytotoxicity. Because electrons of this energy range will deposit their energy within a millimeter, only the cells taking up the I-131 are affected. In the second decay step, unstable Xe-131 decays to stable xenon, releasing a photon with the energy of 364 keV. This product is therapeutically undesirable, because the photon will travel far from the source where iodine is concentrated. It contributes very little cytotoxicity to thyroid cancer cells and increases the total body dose; however, it is this property that makes RAI useful for diagnostic imaging, forming the foundation for DxWBS and RxWBS.

Goals of Radioactive Iodine Therapy for Differentiated Thyroid Cancer

Broadly speaking, the two basic purposes of adjuvant RAI are (a) thyroid remnant ablation and (b) adjuvant therapy for residual microscopic disease. First, RAI provides potent cytotoxicity by targeting thyroid cancer cells remaining in the operative bed, occult lymph node metastases, and distant metastases. Second, RxWBS provides critical information including staging, prognosis, and determining which patients are likely to require additional treatments. Lastly, ablation of the remaining thyroid tissue facilitates the use of serum Tg as a very sensitive and specific marker for disease persistence after primary therapy. Serum Tg provides a powerful means of monitoring for early disease recurrences that are likely to be amenable to curative retreatment.

RAI therapy has been crucial in making DTC one of the most curable malignancies. There are multiple large retrospective series showing a significant reduction in recurrences and cause-specific mortality with the use of RAI.[16,110–111,112,113] A summary of selected references is provided in Table 50.8, although this does not represent a complete list.

Patient Selection for Radioactive Iodine

Despite the evidence that RAI reduces thyroid cancer recurrences and potentially improves survival, there remain limitations on the indications for RAI for DTCs because these benefits have not been demonstrated in the setting of a randomized controlled trial. Moreover, several institutional series have failed to demonstrate a benefit for certain patients with the lowest risk of disease. Finally, the potential benefits in any individual patient must be weighed against toxicities. At our institution, all patients with DTC >1 cm or those with any size tumor with positive lymph nodes, distant metastases, or extrathyroidal extension are recommended RAI after surgery.

The 2009 ATA guideline recommends RAI for all patients with known distant metastases, gross extrathyroidal extension of the tumor regardless of tumor size, or primary tumor size >4 cm, even in the absence of other higher-risk features. RAI is

TABLE 50.8 SELECTED RETROSPECTIVE SERIES DEMONSTRATING CLINICAL BENEFITS OF RAI

Author (Reference)	Patients (N)	Median Follow-Up	Recurrence	Mortality	Comment
Mazzaferri et al. (16)	1,355 DTC	15.7 yr	30-yr RFS RAI: 85% T_4: 70% P <.001	30-yr CSS RAI: 97% T_4: 94% P <.001	RAI reduced recurrences and cancer mortality despite more patients treated with RAI having adverse pathologic features.
Samaan et al. (110)	1,599 DTC	11 yr	Crude RFS RAI: 93% No RAI: 83%	Not reported	RAI was the single most important prognostic factor for RFS and also improved survival, except in low-risk patients.
DeGroot et al. (111)	269 PTC	12 yr	20-yr RFS[a] RAI: 95% T4: 80%	Not reported	RAI improved survival in patients with tumors >1 cm with positive cervical lymph nodes.
Tsang et al. (112)	382 DTC	10.8 yr	10-yr RFS (stage I only) RAI: 95% T_4: 84% P = .038	10-yr OS RFS (stage I only) RAI: 100% T_4: 100% P = .038	On MVA, RAI was associated with decreased local recurrences (HR 0.3; P = .002). No survival benefit.
Taylor et al. (113)	385 DTC	3.1 yr (mean)	Not reported	Not reported	RAI decreased recurrence (HR = 0.3; P = .01), and cancer specific mortality (HR 0.3; P = .04) on MVA

DTC, differentiated thyroid cancer; HR, hazard ratio; MVA, multivariate analysis; OS, overall survival; PTC, papillary thyroid cancer; RAI, radioactive iodine; RFS, relapse-free survival; CSS, cause specific survival; TSH, thyroid-stimulating hormone; yr, year.
[a]Estimated from figure.

recommended for selected patients with 1- to 4-cm thyroid cancers confined to the thyroid who have lymph node metastases or other high-risk features, such as age >45 years, intrathyroidal vascular invasion, multifocal disease, or aggressive histologic variants (tall cell, columnar cell, or insular carcinoma). Follicular and Hürthle cell variants are considered high risk, and these patients are nearly always recommended RAI, except for those with the smallest unifocal FCs manifesting as only capsular invasion (without vascular invasion). These so-called minimally invasive carcinomas are treated effectively with surgery alone and RAI can be avoided. RAI is not recommended for unifocal PTCs <1 cm and without high-risk features or when all the foci in multifocal disease are <1 cm.[41] The 2011 NCCN guidelines recommend RAI for patients with persistent disease and for thyroid remnant ablation in selected patients without gross residual disease. For patients without residual disease or high-risk histology, RAI is not recommended when postoperative Tg is <1 ng/mL and anti-Tg antibodies and RAI imaging are negative.

Selection of Iodine-131 Activity

Three methods of radioisotope dosing are used in the treatment of DTC with RAI (Table 50.9). There is no consensus on the optimal method of I-131 dosing, and an exhaustive body of literature exists on the matter, but this will not be discussed here because of space limitation. For more information the authors refer readers to *Essentials of Thyroid Cancer Management*.[114] The authors use the empiric system at our institution for simplicity. In general, the dosimetric techniques require the expertise of dedicated physics' support and nuclear medicine technologists with specialization in RAI administration. The current University of Florida empiric dosing regimen is summarized in the Table 50.10 for both initial therapy and retreatment settings.

Preparing Patients for Iodine-131

Appropriate preparation for RAI therapy is critical to obtaining the optimal desired effect of therapy, whether for remnant ablation or adjuvant therapy residual disease. There are several components (Table 50.11) comprising optimal preparation, including (a) a low-iodine diet, (b) avoidance of iodinated contrast agents (or adequate washout period if iodinated contrast has already been administered), (c) measuring of urinary iodine levels, (d) administration of rhTSH, (e) avoidance of thyroid replacement, and (f) administration of lithium for augmentation of I-131. With the exception of the latter, all of these steps will deplete the patient's iodine stores and increase the level of TSH and thereby the activity of the NaIS, in an effort to increase the therapeutic efficacy of I-131. Low-iodine diets, avoidance and washout of iodinated contrast agent, and lithium for augmentation of I-131 biological half-life are useful in nearly all patients. Urinary iodine measurement requires 24-hour collection and is reserved for patients with documented iodine contrast administration within the 6 months preceding RAI.

TABLE 50.9 IODINE-131 DOSIMETRY SYSTEMS

System	Description	Typical Doses	Comment
Empiric method	Everyone in a prognostic group gets the same dose	30 to 50 mCi for remnant ablation only 100 to 150 mCi for standard-risk patients 30 to 50 mCi more for higher risk patients 200 mCi for distant metastases	Most simple and widely used Not based on the individuals iodine metabolism
Dosimetry-guided technique	Calculates the upper limits of safe blood and whole-body doses from I-131	Whole-blood limit set at 2 Gy with total-body retention <120 mCi at 48 hr	Prescribes dose that will result in the maximum acceptable level of bone marrow toxicity Requires measuring total body counts at 2, 24, 48, and 72 hr after a diagnostic dose of I-131 Not widely used because of complexity Ignores the effect of prior RAI
Tumor site dosimetry	Prescribes the dose that delivers a set minimum absorbed dose to target tissue	Target dose: 300 Gy to the thyroid remnant (80% success rate) 80 to 120 Gy to nodal or soft tissue metastases (80% control rate)	Technique for whole-blood dosimetry with added focal measurements Extreme complexity and questionable accuracy limit its current use to a few institutions

RAI, radioactive iodine; hr, hours.

TABLE 50.10 UNIVERSITY OF FLORIDA EMPIRIC DOSING OF IODINE-131 FOR TREATMENT OF DIFFERENTIATED THYROID CANCER

Risk Group	Description	I-131 Dose
De novo I-131		
Low	Stage T1N0M0 (remnant ablation only)	50 mCi
Standard	Not low or high risk cancer	150 mCi
High	Stage T4, M1, or known residual disease (positive margin or gross-positive node by imaging)	200 mCi
I-131 After at Least One Prior I-131 Administration		
Standard	Elevated Tg only (no visible disease)	150 mCi
High	Positive margin or distant metastasis (gross residual disease)	200 mCi

Otherwise, the authors approach patients with two general preparation regimens: T_4 deprivation or rhTSH administration. The authors prefer using rhTSH to avoid the morbidity of hypothyroidism. Some experts believe that the cure rate will be higher when patients are prepared with hypothyroidism, but there are data suggesting equivalent efficacy with hypothyroidism versus rhTSH preparation.[115–117] Both approaches also increase the diagnostic sensitivity of both DxWBS and RxWBS, although T_4 deprivation may be superior in this regard.[118,119]

Outpatient Management of Iodine-131

Grigsby et al.[120] described the pattern of radiation exposure in 65 household members of 30 patients treated with RAI. The mean dose to family members was well below regulatory standards at 0.24 mSv and the maximum dose was 1.11 mSv. The Nuclear Regulatory Commission (NRC) has issued guidance on the release of patients following RAI treatment for thyroid cancer, and a copy of all material related to the issue can be found on the NRC website. Major recommendations were issued in 1997 (NRC Regulatory Guide 8.39) and have largely remained in place. Several minor subsequent recommendations have been issued, most recently in early 2011 under 10 CFR 35.75.[121] Overall, the recommendations are intended to keep the exposure to the public "as low as reasonably achievable (ALARA)." The 1997 regulations permitted patients to be released from the control of the licensee. The regulations state that:

- Providers are discouraged from recommending that patients stay in hotels immediately after treatment.
- Patients should avoid public transportation.
- Outpatient release following treatment is limited to patients when the radiation dose to third parties in not likely to exceed 5 mSv of total effective dose equivalent (TEDE). The TEDE is calculated using three factors: (a) activity of I-131 administered, (b) results of the thyroid uptake study, and (c) the occupancy factor, which takes into account the amount of time the patient will spend around other people for a few days after RAI.
- The patient must be capable of self-care, cannot live in a nursing home or communal living facility, and must prefer to be released after RAI.
- Patients must be given radiation safety instructions.

TABLE 50.11 PREPARATION OF PATIENTS FOR IODINE-131

Component	Description	Rationale/Comments
Low-iodine diet	A diet that is low in iodine (≤50 μg/day) for 2 weeks before, and 2 days after, I-131 Forced diuresis to increase urinary clearance of iodine is not recommended Salt, bread, and most dairy products contain high concentrations of iodine and should be avoided It is not feasible to measure urinary iodine levels to ensure low-iodine-diet compliance	The purpose of a low-iodine diet is to deplete the total-body iodine stores to a degree that maximizes the uptake of RAI by thyroid tissue and thyroid cancer Appropriate iodine restriction doubles the absorbed radiation dose to the thyroid remnant and several studies have shown lower rates of measurable Tg after RAI and an increase in the rate of successful remnant ablation[162,163]
Intravenous iodinated contrast exposure	Iodine contrast should be avoided in all patients with DTC Patients who received iodinate contrast within 6 months of RAI should have therapy delayed for 3 to 6 months and require 24 urinary iodine measurements (see below)	An enormous amount of iodine is administered for contrast enhancement during diagnostic CT studies with typical studies requiring >100 mL with an iodine concentration of 150 mg/mL (>10^6 is the recommended daily allowance). This increases iodine stores in virtually all tissues, reducing the subsequent uptake of I-131
Urinary iodine measurement	Only done in patients with a history of IV iodinated contrast exposure within the past 6 months A 24-hour urinary iodine measurement obtained on day 7 of a low-iodine diet should be ≤150 μg/mL	Urinary iodine measurements provide an accurate estimate of the dietary iodine intake and total body iodine stores
Recombinant human thyroid-stimulating hormone (rhTSH)	A 0.9-mg intramuscular injection twice (2 days and 1 day) before I-131 administration The efficacy and safety of rhTSH in children has not been studied so the authors do not use rhTSH in children rhTSH is contraindicated in the presence of cardiovascular disease, brain or spinal cord metastases, or a paratracheal mass	Increases the uptake of I-131 while avoiding the symptoms of prolonged hypothyroidism rhTSH is approved by the U.S. Food and Drug Administration as an alternative to thyroid hormone withdrawal in preparation for diagnostic studies. Its use in association with thyroid remnant ablation or treatment of thyroid cancer is "off-label"
Stop thyroid hormone replacement	Levothyroxine and other thyroid replacement should be withheld 6 weeks before I-131, unless rhTSH is administered, in which case the authors recommend stopping T_4 and T_3 for 3 days before, and the day of, I-131 administration TSH should be elevated to ≥30 μU/mL before I-131	Increases TSH and, thereby, uptake of I-131 into normal and malignant follicular thyroid cells Decreases urinary clearance of I-131
Lithium carbonate to increase the potency of I-131	Lithium carbonate is administered at ~20 mg/kg/day (usually 300 mg three times a day) for 7 days beginning 5 days before I-131 administration Because of its narrow therapeutic range and potential severe toxicities, serum lithium concentration should be measured on days 4 and 5 of therapy (therapeutic range 0.6–1.2 mEq/L) Contraindications: psychiatric problems, dementia, seizure disorder, cardiac arrhythmia, renal insufficiency, hepatic impairment, hypo- or hypernatremia, and certain medications (diuretics, antidepressant, NSAID, seizure medication, or calcium channel blocker)	Lithium decreased the rate of release of I-131 from thyroid cells without interfering with uptake, effectively increasing I-131 retention time (biological half-life) by 50% to 90% No studies have shown improved outcomes; the potential toxicities and contraindications must be considered when considering its use Use of lithium in this setting is "off label use of an approved medication" and the patient must be apprised of this fact

RAI, radioactive iodine; CT, computed tomography; DTC, differentiated thyroid cancer; IV, intravenous; NSAID, nonsteroidal anti-inflammatory drug.

TABLE 50.12 ADVERSE EFFECTS OF RADIOACTIVE IODINE THERAPY

Temporary Side Effect	Permanent Complications
For Most Patients, the Following is Discussed as Part of the Informed Consent:	
Nausea	Second malignancy
Taste disturbance (>50%)	Dry mouth +/– dental problems
Salivary gland swelling (>30%)	Early menopause
Menstrual cycle disturbance	Male and female reproductive problems
With an Administered Dose of >200 mCi	
Bone marrow suppression	
Facial nerve weakness	
Stomatitis	
With an Administered Cumulative Lifetime Dose of >500 mCi	
Alopecia	Bone marrow suppression
Epistaxis	Salivary or nasolactimal duct obstruction
Conjunctivitis	Chronic dry eye
Pneumonitis (widespread lung metastases)	Pulmonary fibrosis (widespread lung metastases)
Neurological (brain and spinal cord metastases)	Neurological (brain and spinal cord metastases)
Administration for a Large Thyroid Remnant	
Thyroiditis	Recurrent laryngeal nerve injury
Thyrotoxicosis	

Data from Potential side effects and complication of I-131 therapy. In: Amdur RJ, Mazzaferri EL, eds. *Essentials of thyroid cancer management* (Cancer treatment and research). New York: Springer, 2005:265–277, with permission.

In our practice, the patient's living condition is assessed with the assistance of a radiation safety officer to ensure that the radiation exposure to family members, caregivers, and the general public remains ALARA. This usually means that patients return to private residences, with their own room and bathroom available, where they will remain alone for 3 days subsequent to I-131. Family members and caregivers should spend time in those areas with the patient only when necessary. Young children are to avoid all contact. Specific instructions on cleaning clothing, linens, bathrooms, and eating utensils are provided.

In 2011, new ATA guidelines were issued on outpatient I-131 management that reiterated the goal of keeping radiation exposure to third parties ALARA.[122,123] The guidelines were intended, in part, to describe the role of the radiation safety officer, standardize patient instructions, and describe best practices. The authors refer readers to that publication for specific recommendations.

Adverse Effects of Iodine-131

Side effects and complications of RAI therapy are shown in Table 50.12.[124] Patients should be given a prescription for antiemetics and instructed to fill it before arriving for RAI administration. Parotid massage and nonsteroid anti-inflammatory drugs may be useful for acute neck swelling or parotitis. Second-malignancy risk warrants discussion with the patient.[125,126] A well-recognized study estimated the excess absolute risk of second cancers from I-131 therapy to be 14.4 for solid cancers and 0.8 for leukemia per 27 mCi per 100,000 person-years of follow-up.[127]

EXTERNAL BEAM RADIOTHERAPY FOR THYROID CANCER

Indications for External Beam Radiotherapy

There are no randomized control trials defining the indications for external beam radiotherapy (EBRT) in thyroid cancer. The European Multicentre Study on Differentiated Thyroid Cancer trial was planned as a prospective multicenter trial to evaluate the benefit of adjuvant EBRT in locally advanced DTC. Patients with pT4 disease with or without lymph node metastases and no known distant metastases who underwent total thyroidectomy, RAI, and TSH suppression were to be randomized to EBRT or observation. The trial closed prematurely, however, as only 16% of patients consented to be randomized to EBRT. The trial was converted to a prospective cohort study, and subsequent results failed to define the role of EBRT in this population.[128–130] Therefore, recommendations for EBRT are based on institutional retrospective experiences and published clinical guidelines. Patients are approached differently with EBRT depending on whether the treatment plan is for primary, adjuvant, or palliative therapy. In general, only patients with unresectable tumor are treated with primary EBRT. Symptomatic metastatic tumors are well palliated with acceptable toxicity with plans utilizing simple beam arrangements to doses of 20 to 30 Gy in 5 to 10 fractions. For curative patients with nonmetastatic disease, RAI is always the preferred adjuvant therapy to EBRT, especially in young patients. EBRT has a niche role as adjuvant therapy after total thyroidectomy for certain patients at high risk for local recurrence who are not amenable to curative therapy with RAI. Table 50.13 summarizes the indications for EBRT from our institution, the 2009 ATA guidelines, and the 2011 NCCN guidelines.[41,131] The authors find it useful to triage patients for EBRT based on the patient's age, the

TABLE 50.13 INDICATIONS FOR EXTERNAL BEAM RADIOTHERAPY

Age	University of Florida	2009 ATA Guidelines	2011 NCCN Guidelines
Age ≤18 yr	Painful metastases or impending normal tissue damage from a growing tumor not amenable to other therapies.	Metastases that are symptomatic or in critical location that are otherwise untreatable.	No child-specific guidelines. *Consider EBRT for:* T4 primary, tumors not likely to concentrate iodine, or tumors with a high risk of residual disease (T4, positive margins, ECE)
Age 19 to 45 yr	Gross tumor on an imaging study that is unresectable and known to be resistant to I-131 (resistance means recurrence after at least one >100 mCi I-131 treatment under optimal conditions). The authors do not use EBRT if RAI may be curative or elevated Tg is the only sign of disease.	Metastases that are symptomatic or in a critical location and are otherwise untreatable.	
Age >45 yr	*Adjuvant treatment after thyroidectomy: Patients at high risk for local-regional recurrence:* T4 primary, nodal metastases with extensive extracapsular extension, or gross residual disease. *Salvage of recurrent disease following thyroidectomy and RAI:* Gross tumor that on an imaging study is unresectable and known to be resistant to I-131 (resistance means recurrence after at least one >100 mCi I-131 treatment under optimal conditions). The authors do not use EBRT if RAI may be curative or elevated Tg is the only sign of disease.	Gross ETE; high likelihood of microscopic residual gross residual tumor not amenable to further surgery.	

ATA, American Thyroid Association; NCCN, National Comprehensive Cancer Network; RAI, radioactive iodine; EBRT, external beam radiotherapy; ETE, extrathyroidal extension.

TABLE 50.14 RETROSPECTIVE SERIES SHOWING A BENEFIT FROM EXTERNAL BEAM RADIOTHERAPY IN PATIENTS WITH DIFFERENTIATED THYROID CANCER TREATED ROUTINELY WITH RADIOACTIVE IODINE

Author (Reference)	Number of Patients	Receiving EBRT (%)	Benefit of EBRT	Subset Benefiting from EBRT
Farahati et al. 1996 (132)	169	59	Local-regional control	Papillary tumors
			Distant failure	Node positive
Chow et al. 2002 (133)	842	12	Local-regional control	Gross residual tumor after thyroidectomy
Kim et al. 2003 (164)	91	25	Local-regional control	pT4 or node positive
Phlips et al. 1993 (135)	94	40	Local control	Extrathyroidal extension or microscopic/gross residual tumor after thyroidectomy
Brierley et al. 2005 (134)	729	44	Local-regional control	Microscopic residual, ETE
			Cause-specific survival	Age >60, microscopic residual, ETE

EBRT, external beam radiotherapy; DTC, differentiated thyroid cancer; ETE, extrathyroidal extension.

Adapted from ref. 130.

potential to curatively treat with RAI, and the presence of high-risk clinical-pathologic features.

Powell et al.[130] provide an excellent review of EBRT for DTC, including evidence supporting the indications for, and role of, EBRT. Table 50.14 summarizes the results of several retrospective analyses showing a benefit of EBRT in patients treated with thyroidectomy and adjuvant RAI. Even if prior I-131 has been given, at least one additional administration with >100 mCi with adequate preparation should be performed before considering EBRT.[112,132–135]

External Beam Radiotherapy Technique

Techniques for treating metastatic disease will vary by site, tumor burden, and clinical circumstances; therefore, this chapter will only discuss the technique used for treating the primary site and nodal regions. When both RAI and EBRT are indicated, the authors prefer to give RAI first because EBRT may result in thyroid stunning, decreasing the effectiveness of subsequent RAI.

CT simulation is used for treatment planning with patients positioned supine with arms at their side and the neck extended such that the mandible is at 90 degrees with respect to the treatment couch. An Aquaplast (WFR/Aquaplast Corporation, Avondale, PA) mask, custom head holder, and shoulder straps are used to immobilize the head and neck and to depress the level of the shoulders. Bolus material should be applied over scars in the neck. Intravenous contrast may be helpful in defining target volumes and normal-tissue structures, but this is contraindicated if RAI is being considered within the next 6 months. Axial CT images are acquired from above the skull base to the middle of the chest. Although not necessary, preoperative images sets may be fused to treatment planning CT scans to aid in target definitions. Historically, conventional anterior posterior/posterior anterior or lateral fields have been described to treat thyroid cancer, often requiring custom bolus materials to ensure homogenous dose distributions. Because the target volume straddles the level of the shoulder and, in nearly all cases, contains concavities with envaginated critical normal tissues, the authors find it useful to treat patients with intensity-modulated radiotherapy (IMRT).

Target Volumes and Dose

Target contours are delineated according to the definitions from the International Commission on Radiation Units. The gross tumor volume (GTV) will be any residual gross disease. The clinical target volume (CTVs) will define areas at risk for subclinical disease beyond any GTV. Schwartz et al.[136] described an IMRT technique treating four separate CTVs with a single IMRT plan using a simultaneous integrated boost. For simplicity, the authors define two CTVs: the high-risk CTV corresponds to the region at highest risk for residual disease (positive margin, ETE, lymph node with extracapsular disease, or gross residual disease) and the standard-risk CTV, which is the region at moderate risk for residual disease (electively irradiated nodal stations).

Kim et al.[137] analyzed the effect of treatment volume on patients treated with EBRT for nonanaplastic thyroid carcinoma. When limited fields were utilized treating only the primary (involved lobe) or recurrent tumor bed and the positive nodal area, 55% of patients developed local-regional failures compared with only 8% of patients treated with extended fields (including elective nodal irradiation). Another series analyzing patterns of failure after EBRT showed that several recurrences occur in superior mediastinal lymph nodes (level VII) when this area is not included in the treated volume.[138] Therefore, the authors advocate for comprehensive irradiation including elective irradiations of cervical and upper mediastinal lymph node stations when indications for EBRT are present. When including the upper mediastinal lymph nodes in the standard risk CTV, the target volume extends inferiorly to the level of the carina. A contouring atlas showing selected CT slices is provided in Figure 50.6, which shows the high-risk CTV and standard-risk CTV. Normal-tissue organ at risks (OARs) include the spinal cord, brainstem, trachea, esophagus, parotid glands, oral cavity, cochleae, pharyngeal constrictors, brachial plexus, mandible, and lungs. Planning target volumes (PTVs) and planning OAR volume are created by three-dimensional symmetric expansions of the CTVs and OARs, respectively, to account for treatment setup uncertainty and organ motion based on institutional policies and generally range from 3 to 5 mm. Daily image guidance may be used to ensure target localization and reduce the setup uncertainties in the low neck. In general, 7 to 9 coplanar axially oriented intensity-modulated beams are used. The multileaf collimator sequencing, segment, and beam weighting are optimized by the inverse planning system based on parameters specified by the planner to meet specific goals for target coverage, limitations on dose heterogeneity, and normal tissue sparing. The authors prescribe 66 to 70 Gy to the high-risk PTV and 54 to 56 Gy to the standard-risk PTV in 33 to 35 fractions using a single IMRT plan with a simultaneous integrated boost.

External Beam Radiotherapy Outcomes

Several institutions have reported outcomes of patients treated with EBRT for thyroid cancer. When interpreting these data, it is important to consider that these series contain heterogeneous patient populations and are largely comprised of patients at very high risk for recurrence, either because of aggressive histologies, recurrent disease, poor or no response to RAI therapy, or gross unresectable tumor. Table 50.15 summarizes the findings of several recent series.

External Beam Radiotherapy Toxicity

One major reason for avoiding EBRT in patients with DTC is the toxicity associated with this therapeutic modality. The acute toxicities reported include mucositis, taste changes, xerostomia, pharyngitis, dysphagia, hoarseness, radiation dermatitis, weight loss, and malnutrition. One series reported an acute and subacute percutaneous feeding tube rate of 29%.[139] Late complications include fibrosis and atrophy of the skin, lung apices, and neck musculature and tracheal and esophageal stenosis. The most commonly reported severe late complication appears to be esophageal stenosis.[136] Late severe dysphagia requiring a permanent feeding tube is uncommon.[136]

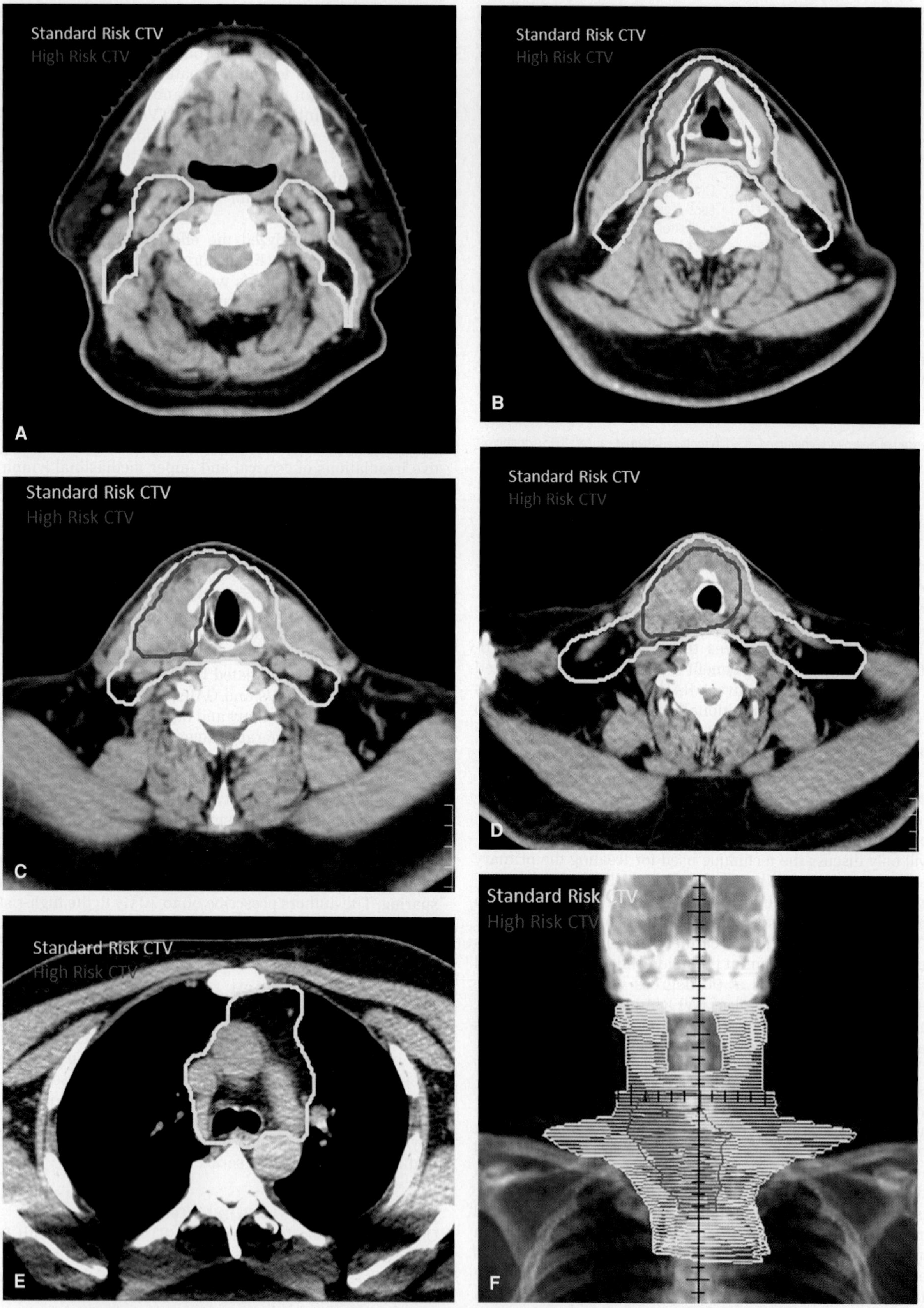

FIGURE 50.6. Intensity-modulated radiation therapy clinical target volume contouring atlas for a patient with T2N0M0 insular thyroid carcinoma status post total thyroidectomy and radioactive iodine. Indications for external beam radiation therapy were insular carcinoma (poorly differentiated) and positive margin.

TABLE 50.15 RETROSPECTIVE SERIES REPORTING OUTCOMES OF PATIENTS TREATED WITH EXTERNAL BEAM RADIATION THERAPY FOR DIFFERENTIATED THYROID CANCER

Author (Reference)	Institution	Years	Number of Patients	Tumor Characteristics	Median EBRT Dose, Gy (range)	Median Follow-Up	Local-Regional Control	Overall Survival
Schwartz et al. 2009 (136)	MD Anderson Cancer Center, Houston, TX	1996–2005	131	ETE: 96%; + margin: 47%	60 (38–72)	38 mo	79% at 4 yr	73% at 4 yr
Terezakis et al. 2009 (139)	Memorial Sloan-Kettering Cancer Center, New York, NY	1989–2006	86	ETE: 79%; + margin: 53%	63 (59–67.5)	35.3 mo	72% at 4 yr	55% at 4 yr
Meadows et al. 2006 (165)	University of Florida, Gainesville, FL	1962–2003	42	Gross residual: 48% Recurrent: 48%	64.9	49 mo	89% at 5 yr	60% at 5 yr

EBRT, external beam radiation therapy; ETE, extrathyroidal extension; yr, years; mo, months.

THYROID-STIMULATING HORMONE SUPPRESSION FOR DIFFERENTIATED THYROID CARCINOMA

A common practice in management of DTC is administration of supratherapeutic doses of T_4 in an effort to drive the TSH below detectable limits (<0.1 mIU/L), thereby decreasing stimulation of residual benign and malignant follicular-derived thyroid cells. There is *in vitro* evidence that TSH-receptor stimulation is sufficient to initiate thyroid tumorigenesis.[140] A large retrospective series of patients with DTC with 30 years of follow-up showed that, compared with no adjunctive therapy, treatment with TSH suppression with T_4 resulted in a 50% reduction in cancer deaths (6% vs. 12%).[16] Another study showed that the degree of TSH suppression (TSH ≤0.05 mIU/L vs. ≥1 mIU/L) was associated with improved relapse-free survival.[141]

A major limitation to TSH suppression is the associated toxicity as these patients experience subclinical and even overt thyrotoxicosis. As such, these patients are prone to bone demineralization and cardiac abnormalities, including tachyarrhythmia, conduction abnormalities, increased contractility, ventricular hypertrophy, systolic and diastolic dysfunction, and even cardiac death.[142] Nevertheless, a meta-analysis with over 4,000 patients with DTC demonstrated that the relative risk of major adverse clinical events was 0.73 (P <.05) favoring a "likely" or "questionable" benefit to TSH suppression in 15 of 17 trials.[143] The authors concluded that TSH suppression is justified following initial therapy for DTC. The authors recommend TSH suppression to just below 0.1 mU/L for high-risk thyroid cancer patients, while maintaining the TSH at or slightly below the lower limit of normal (0.1–0.5 mU/L) in patients at low risk of recurring.

FOLLOW-UP OF A PATIENT WITH DIFFERENTIATED THYROID CARCINOMA

The follow-up of patients with DTC should be placed into the context of whether the patient has a low risk versus a high risk of recurrence. Low-risk patients are those who have no known distant metastases, removal of all macroscopic disease after total thyroidectomy, no evidence of ETE, no aggressive histologic variants, and no evidence of RAI uptake outside of the thyroid bed on an RxWBS. High-risk patients are patients who do not meet the criteria for low risk. All patients require surveillance for recurrent disease because many recurrences are amenable to curative treatment; however, high-risk patients warrant more vigorous follow up and many will require retreatment. The ATA recommends that serum Tg is measured and neck US is performed every 6 to 12 months following primary therapy for DTC.[41] DxWBS and PET-CT scans are utilized only when clinically indicated.

Serum Tg is the most sensitive means of detecting persistent or recurrent tumor after surgery and RAI. Even as an isolated test, an undetectable serum Tg has a negative predictive value of 99%. However, it is important to realize that serum Tg measurement can reflect the level of both normal and malignant thyroid tissue remaining in the body, and that the value is very difficult to interpret in the setting of positive anti-Tg Ab, which is present in approximately 25% of patients with DTCs.

When Tg is elevated, DxWBS can be performed and, if negative, PET-CT may be warranted to assess the extent of disease. Often there is no clear evidence of overt disease on further diagnostic studies. The authors do not recommend proceeding to salvage therapy when an elevated serum Tg is the only evidence of disease.

CHEMOTHERAPY AND TARGETED AGENTS FOR DIFFERENTIATED THYROID CARCINOMA

Traditional systemic cytotoxic therapies have no significant role in the management of DTC because of poor response rates on the order of 25% to 40%.[144] The most commonly utilized agent is doxorubicin, either alone or in combination with cisplatin. Even significant responses are rarely durable for more than a few months. Recent advances in targeted therapeutics have opened new doors for effective systemic therapy for recurrent or metastatic disease that is unresponsive to RAI. Most of the agents currently under investigation target specific pathways involved in cellular proliferation through inhibition of tyrosine kinase (TKI) receptors and angiogenesis through inhibition of vascular endothelial growth factor receptors (VEGFR). Axitinib, an oral TKI that effectively blocks VEGFRs, was studied in a phase II trial for advanced and metastatic thyroid carcinoma (including both follicular-derived and medullary histologies) and resulted in a 31% objective response rate; 38% of patients had stable disease for an average duration of over 16 weeks. Motesanib, another oral TKI, was studied in a similar phase II trial and demonstrated an 81% rate of disease control with a median progression-free survival of 9.3 months. Sorafenib and sunitinib have also been studied in a phase II trial in advanced and metastatic DTC unamenable to RAI with limited success.[145]

MANAGEMENT OF MEDULLARY THYROID CARCINOMA

All patients with MTC should be tested for *RET* mutations, including sporadic cases. Genetic screening and testing is also indicated. Similar to follicular epithelial-derived DTC, initial primary management of localized MTC is total thyroidectomy, which is the only completely effective therapy. Central neck dissection should be performed in all cases and compartment-oriented lateral neck dissection is indicated when clinically involved. There is no role for adjuvant RAI therapy. All patients should be followed with serum calcitonin levels as this presents a sensitive and specific marker for extent of residual disease. The indications for EBRT in a patient with MTC depend on the patient's age. In children (<18 years old), EBRT is reserved for palliation of symptoms from tumors not amenable to other treatment or when tumor progression is likely to cause normal tissue damage. For adults, EBRT is indicated for treatment of unresectable gross disease or when there is a high risk of residual microscopic disease after total thyroidectomy based on pathologic evaluation revealing positive margins, T_4 primary tumors, or nodal metastases with extensive extracapsular extension.

Schwartz et al.[146] reported the outcomes of 34 consecutive patients treated at the M.D. Anderson Cancer Center with EBRT for MTC. Ten patients had recurrent disease, 15 had mediastinal involvement, and 10 had distant metastases; the preradiotherapy serum calcitonin was 556. The median EBRT dose was 60 Gy. The local-regional relapse-free survival, disease-specific survival, and overall survival at 5 years were 87%, 62%, and 56%, respectively, and 9% of patients developed significant late toxicity. Brierley et al.[147] reported the outcomes of 73 consecutive patients treated at Princess Margaret Hospital (Toronto, Ontario, Canada), of which 46 patients were treated with EBRT to a median dose of 40 Gy (range, 20.0–75.5 Gy). EBRT was not associated with improved local-regional relapse-free survival (LRRFS) on multivariate analysis for the overall group, but when the analysis was limited to patients with a high risk of microscopic residual disease (ETE or positive lymph nodes), the 10-year LRRFS was 86% for patients receiving EBRT compared to 52% for patients not receiving EBRT.

Traditional cytotoxic systemic therapies have largely been ineffective in the management of metastatic or recurrent MTC; however, recent advances in therapies targeting the *RET*-tyrosine kinase receptors have shown promising preclinical and early clinical results.[148–151,152]

MANAGEMENT OF ANAPLASTIC THYROID CARCINOMA

Most ATC presents with extraglandular disease and it is not clear that any form of therapy improves outcomes. Complete surgical excision should be the goal of initial therapy, when feasible. However, surgery should be avoided when complete excision is not possible as debulking does not improve outcomes. There is no therapeutic role for RAI. EBRT is the standard of care for palliation of local symptoms from unresectable disease or as adjuvant therapy in the rare case of a completely resected tumor. Even when high doses are administered, however, immediate disease progression is commonly observed.[153] Hyperfractionated therapy may improve outcomes.[154,155] Despite aggressive treatment with concomitant chemoradiotherapy using a variety of agents, including docetaxel, paclitaxel, vincristine, cisplatin, or doxorubicin, outcomes remain grim.[156–159]

SELECTED REFERENCES

A full list of references for this chapter is available online.

4. Boone RT, Fan CY, Hanna EY. Well-differentiated carcinoma of the thyroid. *Otolaryngol Clin North Am* 2003;36:73–90.
9. Siegel R, Ward E, Brawley O, et al. Cancer statistics, 2011: the impact of eliminating socioeconomic and racial disparities on premature cancer deaths. *CA Cancer J Clin* 2011;61:212–236.
10. Aschebrook-Kilfoy B, Ward MH, Sabra MM, et al. Thyroid cancer incidence patterns in the United States by histologic type, 1992–2006. *Thyroid* 2011;21: 125–134.
14. Harach HR, Franssila KO, Wasenius VM. Occult papillary carcinoma of the thyroid. A "normal" finding in Finland. A systematic autopsy study. *Cancer* 1985;56: 531–538.
17. Wood JW, Tamagaki H, Neriishi S, et al. Thyroid carcinoma in atomic bomb survivors Hiroshima and Nagasaki. *Am J Epidemiol* 1969;89:4–14.
18. Parker LN, Belsky JL, Yamamoto T, et al. Thyroid carcinoma after exposure to atomic radiation. A continuing survey of a fixed population, Hiroshima and Nagasaki, 1958–1971. *Ann Intern Med* 1974;80:600–604.
21. Preston DL, Ron E, Tokuoka S, et al. Solid cancer incidence in atomic bomb survivors: 1958–1998. *Radiat Res* 2007;168:1–64.
22. Cardis E, Hatch M. The Chernobyl accident—an epidemiological perspective. *Clin Oncol (R Coll Radiol)* 2011;23:251–260.
23. Cardis E, Krewski D, Boniol M, et al. Estimates of the cancer burden in Europe from radioactive fallout from the Chernobyl accident. *Int J Cancer* 2006;119: 1224–1235.
25. Tucker MA, Jones PH, Boice JD Jr, et al. Therapeutic radiation at a young age is linked to secondary thyroid cancer. The Late Effects Study Group. *Cancer Res* 1991;51:2885–2888.
26. Sadetzki S, Chetrit A, Lubina A, et al. Risk of thyroid cancer after childhood exposure to ionizing radiation for tinea capitis. *J Clin Endocrinol Metab* 2006; 91:4798–4804.
28. Schneider AB, Sarne DH. Long-term risks for thyroid cancer and other neoplasms after exposure to radiation. *Nat Clin Pract Endocrinol Metab* 2005;1:82–91.
29. Acharya S, Sarafoglou K, LaQuaglia M, et al. Thyroid neoplasms after therapeutic radiation for malignancies during childhood or adolescence. *Cancer* 2003;97: 2397–2403.
30. Tuttle RM, Vaisman F, Tronko MD. Clinical presentation and clinical outcomes in Chernobyl-related paediatric thyroid cancers: what do we know now? What can we expect in the future? *Clin Oncol (R Coll Radiol)* 2011;23:268–275.
32. Mortensen JD, Woolner LB, Bennett WA. Gross and microscopic findings in clinically normal thyroid glands. *J Clin Endocrinol Metab* 1955;15:1270–1280.
38. Wong C, Lin M, Chicco A, et al. The clinical significance and management of incidental focal FDG uptake in the thyroid gland on positron emission tomography/computed tomography (PET/CT) in patients with non-thyroidal malignancy. *Acta Radiol* 2011;52:899–904.
39. Nam-Goong IS, Kim HY, Gong G, et al. Ultrasonography-guided fine-needle aspiration of thyroid incidentaloma: correlation with pathological findings. *Clin Endocrinol (Oxf)* 2004;60:21–28.
44. Ko HM, Jhu IK, Yang SH, et al. Clinicopathologic analysis of fine needle aspiration cytology of the thyroid. A review of 1,613 cases and correlation with histopathologic diagnoses. *Acta Cytol* 2003;47:727–732.
49. Stulak JM, Grant CS, Farley DR, et al. Value of preoperative ultrasonography in the surgical management of initial and reoperative papillary thyroid cancer. *Arch Surg* 2006;141:489–494.
52. Ho TY, Liou MJ, Lin KJ, et al. Prevalence and significance of thyroid uptake detected by 18F-FDG PET. *Endocrine* 2011;40:297–302.
56. Samaan NA, Schultz PN, Haynie TP, et al. Pulmonary metastasis of differentiated thyroid carcinoma: treatment results in 101 patients. *J Clin Endocrinol Metab* 1985;60:376–380.
58. Vaisman F, Corbo R, Vaisman M. Thyroid carcinoma in children and adolescents-systematic review of the literature. *J Thyroid Res* 2011;2011:845362.
59. Chow SM, Law SC, Mendenhall WM, et al. Differentiated thyroid carcinoma in childhood and adolescence-clinical course and role of radioiodine. *Pediatr Blood Cancer* 2004;42:176–183.
61. Okada T, Sasaki F, Takahashi H, et al. Management of childhood and adolescent thyroid carcinoma: long-term follow-up and clinical characteristics. *Eur J Pediatr Surg* 2006;16:8–13.
63. Villaret DB, Amdur RJ, Mazzaferri EL. Neck dissections to remove malignant lymph nodes. In: Amdur RJ, Mazzaferri EL, eds. *Essentials of thyroid cancer management (Cancer treatment and research).* New York: Springer, 2005: 131–140.
65. Verburg FA, Mader U, Luster M, et al. Primary tumour diameter as a risk factor for advanced disease features of differentiated thyroid carcinoma. *Clin Endocrinol (Oxf)* 2009;71:291–297.
66. Machens A, Holzhausen HJ, Dralle H. The prognostic value of primary tumor size in papillary and follicular thyroid carcinoma. *Cancer* 2005;103:2269–2273.
67. Baudin E, Travagli JP, Ropers J, et al. Microcarcinoma of the thyroid gland: the Gustave-Roussy Institute experience. *Cancer* 1998;83:553–559.
68. Appetecchia M, Scarcello G, Pucci E, et al. Outcome after treatment of papillary thyroid microcarcinoma. *J Exp Clin Cancer Res* 2002;21:159–164.
70. Kucuk NO, Tari P, Tokmak E, et al. Treatment for microcarcinoma of the thyroid—clinical experience. *Clin Nucl Med* 2007;32:279–281.
71. Lombardi CP, Bellantone R, De Crea C, et al. Papillary thyroid microcarcinoma: extrathyroidal extension, lymph node metastases, and risk factors for recurrence in a high prevalence of goiter area. *World J Surg* 2010;34:1214–1221.
73. Scheumann GF, Seeliger H, Musholt TJ, et al. Completion thyroidectomy in 131 patients with differentiated thyroid carcinoma. *Eur J Surg* 1996;162:677–684.
75. Massin JP, Savoie JC, Garnier H, et al. Pulmonary metastases in differentiated thyroid carcinoma. Study of 58 cases with implications for the primary tumor treatment. *Cancer* 1984;53:982–992.
77. Machens A, Holzhausen HJ, Lautenschlager C, et al. Enhancement of lymph node metastasis and distant metastasis of thyroid carcinoma. *Cancer* 2003;98: 712–719.
78. Chiacchio S, Lorenzoni A, Boni G, et al. Anaplastic thyroid cancer: prevalence, diagnosis and treatment. *Minerva Endocrinol* 2008;33:341–357.
79. Sellers M, Beenken S, Blankenship A, et al. Prognostic significance of cervical lymph node metastases in differentiated thyroid cancer. *Am J Surg* 1992;164: 578–581.
86. Sosa JA, Udelsman R. Total thyroidectomy for differentiated thyroid cancer. *J Surg Oncol* 2006;94:701–707.
87. Bilimoria KY, Zanocco K, Sturgeon C. Impact of surgical treatment on outcomes for papillary thyroid cancer. *Adv Surg* 2008;42:1–12.
88. Haigh PI, Urbach DR, Rotstein LE. Extent of thyroidectomy is not a major determinant of survival in low- or high-risk papillary thyroid cancer. *Ann Surg Oncol* 2005;12:81–89.
91. Hay ID, Grant CS, Taylor WF, et al. Ipsilateral lobectomy versus bilateral lobar resection in papillary thyroid carcinoma: a retrospective analysis of surgical outcome using a novel prognostic scoring system. *Surgery* 1987;102:1088–1095.
92. Haigh PI, Urbach DR, Rotstein LE. AMES prognostic index and extent of thyroidectomy for well-differentiated thyroid cancer in the United States. *Surgery* 2004;136:609–616.
93. Bilimoria KY, Bentrem DJ, Linn JG, et al. Utilization of total thyroidectomy for papillary thyroid cancer in the United States. *Surgery* 2007;142:906–913.
96. Noguchi S, Murakami N, Yamashita H, et al. Papillary thyroid carcinoma: modified radical neck dissection improves prognosis. *Arch Surg* 1998;133:276–280.
99. Dionigi G, Dionigi R, Bartalena L, et al. Surgery of lymph nodes in papillary thyroid cancer. *Expert Rev Anticancer Ther* 2006;6:1217–1229.

100. White ML, Doherty GM. Level VI lymph node dissection for papillary thyroid cancer. *Minerva Chir* 2007;62:383–393.
101. Sadowski BM, Snyder SK, Lairmore TC. Routine bilateral central lymph node clearance for papillary thyroid cancer. *Surgery* 2009;146:696–703.
102. Mulla M, Schulte KM. Central cervical lymph node metastases in papillary thyroid cancer: a systematic review of imaging-guided and prophylactic removal of the central compartment. *Clin Endocrinol (Oxf)* 2011;76:131–136.
103. Moo TA, McGill J, Allendorf J, et al. Impact of prophylactic central neck lymph node dissection on early recurrence in papillary thyroid carcinoma. *World J Surg* 2010;34:1187–1191.
104. Shindo M, Wu JC, Park EE, et al. The importance of central compartment elective lymph node excision in the staging and treatment of papillary thyroid cancer. *Arch Otolaryngol Head Neck Surg* 2006;132:650–654.
106. Shah MD, Hall FT, Eski SJ, et al. Clinical course of thyroid carcinoma after neck dissection. *Laryngoscope* 2003;113:2102–2107.
112. Tsang RW, Brierley JD, Simpson WJ, et al. The effects of surgery, radioiodine, and external radiation therapy on the clinical outcome of patients with differentiated thyroid carcinoma. *Cancer* 1998;82:375–388.
123. Kloos RT. Survey of radioiodine therapy safety practices highlights the need for user-friendly recommendations. *Thyroid* 2011;21:97–99.
126. Sawka AM, Thabane L, Parlea L, et al. Second primary malignancy risk after radioactive iodine treatment for thyroid cancer: a systematic review and meta-analysis. *Thyroid* 2009;19:451–457.
127. Rubino C, de Vathaire F, Dottorini ME, et al. Second primary malignancies in thyroid cancer patients. *Br J Cancer* 2003;89: 1638–1644.
144. Haugen BR. Management of the patient with progressive radioiodine non-responsive disease. *Semin Surg Oncol* 1999;16: 34–41.
148. Lam ET, Ringel MD, Kloos RT, et al. Phase II clinical trial of sorafenib in metastatic medullary thyroid cancer. *J Clin Oncol* 2010;28:2323–2330.
149. Wells SA, Jr., Gosnell JE, Gagel RF, et al. Vandetanib for the treatment of patients with locally advanced or metastatic hereditary medullary thyroid cancer. *J Clin Oncol* 2010;28:767–772.
150. Ye L, Santarpia L, Gagel RF. Targeted therapy for endocrine cancer: the medullary thyroid carcinoma paradigm. *Endocr Pract* 2009;15:597–604.
151. Torino F, Paragliola RM, Barnabei A, et al. Medullary thyroid cancer: a promising model for targeted therapy. *Curr Mol Med* 2010;10: 608–625.
154. Tennvall J, Lundell G, Wahlberg P, et al. Anaplastic thyroid carcinoma: three protocols combining doxorubicin, hyperfractionated radiotherapy and surgery. *Br J Cancer* 2002;86:1848–1853.
155. De Crevoisier R, Baudin E, Bachelot A, et al. Combined treatment of anaplastic thyroid carcinoma with surgery, chemotherapy, and hyperfractionated accelerated external radiotherapy. *Int J Radiat Oncol Biol Phys* 2004;60:1137–1143.
156. Haigh PI, Ituarte PH, Wu HS, et al. Completely resected anaplastic thyroid carcinoma combined with adjuvant chemotherapy and irradiation is associated with prolonged survival. *Cancer* 2001;91: 2335–2342.
158. Troch M, Koperek O, Scheuba C, et al. High efficacy of concomitant treatment of undifferentiated (anaplastic) thyroid cancer with radiation and docetaxel. *J Clin Endocrinol Metab* 2010;95:E54–E57.
161. Xu L, Li G, Wei Q, et al. Family history of cancer and risk of sporadic differentiated thyroid carcinoma. *Cancer* 2011;118:1228–1235.
163. Sawka AM, Ibrahim-Zada I, Galacgac P, et al. Dietary iodine restriction in preparation for radioactive iodine treatment or scanning in well-differentiated thyroid cancer: a systematic review. *Thyroid* 2012;20:1129–1138.

Part E Thorax

Chapter 51 Lung Cancer

Ramesh Rengan, Indrin J. Chetty, Roy Decker, Corey J. Langer, William P. O'Meara, and Benjamin Movsas

EPIDEMIOLOGY

Throughout the world, lung cancer accounts for 13% (1.6 million) of the total cases of cancer and 18% (1.4 million) of the cancer-related deaths based on 2008 estimates.[1] Among males, lung cancer is the most commonly diagnosed cancer and leading cause of cancer death. Among females worldwide, it is the fourth most commonly diagnosed cancer and the second leading cause of cancer death.

In the United States, lung cancer is the second most common cancer and the most common cause of cancer-related death in both men and women. The American Cancer Society estimates 156,940 people in the United States died of lung cancer in 2011, including 85,600 men and 71,340 women.[2] More people in the United States die of lung cancer than from breast, prostate, and colorectal cancer combined. The overall 5-year survival rate for lung cancer is approximately 16%.[3]

The overall incidence and mortality rate for lung cancer rose steadily from the 1930s until peaking in the early 1990s. The incidence and mortality rates for men began to drop around 1990, and the latest analysis demonstrates a drop in the incidence and mortality rates for women for the first time.[4] The lag in the trend of lung cancer rates in women compared with men reflects historical differences in cigarette smoking between the sexes; cigarette smoking in women peaked about 20 years later than in men. Gender and racial disparities exist in the incidence and mortality for lung cancer with rates highest in men, particularly those who are African American.[2,5] In terms of socioeconomics, lung cancer demonstrates the largest disparity of all cancers, with the death rate in men five times higher for the least educated than for the most educated.[2]

Although the lung cancer numbers in the general population are startling, the main risk of lung cancer is based on exposures to carcinogens; most lung cancer cases are attributable to cigarette smoking. Voluntary or involuntary cigarette exposure accounts for 80% to 90% of all cases of lung cancer.[6] Since the 1964 landmark report by U.S. Surgeon General citing smoking as a causal agent for the development of lung cancer,[7] the prevalence of smoking in the United States has declined significantly. More recently, exposure to secondhand smoke has been considered a risk for lung cancer with up to a 30% increase in risk from secondhand smoke exposure associated with living with a smoker.[8] Indoor radon exposure is now considered the second leading cause of lung cancer in the United States.[9] Other known risk factors for lung cancer include exposure to occupational and environmental carcinogens such as asbestos, arsenic, and polycyclic aromatic hydrocarbons.[10–13]

ANATOMY

In the past, a simplified and relatively superficial understanding of thoracic anatomy provided an acceptable framework for the radiation oncologist to design treatment fields in lung cancer patients utilizing conventional techniques with the carina and bony structures as landmarks. As the field of thoracic radiation oncology has moved toward more conformal therapy, however, a more detailed understanding of thoracic anatomy is essential for proper target delineation and treatment design.

The lungs are situated on each side of the mediastinum, which contains the heart, trachea, esophagus, and great vessels. The lungs are conical in shape with an apex projecting upward into the neck for approximately 2 to 3 cm above the clavicle, a base sitting on the diaphragm, a costal surface along the chest wall, and a mediastinal surface that is molded to the heart and other mediastinal structures. Visceral pleura cover the lungs, and parietal pleura cover the inside of the chest cavity. The lungs are freely suspended but are rooted to the mediastinum by the structures emerging from the hilum.

The lungs are divided into distinct lobes—three lobes to the right lung and two to the left. The right lung is divided into the upper, middle, and lower lobes by the oblique (major) and horizontal (minor) fissures. The oblique fissure runs forward and downward from approximately the level of the fifth thoracic vertebral body to the diaphragm, dividing the lungs into upper and lower lobes. The horizontal fissure separates the right middle from the right upper lobe, fanning out forward and laterally from the hilum. The middle lobe is thus a small, triangular lobe bounded by the horizontal and oblique fissures and actually rests on the diaphragm. The left lung is divided by only the oblique fissure into two lobes—the upper and lower lobes. The lingula, located in the left upper lobe, is homologous to the right middle lobe and also touches the diaphragm.

The bronchopulmonary segment is the functional unit of the lung and is defined by the segmental bronchi. The trachea bifurcates at the carina, which lies at the junction between the manubrium and body of the sternum, into the right and left main bronchi. Each main bronchus divides into lobar bronchi, each supplying a lobe of the lung. Although the lingula is located in the left upper lobe, the lingular bronchus is considered by many a lobar bronchus. Each lobar bronchus divides into smaller bronchi that form the bronchopulmonary segments. These segments are pyramidal in shape, with an apex toward the lung root and a base at the pleural surface. Structures entering each bronchopulmonary segment (i.e., bronchus and artery) tend to lie centrally. Structures leaving the segment (i.e., veins and lymphatics) lie in the periphery of the segment within the

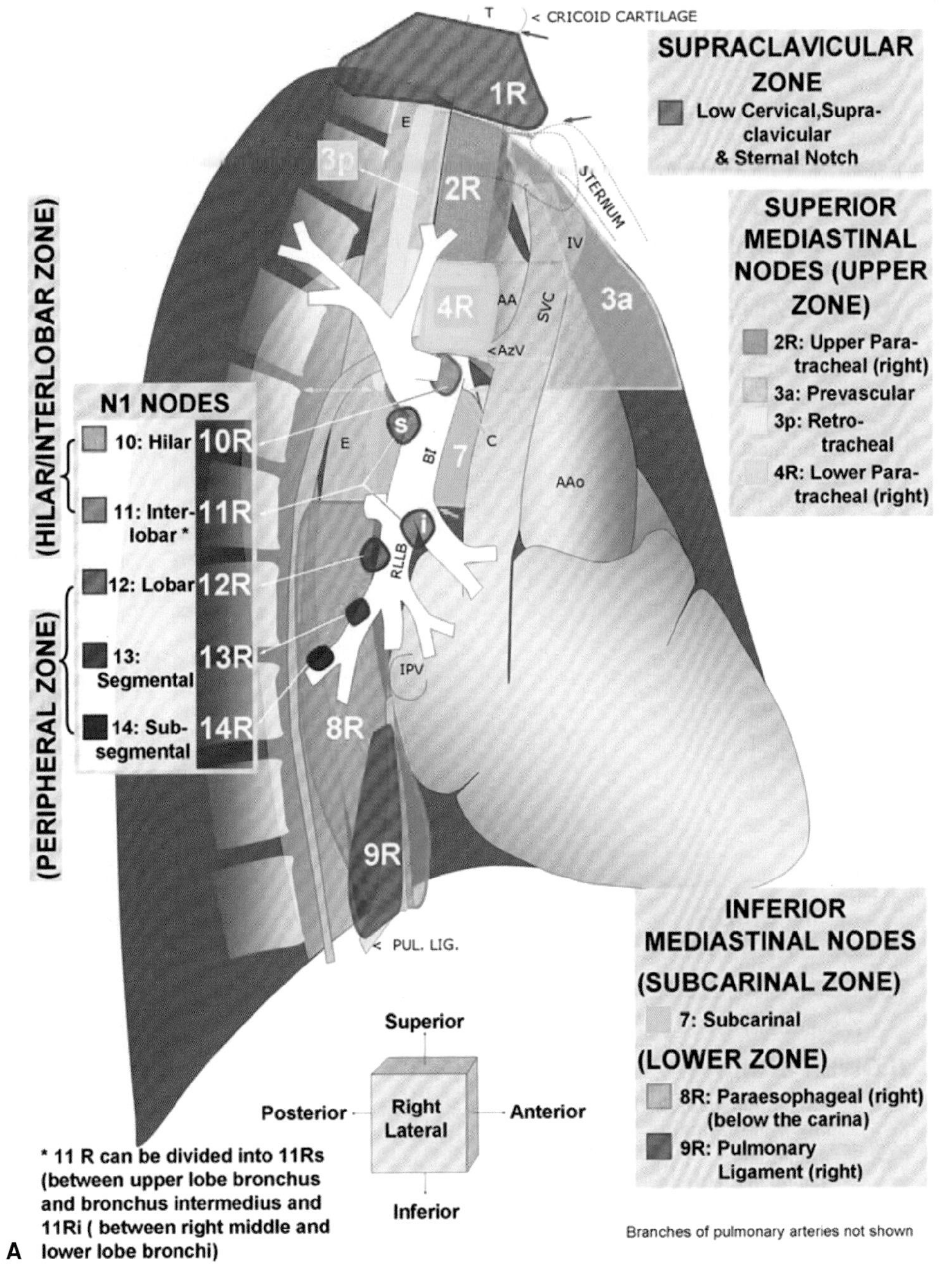

FIGURE 51.1. The International Association for the Study of Lung Cancer lymph node map for lung cancer staging. (From Lababede O, Meziane M, Rice T. Seventh edition of the *Cancer Staging Manual* and stage grouping of lung cancer. *Chest* 2011;139(1):183–189, with permission.) (*continued*)

connective tissue that separates the segments.[14] Segmental bronchi divide into bronchioles, continue to branch, and eventually form the alveoli, where blood-gas exchange occurs.

The main lymphatic drainage for each bronchopulmonary segment follows the vasculature and airways toward the hilum, where it ultimately drains into the mediastinum. However, the rich network of lymphatics within the thorax leads to complex variability in drainage patterns.[15]

For nearly half a century, lymph node maps have been used in lung cancer to describe the clinical and pathologic extent of lymph node involvement.[16] Two such maps—the Naruke lymph node map[17] and the Mountain/Dresler map[18]—have been used the most. Recently, however, the International Association for the Study of Lung Cancer (IASLC) proposed a new lymph node map that reconciles differences among currently used maps and provides precise anatomic definitions for all lymph node stations.[16] The IASLC lymph node map has been endorsed by the American Joint Committee on Cancer (AJCC) and incorporated into the seventh edition of its staging manual. Figure 51.1 shows the IASLC lymph node map, which designates 14 levels of intrapulmonary, hilar, and mediastinal lymph nodes stations. The IASLC also compartmentalized the stations into zones that appear to have prognostic implications and are already utilized in common clinical practice.

CLINICAL PRESENTATION AND PATTERNS OF SPREAD

Lung cancer spreads locally by direct extension of the primary tumor, regionally via involvement of the lymphatics, and distantly via invasion into vascular channels leading to hematogenous spread. In a recent Surveillance Epidemiology and End Results (SEER) analysis involving all lung cancer histologies, 15% of all cases of lung cancer were localized to the primary site at initial diagnosis; 22% had regional lymph node spread, and 56% distant metastasis; and the remaining 7% were stage unknown.[19] In non–small cell lung cancer (NSCLC), half the

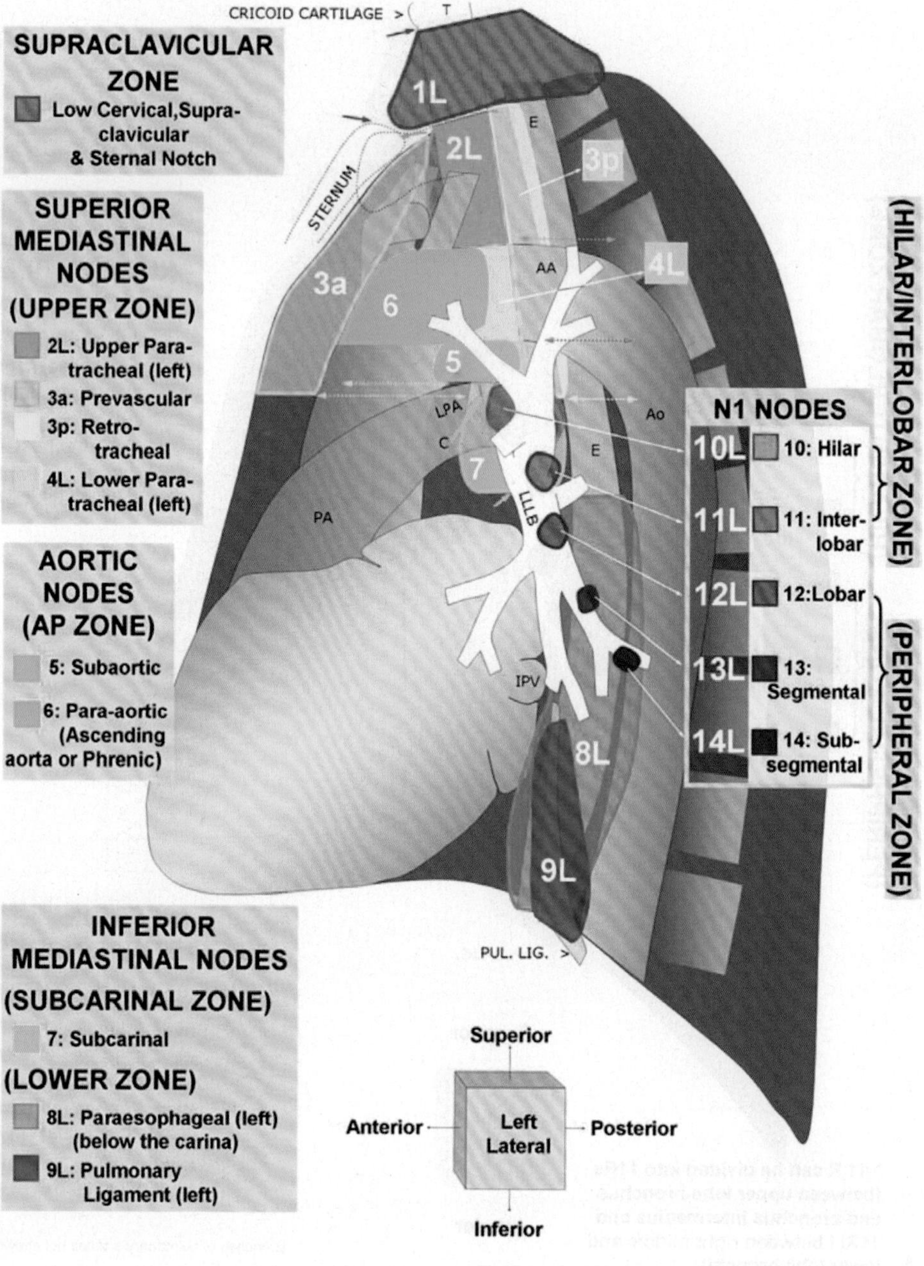

FIGURE 51.1. *(Continued)* **B**

patients present with localized or locally advanced disease and half with advanced disease. In small cell lung cancer (SCLC), 20% to 30% present with locally advanced disease, and 70% to 80% present with advanced disease. Table 51.1 shows the site of metastasis based on histologic type.[20] Signs and symptoms of lung cancer directly reflect the patient's local, regional, or distant pattern of spread.

Intrathoracic Spread

The intrathoracic spread of lung cancer involves direct extension of the primary tumor or lymphatic spread to regional lymph nodes involving the hilum or mediastinum. There is a wide range of symptoms owing to the intrathoracic effects of lung cancer; the most common include cough, dyspnea, hemoptysis, and chest pain.

The central etiology for many symptoms is owing to a growing tumor involving the airway. Cough is present in 50% to 75% of lung cancer patients at presentation and occurs most

TABLE 51.1 SITE OF METASTASIS CORRELATED WITH HISTOLOGIC SUBTYPE IN LUNG CANCER: NECROPSY FINDINGS IN CARCINOMA OF THE BRONCHUS IN 255 PATIENTS WITH METASTASES TO 431 SITES

Site of Metastasis	*Squamous*	*Small Cell*	*Anaplastic*	*Adenocarcinoma*
Lymph nodes	137 (54%)	163 (85%)	135 (76%)	42 (75%)
Liver	58 (23%)	122 (64%)	67 (38%)	26 (47%)
Adrenals	54 (21%)	84 (44%)	69 (39%)	17 (30%)
Bones	59 (23%)	75 (39%)	53 (30%)	23 (41%)
Brain	26 (17%)	45 (42%)	30 (24%)	13 (39%)
Kidney	39 (15%)	28 (15%)	24 (14%)	11 (20%)
Pancreas	9 (4%)	46 (24%)	25 (14%)	3 (5%)
Lung	31 (2%)	13 (7%)	15 (8%)	8 (14%)
Pleura	18 (7%)	21 (11%)	9 (5%)	3 (5%)
Total	**255**	**191**	**179**	**56**

From Line DH, Deeley TJ. The necropsy findings in carcinoma of the bronchus. *Br J Dis Chest* 1971;65(4):238–242, with permission from Elsevier.

frequently in patients with squamous cell and small cell carcinomas because of their tendency to involve central airways.[21,22] As central airway involvement progresses, wheezing may develop. Additionally, tumor eroding into a blood vessel or bleeding from the neovasculature supplying the tumor may lead to hemoptysis, which is a presenting symptom in approximately 25% of patients.[23] If tumor blocks airflow through a portion of the lung, shortness of breath may develop and is identified at presentation in approximately 25% of cases.[21,24] Dyspnea may also be due to the development of atelectasis, postobstructive pneumonia, or a pleural or pericardial effusion.

Chest pain is present in approximately 20% of patients presenting with lung cancer.[21,24] Pain may be attributed to direct extension to the mediastinum, parietal pleura, or chest wall. Pleuritic pain may also be the result of obstructive pneumonitis or a pulmonary embolus related to a hypercoagulable state. Pleural involvement can also manifest as pleural thickening or pleural effusion. During the course of lung cancer, 10% to 15% of all cases will eventually develop a malignant pleural effusion.[25]

Direct extension of a central primary tumor or mediastinal lymph node involvement may lead to nerve involvement. Involvement of the recurrent laryngeal nerve along its course under the arch of the aorta can result in hoarseness. Irritation of the phrenic nerve may initially produce hiccups, and progressive damage can produce unilateral paralysis of the diaphragm with shortness of breath.

Obstruction of the superior vena cava (SVC) from primary tumor or mediastinal lymphadenopathy causes symptoms that commonly include a sensation of fullness in the head and dyspnea. Physical findings include jugular venous distension and occasionally swelling of the face and arms. SVC syndrome is more common in patients with SCLC than NSCLC. The pathophysiology and treatment options for the management of patients with SVC syndrome are discussed in more detail later.

Primary tumors arising within the superior sulcus may produce the classic Pancoast's syndrome manifested by shoulder pain, Horner's syndrome, and brachial plexopathy. Pancoast's syndrome is most commonly caused by NSCLC and only rarely by SCLC. The treatment of patients with superior sulcus tumors (SSTs) will be discussed later.

Distant Extrathoracic Spread

Once vascular or lymphatic invasion occurs, metastatic dissemination to distant sites is common. Contralateral lung, liver, bone, adrenals, and brain are the most frequent sites of distant disease; however, lung cancer can spread to any part of the body (Table 51.1).

Asymptomatic liver metastases may be detected at presentation by liver enzyme abnormalities or on staging workup imaging. Among patients with otherwise resectable NSCLC in the chest, computed tomography (CT) evidence of liver metastasis has been identified in approximately 3% of cases.[26] Positron emission tomography (PET) or integrated PET-CT identifies unsuspected metastases in the liver or adrenal glands in about 4% of patients.[27,28] Autopsy studies have identified hepatic metastases in >50% of patients with either NSCLC or SCLC.[29,30]

Pain in the back, chest, or extremity and elevated levels of serum alkaline phosphatase are usually present in patients with bone metastasis. The serum calcium may be elevated owing to extensive bone disease, although the majority of patients with elevated calcium have paraneoplastic parathyroid hormone (PTH)-like syndrome. Approximately 20% of patients with NSCLC and 30% to 40% of patients with SCLC have bone metastases at presentation.[31,32] An osteolytic radiographic appearance is more frequent than an osteoblastic one, although a mixed picture is common. The most common sites of involvement are the vertebral bodies.

The adrenal glands are a frequent site of metastasis; however, such metastases are only rarely symptomatic. Concern about adrenal metastasis usually occurs when a unilateral mass is found by staging CT in a patient with a known or suspected lung cancer. Most adrenal masses detected on staging scans are benign, as illustrated by a series of 330 patients with operable NSCLC in which 32 (10%) had an isolated adrenal mass.[33] Only 8 of these 32 patients (25%) had a malignancy. Conversely, a negative imaging study does not exclude adrenal metastases. A study of patients with SCLC found that 17% of adrenal biopsies showed metastatic involvement despite having a normal CT scan.[34] The lack of specificity of an initial CT scan in identifying an adrenal mass creates a special problem in patients with an otherwise resectable lung cancer. In this situation, PET may be particularly useful in distinguishing a benign from malignant adrenal mass.[35] Other procedures that may be useful in excluding a metastasis include magnetic resonance imaging (MRI) consistent with a benign adenoma or a negative needle biopsy. Involvement of the adrenal glands is more frequent in patients with widely disseminated disease. In autopsy series, adrenal metastases were identified in about 40% of patients with lung cancer.[30] Patients with an isolated adrenal metastasis but otherwise limited thoracic disease seem to have a much better prognosis than other stage IV disease and may be considered for aggressive definitive management.[36,37]

Symptoms from brain metastasis include headache, vomiting, visual field loss, hemiparesis, cranial nerve deficit, and seizures. In patients with NSCLC, the frequency of brain metastasis is greatest with adenocarcinoma and least with squamous cell carcinoma. The risk of brain metastasis increases with larger primary tumor size and regional node involvement.[38] In patients with SCLC, metastasis to brain is present in approximately 20% to 30% of patients at presentation.[39] Without prophylactic irradiation, relapse in the brain occurs in about one-half of patients within 2 years.[40] An autopsy series of SCLC patients disclosed central nervous system (CNS) metastases in 80% of cases.[41]

Paraneoplastic Syndromes

A paraneoplastic syndrome is a disease or symptom that is the consequence of cancer cells in the body but is not attributable to the local presence of tumor. These phenomena are thought to be mediated by humoral factors secreted by tumor cells or by an immune response against the tumor. Treating the cancer, if successful, usually resolves the syndrome. Some of the more common paraneoplastic syndromes are described next.

Cushing Syndrome

Ectopic production of adrenocorticotropic hormone (ACTH) can cause Cushing's syndrome. Patients typically present with muscle weakness, weight loss, hypertension, hirsutism, and osteoporosis. Hypokalemic alkalosis and hyperglycemia are usually present. Cushing's syndrome is relatively common in patients with SCLC and with carcinoid tumors of the lung. SCLC patients with Cushing's syndrome appear to have a worse prognosis than those without Cushing's syndrome.[42–44]

Syndrome of Inappropriate Antidiuretic Hormone Secretion

The syndrome of inappropriate antidiuretic hormone (SIADH) secretion is frequently caused by SCLC and results in hyponatremia. Approximately 10% of patients who have SCLC exhibit SIADH, and SCLC accounts for approximately 75% of all SIADH.[45,46] Symptoms include headache, muscle cramps, anorexia, and decreased urine output. If left untreated, cerebral edema can develop, leading to mental status changes, coma, seizures, and respiratory arrest. Besides treating the underlying cancer, demeclocycline is the agent of choice.

Hypercalcemia

Hypercalcemia in patients with lung cancer may be attributable to the secretion of a parathyroid hormone–related protein (PTHrP), calcitriol, or other cytokines, including osteoclast activating factors. In one study of 1,149 consecutive lung cancers, 6% of patients had hypercalcemia.[47] Among those with hypercalcemia, squamous cell carcinoma, adenocarcinoma, and SCLC were responsible in 51%, 22%, and 15% of cases, respectively. Symptoms of hypercalcemia include anorexia, nausea, vomiting, constipation, lethargy, polyuria, polydipsia, and dehydration. Renal failure, confusion, and coma are late manifestations.

Lambert-Eaton Myasthenic Syndrome

Lambert-Eaton myasthenic syndrome (LEMS) is an autoimmune disorder characterized by muscle weakness of the limbs that improves with repeated testing, in contrast to myasthenia gravis, which worsens with repetition. Proximal muscles are predominantly affected, and patients complain of difficulty climbing stairs and rising from a sitting position. Approximately 3% of patients with SCLC exhibit LEMS, and SCLC accounts for approximately 60% of all LEMS.[48] The neurologic symptoms of LEMS precede the diagnosis of SCLC in >80% of cases, often by months or years.

Hypertrophic Osteoarthropathy

Hypertrophic pulmonary osteoarthropathy (HPO), most frequently associated with adenocarcinoma, is defined by clubbing and periosteal proliferation of the tubular bones. HPO is further characterized by a symmetrical, painful arthropathy that usually involves the ankles, knees, wrists, and elbows. A radiograph of the long bones shows characteristic periosteal new bone formation. A bone scan or PET typically demonstrates diffuse uptake by the long bones. In a series of 111 lung cancer patients, clubbing was present in 29%.[49]

SCREENING, DIAGNOSTIC STAGING, AND WORKUP

Screening for Lung Cancer

Given the high mortality rate of lung cancer and that the majority of patients are diagnosed at a late stage, lung cancer researchers have theorized that identifying lung cancer at an earlier stage might improve outcomes. Thus, lung cancer has been considered as a candidate for cancer screening. Early screening trials involving chest x-rays and/or sputum failed to demonstrate a survival benefit.[50–52] The role of screening has recently been reinvestigated with the advent of spiral CT scans. Early pilot trials of spiral CT in lung cancer screening looked promising with an increase in the identification of stage I detectable cancer. A subsequent international observational trial using spiral CT screening in a cohort of 31,000 high-risk individuals corroborated the findings, showing that annual spiral CT screening could detect lung cancer at an early, potentially more curable stage, suggesting that the stage I disease detection rate and 10-year survival rate could both exceed 80%.[53] With a possible mortality benefit theorized but not yet proven, some researchers countered that the use of spiral CT screening might not significantly reduce the mortality risk for lung cancer.[54] This set the groundwork for the landmark National Lung Screening Trial (NLST). From August 2002 through April 2004, 53,454 current or former heavy smokers at 33 U.S. medical centers were randomly assigned to three annual screenings with either low-dose CT (26,722 participants) or standard chest x-ray (26,732). Eligible participants were between 55 and 74 years of age with a history of cigarette smoking of at least 30 pack-years and, if former smokers, had quit within the previous 15 years. Persons who had previously received a diagnosis of lung cancer, had undergone chest CT within 18 months before enrollment, had hemoptysis, or had an unexplained weight loss >6.8 kg (15 lb) in the preceding year were excluded. The findings revealed that participants who received low-dose helical CT scans had a 20% relative reduction in risk of death caused by lung cancer compared with the control radiography group ($p = .004$). Additionally, the all-cause mortality was reduced in the CT screening group by 6.7% when compared with the control group ($p = .02$). This is the first randomized trial to demonstrate a reduction in all-cause mortality with screening.[55] This demonstrates that the benefits to screening outweigh the potential risk from biopsy and further diagnostic intervention in patients who had a false-positive screen. Although this is clearly a landmark study, it is unclear at this time whether this trial alone will lead to a paradigm shift in screening for lung cancer with CT. A key issue relates to the cost-benefit ratio of lung cancer screening with low-dose CT. Several similar randomized CT screening trials are under way.[56–60]

Diagnostic Staging and Workup

When a patient presents with suspected lung cancer, testing is indicated to confirm the diagnosis, identify the histologic type, and determine the disease stage, all in an effort to guide management decisions. The process begins with a thorough history and physical examination to identify signs or symptoms suggestive of locally extensive or metastatic disease, assess pulmonary health status, identify significant comorbidities, and assess overall health status. Each impacts the therapeutic options in a more comprehensive manner than stage alone. A detailed history should also elicit tobacco use and past exposure to environmental carcinogens. Weight loss >5% from baseline has direct prognostic implications for survival in lung cancer.[61–63]

Physical examination of the chest may detect signs of partial or complete obstruction of the airways, pneumonia, or pleural effusion. Examination of the neck can reveal evidence of supraclavicular lymphadenopathy. Abdominal examination may detect hepatomegaly. Neurologic examination can detect signs of brain metastasis.

Laboratory studies include complete blood count, liver function tests, and serum electrolytes including calcium. Renal function tests should be performed to assess whether the patient can tolerate intravenous contrast for CT examination or subsequent platinum-based therapy. Liver function test abnormalities could be owing to liver metastasis. Elevation of alkaline phosphatase could be owing to liver or bone metastasis. Calcium elevation could be owing to bone metastasis or paraneoplastic syndrome. Anemia could be owing to metastatic disease.

Radiologic Examinations

Chest X-Ray

Chest x-ray is the initial imaging modality for evaluating a patient with suspected lung cancer. The current x-ray should be compared to prior ones, if available, to determine if a lesion is new, enlarging, or stable.

Computed Tomography

All patients with suspected lung cancer, with or without an abnormal chest x-ray, should undergo a contrast-enhanced CT scan of the chest and upper abdomen to include the entire liver and adrenal glands. Intravenous contrast helps to distinguish vascular structures from mediastinal structures. This not only adds detail to the imaging characteristics of the primary tumor but is also critical to accurately identify suspicious lymph nodes in the mediastinum. CT assessment can establish T-stage by determining tumor size, presence of separate tumor nodules, presence of atelectasis or postobstructive pneumonia, invasion of adjacent structures, and proximal extent of the tumor.

Lymph node enlargement on CT presumes lymph node metastasis in the context of newly diagnosed lung cancer. Most normal mediastinal lymph nodes measure <1 cm, although normal subcarinal lymph nodes can reach a diameter of 1.5 cm. In a patient with known lung cancer, a lymph node is considered suspicious if it measures >1 cm in diameter on its short axis. Unfortunately, many subcentimeter regional lymph nodes may still harbor metastasis. In one study involving pathologic staging, up to 44% of nodes with metastatic deposits were <1 cm in diameter, and 18% of patients with pathologically involved mediastinal nodes did not have any nodes >1 cm.[64]

Positron Emission Tomography or Positron Emission Tomography–Computed Tomography

PET scanning has become standard in the staging workup of lung cancer patients. Although the primary tumor characteristics are usually clearly staged with a CT scan, PET can help distinguish atelectasis from tumor in certain cases.[65] The largest benefit provided by PET is the identification of suspicious lymph nodes or distant metastasis not seen on CT scan. Kalff et al.[66] prospectively evaluated the utility of PET in patients with lung cancer, performing a PET scan on 105 consecutive clinically staged patients with a diagnosis of NSCLC. They found that PET correctly upstaged 26% of patients to palliative from curative intent therapy and appropriately downstaged 10 of 16 patients initially designated for palliative therapy.[66] Additionally, PET can detect malignant disease in lymph nodes of normal size, overcoming one of the major limitations of CT.[67–69] Integrated PET-CT scanners fuse images obtained in tandem from PET and CT, thus providing both anatomic and metabolic information simultaneously. This is superior to CT or PET alone[70,71–72] and can detect malignancy in tumors as small as 0.5 cm.

Although PET has dramatically improved the noninvasive staging of lung cancer patients, it does have some key limitations. On meta-analysis, the sensitivity and specificity of CT for mediastinal nodal metastasis were estimated to be approximately 59% and 79%, respectively, and the sensitivity and specificity of PET were approximately 81% and 90%, respectively.[69] This same meta-analysis also found a difference in the accuracy of PET based on the CT size of a lymph node with a sensitivity of 91% for enlarged mediastinal nodes and 75% for nonenlarged nodes.[69] Because false positives and false negatives are observed with PET, tissue sampling should be pursued to confirm the presence or absence of regional lymph node involvement before a treatment decision is made. A positive PET should not be considered proof of lymph node metastasis, especially if such a conclusion would otherwise exclude surgery.

With highly conformal radiation therapy for lung cancer becoming commonplace, PET is now being used to aid radiation oncologists in the target delineation process for involved-field radiotherapy (IFRT).[73,74] Registration of PET with the planning CT scan at the contouring stage has been shown to enhance the accuracy of defining gross tumor volumes (GTVs).[75] The clinician must be mindful that target volumes based solely on 18F-fluorodeoxyglucose (FDG)-PET positivity have their limitations, with the most notable being a false-negative rate of approximately 25% in mediastinal lymph nodes <1 cm in size.[69] Additionally, the optimal windowing algorithm for the purposes of contouring remains to be determined. Depending on the algorithm employed, the volume that is contoured can vary significantly.[76] When benchmarked against the true pathologic volume, at present the CT-derived contour appears to be more accurate than that derived from FDG-PET regardless of the algorithm employed.[77] Efforts are under way to improve on the accuracy of current PET scanning, and one approach is through the exploration of novel tracers. Standard PET scanning focuses on glucose metabolism with FDG as the radionuclide. Other PET tracers currently being explored for interrogation of distinct components of tumor biology include 18F-fluoromisonidazole (FMISO) and 2-(2-nitro-(1)H-imidazol-1-yl)-N-(2,2,3,3,3-pentafluoropropyl)-acetamide (EF5) for tumor hypoxia; 18F-fluorothymidine (FLT) for tumor proliferation; and 11C-methionine and 11C-tyrosine for amino acid metabolism.[78,79] In addition to potentially improving the accuracy of target delineation, integrating the functional information from these novel tracers into the treatment planning process provides an opportunity for dose escalation to areas of radioresistance.[79]

Special Diagnostic Procedures

Sputum Cytology

Sputum cytology is a rapid, relatively inexpensive but underused means to establish a tissue diagnosis in an individual with a suspected pulmonary carcinoma. Previous reports have indicated that the sensitivity of sputum cytology is 65% in the setting of established cancers.[80] Three specimens increase the diagnostic yield. Sputum samples are considered representative if alveolar macrophages and bronchial epithelial cells are present. The diagnostic yield of sputum cytology is enhanced with centrally located, intraluminal cancers such as squamous cell carcinoma.

Percutaneous Fine Needle Aspiration

CT-guided fine needle aspiration (FNA) is an excellent method for establishing a tissue diagnosis from a suspicious peripheral pulmonary nodule that cannot be reached by bronchoscopy. The risk of a pneumothorax from this procedure is 25%. However, most of these are small, asymptomatic, and resolve without intervention; only approximately 5% require a chest tube. The overall diagnostic yield is 80%.[81] Indeterminate biopsies must be interpreted with caution. FNA cannot rule out malignancy unless another benign diagnosis can clearly be established. Abnormalities involving bone, liver, and adrenal glands can also be confirmed by CT-guided FNA. Frequently, biopsy of one of these suspected metastatic sites simultaneously establishes tissue diagnosis and stage of the disease. Increasingly, as we enter the modern era of molecularly guided therapy, core biopsies are displacing FNAs. This increases the risk but also increases the yield.

Bronchoscopy

Fiberoptic bronchoscopy enables visualization of the tracheobronchial tree to the second or third segmental divisions. Cytologic brushings or biopsy forceps specimens can be obtained from identified lesions. Even when no visible lesion is identified, the bronchus draining the area of suspicion can be lavaged for cytologic analysis. With the use of fiberoptic bronchoscopy combined with special CT imaging techniques, even more peripheral lesions can be reached.[82] The diagnostic yield of fiberoptic bronchoscopy is directly related to the ability of the operator to navigate the scope to the lesion of interest; this can be challenging for peripheral lesions. The superDimension/Bronchus system is a real-time guidance system designed to guide the bronchoscope to specified locations within the bronchial tree. Using this approach, a virtual map of the bronchial tree is generated from a high-resolution CT scan of the chest, enabling the physician to monitor the location of the bronchoscope in real time through feedback from a positional sensor attached to the tip of the bronchoscope. There is evidence that this approach may significantly improve the diagnostic yield for peripheral lesions.[82]

Endoscopic Fine Needle Aspiration

Fiberoptic endoscopy techniques can also be combined with ultrasound to evaluate mediastinal and hilar lymph nodes. Endobronchial ultrasound-guided transbronchial needle aspiration (EBUS-TBNA) involves FNA sampling of ultrasound-suspicious lymph nodes, especially those located in the paratracheal (lymph node levels 2 and 4), subcarinal (level 7), or hilar lymph node stations (level 10).[83] A prospective study comparing EBUS-TBNA with PET-CT scans revealed an accuracy of 98% and a sensitivity and specificity of 92% and 100%, respectively.[84] An esophageal approach known as transesophageal endoscopic ultrasound-guided fine needle aspiration (EUS-FNA) can perform the same function, especially the sampling of mediastinal nodes that are posterior or inferior, such as the retrotracheal (lymph node station 3p), subcarinal (level 7), paraesophageal (level 8), and pulmonary ligament lymph nodes (level 9).[85,86]

Thoracentesis

Most pleural effusions in lung cancer patients are owing to tumor and should be evaluated with thoracentesis. In general, a diagnosis of cancer can be established in 70% to 80% of malignant effusions by thoracentesis.[87] Even if cytology fails to identify cancer cells, repeat thoracenteses improve the diagnostic yield. If on multiple taps the fluid is consistently bloody or exudative, it should be considered malignant. Light's criteria[88] can be used to help classify an effusion as exudative or transudative. As an alternative to repeat thoracentesis, thoracoscopy can be used to simultaneously collect pleural fluid for cytology, visualize the pleural space and biopsy suspicious lesions if present, and perform lymph node biopsies if indicated.

Mediastinoscopy and Mediastinotomy

Mediastinoscopy remains the most accurate technique to assess upper and lower paratracheal (lymph node stations 2 and 4), prevascular (station 3a), retrotracheal (station 3p), subcarinal (station 7), and hilar lymph nodes (station 7) in lung cancer patients. Lymph nodes within the aortopulmonary window (lymph node station 5) and along the ascending aorta (station 6) are not accessible by standard mediastinoscopy techniques; however, they can be evaluated by anterior mediastinotomy (also known as the Chamberlain procedure) or video-assisted thoracoscopic techniques. Although considered the gold standard, mediastinoscopy does have a false-negative rate of approximately 10%.[89] Furthermore, the role of mediastinoscopy for lung cancer has evolved recently. Less invasive techniques such as EBUS-TBNA or EUS-FNA are frequently utilized instead to sample lymph nodes found to be clinically suspicious on imaging.[90] Mediastinoscopy should still be considered in situations where less invasive techniques are nondiagnostic. It is reasonable to forgo invasive staging of the mediastinum in patients with clinical stage I peripheral disease, particularly those with PET-positive primary tumors but no mediastinal uptake and no obviously enlarged nodes on CT. Patients with more locally advanced disease being considered for surgery should undergo mediastinoscopy to rule out N3 disease and to identify those with N2 disease for whom induction therapy should be considered prior to surgery.

Thoracoscopy

Video-assisted thoracoscopy is frequently used for the diagnosis, staging, and resection of lung cancer. Peripheral nodules can be identified and excised using video-assisted, minimally invasive techniques. As discussed previously, this technique is also extremely valuable for evaluation of suspected pleural disease when thoracentesis has been nondiagnostic. Thoracoscopy can also be used to reach mediastinal nodes not accessible by standard mediastinoscopy, EBUS-TBNA, or EUS-FNA techniques.

STAGING

The current seventh edition of the AJCC *Cancer Staging Manual* represents a major change in the developmental process of the staging system. The IASLC established a Lung Cancer Staging Project in 1998 to bring together larger databases available worldwide. The IASLC lung cancer database is comprised of 81,015 cases available for analysis from 46 sources in more than 19 countries, diagnosed between 1990 and 2000, and treated by all therapeutic modalities.[91,92] The results of this project were accepted by the AJCC as the primary source for revisions of the lung cancer staging system in the seventh edition of their staging manual. Definitions of TNM for the seventh edition of the manual are shown in Table 51.2; the stage groupings are shown in Table 51.3. A reference chart can be found in Figure 51.2. This new staging system more

TABLE 51.2 AJCC STAGING OF LUNG CANCER[a]

Tx	Positive cytology only
T1	Tumor that is ≤3 cm in its greatest dimension, does not invade the visceral pleura, and is without bronchoscopic evidence of invasion more proximal than a lobar bronchus
T1a	Tumor is ≤2 cm in its greatest dimension
T1b	Tumor is >2 cm, but ≤3 cm, in its greatest dimension
T2	Tumor with any of the following characteristics: >3 cm but ≤7 cm in its greatest dimension, invades a mainstem bronchus with its proximal extent at least 2 cm from the carina, invades the visceral pleura, or is associated with either atelectasis or obstructive pneumonitis that extends to the hilar region without involving the entire lung
T2a	Tumor is >3 cm, but ≤5 cm, in its greatest dimension
T2b	Tumor is >5 cm, but ≤7 cm, in its greatest dimension
T3	Tumor with any of the following characteristics: >7 cm in greatest dimension; invades the chest wall (including superior sulcus tumors), diaphragm, phrenic nerve, parietal pericardium, mediastinal pleura, main bronchus <2 cm from carina without carina invasion, total atelectasis or obstructive pneumonitis of the entire lung, separate nodule(s) in same lobe as the primary tumor
T4	Tumor of any size that invades the mediastinum, heart, great vessels, carina, trachea, esophagus, vertebral body, or separate tumor nodules in a separate lobe of the ipsilateral lung
N0	No regional lymph node involvement
N1	Involvement of ipsilateral intrapulmonary, peribronchial, or hilar lymph nodes
N2	Involvement of mediastinal or subcarinal lymph nodes
N3	Involvement of contralateral mediastinal or hilar lymph nodes. Involvement of ipsilateral or contralateral scalene or supraclavicular nodes
M0	No distant metastasis
M1a	Malignant pleural effusion, pericardial effusion, pleural nodules, or metastatic nodules in the contralateral lung
M1b	Distant metastasis

[a]The AJCC has adopted the TNM classification, originally proposed by Mountain et al., which is based primarily on surgical findings.

From Goldstraw P, Crowley J, Chansky K, et al. The IASLC Lung Cancer Staging Project: Proposals for the revision of the TNM stage groupings in the forthcoming (seventh) edition of the *TNM Classification of Malignant Tumours*. *J Thorac Oncol* 2007;2(8):706–714, with permission.

TABLE 51.3 STAGE GROUPING: TNM SUBSETS

T and M					
6th ed., TNM (2002)	*7th ed., TNM (2009)*	*N0 Stage*	*N1 Stage*	*N2 Stage*	*N3 Stage*
T1 (≤3 cm)	T1a (≤2 cm)	IA	IIA	IIIA	IIIB
	T1b (>2–3 cm)	IA	IIA	IIIA	IIIB
T2 (>3 cm)	T2a (>3–5 cm)	IB	IIA (IIB)	IIIA	IIIB
	T2b (>5–7 cm)	IIA (IB)	IIB	IIIA	IIIB
	T3 (>7 cm)	IIB (IB)	IIIA (IIB)	IIIA	IIIB
T3 invasion	T3	IIB	IIIA	IIIA	IIIB
T4 (same lobe nodules)	T3	IIB (IIIB)	IIIA (IIIB)	IIIA (IIIB)	IIIB
T4 (extension)	T4	IIIA (IIIB)	IIIA (IIIB)	IIIB	IIIB
M1 (ipsilateral lung)	T4	IIIA (IV)	IIIA (IV)	IIIB (IV)	IIIB (IV)
T4 (pleural effusion)	M1a	IV (IIIB)	IV (IIIB)	IV (IIIB)	IV (IIIB)
M1 (contralateral lung)	M1a	IV	IV	IV	IV
M1 (distant)	M1b	IV	IV	IV	IV

The American Joint Committee on Cancer published edition 7 of its classification system in 2009. The 6th, 5th, 4th, 3rd, 2nd, and 1st editions were published in 2002, 1997, 1992, 1988, 1983, and 1977, respectively. When comparing literature reports from different time periods, including the literature referenced throughout this chapter, remember that staging definitions have slowly changed over time. For example, this table shows how staging nomenclature changed from the 6th to the 7th editions. The 6th edition stage grouping is given in parenthesis.

From Goldstraw P, Crowley J, Chansky K, et al. The IASLC Lung Cancer Staging Project: Proposals for the revision of the TNM stage groupings in the forthcoming (seventh) edition of the *TNM Classification of Malignant Tumours*. *J Thorac Oncol* 2007;2(8):706–714, with permission.

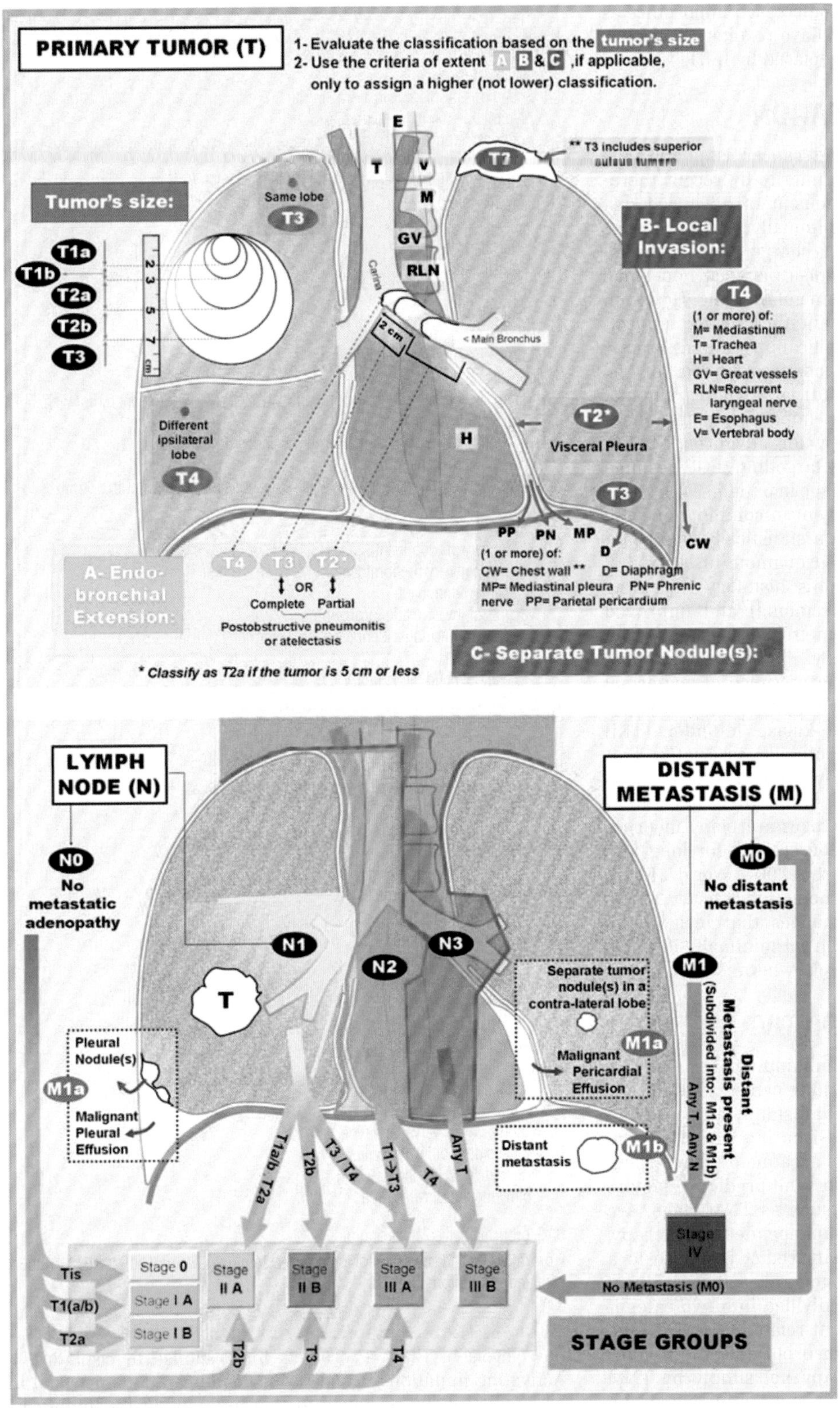

FIGURE 51.2. The American Joint Committee on Cancer released the seventh edition of its lung cancer TNM staging system in 2009. The T classification can be defined by evaluating the size first (upper left), then upgrading the classification (if necessary) based on the other criteria of primary tumor invasion/extent (A, B, and C). The criteria of extent should not be used to assign a lower classification. The lower diagram can be used to define the N and M classification and to determine the corresponding stage. Note that N1, N2, N3, and the separate tumor nodule of M1a were depicted in the lower illustration based on a right-sided tumor (T). For left lung tumors, a mirror image of these descriptors should be used. Additionally, the endobronchial extension and local invasion (A and B of the extent criteria) were shown in the upper illustration based on a left-sided tumor to simplify the drawing. (From Lababede O, Meziane M, Rice T. Seventh edition of the *Cancer Staging Manual* and stage grouping of lung cancer. *Chest* 2011;139(1):183–189, with permission.)

accurately expresses the prognostic significance of both the T and N stages in lung cancer outcome.

Given all of the various ways to assess lymph node status, accuracy in determining the nodal stage is essential.[93] In accordance with IASLC recommendations adopted by the AJCC, when pathologic staging of lymph nodes is pursued, sampling of paratracheal (stations 2R and 4R), subcarinal (station 7), hilar (station 10R), and interlobar lymph nodes (station 11R) should be obtained for right-sided tumors, and aortopulmonary window (station 5), ascending aorta (station 6), subcarinal (station 7), hilar (station 10L), and interlobar (station 11L) lymph nodes for all left-sided tumors. Pulmonary ligament lymph nodes (station 9) should also be evaluated for lower lobe tumors. At least six lymph nodes (three from the mediastinum and three from the hilar region) should be examined. If all resected lymph nodes are negative but the number recommended is not met, the patient is still classified as pN0 in the AJCC staging system.[3] For the radiation oncologist, proper staging of nodal disease has taken on increased importance as advances in conformal radiotherapy have resulted in elective mediastinal nodal irradiation being replaced by IFRT.[94]

PATHOLOGIC CLASSIFICATION

The pathologic classification of lung cancer is undergoing significant transformation, driven primarily by recent therapeutic advancements in the management of advanced disease and the movement toward minimally invasive tissue acquisition procedures. The primary charge of the pathologist in the past had been to distinguish between non–small cell carcinoma and small cell carcinoma of the lung. However, since 2000, there are now important therapeutic implications for each of the four major classifications of lung cancer: (a) squamous cell carcinoma, (b) adenocarcinoma of the lung, (c) small cell carcinoma, and (d) large cell carcinoma. Histology—for the first time—is an important determinant in the selection of systemic therapy for advanced NSCLC. Bevacizumab, a monoclonal antibody targeting VEGF, resulted in grade 4 and 5 pulmonary hemorrhage in patients with squamous cell histology; however, this agent in combination with standard chemotherapy has yielded a statistically significant survival advantage in patients with nonsquamous histology.[95,96] An association between nonsquamous histology (including adenocarcinoma and large cell carcinoma) and improved survival has been observed with pemetrexed in combination with platinum-based chemotherapy.[97,98] Adenocarcinoma histology is often associated with the presence of epidermal growth factor receptor (EGFR) mutations that confer heightened sensitivity to EGFR tyrosine kinase inhibitor (TKI) therapy and with echinoderm microtubule associated protein like 4 (EML4) and anaplastic lymphoma kinase (ALK) translocations that confer sensitivity to the MET/ALK inhibitor crizotinib.[99–102,103] All of these changes are being incorporated into the pathologic classification scheme for lung and have resulted in modifications to the 2004 World Health Organization (WHO) classification scheme for resected specimens[104] (Table 51.4). Additional changes that include the classification of specimens obtained from minimally invasive procedures are reviewed extensively elsewhere.[105,106]

TABLE 51.4 HISTOLOGIC CLASSIFICATION OF LUNG CANCER IN RESECTED SPECIMENS

Preinvasive lesions
Squamous dysplasia/carcinoma in situ
Atypical adenomatous hyperplasia
Adenocarcinoma in situ (nonmucinous, mucinous, or mixed nonmucinous/mucinous)
Diffuse idiopathic pulmonary neuroendocrine cell hyperplasia
Squamous cell carcinoma
Variants
Papillary
Clear cell
Small cell
Basaloid
Small cell carcinoma
Combined small cell carcinoma
Adenocarcinoma
Minimally invasive adenocarcinoma (<3 cm lepidic predominant tumor with <5 mm invasion)
Nonmucinous, mucinous, mixed mucinous/nonmucinous
Invasive adenocarcinoma
Lepidic predominant (formerly nonmucinous BAC pattern, with >5 mm invasion)
Acinar predominant
Papillary predominant
Micropapillary predominant
Solid predominant
Variants of invasive adenocarcinoma
Invasive mucinous adenocarcinoma (formerly mucinous BAC)
Colloid
Fetal (low and high grade)
Enteric
Large cell carcinoma
Variants
Large cell neuroendocrine carcinoma
Combined large cell neuroendocrine carcinoma
Basaloid carcinoma
Lymphoepithelioma-like carcinoma
Clear cell carcinoma
Large cell carcinoma with rhabdoid phenotype
Adenosquamous carcinoma
Sarcomatoid carcinomas
Pleomorphic carcinoma
Spindle cell carcinoma
Giant cell carcinoma
Carcinosarcoma
Pulmonary blastoma
Other
Carcinoid tumor
Typical carcinoid
Atypical carcinoid
Carcinomas of salivary gland type
Mucoepidermoid carcinoma
Adenoid cystic carcinoma
Epimyoepithelial carcinoma

BAC, bronchioloalveolar carcinoma.

From Travis WD. Classification of lung cancer. *Semin Roentgenol* 2011;46(3):178–186, with permission from Elsevier.

PROGNOSTIC AND PREDICTIVE FACTORS

The recent advancements in our understanding of tumor biology have underscored the fact that lung cancer is a heterogeneous cluster of illnesses rather than simply a dual (small cell, non–small cell) disease entity. Given the varied clinical outcomes and significant toxicity of treatment, there is an underlying need for robust prognostic and predictive factors in this disease. Prognostic factors, such as TNM stage, are those that predict clinical outcome independent of therapy, and predictive factors are those that predict response to a particular therapeutic regimen. In general, a discussion of prognostic and predictive factors is divided into two categories: tumor-related factors and patient-related factors. In the near future, these factors may be incorporated into a comprehensive approach to tailor therapy not simply by TNM stage but individualized to the patient and the biology of the patient's tumor.

Tumor-Related Prognostic and Predictive Factors

The past decade has seen significant advances in our understanding of tumor-related prognostic and predictive factors. Excision repair cross-complementation group 1 (ERCC-1)—a key enzyme involved in the pathway that repairs DNA adducts formed with cisplatin—has been identified to be both a positive prognostic factor for survival (ERCC-1 positivity predicts for improved survival after surgical resection) and a negative predictive factor for response to cisplatin-based chemotherapy (low levels of ERCC-1 predicts for response to cisplatin).[107] Activating mutations in the EGFR have been demonstrated to be predictive for response to therapy with EGFR inhibitors, such as gefitinib.[108] Thymidylate synthase (TS), which is an important enzyme in DNA biosynthesis and one of the target enzymes for antifolate drugs, has been proposed as a predictive factor for response to therapy in NSCLC patients receiving pemetrexed, a multitargeted antifolate approved for first-line therapy in combination with cisplatin in advanced lung cancer patients with nonsquamous histology. High levels of TS have been shown in vitro and in vivo to correlate with resistance to pemetrexed, and TS gene expression has been shown to be significantly higher in squamous cell carcinomas than in nonsquamous tumors.[109–111]

Patient-Related Prognostic and Predictive Factors

Given the significant metabolic toll that lung cancer takes on patients, several patient-related factors have been identified as powerful prognostic indicators of clinical outcome. Performance status, as quantified by either the Karnofsky scale or the Eastern Cooperative Oncology Group (ECOG) scale, and weight loss in the 6 months preceding diagnosis have been shown in large trials to be among the factors most predictive of survival (along with TNM stage).[112] Additionally, age, gender, and marital status have been shown to be prognostic for survival in a number of studies.[113] More recently, Movsas et al.[114] reported that baseline quality of life (QOL), as quantified by validated instruments, superseded performance status, age, gender, and other classic prognostic indicators for survival in a prospectively collected data set in patients enrolled on a Radiation Therapy Oncology Group (RTOG) clinical trial, suggesting that QOL may be one of the most important predictors of long-term survival.[114]

GENERAL MANAGEMENT: NON–SMALL CELL LUNG CANCER

The management of NSCLC presents a formidable challenge. Oncologists must not only account for the stage and extent of disease spread at the time of diagnosis but also must carefully weigh the impact of baseline pulmonary functional status and comorbidities on the patient's ability to tolerate treatment. NSCLC is an aggressive tumor of a vital organ that is poorly functioning at baseline in the majority of patients. Therefore, the final therapeutic approach must be tailored to the individual. The treatment principles presented in this section should be viewed as guidelines and not as a cookbook for the management of this disease.

In general, the standard of care for patients with stage I and stage II disease is complete surgical resection with the possible addition of adjuvant chemotherapy. For stage III patients, a significant amount of controversy exists regarding optimal management. For select patients with stage IIIA disease at diagnosis who are candidates for surgical resection, neoadjuvant chemotherapy or chemoradiotherapy is often used. For patients with unresectable stage III disease, the standard approach is concurrent chemoradiotherapy for fit patients or sequential chemotherapy and radiotherapy for patients who cannot tolerate concurrent treatment. Approximately 50% of patients present with evidence of hematogenous dissemination at the time of diagnosis.[115] For stage IV patients without significant local presenting symptoms or need for urgent radiation, systemic chemotherapy is the standard initial treatment approach. For stage IV patients with significant local presenting symptoms requiring urgent radiotherapy, such as SVC obstruction, hemoptysis, or cord compression, palliative radiotherapy followed by systemic chemotherapy is the preferred treatment approach. For patients with stage IV disease, owing to the poor prognosis, a detailed discussion of the goals of care with consideration of early referral to hospice should be part of the initial treatment approach. Recent evidence suggests that early introduction of palliative care into the standard treatment paradigm in this setting not only improves QOL and reduces inappropriate hospitalization at the end of life but may also improve survival.[116]

Resectable Tumors

Preoperative Assessment

Patient selection is critical when an operative approach is being considered for the management of NSCLC. This includes an assessment by the pulmonologist and operating surgeon of the clinical extent of disease, the predicted postresection pulmonary reserve of the patient, and preoperative cardiac clearance for the intended surgical procedure. Although there are no strict guidelines for operability, traditionally patients are considered to be suitable for pneumonectomy if their predicted postoperative forced expiratory volume in 1 second (FEV1) is >1.2 L.[117] Additional contraindications to pneumonectomy are hypercarbia and cor pulmonale.[118,119] Patients are usually referred for preoperative pulmonary function testing, including spirometry, diffusion capacity, and arterial blood gases. Imaging studies include ventilation-perfusion imaging to determine the regional variance in pulmonary function, including the potential loss of functional lung tissue within the planned area of excision.

Stage I and Stage II Non–Small Cell Lung Cancer

The standard of care for a patient with stage I or II lung cancer is surgical resection through either a lobectomy or pneumonectomy with mediastinal lymph node dissection. The Lung Cancer Study Group performed a randomized trial of lobectomy versus limited surgical resection (either through a wedge resection or through segmentectomy) in patients with T1N0 or T2N0 NSCLC. This trial randomized 276 patients to either lobectomy or limited resection and found a 17% risk of local recurrence with limited resection versus 6% with lobectomy ($p = .008$). This observation was associated with a trend toward an increase in all-cause and cancer-specific risk of death in patients randomized to the limited resection (30% and 50% increased risk, respectively [$p = .09$], for both). Additionally, the report did not demonstrate any late functional advantages or decreased perioperative morbidity with limited resection.[120] This study firmly established lobectomy as the standard of care for early-stage lung cancer. The 5-year survival with lobectomy or pneumonectomy with mediastinal nodal dissection is approximately 60% for pN0 disease and 40% in pN1 disease.[121]

In a series from Memorial Sloan-Kettering Cancer Center, Martini et al.[122] documented a survival with lobectomy or pneumonectomy with complete mediastinal nodal dissection of 82% in T1N0 tumors at 5 years and 74% at 10 years, and 68% at 5 years and 60% at 10 years for patients with T2N0 tumors ($p < .0004$). They reported a decreased 5- and 10-year survival rate of 59% and 32%, respectively, in 38 patients who did not undergo lymph node dissection. Additionally, they observed poorer 5- and 10-year survival with wedge resection or segmentectomy of 59% and 35%, respectively, compared with 77% and 70% for patients who underwent lobectomy, corroborating the findings of the Lung Cancer Study Group report. The authors additionally documented second primary cancers in 206 of 598 (34%) patients; 70 of these were lung cancers (34% of second primary cancers). Martini et al.[122] concluded that "(1) Systematic lymph node dissection is necessary to ensure that the disease is accurately staged; (2) lesser resections (wedge/segment) result in high recurrence rates and reduced survival regardless of histologic type; and (3) second primary lung cancers are prevalent in long-term survivors." However, some controversy remains regarding their assertions in the role of mediastinal lymph node dissection in early-stage NSCLC as well as the contention that a sublobar resection is a "compromised" surgical procedure. The American College of Surgeons Oncology Group (ACOSOG) Z0030 trial was a randomized trial of 1,111 patients with N0 or N1 (less than hilar) early-stage NSCLC to either mediastinal lymph node sampling or complete lymphadenectomy during pulmonary resection. The 5-year disease-free survival was 69% in the mediastinal lymph node sampling group and 68% in the mediastinal lymph node dissection group ($p = .92$). There was no difference in local ($p = .52$), regional ($p = .10$), or distant ($p = .76$) recurrence between the two groups, suggesting that complete lymphadenectomy does not improve survival in patients with early-stage NSCLC.[123] There have been several recent series comparing sublobar resection in appropriately selected early-stage NSCLC with lobectomy, showing comparable oncologic outcomes with the more limited resection. Okada et al.[124] performed a retrospective multi-institutional comparison of 567 patients undergoing either a sublobar (N = 305) or a lobar (N = 262) resection for cT1N0M0 (tumor size

<2 cm) disease. With a median follow-up >5 years, they reported a 5-year overall survival (OS) of 89.6% for the sublobar resection group and 89.1% for the lobar resection group. The recurrence rate with sublobar resection was not inferior to those obtained with lobar resection, and postoperative lung function was significantly better in patients who underwent sublobar resection.[124] Two currently active prospective randomized trials are examining the role of sublobar resection in early-stage disease: the Cancer and Leukemia Group B (CALGB) 140503, a randomized trial of sublobar resection versus lobectomy in small, peripheral early-stage operable NSCLC, and ACOSOG Z4032, a prospective randomized trial of sublobar resection with or without brachytherapy for high-risk early-stage NSCLC. These trials will delineate the role of sublobar resection in the management of early-stage NSCLC.

Stage III Non–Small Cell Lung Cancer

Considerable controversy exists regarding the role of surgery in stage III NSCLC. In the 1960s and 1970s, patients with documented N2 disease were generally regarded as incurable and referred for nonoperative approaches. In 1981, Martini et al.[125] reported the outcome of 80 patients with documented N2 disease who underwent complete surgical resection and mediastinal lymph node dissection. Most patients also received postoperative mediastinal irradiation. Survival was 47% at 3 years and 38% at 4 years, with better survival associated with adenocarcinoma histology. Additionally, patients who had small primary tumors and nonbulky mediastinal nodes (i.e., no evidence of mediastinal enlargement on preoperative chest x-ray) had better survival. This study suggested a potential role for surgical resection in select patients with N2 disease.[125] Martini et al.[126] extended this observation in a second report in an expanded cohort of 1,598 patients who underwent surgical resection, 706 of whom had mediastinal nodal involvement. Of these, 151 patients underwent complete surgical resection with mediastinal node dissection. They reported an OS rate of 74% at 1 year, 43% at 3 years, and 29% at 5 years. Survival in patients with clinical stage I or II (pathologic N2) was favorable at 50% at 3 years. Survival in patients with obvious clinical N2 disease was extremely poor at 8% at 3 years. Martini et al.[126] stated: "Very few patients with gross mediastinal nodal involvement benefit from resection. We believe that this group of patients should not be considered for thoracotomy unless innovative forms of treatment can be offered."

Based, in part, on these and similar results with surgical resection alone in stage III disease, neoadjuvant approaches—either preoperative chemotherapy or chemoradiotherapy—were explored in an attempt to facilitate surgical resection. However, significant controversy still exists regarding the role of surgical resection in stage III disease. Van Meerbeeck et al.[127] reported the results of a European Organisation for Research and Treatment of Cancer (EORTC) phase III randomized trial of surgical resection versus radiotherapy after induction chemotherapy in patients with pathologically proven N2 disease. In this study, 579 eligible patients were enrolled and received three cycles of cisplatin-based induction chemotherapy. The 332 patients who responded to induction chemotherapy were then randomized to surgery (167 patients) or radiotherapy (165 patients). Median and 5-year OS for patients randomly assigned to resection versus radiotherapy were 16.4 versus 17.5 months and 15.7% versus 14%, respectively (hazard ratio [HR] 1.06, 95% confidence interval [CI] 0.84 to 1.35). Rates of progression-free survival (PFS) were also similar in both groups. The authors concluded that radiotherapy is the preferred approach in these patients owing to lower rates of treatment-related morbidity and mortality.[127]

Neoadjuvant (Induction) Therapy

Preoperative Chemotherapy

The primary rationale for induction chemotherapy is similar to the rationale for preoperative radiotherapy: to facilitate complete surgical resection of disease. Additionally, induction chemotherapy may potentially sterilize micrometastatic disease beyond the thorax. In 1988, Martini et al.[128] reported on a series of 41 patients with bulky mediastinal nodal involvement, so-called clinical N2 disease, who had evidence of mediastinal nodal enlargement on chest x-ray. Patients received two or three cycles of high-dose cisplatin with vindesine or vinblastine, with or without mitomycin C. Thirty-one (73%) patients had a major radiographic response, 28 patients underwent thoracotomy, and 21 patients (75%) had complete resection of the disease. Eight patients had a pathologic complete response, with an additional 4 patients having "limited microscopic foci of either residual primary or nodal disease." The 3-year survival was 34% for all patients and 54% for those who had complete resection with a median follow-up of 44 months.[128] These promising early results prompted several randomized trials comparing preoperative chemotherapy versus surgical resection alone in stage III NSCLC (Table 51.5). Pass et al.[129] reported the results of a small trial randomizing 27 patients with histologically confirmed N2 disease to preoperative etoposide and cisplatin (EP) followed by surgical resection versus immediate surgical resection with postoperative mediastinal radiation. The initial report showed a trend toward increased survival time for the patients who received preoperative chemotherapy (median, 28.7 months) versus the immediate surgery group (median, 15.6 months) (p = .095). Two separate randomized trials were reported in 1994, both of which were terminated early after enrollment of only 60 patients. Roth et al.[130] randomized 60 patients with resectable, pathologically confirmed IIIA NSCLC between 1987 and 1993 to receive either six cycles of perioperative chemotherapy (cyclophosphamide, EP) and surgery (28 patients) or immediate surgery alone (32 patients). Patients who had a pathologically confirmed tumor response after three cycles of preoperative chemotherapy received three additional cycles of postoperative chemotherapy for a total of six cycles. Patients randomized to perioperative chemotherapy and surgery had an estimated median survival of 64 months compared with 11 months for patients who had immediate

TABLE 51.5 SURGERY ALONE VERSUS NEOADJUVANT CHEMOTHERAPY FOLLOWED BY SURGERY IN STAGE III NON–SMALL CELL LUNG CANCER

Author	Patients	CT	Stages	Resection Rates PCT/Surgery (%)	OR Rates (%)	pCR	Operative Mortality PCT/Surgery (%)	Median Survival PCT/Surgery (Months)
Dautzenberg et al.[459]	26	C/V/P	I, II, IIIA	–	45	–	0	23 vs. 21
Depierre et al.[133]	375	M/I/P	IB, II, IIIA	92 vs. 86	64	11	7.8 vs. 4.5	37 vs. 26 (p = 0.09)
Pass et al.[129]	27	E/P	IIIA N2	85 vs. 86	61	7.6	0	28.7 vs. 15.6 (p = .09)
Rosell et al.[131]	60	M/I/P	IIIA	85 vs. 90	53	3.3	6.6 vs. 6.6	26 vs. 8 (p = .001)
Roth et al.[130]	60	C/E/P	IIIA	61 vs. 66	35	3.6	3 vs. 6	21 vs. 14 (p = .056)

CT, chemotherapy; PCT, preoperative chemotherapy group; OR, objective response; pCR, pathologic complete response rate; C, cyclophosphamide; V, vinblastine; P, cisplatin; M, mitomycin; I, ifosfamide; E, etoposide.

From Depierre A, Westeel V, Jacoulet P. Preoperative chemotherapy for non-small cell lung cancer. *Cancer Treat Rev* 2001;27:119–127, with permission from Elsevier.

surgical resection (P <.008). The estimated 2- and 3-year survival rates were 60% and 56% for the perioperative chemotherapy patients and 25% and 15% for those who had surgery alone. The trial was terminated early because of the magnitude of the treatment benefit for perioperative chemotherapy after an unplanned interim analysis.[130]

Similarly, Rosell et al.[131] randomized 60 patients with pathologically confirmed IIIA NSCLC to either immediate surgical resection or three cycles of mitomycin C, ifosfamide, and cisplatin (MIP) chemotherapy followed by surgical resection. All patients received postoperative mediastinal irradiation. The median survival was 26 months in the patients treated with chemotherapy plus surgery, compared with 8 months in the patients treated with surgery alone (P <.001).[131] The updated 3- and 5-year survival rates for the preoperative chemotherapy arm were 20% and 17%, respectively, compared to 5% and 0%, respectively, for the surgery arm. Additionally, Rosell et al.[132] observed a survival plateau in the preoperative chemotherapy group and interpreted this to imply that preoperative chemotherapy altered the natural progression of stage III disease. Depierre et al.[133] reported the results of the largest randomized trial examining the role of preoperative chemotherapy in 2002. In this study, 355 patients with stage I through stage IIIA (with the exception of T1N0) were randomized to immediate surgical resection versus two cycles of mitomycin, ifosfamide, and cisplatin and two additional postoperative cycles for responding patients. In both arms, patients with pT3 or pN2 disease received thoracic radiotherapy. The median survival was 26 months in the immediate surgery arm versus 37 months with preoperative chemotherapy (p = .15, not significant [NS]). On subgroup analysis, however, a survival benefit was observed in patients with N0 or N1 disease (relative risk [RR] 0.68; p = .027), whereas there was no observed benefit to preoperative chemotherapy in the 122 patients with N2 disease (52 patients in the immediate surgery arm, 70 patients in the preoperative chemotherapy arm; RR = 1.04; p = .85). Betticher et al.[134] reported the results of a multicenter phase II trial of preoperative chemotherapy in 90 patients with previously untreated, potentially operable stage IIIA (mediastinoscopically pN2) NSCLC. Patients received three cycles of docetaxel and cisplatin, with subsequent surgical resection. The pathologic complete response rate was 19% in patients undergoing tumor resection. Interestingly, 31% of patients achieved mediastinal and hilar nodal clearance (downstaged to ypN0) with this regimen. The median survival for these patients was not reached with a median follow-up of 32 months.[134] In an updated report after 5 years of follow-up, the median survival still had not been reached for these patients.[135] Although the data are somewhat divergent, most would recommend preoperative chemotherapy if surgical resection is planned in potentially resectable stage IIIA (pN2) disease.

Preoperative Chemoradiotherapy

Local control rates in stage III disease with chemoradiotherapy alone are inadequate. Le Chevalier et al.[136] observed that the histologic 1-year local control rate was only 15% for patients with unresectable NSCLC treated to 65 Gy. A relationship has been shown between local failure and the subsequent appearance of distant metastases.[137] Furthermore, improved local control in stage III NSCLC has been shown to result in a significant improvement in OS.[138] The rationale for preoperative chemoradiotherapy is that surgical resection after chemoradiotherapy will optimize local control, thereby improving clinical outcomes in locally advanced disease. A phase II trial by the Southwest Oncology Group (SWOG) of induction chemoradiotherapy followed by surgical resection in 126 patients with stage IIIA/IIIB disease showed a promising 3-year survival of 26%.[139] An exploratory analysis of the 27 patients with N3 disease revealed the 2-year survival rate to be 35% for the subgroup with supraclavicular nodes and 0% for the group with contralateral mediastinal nodes. Motivated by these results, an intergroup randomized phase III trial was initiated to determine the value of adding surgery to chemoradiotherapy in stage III disease with a primary end point of OS. Patients with stage T1-3 pN2 M0 NSCLC were randomly assigned to concurrent induction platin-based chemotherapy plus radiotherapy (45 Gy). If no progression, patients either underwent resection or continued radiotherapy to 61 Gy.[140] A total of 202 patients were randomized to surgery and 194 to concurrent chemoradiotherapy. The median OS was 23.6 months in the trimodality arm and 22.2 months in the bimodality group (p = 0.24). For those with pN0 status at thoracotomy, the median OS was 34.4 months. PFS was better in the trimodality arm, median 12.8 months (5.3 to 42.2 months) versus 10.5 months (p = .017). An unplanned, exploratory analysis suggested that patients who underwent lobectomy in the trimodality arm had improved survival compared to matched patients receiving chemoradiotherapy; however, this result is hypothesis-generating only. One of the most important findings from this trial was the significant toxicity of right-sided pneumonectomy after induction chemoradiotherapy. Among the 29 patients who underwent a right pneumonectomy, there were 11 postoperative deaths (38%).[141] Overall, this trial did not demonstrate a survival benefit for the addition of surgery to chemoradiotherapy in patients with stage IIIA NSCLC. In conclusion, the role of neoadjuvant chemoradiotherapy in stage III NSCLC remains unclear. Using a multidisciplinary approach, this strategy should be carefully tailored to the individual patient, accounting for his or her performance status, pulmonary function, extent of disease, extent of surgical resection required, and experience of the clinical team.

Adjuvant Therapy

Postoperative Radiotherapy

Locoregional recurrence after resection of NSCLC is common, occurring in approximately 20% of patients with stage I disease[142,143] and in up to 50% of patients with stage III disease.[135,144,145] The predominant pattern of intrathoracic failure after surgical resection is along the surgical stump or in the mediastinal nodes (Fig. 51.3). Concern over locoregional failure led to the idea that PORT in completely resected stages II and IIIA NSCLC might be beneficial because of evidence that it reduced local recurrence.[146] However, the role of PORT was called into question in 1998 when the Medical Research Council published a meta-analysis of nine randomized controlled trials assessing the effect of PORT after resection.[147] The PORT meta-analysis included information on 2,128 patients and 1,368 deaths. PORT was associated with a decrease in survival for patients with pN1 disease. Given the theoretical benefit of radiotherapy on local control, the detriment in survival was attributed to excessive radiotherapy-induced morbidity exceeding any benefit. There was no survival difference for pN2 patients. This analysis has been criticized for many reasons. Twenty-five percent of the patients were pN0 who did not need adjuvant therapy. There was no quality control in the radiotherapy arms, and it was felt to be inferior to modern standards; many of the patients were treated to large volumes using older Cobalt-60 equipment to fields designed under fluoroscopy. A subsequent SEER analysis provided insight to counter some of the findings from the PORT meta-analysis. In this study, over 7,400 patients with stage II/III resected NSCLC were evaluated. PORT showed an improved 5-year OS for pN2 patients (27 vs. 20%) but reduced OS for pN0 and pN1 patients.[148]

Additional support for the use of PORT in the modern era can be found in the Adjuvant Navelbine International Trialist Association (ANITA) trial.[149] This trial randomized 840 patients at stage IB through stage IIIA between 1994 and 2000 to adjuvant chemotherapy or observation. The use of radiotherapy was not randomized; however, each center decided whether to use PORT before initiation of the study. Radiotherapy doses

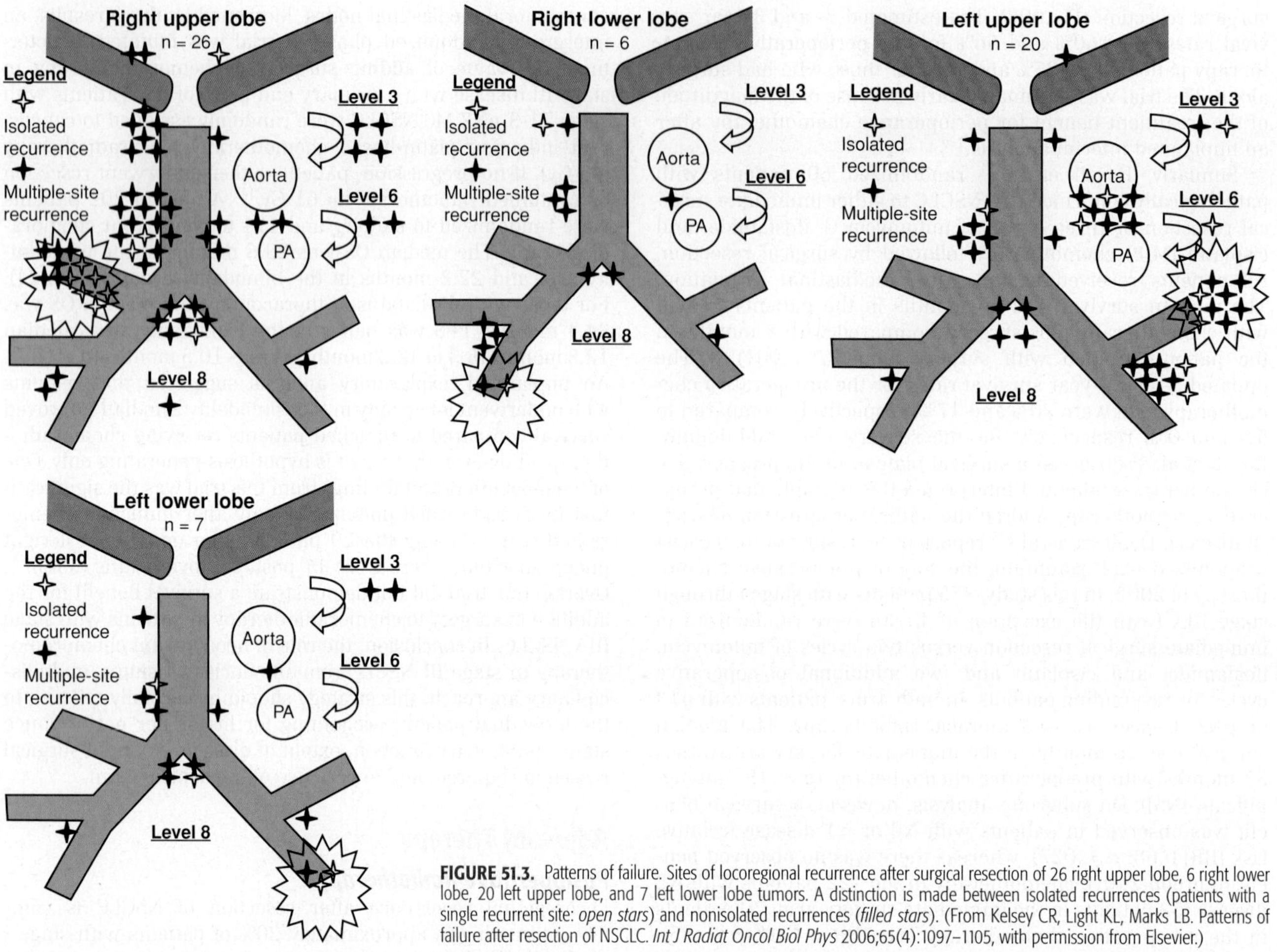

FIGURE 51.3. Patterns of failure. Sites of locoregional recurrence after surgical resection of 26 right upper lobe, 6 right lower lobe, 20 left upper lobe, and 7 left lower lobe tumors. A distinction is made between isolated recurrences (patients with a single recurrent site: *open stars*) and nonisolated recurrences (*filled stars*). (From Kelsey CR, Light KL, Marks LB. Patterns of failure after resection of NSCLC. *Int J Radiat Oncol Biol Phys* 2006;65(4):1097–1105, with permission from Elsevier.)

ranged from 45 to 60 Gy in 2 Gy fractions and were given after completion of chemotherapy. In patients with pN1 disease, PORT had an improved survival in the observation arm (median survival 25.9 vs. 50.2 months) but a detrimental effect in the chemotherapy group (median survival 93.6 months and 46.6 months). In contrast, in patients with pN2 disease, survival was improved both in the chemotherapy (median survival 23.8 vs. 47.4 months) and observation arm (median survival 12.7 vs. 22.7 months). The retrospective evaluation of the ANITA trial supports the findings from the SEER analysis that PORT may confer a benefit in pN2 NSCLC. The Lung Adjuvant Radiotherapy trial (Lung-ART) is an intergroup collaborative effort in Europe, randomizing patients with completely resected locally advanced NSCLC with mediastinal nodal involvement to observation or PORT to 54Gy. Adjuvant chemotherapy is allowed on the control arm, and pre- and/or postoperative chemotherapy is allowed on the radiotherapy arm. The trial is ongoing, and results are not yet available.

Postoperative Chemotherapy

Historically, there was little evidence to support the routine use of adjuvant chemotherapy in completely resected lung cancer patients. However, benefits to chemotherapy began to emerge from clinical trials, as doubt was cast on the role for PORT. In 1995, the Non–Small Cell Lung Cancer Collaborative Group[150] published a meta-analysis that showed mixed results based on the class of chemotherapeutic regimen utilized. There was decreased survival with alkylating agents, no change in survival with fluorouracil (5-FU)-based regimens, and a trend toward improved survival by 5% with cisplatin-based chemotherapy.[150] This benefit was not statistically significant ($p = .08$); however, this publication led to numerous prospective, randomized trials investigating the role of platinum-based adjuvant chemotherapy in NSCLC.

The International Adjuvant Lung Cancer Trial (IALT) reported a statistically significant survival benefit with cisplatin-based adjuvant therapy in patients with completely resected stage I, II, or III NSCLC.[151] In this trial, 1,867 patients were randomized to cisplatin-based adjuvant chemotherapy or observation. With a median follow-up duration of 56 months, patients receiving chemotherapy had a statistically significant higher survival rate (44.5% vs. 40.4% at 5 years) and disease-free survival rate (39.4% vs. 34.3% at 5 years) compared with observation. However, after 7.5 years of follow-up, there were more deaths in the chemotherapy group, and the benefit of chemotherapy decreased over time ($p = .10$).[152]

The National Cancer Institute of Canada JBR.10 trial tested effectiveness of adjuvant vinorelbine plus cisplatin versus observation in 482 patients with completely resected stage IB and II NSCLC.[153] Adjuvant chemotherapy significantly prolonged OS (94 vs. 73 months) and relapse-free survival (not reached in chemo arm vs. 46.7 months) compared to observation alone. Like the IALT trial, some of the benefit diminished with longer follow-up; however, unlike IALT, the survival difference remained statistically significant. After 9 years of follow-up, adjuvant chemotherapy was found beneficial for stage II (median survival 6.8 vs. 3.6 years), although not for stage IB patients.[154]

In the ANITA trial, 840 patients with stage IB through stage IIIA NSCLC were randomized to adjuvant vinorelbine plus cisplatin or to observation.[155] Median and 5-year OS with chemotherapy improved compared with observation. On subset analysis, this benefit was limited to node-positive patients (stage II through stage IIIA). The Lung Adjuvant Cisplatin Evaluation (LACE) meta-analysis showed similar results by pooling data from five large randomized trials enrolling 4,584 patients to examine the role of cisplatin-based adjuvant chemotherapy in completely resected patients. They demonstrated a statistically significant 5.4% absolute survival benefit favoring adjuvant cisplatin.[156]

Postoperative Chemoradiotherapy

With the positive early results from adjuvant chemotherapy trials and prior to the publication of the PORT meta-analysis, a few groups began to explore the role of chemoradiotherapy in the postoperative setting.

One of the first multi-institutional randomized trials to investigate postoperative chemoradiotherapy was led by the ECOG. The ECOG 3590 trial randomized 488 patients with stage II through IIIA NSCLC and negative margins after surgery to either radiotherapy alone or radiotherapy plus four cycles of EP chemotherapy. Radiotherapy in both arms consisted of 50.4 Gy in 28 daily fractions. There was no difference in local recurrence or survival between the two arms.[157]

Before the results of ECOG 3590 were published, the RTOG embarked on a phase II combined modality study using a newer chemotherapy regimen consisting of carboplatin and paclitaxel. RTOG 9705 included 88 patients with stage II and IIIA NSCLC after surgery who received PORT with concurrent carboplatin and paclitaxel. Radiotherapy consisted of 50.4 Gy in 28 fractions with a boost of 10.8 Gy in extranodal extension or T3 lesions. The radiotherapy was administered during cycles 1 and 2. At a median follow-up of 56.7 months, median OS time was 56.3 months, with 1-, 2-, and 3-year survival rates of 86%, 70%, and 61%, respectively. The 1-, 2-, and 3- year PFS rates were 70%, 57%, and 50%, respectively. Toxicities were acceptable. When compared to previously reported studies, the RTOG concluded that these results might portend an improvement in OS and PFS with postoperative chemoradiotherapy in resected NSCLC patients.[158] Promising findings were also noted in a similar study design at Fox Chase Cancer Center,[132] supporting the concept that concurrent chemoradiotherapy should be formally investigated with a modern chemotherapy regimen in node-positive patients in the postoperative setting.

Summary

Adjuvant chemotherapy is accepted as standard of care for patients with node-positive (stages IIA, IIB, and IIIA) NSCLC. PORT might be beneficial in stage IIIA but is not indicated in completely resected stage I and stage II NSCLC. In practice, a patient who clinically appears to have early-stage NSCLC undergoes a gross total resection with pathology-confirmed clear margins but is unexpectedly found to have pN2 disease should receive adjuvant chemotherapy first (because of the known survival benefit) and may subsequently be considered for PORT (because of the reported local control benefit) on completion of chemotherapy.

The role of postoperative therapy for NSCLC patients at high risk for local recurrence has not been clearly established. If a patient who is clinically felt to have early-stage NSCLC undergoes surgery that results in a positive microscopic margin or residual macroscopic disease, the radiation therapy should start earlier, as local recurrence is the most common cause of failure in this group of patients.[159] Chemoradiotherapy should be considered in this setting if the patient is medically fit.[158,160,161]

INOPERABLE TUMORS

Stage I/II Non–Small Cell Lung Cancer

The standard of care for a patient with operable early-stage lung cancer remains lobectomy or pneumonectomy with mediastinal lymph node dissection. However, a significant percentage of these patients cannot tolerate invasive procedures because of the comorbidities prevalent in patients with lung cancer, such as chronic obstructive pulmonary disease and poor cardiovascular health. Historically, the standard therapeutic approach for these patients has been conventionally fractionated definitive radiotherapy alone, with daily fractions delivered over a period of 6 to 8 weeks.[162] More recently, a hypofractionated approach with delivery of a small number of large fractions over a short period of time has gained acceptance. This approach has most commonly been referred to as stereotactic body radiation therapy (SBRT), although recently there has been a move to rename this approach stereotactic ablative radiotherapy (SABR) to emphasize its distinct radiobiology.[163]

Conventionally Fractionated External-Beam Radiotherapy

The RTOG performed a multi-institutional dose escalation study for inoperable NSCLC using three-dimensional conformal radiotherapy (3D-CRT). Patients with small, early-stage tumors were escalated to doses as high as 83.8Gy with acceptable toxicity. The 1-year local control rate for patients treated to this dose was 76%.[164] Hayman et al.[165] performed an adaptive dose escalation trial allowing safe delivery of doses up to 102.9 Gy to small peripheral tumors.[165] However, the OS rates for patients with medically inoperable early-stage NSCLC remain poor when compared to surgery. The 5-year survival for patients treated with definitive radiotherapy range from 10% to 30% and are approximately one-half that reported in surgical series[166–169] (Table 51.6). Several possible explanations exist for this disparity in outcomes, including the poorer

TABLE 51.6 OUTCOME BY RADIATION THERAPY DOSE AND TREATMENT VOLUME FOR PATIENTS WITH EARLY-STAGE NON–SMALL CELL LUNG CANCER

Authors (Reference)	Patients	Dose (Gy)	Local Field (%)	Grade 3–5 Toxicity	Intercurrent Death (%)	Overall Survival (%) 3 Year	Overall Survival (%) 5 Year	Cause-Specific Survival (%) 3 Year	Cause-Specific Survival (%) 5 Year
Dosoretz et al. (436)	152	76%, 60–69	Minority	0%	11	–	10	–	–
Graham et al. (437)	103	Median, 60	20	1%	28	–	13	–	–
Haffty et al. (438)	43	59 continuous or 54 split	–	0%	–	36	21	–	–
Kaskowitz et al. (439)	53	Median, 63	<10	8%	27	19	6	33	13
Krol et al. (440)	108	60 or 65	100	0%	34	31	15	42	31
Noordijk et al. (441)	50	60 split	100	0%	40	33	17	–	–
Rosenzweig et al. (442)	55[a]	≥80	100	7%	2	–	36	–	–
Sandler et al. (443)	77	Median, 60	10	Minimal	16	17	14	22	17
Sibley et al. (444)	141	Median, 64	27	1.5%	43	24	13	–	–
Talton et al. (445)	77	60	0	0%	–	21	17	–	–
Zhang et al. (446)	44	50%, 55–61, 50%, 69–70	0	1 myelitis	20	55	32	–	–

[a]Rosenzweig separately studied 55 stage I and II patients and 27 stage III patients. Overall survival is reported for the 55 stage I/II patients. However, incidence of toxicity is reported over the entire group of 82 patients. All patients regardless of stage were treated with similar prescription doses.

overall health of the medically inoperable patient and the fact that most of these patients are clinically, rather than surgically, staged. An additional limitation is the maximum dose that can be delivered to the tumor through conventionally fractionated external-beam radiotherapy (EBRT) utilizing currently available techniques. Based on fundamental radiobiologic principles, Fletcher[170] predicted that using conventional fraction sizes of 1.8 to 2 Gy, doses of 100 Gy or higher might be required for the sterilization of most NSCLC tumors. These doses are not routinely achievable with conventionally fractionated radiotherapy in the medically inoperable patient without excessive toxicity.

Stereotactic Body Radiotherapy

SBRT refers to the delivery of large doses of radiation to a small treatment volume, usually employing multiple beams, using a small number of fractions (usually five fractions or less). It has been known for quite some time that this approach is remarkably effective at tumor sterilization, presumably due to greater radiobiologic efficacy.[171] This treatment approach was initially put to clinical use over a half-century ago by a Swedish neurosurgeon, Lars Leksell, for the treatment of intracranial metastases.[172] However, unlike the cranial vault, the lung is a highly mobile structure. Thus, application of SBRT in lung cancer was impractical until advanced imaging treatment delivery techniques were developed (Fig. 51.4).

A phase I dose escalation trial enrolled patients with T1–2 N0 NSCLC, stratified into three dose escalation groups based on T-stage and size (T1, T2 <5 cm, and T2 5–7 cm). This trial reported a maximally tolerated dose for T2 tumors >5 cm of 22 Gy $\times$ 3 and was not reached at 20 Gy $\times$ 3 for T1 tumors or at 22 Gy $\times$ 3 for T2 tumors <5 cm.[173] There was a loose association between total delivered dose and likelihood of local failure, with 9 of 10 local failures observed in patients treated to the lower dose levels (<16 Gy $\times$ 3). Based on these results, this group moved forward with a phase II trial, utilizing the dose levels identified in the phase I trial. They were able to duplicate the excellent local control results in this expanded cohort of 70 patients. With a median follow-up of 17.5 months, the local control rate was 95%. However, with such large fraction sizes (of approximately 20 Gy), the group also identified an association between tumor location and toxicity, with severe toxicity occurring at a median of 10.5 months in 17% of those patients with peripheral lesions versus 46% with central lesions.[174] Preliminary data from other institutions suggest that early, central lesions can be treated safely and effectively using a lower dose per fraction (e.g., 7 to 12 Gy).[175] To this end, the RTOG has recently opened a phase I dose escalation trial for patients with centrally located, medically inoperable stage I NSCLC.

Several other institutions have published their experience applying SBRT to early (primarily peripheral) lung cancer with a variety of dose fractionation and prescription schemes (Table 51.7). The initial data appear promising with 80% to 100% local control, 40% to 100% 2- to 3-year survival, and 0% to 4% grade 3 toxicity, although in general the median follow-up for these studies is relatively short.[176–182] Timmerman et al.[174] reported the results of RTOG 0236, a phase II trial of SBRT in medically inoperable patients with T1 or T2 tumors treated to 54 Gy in three 18-Gy fractions. In this study, 59 patients were enrolled, with 55 patients having evaluable disease. At a median follow-up of 34 months, they reported a 3-year primary tumor control rate of 97.6% and a 3-year primary tumor and involved lobe (local) control rate of 90.6%. Two patients experienced regional failure; the locoregional control rate was 87.2%. Eleven patients experienced distant recurrence with a 3-year rate of distant failure of 22.1%. The rates for disease-free survival and OS at 3 years were 48.3% and 55.8%, respectively. The median OS was 48.1 months. Protocol-specific treatment-related grade

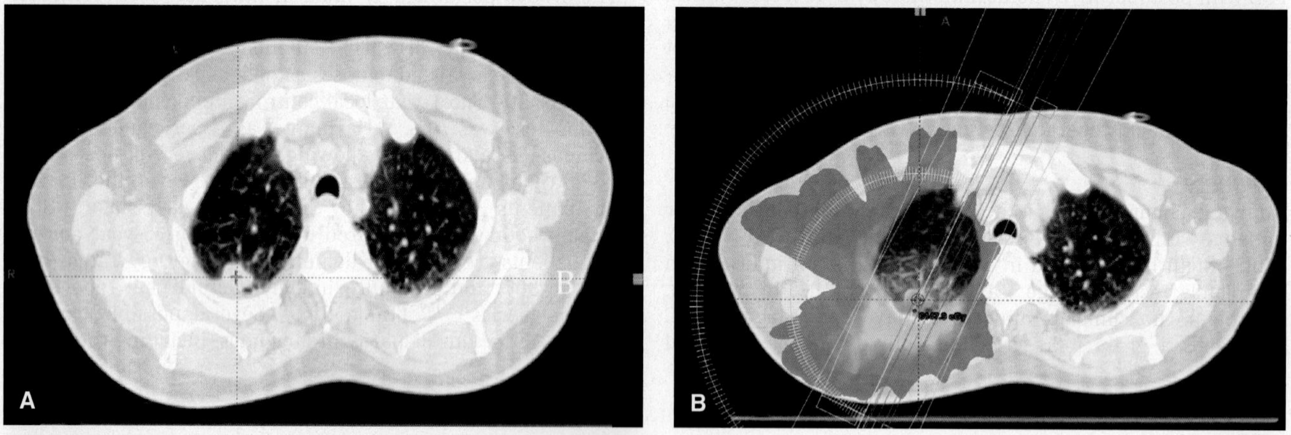

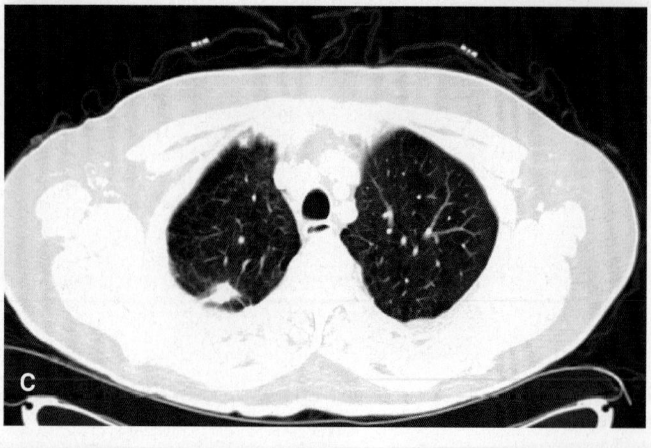

FIGURE 51.4. Stereotactic body radiation therapy (SBRT) in stage I non–small cell lung carcinoma (NSCLC). The patient was diagnosed as having T1N0M0 right upper lobe NSCLC and was treated with SBRT. **A:** Pretreatment tumor volume. **B:** Treatment plan with dose color-wash **C:** CT showing response 6 weeks after treatment.

TABLE 51.7 OUTCOME FOR PATIENTS WITH EARLY-STAGE NON–SMALL CELL LUNG CANCER RECEIVING STEREOTACTIC BODY RADIATION THERAPY

Authors (Reference)	Patient	Dose (Gy)	Stage	Local Control 3 Years (%)	Overall Survival 3 Years (%)
Prospective SBRT Trials					
Baumann et al. (447)	57	15 Gy × 3 to 67%	IA/B	92	60
Fakiris et al. (448)	70	T1: 20 Gy × 3 T2: 22 Gy × 3	T1-T2N0M0	88	43
Koto et al. (449)	31	15 Gy × 3 7.5 Gy × 8	IA/B	T1: 78 T2: 40	72
Ricardi et al. (450)		15 Gy × 3	IA/B	88	73
Timmerman et al. (RTOG 0236) (192)	55	18 Gy × 3	T1-T2N0M0	98	56
Nagata et al. (451)	45	12 Gy × 4	IA/B	98 (30 m)	83
Retrospective SBRT Studies					
Nyman et al. (181)	45	15 Gy × 3	IA/B	80 (43 m)	55
Onishi et al. (452)	257	4.4–35 Gy × 1–14	IA/B	84.2	56.8
Timmerman et al. (174)	70	20–22 Gy × 3	IA/B	95 (2 y)	55 (2 y)
Uematsu et al. (453)	50	7.2 Gy × 10	IA/B	94 (5 y)	66

SBRT, stereotactic body radiation therapy.

All studies are phase II.

Adapted from Onishi H, Shirato H, Nagata Y, et al. Hypofractionated stereotactic radiotherapy (HypoFXSRT) for stage I non-small cell lung cancer: updated results of 257 patients in a Japanese multi-institutional study. *J Thorac Oncol* 2007;2(7 Suppl 3):S94–S100.

3 adverse events were reported in 7 patients; grade 4 adverse events were reported in 2 patients. No grade 5 adverse events were reported. The RTOG (RTOG 0618) initiated a phase II study of SBRT in operable patients with early-stage NSCLC, and, together with the ACOSOG, a randomized trial of SBRT versus sublobar resection for high-risk early-stage NSCLC. SBRT, with its advantage of patient convenience and promising local control results, has largely replaced conventionally fractionated radiotherapy as the standard approach in the medically inoperable patient.

Stage III Non–Small Cell Lung Cancer

Definitive Radiotherapy

The majority of patients with inoperable locally advanced NSCLC will receive definitive thoracic radiotherapy as a part of their treatment strategy. The rationale for definitive radiotherapy in patients with inoperable NSCLC is to provide intrathoracic control of disease. Kubota et al.[183] performed a prospective randomized trial in 63 patients with stage III NSCLC comparing chemotherapy alone to chemotherapy plus thoracic radiotherapy. The survival rate in the thoracic radiotherapy group was 58% at 1 year, 36% at 2 years, and 29% at 3 years, compared with 66%, 9%, and 3% at 1, 2, and 3 years, respectively, in the chemotherapy-alone group. The investigators concluded that thoracic radiotherapy "significantly increases the number of long-term survivors as compared with chemotherapy alone and that radiotherapy to bulky disease in the thorax is an important part of combined modality therapy, and a necessary part of further studies in locally advanced disease." At present, definitive thoracic radiotherapy is part of the standard therapeutic approach for patients with unresectable locally advanced NSCLC. However, because of high local failure rates and the significant toxicity associated with this treatment, the optimal dose, treatment volume, and optimal integration scheme with chemotherapy remain to be defined.

Dose and Fractionation with Radiotherapy Alone

The RTOG launched a prospective randomized trial in 1973 to determine the most effective dose and fractionation schedule in patients with inoperable NSCLC. In the initial report of RTOG 7301, 365 patients with T1-3, N0-2, M0 unresectable NSCLC were randomized to one of four treatment regimens: 40 Gy given in a split course of 20 Gy in five fractions in 1 week, a 2-week rest, and then an additional 20 Gy in 1 week; or 40 Gy, 50 Gy, or 60 Gy given in 2 Gy per fraction continuous course 5 days per week. The split-course group had the poorest survival: 10% at 2 years.[184] The incidence of tumor recurrence in the irradiated volume was 58% for the patients receiving 40 Gy continuous course, 53% for those treated with 40 Gy split course, 49% with 50 Gy continuous irradiation, and 35% in the patients receiving 60 Gy.[185] There were no differences in 5-year survival rates between the four arms. However, based on the differences in local tumor control and short-term survival, this study established 60 Gy as the standard of care.

Motivated by these results, the RTOG moved to explore methods of escalating radiation dose while maintaining the therapeutic ratio through altered fractionation schedules or improved treatment delivery techniques. RTOG 8311 was a randomized phase I/II trial that delivered thoracic radiation at a dose of 1.2 Gy with twice daily fractions escalating from a starting point of 60.0 Gy to 79.2 Gy. A total of 848 patients were enrolled and analyzed for outcome. No significant differences in the risks of acute or late effects in normal tissues were found in the five arms. In a subset analysis of good performance status patients (stage III, Karnofsky performance scale [KPS] ≥70, <6% weight loss), there was a dose response identified for survival with 69.6 Gy yielding improved survival over the lower-dose arms ($p = .02$). There were no differences in survival among the three high-dose arms; therefore, 69.6 Gy became the standard altered fractionation regimen for subsequent RTOG trials.[186]

The development of 3D-CRT in the early 1990s allowed the radiation oncologist to increase the dose distribution to the tumor while restricting the dose to surrounding critical normal structures.[187] This approach had immediate applications in the treatment of NSCLC, and preliminary data suggested that 3D-CRT might allow for safe escalation of dose to the tumor bed.[188] However, it is unclear whether this approach to dose escalation can be broadly applied to all lung cancer patients. Bradley et al.[189] examined 207 patients with inoperable NSCLC and demonstrated by multivariate analysis that GTV was strongly predictive of overall and cause-specific survival, suggesting that large-volume disease might require escalated doses of radiotherapy, if feasible without significantly increased toxicity risk.[189] Rengan et al.[190] examined the value of dose escalation in patients with large-volume stage III disease and found that even in patients with large tumor volumes, local failure rates were significantly reduced when treated to ≥64 Gy. Taken together, these data suggest that dose escalation can be achieved safely in locally advanced NSCLC via novel fractionation or treatment delivery approaches.

Volume of Radiation with Definitive Radiotherapy: Involved-Field Versus Elective Nodal Irradiation in Inoperable Stage III Non–Small Cell Lung Cancer

In the era of two-dimensional (2D) radiation therapy for NSCLC, it was customary to include the elective nodal basin in the radiation portals for any patient receiving curative intent radiotherapy, regardless of stage. There is ample evidence that the elective nodal basins can be safely omitted in stage I NSCLC, as there is low risk of nodal failure after IFRT either with conventionally fractionated radiotherapy or SBRT in this setting in patients who have undergone modern clinical staging.[191,192] The rationale for IFRT in locally advanced disease is to allow for safe dose escalation. Although there are limited data to suggest that escalating radiation dose could improve local control and that this approach would be feasible in locally advanced NSCLC, this increased dose is associated with an increased risk of radiation toxicity when larger treatment volumes are employed.[190] One technique for facilitating dose escalation while maintaining the therapeutic ratio is to utilize IFRT; this approach has been widely adopted. However, there is clear evidence to suggest that the untreated nodal basin may harbor occult disease. Surgical studies report that 10% to 35% of patients with clinically node negative NSCLC have evidence of occult mediastinal metastasis on lymph node dissection.[193] Additionally, although ^{18}FDG-PET/CT has become an indispensible tool for noninvasive staging of the mediastinum, studies have shown that FDG-PET may carry up to a 25% false-negative rate in lymph nodes <1 cm in the short axis.[69] Therefore, some have argued that while IFRT may allow for dose escalation, this may come at the expense of clinical outcome in this disease.[194]

Motivated by this concern, several studies have examined the rate of elective nodal failure in patients treated with IFRT and have shown this to be a relatively rare event.[195] In a study of 524 inoperable patients treated with IFRT, Rosenzweig et al.[196] reported a 2-year elective nodal control rate of 92.4%. Kepka et al.[197] studied 207 unresectable patients, staged without ^{18}FDG-PET and treated with elective nodal irradiation (ENI). This study reported a 2-year elective nodal control rate of 88%. In a separate study, Kepka et al.[198] performed a comparative analysis of IFRT, limited ENI, and extended ENI and reported that substantial incidental radiation dose was delivered to the elective nodal basins even with IFRT; the median dose delivered to these areas ranged from 18 Gy to 45 Gy, depending on the location of the primary tumor and involved nodes as well as the technique employed. Further, there was no significant difference in dose delivered to much of the elective nodal basin between extended and limited ENI. In the only prospective study of ENI versus IFRT, Yuan et al.[199] demonstrated an increase in local control with IFRT of 8% and 15% at 2 and 5 years, respectively. This increase, however, was only statistically significant at the 5-year time point. Additionally, Yuan et al.[199] demonstrated an improved OS rate at 2 years with IFRT (39.4% vs. 25.6%, p = .048) and significantly higher pneumonitis rates in patients treated with ENI (29% vs. 17%, p = .044). Although interesting, this study has been criticized for the imbalances in several factors, including the radiation dose delivered (68 to 74 Gy for IFRT vs. 60 to 64 Gy for ENI) and V_{20} between the two arms, making attribution of the results observed solely to IFRT or ENI problematic. In a recently published single-institution retrospective cohort comparison of patients receiving definitive 3D-CRT for locally advanced NSCLC, Fernandes et al.[200] analyzed 108 consecutive patients treated with either ENI or IFRT. The median follow-up time for survivors was 18.9 months. The median dose for patients treated with IFRT was 69.9 Gy versus 63.6 Gy for ENI. In a multivariable logistic regression analysis, patients treated with IFRT demonstrated a significantly lower risk of high-grade esophagitis (odds ratio 0.31, p = .036). There was a suggestion of improved 2-year local control with IFRT (59.6% IFRT vs. 39.2% ENI); however, this was not significant (p = .23). There were no significant differences in elective nodal control (84.3% vs. 84.3%), distant control (52.7 IFRT vs. 47.7% ENI), and OS (43.7% IFRT vs. 40.1% ENI) rates between ENI and IFRT. The authors concluded that IFRT had a favorable therapeutic ratio compared with ENI owing to reduced acute toxicity. Taken together, these data suggest that IFRT can be employed in patients with locally advanced NSCLC without risk of significant compromise in clinical outcome.

Combined Modality Therapy for Inoperable Stage III Non–Small Cell Lung Cancer

Sequential Chemoradiotherapy

Although dose escalation was achievable and appeared to be associated with improvements in local control in locally advanced NSCLC, the dominant pattern of failure in these patients is through distant dissemination in about 75% to 80% of patients.[185] To address the issue of systemic disease in locally advanced cases, the CALGB initiated a phase III randomized trial of 155 patients with unresectable stage III NSCLC with excellent performance status and minimal weight loss to either radiotherapy alone to 60 Gy or to induction chemotherapy with cisplatin (100 mg/m^2 given intravenously on days 1 and 29) and vinblastine (5 mg/m^2 given intravenously on days 1, 8, 15, 22, and 29) followed by radiotherapy to 60 Gy. Median survival was improved with induction chemotherapy to 13.7 months versus 9.6 months with radiotherapy alone (p = .0066). The 5-year survival was improved from 6% to 17% with induction chemotherapy.[201] A subsequent intergroup trial was launched randomizing 490 patients with inoperable locally advanced NSCLC to one of the following regimens: (a) standard radiation therapy to 60 Gy, (b) induction chemotherapy followed by standard radiation therapy to 60 Gy, and (c) twice-daily radiation therapy to 69.6 Gy as 1.2 Gy given twice daily. Median survival was improved to 13.8 months with induction chemotherapy compared to 11.4 months with standard radiotherapy and 12.3 months with hyperfractionated radiotherapy (p = .03).[202] A third prospective randomized trial reported by Le Chevalier et al.[136] examined a total of 325 patients with unresectable locally advanced NSCLC who were randomized to either radiotherapy alone to 65 Gy delivered in a split course in 26 fractions over 45 days or 3 monthly cycles of VCPC therapy: vindesine, 1.5 mg/m^2 on days 1 and 2; lomustine, 50 mg/m^2 on day 2 and 25 mg/m^2 on day 3; cisplatin, 100 mg/m^2 on day 2; and cyclophosphamide, 200 mg/m^2 on days 2 through 4 followed by radiotherapy to 65 Gy in 26 fractions delivered in a split-course fashion over 45 days starting 2 to 3 weeks after the third cycle of chemotherapy. The 2-year survival rate was 14% in patients receiving radiotherapy alone and 21% in the chemoradiotherapy group (P = .08). The distant metastasis rate was significantly lower in patients receiving induction chemotherapy, with the relative risk of metastasis twofold higher in the radiotherapy-alone arm compared to the chemoradiotherapy group (p <.001). Overall, these trials established the role of chemotherapy, in addition to radiation, in the management of inoperable stage III NSCLC (Table 51.8).

Concurrent Chemoradiotherapy

The EORTC performed a phase III randomized trial comparing concurrent cisplatin-based chemoradiation to radiotherapy alone and demonstrated a clear survival benefit to this approach.[138] Of note, there was no difference in rate of distant metastases; thus, the authors concluded that the benefit in OS was attributable to an improvement in local control secondary to enhanced radiosensitization of the tumor by low-dose cisplatin. A meta-analysis performed in 2010 to examine the value of concurrent chemotherapy in definitive management of NSCLC by O'Rourke et al.[203] included 19 randomized studies with a total of 2,728 patients with NSCLC (stages I through III), who were randomized to receive either concurrent chemoradiotherapy or radiotherapy alone. Concurrent chemotherapy significantly reduced overall risk of death (HR 0.71) and improved overall PFS at any site (HR 0.69). However, this clinical benefit came at the expense of increased acute toxicity, especially severe esophagitis with concurrent treatment (RR 4.96).

TABLE 51.8 SEQUENTIAL CHEMOTHERAPY VERSUS RADIATION THERAPY ALONE FOR LOCALLY ADVANCED NON–SMALL CELL LUNG CANCER

Author (Reference)	RT (Gy)	CT	Sequence	Number of Patients	Median Survival (Months)	Overall Survival (%) 1 Year	2 Year	3 Year	5 Year
Le Chevalier et al. (454)	65	–	–	177	10	41	14	4	–
	65	VCPC	CT → RT → CT	176	12	51	21	12	–
Morton et al. (455)	60	–	–	58	9.6	43	12	–	7
	60	MACC	CT → RT	56	10.4	47	23	–	5
Sause et al. (202)	60	–	–	149	11.4	46	19	6	5
	60	PV	CT → RT	151	13.2	60	32	15	8
	69.6	–	–	152	12	51	24	13	6
Dillman et al. (201)	60	–	–	77	9.7	40	13	11	7
	60	PV	CT → RT	79	13.8	55	26	23	19
NSCLC Collaborative Group meta-analysis (150)	32–65	Various	Neoadjuvant CT; no concurrent CT	3,033	–	41 45	15.7 17.7	6.7 10.1	2.7 4.8

RT, radiation therapy; CT, chemotherapy; VCPC, vindesine, cyclophosphamide, cisplatin, lomustine; MACC, methotrexate, doxorubicin, cyclophosphamide, lomustine; PV, cisplatin, vinblastine; NSCLC, non–small cell lung cancer.

Concurrent Versus Sequential Chemoradiotherapy

Initial phase II trials suggested that concurrent chemoradiotherapy might be an even more effective treatment than sequential chemoradiotherapy.[204] Therefore, Furuse et al.[205] performed a phase III randomized trial comparing concurrent chemoradiotherapy with mitomycin, vindesine, and cisplatin (MVP) to sequential chemotherapy and radiation therapy. They demonstrated a statistically significant survival advantage to the concurrent approach (median survival of 16.5 months vs. 13.3 months and 5-year survival of 15.8% vs. 8.9%). RTOG 9410 compared two different concurrent regimens (cisplatin and vinblastine with conventional radiotherapy, arm 1, or cisplatin and oral etoposide with hyperfractionated radiotherapy, arm 2) with a "standard" sequential regimen of cisplatin followed by conventional radiotherapy (arm 3). Comparing arm 1 to arm 3 (as per the study design), median survival times improved significantly (17 vs. 14.6 months), as did 5-year survival (15% vs. 10%) with an increase in acute grade 3 through grade 5 nonhematologic toxicities.[206,207] The survival in arm 2 was not significantly better than arm 1, although this intensive regimen was associated with much higher esophageal toxicity. Fournel et al.[208] reported the results of a smaller randomized trial that did not show a statistically significant survival advantage for concurrent chemoradiotherapy, with a median survival of 14 months with sequential chemoradiotherapy versus 16 months with concurrent chemoradiotherapy ($p = .24$). Nevertheless, a consistent trend favoring concurrent chemoradiotherapy in median, 2-, 3-, and 4-year survival rates was observed.[208] More recently, a meta-analysis performed by Auperin et al.[209] analyzed data from six clinical trials involving 1,205 patients. The median follow-up was 6 years. They observed a significant benefit favoring concurrent over sequential chemotherapy and radiotherapy with respect to OS (HR 0.84, $p = .004$), with an absolute benefit of 5.7% (from 18.1% to 23.8%) at 3 years and 4.5% at 5 years. PFS was also improved with concurrent chemoradiotherapy (HR 0.90, $p = .07$). Concurrent chemoradiotherapy decreased locoregional progression (HR 0.77, $p = .01$), although not distant progression. Again, this improvement in locoregional control came at the expense of greater acute toxicity for the patient receiving concurrent chemoradiotherapy, with an increase in acute esophageal toxicity (grades 3 and 4) from 4% to 18% with a relative risk of 4.9 ($p < .001$).[209]

Because of the increased toxicity with concurrent chemoradiation, especially acute esophagitis, there are often treatment delays that are potentially detrimental in terms of radiobiologic efficacy. Cox et al.[210] examined the impact of prolonged treatment time in stage III NSCLC treated with radiotherapy alone and documented an association with decreased locoregional control and 5-year survival (15% vs. 0%). To determine whether treatment time had a similar impact in the setting of concurrent chemoradiation, Machtay et al.[211] performed a retrospective study of three prospective RTOG trials (RTOG 9106, 9204, and 9410), all of which included good performance status stage III NSCLC patients treated with cisplatin-based concurrent chemoradiotherapy. The authors defined "short" treatment time as finishing treatment within 5 days of the projected end date. They found that "long" treatment time was significantly associated with acute esophagitis. They also found a nonsignificant trend toward improvement in median survival in the "short" (19.5 months) versus "long" treatment time (14.8 months). This study, although retrospective, indicated that even with concurrent chemoradiation, there could be a detrimental effect on survival with delayed treatment time.[211] Thus, appropriate patient selection and maneuvers to minimize toxicity are increasingly important to minimize the likelihood of treatment delays that can compromise the efficacy of concurrent therapy.

In summary, these data strongly support concurrent chemoradiotherapy as the standard approach for patients with good performance status and minimal weight loss. This therapeutic strategy results in improved OS, likely driven by an improvement in locoregional control in patients with locally advanced NSCLC. Of note, this comes at the expense of greater toxicity to the patient, and therefore patient selection is critical when using this approach.

Cytotoxic Platforms for Concurrent Chemoradiotherapy in Locally Advanced Non–Small Cell Lung Cancer

The management of patients with locally advanced NSCLC remains a therapeutic challenge. The era of combined modality therapy was ushered in by Dillman et al.[201] when the CALGB demonstrated superior survival for chemotherapy with vinblastine and cisplatin followed by definitive radiation (XRT) versus radiation alone. The benefits of sequential chemotherapy followed by radiation were reinforced by subsequent trials by the RTOG and in France.[212–213,214] In fit patients with minimal weight loss (<5% to 10% from baseline) and intact performance status (ECOG performance status 0 to 1), concurrent chemoradiation with a platinum-based combination has demonstrated clear superiority to radiation alone and to sequential chemotherapy followed by radiation.[138,205,207,208,215,216] A meta-analysis by Auperin[217] reinforced this observation, demonstrating a 5% absolute increase in long-term survival. Multiple studies in this arena have confirmed 4- to 5-year survival rates of 10% to 20%, which are clearly better than the 5% to 7% observed with XRT alone in this setting[205,207,208,217,218–219,220,221] (Table 51.9). In the absence of significant comorbidity, hearing loss, or renal compromise in patients who can readily tolerate an acute fluid load, cisplatin-based therapy is considered the

TABLE 51.9 CONCURRENT CHEMORADIOTHERAPY FOR STAGE III NON-SMALL CELL LUNG CANCER

Trial (Reference)	Phase	Number of Patients	Additional Nonconcomitant Agents	Concomitant Chemotherapy	XRT Dose (Gy)	Median PFS (Months)	Median OS (Months)	2-Year OS	4-Year OS	5-Year OS
RTOG 9801 (230)	III	243	± Amifostine	Carbo + Pac	69.6 bid	9	17.9	39%	21%	16%
CALGB 9431 (219)	II	62	DDP + Gem	DDP + Gem	66	8.4	18.3	37%	17%	9%
		58	DDP + Pac	DDP + Pac	66	9.1	14.8	29%		
		55	DDP + Vinorelbine	DDP + Vinorelbine	66	11.5	17.7	40%		
Hoosier (224)	III	203	± Docetaxel	DDP + VP-16	59.4	11	21.7	33%	20%	20%
CALGB 39801 (220)	III	182	–	Carbo + Pac	66	7	12	29%	14%	11%
		184	Carbo + Pac	Carbo + Pac	66	8	14	31%	17%	14%
LAMP (456)	II	74	Carbo + Pac (induction)	Carbo + Pac	63	6.7	12.7	25%	NR	NR
		92	Carbo + Pac (adjuvant)	Carbo + Pac	63	8.7	16.3	31%	NR	NR
RTOG 9410 (207)	III	≈198	DDP + Vinblastine	–	63	NR	14.6	31%	12%	10
		≈198	–	DDP + Vinblastine	63	NR	17.0	37%	21%	16
		≈198	–	VP-16 + DDP	69.6 bid	NR	15.2	32%	17%	13
West Japan (205)	III	156	–	MMC + Vindesine + DDP	56	10	15	35%	17%	15.8%
Czech (457)	III	102	–	DDP + Vinorelbine	60	11.9	16.6	NR	NR	NR
WJTOG0105 (221)	III	153	DDP + Vindesine + MMC	DDP + Vindesine + MMC	60 split	8.2	20.5	45%	28%	17.5%
		152	Carbo + CPT-11	Carbo + CPT-11	60	8.0	19.8	40%	20%	17.8%
		156	Carbo + Pac	Carbo + Pac	60	9.5	22.0	45%	22%	19.5%
OLCSG 0007 (218)	III	99		DDP + Docetaxel	60	13.4	26.8	60.3%	30%	23%
		101		MMC + Vindesine + DDP	60	10.5	23.7	48.1%	23%	16%

XRT, radiotherapy; PFS, progression-free survival; OS, overall survival; Carbo, carboplatin; Pac, paclitaxel; bid, twice daily; DDP, cisplatin; Gem, gemcitabine; VP-16, etoposide; NR, not reached; MMC, mitomycin C; CPT-11, irinotecan.

standard of care. Most North American clinicians have opted for the EP combination. Unlike limited SCLC, where cisplatin is dosed at 60 mg/m^2 every 3 weeks and etoposide at 80 to 120 mg/m^2 daily × 3 both during and after radiation, an alternative dose and schedule is generally used.[222] There are abundant data from the SWOG and RTOG for a schedule that was ultimately phase III tested in RTOG 9309 and later by the Hoosier Oncology Group: cisplatin 50 mg/m^2 days 1 and 8, 29 and 36; and etoposide 50 mg/m^2 intravenously days 1 through 5 and days 19 through 33.[139,140,223,224] This schedule, while inconvenient, is tried and tested and usually safe. Ideally, radiation to a minimum total dose of 60 Gy is given concurrently day 1 with chemotherapy.

In frailer patients or older patients, and in those with significant comorbidity including renal insufficiency (creatinines of 1.5 to 3.0), hearing loss, congestive heart failure, or severe COPD, a carboplatin combination is clearly better tolerated compared to cisplatin, and paclitaxel is often substituted for etoposide. Pilot trials by Belani[225] and Choy[226] clearly demonstrated the safety and efficacy of carboplatin (area under the concentration-time curve [AUC] 2 weekly) and paclitaxel (45 to 50 mg/m^2 weekly) both initiated day 1 of thoracic radiation, followed by two cycles of full-dose "consolidative" chemotherapy once radiation is completed.[227,228] Conventionally, during the consolidation phase, carboplatin AUC 6 and paclitaxel 200 mg/m^2 are administered for two cycles at 3-week intervals. This regimen has become the platform for multiple cooperative group phase II and phase III trials, most notably RTOG 0617.

Many have argued that carboplatin-based therapy is inferior to cisplatin in the treatment of locally advanced NSCLC. However, recent data from Japan in a combined modality trial (West Japan Oncology Group Trial WJTOG 0105) evaluating various concurrent chemoradiation regimens failed to show superiority for cisplatin over carboplatin in the context of concurrent chemoradiation.[221] Investigators led by Nobuyuki Yamamoto compared their erstwhile standard of MVP to weekly carboplatin in combination with either irinotecan or paclitaxel during XRT; in each arm, those without disease progression or untoward toxicity went on to receive two cycles of full-dose chemotherapy during the "consolidation" period using the same agents administered during XRT. The paclitaxel-carboplatin regimen resulted in less toxicity, fewer dose reductions or omissions, and equivalent if not superior survival at 5 years: 19.5% versus 17.5% for MVP and 17.8% for irinotecan-carboplatin. In fairness, this study also compared second-generation to third-generation chemotherapy; to date, this study is the only phase III trial to attempt to address the platinum question, which arises continually in the clinic. There are additional data to suggest that third-generation regimens are superior to second-generation therapy. Segawa et al.[218] form the Okayama Lung Cancer Study Group in Japan that demonstrated therapeutic superiority for docetaxel in combination with cisplatin compared with MVP in combination with XRT. An ongoing, pharmaceutical-based, randomized phase III trial in the context of chemoradiation is comparing pemetrexed-cisplatin (another third-generation regimen) followed by single-agent pemetrexed during the consolidation period to EP during XRT followed by investigator's choice during the consolidation period.[229]

In patients with baseline V20s (percentage of normal lung that will receive >20 Gy) >35% or in those with borderline pulmonary function or other comorbidities, many clinicians consider administration of chemotherapy first for two or even three cycles, followed by radiation alone or concurrent chemoradiation if there has been sufficient tumor shrinkage to allow a more reasonable radiotherapy treatment field. In those with minimal or no tumor shrinkage using this approach, some investigators omit concurrent chemotherapy during XRT to avoid untoward toxicity, proceeding with XRT alone. These patients are often much more symptomatic than those with smaller-volume tumors, with postobstructive symptoms including wheezing, pneumonitis, and hypoxia, and often have compromised performance status. However, the one study to isolate the role of induction therapy prior to concurrent chemoradiation with paclitaxel and carboplatin failed to show a survival advantage compared to concurrent chemoradiation alone.[220]

Toxicity mitigation is another major challenge that has been inadequately addressed. Both acute esophagitis and long-term pneumonitis and pulmonary fibrosis are common complications of combined-modality therapy. A recent meta-analysis by

Auperin et al.[217] demonstrated a sixfold increase in short-term esophagitis, grade 3 or worse (18% vs. 3%) in those receiving concurrent chemoradiation as opposed to asynchronous or sequential chemotherapy and radiation. A phase III study evaluating amifostine as an esophageal protectant failed to show a significant reduction in esophagitis rates, as determined by objective measures, compared to a control arm that did not feature this agent[26]; however, a subsequent analysis based on patient-reported outcomes suggested a modest benefit with reduction in pain and weight loss.[114,230] There is continued interest in evaluating mucosal protectants, including palifermin and other agents, although to date, no prospective randomized phase III trial has demonstrated a palliative benefit. Consequently, the approach to in-field toxicity has generally been reactive rather than pre-emptive. Newer technologies including proton beam may help to reduce the severity and duration of acute and late esophageal and pulmonary effects. This is currently under investigation.

Consolidative Chemotherapy

Consolidative chemotherapy remains highly controversial. A SWOG trial using the EP/XRT regimen as a platform investigated the role of consolidation docetaxel in stage IIIB patients, yielding a 5-year survival rate of nearly 30%, which is virtually unprecedented in the realm of locally advanced NSCLC.[139] However, in a phase III randomized Hoosier Oncology Group trial, docetaxel consolidation failed to yield a survival advantage compared to standard "observation" in patients who had completed concurrent chemoradiation with EP, in part because the reference arm "outperformed" its historic controls.[224] These results were disappointing. However, there was a borderline significant imbalance in baseline pulmonary function favoring the control arm: nearly 60% of patients on the arm featuring no consolidation had an FEV1 ≥2 L, compared to slightly >40% in the investigational arm. Similarly, empiric use of gefitinib as maintenance therapy in a SWOG trial led to a paradoxical survival decrement compared to placebo after completion of docetaxel consolidation.[231] Hence, based on these trials, there is no proven role for consolidative chemotherapy in patients who have already received systemically dosed chemotherapy during thoracic XRT. In those who receive a radiosensitizing schedule of chemotherapy during XRT, the general consensus favors at least two cycles of full-dose chemotherapy after chemoradiation is completed. Despite the disappointments with docetaxel and empiric gefitinib in this setting, the role of consolidation or maintenance therapy after chemoradiation remains an open question.

Targeted Agents in Locally Advanced Disease

There are no data as yet to support the empiric use of EGFRs, TKIs, EGFR monoclonal antibodies (MAbs), or angiogenesis inhibitors either during or after chemoradiation. The CALGB mounted a randomized phase II trial of concurrent radiation and chemotherapy with carboplatin and pemetrexed followed by "consolidative" pemetrexed with or without cetuximab.[232] The latter did not appear to exacerbate typical in-field toxicities, nor did it yield a significant improvement in long-term survival. The RTOG separately spearheaded a phase II study evaluating cetuximab in combination with standard thoracic radiotherapy and weekly paclitaxel-carboplatin, demonstrating feasibility as well a promising median survival approaching 2 years.[233] The phase III trial comparing higher dose XRT (74 Gy) to standard dose (60 Gy) was amended early on to address the role of cetuximab in a 2 × 2 design. Although the component of the trial testing higher versus standard dose XRT was closed because of futility, the C225 question remains open and RTOG 0617 continues to accrue; enrollment completed in November of 2011 and results are eagerly awaited. In higher-risk patients with >5% weight loss or compromised performance status, the CALGB is evaluating induction therapy with nab-paclitaxel and carboplatin followed by concurrent XRT and erlotinib. A previous, analogous phase II CALGB study in higher-risk patients evaluating induction carboplatin and paclitaxel followed by concurrent XRT and gefitinib yielded a median OS of 19 months.[234] Attempts to integrate bevacizumab into the combined-modality approach have been unsuccessful, with adverse events including tracheoesophageal fistulas and pulmonary hemorrhages.[235,236]

Dose Escalation with Concurrent Chemoradiotherapy

Although concurrent chemoradiotherapy has emerged as the standard therapeutic approach for fit patients with unresectable locally advanced disease, this has come at the cost of increased toxicity to the patient. It is therefore unclear whether dose escalation in the setting of concurrent chemotherapy will provide meaningful clinical benefit. The Lineberger Comprehensive Cancer Center group reported the results of a single-institution phase I dose escalation study with concurrent chemoradiation. They performed a stepwise escalation of thoracic radiation dose from 60 to 74 Gy in conjunction with paclitaxel-carboplatin without a clinically significant increase in toxicity.[237] The median survival of 24 months and 5-year survival of 25% in this study were promising, although patient numbers are small. In 2006, the RTOG opened a 2 × 2 phase III randomized trial to simultaneously examine the question of 60 Gy versus 74 Gy and concurrent chemoradiotherapy with or without cetuximab for patients with inoperable stage III NSCLC. After a planned interim analysis, the high-dose radiation therapy (74 Gy) arms of RTOG 0617 were closed to accrual effective June 17, 2011. In a communication to all RTOG trial investigators, Bradley[238] stated that the "high dose arms crossed a futility boundary, meaning that high dose radiation therapy cannot result in a survival benefit with further accrual or follow up of patients on these 2 arms." At the 2011 American Society of Therapeutic Radiology and Oncology (ASTRO) annual meeting, the initial results of this trial were presented, actually demonstrating a statistically significant detriment to survival with 74 Gy ($p = .02$). The interim analysis did not identify patient safety concerns and gave no indication of a statistical difference in high-grade toxicity between arms, nor any clear explanation for the observed decrement in survival. Regardless, the 74-Gy arm for this trial has been closed and 60 Gy remains the standard dose in all RTOG lung cancer trials going forward.[239]

Superior Sulcus Tumors and Pancoast's Syndrome

SSTs were first described in 1838 and the characteristic accompanying neurologic symptoms in 1932 by Dr. Henry Pancoast.[240] The most common tumors of the superior sulcus are bronchogenic, primarily squamous cell, followed by adenocarcinoma, and less likely small cell. SSTs account for <5% of all lung cancer.[241]

Signs and Symptoms

The most common symptom among patients with SST is pain in the shoulder, which may radiate down the arm. This can be attributable to direct tumor invasion of the parietal pleura, vertebral body, ribs one through three, or the brachial plexus (Fig. 51.5). Pain radiating down the ulnar aspect of the arm past the elbow indicates involvement of the T1 nerve root, whereas extension to the fourth and fifth digits indicates involvement of the C8 nerve root or more distally the ulnar nerve. There may be weakness or atrophy of the intrinsic muscles of the hand. SSTs that invade the neural foramina may cause spinal cord compression, which can ultimately occur in up to 25% of patients. Involvement of the stellate ganglion may manifest as Horner's syndrome: the triad of ptosis, papillary miosis, and facial anhidrosis. Irritation or compression of the adjacent sympathetic chain may cause ipsilateral flushing and sweating of the face or reflex sympathetic dystrophy, a regional syndrome of burning neuropathic pain. Pancoast's syndrome

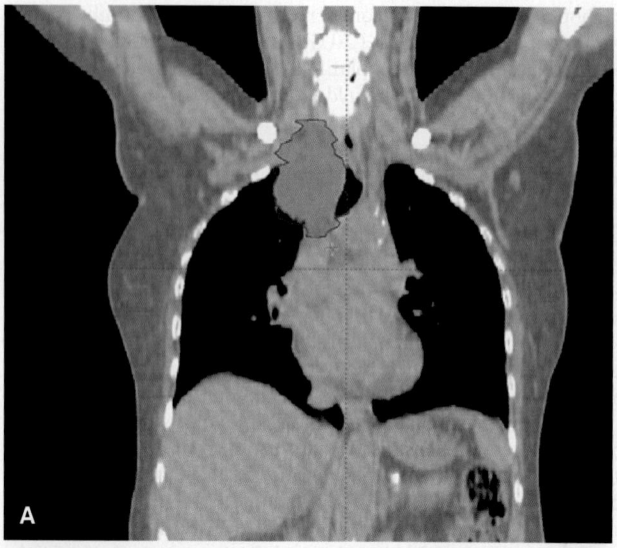

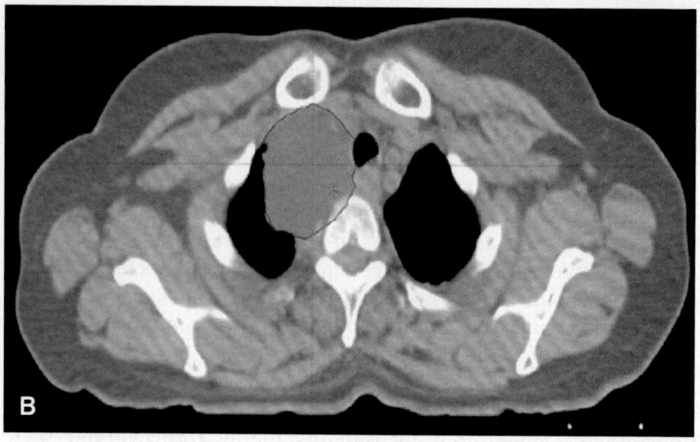

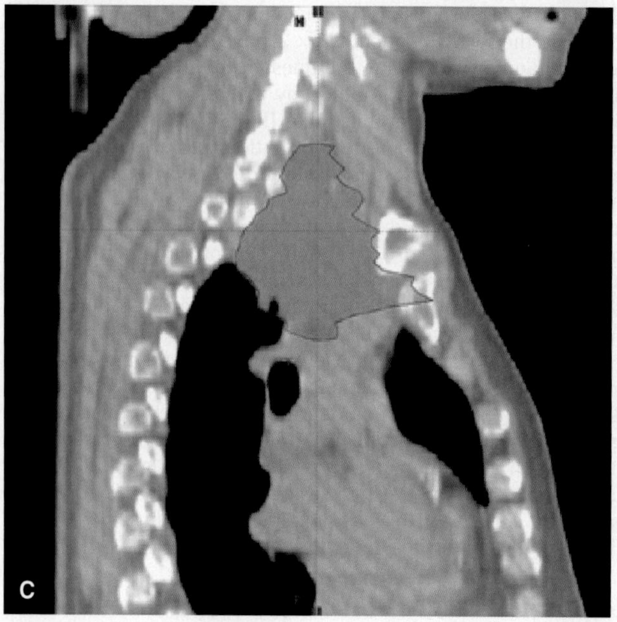

FIGURE 51.5. A 51-year-old former smoker presented with right shoulder pain and right-sided Horner's syndrome and was found to have an adenocarcinoma in the right superior sulcus. **A:** Coronal view with gross tumor volume (GTV) contoured. **B:** An axial view with GTV contoured. A 4-cm tumor is seen invading the mediastinum with displacement of the trachea. He underwent a staging evaluation including mediastinoscopy and was staged as T4N0M0. **C:** Sagittal view with GTV contoured showing vertebral body impingement. The patient was treated with radiotherapy with concurrent cisplatin and etoposide to 50 Gy and underwent resection with negative margins.

is a constellation of signs and symptoms including shoulder/arm pain, Horner's syndrome, and unilateral upper extremity weakness.

Diagnosis and Staging

SSTs are staged in the same way that SCLC and NSCLC are staged elsewhere in the thorax. For patients without metastatic disease, it is important to assess resectability. Surgery typically involves lobectomy with en bloc resection of the chest wall, which may be accompanied by resection of portions of the parasympathetic chain, stellate ganglion, lower trunks of the brachial plexus, subclavian artery, and portions of vertebral bodies.

Management

Determining the feasibility of resection is a critical decision point in the management of NSCLC SSTs. Because of the apical location of the tumor, invasion of the brachial plexus, vertebral bodies, and subclavian vessels is not uncommon and may eliminate surgical resection as an option, depending on the extent of invasion. In addition to CT, PET, and bone scan, MRI is useful in documenting the extent of involvement of the brachial plexus, spinal nerve roots, vertebral bodies, and subclavian vessels and is more sensitive than CT for this purpose.[242] Small cell SSTs in patient with good performance status are treated with concurrent chemoradiotherapy for limited-stage disease or chemotherapy for extensive-stage disease.

Multimodality Therapy for Superior Sulcus Tumors

Several large retrospective series and prospective trials have investigated outcomes of multimodality treatment of SSTs. SWOG 9416/Intergroup 0160 included 110 patients with T3-4, N0-1 SSTs. All patients were treated with two cycles of EP with radiotherapy (45 Gy in 25 fractions), followed by surgery within 3 to 5 weeks, and then two further cycles of chemotherapy.[243] The study included patients with apical tumors and Pancoast's syndrome, or SSTs with chest wall invasion, or involvement of the vertebrae or subclavian vessels. In this study, 88 patients (80%) underwent surgery, and 83 (76%) had complete resection. The 5-year OS was 44%. As well, 61 resected patients (56%) had a pathologic complete response to induction therapy, and their 5-year survival was significantly better at 54%. A Japan Clinical Oncology Group (JCOG) study enrolled 76 patients and used induction mitomycin, vindesine, and cisplatin with 45 Gy in 27 fractions (split course) followed by surgery.[244] The study included patients with SSTs, staged

T3-4, N0-1, and nonbulky N2 disease; 76% of patients underwent resection, and 68% had complete resection. The 5-year OS was 56%. A single-institution French study enrolled 107 patients with SSTs in a prospective trial of induction chemoradiotherapy.[245] The study excluded those with bulky N2 or N3 disease. All patients received EP concurrently with radiotherapy to 45 Gy; 72 patients underwent resection, unresectable patients received an additional 25 Gy. The 3-year OS was 40%.

In patients who are resectable at diagnosis, surgery may be offered as initial therapy. A prospective trial at the University of Texas MD Anderson Cancer Center enrolled 32 patients with resectable or marginally resectable SSTs.[246] All patients had gross total resection initially; 28% had microscopic residual disease. Postoperatively, patients were treated with radiotherapy to 60 Gy in 1.2-Gy fractions (for negative margins) or 64.8 Gy in 1.2-Gy fractions (for positive margins) with concurrent EP. The 5-year locoregional control was 76%, and 5-year OS was 50%.

Chemoradiotherapy

Retrospective evidence suggests that patients who undergo surgery have better local control and survival than those treated with radiation therapy, although such data is subject to significant selection bias.[247] Patients with unresectable localized SSTs and those with stage III disease and bulky N2 (or N3) lymph nodes should be treated with definitive chemotherapy and radiation. Early studies of radiotherapy alone for SSTs show acceptable local control and survival. In a series of 32 patients treated with definitive radiation, 91% of patients with pain reported relief, and 75% of patients with Horner's syndrome had symptomatic improvement.[248] The addition of concurrent chemotherapy improves local control and survival in patients with stage III NSCLC—an observation that has led to the widespread use of concurrent therapy in SSTs. Small series in patients with SSTs appear to support this. A retrospective analysis from the Netherlands examined the outcome of patients treated with chemoradiotherapy.[249] In this study, 49 patients with stage II or III SST received 66 Gy with daily cisplatin (6 mg/m^2); 19 patients had sufficient response to undergo resection, and in these patients there was a 53% pathologic complete response rate. The 5-year OS was 18% in patients who received chemoradiotherapy and 33% in patients who were able to undergo surgery.

RADIOTHERAPY TECHNIQUES AND FUTURE DIRECTIONS

Gross Tumor Volume

The clinically macroscopic disease, as typically identified on any imaging modality, is defined as the GTV. The GTV in the lung cancer patient is usually derived from a treatment planning CT or PET-CT obtained during quiet respiration. Intravenous contrast is usually not required for identification of the primary tumor unless it is located adjacent to the hilum or mediastinum. Studies have shown that the size of the contoured GTV is highly sensitive to the windowing of the CT data set.[250] Harris et al.[250] reported that measurements of pulmonary nodules using the standard "lung" windowing width of 850 Hounsfield units, with a windowing length of –750 Hounsfield units resulted in highly accurate sizing of the parenchymal tumor. Therefore, lung windowing should be used for delineation of the primary tumor GTV. An FDG-PET may be of additional value in the setting of atelectasis.[65] However, the optimal standardized uptake value threshold for defining tumor edge remains to be defined.

Identification of the mediastinal nodal GTV may prove more challenging. Intravenous contrast may be valuable in identifying nodal disease and may be used if there are no contraindications such as allergy or renal insufficiency. Chapet et al.[251] at the University of Michigan developed an axial CT-based definition of the thoracic nodal stations for use in radiation treatment planning and nodal identification. On CT, a short-axis diameter ≥1 cm is often employed for identification of pathologically involved nodes.[252] However, this cutoff is unsatisfactory, having a relatively poor accuracy of approximately 60% for correctly identifying the location and size of nodal disease.[253] FDG PET-CT can add significant value to CT alone in the identification of mediastinal nodal disease. Dwamena et al.[254] performed a meta-analysis of FDG-PET and CT for the identification of mediastinal nodal disease in lung cancer. They reported a mean sensitivity and specificity of 0.79 and 0.91, respectively, for PET and 0.60 and 0.77, respectively, for CT.[254] Although this represents a significant improvement, the gold standard for identification of mediastinal nodal disease is through invasive staging. When feasible, the mediastinum should be pathologically staged through either cervical mediastinoscopy or endobronchial ultrasound with transbronchial needle aspiration; this information should be incorporated into delineating the nodal GTV.

Clinical Target Volume

The clinical target volume (CTV) represents a volumetric expansion of the GTV to encompass microscopic disease. For the primary tumor, pathologically derived correlative data have shown that a 9-mm margin would encompass all microscopic disease in approximately 90% of lung adenocarcinomas.[255] Others have advocated the use of a differential margin based on histology of 8 mm for adenocarcinoma and 6 mm for squamous cell carcinomas to account for 95% of the microscopic extension of disease.[256] For nodal disease, surgical series have shown that a 3-mm margin will encompass 95% of the microscopic extranodal extension of disease in lymph nodes <2 cm. However, larger margins may be required for lymph nodes >2 cm.[257]

Internal Target Volume

The internal target volume (ITV) is defined by International Commission on Radiation Units and Measurements (ICRU) 62 as an expansion of the CTV to account for tumor motion. However, as the CTV includes subclinical disease whose motion cannot be visualized, most clinicians will create an "IGTV," which represents the summation of the contoured GTV on all CT data sets obtained in a respiratory-correlated (or four-dimensional [4D]) CT using established methodologies for image acquisition and correlation.[258] In the absence of a 4D-CT, a "slow" CT may be used with an extended image acquisition time to encompass a full breathing cycle.[259] The IGTV can then be expanded with a uniform volumetric margin to account for microscopic extension of disease and generation of a CTV.

Planning Target Volume

The planning target volume (PTV) is a volumetric expansion of the CTV to account for setup variability. In the past, empiric margins have been used to account for daily variations in patient positioning. However, with the incorporation of image guidance to aid in patient positioning and daily setup, these margins can likely be reduced. Grills et al.[261] showed that calculated population setup margins were reduced from 9 to 13 mm for patients immobilized with a stereotactic body frame and positioned without cone-beam CT to 1 to 2 mm with cone-beam CT. Ideally, with greater integration of image guidance into lung cancer treatment delivery, patient specific margins will be employed to account for tumor setup uncertainty.[260,261]

Dose Constraints

Normal tissue organs at risk (OARs) should be defined using guidelines outlined in prospective protocols, or using a consensus contouring atlas,[262] so that consistent data can be collected and analyzed. The bilateral lungs excluding the GTV, esophagus, and spinal cord should be defined for all patients undergoing 3D

Clinical Radiation Oncology

planning. The heart, pericardium, and brachial plexus should be defined when clinically indicated. For all patients, normal tissue dose limits should be considered in balance with adequate coverage of the target volume. There are multiple, valid models of normal tissue toxicity, including normal tissue complication probability (NTCP) modeling, threshold dose (V_{dose}), and mean dose. Recently, a multidisciplinary effort was undertaken—the Quantitative Analysis of Normal Tissue Effects in the Clinic (QUANTEC)—to summarize the published 3D dose-volume/toxicity data in the literature, review NTCP modeling, and provide practical guidance for the clinician.[263,264]

From collected data in the QUANTEC effort, the risk of radiation pneumonitis (RP) is <20% when the mean lung dose (MLD) is less than approximately 20 Gy, or for V_{20} <30 to 35 Gy, or V_5 <60% with conventional fractionation.[265] Caution is warranted when using IMRT and absolute dose-volume thresholds, because planning algorithms may meet strict dosimetric constraints at the cost of higher dose at other, unconstrained cut points. For esophagus, the collected data suggest that volumes treated at >40 to 50 Gy correlate with acute symptoms and that no dose above prescription be allowed to even small volumes of esophagus. This latter is especially important for heterogeneous IMRT planning.[266] For heart and pericardial dose, the conclusions of QUANTEC reflect a conservative interpretation of the existing literature: if the V_{25} is <10%, then the excess risk of cardiac mortality attributable to ischemic changes is <1% at 15 years. The risk of pericarditis can be minimized by keeping the mean pericardial dose <26 Gy or the pericardial V_{30} <46%. Heart and pericardial exposure should otherwise be minimized, without compromise of target coverage.[267] Brachial plexopathy is rare in patients who have received ≤60 Gy, and proposed brachial plexus dose limits for radiotherapy planning vary considerably; RTOG 0617 suggests a point maximum limit of 66 Gy. RTOG 0972/CALGB 36050 limits the V_{20} to ≤35%.

THREE-DIMENSIONAL CONFORMAL RADIOTHERAPY AND INTENSITY MODULATED RADIOTHERAPY FOR LUNG CANCER PLANNING AND DELIVERY

Introduction

Accurate treatment planning and delivery of radiation for the treatment of lung cancer is confounded by several technical factors, including proper patient setup and localization, the mobility of lung tumors, and tissue inhomogeneity in the vicinity of the lung, as well as the physical and biologic dose implications of delivering dose in >30 fractions versus ≤5 fractions, as in the case of SBRT. To understand the effects of these factors on the accuracy of treatment, one must look more closely at each of the procedures involved in treatment planning and delivery, including treatment simulation, treatment planning, plan evaluation and quality assurance, and treatment delivery. Among other studies, comprehensive reviews of current techniques for lung cancer treatment planning and delivery have been presented by Martel,[268] Senan et al.,[269] and Slotman et al.[270]

Treatment Simulation

The goal of treatment simulation is to acquire an image-based representation of the patient for the purposes of tumor and normal organ delineation for treatment planning. The imaging study is traditionally performed with CT. Serial CT images are acquired of the patient in the same treatment position, using the same immobilization devices as those used during radiation treatment. Slice thickness is typically ≤5 mm; smaller slice thicknesses allow for reconstruction of higher-resolution digitally reconstructed radiographs (DRRs),[269] which may improve localization accuracy during treatment. The anatomic region scanned should include both lungs and often extends from the level of the cricoid cartilage to the second lumbar vertebra.[269] Immobilization refers to the process of "patient fixation" to ensure reproducible patient setup during treatment and between treatment fractions. Custom devices, composed of Styrofoam or other materials that mold to the patient surface, are often fabricated for immobilization. Examples include the Alpha Cradle (KGF Enterprises, Chesterfield, MI) and BodyFIX (Elekta Oncology Systems, Norcross, GA) immobilization systems. In the context of SBRT, the American Association of Physicists in Medicine (AAPM) Task Group Report No. 101[271] recommends the use of 1- to 3-mm axial slice thickness during CT acquisition and the use of standard-of-care immobilization/fixation systems (including stereotactic body frames[272]) for reproducible treatment setup.

Management of Tumor Motion

Motion can result in significant distortion of axial or helical CT scans, manifested as artifacts in the vicinity of the tumor in the 3D image data set.[273] Motion-related artifacts not only render it difficult to assess the full extent of motion but also confound the ability to contour the target accurately on the planning CT data set. As a result of this, the AAPM Task Group Report No. 76[273] recommends that motion management strategies be considered when the range of tumor motion is >5 mm in any direction. The recommended 5-mm criterion may be reduced for techniques, such as SBRT, where tumor motion may become an accuracy-limiting factor.[273] Several different techniques have been proposed to manage and mitigate the effects of tumor motion.[269,270,273] To assess the range of mobility of tumors in the coronal plane, investigators have employed fluoroscopy.[269] Information from fluoroscopy cannot be directly linked to the volumetric simulation CT scan and is also limited by visualization of the target, although the use of implanted markers may overcome this problem.[274] Motion-encompassing methods are utilized to manage the effects of motion during the planning process. These include the generation of 4D-CT scans, which contain spatial and temporal information during the CT acquisition process. 4D-CT scans are typically reconstructed to generate multiple data sets at different phases of the respiratory cycle, ultimately generating an "envelope" of the moving tumor for treatment planning.[275–277] The use of "slow" CT scans (4 seconds per slice) acquired during quiet respiration has also been shown to capture reproducible target volumes for peripheral lung cancers.[259] Methods to limit motion, such as shallow breathing that is forced using abdominal compression devices, have shown to be effective in patients who can tolerate these devices.[278] Techniques such as deep inspiration breath-hold,[279] automatic breathing control,[280] respiratory gating,[281–283] and tumor tracking,[284] although technically challenging to implement, can afford improvement in normal lung sparing, particularly in circumstances where the magnitude of motion is large.[269,273]

With regard to motion-encompassing approaches, automatic tools have been developed to improve efficiency in the contouring of GTVs on multiple data sets to form an ITV. The maximum intensity projection (MIP) represents the highest intensity value encountered along the viewing ray for each pixel in the volumetric data set for the respective breathing phase. The summation of MIP images for each breathing phase therefore results in a composite view of the tumor incorporating all phases of motion. Other techniques, such as a color intensity projection (CIP) technique, in which the motion information from the cumulative 4D data sets are composited into a single color image, have also been proposed.[285] Figure 51.6 provides views of variance in GTV position in different phases of the breathing cycle.

Treatment Planning

The goal of treatment planning is to optimize the therapeutic ratio—that is, to maximize the dose to the target while minimizing dose to surrounding normal organs[286,287] (Fig. 51.7). As

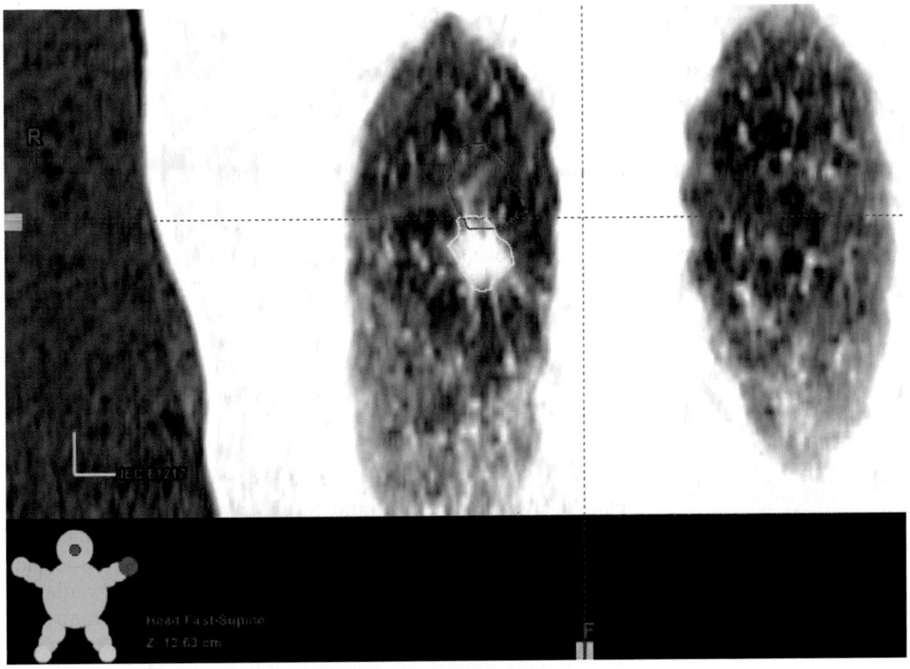

FIGURE 51.6. Tumor motion during a patient's normal respiratory cycle. The yellow wireframe shows the tumor position at full inspiration. The blue wireframe shows the tumor position at full expiration.

described earlier, target and OAR volumes are defined based on imaging studies, primarily CT and PET. PET can be used to differentiate atelectasis from tumor and to determine nodal involvement for central disease.[268] Respiratory-induced mobility of the tumor is accounted for using the internal margin, which represents the "envelope" encompassing tumor movement determined during the simulation 4D-CT acquisition. The internal margin is expanded to form the PTV, which accounts for geometric variation in the CTV owing to day-to-day (interfraction) uncertainties in the patient setup. According to ICRU Report No. 62,[288] a margin (planning risk volume [PRV]) should also be added to an OAR to account for interfraction variation in the OAR position. Margins for the PTV must be designed with an understanding of the random and systematic errors

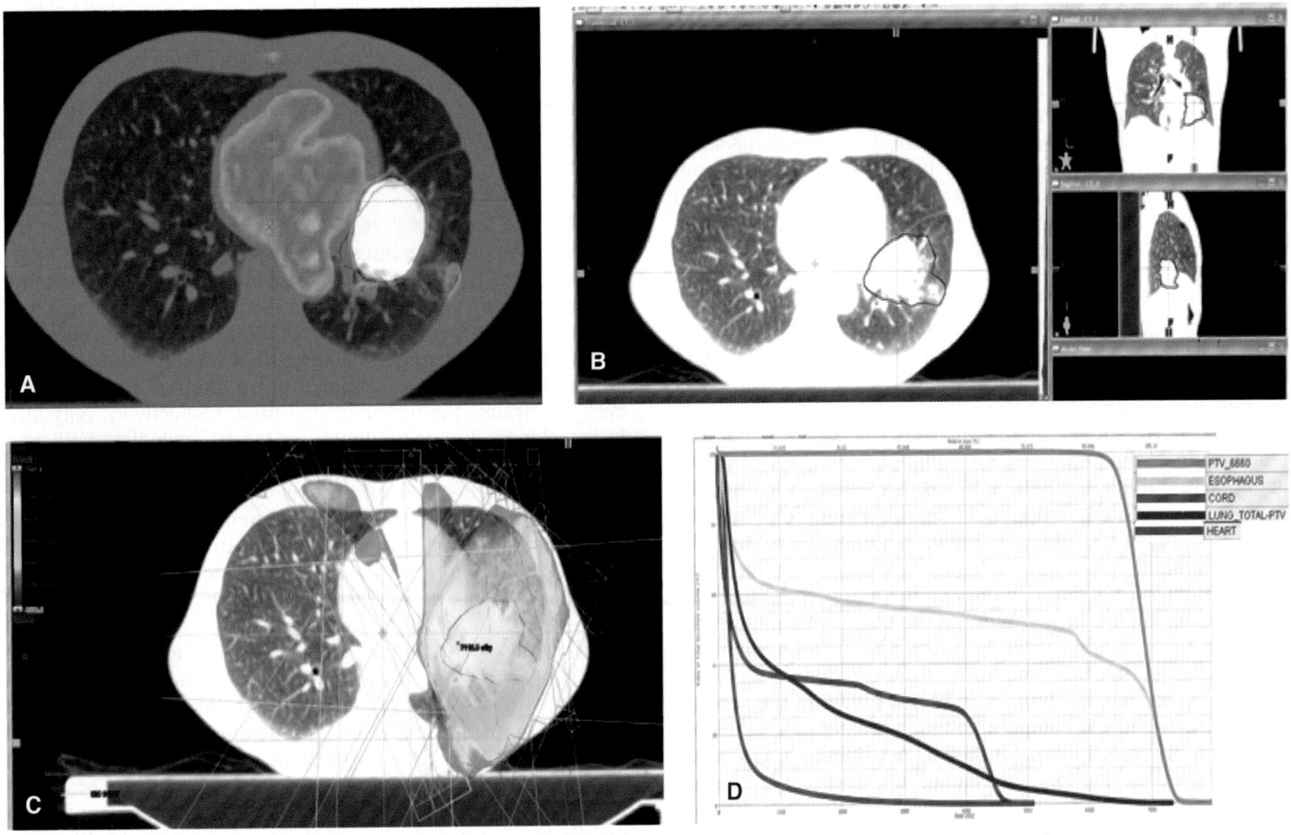

FIGURE 51.7. **A:** CT and PET fused image showing FDG-avid primary tumor. **B:** Axial, coronal, and sagittal views of gross tumor volume contour **C:** Transverse CT image of field arrangement and dose color wash of treatment plan. **D:** Dose volume histogram showing coverage of the planning target volume (*orange*) and dose to the esophagus (*light blue*), spinal cord (*dark blue*), total lung (*purple*), and heart (*red*).

associated with patient setup.[289] For advanced-stage NSCLC, typical margins for the PTV are on the order of 5 to 10 mm if an ITV is used for motion compensation and daily image-guided radiotherapy (IGRT) is employed during treatment. In the absence of motion compensation or IGRT, margins should typically be larger (10 to 20 mm) to minimize the chance of missing the target as a result of motion. Daily IGRT-based setup has been shown to significantly reduce residual errors and, consequently, planning margins.[288–290] For SBRT-based treatments, where motion management and IGRT are the recommended standard of care,[271] PTV margins can range from 3 to 6 mm.[270,272,290,291]

Beam arrangements for treatment planning can range from simple two-field, parallel opposed fields (e.g., anterior-posterior, opposed, anterior-posterior/posterior-anterior [AP/PA]) for late-stage NSCLC to complex multiple gantry angle, modulated beams for more focal treatments. Beams are shaped with a multileaf collimator (MLC), which enables conformation of radiation to the target. Treatment plans should be designed to minimize dose to surrounding normal organs and thereby limit the risk of treatment toxicity, implying sharp gradients in the dose falloff outside the target.[271] AP/PA fields may be considered when disease is more extensive and located centrally. The goal in such cases is to produce a homogeneous dose distribution across the treated volume to encompass the extent of the disease. However, AP/PA beams can only be used for cumulative PTV doses in the range of 40 to 45 Gy (in 1.8 to 2 Gy per fraction) because of spinal cord tolerance. "Off-cord" fields are typically required beyond this dose. When treating large volumes of lung, it is especially important to design treatment plans that adhere to normal lung tolerance doses; dose indices, such as V_{20}, V_5, and MLD, must be closely observed to avoid possible treatment complications.[292] For treatment planning of localized disease, more conformal dose distributions employing multiple beam angles are warranted. Treatment plans can be developed using 3D-CRT or IMRT techniques and should include beams from multiple gantry angles, particularly in the context of SBRT.

For IMRT-based planning, one must bear in mind the interplay effect, which describes the interplay between a given MLC position and instance of radiation delivery with the position of the tumor in the respiratory-induced motion cycle at the same instance.[293] The interplay effect has been shown to average out over the course of ≥30 treatment fractions.[293,294] However, in the SBRT setting, where 3 to 5 dose fractions are delivered, the interplay effect may compromise the planned dose distribution, suggesting that IMRT must be used cautiously for SBRT. Planning for SBRT must be done with an understanding of the dose gradients so as to develop dose distributions with sharp gradients. This is typically achieved using multiple nonoverlapping and noncoplanar beams as necessary and a MLC with ≤5 mm leaf width.[271] The dose prescription line can be low (e.g., 80%) with much smaller margins for beam penumbra ("block edge") than conventional radiotherapy; the motivation is to produce a faster dose falloff and thereby improve sparing of surrounding healthy tissues.[271] The AAPM Task Group No. 101 discourages the use of calculation grid sizes >3 mm for SBRT planning.[271]

Low-density lung tissue in the vicinity of or surrounding thoracic tumors significantly confounds the radiation dose computation problem in lung cancer treatment planning. Conditions of loss of charged-particle equilibrium are produced when the field size is reduced such that the lateral ranges of the secondary electrons become comparable to (or greater than) the field size; such conditions occur for larger field sizes in lung than in water-equivalent tissues because of the increased electron range in lung. Under such circumstances, the dose to the target is determined primarily by the secondary electron interactions and dose deposition. Because conventional dose algorithms do not account explicitly for transport of secondary electrons, they can be severely limited in accuracy under nonequilibrium conditions. Moreover, in low density, lung-equivalent tissues, the range of the secondary electrons contributes to the dose "build-down" effect at the edges of the tumor (at the lung-tumor interface), an effect that increases with beam energy. The article by Reynaert et al.[295] and AAPM Task Group No. 105[295] provide examples of numerous studies reporting on the inaccuracies associated with conventional algorithms for dose calculations in the lung. Therefore, for lung cancer treatment planning in general, and especially when dealing with smaller tumors, where the field sizes are less than 5×5 cm^2, more advanced dose algorithms such as convolution/superposition or the Monte Carlo method are necessary—the latter accounts explicitly for electron transport.[271,297] The AAPM TG Report No. 101[271] and other articles[298] recommend that pencil-beam algorithms not be utilized for SBRT-based lung dose calculations.

Plan Evaluation and Quality Assurance

Plan evaluation of IMRT and SBRT treatment plans requires careful evaluation of DVHs and the entire 3D dose distributions.[271,299] The following items, among others, must be considered to properly evaluate a treatment plan prior to radiation delivery:[271] organ contours and dose-volume–based organ constraints; planning margins for targets and OARs; intrafraction motion and impact on margins; inhomogeneity corrections; dose uniformity and "hot" or "cold" spots in the target region; normal tissue tolerance doses; plan deliverability—that is, the presence of many low-intensity segments that could possibly be removed without compromising plan quality; and unusual beam orientations that might involve collision during gantry rotation. In accordance with national practice guidelines for IMRT[300] and SBRT,[271] redundant verification of the patient-specific treatment plan monitor units and verification measurements of the planned isocenter and 2D dose distributions are necessary. When performing patient-specific verification measurements of highly modulated IMRT fields or SBRT plans, special consideration must be given to the detector size and performance under nonequilibrium conditions.[297] A properly commissioned Monte Carlo dose algorithm may prove valuable for patient-specific verification of IMRT and SBRT treatment plans, given the complexities with accurate measurements under nonequilibrium conditions.[271,297]

Treatment Delivery Technologies

Radiation delivery for lung cancer treatment is generally performed using IGRT-based systems, which can be acquired using megavoltage (MV)- or kilovoltage (kV)-based planar imaging, as well as volumetric, cone-beam CT imaging to localize the patient prior to treatment. Gating or tracking systems, which aim to deliver radiation during a given phase of the breathing cycle or "track" the tumor in real time, respectively, may also be employed. Image-guidance protocols, including type and frequency of imaging, as well as the need for gating or tracking should be decided by the treatment planning team after consideration of factors such as stage of the disease, location of the tumor, degree of tumor mobility, and quality of the IMRT or SBRT treatment plan. Reviews of technologies utilized in the treatment of lung cancer using IMRT and SBRT are provided elsewhere.[268,273,285,301] More recently, volumetric modulated arc therapies (VMATs) have become available for treatment of lung cancers. In one study, an SBRT lung treatment plan performed with VMAT was compared with that of a conventional IMRT plan using the same optimization objective function and constraints.[302] The VMAT plan consisted of a single arc, with partial angles to spare the contralateral lung. The VMAT plan yielded improved target coverage and comparable normal tissue doses compared with the conventional IMRT plan while reducing treatment time by approximately 60%.[302] The faster delivery of radiation with VMAT is likely to substantially mitigate patient movement on the treatment table as a result of discomfort during a long treatment procedure, thereby improving delivery quality. However, as with conventional IMRT, VMAT-based plans are also subject to the interplay effect, which must be considered depending on the mobility of the tumor and the degree of modulation of the MLC fields. Further investigation of the interplay between MLC leaves and tumor motion in the context of VMAT is warranted.

Particle Beam Radiotherapy for Non–Small Cell Lung Cancer

Because of their physical properties and method of interaction with matter, particle beams, such as protons, neutrons, and heavy ions, have the potential to offer improved dose deposition profiles in tissue when compared with photon beam radiation. Although protons have a similar biologic potency to photons, neutrons and heavy ions such as carbon ions deliver a more biologically effective dose than either photons or protons. Limited data on particle beam radiotherapy for lung cancer are available; however, clinical data are emerging on the application of proton beam radiotherapy in these patients. The favorable dose deposition profile of particle beam radiotherapy has generated interest in the potential for this modality to deliver tumoricidal doses in the lung cancer patient while maintaining or improving the therapeutic ratio. Proton beam radiotherapy for the treatment of cancer was originally described by Wilson[303] in 1946, and there has been growing interest over the past decade in clinical application of this modality in a variety of solid tumors, including lung cancer. In a dosimetric comparative study between protons and photons in patients with inoperable NSCLC, Chang et al.[304] reported that proton beam radiotherapy significantly reduced dose to critical normal structures including the esophagus, spinal cord, and heart, even with dose escalation, when compared with photon therapy delivered with advanced treatment delivery techniques such as 3D-CRT or IMRT. Further studies are emerging to assess the potential role of particle therapy in the management of lung cancer.

Early-Stage Disease

Considering the relative unavailability of particle beam radiotherapy and the complexities of delivery of this treatment to a mobile lung tumor, prospective data on the clinical efficacy of this approach in early-stage NSCLC are limited. Bush et al.[305] reported on a series of 68 patients with unresectable stage I NSCLC: the first 22 patients were treated to 51 cobalt gray equivalent (CGE) protons in 10 fractions, and an additional 46 patients were treated to 60 CGE. With a median follow-up of 30 months, the 3-year local control rate was 74% in all patients with 87% local control in T1 (87%) and 49% in T2 tumors. The treatment was well tolerated, with no cases of RP or esophageal or cardiac toxicity. In a smaller series, Hata et al.[306] reported on 21 patients with stage IA/IB treated with a total dose of 50 to 60 CGE at a dose per fraction of 5 to 6 CGE over a median time of 15 days. The 2-year local control and cause-specific survival were 95% and 86%, respectively. There were no grade 3 through grade 5 toxicities in this patient population.[306] Chang et al.[307] reported on a series of 18 patients with centrally located medically inoperable stage I NSCLC treated to 87.5 CGE in 2.5 CGE per fraction with proton beam radiotherapy. With a median follow-up time of 16.3 months, no grade 4 or 5 toxicities were observed. The most common toxicities observed were dermatitis (grade 2, 67%; grade 3, 17%), followed by grade 2 fatigue (44%), grade 2 pneumonitis (11%), grade 2 esophagitis (6%), and grade 2 chest wall pain (6%). The crude local control in these 18 patients was 88.9%, with 11.1% experiencing regional lymph node failure and 27.8% experiencing distant metastasis. At the time of last follow-up, 12 patients (67%) were still alive with 5 patients dying of distant metastatic disease and 1 patient dying of a cardiopulmonary event unrelated to treatment.[307] Miyamoto et al.[308] reported the results of a four-fraction phase II trial of carbon ion radiotherapy in early-stage NSCLC; 79 patients were enrolled and received either 52.8 cGE (stage IA) or 60 CGE (stage IB). The local control rate for all patients was 90% (T1: 98%, T2: 80%). The patients' 5-year lung cancer–specific survival rate was 68% (IA: 87%, IB: 42%). The OS was 45% (IA: 62%, IB: 25%). Half of the deaths were attributable to intercurrent disease. No toxic reactions in the lung greater than grade 3 were detected. Although these results are promising, whether particle beam therapy provides an advantage over photon-based SBRT is not known at this time.

Locally Advanced Disease

Because of the requirement of delivery of tumoricidal doses of radiation to the mediastinal nodes in locally advanced NSCLC, particle beam radiotherapy may be of particular value in this patient population. There are no prospective data to date examining carbon ion radiotherapy in locally advanced disease; however, there are emerging data with proton beam radiotherapy in this setting. Chang et al.[309] recently reported the results of the first 44 patients enrolled on a phase II trial of weekly concurrent carboplatin and paclitaxel with proton beam radiotherapy to 74 CGE in patients with inoperable stage IIIA/IIIB NSCLC. With a median follow-up of 19 months, they observed a promising median OS of 29.4 months in these patients. No patient experienced grade 4 or 5 proton-related adverse events. The most common nonhematologic grade 3 toxicities were dermatitis (n = 5), esophagitis (n = 5), and pneumonitis (n = 1). Nine patients (20.5%) experienced local disease recurrence; 4 patients (9.1%) had isolated local failure. Four patients (9.1%) had regional lymph node recurrence; 1 patient (2.3%) had isolated regional recurrence. Nineteen patients (43.2%) developed distant metastasis. The OS and PFS rates were 86% and 63% at 1 year. Although preliminary, these results suggest that proton beam radiotherapy with concurrent chemotherapy may potentially be of benefit in patients with inoperable locally advanced NSCLC.[309] More clinical trials are needed.

METASTATIC NON–SMALL CELL LUNG CANCER

Basic Therapeutic Precepts

The treatment of advanced NSCLC has evolved over the past 25 years. In the late 1980s, debate centered on the basic efficacy of systemic therapy in patients with metastatic or recurrent disease. The toxicity of cisplatin-based treatment was considerable, and the survival benefits were marginal at best. Many clinicians felt that the side effects exceeded any putative benefit.

By the early 1990s, however, it was clear that platinum-based chemotherapy could prolong survival, improve symptom control, and yield superior QOL compared with best supportive care.[310,311–313] In the 1990s, new agents emerged with enhanced therapeutic index. Carboplatin, although no more effective than cisplatin, was considerably safer with less nephrotoxicity, neurotoxicity, and gastrointestinal toxicity.[314–316] In addition, several new agents, including paclitaxel, docetaxel, gemcitabine, vinorelbine, and irinotecan, were tested and proved compatible with either carboplatin or cisplatin. Phase III studies of these agents partnered with platinum demonstrated survival advantages compared to platinum alone or older, more toxic platinum-based combinations, and the benefits of these platinum-based combinations extended to those >70 years of age, as long as they were fit.[317–323,324,325–328,329,330–331] By the late 1990s, in addition to frontline therapy, phase III trials had clearly demonstrated the efficacy of "salvage" treatment. Docetaxel was approved as second-line treatment based on two randomized trials: one showing a survival advantage compared to best supportive care and the other showing an advantage compared to either vinorelbine or ifosfamide.[332–333] BR10 demonstrated a statistically significant and clinically meaningful response, PFS, and OS benefit for erlotinib compared to placebo in the second- and third-line setting in unselected patients, including those with compromised performance status.[334] Finally, a phase III trial led by Hanna et al.[335] showed therapeutic equivalence between pemetrexed and docetaxel in the second-line setting, with less toxicity for pemetrexed.

As mentioned previously, histology, for the first time, has become an important determinant in the selection of systemic therapy for advanced NSCLC. An association between nonsquamous histology and both improved response and survival has also been observed with pemetrexed in combination with platinum-based chemotherapy, compared with gemcitabine and a platinum agent.[97,98] In contrast, gemcitabine has proven more effective than pemetrexed in the first-line treatment of patients with squamous NSCLC.[97] In patients with adenocarcinoma, pemetrexed has demonstrated activity and garnered U.S. Food and Drug Administration (FDA) approval in the first-line, second-line, and maintenance therapy settings and has been tested in phase II trials in combination with carboplatin and bevacizumab in nonsquamous histology, generating a median PFS of 7.8 months and median survival of 14.1 months.[97,98,335–337]

Additionally, maintenance chemotherapy has now entered into the therapeutic lexicon. Based on recent large phase III randomized trials, both pemetrexed (for nonsquamous histology) and erlotinib (for any histologic subtype) are approved for use as maintenance therapy for those patients who have not progressed on standard platinum-based treatment.[338,339]

Molecular Determinants of Therapy

The presence of EGFR activating mutations in approximately 10% to 15% of lung cancer patients and their association with heightened sensitivity to EGFR TKIs were first recognized by Lynch et al.[108] and Paez et al.[340] in 2004. Multiple retrospective analyses and single-arm phase II trials have confirmed this correlation.[102,341] However, it is only since 2009 that the association between EGFR mutations and improved response rate and PFS have been confirmed in prospective phase III trials in advanced NSCLC.[342,343–345,346,347–349] The Iressa Pan-Asia Study (IPASS), a phase III, multicenter, randomized, open-label, parallel-group study in patients with advanced adenocarcinoma of the lung, was the first trial to demonstrate the potential for EGFR TKIs as first-line therapy in patients with specified clinical and demographic characteristics.[342] Treatment-naive East Asian patients (n = 1,217), either nonsmokers or former light smokers, with adenocarcinoma of the lung were randomized to gefitinib monotherapy 250 mg per day orally or to combination paclitaxel 200 mg/m^2 and carboplatin (AUC, 5 to 6 mg/mL per minute) every 3 weeks for up to six cycles. Among the overall study population, tumors from 437 patients (35.9%) were evaluable for mutation analysis; approximately 60% carried EGFR mutations. Of those with mutations randomized to gefitinib, the response rate exceeded 70%, whereas wild-type patients randomized to gefitinib had a response rate of roughly 1%. At 12 months, PFS was significantly longer in mutation-positive patients in the gefitinib group compared to patients in the paclitaxel/carboplatin (P/C) group (HR 0.48, 95% CI 0.36 to 0.64, p <.001). Conversely, PFS was significantly shorter for gefitinib compared to chemotherapy in patients whose tumors did not harbor mutations (HR 2.85, 95% CI 2.05 to 3.98, p <.001). However, final OS results for the gefitinib and P/C treatment groups were not significantly different for the overall population: 18.6 months for the gefitinib cohort; 17.3 months for the control group (HR 0.901, 95% CI 0.793 to 1.023, p = .109). Similarly, final OS results between the two treatment groups were not significantly different in the EGFR mutation-positive cohort (HR 1.002, 95% CI 0.756 to 1.328, p = .990) or in the EGFR mutation-negative subgroup of patients (HR 1.181, 95% CI 0.857 to 1.628, p = .309), presumably because of crossover to an EGFR TKI in mutation-positive patients randomized to chemotherapy. Despite the absence of a survival benefit, this trial has irrevocably altered the therapeutic paradigm in advanced NSCLC and has laid the groundwork for subsequent phase III trials comparing EGFR TKIs to standard chemotherapy conducted exclusively in patients with the EGFR mutation (Table 51.10).

TABLE 51.10 PHASE III TRIALS COMPARING EGFR TKI TO STANDARD CHEMOTHERAPY IN EGFR MUTANT POSITIVE COHORTS

Author (Reference)	*Study*	*Number of Patients*	*RR (%)*	*Median PFS (Months)*
Mok et al. (342)	IPASS	261	71.2 vs. 47.3	9.8 vs. 6.4
Lee et al. (349)	First-SIGNAL	42	84.6 vs. 37.5	8.4 vs. 6.7
Mitsudomi et al. (348)	WJTOG 3405	177	62.1 vs. 32.2	9.2 vs. 6.3
Maemondo et al. (343)	NEJGSG002	230	73.7 vs. 30.7	10.8 vs. 5.4
Zhou et al. (345)	OPTIMAL	154	83 vs. 36	13.1 vs. 4.6
Rosell et al. (347)	EURTAC	154	54.5 vs. 10.5	9.2 vs. 5.4

EGFR, epidermal growth factor receptor; TKI, tyrosine kinase inhibitor; RR, response rate; PFS, progression-free survival.

Taken together, the results of these trials, particularly with respect to response rate and PFS, support the use of EGFR TKIs in the first-line setting in patients harboring EGFR-activating mutations. To date, however, largely because of crossover at the time of disease progression, this response rate and PFS benefit has not yet translated into an OS advantage. However, it is clear that patients who harbor this mutation live longer than wild-type patients as long as they receive an oral EGFR TKI at some point in their disease course.

Burgeoning Understanding of EML4/ALK in Advanced Non–Small Cell Lung Cancer

ALK positivity defines a distinct molecular subset of NSCLC. Phenotypically, patients whose tumors are likely to prove positive for this molecular marker look similar to those who harbor EGFR mutations. Nearly all have adenocarcinoma, and they are more likely to be nonsmokers. However, ALK translocation (3% to 7%) and EGFR mutation (10% to 15%) are virtually mutually exclusive, and those patients whose tumors harbor ALK translocations do not typically respond to treatment with EGFR TKI.[103,350] Crizotinib, a selective inhibitor of the ALK and MET tyrosine kinases, resulted in preliminary activity in a phase I dose escalation study in previously treated patients with NSCLC whose tumors expressed EML4-ALK. Among 113 evaluable ALK-positive patients receiving this agent, the overall response rate was 56% and median PFS 9.2 months.[103,350] The most common adverse events were mild to moderate and gastrointestinal in nature and included nausea (54%), diarrhea (48%), and vomiting (44%). Other adverse events included liver function test elevations and transient difficulty with light-dark accommodation. Camidge et al.[351] more recently have updated the results of this study; this report included a total of 119 patients treated with crizotinib. The response rate rose to 61% with a median PFS of 10 months. The 1- and 2-year survival rates were 74% and 54%, respectively, and the median survival had not been reached.

During the American Society of Clinical Oncology meeting in 2011, Crino et al.[352] reported a preliminary analysis of enrollees in the phase II trial in NSCLC patients positive for EML4-ALK who had been exposed to multiple lines of therapy. Of 133 patients enrolled, the median age was 52 years, 94% had adenocarcinoma, 68% were never smokers, and 53% were female. The overall response rate was 51.1%; the disease control rate was 74%. Toxicities matched those observed in the original phase I trial. PFS and OS data were not yet available. In addition, there were clinically meaningful improvements in symptoms such as cough, pain, dyspnea, and fatigue. This study is ongoing with a planned sample size of 400 patients. An ongoing phase III trial (NCT00932893) compares crizotinib to standard second-line chemotherapy with either docetaxel or pemetrexed in patients with NSCLC harboring a translocation at the ALK locus whose disease has progressed after one prior chemotherapy regimen. In addition, a first-line trial compared crizotinib to combination pemetrexed and cisplatin in chemotherapy-naive patients with ALK-positive advanced NSCLC. As time goes on, it seems apparent that crizotinib may prolong OS and fundamentally alter the natural history of ALK-positive NSCLC. The FDA granted accelerated approval of this agent on August 26, 2011.

Conclusion

The era of customized care in advanced NSCLC has clearly arrived. The previous "one size fits all" approach has been discarded. Therapeutic decisions are now based on both histology and molecular markers. It is anticipated that other markers will emerge over the next 5 to 10 years. KRAS mutations are present in 20% to 25% of all patients with advanced NSCLC; however, to date, no agent has been identified that can adequately target this marker. Other markers, including BRAF and HER-2/neu are present in 1% to 3% of patients with advanced adenocarcinoma and may prove "actionable" in the small percentage who harbor them. Finally, fibroblast growth factor receptor is present in 20% to 25% of those with squamous histology; molecularly driven studies are now addressing the squamous cell carcinoma cohort for which no specific targeted agent has yet been identified.

PALLIATIVE RADIOTHERAPY

Given the propensity of lung cancer for locoregional recurrence and/or distant metastatic disease, radiotherapy plays an important role in the palliation of symptomatic disease in many lung cancer patients.[353,354] The most common sites of disease that require palliative radiotherapy include the thorax, bone, and brain. Intrathoracic disease and bone metastasis will be covered here. The reader is referred to the CNS section (see Chapter 93).

Palliation of Intrathoracic Disease

Symptoms from progression of intrathoracic lung cancer that may benefit from a course of palliative radiotherapy include cough, hemoptysis, chest wall pain, SVC syndrome, dyspnea from airway obstruction, and hoarseness from involvement of the recurrent laryngeal nerve. In one prospective study following 134 inoperable patients with lung cancer, immediate chest radiotherapy was necessary in 86 patients (64%) because of significant presenting symptoms from intrathoracic disease, and of the remaining 48 patients not receiving initial radiotherapy, 26 patients (54%) required chest radiotherapy later because of symptoms from intrathoracic disease.[355] The rate of palliation of local symptoms is high for chest pain and hemoptysis at 60% to 80%, whereas cough and dyspnea are improved in only 50% to 70%.[356] For intrathoracic disease with an obstructive component, 30 to 45 Gy in 2.5- to 3-Gy fractions over 2 to 3 weeks is generally recommended.[357] For patients with poor performance status or for whom daily radiotherapy over 2 to 3 weeks is logistically difficult, hypofractionated regimens (of 1 to 2 fractions) have been utilized with good palliative results.[358,359] An ASTRO evidence-based guideline for palliative thoracic radiation in lung cancer has recently been published that emphasized either short- or long-course EBRT as the first-line radiation option in the palliative setting and that use of concurrent chemotherapy in the palliative setting is not supported by the current medical literature.[360]

Endobronchial brachytherapy provides relief for patients with endobronchial lesions causing obstruction or hemoptysis.[361,362] The lesion to be treated should be visible by bronchoscopy and generally located in the trachea, main stem, or lower lobe bronchi. This procedure requires the combined efforts of an interventional pulmonologist and brachytherapist. The pulmonologist performs fiberoptic bronchoscopy, placing an afterloading catheter within the airway adjacent to the tumor under direct visualization. In a retrospective study from MD Anderson Cancer Center involving 175 patients with lung cancer who received high dose rate brachytherapy for metastatic or locally recurrent lung cancer, 115 patients (66%) demonstrated symptomatic improvement.[363] A more recent study corroborates the low morbidity and high symptomatic improvement.[364] Endobronchial brachytherapy is primarily indicated in patients with obstructive endobronchial lesions who have already received EBRT.[360] It can also be combined with other interventions that can acutely relieve symptoms related to airway obstruction such as stenting or debulking procedures.

Superior Vena Cava Syndrome

Lung cancer is the most common cause of SVC syndrome and accounts for approximately 80% of cases at diagnosis.[365] If the SVC becomes obstructed because of an extrinsic mass, blood returns to the heart through collateral vessels to the azygous vein or inferior vena cava. Venous collaterals dilate over weeks so that the upper body venous pressure and resulting edema of the arm and face decrease over time. The severity of the symptoms is therefore attributable not only to the degree of SVC narrowing but also to the rapidity with which it develops. The characteristic signs include cyanosis; plethora; distention of subcutaneous veins; and edema of the head, neck, and arm. Patients may report dyspnea or cough. Rarely, severe and acute obstruction can result in cerebral edema or laryngeal stridor. The clinical course may be exacerbated by the development of a thrombus or the simultaneous tumor mass effect on the bronchi or heart.

Traditionally, SVC syndrome was viewed as a medical emergency. Accumulating experience, however, demonstrates that the course of SVC is rarely life threatening. In a review of 107 patients in whom intervention was withheld during evaluation, there were no serious clinical consequences to deferring treatment until diagnosis and staging was completed.[366] Symptoms often improve without active intervention, as collateral vessels dilate.[367] In malignant SVC syndrome, immediate intervention is warranted when the symptoms are life threatening (e.g., cerebral edema leading to altered mental status, stridor, or clinically significant hemodynamic compromise). When urgent intervention is indicated, intravascular stenting provides the most immediate relief and can be accomplished even when there is complete obstruction. In the absence of life-threatening symptoms, the patient should be appropriately staged and biopsied and the underlying malignancy treated in a manner appropriate for its stage and presentation. The majority of patients with SVC syndrome attributed to SCLC will respond to systemic therapy, and patients with extensive-stage SCLC and SVC syndrome should start chemotherapy after a staging evaluation. Similarly, patients with limited-stage SCLC and SVC syndrome with bulky disease should respond rapidly to a cycle of chemotherapy, after which radiation can be added, treating the smaller, postchemotherapy volume to spare normal lung tissue. Patients with NSCLC and SVC syndrome are less likely to respond to chemotherapy, thus the threshold for starting radiation or placing an endovascular stent should be lower.[368] In patients with metastatic NSCLC, palliative radiotherapy is commonly recommended as part of initial therapy.

SMALL CELL LUNG CARCINOMA

In the United States in 2011, approximately 28,000 patients were diagnosed with SCLC, constituting approximately 13% of all lung cancer diagnoses.[2] Over the past several decades, the proportion of SCLC among all lung cancer histologies has been decreasing, perhaps because of smoking cessation and the proliferation of low-tar cigarettes.[369] Although there has been a modest but statistically significant improvement in 2- and 5-year survival in both limited- and extensive-stage disease in recent decades, the outcomes are still extremely poor, particularly since the majority (approximately 60%) of patients present with extensive-stage disease with an expected 2-year survival of only 4%.

Pathology

The establishment of a firm pathologic diagnosis distinguishing SCLC from NSCLC variants such as carcinoma with neuroendocrine features and carcinoid is extremely important in this disease, as it can have a significant impact on management and clinical outcome. Histologically, SCLC is one of the small, round, blue cell tumors (along with neuroblastoma, rhabdomyosarcoma, Merkel cell carcinoma, etc.) with scant cytoplasm and indistinct nucleoli. Cells are often molded together, and crush artifact is commonly noted after needle biopsy but is not pathognomonic. Almost all SCLC samples are immunoreactive to keratin and epithelial membrane antigen, and approximately 80% express thyroid transcription factor-1 (TTF-1).[370] The majority of tumors will stain for neuroendocrine markers including synaptophysin, chromogranin A, neuron-specific enolase, and CD56. Immunohistochemistry alone, however, cannot distinguish SCLC from small cell cancer of nonthoracic origin or from NSCLC with neuroendocrine differentiation. The WHO recognizes that SCLC can occur in a pure type or mixed with NSCLC in up to 30% of cases.

Prognostic Factors in Small Cell Lung Cancer

The most clinically important prognostic factor in SCLC is stage (limited vs. extensive), with a median survival of approximately 23 months for patients with limited disease versus 8 to 9 months for those with extensive disease.[222,371] Other clinical factors consistently reported to correlate with improved survival include good performance status, female gender, and normal lactate dehydrogenase levels at baseline.[372]

Staging Workup

As in patients with NSCLC, patients with SCLC should undergo a timely and efficient history, physical exam, and laboratory and radiographic evaluation. The history and physical should be performed with particular attention to signs and symptoms of paraneoplastic syndromes, including SIADH and elevated ACTH. Laboratory evaluation should include a complete blood count and comprehensive chemistry panel. Radiographic studies should include a CT scan of the chest and abdomen with intravenous contrast and a bone scan.[373] All patients with SCLC, regardless of stage, should undergo a brain MRI with gadolinium or a head CT with contrast to evaluate for brain metastases. A diagnostic thoracentesis should be performed for any identified pleural effusion to determine the presence of malignant cells. If limited-stage disease is suspected, an FDG-PET scan is recommended because it has significant value in identifying distant metastatic dissemination as well as additional regional nodal dissemination beyond that typically seen on CT alone.[374] The TNM staging system adopted by the American Joint Commission for Cancer (AJCC) in the seventh edition of the *Cancer Staging Manual* is applicable to both NSCLC and SCLC. Most historical studies and ongoing prospective trials, however, classify patients as having limited or extensive disease based on the 1973 Veteran's Administration Lung Group staging scheme.[375] In this system, limited stage is defined as disease confined to the ipsilateral hemithorax, which can be safely encompassed within a tolerable radiation portal. Virtually all studies in limited disease exclude malignant pleural effusions. From a practical standpoint, hemithoracic radiotherapy to encompass the entire ipsilateral pleura has little justification because it would confer a significant risk of pulmonary toxicity in a high-risk patient population with little chance of cure. As such, patients with malignant pleural effusions are almost always classified as having extensive-stage disease.

Paraneoplastic Syndromes

Paraneoplastic syndromes are commonly encountered in lung cancer; however, the spectrum of paraneoplastic syndromes in SCLC is distinct from that observed in NSCLC. Neurologic paraneoplastic syndromes are more commonly encountered in SCLC and are thought to be primarily autoimmune in nature. LEMS is seen in 3% of all SCLC patients at presentation and is characterized by proximal muscle weakness that improves with continued activity. This syndrome occurs when autoantibodies are generated against voltage-gated calcium channel receptors on the presynaptic membrane, impeding release of acetylcholine into the neuromuscular junction and resulting in muscular weakness. A wide variety of other rare autoimmune neurologic paraneoplastic syndromes have been described in SCLC, including encephalomyelitis, cerebellar degeneration, and retinopathy.[376] SCLC can also elaborate hormonally active peptides including ACTH and vasopressin leading to Cushing's syndrome and SIADH, respectively. Although SCLC is the most common tumor associated with SIADH, only 10% of patients meet the clinical criteria for SIADH. Similarly, only 5% of SCLC patients present with Cushing's syndrome. Despite the fact that paraneoplastic syndromes may lead to early identification and diagnosis of SCLC, some of these syndromes, such as Cushing's, have been associated with poorer survival.[44] Treatment of the cancer will often, although not always, ameliorate the paraneoplastic syndromes.

General Therapeutic Precepts

Early-stage (i.e., T1-2, N0) SCLC is diagnosed in <5% of incident cases. For these patients, definitive surgical resection is a potential therapeutic option. In a population-based study, lobectomy without adjuvant radiation was associated with an approximately 50% OS.[377] Given the propensity for early nodal dissemination with SCLC, invasive staging of the mediastinum should be performed prior to surgical resection. After surgical resection, the primary mode of failure for these patients is distant dissemination. Tsuchiya et al.[378] reported the results of JCOG9101, a JCOG Lung Cancer Study Group multi-institutional phase II prospective trial evaluating adjuvant EP after complete surgical resection of stage I through stage IIIA SCLC. The majority of patients enrolled had clinical stage I disease (44/62). Three-year survival was 61% overall, 68% in patients with clinical stage I disease, 56% in patients with stage II disease, and 13% in patients with stage IIIa disease.[378] These data suggest a possible role for surgical resection in select patients with pathologically proven stage I or II SCLC.

The majority of patients present with evidence of nodal or distant dissemination at the time of diagnosis. Multiagent chemotherapy, usually etoposide in combination with carboplatin or cisplatin, is an essential part of therapy for these patients. For patients with limited-stage disease, the addition of thoracic radiation significantly improves survival and therefore is an integral part of their treatment regimen. Two meta-analyses have demonstrated not only an improvement in thoracic control but also a significant improvement in absolute survival of about 5% (and relative improvement of about 50%) in patients with limited-stage disease treated with combined modality therapy compared to those treated with chemotherapy alone.[379,380] Patients with extensive-stage disease are usually treated with systemic chemotherapy alone. For select good performance status patients with extensive stage disease who have complete resolution of their extrathoracic tumor burden, consolidative thoracic radiotherapy may be of benefit to reduce the risk of intrathoracic failure.[381] Patients with limited-stage disease (and selected patients with extensive-stage disease) who respond to initial therapy should be offered prophylactic cranial irradiation (PCI), as this has been shown to provide a significant improvement in absolute survival for these patients.[371,382]

Combining Radiation and Chemotherapy for Limited-Stage Disease

A randomized trial by the JCOG evaluated concurrent versus sequential chemotherapy and thoracic radiation in patients with limited-stage SCLC.[383] All patients received 45 Gy in 1.5-Gy fractions twice daily and were randomized to receive four cycles of cisplatin (80 mg/m^2 on day 1) and etoposide (100 mg/m^2 days 1, 2, and 3) every 4 weeks concurrent with radiotherapy (beginning day 2) or every 3 weeks sequentially before radiotherapy. Patients treated concurrently had longer median survival compared to patients treated sequentially: 27 months versus 20 months. A second randomized trial by the National Cancer Institute of Canada compared early with late concurrent chemoradiotherapy.[384] In this trial, 308 patients received cyclophosphamide, doxorubicin, and vincristine alternating with EP and were randomized to 40 Gy in 15 daily fractions given with either the first cycle of EP (week 3) or the last (week 15). The median survival improved to 21 months with early radiotherapy versus 16 months with late treatment (p = .008).[384] These two trials were included in a meta-analysis by Fried et al.[385] that included >1,500 patients from seven randomized trials evaluating the timing of radiotherapy when given concurrently with multiagent chemotherapy. The use of early thoracic radiotherapy, with cycle 1 or 2 of chemotherapy, was associated with improved 2-year OS compared to delayed or sequential chemotherapy and radiation. The benefit was more pronounced when the radiotherapy was given with platinum-based chemotherapy.

The EP combination is the most commonly used first-line chemotherapy regimen in patients with SCLC, either alone (in patients with extensive disease) or in combination with thoracic radiation (in patients with limited-stage disease). In patients with extensive disease, alternative combinations including cisplatin and irinotecan (IP), the addition of an anthracycline or taxane to EP, and higher-dose therapy have been investigated; however, to date, they have not proven superior to EP. The only exception is Japan, where IP has displaced EP. Carboplatin as a substitute for cisplatin is an equivalent regimen to EP in extensive-stage disease with a lower risk of nephropathy. In limited-stage disease, in those fit enough to tolerate it, combination EP administered concurrently with thoracic radiation remains the standard regimen.

Dose and Fractionation

The optimal dose and fractionation scheme for concurrent chemoradiation for limited-stage small cell is an area of active investigation. SCLC is highly radiosensitive, suggesting that hyperfractionation could be employed to reduce late normal tissue toxicity. It also has a high proliferative rate, arguing for accelerated treatment to counteract repopulation. Between 1989 and 1992, 417 patients were enrolled in a randomized, intergroup trial of concurrent accelerated hyperfractionated radiotherapy versus standard daily radiotherapy in patients with limited-stage SCLC.[386] All patients received four cycles of cisplatin (60 mg/m^2 on day 1) and etoposide (120 mg/m^2 on days 1, 2, and 3), and radiotherapy began with cycle 1. In the once-daily arm, patients received 45 Gy in 1.8-Gy fractions over 5 weeks. In the twice-daily arm, patients received 45 Gy in 1.5-Gy fractions over 3 weeks. Patients who achieved a complete response were offered PCI. OS was significantly higher in the twice-daily arm, 26% versus 16% at 5 years, and local recurrence was significantly lower, 36% versus 52%. There was a significant increase in grade 3 acute esophagitis, 26% versus 11%, in the twice-daily arm, with no difference in late toxicity. The 5-year survival rate observed in this study is among the best reported for limited-stage disease; consequently, this treatment approach is considered by many the current standard of care for the management of limited-stage disease.

The perceived radiosensitivity of SCLC led to the initial utilization of modest dose approaches to treat this disease (45 to 50 Gy). However, the intrathoracic relapse rate observed in the once-daily arm of the Turrisi study was 75%, highlighting the inadequacy of these modest doses to achieve meaningful local control.[222] The observed improved survival in the twice-daily arm in this study highlighted the importance of local control in this disease. Therefore, dose escalation, either through an altered fractionation or conventionally fractionated approach, has been explored with a goal of improving intrathoracic control of disease. In 2005, the RTOG reported the results of a phase I dose escalation trial in which 64 patients were enrolled and dose escalated in a stepwise fashion from 50.4 Gy to 64.8 Gy in 1.8 Gy per fraction.[387] The lowest dose cohort received 1.8 Gy once daily for 20 fractions, followed by 1.8 Gy twice daily on the final 3 days. Dose escalation was achieved by the addition of a second daily fraction on the last 5, 7, 9, or 11 days, retaining the 5-week treatment duration. The maximum tolerated dose was determined to be 61.2 Gy in 5 weeks using this scheme. In a follow-up phase 2 study, RTOG 0239,[388] 72 patients were treated to 61.2 Gy in 5 weeks, with twice-daily radiotherapy for the last 9 treatment days. With 19 months median follow-up, 2-year OS was 37% and 2-year locoregional control was 80%.

Dose escalation has also been examined utilizing a daily fractionation scheme. Choi et al.[389] conducted a phase I dose escalation study with both twice-daily and once-daily arms. In the twice-daily arm, 45 Gy in 30 fractions over 3 weeks was the maximum tolerated dose. In the once-daily arm, the dose was escalated to the maximum of 70 Gy in 35 fractions over 7 weeks without dose-limiting toxicity. CALGB 39808 tested the feasibility of this approach with concurrent platinum and etoposide.[390] In this study, 63 patients were treated with two cycles of induction paclitaxel (175 mg/m^2 day 1) and topotecan (1 mg/m^2 days 1 through 5), followed by concurrent thoracic radiation with carboplatin (AUC 5) and etoposide (100 mg/m^2 days 1 through 3). Thoracic radiation consisted of 44 Gy to the mediastinum and primary tumor delivered in 2 Gy per fraction, followed by a cone-down to encompass the involved nodes and primary tumor alone for an additional 26 Gy, totaling 70 Gy in 35 fractions over 7 weeks. Grade 3 or 4 esophagitis was noted in 21% of patients. The OS at 2 years was 48%. Intriguingly, 10 of 63 patients had local relapse within the high-dose field with no relapses within the lower-dose 44-Gy volume, suggesting that a relatively radioresistant subpopulation of tumor cells may exist in some small cell tumors.[390]

In summary, the optimal dose and fractionation approach for SCLC remains to be defined. An ongoing intergroup effort (CALGB 30610, RTOG 0538, NCT00632853) seeks to determine the optimal radiation schedule. Patients are randomized to one of three arms: (a) 45 Gy in 30 fractions over 3 weeks, (b) 61.2 Gy in 5 weeks per RTOG 0239, or (c) 70 Gy in 35 fractions over 7 weeks per CALGB 39808. All patients receive concurrent EP, and radiotherapy begins with cycle 1 or cycle 2. A similar effort is under way in Europe. The Concurrent Once-daily Versus Twice-daily Radiotherapy (CONVERT) trial is a 2-arm randomized phase III study: patients receive either 45 Gy in 30 fractions twice daily or 66 Gy in 33 fractions once daily. All patients receive EP; radiotherapy begins with cycle 2.

Radiotherapy Volume

Limited-stage SCLC is frequently bulky at presentation, requiring large treatment fields to encompass all sites of intrathoracic disease. Therefore, induction chemotherapy has been employed to achieve cytoreduction of disease prior to initiation of thoracic radiotherapy. This approach raises the concern of potentially increasing the risk of marginal treatment failure if the postchemotherapy volume alone is included in the radiation portal. To address this question, the SWOG conducted a randomized study, enrolling 191 patients who had a partial response or stable disease after 6 weeks of induction chemotherapy. They were randomized to receive radiotherapy (48 Gy split course) to either the preinduction or postinduction volume.[391] There was no difference in local recurrence rates: 32% in the preinduction versus 28% in the postinduction arm. Careful retrospective studies of patients treated with preinduction or postinduction thoracic radiotherapy show that local failure is not significantly higher if smaller fields are used. Furthermore, most intrathoracic failures occur in the smaller postchemotherapy radiation field, arguing, as in locally advanced NSCLC, against the use of ENI.[392,393]

Thoracic Radiotherapy for Extensive-Stage Disease

Systemic therapy is the essential element in the treatment of patients with extensive-stage SCLC with good performance status; however, thoracic radiotherapy may play a role in selected patients. Based on the observation that patients have high rates of thoracic relapse after systemic therapy alone, a single-institution prospective randomized trial was undertaken in Yugoslavia.[381] In this trial, 209 patients with extensive disease were enrolled and treated with three cycles of EP. Of those, 110 patients who had a partial response in the chest and a complete response outside the chest were randomized to receive thoracic radiation with concurrent carboplatin and etoposide, followed by two cycles of EP, versus four further cycles of EP alone. All eligible patients received PCI. The thoracic radiation was delivered in 54 Gy in 36 fractions over 12 days. At 5 years, the OS was higher in the arm that featured thoracic radiation: 9% versus 4%. Thoracic radiotherapy in extensive-stage disease is currently the subject of at least two prospective trials. RTOG 0937 is a randomized phase II study in patients with extensive disease who have no more than three extrathoracic sites of disease; patients are randomized to receive 45 Gy of thoracic radiation in 30 twice-daily fractions followed by PCI, versus PCI alone, after chemotherapy. In the Chest Irradiation in Extensive Stage Small Cell Lung Cancer (CREST) trial conducted by the Dutch Lung Cancer Study Group, patients with extensive-stage disease who respond to chemotherapy are randomized to thoracic radiotherapy (30 Gy in 10 fractions) and PCI versus PCI alone. The results of these trials will help to clarify the role of thoracic radiotherapy in extensive-stage disease.

Prophylactic Cranial Irradiation

Brain metastases are present at diagnosis in approximately 20% of patients with SCLC. The brain is also a frequent site of failure after chemotherapy for extensive disease or chemoradiotherapy for limited-stage disease. Several randomized trials have addressed the value of PCI following a response to initial therapy and have consistently demonstrated a decrease in the incidence of brain metastases. A meta-analysis reported the results of 987 patients treated in seven randomized trials enrolling between 1977 and 1995.[394] Here, 85% of these patients had limited stage and 15% extensive. All were randomized to either PCI or to observation following a complete response to initial therapy, although response was most commonly assessed by chest x-ray rather than CT scan. PCI regimens varied from 8 Gy in a single fraction to 40 Gy in 20 fractions. At 3 years, PCI was found to significantly decrease the incidence of brain metastases (59% vs. 33%) and significantly improve OS (21% vs. 15%). There was trend toward improved brain control when PCI was administered earlier and at higher dose. The publication of this study demonstrated the value of PCI in limited-stage SCLC. PCI in extensive-stage SCLC was specifically addressed in a more recent randomized trial conducted by the EORTC. In this trial, 286 patients with extensive-stage SCLC were randomized to either PCI or observation after any response to four to six cycles of chemotherapy. Those assigned to the PCI arm were treated within 4 to 6 weeks of completing systemic therapy. Of note, this study did not require baseline brain imaging, nor did it require repeat brain imaging prior to initiation of PCI. The 1-year cumulative incidence of brain metastases was significantly decreased in the PCI arm at 15% versus 40%, and 1-year OS was significantly increased in the PCI arm at 27% versus 13%. Six different PCI regimens were permitted, with biologically effective dose ranging from 25 to 39 Gy.

Despite the survival benefit reported in the Auperin meta-analysis and the EORTC trial in extensive-stage disease, a variety of dose and fractionation schemes were employed to treat the patients enrolled in the trials. To help define the optimal dose and fractionation for PCI, a multi-institutional intergroup trial was launched to examine standard-dose PCI versus high-dose PCI. Patients with limited-stage SCLC who had achieved a complete response to chemoradiotherapy were randomized to receive PCI in standard dose, 25 Gy in 10 daily fractions, or high-dose, 36 Gy in either 18 daily fractions or 24 twice-daily fractions.[395] In this study, 720 patients were randomized; at 2 years, the cumulative incidence of brain metastases was not significantly different between the two arms: 29% in the standard dose arm versus 23% for high dose. Surprisingly, there was poorer OS in the high-dose arm: 2-year survival was 42% in the standard dose arm versus 36% for high dose. This was attributed to a higher cancer-related mortality in the high-dose arm. Patients enrolled in this trial participated in baseline and follow-up neuropsychological test batteries along with QOL assessments. Wolfson et al.[396] recently reported the results of these assessments and observed an increased incidence of chronic neurotoxicity at 12 months after PCI in the 36-Gy cohort ($p = .02$). Taken together, these results establish 2.5 Gy in 10 fractions as the current preferred regimen to deliver PCI.

NORMAL TISSUE TOXICITY

The risk and severity of radiation toxicity in normal tissue are related to the dose and volume irradiated, as well as the functional organization of the OAR. In serial tissue such as spinal cord, esophagus, and trachea and bronchi, injury of any one organ subunit may result in total organ dysfunction. Therefore, high dose to even small volumes can lead to significant toxicity. In parallel tissues, such as lung, dysfunction of any one organ subunit leads to partial organ dysfunction. In this case, the volume irradiated, even to lower doses, plays a larger role.

Emami et al.[397] published partial-volume organ tolerances for normal tissue that served for more than a decade as the standard source for radiation dose limits. Dose limits were defined for specific toxicity end points, using a 5% complication rate at 5 years ($TD_{5/5}$) or 50% complication rate at 5 years ($TD_{50/5}$). These parameters were based predominantly on clinical data from 2D radiotherapy planning. Recently, a multidisciplinary effort was undertaken, the Quantitative Analysis of Normal Tissue Effects in the Clinic (QUANTEC), to summarize the published 3D dose-volume/toxicity data in the literature, review NTCP modeling, and provide practical guidance for the clinician[263,264] (Table 51.11).

Lung

Clinically significant pneumonitis occurs in 5% to 20% of patients receiving radiation for lung cancer and is one of the key dose-limiting factors in radiation planning for patients with locally advanced disease. RP may occur during fractionated treatment or up to 18 months afterward, with a peak incidence at 2 to 6 months posttreatment. The most common clinical

TABLE 51.11 DOSE-VOLUME CONSTRAINTS FOR NORMAL TISSUES USING STANDARD FRACTIONATION TO TARGET VOLUME AND TRADITIONAL ESTIMATES OF NORMAL TISSUE TOLERANCE OF THERAPEUTIC IRRADIATION

		SBRT[a]						$TD_{5/5}$ Volume[b] (Gy)		$TD_{50/5}$ Volume[b] (Gy)				
Organ	*Conventional RT Alone*	*Number Fx*	*Vol (mL)*	*Vol Max (Gy)*	*Point Max (Gy)*	*Chemo/RT*	*Chemo/RT, Then Surgery*	*1/3*	*2/3*	*3/3*	*1/3*	*2/3*	*3/3*	*Selected TD End Point*
Brachial plexus	–	1	3	14.4	16	–	–	62	61	60	77	70	75	Clinical nerve damage
		3		7.5/fx	8/fx									
		5		6/fx	6.4/fx									
Cord[c]	50 Gy	1	0.25	10	14	45 Gy	45 Gy	50	50	47	70	70	-	Myelitis
		3		6/fx	7.3/fx									
		5		4.5/fx	6/fx									
Esophagus	D_{max} <75 Gy V_{60} <50%	1	5	14.5	19	D_{max} <75 Gy V_{55} <50%	D_{max} <75 Gy V_{55} <50%	60	58	55	72	70	68	Stricture/perforation/fistula
		3		7/fx	9/fx									
		5		5.5/fx	7/fx									
Heart	V_{40} <50%	1	15	16	22	Same as RT alone	Same as RT alone	60	45	40	70	55	50	Pericarditis
		3		8/fx	10/fx									
		5		6.4/fx	7.6/fx									
Kidney[d]	20 Gy[e]	1	<66% (200)[f]	10.6 (8.4)		Same as RT alone	Same as RT alone	50	30	23	-	40	28	Clinical nephritis
		3		6.2/fx (4.8/fx)										
		5		4.6/fx (3.5/fx)										
Liver	30 Gy (<40%)	1	700	9.1		Same as RT alone	Same as RT alone	50	35	30	55	45	40	Liver failure
		3		5.7/fx										
		5		4.2/fx										
Lung[g]	MLD <20 Gy V_{20} <40%	1	1,000	7.4		MLD <20 Gy V_{20} <35% V_{10} <45% V_5 <65%	MLD <20 Gy V_{20} <20% V_{10} <40% V_{40} <55%	45	30	17.5	65	40	24.5	Pneumonitis
		3		3.8/fx										
		5		2.7/fx										

RT, radiation therapy; SBRT, stereotactic body radiation therapy; Fx, fractions; Vol, volume; Max, maximum; Chemo, chemotherapy; TD, tolerance dose; MLD, mean lung dose.

[a]Hypofractionation dose constraints not validated by long-term follow-up.[458]

[b]$TD_{5/5}$ and $TD_{50/5}$ represent the estimated dose for each organ volume or partial organ volume resulting in a 1% to 5% risk and a 50% risk, respectively, at 5 years.[397]

[c]The chance of spinal cord damage is increased as treated volume is increased. Physicians should consider off cord earlier if a significant amount of spinal cord has received constraints dose. In general, spinal cord should not receive dose >60 Gy even in very limited volume. Higher fraction size of radiation or higher daily dose will decrease the tolerance. If the patient is treated with 3 Gy per fraction, the cord constraint should be around 40 Gy (based on biologic effective dose calculation).

[d]Consider a kidney scan if the large volume of one kidney will be treated to a high dose.

[e]Less than 50% of combined both kidneys, or <75% of one side of kidney if another kidney is not functional.

[f]First constraint applies to bilateral kidney hilum and vascular trunk. Second parenthetical constraint applies to bilateral kidney cortices.

[g]For patients receiving concurrent chemo/RT, V_{15} may also be an important parameter to be considered. V_{20} = effective lung volume (total lung volume – GTV) received ≥20 Gy.

presentation includes a persistent nonproductive cough, dyspnea, low-grade fever, and fatigue. Chest x-ray or CT scan may be normal, or, depending on the time course, there may be ground glass opacification (within 2 to 6 months), patchy consolidation (4 to 12 months), or fibrosis (10 months or more) that loosely corresponds to the radiation field. Pulmonary function testing shows reduced lung volumes, tidal volumes, and diffusion capacity.

A variety of dose-volume models have been evaluated as predictive metrics of RP, including threshold volumes (i.e., V_{dose}), MLD, and Lyman-Kutcher-Burman NTCP models. MLD and dose-volume threshold models are more widely used because of their simplicity, and MLD-based risk assessment for RP correlates closely to that calculated using NTCP modeling. A logistic regression of RP versus MLD and the cross-correlation of various V_{dose} parameters suggest a gradual increase in dose response, with no safe threshold dose below which the risk of RP is zero.[265]

From collected data in the QUANTEC effort, the risk of RP is <20% when the MLD is less than approximately 20 Gy with conventional fractionation. With regard to V_{dose} threshold models, where the volume of lung outside of the GTV or PTV receiving a threshold dose is quantified, individual data sets have found different thresholds to be optimal, reflecting the interdependence of the dosimetric parameters as well as differences in technique and the specific clinical end point used. The risk of RP is <20% for V_{20} <30 to 35 Gy or V_5 <60% with conventional fractionation.

All models of conventional fractionation are extrapolated from data sets using standard, simple planning techniques and may have lower predictive power for IMRT, proton therapy, or hypofractionated radiotherapy. Several reports indicate a lower risk of pneumonitis than dose-volume metrics would predict when IMRT is used.[398,399] Caution is warranted when using IMRT and absolute dose-volume thresholds, because planning algorithms may meet strict dosimetric constraints at the cost of higher dose at other, unconstrained cut points. IMRT for the treatment of mesothelioma after pneumonectomy has been associated with an unexpectedly high risk of severe RP and therefore warrants particular care.[400]

RP occurs less commonly after SBRT in comparison to conventionally fractionated radiation.[401] The risk of symptomatic RP does seem to follow a similar relationship to dose and volume irradiated as seen in conventionally fractionated treatment,[402] although specific dose thresholds corresponding to risk thresholds have not yet been fully elucidated. In one large series, the risk of grade 2 or greater RP was 17% when the MLD was >4 Gy versus 4% for lower values and 16% when the V20 was >4% versus 4% for lower values.[403] The AAPM Task Group 101 report included a first approximation of tissue dose tolerances for SBRT.[271] For bilateral lung, they recommended maximum dose to 10 and 15 cc of lung of 7.4 and 7 Gy for single-fraction SBRT, 12.4 and 11.6 Gy for three-fraction SBRT, and 13.5 and 12.5 Gy for five-fraction SBRT.

Radiotherapy-induced dyspnea may have several contributing causes, including not only RP but also radiotherapy to other thoracic OARs. Emerging evidence suggests an interaction between cardiac dose and RP,[404] or there may be additive dyspnea owing to pleural and pericardial effusions, restrictive pericarditis, cardiomyopathy, and bronchial stenosis or bronchiectasis. Bronchial toxicity has been reported with conventional radiotherapy after dose escalation,[405] and QUANTEC recommendations include the caution that doses >80 Gy to the major airways should be avoided.[265] For SBRT, the risk of bronchial stenosis is felt to be higher because of the higher biologically effective dose delivered, and this may be one cause of the reported higher risk of pulmonary toxicity when lesions near the proximal bronchi are being treated.[174] The AAPM Task Group 101 recommends maximum doses to 4 cc and maximum point doses to the proximal tracheobronchial tree of 10.5 and 20.2 Gy for single-fraction SBRT, 15 and 30 Gy for three-fraction SBRT, and 16.5 and 40 Gy for five-fraction SBRT.

Several patient- and treatment-related factors impact the risk of RP, independent of dose and volume. In a large data set derived from patients treated on RTOG trials, the risk of RP was significantly higher for tumors in the lower lung fields.[406] Older age may increase the risk of RP, and patients who continue to smoke through their radiotherapy may be at decreased risk, although the benefits of smoking cessation far outweigh any potential benefit in terms of reduction of risk of RP.[265] Several chemotherapy agents that are commonly administered to lung cancer patients are associated with an increased risk of RP, including docetaxel and gemcitabine.

Glucocorticoids are commonly used to treat developing RP, although this has not been evaluated in a prospective fashion, and the starting dose and tapering schedule are undefined. A starting dose of approximately 60 mg or 1 mg/kg of prednisone may be given for 1 to 2 weeks, followed by a slow taper over 4 to 8 weeks. Symptoms may recur when steroids are discontinued, and although it is hoped that treatment may mitigate the development of lung fibrosis, this has not been established. Prophylactic antibiotics or anticoagulants do not appear to effect the development of RP. Pentoxifylline is a xanthine derivative that improves microvascular blood flow; it was used in a single randomized trial of 40 patients undergoing breast or lung irradiation.[407] The number of patients with grade 2 or 3 pulmonary toxicity was significantly lower in the patients who received pentoxifylline (20% vs. 50%), as was the measured diffusion capacity. Amifostine has been tested in several randomized trials, with mixed results.[230,408] Captopril is an angiotensin-converting enzyme inhibitor that has been shown to reduce the development of radiation-induced fibrosis in rats, although no such protective effect has been demonstrated in humans.[409]

Esophagus

Acute esophagitis is often the most prominent symptom during fractionated radiotherapy for thoracic malignancy, leading to inpatient admissions, dehydration, weight loss, and treatment interruption. Late esophageal toxicity may include stricture, perforation, or fistula formation. Grade 3 or greater acute esophagitis (symptoms requiring hospitalization, endoscopic intervention, surgery, or treatment breaks) occurs in 15% to 25% of patients during or shortly after chemoradiation. Acute esophagitis may coexist with, and be exacerbated by, comorbid conditions such as candidiasis or reflux disease. Severe late toxicity is less common, occurring in <5% of patients,[410,411] and manifests as stenosis or, more rarely, fistula formation.

Several dose-volume metrics have been evaluated as predictors of severe esophagitis. The maximum esophageal dose correlates with symptoms, as do multiple absolute dose and volume thresholds. These are highly cross-correlated, and no consensus has been reached regarding the optimum parameter for radiotherapy planning. Circumferential measures (i.e., limits to the length of entire esophageal circumference treated to threshold dose) have also been significantly correlated with symptoms, as has the mean esophageal dose.[412,413] Two studies independently established consistent parameters for NTCP modeling of grade 2 or greater esophagitis,[412,414] suggesting that this method may be clinically useful. The QUANTEC analysis concludes that volumes treated above 40 to 50 Gy correlate with acute symptoms and suggests that no dose above prescription be allowed to even small volumes of esophagus. This latter information is especially important for heterogeneous IMRT planning.[266]

Esophageal toxicity is related to both dose and volume of irradiation, and the risk and severity are therefore also a function of the size, anatomic arrangement, and proximity of target structures. Other factors identified as increasing the risk or severity of acute esophagitis include the use of accelerated fractionation,[222] older patient age, and the use of concurrent chemotherapy.[201,205,415] Recently, an unexpectedly high risk of tracheoesophageal fistula formation was reported after radiotherapy with concurrent chemotherapy and bevacizumab.[235]

Treatment of acute esophagitis is primarily supportive care, frequently requiring topical agents, dietary changes, and narcotic pain medication. It is often prudent to evaluate patients for viral or candidal esophagitis. Patients may be treated empirically with antifungal agents or with proton pump inhibitors for comorbid reflux disease. The radioprotectant amifostine has been evaluated in several prospective trials in an effort to reduce the risk and severity of acute esophagitis. Although several small trials showed promising results,[408,416,417] no "objective" benefit (in physician-reported esophageal toxicity) was noted in a large cooperative group trial.[230] However, patient-reported outcomes suggested a significant benefit when "subjective" measures centering on swallowing function and pain control were analyzed, suggesting a key "disconnect" between physician and patient perspectives.[418] When esophageal stricture develops, it is usually reversible with repeated dilations. An esophageal fistula can be life threatening, although stenting or surgical management may restore function.

Heart

The cardiotoxicity of radiotherapy has been primarily studied after treatment for breast cancer or mediastinal lymphoma. The overall excess risk of cardiac mortality after thoracic radiotherapy is low but depends on the dose, volume, and the patient's existing cardiac risk factors.[267] Reported toxicities include acute pericarditis, which can progress to chronic pericardial fibrosis, effusion, or rarely constrictive pericarditis. Ischemic changes in the cardiac muscle can manifest after a long latency and may lead to congestive heart failure or ultimately a higher cardiac mortality. Valvular abnormalities have been reported, presumably owing to late fibrotic changes.

Most of the data regarding dose and volume tolerances for the heart are derived from patients treated for breast cancer or lymphoma, typically with distinct beam arrangements that have limited application to 3D conformal or IMRT treatment of lung malignancies. The risk of pericardial toxicity has been correlated with treatment of >50% of the heart contour in 2D planning[419] and to the volume receiving ≥30 Gy in 3D planning.[420] Perfusion studies demonstrate that late ischemic changes to cardiac tissue are also volume dependent,[421] although this has not been directly correlated to clinical outcomes. NTCP modeling has been done using both breast and lymphoma patient data; the derived parameters differ, reflecting the significant differences in technique-related cardiac exposure and underlying patient risk factors. Recommendations made as part of the QUANTEC effort reflect a conservative interpretation of the existing literature: if the V_{25} is <10%, then the excess risk of cardiac mortality attributable to ischemic changes is <1% at 15 years. The risk of pericarditis can be minimized by keeping the mean pericardial dose <26 Gy or the pericardial V_{30} <46%. Heart and pericardial exposure should otherwise be minimized without compromise of target coverage.[267]

Other clinical risk factors for cardiac mortality increasing the risk of radiotherapy-induced cardiac toxicity[422] include hypertension, diabetes, obesity, and genetic predisposition.

The risk of cardiac mortality from radiotherapy has been specifically demonstrated to be increased in patients >60 years old and by tobacco use.[423,424] The sequential use of anthracyclines increases cardiac risk in breast cancer patients, and there are some reports that concurrent paclitaxel may increase the risk.[425,426]

Brachial Plexus

Radiation brachial plexopathy is relatively poorly described with a low incidence. There are case reports of an early, transient plexopathy that occurs during or within weeks to months of radiation at relatively low dose and may resolve spontaneously.[427] Late radiation plexopathy is more clinically significant; it manifests years after radiation to the supraclavicular area with hypesthesia, paresthesia, and weakness of the affected arm and shoulder. It may progress to total paralysis of the affected arm and severe pain.

The dose tolerance of the brachial plexus is less defined than other thoracic organs, partly because of the difficulty in contouring and defining the OAR. A contouring atlas has been proposed so that more robust clinical data can be collected.[262] Peripheral nerves respond as a serial organ, thus it is thought that the maximum point dose should be predictive of plexopathy. Late plexopathy is rare in patients who have received ≤60 Gy. Proposed brachial plexus dose limits for standard, fractionated radiotherapy planning vary considerably; RTOG 0617 suggests a point maximum limit of 66 Gy. RTOG 0972/CALGB 36050 limits the V_{20} to ≤35%.

For SBRT, brachial plexopathy has been reported after treatment of apical tumors. In a series of 37 apical tumors in 36 patients treated with SBRT at Indiana University, 7 patients developed plexopathy at a median of 7 months posttreatment.[428] The cumulative risk of grade 2 to 4 plexopathy was 46% when the plexus received >26 Gy versus 8% when the plexus received ≤26 Gy. AAPM Task Group 101 recommends maximum dose to 3 cc and maximum point dose of 14 and 17.5 Gy for single-fraction SBRT, 20.4 and 24 Gy for three-fraction SBRT, and 27 and 30.5 Gy for five-fraction SBRT.[271]

Quality of Life in Lung Cancer

There has been an increased interest in health-related QOL as a clinically meaningful end point for patients with lung cancer.[429] QOL is a type of patient-reported outcome, defined as any report of the status of a patient's health condition provided directly by the patient, without interpretation of the patient's response by others. Two validated QOL instruments that include both generic and site-specific lung modules are the Functional Assessment of Cancer Therapy-Lung (FACT-L) and the EORTC QOL Questionnaire Core-30 (QLQ-C30) and QLQ-LC13.[430,431] The Lung Cancer Symptom Scale (LCSS) is a shorter (9-item) QOL instrument that is specific for lung cancer.[432]

There are many compelling reasons to study QOL in lung cancer patients. QOL end points, when used to assess the impact of palliative regimens, can identify important differences that may not have been anticipated. Recently, Temel et al.[116] assessed the impact of early palliative care on QOL (using FACT-L) among patients with newly diagnosed metastatic NSCLC[116] randomized to early palliative care or to standard care. They found that patients in the early palliative care arm not only had significant improvement in QOL, with less depression or anxiety, but also had longer median survival (p = .02), despite receiving less therapy.[116]

Another clinically relevant aspect of QOL is its ability to serve as an independent prognostic factor for survival. Movsas et al.[114] reported that the baseline QOL score independently predicted for 5-year survival in patients with stage III NSCLC treated with chemoradiation on RTOG 9801. Studies are beginning to elucidate the biologic underpinnings supporting the relationship between QOL and survival.[433] Importantly, studies have highlighted a critical "disconnect" between patient-reported outcomes and the physician-reported observations.[418] For example, RTOG 9801 was a phase III study testing whether the radioprotector amifostine would reduce the rate of chemoradiation esophagitis in patients with locally advanced NSCLC.[230] Although there was no significant difference in grade ≥3 esophagitis rates, amifostine significantly lowered patient reported swallowing dysfunction (p = .03) and pain (p = .003). To help address this "disconnect," the National Cancer Institute initiated the Patient-Reported Outcomes version of the Common Terminology Criteria for Adverse Events (PRO-CTCAE) project to create patient-reported versions of symptom criteria.

Perhaps the most important reason to study QOL is simply because patients want to be asked about their QOL. Detmar et al.[434] reported on 273 patients receiving palliative chemotherapy, as well as 10 physicians. Almost all patients wanted to discuss QOL issues; however, 25% would discuss emotional or social functioning only if the physician initiated the discussion. Patients have a clear desire to discuss QOL issues.[434,435] Ultimately, QOL should become a routine tool in the clinical care for our patients with lung cancer.

ACKNOWLEDGMENTS

The authors thank Mindy Langer for her exhaustive and critical review of the chapter. They also thank Eric Xanthopoulos for his input and assistance in the preparation of the figures and tables.

SELECTED REFERENCES

A full list of references for this chapter is available online.

38. Mujoomdar A, Austin JH, Malhotra R, et al. Clinical predictors of metastatic disease to the brain from non-small cell lung carcinoma: primary tumor size, cell type, and lymph node metastases. *Radiology* 2007;242(3):882–888.
55. Aberle DR, Adams AM, Berg CD, et al. Reduced lung-cancer mortality with low-dose computed tomographic screening. *N Engl J Med* 2011;365(5):395–409.
65. Nestle U, Walter K, Schmidt S, et al. 18F-deoxyglucose positron emission tomography (FDG-PET) for the planning of radiotherapy in lung cancer: high impact in patients with atelectasis. *Int J Radiat Oncol Biol Phys* 1999;44(3):593–597.
70. Fischer B, Lassen U, Mortensen J, et al. Preoperative staging of lung cancer with combined PET-CT. *N Engl J Med* 2009;361(1):32–39.
75. Fox JL, Rengan R, O'Meara W, et al. Does registration of PET and planning CT images decrease interobserver and intraobserver variation in delineating tumor volumes for non-small-cell lung cancer? *Int J Radiat Oncol Biol Phys* 2005;62(1):70–75.
89. Detterbeck FC, Jantz MA, Wallace M, et al. Invasive mediastinal staging of lung cancer: ACCP evidence-based clinical practice guidelines (2nd edition). *Chest* 2007;132(3 Suppl):202S–220S.
96. Sandler A, Gray R, Perry MC, et al. Paclitaxel-carboplatin alone or with bevacizumab for non-small-cell lung cancer. *N Engl J Med* 2006;355(24):2542–2550.
97. Scagliotti GV, Parikh P, von Pawel J, et al. Phase III study comparing cisplatin plus gemcitabine with cisplatin plus pemetrexed in chemotherapy-naive patients with advanced-stage non-small-cell lung cancer. *J Clin Oncol* 2008;26(21):3543–3551.
103. Kwak EL, Bang YJ, Camidge DR, et al. Anaplastic lymphoma kinase inhibition in non-small-cell lung cancer. *N Engl J Med* 2010;363(18):1693–1703.
107. Olaussen KA, Dunant A, Fouret P, et al. DNA repair by ERCC1 in non-small-cell lung cancer and cisplatin-based adjuvant chemotherapy. *N Engl J Med* 2006;355(10):983–991.
108. Lynch TJ, Bell DW, Sordella R, et al. Activating mutations in the epidermal growth factor receptor underlying responsiveness of non-small-cell lung cancer to gefitinib. *N Engl J Med* 2004;350(21):2129–2139.
114. Movsas B, Moughan J, Sarna L, et al. Quality of life supersedes the classic prognosticators for long-term survival in locally advanced non-small-cell lung cancer: an analysis of RTOG 9801. *J Clin Oncol* 2009;27(34):5816–5822.
116. Temel JS, Greer JA, Muzikansky A, et al. Early palliative care for patients with metastatic non-small-cell lung cancer. *N Engl J Med* 2010;363(8):733–742.
120. Ginsberg RJ, Rubinstein LV. Randomized trial of lobectomy versus limited resection for T1 N0 non-small cell lung cancer. Lung Cancer Study Group. *Ann Thorac Surg* 1995;60(3):615–623.
123. Darling GE, Allen MS, Decker PA, et al. Randomized trial of mediastinal lymph node sampling versus complete lymphadenectomy during pulmonary resection in the patient with N0 or N1 (less than hilar) non-small cell carcinoma: results of the American College of Surgery Oncology Group Z0030 Trial. *J Thorac Cardiovasc Surg* 2011;141(3):662–670.
127. Van Meerbeeck JP, Kramer GW, Van Schil PE, et al. Randomized controlled trial of resection versus radiotherapy after induction chemotherapy in stage IIIA-N2 non-small-cell lung cancer. *J Natl Cancer Inst* 2007;99(6):442–450.
130. Roth JA, Fossella F, Komaki R, et al. A randomized trial comparing perioperative chemotherapy and surgery with surgery alone in resectable stage IIIA non-small-cell lung cancer. *J Natl Cancer Inst* 1994;86(9):673–680.
131. Rosell R, Gomez-Codina J, Camps C, et al. A randomized trial comparing preoperative chemotherapy plus surgery with surgery alone in patients with non-small-cell lung cancer. *N Engl J Med* 1994;330(3):153–158.

134. Betticher DC, Hsu Schmitz SF, Totsch M, et al. Mediastinal lymph node clearance after docetaxel-cisplatin neoadjuvant chemotherapy is prognostic of survival in patients with stage IIIA pN2 non-small-cell lung cancer: a multicenter phase II trial. *J Clin Oncol* 2003;21(9):1752–1759.
138. Schaake-Koning C, van den Bogaert W, Dalesio O, et al. Effects of concomitant cisplatin and radiotherapy on inoperable non-small-cell lung cancer. *N Engl J Med* 1992;326(8):524–530.
140. Albain KS, Swann RS, Rusch VW, et al. Radiotherapy plus chemotherapy with or without surgical resection for stage III non-small-cell lung cancer: a phase III randomised controlled trial. *Lancet* 2009;374(9687):379–386.
148. Lally BE, Zelterman D, Colasanto JM, et al. Postoperative radiotherapy for stage II or III non-small-cell lung cancer using the surveillance, epidemiology, and end results database. *J Clin Oncol* 2006;24(19):2998–3006.
149. Douillard JY, Rosell R, De Lena M, et al. Impact of postoperative radiation therapy on survival in patients with complete resection and stage I, II, or IIIA non-small-cell lung cancer treated with adjuvant chemotherapy: the Adjuvant Navelbine International Trialist Association (ANITA) randomized trial. *Int J Radiat Oncol Biol Phys* 2008;72(3):695–701.
155. Douillard JY, Rosell R, De Lena M, et al. Adjuvant vinorelbine plus cisplatin versus observation in patients with completely resected stage IB-IIIA non-small-cell lung cancer (Adjuvant Navelbine International Trialist Association [ANITA]): a randomised controlled trial. *Lancet Oncol* 2006;7(9):719–727.
156. Pignon JP, Tribodet H, Scagliotti GV, et al. Lung Adjuvant Cisplatin Evaluation: a pooled analysis by the LACE Collaborative Group. *J Clin Oncol* 2008;26(21): 3552–3559.
158. Bradley JD, Paulus R, Graham MV, et al. Phase II trial of postoperative adjuvant paclitaxel/carboplatin and thoracic radiotherapy in resected stage II and IIIA non-small-cell lung cancer: promising long-term results of the Radiation Therapy Oncology Group—RTOG 9705. *J Clin Oncol* 2005;23(15):3480–3487.
164. Bradley J, Graham MV, Winter K, et al. Toxicity and outcome results of RTOG 9311: a phase I-II dose-escalation study using three-dimensional conformal radiotherapy in patients with inoperable non-small-cell lung carcinoma. *Int J Radiat Oncol Biol Phys* 2005;61(2):318–328.
174. Timmerman R, McGarry R, Yiannoutsos C, et al. Excessive toxicity when treating central tumors in a phase II study of stereotactic body radiation therapy for medically inoperable early-stage lung cancer. *J Clin Oncol* 2006;24(30):4833–4839.
187. Fuks Z, Leibel SA, Kutcher GJ, et al. Three-dimensional conformal treatment: a new frontier in radiation therapy. *Important Adv Oncol* 1991:151–172.
190. Rengan R, Rosenzweig KE, Venkatraman E, et al. Improved local control with higher doses of radiation in large-volume stage III non-small-cell lung cancer. *Int J Radiat Oncol Biol Phys* 2004;60(3):741–747.
192. Timmerman R, Paulus R, Galvin J, et al. Stereotactic body radiation therapy for inoperable early stage lung cancer. *JAMA* 2010;303(11):1070–1076.
196. Rosenzweig KE, Sura S, Jackson A, et al. Involved-field radiation therapy for inoperable non small-cell lung cancer. *J Clin Oncol* 2007;25(35):5557–5561.
200. Fernandes AT, Shen J, Finlay J, et al. Elective nodal irradiation (ENI) vs. involved field radiotherapy (IFRT) for locally advanced non-small cell lung cancer (NSCLC): a comparative analysis of toxicities and clinical outcomes. *Radiother Oncol* 2010;95(2):178–184.
201. Dillman RO, Herndon J, Seagren SL, et al. Improved survival in stage III non-small-cell lung cancer: seven-year follow-up of Cancer and Leukemia Group B (CALGB) 8433 trial. *J Natl Cancer Inst* 1996;88(17):1210–1215.
202. Sause WT, Scott C, Taylor S, et al. Radiation Therapy Oncology Group (RTOG) 88–08 and Eastern Cooperative Oncology Group (ECOG) 4588: preliminary results of a phase III trial in regionally advanced, unresectable non-small-cell lung cancer. *J Natl Cancer Inst* 1995;87(3):198–205.
204. Furuse K, Kubota K, Kawahara M, et al. Phase II study of concurrent radiotherapy and chemotherapy for unresectable stage III non-small-cell lung cancer. Southern Osaka Lung Cancer Study Group. *J Clin Oncol* 1995;13(4):869–875.
207. Curran W, Paulus R, Langer CJ, et al. Sequential vs. concurrent chemoradiation for stage III non-small cell lung cancer (NSCLC): randomized phase III trial RTOG 9410. *J Natl Cancer Inst* 2011;103(19):1452–1460.
208. Fournel P, Robinet G, Thomas P, et al. Randomized phase III trial of sequential chemoradiotherapy compared with concurrent chemoradiotherapy in locally advanced non-small-cell lung cancer: Groupe Lyon-Saint-Etienne d'Oncologie Thoracique-Groupe Francais de Pneumo-Cancerologie NPC 95–01 Study. *J Clin Oncol* 2005;23(25):5910–5917.
214. Sause W, Kolesar P, Taylor S, et al. Final results of phase III trial in regionally advanced unresectable non-small cell lung cancer—Radiation Therapy Oncology Group, Eastern Cooperative Oncology Group, and Southwest Oncology Group. *Chest* 2000;117(2):358–364.
217. Auperin A, Le Pechoux C, Rolland E, et al. Meta-analysis of concomitant versus sequential radiochemotherapy in locally advanced non-small-cell lung cancer. *J Clin Oncol* 2010;28(13):2181–2190.
220. Vokes EE, Herndon JE II, Kelley MJ, et al. Induction chemotherapy followed by chemoradiotherapy compared with chemoradiotherapy alone for regionally advanced unresectable stage III non-small-cell lung cancer: Cancer and Leukemia Group B. *J Clin Oncol* 2007;25(13):1698–1704.
222. Turrisi AT III, Kim K, Blum R, et al. Twice-daily compared with once-daily thoracic radiotherapy in limited small-cell lung cancer treated concurrently with cisplatin and etoposide. *N Engl J Med* 1999;340(4):265–271.
223. Gandara DR, Chansky K, Albain KS, et al. Consolidation docetaxel after concurrent chemoradiotherapy in stage IIIB non-small-cell lung cancer: phase II Southwest Oncology Group Study S9504. *J Clin Oncol* 2003;21(10):2004–2010.
224. Hanna N, Neubauer M, Yiannoutsos C, et al. Phase III study of cisplatin, etoposide, and concurrent chest radiation with or without consolidation docetaxel in patients with inoperable stage III non-small-cell lung cancer: the Hoosier Oncology Group and U.S. Oncology. *J Clin Oncol* 2008;26(35):5755–5760.
226. Choy H, Akerley W, Safran H, et al. Multiinstitutional phase II trial of paclitaxel, carboplatin, and concurrent radiation therapy for locally advanced non-small-cell lung cancer. *J Clin Oncol* 1998;16(10):3316–3322.
230. Movsas B, Scott C, Langer C, et al. Randomized trial of amifostine in locally advanced non-small-cell lung cancer patients receiving chemotherapy and hyperfractionated radiation: Radiation Therapy Oncology Group trial 98–01. *J Clin Oncol* 2005;23(10):2145–2154.
232. Govindan R, Bogart J, Stinchcombe T, et al. Randomized phase II study of pemetrexed, carboplatin, and thoracic radiation with or without cetuximab in patients with locally advanced unresectable non-small-cell lung cancer: Cancer and Leukemia Group B trial 30407. *J Clin Oncol* 2011;29(23):3120–3125.
233. Blumenschein GR Jr, Paulus R, Curran WJ, et al. Phase II study of cetuximab in combination with chemoradiation in patients with stage IIIA/B non-small-cell lung cancer: RTOG 0324. *J Clin Oncol* 2011;29(17):2312–2318.
237. Rosenman JG, Halle JS, Socinski MA, et al. High-dose conformal radiotherapy for treatment of stage IIIA/IIIB non-small-cell lung cancer: technical issues and results of a phase I/II trial. *Int J Radiat Oncol Biol Phys* 2002;54(2): 348–356.
239. Bradley J, Paulus R, Komaki R, et al. A randomized phase III comparison of standard-dose (60 Gy) versus high-dose (74 Gy) conformal chemoradiotherapy +/− cetuximab for stage IIIA/IIIB non-small cell lung cancer: preliminary findings on radiation dose in RTOG 0617. ASTRO Annual Meeting, October 2–6, 2011, Miami, FL.
243. Rusch VW, Giroux DJ, Kraut MJ, et al. Induction chemoradiation and surgical resection for superior sulcus non-small-cell lung carcinomas: long-term results of Southwest Oncology Group Trial 9416 (Intergroup Trial 0160). *J Clin Oncol* 2007;25(3):313–318.
255. Grills IS, Fitch DL, Goldstein NS, et al. Clinicopathologic analysis of microscopic extension in lung adenocarcinoma: defining clinical target volume for radiotherapy. *Int J Radiat Oncol Biol Phys* 2007;69(2):334–341.
261. Grills IS, Hugo G, Kestin LL, et al. Image-guided radiotherapy via daily online cone-beam CT substantially reduces margin requirements for stereotactic lung radiotherapy. *Int J Radiat Oncol Biol Phys* 2008;70(4):1045–1056.
264. Bentzen SM, Constine LS, Deasy JO, et al. Quantitative analyses of normal tissue effects in the clinic (QUANTEC): an introduction to the scientific issues. *Int J Radiat Oncol Biol Phys* 2010;76(3 Suppl):S3–S9.
274. Seppenwoolde Y, Shirato H, Kitamura K, et al. Precise and real-time measurement of 3D tumor motion in lung due to breathing and heartbeat, measured during radiotherapy. *Int J Radiat Oncol Biol Phys* 2002;53(4):822–834.
286. Kong FM, Ten Haken RK, Schipper MJ, et al. High-dose radiation improved local tumor control and overall survival in patients with inoperable/unresectable non-small-cell lung cancer: long-term results of a radiation dose escalation study. *Int J Radiat Oncol Biol Phys* 2005;63(2):324–333.
289. Van Herk M, Remeijer P, Rasch C, et al. The probability of correct target dosage: dose-population histograms for deriving treatment margins in radiotherapy. *Int J Radiat Oncol Biol Phys* 2000;47:1121–1135.
292. Allen AM, Czerminska M, Janne PA, et al. Fatal pneumonitis associated with intensity-modulated radiation therapy for mesothelioma. *Int J Radiat Oncol Biol Phys* 2006;65(3):640–645.
296. Chetty IJ, Curran B, Cygler JE, et al. Report of the AAPM Task Group No. 105: issues associated with clinical implementation of Monte Carlo-based photon and electron external beam treatment planning. *Med Phys* 2007;34(12): 4818–4853.
304. Chang JY, Zhang X, Wang X, et al. Significant reduction of normal tissue dose by proton radiotherapy compared with three-dimensional conformal or intensity-modulated radiation therapy in stage I or stage III non-small-cell lung cancer. *Int J Radiat Oncol Biol Phys* 2006;65(4):1087–1096.
305. Bush DA, Slater JD, Shin BB, et al. Hypofractionated proton beam radiotherapy for stage I lung cancer. *Chest* 2004;126(4):1198–1203.
307. Chang JY, Komaki R, Wen HY, et al. Toxicity and patterns of failure of adaptive/ablative proton therapy for early-stage, medically inoperable non-small cell lung cancer. *Int J Radiat Oncol Biol Phys* 2011;80(5):1350–1357.
309. Chang JY, Komaki R, Lu C, et al. Phase 2 study of high-dose proton therapy with concurrent chemotherapy for unresectable stage III nonsmall cell lung cancer. *Cancer* 2011 Mar 22. doi:10.1002/cncr.26080. [Epub ahead of print]
310. Azzoli CG, Baker S Jr, Temin S, et al. American Society of Clinical Oncology Clinical Practice Guideline update on chemotherapy for stage IV non-small-cell lung cancer. *J Clin Oncol* 2009;27(36):6251–6266.
324. Schiller JH, Harrington D, Belani CP, et al. Comparison of four chemotherapy regimens for advanced non-small-cell lung cancer. *N Engl J Med* 2002;346(2): 92–98.
329. Langer CJ, Manola J, Bernardo P, et al. Cisplatin-based therapy for elderly patients with advanced non-small-cell lung cancer: implications of Eastern Cooperative Oncology Group 5592, a randomized trial. *J Natl Cancer Inst* 2002; 94(3):173–181.
332. Shepherd FA, Dancey J, Ramlau R, et al. Prospective randomized trial of docetaxel versus best supportive care in patients with non-small-cell lung cancer previously treated with platinum-based chemotherapy. *J Clin Oncol* 2000;18(10): 2095–2103.
334. Shepherd FA, Rodrigues Pereira J, Ciuleanu T, et al. Erlotinib in previously treated non-small-cell lung cancer. *N Engl J Med* 2005;353(2):123–132.
335. Hanna N, Shepherd FA, Fossella FV, et al. Randomized phase III trial of pemetrexed versus docetaxel in patients with non-small-cell lung cancer previously treated with chemotherapy. *J Clin Oncol* 2004;22(9):1589–1597.
336. Ciuleanu T, Brodowicz T, Zielinski C, et al. Maintenance pemetrexed plus best supportive care versus placebo plus best supportive care for non-small-cell lung cancer: a randomised, double-blind, phase 3 study. *Lancet* 2009;374(9699): 1432–1440.
337. Patel JD, Hensing TA, Rademaker A, et al. Phase II study of pemetrexed and carboplatin plus bevacizumab with maintenance pemetrexed and bevacizumab as first-line therapy for nonsquamous non-small-cell lung cancer. *J Clin Oncol* 2009;27(20):3284–3289.
338. Fidias PM, Dakhil SR, Lyss AP, et al. Phase III study of immediate compared with delayed docetaxel after front-line therapy with gemcitabine plus carboplatin in advanced non-small-cell lung cancer. *J Clin Oncol* 2009;27(4):591–598.
342. Mok TS, Wu YL, Thongprasert S, et al. Gefitinib or carboplatin-paclitaxel in pulmonary adenocarcinoma. *N Engl J Med* 2009;361(10):947–57.
346. Zhou C, Wu YL, Chen G, et al. Erlotinib versus chemotherapy as first-line treatment for patients with advanced EGFR mutation-positive non-small-cell lung cancer (OPTIMAL, CTONG-0802): a multicentre, open-label, randomised, phase 3 study. *Lancet Oncol* 2011;12(8):735–742.
350. Shaw AT, Yeap BY, Mino-Kenudson M, et al. Clinical features and outcome of patients with non-small-cell lung cancer who harbor EML4-ALK. *J Clin Oncol* 2009;27(26):4247–4253.
358. Reinfuss M, Mucha-Malecka A, Walasek T, et al. Palliative thoracic radiotherapy in non-small cell lung cancer. An analysis of 1250 patients. Palliation of symptoms, tolerance and toxicity. *Lung Cancer* 2011;71(3):344–349.
360. Rodrigues G, Videtic G, Sur R, et al. Palliative thoracic radiotherapy in lung cancer. An American Society for Radiation Oncology evidence-based clinical practice guideline. *Pract Radiat Oncol* 2011;1(2):60–71.

362. Ung YC, Yu E, Falkson C, et al. The role of high-dose-rate brachytherapy in the palliation of symptoms in patients with non-small-cell lung cancer: a systematic review. *Brachytherapy* 2006;5(3):189–202.
365. Wilson LD, Detterbeck FC, Yahalom J. Clinical practice. Superior vena cava syndrome with malignant causes. *N Engl J Med* 2007;356(18):1862–1869.
366. Schraufnagel DE, Hill R, Leech JA, et al. Superior vena caval obstruction. Is it a medical emergency? *Am J Med* 1981;70(6):1169–1174.
369. Govindan R, Page N, Morgensztern D, et al. Changing epidemiology of small-cell lung cancer in the United States over the last 30 years: analysis of the surveillance, epidemiologic, and end results database. *J Clin Oncol* 2006;24(28):4539–4544.
371. Slotman B, Faivre-Finn C, Kramer G, et al. Prophylactic cranial irradiation in extensive small-cell lung cancer. *N Engl J Med* 2007;357(7):664–672.
374. Bradley JD, Dehdashti F, Mintun MA, et al. Positron emission tomography in limited-stage small-cell lung cancer: a prospective study. *J Clin Oncol* 2004; 22(16):3248–3254.
378. Tsuchiya R, Suzuki K, Ichinose Y, et al. Phase II trial of postoperative adjuvant cisplatin and etoposide in patients with completely resected stage I-IIIa small cell lung cancer: the Japan Clinical Oncology Lung Cancer Study Group Trial (JCOG9101). *J Thorac Cardiovasc Surg* 2005;129(5):977–983.
380. Arriagada R, Pignon JP, Ihde DC, et al. Effect of thoracic radiotherapy on mortality in limited small cell lung cancer. A meta-analysis of 13 randomized trials among 2,140 patients. *Anticanc Res* 1994;14(1B):333–335.
381. Jeremic B, Shibamoto Y, Nikolic N, et al. Role of radiation therapy in the combined-modality treatment of patients with extensive disease small-cell lung cancer: a randomized study. *J Clin Oncol* 1999;17(7):2092–2099.
382. Auperin A, Arriagada R, Pignon JP, et al. Prophylactic cranial irradiation for patients with small-cell lung cancer in complete remission. Prophylactic Cranial Irradiation Overview Collaborative Group. *N Engl J Med* 1999;341(7):476–484.
385. Fried DB, Morris DE, Poole C, et al. Systematic review evaluating the timing of thoracic radiation therapy in combined modality therapy for limited-stage small-cell lung cancer. *J Clin Oncol* 2004;22(23):4837–4845.
386. Turrisi AT III. Limited-disease small-cell lung cancer research: sense and nonsense. *Int J Radiat Oncol Biol Phys* 2004;59(4):925–927.
396. Wolfson AH, Bae K, Komaki R, et al. Primary analysis of a phase ii randomized trial Radiation Therapy Oncology Group (RTOG) 0212: impact of different total doses and schedules of prophylactic cranial irradiation on chronic neurotoxicity and quality of life for patients with limited-disease small-cell lung cancer. *Int J Radiat Oncol Biol Phys* 2011;81(1):77–84.
397. Emami B, Lyman J, Brown A, et al. Tolerance of normal tissue to therapeutic irradiation. *Int J Radiat Oncol Biol Phys* 1991;21(1):109–122.
400. Miles EF, Larrier NA, Kelsey CR, et al. Intensity-modulated radiotherapy for resected mesothelioma: the Duke experience. *Int J Radiat Oncol Biol Phys* 2008; 71(4):1143–1150.
407. Ozturk B, Egehan I, Atavci S, et al. Pentoxifylline in prevention of radiation-induced lung toxicity in patients with breast and lung cancer: a double-blind randomized trial. *Int J Radiat Oncol Biol Phys* 2004;58(1):213–219.
449. Koto M, Takai Y, Ogawa Y, et al. A phase I/II study on stereotactic body radiotherapy for stage I non-small cell lung cancer. *EJC Suppl* 2007;5(4):380.
454. Le Chevalier T, Arriagada R, Quoix E, et al. Radiotherapy alone versus combined chemotherapy and radiotherapy in nonresectable non-small-cell lung cancer: first analysis of a randomized trial in 353 patients. *J Natl Cancer Inst* 1991;83 (6):417–423.
456. Belani CP, Choy H, Bonomi P, et al. Combined chemoradiotherapy regimens of paclitaxel and carboplatin for locally advanced non-small-cell lung cancer: a randomized phase II locally advanced multi-modality protocol. *J Clin Oncol* 2005; 23(25):5883–5891.

Chapter 52
Mediastinal and Tracheal Cancer

Daniel R. Gomez, C. David Fuller, Sravana Chennupati, and Charles R. Thomas, Jr.

MEDIASTINAL TUMORS

Mediastinal malignancies are quite heterogenous in scope. Invasive thymomas and thymic carcinomas are relatively rare tumors, together representing about 0.2% to 1.5% of all malignancies.[1] Thymic carcinomas are rare, accounting for only 0.06% of all thymic neoplasms.[2] Arising from thymic, neurogenic, lymphatic, germinal, and mesenchymal tissues, mediastinal tumors are usually located in the anterior mediastinum but can also appear in the posterior and middle mediastinum or neck. Lymphomas, the most common type of mediastinal tumor, are discussed in detail in Chapter 89.

Anatomically, the mediastinum is trapezoidal in shape and is essentially the center of the thoracic cavity. It extends from the sternum anteriorly to the vertebral column posteriorly. The lungs and parietal pleurae are the lateral borders, the diaphragm is the floor, and the thoracic outlet of T1, its rib, and the manubrium form the roof of the mediastinum.[3] Conceptually, the mediastinum can be subdivided into three compartments (Fig. 52.1), but no anatomic barriers physically separate the compartments.[4–5,6] The anterior mediastinum is the space anterior to the pericardium and great vessels and is occupied by the thymus, lymph nodes, and small vessels. The middle mediastinum is comprised of the heart, proximal great vessels, central airway structures, and lymph nodes. Tracheal anatomy is depicted in Figure 52.2. The posterior mediastinum is posterior to the heart and great vessels and contains the sympathetic chain ganglia, vagus nerve, thoracic duct, and esophagus. Neoplastic masses that occur within the various compartments in the mediastinum are listed in Table 52.1.

Incidence of Primary Mediastinal Tumors

The frequency and prevalence of primary mediastinal tumors seem to be increasing over time.[7–10] Adults generally develop thymic tumors and lymphomas, but they can also develop germ cell tumors and carcinomas.[10,11] Neurogenic tumors are usually seen in children.[8,12,13]

THYMOMAS

The thymus gland is an irregular lobulated lymphoepithelial organ in the anterior mediastinum. Embryologically, the thymus is derived from the endoderm of the lower portion of the

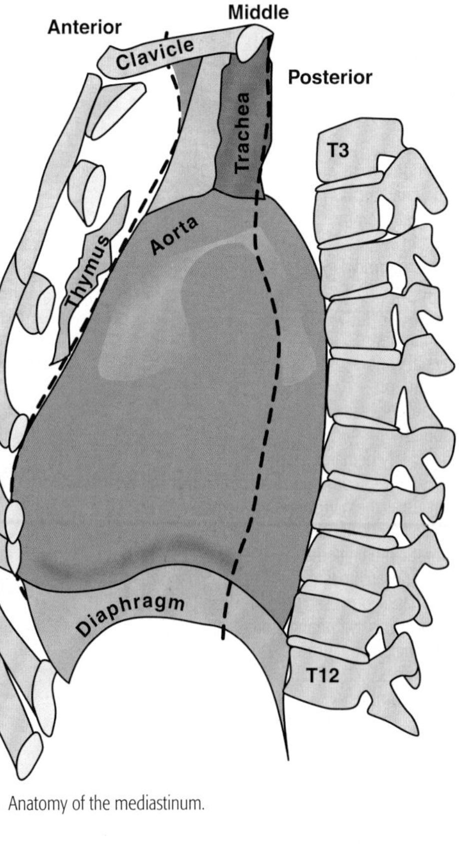

FIGURE 52.1. Anatomy of the mediastinum.

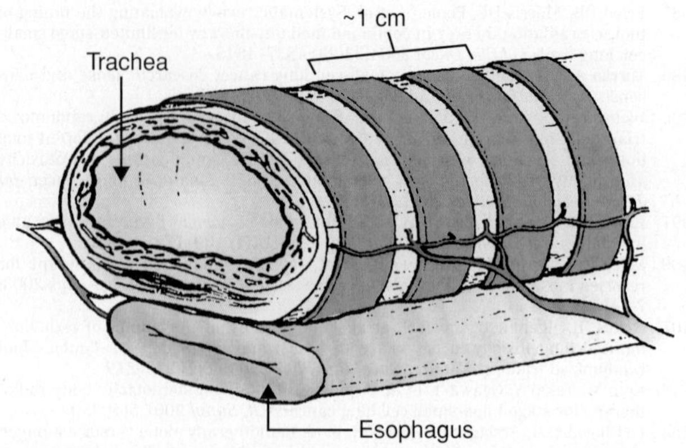

FIGURE 52.2. Representative schema of the trachea. Note the lateral longitudinal anastomotic artery running parallel to the organ and the intercartilaginous branches feeding each tracheal segment. The trachea resides in close proximity to the esophagus.

third pharyngeal pouch and involutes during adulthood, gradually being replaced by adipose tissue. The blood supply is from the internal mammary arteries. The venous drainage is to the innominate and internal thoracic veins. The lymphatics drain into the lower cervical, internal mammary, and hilar nodes.

The vast majority of thymic tumors are thymomas, 90% of which are found in the anterosuperior mediastinum; other variants occur in the middle and posterior mediastinum or neck.[14] Thymomas are epithelial tumors associated with an exuberant lymphoid component composed of immature cortical thymocytes. Although lymphomas, carcinoid tumors, and germ cell tumors can all arise within the thymus, only thymomas, thymic carcinomas, and thymolipomas arise from true thymic elements.

Epidemiology

Thymomas are exceedingly rare. The Surveillance, Epidemiology, and End Results (SEER) project reported the thymoma incidence to be 0.15 per 100,000 person-years.[15] For patients with associated myasthenia gravis, the peak age is in the fourth decade, whereas for patients without myasthenia gravis, the peak age is in the seventh decade or later.[16,17–18,19–21] According to the SEER data, the incidence of thymoma increases into the eighth decade of age and then decreases.[15] Thymomas are more common in men than in women (P = .007) and are most common among Asians or Pacific Islanders (0.49 per 100,000 person-years).

Thymomas are the most common of the anterior mediastinal masses, accounting for about 30% of all such masses.[8,9–10,14,22,23] Of all mediastinal masses, thymomas represent 20% of the tumors in adults[6,11,24,25] and 15% in pediatric populations.[14] Associations of thymomas with Epstein-Barr virus, lymphoepitheliomas, radiation exposure, and cytogenetic abnormalities have been suggested.[26–32]

Natural History

Thymomas are generally characterized by an indolent growth pattern that can be locally invasive. Thirty percent to 40% of patients with a thymoma also have myasthenia gravis.[33] The vast majority of thymomas are cytologically bland tumors and approximately half of them are noninvasive.[10,21,34–36,37,38–44] Roughly one-third of thymomas are asymptomatic and found incidentally on chest x-rays.[40,41,45] Of the symptomatic thymomas, about 40% of cases present with symptoms relating to impingement by the intrathoracic mass, ranging from cough, chest pain, dyspnea, hoarseness, superior vena cava obstruction, and even tumor hemorrhage.[46] Another 30% present with systemic signs and the remainder present with signs of myasthenia gravis.

Thymomas are associated with several parathymic syndromes, the most common of which is myasthenia gravis[47,48]; other autoimmune conditions such as benign cytopenia, hypogammaglobulinemia, and polymyositis have been reported in 2% to 5% of patients.[16,19,47,48–50] Myasthenia gravis is characterized by the presence of antibodies that react with nicotinic acetylcholine receptors in muscle and disrupt transmission at the neuromuscular junction.[51] The cardinal features are weakness and fatigability of skeletal muscles, with most patients first experiencing fatigue in the ocular

TABLE 52.1 HISTOLOGIES OF TUMORS APPEARING IN THE VARIOUS COMPARTMENTS OF THE MEDIASTINUM

Anterior (Anterosuperior)	*Middle*	*Posterior*
Thymic tumors	Lymphomas	Lymphomas
Thymomas	Cysts	Neurogenic tumors
Thymic carcinomas	Bronchogenic	Peripheral nerves
Thymic cysts	Foregut	Malignant peripheral nerve sheath tumors
Carcinoids	Pericardial	
Thymolipomas	Thoracic duct	Schwannomas
Lymphomas	Meningoceles	Neurosarcomas
Hodgkin lymphoma	Mesenchymal tumors	Sympathetic ganglia
Non-Hodgkin lymphoma	Tracheal tumors	Ganglioneuroblastomas
Undifferentiated	Carcinomas	Ganglioneuromas
Germ cell tumors	Cardiac and pericardial tumors	Neuroblastomas
Seminomas		Paraganglia
Nonseminomas	Hernias	Paragangliomas
Embryonal carcinomas	Hiatal	Mesenchymal tumors
Choriocarcinomas	Morgagni	Endocrine tumors
Mixed germ cell tumors	Vascular tumors	Esophageal tumors and cysts
Teratomas (dermoid cysts)	Ascending aortic	Hiatal hernias
Endocrine tumors	Transverse arch	Lateral thoracic meningoceles
Parathyroid adenomas	Descending aortic	
Thyroid tumors	Great vessels	
Mesenchymal tumors	Lymphadenopathy	
Amyloid tumors	Inflammatory	
Castleman's disease	Granulomatous	
Chordomas	Sarcoidosis	
Extramedullary hematopoesis		
Fibromas, fibrosarcomas, malignant fibrous histiocytoma		
Hemangiomas, hemangioendotheliomas, hemangiopericytomas		
Intrathoracic meningioma		
Lipomas, liposarcomas		
Leiomyomas, leiomyosarcomas, leiomyoblastomas		
Lymphangiomas, lymphangiosarcoma, lymphangiomyomatosis		
Mesotheliomas		
Mesenchymomas		
Myxomas		
Rhabdomyosarcomas, rhabdomyomas		
Xanthogranulomas		
Morgagni hernias		

muscles followed by ptosis and diplopia and later developing generalized weakness. More severe cases involve the proximal limb girdle muscles and, in the worst cases, can even affect respiration.[52–53,54] Myasthenia gravis occurs in approximately 45% of patients with thymomas, with the reported prevalence in studies involving more than 100 patients ranging from 10% to 67%.[17,18,20,21,55,56] Conversely, only 10% to 15% of patients with myasthenia gravis have a thymoma.[18,51,57] Roughly one-fourth of patients with myasthenia gravis will have a normal thymus.[58] Of the 75% who have an abnormal thymus, only 15% to 20% will have a thymoma and 60% will have thymic lymphoid hyperplasia.[59] Thymectomy results in clinical improvement in most cases even when the thymus is normal.[60]

Other systemic symptoms occur in 5% to 10% of patients with thymomas as part of a constellation of autoimmune disorders. Souadjian et al.,[47] in reviewing more than 500 cases of thymoma, noted that 71% were associated with systemic disease. These include erythroid and neutrophil hypoplasia, pancytopenia, Cushing syndrome, DiGeorge syndrome, carcinoid syndrome, Lambert-Eaton syndrome, pernicious anemia, nephrotic syndrome, syndrome of inappropriate antidiuretic hormone hypersecretion, Whipple's disease, lupus erythematosus, pemphigus, myotonic dystrophy, scleroderma, polymyositis, polyneuritis, myocarditis polyarthropathy, myotonic dystrophy, Sjogren syndrome, Addison's disease, panhypopituitarism, sarcoidosis, hypogammaglobulinemia, ulcerative colitis, rheumatoid arthritis, Hashimoto's thyroiditis, hyperthyroidism, hyperparathyroidism, and thyroid carcinoma.[14,61–63,64] Other miscellaneous diseases include hypertrophic osteoarthropathy and chronic mucocutaneous candidiasis.[63]

Several studies have also reported an average excess risk of developing a second primary malignancy of 15% for patients with thymomas over that expected in the normal population.[47,49,50,65–67] In one study, the most notable excess risk of subsequent malignancy was for non-Hodgkin lymphoma, with digestive system and soft tissue sarcomas being elevated as well.[15]

The vast majority of thymomas are indolent, but if the tumors spread, they most commonly implant on regional pleural surfaces and can cause pleural plaques, diaphragmatic masses, and malignant pleural effusions.[16] The rate of lymphogenous metastasis in one of the largest databases of 1,093 patients with thymomas was 1.8%, with 90% of positive lymph nodes located in the anterior mediastinum.[68] Only rarely do thymomas spread hematogenously, but metastases have been reported in the liver, lung, and bone.[69]

Diagnosis

Thymic tumors account for 50% of all anterior mediastinal masses, another 25% are lymphomas, and the remainder are various other tumors (see Table 52.1).[10] The latter group often has characteristic radiographic findings (e.g., teratomas). Lymphomas often have other suggestive systemic symptoms or clinical findings such as weight loss, fevers, and lymphadenopathy.

Biopsy can be performed via a fine-needle aspiration, bronchoscopy, mediastinoscopy, video-assisted thoracoscopy, or open biopsy. Often a clinical diagnosis is sufficient for a small thymoma in a patient with a parathymic syndrome. Traditionally, biopsies were avoided because of concern about tumor spillage into the pleural space when the capsule was breached.[70,71] However, no cases of seeding of a needle tract or the biopsy site have been reported, and only three recurrences in thoracotomy scars have been reported.[72,73] A multivariate analysis in one series of 136 patients being treated for thymomas showed better survival among patients who underwent biopsy before surgery (P = .056).[50] Many centers routinely obtain biopsy samples of larger tumors.[18,49,72,74,75–77]

The diagnostic workup begins with a careful evaluation for myasthenia gravis. Routine blood work for common associated syndromes should be done, with serum α-fetoprotein and β-human chorionic gonadotropin in men to rule out a germ cell tumor.[78] Computed tomography (CT) often allows visualization of an anterior mediastinal mass.[43,79–81] Magnetic resonance imaging (MRI) can provide more detail when needed, delineating the musculoskeletal anatomy and neurovascular structures of the mediastinum.[82,83,84] The use of 18 fluorodeoxyglucose (^{18}F) positron emission tomography (PET) is expanding for visualizing several types of malignancies, including thymoma. However, results of PET can be confounded by the physiologic uptake of fluorodeoxyglucose by the thymus in children and young adults.[85,86,87] Nevertheless, this imaging modality has continued to show promise for disease detection and for evaluating prognosis. Recent studies have shown that not only can PET improve the sensitivity of diagnosis, but it also can be helpful for establishing the grade of the disease.[88–89,90,91] In one provocative study in which 49 patients with thymic tumors underwent PET imaging, the rate of fluorodeoxyglucose uptake was compared with the expression of several biologic markers, including glucose transporter-1 (GLUT-1), GLUT-3, hypoxia-inducible factor-1α (HIF-1α), vascular endothelial growth factor (VEGF), microvessel density, CD31 and CD34, p53, and B-cell lymphoma-2 (bcl-2). The authors found a direct correlation between fluorodeoxyglucose uptake on PET and expression of GLUT1, HIF-1α, VEGF, and p53 as well as microvessel density, and several of these markers also correlated with tumor grade.[92] These findings are important because they imply that treatment efficacy could be monitored in terms of metabolic response. Figure 52.3 demonstrates PET findings from a patient with locally advanced thymoma treated with trimodality therapy. Imaging such as this, in conjunction with contrast-enhanced CT scans of the chest, clearly can help in precisely delineating the extent of disease.

In addition to PET, octreotide scanning has shown some efficacy for diagnosing thymic malignancies in small series.[93] MRI was also found to offer improved sensitivity and to provide information regarding tumor grade and invasiveness beyond that which can be gleaned from CT. Common features indicative of a high-grade tumor include low T2-signal foci within the mass, the presence of mediastinal lymphadenopathy, an incomplete capsule, and inhomogenous enhancement.[94,95]

Pathologic Classification

Thymomas have been extensively studied by pathologists because of their varied appearance and the frequent lack of classic malignant features. Several classification systems have been proposed and are in use (Table 52.2). Indeed, even the terminology used to describe thymomas has been inconsistent and imprecise. Thymomas have most often been considered invasive versus noninvasive or alternatively "benign" versus malignant. However, recurrences and metastases after resection have been reported in all large series,[17,18,100–102] regardless of disease stage or histologic subtype.[16,17–18,20,21,42,49,50,101–102,103,104–105,106,107–109] Even bland-appearing, noninvasive thymomas have the fundamental

TABLE 52.2 THYMOMA CLASSIFICATION SYSTEMS

Bernatz et al., 1961[96]	*Müller-Hermelink et al., 1985*[97]	*Suster and Moran, 1999*[98]	*Rosai and Sobin, 1999*[99]
Spindle Cell	Medullary	Thymoma, well-differentiated	Type A
–	Mixed		Type AB
–	Predominantly cortical		Type B1
Lymphocyte–rich Lymphoepithelial	Cortical		Type B2
Epithelial–rich	Well-differentiated thymic carcinoma	Atypical thymoma	Type B3
–	High-grade thymic carcinoma	Thymic carcinoma	Type C

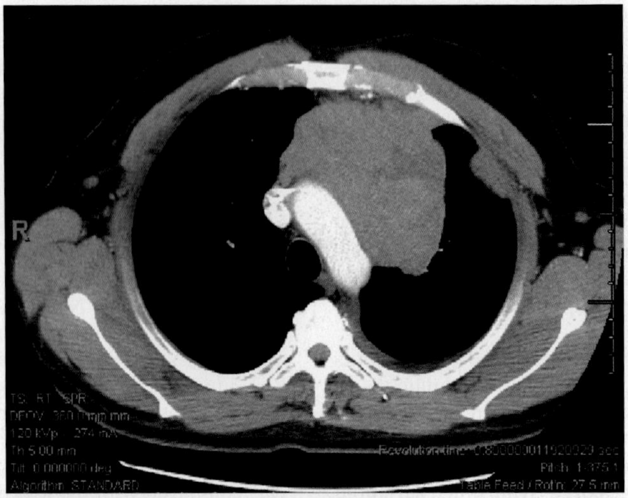

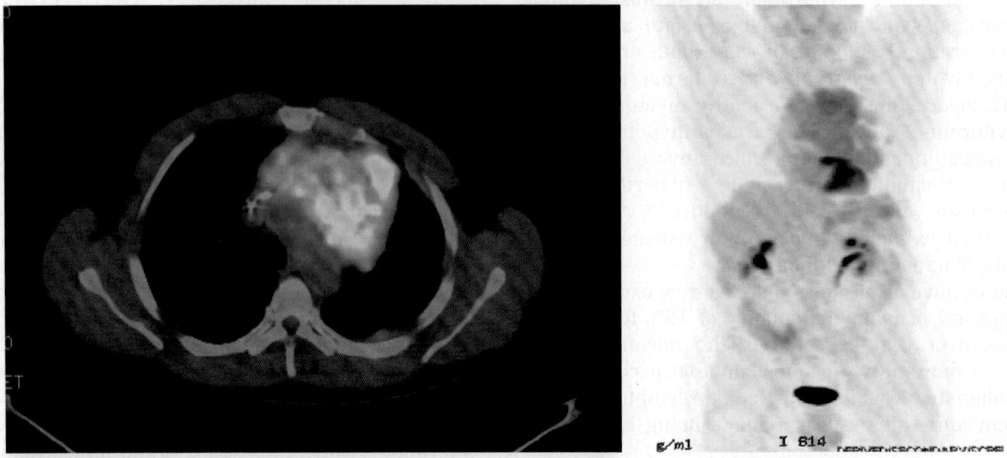

FIGURE 52.3. Positron emission tomography (PET) scanning in thymic malignancies. PET imaging has been shown to aid in delineating the extent of disease and assessing for metastases.

characteristics of a malignant tumor in their ability to recur and metastasize.

The most recent classification was proposed in 1999 and updated in 2004 by the World Health Organization (WHO).[99,110] However, a historical perspective of thymoma classification systems is necessary to interpret the literature. The earliest system, proposed by Bernatz et al.,[96] identified four categories based on predominant cell type: lymphocytic, epithelial, mixed, and spindle cell. The predominant problem with this classification system, as is true of all systems, is its poor correlation with clinical prognosis. Verley and Hollmann[101] also identified four categories: spindle or oval, lymphocyte-rich, differentiated epithelial cell–rich, and undifferentiated epithelial. The first three types are cytologically bland, whereas the fourth category includes pleomorphic tumors with high numbers of mitoses and atypia, which are also considered thymic carcinoma. Unfortunately, this categorization also does not correlate well with prognosis.

Müller-Hermelink et al.[97] based their classification system on the fact that the thymus consists of different subsets of epithelial cells: cortical, medullary, mixed cortical and medullary, and well-differentiated. Although this has been the most widely used system, little association has been found between epithelial cell morphology and prognosis.[111] Although some associations have been found, such as cortical thymomas behaving more aggressively and being more often associated with myasthenia gravis,[75,101,105,112–114] the relationship between histologic types and prognosis is not consistent.[19,76,111,115] Several multivariate analyses of large numbers of patients have shown that the Müller-Hermelink classification system is not an independent predictor of survival.[16,19,74]

Thymic carcinomas can be readily subclassified into well or poorly differentiated. Well-differentiated thymic carcinomas have features typical of thymomas but also contain areas of atypia and mitoses, but usually fewer than 2 per 10 high-power field.[116] The incidence of these tumors and the prognosis associated with them vary among studies. Poorly differentiated thymic carcinomas are clearly recognized as a distinct group. The virtual absence of parathymic syndromes and clear-cut cellular atypia are consistently associated with poor prognosis. Thymic carcinomas can be subdivided into squamous cell, mucoepidermoid, basaloid, lymphoepithelioma-like, small cell or neuroendocrine, sarcomatoid, clear cell, and undifferentiated or anaplastic subtypes.[117] Thymic carcinoid is sometimes referred to as a neuroendocrine thymic tumor because of the presence of neuroendocrine granules, but thymic carcinomas can also contain these granules.

Another problem confounding the use of these classification schemes is that they do not consistently correlate with other schemes.[111] Concordance rates for thymomas classified independently by a panel of pathologists were often as low as 35% within one system, although two small studies demonstrated 78% concordance when using the Müller-Hermelink classification system.[118,119] Considering the persistent problem of the poor correlation between the histopathology of thymomas and their malignant potential and the lack of correlation with systemic syndromes,[43] the demand for a more consistent classification is obvious.

The WHO classification is similar to the Müller-Hermelink system but recognizes six different types of thymic tumors (A, AB, B1, B2, B3, C; see Table 52.2).[110,120] Type A tumors are

TABLE 52.3 MASAOKA STAGING SYSTEM FOR THYMOMAS

Stage		Description
I		Macroscopically completely encapsulated, with no microscopic capsular invasion
II	a	Macroscopic invasion into surrounding mediastinal fatty tissue or mediastinal pleura
	b	Microscopic invasion into the capsule
III		Macroscopic invasion into surrounding organs
IV	a	Pleural or pericardial implants/dissemination
	b	Lymphagenous or hematogenous metastases

Adapted from Masaoka A, Monden Y, Nakahara K, et al. Follow-up study of thymomas with special reference to their clinical stages. *Cancer* 1981;48(11):2485–2492.

composed of neoplastic oval or spindle-shaped epithelial cells without atypia or lymphocytes. Type AB is similar to type A, but with foci of lymphocytes. Type B tumors consist of plump epithelioid cells that can be subdivided into three subtypes defined by increasing proportions of epithelial cells and increasing atypia. Type B1 tumors resemble normal thymic cortex with areas similar to thymic medulla. Type B2 have scattered neoplastic epithelial cells with vesicular nuclei and distinct nucleoli among a heavy population of lymphocytes; perivascular spaces are prominent and a palisading effect of tumor cells along the perivascular spaces may be present. Type B3 is composed of predominantly round or polygonal epithelial cells exhibiting mild atypia admixed with a minor component of lymphocytes; thus, this type resembles what others have described as well-differentiated thymic carcinoma. Thymic carcinomas are designated type C tumors and have clear-cut cytologic atypia and a cytoarchitecture resembling carcinoma that is distinctively unlike normal thymus tissue.[116]

The WHO classification has been evaluated by multiple groups since it was proposed. Concordance rates among different pathologists using the WHO system were 90% and 95% in two studies.[121,122] However, comparison of the WHO subtypes across studies demonstrated that the varying incidence of A and B subtypes was greater than could be ascribed to chance alone.[116] The most clinically distinct subtypes are type B3, formerly known as well-differentiated thymic carcinoma, and type C, thymic carcinomas. The clinical characteristics associated with the other WHO subtypes still vary considerably, but the WHO system seems to correlate well with Masaoka stage (Table 52.3) in studies in which patients were analyzed with the WHO system.[116] The vast majority of type A and AB tumors are Masaoka stage I or II, and the B subtypes tend to resemble the higher Masaoka stages.[116]

The WHO system has been found to have independent prognostic value for disease-specific survival, with only two small studies indicating that stage was the only prognostic variable.[116] Most of the prognostic value of the WHO classification is attributable to type C, having distinctly worse survival,[123–125] but even studies that excluded type C could demonstrate WHO type as having independent prognostic value.[125,126]

More recent pathologic studies have provided intriguing insights on prognostic histologic features. In one such study by Shim et al.[127] that involved assessing the effect of stromal lymphocytic infiltration in thymic carcinoma, patients with low levels of CD4+ lymphocytes and CD20+ lymphocytes within the tumor stroma were found to have lower survival rates, and various combinations of CD4+, CD8+, and CD20+ cells were particularly predictive of worse survival outcomes. These authors concluded that these lymphocytes may work together to suppress cancer progression, and that combinations of them may be useful for stratifying patients in terms of long-term prognosis.[127]

Molecular Characterization

During the past several years, pathologic classification systems for several thoracic malignancies have been improved by molecular characterization of tumors, and this innovation is relevant in thymomas as well. Several studies have shown elevated expression of the epidermal growth factor receptor (EGFR) in large percentages of thymic malignancies, as is also true for non–small cell lung cancer and other epithelial cancers.[128,129–131] However, EGFR mutations are rare in thymic malignancies,[132,133] and as a result, targeted EGFR inhibitors have not shown consistent improvements in thymic tumor response or control rates.[134,135–136] Other signaling pathways that often show overexpression are the VEGF,[137] insulin-like growth factor-1R (IGF-1R),[138] and KIT pathways,[139,140] although in most circumstances the overexpression takes place mainly in thymic carcinomas rather than thymomas. Phase I and II trials with agents targeting receptors in these pathways, like those with EGFR-targeted agents, have been largely disappointing,[141,142] although figitumumab, an anti-IGF-1R antibody, has shown efficacy in early clinical trials for advanced or refractory thymomas,[143,144] and phase II studies are ongoing. In addition, a phase II study evaluating the efficacy of the histone deacetylase inhibitor belinostat in patients with recurrent or refractory advanced thymic epithelial tumors showed that of 41 patients enrolled (25 with thymoma, 16 with thymic carcinoma), the response rate was 8%, with median times to progression and survival of 5.8 and 19.1 months, respectively. These investigators concluded that this agent had "modest" antitumor activity in this setting, but the prolonged duration of the response warranted further study.[145]

Although steroid receptor expression has been thoroughly studied in other malignancies such as breast cancer, less research on this topic has been done in thymic malignancies. Glucocorticoid receptors are known to be expressed in epithelial cells, and the delivery of glucocorticoids can induce apoptosis in thymocytes.[146,147] Indeed, prednisone has been shown to produce significant responses in patients who had not responded to other agents. A recent study evaluating the presence of glucocorticoid, estrogen, and progesterone receptors in thymomas and thymic carcinomas showed that glucocorticoid and estrogen receptors were overexpressed in 83% and 76% of thymic malignancies, and progesterone receptors were overexpressed in <1%. Glucocorticoid receptor expression was also associated with better prognosis among patients who underwent resection.[148] Studies such as these may lead to the discovery of novel, less-toxic therapies for patients with primary, metastatic, or refractory disease.

Staging

The most commonly used staging system for thymomas was published by Masaoka et al.[103] in 1981 (see Table 52.3). Staging is based on the extent of either macroscopic or microscopic invasion into mediastinal structures at the time of surgery. Other groups have tried to improve upon the Masaoka system. For example, the French Groupe d'Etudes des Tumeurs Thymiques classification (Table 52.4) incorporates completeness of resection,

TABLE 52.4 GROUPE D'ETUDES DES TUMEURS THYMIQUESTHYMOMA STAGING SYSTEM

Stage		Description
I	a	Encapsulated tumor, completely resected
	b	Macroscopically encapsulated tumor, completely resected Surgeon suspects mediastinal adhesions and potential capsular invasion
II		Invasive tumor, completely resected
III	a	Invasive tumor, subtotal resection
	b	Invasive tumor, biopsy only
IV	a	Distant pleural implants or supraclavicular metastasis
	b	Distant metastasis

From Gamondes JP, Balawi A, Greenland T, et al. Seventeen years of surgical treatment of thymoma: factors influencing survival. *Eur J Cardiothorac Surg* 1991;5(3):124–131.

TABLE 52.5 OVERALL SURVIVAL RATES FOR PATIENTS WITH THYMOMAS AT 5 AND 10 YEARS

					5-Year Survival				*10-Year Survival*			
Study (Reference)	*Institution*	*Study Years*	*n*	*% R0*	*I*	*II*	*III*	*IV*	*I*	*II*	*III*	*IV*
Kondo and Monden (55)	JACS	1990–1994	924	92	100	98	89	71	100	98	78	47
Regnard et al. (156)	ML, Paris	1955–1993	307	85	89	87	68	66	80	78	47	30
Maggi et al. (18)	Torino	Before 1991	241	88	89	71	72	59	87	60	64	40
Rena et al. (125)	Torino	1988–2000	175	84	100	100	100	100	100	100	85	–
Zhu et al. (157)	Fudan, Shanghai	1989–2002	175	89	100	96	78	57	–	–	–	–
Nakahara et al. (21)	Osaka	Before 1988	141	80	100	92	88	47	100	84	77	47
Wilkins et al. (50)	Johns Hopkins	1957–1997	136	68	84	66	63	40	75	50	44	40
Rea et al. (158)	Padua	1970–2001	132	82	93	93	60	36	84	82	51	0
Blumberg et al. (49)	MSKCC	1949–1993	118	73	95	70	50	100	86	54	26	0
Quintanilla-Martinez et al. (115)	MGH	Before 1994	116	94	100	100	70	70	100	100	60	0
Pan et al. (19)	Taipei	1961–1991	112	80	94	85	63	41	87	69	58	22
Elert et al. (159)	Wurzburg	1957–1988	102	–	83	90	46	–	–	–	–	–

R0, complete resection; JACS, Japanese Association for Chest Surgery; ML, Marie Lannelongue Hospital, Le Plessis-Robinson, France; MSKCC, Memorial Sloan-Kettering Cancer Center; MGH, Massachusetts General Hospital.

which may be of prognostic value but does not allow patients to be compared independent of treatment factors.[149]

Prognostic Factors

The two factors that have consistently demonstrated prognostic value in multivariate analyses in large studies are tumor invasiveness (i.e., disease stage) and completeness of resection.[16,17,19,20,34–36,41,49,50,74,100,103,150,151–154] Disease stage has proven important for prognosis in every large study.[16,17–18,20,21,42,49,50,100,103,155] Mean overall survival rates at 15 years are 78% for those with stage I disease, 73% stage II, 30% stage III, and 8% for stage IV (Table 52.5).[17] At 10 years, mean disease-free survival rates are 92% for those with stage I disease, 87% stage II, 60% stage III, and 35% for stage IV (recurrence rates are summarized in Table 52.6).[17,20,100,115,154]

The extent of resection is the other major factor consistently identified as being prognostic in thymic malignancies.[17,49,50,161–163] Patients for whom complete (R0) resections can be done have significantly better survival than do those with R1 or R2 resections.[103,164] R0 resections are almost always possible for stage I tumors, but resectability rates decrease on average to 50% for stage III tumors.[18,21,42,103] The WHO histology classification also was recently found to be independently associated with prognosis. Major studies reporting analyses of stage, histology, and resection status as independent predictors of survival in thymic tumors are summarized in Table 52.7.

Other potential prognostic factors are tumor size (>10 cm) and the presence of symptoms.[16,49,105] In older series, patients with parathymic syndromes such as myasthenia gravis and other autoimmune diseases fared worse than those without such syndromes,[44,49,154] but this finding has not been replicated in newer series.[17,20,21,50,75,76,103,105,152,168–170] Indeed, some studies have found survival to be better for patients with myasthenia gravis,[18,50,171] perhaps because of earlier detection of thymomas.[49,172–173,174] A study published in 2005 indicated that myasthenia gravis, present in 25% of 1,089 patients from Japan,[56] did not affect 5-year overall survival rates among patients with stage III disease. For patients with stage IV disease, 5-year overall survival rates were 85.1% for patients with myasthenia gravis versus 63.9% for patients without. R0 resection was accomplished in a significantly higher proportion of patients with myasthenia gravis (60%) than those without it (38%).

Another potential prognostic factor is patient age. Patients older than 30 to 40 years may have a better prognosis than younger patients.[16,74,154] Thymomas in children seem to follow a more malignant course than those in adults.[175] Fortunately, malignant thymomas in children are extremely rare.[176]

General Management

Surgery

Surgical resection is the mainstay of treatment for thymomas. A complete *en-bloc* surgical resection (R0) remains the treatment of choice for all thymomas regardless of invasiveness, except in rare advanced cases with extensive intrathoracic or extrathoracic metastasis. Fortunately, the vast majority (90% to 95%) of thymomas are localized.[177] Operative mortality rates average 2.5% (range, 0.7% to 4.9%).[16,17–18,21,42,49,96,159] Resectability rates for stage I thymomas should approximate

TABLE 52.6 RECURRENCE RATES OF THYMOMAS

				% Receiving			*5-Year Recurrence Rates by Stage*			
Study (Reference)	*Study Years*	*Institution*	*n*	*R0*	*Chemo*	*RT*	*I*	*II*	*III*	*IVa*
Kondo and Monden (55)	1990–1994	JACS institutions	862	100	12	32	1	4	28	34
Regnard et al. (156)	1955–1993	ML, Paris	307	85	few	half	4	7	16	58
Maggi et al. (18)	Before 1991	Torino	241	88	7	12	2	13	30	25
Wright et al. (160)	1972–2003	MGH	179	90	–	–	0	0	22	41
Rena et al. (125)	1988–2000	Torino	178	84	13	43	1.6	8.6	28	40
Zhu et al. (157)	1989–2002	Fudan, Shanghai	175	80	14	97	4	2.4	43	57
Cowen et al. (22)	1979–1990	FNCLCC	149	42	100	50	0	7	23	25
Wilkins and Castleman (44)	1957–1997	Johns Hopkins	136	68	7	37	8	10	24	0
Blumberg et al. (49)	1949–1993	MSKCC	118	73	32	58	4	21	47	80
Ruffini et al. (102)	1974–1993	Torino	114	100	–	25	5	10	30	33

R0, complete resection; RT, radiation therapy, JACS, Japanese Association for Chest Surgery; ML, Marie Lannelongue Hospital, Le Plessis-Robinson, France; FNCLCC, Federation Nationale des Centres de Lutte Contre le Cancer; MSKCC, Memorial Sloan-Kettering Cancer Center; MGH, Massachusetts General Hospital.

TABLE 52.7 RESULTS OF MULTIVARIATE ANALYSES OF FACTORS PREDICTING THYMOMA-SPECIFIC SURVIVAL

				P Value		
Study (Reference)	*Institution*	*Study Years*	*n*	*Histology*	*Stage*	*R0*
Okamura et al. (165)	Osaka	1967–2000	273	.05	.0001	NS
Rieker et al. (166)	Heidelberg	1967–1998	218	<.0024	<.001	–
Wright et al. (160)	MGH	1972–2003	179	.004	.002	NS
Rena et al. (125)[a]	Torino	1988–2000	178	.014	.012	.0001
Park et al. (122)[b]	Yonsei	1992–2002	150	.019	<.001	.947
Rea et al. (158)[b]	Padua	1970–2001	132	.0001	.003	NS
Kondo et al. (167)[b]	Tokushima	1973–2001	100	NS	.04	<.05

NS, not statistically significant; R0, complete resection, MGH, Massachusetts General Hospital.

[a]Type C excluded.

[b]Overall survival instead of disease-free survival.

100%, but those rates vary widely for higher-stage thymomas: 43% to 100% (mean, 85%) for stage II, 0% to 89% (mean, 47%) for stage III, and 0% to 78% (mean, 26%) for stage IV.[100]

Because the completeness of resection is such an important prognostic factor, an aggressive surgical approach is justified to remove as much of the lesion as possible at surgery. If residual microscopic disease is suspected of being present (an R1 operation), metallic clips should be placed to help delineate the radiation field. Whether subtotal resections are beneficial is controversial, with some authors demonstrating better survival when debulking takes place before adjuvant radiation therapy[18,21,55,103,104,154] and others finding no benefit from debulking over biopsy alone.[17,18,21,49,74,149,154,171,178] Another large study found significant differences in 5-year survival rates among patients undergoing subtotal resection versus biopsy only (64% vs. 36%) but little difference in 10-year survival rates, suggesting that any benefit may be only in intermediate-term survival.[55] Because of the difficulties in controlling for selection bias and confounding influences of other treatments or disease-related variables, no consensus has been reached as to whether subtotal resections in general are beneficial or not. It is quite possible that a planned incomplete resection that leaves minimal residual disease will be advantageous, especially in the context of adjuvant radiation or chemotherapy.

Advances in surgical techniques for thymectomy have included the use of robotics. Potential advantages of robotic techniques include increased rates of preserved pulmonary function, improved cosmesis, and higher rates of patient compliance because of the minimally invasive nature of the surgery.[179] Several institutions are exploring the use of robotics in thymectomy, and a few studies have been published. Rückert et al.[180] demonstrated the feasibility of this technique for patients undergoing thymectomy for myasthenia gravis. That same group of investigators then published a retrospective cohort study comparing robotic and nonrobotic thoracoscopic thymectomy and found that rates of remission of myasthenia gravis were actually higher for patients who had received a robotic thymectomy; the authors attributed this finding to the potential for improved mediastinal dissection with the robotic technique.[181]

Another minimally invasive procedure is video-assisted thoracoscopic extended thymectomy (VATET). A group in Japan used this procedure to treat 35 patients with clinical stage I thymoma from 1998 to 2009.[182] The authors reported the technique to be safe, with no perioperative deaths and three minor complications. Disease in 20 of the 35 patients was upstaged to Masaoka stage II or III at the time of surgery. At an average follow-up time of 65 months, one patient had experienced recurrence in the bilateral lung.[182] Future studies will need to examine the efficacy and safety of both robotic surgery and VATET for thymic malignancies.

Traditional surgical techniques for patients with stage I thymic tumors produce 5-year survival rates in excess of 90%, with survival rates decreasing slightly at 10 years[18,21,64] and with local recurrence rates of <5%. For stage II and III disease, recurrence rates after surgery alone range from 10% to 47%. In a study of more than 100 patients previously treated for thymoma, causes of death were as follows: 38% were related to thymoma (range, 19% to 58%), 9% to postoperative causes (range, 2% to 19%), 22% to myasthenia gravis (range, 16% to 27%), 9% to other autoimmune diseases (range, 2% to 19%), and 29% to unrelated causes (including other cancers) (range, 8% to 47%).[16,17–18,20,21,42,50,101,104,115,154] Recurrence rates are summarized in Table 52.6.

Patterns of Failure

The pattern of failure in the overwhelming majority of thymomas is locoregional: 81% of recurrences are local, 9% are distant, and 11% are both.[16,17,42,49,101,102] Most recurrences arise within 3 to 7 years,[16,17–18,49,50,102] but recurrence has been documented as late as 32 years after the initial resection.[42,57,169,183,184] The treatment for recurrence is usually surgery and adjuvant radiation.[73,102,185] Most recurrences (50% to 75%) are operable, and of those that are operable, the reported rates of a successful R0 resection range from 45% to 71%.[49,73,100,102,186] Patients with a recurrence after an R0 resection generally experience acceptable short-term and long-term results,[73,185] with 10-year actuarial survival rates ranging from 53% to 72%[73,100,102,187]; 10-year survival rates after an incomplete resection, by contrast, range from 0% to 35%.[17,73,100,102,187] In one recent study from Memorial Sloan-Kettering Cancer Center, of 25 patients who experienced recurrent disease after initial resection, 11 (44%) had disease that was amenable to re-resection. In that same study, 50% of patients undergoing surgery for recurrent disease had an R0 resection, but 82% of these patients experienced a second recurrence. The authors concluded that "despite the historical enthusiasm for re-resection . . . reoperation should be considered only in selected patients."[188]

When recurrent disease is unresectable, radiation and chemotherapy have been used with modest results: 5-year overall survival rates reportedly range from 25% to 50%, with poorer longer-term survival.[18,49,100,102,186,189]

Radiation Therapy

Adjuvant Radiation After Complete Resection

Radiation therapy can be considered as an adjuvant treatment for patients with resected stage II and III thymomas, although recurrence rates for stage I thymomas after an R0 resection are so low that radiation is considered unlikely to offer improvement. The indications for radiation are controversial, with some recommending adjuvant radiation for all patients,[21,104] others recommending adjuvant radiation for stage II and III thymomas,[17,64,77,149,154] and still others recommending radiation only after an incomplete resection.[55,149,154] All of the reported findings regarding adjuvant radiation are retrospective and, because of the rarity of thymoma, they span many decades. Because disease stage and completeness of resection are such important prognostic factors, any analysis of adjuvant radiation must be considered in light of these factors.

Several studies have shown trends toward better local control after adjuvant radiation for completely resected stage II thymoma; one of the largest studies found no difference in recurrence rates,[55] and another series reported worse results with adjuvant radiation.[102] Haniuda et al.[190] found that patients with fibrous adhesion to the mediastinal pleura without microscopic invasion benefited the most from postoperative therapy: recurrence rates among patients with such adhesion were 36.4% versus 0% among those without adhesion. Thus, mediastinal pleura invasion may be another factor to consider. Another study by Chang et al.[191] of patients with completely resected stage II or III thymoma demonstrated similar overall survival rates but improved disease-free survival rates with adjuvant radiation therapy (93% with radiation vs. 70% without). However, several other studies have shown that radiation after resection of stage II thymomas is not beneficial. In one such study, Berman et al.[192] found that the local recurrence rate among 74 patients after complete resection for stage II disease was only 3% and was not affected by receipt of adjuvant radiation. Utsumi et al.[193] reported similar findings in a study of patients with stage I or II completely resected disease. Finally, a SEER analysis of 901 patients showed no clear benefit from adjuvant radiation for patients with completely resected disease.[194]

Unlike these studies, many others (most with fewer than 50 patients) have reported that adjuvant radiation, after R0 resection for stage III thymoma, produces high rates of local control. Urgesi et al.,[152] in a study of 33 patients, reported no in-field recurrences and only 3 out-of-field recurrences, but others have found that adding radiation therapy did not affect local or distant recurrence rates.[49,55,195–197] On the other hand, some studies of completely resected stage II and III thymomas have demonstrated marginal benefits from the use of postoperative treatment.[18,37] The authors recommend that the choice of whether to use adjuvant treatment for stage II or III disease should be made on an individual basis and should consider risk factors such as frank pleural or pericardial invasion, tumor grade, and comorbid conditions. The authors further strongly encourage that proposed treatment strategies be discussed in a multidisciplinary setting before the final recommendation is made.

Adjuvant Radiation After Incomplete Resection

Radiation is often considered when complete resection is not possible. Two studies have suggested that adjuvant radiation can be beneficial for patients with subtotally resected thymomas.[18,37] Unfortunately both studies were small and, as always, subject to selection bias. Another study of 44 patients who had had R0 or R1,2 resections of stage III thymoma showed that adjuvant radiation produced lower recurrence rates (40% vs. 24% without radiation) and may have reduced the recurrence rates among patients with stage IV disease as well.[37] Curran et al.[37] reported no mediastinal failures after radiation in 26 patients with incompletely resected stage III thymoma compared with 79% at 5 years among patients who did not receive radiation. Other investigators have concurred, reporting very low rates of mediastinal failure among patients with gross residual disease treated with adjuvant radiation.[152,198]

Radiation as Neoadjuvant Therapy

Radiation has been proposed as a neoadjuvant strategy to reduce tumor burden and improve resectability, especially for cases involving gross invasion of critical structures.[34,106,155,199–203] Response rates of up to 80% have been reported, and a theoretical decrease in the potential for tumor seeding during surgery has been proposed as well.[18,37,154,199] The rates of R0 resections after neoadjuvant radiation for stage III thymoma can be as high as 53% to 75%,[106,203] which are favorable compared with the typical 50% rate of R0 resections of stage III thymomas.[17,20,21,37,49,77,103,149] Ten-year survival rates do not seem to be better after preoperative radiation, but to date the studies evaluating this approach have been small.[106,202,203]

Radiation as Definitive Therapy

Radiation therapy alone has been used for patients who cannot undergo surgery because of medical conditions or those for whom surgical resection is not possible, with modest results. Arakawa et al.[204] reported that 7 of 12 patients presenting with unresectable tumors treated with primary radiation therapy were still alive at follow-up times ranging from 1 to 5 years. Ciernik et al.[198] reported a 5-year survival rate of 87% for a small group of patients with stage III and IV disease who underwent radiation without resection, and Jackson and Ball[205] found 10-year survival rates of 44% for patients who received radiation after biopsies or incomplete resections. As for the use of radiation for recurrent disease, Urgesi et al.[186] reported outcomes of 21 patients given radiation alone after intrathoracic recurrences of thymoma. The 7-year survival rate of 70% was similar for those treated with radiation alone as for those treated with surgery and adjuvant therapy. Although these results are informative, in the era of combined-modality therapy, the use of preoperative and definitive radiation therapy without chemotherapy is no longer a primary consideration in the management of difficult thymomas.

Chemotherapy

Thymomas are quite sensitive to chemotherapy, with approximately two-thirds of patients showing a clinical response and one-third experiencing a complete response.[67,170,206–211,212–213] The duration of response ranges from 12 to 93 months. Whether chemotherapy influences long-term survival is more difficult to assess. In one retrospective analysis of 90 patients, chemotherapy reduced the rates of metastases to the lung, pleura, or other sites by half (17% vs. 38%; $P < .05$). All of those patients had stage III or IV tumors and were treated with radiation and partial or no resection.[154] Another study reported a nonsignificant trend toward better disease-free survival from the addition of chemotherapy.[178]

The most promising use of chemotherapy is in the neoadjuvant setting. Like preoperative radiation, chemotherapy seems to render tumors more suitable for complete resection. One study demonstrated that neoadjuvant chemotherapy was associated with improved survival for patients with stage III or IVa thymomas.[174]

As is true for the literature on the effects of radiation, most of the series describing the use of chemotherapy are small and retrospective. Drugs commonly used in combination chemotherapy include cisplatin, doxorubicin, and cyclophosphamide. One prospective intergroup study reported disappointing results with combined etoposide, ifosfamide, and cisplatin.[207] A more recent study of patients with advanced disease showed that the combination of carboplatin and paclitaxel produced response rates of 43%, with a median survival time of 20 months. The authors of that report concluded that the clinical activity of that combination was less than that of anthracycline-based therapy.[214]

Aside from cytotoxic agents, somatostatin analogs (e.g., octreotide) and high-dose corticosteroids have shown promise in thymomas.[215,216] In one prospective study, two courses of glucocorticoid therapy before surgery led to a 47% response rate among 17 patients with resectable thymomas.[217] This therapy seems to work by exploiting the ability of corticosteroids to induce apoptosis in CD4+CD8+ immature thymocytes. Another prospective study by the Eastern Cooperative Oncology Group enrolled 42 patients with unresectable, advanced thymic malignancies for whom octreotide scans were positive. Patients were treated with octreotide with or without prednisone. Two patients had complete responses and 10 had partial responses, which led the investigators to conclude that octreotide alone had modest activity and prednisone improved the overall response rate.[218] More recent molecular-level studies of signaling pathway activation have implicated c-KIT and EGFR in thymic malignancies,[142] and some isolated observations of response to targeted therapy such as cetuximab have been noted, but the therapeutic implications of these observations remain to be determined.

Combined Modality Therapy

Some evidence exists to suggest that multimodality treatment can improve resectability and survival among patients with stage III or IV thymomas; typical combinations include neoadjuvant

TABLE 52.8 OUTCOMES AFTER COMBINED MODALITY THERAPY FOR THYMOMAS

Study (Reference)	Institution	n	Preop Chemo	Adjuvant Therapy	% Response	% R0	% pCR	% 5-Year Survival
Lucchi et al. (174)	Pisa	36	cisplatin, vp, epi	RT and chemo	67	78	6	65 (est)
Venuta et al. (74)	Rome	25	cisplatin, vp, epi	RT and chemo	–	80	4	80
Kim et al. (213)	MD Anderson	22	cyclo, doxo, cisplatin, pred	RT and chemo	77	82	18	95
Rea et al. (211)	Padua	16	cyclo, doxo, cisplatin, vin	RT or chemo	100	69	31	57
Yokoi et al. (220)	Tochigi	17	cyclo, doxo, pred	RT and chemo	93	12	7	81

RT, radiation therapy; chemo, chemotherapy; R0, complete resection; pCR, partial complete remission; vp, etoposide; epi, epirubicin; doxo, doxorubicin; vin, vincristine; pred, prednisone; cyclo, cyclophosphamide.

chemotherapy followed by surgery and postoperative radiation, chemotherapy, or both. Prospective trials of preoperative combination chemotherapy have been undertaken at several institutions[74,211,213,219]; the regimens in all cases included cisplatin with some combination of cyclophosphamide, doxorubicin, vincristine, prednisone, or epirubicin. Reported response rates to these regimens range from 77% to 100% (Table 52.8); R0 resections were possible in 57% to 82% of cases; and pathologic complete response rates ranged from 4% to 31%. Overall survival rates at 5 years (57% to 95%) were quite favorable for unresectable stage III or IV thymoma.[74,211,213,219,221] In many of these studies, most if not all patients received postoperative radiation (see Table 52.8), and the results seem superior to historical results from patients who underwent surgical resection alone. In summary, multimodality therapy consisting of preoperative combination cisplatin-based chemotherapy followed by surgery and postoperative radiation can produce excellent results.

Reasonable results have also been obtained from the combination of chemotherapy plus definitive radiation therapy for limited-stage, unresectable thymoma. A prospective intergroup study[206] reported a 5-year survival rate of 52% for 26 patients who were treated with cisplatin, doxorubicin, and cyclophosphamide followed by radiation therapy for patients with unresectable thymomas. The median survival time was 93 months.

Management of Myasthenia Gravis

Thymectomy has been used effectively to induce remission or reduce symptoms of myasthenia gravis. Removal of even normal-appearing thymuses improves symptoms in about half of patients with myasthenia gravis,[222,223,224] which may be related to the associated high acetylcholine receptor activity and the presence of antibodies to striated muscle within the thymus.[225] The mortality rate associated with such surgery, at centers with experience in the preoperative and postoperative management of myasthenia gravis, is essentially the same as that associated with general anesthesia.[51]

Radiation therapy to the thymus has also been reported to be effective for treating myasthenia gravis, with symptom improvement or response noted in about 50% of patients.[226–228] However, radiation treatment alone for myasthenia gravis is mostly of historical interest given the advances in surgical expertise and perioperative management of this syndrome.

Radiation Therapy Techniques

Radiation doses given for thymoma have ranged from 30 to 60 Gy, most often given in standard 1.8- to 2.0-Gy fractions. Typical postoperative doses are 45 to 50 Gy, with higher doses for positive surgical margins or frank invasion. Dose–response effects have been difficult to determine due to the retrospective nature of most published studies; one study did not identify a dose response,[229] but two others did.[178,230]

CT-based treatment planning is essential for targeting the tumor and for accurate dosimetry of critical structures. As is true for all thoracic and mediastinal tumors, the major critical structures include the spinal cord, lung parenchyma, pericardium, heart, and esophagus. The guidelines to be followed to minimize dose to these structures are the same as those used in the treatment of lung cancer. Table 52.9 lists common dose constraints for radiation therapy, with or without chemotherapy, for mediastinal malignancies. These constraints were derived from a Quantitative Analysis of Normal Tissue Effects in the Clinic Consensus analysis published in 2010.[231,232–233,234] Any deviations from these dose constraints should be reviewed in a radiation quality-assurance setting and discussed with the patient before treatment is begun.

Radiation Fields

As radiation planning techniques have evolved, the trend in treating thymic tumors, like non–small cell lung cancer, has been toward use of involved-field techniques. Because thymomas do not routinely spread via the lymphatic system, the draining nodal distributions do not need to be included in the radiation fields.[102] In general, neoadjuvant or definitive radiation therapy is delivered to the entire extent of disease as visualized on CT or PET. When radiation is to be given as adjuvant therapy, the radiation treatment fields are designed based on the pretreatment images, with the field generally encompassing the surgical bed and the superior-inferior extent of disease before treatment (to address "infiltrating" borders); regions of extension into lung parenchyma that likely represent a "pushing" border are omitted.

In theory, hemithoracic radiation could be beneficial in thymic malignancies because of their tendency for pleural metastases. This technique has been assessed in several studies. In one such study, Sugie et al.[235] reported findings from 60 patients with stage I to IV invasive thymoma, 48 of whom had been treated with fields limited to the mediastinum to a dose of

TABLE 52.9 STANDARD DOSE CONSTRAINTS USED IN RADIATION THERAPY FOR THORACIC MALIGNANCIES

Organ at Risk	RT Alone	Chemo and RT	Chemo and RT Before Surgery
Spinal cord	D_{max} <45 Gy	D_{max} <45 Gy	D_{max} <45 Gy
Lung	Mean dose ≤20 Gy V_{20} ≤40%	Mean dose ≤20 Gy V_{20} ≤35% V_{10} ≤45% V_5 ≤65%	Mean dose ≤20 Gy V_{20} ≤30% V_{10} ≤40% V_5 ≤55%
Heart	V_{30} ≤45% Mean dose <26 Gy	V_{30} ≤45% Mean dose <26 Gy	V_{30} ≤45% Mean dose <26 Gy
Esophagus	D_{max} ≤ 80 Gy V_{70} <20% V_{50} <50% Mean dose<34 Gy	D_{max} ≤80 Gy V_{70} <20% V_{50} <40% Mean dose<34 Gy	D_{max} ≤80 Gy V_{70} <20% V_{50} <40% Mean dose <34 Gy
Kidney	20 Gy <32% of bilateral kidney	20 Gy <32% of bilateral kidney	20 Gy <32% of bilateral kidney
Liver	V_{30} ≤40% Mean dose <30 Gy	V_{30} ≤40% Mean dose <30 Gy	V_{30} ≤40% Mean dose <30 Gy

chemo, chemotherapy, RT, radiation therapy; D_{max}, maximum dose; V_x, percent volume of organ receiving x dose.

From Marks LB, Bentzen SM, Deasy JO, et al. Radiation dose-volume effects in the lung. *Int J Radiat Oncol Biol Phys* 2010;76(3 Suppl):S70–S706, with permission from Elsevier.

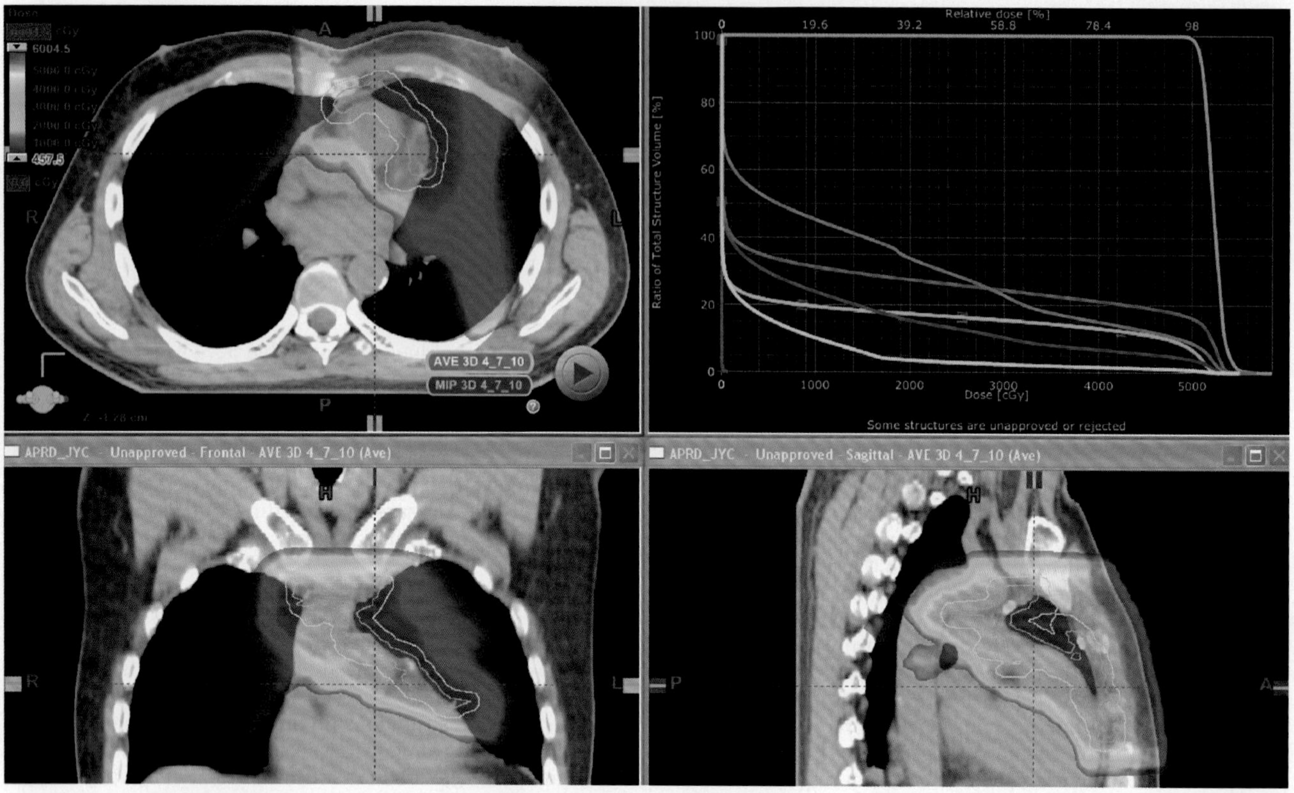

FIGURE 52.4. Representative patient treated with proton beam therapy for invasive thymoma in the postoperative setting. It is evident that proton beam therapy allows for sparing of posterior structures, such as the heart and esophagus.

30 to 64 Gy and the other 12 given hemithoracic radiation therapy to a dose of 11.2 to 16 Gy. Although the toxicity of the extended-field (hemithoracic) radiation was acceptable and seemed to produce modest improvements in pleural dissemination rates, no differences were found in overall survival between the two techniques. Other small studies have also tested hemithoracic radiation to doses of 15 to 20 Gy, and some have had promising results.[236,237,238] However, these studies were small and primarily retrospective. Ultimately, the dose that can be delivered safely in hemithoracic therapy is probably not sufficient for controlling microscopic disease, which typically requires 40 to 45 Gy. However, conformal techniques such as those noted below may allow further dose escalation.

Radiation Modalities and Simulation Techniques

Major advances in radiation technology over the past decade have led to great improvements in both conformality and therapeutic ratio of radiation for thoracic malignancies. The use of four-dimensional CT (4D CT) in treatment simulation and delivery via modalities such as intensity-modulated radiation therapy (IMRT) has been shown to allow the dose to normal structures to be reduced relative to that from 3D conformal radiation and to allow accurate target localization.[239–245] Indeed, a recent study of 496 patients with locally advanced, unresectable non–small cell lung cancer demonstrated that the more advanced technique (4D CT with IMRT) led to lower rates of high-grade radiation pneumonitis and better overall survival compared with 3D simulation and 3D conformal therapy.[246] Similar comparisons for thymic malignancies have not been done because of the rarity of this disease. However, similar paradigms would be expected to apply given the mediastinal location of these tumors and hence their close proximity to the lungs, heart, and esophagus.

Another treatment modality, proton beam therapy, has shown promise for reducing the dose to normal structures while maintaining adequate doses to the tumor target in non–small cell lung cancer.[239,247–251,252,253–254] Indeed, the dose distribution properties of proton therapy, specifically the Bragg peak that minimizes dose distal to the tumor, are well suited for anteriorly located thymic tumors. Proton therapy has been shown to produce greatly reduced doses to critical structures in mediastinal lymphoma, which often presents in the same anterior location as thymic malignancies, compared with photon-based techniques.[255] The dosimetric and clinical effectiveness of proton therapy versus that of photon techniques such as IMRT for thoracic malignancies is currently being evaluated in clinical trials. The findings from these trials will be essential in determining if the dosimetric benefits of proton beam therapy (Fig. 52.4) translate to clinical benefits.

Regardless of treatment modality, the authors recommend that all treatment simulations for patients with thymic tumors take place while the patients are supine and well immobilized with their arms above their head, to maximize the number of potential beam arrangements. The authors recommend that 4D CT scans be obtained at the time of simulation to assess the motion of the tumor during respiration. If 4D CT scanning is not available, the authors recommend either a slow helical scan to encompass all phases of the breathing cycle or that CT images be obtained at full inspiration and expiration to assess the extremes of respiratory motion. Full descriptions of radiation techniques for thymic malignancies are available elsewhere.[256,257]

THYMIC CARCINOMA

Thymic carcinomas are considerably less common than thymomas. Like thymomas, thymic carcinomas are thought to arise from thymic epithelium and typically appear in the anterosuperior mediastinum. The clinical behavior of thymic carcinoma is quite different from that of thymoma, being more aggressive and having a higher propensity for capsular invasion. Thymic carcinoma often presents as advanced disease, the 5-year survival rates for which are much poorer than for thymomas.[55,258,259]

Clinically, thymic carcinoma can present as cough, dyspnea, pleuritic chest pain, phrenic nerve palsy, or superior vena cava syndrome.[258,260,261] Associated paraneoplastic syndromes have been observed occasionally as well.[261–263] CT scans often demonstrate an irregular mass with necrotic, cystic, or calcified regions.[260,264,265,266] In about 80% of cases, thymic carcinoma shows radiographic evidence of invasion into adjacent structures in the mediastinum, with mediastinal lymphadenopathy evident at presentation in about 40%.[261,267,268–269] Distant metastases to regional lymphatics, bone, liver, kidney, and lung are common clinical features.[261,270–272] Bone scanning, MRI, PET with ^{18}F-flourodeoxyglucose or carbon-11–labeled methionine, and single photon emission computed tomography have been used for both diagnosis and evaluation of response to therapy.[85,273,274,275–276]

Historically, thymic carcinomas have been classified as type C thymic tumors in the WHO classification, and disease staging is most often done with the Masaoka clinical staging system for thymomas.[103,277] Because histologic grade is one of the most significant indicators of prognosis, a revised histologic classification has been proposed that broadly divides thymic carcinomas into high- or low-grade lesions.[117] Most thymic carcinomas are undifferentiated high-grade lesions with anaplasia and marked cellular atypia, lacking the histologic features of a normal thymus[278]; others may be of adenocarcinomatous, sarcomatous, squamous, basoloid, mucoepidermoid, or lymphoepithelial-like histology.[260,279,280] Some thymic carcinomas are associated with the multilocular thymic cysts, which are acquired lesions of the thymic gland associated with an inflammatory reaction. Recent studies have demonstrated the importance of thorough sampling of thymic cysts to rule out underlying carcinoma.[281] Most variants of thymic carcinoma are highly lethal, with frequent metastases to regional lymph nodes, bone, liver, and lung.[266,282] Tumors in the low-grade histologic group are characterized by a relatively favorable clinical course and a low incidence of local recurrence and metastasis.[283–285]

Owing to the paucity of experience with this rare tumor, the ideal therapeutic regimen is unknown. Current management strategies involve an aggressive multimodality approach including primary surgical resection and adjuvant cisplatin-based chemotherapy, often coupled with postoperative radiation therapy. Although incomplete resection does not necessarily preclude long-term survival if multimodality platinum-based therapy is used,[286] complete resection is nevertheless the cornerstone of treatment. Takeda et al.[287] observed a median survival time of 57 months for patients with completely resected thymic carcinomas versus 13 months for those with incomplete resection. Most studies have used adjuvant radiation therapy to a dose of 40 to 70 Gy delivered in standard fractionation (1.8- to 2.0-Gy fractions).[229,284,287,288,289–290,291] In one series of 26 patients treated with surgery and postoperative radiation without chemotherapy, Hsu et al.[291] observed a 5-year overall survival rate of 77% for all patients, 82% for patients with completely resected tumors, and 66% for those with subtotally resected tumors. The 5-year local control rate was 91% with a median radiation dose of 60 Gy.

In another study of 40 patients given either surgery and adjuvant radiation or definitive radiation therapy with or without chemotherapy, Ogawa et al.[284] reported complete resections in 16 patients; moreover, patients with complete resection who had received adjuvant radiation of at last 50 Gy had no local disease recurrence. Kondo and Monden[55] observed no survival benefit from adding adjuvant radiation to surgical resection in a retrospective multi-institutional study of 186 patients, although the authors did note that the retrospective nature of the study and its small subgroup sizes precluded any definitive conclusions. These studies seem to indicate that local control is improved with radiation, but a survival benefit remains to be demonstrated.

Thymic carcinoma generally is less responsive to chemotherapy than thymoma,[292] and outcomes after chemotherapy alone are dismal. However, the use of adjuvant cisplatin-based chemotherapy has shown significantly beneficial effects in several studies.[206,293,294] In one such study, Nakamura et al.[294] treated 10 patients with unresectable thymic carcinoma with platinum-based protocols, with or without radiation therapy, and observed a median survival time of 11 months. Yoh et al.[295] reported excellent preliminary results (i.e., a 42% response rate) from the use of weekly cisplatin, vincristine, doxorubicin, and etoposide for the treatment of advanced tumors. Other studies have showed favorable responses from various combinations of cisplatin, etoposide, ifosfamide, doxorubicin, nedaplatin, cyclophosphamide, and vincristine.[206,207,293,294,295–297]

The key to longer survival for thymic carcinoma, like thymoma, is the resectability of the disease. A large multi-institutional study of patients with totally resected thymic carcinoma showed 5-year survival rates of 81.5% for those given chemotherapy, 46.6% for those given chemoradiation, 73.6% for those given radiotherapy alone, and 72.2% for those given no adjuvant treatment[55]; however, the numbers of patients in each subgroup were quite small. Because of the rarity of thymic carcinoma, few treatment recommendations can be made; however, it seems clear that for patients with resectable disease, complete surgical resection is the preferred initial therapeutic intervention.[55,100,287,298,299] For patients with unresectable lesions, neoadjuvant chemotherapy, with or without thoracic radiotherapy, seems reasonable. Ultimately, after complete resection, the most important prognostic factors are initial disease stage and tumor grade. Five-year survival rates for patients with higher disease stage and higher-grade neoplasms range from 15% to 20%, whereas for patients with low-grade, localized disease those rates can range from 80% to 90%.[117,282]

THYMIC CARCINOID

Thymic carcinoid (neuroendocrine) tumors of the thymus are very rare, accounting for <5% of all neoplasms of the anterior mediastinum. They originate from normal thymic Kulchitsky cells, which belong to the amine-precursor-uptake and decarboxylation group.[300] Thymic carcinoid tumors are often confused with thymomas because of similarities in their clinical behavior. Most patients with thymic carcinoid are men aged 30 to 50 years; the male-to-female ratio is 3 to 1.[301] Roughly half of thyroid carcinoids are associated with endocrine disorders such as multiple endocrine neoplasia type-1 (MEN-1) or secondary Cushing syndrome.[302–304] Thymic carcinoids can present with symptoms related to compression of normal structures (chest pain, dyspnea, cough, hoarseness, superior vena cava syndrome)[300,305] or with no symptoms.[304] Thymic carcinoids are best evaluated by CT or MRI for visualizing local invasion of the surrounding structures (pericardium, great vessels, pleura, sternum) and metastases within or outside the thorax. Most thymic carcinoids detected on radiographic studies are already advanced, commonly metastasizing to regional lymph nodes. Metastases are present in up to 70% of patients within 8 years of the initial diagnosis,[306] which may explain the poor prognosis associated with these tumors.

The Masaoka staging system for thymoma has been used for staging thymic carcinoids.[103,301] The WHO system classifies thymic carcinoids as typical carcinoid, atypical carcinoid, large cell neuroendocrine carcinoma, or small cell carcinoma,[99,110] and a system proposed by Klemm and Moran[307] classifies these tumors as well differentiated (low grade), moderately differentiated (intermediate grade), or poorly differentiated (high grade). However, neither grading nor other histologic variables has shown a consistent association with prognosis.[301]

Complete surgical resection is the preferred method of treatment, although recurrence is common. Incomplete resections followed by adjuvant radiation, chemotherapy, or both seem to provide some benefit without increasing morbidity or mortality.[304,306,308,309] Distant metastases to bone, liver, or skin occur in 30% to 40% of cases.[310] Despite aggressive treatment, the prognosis in most cases is poor; according to one report, the overall 5-year survival rate was 31% and all 14 patients were dead after 9 years.[305] Thymic carcinoids associated with MEN-1 are especially lethal; in one study, the 5-year survival rate for patients with thymic carcinoid without associated endocrinopathy was about 70% but was only 35% for those with an endocrinopathy.[304,305,311]

OTHER RARE TUMORS OF THE THYMUS

Thymoliposarcoma was first described by Havlicek and Rosai[312] in 1984. This rare and distinctive entity is considered the malignant counterpart of thymolipoma. Thymoliposarcomas have appeared in adults aged 36 to 77 years, with a slight female predominance. Unlike its thymolipoma counterpart, thymoliposarcoma is not associated with myasthenia gravis. It grows by expansion and has a relatively low risk of distant metastasis in the absence of histologic dedifferentiation. Complete surgical resection or subtotal resection with adjuvant radiation therapy has been used for local control.[312,313]

MALIGNANT MEDIASTINAL GERM CELL TUMORS

Epidemiology

Primary extragonadal germ cell tumors account for 2% to 5% of all germ cell tumors.[314] About two-thirds of these tumors occur in the mediastinum,[315–317] making the mediastinum the most common site of primary extragonadal germ cell tumors among young adults.[318] Germ cell tumors contribute to about 10% of all malignant mediastinal tumors and about 2% of mediastinal neoplasms.[151,319] In a pooled analysis of 341 patients with mediastinal germ cell tumors treated at 11 cancer centers over a 20-year period, the median age of presentation was 33 years for seminomatous tumors and 28 years for nonseminomatous tumors.[320]

Primary extragonadal germ cell tumors have several unexplained associations. Klinefelter syndrome has been documented in patients with mediastinal germ cell tumors but not in patients with testicular germ cell tumors.[321–324] In one study, up to 20% of patients with mediastinal germ cell tumors were found to have the Klinefelter karyotype (47,XXY).[325,326] Several unusual malignant processes are associated with nonseminomatous germ cell tumors, including hematologic malignancies such as acute myeloid leukemia, acute nonlymphocytic leukemia, acute megakaryocytic leukemia, myelodysplastic syndrome, and malignant histiocytosis.[326,327,328–330] In another pooled analysis of primary extragonadal germ cell tumors, 1 in 17 patients with primary mediastinal nonseminomatous germ cell tumors developed a fatal hematologic disorder after the diagnosis of the germ cell tumor.[331]

Natural History

Primary extragonadal germ cell tumors arise along the midline of the body from the pineal gland, through the mediastinum and retroperitoneum, and to the presacral areas. The origin of these primary extragonadal germ cell tumors remains controversial,[332–334] but presumably they arise from germ cells that migrate along the urogenital ridge during embryonic development.[326,335] Because the embryologic urogenital ridge extends from C-6 to L-4, malignant transformation of displaced germ cells can give rise to primary germ cell tumors outside the gonads.

Because primary gonadal germ cell tumors can spread to the retroperitoneum and mediastinum,[316,326] the diagnostic workup must be thorough and meticulous to avoid overlooking an occult gonadal primary. Although primary mediastinal germ cell tumors have the same morphologic and histologic appearance as those of the testes, primary germ cell tumors of the mediastinum are both more aggressive and have a poorer prognosis.[336–338] Like testicular germ cell tumors, mediastinal germ cell tumors can be seminomatous or nonseminomatous. Benign teratomas arise from germ cell elements, but they are not included in this discussion because they are not malignant and surgical resection is often curative.

Primary mediastinal seminomatous germ cell tumors are sensitive to radiation and chemotherapy, but the analogous nonseminomatous tumors are considered poor-risk disease in all staging systems.[338] Nonseminomatous tumors are often invasive at the time of diagnosis, and approximately half of such tumors will present with distant metastases, most often to the lung.[320] Tumor markers can aid in the diagnosis of mediastinal germ cell tumors; serum α-fetoprotein levels are elevated in 75% of patients (median, 2,500 ng/mL) at diagnosis, but β-human chorionic gonadotropin and lactate dehydrogenase levels are elevated in about 50% of patients at presentation.[320]

Clinical Presentation

As is true for many mediastinal tumors, local symptoms are usually caused by tumor compression or invasion of adjacent structures. Primary extragonadal germ cell tumors present with clinical symptoms in 90% to 100% of cases,[339] with dyspnea (25%), chest pain (23%), cough (17%), fever (13%), weight loss (11%), vena cava occlusion syndrome and fatigue or weakness (6% each) being the most common.[320,340,341] Nevertheless, these tumors are asymptomatic in many cases, and a mass is found incidentally on chest x-ray.[342,343] Roughly one-third of seminomatous mediastinal germ cell tumors present with metastases at diagnosis. The cervical lymph nodes are enlarged in about 25% of such cases, but abdominal lymphadenopathy has also been present. Distant metastases from nonseminomatous germ cell tumors are much more common, with rates of 85% to 90% in prior series but in more recent series about 50% at diagnosis.[320,344–345,346,347]

Diagnostic Workup

Mediastinal germ cell tumors are usually readily detected on chest x-rays, with most masses noted in the anterosuperior mediastinum. CT scans of the chest, abdomen, and pelvis are essential to evaluate the mass and to screen for metastases and lymphadenopathy. A careful physical examination and testicular sonography should be performed to rule out an occult primary gonadal tumor. Levels of tumor markers such as α-fetoprotein, β-human chorionic gonadotropin, and lactate dehydrogenase can be helpful for diagnosis, for evaluating treatment efficacy, and for monitoring recurrence.[10,348,349,350] Thus the determination of baseline tumor-marker levels both before treatment has begun and after treatment is completed is essential.

The initial diagnosis of mediastinal germ cell tumors is usually reached through a combination of findings from CT, radiography, sonography, and tumor-marker measurements. Whether PET has a place in the management of these tumors is unclear. In some instances, the tumor marker findings are sufficient to classify the lesion as an extragonadal nonseminomatous germ cell tumor without histologic confirmation, but false-positive β-human chorionic gonadotropin levels have been reported.[351,352] Histopathologic analysis can often be done easily via fine-needle aspiration and cytologic staining for tumor markers. Biopsy samples should be obtained whenever possible because both choice of treatment and prognosis depend greatly on histology.[351,352]

Prognostic Factors

The most important prognostic factor for mediastinal germ cell tumors is histologic type. Seminomas are highly curable, but nonseminomatous germ cell tumors, despite advances in therapy, are associated with poor progression-free and overall survival. The presence of metastases with tumors of either histologic type is also associated with adverse progression-free and overall survival. In nonseminomatous tumors, elevated β-human chorionic gonadotropin levels are associated with inferior overall survival.[320]

General Management

Seminomatous Tumors

Seminomas are quite sensitive to both radiation therapy and chemotherapy, and thus all patients with tumors of seminomatous histology should be treated with curative intent even in the presence of widely metastatic disease. The choice of treatment has definitely evolved with the development of cisplatin-based chemotherapy regimens, and most patients should be initially treated with chemotherapy.[353]

Historically, mediastinal seminomatous tumors (like all mediastinal tumors) were treated surgically.[326,354] Complete radical resection can be considered in some cases if it is technically feasible and if the patients do not want radiation or chemotherapy. Definitive radiation replaced surgical resection for localized mediastinal seminomatous germ cell tumors, with long-term survival rates of 60% to 80% achieved even for those with bulky tumors.[314,326,329,354] Before the advent of platinum-based chemotherapy, radiation therapy had the advantage of being more tolerable and less toxic, and relapses could be effectively treated with systemic chemotherapy.[314] However, cisplatin-based chemotherapy soon eclipsed radiation; in an early application of this approach, Einhorn and Williams[355] at the University of Indiana reported a complete response rate of 63% lasting a median duration of 18 months for 19 patients with disseminated seminoma treated with cisplatin-based chemotherapy. In more modern series, the response to primary therapy is favorable for 92% of patients, and 5-year overall survival rates exceeding 90% are standard.[353]

Residual radiographic abnormalities after the completion of chemotherapy for bulky mediastinal seminomas are not uncommon, but the management strategy in such cases is still controversial. In the vast majority (80% to 90%) of such cases, the residual masses represent dense fibrosis with no viable tumor.[326,356–357,358] Some clinicians have advocated surgical resection or biopsy of all postchemotherapy masses larger than 3 cm,[82,357–359] and others recommend close follow-up in such cases, with early intervention if the mass enlarges on chest x-ray or CT scan and with resection, radiation, or salvage chemotherapy reserved for progressive disease.[326,329,358,360] Whether ^{18}F-FDG-PET is useful for predicting viable tumor is debatable and under investigation.[361,362] Although seminomas are extremely sensitive to radiation therapy, radiation therapy delivered to residual masses after chemotherapy has not shown a significant benefit.

Radiation doses and treatment techniques for mediastinal seminomatous germ cell tumors have varied.[363,364,365–368] Doses as low as 30 Gy and as high as 50 Gy have been recommended.[319,365] The radiation dose should be adjusted based on the size of the lesion, the history of chemotherapy exposure, and the clinical circumstances. The entire mediastinum should be encompassed with anteroposterior-posteroanterior fields with CT guidance. In the prechemotherapy era, use of smaller portals was associated with marginal relapse,[364] and the clinical target volume for definitive radiation alone often covered the supraclavicular, cervical, and para-aortic lymph nodes.[349,363,366,369] Extrapolating from the experience with prophylactic treatment of para-aortic nodes in testicular seminomas, one could assume that the contiguous lymphatic drainage sites for a mediastinal primary could be treated effectively with 20 Gy with minimal morbidity.[370]

In conclusion, cisplatin-based combination chemotherapy can consistently produce 5-year overall survival rates in excess of 90% for mediastinal seminomas. However, for patients who are not candidates for chemotherapy, definitive radiation therapy has produced local tumor control rates of 89% to 100% and long-term survival rates of 60% to 80%.[319,326,364,366,371]

Nonseminomatous Germ Cell Tumors

The primary treatment for nonseminomatous germ cell tumor is intensive cisplatin-based chemotherapy, but surgical resection of all residual masses after first-line chemotherapy is recommended whenever technically possible, either as a one-stage or as a sequential procedure.[372,373,374–375] Chemotherapy regimens should include either cisplatin and etoposide or cisplatin, etoposide, and bleomycin. Patients whose tumors respond well to initial chemotherapy followed by complete resection of any residual mass can have excellent outcomes, but the outcome for patients who do not respond to primary therapy is poor, as salvage therapy is rarely effective.[338]

The role of radiation therapy in nonseminomatous germ cell tumors is not clear. Radiation may be useful for unresectable residual masses given the relatively high rate of persistent viable tumor and the poor success rates of salvage therapy. Nonseminomatous germ cell tumors are also radiation sensitive, but they require higher doses than seminomatous tumors, and doses of 60 Gy or more may be necessary to achieve control.[376]

Before the cisplatin-based chemotherapy era, fewer than 5% of patients with mediastinal nonseminomatous germ cell tumors survived.[349] Since that time, long-term disease-free survival rates have varied from 45% to 72% in studies using cisplatin-based combination chemotherapy followed by surgery.[320,338,377] Several salvage regimens have been used for disease that progresses during or after initial chemotherapy, but unfortunately long-term survival rates for patients with relapsed mediastinal germ cell tumors are <10%.[320,338,378,379] Thus surgical resection and even radiation therapy may be appropriate when no further effective chemotherapy is available.

MEDIASTINAL MESENCHYMAL TUMORS

Epidemiology

True mediastinal mesenchymal lesions are exceedingly rare tumors. Retrospective series suggest that 2% to 8% of all mediastinal lesions are primary mesenchymal tumors; extrapolation of these values puts the estimated incidence at approximately 0.1 to 0.2 per million.[10,380–382] Approximately three-quarters of mediastinal mesenchymal tumors are of lipomatous, lymphangitic, or vascular histology, with the rest composed of unusual histologic variants.[383] The age predilection depends the specific histologic subtype.[49,343,380–382,384]

Clinical Presentation and Workup

Mesenchymal lesions can arise in any of the three mediastinal compartments. Mesenchymal tumors that present in children seem to be more malignant than those presenting in adults.[384,385]

Mediastinal mesenchymal lesions can reach impressively large sizes before detection, typically presenting with symptoms such as chest pain and dyspnea. At least one series suggests that symptomatic presentation is a harbinger of malignant character, with 80% of patients with malignant disease presenting with symptoms versus 44% of patients with benign masses.[10] An accurate histopathologic diagnosis is critical.[384] Tissue for these analyses can be obtained via mediastinoscopic biopsy, fine-needle aspiration, or endoscopy. Disease can be staged according to the American Joint Committee on Cancer staging system for soft tissue tumors.

Tumors of Adipose Tissue

Mediastinal lipomas are the most common of the mediastinal mesenchymal lesions; they represent 1% to 5% of all lipomas.[383,386–388] Mediastinal lesions can occur in isolation or in

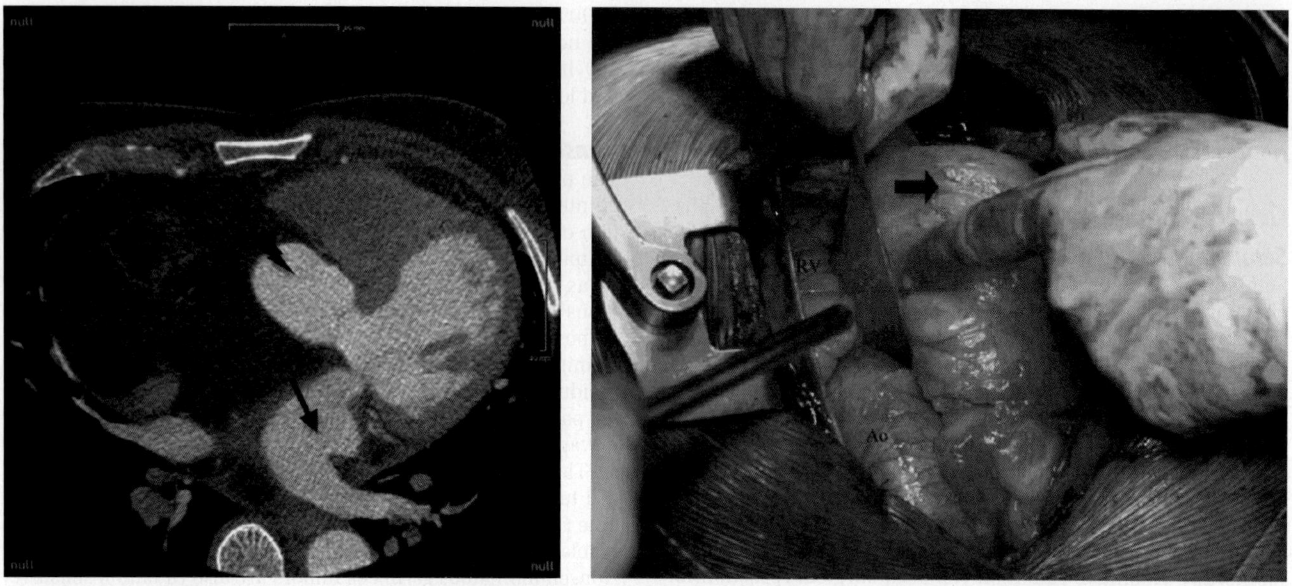

FIGURE 52.5. CT scan (*left*) and intraoperative photograph (*right*) of a primary mediastinal liposarcoma filling right thoracic cavity. The recommended treatment for this malignancy is aggressive surgical resection with adjuvant radiation therapy and consideration of systemic therapy. (From Wiedemann D, Schistek R, Gassner E, et al. Mediastinal liposarcoma. *J Card Surg* 2011;26(2):162–164, with permission form Blackwell Scientific.)

multiples and may mimic cardiomegaly or pleural effusion on a chest x-ray. They are usually well circumscribed and encapsulated but can grow to 20 cm in diameter before detection.[389,390] Although tumors can be quite large and cause significant compressive symptoms,[391–393] gross total resection is almost always curative.[12,394,395–396,397] Technically, lipomas are considered "benign" tumors, but those that are growing or causing symptoms should be referred for surgical resection.

In contrast to lipomas, liposarcomas consist of immature fat cells with malignant histology and behavior. Distinguishing lipomas from liposarcomas can be difficult histologically; liposarcomas are distinguished by size heterogeneity, hyperchromatic nuclei, and eosinophilic cytoplasm.[398] Primary mediastinal liposarcomas often appear in the posterior portion of the mediastinum, but anterior mediastinal liposarcomas are very rare.[399] Tumors often appear to be encapsulated and well circumscribed, even when invasion is present (Fig. 52.5), giving rise to the term "pseudocapsule." In one historical review, survival times for patients with well-circumscribed lesions ranged from 3 to 17 years, whereas patients with grossly invasive tumors died within 2 years.[400] As is true for all sarcomas, the prognosis depends on the histologic grade.[401,402] Optimal treatment consists of surgical resection and adjuvant radiation therapy.[403] Because well-differentiated tumors have little propensity for distant metastases, adjuvant radiation may be withheld after an R0 resection, but the significant local recurrence rates of 20% to 30% should be acknowledged.[401,402,404–407]

Tumors of Lymph Tissue

Tumors arising from the vascular or lymphatic components of the mediastinum make up the bulk of the remaining mediastinal mesenchymal lesions.[380–382] Lymphangiomas and hemangiomas are morphologically similar under light microscopy, and the presence of red blood cells or chyle within the tumor lumen often serves as a primary diagnostic aid.[394] Localized lymphangiomas are rare; more than 90% will have some degree of cervical extension.[408] A cystic lymphangioma is illustrated in Figure 52.6.[409] Lymphangiomatosis is usually seen in children and is characterized by synchronous widespread lymphangiomas[410]; mediastinal or pulmonary involvement carries a poor prognosis.[394,411–419] Lymphangiosarcoma seems to be a malignant variant of lymphangiomas and should probably be treated like other soft tissue sarcomas, with the optimal treatment being full extirpation.[420] In the largest reported retrospective series of 25 patients with mediastinal and cervicomediastinal lymphangiomas, survival rates were excellent after surgical resection alone, and only one patient died of a complication from lymphangioma.[421] Adjuvant radiation has little to offer and may actually be detrimental; in one study, radiation transformed a benign lymphangioma into a malignant lymphangiosarcoma.[422,423–424] However, radiation may be helpful for controlling symptomatic unresectable disease; Johnson et al.[422] described a young patient with surgically refractory chylothorax and lymphangioma who experienced prompt resolution after mediastinal radiation to 20 Gy in 10 fractions. In another report, radiation produced complete local control of large, unresectable lymphangiomas in three patients, findings that are consistent with other anecdotal reports of lymphangiomyomatosis.[414,423]

Tumors of Vascular Tissue

Mediastinal mesenchymal lesions of endothelial origin include hemangiomas, hemangioendotheliomas, and hemangiopericytomas. Many of these tumors have an indolent course, but hemangiopericytomas are notable for high rates of metastasis at presentation.[425–428] Hemangiomas can be capillary or cavernous; cavernous hemangiomas (i.e., angiomyomas or hamartomas) are distinguished from capillary hemangiomas by the presence of smooth muscle. Hemangiomas and hemangioendotheliomas are typically well circumscribed. Hemangioendotheliomas contain the hallmark cytoplasmic Weibel-Palade bodies.[429,430]

Hemangiopericytomas arise from the capillary contractile pericytes of Zimmerman.[425] Although most are indolent, recurrence and metastases have been observed many years after resection.[431] Retrospective studies suggest that high mitotic rates and proliferative indices may portend malignant behavior.[432,433] Nevertheless, long-term survival is still possible with aggressive treatment of metastatic disease.[434] Surgery remains the mainstay of therapy and is often curative.[435] Because of their benign nature, hemangiomas or hemangioendotheliomas should not be treated with radiation.[435] An endoscopic approach has been proposed for several types of intrathoracic tumors including benign hemangiomas and should be explored further.[436] Radiation remains an option for incompletely resected hemangiopericytomas.

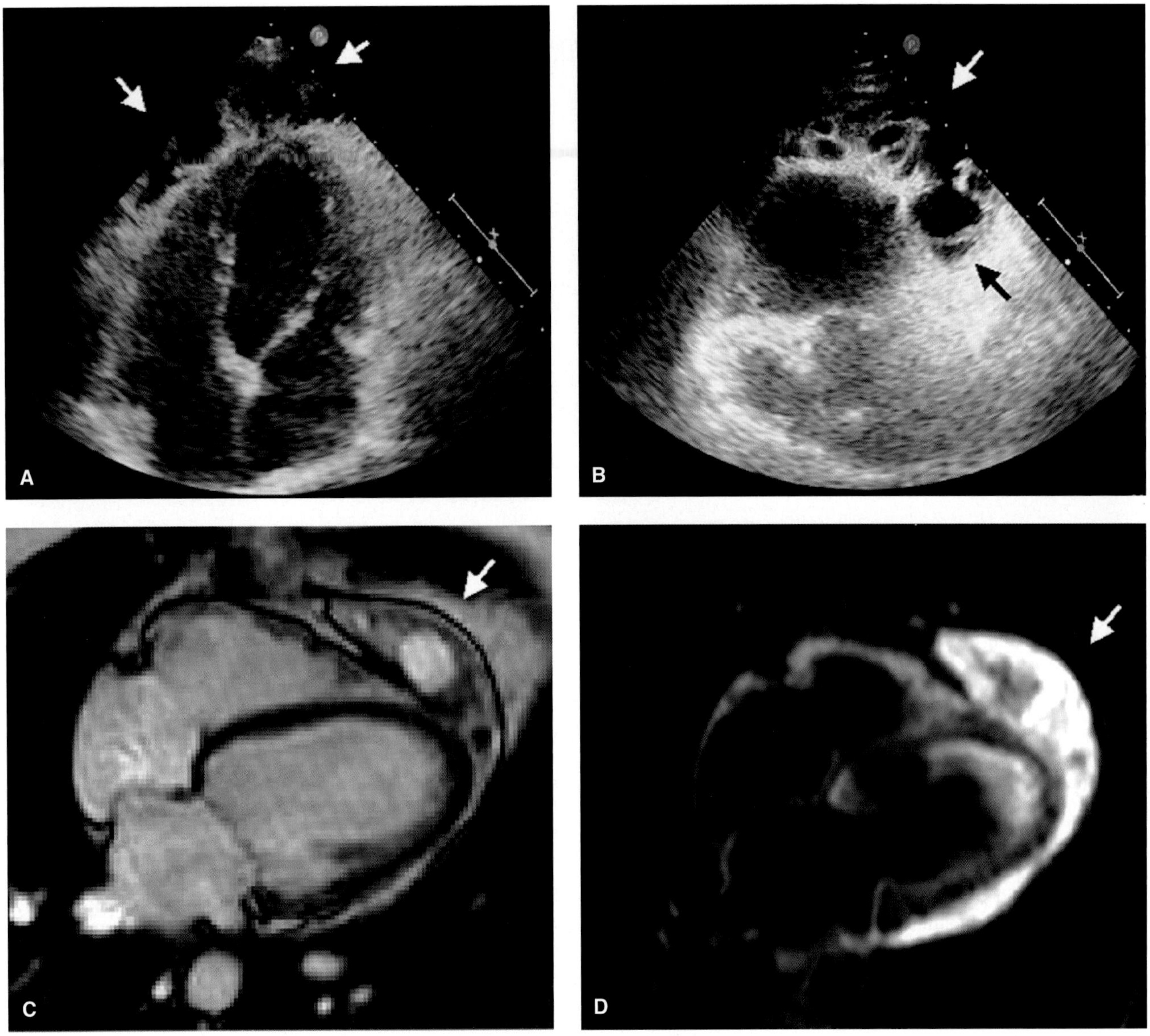

FIGURE 52.6. Echocardiographs (**A** and **B**) and cardiac magnetic resonance images (**C** and **D**) of a mediastinal lymphangioma, involved with the ventricles and the apex of the heart and measuring 7 cm in greatest dimension. (From Conte G, Aldrovandi A, Reverberi C, et al. Mediastinal cystic lymphangioma. *J Am Coll Cardiol* 2011;57(16):e207, with permission from Elsevier.)

Miscellaneous Mediastinal Mesenchymal Lesions

A mélange of other mediastinal mesenchymal lesions have been occasionally encountered; usually of musculoskeletal or connective tissue origin, these lesions typically appear within the posterior mediastinum.[383] These lesions have been treated with surgical excision and occasionally postoperative radiation therapy, depending on the histology and clinical presentation.[380–383,437,438,439–441]

MEDIASTINAL NEUROGENIC TUMORS

Epidemiology

Neurogenic tumors of the thorax are generally classified by their neural cell of origin, including tumors of the nerve sheath (schwannomas and neurofibromas), autonomic ganglion (ganglioneuromas and neuroblastomas), and paraganglion (paragangliomas and pheochromocytomas). Most neurogenic lesions arise in the posterior mediastinum; indeed, they are the most common cause of a posterior mediastinal mass and account for roughly one-quarter to one-third of all mediastinal neoplasms.[8,10,442,443] Neurogenic neoplasms are extremely rare, with an incidence of 0.5 per million in adults.[10] Neuroblastoma, an aggressive variant of neurogenic tumors, occurs primarily in children[444] and appears in the mediastinum in about 20% of cases. Neuroblastoma is covered in the pediatric malignancy section of this book in Chapter 86. Neuroblastomas are more common in white males, and other malignant neurogenic tumors occur at equal rates in both sexes.[445–446,447]

Paragangliomas are rare tumors that arise from extra-adrenal paraganglia and can be either functional (catecholamine secreting) or nonfunctional.[448,449] Most of these tumors are benign, and surgical resection is usually curative, but some studies have suggested that the risk of the tumor being malignant is >10%.[450,451]

The most common neurogenic tumors in adults are benign schwannomas and neurofibromas, often presenting in the setting of neurofibromatosis type-1 (NF-1; described further below). Schwannomas often originate from the intercostal or sympathetic nerves and can become quite large before being

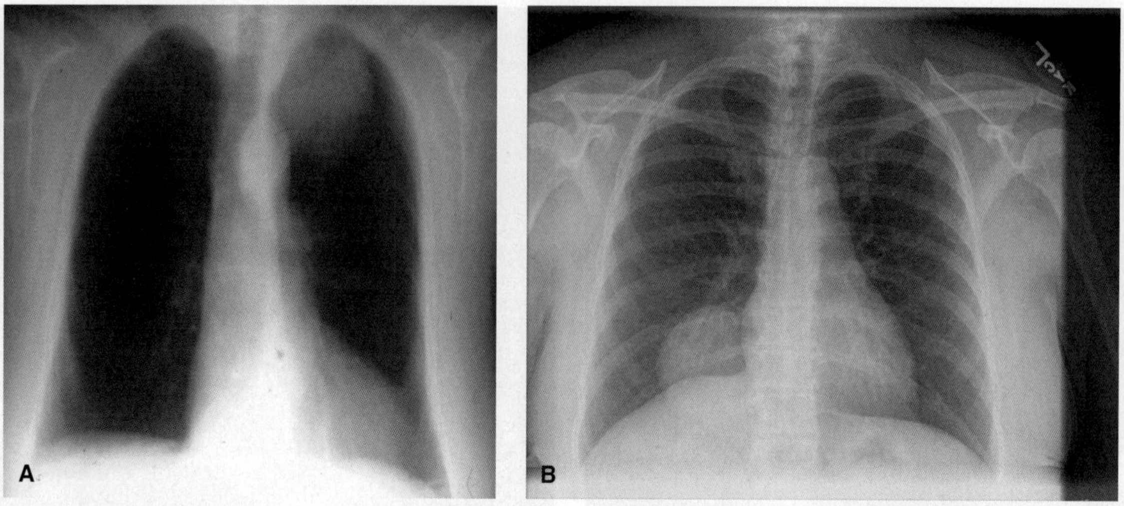

FIGURE 52.7. Posteroanterior chest radiographs of a mediastinal schwannoma **(A)** and a mediastinal neurofibroma **(B)**. (Courtesy of Steve Primack, MD.)

detected,[394] the possibility of achieving a R0 resection depends on the extent of locoregional disease. Long-term local control rates range from 90% to 100%.[443,445,452,453]

NF-1 is an autosomal-dominant neurocutaneous disorder, with an estimated birth incidence of 1 in 2,500.[454] Individuals affected with NF-1 are at increased risk of developing both benign and malignant tumors. The most common benign tumor in individuals with NF-1 is neurofibroma, a heterogeneous benign peripheral nerve sheath tumor.[455,456] Neurofibromas can occur as discrete, focal cutaneous or subcutaneous growths, intraforaminal spinal tumors, or as plexiform tumors. Plexiform neurofibromas are composed of the same cell types as dermal neurofibromas but have an expanded extracellular matrix and a rich vascular supply.[456] In one study of 125 patients with NF-1, plexiform neurofibromas were clinically visible in 30%.[457] Individuals with NF-1 are also at significantly increased risk of developing malignant peripheral nerve sheath tumors (MPNSTs), with a lifetime risk of almost 10%.[458,459] Because most NF-1–associated MPNSTs arise within pre-existing plexiform neurofibromas, individuals with NF-1 and plexiform neurofibromas warrant increased surveillance.

In adults, most malignant mediastinal neurogenic tumors are MPNSTs. In one single-institution experience, MPNSTs were located in the trunk in half of the patients studied.[447] These authors did not distinguish between mediastinal and retroperitoneal locations, but this distinction can be difficult given the lack of an anatomical barrier. Roughly one-third of the patients in that study had NF-1. The median age at presentation of the MPNST was 37 years overall (27 years for patients with NF-1 and 40 for patients without).

MPNSTs have also been linked with prior radiation exposure.[460–463] In one series from the Mayo Clinic, almost 10% of the patients treated there over a 20-year period had a history of radiation exposure.[463]

Natural History and General Management

In up to 80% of cases, mediastinal neurogenic tumors present as an asymptomatic mass on a routine chest x-ray (Figs. 52.7 and 52.8) and can sometimes involve nearly the entire hemithorax.[446,464,465] Large or rapidly growing lesions can cause chest pain and nerve dysfunction (including Horner

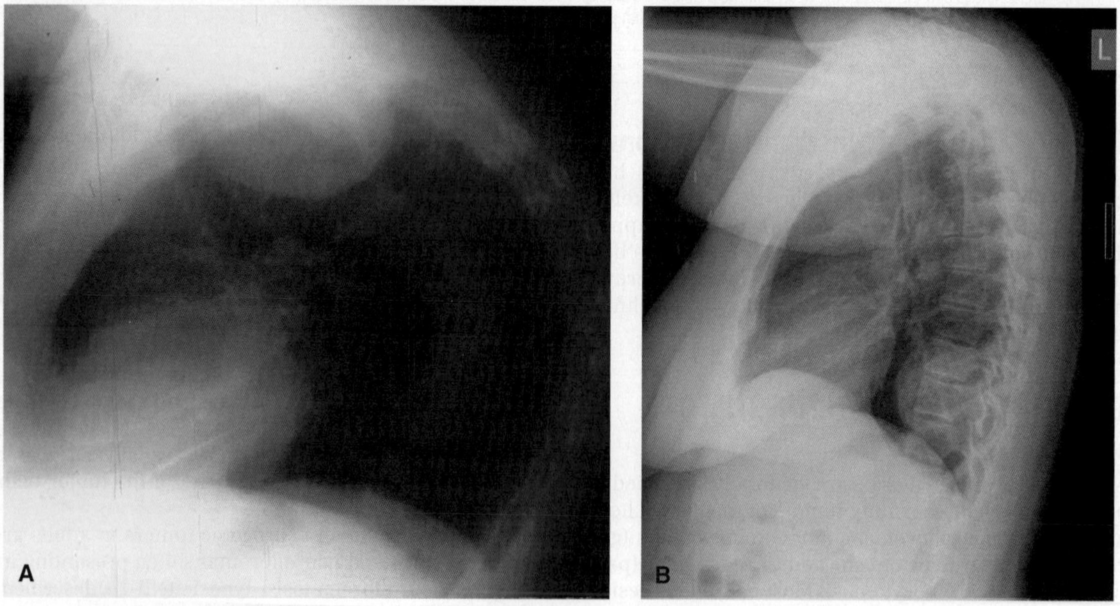

FIGURE 52.8. A: Lateral chest radiograph of a mediastinal schwannoma. **B:** Posteroanterior chest radiograph of a mediastinal neurofibroma. (A and B, courtesy of Steve Primack, MD.)

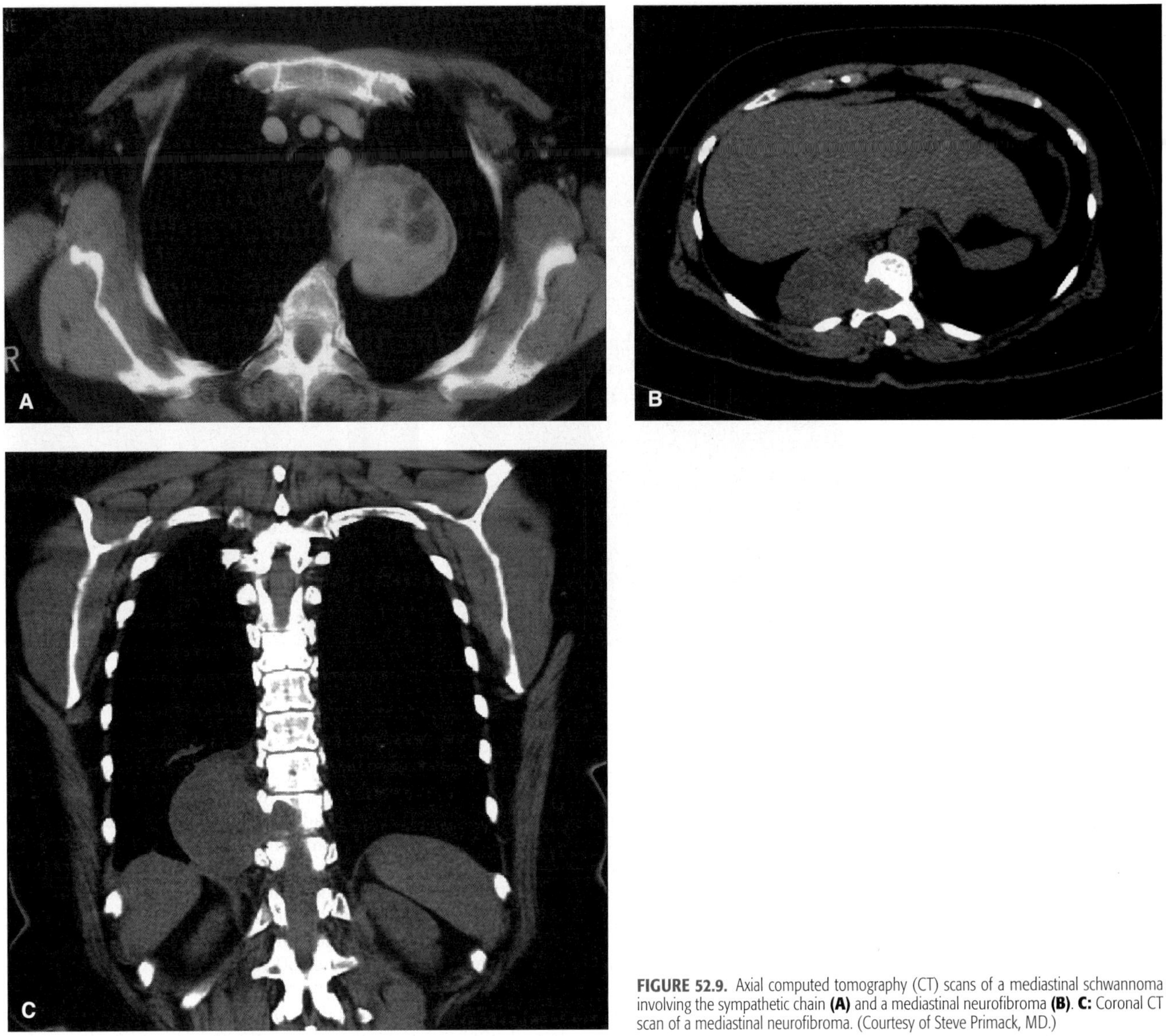

FIGURE 52.9. Axial computed tomography (CT) scans of a mediastinal schwannoma involving the sympathetic chain **(A)** and a mediastinal neurofibroma **(B)**. **C:** Coronal CT scan of a mediastinal neurofibroma. (Courtesy of Steve Primack, MD.)

syndrome) from compression.[466] Proximal organs such as the vagus or phrenic nerves, esophagus, trachea, and cardiac chambers may be involved by direct extension or via the nerve sheath.[467,468,469–473,474] Because MPNSTs are difficult to detect and they metastasize rapidly, they carry a poor prognosis.[475] Local invasion and bony destruction are common.[476] Distant metastases are present in up to one-third of patients at diagnosis.[462]

Management of malignant mediastinal neurogenic tumors entails a multidisciplinary approach similar to the management of adult soft tissue sarcomas. High-resolution CT (Fig. 52.9) is essential, as is MRI (Fig. 52.10), to evaluate the neural and spinal anatomy if involvement is suspected.[477] A definitive pathologic diagnosis is often reached after surgical intervention; examples of histologic slides of a schwannoma and a neurofibroma are shown in Figures 52.11 and 52.12. Histologic examination often reveals nuclear atypia, mitotic figures, cellularity, typical Antoni's A and B areas, and tumor necrosis; these findings, in combination with positive immunohistochemical staining for S-100 protein and negative staining for smooth muscle markers such as desmin, are suggestive of a nerve sheath origin. Of these features, the factor most reliably correlated with malignancy is a mitotic figure of 5 or more in 50 high-power fields. Surgical resection is the mainstay of therapy. An R0 resection should be attempted but is often difficult for mediastinal tumors because of impingement on surrounding structures and, in the case of neurofibromas, the risk of drastic neurologic deficits. Advances in surgical technique, including minimally invasive approaches such as video-assisted thoracoscopic surgery, are available but should be undertaken only by experienced thoracic surgeons.[478–480]

As is true for the treatment of soft tissue sarcomas, adjuvant radiation is part of the treatment of localized MPNSTs. The largest published series to date describes findings from 134 patients with NPNSTs treated at the Mayo Clinic between 1975 and 1993.[463] Only 25 of those patients had mediastinal tumors, and an R0 operation was possible for 70%. This was an improvement over an earlier study showing an R0/R1 rate of only 55% for mediastinal MPNSTs.[481] A variety of radiation techniques were used in the Mayo series. About half of the patients received adjuvant radiation to a mean dose of 51 Gy. At 10 years, the overall survival rate was 42% and local tumor control rate was 50% for the entire group of patients. Prognostic factors for overall survival found to be significant in multivariate analyses were surgical margin status and history of radiation; prognostic factors for local control were surgical margin status, radiation dose, and use of intraoperative radiation or brachytherapy. Use of adjuvant radiation nearly doubled local control rates from 40% to 73% at 3 years and from 34% to 65%

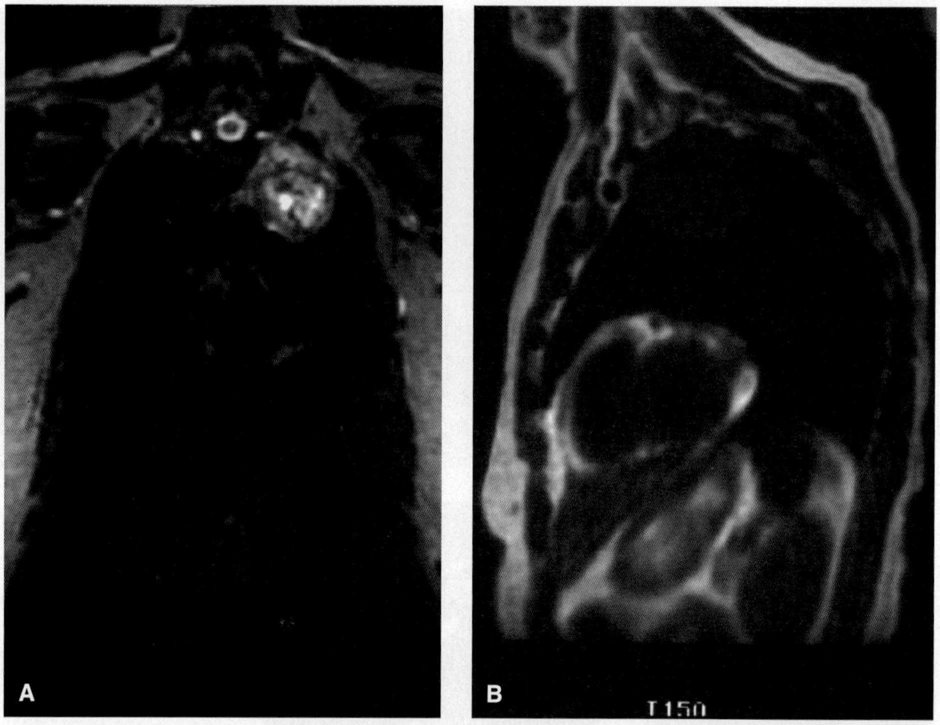

FIGURE 52.10. Coronal **(A)** and sagittal **(B)** magnetic resonance images of a mediastinal schwannoma involving the sympathetic chain. (Courtesy of Steve Primack, MD.)

at 5 years (= .0004), but an apparent benefit in survival (43% vs. 58% at 5 years) was not statistically significant.

Other findings that support the use of radiation after surgery for MPNSTs come from a review of 205 patients with localized MPNSTs at all body sites treated over a 25-year period at the Istituto Nazionale per lo Studio e la Cura dei Tumori in Milan, Italy.[447] That study reported a disease-specific mortality rate of 43% at 10 years, but less than half of the patients received radiation therapy. Variables found to be significant in multivariate analyses for survival included tumor site, tumor size (>12 cm), surgical margin status, and the use of adjuvant radiation ($P = .016$). All of the same factors except for radiation were significantly associated with local control. Patients who received radiation seemed to have had fewer recurrences, but this was not statistically significant. About 30% of patients eventually developed distant metastases, the vast majority of which were pulmonary.

Planning and delivery of external-beam radiation therapy for MPNSTs is facilitated with the use of modern approaches, including 3D conformal radiation, IMRT, and image-guided radiation using cone-beam onboard imaging approaches. Patients with these tumors, which are complicated to manage, should be treated at centers with extensive multidisciplinary experience in thoracic and paraspinal neoplasms. Radiation treatment after surgery for microscopic disease should be given at a minimum dose of 60 Gy in 30 fractions. Given the close proximity of the posterior mediastinum to the spinal cord, careful attention should be paid to immobilization and use of dual image-guidance techniques. Although placing the patient in the prone position may reduce the distance from the

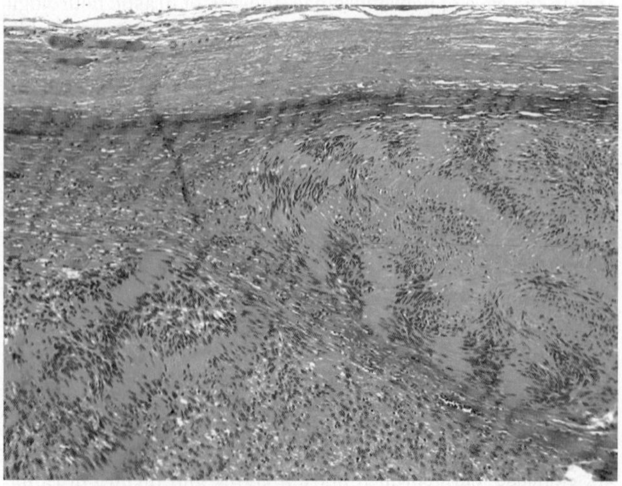

FIGURE 52.11. Hematoxylin-and-eosin–stained section of a schwannoma shows a circumscribed and encapsulated neoplasm composed of low-grade spindled and wavy Schwann cells with alternating palisaded cellular and stroma-rich areas (Verocay bodies) with nonpalisaded cellular foci (Antoni A areas) and hypocellular foci (Antoni B areas). Original magnification 100X. (Courtesy of David Sauer, MD.)

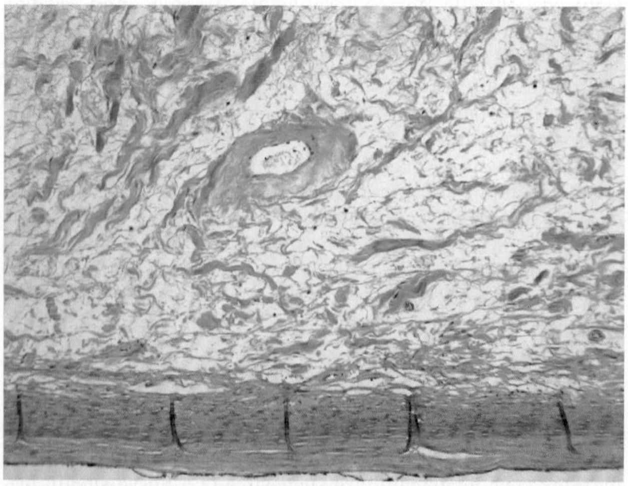

FIGURE 52.12. Hematoxylin-and-eosin–stained section of a neurofibroma shows a circumscribed and encapsulated neoplasm composed of a disorganized proliferation of low-grade spindled fibroblastic and Schwann cells within a myomatous and collagenous stroma (fibrils resembling shredded carrots). Scattered background mast cells and entrapped axons are also present. Original magnification 100X. (Courtesy of David Sauer, MD.)

localization points to the treatment volume, the patient must be able to rest comfortably in the same position throughout the treatments. Daily onboard imaging with stereoscopic guidance can ensure daily accuracy. IMRT is often necessary to provide a concave dose distribution around the spinal cord. In cases of gross residual disease, higher doses may be beneficial but can be challenging to deliver given the constraints on exposure of normal tissues.

For patients with unresectable disease, radiation can be delivered either alone or with chemotherapeutic agents that are typically used for soft tissue sarcomas. Few agents are effective for MPNSTs, and treatment regimens usually include doxorubicin or ifosfamide.[482]

Significant progress has been made in recent years in elucidating the molecular genetics and biology of MPNSTs, especially in patients with NF-1. A variety of genetic alterations have been reported in MPNSTs, but whether any of them are causally related to tumorigenesis or malignant progression is unclear.[483]

TRACHEAL CARCINOMAS

Tracheal neoplasms are quite rare, contributing to fewer than 0.5% of all tumors.[484] Most of the information available to date has been derived from pooled population-based datasets or single-institution series involving a variety of treatment regimens. Review of the largely retrospective data has revealed several patterns: first, surgical resection is the mainstay of therapy; second, local recurrence is a major pattern of failure; and third, adjuvant radiation seems to have some positive effect on outcomes.

Demographics

Primary tracheal malignancy is exceedingly uncommon, accounting for approximately 0.1% to 0.4% of all diagnosed malignancies.[485] Epidemiologic data from the SEER project estimate an incidence of 0.2 per 100,000 persons in the United States; the true incidence of tracheal carcinomas is likely even lower.[486] Traditionally, adenoid cystic carcinomas (formerly known as cylindromas) were considered the most common tracheal neoplasms, but recent reports suggest that the most prevalent histology worldwide is squamous cell (60% to 90%), although adenoid cystic carcinoma seems to be more common among nonsmokers.[487] Tracheal cancer affects roughly twice as many men as women; estimates of incidence from SEER database are 0.2 per 100,000 for men and 0.1 per 100,000 for women.[486] The male-to-female ratio is 2 or 3 to 1 for squamous cancer but is closer to 1 to 1 for adenoid cystic carcinomas.[488] Use of tobacco is associated with squamous cell carcinoma of the trachea but generally not with adenoid cystic carcinoma.[487] Squamous cell variants typically present during the sixth decade of life, whereas adenoid cystic carcinomas seem to present at younger ages. Other histologies include carcinoid, carcinosarcoma, granular cell tumor, hemangioma, neurogenic tumors, chondroma, and chondrosarcoma.[489–535]

Anatomy

The trachea is a fibrocartilaginous tube connecting the larynx superiorly and the mainstem bronchi inferiorly. The esophagus, thyroid, parathyroids, and trachea are derived from the same out-pouching of the embryonic foregut; the lungs arise from terminal tracheal buds. The inferior thyroidal arteries supply the superior trachea, and branches of the bronchial arteries supply the inferior portion. Arterial branches interdigitate between each cartilaginous ring (see Fig. 52.2). In adults, the trachea is 12 cm long; its diameter is slightly larger in men (2.3 cm) than in women (2.0 cm). In cross-section, the organ is "C" or "U" shaped. The upper border lies around the sixth or seventh cervical vertebra, and the lower border around the fourth (full expiration) or sixth (full inspiration) thoracic vertebra. Each centimeter of trachea contains about two cartilaginous rings. The posterior aspect of the trachea is membranous and is intimately associated with the esophagus. Three branches of the inferior thyroid artery supply blood to the upper half of the trachea and connect to the superior thyroid artery, which contributes small vessels that run from the tracheal wall adjacent to the thyroid isthmus. The bronchial arteries supply blood to the lower trachea and carina.

Natural History

Tracheal carcinomas can present with a variety of symptoms, including cough, dyspnea, dysphagia, and hemoptysis.[517,536] Yang et al.[537] reported cough to be the most common symptom (present in 72% of patients), followed by dyspnea (66%), stridor (39%), hemoptysis (39%), and dysphonia (31%). Adenoid cystic carcinomas in particular are often first mistaken for asthma, which is often treated as such until "refractory" obstructive symptoms are evaluated with bronchoscopy, typically after numerous "normal" chest radiographs.[535,536,538–547] Hemoptysis is more likely to be the presenting symptom of squamous cell carcinoma.[537,548] and dysphagia is considered an ominous sign.[549] In one study of nonadenoid cystic/nonsquamous tracheal tumors, benign tumors presented with dyspnea, whereas malignant tumors were associated with hemoptysis.[492]

In 40% to 50% of cases, adenoid cystic carcinomas are diagnosed with synchronous metastases,[550] but survival is relatively long despite the presence of such metastases.[548,550,551–552,553–554] In one series, the median survival time for such patients was 37 months,[488] and median reported survival from the time of diagnosis was approximately 5 years.[487,537] When these tumors spread, they almost always do so in distant nodes rather than in the locoregional paratracheal lymph nodes. Local recurrence is the predominant form of treatment failure and can appear 10 or more years after treatment.[555–557]

Unlike adenoid cystic carcinoma, squamous cell carcinoma has a much more aggressive course, with reported median survival times of only 6 to 12 months depending on resectability.[17,548,552,553,558–562] The disease often presents with local extension via paratracheal lymph nodes (in approximately 30% of cases) and distant metastases.[563]

The clinical course and natural history of other pathologic variants of tracheal tumors are difficult to accurately characterize because of the scarcity of reported findings. Adenocarcinomas and sarcomas are thought to have poor prognoses.[492,528,530,534,564–577] Granular cell tumor, carcinoid, lymphoma, leiomyoma, and small cell carcinoma all have variable prognoses, yet they seem to be less aggressive than the squamous carcinomas, adenocarcinomas, or sarcomas.[492]

Staging and Prognostic Factors

No system for staging tracheal neoplasms has been universally accepted or adopted. One staging system proposed by Licht et al.[45] does not seem to have predictable prognostic value. In some studies, lymph node involvement does not seem to have a significant adverse effect on prognosis,[17,537,563] although an epidemiologic analysis showed an association between nodal status and survival outcomes.[578] The size and location of the tumor seem to be important because of the extent of surgical resection necessary to remove the tumor and higher postoperative mortality associated with carinal resection.[538,578,579] In 2004, Bhattacharyya[578] proposed a staging system wherein stage I is defined as T1N0 disease, stage II as T2N0, stage III as T3N0, and stage IV as T4N0 or any N1 disease (Table 52.10). A similar system, with minor modifications, was used by Webb et al.[487] in evaluating the experience at MD Anderson Cancer Center. Subsequently, Macchiarini[484] proposed a more elaborate staging model that draws from experience with other thoracic malignancies (see Table 52.10). However, at this time it

TABLE 52.10 STAGING SYSTEMS FOR TRACHEAL CARCINOMA

Bhattacharyya Staging System[a]			
Primary Tumor (T)			
T1	Primary tumor confined to trachea; size <2 cm		
T2	Primary tumor confined to trachea; size >2 cm		
T3	Spread outside the trachea but not to adjacent organs or structures*		
T4	Spread to adjacent organs or structures[b]		
Tx	Unknown or cannot be assessed		
Regional Lymph Nodes (N)			
N0	No evidence of regional nodal disease		
N1	Positive regional nodal disease		
Nx	Unknown or cannot be assessed		
Anatomic Stage/Prognostic Groups			
Stage			
I	T1	N0	
II	T2	N0	
III	T3	N0	
IV	Any	N1	
IV	T4	Any	
Macchiarini Staging System[c]			
Primary Tumor (T)			
Tx	Cannot be assessed		
Tis	Any tumour without invasion		
T1a	<3 cm limited to mucosa		
T1b	≥3 cm limited to mucosa		
T2*	Any tumour that invades cartilage or adventitia		
T3	Any tumour that invades trachea or larynx		
T4a	Any tumour that invades carina or main bronchus		
T4b	Any tumour that invades neighbouring structures		
Regional Lymph Nodes (N)			
Nx	Regional lymph nodes cannot be assessed		
N0	No evidence of node metastasis		
N1	Local nodes positive (N1a <3 cm; N1b ≥3 cm)		
Upper third	Highest mediastinal nodes; upper paratracheal nodes, prevascular and retrotracheal		
Middle third	Upper paratracheal nodes; prevascular and retrotracheal; lower paratracheal nodes; para-aortic nodes (ascending aorta or phrenic)		
Lower third	Upper paratracheal nodes; prevascular and retrotracheal; subaortic nodes (aorto-pulmonalis window)		
N1A	1–3 positive nodes in upper third		
N1B	>3 positive nodes in upper third		
N2	Regional nodes positive		
Upper third	Lower paratracheal nodes; subaortic nodes (aortopulmonalis window)		
Middle third	Highest mediastinal nodes; subaortic nodes (aortopulmonalis window)		
Lower third	Upper paratracheal nodes; pulmonary ligament		
Distant Metastasis (M)			
Mx	Distant metastasis cannot be assessed		
M0	No distant metastasis		
M1	Metastasis to nodes other than N1 and N2		
M2	Distant metastasis (e.g., lung)		
Anatomic Stage/Prognostic Groups			
Stage			
0	Tis	N0	M0
Ia	T1a	N0	M0
Ib	T1b–2	N0	M0
IIa	T1b–2	N1	M0
IIb	T1b–2	N2	M0
IIIa	T3	N0	M0
IIIb	T3	N1–2	M0
IVa	Any	N1–2	M1
IVb	Any	N1–2	M2

[a]From ref. (578).

[b]The MD Anderson Cancer Center system denotes "arising from but extending outside of trachea" as T3 disease and does not use T4. From ref. (487).

[c]From ref. (484).

remains to be seen which system will be broadly implemented by clinicians or validated with large-scale clinical datasets.

General Management

Bronchoscopy is essential for diagnosis of tracheal malignancies and for preoperative surgical planning.[536,580–582] In acute respiratory compromise, rigid bronchoscopy (see Fig. 52.2) may be indicated to "core out" the tracheal neoplasm.[538,583,584] In one series of 56 patients reported by Mathisen and Grillo,[585] rigid bronchoscopy led to improved airway symptoms in 90% of cases, with 5% experiencing mild, easily controlled bleeding. Esophagoscopy is suggested for all patients to rule out esophageal invasion. A CT scan of the chest is indicated to aid in evaluation of tumor extension, resectability, involvement of lymph nodes, and pulmonary metastases,[517,536,582,586–590] and coronal reconstruction can be helpful to evaluate tracheal wall thickening and extraluminal extension.[591]

Treatment Approaches

Resectability is universally associated with lower mortality in reported series[17,553,580,592] and as such is the initial strategy for most tracheal primaries.[484,562,563,580,587,593–595] Resection rates vary, however, by institutional and national practice, from 10% to over 65% based on the above cited studies. Historic registry data from the Netherlands demonstrated a resection rate of 12%[558]; however, a recent update[596] suggests that 24% underwent resection in 2000 to 2005 (vs. 58% who received radiotherapy). Contraindications to resection depend in large part on the preference of the surgeon; for example, some authors recommend tracheal resection for at least some patients with adenoid cystic carcinoma with low-burden pulmonary metastases, yet many would consider such cases unresectable.[488,550,597] Regardless, many tracheal carcinomas are either improperly classified (e.g., nontracheal primaries with tracheal extension) or are systematically undertreated surgically.[596]

Most patients undergoing surgery have a median sternotomy and cervical collar excision, although extensive subglottic or high tracheal disease may require cervical exenteration with mediastinal tracheostomy.[550,556,563] Margins may of necessity be compromised to ensure a functioning airway. Technical advances in surgical procedures such as complete mobilization of the right hilar ligament, detachment or implantation of the left hilum, mobilization of the cervical trachea, and techniques for carinal resection or reconstruction and intrapericardial dissection have improved the likelihood of an R0 resection.[293,579,592,598] Gaissert et al.[552,593] reported improvements in both complete resection rates (from 68% to 82%) and in-hospital mortality (declining from 21% to 3%) with the increasing use of such techniques over a 40-year period.

After resection, postoperative radiation is usually recommended.[487,552,553,580,581,584,593] Pathologic features such as completeness of resection, involvement of the thyroid gland, and lymphatic invasion have clearly been shown to have prognostic value,[599] and postoperative radiotherapy is routinely recommended for all patients at many institutions.[487] Preoperative radiotherapy has also been attempted, but fewer reports of this experience have been published. In aggregate, several small retrospective series seem to show a benefit for adjuvant radiation (Table 52.11). Chow et al.[600] found that patients who underwent resection plus adjuvant radiation had a median survival time of 61 months versus 16 months for those who received only surgery. Regnand et al.[17] found that 31 patients who had had a complete resection with adjuvant radiation had seemingly better 5-year survival rates than did 27 patients without adjuvant radiation (74% vs. 53%), but this apparent difference was not statistically significant.

Postoperative radiation seems to be effective for incompletely resected disease as well, with 5-year survival rates of 45% for such patients versus 0% for patients who did not

TABLE 52.11 RESULTS OF RESECTION WITH ADJUVANT IRRADIATION FOR PRIMARY TRACHEAL CARCINOMA

Study (Reference)	Histology	Treatment	Median Survival Times or Rates
Grillo and Mathisen (553)	Squamous (n = 70)	Surgery ± RT[a]	34 mo
		RT	10 mo
	Adenoid cystic (n = 80)	Surgery ± RT[a]	118 mo
		RT	28 mo
Licht et al. (45)	–	Surgery alone (n = 6)	48% (5-yr actuarial)
		RT alone (n = 35)	7%
		Laser/cautery ± RT (n = 24)	28%
			0%
		RT + chemo (n = 2)	
Chow et al. (600)	–	Surgery alone (n = 5)	16 mo
		RT alone (n = 12)	26 mo
		Surgery + RT (n = 5)	61 mo
Regnard et al. (17)	–	R0 + RT (n = 31)	74% (5-year actuarial)
		R0 (n = 27)	53% (*P* = NS)
		R1,2 + RT (n = 15)	47%
		R1,2 (n = 6)	0% (*P* <.05)
Maziak et al. (488)	Adenoid cystic (n = 35)	R0 ± RT (n = 14)[a]	9.8 yr
		R1,2 + RT (n = 15)	7.5 yr
		RT alone (n = 6)	6.2 yr

RT, radiation therapy; chemo, chemotherapy; R0, complete resection; R1,2, incomplete resection.

[a]A minority of these patients received surgery alone.

receive radiation (*P* <.05).[17] Webb et al.,[487] describing the experience at MD Anderson Cancer Center, demonstrated a statistically significant improvement in survival for patients given adjuvant radiotherapy rather than chemoradiation; however, no difference in survival was found between adjuvant radiotherapy and surgery alone. The results of studies of definitive therapy for tracheal tumors are summarized in Table 52.12.

Radiation has also been used as monotherapy for unresectable tumors. Results are best when doses have exceeded 60 Gy.[559,602,604] Mornex et al.[606] found that the 5-year survival rate decreased from 12% for those receiving at least 56 Gy to 5% for those receiving lower doses. However, Chow et al.[600] caution against giving doses higher than 60 Gy, as three of six patients in their study given doses in excess of 60 Gy had severe complications requiring surgical intervention (e.g., tracheoesophageal fistula, esophageal stricture, and severe tracheal crusting), whereas none of the six patients treated with <60 Gy in that study had late side effects. Other authors have corroborated the concern of high doses contributing to the risk of complications.[607] Still, Chow et al.[600] noted significantly better local control among patients who received >50 Gy as adjuvant therapy and >60 Gy as definitive therapy. By way of comparison, Fuwa et al.[605] reported reasonable results with a novel endoluminal-centering catheter; the median dose delivered to the group as a whole was 91 Gy (given as external-beam radiation with low-dose-rate iridium-192 brachytherapy). Only one treatment-related death was reported 1 year after therapy in a patient who had received a total dose of 113 Gy. Harms et al.,[608] using median doses of 60 Gy delivered by external-beam radiation plus 15- to 18-Gy brachytherapy boosts, reported minimal rates of severe (grade 3 or 4) toxicity (8% of 25 patients). Exploratory studies of fast neutrons for locally advanced adenoid cystic carcinomas have been reported; in the University of Washington experience with endoluminal brachytherapy, fast neutrons were considered feasible and toxicity acceptable.[609] A summary of the experience with radiation as monotherapy for primary tracheal neoplasms is given in Table 52.11.

Combined chemoradiotherapy without resection has been attempted at some institutions, usually for nonsquamous tumors, with mixed results.[487,548,610,611] In general, patients with squamous cell carcinoma have fared poorly, and those with small cell carcinoma or lymphoma have done better.[45,487,537,612]

Radiation Techniques

No evidence is available to suggest that adjuvant radiation therapy is not beneficial in tracheal malignancies; however, any postoperative radiation should not begun before 30 to 45 days after surgery to allow sufficient wound healing. Modern CT-based 3D conformal or IMRT techniques should be used. Aggressive treatment is warranted to prevent airway obstruction, even when the intent is palliative.[606] External-beam doses should be about 60 Gy for fully resected disease,[487] with a boost considered for squamous cell lesions with high-risk features.[599] An intraluminal boost technique allows the dose to be increased (and, theoretically, local control to be increased as well) with minimal added acute or late side effects.[561,600,608,613,614–615] Standard constraints on organs at risk should be observed in all cases.[231,232,234,616]

Intraluminal brachytherapy is also useful for palliative treatment. Skowronek et al.,[615] in a study of patients treated with 10 to 30 Gy in 1 to 3 fractions, found that high-dose brachytherapy as monotherapy led to prolonged survival and improved quality of life. In patients with locally extensive disease, the gravest complication of radiation therapy is the development of a tracheoesophageal fistula, which can be difficult if not impossible to avoid. For patients with emergent airway obstruction, rigid bronchoscopy should be performed instead of urgent radiotherapy.

The role of elective nodal irradiation for tracheal carcinoma is uncertain. As mentioned earlier, nodal status does not seem to have prognostic significance; even cervical

TABLE 52.12 RETROSPECTIVE SERIES EXAMINING RADIOTHERAPY ALONE FOR PRIMARY TRACHEAL CARCINOMA

Study (Reference)	Histology	Treatment	Local Control	Survival
Schraube et al. (561)	Squamous (n = 11)	46–60 Gy RT + 15–20 Gy HDR	6/11	31-mo median
Cheung (601)	Squamous (n = 20)	40–60 Gy		5-mo median
	Adenoid cystic (n = 4)	40–60 Gy		12-mo median
Fields et al. (602)	Squamous (n = 17)	>60 Gy	5/6	25% at 5 yr (n = 18)
	Adenoid cystic (n = 1)	40–60 Gy	1/7	
		<40 Gy	0/4	
		>60 Gy	1/1	
Rostom and Morgan (603)	Squamous (n = 28)	60–70 Gy	16/24	11% (4-yr actuarial)
	Adenoid cystic (n = 3)	<60 Gy	0/4	67% at 4 yr
		50–70 Gy		
Makarewick and Mross (604)		60 Gy RT + 6–12 Gy HDR (n = 8)	6/8	9.5-mo median (n = 23)
		40–60 Gy RT (n = 3)	1/3	
		<40 Gy (n = 12)	0/12	
Fuwa et al. (605)		RT + LDR (n = 4) (80–128 Gy)[a]	3/4	75% at 3 yr

HDR, high-dose rate brachytherapy; LDR, low-dose rate brachytherapy; RT, external-beam radiotherapy.

[a]One treatment-related death in patient receiving 60 Gy RT + 53 Gy LDR iridium-192.

adenopathy was not associated with poorer outcome.[537] Given the low proclivity for lymphatic spread of adenoid cystic carcinomas, the choice to avoid elective nodal irradiation for this variant is certainly reasonable. Because local recurrence is the major factor influencing survival, nodal and regional failure patterns are not a main concern. Yet if mediastinal or cervical nodes are seen on radiographic or pathologic examination, or if worrisome pathologic risk features[599] are discovered at surgery, radiation to these regions should be considered.

CONCLUSION

Primary tracheal cancer is quite rare and in most cases is of squamous or adenoid cystic histology. The optimal management strategy for these tumors seems to be a combined-modality approach incorporating surgical resection and postoperative radiation. For localized disease, the role of chemotherapy, either alone or concurrent with radiation, is unknown.

SELECTED REFERENCES

A full list of references for this chapter is available online.

2. Greene MA, Malias MA. Aggressive multimodality treatment of invasive thymic carcinoma. *J Thorac Cardiovasc Surg* 2003;125(2):434–436.
6. Strollo DC, Rosado-de-Christenson ML, Jett JR. Primary mediastinal tumors: part II. Tumors of the middle and posterior mediastinum. *Chest* 1997;112(5):1344–1357.
8. Azarow KS, Pearl RH, Zurcher R, et al. Primary mediastinal masses. A comparison of adult and pediatric populations. *J Thorac Cardiovasc Surg* 1993;106(1):67–72.
11. Whooley BP, Urschel JD, Antkowiak JG, et al. Primary tumors of the mediastinum. *J Surg Oncol* 1999;70(2):95–99.
14. Mullen B, Richardson JD. Primary anterior mediastinal tumors in children and adults. *Ann Thorac Surg* 1986;42(3):338–345.
17. Regnard JF, Fourquier P, Levasseur P. Results and prognostic factors in resections of primary tracheal tumors: a multicenter retrospective study. The French Society of Cardiovascular Surgery. *J Thorac Cardiovasc Surg* 1996;111(4):808–813.
18. Maggi G, Casadio C, Cavallo A, et al. Thymoma: results of 241 operated cases. *Ann Thorac Surg* 1991;51(1):152–156.
23. Thomas CR, Wright CD, Loehrer PJ. Thymoma: state of the art. *J Clin Oncol* 1999;17(7):2280–2289.
28. Teoh R, McGuire L, Wong K, et al. Increased incidence of thymoma in Chinese myasthenia gravis: possible relationship with Epstein-Barr virus. *Acta Neurol Scand* 1989;80(3):221–225.
33. Lara PN Jr. Malignant thymoma: current status and future directions. *Cancer Treat Rev* 2000;26(2):127–131.
37. Curran WJ Jr, Kornstein MJ, Brooks JJ, et al. Invasive thymoma: the role of mediastinal irradiation following complete or incomplete surgical resection. *J Clin Oncol* 1988;6(11):1722–1727.
47. Souadjian JV, Enriquez P, Silverstein MN, et al. The spectrum of diseases associated with thymoma. Coincidence or syndrome? *Arch Intern Med* 1974;134(2):374–379.
52. Drachman DB. Myasthenia gravis (first of two parts). *N Engl J Med* 1978;298(3):136–142.
53. Drachman DB. Myasthenia gravis (second of two parts). *N Engl J Med* 1978;298(4):186–193.
64. Wilkens EW, Grillo HC, Scannell Gea. Role of staging in prognosis and management of thymoma. *Ann Thorac Surg* 1991;51:888–892.
68. Kondo K, Monden Y. Lymphogenous and hematogenous metastasis of thymic epithelial tumors. *Ann Thorac Surg* 2003;76(6):1859–1864.
74. Venuta F, Rendina EA, Pescarmona EO, et al. Multimodality treatment of thymoma: a prospective study. *Ann Thorac Surg* 1997;64(6):1585–1591.
84. Thompson BH, Stabford W. MR imaging of pulmonary and mediastinal malignancies. *MRI Clin North Am* 2000;8(4):729–739.
86. Liu RS, Yeh SH, Huang MH, et al. Use of fluorine-18 fluorodeoxyglucose positron emission tomography in the detection of thymoma: a preliminary report. *Eur J Nucl Med* 1995;22(12):1402–1407.
90. Kumar A, Regmi SK, Dutta R, et al. Characterization of thymic masses using (18) F-FDG PET-CT. *Ann Nucl Med* 2009;23(6):569–577.
92. Kaira K, Endo M, Abe M, et al. Biologic correlation of 2-[18F]-fluoro-2-deoxy-D-glucose uptake on positron emission tomography in thymic epithelial tumors. *J Clin Oncol* 2010;28(23):3746–3753.
103. Masaoka A, Monden Y, Nakahara K, et al. Follow-up study of thymomas with special reference to their clinical stages. *Cancer* 1981;48(11):2485–2492.
106. Akaogi E, Ohara K, Mitsui K, et al. Preoperative radiotherapy and surgery for advanced thymoma with invasion to the great vessels. *J Surg Oncol* 1996;63(1):17–22.
110. Travis WD, Brambilla E, Müller-Hermelink HK, et al. *World Health Organization Classification of Tumours: Pathology & Genetic: Tumours of the Lung, Pleura, Thymus and Heart.* Lyon, Oxford: IARC Press, 2004.
115. Quintanilla-Martinez L, Wilkins EW Jr, Choi N, et al. Thymoma. Histologic subclassification is an independent prognostic factor. *Cancer* 1994;74(2):606–617.
116. Detterbeck FC. Clinical value of the WHO classification system of thymoma. *Ann Thorac Surg* 2006;81(6):2328–2334.
118. Dawson A, Ibrahim NB, Gibbs AR. Observer variation in the histopathological classification of thymoma: correlation with prognosis. *J Clin Pathol* 1994;47(6):519–523.
128. Gilhus NE, Jones M, Turley H, et al. Oncogene proteins and proliferation antigens in thymomas: increased expression of epidermal growth factor receptor and Ki67 antigen. *J Clin Pathol* 1995;48(5):447–455.
132. Girard N, Shen R, Guo T, et al. Comprehensive genomic analysis reveals clinically relevant molecular distinctions between thymic carcinomas and thymomas. *Clin Cancer Res* 2009;15(22):6790–6799.
133. Yoh K, Nishiwaki Y, Ishii G, et al. Mutational status of EGFR and KIT in thymoma and thymic carcinoma. *Lung Cancer* 2008;62(3):316–320.
134. Christodoulou C, Murray S, Dahabreh J, et al. Response of malignant thymoma to erlotinib. *Ann Oncol* 2008;19(7):1361–1362.
138. Girard N, Teruya-Feldstein J, Payabyab EC, et al. Insulin-like growth factor-1 receptor expression in thymic malignancies. *J Thorac Oncol* 2010;5(9):1439–1446.
141. Giaccone G, Rajan A, Ruijter R, et al. Imatinib mesylate in patients with WHO B3 thymomas and thymic carcinomas. *J Thorac Oncol* 2009;4(10):1270–1273.
144. Karp DD, Paz-Ares LG, Novello S, et al. Phase II study of the anti-insulin-like growth factor type 1 receptor antibody CP-751,871 in combination with paclitaxel and carboplatin in previously untreated, locally advanced, or metastatic non-small-cell lung cancer. *J Clin Oncol* 2009;27(15):2516–2522.
150. Cameron R, Loeher P, Thomas C. Neoplasms of the Mediastinum. In: DeVita V, Hellman S, Rosenberg S, eds. *Cancer: principles and practice of oncology,* 6th ed. Philadelphia: Lippincott-Raven, 2000:1019–1036.
155. Myojin M, Choi NC, Wright CD, et al. Stage III thymoma: pattern of failure after surgery and postoperative radiotherapy and its implication for future study. *Int J Radiat Oncol Biol Phys* 2000;46(4):927–933.
165. Okumura M, Ohta M, Tateyama H, et al. The World Health Organization histologic classification system reflects the oncologic behavior of thymoma: a clinical study of 273 patients. *Cancer* 2002;94(3):624–632.
174. Lucchi M, Ambrogi MC, Duranti L, et al. Advanced stage thymomas and thymic carcinomas: results of multimodality treatments. *Ann Thorac Surg* 2005;79(6):1840–1844.
181. Ruckert JC, Swierzy M, Ismail M. Comparison of robotic and nonrobotic thoracoscopic thymectomy: a cohort study. *J Thorac Cardiovasc Surg* 2011;141(3):673–677.
182. Takeo S, Tsukamoto S, Kawano D, et al. Outcome of an original video-assisted thoracoscopic extended thymectomy for thymoma. *Ann Thorac Surg* 2011;92(6):2000–2005.
187. Okumura M, Shiono H, Inoue M, et al. Outcome of surgical treatment for recurrent thymic epithelial tumors with reference to world health organization histologic classification system. *J Surg Oncol* 2007;95(1):40–44.
188. Bott MJ, Wang H, Travis W, et al. Management and outcomes of relapse after treatment for thymoma and thymic carcinoma. *Ann Thorac Surg* 2011;92(6):1984–1992.
191. Chang JH, Kim HJ, Wu HG, et al. Postoperative radiotherapy for completely resected stage II or III thymoma. *J Thorac Oncol* 2011;6(7):1282–1286.
194. Forquer JA, Rong N, Fakiris AJ, et al. Postoperative radiotherapy after surgical resection of thymoma: differing roles in localized and regional disease. *Int J Radiat Oncol Biol Phys* 2010;76(2):440–445.
212. Giaccone G, Ardizzoni A, Kirkpatrick A, et al. Cisplatin and etoposide combination chemotherapy for locally advanced or metastatic thymoma. A phase II study of the European Organization for Research and Treatment of Cancer Lung Cancer Cooperative Group. *J Clin Oncol* 1996;14(3):814–820.
213. Kim ES, Putnam JB, Komaki R, et al. Phase II study of a multidisciplinary approach with induction chemotherapy, followed by surgical resection, radiation therapy, and consolidation chemotherapy for unresectable malignant thymomas: final report. *Lung Cancer* 2004;44(3):369–379.
218. Loehrer PJ Sr, Wang W, Johnson DH, et al. Octreotide alone or with prednisone in patients with advanced thymoma and thymic carcinoma: an Eastern Cooperative Oncology Group phase II trial. *J Clin Oncol* 2004;22(2):293–299.
220. Yokoi K, Matsuguma H, Nakahara R, et al. Multidisciplinary treatment for advanced invasive thymoma with cisplatin, doxorubicin, and methylprednisolone. *Chest* 2005;128(4):145S-b-146S.
223. Evoli A, Batocchi AP, Provenzano C, et al. Thymectomy in the treatment of myasthenia gravis: report of 247 patients. *J Neurol* 1988;235(5):272–276.
232. Marks LB, Bentzen SM, Deasy JO, et al. Radiation dose-volume effects in the lung. *Int J Radiat Oncol Biol Phys* 2010;76(3 Suppl):S70–S76.
233. Marks LB, Yorke ED, Jackson A, et al. Use of normal tissue complication probability models in the clinic. *Int J Radiat Oncol Biol Phys* 2010;76(3 Suppl):S10–S19.
235. Sugie C, Shibamoto Y, Ikeya-Hashizume C, et al. Invasive thymoma: postoperative mediastinal irradiation, and low-dose entire hemithorax irradiation in patients with pleural dissemination. *J Thorac Oncol* 2008;3(1):75–81.
237. Uematsu M, Yoshida H, Kondo M, et al. Entire hemithorax irradiation following complete resection in patients with stage II–III invasive thymoma. *Int J Radiat Oncol Biol Phys* 1996;35(2):357–360.
246. Liao ZX, Komaki RR, Thames HD Jr, et al. Influence of technologic advances on outcomes in patients with unresectable, locally advanced non-small-cell lung cancer receiving concomitant chemoradiotherapy. *Int J Radiat Oncol Biol Phys* 2010;76(3):775–781.
252. Sejpal S, Komaki R, Tsao A, et al. Early findings on toxicity of proton beam therapy with concurrent chemotherapy for nonsmall cell lung cancer. *Cancer* 2011;117(13):3004–3013.
256. Gomez D, Komaki R. Technical advances of radiation therapy for thymic malignancies. *J Thorac Oncol* 2010;5(10 Suppl 4):S336–S343.
257. Gomez D, Komaki R, Yu J, et al. Radiation therapy definitions and reporting guidelines for thymic malignancies. *J Thorac Oncol* 2011;6(7):S1743–S1748.
265. Seto H, Kageyama M, Shimizu M, et al. Assessment of residual tumor viability in thymic carcinoma by sequential thallium-201 SPECT: comparison with CT and biopsy findings. *J Nucl Med* 1994;35(10):1659–1661.
267. Do YS, Im JG, Lee BH, et al. CT findings in malignant tumors of thymic epithelium. *J Comput Assist Tomogr* 1995;19(2):192–197.
274. Sasaki M, Kuwabara Y, Ichiya Y, et al. Differential diagnosis of thymic tumors using a combination of 11C-methionine PET and FDG PET. *J Nucl Med* 1999;40(10):1595–1601.
277. Dadmanesh F, Sekihara T, Rosai J. Histologic typing of thymoma according to the new World Health Organization classification. *Chest Surg Clin North Am* 2001;11(2):407–420.
280. Suster S. Thymic carcinoma: update of current diagnostic criteria and histologic types. *Semin Diagn Pathol* 2005;22(3):198–212.
288. Nonaka T, Tamaki Y, Higuchi K, et al. The role of radiotherapy for thymic carcinoma. *Jpn J Clin Oncol* 2004;34(12):722–726.
291. Hsu HC, Huang EY, Wang CJ, et al. Postoperative radiotherapy in thymic carcinoma: treatment results and prognostic factors. *Int J Radiat Oncol Biol Phys* 2002;52(3):801–805.

294. Nakamura Y, Kunitoh H, Kubota K, et al. Platinum-based chemotherapy with or without thoracic radiation therapy in patients with unresectable thymic carcinoma. *Jpn J Clin Oncol* 2000;30(9):385–388.
307. Klemm KM, Moran CA. Primary neuroendocrine carcinomas of the thymus. *Semin Diagn Pathol* 1999;16(1):32–41.
310. Wick MR, Rosai J. Neuroendocrine neoplasms of the mediastinum. *Semin Diagn Pathol* 1991;8(1):35–51.
327. Nichols CR, Hoffman R, Einhorn LH, et al. Hematologic malignancies associated with primary mediastinal germ-cell tumors. *Ann Intern Med* 1985;102(5):603–609.
331. Hartmann JT, Nichols CR, Droz JP, et al. Hematologic disorders associated with primary mediastinal nonseminomatous germ cell tumors. *J Natl Cancer Inst* 2000;92(1):54–61.
340. Lemarie E, Assouline PS, Diot P, et al. Primary mediastinal germ cell tumors. Results of a French retrospective study. *Chest* 1992;102(5):1477–1483.
346. Israel A, Bosl GJ, Golbey RB, et al. The results of chemotherapy for extragonadal germ-cell tumors in the cisplatin era: the Memorial Sloan-Kettering Cancer Center experience (1975 to 1982). *J Clin Oncol* 1985;3(8):1073–1078.
349. Economou JS, Trump DL, Holmes EC, et al. Management of primary germ cell tumors of the mediastinum. *J Thorac Cardiovasc Surg* 1982;83(5):643–649.
352. Rotmensch S, Cole LA. False diagnosis and needless therapy of presumed malignant disease in women with false-positive human chorionic gonadotropin concentrations. *Lancet* 2000;355(9205):712–715.
358. Schultz SM, Einhorn LH, Conces DJ Jr, et al. Management of postchemotherapy residual mass in patients with advanced seminoma: Indiana University experience. *J Clin Oncol* 1989;7(10):1497–1503.
364. Uematsu M, Kondo M, Dokiya T, et al. The role of radiotherapy in the treatment of primary mediastinal seminoma. *Radiother Oncol* 1992;24(4):226–230.
370. Jones WG, Fossa SD, Mead GM, et al. Randomized trial of 30 versus 20 Gy in the adjuvant treatment of stage I testicular seminoma: a report on Medical Research Council Trial TE18, European Organisation for the Research and Treatment of Cancer Trial 30942 (ISRCTN18525328). *J Clin Oncol* 2005;23(6):1200–1208.
373. Kay PH, Wells FC, Goldstraw P. A multidisciplinary approach to primary nonseminomatous germ cell tumors of the mediastinum. *Ann Thorac Surg* 1987; 44(6):578–582.
378. Saxman SB, Nichols CR, Einhorn LH. Salvage chemotherapy in patients with extragonadal nonseminomatous germ cell tumors: the Indiana University experience. *J Clin Oncol* 1994;12(7):1390–1393.
394. Weiss SW, Goldblum JR, Enzinger FM. *Enzinger and Weiss's soft tissue tumors*, 4th ed. St. Louis: Mosby, 2001.
397. Takeo S, Fukuyama S. Video-assisted thoracoscopic resection of a giant anterior mediastinal tumor (lipoma) using an original sternum-lifting technique. *Jpn J Thorac Cardiovasc Surg* 2005;53(10):565–568.
401. Burt M, Ihde JK, Hajdu SI, et al. Primary sarcomas of the mediastinum: results of therapy. *J Thorac Cardiovasc Surg* 1998;115(3):671–680.
422. Johnson DW, Klazynski PT, Gordon WH, et al. Mediastinal lymphangioma and chylothorax: the role of radiotherapy. *Ann Thorac Surg* 1986;41(3):325–328.
435. Cohen AJ, Sbaschnig RJ, Hochholzer L, et al. Mediastinal hemangiomas. *Ann Thorac Surg* 1987;43(6):656–659.
438. Suster S, Moran CA. Malignant cartilaginous tumors of the mediastinum: clinicopathological study of six cases presenting as extraskeletal soft tissue masses. *Hum Pathol* 1997;28(5):588–594.
447. Anghileri M, Miceli R, Fiore M, et al. Malignant peripheral nerve sheath tumors: prognostic factors and survival in a series of patients treated at a single institution. *Cancer* 2006;107(5):1065–1074.
458. Tucker T, Wolkenstein P, Revuz J, et al. Association between benign and malignant peripheral nerve sheath tumors in NF1. *Neurology* 2005;65(2):205–211.
468. Eguchi T, Yoshida K, Kobayashi N, et al. Multiple schwannomas of the bilateral mediastinal vagus nerves. *Ann Thorac Surg* 2011;91(4):1280–1281.
474. Wang S, Zheng J, Ruan Z, et al. Long-term survival in a rare case of malignant esophageal schwannoma cured by surgical excision. *Ann Thorac Surg* 2011;92 (1):357–358.
477. Reeder LB. Neurogenic tumors of the mediastinum. *Semin Thorac Cardiovasc Surg* 2000;12(4):261–267.
487. Webb BD, Walsh GL, Roberts DB, et al. Primary tracheal malignant neoplasms: the University of Texas MD Anderson Cancer Center experience. *J Am Coll Surg* 2006;202(2):237–246.
488. Maziak DE, Todd TR, Keshavjee SH, et al. Adenoid cystic carcinoma of the airway: thirty-two-year experience. *J Thorac Cardiovasc Surg* 1996;112(6): 1522–1531.
551. Douglas JG, Laramore GE, Austin-Seymour M, et al. Treatment of locally advanced adenoid cystic carcinoma of the head and neck with neutron radiotherapy. *Int J Radiat Oncol Biol Phys* 2000;46(3):551–557.
552. Gaissert HA, Grillo HC, Shadmehr MB, et al. Long-term survival after resection of primary adenoid cystic and squamous cell carcinoma of the trachea and carina. *Ann Thorac Surg* 2004;78(6):1889–1896.
578. Bhattacharyya N. Contemporary staging and prognosis for primary tracheal malignancies: a population-based analysis. *Otolaryngol Head Neck Surg* 2004; 131(5):639–642.
583. Wood DE. Management of malignant tracheobronchial obstruction. *Surg Clin North Am* 2002;82(3):621–642.
596. Honings J, Gaissert HA, Verhagen AF, et al. Undertreatment of tracheal carcinoma: multidisciplinary audit of epidemiologic data. *Ann Surg Oncol* 2009;16(2): 246–253.
599. Honings J, Gaissert HA, Ruangchira-Urai R, et al. Pathologic characteristics of resected squamous cell carcinoma of the trachea: prognostic factors based on an analysis of 59 cases. *Virchows Arch* 2009;455(5):423–429.
605. Fuwa N, Ito Y, Matsumoto A, et al. The treatment results of 40 patients with localized endobronchial cancer with external beam irradiation and intraluminal irradiation using low dose rate (192)Ir thin wires with a new catheter. *Radiother Oncol* 2000;56(2):189–195.
613. Carvalho Hde A, Figueiredo V, Pedreira WL Jr, et al. High dose-rate brachytherapy as a treatment option in primary tracheal tumors. *Clinics* 2005;60(4): 299–304.

Chapter 53 Esophageal Cancer

Brian G. Czito, Albert S. DeNittis, Manisha Palta, and Christopher G. Willett

Less than 15% of patients diagnosed with esophageal cancer are cured, with approximately half of patients presenting with unresectable or metastatic disease. This chapter reviews the natural history and treatment of esophageal cancer, including anatomy, risk factors, patterns of spread and failure, staging, results of current therapeutic approaches, radiation planning techniques, toxicity data, and future treatment strategies.

ANATOMY

The esophagus is a thin-walled, hollow tube approximately 25 cm in length. It is lined with stratified keratinized squamous epithelium, extending from the cricopharyngeus muscle at the level of the cricoid cartilage superiorly to the gastroesophageal junction inferiorly. The lower one-third (5 to 10 cm) of the esophagus may contain glandular elements. Replacement of the stratified squamous epithelium with columnar epithelium is referred to as Barrett's esophagus, often occurring in the lower one-third. The Z-line refers to the endoscopically visible junction of the squamous and glandular epithelium. The esophageal wall is composed of three layers: the mucosa, submucosa, and muscularis propria (Fig. 53.1). The mucosal layer contains the epithelium, lamina propria, and muscularis mucosae. The epithelium is separated from the lamina propria by a basement membrane. In the portion of esophagus containing columnar-type epithelium, the muscularis mucosae may consist of two layers. The mucosa may be divided into distinct layers, including M1 (epithelium), M2 (lamina propria), and M3 (muscularis mucosae). Similarly, the submucosal layer may be divided into inner (SM1), middle (SM2), and outer (SM3) layers. The muscularis propria consists of a circular inner layer and longitudinal outer layer. The adventitia (periesophageal connective tissue) lies directly on the muscularis propria.[1] No serosa is present, facilitating extraesophageal spread of disease.

Although somewhat arbitrary, the esophagus is frequently divided into cervical and thoracic components. The most recent American Joint Committee on Cancer (AJCC) report divides the esophagus into four regions: cervical, upper thoracic, midthoracic, and lower thoracic (Fig. 53.2).[1] The cervical esophagus begins at the cricopharyngeus muscle (approximately the C7 level or 15 cm from the incisors) and extends to the thoracic inlet (at approximately the T3 level or at approximately 20 cm from the incisors, at the level of the suprasternal notch), and therefore lies within the neck. The thoracic esophagus extends from approximately the level of T3 (beginning at about 20 cm) to T10 or T11.[1,2] The upper thoracic esophagus is bordered superiorly by the thoracic inlet and inferiorly by the lower border of the azygos vein, extending from approximately 20 to 25 cm. Radiographically,

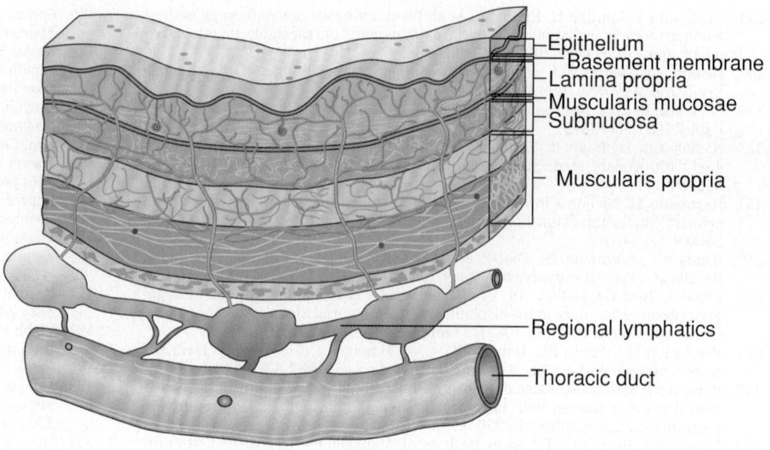

FIGURE 53.1. Diagram of esophageal wall. (Used with the permission of the American Joint Committee on Cancer, Chicago, Illinois. The original source for this material is American Joint Committee on Cancer. *AJCC cancer staging handbook,* 7th ed. New York: Springer, 2010, published by Springer Science and Business Media LLC, www.springerlink.com.)

tumors in this location would be located between the sternal notch and azygos vein. The middle thoracic esophagus extends from the lower border of the azygos vein to the inferior pulmonary veins, extending from approximately 25 to 30 cm. The lower thoracic esophagus extends from the inferior pulmonary veins and to the stomach and is inclusive of the gastroesophageal junction, typically extending from approximately 30 to 40 cm. Endoscopically, the gastroesophageal (GE) junction is often defined as the point where the first gastric fold is encountered, although this may be a "theoretical" landmark. The location of the GE junction can be accurately defined histologically as the squamocolumnar junction. In the most recent AJCC staging system, cancers with an epicenter in the lower thoracic esophagus, gastroesophageal junction, or within the proximal 5 cm of the stomach (i.e., cardia) and extending up to the GE junction or esophagus are staged as an adenocarcinoma of the esophagus. If the epicenter is >5 cm distal to the gastroesophageal junction or within 5 cm of the gastroesophageal junction but does not extend to the junction/esophagus, tumors are classified as stomach cancers. Useful landmarks in reference to endoscopy include the carina (~25 cm from the incisors) and gastroesophageal junction (~40 cm from the incisors).

Siewert et al.[3,4] characterized cancer involving the gastroesophageal junction according to the location of the tumor (Fig. 53.3). If the tumor center is located from >1 cm up to 5 cm above the gastroesophageal junction (Z-line), the tumor is classified as a type I adenocarcinoma of the distal esophagus. If the tumor center is located within 1 cm cephalad to 2 cm caudad to the gastroesophageal junction, it is classified as type II. If the tumor center is located >2 cm below the gastroesophageal junction, the tumor is classified as type III. However, locally advanced/bulky tumors can make it difficult to accurately distinguish where tumors originated in relationship to the GE junction.

Lymphatic Drainage

The esophagus has an extensive, longitudinal interconnecting system of lymphatics. The esophageal lymphatic network is primarily located within the submucosa; however, channels are also

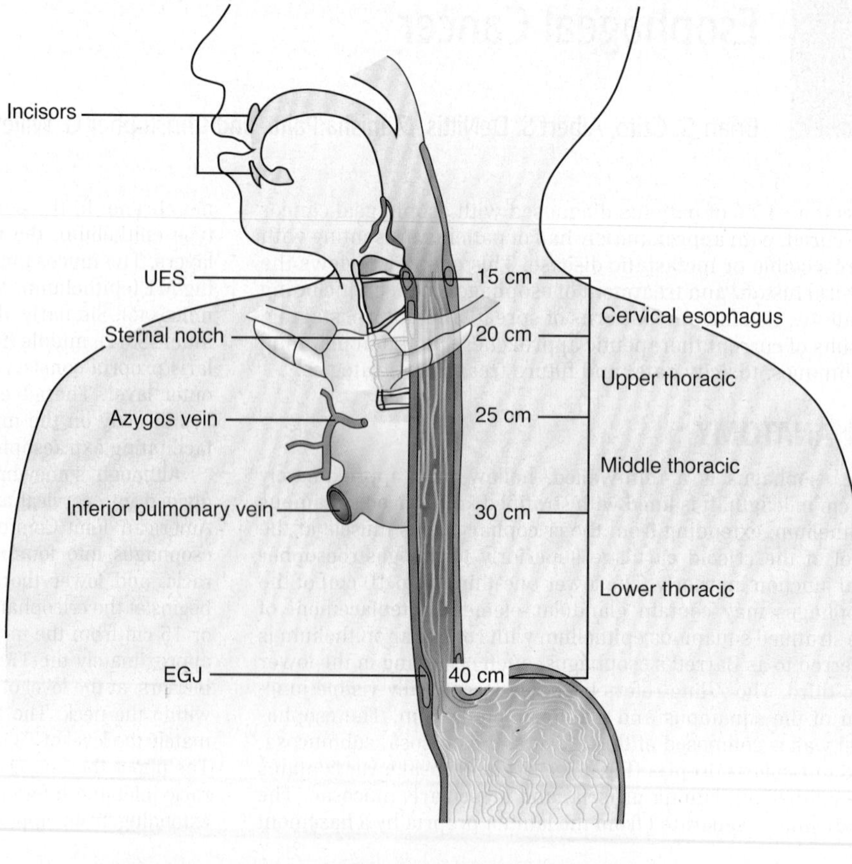

FIGURE 53.2. Anatomy of the esophagus. Note the lengths of various segments of the esophagus as measured from the upper central incisors. (Used with the permission of the American Joint Committee on Cancer, Chicago, Illinois. The original source for this material is American Joint Committee on Cancer. *AJCC cancer staging handbook,* 7th ed. New York: Springer, 2010, published by Springer Science and Business Media LLC, www.springerlink.com.)

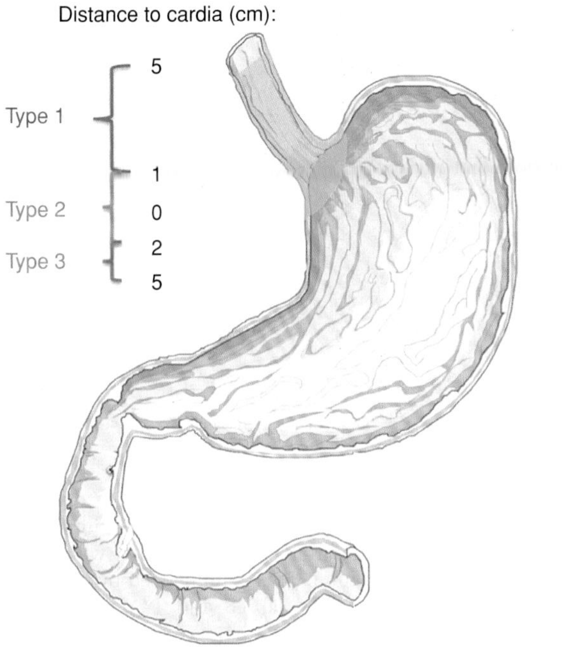

FIGURE 53.3. Siewert classification of the gastroesophageal junction cancers according to the location of the tumor. (From Matzinger O, Gerber E, Bernstein Z, et al. EORTC-ROG expert opinion: radiotherapy volume and treatment guidelines for neoadjuvant radiation of adenocarcinomas of the gastroesophageal junction and the stomach. *Radiother Oncol* 2009;92:164–175; copyright 2009, with permission from Elsevier.)

present within the lamina propria, facilitating spread of even superficial cancers of the esophagus involving the mucosa. In addition to these longitudinal lymphatics, intramural lymphatics may traverse the muscularis propria, facilitating tumor spread to regional lymphatic channels and paraesophageal nodes. Supporting this, autopsy series have demonstrated a relatively high incidence of directly draining channels extending from the submucosa lymphatics into the thoracic duct (Fig. 53.1), facilitating systemic spread. Lymph can travel the entire length of the esophagus before draining into lymph nodes,[2] and thus the entire esophagus is at potential risk for lymphatic involvement. Up to 8 cm or more of 'normal' tissue can exist between gross tumor and micrometastases "skip areas" secondary to this extensive lymphatic network.[5] In addition, as many as 71% of frozen tissue sections scored as margin negative by conventional histopathology show involvement by lymphatic micrometastases with immunohistochemistry.[6] Lymphatics of the esophagus drain into nodes that usually follow arteries, including the inferior thyroid artery, the bronchial and esophageal arteries, and the left gastric artery (celiac axis).[7]

Epidemiology and Risk Factors

Esophageal carcinoma accounts for approximately 6% of all gastrointestinal malignancies. In 2012, there will be an estimated 17,460 new patients diagnosed with esophageal cancer in the United States and 15,070 deaths. Most cases occur in males, at a rate of 4:1 relative to females.[8,9]

The incidence of esophageal carcinoma varies according to geography. The highest incidence occurs in Linxian, China, Russia, and the Caspian region of Iran. The incidence there is 100/100,000 persons. In addition, there are many differences within regions within those countries. In areas such as northern France, Kazakhstan, and South Africa incidence can be as high as 50 to 99/100,000. Although the reasons for the geographic discrepancy are unknown, some reports have linked the arid climate and alkaline soil with these high-risk areas, as well as the ingestion of nitrosamines, and inversely to the consumption of riboflavin, nicotinic acid, magnesium, and zinc.[10,11] In the United States, the incidence rate among males is <5/100,000. Over the last 20 years, there has been an increase in the incidence of adenocarcinoma at a rate of 5% to 10% per year. This is a more rapid increase than that for any other cancer.[12] In 1987, adenocarcinoma was reported to represent 34% and 12% of esophageal cancers in White men and women versus 3% and 1% for African American men and women, respectively.[12] As of 1998, esophageal adenocarcinoma accounted for almost 55% of all diagnosed cases in White men. African American men are more frequently diagnosed with squamous cell carcinoma.[12–14]

In North America and Western Europe, alcohol and tobacco use are the major risk factors for squamous cell carcinoma, accounting for 80% to 90% of cases.[15] Reports have described the relative risk of esophageal cancer by the amount of alcohol and tobacco consumed, including a relative risk of 155:1 when consuming >30 g/day of tobacco along with 121 g/day of alcohol.[16]

Diets of scant amounts of fruits, vegetables, and animal products are associated with increases in squamous cell carcinoma.[17] Patients with Plummer-Vinson (Paterson-Kelly) syndrome, a condition characterized by iron-deficiency anemia and low riboflavin levels, are at an increased risk for oral cavity, hypopharyngeal, and esophageal cancer. In addition, dietary intake of nitrosamines, nitrosamides, and *N*-nitroso compounds has been implicated in esophageal carcinoma. Examples of nitrate-rich foods include pickled vegetables, alcoholic beverages, cured meats, and fish.[18,19]

Other risk factors associated with esophageal carcinoma include achalasia and tylosis. Achalasia of long duration (25 years) is associated with a 5% incidence of squamous cell carcinoma.[20,21] Patients with tylosis (hyperkeratosis of the palms and soles and papilloma of the esophagus) have a reported 38% risk in developing esophageal cancer at a mean age of 45 years.[22] In addition, carcinoma of the esophagus occurs in 2% to 4% of patients with head and neck cancer.

Risk factors leading to the development of adenocarcinoma of the esophagus are being increasingly understood. Most esophageal adenocarcinomas tend to arise from the metaplastic columnar-lined epithelium known as Barrett's esophagus.[23] Severe and long-standing gastroesophageal reflux disease has clearly been shown to be a significant risk factor for Barrett's esophagus, which may lead to adenocarcinoma. It has been estimated that patients with long-standing severe reflux have a 44-fold risk of developing adenocarcinoma.[24] Tobacco use is a more moderate risk factor for adenocarcinoma development. Smokers appear to have a twofold to threefold greater risk for developing esophageal adenocarcinoma than nonsmokers.[25,26] The relative risk of esophageal adenocarcinoma persists to three decades following smoking cessation, in contrast to a significant decline in similar patients with squamous cell carcinoma.[27] Obesity has also been linked to a threefold to fourfold risk of adenocarcinoma, possibly due to an increased risk of reflux.[28] It has been estimated that a middle-aged patient with Barrett's esophagus has a 10% to 15% risk of developing esophageal adenocarcinoma during his or her lifetime.[29]

Although many risk factors are associated with esophageal carcinoma, few studies have demonstrated a causal relationship leading to pathogenesis. Motesano et al.[30] reported possible genetic abnormalities involved in the genesis of esophageal cancer. In addition, possible differences in mechanisms of pathogenesis for squamous cell carcinoma and adenocarcinoma were described. Genetic abnormalities in squamous cell carcinoma include p53 mutations and multiple allelic losses at 3p and 9q, with amplification of cyclin D1 and epidermal growth factor receptor (EGFR). These mutations lead to cell hyperplasia, low- and high-grade dysplasia, and, ultimately, squamous cell carcinoma. In contrast, genetic abnormalities in adenocarcinoma include overexpression of p53, multiple allelic losses at 17p, 5q, and 13q, and amplification and overexpression of EGFR and human epidermal growth factor receptor 2 (HER-2). These abnormalities may be involved in the stepwise development of Barrett's esophagus, dysplasia, and, ultimately, adenocarcinoma. These differences suggest that squamous cell carcinoma and adenocarcinoma have different series of genetic mutations as etiologies, but these abnormalities occur in 23% to 94% of tumors studied.

NATURAL HISTORY AND PATTERNS OF SPREAD

Squamous cell carcinoma is characterized by extensive local growth and proclivity to lymph node metastases. Because the esophagus has no covering serosa, direct invasion of contiguous structures may occur early. Lesions in the upper esophagus can impinge on or invade the recurrent laryngeal nerves, carotid arteries, and trachea. If extraesophageal extension occurs in the mediastinum, tracheoesophageal or bronchoesophageal fistula may occur. Tumors in the lower one-third of the esophagus can invade the aorta or pericardium, resulting in mediastinitis, massive hemorrhage, or empyema.

A review correlating the incidence of lymph node metastases with depth of penetration revealed that 18% of patients with spread to the submucosa had lymph node involvement.[31] For T1 lesions, the reported incidence of nodal spread is 14% to 21%; for T2 lesions, this rises to 38% to 60%.[32,33] The location of involved lymph nodes is influenced by the origin of the primary tumor. At autopsy, lymph node metastases are found in approximately 70% of patients.[34,35–36] In patients with cervical lesions, lymph node metastases to the abdominal lymph nodes are rare. Distant metastasis can occur at almost any site (Table 53.1).[37]

A review of 1,077 patients with squamous cell carcinoma of the thoracic esophagus undergoing esophagectomy further characterized patterns of nodal spread. Primary disease was located in the upper (5%), middle (63%), and lower (32%) thoracic esophagus. In total, 47% of patients had lymph node metastases. On multivariate analysis, T stage, tumoral length, and degree of differentiation significantly correlated with incidence of lymph node metastases. In approximately 6% of cases, skip metastasis (distant lymph node metastases without regional lymph node metastasis) occurred, usually in patients with poorly differentiated, large and deeply invasive tumors. Of involved nodes, 37% were macroscopically involved versus 63% microscopically involved, indicating that most lymph node metastases would be below the resolution of detection using contemporary imaging tools. Lymph node involvement was grouped into five categories; cervical, thoracic upper mediastinum, thoracic middle mediastinum, thoracic lower mediastinum, and abdominal lymph nodes. Figure 53.4 shows the incidence of nodal metastases based on primary tumor location.[38]

TABLE 53.1 DISTRIBUTION OF METASTASES BY ANATOMIC SITE

Site	(n = 79)	Percentage
Lymph nodes	58	73
Lung	41	52
Liver	37	47
Adrenals	16	20
Diaphragm	15	19
Bronchus	13	17
Pleura	13	17
Stomach	12	15
Bone	11	14
Kidneys	10	13
Trachea	10	13
Pericardium	9	11
Pancreas	9	11

From Anderson LL, Lad TE. Autopsy findings in squamous-cell carcinoma of the esophagus. *Cancer* 1982;50:1587–1590, with permission.

For lower esophageal and gastroesophageal junctional adenocarcinomas, approximately 70% of patients will have nodal metastases at presentation. This is influenced by tumoral depth of penetration, with nearly all T3 and T4 lesions exhibiting metastases in surgical series. Pathologic resection data demonstrated rates of lymphatic involvement for lower esophageal and GE junctional tumors of 45%, 85%, and 100% for T2, T3, and T4 tumors, respectively (Fig. 53.5).[33] In patients with lower esophageal cancer, involvement of both mediastinal and abdominal lymph nodes is common (Fig. 53.6).[33] The primary direction for lymphatic flow for the lower esophagus is toward the abdomen. According to the classification by Siewert, nodal metastases are often seen in the mediastinum and abdomen for type I tumors, whereas type III tumors metastasize almost exclusively inferiorly, toward the celiac axis. Type II tumors are intermediate, preferentially spreading inferiorly and less frequently into the mediastinum. The primary value in the Siewert classification is to the guidance of appropriate type surgery (i.e., type I tumors are generally treated with esophagectomy and mediastinal lymph node resection, with types II and III approached through the abdomen), although it may be useful in radiation field design as well.[3] Generally speaking, the incidence of abdominal nodal involvement increases as one proceeds distally in the esophagus to the gastroesophageal junction. For patients with tumors arising from the gastroesophageal junction, mediastinal involvement is less common. Nodal metastases above the level of the carina are rare in lower esophageal and junctional tumors.[39] In addition, histologic analyses of lower esophagus and gastroesophageal junction adenocarcinoma specimens suggest that many patients without nodal involvement on conventional

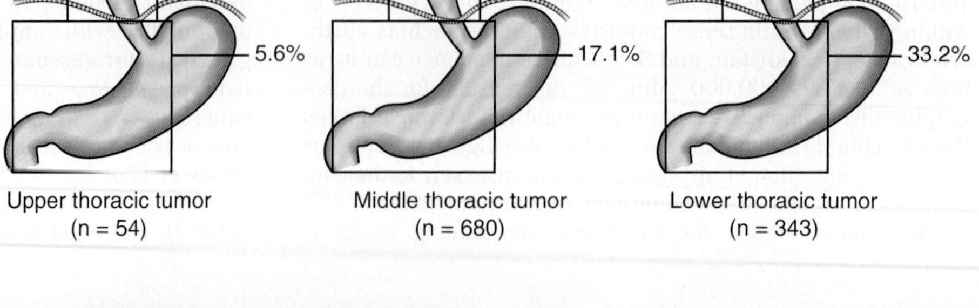

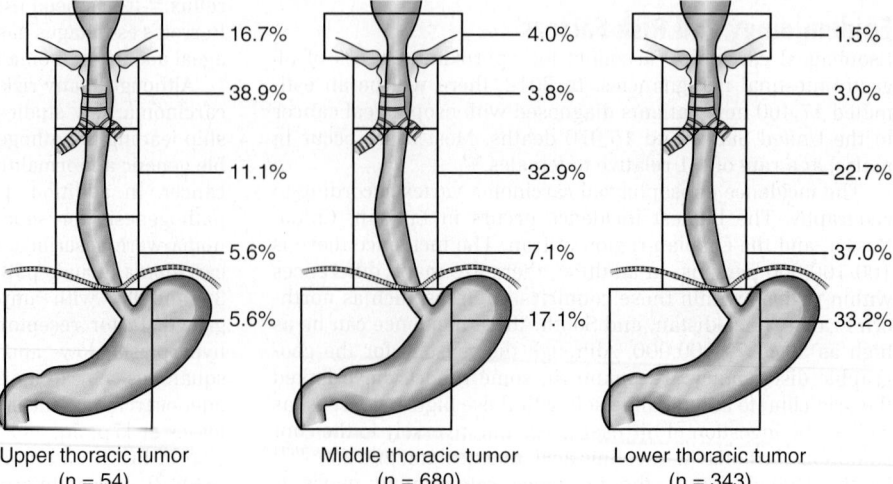

FIGURE 53.4. Positive lymph node distribution according to the location of the primary tumor, squamous cell carcinoma. (From Huang W, Li B, Gong H, et al. Pattern of lymph node metastases and its implication in radiotherapeutic clinical target volume in patients with thoracic esophageal squamous cell carcinoma: a report of 1077 cases. *Radiother Oncol* 2010;95:229–233; with permission from Elsevier.)

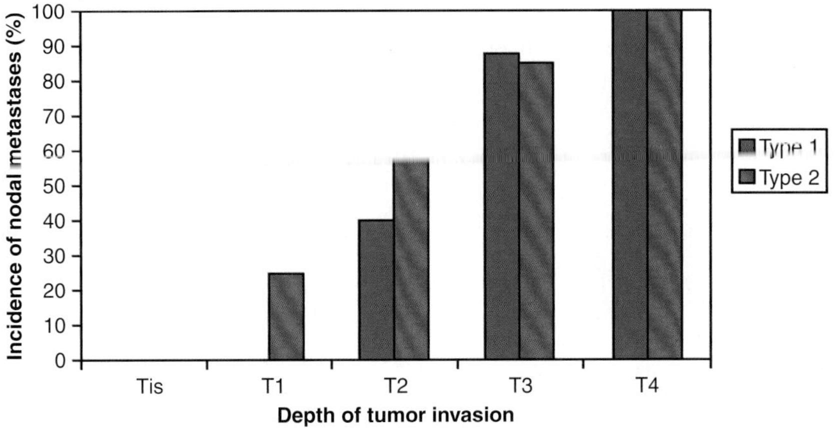

FIGURE 53.5. The incidence of nodal metastases related to depth of tumor invasion, adenocarcinoma. (From Dresner SM, Lamb PJ, Bennett MK, et al. The pattern of metastatic lymph node dissemination from adenocarcinoma of the esophagogastric junction. *Surgery* 2001;129:103–109; with permission form Elsevier.)

histopathology actually have involvement when assessed by immunohistochemistry.[40]

Extensive nodal mapping has been performed by Japanese investigators, who have devised the Japanese Gastric Cancer Association Classification (Fig. 53.7).[41] Using this system of nodal classification, investigators from Erlangen evaluated 326 patients with esophagogastric junction carcinoma undergoing primary resection. Tumors were stratified as AEG type I (distal esophagus), II (gastric cardia), and III (subcardia). Note there was significant overlap in the majority of tumors for all stages, with an overall incidence of lymph node metastasis of 71%. In T1 patients, only 17% exhibited lymph node metastasis, whereas 78%, 86%, and 90% of T2, T3, and T4, respectively, had involved nodes. Figure 53.8 shows varying patterns of nodal spread based on T stage as well as AEG location. Additional generalizations from this study include the following: (a) lymph vascular invasion was highly predictive of nodal spread and (b) proximal extension of type II and III tumors into the distal esophagus (particularly beyond the Z-line) predicted an increasing incidence of paraesophageal lymph node involvement.[42]

LOCAL FAILURE

Aisner et al.[43] and LePrise et al.[44] reviewed the patterns of failure in esophageal cancer after radical irradiation, radical surgery, or a combination of both (Table 53.2). These data suggest that high rates of local recurrence occur when either radiation therapy or surgery alone is used. In a series at the University of Pennsylvania and Fox Chase Cancer Center of patients with adenocarcinoma of the esophagus and gastroesophageal junction treated with surgery alone, the local-regional recurrence rate was 77%.[45] In contemporary randomized trials, local failure rates with surgery alone range from 32% to 45%.[46–49] Similarly, data from recent randomized trials of esophageal cancer using "definitive" chemoradiation also indicates that local failure is a major cause of failure, with approximately 50% of patients failing locally (Table 53.3). In many trials, patterns of failure are reported as first site of recurrence. This fact, along with infrequent posttherapy imaging and inability to detect subclinical recurrences, likely leads to underestimates of local recurrence rates. These data clearly emphasize the need for improvements in local treatment modalities.

CLINICAL PRESENTATION

Symptoms of esophageal cancer often start 3 to 4 months before diagnosis. Location of the primary tumor in the esophagus may influence presenting symptoms. Dysphagia is seen in >90% of patients regardless of location. Odynophagia is present in up to 50% of patients.[50] Weight loss is common, with 40% to 70% of patients reporting a loss of >5% of total body weight. This extent of weight loss has been associated with a worse prognosis. Less

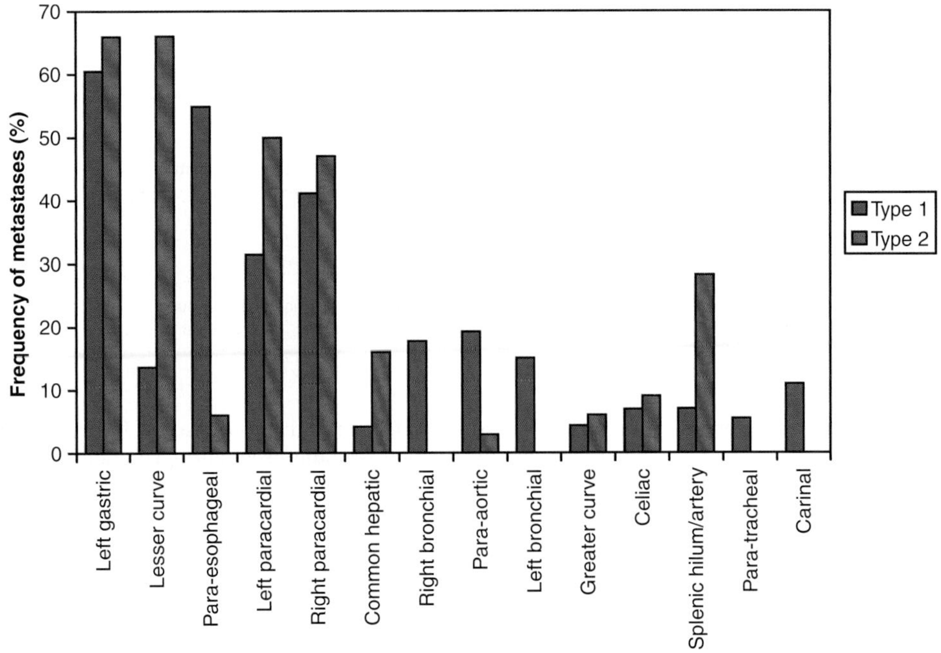

FIGURE 53.6. Distribution of nodal metastases by frequency of site involved for adenocarcinoma. (From Dresner SM, Lamb PJ, Bennett MK, et al. The pattern of metastatic lymph node dissemination from adenocarcinoma of the esophagogastric junction. *Surgery* 2001;129:103–109; with permission form Elsevier.)

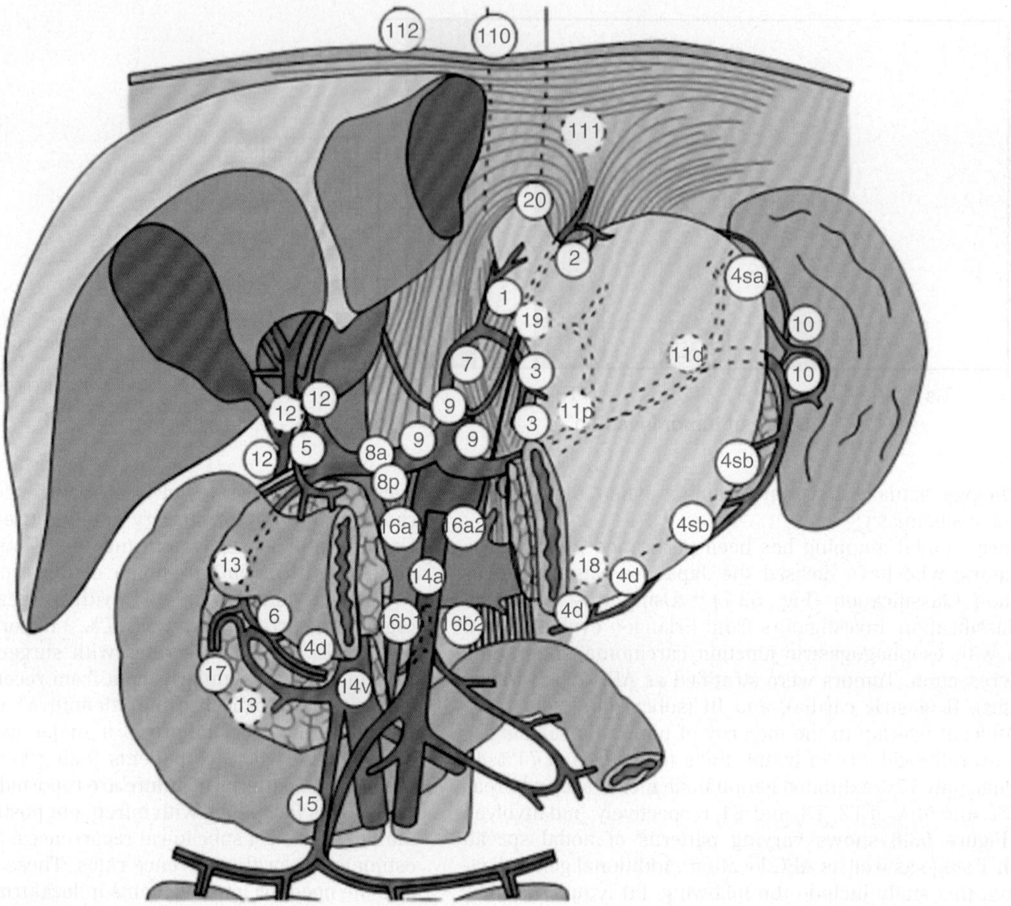

No. 1	Right paracardial LN
No. 2	Left paracardial LN
No. 3	LN along the lesser curvature
No. 4sa	LN along the short gastric vessels
No. 4sb	LN along the left gastroepiploic vessels
No. 4d	LN along the right gastroepiploic vessels
No. 5	Suprapyloric LN
No. 6	Infrapyloric LN
No. 7	LN along the left gastric artery
No. 8a	LN along the common hepatic artery (Anterosuperior group)
No. 8p	LN along the common hepatic artery (Posterior group)
No. 9	LN around the celiac artery
No. 10	LN at the splenic hilum
No. 11p	LN along the proximal splenic artery
No. 11d	LN along the distal splenic artery
No. 12a	LN in the hepatoduodenal ligament (along the hepatic artery)
No. 12b	LN in the hepatoduodenal ligament (along the bile duct)
No. 12p	LN in the hepatoduodenal ligament (behind the portal vein)
No. 13	LN on the posterior surface of the pancreatic head
No. 14v	LN along the superior mesenteric vein
No. 14a	LN along the superior mesenteric artery
No. 15	LN along the middle colic vessels
No. 16a1	LN in the aortic hiatus
No. 16a2	LN around the abdominal aorta (from the upper margin of the celiac trunk to the lower margin of the left renal vein)
No. 16b1	LN around the abdominal aorta (from the lower margin of the left renal vein to the upper margin of the inferior mesenteric artery)
No. 16b2	LN around the abdominal aorta (from the upper margin of the inferior mesenteric artery to the aortic bifurcation)
No. 17	LN on the anterior surface of the pancreatic head
No. 18	LN along the inferior margin of the pancreas
No. 19	Infradiaphragmatic LN
No. 20	LN in the esophageal hiatus of the diaphragm
No. 110	Paraesophageal LN in the lower thorax
No. 111	Supradiaphragmatic LN
No. 112	Posterior mediastinal LN

FIGURE 53.7. Locations of lymph node stations. (From Matzinger O, Gerber E, Bernstein Z, et al. EORTC-ROG expert opinion: radiotherapy volume and treatment guidelines for neoadjuvant radiation of adenocarcinomas of the gastroesophageal junction and the stomach. *Radiother Oncol* 2009;92:164–175; with permission from Elsevier.)

frequent symptoms may include vague chest pain, hoarseness, cough, and glossopharyngeal neuralgia.[51]

Advanced lesions can produce signs and symptoms from tumor invasion into local structures. Hematemesis, hemoptysis, melena, dyspnea, and persistent cough secondary to tracheoesophageal or bronchoesophageal fistula may occur. Compression or invasion of the left recurrent laryngeal nerve or the phrenic nerves can cause dysphonia or hemidiaphragm paralysis. Superior vena cava syndrome and Horner's syndrome can also occur for very advanced lesions. Pleural effusion and exsanguination resulting from aortic communication may also be seen.[50] Abdominal and back pain may occur with celiac axis nodal involvement with lower esophageal tumors.

DIAGNOSTIC WORKUP

After a thorough history and physical examination, all patients with suspected esophageal cancer should have a workup

TABLE 53.2 PATTERNS OF FAILURE IN ESOPHAGEAL CANCER

		Recurrence (%)					
Modality	Number of Patients	Local	Marginal	Neck	Mediastinal	Local and Distant	Distant
Irradiation alone (30–80 Gy)	517	25–84	25	10–43			23–65
Radical surgery alone	266	21–50		44	33		17–65 33 Abdominal nodes 17 Liver 6 Lung
Combined radiation therapy and surgery (primarily preoperative irradiation, 35–50 Gy usual dose)	2,078	22–87	53[a]		20[a]		7–43[b]
Radiation therapy and chemotherapy alone[c]	254	15–39				5–25	6–25
Preoperative radiation therapy and chemotherapy[c]	150	2–36				5–38	16–29

[a]From one study.

[b]From two studies.

[c]Data from LePrise EA, Meunier BC, Etienne PL, et al. Sequential chemotherapy and radiotherapy for patients with squamous cell carcinoma of the esophagus. *Cancer* 1995;75:2.

Modified from Aisner J, Forastiere A, Aroney R. Patterns of recurrence for cancer of the lung and esophagus. In: Wittes RE, ed. *Cancer treatment symposia: proceedings of the Workshop on Patterns of Failure after Cancer Treatment,* Vol. 2. Washington, DC: U.S. Department of Health and Human Services, 1983:87.

similar to that outlined in Table 53.4. Attention should be paid to cervical and supraclavicular lymph nodes. Basic blood counts and a metabolic panel with liver function tests should be obtained.

Although the esophagogram may be used to define lesion extent, endoscopy is the best tool to diagnose and define the extent of the lesion. During flexible endoscopy, biopsies and brushings should be taken of the primary site and suspicious areas harboring satellites or submucosal spread. In addition, accurate endoscopic measurement and characterization of tumor and gastroesophageal junction in relation to the incisors facilitates radiation treatment planning. Examination with panendoscopy of the oral cavity, pharynx, larynx, and tracheobronchial tree may also be performed at the time of esophagoscopy in patients with squamous cell carcinomas, given the high incidence of second tumors in the head and neck and

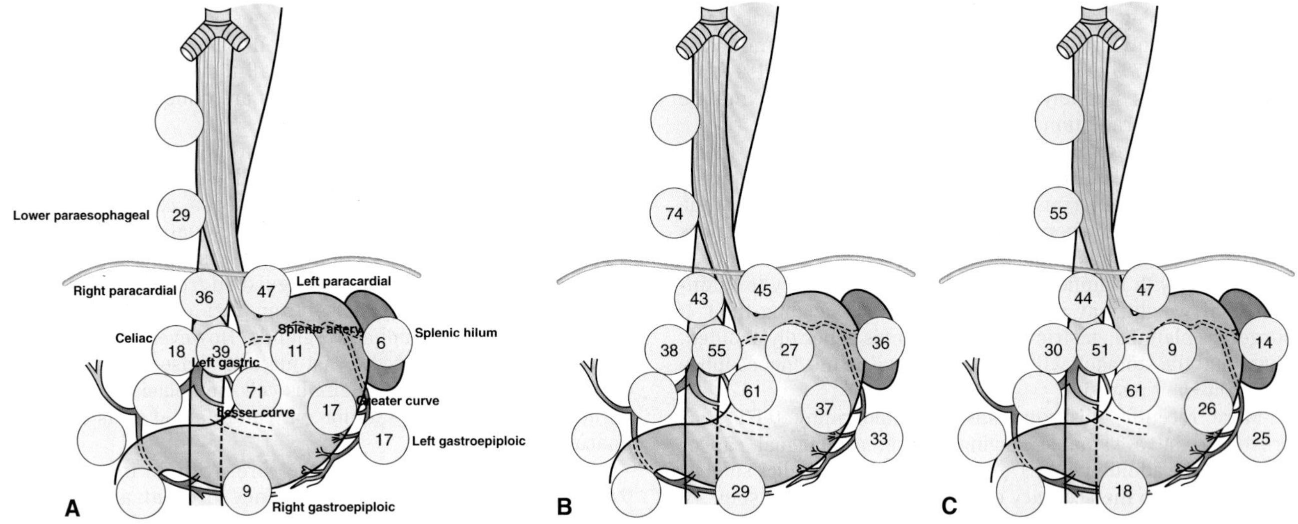

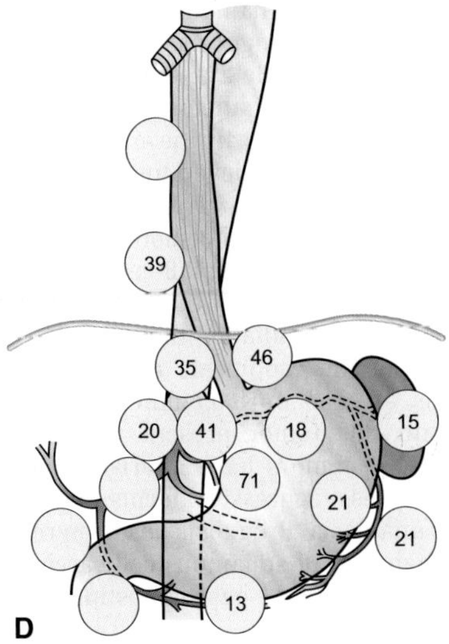

FIGURE 53.8. A: Frequency of nodal involvement for T2 tumors. **B:** Frequency of nodal involvement for T3-4 tumors. **C:** Frequency of involvement for AEG type I tumors. **D:** Frequency of nodal involvement for AEG type II/III tumors. (Based on data from Meier et al.[42])

TABLE 53.3 LOCAL FAILURE RATES FROM RANDOMIZED TRIALS EVALUATING CHEMORADIATION ALONE IN ESOPHAGEAL CANCER

	Dose (Gy)	Local Failure (Crude) (%)	Local Failure (2 Year) (%)
RTOG 85-01[146]	50	45	47
INT 0123[115]	50	55	52
INT 0123[115]	64	50	56
German[152]	> 60	51	58

INT, Intergroup; RTOG, Radiation Therapy Oncology Group.

upper airway.[2] In addition, bronchoscopy should generally be performed in patients with proximal malignancies to evaluate for the presence of tracheal or carinal invasion, particularly for patients with tumors abutting these structures on computed tomography (CT). CT of the thorax and abdomen is critical to identify metastases to the liver, upper abdominal nodes, or adrenals. However, CT may not adequately assess periesophageal lymph node involvement or accurately define the true extent of the primary tumor.[52,53] Conventional CT scan can accurately determine resectability in only 65% to 85% of cases. Furthermore, CT accurately predicts T stage in approximately 70% of cases and nodal involvement in only 50% to 70% of cases.[54–56]

To more accurately assess periesophageal and celiac lymph node involvement and transmural extent of disease, endoscopic ultrasonography (EUS) should be performed. EUS provides accuracy rates of 85% to 90% for tumor invasion (T stage) and 75% to 80% for lymph node metastases when matched to surgical pathology.[57–60] However, the accuracy of endoscopic ultrasound following neoadjuvant therapy is significantly less, ranging from 27% to 48% for T staging and 38% to 71% for N staging. This is possibly due to the failure to discriminate tumor from postradiation inflammation and fibrosis.[61–63]

Surgical staging procedures, including thoracoscopy, mediastinoscopy, and laparoscopy, may provide additional staging information and are considered in selected patients at some institutions.[64] Laparoscopy would primarily be used for tumors at the gastroesophageal junction.

Patients with significant obstruction with inability to maintain their weight may require placement of a feeding tube. If surgery is planned, gastric tube placement is generally avoided, given that the stomach will ultimately serve as the "neoesophagus" following resection.

More recently, positron emission tomography (PET) has proven to be a valuable staging tool in esophageal cancer patients. The addition of PET to standard staging studies such as CT can improve the accuracy of detecting stage III and stage IV disease by 23% and 18%, respectively.[65,66] Overall, it is estimated that PET will detect distant metastatic disease in approximately 20% of patients who are considered to have local regional disease only by CT. However, PET also appears to have a lower accuracy in detecting local nodal disease compared to CT alone or in combination with endoscopic ultrasound. Of importance, emerging data suggest that PET can be used to predict response to therapy, with "PET responders" experiencing significantly improved outcomes compared to "nonresponders."[67] In addition, PET has been used to predict response to treatment early during the treatment course. This has led to ongoing investigation of early treatment response as measured by PET as a surrogate for therapeutic efficacy and clinical outcomes.[68]

TABLE 53.4 DIAGNOSTIC WORKUP FOR ESOPHAGEAL CANCER

Multidisciplinary evaluation (surgical, radiation, and medical oncology)
History and physical
Complete blood count and chemistry profile
Upper gastrointestinal endoscopy and biopsy
Chest, abdomen, and pelvic computed tomography (CT) with oral and intravenous contrast (combined positron emission tomography [PET]-CT optimal)
PET evaluation (combined PET-CT optimal)
Endoscopic ultrasound, with fine needle aspiration if indicated (if no evidence of distant metastases)
Bronchoscopy if tumor is located at or above the carina or there is suspected airway involvement
Nutritional assessment and consideration of feeding tube (nasogastric or feeding jejunostomy) in selected situations

STAGING SYSTEMS

Esophageal staging can be based on pathologic or clinical criteria. Pathologic staging is performed after invasive procedures, including esophagectomy, mediastinotomy, or thoracotomy. Clinical staging is often employed with "definitive" and neoadjuvant chemoradiation approaches and is less accurate. With the combination of CT, PET, and EUS, clinical staging closely correlates with pathologic stage. Note that the most recent AJCC staging system takes into consideration tumor type and grade, as well as involved number of lymph nodes (Table 53.5).

PATHOLOGIC CLASSIFICATION

Squamous cell carcinoma and adenocarcinoma comprise 95% of all esophageal tumors, although other rare histologic subtypes are occasionally seen (Table 53.6).[69]

Given that there has been a rise in adenocarcinoma compared to squamous cell carcinoma, examinations of outcomes by histology have been performed. Some series have reported that patients with squamous cell carcinomas have improved survival,[70] whereas others have suggested that patients with adenocarcinoma have an improved survival[71] and others report no survival differences. Overall there can be no direct comparison until randomized studies are done with stratification based on histology.

Pseudosarcoma is a variant of a poorly differentiated squamous cell carcinoma with spindle-shaped cells in the stroma resembling fibroblasts. Verrucous carcinoma is a well-differentiated, papillary variant of squamous cell carcinoma.[2] Squamous cell carcinoma *in situ* is rarely seen in the United States and should be distinguished from dysplasia.[72–74]

Adenocarcinoma may arise from foci of ectopic gastric mucosa or intrinsic esophageal glands. However, as described previously, it is believed the vast majority arise from Barrett's esophagus. If a focus of squamous cell metaplasia is found in an adenocarcinoma, the tumor may be referred to as an adenoacanthoma.[75]

Adenoid cystic carcinomas are rare, with an incidence of 0.75%. Patients with this malignancy present around the sixth decade of life and have a poor median survival.[76] Mucoepidermoid tumors (adenosquamous carcinomas) are more aggressive and carry a poor prognosis.[77] The incidence of small-cell carcinoma is approximately 2%. Patients with these malignancies often present in the sixth to eighth decades of life, and the lesion is usually located in the middle to lower esophagus in males.[78,79] These are believed to originate in the argyrophilic cells in the esophagus and may produce paraneoplastic syndromes, such as antidiuretic hormone secretion and hypercalcemia.[80] The clinical course of small-cell carcinoma is similar to that of small-cell carcinoma of the lung and may be responsive to chemotherapy and radiation therapy.[77,79]

Nonepithelial tumors of the esophagus are rare. Among these, leiomyosarcomas are the most common. Twenty-five percent of patients with this tumor present with metastases.[81–83] Histologically, these tumors have interlacing bundles of spindle-shaped cells. Less aggressive forms have fewer mitotic figures and less anaplasia. Prognosis has been reported to be more favorable than that of squamous cell carcinoma.[77] In patients with Kaposi's sarcoma, gastrointestinal involvement of the esophagus can be seen.[84]

TABLE 53.5 AMERICAN JOINT COMMITTEE ON CANCER 2010 ESOPHAGEAL CANCER STAGING SYSTEM

Clinical Extent of disease before any treatment	*Stage Category Definitions*	*Pathologic* Extent of disease through completion of definitive surgery
y clinical–staging completed after neoadjuvant therapy but before consequent surgery		y pathologic–staging completed after neoadjuvant therapy AND consequent surgery
	Primary Tumor (T)	
TX	Primary tumor cannot be assessed	TX
T0	No evidence of primary tumor	T0
Tis	High-grade dysplasia[a]	Tis
T1	Tumor invades lamina propria, muscularis mucosae, or submucosa	T1
T1a	Tumor invades lamina propria or muscularis mucosae	T1a
T1b	Tumor invades submucosa	T1b
T2	Tumor invades muscularis propria	T2
T3	Tumor invades adventitia	T3
T4	Tumor invades adjacent structures	T4
T4a	Resectable tumor invading pleura, pericardium, or diaphragm	T4a
T4b	Unresectable tumor invading other adjacent structures, such as aorta, vertebral body, trachea, etc.	T4b
	Regional Lymph Nodes (N)	
NX	Regional lymph nodes cannot be assessed	NX
N0	No regional lymph node metastasis	N0
N1	Regional lymph node metastases involving 1–2 nodes	N1
N2	Regional lymph node metastases involving 3–6 nodes	N2
N3	Regional lymph node metastases involving ≥7 nodes	N3
	Distant Metastasis (M)	
M0	No distant metastasis (no pathologic M0; use clinical M to complete stage group)	M0
M1	Distant metastasis	M1

Anatomic Stage–Prognostic Groups

Squamous Cell Carcinoma,[b] Clinical or Pathologic

Group	T	N	M	Grade	Tumor Location[c]
0	Tis(HGD)	N0	M0	1	Any
IA	T1	N0	M0	1, X	Any
IB	T1	N0	M0	2–3	Any
	T2–3	N0	M0	1, X	Lower, X
IIA	T2–3	N0	M0	1, X	Upper, middle
	T2–3	N0	M0	2–3	Lower, X
IIB	T2–3	N0	M0	2–3	Upper, middle
	T1–2	N1	M0	Any	Any
IIIA	T1–2	N2	M0	Any	Any
	T3	N1	M0	Any	Any
	T4a	N0	M0	Any	Any
IIIB	T3	N2	M0	Any	Any
IIIC	T4a	N1–2	M0	Any	Any
	T4b	Any	M0	Any	Any
	Any	N3	M0	Any	Any
IV	Any	Any	M1	Any	Any

Adenocarcinoma, Clinical or Pathologic

Group	T	N	M	Grade
0	Tis(HGD)	N0	M0	1, X
IA	T1	N0	M0	1–2, X
IB	T1	N0	M0	3
	T2	N0	M0	1–2, X
IIA	T2	N0	M0	3
IIB	T3	N0	M0	Any
	T1–2	N1	M0	Any
IIIA	T1–2	N2	M0	Any
	T3	N1	M0	Any
	T4a	N0	M0	Any
IIIB	T3	N2	M0	Any
IIIC	T4a	N1–2	M0	Any
	T4b	Any	M0	Any
	Any	N3	M0	Any
IV	Any	Any	M1	Any
Stage unknown				

General Notes:

For identification of special cases of TNM or pTNM classifications, the "m" suffix and "y," "r," and "a" prefixes are used. Although they do not affect the stage grouping, they indicate cases needing separate analysis.

m suffix indicates the presence of multiple primary tumors in a single site and is recorded in parentheses: pT(m)NM.

y prefix indicates those cases in which classification is performed during or following initial multimodality therapy. The cTNM or pTNM category is identified by a y prefix. The ycTNM or ypTNM categorizes the extent of tumor actually present at the time of that examination. The y categorization is not an estimate of tumor prior to multimodality therapy.

r prefix indicates a recurrent tumor when staged after a disease-free interval and is identified by the r prefix: rTNM.

a prefix designates the stage determined at autopsy: aTNM.

Surgical margins is a data field recorded by registrars describing the surgical margins of the resected primary site specimen as determined only by the pathology report.

Neoadjuvant treatment is radiation therapy or systemic therapy (consisting of chemotherapy, hormone therapy, or immunotherapy) administered prior to a definitive surgical procedure. If the surgical procedure is not performed, the administered therapy no longer meets the definition of neoadjuvant therapy.

Additional descriptors:

- ❑ **Lymphatic Vessel Invasion (L) and Venous Invasion (V)** have been combined into Lymph-Vascular invasion (LVI) for collection by cancer registrars. The College of American Pathologists (CAP) checklist should be used as the primary source. Other sources may be used in the absence of a checklist. Priority is given to positive results.
- ❑ Lymph-Vascular Invasion Not Present (absent)/Not Identified; Lymph-Vascular Invasion Present/Identified; Not Applicable; Unknown/Indeterminate.
- ❑ **Residual Tumor (R)** refers to the absence or presence of residual tumor after treatment. In some cases treated with surgery and/or with neoadjuvant therapy there will be residual tumor at the primary site after treatment because of incomplete resection or local and regional disease that extends beyond the limit of ability of resection.
- ❑ RX, presence of residual tumor cannot be assessed; R0, no residual tumor; R1, microscopic residual tumor; R2, macroscopic residual tumor.

[a]High-grade dysplasia includes all noninvasive neoplastic epithelium that was formerly called carcinoma *in situ,* a diagnosis that is no longer used for columnar mucosae anywhere in the gastrointestinal tract.

[b]Or mixed histology including a squamous component or not otherwise specified.

[c]Location of the primary cancer site is defined by the position of the upper (proximal) edge of the tumor in the esophagus.

Used with the permission of the American Joint Committee on Cancer, Chicago, Illinois. The original source for this material is American Joint Committee on Cancer. *AJCC cancer staging handbook,* 7th ed. New York: Springer, 2010, published by Springer Science and Business Media LLC, www.springerlink.com.

TABLE 53.6 PATHOLOGIC CLASSIFICATION OF MALIGNANT ESOPHAGEAL TUMORS

Epithelial Tumors
Squamous cell carcinoma
Variants of squamous cell carcinoma
Basaloid squamous cell carcinoma
Squamous cell carcinoma with sarcomatoid features
Undifferentiated carcinoma
Spindle cell carcinoma
Pseudosarcoma and carcinosarcoma
Verrucous carcinoma
In situ carcinoma
Adenocarcinoma
Adenoacanthoma
Adenoid cystic carcinoma (cylindroma)
Mucoepidermoid carcinoma
Adenosquamous carcinoma
Carcinoid
Small-cell carcinoma
Nonepithelial Tumors
Sarcoma, 13 variants reported, most common is leiomyosarcoma
Malignant melanoma
Myoblastoma
Choriocarcinoma
Lymphoma

Malignant melanoma is rare and can occur as a primary esophageal tumor or as a metastasis. These lesions are usually large and often covered by intact squamous mucosa with focal areas of ulceration. Spread is usually submucosal. Mean survival is approximately 7 months.[85,86] Lymphoma comprises approximately 1% of esophageal malignancies. It is usually associated with direct extension from other organs, although primary esophageal lymphoma has been reported.[87]

PROGNOSTIC FACTORS

According to the Union Internationale Contre le Cancer/American Joint Cancer Committee seventh-edition staging system, R-status, age, and histologic subtype were independent prognostic factors of survival, whereas tumor grade and site were not.[88] It should be recalled that these data consider patients treated with surgery alone and as such do not apply to patients receiving chemotherapy or radiotherapy. A study published by Nomura et al.[89] evaluated 301 patients treated with chemoradiotherapy showed that T stage, M stage, and gender were prognostic factors in multivariate analysis.

In addition to stage, other factors portend outcome. Tumor length/size may also impact outcome. In a study of 582 patients undergoing surgical resection as primary treatment, tumoral length adversely affected survival, with 5-year survival rates of 77%, 48%, 38%, and 23% for tumor lengths of 1, 2, 3, or >3 cm, respectively ($p < .001$).[90] Of note, length was not prognostic if patients were N+ or M+. Similarly, in adenocarcinoma patients, 5-year survival rates have been shown to be significantly higher for patients with tumors ≤2 cm compared to those >2 cm.[91]

In another large study from the Mayo Clinic, clinicopathologic factors that affected prognosis included T and N status, tumor grade, age >76 years, extracapsular lymph node extension, and the absence of chemotherapy or radiotherapy; anatomic location did not influence survival.[92] In addition, weight loss and low overall performance status also indicate poor prognosis.[93] Deep ulceration of the tumor, sinus tract formation, and fistula formation are other poor prognostic factors.[50]

Obtaining uninvolved pathologic margins at resection is of significant importance with regard to long-term outcome. An Intergroup study (discussed later) evaluating chemotherapy preceding and following esophagectomy showed that outcomes were similar in patients undergoing R1 resection (positive microscopic margins) or R2 resection (gross residual disease) or patients not undergoing resection at all. Only patients undergoing R0 resection (uninvolved margins) had a substantial chance of long-term disease-free survival.[47] A patterns-of-care survey examined the outcomes of patients with adenocarcinoma and squamous cell carcinoma of the esophagus between 1996 and 1999. Patients were treated with radiation therapy across 59 institutions. On multivariate analysis, significant improvements in survival were seen in patients treated at centers with ≥500 new cancer patients per year compared to centers seeing <500 (hazard ratio 1.32; $p = 0.03$).[94]

GENERAL MANAGEMENT

Treatment for esophageal carcinoma is characterized as curative or palliative. According to one historical study,[95] only 20% patients present with cancer of the esophagus that is truly localized to the esophagus, indicating that at the time of diagnosis, approximately 80% patients have either locally advanced or distant disease.

Surgery with Curative Intent

Surgery of the thoracic esophagus usually requires a subtotal or total esophagectomy and is usually undertaken for lesions of the middle to lower one-third of the thoracic esophagus and gastroesophageal junction. Patients with stage I to III are often considered for potentially curative resection; however, aortic, tracheal, heart, or great vessel invasion may preclude resection. Esophagectomy may be accomplished by a number of techniques, including a transhiatal esophagectomy, right thoracotomy with laparotomy with intrathoracic anastomosis (Ivor-Lewis esophagogastrectomy), right thoracotomy with laparotomy with cervical anastomosis (McKeown esophagogastrectomy), left thoracotomy, or radical esophagectomy via open or laparoscopic approaches. Each technique has its advantages and disadvantages. In general, advantages of the transthoracic approach include better visualization with access and resection of the upper two-thirds of the esophagus and mediastinal lymph nodes. Alternatively, the transhiatal approach has less morbidity than thoracotomy (including respiratory compromise) with easier access to anastomotic leaks (neck vs. thorax). In any instance, achievement of negative margins at resection has been reported to be a significant prognostic factor and should be the goal of esophageal resection. Exemplifying this, in a study of 500 patients undergoing transthoracic resection, patients undergoing margin-negative resection had a 5-year survival rate of 29% versus no 5-year survivors in patients with involved margins.[96]

The Ivor-Lewis procedure is the classic approach to expose mid-esophageal lesions. A left thoracotomy procedure exposes lesions of the gastroesophageal junction. Transhiatal esophagectomy is performed without a thoracotomy and is useful in lower esophageal lesions, although direct visualization and dissection of varying mediastinal lymph nodes cannot be achieved. The optimal surgical approach is unknown. A randomized trial comparing transhiatal versus transthoracic approaches in patients with adenocarcinoma showed no significant survival advantage to the latter, although a possible trend was noted (5-year survival, 29% vs. 39%). However, perioperative mortality was also increased with the transthoracic approach.[46]

Laparotomy can be performed before or concurrently with esophagectomy to rule out any disease below the diaphragm. Multiple reconstruction options are available following definitive surgery; esophagogastrostomy is the most widely used, using the stomach as a conduit to replace the esophagus. Patients with significant obstruction and inability to maintain their weight often require placement of feeding jejunostomy. If possible surgery is planned, gastric tube placement is generally avoided, given that the stomach will ultimately serve as the "neoesophagus" following resection. Colon interposition, preferably with the left colon, can also be used; however, this approach is generally reserved for patients who have previously undergone gastric surgery or other procedures that have devascularized the stomach.

Squamous cell carcinoma of the cervical esophagus presents a difficult management situation. Proximal esophageal tumors <5 cm from the cricopharyngeus are generally treated with definitive chemoradiotherapy. If surgery is performed, resection of portions of the pharynx, the entire larynx, thyroid gland, and the proximal esophagus is often required. Radical neck dissections are also carried out.[50] Because of the significant morbidity and loss of organ function with surgery, chemoradiation alone has been frequently employed. The survival probability with definitive chemoradiotherapy is similar, without the major functional impairments, morbidity, and mortality associated with surgery.[97]

Curative Combination Therapy

In the treatment of patients with esophageal cancer, an approach of radiation therapy with concurrent chemotherapy, with or without surgery, is frequently adopted. Multiagent chemotherapy with cisplatin and 5-fluorouracil (5-FU) is used most frequently, although combinations of other agents (e.g., paclitaxel and carboplatin) are being increasingly used. Additional taxanes, topoisomerase inhibitors, and anti-epidermal growth factor receptor inhibitors with radiation therapy are under investigation.

Palliative Treatment

Palliative treatment is frequently used for the relief of symptoms of esophageal carcinoma, especially dysphagia.[98] Surgical palliation involves resection and reconstruction, if possible, removing the bulk of the disease, potentially preventing abscess and fistula formation, as well as bleeding. Substernal bypass with the colon or entire stomach has also been carried out.[98] However, given the poor prognosis in patients with advanced disease and morbidity associated with resection, a surgical approach is not commonly adopted and should be avoided in patients who can be managed with nonsurgical modalities.

Endoscopic dilatation is a reasonable alternative. When the lumen of the esophagus is dilated to 15 mm, dysphagia is often no longer experienced. Repeat dilatation is often required.[50] Esophageal stenting with either conventional plastic stents or metallic self-expanding stents can also be used to maintain patency.[99]

Palliative irradiation is frequently used to control the primary disease, as well as distant metastases. Resolution of symptoms, especially pain and dysphagia, can be accomplished in up to 80% of patients. Palliative treatment regimens range from 30 Gy over 2 weeks[51] to 50 Gy over 5 weeks. Laser ablation with or without intraluminal brachytherapy can be used. The addition of 3 fractions of 7 Gy each can improve the stenosis-free interval and prevent obstruction.[99]

RADIATION THERAPY TECHNIQUES

Simulation

When patients are simulated, the radiation oncologist should know the extent of disease based on imaging (barium swallow, CT, PET), as well as on endoscopy. CT simulation is appropriate for treatment planning. During simulation, the patient is positioned, straightened, and immobilized on the simulation table. An immobilization device is used to minimize variation in daily setup. Arms are generally placed overhead and knee support underneath the legs. Palpable neck disease should be marked with a radiopaque wire. The administration of oral contrast to delineate the esophagus is generally used and helps to define the extent of mucosal irregularity. For GE junctional tumors (particularly with significant gastric involvement), it may be advisable to have the patient come in with an empty stomach. For cervical and upper thoracic lesions, an immobilization mask may assist in creating a reproducible position. Some authors have also advocated that mid-esophageal primaries be simulated in prone position to maximize distance between the target volumes and spinal cord. The patient is placed on the CT simulator in the treatment position, and a scan of the entire area of interest with margin is obtained. At minimum, 3- to 5-mm slices should be used, allowing accurate tumor characterization, as well as improved quality of digitally reconstructed radiographs. If patients lose >10% of their body weight during therapy, consideration should be given to repeat CT planning. Arterial phase intravenous contrast is generally used to delineate mediastinal and abdominal vascular nodal basins, including the celiac axis and to allow the radiation oncologist to discern normal vasculature from other adjacent normal structures, and potential adenopathy. The tumor and vital structures are then outlined on each slice on the treatment planning system, enabling a three-dimensional treatment plan to be generated. The use of respiratory gating or breath-hold techniques may help to reduce target motion with respiration and, therefore, avoid normal-tissue irradiation associated with larger margins used in free-breathing approaches, particularly for lower esophageal cancers. Additional techniques to minimize physiologic motion include abdominal compression devices. Four-dimensional CT scan may be appropriate to assess tumoral motion, facilitating appropriate margin placement on the target volumes, particularly in lower esophageal tumors and/or disease involving the stomach.

Treatment Planning

Target Design

In the design of radiation fields for esophageal cancer, it is important to define varying target volumes, including gross disease as well as potential areas of subclinical involvement (i.e., the gross tumor volumes [GTVs] and clinical target volumes [CTVs], respectively). Definition of gross tumor volume is based on multiple studies, including endoscopic descriptions (from both esophagogastroduodenoscopy [EGD] and EUS). The proximal and distal aspects of the tumor should be standardly defined by the gastroenterologist based on distance from the incisors, as well as relationship to varying landmarks as measured from the incisors (e.g., the GE junction). The radiation oncologist is able to use these measurements to help correlate with disease extent visualized on planning CT scan, using varying anatomic landmarks (e.g., the GE junction, which is frequently located ~40 cm from the incisors in many patients), as well as carina (which is frequently located at ~25 cm in most patients) to help more accurately define the GTV. Esophageal wall thickening correlating to the gross tumor volume can frequently be visualized on diagnostic and radiation planning CT. Similarly, EUS appears to be the most reliable test in detecting lymphadenopathy related to nodal spread. As in EGD, the endoscopist should be encouraged to accurately define not only the primary disease extent on EUS as measured by distances from the incisors, but also depth of penetration and potential involvement of adjacent structures, which can also be used to help guide GTV delineation. Similarly, EUS may detect lymph nodes that may not be appreciated on CT or PET imaging, and the endoscopist should describe the size as well as the location (e.g., distance from incisors, relationship to adjacent mediastinal structures, etc.) of these, further facilitating accurate definition of potentially involved lymph nodes, either adjacent to or well removed from the primary tumor itself. In addition, radiographic areas of lymphadenopathy should similarly be included in the GTV.

Although the utility of PET in esophageal cancer staging primarily lies in its ability to detect distant metastases not fully appreciated on CT imaging (and thereby alter treatment approach of these patients),[100,101] diagnostic PET/CT has more recently been integrated into radiation planning of esophageal cancer patients and definition of GTV. Generally, gross disease as defined on PET is characterized by a standard uptake value of >2 to 2.5.[102] Generally speaking, PET-avid nodes should be included within the GTV volume. In a study from Fox Chase Cancer Center, the mean GTV length as determined by PET/CT closely correlated with endoscopy findings.[59] Another study from Australian investigators reported that CT-alone–based definition of GTV excluded PET-avid disease in a majority of patients, resulting in a potential geographic miss of disease in a significant minority of patients.[103] Similarly, the fusion of CT-PET has been shown to prompt GTV and planning target volume (PTV) modification in a majority of patients.[104] Recent analysis of PET/CT-based (as compared to CT alone) radiotherapy planning of esophageal cancer patients indicated a reduction of intraobserver and interobserver variability in GTV delineation.[105]

Finally, although the routine use of fluoroscopic barium swallow in esophageal cancer has decreased, this study may still be useful to the radiation oncologist for field design. A study by Chinese investigators suggested that, as compared to CT, endoscopy with barium swallow more accurately defines the true length of middle and lower esophageal tumors, although CT appeared to better determine this for tumors located at the GE junction.[106]

In summary, accurate definition of primary and nodal gross disease is paramount in radiation esophageal cancer planning. It is important to rely on all diagnostic studies, including barium swallow (when available), EGD, EUS, and CT, as well as PET scan.

The identification of potential direct and nodal pathways for spread of subclinical disease (i.e., CTV definition) in esophageal cancer is also of paramount importance. These areas vary significantly, depending on site of origin of disease, making esophageal cancer planning somewhat complex. In terms of direct disease extension along the esophagus itself, varying reports have assessed the histologic findings at primary esophagectomy to determine subclinical extent of disease. One prospective analysis of 66 resection specimens showed that placement of a 3-cm margin proximally and distally on the primary tumor would cover microscopic disease extension in 94% of squamous cell carcinomas. Similarly, in GE junctional carcinomas, a 3-cm proximal margin included subclinical disease extension in 100% of patients, and 5 cm distally covered 94% of subclinical spread.[106]

As described previously, the esophagus is characterized by a rich submucosal network of lymphatics that facilitates early lymph node spread of disease, even for superficial esophageal cancers. The appropriate cranial and caudal margins remain a matter of debate in the treatment of esophageal cancer. Historically, very large fields were treated, encompassing potential pathways and lymphatic spread from the thoracic inlet down to the celiac axis region; however, such fields are potentially fraught with treatment-related toxicity and may be difficult for patients to tolerate, particularly in the context of concurrent chemotherapy delivery. Most contemporary radiation trials used margins of 3 to 5 cm cranially and caudally on the GTV, along with an approximate 2-cm radial margin. With disease located at or above the carina (or middle/upper one-third of the esophagus in some instances), many of these trials recommended fields inclusive of the supraclavicular lymph node basins, whereas celiac axis nodal basin coverage was recommended for disease of the distal esophagus.[107] Further description of lymph node basin coverage follows.

Field Design

Historically, the treatment of very proximal (cervical) esophageal cancers has been challenging. Because of the changing contour from the neck to the thoracic inlet, treatment of lesions in the upper one-third of the esophagus may present a difficult technical problem. Lesions in the upper cervical or postcricoid esophagus are treated from the laryngopharynx to the carina, depending on extent of disease. Supraclavicular and superior mediastinal nodes are irradiated electively. Using older/conventional methods, this was achieved with lateral parallel opposed or oblique portals to the primary tumor and a single anterior field for the supraclavicular and superior mediastinal nodes.[93] Another historical technique treated lesions in this region by means of a four-field box approach, using a wax bolus to build up the lack of tissue above the shoulders, acting as a compensator. A high-energy beam (>15 MV) is used, and both sides of the neck are treated prophylactically. Other methods of treating lesions at the thoracic inlet include 140-degree arc rotations, anterior wedged pairs, and three- or four-field techniques using posterior oblique portals combined with a single anterior portal or anteroposterior–posteroanterior (AP/PA) fields.[93] Using three-dimensional (3D) approaches, varying techniques have been implemented, including treatment of the primary tumor and lymph nodes using an AP/PA approach to 39.6 to 41.4 Gy at 1.8 Gy per fraction, followed by a left or right opposed oblique pair to bring the total dose to 50.4 Gy, thereby limiting the spinal cord dose. This technique will generally exclude the supraclavicular fossa, and a separate electron field is often added, treating to a depth of 2 to 3 cm, depending upon individual anatomy. More recently, however, intensity-modulated radiation therapy (IMRT)–based planning has facilitated the treatment of upper esophageal lesions and is our preferred method for treating these tumors (Fig. 53.9) Strict normal tissue constraints, including normal lung and spinal cord, are important considerations in using these techniques (discussed later).

Based on the previously described and other pathologic patterns of spread data in squamous cell carcinoma of the esophagus, general guidelines in terms of field design can be made as follows: For cervical and upper thoracic squamous cell carcinoma, the CTV should generally include nodal basins extending from the lower cervical and supraclavicular region superiorly to the subcarinal lymph node basin inferiorly, inclusive of the upper paraesophageal lymph nodes (Fig. 53.9). For lower esophageal squamous cell carcinomas, lymph node basins from the subcarinal region superiorly to the left gastric and common hepatic artery/celiac lymph nodal basins inferiorly should generally be included (described further later in this chapter). For tumors of the middle esophagus, we recommend individual field design according to clinical scenarios, with a more complete coverage of paraesophageal mediastinal lymph nodes, particularly in patients with a good performance status (Fig. 53.10).[37] These are general guidelines, and all plans should be individualized based on available imaging and endoscopic findings.

In field design, potential nodal involvement (and therefore target volumes) on nodal size is problematic, given that some reports demonstrated that <15% of metastatic nodes are >1 cm and that average size differences between involved and uninvolved nodes are frequently not significantly different.[108] In addition, fluorodeoxyglucose-PET scanning has an estimated sensitivity of only 67% of detecting nodal metastases.[8] Even endoscopic ultrasound, generally considered the most sensitive test for detecting lymph node metastases, is only able to detect such disease in approximately 75% of patients.[109] Therefore, it is not appropriate to rely exclusively on varying imaging modalities to define areas of subclinical spread for esophageal cancer, realizing that patterns-of-spread data are important in determining radiation field design.

The design of radiation fields for the treatment of adenocarcinoma of the esophagus is similar to that of lower thoracic squamous cell carcinomas but deserves special mention. Periesophageal lymph nodes are generally included in all patients. Given that lymph node involvement is clearly associated with depth of tumor penetration (T stage) and the fact that most patients in the United States and Europe presenting with

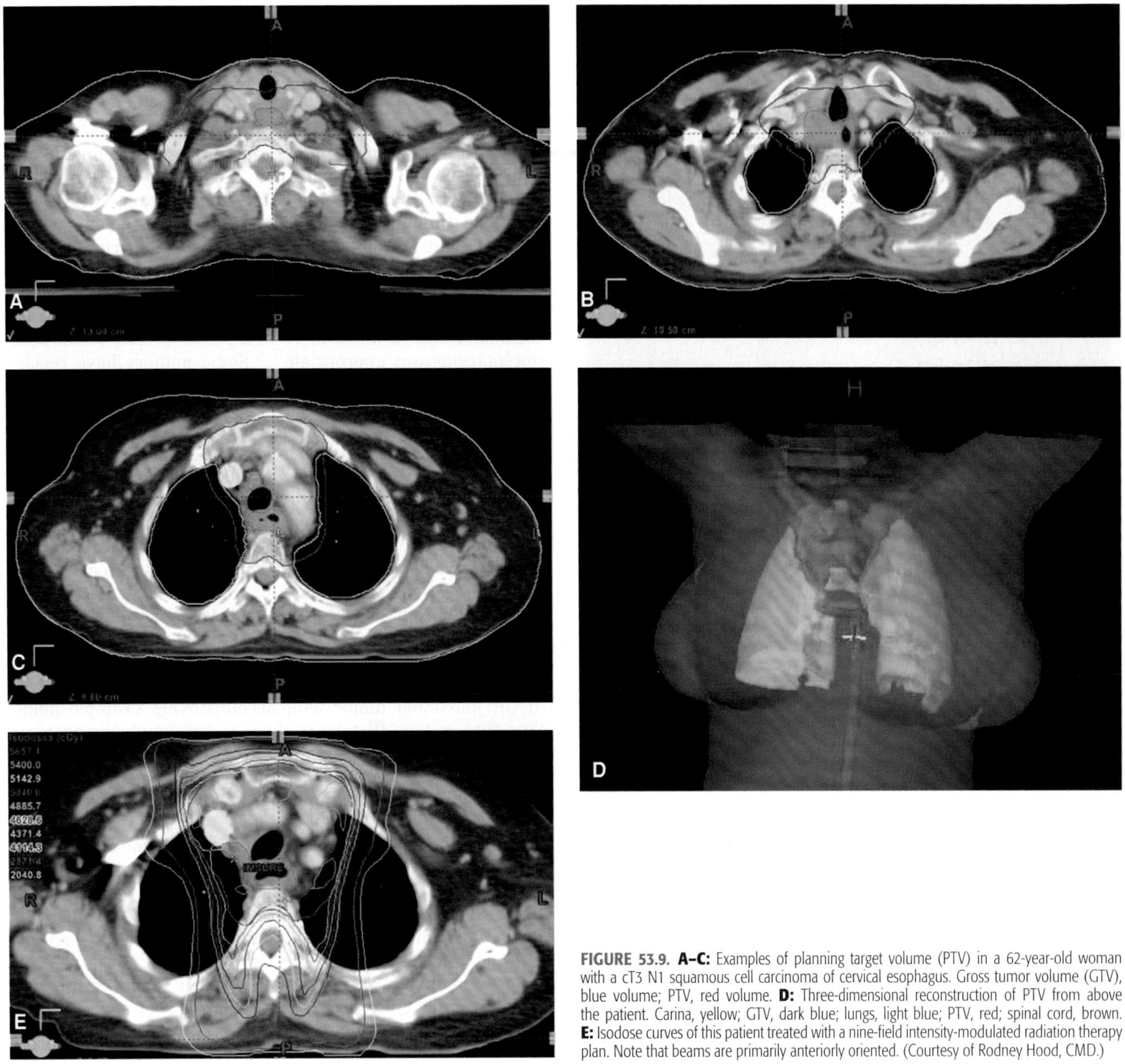

FIGURE 53.9. A–C: Examples of planning target volume (PTV) in a 62-year-old woman with a cT3 N1 squamous cell carcinoma of cervical esophagus. Gross tumor volume (GTV), blue volume; PTV, red volume. **D:** Three-dimensional reconstruction of PTV from above the patient. Carina, yellow; GTV, dark blue; lungs, light blue; PTV, red; spinal cord, brown. **E:** Isodose curves of this patient treated with a nine-field intensity-modulated radiation therapy plan. Note that beams are primarily anteriorly oriented. (Courtesy of Rodney Hood, CMD.)

GE junctional carcinoma will have more advanced disease, inclusion of celiac lymph basins for adenocarcinoma of the distal esophagus/GE junction is usually indicated. Based on the previously described patterns of spread data from Erlangen and others, specific considerations include the following: Lymph vascular invasion is highly predictive of nodal spread. Proximal extension of tumors (particularly beyond the Z-line into the distal esophagus for type II and III tumors) predicts an increasing incidence of paraesophageal lymph node involvement. Based on an estimated nodal incidence cutoff of 20% for inclusion, specific considerations include the following: (a) The lower paraesophageal, paracardial, lesser curvature, and left gastric artery nodes should be included in the CTV. (b) The presence of lymph vascular invasion predicts a nodal positivity rate of >20% in the left and right gastroepiploic, greater curvature, celiac trunk, and splenic hilar regions. (c) In T3/4 disease, the gastroepiploic, greater curvature, celiac trunk, splenic hilar, splenic artery, and common hepatic artery should be included. (d) High-grade tumors should also include the left gastroepiploic, greater curvature, and celiac trunk nodes in CT design. (e) Larger and more deeply penetrating tumors should also include the splenic artery and splenic hilar nodes, as well as those along the greater curvature. (f) Tumors extending above the diaphragm and those extending >1.5 cm beyond the Z-line should include the mid paraesophageal nodes, treating up to the carina. Of note, significant involvement of the distal esophagus by GE junctional tumors (>1.5 cm beyond the Z-line) should lead to inclusion of not only lower, but also middle paraesophageal nodes based on patterns of spread. However, treating these more extensive fields must be weighed against potential side effects of increased normal-tissue irradiation. In summary, middle and lower paraesophageal nodes should be included in patients with T2-T4 type I and T2-T4 type II tumors extending >1.5 cm above the Z-line and T3-T4 type II patients. The splenic hilar and artery nodes are considered “spareable” in T2 tumors, notably type I.[42]

Although, historically, two-dimensional–based radiation planning has been carried out primarily using anatomic landmarks such as bone and carina, as well as fluoroscopic barium swallow, to determine field borders, contemporary treatment planning using CT-based planning allows improved visualization of both target and nontarget structures, along with

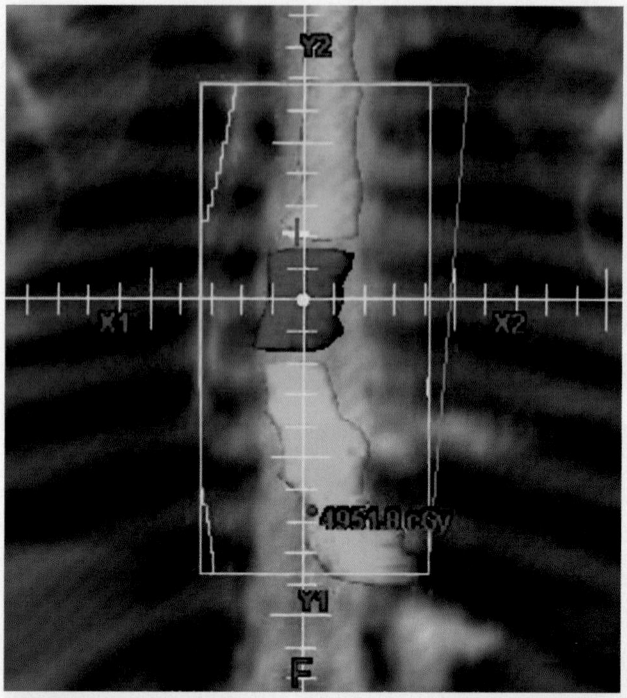

FIGURE 53.10. Example field for a midesophageal squamous cell carcinoma. Note that the field is inclusive of adjacent mediastinal/paraesophageal nodes, with approximately 5 cm margin superiorly on the gross tumor volume (GTV), as well as slightly larger margin on the inferior aspect of the GTV based on concern of previously unappreciated spread at time of endoscopy.

three-dimensional reconstruction and creation of a "beam's-eye" view of varying fields, allowing improved conformality around target structures and improvements in normal-tissue sparing. Because volumetric data can be obtained by CT scans, dose–volume histogram data can also be generated. A variety of three-dimensional techniques are being used and are described later.

Potential beam orientations for the treatment of thoracic esophageal and gastroesophageal junction tumors (again defined as tumors involving the gastroesophageal junction with an epicenter within 5 cm proximal or distal to the GE junction) include an AP/PA-alone approach, an initial AP/PA approach followed by AP/right posterior oblique (RPO)/left posterior oblique (LPO) fields with or without boost, an initial APPA approach followed by RAO/LPO fields with or without boost, and a three-field technique (AP/PA with left lateral or oblique field). One of our preferred approaches in lesions of the thoracic esophagus or GE junction is to use an initial AP/PA/RAO/LPO fields, with boost fields using laterally oriented beams. The inferior margin of the initial fields includes the gastroesophageal junction and, for lower or middle one-third lesions, the celiac axis nodal basins (generally located at the level of T12 and identifiable on CT), as well as gastrohepatic ligament. Initial fields are treated to a dose of 45 Gy, taking care to avoid as much of the heart as reasonably possible while continuing to minimize the kidney volume in the radiation field, inclusive of the above nodal basins. Reduced fields encompassing gross disease with an approximate 2-cm margin through oblique or lateral fields may then be used for an additional 5.4 Gy. Doses usually do not exceed 50 Gy (discussed later).

A margin of 5 cm above and below the GTV is generally recommended to cover subclinical submucosal/nodal disease, as well as an approximate 2.0- to 2.5-cm radial margin, although individual margins are case dependent. Because it is imperative to account for daily setup uncertainty as well as physiologic internal organ motion (secondary to respiration, peristalsis, cardiac motion, etc.), additional margin must be added to a clinical target volume, particularly to the more mobile distal esophagus. More recently, the internal target volume (ITV) has been used to account for physiologic motion of the target volume, which is included in the PTV. Varying reports analyzing esophageal motion have shown average anterior and posterior motion ranges from 0.1 to 4 mm, lateral motion from 0.3 to 4.2 mm, and superior-to-inferior motion from 3.7 to 10 mm.[107] An analysis evaluating interfraction esophageal motion in the right–left and AP direction showed average right–left motion of 1.8 ± 5.1 mm (favoring leftward movement) and average AP motion of 0.6 ± 4.8 mm (favoring posterior movement), with an average absolute motion of 4.2 mm or less in the right–left and AP directions. The authors concluded that 12-mm left, 10-mm posterior, and 9-mm anterior margins are appropriate.[110] Some authors have recommended defining 1-cm radial, 1.5-cm distal, and 1-cm proximal margins from CTV to ITV if target motion data are not available. Image-guided radiation therapy, including cone beam CT, may also be useful in localizing tumor and establishing physiologic variability between daily treatments.

Figure 53.11 shows general recommendations for elective target nodal station coverage in a patient with a type I GE junctional tumor with an accompanying example field. Figure 53.12 shows general recommendations for elective target nodal station coverage in a patient with a type II GE junctional tumor. Nodal basins are similar to type I tumors with the exception of inclusion of nodal basins along the splenic artery course. Figure 53.13 shows general recommendations for elective target nodal station coverage in a patient with a type III GE junctional tumor with accompanying example fields. Note that in type III tumors there is less emphasis on more proximal (lower mediastinal) nodes and more comprehensive coverage of the splenic artery course, including splenic hilum. Figure 53.14 shows examples of varying nodal locations on axial CT images.

Another potential approach in the treatment of thoracic esophageal cancer is the use of IMRT. IMRT also uses CT-based planning, again allowing 3D reconstruction of varying structures. However, IMRT differs from 3D planning through the delivery of radiation dose by partitioning a radiation field into multiple smaller fields of varying shapes and sizes, varying the dose intensity between each area. This is carried out with either dynamic IMRT (in which collimating leaves move in and out of the radiation beam path during treatment) or "step-and-shoot" IMRT (in which the leaves change the radiation field shape while the beam is turned off). Either method is particularly effective at conforming radiation dose to the target structures while avoiding dose to normal tissue. Radiation oncologists must determine which structures are most critical and weight their importance during the treatment planning process. Of importance, the greater the number of "avoidance" normal structures, the more difficult it is to meet all dose constraints. IMRT use "inverse planning," in which an intended prescription dose is placed on target volumes and dose constraints are placed on normal-tissue structures. Thereafter, computer software algorithms allow design of unconventional treatment fields that would not otherwise be possible with standard planning methods. Radiation oncologists and medical physicists critically evaluate numerous plans until dose constraints are satisfactorily met. The result should be a series of radiation doses that closely conform to the target volumes while minimizing dose to normal tissues. Dosimetric comparisons of IMRT versus 3D conformal therapy in cervical esophageal cancer have demonstrated superior target volume coverage and conformality with decreased normal-tissue dose.[111] A potential disadvantage of IMRT is the possibility of delivering low doses of radiation therapy to normal tissue areas that might not normally be irradiated using 2D or 3D techniques. The influence of this on toxicity (e.g.,

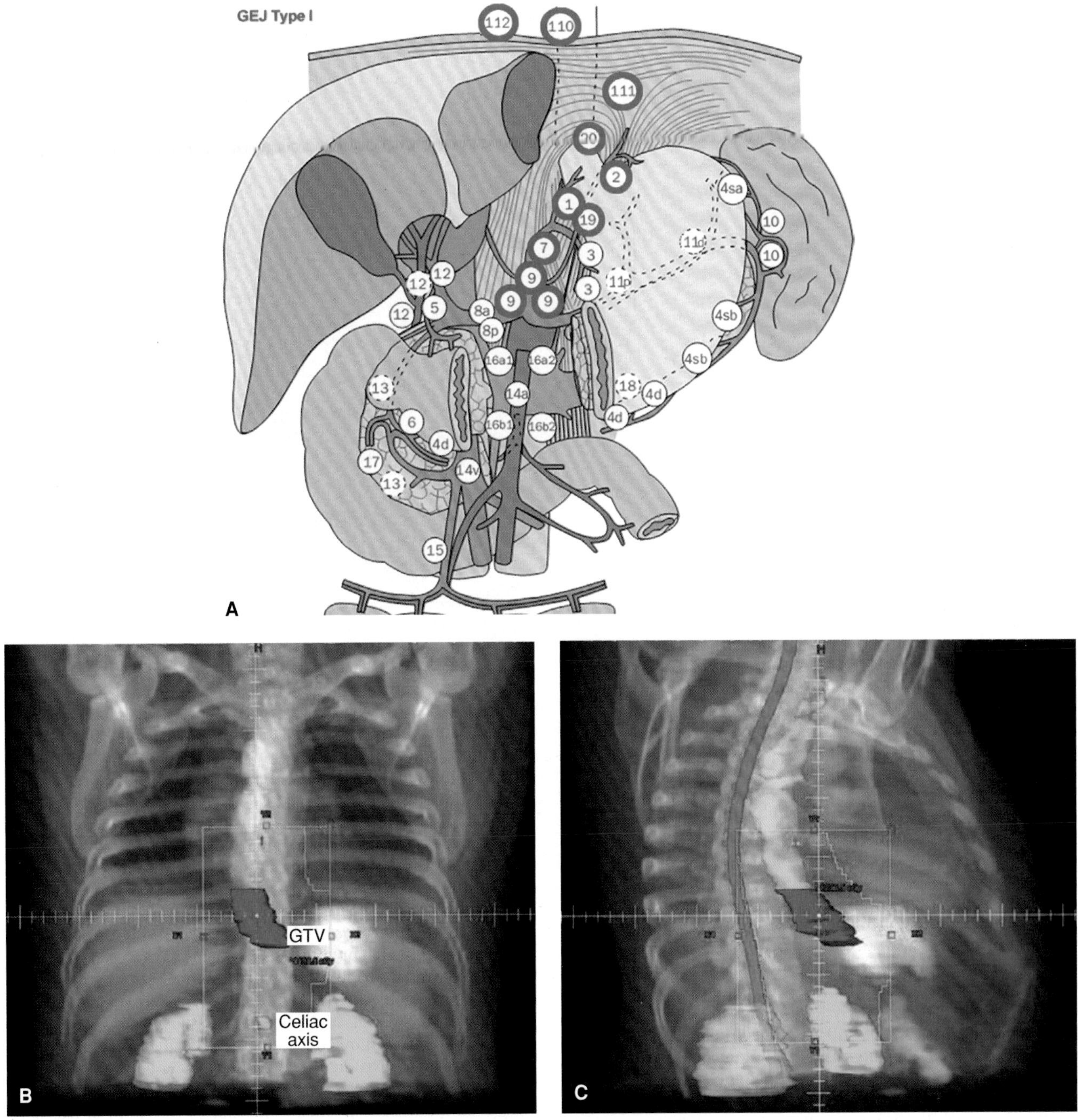

FIGURE 53.11. A: Recommended nodal basins to be included for type I gastroesophageal (GE) junctional tumors based on Japanese Gastric Cancer Association lymph node stations. (From Matzinger O, Gerber E, Bernstein Z, et al. EORTC-ROG expert opinion: radiotherapy volume and treatment guidelines for neoadjuvant radiation of adenocarcinomas of the gastroesophageal junction and the stomach. *Radiother Oncol* 2009;92:164–175; with permission from Elsevier.) **B:** Example field for a type I GE junctional adenocarcinoma. **C:** Example oblique field for a type I GE junctional tumor, inclusive of the above nodal basins.

low-dose pulmonary irradiation and development of postoperative pulmonary complications) remains uncertain. Another potential disadvantage to IMRT is possible dose inhomogeneity, leading to potential hot spots in normal organs. Because IMRT requires precise target definition, the potential for marginal miss increases, and careful target delineation is of paramount importance. With setup uncertainty, physiologic organ motion, and so on, care must be taken to ensure accurate and reproducible setup, including the use of immobilization devices, possible respiratory gating/breath-hold techniques, and so on. Generally, high-energy photons (4 to 18 MV) are recommended when using 3D conformal or IMRT therapy, potentially facilitating a reduction the integral lung dose.

Dose Constraints

In radiation therapy planning of esophageal cancer, normal-tissue tolerance should always be considered. The spinal cord dose is generally limited to 45 Gy using 1.8-Gy fractions (and potentially less when delivered with novel systemic agents). Efforts to minimize radiation to the heart (in particular the left ventricle in lower esophageal/gastroesophageal junction lesions) should be made. Adopting an off-heart approach using oblique orientations (including right anterior and left posterior, described earlier) is one potential way of achieving this, although multiple approaches exist, including IMRT-based techniques. Similarly, efforts to minimize dose to normal pulmonary tissues should be made, based on data suggesting

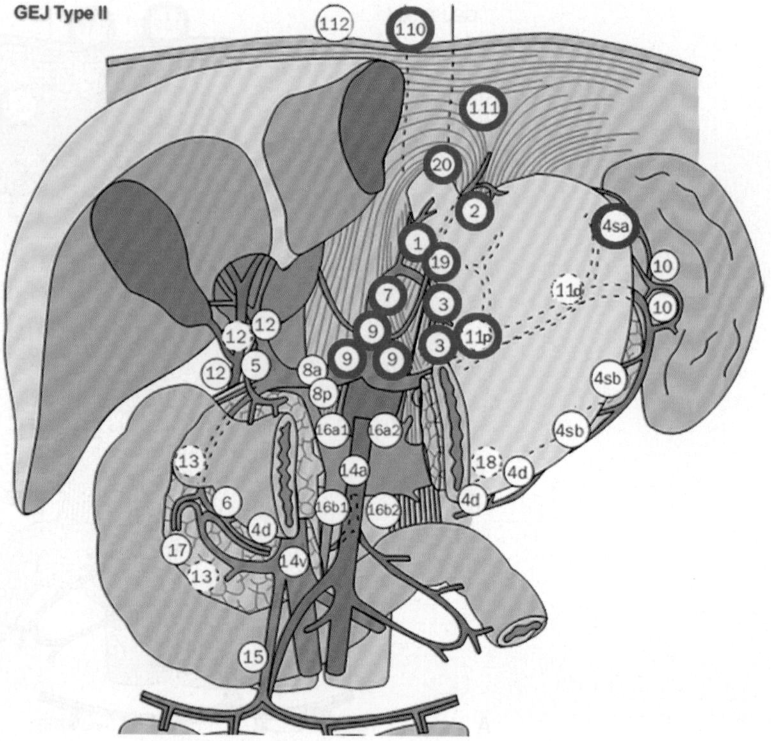

FIGURE 53.12. Recommended nodal basins to be included for type II gastroesophageal junctional tumors based on Japanese Gastric Cancer Association lymph node stations. (From Matzinger O, Gerber E, Bernstein Z, et al. EORTC-ROG expert opinion: radiotherapy volume and treatment guidelines for neoadjuvant radiation of adenocarcinomas of the gastroesophageal junction and the stomach. *Radiother Oncol* 2009;92:164–175; with permission from Elsevier.)

that the volume of irradiated lung may correspond to postoperative complications and worsened pulmonary function (described later). Frequently, the volume of irradiated lung can be minimized using a simple AP/PA approach. However, this sometimes results in significant cardiac dose, particularly in lower esophagus and gastroesophageal junction tumors. Therefore, oblique orientations are sometimes used, resulting in increased volumes of normal lung being irradiated. When giving concurrent chemotherapy, we generally limit these fields to 13 to 15 Gy.

Accurate delineation of adjacent organs, including lungs, liver, kidneys, heart, and spinal cord, is important. Varying dose–volume normal-organ constraints have been suggested, including achieving a lung V_{20} of <20%, limiting >2,300 cc of normal lung tissue to <5 Gy, and using mean lung dose of <18 Gy. Similarly, a V_{10} of ≤60% has been proposed to reduce the incidence of postoperative pulmonary complications. Historically, heart dose constraints have included maintaining one-third, two-thirds, and total heart volumes of <45, 40, and 30 Gy, respectively. Recommended heart constraints include keeping <30% of the cardiac volume to a total dose of 40 Gy and <50% receiving 25 Gy, minimizing dose to the left ventricle. In the setting of potentially significant volumes of heart in the radiation field, consideration of 4D CT and/or breath-hold techniques can be made. For lower esophageal and gastroesophageal cancers, it is recommended that at least 70% of one physiologically functioning kidney receive a total dose of <20 Gy, and that, collectively, no more than 50% of the combined functional renal volume should receive >20 Gy.[41] One should also consider the possibility of impaired kidney function in the context of varying comorbidities, using nuclear medicine renal studies to assess individual renal function in such situations or where significant volumes of kidneys are anticipated to be within the radiation field. Generally, 70% of the liver parenchyma should be kept to a dose of <30 Gy. Many of these constraints can be achieved through the use of three-dimensional planning with appropriate and careful design of shielding blocks/multileaf collimation and dose-volume histogram analysis, with the use of IMRT in select cases.

Doses of Radiation

Because local-regional failure is common after conventional chemoradiation, investigators have evaluated dose escalation techniques. Varying series using doses beyond 50 Gy have shown local control rates ranging from approximately 77% to 88%.[112,113] However, Minsky et al.[114,115] reported the results of a randomized trial in which 236 patients with clinical stage T1-4, N0/1, M0 squamous cell or adenocarcinoma of the esophagus were selected for nonsurgical therapy. Patients were randomized to receive 64.8 versus 50.4 Gy, both with concurrent 5-fluorouracil and cisplatin chemotherapy. Patients with cervical, mid, or distal esophageal cancer were eligible, with the exception of those with tumors within 2 cm of the gastroesophageal junction, with approximately 85% of patients with squamous cell histology. This study was closed after interim analysis showed no probability of superiority in the high-dose arm. No significant difference in median survival (13 vs. 18.1 months), 2-year survival (31% vs. 40%), or local-regional failure/persistence of disease (56% vs. 52%) was seen between the high-dose and standard-dose arms. Eleven treatment-related deaths occurred in the high-dose arm compared with 2 in the standard-dose arm, with 7 of the 11 high-dose arm deaths occurring in patients who received 50.4 Gy or less. The authors performed a separate survival analysis including only patients receiving the assigned radiation dose. Despite this, no survival advantage was noted in the high-dose arm. These authors concluded that higher radiation doses did not increase survival or local/regional control, and that the standard radiation dose for patients treated with concurrent 5-FU and cisplatin chemotherapy is 50.4 Gy. Based on these data, standard dose of radiation therapy for esophageal cancer is usually 50 to 50.4 Gy at 1.8 to 2 Gy per fraction, including delivery of similar doses in the both the definitive, adjuvant (45 to 50 Gy) or neoadjuvant (45 to 50 Gy) settings.

Brachytherapy

In addition to external-beam radiation therapy (EBRT), intracavitary therapy can be used with curative or palliative

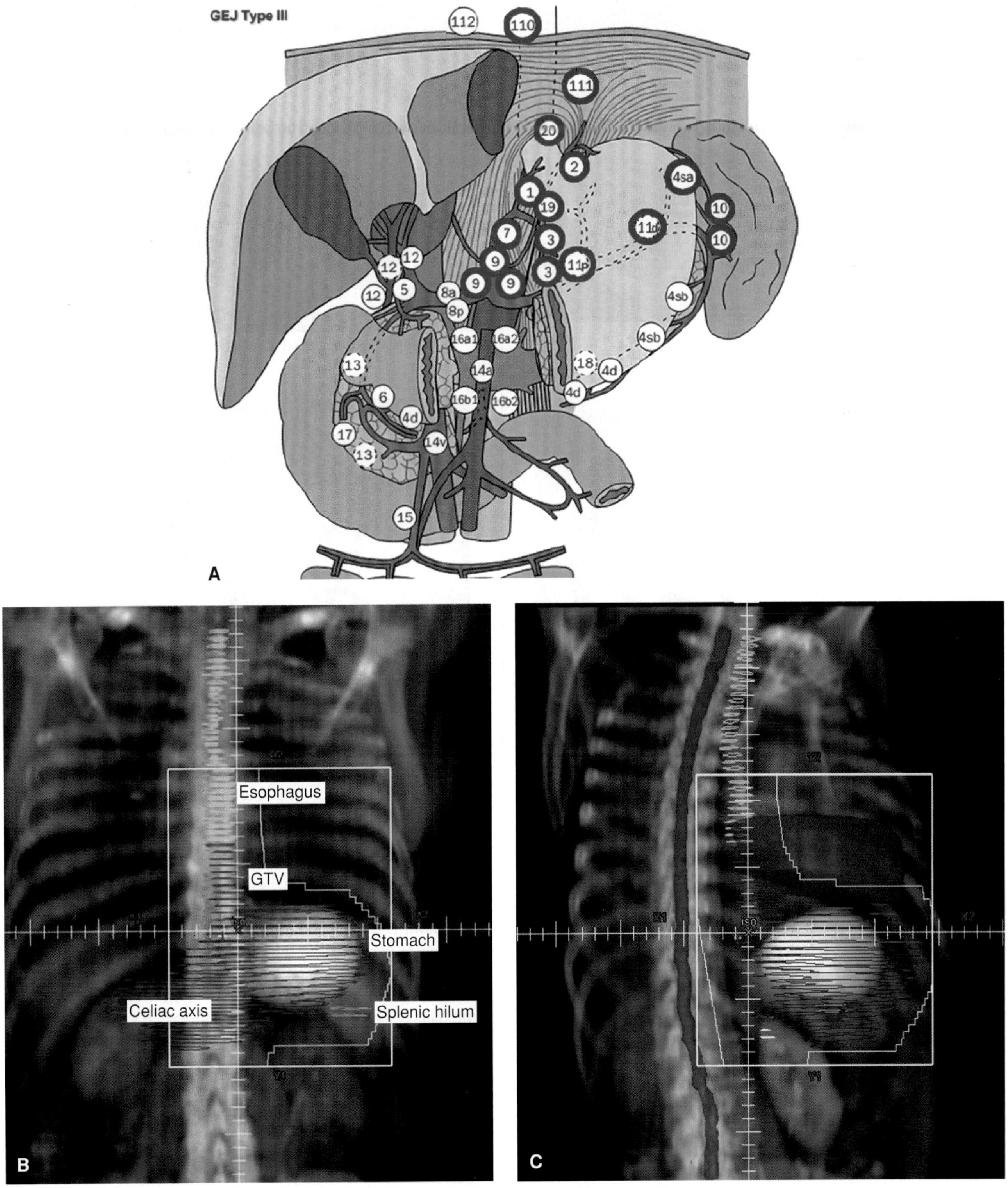

FIGURE 53.13. A: Recommended nodal basins to be included for type III gastroesophageal (GE) junctional tumors based on Japanese Gastric Cancer Association lymph node stations. (From Matzinger O, Gerber E, Bernstein Z, et al. EORTC ROG expert opinion: radiotherapy volume and treatment guidelines for neoadjuvant radiation of adenocarcinomas of the gastroesophageal junction and the stomach. *Radiother Oncol* 2009;92:164–175; with permission from Elsevier.) **B:** Example field for a type III gastroesophageal junctional adenocarcinoma. **C:** Example oblique field for a type III GE junctional tumor, inclusive of the above nodal basins.

intent. Brachytherapy has also been used as a dose escalation tool in addition to EBRT. The advantage of brachytherapy centers on exploitation of the inverse-square law and quick dose fall-off, thus sparing surrounding tissues from radiation while providing focal dose escalation. The radioactive source of choice is usually ^{192}Ir. High-dose-rate (HDR) techniques can deliver 100 to 400 Gy/hour, allowing treatment to be given in 5 to 10 minutes.

With brachytherapy, an afterloading catheter is introduced through the nose into the esophagus to the primary tumor site under fluoroscopic guidance. This is often performed with the patient on the simulation table. Contrast may be used to define

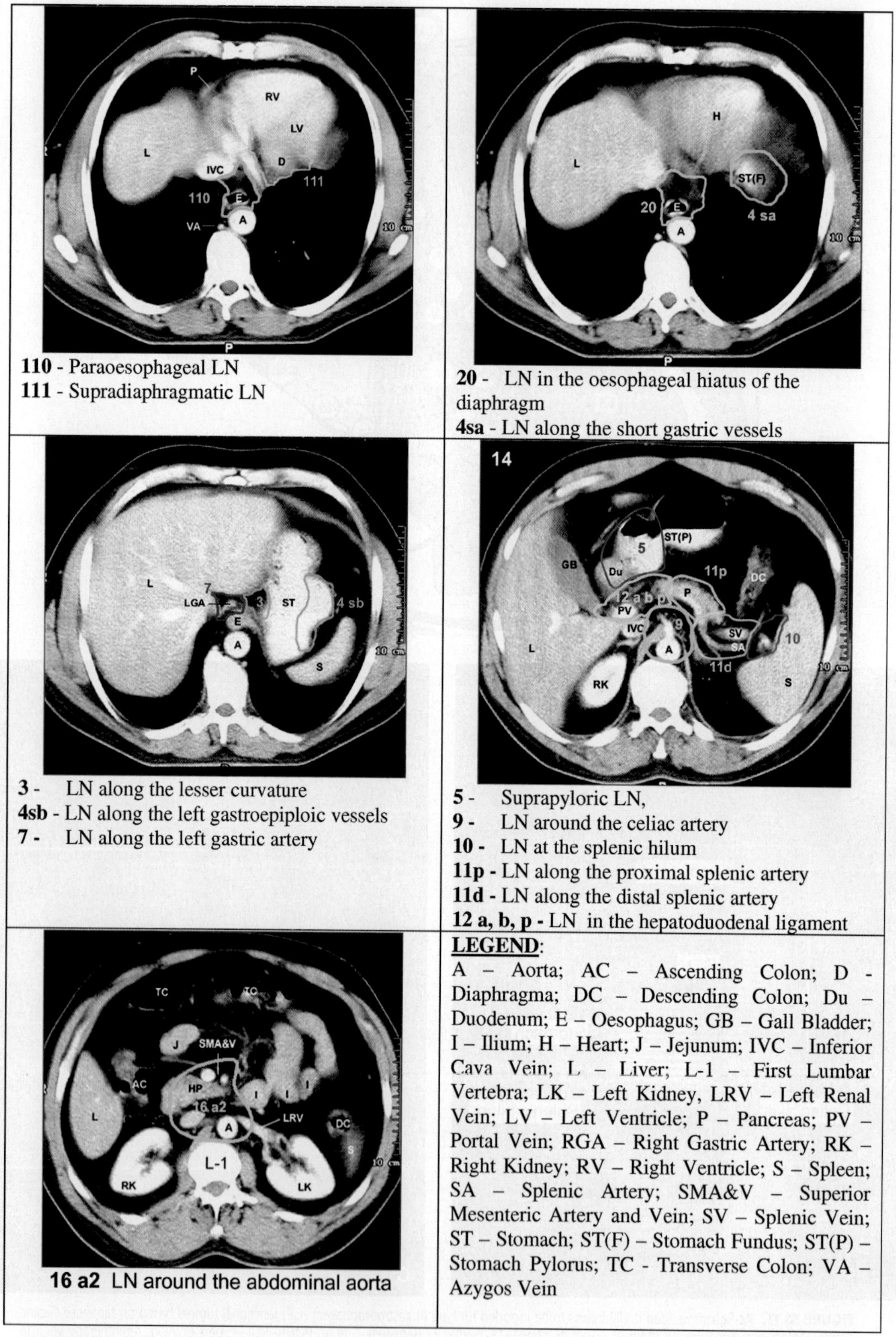
110 - Paraoesophageal LN
111 - Supradiaphragmatic LN
20 - LN in the oesophageal hiatus of the diaphragm
4sa - LN along the short gastric vessels
3 - LN along the lesser curvature
4sb - LN along the left gastroepiploic vessels
7 - LN along the left gastric artery
5 - Suprapyloric LN,
9 - LN around the celiac artery
10 - LN at the splenic hilum
11p - LN along the proximal splenic artery
11d - LN along the distal splenic artery
12 a, b, p - LN in the hepatoduodenal ligament
16 a2 LN around the abdominal aorta
LEGEND:
A – Aorta; AC – Ascending Colon; D - Diaphragma; DC – Descending Colon; Du – Duodenum; E – Oesophagus; GB – Gall Bladder; I – Ilium; H – Heart; J – Jejunum; IVC – Inferior Cava Vein; L – Liver; L-1 – First Lumbar Vertebra; LK – Left Kidney, LRV – Left Renal Vein; LV – Left Ventricle; P – Pancreas; PV – Portal Vein; RGA – Right Gastric Artery; RK – Right Kidney; RV – Right Ventricle; S – Spleen; SA – Splenic Artery; SMA&V – Superior Mesenteric Artery and Vein; SV – Splenic Vein; ST – Stomach; ST(F) – Stomach Fundus; ST(P) – Stomach Pylorus; TC - Transverse Colon; VA – Azygos Vein

FIGURE 53.14. Examples of lymph node stations on corresponding computed tomography slices. (From Matzinger O, Gerber E, Bernstein Z, et al. EORTC-ROG expert opinion: radiotherapy volume and treatment guidelines for neoadjuvant radiation of adenocarcinomas of the gastroesophageal junction and the stomach. *Radiother Oncol* 2009;92:164–175; with permission from Elsevier.)

the tumor site. CT scan can also be used to discern tumor location. After localization films are taken and dosimetry generated, the catheter is then attached to a remote afterloader through a guide cable and the ^{192}Ir source inserted through remote control. Doses of 5 to 20 Gy are usually delivered to a depth of 1 cm from the center of the catheter. Dose can be shaped and modified through the use of dwell times.

RESULTS OF THERAPY

The best survival results have been reported in patients who have esophageal tumors that are truly localized. Survival rates range from 25% to >35% at 5 years, and these results have been attained using an array of treatment approaches. Problems arise in comparisons of various modalities, however, because of patient selection factors. A review of the Princess Margaret Hospital data[116] supported the concept that extent of tumor, rather than therapy, is the most important factor influencing survival. They found a significant correlation between T stage and response to treatment: T1 lesions showed a 100% response rate, whereas T2 and T3 lesions had response rates of 68% and 58%, respectively. Not unexpectedly, they also found differences in survival according to T stage, M stage, and overall stage. Almost 20% of patients with stage I disease were alive at 3.5 years, whereas only 11% of stage II patients were alive after the same interval, and all patients with stage III died of disease by approximately 1.5 years following therapy.

Surgery Alone

Surgery remains a benchmark to which other modalities are compared. Surgery removes the tumor, a length of normal esophagus, and lymph nodes. Although multiple techniques exist for the resection of esophageal cancer, no one surgical approach has clearly been shown to be superior with regard to complications or outcomes. Proponents of more extended resection (including transthoracic approaches) have advocated that such procedures result in a superior nodal clearance and therefore offer a more complete "oncologic" resection. A trial from the Netherlands randomized 220 patients with esophageal adenocarcinoma to transhiatal esophagectomy alone or transthoracic esophagectomy with extended lymph node dissection. Patients undergoing transhiatal resection experienced significantly fewer pulmonary complications and chylous leaks, as well as significantly reduced ventilator dependence and intensive care unit and hospital stays. At a median 4.7-year follow-up, no significant difference in local-regional recurrence was seen between the two groups (32% transhiatal vs. 31% transthoracic). Furthermore, no significant differences were seen in median disease-free survival (1.4 vs. 1.7 years; $p = .15$) or median overall survival (1.8 vs. 2.0 years; $p = .38$). However, there did appear to be a nonsignificant trend favoring the transthoracic approach in improved disease-free survival (5-year, 27% vs. 39%) and overall survival (5-year, 29% vs. 39%) The authors concluded that a transhiatal approach was associated with less morbidity relative to transthoracic surgery, with no apparent survival advantage with either technique, although a trend toward improved survival with longer follow-up was seen.[46] In summary, none of the surgical approaches to localized esophageal cancer has clearly been shown to be superior with regard to complications or outcomes, and no one standard surgical approach exists for esophageal cancer resection.

After resection alone, however, local-regional relapse is a common mode of failure. Contemporary randomized trials with surgery alone arms have reported local regional failure rates of 32% to 45%.[46–49] It should be remembered that patterns of failure reports often describe first site of failure only and may include only patients undergoing R0 resection, potentially underreporting the true incidence of local-regional recurrence. These and other data suggest that even with modern surgical techniques, local-regional persistence of disease after resection remains a major problem. Prospective, randomized trials using surgery alone in the treatment of esophageal cancer have reported 3-year survival rates ranging from 6% to 48%, with more favorable rates likely reflecting inclusion of patients with earlier-stage disease[117–121] (Table 53.7). Given these high rates of relapse and poor long-term survival, the integration of adjuvant or neoadjuvant chemoradiation approaches into the treatment of esophageal cancer is rational and indicated.

Radiation Therapy Alone

There are no randomized studies comparing surgery alone with radiation alone, and radiation therapy alone has been usually delivered when lesions are deemed inoperable because of tumor extent, medical contraindications, and/or palliative treatment is indicated. In general, patients receiving radiation as a sole treatment modality have a median survival of 6 to 12 months and 5-year survival of <10%.

A large review analyzing 49 series involving >8,400 patients treated primarily with radiation therapy alone found overall survival rates at 1, 2, and 5 years to be 18%, 8%, and 6%, respectively.[122] Hancock and Glatstein[97] reviewed 9,511 patients and found only 5.8% were alive at 5 years. Okawa et al.[123] reported 5-year survival rates by stage. For patients with stage I disease, the 5-year survival rate was 20%; stage II, 10%; stage III, 3%; and stage IV, 0%. Overall, the 5-year survival rate was 9%. For cervical esophageal lesions treated with radiation alone, the cure rates are comparable with those in patients treated with surgery alone. Lederman[124] treated 263 patients with radiation therapy alone and reported 3- and 5-year survival rates of 11% and 7%, respectively. In a more contemporary series, an Intergroup randomized study (discussed later) comparing combined chemotherapy with 5-FU and cisplatin with radiotherapy (50 Gy) versus radiotherapy only (64 Gy) showed that 3-year survival with radiotherapy alone was 0%. These and other data suggest that treatment with radiation therapy alone for esophageal cancer patients is palliative in the vast majority of patients.

TABLE 53.7 COMPARISON OF SURGICAL ARMS IN RANDOMIZED STUDIES

Trial	Year	Patients (Total)	Patients (Surgical)	Median Survival (Months)	Two-Year Survival	Three-Year Survival
Walsh et al.[117]	1996	110	55	11	26	6
Urba et al.[49]	2001	100	50	18	NA	15
Bosset et al.[119]	1997	282	139	19	40	35
Kelsen et al.[47]	1998	440	227	16	37	23
MRC[118]	2002	802	402	13	34	NA
Burmeister[141]	2005	256	128	19	NA	31
van Hagen et al.[120]	2010	363	188	26	NA	48
Mariette et al.[121]	2010	195	98	44	NA	NA

MRC, Medical Research Council Oesophageal Cancer Working Group; NA, not applicable.

Preoperative Radiation Therapy

The use of preoperative radiation therapy has potential biologic and physical advantages, including increased resectability of tumors, increased tumor radioresponsiveness secondary to improved tumor oxygenation, a theoretical decreased likelihood of dissemination at the time of surgery, and avoidance of surgery in patients with rapidly progressive disease.

There are multiple, largely historical randomized studies comparing preoperative irradiation followed by surgery with surgery alone. These studies demonstrate no clinical benefit to the use of preoperative radiation therapy alone (Table 53.8). Launois et al.[125] reported delivering 40 Gy over 8 to 12 days with surgery 8 days later versus surgery alone. Resection rates were similar—70% and 58% for preoperative irradiation and for surgery alone, respectively. The 5-year survival rate after resection was 11.5% for those treated with surgery alone, compared with 9.5% for those treated with irradiation and surgery. The second randomized study, published by the European Organisation for Research and Treatment of Cancer (EORTC), used 33 Gy over 12 days.[126] There was no significant difference in survival between those receiving preoperative irradiation and those receiving surgery alone. Arnott et al.[127] reported on 176 patients, 86 of whom were treated with esophagectomy alone versus 90 who were treated with preoperative radiation therapy. Preoperative radiation therapy was delivered with 4-MV photons using opposed fields, delivering 20 Gy at 2 Gy per fraction. Resectability and local failure were not reported.

TABLE 53.8 RANDOMIZED TRIALS OF PREOPERATIVE RADIATION THERAPY FOR ESOPHAGEAL CANCER

				Local Failure		Survival (5-Year)	
Author	Patients	Dose (Gy)	Fraction (Gy)	Surgery	RT + Surgery	Surgery	RT + Surgery
Launois et al.[125]	109	40	NA	NA	NA	12	10
Gignoux et al.[126]	229	33	3.3	67	46	8	10
Arnott et al.[a127]	176	20	2	NA	NA	17	9
Wang et al.[128]	160	40	2	NA	NA	30	35

NA, not applicable; RT, radiation therapy
[a]Both squamous and adenocarcinoma.

Patients receiving low-dose radiation therapy did not demonstrate a benefit in 5-year overall survival rates (17% vs. 9% for surgery and preoperative radiation, respectively; $p = .4$). Wang et al.[128] randomized 206 patients to surgery alone versus 40 Gy in 2-Gy fractions delivered preoperatively. No significant survival advantage was seen for patients receiving radiation therapy (35% vs. 30%; $p > .05$).

A meta-analysis from the Oeosophageal Cancer Collaborative Group updated data from five randomized trials of >1,100 patients comparing preoperative radiotherapy alone versus surgery alone. The majority of patients had squamous cell carcinoma. At a median follow-up of 9 years, the hazard ratio was 0.89, suggestive of an overall reduction in the risk of death of 11% and absolute survival benefit of 4% at 5 years with the use of preoperative radiotherapy. However, this was not statistically significant ($p = .06$). The authors concluded that there was no clear evidence that preoperative radiotherapy improves survival of patients with potentially resectable esophageal cancer.[4]

In general, there were no differences in resectability rates or survival in almost all of the individual studies. Interpretation of these varying studies is complicated by differences in radiation techniques, suboptimal radiation doses, and inadequate radiation volumes. Nonetheless, although preoperative radiation therapy alone may improve local control, there is no convincing data that it results in improved survival in esophageal cancer patients.

Postoperative Radiation Therapy

The main advantage to adjuvant versus neoadjuvant approaches is knowledge of the pathologic staging for appropriately selected patients for therapy. Postoperative therapy may allow the radiation oncologist to treat areas at risk for recurrence while sparing otherwise normal radiosensitive structures, thereby decreasing toxicity. In addition, patients with pathologic T1, N0, M0 or metastatic disease may be spared treatment. Postoperative irradiation has historically been delivered to patients with esophageal cancer who have bulky tumors with gross residual disease or histologically proven microscopic residual disease. Potential disadvantages of postoperative radiation include limited tolerance of normal tissues after gastric pull-up or intestinal interposition and irradiation of a devascularized tumor bed, potentially larger fields compared to a preoperative approach, and potential delays in adjuvant treatment delivery.

Three randomized trials have assessed surgery alone versus surgery followed by postoperative radiation therapy.[129–131] In a French trial, 221 patients with squamous cell carcinoma of the mid-lower esophagus undergoing esophagectomy were randomized to postoperative radiation therapy or no further treatment. Patients were stratified by extent of nodal involvement. Total dose was 45 to 55 Gy at 1.8 Gy per fraction, beginning within 3 months of surgery. Five-year survival in node-negative patients was 38% versus 7% with involved nodes. No significant survival difference was seen in patients receiving postoperative radiation versus surgery alone. Rates of local regional recurrence were lower in patients receiving radiation therapy (85% vs. 70%; p = NS). However, in patients without nodal involvement, local-regional recurrence was significantly improved in patients receiving postoperative therapy (90% vs. 65%; $p < .2$). The authors concluded that postoperative radiation therapy did not improve survival after resection for squamous cell carcinoma.[129]

Investigators from the University of Hong Kong reported the results of a randomized trial of 130 patients treated with postoperative radiation therapy versus surgery alone. Patients who underwent either curative or palliative resections were included in this trial. Radiation therapy was delivered to a total dose of 49 Gy (curative patients) or 52.5 Gy (palliative patients) using 3.5-Gy fractions. Most patients had squamous cell histology. Local recurrence was noted in 15% of patients receiving radiation and 31% of patients with surgery only ($p = .06$). In patients with squamous cell carcinoma, the local recurrence rate was 15% with radiation therapy versus 36% with surgery alone ($p = .02$). Median survival in patients was worse in patients receiving postoperative radiotherapy versus control patients (8.7 vs. 15.2 months; $p = .02$). Ten patients undergoing surgery alone had tracheal bronchial recurrence resulting in death versus 3 patients receiving adjuvant radiation therapy ($p = .07$). The authors concluded that postoperative radiation therapy was associated with increased morbidity and death caused by irradiation injury, as well as with the early appearance of metastatic disease and a reduced overall survival, although patients receiving radiation therapy were less likely to have a tracheobronchial recurrence. However, it should be noted the high rate of complications associated with radiation therapy in this study may possibly be related to the high dose per fraction and large total dose delivered.[130]

Last, a study conducted by Xiao et al.[131] randomized 549 patients to radical resection versus radical resection followed by radiation therapy. All patients had squamous cell carcinoma. The radiation dose delivered was 60 Gy in 6 weeks. Patients were classified into three groups: group 1, no lymph node involvement; group 2, one to two lymph nodes involved; group 3, three or more lymph nodes involved. Results showed T stage, stage group, and the number of lymph nodes involved by tumor were highly predictive of survival. The 5-year survival for groups 1, 2, and 3 were 58.1%, 30.6%, and 14.4%, respectively. Local control and survival were improved in patients receiving postoperative irradiation. For patients with involved lymph nodes, 5-year survival for resection-only patients versus patients receiving resection and radiation therapy were 17.6% and 34.1%, respectively ($p = .04$).

In summary, postoperative radiation therapy may decrease local recurrence, particularly in the setting of involved margins, although the impact of this adjuvant treatment on overall survival remains less clear.

Postoperative Combined Chemoradiation

A large randomized Intergroup trial evaluating the role of adjuvant chemoradiation after surgery versus surgery alone for patients with adenocarcinoma of the stomach and GE junction was reported. In this study, patients with resected, margin-negative gastric or gastroesophageal junction adenocarcinoma were randomly assigned to surgery alone versus surgery with postoperative chemoradiotherapy. Approximately 20% of patients had lesions in the gastroesophageal junction.

A significant survival advantage was seen in the adjuvantly treated group (median survival 27 vs. 36 months; $p = .005$). On subset analysis, this benefit was detected in patients with gastroesophageal cancer.[132] Long-term results at >10-year median follow-up continued to show significant improvement in overall and disease-free survival in the chemoradiation group, benefiting all T- and N-stage patients included in the trial.[133] Therefore, in patients with resected-stage group Ib-IV, nonmetastatic GE junctional carcinoma, it is appropriate to advise adjuvant chemoradiotherapy in efforts to potentially improve upon local control and survival.

Preoperative Chemotherapy

Five randomized trials showed conflicting results with the use of neoadjuvant chemotherapy alone in the treatment of esophageal cancer, with two of these trials also including gastric cancers. Kelsen et al.[47] reported the results of an Intergroup study randomizing 440 patients with squamous cell carcinoma and adenocarcinoma to receive either combined cisplatin or 5-FU chemotherapy for three cycles followed by resection, followed by a similar regimen of adjuvant chemotherapy, versus immediate resection with no chemotherapy. No apparent survival advantage (3-year survival of 23% vs. 26%) was seen in patients receiving chemotherapy. In addition, rates of local failure (32% vs. 31%) and distant metastasis development (41% vs. 50%) were not significantly different between the two groups. The authors concluded that neoadjuvant chemotherapy with cisplatin and 5-FU did not improve survival in patients with resectable esophageal cancer. Long-term results from a follow up analysis reported that only 59% and 63% of patients undergoing preoperative chemotherapy and surgery alone, respectively, underwent R0 resection, and patients undergoing less than R0 resection had an ominous prognosis, with only 5% of patients undergoing R1 resection surviving >5 years and no difference in median survival rates for patients with R1, R2, or no resection. In this follow-up study, patients with objective tumor regression after preoperative chemotherapy did have improved survival. An important caveat from this study is that all long-term R1 survivors received adjuvant RT, and the authors concluded that after R1 resection, postoperative chemoradiotherapy offers the possibility of long-term disease-free survival to a small percentage of patients.[134]

In contrast to the Intergroup study, a similar trial from the Medical Research Council (MRC) randomized 802 patients with squamous cell carcinoma or adenocarcinoma of the esophagus to either two cycles of combined cisplatin/5-FU chemotherapy or surgery alone. Patients receiving neoadjuvant chemotherapy had a statistically improved 2-year survival (43% vs. 34%).[118] Follow-up analysis at a median follow-up of 6 years showed a persistent, significant survival benefit in the chemotherapy group (5-year survival 23% vs. 17%), with the effect maintained for both squamous cell carcinoma and adenocarcinoma patients.[135] The reason for outcomes differences between these trials is not clear.

A smaller trial of 169 patients with squamous cell carcinoma of the esophagus randomized patients to receive preoperative chemotherapy alone with two to four cycles of etoposide and cisplatin–based chemotherapy versus surgery alone. Median and 5-year survival rates significantly favored the chemotherapy group at 16 versus 12 months and 26 versus 17%, respectively. The authors concluded that preoperative chemotherapy with a combination of etoposide and cisplatin improves survival in patients with squamous carcinoma of the esophagus.[136]

A more heterogeneous European study (the Medical Research Council Adjuvant Gastric Infusional Chemotherapy trial) randomly assigned patients with resectable adenocarcinoma of the stomach, gastroesophageal junction, or lower esophagus to preoperative and postoperative chemotherapy with epirubicin, cisplatin, and 5-FU versus surgery alone. Although originally designed to include patients with only tumors of the stomach, eligibility was later expanded to include tumors of the lower one-third of the esophagus. Approximately one-fourth of patients had adenocarcinoma involving the lower esophagus or gastroesophageal junction. No patient achieved pathologic complete response. However, patients receiving perioperative chemotherapy had a hazard ratio for death of 0.75, which was highly significant. Five-year survival in patients receiving chemotherapy was 36% versus 23% in patients undergoing surgery alone ($p = .009$). Subgroup analysis of patients with lower esophageal or gastroesophageal junction tumors showed benefit to the delivery of perioperative chemotherapy.[137] A follow-up study is evaluating the role of the vascular endothelial growth factor inhibitor bevacizumab with a similar backbone regimen.

French investigators reported the results of a similar randomized trial of 224 patients assigned to perioperative chemotherapy (cisplatin and 5-FU) versus surgery alone. Although originally designed to include only patients with tumors of the lower one-third of the esophagus or gastroesophageal junction, eligibility was later expanded to include gastric cancers. Most patients (75%) had disease of the lower esophagus or gastroesophageal junction. Chemotherapy consisted of planned two or three preoperative and three or four postoperative cycles. This study was prematurely terminated because of low accrual. Patients receiving chemotherapy had improved overall survival (5-year, 38% vs. 24%; $p = .02$), disease-free survival (5-year, 34% vs. 19%, $p = .003$), and R0 resection rates (84% vs. 73%; $p = .04$). Only 50% of patients received postoperative chemotherapy. T0 disease (complete pathologic response at the primary site) was seen in 3% of neoadjuvantly treated patients. Total local regional recurrence rates were 24% and 26%, respectively in the chemotherapy versus surgery group, with distant recurrence rates of 42% versus 56%, respectively.[138] In addition to the foregoing studies, two recent meta-analyses suggested that neoadjuvant chemotherapy resulted in absolute 2- and 5-year survival benefit of 7% and 4%, respectively.[139,140]

Preoperative Chemoradiation Versus Surgery Alone

Walsh et al.[117] reported a randomized study to evaluate the role of concurrent preoperative chemoradiation combined with surgery. A total of 110 patients with adenocarcinoma of the esophagus were randomized to receive cisplatin, 5-FU, and concurrent radiation therapy followed by surgery versus surgery alone. Combined-modality patients received two courses of chemotherapy at weeks 1 and 6. Patients were treated using anteroposterior–posteroanterior fields (later changed to a three-field technique) to a total dose of 4,000 cGy in 15 fractions. Surgery was performed 4 to 6 weeks later, using five separate approaches. Median survival was 16 months with preoperative chemoradiation therapy compared to 11 months for the patients treated with surgery alone ($p = .01$). The 1-, 2-, and 3-year survival rates were 52%, 37%, and 32%, respectively, for patients who received multimodality therapy and 44%, 26%, and 6%, respectively, for those patients assigned to surgery. These results were significant at 3 years ($p = .01$). The authors concluded that neoadjuvant chemoradiation was superior to surgery alone in patients with resectable esophageal adenocarcinoma. This trial has been criticized for its poor surgery-alone results, short follow-up, and lack of prerandomization CT staging.

Urba et al.[49] reported the results of 100 patients with nonmetastatic esophageal carcinoma (squamous and adenocarcinoma histology) randomized to receive preoperative chemoradiation followed by surgery versus transhiatal esophagectomy alone. Chemotherapy consisted of cisplatin, 5-FU, and vinblastine. Only 69% of the patients were able to receive the intended chemotherapy dose. Radiation was delivered at 1.5 Gy twice daily for 3 weeks to a total dose of 4,500 cGy. No elective nodal irradiation was performed. Surgery was performed on day 42. Tumors >5 cm, patient age >70 years, and squamous cell histology were associated with inferior survival. At median follow-up of 8 years, no significant difference in survival was seen between treatment arms, with a median survival of 17 months. However, 3-year survival rate was 16% in the surgery-alone arm versus 30% in the combined-modality arm (p = .15). A higher incidence of locoregional failure as first site of failure was seen in surgery-alone patients (42% vs. 19%, p = .02). In patients experiencing pathologic complete response, a median survival of 50 months and a 3-year survival rate of 64% was seen versus patients with residual tumor in the surgical specimen, where median survival was 12 months with a 3-year survival rate of 19% (p = .01). The investigators stated that "Although this is not statistically significant, this suggests a possible trend to the benefit of multimodality therapy, but the sample size was too small to detect a more subtle survival difference," and that surgery should be continued as a standard of care.

Bosset et al.[119] reported an EORTC trial randomizing 282 patients with squamous cell carcinoma of the esophagus to either immediate surgical resection or preoperative therapy using concurrent cisplatin chemotherapy with radiation therapy. Patients were treated with split-course radiotherapy with a 2-week interval, using 3.7 Gy per fraction to a total of 37 Gy. Postoperative mortality was significantly higher in patients receiving preoperative therapy (12% vs. 4%). Outcomes showed patients receiving neoadjuvant therapy experienced a significant improvement in disease-free survival, cancer-related mortality, margin-negative resection, and local control; however, no improvement in overall survival was seen versus patients undergoing surgery alone (median survival was 18.6 months for both groups). The authors concluded that neoadjuvant chemoradiation improved disease-free survival and local control in patients with squamous cell carcinoma of the esophagus but had no impact on overall survival. They judged that the increase in postoperative mortality in the combined group "could be due to deleterious effects of the high-dose of radiation per fraction," among other factors, and believed that the dose of 3.7 Gy per fraction "probably had a detrimental effect." This trial has also been criticized for the split-course treatment approach, as well as for potential delivery of suboptimal chemotherapy.

Burmeister et al.[141] reported an Australian study randomizing 257 patients with adenocarcinoma and squamous cell carcinoma of the esophagus to surgery alone versus neoadjuvant therapy using concomitant 5-FU and cisplatin. Patient received 2.33 Gy per fraction to a total dose of 35 Gy. Patients undergoing neoadjuvant therapy had a 16% pathologic complete response rate at resection. Patients receiving neoadjuvant therapy were more likely to undergo curative resection and have negative lymph nodes on histologic examination. However, no significant improvement in median survival was seen (19 vs. 22 months; hazard ratio 0.89; p = .57). On subset analysis, there appeared to be a trend toward improved survival in patients with squamous cell carcinoma undergoing neoadjuvant therapy versus surgery alone (progression-free survival hazard ratio, 0.47; p = .01; overall survival hazard ratio, 0.69; p = .16). The authors concluded that neoadjuvant chemoradiation as delivered in their study provided no obvious survival benefit in patients with esophageal cancer, although further study was warranted in patients with squamous cell carcinoma. Potential criticisms of this trial include delivery of a single chemotherapy cycle, as well as delivery of lower radiation doses.

Results of a Cancer and Leukemia Group B study described 56 patients (75% with adenocarcinoma) randomized to either surgery alone or neoadjuvant chemoradiation followed by surgical resection. Patients in the neoadjuvant therapy arm received cisplatin/5-FU–based chemotherapy and 50.4 Gy of external beam radiation therapy at 1.8 Gy per fraction. This trial was closed prematurely due to poor accrual. In patients undergoing neoadjuvant therapy, pathologic complete response rate was 40%. A significant improvement in local control and survival was seen in patients receiving neoadjuvant combined-modality therapy (5-year survival, 39% vs. 16%). The authors concluded that neoadjuvant chemoradiation in patients with esophageal cancer significantly improves progression-free and overall survival.[142]

Results of the largest randomized trial (the Chemoradiotherapy for Oesophageal Cancer Followed by Surgery Study, or CROSS trial) assessing neoadjuvant chemoradiotherapy in the treatment of esophageal cancer showed a significant survival benefit in patients receiving preoperative therapy, with the majority of patients included in this trial having locally advanced adenocarcinoma.[120] Patients with resectable T1N1 or T2-3 N0-1 tumors received preoperative chemoradiotherapy consisting of weekly paclitaxel and carboplatin with concurrent radiotherapy to a dose of 41.4 Gy versus surgery alone. R0 resection rates were 92% in patients receiving neoadjuvant chemoradiotherapy versus 69% for surgery alone, with a pathologic complete response rate of 29% in patients receiving preoperative therapy. No significant differences were seen in in-hospital mortality (4% vs. 4%). Median survival was 49 months in patients receiving chemoradiotherapy versus 24 months in surgery alone, with a significant improvement in 3-year survival (58% vs. 44%). The authors concluded that weekly administration of carboplatin and paclitaxel with concurrent radiotherapy improves overall survival compared to surgery alone and that this regimen can be considered the standard of care for patients with resectable esophageal or esophagogastric junction cancer.

In contrast, a preliminary report from France evaluating primarily early-stage squamous cell esophageal cancer patients randomized to receive preoperative chemoradiotherapy versus surgery alone showed no significant difference in outcomes.[121] In this study, patients with early-stage disease (stage I-II) were randomized to receive surgery alone versus neoadjuvant chemoradiotherapy using concurrent 5-FU and cisplatin with 45 Gy. Thirty-day postoperative mortality rates were 1% in the surgery-alone group versus 7% in the neoadjuvant group (p = .054). Median survival was not significantly different between the groups (44 vs. 32 months; p = .66). The authors concluded that neoadjuvant chemoradiotherapy with cisplatin and 5-FU did not improve survival but increased postoperative mortality for patients with early-stage esophageal cancer. Outcomes of these trials are shown in Table 53.9.

Given these conflicting results of contemporary trials, multiple meta-analyses have been performed. Two of the largest and most contemporary of these demonstrated an absolute 2- and 5-year overall survival benefit of 13% and 6.5% with the use of neoadjuvant chemoradiotherapy, respectively, when compared to surgery-alone approaches, also suggesting a larger benefit of preoperative chemoradiotherapy as compared to a chemotherapy alone.[139,140] It should be kept in mind that some of the included trials used sequential (vs. concurrent) chemotherapy, delivered what would be considered suboptimal doses of radiation therapy, used antiquated radiation therapy techniques, delivered (arguably) inadequate chemotherapy, and so on, potentially underestimating the effect of neoadjuvant combined-modality therapy. That being said, an updated meta-analysis including a total of 24 randomized trials evaluating the role of neoadjuvant chemoradiotherapy, neoadjuvant chemotherapy, or comparison of the two in patients with resectable esophageal cancer was recently reported,[143] evaluating the outcomes of >4,000 patients. All-cause mortality for neoadjuvant chemoradiotherapy trials estimated an absolute survival benefit at 2 years of 8.7%, with survival benefits similar between squamous cell carcinoma and adenocarcinoma patients. By comparison, estimated absolute survival difference at 2 years was 5.1% in patients receiving neoadjuvant

TABLE 53.9 RESULTS OF PREOPERATIVE COMBINED CHEMORADIATION VERSUS SURGERY ALONE–PHASE III TRIALS

Study	*Median Follow-up (Year)*	*Pathology*	*Regimen*	*Number of Patients*	*Pathologic Complete Response*	*Three-Year Survival*	*Survival Difference*
Urba et al.[49]	8.2	SCC + adeno	5-FU-CDDP- Vinb/45 Gy Surg	50	28	CMT/Surg: 30%	$p = .15$
(Michigan)				50	–	Surg alone: 16%	
Bosset et al.[119]	4.6	SCC	CDDP/37 Gy Surg	143	20	CMT/Surg: 33%	NS
(EORTC)				138	–	Surg alone: 36%	
Walsh et al.[117]	1.5	Adeno	5-FU-CDDP/40 Gy Surg	58	22	CMT/Surg: 32%	$p = .01$
(Ireland)				55	–	Surg alone: 6%	
Burmeister et al.[141]	5.4	SCC + adeno	5-FU-CDDP/35 Gy Surg	128	16	CMT/Surg: 35%	NS
(Austria)				128	–	Surg alone: 31%	
Tepper et al.[142]	6.0	SCC + adeno	5-FU-CDDP/50 Gy Surg	30	40	CMT/Surg: 39% (5 yr)	$p = .008$
(USA)				26	–	Surg alone: 16% (5 yr)	
van Hagen et al.[120]	3.8	SCC + adeno	Pac-Carbo/41.4 Gy Surg	180	29	CMT/Surg: 58%	$p = .003$
(Netherlands)				188	–	Surg alone: 44%	
Mariette et al.[121]	5.7	SCC + adeno	5-FU-CDDP/45 Gy	97	29	CMT/Surg: 32 mo (med OS)	NS
(France)				98	–	Surg alone: 44 mo (med OS)	

adeno, adenocarcinoma; Carbo, carboplatin; CDDP, cisplatin; CMT, combined-modality therapy; EORTC, European Organisation for Research and Treatment of Cancer; 5-FU, 5-fluorouracil; med OS, median overall survival; Pac, paclitaxel; SCC, squamous cell carcinoma; Surg, surgery; Vinb, vinblastine.

chemotherapy and was significant only for adenocarcinoma patients. The authors concluded that neoadjuvant chemoradiotherapy improves survival compared with surgery alone in operable patients, as does neoadjuvant chemotherapy, although the benefit of neoadjuvant chemotherapy was not as great as with neoadjuvant chemoradiotherapy, that a clear advantage is not established, and further randomized trials comparing these two strategies are warranted.

In summary, the above data suggest that neoadjuvant concurrent chemoradiation improves local control and modestly improves survival versus surgery alone in patients with resected esophageal cancer.

Preoperative Chemoradiation Versus Preoperative Chemotherapy

A randomized trial comparing neoadjuvant chemotherapy alone versus neoadjuvant combined-modality therapy was conducted by German investigators (Preoperative Chemotherapy, or Radiochemotherapy in Esophagogastric Adenocarcinoma, or POET, Trial).[144] Patients with advanced esophagogastric adenocarcinoma were randomized to receive (a) cisplatin/5-FU–based chemotherapy alone versus (b) a similar induction chemotherapy, followed by concurrent cisplatin/etoposide with 30 Gy of radiation therapy. Both groups went on to receive surgery. Although this study was closed early due to poor accrual, patients receiving preoperative chemoradiotherapy had significantly higher N0 rates (37% vs. 64%; $p = .04$) and pathologic complete response rates (2% vs. 16%; $p = .03$), as well as significant trends toward improved local control (59% vs. 76%; $p = .06$) and overall survival (3-year survival, 28% vs. 47%; $p = .07$; hazard ratio, .67). The authors concluded that preoperative combined modality improves overall survival as compared to chemotherapy alone in patients with locally advanced esophagogastric adenocarcinoma.

A smaller phase II study from Australian investigators randomized 75 patients to receive either preoperative chemotherapy with cisplatin and infusional 5-FU versus preoperative chemoradiotherapy with the same drugs with radiation therapy commencing day 21 of chemotherapy, delivering 35 Gy in 15 fractions.[145] Histopathologic response rate and noncurative resection rates were significantly improved in the radiation-containing arm (8% vs. 31% and 11% vs. 0%, respectively). However, median overall survival was not significantly different between the groups (29 vs. 32 months). The authors concluded that despite their being no difference in survival, the potential advantage of achieving negative margins made preoperative chemoradiotherapy a reasonable option for bulky, locally advanced resectable adenocarcinoma of the esophagus.

Radiation Therapy Alone Versus Chemoradiation

There are multiple randomized studies comparing radiation therapy alone with concurrent radiation and chemotherapy[146–148] as definitive therapy. However, many of these studies are handicapped by small patient numbers, substandard chemotherapy delivery, and the use of suboptimal radiotherapy techniques. This makes treatment results difficult to interpret. The landmark trial establishing the superiority of concurrent chemoradiation to radiation therapy alone was Radiation Therapy Oncology Group (RTOG) 85-01. Herskovic et al.[149] reported results of this two-arm trial that treated 60 control patients with radiation alone to a total dose of 64 Gy versus 61 patients with 50 Gy of radiation therapy with concurrent 5-FU and cisplatin. The chemotherapy protocol consisted of four planned courses of infusional 5-FU and cisplatin. Although less radiation was delivered in the concurrent-therapy arm, the results demonstrated a significant advantage of the combined-modality arm over the radiation-alone arm. The median survival in patients treated by radiation alone was 8.9 months compared with 12.5 months for those treated with combined therapy, with 2-year survival rate 10% versus 38%; the incidence of local recurrence decreased from 24% to 16%, and the 2-year distant metastasis rate decreased from 26% to 12%. Because of this highly significant survival difference, the randomization was stopped, and 69 additional patients were treated on the chemoradiation arm. Updated trial results[146,150] showed that at 5 years, survival rates were 26% and 0%, respectively, for chemoradiation and radiation therapy alone. Local recurrence rates were also decreased with the use of combined-modality therapy versus radiation alone (45% vs. 69%), and distant metastases were more frequent in the radiation-alone arm at 40% versus 12% for the combined-modality group. The incidence of acute toxicity, however, was higher for the combined-modality arm versus the radiation-alone arm (44% vs. 25%). Similarly, the incidence of life-threatening side effects, including hematologic toxicity and fistula formation, was increased from 3% to 20%. In conclusion, this study demonstrated a significant improvement in local control, median and overall survival, and distant metastasis development with the addition of chemotherapy, at the cost of increased side effects.

Comparison of outcomes data from "definitive" chemoradiation approaches suggests that survival with combined chemoradiation is similar to that achieved by surgery alone. In previously discussed studies, median survivals of 14 to 20 months and

5-year survival rates of 20% to 30% were achieved with chemoradiation alone; in comparison, in the MRC trial and Intergroup trial evaluating surgery alone, median survivals were 13 to 16 months, with 5-year survivals of approximately 20%. In addition, local failure rates appear similar. For example, in the RTOG/Intergroup studies using chemoradiation therapy alone, local failure rates as a first site of failure range from 39% to 45%. In comparison, local failure rate for the Intergroup study evaluating surgery alone was 31%. However, this analysis was limited to patients undergoing R0 resection only (59% of patients).[134] This would undoubtedly be higher if all patients were considered. Therefore, local failure and survival rates appear similar between "definitive" chemoradiation and surgical approaches.

Chemoradiation Versus Chemoradiation Followed by Surgery

Two randomized trials examined whether surgery is necessary after combined-modality therapy. A report from French investigators randomized 445 patients with clinically resectable squamous cell or adenocarcinoma of the esophagus.[151] All patients received concurrent 5-fluorouracil and cisplatin–based chemoradiation. Patients were treated with one of two radiation regimens: 46 Gy over 4.5 weeks (continuous) or 30 Gy at 15 Gy per week (split course). Two hundred fifty-nine patients who had at least a partial response were then randomized to either surgery or additional combined-modality therapy of 5-FU and cisplatin delivered concurrent with radiation (either an additional 20 Gy at 2 Gy per day or a split course of 15 Gy). No significant difference in 2-year survival (34% vs. 40%; $p = .56$) or median survival (18 vs. 19 months) was seen between the groups, although 2-year local control results favored the surgical arm (66% vs. 57%). The death rate at 3 months following treatment was 9% in the surgery group versus 1% in the combined-modality therapy–alone group. In addition, patients undergoing surgery were found to have a worse quality of life. However, the rate of stent and dilatation requirement was higher in the nonsurgical arm. The results of this trial suggest that surgery after chemoradiation in responding patients does not further enhance survival.

In another study, from Germany, patients with potentially resectable squamous cell carcinoma of the esophagus received induction chemotherapy with 5-FU, leucovorin, etoposide, and cisplatin for three cycles, followed by concurrent etoposide and cisplatin with 40 Gy of external-beam radiation therapy.[152] Patients were then randomized to receive surgery versus continuing with combined chemoradiation (total radiation dose increased to 60 to 65 Gy, with or without brachytherapy). Local control was significantly improved in patients undergoing surgery (2-year local control, 64% vs. 41%; $p < .05$). Despite this, no significant difference in survival was seen (median survival, 16 vs. 15 months; 3-year survival; 31% vs. 24%; $p =$ NS). The "severe" postoperative complication rate (including infection, leak) was 70%, and the hospital mortality rate was 11%. Overall treatment-related mortality was significantly higher in patients undergoing surgery (13% vs. 3.5%). In patients who did not respond to induction chemotherapy, 3-year survival was improved in patients undergoing surgery (18% vs. 9%). On regression analysis, only tumor response to induction chemotherapy was found to be a significant prognostic factor. An important caveat to this trial was that only approximately two-thirds of patients in the surgery arm actually had surgery. The authors concluded that (a) surgery after combined-modality therapy improves local control but had no impact on overall survival and (b) nonresponders to induction chemotherapy may benefit from surgery, and it may be appropriate to individualize therapy based on response to induction treatment. Although it has not been well studied, retrospective experience suggested that definitive chemoradiation in patients with adenocarcinoma of the esophagus results in median survival of 21 months and 2-, 3-, and 5-year survival rates of 44%, 33%, and 20% respectively.[153]

In summary, although surgery after combined chemoradiation for esophageal cancer appears to improve local control, its effect on ultimate survival is unclear.

Brachytherapy

Gaspar et al.[154,155] reported the results of a prospective trial evaluating intraluminal brachytherapy in patients with nonoperable esophageal cancer. Patients initially received 50 Gy of external irradiation with concurrent chemotherapy, followed by a 2-week break and brachytherapy administration. Patients received either 15 Gy using HDR techniques over three consecutive weeks (5 Gy/fraction) or a single administration of 20 Gy using low–dose-rate (LDR) techniques. Dose was prescribed to 1 cm from the source axis. Treatments were accomplished by placement of a 10- to 12-French applicator inserted transnasally or transorally. The target length was defined as the pretreatment tumor length with 1-cm margin proximally and distally as determined by CT, barium swallow, and endoscopy. Both external irradiation and brachytherapy were given concurrently with 5-FU chemotherapy. After the development of fistulas in six patients, the HDR dose was reduced to 10 Gy in two fractions, and the LDR arm was ultimately closed because of poor accrual. Results showed a median survival of 11 months in all patients. Local disease persistence/recurrence was observed in 63% of 49 eligible patients receiving HDR therapy. Six patients developed esophageal fistulas, resulting in three deaths. These fistulas were deemed treatment related. The 1-year actuarial fistula development rate was 18%. The investigators concluded that esophageal brachytherapy, particularly in conjunction with chemotherapy, should be approached with caution. Review of other combined brachytherapy/EBRT series suggests that fistula formation rates range from 0% to 12%, with a possible trend toward a higher incidence in patients receiving concurrent chemotherapy with brachytherapy. The incidence of brachytherapy related mortality varies from 0% to 8%, with most series reporting rates of 4% or less.[156]

Other studies have suggested that HDR brachytherapy is effective for palliation of dysphagia in up to 90% of patients.[156] Danish investigators reported the results of a randomized trial of 209 patients with dysphagia due to inoperable esophageal or gastroesophageal junctional tumors.[157] Patients were randomized to either endoscopic stent placement or single-dose HDR brachytherapy. Patient exclusion criteria included tumors >12 cm, tumors within 3 cm of the upper esophageal sphincter, deeply ulcerated tumors, tracheoesophageal fistula/tracheal involvement, presence of a pacemaker, and previous radiation treatment or stent placement. Brachytherapy was delivered through a flexible 1-cm applicator delivering a dose of 12 Gy prescribed to 1 cm from the source axis. The treatment length was defined as gross disease plus 2 cm proximally and distally. Although trial results showed a more rapid improvement in dysphagia after stent insertion, long-term dysphagia relief was significantly improved in the group receiving brachytherapy. Patients undergoing brachytherapy experienced more days with low-grade or no dysphagia versus patients with stent placement. Complications rates were higher following stent placement (33% vs. 21%), primarily due to an increased incidence of late hemorrhage in the stent group. The authors concluded that single-dose brachytherapy is preferable to stent placement as the initial treatment for patients with progressive dysphagia due to inoperable esophageal or gastroesophageal junction carcinoma.

For patients treated with curative intent (unifocal thoracic tumors <10 cm, no distant metastases, no airway involvement or cervical esophageal location), the American Brachytherapy Society recommends a brachytherapy dose of 10 Gy in two weekly fractions of 5 Gy each (HDR) or 20 Gy in a single course

TABLE 53.10 SELECTION CRITERIA FOR BRACHYTHERAPY IN THE TREATMENT OF ESOPHAGEAL CANCER

Good Candidates	Poor Candidates	Contraindications
Primary tumor ≤10 cm length	Extra esophageal extension	Esophageal fistula
Tumor confined to the esophageal wall	Tumor >10 cm in length	Cervical esophageal location
Thoracic esophagus location	Regional lymphadenopathy	Stenosis that cannot be bypassed
No regional lymph node or systemic metastases	Tumor involving gastroesophageal junction or cardia	

at 0.4 to 1 Gy/hour (LDR). The dose is prescribed to 1 cm from mid source and delivered through a 6- to 10-mm applicator. The recommended active length is the visible mucosal tumor with a 1- to 2-cm proximal and distal margin. Ideally, brachytherapy is started 2 to 3 weeks after completion of concurrent external irradiation/chemotherapy to allow mucositis resolution. Concurrent chemotherapy with brachytherapy is not recommended. In palliative cases, a similar approach is recommended, with delivery of 10 to 14 Gy in one or two fractions (HDR) or 20 to 25 Gy in a single course (LDR). In previously untreated patients with a short life expectancy (<3 months), a dose of 15 to 20 Gy in two to four fractions (HDR) or of 25 to 40 Gy (LDR) without external irradiation is recommended (Tables 53.10 to 53.12).[158] In summary, the use of brachytherapy in the curative approach to esophageal cancer does not appear to significantly improve results achieved with combined external-beam radiation therapy with chemotherapy alone.

Palliative Treatment

Although treatment advances have occurred in esophageal cancer over the last 20 years, the majority of patients diagnosed with esophageal cancer will die of their malignancy. Therefore, palliation remains an important goal. Dysphagia is a common presenting symptom, and may significantly impair patient's quality of life. Many studies report a 60% to >80% rate of relief from dysphagia with radiation.[159] Coia et al.[159] reported that nearly half of patients with baseline dysphagia experienced an improvement in swallowing within 2 weeks of treatment initiation. By the completion of the sixth week, >80% experienced improvement. A median time to maximal improvement was approximately 1 month. Given the superior outcomes of patients receiving concurrent chemotherapy with radiation therapy in nonmetastatic disease, palliative chemoradiation is likely preferable to radiation alone for patients with advanced-stage esophageal carcinoma who have a good performance status. As described earlier, intraluminal brachytherapy has also been used for palliation of dysphagia. The previously described randomized trial from the Netherlands comparing intraluminal brachytherapy to stent placement showed that although patients undergoing stenting experienced a more rapid improvement in dysphagia, long-term palliation was significantly improved in patients treated with brachytherapy.[157]

TABLE 53.11 SUGGESTED SCHEMA FOR DEFINITIVE EXTERNAL BEAM RADIATION AND ESOPHAGEAL BRACHYTHERAPY

External-Beam Radiation
From 45 to 50 Gy in 1.8- to 2.0-Gy fractions, 5 fractions/wk, wk 1 to 5

Brachytherapy
High dose rate: total dose of 10 Gy, 5 Gy/fraction, 1 fraction/wk, starting 2 to 3 wk after completion of external beam
Low dose rate: total dose of 20 Gy, single course, 0.4 to 1.0 Gy/hr, starting 2 to 3 wk from completion of external beam

All doses are specified 1 cm from the midsource or mid-dwell position.

TABLE 53.12 SUGGESTED SCHEMA FOR EXTERNAL BEAM RADIATION AND BRACHYTHERAPY IN THE PALLIATIVE TREATMENT OF ESOPHAGEAL CANCER

(a) Recurrent after external-beam radiation and short life expectancy
Brachytherapy:
HDR: total dose of 10 to 14 Gy, one or two fractions
LDR: total dose of 20 to 40 Gy, one or two fractions, 0.4 to 1.0 Gy/hr

(b) No previous external-beam radiation
External-beam radiation:
From 30 to 40 Gy in 2- to 3-Gy fractions
Brachytherapy
HDR: 10 to 14 Gy, one or two fractions
LDR: total dose of 20 to 25 Gy, single course, 0.4 to 1.0 Gy/hr

(c) No previous external beam radiation, life expectancy >6 mo
External-beam radiation:
From 45 to 50 Gy in 1.8- to 2.0-Gy fractions, 5 fractions/wk, wk 1 to 5
Brachytherapy
HDR: total dose of 10 Gy, 5 Gy/fraction, 1 fraction/wk, starting 2 to 3 wk after completion of external beam
LDR: total dose of 20 Gy, single course, 0.4 to 1.0 Gy/hr, starting 2 to 3 wk after completion of external beam

All doses are specified 1 cm from the midsource or mid-dwell position.
HDR, high dose rate; LDR, low dose rate.

The palliative management of patients with tracheoesophageal fistula presents a clinical dilemma. Fistulization usually precludes surgery. These patients are often treated effective with the placement of silicone-covered, self-expanding metal stents, often obviating palliative surgery. In addition, placement of feeding gastrostomy or jejunostomy may be appropriate. Although considered a "relative" contraindication to radiation therapy, limited data from a Mayo Clinic series suggests that radiation therapy may not increase fistula severity and can be administered safely in this setting; however, the presence of fistula is a poor prognostic factor.[160]

TREATMENT SEQUELAE

Advances in surgical technique, as well as improved preoperative and postoperative management, have decreased treatment-related mortality. Contemporary operative mortality rates are generally <10%.[152,161] Complication rates can exceed 75%, including pulmonary and cardiac complications, anastomotic leak, and recurrent laryngeal nerve paralysis. Stricture formation can occur in 14% to 27% of patients. The addition of preoperative radiation therapy and chemotherapy may enhance surgical complication rates.

More than 75% of patients receiving radiation experience transient esophagitis and dysphagia, sometimes requiring some type of nutritional support. Chemotherapy-related leukopenia and thrombocytopenia are common. Additional acute toxicities of radiation therapy include esophagitis, epidermitis, fatigue, and weight loss in most patients. Nausea and vomiting are relatively common, particularly in patients with lower esophageal and gastroesophageal junction tumors. Many symptoms resolve within 1 to 2 weeks of treatment completion. A perforated esophagus is life-threatening and can be characterized by substernal chest pain, a high pulse rate, fever, and hemorrhage.[93] The addition of chemotherapy can significantly increase acute complications. Moderate-to-severe and even life-threatening toxicities have been reported in 50% to 66% of patients.[71,149,162] In the previously discussed RTOG study of chemoradiation alone, patients treated with combined therapy had a higher incidence of acute grade 3 (44% vs. 25%) and grade 4 toxicity (20% vs. 3%) compared to patients receiving radiation therapy alone.[146] Chemoradiation treatment–related mortality rates range from 0% to 3%.[71,117,141,149,152]

The most common late effects following radiation therapy are stenosis and stricture formation. Stenosis can occur in

>60% of patients. Stricture requiring dilatation has been reported to occur at least 15% to 20% of the time. Dysphagia may be relieved with two to three dilatations.[71] Long-term results from the RTOG study showed that late grade 3 or greater toxicity was similar in the combined versus radiation-alone arms (29% vs. 23%). However, grade 4 or greater toxicity was higher in patients receiving combined-modality therapy (10% vs. 2%).[150] Other complications include clinically apparent damage to organs within the radiation therapy volume, although this is uncommon. Chemotherapy may further increase the risk of late treatment-related toxicities.

The effects of radiation on pulmonary and cardiac function deserve special mention. Pulmonary complications associated with either the definitive or neoadjuvant treatment of esophageal cancer patients can be broadly broken up into symptomatic pneumonitis following treatment completion and postoperative pulmonary complications in patients undergoing resection. Although they are still ill defined, various institutional series have described predictive factors for these complications (which are not mutually exclusive), which are described in the following.

Radiation pneumonitis is a relatively common complication in the treatment of thoracic (lung) malignancies, with can range from minimally symptomatic to fatal. Common symptoms include nonproductive cough, dyspnea, and, more uncommonly, respiratory distress. Generally, this occurs 2 to 6 months after radiation therapy completion. The ability to predict radiation pneumonitis has been a significant topic of investigation. However, most data come from patients with lung cancer, who may have more underlying intrinsic pulmonary/smoking-related disease. A variety of predictive parameters have been suggested, including V_{20} of >25%–30%, mean lung dose of >15 to 20 Gy, V_5 of >42%, and absolute V_5 of >3,000 cm^3.[107]

In nonoperative patients, an analysis of esophageal cancer patients from Japan treated definitively to a dose of 60 Gy with concurrent 5-FU and cisplatin showed a radiation pneumonitis incidence of 27%.[163] The authors concluded that an optimal V_{20} threshold to predict symptomatic pneumonitis was approximately 30%. In a study of 101 both operative and nonoperative patients (88% distal esophagus/GE junction) from the MD Anderson Cancer Center undergoing a mix of 3D and IMRT radiation therapy, 59%, 5%, and 1% of patients experienced grade 2, 3, and 5 radiation pneumonitis, respectively.[164] An analysis from Japan using fields inclusive of supraclavicular, mediastinal, and celiac regions up to a dose of 60 Gy with concurrent cisplatin and 5-FU showed a 2-year cumulative incidence of late, high-grade cardiopulmonary toxicities for patients ≥75 years of 29% versus 3% in younger patients. They concluded that older patients may not tolerate extensive radiation fields.[165] Other studies have shown that significant declines in diffusion capacity and total lung capacity may occur in patients irradiated for esophageal cancer.[166]

In operative patients, a study of 110 patients treated with preoperative chemoradiotherapy followed by resection at the MD Anderson Cancer Center showed that mean lung dose, effective dose, and absolute lung dose receiving ≤5 Gy were predictors of development of postoperative pulmonary complications.[167] In a report on patients from the same institution describing complications in patients receiving neoadjuvant combined modality therapy,[168] 18% experienced pulmonary complications, with higher rates when the V_{10} was ≥40% (35% vs. 8%) and V_{15} was ≥30% (33% vs. 10%), leading the authors to conclude that minimization of lung volume irradiation was important in the preoperative planning of these patients. This increase in postoperative pulmonary complications (pneumonia, acute respiratory distress syndrome) when the V_{10} was >40% suggests that the volume of remaining/undamaged functional lung may determine postoperative pulmonary function, that is, patients with a small lung volume initially may be at higher risk of experiencing pulmonary complications, even if the relative V_5 is low, and that patients with small lung volume with less functional reserve may be more susceptible to postoperative pulmonary complications. Therefore, it is important to consider not only the dose–volume histogram of the lung, but also the total lung volume.

A study from China evaluating patients receiving chemoradiotherapy followed by resection showed that the volume of lung spared from doses of ≥5 Gy was the only independent dosimetric factor on multivariate analysis in predicting postoperative pulmonary complications.[169] Wang et al.[170] similarly described that the relative V_5 and all spared volumes from 5 to 35 Gy significantly correlated with the incidence of postoperative pulmonary complications, although on multivariate analysis, V_5 was the only significant independent predictive factor, indicating that the volume of "unexposed" lung during induction therapy was predictive. Of note in this study was that the majority of patients were treated with induction chemotherapy alone initially (most paclitaxel), which has been shown to increase rates of pneumonitis in other disease sites. A significant association of induction chemotherapy alone prior to concurrent chemoradiotherapy was seen as a predictor of grade 2 or greater pneumonitis (49% vs. 14%; $p = .003$), leading the authors to conclude that induction chemotherapy alone may sensitize lung tissue to radiation damage. In contrast to the foregoing studies, however, another analysis of 98 patients receiving preoperative chemoradiotherapy with 5-FU and cisplatin showed no difference in pulmonary complications versus patients undergoing surgery alone, with no correlation of any lung dose–volume histogram findings with development of postoperative pulmonary complications seen, leading the authors to conclude that neoadjuvant chemoradiotherapy had no detrimental impact on postoperative course.[171] Finally, an analysis from Taiwan of neoadjuvantly, IMRT-treated esophageal cancer patients undergoing resection suggested that preoperative (not prechemoradiation) forced expiratory volume in 1 second was an independent factor associated with postoperative pulmonary complications and that reducing the absolute volume of the right lung irradiated might decrease the risk of postoperative pulmonary complications.[172]

Radiation-induced cardiac toxicity is a broad term describing potential radiation injury to a number of cardiac structures, including pericardium (as manifested by effusion, pericarditis), coronary arteries, the heart muscle itself, and cardiac valves, as well as nerve/conduction injury. Radiation injury primarily consists of fibrosis and/or small-vessel injury. "Classic" radiation tolerance (TD5/5) of the heart is about 60 Gy when 25% or less of the heart is irradiated and 45 Gy if 65% of the heart is irradiated, assuming 2 Gy per fraction. The mechanism of radiation-induced cardiac injury is relatively poorly defined, particularly in the context of esophageal cancer. Historical data from the treatment of Hodgkin's disease patients suggest that a dose of >40 Gy may increase the risk of cardiac death, as well as of pericarditis.[173,174] Several studies of cardiac toxicity and esophageal cancer patient demonstrated that a V_{30} of >46% predicted a significant increase in pericardial effusion, and increasing fraction size (particularly ≥3.5 Gy) also predicted the same. In addition, some authors have shown a possible trend for decrease in ejection fraction in patients with increasing V_{20} of the left ventricle.[107] In a study of 150 esophageal cancer patients receiving chemoradiotherapy (49 neoadjuvantly), the incidence of pericardial effusion was 28%, usually developing within 15 months of radiation therapy, with median onset time of approximately 5 months. The risk of pericardial effusion was associated with mean pericardial doses over an array of dose–volume points to the pericardium from 5 to 45 Gy. A matched-pair analysis of nonradiation patients receiving surgery versus those treated neoadjuvantly was performed, with 42% of patients in the radiation group demonstrating ischemia/scarring on single-photon emission computed tomography images versus 4% in the surgical group, with a median onset to abnormality of 3 months.[175] In a Japanese study, long-term analysis of 139 patients treated with definitive chemoradiotherapy (cisplatin/5-FU with 60 Gy EBRT) for squamous cell carcinoma revealed grade 2, 3, and 4 late pericarditis occurring in 6%, 5%, and 1% of patients, respectively; grade 4 heart failure in 2 patients; grade 2, 3, and 4 pleural effusion development in 5%, 6%, and 0% of patients, respectively; and grade 2, 3, and 4 radiation pneumonitis development in 1%, 2%, and 0% of patients, respectively.[176]

FUTURE CONSIDERATIONS

Although modest improvements in survival have been achieved by combining neoadjuvant chemoradiation and surgery, patients treated with chemoradiation alone or with surgery have unacceptably high local-regional relapse rates and mortality rates. Ultimately, approximately 75% of patients succumb to metastatic disease. As described previously, efforts at radiation dose escalation have not resulted in significant gains for this disease. Given these data, clinical trials have turned to studies evaluating new and potentially more effective chemotherapeutic agents with radiation therapy. Agents such as irinotecan, oxaliplatin, capecitabine, epirubicin, gemcitabine, and docetaxel have been or are being investigated in the metastatic setting, as well as "curative" settings in combination with radiation therapy. Furthermore, there is ongoing investigation of the use of the vascular endothelial growth factor inhibitor bevacizumab, the HER2/neu receptor antagonist trastuzumab, and inhibitors of the epidermal growth factor receptors, including the antibodies cetuximab and panitumumab, in the treatment of esophageal cancer. All of these agents have radiosensitizing properties. The investigation of these agents with radiation therapy is the subject of ongoing and future trials.

SUMMARY

The prognosis for patients with carcinoma of the esophagus remains poor despite recent advances in combined-modality therapies. No firm recommendation can be made for managing locally advanced disease. The data suggest that neoadjuvant chemoradiation improves outcomes in patients who are candidates for surgery. Alternatively, randomized trials have also suggested that perioperative chemotherapy improves outcomes in these patients. However, many patients are not able to tolerate surgery, and combined chemoradiation may be more appropriate in selected patients because definitive chemoradiation has resulted in survival rates comparable to those from surgery alone. Locoregional failure remains a significant pattern of relapse. For patients with stage IV disease, palliation with single-modality therapy or several modalities should be used and tailored to the patient's specific symptoms. Current unresolved issues include the following:

1. Which subsets of patients are more likely to benefit from the addition of surgery than others?
2. Which subsets of patients are more likely to benefit from the addition of neoadjuvant and/or perioperative therapies?
3. Can introduction of newer chemotherapy/targeted agents in the neoadjuvant or concurrent setting improve the results over "standard" chemoradiation with cisplatin and 5-FU?
4. Will new technologies such as 3D conformal therapy, PET-based planning, intensity-modulated radiation therapy, proton therapy, and image-guided radiation therapy decrease complication rates and influence cure rates?
5. Will PET scan allow early prediction of both response to treatment and ultimate outcomes and potentially allow avoidance of delivery of ineffective treatments early on during the course of therapy?
6. Will the identification of molecular prognostic markers allow "individualization" of treatments among patients?
7. In surgical patients, is there a superiority of a neoadjuvant chemoradiation versus a perioperative chemotherapy approach, and will some patients benefit from one particular treatment approach?

SELECTED REFERENCES

A full list of references for this chapter is available online.

1. American Joint Committee on Cancer. *Esophagus.* New York: Springer-Verlag, 2010.
3. Rudiger Siewert J, Feith M, Werner M, et al. Adenocarcinoma of the esophagogastric junction: results of surgical therapy based on anatomical/topographic classification in 1,002 consecutive patients. *Ann Surg* 2000;232:353–361.
4. Arnott SJ, Duncan W, Gignoux M, et al. Preoperative radiotherapy for esophageal carcinoma. *Cochrane Database Syst Rev* 2005;CD001799.
6. Hosch SB, Stoecklein NH, Pichlmeier U, et al. Esophageal cancer: the mode of lymphatic tumor cell spread and its prognostic significance. *J Clin Oncol* 2001;19:1970–1975.
24. Lagergren J, Bergstrom R, Lindgren A, et al. Symptomatic gastroesophageal reflux as a risk factor for esophageal adenocarcinoma. *N Engl J Med* 1999;340:825–831.
33. Dresner SM, Lamb PJ, Bennett MK, et al. The pattern of metastatic lymph node dissemination from adenocarcinoma of the esophagogastric junction. *Surgery* 2001;129:103–109.
34. Akiyama H, Tsurumaru M, Kawamura T, et al. Principles of surgical treatment for carcinoma of the esophagus: analysis of lymph node involvement. *Ann Surg* 1981;194:438–446.
37. Anderson LL, Lad TE. Autopsy findings in squamous-cell carcinoma of the esophagus. *Cancer* 1982;50:1587–1590.
38. Huang W, Li B, Gong H, et al. Pattern of lymph node metastases and its implication in radiotherapeutic clinical target volume in patients with thoracic esophageal squamous cell carcinoma: a report of 1077 cases. *Radiother Oncol* 2010;95:229–233.
39. Monig SP, Baldus SE, Zirbes TK, et al. Topographical distribution of lymph node metastasis in adenocarcinoma of the gastroesophageal junction. *Hepatogastroenterology* 2002;49:419–422.
40. Schurr PG, Yekebas EF, Kaifi JT, et al. Lymphatic spread and microinvolvement in adenocarcinoma of the esophago-gastric junction. *J Surg Oncol* 2006;94:307–315.
41. Matzinger O, Gerber E, Bernstein Z, et al. EORTC-ROG expert opinion: radiotherapy volume and treatment guidelines for neoadjuvant radiation of adenocarcinomas of the gastroesophageal junction and the stomach. *Radiother Oncol* 2009;92:164–175.
42. Meier I, Merkel S, Papadopoulos T, et al. Adenocarcinoma of the esophagogastric junction: the pattern of metastatic lymph node dissemination as a rationale for elective lymphatic target volume definition. *Int J Radiat Oncol Biol Phys* 2008;70:1408–1417.
43. Aisner J, Forastiere A, Aroney R. Patterns of recurrence for cancer of the lung and esophagus. *Cancer Treat Symp* 1983;2:87–105.
44. LePrise E, Meunier B, Etienne P, et al. Sequential chemotherapy and radiotherapy for patients with squamous cell carcinoma of the esophagus. *Cancer* 1995;75:2.
45. Whittington R, Coia LR, Haller DG, et al. Adenocarcinoma of the esophagus and esophago-gastric junction: the effects of single and combined modalities on the survival and patterns of failure following treatment. *Int J Radiat Oncol Biol Phys* 1990;19:593–603.
46. Hulscher JB, van Sandick JW, de Boer AG, et al. Extended transthoracic resection compared with limited transhiatal resection for adenocarcinoma of the esophagus. *N Engl J Med* 2002;347:1662–1669.
47. Kelsen DP, Ginsberg R, Pajak TF, et al. Chemotherapy followed by surgery compared with surgery alone for localized esophageal cancer. *N Engl J Med* 1998;339:1979–1984.
48. Law SY, Fok M, Wong J. Pattern of recurrence after oesophageal resection for cancer: clinical implications. *Br J Surg* 1996;83:107–111.
49. Urba SG, Orringer MB, Turrisi A, et al. Randomized trial of preoperative chemoradiation versus surgery alone in patients with locoregional esophageal carcinoma. *J Clin Oncol* 2001;19:305–313.
65. Blackstock AW, Farmer MR, Lovato J, et al. A prospective evaluation of the impact of 18-F-fluoro-deoxy-D-glucose positron emission tomography staging on survival for patients with locally advanced esophageal cancer. *Int J Radiat Oncol Biol Phys* 2006;64:455–460.
66. Flamen P, Lerut A, Van Cutsem E, et al. Utility of positron emission tomography for the staging of patients with potentially operable esophageal carcinoma. *J Clin Oncol* 2000;18:3202–3210.
67. Monjazeb AM, Riedlinger G, Aklilu M, et al. Outcomes of patients with esophageal cancer staged with $^{[18F]}$fluorodeoxyglucose positron emission tomography (FDG-PET): can postchemoradiotherapy FDG-PET predict the utility of resection? *J Clin Oncol* 28:4714–4721.
70. Gill PG, Denham JW, Jamieson GG, et al. Patterns of treatment failure and prognostic factors associated with the treatment of esophageal carcinoma with chemotherapy and radiotherapy either as sole treatment or followed by surgery. *J Clin Oncol* 1992;10:1037–1043.
88. Gertler R, Stein HJ, Langer R, et al. Long-term outcome of 2920 patients with cancers of the esophagus and esophagogastric junction: evaluation of the New Union Internationale Contre le Cancer/American Joint Cancer Committee staging system. *Ann Surg* 2011;253:689–698.
89. Nomura M, Shitara K, Kodaira T, et al. Prognostic impact of the 6th and 7th American Joint Committee on Cancer TNM staging systems on esophageal cancer patients treated with chemoradiotherapy. *Int J Radiat Oncol Biol Phys* 2012;82:946–952.
90. Wang BY, Goan YG, Hsu PK, et al. Tumor length as a prognostic factor in esophageal squamous cell carcinoma. *Ann Thorac Surg* 2011;91:887–893.
91. Gaur P, Sepesi B, Hofstetter WL, et al. Endoscopic esophageal tumor length: a prognostic factor for patients with esophageal cancer. *Cancer* 2011;117:63–69.

92. Yoon HH, Khan M, Shi Q, et al. The prognostic value of clinical and pathologic factors in esophageal adenocarcinoma: a Mayo cohort of 796 patients with extended follow-up after surgical resection. *Mayo Clin Proc* 2010;85:1080–1089.
94. Suntharalingam M, Moughan J, Coia LR, et al. Outcome results of the 1996–1999 patterns of care survey of the national practice for patients receiving radiation therapy for carcinoma of the esophagus. *J Clin Oncol* 2005;23:2325–2331.
97. Hancock SL, Glatstein E. Radiation therapy of esophageal cancer. *Semin Oncol* 1984;11:144–158.
98. Skinner DB. En bloc resection for neoplasms of the esophagus and cardia. *J Thorac Cardiovasc Surg* 1983;85:59–71.
101. van Westreenen HL, Westerterp M, Bossuyt PM, et al. Systematic review of the staging performance of 18 F-fluorodeoxyglucose positron emission tomography in esophageal cancer. *J Clin Oncol* 2004;22:3805–3812.
103. Leong T, Everitt K, Yuen K, et al. A prospective study to evaluate the impact of coregisted PET/CT images in radiotherapy treatment planning for esophageal cancer. *Int J Radiat Oncol Biol Phys* 2004;60:S139–S140.
104. Zobotto L, Toubouol E, Lerouge D, et al. Impact of Ct and 18 F-deoxyglucose positron emission tomography image fusion for conformal radiotherapy in esophageal carcinoma. *Int J Radiat Oncol Biol Phys* 2005;63:340.
105. Vesprini D, Ung Y, Kamra J, et al. The addition of 18-fluodeoxglucose positron emission tomography (FDG-PET) to CT based radiotherapy planning of carcinoma of the esophagus decreases both the intra- and interobserver variability of GTV dlineation. *Int J Radiat Oncol Biol Phys* 2006;66:S299–S300.
106. Gao XS, Qiao X, Wu F, et al. Pathological analysis of clinical target volume margin for radiotherapy in patients with esophageal and gastroesophageal junction carcinoma. *Int J Radiat Oncol Biol Phys* 2007;67:389–396.
107. Hazard L, Yang G, McAleer M, et al. Principles and techniques of radiation therapy for esphageal and gastroesophageal junction cancers. *J Natl Compr Canc Netw* 2008;6:870–878.
108. Schroder W, Baldus SE, Monig SP, et al. Lymph node staging of esophageal squamous cell carcinoma in patients with and without neoadjuvant radiochemotherapy: histomorphologic analysis. *World J Surg* 2002;26:584–587.
109. Lightdale CJ, Kulkarni KG. Role of endoscopic ultrasonography in the staging and follow-up of esophageal cancer. *J Clin Oncol* 2005;23:4483–4489.
110. Cohen RJ, Paskalev K, Litwin S, et al. Esophageal motion during radiotherapy: quantification and margin implications. *Dis Esophagus* 2010;23:473–479.
112. Burmeister BH, Dickie G, Smithers BM, et al. Thirty-four patients with carcinoma of the cervical esophagus treated with chemoradiation therapy. *Arch Otolaryngol Head Neck Surg* 2000;126:205–208.
113. Murakami M, Kuroda Y, Okamoto Y, et al. Neoadjuvant concurrent chemoradiotherapy followed by definitive high-dose radiotherapy or surgery for operable thoracic esophageal carcinoma. *Int J Radiat Oncol Biol Phys* 1998;40:1049–1059.
114. Minsky BD, Pajak TF, Ginsberg RJ, et al. INT 0123 (Radiation Therapy Oncology Group 94-05) phase III trial of combined-modality therapy for esophageal cancer: high-dose versus standard-dose radiation therapy. *J Clin Oncol* 2002;20:1167–1174.
115. Minsky BD, Neuberg D, Kelsen DP, et al. Final report of Intergroup Trial 0122 (ECOG PE-289, RTOG 90-12): phase II trial of neoadjuvant chemotherapy plus concurrent chemotherapy and high-dose radiation for squamous cell carcinoma of the esophagus. *Int J Radiat Oncol Biol Phys* 1999;43:517–523.
117. Walsh TN, Noonan N, Hollywood D, et al. A comparison of multimodal therapy and surgery for esophageal adenocarcinoma. *N Engl J Med* 1996;335:462–467.
118. Medical Research Council Oesophageal Cancer Working Group. Surgical resection with or without preoperative chemotherapy in oesophageal cancer: a randomized controlled trial. *Lancet Oncol* 2002;359:1727–1733.
119. Bosset JF, Gignoux M, Triboulet JP, et al. Chemoradiotherapy followed by surgery compared with surgery alone in squamous-cell cancer of the esophagus. *N Engl J Med* 1997;337:161–167.
120. van Hagen P, Hulshof M, van Lanschot JJB, et al. Preoperative Chemoradiotherapy for Esophageal or Junctional Cancer. *N Engl J Med* 2012;366:2074–2084.
121. Mariette C, Seitz J, Maillard E, et al. Surgery alone versus chemoradiotherapy followed by surgery for localized esophageal cancer: analysis of a randomized controlled phase III trial FFCD 9901. *J Clin Oncol* 2010;28:15s.
122. Earlam R, Cunha-Melo JR. Oesophageal squamous cell carcinoma: I. A critical review of surgery. *Br J Surg* 1980;67:381–390.
125. Launois B, Delarue D, Campion JP, et al. Preoperative radiotherapy for carcinoma of the esophagus. *Surg Gynecol Obstet* 1981;153:690–692.
126. Gignoux M, Roussel A, Paillot B, et al. The value of preoperative radiotherapy in esophageal cancer: results of a study of the E.O.R.T.C. *World J Surg* 1987;11:426–432.
127. Arnott SJ, Duncan W, Kerr GR, et al. Low dose preoperative radiotherapy for carcinoma of the oesophagus: results of a randomized clinical trial. *Radiother Oncol* 1992;24:108–113.
128. Wang M, Gu XZ, Yin WB, et al. Randomized clinical trial on the combination of preoperative irradiation and surgery in the treatment of esophageal carcinoma: report on 206 patients. *Int J Radiat Oncol Biol Phys* 1989;16:325–327.
129. Teniere P, Hay JM, Fingerhut A, et al. Postoperative radiation therapy does not increase survival after curative resection for squamous cell carcinoma of the middle and lower esophagus as shown by a multicenter controlled trial. French University Association for Surgical Research. *Surg Gynecol Obstet* 1991;173:123–130.
130. Fok M, Sham JS, Choy D, et al. Postoperative radiotherapy for carcinoma of the esophagus: a prospective, randomized controlled study. *Surgery* 1993;113:138–147.
131. Xiao ZF, Yang ZY, Miao YJ, et al. Influence of number of metastatic lymph nodes on survival of curative resected thoracic esophageal cancer patients and value of radiotherapy: report of 549 cases. *Int J Radiat Oncol Biol Phys* 2005;62:82–90.
132. Macdonald JS, Smalley SR, Benedetti J, et al. Chemoradiotherapy after surgery compared with surgery alone for adenocarcinoma of the stomach or gastroesophageal junction. *N Engl J Med* 2001;345:725–730.
133. Macdonald JS, Benedetti J, Smalley SR, et al. Chemoradiation of resected gastric cancer: a 10-year follow-up of the phase III trial INT0116 (SWOG 9008). *J Clin Oncol* 2009;27.
134. Kelsen DP, Winter KA, Gunderson LL, et al. Long-term results of RTOG trial 8911 (USA Intergroup 113): a random assignment trial comparison of chemotherapy followed by surgery compared with surgery alone for esophageal cancer. *J Clin Oncol* 2007;25:3719–3725.
135. Allum WH, Stenning SP, Bancewicz J, et al. Long-term results of a randomized trial of surgery with or without preoperative chemotherapy in esophageal cancer. *J Clin Oncol* 2009;27:5062–5067.
136. Boonstra JJ, Kok TC, Wijnhoven BP, et al. Chemotherapy followed by surgery versus surgery alone in patients with resectable oesophageal squamous cell carcinoma: long-term results of a randomized controlled trial. *BMC Cancer* 2011;11:181.
137. Cunningham D, Allum WH, Stenning SP, et al. Perioperative chemotherapy versus surgery alone for resectable gastroesophageal cancer. *N Engl J Med* 2006;355:11–20.
138. Ychou M, Boige V, Pignon JP, et al. Perioperative chemotherapy compared with surgery alone for resectable gastroesophageal adenocarcinoma: an FNCLCC and FFCD multicenter phase III trial. *J Clin Oncol* 2011;29:1715–1721.
139. Gebski V, Burmeister B, Smithers BM, et al. Survival benefits from neoadjuvant chemoradiotherapy or chemotherapy in oesophageal carcinoma: a meta-analysis. *Lancet Oncol* 2007;8:226–234.
140. Thirion P, Michiels S, Le Maitre A, et al. Individual patient data-based meta-analysis assessing pre-operative chemotherapy in resectable oesophageal carcinoma. *J Clin Oncol* 2007;25:200s.
141. Burmeister BH, Smithers BM, Gebski V, et al. Surgery alone versus chemoradiotherapy followed by surgery for resectable cancer of the oesophagus: a randomised controlled phase III trial. *Lancet Oncol* 2005;6:659–668.
142. Tepper J, Krasna MJ, Niedzwiecki D, et al. Phase III trial of trimodality therapy with cisplatin, fluorouracil, radiotherapy, and surgery compared with surgery alone for esophageal cancer: CALGB 9781. *J Clin Oncol* 2008;26:1086–1092.
143. Sjoquist KM, Burmeister BH, Smithers BM, et al. Survival after neoadjuvant chemotherapy or chemoradiotherapy for resectable oesophageal carcinoma: an updated meta-analysis. *Lancet Oncol* 2011;12:681–692.
144. Stahl M, Walz MK, Stuschke M, et al. Phase III comparison of preoperative chemotherapy compared with chemoradiotherapy in patients with locally advanced adenocarcinoma of the esophagogastric junction. *J Clin Oncol* 2009;27:851–856.
145. Burmeister BH, Thomas JM, Burmeister EA, et al. Is concurrent radiation therapy required in patients receiving preoperative chemotherapy for adenocarcinoma of the oesophagus? A randomised phase II trial. *Eur J Cancer* 2011;47:354–360.
146. al-Sarraf M, Martz K, Herskovic A, et al. Progress report of combined chemoradiotherapy versus radiotherapy alone in patients with esophageal cancer: an intergroup study. *J Clin Oncol* 1997;15:277–284.
147. Araujo CM, Souhami L, Gil RA, et al. A randomized trial comparing radiation therapy versus concomitant radiation therapy and chemotherapy in carcinoma of the thoracic esophagus. *Cancer* 1991;67:2258–2261.
148. Roussell A, Jacob J, Haegele P, et al. Controlled clinical trial for the treatment of patients with inoperable esophageal carcinoma: a study of EORTC Gastrointestinal Tract Cancer Cooperative Group. *Rec Results Cancer Res* 1988;110–121.
149. Herskovic A, Martz K, al-Sarraf M, et al. Combined chemotherapy and radiotherapy compared with radiotherapy alone in patients with cancer of the esophagus. *N Engl J Med* 1992;326:1593–1598.
150. Cooper JS, Guo MD, Herskovic A, et al. Chemoradiotherapy of locally advanced esophageal cancer: long-term follow-up of a prospective randomized trial (RTOG 85-01). Radiation Therapy Oncology Group. *JAMA* 1999;281:1623–1627.
151. Bedenne L, Michel P, Bouche O, et al. Chemoradiation followed by surgery compared with chemoradiation alone in squamous cancer of the esophagus: FFCD 9102. *J Clin Oncol* 2007;25:1160–1168.
152. Stahl M, Stuschke M, Lehmann N, et al. Chemoradiation with and without surgery in patients with locally advanced squamous cell carcinoma of the esophagus. *J Clin Oncol* 2005;23:2310–2317.
153. Gwynne S, Hurt C, Evans M, et al. Definitive chemoradiation for oesophageal cancer—a standard of care in patients with non-metastatic oesophageal cancer. *Clin Oncol (R Coll Radiol)* 2011;23:182–188.
155. Gaspar LE, Winter K, Kocha WI, et al. A phase I/II study of external beam radiation, brachytherapy, and concurrent chemotherapy for patients with localized carcinoma of the esophagus (Radiation Therapy Oncology Group Study 9207): final report. *Cancer* 2000;88:988–995.
156. Vuong T, Szego P, David M, et al. The safety and usefulness of high-dose-rate endoluminal brachytherapy as a boost in the treatment of patients with esophageal cancer with external beam radiation with or without chemotherapy. *Int J Radiat Oncol Biol Phys* 2005;63:758–764.
157. Homs MY, Steyerberg EW, Eijkenboom WM, et al. Single-dose brachytherapy versus metal stent placement for the palliation of dysphagia from oesophageal cancer: multicentre randomised trial. *Lancet* 2004;364:1497–1504.
158. Gaspar LE, Nag S, Herskovic A, et al. American Brachytherapy Society (ABS) consensus guidelines for brachytherapy of esophageal cancer. Clinical Research Committee, American Brachytherapy Society, Philadelphia, PA. *Int J Radiat Oncol Biol Phys* 1997;38:127–132.
159. Coia LR, Soffen EM, Schultheiss TE, et al. Swallowing function in patients with esophageal cancer treated with concurrent radiation and chemotherapy. *Cancer* 1993;71:281–286.
160. Gschossmann JM, Bonner JA, Foote RL, et al. Malignant tracheoesophageal fistula in patients with esophageal cancer. *Cancer* 1993;72:1513–1521.
163. Asakura H, Hashimoto T, Zenda S, et al. Analysis of dose-volume histogram parameters for radiation pneumonitis after definitive concurrent chemoradiotherapy for esophageal cancer. *Radiother Oncol* 95:240–244.
164. Hart JP, McCurdy MR, Ezhil M, et al. Radiation pneumonitis: correlation of toxicity with pulmonary metabolic radiation response. *Int J Radiat Oncol Biol Phys* 2008;71:967–971.
165. Morota M, Gomi K, Kozuka T, et al. Late toxicity after definitive concurrent chemoradiotherapy for thoracic esophageal carcinoma. *Int J Radiat Oncol Biol Phys* 2009;75:122–128.
166. Gergel TJ, Leichman L, Nava HR, et al. Effect of concurrent radiation therapy and chemotherapy on pulmonary function in patients with esophageal cancer: dose-volume histogram analysis. *Cancer J* 2002;8:451–460.
167. Tucker SL, Liu HH, Wang S, et al. Dose-volume modeling of the risk of postoperative pulmonary complications among esophageal cancer patients treated with concurrent chemoradiotherapy followed by surgery. *Int J Radiat Oncol Biol Phys* 2006;66:754–761.
168. Lee HK, Vaporciyan AA, Cox JD, et al. Postoperative pulmonary complications after preoperative chemoradiation for esophageal carcinoma: correlation with pulmonary dose-volume histogram parameters. *Int J Radiat Oncol Biol Phys* 2003;57:1317–1322.

169. Wang SL, Liao Z, Vaporciyan AA, et al. Investigation of clinical and dosimetric factors associated with postoperative pulmonary complications in esophageal cancer patients treated with concurrent chemoradiotherapy followed by surgery. *Int J Radiat Oncol Biol Phys* 2006;64:692–699.
170. Wang S, Liao Z, Wei X, et al. Association between systemic chemotherapy before chemoradiation and increased risk of treatment-related pneumonitis in esophageal cancer patients treated with definitive chemoradiotherapy. *J Thorac Oncol* 2008;3:277–282.
171. Dahn D, Martell J, Vorwerk H, et al. Influence of irradiated lung volumes on perioperative morbidity and mortality in patients after neoadjuvant radiochemotherapy for esophageal cancer. *Int J Radiat Oncol Biol Phys* 77:44–52.
172. Hsu FM, Lee YC, Lee JM, et al. Association of clinical and dosimetric factors with postoperative pulmonary complications in esophageal cancer patients receiving intensity-modulated radiation therapy and concurrent chemotherapy followed by thoracic esophagectomy. *Ann Surg Oncol* 2009;16:1669–1677.
173. Cosset JM, Henry-Amar M, Pellae-Cosset B, et al. Pericarditis and myocardial infarctions after Hodgkin's disease therapy. *Int J Radiat Oncol Biol Phys* 1991; 21:447–449.
174. Hancock SL, Donaldson SS, Hoppe RT. Cardiac disease following treatment of Hodgkin's disease in children and adolescents. *J Clin Oncol* 1993;11:1208–1215.
175. Gayed IW, Liu H, Yusuf SW, et al. The prevalence of myocardial ischemia after concurrent chemoradiation therapy as detected by gated myocardial perfusion imaging in patients with esophageal cancer. *J Nucl Med* 2006;47:1756–1762.
176. Ishikura S, Nihei K, Ohtsu A, et al. Long-term toxicity after definitive chemoradiotherapy for squamous cell carcinoma of the thoracic esophagus. *J Clin Oncol* 2003;21:2697–2702.

Chapter 54
Tumors of the Heart, Pericardium, and Great Vessels

Lawrence J. Sheplan Olsen, Gregory M.M. Videtic, and Roger M. Macklis

ANATOMY

The heart is a hollow, conical [MB1]organ with muscular walls. In the adult, it measures approximately 12 cm in length, 8 to 9 cm in width, and 6 cm in thickness. It is located in the inferior aspect of the middle mediastinum, with two-thirds lying to the left of midline and one-third to the right. The heart lies posterior to the sternum and rib cage, and anatomic landmarks on the chest wall may be used to approximate its position. The apex is located roughly 8 cm to the left of midline in the fifth intercostal space, and the base is at the level of the third costal cartilage. It rests on the diaphragm inferiorly. The heart receives its blood supply from the coronary arteries, which are located in the space between the myocardium and epicardium. The pericardial fat provides a smooth contour and is also located in this space. The heart has four chambers: two ventricles with thick muscular walls and two atria with thin muscular walls. Although the heart is not attached to surrounding organs, it is held in position by its association with the great vessels (GV) and the pericardium. The GV include the aorta, superior and inferior venae cava (IVC), pulmonary artery, and pulmonary veins, which arise from (or terminate in) the left ventricle, right atrium, right ventricle, and left atrium, respectively. The roots of the GV, along with the heart, are encompassed by the parietal pericardium. In combination with the epicardium, this fibrous layer provides a smooth cavity in which the heart can pump freely. Externally the pericardium is adherent to, but separate from, the mediastinal pleura, creating a potential space through which the phrenic nerve traverses.[1]

INCIDENCE AND EPIDEMIOLOGY

Tumors of the heart, GV, and pericardium are rare and include a range of disease presentations: primary neoplasms; secondary metastases from a known malignancy; or direct tumor invasion into the structures, which is seen in certain cancers such as Hodgkin or non-Hodgkin lymphoma, lung cancer, or malignant thymoma. The focus of this chapter will be to review the epidemiology, diagnosis, natural history, and management of primary tumors arising from the heart, pericardium, and GV, as well as metastatic disease to these sites.

The first described case of a primary cardiac tumor was by Albers in 1835.[2] Reynen[3] performed a compilation of autopsy series consisting of over 700,000 cases and found 157 primary cardiac tumors. The overall incidence of primary tumors is 0.021%, with a range from 0% to 0.19%. Approximately 75% of primary tumors of the heart are benign, and about half of those are atrial myxomas arising from the interatrial septum.[4-6] Lipomas, papillary fibroelastomas, and rhabdomyomas each account for approximately 10% of cases. Fibromas, hemangiomas, and teratomas are less common benign cardiac tumors.[7] Cystic atrioventricular node tumors are extremely rare but may lead to sudden death, despite their small size.[8] There is an increased incidence of cardiac myxomas among females and in patients with Carney complex, an inherited autosomal dominant disorder that also shows hyperpigmented lentigines, blue nevi, schwannomas, endocrine tumors, and endocrinopathies.[9,10] The syndrome is most commonly caused by an inactivating germline mutation of the *PRKAR1 A* tumor-suppressor gene on chromosome 17q23-q24.[9,11,12] Variants include the LAMB (*l*entigines, *a*trial myxoma, *m*ucocutaneous myxoma, and *b*lue nevi) and NAME (*n*evi, *a*trial myxoma, *m*yxoid neurofibroma, and *e*phelides) syndromes.[8] Myxomas in patients with Carney complex account for 7% of all cardiac myxomas, are typically found at a younger age, and may have higher recurrence rates.[4,13] Hamartomas, rhabdomyomas, and fibromas are diagnosed almost exclusively in children.[14] Rhabdomyomas are the most common pediatric cardiac tumor and are associated with tuberous sclerosis.

Malignant primary tumors comprise the remaining 25% of cardiac neoplasms. Primary malignancies of the myocardium comprise the bulk of the remaining cases, of which sarcomas account for the vast majority. Malignant fibrous histiocytoma, angiosarcoma, fibrosarcoma, and rhabdomyosarcoma are among the more common histologic types.[15] Table 54.1 summarizes the relative frequency of specific subtypes of sarcoma that may be diagnosed. The median age at diagnosis is 30 to 40 years, slightly younger than that for benign

TABLE 54.1 DISTRIBUTION OF HISTOLOGIC SUBTYPES OF CARDIAC SARCOMA

Subtype of Sarcoma	*Number of Cases*	*Percentage of Cases*
Angiosarcoma	105	28
Rhabdomyosarcoma	43	12
Undifferentiated/NOS	43	12
Fibrosarcoma	39	10
Malignant fibrous histiocytoma	33	9
Leiomyosarcoma	26	7
Liposarcoma	20	5
Other	64	17
Total	**373**	**100**

NOS, not otherwise specified.
Data compiled from refs. 7, 15, 27, 44, 45.

tumors, and there is no sex predilection as seen in myxoma.[15] Lymphomas account for only about 2% of primary cardiac tumors, but the incidence appears to be increasing.[16] Melanoma and carcinoma may also occur infrequently.

Primary malignant tumors of the pericardium are exceedingly rare and include mesothelioma, fibrosarcoma, angiosarcoma, and malignant teratoma.[17] An American Medical Association survey of nearly 500,000 autopsies revealed a 0.0022% incidence of primary malignant pericardial neoplasms.[18] It appears that malignant mesothelioma is the most common primary malignancy of the pericardium, accounting for 50% of primary pericardial tumors. Asbestos has well-established associations with pleural and peritoneal mesothelioma, and there appears to be some correlation in pericardial mesothelioma.[19] Unfortunately, due to the low incidence, this association has been inconsistent, and no other risk factors have been identified.[20–22] There have been very few cases reported since 1994, when 140 cases had been reported in the literature.[17,18,20–26] Fibrosarcoma, angiosarcoma, synovial sarcoma, and teratoma of the pericardium have also been documented.[17,21,26]

With advances in echocardiography, computed tomography (CT), and magnetic resonance imaging (MRI), the postmortem diagnosis of cardiac tumors is becoming less common. Surgical series seem to demonstrate an increase in the ratio of benign to malignant tumors, with malignant tumors accounting for only 10% of cases in a narrow range of 6% to 20%.[14,27–32] This is likely the result of surgical management of benign myxoma, which accounts for over 80% of patients in some series, combined with changes in patient selection.[27,28,31]

The majority of primary cardiac tumors arise in adults with a median age of 45 to 55 years, but can be seen at any age.[14,27–32] Among 533 cases in the database of the Armed Forces Institute of Pathology, McAllister and Fenoglio[7] noted that 83% of patients were adults. Infants (<1 year of age) comprised 9% of the patients and, in this group, 96% of tumors were benign and only 4% were malignant. In a review of the data from the National Cancer Institute Surveillance, Epidemiology, and End Results from 1973 to 1987, Mack[15] reported no sex predilection for the incidence of sarcoma of the mediastinum and heart.

Metastatic disease to the heart and pericardium occurs at a frequency much greater than that of primary tumors.[33–39] In a review of more than 12,000 autopsies in Hong Kong, Lam et al.[37] noted that cardiac metastases were over 20 times more common than primary tumors and may be present in up to 20% of patients dying of disease. The majority of cases have involvement of the pericardium, whereas myocardial involvement is uncommon. In a review of autopsy series of patients with a known malignancy, Hanfling[35] noted the rate of reported cardiac involvement increased steadily from 1.5% in the late 1800 s to 18.3% in 1960. Contemporary series indicate the rate of cardiac metastases in patients dying of cancer may be as high as 20%.[7,35–38,40,41]

The sites of origin of cardiac metastases from solid tumors are summarized in Table 54.2. Lung cancer is the most common cause of cardiac metastases and accounts for nearly one-half of all cases. Upper gastrointestinal malignancies and breast cancer are also common causes of cardiac metastases, accounting for one-fourth of all cases. The remaining one-fourth of cases arise from a wide variety of other malignancies.[33–38] Melanoma is purported to have the highest propensity for metastatic spread to the heart and tends to involve the endocardium or myocardium, with some series showing its incidence of cardiac metastases rivaling or exceeding that of lung cancers.[2,41] Cardiac metastases may also originate from lymphoma or leukemia. In 1960, Hanfling[35] reported that the proportion of cardiac metastases arising from these malignancies rivals that arising from solid tumors. However, multiple medical advances in both chemotherapy and diagnosis have occurred since then, and modern series consistently report that these histologies account for approximately 17% of cardiac metastases.[33,34,36,37]

Tumors of the GV are extremely rare. The literature on these consists mainly of case reports, and approximately 130 cases have been documented. As a whole, tumors of the GV are about as common as primary malignant pericardial mesothelioma. The largest series has been reported by Burke and Virmani.[42] They evaluated 45 tumors on the files of the Armed Forces Institute of Pathology and found that all of the tumors were sarcomas, including intimal (undifferentiated) sarcoma, angiosarcoma, leiomyosarcoma, and synovial sarcoma. There appeared to be no sex predilection for tumors of the aorta or pulmonary artery, although the female-to-male ratio was 3 to 1 among patients with tumors of the IVC.

TABLE 54.2 SITE OF ORIGIN FOR CARDIAC METASTASES

Primary Tumor	*Number of Patients*	*Percentage of Cases*
Lung	271	47
Upper gastrointestinal[a]	107	19
Breast	42	7
Genitourinary (nonprostate)	37	6
Melanoma	28	5
Other	93	16
Total	**578**	**100**

[a]Includes esophagus, stomach, small bowel, pancreas, and hepatobiliary primary tumors.

Data compiled from refs. 33–38.

NATURAL HISTORY

Tumors of the Myocardium

Myxomas, as discussed previously, are the most common benign tumors of the heart, are seen in women twice as frequently as men, and are diagnosed at a mean age of 45 to 55 years, but have been documented in infants and octogenarians.[27–32,43] Benign myxomas tend to be slow growing and are minimally invasive and as such may have a long duration of symptoms before diagnosis. Typically, these tumors arise from the interatrial septum and grow into the adjacent chamber. The left atrium is the most common site of involvement for myxoma, and this is 6 to 7 times more common than myxoma of the right atrium. The tumor may also be located in the ventricles or the valves and can be bilateral. Although they are considered benign, the tumor can elicit dramatic symptoms from valvular insufficiency, congestive heart failure, and embolic phenomena. Surgical excision is the treatment of choice, with local recurrence rates ranging from 0% to 5.4%.[8]

Primary malignant tumors of the myocardium, most commonly sarcomas, do not show a predilection for site of the tumor in the heart, except for angiosarcomas, which tend to occur more frequently in the right atrium, and often present late with advanced disease and lung metastases.[14,27,28,30,31] The duration of symptoms is on the order of months, and survival is poor. Even after attempts at curative resection, recurrences are common, and the median survival ranges from 6 to 18 months.[14,27–32,44,45] The cause of death is most often complications of locally recurrent disease with invasion of adjacent chambers, valves, or pericardium. Tamponade, hemopericardium, and distant metastases are common.[45] About 30% of primary cardiac sarcomas have distant metastases at the time of diagnosis.[2] The high incidence of hematogenous dissemination of a cardiac sarcoma may be explained by the high rate of blood flow through the heart.[46]

Tumors of the Pericardium

Mesothelioma is the most common pericardial neoplasm and may either be confined to the pericardial sac at diagnosis or extend beyond it, involving the myocardium or mediastinal structures.[20–22] Of 140 primary malignant pericardial mesotheliomas reported in the literature, only 28% of cases were diagnosed antemortem.[21] These tumors have been documented to metastasize by lymphatic and hematogenous routes to involve regional lymph nodes, lung, liver, brain, bone, and adrenal glands.[17,18,20–25] Despite the metastatic potential, pericardial tumors are more often fatal because of local complications, such as restrictive pericarditis with resultant cardiac tamponade, arrhythmia due to myocardial invasion, or vena caval obstruction. Even if the tumor can be diagnosed antemortem, survival is poor. Typically, the onset of symptoms does not occur until the tumor is well advanced, and from that time the median survival is <6 months, with only a handful of patients surviving beyond 1 year.[23–25]

Tumors of the Great Vessels

The median age at presentation is 40 to 60 years for tumors of the GV.[42] The natural history and clinical presentation depend on the exact location of the primary tumor. Depending on the location, symptoms may include dyspnea, cough, hemoptysis, pain, and thromboembolic phenomena, including pulseless extremities, stroke, peripheral edema, and superior vena cava (SVC) syndrome. In the series by Burke and Virmani,[42] they found that in contrast to the tumors of the aorta and pulmonary artery that were aggressive sarcomas arising from the vessel lumen, tumors of the inferior vena cava (IVC) were mostly low-grade leiomyosarcomas originating from the medial layer of smooth muscle in the vessel wall.

DIAGNOSIS

Tumors of the heart have been referred to as the "great imitators" of the cardiovascular system, and although there are no pathognomonic signs or symptoms, cardiac tumors can often be detected through careful attention to both cardiac and extracardiac manifestations of the disease.[47,48] It is not surprising that tumors of the heart are often asymptomatic until they become advanced enough to affect blood flow or cardiac function.[35] As the tumor enlarges, disturbances in normal heart function produce different signs and symptoms depending on the location of the tumor. The scope of clinical presentation is summarized in Table 54.3. Tumors involving the right heart may result in pulmonary emboli, pulmonary hypertension, tricuspid valve disease, or SVC or IVC obstruction. Left-sided tumors can cause mitral valve disease, thromboembolic phenomena, and rapidly progressive congestive heart failure, which may be refractory to treatment. A characteristic auscultation finding referred to as a tumor plop may be heard during early diastole in 30% of patients.[49] Arrhythmias are very common and are predominantly supraventricular tachycardia or nonspecific conduction anomalies.[48] Specific presenting complaints are equally varied. Dyspnea is the most common presenting complaint and is noted in 59% to 88% of patients.[33,44,50,51] Palpitations or syncope is also seen frequently, may be positional, and, if the tumor obstructs a valve orifice, sudden death may result. Chest pain can be anginal, resulting from direct myocardial invasion or obstruction of the main coronary ostia. It can also be sharp, due to invasion of the pericardium, with resulting pericarditis. Constitutional symptoms also occur, with fever, malaise, anemia, and weight loss.[33,35,44,48,50,51] Tumors of the pericardium and GV show a similarly variable constellation of symptoms, and as such, they pose the same diagnostic difficulties as tumors of the myocardium.

Physical examination may reveal tachycardia, murmur (which may be positional), pericardial rub, gallops, peripheral edema, jugular venous distention, rales, and stigmata of thromboembolic disease. Electrocardiography (ECG) most often reveals nonspecific ST- and T-wave changes, although low-voltage ECG, supraventricular tachycardia, bundle-branch block, or second-degree (type II) or third-degree atrioventricular node block may also be noted. Laboratory studies may reveal anemia, erythrocytosis, thrombocytosis, thrombocytopenia, leukocytosis, and elevated erythroid sedimentation rate.[44,48,51,52]

TABLE 54.3 SCOPE OF CLINICAL MANIFESTATIONS OF CARDIAC TUMORS

Cardiovascular Manifestations	*Extracardiac Manifestations*
Electrocardiogram findings	Pulmonary
Low voltage	Rales
Atrial fibrillation or flutter	Dyspnea
Supraventricular tachycardia	Hemoptysis
Conduction anomalies	Pulmonary hypertension
Bundle branch block	Upper digestive tract
Atrioventricular block (2 nd or 3rd degree)	Hematemesis
Ventricular tachycardia	Dysphagia
Ventricular fibrillation	Embolic phenomena
Pericardial signs	Right-sided tumors
Friction rub	Pulmonary emboli
Pericarditis	Left-sided tumors
Effusion	Stroke
Tamponade	Splinter hemorrhages
Congestive heart failure	Peripheral arterial occlusion
Peripheral edema	Raynaud's phenomenon
Jugular venous distention	Peripheral findings
Valvular insufficiency	Clubbing
Chest pain	Ascites
Palpitations	Constitutional symptoms
Syncope	Anemia
Sudden death	Fatigue
Superior or inferior vena caval obstruction	Fever
Myalgia	Weight loss
	Arthralgia

DIAGNOSTIC WORKUP

Before the advent of echocardiography and angiography, 66% of tumors were diagnosed intraoperatively during exploration for suspected valvular disease. With current techniques, the diagnosis can be made reliably in the preoperative setting in almost 90% of cases.[27] The diagnostic evaluation of patients with suspected cardiac tumors is presented in Table 54.4.

Physical examination and ECG findings have been described above. The imaging techniques used in the diagnosis and evaluation of cardiac tumors include chest radiography, CT, MRI, echocardiography, radionuclide scintigraphy, and cardiac catheterization. Although there is considerable overlap among these studies, each modality is unique and complements the others in evaluating the tumor. Chest radiography shows abnormalities in over 80% of patients. Unfortunately, abnormalities are usually nonspecific and therefore of limited usefulness. Findings include cardiomegaly, an abnormal cardiac contour, mediastinal widening, or evidence of congestive heart failure.[48,53,54] Calcifications

TABLE 54.4 DIAGNOSTIC EVALUATION FOR A SUSPECTED OR KNOWN CARDIAC TUMOR

Required Studies	*Optional Studies*
History	Cardiac catheterization, right or left sided
Physical examination	Pressure and output measurements
Blood work	Coronary angiography
Complete blood count	Endomyocardial biopsy
Liver function tests	Transesophageal echocardiography
Renal profile	ECG-gated MRI
Electrolytes	Radionuclide scintigraphy, including PET
ECG	Pericardiocentesis
Imaging	Staging for malignant tumors
Chest radiography	CT of the abdomen, pelvis, and brain
Transthoracic echocardiography	Bone scan
Contrast-enhanced dynamic CT	

CT, computed tomography; ECG, electrocardiography; MRI, magnetic resonance imaging; PET, positron emission tomography.

are present in up to 20% of cases, perhaps relating to the presence of valvular or pericardial disease.[53,55] Calcifications on imaging may also suggest the presence of a fibroma. In the setting of a malignant tumor, chest radiography may also reveal hilar nodal, pulmonary, or osseous metastatic disease.

Echocardiography, M-mode and two-dimensional, is the diagnostic procedure of choice among patients with suspected cardiac tumors. Either transthoracic (TTE) or transesophageal (TEE) techniques can be performed, yielding valuable information regarding size, shape, location, mobility, and areas of attachment.[48] In a review of 533 primary cardiac tumors, Blondeau[27] found echocardiography provided a 98% diagnostic accuracy rate among the 437 patients for whom it was used. Bogren et al.[54] found that echocardiography detected abnormalities in 63 of 65 (97%) patients with primary cardiac tumors. With this high level of diagnostic yield, and because the use of TTE has no known side effects, it should be performed for all patients. TEE is a complementary procedure to TTE. It is a more invasive procedure and is not required in all patients, but it may be used for guidance during endomyocardial biopsy and may also provide better evaluation of the left atrial appendage and right-sided tumors.[56–58]

Cross-sectional imaging has also become indispensable in the evaluation of nonmyxomatous cardiac tumors. With the development of contrast-enhanced dynamic CT (Fig. 54.1B) and ECG-gated MRI (Fig. 54.1A, 54.1C), real-time imaging of the heart provides fine details of the tumor, with delineation of intraluminal, intramyocardial, and extracardiac extension.[48,59–62] The findings may be used to plan the surgical approach and, should adjuvant therapy be required, could also be used for radiotherapy treatment planning. Compared to chest radiographs, both CT and MRI are more sensitive in

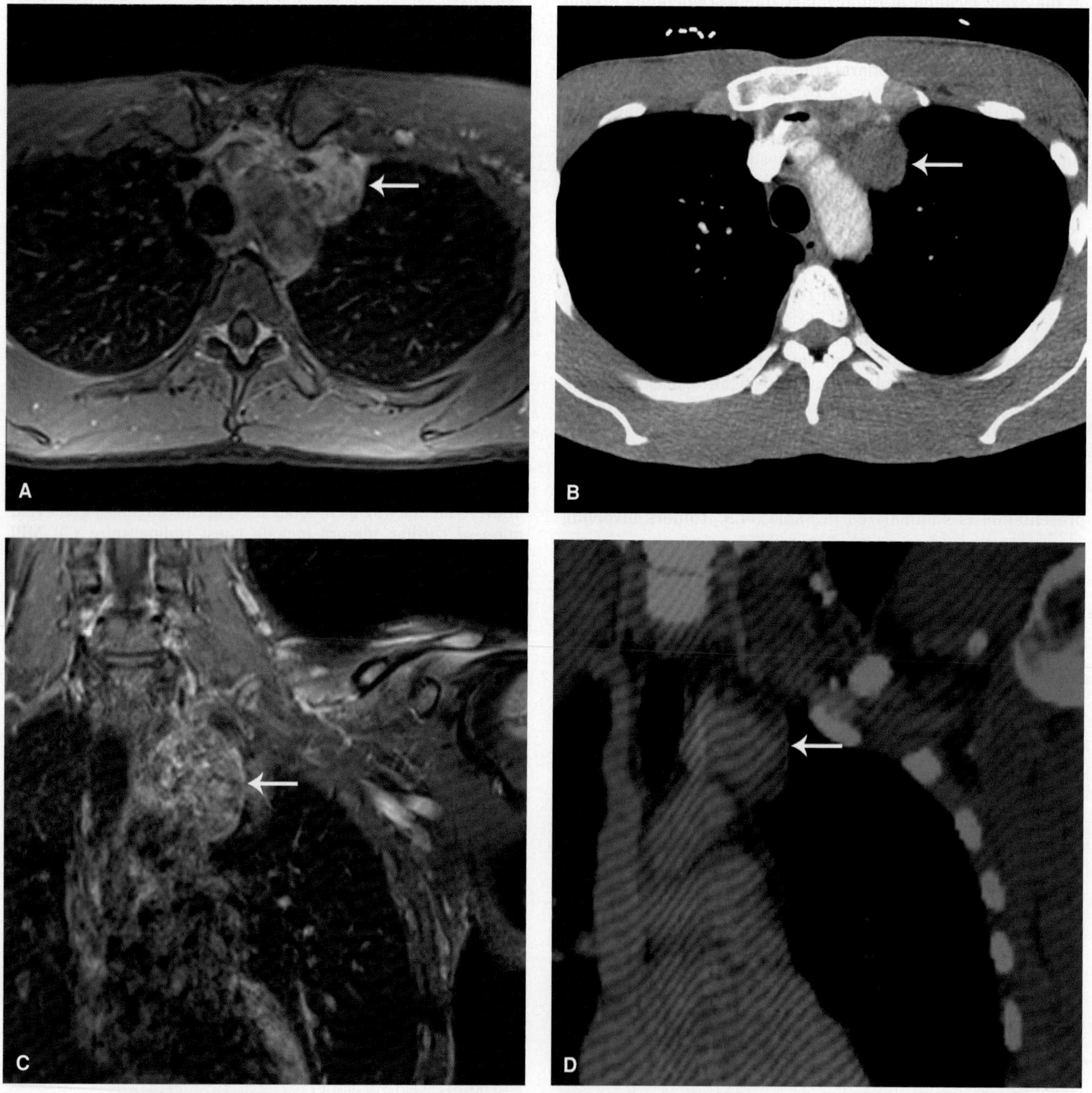

FIGURE 54.1 Axial contrast-enhanced fat-saturated T1 magnetic resonance image (MRI) of a primary cardiac neoplasm arising from the left atrium **(A)**; corresponding axial contrast-enhanced computed tomography (CT) **(B)**, coronal contrast-enhanced fat-saturated T1 MRI **(C)**, and coronal fluorodeoxyglucose positron emission tomography CT **(D)** images. Tumor indicated by *white arrows*.

detecting metastatic disease. If these studies are positive, tissue diagnosis may be made without the need for endomyocardial biopsy or thoracotomy. If they have not been performed before surgery, CT of the brain, chest, and upper abdomen and a bone scan are recommended in the staging of malignant cardiac tumors.

Radionuclide imaging has been used in the evaluation of cardiac tumors. Gated cardiac blood pool scintigraphy has limited resolution, but it may be able to detect tumors when other modalities have failed. Gallium-67 and thallium-201 scans may reveal intramyocardial invasion.[48,54] Positron emission tomography (PET), with or without CT fusion (PET-CT) (Fig. 54.1D), is rapidly gaining favor in the staging of many cancers, and there are scattered case reports on its usefulness in evaluating cardiac tumors.[63,64]

Cardiac catheterization was heavily utilized in the past, but its usefulness has diminished with the emergence of the noninvasive techniques noted previously. Catheterization may reveal wall structural or motion abnormalities, intracavitary filling defects, or evidence of neovascularization of the tumor.[48,54] If a malignant tumor is suspected, endocardial biopsy may provide tissue for pathologic diagnosis. For patients who may undergo surgical resection of their tumor, catheterization is still recommended for the detection of coronary artery disease and pulmonary hypertension.

STAGING SYSTEM AND PATHOLOGIC CLASSIFICATION

There is no accepted staging system available for cardiac tumors. With respect to pathologic classification, tumors of the heart and pericardium may be classified as primary (originating from the heart) or metastatic (originating from malignancies of other organs). Primary cardiac tumors can be further subclassified by the site of origin and by malignant potential (Table 54.5).

PROGNOSTIC FACTORS

In general, the prognosis for patients with either primary or secondary malignant tumors of the heart is poor. The median survival of patients with malignant primary tumors is approximately 1 year, and both local and distant relapses are common. Blondeau[27] reported that angiosarcoma had a median survival of 2.14 years, compared with only 0.75 years for fibrosarcoma. Llombart-Cussac et al.,[65] on the other hand, noted a worse survival for angiosarcomas due to their propensity to present late with advanced disease. The series from Burke et al.[44] and Putnam et al.[45] indicate that the histologic subtype does not appear to have prognostic value, although the microscopic finding of more than 10 mitoses per high-power field does portend a worse prognosis. Tazelaar et al.[66] also noted a worse outcome for tumors with high mitotic activity and necrosis. Conversely, the ability to resect all gross tumor and a left atrial site of origin predict for longer survival.[44,45] Although the duration of symptoms is typically short, some patients have a more protracted course, and outcome may be better in those with symptoms for more than 3 months before diagnosis.[67] The use of adjuvant radiotherapy has been associated with longer median survival (22.7 vs. 9.6 months), whereas adjuvant chemotherapy has provided mixed results.[44,67] Given the retrospective nature of these studies, patient selection may be a source of bias. If a controlled, prospective study could be completed, it is unclear if it would confirm an improved prognosis with either type of adjuvant therapy.

The discovery and diagnosis of metastatic disease in the myocardium is rare in the antemortem setting, and hence prognostic factors have not been elucidated. Malignant pericardial effusion, on the other hand, is more easily diagnosed in life and can be appropriately palliated with pericardiocentesis, pericardiotomy, or pericardial sclerosis. Among patients with metastases from a solid tumor, the median survival after the procedure is approximately 3 to 4 months, and it appears to be improved with better performance status.[68,69]

TABLE 54.5 PATHOLOGIC CLASSIFICATION OF CARDIAC TUMORS

Pericardial Tumors	*Myocardial Tumors*
Benign Subtypes	***Benign Subtypes***
Teratoma	Myxoma
Pericardial cysts	Lipoma
Fibroma	Papillary fibroelastoma
Angioma	Rhabdomyoma
Lipoma	Fibroma
Malignant Subtypes	Hamartoma
Mesothelioma	Hemangioma
Angiosarcoma	Teratoma
Fibrosarcoma	***Malignant Subtypes***
Malignant teratoma	Sarcoma
	Lymphoma
	Malignant teratoma
	Melanoma
	Carcinoma

MANAGEMENT

Primary Pericardial Tumors

Fewer than 200 primary pericardial malignant tumors have been reported in the literature to date, and less than one-third of these were diagnosed during life.[17,18,20–25,70–73] Among those diagnosed before autopsy, locally advanced or metastatic disease is common, and palliative treatment may be the most appropriate option. Relief of pericardial tamponade can be achieved rapidly through pericardiocentesis. Palliative surgical approaches include pericardiectomy or pericardial sclerosis to alleviate the symptoms of effusion and potentially prevent its recurrence. In keeping with the contemporary data supporting the use of radiotherapy in cases of primary pleural mesothelioma, it is appropriate to consider its use in the setting of primary pericardial mesothelioma, although there are few clinical data defining its use.[74] Both external-beam radiotherapy and instillation of radiopharmaceuticals (phosphorus-32, gold-198) have been reported in the palliative setting for this disease.[6,17]

Surgical resection of all gross disease is the treatment of choice in the definitive setting. As with pleural mesothelioma, a high rate of local recurrence should be expected without adjuvant therapy, and postoperative radiotherapy and chemotherapy should be considered. The radiation treatment volume should include the entire pericardial surface and likely would include the mediastinal lymph nodes.

Benign Cardiac Tumors

The most common benign cardiac tumors are atrial myxomas in adults and rhabdomyomas in children. These are both treated surgically with low mortality rates and local control rates in excess of 95%.[14,27–31,50,67] Endo et al.[29] reported a 5-year overall survival rate of 86% after resection of atrial myxoma. Bogren et al.[54] found the 5-year survival rate was 87% for patients with myxoma and 76% for all patients treated for a benign cardiac tumor. Blondeau[27] reported 444 patients had resection of a myxoma with a 4% 30-day surgical mortality rate, a 1% late tumor- or treatment-related mortality rate, and only a 2% risk of local relapse. Given the high rate of cure, with an acceptable rate of morbidity, surgical resection without adjuvant chemotherapy or radiotherapy is generally appropriate for benign primary cardiac neoplasms. Some rhabdomyomas may even regress spontaneously without the need for aggressive resection.[75]

Malignant Primary Cardiac Tumors

Surgical resection is the primary treatment of choice for patients with primary malignant cardiac tumors. Unfortunately, local resection is often incomplete because of the extent and invasiveness of the tumor and lack of experience with extended cardiac resection and partly because of uncertainty of diagnosis at the time of initial surgery.[76] In experienced hands, even tumors requiring complete reconstruction of the entire right and left atria and up to 30% of the right ventricle may be resectable and still retain adequate cardiac function.[76] Even in the presence of a complete excision, local relapse is common and accounts for as much as one-third of deaths. Sarcomas account for almost all primary malignant cardiac neoplasms, and the treatment principles should be similar to those for soft tissue sarcoma arising from other areas of the body.[77] After complete or incomplete resection of the tumor, adjuvant radiotherapy and chemotherapy may be used in an attempt to gain control of local and distant disease, respectively. There are conflicting reports on the effectiveness of chemotherapy, and given the small sample sizes it is difficult to draw conclusions, but it seems to be less beneficial if patients are not able to obtain a complete resection.[44,45,76] Combination chemotherapy appears to have greater efficacy than single-agent therapy, with different combinations of agents such as cyclophosphamide, ifosfamide, doxorubicin, and paclitaxel in use.[45,78–81]

Anecdotal cases of orthotopic heart transplantation for patients with malignant neoplasms of the heart were first described in 1981 by Jamieson et al.[82] and in several reports in the literature since then, with some promising results in selected cases.[83–92] Although this technique should ideally achieve a complete tumor resection, the results have been mixed. There have been some case reports of long-term survivors, while many other patients have developed distant metastases and subsequent death within months of transplant. Some have attempted cardiac explantation, tumor removal, and autotransplantation.[81] Although orthotopic heart transplantation has promise, theoretical dangers exist, including the potential protumor effect of immune suppression and a decreased ability to tolerate adjuvant radiotherapy or chemotherapy.

Metastatic Tumors of the Heart and Pericardium

There is no known curative therapy for patients with metastatic disease to the heart. Appropriate management of the primary metastatic tumor with systemic therapy may be indicated as a first-line approach for cardiac, pericardial, or GV metastases. Surgery may have a role in both diagnosis and palliation for patients with malignant pericardial disease.[68,69] Emergency pericardiocentesis or pericardiotomy can alleviate cardiac tamponade and yield the diagnosis, and the instillation of a sclerosing agent, such as tetracycline, can often effectively prevent the reaccumulation of the pericardial effusion. Palliative radiotherapy may be used to relieve symptoms of life-threatening outflow obstruction or pericardial disease.

Tumors of the Great Vessels

Resection of the tumor with graft reconstruction of the vessel is the treatment of choice. As with sarcomas of the heart, sarcomas of the GV are treated based on the same philosophy as used for treatment of soft tissue sarcoma.[77] Postoperative radiotherapy should be considered for all patients, even those with low-grade tumors, because local recurrence would likely not be amenable to salvage surgical resection.[31,42,44]

RADIOTHERAPY

In general, the most common indications for radiotherapy will be for any primary malignant cardiac tumors and as adjuvant therapy after resection. Less common would be the use of radiotherapy in the definitive setting for a tumor that is not resectable.

Given that sarcomas are the most common malignant cardiac tumors seen, treatment approaches have been extrapolated from the management approach for sarcomas at other body sites. Thus, for completely resected tumors with negative margins, postoperative doses of 45 to 50 Gy at 1.8 to 2 Gy per fraction have been used.[77] The initial target should include all areas known to harbor tumor before surgery with a margin of about 2 cm. This target should be derived from diagnostic imaging and other investigations and also by the operative description of the surgeon. In the setting of incomplete resection (involved microscopic margins or gross residual disease), an additional 10 to 20 Gy boost should be considered to the volume at risk. For GV tumors, the target volume will vary depending on the tumor origin, but as with cardiac primaries, should include a minimum expansion of 2 cm around the preoperative mass. Doses from 45 to 50 Gy are suggested for microscopic residual disease and 60 to 70 Gy for gross residual or unresectable disease.[93–96] For patients with pericardial mesothelioma, the entire pericardium will need to be included in the initial target volume, but the total dose deliverable will be limited by the tolerance of the myocardium itself. For tumors with a high propensity for nodal involvement (i.e., mesothelioma, angiosarcoma, rhabdomyosarcoma, carcinoma, or lymphoma), coverage of the mediastinal lymph nodes is also recommended.

Although historical practice has involved two-dimensional planning and static beam arrangements, such as anteroposterior parallel-opposed techniques to cover the desired initial target volume, contemporary radiotherapy should be planned using a three-dimensional (3D) conformal approach in most cases, with careful delineation of gross tumor volumes, clinical target volumes, and planning target volumes as defined by the nature of the primary tumor, its expected natural history, and the management approach (definitive or adjuvant). When planning radiotherapy, normal tissue constraints should be observed for each case, with an emphasis on cardiac, lung, spinal cord, and esophageal tolerances. If required, advanced techniques such as intensity-modulated radiotherapy (IMRT) may be of use for the boosting target volumes to obtain the desired dose to the target while limiting dose to normal structures. IMRT techniques allow for the selective intensification or reduction of dose to areas of specific concern and may allow for greater sparing of normal tissues without sacrificing tumor coverage or dosing. Late toxicities of interest after radiotherapy include not only radiation-induced heart disease (RIHD) but also radiation pneumonitis and fibrosis. There are otherwise few reports on variations to improve the efficacy of conventional radiotherapy. One example was the use of hyperfractionation to a dose of 70.5 Gy at 1.5 Gy per fraction with a radiosensitizer, iododeoxyuridine.[46]

There have been a number of recent advances in the technology of delivering radiation that allow clinicians to deliver extremely high doses while strictly minimizing normal tissue injury. Two recent clinical reports are examples of this, with one describing the use of carbon-ion radiotherapy and the other stereotactic body radiotherapy (SBRT) for cases of cardiac sarcomas, using a dose of 64 Gy in 16 fractions over 4 weeks for the former.[97,98] Such dose schedules have been extrapolated from SBRT data used for lung cancer[99,100] and typically employed the critical organ dose constraints used in these approaches.[101] Mindful of the limited reported use of such high-dose, highly conformal techniques, it is conceivable that they may offer a means to safely escalate doses to those which would theoretically be optimal for tumor control. This is attractive given the poor outcomes seen with current therapies.[97,98] Patients who may be the best candidates for using such novel approaches may also be those who have received prior radiotherapy and suffer an isolated in-field recurrence. Because using conventional radiotherapy techniques would likely exceed critical structure dose constraints, SBRT may make high-dose therapy

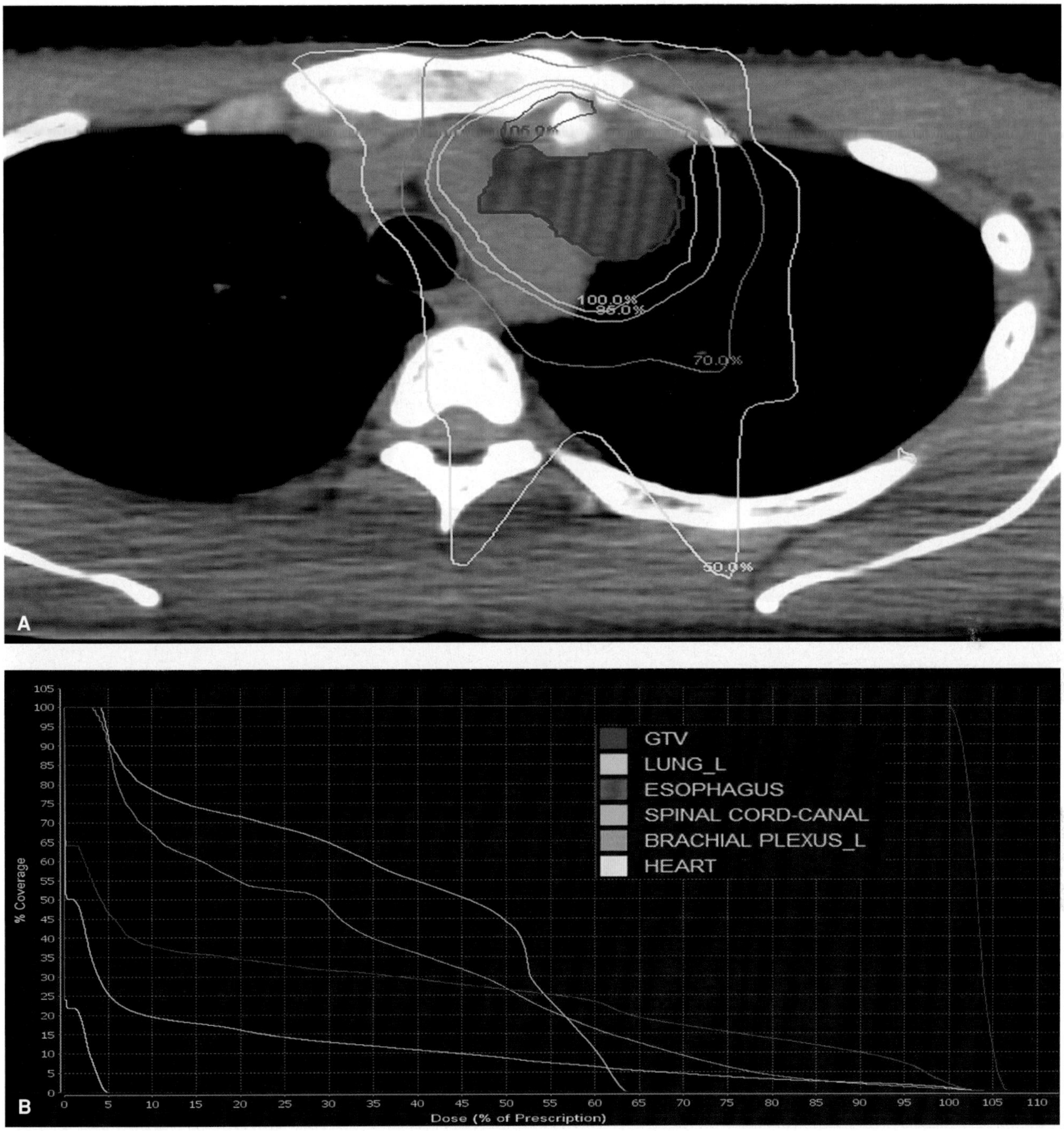

FIGURE 54.2. Sample three-dimensional conformal plan developed for a patient with an unresectable epithelioid hemangioendothelioma of the aortic arch **(A)** and corresponding dose–volume histogram data **(B)**. GTV, gross tumor volume.

feasible in the setting where otherwise anything other than palliative doses might not have been possible. Advanced technologies must be used with caution, however, because cardiac and respiratory motions introduce considerable uncertainty in tumor localization and predictability of dose delivery. Alternatively, gating procedures may be instituted to decrease positioning uncertainty and thus decrease the necessary target expansions.[102] Normal tissue and tumor motion can be evaluated using fluoroscopy or utilizing four-dimensional CT scanning when available. Image guidance to further improve targeting accuracy is of interest, but at present it remains only an investigational question. Representative isodose distributions, and their corresponding DVH data, are shown in Figure 54.2 for a 3D conformal radiotherapy plan and in Figure 54.3 for an SBRT plan.

As noted, the total dose to be delivered is primarily limited by cardiac and lung tolerance. Much of the available evidence on tolerance of the heart is based on patients previously treated for malignancies such as Hodgkin lymphoma or breast cancer. In general, RIHD may manifest as pericarditis, myocarditis, conduction defects, or coronary vascular disease.[103,104] Damage to the pericardium is most often observed clinically. Risk factors for developing RIHD include total dose, dose per fraction, irradiated volume, radiation technique, age at exposure, and use of concurrent or anthracycline-based chemotherapy. Emami et al.[93] estimated the tolerance dose that within 5 years will cause a minimal 5% complication rate (TD5/5) for developing pericarditis to be 40 Gy for the whole heart and 60 Gy for one-third of the heart. However, current estimates of normal tissue tolerances tend to be conservative,

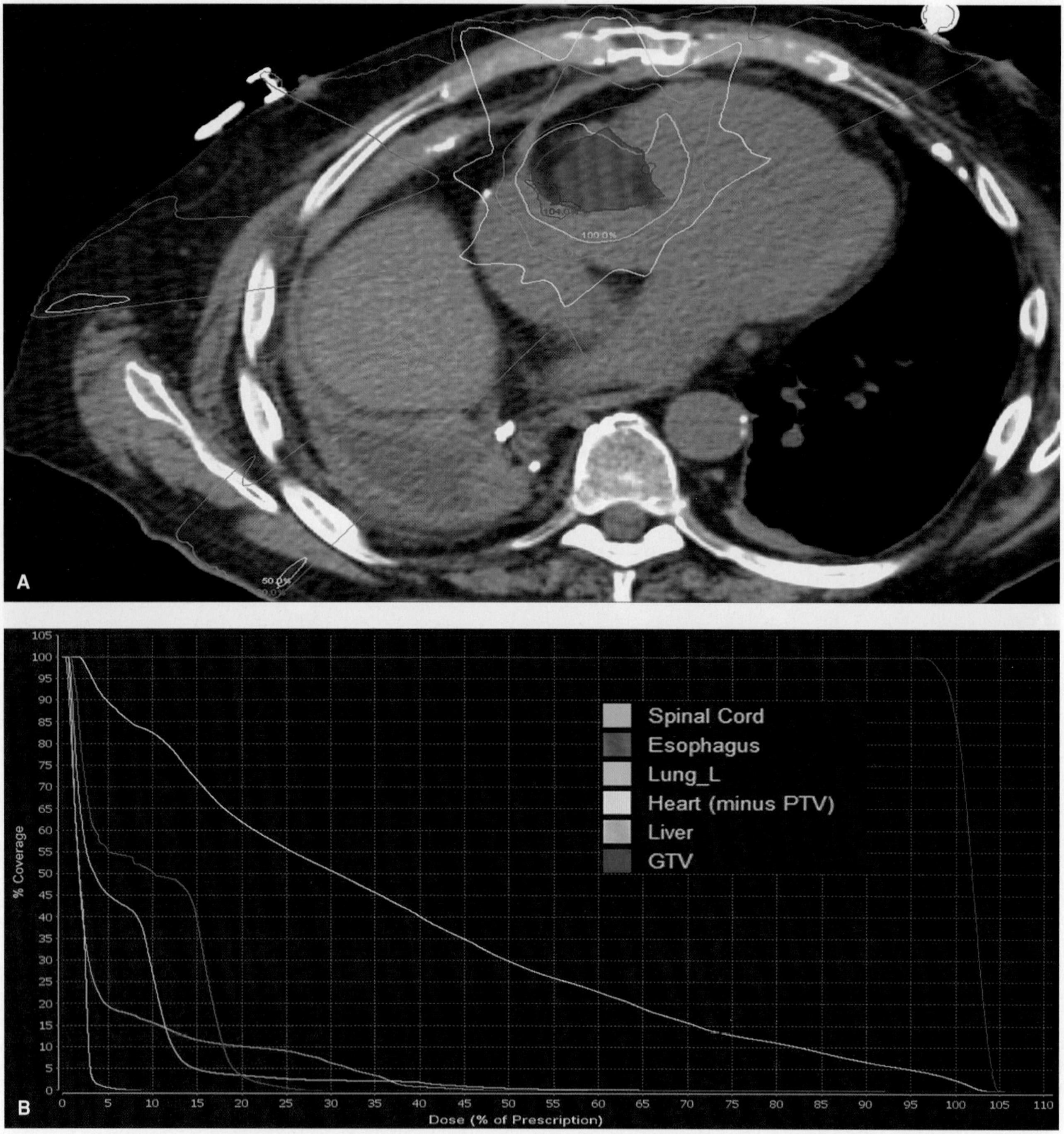

FIGURE 54.3. Sample stereotactic body radiotherapy plan developed for a patient with a local recurrence of a pleomorphic sarcoma of the pulmonary artery **(A)** and corresponding dose–volume histogram data **(B)**. GTV, gross tumor volume.

and administration of chemotherapeutic agents must also be taken into account.[105] Most recently Gagliardi et al.[94] reviewed all the available data on cardiac toxicities and concluded that the whole-organ dose at which toxicity occurs in 50% of cases (TD50) is on the order of 48 to 50.6 Gy, but that side-effect profiles must be considered in relation to the probability of tumor control in the specific patient. Certainly, in these aggressive tumors with poor outcomes, recurrence is equally or more morbid than the potential toxicities, and this must be balanced and discussed with the individual patient. With respect to other structures relevant to target planning for cardiac or GV tumors, Werner-Wasik et al.[96] have reported that doses as high as 74 Gy with concurrent chemotherapy can be delivered safely to segments of the esophagus, but that no single best threshold is identifiable for limiting esophageal toxicity. In a comprehensive literature review on lung tolerances performed by Marks et al.,[95] the authors recommended limiting the volume of lung receiving 20 Gy (V20) to ≤30% to 35%, and the mean lung dose to ≤20 to 23 Gy in order to minimize lung toxicity.

RESULTS

Case reports and small retrospective series have been the primary means of understanding outcomes for this rare class of tumors. A classic example is the report by Sagerman et al.,[106] who published in 1964 one of the earliest reports of adjuvant radiotherapy for attempted cure. The patient was a 55-year-old woman with a primary cardiac fibromyxosarcoma. After incomplete resection, she underwent external-beam radiotherapy to a dose of 63 to 75 Gy to the primary site, with proper shielding of the spinal cord. As a result of the use of lateral fields, the left lung received 35 Gy to a large volume. The patient was treated with prophylactic steroids to prevent radiation pneumonitis and fibrosis. She died 8 months later with brain and lung metastases. Autopsy revealed complete sterilization of the primary tumor.

Despite the most aggressive treatment regimens with surgical resection, postoperative radiotherapy, and chemotherapy, the overall survival for patients with primary malignant cardiac tumors is poor, and this is true even in light of more recent reports that have suggested better outcomes with contemporary adjuvant radiotherapy or chemoradiotherapy.[44,78,79,81] Operative mortality is relatively common, at 8% to 9%, and is twice as high compared to that following resection of benign tumors.[76,107] The median survival in most surgical series is in the range of 9 to 12 months,[14,27,28,30,45,65,78,107,108] with outliers as low as 6 months.[31,44,109] and as high as 23.5 months among patients who survived surgery in one of the most recent reports.[76] Putnam et al.[45] reported a median survival of 11 months and a 2-year overall survival rate of only 14%. In this series, the authors also noted the importance of complete resection. For patients in whom complete resection was possible, the median survival was 24 months, compared with only 10 months for those with incomplete resection. Llombart-Cussac et al.[65] also noted improved survival with complete resection (22 vs. 7 months). Burke et al.[44] reported significantly improved median survival of 12 months among patients who underwent adjuvant radiotherapy, chemotherapy, or both, compared with 3 months in those who did not have adjuvant therapy.

A group from Japan reported the first use of definitive carbon-ion radiotherapy in the treatment of a patient with cardiac angiosarcoma.[97] After treatment, the tumor volume reduced by 86% and became negative on PET scan. After 18 months, the primary tumor remained controlled, but the patient had developed bilateral lung metastases 4 months after treatment. Selected patients who develop recurrence after undergoing combined modality therapy may still benefit from aggressive management of their disease, with one author reporting an improved median survival from 25 months with no treatment, compared with 47 months with resection, radiofrequency ablation, or radiotherapy.[76] Others have shown similar benefits to this approach at the time of recurrences.[81]

The median survival for patients with metastatic disease to the heart is approximately 3 to 4 months, but rare cases of long-term survival, as long as 3 years, have been documented and may be related to primary tumor histologic type and performance status.[68,69,110] Pericardiotomy or pericardial sclerosis appears to offer at least temporary control of tamponade and effusion in up to 90% of cases.[68,69] Palliative treatment with radiation is well tolerated and is effective in controlling cardiac tamponade in approximately 60% of patients. Cham et al.[110] reported the results of radiotherapeutic palliation for 38 patients with secondary tumors of the heart and pericardium. Thirty-seven patients were noted to have pericardial involvement, nine also had invasion of the myocardium, and one had only endocardial involvement. The radiation dose was 25 to 30 Gy in 3 to 4 weeks for 32 patients. The dose was 15 to 20 Gy in 1.5 to 2 weeks for the remaining six patients, all of whom had lymphoreticular tumors. The overall response rate was 61%, with a median duration of response of 3 to 4 months. Lymphoreticular tumors had the best response rate (6 of 7 cases) followed by breast cancer (11 of 16 cases). Only 6 of the remaining 15 cases showed a response. Although the median survival among patients with metastases to the heart and pericardium is short, palliative efforts are not in vain because tamponade appears to be effectively controlled with these measures.

Among patients treated for GV tumors, median survival depends on the location, resectability, and grade of the primary tumor. Burke and Virmani[42] reported the median survival was 5 months for aortic sarcoma, 23 months for sarcoma of the pulmonary artery, and 37 months for sarcoma of the IVC. Two patients with sarcoma of the SVC were alive and without disease 10 and 72 months posttreatment. Local relapse was documented in 2 patients, although metastatic disease occurred in 19 of 45 patients. The sites most commonly involved by metastases were the lung, liver, and bone. Involvement of the peritoneum, adrenals, kidneys, skin, and lymph nodes was also noted.

Treatment Sequelae

Late radiation-induced cardiac or pulmonary sequelae after the definitive treatment of cardiac tumors have not been well documented, probably as a result of the poor overall survival. The cardiotoxic effects of doxorubicin have been well documented, and there is evidence for increased risk when it is given in conjunction with radiotherapy[105]; therefore, concurrent therapy should be avoided to the degree possible.

ACKNOWLEDGMENTS

Dedicated to the love of my life, Lizbeth Robles. The authors thank Nicole Pavelecky, CMD, Rahul Tendulkar, MD, and Mark Chidel, MD.

REFERENCES

1. Gray H, Clemente CD. *Anatomy of the human body.* 30th American ed. Philadelphia: Lea & Febiger, 1985.
2. Burke AP, Virmani R. *Tumors of the heart and great vessels. Atlas of tumor pathology.* 3rd series. Vol. 16. Washington, DC: Armed Forces Institute of Pathology, 1996.
3. Reynen K. Frequency of primary tumors of the heart. *Am J Cardiol* 1996; 77(1):107.
4. Reynen K. Cardiac myxomas. *N Engl J Med* 1995;333(24):1610–1617.
5. Sarjeant JM, Butany J, Cusimano RJ. Cancer of the heart: epidemiology and management of primary tumors and metastases. *Am J Cardiovasc Drugs* 2003; 3(6):407–421.
6. Lokich JJ. The management of malignant pericardial effusions. *JAMA* 1973; 224(10):1401–1404.
7. McAllister HA, Fenoglio JJ. *Tumors of the cardiovascular system. Atlas of tumor pathology.* Washington, DC: Armed Forces Institute of Pathology, 1978.
8. Butany J, et al. Cardiac tumours: diagnosis and management. *Lancet Oncol* 2005;6(4):219–228.
9. Carney JA, et al. Dominant inheritance of the complex of myxomas, spotty pigmentation, and endocrine overactivity. *Mayo Clin Proc* 1986;61(3):165–172.
10. Nwokoro NA, et al. Spectrum of malignancy and premalignancy in Carney syndrome. *Am J Med Genet* 1997;73(4):369–377.
11. Wilkes D, McDermott DA, Basson CT. Clinical phenotypes and molecular genetic mechanisms of Carney complex. *Lancet Oncol* 2005;6(7):501–508.
12. Kirschner LS, et al. Genetic heterogeneity and spectrum of mutations of the PRKAR1 A gene in patients with the carney complex. *Hum Mol Genet* 2000;9(20): 3037–3046.
13. Vidaillet HJ Jr, et al. "Syndrome myxoma": a subset of patients with cardiac myxoma associated with pigmented skin lesions and peripheral and endocrine neoplasms. *Br Heart J* 1987;57(3):247–255.
14. Murphy MC, et al. Surgical treatment of cardiac tumors: a 25-year experience. *Ann Thorac Surg* 1990;49(4):612–618.
15. Mack TM. Sarcomas and other malignancies of soft tissue, retroperitoneum, peritoneum, pleura, heart, mediastinum, and spleen. *Cancer* 1995;75(1 Suppl):211–244.
16. Petrich A, Cho SI, Billett H. Primary cardiac lymphoma: an analysis of presentation, treatment, and outcome patterns. *Cancer* 2011;117(3):581–589.
17. Kralstein J, Frishman W. Malignant pericardial diseases: diagnosis and treatment. *Am Heart J* 1987;113(3):785–790.
18. Strauss R, Merliss R. Primary tumor of the heart. *Arch Pathol* 1945;39:74–78.
19. Mensi C, et al. Pericardial mesothelioma and asbestos exposure. *Int J Hyg Environ Health* 2011;214(3):276–279.
20. Aggarwal P, Wali JP, Agarwal J. Pericardial mesothelioma presenting as a mediastinal mass. *Singapore Med J* 1991;32(3):185–186.
21. Kaul TK, Fields BL, Kahn DR. Primary malignant pericardial mesothelioma: a case report and review. *J Cardiovasc Surg (Torino)* 1994,35(3).261–267.
22. Thomason R, et al. Primary malignant mesothelioma of the pericardium. Case report and literature review. *Tex Heart Inst J* 1994;21(2):170–174.
23. Norman MG. Primary mesothelioma of the pericardium. *Can Med Assoc J* 1965; 92:129–133.
24. Sytman AL, MacAlpin RN. Primary pericardial mesothelioma: report of two cases and review of the literature. *Am Heart J* 1971;81(6):760–769.
25. Andersen JA, Hansen BF. Primary pericardial mesothelioma. *Dan Med Bull* 1974;21(5):195–200.
26. Yokouchi Y, et al. Primary cardiac synovial sarcoma: a case report and literature review. *Pathol Int* 2011;61(3):150–155.
27. Blondeau P. Primary cardiac tumors—French studies of 533 cases. *Thorac Cardiovasc Surg* 1990;38(Suppl 2):192–195.
28. Centofanti P, et al. Primary cardiac tumors: early and late results of surgical treatment in 91 patients. *Ann Thorac Surg* 1999;68(4):1236–1241.
29. Endo A, et al. Characteristics of 161 patients with cardiac tumors diagnosed during 1993 and 1994 in Japan. *Am J Cardiol* 1997;79(12):1708–1711.

Clinical Radiation Oncology

30. Miralles A, et al. Cardiac tumors: clinical experience and surgical results in 74 patients. *Ann Thorac Surg* 1991;52(4):886–895.
31. Molina JE, Edwards JE, Ward HB. Primary cardiac tumors: experience at the University of Minnesota. *Thorac Cardiovasc Surg* 1990;38(Suppl 2):183–191.
32. Perchinsky MJ, Lichtenstein SV, Tyers GF. Primary cardiac tumors: forty years' experience with 71 patients. *Cancer* 1997;79(9):1809–1815.
33. Adenle AD, Edwards JE. Clinical and pathologic features of metastatic neoplasms of the pericardium. *Chest* 1982;81(2):166–169.
34. Fabian JT, Rose AG. Tumours of the heart. A study of 89 cases. *S Afr Med J* 1982;61(3):71–77.
35. Hanfling SM. Metastatic cancer to the heart. Review of the literature and report of 127 cases.*Circulation* 1960;22:474–483.
36. Klatt EC, Heitz DR. Cardiac metastases. *Cancer* 1990;65(6):1456–1459.
37. Lam KY, Dickens P, Chan AC. Tumors of the heart. A 20-year experience with a review of 12,485 consecutive autopsies. *Arch Pathol Lab Med* 1993;117(10):1027–1031.
38. Lockwood WB, Broghamer WL Jr. The changing prevalence of secondary cardiac neoplasms as related to cancer therapy. *Cancer* 1980;45(10):2659–2662.
39. Reynen K, Kockeritz U, Strasser RH. Metastases to the heart. *Ann Oncol* 2004;15(3):375–381.
40. Salcedo EE, et al. Cardiac tumors: diagnosis and management. *Curr Probl Cardiol* 1992;17(2):73–137.
41. Silvestri F, et al. Metastases of the heart and pericardium. *G Ital Cardiol* 1997;27(12):1252–1255.
42. Burke AP, Virmani R. Sarcomas of the great vessels. A clinicopathologic study. *Cancer* 1993;71(5):1761–1773.
43. St John Sutton MG, et al. Atrial myxomas: a review of clinical experience in 40 patients. *Mayo Clin Proc* 1980;55(6):371–376.
44. Burke AP, Cowan D, Virmani R. Primary sarcomas of the heart. *Cancer* 1992;69(2):387–395.
45. Putnam JB Jr, et al. Primary cardiac sarcomas. *Ann Thorac Surg* 1991;51(6):906–910.
46. Movsas B, et al. Primary cardiac sarcoma: a novel treatment approach. *Chest* 1998;114(2):648–652.
47. Goodwin JF. The spectrum of cardiac tumors. *Am J Cardiol* 1968;21(3):307–314.
48. Thomas CR Jr, et al. Primary malignant cardiac tumors: update 1992. *Med Pediatr Oncol* 1992;20(6):519–531.
49. Keren A, et al. The etiology of tumor plop in a patient with huge right atrial myxoma. *Chest* 1989;95(5):1147–1149.
50. Livi U, et al. Cardiac myxomas: results of 14 years' experience. *Thorac Cardiovasc Surg* 1984;32(3):143–147.
51. Peters MN, et al. The clinical syndrome of atrial myxoma. *JAMA* 1974;230(5):695–701.
52. Becker RC, Hobbs RE, Ratliff NB. Cardiac rhabdomyosarcoma: case report with review of clinical and pathologic features. *Cleve Clin Q* 1984;51(1):83–88.
53. Abrams HL, Adams DF, Grant HA. The radiology of tumors of the heart. *Radiol Clin North Am* 1971;9(2):299–326.
54. Bogren HG, DeMaria AN, Mason DT. Imaging procedures in the detection of cardiac tumors, with emphasis on echocardiography: a review. *Cardiovasc Intervent Radiol* 1980;3(3):107–125.
55. Steiner RE. Radiologic aspects of cardiac tumors. *Am J Cardiol* 1968;21(3):344–356.
56. Mugge A, et al. Diagnosis of noninfective cardiac mass lesions by two-dimensional echocardiography. Comparison of the transthoracic and transesophageal approaches. *Circulation* 1991;83(1):70–78.
57. Lynch M, et al. Right-sided cardiac tumors detected by transesophageal echocardiography and its usefulness in differentiating the benign from the malignant ones. *Am J Cardiol* 1997;79(6):781–784.
58. Fye WB, Molina JE. Right atrial angiosarcoma: echocardiographic diagnosis and surgical correlation. *Johns Hopkins Med J* 1980;147(3):111–116.
59. Freedberg RS, et al. The contribution of magnetic resonance imaging to the evaluation of intracardiac tumors diagnosed by echocardiography. *Circulation* 1988;77(1):96–103.
60. Lipton MJ, et al. Clinical applications of dynamic computed tomography. *Prog Cardiovasc Dis* 1986;28(5):349–366.
61. Lund JT, et al. Cardiac masses: assessment by MR imaging. *AJR Am J Roentgenol* 1989;152(3):469–473.
62. Restrepo CS, et al. CT and MR imaging findings of malignant cardiac tumors. *Curr Probl Diagn Radiol* 2005;34(1):1–11.
63. Lee JC, et al. Positron emission tomography combined with computed tomography as an integral component in evaluation of primary cardiac lymphoma. *Clin Cardiol* 2010;33(6):E106–E108.
64. Probst S, et al. The appearance of cardiac metastasis from squamous cell carcinoma of the lung on F-18 FDG PET/CT and post hoc PET/MRI. *Clin Nucl Med* 2011;36(4):311–312.
65. Llombart-Cussac A, et al. Adjuvant chemotherapy for primary cardiac sarcomas: the IGR experience. *Br J Cancer* 1998;78(12):1624–1628.
66. Tazelaar HD, Locke TJ, McGregor CG. Pathology of surgically excised primary cardiac tumors. *Mayo Clin Proc* 1992;67(10):957–965.
67. Poole GV Jr, et al. Tumors of the heart: surgical considerations. *J Cardiovasc Surg (Torino)* 1984;25(1):5–11.
68. Davis S, Rambotti P, Grignani F. Intrapericardial tetracycline sclerosis in the treatment of malignant pericardial effusion: an analysis of thirty-three cases. *J Clin Oncol* 1984;2(6):631–636.
69. Appelqvist P, Maamies T, Grohn P. Emergency pericardiotomy as primary diagnostic and therapeutic procedure in malignant pericardial tamponade: report of three cases and review of the literature. *J Surg Oncol* 1982;21(1):18–22.
70. Lee MJ, et al. A case of malignant pericardial mesothelioma with constrictive pericarditis physiology misdiagnosed as pericardial metastatic cancer. *Korean Circ J* 2011;41(6):338–341.
71. Morita S, et al. Multicystic mesothelioma of the pericardium. *Pathol Int* 2011;61(5):319–321.
72. Terada T. Primary sarcomatoid malignant mesothelioma of the pericardium. *Med Oncol* 2012;29(2):1345–1346.
73. Marinaccio A, et al. Incidence of extrapleural malignant mesothelioma and asbestos exposure, from the Italian national register. *Occup Environ Med* 2010;67(11):760–765.
74. Raja S, Murthy SC, Mason DP. Malignant pleural mesothelioma. *Curr Oncol Rep* 2011;13(4):259–264.
75. Nir A, et al. Tuberous sclerosis and cardiac rhabdomyoma. *Am J Cardiol* 1995;76(5):419–421.
76. Bakaeen FG, et al. Outcomes after surgical resection of cardiac sarcoma in the multimodality treatment era. *J Thorac Cardiovasc Surg* 2009;137(6):1454–1460.
77. O'Sullivan B, et al. Preoperative versus postoperative radiotherapy in soft-tissue sarcoma of the limbs: a randomised trial. *Lancet* 2002;359(9325):2235–2241.
78. Pessotto R, et al. Primary cardiac leiomyosarcoma: seven-year survival with combined surgical and adjuvant therapy. *Int J Cardiol* 1997;60(1):91–94.
79. Antunes MJ, et al. Primary cardiac leiomyosarcomas. *Ann Thorac Surg* 1991;51(6):999–1001.
80. Loffler H, Grille W. Classification of malignant cardiac tumors with respect to oncological treatment. *Thorac Cardiovasc Surg* 1990;38(Suppl 2):173–175.
81. Mery GM, et al. A combined modality approach to recurrent cardiac sarcoma resulting in a prolonged remission: a case report. *Chest* 2003;123(5):1766–1768.
82. Jamieson SW, et al. Operative treatment of an unresectable tumor of the left ventricle. *J Thorac Cardiovasc Surg* 1981;81(5):797–799.
83. Coelho PN, et al. Long-term survival with heart transplantation for fibrosarcoma of the heart. *Ann Thorac Surg* 2010;90(2):635–636.
84. Armitage JM, et al. Heart transplantation in patients with malignant disease. *J Heart Transplant* 1990;9(6):627–630.
85. Aufiero TX, et al. Heart transplantation for tumor. *Ann Thorac Surg* 1993;56(5):1174–1176.
86. Crespo MG, et al. Heart transplantation for cardiac angiosarcoma: should its indication be questioned? *J Heart Lung Transplant* 1993;12(3):527–530.
87. Goldstein DJ, et al. Experience with heart transplantation for cardiac tumors. *J Heart Lung Transplant* 1995;14(2):382–386.
88. Grandmougin D, et al. Total orthotopic heart transplantation for primary cardiac rhabdomyosarcoma: factors influencing long-term survival. *Ann Thorac Surg* 2001;71(5):1438–1441.
89. Michler RE, Goldstein DJ. Treatment of cardiac tumors by orthotopic cardiac transplantation. *Semin Oncol* 1997;24(5):534–539.
90. Siebenmann R, et al. Primary synovial sarcoma of the heart treated by heart transplantation. *J Thorac Cardiovasc Surg* 1990;99(3):567–568.
91. Talbot SM, et al. Combined heart and lung transplantation for unresectable primary cardiac sarcoma. *J Thorac Cardiovasc Surg* 2002;124(6):1145–1148.
92. Uberfuhr P, et al. Heart transplantation: an approach to treating primary cardiac sarcoma? *J Heart Lung Transplant* 2002;21(10):1135–1139.
93. Emami B, et al. Tolerance of normal tissue to therapeutic irradiation. *Int J Radiat Oncol Biol Phys* 1991;21(1):109–122.
94. Gagliardi G, et al. Radiation dose-volume effects in the heart. *Int J Radiat Oncol Biol Phys* 2010;76(3 Suppl):S77–S85.
95. Marks LB, et al. Radiation dose-volume effects in the lung. *Int J Radiat Oncol Biol Phys* 2010;76(3 Suppl):S70–S76.
96. Werner-Wasik M, et al. Radiation dose-volume effects in the esophagus. *Int J Radiat Oncol Biol Phys* 2010;76(3 Suppl):S86–S93.
97. Aoka Y, et al. Primary cardiac angiosarcoma treated with carbon-ion radiotherapy. *Lancet Oncol* 2004;5(10):636–638.
98. Soltys SG, et al. Stereotactic radiosurgery for a cardiac sarcoma: a case report. *Technol Cancer Res Treat* 2008;7(5):363–368.
99. Timmerman R, et al. Extracranial stereotactic radioablation: results of a phase I study in medically inoperable stage I non-small cell lung cancer. *Chest* 2003;124(5):1946–1955.
100. Timmerman R, et al. Excessive toxicity when treating central tumors in a phase II study of stereotactic body radiation therapy for medically inoperable early-stage lung cancer. *J Clin Oncol* 2006;24(30):4833–4839.
101. Bezjak A. RTOG 0831: Seamless phase i/ii study of stereotactic lung radiotherapy (SBRT) for early stage, centrally located, non-small cell lung cancer (NSCLC) in medically inoperable patients. 2011. Available at: http://www.rtog.org/ClinicalTrials/ProtocolTable/StudyDetails.aspx?study = 0813.
102. Li G, et al. Advances in 4D medical imaging and 4D radiation therapy. *Technol Cancer Res Treat* 2008;7(1):67–81.
103. Gaya AM, Ashford RF. Cardiac complications of radiation therapy. *Clin Oncol (R Coll Radiol)* 2005;17(3):153–159.
104. Prosnitz RG, Chen YH, Marks LB. Cardiac toxicity following thoracic radiation. *Semin Oncol* 2005;32(2 Suppl 3):S71–S80.
105. Billingham ME, et al. Adriamycin cardiotoxicity: endomyocardial biopsy evidence of enhancement by irradiation. *Am J Surg Pathol* 1977;1(1):17–23.
106. Sagerman RH, Hurley E, Bagshaw MA. Successful sterilization of a primary cardiac sarcoma by supervoltage radiation therapy. *Am J Roentgenol Radium Ther Nucl Med* 1964;92:942–946.
107. Bakaeen FG, et al. Surgical outcome in 85 patients with primary cardiac tumors. *Am J Surg* 2003;186(6):641–647.
108. Bear PA, Moodie DS. Malignant primary cardiac tumors. The Cleveland Clinic experience, 1956 to 1986. *Chest* 1987;92(5):860–862.
109. Herrmann MA, et al. Primary cardiac angiosarcoma: a clinicopathologic study of six cases. *J Thorac Cardiovasc Surg* 1992;103(4):655–664.
110. Cham WC, et al. Radiation therapy of cardiac and pericardial metastases. *Radiology* 1975;114(3):701–704.

Part F Breast

Chapter 55
Breast Cancer: Stage Tis

David E. Wazer and Douglas W. Arthur

Noninvasive carcinoma of the breast (stage Tis) includes Paget's disease of the nipple and two histopathologic entities that are distinct in both their clinical presentation and biologic potential: lobular carcinoma in situ (LCIS) and ductal carcinoma in situ (DCIS). As a result of the increase in the use of mammography, these three histopathologic entities comprise a larger percentage of all breast cancer cases seen today. There remains considerable controversy regarding the optimal treatment approach and, as a consequence, treatment recommendations range from observation to breast conservation therapy to mastectomy. It is, therefore, important to understand the distinguishing pathologic appearances, biologic characteristics, and natural history of these three noninvasive breast disease entities to appropriately formulate coherent treatment recommendations.

LOBULAR CARCINOMA IN SITU

LCIS is characterized by multicentric breast involvement and consists of loose, discohesive epithelial cells that are large in size, variable in shape, and contain a normal cytoplasm to nucleus ratio.[1] The extent of involvement of the lobular lumen ranges from simple filling to moderate to severe distention with extension into the adjacent extralobular ducts.[2] As such, the lines of histologic delineation can become blurred between atypical ductal hyperplasia, LCIS, and, when ductal extension is seen, DCIS. This overlap of histologic morphology may complicate the interpretation of studies from different institutions.[1–4]

LCIS has been reported to present with a multicentric distribution in up to 90% of mastectomy specimens, with bilateral involvement in 35% to 59%.[5,6–7] LCIS cells are commonly estrogen-receptor positive, although overexpression of c-erbB-2 and p53 are uncommon.[4,8,9–10] The loss of E-cadherin is often observed,[8,11,12] and the absence of this adhesion molecule may explain the growth pattern seen with LCIS.

LCIS represents <15% of all noninvasive breast cancer.[13–15] The majority of women are premenopausal at diagnosis, with an average age of 45 years.[1,3,16] Risk factors for the development of LCIS correspond to those identified for invasive carcinoma.[17] Because the male breast lacks lobular elements, this entity has not been described in men.[3] As there are no clinical or mammographic indicators that are characteristic of LCIS, it is often detected as an incidental biopsy finding.[1,4] In a minority of cases, LCIS can be detected with mammographic calcifications; however, more commonly, calcifications are in adjacent tissue and are not histologically associated with LCIS.[18–20] In excisional biopsy specimens, DCIS or invasive carcinoma are frequently identified even when LCIS is the sole histologic entity seen on core biopsy.[21–23]

LCIS is considered a marker of increased risk for the subsequent development of invasive (usually ductal) carcinoma[3,13,14,16] that may be greatest for high-grade or more extensive lesions.[1,24] This risk appears to be nearly equal for both breasts.[25]

The question as to whether LCIS can serve as a direct precursor lesion to the subsequent development of invasive lobular carcinoma is unresolved. Some studies have suggested a clonal link of synchronously detected LCIS and invasive lobular carcinoma,[26] whereas others have not.[27] In an analysis of 182 patients with LCIS who were inadvertently enrolled on the National Surgical Adjuvant Breast and Bowel Project (NSABP) B-17 trial for DCIS and treated with lumpectomy only, there was a 14.4% in-breast tumor recurrence (IBTR) rate and a 7.8% contralateral breast tumor recurrence rate after a median follow-up of 12 years.[28] Nine IBTRs (5% of the total cohort) were invasive carcinoma, and 17 (9% of the total cohort) were DCIS. Although the frequency of contralateral breast tumor recurrence rate was less than that of IBTR, the frequency of invasive contralateral breast tumor recurrence rate (5.6% of total cohort) was similar to invasive IBTR (5% of total cohort). Of note, all of the IBTR were documented to be at the site of the index lesion except for one, characterized as pure LCIS, that was found at a remote site.

The evidence associating LCIS with the subsequent development of invasive disease raises the question as to whether magnetic resonance imaging (MRI) would be a useful screening tool. Limited data exists to formulate a firm recommendation. In 2007, the American Cancer Society stated there was insufficient data; however, in 2009, the National Comprehensive Cancer Network published guidelines reflecting a panel consensus opinion that annual breast MRI should be considered in patients with LCIS. Since 2007, three studies have been published evaluating the role of MRI in patients with LCIS.[29–30,31] Each document revealed a small but defined 3.8% to 4.5% breast cancer detection rate supporting consideration for an annual MRI in this subset of patients.

Management for LCIS depends on whether it is associated with another malignancy (DCIS or invasive carcinoma) or if LCIS is the sole histologic diagnosis. Approximately 10% of early-stage breast cancers have an associated component of LCIS.[32–34] The effect that LCIS has on the outcome of conservative management of early-stage breast cancer has only recently been evaluated. Limited studies suggest that the presence of LCIS should influence treatment approach[35]; however, the most widely accepted treatment approach is to manage the breast according to the dominant malignant histology (DCIS or invasive carcinoma) and disregard the LCIS. In such circumstances, it is not necessary to pursue additional surgery to obtain clear margins for LCIS.[27,32,33,36,37]

If LCIS is the sole histologic diagnosis, treatment recommendations range from conservative to radical. When first described as an entity, the significance of LCIS was unknown and mastectomy was often performed.[38] The high frequency of contralateral breast involvement was subsequently used to justify contralateral biopsy and even bilateral mastectomy.[16,38] Observational studies after wide local excision alone have led to a better understanding of the natural history of this condition, and a more conservative approach is now commonly practiced.[3,13,14] In patients with LCIS as the sole histologic diagnosis, the most widely accepted clinical practice is close observation with regular physical examination and mammographic surveillance.[3,13–15,28] There is no role for radiotherapy in the management of LCIS. The fact that LCIS commonly involves both breasts makes treatment with unilateral mastectomy both inadequate and illogical. Bilateral prophylactic mastectomy is likely excessive in all but those patients believed to be at highest risk: young age, diffuse high-grade lesion, and significant family history. A less radical prophylactic approach in high-risk patients is to consider the use of tamoxifen. Tamoxifen has demonstrated efficacy in the prevention of invasive carcinoma and, in the context of LCIS, has been shown to reduce risk by 56%.[39,40]

PAGET'S DISEASE

The clinical presentation of crusting and eczematous changes of the nipple–areola complex were first described in 1856. However, it was not until 1874 that the association with an underlying breast cancer was reported by Sir James Paget.[41] Paget's disease of the nipple is characterized by the presence of Paget's cells that are located throughout the epidermis.[42] Paget's cells are large and have hyperchromatic, round to oval nuclei with abundant amphophilic to clear cytoplasm. Mitoses are commonly seen, and the cells can be found in clusters or individually in the basal layers. The fact that Paget's disease is associated with an underlying malignancy in >95% of cases has generated discussion regarding the origin of these malignant cells. The epidermotropic theory appears to be the prevailing opinion, with the belief that the disease originates from the underlying in situ or invasive disease. This is supported by histologic evidence of intraepithelial extension, immunohistochemical studies, and evidence suggesting that the epidermal keratinocytes release a motility factor, heregulin-α, that results in the chemotaxis of Paget's cells that migrate to the overlying nipple epidermis.[43,44]

Paget's disease is a rare entity representing <5% of all breast cancer cases[45,46] and is typically diagnosed in the fifth or sixth decade of life. Synchronous bilateral and male Paget's disease have been reported.[43,47,48]

Patients with Paget's disease describe itching and burning of the nipple and areola. There is a slow progression toward a crusting eczematoid appearance that can extend to the periareolar skin. If neglected, bleeding, pain, and ulceration can occur.[46,49] Alternatively, Paget's disease can be asymptomatic and present as a pathologic finding after incidental surgical removal of the nipple–areolar complex.[50] The differential diagnosis includes superficial spreading melanoma, pagetoid squamous cell carcinoma in situ, and clear cells of Toker.[42,51] A palpable mass is detected in approximately 50% of patients at diagnosis; in >90% of cases, this will be an invasive carcinoma. In contrast, if no palpable mass is detected, 66% to 86% will have an underlying DCIS. These associated malignancies are usually located centrally, although they can occur elsewhere in the breast.[43,46,52] Mammographic findings are frequent in the presence of a palpable mass; however, normal mammograms are reported in as many as 50% of cases.[46,53]

At presentation, clinical evaluation includes bilateral breast examination, mammography, and biopsy to confirm the diagnosis of Paget's disease and to fully evaluate the extent of the associated malignancy. The prognosis does not depend on the diagnosis of Paget's disease but rather on the associated malignancy. Therefore, local treatment, as well as systemic and regional nodal disease risk management, should be based on the associated disease.

Management of Paget's disease continues to evolve. Mastectomy was employed in the past, although this has been increasingly supplanted by breast-conserving treatment.[54–57] The infrequent occurrence of this disease entity, the range of disease presentations (nipple involvement with or without an underlying mass and association with invasive vs. noninvasive disease), and the variable extent of surgical resection has made the evaluation of treatment options difficult. Small series have described results with various forms of breast-conserving treatment, including wide local surgical resection alone, radiotherapy alone, and wide excision followed by whole-breast radiotherapy. Conservative surgery alone for Paget's disease appears to be inadequate, with reported local recurrence rates of 25% to 40%.[5,58,59,60,61,62] The use of radiotherapy alone has been reported as achieving an 85% local control rate in a small series of patients with Paget's disease of the nipple who presented without an associated palpable mass.[63] However, this approach has not been widely adopted because of the undefined histologic type and extent of the underlying disease leading to uncertainty in field design and total radiation dose.

The combination of limited surgical resection and postoperative radiotherapy appears to be the most practical breast-conserving approach. Two studies have evaluated the combined use of surgery and radiotherapy in Paget's disease of the nipple. The European Organisation for Research and Treatment of Cancer (EORTC) Study 10873 was a multi-institutional registry trial that reported a 5-year local recurrence rate of 5.2%.[64] In this study, a complete excision with tumor-free margins of the nipple–areolar complex and underlying breast tissue was followed by whole-breast radiotherapy. The median follow-up was 6.4 years, and the majority of these patients were found to have an underlying DCIS without a palpable mass. A separate study consisted of a seven-institution collaborative review of 36 patients with Paget's disease without a palpable mass or mammographic density.[65,66] Patient follow-up was a median of 9.4 years. The extent of surgical resection varied as patients underwent complete (69%) or partial (25%) excision of the nipple–areolar complex and underlying breast tissue, with 6% reported as biopsy only. The final margin status was documented as negative in 56%, positive in 6%, and unknown in 39%. All received whole-breast irradiation, and most received an additional boost dose to the tumor bed. The actuarial rate of local failure as the only site of first recurrence was 9% at 5 years and 13% at both 10 and 15 years. Two additional patients recurred in the treated breast simultaneously with regional and distant metastasis at 69 and 122 months. Despite the differences in clinical, pathologic, and treatment factors, statistical evaluation did not identify any factors that significantly predicted for risk of local recurrence.

Current data suggest that a combined-modality approach that conserves the breast is an appropriate alternative to mastectomy in properly selected patients with underlying noninvasive or invasive carcinoma of limited extent. As with any breast-conserving approach, patients with multicentric disease extension should be excluded. Surgical resection should include the nipple–areolar complex with microscopically clear margins surrounding both the Paget's disease and the associated malignancy. Whole-breast radiotherapy is delivered with standard techniques. Management of regional nodes and the risk of systemic disease are dictated by the associated malignancy.

DUCTAL CARCINOMA IN SITU

Clinical Presentation and Epidemiology

DCIS is a neoplastic process that is confined to the ductal system of the breast and lacks histologic evidence of invasion.

These cells neither disrupt the basement membrane nor involve the surrounding breast stroma. This entity lacks the ability to metastasize and is confined to the breast.[67–70] Axillary node involvement is rare (0% to 5%) and most likely is associated with an undetected focus of invasive carcinoma.[71] Risk factors for the development of DCIS are the same as those identified for invasive carcinoma,[17] including family history, reproductive events such as delayed age of first live birth and nulliparity, history of benign breast biopsy, and dietary factors such as alcohol consumption. Before the use of screening mammography, DCIS typically presented as a palpable mass or nipple discharge. An invasive component commonly was found, and pure DCIS rarely was encountered. The widespread use of mammography now routinely detects DCIS <1 cm in diameter and results in breast cancer–free survival rates that approach 100%.[71]

With the increased use of mammography and as pathologists began to recognize DCIS as a pathologic entity, the incidence of DCIS has markedly increased.[72–74] The incidence of DCIS in the United States rose from 4,800 cases in 1983 to >50,000 cases in 2004, representing a 10-fold increase in only 20 years.[75] Of the nearly 290,000 new breast cancers that occur annually, approximately 58,000 are anticipated to be noninvasive, of which 85% will be DCIS.[76] Of these, 90% are expected to be nonpalpable.[44] Studies have shown that the rate of screen-detected DCIS increases with age despite that it accounts for a progressively smaller proportion of the total breast cancers detected.[77] The rate of DCIS detection has been reported to increase from 0.56 per 1,000 mammograms among women aged 40 to 49 years to 1.07 per 1,000 mammograms among women aged 70 to 84 years.[77]

Imaging

Ninety-five percent of new cases of DCIS present with mammographic abnormalities, of which microcalcifications are most typical.[78] Noncalcified mammographic abnormalities make up the remaining findings, with asymmetric densities identified in 10%, dominant masses in 8%, and abnormal galactograms (performed for evaluation of nipple discharge) in 6%. Amorphous, coarse, fine pleomorphic, and fine linear are all forms of calcifications that that can be related to DCIS. Linear and segmental calcifications are considered suspicious distribution and can be associated with DCIS in up to 80% of cases.[79] Linear and branching calcifications frequently are associated with high-grade DCIS and necrosis, whereas fine and granular calcifications are associated more commonly with low-grade DCIS[80–83] (Fig. 55.1A,B).

Initial evaluation should include magnification views that allow for complete characterization of mammographic findings and determination of the need for biopsy. The extent of the lesion as determined mammographically may be used as a guide for excision; however, the size typically is underestimated by 1 to 2 cm when compared with pathologic measurements.[81,84,85] Prior to 2000, MRI was not considered a useful imaging modality for DCIS. However, change in MRI imaging acquisition and an improved understanding of non-masslike malignant lesion imaging characteristics now has MRI considered a valuable imaging tool for DCIS.[86] MRI now presents as the imaging modality with the highest sensitivity to detect DCIS, particularly high-grade DCIS. MRI has additionally been shown to better establish the extent of DCIS, thus aiding treatment planning.[87] In cases that present with nipple discharge and a negative mammogram, galactography may be helpful in determining the likelihood of underlying DCIS versus papilloma[88] (Fig. 55.1C).

Pathology and Biology

The histologic diversity of DCIS can lead to difficulty in distinguishing it from other pathologic entities.[69,70] The spectrum of DCIS extends from noncomedo, low-grade DCIS that can be similar in appearance to atypical ductal hyperplasia to comedo, high-grade DCIS. In addition, DCIS can extend into lobules, making it difficult to distinguish from LCIS.[89] Traditionally, classification of DCIS has followed its architectural or morphologic appearance. The five subtypes of DCIS are comedo, solid, cribriform, micropapillary, and papillary,[69,70,90] and it is common to encounter a mixture of subtypes within the same specimen.[88] The characteristic features of each type are shown in Figure 55.2. Less common subtypes have been described and include apocrine, neuroendocrine, signet-cell cystic hypersecretory carcinoma, and clinging DCIS.[91]

In 1997, a consensus conference committee was convened to reach an agreement on the pathologic classification of DCIS and the identification of specific features that may convey prognostic significance.[68] Methods of processing and evaluating the pathologic specimen were also addressed. Rather than endorsing any specific classification system, the committee recommended and described features that should be documented for each case of DCIS, thus separating out important pathologic components and providing a comprehensive evaluation of the pathologic findings. These features include nuclear grade, presence of necrosis, polarization, and architectural pattern(s). The committee extended its recommendations to include margin status, lesion size, extent of microcalcifications, and correlation between specimen x-ray and mammographic findings. The DCIS Working Party of the EORTC arrived at similar conclusions and emphasized the importance of cytonuclear and architectural differentiation.[92]

Three-dimensional examination and reconstruction techniques have resulted in a better understanding of the enormously complex structure of the mammary duct–lobular system and the patterns by which DCIS can spread within the breast[6,84,93] (Fig. 55.3). Knowledge of the anatomy and distribution of DCIS within the mammary ductal tree can be useful in selecting patients for breast conservation and assuring maximal surgical clearance of the lesion while preserving an acceptable cosmetic result. For example, Ohtake et al.[6,84] studied the duct–lobular system with computer graphic reconstruction and found that the breast consists of 16 to 24 duct–lobular systems, each culminating in a corresponding collecting duct at the nipple. They also identified ductal anastomoses that established a connection between the various ductal–lobular units and provided a potential pathway for tumor extension and subsequent diffuse involvement.[6,84] Their proposed model for the development of widespread intraductal tumor extension within the breast is seen in Figure 55.4.

Faverly et al.[94] have described the DCIS growth pattern within the ductal tree and the implications for surgical excision. The growth patterns documented include unicentric (one area only), multicentric (two distinct areas separated by >4 cm), continuous (extension along ductal system without gaps), and discontinuous or multifocal (two or more areas separated by <4 cm). They found that in mammographically detected DCIS, a multicentric growth pattern was rare (<2%), with most cases showing an even distribution between discontinuous and continuous growth patterns. Of cases with a discontinuous growth pattern, 63% had foci separated by gaps that measured <5 mm, 83% had foci separated by <10 mm, and only 8% had foci separated by >10 mm. There was a correlation between differentiation and growth pattern such that 90% of poorly differentiated DCIS showed a continuous growth pattern, whereas 70% of well-differentiated DCIS had a discontinuous growth pattern. Based on these findings, the authors concluded that a 1-cm margin of normal tissue around the lesion would lead to complete surgical clearance of histologically evident DCIS in 90% of cases. DCIS is a precursor lesion to invasive ductal carcinoma and exists along an evolutionary continuum that starts with benign breast tissue and ends with an invasive breast carcinoma.[95] This concept has been validated in several ways. For years, pathologists have recognized and documented confirmation of a histologic progression from

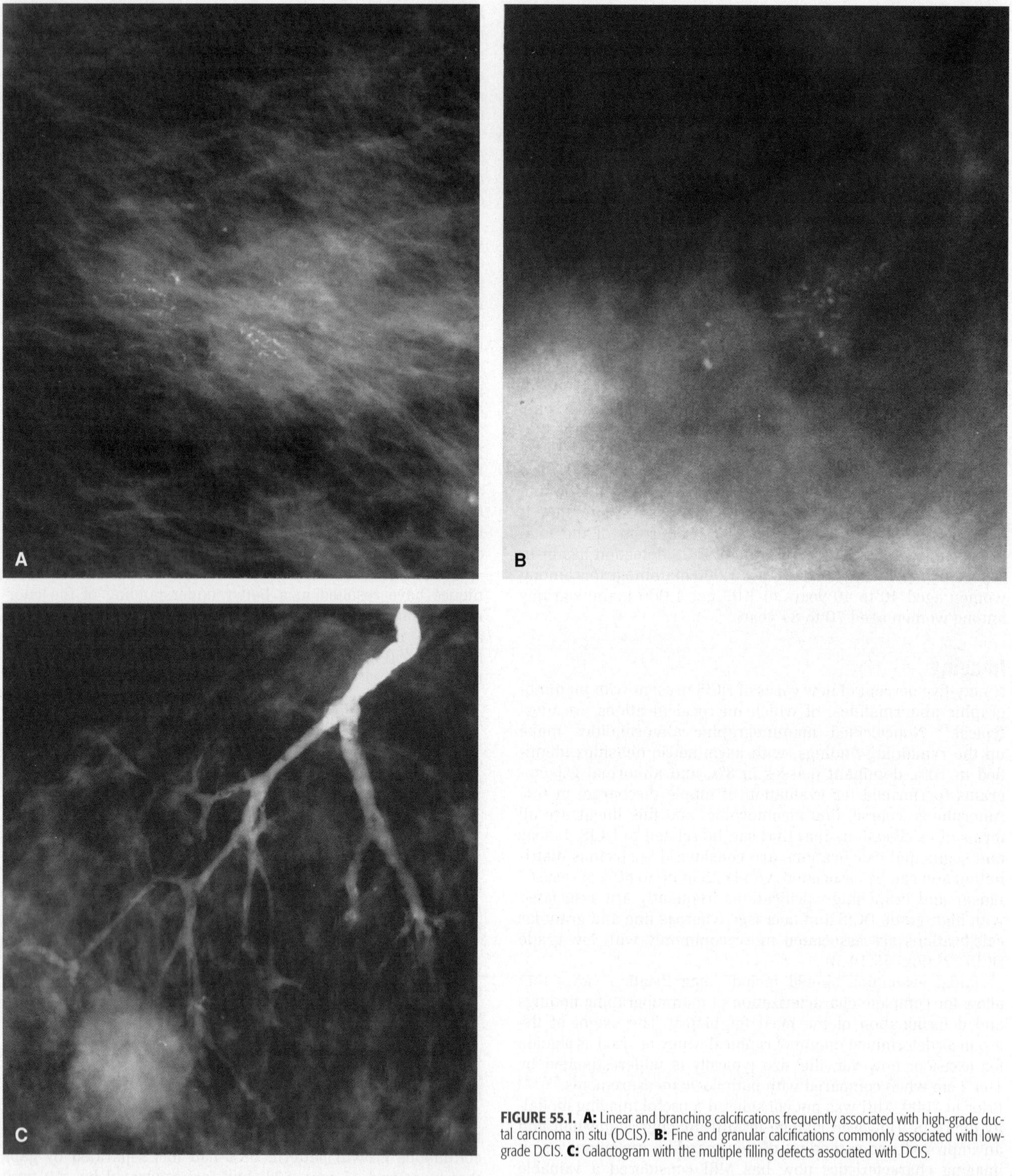

FIGURE 55.1. A: Linear and branching calcifications frequently associated with high-grade ductal carcinoma in situ (DCIS). **B:** Fine and granular calcifications commonly associated with low-grade DCIS. **C:** Galactogram with the multiple filling defects associated with DCIS.

benign breast cells to invasive breast cancer. The evolutionary concept is supported by the recognized association between the presence of DCIS and the subsequent increased risk of developing an invasive breast cancer.[75,96,97] In some series, a 10-fold risk of developing an invasive lesion has been reported. At the biologic and molecular level, many studies have demonstrated that DCIS and invasive breast cancer are highly similar at the cellular and molecular levels.[95,98–100,101–102] These similarities have now been shown to extend to global gene expression profiles as DCIS has been classified under luminal, basal, and erbB2 intrinsic molecular subtypes.[98,103] Additionally, these shared identical genetic abnormalities between DCIS and synchronous invasive breast cancer demonstrate a clonal relationship of biologic progression.[75,96,97,104] The biologic evolution from benign breast cells to invasive breast cancer occurs through highly diverse genetic mechanisms.

Genetic and molecular differences have been documented that differentiate DCIS from normal breast tissue. Genetic alterations have been evaluated with an analysis of loss of heterozygosity that has demonstrated gain or loss of multiple loci.[96,97,104–106] Loss of heterozygosity is not seen in normal breast tissue. The frequency of loss of heterozygosity correlates with histologic progression of breast tissue from benign to malignant. Loss of heterozygosity is seen in approximately

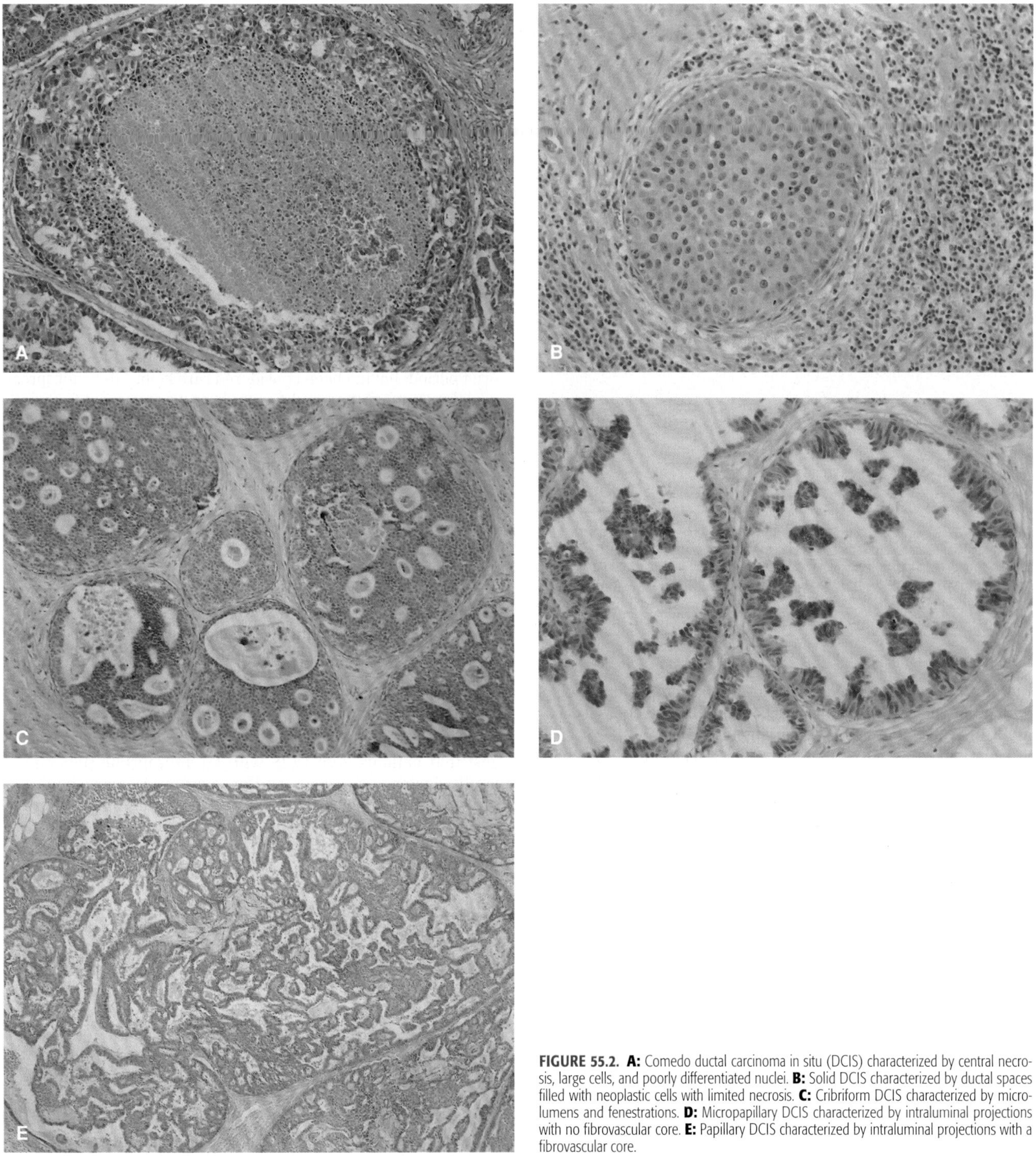

FIGURE 55.2. A: Comedo ductal carcinoma in situ (DCIS) characterized by central necrosis, large cells, and poorly differentiated nuclei. **B:** Solid DCIS characterized by ductal spaces filled with neoplastic cells with limited necrosis. **C:** Cribriform DCIS characterized by microlumens and fenestrations. **D:** Micropapillary DCIS characterized by intraluminal projections with no fibrovascular core. **E:** Papillary DCIS characterized by intraluminal projections with a fibrovascular core.

50% of atypical ductal hyperplasia. Among specimens harvested from cancerous breasts, 77% of noncomedo and 80% of comedo DCIS lesions share loss of heterozygosity with the synchronous invasive lesion in at least one locus.[104]

Molecular markers have been studied in DCIS and are found to have a heterogeneous distribution of expression.[75] The estrogen receptor is present in 70% of DCIS; however, the rate of expression is higher in low-grade lesions (90%) than in high-grade lesions (25%). This association with histologic grade is reversed for the rate of overexpression of HER2/neu proto-oncogene and the p53 tumor suppression gene. Approximately 50% of all DCIS lesions have overexpression of HER2/neu, and in 25% the p53 tumor suppressor gene is also detected. Both of these molecular markers are noted in <20% of low-grade lesions but are present in approximately two-thirds of high grade lesions.

Alterations in the surrounding breast parenchyma may also be seen with DCIS. High-grade DCIS, in particular, has been associated with the breakdown of the myoepithelial cell layer and basement membrane surrounding the ductal lumen,[107] proliferation of fibroblasts, lymphocyte infiltration, and angiogenesis in the surrounding stromal tissues.[108,109] Whether these stromal changes reflect important steps that facilitate primary tumor transformation or secondary alterations in response to ductal epithelium that is being transformed is unknown. Quantitative changes in the expression of genes related to cell

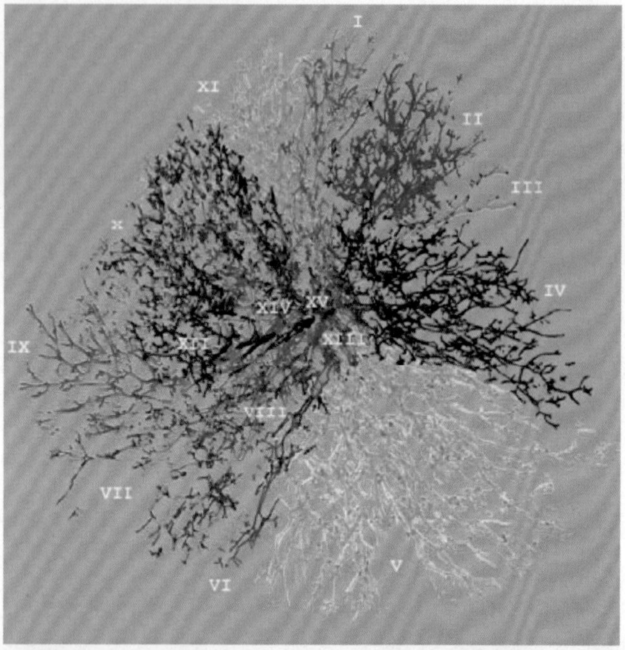

FIGURE 55.3. All ducts and their branches in an autopsy breast, viewed en face. Each Roman numeral refers to a different independent duct system. (From Going JJ, Moffat DF. Escaping from flatland: clinical and biological aspects of human mammary duct anatomy in three dimensions. *J Pathol* 2004;203:538–544. Reprinted by permission of Wiley-Liss, Inc., a subsidiary of John Wiley & Sons, Inc.)

motility, adhesion, and extracellular-matrix composition—all of which may be related to the acquisition of invasiveness—occur as DCIS evolves into invasive carcinoma.[110]

Data suggest that DCIS represents a stage in the development of breast cancer in which most of the molecular changes that characterize invasive breast cancer are already present, although the lesion has not yet assumed a fully malignant phenotype. A final set of events, which probably includes gain of function by malignant cells and loss of function and integrity by surrounding normal tissues, is associated with the transition from a preinvasive DCIS lesion to invasive cancer. Most, if not all, clinically relevant features of breast cancer, such as hormone-receptor status, the level of oncogene expression, and histologic grade, are probably determined by the time that DCIS has evolved.[111–114]

An occult microinvasive tumor (one that does not exceed 0.1 cm in diameter) may be seen with some cases of DCIS. Such cases are classified as *microinvasive breast cancer*[115] and are generally treated according to the guidelines for invasive disease. Occult microinvasive tumors are most common in patients with DCIS lesions that are >2.5 cm in diameter,[116] those presenting with palpable masses or nipple discharge, and those with high-grade DCIS or comedonecrosis.[88,117]

Natural History of Ductal Carcinoma in Situ

The overall incidence of DCIS in the general population is unclear. In an attempt to address this incidence, a small number of autopsy studies have been reported. One series examined 185 randomly selected breasts from 101 women in which a subgross sampling technique was used[118] and one or more foci of DCIS were found in 6% of cases. A review of seven autopsy series of women not known to have breast cancer during life showed a median prevalence of DCIS of 8.9% (range, 0% to 14.7%).[119] The fact that some autopsy series document a greater incidence of DCIS in asymptomatic women than most clinical series suggests either the possibility that DCIS is either underdiagnosed or that many cases are not clinically significant.

A primary consideration in the natural history of DCIS is the risk of progression to invasive carcinoma. The published evidence on the clinical course of untreated DCIS is sparse because it has been recognized as a distinct entity for only a relatively brief period, having been considered rare before the widespread use of mammography and having been treated most frequently by mastectomy. Those cases for which long-term follow-up data are available were grossly palpable DCIS—a form that may not be equivalent to the mammographic DCIS that is seen more commonly today. The few published long-term follow-up studies of DCIS after only biopsy document an overall incidence of subsequent invasive carcinoma of >36%.[7,120–122] Most of these subsequent malignancies occur within 10 years, although as many as one-third may develop after 15 years.[7,120]

Women with DCIS in one breast are at risk for a second tumor (either invasive or in situ) in the contralateral breast[123]; the rate at which such tumors develop is similar to that among women with primary invasive breast cancer at approximately 0.5% to 1% per year.

DCIS is a part of the breast/ovarian cancer syndromes defined by BRCA1 and BRCA2, with mutation rates similar to those found for invasive breast cancer.[124] These findings suggest that patients with DCIS with an appropriate personal or family history of breast and/or ovarian cancer should be screened and followed according to the same high-risk protocols as developed for invasive breast cancer.

Treatment Options for Ductal Carcinoma in Situ

Prognostic Factors and Their Interpretation

The goal of treatment with DCIS is prevention of local recurrence, with particular emphasis on the prevention of invasive breast cancer. Treatment decisions are largely based on information provided by mammography and, most especially, pathologic evaluation of the biopsy specimen. As such, in the consideration of treatment options, it is important for the clinician to be aware of some of the technical limitations associated with the clinical and histopathologic assessment of DCIS.

Studies performed during the past two decades clearly have suggested that DCIS is not a single disease. Rather, DCIS encompasses a diverse group of lesions that differ with regard to their clinical presentation, mammographic features, extent

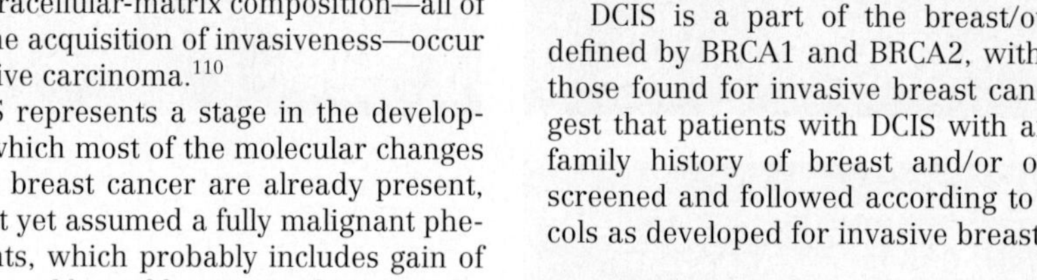

FIGURE 55.4. Models for the formation of widespread intraductal tumor extension over multiple mammary duct–lobular systems. *Narrow line,* normal mammary duct–lobular systems; *bold line,* intraductal tumor extension; *closed circle,* invasive tumor foci. **Left:** Multicentric development. **Middle:** Unicentric development with continuous intraductal tumor extension. **Right:** Unicentric development with continuous intraductal tumor extension through ductal anastomoses connecting adjacent duct–lobular systems. (From Ohtake T, Abe R, Kimijima I, et al. Intraductal extension of primary invasive breast carcinoma treated by breast-conservation surgery. *Cancer* 1995;76:32–45, with permission. Reprinted by permission of Wiley-Liss, Inc., a subsidiary of John Wiley & Sons, Inc.)

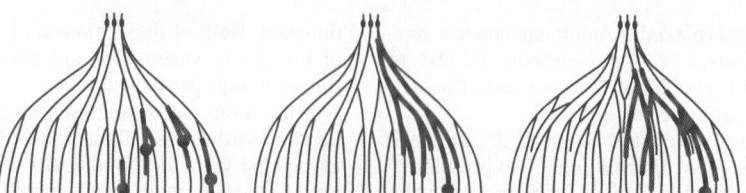

and distribution within the breast, histologic characteristics, and biologic markers. Moreover, clinical follow-up studies have indicated that these lesions vary in their propensity to recur or progress to invasive breast cancer. As a consequence, a significant proportion of patients diagnosed with DCIS can be treated adequately with breast-conserving therapy (i.e., excision with or without radiation therapy). Which patients with DCIS can be treated safely with excision alone and which patients require radiation therapy after excision are pressing clinical questions. Attempts to resolve this issue have focused on the identification of risk factors for local recurrence after breast-conservation therapy for DCIS. Through multiple retrospective studies, several factors have been identified that may be important in defining local failure risk. These include symptomatic presentation,[125,126–127] lesion size,[127,128] histopathologic subtype,[125] nuclear/cytologic grade,[126,127,129] central necrosis,[126,127,129] margin status,[127,130,131] and patient age.[125,131,132,133]

The relative importance of any histopathologic factor in predicting the probability of local recurrence and, in turn selecting the appropriate therapeutic option for a given patient, is unclear. This is partly the result of the inherent difficulty associated with the establishment of standardized and reproducible systems of pathologic classification, including such apparently straightforward assessments of grade, margin width, and lesion size.

Efforts to classify DCIS have been based primarily on the nuclear grade of the lesion and/or the presence or absence of necrosis. Several studies have shown that there is an association between high nuclear grade and/or necrosis and the risk of local recurrence and progression to invasion.[126,127,129] Although the criteria for histologic grading systems have been published, there are limited data regarding the ability of pathologists to apply them in a reproducible manner.

Several studies have shown that the status of the microscopic margins appears to be important in predicting the likelihood of recurrence in the breast for patients with both invasive breast cancer and DCIS treated with breast-conserving therapy.[127,130,131] However, there are numerous technical problems in the evaluation of margins of breast-excision specimens. First, if a specimen is removed in more than one fragment, the margins cannot be evaluated. Second, there is no standardized method for sampling or reporting margins, and this process is subject to sampling error. Finally, it is often difficult to provide an accurate assessment of the margin width for patients who undergo a re-excision because the initial biopsy site can be eccentrically located in the surgical specimen.

Most DCIS lesions present as a nonpalpable, grossly inapparent mammographic abnormality, which can make accurate determination of the size or extent of the lesion difficult (Fig. 55.5). The modalities available to assess the size of the lesion are mammography, MRI, and pathologic examination. Mammography frequently will underestimate the pathologic extent of DCIS, particularly for well-differentiated lesions in which substantial areas of the tumor may not contain microcalcifications. MRI has been demonstrated to more accurately estimate the disease extent; however, it should be recognized that pathologic assessment of lesion size can be difficult. Macroscopic examination of a specimen containing DCIS rarely reveals a grossly evident tumor that can be measured. Therefore, the assessment of the size of the lesion must be estimated from histologic sections.

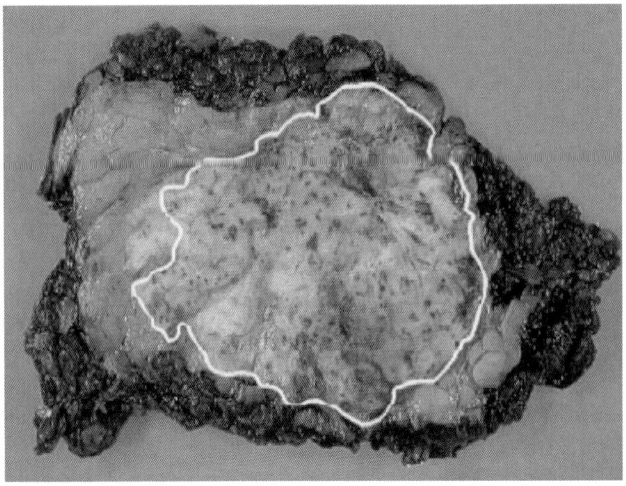

FIGURE 55.5. Extensive ductal carcinoma in situ (DCIS) in a mastectomy breast sectioned in the coronal plane. Every parenchymal structure (duct or lobule) within the marked perimeter is colonized by DCIS; outside that boundary there is none. (From Going JJ, Moffat DF. Escaping from flatland: clinical and biological aspects of human mammary duct anatomy in three dimensions. *J Pathol* 2004;203:538–544. Reprinted by permission of Wiley-Liss, Inc., a subsidiary of John Wiley & Sons, Inc.)

Mastectomy for Ductal Carcinoma in Situ

Mastectomy was the standard treatment of DCIS through the first four decades of its recognition as a distinct histopathologic entity. Mastectomy is a highly effective treatment for DCIS, with a locoregional control rate of 96% to 100% and cancer-specific mortality rates of ≤4%.[134] No randomized study has compared mastectomy with breast-conservation treatment for DCIS. Therefore, the relative outcomes for mastectomy and breast-conservation treatment can be estimated only by reviewing nonrandomized, retrospective studies. Local treatment failure after mastectomy[134] may occur because of unrecognized invasive carcinoma that results in local recurrence or distant metastasis, or it may be the result of incomplete removal of breast tissue with the subsequent formation of a new primary tumor.

Data from some surgical trials[135] and large treatment registries[136] suggest that the rates of local or regional recurrence are significantly lower after mastectomy than after breast-conserving surgery, although there have been no significant differences in overall survival. Metastatic breast cancer can follow the recurrence of an invasive tumor or the development of cancer in the contralateral breast. However, death related to breast cancer within 10 years after the diagnosis of DCIS occurs in only 1% to 2% of all patients, irrespective of whether mastectomy or breast-conserving surgery was performed.[136]

The role of postmastectomy chest wall radiation following mastectomy or skin-sparing mastectomy and close pathologic margins has been debated in the literature but is not presently considered the standard of care. Some studies show an increased risk of chest wall failure in selected cases of high-grade DCIS undergoing mastectomy with pathologic margins <1 mm, leading to a routine recommendation of postmastectomy radiation in these cases.[137] The empiric use of a close or positive margins as a trigger for postmastectomy radiation has been challenged, providing a strong argument against postmastectomy radiation.[138] This retrospective review evaluated the risk of chest wall recurrence following mastectomy, specifically looking at skin-sparing mastectomy and high-risk features of high-grade and close margins. In this series, the overall risk of chest wall recurrence was rare at 1.7% and only 3.3% for high-grade DCIS. Margins <5 mm were not at increased risk. It was concluded that the chest wall failure rate was sufficiently low that a routine recommendation of postmastectomy radiation DCIS with high-risk features was not warranted.

Breast Conservation for Ductal Carcinoma in Situ

Four prospective randomized studies of excision only versus excision plus breast irradiation for DCIS have been performed with reported results, and all have shown that the rate of local recurrence was reduced with the addition of radiation (Table 55.1). The NSABP B-17 trial[139–141] consisted of 813 patients who were stratified by age (≤49 years vs. >49 years), DCIS versus DCIS plus

TABLE 55.1 LUMPECTOMY VERSUS LUMPECTOMY AND WHOLE-BREAST RADIOTHERAPY: RANDOMIZED CLINICAL TRIALS FOR DUCTAL CARCINOMA IN SITU

Trial Group	Number of Patients	Follow-Up	Local Recurrence (Cumulative %) DCIS + Invasive Carcinoma		
			L	L + XRT	p Value
NSABP B-17	818	12-y actuarial	31.7	15.7	<.000005
		17.25-y median	35.0	19.8	–
EORTC 10853	1,010	10.2-y median	25.0	15.0	<.0001
UK/ANZ	1,030	12.7-y median	19.4	7.1	<.00001
SweDCIS	1,046	8-y mean	27.1	12.1	–

DCIS, ductal carcinoma in situ; L, lumpectomy; L + XRT, lumpectomy and postoperative radiotherapy; NSABP, National Surgical Adjuvant Bowel and Breast Project; EORTC, European Organisation for Research and Treatment of Cancer; UK/ANZ, United Kingdom, Australia, and New Zealand; SweDCIS, Swedish Breast Cancer Group DCIS study.

LCIS, method of detection, and whether an axillary dissection was performed. Tumor size was determined by mammogram, gross pathologic measurement, or clinical examination. Of the patients enrolled, 83% had nonpalpable tumors. The 17.5-year rate of local recurrence was 19.8% with radiation and 35.9% without radiation. The average annual incidence rates of ipsilateral noninvasive recurrences and ipsilateral invasive recurrences were reduced with breast irradiation by 47% and 52%, respectively.[141] An analysis of clinical variables showed that microcalcifications extending beyond a maximum dimension >1 cm were associated with an elevated risk of breast recurrence. A central pathology review was performed, including a multivariate analysis of histopathologic variables (Table 55.2). Comedonecrosis in patients treated on NSABP B-24 did not correlate with an increased risk of IBTR; however, comedonecrosis did relate to the risk of DCIS-IBTR. The prognostic value of margin status (free vs. unknown/involved) depended on the treatment group and was greater among those treated with lumpectomy and radiotherapy alone as compared to those that also received tamoxifen.[132,140,141]

The EORTC 10853 trial[142,143] randomly allocated 1,010 patients with ≤5 cm DCIS and negative margins to excision versus excision plus breast irradiation. Lesions were nonpalpable in 79% of patients, and the mean maximal tumor diameter was approximately 2 cm. The 10-year rate of local recurrence was 15% for patients treated with radiation, as compared with 25% for patients treated without radiation (p <.0001). At a median follow-up of 10.2 years, radiation therapy resulted in risk reduction for both invasive and noninvasive breast relapse of

TABLE 55.2 HAZARD RATIOS FOR INVASIVE IPSILATERAL BREAST TUMOR (I-IBTR) RECURRENCE OR DUCTAL CARCINOMA IN SITU (DCIS-IBTR) BASED ON COMEDONECROSIS AND MARGIN STATUS ADAPTED FROM NSABP B-17 AND B-24

Histopathologic Variable	I-IBTR HR (95% CI)	DCIS-IBTR HR (95% CI)
Comedonecrosis		
Absent	1.00	1.00
Present	0.87 (0.62–1.21) p = .41	2.21 (1.52–3.2) p = <.001
Margin status		
LRT, margin-free	1.00	1.00
LRT, involved/uncertain	2.61 (1.68–4.05) p = <.001	1.65 (1.00–2.73) p = .05
LRT + TAM, margin free	1.00	1.00
LRT + TAM, involved/uncertain	1.27 (0.73–2.20) p = .40	1.32 (0.77–2.28) p = .31

I-IBTR, ipsilateral in-breast tumor recurrence; DCIS-IBTR, ductal carcinoma in situ–in-breast tumor recurrence; NSABP, National Surgical Adjuvant Breast and Bowel Project; HR, hazard ratio; CI, confidence interval; LRT, lumpectomy + radiotherapy; TAM, tamoxifen.

42%. As with the NSABP B-17 study, a central pathology review was performed.[125,142] In a multivariate analysis, factors associated with an increased risk of local recurrence were ≤40 years of age, clinically symptomatic presentation (nipple discharge or palpable mass), intermediate or poorly differentiated DCIS, solid/comedo and cribriform histologic growth pattern, involved or uncertain margins, and treatment by local excision alone. The risk of DCIS recurrence was documented to be less following treatment of well-differentiated DCIS as compared to intermediate and poorly differentiated DCIS; however, there was no difference seen in invasive recurrence. Although early publications suggested a relationship between histologic type and risk of distant metastasis and death, with additional follow-up no statistically significant relationship is now appreciated.

The EORTC 10853 trial did not allow the identification of an appropriate margin width for treatment with or without radiotherapy because the eligibility criteria did not require reporting of the margin status. Nonetheless, the central review of cases did provide some information regarding the relative importance of surgical margin as related to local failure risk. A recurrence rate of 24% at 4 years was observed in cases with close/involved margins after excision alone. Radiotherapy was not adequate to compensate for involved margins because even with the application of irradiation, the recurrence rate was 20% in this group. These data and others[127,128,130,131] are strongly suggestive that obtaining a microscopic complete excision is essential for optimal local control in breast-conserving therapy for DCIS. Of further note, even in the group of DCIS cases for which margins could be considered optimal (i.e., those patients who underwent a surgical re-excision in which no residual DCIS was found), a 4-year local recurrence rate of 18% was observed when these patients were treated with surgery alone.[125]

The United Kingdom, Australia, and New Zealand (UK/ANZ) DCIS trial is a randomized trial investigating the role of adjuvant radiotherapy.[144,145] With a 2 × 2 factorial protocol design, the aim of this study was to compare excision alone versus excision plus tamoxifen versus excision plus radiotherapy versus excision plus radiotherapy and tamoxifen. Tamoxifen was prescribed as 20 mg per day, and radiotherapy was delivered through whole-breast tangential fields to a total dose of 50 Gy. Boost was not recommended, and elective decision to withhold or provide one of the treatments was permitted. Data has been reported with a median follow-up of 12.7 years. The addition of radiotherapy was demonstrated to reduce the risk of IBTR. Of the 1,030 patients randomized between no radiotherapy versus radiotherapy, ipsilateral IBTR was 19.4% versus 7.1%, respectively (p <.0001). The addition of tamoxifen offered no benefit toward overall ipsilateral local control when administered in addition to radiotherapy; however, tamoxifen did appear to reduce the ipsilateral recurrence rate of DCIS (but not invasive carcinoma) in the absence of radiotherapy.[144,145]

The Swedish Breast Cancer Group SweDCIS study was a randomized trial that enrolled 1,067 patients from 1987 to 1999, with 1,046 of these patients followed for a mean of 8 years. Patients were randomized between lumpectomy followed by radiotherapy and lumpectomy only for treatment of DCIS.[146] Following a sector resection, microscopic clear resection was not required, and 50 Gy in 25 fractions to the whole breast was delivered in the majority of patients. A split course, 54 Gy in 2-Gy fractions, delivered in two treatment series separated by a 2 week break was allowed. No boost dose was delivered. The in-breast failure risk reduction is reported as 16% at 10 years (95% confidence interval [CI] 10.3% to 21.6%) with a relative risk of 0.40 (95% CI 0.30 to 0.54). Detailed analysis did not identify any patient or tumor characteristic subgroups that did not benefit in risk reduction from the addition of postoperative radiotherapy. Additionally, despite combining factors entailing a low risk of recurrence without radiotherapy, a low-risk group that did not significantly benefit from the addition of radiotherapy could not be identified.

A meta-analysis was completed utilizing the individual patient data from each of the four randomized trials mentioned, and an overview of results was reported by the Early Breast Cancer Trialists' Collaborative Group (EBCTCG).[147] With a total of 3,729 women eligible for analysis, it was demonstrated that radiotherapy reduced the absolute 10-year risk of any ipsilateral breast event (recurrent DCIS or invasive disease) by 15.2% (standard error [SE] 1.6%, 12.9% vs. 28.1%, 2 p <.00001). This analysis further establishes strong and consistent evidence that the addition of radiotherapy following breast-conserving surgery for DCIS approximately reduces the risk of IBTR by 50%. Subgroup analyses from these randomized trials have demonstrated that the absolute benefits of radiotherapy are greater in women at increased risk for tumor recurrence, such as women with involved surgical margins (identified on retrospective pathologic review), younger women, and those with tumors that have high-grade or comedonecrotic features.[125,139,140,142,147] However, this meta-analysis confirms that no matter what the underlying rate of ipsilateral IBTR is within subgroups evaluated, the risk reduction of approximately 50% remained. This was demonstrated across categories defined by patient age, type of excision, use of tamoxifen, method of detection, margin status, tumor focality, and histologic or nuclear grade. There was little impact of radiotherapy on contralateral or distant events and a difference in the risk of death from breast cancer was not appreciated.

Patient age is an important prognostic variable for local recurrence after breast conservation for DCIS.[125,131,132,133] In younger patients, DCIS more frequently contains adverse prognostic pathologic features and extends over a greater distance in the breast than in older patients.[133] In series with adequate follow-up, younger patients treated with lumpectomy and radiation therapy had a significantly higher rate of local recurrence than older patients, especially for invasive local recurrences.[133] Some studies have suggested that careful attention to margin status and excising larger volumes of tissue can reduce this difference substantially.[131,133] No available data show that younger patients have better long-term cancer-free survival rates if treated by mastectomy rather than lumpectomy and radiation therapy. Successful treatment of younger patients with DCIS with lumpectomy and radiation therapy requires careful attention to patient evaluation, selection, and surgical technique. When this is done, age at diagnosis should not be a contraindication to breast-conserving therapy.

The randomized trials discussed were designed and conducted over a decade ago. Since then, imaging technology, surgical techniques, and pathologic evaluation have continued to advance, suggesting that the patients encountered with DCIS presently may represent a group a patients with smaller, less extensive disease that is better surgically cleared as compared to those included in the randomized trials. As a result, the value of adjuvant radiotherapy has been hypothesized to be lower than indicated in previous trials. However, it should be noted that the tumor characteristics of those included in the randomized trials represented limited and mammographically detected disease. Despite this, several recent studies have attempted to identify and treat patients with highly selected favorable tumor characteristics with excision alone (i.e., without whole-breast irradiation) and report 10-year local failure rates of 3% to 25%.[130,134] One of these studies[128] has proposed a scoring system using histopathologic features including tumor size, grade, and margin width in an attempt to stratify patients according to local failure risk after excision plus or minus whole-breast irradiation. Each variable was assigned a score of 1 to 3, and the sum total defined the Van Nuys Prognostic Index. Although appealingly simple, this scheme[128] is drawn from the retrospective analysis of a patient cohort in which there exist several methodologic shortcomings, and it has not been independently validated.[148]

Wong et al.[149] performed a prospective study that attempted to identify patients with "low-risk" DCIS who can be spared whole-breast radiation therapy. This trial enrolled 158 patients with lesions that were mostly grade 1 or 2 and with a mammographic extent of ≤2.5 cm who were treated with wide excision, with final margins of ≥1 cm or a re-excision without residual DCIS. Tamoxifen was not permitted. The median age was 51 years. The most recent data, with a median follow-up of 10 years,[150] reports an estimated annual percentage rate of 2.1% local recurrence. Of those with an IBTR, 68% had a DCIS recurrence and 32% experienced recurrence with invasive carcinoma. These data provide prospective evidence that despite margins of >1 cm, the local recurrence rate is substantial even in patients with small grade 1 or 2 DCIS following treatment with wide excision alone.

In an intergroup trial run by the Eastern Cooperative Oncology Group and North Central Cancer Treatment Group, wide excision only in a population of conservatively selected patients with DCIS was evaluated.[151] Eligibility included patients with low- or intermediate-grade DCIS measuring ≤2.5 cm or high-grade DCIS measuring ≤1 cm. Microscopic margin width was required to be ≥3 mm with no residual calcifications on postoperative mammograms. The majority of these patients had a more favorable profile than that reflected by the eligibility criteria with median lesion size of 6 mm and the majority having margins >5 mm. Additionally, after 2000, patients had the choice of taking tamoxifen, potentially impacting recurrence rates and/or time to recurrence intervals. In the study, 565 patients were evaluable, and with a median follow-up of 6.2 years, the 5-year rate of ipsilateral in-breast failure was 6.1% in the low-intermediate grade group and 15.3% in the high-grade group. Whether this identifies the low-intermediate grade group as a group that could avoid radiotherapy remains to be demonstrated, as this may represent a group with a delayed IBTR pattern. The Radiation Therapy Oncology Group conducted a prospective randomized trial to further assess the need for radiotherapy in low-risk DCIS. Following lumpectomy with ≥3-mm clear margins of resection, patients were stratified according to age (<50 vs. ≥50 years), tumor size (≤1 vs. >1 to 2.5 cm), margin status (negative re-excision vs. 3 to 9 mm vs. ≥10 mm), grade, and the use of tamoxifen (at the discretion of the managing physician). Following stratification, patients were randomized to whole-breast irradiation versus observation. This trial closed early due to accrual rate, enrolling 636 of the planned 1,800 patients. Meaningful results may be possible but have not yet been presented to date. The NSABP and Radiation Therapy Oncology Group have jointly launched a phase III accelerated partial-breast irradiation trial that randomly allocates patients between standard whole-breast irradiation following lumpectomy versus accelerated partial-breast irradiation to determine if in-breast control rates are comparable. As the in-breast failure patterns for DCIS suggest that treatment directed to the primary lesion plus a 2-cm margin should achieve local control rates that equate to whole-breast treatment approaches, patients with pure DCIS or DCIS and LCIS are eligible for stratified randomization.

Follow-Up and Management of Recurrence

Ipsilateral tumor recurrences in patients with DCIS are usually detected on surveillance mammography, although one-quarter may be detected on the basis of changes on physical examination of the breast or chest wall.[152,153] For this reason, patients should be scheduled for a baseline mammogram 6 to 12 months after initial therapy and at least annually thereafter. Distant breast cancer metastases in the absence of regional recurrence are unusual. Local recurrences after breast-conserving surgery and radiotherapy are generally treated with mastectomy. Selected patients with local recurrences who have not previously received radiotherapy may be candidates for local excision and radiotherapy. The clinical outcome of

TABLE 55.3 TAMOXIFEN VERSUS NO TAMOXIFEN: RANDOMIZED CLINICAL TRIALS FOR DUCTAL CARCINOMA IN SITU

Trial Group	Number of Patients	Follow-Up	Local Recurrence (Cumulative %) DCIS + Invasive Carcinoma – Tam	+ Tam	p Value
NSABP B-24	1,798	13.6-y median	16.6	13.2	–
UK/ANZ					
No radiotherapy	1,053	12.7-y median	17.0	13.2	.04
Radiotherapy	523		2.6	2.4	.8

DCIS, ductal carcinoma in situ; Tam, tamoxifen; NSABP, National Surgical Adjuvant Bowel and Breast Project; UK/ANZ, United Kingdom, Australia, and New Zealand.

ipsilateral tumor recurrence is governed by the nature of the recurrence. Patients with recurrent DCIS have an excellent prognosis, with <1% risk of further recurrence after salvage mastectomy. Patients with invasive recurrence after breast-conserving surgery for DCIS have a prognosis similar to those with early-stage breast cancer, with a 15% to 20% risk of metastatic recurrence at 8 years.[153]

The Role of Tamoxifen for Ductal Carcinoma in Situ

The use of tamoxifen in the treatment of DCIS has been studied; however, results have been conflicting. Therefore, its role is not yet clearly defined. Additional studies are being conducted evaluating the role of aromatase inhibitors,[154,155] and Her2Neu targeted treatment is presently being investigated in the NSABP B-43 trial. In this prospective randomized trial, patients with Her2Neu-positive DCIS are treated with postlumpectomy radiotherapy and randomized between herceptin or observation. The NSABP B-24 trial[132,141] compared excision plus radiotherapy to excision, radiotherapy, and tamoxifen. Patients who received tamoxifen had a decreased incidence of breast cancer events (invasive or noninvasive ipsilateral or contralateral breast cancer) compared with patients who did not receive tamoxifen. With a median follow-up of 163 months, the addition of tamoxifen translated into a significant 32% reduction in invasive IBTR (9.0% vs. 6.6%, $p = .025$), a nonsignificant 16% reduction in DCIS-IBTR (7.6% vs. 6.7%, $p = .33$), and a 32% reduction in contralateral breast cancer (8.1% vs. 4.9%, $p = .023$); however, no survival benefit was found (Table 55.3). Positive tumor margins were significantly associated with breast recurrence. The 15-year cumulative incidence of invasive IBTR was reduced from 17.4% in patients with positive margins to 11.5% with the addition of tamoxifen. In those with tumor-free margins, tamoxifen did not improve in-breast disease control with a 7.4% and 7.5% incidence of invasive IBTR with and without tamoxifen, respectively.

In contrast to the findings of the NSABP B-24 trial, the UK/ANZ DCIS trial found that tamoxifen had no effect in reducing local recurrence rate when combined with whole-breast radiation therapy (Table 55.3). When used as single agent without radiation therapy after lumpectomy, tamoxifen had no effect on the incidence of invasive recurrence but did show a statistically significant reduction in the risk of DCIS recurrence (10.4% vs. 7.4%, $p = .04$).[144,145] As such, the role of tamoxifen for DCIS in the absence of whole-breast radiotherapy remains to be defined.

Because DCIS is a precursor to invasive breast cancer and shares many biologic features of invasive carcinoma, it is increasingly recognized as a target for preventive measures. In the largest trials of the prevention of primary breast cancer among women at high risk for breast cancer by virtue of age, family history, or prior benign breast disease, tamoxifen reduced the risk of DCIS by 50% to 70%.[39,156]

A Decision Tree for Ductal Carcinoma in Situ

The management of DCIS requires the coordinated, multidisciplinary interaction of radiologists, surgeons, pathologists, and oncologists. Patients are first assessed to determine if they are candidates for breast-conserving surgery. Women with multicentric DCIS, as defined by the presence of two or more tumors in separate quadrants of the breast, and those with extensive or diffuse DCIS or suspicious-appearing microcalcifications throughout the breast are candidates for mastectomy, as are women in whom negative margins or acceptable cosmesis cannot be achieved with the use of breast-conserving surgery. Some women may prefer mastectomy to breast conservation to minimize the chance of ipsilateral recurrence or for other reasons.

Patients deemed to be appropriate candidates for breast conservation require complete surgical excision of the affected area. The extent of DCIS in the breast and the existing margin determine the likelihood of identifying residual disease on re-excision. Nearly half of patients with margins <1 mm have residual DCIS on re-excision.[37] However, the optimal margin width for the management of DCIS is not known. At a minimum, there should be no tumor at the margin.

Neither dissection of axillary lymph nodes nor mapping of sentinel lymph nodes is routinely warranted in patients with DCIS because of the very low incidence of axillary metastases.[157] Three to 13% of patients with DCIS, and a slightly greater percentage with DCIS and microinvasion, have isolated tumor cells in sentinel axillary lymph nodes.[158] The prognostic significance of these cells is not clear. Clinical experience suggests that patients have a much better outcome than would be predicted by such rates of nodal metastases, and most instances represent micrometastases of unclear metastatic potential. However, sentinel lymph node mapping may be used in selected patients with a higher likelihood of occult invasive cancer—those with extensive, high-grade DCIS or palpable masses—and those undergoing mastectomy as sentinel node mapping cannot be performed afterward if invasive tumor is identified.[159]

After breast-conserving surgery, radiotherapy is administered using tangential fields to the whole breast with a standard dose of 45 to 50 Gy delivered in daily fractions of 180 to 200 cGy. On the basis of extrapolation from data on the treatment of invasive breast cancer,[160] a radiation boost to the tumor bed may be added to whole-breast treatment, particularly for women with close surgical margins, although the benefit of a boost in the management of DCIS is not established. There is no role for postmastectomy or nodal irradiation in the treatment of DCIS.

It is not yet possible to prospectively identify women who are at sufficiently low risk that radiotherapy may not be of some clinical advantage in preventing recurrences. After discussing the various options, patients may elect not to receive radiation treatment; however, they must understand and accept the increased risk of recurrence that this choice probably entails.

In summary, despite considerable advances in our clinical knowledge base, the answer to the question "when should radiotherapy be used for DCIS?" remains complex and surrounded by considerable controversy. Two fundamental considerations must be emphasized:

1. A primary goal of breast-conserving therapy for DCIS is to achieve the best possible cosmetic outcome. Attempts to obtain wide surgical margins through deforming, large-volume breast excisions represent cosmetic failures and defeat the purpose of breast conservation.
2. Breast irradiation reduces the risk of subsequent invasive or noninvasive carcinoma in the treated breast and thus reduces the risk of the ultimate cosmetic failure— mastectomy.

According to prospectively randomized trials of breast-conserving therapy for DCIS, radiotherapy reduces subsequent breast recurrence in all patient groups irrespective of prognostic risk factors. That is not to say, however, that radiotherapy must be used for all patients with DCIS. In all cases, a realistic and balanced discussion of the relative risks and

TABLE 55.4 MANAGEMENT SCHEME FOR DUCTAL CARCINOMA IN SITU

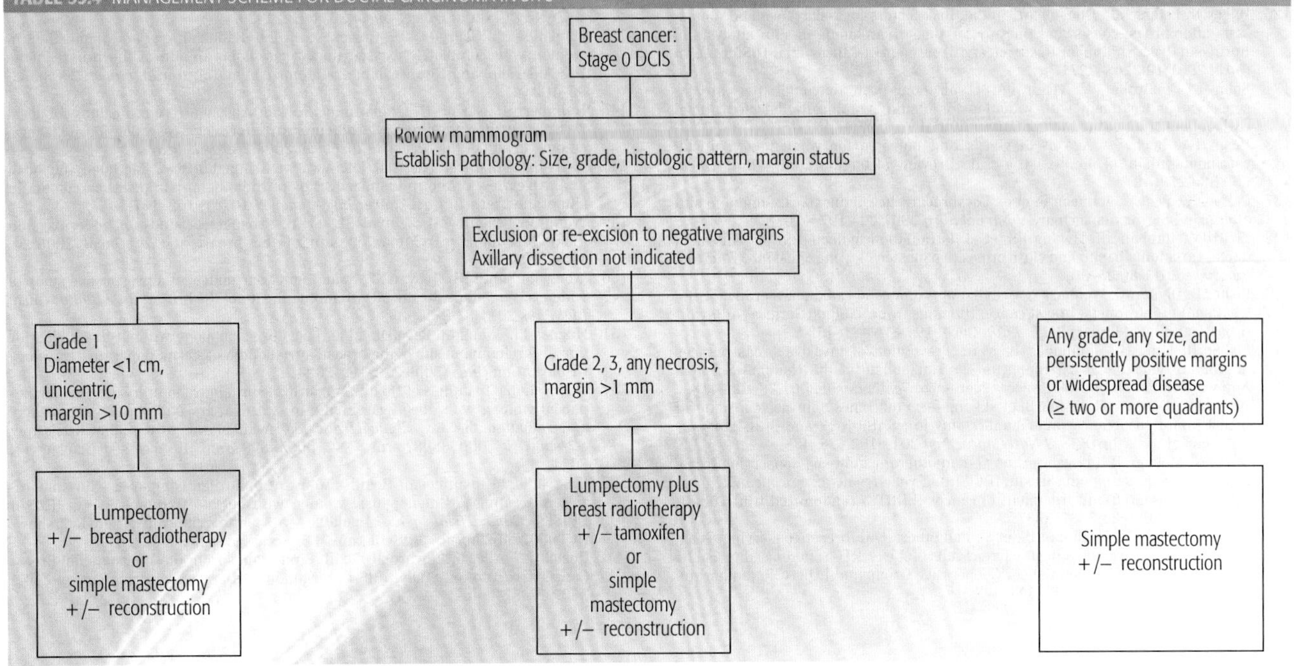

DCIS, ductal carcinoma in situ.

benefits of treatment options should be presented to the patient. Reasonable estimates of breast recurrence during the ensuing decade with or without radiotherapy are available based on level I evidence from prospective clinical trials. A decision tree to assist in the selection of treatment options is presented in Table 55.4.

SELECTED REFERENCES

A full list of references for this chapter is available online.

6. Ohtake T, Abe R, Kimijima I, et al. Intraductal extension of primary invasive breast carcinoma treated by breast—conservation surgery. *Cancer* 1995;76:32–45.
7. Sanders ME, Schuyler PA, Dupont WD, et al. The natural history of low-grade ductal carcinoma in situ of the breast in women treated by biopsy only revealed over 30 years of long-term follow-up. *Cancer* 2005;103:2481–2484.
8. Acs G, Lawton TJ, Rebbeck TR, et al. Differential expression of E-cadherin in lobular and ductal neoplasms of the breast and its biologic and diagnostic implications. *Am J Clin Pathol* 2001;115:85–98.
12. Vos CB, Cleton-Jansen AM, Verx G, et al. E-cadherin inactivation in lobular carcinoma in situ of the breast: an early event in tumorigenesis. *Br J Cancer* 1997; 76:1131–1133.
25. Chuba PJ, Hamre MR, Yap J, et al. Bilateral risk for subsequent breast cancer after lobular carcinoma-in-situ: analysis of surveillance, epidemiology, and end results data. *J Clin Oncol* 2005;23:5534–5541.
27. Ben-David MA, Kleer CG, Paramagul C, et al. Is lobular carcinoma in situ as a component of breast carcinoma a risk factor for local failure after breast-conserving therapy? *Cancer* 2006;106:28–34.
28. Fisher ER, Land SR, Fisher B, et al. Pathologic findings from the National Surgical Adjuvant Breast and Bowel Project—twelve-year observations concerning lobular carcinoma in situ. *Cancer* 2004;100:238–244.
29. Friedlander LC, Roth SO, Gavenonis SC. Results of MR imaging screening for breast cancer in high-risk patients with lobular carcinoma in situ. *Radiology* 2011;261(2):421–427.
30. Port ER, Park A, Borgen PI, et al. Results of MRI screening for breast cancer in high risk patients with LCIS and atypical hyperplasia *Ann Surg Oncol* 2007,14: 1051–1057.
32. Abner AL, Connolly JL, Recht A, et al. The relationship between the presence and extent of lobular carcinoma in situ and the risk of local recurrence for patients with infiltrating carcinoma of the breast treated with conservative surgery and radiation therapy. *Cancer* 2000;88:1072–1077.
33. Moran M, Haffty B. Lobular carcinoma in situ as a component of breast cancer: the long-term outcome in patients treated with breast-conservation therapy. *Int J Radiat Oncol Biol Phys* 1998;40:353–358.
34. Sasson AR, Fowble B, Hanlon AL, et al. Lobular carcinoma in situ increases the risk of local recurrence in selected patients with stages I and II breast carcinoma treated with conservative surgery and radiation. *Cancer* 2001;91: 1862–1869.
35. Jolly S, Kestin LL, Goldstein NS, et al. The impact of lobular carcinoma in situ in association with invasive breast cancer on the rate of local recurrence in patients with early-stage breast cancer treated with breast-conserving therapy *Int J Radiat Oncol Biol Phys* 2006;66:365–371.
36. Ciocca RM, Li T, Freedman GM, et al. Presence of lobular carcinoma in situ does not increase local recurrence in patients treated with breast-conserving therapy. *Ann Surg Oncol* 2008;15:2263–2271.
37. Neuschatz AC, DiPetrillo T, Steinhoff M, et al. The value of breast lumpectomy margin assessment as a predictor of residual tumor burden in ductal carcinoma in situ of the breast. *Cancer* 2002;94:1917–1924.
39. Fisher B, Costantino J, Wickerham DL, et al. Tamoxifen for prevention of breast cancer: report of the National Surgical Adjuvant Breast and Bowel Project P-1 study. *J Natl Cancer Inst* 1998;90:1371–1388.
40. Vogel VG, Costantino JP, Wickerham DL, et al. National Surgical Adjuvant Breast and Bowel Project update: prevention trials and endocrine therapy of ductal carcinoma in situ. *Clin Cancer Res* 2003;9:495S–501S.
55. Kawase K, DiMaio DJ, Tucker SL, et al. Pagets disease of the breast: there is a role for breast conserving therapy *Ann Surg Oncol* 2005;12:1–7.
59. Fischer B, Anderson S, Bryant J, et al. Twenty-year follow-up of a randomized trial comparing total mastectomy, lumpectomy, and lumpectomy plus irradiation for the treatment of invasive breast cancer. *N Engl J Med* 2002;347:1233–1241.
61. Polgar C, Orosz Z, Kovacs T, et al. Breast-conserving therapy for Paget disease of the nipple. *Cancer* 2002;94:1904–1905.
64. Bijker N, Rutgers EJT, Duchateau L, et al. Breast-conserving therapy for Paget disease of the nipple. *Cancer* 2001;91:472–477.
65. Marshall JK, Griffith KA, Haffty BG, et al. Conservative management of Paget disease of the breast with radiotherapy. *Cancer* 2003;97:2142–2149.
66. Pierce LJ, Haffty BG, Solin LJ, et al. The conservative management of Paget's disease of the breast with radiotherapy. *Cancer* 1997;80:1065–1072.
68. Consensus conference on the classification of ductal carcinoma in situ. *Cancer* 1997;80:1798–1802.
71. Silverstein MJ. Current management of noninvasive (in situ) breast cancer. *Adv Surg* 2000;34:17–41.
76. American Cancer Society. *Cancer facts and figures*. Atlanta, GA: American Cancer Society, 2011.
77. Ernster VL, Ballard-Barbash R, Barlow WE, et al. Detection of ductal carcinoma in situ in women undergoing screening mammography. *J Natl Cancer Inst* 2002;94:1546–1554.
79. D'Orsi CJ. Imaging for the diagnosis and management of ductal carcinoma in situ. *J Natl Cancer Inst Mongr* 2010;2010(4):214–217.
84. Ohtake T, Kimijima I, Fukushima T, et al. Computer-assisted complete three-dimensional reconstruction of the mammary ductal/lobular systems. *Cancer* 2001;91:2263–2272.
86. Lehman CD. Magnetic resonance imaging in the evaluation of ductal carcinoma in situ. *J Natl Cancer Inst Monogr* 2010;(4):214–217.
87. Berg WA, Gutierrez L, Nessairer MS, et al. Diagnositic accuracy of mammography, US, and MR imaging in preoperative assessment of breast cancer. *Radiology* 2004;133:830–849.
91. Lagios MD. Ductal carcinoma in situ: controversies in diagnosis, biology, and treatment. *Breast J* 1995;1:68–78.
94. Faverly DRG, Burgers L, Bult P, et al. Three dimensional imaging of mammary ductal carcinoma in situ; clinical implications. *Semin Diagn Pathol* 1994;11: 193–198.
98. Allred DC. Ductal carcinoma in situ: terminology, classification and natural history. *J Natl Cancer Inst Monogr* 2010;2010(41):134–138.
99. Hannemann J, Velds A, Halfwerk JB, et al Classification of ductal carcinoma in situ by gene expression profiling. *Breast Cancer Res* 2006;8(5):R61.
100. Kuerer HM, Albarracin CT, Yang WT, et al. Ductal carcinoma in situ: state of the science and roadmap to advance the field. *J Clin Oncol* 2009;27:279–288.
103. Allred DC, Wu Y, Mao S, et al. Ductal carcinoma in situ and the emergence of diversity during breast cancer evolution. *Clin Cancer Res* 2008;14:370–378.

124. Claus EB, Petruzella S, Matloff E, et al. Prevalence of BRCA1 and BRCA2 mutations in women diagnosed with ductal carcinoma in situ. *JAMA* 2005;293:553–554.
125. Bijker N, Peterse JL, Duchateau L, et al. Risk factors for recurrence and metastasis after breast-conserving therapy for ductal carcinoma-in-situ: analysis of European Organization for Research and Treatment of Cancer Trial 10853. *J Clin Oncol* 2001;19:2263–2271.
131. Solin LJ, Fourquet A, Vicini FA, et al. Long-term outcome after breast-conservation treatment with radiation for mammographically detected ductal carcinoma in situ of the breast. *Cancer* 2005;103:1137–1146.
133. Vicini FA, Recht A. Age at diagnosis and outcome for women with ductal carcinoma-in-situ of the breast: a critical review of the literature. *J Clin Oncol* 2002;20:2736–2744.
137. Carlson G, Page A, Johnson E, et al. Local recurrence of ductal carcinoma in situ after skin-sparing mastectomy. *J Am Col Surg* 2007;204:1074–1078.
138. Chan LW, Rabban JR, Hwang ES, et al. Is radiation indicated in patients with ductal carcinoma in situ and close or positive mastectomy margins. *Int J Rad Onc Biol Phys* 2011;80:25–30.
139. Fisher B, Dignam J, Wolmark N, et al. Lumpectomy and radiation therapy for the treatment of intraductal breast cancer: findings from National Surgical Adjuvant Breast and Bowel Project B-17. *J Clin Oncol* 1998;16:441–452.
140. Fisher B, Land S, Mamounas E, et al. Prevention of invasive breast cancer in women with ductal carcinoma in situ: an update of the National Surgical Adjuvant Breast and Bowel Project experience. *Semin Oncol* 2001;28:400–418.
141. Wapnir IL, Dignam JJ, Fisher B, et al Long-term outcomes of invasive ipsilateral breast tumor recurrences after lumpectomy in NSABP B-17 and B-24 randomized clinical trials for DCIS. *J Natl Cancer Inst* 2011;103:478–488.
142. Bijker N, Meijnen PH, Bogaerts J, et al. Radiotherapy in breast-conserving treatment for ductal carcinoma in situ (DCIS): ten-year results of European organization for research and treatment of cancer (EORTC) randomized trial 10853. *J Clin Oncol* 2006;24:3381–3387.
143. Julien JP, Bijker N, Fentiman IS, et al. Radiotherapy in breast-conserving treatment for ductal carcinoma in situ: first results of the EORTC randomised phase III trial 10853. EORTC Breast Cancer Cooperative Group and EORTC Radiotherapy Group. *Lancet* 2000;355:528–533.
144. Cusck J, Sestak I, Pinder SE, et al. Effect of tamoxifen and radiotherapy in women with locally excised ductal carcinoma in situ: long-term resulrs from the UK/ANZ DCIS trial *Lancet Oncol* 2011;12:21–29.
145. Houghton J, George WD, Cuzick J, et al. Radiotherapy and tamoxifen in women with completely excised ductal carcinoma in situ of the breast in the UK, Australia, and New Zealand: randomized controlled trial. *Lancet* 2003;362: 95–102.
146. Holmberg L, Garmo H, Granstrand B, et al. Absolute risk reductions for local recurrence after postoperative radiotherapy after sector resection for ductal carcinoma in situ of the breast *J Clin Oncol* 2008;26:1247–1252.
147. Early Breast Cancer Trialists' Collaborative Group, Correa C, McGale P, Taylor C, et al. Overview of the randomized trials of radiotherapy in dictal carcinoma in situ of the breast. *J Natl Cancer Inst Mongr* 2010;(41):162–167.
149. Wong JS, Kaelin CM, Troyan SL, et al. Prospective study of wide excision alone for ductal carcinoma in situ of the breast. *J Clin Oncol* 2006;24: 1031–1036.
150. Wong JS, Smith BL, Troyan SL, et al. Eight-year update of a prospective study of wide excision alone for ductal carcinoma in situ of the breast. *Int J Radiat Oncol Biol Phys* 2011;81:S31.
151. Hughes LL, Wang M, Page DL, et al. Local excision alone without irradiation for ductal carcinoma in situ of the breast: a trial of the Eastern Cooperative Oncology Group. *J Clin Oncol* 2009;27:5319–5324.
154. U.S. National Institutes of Health. Anastrozole or tamoxifen in treating postmenopausal women with ductal carcinoma in situ who are undergoing lumpectomy and radiation therapy. *ClinicalTrials.gov.* Available at: http://clinicaltrials.gov/ct2/show/NCT00053898?term = NCT00053898&rank=1. Accessed October 11, 2011.
155. U.S. National Institutes of Health. Adjuvant tomoxifen compared with anastrozole in treating postmenopausal women with ductal carcinoma in situ (IBIS-II DCIS). *ClinicalTrials.gov.* Available at: http://clinicaltrials.gov/ct2/show/NCT00072462?term = IBIS+II&rank = 2. Accessed October 11, 2011.
156. Cuzick J, Forbes J, Edwards R, et al. First results from the International Breast Cancer Intervention Study (IBIS-I): a randomised prevention trial. *Lancet* 2002; 360:817–824.

Chapter 56
Breast Cancer: Early Stage

Sharad Goyal, Thomas A. Buchholz, and Bruce G. Haffty

Radiation therapy plays an essential and critical role in the management of breast cancer. In a general radiation oncology practice, breast cancer typically comprises approximately 25% of total patient caseload. This chapter will provide an overview of general concepts in breast cancer and will then focus on management of early-stage invasive disease. The conservative management of early-stage disease by lumpectomy with or without radiation is a major focus of this chapter. Postmastectomy radiation, as well as advanced invasive disease and local-regional recurrence, will be covered in the advanced disease chapter that follows. Management of ductal carcinoma *in situ* and lobular carcinoma *in situ* are the focus of the previous chapter.

ANATOMY

The female breast lies on the anterior chest wall superficial to the pectoralis major muscle.[1] The breast can extend from the midline to near the midaxillary line and cranial caudally from the second anterior rib to the sixth anterior rib. The upper-outer quadrant of the breast extends into the region of the low axilla and is frequently referred to as the axillary tail of Spence. This anatomical feature results in the upper outer quadrant of the breast containing a greater percentage of total breast tissue compared with the other quadrants, and, therefore, a greater percentage of breast cancers occur in this anatomical location.

The breast is made up of the mammary gland, fat, blood vessels, nerves, and lymphatics[2] (Fig. 56.1). The surface of the breast has deep attachments of fibrous septa, called Cooper's ligament, which run between the superficial fascia (attached to the skin) and the deep fascia (covering the pectoralis major and other muscles of the chest wall). Skin dimpling may be caused by tumors affecting these supporting structures. It is important to realize, from a staging perspective, that the chest wall includes the ribs, intercostal muscles, and the serratus anterior muscle, but not the pectoral muscles.

The breast parenchyma is composed of lobules and ducts. The function of the lobules is to produce milk and the function of the ducts is to transport lactation products to the nipple. The peripheral ducts converge into major lactiferous ducts, which then communicate with the nipple–areola complex. Most breast cancers develop at the interface between the ductal system and the lobules, a region called the terminal ductal lobular unit.

The breast parenchyma is intermixed with connective tissue, which has a rich vascular and lymphatic network. Mammary gland lymphatics begin in the interlobular or prelobular spaces, follow the ducts, and end in the subareolar network of lymphatics of the skin. The predominant lymphatic drainage of the breast is to axillary lymph nodes, which is commonly described in three levels, based on the relation of the lymph node regions to the pectoralis minor muscle (Fig. 56.2). The level I axilla is caudal and lateral to the muscle, level II is beneath the muscle, and level III (also known as the infraclavicular region) is cranial and medial to the muscle. A standard axillary lymph node dissection resects the tissue and lymph nodes within levels I and II. It is very unusual to have involvement of level III of the axilla without disease in level I or II. The axillary lymph nodes continue underneath the clavicle to become the supraclavicular lymph nodes, which can be involved in locally advanced breast cancers.

Lymphatics can also drain directly into the internal mammary lymph node chain (IMC), which are intrathoracic structures located in the parasternal space. Although these nodes are not usually visualized on computed tomography (CT), the anatomical region of the IMC can be determined by the internal mammary artery and vein, which are easily visualized by CT

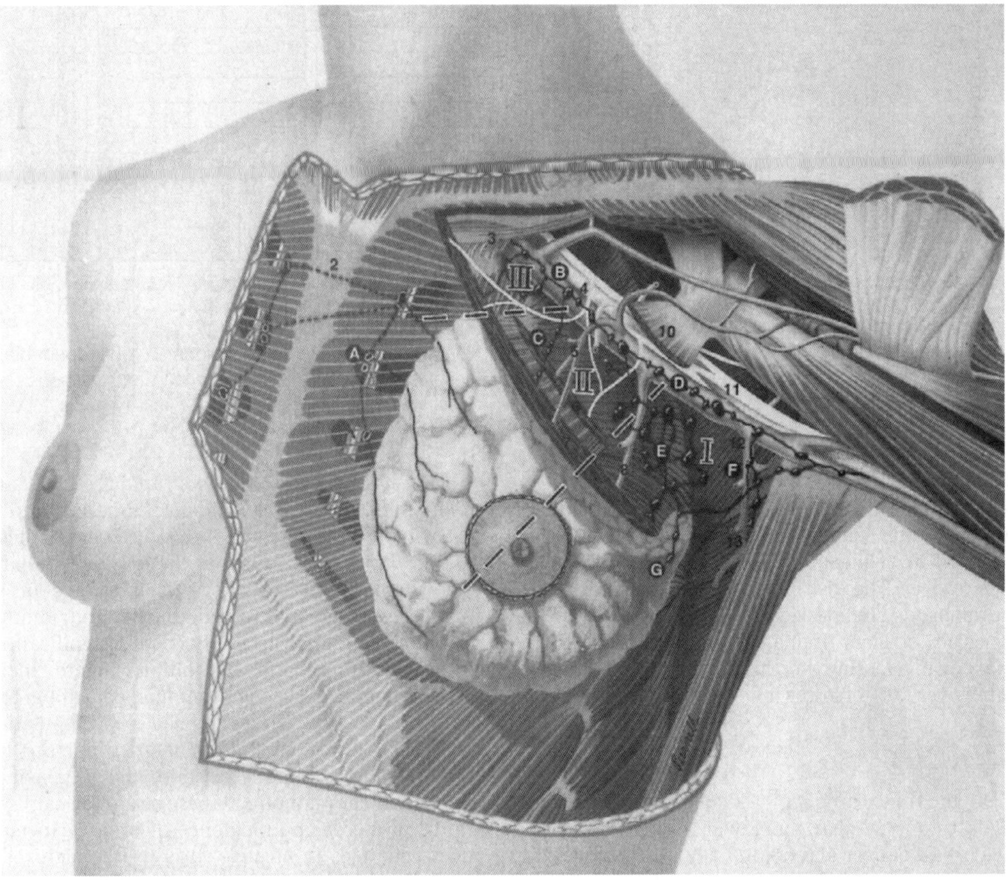

FIGURE 56.1. Anatomy of the breast and lymphatic drainage. (From Osborne MP. Breast development and anatomy. In: Harris JR, Hellman S, Henderson IC, et al., eds. *Breast diseases.* Philadelphia: JB Lippincott, 1987:1–14, with permission.)

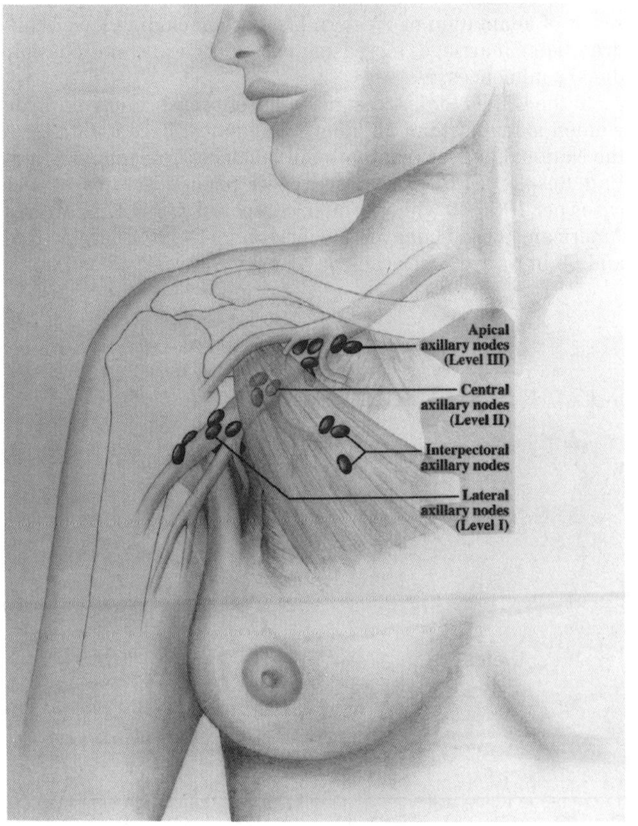

FIGURE 56.2. Location of the three levels of axillary lymph nodes. (Redrawn from Morrow M. Axillary node dissection: what role in managing BCa? *Contemp Oncol* 1994;8(4):16–27, copyright Medical Economics. Adapted from an illustration by John Daughterty, copyright 1994.)

(Fig. 56.3) and usually lie 3 to 4 cm lateral to midline. When breast cancer involves the IMC, the majority of patients will have disease that is limited to lymph nodes in the first three interspaces. Regardless of location in the breast, the axilla is the most common site of lymphatic involvement. However, breast cancers that develop in the medial, central, or lower breast more commonly drain to the IMC (in addition to the axilla) than those occurring in the lateral and upper quadrants.

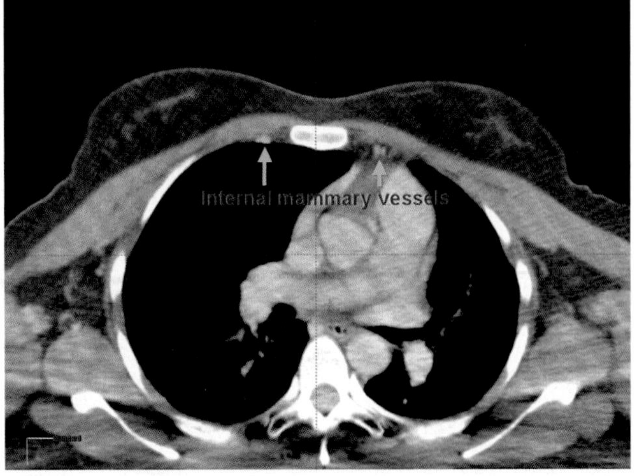

FIGURE 56.3. Treatment planning computed tomography scan of the chest demonstrating the location of the internal mammary vessels, which are typically located approximately 3 to 4 cm lateral to midline and approximately 3 cm deep to the surface. The internal mammary nodes are in close proximity to the vessels, with the most critical nodes being located in the first three intercostal spaces.

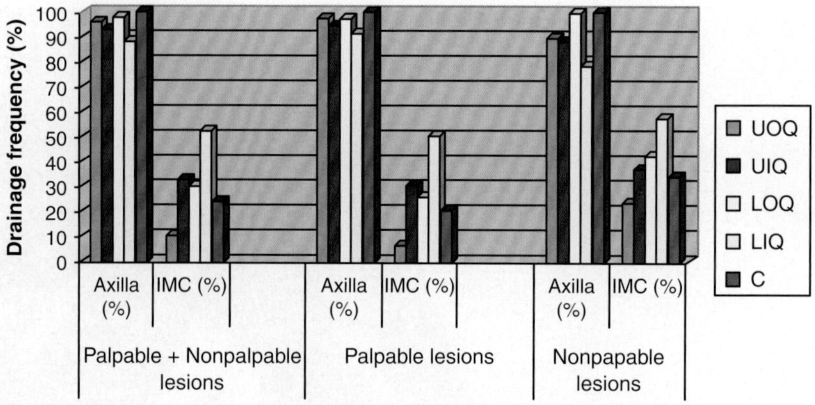

FIGURE 56.4. Distribution of lymphatic drainage of the breast to axillary and internal mammary chains according to the location within the breast. (Data extracted from study of 700 patients undergoing sentinel lymph node mapping by Estourgie et al. Lymphatic drainage patterns from the breast. *Ann Surg* 2004;239(2):232–237.)

The use of lymphoscintigraphy, by injecting technicium-99 radiocolloid into the peritumoral region followed by scintillation scanning, is used now for sentinel lymph node imaging. This technique has helped to delineate primary lymphatic drainage patterns of breast cancer. The distribution of axillary and internal mammary drainage is summarized in Figure 56.4.[3] Even in inner quadrant lesions, axillary drainage is more common than internal mammary drainage. However, internal mammary drainage was present in over 50% of lower inner quadrant lesions.

EPIDEMIOLOGY

Breast cancer is the most frequently diagnosed cancer in women, and it is estimated that there will be 229,060 new cases of invasive breast cancer and 63,300 new cases of *in situ* breast cancers among women in the United States in 2012.[4] Primarily due to increased utilization of screening mammography, breast cancer incidence rates increased rapidly in the 1980s. It is estimated that 39,920 breast cancer deaths will occur in 2012, with breast cancer ranking second among cancer deaths in women (after lung cancer). In contrast to the significant number of breast cancer cases in women, it is expected that 2,190 cases of breast cancer will be diagnosed in men in 2012, with approximately 410 breast cancer deaths in men. Due to a combination of early detection, increased awareness, and improvements in therapy, death rates from breast cancer actually declined by approximately 2.3% per year from 1990 to 2007. The decrease in breast cancer mortality is demonstrated in Figure 56.5.

There is considerable geographic, ethnic, and racial variability in breast cancer incidence. Ethnicity and national origin rank highly as predictors of risk for breast cancer, with up to a 10-fold variation throughout the world.[5] Compared with other well-established risk factors such as age of menarche and menopause, age at first childbirth, and family history, geographic and ethnic variability is quite significant. It is likely that a complex interaction of multiple factors, including genetic, environmental, and socioeconomic, contribute to the wide variability in age-adjusted incidence across populations.

The potential contribution of environmental factors and lifestyle is clearly demonstrated in the increasing incidence of breast cancers among Japanese American women and in trends of increasing incidence of breast cancer in Japan with recent changes in lifestyle. It is well recognized that the relatively low incidence of breast cancer in Asian immigrants to the United States has gradually increased as these immigrants have adapted to Western lifestyles.[6] In Japan, incidence rates have more than doubled from 1960 to 1990. This is likely a result of adaptation of Western lifestyles, including fewer children, later marriage, increasing rates of obesity, and possibly dietary influences.[7]

In the United States, the incidence of breast cancer in white women is higher than all other populations. Recent data from the National Cancer Institute's Surveillance, Epidemiology, and End Results (SEER) program report incidence rates of 141 cases per 100,000 white women, compared with 122 in African American, 97 in Asian or Pacific Islanders, 90 in Hispanics, and 58 in Native Americans or Alaskan Natives.[8]

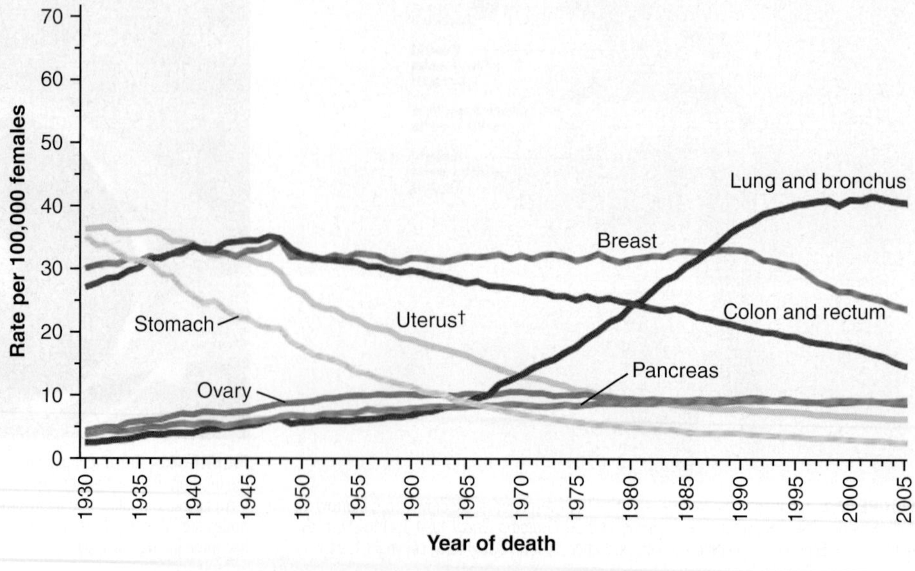

FIGURE 56.5. Age-adjusted cancer death rates for women. Statistics show a recent decrease in breast cancer mortality due to an increase in screening detected malignancies and improvements in treatment. (From Jemal A, Siegel R, Xu J, et al. Cancer statistics, 2010. *CA Cancer J Clin* 2010;60:277–300, with permission.)

TABLE 56.1 RISK FACTORS FOR BREAST CANCER IN WOMEN

Risk Factors	Category at Risk	Comparison Category
Established Risk Factors		
Older age	Older than 50	Younger than 50
Country of residence	North America or Northern Europe	Asia or Africa
Germ-line mutation	With *BRCA1* or *BRCA2* mutations	Without *BRCA1* or *BRCA2* mutations
Personal history of breast cancer	With history of invasive breast carcinoma	No history of invasive breast carcinoma
High radiation exposure to chest area	With high radiation exposure to chest	Without radiation exposure
Atypical hyperplasia in breast biopsy	With atypical hyperplasia	Without hyperplasia
Cytological findings (fine-needle aspiration; nipple aspiration fluid)	Proliferation with atypia	No abnormality detected
Family history of breast cancer	With one or more close relatives with breast cancer	No close relatives with breast cancer
Early menarche	Menarche before age 12	Menarche after age 14
Late menopause	Menopause after age 55	Menopause before age 55
Older age at 1st full-term birth	Older than 30 years when first child was born	Younger than 20 years when first child was born
Not having children	Without children	With one or more children
Using menopausal hormone therapy	With hormone treatment after menopause	Without hormone treatment after menopause
Obesity after menopause	Obese after menopause	Not obese after menopause
Other Reported Risk Factors		
Using birth control pills	Current use	None
Tall height	Taller than 5 ft 9 inches	Shorter than 5 ft 3 inches
Regular alcohol consumption	Regularly consume alcoholic beverages	No alcoholic beverages consumption
Breast-feeding	None	Longer than 1 year
Postmenopausal body mass index (BMI)	Higher BMI	Lower BMI
Jewish heritage	Yes	No
Possible Risk		
High-density breasts on mammograms	With high-density mammograms	With low-density mammograms
High socioeconomic position	Have high socioeconomic position	Have low socioeconomic position
Physical activity	Lower	>3 hr/wk
Dietary factors	High-fat, low-fiber	Low-fat, high fiber

Although incidence is lower in African American women, the age of onset is younger and African American women are more likely to be diagnosed at a more advanced stage. Several studies have reported an earlier onset of breast cancer in African American, compared with white women, by approximately 10 years; other studies have indicated that after correcting for stage, African American women have more aggressive biology and a poorer overall prognosis.[9,10]

Risk Factors

Table 56.1 summarizes the major risk factors associated with development of breast cancer. With the exception of female gender, increasing age is the most consistent and significant risk factor, with most populations demonstrating increasing incidence rates with age. Other risk factors include personal history and family history of breast cancer, nulliparity or late age at first childbirth, early menarche and late menopause, prior breast biopsy with hyperplasia or atypical hyperplasia, high breast tissue density, radiation exposure at a young age, alcohol consumption, and use of postmenopausal hormone therapy. Some of the national origin or ethnicity variability discussed above may be explained in part by differences in established risk factors, such as age of menarche, parity, and age at first childbirth. However, these factors explain only part of the variability observed in national origin, indicating underlying genetic, environmental, and dietary factors are likely to contribute to the differences in the worldwide incidence of breast cancer.[11] Breastfeeding, physical activity, and maintaining a healthy body weight have been demonstrated in various studies to be associated with a lower risk of breast cancer.[11]

Age

The risk of breast cancer increases exponentially up to the age of menopause, at which time the rate of increase in the risk slows significantly. After the age of 80, the incidence of breast cancer begins to show a slight decline. For women in their late 30s, the annual increase in risk of developing breast cancer is approximately 0.07% per year. This increases to 0.44% per year for women in their late 70s. Although these percentages may seem low, they represent only the risk for a given year; the lifetime risk is a summation of the annual breast cancer risks. Because younger women have a longer life expectancy than older women, younger women have a greater lifetime risk. Only 0.43% of women develop breast cancer before the age of 40, whereas 4% of women develop breast cancer between the ages of 40 and 59 and 6.88% of women develop breast cancer between the ages of 60 and 79.[8]

Child Bearing/Parity/Breastfeeding

The protective effect of child bearing at younger ages on breast cancer risk is well established. In a worldwide case control study, MacMahon et al.[5,12] demonstrated a nearly linear relation between relative risk of breast cancer and age at first birth, with women aged 20 to 25 having nearly a 50% reduction in the relative risk of breast cancer compared with nulliparous women. Interestingly, for women whose first childbirth occurred over age 35, the risk appears greater than nulliparous women. Data on the effect of breastfeeding are not as strong as the data on age at first childbirth, but they do suggest a protective effect. The Oxford Collaborative Group conducted an analysis of 47 studies evaluating breastfeeding and breast cancer risk and reported a decrease in relative risk of breast cancer by 4.3% for each 12 months of breastfeeding.[13]

Ovarian Function

The relation between ovarian function and breast cancer risk has long been recognized, with long menstrual history (early menarche and late menopause) contributing significantly to breast cancer risk. In experimental models and observational studies, removal of the ovaries reduces the risk of breast cancer.[5] Women with surgically induced menopause have been shown to have significantly reduced risks of breast cancer compared with women whose menopause occurred naturally. In comparison with women whose menopause occurs between the ages of 45 and 54 (relative risk = 1), women with early menopause before age 45 have a relative risk of breast cancer of 0.73 and women with late menopause at age 55 or older have a relative risk of 1.48. The data on early onset of menses and its association with breast cancer risk are also well established.[5]

Exogenous Hormone

The risk of breast cancer associated with hormonal therapy has been controversial. A collaborative meta-analysis from 51 epidemiological studies of over 150,000 women did show an increased relative risk of 1.35 for current or recent users of hormonal replacement therapy.[14] The authors reported that postmenopausal hormone replacement therapy increased the annual relative risk of developing breast cancer by 2.3% for each year of hormonal therapy. A randomized trial of postmenopausal hormone therapy from the Women's Health Initiative Study comparing estrogen and progestin with placebo was closed prematurely, demonstrating a 24% increase in breast cancer, coronary heart disease, stroke, and pulmonary emboli. This study of 46,000 women reported that the combined use of estrogen and progesterone increased the relative risk of breast cancer 8% compared with the risk in nonusers, whereas the use of estrogen alone increased the relative risk only 1%.[15] After publication of this study, a dramatic decrease of almost 7% between 2002 to 2003 was primarily attributed to the reduction in the use of hormone replacement therapy following the publication of results from the Women's Health Initiative in 2002. Since then, breast cancer incidence rates have been generally stable.[4] Other studies have also demonstrated increased risks of breast cancer with long-term use of hormonal replacement therapy.[16] However, short-term use of hormonal replacement, particularly in women with severe menopausal symptoms, has not been consistently associated with breast cancer risk. For women who have undergone hysterectomy, it seems that hormone replacement therapy with estrogen alone rather than estrogen and progesterone has a minimal effect on breast cancer risk. For women who have not undergone hysterectomy and who elect to be treated with hormone replacement therapy, combined estrogen and progesterone remains the standard for hormone replacement therapy to avoid the risk of endometrial cancer that is associated with unopposed estrogen replacement.[16]

The use of oral contraceptives has not been consistently shown to increase the risk of breast cancer. There is some evidence that use of oral contraceptives for more than 4 years prior to first pregnancy increases the risk of breast cancer. Other studies, however, have not demonstrated increased risks of breast cancer, even with long-term exposures of more than 15 years.[17,18]

Family History

The increased risk of breast cancer as a function of family history is well established. For women with a second-degree relative (aunt, grandmother) with breast cancer, the risk is about 1.5, and for women with a history in first-degree relatives (mother or sister), the risk is 1.7 to 2.5.[19] This may be explained in part by inheritance of a genetic condition that predisposes an individual to breast cancer development (e.g., mutations in *BRCA1* or *BRCA2*); shared lifestyle; and inheritance of genes that affect risk factors, such as body habitus and age at menarche. Between 20% and 25% of women diagnosed with breast cancer have a positive family history of the disease, and approximately 10% of women with breast cancer are from families who display an autosomal dominant pattern of breast cancer inheritance.[20] The actual risk that family history conveys depends on the number of relatives affected and their age at diagnosis (having a first-degree relative with premenopausal breast cancer conveys a greater risk than does having a first-degree relative with postmenopausal cancer). Women with one first-degree relative affected by the disease have an increased relative risk of developing breast cancer two to three times that of women with no family history. Women with two or more first-degree relatives with a diagnosis of breast cancer have a still greater risk, four to six times that of women with no family history.[19]

Women with a strong family history, particularly those with multiple first- and second-degree relatives diagnosed with breast cancer in the premenopausal years, are at risk for carrying mutations in the breast cancer susceptibility genes, *BRCA1* or *BRCA2*. Although these mutations are present in <1% of the population and account for approximately 5% to 10% of all breast cancer cases, women carrying these mutations have a lifetime risk of developing breast cancer of up to 70% to 80%.[20] Genetic counseling or testing should be considered in women at risk for carrying these mutations. Recently, the National Comprehensive Cancer Network (NCCN) published guidelines for genetic testing.[21,22] In the context of pre- and posttest counseling, the NCCN recommends that genetic testing be offered when:

1. The individual has a family history of a known *BRCA1/BRCA2* mutation,
2. Personal history of breast cancer plus one of the following:
   a. Diagnosed age 45 years or younger
   b. Diagnosed age ≤50 years with *one or more* close blood relatives with breast cancer ≤50 years
   c. Two breast primaries when first breast primary occurred before age 50
   d. Diagnosed at any age, with two or more close blood relatives with breast and/or epithelial ovarian/fallopian tube/primary peritoneal cancer at any age
   e. Close male relative with breast cancer
   f. An individual of ethnicity associated with higher mutation frequency (e.g., Ashkenazi Jewish).
3. Personal history of epithelial ovarian/fallopian tube/primary peritoneal cancer, or
4. Personal history of male breast cancer.

Personal History of Breast Cancer and History of "Benign" Breast Biopsy

Women with a prior history of breast cancer are at an elevated risk to develop a second contralateral breast cancer.[1] Studies with long-term follow-up have demonstrated a risk of breast cancer in the contralateral breast of approximately 10% to 15%, depending on the patient population and length of follow-up.[23] Patients treated for invasive breast cancer or ductal carcinoma *in situ* (DCIS) have similar risks of developing a contralateral breast cancer, which does not appear to be effected by the type of local therapy for the initial lesion. A recent analysis of DCIS patients from the Connecticut Tumor Registry demonstrated a relative risk of developing contralateral breast cancer of 3.35 compared with women without a diagnosis of breast cancer.[24] The risk of contralateral breast cancer as a function of prior radiation treatment is discussed in detail later.

Although women with a history of fibrocystic changes have been reported to have an elevated risk of breast cancer, recent evidence suggests that the majority of the elevated risk is due to the smaller proportion of women whose biopsy reveals atypical hyperplasia. Results from the Breast Cancer Detection Demonstration Project, which included over 280,000 women in 29 centers, demonstrated that women with atypical hyperplasia had 4.3 times the breast cancer risk of women without proliferative disease (95% confidence interval [CI], 1.7 to 11.0). In women with proliferative disease lacking atypical hyperplasia the relative risk was 1.3 (95% CI, 0.77 to 2.2). In that study the joint occurrence of family history and atypical hyperplasia had a strong synergistic effect on breast cancer risk.[25]

Radiation Exposure

Exposure to ionizing radiation during or after puberty increases the risk for development of carcinoma of the breast. Land et al.[26,27] reviewed reports on three populations of patients exposed to ionizing radiation by atomic bombings, multiple fluoroscopic examinations for tuberculosis, and multiple examinations for mastitis. They concluded that the risk of radiation-induced cancer of the breast increased approximately linearly with increasing dose and was heavily dependent on age at exposure.

In a study of 31,710 women who had tuberculosis and were examined with repeated fluoroscopic studies, a substantial proportion (26.4%) received doses to the breast of ≥0.1 Gy; the breast cancer risk was greatest among women who had radiation exposure between the ages of 10 and 14 years (relative risk [RR] 4.5 per 0.01 Gy and an additive risk of 6.1 per 104 person-years per 0.01 Gy); there was substantially less excess risk with increasing age at first exposure.[28]

A high risk of solid tumors, especially breast cancer, has been described in women treated with radiation therapy at a young age for Hodgkin lymphoma. In a review of 1,380 women treated at 15 institutions before the age of 16 years, breast cancer developed in 17 women; 7 after radiation therapy alone and in 10 after irradiation and chemotherapy. Sixteen breast cancers appeared within or at the margin of the irradiation fields. The cumulative probability of breast cancer at 40 years of age was 35%. Women in this cohort of survivors had a risk of breast cancer 70 times higher than that of the general population.[29]

In a recent study, relative risks of breast cancer were defined by radiation dose to the chest (0, 20 ≤ 40 Gy, or ≥ 40 Gy). Estimates were from this case-control study conducted within an international population-based cohort of 3,817 female survivors of Hodgkin lymphoma diagnosed at age 30 years or younger. For a survivor who was treated at age 25 years with a chest radiation dose of at least 40 Gy without alkylating agents, estimated cumulative absolute risks of breast cancer by age 35, 45, and 55 years were 1.4% (95% CI, 0.9% to 2.1%), 11.1% (95% CI, 7.4% to 16.3%), and 29.0% (95% CI, 20.2% to 40.1%), respectively.[30] A reduced volume of radiation fields has also been shown to reduce the breast cancer risk associated with treatment of Hodgkin lymphoma. The current practice of limiting radiation fields to involved nodal regions should help to further reduce the risk of radiation related breast cancers in Hodgkin's survivors.[31]

Body Mass Index, Physical Activity, and Dietary Factors

The inherent complex interaction between body mass, physical activity, and diet complicates interpretation of epidemiologic studies correlating these factors with breast cancer risk. Body mass index (BMI) has been clearly associated with breast cancer risk in a number of studies, but it appears to influence breast cancer risk predominantly in postmenopausal women. In premenopausal women, most studies have not observed a strong relation between BMI and breast cancer risk. In postmenopausal women, a pooled analysis of prospective studies demonstrated the risk of breast cancer to be 30% higher in postmenopausal women with a BMI over 31 kg/m^2 compared with women with a BMI of 20 kg/m^2.[32] The higher risk of breast cancer with increased BMI in postmenopausal women is likely due to higher estradiol levels associated with increased adipose tissue and increased aromatase, which is involved in the conversion of androgens to estradiol. In postmenopausal women, this is the primary source of estradiol, whereas in premenopausal women estradiol is predominantly from the ovaries so there is little association with BMI and estradiol levels.

Physical activity can have a significant impact on BMI, so it is sometimes difficult to separate these two effects in interpreting breast cancer risk. A majority of studies, however, have observed a lower risk of breast cancer among women who are more physically active compared with women who are sedentary.

Although it has been suggested that obesity and high intake of meat, dairy products, and fat may increases risk and fiber, fruits and vegetables, and phytoestrogens (soy products) may reduce risk, strong links between diet and breast cancer risk have not been clearly established.[33] Accurate data regarding nutritional factors are difficult to evaluate in most epidemiologic studies. A pooled analysis of eight prospective studies did not conclude a relation between dietary fat intake and breast cancer risk. Similarly, large prospective studies have failed to demonstrate an association between dietary fiber intake and breast cancer risk.[34] Phytoestrogens found in soy products and many cereals, tea, and vegetables may reduce the effects of estrogens. Given the lower incidence of breast cancer in Asian countries with high soy intake, one might hypothesize a relation between this dietary factor and breast cancer risk. Although animal studies suggest that high soy intake is protective, human studies have not been as conclusive.

Alcohol Consumption

In an analysis by the Oxford Group of 53 epidemiological studies, including 58,515 women with breast cancer and 95,067 women without breast cancer, women with daily consumption of four or more drinks a day had a 50% higher breast cancer risk.[35] The average consumption of alcohol reported was 6.0 g per day (about half a unit or drink of alcohol per day). Compared with women who reported drinking no alcohol, the relative risk of breast cancer was 1.32 (1.19 to 1.45; P <.00001) for an intake of 35 to 44 g per day alcohol, and 1.46 (1.33 to 1.61; P <.00001) for ≥45 g per day or more of alcohol. The relative risk of breast cancer increased by 7.1% (95% CI, 5.5 to 8.7%; P <.00001) for each additional drink of alcohol consumed on a daily basis. Chen et al.[36] reported on a prospective observational study of 105,986 women enrolled in the Nurses' Health Study between 1980 and 2008. With 2.4 million person-years of follow-up, 7,690 cases of invasive breast cancer were diagnosed. They found that increasing alcohol consumption was associated with increased breast cancer risk that was statistically significant at levels as low as three to six drinks per week (RR 1.15; 95% CI, 1.06 to 1.24). Moreover, binge drinking, but not frequency of drinking, was associated with breast cancer risk after controlling for cumulative alcohol intake. They concluded that low levels of alcohol consumption were associated with a small increase in breast cancer risk, with the most consistent measure being cumulative alcohol intake throughout adult life.

Although the relation among physical activity, BMI, and dietary factors may be difficult to separate, it is apparent that maintaining a sound, varied diet, limiting alcohol intake, avoidance of obesity, and moderate physical activity are modifiable behaviors that can impact breast cancer risk (as well as other health-related issues) and should be encouraged.

Mammographic Density

There is a large body of evidence suggesting a correlation between mammographic breast density and breast cancer risk.[37,38–39] The risk of breast cancer associated with the highest category of density has been estimated to be two to six times greater than in the lowest category. Although the causal link between mammographic density remains poorly understood, breast density is in part attributable to genetic factors.

Boyd et al.[40] and Byrne et al.[41] noted that women with 75% or greater breast density parenchymal patterns on the mammogram had a fivefold greater risk of breast cancer. This parameter was independent of other prognostic factors, such as family history, age at first birth, or alcohol consumption.

Determining an Individual's Risk

It is important to consider the combination of risk factors when a generalized risk profile is determined. Gail et al.[42] have used these epidemiologic risk factors to derive a model for predicting an individual's annual and lifetime risks of breast cancer. In the Gail model, an individual's annual risk of breast cancer is based on her present age, number of first-degree relatives

TABLE 56.2 GENES ASSOCIATED WITH HEREDITARY BREAST CANCER

Gene/Syndrome	Approximate Relative Breast Cancer Risk
BRCA1/BRCA2	10–20 times relative risk
P53-Li-Fraumeni	2–6 times relative risk
PTEN Cowden's	2–4 times risk
STK11 Peutz-Jeghers	10–15 times risk
ATM (ataxia-telangiectasia)	3–4 times risk
CHEK2	2 times risk
BRIP1–Fanconi's anemia	2 times risk
PALB2	2–3 times risk

TABLE 56.3 PROBABILITY OF *BRCA1* GERMLINE MUTATIONS IN VARIOUS CLINICAL SCENARIOS

Scenario	Probability
Mother or father proven carrier	50%
40-year-old with breast cancer and a first-degree relative with breast cancer	
Ashkenazi	20%
Non-Ashkenazi	5%
60-year-old with bilateral breast cancer and a first-degree relative with breast cancer	
Ashkenazi	20%
Non-Ashkenazi	5%
30-year-old with breast cancer and a first-degree relative with ovarian cancer	
Ashkenazi	50%
Non-Ashkenazi	20%

Data from Shattuck-Eidens D, Oliphant A, McClure M, et al. BRCA1 sequence analysis in women at high risk for susceptibility mutations. Risk factor analysis and implications for genetic testing. *JAMA* 1997;278:1242–1250.

with breast cancer, age at first birth, age at menarche, number of breast biopsies, and history of atypical ductal hyperplasia. The use of exogenous hormones is not considered in this model, and many of the other risk factors discussed above are not incorporated into this specific model.

PREVENTION AND GENETIC SCREENING

Approximately 10% of breast cancer patients have familial breast cancer, typically defined as breast cancer showing an autosomal dominant inheritance pattern.[20] During the 1990s, germline mutations in three important tumor suppressor genes—*p53*, *BRCA1*, and *BRCA2*—were discovered in family members of individuals with familial breast cancer.[43–45] All three genes have been shown unequivocally to predispose to breast cancer. A number of genetic conditions associated with increased risk of breast cancer are summarized in Table 56.2.

Mutations in *p53*

Germline mutations in the *p53* gene are very rare and result in Li-Fraumeni syndrome, named after two investigators who made significant contributions to the understanding of this condition.[45] The *p53* gene is one of the most important tumor suppressor genes and has been called the "guardian of the genome" because of its critical role in cellular pathways that recognize and direct a response to DNA injury. One consequence of a germline mutation in *p53* is an increased risk for a variety of cancers, including childhood sarcomas, gynecologic tumors, and breast cancer. Breast cancer is the most common malignancy in patients with Li-Fraumeni syndrome; the lifetime risk is estimated to be 90%.[45]

Mutations in *BRCA1* and *BRCA2*

Studies of patients with familial breast cancer led to the discovery of *BRCA1* in 1995 and *BRCA2* in 1996. Similar to *p53*, both *BRCA1* and *BRCA2* are tumor suppressor genes that contribute to the stability of the genome by mediating the effects of the cellular response to DNA injury. Individuals with a germline mutation in *BRCA1* have a lifetime risk of breast cancer of 65% to 85%. In addition, these individuals have an elevated lifetime risk of ovarian cancer, which may approach 50%. Other types of cancer that develop more frequently in *BRCA1* carriers include colon and prostate cancers. The lifetime risk of breast cancer for women with germline *BRCA2* mutations mirrors that for women with *BRCA1* mutations. *BRCA2* mutation carriers are also at increased risk for ovarian cancer compared with the general population, but their risk is much less than the risk in women with *BRCA1* mutations. *BRCA2* is also associated with male breast cancer and pancreatic cancer. Genetic screening for germline mutations in *BRCA1* and *BRCA2* is now possible. Testing should be performed in centers equipped with genetic counseling programs designed to properly inform individuals of the social, economic, and legal consequences associated with genetic testing. Germline mutations in *BRCA1* and *BRCA2* are rare, occurring in fewer than 7% of patients with breast cancer. Thus, only a minority of breast cancer patients with a family history of the disease would be predicted to carry a mutation in one of these genes. Table 56.3 contains data concerning the probability of carrying a *BRCA1* mutation based on an individual's age at cancer diagnosis, personal cancer history, and family cancer history and whether the individual is of Ashkenazi Jewish descent.[46]

No definitive data exist on which to base screening recommendations for individuals with a proven germline mutation in a gene predisposing to the development of breast cancer. The NCCN has published a guideline recommending that individuals with a genetic predisposition undergo annual clinical and self-breast examination prior to age 25 and annual mammography or magnetic resonance imaging (MRI) and semiannual clinical and self-breast examination after age 25.[47] In addition, annual pelvic examinations with transvaginal sonography, color Doppler examinations of the ovaries, and measurement of serum cancer antigen (CA-125) levels are recommended beginning at age 25 to 35 years. For those women over the age of 35, a risk-reducing bilateral salpingo-oophorectomy is recommended, with possible short-term hormone replacement therapy.

Breast Cancer Prevention Strategies

Tamoxifen

Understanding of the role of estrogens and progesterones in breast cancer development has led to the development of pharmacologic strategies that could significantly decrease the incidence of breast cancer over the next two decades.

Several pharmaceuticals that affect the estrogenic pathways have been studied as chemopreventive agents, but the only agent for which mature data from clinical trials are available is tamoxifen.[48,49–50,51–52,53] Interest in tamoxifen as a chemopreventive agent arose after a number of randomized trials designed to test the efficacy of hormonal therapy for invasive breast cancer reported that tamoxifen reduced the incidence of contralateral breast cancer. On the basis of these data, in 1992 the National Surgical Adjuvant Breast and Bowel Project (NSABP) began a randomized, placebo-controlled study (the P-1 trial) to test the efficacy of 5 years of tamoxifen in the prevention of breast cancer.[53] Between 1992 and 1997, 13,388 women with a 1.67% or greater predicted risk of developing breast cancer within 5 years were enrolled in this trial. Risk was assessed using a modification of the Gail model, which permitted enrollment of any woman older than 60 years of age and selected women younger than 60 years with additional risk factors that increased their annual risk to at least that of a

TABLE 56.4 RESULTS OF CHEMO-PREVENTION TRIALS

	Royal Marsden (Tamoxifen vs. Placebo)[55]	NSABP-P1 (Tamoxifen vs. Placebo)[53]	Italian (Tamoxifen vs. Placebo)[56]	IBIS-1 (Tamoxifen vs. Placebo)[50]	MORE (Raloxifene vs. Placebo)[49]	STARR (Tamoxifen vs. Raloxifene)[54]
Entry dates	1986–1996	1992–1997	1992–1997	1992–2001	1994–1999	1999–2005
Number randomized	2,494 (1,238 vs. 1.233)	6,681 vs. 6,707	2,700 vs. 2,708	3,573 vs. 3,566	2,557 + 2,572 vs. 2,576	9,726 vs. 9,745
Age (yr)	30–70	≥35	35–70	35–70	66.5 (median)	≥35
Agent dose	Tamoxifen 20 mg	Tamoxifen 20 mg	Tamoxifen 20 mg	Tamoxifen 20 mg	Raloxifene 60 mg or 120 mg	Tamoxifen 20 mg, raloxifene 60 mg
Planned length (yr) of treatment	5–8	5	5	5	4	5
Breast Cancers						
Total	62 vs. 75	124 vs. 244	34 vs. 45	69 vs. 101	31/2 vs. 43	220 vs. 248
Invasive	54 vs. 64	89 vs. 175	28 vs. 40	64 vs. 85	22/2 vs. 39	163 vs. 168
Noninvasive	7 vs. 7	35 vs. 69	5 vs. 4	5 vs. 16	9/2 vs. 4	57 vs. 80
Unknown	1 vs. 4	–	1 vs. 1	–	–	–
ER Status (Invasive Only)						
Positive	31 vs. 44	41 vs. 130	–	44 vs. 63	10/2 vs. 31	115 vs. 109
Negative	17 vs. 10	38 vs. 31	–	19 vs. 19	9/2 vs. 4	44 vs. 51

60-year-old. In addition, women with a history of lobular carcinoma *in situ* (LCIS) were included. Women were not allowed to use estrogen replacement therapy during their participation in the trial. The results of the NSABP P-1 trial indicated that tamoxifen reduced the rates of invasive and noninvasive breast cancer by 49% and 50%, respectively. The benefit of tamoxifen was seen in all age groups (≤49 years, 50 to 59 years, ≥60 years). In addition, women with a history of atypical ductal hyperplasia had an 86% risk reduction, and women with a history of LCIS had a 56% risk reduction. Finally, the benefit was seen across all subgroups specified according to family history of breast cancer. Tamoxifen selectively reduced the incidence of estrogen receptor–positive tumors; estrogen receptor–negative tumors developed at an equal rate in the tamoxifen and placebo groups. No evidence was shown of a cardioprotective effect of tamoxifen in this trial, but the number of osteoporosis-related fractures was reduced in the tamoxifen-treated cohort. Tamoxifen increased the risk of developing stage I endometrial cancer (risk ratio of 2.53).

More recently, a landmark study was published that compared tamoxifen to raloxifene as a preventative agent in postmenopausal women with breast cancer. Raloxifene, a drug that is primarily used in prevention of osteoporosis, had been shown in prior studies to decrease the incidence of breast cancers. The NSABP study of tamoxifen and raloxifene was a prospective, double-blind, randomized clinical trial.[54] There were 19,747 postmenopausal women of mean age 58.5 years with increased 5-year breast cancer risk. Patients were randomized to oral tamoxifen (20 mg per day) or raloxifene (60 mg per day) for 5 years. There were 163 cases of invasive breast cancer in women assigned to tamoxifen and 168 in those assigned to raloxifene, which was not significantly different between the two arms. The main benefit of raloxifene was in toxicity. There were 36 cases of uterine cancer with tamoxifen and 23 with raloxifene. No differences were found for other invasive cancer sites, for ischemic heart disease events, or for stroke. Thromboembolic events also occurred less often in the raloxifene group. The number of osteoporotic fractures in the groups was similar and there were fewer cataract surgeries with raloxifene. There was no difference in the total number of deaths (101 vs. 96 for tamoxifen vs. raloxifene) or in causes of death. It appears from this study that raloxifene is as effective as tamoxifen in reducing the risk of invasive breast cancer and has a lower risk of thromboembolic events. Of note there were slightly more noninvasive cancers in the raloxifene group, but that was not statistically significant

A comparison of the tamoxifen P-1, P-2, and other tamoxifen prevention trials is outlined in Table 56.4.[48,49–50,51–52,55,56]

Prophylactic Surgery

An alternative strategy used to prevent breast cancer development is prophylactic surgical intervention. Hartmann et al.[57] analyzed outcomes in women with a family history of breast cancer who underwent bilateral prophylactic mastectomy at the Mayo Clinic between 1960 and 1993. With a median follow-up time of 14 years, only 4 of the 639 treated patients developed breast cancer. According to the Gail model, 37.4 cases of breast cancer would have been expected to develop in this population, so the prophylactic surgery resulted in an 89.5% risk reduction ($P < .001$).[57]

Breast cancer prevention strategies will continue to be a dynamic area of preclinical and clinical research.

NATURAL HISTORY AND ORIGINS

All forms of breast cancer are believed to develop as a consequence of unregulated cell growth and the development of phenotypic changes such as the ability to invade, recruit a new blood supply, and metastasize. These changes in phenotypes are secondary to the development of aberrations in genetic pathways. Some of these aberrations are inherited (germline mutations), whereas others develop during the life of a breast cell (somatic mutations). It is currently believed that most breast cancer is a consequence of a series of somatic mutations. As previously noted, only 20% to 25% of breast cancer patients have a history of breast cancer in a first-degree relative. However, it is possible that some women without a first-degree relative with breast cancer still inherit a genetic background that predisposes to breast cancer. These mutations may be insufficient to cause breast cancer unless accompanied by other mutations and, therefore, would be predicted to have a low penetrance. Historically, it has been much more difficult to discover low-penetrance mutations than to discover germline mutations that result in an autosomal dominant pattern of breast cancer development. However, with newer molecular techniques, such as DNA-array assays, the identification of low-penetrance predisposing mutations may be more feasible.

Left untreated, breast cancer can have a variable clinical course. A classic article by Bloom et al.[58] outlined the natural history of breast cancer patients, seen between 1805 and 1933, not treated by surgery or irradiation, 250 of whom had a pathologic diagnosis of cancer. There were no patients with stage I disease, 2.4% with stage II, 23% with stage III, and 74% with stage IV. Survival in the untreated group was 3.6% compared with an overall survival of 34% in patients treated with radical or modified radical mastectomy with or without radiation.

Concepts regarding the natural history of breast cancer have undergone great evolution over the past 100 years, with a profound impact on the management of these patients. The Halsted[59] model was based on an orderly progression to the regional lymph nodes and from there to distant metastatic sites. Later, Keynes[60] and Crile et al.[61] suggested that breast cancer is a systemic disease and that extensive surgery to achieve local tumor control was not as important as originally believed. This alternative hypothesis was fully demonstrated in both laboratory and clinical studies by Fisher,[62] who advanced the concept that breast cancer, as a systemic process involving host–tumor interactions, would not show substantial effects on survival with variations in locoregional treatment. A third hypothesis put forward by Hellman[63] considers breast cancer as a heterogeneous disease with a spectrum extending from a tumor that remains localized throughout its course to one that disseminates systemically, even when detected as a small lesion, suggesting that metastases are a function of tumor growth and progression factors.

The growth rate of a tumor in the breast is thought to be constant from the date of origin. Using estimates of doubling time, it would take an average of approximately 5 years for a tumor to reach palpable size, and those lesions with slower doubling time would have an even longer latent period.[64]

The most common site of origin of breast cancer is the upper outer quadrant (38.5%), followed by the central area (29%), the upper inner quadrant (14.2%), the lower outer quadrant (8.8%), and the lower inner quadrant (5%).[64] These rates correlate with the amount of breast tissue in the various quadrants. Cancer is somewhat more common in the left than in the right breast and may appear in both breasts simultaneously (1% to 2%). As noted above, women with a history of breast cancer have a 10% to 15% risk of developing a new primary in the contralateral breast.

As the cancer grows, it travels along the ducts, eventually breaking through the basement membrane of the duct, invading adjacent lobules, ducts, fascial strands, and the mammary fat, spreading through the breast lymphatics and into the peripheral lymphatics. The tumor can grow through the wall of blood vessels, spread into the deep lymphatics of the dermis, and eventually produce edema of the skin (*peau d'orange*), which usually indicates that the superficial as well as the deep lymphatics are involved. Skin dimpling can be caused by involvement of Cooper's ligament. Ulceration and infiltration of overlying skin, which may develop late in the course of the disease, are usually preceded by fixation and localized redness of the skin over the tumor and are less frequently seen because of the current emphasis on screening and early diagnosis.[64]

Axillary Spread

A common route of spread of breast carcinoma is first through the axillary lymph nodes, with the incidence increasing with larger tumors. Depending on mode of detection, tumor size, histology, and other clinical or pathological factors, between 10% and 40% of newly diagnosed stage T1 and T2 breast cancers have pathologic evidence of axillary nodal metastases. Voogd et al.[65] assessed 7,680 patients with documented invasive breast cancer; of 5,125 patients known to have clinically negative lymph nodes who underwent axillary dissection, 1,748 (34%) had positive lymph nodes at pathologic examination. Univariate analysis showed that lymph node metastases were associated with tumors larger than 1 cm ($P = .001$), moderate or poorly differentiated nuclear grade ($P = .005$), high fraction of cells in the growth phase (S phase) of the cell cycle ($P = .041$), presence of lymphatic vascular invasion ($P < .001$), and age younger than 60 years ($P = .01$).

Multiple studies have shown a strong relation between primary tumor size and axillary nodal involvement.[66–70] Even patients with T1a and T1b disease have significant nodal involvement. Mustafa et al.[71] noted an overall frequency of axillary lymph node metastases in T1a and T1b lesions of 16%; integrating age, tumor size, and grade predicted the frequency of nodal metastases. Overall, patients with all three poor prognostic indicators had a 34% incidence of nodal involvement, and those with no poor prognostic factors had a ≤7% probability of nodal metastases. Gann et al.[72] reviewed 18,025 patients with a diagnosis of breast carcinoma from the American College of Surgeons database. On multivariate analysis, the following factors were independently associated with a greater likelihood of one or more positive lymph nodes: larger tumor size, young age, African American or Hispanic race, outer-half tumor location, poor or moderate differentiation, aneuploidy, and infiltrating ductal histologic type.

Although up to 30% to 40% of T1 or T2 clinically node-negative breast cancers may have pathologically involved lymph nodes, data from NSABP-04 suggest that less than half of clinically negative but pathologically positive axilla will experience a clinical relapse in the axilla.[73] In this study, operable breast cancer patients, who were primarily diagnosed with palpable breast tumors in the premammography era, were randomized to one of three arms: simple mastectomy without axillary dissection, simple mastectomy with axillary dissection, or simple mastectomy with comprehensive chest wall and regional nodal irradiation. In the arm undergoing axillary dissection, nodal positivity was approximately 40%. Nodal control was excellent (>97%) in this arm as well as in the arm treated with radiation. In the simple mastectomy arm, where no nodal treatment by radiation or dissection was administered, the axillary failure rate was approximately 20%. Assuming equal distribution among the arms, it is presumed the pathological involvement was approximately 40%, indicating that less than half of those with pathological involvement eventually failed clinically.

Internal Mammary Spread

Metastases to the internal mammary nodes (IMNs) are correlated with tumor size, are more frequent from medial half and central lesions, and occur more frequently when there is axillary node involvement (Table 56.5).[74] A table with more detailed analysis of internal mammary involvement by tumor size, location and number of positive nodes is found in

TABLE 56.5 INTERNAL MAMMARY NODE INVOLVEMENT RELATED TO LOCATION OF PRIMARY TUMOR AND TO AXILLARY NODE INVOLVEMENT[a]

	Location of Primary Tumor				
Axillary Involvement	*Upper Inner Quadrant (%)*	*Lower Inner Quadrant (%)*	*Central (%)*	*Upper Outer Quadrant (%)*	*Lower Outer Quadrant (%)*
Axilla not involved	20/143 (14)	2/36 (6)	5/76 (7)	7/170 (4)	2/40 (5)
Axilla involved	47/105 (45)	18/25 (72)	65/140 (46)	47/212 (22)	10/53 (19)
Total	**67/248 (27)**	**20/61 (33)**	**70/216 (32)**	**54/382 (14)**	**12/93 (13)**

[a]Number of patients with internal mammary node involvement/total number of patients.

From Handley RS. Carcinoma of the breast. *Ann R Coll Surg Engl* 1975;57:59–66. Copyright The Royal College of Surgeons of England. Reproduced with permission.

Chapter 57. Veronesi et al.[75] found that, among women with tumors larger than 2 cm who were younger than 40 years of age and had positive axillary nodes, there was a 41% risk of having positive IMNs on IMN dissection; the corresponding risk for patients of that age with negative nodes was 16%. Sugg et al.[76] reviewed 286 patients with breast cancer who underwent IMN dissection. Positive IMNs were associated with primary tumor size (P <.0001) and the number of positive axillary nodes (P <.0001), but not with age or primary tumor location. Patients who had positive IMNs (25% of all patients) had a significantly worse overall 20-year disease-free survival rate than did patients with negative IMNs (P <.0001). Clinical failure of the internal mammary nodes is extremely rare, despite the evidence of pathological involvement from these studies. Most studies looking at nodal failure patterns report failure in the internal mammary region of <1%.[77–81]

Supraclavicular Spread

Spread to supraclavicular lymph nodes usually follows involvement in the high axillary lymph nodes or IMNs depending on the location of the primary lesion. Chen et al.[82] reviewed 2,658 patients with invasive breast cancer who underwent surgery and adjuvant therapy. With a median follow-up period of 39 months, supraclavicular lymph node metastasis developed in 113 (4.3%). Young age (≤40 years), tumor size >3 cm, angiolymphatic invasion, negative estrogen-receptor status, and DNA synthetic phase fraction >4% were significant for predicting supraclavicular metastasis on univariate analysis. Three predictive factors were significant after multivariate analysis: high histologic grade, more than four positive nodes, and axillary level II or III involved nodes. In patients with axillary level I involved nodes and four or fewer positive nodes, the incidence of supraclavicular lymph node metastasis was 4.4%, but if axillary level III was involved, it increased to 15.1%.

Clinical failure in the supraclavicular fossa is relatively rare in patients with early-stage breast cancer and is dependent on the degree of axillary involvement. For patients with no or minimal nodal involvement (less than three involved axillary nodes), supraclavicular failure is extremely rare. In an analysis of 691 patients with zero to three nodes involved undergoing breast-conserving surgery and radiation therapy to tangential fields only without regional nodal irradiation, Galper et al.[78] reported failure in the supraclavicular fossa in 1.3% of patients.

Several studies have demonstrated that the failure rate in supraclavicular nodes, left untreated, may be as high as 20% in patients with advanced disease or more than four lymph nodes involved.[83–86,87] In a cohort of 1,031 patients with operable breast cancer treated with mastectomy and level I or II node dissection plus adriamycin-based chemotherapy, but no radiation, Strom et al.[87] reported failure in the supraclavicular fossa was 8% at 10 years. Predictors of supraclavicular failure included four or more involved nodes and gross extranodal extension. In these subgroups, supraclavicular failure ranged from 14% to 19%. Radiation to the supraclavicular fossa in these higher risk patients results in high local control rates, with isolated supraclavicular failures occurring in less that 1% of prophylactically treated nodes.

Systemic Spread

Using monoclonal antibodies to epithelial cytokeratins or tumor-associated cell membrane glycoproteins, carcinoma cells can be detected on cytologic bone marrow (or lymph node) preparations. Braun et al.[88] combined patient data from nine studies involving 4,703 patients with stage I, II, or III breast cancer. Micrometastasis was detected in 30.6% of the patients. With a median follow-up of 5.2 years, patients with bone marrow micrometastasis had larger tumors and tumors with a higher histologic grade and more often had lymph node metastases and hormone receptor–negative tumors, compared with those without bone marrow micrometastasis. The presence of micrometastasis was a significant prognostic factor for poorer overall survival (RR 2.15; P <.001), breast cancer–specific survival (RR 2.44; P <.001), disease-free survival (RR 2.13), and distant disease-free survival (RR 2.33; P <.001 for all outcomes measures). In multivariable analysis, micrometastasis was an independent predictor of a poor outcome.

Local Control and Systemic Metastasis

Patients treated for breast cancer are at risk for local-regional failure, as well as systemic metastasis. It is evident from the available literature that optimizing local control can impact systemic metastasis and survival, and similarly, systemic therapy can impact local control.[89–91,92] Integration of systemic therapy with radiation will be discussed in detail later, but numerous studies have clearly demonstrated a significant improvement in local control with the use of radiation therapy and systemic therapy (both cytotoxic and hormonal) compared with radiation therapy without the use of systemic therapy.[92–97] Appropriate integration of both local and systemic treatments through a multidisciplinary approach is thus essential to optimize outcome. Although there is some overlap, prognostic factors for local-regional control and systemic metastasis often differ.

For patients with early-stage invasive breast cancer, even with appropriate systemic therapy, development of metastasis can vary from <5% in women with T1a disease and favorable histology, to >40% for women with T2 tumors and pathologically involved lymph nodes. Similarly, local-regional failure rates can vary from <5% to over 40% depending on local treatment and prognostic factors for local failure.[93–95,96,98–100,101–102]

The impact of local control on systemic metastasis in breast cancer as well as other malignancies has been the subject of considerable debate and controversy. Although the benefits of local control with respect to cosmesis and quality of life are apparent, the independent effect of local control on systemic disease and survival has been questioned. Several studies have identified local control as an independent predictor of disease-free or overall survival.[99,102,103–106] Fisher et al.,[103] in an analysis of patients treated in NSABP protocol B-06, concluded that ipsilateral breast tumor recurrence was a harbinger, but not a cause, of distant metastases. Although mastectomy or breast irradiation after lumpectomy prevented expression of the marker (breast relapse), neither lowered the risk of distant metastases, which was determined by a host of prognostic factors.

More recent meta-analyses, however, have demonstrated a small but significant impact of local control on systemic metastasis and overall survival.[89,90] A meta-analysis of randomized trials by Vinh-Hung and Verschraegen[90] comparing breast-conserving surgery without radiation to breast-conserving surgery with radiation confirms an approximate threefold reduction in local relapse with radiation therapy and an 8.6% improvement in mortality in the radiated cohorts.

One of the most convincing and authoritative studies related to this subject is the recent analysis of the Early Breast Cancer Trialists Collaborative Group (EBCTCG).[89] In this analysis, over 42,000 women were enrolled in 78 randomized trials that compared 24 types of local treatment (radiotherapy vs. no radiotherapy, more vs. less surgery, or more surgery vs. radiotherapy). The EBCTCG attempted to relate the effect on local control to breast cancer mortality by grouping studies into whether the 5-year local relapse risk difference between the two comparisons of local therapy exceeded 10%. In those comparisons in which the difference in 5-year local recurrence risk was <10%, there was no impact on 15-year breast cancer mortality. However, there were 25,000 women enrolled in trials in whom the comparisons involved >10% differences in local control. In those studies, the difference in local recurrence risks at 5 years were 7% versus 26%, and the 15-year mortality risks were 44.6% versus 49.5% (P <.00001). Figure 56.6 summarizes the results of this meta-analysis with respect to the impact of radiation on breast cancer mortality in both breast conservation and

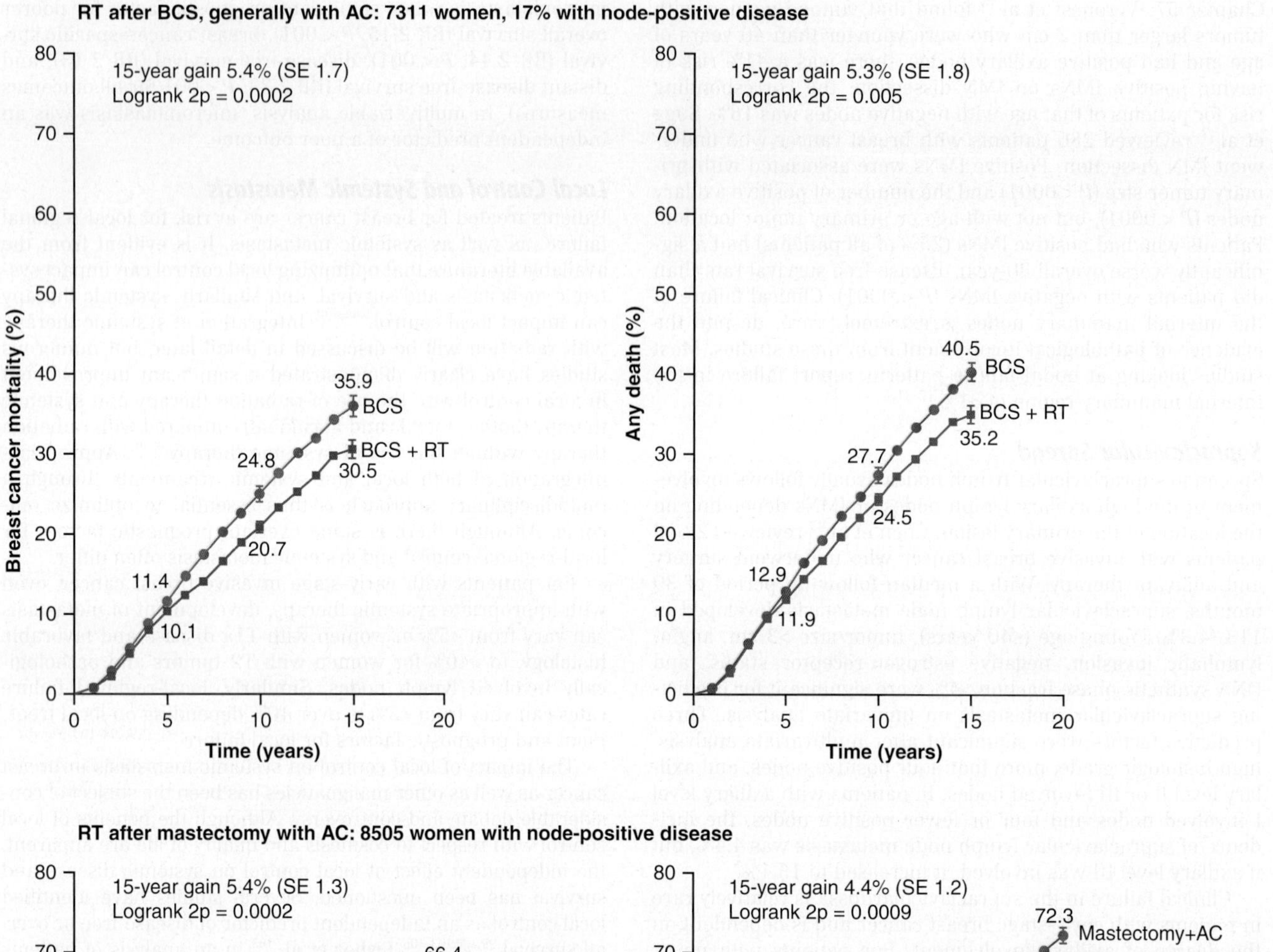

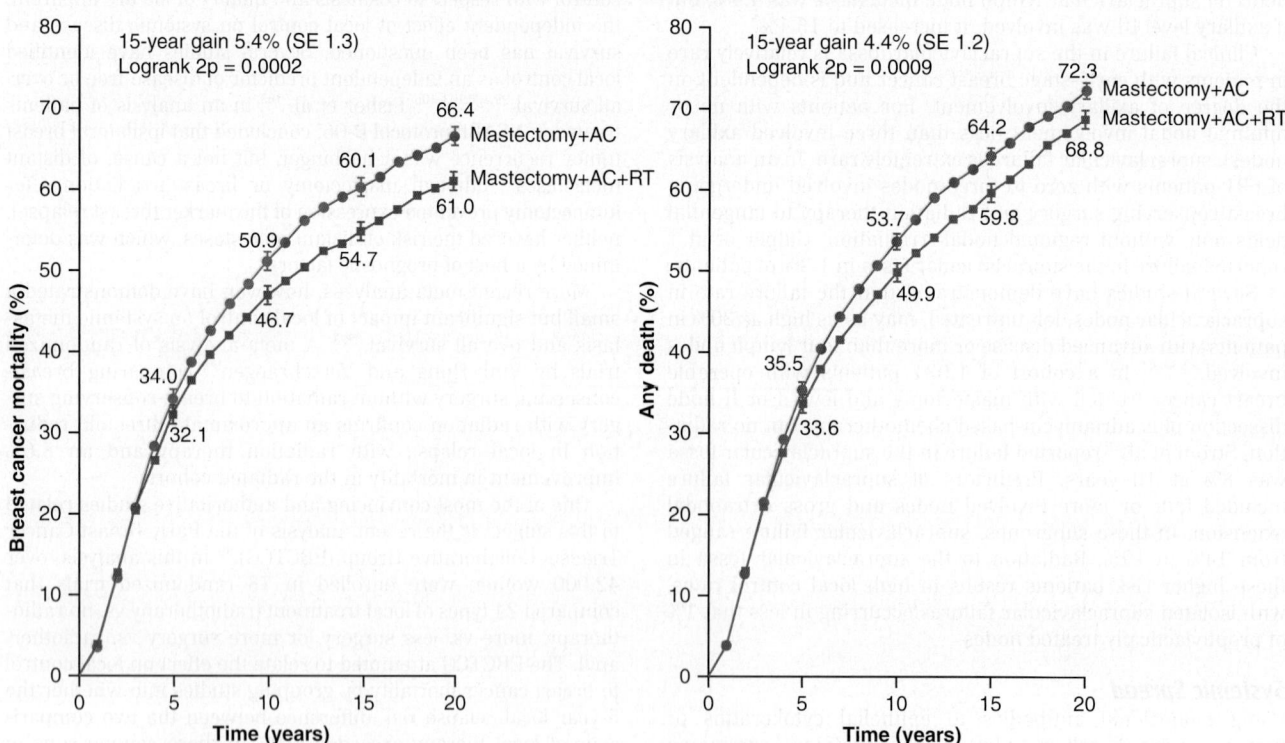

FIGURE 56.6. Effect of radiotherapy on breast cancer mortality and on all-cause mortality after breast-conservation surgery or after mastectomy with axillary clearance: 15-year or 20-year probabilities. (From Clarke M, Collins R, Darby S, et al. Effects of radiotherapy and of differences in the extent of surgery for early breast cancer on local recurrence and 15-year survival: an overview of the randomised trials. *Lancet* 2005;366: 2087–2106, with permission from Elsevier.)

TABLE 56.6 BREAST CANCER SCREENING GUIDELINES

Age Group	ACS (2003)	ACR (2000)	NCI (2002)
20–39	BSE optional; CBE every 3 years.	Monthly BSE; CBE every 3 years	No recommendation.
40–49	Annual mammography and CBE from 40 years.	Annual mammography and CBE from 40 years.	Mammography every 1–2 years.
>49	Annual mammography and CBE as long as a woman is in reasonably good health.	Annual mammography and monthly CBE as long as a woman is in reasonably good health.	Mammography every 1–2 years.
At increased risk	Consult with their doctors about the benefits and limitations of starting mammography screening earlier, having additional tests (i.e., breast ultrasound and MRI), or having more frequent exams.	Consult with their physician about beginning mammography screening before age 40.	Seek expert medical advice about whether they should begin screening before age 40 and the frequency of screening.

ACR, American College of Radiology; ACS, American College of Surgeons; BSE, breast self-examination; CBE, clinical breast examination; NCI, National Cancer Institute; MRI, magnetic resonancy imaging.

following mastectomy. An update from the EBCTCG focused on 10,801 women enrolled in 17 randomized trials of radiotherapy versus no radiotherapy after breast-conserving surgery and relates the absolute reduction in 15-year risk of breast cancer death to the absolute reduction in 10-year recurrence risk.[107] Overall, radiotherapy reduced the 10-year risk of any first recurrence from 35.0% to 19.3% (*P* <00001) and reduced the 15-year risk of breast cancer death from 25.2% to 21.4% (*P* <0001). In women with pN+ disease (n = 1,050), radiotherapy reduced the 10-year recurrence risk from 63.7% to 42.5% (*P* <00001) and the 15-year risk of breast cancer death from 51.3% to 42.8% (*P* = 01). Overall, about one breast cancer death was avoided by year 15 for every four recurrences avoided by year 10.

CLINICAL PRESENTATION

The majority of patients with T1 or T2 breast cancers present with a painless or slightly tender breast mass or have an abnormal screening mammogram. Patients with more advanced tumors may have breast tenderness, skin changes, bloody nipple discharge, or occasionally change in the shape and size of the breast. Rarely, patients may present with axillary lymphadenopathy or even distant metastasis. As noted previously, however, depending on tumor size, method of detection, and pathologic factors associated with the primary tumor, up to 30% to 40% of women with a clinically negative axilla may harbor subclinical pathologically involved axillary nodes.

The impact of delays in evaluation or treatment on the survival of patients with breast cancer is controversial. Richards et al.,[108] in a review of 2,964 patients, found 942 (32%) who had symptoms for 12 or more weeks before their first hospital visit. Locally advanced or metastatic disease was detected in 32% of patients with delays compared with 10% of patients with intervals of <12 weeks between the onset of symptoms and hospital referral (*P* <.0001). Multivariate analysis showed that a longer duration of symptoms had a highly significant adverse influence on survival, but this was no longer evident when tumor size and stage were included in the model. Olivotto et al.[109] found that delays in diagnosis of 6 to 12 months led to increased risk of larger tumor size and more lymph node metastases compared with patients diagnosed within 4 to 12 weeks of an abnormal screening mammogram result.

SCREENING IN BREAST CANCER

Mammography

Screening mammography has resulted in a shift in both the incidence and stage of patients presenting with breast cancer. In a simplified model described by Harris et al.,[110] for every 1,000 screening mammograms, 80 women (8%) will be recalled for additional diagnostic imaging, 10 (1%) will require tissue diagnosis, and of those undergoing biopsy only 3 (0.3%) will have a malignancy.

There is a large body of evidence that early detection by mammography, followed by appropriate local, regional, and systemic treatment, is associated with reduced breast cancer mortality rates for women 50 years of age and older.[111–114] Although it remains an active area of debate, several authors agree that screening mammography in women 40 to 49 years of age may reduce mortality from breast cancer,[25,112–118] and mammographic screening beginning at age 40 is encouraged in the majority of published guidelines (Table 56.6). The reader is referred elsewhere for an extensive discussion of screening mammography studies.[112–114] Selected series will be briefly discussed here and a summary of the classic screening mammography trials is summarized in Table 56.7.[70,119–124,125,126–127] Collectively, these studies

TABLE 56.7 RANDOMIZED CONTROLLED TRIALS OF BREAST CANCER SCREENING

Trial (Reference)	Screening Protocol: Approach	Screening Protocol: Frequency	Population: Age Group	Population: Invited	Population: Control	Follow-up (Years)	Relative Risk (95% Confidence Interval)
HIP, 1963–1969 (129)	2 VMM 1 CBE	24 mo 4 rounds	40–49	14,432	14,701	18	0.77 (0.53–1.11)
			50–64	16,568	16,299	18	0.80 (0.59–1.08)
Malmo, 1976–1990 (120)	1 or 2 VMM	18–24 mo 5 rounds	45–49	13,528	12,242	12.7	0.64 (0.45–0.89)
			50–69	17,134	17,165	9	0.86 (0.64–1.16)
Kopparberg, 1977–1985 (125)	1 VMM	24 mo 4 rounds	40–49	9,650	5,009	20	0.76 (0.42–1.40)
			50–74	28,939	13,551	20	1.06 (0.65–1.76)
Ostergotland, 1977–1985 (125)	1 VMM	24 mo 4 rounds	40–49	10,240	10,441	20	0.52 (0.39–0.70)
			50–74	28,229	26,830	20	0.81 (0.64–1.03)
Edinburgh, 1979–1988 (119)	1 or 2 VMM	24 mo 4 rounds	45–49	11,755	10,641	14	0.83 (0.54–1.27)
	CBE (initial)		50–64	11,245	12,359	10	0.85 (0.62–1.15)
CNBSS-1, 1980–1987 (127)	2 VMM CBE	12 mo 4–5 rounds	40–49	25,214	25,216	11–16	1.07 (0.75–1.52)
CNBSS-2, 1980–1987 (122)	2 VMM CBE	12 mo 4–5 rounds	50–59	19,711	19,694	13	1.02 (0.78–1.33)
Stockholm, 1981–1985 (121)	1 VMM	28 mo 2 rounds	40–49	14,185	7,985	11.4	1.01 (0.51–2.02)
			50–64	25,815	12,015	7	0.65 (0.4–1.08)
Gothenburg (126)	2 V MM	18 mo 5 rounds	39–49	11,724	14,217	12	0.56 (0.32–0.98)
			50–59	9,276	16,394	13	0.91 (0.61–1.36)

1 VMM, one-view mammography of each breast; 2 VMM, two-view mammography of each breast; CBE, clinical breast examination.

demonstrate a decrease in mortality and migration of patients from later stages of disease to earlier stages of disease with the use of screening mammography.[25,112–118,120,123,124]

Sixteen-year results are available from the Health Insurance Plan study, which involved two systematically selected, randomly sampled groups of approximately 31,000 women aged 40 to 64 years who were offered screening examinations.[128,129] Compared with the control group, which was observed and monitored, the mortality rate was reduced by approximately one-third in screened women 50 to 59 years of age. The survival difference between mammography-only and clinical examination–only cases appeared in years 7 to 10 after diagnosis. Although the greatest difference in mortality between screened and control group was detected in women 50 to 59 years of age when they entered the study, the differences are in favor of the study group at all ages.

Tabár et al.[123–124,125] demonstrated the benefit from mammography screening in two Swedish counties. In the group of women 20 to 69 years of age, there were 6,807 diagnosed with breast carcinoma over a 29-year period and 1,863 breast carcinoma deaths. The mortality rate from breast carcinoma diagnosed in women 40 to 69 years of age who were screened during the screening period (1988–1996) declined by 63% (RR 0.37) compared with the breast carcinoma mortality rate during the period when no screening was available (1968–1977). The reduction in mortality rate observed during the service-screening period, adjusted for selection bias, was 48%. No significant change in breast carcinoma mortality rate was observed over the three periods in women who did not undergo screening. In a recent long-term update, there has remained a highly significant reduction in breast cancer mortality in women invited to screening (RR 0.69; 95% CI: 0.56 to 0.84; $P = .001$). At 29 years of follow-up there was a reduction in 1 death for every 414 women undergoing screening for 7 years. They conclude that the group invited to screening resulted in a highly significant decrease in breast cancer specific mortality.[130]

In contrast to the above, a Canadian study revealed that in women aged 50 to 59 years, the addition of annual mammography screening to physical examination had no effect on breast cancer mortality. Miller et al.[122] reported a study of 39,405 women (aged 50 to 59 years) randomly assigned to one of two study groups. By December 31, 1993, 622 invasive and 71 *in situ* breast cancers were observed in the mammography plus physical examination group, compared with 610 and 16, respectively, in the physical examination–only group. At 13-year follow-up, the number of deaths from breast cancer was 107 in the mammography plus physical examination group and 105 in the physical examination–only group. The results of the Canadian study may be due to the unbalanced allocation of women with advanced cancers (large tumors, four or more positive nodes) to the screened group, the poor quality of the mammography in the trial, and an insufficient sample size.[116,131]

Screening in Women Under Age 50

Although the majority of studies clearly support the impact of screening mammography on mortality in women over 50 years of age, data on screening younger women are more conflicting. Frisell and Lidbrink[121] presented updated data on breast cancer mortality for women younger than age 50 years from the Stockholm Mammographic Screening Trial. Approximately 40,000 women aged 40 to 64 years (14,842 aged 40 to 49 years) were randomized to a trial of breast cancer screening by single-view mammography alone; 20,000 women (7,103 aged 40 to 49) were randomized to a control group. In the 40- to 49-year age group, 24 and 12 breast cancer deaths were found in the study and control groups, respectively, after 11.4 years of follow-up. The relative risk of breast cancer death in screened versus nonscreened women was 1.08 (95% CI, 0.54 to 2.17).

A large trial was conducted in the United Kingdom involving 45,841 women aged 45 to 64 years who were offered annual screening by clinical examination and mammography; 63,636 were taught breast self-examination, and 127,117, for whom no extra services were provided, constituted a control population.[132] After 16 years of follow-up, the breast cancer mortality rate was 27% lower in the two screening centers combined than in the four comparison centers. A 35% decrease in mortality rate was observed in mammographically screened women in all cohorts aged 45 to 64 years at entry. There was no evidence of less benefit in women aged 45 to 49 years at initial screening compared with a reduction of 25% in women aged 50 to 74 years.[133]

In a Swedish study evaluating women in the 40- to 49-year age group, Hellquist et al.[134] reported 803 breast cancer deaths in a screening study group compared with 1,238 deaths in a control group after 16 years of follow-up. The estimated relative risk for women screened in this younger population was 0.74 (95% CI, 0.66 to 0.83), concluding that screening mammography reduced the breast cancer mortality rate in this younger population.

In the United States, screening mammography beginning at age 40 years is recommended for the general population.[135] For some women at high risk for development of breast cancer, annual screening may be started at an earlier age. These women include those with a personal history of breast cancer, those who have had therapeutic radiation to the breast area especially for Hodgkin lymphoma, *BRCA*-positive women, women with a family history of a first-degree relative with breast cancer at a young age, and women with a biopsy diagnosis of LCIS or atypical ductal hyperplasia.

Despite some conflicting data in the large randomized trials and meta-analyses summarized above, there is general agreement that screening mammography can have a significant impact on stage of presentation of disease and breast cancer mortality. Given the incidence of breast cancer, promotion of screening for breast cancer is a major public health issue. The National Cancer Institute, American Cancer Society, and the American College of Radiology recommend a baseline mammogram at the age of 35 years (30 years in high-risk groups).[135,136] Repeat examinations should be carried out every 2 years beginning at 40 years of age. In women older than 50 years, mammograms should be performed annually. Risk factor information could be used to determine the optimal frequency of screening. The U.S. Preventive Services Task Force (USPSTF) published a controversial recommendation statement on screening breast cancer in the general population.[137] It recommended against routine screening mammography in women aged 40 to 49 years and recommended biennial screening mammography for women between the ages of 50 and 74 years. The group felt there was insufficient evidence to assess the additional benefits and harms of screening mammography in women 75 years or older. The Canadian Task Force on Preventive Health Care recently recommended against any screening in women aged 40 to 49 years and only every 2 or 3 years in women aged 50 to 74.[138]

This issue continues to be controversial and recommendations of the American Cancer Society and American College of Radiology have not been modified.

Digital Versus Screen Film Mammography

There has been increased utilization of digital mammography for screening. This technology utilizes a special detector capable of transforming x-ray images into electronic digital image. Advantages include no film processing, faster image acquisition, and less call-backs due to the ability to manipulate the image digitally. Results of a large-scale American College of Radiology Imaging Network (ACRIN) trial of 49,000 women revealed that digital mammography overall was at least as good as screen film mammography, but was superior in younger women and women with dense breasts.[139] Given the potential efficiencies and advantages of digital mammography, most centers are moving in this direction.

Magnetic Resonance Imaging Screening

The role of MRI screening is rapidly evolving. MRI is unlikely to replace mammography for screening of the general population and is not recommended by the USPSTF in their statement on breast cancer screening.[137,140,141] However, its use in screening high-risk populations has recently been supported in several studies. In a prospective study by Lehman et al.,[142] MRI detected otherwise occult contralateral breast cancers in 4% of women with a recent diagnosis of unilateral breast cancer. In 103 women with unilateral breast cancer, MRI detected four contralateral breast cancers, while mammography detected none. The increased yield was associated with 12% of women having an MRI recommended biopsy, resulting in a 33% positive predictive value.

For women at high risk for breast cancer due to strong family history or positive *BRCA1/BRCA2* status, the standard screening techniques of breast self-examination, clinical breast examination, and mammography may be suboptimal. Nearly half of the cancers in this population are detected by physical examination between routine radiographic surveillance. In this population, increased breast density and rapid proliferative rates likely contribute to the relative insensitivity of mammography. Although MRI has not yet been shown to impact mortality, the sensitivity of MRI over mammography, clinical examination, and ultrasound in this high-risk population has been demonstrated in several studies.[143–146,147] In a surveillance study, 236 women with *BRCA1/BRCA2* mutations underwent one to three annual screenings with breast examination, mammography, MRI, and ultrasound. Of 22 cancers detected, 17 (77%) were detected by MRI, 8 (36%) by mammography, 7 (33%) by ultrasound, and 2 (9.1%) by breast examination. All four screening modalities combined had a sensitivity of 95%, which compared favorably to the 45% sensitivity for mammography and breast examination alone.[145]

In a landmark study by Kriege et al.,[147] 1,909 eligible women (cumulative lifetime risk of breast cancer of 15% or more) at high risk for familial breast cancer, including 358 carriers of germ-line mutations, were screened with an annual MRI and mammography. Within a median follow-up period of 2.9 years, the screening program yielded 51 tumors. The sensitivity of clinical breast examination, mammography, and MRI for detecting invasive breast cancer was 17.9%, 33.3%, and 79.5%, respectively, and the specificity was 98.1%, 95.0%, and 89.8%, respectively. The overall discriminating capacity of MRI was significantly better than that of mammography ($P < .05$). From this study it appears that MRI is more sensitive than mammography in detecting tumors in women at high risk for familial breast cancer.

In a multicenter cohort study of 649 high-risk women aged 35 to 49 with a strong family history and high probability of *BRCA1/BRCA2* mutation, the Magnetic Resonance Imaging in Breast Screening Study detected a total of 35 cancers and found that contrast-enhanced MRI was more effective then mammography in detecting cancers, particularly for women with *BRCA1* cancers.[148]

Ultrasound Screening

Ultrasound is a complementary tool to mammography for the diagnosis of breast cancer. As with MRI, it is unlikely to replace mammography for screening the general population. The NCCN recommends ultrasound for those women presenting with a dominant mass or asymmetric thickening or nodularity.[47,149] In a randomized trial of ultrasound and mammography of 2,809 women with dense breasts from ACRIN, adding a single screening ultrasound yielded an additional 1.1 to 7.2 additional cancers found in high-risk women but substantially increased the number of false positives.[150] The role of screening ultrasound and selection of patients remains controversial and will likely continue to evolve over the next decade.

Screening by Physical Examination

Two studies have evaluated the effectiveness of screening by breast self-examination alone, the United Kingdom and the Canadian trials. Using Breast Cancer Registry data, Constanza and Foster[151,152] found fewer deaths from breast cancer (14% vs. 26%) and improved estimated 5-year survival rates (75% vs. 59%) among women who reported performing breast self-examination compared with those who did not. In the Breast Cancer Detection Demonstration Project, the estimated overall sensitivity of breast self-examination in detecting breast cancer was 26%, compared with 75% for the combination of clinical breast examination and mammography.[153]

Clinical breast examination and self-examination may be complementary to mammography, perhaps detecting interval cancers in the 10% to 12% of cancers not visualized by mammography. Although it is evident that clinical screening is not as sensitive as mammography, the combination of clinical examination and mammography appears to yield optimal results in early detection.

DIAGNOSIS AND WORKUP

The workup of a patient with a breast mass, including complete clinical and family history, is summarized in Table 56.8. The patient should be examined both sitting up and lying down (to confirm masses felt on the sitting-up examination and to detect lesions deeper in the breast or against the chest wall). Careful inspection of both breasts should be made, including size, form, and symmetry, changes in pigmentation, scaling or discharge from the nipple, and dilated veins or edema of the skin in a nonpregnant patient. The location, size, consistency, tenderness, and mobility of the palpable tumor should be recorded. It is useful to draw and photograph the projection of any suspect or palpable masses on the skin of the breast or nodal areas.

In addition to examination of the breast, careful evaluation of the axilla and supraclavicular node areas is mandatory. The number, consistency, tenderness, mobility or fixation, and size of lymph nodes should be noted. Clinically node-negative patients have pathologic involvement in 10% to 40% of cases (depending on primary tumor size), whereas no pathologic

TABLE 56.8 DIAGNOSTIC WORKUP FOR CARCINOMA OF THE BREAST, STAGE T1 AND T2

General
History with emphasis on presenting symptoms, menstrual status, parity, family history of cancer, other risk factors
Physical examination with emphasis on breast, axilla, supraclavicular area, abdomen,
Special Tests
Biopsy (core biopsy directed by physical examination, ultrasound, or mammography as indicated, or needle localization)
Radiologic Studies
Before biopsy
Mammography/ultrasonography
Chest radiographs
Magnetic resonance imaging of breast (selected cases)
After positive biopsy
Bone scan (when clinically indicated, for stage II or III disease or elevated serum alkaline phosphatase levels)
Computed tomography of chest, abdomen and pelvis for stage II or III disease and/or abnormal liver function tests
Laboratory Studies
Complete blood cell count, blood chemistry
Urinalysis
Other Studies
Hormone receptor status (ER, PR)
HER2/neu status
Consider genetic counseling/*BRCA* testing in selected cases

evidence of tumor is found in 25% to 30% of patients with clinically palpable axillary nodes.

Examination of the abdomen for liver enlargement and evaluation for bony pain are also essential. Finally, a complete pelvic examination should be part of the overall evaluation of the patient, if not recently performed by the patient's other physicians.

Laboratory studies include a complete blood count and chemistry profile, including liver function tests (e.g., aspartate aminotransferase, alanine aminotransferase, lactate dehydrogenase, bilirubin).

Imaging in Breast Cancer Diagnosis and Workup

Routine radiographic studies include chest radiography and bilateral mammograms. As clinically indicated, these may be supplemented by CT scanning, MRI, or positron emission tomography (PET) scans, bone scans, and plain radiographs of *symptomatic* bones, if clinically warranted.

Mammography

Mammography remains the most critical component of diagnostic imaging in breast cancer patients, and bilateral mammograms should be performed routinely in the workup of the breast cancer patient. The BIRADS (Breast Imaging Reporting and Data System) classification system, outlined in Table 56.9 has been widely adopted in classifying mammograms with respect to appropriate follow-up and intervention.[154]

The radiation oncologist should be familiar with the difference between diagnostic and screening mammography, because a majority of conservatively treated breast cancer patients will have undergone diagnostic mammography prior to treatment, as well as in follow-up. Screening mammography refers to routine mammographic images in asymptomatic women and consists of two views: craniocaudal and mediolateral oblique of each breast. Diagnostic mammography is used to characterize abnormalities detected at screening or in women with palpable masses, employs additional magnification views, and is generally done with the radiologist present to determine the need for additional views or follow-up studies. Following breast conservation, most patients will undergo diagnostic mammograms, as additional images are often needed to rule out suspicious findings in the previously radiated breast. Some mammographers recommend reverting to screening studies after several years of stable mammography in the conservatively managed breast cancer patient.

Kopans et al.[155] reviewed the advantages and disadvantages of diagnostic imaging techniques for evaluation of patients with breast cancer. Classically, breast carcinoma is seen as an ill-defined mass that may have spiculated margins (Fig. 56.7), although rarely cancers may also be seen with a knobby, lobulated, or even a smooth contour (ultrasonography may distinguish them from cystic masses). Architectural distortion of the breast tissue may be present. The appearance of linear, radiated, or spiculated changes around a central focus should always be considered suspect for carcinoma. The tumor may be hidden by dense parenchyma; review of previous mammogram compression views and sometimes ultrasonograms is very important in detecting subtle interval changes in the appearance of the breast.[110]

Calcifications can be associated with either benign or malignant conditions of the breast. However, calcifications associated with malignant tumors are typically 100 to 300 μm in size and are rod like, tubular, branching, or punctate. Clusters of microcalcifications (more than five) are suggestive of intraductal disease, and in nonpalpable lesions needle localization aids in the diagnosis (Fig. 56.8). For patients undergoing biopsy of a suspicious mass or calcifications, about 30% will yield a diagnosis of malignancy.[110] The average sensitivity of mammography is approximately 90% (60% to 95%) and the specificity is 94% (50% to 98%). The positive predictive value is approximately 8% to 14% for screened patients, but is significantly higher for patients with symptoms or palpable masses.[155] If microcalcifications were initially present, radiographs of the surgical specimen and postlumpectomy mammography are important to rule out residual disease for patients considering breast-conservation therapy.[156] Lally et al.[157] reported on 114 patients with calcifications on mammography diagnosed with breast cancer. Of these cases, 75 breasts at risk had no residual suspicious calcifications and proceeded to radiotherapy without further surgery or mammography. Thirty-six breasts at risk proceeded to radiation with either known suspicious calcifications or with nondocumented removal of calcifications after another excision. Of the 36 breasts there were 7 local failures

TABLE 56.9 AMERICAN COLLEGE OF RADIOLOGY BIRADS ASSESSMENT CATEGORIES: MAMMOGRAPHY

Complete Final Assessment Categories	
Category 1 Negative	There is nothing to comment on. The breasts are symmetric and no masses, architectural disturbances, or suspect calcifications are present.
Category 2 Benign finding	This is also a negative mammogram, but the interpreter may wish to describe a finding. Involuting, calcified fibroadenomas, multiple secretory calcifications, fat-containing lesions such as oil cysts, lipomas, galactoceles, and mixed-density hamartomas all have characteristic appearances, and may be labeled with confidence. The interpreter might wish to describe intramammary lymph nodes, implants, and the like, while still concluding that there is no mammographic evidence of malignancy.
Category 3 Probably benign finding–short-interval follow-up suggested	A finding placed in this category should have a very high probability of being benign. It is not expected to change over the follow-up interval, but the radiologist would prefer to establish its stability. Data are becoming available that shed light on the efficacy of short-interval follow-up. At present, most approaches are intuitive. These will likely undergo future modification as more data accrue as to the validity of an approach, the interval required, and the type of findings that should be followed.
Category 4 Suspicious abnormality–biopsy should be considered	These are lesions that do not have the characteristic morphologies of breast cancer but have a definite probability of being malignant. The radiologist has sufficient concern to urge a biopsy. If possible, the relevant probabilities should be cited so that the patient and her physician can make the decision on the ultimate course of action.
Category 5 Highly suggestive of malignancy–appropriate action should be taken	These lesions have a high probability of being cancer.
Category 0 Need additional imaging evaluation	Finding for which additional imaging evaluation is needed. This is almost always used in a screening situation and should rarely be used after a full imaging workup. A recommendation for additional imaging evaluation includes the use of spot compression, magnification, special mammographic views, ultrasound, and so forth.

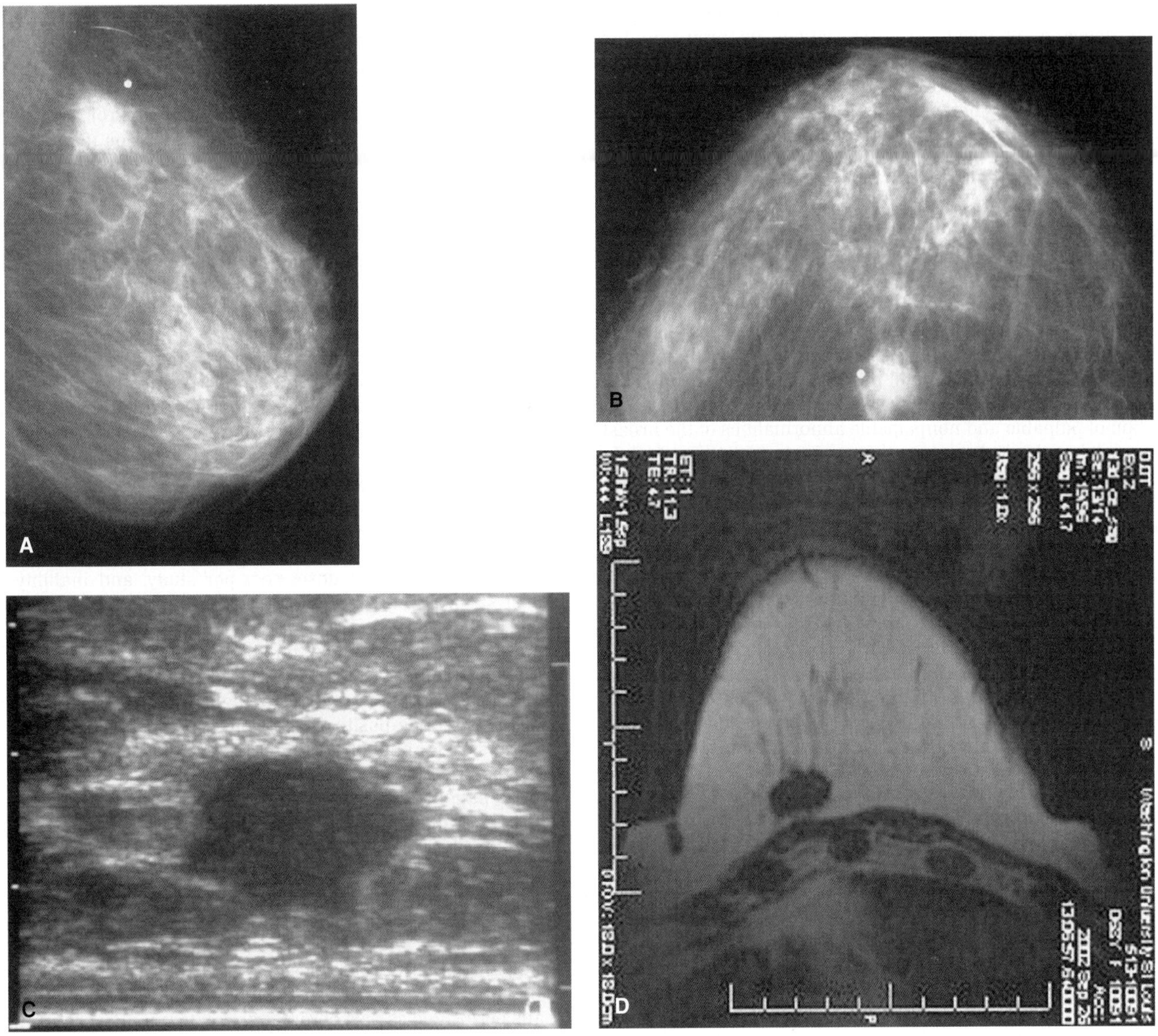

FIGURE 56.7. Medial-lateral **(A)** and cephalad-caudal **(B)** views of mammogram depicting a 1-cm mass with stellate margins deeply located in the upper quadrant of the left breast, histologically proven to be an invasive ductal carcinoma. Example of ultrasonogram of the breast showing a hypoechoic mass with "shadowing" deeper to the lesion, characteristic of invasive carcinoma **(C)**. T1-weighted magnetic resonance image of the breast demonstrating a mass that proved to be an invasive carcinoma **(D)**.

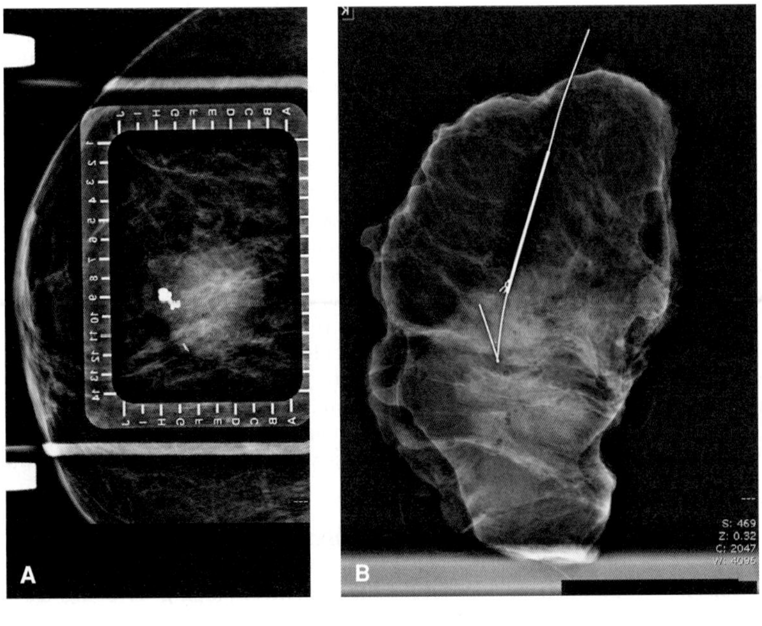

FIGURE 56.8. A: Mammogram demonstrating microcalcifications in the central portion of the breast with needle localization in place. **B:** Radiograph showing microcalcifications in the central portion of the wide excisional biopsy specimen. Pathologic diagnosis was intraductal carcinoma. Postlumpectomy mammogram showed no residual calcifications in the breast. Patient was treated with breast-conservation surgery and irradiation years ago and remains tumor free.

and 1 regional failure. Of 34 breasts that underwent re-excision after detection of suspicious calcifications by preirradiation mammography, 20 (59%) were found to have residual disease. Patients with documented removal of suspicious calcifications were found to have better local control than patients without documented removal. In addition, the presence of calcifications on a preirradiation mammogram was associated with a high probability of detecting residual disease.

Ultrasound

Ultrasound can be a useful tool to complement physical examination and mammography in the diagnosis and treatment of breast cancer. Its use as a screening tool is limited and is the focus of ongoing investigations, as previously noted. Ultrasonography has a reported sensitivity of 73% and specificity of 95%. It is very helpful in differentiating cysts from solid tumors, and its primary use is the identification and characterization of palpable and nonpalpable abnormalities of the breast detected by physical examination or mammography.[110,158] In the evaluation of a palpable mass in 420 patients, if both mammography and ultrasound are negative, Soo et al.[159] reported the negative predictive value to be >99%. This was confirmed in a larger study of 3,516 patients from the Netherlands reported by Flobbe et al.[160]

In addition to complementing physical examination and mammography in diagnosis, ultrasound is often used as a guide for interventional procedures. Ultrasound-guided core biopsies are routinely performed in the diagnosis of breast cancer and have been shown to be more cost-effective than stereotactic biopsy. Ultrasound can also be used for fine-needle aspiration biopsies, cyst aspirations, presurgical localizations, and evaluation of breast tissue surrounding implants.

Magnetic Resonance Imaging

Although controversial for routine use, the use of MRI to supplement mammography in breast cancer diagnosis and treatment is rapidly increasing (see Fig. 56.7). In a review of MRI in the management of breast cancer, Hylton[161] summarized the potential for the current use of MRI: to complement mammography in screening; for differential diagnosis of questionable findings on physical examination, mammography, and ultrasound; and assessment of response in the neoadjuvant treatment of breast cancers. The NCCN recommends breast MRI for those women with early-stage disease whose breasts cannot be imaged adequately by mammography and ultrasound, those women who receive neoadjuvant chemotherapy to assess response to occult breast cancer, or women with genetic mutations leading to a higher risk of bilateral or contralateral breast cancer.[47,162,163]

In a retrospective study of MRI in the management of 441 women with breast cancer, Upponi and Warren[164] reported the indications for MRI studies were diagnostic in 176, monitoring chemotherapy in 126, and study of MRI screening for breast cancer in 139. MRI results were confusing or incorrect in 6% of the diagnostic group, 13% of the chemotherapy group, and 9% of the screening group. The authors report that MRI resulted in an increase in confidence or change in clinical plan in 46% of the diagnostic group, 72% of the chemotherapy group, and 80% of the screening group. In 44 of 283 of these, MRI caused a beneficial change in the clinical plan based on conventional radiology.

Esserman et al.[165] reported that MRI successfully detected cancer in 55 of 58 cases. There were two false-positive and two false-negative results, including a nonsignificant enhancement of one lesion. The anatomic extent of disease was correctly identified in 98% of cases by MRI but in only 55% by mammography. The utility of MRI as an adjunct to mammography in problematic cases was investigated by Lee et al.[166] In 86 lesions with equivocal findings on mammography, positive findings were seen in 38 on MRI. Of these, 26 corresponded to areas of mammographic abnormalities. The remaining 12 sites were in areas where no abnormality had been suspected on mammography. Biopsies were performed on all 38 positive sites, and 10 (26%) were found to be malignant.

MRI has a clear role in the evaluation of patients who present with axillary metastasis with no evidence of a primary tumor in the breast by physical examination or mammography. In an analysis from Memorial Sloan-Kettering Cancer Center, Buchanan et al.[167] reported on 55 patients who presented with axillary adenopathy without evidence of distant disease. MRI revealed suspicious lesions in 76% (42 of 55). In 62% (26 of 42), the MRI finding proved to be the occult primary tumor, of whom 58% (15 of 26) were candidates for breast conservation. MRI did not identify the primary tumor in 25 women. Of these 25, 12 underwent mastectomy, and cancer was found in 4 of these 12. The authors concluded that breast MRI detects mammographically occult cancer in half of women with axillary metastases and is a valuable tool for patients with occult primary breast cancer.

Computed Tomography

There is no established role for CT scans in routine staging of patients with early-stage breast cancer. The need for iodine contrast material to differentiate benign from malignant conditions, high radiation dose, cost per study, and inability to detect small lesions precludes the use of CT for initial evaluation, except under special circumstances. Most patients with node-negative breast cancer do not need to undergo routine CT scans for staging, because the yield is exceeding low. A small percentage of women with very high-risk node-negative disease or with node-positive disease may be upstaged by routine CT scans and, although the yield is low, it is common practice to CT stage high-risk node-negative and node-positive breast cancer patients. At present, the NCCN guidelines on breast cancer recommend an abdominopelvic CT if abnormal lab values or physical examination are present or if the patient is deemed as a stage IIIA (T3N1M0) or greater.[47,168,169]

Many women undergoing breast-conserving surgery and radiation do have CT scans as part of radiation therapy treatment planning. Without the use of contrast and specific diagnostic imaging protocols, these scans should not be considered as part of a staging procedure. In a study of 153 extended CT scans performed as part of radiation treatment, however, Mehta and Goffinet[170] reported 11% revealed unexpected abnormalities, most of which were non-malignant. Only 2 of the 153 were found to have occult disease resulting in a change in stage.

Bone Scans

Routine bone scan at the time of initial treatment of stage I and II breast cancer is of limited value and should be reserved for patients with bone pain.[171] In patients with stage I disease, the incidence of abnormalities on bone scan is approximately 2%, but a greater incidence of abnormalities is found in stages II (10%) and III (>20%).[172] In a group of 7,604 patients who had bone scans, of over 20,000 women operated for breast cancer in Denmark, approximately 5% had abnormal study results.[173] The incidence of abnormal scan results was greater in patients older than 60 years (8%) than in the younger group (3%), most likely because of the many benign bone and joint disorders frequently seen in older women.

Koizumi et al.[174] reviewed records from 5,538 patients with breast cancer. The overall incidence of metastasis to bone was 2.13% (0% in patients with stage 0, 0.08% in stage I, 1.09% in stage II, 9.96% in stage III, and 34.04% in stage IV). Bone scans are more commonly recommended in patients with stage II larger tumors (>3 cm), aggressive histopathologic features, and in stage III or IV cancer.

Positron Emission Tomography Scanning

PET using ^{18}F-labeled fluorodeoxyglucose (FDG) scanning, although not a routine component of staging, is being used more frequently in breast cancer. Its application in patients on initial presentation with early-stage disease has not been established. However, its potential role in patients with metastatic, advanced, and local-regional relapse of disease is rapidly evolving. At present, the NCCN guidelines recommend against routine PET scans in patients with stage 0 to IIIA disease but does state that it may be useful patients with locally advanced disease or in situations where standard imaging results are equivocal or suspicious.[47,168,169]

In an analysis of PET scanning in 165 patients from British Columbia, Weir et al.[175] concluded that there are two clinical situations in which PET appears to be particularly valuable. The first is in the evaluation of patients who are suspected of having a tumor recurrence. The other is in identifying patients with multifocal or distant sites of malignancy who otherwise appear to have an isolated, potentially curable, local-regional recurrence.

Schirrmeister et al.[176] also evaluated FDG-PET scanning and compared it prospectively with standard staging procedures within 2 weeks before surgery in 117 women who had palpable breast tumors or lesions suggestive of cancer on mammography or ultrasonography. On biopsy, 89 patients were determined to have breast cancer and 28 benign tumors. For interpreting results as being breast cancer, FDG-PET had a sensitivity of 93%, a specificity of 78%, an accuracy of 89%, a positive predictive value of 92%, and a negative predictive value of 96%. In detecting multifocal lesions, FDG-PET was twice as sensitive (63%) as the combination of mammography and ultrasonography (32%). Distant metastases in three patients were missed with the standard staging procedures but detected with FDG-PET. Because FDG-PET had a false-negative rate of 20% for detection of lymph node metastases, this imaging method cannot replace histologic evaluation of axillary nodes.

Summary of Imaging for Breast Cancer

All women should undergo history and physical examination, with mammography and liver function tests. Ultrasound or MRI may be useful in selected cases to complement mammography. For women who have operable disease with normal liver function tests, surgical staging of the breast and node sampling is performed. For low-risk patients, no further staging is required. For women with more advanced disease and those being considered for neoadjuvant chemotherapy, preoperative staging would routinely include a bone scan, chest x-ray and CT, or abdominal ultrasound. PET scanning may be considered in selected cases.

Pathologic Studies

Histopathologic diagnosis may be obtained by fine-needle aspiration of cystic or solid masses or biopsies of solid masses; any fluid aspirated from the breast should be examined for malignant cells. Fine-needle aspiration of the breast is a simple, low-cost, accurate diagnostic technique that has been used for many years in Europe and is gaining increasing acceptance in the United States.[177,178] A potential limitation of fine-needle aspiration is that it provides cytology and no tissue architecture. Therefore, while the presence of malignant cells can be detected, cytology from fine-needle aspiration cannot conclusively differentiate invasive from noninvasive disease. However, for lesions that are palpable or easily visualized on ultrasound, this method results in rapid and efficient diagnosis.

Stereotactic core needle biopsy is increasingly used to obtain a histologic diagnosis with high accuracy, particularly in small breast lesions.[179] In 6,152 lesions sampled at multiple institutions, 817 (13.3%) showed infiltrating breast cancer, 167 (2.7%) showed intermediate or high-grade DCIS, and 213 (3.5%) showed atypical hyperplasia or low-grade DCIS. Complete agreement between the core biopsy and subsequent histologic sections was reached in 89.7% of lesions and partial agreement in 9.2%. Clinically significant complications occurred in only 6 of 3,765 cases (0.2%) for which follow-up was available.

Breast biopsy of any suspicious mass is mandatory. The biopsy usually can be done using local anesthesia; the patient should be informed of the nature of the lesion to allow for her greater participation in therapeutic decisions. There has been no evidence that delay in treatment up to 2 weeks after biopsy worsens prognosis.[180]

In nonpalpable lesions, needle localization and radiographic techniques are necessary to identify the tissue to be removed. Failure to remove the mammographic abnormality has been reported in 2% to 8% of patients undergoing needle localization.[181] The localizing wires should be left in place in the specimen and a radiograph obtained to ensure that the area of abnormality has been adequately excised. If the specimen radiograph does not document complete tumor removal, an immediate re-excision of the area at the tip of the wire should be carried out. However, specimen mammography may be of questionable benefit in the management or outcome of most patients undergoing image-guided, needle-localized breast biopsies. Bimston et al.[182] reviewed 164 patients who underwent 165 needle/dye-localized breast biopsies for suspect mammographic abnormalities. In only three (1.8%) cases did the patient clearly benefit from specimen mammography; in no patient was a malignant neoplasm missed.

If there is any question, particularly in patients with microcalcifications, a postbiopsy mammogram should be obtained to determine the completeness of tumor excision.[110] The surgeon should prepare (orient) the specimen accordingly, and the margins of the resected breast tissue should be identified and inked before processing. The pathologist should be made aware of the nature of the lesion for appropriate processing of the specimen.[183] Radiation oncologists should be familiar with the implications of the diagnostic procedures for carcinoma of the breast as active participants in a breast preservation therapeutic approach.

In the United States, estrogen-receptor (ER) and progesterone-receptor (PR) assays are routinely done in the for patients with breast cancer; these parameters are correlated with prognosis and tumor response to chemotherapeutic and hormonal agents.[184,185] Immunohistochemical techniques are commonly employed and correlate well with other hormonal-receptor assays. Cellular assays measure the growth fraction (S-phase fraction [SPF]) of tumors, either by thymidine-labeling index (TLI) or flow cytometry methods, and other tumor markers have prognostic implications, sometimes independent of tumor stage and hormone-receptor status.[186,187] *HER-2/neu* assay is being done routinely because overexpression is associated with poor prognosis, and these patients are currently being offered adjuvant therapy directed at *HER2/neu*.[188,189] *HER2/neu* analysis by fluorescent in situ hybridization techniques has recently evolved as the standard for determining response to therapy directed at the *HER2/neu* oncogene.[188,189]

Staging

Two staging systems are widely used for breast cancer: the American Joint Committee on Cancer (AJCC) (Table 56.10) and the Union Internationale Contre le Cancer systems.[190,191] Major changes made in the seventh edition of the *AJCC Cancer Staging Manual* include:[190]

1. Identified specific imaging modalities that can be used to estimate clinical tumor size, including mammography, ultrasound, and magnetic resonance imaging (MRI).
2. Maintained that the term "inflammatory carcinoma" be restricted to cases with typical skin changes involving a third or more of the skin of the breast. While the histologic presence of invasive carcinoma invading dermal lymphatics is supportive of the diagnosis, it is not required, nor is

TABLE 56.10 AMERICAN JOINT COMMITTEE ON CANCER STAGING OF BREAST CANCER

Primary Tumor (T)	
Definitions for classifying the primary tumor (T) are the same for clinical and for pathologic classification. If the measurement is made by physical examination, the examiner will use the major headings (T1, T2, or T3). If other measurements, such as mammographic or pathologic measurements, are used, the subsets of T1 can be used. Tumors should be measured to the nearest 0.1-cm increment.	
TX	Primary tumor cannot be assessed
T0	No evidence of primary tumor
Tis	Carcinoma *in situ*
Tis (DCIS)	Ductal carcinoma *in situ*
Tis (LCIS)	Lobular carcinoma *in situ*
Tis (Paget's)	Paget's disease of the nipple with no tumor
Note: Paget's disease associated with a tumor is classified according to the size of the tumor.	
T1	Tumor 2 cm or less in greatest dimension
T1mic	Microinvasion 0.1 cm or less in greatest dimension
T1a	Tumor more than 0.1 cm but not more than 0.5 cm in greatest dimension
T1b	Tumor more than 0.5 cm but not more than 1 cm in greatest dimension
T1c	More than 1 cm but not more than 2 cm in greatest dimension
T2	Tumor more than 2 cm but not more than 5 cm in greatest dimension
T3	Tumor more than 5 cm in greatest dimension
T4	Tumor of any size with direct extension to chest wall[f] or skin, only as described below
T4a	Extension to chest wall, not including pectoralis muscle
T4b	Edema (including *peau d'orange*) or ulceration of the skin of the breast or satellite skin nodules confined to the same breast
T4c	Both (T4a and T4b)
T4d	Inflammatory carcinoma
Regional Lymph Nodes (N)	
NX	Regional lymph nodes cannot be assessed (e.g., previously removed)
N0	No regional lymph node metastasis
N1	Metastasis to movable ipsilateral axillary lymph node(s)
N2	Metastasis to ipsilateral axillary lymph node(s) fixed or matted, or in clinically apparent[a] ipsilateral internal mammary nodes in the absence of clinically evident axillary lymph node metastasis
N2a	Metastasis in ipsilateral axillary lymph nodes fixed to one another (matted) or to other structures
N2b	Metastasis only in clinically apparent[a] ipsilateral internal mammary nodes and in the absence of clinically evident axillary lymph node metastasis
N3	Metastasis to ipsilateral mammary lymph node(s) with or without axillary lymph node involvement, or in clinically apparent[a] ipsilateral internal mammary lymph node(s) and in the presence of clinically evident axillary lymph node metastasis; or metastasis in ipsilateral supraclavicular lymph node(s) with or without axillary or internal mammary lymph node involvement
N3a	Metastasis in ipsilateral infraclavicular lymph node(s)
N3b	Metastasis in ipsilateral internal mammary lymph node(s) and axillary lymph node(s)
N3c	Metastasis in ipsilateral supraclavicular lymph node(s)
Pathologic Classification (pN)	
*p*NX	Regional lymph nodes cannot be assessed (e.g., previously removed or not removed for pathologic study)
*P*N0	No regional lymph node metastasis histologically, no additional examination for isolated tumor cells (ITC)
Note: ITC are defined as single tumor cells or small cell clusters not greater than 0.2 mm, usually detected only by immunohistochemical (IHC) or molecular methods but which may be verified on hematoxylin-and-eosin stains. ITCs do not usually show evidence of malignant activity (e.g., proliferation or stromal reaction).	
p N0(i–)	No regional lymph node metastasis histologically, negative IHC
p N0(i+)	No regional lymph node metastasis histologically, positive IHC, IHC cluster no greater than 0.2 mm
p N0(mol–)	No regional lymph node metastasis histologically, negative molecular findings [reverse transcriptase polymerase chain reaction (RT-PCR)]
p N0(mol+)	No regional lymph node metastasis histologically, positive molecular findings (RT-PCR)
p N1	Metastasis in 1 to 3 axillary lymph nodes, and/or in internal mammary nodes with microscopic disease detected by sentinel lymph node dissection but not clinically apparent[b]
p N1mi	Micrometastasis (greater than 0.2 mm, none larger than 2.0 mm)
p N1a	Metastasis in 1 to 3 axillary lymph nodes, one larger than 2.0 mm
p N1b	Metastasis in internal mammary nodes with microscopic disease detected by sentinel node dissection but not clinically apparent[c]
p N1c	Metastasis in 1 to 3 axillary lymph nodes and in internal mammary lymph nodes with microscopic disease detected by sentinel lymph node dissection but not clinically apparent[c] (If associated with greater than 3 positive axillary lymph nodes, the internal mammary nodes are classified as pN3b to reflect increased tumor burden.)
p N2	Metastasis in 4 to 9 axillary lymph nodes, or in clinically apparent[b] internal mammary lymph nodes in the absence of axillary lymph node metastasis
p N2a	Metastasis in 4 to 9 axillary lymph nodes (at least one tumor deposit greater than 2.0 mm)
p N2b	Metastasis in clinically apparent[b] internal mammary lymph nodes in the absence of axillary lymph node metastasis
p N3	Metastasis in 10 or more axillary lymph nodes, or in infraclavicular lymph nodes, or in clinically apparent[b] ipsilateral internal mammary lymph nodes in the presence of 1 or more positive axillary lymph nodes; or in more than 3 axillary lymph nodes with clinically negative microscopic metastasis in internal mammary lymph nodes or in ipsilateral supraclavicular lymph nodes
p N3a	Metastasis in 10 or more axillary lymph nodes (at least one tumor deposit greater than 2.0 mm), or metastasis to the infraclavicular lymph nodes
p N3b	Metastasis in clinically apparent[b] ipsilateral internal mammary lymph nodes in the presence of 1 or more positive axillary lymph nodes; or in more than 3 axillary lymph nodes and in internal mammary lymph nodes with microscopic disease detected by sentinel lymph node dissection but not clinically apparent[c]
p N3c	Metastasis in ipsilateral supraclavicular lymph nodes
Distant Metastasis (M)	
MX Distant metastasis cannot be assessed	
M0 No distant metastasis	
M1 Distant metastasis	

[a]Clinically apparent is defined as detected by imaging studies (excluding lymphoscintigraphy) or by clinical examination or grossly visible pathologically.

[b]Clinically apparent is defined as detected by imaging studies (excluding lymphoscintigraphy) or by clinical examination.

[c]Not clinically apparent is defined as not detected by imaging studies (excluding lymphoscintigraphy) or by clinical examination.

Used with the permission of the American Joint Committee on Cancer (AJCC), Chicago, Illinois. The original source for this material is the *AJCC Cancer Staging Manual,* Seventh Edition (2010) published by Springer Science and Business Media LLC, www.springer.com.

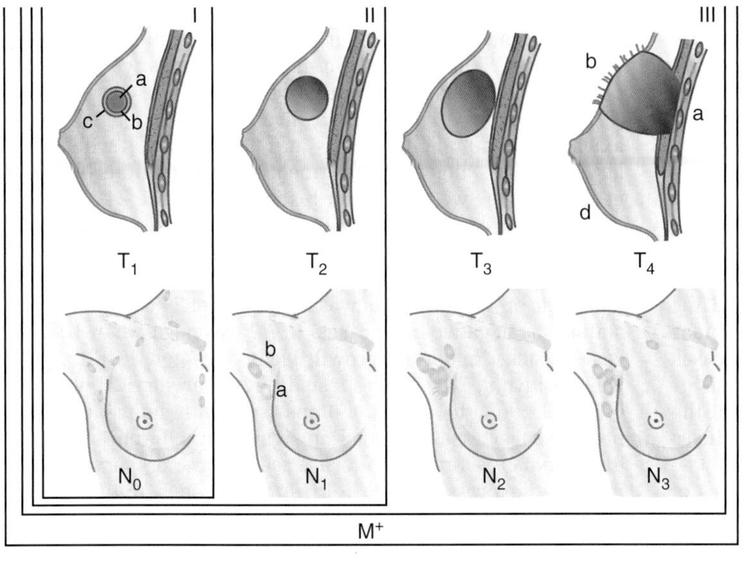

FIGURE 56.9. Clinical staging of carcinoma of the breast. Stages, in part, reflect curability by locoregional treatment modalities prognostically (surgery and radiation therapy). The equivalence of T and N categories are as follows: T2 = N1, T3 = N2, T4 = N3. The American Joint Committee on Cancer and Union Internationale Contre le Cancer classification systems use similar categories and stages. (From Langmuir VK, Poulter CA, Qazi R, et al. Breast cancer. In: Rubin P, ed. *Clinical oncology: a multidisciplinary approach for physicians and students,* 7th ed. Philadelphia: WB Saunders, 1993, with permission.)

dermal lymphatic invasion without typical clinical findings sufficient for a diagnosis of inflammatory breast cancer.

3. Classification of isolated tumor cell clusters and single cells is more stringent. Small clusters of cells not greater than 0.2 millimeters, or nonconfluent or nearly confluent clusters of cells not exceeding 200 cells in a single histologic lymph node cross section are classified as isolated tumor cells.
4. Stage I breast tumors have been subdivided into Stage IA and Stage IB; Stage IB includes small tumors (T1) with exclusively micrometastases in lymph nodes (N1mi).
5. Created new M0(i+) category, defined by presence of either disseminated tumor cells detectable in bone marrow or circulating tumor cells or found incidentally in other tissues (such as ovaries removed prophylactically) if not exceeding 0.2 millimeters. However, this category does not change the stage grouping. Assuming that they do not have clinically and/or radiographically detectable metastases, patients with M0(i+) are staged according to T and N.

The current AJCC staging for breast cancer does not include in the calculation of tumor size additional tumor found at the time of re-excision; this may result in understaging and undertreatment of patients with breast cancer.[192] The Columbia staging system is important both historically and because it clearly identifies prognostic factors affecting operability.[64] Figure 56.9 depicts the various clinical stages according to tumor and nodal characteristics.

Pathologic Classification

The World Health Organization has classified proliferative conditions and tumors of the breast into the following categories: benign mammary dysplasias, benign or apparently benign tumors, carcinoma, sarcoma, carcinosarcoma, and unclassified tumors.[193] The AJCC has developed the alternative system shown in Table 56.11.[190]

Numerous detailed reports and monographs describe the pathologic features and clinical implications of carcinoma of the breast, which are reviewed elsewhere.[110,194–197] The radiation oncologist should be familiar with the histologic characteristics of breast cancer because many of them affect prognosis and may have important therapeutic implications. Brief descriptions of several types of carcinoma of the breast follow.

Microinvasive carcinoma is defined as "the extension of cancer cells beyond the basement membrane into the adjacent tissues with no focus more than 0.1 cm in greatest dimension." Lesions that fulfill this definition are staged as T1mic, a subset of T1 breast cancer. The AJCC staging manual further states that "when there are multiple foci of microinvasion, the size of only the largest focus is used to classify the microinvasion" and that the sizes of the individual foci should not be added together. They also state that "the prognosis of microinvasive carcinoma is generally thought to be quite favorable, although the clinical impact of multifocal microinvasive disease is not well understood at this time." Widely varying definitions of microinvasion have been used, and some differ substantially from that offered here.[190]

Invasive (infiltrating) ductal carcinoma is the most common type of breast cancer, comprising more than 50% of all cases. It appears as solid cords or groups of ductal tumor cells varying in size and cytoplasmic content and degree of differentiation.[198] Necrosis is rare, but lymphatic invasion may be present. An associated *in situ* component is frequently seen.

Tubular carcinoma is composed of tubular structures typically lined by a single layer of well-differentiated epithelium. The tubular cells simulate those of normal ducts or ductules,

TABLE 56.11 AMERICAN JOINT COMMITTEE ON CANCER HISTOPATHOLOGIC CLASSIFICATION OF BREAST TUMORS

In Situ Carcinomas
NOS
Intraductal (*in situ*)
Paget's disease and intraductal
Invasive Carcinomas
NOS
Ductal
Inflammatory
Medullary, NOS
Medullary with lymphoid stroma
Mucinous
Papillary (predominantly micropapillary pattern)
Tubular
Lobular
Paget's disease
Undifferentiated
Squamous cell
Adenoid cystic
Secretory
Cribriform

NOS, not otherwise specified.

Used with the permission of the American Joint Committee on Cancer (AJCC), Chicago, Illinois. The original source for this material is the AJCC Cancer Staging Manual, Seventh Edition (2010) published by Springer Science and Business Media LLC, www.springer.com.

are arranged in multiglandular cribriform or adenocystic configurations, and are frequently associated with other *in situ* carcinomas of the breast.[199] Tubular carcinomas have a nonaggressive growth pattern, with an excellent prognosis. A meta-analysis of 680 women showed an overall frequency of nodal metastasis of 13.8%.[200] In view of the low incidence of axillary node metastases at presentation (7%) in low-risk tubular carcinoma of the breast (≤1 cm), some have advocated that axillary dissection may be omitted. In a retrospective review of 73 cases of tubular carcinoma, Sullivan et al.[201] reported treatment with conservative surgery (CS) plus radiation therapy (RT) in 67%, CS without RT in 18%, and mastectomy in 15%. The published literature of 529 conservatively treated tubular carcinomas was reviewed along with the 62 conservative cases from their series. No patients developed distant metastasis or died from disease. Local failure occurred in three (4%) of the cases. The literature review showed that adjuvant RT reduces local failure following CS for tubular carcinoma.

Medullary carcinoma is composed of cords and masses of large cells with reticular pleomorphic nuclei containing prominent nucleoli. There is a scant fibrous stroma, but lymphoid infiltrate is prominent. These tumors are microscopically and grossly well circumscribed. Prognosis, in general, is better than for other tumors. These tumors are more frequently seen in younger women and are commonly associated with patients with *BRCA1* mutations.[202]

Lobular invasive carcinoma may be interspersed with; the cells appear singly or in small clusters in a targetoid or single-file pattern. Some scirrhous carcinomas probably are invasive lobular lesions; these tumors tend to be aggressive and multicentric and are prone to development of distant metastases. Du Toit et al.[203] reported five subtypes of lobular carcinomas in 171 cases and observed a 12-year actuarial survival rate of 100% for the tubulolobular subtype but of only 47% for the solid variant. Two other characteristics of invasive lobular carcinoma (ILC) is that it is often "mammographically silent," meaning its detection or the full appreciation of extent of disease is often not visualized mammographically. Invasive lobular cancers are much more commonly ER-positive than invasive ductal carcinoma. Infiltrating pleomorphic lobular carcinoma, an aggressive variant of ILC, was described in 38 cases; 29% of the specimens demonstrated signet ring cells.[204]

Mucinous carcinoma, also called mucoid or colloid carcinoma, has been observed in older women with relatively long duration of symptoms.[205] It is more likely to be devoid of a cellular reaction; necrosis and lymphatic invasion are very rare. It is slowly growing with a pushing border and has a low frequency of axillary lymph node metastasis. Survival is appreciably better than with invasive ductal carcinoma.[206] Anan et al.[207] evaluated 76 patients with mucinous carcinoma (52 pure type and 24 mixed type). The incidence of lymphatic vessel invasion (4%) and nodal involvement (4%) was lower in pure mucinous carcinoma than in mixed carcinoma (P <.05). No nodal involvement occurred in patients with pure mucinous carcinoma <3 cm in diameter.

Adenocystic carcinoma is rarely found in the breast. Histologic features and clinical behavior are similar to its counterpart in the salivary gland and the upper respiratory tract.[208] In 28 patients, only 1 had axillary node metastases; 22 were treated with mastectomy and 6 with local excision (with breast irradiation in 5). With a median follow-up of 7 years, there were no local recurrences; the 5-year disease-free survival rate was 95%.[209]

Invasive micropapillary carcinoma of the breast is characterized by growth of tumor cell clusters in prominent clear spaces resembling dilated angiolymphatic vessels. Nasser et al.[210] reported on 83 invasive micropapillary carcinomas; the mean tumor size was 4 cm, 22% invaded skin, 58% were poorly differentiated, and 71% were ER-positive. Axillary node metastases were present in 77% of cases and were typically multiple (51% had three or more positive). Forty-six percent of the patients died from their disease (mean interval to death, 36 months). Skin involvement and nodal status were the only parameters predictive of poor survival (P = .01).

Metaplastic carcinoma is relatively rare. Park et al.[211] noted axillary lymph node metastasis in 6 (40%) of 15 in whom axillary node dissection was performed. A recent analysis by Beatty et al.,[212] of the Swedish Cancer Institute, identified 24 cases that were compared with typical breast cancer cases matched for age, date of diagnosis, stage, and ER, PR, and *HER2* status. The mean metaplastic primary tumor diameter was 2.5 cm. The histologic or nuclear grade was high in 21 of 24 cases. ER or PR status was negative in all cases. *HER2* was negative in 10 of 11 cases tested. Epidermal growth factor receptor (EGFR; *HER1*) was positive in 7 of 7 cases tested. Five-year survival was 83% (95% CI, 66% to 100%). Comparison with matched typical breast cancer cases revealed no significant difference in multidisciplinary treatment patterns, recurrence, or survival. The increased expression of EGFR (*HER1*) provides an opportunity for targeted tumor therapy in these tumors.

In an analysis of the MD Anderson Cancer Center experience and the SEER database, Hennessey et al.[213] identified 100 patients with metaplastic sarcomatoid carcinoma, and 213 patients in the SEER database with similar histology. They conclude that these are aggressive tumors with poor response to therapy and poor outcomes, also suggesting that studies evaluating novel targeted therapy are needed for these patients.

Spindle cell carcinoma of the breast, a variant of metaplastic carcinoma, includes a wide spectrum of lesions with mildly atypical features that may resemble fasciitis, fibromatosis, or myofibroblastic tumors. Unlike spindle cell carcinomas in general, they have no propensity for distant metastasis and should be termed *tumors* rather than *carcinomas.* Sneige et al.[214] studied 24 cases of fibromatosis-like spindle cell breast carcinoma. Treatment consisted of local excision (7 cases) or modified radical mastectomy (13 cases) and was not specified in 4 cases. In patients who underwent axillary nodal dissection, no lymph node metastases were found. Local recurrences developed in two of the six patients who underwent local excision only.

Primary neuroendocrine small cell carcinoma is uncommon. Francois et al.[215] reported seven cases, and Shin et al.[216] described nine cases. Immunohistochemical analysis showed consistent staining for cytokeratin markers but variable staining with neuroendocrine markers. The histologic type and prognosis are identical to those of lung cancer. It is important to distinguish these lesions from metastatic lung tumors or direct invasion of breast by Merkel cell carcinoma, lymphoma, or carcinoid tumor. It is reasonable to treat these patients with aggressive multiagent chemotherapy, excision of the primary tumor, and breast irradiation, although no data are available on the outcome of this approach.

Paget's disease describes involvement of the nipple by tumor. Most investigators agree that it represents extension of neoplasms from subjacent ducts in the nipple or metastases from an underlying carcinoma.[1] The tumor seems to travel linearly down the ducts and may appear to be multicentric. There may be an associated subareolar tumor. Breast-conserving surgery followed by radiation is effective in this disease.[217,218]

Cystosarcoma phyllodes is usually a benign lesion; in broad, fibrous beads that look "leaflike" are cystic clefts lined by a single layer of cells. These tumors are large; usually they are encapsulated, without invasion of the adjacent breast.[64] The lesions frequently develop from pre-existing fibromas and have a long initial period of slow growth followed by a sudden, rapid increase in size. The grade (mitotic rate), surgical margins, and proliferative index have prognostic importance.[219]

Primary mammary lymphomas are rare. In a study of 35 cases, including 16 primary lymphomas, diffuse large cell lymphoma was present in 10 of 16 primary and 14 of 18 secondary cases.[220] Lymphoepithelial lesions in ducts and lobules and frequent vascular involvement were found in both primary and secondary cases. Immunohistochemistry studies of 13 tumors showed that 12 were B cell in origin, and one was a primary T-cell lymphoma. Survival was related to stage and histologic characteristics. Half of the patients with primary lymphoma had recurrent disease. Although some local recurrences were observed, recurrence in other extranodal sites predominated.

Sarcoma

Primary breast sarcomas are occasionally seen. McGowan et al.[221] described 78 cases of primary breast sarcoma without metastatic disease (76 women, 2 men); 32 patients had malignant cystosarcoma phyllodes, and the others had stromal sarcomas (14 patients), angiosarcomas (8 patients), fibrosarcomas (7 patients), carcinosarcomas (5 patients), liposarcomas (4 patients), or other lesions (8 patients). The cause-specific survival rate was 48%, the relapse-free rate was 42%, and the local relapse-free rate was 75% at 10 years. No statistically significant difference in outcome was noted between those treated with conservation surgery and those undergoing mastectomy. Patients with negative margins had a significantly better local relapse-free rate than did those with positive margins (80% vs. 33%; $P = .009$).

PROGNOSTIC FACTORS FOR SURVIVAL AND METASTASIS

Carcinoma of the breast represents a wide spectrum of tumors with a variety of clinical, biological, and genetic characteristics resulting in a considerable variation in prognosis. It is important to understand, particularly from the radiation oncologists' perspective, that prognostic factors for systemic relapses and prognostic factors for local relapse differ significantly. Furthermore, prognostic factors for local relapse after mastectomy differ substantially from prognostic factors for local relapse after lumpectomy and radiation.[222] For example, tumor size and nodal status are clearly among the strongest predictors of overall survival and metastasis and are also strong predictors of postmastectomy chest wall relapse when radiation is not used.[110,223,224] However, these factors have not been consistently reported to be prognostic factors for in breast relapse after cancer surgery. On the other hand, margin status is a strong predictor of relapse in the conservatively treated breast but is not strongly correlated with distant metastasis.[225–227] Young age is also a very strong predictor of local relapse after breast-conserving therapy, and although it has been shown to be predictive of systemic metastasis, the effect of young age on distant metastasis as an independent factor is clearly not as significant as it is for local relapse in the conservatively managed patient.[228] Patients, as well as clinicians, often become confused regarding these issues, resulting in misconceptions regarding appropriate decision making and treatment. Below, prognostic factors for systemic relapse (i.e., distant metastasis and disease-free and overall survival) are discussed. A more in-depth discussion of prognostic factors for local relapse following lumpectomy and radiation is included later in the section on selection factors for the conservative management of breast cancer. Prognostic factors related to postmastectomy chest wall recurrence for patients with early-stage disease are discussed in Chapter 57.

The College of American Pathologists presented a consensus statement in 1999 summarizing prognostic factors in breast cancer.[229] Factors were category I if they were proven to be of prognostic importance and useful in clinical patient management. Category II factors had been extensively studied biologically and clinically, but their importance remains to be validated in studies. Category III included all other factors not sufficiently studied to demonstrate their prognostic value.

Category I included tumor size, lymph node status, micrometastasis, histologic grade, mitotic count, and hormonal-receptor status. Category II included *HER2/neu* expression, *p53* mutations, lymphovascular invasion, and DNA ploidy. Category III included tumor angiogenesis, EGFR, transforming growth factor, *Bcl-2,* and cathepsin D overexpression.

More recently, based on advances in molecular techniques allowing for genetic profiling of tumors, additional molecular prognostic factors have been identified, which can further refine clinical decision making and are already being applied clinically. This section will focus on the category I and II factors and discuss more recently introduced promising prognostic factors that may influence distant metastasis and clinical management.

Tumor Size

The size of the primary tumor ranks among the strongest predictors of distant metastasis and disease-free and overall survival. Although tumor size correlates strongly with the presence and number of involved axillary lymph nodes, it is clearly an independent prognostic factor. Among patients with documented node-negative disease, tumor size remains a strong and independent predictor of disease-free and overall survival. In a classic study with over 20 years of follow-up, Rosen et al.[194] reported a recurrence-free survival of 88% for tumors <1 cm, 72% for tumors 1.1 to 3.0 cm, and 59% for tumors 3.1 to 5.0 cm. In an analysis of 826 women with node-negative breast cancer treated by mastectomy at the University of Chicago with a median follow-up of 13.5 years, Quiet et al.[230] reported a 20-year disease-free survival of 79% for patients with tumors <2 cm, compared with 64% with tumors >2 cm. In multivariate analysis, the strongest predictor of outcome and time to relapse was pathologic tumor size. Survival as a function of primary tumor size in node-negative breast cancer patients is illustrated in Figure 56.10.

Axillary Nodal Status

Of all prognostic factors, nodal status continues to be the strongest predictor of disease-free and overall survival and is the primary factor that governs breast cancer staging. (Fig. 56.11).[190] Although there is a direct relation between the number of axillary nodes involved and the risk of distant metastasis, the most commonly employed schema is to group patients into four prognostic categories (node negative, 1 to 3 involved nodes, 4 to 9 involved nodes, and more than 10 involved nodes). These nodal prognostic categories are

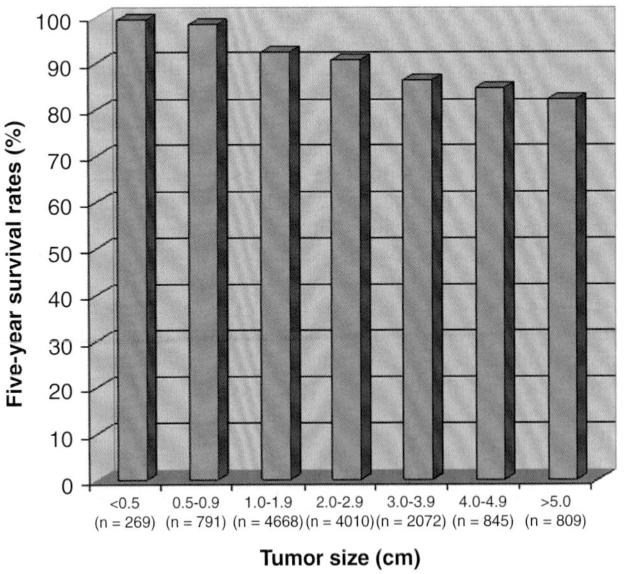

FIGURE 56.10. Five-year survival according to tumor size in node negative breast cancers (Data adapted from Carter CL, Allen C, Henson DE. Relation of tumor size, lymph node status and survival in 24,740 breast cancer cases. *Cancer* 1989;63:181–187.)

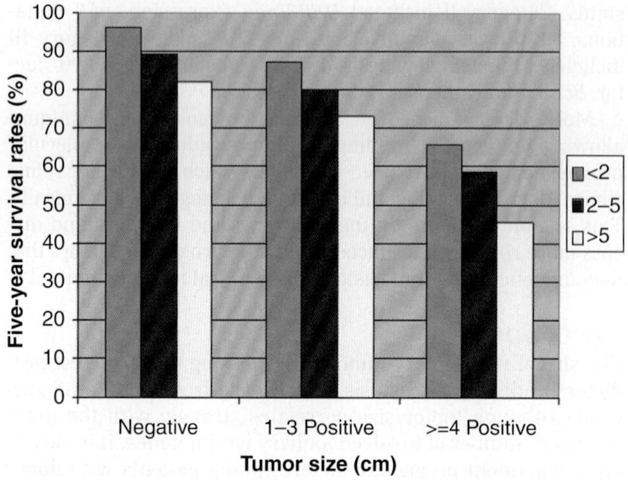

FIGURE 56.11. Five-year survival according to tumor size and nodal status. (Data adapted from Carter CL, Allen C, Henson DE. Relation of tumor size, lymph node status and survival in 24,740 breast cancer cases. *Cancer* 1989;63:181–187.)

employed in the N staging of the current AJCC staging system. Although outcomes will continually improve as systemic therapies advance, data from previous NSABP trials treated primarily with local-regional therapy alone revealed 5-year survival rates of 82.8% for node negative, 73% for 1 to 3 positive nodes, 45.7% for 4 to 12 positive nodes, and 28.4% for more than 13 positive nodes.[73,180,231–233]

Micrometastasis

The influence of microscopic disease in the lymph nodes has been the subject of several recent analyses due to the increased detection of micrometastasis in the era of sentinel lymph node biopsy. Most recent studies have demonstrated that by using a combination of blue dye and radiolabeled colloid techniques the sentinel node can be identified in >95% of cases.[234–235,236] In experienced hands, false-negative sentinel node rates are low (<10%), and prognosis of sentinel node-negative patients is similar to node-negative patients who have undergone a complete axillary dissection. Although the standard of care for sentinel node-positive patients has traditionally been completion axillary dissection, recent results of the American College of Surgeons Oncology Group (ACOSOG) Z0011 trial have challenged the need for completion axillary dissection in selected sentinel node-positive patients.[237] The need for axillary dissection in node-positive patients will likely continue to be highly individualized and will be further evaluated in ongoing clinical trials.[238]

Hansen et al.[239] evaluated the sentinel node in 696 women by hematoxylin and eosin staining and immunohistochemistry. With a median follow-up of 38 months the size of the sentinel node metastasis (<2 mm or >2 mm) was a significant prognostic factor. There was no difference in disease-free or overall survival, however, between true node-negative and immunohistochemistry-only -positive cases. Additional data from large databases will continue to emerge in the coming years to further refine the prognostic significance of micrometastasis and immunohistochemistry-only positive lymph node metastasis in breast cancer patients.

Tumor Type

The histologic subtype of invasive cancer has been shown to be of prognostic value in several studies. The tubular, mucinous, and medullary subtypes have been shown to have a more favorable prognosis, compared with invasive ductal.[194,201,240,241] Invasive lobular tumors appear to have a prognosis similar to invasive ductal tumors.[242] Poor prognostic categories include metaplastic, undifferentiated, and other rarer subtypes.[110,195]

In a classic analysis of 293 T2N0 breast cancers with over 20 years of follow-up treated by mastectomy, Rosen et al.[194] reported more favorable relapse rates in medullary, mucinous, tubular, and papillary subtypes compared with invasive ductal and invasive lobular tumors.

Tumor Grade

Multiple tumor grading systems have been proposed in an effort to standardize and improve interobserver variability. The Scarff-Bloom-Richardson classification system utilizes mitotic index, differentiation, and pleomorphism, each with scores of 1 to 3. Scores of 3 to 5 are well differentiated, 6 to 7 moderately differentiated, and 8 to 9 poorly differentiated. This system is commonly employed and has been shown to be of independent prognostic significance.[243]

Elston and Ellis[244] of the Nottingham group refined this methodology. The revised technique involves evaluation of three morphological features—the percentage of tubule formation, the degree of nuclear pleomorphism, and an accurate mitotic count using a defined field area. A numerical scoring system is used and the overall grade is derived from a summation of individual scores for the three variables: three grades of differentiation are used. Histologic grade, assessed in 1,831 patients, shows a very strong correlation with prognosis; patients with grade I tumors have a significantly better survival than those with grade II and III tumors (P <.0001). If the protocol is followed, reproducible and consistent results regarding prognosis can be obtained.

Estrogen and Progesterone Hormonal Receptors in Tumor Cells

Several studies have indicated that patients with hormonal receptors have a significantly higher survival rate.[245,246] Crowe et al.[247] studied 1,392 patients with carcinoma of the breast treated with modified radical mastectomy. ER-positive tumors (≥3 fmol/mg cytosol protein) were found in 1,063 patients (76.4%). Their 10-year overall survival rate of 65.9% was significantly better than the 56% rate in 329 patients with ER-negative tumors (P = .0001). However, this correlation is not consistent, with conflicting reports regarding the prognostic significance of hormonal receptor status.[248] The apparent discrepancy in some of these reports may be explained by technical nuances. Esteban et al.[249] noted that quantitative immunohistochemistry of ERs provides results with better predictive value than the biochemically procured ones.[250]

Tumors that express both ER and PR have the greatest benefit from hormonal therapy, but those containing only ER or PR still have significant responses. Two types of ERs—ER-α and ER-β—have now been identified. PR also exists in two forms, PRA and PRB.[251] Patients with tumors negative for hormonal receptors have only a small probability of responding to hormonal therapy.[185,251]

Lymphatic and Vascular Invasion

Lymphatic and vascular invasion (LVI) in the peritumoral region has been clearly demonstrated to be of independent prognostic significance in several studies.[252–256] In the study by Rosen et al.,[194] recurrence rate for LVI-positive stage I patients was 38% compared with 22% for LVI-negative patients.

Proliferative Indices, S-Phase, and Thymidine Labeling Index

Various techniques for evaluating the proliferative rate of a tumor have been shown to correlate with distant metastasis and survival. The most common are the fraction of cells in SPF, TLI, mitotic index, or antibodies directed against proliferative markers such as Ki-67 and proliferating cell nuclear antigen.

Thymidine labeling represents the fraction of cells in S phase of the cell cycle and is based on the active incorporation of labeled thymidine into DNA; the TLI of primary breast cancers appears closely related to steroid receptor status and generally unrelated to pathologic stage. Retrospective analyses have shown that TLI is a prognostic indicator, independent of tumor size, steroid receptors, and *p53,* and Bcl-2 protein expression. Together with patient age and tumor size, TLI is able to identify patients at different levels of risk for locoregional or distant metastases.[257]

Wenger and Clark[258] concluded that despite different techniques and cut points, a higher SPF is in general associated with worse tumor grade, absence of steroid receptors, larger tumors, and positive axillary lymph nodes. Higher SPF is usually associated with worse disease-free and overall survival rates in both univariate and multivariate analyses.

Bryant et al.,[259] in over 4,000 patients from NSABP protocol B-14 who had ER-positive tumors and no axillary lymph node involvement, found a strong association between SPF and disease-free and overall survival rate.

DNA Ploidy Index

Most breast cancers exhibit a bimodal distribution of DNA values. DNA ploidy as measured by flow cytometry correlates with nuclear grade, with low-grade tumors being diploid and high-grade tumors being aneuploid.[260] Ploidy was found to be associated with histologic type, tumor grade, and SPF values, but not with patient age, menopausal status, tumor size, axillary nodal status, ER status, or PR status.[261] Diploid tumors tend to be ER-positive, whereas aneuploid tumors are frequently ER-negative. Older patients are more likely to have hyperdiploid tumors.[262] Diploid tumors tend to have a better prognosis than those with an aneuploid DNA distribution.[263,264] Toikkanen et al.,[265] in 351 patients monitored for a minimum of 22 years, observed a 25-year survival rate of 28% for patients with nondiploid tumors, in contrast to 48% for those with a diploid DNA pattern. In a European Organisation for Research on Treatment of Cancer (EORTC) trial evaluation of DNA, proliferative compartment was the most important predicting factor for overall survival and metastasis-free survival in 281 premenopausal, lymph node–negative patients with invasive carcinoma of the breast.[266]

Studies by Ewers et al.[267] and Fallenius et al.[268] also confirm the prognostic significance of DNA ploidy. Keyhani-Rofagha et al.[269] and Witzig et al.[270] reported no statistically significant prognostic significance of DNA ploidy.

HER2/neu

The *HER2/neu* proto-oncogene (also called c-*erbB-2*) located on chromosome 17 codes for a transmembrane glycoprotein, p185, which has tyrosine kinase activity and is homologous to the EGFR.[271] It is amplified or overexpressed in up to 30% of human breast carcinomas. Overexpression of the protein is associated with tumor aggressiveness and decreased disease-free survival in node-positive patients, with variable prognostic significance among node-negative patients. The conflicting reports regarding the prognostic significance of *HER2/neu* may be related to interobserver variability in interpretation of staining and uncertainty regarding the significance of intermediate staining.[188,189,271] Staining for overexpression of *HER2/neu* is interpreted on a 0 to 3+ scale. The available data suggest that the majority of 0 to 1 staining is clearly negative and 3+ is clearly positive, while the classification of those patients with 2+ staining remains uncertain. Amplification of the oncogene identified using fluorescent *in situ* hybridization (FISH) techniques has been found to be of more prognostic value.[188,189,271,272]

Variability in the prognostic value of *HER2/neu* may be related to variability in interpretation of protein expression levels. Birner et al.[273] correlated results of the Hercep Test with *HER-2/neu* oncogene gene amplification assessed by FISH in 303 patients with lymph node–positive breast cancer.[273] Results were compared with FISH analysis performed in all 2+ and 3+ specimens (103 cases) and 104 *HER-2/neu*-negative specimens; 3+ carcinomas were found in 8.9% to 15.7% of specimens. FISH revealed that almost exclusively 3+ positive cases had *HER-2/neu* gene amplification.

In univariate analysis, staining with the HercepTest revealed a worse prognosis in 3+ cases, which were significantly associated with lower ER levels and histologic grade III tumors. More critical than its prognostic significance, however, is its predictive value with respect to response to therapy and its value in identifying patients who may benefit from adjuvant targeted therapy directed at the protein.[274] Several studies have demonstrated that *HER-2/neu* status may be predictive of response to hormonal therapy, resistance to alkylating agent–based chemotherapy, and response to taxanes.[275,276]

p53 Gene

The *p53* tumor suppressor gene encodes a nuclear phosphoprotein that is thought to be important to cell cycle regulation and DNA repair and that also may regulate induction of apoptosis by ionizing radiation.[277,278] The *p53* gene is most frequently mutated in sporadic breast cancer; alterations of this gene were identified in 43 of 192 tumors (22%).[278] Mutations of *p53* were found more often in tumors of younger women ($P = .002$) and African American women ($P = .04$) and in tumors lacking ER ($P = .03$), PR ($P = .04$), or both ($P = .06$). In 843 cases of breast cancer, *p53* mutations were not found in low-grade carcinomas (tubular, mucinous, papillary, and invasive cribriform types), but were observed in 4.2% of ILCs (6 of 140 cases), 15.5% of high-grade IDCs (99 of 640 cases), and 50% of pure medullary carcinomas (5 of 10 cases).[279] The overall survival rates were not significantly different in patients with mutant or wild-type *p53* tumors. In another study of 156 patients with primary invasive breast cancer, overexpression of p53 protein emerged as a reliable and independent predictor for disease recurrence and reduced survival.[280] Jansen et al.,[281] in a study of 345 patients with breast cancer with a median follow-up of more than 10 years, noted that *Bcl-2* expression was not a prognostic factor, but *p53* was an independent prognostic factor for overall survival ($P = .005$) and postrelapse survival ($P = .006$). However, *p53* status was important only in the *Bcl-2*–positive subgroup.

Genetic Profiling

Recent developments in DNA microarray technologies allow for extensive profiling of tumors based on their gene expression signatures.[282] Using this technology, investigators from the Netherlands Cancer Institute screened thousands of genes to develop a 70-gene prognostic signature that in 295 women demonstrated a 10-year disease-free survival of 50.6% in 180 poor prognosis signature patients compared with 85.2% in 115 women with a favorable signature. In a recent validation study, the profiling outperformed classic prognostic criteria, but the magnitude of the prognostic value was not as strong.[283,284,285]

Gene expression profiling has had a marked impact on our understanding of the biology of breast cancers and is routinely used in clinical decision making. Categorizing breast cancer into distinct clinical subtypes of luminal A, luminal B, *HER2/neu,* and basal-like has significant prognostic value and impacts on decisions regarding systemic therapy options.[286,287] Although gene profiling forms the basis of this subtyping, most clinicians rely on common molecular markers of ER, PR, *HER2/neu,* Ki-67, and others as a surrogate to classify patients into these intrinsic subtypes of breast cancer for clinical decision making.[288]

An assay using gene profiling on paraffin-embedded specimens has been developed by Genomics Health Inc (Redwood City, CA, USA) The Oncotype DX assay is based on reverse transcriptase polymerase chain reaction assays to quantify

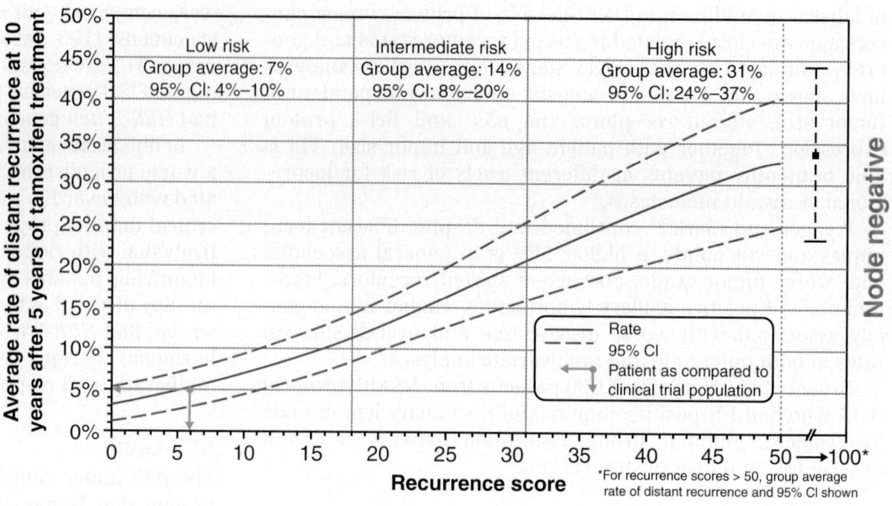

FIGURE 56.12. Risk stratification in patients with receptor positive tumors treated with hormonal therapy broken as a function of recurrence score using the Oncotype DX gene profiling scheme.

expression of selected genes in paraffin embedded tissues. A panel of 16 cancer-related genes and 5 reference genes were employed to compute a recurrence score (0 to 100), which is used to estimate the odds of relapse over 10 years. Specimens from patients in NSABP trials with ER-positive tumors treated with tamoxifen alone were used to validate this scheme in which patients were categorized as low risk (<18 score), intermediate risk (18 to 30), or high risk (31 to 100). As shown in Figure 56.12, the likelihood of distant metastasis is low in those patients with favorable scores treated with tamoxifen alone.[289] These data can be used to determine which patients with ER-positive tumors and otherwise favorable factors may avoid chemotherapy and aid the clinician and patient in clinical decision making.

Age

Although young age has consistently been shown to be a predictor of local relapse following breast-conserving surgery, there are conflicting data regarding its prognostic significance for distant metastasis and overall survival.[8,222,228,290–293] The available data are confounded by the fact that younger women often present with palpable disease and have larger tumors with a higher percentage of positive nodes. Several studies, however, have shown that when corrected for stage, young age remains a significant prognostic factor for distant metastasis. In an analysis of 1,751 patients with nonmetastatic breast cancer, Vanlemmens et al.[294] demonstrated that younger women had a higher proportion of patients with ER-negative and high-grade tumors and lower disease-free and breast cancer–specific survival. In multivariate analysis, young age at diagnosis was an independent poor prognostic factor. Kolias et al.,[295] however, in an analysis of 2,879 patients younger than 70 years old with operable disease in the Nottingham database, demonstrated that the association of young age at diagnosis with a worse prognosis was explained by a higher proportion of poorly differentiated cancers in young women and that young age itself had no influence on the prognosis of the individual. Although clearly not as valid as tumor size and nodal status, young age may be considered in combination with other prognostic factors in clinical decision making as a potential negative prognostic factor.

Race

African American women are commonly diagnosed with more advanced stages of breast cancer than white women.[8] Simon and Severson,[296] in a review of 10,502 women diagnosed with breast cancer (82% white and 18% African American), observed that African American women were more likely to present with regional or distant disease (45%) than white women (37%). White women had a better survival rate than African American women during the first 4 years after diagnosis (P <.0001), but there were no significant differences in survival by race in women who lived longer than 4 years (P = .64). Black women are more likely than whites to report that they have not had a mammogram within 3 years before diagnosis. However, history of mammographic screening accounted for <10% of the observed differences in stage at diagnosis.[297]

In 75 black and 615 white women with stage I and II breast cancer treated with breast-conservation therapy and CMF (cyclophosphamide, methotrexate, and fluorouracil), with or without prednisone and tamoxifen, the 5-year actuarial local-only first failure rates were 5% for black women and 6% for white women (P = .53); regional-only failure, 9% and 1% (P = .002); and regional recurrence as any component of first failure, 16% and 4%, respectively (P = .001).[298] The 5-year overall survival rate for the black patients was 82% versus 91% for the white patients (P = .01); the disease-free survival rates were 64% and 83%, respectively (P = .0002).

Eley et al.[299] reported on a study of 612 black and 518 white women aged 20 to 79 years with primary invasive breast cancer. After controlling for geographic site and age, the risk of dying was 2.2 times greater for blacks than whites. Adjustment for stage reduced risk from 2.2 to 1.7; further adjustment for sociodemographic variables had no effect. They concluded that approximately 75% of the racial difference in survival was explained by prognostic factors. Other studies have also indicated that black women more commonly develop breast cancers that are high grade and negative for ER, PR, and *HER2/neu*.[300,301]

Obesity and Body Mass Index

In a study of 923 women treated by mastectomy and axillary dissection, those who were obese (25% or more over optimal weight for height) at the time of primary breast cancer treatment 10 years after diagnosis were at significantly greater risk for recurrence (42%), compared with nonobese patients (32%; P <.01).[302] On multivariate analysis, obesity remained a statistically significant prognostic factor after controlling for tumor size, number of positive axillary lymph nodes, age at diagnosis, and adjuvant chemotherapy. Recurrent disease developed in 32% of obese patients compared with 19% of nonobese women.

Daling et al.,[303] in a study of 1,177 women 45 years of age and younger who had invasive ductal breast carcinoma, found that women with breast carcinoma who were in the highest quartile of BMI were 2.5 times more likely to die of their disease within 5 years of diagnosis compared with women in the lowest quartile of BMI.[303]

Smoking

High plasma levels of estrogens are associated with increased breast cancer risk. Manjer et al.[304] in an analysis of 792 women in a mammographic screening trial with a mean follow-up of 12.1 years observed that 145 patients died of breast cancer. The RRs for smokers and ex-smokers, compared with those who had never smoked, were 1.44 and 1.13, respectively. The association with smoking remained significant after adjustment for age and stage at diagnosis and other potential confounders.

Pregnancy

Kroman et al.[305] investigated the prognostic effect of age at first birth and total parity in 10,703 women with primary breast cancer. After adjusting for age and stage of tumor, the number of full-term pregnancies had no prognostic value. However, women with primary childbirth between 20 and 29 years experienced a significantly reduced risk of death compared with women with primary childbirth before the age of 20 years (20 to 24 years, RR 0.88; 25 to 29 years, RR 0.80). Psyrri and Burtness[306] reviewed 117 articles and three abstracts referring to breast cancer in pregnancy. They concluded the prognosis of the pregnant breast cancer patient is similar to her stage-matched nonpregnant counterparts in most series. Management of breast cancer during and after pregnancy is discussed in detail later.

Although in the past it was thought that pregnancy after the diagnosis of breast cancer was associated with a worse prognosis, recent evidence suggests the opposite.[307] Women with a history of breast cancer should be reassured that there is not strong evidence to suggest that subsequent pregnancy will increase the risk of recurrence.

Tumor Location

There is some evidence that medially located tumors have a poorer prognosis than laterally located tumors. An analysis of 45,880 patients from the SEER database by Gaffney et al.[308] demonstrated that the hazard ratio for inner quadrant location compared with outer quadrant was 1.27 for breast cancer specific survival and 1.11 for overall survival. Both were significant on multivariate analysis. Lohrisch et al.,[309] in an analysis of 6,781 patients, also demonstrated a twofold risk of relapse and breast cancer death associated with high-risk medial breast tumors compared with lateral tumors. They postulate that this may be due to occult spread to internal mammary nodes. On the other hand, Janni et al.[310] in an analysis of 2,414 patients concluded that there is no sufficient evidence to support any independent prognostic significance of tumor location in early breast cancer. However, medial tumor location may lead to the underestimation of axillary lymph node involvement.

Selected Other Prognostic Factors

A wide variety of other prognostic factors have been extensively evaluated. Although some of these have been promising in initial reports, they have not been applied in routine clinical decision making. However, these markers may help to supplement information obtained with more established prognostic factors. Furthermore, with additional testing and validation, some of these markers may serve as targets for therapeutic interventions. Extensively evaluated and reported potentially useful prognostic factors include cathepsin-D, vascular endothelial growth factor, EGF, *Bcl-2,* carcinoembryonic antigen, prostate specific antigen, E-cadherin and others. The reader is referred elsewhere for an extensive review of molecular prognostic factors in breast cancer.[311,312]

MANAGEMENT OF BREAST CANCER

Management of invasive breast cancer should be based on the clinical extent and pathologic characteristics of the tumor, in addition to the age of the patient (menopausal status), some biologic prognostic factors, and the preference and psychological profile of the individual patient, optimally in a multidisciplinary setting. Although surgical, medical, and radiation oncology remain the primary therapeutic disciplines in the management of breast cancer, the patients management often is dependent on input from diagnostic radiology and pathology, the primary physician involved, and support services such as genetic counseling, social work, nursing, and others.

Chang et al.[313] analyzed the records of 75 women with 77 breast lesions examined in a multidisciplinary breast cancer center; the panel disagreed with treatment recommendations from the outside physicians in 32 cases (43%), and agreed in 41 (55%). For the 32 patients with a disagreement, the treatment recommendations were breast-conservation treatment instead of mastectomy (n = 14; 41%) or re-excision (n = 2; 6%), and further workup instead of immediate definitive treatment in 10 (31%).

Patients with lesions smaller than 5 cm in diameter and some specific characteristics to be discussed later should be offered available options, with each modality thoroughly discussed. In some states, legislation has been enacted requiring treating physicians to comply with this practice.

Surgical Management of Breast Cancer

The surgical management of patients with early-stage operable breast cancer addresses both the primary tumor and regional lymphatics. The primary tumor may be managed by mastectomy or lumpectomy and the nodal regions may be surgically addressed by lymph node dissection or sentinel node biopsy. The radiation oncologist should be aware of the various surgical procedures, as it may influence the radiotherapeutic management. Procedures that remove the bulk of parenchymal breast tissue include the radical mastectomy, extended radical mastectomy, modified radical mastectomy, simple mastectomy (also referred to as total mastectomy), skin-sparing mastectomy, and nipple-sparing mastectomy. Partial mastectomy, lumpectomy, tylectomy, and quadrantectomy are collectively referred to as breast-conserving surgery.

Breast-conserving approaches, as well as the skin-sparing and nipple-sparing mastectomy, used in early-stage breast cancers, are briefly discussed here as they are often used in early-stage disease. Details of the mastectomy procedures are summarized in Chapter 57.

Skin-Sparing Mastectomy

Skin-sparing mastectomy is a standard mastectomy, with minimal skin sacrifice at the mastectomy site.[110] This is often performed when immediate reconstruction is planned. This technique attempts to remove all breast tissue, but the preservation of skin provides cosmetic and reconstructive advantages. The procedure is oncologically sound, and patients undergoing skin-sparing mastectomy do not require postmastectomy radiation unless they have risk factors that place them at higher risk (i.e., positive nodes, positive margins, large primary tumors), as discussed in Chapter 57.

Nipple-Sparing Mastectomy

The nipple-sparing mastectomy is distinct from the skin-sparing mastectomy in that the nipple and/or nipple areola complex are conserved. This procedure is more controversial and is not routinely employed in cancer patients. However, there have been recent studies employing this technique in combination with intraoperative electrons in patients with operable breast cancer.[314]

Lumpectomy

Another treatment of breast cancer, initially described by Keynes in 1929 and 1937, combined breast-conserving surgery

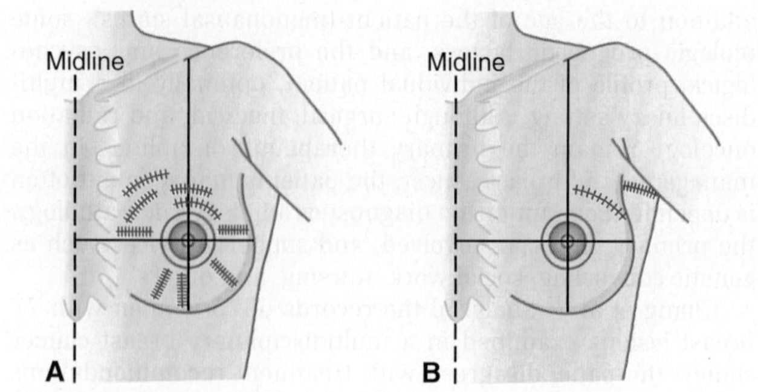

FIGURE 56.13. National Surgical Adjuvant Breast Project recommendations for the direction of incisions used for tumorectomy **(A)** and for axillary node dissection **(B)**. (Courtesy of Bernard Fisher, MD, Chairman, National Surgical Adjuvant Breast Project. From Bedwinek JM. Treatment of stage I and II adenocarcinoma of the breast by tumor excision and irradiation. *Int J Radiat Oncol Biol Phys* 1981;7:1553, with permission from Elsevier.)

by wide local excision of the tumor followed by definitive irradiation to the intact breast.[60,315–317] Various terms have been used to describe the surgical approach, including lumpectomy, wide local excision, breast-conserving surgery, tylectomy, tumorectomy, segmental mastectomy, partial mastectomy, and quadrantectomy. This approach is extensively discussed in this chapter. The NSABP recommends specific types of incisions depending on the location of the tumor (Fig. 56.13). The radiation oncologist may play an advisory role, as in many cases the patient may be evaluated by both the surgeon and the radiation oncologist before the definitive operation.

The optimal extent of breast resection for treatment of T1 and T2 breast cancer has not been defined. Increasing the size of the resection may lower the risk of local recurrence but also has an adverse impact on the cosmetic outcome. Because cosmesis is a critical reason for performing tumor excision and irradiation instead of mastectomy, wide local excision with microscopically negative margins is preferable to segmental mastectomy or quadrantectomy.

Surgical removal of additional breast tissue surrounding the original excision site is indicated when margins are positive and there is a substantial probability that the tumor cell burden exceeds what can be controlled by the usual doses of radiation. The percentage of patients with residual tumor at the time of re-excision varies widely (32% to 62%), depending on the criteria used for taking a patient back to the operating room for more breast surgery. If the initial margins of resection are positive, 55% to 69% of re-excision specimens contain cancer cells, compared with 49% in cases with unknown margins.[318–321] Tumor size alone is not usually considered an indication for re-excision in the absence of other factors.

Some authors have advocated re-excision of the primary site if the biopsy was performed at an outside hospital and margins of resection were unknown. Of 210 patients having surgery at the MD Anderson Cancer Center, 67 underwent re-excision after biopsies performed at other institutions, and invasive carcinoma was identified in 57%.[319] An 8.2% incidence of breast recurrence (12 of 135 patients) was noted when the tumor excision was performed before referral to the MD Anderson Cancer Center, but only 2% (4 of 210) when it was performed at that institution.

Other factors that may have an impact on the rate of positive re-excisions include extensive intraductal carcinoma (EIC) and residual calcifications on a postlumpectomy preirradiation mammogram. At Harvard University, when EIC was detected on the initial biopsy, 88% of the re-excisions were positive, compared with 48% when EIC was absent.[320] At the University of Pennsylvania, when a posttylectomy mammogram detected residual microcalcifications, 86% of the re-excisions contained tumor.[321] In a series from Yale, reported by Lally et al.,[157] of 34 patients with a postlumpectomy mammogram that showed suspicious residual calcification who underwent re-excision, 20 (59%) were found to have residual disease. Patients whose initial tumor was associated with calcifications with questionable, close, or positive margins should be evaluated with a prelumpectomy mammogram with guided re-excision if suspicious residual calcifications are present.

Based on these findings, the authors recommend re-excision at the primary tumor site (a) when the surgical procedure was less than a complete lumpectomy, such as an initial incisional biopsy or core biopsy, (b) when pathologic margins on the initial excisional biopsy are shown to be involved by tumor, and (c) when there are residual suspicious microcalcifications on a postlumpectomy mammogram. As will be discussed later, although re-excision for involved margins is indicated, selected patients with a focally involved margin may be treated with radiation therapy, without re-excision, following lumpectomy with acceptable local control rates.

Choices Between Mastectomy and Breast-Conserving Surgery in Early-Stage Disease

For the majority of patients with early-stage breast cancer, breast-conserving surgery and mastectomy are both reasonable options, and patients are often conflicted regarding the choice. Patients should be reassured that provided they meet the criteria for breast-conserving surgery, all of the available medical evidence demonstrates equivalent long-term survival rates with both modalities.

A modified radical mastectomy may be preferable for some patients who wish to avoid radiation, for those in whom removal of clinical and radiographically apparent disease will result in a suboptimal cosmetic result, for those with diffusely positive margins which cannot be cleared with re-excision, and those with diffuse suspicious microcalcifications. Even patients who are ideally suited for breast-conserving therapy may have a personal preference for mastectomy, based on a number of factors.

Whelen et al.[322] reported on the decision-making process in 82 consecutive node-negative patients presented with a decision board of therapeutic choices. Overall, 95% of women chose lumpectomy and breast irradiation. Kelemen et al.[323] evaluated the choice between breast-conserving surgery and modified radical mastectomy in 7,815 women with early-stage breast cancer. There was a progressive increase from 16% to 47% in the use of breast-conserving therapy to treat tumors of all sizes over the 11 years of the study ($P < .0001$), and it was more frequently used for ≤2 cm tumors with an odds ratio of 2.46. Breast-conserving therapy was used at a slightly higher rate in medical centers than in community hospitals (31% vs. 28%; $P < .0001$); its use varied among geographic regions from a low of 24% in the southwestern United States to 36% in the northeast and 40% in hospitals outside the continental United States ($P < .0001$). Local availability of radiation therapy did not influence choice of treatment.

In response to a questionnaire mailed to 2,405 oncologists from all three disciplines and 60 oncology nurses in the United States, Tannock and Belanger[324] noted that more than 60% thought that modified radical mastectomy and conservation surgery plus irradiation were equivalent options for patients with stage T1 and T2 carcinoma of the breast; 31% of the surgical oncologists favored the former and 35% of the radiation oncologists favored the latter approach. Medical oncologists were equally divided between the two procedures (14% and 18%, respectively).

In an analysis from Canada, Temple et al.[325] prospectively evaluated participants with a first diagnosis of localized unilateral breast cancer who were candidates for breast-conserving therapy or mastectomy. Of 157 patients between 1992 and 1995, 71.3% anticipated having breast-conserving surgery and 28.7% anticipated modified radical mastectomy. The patient, physician, and significant other were perceived to play a role in the decision process. The two top-ranked items perceived to have influenced treatment choice were doctor's advice and possibility of complete cure. Most women (60%) participated in treatment choice to the degree that they preferred, but only 13.6% received the preferred amount of information. The type of planned surgery was predicted by surgeon, contribution of doctor to choice of treatment, importance of breasts to sexuality, self-efficacy, and concerns about cancer recurrence from a multivariable logistic regression model. The authors concluded that both patient and surgeon factors are important predictors of type of planned surgery, but there is a gap between women's preferences and actual experiences with regard to information provided.

Some patients with early-stage breast cancer will choose mastectomy to avoid the course of radiation, either due to the logistics of 6 weeks of therapy or due to fears of radiation therapy. It is likely that more mature results and selection factors for treating women with accelerated partial breast irradiation will become available. For those women in whom the time commitment of treatment is an issue, this option may further impact the choice between mastectomy and breast-conserving surgery.

Patients selecting mastectomy should also be made aware that this procedure does not totally eliminate the need for radiation treatment. For patients with early-stage operable breast cancer treated by modified radical mastectomy, postoperative irradiation of the chest wall and peripheral lymphatics may be indicated in selected patients with high-risk characteristics, positive nodes, or positive resection margins. Indications for postmastectomy radiation are discussed in Chapter 54.

Surgical Management of Axillary Lymph Nodes

An axillary node dissection or sentinel node biopsy are a standard component of the staging process for a majority of women with early-stage invasive breast cancer.[190] Although the role of complete axillary dissection is evolving, currently most patients with positive sentinel nodes will undergo completion axillary dissection. Clearly the procedure is most important for women in whom axillary nodal status will influence subsequent management with respect to adjuvant systemic therapy. The role of axillary dissection and sentinel node sampling, however, continues to evolve and is currently being evaluated in several trials. It is not uncommon for clinicians to avoid axillary staging if it is not going to influence management.[68,326,327] This is relevant in elderly women with receptor-positive tumors who will receive hormonal therapy, regardless of nodal status, and who are not thought to be candidates for cytotoxic chemotherapy. Recent data from the ACOSOG Z0011 trial may obviate the need for axillary dissection for selected woman of any age with a positive sentinel node biopsy.[237,238] As will be discussed later, axillary radiation, as with axillary dissection, results in a high rate of regional control.[68,326,327]

Axillary Node Dissection

The axillary contents are divided into three levels: level I represents tissue between the axillary vein and the latissimus dorsi muscle and the lateral border of the pectoralis minor muscle; level II is located between the lateral and medial borders of the pectoralis minor muscle; and level III is between the medial border of the pectoralis minor and Halsted's ligament (the apex of the axilla).[1] Thorough dissection of levels I and II has traditionally been the most common axillary surgical procedure in patients with clinically node-negative breast cancer. Complete axillary dissection, including level III, may be performed in patients with clinically positive lymph nodes. A higher incidence of breast and arm edema has been noted with level III axillary node dissection, and the benefit of dissecting the level III lymph nodes has not been demonstrated.[328] Pigott et al.[329] reported on 146 patients treated with radical mastectomy (either modified or Halsted) for invasive ductal or lobular carcinoma of the breast. Eighty patients (55%) had histologically proven axillary lymph node metastases. If only the low (level I) axillary lymph nodes had been removed, 18 patients (25%) would have had metastases confined to levels II and III that would have gone undetected. However, only 1.4% of patients showed positive level III lymph nodes if levels I and II were negative.

Approximately 20% to 40% of patients with carcinoma of the breast and clinically negative lymph nodes have pathologic evidence of lymph node metastases.[1,110,233,330,331] Yet, in patients with stage I or II breast cancer and clinically negative axillary lymph nodes, if an axillary dissection is not performed, axillary recurrence develops in only approximately 20%.[73] In patients with clinically positive axilla, 20% to 30% have no histologic evidence of nodal metastatic disease.[73]

The necessity of axillary dissection has been questioned in selected patients with a low probability of nodal involvement by Silverstein et al.,[68] who reported positive axillary lymph nodes in only 3 (3%) of 96 patients with tumors ≤5 mm in diameter and in 27 (17%) of 156 patients with tumors 6 to 10 mm in diameter. Iwasaki et al.,[332] in a group of 823 patients with T1N0M0 invasive breast cancer, also identified a subgroup of patients who may not need to undergo axillary lymph node dissection. Certain tumor types (medullary, mucinous, and tubular carcinoma) had lower positive rates for lymph node involvement. With regard to the histologic grade, lymph node positivity increased significantly with high-grade tumors.

In a randomized trial, evaluating the necessity of axillary dissection in older women, Martelli et al.[333] reported on 219 women, 65 to 80 years of age, with early breast cancer and clinically negative axillary nodes who were randomized to conservative breast surgery with or without axillary dissection. Tamoxifen was prescribed to all patients for 5 years. With a follow-up of 60 months, there were no significant differences in overall or breast cancer mortality or crude cumulative incidence of breast events between the two groups. Only two patients in the no axillary dissection arm (8 and 40 months after surgery) developed overt axillary involvement during follow-up. They conclude that older patients with T1N0 breast cancer can be treated by conservative breast surgery and no axillary dissection without adversely affecting breast cancer mortality or overall survival.

In light of the increased use of primary tumor-related factors, including molecular profiling, for decision making regarding systemic therapy, combined with sentinel node procedures and low rates of regional relapse with radiation therapy or observation in selected patients, it is likely that axillary dissection will be less frequently employed in the future.

Sentinel Lymph Node Biopsies

In recent years there has been a substantial increase in the use of sentinel lymph node biopsies to stage patients with breast cancer. Patients are injected around the tumor with technetium-99m (^{99m}Tc) sulfur colloid and vital blue dye, and a handheld γ-probe is used to identify areas of highest radioisotope uptake in the lymphatic system. The lymph nodes underlying this area (sentinel lymph nodes) are removed.[235,334–336] The sentinel node procedure has been widely embraced as an acceptable standard for women with breast cancer and has a high degree of sensitivity and specificity.[337]

Although the current standard for patients with a positive sentinel node is to undergo completion axillary dissection, the necessity of this has been questioned and was the subject of the ACOSOG Z0011.[237] This was a prospective trial examining survival of patients with sentinel node metastases detected by standard hematoxylin and eosin staining, who were randomized to undergo axillary lymph node dissection (ALND) after sentinel lymph node dissection (SLND) versus SLND alone; all

TABLE 56.12 SUGGESTED APPROACH FOR RADIATION FIELD DESIGN IN SENTINEL NODE POSITIVE PATIENTS NOT UNDERGOING AXILLARY LYMPH NODE DISSECTION

Clinical Scenario	Sentinel Nodes +/Total Sentinel Nodes Sampled	Probability of Additional Nodes MSKCC[341] (%)	Probability of Additional Nodes MDACC[340] (%)	Probability of Four or More Nodes Involved[339] (%)	Field Design
IDC, 1.0 cm, ER+, LVI−	1 (IHC only)/3	3	8	<1	Tangents only
IDC, 1.8 cm, G3, ER+, LVI−, Unifocal	1 (macro)/2	27	24	2	High tangents
IDC, 2.0 cm, ER−, LVI+	2 (macro)/2	63	55	30	High tangents/consider full nodal treatment
ILC, 4.0 cm ER+, multifocal, LVI−	2 (macro)/2	77	64	40	High tangents/consider full nodal treatment
IDC, 3 cm, ER−, LVI+, multifocal	3 (macro with ENE)/3	78	95	80	Full nodal treatment

IDC, infiltrating ductal carcinoma; ER, estrogen receptor; LVI, lymphovascular invasion; ILC, infiltrating lobular carcinoma; G, grade; IHC, immunohistochemistry; macro, macroscopic; ENE, extranodal extension.

patients received whole-breast irradiation. There were 446 patients randomized to SLND alone and 445 to SLND plus ALND. Patients were equally stratified according to multiple factors; those randomized to SLND plus ALND had a median of 17 axillary nodes removed compared with a median of only 2 sentinel nodes removed with SLND alone (P <.001). At a median follow-up time of 6.3 years, there were no statistically significant differences in local recurrence (P = .11) or regional recurrence (P = .45) between the two groups. Interestingly, ALND also removed more positive lymph nodes (P <.001) in 27% of the patients in this group. The patients in this trial all had whole-breast irradiation, but regional nodal irradiation was not allowed. The reason for the low regional relapse rates is likely a combination of factors, including a favorable subset of patients with a low likelihood of a high residual axillary burden of disease, the use of systemic therapy, and incidental radiation to the residual nodes in level I or II from the tangential breast irradiation. Several studies describe an approach to radiation field design based on probability of additional axillary nodal involvement in patients with positive sentinel nodes (Table 56.12).[238,338–341]

The ALMANAC (Axillary Lymphatic Mapping Against Nodal Axillary Clearance) trial is a multicenter randomized trial of 1,031 patients randomly assigned to sentinel node biopsy (n = 515) or standard axillary dissection (n = 516).[335] Mansel et al.[335] reported the primary outcome measures, which were arm and shoulder morbidity and quality of life. Drain usage, length of hospital stay, and resumption of normal activities after surgery were all highly significantly better in the sentinel lymph node group. In addition patient recorded quality of life and arm functioning scores were also significantly better, with no increase in anxiety levels in the sentinel node group. The authors conclude that sentinel node biopsy is the treatment of choice for patients who have early-stage breast cancer and clinically negative nodes.

Veronesi et al.[342] also reported on a randomized trial of 516 patients with T1 tumors, randomized to either sentinel node biopsy or total axillary dissection. Axillary dissection was performed in the sentinel node group if the sentinel node contained metastases. In the axillary dissection group, the overall accuracy of the sentinel node status was 96.9%, the sensitivity 91.2%, and the specificity 100%. There was less pain and better arm mobility in the patients who underwent sentinel node biopsy only than in those who also underwent axillary dissection. There were 15 events associated with breast cancer in the axillary dissection group and 10 such events in the sentinel node group. Among the 167 patients who did not undergo axillary dissection, there were no cases of overt axillary metastasis during follow-up.

Weaver et al.[343] evaluated 443 patients with breast cancer. After sentinel node biopsies, a complete axillary lymph node dissection was performed. Original pathologic material was reviewed for 431 patients enrolled in this study and for 214 patients with node-negative disease. Metastases were detected in 16% of the sentinel lymph nodes and in 4% of the nonsentinel nodes (odds ratio [OR] 4.3; P <.001). Occult metastases were detected in 4% of the sentinel lymph nodes and in 0.3% of the nonsentinel nodes. The probability of detecting metastases in nonsentinel nodes was more than 13 times greater in patients with positive sentinel lymph nodes than in patients with negative sentinel lymph nodes (P <.001).

The role of sentinel lymph node procedures in patients undergoing neoadjuvant chemotherapy is covered in Chapter 57.

SYSTEMIC MANAGEMENT OF BREAST CANCER

Systemic therapy is an essential component of both early-stage node-negative breast cancer as well as advanced-stage disease. Hormonal therapy, cytotoxic chemotherapy, and the more recently introduced biological therapies are routinely employed in the vast majority of patients with early-stage breast cancer. For patients with all stages of breast cancer, systemic therapy has been shown to decrease the relative risk of relapse and mortality. However, there are subsets of patients with a very favorable prognosis and extremely low rate of relapse, in whom the risk reduction results in only a very small absolute benefit. It is beyond the scope of this chapter to discuss all of the issues related to systemic management of breast cancer and the reader is referred to comprehensive reviews on the use of chemotherapy, endocrine therapies, and biologic therapies in the systemic management of breast cancer. These issues are also discussed in more detail in Chapter 57.[344–346]

In the recent 2011 St. Galen consensus meeting, the panel adopted the approach that systemic therapy should be made based on recognition of intrinsic subtypes, and that for practical reasons these intrinsic subtypes could be approximated based on more conventional parameters of estrogen receptor, progesterone receptor, *HER2/neu*, and Ki-67. Endocrine therapy alone is generally adequate for luminal A type cancers, while chemotherapy is typically indicated for luminal B and triple negative cancers, and trastuzumab is generally added for *HER2*-positive disease.[347]

RADIATION THERAPY IN THE MANAGEMENT OF EARLY-STAGE INVASIVE BREAST CANCER

The radiation oncologist plays a critical role in the management of early-stage breast cancer. As noted previously, the role of radiation therapy in postmastectomy radiation and in the neoadjuvant treatment of advanced breast cancers will be discussed in Chapter 57. The remainder of this chapter will primarily be focused on the role of radiation therapy in the conservative management of early-stage invasive breast cancer.

This will include an extensive discussion of the studies establishing breast-conserving surgery and radiation as the preferred standard of care for the majority of women with early-stage invasive disease and studies evaluating the avoidance of radiation therapy in selected patients. Integration of radiation therapy with systemic therapy will be discussed, as will selection of patients for breast-conserving therapy. Risk factors for local relapse and controversies in the management of patients with special circumstances will be discussed. Technical issues in the delivery of radiation therapy for early-stage breast cancer, including dosing and fractionation, matching techniques, and newer technical approaches, will be presented. The rapidly evolving area of partial breast irradiation will also be discussed. Follow-up of the breast cancer patient and sequelae of treatment will be presented. Management of local relapse in the conservatively treated breast and postmastectomy will be covered in Chapter 57. The role of radiation therapy in the management of DCIS and LCIS was discussed Chapter 55.

Breast-Conserving Therapy and Patient Selection

Breast-conserving surgery followed by radiation therapy to the intact breast is now clearly established as the most acceptable standard of care for the majority of women with early-stage invasive breast cancer. In 1992, the *Journal of the National Cancer Institute* published a monograph that stated that breast-conservation treatment is an appropriate method of primary therapy for most women with stage I or II breast cancer and is preferable because it provides survival equivalent to that of total mastectomy and axillary dissection while preserving the breast.[348] Recommended techniques for breast-conservation treatment are wide local excision of the primary tumor, preferably with clear margins, axillary lymph node dissection, and breast irradiation (45 to 50 Gy), usually with a boost (10 to 20 Gy, depending on tumor size and status of the surgical margins). As will be discussed in detail under prognostic factors, while widely negative margins are desirable, patients with focally involved margins can be treated with radiation with excellent local control rates.

In addition to tumor control and survival, conservation of the breast with optimal cosmetic results is a crucial goal of this therapy, which is associated with improved psychoemotional adjustment of the patient to the diagnosis and treatment of carcinoma of the breast. It also enhances the acceptance by women of mammographic screening for early detection of this disease.

The widespread embracement of breast-conserving surgery followed by radiation therapy is based on numerous mature and well-documented studies, both prospectively designed randomized trials and large retrospective series of appropriately selected patients treated with breast conservation followed by radiation therapy.

It is important to select appropriate patients and tumors for breast-conservation therapy, with close consultation between the surgeon, medical oncologist, and the radiation oncologist and after thorough discussion of therapeutic alternatives with the patient. Risks and benefits of breast-conserving therapy compared with mastectomy should be discussed. Despite the clear evidence of equivalence, some patients will still prefer mastectomy, which remains an acceptable standard of care for all women with operable breast cancers. Although avoidance of radiation may be a primary rationale for some patients in choosing mastectomy, patients should realize that even with early-stage operable disease postmastectomy radiation may be indicated based on the pathologic findings at mastectomy. It is likely that over the next several years, long-term results and selection factors for accelerated partial breast irradiation will become available and may further influence patient choices regarding breast-conserving surgery with more rapid radiation compared with mastectomy.[349,350–351]

Ideally, patients electing breast-conserving surgery and radiation will have unicentric primary tumors that are <4 to 5 cm in diameter, as cosmesis is affected by the amount of tissue that must be removed in relation to the size of the breast.[352] For patients in whom the size of the tumor, compared with the size of the breast, will result in an unacceptable cosmetic outcome, neoadjuvant chemotherapy followed by lumpectomy and radiation has been demonstrated to result excellent breast-conservation rates.[353–355] This was discussed in detail in Chapter 54.

With careful attention to surgical margins, radiation technique, and the appropriate use of systemic therapy, local relapse rates in the majority of conservatively managed patients are low, and only a minority of patients with early-stage invasive breast cancer are not suitable for breast-conserving therapy. There are several perceived relative "contraindications" to breast-conserving therapy, including patients with collagen vascular disease, patients with germline mutations that predispose to breast cancer development, and those with positive margins, more advanced disease, multicentric disease, pregnancy, or who have had prior radiation. Although many of these factors require careful consideration and discussion between the treating physicians and the patient, as will be discussed in the section on special circumstances, selected patients faced with breast cancer in the setting of these controversial circumstances can be offered breast-conserving therapy with acceptable outcomes. Although some clinicians believe that patients at higher risk for development of local recurrence should not be treated with conservation surgery, there are relatively few absolute contraindications.

Perhaps with the exception of the patients with persistently positive diffuse margins or gross multicentric disease, where removal of clinically and radiographically apparent disease would result in an unacceptable cosmetic outcome, breast-conserving therapy followed by radiation can be offered to most women with early-stage breast cancer and may be offered to a high percentage of women with advanced cancers following neoadjuvant chemo- or hormonal therapy. The decision regarding breast-conserving therapy compared with mastectomy is often based on personal preference as the available medical and scientific evidence suggests equivalent overall and disease-free survival in all subsets of patients.

Early Reports of Breast-Conserving Therapy

In 1937, Keynes[60] stated that "widespread operations based upon the permeation theory of lymphatics and fascial planes have no real justification and the idea of conservative treatment of cancer of the breast may become less repugnant to us [surgeons]." He treated 325 patients with local removal of the breast tumor and radium implantation at the site of local incision as well as in the axilla. In 250 patients, the 5-year survival rate was 71% for group 1 (disease confined to the breast), 29% for group 2 (disease apparently confined to breast and axilla), and 23.6% for group 3 (advanced disease or inoperable cancer). At the time, the results were comparable with those achieved with radical mastectomy. Other early reports[316,356–359] paved the way for the development of randomized trials that have now clearly established breast-conserving surgery followed by radiation therapy as an accepted standard of care.

Randomized Studies Comparing Breast-Conserving Surgery Plus Radiation Therapy to Mastectomy

There have been numerous randomized trials that have now clearly established breast-conserving surgery followed by radiation therapy as equivalent to mastectomy for appropriately selected patients with early-stage breast cancer. Table 56.13 summarizes these randomized trials. In all of these trials, local tumor excision (tylectomy, lumpectomy), segmental mastectomy, or quadrantectomy combined with irradiation to the breast yielded survival and tumor control rates similar to those achieved with

TABLE 56.13 PROSPECTIVE RANDOMIZED TRIALS COMPARING CONSERVATIVE SURGERY AND RADIATION WITH MASTECTOMY FOR EARLY-STAGE BREAST CANCER

	Institut Gustave-Roussy (1972–84)[370]	*Milan (1973–80)*[102]	*NSABP B-06 (1976–84)*[93]	*NCI (1979–87)*[373]	*EORTC (1980–86)*[362]	*Danish (1983–89)*[364]
Number of patients	179	701	1219	237	874	904
Stage	1	1	1 and 2	1 and 2	1 and 2	1, 2, 3
Surgery	2-cm gross margin	Quadrantectomy	Lumpectomy	Gross excision	1-cm gross margin	Wide excision
Follow-up (yr)	15	20	20	18	10	6
Overall Survival						
CS+RT (%)	73	42	46	59	65	79
Mastectomy (%)	65	41	47	58	66	82
Local Recurrence						
CS+RT (%)	9	9	14	22	20	3
Mastectomy (%)	14	2	10	6	12	4

EORTC, European Organisation for Research and Treatment of Cancer; NCI, National Cancer Institute; NSABP, National Surgical Adjuvant Breast and Bowel Project; RT, Radiation therapy; CS+RT, conservative therapy.

modified or classic radical mastectomy.[93,101,102,360–361,362,363–364] Each of these randomized trials, as well as meta-analyses of the trials, clearly demonstrate equivalent mortality rates in conservatively treated patients compared with mastectomy.[365–367]

The earliest prospective, randomized trial comparing breast conservation with radical mastectomy was conducted at Guy's Hospital in London. Three hundred and seventy women with stage I or II breast cancer were randomly assigned to receive either standard radical mastectomy or wide local excision plus irradiation.[368] Although the rates of survival and distant metastasis were not significantly different for stage I disease, in stage II the recurrence rates in the breast and axilla were higher in the group treated with local excision and irradiation, and survival was significantly lower because of a higher rate of distant metastasis. Major weaknesses of this study were the low doses of irradiation used (35 to 38 Gy to the breast and 25 to 27 Gy to the axilla), probably patient selection, and surgical techniques.

Veronesi et al.[363] reported on 701 patients with tumors <2 cm in diameter and without palpable axillary nodes of whom 352 were randomly assigned to treatment with either quadrantectomy and axillary dissection plus irradiation (50 Gy in 5 weeks to the breast and 10-Gy boost) and 349 to radical (Halsted) mastectomy. Women with positive axillary lymph nodes also received 12 cycles of adjuvant chemotherapy with CMF. Actuarial 20-year overall and disease-free survival rates were comparable in the two groups (58%). The death rates from breast cancer were 26.1% and 24.3%. The incidence of local failure was 2.3% with mastectomy and 8.8% with quadrantectomy and irradiation. There was no difference in the incidence of contralateral breast cancer (10.2% and 8.7%, respectively).[102]

Fisher et al.[93,360] updated the results of the NSABP protocol B-06 in 1,843 women with clinical stage I or II carcinoma of the breast <4 cm in diameter. Patients were randomly assigned to be treated with total mastectomy or lumpectomy (segmental mastectomy), with or without irradiation. Irradiated patients received 50 Gy to the breast through tangential fields irradiation and a boost to the operative site was not given. With 20-year follow-up, there was no significant difference in survival among patients treated with mastectomy, lumpectomy alone, or lumpectomy combined with irradiation (Fig. 56.14). For the patients treated with lumpectomy alone, the ipsilateral breast relapse rates were approximately 40% if the nodes were negative and 50% if they were positive. For patients treated with lumpectomy and irradiation, the corresponding rates were 10% for all patients and those with negative nodes and 5% for those with positive nodes, illustrating the interaction of irradiation and adjuvant chemotherapy in local tumor control. Cumulate incidence of ipsilateral breast tumor relapse in the lumpectomy alone compared with the lumpectomy and radiation arm is shown in Figure 56.15.

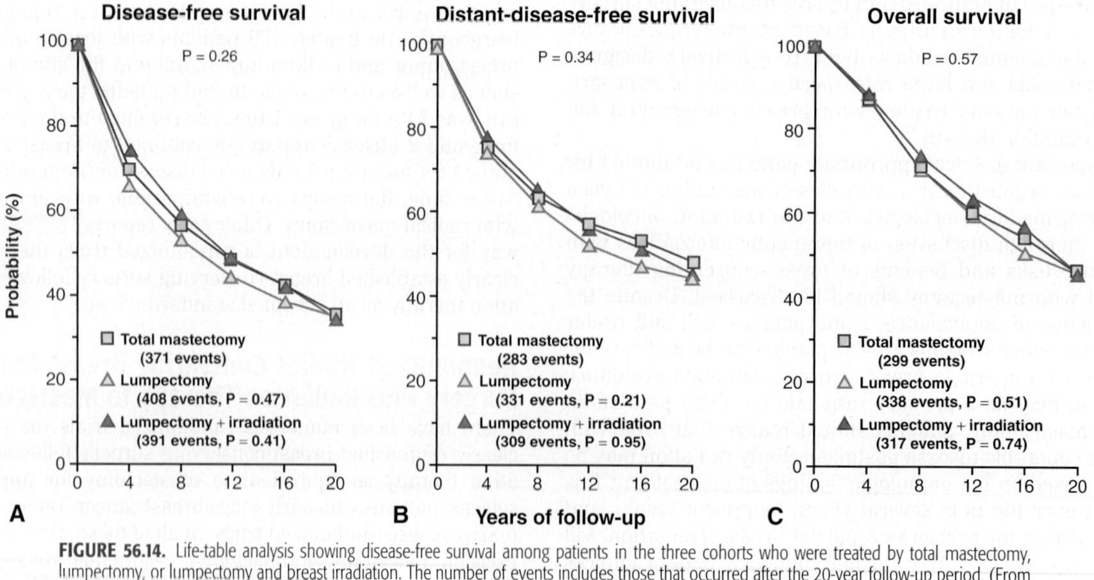

FIGURE 56.14. Life-table analysis showing disease-free survival among patients in the three cohorts who were treated by total mastectomy, lumpectomy, or lumpectomy and breast irradiation. The number of events includes those that occurred after the 20-year follow-up period. (From Fisher B, Anderson S, Bryant J, et al. Twenty-year follow-up of a randomized trial comparing total mastectomy, lumpectomy, and lumpectomy plus irradiation for the treatment of invasive breast cancer. *N Engl J Med* 2002;347:1233–1241, 2002, copyright Massachusetts Medical Society.)

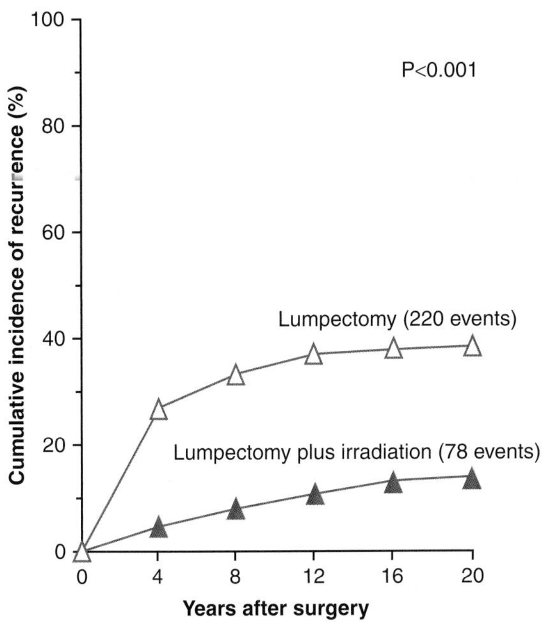

FIGURE 56.15. Cumulative incidence of ipsilateral breast recurrence after lumpectomy (*open diamonds*) or lumpectomy plus breast irradiation (*solid diamonds*) in 1,137 patients in the current-update cohort (cohort B) who had either negative or positive nodes and tumor-negative specimen margins. (From Fisher B, Anderson S, Bryant J, et al. Twenty-year follow-up of a randomized trial comparing total mastectomy, lumpectomy, and lumpectomy plus irradiation for the treatment of invasive breast cancer. *N Engl J Med* 2002;347:1233–1241, 2002, copyright Massachusetts Medical Society.)

The Institut Gustave-Roussy conducted a prospective, randomized trial comparing mastectomy with local excision plus irradiation for women with cancers measuring ≤2 cm.[369,370] The 15-year disease-free survival rate was 55% for the tumorectomy group and 45% for the mastectomy group (*P* = .23). The 15-year local recurrence rate was 9% in the conservation surgery and irradiation group and 14% in the mastectomy group.

The EORTC Breast Cancer Cooperative Group conducted a randomized trial of women with stage I or II breast cancer comparing modified radical mastectomy (420 patients) with breast-conservation therapy (448 patients).[362] The actuarial 8-year local tumor control rate was similar in both arms, 91% in the mastectomy group and 87% in the breast-conservation therapy group. There was one axillary recurrence in the mastectomy group and three in the conservation therapy group.

A Danish Cooperative Study carried out a similar randomized trial in 905 women (another 248 patients were treated with mastectomy or breast-conservation therapy according to preference without randomization).[371] High-risk patients (tumor >5 cm, invasion to skin or deep fascia, metastatic axillary lymph nodes) who were treated with breast-conservation therapy received radiation therapy to the regional lymph nodes. Those who were treated with mastectomy also received irradiation of the same target volume and all high-risk patients received adjuvant CMF. At 6 years, the recurrence-free survival rate in 430 patients treated with breast-conservation therapy was 70%, compared with 66% in 429 patients treated with mastectomy. Overall survival rates were 79% and 82%, respectively. There were 12 breast relapses in the former group (3%) and 19 chest wall recurrences in the latter group (4%). In the breast-conservation therapy group, 31% of patients had excellent and 41% had satisfactory cosmesis.

The U.S. National Cancer Institute reported results of a randomized study in which 122 patients with T1–2N0M0 disease were treated with modified radical mastectomy and 125 with breast-conservation therapy (45 to 50 Gy to breast plus 15- to 20-Gy boost).[372] Recently updated by Poggi et al.[373] with a median follow-up of 18.4 years, there was no detectable difference with regard to overall survival between patients treated with mastectomy and those treated with breast-conserving therapy (58% vs. 54%; *P* = .67 overall). Twenty-seven women in the breast-conserving therapy arm (22%) experienced an in-breast event. After censoring in-breast events in the breast-conserving therapy arm that were salvaged successfully by mastectomy, disease-free survival also was found to be statistically similar (67% in the mastectomy arm vs. 63% in the breast-conserving therapy arm; *P* = .64 overall). There was no statistically significant difference in the incidence of contralateral breast carcinoma between the two treatment groups.

Van Dongen et al.[101,362] reported on an EORTC trial comparing modified radical mastectomy with breast-conserving therapy (lumpectomy, axillary clearance, and irradiation to the breast, 50 Gy in 5 weeks and a 25-Gy boost with iridium implant) in 168 patients with stage I and 734 with stage II disease. Patients with microscopically incomplete excision of the tumor were included. Updated analysis from this trial with a median follow-up period of 13.4 years revealed locoregional recurrence rates were higher in the breast-conservation therapy group (10-year rate, 19.7%) than in the mastectomy group (10-year rate, 12.2%, *P* = .0097). The overall survival rate at 10 years was 66.1% for patients undergoing mastectomies and 65.2% for patients undergoing breast-conservation therapy (*P* = .11).

Additional Experiences with Breast-Conserving Surgery Plus Radiation Therapy

Although the acceptance of breast-conserving surgery plus radiation therapy as an alternative to mastectomy has been established based on the numerous randomized trials outlined above, large retrospective experiences with long-term follow-up have provided additional data regarding the selection of patients for breast-conserving therapy and radiation, prognostic factors for local-regional end points, impact of various treatment policies and techniques, complications, cosmesis, and long-term outcomes.

Mature Retrospective Series of Breast-Conserving Surgery Plus Radiation Therapy

There have been numerous reports of breast-conserving therapy and radiation, now with follow-up exceeding 10 to 15 years. These studies have provided valuable data regarding technical issues related to treatment and have provided additional data regarding outcomes in subsets of patients, prognostic factors for local control, cosmesis, and other sequelae. Lessons learned from these retrospective series have yielded valuable insight into the conservative management of breast cancer and provide the basis for further prospective studies. Selected publications are highlighted below and in the section on prognostic factors for local control. Long-term outcome from some of these experiences are summarized in Table 56.14.[99,104,298,317,356,369,374–391] Collectively these studies clearly show long-term outcomes that are consistent with the randomized trials noted above. Local failure rates will depend on follow-up, selection factors, and treatment, as discussed later, but in general are expected to range between 0.5% and 1% per year.

PROGNOSTIC FACTORS FOR LOCAL RELAPSE FOLLOWING BREAST-CONSERVING SURGERY PLUS RADIATION THERAPY

The retrospective experiences outlined above together with the prospective randomized trials have provided additional data confirming acceptable long-term local control, cosmesis, and toxicities and have identified prognostic factors that lead to higher local relapse rates and impact treatment policies.

Local relapse in the conservatively managed breast is an active area of investigation, with numerous studies dedicated

TABLE 56.14 CONSERVATION SURGERY AND IRRADIATION: NONRANDOMIZED STUDIES STAGE I AND II BREAST CANCER: RESULTS OF SELECTED STUDIES

Study (Reference)	Number of Patients	Stage	Dose (Gy) Breast	Dose (Gy) Boost	Local Tumor Control (%)	Excellent or Good Cosmesis (%)	10-Year Disease-Free Survival (%)
Amalric et al. (356)	1,440	I, II	60	15–20	80	90	74
Barr et al. (374)	411	I, II, III	48.4	20	88	NS	NS
Bartelink et al. (375)	585	T1,T2	50	25	98	NS	T1,92[a] T2,85
Calle et al. (376)	411	I, II	50	10	89	88	78
Clark et al. (377)	1,504	T1–2NO	40/3 wk	5–15	86	NS	70
Clarke et al. (378)	436	T1,T2	45	15	90	NS	–
Delouche et al. (379)	410	T1,T2	50–60	Yes	T1,94 T2,86	93	62.5
Dewar al. (380)	757	TO–2	45	15	92	–	69
Dubois et al. (381)	231	I	45	10–15	1,91	90	1–84
	161	II			84		11–75
Fagundes et al. (382)	425	T1,T2	50	10–15	92	77	74[b]
Fourquet et al. (383)	518	T1,T2	57–62	5–12	90	NS	NS
Fowble et al. (104)	697	I, II	50	10–15	91	93	1–79 II-67
Gage et al. (384)	1,870	I, II	45–50	10–20	87	NS	NS
Haffty et al. (99)	433	I, II	48	10–20	92	NS	81
Kurtz et al. (298)	1,593	I, II	50–60	20	89	–	86
Leborgne et al. (385)	796	I, II	50	10–20	87[b]	NS	82[c]
Osborne et al. (386)	263	T1,T2	45	10	I, 85 11,81	–	I, 54 II, 29
Pierquin et al. (387)	245	I, II	50	10–20	90	82	75[c]
Recht et al. (388)	366	I, II	50	10	I, 96 II, 90	–	–
Sarrazin et al. (369)	179	T1smT2	45	15	95	92	85[b]
Solin et al. (389)	217	T1	45–50	10–15	95	90	T1, 80[b]
	166	T2	45–50	10–15	92	90	T2, 69[b]
van Limbergen et al. (390)	235	T1,T2(3)	40–65	8–20	90	–	T1,75.4 T2, 61.9
Vicini et al. (391)	1,396	I, II	50	10	92	87	NS
Vilcoq et al. (317)	314	T1,T2	50–55	10–20	90	–	84[b]

NS, not stated.
[a]Six-year disease-free survival. [b]Five-year disease-free survival. [c]Fifteen-year disease-free survival.

TABLE 56.15 SUMMARY OF RISK FACTORS FOR LOCAL RELAPSE

Prognostic Factor	Effect	Strength of Data	Comment
Age	Young age increases local relapse	Multiple studies Upheld in multivariate analysis Few conflicting reports	Remains among the strongest factors
Margins	Positive margins increase local relapse	Multiple studies Upheld in multivariate analysis Few conflicting reports	Remains among the strongest factors. Data on "close" margins are less consistent.
Systemic therapy	Systemic therapy (chemo and hormonal) lowers risk of local relapse	Multiple studies support Some conflicting reports	May delay rather than counteract risk
Radiation dose	Higher doses decrease local relapse	Multiple studies support Confirmed in randomized trials (boost vs. no boost) Some conflicting data regarding doses above 50 Gy	Interaction with margins and age Necessity of "boost" in women over 50 and with widely negative margins unclear
Extensive intraductal component (EIC)	EIC positive tumors have higher rates of local relapse	Initial studies supportive Some confirmatory studies Some conflicting studies	Recent data suggest that negative margin status eliminates this as a risk factor
LCIS as a component	LCIS as a component increases risk of local relapse	Conflicting data with no clear consensus	Patients with LCIS are suitable candidates for BCS. Debate remains regarding need for clear LCIS margins.
Lobular histology	Lobular histology has higher local relapse rates	Conflicting data with no clear consensus	Should be treated similar to invasive ductal cancers
BRCA1/2	Higher late local relapses in *BRCA1/2* patients	Several confirmatory studies Some conflicting data	Higher relapse rates related to late "new primaries." This may be minimized by prophylactic hormonal manipulation
Tumor size	Larger tumors result in higher local relapses	Some confirmatory studies Several conflicting studies	Data is confounded by more frequent use of systemic therapy in larger tumors
Nodal status	Higher local relapse rates in node positive patients	Several conflicting studies	As with tumor size, data are confounded by more frequent use of systemic therapy in node positive patients
Receptor status	Higher local relapse rates in triple negative and *HER2*-positive patients	Some confirmatory studies Few conflicting studies Under active investigation	Would offer these patients conventional whole breast irradiation

LCIS, lobular carcinoma *in situ;* BCS, breast-conserving surgery.

TABLE 56.16 IPSILATERAL BREAST RECURRENCE RATES BY AGE

Study (Reference)	Follow-Up (Year)	≤35 Year Number of Patients	≤35 Year Recurrence	>35 Year Number of Patients	>35 Year Recurrence
Clarke and Martinez (392)	5 (mean)	32	3 (9%)	424	21 (5%)
Fowble et al. (293)	8 (actuarial)	61	15 (24%)	916	119 (13%)
Haffty et al. (92)	8.2 (median)	34	5 (15%)	349	38 (11%)
Halverson et al. (393)	7 (actuarial)	37	3 (9%)	474	57 (12%)
Kini et al. (400)	10 (median)		24%		7%
Kurtz et al. (401)	11 (mean)	91	15 (16%)	1,291	129 (10%)
Matthews et al. (396)	≥2	72	11(15%)	306	15 (5%)
Nixon et al. (397)	8.3 (median)	107	15 (14%)	1,026	92 (9%)
Veronesi et al. (398)	6 (median)	95	9 (9%)	1,137	45 (4%)
Vicini et al. (391)	5 (actuarial)	65	14 (21%)	721	65 (9%)

to the evaluation of factors that identify patients at increased risk for local relapse following lumpectomy and radiation therapy. Although prognostic factors for local relapse are not as well evaluated as they have been for systemic relapse, there have been numerous studies demonstrating the prognostic value of molecular and genetic markers for local relapse. Local relapse following breast-conserving surgery and radiation can be governed by a complex array of host, primary tumor, and treatment factors.

Given the complex interaction of these factors, it is sometimes difficult to separate out the independent significance of any one factor. There have, however, been several factors that have been consistently reported in influencing local relapse in the conservatively managed breast cancer patient. Table 56.15 summarizes some of the more commonly reported prognostic factors for local relapse. The factors that most consistently have been reported to influence local relapse, namely, young age, margin status, and the use of systemic therapy, are discussed first, followed by other commonly evaluated prognostic factors.

Age

Young age has been shown in numerous studies to be a risk factor for breast recurrence in conservation surgery and irradiation. These are summarized in Table 56.16.[92,293,392–401]

Different investigators have used various age cutoffs, such as 40, 35, and 30 years. Vilcoq et al.[317] found a locoregional recurrence rate of 35% versus 4% in women younger or older than 30 years. Kurtz et al.[395] reported a 19% incidence of local recurrence in 210 women younger than 40 years of age, compared with 9% in 1,172 older women. This observation correlated with EIC, high tumor grade, and a major mononuclear cell reaction. The Harvard Joint Center's inferior results in younger women also correlated with the presence of EIC.[402] These findings have also been reported by other authors.[379,390,403]

One of the most significant and powerful studies correlating young age with local relapse was the large EORTC boost versus no boost trial.[404] Overall in this study young patient age was a significant predictor of local relapse. As shown in Figure 56.16, the use of a boost, as will be discussed later, was most effective in younger women, although the more recent update found an advantage to the boost in all age groups.[405] In a review of 3,602 women who underwent surgery (breast conservation, 55%, or mastectomy, 45%) for early breast cancer and were rolled in EORTC studies, de Bock et al.[406] clearly demonstrated the impact of young age on local relapse. The results of multivariate analysis showed that younger age and breast conservation were risk factors for isolated locoregional recurrence (breast cancer under 35 years of age vs. over 50 years of age: hazard ratio [HR] 2.80; 95% CI, 1.41 to 5.60; breast cancer age 35 to 50 years vs. over 50 years: HR 1.72; 95% CI, 1.17 to 2.54; breast conservation: HR 1.82; 95% CI, 1.17 to 2.86). After perioperative chemotherapy, less isolated locoregional recurrences were observed (HR 0.63; 95% CI, 0.44 to 0.91). It is concluded that young age and breast-conserving therapy are both independent predictors for isolated locoregional recurrence. The authors note that as an isolated locoregional recurrence is a potentially curable condition, women treated with breast conservation or diagnosed with breast cancer at a young age should be monitored closely to detect local recurrence at an early stage.

Numerous other studies have confirmed in univariate and multivariate analyses a significant correlation between younger age and local relapse rates. Although there is no apparent cutoff age where relapse rates significantly change, most of the studies have selected 35 years of age or 40 years of age to demonstrate the differences.[290,292,293,394,397,407,408] However, one study that compared the outcome of breast conservation in patients under 40 found that those under 35 had a higher risk of recurrence compared with those aged 36 to 40.[409]

Margin Status

Positive margin status has been one of the most consistently reported factors associated with higher local relapse rates. Selected studies are summarized in Table 56.17.[225,226,375,380,392,410–425] Due to the varying definitions of margin status and the complex interaction between margin status and use of systemic therapy, radiation dose, and patient age, there are conflicting conclusions regarding the influence of margin status on local relapse.

TABLE 56.17 IPSILATERAL BREAST RECURRENCE RATES BY MARGINS

Study (Reference)	Follow-Up (Year)	Recurrence Rates with Different Margin Status: Positive (%)	Close (%)	Negative (%)
Anscher et al. (411)	5 actuarial	10	–	2
Bartelink et al. (375)	6 actuarial	7	–	2
Borger et al. (412)	5 actuarial	16	–	2
Clarke and Martinez (392)	5 mean	9	–	4
Dewar et al. (380)	10 actuarial	14	–	6
DiBiase et al. (413)	10 actuarial	33	–	12
Freedman et al. (414)	5 actuarial	12	14	7
Ghossein et al. (415)	7 median	10	–	12
Hartsell et al. (416)	3.4 median	11	–	2
Heimann et al. (417)	5 actuarial	11	–	2
Jobsen et al. (426)	10 actuarial	12	–	5
Obedian and Haffty (225)	10 actuarial	17	2	2
Peterson et al. (419)	8 actuarial	10	17	8
Park et al. (418)	8 crude rate	18	7	7
Pittinger et al. (424)	4.5 crude rate	25	2.9	3
Ryoo et al. (420)	3.5 median	–	13	8
Schnitt et al. (447)	6.2 median	13	4	2
Smitt et al. (226)	–	9	16	2
Solin et al. (422)	5 actuarial	2	11	7
Vicini et al. (423)	12 actuarial	30	18–24	9
Wazer et al. (425)	12 actuarial	17	9	5

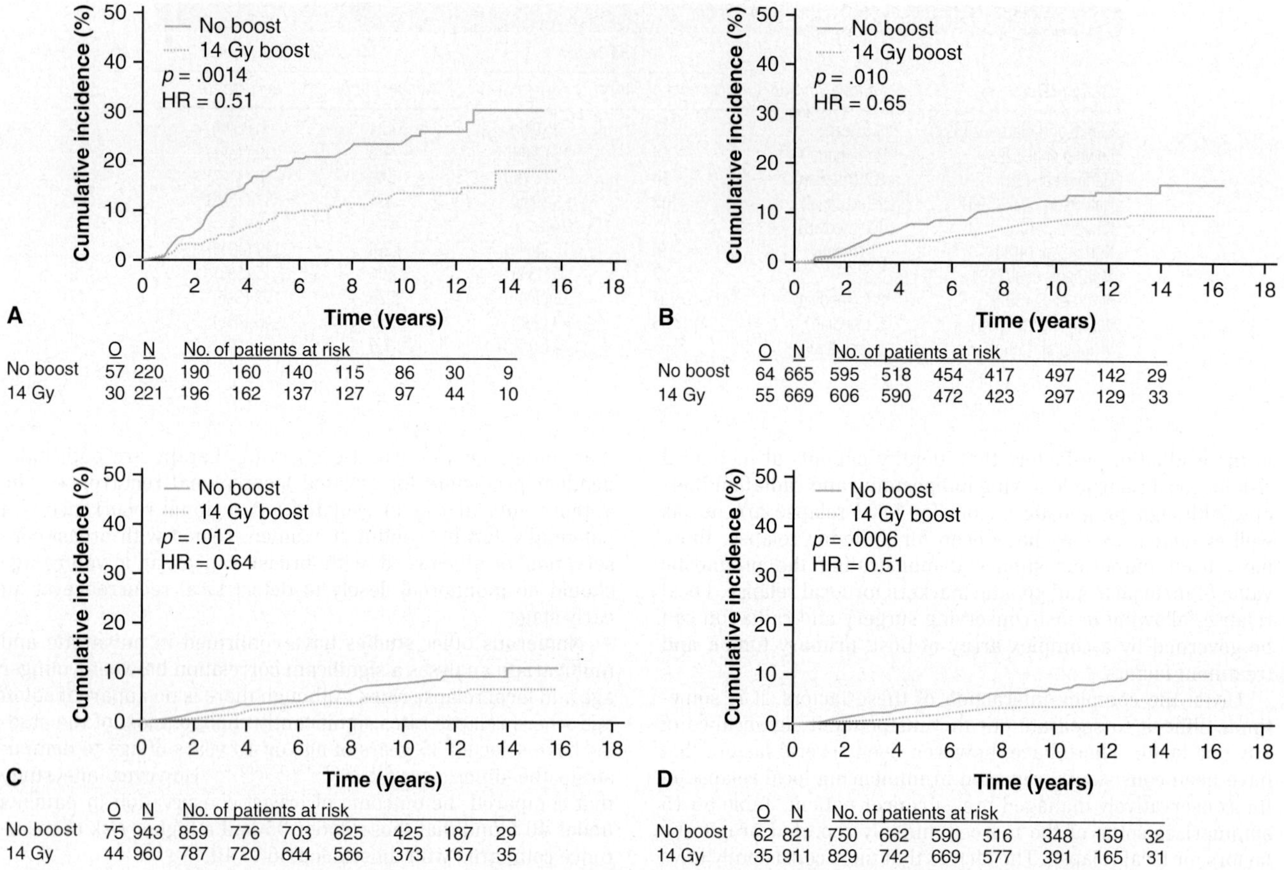

FIGURE 56.16. Cumulative incidence of recurrence of tumor in the ipsilateral breast after whole-breast irradiation at 50 Gy, with or without an additional dose to the tumor bed as a function of age group. (From Bartelink H, Horiot JC, Poortmans PM, et al. Impact of a higher radiation dose on local control and survival in breast-conserving therapy of early breast cancer: 10-year results of the randomized boost versus no boost EORTC 22881–10882 trial. *J Clin Oncol* 2007;25(22):3259–3265, with permission.)

Definition of a negative margin is variable between institutions and in national studies. Although some consider no tumor cells seen on the inked margin definitive, as defined by the NSABP, others consider negative as margins of 1 or 2 mm beyond invasive cancer; of note, many of the studies evaluating margin status utilized pathological reports without a central re-review of the original pathology.

The degree of margin involvement (i.e., whether it is focally involved or more diffusely involved) is also a critical issue in determining the significance of margin involvement and how it should influence management. Although there are clearly conflicting reports, it is evident that obtaining a wide negative margin is desirable. However, a focally involved margin, particularly when re-excision is not technically feasible, as may be the case with a focally involved deep margin at the pectoralis facia, is not a contraindication to breast-conserving therapy.

Interaction Between Margin Status and Other Variables

The complex interaction between margin status and other treatment-related factors is demonstrated in a recent study by Park et al.[418] They demonstrated that local relapse was significantly higher in patients with diffuse margin involvement than in patients with negative margins. Patients with focally involved margins also had a higher risk of local relapse than patients with negative margins. However, in those women with focally involved margins who received systemic therapy, the local relapse rate was similar to those with negative margins. Whether systemic therapy delays or negates the effect of a focally involved margin is a matter of debate, but clearly there are confounding factors that complicate interpretation of the available data.

Freedman et al.[414] studied 1,262 patients with clinical stage I or II breast cancer treated by breast-conserving surgery, axillary node dissection, and radiation therapy. The final margins were negative in 77%, positive in 12%, and close (≤2 mm) in 11%. The 5-year incidence of ipsilateral breast tumor recurrence was not significantly different amoung patients with negative (4%), positive (5%), or close (7%) margins. However, by 10 years, a significant difference in ipsilateral breast tumor recurrence became apparent (negative 7%, positive 12%, close 14%; $P = .04$). The 5-year cumulative ipsilateral breast tumor recurrence rate in patients with close or positive margins was 1% with adjuvant systemic therapy and 13% with no adjuvant therapy. However, by 10 years, the ipsilateral breast tumor recurrence rate was similar (18% vs. 14%), due to more late failures in the patients who received adjuvant systemic therapy.

A study by Jobsen et al.[426] demonstrates some of the difficulties associated with interpretation of studies related to margin status and local relapse as it relates to other prognostic factors. In a study of 1,752 patients with known margin status and a median follow-up of 78 months, the 10-year local relapse rate was 5.6% and 12.2% for negative and positive margins, respectively. An interaction between age category and margin status was noted in relation to local relapse-free survival. The 5-year local relapse rate for women younger than 40 years of age was 8.4% for negative margins and 36.9% for positive margins (P = .005). On the other hand, the 5-year local relapse rate for women over 40 years old was 2.6% for negative and 2.2% for positive margins.

Although it is clear that margin status is a significant risk factor for local relapse, and negative margins are desirable, the available data suggest that patients with a focally involved margin are suitable candidates for breast-conserving therapy followed by radiation therapy to the intact breast.

Effect of Systemic Therapy on Local Control

The use of systemic therapy, in the form of adjuvant tamoxifen or adjuvant chemotherapy, has been clearly shown to impact local control in numerous retrospective and prospective randomized trials. Although it has been clearly demonstrated in randomized trials that chemotherapy and tamoxifen are not appropriate substitutes for radiation therapy, in patients who are treated with radiation therapy, the use of systemic therapy improves local control.[93,94,97,427] As with the other critical prognostic factors, the degree to which systemic therapy influences local control is confounded by other factors.

In the NSABP B-06 trial, patients with lymph node–positive disease who were treated with radiation therapy and chemotherapy had an 8-year local recurrence rate of 5% compared with a local recurrence rate of 12% in lymph node–negative patients treated with surgery and radiation therapy alone.[360] In the NSABP B-21 trial, tamoxifen similarly improved local control rates in patients with lymph node–negative breast tumors smaller than 1 cm. The crude rate of breast tumor recurrence was only 3% in women randomly assigned to undergo lumpectomy, radiation therapy, and tamoxifen compared with 7% in women treated with lumpectomy and radiation therapy alone.[95] A retrospective analysis from the MD Anderson Cancer Center investigating the impact of systemic therapy on local control after breast-conserving therapy in patients with lymph node–negative breast cancer further confirmed these data.[97] In this study, 277 patients treated with systemic therapy had improved 5-year (97.5% vs. 89.8%) and 10-year (95.6% vs. 85.2%) local control rates compared with 207 patients who received no systemic treatment. No statistically significant difference was evident in local control between patients treated with chemotherapy and those treated with tamoxifen alone (P = .219). In a Cox regression analysis, the use of systemic therapy was the most powerful clinical, pathologic, or treatment predictor of local control, producing a 3.3-fold reduction in the risk of local recurrence. Similar results have been reported in series from Yale as well as the Netherlands, where the risk of local relapse was lower among patients treated by breast-conserving surgery and radiation with adjuvant chemotherapy or adjuvant tamoxifen, compared with patients treated without adjuvant systemic therapy.[427,428] Table 56.18 summarizes several of these studies that have evaluated local control as a function of systemic therapy. It is evident that both hormonal therapy as well as cytotoxic chemotherapy influence local relapse rates.[429–431]

TABLE 56.18 IPSILATERAL BREAST RECURRENCE RATES BY SYSTEMIC TREATMENT (SysTx)

Study (Reference)	Number of Patients	Follow-Up (Year)	SysTx	Local Relapse With SysTx	Local Relapse Without SysTx	P
NSABP-13 (431)	760	8	CTX	2.6%	13%	.001
NSABP-14 (430)	1400	10	Tam	3.4%	10.3%	.001
Buchholz (97)	484	8	CTX+Tam	4.4%	14.8%	.004
Haffty et al. (92)	548	7	CTX+Tam	6%	12%	.02
Park et al. (positive margin) (418)	45	8	CTX	7%	18%	.05
Van der Leest (427)	758	8.5	CTX	5%	12%	.002

CTX, chemotherapy; Tam, tamoxifen.

TABLE 56.19 CONSERVATION SURGERY AND IRRADIATION IN BREAST CANCER: LOCAL RECURRENCE AT 5 YEARS CORRELATED WITH INITIAL TUMOR STAGE

Study (Reference)	Stage T1 or I		Stage T2 or II	
	Percent Local Recurrence (Total Number of Patients in Study)			
Barr et al. (374)	12	(101)	12	(255)
Bartelink et al. (375)	2	(360)	2	(197)
Calle et al. (376)	7	(190)	11	(113)
Clarke et al. (392)	6	(305)	3	(95)
Delouche et al. (379)	6	(220)	14	(190)
Dubois et al. (381)	10.8	(231)	16.1	(161)
Eberlein et al. (433)	13	–	12	–
Fisher et al. (434)	7	(306)	12	(257)
Fowble et al. (104)	8	–	8	–
Leung et al. (435)	7.4	(150)	12.8	(335)
Perez et al. (436)	5	(1039)	10	(308)
Pierquin et al. (387)	8	–	12	–
Solin et al. (389)	5	(217)	8	(166)
Stotter et al. (437)	10	(249)	12	(241)
van Limbergen et al. (390)	5	(57)	11.5	(104)

Trastuzumab (Herceptin) is a humanized monoclonal antibody against the human EGFR-2 (*HER2*), which is amplified or overexpressed in about 15% to 20% of invasive breast cancers; these tumors are known to be more aggressive and more susceptible to recurrence than *HER2*-negative tumors. Romond et al.[274] reported on a combine analysis from two large cooperative group studies investigating the utility of trastuzumab in *HER2*-positive patients with operable breast cancer and found that trastuzumab improved disease-free survival by an absolute value of 12% at 3 years and was associated with a 33% reduction in the risk of death (P = .015). Interestingly, they also reported that ipsilateral breast tumor recurrence as a site of first failure was reduced from 57 patients to 27 patients with the use of trastuzumab. Recently, Kiess et al.[432] reported on a series of 197 women with early-stage breast cancer; 70 women did not receive trastuzumab while 102 did receive trastuzumab. They found that the 3-year locoregional recurrence-free survival rate was 90% without trastuzumab and 99% with trastuzumab. Moreover, locoregional recurrences were reduced from 7 to 1 with the use of trastuzumab.

Tumor Size

Although tumor size is clearly a strong predictor of systemic relapse and overall survival, its prognostic value in local relapse has not been consistently reported (Table 56.19).[98,363,374–376,379,381,387,389,390,392,433–437] Differences are probably related to the treatment techniques used (e.g., completeness of tumor excision, use of irradiation boost) and the complex interaction of other prognostic factors, as noted above.

Tumor Location

Location of the primary tumor within the breast is not known to be a contraindication to breast-conserving surgery, and any specific location is not associated with a higher local relapse rate. Haffty et al.,[438] in a review of 1,014 patients with early breast cancer treated with breast-conservation therapy, identified 98 patients who had a central or subareolar tumor. Ten of 98 patients had the nipple–areola complex sacrificed at the time of surgery, whereas the remaining 88 patients had the entire area included in the boost cone–down field. The 10-year actuarial breast recurrence-free survival rate was 84%, the distant disease-free survival rate was 88%, and the overall survival rate was 79%, similar to patients with tumors in other locations. The nipple–areola complex could be preserved in most patients, and there were no significant complications. Thus, a subareolar breast cancer presentation was not a contraindication to breast-conserving therapy in early-stage disease.

However, Gajdos et al.[439] reported on 95 women with tumors located within 2 cm of the border of the areola, considered to be subareolar carcinomas; 62 were treated with breast-conserving surgery and 33 with mastectomies. Radiation therapy was given to 87% of the breast-conserving surgery group and to 13% of the mastectomy group. The nipple–areola complex was removed in 11 women in the breast-conserving group. On univariate analysis, variables significantly related to pathologic involvement of the nipple–areola complex were clinical involvement of the nipple–areola complex (P = .001), mammographic calcifications or Paget's disease (P <.001), pathologic tumor size (P = .019), and the presence of an EIC (P = .098). When radiation therapy was accounted for in multivariate analysis, the only variable significantly related to local recurrence in patients undergoing breast-conserving surgery was clinical involvement of the nipple–areola complex.

Extensive Intraductal Carcinoma

According to the Harvard definition of EIC, 25% or more of the primary tumor is intraductal carcinoma, and intraductal carcinoma is seen outside (adjacent to) the infiltrating tumor border.[440] Fourquet et al.[383] reported a 20% incidence of EIC in 185 women younger than 45 years of age compared with 10.4% in 279 older women. EIC involving the primary tumor and adjacent tissues has been reported by some groups, particularly Harvard University and Marseilles, to be associated with a higher incidence of breast recurrences.[395,441,442] In contrast, others have found no significant impact on local tumor control with EIC.[196,232,378,390] This difference may be related to the definition of EIC, adequacy of tumor excision, doses of irradiation delivered to the boost volume, as well as interactions with other factors. It has been reported by some that a somewhat higher breast relapse rate in EIC-positive patients was seen only in women younger than 40 years of age. Table 56.20 summarizes reports of breast relapse correlated with presence of EIC in selected studies.[98,196,198,375,398,402,433,442–444]

Holland et al.[445] stated that an EIC component is associated with subsequent breast recurrence because of the presence of residual intraductal carcinoma in these patients. In a series of 214 women who underwent mastectomy, 71% of those with EIC had residual intraductal carcinoma, compared with 28% of those without that pathologic feature. In particular, 44% of the EIC-positive patients had prominent residual tumor compared with 3% of those who were EIC negative (P <.00001).

The impact of EIC on local relapse, however, appears to be minimized if negative margins are achieved. Although negative margins are desirable in all patients undergoing breast-conserving surgery, attention to margins in patients with EIC is particularly relevant, as a negative margin may decrease or eliminate the significance of EIC with respect to local failure. In a study from the Harvard group, Gage et al.[446] evaluated clinical stage I or II breast carcinoma treated with radiation therapy as part of breast-conserving therapy, of whom 343 had invasive ductal histology evaluable for an extensive intraductal component, had inked margins that were evaluable for an review of their pathology slides, and received ≥60 Gy to the tumor bed. The 5-year rate of ipsilateral breast recurrence (IBR) for patients with negative margins was 2%; for patients with positive margins, the rate was 16%. Among patients with negative margins, the 5-year rate of IBR was 2% for all patients with close margins (negative ≤1 mm) and 3% for those with negative margins >1 mm. For patients with close margins, the rates were 2% and 0% for EIC-negative and EIC-positive tumors, respectively; the corresponding rates for patients with negative margins greater than 1 mm were 1% and 14%. The 5-year rate of IBR for patients with focally positive margins was 9% (9% for EIC-negative and 7% for EIC-positive patients). The 5-year crude rate of IBR for patients with greater than focally positive margins was 28% (19% for EIC-negative and 42% for EIC-positive patients). The authors conclude that patients with negative margins of excision have a low rate of recurrence in the treated breast, whether the margin is >1 mm or ≤1 mm and whether the carcinoma is EIC-negative or EIC-positive. It appears from this study that although EIC may be a poor prognostic factor for local relapse, achievement of a negative margin eliminates EIC as a risk factor.

From a group of 885 patients treated for clinical stage I or II invasive breast cancer, Schnitt et al.[447] limited their study to 181 patients with invasive ductal carcinoma (IDC) who received a radiation dose to the surgical site of 60 Gy or greater, whose final microscopic margins of resection were evaluable, and who had at least 5 years of follow-up. In 157 patients (87%), the tumor was evaluable for the presence or absence of EIC. The 5-year rates of recurrence among patients with negative, close, focally positive, and more than focally positive margins were 0%, 4%, 6%, and 21%, respectively. Among the 127 patients with EIC-negative tumors, the 5-year recurrence rate was <10% in all margin groups. Among the 30 patients with EIC-positive tumors, the 5-year recurrence rate was 0% when margins were negative or close but 50% when margins were more than focally positive. These results provide support for the use of breast-conserving therapy (including an irradiation boost to the primary site) for patients with EIC-positive tumors and negative margins.

TABLE 56.20 INCIDENCE OF BREAST RELAPSE CORRELATED WITH EXTENSIVE INTRADUCTAL CARCINOMA COMPONENT IN PRIMARY BREAST TUMOR ADJACENT BREAST

	Percent Breast Recurrence at 5 Years (Total Number of Patients in Study)			
Study (Reference)	EIC Present		EIC Absent	
Bartelink et al. (375)	9	(79)	2	(208)
Boyages et al. (443)	24	(166)	6	(418)
Eberlein et al. (433)	27	(166)	7	(418)
Fisher et al. (196)	11	(56)	9	(366)
Fowble et al. (98)	22	(23)	4	(252)
Kurtz et al. (298)	18	(106)	8	(390)
Schnitt et al. (444)	15	(133)	1	(98)
Veronesi et al. (398)				
Quadrantectomy	10	(22)	4	(338)
Tumorectomy	30	(38)	8	(307)
Zafrani et al. (198)	11	(63)	6	(361)

EIC, extensive intraductal carcinoma.

Histology

In general, studies that have evaluated local relapse in relation to histologic subtypes of breast cancer have not demonstrated higher relapse rates associated with specific histologic patterns. Weiss et al.[240] reported on 879 patients with stage I and II breast cancer treated with conservation surgery and irradiation. The patients were divided into 7 groups based on histologic subtype: 368 patients with infiltrating and intraductal ductal carcinoma, 389 with IDC, 41 with ILC, 23 with combined infiltrating ductal and lobular carcinoma, 28 with medullary carcinoma, 12 with colloid carcinoma, and 18 with tubular carcinoma. There were no significant differences in 5-year actuarial overall survival, cause-specific survival, or relapse-free survival rates among the histologic categories. There was, however, a difference among the seven groups in distant metastasis only at first failure, with IDCs having the highest rate.

Thurman et al.,[241] in an analysis of the Harvard series, identified twenty clinical stage I and II patients with mucinous carcinoma, 27 with medullary carcinoma, 28 with tubular carcinoma, and 1,055 with IDC were identified. No significant

TABLE 56.21 LOBULAR CARCINOMA TREATED WITH BREAST CONSERVING SURGERY AND RADIATION (SELECTED SERIES WITH 10-YEAR FOLLOW-UP)

Study (Reference)	Number Lobular/ Number Ductal	Local Relapse Lobular/ Ductal	Contralateral Lobular/ Ductal	Overall Survival Lobular/Ductal
Santiago et al. (449)	55/1093	18% vs. 12% (NS)	12% vs. 8% (NS)	85% vs. 79% (NS)
Vo et al. (450)	04/1120	4% vs. 9% (NS)	11.5% vs. 11.9% (NS)	81% vs. 85% (NS)
Moran et al. (453)	142/1760	20% vs. 13% (NS)	26% vs. 12% (P = .006)	68% v. 78% (P = .08)
Salvadori et al. (452)	286/1903	8% vs. 8% (NS)	NR	NR
Peiro et al. (451)	93/1089	15% vs. 13% (NS)	4% vs. 6% (NS)	NR

NS, not significant; NR, no results.

difference was seen in the site of first failure among the four histologic types within the first 10 years after treatment. Local failure was significantly associated with age <50 years (P = .04), positive surgical margins (P = .007), lymphovascular invasion (P = .04), and presence of an extensive intraductal component (P <.001).

An analysis of medullary carcinomas treated conservatively was performed by the Yale group, who identified 46 cases of conservatively treated patients with medullary histology who were compared with 1,444 patients with infiltrating ductal carcinoma.[202] The medullary cohort presented at a younger age with a higher percentage of patients in the 35 years or younger age group (26.1% vs. 6.6%; P <.00001). Twelve patients with medullary histology underwent genetic screening, and six patients were identified with deleterious mutations. This group showed greater association with *BRCA1/2* mutations compared with screened patients in the control group (50.0% vs. 15.8%; P = .0035). The medullary cohort was also significantly associated with greater T stage and tumor size (37.0% vs. 17.2%; T2 mean size 3.2 vs. 2.5 cm; P = .00097) as well as negative ER (84.9% vs. 37.6%; P <.00001) and PR (87.5% vs. 48.1%; P = .00001) status. Breast relapse-free rates were not significantly different from the invasive ductal cancers (76.7% vs. 85.2%), however, 10-year distant relapse-free survival in the medullary cohort was significantly better than in the control group (94.9% vs. 77.5%; P = .028).

Tubular carcinomas treated with conservative surgery and radiation were reviewed by Sullivan et al.[201] They reviewed 62 of their own cases from the Massachusetts General as well as 529 cases from the literature. They conclude that tubular carcinoma is associated with an excellent prognosis, but long-term follow-up is essential for detecting local failures. Adjuvant RT reduces the incidence of local failure following CS for tubular carcinoma. However, elderly women treated by CS may have a very low risk of local recurrence without adjuvant RT.

Infiltrating Lobular Carcinoma

A review of the literature strongly supports local tumor resection and breast irradiation as appropriate therapy for invasive lobular breast cancer, following the same guidelines used for invasive ductal tumors. Breast tumor control and survival after breast-conserving therapy are equivalent in patients with invasive ductal or lobular carcinoma. Due to the presumed multicentric nature of lobular carcinomas, several groups have attempted to assess whether these subtypes are more prone to local failure with breast-conserving approaches.[242,448–453] Table 56.21 summarizes results of several selected series of patients treated with breast-conserving surgery and radiation comparing outcomes in lobular carcinoma to invasive ductal carcinomas. Although some of the studies show higher contralateral rates in lobular carcinomas, local relapse, disease-free, and overall survival appear to be comparable to invasive ductal carcinomas. The majority of studies show local-regional control, disease-free, and overall survival rates in lobular carcinomas that are comparable to patients with invasive ductal carcinomas.

Lobular Carcinoma In Situ as a Component of Invasive Cancers

Several groups have evaluated whether patients with LCIS as a component of invasive cancer or DCIS was associated with higher local relapse rates. Conflicting results from these studies, as outlined in Table 56.22, preclude firm conclusions.[454–458] Sasson et al.[458] noted that LCIS was present in 65 of 1,274 patients (5%) with stage I or II breast cancer. LCIS was more likely to be associated with an ILC (30 of 59 patients; 51%) than with IDC (26 of 1,125 patients; 2%). The 10-year cumulative incidence rate of ipsilateral breast tumor recurrence was 6% in women without LCIS compared with 29% in women with LCIS (P = .0003). In both groups, the majority of recurrences were invasive. The 10-year cumulative incidence rate of ipsilateral breast tumor recurrence in patients who received tamoxifen was 8% when LCIS was present compared with 6% when LCIS was absent (P = .46). In a series of 56 patients with an LCIS component, Jolly et al.[456] reported a higher risk of local relapse at 10 years (14%) compared with a rate of 7% in cases without an LCIS component. In multivariate analysis a component of LCIS was associated with a higher risk of local relapse.

However, studies from Yale, Harvard, Michigan, and a more recent study from Fox Chase failed to show a higher local relapse rate in patients with a component of LCIS. Abner et al.[454] reviewed 1,181 patients with stage I or II infiltrating ductal, infiltrating lobular, or infiltrating carcinoma with mixed features who had received at least 60 Gy to the tumor bed and

TABLE 56.22 STUDIES EVALUATING LCIS AS A COMPONENT OF BREAST CANCER LOCAL RELAPSE IN BREAST-CONSERVING THERAPY PLUS RADIATION THERAPY

	Number of Patients and Controls			Local relapse		
Study (Reference)	With LCIS	Without LCIS	Follow-Up (Median, Year)	With LCIS (%)	Without LCIS (%)	P
Moran and Haffty (457)	51	1,045	10.6	5	7	NS
Abner et al. (454)	119	1,062	13.4	13	12	NS
Ben-David et al. (455)	64	121	3.9	100	99.1	NS
Jolly et al. (456)	46	551	8.7	14	7	.04
Sasson et al. (458)	65	1,209	6.3	15	5	.001
Ciocca et al. (459)	290	2,604	6.0	4.5	3.8	NS

LCIS, lobular carcinoma *in situ;* NS, not significant

had a minimum follow-up of 8 years. Of the 1,181 patients, 137 had detectable LCIS in or adjacent to the tumor. The 8-year local recurrence rate was not significantly increased for patients with LCIS overall or for the subgroup of patients with LCIS in or adjacent to the tumor. The risk of contralateral disease and of distant treatment failure also was unaffected by the presence or extent of LCIS (5% to 10% in all groups). Similar results were reported by Moran and Haffty[457] in an analysis of the Yale series where there was no statistically significant difference between patients with or without a component of LCIS in the 10-year overall survival (67% vs. 72%), distant disease-free survival (62% vs. 79%), or ipsilateral breast tumor recurrence-free survival (77% LCIS vs. 84% control). Ben-David et al.[455] reported the results on 64 cases treated at University of Michigan and also found no association between local failure and presence of LCIS. The presence of LCIS at the margins and the size and presence of multifocal LCIS did not alter the rate of local control. Ciocca et al.,[459] in an analysis of 290 patients with LCIS as a component compared with 2,604 without LCIS as a component, showed no difference in local control, even if LCIS was present at the final margin.

Other Histologic Features

Clemente et al.,[460] in 506 cases of infiltrating ductal carcinoma (T1-2N0M0), described peritumoral lymphatic infiltration in 6.9% of routinely evaluated specimens, whereas in a randomly selected group of 234 cases the frequency was 20%. Patients with peritumoral lymphatic infiltration had worse disease-free and total survival rates than those without this feature (P = .0001 for each), as well as more local recurrences (P = .0001) and a higher incidence of distant metastases (P = .0576).

Wong et al.,[461] in a study of 234 patients with clinical T1N0 breast cancer treated with breast-conservation surgery and radiation therapy, scored 180 patients as lymphatic vessel invasion negative and 54 as invasion positive (23 focal and 31 extensive). The local first failure rates were 14% and 22%, respectively. The percentages of regional distant failure (without local failure) were 12% and 21%, respectively. At 10 years, 60% of the lymphatic vessel invasion–negative patients remained free of any failure, compared with 50% of the lymphatic vessel invasion–positive patients.

Nodal Status

Although nodal status is the strongest predictor of distant metastasis and overall survival, most studies have not clearly demonstrated an effect of nodal status on local control in the conservatively managed breast cancer patient. This may be because a majority of node-positive patients receive chemotherapy or hormonal therapy, which may counteract any adverse effects on local relapse. There are some data, however, that suggest an effect of nodal status on local relapse in conservatively managed patients. The Primary Therapy of Breast Cancer Study Group and others noted lower survival and a greater incidence of local recurrences in patients with positive axillary nodes after partial mastectomy.[233,462–464] At the Institut Gustave-Roussy, among 356 patients, local recurrence was noted in 26% of those with and 6.5% of those without nodal involvement; the greater the number of nodes involved, the more likely the occurrence of local failure and the lower the survival rate.[242,465] Increased incidence of breast relapse was also observed by van Limbergen et al.[390] in patients with N1b metastasis (8 of 42 patients, or 19%) and in those in whom three or more lymph nodes (4 of 14 patients, or 28.6%) compared with patients with N0 or N1a lymph nodes (14 of 187; 7.5%). However, more recent reports by several investigators noted lower survival rates but fewer breast relapses after breast-conservation therapy in patients with positive nodes. Again, this is likely a result of the interaction of irradiation to the breast with adjuvant chemotherapy. Because most node positive patients receive chemotherapy, which is synergistic with radiation in lowering the local relapse rate, any potential adverse effect of positive nodes on local relapse may be lost.

Molecular Factors and Local Relapse

In comparison with an explosion of data regarding molecular markers as risk factors for overall survival and distant metastasis in breast cancer, there are relatively few data relating molecular markers to local relapse in the conservatively managed breast. There have been several studies, however, that demonstrate the potential application of molecular markers in predicting local-regional relapse in breast cancer patients.[466–468] Particularly exciting is the potential to not only use these markers to identify patients at risk for relapse, but also to consider the molecular markers as potential targets for therapeutic intervention and increasing radiation sensitivity. Several molecular markers have been shown in bench studies to be associated with radiation resistance, including *p53*, *HER2/neu*, insulin-like growth factor-1 receptor, and other markers associated with hypoxia.[467–490] In general, molecular subtypes of breast cancer may be organized into the following general categories: luminal A (ER-positive or PR-positive and Ki-67 <14%), luminal B (ER-positive or PR -positive and Ki-67 ≥14%), luminal-*HER2* (ER-positive or PR-positive and *HER2*-positive), *HER2* enriched (ER-negative, PR-negative, and *HER2*-positive), and basal-like (ER-negative, PR-negative, *HER2*-negative, and EFGR-positive or CK5/6-positive).

Haffty et al.[491] examined patients treated with breast-conserving therapy plus radiation and identified 482 patients with ER, PR, and *HER2* available for analysis. Patients were then stratified into triple negative (TN) and non-TN status. They found that at 5 years, the TN cohort had a poorer distant metastasis-free rate compared with the other subtypes (67% vs. 82%, respectively; P = .002). TN subtype was an independent predictor of distant metastasis (HR 2.14; 95% CI, 1.31 to 3.53; P = .002) and cause-specific survival (HR 1.79; 95% CI, 1.03 to 3.22; P = .047). However, there was no significant difference in local control between the TN and other subtypes (83% vs. 83%, respectively). The authors concluded that although patients classified as TN have a poor prognosis, there was no evidence that these patients are at higher risk for local relapse after conservative surgery and radiation.

Nguyen et al.[492] reported on 793 patients with invasive breast cancer who received breast-conserving therapy and radiation. With a median follow-up of 70 months, the 5-year rate of local recurrence was 1.8%; 0.8% (0.3, 2.2) for luminal A, 1.5% (0.2, 10) for luminal B, 8.4% (2.2, 30) for *HER2*, and 7.1% (3.0, 16) for basal. In addition, on multivariate analysis, *HER2* and basal subtypes were associated with increased local recurrence as compared with luminal A (P <.01). Luminal B and basal subtypes were associated with increased distant metastases as compared with luminal A (P <.04).

Voduc et al.[493] investigated the rate of local and regional relapse in 2,985 patients stratified by molecular subtype. With a median follow-up of 12 years, they found that after breast-conserving therapy and radiation, patients with luminal A tumors had the most favorable prognosis, with local relapse and regional relapse rates of only 8% and 3% at 10 years, respectively. *HER2*-enriched and basal-like groups exhibited the highest rates of LR (21% and 14%, respectively) and regional relapse (16% and 14%, respectively). After mastectomy, patients with luminal A tumors again had the best prognosis, with rates of local relapse and regional relapse (8% and 4%, respectively, at 10 years). All non–luminal A subtypes exhibited a greater risk of local relapse and regional relapse.

A recent analysis of triple negative breast cancers from a large Canadian database revealed an interesting observation. Abdulkarim et al.[494] reported a higher rate of local relapse among T1/T2 node negative mastectomy patients with treated without radiation who had triple negative disease compared with a similar node negative cohort treated with breast-conserving

TABLE 56.23 MOLECULAR MARKERS IN THE LOCAL MANAGEMENT OF EARLY BREAST CANCER TREATED WITH BREAST CONSERVATION SURGERY PLUS RADIATION THERAPY

Markers	*Study (Reference)*	*Patient Population*	*Local Relapse*
ER/PR	Silvestrini, 1995 (485)	970 node negative	No correlation for either ER or PR
	Elkhuizen et al., 1999 (472)	195 case-control IBC	Higher frequency of PR-negative tumors in locally recurrent population (75% vs. 60%; *P* = .03)
	Vrieling et al., 2003 (498)	5,569 cases	Higher recurrence rate was observed in ER-negative or PR-negative tumors
	Grills et al., 2005 (497)	1,500 IBC	Regional nodal failure was associated with ER status on univariate analysis
	Choi et al., 2005 (483)	103 IBC	Neither ER nor PR correlated with local relapse rate. PR negativity was related with distant metastasis
	Santiago et al., 2004 (477)	937 IBC	Negative PR status was related to local relapse rate
HER2/neu	Haffty et al., 1996 (469)	20 case-control IBC	Higher expression of *HER2/neu* in patients experiencing local relapse (19% vs. 10%; *P* = .10)
	Pierce et al., 1994 (474)	137 IBC	*HER2/neu* correlated with extensive intraductal component but did not correlate to local relapse
	Kim et al., 2003 (484)	611 IBC	*HER2/neu* correlated with overall survival but not local relapse
	Choi et al., 2005 (483)	103 IBC	*HER2/neu* was not related with local or distant failure
	Harris et al., 2006 (488)	356 IBC	*HER2/neu* was not related to local failure
Triple negative (TN)	Haffty et al., 2006 (491)	482 IDC	TN was not related to local control
	Nguyen et al., 2008 (492)	793 IDC	Increased local failure with TN or *HER2*+ subtypes
	Voduc et al., 2010 (493)	2985 IDC	Increased local failure with TN or *HER2*+ subtypes
	Mamounas et al., 2010 (496)	1674 IDC	Increased local failure with higher Oncotype DX score
p53	Silvestrini et al., 1997 (482)	496 IBC	No correlation with p53 and local relapse
	Turner et al., 2000 (470)	94 IBC	p53 overexpression more common in locally recurrent group compared to locally controlled group (26% vs. 9%; *P* = .02)
	Elkhuizen et al., 1999 (472)	195 case-control IBC	p53 expression similar in locally recurrent and locally controlled group (21% vs. 23%; *P* = .61)
	Amornmarn et al., 2000 (487)	112 IBC	p53 expression associated with all local recurrence cases (only 4 local relapses in series)
	Choi et al., 2005 (483)	103 IBC	p53 was not related with local or distant failure
Proliferative markers	Choi et al., 2005 (483)	103 IBC	Ki-67 positivity was related with distant but not local failure
	Silvestrini et al., 1997 (481)	496 IBC	Thymidine-labeling index was not related with local failure
ATM mutation	Meyer et al., 2004 (489)	135 IBC	ATM gene alterations were not related to patient outcomes

ER, estrogen receptor; PR, progesterone receptor; IBC, inflammatory breast cancer; IDC, invasive ductal carcinoma; ATM, ataxia telangiectasis mutations.

surgery and radiation. These results emphasize the point that triple negative breast cancers do not necessarily fair better with mastectomy.[495]

Mamounas et al.[496] investigated the risk of locoregional recurrence (LRR) in patients with early-stage, node-negative ER-positive breast cancer treated on the NSABP B14 and B20 based on the Oncotype DX recurrence score (RS). The RS was available in 355 placebo treated patients (B14), 424 chemotherapy plus tamoxifen patients (B20) and 895 tamoxifen patients (B14 and B20). In the tamoxifen-treated patients, the risk of LRR was 4.3% for patients with low RS (<18), 7.2% for those with intermediate RS (18 to 30), and 15.8% for those with high RS (>30). In placebo-treated patients, the risk of LRR was 10.8% for patients with low RS, 20.0% for those with intermediate RS, and 18.4% for those with high RS. In chemotherapy-treated patients, the risk of LRR was 1.6% for patients with low RS, 2.7% for those with intermediate RS, and 7.8% for those with high RS. The authors concluded that the Oncotype DX recurrence score was a significant predictor of LRR.

These analyses, while showing a consistent trend, should be considered exploratory and are not significant enough to base clinical decision making on. This is clearly an area that is an active area of investigation, ideally with molecular studies linked to large clinical trials, to help identify molecular markers predictive of local-regional outcomes and hopefully identify potential targets for improving outcomes. Table 56.23 summarizes selected studies evaluating molecular markers for local-regional relapse in conservatively managed breast cancers.[490,497,498]

BREAST-CONSERVING SURGERY WITHOUT RADIATION

Based on the mature data from the well-conducted randomized trials outlined above and on long-term follow-up from the several large retrospective series, it is apparent that breast-conserving surgery followed by radiation therapy is a safe and effective modality for the majority of women with early-stage invasive breast cancer.[110] Whether subsets of patients can be treated with breast-conserving surgery alone without irradiation has been the subject of considerable debate and several randomized trials. With the possible exception of selected elderly women, which will be discussed in a later section, subsets of patients in whom radiation therapy can be safely avoided have yet to be clearly identified. Collectively, the randomized studies to date consistently demonstrate an approximately threefold greater local relapse rate in the unirradiated cohorts.[90] Although the majority of these trials did not demonstrate an impact on survival, recent pooled analysis of these randomized trials demonstrates a small, but statistically significant impact on mortality as a result of the omission of radiation.

Vinh-Hung and Verschraegen[90] conducted a pooled analysis of published randomized clinical trials that compared radiotherapy versus no radiotherapy after breast-conserving surgery. The outcomes studied were ipsilateral breast tumor recurrence and patient death from any cause. A search of the literature identified 15 trials with a pooled total of 9,422 patients available for analysis. The relative risk of ipsilateral breast tumor recurrence after breast-conserving surgery, comparing patients treated with no radiotherapy or radiotherapy, was 3.00 (95% CI, 2.65 to 3.40). Mortality data were available for 13 trials with a pooled total of 8,206 patients. The relative risk of mortality was 1.086 (95% CI, 1.003 to 1.175), corresponding to an estimated 8.6% (95% CI, 0.3% to 17.5%) relative excess mortality if radiotherapy was omitted (Fig. 56.17A,B).

In an analysis from the EBCTCG, similar conclusions were reached evaluating various forms of local therapy.[89,107] Within this meta-analysis were 10,801 women treated with breast-conserving surgery in trials randomizing patients to radiation therapy versus no radiation therapy. The majority included patients with axillary clearance of node-negative disease and generally were treated with radiation to the conserved breast alone. The reduction in local recurrence (mainly in the conserved breast) in patients treated with radiotherapy was

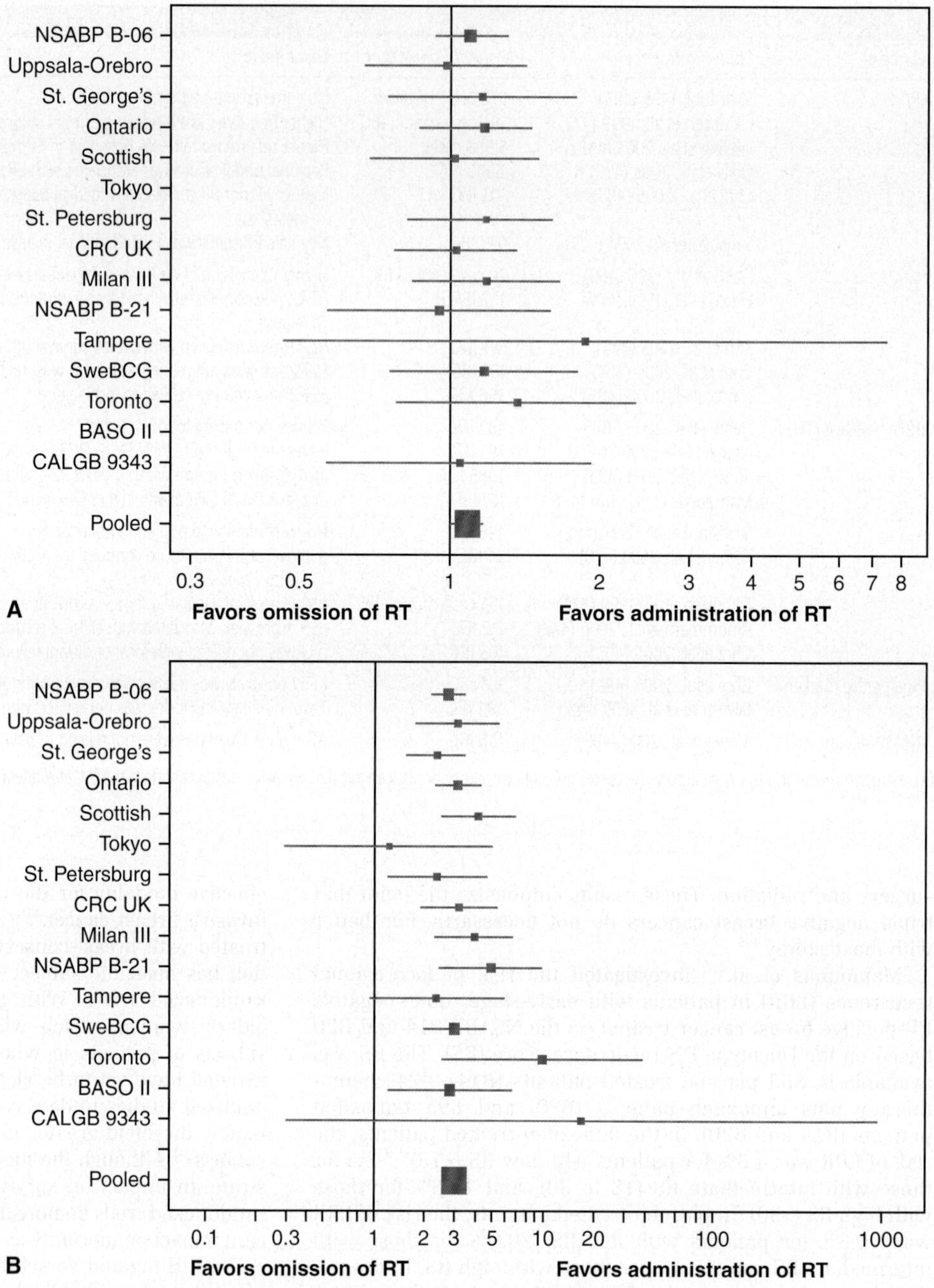

FIGURE 56.17. Meta-analysis of survival and local control in randomized trials comparing breast conserving surgery with or without radiation. This meta-analysis demonstrated a threefold reduction in local relapse and a small but significant increase in survival with the use of radiation therapy following lumpectomy. (From Vinh-Hung V, Verschraegen C. Breast-conserving surgery with or without radiotherapy: pooled-analysis for risks of ipsilateral breast tumor recurrence and mortality. *J Natl Cancer Inst* 2004;96:115–121, with permission.)

highly significant (P <.00001) in every separate trial. As seen in Figure 56.18, the recurrence rate ratio, comparing those allocated radiotherapy with those not, is about 0.3 in every trial, corresponding to a proportional reduction of 70%. Considering all 17 trials together, the 10-year risk of local recurrence is 19% among those allocated radiotherapy and 35% among those not, corresponding to an absolute reduction of 16% in this 10-year risk. The proportional risk reduction for breast cancer mortality is much less than that for local recurrence, and none of the trial-specific breast cancer mortality results are clearly significant on their own. However, collectively there is a significant impact on breast cancer mortality (breast cancer death rate ratio 0.83, standard error [SE] 0.05; 95% CI, 0.75 to 0.912; P =.0002), indicating a reduction of about one-sixth in the annual breast cancer mortality rate. The 15-year risk of death from breast cancer (in the hypothetical absence of other causes) is 30·5% among those allocated post–breast-conserving surgery radiotherapy and 35.9% among those not (corresponding to an absolute reduction of 5.4%; SE 1.7). Figure 56.19 highlights a recent update of the EBCTCG, demonstrating the impact of radiation therapy on outcome in early-stage breast cancer.[107]

Randomized Trials

Selected trials comparing breast-conserving surgery alone to breast-conserving surgery with radiation are summarized in Table 56.24.[93,95,499,500–502] The Uppsala-Orebro Breast Cancer Study group reported on a trial in which women with stage I breast carcinoma were randomly assigned to be treated with either sector resection and axillary dissection plus 54 Gy breast irradiation (184 patients) or the same surgical procedure alone (197 patients).[500] The actuarial local recurrence rates after a median follow-up of 63 to 65 months were 2.3% in the irradiated group and 18.4% with surgery only. The 5-year disease-free survival rates were 91% and 87%, and the 5-year overall survival rates were 91% and 90%, respectively.

Isolated local recurrence (events/woman-years)

Year started and study name	RT sites	Events/woman-years: Allocated BCS + RT	Events/woman-years: Allocated BCS	BCS+RT events: Logrank O–E	BCS+RT events: Variance of O–E	Ratio of annual event rates BCS + RT: BCS
(a) Radiotherapy only to conserved breast: 14% node positive						
1976 NSABP B-06	BW*	125/6862	285/4991	−93.3	84.8	
1981 Uppsala-Örebro	BW	10/1636	43/1511	−17.7	12.7	
1982 St. George's London	BW*	12/1202	31/1047	−11.5	9.6	
1984 Ontario COG	BW+S	53/3543	155/2754	−58.2	48.2	
1987 INT Milan 3	BW+S*	19/2478	60/2005	−25.1	18.2	
1989 NSABP B-21	BW+S*	6/1810	40/1729	−17.3	11.2	
1991 Swedish BCCG	BW	33/3718	92/3429	−30.8	30.5	
(a) Subtotal		258/ 21249	706/ 17466	−254.0	215.3	0.31 (SE 0.04), 2p<0.00001
5-year risk		7.2%	25.6%			
(b) Radiotherapy to conserved breast and other sites: 24% node positive						
1982 St. George's London	BW + AF*	14/620	30/380	−10.9	9.7	
1985 Scottish	BW + S + (AF) + IMC	16/2598	83/2260	−33.0	22.5	
1985 West Midlands, UK	BW + S + AF + IMC	42/2398	104/1929	−36.8	34.2	
1986 CRC, UK	Various	33/1604	77/1454	−24.3	25.7	
(b) Subtotal		105/ 7220	294/ 6023	−105.0	92.1	0.32 (SE 0.06), 2p<0.00001
5-year risk		7.7%	26.7%			
Total (a + b)		363/ 28469	1000/ 23489	−359.0	307.4	0.31 (SE 0.03), 2p<0.00001
5-year risk		7.3%	25.9%			

Heterogeneity between 11 strata: $\chi^2_{10} = 7.8$; p = 0.6

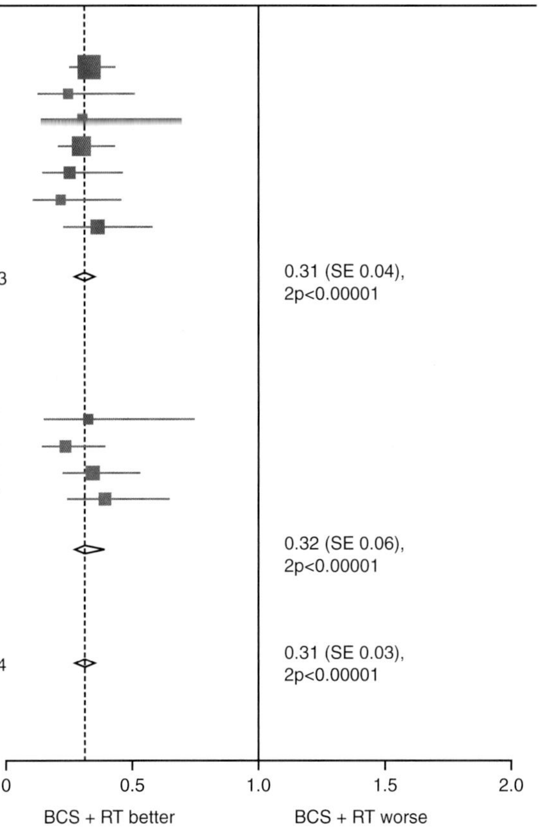

Isolated local recurrence (events/woman-years)

Year started and study name	RT sites	Events/woman-years: Allocated BCS + RT	Events/woman-years: Allocated BCS	BCS+RT deaths: Logrank O–E	BCS+RT deaths: Variance of O–E	Ratio of annual death rates BCS + RT: BCS
(a) Radiotherapy only to conserved breast: 14% node positive						
1976 NSABP B-06	BW*	267/731	305/719	−19.7	135.0	
1981 Uppsala Örebro	BW	37/184	34/197	2.3	16.8	
1982 St. George's London	BW*	24/128	25/122	−2.5	10.9	
1984 Ontario COG	BW+S	91/416	123/421	−16.4	51.5	
1987 INT Milan 3	BW+S*	40/294	51/273	−6.2	21.3	
1989 NSABP B-21	BW+S*	8/337	8/336	0.5	3.9	
1991 Swedish BCCG	BW	32/593	41/594	−3.9	18.0	
(a) Subtotal		499/ 2683	587/ 2662	−45.8	257.4	0.84 (SE 0.06), 2p = 0.004
15-year risk		28.0%	33.2%			
(b) Radiotherapy to conserved breast and other sites: 24% node positive						
1982 St. George's London	BW + AF*	31/80	28/70	−2.1	12.2	
1985 Scottish	BW + S + (AF) + IMC	59/293	78/296	−5.0	30.2	
1985 West Midlands, UK	BW + S + AF + IMC	88/358	107/349	−11.4	45.3	
1986 CRC, UK	Various	76/259	89/261	−8.3	37.6	
(b) Subtotal		254/ 990	302/ 976	−26.9	125.3	0.81 (SE 0.08), 2p = 0.02
10-year risk		28.2%	35.1%			
Total (a + b)		753/ 3673	889/ 3638	−72.7	382.7	0.83 (SE 0.05), 2p = 0.0002
15-year risk		30.5%	35.9%			

Heterogeneity between 11 strata: $\chi^2_{10} = 3.8$; p = 0.96

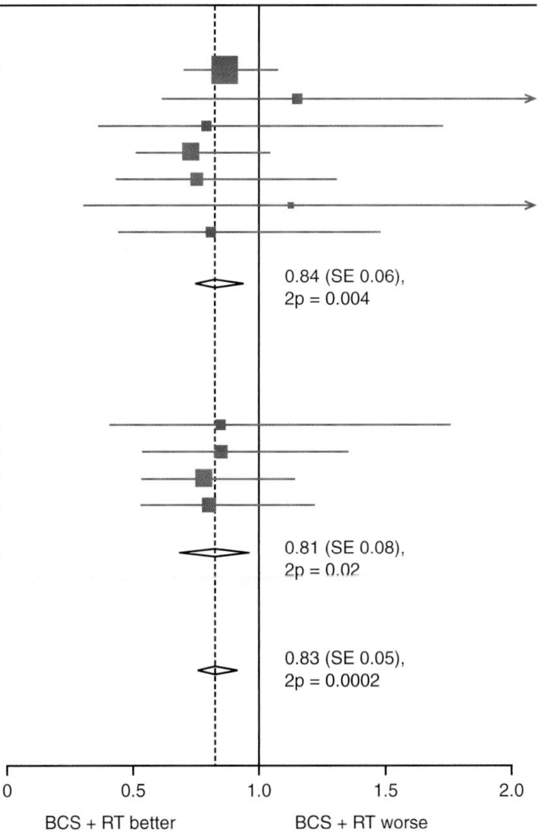

FIGURE 56.18. Meta-analysis of local control and survival from the Early Breast Cancer Trialists Collaborative Group demonstrating the impact of radiation therapy on both local control and survival in the management of breast cancer. (From Clarke M, Collins R, Darby S, et al. Effects of radiotherapy and of differences in the extent of surgery for early breast cancer on local recurrence and 15-year survival: an overview of the randomised trials. *Lancet* 2005;366:2087–2106, with permission from Elsevier.)

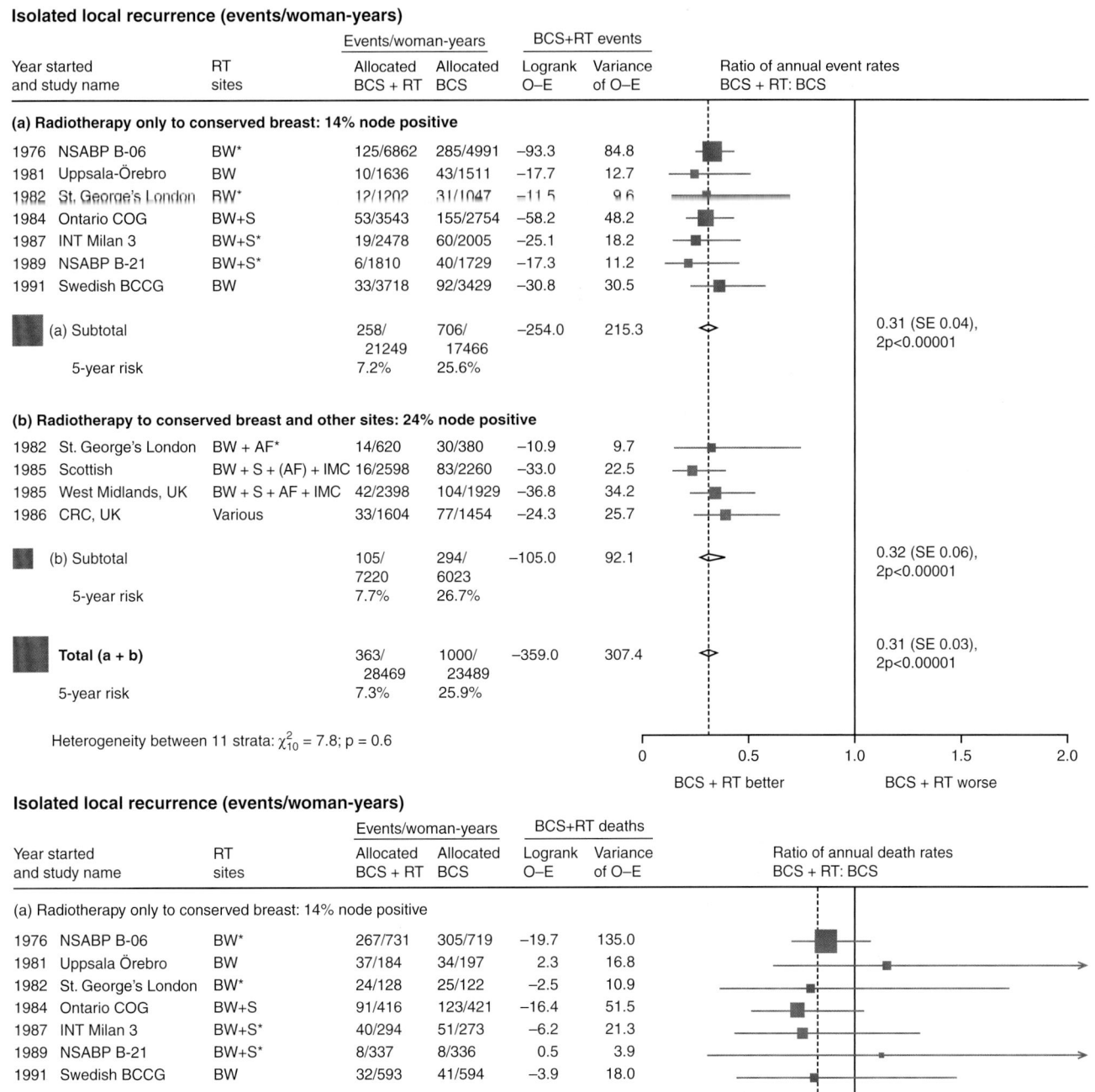

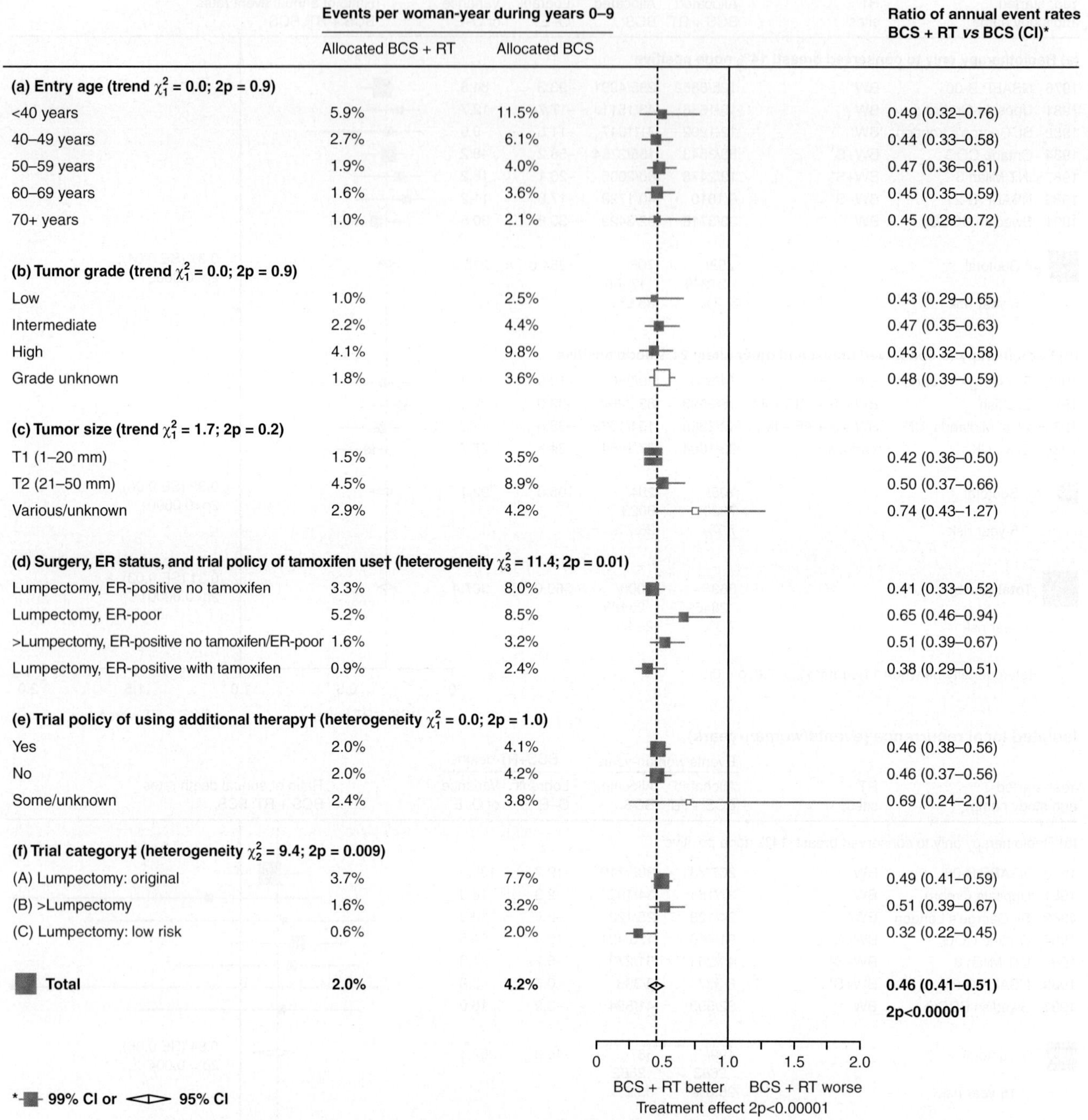

FIGURE 56.19. Updated meta-analysis from the Early Breast Cancer Trialists Collaborative Group comparing breast-conserving surgery alone to breast-conserving surgery with radiation therapy. (From Darby S, McGale P, Correa C, et al. Effect of radiotherapy after breast-conserving surgery on 10-year recurrence and 15-year breast cancer death: meta-analysis of individual patient data for 10,801 women in 17 randomised trials. *Lancet* 2011;378:1707–1716, with permission from Elsevier.)

TABLE 56.24 RESULTS OF SELECTED RANDOMIZED TRIALS OF BREAST CONSERVING SURGERY WITH OR WITHOUT RADIATION

Study (Reference)	Criteria for Eligibility	Number of Patients	Follow-Up (Years)	Radiation Therapy With (%)	Radiation Therapy Without (%)	P
Fisher et al. B-06 (93)	<4 cm node positive/negative	930	10	12.4	40.9	<.001
Liljegren et al. (500)	<2 cm node negative	381	10	8.5	24.0	.0001
Veronesi et al. (501)	<2.5 cm	579	10	5.8	23.5	<.001
Clark et al. (499)	<2 cm node negative	837	3	5.5	25.7	<.001
Fisher et al. B-21 (95)	<2 cm node negative	1,009	8	2.8	16.5	<.001
Winzer et al. (502)	<2 cm node negative	347	5.9	3.2	27.8	.001

Whelan et al.[503] reported on a randomized study of women with stage I or II node-negative breast cancer; 403 had lumpectomy, axillary dissection, and breast irradiation and 396 had the same surgical procedure without irradiation. A dose of 40 Gy was given in 16 fractions to the whole breast, followed by a boost of 12.5 Gy in 5 fractions to the primary site. No patient received adjuvant systemic therapy. The 5-year ipsilateral breast relapse rate was 8% in patients receiving irradiation and 30% in the surgery-alone group (P <.0001). Survival rates at 5 years were 88% and 86%, respectively. Ipsilateral breast relapse correlated with increased incidence of distant metastases and greater mortality from cancer.

Clark et al.[499] reported on a randomized study of 421 patients with tumors 4 cm or smaller and negative nodes who were treated with wide local excision and axillary dissection alone and 416 patients who were treated with the same surgery plus breast irradiation (40 Gy in 3 weeks, 16 fractions, and 12.5-Gy boost in 5 fractions). With 7.6 years' median follow-up, breast recurrences were seen in 148 (35%) of the nonirradiated patients and in 147 (11%) of the irradiated patients (P <.0001); 99 patients (24%) in the former group and 87 (21%) in the latter group died during the study period.

Forrest et al.,[504] after local excision of breast tumors <4 cm in diameter and axillary dissection, randomly assigned 291 patients to receive irradiation of 50 Gy to the breast plus a 10- to 15-Gy boost and 294 to receive no irradiation. Patients received either tamoxifen or 6 cycles of CMF. Overall survival was equivalent in the two groups. The rates of locoregional relapse were 6.1% (18 patients) in the irradiated group and 28.6% (84 patients) in the excision-alone group.

Renton et al.[505] analyzed 418 patients treated by wide local excision and adjuvant chemotherapy (tamoxifen if ER-positive and CMF chemotherapy if ER-negative) who were randomized to have radiation therapy to the breast or not. At a minimum 5-year follow-up, the local recurrence rate in patients receiving irradiation was 13% compared with 35% in those not so treated. When histologically local excision was incomplete and patients received radiation therapy, the local recurrence rate was 17%.

One of the most significant trials addressing the issue of local relapse following lumpectomy alone was from the NSABP-06.[93] This trial included three arms—modified radical mastectomy, lumpectomy with radiation, and lumpectomy without radiation—and included both node-positive and node-negative patients. In this trial, breast irradiation decreased the likelihood of a recurrence in the ipsilateral breast in the group of 1,137 lumpectomy-treated women whose surgical specimens had tumor-free margins. The cumulative incidence of a recurrence in the ipsilateral breast 20 years after surgery was 14.3% among the women who underwent irradiation after lumpectomy and 39.2% among those who underwent lumpectomy without irradiation (P <.001). The benefit of radiation therapy was independent of the nodal status. Among the women with negative nodes, 36.2% of those who did not receive radiation therapy and 17.0% of those who did had a recurrence in the ipsilateral breast within 20 years (P <.001). Among the women with positive nodes, 44.2% of those who did not undergo irradiation and 8.8% of those who did had a recurrence in the ipsilateral breast (P <.001). Among the lumpectomy-treated women whose surgical specimens had tumor-free margins, the hazard ratio for death among the women who underwent postoperative breast irradiation, as compared with those who did not, was 0.91 (95% CI, 0.77 to 1.06; P = .23). Radiation therapy was associated with a marginally significant decrease in deaths due to breast cancer. This decrease was partially offset by an increase in deaths from other causes.

Because of continued uncertainty regarding the need for radiation in more favorable tumors, the NSABP continued to investigate this issue of elimination of irradiation. In the B-21 trial, 1,009 women treated by lumpectomy were randomly assigned to tamoxifen (n = 336), radiation therapy and placebo (n = 336), or radiation therapy and tamoxifen (n = 337).[94] End points were divided rates of breast relapse, distant recurrence, and contralateral breast cancer. Radiation and placebo resulted in a 49% lower hazard rate of local relapse as opposed to tamoxifen alone; radiation and tamoxifen resulted in a 63% lower rate as opposed to radiation and placebo. When compared with tamoxifen alone, radiation plus tamoxifen resulted in an 81% reduction in hazard rate of ipsilateral breast tumor recurrence (IBTR). Cumulative incidences of local relapse through 8 years were 16.5% with tamoxifen, 9.3% with radiation and placebo, and 2.8% with radiation and tamoxifen. The authors concluded that in women with tumors ≤1 cm, local relapse occurs with enough frequency after lumpectomy to justify considering radiation therapy regardless of ER status.

In another landmark trial, Veronesi et al.[398,501] randomly assigned 567 women with small cancers of the breast (<2.5 cm in diameter) to quadrantectomy followed by radiation therapy or to quadrantectomy alone. All patients underwent total axillary dissection. The number of IBTRs was significantly higher in patients treated with surgery alone (59 cases of 273; 10-year crude cumulative incidence of 23.5%) than in patients treated with surgery plus radiotherapy (16 cases of 294; 10-year crude cumulative incidence of 5.8%). The difference in IBTR frequency between the two treatments was high in women up to 45 years of age, tending to decrease with increasing age up to no apparent difference in women older than 65 years. Overall survival curves for the two groups did not differ significantly (P = .326). However, a limited survival advantage was evident after radiotherapy for node-positive women.

Other Nonrandomized Studies of Lumpectomy Alone

Lim et al.[506] recently updated a prospective single arm trial addressing omission of radiation for highly selected favorable patients from the Harvard group. Eighty-seven (of 90 planned) patients enrolled from 1986 until closure in 1992, when a predefined stopping boundary was crossed. Patients were required to have a unicentric, T1, pathologic node-negative invasive ductal, mucinous, or tubular carcinoma without an extensive intraductal component or lymphatic-vessel invasion. Surgery included local excision with margins of at least 1 cm or a negative re-excision. No RT or systemic therapy was given. Nineteen patients (23%) had local recurrence) as a first site of failure (average annual local recurrence: 3.5 per 100 patient-years of follow-up). The authors concluded that even in this highly selected cohort, a substantial risk of local recurrence occurred after breast-conserving therapy alone with margins of ≥1.0 cm.

McCready et al.[507] reported on a postmenopausal group of 244 patients with breast cancer treated with lumpectomy alone. With a median follow-up of 9.1 years, the overall breast relapse rate was 24% (59 of 244). On univariate analysis, smaller tumor size, negative nodes, positive ER status, and no lymphovascular or perineural invasion were associated with significantly lower relapse rates (P <.05). On multivariate analyses, lymphovascular or perineural invasion, age, and amount of DCIS were all significantly associated with greater risk of local relapse. The authors defined a low risk subgroup (node-negative, younger than 65 years of age, no comedo, ER positive, no emboli) with a crude 10-year local recurrence rate of 9%.

Conservative Surgery Alone in Elderly Women

The available evidence clearly establishes lumpectomy followed by radiation as the standard of care for the majority of women with early-stage invasive breast cancer. As noted in the numerous randomized trials reported above, lumpectomy alone results in a threefold increase in local relapse and compromised breast cancer–related survival to a lesser degree.[90] Given the lower reported local relapse rates in elderly women, however, the absolute benefit of radiation therapy following breast-conserving surgery, however, may be less. The question of whether radiation can be eliminated following breast-conserving therapy has been addressed in both retrospective and, more recently, carefully designed prospective randomized trials.

There is evidence from several retrospective and prospective series that elderly women may be spared radiation. Cooke et al.[508] identified 44 women treated with partial mastectomy, breast irradiation, and tamoxifen and compared them with 53 women treated in a similar fashion but without breast irradiation. At 39 months, the breast tumor recurrence rate was 5% with breast irradiation and 21% when irradiation was omitted. Of those not receiving irradiation, no breast relapses were seen in 22 patients older than 70 years of age at diagnosis, in contrast to 8 breast recurrences in 31 patients younger than 70 years.

In the trial of quadrantectomy versus quadrantectomy plus radiation reported by Veronesi et al.,[501] although there was a clear benefit in local control overall, the benefit was significant and apparent only in younger women; for patients over age 65 there was no significant benefit.

Gajdos et al.[509] noted that reported rates of local and distant recurrence for elderly patients were comparable with those for younger patients after both mastectomy and breast conservation. Ninety-eight of 920 patients older than 70 years of age were undertreated by conventional criteria. Undertreated elderly patients were significantly older (78 vs. 76 years; $P = .003$), were diagnosed with excisional biopsy more often (69% vs. 57%; $P = .069$) and had fine-needle aspiration less frequently (22% vs. 38%; $P = .069$), and were more likely to have breast-conservation therapy (90% vs. 73%; $P = .004$). Local and distant disease-free survival rates for both groups were comparable. Tamoxifen treatment significantly reduced the chances for development of distant metastasis in node-negative elderly patients with invasive tumors ($P = .028$). Omission of chemotherapy had no impact on disease control in the elderly. Therefore, elderly women with favorable prognostic factors may be candidates for treatment with tumor resection and tamoxifen without irradiation or chemotherapy and with close follow-up.

Given the apparent biological differences in breast cancers in the elderly, as well as the logistical issues in daily radiation treatment, two randomized trials have addressed the issue of the need for radiation therapy in elderly women with early-stage breast cancer.[175,510] The first trial from the Cancer and Leukemia Group B (CALGB), published by Hughes et al.[510] randomly assigned 636 women with clinical stage I, ER-positive breast carcinoma treated by lumpectomy to receive tamoxifen plus radiation therapy (317 women) or tamoxifen alone (319 women). The only significant difference between the two groups was the rate of local or regional recurrence at 5 years (1% in the group given tamoxifen plus irradiation and 4% in the group given tamoxifen alone; $P < .001$). There were no significant differences between the two groups with regard to the rates of mastectomy for local recurrence, distant metastases, or 5-year rates of overall survival. The authors concluded that lumpectomy plus adjuvant therapy with tamoxifen alone is a reasonable choice for the treatment of women 70 years of age or older who have early, ER-positive breast cancer.

The second trial was a Canadian study published by Fyles et al.[511] of women 50 years of age or older who had T1 or T2 node-negative breast cancer. In this trial, 769 women with early breast cancer with a tumor diameter of ≤5 cm were randomly assigned to receive breast irradiation plus tamoxifen (386 women) or tamoxifen alone (383 women). With a median follow-up of 5.6 years, the rate of local relapse at 5 years was 7.7% in the tamoxifen group and 0.6% in the group given tamoxifen plus irradiation (HR 8.3; 95% CI, 3.3 to 21.2; $P < .001$). The corresponding 5-year disease-free survival rates were 84% and 91% ($P = .004$). A subgroup analysis of 611 women with T1, receptor-positive tumors, similar to the CALGB cohorts, also indicated a benefit from radiotherapy, with the 5-year rates of local relapse of 0.4% with tamoxifen plus radiotherapy and 5.9% with tamoxifen alone ($P < .001$). There was also a significant difference in the rate of axillary relapse at 5 years (2.5% in the tamoxifen group and 0.5% in the group given tamoxifen plus irradiation; $P = .049$), but there were no significant difference in the rates of distant relapse or overall survival. In both of these trials, women were not required to have surgical staging of the axilla, but they did have clinically negative axilla in both, and follow-up remains relatively short. Both studies show that even this favorable subgroup benefits from radiation with respect to local control, but the absolute benefit is small.

As a follow-up to the CALGB study, Smith et al.[511] conducted a detailed analysis of women over age 70 from the SEER-Medicare database. They identified 8,724 women aged 70 years or older treated with conservative surgery for small, lymph node-negative, ER-positive (or unknown receptor status) breast cancer. Using a proportional hazards model, they tested whether radiation therapy was associated with a lower risk of a combined outcome, defined as a second ipsilateral breast cancer reported by SEER, or a subsequent mastectomy reported by Medicare claims. The results, summarized in Figure 56.20, were similar to those reported by the randomized studies above in that radiation therapy, compared with no radiation therapy, was associated with a lower risk of the combined outcome (HR 0.19; 95% CI, 0.14 to 0.28). Radiation therapy was associated with an absolute risk reduction of 4.0 events per 100 women at 5 years (from 5.1 events without radiation therapy to 1.1 with radiation therapy) and 5.7 events per 100 women at 8 years (from 8.0 events without radiation therapy to 2.3 with radiation therapy; $P < .001$).

Using a comorbidity analysis, radiation therapy was most likely to benefit those aged 70 to 79 years without comorbidity (number needed to treat to prevent one event, 21 to 22 patients) and was least likely to benefit those aged 80 years or older with moderate to severe comorbidity (number needed to treat, 61 to 125 patients). The authors conclude that for older women with early breast cancer, radiation therapy was associated with a lower risk of a second ipsilateral breast cancer and subsequent mastectomy. Patients aged 70 to 79 years with minimal comorbidity were the most likely to benefit, and older patients with substantial comorbidity were least likely to benefit.

Collectively, these studies indicate that the benefit of radiation therapy for elderly women is significant in terms of local control, but this absolute benefit is relatively small and must be weighed against comorbidities and other competing risks. The two randomized trials and the SEER-Medicare analysis are summarized in Table 56.25. For women with favorable T1N0 receptor-positive breast cancers, tamoxifen alone is a

TABLE 56.25 FIVE-YEAR OUTCOME OF BREAST-CONSERVING SURGERY WITH OR WITHOUT RADIOTHERAPY IN ELDERLY WOMEN WITH BREAST CANCER

		Number of Patients			*Ipsilateral Relapse*			*Axillary Relapse*			*Distant Relapse*		
Study (Reference)	*Age (Year)*	*CS*	*CS+RT*	*Follow-Up*	*CS (%)*	*CS+RT (%)*	*P*	*CS (%)*	*CS+RT (%)*	*P*	*CS (%)*	*CS+RT (%)*	*P*
Fyles et al. (511)	≥50	383	386	5.6 (median)	7.7	0.6	<.001	2.5	0.5	.049	4.0	4.5	.69
Hughes et al. (510)	≥70	319	317	>8	4.1	0.6	<.01	0.6	0	.08	1.9	2.2	.77
Smith et al. (512)	≥70	2364	6360	5.0 (median)	5.1	1.1	<.001	–	–	–	–	–	–

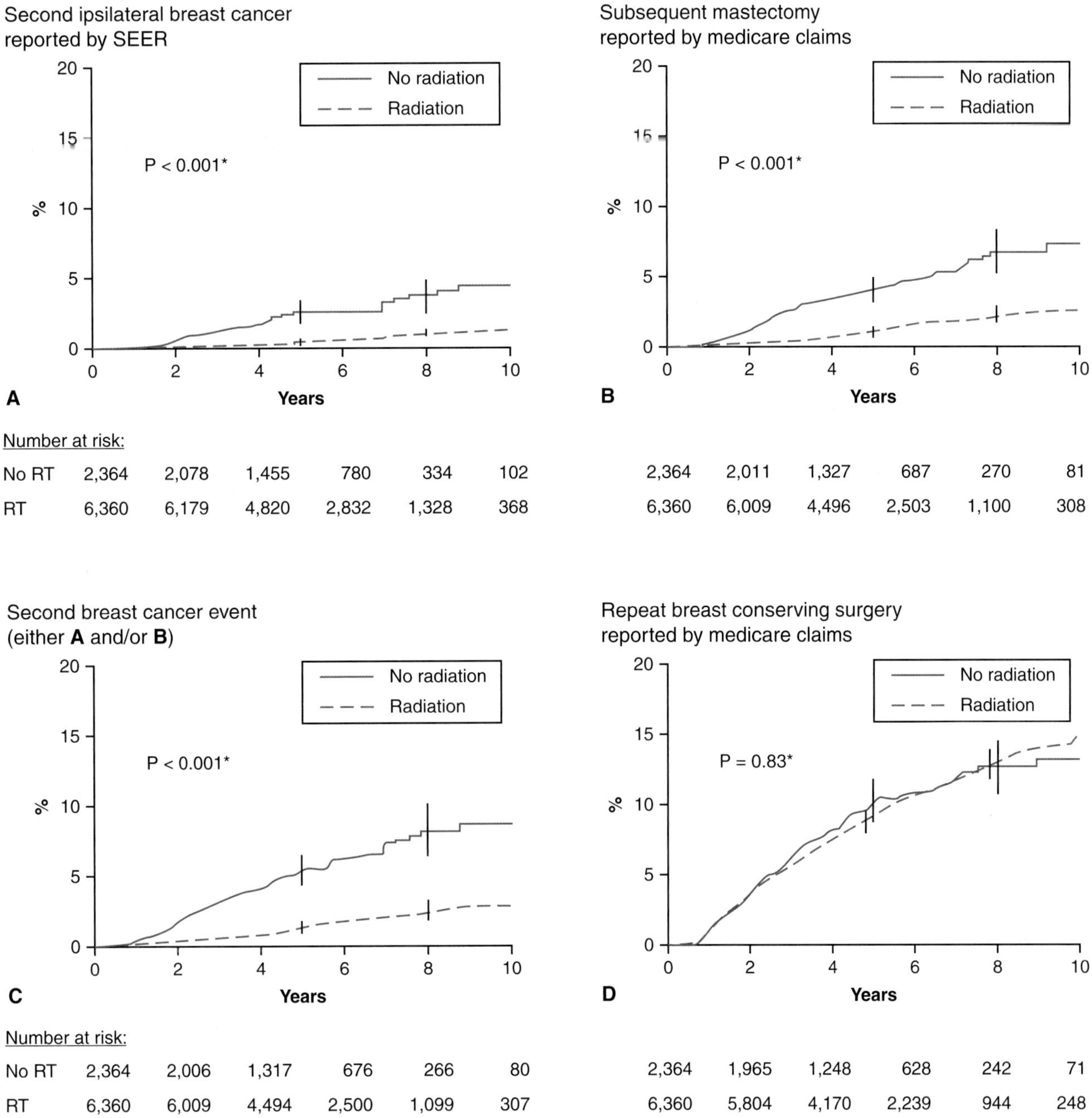

FIGURE 56.20. Association of radiation therapy with outcomes in elderly women. Patients were at risk for all outcomes beginning 9 months after diagnosis. **A:** Second ipsilateral breast cancer reported by Surveillance, Epidemiology, and End Results (SEER). This outcome was defined as a second ipsilateral, pathologically confirmed, invasive breast cancer. **B:** Subsequent mastectomy reported by Medicare claims. **C:** Second breast cancer event defined as a second ipsilateral, pathologically confirmed, invasive breast cancer reported by SEER data or as a subsequent mastectomy reported by Medicare claims. **D:** Repeat breast-conserving surgery as reported by Medicare claims. RT, radiation therapy. Error bars equal 95% confidence intervals. *P* values were calculated from a two-sided log-rank test. (From Smith BD, Gross CP, Smith GL, et al. Effectiveness of radiation therapy for older women with early breast cancer. *J Natl Cancer Inst* 2006;98:681–690, with permission.)

reasonable option that should be discussed. For patients with multiple comorbidities and shorter life expectancies, this option is often chosen. The authors own preference in patients with low comorbidity and long life expectancy is to offer radiation, even in those over age 70 with ER-positive tumors.

HYPOFRACTIONATED WHOLE-BREAST IRRADIATION

In breast cancer, the standard radiation therapy schedule treatment delivers 1.8 to 2.0 Gy per day for 25 to 28 days for a total dose of 45 to 50.4 Gy followed by a 5 to 8 fraction boost (10 to 16 Gy) for a total dose of 60 to 66 Gy delivered for 6 to 7.5 weeks. There has a been a growing trend toward hypofractionation, which involves delivering a higher dose per fraction for a shorter number of fractions for a biologically equivalent dose. This has been shown to be safe and effective as a standard treatment schedule in multiple randomized trials and will be discussed below.

The UK Standardisation of Breast Radiotherapy (START) Trial A randomized patients with early breast cancer (pT1-3a pN0-1 M0); these patients received either 50 Gy in 25 fractions of 2.0 Gy versus 41.6 Gy or 39 Gy in 13 fractions of 3.2 Gy or

3.0 Gy over 5 weeks after surgery.[513] Thus, the overall treatment time was kept constant in all three arms. The trial did allow treatment of regional lymph nodes (supraclavicular and axillary) with additional radiation fields, and these were used in 20% of the patients. With the primary end point of locoregional tumor relapse, 749 women were assigned to the 50 Gy group, 750 to the 41.6 Gy group, and 737 to the 39 Gy group. With a median follow-up of 5.1 years, the rate of local-regional tumor relapse at 5 years was 3.6% (95% CI, 2.2 to 5.1) after 50 Gy, 3.5% (95% CI, 2.1 to 4.3) after 41.6 Gy, and 5.2% (95% CI, 3.5 to 6.9) after 39 Gy. The authors concluded that a lower total dose in a smaller number of fractions could offer similar rates of tumor control as standard fractionation. A major limitation of the study is the use of a conventionally fractionated boost of 14 Gy in 7 fractions. How this boost interacted with the altered fractionation effects is unclear.

The UK START Trial B randomized patients with early breast cancer (pT1-3a pN0-1 M0) at 23 centers in the UK who were assigned after primary surgery to receive 50 Gy in 25 fractions of 2.0 Gy over 5 weeks or 40 Gy in 15 fractions of 2.67 Gy over 3 weeks.[514] In contrast to the START A trial, the overall treatment time was not consistent in both arms. With the primary end point of locoregional tumor relapse, 1,105 women were assigned to the 50 Gy group and 1,110 to the 40 Gy group. With a median follow-up of 6.0 years (interquartile range 5.0 to 6.2) the rate of local-regional tumor relapse at 5 years was 2.2% (95% CI, 1.3 to 3.1) in the 40 Gy group and 3.3% (95% CI, 2.2 to 4.5) in the 50 Gy group, representing an absolute difference of –0.7% (95% CI, –1.7% to 0.9%).

Whelan et al.[515] reported on a study of women with invasive breast cancer who had undergone breast-conserving surgery and were randomized to whole-breast irradiation either at a standard dose of 50.0 Gy in 25 fractions over a period of 35 days (the control group) or at a dose of 42.5 Gy in 16 fractions over a period of 22 days (the hypofractionated radiation group). Notably, women with breast separations >25 cm were excluded. The risk of local recurrence at 10 years was 6.7% among the 612 women assigned to standard irradiation as compared with 6.2% among the 622 women assigned to the hypofractionated regimen (95% CI, –2.5 to 3.5). At 10 years, 71.3% of women in the control group as compared with 69.8% of the women in the hypofractionated radiation group had a good or excellent cosmetic outcome. The authors concluded that hypofractionated whole-breast irradiation was not inferior to standard radiation treatment in women who had undergone breast-conserving surgery for invasive breast cancer with clear surgical margins and negative axillary nodes.

A randomized trial from Hospital Necker in Paris compared 45 Gy in 25 fractions delivered in 5 weeks to 23 Gy delivered as 5 Gy on days 1 and 3 and 6.5 Gy on days 15 and 17. In patients treated by lumpectomy (56 in the conventional arm and 45 in the hypofractionation arm) the local-regional recurrence rate was similar (7% vs. 4%).[516]

In 2011, a task force authorized by the American Society for Radiation Oncology (ASTRO) weighed evidence from a systematic literature review and produced recommendations regarding the use of hypofractionated radiotherapy in patients with breast cancer.[517] They stated that hypofractionated whole-breast irradiation was likely equivalent to conventional fractionation in patients who meet all of the following criteria: (a) age over 50 years, (b) pathologic state T1–2N0 treated with lumpectomy, (c) patient has not received systemic chemotherapy, and (d) the minimum and maximum dose along the central axis is not <93% and not >107% of the prescription dose, respectively. For patients not receiving a radiation boost, the task force favored a dose schedule of 42.5 Gy in 16 fractions when hypofractionated radiotherapy is planned; there was no conclusion regarding the use of a tumor bed boost in patients treated with hypofractionation. Lastly, the task force also recommended that the heart should be excluded from the primary treatment fields when hypofractionated whole-breast irradiation is used due to lingering uncertainty regarding late effects of this treatment on cardiac function.

In the authors institution, every effort is made to follow the ASTRO consensus guidelines. However, patient factors such as distance from the radiotherapy facility, age, and comorbidities all play a role in offering a patient hypofractionated whole-breast radiotherapy. At present, the RTOG-1005 is a phase III randomized trial comparing two fractionation schemes for whole-breast irradiation: hypofractionated radiation with concurrent boost versus standard whole-breast irradiation plus sequential boost for patients with early-stage breast cancer.

RADIATION MANAGEMENT OF THE REGIONAL LYMPHATICS

Radiation therapy of the regional lymphatics remains one of the most variable aspects of breast-conserving therapy.[327,518,519] The role of radiation therapy in management of the regional lymphatics is influenced by the risk of subclinical microscopic disease in regional nodal basins and patterns of failure. This risk is in part determined by disease characteristics and in part determined by the extent of surgical evaluation of the axilla, which has become increasingly relevant as a result of increased use of sentinel node, and whether completion axillary dissections are performed for those patients with sentinel node–positive disease. Furthermore, clinicians differ significantly regarding their philosophy with respect to the treatment of subclinical microscopic disease, particularly as it relates to the internal mammary chain.

The issue of whether one treats the "axilla" in conservatively managed patients is further complicated by both uncertainty and misconceptions about the degree to which the axilla receives radiation from a standard tangential field. Although this will vary considerably, as will be discussed in the section on radiation techniques, tangential radiation ports will likely treat most level I nodes and a portion of level II nodes.[520]

All of this uncertainty, debate, and controversy is well founded as there are little in the way of randomized data to establish a clear standard. Studies are under way randomizing high-risk node-negative and node-positive patients to treatment

TABLE 56.26A TREATMENT POLICY FOR CONSERVATIVE MANAGEMENT OF EARLY STAGE INVASIVE BREAST CANCER

Treatment Volume	Indication	Fraction Size/Technique	Total Dose	Comment
Whole breast	Routinely following BCS	2 (prefer) or 1.8 Gy/ tangents with wedges or dynamic wedges to optimize homogeneity	45–50.4 Gy	Consider omission of RT in elderly with stage I disease and comorbidities
Boost	Routinely following whole breast	2 or 1.8 Gy (prefer 2 Gy)/*en face* electrons	10–16 Gy to bring total dose to >60 Gy	Consider no boost for widely negative margins in women over 60
Accelerated whole breast	On protocol or ASTRO consensus guidelines	2.66 Gy tangents with no nodal fields/no boost	42.5 Gy	
Accelerated partial breast	On protocol or ASTRO consensus guidelines	3.4–3.8 Gy/external beam conformal, interstitial, or MammoSite	34–38.5 Gy	

BCS, breast-conserving surgery; RT, radiation therapy; ASTRO, American Society for Radiation Oncology.

TABLE 56.26B TREATMENT POLICY FOR REGIONAL NODES

Treatment Volume	Indication	Fraction Size/Technique	Total Dose	Comment
Supraclav	• Clinical N2 or N3 disease • >4 +LN after axillary dissection • 1–3 +LN with high risk features • Node + sentinel lymph node with no dissection unless risk of additional axillary disease is very small • High risk[a] no dissection	1.8–2.0 Gy (prefer 200)/AP or AP-PA	45–50.4 Gy	May omit with 1–3 positive nodes in select cases
Axilla	• N+ with extensive ECE • SN+ with no dissection • Inadequate axillary dissection • High risk[a] with no dissection	1.8–2.0 Gy/AP—Consider posterior axillary boost if suboptimal coverage with AP only	45–50.4 Gy	Axilla may be intentionally included with use of high tangents
Internal mammary	Individualized but consider for: • Positive axillary nodes with central and medial lesions • Stage III breast cancer • +SLN in the IM chain • +SLN in axilla with drainage to IM on lymphosintigraphy	1.8–2.0 Gy/Partially wide tangents or separate IM electron/photon	45–50.4 Gy	

LN, lymph node; +, positive; AP, anterior-posterior; PA, posterior-anterior; ECE, extracapsular extension; SN, sentinel node; SLN, sentinel lymph node; IM, internal mammary.
[a]High risk is defined as estimated probability of nodal involvement greater than 10% to 15%.

to the breast or chest wall only compared with the breast or chest wall and regional lymphatics. In the interim, reliance on available retrospective data, calculated risks of subclinical disease, and patterns of failure form the basis for various treatment policies. Current treatment policies and guidelines at the authors institutions are outlined in Table 56.26.

Although in the earlier years of breast-conservation therapy, node-negative as well as node-positive patients often received regional nodal treatment, most authors currently agree that it is not necessary to irradiate the regional lymphatics if the nodes are pathologically negative and an adequate axillary dissection has been performed.[79,327,521] This general practice has now been extended to those patients with a negative sentinel node, because available studies have demonstrated a low rate of pathologically involved nodes after a negative sentinel node procedure performed by an experienced surgeon.[234,335,522]

However, as noted previously, the clinically negative axilla harbors subclinical microscopic disease in up to 40% of patients with early-stage operable breast cancer,[331] and both axillary dissection and axillary radiation result in high rates of regional nodal control.[79,110,327,331,521]

Radiation Compared with Axillary Surgery

Sentinel node sampling, with or without full axillary dissection, is now the most common method of axillary management in women with early-stage breast cancer. For patients in whom full axillary staging will not affect subsequent systemic management, who have not undergone any axillary staging procedure, or who have a positive sentinel node and did not undergo further axillary staging, axillary radiation has been shown to result in high rates of regional nodal control.[79,110,327,521,523] Selected series demonstrating nodal control rates with radiation therapy in breast-conserving therapy are summarized in Table 56.27.[81,379,386,435,524–528] Table 56.28 summarizes results of randomized trials comparing axillary surgery to radiation or observation.[73,333,529–538]

Retrospective Experiences

Haffty et al.[79] reported actuarial nodal control rates of 97% and 96% at 10 years for two groups of patients, 245 receiving irradiation alone without axillary dissection and 187 treated with irradiation to the supraclavicular lymph nodes and IMNs after axillary dissection. Minimal morbidity was associated with this treatment policy. Recently Pejavar et al.[539] updated the Yale experience, demonstrating a 98% 5-year regional nodal control rate in 582 patients with invasive breast cancer treated by regional nodal irradiation without dissection compared with 98% 5-year nodal control rate in 1,440 patients treated by axillary dissection. Within this experience were 16 patients with positive sentinel nodes who did not undergo completion axillary dissection and were treated with radiation therapy. None of those sentinel node–positive patients recurred.

Galper et al.[525] estimated the efficacy of axillary radiation therapy after a positive sentinel node biopsy and evaluated the risk of regional nodal failure for patients with clinical stage I or II,

TABLE 56.27 AXILLARY RECURRENCE AFTER AXILLARY LYMPH NODE DISSECTIONOR AXILLARY RADIATION IN CONSERVATIVELY MANAGED PATIENTS

	Number of Patients				Axillary Failure/Number of Failures (% Failure)	
Study (Reference)	N0	N1 (Clinical)	RT Dose (Gy)	Follow-Up (Year)	N0	N1
Royal Marsden (386)	211	52	50/25	120 (min)	3 (1)	15 (29)
Institut Curie (524)	332	–	50/25	54 (ave)	7 (2)	–
Santiago (528)	171	–	50/25	62 (med)	4 (2)	–
Charlebourg (379)	281	–	50–70	60 (min)	4 (1)	–
Henri Mondor (435)	446	47	69/33	120 (ave)	0 (0)	3 (6)
Groupe European (527)	1,040	181	45–70	>60 (med)	19 (2)	7 (4)
Tufts (526)	73	–	45/25	54	1 (1)	–
JCRT (81)	335	35	44–55/22–30	73 (med)	3 (1)	1 (3)
Yale University (79)	590	–	46	>120	18 (2)	–
JCRT (525)	292	126[a]	64–68	96	3 (1)	3 (2)

RT, radiation therapy.
[a]All the patients received limited axillary dissection; RT dose, radiotherapy dose to axilla, given as total dose in Gy/number of fractions.

TABLE 56.28 AXILLARY FAILURE RATES IN PATIENTS IN RANDOMIZED TRIALS COMPARING AXILLARY TREATMENTS

Trials (Reference)	Study Design	Number of Patients	Follow-Up (Month)	Positive LNs (%)	Axillary Failure Rates AxD (%)	AxRT(%)	OBS (%)
NSABP B-04 (331)	M (AxD vs. AxRT vs OBS)	1079	126 (ave)	40	1	3	19
Institut Curie (532)	CS (AxD vs. AxRT)	658	180 (med))	18	1	3	NA
Edinburgh (531)	M (AxD vs. AxRT)	275	72 (min)	30	1	14	NA
Guy's I (530)	M vs. CS (AxD vs. AxRT)	232	180 (min)	25	1	19	NA
Guy's II (530)	M vs. CS (AxD vs. AxRT)	258	120 (min)	31	1	13	NA
Manchester I (533)	M (AxRT vs. OBS)	714	60 (min)	NA	NA	19	37
Manchester II (534)	CS (AxRT vs. OBS)	708	65 (med)	NA	NA	10	23
International Breast Cancer Study Group (535)	M or CS (AxD vs. OBS)	454	79 (med)	14	0.4	NA	1.3
Italian Oncological Senology Group (537)	CS	435	63 (med)	NA	NA	0.5	1.5
Milan (333)	CS	219	60	23	1	NA	1.8

Positive LNs, incidence of pathologically involved lymph nodes in patients undergoing axillary lymph node dissection; AxRT, axillary radiotherapy; OBS, observation; ave, average length of follow-up; M, simple or radical mastectomy; CS, breast-conserving surgery; min, minimum length of follow-up; med, median length of follow-up; NA, not applicable.

clinically node-negative invasive breast cancer treated with either no dissection or a limited dissection (removal of five nodes or less) followed by axillary radiation therapy. Two hundred ninety-two patients had axillary radiation therapy instead of axillary dissection; 126 underwent axillary radiation therapy following limited node dissection. The median dose to the axilla was 46 Gy and to the supraclavicular fossa 45 Gy. Among patients found to have positive nodes on limited dissection, adjuvant chemotherapy and tamoxifen were administered to 81% and 7% of subjects, respectively. All patients had an 8-year follow-up. Six of the 418 patients (1.4%) had regional nodal failure within 8 years; four had simultaneous regional and distant recurrences; and two had isolated axillary failures. Three of the 292 patients (1%) with no axillary dissection, 0 of 84 patients with pathologically negative nodes, and 3 of 42 patients (7%) with pathologically involved nodes had regional node failure as a first site of failure.

A group of 511 patients with 519 stage I and II breast cancers treated with lumpectomy, with or without axillary dissection, and irradiation were reviewed by Halverson et al.[540] Management of the axilla consisted of irradiation after axillary dissection in 74, irradiation alone in 75, and observation in 21 patients; the extent of nodal irradiation was at the discretion of the attending radiation oncologist. Overall, axillary recurrence was uncommon (1.2%) but was slightly more frequent after irradiation alone (2.7%) than after surgery alone (0.3%; $P = .14$). There was no benefit for supplemental axillary irradiation after an axillary dissection yielding negative nodes or one to three positive nodes. Among the 21 patients in whom the axilla was not treated, axillary recurrence was not observed. Supraclavicular failures were rare in women with negative or one to three positive axillary lymph nodes (0.5%) and were not significantly affected by elective irradiation. IMN recurrence was seen in only one patient and was not influenced by elective internal mammary irradiation.

Randomized Studies

Randomized studies evaluating axillary treatment (dissection vs. observation vs. radiation) are summarized in Table 56.28. One of the largest and earliest comparisons of axillary surgery to radiation was the NSABP-04 study, in which operable clinically node-negative patients were randomly assigned to radical mastectomy, simple mastectomy, or simple mastectomy with radiation to the chest wall and regional lymphatics.[73] The nodal relapse rate approached 20% in those assigned to simple mastectomy without radiation. The nodal control rates in the radical mastectomy arm and simple mastectomy plus radiation arm were comparable, with <3% relapse rate in each of these arms.

A direct comparison of axillary treatment by dissection compared with radiation was recently reported by Louis-Sylvestre et al.,[532] in which 658 patients with a breast carcinoma <3 cm in diameter and clinically uninvolved lymph nodes were randomly assigned to axillary dissection or axillary radiotherapy after breast-conserving surgery with radiation to the breast. Of the group undergoing dissection, 21% of the patients in the axillary dissection group were node positive. At 10 and 15 years, survival rates were identical in both groups (73.8% vs. 75.5% at 15 years). Recurrences in the axilla were less frequent in the axillary dissection group at 15 years (1% vs. 3%; $P = .04$). There was no difference in recurrence rates in the breast or supraclavicular region or distant metastases between the two groups.

Veronesi et al.[537] carried out a study in which women older than 45 years of age with breast cancer up to 1.2 cm were randomized, 214 of whom were treated with breast-conservation surgery and irradiation without axillary treatment and 221 with conservation surgery plus breast and axillary radiation therapy (50 Gy in 5 weeks).After a median follow-up of 63 months, overt axillary metastases were fewer than expected: three cases in the no axillary treatment group (1.5%) and one in the RT group (0.5%). This study suggests that occult axillary metastases might never become clinically overt and axillary dissection might be avoided in patients with small carcinomas and a clinically negative axilla. Axillary RT seems to protect the patients from axillary recurrence almost completely. It is possible that systemic therapy, the undamaged immunocompetent tissue in the axillary lymph nodes, and axillary irradiation may all be factors contributing to the low incidence of axillary failures in these patients. Also, in the patients receiving no axillary irradiation, it is highly likely that the level I lymph nodes were included in the standard tangential fields.[327,520,541]

The European After Mapping of the Axilla Radiation or Surgery Trial is nearing completion. This trial randomizes patients after positive sentinel nodes to axillary dissection or axillary radiation and will help to address issues of local-regional control, survival, and morbidity using these two approaches.[542]

Irradiation of Lymphatics in Patients with Positive Axillary Lymph Nodes

Although there is general consensus that radiation to the regional lymph nodes is not necessary in patients with pathologically node-negative disease, there is considerable variability in radiation to the regional lymphatics in patients with pathologically node-positive disease.[77–79,327,523,543] Many radiation oncologists favor irradiation of the regional lymphatics in addition to the breast in node-positive women, while others favor no nodal irradiation, particularly in women with one to three positive nodes. Based on the potential disease-free and overall survival advantage, as well as the risk of failure in the supraclavicular region, most radiation oncologists favor at least supraclavicular nodal irradiation in patients with four or more nodes. The recent presentation of preliminary results of the National Cancer Institute of Canada's MA.20 trial demonstrates a distant metastasis, disease-free survival, and potential survival advantage to regional nodal irradiaton.[544] The majority of patients in this trial had one to three positive nodes and were randomized after breast-conserving surgery to tangential breast irradiation alone or breast irradiation with regional nodal irradiation to the supraclavicular and internal mammary regions. Full publication of this trial is eagerly awaited. A similar trial of the EORTC, randomizing high-risk node-negative and node-positive patients to treatment to the breast or chest wall alone or breast or chest wall and regional lymphatics, may help to further clarify this important issue.

Acknowledging the lack of definitive data and clear consensus and allowing for flexibility depending on patient and physician preferences, the guidelines that the authors advocate are summarized in Table 56.26. In general, the authors favor treatment of the supraclavicular fossa in patients with positive nodes. Treatment of the axilla and internal mammary will vary, with attention to the indications outlined in the table. Until results of the ongoing MA.20 and EORTC randomized trials are fully available, regional lymphatic irradiation will likely continue to be highly individualized based on physician and patient preferences.

Sarrazin et al.[370] carried out a randomized study comparing 88 patients treated with tumorectomy and irradiation and 91 patients treated with mastectomy. In a second randomization in the study, the patients with positive axillary lymph nodes in the first randomization were randomly assigned to receive or not receive nodal irradiation. There was no significant difference in overall survival between the two groups. Nevertheless, Yarnold[521] advised elective irradiation of the axilla and the supraclavicular fossa in selected patients, such as those with four or more metastatic axillary lymph nodes, involvement of the apex of the axilla, or gross extracapsular tumor extension, even if the patients are to receive adjuvant chemotherapy. These recommendations are supported by reports that document the benefit of postmastectomy irradiation in patients receiving chemotherapy, which are reviewed in more detail in Chapter 54.

Treatment of the axilla varies significantly in patients with positive nodes. For those patients with negative nodes or with one to three positive nodes without extracapsular extension (ECE) who undergo adequate axillary dissection, there does not appear to be a benefit to targeting the full axilla.[77–80,327,540] There is considerable variability regarding treatment of the full axilla, even in patients with multiple positive nodes.[77,81,520,543] The risk of axillary recurrence after full dissection is low in patients with ECE, even without axillary lymph node irradiation. Whether to treat the full axilla following dissection for patients with multiple positive nodes or ECE generally includes consideration of the extent of dissection, the degree of nodal involvement and ECE, and the degree to which the patient and physician are willing to accept some increased risk of lymphedema with full axillary radiation following dissection.[110,327]

Hetelekidis et al.[255] evaluated 368 patients with T1 or T2 breast cancer and pathologically positive lymph nodes treated with breast-conserving therapy. The median number of sampled lymph nodes was 10. Twenty percent of the patients were treated with supraclavicular radiation therapy, and 64% received both axillary and supraclavicular radiation therapy (45 Gy). One hundred twenty-two patients (33%) had ECE. There was no significant correlation of either disease-free or overall survival or local, regional nodal, or distant failure rates in patients with ECE compared with those without it.

Pierce et al.,[545] in a review of 72 women with breast cancer treated with conservation surgery and irradiation, identified 27 patients (37.5%) who had evidence of ECE in the axilla. With a median follow-up of 14 months, 1 of 27 (4%) patients with ECE experienced an axillary failure, compared with 0 of 45 patients without ECE. Several authors concluded that ECE is associated with decreased survival but not with increased axillary failures and that radiation therapy may be omitted in a dissected axilla if the sole indication is extracapsular disease.

Internal Mammary Node Irradiation

The role of internal mammary nodal irradiation in node-positive breast cancer patients remains a controversial issue. Although, ongoing trials from the National Cancer Institute of Canada and EORTC may help to address this, currently there is no clear consensus on the role of internal mammary irradiation.[518,519,546–548]

Several surgical series comparing extended radical mastectomy and radical mastectomy, without adjuvant systemic therapy, have shown that extended radical mastectomy was associated with improved survival rates in patients with medial T1 or T2 tumors and positive axillary nodes.[549,550] These surgical series and selected series evaluating internal mammary irradiation are summarized in Table 56.29.[546–550] In a randomized trial of patients with node-positive breast cancer treated with postmastectomy radiation, randomized to internal mammary radiation or no internal mammary radiation, Romestaing[551] showed no advantage to internal mammary irradiation. The full manuscript of this study has not as yet been published. The majority of randomized trials evaluating postoperative radiation therapy did include radiation to the internal mammary chain. However, it is difficult to distinguish whether the benefit derived from such treatment related specifically to radiation of the internal mammary chain or to the breast or chest wall, supraclavicular, or axillary treatment administered.

Freedman et al.[552] examined data regarding patterns of failure after elective IMN treatment. Although controversial, data from the prospective, randomized trials of IMN treatment did not seem to support elective dissection or irradiation. IMN

Clinical Radiation Oncology

TABLE 56.29 STUDIES EVALUATING IMPACT OF INTERNAL MAMMARY TREATMENT (SURGERY OR RADIATION) ON 10 YEARS SURVIVAL

		Number of Patients			Overall Survival			Distant Metastasis-Free Survival			Disease-Free Survival		
Study (Reference)	Type of IMN Treatment	With IMN Treatment	Without IMN Treatment	Follow-Up (Year)	With IMN Treatment (%)	Without IMN Treatment (%)	P	Without IMN Treatment (%)	With IMN Treatment (%)	P	Without IMN Treatment (%)	With IMN Treatment (%)	P
Meier et al. (550)	dissection	56	56	10	73.6	60.4	.130	–	–	–	–	–	–
Lacour et al. (549)	dissection	750	703	10	56	53	.40	44	49	NS	–	–	–
Fowble et al. (546)	radiation	114	1,269	6	80	81	0.87	–	–	–	82	87	.38
Obedian and Haffty (547)	radiation	535	411	13	72	84	NS	77	87	NS	–	–	–
Stemmer et al.[a] (548)	radiation	67	33	6.4	78	64	.08	–	–	–	73	52	.02
Romestaing (551)	radiation	1,200 Total	10	62.6	59.6	.87	–	–	–	–	–	–	

IMN, internal mammary lymph nodes; NS, not significant.
[a]Survival data documented at the end point of follow-up.

irradiation did not contribute to survival, yet it raised the risk of cardiac toxic effects. Sentinel lymph node mapping provided an opportunity to examine the IMN chain in early breast cancer. It is possible that biopsy of the "hot" nodes could be used to select patients who are most likely to benefit from additional regional therapy to these nodes.

Fowble et al.[546] compared the outcome in 1,383 women with stage I or II breast cancer who underwent wide excision, axillary node dissection with 10 or more nodes removed, and breast irradiation. A total of 114 women had radiation to the IMNs with deep tangents and 1,269 did not. All axillary node-positive women received adjuvant chemotherapy or tamoxifen, or both. There were no significant differences in ipsilateral breast tumor recurrence, regional node recurrence, and initial or total distant metastases for the two groups. No IMN failures were observed among the 114 patients whose IMNs were treated, and only 4 IMN failures were found in the 1,269 other patients (2 of whom had distant metastases). Similarly, 5- and 10-year actuarial overall and cause-specific survival rates were not significantly different.

In a series from Yale, Obedian and Haffty[547] found no difference in the 10-year disease-free survival rate after breast irradiation and excision, regardless of whether IMNs were irradiated. Of 984 patients with invasive breast cancer who were treated with conservative surgery and radiotherapy, patients were divided into two groups: those treated by intentionally targeting the internal mammary nodes (n = 535) and without intentionally targeting the internal mammary nodes (n = 411). The decision not to use a separate internal mammary field was a result of a change in treatment policy over time and generally not based on number of nodes or tumor location. There were no significant differences between the groups with respect to age, ER or PR status, or use of adjuvant chemotherapy or hormone therapy. There were more patients with T2 tumors, positive nodes, medial lesions, indeterminate margins, and slightly longer follow-up in the group treated to the internal mammary chain. There were no significant differences between the groups with respect to overall survival or distant metastasis-free survival.

In a study by Stemmer et al.[548] of 100 node-positive patients scheduled to receive radiation to the internal mammary chain, 67 received the radiation and 33 did not due to technical difficulties. At a median follow-up of 77 months, disease-free survival was significantly prolonged in patients receiving internal mammary radiation compared with those without internal mammary radiation (73% vs. 52%; P =.02). A trend was seen for overall survival (78% vs. 64%; P =.08). Cox regression multivariate analysis found IMN radiotherapy to be significant both for disease-free and overall survival. There was no treatment-related mortality.

It is evident that data are conflicting, and opinions regarding the role of internal mammary radiation remain unresolved. Until more definitive data become available, it is likely that patient and physician biases will dictate practice. The authors approach is summarized in Table 56.26, acknowledging that uncertainties in the available data allow for substantial flexibility. The radiation oncologist, however, must be familiar with the various techniques to treat internal mammary nodes, which are summarized later in the section on techniques.

SEQUENCING CHEMOTHERAPY AND HORMONAL THERAPY

Sequencing Chemoradiation in the Conservative Management of Breast Cancer

With the increasing use of systemic therapy in patients with early-stage breast cancer, the integration of this treatment with surgery and radiation therapy has become an important clinical question. Initial retrospective series evaluating treatment sequencing suggested that a delay in the onset of radiation therapy to permit delivery of chemotherapy increased local recurrence rates.[91,553,554] These data are summarized in a pooled analysis by Huang et al.[91] Ten retrospective studies involving 7,401 patients investigated the association between delay in initiating postoperative RT and local control in breast cancer (after lumpectomy in nine studies and lumpectomy or mastectomy in one study). Eight of these studies compared local control between patients who were treated more than 8 weeks after surgery and those treated within 8 weeks of surgery. The pooled random-effects odds ratio from the combined analysis was 1.62 (95% CI, 1.21 to 2.16), corresponding to an increase in the 5-year LRR from 5.8% in those patients treated within 8 weeks to 9.1% in those patients treated between 9 and 16 weeks after surgery. In a separate analysis exploring the optimum sequencing of adjuvant RT and systemic chemotherapy after surgery for breast cancer from 11 retrospective series, the pooled random-effects odds ratio in these 11 studies was 2.28 (95% CI, 1.45 to 3.57), corresponding to an increase in the 5-year LRR from 6.0% in the RT-first group to 16.0% in the chemotherapy-first group (Fig. 56.21).

Most of these data are subject to criticism due to their retrospective nature, the fact that patients were treated in an earlier era with different surgical techniques and lack of attention to margins, and inclusion of heterogenous groups of patients with these caveats, but there appears to be a trend toward higher local relapse rates with delays in radiation therapy, which appears to have been an appropriate concern with respect to integration of radiation therapy and chemotherapy in the conservatively managed patients.

Initial data regarding these concerns related to the delay in radiation while chemotherapy was being delivered led the Harvard group at Joint Center for Radiation Therapy (JCRT) to investigate the sequencing of radiation therapy and chemotherapy in a randomized prospective clinical trial.[553,554] In this trial, women treated with breast-conserving surgery were randomly assigned to 4 cycles of doxorubicin-based combination chemotherapy, followed by radiation therapy or radiation therapy followed by 4 cycles of the same chemotherapy. In an update of this trial, Bellon et al.[555] reported no statistically significant treatment difference in the rates of freedom from any event, including breast cancer recurrence, contralateral breast cancer, second malignancy, or death (Fig. 56.22). The 10-year rate of any event was 46% for patients in the chemotherapy-first arm compared with 51% in the radiation-first arm. The 10-year rates of distant metastasis were 35% and 36% in the two arms, respectively; and the 10-year rates of death were 28% and 33%, respectively. For the 123 patients with negative margins, the crude local recurrence rates for chemotherapy-first and radiation-first patients were 6% and 13%, respectively. Corresponding rates of distant and regional recurrences were 18% and 26%. Among women with close margins (n = 47), crude local recurrence rates were 32% and 4%, respectively; distant or regional recurrences were 37% and 43%. In the group with positive margins (n = 51), local recurrences occurred in 23% of chemotherapy-first and 20% of radiation-first patients.

Although the JCRT study provided important data concerning treatment sequencing, this study predominantly focused on patients with lymph node–positive disease. Investigators from the MD Anderson Cancer Center performed a retrospective analysis of sequencing of chemotherapy and radiation in 124 patients with lymph node–negative disease treated with breast-conserving therapy.[556] In this series, 79% of the patients had negative margins. The 5-year actuarial rates of local control were 100% for the chemotherapy-first group (most commonly 6 cycles of doxorubicin-based chemotherapy) and 94% for the radiation-first group (P = .351). The 5-year recurrence-free survival rates for the chemotherapy-first and radiation-first groups were 92% and 77% (P = .083), respectively. These data

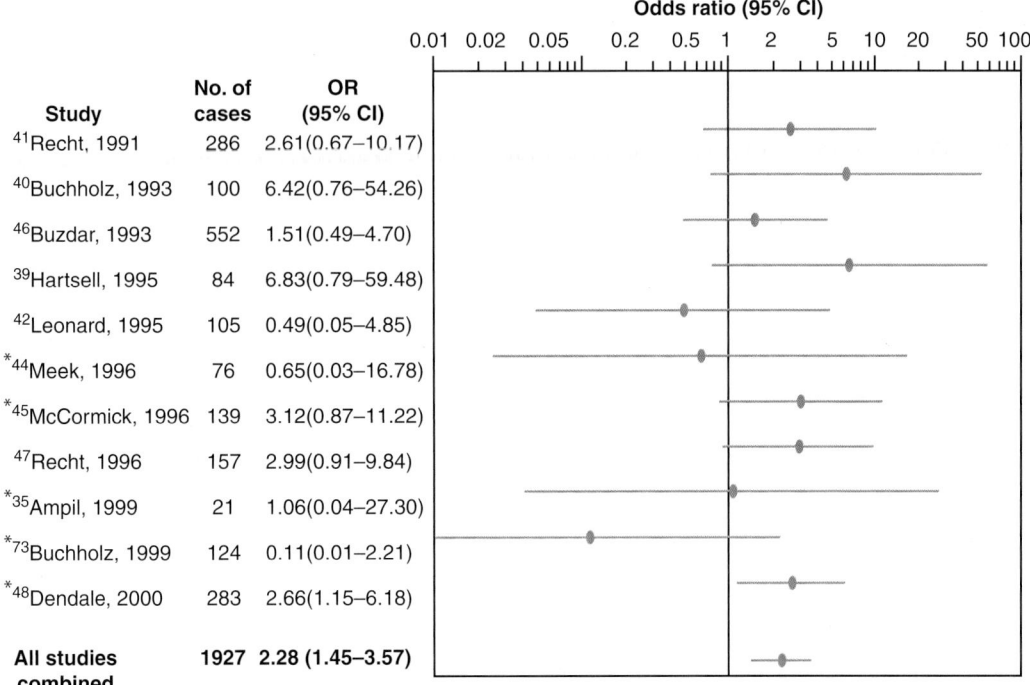

Study	No. of cases	OR (95% CI)
[41]Recht, 1991	286	2.61(0.67–10.17)
[40]Buchholz, 1993	100	6.42(0.76–54.26)
[46]Buzdar, 1993	552	1.51(0.49–4.70)
[39]Hartsell, 1995	84	6.83(0.79–59.48)
[42]Leonard, 1995	105	0.49(0.05–4.85)
*[44]Meek, 1996	76	0.65(0.03–16.78)
*[45]McCormick, 1996	139	3.12(0.87–11.22)
[47]Recht, 1996	157	2.99(0.91–9.84)
*[35]Ampil, 1999	21	1.06(0.04–27.30)
*[73]Buchholz, 1999	124	0.11(0.01–2.21)
*[48]Dendale, 2000	283	2.66(1.15–6.18)
All studies combined	**1927**	**2.28 (1.45–3.57)**

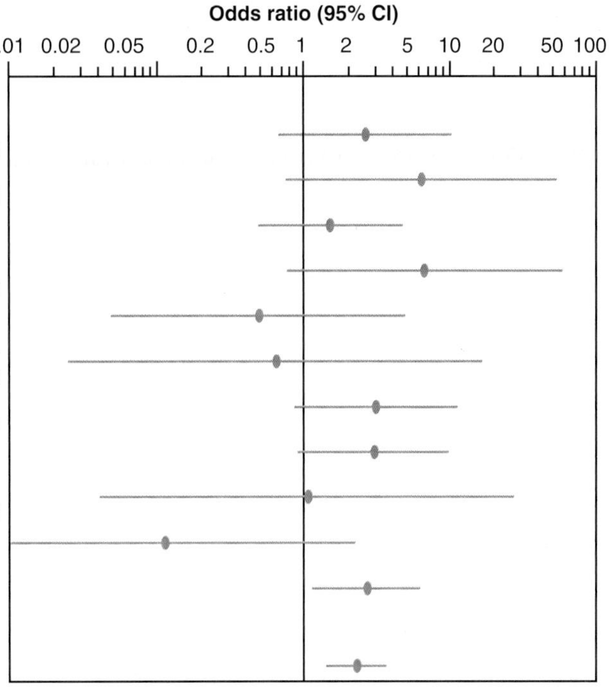

FIGURE 56.21. Associations between delay in postoperative radiotherapy (RT) and local recurrence rates (LRRs) in studies of the sequencing of adjuvant RT and chemotherapy for breast cancer. LRRs in patients who received delayed RT following initial chemotherapy are compared with the rates observed in those patients who received early RT by chemotherapy. Low-quality studies are indicated by an asterisk. (From Huang J, Barbera L, Brouwers M, et al. Does delay in starting treatment affect the outcomes of radiotherapy? A systematic review. *J Clin Oncol* 2003;21:555–563. Reused with permission. © 2012 American Society of Clinical Oncology. All rights reserved.)

again support an adjuvant-therapy schedule in which chemotherapy is delivered first. The median delays in radiation delivery were 6.7 months in the MD Anderson Cancer Center series and 16 weeks in the JCRT series.

More recently, with the addition of taxane-based chemotherapy to adriamycin-based regimens, concerns have arisen regarding the additional delays in initiating radiation therapy in conservatively managed patients. This was addressed in a study by Sartor et al.[557] In this randomized CALGB study evaluating adriamycin and cytoxan versus adriamycin and cytoxan, followed by taxane, there were 345 conservatively managed patients. Although the sequencing of radiation was not randomized, patients in the adriamycin plus taxane arm had radiation delayed by an additional 84 days (4 21-day cycles of taxol). Despite this added delay, local-regional relapses were lower in the adriamycin plus taxane compared with the adriamycin arm (9.7% vs. 3.7%; $P = .04$). (The majority of patients in this randomized trial presumably had negative surgical margins.)

For the majority of patients undergoing breast-conserving surgery with negative margins, these data collectively indicate that administration of chemotherapy prior to radiation therapy does not result in excessive rates of local relapse, provided all modalities are given in a timely fashion without excessive delays. Whether patients with positive or close margins or other risk factors for local relapse would benefit from earlier administration of radiation remains an unresolved issue.

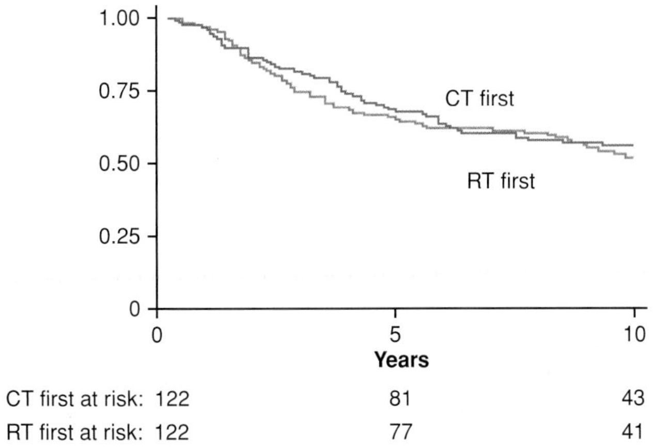

FIGURE 56.22. Event-free survival (including breast cancer recurrence, contralateral breast cancer, second malignancy, or death) by sequencing of chemotherapy and radiation following breast-conserving therapy, from the Harvard randomized trial. (From Bellon JR, Come SE, Gelman RS, et al. Sequencing of chemotherapy and radiation therapy in early-stage breast cancer: updated results of a prospective randomized trial. *J Clin Oncol* 2005;23:1934–1940. Reprinted with permission. © 2005 American Society of Clinical Oncology.)

Concurrent Chemoradiation in Breast-Conserving Therapy

Although the concurrent use of chemoradiation therapy in conservatively managed breast cancer has fallen out of favor, there are data that suggest a high rate of local control in patients treated concurrently. These studies are summarized in Table 56.30.[558–562] (The chemotherapy regimens used in these studies are no longer routinely employed because they are less effective.)

A randomized trial of concurrent versus sequential CMF chemotherapy was reported by Arcangeli et al.[557] A total of 206 patients who had quadrantectomy and axillary dissection for breast cancer and were planned to receive adjuvant CMF chemotherapy were randomized to concurrent or sequential radiotherapy. Radiotherapy was delivered only to the whole breast through tangential fields to a dose of 50 Gy in 20 fractions over 4 weeks, followed by an electron boost of 10 to 15 Gy in 4 to 6 fractions to the tumor bed. No differences in 5-year breast recurrence-free, metastasis-free, disease-free, and overall survival were observed in the two treatment groups. All patients completed the planned radiotherapy. No evidence of an increased risk of toxicity was observed between the two arms. No difference in radiotherapy and in the chemotherapy

TABLE 56.30 SELECTED STUDIES EVALUATION CONCURRENT CHEMORADIATION IN BREAST-CONSERVING SURGERY WITH RADIATION

Study (Reference)	Number of Patients: CON-CRT	Number of Patients: Non-CON-CRT	Follow-Up (Median, Year)	Type of Chemo	Local Control: CON-CRT (%)	Local Control: Non-CON-CRT (%)	P	Toxicity with CON-CRT
Haffty et al. (562)	109	426	8.8	CMF (mainly)	92	83	<.001	Cosmetic results, toxicities, and long-term complications acceptable
Bellon et al. (559)	112	–	7.8	CMF (prospective)	96	–	–	
Markiewicz et al. (560)	210	–	5.2 for node-negative; 7.6 for node-positive	CF during radiation therapy flowed by further CMF	87 (10 yr)	–	–	Cosmesis and complications acceptable
Rouesse et al. (561)	210	206	5.25	FNC for CON-CRT, FEC for sequential RT	97	91	.01	Febrile neutropenia and grade 3–4 leukopenia significantly more frequent
Toledano et al. (563)	107	107	6.7	CNF	–	–	–	Increased incidence of grade 2 or greater late side effects.
Arcangeli et al. (558)	106	100	5.4	CMF	97	96	NS	Late toxicity and cosmesis not available yet

CON-CRT, concurrent chemotherapy; CMF, cyclophosphamide/methotrexate/5-fluofouracil; CF, oral cyclophosphamide/intravenous 5-fluorouracil; CNF, cyclophosphamide/mitoxantrone/5-fluorouracil, NS, not significant.

dose intensity was observed in the two groups. The authors concluded that in patients with negative surgical margins receiving adjuvant chemotherapy, radiotherapy can be delayed to up to 7 months. However, concurrent administration of CMF chemotherapy and radiotherapy was safe, and the authors suggest that such an approach might be reserved for patients at high risk of local recurrence.

Another randomized study of concurrent versus sequential radiation therapy was reported by Rouesse et al.[561] This study supports the concept that concurrent use of chemotherapy with radiation therapy improves local control in breast cancer. This trial compared concurrent chemoradiotherapy with FNC (5-fluourouracil [5-FU] 500 mg/m^2, mitoxantrone 12 mg/m^2, and cyclophosphamide 500 mg/m^2), to sequential FEC (5-fluorouracil 500 mg/m^2, epirubicin 60 mg/m^2, and cyclophosphamide 500 mg/m^2) followed by radiation in node-positive breast cancer in 650 women with operable breast cancer. All patients had node-positive disease and were randomized to sequential or concurrent chemoradiotherapy. Although there were no differences in disease-free or overall survival, local recurrences were significantly lower with concurrent therapy (3% vs. 7%). Of patients undergoing breast conservation, there were 6 local-regional relapses in the concurrent arm compared with 18 local-regional relapses in the sequential arm ($P = .01$). In multivariate Cox analysis, the sequential group had an increased risk of local-regional relapse compared with those in the concurrent group (RR 2.8; 95% CI, 1.1 to 7.2).

Toledano et al.[563] recently reported the results of the ARCOSEIN sequential versus concurrent adjuvant chemotherapy with radiation therapy after breast-conserving surgery. After breast-conserving surgery, patients were treated either with sequential treatment with chemotherapy first followed by RT (arm A) or chemotherapy administered concurrently with RT (arm B). In all patients, the chemotherapy regimen consisted of mitoxantrone (12 mg/m^2), 5-FU (500 mg/m^2), and cyclophosphamide (500 mg/m^2), 6 cycles (day 1 to day 21). Among the 214 evaluable patients, 107 were treated in each arm. Although local control was slightly superior in the concurrent arm, subcutaneous fibrosis, telangiectasia, skin pigmentation, and breast atrophy were significantly increased in arm B. No statistical difference was observed between the two arms of the study concerning grade 2 or greater pain, breast edema, or lymphedema.

Another randomized trial recently reported by Calais et al.,[564] which is similar to the Rouesse et al.[561] study, compared concurrent radiotherapy with mitoxantrone, 5-FU and cyclophosphamide to the same regimen followed by radiation therapy. Although toxicities were higher in the concurrent group, those patients with positive nodes had a significantly lower local relapse rate in the concurrent arm.

The concurrent use of chemotherapy and radiation following breast-conserving therapy has been reported in several nonrandomized studies. A prospective single-arm study by Bellon et al.[559] also demonstrated favorable local control in a high-risk group of patients treated with concurrent CMF chemotherapy and reduced-dose radiation. Several other retrospective series, including one recently conducted from Yale, have demonstrated favorable local control rates and acceptable toxicity in patients at high risk for local relapse using concurrent chemoradiotherapy.[428] In the Yale retrospective series, which compared 109 patients treated with concurrent chemoradiation to 426 patients treated with sequential chemoradiation, the concurrent group had a lower rate of local relapse, despite overall poorer prognostic factors for local control. However, the majority of these studies did not employ the most commonly used current chemotherapy agents such as adriamycin and taxanes. Therefore, it is difficult to extrapolate these results to current practice.

More recently, monoclonal antibodies such as trastuzumab and bevacizumab (Avastin) are being used commonly in the management of breast cancer patients. Romond et al.[274] reported on a combine analysis from two large cooperative group studies investigating the utility of trastuzumab in *HER2*-positive patients with operable breast cancer and found that trastuzumab improved patient outcomes. There was no difference in acute locoregional toxicities, but it should be noted that the use of trastuzumab was associated with an increased risk of congestive heart failure or death from cardiac causes (4.1% vs. 0.8%). Goyal et al.[565] reported on a series of 14 patients receiving bevacizumab in combination with whole-breast irradiation who were then matched to a group of patients who received whole-breast irradiation alone. No patient receiving bevacizumab plus RT experienced grade 3 or higher toxicity; however, three matched control patients experienced a grade 3 skin reaction. There was no difference in fatigue, radiation fibrosis, pneumonitis, or lymphedema between the two groups. Five patients (35%) developed reduction in ejection fraction in the bevacizumab arm; two with right-sided and three with left-sided treatment. Patients with left-sided treatment experienced a persistent reduction in ejection fraction compared with those receiving right-sided treatment. Thus, when treating patients with left-sided breast cancer, exclusion of the heart from the beam's eye view should be undertaken such that no unnecessary radiation dose is delivered to the heart. One challenge moving forward is determining the toxicities of these novel

TABLE 56.31 OUTCOMES OF CONCURRENT OR SEQUENTIAL TAMOXIFEN WITH RADIATION THERAPY IN EARLY-STAGE BREAST CANCER

Study (Reference)	*Number of Patients* CON-TAM	SEQ-TAM	Follow-Up (Median, Year)	*Total Local Relapse* CON-TAM (%)	SEQ-TAM (%)	P	*Distant Metastasis* CON-TAM (%)	SEQ-TAM (%)	P	*Secondary Malignancy* CON-TAM (%)	SEQ-TAM (%)	P	Complications
Ahn et al. (569)	254	241	10.0	5.9	7.5	.59	8.3	12.0	.16	17.3	15.8	.16	
Harris et al. (570)	174	104	8.6	4.0	4.8	.76	–	–	–	–	–	–	No significant difference between the two groups for arm edema, pneumonitis, and rib fracture
Pierce et al. (572)	202	107	10.3	15.8	14.0	.67	–	–	–	–	–	–	No significant differences between two groups for grade 3 or 4 toxicity; one grade 3 pulmonary toxicity observed in CON-TAM group

CON-TAM, concurrent tamoxifen; SEQ-TAM: sequential tamoxifen.

therapies in combination with conventionally fractionated and hypofractionated radiotherapy regimens.

The critical issue that arises with conservatively managed breast cancer is whether the modest gain in local control outweighs the added toxicities and risks of concurrent chemoradiotherapy, using currently available agents. The benefit in local-regional control obtained in the Rouesse et al.[561] study was statistically significant, but it remains debatable whether the added toxicity of the concurrent program is worth the added risk. Potential issues with concurrent chemoradiation, as pointed out in a study by Burstein et al.,[566] include high rates of radiation pneumonitis in patients treated with radiation given in combination with weekly paclitaxel. Although they observed more favorable results with less frequent dosing, this study highlights the importance of prospective evaluation of radiation in combination with newer chemotherapeutic agents. Furthermore, this study highlights the importance of the dosing and scheduling of the chemotherapy agents given in combination with radiation.

The challenge over the next few years will be to identify those patients, who when treated by the traditional approach of surgery followed by chemotherapy followed by radiation therapy, remain at elevated risk of local relapse. Also at risk may be subsets of patients treated with neoadjuvant chemotherapy followed by surgery followed by radiation. Those patients who, when treated by these traditional sequencing approaches, are at high risk of local relapse are ideally suited for prospective evaluation of novel approaches using concurrent chemoradiation strategies. From such trials we can hopefully minimize local-regional relapse and optimize disease-free and overall survival, with acceptable treatment-related morbidity.

Sequencing Tamoxifen/Hormonal Therapy and Radiation Therapy in Conservatively Managed Patients

The question of optimal scheduling of hormonal therapy and radiation has been raised due to theoretical concerns that tamoxifen may decrease the radiation sensitivity of tumors. In cell culture studies, tamoxifen causes arrest of breast cancer cells in culture in the relatively radioresistant G_0/G_1 phases of the cell cycle. Although there are conflicting data, suggesting both no effect and increased radiation sensitivity, clinicians and patients have been in a quandary as to whether it is reasonable to begin tamoxifen during radiation. In addition, clinical studies have suggested increased pulmonary and breast fibrosis, possibly related to increased concentrations of transforming growth factor-β with the concurrent use of tamoxifen.[567] In a retrospective case series, Wazer et al.[568] reported a trend for an adverse cosmetic outcome associated with breast fibrosis in patients treated with tamoxifen and breast irradiation given either concurrently or sequentially ($P = .06$), although this was not confirmed in other series.[569–570,571]

A series of three separate retrospective series, however, performed independently but published simultaneously, reached similar conclusions that sequential or concurrent use of tamoxifen were both acceptable.[569–570,571–572] These studies are summarized in Table 56.31. The largest study, by Ahn et al.[569] from the Yale group compared 254 patients treated with concurrent tamoxifen and radiation therapy to 241 treated by radiation therapy followed by tamoxifen (n = 241). There were no significant differences in the risk of ipsilateral breast tumor recurrence, disease-free survival, or overall survival. The hazard ratio for ipsilateral breast tumor recurrence comparing sequential with concurrent tamoxifen and radiation therapy was 0.93 (95% CI, 0.42 to 2.05; $P = .86$). In this study morbidity outcomes were not reported.

The second study, by Harris et al.,[570] from the group at the University of Pennsylvania compared 174 patients treated with concurrent tamoxifen and radiation therapy with 104 patients treated with radiation therapy followed sequentially by tamoxifen. Similar to the Yale study, patients were accrued throughout a long period between 1980 and 1995, and again no significant differences in ipsilateral breast tumor recurrence, disease-free survival, or overall survival were observed between groups. The hazard ratio for ipsilateral breast tumor recurrence (sequential vs. concurrent) was 1.23 (95% CI, 0.33 to 4.49; $P = .78$). In this study breast edema and arm edema as well as cosmetic outcome and pneumonitis were analyzed and no significant differences were observed.

The third study, by Pierce et al.,[572] evaluated results from a randomized trial, in which patients were randomly assigned to cyclophosphamide, doxorubicin, and fluorouracil (CAF) followed by tamoxifen; CMF; or CMF followed by tamoxifen. Although the sequencing of tamoxifen was not randomized, 202 patients received concurrent tamoxifen and radiation therapy and 107 received radiation therapy followed sequentially by tamoxifen. In this study, no differences were noted in the risk of ipsilateral breast tumor recurrence, disease-free survival, or survival between radiation therapy followed sequentially by tamoxifen and concurrent tamoxifen and radiation therapy group. Patients who received concurrent tamoxifen and radiation therapy were more likely to receive radiation after chemotherapy, with less delay. The hazard ratio for risk of ipsilateral breast tumor recurrence (radiation therapy followed sequentially by tamoxifen vs. concurrent tamoxifen and radiation therapy) was 0.73 (95% CI, 0.26 to 2.04; $P = .54$).

Although these studies are limited by their retrospective design, they do offer some reassurance that the concurrent use of hormonal therapy with radiation therapy does not result in excessive rates of local relapse. Although a large randomized trial would be the appropriate next step in addressing this issue, it is unclear whether this issue will be addressed by such a trial in the near future. Given the lack of more definitive data, it appears that either the concurrent or the sequential use of tamoxifen is acceptable in the conservatively managed breast cancer patient. The majority of available data on the use of hormonal therapy and radiation are with tamoxifen. In a prospective phase II randomized trial evaluating concurrent or sequential letrozole, Azria et al.[573] reported no difference in local relapse (one in each arm) at 26 months of follow-up. In addition, only two patients in each group had grade 2 or worse late effects. These authors conclude that letrozole can be safely delivered concomitantly with radiation, but longer follow-up is awaited from this trial.

BREAST-CONSERVING THERAPY: CONTROVERSIES AND SPECIAL CIRCUMSTANCES

The available evidence from all of the retrospective and prospective trials above suggests that although there are clearly cohorts of patients who are at increased risk of local relapse, there are relatively few contraindications to breast-conserving therapy and there is little evidence that treatment of patients at higher risk for local relapse with breast-conserving therapy compromises overall survival. Careful attention to patient selection, surgical technique, and radiation technique, with the appropriate integration of systemic therapy, should minimize the probability of local relapse. There are several areas of controversy and special circumstances in the selection of patients for breast-conserving therapy that warrant specific discussion.

Breast-Conserving Surgery and Radiation in Familial Breast Cancer and Carriers of *BRCA1/2* Mutations

There is considerable controversy and uncertainty regarding the role of breast-conserving surgery and radiation in carriers of *BRCA1/2* mutations.[466,574,575] It has been just over a decade since these two major breast cancer predisposition genes were identified. Genetic linkage studies from families at high risk for predisposing germline mutations have led to the identification of the *BRCA1/2* genes, and these two genes are thought to account for 5% to 10% of breast cancers.[20,44,576–579] Patients with either mutation have up to an 80% lifetime risk of developing breast cancer depending on variable penetrance of the gene. Inherited mutation of *BRCA1* also confers a 20% to 40% lifetime risk of ovarian cancer. Typical patient characteristics of *BRCA*-associated breast cancer include young age at onset and bilateral involvement. The median age at breast cancer diagnosis is 40 for *BRCA1* carriers and 45 for *BRCA2* carriers.[20,576–579] Tumor characteristics of *BRCA1* carriers have been well described. Histopathologic features are often more aggressive, with high nuclear grade, aneuploidy, and high proliferation indices; tumors with a medullary component are more common. Estrogen and progesterone receptors are more likely to be negative when compared with *BRCA2* or sporadic counterparts. Although there are some conflicting data, *BRCA1/2* carriers with breast cancer appear to have equivalent survival when compared with age and staged matched patients with sporadic disease.[20,44,580,581–582]

The loci for *BRCA1* and *BRCA2* are chromosome 17q21 and chromosome 13q12-13, respectively.[20,576–579] Both function as tumor suppressor genes and are involved in DNA double-strand break repair. The role of *BRCA1/2* in DNA repair suggests the possibility of hypersensitivity to radiation, as well as the potential for radiation-induced complications including second cancers. DNA double-strand breaks caused by ionizing radiation in *BRCA1/2* carriers could theoretically result in increased cell kill secondary to deficient repair mechanisms.[20,46,583–585]

The risk of both contralateral primary breast cancer and ovarian cancer is substantially higher in patients with *BRCA1/2* mutations than sporadic counterparts. An early publication by the Breast Cancer Linkage Consortium estimated a 64% risk of contralateral breast cancer by the age of 70 years in patients who have had *BRCA1*-associated breast cancer.[44,586] The cumulative risk of ovarian cancer in these patients was 44% by age 70 years. Women with *BRCA2* mutations have a risk of breast cancer similar to patients with *BRCA1* mutations. There is a lesser risk of ovarian cancer, with a cumulative risk of <10% by age 70 years. These results have been interpreted with caution, as linkage studies are likely to overestimate the cancer risk associated with *BRCA1/2* mutations. Several studies of known germline *BRCA1/2* carriers have demonstrated a less pronounced increase in the rate of contralateral breast cancer compared with sporadic controls.[20,44,586]

Early study of familiar breast cancer used positive family history as a surrogate for genetic predisposition. Many of the patients included likely did not harbor germline mutations of the *BRCA1/2* genes. Seynaeve et al.[582] for the Dutch Cancer Society investigated local recurrence after breast-conservation therapy in patients with *three or more* first-degree relatives with breast or ovarian cancer or *BRCA1/2* families. Local recurrence rates were initially similar, but with longer follow-up there was a higher rate of recurrence in the hereditary group when compared with age-matched sporadic patients. Other studies of breast-conservation therapy in patients with a family history of breast cancer have not shown an increase in ipsilateral breast recurrence.[407,408,587] Disparate results are expected, as family history is not the sole factor in genetic predisposition.

The risk of local and contralateral breast cancers as a function of *BRCA1* and *BRCA2* status have been evaluated by numerous groups over the past 10 years.[288,575,581,582,588,589,590–591,592–593,594–599] These are summarized in Table 56.32.

Robson et al.[575] studied breast-conservation therapy in Ashkenazi women with the *BRCA* gene founder mutations (*BRCA1* 185delAG, *BRCA1* 5382insC, and *BRCA2* 617delT). Archival tissue samples were retrieved from 305 women, and 28 *BRCA* gene founder mutations were detected. *BRCA1/2* carriers had a nonsignificant trend toward increased ipsilateral

TABLE 56.32 RATE OF IPSILATERAL BREAST TUMOR RELAPSE IN *BRCA* MUTATION CARRIERS COMPARED TO SPORADIC CONTROLS

Study (Reference)	Number of Patients Genetic	Number of Patients Sporadic	Follow-Up (Year)	IBTR Sporadic (%)	IBTR Genetic (%)	P	Notes
Seynaeve et al. (582)	87	174	10	16	30	.05	More recurrences elsewhere? in cancers
Robson et al. (598)	28	277	10	6.9	22	.25	Only tested for founder mutations in Ashkenazi women
Robson et al. (581)	56	440	9.6	7	13	.68	As above
Haffty et al. (589)	23	135	12	21	46	.007	No oophorectomy or Tamoxifen in *BRCA* group
Pierce et al. (592)	160	445	7.9	17	24	.19	HR for IBTR was significant in those carriers who did not undergo prophylactic oophorectomy
Kirova et al. (590)	29	107	13	19	24	.47	
Garcia-Etienne et al. (588)	54	162	5	4	15	.03	

HR, hazard ratio; IBTR, ipsilateral breast tumor recurrence.

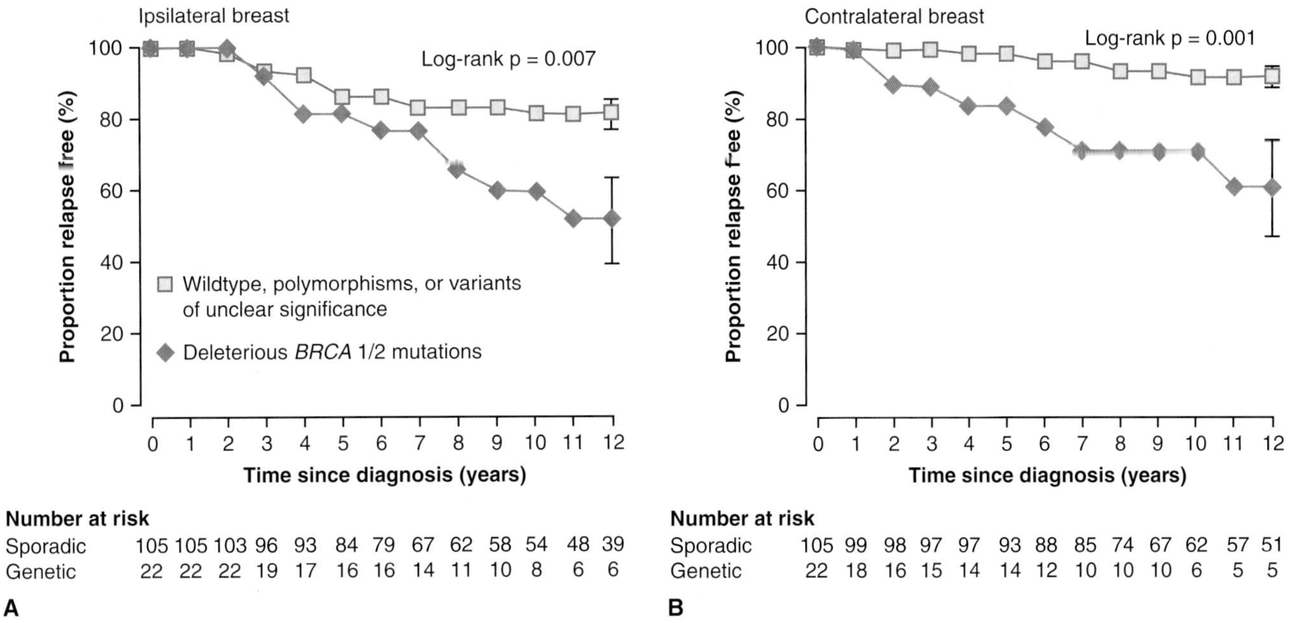

FIGURE 56.23. Risk of ipsilateral and contralateral breast tumor relapse as a function of *BRCA1/BRCA2* mutation status in a cohort of conservatively managed breast cancer patients. (From Haffty BG, Harrold E, Khan AJ, et al. Outcome of conservatively managed early-onset breast cancer by BRCA1/2 status. *Lancet* 2002;359:1471–1477, with permission.)

breast cancer recurrence and decreased overall survival at 5 and 10 years. This trend may be related to the greater likelihood of young age and axillary lymph node involvement in women with *BRCA* founder mutations. On univariate analysis, age but not *BRCA* mutation status was associated with ipsilateral breast tumor recurrence. The significance of age was maintained on multivariate analysis, with a relative risk of 2.5. The risk of contralateral breast cancer at 5 and 10 years was 14.8% and 27.0%, respectively.

This series from Memorial Hospital was later combined with data from McGill University, yielding a total of 56 women with founder mutations. Again, *BRCA1/2* carriers had an increased risk of contralateral breast cancer at a median follow-up of 9.7 years (27% vs. 8%; $P < .001$). Ipsilateral breast cancer recurrence for *BRCA1/2* carriers was similar to noncarriers, and age <50 at diagnosis was the only significant predictor of metachronous ipsilateral disease ($P = .002$).[581] *BRCA1* mutations were an independent predictor of breast cancer mortality on multivariate analysis, but only for women who did not receive chemotherapy. *BRCA2* mutations had no impact on breast cancer-specific survival.

Haffty et al.[589] studied breast-conservation therapy in germline carriers with early-onset breast cancer. One hundred and twenty-seven women diagnosed with breast cancer at age 42 years or younger agreed to undergo genetic testing, and 22 were found to have *BRCA1/2* mutations. Adjuvant tamoxifen or oophorectomy were not used in any of the carriers of *BRCA1/2* mutations. Patients in the genetic group were younger than sporadic patients, and this difference was significant on multivariate analysis. Treatment outcomes were compared with results from patients with sporadic disease. With a median follow-up of 12.7 years, the genetic group had a higher rate of ipsilateral (49% vs. 21%; $P = .007$) and contralateral breast events (42% vs. 9%; $P = .001$). Nine of the 11 ipsilateral breast recurrences were classified as second primary tumors, based on a difference in tumor location (n = 7) or histology (n = 8). The rate of ipsilateral and contralateral events was much higher than those reported in earlier series and may be attributable to both the young age of the patients at diagnosis and longer duration of follow-up. The proportion of relapse free *BRCA1/2* carriers was similar to noncarriers at 5 years and then progressively declined with time (Fig. 56.23). It is promising that all of the second events in *BRCA1/2* carriers were successfully salvaged and remained disease free. Steinmann et al.[600] confirmed the increased risk of developing ipsilateral second primaries in *BRCA1/2* carriers and extended this concern to patients with bilateral breast cancer. Although the high rate of local relapses and contralateral events in these studies might be considered unacceptable, it is likely that the use of risk reduction strategies, such as tamoxifen or oophorectomy, would reduce these events to an acceptable level. Recent similar case control type studies were undertaken by and Garcia-Etienne et al.[588] and Kirova et al.[590] The study by Kirova et al. did not show a statistically higher local relapse rate in *BRCA1/2* carriers. However, the study by Garcia-Etienne et al., comparing 54 genetic cases to 162 sporadic cases, reported a 15% local relapse rate in the genetic group compared with a 4% local relapse rate in the sporadic group ($P = .03$).

Although the data presented above have some apparent conflicting conclusions, a recent study by Pierce et al.[592] helps to resolve some of these issues. In a large collaborative study these authors evaluated a total of 160 *BRCA1/2* mutation carriers with breast cancer matched to 445 controls with sporadic breast cancer (Fig. 56.24). Median follow-up was 7.9 years for mutation carriers and 6.7 years for controls. Although there was no significant difference in IBTR overall between carriers and controls (15-year estimates were 24% for carriers and 17% for controls; HR 1.37; $P = .19$), a subset analysis revealed higher rates of local relapse in those carriers who had not undergone prophylactic oophorectomy. Multivariate analyses for IBTR found *BRCA1/2* mutation status to be an independent predictor of IBTR when carriers who had undergone oophorectomy were removed from analysis (HR 1.99; $P = .04$); the incidence of IBTR in carriers who had undergone oophorectomy was not significantly different from that in sporadic controls ($P = .37$). Contralateral breast cancers were significantly more frequent in carriers versus controls, with 10- and 15-year estimates of 26% and 39% for carriers and 3% and 7% for controls, respectively (HR 10.43; $P < .0001$). Tamoxifen use significantly reduced the risk of contralateral breast cancers in mutation carriers (HR 0.31; $P = .05$). Thus, it appears that this study confirms the findings of Haffty et al.[589] that *BRCA1/2* carriers have a high rate of both contralateral and ipsilateral breast events if they do not undergo specific measures to reduce the risk of subsequent breast cancers by undergoing oophorectomy or tamoxifen.

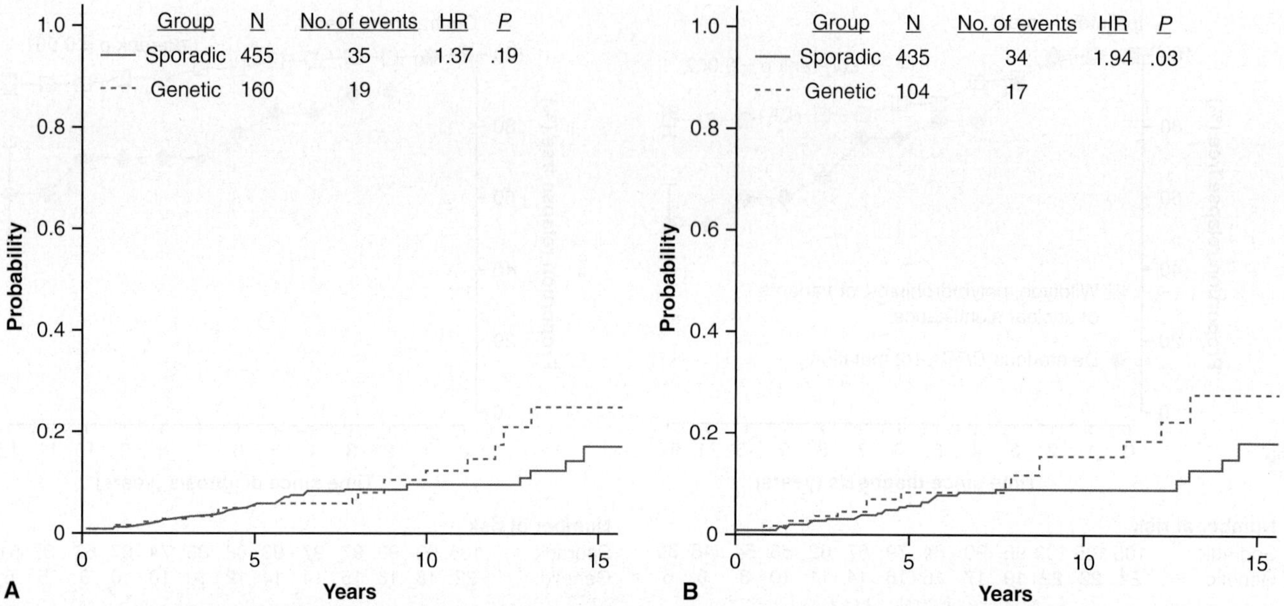

FIGURE 56.24. Risk of ipsilateral breast tumor relapse in *BRCA* carriers as a function of whether carriers had undergone prophylactic oophorectomy. In *BRCA* carriers who did not undergo oophorectomy, the risk of late local relapses was significantly greater than sporadic controls. (From Pierce L, Levin AM, Rebbeck TR, et al. Ten-year multi-institutional results of breast-conserving surgery and radiotherapy in BRCA1/2-associated stage I/II breast cancer. *J Clin Oncol* 2006;24:2437–2443. Reprinted with permission. © 2006 American Society of Clinical Oncology.)

Prophylactic mastectomy has been shown to significantly reduce the incidence of breast cancer in women with a family history of breast cancer and specifically women with *BRCA1/2* mutations.[57] This risk reduction strategy has complex emotional and psychological implications, and there are no data to suggest an improvement in survival when compared with close surveillance. Most preventative strategies have focused on primary prevention, but prophylactic strategies should also be considered at the time of breast cancer diagnosis. Oophorectomy and tamoxifen offer similar risk reduction for breast cancer patients with germline mutations. These agents have not been widely used in studies of conservatively managed breast cancer patients with *BRCA1/2* mutations. Their potential benefits must be weighed against the possible complications of premature menopause following oophorectomy and the side effects of tamoxifen.

In a recent study of 655 women with *BRCA1/2* mutations diagnosed with breast cancer and treated with breast-conserving therapy (n = 302) or mastectomy (n = 353) from a multicenter collaborative group, Pierce et al.[596] reported on local failure, as first failure was significantly more likely in those treated with breast conservation (23.5 vs. 5.5%, respectively), at 15 years (P <.0001). Of note, the in-breast relapse rate appeared to be reduced in the breast-conservation group by chemotherapy, whereas the 15-year estimate in carriers treated with breast-conserving therapy and chemotherapy was 11.9% and did not significantly differ from those treated with mastectomy. There were no differences seen in regional or systemic recurrences between the breast-conserving therapy and mastectomy groups and no difference in overall survival, but contralateral breast cancers were common in both cohorts.

Women with *BRCA1/2* mutations who underwent prophylactic oophorectomy to reduce the risk of ovarian cancer were found to have a decreased incidence of breast cancer. Rebbeck[601] studied the risk of breast cancer in 43 *BRCA1* carriers with no history of breast or ovarian cancer who underwent prophylactic bilateral oophorectomy. When these patients were compared with *BRCA1* controls who did not undergo oophorectomy, there was a significant reduction in breast cancer risk (HR 0.53). A follow-up report from this author identified 551 women with *BRCA1/2* germline mutations and reported the incidence of ovarian and breast cancer in women who had undergone prophylactic oophorectomy and matched controls.[602,603] Six women who underwent prophylactic oophorectomy were diagnosed with stage I ovarian cancer at the time of the procedure. With a median follow-up of 8 years, two women developed papillary serous peritoneal carcinoma after oophorectomy and 58 controls were diagnosed with ovarian cancer. After the exclusion of women who were diagnosed with cancer at surgery, oophorectomy reduced the risk of ovarian cancer by 96%. Oophorectomy also reduced the incidence of breast cancer in the subgroup of 241 women with no history of breast cancer or prophylactic mastectomy. Twenty-one of the 99 (21.2%) women who underwent prophylactic oophorectomy developed breast cancer versus 60 of the 142 (42.3%) women in the control group (HR 0.47).

Kauff et al.[604] conducted a prospective study of the risk of gynecologic cancer and breast cancer in 170 *BRCA1/2* carriers who chose to undergo surveillance or prophylactic oophorectomy. In the 98 women who chose prophylactic oophorectomy, 3 were later diagnosed with breast cancer and peritoneal cancer was diagnosed in 1 patient. The surveillance group of 72 patients yielded 8 breast cancers, 4 ovarian cancers, and 1 peritoneal cancer. With a median follow-up of only 24 months, this prospective study supports an early reduction in breast and ovarian cancer risk with prophylactic oophorectomy.

In prospective trials, tamoxifen has been shown to reduce both the risk of breast cancer in high-risk women and the risk of contralateral breast cancer in patients with breast cancer.[53,605] An analysis of the NSABP-P1 data from the tamoxifen versus placebo prevention trial identified 19 *BRCA1/2* mutations in the 288 women who developed breast cancer.[96] Five of the 8 women with *BRCA1* mutations had taken tamoxifen versus 3 of 11 women with *BRCA2* mutations. This represented a 62% reduction in breast cancer incidence for *BRCA2* carriers, but no benefit for tamoxifen in *BRCA1* carriers. The dataset was small, however, with low power to detect a protective effect.

Narod et al.[585] studied tamoxifen and the risk of contralateral breast cancer in *BRCA1/2* carriers. This collaborative effort compared women with bilateral breast cancer and women with unilateral breast cancer in a case-control study. Sixty-four (13%) *BRCA1* mutation carriers used tamoxifen versus 39 (33%) *BRCA2* carriers. This difference is expected as breast cancers associated with *BRCA1* mutations are typically ER-negative and *BRCA2*-associated breast cancers are commonly ER-positive. Tamoxifen protected against contralateral

TABLE 56.33 STUDIES EVALUATING COLLAGEN VASCULAR DISEASE IN BREAST CONSERVING THERAPY

	CVD			
Study (Reference)	Total Number	Number with Breast Cancer	Design	Findings
De Naeyer et al. (609)	3	1	Case report	Necrosis and progressive fibrosis
Fleck et al. (607)	9	4	Case report	Necrosis, brachial plexopathy, and severe moist desquamation
Robertson et al. (612)	2	2	Case report	Severe breast fibrosis, erythema, and pain
Chen et al. (614)	36	36	Case control	Late complication rates higher only in scleroderma
Morris and Powell (608)	209	19	Retrospective	Increased radiation late effects appear in nonrheumatoid arthritis cases
Ross et al. (613)	61	?	Case control	No differences in acute/chronic complications
Phan et al. (610)	38	?	Case control	No difference was observed in the incidence of acute or late complications between the two groups.
Rakfal and Deutsch (611)	6	4	Case report	No severe acute or late radiation complications

CVD, collagen vascular disease.

breast cancer, with an odds ratio of 0.38 for *BRCA1* carriers and 0.63 for *BRCA2* carriers. The combined risk reduction for *BRCA1* and *BRCA2* carriers was 50%. The benefit of tamoxifen in *BRCA1* carriers was possibly detected due to the larger sample size. This study also noted a reduction in contralateral breast cancer in patients who received oophorectomy. The odds ratio was 0.42, which is similar to the reduction in contralateral breast cancer noted with tamoxifen.

Although the conservative management of breast cancer in patients with *BRCA1/2* germline mutations warrants further study, the available evidence indicates that breast-conserving therapy followed by radiation therapy is an appropriate alternative to bilateral mastectomy in early-stage breast cancer in these women. Theoretical concerns for radiation-induced complications have not been demonstrated.[606] Although development of second primary tumors in the ipsilateral and contralateral breast remains a concern, prophylactic oophorectomy and tamoxifen appear to significantly reduce the probability of these secondary events.[20,585,592,601] Prophylactic oophorectomy is even more critical in the risk-reduction strategy for the development of primary tumors of the ovary. For those women considering breast-conserving surgery and radiation therapy, strategies to reduce secondary events, including prophylactic oophorectomy as soon as child-bearing issues have been addressed and resolved, with or without tamoxifen or other hormonal agents as indicated, appear to be rational and viable options. Despite some evidence that tamoxifen reduces the risk of secondary breast cancers in patients who are carriers of *BRCA1/2* mutations, the use of tamoxifen in *BRCA1* breast cancer patients who are ER-negative remains unresolved and controversial.

Collagen Vascular Disease

Increased acute and late effects of irradiation have been reported in patients with pre-existing collagen vascular disease (CVD). Selected studies addressing this issue are summarized in Table 56.33.[607–614]

Fleck et al.[607] reported on five women in whom CVD developed 3 months to 10 years after radiation therapy and who had no complications. However, in three of four women with pre-existing CVD, severe complications developed, characterized by persistent moist desquamation, paresthesias in the ipsilateral arm, chest wall necrosis requiring surgical resection, and osteonecrosis of the clavicle, sternum, and rib cage. These authors concluded that a history of active CVD appeared to be a contraindication to breast-conservation surgery and irradiation.

On the other hand, Ross et al.[613] evaluated a group of 61 patients with CVD who were compared with a matched control group of 61 patients without CVD. The CVD group included 39 patients with rheumatoid arthritis, 13 with systemic lupus erythematosus, 4 with scleroderma, 4 with dermatomyositis, and 4 with polymyositis. Overall, there was no significant difference between the CVD and control groups in terms of postirradiation acute complications (11% and 7%, respectively) or late complications (10% and 7%, respectively). This was also true when only patients who were treated definitively were considered. Three patients in the CVD group had fatal complications, compared with none in the control group. Rheumatoid arthritis was associated with a slight increase in late complications in definitively treated patients, whereas systemic lupus erythematosus was associated with a slight increase in acute reactions. No significant acute or late reactions were observed in the patients with scleroderma, dermatomyositis, or polymyositis.

Morris and Powell[608] treated 96 patients with documented CVD with breast-conservation therapy (127 sites irradiated). Grade 3 or higher acute complications were seen in 15 of the 127 (11.8%) sites, and the actuarial rate of significant late complications was 24% at 10 years. There was a single in-field sarcoma. Patients with rheumatoid arthritis had less severe late effects than those with other CVD (6% vs. 37% at 5 years; $P = .0001$).

In a study specifically evaluating conservatively treated breast cancer patients, Chen et al.[614] from the Yale group identified 36 patients with documented CVD conservatively treated for early-stage breast cancer between 1975 and 1998. All of these patients were treated with conventional radiation therapy to a median total dose of 64 Gy. Seventeen had rheumatoid arthritis; four, scleroderma; four, Reynaud's phenomenon; five, lupus erythematosus; two, Sjögren disease; and four, polymyositis. Each of these patients was matched to two control patients without a history of CVD. Acute and late complications were assessed using a six-point scale from the toxicity criteria of the RTOG and the EORTC. No significant difference was detected between the CVD and control groups with respect to acute complications (14% vs. 8%). With respect to late complications, a significant difference was observed (17% vs. 3%) between the two groups. However, when patients in the CVD group were analyzed by specific disease, this significance disappeared in all but the scleroderma group.

Collectively these data suggest that with the exception of patients with scleroderma, there does not appear to be a significantly greater late complication rate associated with CVD. Nevertheless, when patients with CVD are irradiated, it is prudent to limit the whole-breast dose to 45 Gy with 1.8-Gy fractions, use 6-MV photons, optimize homogeneity of dose distribution, avoid concurrent chemoirradiation, and discuss with patients the potential increased risks of radiation sequelae. There are small, limited case series of treating breast cancer in patients with CVD with hypofractioned whole-breast or partial-breast radiotherapy.

Pregnancy

Breast Cancer During Pregnancy

Breast cancer is the most common cancer diagnosed during pregnancy and represents a significant therapeutic challenge. Recently, an expert international panel met and published general recommendations for breast cancer developing during pregnancy.[615] The panel noted that the goal for the pregnant women with breast cancer is the same as that of the nonpregnant women: local control of disease and prevention of systemic metastasis. However, due to adverse effects on the fetus, certain treatment modalities, including radiation, must be avoided.

The incidence of breast cancer associated with pregnancy is estimated to be 1.5 to 2 in 10,000 pregnancies. Alberktsen et al.,[616] in a study of 802,457 women from the Cancer Registry of Norway, observed a relative risk of 1.24 for breast cancer in the 3 to 4 years immediately after a pregnancy, followed by a decreased risk thereafter.

The prognosis of patients developing breast cancer during pregnancy, stage for stage, appears to be similar to age-matched controls, although delays in diagnosis may result in higher stages in pregnant women. Several studies have stated that poorer prognosis in breast cancer associated with pregnancy may be related to delay in diagnosis because pregnancy impedes early detection, and possibly to the biology of the tumor.[617] Zemlickis et al.[618] compared 118 women with breast cancer (119 pregnancies) with 269 nonpregnant control patients. The distribution of breast cancer stages among the 118 pregnant women was compared with that among 5,115 cases of breast cancer in nonpregnant women of reproductive age. Women having breast cancer in pregnancy were 2.5 times more likely to have metastatic disease (95% CI, 1.1 to 5.3) and had a significantly lower chance of having stage I disease ($P = .015$). However, stage for stage survival of pregnant women did not differ from that of the control patients. A number of authors have commented on the high percentage of pregnant patients with lymph node involvement, compared with nonpregnant patients. Others have also suggested that the poorer outcome relates to the young age of the patient and not necessarily to the pregnancy.[306,619,620] A single-institution retrospective chart review was performed on 99 patients identified with pregnancy-associated breast cancer (PABC), where non-PABC controls were matched 2 to 1 to PABC cases by year of diagnosis and age.[621] They found that PABC cases were more likely than controls to be negative for estrogen receptor (59% vs. 31%; $P < .0001$) and negative for progesterone receptor (72% vs. 40%; $P < .0001$). Cases were also more likely to have advanced T class ($P = .03$) and N class ($P = .01$) and higher grade tumors ($P = .0115$). With a median follow-up of 6.3 years for cases and 4.7 years for controls, overall survival did not differ between cases and controls ($P = .08$).

As will be discussed below, selected chemotherapy agents can be administered during the second and third trimesters. Although therapeutic abortion is not necessary, women with high-risk disease may find this preferable. They also note that in women with known deleterious mutations in *BRCA1/2*, early pregnancy is not known to decrease subsequent breast cancer risk. In addition, the available evidence suggests that in women with a history of breast cancer, subsequent pregnancy does not increase the risk of recurrence.

In addition to requiring close coordination among multidisciplinary cancer care givers, management of breast cancer during pregnancy also benefits from having obstetricians and pediatricians closely involved in therapeutic decision making. It is likely that as pregnancy in Western society is delayed to older ages, the incidence of breast cancer developing during pregnancy will increase.

Breast cancers during pregnancy are almost universally diagnosed after an abnormal physical examination finding.[306] There frequently may be a delay in diagnosis because the breast mass is thought to represent obstructed milk ducts and inflammatory changes of the breast may be misdiagnosed as cellulitis. For patients who present with a breast mass, a careful history and physical examination should be performed. The overall goal of managing breast cancer during pregnancy requires attention to both the mother and the fetus. Certain diagnostic and therapeutic interventions are known to be teratogenic and therefore are best avoided. Although theoretically a chest radiograph may be safely performed because the maximum dose to the fetus is <0.005 Gy, radiographic and scintigraphic imaging for staging should be minimized or deferred.[292] Mammography is somewhat controversial, although the irradiation dose to the fetus is minimal (<0.5 mrem).[622] Ultrasound evaluations of the breast and lymph nodes can provide diagnostic information and serve as a method of guidance for core biopsy. Pathology of breast cancer during pregnancy is most frequently invasive ductal with high nuclear grade and lower rates of ER and PR positivity.[306]

The management of the patient and the risks of certain interventions are also highly dependent on the week of gestation. In general, potentially harmful interventions carry the greatest risk during the period of organogenesis (first trimester) and are safest during the final trimester. For patients with operable disease, data suggest that surgery can be safely performed after the 12th week of pregnancy. The type of surgical procedure is dependent on the extent of disease and the trimester of the pregnancy.[306,616,618,619] Few data exist concerning the safety and efficacy of sentinel lymph node biopsy. Although the blue dye used in sentinel lymph node surgery is not approved for use in pregnant patients, the estimated radiation dose to the fetus from the radiocolloid tracer is low. Except for radiation, treatment should not be altered or delayed because of pregnancy. Either a modified radical mastectomy or lumpectomy with axillary dissection is acceptable local treatment. Immediate breast reconstruction should not be performed.

Systemic chemotherapy with FAC (5-fluorouracil, doxorubicin, cyclophosphamide) has been used in pregnancy. Investigators from MD Anderson Cancer Center reported a prospective series of 57 pregnant breast cancer patients who were treated on a single-arm, multidisciplinary, protocol with FAC in the adjuvant (n = 32) or neoadjuvant (n = 25) setting.[623] Parents and guardians were surveyed by mail or telephone regarding outcomes of children exposed to chemotherapy *in utero*. All women who delivered had live births. One child has Down syndrome and two have congenital anomalies (club foot; congenital bilateral ureteral reflux). They conclude that breast cancer can be treated with FAC chemotherapy during the second and third trimesters without significant short-term complications for the majority of children exposed to chemotherapy *in utero*. Longer follow-up of the children is needed to evaluate possible late side effects such as impaired cardiac function and fertility. Administration of chemotherapy in the first trimester is associated with a high risk of birth defects (17%, 24 of 139), in terms of probability of intrauterine growth retardation, prematurity, fetal malformation, or death this risk is less in the second and third trimesters (1.3%, 2 of 150).[624]

As a general principle, hormonal therapy and radiation therapy should be avoided until after delivery. In one study the estimated dose to the fetus from breast or chest wall radiation to a dose of 0.5 Gy is 0.02 Gy in the first trimester, 0.022 to 0.246 Gy during the second trimester, and 0.02 to 0.586 Gy during the third trimester. Dose to the fetus in the range of 0.1 to 0.9 Gy during the first trimester have been associated with mental retardation.[625]

When the patient chooses breast-conserving therapy, irradiation should be deferred until the fetus is delivered because 50 Gy delivered to the breast, even with external shielding, exposes the fetus to 0.1 to 0.15 Gy if it is small and contained in the true pelvis. During later gestation, when the fetus is larger and high in the abdomen, some fetal areas may receive as much as 2 Gy.[625] In another study using a phantom (film dosimetry), doses to the pelvis ranged from 0.043 Gy with 4-MV x-rays to 0.158 Gy with cobalt-60 (^{60}Co) to the midpelvis.[626]

Although there is some question whether there is any safe dose of irradiation to the fetus, Brent,[627] in an extensive review of the literature, defined 0.05 Gy as a relatively safe upper limit of fetal exposure. Hall[628] suggested that 0.1 Gy *in utero* exposure be used as a dose beyond which a therapeutic abortion should be considered.

Some authors have suggested therapeutic abortion based on a study by Adair,[629] who reported in the early 1950s a better outcome in patients who terminated their pregnancies. However, in 63 patients treated at Mayo Clinic, the 5-year survival rate was 59% in the women who carried to term and 43% in those who underwent a therapeutic abortion. The latter group had more advanced tumors.[630] Petrek[617] also noted that therapeutic abortion does not alter the outcome in patients with breast cancer. Contrary to popular belief, pregnancy does not appear to stimulate the growth of breast cancer. Therefore, no justification exists for therapeutic abortion, which may be relevant only in the patient who has rapidly progressing disease, such as inflammatory breast cancer or metastatic disease.

Pregnancy After Breast Cancer

Almost one-third of women of reproductive age in whom breast cancer later develops have one or more pregnancies, and 70% of these occur within 5 years of treatment.[631] No data are available to suggest that subsequent pregnancy hastens or induces breast cancer recurrence. When matched by age and stage with nonpregnant patients, pregnant women with breast cancer do not have a worse outcome than nonpregnant patients with comparable stages. However, in patients receiving adjuvant chemotherapy, a minimum of 12 months between treatment and conception is advised. Breastfeeding is contraindicated in patients receiving chemotherapy because antineoplastic agents are excreted in the milk.[306,617,619]

Sutton et al.[632] reviewed 227 women 35 years of age or younger at diagnosis who became pregnant after treatment with CAF adjuvant chemotherapy. Twenty-five patients had 33 pregnancies. The median interval between completion of chemotherapy and pregnancy was 12 months (range, 0 to 87 months). Ten pregnancies were terminated, 2 ended in spontaneous abortion, 2 patients were still pregnant at the time of the report, and 19 produced normal full-term infants. The incidence of recurrence was 46% in patients without pregnancy, compared with 28% in those who had subsequent pregnancies. Similarly, 38% of patients without subsequent pregnancy were dead at the time of the report, compared with 12% of patients who became pregnant after chemotherapy treatment for breast cancer.

A population-based matched survival study assessed the risk of death for patients with breast cancer in relation to whether they delivered a live child subsequent to their cancer diagnosis.[633] Among 2,548 women younger than 40 years of age diagnosed with carcinoma of the breast, 91 experienced subsequent deliveries (10 months or longer after the diagnosis) and 471 control patients were matched for stage, age, and year of breast cancer diagnosis. The control subjects had to survive at least the interval between the cancer diagnosis and the delivery of their matched counterparts. The control subjects had a 4.8-fold greater risk of death compared with those who delivered after the diagnosis of breast cancer. These authors' interpretation of this result was that there was a "healthy mother effect" (only women who felt healthy gave birth, and those who were affected by the disease did not). Nevertheless, 6 of 8 deaths among the 91 patients who did give birth were related to breast cancer.

Dow et al.[634] evaluated treatment outcome and quality of life in 23 patients with subsequent pregnancies in a group of 1,624 patients treated with breast-conservation surgery and irradiation. This group was compared with 23 patients without subsequent pregnancy who were matched by age and stage at diagnosis and by time to pregnancy without recurrence. There were 32 pregnancies and 30 live births. Six of 23 (22%) women having children after breast cancer therapy had locally recurrent tumor, compared with 29% in the case-matched group. Contralateral breast cancer developed in one woman (4%) in the pregnancy group, compared with 11% in the case-matched group.

It may be helpful to suggest a waiting time (2 to 3 years) for the patient to regain health before attempting the physical stress of pregnancy and deferral of childbearing until after the period of greatest risk of recurrence of the tumor.[631] The individual woman's prognosis, well-being, desire for children, support from spouse or significant other, and other sociodemographic factors must be carefully considered in this difficult decision-making process.

Lactation After Breast-Conservation Therapy

Successful breastfeeding, from the untreated as well as the treated breast, is possible after conservation surgery and irradiation. Higgins and Haffty[635] reviewed the records of 890 patients treated with radiation therapy for early-stage (stage I or II) breast cancer. This series was recently updated by Moran et al.[636] Of over 3,000 patients treated from 1965 to 2003, a cohort of 21 premenopausal women who underwent breast-conserving therapy and subsequently sustained full-term pregnancies were identified. Lactation outcome parameters (breast swelling, ability to lactate, and volume of lactation in the treated and untreated breasts) were the main outcome measures. There were 28 pregnancies in 21 patients. One patient underwent bilateral breast treatment; therefore, a total of 22 breasts were irradiated. All patients interviewed reported little or no swelling of the treated breast during pregnancy. Of the patients studied, 4 (18.2%) elected pharmacologic suppression of lactation. Of the remaining 18 breasts, lactation occurred in 10 (55.6%), did not occur in 7 (38.9%), and was unknown for 1 (5.5%). The volume was reported as significantly diminished in 80% of breasts treated. Lactation in the contralateral breast occurred in all patients who did not undergo pharmacologic suppression. The authors confirm that successful lactation in the contralateral, untreated breast after breast-conserving therapy is expressed. In the treated breast, functional lactation is possible but is significantly diminished in the majority of patients. Tralins[637] reported results of a survey describing 53 women who became pregnant after conservation therapy and breast irradiation. Eighteen exhibited some lactation and 13 (24.5%) were able to breastfeed from the involved breast. Pregnancy or lactation had no impact on prognosis; with a 5.4-year mean follow-up, the tumor-free survival rate was 82%.

Breast Irradiation in Patients Previously Irradiated for Hodgkin Lymphoma

There is an increased incidence of breast cancer in female patients who have previously undergone mantle irradiation for Hodgkin lymphoma. Numerous studies have demonstrated a significantly increased relative risk of breast cancer in women treated for Hodgkin lymphoma, with the risk significantly increasing with decreasing age of exposure. Table 56.34 summarizes the findings of several series.[29,30,638–642,643,644–649,650,651–656]

Travis et al.[30] estimated that for a female Hodgkin lymphoma survivor who was treated at age 25 years with a chest radiation dose of at least 40 Gy without alkylating agents, the cumulative absolute risks of breast cancer by age 35, 45, and 55 years were 1.4% (95% CI, 0.9% to 2.1%), 11.1% (95% CI, 7.4% to 16.3%), and 29.0% (95% CI, 20.2% to 40.1%), respectively. In addition to radiation dose, treatment volumes may also play a role in determining a woman's risk of developing breast cancer after radiotherapy for Hodgkin lymphoma. A study by De Bruin et al.[657] reported on a cohort of 1,122 female patients with Hodgkin lymphoma treated between 1965 and 1995. The overall cumulative incidence 30 years after treatment was 19%; for those treated before age 21 years, it was 26%. Moreover, mantle field irradiation was associated with a 2.7-fold increased risk in developing breast cancer compared with similarly dosed (36 to 44 Gy) mediastinal irradiation alone.

TABLE 56.34 RISK OF SECONDARY BREAST CANCER DEVELOPMENT AFTER MANTLE RADIOTHERAPY FOR HODGKIN LYMPHOMA

	Population				*Average Follow-Up*	*Interval to Breast Cancer*	*Breast Cancer Cases*		
Study (Reference)	*Number*	*Sex*	*Age (Year)*	*Treatment*	*(Year)*	*Detection*	*Number*	*Age Range (Year)*	*Relative Risk (95% CI)*
Aisenberg et al. (632)	111	F		RT±CT	18	8.5–25	14	23–49	
			≤19						56 (23.3–107)
			20–29						7.0 (2.3–16.4)
			≥30						0.9 (0–5.3)
Chung et al. (640)	136	F	–	RT±CT	14.8	6–22	11	30–63	AR = 55.1 cases/10,000 patient-years
Carey et al. (639)	164	F	–	RT	–	11–17	4	37.3	5.45
Guibout et al. (642)	1,258	F	≥17	RT±CT	16	16–28	4	30–34	7.01 (22–164)[a]
Hoppe (644)	2,498	F and M	–	RT±CT	–	–	25	–	4.1
Tinger et al. (649)	152	F	–	RT±CT	>5	4–23	10	27–64	2.2
Bhatia et al. (29)	483	F	<16	RT±CT	11.4	–	17	16–42	75.3
Mauch et al. (652)	349	F	3–69	RT±CT	10.7	–	13	–	6.5 (3.5–11.2)
Salloum et al. (647)	144	F	–	RT±CT	13.5	13.9–14	2	39–41	2 (0.6–7.4)
Hancock et al. (643)	885	F	–	RT±CT	10	4.5–23	25	22–75	4.1 (2.6–5.9)
Prior and Pope (653)	777	F	–	RT±CT	6.7	10–19	9	–	2.2
Tucker et al. (655)	1,507	F and M	–	RT±CT	6.2	8	3	–	12 (2.3–35)
Kaldor et al. (654)	11,491	F	–	RT±CT	1–20+	–	62	–	1.4
Travis et al. (650)	3,817	F	≤30	RT±CT	–	7–30	105	27–57	3.2 (1.4–8.2)
Metayer et al. (646)	2,725	F	≤21	RT±CT	10.5	–	52	–	4.9
Swerdlow et al. (648)	2,085	F	–	RT±CT	1–15	–	19	–	14.4 (5.7–29.3)[b]
Van Leeuwen et al. (651)	544	F	<40	RT±CT	14.1	1–20+	27	–	5.2 (3.4–7.6)
Gervais-Fagnou et al. (641)	427	F	≤30	RT±CT	12.3	9–25	15	30–52	10.6 (5.8–17)
Hudson et al. (645)	165	F	–	RT±CT	15.1	3.6–24.9	6	–	33 (12–72)[a]
Wolden et al. (656)	207	F	<21	RT±CT	13.1	8.5–27.9	16	–	26 (15–42)

CI, confidence interval; RT, radiation therapy; CT, chemotherapy; AR, absolute risk; F, female; M, male.
[a]Standardized incidence ratio. [b]For patients treated at ages younger than 25 years.

Mastectomy has been recommended as the preferred treatment option in these women. Lumpectomy followed by breast irradiation has been considered by some to be contraindicated due to the cumulative radiation dose to the breast. However, in selected patients using careful breast irradiation techniques that avoid significant overlap with the previous mantle port, anecdotal and retrospective reports in small numbers of patients suggest that it is possible to offer breast-conservation therapy. Therapeutic options and the potential increased risk of reirradiation sequelae should be thoroughly discussed with the patient. A second issue that should also be considered is the risk of the development of new primary. Similar to patients with *BRCA* mutations, patients who have a history of breast cancer development after irradiation for Hodgkin lymphoma are at risk in the development of subsequent new primaries and may benefit from prevention strategies such as mastectomy.

Elkin et al.[658] reported on a retrospective multicenter, cohort study of 253 patients treated for Hodgkin lymphoma with radiation therapy who developed breast cancer and matched 3 to 1 with 741 patients with sporadic breast cancer. They found that patients had a median time from diagnosis of Hodgkin's to breast cancer of 18 years, with a median age at breast cancer diagnosis of 42 years. Breast cancer after RT for Hodgkin lymphoma was more likely to be detected by screening, was more likely to be diagnosed at an earlier stage, and was more likely to be bilateral at diagnosis. Hodgkin lymphoma survivors had an increased risk of metachronous contralateral breast cancer (HR 4.3; 95% CI, 1.7 to 11.0) and death as a result of any cause (HR 1.9; 95% CI, 1.1 to 3.3).

Cutuli et al.[659] reported on a retrospective multicenter analysis in which 117 women and 2 men treated for Hodgkin lymphoma subsequently developed 133 breast cancers. Hodgkin lymphoma treatment was radiation therapy alone in 74 patients and combined modality with chemotherapy in 43 patients. Breast cancer occurred after a median interval of 16 years. Tumors were treated by mastectomy without (n = 67) or with (n = 10) irradiation. Forty-four tumors were treated with lumpectomy without (n = 12) or with (n = 32) radiation therapy. Sixteen patients had isolated breast relapses, 39 had metastases, and 34 died. Young women treated for Hodgkin lymphoma should be carefully monitored in the long term by clinical examination, mammography, and ultrasonography. The authors suggested that a baseline mammography be performed 5 to 8 years after supradiaphragmatic irradiation (complete mantle or involved field) in patients treated before 30 years of age. Subsequently, mammography should be performed every 2 years or each year, depending on the characteristics of the breast tissue (e.g., density) and especially in the case of an association with other breast cancer risk factors.

Wolden et al.[660] described 71 cases of breast cancer in 65 survivors of Hodgkin lymphoma. Median age at diagnosis was 24.6 years for Hodgkin lymphoma and 42.6 years for breast cancer; the relative risk for invasive breast cancer after Hodgkin lymphoma was 4.7 compared with an age-matched cohort. Cancers were detected by self-examination in 63%, mammography in 30%, and by physical examination alone in 7%. The majority were of invasive ductal histology and 27% had positive axillary nodes. The tumor was ER-positive in 63% of the cases, and 25% of patients had an associated family history. The majority of tumors were smaller than 4 cm. Ninety-five percent of cases were managed by mastectomy because of prior irradiation, and two women underwent excisional biopsy with breast irradiation. One of these patients had tissue necrosis in the region of overlap with the prior mantle field. The incidence of bilateral breast cancer was 10%. The 10-year disease-specific survival rate for DCIS was 100%, stage I, 88%, stage II, 55%, stage III, 60%, and stage IV, 0%.

One of the largest series using breast-conserving therapy plus radiation in patients previously treated for Hodgkin lymphoma is from Deutsch et al.[661] In this retrospective review, 12 women treated with radiotherapy with or without chemotherapy for Hodgkin lymphoma (11 patients) and non-Hodgkin lymphoma (1 patient) in whom breast cancer developed 10 to 29 years later were treated with lumpectomy and breast irradiation. Patients were treated with whole-breast daily

TABLE 56.35 CONSERVATIVE SURGERY AND RADIATION IN THE TREATMENT OF MULTICENTRIC BREAST CANCER

Study (Reference)	Patients		Follow-Up (Year)		Local Relapse Rate			Comment
	Number of SIBC	Controls	SIBC	Controls	SIBC (%)	Controls (%)	P	
Yale (665)	13	1,047	6	6	25	12	.403	Local recurrence rate in SIBC is greater than seen in patients with single lesions.
JCRT (666)	10	707	5.3 (median)	6.3 (median)	40	11	.019	The presence of two or more primary tumors in the breast associated with a high likelihood of local recurrence.
St Luke's (668)	36	19[a]	5	5	3	0	.54	No significant differences in the local or distant disease-free survival between the group treated with breast conservation and the group treated with mastectomy.
Rush (667)	27		4.4 (median)		3.7	–	–	
France (669)	61	525	5.9 (median)	5.9 (median)	25	11	<.005	Macroscopically multiple breast cancers are at higher local failure risk, especially if multiplicity is clinically apparent, or if three or more gross nodules are seen on pathologic examination.

SIBC, synchronous ipsilateral breast cancer.
[a]All are SIBC treated with mastectomy.

irradiation with a fractionation of 2 Gy to 50 Gy with boost to the operative area. Six also received adjuvant chemotherapy for breast cancer. Breast irradiation was well tolerated without any unusual acute or chronic sequelae. They conclude that this may be an option for previously radiated Hodgkin's survivors who develop early-stage breast cancer.

This controversial area will continue to evolve. Given the development of partial breast irradiation programs over the past several years, it is likely that data regarding reirradiation with partial breast programs will be reported.[662,663] Clearly, however, Hodgkin's survivors and others who receive radiotherapy to breast at a young age are at high risk for developing breast cancers and should be carefully monitored. Women who develop breast cancer should be advised that mastectomy remains the treatment of choice. However, for patients highly motivated for breast preservation, anecdotal experiences using a variety of approaches have revealed acceptable toxicity and cosmesis.

Patients with More than One Invasive Carcinoma (Multicentric Disease)

Multicentricity of breast cancer has been considered by some a contraindication to breast-conserving surgery and suggest mastectomy as the preferred option.[664] Conservation surgery and breast radiation therapy as an alternative to mastectomy is controversial in patients with two or more lesions in the same breast. Several studies have addressed this issue, and it appears that the risk of relapse in the conservatively treated patient is slightly higher than if there is one lesion, but the risk may be acceptable in patients with two or perhaps three lesions provided these lesions are surgically excised with negative margins and there are no residual areas of suspicion on physical examination, mammogram, or imaging studies. Selected studies evaluating the conservative management of breast cancer in patients with multicentric disease are summarized in Table 56.35.[665–669]

Kurtz et al.,[669] in an analysis of 586 patients with unilateral stage I or II breast cancer treated with breast-conserving surgery and irradiation, found 61 patients who had two or more microscopic tumor nodules. After a median follow-up of 71 months, 15 patients (25%) had a recurrence in the treated breast, compared with 56 of 525 (11%) patients with single tumors (P <.005). Recurrence was noted more often in patients with multiple tumors diagnosed clinically or mammographically (8 of 22, 36%) than when multicentricity was apparent only on pathologic examination (7 of 39, 18%).

Wilson et al.[665] reviewed their experience in 1,060 patients treated with conservation surgery and breast irradiation of whom 13 (1.2%) presented with synchronous multicentric ipsilateral breast cancer. With a median follow-up of 71 months, 3 of the 13 (23%) had an ipsilateral breast recurrence (72-month actuarial rate of 25%) compared with 12% in the single-lesion population. The use of conservation therapy in patients with more than one primary lesion should be considered with caution, and patients should be forewarned of the need for more extensive resections and the increased risk of breast relapse. Because resection of a larger volume of breast is required, cosmetic results may be compromised, and expectations may not be met. In such instances, a mastectomy may be the preferred approach.

Conservation Surgery and Irradiation After Breast Augmentation

A growing number of breast cancers occur in women with prior augmentation mammoplasty. The stage of breast cancer at diagnosis in women who have undergone augmentation mammoplasty has been examined with conflicting results. In a retrospective review, Clark et al.[670] reported that 24% of 33 patients with augmented breasts and 42% of 1,735 patients with nonaugmented breasts had mammographically detected cancers (P = not significant). The incidence of DCIS in the two groups was similar (18% vs. 15%, respectively). Sizes of the mammographically detected tumors in the two groups were comparable. However, palpable tumors in the augmented group were significantly smaller than those in the nonaugmented group. Axillary lymph node involvement was detected in 19% of the augmented group and 41% of the nonaugmented group. Among those with mammographically detected tumors, there was no significant difference in axillary lymph node metastases between patients with augmented versus nonaugmented breasts (13% vs. 15%, respectively).

Patients with augmentations who have breast cancer are currently being treated with conservation therapy, but no study has investigated the complications and cosmetic results of radiation therapy specifically in this group of women.

Breast-conservation therapy in 17 augmented patients with breast cancer was reported by Handel et al.,[671] where 15 patients were available for follow-up. In 10 patients (67%), significant capsular contracture occurred in the irradiated breast an average of 12 weeks after completion of treatment. Four patients underwent revision surgery to correct symptoms arising from contracture. These authors concluded that irradiation of the breast for cancer in augmented women results in a high incidence of scar tissue contracture and poor cosmetic results.

In contrast, Guenther et al.[672] evaluated 20 women in whom breast cancer developed after augmentation mammoplasty (14 subcutaneous implants and 6 retromuscular implants). Patients were treated with wide local tumor excision and level I and II axillary lymph node dissection. Irradiation was delivered to the breast (45 to 50 Gy), and a boost (14 to 21 Gy) was given to the tumor excision site with either photons, electrons, or iridium-192 (^{192}Ir) implant. With a median follow-up of 3.8 years (range, 6 months to 9.3 years), there were no local recurrences, although distant metastases developed in two patients. Seventeen patients (85%) had good or excellent cosmetic results.

Breast Conservation and Mammoplasty

Women with large, pendulous breasts have been documented to have poorer cosmetic outcomes when undergoing irradiation after breast-conservation surgery (thought to be caused by dose inhomogeneity) compared with women who have small or medium-size breasts. Smith et al.[673] evaluated 10 women who had undergone bilateral reduction mammoplasty for breast malignancy followed by radiation therapy. A variety of reduction techniques were used to include the malignant lesions. Patients received 50 Gy in 25 fractions in 5 weeks after surgery. Radiation therapy was usually initiated within 4 weeks after surgery. With a follow-up of 37 months, no patients have had complications from the surgery or radiation therapy. No local recurrent malignancies have been detected. Cosmesis has been good to excellent in all patients.

Bilateral Carcinoma of the Breast

Among factors reported to be associated with an increased risk of bilateral breast carcinoma are younger age, family history of breast cancer, lobular carcinoma, multicentric disease, histologic differentiation of the primary tumor, parity, and PR-positive status.[674,675,676–679] The appearance may be synchronous (1% to 2%) or metachronous (5% to 8%). Synchronous breast carcinoma was defined as a contralateral cancer diagnosed within 1 year of initial diagnosis.

Patients with bilateral carcinoma have been treated with total or modified radical mastectomy. However, the available evidence clearly supports lumpectomy followed by breast irradiation as an acceptable alternative for appropriately selected women. Solin et al.[680] reported on 30 treated with breast-conservation therapy (11 with concurrent and 19 with metachronous carcinoma). A dose of 45 to 50 Gy was delivered to both breasts with tangential fields, in addition to a boost of 10 to 15 Gy with either iridium implant or electrons. The tangential fields were matched in the midline in 17 patients and overlapped by up to 3 cm in 10 patients. In the 60 treated breasts, the 5-year actuarial local failure rate was 6%. In 25 treated breasts with a minimum of 2 years of follow-up, 68% had excellent and 24% had good cosmetic results. The incidence of arm edema was 6%, similar to that reported in patients with unilateral disease.

Hungness et al.[681] reviewed their experience with 51 patients with bilateral synchronous breast cancer (2.1% of 2,382 treated for breast cancer during the same period). The first cancer was detected by palpation in 81% and by mammography in 14%. The corresponding figures for the contralateral cancer were 24% and 54%, respectively. The histologic type of cancer was identical in the two breasts in 29 patients (57%) and was different in 22 patients (43%). The overall 10-year survival rate was 66%.

Heron et al.[682] compared the outcomes in 1,315 patients (89.9%) with unilateral, 103 (7.1%) with metachronous, and 47 (3.0%) with synchronous breast carcinoma treated with either mastectomy or breast-conservation therapy. Patients with synchronous and metachronous bilateral carcinoma had a worse 8-year disease-free survival rate compared with patients who had unilateral breast carcinoma, as well as increased risk of distant metastasis. In multivariate analysis, differences in local tumor control and overall survival were not statistically significant for patients who had bilateral or metachronous cancer compared with those who had unilateral disease.

Kollias et al.,[683] in 3,210 women age 70 years or younger treated for primary operable breast cancer, identified 106 who had bilateral breast cancer; in 26 (0.8%) the disease was synchronous and in 80 (24%) a contralateral breast cancer developed after treatment for an initial primary breast cancer. There was a significant difference in survival between women with unilateral breast cancer, synchronous bilateral breast cancers, and metachronous contralateral breast cancer, with survival rates at 16 years of 53.8%, 42.4%, and 60.1%, respectively (P <.0001) from the date of the diagnosis of the first primary tumor. There was no difference in survival among the three groups from the date of diagnosis of the second primary in cases of metachronous contralateral breast cancer (P = .31).

Ninety-five patients with bilateral carcinoma of the breast treated with mastectomy (60 patients), conservation of the breast (17 patients), or both (18 patients) were studied by Gustafsson et al.[684] Cumulative 5-year local tumor control rates were 94% for the 138 mastectomy patients and 90% for the 52 patients treated with breast-conservation therapy. Twenty-eight percent of the first carcinomas were stage I, compared with 43% of second carcinomas (P <.05), probably reflecting the close follow-up after initial treatment. The 5-year distant disease-free survival rate from treatment for the second carcinoma was 74%. The 5-year distant recurrence-free survival rate when second carcinomas were diagnosed within 5 years was 58%, compared with 95% for patients diagnosed more than 5 years after the first carcinoma.

De la Rouchefordiere et al.[685] reported on 149 patients with simultaneous bilateral breast cancer (diagnosed within 6 months). Of 298 tumors, 40% were T0 or T1, 45% T2, and 15% were T3 or T4. The majority (83%) were clinically node negative. Treatments were bilateral mastectomy in 43%, irradiation in 16%, and both in 41% of the patients. Fifty-one patients had bilateral breast-conserving therapy and 24 were treated exclusively with irradiation. The 5-year disease-free survival rates were 70% to 86%, respectively, similar to those observed at the same institution in patients with unilateral tumors. Cosmesis was assessed in 48 patients and was acceptable in 37 (77%). These authors advised special attention should be paid to any possible overlap of the supraclavicular and internal mammary fields over the spinal cord; in one patient, spinal cord myelopathy developed at T6.

Freedman et al.[587] reviewed records of 116 patients with bilateral breast cancer and a breast cancer family history. The primary treatment was a breast-conserving procedure in 55 and a mastectomy in 61. Locoregional recurrences occurred in 4 of 46 cases treated with breast-conserving therapy, resulting in a 10-year actuarial locoregional tumor control rate of 83%. Of nine patients who did not receive radiation as a component of their breast-conserving therapy, locoregional recurrences developed in four (10-year locoregional control rate of 49%). The 10-year actuarial rates of locoregional control after mastectomy with and without radiation were 91% and 89%, respectively.

Fung et al.[686] reported on 55 women with stage 0, I, or II concurrent (n = 12) or sequential (n = 43) bilateral breast cancers treated with irradiation after breast-conserving surgery. The tangential fields were matched with no overlap in 40 patients (73%); there was overlap on skin of up to 4 cm in 14 patients (25%). For the 110 treated breast cancers, the 10-year actuarial local failure rate was 15%. Complications included breast edema (28%), arm edema (8%), pneumonitis (4%), cellulitis (3%), rib fracture (1%), and brachial plexopathy (1%). No patient had match line fibrosis. For patients with a minimum of 3 years of relapse-free follow-up, the rate of excellent or good cosmetic outcome for 104 treated breasts was 85%.

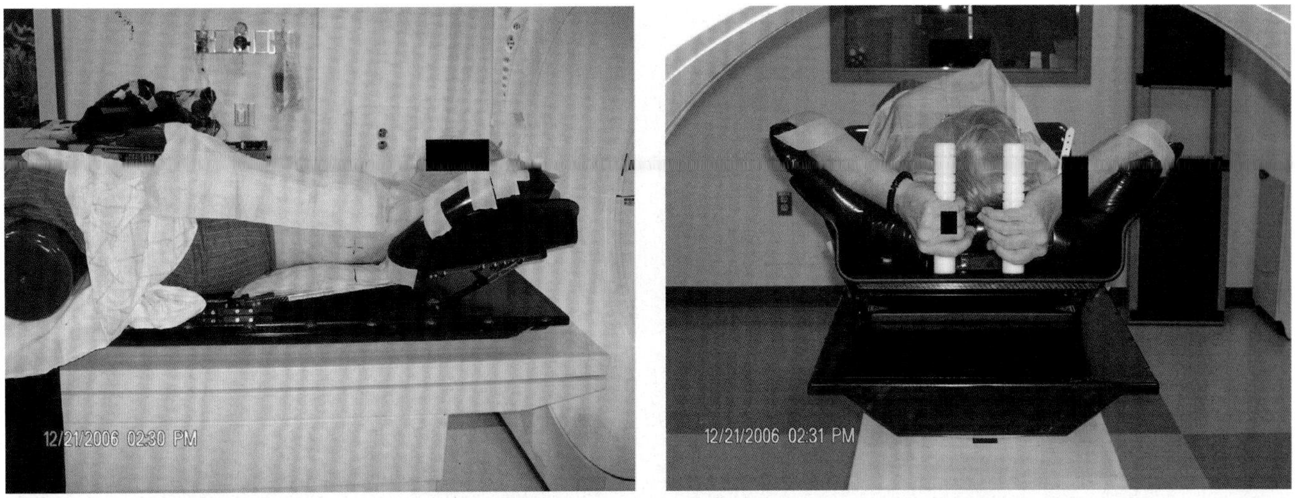

FIGURE 56.25. Patient immobilized for breast irradiation on a slant board with custom mold to minimize day-to-day positioning errors.

TECHNICAL ISSUES IN RADIATION MANAGEMENT OF EARLY-STAGE DISEASE

Treatment Position

Most patients are treated in the supine position, with the arm abducted (90 degrees or greater). Commercially available or custom made breast tilt boards with armrests that maintain the patient's daily position with the slope of the chest wall parallel to the table, often in combination with immobilization devices (e.g., Alpha cradle, plastic molds) are typically used to reproduce daily positioning and minimize day-to-day setup errors (Fig. 56.25).

Other treatment positions have been used to improve the dosimetry in patients with large, pendulous breasts. A lateral decubitus position has been suggested by investigators at the Institut Curie.[687,688]

Irradiation in the prone position has been proposed by Merchant and McCormick,[689] with reduction of dose in the high-dose region to 102% to 103% of the dose to the irradiated breast, as well as reduction of volume and dose to the underlying lung and heart and reduction of scattered dose to the contralateral breast. This technique is being increasingly employed and follow-up data appear to be promising with respect to toxicity and early outcomes.[690] Patient positioning and a corresponding CT image are shown in Figures 56.26 and 56.27.

Treatment Volume

The entire breast and chest wall are included in the irradiated volume as shown in Figures 56.28 and 56.29. Radiopaque surgical clips placed at the margin of the tumor bed may assist in defining the target volume.[691] The upper margin of the portals should be placed at the head of the clavicle to include the entire breast. The medial margin, if no internal mammary portal is used, should be at or 1 cm over the midline. If an internal mammary field is used, the medial tangential portal is located at the lateral margin of the internal mammary field. (See discussion later on regional nodal irradiation.) The lateral-posterior margin should be placed 2 cm beyond all palpable breast tissue, which is usually near the midaxillary line. The inferior margin is drawn 2 to 3 cm below the inframammary fold. Recently, the RTOG published their consensus definitions for breast cancer radiation therapy planning, which are listed in Table 56.36. An illustration of nodal volumes drawn on an axial planning CT scan is shown in Figure 56.30.

In patients treated with 6-MV or lower-energy photons with wide tangential fields in whom separation is >22 cm, there may be significant dose inhomogeneity in the breast; this may correlate with less satisfactory cosmetic results.[352,692] This problem can be minimized by using higher-energy photons (10 tOo 18 MV) to deliver a portion of the breast radiation (approximately 50%) as determined with treatment planning

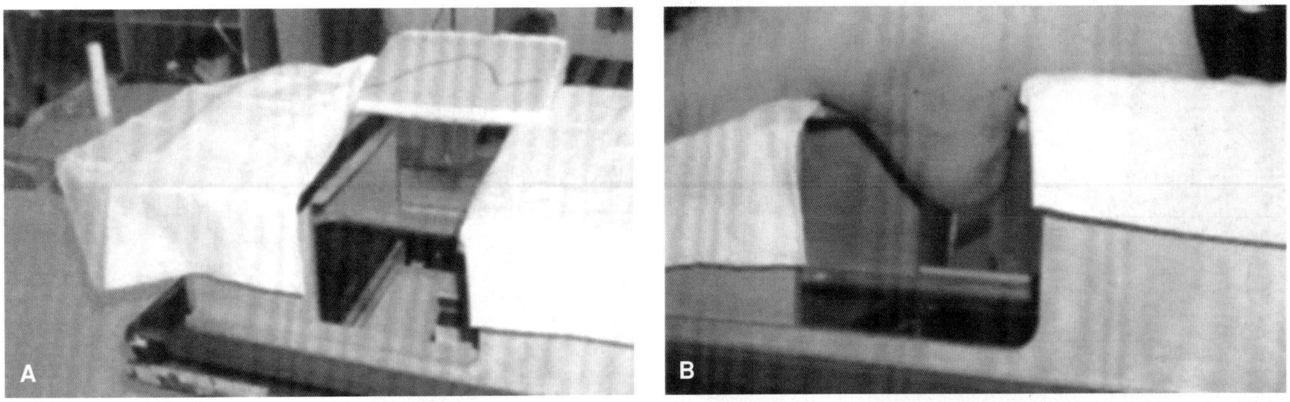

FIGURE 56.26. Prone breast board. **A:** Customized prone breast board with adjustable aperture and wedge for contralateral breast. **B:** Ipsilateral breast and anterior chest wall hang in dependent fashion away from thorax with ipsilateral arm placed above head. (From Goodman K, Hong L, Wagman R, et al. Dosimetric analysis of a simplified intensity modulation technique for prone breast radiotherapy. *Int J Radiat Oncol Biol Phys* 2004;60(1):95–102, with permission form Elsevier.)

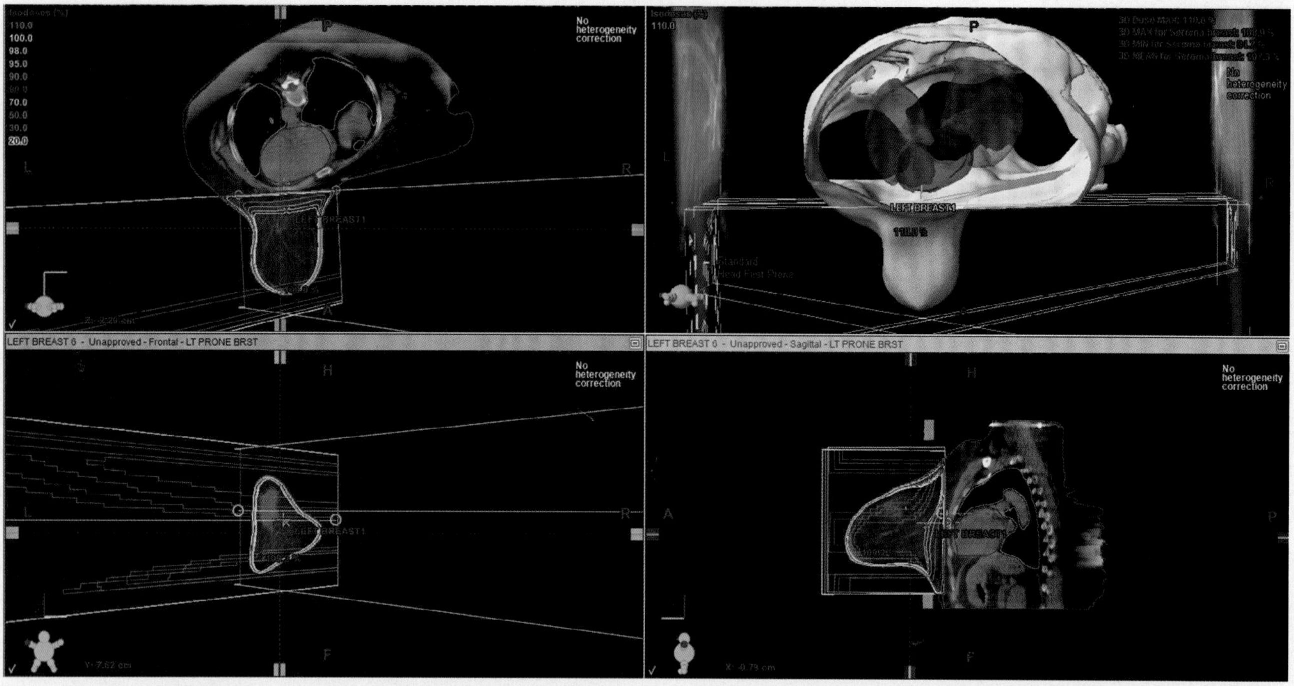

FIGURE 56.27. Computed tomography simulation images used to determine arrangement of tangent beams in prone breast irradiation. (From Goodman K, Hong L, Wagman R, et al. Dosimetric analysis of a simplified intensity modulation technique for prone breast radiotherapy. *Int J Radiat Oncol Biol Phys* 2004;60(1):95–102, with permission form Elsevier.)

to maintain the inhomogeneity throughout the entire breast to between 93 and 105%. If desired, the buildup of the beam may be modified with a "degrader." "Simple intensity-modulated radiation therapy" techniques such as field-in-field or dynamic multileaf collimators (MLCs) to achieve electronic tissue compensation may be utilized to reduce dose inhomogeneity as well. Bolus should be avoided in conservatively managed patients. A variety of immobilizing devices or molds may be constructed to support the breast in the treatment position (Fig. 56.31). A polyvinyl chloride, ring-shaped device, held by a strap has been used around the breast to aid in positioning of patients with large, pendulous or flaccid breasts. Skin reactions where material is in contact with the skin should be closely monitored.[693]

Alignment of the Tangential Beam with the Chest Wall Contour

The anterior chest wall slopes downward from the midchest to the neck. To make the posterior edge of the tangential beam follow this downward-sloping contour, the collimator of the tangential beam may be rotated, or the patient may be placed on a slant so that the slope of the chest wall is parallel to the table. An alternative is to make the deep posterior edge of the tangential beam follow the chest wall contour by means of a rotating beam splitter mounted on a tray without rotation of the collimator or using multileaf collimation. In this way, the superior edge of the tangential beam remains in the true vertical and matches perfectly the vertical inferior edge of the supraclavicular field if used.

Usually up to 2 to 3 cm of underlying lung may be included in the tangential portals. The amount of lung included in the

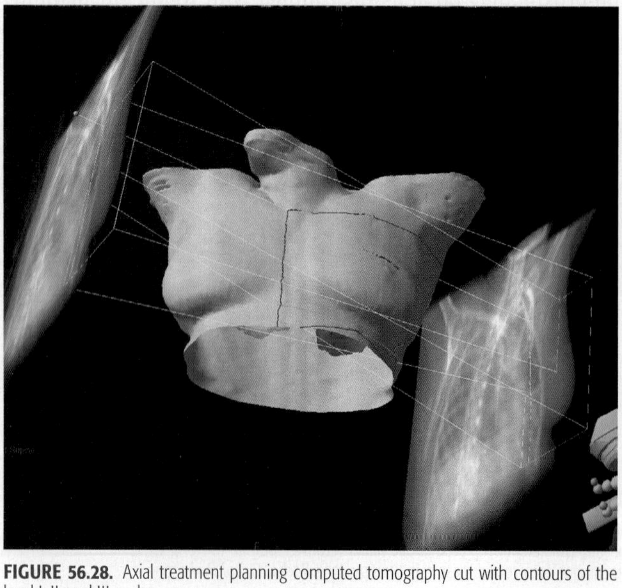

FIGURE 56.28. Axial treatment planning computed tomography cut with contours of the level I, II, and III nodes.

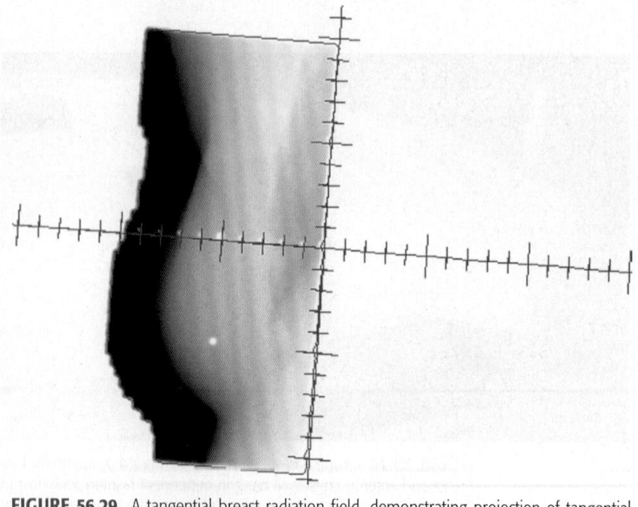

FIGURE 56.29. A tangential breast radiation field, demonstrating projection of tangential field on simulation film and patient surface.

TABLE 56.36 RADIATION THERAPY ONCOLOGY GROUP CONSENSUS DEFINITIONS FOR BREAST CANCER RADIATION THERAPY PLANNING

	Cranial	Caudal	Anterior	Posterior	Lateral	Medial
Breast	Clinical reference + second rib insertion	Clinical reference + loss of CT apparent breast	Skin	Excludes pectoralis muscles, chestwall muscles, ribs	Clinical reference/midaxillary line typically, excludes lattismus dorsi	Sternal–rib junction
Breast + chest wall	Same	Same	Same	Includes pectoralis muscles, chestwall muscles, ribs	Same	Same
Chest wall	Caudal border of the clavicle head	Clinical reference + loss of CT apparent contralateral breast	Skin	Rib–pleural interface. (includes pectoralis muscles, chestwall muscles, ribs)	Same	Same
Supraclavicular	Caudal to the cricoid cartilage	Junction of brachioceph.- axillary vns./caudal edge clavicle head	Sternocleido mastoid (SCM) muscle	Anterior aspect of the scalene m.	Cranial: lateral edge of SCM m. Caudal: junction 1st rib-clavicle	Excludes thyroid and trachea
Axilla: Level I	Axillary vessels cross lateral edge of pec. minor m.	Pec. major muscle insert into ribs	Plane defined by: anterior surface of pec. maj. m. and lat. dorsi m.	Anterior surface of subscapular is m.	Medial border of lat. dorsi m.	Lateral border of pec. minor m.
Axilla: Level II	Axillary vessels cross medial edge of pec. minor m.	Axillary vessels cross lateral edge of pec. minor m.	Anterior surface pec. minor m.	Ribs and intercostal muscles	Lateral border of pec. minor m.	Medial border of pec. minor m.
Axilla: Level III	Pec. minor m. insert on cricoid	Axillary vessels cross medial edge of pec. minor m.	Posterior surface pec. major m.	Ribs and intercostal muscles	Medial border of pec. minor m.	Thoracic inlet
Internal mammary	Superior aspect of the medial 1st rib.	Cranial aspect of the 4th rib				

CT, computed tomography; brachioceph.-axillary vns, brachiocephalic-axillary veins; lat. dorsi m., latissimus dorsi muscle; pec. minor m., pectoralis minor muscle; pec. major m., pectoralis major muscle.

irradiated volume is greatly influenced by the portals used. Bornstein et al.[694] determined the amount of lung irradiated in 40 patients with breast cancer using CT scans for treatment planning in the treatment position. Parameters measured from simulator films included the perpendicular distance from the posterior tangential field edge to the posterior part of the anterior chest wall at the center of the field (central lung distance [CLD]), the maximum perpendicular distance from the posterior tangential field edge to the posterior part of the anterior chest wall (maximum lung distance [MLD]), and the length of lung as measured at the posterior tangential field edge on the simulator film (Fig. 56.32). The best predictor of the percentage of ipsilateral lung volume treated by the tangential fields was the CLD. A CLD of 1.5 cm predicted that approximately 6% of the ipsilateral lung would be included in the tangential field, a CLD of 2.5 cm, approximately 16%, and a CLD of 3.5 cm, approximately 26% of the ipsilateral lung. A typical acceptable dose–volume histogram of a left-sided breast cancer treated with external-beam radiation is given in Figure 56.33.

When the CLD is >3 cm, in treatment of the left breast, a significant volume of heart will also be irradiated. To avoid this, a medial tangential breast port (3- to 5-cm wide), somewhat similar to an internal mammary port, may be designed. The beam is angled 10 to 15 degrees laterally to conform to the angle of the medial breast port. The dose is prescribed to the posterior border of the chest wall as determined by CT scanning.

Special attention should be paid to minimizing the volume of heart irradiated.[695] As will be discussed later in the section on cardiac sequelae, even small amounts of heart in the field can affect cardiac function. Marks et al.[696] have suggested the use of a cardiac block if the heart is in the tangential field, which can be supplemented by an electron field as shown in Figure 56.34. Use of short (10- to 15-second) treatments while the patient holds her breath is also feasible as a way of reducing cardiac radiation during left-sided breast cancer treatment.[697]

Doses of Radiation and Fractionation

Whole-Breast Dose

With whole-breast irradiation, tumor doses of approximately 45 to 50 Gy are delivered to the entire breast over 5 to 6 weeks (1.8- to 2-Gy tumor dose daily, 5 weekly fractions). Some authors have suggested daily fractions of 1.8 Gy for patients

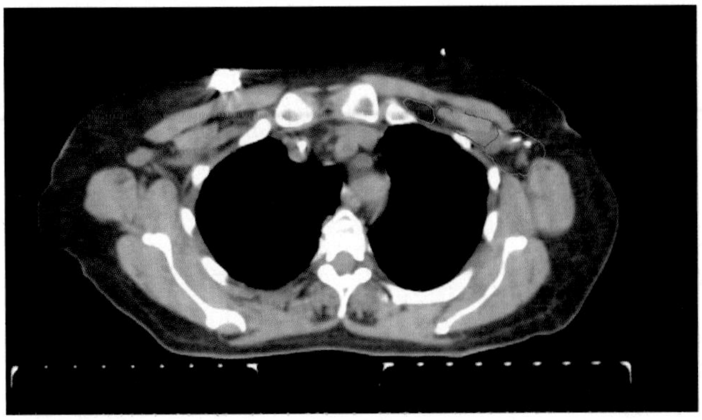

FIGURE 56.30. Nodal volumes drawn on axial planning CT scan.

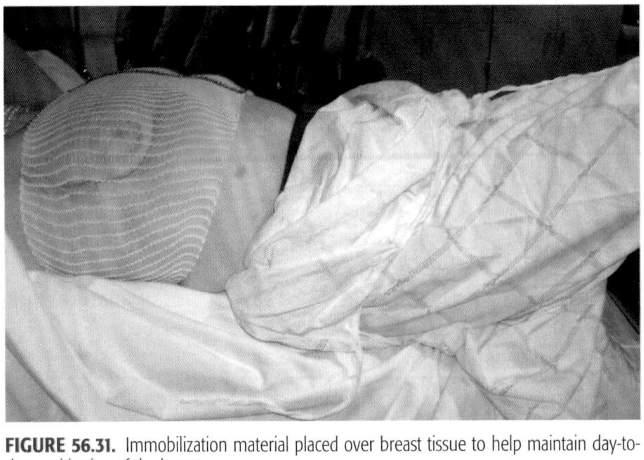

FIGURE 56.31. Immobilization material placed over breast tissue to help maintain day-to-day positioning of the breast.

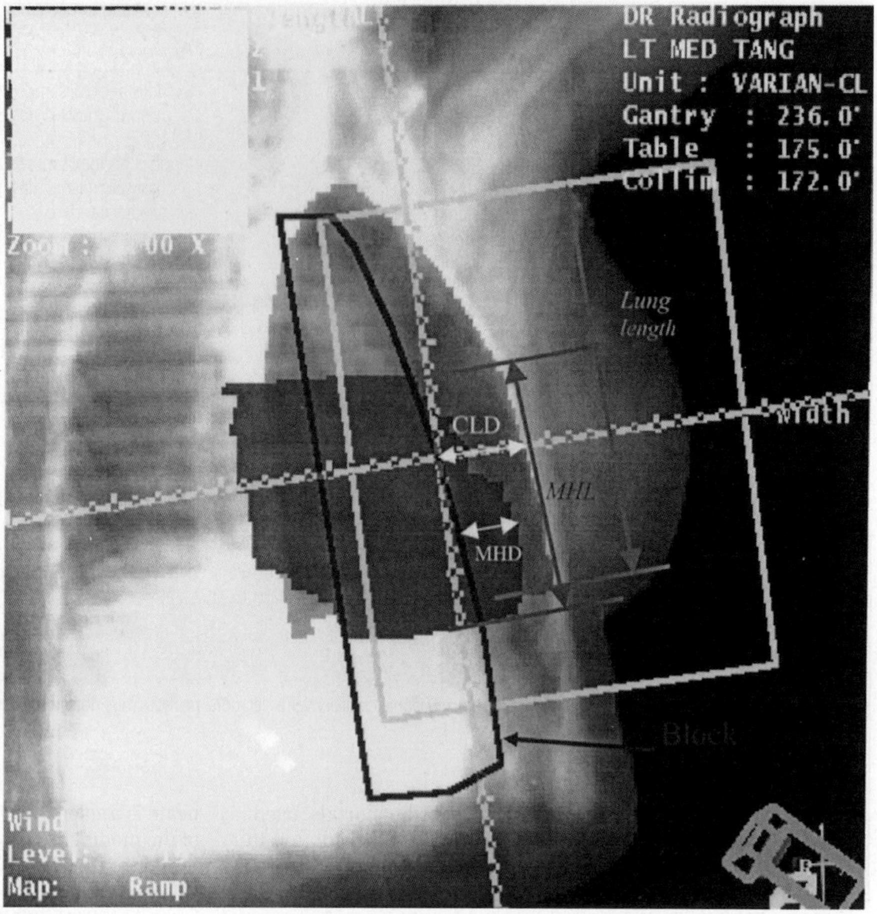

FIGURE 56.32. Measurement of the radiographic parameters using virtual simulator. The contoured heart is shown in *black,* the lung in *gray.* The central lung distance (CLD) is the lung distance in the projection of the tangential fields at the level of the central axis. Lung length is the vertical lung distance included in the radiation port. The maximal heart distance (MHD) is the width of heart in the tangent fields at its maximal level, whereas the maximal heart length (MHL) is the maximal length in tangential fields referring to the heart contour in a digitally reconstructed radiograph (DRR). (From Kong F-M, Klein EE, Bradley JD, et al. The impact of central lung distance, maximal heart distance, and radiation technique on the volumetric dose of the lung and heart for intact breast radiation. *Int J Radiat Oncol Biol Phys* 2002;54:963–971, with permission from Elsevier.)

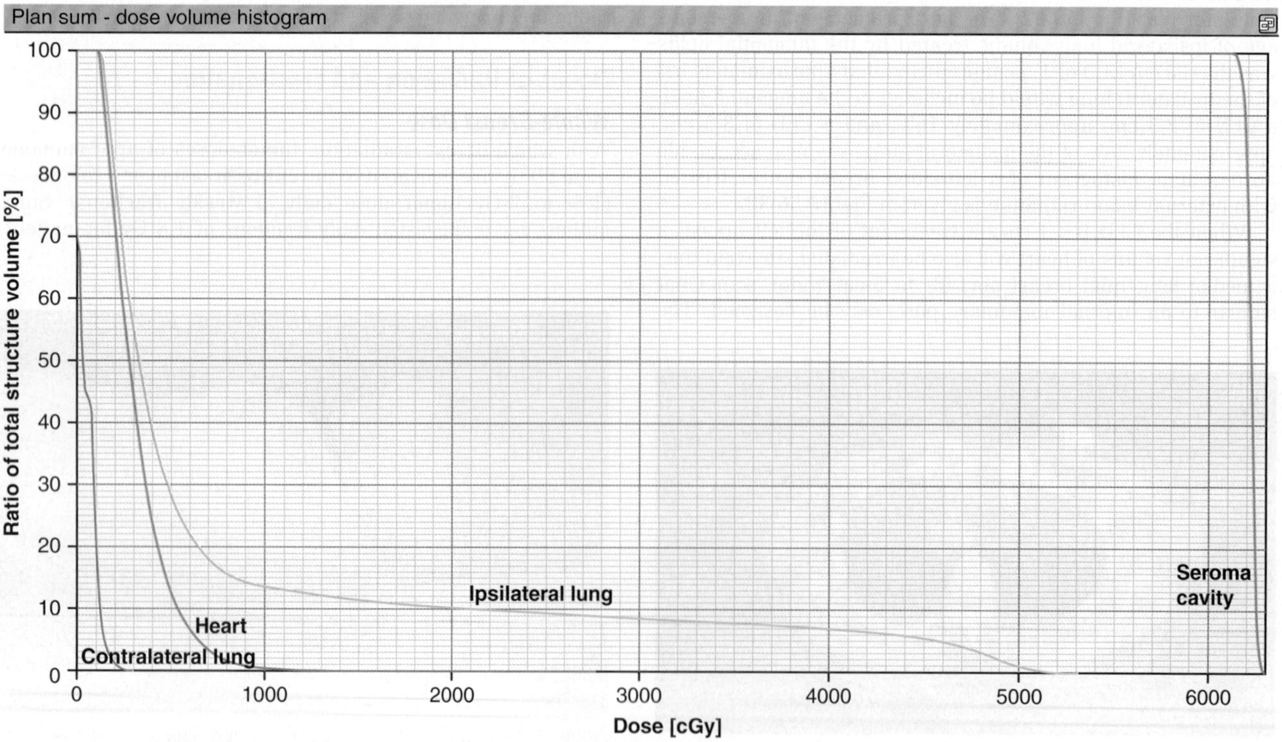

FIGURE 56.33. Dose-volume histogram of left-sided breast cancer treated with external beam radiation.

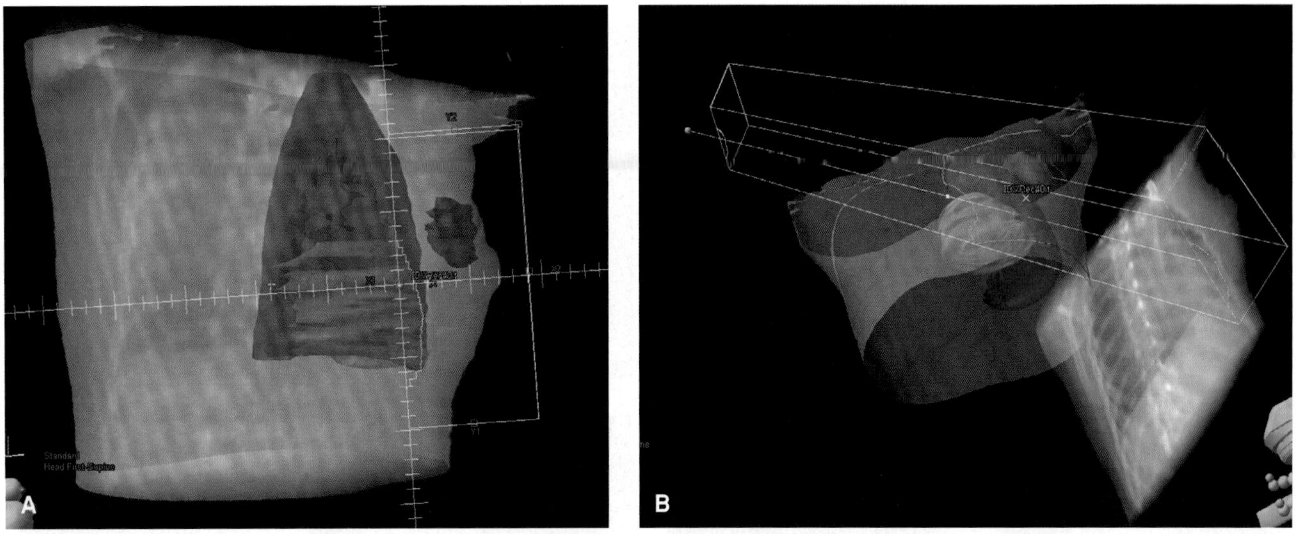

FIGURE 56.34. **A and B:** Left tangential breast field with heart block to shield left ventricle from radiation port. Projection of heart block on breast shields minimal amount of breast tissue. If necessary, a shadow electron field may be added to cover the portion of breast tissue shielded by heart block.

with large, pendulous breasts or when irradiation is combined with chemotherapy.[559,560,698] The authors' preference is to use 2 Gy fractions to 50 Gy because this is the scheme used in the vast majority of randomized trials using whole-breast radiation therapy following conservative surgery.

Alternative fractionation schemes have been employed and have been shown to be acceptable. These are discussed in greater detail in the hypofractionation section.

Radiation Beams

X-ray energies of 4 to 6 MV are preferred to treat the breast. Photon energies >6 MV underdose superficial tissues beneath the skin surface, but higher-energy photons may be helpful in large breasts to decrease the integral breast dose. In these patients the high-energy photon beam may be "degraded" to bring the maximum dose to more superficial tissues. It is not necessary to apply bolus to the breast because the skin is usually not at risk for recurrence after complete excision of a T1 or T2 lesion, as is the skin of the chest wall after a mastectomy. Use of bolus results in impaired cosmetic results.[352]

Wedges or compensating filters must be used for a portion of the treatment to achieve a uniform dose distribution in the breast (5% to 8% dose variance from the chest wall to the apex). Although conventional wedges improve dose homogeneity at the central axis of the breast, significant inhomogeneity can occur in the superior and inferior portions of the breast. Currently, with the use of MLCs and more sophisticated treatment planning techniques, optimization of homogeneity throughout the breast can be achieved through the use of a variety of techniques. Dose homogeneity in a breast plan uncompensated (without wedges), with standard wedges, and with electronic dynamic wedge technique to improve homogeneity in the superior inferior plane are outlined in Figure 56.35. These techniques are discussed in more detail later.

Boost to Tumor Site

The need for a boost to the tumor bed following lumpectomy and whole-breast radiation remains an area of debate. In the earlier years of breast-conserving surgery, status of the surgical margins were not always assessed. Recent retrospective data suggest that patients with known negative margins have high local control rates with no boost following whole-breast irradiation.[699] Fisher et al.[670] have all raised the question of the need for a radiation dose boost at the excision site.

Most authors report that 65% to 80% of breast recurrences after conservation surgery and irradiation occur around the primary tumor site.[104,106,196,298,376,388,671–703] These data provide a strong rationale for a tumor bed boost. Various series suggest that patients treated with higher doses have a greater probability of tumor control. Clark et al.[377] noted in 1,504 patients a greater incidence of failures at 10 years of 17% in those to whom no boost was delivered, compared with 11% in those who received doses of 5 to 15 Gy at the primary excision site ($P = .03$). In other series of patients with unknown surgical margins, patients receiving a boost had roughly half the breast failure rate (6% to 11%) compared with those with no boost (9% to 20%).[110,388,404,704]

Others have advocated tailoring the need for a boost depending on margins. Arthur et al.[699] reported on 205 patients who underwent re-excision prior to radiation. All patients in this cohort had no tumor on re-excision and were treated with whole-breast irradiation to a dose of 50 Gy without a boost. Five failures were documented, resulting in a 15-year local control rate of 92.4%. The authors advocate selective avoidance of the boost in these patients.

Randomized Data

The Lyon Breast Cancer Trial conducted a randomized study to assess the role of the boost in breast-conserving therapy in patients with stage I and II breast cancer (≤3 cm) who were treated with complete local tumor excision, axillary dissection, and 50 Gy to the breast in 20 fractions over 5 weeks and randomly assigned to receive or not a boost of 10 Gy with electrons to the tumor bed.[705] With a median follow-up of 3.3 years, at 5 years 10 of 521 women who received a boost (3.6%) and 20 of 503 (4.5%) who received no further treatment experienced a local breast relapse ($P = .044$). Time to local recurrence is shown in Figure 49.52, with more patients failing after 7 years in the no-boost arm.

Bartelink et al.[404] reported the results of the EORTC trial in which, after complete lumpectomy and axillary dissection, patients with stage I or II breast cancer received 50 Gy of radiation to the whole breast in 2-Gy fractions over a 5-week period and were randomly assigned to receive either no further local treatment (2,657 patients) or a boost of 16 Gy, usually given in 8 fractions by electron beam (2,661 patients). In the initial report, with a median follow-up of 5.1 years, local

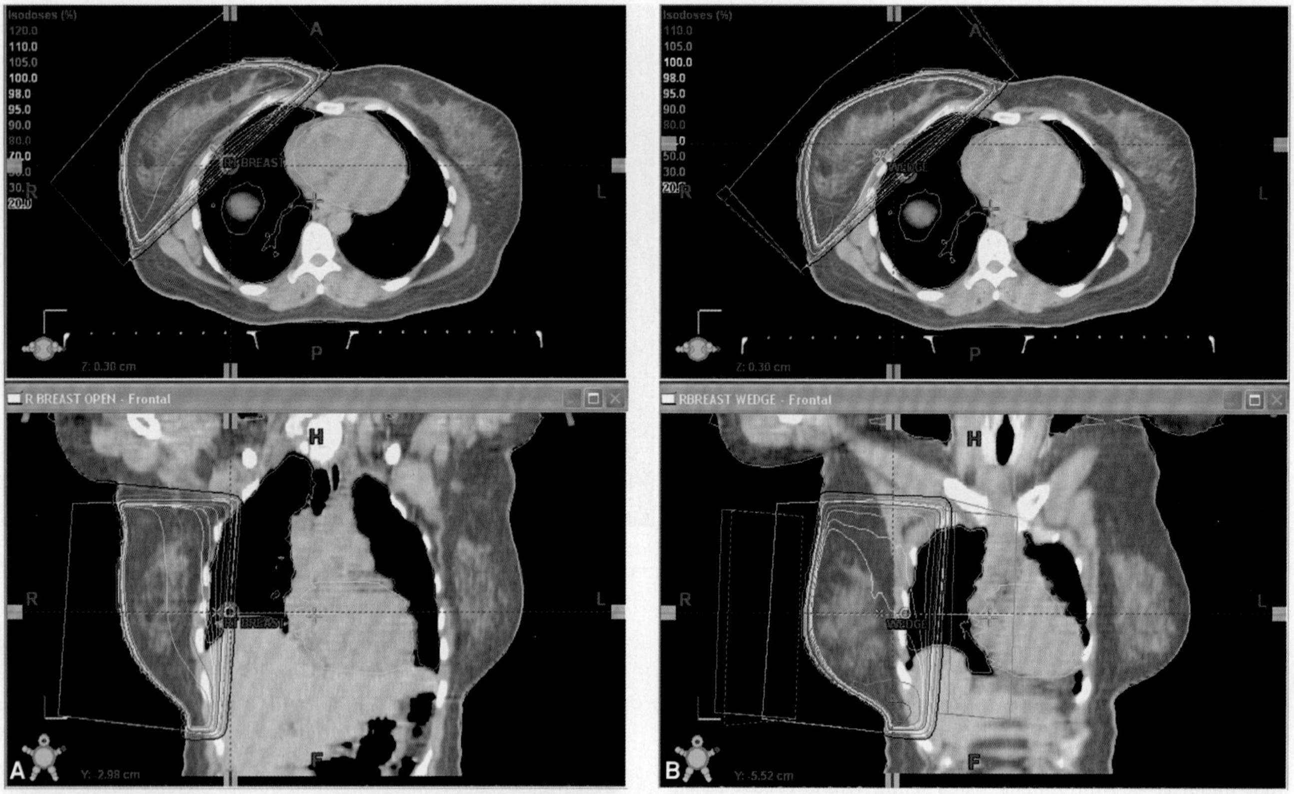

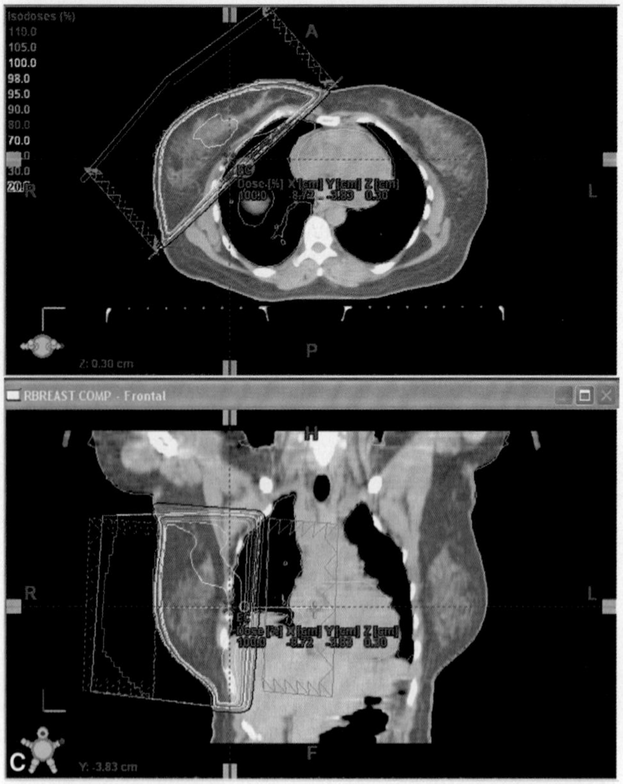

FIGURE 56.35. Isodose distributions from three breast plans. **A:** Open fields demonstrating inhomogeneity. **B:** Standard wedges demonstrating improvement in central axis, but with a hot spot in the superior inferior plane. **C:** Dynamic wedge plan showing improved homogeneity in both the central axis as well as the superior–inferior plane.

recurrences were observed in 182 of the 2,657 patients in the standard-treatment group and 109 of the 2,661 patients in the additional-radiation group. The 5-year actuarial rates of local recurrence were 7.3% and 4.3%, respectively (*P* <.001). Patients 40 years of age or younger benefited most; at 5 years, their rate of local recurrence was 19.5% with standard treatment and 10.2% with additional radiation (RR 0.46; 99% CI, 0.23 to 0.89; *P* = .002). In an update of this study published in 2007, with a median follow-up of 10.8 years, a significant benefit to the boost was noted in all age groups, with an overall hazard ratio of 0.59 in favor of the boost[405] (see Fig. 56.16).

If a decision is made not to use a boost, careful assessment of lumpectomy margins is critical, as discussed in the following section.

Electron Versus Interstitial Boosts

Before the widespread availability of electron beam therapy, interstitial brachytherapy or cone-down photon boost was popular. Experiences with interstitial boosts have been reported by several groups, using both high dose rate after loading and low dose rate temporary implants.[706–715] The reader is referred to these studies and the chapter on brachytherapy for a more extensive discussion of techniques related to interstitial tumor bed boosts. Currently, most institutions prefer electron beam boost because of its relative ease in setup, outpatient setting, lower cost, decreased time demands on the physician, and excellent results compared with ^{192}Ir implants. The introduction of single lumen or multilumen balloon catheters, used primarily in partial breast irradiation, can also be considered an interstitial boost technique. Cosmetic results with either boost technique at various institutions are summarized in Table 56.37.

Electron Boosts

The patient is positioned with the arm toward the head to flatten the breast contour and may be rolled so the tumor bed is parallel to the table and the accelerator head can point straight down onto the target volume. An electron energy is selected that covers the target volume depth (usual range is 9 to 16 MeV electrons), based on review of the physical examination, mammogram, ultrasound, CT, or other imaging used to ascertain the location and depth of the tumor or metallic surgical clips. The 90% prescription isodose line is limited to the chest wall to decrease dose to the lung. The clinical setup for electron boost involves marking the projection of the postlumpectomy volume on the skin and adding 2 to 3 cm in all directions.

Accurate target volume definition is critical with any boost technique. Methods vary from simple and unsophisticated (as described in the previous paragraph) to complex and expensive, such as ultrasound and CT definition of the target volume.[716,717] The accuracy of using the scar to define the lumpectomy cavity has been questioned. In a study by Oh et al.,[716] 30 women consecutively treated for 31 breast cancers had simulation CT scans performed before and after whole-breast irradiation. CT breast volumes were delineated using clinically defined borders, and excision cavity volumes were contoured based on surgical clips, the presence of a hematoma, or other surgical changes. Hypothetical electron boost plans were generated using the surgical scar with a 3-cm margin and analyzed for coverage. The volume reduction (R) in the excision cavity was inversely correlated with time elapsed since surgery ($R = 0.46$; $P < .01$) and body weight ($R = 0.50$; $P < .01$). The scar-guided hypothetical plans failed to cover the excision cavity adequately in 62% and 53.8% of cases using the pretreatment and postradiation CTs, respectively.

Surgical clips are ideal for the localization of the tumor bed.[691,717,718] The surgical clip method requires the cooperation of the surgical team. Despite the fact that it would theoretically take an infinite number of clips to define every extension of a typical tylectomy cavity, in practice six clips suffice (superficial, deep, medial, lateral, cephalad, and caudal). In a study reported by Denham et al.,[719] surgical hemoclips were left *in situ* in 27 patients to demarcate the limits of the excision cavity. The position of these clips varied widely in relation to the patient's recollection of the position of the original lump, the surgical notes, and the surgical scar. Incomplete coverage of the excision cavity in the "coronal" (*en face*) plane using an electron field could have occurred in an estimated 10 of 24 (42%) cases had surgical clips not been left *in situ*. Depth of the surgical clips below the skin surface also varied markedly; in 19 of 26 (73%) cases, the clips were observed to be ≥3 cm below the skin surface, whereas in only 5 of 26 (19.2%) cases were the clips found to be ≤2 cm deep to the surface. Had a 9-MeV electron beam been used to treat all of the patients, a major underdose of the excision cavity would have been likely in 21 of 26 (81%) evaluable cases. Coverage would have improved to 11 of the 26 (42%) had a 12-MeV beam been used.

TABLE 56.37 EXCELLENT OR GOOD COSMETIC RESULTS WITH ELECTRON BEAM OR INTERSTITIAL BRACHYTHERAPY BOOST IN BREAST CONSERVATION THERAPY

Study (Reference)	Electron Beam	Brachytherapy	Follow-Up
Fourquet et al. (710)	39/52 (75%)	48/68 (71%)	3–7.3 yr
Mansfield et al. (704)	357/376 (95%)	575/629 (91%)	1 mo to 12 yr
Olivotto et al. (711)	36/36 (100%)	298/497 (60%)	5 yr
Perez et al. (712)	366/449 (81%)	97/129 (75%)	3–20 yr
Ray and Fish (713)	97/107 (91%)	12/23 (52%)	6–120 mo
Touboul et al. (707)	104/126 (82%)	91/148 (61%)	29–1 39 mo
Vicini et al. (708)	(90%)	(88%)	59.3 mo (median)

Fein et al.[718] described a study in patients with stage I or II breast cancer treated with breast-conservation therapy; surgical clips were placed in the excision cavity in 556 patients, and no clips were placed in 808. After breast irradiation with tangential fields, the primary tumor incision site was boosted with electron beam (14 to 20 Gy). The actuarial breast recurrence rates at 10 years were 11% in patients with clips and 5% in patients without clips ($P = .01$). Increased rates of breast recurrence were noted for patients with clips who had some of the following: no adjuvant treatment, unknown surgical margins, no re-excision, pathologic negative nodes, and outer location of primary tumor. The higher incidence of breast relapse may be related to a specific surgeon who had a breast recurrence rate of 21%, compared with 6% for the remainder of the surgeons ($P = .01$); the status of the margins was unknown in 48% of these patients, compared with 10% overall ($P = .001$). The authors concluded that failure to ink the surgical specimen and inadequate assessment of margins cannot be compensated by placement of surgical clips or treatment planning using CT to delineate the surgical bed. On the other hand, this study failed to show any benefit from use of surgical clips at the tumor excision margins to design the boost volume.

Ultrasonography can provide the depth of the biopsy cavity, as well as the other dimensions, for use in designing electron portal borders and selection of electron energy.[717,720] Ultrasonography was used in 30 patients to measure breast thickness for determination of the most appropriate electron beam energy for the boost. In most patients the depth was ≤4 cm, but in eight patients (32%), energy higher than 12 MeV should have been used to cover adequately the depth of the target volume.

CT-guided portal design should be done in the treatment position. This technique gives good definition of the depth of the chest wall and has been shown to be similar to ultrasound in delineating the lumpectomy cavity.[717,720] Delineation of the biopsy cavity becomes more difficult with increased interval from surgery. The combination of surgical clips with a treatment planning CT scan to define the lumpectomy site for electron boost is most ideal. In the absence of surgical clips, the CT scan evaluation of the biopsy cavity or postsurgical changes, in combination with clinical information including mammography findings, scar location, operative reports, and patient input, will provide accurate information regarding placement of the field and energy of the electron boost.

A recent multi-institutional study reported interobserver variabilities in the delineation of the seroma cavity and organs at risk in breast cancer patients undergoing breast-conserving surgery and whole-breast irradiation.[721] Nine radiation oncologists specializing in breast radiotherapy from eight institutions independently delineated target volumes on the same three breast cancer patients. They concluded that "variations in delineating the targets and OAR's [organs at risk] for breast RT by well-experienced observers from different institutions are substantial for all relevant structures."

To reduce these variations, guidelines for contouring the seroma cavity have been established; the Seroma Clarity Scale (SCS), developed by the British Columbia Cancer Agency and the

Cavity Visualization Score (CVS), developed by a Stanford group.[717,722] Both scoring systems are remarkably similar with the distinction being the SCS is a scale from 0 to 5, with 0 being no visible seroma cavity and 1 being a scar or shadow; the CVS is a scale from 1 to 5, with 1 being no visible seroma cavity, and omits the presence of a scar or shadow on the scale. The scores of 2 to 5 are relatively consistent between the two classification methods.

It is pertinent to note that each of these classification systems were developed without noting the presence of surgical clips or fiducial markers with respect to the seroma cavity. However, the authors, along with other investigators, have previously published that the presence of surgical clips or fiducial markers in the surgical bed improve the interphysician accuracy in the delineation of the seroma cavity in early-stage breast cancer patients.[723,724] In a study by Shaikh et al.,[725] the presence of fiducial markers improved the mean CVS score (from 2.5 to 3.5) and accuracy of physician contours compared with patients without fiducial markers. The use of titanium clips in patients treated with accelerated partial breast irradiation (APBI) is a focus of the United Kingdom IMPORT LOW (Intensity Modulated and Partial Organ Radiotherapy) trial.[726] An audit of the trial was performed to determine inter- and intraphysician variation for tumor bed localization for radiotherapy planning. Although no control group was used, clips were essential for the localization of the surgical cavity in 22 of 30 (73%) patients and led to modifications in radiotherapy field borders in 18 of 30 (60%) patients. A recent study by Dzhugashivili et al.[724] found that the visualization of the lumpectomy cavity was greatly improved in treatment-planning CT scans when clips were present; this was found to be even more pronounced in patients with very dense mammary glands, regardless of the physician reading the CT image.

Irradiation of Regional Lymphatics

Radiation therapy to the breast or chest wall and regional lymphatics can be technically challenging and, as previously discussed, remains one of the more variable and controversial aspects in management. A wide variety of available techniques, in combination with difficulties associated with matching fields, anatomic variability between patients, and lack of clear evidence regarding the superiority of any single approach, has resulted in a lack of consensus in regional nodal management.

Anatomic variation was highlighted in a study by Mansur et al.[727] They reported on 65 patients with breast cancer who had volumetric CT scanning in the treatment position. The IMNs and axillary lymph node regions were delineated according to a cross-sectional nodal atlas. The variable depths of IMNs at different intercostal spaces result in dose variations if the internal mammary port is treated with a single or inadequate electron beam energy. Axillary lymph nodes frequently overlapped the head of the humerus anteriorly when the arm was angled more than 90 degrees, but did not when the arm was angled 90 degrees or less. The larger the angle, the less head of the humerus could be spared in the supraclavicular port.

Arthur et al.[728] evaluated treatment techniques for coverage of the intact breast and ipsilateral lymph node regions. Anatomic outlines were obtained from five randomly selected patients with CT scanning in treatment position (three with cancer of the left breast and two of the right). Three techniques used to treat ipsilateral breast and internal mammary and supraclavicular nodes (extended tangents, five-field, partially wide tangents) were configured and compared with a supraclavicular field matched to standard tangential fields. All of the treatment techniques covering IMNs included at least 10% more lung and heart volume than that covered by standard tangential fields. Because of increased chest wall thickness and depth of IMNs superiorly, complete coverage was not achieved with any technique if the IMN target extended superiorly into the medial supraclavicular field.

Goodman et al.[729] examined the relation between tangential, anterior, and posterior radiation fields and regional lymph nodes, including level I to III axillary and supraclavicular lymph nodes in 55 patients who underwent CT scanning in the supine position. The mean depths of the level I to III axillary nodes were 4.6, 5.1, and 3.6 cm, respectively. The mean depth of the supraclavicular nodes was 3.9 cm. With the treatment using two tangential fields, level I axillary nodes appeared in the tangential portals in nine of nine patients, either alone or with other lymph node groups. In the three-field group, level I axillary nodes were in 16 of 16 tangential fields either alone or with level II nodes (8 patients). In eight patients, level III and the supraclavicular nodes were included in the anterior field, and in the other eight, levels II and III and the supraclavicular nodes were in the anterior field. There was considerable variation in the depth of supraclavicular and axillary lymph nodes in the fields in which these nodal groups appear and in the nodal group present in the posterior axillary boost field. To be certain that nodal groups to be treated are actually treated, as well as to minimize tissue irradiated, these authors recommended that before the placement of radiation fields, the nodal groups be outlined on a CT scan. From a practical standpoint, whether this results in better tumor control than standard techniques has not been demonstrated.

Supraclavicular Lymph Nodes

The inferior border of the supraclavicular field is matched to the tangential field usually just below the clavicular head. The medial border is 1 cm across the midline, extending upward, following the medial border of the sternocleidomastoid muscle to the thyrocricoid groove. The lateral border is a vertical line at the level of the coracoid process, just medial to the humeral head. This field is angled approximately 10 to 15 degrees laterally to spare the cervical spine (Fig. 56.36). The typical width of the supraclavicular field is 7 to 9 cm. The supraclavicular field is extended laterally to treat the full axilla, as clinically indicated. Figure 56.36 demonstrates a supraclavicular field with the supraclavicular and level I, II, and III nodes outlined. Level I as well as a portion of level II nodes will often be included in the tangential field; level III and supraclavicular nodes are covered in the supraclavicular field.

The total dose delivered to the supraclavicular field is 46 to 50.4 Gy at 1.8 to 2 Gy per day (calculated at a depth of 3 cm) in 5 fractions per week. For obese patients, an assessment of the depth of lymph nodes with ultrasound or CT treatment planning is useful to ensure adequate dose is delivered to the target.

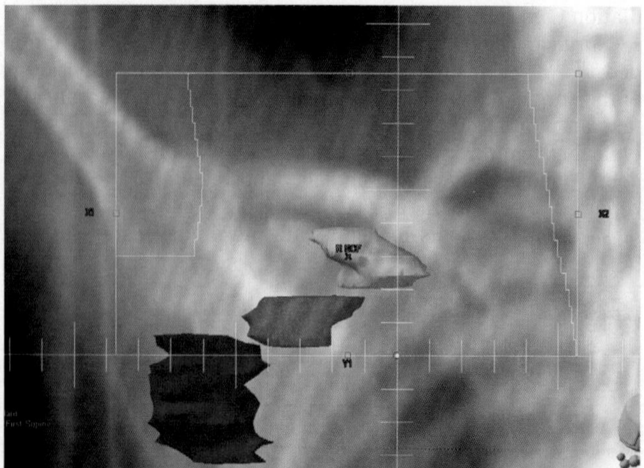

FIGURE 56.36. Supraclavicular and axillary field and field borders. Level I, II, and III nodes are demonstrated on the film. Note that level I nodes are included primarily in the tangential field in this case.

For patients in whom the target is deeper than 3 cm, higher energy photons should be considered.

Axillary Lymph Nodes

When the axilla is treated in patients with positive nodes, or in patients with inadequate or undissected axillae, the supraclavicular field is extended laterally to cover at least two-thirds of the humeral head, as demonstrated in Figure 56.36. The dose to the midplane of the axilla from the supraclavicular field is calculated at a point approximately 2 cm inferior to the midportion of the clavicle. Depending on the dose distribution and patient's anatomy, a posterior axillary boost may be considered or anterior axillary boost, as suggested by Wang et al.,[730] may be considered.

Posterior Axillary Boost

There is considerable debate regarding the necessity of a posterior axillary boost. Bentel et al.[731] questioned its necessity in a majority of patients. In 49 patients undergoing treatment-planning CT scanning in the treatment position, the maximum depth of the supraclavicular and axillary lymph nodes was measured on CT images and the relation between the supraclavicular and axillary lymph node depth and patient diameter was determined. For an anterior field, the relative dose to the supraclavicular and axillary lymph nodes were calculated for a 6-MV photon beam. If an anterior 6-MV beam only is used to treat both supraclavicular and axillary lymph nodes, the dose to the axilla is within ± 5% of the supraclavicular dose in 53% (26 of 49) patients and is 90% or more of the dose delivered to the supraclavicular nodes in 90% (44 of 49) of patients. These authors concluded that higher energy beams or anterior-posterior/posterior-anterior supraclavicular axillary fields may be reasonable when the axillary and supraclavicular nodes are deep.

The posterior axillary boost has been employed to supplement axillary dose. At the end of the treatments to the supraclavicular field, the dose to the midplane of the axilla may be supplemented by a posterior axillary field, as shown in Figure 56.37. Alternatively, the axilla should be contoured in CT-treatment planning as variation of the depth of the axilla from the anterior-posterior skin surface varies from patient to patient and the supplement prescription point can be adjusted accordingly. If the dose is determined to be inadequate, a posterior boost or anterior boost, as suggested by Wang et al.,[730] may be employed. When a posterior axillary boost is used, the borders are as follows: medially, the border is drawn to allow 1.5 to 2 cm of lung to show on the portal film; inferiorly, the border is at the same level as the inferior border of the supraclavicular field; laterally, the border just blocks fall-off across the posterior axillary fold; lastly, the superior border splits the clavicle and the superolateral border shields or splits the humeral head. Additional dose to the axilla midplane is usually administered to complete 46 to 50 Gy (2 Gy daily). When indicated, a boost of 10 to 15 Gy is delivered with reduced portals.

If the supraclavicular nodes are not felt to be at risk, a separate axillary field may not always be necessary to treat the axilla. In a study of 39 women with surgical clips in the axilla, Schlembach et al.[520] demonstrated that with tangential fields, placing the caudal border of the field within 2 cm of the humeral head and 2 cm deep to the chest wall–lung interface includes the majority of level I and level II lymph nodes (Fig. 56.38).

Internal Mammary Lymph Nodes

The benefit of irradiation of the IMNs is an unresolved issue because clinical failures at this site are very rare and the majority of patients at risk receive adjuvant therapy.[547,552] However, the IMNs are difficult to treat because their exact location is often uncertain and the radiation fields that include them irradiate more normal tissue.[732,733] Several techniques are used, the most common of which is a direct anterior field matched to tangential fields, which was developed for postmastectomy radiation therapy and increases the volume of heart and lung tissue in the field. With this technique, the rising contour of the intact breast interferes with dosimetry, which may affect the traditional dose prescription point at depths of 4 to 5 cm and may prevent an easy match to the breast tangential fields. Including the IMNs in the tangential fields (wide or deep tangents) may significantly increase the volume of irradiated lung and heart tissue and often includes a portion of the contralateral breast as well.

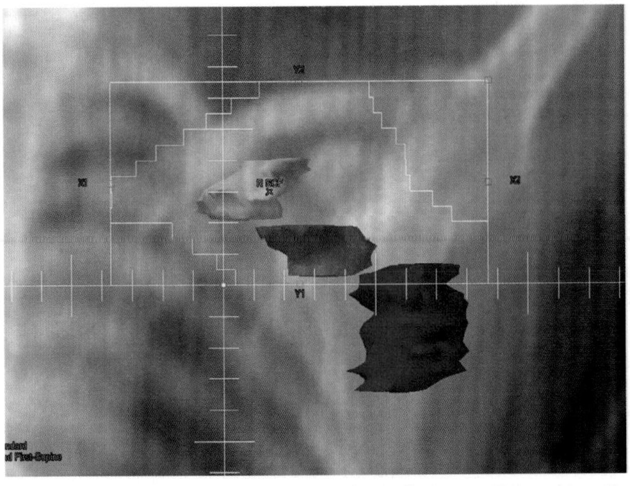

FIGURE 56.37. Posterior axillary field used to supplement the dose at midplane of the axilla. Note the small amount of lung included and the shielding of the humeral head (whenever possible).

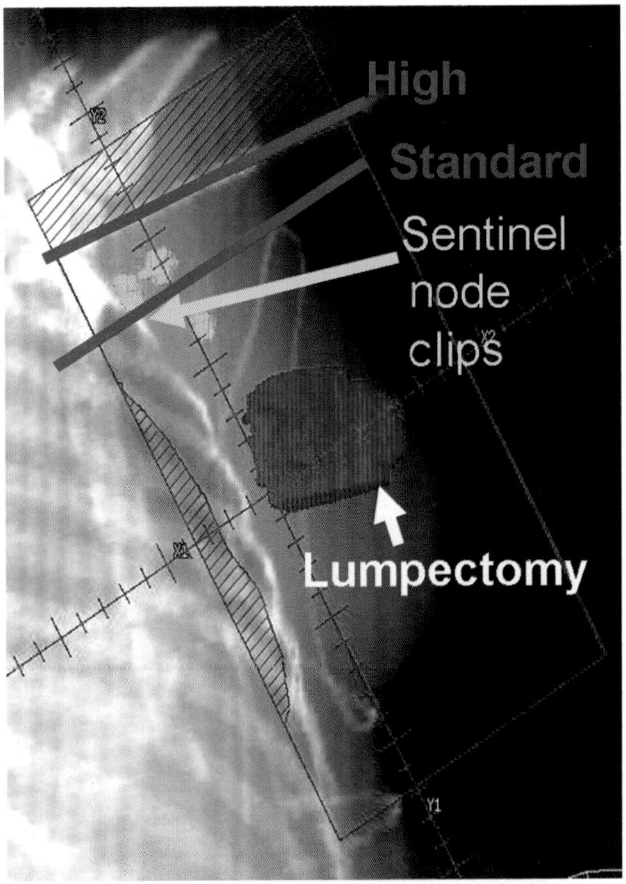

FIGURE 56.38. "High" tangential field shown coverage of level I and portion of level II nodes. With caudal edge of the field within 2 cm of the humeral head and leading edge approximately 2 cm from lung–chest wall interface, the majority of nodes in level I and level II will be covered by this technique.

The medial border of the IMN field is the midline. The lateral border is usually 5 to 6 cm lateral to the midline. The superior border abuts the inferior border of the supraclavicular field and the inferior border is at the xiphoid or higher. If only the IMNs are to be treated, the superior border of the field is at the first intercostal space (superior border of the head of the clavicle). The field is set, as described previously, with an oblique incidence to match the medial tangential portal (Fig. 56.39).

The dose to the IMN field (45 to 50 Gy at 1.8 to 2 Gy per day) is calculated at a point 4 to 5 cm beneath the skin surface (depending on the thickness of anterior chest wall and ideally based on CT localization). Careful individualized planning and use of electrons of appropriate energy for all or a major portion of the IMN irradiation are necessary to minimize dose to the lung. To spare underlying lung, mediastinum, and spinal cord, electrons in the range of 12 to 16 MeV are preferred for a portion of the treatment, for example 14.4 to 16.2 Gy delivered with 4- to 6-MV photons and 30.6 to 32.4 Gy with electrons.

A solution that avoids matching of fields is the use of partially wide tangential fields to treat the internal mammary chain.[734] Although IMNs can be imaged more clearly by radionuclide techniques, the nodes are typically located by identification of the internal mammary vessels, which can be seen on the CT simulator. The nodes in the first three intercostal spaces are thought to be most clinically significant. The medial border of the tangential field is moved 3 to 5 cm across the midline to cover the internal mammary nodes in the first three intercostal spaces. To minimize lung and cardiac exposure, a block is drawn in, as demonstrated in Figure 56.40, to block the inferior mediastinal nodes. The portal films should be inspected carefully to ensure that an excessive amount of lung or heart is not being irradiated. It is important to verify on the clinical setup that targeted breast tissue is not covered by the block.

Severin et al.[734] compared the partially wide tangent technique (PWT) of breast and internal mammary chain irradiation with photon/electron (P/E) and standard tangent (ST) techniques in terms of dose homogeneity within the breast and the dose to critical structures such as the heart and lung in 16 patients who underwent CT simulation for left-sided breast cancers. The mean dose to the left breast with the ST, P/E, and PWT techniques was 94.7%, 98.4%, and 96.5%, respectively ($P = .029$). The left lung received the lowest mean dose with the ST technique (13.9%) compared with PWT (22.8%) and P/E (24.3%). The internal mammary chain volume was most consistently treated with the PWT (mean dose 99%) versus P/E (86%) and ST (38.4%) techniques, although this technique was associated with the greatest amount of contralateral breast (mean dose 5.8%) versus ST (3.2%) versus P/E (2.8%). The heart received the least dose with ST (mean dose 6.7%) versus PWT (10.3%) and P/E (19%). Pierce et al.,[733] evaluating seven techniques of treating postmastectomy chest wall and lymphatics, also reported that the PWT technique was the most appropriate balance of target coverage and normal tissue sparing when irradiating the chest wall and internal mammary chain.

CT treatment planning is useful for irradiation of the IMN. Although the lymph nodes are most often not visible, the internal mammary vessels can be clearly seen and contoured on axial CT slices. This anatomic region can then be visualized in treatment field design and in dosimetry planning.

Matching the Tangential Fields with the Supraclavicular Field

A hot spot caused by divergence of the tangential beams into the supraclavicular field and of the supraclavicular beam into the tangential fields can exist just beneath the skin surface at the junction of the inferior border of the supraclavicular field and the superior border of the tangential fields.[735] The sharp beam of a linear accelerator and the "horns" at the edge of this beam produce a marked increase in dose beneath the match line if these divergences are not corrected. This

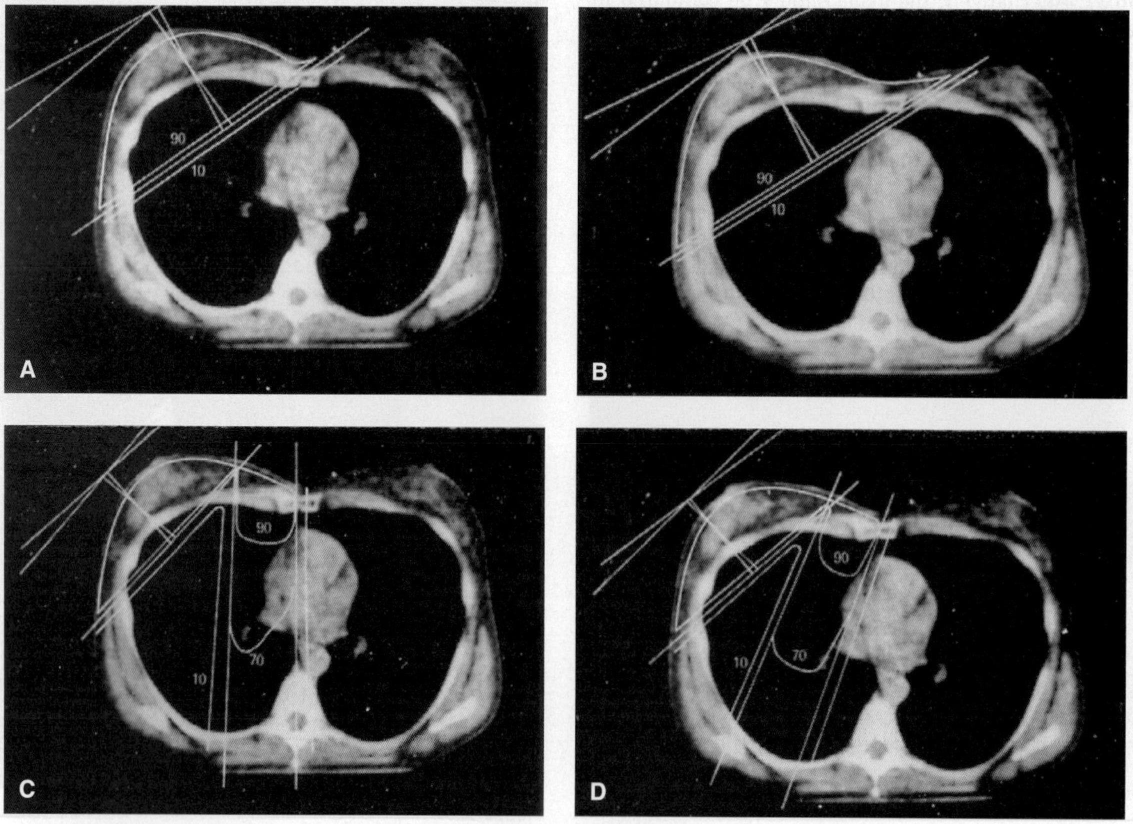

FIGURE 56.39. Irradiation of the breast: field configurations and isodose lines for 6-MV photons. **A:** "Standard tangents" technique. **B:** Deep tangents technique. **C:** *En face* internal mammary field (IMF) technique. **D:** Twenty-degree IMF technique. (From Roberson PL, Lichter AS, Bodner A, et al. Dose to lung in primary breast irradiation. *Int J Radiat Oncol Biol Phys* 1982;9:97–102, with permission from Elsevier.)

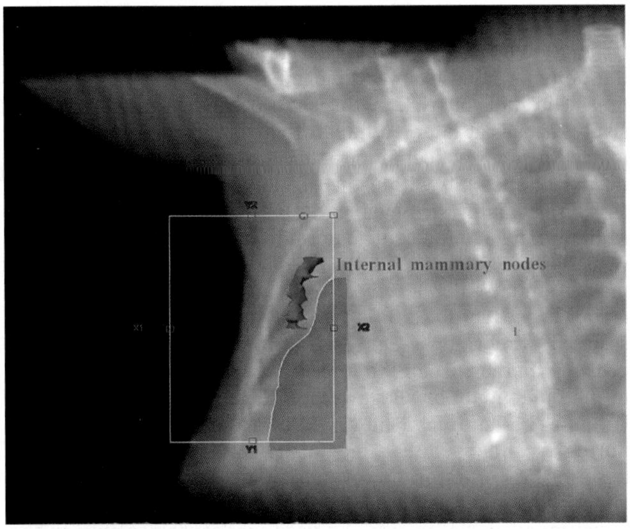

FIGURE 56.40. Partially wide tangential field covering internal mammary chain. The medial border of the tangential field is set 2 to 3 cm to the contralateral side to include the internal mammary chain. Below the fourth intercostals space, the field is blocked to minimize dose to the lungs and heart. Projection of the field on the patient's surface demonstrates adequate coverage of the involved breast–chest wall with this technique. With this technique, there may be a small amount of overlap onto the superior contralateral breast.

increased dose may result in severe match line fibrosis or even rib fracture.

There are numerous methods to adjust for divergence of the beams and minimize match line fibrosis. The divergence of the tangential fields can be eliminated by angling the foot of the treatment couch away from the radiation source to direct the tangential beams inferiorly so that the superior edges of these beams line up perfectly with the inferior border of the supraclavicular field (Fig. 56.41).[736] In addition, the collimator may be rotated to geometrically eliminate overlap at this junction. Alternatively, the "hanging block" technique, in which a vertical block is affixed to the superior portion of the collimator to block off the nonvertical portion of the tangential beam, can be used (Fig. 56.42).

The inferior divergence of the supraclavicular beam can be eliminated by blocking the inferior half of the beam. This can be accomplished with a beam splitter or with multileaf collimation so that the central, nondiverging portion of the beam becomes the inferior border of this field (see Fig. 56.44B). The combination of the half-beam block supraclavicular field and the couch kick technique for the tangential field results in minimal overlap and has essentially eliminated the problem of match line fibrosis.

The Single Isocenter Technique for Matching Supraclavicular and Tangential Fields

An alternative and attractive method for minimizing field matching problems between the supraclavicular and tangential fields is to use a technique that employs a single isocenter placed at the junction of the supraclavicular and tangential fields, as demonstrated in Figure 56.43. This single isocenter serves as the isocenter for both the supraclavicular/axillary axillary field and the tangential field, such that the nondivergent central axis single isocenter results in a perfect match of the supraclavicular and tangential fields.[737] As demonstrated, when treating the supraclavicular field, the beam below the isocenter is completely blocked. The supraclavicular field is typically angled 5% to 10% away from the spinal cord. Without moving the isocenter or patient, the tangential field is treated by closing the field above the isocenter and angling the beam to treat the tangential fields. Using this technique, there is not an option for rotating the collimator. If the patient's anatomy and positioning is ideal, the tangential field is closed down to the central axis, an acceptable amount of lung is exposed (<3 cm), and no block may be required. In some cases the

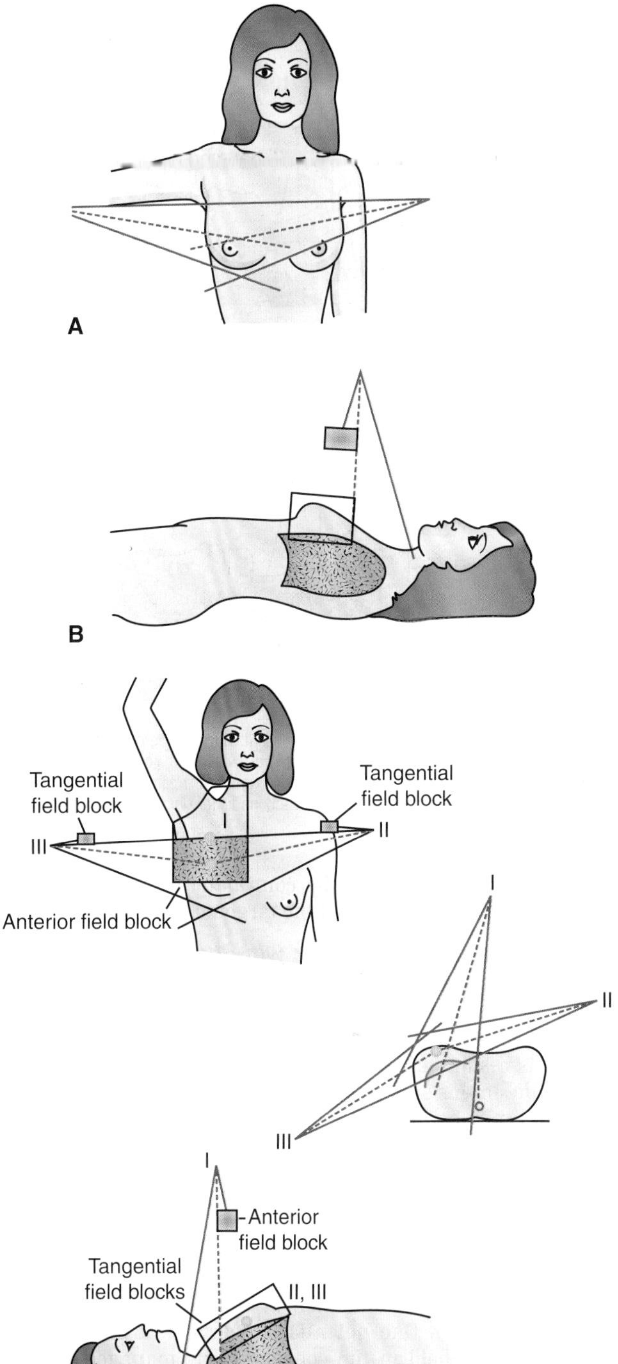

FIGURE 56.41. **A:** Inferior angulation of the tangential beams eliminates their divergence into the supraclavicular field. **B:** Splitting the supraclavicular beam eliminates its divergence down into the tangential field. (A and B from Bedwinek JM. Treatment of stage I and II adenocarcinoma of the breast by tumor excision and irradiation. *Int J Radiat Oncol Biol Phys* 1981;7:1553, with permission from Elsevier.) **C:** Three-field treatment beam geometry in irradiation of the intact breast and supraclavicular fields illustrated in coronal, cross-sectional, and sagittal projections. The supraclavicular and tangential field blocks are shaded. (C from Svensson GK, Chin LM, Siddon RL, et al. Breast treatment techniques at the Joint Center for Radiation Therapy. In: Harris JR, Hellman S, Silen W, eds. *Conservative management of breast cancer: new surgical and radiotherapeutic techniques.* Philadelphia: JB Lippincott, 1983, with permission.)

tangential field needs to be opened up beyond the central axis and a block drawn to minimize lung exposure while maintaining coverage of the breast. Because much of the setup is performed on the CT simulator, it is critical when using this technique to clinically view the medial and lateral setups on the patient to ensure that the entire breast is covered, the medial

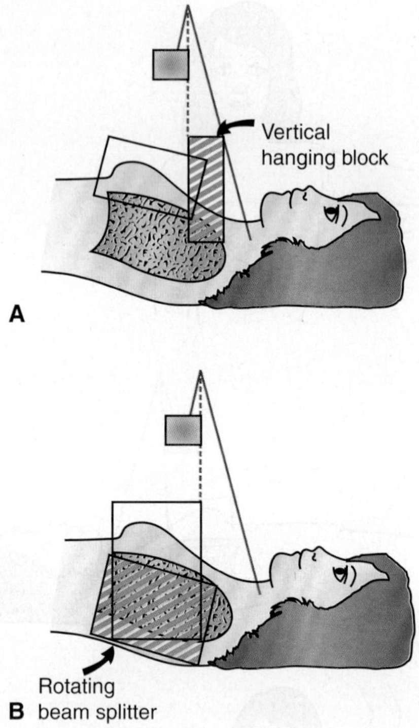

FIGURE 56.42. The superior edge of the tangential beams can be made perfectly vertical by means of the "hanging block" technique **(A)** or by avoiding collimator rotation with the use of a rotating beam splitter **(B)**. (From Bedwinek JM. Treatment of stage I and II adenocarcinoma of the breast by tumor excision and irradiation. *Int J Radiat Oncol Biol Phys* 1981;7:1553, with permission from Elsevier.)

border is not extending to the contralateral breast, and the blocks are not covering any of the targeted breast tissue.

Matching the Tangential Fields with the Internal Mammary Field

When an internal mammary field is required, the match between it and the medial tangential field can be a problem if there is a significant amount of breast tissue beneath the match line. In this situation, a cold spot can exist (Fig. 56.44). The effect may be negligible if the breast tissue beneath this match line is thin (see Fig. 56.44B), or it can be avoided by including the internal mammary nodes in the tangential field, as described above (see Fig. 56.44C). Woudstra and van der Werf[738] described a technique using an oblique incidence of the internal mammary portal to match the orientation of the adjacent medial tangential portal; this results in a more homogeneous dose distribution at the junction of the two fields (Fig. 56.45). One potential advantage of the partially wide tangential field in the conservatively managed patient is that it avoids the problem of matching over breast tissue.

Irradiation Dose to the Contralateral Breast

Irradiation dose to the contralateral breast is of concern due to the potential long-term carcinogenic effect of scattered radiation. The data on risk of the contralateral breast are extensively discussed later. Although this risk appears to be minimal with modern techniques, the goal must be to expose all normal tissues not within the target volume to as low a dose as is reasonably achievable. Fraass et al.[739] measured the radiation dose to the contralateral breast in 16 women treated with 6-MV photon tangential fields and performed phantom measurements. For a typical treatment of 50 Gy, the contralateral breast received 0.5 to 2 Gy. Use of tangential fields only resulted in more dose delivered to the surface of the opposite breast, whereas use of the internal mammary field in addition to the tangential portals gave more dose deeper in the breast. Use of a 2.5-cm-thick lead shield over the contralateral breast during treatment with a medial tangential field reduced the dose to 35% of its original value. Similar shields used on the lateral tangential field had no protective effect. These authors recommended that wedges be used whenever possible on the lateral tangential fields rather than on the medial to decrease the dose to the contralateral breast.

A dosimetric study demonstrated that most of the scatter dose received by the opposite breast originates in the collimator and accessories of the accelerator, and it can be significantly decreased by increasing the distance between the source and the patient's skin.[740] Therefore, an isocentric source–skin distance technique may be desirable. The use of half-field blocks (beam splitter) or, even better, independent jaws combined with tailored beam splitters or a MLC following the contour of the chest wall of the patient is very helpful in decreasing the dose to the contralateral breast.

Kelly et al.[741] reviewed the dose to the contralateral breast from breast irradiation with tangential fields using four different techniques. The highest dose was delivered with the use of Cerrobend half-beam blocks (regardless of the proportion of wedge used). Remaining techniques gave similar dose ranges, with the lowest total dose produced by the asymmetric jaw with no medial wedge.

The clinical significance of this inadvertent radiation dose to the opposite breast is uncertain, as various investigators have shown no increased risk of contralateral breast malignancy after treatment of the original breast by radiation therapy.[23,93,678,742]

Three-Dimensional Conformal or Intensity-Modulated Radiation Therapy

Standard opposed tangential fields with appropriate use of wedges to optimize dose homogeneity remains the most commonly employed method for delivery of whole-breast irradiation. A number of publications have explored the potential advantages of three-dimensional conformal radiation therapy

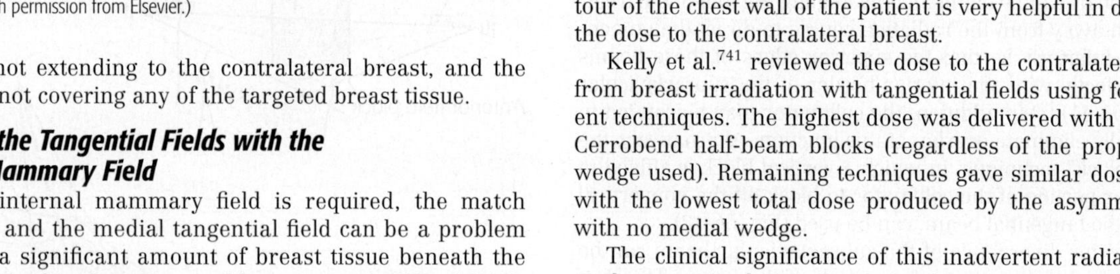

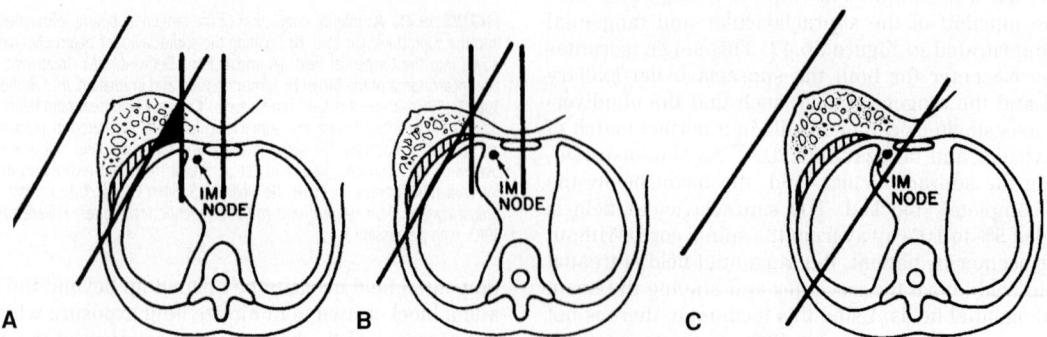

FIGURE 56.43. Diagrams showing several relationships between internal mammary and tangential fields. **A:** A significant cold region exists if the internal mammary (IM) tangential matchline overlies a large amount of breast tissue. **B:** The cold area may be negligible if the breast tissue beneath the matchline is thin. **C:** The lack of a separate IM field can result in irradiation of an excessive volume of lung, particularly in large-chested patients. (From Bedwinek JM. Treatment of stage I and II adenocarcinoma of the breast by tumor excision and irradiation. *Int J Radiat Oncol Biol Phys* 1981;7:1553, with permission from Elsevier.)

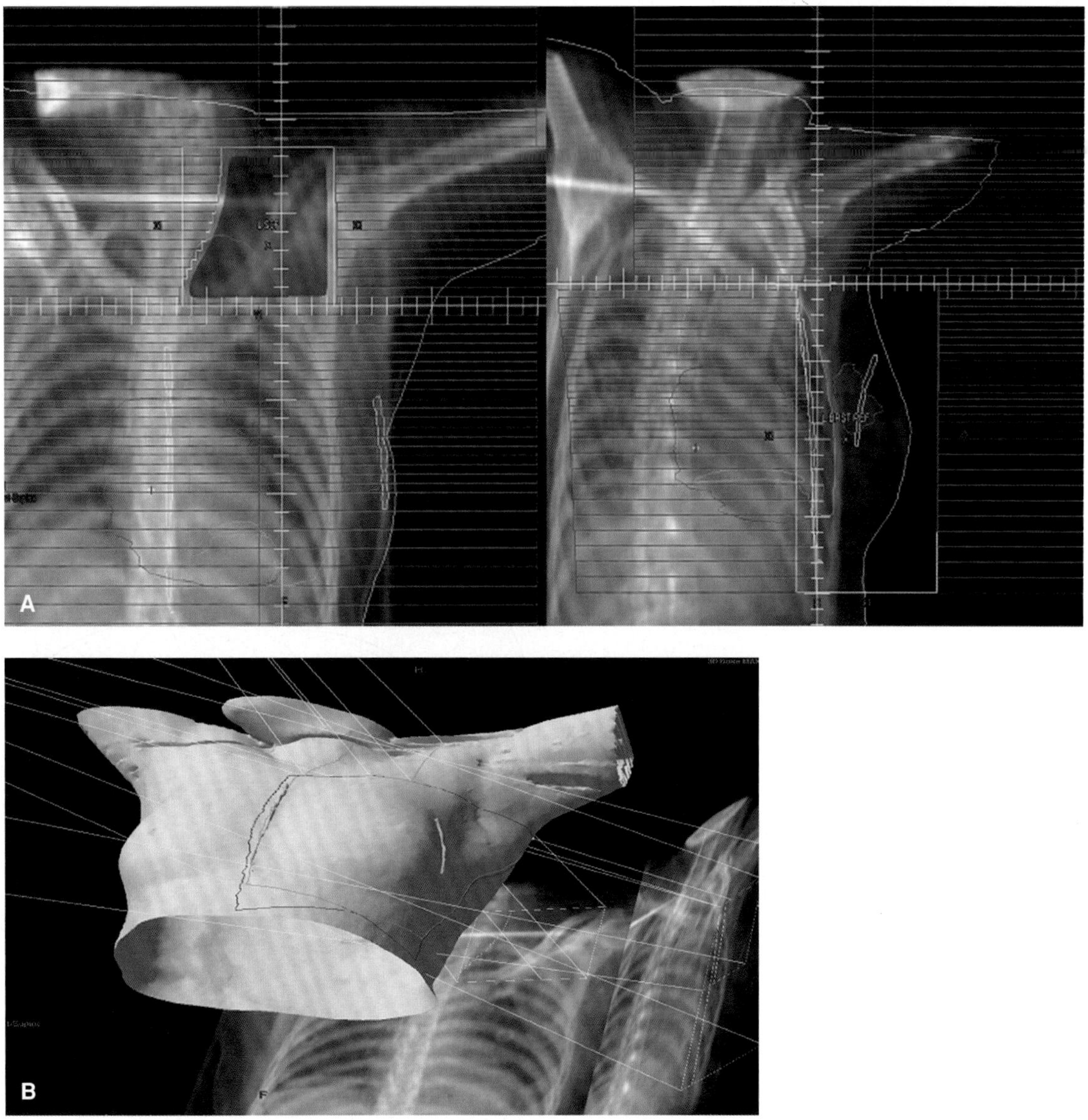

FIGURE 56.44. A and B: Monoisocentric matching technique. Single isocenter is set at the match between the supraclavicular and tangential fields. The inferior portion of the beam is blocked for the supraclavicular treatment and the superior blocked for the tangential field, with no movement of the isocenter, resulting in an ideal match. Blocks are drawn as indicated to shield lung and heart. The field should be viewed clinically to ensure that the blocks drawn to shield the heart and lungs to not block target tissue on the breast–chest wall. Projection of fields onto patient surface demonstrates perfect match of the supraclavicular and tangential fields.

(3D-CRT) or intensity-modulated radiation therapy (IMRT) to treat patients with breast cancer. Theoretically, 3D-CRT involves a reduction in the volume of normal tissues receiving a high dose, with an increase in dose to the target volume that includes the tumor and a limited amount of normal tissue. IMRT potentially can further improve the dose distribution between the target and nontarget tissue, but may also increase the volume of tissue exposed to lower doses of radiation. As suggested in a review by Hall and Wuu,[628] this may increase the risk of second malignanciesthe potential gains and limitations of advanced planning techniques must be weighed carefully.

Solin et al.[743] devised 38 3D treatment plans in two patients using multiple CT scan sections and compared various dose distributions. Breast inhomogeneity doses ranged from 5% to 10%. Cobalt-60 produced greater inhomogeneities than 6-MV photons, with minimal improvement in tumor dose coverage. In contrast, 15-MV photons had significantly worse tumor coverage at shallow depths, although there was a slight reduction in hot spots. These authors were unable to identify any beam arrangement that improved dose distributions compared with standard tangential fields.

Vicini et al.[744] reported on 281 patients treated with whole-breast IMRT using multiple static MLC segments. Figure 56.46 shows a representative dose distribution. The median volume of breast receiving 105% of the prescribed dose was 11% (range, 0% to 67.6%). The median breast volume receiving 110% of the prescribed dose was 0% (range, 0% to 39%), and the median breast volume receiving 115% of the prescribed dose was also 0%. Only three (1%) experienced grade III toxicity. The cosmetic results at 12 months (95 patients analyzable) were rated as excellent or good in 94 patients (99%). No skin telangiectasias, significant fibrosis, or persistent breast pain was noted. These authors concluded that the use of intensity modulation with a static MLC technique for tangential whole-breast RT is an efficient method for achieving a uniform and standardized dose throughout the whole breast, and widespread implementation of this technology can be achieved with minimal imposition on clinic resources and time constraints. As demonstrated in Figure 56.47, Dunst et al.[745] compared optimized IMRT with 3D-CRT and reported a small reduction in does to the heart, lungs, and contralateral breast with IMRT.

In a trial of patients undergoing breast-conserving therapy, 358 patients undergoing whole-breast irradiation were

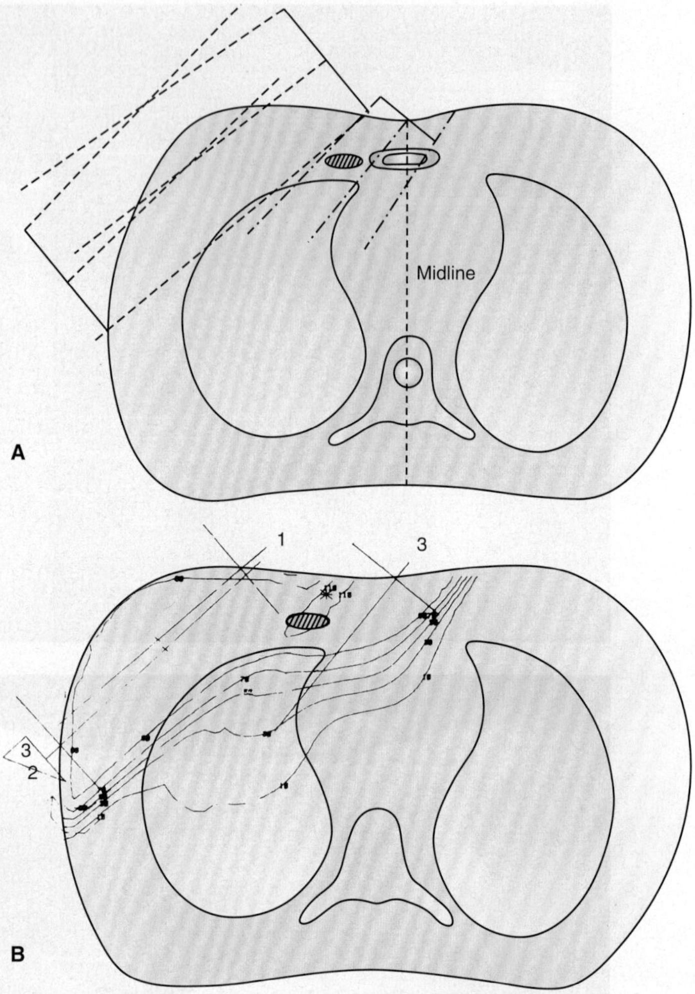

FIGURE 56.45. A: An obliquely incident electron beam matched to the usual tangential beams. **B:** Isodose presentation of optimal matching of an obliquely incident electron beam to the tangential beams. The target volume is enclosed by the 90% isodose line (= 40.5 Gy). Electron beam, 16 MeV; photon beam, 6 MV. (From Woudstra E, van der Werf H. Obliquely incident electron beams for irradiation of the internal mammary lymph nodes. *Radiother Oncol* 1987;10:209–215, with permission from Elsevier.)

randomized to radiation to the breast with standard wedges or with IMRT. Those randomized to IMRT experienced significantly lower degrees of moist desquamation due to the improved homogeneity with the IMRT techniques employed.[746,747] In another randomized trial of IMRT in breast cancer, 306 women were randomized to standard treatment with tangential fields with wedge compensators compared with IMRT. The standard control patients were 1.7 times more likely to have a change in photographic appearance compared with those in the IMRT arm.[748] Further follow-up and additional studies relating to the technical delivery of radiation therapy in early-stage breast cancer will evolve rapidly in the next several years due to the rapid advances in technology.

It is important to recognize that the term intensity-modulated radiation therapy has been used in various ways to describe breast cancer treatment. In some studies, IMRT is described as a method of 3D dose compensation without a change in the gantry angles of predesigned tangential fields. In such instances, dose distribution has been improved but the fields are not more conformal. Accordingly, low dose to other organs is not an issue. For others, IMRT attempts to improve conformality of the high-dose region by using multiple field angles that increase the volume of normal tissues that receive low radiation doses.

ACCELERATED PARTIAL BREAST IRRADIATION

The current standard of care for women with invasive breast cancer remains whole-breast irradiation following breast-conserving surgery.[749] With the notable exception of selected elderly women, omission of radiation therapy has now been proven in numerous randomized trials and meta-analysis to compromise local control and to a lesser extent breast cancer–related mortality. For some women, the 6-week course of daily radiation with its associated time and travel issues is not feasible. In response to this, a wide variety of accelerated forms of treatment have been developed and have been proven safe and effective in short-term studies.[663] These approaches include multicatheter interstitial implants placed around the excision cavity, a single balloon catheter that can be after loaded with a central radiation source (MammoSite) that is placed into the excision cavity, external-beam conformal partial breast irradiation, and intraoperative single-dose irradiation. Although these techniques vary considerably, they share the common strategy of delivering the radiation to a smaller volume of breast tissue around the lumpectomy site, using fewer larger fractions delivered over a shorter time. The rationale behind this approach is that the majority of breast relapses occur at or near the lumpectomy site. Pathological studies from mastectomy specimens have demonstrated a lower probability of subclinical microscopic disease with increasing distance from the primary tumor.[102,103,222,298,391,663,750–752] Although the early results clearly demonstrate the feasibility and acceptable toxicity of accelerated partial breast irradiation, this approach has not yet been demonstrated in a randomized trial to be equivalent to whole-breast irradiation. There are several randomized ongoing trials that will attempt to answer the question of whether this approach is equivalent to whole-breast irradiation for selected patients. The current NSABP-39/RTOG-0413 is well under way with high enrollment.[753] Although the mature results of

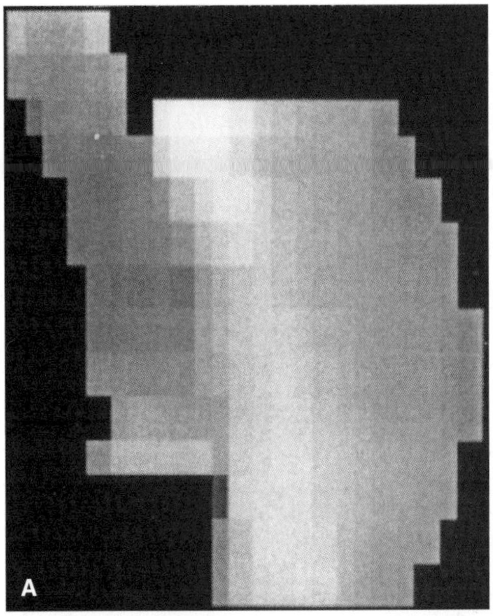

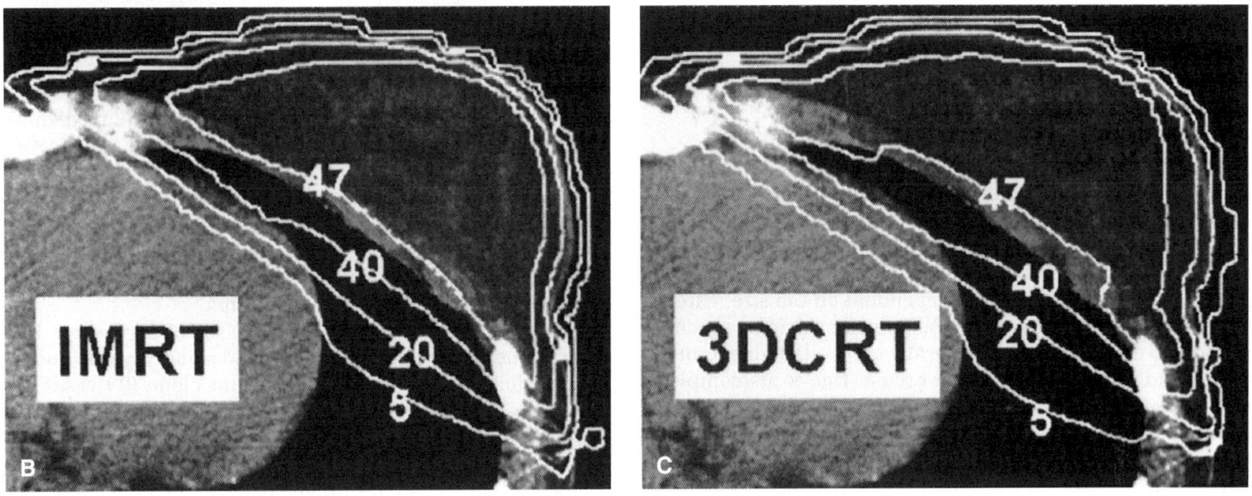

FIGURE 56.46. A: Beam intensity profile over the breast (*lighter*) and the internal mammary nodes (*darker*) to minimize dose to the heart. (A from Cho BCJ, Hurkmans CW, Damen EMF, et al. Intensity modulated versus non-intensity modulated radiotherapy in the treatment of the left breast and upper internal mammary lymph node chain: a comparative planning study. *Radiother Oncol* 2002;62:127–136, with permission from Elsevier.) **B:** Dose distribution to the breast with intensity modulated radiation therapy. **C:** Dose distribution to the breast with three-dimensional conformal radiation therapy. (B and C from Keall PJ, Arnfield MR, Arthur DW, et al. An IMRT technique to reduce the heart and lung dose for early stage breast cancer. *Int J Radiat Oncol Biol Phys* 2001;51(Suppl 1):247(abstr), with permission from Elsevier.)

this trial will not be available for several years, it should help to identify appropriate patients for this approach. Ongoing randomized trials investigating partial breast irradiation are summarized in Table 56.38. The NSABP-RTOG trial will randomize 4,300 women with early-stage breast cancer (including DCIS) to whole-breast versus accelerated partial breast irradiation. This trial allows for any one of the three techniques of partial breast irradiation, namely, interstitial brachytherapy, MammoSite, or 3D-CRT.[663] The techniques are selected based on physician or patient preference prior to randomization. Fraction size is slightly higher for the external-beam conformal (3.85 Gy vs. 3.4 Gy) but all three employ twice daily radiation

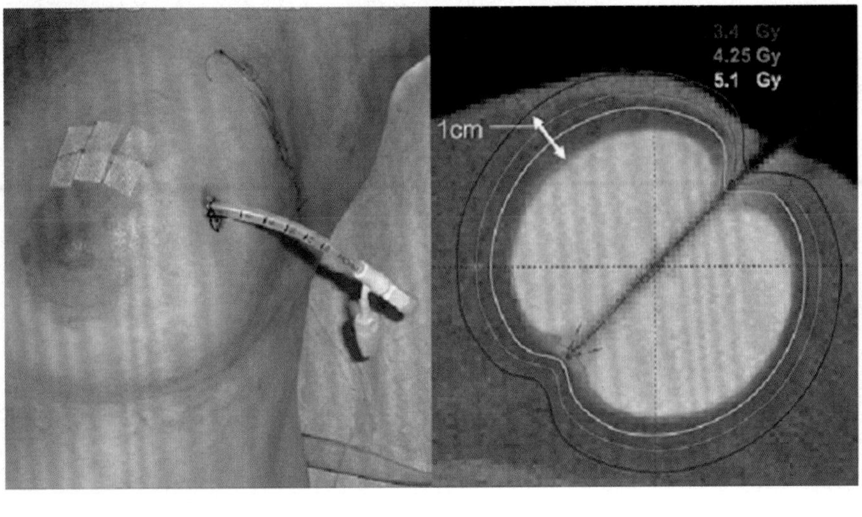

FIGURE 56.47. Partial breast irradiation demonstrating the MammoSite breast brachytherapy device. (From Arthur DW, Vicini FA. Accelerated partial breast irradiation as a part of breast conservation therapy. *J Clin Oncol* 2005;23:1726–1735. Reused with permission. © 2012 American Society of Clinical Oncology. All rights reserved.)

TABLE 56.38 RANDOMIZED TRIALS OF ACCELERATED PARTIAL BREAST IRRADIATION

Institution/Trial	Number of Cases	Control Arm	Experimental Arm
NSABP B 39 RTOG 0413	3,000	50–50.4 Gy WB +/– 10–16 Gy boost	1. Interstitial Brachytx, or 2. MammoSite™, or 3. 3D Conformal EBRT
National Institute of Oncology Budapest, Hungary	570	50 Gy WB	1. Interstitial Brachytx (5.2 Gy × 7) or 2. Electrons (50 Gy)
European Brachytherapy GEC-ESTRO Working Group	1,170	50–50.4 Gy WB + 10 Gy boost	Brachytherapy only 32.0 Gy 8 fractions HDR 30.3 Gy 7 fractions HDR 50 Gy PDR
European Institute of Oncology (ELIOT)	824	50 Gy WB + 10 Gy boost	Intraoperative Single fraction EBRT 21 Gy × 1
University College of London (TARGIT)	1,600	WBRT (per center) + boost	Intra-operative Single fraction EBRT 5 Gy × 1
Canadian Trial (RAPID)	2,128	WBRT 42.5 in 16 or 50 in 25	3 CRT 38.5 Gy in 10
Medical Research Council-UK Import Low	1,935	WB 2.67 Gy × 15	PBI 2.67 Gy × 15

WB, whole breast; EBRT, external-beam radiation therapy; HDR, high-dose rate; PDR, pulsed-dose rate; CRT, conformal radiation therapy; PBI, partial breast irradiation.

for a total of 10 treatments for a total dose of 38.5 or 34 Gy, respectively, over 5 days. Each of the various techniques of partial breast irradiation is discussed below.

Multicatheter Interstitial Techniques

Experience is greatest with the multicatherter interstitial technique, as it was initially developed (and is still employed) as a boost technique following whole-breast irradiation.[754–756] As demonstrated in Figure 56.48, multiple catheters are generally position at 1.0- to 1.5-cm intervals, with the total number of catheters and planes employed dependent on the size, extent, and shape of the target. With refinements in image-guided techniques, this approach is generally quite adaptable to most cavities and locations within the breast. Due to its complexity, user dependence, and logistics, however, the use of this technique has been less widely embraced, compared with the MammoSite (described below) and external-beam techniques.

Kuske et al.[757] recently reported the results of RTOG-95-17, a phase I and II study employing APBI using multiplane interstitial catheters in 99 women with early-stage breast cancer. The inclusion criteria for this study included invasive nonlobular tumors ≤3 cm after lumpectomy with negative surgical margins and axillary dissection with zero to three positive axillary nodes without extracapsular extension. The patients were treated with either low-dose rate (LDR) APBI (45 Gy in 3.5 to 5 days) or high-dose rate (HDR) APBI (34 Gy in 10 twice-daily fractions within 5 days). Chemotherapy and/or tamoxifen were administered at the discretion of the treating physicians. Of the 99 women, 33 were treated with LDR and 66 with HDR APBI. Of the 66 patients treated with HDR APBI, 2 (3%) had grade 3 or 4 toxicity. Of the 33 patients treated with LDR, 3 (9%) had grade 3 or 4 toxicity during brachytherapy. No patient experienced late grade 4 toxicity; the rate of grade 3 toxicity was 18% for the LDR and 4% for the HDR groups.

Vicini et al.[227] reported on 133 cases of early-stage breast cancer managed with lumpectomy and axillary lymph node dissection followed by interstitial implant alone (99 cases using LDR and 34 with HDR implant) to the tumor bed, matched to a control group treated with external beam from the same institution. The number of catheters per patient ranged from 11 to 18 (median, 16). Tumor size ranged from 0.1 to 3 cm (median, 1.1 cm), with margins of excision >2 mm. Patients treated with LDR implants received 50 Gy over 96 hours as an inpatient procedure and those treated with HDR implants received 32 Gy in 8 fractions over 4 days (twice daily) as an outpatient procedure. The median follow up for the external beam radiation therapy

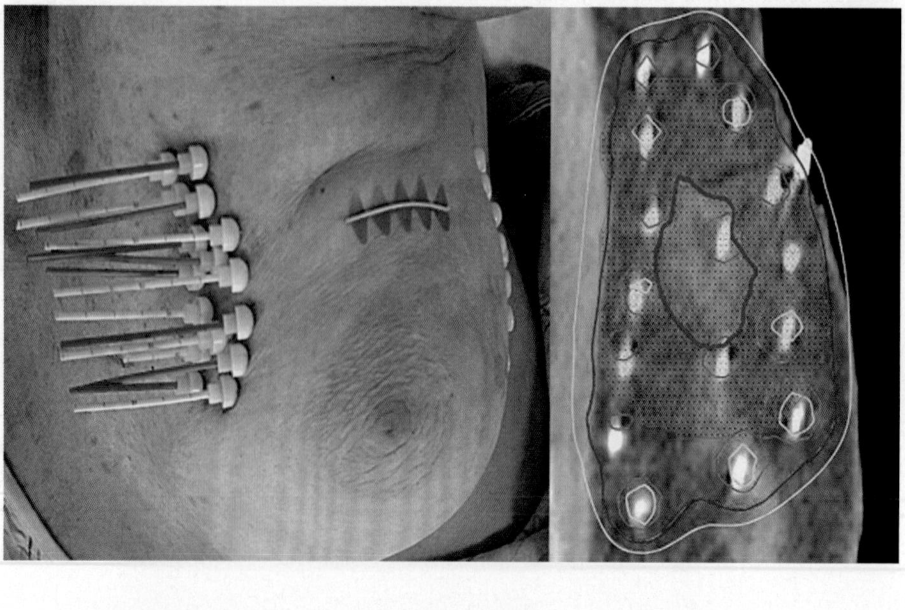

FIGURE 56.48. Partial breast irradiation demonstrating the with multiplane interstitial implant technique. (From Arthur DW, Vicini FA. Accelerated partial breast irradiation as a part of breast conservation therapy. *J Clin Oncol* 2005;23:1726–1735. Reused with permission. © 2012 American Society of Clinical Oncology. All rights reserved.)

group was 5.7 years versus 3.2 years for brachytherapy. No local or regional failures have been detected and only one patient failed distantly in the HDR group. No significant adverse sequelae were noted, and cosmetic results were judged to be good or excellent in 98% of patients. No statistically significant differences were noted in the 5-year actuarial rates of ipsilateral breast (3% vs. 0%; $P = .17$) or locoregional failure (4% vs. 0%; $P = .37$) between patients treated with external-beam radiation therapy and those treated with brachytherapy alone. In a recent update of this study with 12 years follow-up, there was no difference in the rate of local recurrence (3.8% vs. 5.0%; $P = .40$), regional recurrence (0% vs. 1.1%; $P = .15$), disease-free survival (87% vs. 91%; $P = .30$), cause-specific survival (93% vs. 95%; $P = .28$), or overall survival (78% vs. 71%; $P = .06$) between the WBI and APBI groups, respectively.[758]

Arthur et al.[759] used HDR brachytherapy (34 Gy in 10 fractions twice a day over 5 days) in 26 patients or LDR (45 Gy given at a dose rate of 0.45 to 0.50 Gy per hour) in 18 patients. After a median follow-up of 31 months (range, 11 to 61 months), all patients remain locally controlled. Among patients receiving doxorubicin after brachytherapy, at a median follow-up of 12 months, recall reactions involving the skin overlying the implant site were observed in 42% of patients (6 of 14). On multivariate analysis, a recall reaction ($P = .0007$) and LDR brachytherapy ($P = .04$) were significant predictors of fibrosis and telangiectasis.

Wazer et al.[760] reported the results of APBI using high-dose rate interstitial brachytherapy in a phase I or II single multi-institutional study in 33 women with early-stage breast cancer. Eligible patients included those with T1, T2, N0, N1 (≤3 nodes positive), and M0 tumors of nonlobular histologic features with negative surgical margins, no extracapsular lymph node extension, and a negative postexcision mammogram. High-activity ^{192}Ir (3 to 10 Ci) was used to deliver 3.4 Gy per fraction, 2 fractions per day, for 5 consecutive days, to a total dose of 34 Gy to the target volume. The mean tumor size was 1.3 cm, and 55% had an extensive intraductal component. Three patients had positive axillary nodes. The RTOG late radiation morbidity scoring scheme was applied. Clinically evident fat necrosis occurred in eight patients at a median of 7.5 months after HDR brachytherapy completion. The only variables significantly associated with grade 3 or 4 toxicity were the number of source dwell positions and the volume of tissue encompassed by the prescription isodose shell. The global cosmetic scores after a minimum of 18 months' follow-up were 0 cases with poor, 4 with fair, 5 with good, and 24 with excellent scores. One case of ipsilateral breast tumor recurrence was diagnosed.

MammoSite

MammoSite as an alternative method of delivering accelerated partial breast irradiation has been widely embraced due to its simplicity and less dependence on user experience.[351,663,761,762] The technique employs a single balloon catheter introduced into the lumpectomy site either at the time of lumpectomy or percutaneously after the procedure. In the current NSABP/RTOG clinical trial, patients cannot be randomized until after the lumpectomy procedure when final margins and nodal status are known, and hence the device must be placed after the lumpectomy procedure. As shown in Figure 56.48, the catheter is located centrally within a distal balloon, which is inflated once the catheter is placed in the lumpectomy cavity. Adequacy of placement requires symmetry of the balloon, conformance of the balloon surface to the lumpectomy cavity, and a minimum distance between the surface of the balloon and skin of >5 mm (ideally >7 mm). Treatment is delivered via a high-dose rate remote after-loading system to a circumferential 1-cm distance from the balloon surface. This technique is one of the three methods employed in the ongoing randomized trial, with a dose prescription of 3.4 Gy delivered at 1 cm twice daily to a total dose of 34 Gy over 5 days.

Although early experiences with this technique are promising, the results of the ongoing randomized trial will help to identify suitable patients. The most extensive experience with this technique has been reported by the American Society of Breast Surgeons MammoSite Registry Trial, which included 1,419 patients treated in 87 institutions.[351,763,764] This was a nonrandomized single-arm registration trial in which data were collected prospectively on clinical use of the MammoSite breast brachytherapy catheter for delivering breast irradiation. They reported on 1,237 patients (87% of enrolled patients) who received APBI (34 Gy to 1.0 cm in 10 fractions; 91% of the patients with invasive carcinoma (977 of 1,068 patients) had negative lymph node status, and 99% of all patients had negative margins. The median patient age was 65 years. Five hundred fifty-four catheters (45%) were placed with an open cavity at the time of lumpectomy, and 683 catheters (55%) were placed after lumpectomy. Skin spacing ranged from 2 to 75 mm (median, 10 mm). At 5 years, 37 cases (2.6%) developed an IBTR, for a 5-year actuarial rate of 3.80% (3.86% for inflammatory breast cancer [IBC] and 3.39% for DCIS). Negative ER status ($P = .0011$) was the only clinical, pathologic, or treatment-related variable associated with IBTR for patients with IBC and young age (<50 years; $P = .0096$) and positive margin status ($P = .0126$) in those with DCIS. The percentage of breasts with good or excellent cosmetic results at 60 months (n = 371) was 90.6%.The authors concluded that treatment efficacy, cosmesis, and toxicity 5 years after treatment with APBI using the MammoSite device are good and similar to those reported with other forms of APBI with similar follow-up.

External-Beam Conformal Radiation

Although external-beam conformal radiation has been developed only recently, it is the one that is most widely employed in the ongoing randomized trial.[217,765,766] Recent data suggest that over 70% of patients in the randomized trial are opting for the 3D-CRT. Its widespread acceptance is likely because it is totally noninvasive and delivers a homogenous dose distribution. Although the ongoing trial mandates supine position, some authors have advocated prone accelerated breast irradiation.[217,765,766]

Three-dimensional-CRT, as shown in Figure 56.49, generally employs multiple conformal fields, although plans as simple as two opposing small conformal fields may be adequate. Challenges with this technique include daily positioning of the target, movement with breathing, and delivery of higher doses to surrounding normal breast tissue than with the brachytherapy. Nonetheless this approach has been widely embraced and has been shown to be reproducible. In the phase I and II RTOG-0319 trial of external-beam conformal radiation, Vicini et al.[766] examined the use of 3D-CRT to deliver accelerated partial breast irradiation. Reproducibility, as measured by technical feasibility, was the primary end point. This study was designed such that if fewer than 5 cases in the first 42 patients evaluable were scored as unacceptable, the treatment would be considered reproducible. Patients received 38.5 Gy in 3.85 Gy per fraction delivered twice daily. The clinical target volume included the lumpectomy cavity plus a 10- to 15-mm margin bounded by 5 mm within the skin surface and the lung–chest wall interface. The planning target volume included the clinical target volume plus a 10-mm margin. A total of 58 patients were enrolled on this study over an 8-month period, 5 of whom were ineligible or did not receive protocol treatment. There were 4 cases with major variations and a total of 32 cases with minor variations in treatment plans. Based on this analysis, the authors concluded that accelerated partial breast irradiation using 3D conformal external-beam radiation therapy was technically feasible and reproducible in a multi-institutional trial using exceptionally strict dosimetric criteria. An update of this study found that the ipsilateral breast failure rate was 6%, in-field failure rate was 2%, and contralateral breast failure rate was 0%.[767] Only two (4%) grade 3 toxicities were observed.

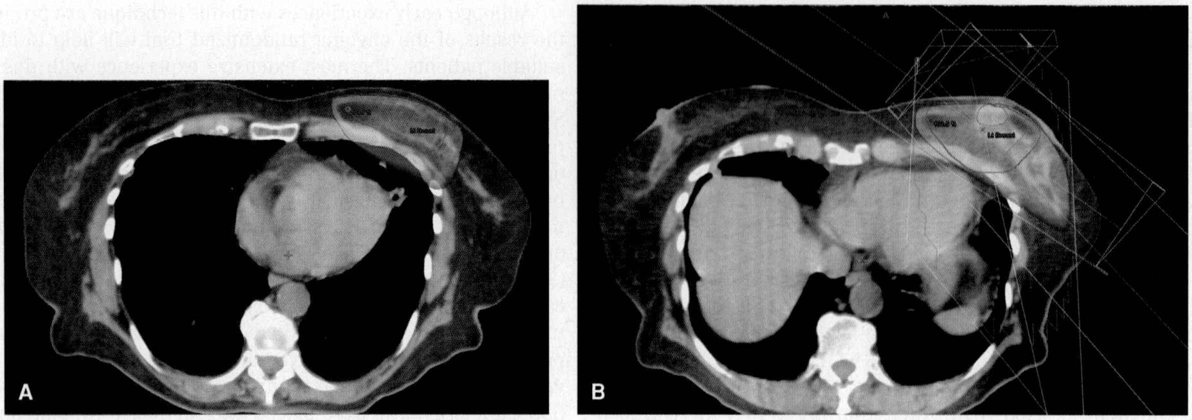

FIGURE 56.49. A and B: Partial breast irradiation demonstrating the external-beam conformal radiation technique.

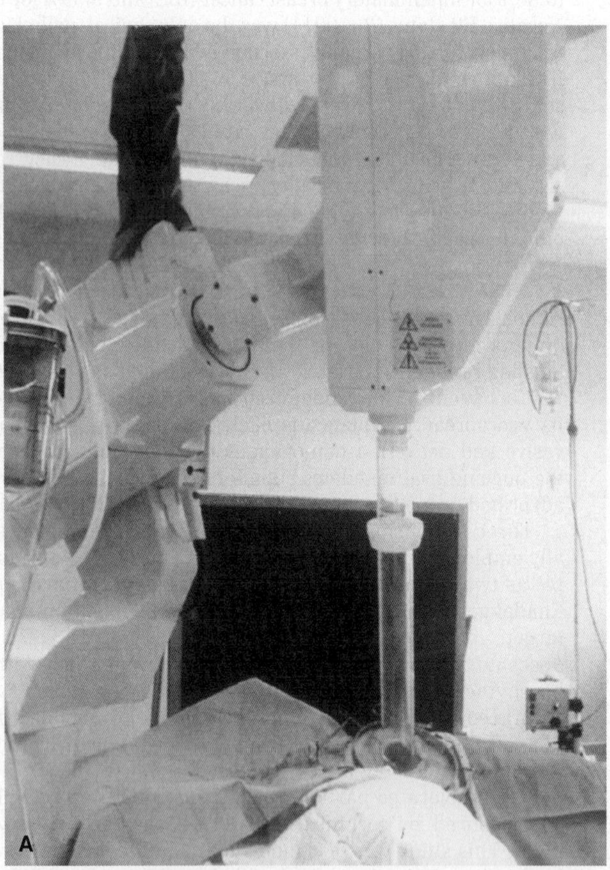

FIGURE 56.50. A: Linear electron beam accelerator in operating room during intraoperative radiation therapy. **B:** Proper placement of applicator in the breast. **C:** Before intraoperative radiation therapy delivery, an aluminum-lead disc (4 mm Al and 5 mm Pb thick) is placed between the deep face of residual breast and pectoralis muscle. (From Veronesi U, Oreechia R, Luini A, et al. A preliminary report on intraoperative radiotherapy (IORT) in limited-stage breast cancers that are conservatively treated. *Eur J Cancer* 2001;37:2178–2183, with permission.)

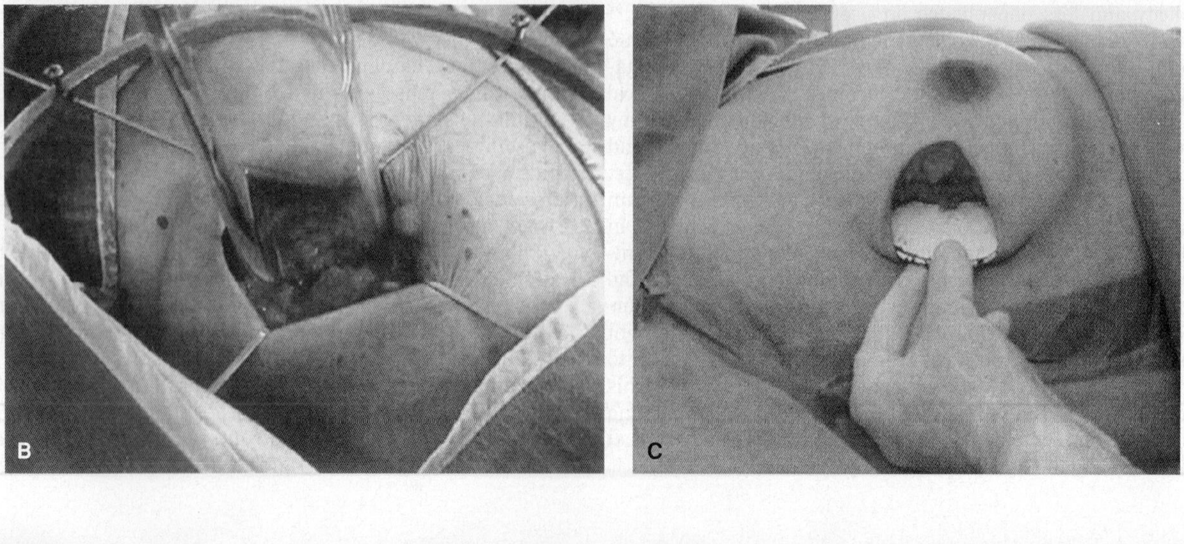

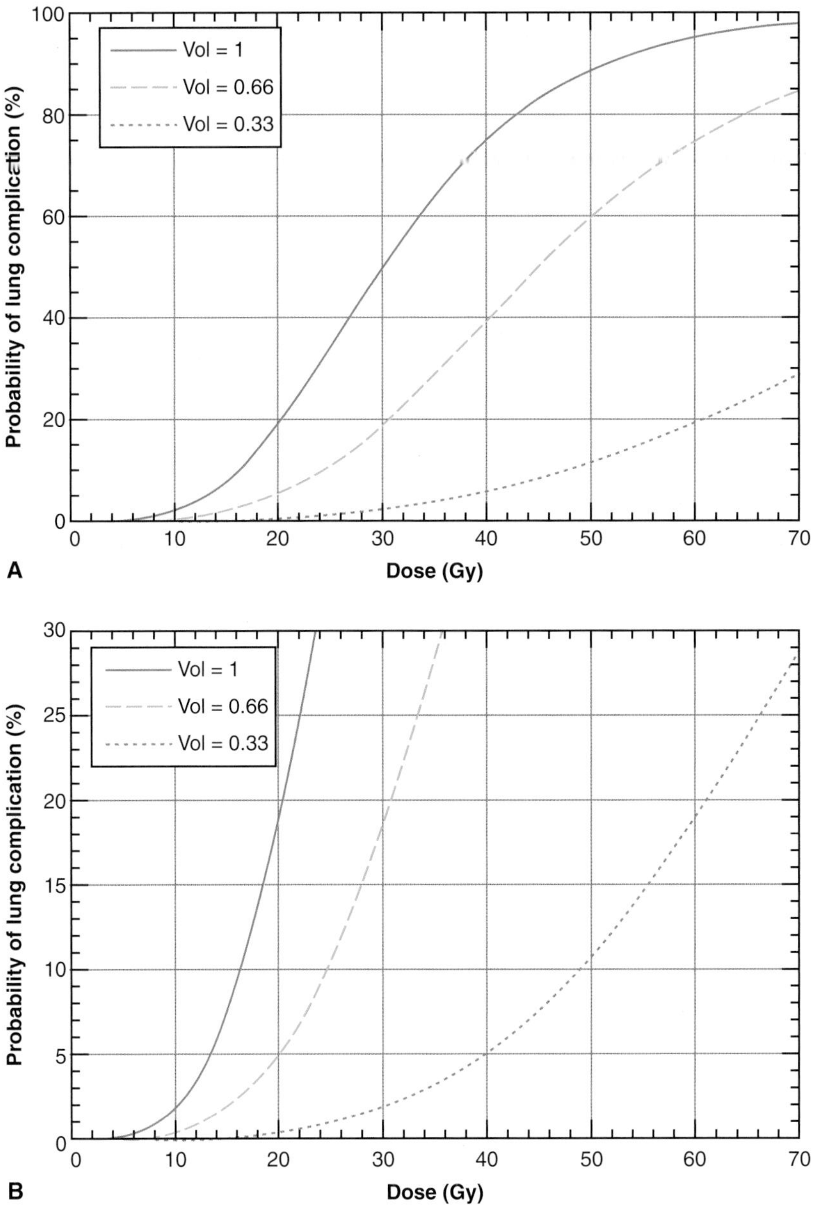

FIGURE 56.51. Probability of radiation pneumonitis versus dose. The relative lung volumes are 100%, 66%, and 33%. The curve parameters are $D_{50} = 30$ Gy, $\gamma = 1.01$, $s = 0.01$. The curve covers the probability range up to 100% **(A)**, and up to 30% (i.e., within the interval of the clinical data) **(B)**. (From Gagliardi G, Bjohle J, Lax I, et al. Radiation pneumonitis after breast cancer irradiation: analysis of the complication probability using the relative seriality model. *Int J Radiat Oncol Biol Phys* 2000;46:373–381, with permission from Elsevier.)

There have, however, been some reports of increased toxicity with external-beam radiation using the fractionation schedule of 3.85 Gy per fraction, twice daily for 10 fractions.[768,769] Longer follow-up and detailed outcomes from the ongoing NSABP/RTOG randomized trial will help to shed further light on this issue.

Again, the ongoing randomized trial will help to further define acceptability and reproducibility of 3D conformal external-beam radiation as an option for women with early-stage invasive breast cancer.

Intraoperative Accelerated Partial Breast Irradiation

APBI has been most widely employed outside of the United States.[770,771] The radiation is delivered in a single intraoperative dose to the lumpectomy site at the time of surgery, using intraoperative electrons or intraoperative photons (Fig. 56.50). Vaidya et al.[772] describe a preliminary report using a 50 kV spherical source to deliver a dose of 20 Gy at a depth of 1 cm, with acceptable toxicity. This group recently published the results of a phase III study that randomized over 2,200 women to either targeted intraoperative RT (IORT) or whole-breast irradiation.[773] At 4 years, there were six local recurrences in the IORT cohort and five in the whole-breast irradiation cohort. The 4-year estimate of local recurrence in the conserved breast was 1.2% and 0.95% in the IORT and whole-breast irradiation cohorts, respectively. There were no differences in complications between the two groups.

Veronesi et al.[770] developed an intraoperative radiation therapy (IORT) technique for a breast quadrant after the removal of the primary carcinoma using a mobile linear accelerator with a robotic arm to deliver electron beams with energies from 3 to 9 MeV. Through a Perspex applicator, the radiation is delivered directly to the mammary gland, and to spare the skin from radiation, the skin margins are stretched out of the radiation field (Fig. 56.51A,B). To protect the thoracic wall, an aluminum–lead disc is placed between the gland and the pectoralis muscle (see Fig. 56.52C). Different dose levels were tested from 10 to 21 Gy without important side effects. They estimated that a single fraction of 21 Gy is equivalent to 60 Gy delivered in 30 fractions at 2 Gy per fraction. Seventeen patients received an IORT dose of 10 to 15 Gy as a boost to external radiation therapy, whereas 86 patients received 17,

TABLE 56.39 ASTRO CONSENSUS GUIDELINES FOR SUITABILITY OF PATIENTS TO RECEIVE ACCELERTATED PARTIAL BREAST IRRADIATION OFF TRIAL

Patients "Suitable" for APBI if all Criteria Are Present	
Patient Factors	
Age (years)	≥60
BRCA1/2 mutation	Not present
Pathologic Factors	
Tumor size	≤2 cm
T stage	T1
Margins	Negative by at least 2 mm
Grade	Any
LVSI	No
ER status	Positive
Multicentricity	Unicentric only
Multifocality	Clinically unifocal with total size ≤2.0 cm
Histology	Invasive ductal or other favorable subtypes¶
Pure DCIS	Not allowed
EIC	Not allowed
Associated LCIS	Allowed
Nodal Factors	
N stage	pN0 (i⁻, i⁺)
Nodal surgery	SN Bx or ALND
Treatment Factors	
Neoadjuvant therapy	Not allowed
"Cautionary" Group: Any of These Criteria Should Invoke Caution and Concern When Considering APBI	
Patient Factors	
Age (years)	50 to 59
BRCA1/2 mutation	NA
Pathologic Factors	
Tumor size	2.1–3.0 cm
T stage	T0 or T2
Margins	Close (<2 mm)
Grade	NA
LVSI	Limited/focal
ER status	Negative
Multicentricity	NA
Multifocality	Clinically unifocal with total size 2.1–3.0 cm
Histology	Invasive lobular
Pure DCIS	≤3 cm in size
EIC	≤3 cm in size
Associated LCIS	NA
Nodal Factors	
N stage	NA
Nodal surgery	NA
Treatment Factors	
Neoadjuvant therapy	NA
Patients "Unsuitable" for APBI Outside of a Clinical Trial if any of These Criteria Are Present	
Patient Factors	
Age (years)	<50
BRCA1/2 mutation	Present
Pathologic Factors	
Tumor size	>3 cm
T stage	T3–4
Margins	Positive
Grade	NA
LVSI	Extensive
ER status	NA
Multicentricity	Present
Multifocality	If microscopically multifocal >3 cm in total size or if clinically multifocal
Histology	NA
Pure DCIS	If >3 cm in size
EIC	If >3 cm in size
Associated LCIS	NA
Nodal Factors	NA
N stage	pN1, pN2, pN3
Nodal surgery	None performed
Treatment Factors	NA
Neoadjuvant therapy	If used

APBI, accelertated partial breast irradiation; LVSI, lymphovascular space involvement; DCIS, ductal carcinoma *in situ;* EIC, extensive intraductal carcinoma; LCIS, lobular carcinoma *in situ;* SN, sentinel node; ALND, axillary lymph node dissection; NA, not applicable.

19, or 21 Gy intraoperatively as their whole treatment. The follow-up time of the 101 patients ranged from 1 to 17 months (mean, 8 months). The IORT treatment was very well accepted by all patients. The authors believe that single-dose IORT after breast resection for small mammary carcinomas may be an excellent alternative to the traditional postoperative radiation therapy. Based on these data the European Institute of Oncology has conducted a randomized trial comparing this option to whole-breast irradiation for selected patients, and results of this trial are eagerly awaited.[771]

In 2009, a task force of experts in the field of breast cancer developed a consensus statement on behalf of ASTRO on the use of APBI. They reported their recommendations on the suitability of patients receiving APBI outside the context of a clinical trial and divided patients into three categories: suitable, cautionary, and unsuitable (Table 56.39).[774,775] In general, patients ≥60 years, with node-negative, invasive ductal tumors ≤2 cm, with negative margins, ER positivity, and no lymphovascular space involvement were deemed suitable for use of APBI off trial. The task force hoped their recommendations would provide guidance regarding the use of APBI outside a clinical trial and serve as a framework to promote additional research into the optimal role of APBI in the treatment of breast cancer.

COSMETIC OUTCOMES AND SEQUELAE

Cosmesis

Surgical, radiotherapeutic, chemotherapeutic, and host factors may influence cosmetic outcome.[352] Surgical factors to be considered include extent of surgical resection, re-excision, orientation and length of the scar, closure or not of the tylectomy cavity, separate or continuous axilla–tylectomy scars, extent of the axillary dissection, and whether an ellipse of skin over the tumor was removed. Radiation therapy factors are doses to the whole breast with tangential portals, homogeneity of dose throughout the breast (use of wedge or compensating filters), use of bolus, fractionation, overall duration of therapy including breaks, type and dose of boost, beam energy, and volume treated (whether peripheral lymphatic irradiation is administered). Chemotherapy issues include cytotoxic agents used, timing and sequence relative to radiation therapy, and doses and combinations of drugs. Host factors include size and shape of the breast, age, race, compliance with care and hygiene, concurrent medical illnesses (e.g., hypertension, diabetes, CVD), and intrinsic sensitivity to radiation.

Different methods have been used to evaluate breast cosmesis after breast-conservation therapy. Some are flawed because they do not establish strict guidelines or criteria for objectively judging cosmetic outcome. Pezner et al.[776] used scales and

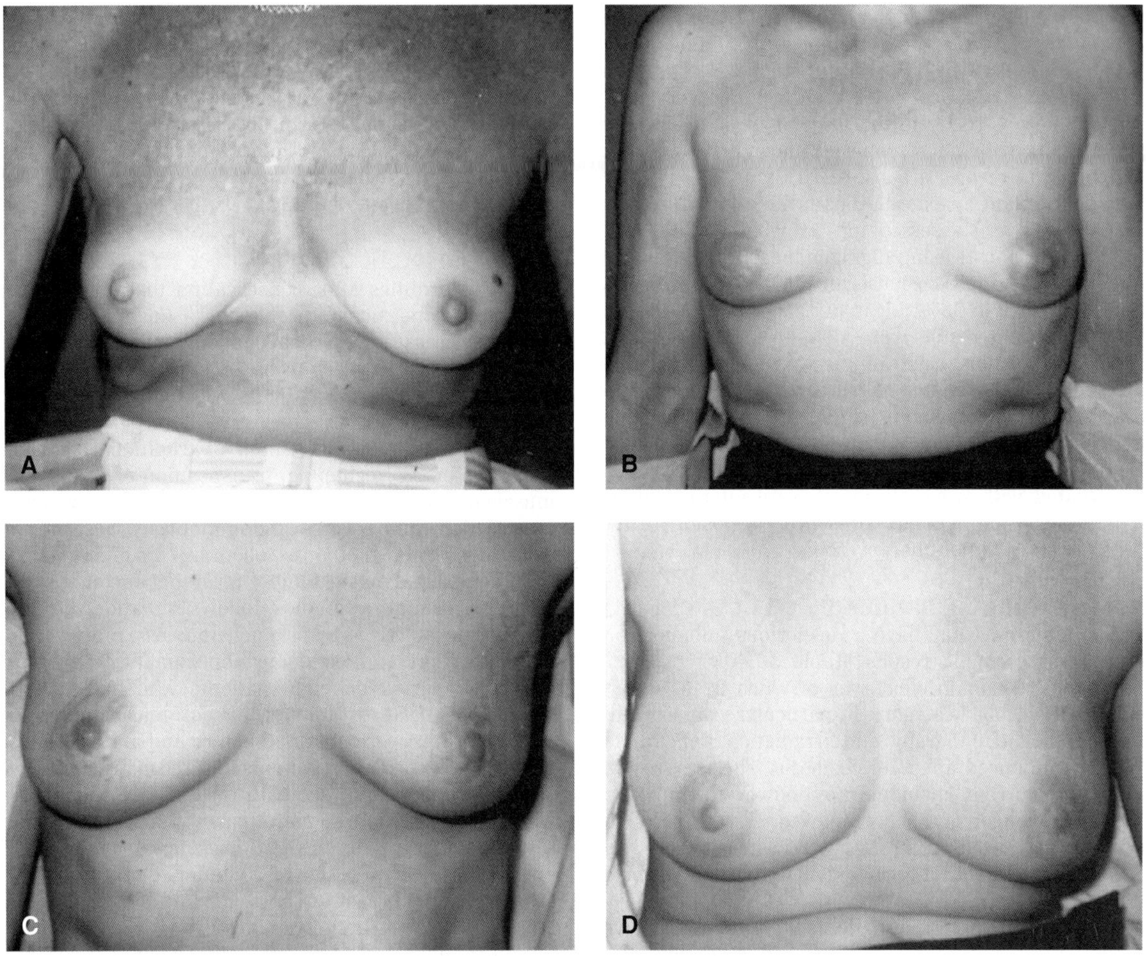

FIGURE 56.52. **A** through **D:** Photographs of patients showing excellent cosmetic results obtained with conservation surgery and irradiation for patients with T1 and T2 carcinomas of the breast. The patient in **(C)** has minimal telangiectasia in the area treated with a boost (upper region of left breast).

standard procedures for obtaining color slides to assess the cosmetic results of breast-conservation therapy and other scales designed by various investigators were given to patients for comparison. The study demonstrated that observer-based consensus of cosmetic results is difficult to obtain with two commonly used scales, but by changing the scale gradations from four to two (zero to one vs. two to three satisfactory results), consensus exceeding 85% of observers can be obtained.

A commonly employed simple scale, developed by the Harvard group, employs a 4-point scale: excellent, good, fair, and poor.[777] At Washington University, questionnaires were completed by 458 patients and their radiation oncologists at regular 6-month intervals after treatment. Cosmetic outcome analysis of these patients was done for clinical and treatment-related factors.[352] Approximately 80% of patients had excellent or good cosmesis (Fig. 56.52). Clinical factors at presentation were analyzed by age, menopausal status, race, and tumor-related parameters of size, palpable status, and location. Patients older than 60 years of age had lower excellent cosmetic scores compared with patients 60 years of age or younger. Tumor size significantly influenced cosmetic outcome, most likely related to the volume of breast removed and perhaps boost dose. Cosmetic outcome by race indicated 40% of whites had an excellent cosmetic rating, compared with only 18% for African Americans. Thirty percent of African American patients received concurrent chemotherapy or hormonal therapy with irradiation, compared with 23% of white patients. Of African American patients, 14% were obese, 17% were hypertensive, 25% had both obesity and hypertension, and 4% had diabetes.

Poorer cosmetic outcomes in African American women have also been reported by Pierce et al.[490] and Tuomokuomo and Haffty.[301] In the study by Tuomokomo and Haffty,[301] a detailed cosmetic analysis was performed on a subset of 20 African American patients and 20 white patients from the Yale database. The two groups were intentionally matched by age, follow-up, adjuvant therapy, and breast size and were asked to participate in a detailed cosmetic evaluation. With respect to overall cosmetic outcome and all specific cosmetic measures (edema, fibrosis, and pigmentation), African American patients fared more poorly than white patients. Overall cosmesis was good to excellent in 55% of African Americans, compared with 90% of whites.

Cosmesis may be affected by multiple breast and axillary surgical factors.[352] The type of breast surgery is important, with patients undergoing excisional biopsy having the highest rate of excellent cosmesis (56%) compared with wide excision (35%) or quadrantectomy (13%; $P = .0001$). Scar orientation compliance with NSABP guidelines was a significant factor, with a 44% excellent cosmetic rating compared with 27% for patients with noncompliant scar orientations ($P = .0034$). Re-excision of the primary site also resulted in a lower rate of excellent cosmesis ($P = .0002$). Breast tissue resection of >100 cm^3 was associated with lower rates of excellent or good cosmesis, independent of breast size ($P = .0001$). Similarly, a resected skin area of >20 cm^2 was correlated with a lower excellent cosmetic result ($P = .045$). Extent of axillary surgery did not significantly affect breast cosmesis.

Radiation factors affecting cosmesis included treatment volume (tangential breast fields only vs. three fields or more; $P = .034$), whole-breast dose >50 Gy ($P = .024$), total dose to the tumor site >65 Gy ($P = .06$), and optimum dose distribution created with use of compensating filters. Daily fraction size of 1.8 Gy versus 2 Gy, boost versus no boost, type of boost (brachytherapy vs. electrons), total irradiation dose, and use of bolus were not significant factors. Vrieling et al.[486] published a report of the randomized EORTC trial in which 5,318 women with early-stage breast cancer after tumorectomy were randomized to a boost of 16 Gy to the tumor bed or no further treatment. Patients with microscopically incomplete excision were randomized to receive a boost of 10 Gy or 25 or 26 Gy with interstitial implant or external-beam radiation. Cosmetic results at 3 years were assessed in 731 women (364 with boost, 367 without boost) using digitizer measurements, and displacement of the nipple cosmesis in the boost group was excellent in 33%, good in 38%, fair in 26%, and poor in 3%. In the no-boost group, the results were 42%, 44%, 13%, and 1%, respectively. The position of the nipple was the only moderately representative parameter of the overall cosmetic outcome. Other measurements had no significant correlation with cosmesis. A global assessment of the appearance of the breast was thought to be a reliable method to assess cosmetic results. Factors associated with worse cosmesis were inferior tumor location, large excision volume, presence of postoperative complications, and radiation therapy boost.

Impact of Adjuvant Chemotherapy on Cosmesis

Adjuvant chemotherapy may have a deleterious influence on excellent to good cosmetic results (Table 56.40).[328,352,777–779] In several studies, the main effect was a switch from "excellent" results to the "good" category. In particular, concomitant administration of chemotherapy and irradiation appears to have a more pronounced affect on cosmesis. The majority of studies using concurrent chemotherapy, however, employed agents that are no longer routinely employed.

Rose et al.,[777] reported on the Harvard cosmesis data and found that 68% of women not receiving chemotherapy had an excellent result at 3 years, compared with 37% who did receive chemotherapy. Conversely, 9% of patients who did not receive chemotherapy were judged to have fair or poor cosmetic results, compared with 24% of those who received chemotherapy. These differences were mostly the result of an increase in breast retraction and, to a lesser extent, development of telangiectasia.

Taylor et al.[352] also reported impaired cosmetic outcome with concurrent administration of chemoirradiation. Excellent cosmetic outcome was observed in 43% of patients receiving sequential chemotherapy, in 25% receiving concomitant chemoirradiation, and in 41% receiving no adjuvant therapy ($P = .02$). The specific effect of methotrexate on cosmetic outcome was evaluated, and the proportion of excellent cosmetic outcomes with methotrexate omitted was 41% versus 16% with methotrexate included. Good results were obtained in 23% versus 58%, fair results in 23% versus 26%, and poor results in 12% versus 0%, respectively ($P = .14$). Similarly, studies by Markiewicz et al.[560,779] and Danoff et al.[780] report no compromise of cosmesis in patients receiving concurrent chemoradiation if methotrexate was held during the radiation.

In a randomized trial of concurrent versus sequential radiation therapy, using fluorouracil, Cytoxan, and mitoxantrone, Rouesse et al.[561] also reported comparable and acceptable cosmetic outcomes, whether patients were treated with sequential or concurrent chemotherapy.

TABLE 56.40 IMPACT OF ADJUVANT CHEMOTHERAPY ON COSMESIS IN BREAST CONSERVATION THERAPY

		Good to Excellent Cosmesis (%)	
Institution (Reference)	Chemotherapy	Radiation Therapy without Chemotherapy	Radiation Therapy with Chemotherapy
Harvard University (778)	CMF, A	92	67
Palo Alto (328)	CMF	88	73
National Cancer Institute (780)	AC	80	70
University of Pennsylvania (560)	CMF ± P	89	81
Washington University (352)	CMF	81	78

CMF, cyclophosphamide, methotrexate, 5-fluorouracil; A, doxorubicin; AC, doxorubicin, cyclophosphamide; P, prednisone.

Breast Cosmetic Surgery After Irradiation

Breast deformities after conservation therapy may represent difficult reconstructive problems.[781] Correction of a locally damaged breast is a surgical challenge that can result in a fully restored breast if selection of the surgical procedure is properly carried out. In 37 patients who underwent correction of deformities after breast-conservation surgery, which included simple submuscular placement of traditional or expandable implants, breast reshaping, transposition of a latissimus dorsi muscle or musculocutaneous flap, transverse rectus abdominis muscle flap, and reverse abdominoplasty, aesthetic outcome was judged to be good or excellent in 78% of patients.

When partial mastectomy, a term that encompasses a diversity of excisional techniques, follows radiation therapy, breast defects characterized by parenchymal loss, nipple–areola complex distortion, and cutaneous abnormalities can occur. Slavin et al.[782] reported on eight patients who had reconstructive correction of an irradiated partial mastectomy deformity. Mammograms were obtained before and after the myocutaneous flap procedure. Six patients had reconstructions with latissimus dorsi flaps and two with rectus flaps. No patient underwent reconstruction sooner than 1 year after completion of radiation therapy for the entire group; a mean of 2.6 years elapsed from completion of radiation therapy to flap reconstruction of the breast. An aesthetic improvement of the partial mastectomy deformity was achieved in all eight patients. Complications consisted only of seroma formation in two patients after latissimus flap reconstruction. Mammographic evaluation revealed degeneration of the soft tissues of both types of flaps, a change that occurs as early as 6 months after operation and appears as a radiolucent area.

In a review of the MD Anderson Cancer Center experience, Kronowitz et al.[783] evaluated results of 69 patients who underwent repair of a partial mastectomy defect after radiation. They concluded that immediate repair of partial mastectomy defects with local tissues results in a lower risk of complications and better aesthetic outcomes than immediate repair of partial mastectomy defects with a latissimus dorsi flap.

Follow-Up of Patients Treated with Breast-Conservation Surgery and Irradiation

It is important to closely monitor patients treated with conservation surgery and irradiation because early detection of a local recurrence may allow for another wide local excision or a total mastectomy, without significantly compromising the overall survival of the patient.[103,222,348,750,784–786] Although the optimal interval for follow-up mammography has not been determined, a postradiation bilateral diagnostic mammogram should be obtained within the first year following radiation therapy.[156,787–789]

A careful history and physical examination are indicated every 3 to 6 months for 3 years and every 6 months for the following 2 years and annually thereafter. In patients who underwent breast-conservation therapy, a diagnostic mammogram every 6 to 12 months for the first 2 years and yearly thereafter is sufficient unless the radiologist recommends more frequent examinations.[156,788,789] Monthly breast self-examination should be emphasized to every patient, including demonstration of the examination in the upright and supine positions. At least yearly evaluation is mandatory even 10 years after therapy because of the possibility of late breast relapses and occasional distant metastases. According to the American Society of Clinical Oncology's surveillance guidelines, intensive follow-up should be limited to high-risk patients with breast cancer, especially those who enter randomized clinical trials.[790]

If there is strong evidence of suspect microcalcifications, masses, or architectural distortions of the breast after conservation surgery and irradiation, a biopsy should be obtained to rule out a recurrence. At times, these patients are difficult to evaluate. Posttreatment hematomas, fat necrosis, seromas, cysts, and scar tissue pose frequent dilemmas. Consultation with an experienced mammographer is essential.

Kollias et al.[791] in the United Kingdom evaluated 5,102 contralateral screening mammograms performed biennially on 2,511 women aged ≤70 years after treatment for primary operable breast cancer. Sixty-five metachronous contralateral breast cancers were identified: 21 (32%) at routine clinical examination, 24 (37%) at mammography, and 20 (31%) by patients between routine follow-up appointments. The prognostic features of metachronous cancers were better than or similar to those of the first cancer in 59 of 65 (91%) cases. Mammography may have contributed to the long-term survival of 16 of 26 women in whom the histologic characteristics of the first cancer predicted a good prognosis. The cancer detection rate with mammography for these women was 6.5 per 1,000 contralateral mammograms at a cost of 3,852 pounds sterling (6,108 dollars) per cancer detected, suggesting that surveillance mammography of the contralateral breast is of value in women whose first cancer predicted a favorable prognosis.

Kramer et al.[792] assessed the efficacy of contrast-enhanced dynamic MRI compared with palpation, mammography, and ultrasonography in 33 patients after breast-conservation therapy. The sensitivities for the diagnosis of local recurrences were 51% for palpation, 67% for mammography, 85% for ultrasonography, and 91% for MRI. All multicentric local recurrences were diagnosed by MRI. Mammography did not diagnose 11 local recurrences in radiodense breast, and ultrasonography was able to diagnose 8 of the 11, whereas MRI diagnosed 10 of the 11 recurrences. MRI may be useful as a complement to mammography and ultrasonography in the radiodense breast.[788]

It is important to define the cost–benefit ratio of follow-up procedures. In a controlled trial in Italy, 655 women were randomly assigned to be monitored with an intensive surveillance program including physician visits, bone scan, liver ultrasonography, chest radiography, and laboratory tests after initial treatment for breast cancer.[793] A control group of 665 women was monitored by their physicians with physical examination and only the clinically indicated tests. Both groups received a yearly mammogram. Compliance in both protocols was more than 80%. With a median follow-up of 71 months, there was no difference in overall survival between the two groups. There were 132 deaths (20%) in the intensive surveillance group and 122 deaths (18%) in the control group. Time to detection of recurrence and parameters related to quality of life were similar in both groups. Therefore, unnecessary tests are discouraged in the follow-up of patients treated for breast cancer.

Radiographic Findings After Breast-Conservation Therapy

Dershaw[156] summarized the most frequent mammographic findings: parenchymal distortion and fibrosis at the tumor excision site (secondary to surgical scar and irradiation); skin thickening, seen in 90% of patients, which may be diffuse or more prominent at the surgical excision site; and calcifications, due to fat necrosis, which are coarse and round and have radiolucent centers. Dershaw et al.[789] retrospectively reviewed the mammograms of 22 patients with local tumor recurrence that were usually associated with 10 or more calcifications (17 patients, 77%). Recurrences commonly contained very suspect patterns of calcification, with linear forms in 15 cases (68%) and pleomorphic forms in 17 cases (77%). The distribution of calcifications was usually clustered (73%, 16 of 22) or segmental (18%, 4 of 22). Recurrences were characterized as obviously malignant in 77% of cases. The remainder were indeterminate, requiring biopsy. Therefore, women without worrisome mammographic patterns need not undergo breast biopsy. If the findings are stable, mammographic follow-up is sufficient. However, a change in number or characteristic pattern warrants a biopsy to rule out recurrent tumor. Mammographic findings were correlated with clinical observations in several studies.[388,701,704,750,785,788,794–796] Most changes are observed in the first 12 months after therapy, with stabilization achieved at 12 to 36 months after completion of therapy. Breast edema is mammographically present in virtually all patients at completion of therapy, with a steady increase over 36 months and stabilization by 42 months.

Pretreatment and posttreatment mammograms were reviewed in 103 patients undergoing conservation therapy.[797] The main posttreatment findings were a diffuse increase in parenchymal density with coarse stromal pattern, some parenchymal distortion, and thickening of the skin. Changes reached a peak at 9 months and slowly resolved over the next 2 years. At 31 to 33 months, 3 of 15 patients still had dense parenchyma and 6 had skin thickening. Sixty-nine patients had fibroadenosis. Scar with retraction in the surgical area was observed on the mammograms of 71 patients. Fat necrosis was noted in two patients. During the 3-year follow-up, recurrent cancer was noted in two treated breasts, and contralateral breast cancer developed in three women.

Orel et al.[798] reported on 1,145 women with early breast cancer treated with lumpectomy and irradiation. One hundred two women with various mammographic and clinical findings later required biopsy at the treated site, and 58 had two sets of mammograms available for review (one within 3 months of the biopsy). Recurring cancer was documented in 38 (66%) of 58 patients. Thirteen (34%) of the recurrences were detected solely with mammography, and eight others were detected both mammographically and clinically. The positive predictive value for mammographic abnormalities was 72% (76% for soft tissue microcalcifications and 62% for other findings). Twenty-one recurrences (55%) were within the lumpectomy quadrant. Within the lumpectomy site, sensitivity was substantially better for physical examination (71%) than for mammography (43%). In the remaining breast outside the lumpectomy quadrant, mammography had a significantly higher sensitivity (71%) and positive predictive value (86%). The most common posttreatment findings reported by Orel et al.[798,799] and Stomper et al.[800] were calcifications alone (48%) or with a mass (29%), distortion of the breast parenchyma (20%), and inflammatory thickening of the breast skin.

Stomper et al.[800] reported on 50 of 1,600 patients with stage I or II invasive breast cancer treated with conservation surgery and irradiation on whom biopsies were performed within 4 months of a mammogram for suspected recurrence in the irradiated breast. The tumor was suspected based on mammography in only eight patients (35%), on physical examination in nine (39%), and on both in six (26%). The most common radiographic findings were calcifications with or without a mass. Histologic evidence of recurrent cancer was found in 23 of 45 (51%) biopsy specimens. Sixty-five percent of patients had recurrences at the primary site and 22% in other sites; 13% were multifocal.

MRI is increasingly used in the evaluation of patients with equivocal mammographic findings. Viehweg et al.[801] followed 207 patients with breast cancer treated with breast-conservation therapy; 40 patients were examined 0 to 12 months and 167 patients later than 12 months after radiation therapy. Suspect or indeterminate findings were suggested by clinical examination or conventional imaging in 80 studies. In 127 women, MRI was performed in breast tissue that was difficult to assess due to scarring or dense breast tissue. Recurrent carcinoma was confirmed in 27 patients by surgical biopsy. All 27 carcinomas, except for one with a slow signal increase, demonstrated early rise of signal intensity on dynamic T1-weighted, contrast-enhanced images. During the first year after therapy, the diagnostic accuracy was not improved by additional use of contrast-enhanced MRI because of strong and sometimes early and ill-circumscribed enhancement. Later than 12 months after therapy, enhancement decreased significantly and the false-positive calls could be reduced from 49 (conventional imaging) to 12 (conventional imaging plus MRI). A total of 12 of 26 recurrences and multifocality in four of five cases were diagnosed by MRI alone at this time.

Dao et al.[802] evaluated 35 women with breast carcinoma treated with conservation therapy who underwent posttreatment MRI. Nine patients had recurrent tumors, and 26 had a benign fibrotic mass confirmed at biopsy. In all cases, a localized hypointense area was present on plain spin-echo T1-weighted images. In all recurrent tumors, dynamic gadolinium-enhanced T1-weighted images demonstrated early increased signal intensity of the lesion within 3 minutes after bolus injection.

Drew et al.[803] also investigated MRI for screening for local recurrence after breast-conserving therapy. One hundred five patients were recruited for the study. Sixteen biopsies were performed and nine recurrences were confirmed histologically. The sensitivity for clinical examination, mammography, examination combined with mammography, and MRI alone for the detection of recurrent cancer were 89%, 67%, 100%, and 100%, respectively, and the specificity was 76%, 85%, 67%, and 93%. The authors concluded that when combined, clinical examination and mammography are as sensitive as MRI of the breast for the detection of locoregional recurrence, but MRI has greater specificity.

SEQUELAE OF IRRADIATION IN BREAST CANCER

The most frequent complications associated with conservation surgery plus irradiation are arm or breast edema, breast fibrosis, painful mastitis or myositis, pneumonitis, and rib fracture. Apical pulmonary fibrosis is occasionally noted when the regional lymph nodes are irradiated.[1,110,318,352,804,805]

Lymphedema and Breast Edema

Complications from axillary surgery, regardless of breast surgical procedure, have been reported by several authors. It should be emphasized that before the treatment of arm lymphedema after breast carcinoma, it is mandatory to differentiate between treatment-associated complications and tumor recurrence in the regional lymphatics.

An extensive review of the literature related to arm edema following breast surgery was conducted by Erickson et al.[806] They found that arm edema is a common complication of breast cancer therapy that can result in substantial functional impairment and psychological morbidity. The risk of arm edema increases when axillary dissection and axillary radiation therapy are used. Preventive measures have not been well studied. Nonpharmacologic treatments, such as massage and exercise, have been shown to be effective therapies for lymphedema, but the effect of pharmacologic interventions remains uncertain. They conclude that as arm edema becomes more prevalent with the increasing survival of breast cancer patients, further research is needed to evaluate the efficacy of preventive strategies and therapeutic interventions.[44]

Maunsell et al.[807] evaluated frequency of upper extremity problems from axillary surgery in 223 patients. At 3 months after surgery, 82% of patients reported at least one arm problem: swelling (24%), weakness (26%), some limitation in range of movement (32%), stiffness (40%), pain (55%), and numbness (58%). The severity of these problems changed little 15 months later. Regardless of the type of mastectomy, women who underwent axillary dissection had more problems.

Clarke et al.[403] observed breast edema in approximately 20% of patients not undergoing axillary dissection, compared with 80% of those in whom this procedure was performed. The extent of the axillary dissection (medial or lateral to the tendon of the pectoralis minor) influences the incidence of breast or arm edema, with this complication being more frequent when more extensive axillary dissections are carried out (beyond level II—middle). On the other hand, Dewar et al.[808] reported a greater incidence of upper limb sequelae in patients undergoing axillary surgery and irradiation (33.7%) or irradiation alone (26%) than in patients treated with axillary dissection only (7.2%). The most frequently noted complications were edema, impaired shoulder mobility, pain on movement, sensory or motor deficit, and pectoral muscle fibrosis.

Pain and discomfort after axillary lymph node dissection were significantly related to quality of life. Hack et al.,[809] in 220 women with breast cancer who had undergone axillary lymph node dissection, noted that 73% had sensation of pain or discomfort or the point of maximum arm–shoulder movement was different between the affected and nonaffected side. Although more than half of the patients experienced pain-related discomfort and disability, patients in general reported a good quality of life and mental health. Younger women had significantly greater pain than older women. Patients with more than 13 lymph nodes dissected and patients receiving chemotherapy reported more pain.

Sentinel node sampling appears to be associated with a much lower degree of lymphedema.[335] Sener et al.[810] reported that 9 of 303 patients (3%) who underwent only sentinel lymphadenectomy had lymphedema, compared with 20 of 117 patients (17%) who underwent sentinel lymphadenectomy combined with axillary dissection ($P < .0001$). Among 303 patients who underwent sentinel lymphadenectomy only, lymphedema developed in 8 of 155 patients (5%) who had tumors in the upper-outer quadrant and in 1 of 148 patients (0.7%) whose tumors were in other locations. The ALMANAC randomized trial also confirms lower morbidity and improved quality of life following sentinel node biopsy compared with axillary dissection.[335] Various treatment regimens have been used to treat lymphedema.[811] The compression pump, along with skin care, exercise, and compression garments, is one. A second treatment is known as *complex decongestive physiotherapy* or *complex physical therapy*. Arm care, therapeutic exercises, manual lymph node drainage, and compression bandages or garments comprise this treatment regime. Decreases in lymphedema are noted if women are compliant with the prescribed treatment program.

Brorson et al.[812] reported on 20 patients with arm lymphedema after breast cancer treatment who underwent liposuction combined with controlled compression therapy or controlled compression therapy alone. Liposuction combined with controlled compression therapy reduced arm edema volume by (median) 115% (range, 92% to 179%), whereas controlled compression therapy alone decreased arm edema volume by only 54% (range, 7% to 81%; $P = .008$).

In general the incidence of breast or arm edema after conservation therapy varies, and it is related to performance and technique of axillary dissection, whether the axillary lymph nodes were irradiated, and the dose of radiation delivered.

Skin and Breast Complications

A wide variety of symptoms may occur following radiation treatment to the conservatively treated breast. McCormick et al.[318] showed that breast swelling was the most frequently noted symptom (31% of patients), followed by muscle pain (on motion), incision site pain, and general breast discomfort (approximately 20%). Rib pain was noted by 13%. Forty-eight percent of patients reported more breast discomfort in the treated breast compared with the untreated breast during sexual activity (64 sexually active patients).

In addition to host factors such as such as CVS and diabetes, underlying genetic factors may play a role in radiation complications. Iannuzzi et al.[813] evaluated 46 patients with early-stage breast carcinoma who underwent limited surgery and breast irradiation. DNA was isolated from blood lymphocytes. Nine ataxia telangiectasis mutations were identified in six patients (eight novel and one rare). The median follow-up was 3.2 years (range, 1.3 to 19.3 years). All three of the patients (100%) who manifested grade 3 or 4 subcutaneous late sequelae possessed ataxia telangiectasis mutations, whereas only 3 of the 43 patients (7%) who did not have this form of severe toxicity harbored an ataxia telangiectasis mutation ($P = .001$).

Skin effects after postlumpectomy radiation therapy may be affected more significantly by the increase in the dose of radiation per fraction than by the total dose. Gorodetsky et al.[814] studied 110 women with breast cancer who had been treated with lumpectomies and radiation therapy and normal controls using a viscoelasticity skin analyzer. With increasing age, the viscoelasticity of the skin decreased and anisotropy increased significantly. A small but significant increase in skin stiffness was noted with radiation therapy in the range of 45 to 50 Gy given in fractions of 1.8 Gy. A dose of 50 Gy given in fractions of 2.5 Gy produced a more pronounced effect.

Pseudosclerodermatosus panniculitis is an unusual variant of panniculitis seen as a complication of radiation therapy. Carrasco et al.[815] described four women in whom this unusual entity developed on the anterior chest and abdominal skin after they received radiation therapy for either breast carcinoma or painful bone metastases from breast carcinoma. Histopathologically, the epidermis and dermis of the involved area showed little or no evidence of radiodermatitis. The main findings were in subcutaneous tissue and consisted of thickened sclerotic septa, composed of both thick and thin collagen bundles, and a lobular panniculitis characterized by lipophagic granulomas and scattered lymphocytes and plasma cells. This sequela should be distinguished from subcutaneous metastatic disease, cellulitis, or connective tissue diseases involving the subcutaneous fat.

Rayan et al.[816] reported on a randomized clinical trial of breast-conserving surgery and tamoxifen with or without radiation therapy in women 50 years of age and older treated for stage T1 or T2, node-negative breast cancer. A companion study to assess breast pain was carried out during the past 2 years of accrual to the trial, in which 86 patients participated. Forty-one received radiation therapy and tamoxifen and 45 tamoxifen alone. The median age was 70 years. Baseline pain and quality-of-life scores were similar for the two groups. At 3 months, patients receiving radiation therapy experienced more breast pain compared with those receiving tamoxifen alone, but this did not reach statistical significance. At 3 months, the pain scores for the radiation therapy and tamoxifen and tamoxifen alone groups were 2.39 and 1.83, respectively ($P = .47$). At 12 months, pain scores were lower and fairly similar in both groups, with a difference of 0.20 ($P = .71$).

Tamoxifen has been shown to induce secretion of tumor growth factor-β, which has been implicated in pathogenesis of radiation fibrosis. Li et al.,[719] in a study of 91 patients with T1 or T2 breast cancer, noted that tumor growth factor-β and the receptor–ligand complex appeared to be of clinical value in identifying patients at risk for development of postirradiation fibrosis of the breast. Wazer et al.[568] showed a trend toward decreased cosmesis in patients receiving tamoxifen. In a randomized study, pulmonary fibrosis developed in 15 of 24 (63%) women treated with 36.6 Gy in 12 fractions and tamoxifen, compared with 10 of 30 (33%) receiving irradiation alone. Also, 5 of 14 (36%) women treated with 40.9 Gy in 22 fractions and tamoxifen had lung fibrosis, compared with 2 of 16 (13%) receiving irradiation alone.[567] In contrast, Fowble et al.[817] observed no difference in cosmetic results or complications in 154 patients who received tamoxifen in combination with breast-conservation therapy compared with 337 patients who did not receive tamoxifen. The incidences of radiation pneumonitis were 0.2% and 0.3%, respectively. The sequence of tamoxifen, given concurrently or following radiation, has not been clearly shown to correlate with complications or cosmesis.[569–570,571]

Markiewicz et al.[779] analyzed complications in 1,053 women with stage I or II breast cancer treated with breast-conserving therapy. Of this group, 206 received chemotherapy alone, 141 had hormonal therapy alone, 94 had both, and 612 received no adjuvant therapy. The incidence of grade 4 or 5 arm edema (≥2 cm difference in arm circumference) was 2% without chemotherapy and 8% with chemotherapy ($P = .00002$). However, the incidence of arm edema was not affected by sequencing or type of chemotherapy; it occurred in 10% and 7% of patients with sequential or concurrent treatment, respectively, and in 8% and 18% of patients treated with CMF or CAF, respectively. The incidence of clinical pneumonitis and rib fracture was not influenced by use of chemotherapy, sequencing of drugs, or use of hormonal therapy. These authors concluded that some chemotherapy could be given concurrently with radiation therapy to the breast without significant compromise of cosmetic results or sequelae of treatment.

Hyperbaric oxygen therapy has been shown to be effective in the treatment of some late radiation sequelae. Carl et al.[818] reported on 44 patients with persistent local symptoms after breast-conserving therapy. Hyperbaric oxygen therapy (100% oxygen at 240 kPa for 90-minute sessions) was administered to 32 patients for a median of 25 sessions (range, 7 to 60 sessions). The remaining 12 patients declined hyperbaric treatment and acted as control subjects. The patients given hyperbaric oxygen therapy demonstrated a significant reduction in pain, edema, and erythema scores compared with untreated control subjects ($P < .001$). Seven of the 32 women who were treated with hyperbaric oxygen therapy were free of symptoms after treatment, whereas all 12 patients in the control group had persistent complaints. However, hyperbaric oxygen therapy did not have a significant effect on fibrosis and telangiectasia in the irradiated breast.

Brachial Plexopathy

Brachial plexus dysfunction is a possible complication of regional nodal radiation therapy. In a review of 1,624 patients, brachial plexus sequelae were observed in 1.8% of patients.[819] Pierce et al.[819] found that the incidence of brachial plexopathy was significantly higher when the axillary dose was >50 Gy ($P = .004$). However, dose alone did not determine whether radiation damage would develop in a given patient. Treatment technique (two vs. three fields; $P = .0009$) and concomitant chemotherapy were also risk factors. Other investigators have found the incidence of this complication to be ≤1%.[98,379] It is very important but difficult to distinguish between metastatic and radiation-induced brachial plexopathy.

Treatment for radiation brachial plexopathy consists of transdermal electrical nerve stimulation, dorsal column stimulators, neurolysis, and neurolysis with omentoplasty. Physical therapy, tricyclics, antiarrhythmics, anticonvulsives, nonsteroidal anti-inflammatory drugs, and steroids are helpful in therapy of both radiation-induced and metastatic brachial plexopathies.[820]

Pritchard et al.[821] used hyperbaric oxygen in 34 volunteers with radiation-induced brachial plexopathy who were randomized to hyperbaric oxygen or a control group. The hyperbaric oxygen group breathed 100% oxygen for 100 minutes in a hyperbaric chamber (30 sessions over 6 weeks). The control group breathed a gas mixture equivalent to breathing 100% oxygen at surface pressure. Normalization of the warm sensory threshold was seen in two of the patients receiving hyperbaric oxygen therapy. Two cases with marked chronic arm lymphedema reported major improvement in arm volume. These authors concluded that there is no reliable evidence to support hyperbaric oxygen therapy to slow or reverse radiation-induced brachial plexopathy, although improvements in warm sensory threshold suggest a therapeutic effect improvement in long-standing arm lymphedema and justify further investigation.

Pulmonary Sequelae

Symptomatic pneumonitis is infrequent. This clinical syndrome is noted one to several months after irradiation.[822] Patients present with dry cough (88%), shortness of breath (35%), or fever (53%), and on radiographic studies a pulmonary infiltrate is observed in the irradiated volume.[804] The risk for development of radiation pneumonitis may be related to the volume of lung irradiated.[804,823]

The addition of regional nodal radiation therapy to breast irradiation significantly increase the incidence of symptomatic pneumonitis (1% without and 4% with regional node radiation therapy; P <.001). Combined axillary dissection and nodal irradiation result in a significantly higher incidence of arm edema compared with either alone (9.5% with axillary dissection, 6.1% with radiation therapy to the axilla and supraclavicular fossa, and 31% with combined modality therapy; P <.001).[823]

Lingos et al.[804] reported on radiation pneumonitis in a retrospective review of 1,624 patients treated with conservation surgery and irradiation. Overall, pneumonitis developed in 1% of patients. No patient had late or persisting pulmonary symptoms. The incidence of radiation pneumonitis was correlated with the combined use of chemotherapy and a supraclavicular field (P = .0001). Fourteen of 17 patients who had radiation pneumonitis also had IMNs treated. When patients treated with the three-field technique received chemotherapy concurrently with irradiation, the incidence of radiation pneumonitis was 8.8% (8 of 92) compared with 1.3% (3 of 236) for those who received sequential chemotherapy and irradiation to the breast only and 0.5% (6 of 1,296) for those treated with irradiation to the breast only without chemotherapy (P = .002). In this study, the volume of lung irradiated did not correlate with the risk for development of radiation pneumonitis.

Taghian et al.,[824] in 41 patients treated with radiation therapy and paclitaxel (21 concurrent, 20 sequential), also described a higher incidence of pneumonitis (14.6%) compared with control patients irradiated and not receiving chemotherapy (1.1%; P <.0001). Burstein et al.[566] also recently reported that the concurrent use of weekly paclitaxel with radiation result in high rates of pneumonitis. However, an analysis of patients treated with radiation as a component of a randomized trial, in which 50% of the patients were treated with paclitaxel and 50% were treated with a nontaxane regimen, found that the rates of pneumonitis were very low and not significantly different between the two arms.[825]

The effect of tangential field technique on pulmonary function was reported by Lund et al.[826] in 25 patients treated with conservation surgery and irradiation. Dynamic and static lung volumes, distribution of ventilation, and gas transfer were measured before irradiation and at varying intervals up to 1 year after completion of therapy. There was a small but statistically significant decrease in the forced vital capacity and forced expired volume in 1 second 3 months after irradiation (P <.05). These changes normalized within 1 year. The reduction in total lung capacity after 3 months almost achieved statistical significance (P = .06). These slight restrictive ventilatory changes are reversible and have no clinical importance.

Radiation pneumonitis was retrospectively assessed on the basis of clinical symptoms and radiologic findings using a serial organ model by Gagliardi et al.[827] As demonstrated in Figure 56.52, a lung volume effect was relevant in the description of radiation pneumonitis. Lind et al.[828] measured pulmonary function 5 months after radiation therapy in 144 patients with node-positive stage II breast cancer. No deterioration of pulmonary function was detected among the patients who were treated with local radiation therapy. Patients undergoing locoregional radiation therapy showed a 5% mean reduction in diffusion capacity (P <.001) and a 3% mean reduction in vital capacity (P = .001).

Cardiac Sequelae

The potential for excess cardiac morbidity associated with the use of radiation therapy in breast cancer has been extensively evaluated. It has been clearly demonstrated, based on data from randomized trials, overview, and meta-analyses, that when using older techniques, excess cardiac mortality from radiation offsets some of the benefits that radiation therapy clearly produced with respect to breast cancer mortality.[70,365,829] Although the evidence from more modern trials, using techniques that minimize exposure to the normal cardiac and pulmonary structures, have reduced cardiac toxicity, the radiation oncologist must be cognizant of the potential for adverse cardiac effects of incidental irradiation, particularly in the setting of left-sided breast cancers in patients receiving other cardiotoxic therapies, including adriamycin, epirubicin, and trastuzumab.[830,831]

Earlier techniques of radiation therapy from large pools of randomized data have clearly been implicated in excess cardiac mortality. In an analysis of over 90,000 Swedish women, comparing left- to right-sided cancers, Darby et al.[832] from the Oxford group reported excess ischemic heart disease mortality more than 10 years after initial treatment in the left-sided cancer group (HR 1.13; 95% CI, 1.03 to 1.25; P = .01). The majority of cardiovascular deaths were from earlier studies using techniques that are no longer used. However, for patients treated after 1980, although the ratio was still 1.11, the confidence intervals were much larger (0.95 to 1.29), so the hazard remains uncertain for the more modern techniques.

Gyenes et al.[833] reported on the incidence of ischemic heart disease 15 to 20 years after adjuvant radiation therapy in 960 patients with breast cancer enrolled in the Stockholm Breast Cancer Trial. Of 37 long-term survivors, 20 received left-sided therapy and 17 received right-sided therapy or no therapy. Radiation therapy consisted of tangential fields for preoperative treatment and electron beam portals, which included the IMNs, for postoperative therapy (45 to 50 Gy). Evaluation consisted of echocardiography, exercise stress tests with ^{99m}Tc myocardial perfusion scan, and careful history for cardiac risk factors. Results showed that 5 of 20 (25%) patients treated with left-sided radiation had defects on ^{99m}Tc scan, compared with 0 of 17 control patients (P = .05).

Paszat et al.[834] conducted a study of 25,570 cases of invasive female breast cancer that were linked to radiation therapy records from Ontario cancer centers. Postlumpectomy radiation therapy was administered to 1,555 patients on the left side and to 1,451 on the right side. Two percent of women with left-sided radiation therapy had a fatal myocardial infarction compared with 1% of women with right-sided radiation therapy (P = .02). Adjusting for age at diagnosis, the relative risk for fatal myocardial infarction with left-sided postlumpectomy radiation therapy was 2.10.

Rutqvist et al.[835] followed 684 patients with breast cancer treated with breast-conserving surgery and radiation therapy using tangential photon fields (48 to 52 Gy in 4.5 to 5.5 weeks). The median follow-up was 9 years. In 88% of patients, the target volume involved the breast only; in the remaining patients, regional nodes were irradiated. A control group included 4,996 patients with breast cancer who underwent mastectomies without postoperative radiation therapy. Twelve patients (1.8%) in the irradiated group had myocardial infarctions and five patients (0.7%) died as a result of myocardial infarctions. The relative risk for a myocardial infarction between the irradiated group and the control group was 0.6, and the relative risk for death was 0.4. The study presents no evidence that the risk for myocardial infarction is increased with radiation therapy after breast-conserving surgery regardless of which side the tumor was located. However, because the number of myocardial infarctions in the study was small, there is no way to rule out the possibility of cardiac problems in patients with left breast carcinomas.

Shapiro et al.[830] assessed the cardiac effects in 299 patients with breast cancer prospectively randomized to receive either 5 cycles or 10 cycles of cyclophosphamide and a doxorubicin intravenous bolus every 21 days. Of the 299 patients, 122 received radiation therapy. The risk of major cardiac events (congestive heart failure, acute myocardial infarction) was assessable in 276 patients, with a median follow-up of 6 years (range, 0.5 to 19.4 years). The estimated risk of cardiac events per 100 patient-years was significantly higher for 10 cycles than for 5 cycles of chemotherapy (1.7 vs. 0.5; $P = .02$). The risk of cardiac events in the 5-cycle patients, regardless of the cardiac radiation therapy dose volume, did not differ significantly from rates of cardiac events predicted for a general female population. For patients receiving 10 cycles, the incidence of cardiac events was significantly increased (RR 3.6; $P < .00003$) compared with the general population, particularly in groups that also received moderate- and high–dose-volume cardiac radiation therapy.

Cuzick et al.[829] updated cardiac toxicity data from eight randomized trials initiated before 1975 in which radiotherapy was the randomized option and surgery was the same for both treatment arms. An initial analysis of these trials demonstrated an increased all-cause mortality rate in 10-year survivors associated with radiation, but in the update this was no longer present. The initial increase in mortality in the radiation arms was strongly influenced by the earliest trials, and more recent trials have found a nonsignificant net benefit in overall mortality associated with radiation therapy. However, an excess of cardiac deaths was apparent in both early and more recent trials ($P < .001$), but this was offset by a reduced number of deaths due to breast cancer, especially in more recent trials. Based on this it is clearly prudent to use techniques that minimize cardiac dose.

Although clinical evidence of cardiac morbidity has decreased with modern techniques, care should be taken to exclude heart from the tangential radiation field. In an analysis of 114 patients, Marks et al.[696] assessed RT-induced left ventricular perfusion defects and whether these perfusion defects are related to changes in cardiac wall motion or alterations in ejection fraction. Patients were imaged 30 to 60 minutes after injection of ^{99m}Tc sestamibi or tetrofosmin. Post-RT perfusion scans were compared with the pre-RT studies to assess for RT-induced perfusion defects as well as functional changes in wall motion and ejection fraction. The incidence of new perfusion defects 6, 12, 18, and 24 months after RT was 27%, 29%, 38%, and 42%, respectively. New defects occurred in approximately 10% to 20% and 50% to 60% of patients with <5% and >5% of their left ventricle included within the RT fields, respectively. The rates of wall motion abnormalities in patients with and without perfusion defects were 12% to 40% versus 0% to 9%. These authors note that RT causes volume-dependent perfusion defects in approximately 40% of patients within 2 years of RT, and that these perfusion defects are associated with corresponding wall-motion abnormalities. However, additional study is necessary to determine if these defects are associated with functional consequences.

Given these findings, the authors suggest the use of a heart block if needed to reduce or eliminate cardiac irradiation. CT-based 3D treatment planning is used to design such cardiac blocks and select the optimal gantry angle to minimize the need for a heart block. There may be a small amount of breast tissue underdosed if the block overlies the medial inferior breast, but this tissue is typically <5%. In situations where the heart block may underdose the high-risk volume of the breast or chest wall, an "electron patch" can be used to treat the target tissue in the shadow of the heart block. A tangential field with a heart block is demonstrated in Figure 56.33.

Although it is clearly prudent to minimize exposure of the heart during radiation therapy, using modern techniques, the available evidence does not suggest a higher incidence of cardiac mortality in left-sided radiation therapy.

Analysis of the randomized postmastectomy Danish trials, with over 10 years of follow-up, showed no excess cardiac mortality with the use of postmastectomy radiation. Hojris et al.[277] reported that the relative hazard of morbidity from ischemic heart disease among patients in the radiotherapy compared with the no-radiotherapy group was 0.86 (95% CI, 0.6 to 1.3), and that for death from ischemic heart disease was 0.84 (0.4 to 1.8). The hazard rate of morbidity from ischemic heart disease in the radiotherapy group compared with the no-radiotherapy group did not increase with time from treatment.

Patt et al.[836] analyzed data from the SEER-Medicare database for women who were diagnosed with nonmetastatic breast cancer from 1986 to 1993, had known disease laterality, underwent breast surgery, and received adjuvant radiotherapy; 8,363 patients had left-sided breast cancer and 7,907 had right-sided breast cancer. With a mean follow-up of 9.5 years (range, 0 to 15 years), there were no significant differences in patients with left- versus right-sided cancers for hospitalization for ischemic heart disease (9.9% vs. 9.7%), valvular heart disease (2.9% vs. 2.8%), conduction abnormalities (9.7% vs. 9.6%), or heart failure (9.7% vs. 9.7%). The adjusted hazard ratio for left- versus right-sided breast cancer was 1.05 (95% CI, 0.94 to 1.16) for ischemic heart disease, 1.07 (95% CI, 0.89 to 1.30) for valvular heart disease, 1.07 (95% CI, 0.96 to 1.19) for conduction abnormalities, and 1.05 (95% CI, 0.95 to 1.17) for heart failure.

Similar conclusions were reached by Nixon et al.[837] who reviewed 365 patients with 12-year follow-up who received irradiation to the left breast and 380 who received irradiation to the right breast as part of conservation therapy. Equivalent proportions from each group died of non–breast cancer causes (11%), including nine patients (2%) from each group who died from cardiac causes. Also, Vallis et al.,[838] in a retrospective review of 2,128 women treated with lumpectomy and breast irradiation with a median follow-up of 10.2 years, noted that the incidence of myocardial infarction in the study cohort was comparable with that in an age-matched general population of women in Ontario.

The potential for cardiac vessel injury from radiation was recently explored in an elegant study by Nilsson et al.[839] who analyzed radiation fields and subsequent coronary angiograms in a Swedish breast cancer cohort study. For right-sided compared with left-sided breast cancers, the odds ratio for grade 3 to 5 stenosis in arteries likely to be within the tangential radiation port was 4.38 (95% CI, 1.64 to 11.7) and was 7.22 (95% CI, 1.64 to 31.8) for grade 4 or 5 stenosis. They conclude there is an increased risk and direct link between radiation and the location of the coronary stenosis. In a related editorial Zagar and Marks[840] emphasize the potential effects of radiation on the heart but point out that improved radiation techniques, including custom blocking of the heart and other techniques to manipulate the radiation dose, are likely to minimize these risks and improve the therapeutic ratio.

Collectively, these data suggest that although there may be excess cardiac morbidity using tangential fields to treat left-sided breast cancers, these effects can be minimized through careful treatment planning. It remains prudent to minimize cardiac exposure in all patients, and particularly in those receiving left-sided radiation in combination with other potentially cardiotoxic drugs.

Risk of Stroke with Supraclavicular Radiation

For patients with node-positive disease undergoing supraclavicular radiation, there is a theoretical concern regarding the potential for development of accelerated carotid artery stenosis. In a study by Jagsi et al.,[841] rates of stroke in 820 eligible early-stage breast cancer patients treated with radiation therapy were compared with expected rates. The relation between potential risk factors and actuarial rate of first stroke was analyzed. On multivariate analysis, only age (P <.001) and hypertension (P = .003) remained significant predictors of cardiovascular accident or transient ischemic attack. Age was the only significant predictor of cardiovascular accident alone (P <.001). This study found no significant association between supraclavicular RT and stroke after controlling for other factors. This study is in agreement with the findings of the EBCTCG who reported the causes of nonbreast cancer death in 32,800 patients treated in trials of surgery with and without RT. Although the incidence of heart disease was found to be significantly greater in those women who received RT, no significant excess mortality from RT was observed due to stroke. However, a recent nested case-control study by Nilsson et al.[842] showed a significant increase in stroke (OR 1.8; 95% CI, 1.1 to 2.8) when comparing patients treated to the supraclavicular and internal mammary regions with those not treated to these regions. In addition, a study by Woodward et al.[843] of the SEER database comparing 5,281 women presumably without supraclavicular radiation with negative nodes to 482 women presumably treated to the supraclavicular region with more than four nodes did not find any increased rate of hospitalization for stroke in the treated population.

Contralateral Breast Cancer and Irradiation

Although all patients with a diagnosis of breast cancer are at increased risk for developing a contralateral breast cancer, the additional risk contributed by radiation treatment appears to be minimal, particularly when one uses modern techniques and maintains a dose to the contralateral breast that is as low as is reasonably achievable. Although this issue is often a concern raised by patients, the available data using modern radiation techniques do not suggest a significant increase of risk for contralateral breast cancers in breast cancer patients who have been irradiated, in comparison to similar cohorts of breast cancer patients who have not undergone radiation.[1,23,93,110,678,742,844,845,846,847] Although there is some evidence suggesting a slight excess risk in women who are irradiated at a relatively young age (i.e., <45 years at diagnosis), the risk is extremely small and may be related to use of older techniques, and most experts would agree that the benefit of radiation far outweighs the risk.[844] Nonetheless, it appears prudent to be aware of these potential risks and employ techniques that minimize scattered dose to the contralateral breast. As demonstrated in Table 56.41, the reported incidence of contralateral cancer in the majority of these studies of patients treated with conservative surgery and radiation do not appear to be elevated compared with those treated by mastectomy without radiation.

However, the EBCTCG overview analysis does suggest an elevated incidence of contralateral breast cancer in patients receiving radiation compared with those who did not receive radiation.[89] This overview analysis of all randomized trials comparing radiation to surgery demonstrated an increased relative risk of contralateral breast cancers of 1.18 (=.002). Although the excess risk appears to be driven primarily by older trials using antiquated techniques, these data do demonstrate the potential long-term effects of radiation-related secondary cancers and highlight the need to maintain dose to the contralateral breast as low as possible.

TABLE 56.41 INCIDENCE OF CONTRALATERAL BREAST CANCER IN CARCINOMA OF THE BREAST TREATED WITH CONSERVATION SURGERY AND IRRADIATION OR MASTECTOMY

Study (Reference)	*Conservation Therapy*	*Mastectomy*
Arriagada et al. (845)[a]	88 (14%)	91 (11%)
Broët et al. (736)	1,819 (3.8%)	1,815 (3.9%)
Clark et al. (377)	1,504 (3%)	–
Dewar et al. (380)	757 (6%)[b]	–
Hill-Keyser et al. (852)	1,801 (15.4%)[c]	–
Montague (319)	316 (1.9%)[d]	576 (5.2%)
Nielsen et al. (847)	–	No RT 1,545 (4%) RT 1,538 (5%)
Obedian et al. (23)	1,029 (10%)[e]	1,387,(10%)[e]
Recht et al. (388)	366 (9%)[f]	–
Rosen et al. (197)	– –	RT, 76(10.7%) No RT, 47 (9.4%)
Sarrazin et al. (370)	88 (9%)	91 (9%)
Veronesi et al. (102)	349 (5%)[g]	352 (5%)[g]
Hooning et al. (846)	RR 1.5[h]	RR 1.0

RT, radiation therapy.
[a]Risk at 15 years [update of Sarrazin data (862)].
[b]Actuarial relapse at 10 years.
[c]Actuarial risk at 20 years.
[d]Excludes simultaneous bilateral cancer.
[e]Actuarial risk at 15 years
[f]Actuarial risk at 5 years.
[g]Actuarial risk at 12 years.
[h]Relative risk of tangential fields increased compared to mastectomy with electron fields.

A report by Hankey et al.,[848] involving 27,175 women treated for breast cancer between 1960 and 1975, disclosed a relative risk of 1.2 to 1.4 for development of cancer in the contralateral breast in irradiated patients compared with those who did not receive irradiation. These authors, however, concluded that the data did not indicate a pattern of relative risk consistent with an increased incidence of carcinoma in the opposite breast.

Boice et al.[844] evaluated the risk of second cancers associated with radiation therapy to the breast in 41,109 women with breast cancer who were registered in the Connecticut Tumor Registry between 1935 and 1982. They reviewed the records of 655 women in whom a second breast cancer developed 5 years or longer after initial treatment and compared the radiation exposure in these patients with the exposure in 1,189 matched control patients who did not have a second cancer. The average dose to the contralateral breast in women exposed to radiation was 2.82 Gy. The relative risk for development of a second breast cancer was 1.9 in the women who received radiation therapy, and among patients who survived for 10 years or longer, the relative risk was 1.33. Women <45 years of age had a relative risk of 1.59 for development of a second breast cancer, compared with 1.01 for older women. According to these authors, younger patients should be informed that, based on the results of this study, after 10 years the risk for development of a second cancer increases from 14% if they do not receive irradiation to 22% if they choose treatment involving irradiation.

On the other hand, Levitt and Mandell[849] estimated the dose delivered to the contralateral breast to be between 1 and 4 Gy. Assuming that 20,000 women undergo radiation therapy after conservation surgery and using data on the risk for development of breast cancer after various doses of ionizing radiation, they concluded that fewer than one additional case of breast cancer would occur after 10 years. Storm et al.,[850] in a case-controlled study of a registry-based cohort of patients with breast cancer in Denmark, also concluded there was little, if any, risk of radiation-induced breast cancer associated with exposure of adult breast tissue to low-dose irradiation.

Obedian et al.[23] compared 1,029 breast cancer patients treated with conservative surgery and radiation to a cohort of 1,387 breast cancer patients who underwent surgical treatment by mastectomy and who did not receive postoperative radiation during the same time period. The median follow-up was 14.6 years for the conservatively treated group and 16 years for the mastectomy group. The 15-year risk of any second malignancy was nearly identical for both cohorts (17.5% vs. 19%, respectively). The second breast malignancy rate at 15 years was 10% for both groups. In the subset of patients ≤45 years of age at the time of treatment, the second breast and nonbreast malignancy rates at 15 years were 10% and 5% for patients undergoing breast-conserving therapy versus 7% and 4%,respectively, for patients undergoing mastectomy (probability not statistically significant).

To address whether the radiation administered may influence the development of breast cancers on the contralateral side, Khan and Haffty[851] evaluated the location of contralateral breast cancers developing after radiation. There was not a preponderance of medial lesions developing in the contralateral group (where radiation dose would be higher), suggesting that there was no cause–effect relation with respect to the prior radiation. In a study by Hill-Kayser et al.[852] the 20 year risk of contralateral breast cancer in 1801 patients treated with breast-conserving surgery and radiation was 15.4%. They also demonstrated that the distribution of location of the contralateral tumors did not appear to be influenced by the prior irradiation.

In a recent update of the Danish randomized trials of postmastectomy radiation, Nielsen et al.[741] also reported no excess risk of second malignancies in the contralateral breast in patients randomized to receive radiation. In this long-term follow-up performed among the 3,083 patients from the Danish Breast Cancer Cooperative Group 82B and 82C, randomized to postmastectomy radiation or not, there was no significant difference in the risk of contralateral breast cancers (6% RT vs. 5% no RT) between the two groups.

Hooning et al.,[846] in a study from Amsterdam of over 7,000 predominantly young women treated with or without radiation, did note an increase in contralateral breast cancer with decreasing age with tangential breast irradiation, particularly in young women with a strong family history. Of note, patients treated with mastectomy and chest wall electrons, where scattered dose to the contralateral breast was less, did not experience an increased contralateral breast cancer risk. The joint effects of tangential breast irradiation following lumpectomy and strong family history on contralateral breast cancer resulted in a hazard ratio of 3.52 (95% CI, 2.07 to 6.02; $P = .043$).

With modern technology scattered dose to the contralateral breast is lower and should minimize this issue, but care should be taken, particularly in younger women, to ensure that the dose to the contralateral breast is as low as possible.

Incidence of Other Second Malignancies

The incidence of secondary malignancies, as with the issue of contralateral breast cancer, appears to be very low, and it is evident that the appropriate use of radiation therapy far outweighs the risk of radiation induced malignancy. Nonetheless, there is some evidence, with very long-term follow-up, of higher rates of secondary cancers. Although this may be more prevalent with older techniques, it is an important component of treatment planning to minimize dose to nontarget normal tissues. In addition to the excess risk of contralateral breast cancers discussed previously, the EBCTCG overview analysis did demonstrate an excess risk of secondary cancers of the lung and esophagus as well as leukemia and sarcoma in all randomized trials of breast cancer that compared patients treated with and without radiation. The increased relative risk for each of these secondary malignancies as a function of radiation treatment for breast cancer was: lung cancer, 1.61 (± 0.18; $P = .007$); esophagus cancer, 2.06 (± 0.53; $P = .05$), leukemia, 1.71 (± 0.36; $P = .03$), and sarcoma, 2.34 (± 0.62; $P = .03$). The total relative risk for all secondary nonbreast malignancies was 1.20 (± 0.06; $P = .001$). Although the increased risk of secondary malignancies may be driven primarily by trials using older techniques, they highlight the importance of limiting dose to nontarget tissues.

Huang and Mackillop,[853] in an analysis of 194,798 women from the SEER database who were diagnosed with invasive breast carcinoma (exclusive of those with distant metastasis) between 1973 and 1995, identified 54 women in a radiation therapy cohort and 81 women in a non–radiation therapy cohort in whom soft tissue sarcoma subsequently developed. In the radiation therapy cohort, the standardized incidence ratio was 26.2 for angiosarcoma and 2.5 for other sarcomas; in the non–radiation therapy cohort, the standardized incidence ratios were 2.1 and 1.3 (95% CI, 1.0 to 1.7), respectively. The largest increase was observed in the chest wall breast. The elevated relative risk was significant even within 5 years of radiation therapy, but it reached a maximum between 5 to 10 years.

Karlsson et al.[854] quantified the risk of posttreatment sarcoma in 122,991 women with breast cancer in the Swedish Cancer Register. One-hundred and sixteen cases were found, giving a standardized incidence ratio of 1.9 per 10^4 women. The absolute risk was 1.3 per 10^4 person-years. There were 40 angiosarcomas and 76 sarcomas of other types. The sarcomas were located in the breast region or on the ipsilateral arm in 63% (67 of 106). In a case-control study, angiosarcoma correlated significantly with lymphedema of the arm (OR 0.5), but no correlation with previous irradiation was observed. However, for other histologic types of sarcomas, the risk increased linearly with the integral dose to 150 to 200 J and stabilized at higher energies. The risk was 2.4 for an energy of 50 J, approximately corresponding to the radiation of the breast after breast-conserving surgery.

More contemporary retrospective series have not reported an excess risk of secondary malignancies. However, interpretation of these series is limited by follow-up periods of less than 20 years, which may not be adequate. A study by Fowble et al.[855] evaluated nonbreast malignancies with approximately 9 years of follow-up and reported the 10-year risk of second malignancy was 16% for all cancers, 7% for contralateral breast cancer, and 8% for all second non–breast cancer malignancies. Obedian et al.[23] also reported no increased risk of second nonbreast malignancies in patients treated with conservative surgery and radiation compared with a cohort treated with mastectomy without radiation during the same time interval. The 15-year risk of a second nonbreast malignancy was 11% for the radiation group and 10% for the mastectomy group.

Galper et al.[856] analyzed the risk for development of second nonbreast malignancies in 1,884 patients with clinical stage I or II breast cancer treated with excision and radiation therapy. By 8 years of follow-up, 147 (8%) had a second nonbreast malignancy compared with the 127.7 expected from SEER. This corresponds to an absolute excess of 1% of the study population and a relative increase of 15% greater than expected from SEER ($P = .05$). Lung as a second nonbreast malignancy was observed in 33 women, 50% more than the 21.67 predicted by SEER ($P = .01$), although most of the lung malignancies occurred <5 years after treatment. Of seven sarcomas, three developed in the radiation field. Second nonbreast malignancies occurred in a substantial minority (8%) of patients treated with conservation surgery and radiation therapy. However, the absolute excess risk compared with the general population was very small (1%) and only evident after 5 years.

Ahsan and Neugut[857] reviewed SEER data in 220,806 women in whom breast cancer was diagnosed between January 1, 1973, and December 31, 1993. In women who had received radiation therapy for breast cancer, the relative risk for esophageal squamous cell carcinoma increased to 5.42 and the relative risk for esophageal adenocarcinoma increased to 4.22 10 years or more after radiation therapy. No increased risk was seen for either type of carcinoma among patients with breast cancer who did not receive radiation therapy.

The available evidence of the risk of lung cancer in patients undergoing radiation suggests that smoking and radiation may be synergistic in contributing to the risk of lung cancer. Ford et al.[858] analyzed smoking, radiation, and both exposures on lung carcinoma development in women who were treated previously for breast carcinoma in a case-control study of 280 female patients with a diagnosis of breast cancer prior to lung cancer. Smoking increased the odds of lung carcinoma in women without radiation (odds ratio 6.0; 95% CI, 3.6 to 10.1), but radiation did not increase lung carcinoma risk in nonsmoking women (OR 0.5; 95% CI, 0.3 to 1.1). Overall, the odds ratio for both radiation and smoking, compared with no radiation or smoking, was 9.0 (95% CI, 5.1 to 15.9). The authors conclude that smoking is a significant independent risk factor for lung carcinoma after breast carcinoma, but radiation alone was not. Smoking and radiation combined enhanced the effect of either alone.

Deutsch et al.,[859] in a long-term analysis of the NSABP-04 and NSABP-06 trials, suggest an excess risk of lung cancers associated with the extent of radiation. The records of all patients who developed a recurrence in the lung or a new primary lung tumor were reviewed to determine the incidence and laterality of confirmed and probable primary lung carcinoma. For the NSABP-04 trial, which employed more comprehensive radiation with larger lung volumes, there were a total of 23 subsequent confirmed and probable ipsilateral or contralateral primary lung carcinomas. In those patients who had received comprehensive postmastectomy radiotherapy, there was a statistically significant increase in the incidence of these new primary tumors ($P = .029$). With regard to the development of confirmed new primary ipsilateral lung carcinoma alone, the incidence was statistically significantly increased ($P = .013$) in those patients who had received radiotherapy as part of their treatment, and when confirmed and probable ipsilateral lung carcinomas were analyzed, there was a strong trend toward a statistically significant increase in those patients who had received radiotherapy ($P = .066$). For the NSABP-06 (mean follow-up of 19.0 years), there was a total of 30 second primary lung carcinomas but no increase in either ipsilateral or contralateral primary tumors of the lung in those patients who had received radiotherapy. They conclude that extensive postmastectomy irradiation of the chest wall and regional lymphatic node areas, with consequent exposure of a greater volume of lung to higher doses as administered in the NSABP-04 trial, compared with postlumpectomy breast irradiation in the NSABP-06 trial, was associated with an increased incidence of subsequent primary lung tumors, both ipsilateral and contralateral. Unfortunately, data regarding smoking were not available in this analysis.

Postirradiation Angiosarcoma of the Breast

Special attention should be paid to uncommon skin changes of the treated breast because clinical suspicion is the main clue to the diagnosis of postirradiation angiosarcoma. The primary therapy is simple mastectomy if wide tumor-free margins can be achieved. At this time, there is no clear indication for standard adjuvant chemotherapy or irradiation. Angiosarcomas arising in the field of radiation therapy are rare. Unlike other radiation-induced sarcomas, cutaneous angiosarcoma often occurs within a short time after irradiation. It is important to differentiate atypical vascular lesions from angiosarcoma, but currently there is no evidence that they represent a precursor to radiation-induced angiosarcoma. Deutsch and Rosenstein[860] reported an angiosarcoma arising in the breast more than 7 years after lumpectomy and breast irradiation. The initial appearance was very similar to late radiation dermatitis, and the true nature of the malignant lesion was not known for 23 months. Fineberg and Rosen[861] studied three patients with cutaneous angiosarcoma and four patients with atypical vascular lesions. All had breast-conserving surgery and axillary lymph node dissection, and six patients received conventional high-energy postoperative doses of external-beam radiation to the breast. Angiosarcoma was diagnosed 3.5, 3.7, and 5.25 years after radiation therapy. The three angiosarcomas were multifocal or diffuse and high grade, with solid cellular foci located mainly in the dermis. Two patients with angiosarcoma underwent mastectomy; one died 10 months after diagnosis with recurrent local angiosarcoma, and the other was alive and tumor free 2 months after diagnosis.

Feigenberg et al.[862] reported results of hyperfractionated radiation therapy in conjunction with surgery for angiosarcoma occurring after breast-conserving therapy in three patients. All three patients were treated initially with radical surgery for the angiosarcoma, but extensive recurrences were noted within 1 to 2 months of surgery. Because of the extremely rapid growth before and after surgery, hyperfractionated radiation therapy was used. Two of the patients underwent resection of the recurrence after radiation therapy, and neither specimen demonstrated any evidence of high-grade angiosarcoma. All three patients were alive without any recurrent disease 22, 38, and 39 months, respectively, after treatment. For previously untreated angiosarcoma, the authors recommend hyperfractionated radiation therapy followed by surgery to enhance disease control and, in recurring tumors, removing as much reirradiated tissue as possible.

Thirty-six cases of angiosarcoma after irradiation had been reported in the literature, and Edeiken et al.[863] presented two additional patients treated with breast-conserving treatment in whom angiosarcoma developed in the field of prior irradiation. Seven cases of angiosarcoma after radiation therapy for breast-conserving treatment of breast carcinoma had been reported, and the average time between the administration of radiation therapy and development of angiosarcoma was 8.6 years.

Marchal et al.[864] reported on nine breast angiosarcomas identified in a review of 18,115 patients who underwent breast-conserving treatment for carcinomas at 11 French cancer centers over a 20-year period ending in 1997. The estimated prevalence of angiosarcomas after breast-conserving therapy for carcinomas was 5 per 10,000, which is approximately the same as for primary angiosarcomas in healthy breasts. The patients had a mean age of 62.5 years when the primary breast cancer was treated and 69 years when the angiosarcoma was diagnosed. Most angiosarcomas were stage T1N0M0 and were treated with radical mastectomy; two patients underwent reirradiation, and two patients were given adjuvant chemotherapy. The median time to the median survival after diagnosis of an angiosarcoma was 15.5 months. One patient was alive without progression of disease 32 months after a salvage mastectomy and the rest had died.

In a series of 3,295 patients treated with conservative surgery and irradiation for breast cancer, Zucali et al.[865] observed three cases of soft tissue sarcoma in irradiated breasts. It appears from these collective experiences that the risk of a second primary tumor in the irradiated breast is too low to justify modification of current policies of conservation therapy of breast cancer.

A rare complication after radical mastectomy is development of lymphangiosarcoma. It is associated with the development of lymphedema in the affected extremity and occurs in approximately 5 of 1,000 patients who had radical mastectomy and survived 5 years.[866]

Cost Versus Benefit in Breast Cancer Treatment

Barlow et al.[867] compared the total medical care costs from a regional nonprofit health management organization of breast-conservation therapy versus a mastectomy 5 years after diagnosis in 1,675 women with early-stage breast cancer who had initial diagnoses between 1990 and 1997 and were 35 years of age or older. These women were classified into four groups according to treatment: mastectomy only (group 1, n = 183), mastectomy plus adjuvant therapy (group 2, n = 417), breast-conservation therapy plus radiation therapy (group 3, n = 405), and breast-conservation therapy plus radiation therapy and adjuvant therapy (group 4, n = 670). At 6 months, the costs of the treatments differed significantly (P <.001). Breast-conservation therapy was more expensive than mastectomy. At 1 year, costs still differed significantly (P <.001) but were influenced more by the use of adjuvant therapy. By 5 years, the overall cost for breast-conservation therapy was lower than for a mastectomy, presumably due to costs of reconstruction or complications of mastectomy.

Warren et al.[868] linked data of women with breast cancer from the SEER cancer registries with their Medicare claims from 1990 through 1998. Initial care costs for the 6 months after diagnosis for women who underwent breast-conservation therapy and irradiation were approximately $450 per month higher than for women with modified radical mastectomy in the continuing-care phase; costs for women undergoing breast-conserving surgery with radiation therapy were significantly less than for modified radical mastectomy cases. The two groups had similar costs in the terminal-care phase. Long-term costs for women undergoing breast-conserving therapy with radiation therapy were not statistically different from those for women undergoing modified radical mastectomy.

Liljegren et al.[869] evaluated the cost-effectiveness of radiation therapy in a prospective, randomized trial of 381 women treated with sector resection plus axillary dissection with or without radiation therapy in stage I breast cancer. After a median follow-up of 5 years, 43 local recurrences, 6 of them in the radiation therapy group, had occurred (P <.0001). No differences in regional and distant metastases or survival rate were observed. Direct medical costs as well as indirect costs, in terms of production lost during the treatment period and travel expenses, were estimated from data in the medical records and the Swedish National Insurance Registry of each patient. Taking into account the cost of primary treatment, follow-up, cost of treatment of a local recurrence, travel expenses, and indirect costs (production lost) and excluding costs for treatment of regional and distant recurrence, the cost per avoided local recurrence at 5 years was $44,438. Adjustment of quality of life showed a cost for every gained quality-adjusted life-year (QALY) to be approximately $210,526. These results stress the importance of identifying risk factors for local recurrence, a better understanding of the impact on quality of life of a local recurrence, and adding cost evaluations to clinical trials in early breast cancer.

Hayman et al.[870] performed a cost-utility analysis of electron beam boost using a Markov model. From a societal perspective, outcomes were measured in QALYs. On the basis of the Lyon trial, the electron-beam boost was assumed to reduce local recurrences by approximately 2% at 10 years but to have no impact on survival. Direct medical, time, and travel costs were considered. The electron-beam boost led to an additional cost of $2,008, an increase of 0.0065 QALY, and an incremental cost-effectiveness ratio of over $300,000 QALY. Even if patients do value a small cancer risk reduction, the mean cost-effectiveness ratio remains high, at $70,859 QALY, which is well above the commonly cited threshold for cost-effectiveness care ($50,000 QALY). The electron beam boost is cost-effective only if patients place an unexpectedly high value on the small absolute reduction in local tumor recurrences achievable with it.

The development of accelerated partial breast irradiation, with its associated reduced number of treatments, has recently been evaluated with respect to its costs by Suh et al.[571] Treatment planning and delivery utilization data were modeled for eight different breast RT techniques: (a) whole-breast radiation: 60 Gy in 30 fractions; (b) WBRT: 50 Gy in 25 fractions; (c) accelerated whole-breast radiation: 42.5 Gy in 16 fractions; (d) whole-breast IMRT: 60 Gy in 30 fractions; (e) accelerated partial breast irradiation, MammoSite: 34 Gy in 10 twice-daily fractions; (f) accelerated partial breast HDR interstitial: 34 Gy in 10 twice-daily fractions; (g) accelerated partial breast 3D-CRT: 38.5 Gy in 10 twice-daily fractions; or (h) accelerated partial breast IMRT: 38.5 Gy in 10 twice-daily fractions. Costs incurred by payer and patient (i.e., direct nonmedical costs; time and travel) were estimated and total societal costs were then calculated. The least expensive partial breast-based RT approaches were the external-beam techniques (APBI 3D-CRT, APBI-IMRT). Any reduced cost to patients for the HDR brachytherapy-based APBI regimens were overshadowed by substantial increases in cost to payers, resulting in higher total societal costs; the cost of HDR treatment delivery was primarily responsible for the increased direct medical cost. For the whole-breast–based RT approaches, treating without a boost or with accelerated whole-breast irradiation reduced total costs. Overall, accelerated whole-breast irradiation was the least costly of all the regimens, in terms of costs to society; APBI approaches, in general, were favored over whole-breast techniques when only considering costs to patients.

Psychoemotional Aspects and Quality of Life in Patients with Breast Cancer

Approximately 25% to 35% of patients diagnosed with breast cancer have significant psychosocial distress manifested by anxiety or depression and some level of sexual dysfunction. These disruptive consequences of treatment remain bothersome for at least 2 years after initial therapy. Jensen,[871] in a review of the literature studying psychosocial factors and their relation to breast cancer, revealed major methodologic problems in evaluation of the data, including small sample size, retrospective design, lack of cross-referencing for other important factors, cross-referencing studies instead of longitudinal studies, and insufficient statistical analysis. Regarding psychosocial factors, some of the most valid studies indicate that the risk of getting breast cancer may be connected with difficulties in expressing feelings, especially ones of aggression-coping strategy, amount of stress, and level of activity, which seem to be of possible influence on the prognosis. A possible connection between psyche and the immunologic system has been proposed, but there have been few data to support it.

The specific types, magnitude, and duration of emotional dysfunction of women undergoing breast-conservation therapy compared with those treated with mastectomy are highly variable, and although somewhat different, they require the attention and psychotherapeutic support of the treating physicians.[872,873] Radical surgery produces more psychoemotional disruption in terms of feelings about body image, physical attractiveness, and sexuality, whereas lumpectomy and irradiation may interfere temporarily with the patient's lifestyle and may cause worries about cancer and the perceived adverse effects of irradiation. However, at present this assumption is not supported by research findings; the fear of recurrence has been reported to be similar in women undergoing mastectomy or breast-conservation therapy.

A clinical decision analysis on the quality-adjusted life expectancy of patients with breast cancer, comparing a group treated with mastectomy and one treated with breast-conservation therapy, showed that breast-conservation therapy yields better quality-adjusted life expectancy than mastectomy. However, there are selected subgroups of patients who should preferably undergo mastectomy.[874] Lasry and Margolese,[875] in a comparison of psychological effects on some patients randomly assigned to NSABP protocol B-06, noted that patients who underwent more radical surgery did not express less fear of cancer recurrence than those treated with lumpectomy. The expected tradeoff between breast conservation and increased fear of cancer recurrence did not occur.

Body image, as a component of self-concept, was compared through mailed questionnaires sent to 257 patients treated with mastectomy, mastectomy with delayed reconstruction, mastectomy with immediate reconstruction, or conservation therapy.[876] When analysis of covariance with age was used, body image in the conservation therapy group was significantly more positive than in either the mastectomy group or the mastectomy with immediate reconstruction group. No differences in self-concept were evident among the four groups.

The advantage of breast-conservation therapy is psychological because preservation of the configuration of the body maintains the sensation of female identity and body image to a better extent than mastectomy.[371] Breast-conservation therapy does not, however, reduce the high frequency of anxiety phenomena, mental instability, and depression. Psychosocial adjustment, body image, and sexual function were retrospectively assessed in 72 women who had partial and 147 women who had total mastectomy and immediate breast reconstruction.[877,878] Questionnaires completed at a mean of 4 years after surgery (44% of questionnaires returned) showed that fewer than 20% of women reported good adjustment in the areas measured. There was no significant difference between the two groups with regard to body image, sexual attractiveness, or marital happiness. Of 184 women who answered the question, 109 (59%) believed that cancer had brought them closer to their partner, 44 (24%) saw no significant impact, and 31 (17%) believed that cancer had interfered with their relationships. There was no significant differences between the two surgery groups with regard to frequency of sexual expression, desire for sex, or actual sexual activity. Pleasure with breast caressing had decreased since cancer treatment for 44% of women with partial mastectomy and for 83% of those with mastectomy and breast reconstruction. With regard to satisfaction with appearance of the breast, there was no significant difference between the surgical groups.

Schain et al.[873] prospectively studied 142 women participating in clinical trials who were randomly assigned to undergo mastectomy or lumpectomy and radiation therapy. Baseline assessments were made before randomization and at 6, 12, and 24 months after treatment. At 6 months, patients receiving mastectomy reported significantly less control of events in their lives (P = .003) and more problems with sexual relations (P = .021) than did their conservatively treated counterparts. In addition, there were marked differences between patients receiving mastectomy and those undergoing lumpectomy or irradiation in the degree of distress over body image (P = .059 at 24 months). This study concluded that breast-conservation therapy protects a woman's perception of her body but does not, over time, contribute to more positive sexual adjustment.

Despite numerous studies of partial mastectomy and psychological morbidity in the first 24 months after surgery, little is known about the long-term psychosocial repercussions. Dorval et al.[879] assessed the effect of the type of mastectomy on psychological adjustment in 124 breast carcinoma survivors, 47 of whom underwent partial mastectomy and 77 total mastectomy, 8 years after initial treatment. Interviews were also conducted 3 and 18 months after surgery. Psychological distress was assessed using the Psychiatric Symptom Index. No statistically significant differences between partial and total mastectomy were observed with respect to long-term quality of life. Among women younger than 50 years of age, partial mastectomy appeared to be protective against distress compared with total mastectomy (P = .04). In contrast, among women 50 years of age or older, partial mastectomy was associated with higher psychological distress.

With the increasing use of adjuvant chemotherapy in younger women with early-stage breast cancer, the long-term impact on quality of life, effects of premature menopause, and changes in perceived sexual attractiveness must be given a high priority for research to improve posttreatment adjustment and satisfaction in these patients.[877,880,881] Women who received chemotherapy were more likely to worry about breast cancer recurrence (P = .001), had sex less frequently (P = .013), tended to desire sex less frequently (P = .032), and had more vaginal dryness (P <.001) and dyspareunia (P <.001). Their ability to reach orgasm through intercourse tended to be reduced (P = .043), and their sexual satisfaction was significantly poorer (P = .001). The ability to have orgasm through noncoital caressing did not differ from that of other women. There was a significant correlation between the age of the patient and the frequency of sexual desire and activity.

In two large-scale clinical trials in Switzerland, adjuvant chemotherapy had a measurable effect on health-related quality of life, but this effect was transient and minor compared with the effect of patients' adjustment and coping after diagnosis and surgery.[882]

Ganz et al.[880] conducted a survey of 864 breast cancer survivors. RAND Health Survey scores were as good or better than those of healthy, age-matched women, and the frequency of depression was similar to general population samples. Marital or partner adjustment was similar to that in normal healthy samples, and sexual functioning mirrored that of healthy, age-matched postmenopausal women. However, these breast cancer survivors reported higher rates of physical symptom (e.g., joint pains, headaches, and hot flashes) than healthy women. Sexual dysfunction occurred more frequently in women who had received chemotherapy (all ages) and in younger women who were no longer menstruating. In women 50 years of age and older, tamoxifen therapy was unrelated to sexual functioning. Clinicians should inquire about common symptoms to provide symptomatic management or counseling for these women.

Ganz et al.[881] also surveyed 1,096 women diagnosed with early-stage breast cancer between 1 and 5 years earlier in two large metropolitan centers in the United States; 356 had received tamoxifen alone, 180 chemotherapy alone, 395 chemotherapy and tamoxifen, and 265 received no adjuvant therapy. No significant differences in global quality-of-life or in depression scores were observed among the four treatment groups. The group receiving no adjuvant therapy had a physical functioning composite score that was at the mean for a normal population of healthy women, whereas those in the adjuvant treatment groups scored slightly lower. The mental health score was not significantly different among the four treatment groups and approximated scores from the normal population of healthy women. Overall, breast cancer survivors function at a high level, similar to healthy women without cancer. However, compared with survivors with no adjuvant therapy, those who received chemotherapy have significantly more sexual problems, and those treated with tamoxifen experience more vasomotor symptoms.

Nissen et al.[883] carried out a quality-of-life study in women 30 to 85 years of age with newly diagnosed breast carcinoma who underwent breast-conserving surgery (n = 103), mastectomy alone (n = 55), or mastectomy with reconstruction (n = 40). Quality of life was assessed after diagnosis (baseline) and at 1, 3, 6, 12, 18, and 24 months. Women who underwent mastectomy with reconstruction had greater mood disturbance (P = .002) and poorer well-being (P = .002) after baseline than women who had mastectomy alone, and these differences remained 18 months after surgery. The breast-conserving surgery and mastectomy-only groups did not differ significantly regarding well-being.

CONCLUSION

Radiation therapy plays an essential and critical role in the management of breast cancer, the most common cancer diagnosed in women. Early detection by mammography, followed by appropriate oncologic therapy, may be associated with reduced breast cancer mortality rates for women aged 50 years and older. After breast-conserving surgery, whole breast irradiation improves local control and survival rates in appropriately selected patients and therefore should be considered for all patients. The development of molecular signatures predictive for locoregional recurrence may revolutionize how we select patients for radiotherapy; significant progress has been made in this area with systemic therapy but similar work is needed with regard to locoregional therapies. Accelerated forms of treatment including hypofractionated whole breast irradiation and accelerated partial breast irradiation may increase the utilization rate of radiotherapy after breast-conserving surgery. Ongoing research will help to further define the safety and acceptability of these techniques in women with early stage breast cancer.

SELECTED REFERENCES

A full list of references for this chapter is available online.

5. MacMahon B. Epidemiology and the causes of breast cancer. *Int J Cancer* 2006;118(10):2373–2378.
14. Breast cancer and hormone replacement therapy: collaborative reanalysis of data from 51 epidemiological studies of 52,705 women with breast cancer and 108,411 women without breast cancer. Collaborative Group on Hormonal Factors in Breast Cancer. *Lancet* 1997;350(9084):1047–1059.
15. Rossouw JE, Anderson GL, Prentice RL, et al. Risks and benefits of estrogen plus progestin in healthy postmenopausal women: principal results From the Women's Health Initiative randomized controlled trial. *JAMA* 2002;288(3): 321–333.
21. Ready K, Arun B. Clinical assessment of breast cancer risk based on family history. *J Natl Compr Canc Netw* 2010;8(10):1148–1155.
30. Travis LB, Hill D, Dores GM, et al. Cumulative absolute breast cancer risk for young women treated for Hodgkin lymphoma. *J Natl Cancer Inst* 2005; 97(19):1428–1437.
37. Boyd NF, Dite GS, Stone J, et al. Heritability of mammographic density, a risk factor for breast cancer. *N Engl J Med* 2002;347(12):886–894.
47. Bevers TB, Anderson BO, Bonaccio E, et al. NCCN clinical practice guidelines in oncology: breast cancer screening and diagnosis. *J Natl Compr Canc Netw* 2009;7(10):1060–1096.
49. Cummings SR, Eckert S, Krueger KA, et al. The effect of raloxifene on risk of breast cancer in postmenopausal women: results from the MORE randomized trial. Multiple Outcomes of Raloxifene Evaluation. *JAMA* 1999;281(23):2189–2197.
50. Cuzick J, Forbes J, Edwards R, et al. First results from the International Breast Cancer Intervention Study (IBIS-I): a randomised prevention trial. *Lancet* 2002;360(9336):817–824.
53. Fisher B, Costantino JP, Wickerham DL, et al. Tamoxifen for prevention of breast cancer: report of the National Surgical Adjuvant Breast and Bowel Project P-1 Study. *J Natl Cancer Inst* 1998;90(18):1371–1388.
57. Hartmann LC, Schaid DJ, Woods JE, et al. Efficacy of bilateral prophylactic mastectomy in women with a family history of breast cancer. *N Engl J Med* 1999;340(2):77–84.
59. Halsted WS. The results of operations for the cure of cancer of the breast performed at Johns Hopkins Hospital from June 1889 to January 1894. *Johns Hopkins Hosp Bull* 1894;4:297.
63. Hellman S. Karnofsky Memorial Lecture. Natural history of small breast cancers. *J Clin Oncol* 1994;12(10):2229–2234.
74. Handley RS. Carcinoma of the breast. *Ann R Coll Surg Engl* 1975;57(2):59–66.
75. Veronesi U, Cascinelli N, Bufalino R, et al. Risk of internal mammary lymph node metastases and its relevance on prognosis of breast cancer patients. *Ann Surg* 1983;198(6):681–684.
87. Strom EA, Woodward WA, Katz A, et al. Clinical investigation: regional nodal failure patterns in breast cancer patients treated with mastectomy without radiotherapy. *Int J Radiat Oncol Biol Phys* 2005;63(5):1508–1513.
89. Clarke M, Collins R, Darby S, et al. Effects of radiotherapy and of differences in the extent of surgery for early breast cancer on local recurrence and 15-year survival: an overview of the randomised trials. *Lancet* 2005;366(9503):2087–2106.
90. Vinh-Hung V, Verschraegen C. Breast-conserving surgery with or without radiotherapy: pooled-analysis for risks of ipsilateral breast tumor recurrence and mortality. *J Natl Cancer Inst* 2004;96(2):115–121.
91. Huang J, Barbera L, Brouwers M, et al. Does delay in starting treatment affect the outcomes of radiotherapy? A systematic review. *J Clin Oncol* 2003;21(3):555–563.
93. Fisher B, Anderson S, Bryant J, et al. Twenty-year follow-up of a randomized trial comparing total mastectomy, lumpectomy, and lumpectomy plus irradiation for the treatment of invasive breast cancer. *N Engl J Med* 2002;347(16):1233–1241.
94. Fisher B, Anderson S, Tan-Chiu E, et al. Tamoxifen and chemotherapy for axillary node-negative, estrogen receptor-negative breast cancer: findings from National Surgical Adjuvant Breast and Bowel Project B-23. *J Clin Oncol* 2001; 19(4):931–942.
95. Fisher B, Bryant J, Dignam JJ, et al. Tamoxifen, radiation therapy, or both for prevention of ipsilateral breast tumor recurrence after lumpectomy in women with invasive breast cancers of one centimeter or less. *J Clin Oncol* 2002;20(20): 4141–4149.
101. van Dongen JA, Voogd AC, Fentiman IS, et al. Long-term results of a randomized trial comparing breast-conserving therapy with mastectomy: European Organization for Research and Treatment of Cancer 10801 trial. *J Natl Cancer Inst* 2000;92(14):1143–1150.
102. Veronesi U, Cascinelli N, Mariani L, et al. Twenty-year follow-up of a randomized study comparing breast-conserving surgery with radical mastectomy for early breast cancer. *N Engl J Med* 2002;347(16):1227–1232.
107. Darby S, McGale P, Correa C, et al. Effect of radiotherapy after breast-conserving surgery on 10-year recurrence and 15-year breast cancer death: meta-analysis of individual patient data for 10,801 women in 17 randomised trials. *Lancet* 2011;378(9804):1707–1716.
125. Tabár L, Vitak B, Chen HH, et al. The Swedish Two-County Trial twenty years later. Updated mortality results and new insights from long-term follow-up. *Radiol Clin North Am* 2000;38(4):625–651.
130. Tabar L, Vitak B, Chen TH, et al. Swedish two-county trial: impact of mammographic screening on breast cancer mortality during 3 decades. *Radiology* 2011;260(3):658–663.
132. UK Trial Group. 16-year mortality from breast cancer in the UK Trial of Early Detection of Breast Cancer. *Lancet* 1999;353(9168):1909–1914.
147. Kriege M, Brekelmans CT, Boetes C, et al. Efficacy of MRI and mammography for breast-cancer screening in women with a familial or genetic predisposition. *N Engl J Med* 2004;351(5):427–437.
148. Leach MO, Boggis CR, Dixon AK, et al. Screening with magnetic resonance imaging and mammography of a UK population at high familial risk of breast cancer: a prospective multicentre cohort study (MARIBS). *Lancet* 2005;365(9473):1769–1778.
149. Bevers TB. Ultrasound for the screening of breast cancer. *Curr Oncol Rep* 2008;10(6):527–528.
150. Berg WA, Blume JD, Cormack JB, et al. Combined screening with ultrasound and mammography vs mammography alone in women at elevated risk of breast cancer. *JAMA* 2008;299(18):2151–2163.
162. Bevers TB, Anderson BO, Bonaccio E, et al. Breast cancer screening and diagnosis. *J Natl Compr Canc Netw* 2006;4(5):480–508.
168. Carlson RW, Allred DC, Anderson BO, et al. Invasive breast cancer. *J Natl Compr Canc Netw* 2011;9(2):136–222.
169. Carlson RW, Allred DC, Anderson BO, et al. Breast cancer. Clinical practice guidelines in oncology. *J Natl Compr Canc Netw* 2009;7(2):122–192.
224. Recht A, Edge SB, Solin LJ, et al. Postmastectomy radiotherapy: clinical practice guidelines of the American Society of Clinical Oncology. *J Clin Oncol* 2001; 19(5):1539–1569.
236. Krag DN, Julian TB, Harlow SP, et al. NSABP-32: phase III, randomized trial comparing axillary resection with sentinel lymph node dissection: a description of the trial. *Ann Surg Oncol* 2004;11(3 Suppl):208S–210S.
237. Giuliano AE, Hunt KK, Ballman KV, et al. Axillary dissection vs no axillary dissection in women with invasive breast cancer and sentinel node metastasis: a randomized clinical trial. *JAMA* 9 2011;305(6):569–575.
238. Haffty BG, Hunt KK, Harris JR, et al. Positive sentinel nodes without axillary dissection: implications for the radiation oncologist. *J Clin Oncol* 2011;29(34): 4479–4481.
274. Romond EH, Perez EA, Bryant J, et al. Trastuzumab plus adjuvant chemotherapy for operable HER2-positive breast cancer. *N Engl J Med* 2005;353(16):1673–1684.
284. van't Veer LJ, Paik S, Hayes DF. Gene expression profiling of breast cancer: a new tumor marker. *J Clin Oncol* 2005;23(8):1631–1635.
286. Perou CM, Sorlie T, Eisen MB, et al. Molecular portraits of human breast tumours. *Nature* 2000;406(6797):747–752.
289. Paik S, Shak S, Tang G, et al. A multigene assay to predict recurrence of tamoxifen-treated, node-negative breast cancer. *N Engl J Med* 2004;351(27):2817–2826.
327. Recht A, Houlihan MJ. Axillary lymph nodes and breast cancer: a review. *Cancer* 1995;76(9):1491–1512.
331. Fisher B, Jeong JH, Anderson S, et al. Twenty-five-year follow-up of a randomized trial comparing radical mastectomy, total mastectomy, and total mastectomy followed by irradiation. *N Engl J Med* 2002;347(8):567–575.
335. Mansel RE, Fallowfield L, Kissin M, et al. Randomized multicenter trial of sentinel node biopsy versus standard axillary treatment in operable breast cancer: the ALMANAC Trial. *J Natl Cancer Inst* 2006;98(9):599–609.
337. Krag D, Weaver D, Ashikaga T, et al. The sentinel node in breast cancer—a multicenter validation study. *N Engl J Med* 1998;339(14):941–946.
342. Veronesi U, Paganelli G, Viale G, et al. A randomized comparison of sentinel-node biopsy with routine axillary dissection in breast cancer. *N Engl J Med* 2003; 349(6):546–553.
347. Goldhirsch A, Wood WC, Coates AS, et al. Strategies for subtypes—dealing with the diversity of breast cancer: highlights of the St. Gallen International Expert Consensus on the Primary Therapy of Early Breast Cancer 2011. *Ann Oncol* 2011; 22(8):1736–1747.
349. Arthur DW, Vicini FA, Kuske RR, et al. Accelerated partial breast irradiation: an updated report from the American Brachytherapy Society. *Brachytherapy* 2003;2(2):124–130.
354. Chen AM, Meric-Bernstam F, Hunt KK, et al. Breast conservation after neoadjuvant chemotherapy: the MD Anderson cancer center experience. *J Clin Oncol* 2004;22(12):2303–2312.
362. van Dongen JA, Bartelink H, Fentiman IS, et al. Randomized clinical trial to assess the value of breast-conserving therapy in stage I and II breast cancer, EORTC 10801 trial. *J Natl Cancer Inst Monogr* 1992(11):15–18.
373. Poggi MM, Danforth DN, Sciuto LC, et al. Eighteen-year results in the treatment of early breast carcinoma with mastectomy versus breast conservation therapy: the National Cancer Institute Randomized Trial. *Cancer* 2003;98(4):697–702.
404. Bartelink H, Horiot JC, Poortmans P, et al. Recurrence rates after treatment of breast cancer with standard radiotherapy with or without additional radiation. *N Engl J Med* 2001;345(19):1378–1387.
427. van der Leest M, Evers L, van der Sangen MJ, et al. The safety of breast-conserving therapy in patients with breast cancer aged < or = 40 years. *Cancer* 2007;109(10):1957–1964.
432. Kiess AP, McArthur HL, Mahoney K, et al. Adjuvant trastuzumab reduces locoregional recurrence in women who receive breast-conservation therapy for lymph node-negative, human epidermal growth factor receptor 2-positive breast cancer. *Cancer* 2012;118(8):1982–1988.
491. Haffty BG, Yang Q, Reiss M, et al. Locoregional relapse and distant metastasis in conservatively managed triple negative early-stage breast cancer. *J Clin Oncol* 2006;24(36):5652–5657.
492. Nguyen PL, Taghian AG, Katz MS, et al. Breast cancer subtype approximated by estrogen receptor, progesterone receptor, and HER-2 is associated with local and distant recurrence after breast-conserving therapy. *J Clin Oncol* 2008; 26(14):2373–2378.
493. Voduc KD, Cheang MC, Tyldesley S, et al. Breast cancer subtypes and the risk of local and regional relapse. *J Clin Oncol* 2010;28(10):1684–1691.
494. Abdulkarim BS, Cuartero J, Hanson J, et al. Increased risk of locoregional recurrence for women with T1-2N0 triple-negative breast cancer treated with modified radical mastectomy without adjuvant radiation therapy compared with breast-conserving therapy. *J Clin Oncol* 2011;29(21):2852–2858.
496. Mamounas EP, Tang G, Fisher B, et al. Association Between the 21-gene recurrence score assay and risk of locoregional recurrence in node-negative,

Clinical Radiation Oncology

estrogen receptor-positive breast cancer: results from NSABP B-14 and NSABP B-20. *J Clin Oncol* 2010;28(10):1677–1683.
500. Liljegren G, Holmberg L, Adami HO, et al. Sector resection with or without postoperative radiotherapy for stage I breast cancer: five-year results of a randomized trial. Uppsala-Orebro Breast Cancer Study Group. *J Natl Cancer Inst* 1994;86(9):717–722.
501. Veronesi U, Marubini E, Mariani L, et al. Radiotherapy after breast-conserving surgery in small breast carcinoma: long-term results of a randomized trial. *Ann Oncol* 2001;12(7):997–1003.
502. Winzer KJ, Sauer R, Sauerbrei W, et al. Radiation therapy after breast-conserving surgery; first results of a randomised clinical trial in patients with low risk of recurrence. *Eur J Cancer* 2004;40(7):998–1005.
503. Whelan T, Clark R, Roberts R, et al. Ipsilateral breast tumor recurrence postlumpectomy is predictive of subsequent mortality: results from a randomized trial. Investigators of the Ontario Clinical Oncology Group. *Int J Radiat Oncol Biol Phys* 1994;30(1):11–16.
506. Lim M, Bellon JR, Gelman R, et al. A prospective study of conservative surgery without radiation therapy in select patients with stage I breast cancer. *Int J Radiat Oncol Biol Phys* 2006;65(4):1149–1154.
511. Fyles AW, McCready DR, Manchul LA, et al. Tamoxifen with or without breast irradiation in women 50 years of age or older with early breast cancer. *N Engl J Med* 2004;351(10):963–970.
512. Smith BD, Gross CP, Smith GL, et al. Effectiveness of radiation therapy for older women with early breast cancer. *J Natl Cancer Inst* 2006;98(10):681–690.
513. Bentzen SM, Agrawal RK, Aird EG, et al. The UK Standardisation of Breast Radiotherapy (START) Trial A of radiotherapy hypofractionation for treatment of early breast cancer: a randomised trial. *Lancet Oncol* 2008;9(4):331–341.
514. Bentzen SM, Agrawal RK, Aird EG, et al. The UK Standardisation of Breast Radiotherapy (START) Trial B of radiotherapy hypofractionation for treatment of early breast cancer: a randomised trial. *Lancet* 2008;371(9618):1098–1107.
515. Whelan TJ, Pignol JP, Levine MN, et al. Long-term results of hypofractionated radiation therapy for breast cancer. *N Engl J Med* 2010;362(6):513–520.
517. Smith BD, Bentzen S, Correa C, et al. Fractionation for whole breast irradiation: an American Society for Radiation Oncology (ASTRO) evidence-based guideline. *Int J Radiation Oncol Biol Phys* 2011;81(1):59–68.
520. Schlembach PJ, Buchholz TA, Ross MI, et al. Relationship of sentinel and axillary level I–II lymph nodes to tangential fields used in breast irradiation. *Int J Radiat Oncol Biol Phys* 2001;51(3):671–678.
532. Louis-Sylvestre C, Clough K, Asselain B, et al. Axillary treatment in conservative management of operable breast cancer: dissection or radiotherapy? Results of a randomized study with 15 years of follow-up. *J Clin Oncol* 2004;22(1):97–101.
537. Veronesi U, Orecchia R, Zurrida S, et al. Avoiding axillary dissection in breast cancer surgery: a randomized trial to assess the role of axillary radiotherapy. *Ann Oncol* 2005;16(3):383–388.
544. Whelan T. NCIC CTG MA.20: an intergroup trial of regional nodal irradiation in early breast cancer. *J Clin Oncol* 2011;9(Suppl):(abstr LBA1003).
555. Bellon JR, Come SE, Gelman RS, et al. Sequencing of chemotherapy and radiation therapy in early-stage breast cancer: updated results of a prospective randomized trial. *J Clin Oncol* 2005;23(9):1934–1940.
563. Toledano A, Garaud P, Serin D, et al. Concurrent administration of adjuvant chemotherapy and radiotherapy after breast-conserving surgery enhances late toxicities: long-term results of the ARCOSEIN multicenter randomized study. *Int J Radiat Oncol Biol Phys* 2006;65(2):324–332.
569. Ahn PH, Vu HT, Lannin D, et al. Sequence of radiotherapy with tamoxifen in conservatively managed breast cancer does not affect local relapse rates. *J Clin Oncol* 2005;23(1):17–23.
570. Harris EE, Christensen VJ, Hwang WT, et al. Impact of concurrent versus sequential tamoxifen with radiation therapy in early-stage breast cancer patients undergoing breast conservation treatment. *J Clin Oncol* 2005;23(1):11–16.
573. Azria D, Belkacemi Y, Romieu G, et al. Concurrent or sequential adjuvant letrozole and radiotherapy after conservative surgery for early-stage breast cancer (CO-HO-RT): a phase 2 randomised trial. *Lancet Oncol* 2010;11(3):258–265.
581. Robson ME, Chappuis PO, Satagopan J, et al. A combined analysis of outcome following breast cancer: differences in survival based on BRCA1/BRCA2 mutation status and administration of adjuvant treatment. *Breast Cancer Res* 2004;6(1):R8–R17.
582. Seynaeve C, Verhoog LC, Van De Bosch LM, et al. Ipsilateral breast tumour recurrence in hereditary breast cancer following breast-conserving therapy. *Eur J Cancer* 2004;40(8):1150–1158.
589. Haffty BG, Harrold E, Khan AJ, et al. Outcome of conservatively managed early-onset breast cancer by BRCA1/2 status. *Lancet* 2002;359(9316):1471–1477.
592. Pierce LJ, Levin AM, Rebbeck TR, et al. Ten-year multi-institutional results of breast-conserving surgery and radiotherapy in BRCA1/2-associated stage I/II breast cancer. *J Clin Oncol* 2006;24(16):2437–2443.
593. Pierce LJ, Phillips KA, Griffith KA, et al. Local therapy in BRCA1 and BRCA2 mutation carriers with operable breast cancer: comparison of breast conservation and mastectomy. *Breast Cancer Res Treat* 2010;121(2):389–398.
643. Hancock SL, Tucker MA, Hoppe RT. Breast cancer after treatment of Hodgkin's disease. *J Natl Cancer Inst* 1993;85(1):25–31.
650. Travis LB, Hill DA, Dores GM, et al. Breast cancer following radiotherapy and chemotherapy among young women with Hodgkin disease. *JAMA* 2003;290(4):465–475.
663. Arthur DW, Vicini FA. Accelerated partial breast irradiation as a part of breast conservation therapy. *J Clin Oncol* 2005;23(8):1726–1735.
675. Recht A. Radiotherapy and surgery in early breast cancer. *N Engl J Med* 1996;334(15):989.
705. Romestaing P, Lehingue Y, Carrie C, et al. Role of a 10-Gy boost in the conservative treatment of early breast cancer: results of a randomized clinical trial in Lyon, France. *J Clin Oncol* 1997;15(3):963–968.
742. Nielsen HM, Overgaard M, Grau C, et al. Study of failure pattern among high-risk breast cancer patients with or without postmastectomy radiotherapy in addition to adjuvant systemic therapy: long-term results from the Danish Breast Cancer Cooperative Group DBCG 82 B and C randomized studies. *J Clin Oncol* 2006;24(15):2268–2275.
746. Pignol J. A multicentre randomized trial of breast IMRT to reduce acute radiation dermatitis. *J Clin Oncol* 2008;26(13):2085–2092.
748. Donovan E, Bleakley N, Denholm E, et al. Randomised trial of standard 2D radiotherapy (RT) versus intensity modulated radiotherapy (IMRT) in patients prescribed breast radiotherapy. *Radiother Oncol* 2007;82(3):254–264.
768. Jagsi R, Ben-David MA, Moran JM, et al. Unacceptable cosmesis in a protocol investigating intensity-modulated radiotherapy with active breathing control for accelerated partial-breast irradiation. *Int J Radiat Oncol Biol Phys* 2010;76(1):71–78.
769. Hepel JT, Tokita M, MacAusland SG, et al. Toxicity of three-dimensional conformal radiotherapy for accelerated partial breast irradiation. *Int J Radiat Oncol Biol Phys* 2009;75(5):1290–1296.
774. Smith BD, Arthur DW, Buchholz TA, et al. Accelerated partial breast irradiation consensus statement from the American Society for Radiation Oncology (ASTRO). *J Am Coll Surg* 2009;209(2):269–277.
790. American Society of Clinical Oncology. Recommended breast cancer surveillance guidelines. *J Clin Oncol* 1997;15:2149–2156.
824. Taghian AG, Assaad SI, Niemierko A, et al. Risk of pneumonitis in breast cancer patients treated with radiation therapy and combination chemotherapy with paclitaxel. *J Natl Cancer Inst* 2001;93(23):1806–1811.
839. Nilsson G, Holmberg L, Garmo H, et al. Distribution of coronary artery stenosis after radiation for breast cancer. *J Clin Oncol* 2012;30(4):380–386.
841. Jagsi R, Griffith KA, Koelling T, et al. Stroke rates and risk factors in patients treated with radiation therapy for early-stage breast cancer. *J Clin Oncol* 2006;24(18):2779–2785.
842. Nilsson G, Holmberg L, Garmo H, et al. Radiation to supraclavicular and internal mammary lymph nodes in breast cancer increases the risk of stroke. *Br J Cancer* 2009;100(5):811–816.
844. Boice JD Jr, Harvey EB, Blettner M, et al. Cancer in the contralateral breast after radiotherapy for breast cancer. *N Engl J Med* 1992;326(12):781–785.
846. Hooning MJ, Aleman BM, Hauptmann M, et al. Roles of radiotherapy and chemotherapy in the development of contralateral breast cancer. *J Clin Oncol* 2008;26(34):5561–5568.
870. Hayman JA, Hillner BE, Harris JR, et al. Cost-effectiveness of adding an electron-beam boost to tangential radiation therapy in patients with negative margins after conservative surgery for early-stage breast cancer. *J Clin Oncol* 2000;18(2):287–295.

Chapter 57
Breast Cancer: Locally Advanced and Recurrent Disease, Postmastectomy Radiation, Systemic Therapies

Thomas A. Buchholz, David E. Wazer, and Bruce G. Haffty

Patients who present with locally advanced breast cancer require care from a multidisciplinary team that incorporates diagnostic imaging, chemotherapy, surgery, and careful pathology assessment, including molecular-based studies, radiation, and, if indicated, biologic and hormonal therapies. The treatment outcome for an individual patient may depend on the degree to which this multidisciplinary approach is integrated and the expertise of the treatment team. The input and coordination from each multidisciplinary discipline is especially important in the management of patients with locally advanced disease because such patients have the highest risk of disease recurrence without optimal treatment and require the most complex decision making.

Fortunately, the outcome for patients with locally advanced breast cancer has improved dramatically. Before the routine use of chemotherapy, patients treated with mastectomy, radiation, or a combination of the two had high rates of distant metastases and death.[1–2,3] The introduction of adjuvant and neoadjuvant chemotherapy and hormone therapy regimens has significantly improved the prognosis. Furthermore, new systemic regimens and introduction of biologic therapies have offered additional improvements and further increased the importance of local-regional disease eradication.

This chapter focuses on the management of locally advanced breast cancer, with a focus on local-regional control and radiation therapy. There is no consensus on the definition of "locally advanced breast cancer," but most commonly this term refers to stage III disease, meaning advanced primary or nodal disease without clinically evident systemic metastases. In addition to reviewing management strategies for stage III breast cancer, this chapter also reviews the role of postmastectomy radiation and systemic treatments for patients with all stages of invasive breast cancer. Management and outcome of locally recurrent breast cancer and selected unusual presentations of breast cancers are also discussed.

EPIDEMIOLOGY OF LOCALLY ADVANCED BREAST CANCER

Between 1980 and 1987, the incidence of breast cancer increased by approximately 4% each year, in part because of the increase in use of screening mammography. Between 1987 and 1994 the incidence was constant and then increased again at a 1.6% rate up until 1999, after which time breast cancer incidence has decreased by 2% per year.[4] Between 1988 and 2000 there was a steady increase in tumors diagnosed at a size of 2.0 cm or less, but since 2000 this incidence rate has decreased by 3.3% per year, and the rate of tumors of >5.0 cm has increased by 2% per year since 1992.[4] A few reasons undoubtedly contributed to the decline in the percentage of cases of locally advanced disease at diagnosis during the late 1980s. First, mammographic screening resulted in a larger proportion of patients being diagnosed with earlier disease stages. A second important contribution was women's health initiatives and public education efforts that prompted women to seek medical care at the first sign of a breast mass. Finally, the medical community has become better educated about appropriate standards for evaluating a breast mass.

Table 57.1 gives estimates of the percentage of breast cancers diagnosed as T3 disease or with lymph node involvement according to data from the Surveillance, Epidemiology and End Results (SEER) Program, as reported by the American Cancer Society. Estimates indicate that 230,480 new cases of invasive breast cancer will be diagnosed in 2011.[5] Using the percentages in Table 57.1 would yield an estimated 16,134 new cases with primary tumors of >5.0 cm and 69,144 new cases with lymph node–positive disease at diagnosis.

Table 57.1 also includes data concerning the distribution of disease in Whites and in African Americans. African-American women with breast cancer more commonly present with advanced primary disease and lymph node–positive disease than do White women with breast cancer.[4] This has been explained on the basis of both socioeconomic factors and biology. Specifically, African-American women with breast cancer reportedly have less access to medical care and undergo screening mammography less often than do White women. African-American women also more often have breast cancers that are of higher nuclear grade and more frequently have estrogen receptor (ER)-negative disease compared with white women.[6,7]

Inflammatory breast cancer is an important subcategory of locally advanced breast cancer that has a unique epidemiology, presentation, and biology. Inflammatory breast cancers are rare, accounting for only 2% of all breast cancers in the United States.[8] Estimates indicate that approximately 4,000 cases of inflammatory breast cancer would be diagnosed in the United States in 2010. During the 1990 s, the incidence of inflammatory breast cancer increased slightly. No known risk factors have been identified that are unique for the development of this form of breast cancer. However, the disease tends to occur in a younger population than does noninflammatory breast cancer. The proportion of African-American women with breast cancer diagnosed with inflammatory breast cancer is higher than the proportion of White women with breast cancer. Lymph node involvement at the time of diagnosis is much more common in patients with inflammatory breast cancer than in those with noninflammatory breast cancer, and it is more common for patients with inflammatory breast cancer to have distant metastases at diagnosis.[8]

TABLE 57.1 ESTIMATES OF BREAST CANCER EXTENT OF DISEASE AT DIAGNOSIS FOR 2005–2006

	All Races (%)	White (%)	African American (%)
Tumor ≤2.0 cm	64	66	52
Tumor 2.1–5.0 cm	29	28	36
Tumor >5.0 cm	7	6	12
Lymph node–negative	64	65	55
Lymph node–positive	30	30	35
Distant metastasis	6	5	10

Percentages are calculated from the respective incidence values provided from Figure 5 of American Cancer Society. *Breast cancer facts and figures 2009–2010.* Atlanta, GA: Author, 2009.

NATURAL HISTORY

Natural History of Locally Advanced Breast Cancer

The outcomes of patients who present with locally advanced breast cancer were once poor, but improvements in treatments have changed the prognosis considerably. Currently, many patients with locally advanced disease can be cured. As the disease grows within the breast, the tumor may infiltrate or invade the dermis or the chest wall. Skin retraction may occur because of tumor invasion of Cooper's ligaments, although this process can also be present in early-stage disease. Tumor growth can also lead to infiltration or obstruction of the lymphatic drainage of the breast and breast skin, causing edema of the breast, known as peau d'orange. In addition, primary tumor growth increases the risk of spread through the lymphatics to involve regional lymph nodes and/or spread hematogenously to involve distant sites such as the liver, lung, bone, and brain.

Most advanced primary tumors are associated with axillary lymph node involvement at the time of diagnosis. The axillary lymph node region is divided into three levels, defined according to their relationship to the pectoralis minor muscle: level I lymph nodes are inferolateral to the muscle, level II are beneath the muscle, and level III are superomedial to the pectoralis muscle (these lymph nodes are also called infraclavicular lymph nodes). Additional lymph nodes that may be involved in locally advanced breast cancer include Rotter's nodes, which are located between the pectoralis minor and pectoralis major muscles, and the supraclavicular and internal mammary lymph nodes. Figure 57.1 shows computed tomography (CT) scans from patients with locally advanced breast cancer presenting with involvement of the level II axilla (Fig. 57.1A), an infraclavicular lymph node (Fig. 57.1B), a Rotter's lymph node (Fig. 57.1C), and an internal mammary lymph node (Fig. 57.1D).

The clinical course of locally advanced breast cancer depends on several factors, including the specific disease characteristics at presentation, the biologic features of the disease, and the treatment given. Without treatment, almost all locally advanced breast cancers eventually metastasize to visceral organs and become life-threatening.[1,2] Local disease progression can lead to ulceration of the breast skin, pain, bleeding,

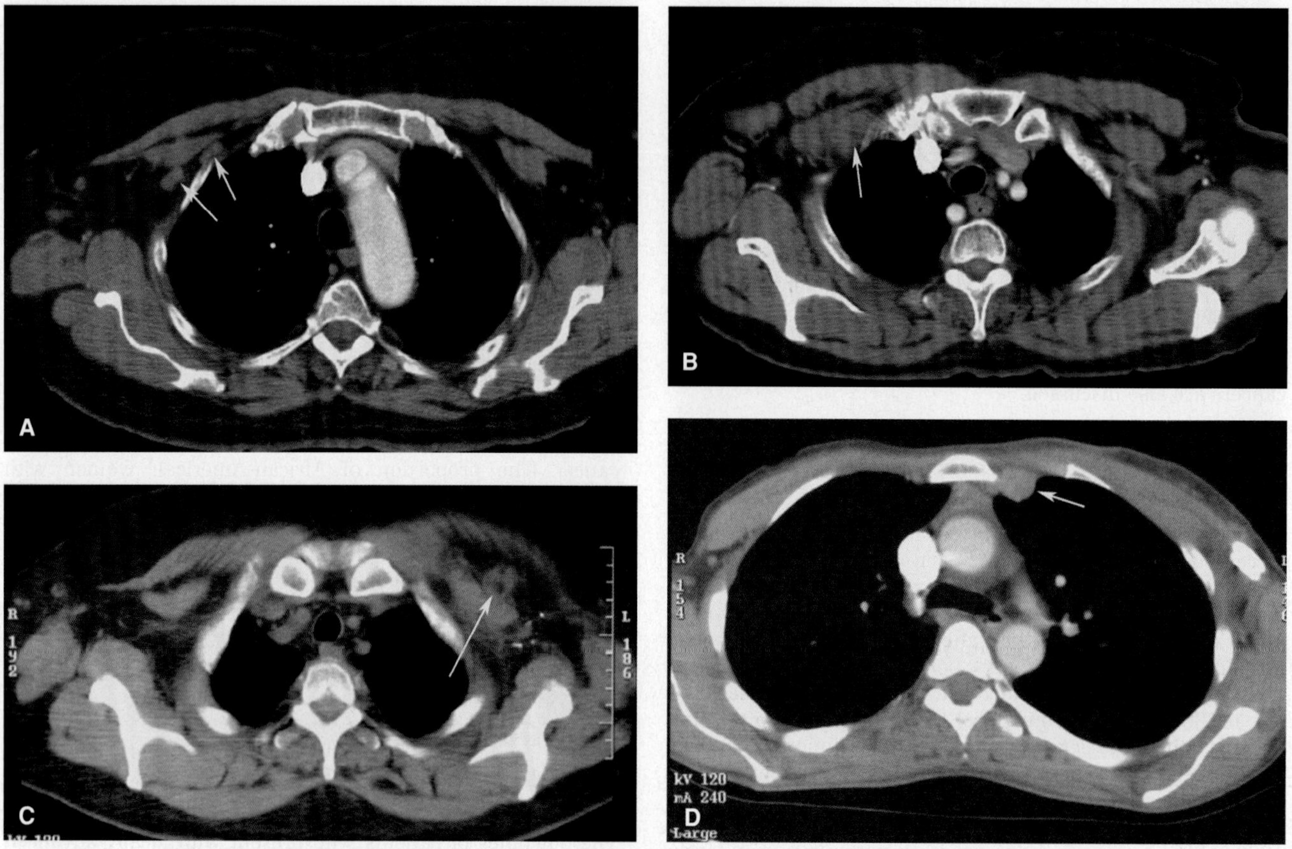

FIGURE 57.1. Computed tomography images of patients with lymph node involvement at the time of diagnosis. **A:** Image from a patient with involvement of axillary lymph nodes in the level II axilla. The white arrows show the involved lymph nodes, which are just beneath the pectoralis minor muscle. **B:** An involved level III axillary lymph node (white arrow) that extents superomedially to the pectoralis minor muscle. **C:** An involved Rotter's lymph node (*white arrow*), which is anterior to the pectoralis minor and beneath the pectoralis major muscle. **D:** Image from a patient with an involved internal mammary lymph node (*white arrow*).

and infection. Progression of untreated regional lymphatic disease can cause pain, brachial plexopathy, arm edema, obstruction and thrombosis of the brachial vasculature, and skin ulceration.

Treatment advances have improved survival rates for women with locally advanced breast cancer. Before the use of systemic treatment became routine, patients with advanced disease treated with mastectomy, radiation therapy, or both had 5-year survival rates of only 25% to 45%.[1–2,3] After the introduction of combined-modality treatments including surgery, radiation therapy, and chemotherapy, the 5-year survival rates approach 80% for patients with stage IIIA disease and 45% for patients with stage IIIB disease.[9] More recent data suggest continued improvement with the addition of more-effective systemic regimens. For example, a recent SEER study examining patients with IIIB/C disease reported a 2-year breast cancer death rate of only 10%.[10] The subset of patients with inflammatory breast cancer had a worse outcome than those with noninflammatory IIIB/C disease. In addition to stage, survival of locally advanced disease is dependent on other factors. For example, an elderly woman with a neglected ER-positive, hormonally responsive, stage III breast cancer that did not metastasize over a 1- to 2-year period of growth will have a much more favorable prognosis compared to a young woman with an ER-negative T4 tumor that presented with a history of rapidly progressive disease.

When considering improvements in the outcome of patients with stage III disease over time, it is important to recognize the effect of stage migration. Improvements in diagnostic imaging over time increase the likelihood of detecting metastatic disease, which results in some cases of stage III disease being reclassified as stage IV, which can have the effect of improving the outcome statistics for both stage III and stage IV disease. A similar effect was introduced by the 2003 change in the American Joint Commission of Cancer (AJCC) breast cancer staging system, which incorporated the number of positive lymph nodes in the pathologic disease stage. Specifically, many patients with four or more positive lymph nodes in the past would have had stage II disease but are classified as having stage III disease in the 2003 staging system. Indeed, a study that compared the stage-specific survival of 1,350 patients staged according to the 1988 AJCC staging system to the stage-specific survival of the same patients restaged according to the 2003 AJCC system found that the 10-year overall survival rates were significantly higher when the 2003 system was used, both for patients with stage II disease (76% [2003] vs. 65% [1988], $p < .0001$) and for those with stage IIIA disease (59% [2003] vs. 45% [1988], $p < .0001$).[11] The reason for the better stage-specific outcome was that restaging into the 2003 system led to most of the patients with four or more positive lymph nodes being moved from the stage II to the stage III category.

Natural History of Inflammatory Breast Cancer

Inflammatory breast cancer is a clinically defined subcategory of locally advanced breast cancer. The hallmarks of inflammatory breast cancer are rapid disease onset and the clinical findings of skin erythema, edema (peau d'orange), brawny breast induration, warmth, and asymmetric enlargement. Typically, extensive lymphovascular invasion by tumor emboli is present that involves the superficial dermal plexus of vessels in the papillary and high reticular dermis.[12] It is critical to distinguish inflammatory breast cancers from locally advanced breast cancer with secondary lymphatic congestion. Neglected primary tumors can also lead to breast erythema, edema, warmth, and asymmetric enlargement, particularly when bulky axillary adenopathy impedes the normal lymphatic flow from the breast. However, the former has a history of rapid onset, whereas the latter tends to have a long interval between the first symptom and the presentation for medical treatment.

Despite the natural history of inflammatory breast cancer being one of rapid disease progression and early distant dissemination,[12,13] in the United States, approximately 70% of patients with inflammatory breast cancer have only evidence of local-regional disease at the time of diagnosis.[14] Patients with inflammatory breast cancer typically have a worse clinical outcome than do other patients with T4 disease, suggesting that inflammatory breast cancer is a distinct biologic entity.[10] However, the prognosis for patients with inflammatory breast cancer has improved. Before the availability of combination chemotherapy, inflammatory breast cancer was almost uniformly fatal. Fewer than 5% of patients treated with surgery, radiation therapy, or both survived past 5 years, and the expected median survival time for such patients was <15 months.[13] Local recurrence rates after surgery or radiation therapy were also high at approximately 50%.[15,16] The introduction of doxorubicin-based chemotherapy improved outcomes.[17,18] An evaluation of the outcome of patients with inflammatory breast cancer registered in the SEER Program found that breast cancer–specific survival rates for patients with inflammatory breast cancer improved continuously throughout the 1990s.[19] Currently, local control rates for patients treated with chemotherapy, mastectomy, and postmastectomy radiation approach 70% to 80%, and 5-year survival rates are approximately 40%.[17,18]

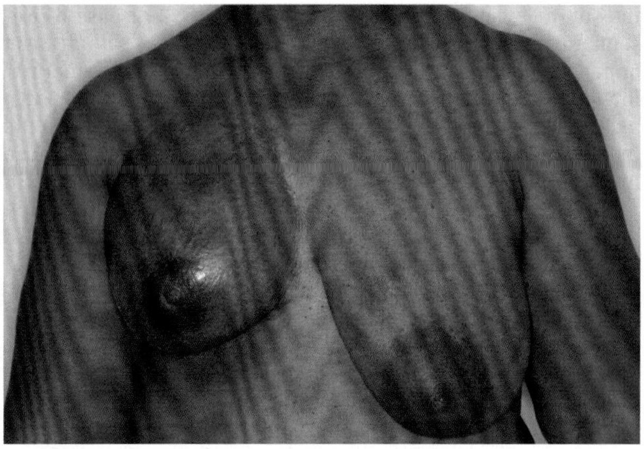

FIGURE 57.2. Photograph of a patient with a locally advanced noninflammatory right breast cancer at the time of diagnosis.

CLINICAL PRESENTATION OF LOCALLY ADVANCED BREAST CANCER

Locally advanced breast cancer most commonly is diagnosed after a palpable mass is detected within the breast. Advanced disease can cause symptoms such as local or regional pain, bleeding, paresthesia, and paresis. As previously indicated, it is critically important to determine the onset of symptoms and the rate of disease progression to reach an accurate diagnosis as to whether an advanced breast cancer represents an inflammatory carcinoma.

Diagnostic Workup

For patients with locally advanced breast cancer, the workup should start with a careful history and physical examination. The breast examination should include note of the breast symmetry, as well as careful inspection for involvement or edema of the skin. Peau d'orange can sometimes be subtle and at times can be best detected through gentle compression of the dermis between two fingers, which can elicit an increased prominence of the hair follicles and skin thickening compared with the skin overlying the contralateral breast. This finding may be missed on a quick visual inspection. Other times, physical examination findings are more obvious. Figure 57.2 shows a photograph of a patient with a neglected locally advanced breast cancer presenting with peau d'orange, inflammatory changes, breast retraction and involution, and effacement of the nipple–areola complex. Medical photographs are helpful to document the extent of visible abnormalities before treatment is begun and can be used to assess disease response to treatments.

The extent of palpable disease should also be measured and documented. Fixation of a breast mass to the pectoralis muscle or chest wall should be determined by assessing the mobility of the mass with the pectoralis muscle relaxed and contracted. Regional lymph nodes should be thoroughly evaluated by careful clinical examination with the patient in both supine and sitting positions. Clinical nodal evaluation may be supplemented with ultrasonographic imaging.

All cases of locally advanced disease require complete staging before initiation of therapy. Laboratory studies should include a complete blood cell count and serum chemistry profile with liver function tests. Radiographic studies should include a chest radiograph, a CT scan of the abdomen, a bone scan, and plain radiographs of symptomatic regions or areas of increased uptake on bone scans. Bone scans are recommended for all patients with locally advanced disease; up to 35% of patients with clinical stage III cancer can show abnormal bone scan results.[20] If any neurologic symptoms suggestive of cerebral metastases are present, a contrast-enhanced CT scan or gadolinium-enhanced magnetic resonance imaging (MRI) scan of the brain should be obtained. Gadolinium-enhanced MRI is the preferred imaging technique if leptomeningeal carcinomatosis is suspected.

There is increasing interest in the use of [^{18}F]fluorodeoxyglucose positron emission tomography (PET)/CT for disease staging of patients with locally advanced breast cancer, particularly those with inflammatory breast cancer. In a study of 41 women presenting with inflammatory breast cancer, PET/CT was able to detect distant metastases that were not found with other staging studies in 17% of the patients.[21]

Staging of Locally Advanced Breast Cancer

A comprehensive discussion of disease staging systems for breast cancer is provided in Chapter 56. Some staging considerations are particularly relevant to patients with stage III disease. Stage III breast cancer can represent either T3 disease (tumors >5.0 cm) with involved lymph nodes, N2 or N3 disease, or T4 disease.[22]

Specific aspects of both primary tumor and nodal staging in locally advanced breast cancer warrant additional consideration. Specifically, T4 disease may represent invasion into the chest wall (T4a), tumors associated with breast edema or skin ulceration or satellite nodules (T4b), both invasion and T4b characteristics (T4c), or inflammatory breast cancer (T4d). Invasion of disease into the pectoralis major muscle without chest wall invasion and dimpling or fixation of the overlying skin does not qualify as T4 disease. Both clinical and pathologic staging systems have been established for N2 and N3 disease. Clinical N2 disease signifies either involved axillary lymph nodes that are fixed to one another or to surrounding structures (N2a) or involved internal mammary lymph nodes without concurrent disease in the axilla (N2b), as determined by physical examination or imaging studies. Clinical N3 disease is disease that involves the infraclavicular region (N3a), both the axilla and internal mammary lymph nodes (N3b), or the supraclavicular region (N3c). Pathologic N2 disease represents involvement of 4 to 9 axillary lymph nodes with at least one focus measuring >2.0 mm (N2a) or clinical involvement of internal mammary lymph nodes with pathologically negative axillary lymph nodes (N2b). Pathologic N3 disease represents involvement of an infraclavicular lymph node or 10 or more involved lymph nodes with at least one focus measuring >2.0 mm (N3a), clinical involvement of internal mammary lymph nodes with 1 to 9 axillary lymph nodes involved, pathologic involvement of a sentinel internal mammary lymph node with four or more axillary lymph nodes involved (N3b), or a metastasis in the supraclavicular region (N3c).[22]

Neoadjuvant chemotherapy is recommended for most patients with locally advanced breast cancer. The initial extent of disease is an important factor for later local-regional treatment decisions and will be known only from the initial physical examination and radiographic findings. It is therefore imperative that disease in all patients be carefully assigned a clinical stage before any treatment is begun.

PATHOLOGY AND BIOLOGY OF LOCALLY ADVANCED BREAST CANCER

The histopathology of locally advanced disease is relatively similar to that of early-stage disease. Both infiltrating ductal carcinoma and lobular carcinoma can present as locally advanced disease. However, it is unusual for histologically "favorable" tumor types (e.g., tubular carcinoma, mucinous carcinoma, and medullary carcinoma) to present at advanced clinical stages unless the breast mass has been present for a long time.

The term "locally advanced breast cancer" encompasses a biologic spectrum of diseases. Locally advanced disease that has developed between interval (annual) screening mammograms is most often ER-negative, with high nuclear grade and high proliferative index. In contrast, patients who present with extensive local-regional disease after years of medical neglect more often are found to have ER-positive disease with low nuclear grade and low proliferative index.

Inflammatory breast cancer also has biologic characteristics that differ from those of noninflammatory breast cancer. Specifically, inflammatory cancer more often is of high histologic grade, shows high percentages of cells in S phase and aneuploidy, does not express the ER, and expresses high levels of p53 and epidermal growth factor.[23,24] Of interest, most investigators have found that HER2/neu overexpression is no more common in inflammatory breast cancer than in noninflammatory advanced disease.[23,25] Other, more recently discovered markers include the propensity of inflammatory tumors to overexpress RhoC GTPase and to not express the tumor suppressor gene WIPS3.[26,27] Finally, others have described that inflammatory breast cancers with loss of MUC-1 may be associated with poorer survival than tumors that express MUC-1. If these findings are confirmed and validated, markers such as these may prove to be useful for diagnosis and possibly as future therapeutic targets.[26,27] More recently, investigators have noted that overexpression of E-cadherin may play an important role in the tumor emboli formation that is typically noted in the dermal lymphatics, and preclinical work suggests that targeting E-cadherin may decrease invasiveness.[28,29]

GENERAL MANAGEMENT AND TREATMENT RESULTS FOR LOCALLY ADVANCED BREAST CANCER

Locally advanced disease requires multimodality therapy aimed at eradicating all disease in the local-regional area and preventing distant disease recurrence. These goals are best achieved through the use of combined-modality treatments that include chemotherapy, surgery, and radiation. In addition, ER-positive disease should be treated with hormonal therapy, and HER2/neu–positive disease should be treated with trastuzumab. Combined-modality therapy has significantly improved the prognosis for patients with advanced breast cancer. As previously noted, the prognosis of patients with locally advanced disease treated in the era before chemotherapy was available was very poor, with 5-year survival rates of only 25%.[1–2,3] In contrast, more recent single-institution studies have reported 5-year survival rates approaching 80% for patients with stage IIIA disease and 45% for patients with stage IIIB disease.[9] National database studies also reflect improvements in survival over time. For example, a study evaluating the outcome of patients with lymph node–positive breast cancer demonstrated that 5-year survival rates were significantly better in the group treated in 1995–1999 than in the group treated in 1975–1979 (Fig. 57.3).[30] The most recent data from the American Cancer Society estimated an 84% 5-year survival for patients diagnosed between 1999–2005 who had lymph node–positive disease without distant metastases.[4] These survival statistics are likely to show continued improvement over time because since 1999 several positive phase III clinical trials have shown that a new systemic treatment strategy may improve outcome among patients with lymph node–positive breast cancer. What is particularly exciting is that some of these advances represent incremental improvements in outcome over previous advances, so that when the benefits are added together the improvements over time become quite significant. As evidence of this improvement, an interesting study recently reported that between 1950 and 1980, the U.S. Food and Drug Administration approved fewer than 5 new systemic treatments for breast cancer during each decade; in contrast, 6 new agents were approved during the 1980s, and 12 new agents were approved during the 1990s.[31] The pace

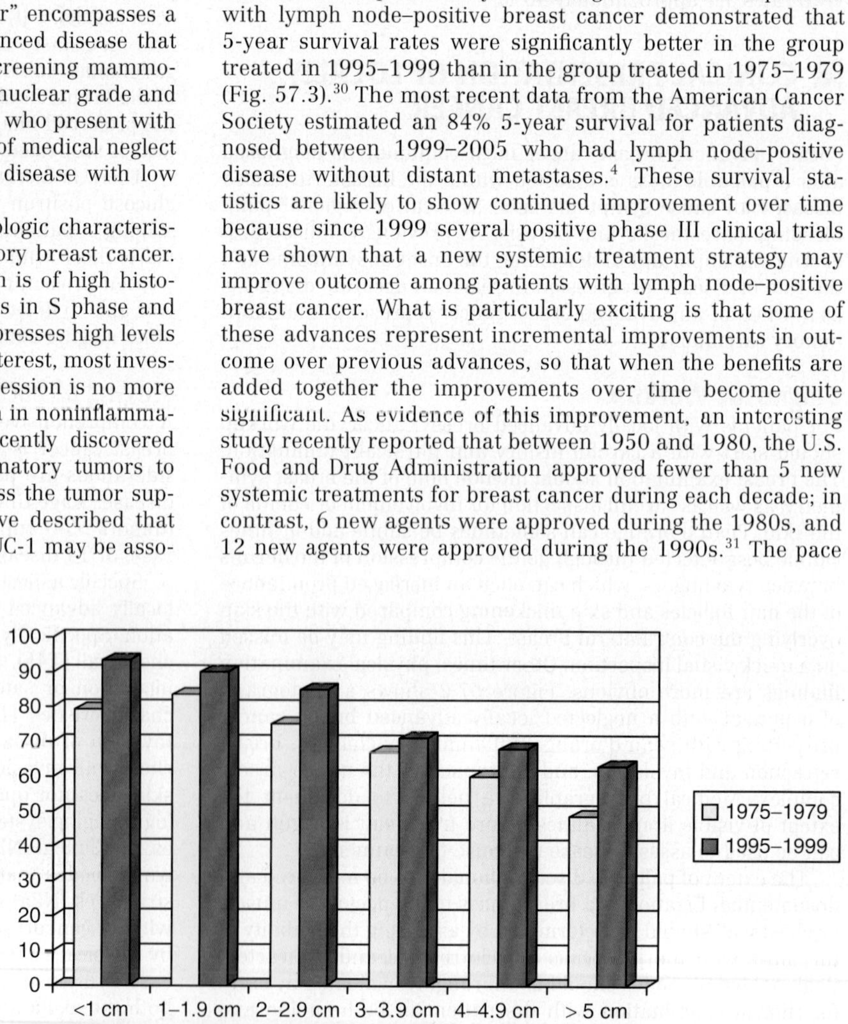

FIGURE 57.3. Five-year survival rates for patients with positive axillary lymph nodes according to tumor size and year of diagnosis. (Data from Elkin et al.[30]; reprinted from Buchholz TA Locally advanced breast cancer. In: Haffty BG, Wilson L, eds. *Handbook of radiation oncology*. Sudbury, MA: Jones and Bartlett, 2008.)

of change in available therapeutics has been even greater in the last decade. These new treatments are likely to continue to improve the prognosis for patients with advanced breast cancer during the decades to come, and the rate at which new agents for breast cancer treatment are introduced is expected to accelerate with identification of new therapeutic targets.

Overview of Treatment

Locally advanced breast cancer can present as either operable disease or inoperable disease. The current standard of treatment for all patients with inoperable breast cancer is to proceed with neoadjuvant chemotherapy as the initial therapy. Approximately 80% to 90% of patients with advanced breast cancer will show partial or complete clinical response to neoadjuvant chemotherapy,[32,33] and most patients presenting with inoperable breast cancer become candidates for surgery after neoadjuvant treatment.

No criteria have been agreed upon to distinguish inoperable from operable disease. In general, neoadjuvant chemotherapy is preferred if an initial surgical procedure is not likely to completely resect all gross disease with achievement of negative surgical margins. This includes most patients with T4 disease and all patients with inflammatory breast cancer, and for such patients neoadjuvant chemotherapy can allow primary closure of the skin flaps of the mastectomy. For patients with operable stage IIIA disease, initial surgery followed by adjuvant chemotherapy or neoadjuvant chemotherapy are equally good options. The advantages of each are highlighted in the following.

Neoadjuvant Chemotherapy–Advantages and Disadvantages

Neoadjuvant chemotherapy has become an increasingly popular treatment strategy for patients with stage II or III breast cancer. The use of neoadjuvant chemotherapy has several potential advantages over the traditional sequence of surgery followed by adjuvant chemotherapy, but it also carries some disadvantages (Table 57.2). Several trials have clearly shown that neoadjuvant chemotherapy substantially reduces the size of the primary tumor and nodal metastases in >80% of cases. Accordingly, for patients with large primary tumors, the approach of using chemotherapy as the initial treatment has been shown to increase the probability that breast-conserving surgery can be performed.[32,34–36] A second advantage of using chemotherapy first is that this sequence allows the response of the disease to a particular chemotherapy regimen to be assessed, which in turn could provide an opportunity to "cross over" to a different treatment regimen if disease in an individual patient shows little or no response to the first regimen. By doing so, a potentially effective second-line agent can be given rapidly, and the toxicity of an ineffective first regimen can be avoided.

Neoadjuvant chemotherapy has also been proven to be extremely valuable for clinical research. After several studies showed a strong correlation between the achievement of a pathologic complete response (pCR; defined as no residual cancer being found in the postchemotherapy surgical specimen) and survival,[32–34] investigators began using pCR rates as a short-term surrogate of the success of a chemotherapy regimen. Phase III randomized trials in which pCR rates were used as the primary endpoint have allowed the activity of two chemotherapy regimens to be compared with relatively small study populations and very short follow-up times relative to studies comparing two chemotherapy regimens used in an adjuvant setting. Neoadjuvant chemotherapy can also facilitate translational research to investigate the mechanisms of chemotherapy-induced cell death and chemotherapy resistance. For example, it has proven feasible to study changes in tumor genomes in response to treatment and how such changes correlate with chemotherapy response through the use of cDNA microarrays from serial biopsy specimens.[37] Such studies are likely to provide significant insights into the heterogeneity of tumor response and to identify new targets for therapies.

Some have asserted that treatment with neoadjuvant chemotherapy also provides additional prognostic information. Clearly the prognosis for patients with a pCR (defined as complete eradication of invasive disease and negative axillary lymph nodes at the time of surgical treatment) is better than the prognosis would have been before treatment. However, an equal percentage of patients will be found to have residual disease after chemotherapy, which confers a worse prognosis than originally anticipated. Therefore, the true value of the additional prognostic information from the use of neoadjuvant chemotherapy will come only when additional treatments become available that can positively influence prognosis for those with a high residual disease burden. Currently, there are a number of clinical protocols to evaluate new therapeutics specifically in patients who exhibit a poor response to neoadjuvant treatment.

One theoretical advantage of neoadjuvant chemotherapy that has not been borne out in practice was the hope that earlier delivery of chemotherapy might improve survival for patients with locally advanced breast cancer. Clearly most of the patients who present with advanced disease and subsequently die of that disease do so as a consequence of the progression of metastatic disease that was present at a microscopic level at the time of diagnosis. Therefore, the suggestion that initiating chemotherapy at diagnosis (when the micrometastatic tumor burden would be lowest) would improve outcome relative to delaying chemotherapy until after surgical resection was a rational one. This was further supported by preclinical animal studies showing that removal of the primary tumor could increase the growth rate of existing micrometastases and that treating animals with either chemotherapy or tamoxifen before resection of the primary tumor abrogated this adverse effect.[38]

Two large randomized trials have been conducted to test the hypothesis that neoadjuvant chemotherapy could improve survival in patients with operable breast cancer. The first of these trials was the National Surgical Adjuvant Breast and Bowel Project (NSABP) B-18 study, in which 1,523 patients with operable breast cancer were randomly assigned to receive

TABLE 57.2 CONSIDERATIONS REGARDING THE SEQUENCING OF SURGERY AND CHEMOTHERAPY FOR PATIENTS WITH OPERABLE LOCALLY ADVANCED BREAST CANCER

Advantages of Performing Surgery First	*Advantages of Neoadjuvant Chemotherapy*
Removes the source of distant metastases	May allow breast conservation after effecting a disease response
Reduces the interval between diagnosis and effective treatment for patients with disease that is resistant to chemotherapy	Allows an *in vivo* assessment of sensitivity to a chemotherapy regimen
Provides clear information concerning the original extent of disease	Allows chemotherapy to be changed if the disease proves resistant
Provides clear prognostic information concerning the risk of recurrence after mastectomy and therefore the indications for using postmastectomy radiation	Permits an assessment of pathologic disease response, which allows for the further stratification of an individual patient's prognosis
	Allows direct comparison of different treatment regimens in clinical trials with a short-term study endpoint (pathologic complete response)
	Allows serial biopsies and images of tumor to be obtained during treatment to gain insight into the molecular mechanisms of tumor sensitivity and resistance

four cycles of doxorubicin and cyclophosphamide (AC) either before or after surgical treatment.[32,34] After 16 years, the overall survival rates and disease-free survival rates were nearly identical between the two groups ($p = .99$ and $p = .93$, respectively).[39] However, in an unplanned subgroup analysis the authors found an interaction between age and sequencing of chemotherapy. Patients younger than 50 years of age had a 16-year overall survival of 61% with neoadjuvant chemotherapy versus 55% with adjuvant chemotherapy. An opposite trend noting an improvement with adjuvant chemotherapy was noted in the patients 50 years old and older.[39] A second randomized prospective trial, conducted by the European Organization for Research and Treatment of Cancer (EORTC), confirmed these results and again found equivalent rates of 10-year survival and distant metastases between the neoadjuvant chemotherapy and adjuvant chemotherapy treatment groups.[40] A meta-analysis of data from 3,946 patients treated in nine randomized trials comparing neoadjuvant with adjuvant chemotherapy in breast cancer found no statistical difference in the risk of death (risk ratio, 1.00), disease progression (risk ratio, 0.99), or distant disease recurrence (risk ratio, 0.94).[41]

The increasing use of neoadjuvant chemotherapy in patients with clinically negative lymph nodes has also created a controversy with respect to the sequencing of chemotherapy and sentinel lymph node surgery. It is clear from the B-18 trial and other institutional studies that neoadjuvant chemotherapy leads to complete eradication of disease within lymph nodes in roughly 20% to 40% of patients.[32,42] If this eradication occurs selectively within the sentinel lymph node but not in other involved axillary lymph nodes, there is the potential that the false-negative rate of sentinel lymph node surgery after chemotherapy may be higher than sentinel lymph node surgery performed prior to chemotherapy. In addition, the original extent of axillary disease is unknown when sentinel lymph node surgery is performed after chemotherapy. This can have implications with respect to radiation treatment field design or recommendations concerning whether to use postmastectomy radiation. In some instance, this can also have implications with respect to adjuvant chemotherapy treatment decisions.

There are some advantages to performing the sentinel lymph node surgery after rather than before neoadjuvant chemotherapy. Of importance, with this strategy, most commonly patients only have to go one surgery rather than two. Second, if a component of disease is removed prior to surgery, then the prognostic value of achieving a pCR is less certain. Finally, performing surgery prior to chemotherapy delays the administration of systemic treatments, particularly if an axillary metastasis is found and the patient then undergoes an axillary dissection. Finally, because patients will more commonly have pathologically lymph node–negative disease after neoadjuvant chemotherapy, they more commonly will not require a completion axillary dissection.[43]

A number of groups have studied the identification rates and false-negative rates associated with sentinel lymph node surgery. The largest experience has been from the NSABP B-27 trial, which randomized 2,411 patients to one of three neoadjuvant chemotherapy regimens. A total of 428 of these patients had lymphatic mapping attempted. Successful identification of a sentinel lymph node was made in 85%, and the false-negative rate was 11% (defined as the number of patients with positive nonsentinel lymph nodes with a negative sentinel lymph node divided by the total number of patients with positive axillary lymph nodes).[44]

A meta-analysis investigated 1,273 patients (21 published studies) treated with a sentinel lymph node biopsy with subsequent axillary dissection following neoadjuvant chemotherapy.[45] These authors reported a pooled identification rate of 90% and false-negative rate of 12%. Because these outcomes are similar to those reported in multicenter studies in which sentinel lymph node surgery was performed prior to systemic therapy, delaying sentinel lymph node surgery until after chemotherapy appears acceptable.

Neoadjuvant Hormonal Therapy

There are fewer data concerning the long-term outcome of patients treated with hormone therapy prior to surgery. In part this is because most patients treated with neoadjuvant systemic treatments for an ER-positive breast cancer have disease extent that necessitates both chemotherapy and hormonal treatments. However, interest in neoadjuvant hormonal therapy increased after reports from studies that found that patients with ER-positive disease have a lower probability of achieving a pCR compared to those with ER-negative disease.[46] For example, patients with lobular breast cancer, in whom >90% of tumors are ER-positive, have particularly low rates of pCR.[47] In addition, some patients with ER-positive breast cancer that is locally advanced and/or lymph node–positive at presentation are not candidates for neoadjuvant chemotherapy due to comorbid medical conditions. For such patients, treatment with neoadjuvant hormonal therapy is a reasonable option.[48]

Responses to neoadjuvant hormonal therapy occur over a slower period of time than those to neoadjuvant chemotherapy, and the rates of pCR with hormonal therapy are lower than those achievable with neoadjuvant chemotherapy. After aromatase inhibitors became available for postmenopausal patients with ER-positive disease, neoadjuvant hormone therapy trials were developed to directly compare the activities of various agents. A 330-patient randomized trial run in the United Kingdom compared 3 months of anastrozole, tamoxifen, or combined anastrozole/tamoxifen and found response rates of 36% to 39%, with only 1% to 3% achieving a clinical complete response.[49] In the subgroup of 124 patients who were not candidates for breast conservation at diagnosis, the rates of breast conservation after 3 months of neoadjuvant hormone treatment were highest in the anastrozole-alone arm. An Italian trial randomized patients to 3 months of anastrozole versus tamoxifen and also noted a higher rate of breast conservation after treatment with anastrozole alone versus tamoxifen alone.[50] The overall response rates were similar to those in the United Kingdom study.

Breast Conservation Therapy After Neoadjuvant Chemotherapy

As noted, one of the potential benefits of neoadjuvant chemotherapy is that a large primary tumor will respond favorably to neoadjuvant chemotherapy, thereby rendering the disease amenable to a breast conservation surgical approach. One important consideration for performing breast-conserving surgery after neoadjuvant chemotherapy concerns the volume of surgical resection. This is less of a problem for patients with small initial primary tumors that shrink still further after neoadjuvant chemotherapy. However, for patients with T3 disease for whom initial breast-conserving surgery would be deforming, the volume of resection after neoadjuvant chemotherapy must be directed at the residual nidus rather than the original extent of disease. In some instances, neoadjuvant chemotherapy successfully shrinks large primary tumors to smaller residual niduses that can easily be resected in small volumes of tissue with good or excellent aesthetic outcomes. However, breast cancers can respond to neoadjuvant chemotherapy in a variety of ways, as shown in Figure 57.4. For tumors that shrink to a residual nidus, limited surgery would successfully resect the volume of residual disease, and the outcome, particularly for those with a pCR, would be expected to be excellent. However, in other cases, tumors respond favorably to neoadjuvant chemotherapy, but the residual disease is diffuse, multifocal, and scattered throughout the original tumor volume. In such cases,

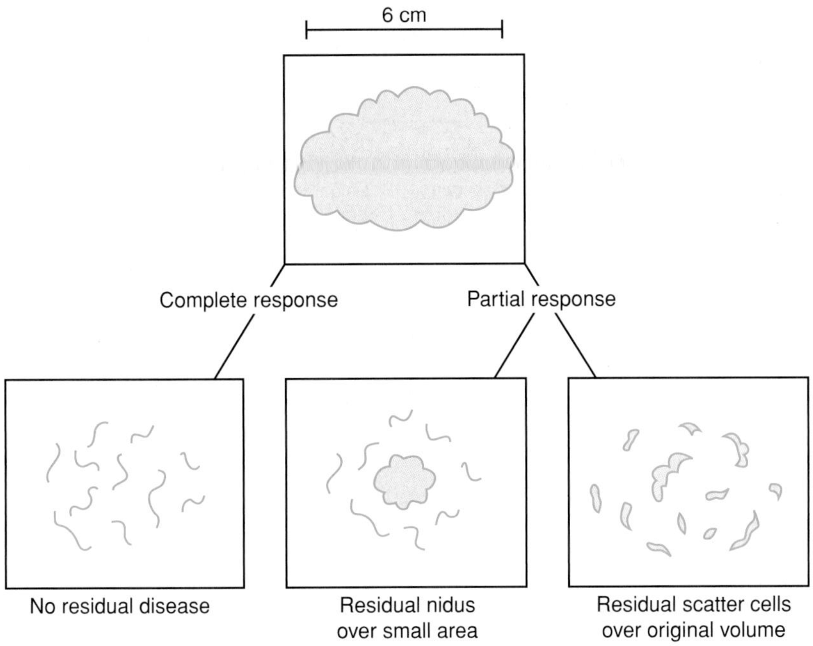

FIGURE 57.4. Three potential pathologic outcomes of a primary tumor that responds to neoadjuvant chemotherapy. (From Buchholz TA, Hunt KK, Whitman GJ, et al. Neoadjuvant chemotherapy for breast carcinoma: multidisciplinary considerations of benefits and risks. *Cancer* 2003;98:1150–1160.)

a small surgical resection carries the risk of leaving a residual disease burden within the breast. Careful selection of cases for breast conservation is therefore critical.

One of the first studies to provide findings regarding appropriate selection criteria for breast conservation after neoadjuvant chemotherapy examined 143 mastectomy specimens from patients given neoadjuvant chemotherapy to determine patterns of residual disease and their relationships to clinical factors.[51] Only 23% of tumors had clinical and pathologic features that would have predicted success with breast conservation. Important selection criteria included resolution of skin edema, favorable clinical response to neoadjuvant treatment, lack of multicentricity, and lack of extensive lymphovascular space invasion.

Since those findings were published, several groups have studied the clinical outcome of patients treated with breast conservation after neoadjuvant chemotherapy. In general, the outcome results have varied considerably across series, for several possible reasons. First, the selection criteria vary considerably across studies, and not surprisingly studies that include patients with positive surgical margins or inflammatory breast cancer tended to report higher rates of local recurrence.[52,53] Similarly, some studies in which patients who achieved complete clinical resolution of disease could elect to forgo surgery showed higher recurrence rates.[54] Other studies, however—predominantly from institutions with well-coordinated multidisciplinary teams and careful pathologic analysis of the surgical specimen—reported excellent outcomes.[55,56]

Two of the most influential publications that addressed breast conservation after neoadjuvant chemotherapy were from the two largest randomized trials (NSABP B-18 and EORTC) comparing neoadjuvant chemotherapy with adjuvant chemotherapy for patients with stage II or stage III breast cancer. The conclusion in both studies was that neoadjuvant chemotherapy offered an advantage because breast conservation rates were higher in the neoadjuvant chemotherapy groups.[32,34,36] However, it is important to recognize that approximately 60% of the patients enrolled in these studies were considered candidates for breast conservation at the time of diagnosis. Therefore in the B-18 study, the improvement in breast conservation rates from 60% to 68% for patients treated with neoadjuvant chemotherapy essentially showed that 20% of initial mastectomy candidates (8 of 40 patients) could undergo breast conservation surgery instead after neoadjuvant chemotherapy. Not surprisingly, this increase was directly due to a higher percentage of patients with T3 disease being offered breast conservation after first responding to chemotherapy. Both studies reported that the overall breast recurrence risk in patients treated with neoadjuvant chemotherapy was not statistically different from that in patients treated with surgery first.[32,34,36] However, in the B-18 study, the breast recurrence rate in a subset of patients who initially would have required a mastectomy but were treated with breast conservation after a favorable response to neoadjuvant chemotherapy was twice that of the patients with smaller tumors who were treated with surgery first (15.7% vs. 7.6%, respectively).[34]

A meta-analysis of the nine randomized studies comparing neoadjuvant and adjuvant chemotherapy reported that the use of neoadjuvant chemotherapy was associated with an increase in the relative risk of local-regional recurrence relative to adjuvant chemotherapy (relative risk, 1.22; 95% confidence interval [CI], 1.04 to 1.43).[41] This difference was largely influenced by the trials in which surgery was not performed and breast conservation after neoadjuvant chemotherapy was achieved with the use of radiation therapy alone (in those trials the relative risk was 1.53 and the 95% CI was 1.11 to 2.10).[41] These findings indicate that patients who achieve a complete clinical response would still benefit from a surgical procedure in addition to radiation.

Two of the largest studies showing acceptable outcomes for breast conservation after neoadjuvant chemotherapy have been from the Istituto Nazionale Tumori in Milan, Italy, and the University of Texas MD Anderson Cancer Center.[55,56] The Milan experience consisted of 536 patients treated with neoadjuvant chemotherapy for a primary tumor 2.5 cm in diameter or larger. Eighty-five percent of these patients subsequently had breast-conserving surgery. However, it is important to note that the initial tumor size in more than half of these women was <4 cm, and thus these women may have been candidates for breast conservation at diagnosis. The 8-year rate of breast recurrence as a first site of failure in those treated with breast conservation was 6.8%.[55] In the MD Anderson series, 340 carefully selected patients were treated with breast conservation therapy after showing a favorable response to chemotherapy.[56]

Patient selection criteria for the breast-conserving approach included having no residual T4 breast skin abnormalities, negative surgical margins, no multicentric disease, no residual malignant calcifications on postoperative mammogram, and the willingness and ability to undergo both surgery and radiation therapy. With these criteria, the outcome was favorable, with 5- and 10-year local recurrence rates of 5% and 10%, respectively, despite the fact that 72% of patients in the study had clinical stage IIB or III disease. Four factors were found to be independently associated with breast cancer recurrence and local-regional recurrence: clinical N2 or N3 disease, lymphovascular space invasion, a multifocal pattern of residual disease, and residual disease >2 cm in diameter.[56] Eighty-four percent of patients had none or just one of these factors, and the recurrence rate at 10 years in this group was only 4%.[57] In contrast, the 4% of patients with three of these factors had a recurrence rate of 45%. Women with primary clinical T3 or T4 disease were at very low risk of recurrence if the tumor shrank to a solitary nidus or showed a pCR, but among patients with T3/T4 tumors that broke up and left a multifocal pattern of residual disease the breast cancer recurrence rate was 20%.[56] More recently this same group validated this prognostic index in a more recent cohort of patients. The patients had respective 5-year locoregional recurrence–free survival rates of 92% (score, 0, $n = 91$), 92% (score, 1; $n = 82$), 84% (score, 2; $n = 38$), and 69% (score, 3 to 4; $n = 13$) ($p = .01$).[58]

The investigators from MD Anderson recently updated their experience and compared how treatment with neoadjuvant versus adjuvant chemotherapy affected rates of local-regional failures in 2,984 patients treated with breast conservation therapy between 1987 and 2005. After adjusting for differences in clinical stage, their multivariate analysis demonstrated no differences in local-regional recurrence between surgery-first and chemotherapy-first patients.[59]

When considering the outcome of breast conservation therapy for patients with locally advanced breast cancer, it is important to consider that patients with stage III breast cancer are at risk for local-regional recurrence even when mastectomy is performed. In addition, patients with advanced disease are at significant risk for distant metastases, which is an additional incentive to avoid removing the entire breast when breast-conserving surgery can be done with acceptably low recurrence rates. The investigators from MD Anderson applied the four prognostic criteria associated with breast recurrence in patients treated with neoadjuvant chemotherapy and breast conservation to a cohort of patients treated with neoadjuvant chemotherapy, mastectomy, and postmastectomy radiation.[60] These investigators found that for patients who had none or one of these factors, the results with either local-regional treatment approach were excellent and equivalent. Among patients with two factors, a nonsignificant trend was evident toward fewer local-regional recurrences with mastectomy, and for the small cohort of patients with three or four factors, mastectomy provided a statistically significant benefit. This trend was also noted in their updated validation paper.[58]

Mastectomy

In the United States, mastectomy continues to be the most common local-regional treatment for breast cancer, particularly for patients with locally advanced disease. Several alternative mastectomy approaches are available for women with breast cancer (Table 57.3). A simple or total mastectomy resects the breast but not the axillary contents. For patients with clinical stage T1/T2 N0 disease who are not interested in breast conservation, a total mastectomy with a sentinel lymph node dissection may be the treatment of choice. A modified radical mastectomy (removal of the breast plus a level I/II axillary dissection) remains the standard of care for patients with clinically positive lymph nodes or locally advanced disease.

TABLE 57.3 TYPES OF MASTECTOMIES USED AS TREATMENTS FOR BREAST CANCER

Surgical Therapies for Breast Cancer	*Definition*
Segmental mastectomy, lumpectomy, tylectomy	Removal of the primary tumor with a surrounding margin of breast tissue
Total or simple mastectomy	Removal of the breast but not the axillary contents
Modified radical mastectomy	Removal of the breast plus an axillary level I/II dissection
Radical mastectomy	Removal of the parenchyma breast tissue and pectoralis major muscle plus an axillary level I/II dissection
Extended radical mastectomy	Removal of the breast and pectoralis major muscle plus an axillary level I/II and internal mammary lymph node dissection; may also include a level III axillary lymph node dissection
Skin-sparing mastectomy	Total or modified radical mastectomy with preservation of a significant component of the native skin of the breast to optimize the aesthetic result of an immediate reconstruction

Postmastectomy Radiation Therapy

Meta-Analyses of Postmastectomy Radiation Therapy Trials

Adjuvant radiation has been used after mastectomy for many decades. Indeed, some of the first randomized, prospective trials in medicine were done to investigate the efficacy of postmastectomy radiation. Despite this, significant controversy remains over the indications for its use. It is clear that mastectomy without radiation offers excellent local-regional control rates for most patients with noninvasive or early-stage, lymph node–negative disease. In contrast, patients with stage III breast cancer (four or more positive lymph nodes or T3/T4 primary tumors) have a clinically relevant risk of local-regional recurrence after mastectomy and thus would benefit from adjuvant radiation. What is less clear is whether radiation provides a survival advantage for patients with stage II breast cancer and one to three positive lymph nodes.

In 1987, Cuzick et al.[61] published the first meta-analysis of data from postmastectomy radiation therapy trials and reported that radiation use was associated with a poorer overall survival rate. In a subsequent analysis, the same group reported that postmastectomy radiation therapy decreased the breast cancer death rate but increased the non–breast cancer death rate,[62] which resulted in equivalent overall survival rates in the radiation and no-radiation groups. These analyses are mostly of historical interest because of the considerable heterogeneity in the surgical and radiation therapy treatments used in these trials as compared with modern treatment approaches. Moreover, these early trials often enrolled patients with early-stage disease, who would not be predicted to derive any benefit from radiation therapy. Finally, the early studies of postmastectomy radiation predated the use of systemic therapy.

After the Cuzick meta-analyses, the Early Breast Cancer Trialists' Collaborative Group obtained the raw data from every randomized trial that investigated the role of radiation in breast cancer. Through the years, this group has published a series of meta-analyses that have provided important insights into the risks and benefits of postmastectomy radiation therapy.[63] In the most recently published analysis, based on data from 9,933 patients, postmastectomy radiation therapy reduced the 15-year isolated local-regional recurrence rates for patients with lymph node–positive disease from 29% to 8%.[64] Of importance, this reduction led to a 5% decrease in the 15-year breast cancer mortality rate (60% vs. 55%). In 2005, the group reanalyzed updated data, with the resulting publication expected in 2012. This updated further subdivided patients according to pathologic lymph node status, and the provisional

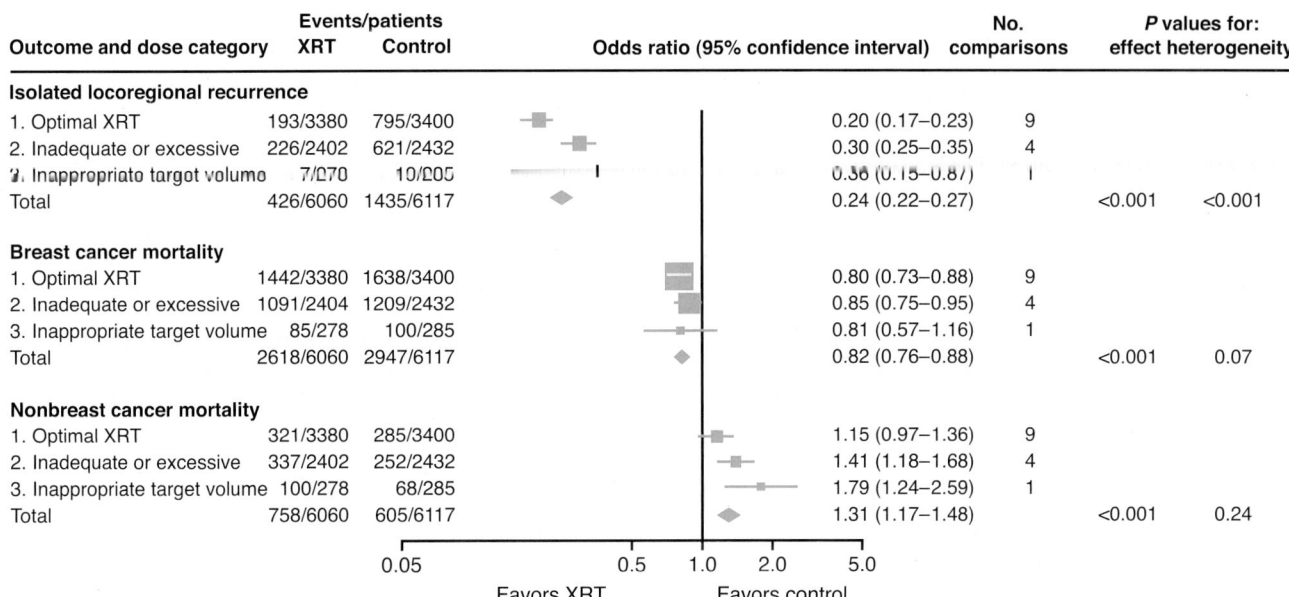

Outcome and dose category	Events/patients XRT	Events/patients Control	Odds ratio (95% confidence interval)	No. comparisons	*P* values for: effect	*P* values for: heterogeneity
Isolated locoregional recurrence						
1. Optimal XRT	193/3380	795/3400	0.20 (0.17–0.23)	9		
2. Inadequate or excessive	226/2402	621/2432	0.30 (0.25–0.35)	4		
3. Inappropriate target volume	7/270	10/265	0.36 (0.15–0.87)	1		
Total	426/6060	1435/6117	0.24 (0.22–0.27)		<0.001	<0.001
Breast cancer mortality						
1. Optimal XRT	1442/3380	1638/3400	0.80 (0.73–0.88)	9		
2. Inadequate or excessive	1091/2404	1209/2432	0.85 (0.75–0.95)	4		
3. Inappropriate target volume	85/278	100/285	0.81 (0.57–1.16)	1		
Total	2618/6060	2947/6117	0.82 (0.76–0.88)		<0.001	0.07
Nonbreast cancer mortality						
1. Optimal XRT	321/3380	285/3400	1.15 (0.97–1.36)	9		
2. Inadequate or excessive	337/2402	252/2432	1.41 (1.18–1.68)	4		
3. Inappropriate target volume	100/278	68/285	1.79 (1.24–2.59)	1		
Total	758/6060	605/6117	1.31 (1.17–1.48)		<0.001	0.24

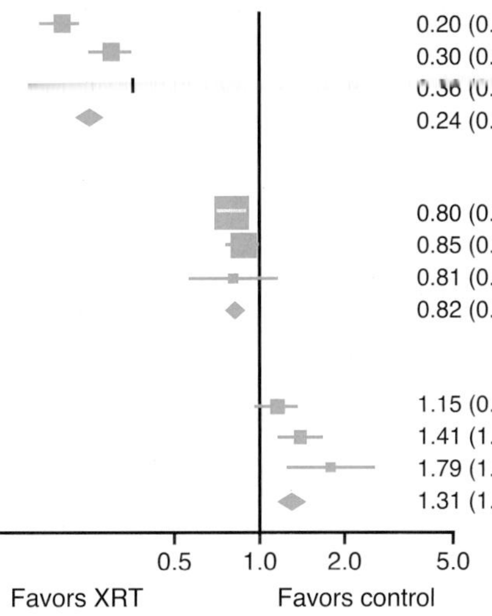

FIGURE 57.5. Data from a meta-analysis showing the association between postmastectomy radiation therapy and locoregional recurrence, breast cancer mortality, and mortality from other causes. The trials were analyzed and divided according the appropriateness of the radiation dose (labeled in the figure as "inadequate or excessive") and design of the radiation treatment fields. This figure shows that the trials with the highest quality of radiation therapy achieved the greatest proportional reduction in locoregional recurrences, were the only trials associated with an improvement in breast cancer mortality, and were the only trials that did not find an association between radiation use and increased mortality from other causes. (From Gebski V, Lagleva M, Keech A, et al. Survival effects of postmastectomy adjuvant radiation therapy using biologically equivalent doses: a clinical perspective. *J Natl Cancer Inst* 2006;98(1):26–38.)

findings have been presented.[65] In this update postmastectomy radiation reduced 15-year rates of isolated local recurrences in pN0 patients from 5.8% to 2.4% (n = 1,277), in patients with one to three positive lymph nodes by 24.7% versus 5.3% (n = 3,316), and in patients with four or more positive lymph nodes by 40.6% versus 12.9% (n = 2,813). The improvement in local-regional recurrence with postmastectomy radiation was associated with a statistically significant improvement in death from breast cancer and overall survival for the patients with one to three positive lymph nodes and those with four or more positive lymph nodes but not for the patients with lymph node–negative disease.[65]

It is important to recognize the limitations of meta-analyses when considering the relevance of these reports to modern treatments for breast cancer. One problem with including trials dating back to the 1950s is that the radiation doses, fractionation patterns, treatment units, and field designs differ significantly from current standards. To minimize these confounding effects, Van de Steene et al.[66] conducted a similar meta-analysis but excluded trials that began before 1970, trials with small sample sizes, trials with relatively poor survival rates, and trials that used radiation fractionation schedules that are no longer in standard practice. When these studies were excluded, use of postmastectomy radiation therapy was associated with an even greater overall survival advantage. Moreover, adjuvant radiation probably can improve survival even further if the risk of dying from micrometastatic disease is minimized through the use of systemic therapy. To investigate this question, Whelan et al.[67] performed a meta-analysis of postmastectomy radiation trials that included systemic therapy for both treatment groups. In this analysis, the addition of radiation after mastectomy led to an even greater reduction in the risk of any recurrence (odds ratio, 0.69) and the risk of death (odds ratio, 0.83). Finally, another meta-analysis attempted to account for the quality of radiation delivery in these trials.[68] In this study, the authors defined optimal dose as a between 40 and 60 Gy delivered in 2-Gy fractions and optimal treatment field arrangements as ones that included both the chest wall and the regional lymphatics. They then reanalyzed the data from the Early Breast Cancer Trialists' Collaborative Group according to the quality of radiation treatments and demonstrated that proportional reduction in local-regional recurrence was 80% for trials with optimal dose and treatment fields, compared to 70% and 64% for trials that were suboptimal with respect to dose or field arrangements, respectively. In addition, there was a statistically significant improvement in breast cancer mortality in the trials that used optimal radiation dose and treatment fields but not in the other trials (Fig. 57.5).

In summary, these meta-analyses conclusively demonstrated that radiation has an important role in the management of locally advanced breast cancer. By reducing the risk of recurrence after mastectomy, radiation offers an incremental improvement in overall survival. Radiation seems to offer the greatest benefit when given using modern treatment techniques that minimize the risk of normal-tissue injury and maximize the probability of tumor control and when given to patients who also receive systemic treatments.

Phase III Randomized Trials Investigating Postmastectomy Radiation Therapy

The three most recently completed randomized trials investigating the efficacy of postmastectomy radiation for patients with stage II or III breast cancer were conducted in the 1980s and have 15- to 20-year outcome data. The largest of these studies was the Danish Breast Cancer Cooperative Group 82b trial, which randomly assigned 1,708 premenopausal women with stage II or III breast cancer to receive mastectomy followed by nine cycles of cyclophosphamide, methotrexate, and fluorouracil (CMF) chemotherapy or mastectomy, radiation therapy, and eight cycles of CMF chemotherapy.[69] At the same time, this group also conducted the 82c trial, in which >1,300 postmenopausal women were randomly assigned to undergo mastectomy and 1 year of tamoxifen or mastectomy, tamoxifen, and radiation therapy.[70] Finally, a smaller trial, conducted in Vancouver, Canada, randomly assigned 318 premenopausal women with lymph node–positive disease to undergo mastectomy and CMF chemotherapy with or without postmastectomy radiation therapy.[71] In all three of these studies, patients

TABLE 57.4 LOCAL-REGIONAL RECURRENCE, RATES OF DISTANT METASTASIS, AND OVERALL SURVIVAL IN RANDOMIZED TRIALS COMPARING THE USE OF POSTMASTECTOMY RADIATION FOR PATIENTS TREATED WITH MASTECTOMY AND SYSTEMIC THERAPY[69-72]

Trial	Local-Regional Recurrence Rates (First Events Only)	Rates of Distant Metastasis	Survival Rate
Danish 82b (10 yr)			
Radiation	9%	Not provided	45%
No radiation	32%		54%
	$p < .0001$		$p < .0001$
Danish 82c (10 yr)			
Radiation	8%	Not provided	45%
No radiation	35%		36%
	$p < .0001$		$p = .03$
Danish 82b and 82c (18 yr)			
Radiation	14%	53%	Not provided
No radiation	49%	64%	
	$p < .0001$	$p < .0001$	
Vancouver, Canada (20 yr)	13%	52%	47%
Radiation	39%	69%	37%
No radiation	$p < .0001$	$p = .004$	$p = .03$

treated with radiation had a lower long-term risk of isolated local-regional recurrence than did patients randomized to no radiation therapy. Of importance, these improvements led to fewer patients developing metastatic disease and an improvement in overall survival.[71,72] The results from these three trials are shown in Table 57.4.

Several important concepts can be ascertained from these studies. First, these studies, together with the Oxford meta-analyses, clearly demonstrate that by reducing local-regional recurrence, postmastectomy radiation therapy could improve overall survival. Second, these trials demonstrated that these patients had a clinically relevant risk of local-regional recurrence despite the use of either CMF chemotherapy or tamoxifen. These findings imply that the benefits of systemic treatments are predominantly to lower the competing risk of distant metastases, which makes the achievement of local-regional control more important.

One controversy that arose after the publication of these studies concerns the most appropriate indications for postmastectomy radiation. Specifically, these trials led to a debate as to whether postmastectomy radiation therapy is indicated for patients with stage II breast cancer with one to three positive lymph nodes. Most of the patients enrolled in the Danish and British Columbia trials had stage II disease with one to three positive lymph nodes.[69-71] Accordingly, many have argued that these findings suggest that all patients with lymph node–positive disease should receive radiation after mastectomy. This argument is further supported by the recent analysis from the Early Breast Cancer Trialists' Collaborative Group, which also noted a survival advantage in the patients with one to three positive lymph nodes.[65] The difficulty in interpreting these data, however, is that many patients in these trials did not undergo a formal level I/II axillary dissection. In the Danish studies, the median number of axillary lymph nodes resected was only seven,[69] which is approximately 50% of the number reported from studies conducted in the United States. In addition, 76% of the patients had <10 lymph nodes removed, and 15% had three or fewer lymph nodes removed.[69] In the Vancouver trial, the median number of resected lymph nodes was 11.[73] Given the less extensive axillary surgery done in these studies, it is highly probable that some of the patients in these studies reported as having had one to three positive lymph nodes would have had four or more positive lymph nodes if a standard axillary dissection had been performed. Correspondingly, their risk of a chest wall or supraclavicular recurrence would be higher than that usually estimated for patients with one to three positive nodes. Moreover, failure to remove these additional involved axillary lymph nodes would predispose patients to axillary recurrence, which could be avoided by a more complete axillary dissection. Indeed, the most recent update of the Danish studies reported that 43% of all local-regional recurrences included recurrence in the axilla.[72] To further investigate this question, the Danish investigators reanalyzed their trial results specifically with regard to the patients who had eight or more lymph nodes resected. For the patients with one to three positive lymph nodes, there continued to be significant improvements in local-regional control (96% vs. 73%) and overall survival (57% vs. 48%) in the patients randomized to receive postmastectomy radiation.[74]

Risks of Local-Regional Recurrence After Modified Radical Mastectomy and Systemic Treatment

Another aspect to consider concerning the data of the patients with one to three positive lymph nodes treated in these trials is that the local-regional recurrence rates appear much higher than for patients treated in the United States with standard modified radical mastectomy and systemic treatments. Specifically, the 18-year rate of isolated local-regional recurrence for the patients in the Danish studies treated with mastectomy and systemic treatment was 41% and the 18-year rate for the subgroup with one to three positive lymph nodes was 37%.[72] Even in limiting the analysis to patients with eight or more lymph nodes resected, the local-regional recurrence rate was 27%.[74] In the updated Oxford analysis, the 15-year overall rate of local-regional recurrence was 25%, although it is important to note the a majority of patients included in this subset of the meta-analysis were the patients treated in the Danish trials.[65]

The risks of recurrence in the Danish and Vancouver trials after mastectomy and chemotherapy were high relative to those reported from large series from the United States and from a European cooperative group. To help define the indications for radiation, several groups recently conducted studies to assess which patients are at risk for local-regional recurrence after treatment with a mastectomy that included a level I/II axillary dissection, systemic treatment, and no radiation. The results from the largest of these studies are summarized in Table 57.5.[75-78] In general, the findings suggest that the 10-year local-regional recurrence risk for patients with one to three positive lymph nodes was approximately 12% to 15%, which is nearly one-third of the local-regional recurrence rate in the no-radiation group of the Vancouver and Danish trials and one-half that of the Oxford overview. The reasons for these lower risks are not clearly known but probably reflect differences in the surgical procedure performed. In addition, these patterns-of-failure studies reported outcomes at 10 years, whereas the

TABLE 57.5 LOCAL-REGIONAL RECURRENCE RATES IN PATIENTS NOT TREATED WITH RADIATION AFTER MASTECTOMY IN RANDOMIZED CLINICAL TRIALS[75-78]

Patterns-of-Failure Studies	Number of Patients	Local-Regional Recurrence Rate at 10 Years (%)
ECOG		
1–3 positive lymph nodes	1,018	13
≥4 positive lymph nodes	998	29
MD Anderson		
1–3 positive lymph nodes	466	12
≥4 positive lymph nodes	419	27
NSABP		
1–3 positive lymph nodes	2,957	6–11
≥4 positive lymph nodes	2,784	14–25
IBCSG		
1–3 positive lymph nodes	2,408	14–27
≥4 positive lymph nodes	1,659	24–35

ECOG, Eastern Cooperative Oncology Group; IBCSG, International Breast Cancer Study Group; NSABP, National Surgical Adjuvant Breast and Bowel Project.

randomized, prospective studies reported outcome data at 18 and 20 years. In the Danish studies, the local-regional recurrence rate rose relatively consistently by 1% per year between the 10th and 25th follow-up years.[72] Similarly, in the Vancouver randomized trial, approximately 20% of local-regional recurrences in the group that did not receive postmastectomy radiation developed after 10 years of follow-up.[71]

Stage II breast cancer with one to three positive lymph nodes is also heterogeneous with respect to other prognostic factors that affect local-regional recurrence risk. Table 57.6 shows various cofactors that have been found to increase the risk of local-regional recurrence within this subgroup. Cheng et al.[80] analyzed 110 patients with a minimum follow-up of 25 months who were treated with modified radical mastectomy without radiation and had one to three positive axillary nodes (median number of nodes examined, 17). Sixty-nine patients received adjuvant chemotherapy and 84 received adjuvant hormonal therapy with tamoxifen. These investigators defined four factors (age <40 years, tumor ≥3 cm, ER-negative disease, and lymphovascular invasion) that segregated the patients into a high-risk group (with three or four factors) and a low-risk group (with two or fewer factors). Tumor size was also found to be an important cofactor in work from MD Anderson, but those authors found a size of 4 cm to increase the risk. Finally, findings from the International Breast Cancer Study Group Trials I through VII found that premenopausal women with one to three positive lymph nodes had local-regional recurrence risks ranging from 19% to 27% if they had G2-3 disease with vascular invasion but that risk was <15% if they had G1 disease with no vascular invasion.[77] Among postmenopausal women with one to three positive lymph nodes, those with G3 disease and tumors >2 cm had a local-regional recurrence risk of 24% as compared with less than 15% for those with G1–2 disease with tumors <2 cm.

Margin status is another important co-risk factor in this cohort. In an analysis of the 34 of patients with close or positive margins whose primary tumor was smaller than 5 cm with zero to three positive axillary nodes and who received no postoperative radiation, Freedman et al.[81] reported a relatively high risk of local relapse, but only among younger women. Five chest wall recurrences appeared at a median interval of 26 months (range, 7 to 127 months), resulting in an 8-year cumulative incidence of a chest wall recurrence of 18%. Patient age correlated with the cumulative incidence of chest wall recurrence at 8 years; the rate for women of age ≤50 years was 28% versus 0% for women older than 50 years ($p = .04$). Katz et al.[82] also found close or positive margins to be an independent risk factor for the development of local-regional recurrence after mastectomy, but in that series age did not affect this risk. The 10-year risk for the 29 patients with close or positive margins was 45%; the risk was 33% for those with pectoralis fascia invasion even when negative margins were achieved.

The presence of multicentric disease is strongly associated with other risk factors for local-regional recurrence, such as tumor size and nodal involvement. However, in patients with stage II disease with one to three positive lymph nodes, multicentric disease does not seem to elevate the risk of local-regional recurrence. Fowble et al.[83] reported that patients with multicentric disease without other strong risk factors for postmastectomy chest wall relapse had a 5-year actuarial risk of an isolated local-regional recurrence of 8%. By comparison, Katz et al.[82] found a 10-year recurrence risk of 37% for patients with multicentric disease, but limiting the analysis to only patients with one to three positive lymph nodes eliminated any association between multicentric or multifocal disease and local-regional recurrence.

The MD Anderson group recently re-evaluated their local-regional recurrence risk in a more contemporary era of patients with zero to three positive lymph nodes treated after publication of the Danish trial results.[84] Since that time, the institutional philosophy was to consider postmastectomy radiation for the subgroups of patients with one to three positive lymph nodes: age <40 years, lymphovascular space invasion, tumor size <4 cm, three positive lymph nodes or a positive lymph node ratio of 20% or greater, or extensive extracapsular extension. In general, patients without these features and those with T1,2 N0 disease were not offered postmastectomy treatment. The authors analyzed >1,000 patients treated for a pT1 or pT2 tumor between 1997 and 2002 with mastectomy, a modern chemotherapy regimen, and no radiation. They analyzed the locoregional outcome of 753 patients with negative lymph nodes, 176 with one positive lymph node, 69 with two positive lymph nodes, and only 21 patients with three positive lymph nodes. The 10-year locoregional recurrence rates were low overall, with respective rates of 2.1% (node negative), 3.3% (one positive node), and 7.9% (two positive nodes). The group with three positive lymph nodes was too small to provide meaningful data. These data suggest that the selection criteria used were effective in selecting a cohort of patients with early-stage, lymph node–positive disease who are at very low risk of having a local-regional recurrence.

Even if the risk of local-regional recurrence for most patients with one to three positive lymph nodes is relatively low after a modified radical mastectomy and chemotherapy, radiation could still provide a benefit. Indeed, Woodward et al.[85] found that the risk of local-regional recurrence after mastectomy and anthracycline-based chemotherapy was only 13% for patients with stage II disease and one to three positive lymph nodes. However, at the same institution, patients with similarly staged disease treated with postmastectomy radiation had a local-regional recurrence risk of only 3%.[85] Whether this degree of benefit is clinically meaningful with respect to patient survival is unknown. A recent investigation of this question evaluated data from the SEER Program concerning patients with T1 or T2 primary tumors treated with mastectomy. In that study, radiation use led to a 15% to 20% relative reduction in breast cancer mortality, but this reduction only became significant in a multivariate analysis of patients with seven or more positive lymph nodes.[86] Because the treating physicians made the decisions concerning the use of radiation for the patients included in that database, unidentified biases could be present

TABLE 57.6 COFACTORS ASSOCIATED WITH A >15% LOCAL-REGIONAL RECURRENCE AFTER MASTECTOMY AND CHEMOTHERAPY IN PATIENTS WITH ONE TO THREE POSITIVE LYMPH NODES

Study	Number of Patients	Cofactors
Katz et al.[75]	466	Tumor size >4 cm Extracapsular extension >2 mm Less than 10 lymph nodes removed 20% of lymph nodes involved Invasion of skin/nipple Invasion of pectoralis fascia Close or positive margins
Wallgren et al.[77]	2,408	Premenopausal, G2 or G3, LVSI Postmenopausal, G3 Postmenopausal, G2, T2 disease
Taghian et al.[78]	2,957	Age <50 yr, T2 disease
Truong et al.[79]	821	Age <45 yr Twenty-five percent of lymph nodes involved ER-negative disease G3 disease Medial tumor location
Cheng et al.[80]	110	Age <40 yr Tumor size ≥3 cm Presence of LVSI No tamoxifen use

ER, estrogen receptor; LVSI, lymphovascular space invasion.

that affected these results. Indeed, other investigators, evaluating data from the same program on patients with T1 or T2 primary tumors with one to three positive lymph nodes, compared the outcome of those treated with breast-conserving surgery with radiation versus mastectomy without radiation.[87] In that study, multivariate analyses showed that patients treated with breast conservation plus radiation had significantly improved survival compared with those treated with mastectomy without radiation. Again, unaccounted biases probably affected these results to some degree.

It is also important to recognize that the patients at lowest risk for local-regional recurrence may be the cohort who achieve the greatest relative survival advantage from avoidance of a local-regional recurrence. This is because the risk factors for local-regional recurrence overlap with those for the development of distant metastases. For example, extensive lymph node involvement leads to a high risk of local-regional recurrence but also predicts for a high competing risk of distant metastases that may not be avoided through the use of postmastectomy radiation. In an interesting analysis conducted using data from the Danish randomized trials, investigators demonstrated that the greatest proportional survival advantage associated with postmastectomy radiation was found in the subgroups of patients with the most favorable prognostic features (fewer than three positive lymph nodes, small tumor sizes, ER-positive disease).[88]

Another cohort of patients in whom the use of postmastectomy radiation is controversial are those with pathologic T3 N0 disease. One reason for this controversy is that there are limited data regarding the risk of local-regional recurrence after mastectomy and systemic treatments in such patients. This lack of data is a consequence of the fact that the majority of breast cancers that are 5 cm or greater will have lymph node–positive disease and that a large percentage of patients with clinical T3 N0 disease are currently treated with neoadjuvant chemotherapy. Historically, patients with pathologic T3 N0 disease who were treated with an initial mastectomy were recommended to receive postmastectomy radiation. However, two recent publications indicated that the risk of local-regional recurrence is relatively low. Floyd et al.[89] published data concerning a multicenter study of 70 patients treated with mastectomy, systemic therapy, and no radiation for patients with pathologic T3 N0 disease and reported a 5-year local-regional recurrence of only 8%. Those who had lymphovascular space invasion had a 21% local-regional recurrence compared to a rate of only 4% for those without lymphovascular space invasion. Finally, of the patients who experienced a local-regional recurrence, 89% had the chest wall as their only site of recurrence. In addition, Taghian et al.[90] analyzed the outcome of 313 patients with pathologic stage T3 N0 disease who were treated with mastectomy, systemic treatments, and no radiation on NSABP clinical trials. The 10-year LRR for this series was only 7%, with 24 of the 28 local-regional recurrences developing only on the chest wall.

Both the American Society for Therapeutic Radiology and Oncology and the American Society of Clinical Oncology have published consensus statements recommending postmastectomy radiation therapy for women with four or more positive lymph nodes or advanced primary disease. Both statements included the recommendation that an additional trial be performed to further clarify the benefit of postmastectomy radiation therapy for women with stage II disease and one to three positive lymph nodes.[91,92] Unfortunately, an Intergroup trial designed to determine the benefits of postmastectomy radiation therapy for such patients closed owing to poor accrual. However, the Selective Use of Postoperative Radiotherapy after Mastectomy trial is accruing patients in the United Kingdom, through EORTC, and in Asia and may in the future provide answers to this question.

In summary, it is clear that postmastectomy radiation offers a significant benefit for patients in terms of a 20% to 40% risk of local-regional recurrence, and therefore it should be recommended for all such patients. It is reasonable to discuss the risks and benefits of radiation for patients with intermediate-risk disease, such as those with pathologic stage II breast cancer. It is hoped that ongoing studies will further refine risk stratification within this subset by considering other cofactors, such as margin status, lymphovascular space invasion, patient age, extent of axillary dissection, and presence of extracapsular disease. In the future, this may be a cohort of patients in whom molecular predictive tests may further stratify treatment decisions.

Postmastectomy Radiation Therapy After Neoadjuvant Chemotherapy

Neoadjuvant chemotherapy has now become a standard initial therapy for most patients with locally advanced breast cancer. As the use of neoadjuvant chemotherapy has become more common, new questions regarding the indications for postmastectomy radiation therapy have arisen. This is because historically the decision to administer radiation therapy was made predominantly on the basis of the pathologic extent of disease. However, neoadjuvant chemotherapy changes the extent of pathologic disease in 80% to 90% of cases, and it is unclear whether and how the posttreatment pathologic information should guide decisions regarding radiation treatment. What has been learned is that the correlations between pathologic extent of disease and local-regional recurrence after mastectomy are different for patients treated with chemotherapy first compared with those treated with surgery first.[93] Specifically, one study found that the local-regional recurrence rate associated with a particular pathologic extent of disease after surgery was higher among patients treated with chemotherapy first than among patients treated with surgery first. This is not particularly surprising, in that in the neoadjuvant chemotherapy group, the pathologic examination represented residual disease after treatment, whereas in those treated with surgery first, the extent of disease represented untreated cancer. However, these findings imply that the risk of local-regional recurrence for patients given neoadjuvant chemotherapy is determined by both the pretreatment clinical stage and the extent of pathologically residual disease after chemotherapy.

Information on the efficacy of postmastectomy radiation therapy for patients treated with neoadjuvant chemotherapy is limited. One of the first published studies investigating this issue compared the outcomes of 579 patients who received neoadjuvant chemotherapy, mastectomy, and radiation therapy with those of 136 patients who were treated with neoadjuvant chemotherapy and mastectomy.[94] Patients in this study had been treated in prospective chemotherapy trials in which radiation therapy was given on the basis of physician recommendations and patient preferences. Therefore, the patients with worse disease characteristics were more often treated with radiation therapy. Despite this, the local-regional recurrence rate was found to be significantly lower in the group treated with postmastectomy radiation therapy than in the group treated with neoadjuvant chemotherapy and mastectomy (10-year local-regional recurrence rates were 8% and 22%, respectively; $p = .001$). For patients with clinical stage III disease or extensive disease after chemotherapy, radiation led to significant improvements in local-regional recurrence and overall and cause-specific survival rates. Multivariate analyses indicated that radiation was independently associated with a lower risk of local-regional recurrence (hazard ratio for not receiving radiation therapy, 7.0; $p < .0001$) and a lower risk of breast cancer death (hazard ratio for not receiving radiation therapy, 2.03; $p < .0001$).[94]

The same group of investigators has also shown that among patients with stage III disease who achieved a pCR, the local-regional recurrence rate for those treated with radiation therapy was 7% versus 33% for those who did not receive radiation therapy ($p = .040$). Radiation use in these patients was also associated with an improvement in survival. Finally, this group also tried to address which patients given neoadjuvant chemotherapy for clinical stage II breast cancer should receive radiation therapy. In a recent publication, they examined patients with clinical T3 N0 disease and reported a 4% 5-year local-regional recurrence rate in 119 patients who received postmastectomy radiation compared to a 24% rate in the 43 patients who did not ($p < .001$).[95]

There remains significant controversy as to which patients with clinical stage T1 2N1 disease treated with neoadjuvant chemotherapy and mastectomy benefit from radiation. It may be that response to the chemotherapy may help to guide such treatment decisions. Retrospective analyses from the MD Anderson Cancer Center and the NSABP suggested that patients with clinical stage IIA/IIB disease who have lymph node–negative disease after neoadjuvant chemotherapy and who do not receive radiation have a <10% risk of local-regional recurrence.[96,97] This cohort is estimated to represent 40% of the original population. In contrast, for the remaining 60% of the patients who have residual lymph node–positive disease after neoadjuvant chemotherapy, the risk of local-regional recurrence is >15%.[96,97] Therefore, the use of neoadjuvant chemotherapy for patients with stage II disease may further risk-stratify patients and permit avoidance of postmastectomy radiation in 30% to 40% of this population. This would permit avoidance of the toxicities and costs in this cohort.

In summary, the use of postmastectomy radiation therapy is reasonable for all patients with clinical T3 or T4 tumors or clinical stage III disease regardless of their response to the chemotherapy regimen. In terms of clinical stage I or II breast cancer, postmastectomy radiation therapy should be recommended for patients with four or more positive lymph nodes after chemotherapy and for the unusual patient in whom the disease progresses and the primary tumor exceeds 5 cm in diameter. Clearly, however, additional studies are needed to quantify the local-regional recurrence risk for patients who present with T1 or T2 N1 disease and have zero to three positive lymph nodes after neoadjuvant chemotherapy.

Systemic Therapy

Systemic treatments play a critical role in the multidisciplinary management of both early-stage and locally advanced breast cancer. After tamoxifen and anthracyclines were established as important components of adjuvant treatments in the late 1980s, there were few significant advances for nearly two decades. However, in the recent past the landscape of breast cancer adjuvant and neoadjuvant systemic treatments has rapidly changed. These recent advances in the systemic management of breast have contributed to the decreasing breast cancer death rates recently noted. A full description of the vast array of systemic chemotherapy, hormone therapy, and molecular therapies is beyond the scope of this chapter. However, we will review the current state of these therapeutics.

Meta-Analyses

Similar to their meta-analyses of radiotherapy trials in breast cancer, the Early Breast Cancer Trialists' Collaborative Group has analyzed overviews of trials investigating chemotherapy and hormonal therapy for breast cancer. Their most recent complete meta-analysis was published in 2005 and evaluated data from almost 150,000 patients treated on 194 randomized trials that investigated chemotherapy or hormonal therapy.[98] Only trials that began by 1995 were included, so no data were available concerning the efficacy of taxanes or trastuzumab. More recently, they published an update on the efficacy of adjuvant tamoxifen using data from 21,457 patients treated in 20 randomized trials[99] and an analysis of trials comparing aromatase inhibitors versus tamoxifen.[100]

The use of chemotherapy was found to reduce the probability of recurrence and the risk of death both for patients with lymph node–positive disease and those with lymph node–negative disease.[98] The proportional reduction in recurrence and breast cancer mortality achieved with chemotherapy was very similar for both groups. However, because patients with positive lymph nodes have a much greater risk of recurrence and death from disease, the absolute percentage who benefit from chemotherapy is greatest in this cohort. Use of multiagent chemotherapy resulted in an improved outcome compared to single-agent chemotherapy. In addition, there was a significant benefit in using anthracycline (fluorouracil, doxorubicin, and cyclophosphamide [FAC] or fluorouracil, epirubicin, and cyclophosphamide [FEC]) chemotherapy compared to CMF chemotherapy. Finally, the benefits of chemotherapy varied according to patient age, with patients younger than 50 years of age achieving a greater proportional reduction in the risk of recurrence (proportional reduction of 36%) than patients 50 to 69 years old (proportional reduction of 29%). The respective proportional reduction in the annual death rates for these cohorts was 38% and 20%. Based on data from this analysis, Table 57.7 estimates the 5-year risk of recurrence and the absolute magnitude of benefit polychemotherapy by age and lymph node status.[98]

TABLE 57.7 BENEFITS OF POLYCHEMOTHERAPY VERSUS NO CHEMOTHERAPY IN REDUCING THE 5-YEAR RISK OF BREAST CANCER RECURRENCE

Cohort	Rates of Recurrence With and Without Chemotherapy (%)	Absolute Benefit (%)
Age <50 yr, LN–	17.5 vs. 27.4	9.9
Age <50 yr, LN+	40.6 vs. 55.2	14.6
Age 50–69 yr, LN–	14.3 vs. 19.6	5.3
Age 50–69 yr, LN+	36.7 vs. 42.6	5.9

LN–, lymph node–negative; LN+, lymph node–positive. Data were obtained from Figure 3 of the 2005 Early Breast Cancer Trialists' Collaborative Group meta-analysis.[98]

Five years of tamoxifen therapy also provide a significant benefit in reducing recurrence (reduced by 47% through 10 years) and improving survival for patients with ER-positive disease (~33% proportional reduction in breast cancer death rate).[99] Tamoxifen provided a benefit for both younger and older patients with ER-positive or ER-unknown disease but did not provide a benefit for patients with ER-negative disease. The data indicate that 5 years of tamoxifen therapy provided better outcomes than 1 to 2 years of treatment. For patients with ER-positive, lymph node–negative disease not treated with chemotherapy, tamoxifen treatment reduced the 10-year risk from 34.8% (no tamoxifen) to 19.1% (tamoxifen). In the lymph node–positive cohort, the 10-year risk of recurrence was 57.0% versus 41.5%, respectively. Tamoxifen continued to provide clinically and significant improvements in similar patients also treated with chemotherapy.[99]

More Recent Advances: Chemotherapy

There have been important incremental advances beyond the standard of anthracycline chemotherapy in more recent years, most notably the introduction of taxanes. Three of the most important recent trials that have shown a benefit for adjuvant taxanes after anthracycline chemotherapy are the CALGB 9344/Intergroup 0148 trial,[101] the NSABP B-28 trial,[102] and the BCIRG 001 trial.[103] The design and results of these trials are given in Table 57.8. In aggregate, these trials indicated that the addition of taxanes to anthracycline chemotherapy provides an additional reduction in the risk of recurrence in the adjuvant treatment of breast cancer.

These individual trial results have been confirmed in meta-analyses of adjuvant taxane trials in breast cancer. The most recent analysis revealed that incorporating a taxane into anthracycline-based chemotherapy improved disease-free survival (hazard ratio, 0.83) and overall survival (hazard ratio, 0.85). The improvement was not affected by type of taxane, ER

TABLE 57.8 REVIEW OF ADJUVANT TAXANE CHEMOTHERAPY TRIALS

Trial	Study Population	Randomization	Outcome
CALGB 9344[101]	3,121 patients with lymph node–positive breast cancer	AC × 4 vs. AC × 4 followed by paclitaxel × 4	5-yr DFS improved from 65% to 70%
NSABP B-28[102]	3,060 patients with lymph node–positive breast cancer	AC × 4 vs. AC × 4 followed by paclitaxel × 4	5-yr DFS improved from 72% to 76%
BCIRG 001[103]	1,491 patients with lymph node–positive breast cancer	FAC × 6 vs. TAC × 6	5-yr DFS improved from 68% to 75%

AC, doxorubicin and cyclophosphamide; DFS, disease-free survival; FAC, fluorouracil, doxorubicin, and cyclophosphamide; TAC, docetaxel, doxorubicin, and cyclophosphamide.

expression, number of positive lymph nodes, or menopausal status.[104]

Once taxanes became established as important components of adjuvant treatment of breast cancer, new trials began investigating the administration schedule of treatments. The CALGB 9741/Intergroup trial randomized patients receiving doxorubicin/cyclophosphamide (AC) × 4 followed by paclitaxel × 4 or A × 4, paclitaxel × 4, and C × 4 to a schedule that delivered the drugs every 3 weeks versus a "dose-dense" schedule of giving the chemotherapy with growth factor support every 2 weeks.[105] The finding from this trial indicated that the dose-dense therapy further improved disease-free survival (4-year disease-free survival rate was 82% [dose dense] vs.75% [every-3-week administration]).

Many oncologists want a less intensive chemotherapy regimen for patients with low-risk disease and for patients with comorbidities. For such patients, a practice changing trial from the US Oncology group compared four cycles of AC to four cycles of docetaxel/cyclophosphamide (TC). With 7-years of follow-up, the TC arm had statistically significant improvements in both disease-free rate (81% vs. 75%; p = .03) and overall survival (87% vs. 82%; p = .03).[106]

More Recent Advances: Hormonal Therapy

In addition to chemotherapy, hormonal therapy is indicated for all patients with ER- or progesterone receptor (PR)–positive disease. Tamoxifen is the preferred hormonal treatment for all premenopausal women who continue to have ovarian function after chemotherapy. For postmenopausal women, the use of an aromatase inhibitor is equally appropriate. Aromatase inhibitors have proven to be a significant advance in hormonally responsive breast cancer. Unlike tamoxifen, which directly blocks the estrogen receptor on tumor cells, aromatase inhibitors provide beneficial effects by decreasing circulating estrogen by inhibiting the conversion of adrenal testosterone–like hormones into estrogen. Accordingly, aromatase inhibitors do not carry some of the same proestrogenic effects that have been associated with tamoxifen, such as its potentially beneficial effects against osteoporosis and its potentially harmful effects of stimulating the endometrial lining.

After the safety and efficacy of aromatase inhibitors were established in postmenopausal women with ER-positive metastatic disease, these agents were studied in the adjuvant setting and also proved to be of clinical value. Table 57.9 reviews the results of three important recent adjuvant studies in which the use of an aromatase inhibitor was found to be superior to the previously established standard of 5 years of tamoxifen therapy. Based on the results of these trials, there are a number of options for postmenopausal patients, including anastrozole for 5 years, letrozole for 5 years, initial tamoxifen for 2 to 3 years followed by exemestane, or tamoxifen for 5 years followed by 5 years of letrozole.[107–110]

The Oxford group conducted a meta-analysis of trials comparing aromatase inhibitors versus tamoxifen.[100] Aromatase inhibitors provided a 2.9% absolute decrease in the risk of recurrence in a cohort of 9,856 patients treated on trials directly comparing an aromatase inhibitor to tamoxifen. In addition, in trials that tested sequential tamoxifen/aromatase inhibitor versus tamoxifen alone, a 3.1% absolute decrease in recurrence was noted. Based on such data, American Society of Clinical Oncology published a clinical practice guideline recommending that postmenopausal women with hormone receptor–positive tumor receive a treatment that incorporates an aromatase inhibitor.[111]

More Recent Advances: Trastuzumab

One of the most significant recent advances in breast cancer treatment has been the introduction of trastuzumab into the adjuvant treatment for patients with tumors that have gene amplification of the HER2/neu gene. In 2005, the initial results of a series of randomized, prospective trials designed to evaluate whether the addition of trastuzumab increased the efficacy of adjuvant chemotherapy of patients with HER2/neu overexpression were published. The results of these studies were dramatic and indicated a significant incremental benefit for the use of trastuzumab over chemotherapy alone. Table 57.10 reviews the preliminary results of three of these studies.[113–114,115,116] In the United States, the results of two similarly designed trials from the NSABP and the North Central Cancer Treatment Group were combined and after a median follow-up of 3.9 years indicated a 48% reduction in the relative risk of recurrence and a 31% reduction in the risk of death compared to anthracycline and taxane chemotherapy alone.[112] In all trials, trastuzumab increased the risk for a decrease in cardiac

TABLE 57.9 REVIEW OF ADJUVANT AROMATASE INHIBITOR TRIALS

Trial	Study Population	Randomization	Outcome
ATAC[107]	9,356 postmenopausal patients	Arimidex × 5 yr vs. tamoxifen × 5 yr vs. both	Arimidex reduced the relative risk of recurrence over tamoxifen by 23% (3.7% absolute reduction of the risk at 6 yr); fewer contralataral breast cancers, fewer serious side effects
NCIC MA.17[108]	5,187 postmenopausal patients	Letrozol vs. placebo × 5 yr after 5 yr of tamoxifen	Letrozole reduced the risk of distant recurrence and the risk of contralataral breast cancers; absolute benefit was 2.4% after 30 mo median follow-up
Intergroup Exemestane Trial[109]	4,742 postmenopausal patients	2–3 yr of tamoxifen, then switching to exemestane vs. continuing tamoxifen × 5 yr	Exemestane reduced the relative risk of recurrence over tamoxifen by 32% (4.7% absolute reduction of the risk at 3 yr)
BIG 1-98 trial[110]	8,010 postmenopausal patients	Letrozole vs. letrozole + tamoxifen vs. tamoxifen vs. tamoxifen + letrozole	Comparing two letrozole-first arms against 2 tamoxifen arms: 5-yr recurrences were reduced by 19% and distant metastases reduced by 27% (2.6% absolute improvement in 5-yr disease-free survival)

TABLE 57.10 REVIEW OF TRIALS EVALUATING ADJUVANT TRASTUZUMAB WITH CHEMOTHERAPY FOR PATIENTS WITH HER2/NEU-POSITIVE BREAST CANCER

Trial	*Study Population*	*Randomization*	*Outcome*
NSABP B-31, NCCTG N9831[112]	3,351 patients with HER2/neu–positive disease; 94% had lymph node–positive disease	AC × 4 followed by paclitaxel × 4 with or with trastuzumab given concurrently with paclitaxel and as adjuvant therapy × 1 yr	Trastuzumab reduced the relative risk of recurrence over chemotherapy alone by 48% (9% absolute reduction of the risk at 3 yr); there was a 31% proportional reduction in the risk of death
HERA trial[113]	5,081 patients with HER2/neu–positive disease; 68% had lymph node–positive disease	Minimum of four cycles of chemotherapy and then randomized to no trastuzumab vs. trastuzumab × 1 yr vs. trastuzumab × 2 yr	Trastuzumab × 1 yr reduced the relative risk of recurrence over chemotherapy alone by 46% (8.4% absolute reduction of the risk at 3 yr); there was insufficient follow-up to assess the trastuzumab × 2 yr arm
FinHer Study[114]	232 patients with HER2/neu–positive; 84% had lymph node–positive disease	Docetaxel or vinorelbine × 3, FEC × 3, then randomized to no trastuzumab vs. trastuzumab × 9 wk	Trastuzumab reduced the relative risk of recurrence or death over chemotherapy alone by 58% (11% absolute reduction of the risk at 3 yr)
BCIRG 006[115]	3174 patients with HER2/neu–positive; 71% had lymph node-positive disease	AC × 4 + docetaxel × 4, with or with trastuzumab given concurrently with docetaxel and as adjuvant therapy × 1 yr, third arm of docetaxel/carboplatinum/trastuzumab × 6, then as adjuvant therapy × 1 yr	Trastuzumab reduced the relative risk of recurrence or death over chemotherapy alone by 39%

AC, doxorubicin and cyclophosphamide; FEC, fluorouracil, epirubicin, and cyclophosphamide.

ejection fraction, and it became more fully appreciated that patients treated with this agent require careful cardiac supervision. For most of these trials, patients who required radiation received trastuzumab concurrently during radiation treatments. No increase in cardiac events or other serious sequelae has been reported as a consequence of the concurrent use of trastuzumab and radiation.[117]

Treatment Algorithms for Locally Advanced Breast Cancer

Figure 57.6 shows an algorithm for the management of patients with locally advanced operable cancer and patients who present with either operable or inoperable disease. Neoadjuvant chemotherapy is the preferred initial treatment for patients with inoperable disease and for selected patients with advanced but operable disease who are interested in being treated with breast conservation therapy. For such patients, neoadjuvant chemotherapy should consist of a regimen that contains anthracyclines and taxanes, given in either a sequential or concurrent fashion. The rationale of using all agents "up front" rather than splitting the course of treatment is to give the therapy in the most dose-dense fashion. Patients with HER2/neu–positive disease are recommended to receive trastuzumab concurrent with the neoadjuvant taxane.

After neoadjuvant chemotherapy, all patients should undergo surgical resection. Mastectomy remains the standard of care for most patients with locally advanced disease, but breast-conserving surgery can be considered for carefully selected patients. Axillary lymph node dissection should be performed for all patients with involved axillary lymph nodes at the time of presentation, regardless of the clinical response of axillary disease to neoadjuvant treatment. Sentinel lymph node surgery is appropriate for patients who present with a clinical negative axilla prior to neoadjuvant chemotherapy. After surgery, adjuvant radiation to the breast, chest wall, and draining lymphatics should be offered to all patients with clinical stage III disease.

Some cases of advanced disease fail to respond to neoadjuvant chemotherapy, and such patients have a poor outcome. However, a small percentage of patients can achieve long-term survival with aggressive local-regional therapies. A study of

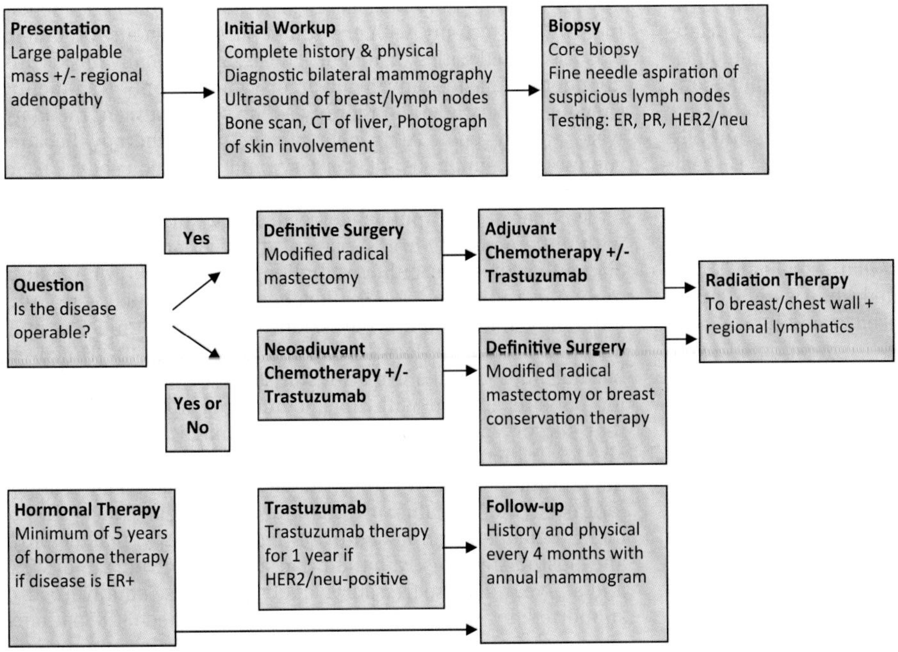

FIGURE 57.6. Flow diagram of workup and treatment recommendations for patients who present with locally advanced breast cancer.

177 patients with advanced disease that was refractory to neoadjuvant chemotherapy reported a 10-year survival rate of 33% after aggressive local-regional treatments.[118] Not surprisingly, patients with ER-positive disease had the best outcome, in part because effective systemic therapies were still available to them.

For patients in whom the disease remains inoperable after neoadjuvant chemotherapy, preoperative or definitive radiation remains the treatment of choice. Surgeons and radiation oncologists need to carefully coordinate the care of such patients, and the future operability of the breast needs to be considered early in the treatment course because radiation-induced breast edema and erythema can mimic the clinical findings of advanced breast cancer. A study of 38 patients who underwent radiation therapy with or without mastectomy after the disease remained inoperable after neoadjuvant chemotherapy found that 46% were alive and 33% were free of distant disease at 5 years after treatment.[119] Those patients who were able to undergo mastectomy after preoperative radiation had the best local-regional control. Preoperative radiation led to surgical complications in 9% of patients treated with <54 Gy but in 70% of the patients treated to doses of ≥54 Gy.

Some centers have piloted concurrent chemoradiation strategies as neoadjuvant approaches. In one recent study of the use of neoadjuvant paclitaxel followed by concurrent paclitaxel–radiation for patients with operable stage II/III breast cancer, 13 of the 38 patients (34%) experienced pCR and acceptably low treatment toxicity.[120] Another group of investigators also completed a phase I/II multi-institutional study of concurrent paclitaxel–radiation for 105 patients with locally advanced breast cancer and also found a pCR rate of 23%.[121] Again, acceptable treatment toxicity was noted. However, because other investigators have found significant rates of pulmonary injury when paclitaxel and radiation were given concurrently to women with breast cancer, this approach is best taken within the context of a clinical research protocol.

Treatment Results for Locally Advanced Breast Cancer

As noted earlier in this chapter, stage III breast cancer historically has been associated with a very poor prognosis, with high rates of local-regional recurrence, distant metastases, and death. However, advances in all of the disciplines involved in breast cancer treatment have improved the outcome of such patients. With modern treatment strategies that include systemic therapy with taxanes and anthracyclines, appropriate surgical intervention, and local-regional irradiation, outcomes have significantly improved. With respect to local-regional control, a recent study evaluating outcome after mastectomy and radiation for patients with advanced disease that was initially treated with neoadjuvant chemotherapy reported a 10-year local-regional control rate of 89%.[94] Patients with ER-negative disease and significant residual disease burden or skin invasion had rates of local-regional recurrence approaching 20%, whereas those without these features had excellent local-regional outcomes. As previously indicated, the risk of distant metastases has also significantly decreased over time. A reasonable estimate of 10-year survival rates for patients given modern treatments for stage III breast cancer is approximately 50%.[9]

Patients with supraclavicular lymph node disease at diagnosis have a poorer outcome than do other patients with stage III disease. However, because some studies of patients treated with chemotherapy have reported 10-year survival rates of 25%, the AJCC recategorized this stage of disease from stage IV to stage IIIC.[122] The local-regional management of such disease should be the same as for stage III disease. A recent study investigating the outcome of 70 patients with supraclavicular disease who were treated with neoadjuvant chemotherapy, surgery, and radiation reported a 5-year local-regional control rate of 77% and a 5-year overall survival rate of 47%.[94] Patients in whom the supraclavicular disease showed a CR to neoadjuvant chemotherapy had better outcomes than did those with persistent disease after chemotherapy.

GENERAL MANAGEMENT AND TREATMENT RESULTS FOR INFLAMMATORY BREAST CANCER

Because inflammatory breast cancer is relatively uncommon, no data from randomized studies are available regarding the optimal therapeutic approach for this disease. In general, however, it is clear that management of inflammatory breast cancer requires carefully integrated care by a multidisciplinary team. Ideally, such patients should be evaluated in a multidisciplinary center by all specialists at the time of presentation to confirm the diagnosis of inflammatory disease, document the extent of disease (including photographs of areas of involved skin), and agree on a treatment plan. Inflammatory breast cancer is considered inoperable at presentation and should be treated initially with neoadjuvant chemotherapy (with consideration of trastuzumab if the tumor is HER2/neu–positive). Patients should be carefully monitored for response, and after achievement of the maximal clinical response, patients should be reevaluated for mastectomy. About 80% of patients with inflammatory breast cancer will achieve a clinical response, and their disease will become operable.[123] All patients should receive postmastectomy radiation therapy delivered to the chest wall and the draining lymphatics.

The optimal chemotherapy regimen for patients with inflammatory breast cancer includes both anthracyclines and taxanes. The introduction of anthracycline chemotherapy, when combined with local-regional treatments, provided the first evidence of treatment efficacy in this disease. Investigators at MD Anderson conducted a series of single-group prospective trials for patients with inflammatory breast cancer and found that neoadjuvant chemotherapy with FAC followed by local-regional therapy led to a 5-year survival rate of 25%. Subsequently, these investigators introduced sequential FAC or FEC followed by weekly paclitaxel and reported that the addition of taxanes improved the progression-free and overall survival of patients with inflammatory disease.[123]

Local-regional treatment is an essential component of therapy for inflammatory disease. Before the routine use of chemotherapy, mastectomy, with or without postmastectomy radiation, was associated with a dismal prognosis, and so many physicians abandoned mastectomy in favor of radiation-only treatments. Outcomes after radiation therapy as the sole treatment modality were equally poor. After neoadjuvant chemotherapy became routine, combinations of surgery and radiation have been reevaluated.

De Boer et al.[124] published results of a study of 54 patients with inflammatory breast cancer treated after neoadjuvant chemotherapy with either radiation only (n = 35) or mastectomy plus radiation (n = 19). For the patients treated with radiation only, the median progression-free survival time was only 16 months and the local recurrence rate was 34%. However, because these results were not statistically different from those for patients treated with mastectomy, the authors concluded that surgery provided no clinical advantage over chemotherapy and radiation alone. In contrast, Perez et al.[125] found that the addition of mastectomy to local treatment significantly improved the outcome of inflammatory breast cancer treatment. Patients given neoadjuvant chemotherapy, mastectomy, and postmastectomy radiation had a local control rate of 79% and a 5-year disease free survival of 40%. These data were also supported by Panades et al.,[126] who evaluated 308 patients given chemotherapy as a component of their treatment and found that the 10-year local-recurrence-free survival rates were significantly better for patients who underwent mastectomy than for those who did not (about 60% vs. 34%, respectively; $p = .0001$), as were the 10-year breast cancer–specific survival rates (about 34% with mastectomy vs. 23% without, $p = .005$). A multivariate analysis that considered other potential prognostic factors found that the use of mastectomy remained a significant factor for improved local recurrence–free survival ($p = .04$). Results from an MD Anderson study also confirmed these results, with multivariate analysis revealing that a complete or partial response to neoadjuvant chemotherapy, the use of radiotherapy, and the addition of mastectomy to the therapeutic regimen all significantly improved disease-specific survival.[127]

More recent studies have focused on whether breast conservation can be safely performed for patients who achieved a CR to neoadjuvant chemotherapy.[125,128,129,130] Some series reported favorable control rates.[130] However, Swain and Lippman[131] reported a local recurrence rate of 30% despite their patients having achieved a clinical CR to neoadjuvant chemotherapy and multiple negative biopsies before irradiation. Low and colleagues[128] also reported a 40% local recurrence rate in 15 patients with inflammatory breast cancer treated with radiation therapy alone after a biopsy-proven CR. Finally, Brun and colleagues[129] reported a 54% local failure rate with attempts at breast conservation, and Chevallier and colleagues[132] reported a 61% local failure rate in patients treated with breast conservation after they had achieved a CR to neoadjuvant chemotherapy.

Radiation therapy also has an important role in the management of inflammatory breast cancer. After neoadjuvant chemotherapy and mastectomy, radiation use can be associated with local-regional control rates of >80%.[133] However, these results have been achieved with high-dose, aggressive treatments. Because inflammatory breast cancer has a rapid doubling time, investigators from MD Anderson investigated an accelerated hyperfractionated radiation delivery schedule in which 51 Gy is delivered to the chest wall and draining lymphatic fields by giving 1.5 Gy twice a day.[133] Subsequently, the chest wall is boosted to an additional 15 Gy, given in ten 1.5-Gy fractions twice daily. That approach was found to significantly improve local-regional disease control among patients treated to the 66-Gy total dose compared with a group treated only to 60 Gy on this schedule, with the respective 10-year local-regional control rates being 77% versus 58% ($p = .04$). Statistically significant improvements were also seen in 5- and 10-year overall survival rates between these two groups ($p = .03$), and a trend toward improvement in 5- and 10-year disease-free survival rates was noted as well ($p = .06$). In a more recent update from these investigators in which the outcome of 192 patients treated with neoadjuvant chemotherapy, mastectomy, and postmastectomy radiation was evaluated, the authors reported a 5-year local-regional control rate of 84%.[134] Factors associated with higher rates of local-regional control included partial response to chemotherapy, negative margins, three or fewer positive lymph nodes, and the use of taxane chemotherapy.[134]

Inflammatory breast cancer outcome is also affected by biologic subtype, as determined by ER, PR, and HER2/neu status. An update of the MD Anderson inflammatory breast cancer experience analyzed 316 patients with nonmetastatic inflammatory breast cancer treated with curative intent between 1974 and 2008 who had known ER, PR, and HER2/neu status.[135] The 5-year rate of locoregional recurrence in patients with triple-negative disease was much higher than that for other subtypes—39% despite aggressive local-regional treatments—and the 5-year rate of distant metastasis was 57%.[135] New therapeutic targets are needed in such patients, and recent research has identified potential biologic roles of NF-κB, Rho C GTPase, WISP3, and E-cadherin.[136]

In summary, all patients with inflammatory breast cancer require management by a multidisciplinary team. After initial staging and careful documentation of the extent of disease, patients should receive initial chemotherapy. The chemotherapy course should include both an anthracycline and a taxane, which can be given either concurrently or sequentially. Anti-HER2 therapy (trastuzumab) should given with chemotherapy for patients with HER2/neu–positive disease. The majority of patients who exhibit a disease response and become operable should then undergo a modified radical mastectomy. Postmastectomy radiation treatments to the chest wall and draining lymphatics should be given as adjuvant therapy. This approach was recently endorsed by a consensus panel of inflammatory breast cancer experts.[137] The dose of radiation to the initial fields should be 50 Gy in 25 fractions given once a day or 51 Gy in 1.5-Gy fractions given twice a day. Subsequently, the chest wall and any areas of gross disease that has not be resected should be boosted to 60 to 66 Gy. Patients with ER-positive disease should also receive hormonal therapy. Some patients will continue to have inoperable disease after neoadjuvant chemotherapy. These patients should receive either preoperative radiation to the breast and draining lymphatics to a dose of 50 to 51 Gy, or, if the disease is unlikely to become resectable, high-dose (72 Gy) definitive radiation is indicated using a reduced-field technique.

Clearly great strides have been made over the last two decades in the management of inflammatory breast cancer, and patients whose disease is managed with trimodality therapy can have local-regional control rates >80% and 5-year survival rates of ≥40% or more. Improvements in systemic therapy will, it is hoped, further augment these results.

GENERAL MANAGEMENT AND TREATMENT RESULTS FOR LOCALLY OR REGIONALLY RECURRENT BREAST CANCER

The development of a local-regional recurrence after primary treatment of an invasive breast cancer, particularly for those treated with an initial mastectomy, often develops into life-threatening condition. Accordingly, all patients should undergo disease restaging at the time of recurrence to rule out metastatic disease. All patients with local-regional recurrence should also have a biopsy for histopathologic confirmation and for re-evaluation of hormone receptor and HER2/neu status.

Local-regional recurrences are relatively uncommon, and patients with local-regional recurrences represent a heterogeneous group. Therefore, treatment strategies must be tailored to individual cases.

Recurrence in the Breast After Breast Conservation Therapy

Mastectomy remains the standard salvage treatment for disease that recurs in the breast after breast-conserving treatment. Most such patients will have been previously treated with breast irradiation and therefore would not be candidates for a breast-conserving approach. However, some single-institutional studies investigated additional breast-conserving surgery with or without radiation. Salvadori et al.[138] compared the outcome of 134 patients treated with mastectomy for a localized breast recurrence to 54 highly selected patients treated with a second breast-conserving surgery alone. They found that a second breast recurrence was more common at 5 years in the re-excision group (19% vs. 4%). Komoike et al.[139] also reported a relatively high rate (30%) of a second breast relapse after local surgery only for recurrent disease. Experience with giving a second course of radiation therapy following local resection of a breast recurrence has also been limited, with most approaches being limited to a partial breast reirradiation strategy. Deutsch et al.[140] treated 39 women with 50 Gy to the operative area using electrons after a repeat lumpectomy for an intact breast recurrence but reported a rate of second recurrence of 23%. Resch et al.[141] treated 17 ipsilateral breast tumor recurrence patients with pulse-dose-rate brachytherapy following repeat lumpectomy and noted a second breast recurrence in 5. Finally, in the largest series to date, Hannoun-Levi et al.[142] treated 69 highly selected patients with interstitial brachytherapy after a second lumpectomy for an intact breast recurrence and after a median follow-up of 50 months reported that 11 (16%) developed a second recurrence. Grade 2-3 late complications developed in 0% to 32% of the patients, depending on the radiation dose.

Patients with recurrence in the breast are also at risk of axillary metastases. Patients who initially underwent sentinel lymph node surgery should have an axillary lymph node dissection at the time of recurrence. The use of systemic therapy after breast recurrence needs to be decided on an individual basis according to the risk of metastatic disease, the previous systemic treatments used, and hormone receptor status.

Several investigators have investigated prognostic factors associated with outcome for patients with breast recurrence after treatment for an invasive breast cancer. Quite consistently through these studies is the finding that patients with an interval to development of recurrence of <2 years have a worse outcome than those who develop recurrent disease many years after treatment. In part, this may be explained by the hypothesis that early breast recurrences develop from repopulation of persistent microscopic disease, whereas some late breast recurrences represent a new primary tumor. Investigators from Yale University were among the first to provide insights into the prognostic importance of this distinction. These authors evaluated a series of 136 such patients and used clinical criteria to classify recurrences as either true recurrences or new primary tumors.[143] New primary tumors were defined by one of the following: location in the breast remote from the original tumor bed site, a change in histology, or a change from aneuploid to diploid status. Subsequently, investigators from MD Anderson undertook a similar analysis of 139 patients with in-breast recurrences. Both studies found that patients considered to have new primary tumors had significantly longer intervals between their initial primary tumor and the recurrence and had significantly lower rates of distant metastasis and death after the recurrence.[144] These data were later validated by this group in a study of 447 patients.[145] These findings may be valuable in decisions regarding systemic treatments.

Reconstructive surgery can also be considered for patients treated with mastectomy, but the previous history of breast radiation may limit the success of implant-based procedures. Forman et al.[146] reported significant complications in 6 of the 10 patients in whom a tissue expander and implant was attempted after mastectomy in the setting of an ipsilateral breast recurrent treatment. Autologous tissue reconstruction may provide better outcomes. Moran et al.[147] reported on 14 patients who underwent free TRAM flaps with anastomosis to the thorocodorsal vessels in patients being treated for a breast recurrence. The complication rate was only 14%, and the aesthetic result was rated as excellent.

Local-Regional Recurrence After Mastectomy

Patients with recurrent disease after initial mastectomy have a worse prognosis than those with recurrent disease after initial breast conservation therapy. In the Canadian and the Danish prospective studies that evaluated postmastectomy radiation, patients who developed local-regional recurrence had very high rates of subsequently developing metastatic disease.[71,148] In the Danish trial, the 5-year rate of distant metastatic disease development after an isolated local-regional recurrence was 73%, and the rate was no different for those in whom disease recurred after mastectomy only versus those with recurrent disease after mastectomy and radiation.[148] Similarly, in the Vancouver trial, of the 39 patients who developed a local-regional recurrence, 37 eventually developed metastatic disease.[71]

Several publications have provided insights into the factors of prognostic significance for patients with local-regional recurrence after mastectomy. One of the largest series was an analysis of the 535 patients who developed a postmastectomy recurrence after treatment in the Danish 82b and 82c randomized trials.[148] In multivariate analyses, the investigators found the following factors to be associated with a poorer outcome: large initial primary tumor and high number of positive lymph nodes, extracapsular extension, recurrence in the infraclavicular or supraclavicular regions, and a disease-free interval of <2 years. Other series have reported similar findings. In general, patients who present with chest wall recurrence, particularly those who have resectable disease and have not undergone radiation, have a greater probability of disease control and improved outcome. Investigators from MD Anderson found that initial nodal status, time to recurrence, and ability to use radiation to treat the recurrence were all independent predictors of outcome for patients with a chest wall recurrence.[149] The 19 patients in whom these three factors were favorable had a 5-year overall survival of 86% (median survival time, 141 months). The 5-year survival rate for the 89 patients who had one or two unfavorable features was 48% (median survival time, 54 months), and all 22 of the patients who had all three unfavorable factors died within 5 years of the recurrence (median survival, 16 months). Outcome for patients with T1/T2 disease with one to three positive lymph nodes was as poor after a local-regional recurrence as was the outcome for patients with four or more positive lymph nodes.[150] In contrast, patients with initial lymph node–negative disease had a significantly better outcome.

Few data are available to quantify the benefits of systemic therapy for patients with local-regional recurrence. In one of the few series evaluating this issue, authors from British Columbia found in a nonrandomized study that use of chemotherapy at the time of recurrence reduced the probability of death from breast cancer, but this difference was not statistically significant compared with those who did not have chemotherapy at recurrence ($p = .07$). Finally, a randomized trial that investigated tamoxifen use versus no systemic therapy after salvage local therapy for patients with recurrent disease after mastectomy found improvement in 5-year disease-free survival from 36% to 59% ($p = .007$),[151] supporting the use of systemic treatments in the management of patients with recurrent disease.

Investigators from MD Anderson conducted a series of four prospective single-group protocols evaluating systemic therapies for patients with either local-regional recurrence or metastatic disease that was converted to "no evidence of disease" after surgery, radiation, or both.[152] The findings suggest that for patients with anthracycline-naive disease, the introduction of doxorubicin at the time of recurrence can lead to improved survival, and more recently the use of docetaxel also seemed to lead to favorable outcome for patients who had previously had anthracycline treatment. The 3-year disease-free survival rate for such patients was 58%.[152]

The general management strategy for an isolated local-regional recurrence after mastectomy requires input from a multidisciplinary team. The initial evaluation should define the sites of disease involvement and determine whether the patient is able to undergo resection of all gross disease with negative surgical margins. Surgical therapy is recommended for patients with resectable disease, provided the patients can tolerate the surgery and the morbidity of the surgery is acceptable. After surgery, if the patients had not previously been given radiation therapy, they should receive comprehensive local-regional radiation. A study from Washington University found that patients who had radiation therapy to the chest wall and regional lymphatics had better outcomes than those in whom radiation fields were limited to the site of the recurrent disease.[153] Finally, because patients with recurrent disease after mastectomy are at high risk of developing distant metastatic disease, those who have not been previously treated with anthracyclines or taxanes (or trastuzumab if the tumor is HER2/neu–positive) should strongly consider treatment with these agents.[154] Patients with ER-positive disease should receive appropriate second-line endocrine therapy.

Patients presenting with bulky, unresectable disease should be considered for neoadjuvant chemotherapy if active systemic agents are available. If the disease responds favorably, some of these patients may become candidates for surgical resection, which then can be consolidated with comprehensive radiation. The prognosis for those whose disease fails to respond is very poor, and radiation treatments alone are unlikely to render such patients free of disease. Nevertheless, aggressive local-regional radiation is often used to help stabilize the disease and to avoid the significant adverse consequences of uncontrolled growth of local-regional disease. The dose of radiation to be used depends on the presence or absence of gross disease and whether patients have previously undergone radiation therapy. For patients who have not had radiation therapy and do not have gross disease, we recommend comprehensive treatment to the chest wall and draining lymphatics to a dose of 50 to 54 Gy followed by a boost to the chest wall to 60 to 66 Gy. Hyperfractionated chest wall irradiation does not seem to provide any benefit over that of conventional therapy given once daily.[155] For patients who develop recurrences in a chest wall that has been previously irradiated, the treatment options are more difficult. Investigators from Duke University have had some success with combining a second course of radiation with chemotherapy and hyperthermia.[156]

Regional Nodal Relapse

Patients with regional relapse have a less favorable prognosis than patients with intact breast or chest wall recurrences. In general, patients with isolated resectable disease in the low axilla should be treated with axillary dissection, comprehensive radiation to sites not previously treated, including the chest wall, and systemic therapy. Most patients with recurrence in the supraclavicular fossa or internal mammary lymph nodes have unresectable disease. If active chemotherapy agents are available, it is reasonable to consider using neoadjuvant systemic treatment and consolidating with radiation at the point of maximal response. Woodward et al.[157] investigated the outcome of 140 patients with local-regional recurrence after mastectomy and doxorubicin chemotherapy and found that the 47 who had supraclavicular disease at the time of recurrence had a worse outcome than the remaining patient with recurrences in other sites (3-year distant disease-free survival of 40% vs. 54%, respectively; $p = .003$).

GENERAL MANAGEMENT AND TREATMENT RESULTS FOR UNUSUAL PRESENTATIONS OF BREAST CANCER

Axillary Metastases with Unknown Primary

The presentation of metastatic disease within axillary lymph nodes without an identifiable primary source is unusual, accounting for <1% of newly diagnosed breast cancer cases.[158–160] Workup for patients who present with axillary disease with an occult primary should initially be aimed at establishing the diagnosis and whether the disease represents a distant metastasis from a different site. Initial evaluation should include a history and physical examination (with particular attention to a skin exam to rule out an unsuspected truncal melanoma), routine serum studies, bilateral mammography, chest radiography, liver imaging, and bone scan. If no primary disease is detected with mammography, ultrasound and MRI scan of the breast is indicated. Cytologic confirmation of disease within axillary lymph nodes can be obtained with ultrasound-guided fine needle aspiration. Tumor markers, including ER, PR, and HER2/neu, can and should be performed on the cytologic specimens. Most individuals present with advanced nodal disease at presentation and are clinically staged as having T0 N2-3 disease.

Modified radical mastectomy and postmastectomy radiation have been the historical local-regional treatments for patients with an occult breast primary and axillary metastases. Studies vary significantly with respect to the frequency with which a primary is found within the breast during pathologic examination. In addition, most of these studies predate the use of MRI screening or other improvements in diagnostic imaging. In general however, approximately two-thirds of the cases are found to have an invasive breast cancer on pathologic examination of a mastectomy specimen.[158] Patients with inoperable nodal disease at presentation are treated with neoadjuvant chemotherapy prior to mastectomy. For such individuals, the probability of finding disease within the breast is likely even lower.

More recently, a number of investigators have investigated the safety of breast conservation therapy for patients with occult primary disease. An optimal treatment strategy for such patients can consist of neoadjuvant chemotherapy, reimaging of the breast to evaluate for calcifications resulting from tumor cell death, axillary dissection, and irradiation of the breast and draining lymphatics. Early attempts at breast conservation without breast irradiation resulted in high subsequent breast recurrence rates.[161,162] More recent studies that incorporate breast irradiation have yielded better results. In one of the largest series, investigators from MD Anderson evaluated 45 patients treated over a 47-year period and compared the outcome of those treated with mastectomy (n = 13) to those treated with breast conservation (n = 32).[159] These authors found equivalent rates of local-regional control, disease-free survival, and overall survival between the mastectomy and breast conservation cohorts. With a median follow-up of 7 years, only 2 of the 25 breast conservation patients who received breast irradiation developed a local recurrence. Similar results have been reported from the Royal Marsden Hospital. In a series of 48 patients, they found a 14% local-regional recurrence rate after breast radiation and an unacceptable rate of 80% if breast radiation was omitted.[163]

Male Breast Cancer

Breast cancer developing in males is unusual. The American Cancer Society estimated that there would be 2,140 new cases of male breast cancer in the United States in 2011, which would account for only 0.9% of the total new breast cancer cases. It is also estimated that 450 men would die of breast cancer during 2011.[5] The ratio of the number of deaths to new cases is 21% for males, compared to a ratio of 17% for females.[5]

There are several known risk factors for male breast cancer. Similar to female breast cancer, breast cancer is more common in elderly men than in young men. Some conditions that affect testosterone and estrogen levels can increase the risk of breast cancer in men. Examples of some of such conditions include a history of an undescended testicle, history of orchiectomy, and Klinefelter's syndrome.[164] In addition, genetic conditions also can contribute, and men with a family history of female breast cancer have an increased risk. Germline mutations in the BRCA2 gene have been reported in 4% to 16% of men with breast cancer, and, unlike the situation for females, are more common than germline mutations in BRCA1.[165,166]

Males have a similar histopathologic spectrum of breast cancers, with the exception of having lower rates of invasive lobular disease. In addition, male breast cancers more frequently are ER-positive (estimated rate of 90%) and HER2/neu–negative compared to female breast cancer.[167] The presenting symptom for male breast cancer patients is typically a breast mass or axillary adenopathy. Most male breast cancer patients present with locally advanced disease. Diagnostic workup is similar to that for female breast cancer and should include bilateral mammography. Treatment decisions are also similar to those used in women. Men tend to present with more advanced clinical stage disease than females and correspondingly have worse outcome as a population. A study evaluating 1988–2003 SEER Program data found that although men were noted to have more advanced disease compared to females, when comparing outcome specifically for those with stage II or stage III disease there were no gender-specific differences.[167]

Mastectomy with or without postmastectomy radiation is the most common local-regional treatment approach. Investigators at MD Anderson reviewed 142 patients treated with mastectomy without radiation therapy and found that, similar to female patients, margin status, number of positive nodes, and tumor size predicted local-regional failure.[93] Accordingly, decisions concerning postmastectomy radiation should be based on similar criteria used in the treatment of female breast cancer.

Similarly, systemic treatments are indicated for male breast cancer patients who have a clinically relevant risk of distant metastases. Data supporting the use of particular chemotherapy regimens are lacking, given the rarity of the disease. In addition to chemotherapy, because most male breast cancers are hormonally responsive, tamoxifen is indicated for the majority of cases. Retrospective series suggested that tamoxifen use can reduce the risk of recurrence and death.[168] The role of aromatase inhibitors in males is under investigation.

RADIATION TREATMENT TECHNIQUES AFTER MASTECTOMY

Target Definitions

Traditionally, postmastectomy radiation therapy included treatment to the chest wall and draining lymphatics in the undissected axillary apex/supraclavicular fossa. It is clear from pattern-of-failure studies from patients treated with mastectomy without radiation that the chest wall is the most common site of recurrent disease, accounting for two-thirds to three-fourths of all local-regional recurrences. It is also clear that patients with stage III disease (T3 N1, T4, or pathologic N2-3 disease) have a clinically relevant risk of recurrence in the axillary apex/supraclavicular fossa. A study of >1,000 patients who did not receive radiation after treatment with mastectomy and chemotherapy found the 10-year risk of recurrence in the axillary apex/supraclavicular fossa to be 14% to 19% for patients with four or more positive lymph nodes, 20% or greater positive lymph nodes, or extracapsular extension of disease that measured >2 mm.[169]

The benefit or radiation for treatment of the dissected level I/II axilla is less clear. In this same study, in which all patients had a standard axillary lymph node dissection (median number of lymph nodes recovered, 17), the 10-year risk of recurrence in this region was only 3% and not predicted by the extent of axillary disease or extracapsular extension.[169] In contrast, 43% of the patients treated in the no-radiation arms of the Danish postmastectomy radiation trials and who developed a local-regional recurrence had the axilla as a component of their local-regional recurrence.[72] The higher recurrence rate in the axilla likely was a consequence of a less extensive axillary level I/II dissection (median number of lymph nodes recovered was 7) in the Danish studies. These data, taken together, suggest that the decision to include the level I/II as a target for postmastectomy radiation in large part is determined by the completeness of the axillary dissection.

The treatment of the internal mammary lymph nodes for patients treated with postmastectomy radiation is controversial and the subject of ongoing phase III studies. The justification for including this region is based on previous experiences of dissecting the internal mammary chain, which found that up to 35% to 50% of patients with clinically advanced disease will have microscopic involvement of lymph nodes within this region.[170,171] Table 57.11 shows the rates of internal mammary lymph nodes involvement from a more recent study of 2,269 patients from China who underwent resection of these nodes as a component of an extended radical mastectomy.[172] The randomized trials that have shown a survival advantage for postmastectomy radiation included the internal mammary lymph nodes within their treatment target volume.[69,70,73] Finally, inclusion of the internal mammary lymph nodes provides a broader coverage of the chest wall, which may prove to be secondary benefit in avoiding marginal misses.

TABLE 57.11 RATE OF PATHOLOGIC INVOLVEMENT OF INTERNAL MAMMARY LYMPH NODES IN PATIENTS WHO UNDERWENT EXTENDED RADICAL MASTECTOMY[172]

Subgroup	*Rate of Involvement of the Internal Mammary Lymph Nodes (%)*
Patients with 4–6 positive axillary lymph nodes	28
Patients with 7 or more positive axillary lymph nodes	42
Medial tumors with 1–3 positive axillary lymph nodes	24
Medial tumors with 4–6 positive axillary lymph nodes	48
T3 tumors in patients of age 35 yr or younger	25
T2 tumors with 1–3 positive axillary lymph nodes	20
T2 tumors with 4–6 positive axillary lymph nodes	32
T2 tumors with 7 or more positive axillary lymph nodes	42
T2 medial tumors overall	21

When radiation is used after mastectomy for patients with stage II breast cancer, the appropriate target volumes are less clear. Patients with stage II breast cancer with one to three positive lymph nodes fail predominantly on the chest wall and have a much lower risk of recurrence in the axillary apex/supraclavicular fossa. In a site of failure analysis cited earlier, the risk of recurrence in the axilla/supraclavicular fossa for patients with one to three positive lymph nodes and no extracapsular extension was only 4%.[169] For these reasons, some have advocated treatment of the chest wall only in such patients. However, the trials showing a survival advantage for the use of postmastectomy radiation included the axillary apex/supraclavicular fossa within the treatment fields, and more recent data of the MA-20 trial discussed in Chapter 56, suggests some benefits of lymphatic drainage for patients with stage II disease.

CT simulation is very useful to precisely delineate target volumes. For example, the internal mammary vessels within the first three intercostal interspaces, which are where lymph nodes at risk within this region are located, can be easily identified and contoured. Likewise, the depth of the level III axilla and supraclavicular fossa varies greatly according to individual anatomy and patient weight. Contouring the region helps to ensure that these targets fall within the desired isodose lines. A recent analysis that evaluated various dose prescriptions used for supraclavicular field treatments found that 6-MV photons prescribed to D_{max} or a depth of 3 cm significantly underdosed contoured lymph node regions at risk in overweight and obese patients (defined according to patient body mass index).[173] Finally, for patients who require treatment to the low axilla, contouring the region at risk also helps to more precisely conform the dose distribution to the area in need of treatment.

Technique

Patients should be immobilized with their ipsilateral arm abducted (90 to 120 degrees) and externally rotated. In assessing arm position, it is important to have the soft tissues of the arm cranial to the junction of the tangent and supraclavicular fossa field. In addition, skin folds within the supraclavicular fossa should be avoided if possible. Patients are placed on a 10- to 15-degree angle board to flatten the slope of the chest wall in the region of the sternum. Radiopaque wires are placed on the mastectomy scar, and the patient undergoes a treatment-planning noncontrast CT scan. The border between the chest wall and the supraclavicular fields is typically placed at the bottom of the clavicular head. Appropriate isocenters and setup points are determined and marked. Targeted areas of interest are then contoured on the CT slices.

Several techniques are available treat the chest wall and internal mammary lymph nodes. One of the more common methods is to use a 15- to 25-degree obliqued electron field to treat the medial chest wall and internal mammary lymph nodes. The lateral border of this field is then matched on the skin to a pair of photon tangent fields that treat the lateral chest wall and are created with matched nondivergent deep and cranial borders. A nondivergent cranial border is created through rotation of the couch, and a nondivergent deep border is achieved by overrotating the gantry or a half-beam block. The collimators are rotated to match the chest wall slope, and any volume that extends into the supraclavicular field is blocked. An alternative technique that is particularly of benefit for patients with very little tissue between the lung and skin is to use three electron fields. The junction of such fields should be moved every week to minimize the consequences of the required gantry rotation necessary to make the fields apposition for the lateral chest wall. These fields are then match to a supraclavicular/axillary apex field, which has been described in Chapter 56. For patients with advanced disease, the supraclavicular lateral field edge is often extended to give margin on the superior-lateral chest wall and to provide treatment of the anterior interpectoral Rotter's lymph nodes.

Figures 57.7 to 57.9 show examples of matched electron, tangent fields; chest wall electron-only fields; and a supraclavicular/axillary apex field. All chest wall radiation fields should be designed to avoid irradiating the heart. The advantages of the field designs described here is that with the use of CT treatment planning, the beam arrangement and selection of electron energies can be determined so that cardiac irradiation is avoided or minimized.

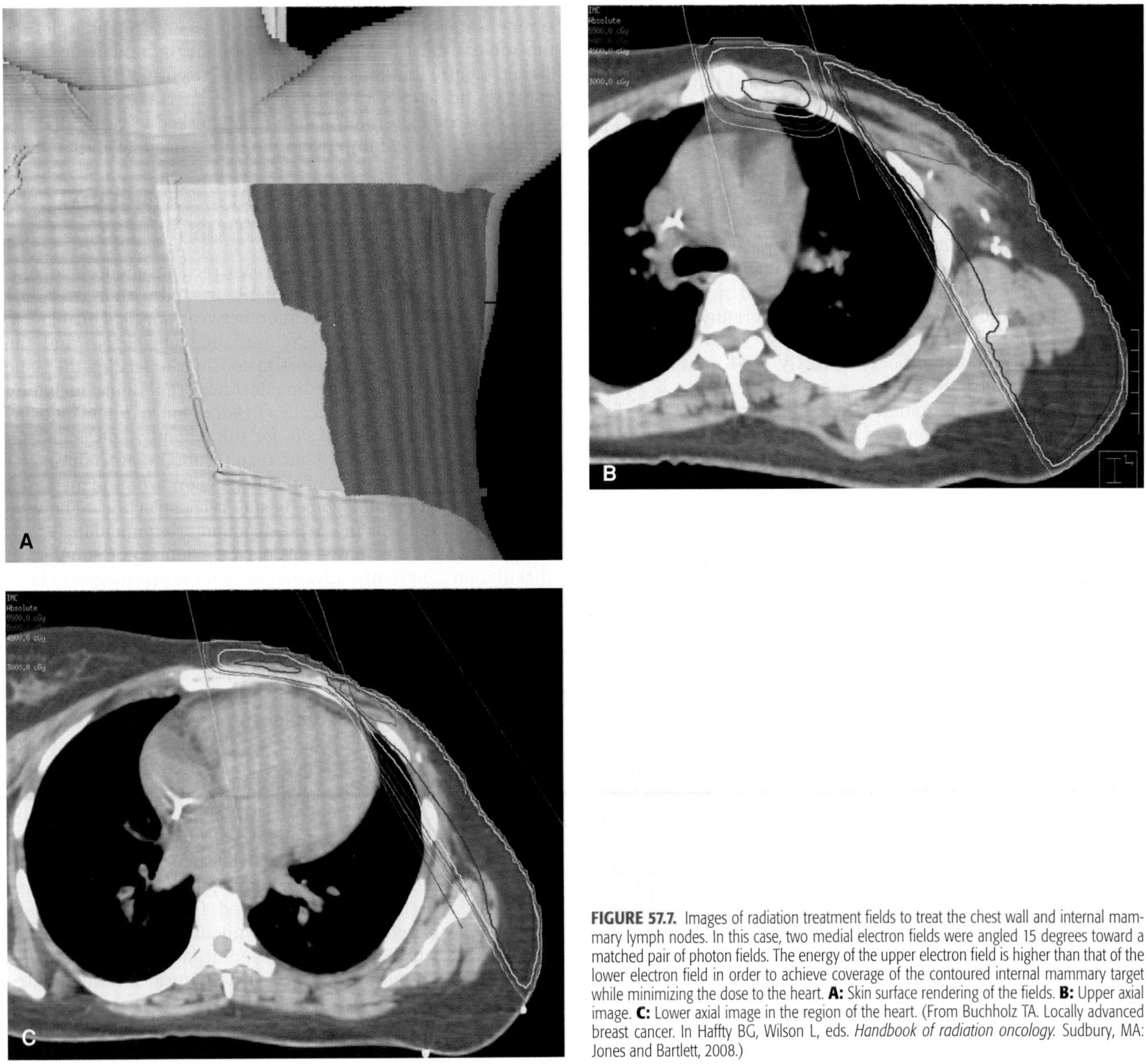

FIGURE 57.7. Images of radiation treatment fields to treat the chest wall and internal mammary lymph nodes. In this case, two medial electron fields were angled 15 degrees toward a matched pair of photon fields. The energy of the upper electron field is higher than that of the lower electron field in order to achieve coverage of the contoured internal mammary target while minimizing the dose to the heart. **A:** Skin surface rendering of the fields. **B:** Upper axial image. **C:** Lower axial image in the region of the heart. (From Buchholz TA. Locally advanced breast cancer. In Haffty BG, Wilson L, eds. *Handbook of radiation oncology.* Sudbury, MA: Jones and Bartlett, 2008.)

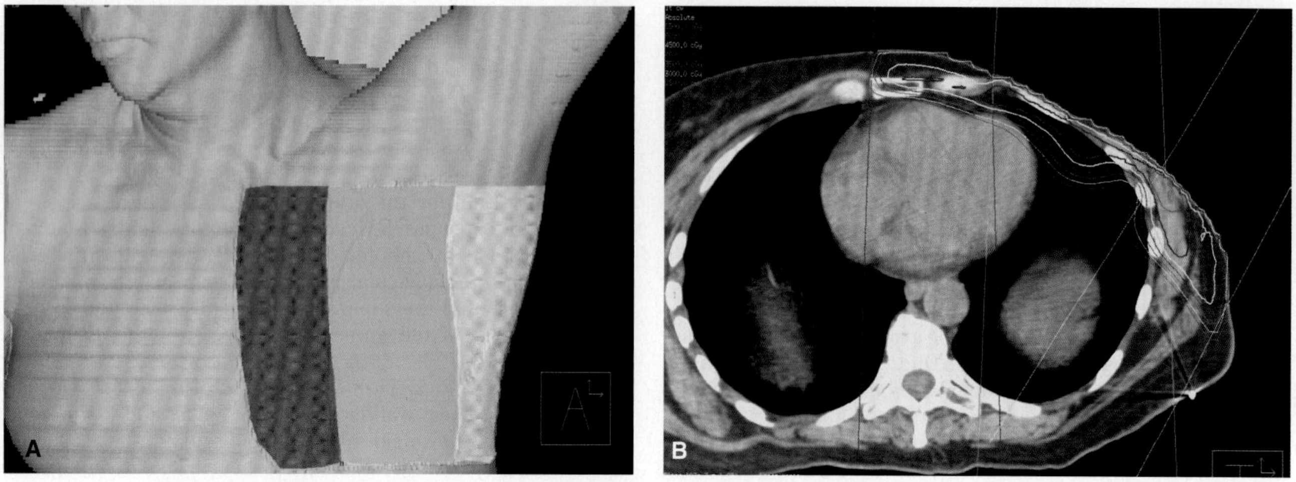

FIGURE 57.8. Images of radiation treatment fields using a matched electron field technique to treat the chest wall and internal mammary lymph nodes. Three medial electron fields are matched on the skin. The junction between the middle and lateral fields is shifted weekly due to the differences in gantry angle. **A:** Skin surface rendering of the fields. **B:** Axial image of the fields.

Dosimetry and Dose

Initial fields and target volumes should be treated to a total dose of 50 Gy in 25 fractions over 5 weeks. A 3- to 5-mm bolus is used over the chest wall every other day or every day for 2 weeks (20 Gy total dose) and then as needed to ensure that a brisk radiation dermatitis develops. However, this dermatitis should not lead to a treatment interruption. There are no studies evaluating the optimal total dose, but in our institution we boost the chest wall with electron fields (5 to 10 cm beyond the mastectomy scar and covering the tumor bed location of the original primary) for an additional 10 Gy in 5 fractions over 1 week beyond the initial 50-Gy course. In addition, we boost all sites of unresected but initially involved adenopathy in the internal mammary, infraclavicular, and supraclavicular regions with a radiation boost. If ultrasonography has shown a resolution of disease in these areas to ≤1 cm, we treat this region with an additional boost of 10 Gy. If >1 cm of disease persists, we increase the boost dose to 16 Gy.

Three-dimensional treatment-planning systems allow for evaluation of dose distributions in multiple off-axis slices and calculations of dose using heterogeneity correction factors. Dose distributions can be modulated through standard wedge compensators or field-in-field techniques. Electron energies for the medial chest wall/internal mammary lymph node fields should ensure that the 90% isodose curve covers the contoured volume and avoids irradiation of the heart. In addition, the supraclavicular dosimetry should be checked to verify that the 90% isodose curve fully covers the undissected level III axilla.

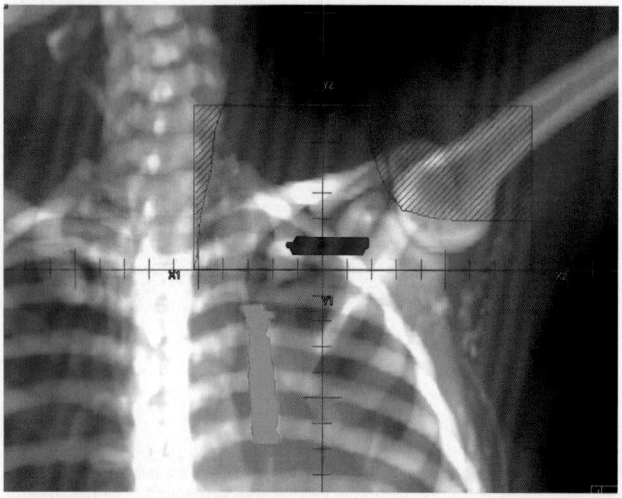

FIGURE 57.9. Images of a radiation treatment field used to treat the axillary apex/supraclavicular fossa. The level III region of the axillary and the upper internal mammary vessels have been contoured on axial computed tomography images and reconstructed on this image. These contours are used to determine depth of dose prescription. (From Buchholz TA. Locally advanced breast cancer. In Haffty BG, Wilson L, eds. *Handbook of radiation oncology.* Sudbury, MA: Jones and Bartlett, 2008.)

POSTMASTECTOMY RADIATION AND BREAST RECONSTRUCTION

Coordination of radiation and breast reconstruction is a commonly encountered issue for patients treated with mastectomy and requires clear communication between surgical oncologist, reconstructive/plastic surgeon, radiation oncologist, and the patient. There are many factors to consider regarding the issue of reconstruction and postmastectomy radiation, including ensuring the safety and efficacy of radiation treatments, ensuring the maximal quality of life for the patients, and achieving the optimal long-term aesthetic result from the procedure.

The two major classes of reconstruction are implant-based approaches and autologous tissue reconstruction. The two options for timing for the reconstruction are immediate—done at the time of mastectomy—or delayed—done after completion of radiation. There are advantages and disadvantages of both approaches and both timings. Implant-based approaches are simpler surgical procedures that avoid the donor-site morbidities of autologous tissue transfers. In addition, implants can be used in thin women who do not have adequate volume of autologous tissue in donor sites. Typically, for this procedure, a tissue expander is placed under the pectoralis major muscle and, after full expansion is achieved, replaced with an implant. Most women treated with postmastectomy radiation who undergo implant-based reconstruction require an immediate reconstruction procedure. This is because after radiation the normal tissues are less compliant, and tissue expanders are often unsuccessful and may cause rib fractures and other injuries. For women treated with autologous tissues, the reconstruction can be immediate or delayed. Immediate reconstruction has the benefit of being accompanied by a skin-sparing mastectomy, which preserves a significant component of the normal breast skin and preserves the natural inframammary sulcus and other skin envelopes. These elements are important to achieving the optimal cosmetic outcome. The downsides of immediate reconstruction relative to delayed reconstruction are twofold: radiation has adverse effects on the long-term aesthetics of breast reconstructions, particularly implant-based reconstruction, and reconstruction has a negative effect on the design and delivery of radiation treatment fields.

Effects of Radiation on Reconstruction

The majority of patients who undergo an immediate reconstruction and require postmastectomy radiation will have an aesthetic change as a consequence of treatments. In general, implant-based reconstruction has high rates of late contraction, fibrosis, implant fixation, and poor aesthetic outcome. Many of these changes begin 6 months after treatment and insidiously progress over time. Spear et al.[174] reviewed the data on breast reconstruction with implants and found that 53% complication rate after radiation compared to a 10% rate in those who did not require radiation ($p < .001$). Fox Chase investigators reported a 27% rate of significant complication after irradiation of tissue expander or implant.[175] MD Anderson investigators reported and even higher rate of 40% to 50% unless the implant was combined with an autologous tissue flap.[176]

Complications also develop for patients treated with an immediate autologous tissue reconstruction followed by radiation, although the effects, although common, may be less severe than implant-based approaches. Investigators from MD Anderson compared complications in patients treated with radiation and autologous tissue reconstruction. Those with an immediate reconstruction had a higher rate of complications compared to those with a delayed reconstruction (87.5% vs. 8.6%, respectively; $p < .001$).[177] Furthermore, 28% of the patients with immediate reconstruction required an additional flap to improve aesthetics.

Effects of Reconstruction on Radiation Treatment and Delivery

Reconstruction affects the contour of the chest and can make the delivery of radiation to the appropriate targeted areas more challenging. Overinflated tissue expanders can cause significantly sloping contours at field junction between chest wall and internal mammary fields and between chest wall and supraclavicular/axillary apex fields. As a consequence, compromises are sometimes necessary in order to deliver the treatment safely. A study evaluated the effects reconstruction had in radiation treatment field designs in 112 postmastectomy radiation plans.[178] These authors reported that compromises in the field design were made in 52% of these cases because of the geometric constraints caused by the reconstruction (33% were considered moderate compromises and 19% major compromises). In a matched control set treated with mastectomy without reconstruction, only 7% of cases had compromises in plans due to patient anatomy.[179,180]

SELECTED REFERENCES

A full list of references for this chapter is available online.

1. Haagensen CD, Cooley E. Radical mastectomy for mammary carcinoma. *Ann Surg* 1969;170:884.
2. Haagensen CD, Stout AP. Carcinoma of the breast: criteria of inoperability. *Ann Surg* 1943;118:859–870.
10. Dawood S, et al. Differences in survival among women with stage III inflammatory and noninflammatory locally advanced breast cancer appear early: a large population-based study. *Cancer* 117(9):1819–1826.
15. Zucali R, et al. Natural history and survival of inoperable breast cancer treated with radiotherapy and radiotherapy followed by radical mastectomy. *Cancer* 1976;37(3):1422–1431.
29. Tomlinson JS, Alpaugh ML, Barsky SH. An intact overexpressed E-cadherin/alpha,beta-catenin axis characterizes the lymphovascular emboli of inflammatory breast carcinoma. *Cancer Res* 2001;61(13):5231–5241.
32. Fisher B, et al. Effect of preoperative chemotherapy on local-regional disease in women with operable breast cancer: findings from National Surgical Adjuvant Breast and Bowell Project B-18. *J Clin Oncol* 1997;15:2483–2493.
33. Kuerer HM, et al. Clinical course of breast cancer patients with complete pathologic primary tumor and axillary lymph node response to doxorubicin-based neoadjuvant chemotherapy. *J Clin Oncol* 1999;17:460–469.
34. Wolmark N, et al. Preoperative chemotherapy in patients withoperable breast cancer: nine-year results from National Surgical Adjuvant Breast and Bowel Project B-18. *Cancer* 2001;30:96–102.
35. Fisher ER, et al. Pathobiology of preoperative chemotherapy: findings from the National Surgical Adjuvant Breast and Bowel (NSABP) protocol B-18. *Cancer* 2002;95:681–695.
36. van der Hage JA, et al. Preoperative chemotherapy in primary operable breast cancer: results from the European Organization for Research and Treatment of Cancer trial 10902. *J Clin Oncol* 2001;19:4224–4237.
37. Buchholz TA, et al. Global gene expression changes during neoadjuvant chemotherapy for human breast cancer. *Cancer J* 2002;8(6):461–468.
38. Fisher B, et al. Effect of local or systemic treatment prior to primary tumor removal on the production and response to a serum growth-stimulating factor in mice. *Cancer Res* 1989;49(8):2002–2004.
39. Rastogi P, et al. Preoperative chemotherapy: updates of National Surgical Adjuvant Breast and Bowel Project Protocols B-18 and B-27. *J Clin Oncol* 2008;26(5):778–785.
40. van Nes JG, et al. Preoperative chemotherapy is safe in early breast cancer, even after 10 years of follow-up; clinical and translational results from the EORTC trial 10902. *Breast Cancer Res Treat* 2009;115(1):101–113.
41. Mauri D, Pavlidis N, Ioannidis JP. Neoadjuvant versus adjuvant systemic treatment in breast cancer: a meta-analysis. *J Natl Cancer Inst* 2005;97(3):188–194.
42. Kuerer HM, et al. Incidence and impact of documented eradication of breast cancer axillary lymph node metastases before surgery in patients treated with neoadjuvant chemotherapy. *Ann Surg* 1999;230(1):72–78.
43. Hunt KK, et al. Sentinel lymph node surgery after neoadjuvant chemotherapy is accurate and reduces the need for axillary dissection in breast cancer patients. *Ann Surg* 2009;250(4):558–566.
44. Mamounas EP, et al. Sentinel node biopsy after neoadjuvant chemotherapy in breast cancer: results from National Surgical Adjuvant Breast and Bowel Project Protocol B-27. *J Clin Oncol* 2005;23(12):2694–2702.
45. Xing Y, et al. Meta-analysis of sentinel lymph node biopsy after preoperative chemotherapy in patients with breast cancer. *Br J Surg* 2006;93(5):539–546.
46. Rouzier R, et al. Nomograms to predict pathologic complete response and metastasis-free survival after preoperative chemotherapy for breast cancer. *J Clin Oncol* 2005;23(33):8331–8339.
47. Cristofanilli M, et al. Invasive lobular carcinoma classic type: response to primary chemotherapy and survival outcomes. *J Clin Oncol* 2005;23(1):41–48.
48. Kaufmann M, et al. Recommendations from an international expert panel on the use of neoadjuvant (primary) systemic treatment of operable breast cancer: an update. *J Clin Oncol* 2006;24(12):1940–1949.
49. Smith IE, et al. Neoadjuvant treatment of postmenopausal breast cancer with anastrozole, tamoxifen, or both in combination: the Immediate Preoperative Anastrozole, Tamoxifen, or Combined with Tamoxifen (IMPACT) multicenter double-blind randomized trial. *J Clin Oncol* 2005;23(22):5108–5116.
50. Cataliotti L, et al. Comparison of anastrozole versus tamoxifen as preoperative therapy in postmenopausal women with hormone receptor-positive breast cancer: the Pre-Operative "Arimidex" Compared to Tamoxifen (PROACT) trial. *Cancer* 2006;106(10):2095–2103.
53. Rouizer R, et al. Primary chemotherapy for operable breast cancer: incidence and prognostic significance of ipsilateral breast tumor recurrence after breast-conserving surgery. *J Clin Oncol* 2001;19:3828–3835.
54. Swain SM, et al. Neoadjuvant chemotherapy in the combined modality approach of locally advanced nonmetastatic breast cancer. *Cancer Res* 1987;47(14):3889–3894.
55. Bonadonna G, et al. Primary chemotherapy in operable breast cancer: eight-year experience at the Milan Cancer Institute. *J Clin Oncol* 1998;16(1):93–100.
56. Chen AM, et al. Breast-conserving therapy after neoadjuvant chemotherapy: the M. D. Anderson Cancer Center experience. *J Clin Oncol* 2004;22:2303–2312.
57. Chen AM, et al. Breast conservation after neoadjuvant chemotherapy: a prognostic index for clinical decision-making. *Cancer* 2005;103(4)689–695.
58. Akay CL, et al. Evaluation of the MD Anderson prognostic index for local-regional recurrence after breast conserving therapy in patients receiving neoadjuvant chemotherapy. *Ann Surg Oncol* 2012;19(3):901–907.
60. Huang EH, et al. Comparison of risk of local-regional recurrence after mastectomy or breast conservation therapy for patients treated with neoadjuvant chemotherapy and radiation stratified according to a prognostic index score. *Int J Radiat Oncol Biol Phys* 2006;66(2):352–357.
61. Cuzick J, et al. Overview of randomized trials of postoperative adjuvant radiotherapy in breast cancer. *Cancer Treat Rep* 1987;71(1):15–29.
62. Cuzick J, et al. Cause-specific mortality in long-term survivors of breast cancer who participated in trials of radiotherapy. *J Clin Oncol* 1994;12(3):447–453.
63. Early Breast Cancer Trialists' Collaborative Group. Favourable and unfavourable effects on long-term survival of radiotherapy for early breast cancer: an overview of the randomised trials. *Lancet* 2000;355(9217):1757–1770.
64. Early Breast Cancer Trialists' Collaborative Group. Effects of radiotherapy and of differences in the extent of surgery for early breast cancer on local recurrence and 15-year survival: an overview of the randomised trials. *Lancet* 2005;366(9503):2087–2106.
67. Whelan TJ, et al. Does locoregional radiation therapy improve survival in breast cancer? A meta-analysis. *J Clin Oncol* 2000;18(6):1220–1229.
68. Gebski V, et al. Survival effects of postmastectomy adjuvant radiation therapy using biologically equivalent doses: a clinical perspective. *J Natl Cancer Inst* 2006;98(1):26–38.
69. Overgaard M, et al. Postoperative radiotherapy in high-risk premenopausal women with breast cancer who receive adjuvant chemotherapy. *N Engl J Med* 1997;337:949–955.
70. Overgaard M, et al. Randomized trail evaluating postoperative radiotherapy in high risk postmenopausal breast cancer patients given adjuvant tamoxifen: results from the DBCG 82 c trial. *Lancet* 1999;353:1641–1648.
71. Ragaz J, et al. Locoregional radiation therapy in patients with high-risk breast cancer receiving adjuvant chemotherapy: 20-year results of the British Columbia randomized trial. *J Natl Cancer Inst* 2005;97(2):116–126.
72. Nielsen HM, et al. Study of failure pattern among high-risk breast cancer patients with or without postmastectomy radiotherapy in addition to adjuvant systemic therapy: long-term results from the Danish Breast Cancer Cooperative Group DBCG 82 b and c randomized studies. *J Clin Oncol* 2006;24(15):2268–2275.
73. Ragaz J, et al. Adjuvant radiotherapy and chemotherapy in node-positive premenopausal women with breast cancer. *N Engl J Med* 1997;337(14):956–962.

74. Overgaard M, Nielsen HM, Overgaard J. Is the benefit of postmastectomy irradiation limited to patients with four or more positive nodes, as recommended in international consensus reports? A subgroup analysis of the DBCG 82 b&c randomized trials. *Radiother Oncol* 2007;82(3):247–253.
75. Katz A, et al. Loco-regional recurrence patterns following mastectomy and doxorubicin-based chemotherapy: implications for postoperative irradiation. *J Clin Oncol* 2000;18:2817–2827.
76. Recht A, et al. Locoregional failure ten years after mastectomy and adjuvant chemotherapy with or without tamoxifen without irradiation: experience of the Eastern Cooperative Oncology Group. *J Clin Oncol* 1999;17:1689–1700.
77. Wallgren A, et al. Risk factors for locoregional recurrence among breast cancer patients: results from International Breast Cancer Study Group Trials I through VII. *J Clin Oncol* 2003;21(7):1205–1213.
78. Taghian A, et al. Patterns of locoregional failure in patients with operable breast cancer treated by mastectomy and adjuvant chemotherapy with or without tamoxifen and without radiotherapy: results from five National Surgical Adjuvant Breast and Bowel Project randomized clinical trials. *J Clin Oncol* 2004;22(21):4247–4254.
80. Cheng JC, et al. Locoregional failure of postmastectomy patients with 1-3 positive axillary lymph nodes without adjuvant radiotherapy. *Int J Radiat Oncol Biol Phys* 2002;52(4):980–988.
81. Freedman GM, et al. A close or positive margin after mastectomy is not an indication for chest wall irradiation except in women aged fifty or younger. *Int J Radiat Oncol Biol Phys* 1998;41(3):599–605.
82. Katz A, et al. The influence of pathologic tumor characteristics on locoregional recurrence rates following mastectomy. *Int J Radiat Oncol BIol Phys* 2001;50(3): 735–742.
85. Woodward WA, et al. Locoregional recurrence after doxorubicin-based chemotherapy and postmastectomy radiation: implications for patients with early stage disease and predictors for recurrence after radiation. *Int J Radiat Oncol BIol Phys* 2003;57:336–344.
86. Smith BD, Smith GL, Haffty BG. Postmastectomy radiation and mortality in women with T1-2 node-positive breast cancer. *J Clin Oncol* 2005;23(7):1409–1419.
87. Buchholz TA, et al. Radiation use and long-term survival in breast cancer patients with T1,T2 primary tumors and 1-3 positive axillary lymph nodes. *Int J Radiat Oncol BIol Phys* 2006 (in press).
88. Kyndi M, et al. High local recurrence risk is not associated with large survival reduction after postmastectomy radiotherapy in high-risk breast cancer: a subgroup analysis of DBCG 82 b&c. *Radiother Oncol* 2009;90(1):74–79.
90. Taghian AG, et al. Low locoregional recurrence rate among node-negative breast cancer patients with tumors 5 cm or larger treated by mastectomy, with or without adjuvant systemic therapy and without radiotherapy: results from five national surgical adjuvant breast and bowel project randomized clinical trials. *J Clin Oncol* 2006;24(24):3927–3932.
92. Recht A, et al. Postmastectomy radiotherapy: clinical practice guidelines of the American Society of Clinical Oncology. *J Clin Oncol* 2001;19(5):1539–1569.
93. Buchholz TA, et al. Pathologic tumor size and lymph node status predict for different rates of locoregional recurrence after mastectomy for breast cancer patients treated with neoadjuvant versus adjuvant chemotherapy. *Int J Radiat Oncol Biol Phys* 2002;53(4):880–888.
98. Early Breast Cancer Trialists' Collaborative Group, et al. Effects of chemotherapy and hormonal therapy for early breast cancer on recurrence and 15-year survival: an overview of the randomised trials. *Lancet* 2005;365(9472):1687–1717.
99. Davies C, et al. Relevance of breast cancer hormone receptors and other factors to the efficacy of adjuvant tamoxifen: patient-level meta-analysis of randomised trials. *Lancet* 2011;378(9793):771–784.
100. Dowsett M, et al. Meta-analysis of breast cancer outcomes in adjuvant trials of aromatase inhibitors versus tamoxifen. *J Clin Oncol* 2010;28(3):509–518.
102. Mamounas EP, et al. Paclitaxel after doxorubicin plus cyclophosphamide as adjuvant chemotherapy for node-positive breast cancer: results from NSABP B-28. *J Clin Oncol* 2005;23(16):3686–3696.
103. Martin M, et al. Adjuvant docetaxel for node-positive breast cancer. *N Engl J Med* 2005;352(22):2302–2313.
104. De Laurentiis M, et al. Taxane-based combinations as adjuvant chemotherapy of early breast cancer: a meta-analysis of randomized trials. *J Clin Oncol* 2008; 26(1):44–53.
113. Piccart-Gebhart MJ, et al. Trastuzumab after adjuvant chemotherapy in HER2-positive breast cancer. *N Engl J Med* 2005;353(16):1659–1672.
114. Joensuu H, et al. Adjuvant docetaxel or vinorelbine with or without trastuzumab for breast cancer. *N Engl J Med* 2006;354(8):809–820.
116. Romond EH, et al. Trastuzumab plus adjuvant chemotherapy for operable HER2-positive breast cancer. *N Engl J Med* 2005;353(16):1673–1684.
128. Low JA, et al. Long-term follow-up for locally advanced and inflammatory breast cancer patients treated with multimodality therapy. *J Clin Oncol* 2004;22(20):4067–4074.
130. Arthur DW, et al. Accelerated superfractionated radiotherapy for inflammatory breast carcinoma: complete response predicts outcome and allows for breast conservation. *Int J Radiat Oncol Biol Phys* 1999;44(2):289–296.
135. Li J, et al. Triple-negative/basal subtype predicts poor overall survival and high locoregional relapse in inflammatory breast cancer. *Oncologist* 2011 (in press).
144. Huang E, et al. Classifying local disease recurrences after breast conservation therapy based on location and histology: new primary tumors have more favorable outcomes than true local disease recurrences. *Cancer* 2002;95(10): 2059–2067.
148. Nielsen HM, et al. Loco-regional recurrence after mastectomy in high-risk breast cancer–risk and prognosis. An analysis of patients from the DBCG 82 b&c randomization trials. *Radiother Oncol* 2006;79(2):147–155.
153. Halverson KJ, et al. Isolated local-regional recurrence of breast cancer following mastectomy: radiotherapeutic management. *Int J Radiat Oncol Biol Phys* 1990; 19(4):851–858.

Part G Gastrointestinal

Chapter 58
Stomach Cancer

Brian G. Czito, Manisha Palta, and Christopher G. Willett

ANATOMY

The stomach begins at the gastroesophageal (GE) junction and ends at the pylorus. The stomach is generally divided into anatomic regions, including the gastric cardia (the region surrounding the superior opening of the stomach where it connects with the GE junction/level of the lower esophageal sphincter), the fundus (situated superiorly, a rounded portion superior to the body and to the left of the cardia), the body (a large, central portion of the stomach), and the pyloric canal (distally, connecting to the duodenum). The pylorus is composed of two parts: the pyloric antrum, which connects to the body of the stomach, and the pyloric canal, which empties into the duodenum (Fig. 58.1). The pylorus communicates with the duodenum of the small intestine via the pyloric sphincter (valve). This valve regulates the passage of chyme from stomach to duodenum and prevents backflow of chyme from duodenum to stomach. A plane passing through the incisura angularis on the lesser curvature divides the stomach into the body and the pyloric portion (antrum). The anterior surface of the stomach is covered with peritoneum of the greater sac. At the left and cranially, it abuts the diaphragm. In view of the increasing incidence of gastric cancer at the GE junction, it is important to note that there is either no or variable visceral peritoneal covering at the most proximal portion of the GE junction.[1] Positive radial margins at this site are often "true" positive margins, whereas many other positive margins in the stomach are free serosal margins unless the tumor is adherent to an adjacent organ or structure. The right portion of the anterior gastric surface is adjacent to the left lobe of the liver and the anterior abdominal wall. Posteriorly, the stomach is covered with peritoneum of the lesser sac or omental bursa. The stomach contacts many visceral structures; from superior to inferior, it is adjacent to the spleen, left adrenal gland, superior portion of the left kidney, ventral portion of the pancreas, and transverse colon. The hepatogastric ligament or lesser omentum is attached to the lesser curvature and contains the left gastric artery and the right gastric branch of the hepatic artery. Histologically, the wall of the stomach has five layers: the mucosa, the submucosa, muscular layer, subserosa, and serosa. The muscularis layer is composed of an outer longitudinal layer, a middle circular layer, and inner oblique layer.

The stomach's vascular supply is derived from the celiac axis. The celiac artery usually has three branches: the left gastric artery, which supplies the upper right portion of the stomach; the common hepatic artery, which gives rise to the right gastric artery supplying the lower right portion of the stomach, and the right gastroepiploic branch supplying the lower portion of the greater curvature; and the splenic artery, which gives rise to the left gastroepiploic supplying the upper portion of the greater curvature and the short gastric arteries supplying the fundus. Variations in this normal vascular supply are common. The celiac axis originates at or below the pedicle of T12 in approximately 75% of patients and at or above the pedicle of L1 in 25% of patients.[2] The lymphatic drainage of the stomach follows the arterial supply. Although most lymphatics ultimately drain to the celiac nodal basin, lymph drainage sites can include the splenic hilum, suprapancreatic nodal groups, porta hepatis, and gastroduodenal areas.

EPIDEMIOLOGY

Gastric cancer is estimated to afflict 21,320 people in the United States in 2012 and result in 10,540 deaths.[3] Worldwide, gastric cancer remains a significant cause of cancer-related mortality, with nearly one million new cases annually and an estimated 700,000 deaths, making it the second-leading cause of cancer-related deaths. During the past 70 years, there has been a significant decline in the incidence of gastric cancer in both sexes in Western countries. The causes of this decline are unknown.[4,5] Although the overall decrease in gastric cancer incidence is encouraging, there has been a steady and dramatic increase in the incidence of proximal lesser curvature, cardia, and GE junction tumors over the past 20 years, especially in White males.[6] In contrast to the increasing incidence of more proximal gastric cancers seen in the Western Hemisphere and parts of Europe, distal tumors continue to comprise most gastric cancers in the Far East and other parts of the world.

Risk factors implicated in gastric cancer development include consumption of smoked, pickled, and salted foods; low intake of fruits and vegetables; low socioeconomic status; smoking; decreased use of refrigeration; and dried meat/fish consumption.[4,7] Pernicious anemia is associated with gastric cancer, with 5% to 10% of patients with pernicious anemia developing gastric cancer. Prior subtotal gastrectomy for benign lesions also carries a 25% risk for subsequent malignancies, with latency periods of 15 to 40 years.[8] Villous adenomas are clearly premalignant; hyperplastic or hamartomatous polyps occur more frequently and are apparently benign. Gastric ulcers carry no increased risk, although previous distal gastrectomy for benign disease confers a 1.5- to 3-fold relative risk for development of gastric cancer, with a latency period of 15 to 20 years. Additionally, patients with a family history of nonhereditary gastric cancer have a higher risk for developing similar disease, with a very small percentage of patients developing gastric cancer in the context of an inherited syndrome. The presence of

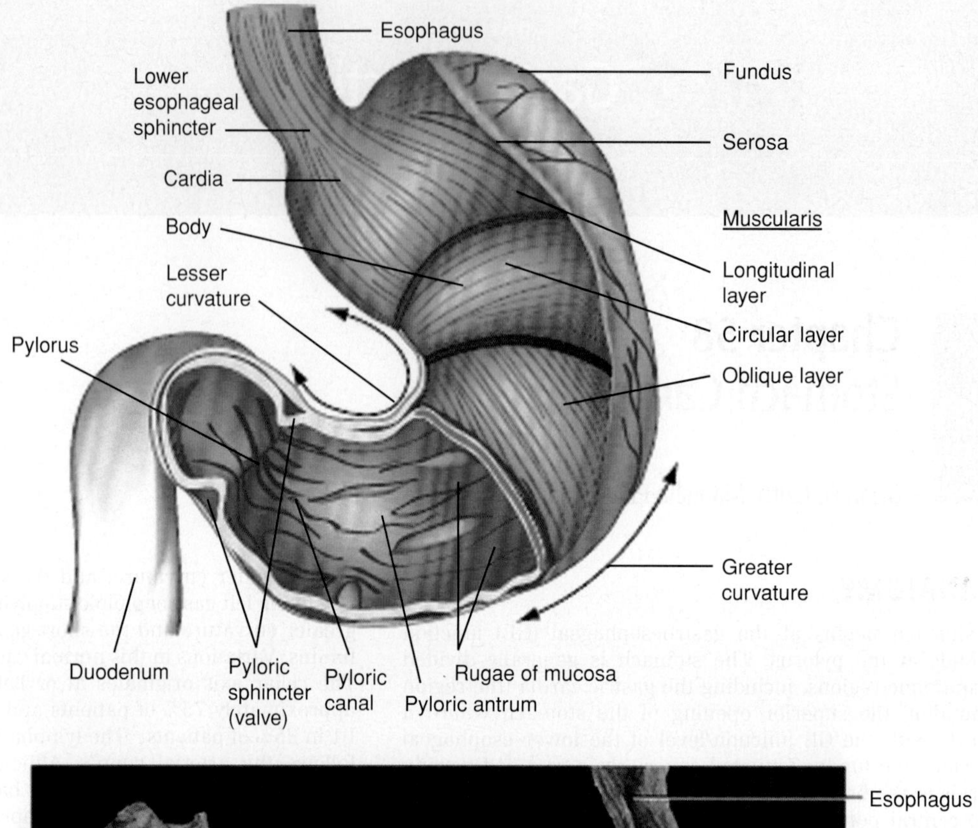

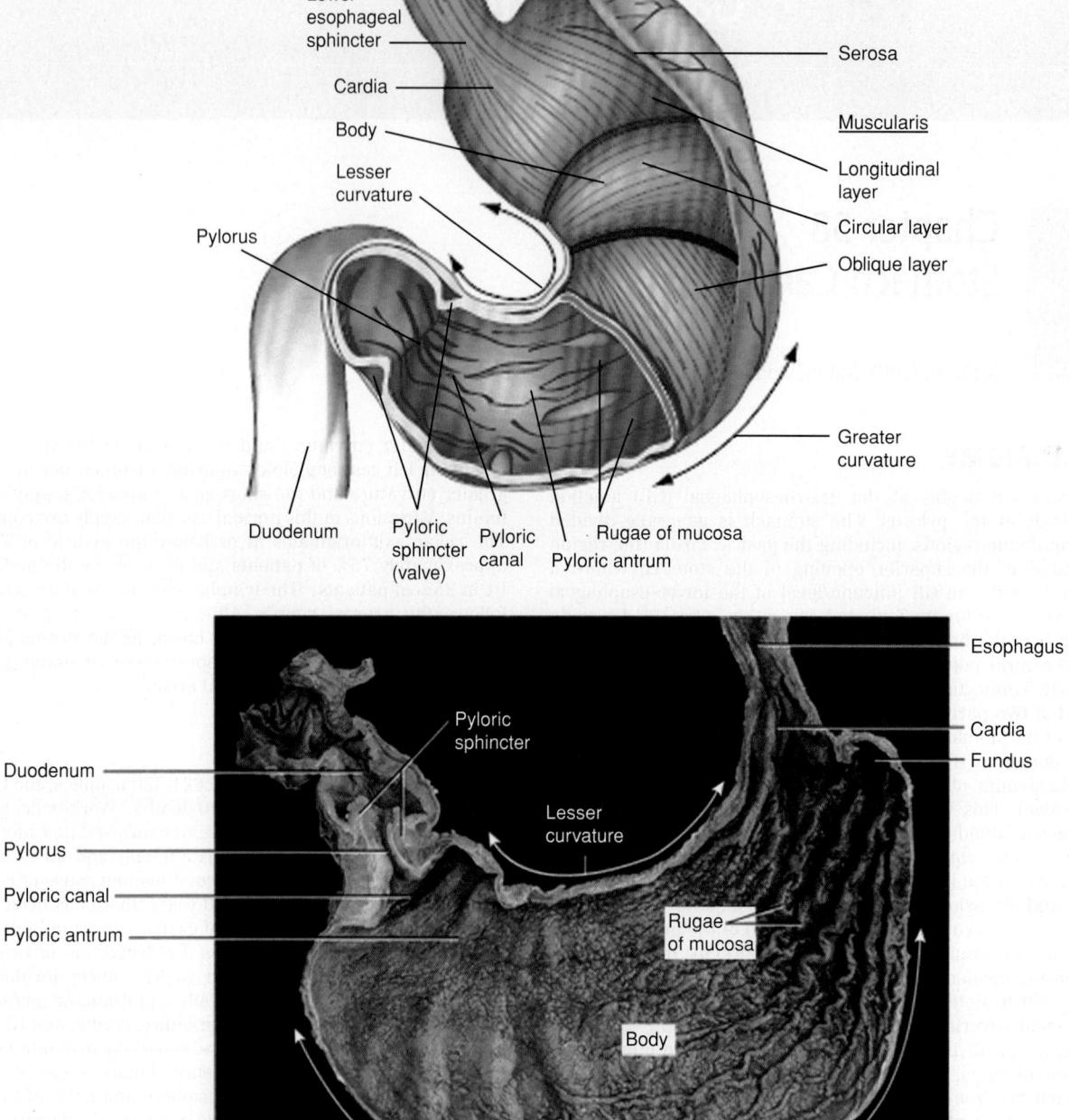

FIGURE 58.1. Gastric anatomy. (From Tortora GJ, Grabowski SR. *Principles of anatomy and physiology*, 9th ed. New York: John Wiley & Sons, Inc. Copyright 1996. Reprinted with permission of John Wiley & Sons, Inc.)

Helicobacter pylori is associated with a three to six times greater risk of gastric cancer than if infection is absent. The increased association of *H. pylori* appears to be confined to those with distal gastric cancer and intestinal-type malignancy.[9] Although this association of *H. pylori* infection with gastric cancer may provide new insight into the pathogenesis of this tumor, only a small minority of infected people develop gastric carcinoma, and there are no firmly established data regarding the screening of infected patients or the effect of treatment for infection on subsequent malignancy.

Historically, gastric adenocarcinomas have been diagnosed as intestinal or diffuse types. Intestinal types are more prevalent in high-incidence areas and responsible for much of the observed global ethnic variation of disease.[10] In contrast, diffuse gastric cancer incidence is fairly uniform among geographic regions or race and more uncommon than intestinal type. More recently, there has been an emergence of another distinct subtype—proximal gastric cancers. These are often grouped with GE junction and distal esophageal adenocarcinomas, with a rapidly rising incidence in industrialized nations.

The risks factors for these individual types appear to vary significantly. Risk factors of intestinal, noncardia gastric cancers appear to center around inflammatory causes and environmental factors, including *H. pylori,* chronic gastritis, tobacco, high salt intake, and alcohol consumption. The less common diffuse gastric cancer subtype appears to be distinct, with E-cadherin mutations/silencing thought to be a common precursor event with this histology. Hereditary diffuse gastric cancer is a genetic syndrome in which there is loss of function/mutation in the E-cadherin gene. In proximal gastric cancer (and in contrast to intestinal types), *H. pylori* infection has been found to be potentially protective, possibly through associated atrophic gastritis and reduced acid production with subsequent reduction in gastroesophageal reflux disease (GERD). This possible association remains an ongoing area of study.[10]

PATTERNS OF SPREAD

Cancer of the stomach may extend directly into the omenta, pancreas, diaphragm, transverse colon or mesocolon, and duodenum. Peritoneal contamination with carcinomatosis is possible after a lesion extends beyond the gastric wall to a free peritoneal (serosal) surface.[11]

Microscopic or subclinical spread beyond the visible gross lesion occurs frequently because of the abundant lymphatic channels within the submucosal and subserosal layers of the gastric wall. The submucosal plexus in the esophagus and subserosal plexus in the duodenum allow proximal and distal spread.

It is difficult to perform a complete node dissection because of the numerous pathways of lymphatic drainage from the stomach (Fig. 58.2). Initial drainage is to lymph nodes along the lesser and greater curvatures (i.e., gastric and gastroepiploic nodes) but also includes the celiac axis, porta hepatis, splenic, suprapancreatic, pancreaticoduodenal, adjacent para-aortics, and distal paraesophageal system. The relative risks for nodal involvement in gastric cancer depend on the location of the primary tumor as well as extent of gastric wall involvement.

Gastric venous drainage is primarily to the liver by the portal system. Liver involvement is found in as many as 30% of patients at initial exploration, and it can occur as a result of venous metastasis, peritoneal-based spread, and direct extension (Fig. 58.3).

CLINICAL PRESENTATION

The most common presenting symptoms of stomach cancer are loss of appetite, early satiety, abdominal discomfort, unintentional weight loss, anemia-related weakness, nausea and vomiting, and tarry stools. Duration of symptoms is <3 months in almost 40% of patients and >1 year in 20%. Physical examination can reveal advanced disease, for which the presentation may include an abdominal mass (epigastric or liver mass as well as a periumbilical node [i.e., Sister Mary Joseph node]), palpable left supraclavicular nodes (i.e., Virchow's node), or a rectal shelf (representing peritoneal seeding [i.e., Blumer's shelf]).

DIAGNOSTIC WORKUP

Diagnosis is usually confirmed by upper gastrointestinal endoscopy as well as imaging studies in some instances. Double-contrast x-ray studies may reveal small lesions limited to the inner layers of the gastric wall. Endoscopy with direct visualization, cytology, and biopsy yields the diagnosis in ≥90% of exophytic lesions; however, infiltrative (linitis plastica), small (<3 cm), or cardia lesions may be more difficult to diagnose endoscopically. Endoscopic ultrasonography is the most accurate method of determining depth of tumor invasion (intramural vs. extramural extension) prior to resection but is less accurate in detecting regional nodal metastases.[12,13] In some institutions, needle biopsies of suspicious nodes are performed at the time of endoscopic ultrasound.

Abdominal computed tomography (CT) is useful in determining the abdominal extent of disease and may help to determine which lesions extend to surgically unresectable structures but are of lesser value in detecting small lymph node metastases or peritoneal spread. Distant metastases should be ruled out with contrast-enhanced CT of the chest, abdomen, and pelvis. CT may provide valuable tumor localization information if irradiation is indicated. If a proximal gastric cancer extends to involve the esophagus, CT of the chest will help to rule out involvement of mediastinal nodes or the lung parenchyma.

Helical CT may be more useful than conventional CT in identifying smaller lymph nodes, which are particularly relevant to staging of gastric cancer patients. In a single-institution experience, 58 patients underwent nodal dissection for gastric cancer.[14] A total of 1,082 nodes were resected, and 138 were metastatic. Helical CT was able to identify 1.1% of the 649 lymph nodes that were 1 to 4 mm in diameter, 45.1% of the 355 nodes of 5 to 9 mm, and 72% of the nodes >9 mm. For nodes ≥5 mm, the sensitivity for identifying metastatic nodes was greater than for nonmetastatic nodes (75.2% vs. 41.8%, respectively).

The value of laparoscopy in the staging of gastric cancer remains a subject of study. In one study of 71 patients with CT criteria of resectable disease, 69 completed laparoscopic evaluation.[15] Forty-one of the 69 patients proceeded to laparotomy with curative intent, and 38 of 41 patients had resection of all gross tumor. Pathologic evidence documented hepatic metastasis in three patients with a negative CT scan of the liver, and one of them was detected by laparoscopy. Laparoscopy confirmed disease in 16 of 17 patients with peritoneal metastases (avoiding 12 laparotomies, 17%). The combination of CT scan and laparoscopy for staging information yielded a resectability rate of 93% in patients defined as potential candidates for curative gastric cancer surgery. Similarly, a large series from Memorial Sloan-Kettering Cancer Center of >600 patients with potentially resectable gastric adenocarcinoma by conventional imaging underwent laparoscopic staging, resulting in distant metastases being detected in 31% of patients.[16] A systematic review on the role of diagnostic laparoscopy showed that change in patient management occurred in 9% to 60% of patients initially deemed resectable by preoperative imaging, predominantly through the identification of patients with metastatic disease who would not benefit from either laparotomy or neoadjuvant therapy, thereby avoiding unnecessary interventions. This primarily related to patients with advanced (T3, T4) gastric cancer, with relatively minimal benefit in early-stage patients, prompting the authors to recommend diagnostic laparoscopy for patients with locally advanced-stage disease.[17] In addition, peritoneal fluid can be sampled for cytology at laparoscopy. If positive, this is a poor prognostic indicator and the patient should be considered as having M1 disease.

Overall treatment planning in gastric cancer may be improved by accurate preoperative classification of key prognostic factors, namely depth of invasion (T category) and lymph node involvement (N category). A prospective study in 108 patients evaluated endogastric ultrasonography (EUS), CT, and intraoperative surgical assessment for T and N classification.[18] T-staging was accurately characterized by CT in 43% of the cases, EUS in 86% of cases, and intraoperative assessment in 56% of cases. Staging of N1 and N2 lymph nodes was correct with CT in 51% of the cases, 74% with EUS, and 54% with intraoperative assessment. Advanced gastric tumors tended to be more accurately staged with CT, although CT, in general, overstages the T-category and understages the N category. EUS showed a high accuracy for all the T-categories, although it also tends to understage N-categories. Finally, intraoperative assessment was equally accurate for all N-categories but tended to overstage early T-stages and to understage N-categories. A meta-analysis and systematic review of the

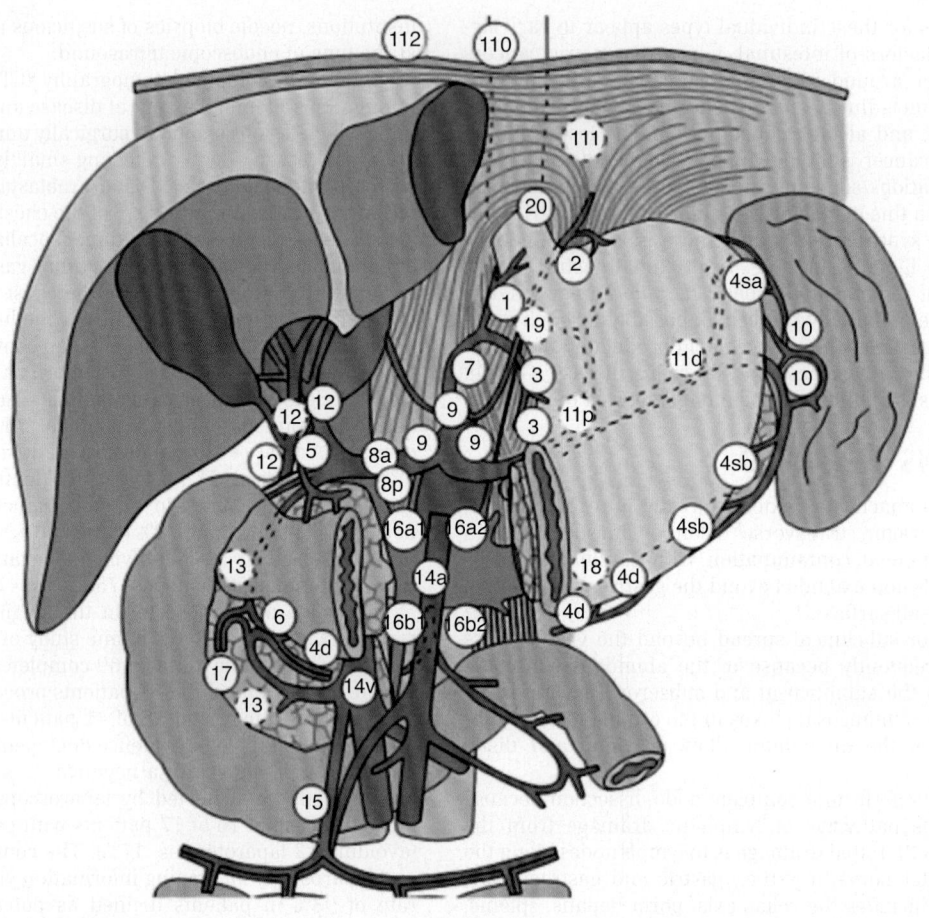

No. 1	Right paracardial LN
No. 2	Left paracardial LN
No. 3	LN along the lesser curvature
No. 4sa	LN along the short gastric vessels
No. 4sb	LN along the left gastroepiploic vessels
No. 4d	LN along the right gastroepiploic vessels
No. 5	Suprapyloric LN
No. 6	Infrapyloric LN
No. 7	LN along the left gastric artery
No. 8a	LN along the common hepatic artery (Anterosuperior group)
No. 8p	LN along the common hepatic artery (Posterior group)
No. 9	LN around the celiac artery
No. 10	LN at the splenic hilum
No. 11p	LN along the proximal splenic artery
No. 11d	LN along the distal splenic artery
No. 12a	LN in the hepatoduodenal ligament (along the hepatic artery)
No. 12b	LN in the hepatoduodenal ligament (along the bile duct)
No. 12p	LN in the hepatoduodenal ligament (behind the portal vein)
No. 13	LN on the posterior surface of the pancreatic head
No. 14v	LN along the superior mesenteric vein
No. 14a	LN along the superior mesenteric artery
No. 15	LN along the middle colic vessels
No. 16a1	LN in the aortic hiatus
No. 16a2	LN around the abdominal aorta (from the upper margin of the celiac trunk to the lower margin of the left renal vein)
No. 16b1	LN around the abdominal aorta (from the lower margin of the left renal vein to the upper margin of the inferior mesenteric artery)
No. 16b2	LN around the abdominal aorta (from the upper margin of the inferior mesenteric artery to the aortic bifurcation)
No. 17	LN on the anterior surface of the pancreatic head
No. 18	LN along the inferior margin of the pancreas
No. 19	Infradiaphragmatic LN
No. 20	LN in the esophageal hiatus of the diaphragm
No. 110	Paraesophageal LN in the lower thorax
No. 111	Supradiaphragmatic LN
No. 112	Posterior mediastinal LN

FIGURE 58.2. Locations of gastric lymph node stations. (From Matzinger O, Gerber E, Bernstein Z, et al. EORTC-ROG expert opinion: radiotherapy volume and treatment guidelines for neoadjuvant radiation of adenocarcinomas of the gastroesophageal junction and the stomach. *Radiother Oncol* 2009;92:164–175, with permission from Elsevier.)

role of EUS in T- and N-staging in nearly 2,000 patients with gastric cancers suggested the sensitivity for detecting T1, 2, 3, and 4 disease was 88, 82, 90, and 99%, respectively, with nodal staging sensitivity for N1 and N2 disease 58 and 65%, respectively, also suggesting that accuracy was higher with more advanced disease.[19] Another systematic review concluded that EUS, multidetector CT, and MRI achieve similar results in terms of diagnostic accuracy of T-staging and assessing serosal involvement. Given that most experience has been gained with EUS, this was felt to remain as the first-choice imaging modality in the preoperative T-staging of gastric cancer.[20] However, it should be remembered that EUS accuracy highly depends on the experience and expertise of the operating physician.

The positron emission tomography (PET) scan has a lower detection rate in some cases of gastric cancers owing to the low fluorine-18 fluorodeoxyglucose (FDG) accumulation in patients with diffuse or mucinous tumors.[21] Approximately 40% of gastric carcinomas, notably above histologies, may not be detected

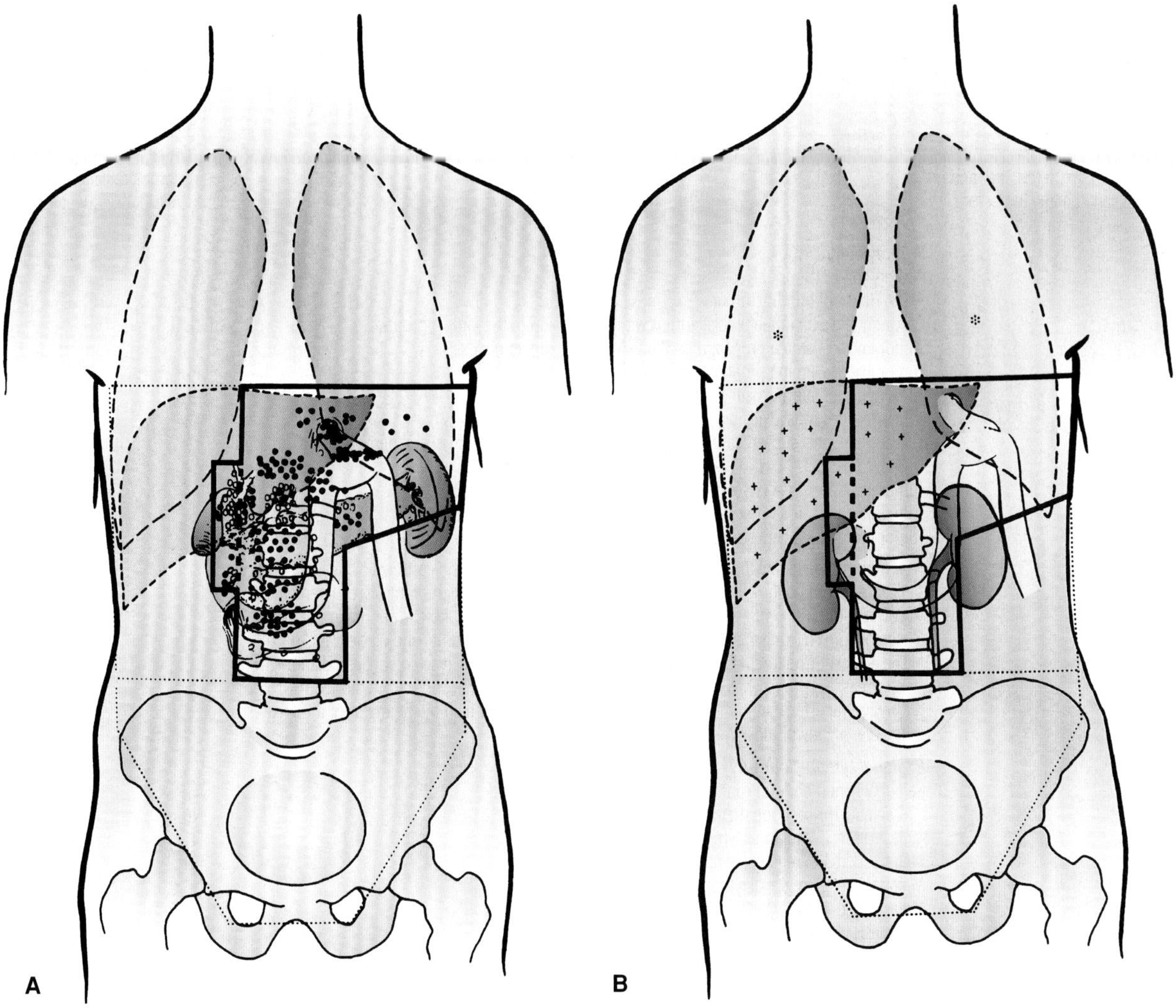

FIGURE 58.3. Patterns of failure in 82 evaluable patients in the University of Minnesota Reoperation series. **A:** Large bold circles indicate local failures in surrounding organs or tissues; large open circles indicate lymph node failures. **B:** Asterisk (*) indicates lung metastasis; plus (+) indicates liver metastasis. Superimposed irradiation portals encompass postsurgical gastric remnant, anastomoses, duodenal stump, gastric bed structures, and primary and secondary areas of lymph node drainage; broken lines represent upper and total abdomen fields. (From Gunderson LL, Sosin H. Adenocarcinoma of the stomach: areas of failure in a reoperation series [second or symptomatic looks]. Clinicopathologic correlation and implications for adjuvant therapy. *Int J Radiat Oncol Biol Phys* 1982;8:1, with permission from Elsevier.)

with PET scan.[22] PET alone has been described as displaying a lower sensitivity when compared to CT in detecting nodal involvement, although specificity is improved.[23] Given this, PET alone is likely not an adequate diagnostic procedure for evaluation of gastric cancer and generally should be used in conjunction with CT scan for correlation, allowing more accurate preoperative staging than either modality alone. A suggested diagnostic evaluation for gastric cancer is shown in Table 58.1.

A prospective report analyzed the potential involvement of bone marrow at the time of radical surgery after obtaining material through aspiration and the use of monoclonal antibody CK-2 directed to component 18 of the intracellular cytokeratin.[24] Among the 180 patients evaluated, 53% had a positive test showing malignant cells in the bone marrow. The finding was correlated with pT ($p = .07$) and Borrmann's classification ($p = .02$) (see later discussion).[25] The estimation of tumor cell contents in the bone marrow ($<3 \times 10^6$) was related significantly to overall and disease-free survival ($p = .04$ and $p < .007$, respectively). The multivariate analyses detected that bone marrow malignant involvement was an independent prognostic factor for disease-free survival in pT1 to pT2 stages ($p = .004$), intestinal histologic subtypes ($p < .008$), and N0 patients ($p = .004$).

TABLE 58.1 DIAGNOSTIC WORKUP FOR GASTRIC CANCER

History and physical
Upper gastrointestinal endoscopy and biopsy
Chest, abdomen, pelvic CT with oral and intravenous contrast (preferably correlated with PET when PET is performed)
Complete blood count (CBC) and comprehensive metabolic panel
Endoscopic ultrasound if no evidence of metastases with fine-needle aspiration (FNA) as indicated
Biopsy confirmation of suspected metastatic gastric cancer
H. pylori testing performed and treatment delivered where clinically indicated

STAGING

The current tumor-node-metastasis (TNM) system is depicted in Table 58.2.[26] In the most recent American Joint Committee on Cancer (AJCC) staging of gastric cancers, cancers whose midpoint is in the lower thoracic esophagus, GE junction, or within the proximal 5 cm of the stomach (cardia) *and* extending to the GE junction or esophagus are staged as esophageal neoplasms. All other cancers with a midpoint in the stomach lying more than 5 cm distal to the GE junction or those within 5 cm of the GE junction (but not involving the GE junction or esophagus) are staged using the gastric cancer staging system. Potential drawbacks of this system are that it is based primarily

TABLE 58.2 AMERICAN JOINT COMMITTEE ON CANCER 2010 GASTRIC CANCER STAGING

Clinical *Extent of Disease Before any Treatment*	*Stage Category Definitions*	*Pathologic* *Extent of Disease During and from Surgery*
(Note y indicates clinical–staging completed after neoadjuvant therapy but before subsequent surgery)		(Note y indicates pathologic–staging completed after neoadjuvant therapy AND subsequent surgery)
	Primary Tumor (T)	
Tx	Primary tumor cannot be assessed	TX
T0	No evidence of primary tumor	T0
Tis	Carcinoma in situ: intraepithelial tumor without invasion of the lamina propria	Tis
T1	Tumor invades lamina propria, muscularis mucosae, or submucosa	T1
T1a	Tumor invades lamina propria or muscularis mucosae	T1a
T1b	Tumor invades submucosa	T1b
T2	Tumor invades muscularis propria	T2
T3	Tumor penetrates subserosal connective tissue without invasion of visceral peritoneum or adjacent structures*,**,***	T3
T4	Tumor invades serosa (visceral peritoneum) or adjacent structures**,***	
T4a	Tumor invades serosa (visceral peritoneum)	
T4b	Tumor invades adjacent structures	
	*A tumor may penetrate the muscularis propria with extension into the gastrocolic or gastrohepatic ligaments, or into the greater or lesser omentum, without perforation of the visceral peritoneum covering these structures. In this case, the tumor is classified T3. If there is perforation of the visceral peritoneum covering the gastric ligaments or the omentum, the tumor should be classified T4. **The adjacent structures of the stomach include the spleen, transverse colon, liver, diaphragm, pancreas, abdominal wall, adrenal gland, kidney, small intestine, and retroperitoneum. ***Intramural extension to the duodenum or esophagus is classified by the depth of the greatest invasion in any of these sites, including the stomach.	
	Regional Lymph Nodes (N)	
NX	Regional lymph node(s) cannot be assessed	NX
N0	No regional lymph node metastasis*	N0
N1	Metastasis in 1–2 regional lymph nodes	N1
N2	Metastasis in 3–6 regional lymph nodes	N2
N3	Metastasis in ≥7 regional lymph nodes	N3
N3a	Metastasis in 7–15 regional lymph nodes	N3a
N3b	Metastasis in ≥16 regional lymph nodes	N3b
	*A designation of pN0 should be used if all examined lymph nodes are negative, regardless of the total number removed and examined.	
	Distant Metastasis (M)	
M0	No distant metastasis (no pathologic M0; used clinical M to complete stage group)	M1
M1	Distant metastasis	

Group	*Stage* *T*	*N*	*M*
0	Tis	N0	M0
IA	T1	N0	M0
IB	T2	N0	M0
	T1	N1	M0
IIA	T3	N0	M0
	T2	N1	M0
	T1	N2	M0
IIB	T4a	N0	M0
	T3	N1	M0
	T2	N2	M0
	T1	N3	M0
IIIA	T4a	N1	M0
	T3	N2	M0
	T2	N3	M0
IIIB	T4b	N0	M0
	T4b	N1	M0
	T4a	N2	M0
	T3	N3	M0
IIIC	T4b	N2	M0
	T4b	N3	M0
	T4a	N3	M0
IV	Any T	Any N	M1
Stage unknown			

General Notes

For identification of special cases of TNM or pTNM classifications, the "m" suffix and "y," "r," and "a" prefixes are used. Although they do not affect the stage grouping, they indicate cases needing separate analysis:

m suffix indicates the presence of multiple primary tumors in a single site and is recorded in parentheses: pT(m)NM. **y prefix** indicates those cases in which classification is performed during or following initial multimodality therapy. The cTNM or pTNM category is identified by a "y" prefix. The ycTNM or ypTNM categorizes the extent of tumor actually present at the time of that examination. The "y" categorization is not an estimate of tumor prior to multimodality therapy.

TABLE 58.2 (Continued)

(Footnote continued)

r prefix indicates a recurrent tumor when staged after a disease-free interval and is identified by the "r" prefix: rTNM.

a prefix designates the stage determined at autopsy: aTNM.

surgical margins is data field recorded by registrars describing the surgical margins of the resected primary site specimen as determined only by the pathology report.

neoadjuvant treatment is radiation therapy or systemic therapy (consisting of chemotherapy, hormone therapy, or immunotherapy) administered prior to a definitive surgical procedure. If the surgical procedure is not performed, the administered therapy no longer meets the definition of neoadjuvant therapy.

Additional Descriptors

Lymphatic vessel invasion (L) and venous invasion (V) have been combined into lymph-vascular invasion (LVI) for collection by cancer registrars. The College of American Pathologists' (CAP) Checklist should be used as the primary source. Other sources may be used in the absence of a checklist. Priority is given to positive results:

Lymph-Vascular Invasion Not Present (absent)/Not Identified

Lymph-Vascular Invasion Present/Identified

Not Applicable

Unknown/Indeterminate

Residual Tumor (R)

The absence or presence of residual tumor after treatment. In some cases treated with surgery and/or with neoadjuvant therapy, there will be residual tumor at the primary site after treatment because of incomplete resection or local and regional disease that extends beyond the limit of ability of resection:

RX Presence of residual tumor cannot be assessed, R0 No residual tumor, R1 Microscopic residual tumor, R2 Macroscopic residual tumor

on surgical outcomes and not entirely suitable in considering clinical baseline staging and preoperative therapy.

PATHOLOGY

Adenocarcinomas account for 90% to 95% of all gastric malignancies. Lymphomas, including both favorable and unfavorable histologies, are the second most common malignancies. Rarely, leiomyosarcomas (2%), carcinoid tumors (1%), adenoacanthomas (1%), and squamous cell carcinomas (1%) occur.

The site of origin of gastric cancers within the stomach has changed in the United States over recent decades, and proximal lesions are being diagnosed and treated more frequently. Although the highest frequency is still in the antrum/distal stomach (approximately 40%), the lowest frequency is now in the body rather than proximal portion of the stomach (approximately 25%), with intermediate frequency in the proximal stomach and GE junction (approximately 35%). Several investigators have reported an increased frequency of cardia lesions. As described previously, cardia lesions appear to have different epidemiologic factors, exhibit different tumor biology, and have an inferior prognosis from lesions in the other sites.[27–28,29–31] Gastric cancers sometimes are categorized according to Borrmann's five types. Type I tumors are polypoid or fungating; type II are ulcerating lesions surrounded by elevated borders; type III have ulceration with invasion of the gastric wall; type IV are diffusely infiltrating (linitis plastica); and type V are unclassifiable.[25]

PROGNOSTIC FACTORS

The most important prognostic indicators reflect tumor extent. If hematogenous or transperitoneal spread is present, the outcome is, essentially, uniformly fatal. Survival rates decrease with progressive tumor extension within or beyond the gastric wall.[27,32,33,34] The number of involved lymph nodes also has a significant impact on survival. Lymph node involvement is important, as are the number and locations of nodes affected.[27,34,35,36] Minimal node involvement adjacent to the primary lesion only moderately affects prognosis.[32,36,37] The finding of either involved lymph nodes or complete wall penetration is usually not as ominous as the presence of both[32,34,36,38] (Table 58.3). Additional prognostic indicators include a poor performance status, elevated alkaline phosphatase levels, and ethnicity.[39] In one study, Asian-Pacific Islanders born in the United States were compared to those born abroad, finding that only foreign-born Asian-Pacific Islanders had a more favorable survival compared to indigenous Caucasians.[40]

Flow cytometry is also prognostically valuable; aneuploidy is associated with unfavorable tumor location, lymph node metastasis, and primary tumor invasion.[41–43] Unfavorable DNA flow cytometry correlates with a poor prognosis.[41] The prognosis is worse for cardia lesions, and flow cytometry reveals a greater incidence of aneuploidy.[43] The gross pathologic appearance of the primary lesion also reveals prognostic information, although it is not known whether this factor is independent of

TABLE 58.3 EXTENT OF INITIAL DISEASE COMPARED WITH SURVIVAL RATES FOR CANCER OF THE STOMACH

	5-Year Survival Rate (%)		*≥5-Year Disease-Free Survival Rate (%)*
Extent of Disease	*Dockerty*[32a]	*Kennedy*[34]	*University of Minnesota Reoperation Series*[33]
Negative Lymph Nodes			
Mucosa only	100	85	–
Beyond mucosa but within wall	61	52	–
Through wall	44	47	–
Positive Lymph Nodes			
Nodal extent	15	–	19
Regional only	–	17	–
Nonregional	–	6	–
Extent of Primary			
Within wall	–	–	40
Through wall	–	–	12

[a]Percentages are of those patients who left the hospital.

Clinical Radiation Oncology

tumor stage. Patients with Borrmann type I and II tumors have relatively favorable 5-year survival rates, although patients with type IV (linitis plastica) fare poorly.[37,44–46]

The molecular biology of gastric cancer reflects the heterogeneity of its causes and its histologic subtypes. Identification of the genetic and phenotypic variables existing among gastric cancers may lead to more directed therapeutic approaches and a more accurate prediction of clinical outcome. Changes that may affect the behavior of gastric tumor cells involve four major types of alterations. Loss of tumor suppressor gene function, especially inactivation of the p53 gene, appears to play a critical role. The p53 gene is located on the short arm of chromosome 17 and plays a key role in tumor suppression and cell-cycle regulation.[47] The p53 gene halts DNA replication and triggers programmed cell death in response to DNA damage.[48] Loss of p53 function allows malignancy to develop, affects the effectiveness of chemotherapy and irradiation, and predisposes cells to genetic instability.[49,50] The latter is particularly important because p53 mutations occur early in tumorogenesis.[51]

A second major aberration affecting gastric epithelial cells is the impact of alterations in mismatch repair genes. Two such genes, hMSH3 and hMLH1, on chromosome 2 and 3, respectively, account for replication errors throughout the genome. Mutations in these genes are implicated in cancer family syndromes and hereditary nonpolyposis colorectal cancer, which is a disease associated with an increased tendency for the development of gastric tumors.[52] Mutations in these genes generate genetic instability and have the potential to lead to further alterations in oncogenes.

Two proto-oncogenes, c-met and k-sam, are associated with scirrhous carcinoma of the stomach. The former encodes hepatocyte growth factor, which is a potent endogenous promoter of gastric epithelial cell growth.[53] Its overexpression correlates with tumor progression and metastasis.[54] The latter encodes a tyrosine kinase receptor family.[54] In scirrhous carcinoma, c-met and k-sam amplification may occur independently. There is a tendency for k-sam to be activated in women <40 years of age and c-met to be amplified in men >50 years of age.[51,55]

Peptide receptors, including estrogen receptors and epidermal growth factor receptors, are associated with adverse prognoses.[56,57] Epidermal growth factor receptors and levels correlate with higher rates of primary tumor infiltration, poorer histologic differentiation, and linitis plastica.[58] The pathophysiologic relation between these peptide receptors and their association with poor prognoses is not well understood.

Modern molecular biology observations confirm the heterogeneity of human gastric cancer. Genetic alterations detected and potentially associated with a worse prognosis include CD44 expression; telomerase reactivation; p53 gene inactivation; dysfunction of repair genes such as hMSH3 and hMLH1; overexpression of proto-oncogenes such as erb-B2, bcl-2, c-met, and k-sam; estrogenic receptor expression; and presence of viral genomes.[59] Gastric cancers with class II major histocompatibility complex antigen expression have a better prognosis; however, the loss of expression is not an independent prognostic factor.[58] Illustrating the importance of understanding and potential exploitation of these genetic alterations, a recent randomized study was conducted in patients with HER2 overexpression. Patients with locally advanced or metastatic gastric or GE cancer (the ToGA trial) were randomized to determine whether trastuzumab (an antibody against the HER2 gene product/receptor) enhanced treatment efficacy when added to cisplatin and 5-fluorouracil (5-FU)/capecitabine therapy. This study showed that the addition of trastuzumab achieved a significant improvement in overall and progression-free survival.[59a] These and other data have led to the initiation of the Radiation Therapy Oncology Group (RTOG) 1010 trial, which randomized patients with esophageal/GE junction tumors to receive preoperative radiation therapy concurrent with paclitaxel/carboplatin, with or without trastuzumab, followed by resection.

GENERAL MANAGEMENT

Surgical Management

Operative attempts are highly successful if disease is limited to the mucosa; however, the incidence of such early lesions at diagnosis is <5% in most U.S. series. In Japan, the incidence of lesions initially confined to the mucosa or submucosa was only 3.8% in 1955 and 1956, although by 1966, as a result of screening procedures, this figure had increased to 34.5%, with corresponding survival rates of 90.9%.[60] For very early gastric cancer, endoscopic mucosal resection and endoscopic submucosal dissection have been successfully used as less radical alternatives to standard surgery. Endoscopic laser surgery has been applied successfully to patients with very early gastric cancer whose tumors are inoperable because of complicating medical illness. Small lesions that are pedunculated, noninvasive, and well differentiated have lymph node metastasis in <5% of cases and can be completely removed endoscopically in 75% of cases.[61] Radiation therapy with chemotherapy may be considered as adjuvant therapy in selected situations. These approaches in early gastric cancer (uncommonly seen in Western society) require meticulous patient selection and remain a topic of investigation.

Curative or palliative surgical resection is possible for 50% to 60% of patients at the time of initial disease presentation. However, only approximately 25% to 40% are eligible for potentially curative resection. Generally, patients with evidence of peritoneal involvement, distant metastases, or locally advanced disease (including encasement of unresectable/major blood vessels) are generally considered to have unresectable disease. Palliative resection is usually reserved for rare cases, including symptomatic palliation of bleeding uncontrolled by other methods. In some instances, unresectable tumors may be debulked successfully, with sites of minimal residual disease marked judiciously with clips. This may palliate and permit accurate delivery of postoperative radiation therapy. In patients with gastric outlet obstruction, gastrojejunostomy may be performed and preferable to endoscopic placement of stents in patients with expected longer survival.

No prospective randomized trials have definitively established optimal surgical therapy.[62] Generally, it is recommended that gastric cancer surgery be performed by experienced surgeons in high-volume centers, entailing removal of the perigastric lymph nodes (D1) as well as those along the main vessels of the celiac trunk (D2), with the goal of examining ≥15 lymph nodes (discussed later).[6] The preferred treatment for gastric carcinoma, especially for lesions arising in the body and antrum, is a radical subtotal gastrectomy. This operation removes approximately 80% of the stomach along with the node-bearing tissue, the gastrohepatic and gastrocolic omenta, and the first portion of the duodenum. Larger lesions may require total gastrectomy. For more proximal tumors, both proximal and total gastrectomy may be appropriate depending on extent of disease. There appears to be no advantage to performing total gastrectomy if subtotal gastrectomy produces satisfactory margins (i.e., 5 cm). Patients treated with total gastrectomy characteristically have 5-year survival rates of 10% to 15%, and those undergoing radical subtotal gastrectomy have 5-year survival rates of 25% to 45%.[35,63,64] The inferior survivorship of patients undergoing total gastrectomy probably reflects larger tumors and unfavorable proximal lesions that prompt such a procedure. The value of splenectomy has not been addressed in prospective randomized trials; however, retrospective Japanese data do not support a survival benefit.[47,65] Because routine splenectomy has not shown significant improved outcomes and potentially increases complication rates, complete removal of splenic nodes is not commonly performed by Western surgeons. The use of laparoscopic approaches in gastric cancer resection may reduce blood loss while potentially decreasing length of postoperative hospital

TABLE 58.4 POSITIVE MARGINS IN RESECTED LONGITUDINAL GASTRIC SPECIMENS

Study (Reference)	Number of Margins Positive/ Number Resected	Percentage
Whittington et al. (73)	34/106	32
Bleiberg et al. (67)	22/111	20
Regine & Mohiuddin (70)	31/120	26
Slot et al. (72)	16/58	28
Gez et al. (68)	7/22	32
Siewert et al. (71)	71/307	23
Gill et al. (69)	1/14	7
Allum et al. (74)	78/436	16
Total	**260/1,074**	**24**

stay and remains the subject of ongoing investigation. In patients who undergo adjuvant chemoradiotherapy, it may be prudent to place feeding jejunostomy at the time of resection.

The propensity for gastric carcinoma to spread via the submucosal lymphatics suggests that a 5-cm margin of normal tissue proximally and distally may be optimal. It may be necessary to include a portion of esophagus or duodenum to achieve adequate margins. Frozen-section pathologic evaluation of surgical margins has been advocated to confirm their adequacy.[35] The importance of careful evaluation of longitudinal margins is emphasized in several series (Table 58.4) with documented positive pathologic margins in approximately one-quarter of "curatively" resected specimens.[66–68,69,70–73] The approximate 25% positive longitudinal margin correlates almost precisely with the incidence of locoregional recurrence in the anastomosis or stump, as discussed later in this chapter.

Although R0 resection with adequate lymph node sampling is a primary goal for gastric cancer surgery, approximately half of patients end up with uninvolved margins. Although the longitudinal margin is routinely evaluated, equally important but frequently not assessed are the radial or circumferential margins. The incidence of radial margin positivity is not well reported in the literature (most of the series referenced in Table 58.4 addressed longitudinal margins alone). The rising incidence of T3 and T4 GE tumors will likely result in an increasing rate of microscopically positive radial margins. Because the perigastric tissue surrounding the GE junction and distal esophagus has no serosa, lesions that extend to the pathologic radial margin represent a true positive margin in a large percentage of cases.

The extent of lymph node dissection is controversial. At resection, it is recommended at least 15 lymph nodes be retrieved to reduce stage migration. In a D0 dissection, there is generally incomplete removal of the lymph nodes along the greater and lesser curvature. D1 dissection refers to removal of nodes along the lesser curvature (nodal stations 1, 3, and 5) and greater curvature (nodal stations 2, 4, and 6) (Fig. 58.2). In addition, more extensive lymph node dissection, including removal of nodes along the left gastric artery (nodal station 7), common hepatic artery (nodal station 8), celiac trunk (nodal station 9), and splenic artery (nodal stations 10 and 11) are referred to as a D2 dissection. In series with rigorous pathologic evaluation of these nodes,[74] the likelihood of discovering lymph node metastasis increases markedly in both D1 and D2 procedures. There appears to be a small subset of patients who have limited metastasis in the celiac axis, superior pancreatic, or retroduodenal chains and may be cured by a D2 lymph node resection.[75] Data from the Surveillance Epidemiology and End Results (SEER) database show that the number of nodes examined correlated with overall survival, potentially reflecting improved staging in these patients.[76] Japanese researchers advocate complete lymph node removal to improve the rates of local control and survival. Several nonrandomized clinical trials suggested that extended lymphadenectomy may improve survival.[77–78,79–80] Others[81] reported that increasingly radical lymphadenectomies failed to improve survival or reduce the risk of locoregional failure. At least four prospective randomized trials of lymphadenectomies have been reported[74,82–86,87] and show no survival advantage with more extensive lymph node dissection. Additionally, morbidity and mortality rates have been significantly higher for patients undergoing more extensive nodal dissection. An even more extensive lymph node dissection may entail para-aortic nodal dissection. However, a Japanese trial comparing D2 lymphadenectomy versus the same with para-aortic nodal dissection did not show any differences in overall or relapse-free survival between the groups, indicating the later approach should not be used in patients with curable gastric cancer.[88] However, other important principles of lymph node dissection have been elucidated through these trials. The first is that as more lymph node areas are dissected and as pathologic lymph node evaluation is more rigorous, considerable stage migration occurs. This stage migration produces an apparent improvement in stage-specific survival without improvement in survival in the group overall.

TABLE 58.5 PATTERNS OF FAILURE AFTER "CURATIVE" RESECTION OF GASTRIC CANCER

Pattern of Failure	Incidence in Total Patient Group (%)		
	Clinical[94]	University of Minnesota Reoperation[38a]	Autopsy[90,91,93,96]
Locoregional[b]	38	67	80–93
Peritoneal seeding	28	41	30–43
Localized	–	19	–
Diffuse	–	22	–
Distant metastases	52	22	49

[a]107 patients at risk.

[b]Local or regional failure based on direct extension of tumor, lymphatic spread, or operative wound implant; one or more distant metastases on hematologic basis; abdominal involvement on basis of peritoneal seeding or peritoneal lymphatics.

Failure Patterns After Surgical Resection

Local failures in the tumor bed and/or regional lymph nodes and distant failures by hematogenous or peritoneal routes are common mechanisms of failure after "curative" resection in clinical, reoperative, and autopsy series[38,89, 90–92,93] (Tables 58.5 and 58.6). For GE junction lesions, the liver and lungs are common sites of distant metastases. With gastric lesions that do not extend to the esophagus, the initial site of distant metastasis is usually the liver, and many failures could be prevented if an effective abdominal treatment could be combined with treatment to the primary site. In the series of Landry et al.,[94] 50 of 88 (57%) failing patients had disease progression within the abdomen only. Abdominal treatment also could address peritoneal seeding, which occurs in 23% to 43% of postgastrectomy patients.[89–92,93,94,95,96,97]

TABLE 58.6 PATTERNS OF LOCOREGIONAL FAILURE AFTER RESECTION OF GASTRIC CANCER

Failure Area	Incidence (%)		
	Clinical[a]	Reoperation[b]	Autopsy[c]
Gastric bed	21	54	52–68
Anastomosis or stumps	25	26	54–60
Abdominal or stab wound	–	5	–
Lymph node(s)	8	42	52

[a]130 patients at risk [97].

[b]107 patients at risk [38].

[c]92 patients at risk [93] and 28 patients at risk [96].

Locoregional failures occur commonly in organs and structures of the gastric bed and in lymph nodes (Table 58.6). Clinically detectable locoregional recurrence following surgical resection alone generally exceeds 25%. However, reoperation and autopsy series have suggested that these rates are much higher.[98] Failures in the anastomoses, gastric remnant, or duodenal stump also are frequent, as suggested by the incidence of positive longitudinal resection margins (Tables 58.4 and 58.6). As is true for most sites, clinical series underestimate the true incidence of locoregional failure when compared with reoperative or autopsy series (Table 58.5). Progressive extension of the operative procedure to include routine splenectomy, omentectomy, and radical lymph node dissection neither improved survival nor decreased the incidence of locoregional failures in the University of Minnesota series.[38,96] Subsequent failure in areas of initial node dissection occurred frequently, even with radical node dissections[38] (Fig. 58.3). The high rate of regional node relapse provides a partial explanation for the lack of survival benefit with a D2 (extended lymphadenectomy) versus D1 (limited lymphadenectomy) node dissection in the phase III surgical trials discussed previously.

Indications for Radiation Therapy

The results of the U.S. Gastrointestinal Intergroup Gastric Adjuvant Trial has changed the standard of care in the United States to the use of both chemotherapy and radiation therapy in the postoperative setting for patients with disease extension through the gastric wall and/or with nodes positive for tumor (discussed later).[99] Postoperative irradiation plus concurrent and maintenance 5-FU–based chemotherapy is recommended for patients with stage IB-IV and M0 gastric cancer.[99] Quality control of irradiation field design was conducted during the cycle of chemotherapy given before the start of concurrent chemoirradiation. The up-front quality control provided the mechanism to correct most of the major or minor deviations (35% incidence) in irradiation field design before the start of treatment and resulted in only a 6.5% final major deviation rate.

Radiation therapy, usually administered with concomitant 5-FU–based chemotherapy, is also indicated for locally confined gastric cancer that either is not technically resectable or occurs in medically inoperable patients. In this setting, therapy can be administered with curative or palliative intent, depending on the clinical situation. Those who undergo gastric resection with incomplete tumor resection or have truly positive margins of resection also are managed appropriately by combined-modality postoperative therapy.

RADIATION THERAPY TECHNIQUES

Simulation

When gastric cancer patients are simulated, the radiation oncologist should know the extent of disease based on imaging (barium swallow, CT, PET) as well as endoscopic procedures. CT simulation is appropriate for treatment planning. During simulation, the patient is positioned, straightened, and immobilized on the simulation table. An immobilization device is used to minimize variation in daily setup. Arms are generally placed overhead, and knees are supported underneath the legs. The administration of oral contrast to delineate the stomach is generally used and may help define the extent of mucosal irregularity. It may be advisable to have the patient come in with an empty stomach. The patient is placed on the CT simulator in the treatment position, and a scan of the entire area of interest with margin is obtained. At minimum, 3- to 5-mm slices should be used, allowing accurate tumor characterization as well as improved quality of digitally reconstructed radiographs. If patients lose >10% of their body weight during therapy, consideration should be given to repeat CT planning. Arterial phase IV contrast is generally used to delineate mediastinal and abdominal vascular nodal basins, including the celiac axis, and to allow the radiation oncologist to discern normal vasculature from other adjacent normal structures, potential adenopathy, and so forth. The tumor (if the patient is surgically naïve) and vital structures are then outlined on each slice on the treatment-planning system, enabling a three-dimensional (3D) treatment plan to be generated. The use of respiratory gating or breath-hold techniques may help to reduce target motion with respiration and, therefore, avoidance of normal tissue irradiation associated with larger margins used in free-breathing approaches. Four-dimensional (4D) CT scan may be appropriate to assess tumoral motion, facilitating appropriate margin placement on the target volumes.

Treatment Planning

Target Design

For a detailed description of target and field design in proximal gastric cancer involving the GE junction, the reader is referred to Chapter 53. In the design of radiation fields for neoadjuvantly treated or locally unresectable gastric cancer (as well as in the re-creation of tumoral volumes in adjuvantly treated patients), it is important to define varying target volumes, including gross disease as well as potential areas of subclinical involvement (i.e., the gross tumor volume [GTV] and clinical target volume [CTV], respectively). Defining GTV (including re-creation of volumes in the adjuvant setting) is based on multiple studies, including endoscopic descriptions (from both esophagogastroduodenoscopy and endoscopic ultrasound) as well as cross-sectional imaging. Gastric wall thickening correlating to the GTV can frequently be visualized on diagnostic and radiation planning CT. Similarly, EUS appears to be the most reliable test in detecting lymphadenopathy related to nodal spread. The endoscopist should be encouraged to accurately define not only the primary disease extent on EUS but also depth of penetration and potential involvement of adjacent structures, which can also be used to help guide GTV delineation. Similarly, EUS may allow detection of lymph nodes that may not be appreciated on CT or PET imaging, and the endoscopist should describe the size as well as location (e.g., relationship to tumor or adjacent structures). Additionally, radiographic areas of lymphadenopathy should similarly be included in the GTV. In GTV design, basing potential nodal involvement (and therefore target volumes) on nodal size is problematic given that metastatic nodes may frequently be below the resolution of conventional imaging. Therefore, it is not appropriate to rely exclusively on imaging modalities to define areas of subclinical spread for gastric cancer, realizing established pathologic patterns of spread data is important in determining radiation field design.

The identification of potential direct and nodal pathways for spread of subclinical disease (i.e., CTV definition) in gastric cancer is also of paramount importance. These areas vary significantly depending on site of origin of disease, making gastric cancer planning somewhat complex. As described previously, the stomach is characterized by a rich network of lymphatics that facilitates early lymph node spread of disease. Some authors have recommended dividing the stomach into three equal lengths (upper/proximal, middle, and distal), with tumors classified by location of the bulk of their masses in these respective sites. Therefore, practically speaking, the stomach can be divided into proximal (remembering that in the AJCC seventh edition staging system, involvement of the GE junction by proximal third tumors would be classified as an esophageal tumor), middle, or distal segments (Fig. 58.4).

Primarily based on extensive analysis of patterns of nodal spread from surgical series, Japanese investigators have developed lymph node station classifications (the Japanese classification of gastric carcinoma of the Japanese Gastric Cancer Association) that have been validated in other series (Fig. 58.2).

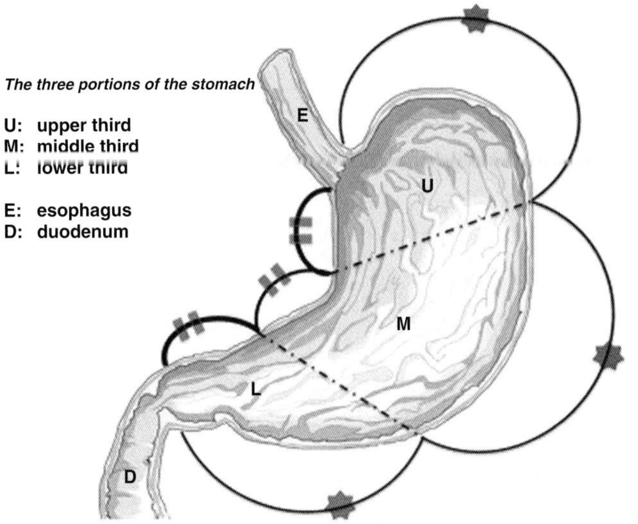

FIGURE 58.4. Subdivision of the stomach into equal lengths along greater and lesser curves. (From Matzinger O, Gerber E, Bernstein Z, et al. EORTC-ROG expert opinion: radiotherapy volume and treatment guidelines for neoadjuvant radiation of adenocarcinomas of the gastroesophageal junction and the stomach. *Radiother Oncol* 2009;92:164–175, with permission from Elsevier.)

Based on this system, general recommendations for CTV definition for tumors in varying parts of the stomach are as follows. Proximal third stomach tumors should include the contour of the stomach with exclusion of the pylorus and antrum (keeping a minimal margin of 5 cm from the GTV). Middle third tumors should include the contour of the stomach from the cardia to the pylorus. Distal third tumor CTVs should include the stomach except for the cardia/fundus, again keeping a minimal margin of 5 cm from the GTV. If pyloric/duodenal invasion is present, the CTV would be expanded along the duodenum with a margin of 3 cm from the tumor. Nodal volumes to be included are further described later, and it has been recommended that the CTV consist of a 5-mm margin around corresponding vessels. If target motion is not accounted for, the minimal recommended 3D margins to the CTV to obtain the internal target volume (ITV) are 1.5 cm in all directions, taking into account physiologic organ motion, particularly respiratory motion. The PTV can then be defined as the ITV volume plus a 3D margin of 5 mm.[101]

Field Design

Based on the likely sites of locoregional failure (Table 58.6), in resected patients, the gastric/tumor bed, anastomosis and gastric remnant, and regional lymphatics should be included in most patients.[38,93,96,97,100] Major nodal chains at risk include the lesser and greater curvature, celiac axis, pancreaticoduodenal, splenic, suprapancreatic, porta hepatis, and, in some, para-aortics to the level of mid-L3.

The relative risk of nodal metastases at a specific nodal location depends on both the site of origin of the primary tumor[102,103] and other factors including width and depth of invasion of the gastric wall. On the basis of previously described patterns of failure data, general guidelines in terms of field design can be made as illustrated in Figures 58.5 through 59.7 and discussed later. These are general guidelines, and all plans should be individualized according to available imaging and endoscopic data, and generalized portals based on patterns of failure data frequently need to be modified on the basis of the individual patient's initial extent of disease.[102,103] As seen in Figures 58.5 to 58.7, gastric tumors (i.e., without GE junction involvement) that originate in the proximal portion of the stomach have a higher propensity of spread to nodes in the

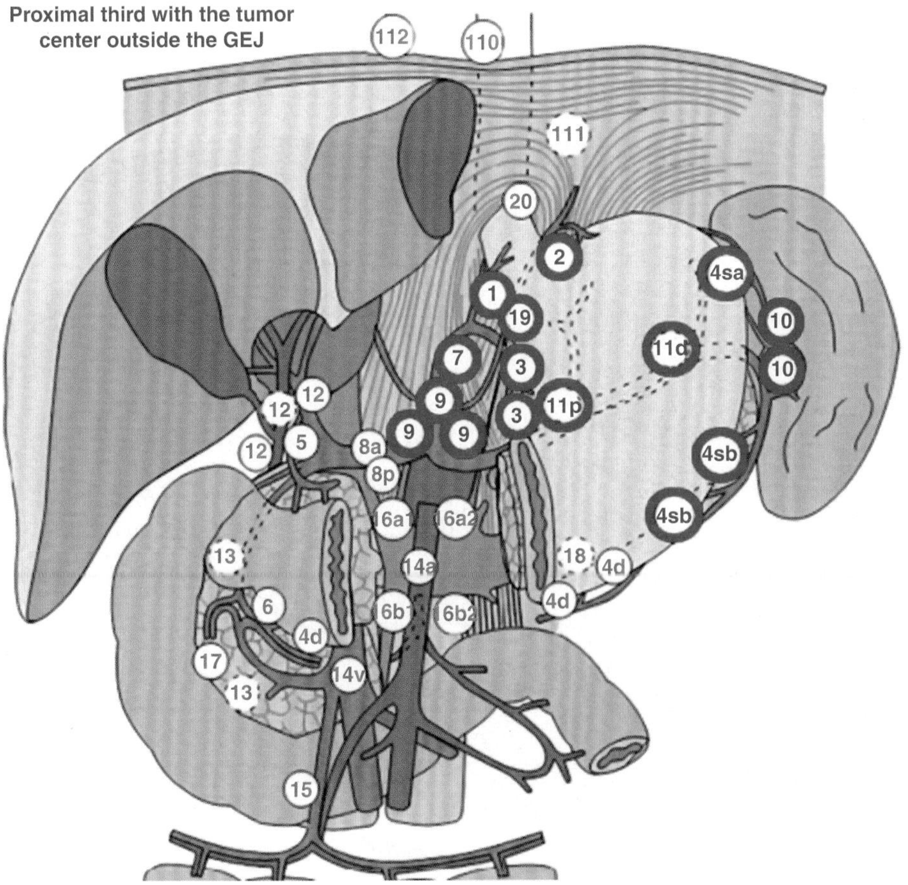

FIGURE 58.5. Suggested lymph node station coverage for tumors of the proximal third of the stomach without involvement of the GE junction. (From Matzinger O, Gerber E, Bernstein Z, et al. EORTC-ROG expert opinion: radiotherapy volume and treatment guidelines for neoadjuvant radiation of adenocarcinomas of the gastroesophageal junction and the stomach. *Radiother Oncol* 2009;92:164–175, with permission from Elsevier.)

Middle third

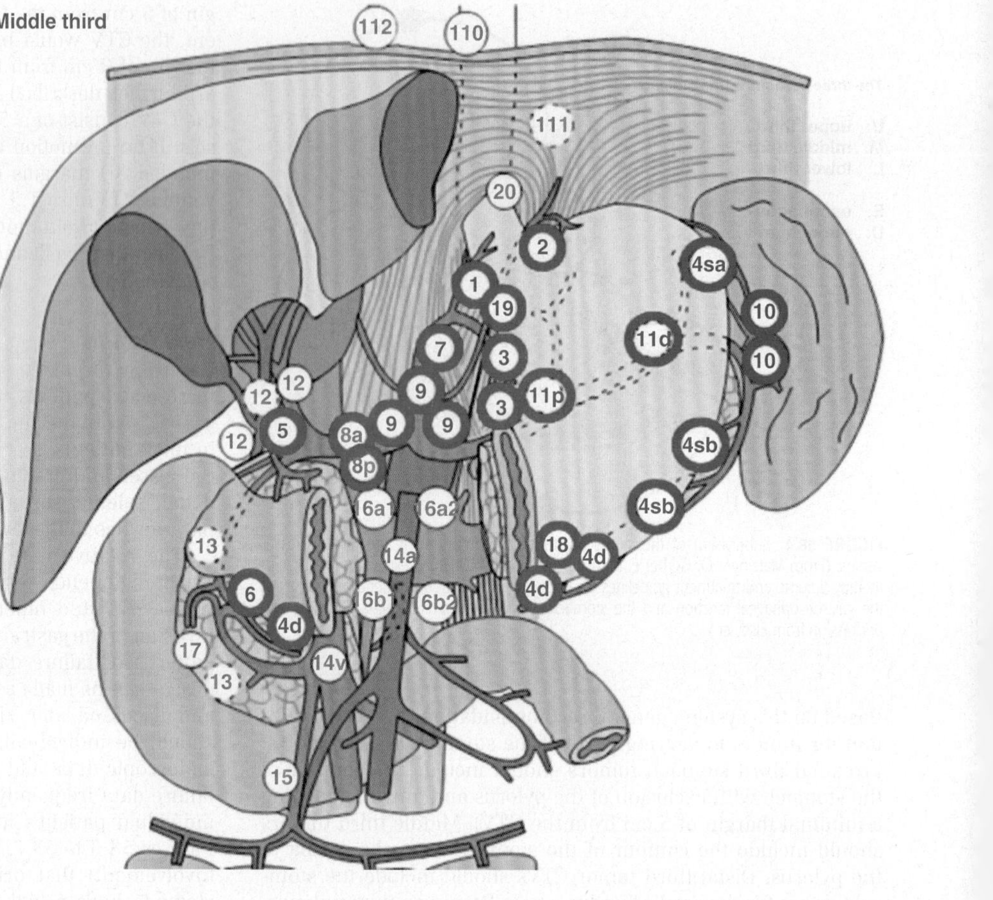

FIGURE 58.6. Suggested lymph node nodal coverage of patients with middle third gastric carcinomas. (From Matzinger O, Gerber E, Bernstein Z, et al. EORTC-ROG expert opinion: radiotherapy volume and treatment guidelines for neoadjuvant radiation of adenocarcinomas of the gastroesophageal junction and the stomach. *Radiother Oncol* 2009;92:164–175, with permission from Elsevier.)

Distal third:

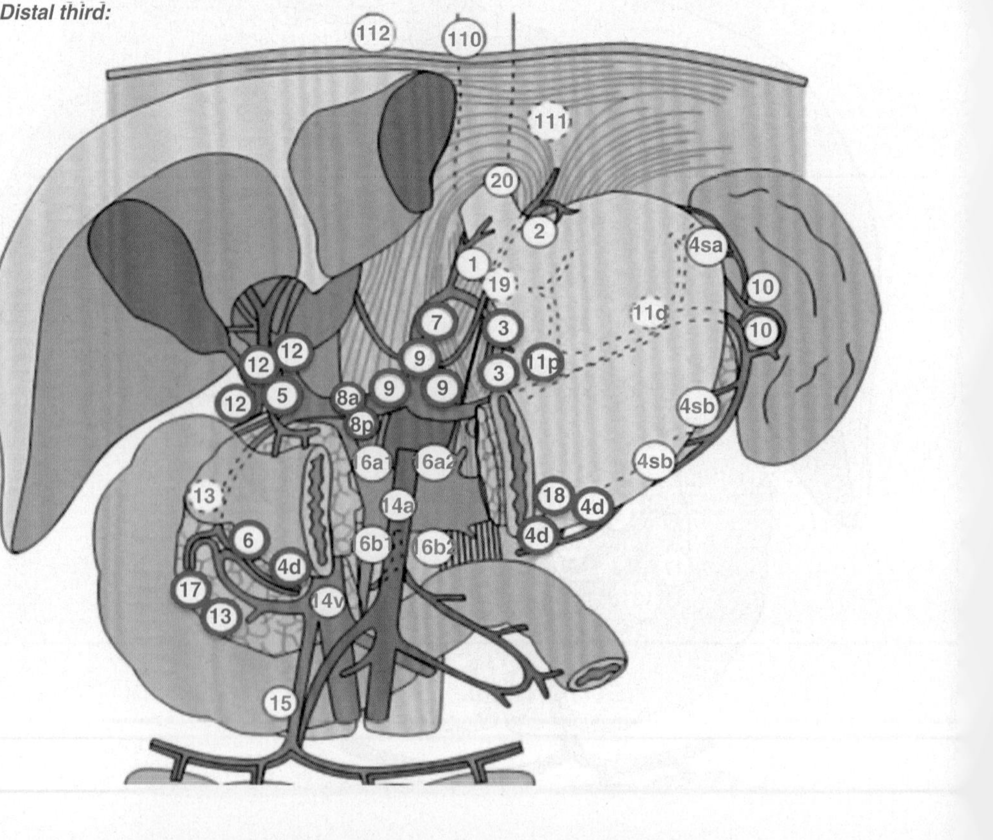

FIGURE 58.7. Suggested nodal coverage for primary gastric cancers of the distal third of the stomach. (From Matzinger O, Gerber E, Bernstein Z, et al. EORTC-ROG expert opinion: radiotherapy volume and treatment guidelines for neoadjuvant radiation of adenocarcinomas of the gastroesophageal junction and the stomach. *Radiother Oncol* 2009;92:164–175, with permission from Elsevier.)

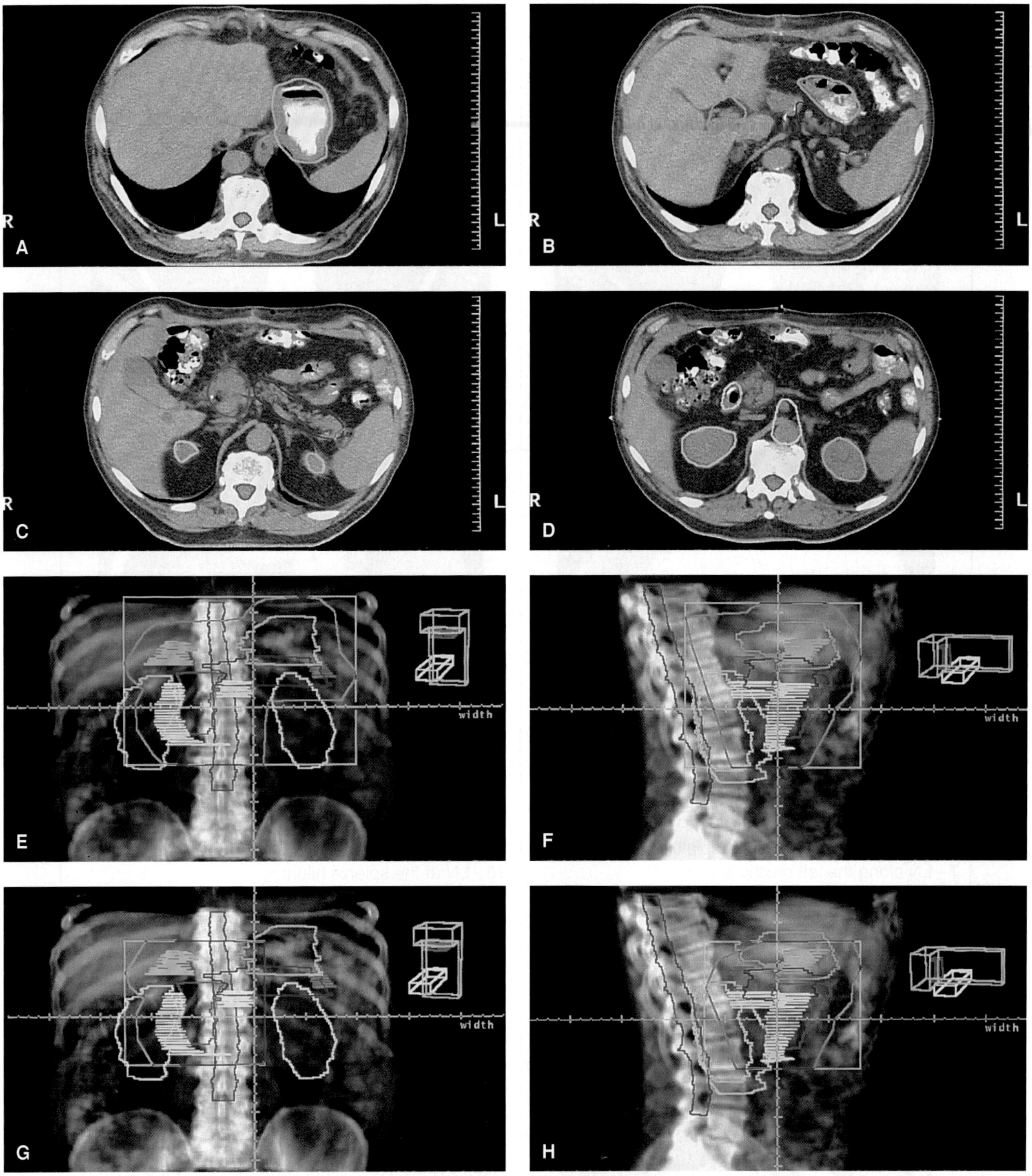

FIGURE 58.8. Optimized postoperative irradiation fields for patient with T3N1 antral primary. Structures of interest were delineated at time of computed tomography simulation (*A–D*), and irradiation fields were designed with the aid of digitally reconstructed radiographs (*E–H*). **A:** Gastric remnant (*teal*). **B:** Gastric remnant plus body/tail of pancreas (*dark blue*), splenic hilum (*salmon*), and porta hepatis (*medium blue*). **C:** Head of pancreas (*magenta*) and kidneys (*left, orange; right, light green*) are delineated in addition to body/tail of pancreas and splenic hilum. **D:** Celiac artery (*yellow*) and duodenum (*yellow–green*) are shown together with head of pancreas and kidneys. A four-field technique of AP (anteroposterior), PA (posteroanterior), and paired laterals was designed to include the gastric remnant (*teal*), tumor bed (head of pancreas [*magenta*], first and second part of duodenum [*yellow–green cross hatched*]), pertinent nodal volumes (perigastric, pancreaticoduodenal, porta hepatic [*medium blue cross hatched*], celiac [*yellow cross hatched*], and suprapancreatic) and the optional nodal volume of splenic hilum (*salmon cross hatched*). **E:** Initial AP field (field margins as shown in *medium blue* exclude approximately two-thirds of the left kidney while including about 50% of the right kidney). Exclusion of the optional splenic hilar nodes would have allowed additional but minimal sparing of the left kidney in view of the adjacency of gastric antrum and splenic hilum. **F:** Initial right lateral field demonstrated exclusion of the spinal cord. **G:** Reduced AP field with exclusion of splenic hilar nodes and most of the gastric remnant. **H:** Reduced right lateral field.

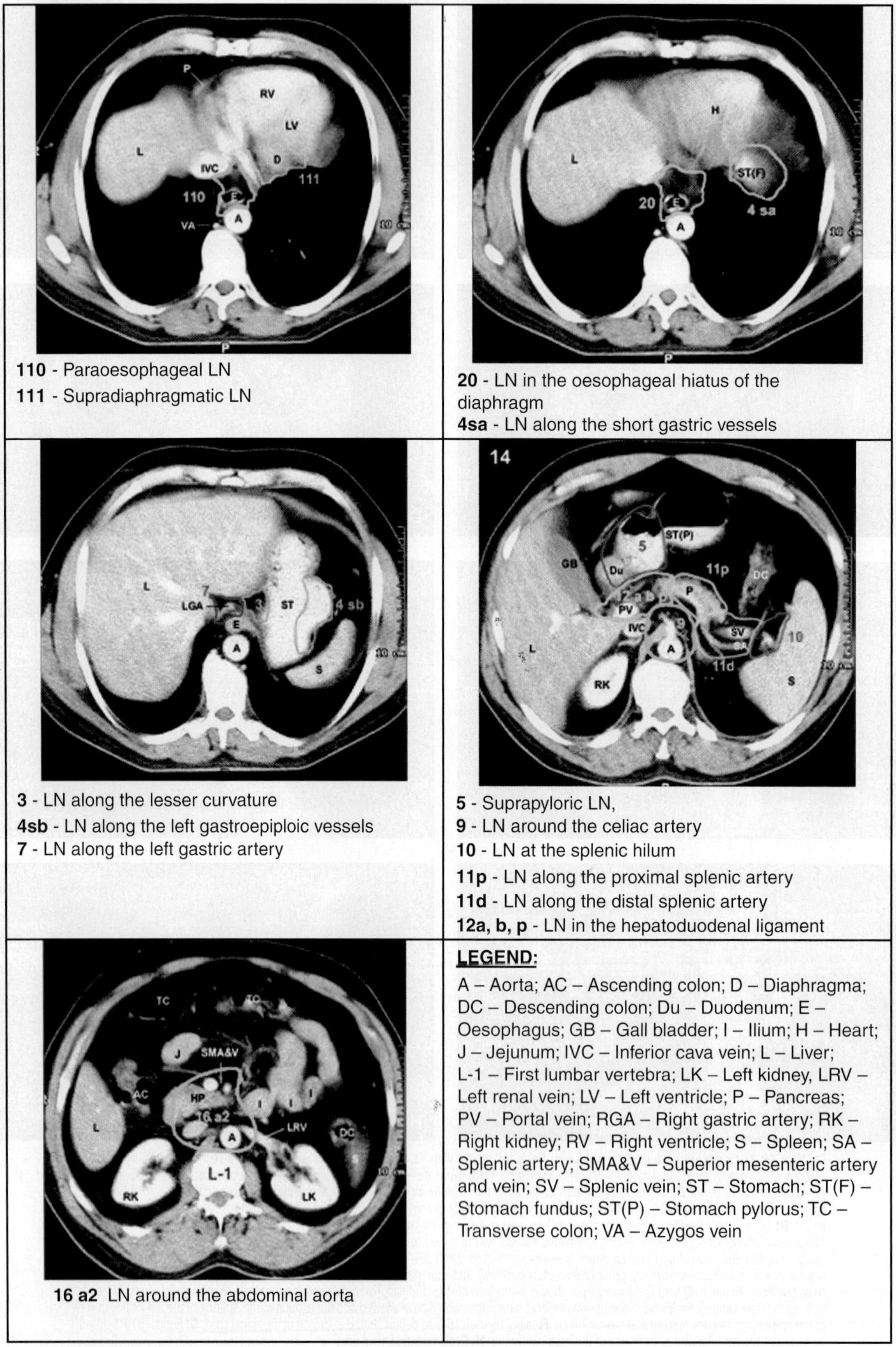

FIGURE 58.9. Examples of locations of varying nodal stations and anatomic structures on axial CT slices. (From Matzinger O, Gerber E, Bernstein Z, et al. EORTC-ROG expert opinion: radiotherapy volume and treatment guidelines for neoadjuvant radiation of adenocarcinomas of the gastro-esophageal junction and the stomach. *Radiother Oncol* 2009;92:164–175, with permission from Elsevier.)

pericardial region but a lower likelihood of involvement of nodes in the region of the gastric antrum, periduodenal area, and porta hepatis. Tumors that originate in the body of the stomach can spread to all nodal sites but have the highest likelihood of spreading to nodes along the greater and lesser curvature near the location of the primary tumor mass. Nodal basins are similar to upper-third tumors with the exception of inclusion of nodal basins along the pyloric region, common hepatic artery, and additional coverage along the greater curvature. Tumors that originate in the distal stomach, in the region of the gastric antrum, have a high likelihood of spread to the periduodenal, peripancreatic, and porta hepatis nodes, whereas they have a lower likelihood of spread to the nodes near the cardia of the stomach, the periesophageal and mediastinal nodes, or to the splenic hilar nodes—that is, there is less emphasis placed on more proximal nodes (including coverage of the splenic artery course, including splenic hilum) and more comprehensive coverage of pancreaticoduodenal nodal basins. Figure 58.8 shows an example of 3D fields for a T3N1 antral tumor. Figure 58.9 shows examples of varying nodal locations on axial CT images. Any tumor originating in the stomach has a high propensity of spread to nodes along the greater and lesser curvature, although they are most likely to spread to those sites in close anatomic proximity to the primary tumor mass.

Additional guidelines for defining the CTV for postoperative irradiation fields have been developed based on location and extent of the primary tumor (T-stage) and location and extent of known nodal involvement (N-stage).[103] Table 58.7 presents general guidelines on the impact of T- and N-stages on inclusion of the remaining stomach (gastric remnant), tumor bed, and nodal sites, whereas Tables 58.8–58.10 present treatment guidelines based on TN-stage within each of three primary sites (proximal, mid, and distal stomach). With proximal gastric lesions or lesions at the GE junction, a 3- to 5-cm margin of distal esophagus should be included; if the lesion extends through the entire gastric wall, a major portion of the left hemidiaphragm should be included. In these circumstances, blocking can decrease the volume of irradiated heart. For unresectable lesions with moderate periesophageal extension, it may not be possible to exclude an adequate amount of heart with anteroposterior/posteroanterior (AP/PA) fields, and the use of lateral or oblique fields for a portion of treatment is likely indicated. In general, for patients with node-positive disease, there should be wide coverage of tumor bed, remaining stomach, resection margins, and nodal drainage regions. For node-negative disease, if there is a good surgical resection with pathologic evaluation of at least 15 nodes, and there are wide surgical margins on the primary tumor (at least 5 cm), treatment for the nodal beds may be optional. Treatment for the remaining stomach should depend on a balance of the likely normal tissue morbidity and the perceived risk of local relapse in the residual stomach.

Although parallel-opposed AP/PA fields are a practical arrangement for tumor bed and nodal irradiation, multifield techniques should be used if they can improve long-term tolerance of normal tissues. Tightly contoured AP/PA fields should be designed to spare as much normal tissue as possible (Figs. 58.10 and 58.11). In institutional series, the average

TABLE 58.7 GENERAL GUIDELINES OF IMPACT OF T- AND N-STAGE ON INCLUSION OF REMAINING STOMACH, TUMOR BED, AND NODAL SITES WITHIN IRRADIATION FIELDS

TN Stage	*Remaining Stomach*[a]	*Tumor Bed*	*Nodes*
T1-2 (not into subserosa) N0	N	N	N
T2N0 (into subserosa)[b]	Variable	Y	N
T3N0	Variable	Y	N
T4N0	Variable	Y	Variable
T1-2N+	Y	N	Y
T3-4N+	Y	Y	Y

N, no; Y, yes.

[a]Inclusion of the remaining stomach is preferable in most patients if two-thirds of one kidney can be excluded. This depends on the extent of surgical resection and uninvolved margins (in centimeters).

[b]Posterior wall T2N0 lesions, or those that extend beyond the muscularis propria, especially tumors located in the proximal or distal stomach, are at risk for local relapse. In addition, patients with low-stage disease with close or positive surgical margins should be considered for treatment to the tumor bed.

From Smalley SS, Gunderson L, Tepper J, et al. Gastric surgical adjuvant radiotherapy consensus report: rationale and treatment implementation. *Int J Radiat Oncol Biol Phys* 2002;52:283–293, with permission from Elsevier.

TABLE 58.8 IMPACT OF SITE OF PRIMARY GASTRIC LESION AND TN STAGE ON IRRADIATION VOLUMES: CARDIA/PROXIMAL ONE-THIRD OF STOMACH (GENERAL GUIDELINES)

Site of Primary and TN Stage	*Remaining Stomach*	*Tumor Bed Volumes*[a]	*Nodal Volumes*	*Tolerance Organ Structures*
Cardia/proximal one-third of stomach	Preferred, but spare two-thirds of one kidney (usually right)	T-stage dependent	N-stage dependent	Kidneys, spinal cord, liver, heart, lung
T2N0 with invasion of subserosa	Variable dependent on surg-path findings[b]	Medial left hemidiaphragm, adjacent body of pancreas (± tail)	None or perigastric[c]	
T3N0	Variable dependent on surg-path findings[b]	Medial left hemidiaphragm, adjacent body of pancreas (± tail)	None or perigastric; optional: periesophageal, mediastinal, celiac[c]	
T4N0	Variable dependent on surg-path findings[b]	As for T3N0 plus site(s) of adherence with 3–5 cm margin	Nodes related to site of adherence, ± perigastric, periesophageal, mediastinal, celiac	
T1-2N+	Preferable	Not indicated for T1, as above for T2 into subserosa	Perigastric, celiac, splenic, suprapancreatic ± periesophageal, mediastinal, pancreaticoduodenal, porta hepatis[d]	
T3-4N+	Preferable	As for T3, T4N0	As for T1-2N+ and T4N0	

surg-path, surgical-pathologic.

[a]Use preoperative imaging (computed tomography [CT], barium swallow), surgical clips, and postoperative imaging (CT, barium swallow).

[b]For tumors with wide (>5 cm) surgical margins confirmed pathologically, treatment of residual stomach may not be necessary, especially if this would result in substantial increased normal tissue morbidity.

[c]Optional node inclusion for T2–3N0 lesions if adequate surgical node dissection (D2 dissection) and at least 10–15 nodes are examined pathologically.

[d]Pancreaticoduodenal and porta hepatis nodes are at low risk if nodal positivity is minimal (i.e., 1–2 positive nodes with 10–15 nodes examined) and this region may not need to be irradiated. Periesophageal and mediastinal nodes are at risk if there is esophageal extension.

From Smalley SS, Gunderson L, Tepper J, et al. Gastric surgical adjuvant radiotherapy consensus report: rationale and treatment implementation. *Int J Radiat Oncol Biol Phys* 2002;52:283–293, with permission from Elsevier.

TABLE 58.9 IMPACT OF SITE OF PRIMARY GASTRIC LESION AND TN STAGE ON IRRADIATION VOLUMES: BODY/MIDDLE ONE-THIRD OF STOMACH (GENERAL GUIDELINES)

Site of Primary and TN Stage	*Remaining Stomach*	*Tumor Bed Volumes*[a]	*Nodal Volumes*	*Tolerance Organ Structures*
Body/middle one-third of stomach	Yes—but spare two-thirds of one kidney	T-stage dependent	N-stage dependent—spare two-thirds of one kidney	Kidneys, spinal cord, liver
T2N0 with invasion of subserosa, especially post wall	Yes	Body of pancreas (± tail)	None or perigastric; optional: celiac, splenic, suprapancreatic, pancreaticoduodenal, porta hepatis[b]	
T3N0	Yes	Body of pancreas (± tail)	None or perigastric; optional: celiac, splenic, suprapancreatic, pancreaticoduodenal, porta hepatis[b]	
T4N0	Yes	As for T3N0 plus site(s) of adherence with 3–5 cm margin	Nodes related to site of adherence ± perigastric, celiac, splenic, suprapancreatic, pancreaticoduodenal, porta hepatis	
T1-2N+	Yes	Not indicated for T1; as for T2N0 with invasion of subserosa	Perigastric, celiac, splenic, suprapancreatic pancreaticoduodenal, porta hepatis	
T3-4N+	Yes	As for T3, T4N0	As for T1-2N+ and T4N0	

[a]Use preoperative imaging (computed tomography [CT], barium swallow), surgical clips, and postoperative imaging (CT, barium swallow).

[b]Optional node inclusion for T2-3N0 lesions if adequate surgical node dissection (D2 dissection) and at least 10–15 nodes examined pathologically.

From Smalley SS, Gunderson L, Tepper J, et al. Gastric surgical adjuvant radiotherapy consensus report: rationale and treatment implementation. *Int J Radiat Oncol Biol Phys* 2002;52: 283–293, with permission from Elsevier.

irradiation field measured 15 cm × 15 cm.[33,104,105] More routine use of multifield techniques should be considered when preoperative imaging exists to allow accurate reconstruction of target volumes. Single-institution data suggest that multifield arrangements may produce less toxicity. Although AP/PA fields can be weighted anteriorly to keep the spinal cord dose at acceptable levels, a four-field technique, if feasible, can spare spinal cord with improved dose homogeneity. Depending on the posterior extent of the gastric fundus, either obliqued or more routine lateral portals can be used to deliver a 10- to 20-Gy component of irradiation to spare spinal cord or kidney. When lateral fields are used, liver and kidney tolerance limits the use of lateral fields to ≤20 Gy. Patients should be treated with high-energy photons when possible. With the wide availability of 3D treatment-planning systems, it may be possible to more accurately target the high-risk volume and to use unconventional field arrangements to produce superior dose distributions. To accomplish this without marginal misses, it will be necessary to both carefully define and encompass the various target volumes because the use of oblique or noncoplanar beams could exclude target volumes that would be included in AP/PA fields or nonoblique four-field techniques (AP/PA and laterals). Although, historically, two-dimensional (2D)-based radiation planning has been carried out primarily using anatomic landmarks as well as fluoroscopic barium swallow to determine field borders (Figs. 58.10 and 58.11), contemporary treatment planning using CT-based planning allows improved visualization of both target and nontarget structures, along with 3D reconstruction and creation of a "beams eye" view of varying fields, allowing improved conformality around target structures and improvements in normal tissue sparing. Because volumetric data can be obtained by CT scans, dose-volume histogram data can also be generated. A variety of 3D techniques are presently used and described later.

Because it is important to account for daily setup uncertainty as well as physiologic internal organ motion (secondary to respiration, peristalsis, cardiac motion, etc.), an additional margin must be added to a CTV. Interfraction variability in stomach location occurs, often owing to variations in gastric filling. Intrafraction changes in target shape and location may be attributable to respiratory motion, which, particularly in the superior to inferior direction, may frequently exceed 1 to 1.5 cm.[98]

TABLE 58.10 IMPACT OF SITE OF PRIMARY GASTRIC LESION AND TN STAGE ON IRRADIATION VOLUMES: ANTRUM/PYLORUS/DISTAL ONE-THIRD OF STOMACH (GENERAL GUIDELINES)

Site of Primary and TN Stage	*Remaining Stomach*	*Tumor Bed Volumes*[a]	*Nodal Volumes*	*Tolerance Organ Structures*
Antrum/pylorus/distal one-third of stomach	Yes—but spare two-thirds of one kidney, usually left	T-stage dependent	N-stage dependent	Kidneys, liver, spinal cord
T2N0 with invasion of subserosa	Variable dependent on surg-path findings[b]	Head of pancreas (± body), 1st and 2nd part of duodenum	None or perigastric; optional: pancreaticoduodenal, porta hepatis, celiac, suprapancreatic[c]	
T3N0	Variable dependent on surg-path findings[b]	Head of pancreas (± body), 1st and 2nd part of duodenum	None or perigastric; optional: pancreaticoduodenal, porta hepatis, celiac, suprapancreatic[c]	
T4N0	Preferable but dependent on surg-path findings[b]	As for T3N0 plus site(s) of adherence with 3–5 cm margin	Nodes related to site(s) of adherence ± perigastric, pancreaticoduodenal, porta hepatis, celiac, suprapancreatic	
T1-2N+	Preferable	Not indicated for T1; as for T2N0 with invasion of subserosa	Perigastric, pancreaticoduodenal, porta hepatis, celiac, suprapancreatic, optional—splenic hilum	
T3-4N+	Preferable	As for T3, T4N0	As for T1-2N+ and T4N0	

surg-path, surgical-pathologic.

[a]Use preoperative imaging (computed tomography [CT], barium swallow), surgical clips, and postoperative imaging (CT, barium swallow).

[b]For tumors with wide (>5 cm) surgical margins confirmed pathologically, treatment of residual stomach is optional if this would result in substantial increased normal tissue morbidity.

[c]Optional node inclusion for T2–3N0 lesions if adequate surgical node dissection (D2 dissection) and at least 10–15 nodes examined pathologically.

From Smalley SS, Gunderson L, Tepper J, et al. Gastric surgical adjuvant radiotherapy consensus report: rationale and treatment implementation. *Int J Radiat Oncol Biol Phys* 2002; 52:283–293, with permission from Elsevier.

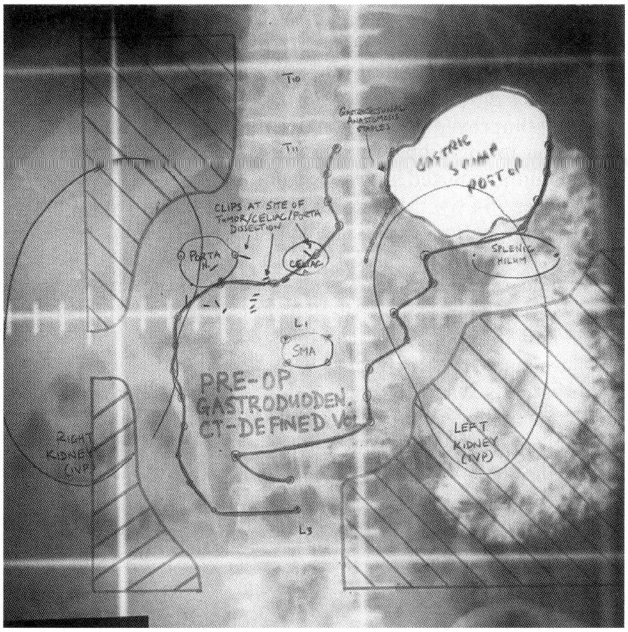

FIGURE 58.10. Simulation film for T3 antral tumor with two of five peritumoral lymph nodes metastatically involved (radical subtotal gastrectomy with D1 node dissection). Simulation film identifies areas at risk for recurrence, including preoperative gastric/tumor bed (defined by preoperative computed tomography [CT] scan), anastomotic sites and gastric stump (staple line seen on precontrast simulation films and marked on postintravenous pyelogram/postcontrast film), and regional lymphatics (celiac, porta hepatis, superior mesenteric artery, and splenic nodes identified on CT, and pancreaticoduodenal nodes lie in C-loop of duodenum identified by preoperative CT). The right kidney is spared for approximately three-fourths of its volume, whereas the left kidney has about one-third of its volume blocked. (From Smalley SS, Gunderson L, Tepper J, et al. Gastric surgical adjuvant radiotherapy consensus report: rationale and treatment implementation. *Int J Radiat Oncol Biol Phys* 2002;52:283–293, with permission from Elsevier.)

In effort to reduce this, kilovoltage radiographic matching can be used with particular emphasis on matching of surgical clips. An additional technique that may improve treatment accuracy is cone-beam CT, which allows direct target matching within a given fraction. Similarly, movement related to respiratory motion can be assessed using 4D CT, which images the patient in all phases of respiration (similar to what is performed fluoroscopically but using CT). Similarly, respiratory gating techniques may allow reduction in the target volume/smaller margins, allowing for treatment during a more stationary phase of the respiratory cycle (either in expiration or breath-hold).[98]

Another potential approach in the treatment for gastric cancer is the use of intensity-modulated radiation therapy (IMRT). IMRT also uses CT-based planning, again allowing 3D reconstruction of varying structures. However, IMRT differs from 3D planning through the delivery of radiation dose by partitioning a radiation field into multiple smaller fields of various shapes and sizes, varying the dose intensity between each area. This is carried out with either dynamic IMRT (where collimating leaves move in and out of the radiation beam path during treatment) or "step-and-shoot" IMRT (where the leaves change the radiation field shape while the beam is turned off). Either method is particularly effective at conforming radiation dose to the target structures while avoiding dose to normal tissue. Radiation oncologists must determine which structures are most critical and weight their importance during the treatment-planning process. Importantly, the greater the number of "avoidance" normal structures, the more difficult it is to meet all dose constraints. IMRT utilizes "inverse planning," where an intended prescription dose is placed on target volumes and dose constraints are placed on normal tissue structures. Thereafter, computer software algorithms allow design of unconventional treatment fields that would not otherwise be possible with standard planning methods. Radiation oncologists and medical physicists critically evaluate numerous plans until dose constraints are satisfactorily met. The result should be a series of radiation doses that closely conform to the target volumes while minimizing dose to normal tissues. IMRT may be appropriate in selected cases to reduce doses to normal structures, including heart, liver, and kidneys. A potential disadvantage of IMRT is the possibility of delivering low doses of radiation therapy to normal tissue areas that might not normally be irradiated using 2D or 3D techniques. Another potential disadvantage to IMRT is possible dose inhomogeneity, leading to potential "hot spots" in normal organs. Because IMRT requires precise target definition, the potential for "marginal miss" increases and careful, accurate target delineation is of paramount importance. With setup uncertainty and physiologic organ motion, care must be taken to ensure accurate and reproducible setup, including, with the use of immobilization devices, possible respiratory gating/breath-hold techniques. Block margins may be minimized with efforts to reduce intrafractional position variability, including breath-hold techniques. Generally, high-energy photons (10 to 18 MV) are recommended when using 3D conformal or IMRT therapy, potentially facilitating a reduction in the integral dose.

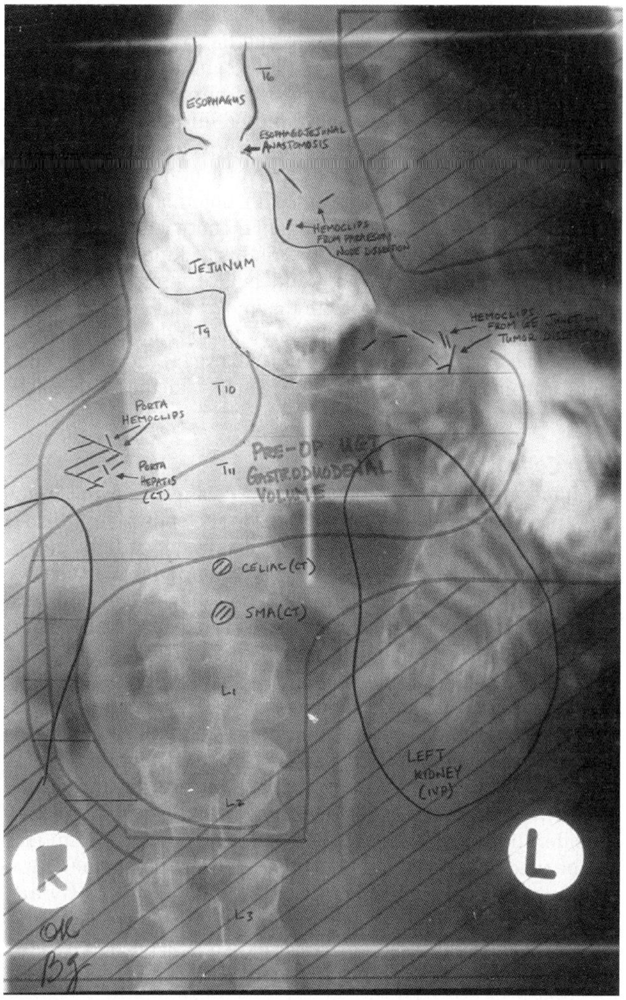

FIGURE 58.11. Simulation film for a T4 (diaphragm invasion) gastroesophageal junction tumor with 4 of 15 involved lymph nodes (total gastrectomy with modified R3 node dissection). Areas at risk for recurrence include preoperative gastric/tumor bed (defined by preoperative upper gastrointestinal radiographs and hemoclips placed at time of resection to mark tumor bed and diaphragm invasion), anastomotic sites and stump (anastomosis visualized at juncture of residual distal esophagus and jejunum), and regional lymphatics (including the celiac, porta hepatis, and pancreaticoduodenal areas as well as the distal paraesophageal nodes). (From Smalley SS, Gunderson L, Tepper J, et al. Gastric surgical adjuvant radiotherapy consensus report: rationale and treatment implementation. *Int J Radiat Oncol Biol Phys* 2002;52:283–293, with permission from Elsevier.)

Multiple dosimetric studies comparing IMRT to two-field and 3D conformal radiation therapy plans have shown significant reductions in kidney, liver, heart, lung, and spinal cord dose. Although IMRT may result in improved normal tissue sparing, many of the acute toxicities encountered during radiation may persist given that many symptoms arise from radiation of the target, including gastric mucosa. The value of IMRT may lie primarily in normal organ sparing with potential reductions in long-term toxicity in surviving patients. There is ongoing investigation into further enhancements of this technique using volumetric modulated arc therapy and helical tomotherapy. This may also become important with the integration of newer/novel systemic agents, in conjunction with radiation therapy, of which many act as potent tumoral (and normal organ) radiation sensitizers and may reduce treatment-related toxicities as well as avoidance of treatment interruptions.[98]

Dose Constraints

In radiation therapy planning of gastric cancer, normal tissue tolerance should always be considered. The spinal cord dose is generally limited to 45 Gy using 1.8-Gy fractions (and potentially less when delivered with novel systemic agents). Accurate delineation of adjacent organs including lungs, liver, kidneys, heart, and spinal cord are important. Varying dose-volume normal organ constraints have been suggested. Historically, heart dose constraints have included include maintaining one-third, two-thirds, and total heart volumes <45, 40, and 30 Gy, respectively. Recommended heart constraints include keeping <30% of the cardiac volume to a total dose of 40 Gy and <50% receiving 25 Gy, minimizing dose to the left ventricle. In the setting of potentially significant volumes of heart in the radiation field, consideration of 4D CT and/or respiratory gating techniques can be made. It is recommended that at least 70% of one physiologically functioning kidney receive a total dose <20 Gy and that collectively ≤50% of the combined functional renal volume should receive >20 Gy.[100] In some patients, a portion of both kidneys will fall within the treatment field; however, at least two-thirds to three-fourths of one kidney should be excluded beyond a dose of 20 Gy. For proximal gastric lesions, ≥50% of the left kidney is commonly within the irradiation portal, and the right kidney must be appropriately spared. For distal lesions with narrow or positive duodenal margins, a similar amount of right kidney often is included, and every effort must be taken to spare enough left kidney to maintain function. Late renal sequelae have not been encountered with these techniques.[33,70,106] One should also consider the possibility of impaired kidney function in the context of varying comorbidities, using nuclear medicine renal studies to assess individual renal function in such situations or where significant volumes of kidneys are anticipated to be within the radiation field. Generally, 70% of the liver parenchyma should be kept to a dose <30 Gy. Many of these constraints can be achieved through the use of 3D planning with appropriate and careful design of shielding blocks/multileaf collimation and dose-volume histogram analysis, with the use of IMRT in select cases.

Doses of Radiation

Generally, doses in the range of 45 to 50.4 Gy should be delivered at 1.8 Gy per fraction. Although primarily limited by normal tissue contrasts in the upper abdomen, several series have reported improved locoregional control with radiation dose escalation in the adjuvant setting. A report from Mayo Clinic investigators reported high locoregional control rates with radiation doses >54 Gy.[105] Similarly, a report from Italian investigators treating patients adjuvantly with hyperfractionated radiation therapy to a dose of 55 Gy, with concurrent 5-FU, showed an in-field recurrence rate of only 7.5% and survival rate of 52% with a median follow-up >5 years.[107] With regimens using single daily fractions, the usual dose is 45 delivered in 1.8- to 2-Gy fractions over 5 weeks, with a field reduction after 45 Gy in patients receiving boost-field treatments. Reduced boost fields to small areas of residual disease and a small volume of stomach or small intestine sometimes can be cautiously carried to doses of 55 to 60 Gy with multifield techniques. In such instances, informed consent should include a discussion of an increased risk of grade 3 to 4 gastrointestinal toxicity.

RESULTS OF THERAPY

Locally Advanced Unresectable or Subtotally Resected Gastric Cancer

For patients with locally advanced unresectable or subtotally resected gastric carcinoma, radiotherapeutic approaches both with and without chemotherapy have been used because these tumors appear localized without clinically detectable metastases. Combined treatment with radiation therapy and chemotherapy appears to prolong survival but rarely results in long-term cure.[108] Although only a modest effect on survival is seen, these studies have established, importantly, the foundation of contemporary combined modality therapy and have served as a stimulus to further clinical investigation in gastric cancer as well as other gastrointestinal disease sites. The results of these phase III studies have had a significant impact on clinical trial development in gastrointestinal malignancies (Table 58.11).

In a historical trial from 1969, Moertel et al.[108] reported the results of a prospective, controlled double-blind study of patients with locally advanced unresectable gastric cancer. In this study, 48 patients were randomized to 35 to 40 Gy of radiation therapy over 4 weeks with and without 5-FU. Mean survival was 13 months in patients receiving radiation therapy and 5-FU versus 5.9 months for the radiation therapy patients (p <.01). These results demonstrated for the first time the clinical benefit of combining concurrent 5-FU with radiation therapy and encouraged further investigation of combination therapy in gastric cancer and other gastrointestinal disease sites (esophageal, pancreatic, rectal, and anal carcinomas).

As a follow-up to this study, the Gastrointestinal Tumor Study Group (GITSG) examined the combination of 5-FU/MeCCNU, or 1-(2-chloroethyl)-3-(4-methylcyclohexyl)-1 nitrosourea, and radiotherapy (RT; 50 Gy/split course/8 weeks)

TABLE 58.11 UNRESECTABLE OR RESIDUAL GASTRIC CANCER: TREATMENT RESULTS OF RANDOMIZED TRIALS

Group or Institution (Reference)	Treatment Arms	Number of Patients	EBRT Dose	Chemotherapy	Survival Results
Mayo Clinic (108)	EBRT + ChT vs. EBRT	48	35–40 Gy	5-FU	Increased survival for EBRT + 5-FU with mean survival 13 mo vs. 5.9 mo and 3/25 (12%) vs. 0/23 5-y survival
GITSG (109)	EBRT + ChT vs. ChT	90	50-Gy split course	5-FU + MeCCNU	Advantage in long-term survival with EBRT + ChT at 18% vs. 7% (p <.05)

EBRT, external-beam radiation therapy; ChT, chemotherapy; 5-FU, 5-fluorouracil; GITSG, Gastrointestinal Tumor Study Group; MeCCNU, 1-(2-chloroethyl)-3-(4-methylcyclohexyl)-1 nitrosourea.

versus the same chemotherapy alone in locally advanced gastric cancer.[109] Patients were eligible if the tumor involved regional lymph nodes or adjacent structures that could be completely resected en bloc. Of the 90 patients entered, 66 patients had a resection of the primary tumor. Of these, 23 patients had gross residual disease, 36 patients had microscopic residual and 7 patients had no documented residual disease. The study was closed prematurely because of an excess of early deaths in the combined chemotherapy–RT arm. The excessive early mortality of the combined-modality arm was attributed to early tumor progression and poor tolerance of the combined-modality regime. However, further follow-up beyond 3 years indicated continuing mortality among the chemotherapy-alone arm, whereas the combined chemoradiotherapy arm exhibited a plateau with 18% of patients surviving 5 years. Thus, despite an excess of early mortality, the combined-modality arm exhibited an overall superiority in 5-year survival. It is important to note that patients who had had their primary tumor resected experienced superior survival to those without resection. All of the survival benefit in patients receiving combined modality was in patients whose primary tumor had been resected. This trial showed that combined chemoradiation therapy is capable of rendering a substantial percentage of patients with microscopic residual gastric cancer free from disease. It furthermore supported the rationale of exploring chemoradiation adjuvant trials in completely resected patients at high risk for locoregional relapse because control of microscopic disease was able to cure a significant number of these patients.

Resectable Gastric Cancer

The recognition of the high rates of local and regional failure following surgery in patterns of failure analyses has served as the basis for clinical trials assessing the value of radiation therapy both with and without chemotherapy as an adjuvant treatment (Table 58.5). Although these studies have all addressed the important question of whether clinical outcome is enhanced by adjuvant radiation therapy, there has been marked variability in radiation dose and schedule, sequence with surgery (preoperatively, intraoperatively, or postoperatively), and the use of concurrent and maintenance chemotherapy (Table 58.12). These differences in study design may explain in part the conflicting results observed in phase III studies.

Adjuvant Radiation Therapy

Two randomized phase III studies have studied the use of external-beam radiation therapy alone (EBRT) with surgery.[66,110,111] Although both studies used similar radiation dose and schedule, sequence with surgery differed. In the British Stomach Cancer Group study, 436 patients were randomized to surgery alone; postoperative radiation therapy (45 to 50 Gy in 25 to 28 fractions); or cytotoxic chemotherapy with mitomycin, doxorubicin, and fluorouracil (FAM).[66,110] The 5-year survival for surgery alone was 20%, for surgery plus radiation therapy 12%, and for surgery plus chemotherapy 19%. In this study, no survival advantage was observed for patients who received postoperative EBRT, although there was an apparent improvement in local control, demonstrating that local disease could be affected by adjuvant radiation therapy. Locoregional failure was documented in only 15 of 153 patients (10%) in the irradiation arm versus 39 of 145 patients (27%) in the surgery-alone arm and 26 of 138 patients (19%) in the FAM group. Interpretation of the results is complicated by the inclusion of 171 patients undergoing resection with gross or microscopic residual carcinoma. These patients would not be candidates for contemporary gastric surgical adjuvant trials in the United States. In addition, approximately one-third of patients randomized to receive adjuvant treatment did not receive the assigned therapy. Of 153 patients randomized to the irradiation arm, only 104 (68%) received a dose ≥40.5 Gy, and 36 (24%) received none.

Neoadjuvant Radiation Therapy

In contrast, the results of a phase III study from Beijing demonstrated a survival benefit for patients with gastric cardia carcinoma receiving preoperative irradiation and surgery versus surgery only.[111] In this study, 370 patients with gastric cardia carcinoma were randomized to 40 Gy in 20 fractions over 4 weeks of preoperative irradiation and surgery or surgery only. The 5-year survival rates of preoperative irradiation and surgery and the surgery-alone group were 30% and 20%, respectively (10-year, 20% and 13%, respectively). These differences were statistically significant (p = .009). Further, local and regional nodal control was improved in patients undergoing preoperative irradiation and surgery (61% and 61%) versus surgery (48% and 45%) only. Morbidity and mortality rates were not increased in patients receiving preoperative irradiation and surgery.

Intraoperative Radiation Therapy

An alternative approach to postoperative or preoperative irradiation is intraoperative radiation therapy (IORT).[112,113] The advantage of this technique is the ability to deliver a single large fraction (10 to 35 Gy) of radiation to the tumor or tumor bed while excluding or protecting surrounding normal tissue from the high-dose field. This approach permits high-dose irradiation with minimal normal tissue treatment. Two randomized trials have examined the efficacy of IORT in combination with surgery for patients with gastric carcinoma. Abe et al.[113]

TABLE 58.12 ADJUVANT IRRADIATION WITH AND WITHOUT CHEMOTHERAPY FOR RESECTED GASTRIC CANCER: TREATMENT RESULTS OF RANDOMIZED TRIALS

			Survival		Locoregional Relapse		
Series/Treatment Method	Patients	Median (Months)	Long Term[a] (%)	p Value	N	%	p Value
1. Mayo Clinic [95]							
a. Surgery alone	23	15	4	–	–	54	–
b. Postop EBRT + 5-FU	39	24	23	.05		39	–
2. British Stomach Group [110]							
a. Surgery alone	145	–	20	–	39	27 (3 y)	–
b. Postop ChT	138	–	19	–	26	19 (3 y)	–
c. Postop EBRT	153	–	12	–	15	10 (3 y)	–
3. China–Beijing [111]							
a. Surgery alone	199	–	20	–	–	52	–
b. Preop EBRT	171	–	30	.009	–	39	<.025
4. Intergroup 0116 [99]						Disease-free survival (3 y)	
a. Surgery alone	275	27	41	–		31	–
b. Postop EBRT + ChT	281	36	50	.005		48	<.001

N, patient number; postop, postoperative; EBRT, external-beam radiation therapy; 5-FU, 5-fluorouracil; ChT, chemotherapy; preop, preoperative.

[a]Long-term survival is 5-year data for Mayo Clinic and Beijing series, and 3-year data is for British and Intergroup 0116.

from Kyoto University performed a randomized trial of 211 patients with gastric cancer comparing surgery alone with surgery and intraoperative radiation (28 to 35 Gy). Patients were randomized based on hospital day of admission for surgery. For patients with tumor confined to the gastric wall, 5-year survival rates were similar for IORT and for resection alone. However, patients with Japanese stages II to IV disease who received IORT in conjunction with resection showed improved survival over patients who underwent resection without irradiation. Among patients with stage IV disease (who usually had local residual disease after maximal resection), there were no 5-year survivors who received surgery alone; however, 15% of the patients who received IORT were alive at 5 years. The experience with IORT in gastric cancer at Kyoto University suggested that IORT may be beneficial in the treatment for locally advanced malignancies of the stomach.

To further evaluate this approach, Sindelar et al.[114] at the National Cancer Institute conducted a prospectively randomized controlled trial comparing surgical resection and IORT with conventional therapy in gastric carcinoma. Patients in the experimental group underwent gastrectomy, and IORT was administered to the gastric bed (20 Gy). Patients in the control group underwent resection and postoperative EBRT to the upper abdomen (50 Gy in 25 fractions) for advanced-stage lesions extending beyond the gastric wall. Of the 100 patients screened for the study, 60 patients were randomized and underwent exploratory surgery. Nineteen patients were excluded intraoperatively because of unresectability or metastases, leaving 41 patients in the study. The median survival for patients with tumors of all stages was 25 months for the IORT group and 21 months for the control group (p = not significant [NS]). Locoregional disease relapse occurred in 7 of 16 IORT patients (44%) and in 23 of 25 control patients (92%) ($p < .001$). Complication rates were similar between IORT and control patients. Although IORT failed to afford a significant advantage over conventional therapy in overall survival, IORT significantly improved control of locoregional disease. The use of IORT in gastric cancer remains a topic of investigation.

Adjuvant Chemotherapy

A randomized trial from Japan evaluated 579 patients undergoing resection to receive adjuvant chemotherapy alone versus observation alone. Primarily, early T-stage patients in the treatment group received a combination of mitomycin and fluorouracil twice weekly for 3 weeks following surgery, followed by delivery of UFT (uracil + tegafur [an oral 5-FU prodrug]). No survival benefit was seen with adjuvant chemotherapy.[115] However, a more recent follow-up study from Japan evaluated the efficacy of adjuvant chemotherapy in patients with stage II/III gastric cancer undergoing R0, D2 dissection (excluding T1 patients). This study randomized 1,059 patients to surgery alone versus treatment with S-1, an oral fluoropyrimidine combining tegafur and oxonic acid. Three-year survival was significantly improved in patients receiving adjuvant chemotherapy (80%) versus surgery alone (70%).[116] Whether the impact of S-1 in the Asian population can be extrapolated to Western patients remains less clear and the subject of investigation, including potential biologic differences among populations regarding how this drug is metabolized.

A meta-analysis of 17 randomized controlled trials using individual patient data comparing surgery alone to surgery with adjuvant chemotherapy in patients with resectable gastric cancer was performed. In this study, adjuvant chemotherapy was associated with a significant survival benefit in terms of overall survival (hazard ratio [HR] 0.82, confidence interval [CI] 0.76 to 0.90, $p < .001$) and disease-free survival. Estimated 5-year overall survival was increased from approximately 50% to 55% with the use of chemotherapy. The authors[117] concluded that adjuvant chemotherapy with fluorouracil-containing regimens reduce the risk of death in gastric cancer compared to surgery alone. As discussed previously, how these varying studies apply to Western patients remains unclear.

Adjuvant Chemoradiation Therapy

Because of the promising results in the early studies of combined-modality therapy for locally advanced unresectable or subtotally resected gastric cancer, investigators also have studied this combination in resectable gastric carcinoma. A small study from South Africa randomized 66 patients with resected gastric cancer (T1 to T3, N1 or N2, M0) to low-dose postoperative irradiation (20 Gy in eight fractions over 10 days) and 5-FU or no further therapy.[86] No difference in survival was observed between the patients undergoing surgery and adjuvant therapy and those undergoing surgery alone. Given the subtherapeutic doses of radiation used in this study, it is difficult to draw any conclusions as to the efficacy of adjuvant radiation therapy and 5-FU.

In 1984, Moertel et al.[95] reported the results of a prospective randomized trial conducted at the Mayo Clinic of 62 patients with poor prognosis but completely resected gastric cancers who were randomized to either surgery alone or surgery followed by irradiation (37.5 Gy in 24 fractions over 4 to 5 weeks) with concurrent 5-FU. A nonstratified, prerandomization scheme was used with a 2:3 ratio favoring treatment. Informed consent was requested of only the 39 patients randomized to treatment. Ten of the 39 patients refused further therapy and were observed. When analyzed by intent to treat, the adjuvant arm had statistically significant improvement in both relapse-free and overall survival (overall 5-year survival 23% vs. 4%, $p < .05$). When patient outcome was compared with actual treatment received (29 adjuvant treatment, 33 surgery alone), 5-year survival still favored the adjuvant group (20% vs. 12%), although the differences were not statistically significant in view of the small patient numbers. The 10 patients who refused assignment to adjuvant treatment had more favorable prognostic findings than the other two groups of patients. When the two groups with equally poor prognostic factors were compared, the 5-year overall survival was 20% versus 4%, with an advantage to those receiving adjuvant treatment. When analyzed by treatment delivered, locoregional relapse was decreased with adjuvant treatments (54% incidence with surgery alone vs. 39% with irradiation and 5-FU).

Because of these conflicting results, an Intergroup trial (INT 0116) was initiated to evaluate postoperative combined 5-FU–based chemotherapy and irradiation to the gastric bed and regional nodes versus surgery only following resection of gastric cancer.[99] Eligibility included patients with stage group IB through IV nonmetastatic adenocarcinoma of the stomach or GE junction. After an en bloc resection, 556 patients were randomized to either observation alone or postoperative 5-FU/leucovorin for one cycle followed by combined-modality therapy consisting of 45 Gy in 25 fractions plus concurrent 5-FU and leucovorin (4 days in week 1, 3 days in week 5) followed by two monthly 5-day cycles of 5-FU and leucovorin. Minor or major errors in field design were discovered in 35% during preirradiation quality assurance review, allowing most deviations to be corrected prior to radiation therapy initiation, resulting in a 6.5% final major deviation rate. Nodal metastases were present in 85% of the cases. With 5 years of median follow-up, 3-year relapse-free survival was 48% for adjuvant treatment and 31% for observation ($p = .001$); 3-year overall survival was 50% for treatment and 41% for observation ($p = .005$). The median overall survival in the surgery-only group was 27 months, compared with 36 months in the chemoradiotherapy group; the HR for death was 1.35 (95% CI 1.09 to 1.66, $p = .005$). The HR for relapse in the surgery-only group as compared with the chemoradiotherapy group was 1.52 (95% CI 1.23 to 1.86, $p < .001$). The median duration of relapse-free survival was 30 months in the chemoradiotherapy group and 19 months in the surgery-only group. Patterns of failure were based on the site of first relapse only and were categorized as local, regional, or distant. Local recurrence occurred in 29% of patients who relapsed in the surgery-only group and 19% of those who relapsed in the chemoradiotherapy group. Regional relapse—typically abdominal carcinomatosis—was reported in 72% of those who relapsed in the surgery-only group and 65% of those who relapsed in the chemoradiotherapy group. Extra-abdominal distant metastases were diagnosed in 18% of those who relapsed in the surgery-only group and 33% of those who relapsed in the chemoradiotherapy group. Treatment was tolerable, with three (1%) toxic deaths. Grades 3 and 4 toxicity occurred in 41% and 32% of cases, respectively, and 17% of patients assigned to the chemoradiotherapy group stopped treatment owing to toxicity from therapy. Long-term results at >10-year median follow-up continued to show significant improvement in overall and disease-free survival in the chemoradiation group, benefiting all T- and N-stage patients included in the trial.[118] The results of this large study demonstrate a clear survival advantage for the use of postoperative chemoradiation and strongly support its integration into the routine care of patients with curatively resected high-risk carcinoma of the stomach and GE junction.[119]

The follow up Intergroup trial CALGB 80101 randomized patients with resected gastric or GE junction adenocarcinoma to receive either (a) one cycle of 5-FU/leucovorin, followed by 45 Gy with concurrent continuous infusion 5-FU, followed by two additional cycles of 5-FU/leucovorin; or (b) one cycle of ECF (epirubicin, cisplatin, 5-FU), followed by 45 Gy with concurrent, continuous infusional 5-FU, followed by two additional cycles of reduced dose ECF. Preliminary trial results showed that grade 4 toxicity was significant higher in arm 1 at 40% versus 26% (p <.001), including higher rates of neutropenia, diarrhea, and mucositis. Median overall survival was 37 months versus 38 months (p = .8), 3-year overall survival 50% versus 52%, and 3-year disease-free survival 46% versus 47%. The conclusions from these preliminary results were that following curative resection of gastric or GE junction adenocarcinoma, postoperative chemoradiotherapy using ECF before and after 5-FU–based radiation does not improve survival compared to bolus 5-FU/leucovorin given in the same manner.[120]

A large retrospective study from Korea evaluated the role of adjuvant chemoradiation in patients undergoing D2 gastric cancer resection, a group that was not adequately represented in the aforementioned Intergroup trial. In the Korean study, 544 patients treated with D2 dissection and postoperative chemoradiation therapy were compared to 446 patients with similar characteristics treated with D2 dissection alone. Overall survival was significantly higher in patients treated with adjuvant chemoradiation (median survival 95 vs. 63 months, p = .02) as well as significant improvement in relapse-free survival.[81] Additionally, a recent collective review of nine randomized trials incorporating radiation therapy approaches with surgery alone also demonstrated a significant 5-year survival benefit with the addition of radiation therapy in resectable gastric cancer patients.[121]

A Korean phase III trial (the Adjuvant Chemoradiation Therapy in Stomach Cancer [ARTIST] study) compared the effects of adjuvant chemoradiation (capecitabine/cisplatin [XP] + RT) to adjuvant chemotherapy alone (capecitabine/cisplatin) following D2 resection of gastric cancer in 458 patients.[121a] Treatment was completed as planned by 75.4% of patients (172 of 228) in the XP arm and 81.7% (188 of 230) in the XP/RT/XP arm. The addition of radiation to XP chemotherapy did not significantly prolong disease-free survival (p = .086). However, in the subgroup of patients with pathologic lymph node metastasis at the time of surgery (n = 396), patients randomly assigned to the XP/RT/XP arm experienced superior disease-free survival when compared with those who received XP alone (p = .0365), and the statistical significance was retained at multivariate analysis (estimated HR 0.69, p = .047). The authors[121a] concluded that the addition of RT to XP chemotherapy did not significantly reduce recurrence after curative resection and D2 lymph node dissection in gastric cancer, although a subsequent trial (ARTIST-II) in patients with lymph node–positive gastric cancer is planned. Additionally, a study by the Dutch Colorectal Cancer Group (the Chemoradiotherapy after Induction Chemotherapy in Cancer of the Stomach [CRITICS] trial) is randomizing patients to receive preoperative chemotherapy (epirubicin, cisplatin, capecitabine) for three cycles followed by D1+ resection, followed by a similar postoperative chemotherapy regimen, with or without radiotherapy concurrent with cisplatin/capecitabine.

Preoperative Chemoradiation Therapy

Because preoperative radiation therapy and chemotherapy have improved the surgical outcome in patients with rectal and esophageal cancer, this treatment is a logical approach to explore in gastric cancer as well. Although no phase III trials have tested the value of preoperative radiation plus chemotherapy for patients with gastric cancer, two phase III trials for patients with esophagus cancer have included either lesions of the gastric cardia[122] or the esophagogastric junction.[123] In both trials, the trimodality arm demonstrated an improvement in survival when compared with the control arm of surgery alone. The series by Walsh et al.[122] (adenocarcinoma of the esophagus or gastric cardia) demonstrated a median survival of 16 versus 11 months and 3-year survival of 32% versus 6% (p = .01), with the advantage to trimodality treatment. The U.S. Gastrointestinal Intergroup phase III trial (adenocarcinoma or squamous cell of the esophagus or GE junction), which closed prematurely owing to low accrual, resulted in a median survival of 54 months versus 21.6 months and 5-year survival of 39% versus 16% (p = .008), with an advantage to the trimodality arm.

Preoperative chemoradiation data for patients with gastric cancer is limited to phase II studies from single institutions and cooperative groups. MD Anderson Cancer Center has reported a study in which 33 patients completed a preoperative protocol that started with induction chemotherapy of 5-FU, leucovorin, and cisplatin, followed by 45 Gy of radiation therapy in 25 fractions over 5 weeks. Infusional 5-FU was administered concurrently with radiation therapy. In 28 patients (85%), a gastrectomy was performed and D2 lymph node dissection was attempted. Pathologic complete and partial response was found in 64% of all operated patients. These patients showed a significantly longer median survival of 64 months in comparison with 13 months in patients with tumors not pathologically responding.[124a] In a study from the same institution, 41 patients with operable gastric cancer received two cycles of continuous 5-FU, paclitaxel, and cisplatin followed by 45 Gy of radiation therapy with concurrent 5-FU and paclitaxel. An R0 resection was achieved in 78% of patients, pathologic complete response in 25%, and pathologic partial response in 15%. Pathologic response, R0 resection, and postoperative T- and N-stage were correlated with overall and disease-free survival.[124b] The Radiation Therapy Oncology Group reported the results of a phase II study of 49 patients undergoing induction 5-FU, leucovorin, and cisplatin followed by concurrent radiation therapy and infusional 5-FU and paclitaxel.[124c] Resection was attempted 5 to 6 weeks after radiation therapy and chemotherapy. The pathologic complete response and R0 resection rates were 26% and 77%, respectively. At 1 year, more patients with tumors exhibiting a pathologic complete response (89%) were living than patients with tumors exhibiting a less favorable response (66%). Grade 4 toxicity occurred in 21% of patients. These data appear to support a randomized phase III study evaluating preoperative versus postoperative radiation therapy and chemotherapy.[124c]

Preoperative Chemoradiation Versus Preoperative Chemotherapy

A randomized trial comparing neoadjuvant chemotherapy alone versus neoadjuvant combined modality therapy was conducted by German investigators (the Preoperative Chemotherapy or Radiochemotherapy in Esophago-gastric Adenocarcinoma Trial [POET]).[125] Patients with advanced esophagogastric adenocarcinoma were randomized to receive (a) cisplatin/5-FU–based chemotherapy alone versus (b) a similar induction chemotherapy followed by concurrent cisplatin/etoposide with 30 Gy of radiation therapy. Both groups went on to receive surgery. Although this study closed early owing to poor accrual, patients receiving preoperative chemoradiotherapy had significantly higher N0 rates (37 vs. 64%, $p = .04$) and pathologic complete response rates (2% vs. 16%, $p = .03$), as well as statistical trends toward improved local control (59% vs. 76%, $p = .06$) and overall survival (3-year survival 28% vs. 47%, $p = .07$, HR 0.67). The authors concluded that preoperative combined modality improves overall survival as compared to chemotherapy alone in patients with locally advanced esophagogastric adenocarcinoma.[125] Along these lines, a randomized phase II/III trial of preoperative chemoradiotherapy versus preoperative chemotherapy alone for resectable gastric and GE junction cancer (the TOPGEAR study) was recently initiated in Australia.

Perioperative Chemotherapy

Various combinations of active drugs have been reported to improve the response rate among patients with metastatic or locally unresectable gastric carcinoma.[9] A combination of FAM has been associated with a 30% to 40% response rate and was the most widely prescribed regimen for patients with advanced disease in the 1980s.[9] Despite an initial response rate of 64% when a combination of etoposide, doxorubicin, and cisplatin (EAP) was used by German investigators, in subsequent trials this regimen was considerably less effective and extremely toxic.[126,127–128] A combination of fluorouracil, doxorubicin, and high-dose methotrexate (FAMTX) was associated with a significant improvement in response rate compared with either EAP or FAM. As a result of these studies, FAMTX became standard therapy for metastatic disease.

In a British study of patients with unresectable or metastatic gastric and esophageal adenocarcinoma, 274 patients were randomized to either 5-FU, doxorubicin, and methotrexate (FAMTX) or epirubicin, cisplatin, and continuous infusion 5-FU (ECF).[129,130] ECF was associated with a superior response rate (45% vs. 21%, $p = .0002$), median survival (8.7 months vs. 5.7 months, $p = .0006$ vs. .006), and 1-year survival (36% vs. 21%). Moreover, ECF was associated with a superior quality of life and less toxicity.

The Medical Research Council (MRC) subsequently initiated a trial (the Medical Research Council Adjuvant Gastric Infusional Chemotherapy [MAGIC] trial) to address the question of perioperative chemotherapy (pre- and post-) in operable gastric cancer patients. Patients with resectable adenocarcinoma of the stomach, GE junction, or lower esophagus were randomized to preoperative and postoperative chemotherapy with epirubicin, cisplatin, and 5-FU (ECF) versus surgery alone. Although originally designed to include patients with only tumors of the stomach, eligibility was later expanded to include tumors of the lower third of the esophagus, with approximately one-fourth of patients having adenocarcinoma involving the lower esophagus or GE junction. The resected tumors were significantly smaller and less advanced in the perioperative chemotherapy group. With a median follow-up of 4 years, 149 patients in the perioperative chemotherapy group and 170 patients in the surgery group had died. As compared with the surgery group, the perioperative chemotherapy group had statistically improved progression-free and overall survival rates. No patient achieved pathologic complete response. However, patients receiving perioperative chemotherapy had a HR for death of 0.75, which was highly significant, with 5-year survival in patients receiving chemotherapy 36% versus 23% in patients undergoing surgery alone ($p = .009$).[131] A follow-up MRC study is evaluating the role of the vascular endothelial growth factor inhibitor bevacizumab with this regimen (MAGIC B).

French investigators reported the results of a similar randomized trial of 224 patients assigned to perioperative chemotherapy (cisplatin and 5-FU) versus surgery alone. Although originally designed to include only patients with tumors of the lower third of the esophagus or GE junction, eligibility was later expanded to include gastric cancers, although most (75%) of patients had disease of the lower esophagus or GE junction. Chemotherapy consisted of a planned two to three preoperative and three to four postoperative cycles. This study was prematurely terminated because of low accrual. Nonetheless, patients receiving chemotherapy had improved overall survival (5-year 38% vs. 24%, $p = .02$), disease-free survival (5-year 34% vs. 19%, $p = .003$), and R0 resection rates (84% vs. 73%, $p = .04$). Only 50% of patients received postoperative chemotherapy. T0 disease (complete pathologic response at the primary site) disease was seen in 3% of neoadjuvantly treated patients. Total locoregional recurrence rates were 24% and 26%, respectively, in the chemotherapy versus surgery group, with distant recurrence rates of 42% versus 56%, respectively.[132]

Palliative Radiation Therapy

Radiation therapy is capable of providing substantial palliation of local gastric cancer symptoms.[133–135,136,137,138] It appears that 50% to 75% of patients can expect improvement of symptoms such as gastric outlet obstruction, pain from local tumor extension, bleeding, or biliary obstruction.[136] The likelihood of benefit may increase with concomitant 5-FU administration, with less tumor bulk, and if the patient's performance score is better before therapy.[105,134,139,140] The median duration of palliation varies from 4 to 18 months in reports addressing this issue.[134,139–141]

SEQUELAE OF THERAPY

Anorexia, nausea, and fatigue are very common complaints during gastric radiation therapy; however, the understanding of these problems is quite limited.[122,142–144,145] Although visceral afferents may play some role in the acute emetogenic effects of radiation, other unknown factors, possibly chemical in nature and mediated by the chemoreceptor trigger zone, appear to be more important. Although selective serotonin ($5\text{-}HT_3$) antagonists effectively treat radiation-induced emesis, it is not clear whether the mechanism of action is directed at the $5\text{-}HT_3$ receptor alone or has an effect on inhibition of serotonin release.[146] Other compounding factors may include the altered gastric motility and prolonged gastric emptying time observed in animal experiments as a response to irradiation.[93,142,143,147] Chemotherapy-related leukopenia and thrombocytopenia may occur. If chemotherapy is used with irradiation, blood counts are generally obtained once to twice weekly. Additional acute toxicities of radiation therapy include esophagitis, epidermitis, fatigue, and weight loss in most patients. Nausea, vomiting, dehydration, and anorexia are relatively common, particularly in patients with lower esophageal and GE junction tumors. During therapy, patient tolerance, weight, and blood counts are checked at least weekly. Many symptoms resolve within 1 to 2 weeks of treatment completion. Because of potential toxicities in the treatment for gastric cancer patients (dehydration, weight loss, anorexia, etc.), aggressive supportive measurements and symptom management are indicated in efforts to avoid treatment-related interruptions, hospitalizations, or failure to complete the intended treatment course. Varying antiemetics should be used liberally, including on a prophylactic basis. Antacids including proton pump inhibitors are frequently implemented, and antidiarrheal medications may be appropriate. Additionally, nutritional supportive measurements are paramount and, when appropriate, the use of enteral methods implemented. In selected cases, the use of feeding jejunostomy may be appropriate. Patients may require intermittent hydration both during and shortly following the treatment course. Postoperatively, B_{12}, iron, and calcium levels should be monitored and supplemented as appropriate.

Nutritional complications of treatment and myelosuppression, if concurrent chemotherapy is used during irradiation, can carry substantial morbidity and even occasional mortality from therapy. The GITSG reported a minimum 13% treatment-related mortality from nutritional problems or septic events on their concurrent chemoradiation arm,[109] and almost 20% of the patients of Caudry et al.[148] were unable to complete therapy because of nutritional problems. However, others reported no severe or life-threatening nutritional compromise with aggressive chemoradiation.[104,105,149] Toxic gastrointestinal effects usually are managed with careful nutritional support and antiemetic therapy. It may be prudent to proactively prescribe antiemetics at the initiation of therapy in patients undergoing aggressive upper abdominal irradiation.

Myelosuppression causing serious or, rarely, lethal toxicity also is reported in many of the combined-modality trials.[104,105,112,149] If blood counts are monitored weekly during combined-modality therapy, serious problems with sepsis or bleeding should be uncommon.[104,105,112]

Moderate doses of 16 to 36 Gy reduce secretion of pepsin and hydrochloric acid.[1,13,93,150] For this reason, radiation therapy was once a common and successful therapy for peptic ulcer disease. Most of the gastric ulcers healed, although they recurred in approximately 40% of patients.[1,93,150] Gastric acid secretion decreased in almost all cases, with achlorhydria in 25% to 40%.[61] The gastric acid decrease usually persisted from 1 to 6 months; however, 25% showed persistent decrease in acid production for 1 to 5 years or more.

Gastric late effects were categorized by the Walter Reed Group as dyspepsia, radiation gastritis, uncomplicated gastric ulcer, or gastric ulcer with perforation or obstruction.[151–153] The associations between dose and these late effects are described in Table 58.13. These data suggest a 20% to 30% incidence of ulceration with doses of 45 to 59 Gy, with complications of these ulcers in 30% to 50% of the treated patients. Some caution is necessary in interpreting this experience because the Walter Reed cohort was treated with 200-keV photons or 1-MV photons using a 70-cm target-skin distance, usually using only one field each day with daily fraction sizes of 3 Gy to midline, which sometimes produced daily given doses of 4 to 6 Gy.[152,153]

Most data suggest that gastric late effects are rare with doses of 40 to 52 Gy using conventional fractionation of 1.8 to 2 Gy. The relatively low risk of gastric late effects with doses <50 Gy is corroborated by many series using radiation therapy with or without chemotherapy for locally advanced gastric cancer.[36,42,56,64,71,122] However, doses in the range of 50 to 55 Gy may produce variable gastric late effects, which have been reported to reach 9% in some series. Doses of 60 Gy carried a 5% to 15% risk of gastric late effects.[1–3,46,56,61,90,106,122,134,135,140,148,150–156,157,158]

The ability of histamine (H_2) blockers and sucralfate to prevent the later development of radiation-induced gastric ulcerations is unproven. It may be reasonable to administer H_2 blockers or proton pump inhibitors prophylactically to patients receiving >45 Gy to any significant volume of the stomach or proximal duodenum.

Several series have described a gradual decline in renal function occurring ≥18 to 24 months following postoperative radiation therapy for gastric cancer. However, it is unclear that this is of clinical significance, and long-term renal function among gastric cancer survivors has not been reliably reported. Nonetheless, advanced techniques may enhance renal sparing and also allow potential dose escalation as well as integration of novel (and potentially nephrotoxic) systemic agents.[98] Radiation-induced cardiac toxicity is a broad term describing potential radiation injury to a number of cardiac structures, including pericardium (as manifested by effusion, pericarditis), coronary arteries, the heart muscle itself, and cardiac valves as well as nerve/conduction injury. Radiation injury primarily consists of fibrosis and/or small vessel injury. The mechanism of radiation-induced cardiac injury is relatively poorly defined, particularly in the context of gastric cancer. Historical data from the treatment for Hodgkin's disease patients have suggested that dose >40 Gy may increase the risk of cardiac death as well as pericarditis.[159,160] Several studies of cardiac toxicity and esophageal cancer patients have demonstrated that an increasing V_{30} predicted for a significant increase in pericardial effusion, and increasing fraction size (particularly ≥3.5 Gy) also predicted for the same. Additionally, some authors have shown a possible trend for decrease in ejection fraction in patients with increasing V_{20} of the left ventricle.[161] A more detailed discussion on potential long-term cardiac sequelae of radiation therapy can be found in Chapter 53.

TABLE 58.13 RADIATION DOSE COMPARED WITH LATE EFFECTS IN THE WALTER REED EXPERIENCE[151–153]

		Radiation Late Effects (%)[a]			
Dose (Gy)	Number of Patients[b]	Dyspepsia	Gastritis	Ulcer	Complicated Ulcer[c]
<40	111	5	2	3	0
40–44.99	23	0	22	0	0
45–49.99	27	4	19	11	11
50–54.99	34	0	24	18	12
55–59.99	14	0	50	14	7
>60	8	0	0	13	38

[a]Results reported as number of patients with injury/total number of patients treated with this dose.

[b]Total number of patients treated at this dose.

[c]Ulcers complicated by obstruction or perforation.

CONCLUSIONS AND RECOMMENDATIONS

Radiation therapy, usually administered with concomitant 5-FU–based chemotherapy, is indicated for locally confined gastric cancer that either is not technically resectable or occurs in medically inoperable patients. In this setting, therapy can be administered with curative or palliative intent, depending on the clinical situation. Those who undergo gastric resection with incomplete tumor resection or have truly positive margins of resection are also appropriately managed by combined-modality therapy. Preferably, patients with locally advanced disease that is unresectable with negative margins would be identified preoperatively with endoscopic ultrasonography and CT staging. Preoperative chemoradiation then could precede an attempt at gross total resection, alone or in combination with IORT, and maintenance chemotherapy.

The results of the U.S. Gastrointestinal Intergroup Gastric Adjuvant Trial have changed the standard of care in the United States to the use of both chemotherapy and radiation therapy in the postoperative setting for patients with disease extension through the gastric wall and/or with nodes positive for tumor. Postoperative irradiation and concurrent and maintenance 5-FU–based chemotherapy are recommended for patients with stage IB, II, IIIA, IIIB, or IV and M0 gastric cancer. The role of postoperative chemoradiation in patients with T2N0 tumors remains more controversial. In patients with high-risk features (i.e., poorly differentiated or higher-grade cancers, lymph vascular invasion, perineural invasion, age <50 years, or suboptimal resection including lymph node resection), postoperative chemoradiotherapy may be indicated.

Clinical Radiation Oncology

Because extended node dissections were not commonly performed as a component of surgery in the Intergroup trial, some have questioned whether postoperative chemoradiation would give added benefit following a D2 nodal resection. Similarly, given the survival benefit from the use of perioperative chemotherapy alone in European esophagogastric patients, ongoing trials are examining the role of adjuvant chemoradiation in both the settings of perioperative chemotherapy as well as D2 lymph node dissection. Additionally, further trials are investigating new systemic agents with radiation therapy to establish efficacy compared with 5-FU and leucovorin. Given the poor prognosis with patients receiving either perioperative chemotherapy or adjuvant chemoradiotherapy, integration of the approaches has the potential to improve disease-related outcomes compared to either alone. Similarly, on the basis of encouraging outcomes with phase II preoperative chemoradiation trials in patients with gastric cancer and phase III esophagus cancer trials, it would be appropriate to continue to evaluate this approach in patients with both potentially resectable and unresectable lesions.

The irradiation field design from the current phase III U.S. Gastrointestinal Intergroup trial was based on optimized field design related to both site of the primary lesion and T- and N-stage of disease.[103] With the wide availability of 3D conformal treatment-planning systems, it may be possible to more accurately target the high-risk volume and to use unconventional field arrangements and/or IMRT to produce superior dose distributions. To accomplish this without marginal misses, however, it will be necessary to both carefully define and encompass the various target volumes (tumor bed, nodal sites at risk) because target volumes that would be included in AP/PA fields may be missed with other field arrangements (oblique, lateral, noncoplanar).

SELECTED REFERENCES

A full list of references for this chapter is available online.

1. Goss CM. *Anatomy of the human body.* Philadelphia, PA: Lea & Febiger, 1973.
2. Kao GD, Whittington R, Coia L. Anatomy of the celiac axis and superior mesenteric artery and its significance in radiation therapy. *Int J Radiat Oncol Biol Phys* 1993;25:131–134.
3. Siegel R, Naishadham D, Jemal A. Cancer statistics, 2012. *CA Cancer J Clin* 2012;62(1):10–29. doi:10.3322/caac.20138. Epub 2012 Jan 4.
6. Ajani JA, Barthel JS, Bekaii-Saab T, et al. Gastric cancer. *J Natl Compr Canc Netw* 2010;8:378–409.
9. Fuchs CS, Mayer RJ. Gastric carcinoma. *N Engl J Med* 1995;333:32–41.
10. Shah MA, Kelsen DP. Gastric cancer: a primer on the epidemiology and biology of the disease and an overview of the medical management of advanced disease. *J Natl Compr Canc Netw* 2010;8:437–447.
14. Fukuya T, Honda H, Hayashi T, et al. Lymph-node metastases: efficacy for detection with helical CT in patients with gastric cancer. *Radiology* 1995;197:705–711.
16. Sarela AI, Lefkowitz R, Brennan MF, et al. Selection of patients with gastric adenocarcinoma for laparoscopic staging. *Am J Surg* 2006;191:134–138.
17. Leake PA, Cardoso R, Seevaratnam R, et al. A systematic review of the accuracy and indications for diagnostic laparoscopy prior to curative-intent resection of gastric cancer. *Gastric Cancer* 2011 Jun 11. [Epub ahead of print]
19. Puli SR, Batapati Krishna Reddy J, Bechtold ML, et al. How good is endoscopic ultrasound for TNM staging of gastric cancers? A meta-analysis and systematic review. *World J Gastroenterol* 2008;14:4011–4019.
20. Kwee RM, Kwee TC. Imaging in local staging of gastric cancer: a systematic review. *J Clin Oncol* 2007;25:2107–2116.
21. Stahl A, Ott K, Weber WA, et al. FDG PET imaging of locally advanced gastric carcinomas: correlation with endoscopic and histopathological findings. *Eur J Nucl Med Mol Imaging* 2003;30:288–295.
22. Das P, Jiang Y, Lee JH, et al. Multimodality approaches to localized gastric cancer. *J Natl Compr Canc Netw* 2010;8:417–425.
23. Chen J, Cheong JH, Yun MJ, et al. Improvement in preoperative staging of gastric adenocarcinoma with positron emission tomography. *Cancer* 2005;103:2383–2390.
26. Edge S, Byrd D, Compton C, et al. *Stomach.* New York: Springer-Verlag, 2010.
29. MacDonald J, Cohn I, Gunderson LL. *Carcinoma of the stomach.* Philadelphia, PA: JB Lippincott, 1985.
30. Meyers WC, Damiano RJ Jr, Rotolo FS, et al. Adenocarcinoma of the stomach. Changing patterns over the last 4 decades. *Ann Surg* 1987;205:1–8.
31. Yamada Y, Kato Y. Greater tendency for submucosal invasion in fundic area gastric carcinomas than those arising in the pyloric area. *Cancer* 1989;63:1757–1760.
33. Gunderson LL, Sosin H. Adenocarcinoma of the stomach: areas of failure in a re-operation series (second or symptomatic look) clinicopathologic correlation and implications for adjuvant therapy. *Int J Radiat Oncol Biol Phys* 1982;8:1–11.
35. Douglass HO Jr, Nava HR. Gastric adenocarcinoma—management of the primary disease. *Semin Oncol* 1985;12:32–45.
37. Maruta K, Shida H. Some factors which influence prognosis after surgery for advanced gastric cancer. *Ann Surg* 1968;167:313–318.
38. Gunderson LL. Gastric cancer—patterns of relapse after surgical resection. *Semin Radiat Oncol* 2002;12:150–161.
39. Chau I, Norman AR, Cunningham D, et al. Multivariate prognostic factor analysis in locally advanced and metastatic esophago-gastric cancer—pooled analysis from three multicenter, randomized, controlled trials using individual patient data. *J Clin Oncol* 2004;22:2395–2403.
40. Byfield SA, Earle CC, Ayanian JZ, et al. Treatment and outcomes of gastric cancer among United States-born and foreign-born Asians and Pacific Islanders. *Cancer* 2009;115:4595–4605.
48. Lane DP. Worrying about p53. *Curr Biol* 1992;2:581–583.
49. Kastan MB, Onyekwere O, Sidransky D, et al. Participation of p53 protein in the cellular response to DNA damage. *Cancer Res* 1991;51:6304–6311.
52. Lynch HT, Smyrk TC, Watson P, et al. Genetics, natural history, tumor spectrum, and pathology of hereditary nonpolyposis colorectal cancer: an updated review. *Gastroenterology* 1993;104:1535–1549.
59a. Bang YJ, Van Cutsem E, Feyereislova A, et al. Trastuzumab in combination with chemotherapy versus chemotherapy alone for treatment of HER2-positive advanced gastric or gastro-oesophageal junction cancer (ToGA): a phase 3, open-label, randomised controlled trial. *Lancet* 2010;376(9742):687–697. Erratum in: *Lancet* 2010;376(9749):1302.
66. Allum WH, Hallissey MT, Ward LC, et al. A controlled, prospective, randomised trial of adjuvant chemotherapy or radiotherapy in resectable gastric cancer: interim report. British Stomach Cancer Group. *Br J Cancer* 1989;60:739–744.
67. Bleiberg H, Goffin JC, Dalesio O, et al. Adjuvant radiotherapy and chemotherapy in resectable gastric cancer. A randomized trial of the gastro-intestinal tract cancer cooperative group of the EORTC. *Eur J Surg Oncol* 1989;15:535–543.
68. Gez E, Sulkes A, Yablonsky-Peretz T, et al. Combined 5-fluorouracil (5-FU) and radiation therapy following resection of locally advanced gastric carcinoma. *J Surg Oncol* 1986;31:139–142.
70. Regine WF, Mohiuddin M. Impact of adjuvant therapy on locally advanced adenocarcinoma of the stomach. *Int J Radiat Oncol Biol Phys* 1992;24:921–927.
71. Siewert JR, Lange J, Bottcher K, et al. [Stomach cancer—the current situation from the surgical viewpoint]. *Dtsch Med Wochenschr* 1987;112:622–628.
72. Slot A, Meerwaldt JH, van Putten WL, et al. Adjuvant postoperative radiotherapy for gastric carcinoma with poor prognostic signs. *Radiother Oncol* 1989;16:269–274.
73. Whittington R, Coia LR, Haller DG, et al. Adenocarcinoma of the esophagus and esophago-gastric junction: the effects of single and combined modalities on the survival and patterns of failure following treatment. *Int J Radiat Oncol Biol Phys* 1990;19:593–603.
74. Bunt AM, Hogendoorn PC, van de Velde CJ, et al. Lymph node staging standards in gastric cancer. *J Clin Oncol* 1995;13:2309–2316.
75. Douglass HO, Clark JL, Barcewicz P, et al. Importance of the R_2 lymph node dissection in the surgical treatment of gastric cancer. *Proc Am Soc Clin Oncol* 1989;8:101.
76. Smith DD, Schwarz RR, Schwarz RE. Impact of total lymph node count on staging and survival after gastrectomy for gastric cancer: data from a large US-population database. *J Clin Oncol* 2005;23:7114–7124.
77. Soga J, Ohyama S, Miyashita K, et al. A statistical evaluation of advancement in gastric cancer surgery with special reference to the significance of lymphadenectomy for cure. *World J Surg* 1988;12:398–405.
78. Dupont JB Jr, Lee JR, Burton GR, et al. Adenocarcinoma of the stomach: review of 1,497 cases. *Cancer* 1978;41:941–947.
81. Kim S, Lim DH, Lee J, et al. An observational study suggesting clinical benefit for adjuvant postoperative chemoradiation in a population of over 500 cases after gastric resection with D2 nodal dissection for adenocarcinoma of the stomach. *Int J Radiat Oncol Biol Phys* 2005;63:1279–1285.
82. Bonenkamp JJ, Hermans J, Sasako M, et al. Extended lymph-node dissection for gastric cancer. *N Engl J Med* 1999;340:908–914.
83. Bonenkamp JJ, Songun I, Hermans J, et al. Randomised comparison of morbidity after D1 and D2 dissection for gastric cancer in 996 Dutch patients. *Lancet* 1995;345:745–748.
84. Bunt AM, Hermans J, Smit VT, et al. Surgical/pathologic-stage migration confounds comparisons of gastric cancer survival rates between Japan and Western countries. *J Clin Oncol* 1995;13:19–25.
85. Cuschieri A, Weeden S, Fielding J, et al. Patient survival after D1 and D2 resections for gastric cancer: long-term results of the MRC randomized surgical trial. Surgical Co-operative Group. *Br J Cancer* 1999;79:1522–1530.
86. Dent DM, Madden MV, Price SK. Randomized comparison of R1 and R2 gastrectomy for gastric carcinoma. *Br J Surg* 1988;75:110–112.
88. Sasako M, Sano T, Yamamoto S, et al. D2 lymphadenectomy alone or with para-aortic nodal dissection for gastric cancer. *N Engl J Med* 2008;359:453–462.
89. Gunderson LL, Hoskins RB, Cohen AC, et al. Combined modality treatment of gastric cancer. *Int J Radiat Oncol Biol Phys* 1983;9:965–975.
90. Gunderson LL, Willett C, Harrison LB, et al. *Intraoperative irradiation: techniques and results.* Totowa, NJ: Humana Press, 1999.
91. Horn RC Jr. Carcinoma of the stomach; autopsy findings in untreated cases. *Gastroenterology* 1955;29:515–523; discussion 523–515.
92. Papachristou DN, Fortner JG. Local recurrence of gastric adenocarcinomas after gastrectomy. *J Surg Oncol* 1981;18:47–53.
94. Landry J, Tepper JE, Wood WC, et al. Patterns of failure following curative resection of gastric carcinoma. *Int J Radiat Oncol Biol Phys* 1990;19:1357–1362.
95. Moertel CG, Childs DS, O'Fallon JR, et al. Combined 5-fluorouracil and radiation therapy as a surgical adjuvant for poor prognosis gastric carcinoma. *J Clin Oncol* 1984;2:1249–1254.
96. Gilbertsen VA. Results of treatment of stomach cancer. An appraisal of efforts for more extensive surgery and a report of 1,983 cases. *Cancer* 1969;23:1305–1308.
97. McNeer G, Vandenberg H, Donn F, et al. A critical evaluation of subtotal gastrectomy for the cure of cancer of the stomach. *Ann Surg* 1957;134:2.
98. Callister MD, Gunderson LL. Advancements in radiation techniques for gastric cancer. *J Natl Compr Canc Netw* 2010;8:428–435; quiz 436.
99. MacDonald JS, Smalley SR, Benedetti J, et al. Chemoradiotherapy after surgery compared with surgery alone for adenocarcinoma of the stomach or gastroesophageal junction. *N Engl J Med* 2001;345:725–730.
100. Matzinger O, Gerber E, Bernstein Z, et al. EORTC-ROG expert opinion: radiotherapy volume and treatment guidelines for neoadjuvant radiation of adeno-

carcinomas of the gastroesophageal junction and the stomach. *Radiother Oncol* 2009;92:164–175.
102. Smalley SR, Gunderson L, Tepper J, et al. Gastric surgical adjuvant radiotherapy consensus report: rationale and treatment implementation. *Int J Radiat Oncol Biol Phys* 2002;52:283–293.
103. Tepper JE, Gunderson LL. Radiation treatment parameters in the adjuvant postoperative therapy of gastric cancer. *Semin Radiat Oncol* 2002;12:187–195.
104. Thirlwell M, Keable H, Kost K, et al. Combination of 5-fluorouracil (5 FU) plus semustine (MECCNU) with and without radiotherapy (RT) in advanced gastric and pancreatic carcinoma. *Proc Am Soc Clin Oncol* 1981;22:449.
105. Henning GT, Schild SE, Stafford SL, et al. Results of irradiation or chemoirradiation following resection of gastric adenocarcinoma. *Int J Radiat Oncol Biol Phys* 2000;46:589–598.
106. Willett CG, Tepper JE, Orlow EL, et al. Renal complications secondary to radiation treatment of upper abdominal malignancies. *Int J Radiat Oncol Biol Phys* 1986;12:1601–1604.
107. Arcangeli G, Saracino B, Angelini F, et al. Postoperative adjuvant chemoradiation in completely resected locally advanced gastric cancer. *Int J Radiat Oncol Biol Phys* 2002;54:1069–1075.
108. Moertel CG, Childs DS, Reitemeier R, et al. Combined 5 fluorouracil and supervoltage radiation therapy of locally unresectable gastrointestinal cancer. *Lancet* 1969;865:867.
109. A comparison of combination chemotherapy and combined modality therapy for locally advanced gastric carcinoma. Gastrointestinal Tumor Study Group. *Cancer* 1982;49:1771–1777.
110. Hallissey MT, Dunn JA, Ward LC, et al. The second British Stomach Cancer Group trial of adjuvant radiotherapy or chemotherapy in resectable gastric cancer: five-year follow-up. *Lancet* 1994;343:1309–1312.
111. Zhang ZX, Gu XZ, Yin WB, et al. Randomized clinical trial on the combination of preoperative irradiation and surgery in the treatment of adenocarcinoma of gastric cardia (AGC)—report on 370 patients. *Int J Radiat Oncol Biol Phys* 1998;42:929–934.
113. Abe M, Takahashi M, Ono K, et al. Japan gastric trials in intraoperative radiation therapy. *Int J Radiat Oncol Biol Phys* 1988;15:1431–1433.
114. Sindelar WF, Kinsella TJ, Tepper JE, et al. Randomized trial of intraoperative radiotherapy in carcinoma of the stomach. *Am J Surg* 1993;165:178–186; discussion 186–177.
115. Nakajima T, Nashimoto A, Kitamura M, et al. Adjuvant mitomycin and fluorouracil followed by oral uracil plus tegafur in serosa-negative gastric cancer: a randomised trial. Gastric Cancer Surgical Study Group. *Lancet* 1999;354:273–277.
116. Sakuramoto S, Sasako M, Yamaguchi T, et al. Adjuvant chemotherapy for gastric cancer with S-1, an oral fluoropyrimidine. *N Engl J Med* 2007;357:1810–1820.
117. Paoletti X, Oba K, Burzykowski T, et al. Benefit of adjuvant chemotherapy for resectable gastric cancer: a meta-analysis. *JAMA* 2010;303:1729–1737.
118. Macdonald JS, Benedetti J, Smalley SR, et al. Chemoradiation of resected gastric cancer: a 10-year follow-up of the phase III trial INT0116 (SWOG 9008). *J Clin Oncol* 2009;27:15S.
119. Rudiger Siewert J, Feith M, Werner M, et al. Adenocarcinoma of the esophagogastric junction: results of surgical therapy based on anatomical/topographic classification in 1,002 consecutive patients. *Ann Surg* 2000;232:353–361.
120. Fuchs C, Tepper J, Niedzwiecki D, et al. Postoperative adjuvant chemoradiation for gastric or gastroesophageal junction (GEJ) adenocarcinoma using epirubicin, cisplatin, and infusional (CI) 5-FU (ECF) before and after CI 5-FU and radiotherapy (CRT) compared with bolus 5-FU/LV before and all CRT: intergroup trial CALGB80101. *J Clin Oncol* 2011;29:4003.
121. Valentini V, Cellini F, Minsky BD, et al. Survival after radiotherapy in gastric cancer: systematic review and meta-analysis. *Radiother Oncol* 2009;92:176–183.
121a. Lee J, Lim DH, Kim S, et al. Radiotherapy in completely resected gastric cancer with D2 lymph node dissection: the ARTIST trial. *J Clin Oncol* 2011 December 19. [Epub ahead of print]
122. Walsh TN, Noonan N, Hollywood D, et al. A comparison of multimodal therapy and surgery for esophageal adenocarcinoma. *N Engl J Med* 1996;335:462–467.
123. Krasna M, Tepper J, Niedzwiecki D, et al. *Trimodality therapy is superior to surgery alone in esophageal cancer: results of CALGB 9871*. ASCO Gastrointestinal Cancer Symposium, January 26–28, 2006, San Francisco, CA.
124a. Ajani J, Mansfield P, Janjan N, et al. Multiinstitutional trial of preoperative chemoradiotherapy in patients with potentially resectable gastric carcinoma. *J Clin Oncol* 2004;22:2774–2780.
124b. Ajani J, Mansfield P, Crane C, et al. Paclitaxel-based chemoradiotherapy in localized gastric carcinoma: degree of pathologic response and not clinical parameters dictated patient outcome. *J Clin Oncol* 2005;23:1237–1244.
124c. Ajani J, Winter K, Okawara A, et al. Phase II trial of preoperative chemoradiation in patients with localized gastric adenocarcinoma (RTOG 9904): quality of combined modality therapy and pathologic response. *J Clin Oncol* 2006;24:3953–3958.
125. Stahl M, Walz MK, Stuschke M, et al. Phase III comparison of preoperative chemotherapy compared with chemoradiotherapy in patients with locally advanced adenocarcinoma of the esophagogastric junction. *J Clin Oncol* 2009;27:851–856.
126. Kelsen D, Atiq OT, Saltz L, et al. FAMTX versus etoposide, doxorubicin, and cisplatin: a random assignment trial in gastric cancer. *J Clin Oncol* 1992;10:541–548.
131. Cunningham D, Allum WH, Stenning SP, et al. Perioperative chemotherapy versus surgery alone for resectable gastroesophageal cancer. *N Engl J Med* 2006;355:11–20.
132. Ychou M, Boige V, Pignon JP, et al. Perioperative chemotherapy compared with surgery alone for resectable gastroesophageal adenocarcinoma: an FNCLCC and FFCD multicenter phase III trial. *J Clin Oncol* 2011;29:1715–1721.
136. Klaassen DJ, MacIntyre JM, Catton GE, et al. Treatment of locally unresectable cancer of the stomach and pancreas: a randomized comparison of 5-fluorouracil alone with radiation plus concurrent and maintenance 5-fluorouracil—an Eastern Cooperative Oncology Group study. *J Clin Oncol* 1985;3:373–378.
138. Moertel CG, Rubin J, O'Connell MJ, et al. A phase II study of combined 5-fluorouracil, doxorubicin, and cisplatin in the treatment of advanced upper gastrointestinal adenocarcinomas. *J Clin Oncol* 1986;4:1053–1057.
145. Smalley S, Evans R. *Radiation morbidity to the gastrointestinal tract and liver.* London: Butterworth, 1989.
157. Rubin P, Casarett G. *Clinical radiation pathology.* Philadelphia, PA: WB Saunders, 1968.
159. Cosset JM, Henry-Amar M, Pellae-Cosset B, et al. Pericarditis and myocardial infarctions after Hodgkin's disease therapy. *Int J Radiat Oncol Biol Phys* 1991;21:447–449.
160. Hancock SL, Donaldson SS, Hoppe RT. Cardiac disease following treatment of Hodgkin's disease in children and adolescents. *J Clin Oncol* 1993;11:1208–1215.
161. Hazard L, Yang G, McAleer M, et al. Principles and techniques of radiation therapy for esophageal and gastroesophageal junction cancers. *J Natl Compr Cancer Netw* 2008;6:870–878.

Chapter 59
Pancreatic Cancer

Manisha Palta, Christopher G. Willett, and Brian G. Czito

ANATOMY AND PATHWAYS OF SPREAD

The pancreas lies in the retroperitoneal space of the upper abdomen at about the level of the first two lumbar vertebrae. It is divided into head (including the uncinate process), neck, body, and tail (Fig. 59.1). It has intimate contact with surrounding organs, including stomach, duodenum, jejunum, kidneys, spleen, and major vessels, which can be involved by direct tumor extension. Tumors in the pancreatic head often invade or compress the common bile duct, causing jaundice and dilatation of the bile and pancreatic ducts and gallbladder.

The rich lymphatic drainage of the pancreas is interconnected with duodenal lymphatics. Regional drainage of the pancreatic head is to pancreaticoduodenal, porta hepatis, celiac, and superior mesenteric lymph nodes. The pancreatic body and tail drains to splenic artery, inferior pancreatic, celiac, superior mesenteric, and para-aortic nodal basins.[1] With posterior, retroperitoneal tumor extension, para-aortic nodes are at risk. The main venous channels drain via the portal system to the liver. The lungs and pleura may be involved with posterior tumor extension into tissues with venous drainage by the vena cava or its tributaries. Generalized peritoneal involvement is more common with carcinoma of the body and tail than with carcinoma of the head of the pancreas.

EPIDEMIOLOGY AND RISK FACTORS

In 2012 an estimated 43,920 new cases of pancreatic cancer were diagnosed in the United States, with 37,390 estimated deaths from the disease, making pancreatic cancer the fourth leading cause of cancer-related death in the United States.[2] At present, surgery offers the only means of cure. Unfortunately, only 10% to 20% of patients present with tumors amenable to resection. Even among patients who present with localized disease, the 5-year overall survival (OS) is approximately 20%, and median survival ranges from approximately 13 to 20 months.[3] Contemporary survival rates have reported improved results, particularly in patients with complete surgical resection (R0) and node negative (N0) disease.[4–6] Patients who present with locally advanced, unresectable pancreatic cancer have a median survival of approximately 8 to 14 months, with rare long-term survival. Up to 60% of patients present with

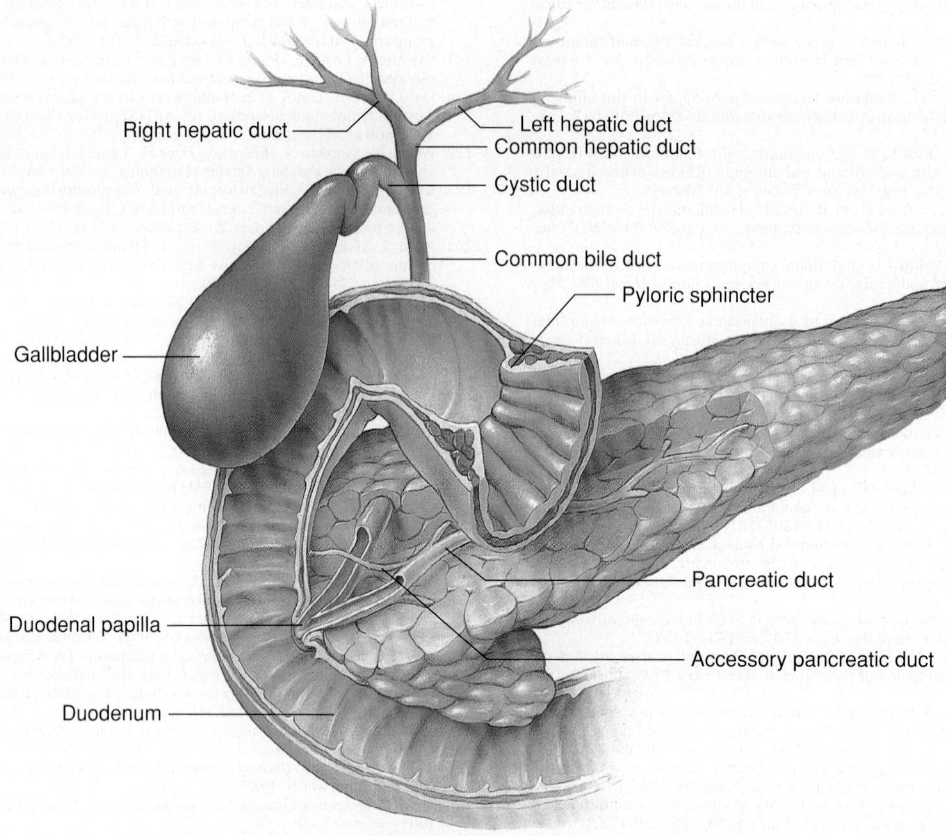

FIGURE 59.1. Pancreas and gallbladder duct anatomy. (Provided by the Anatomical Chart Company.)

metastatic disease, which carries a shorter median survival of 4 to 6 months.[7]

The incidence of pancreatic cancer rises sharply after age 45, with higher rates in males than females (1.3:1) and in black males compared with the general population (14.8/100,000:8.8/100,000).[8] Familial aggregation of pancreatic cancer is estimated in 5% to 10% of newly diagnosed cases. It is associated with *BRCA1/2* mutations, familial atypical multiple mole melanoma syndrome, Peutz-Jeghers syndrome, familial adenomatous polyposis, hereditary nonpolyposis colorectal cancer, hereditary pancreatitis, ataxia telangiectasia, and Li-Fraumeni syndrome, with lifetime risk ranging from 5% to 40%.[9,10] Described risk factors for pancreatic cancer include chronic pancreatitis, smoking, alcohol consumption, *Helicobacter pylori* infection, and factors associated with metabolic syndrome such as obesity and glucose intolerance.[11,12]

CLINICAL PRESENTATION

Most patients with pancreatic cancer experience pain, weight loss, or jaundice. Classically, pain from pancreatic cancer is characterized by radiation to the back, given the organ's retroperitoneal location. Jaundice, due to biliary obstruction, is often accompanied by pruritus, acholic stools, and dark urine color. The initial presentation varies according to tumor location. Patients with tumors in the pancreatic body or tail usually present with pain and weight loss, while those in the head of the gland typically present with jaundice, steatorrhea, weight loss, and pain. Recent onset of atypical diabetes mellitus, unexplained thrombophlebitis, or history of pancreatitis is often noted. Patients with pancreatic cancer frequently present with unresectable or metastatic disease, in part due to these nonspecific presenting symptoms and the tendency for early invasion and metastases. No effective screening method to detect disease at the localized stage has been identified. Positive physical findings, if any, generally reflect incurable disease. These may include a palpable abdominal mass (i.e., pancreas, liver, or gallbladder due to biliary obstruction), ascites, supraclavicular nodes, or palpable rectal shelf (i.e., peritoneal seeding).

EVALUATION

In recent years, significant advances have been achieved in the imaging and staging of pancreatic cancer.[13] Currently, the principal diagnostic tools are helical computed tomography (CT) scan, endoscopic ultrasound (EUS), and laparoscopy. Magnetic resonance imaging (MRI) and positron emission tomography (PET) are emerging imaging techniques in initial evaluation of pancreatic malignancies. These tools have facilitated the characterization of the primary tumor (resectable or borderline resectable vs. unresectable) as well as the identification of metastatic disease so patients can be appropriately and reliably triaged to operative and nonoperative therapies.

The most commonly used staging and diagnostic examination tool is abdominal CT scan. Newer generation, multidetector, high-speed helical CT performed with contrast enhancement and thin section imaging allows high resolution, motion-free images of the pancreas and its surrounding structures to be obtained at varying phases of enhancement. This allows for adequate imaging of the pancreas and assessment of metastatic deposits in other intra-abdominal organs such as the liver.[14] Over 90% of patients deemed unresectable due to vascular involvement by CT are truly inoperable at time of surgery.[15] CT staging is limited, however, in detection of nodal involvement and peritoneal disease. Pathologic confirmation of malignancy is a necessary step prior to initiating therapy for patients with locally advanced tumors; CT can be utilized to facilitate fine-needle aspiration (FNA).

Another tool for staging and diagnosis is EUS. In this procedure, an endoscope with an ultrasound transducer at its tip is passed into the stomach and duodenum, where it provides high-resolution images of the pancreas and surrounding vessels. EUS facilitates FNA without exposing the peritoneum to potential tumor seeding, as may occur with CT-guided biopsy. Sensitivity for EUS is at least comparable to CT, with tumor detection reported as high as 97%.[16] An advantage of EUS over CT is the ability to detect small lesions, which might not be well visualized on cross-sectional imaging.[17] Interpretation of EUS is highly operator dependent. Frequently, endoscopic ultrasound is performed in conjunction with endoscopic retrograde cholangiopancreatography.[18] This combined diagnostic approach allows for staging, therapeutic stenting of the common bile duct when indicated, and diagnostic FNA simultaneously.

A limitation of current imaging techniques is the inability to visualize small (1 to 2 mm) liver and peritoneal implants. Staging laparoscopy has been used preoperatively to assess for intraperitoneal metastases. A recent meta-analysis demonstrated that the adoption of staging laparoscopy and laparoscopic ultrasound will prevent up to 50% of patients from undergoing unnecessary laparotomy.[19] Patients with locally advanced disease and involved peritoneal washings or positive peritoneal biopsies have the same prognosis as those with metastatic disease; these patients are more appropriately treated with systemic therapies.[20]

Advances in MRI, including high-resolution imaging, faster acquisition time, three-dimensional (3D) reconstruction, functional imaging, and MR cholangiopancreatography have led to an improved ability of MRI to diagnose and stage pancreatic cancer.[14] This modality can be used in patients with poor renal function to assess the primary tumor and determine resectability; however, studies suggest that MRI is not as sensitive as EUS or CT in tumor detection.[21] A potential advantage of MRI is identification of small foci of hepatic metastatic disease difficult to appreciate by CT or to further characterize ill-defined lesions seen on CT.[22]

Initial studies showed that PET has a higher sensitivity, specificity, and accuracy than CT in diagnosing pancreatic carcinomas.[23–24,25] More recent studies have compared integrated PET-CT with PET or CT alone in pancreatic cancers. Lemke et al.[23] evaluated 104 patients, with suspected pancreatic lesions. Integrated PET-CT had a higher sensitivity for malignancy detection than either PET or CT alone (96% vs. 84% vs. 77%) but did not improve specificity (64%). PET may also be a useful adjunct in the identification of benign versus malignant lesions and presence of metastatic disease. Although PET-CT may be useful in initial diagnosis, its role in determining resectability has been questioned as coregistration is often performed with lesser resolution CT images and high metabolism can obscure peripancreatic planes.[26]

High-resolution pancreatic CT and EUS remain the current standard for diagnosis and staging of pancreatic malignancies. Staging laparoscopy is useful in assessing for intraperitoneal and liver disease. MRI and PET-CT are emerging technologies that require further investigation. All image modalities are inadequate to stage lymph node involvement, and further advances may improve the ability to diagnose, stage, and appropriately select further therapies.

TUMOR STAGING

Staging is rarely used in published series, and tumors are instead characterized as resectable, unresectable, or metastatic. A new subclassification of localized pancreatic cancer (borderline resectable) has emerged.

The current American Joint Committee on Cancer 2010 tumor, node, and metastasis staging system is described in Table 59.1. Common criteria of resectability are outlined in Table 59.2.

TABLE 59.1 AMERICAN JOINT COMMITTEE ON CANCER STAGING 2010 CLASSIFICATION FOR PANCREATIC CANCER

American Joint Committee on Cancer (AJCC) TNM Staging of Pancreatic Cancer (2010)

Because only a few patients with pancreatic cancer undergo surgical resection of the pancreas (and adjacent lymph nodes), a single TNM classification must apply to both clinical and pathologic staging.

Primary Tumor (T)

TX	Primary tumor cannot be assessed
T0	No evidence of primary tumor
Tis	Carcinoma *in situ**
T1	Tumor limited to the pancreas, 2 cm or less in greatest dimension
T2	Tumor limited to the pancreas, more than 2 cm in greatest
T3	Tumor extends beyond the pancreas but without involvement of the celiac axis or the superior mesenteric artery
T4	Tumor involves the celiac axis or the superior mesenteric artery (unresectable primary tumor)

*This also includes the "PanIn III" classification.

Regional Lymph Nodes (N)

NX	Regional lymph nodes cannot be assessed
N0	No regional lymph node metastasis
N1	Regional lymph node metastasis

Distant Metastasis (M)

M0	No distant metastasis
M1	Distant metastasis

Stage Grouping

Stage 0	Tis	N0	M0
Stage IA	T1	N0	M0
Stage IB	T2	N0	M0
Stage IIA	T3	N0	M0
Stage IIB	T1	N1	M0
	T2	N1	M0
	T3	N1	M0
Stage III	T4	Any N	M0
Stage IV	Any T	Any N	M1

Used with the permission of the American Joint Committee on Cancer (AJCC), Chicago, Illinois. The original source for this material is the *AJCC Cancer Staging Manual*, 7th ed (2010) published by Springer Science and Business Media LLC, www.springer.com.

PATHOLOGIC CLASSIFICATION

Approximately 85% to 90% of pancreatic cancers are adenocarcinomas. Other neoplasm histological cell types include intraductal papillary mucinous neoplasm, mucinous cystic, solid pseudopapillary, acinar cell, pancreaticoblastoma, neuroendocrine,

TABLE 59.2 CRITERIA DEFINING RESECTABILITY STATUS

Resectable (Head, Body, and Tail)
- No distant metastases
- Clear fat planes around celiac axis, hepatic artery, and superior mesenteric arteries (SMA)
- No radiographic evidence of superior mesenteric vein (SMV)/portal vein abutment, distortion, tumor thrombus, or venous encasement

Borderline Resectable (Head and Body)
- No distant metastases
- Venous involvement of the SMV/portal vein demonstrating tumor abutment with impingement and narrowing of the lumen, encasement of the SMV/portal vein but without encasement of nearby arteries, or short segment venous occlusion resulting from either tumor, thrombus, or encasement but with suitable vessel proximal and distal to the area of venous involvement, allowing for safe resection and reconstruction
- Tumor abutment on SMA not to exceed greater than 180 degrees of the circumference of the vessel wall
- Gastroduodenal artery encasement up to origin at hepatic artery with either short segment encasement or direct abutment of the hepatic artery, without extension to the celiac axis

Unresectable
- Distant metastases
- Greater than 180 degree encasement of SMA or celiac abutment
- Unreconstructable SMV/portal occlusion
- Aortic invasion or encasement

Note: nodal metastases beyond the field of resection denotes unresectability.

Adapted and reproduced with permission from the NCCN Clinical Practice Guidelines in Oncology (NCCN Guidelines®) for Pancreatic Adenocarcinoma (V.2.2012) © 2012 National Comprehensive Cancer Network, Inc. Available at NCCN.org. To view the most recent and complete version of the NCCN Guidelines®, go on-line to NCCN.org.

squamous cell, serous cystadenocarcinoma, and lymphoma. Management and treatment sections will focus on pancreatic adenocarcinomas, given this is the predominate histologic subtype. The histopathology of lesions in the periampullary region of the head of the pancreas is of particular importance as different types of adenocarcinomas, originating from the pancreas, bile duct, ampullary region, or duodenum, respectively, portend different prognoses.[27]

Pancreatic adenocarcinomas evolve from noninvasive pancreatic intraepithelial neoplasias, acquiring various genetic and epigenetic mutations. Several molecular abnormalities have been implicated in contributing to the development of pancreatic cancer. The most frequent genetic alterations are activation of the oncogene *KRAS* and inactivation of tumor suppressor genes including *TP53*, p16 (*CDKN2*), *DPC4* (*SMAD4*), and *BRCA2*, with reported incidences ranging from 50% to 95% in pancreatic tumors.[28] These molecular changes have the potential to help in identifying precursor lesions with a high likelihood of progressing into carcinomas, characterizing pathologically ambiguous lesions, and useful in development of screening regimens.

GENERAL MANAGEMENT

Operative Considerations

Surgery, as part of a multimodality treatment approach for patients with resectable pancreatic cancer, represents the only potentially curative treatment strategy.[29] More than 80% of patients present with advanced disease that is not amenable to curative resection, with roughly two-thirds presenting in the pancreatic head. The standard surgical treatment for pancreatic cancer of the head or uncinate is pancreaticoduodenectomy, first described by Whipple et al.[30] in 1935. For pancreatic tail lesions, distal pancreatectomy is employed, frequently with splenectomy. Initially, high operative morbidity and mortality rates led to technical modifications of the operation that, combined with improvements in anesthesia and critical care, have resulted in current perioperative mortality rates of ≤2% at high-volume centers.[31–32,33] With reduced morbidity from the Whipple procedure, there is no age limitation, and selected patients, even at ages >80 years, may undergo pancreaticoduodenectomy.[34–36]

Several studies report low postoperative mortality rates and appropriate patient selection at high-volume institutions, highlighting the importance of performing such procedures at institutions with extensive experience.[37–40] In addition, the definition of resectable lesions has broadened with the ability to perform venous reconstructions with minimal increase in morbidity or mortality.[41,42] There are no universally accepted criteria for resectability other than absence of distant lymph node involvement or visceral, peritoneal, or extra-abdominal metastases, although the high likelihood of achieving R0 resection should be the ultimate goal.

The prognosis, even among resectable patients, remains poor, with 5-year survival rates of 10% to 25%. The number of nodes harvested appears to impact outcomes; data suggest that 12 to 15 lymph nodes constitutes an adequate assessment, although impact on outcomes may simply reflect accurate staging.[43,44] Although appropriate lymph node dissection is desirable, trials of extended lymphadenectomy conveyed no survival benefit and compromised quality of life.[45,46] Pathologic assessment provides important prognostic information, including margin status, tumor grade, tumor size, lymphovascular invasion, and lymph node involvement. The presence of positive operative margins, poor histologic grade, larger tumor size, lymphovascular invasion, and lymph node involvement portends a poorer prognosis.[47–48,49,50–51] Similarly, patients with elevated pre- and postoperative carbohydrate antigen 19-9 (CA19-9) have inferior disease-free survival (DFS) and OS.[51,52,53–54]

In an effort to minimize surgical morbidity, pylorus-preserving pancreaticoduodenectomy and laparoscopic resection techniques have developed. Pylorus-sparing pancreaticoduodenectomy potentially improves gastrointestinal function without compromising oncologic management.[55,56] Laparoscopic pancreatic resection was first explored in the late 1990s, and its use has increased dramatically.[57,58] Although most experiences are small, retrospective, single-institution series, laparoscopic resection, in experienced hands, appears a reasonable option for distal pancreatic resections.[59–62] The data on laparoscopic pancreaticoduodenectomy are more limited; the difficulty with this procedure arises from more complex dissection and the need for reconstruction.[42,58] However, preliminary data suggest that despite prolonged operative times and potential increase in postoperative fistula formation, laparoscopic resection offers shortened hospitalization and equivalent oncologic results.[58,63–65]

Cause of Death and Patterns of Failure

For patients with locally unresectable tumors or metastatic disease, death usually results from hepatic failure secondary to biliary obstruction by local tumor extension or hepatic replacement by metastases. For the 10% to 20% of patients undergoing a potentially curative pancreaticoduodenectomy, three major sites of disease relapse dominate: locoregional, peritoneal cavity, and liver (Table 59.3). High local failure rates of 50% to 86% occur despite resection because of frequent lymphatic and perineural involvement and cancer invasion into the retroperitoneal soft tissues, with an inability to achieve wide retroperitoneal soft tissue margins due to anatomic constraints (SMA and SMV, portal vein, and inferior vena cava).[50,66,67] The incidence of microscopic residual disease after careful evaluation of the posterior peripancreatic soft tissue margin is as high as 40%.[67] Therefore, tumor stage, grade, and resection margin status are the best predictors of survival after surgery.[66,67] The use of adjuvant therapy after surgery can reduce the incidence of local failure, but distant disease recurrence rates remain high.

RADIATION THERAPY TECHNIQUES

Dose-Limiting Tissues

The dose-limiting organs for irradiation of upper abdominal malignancies include the small bowel, stomach, liver, kidneys,

TABLE 59.3 PATTERNS OF FAILURE AFTER RESECTION OF PANCREATIC CANCER WITHOUT ADJUVANT RADIATION THERAPY OR CHEMOTHERAPY

Author (Reference)	Number of Patients	Local (%)	Incidence of Failure (%) Peritoneal	Liver
Patterns of Failure After Surgery				
Tepper et al. (71)	26	13 (50)	NA	NA
Griffin et al. (69)	36[a]	19 (53)	11 (31)	16 (44)
Whittington et al. (155)	29	22 (85)	6 (23)	6 (23)
Ozaki (70)	14	12 (86)	5 (36)	11 (79)
Westerdahl et al. (72)	74	64 (86)	NA	68 (92)
Patterns of Failure With Surgery and Adjuvant Therapy				
Foo et al. (156)	29	3 (10)	12 (41)	12 (41)
Abrams et al. (87)[b]	29	10 (34)	4 (14)	9 (31)
Paulino and Latona (157)	38	– (25)	– (33)	– (80)
Hattangadi et al. (158)	86	– (31)	– (55)	– (53)
Regine (84)[b]				
Gemcitabine CRT	184	56 (30)	138 (75)[c]	
5-FU CRT	197	70 (36)	140 (71)[c]	

NA, not available; CRT, chemoradiation; 5-FU, 5-fluorouracil.

[a]Ten patients received external-beam irradiation.

[b]First site of failure only.

[c]distant failure.

and spinal cord. Various techniques, such as 3D conformal radiotherapy (3DCRT) and intensity-modulated radiotherapy (IMRT), can spare these organs. Given long-term survival is low, the actual number of patients at risk for late complications is small. Late small bowel and gastric effects may also be decreased through reduction of the volume of these organs within the high-dose field.

Treatment Volumes, Fields, and Doses

In patients undergoing surgery, clips should be placed to mark the extent of the lesion for postoperative irradiation. Used sparingly (e.g., a single small vascular clip placed to mark superior, inferior, lateral, and medial margins), small clips produce only minimal interference on CT scans.

The patient should be positioned supine during simulation and treatment. Until the mid-1990s, conventional simulation was the standard for radiotherapy treatment planning in pancreatic malignancies. During conventional simulation, an initial set of anterior-posterior/posterior-anterior (AP/PA) and cross-table lateral films is obtained after injection of renal contrast medium to identify both operative clips and renal position relative to the field center. Additional films can be obtained with contrast medium in the stomach and duodenal loop in unresected patients.

Three-dimensional conformal radiotherapy represents a major paradigm shift in radiation oncology treatment planning with better visualization of internal organs and target delineation. CT-based treatment planning allows the construction of normal tissue dose–volume histograms and the generation of treatment plans that optimize radiation dose delivery to tumor while sparing critical normal tissues. Despite this advancement, the intent of treatment remains the same. Multiple field, fractionated, external-beam techniques utilizing high-energy photons deliver 45 to 50 Gy in 1.8 Gy fractions to tumor bed, unresected or residual tumor, and lymph node–bearing areas at risk. After 45 to 50.4 Gy, a boost field can be designed to include unresected or gross residual disease, as defined by CT scans and clips, while excluding most of the stomach and small bowel.

With lesions in the head of the pancreas, major node groups include the pancreaticoduodenal, porta hepatis, celiac, and superior mesenteric nodes. Approximately two-thirds of the left kidney must be excluded from the AP/PA field because the right kidney is often in the field due to duodenal (bed) inclusion. The entire duodenal loop with margin is generally included, as pancreatic head lesions may invade the medial wall of the duodenum and place the entire circumference at risk, including the pancreaticoduodenal nodal basins. The superior field extent is often at the middle or upper portion of the T11 vertebral body for adequate margins on the celiac vessels (T12, L1) and the inferior limit at the level L2–3 to include the superior mesenteric lymph nodes and third portion of the duodenum. The upper field extent is sometimes more superior with body lesions to obtain adequate margin on the primary lesion. With lateral fields, the anterior field margin is 1.5 to 2.0 cm beyond gross disease. The posterior margin is often 1.5 cm behind the anterior portion of the vertebral body to allow adequate margins on para-aortic nodes, which are at risk with posterior tumor extension in head or body lesions. The lateral contribution usually is limited to 15 to 18 Gy because a moderate volume of kidney or liver may be in the irradiated volume (Fig. 59.2).

With pancreatic body or tail lesions, at least 50% of the left kidney may need to be included to achieve adequate margins on node groups at risk (i.e., lateral suprapancreatic, splenic artery, and splenic hilum nodes). Inclusion of the entire duodenal loop is often not indicated with body or tail lesions, and at least two-thirds of the right kidney can be preserved. With customized multileaf collimator (MLC) blocking, it is usually possible to cover pancreaticoduodenal and porta hepatis nodes adequately (Fig. 59.3).

After resection, AP/PA and lateral fields are designed on the basis of preoperative CT primary tumor volumes, preoperative duodenal loop location, operative clip placement, and postoperative CT nodal volumes (Radiation Therapy Oncology Group [RTOG] contouring atlas accessible on their website). The anterior border is determined by vascular or nodal boundaries (porta hepatis, superior mesenteric, and celiac), as demonstrated on CT, as well as preoperative tumor location.

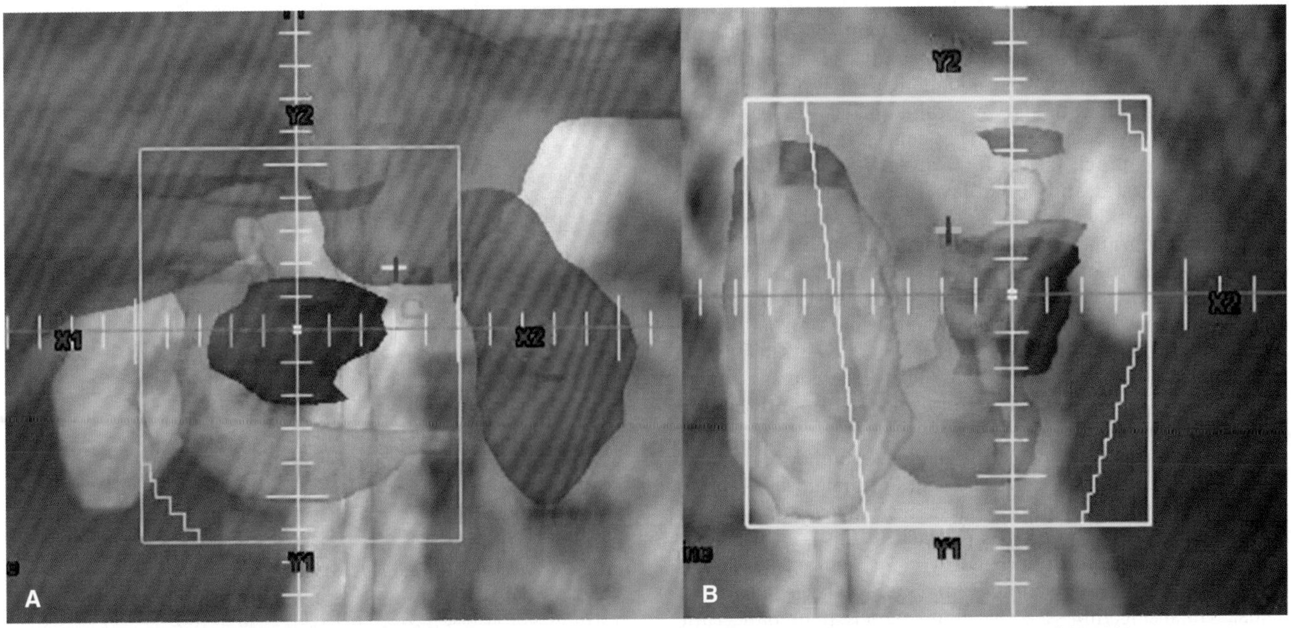

FIGURE 59.2. External-beam four-field technique for pancreatic head lesion. **A:** The anteroposterior/posteroanterior (AP/PA) field, which includes gross tumor (*red*), duodenal loop (*pink*) (plus approximately 50% of the right kidney [*light green*]), liver (*brown*), and nodal areas at risk (porta hepatis: *orange*, superior mesenteric arteries: *green*, celiac: *magenta*). Most of the left kidney (*blue*) is excluded from the AP/PA field. **B:** The right lateral field with an anterior margin beyond gross disease and a posterior margin behind front edge of vertebral body. The liver contour (*brown*) has been removed from lateral field for visualization of other structures.

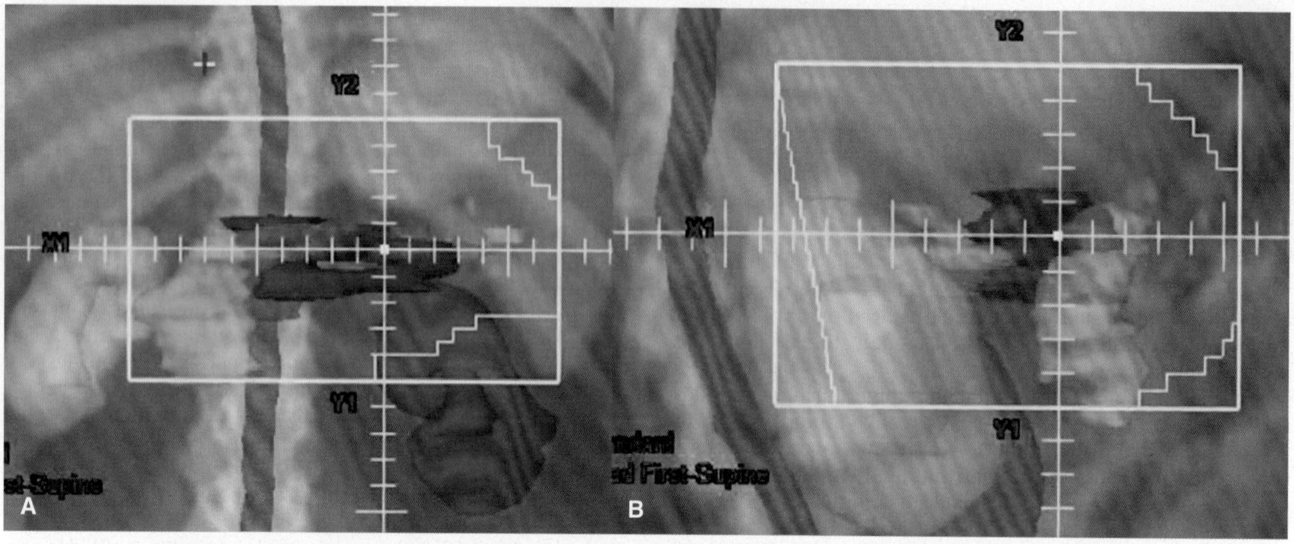

FIGURE 59.3. External-beam four-field technique for unresectable tail of pancreas lesion. **A:** The anteroposterior/posteroanterior (AP/PA) field showing lesion (*red*) and head of pancreas (*green*). The field is extended to the patient's left to include coverage of the splenic hilum (*cyan*). Much of the right kidney (*light green*) is excluded from the field and multileaf collimators block most of the left kidney (*blue*). **B:** The right lateral field with an anterior margin beyond gross disease and a posterior margin at least 1.5 cm behind front edge of vertebral body.

RADIATION THERAPY RESULTS

Resectable Tumors: Adjuvant Therapy

After surgical resection of pancreatic cancer, local recurrence rates range from 50% to 86% and distant recurrence rates from 40% to 90%, most commonly to the liver or peritoneum.[50,67–68,69–72] This provides the rationale for adjuvant therapy, including adjuvant external-beam radiation therapy (EBRT), chemotherapy, and chemoradiotherapy (CRT), which have been employed in an effort to improve patient outcomes (Table 59.4). Despite multiple randomized trials, a definitive role for adjuvant therapy for resected pancreatic cancer has not been established.

Prospective Trials

The Gastrointestinal Tumor Study Group (GITSG) conducted the first multicenter prospective trial of adjuvant CRT for patients with resected pancreatic cancer and negative surgical margins, laying the foundation for the adoption of CRT in the United States. Forty-three patients were randomized to observation or CRT to 40 Gy delivered in split-course fashion with concurrent 5-fluorouracil (5-FU) (500 mg/m^2) as an intravenous bolus on the first 3 and last 3 days of radiation, followed by maintenance weekly 5-FU for 2 years or until disease progression. At interim analysis, improvements in median DFS and OS with CRT were observed: 11 versus 9 months and 20 versus 11 months, respectively. Two-year OS was 42% in the CRT group versus 15% in the surgery-alone arm.[73] An additional 30 patients were later enrolled to receive adjuvant CRT. These additional patients confirmed the survival outcomes seen in the original trial, with median survival of 18 months and a 2-year survival of 46%.[74]

The GITSG trial has been criticized for a number of reasons. The trial closed prematurely following enrollment of 43 of an intended 100 patients due to slow accrual over the 8-year enrollment period. The EBRT approach in this trial was considered low dose and antiquated by contemporary standards due to a split-course technique and use of large treatment fields, which encompassed the entire pancreas or pancreatic bed and the celiac, pancreaticosplenic, peripancreatic, and retroperitoneal regional lymph nodes. Additionally, the inclusion of both CRT and adjuvant chemotherapy after surgery evaluated two treatment variables, making it difficult to discern the true effect of either treatment alone. In the CRT arm, there were issues of compliance, with 32% of patients assigned to CRT receiving inappropriate radiation and 25% of patients failing to initiate treatment within 10 weeks postsurgery, the

TABLE 59.4 PROSPECTIVE, RANDOMIZED TRIALS FOR ADJUVANT THERAPY FOR PANCREATIC CANCER

Series (Reference)	Number of Patients	Median Survival (Month)	2-Year Survival (%)	5-Year Survival (%)
GITSG (73)				
Chemoradiation	21	20.0	42	15
Observation	22	10.9	15	5
Chemoradiation (expanded cohort) (74)	30	18.0	46	17
EORTC (75,76)				
Chemoradiation	110	21.6	51	25
Observation	108	19.2	41	22
ESPAC-1 Pooled Data (78)				
Chemotherapy	238	19.7	NA	NA
No chemotherapy	235	14.0	NA	NA
Chemoradiation	175	15.5	NA	NA
No chemoradiation	178	16.1	NA	NA
ESPAC-1 2×2 analysis (79)				
Chemotherapy	147	20.1	40	21
No chemotherapy	142	15.5	30	8
Chemoradiation	145	15.9	29	10
No chemoradiation	144	17.9	41	20
CONKO (80,81)				
Chemotherapy (gemcitabine)	186	23	30.5	21
Observation	182	20	14.5	9
ESPAC-3 (83)				
Chemotherapy (5-FU)	551	23	48	NA
Chemotherapy (gemcitabine)	537	23.6	49	NA
RTOG-9704 (Pancreatic Head) (84–86)				
Gemcitabine then chemoradiation	187	20.5	31 (3 year)	22
5-FU then chemoradiation	201	17.2	22 (3 year)	18

EORTC, European Organisation for Research and Treatment of Cancer; ESPAC, European Study Group for Pancreatic Cancer; GITSG, Gastrointestinal Tumor Study Group; NA, not available; CONKO, Charite Onkologie; 5-FU, 5-fluorouracil; RTOG, Radiation Therapy Oncology Group.

protocol-specified time limit. Only 9% of patient completed the planned 2-year maintenance chemotherapy course. In addition, survival in the control arm was low compared to historical controls. Despite these limitations and the failure to reach the desired patient accrual, the GITSG trial demonstrated a benefit for CRT, which became standard adjuvant therapy, particularly in the United States.

A second study sponsored by the European Organisation for Research and Treatment of Cancer (EORTC) sought to confirm the findings of the original GITSG study. Two hundred eighteen patients with resected pancreas (n = 114) or nonpancreas periampullary cancers (n = 104) were randomly assigned to observation or CRT to 40 Gy in a split-dose fashion with concurrent continuous infusional 5-FU (25 mg/kg) without further adjuvant chemotherapy. This study showed no significant improvement (P = .208) in median survival (19 months [observation] vs. 24.5 months [CRT]) or 2-year survival (41% [observation] vs. 51% [CRT]).[75] Long-term follow-up of the EORTC trial demonstrated no difference in 5-year OS with CRT use: 22% (surgery alone) versus 25% (CRT). *Post hoc* analysis of pancreatic head lesions failed to demonstrate a benefit with CRT, with a median OS of 1.3 years for CRT versus 1 year for surgery alone.[76]

This trial has been criticized for its heterogeneous patient population, which included patients with both pancreatic and other periampullary primary tumors. Periampullary carcinomas have a significantly better prognosis compared with pancreatic cancer; the two entities thus represent truly different diseases and potentially dilutes any evidence of benefit for adjuvant CRT.[77] Similar to the GITSG trial, older EBRT techniques—split course and low total dose—were used. Also, >20% of patients in the CRT arm did not receive the intended treatment due to postoperative complications or patient refusal. The trial did not include maintenance chemotherapy in the treatment arm. Finally, although a small subset, patients undergoing noncurative resection and patients with positive surgical margins were still eligible for enrollment. The discordant results of the EORTC and GITSG trials have led some investigators to attribute the OS benefit seen in the GITSG trial to maintenance chemotherapy administration rather than to EBRT.

An additional European trial conducted by the European Study Group for Pancreatic Cancer (ESPAC) aimed to further explore the question of appropriate adjuvant therapy for "macroscopically" resected pancreatic cancers. Treating physicians were allowed to enroll patients into one of three parallel randomized studies:

1. Chemoradiation versus no chemoradiation (n = 68), consisting of 20 Gy over 2 weeks with 5-FU (500 mg/m^2) on days 1 through 3, then repeated after a 2-week break;
2. Chemotherapy versus no chemotherapy (n = 188), consisting of bolus 5-FU (425 mg/m^2) and leucovorin (20 mg/m^2) given for 5 days every 28 days for 6 cycles; or
3. A 2-by-2 factorial design of 285 patients enrolled on chemoradiotherapy (n = 70), chemotherapy (n = 74), chemoradiotherapy with maintenance chemotherapy (n = 72), or observation (n = 69).

The data from the treatment groups from all three parallel trials were then pooled for analysis. There was no survival difference between the 175 patients who received adjuvant chemoradiation and the 178 patients who did not receive therapy (median survival, 15.5 vs. 16.1 months; P = .24). In the chemotherapy arm, however, a 35% reduction in death was seen in the group who received adjuvant chemotherapy (n = 238) compared with those who received no chemotherapy (n = 235), with a difference in median survival of 19.7 versus 14 months (P = .0005).[78] On further follow-up of patients randomized using the 2-by-2 factorial design, the 5-year survival rate for the patients who received chemotherapy was 21% versus 8% for those who did not. Additionally, adjuvant CRT was associated with a deleterious effect on survival.[79]

A number of problems are associated with the interpretation of these data. First, the complex trial design has the potential for bias, because patients or physicians could select randomization for one treatment variable. Also, as in the aforementioned trials, the EBRT technique used was, by contemporary standards, considered outdated, using split course and low total dose. No details of EBRT delivery or central quality assurance for EBRT, surgery, or pathology are available. In addition, many treatment violations occurred, as only 62% of patients received full CRT treatment and only 42% of patients in the chemotherapy arms completed the predefined regimen. Although many have attempted to draw conclusions from the updated publication, the 2-by-2 factorial cohort of the study was not powered to detect OS differences. Additionally, patients receiving CRT in the ESPAC trial experienced poorer survival outcomes compared with those in other reported CRT series. Also, patients who had received prior "background" chemotherapy or radiation therapy were still eligible for enrollment. As in the EORTC trial, no maintenance chemotherapy was administered. Despite these critiques, some have speculated that the detriment seen in the CRT group may have resulted from delayed administration of systemic therapy shown to improve survival in the ESPAC trial.

A common critique of the aforementioned trials of adjuvant therapy is the lack of restaging to evaluate for the presence of persistent or metastatic disease after surgical resection and prior to the initiation of adjuvant therapy. The time between initial staging and the commencement of adjuvant treatment can be as long as 3 to 4 months, during which a significant number of patients would be expected to develop radiographically apparent metastases. Without interval restaging, these patients may inappropriately receive CRT. Although these three trials formed the foundation for adjuvant treatment approaches to resectable pancreatic cancer, perhaps because each trial was fraught with flaws, there continues to be little consensus regarding the "most appropriate" treatment. A relative dichotomy in adjuvant treatment approaches for resectable pancreatic cancer has emerged between the United States and parts of Europe, with adjuvant CRT frequently implemented in the United States and adjuvant chemotherapy alone administered in parts of Europe.

Building from the data showing potential benefit to adjuvant chemotherapy, investigators in Europe conducted a randomized phase III trial of observation versus adjuvant gemcitabine in patients with resected pancreatic cancer. Three hundred sixty-eight patients were enrolled on the Charite Onkologie (CONKO) trial and randomized to observation or adjuvant gemcitabine (1,000 mg/m^2) intravenous days 1, 8, and 15 every 4 weeks for 6 months.[80] The primary end point was DFS, and patients treated with gemcitabine achieved a statistically significantly longer DFS (14.2 vs. 7.5 months) than those observed after surgery. This improvement was seen in both the R0 and R1 subgroups. At initial publication, there was no difference in OS. With longer follow-up, median and 5-year OS were both improved in patients receiving gemcitabine (23 vs. 20 months, and 21% vs. 9%, respectively).[81] These findings were supported by a smaller randomized study from Japan, which again demonstrated a DFS benefit for gemcitabine compared to surgery alone.[82] At the same time the CONKO trial was enrolling patients, ESPAC-3, the largest randomized controlled trial in pancreatic cancer to date, enrolled 1,088 patients with pancreatic adenocarcinoma who underwent R0 or R1 resection. Patients were randomly assigned to 6 cycles of adjuvant gemcitabine (3 weekly infusions of 1,000 mg/m^2) or 6 cycles of bolus 5-FU (425 mg/m^2)/leucovorin (LV) (20 mg/m^2). Patients receiving 5-FU/LV experienced significantly higher rates of grade 3 or 4 gastrointestinal toxicity (stomatitis and diarrhea), whereas patients receiving gemcitabine experienced significantly higher rates of grade 3 or 4 hematologic toxicity. At a median follow-up of 34.2 months, there was no difference between the two groups in the primary end point of OS. Given its favorable toxicity profile, in many parts of Europe, gemcitabine alone is considered the standard adjuvant treatment in patients with resectable pancreatic cancer.[83] The focus of future European adjuvant therapies for resectable pancreatic cancer has centered on finding the ideal combination of systemic agents. The ongoing ESPAC-4 trial is accruing patients with resected pancreatic cancer for randomization to gemcitabine alone versus gemcitabine/capecitabine; the trial is expected to close in 2014.

In the United States, however, the GITSG trial laid the foundation for CRT as the predominate adjuvant treatment modality. The RTOG/Gastrointestinal Intergroup trial 9704 was a phase III randomized study comparing adjuvant 5-FU–based chemotherapy to gemcitabine-based chemotherapy, with both regimens followed by CRT. Four hundred fifty-one patients with resected pancreatic cancer were randomized to continuous infusion 5-FU (250 mg/m^2/day) or gemcitabine (1,000 mg/m^2 weekly) for 3 weeks prior to CRT and 12 weeks after CRT. CRT in both groups consisted of 50.4 Gy delivered with continuous infusion 5-FU (250 mg/m^2/day).[84] Prospective quality assurance of all radiation therapy plans was required. This trial was powered to demonstrate a survival benefit for the entire cohort and for the subgroup of patients with pancreatic head lesions. On initial analysis of the pancreatic head subgroup (n = 388), a nonsignificant trend toward improved median and 3-year OS was seen in the gemcitabine arm: 20.5 versus 16.9 months and 31% versus 22%, respectively. However, a higher incidence of grade 3 or higher hematologic toxicity was also seen in the gemcitabine group, with no significant differences seen in severe nonhematologic toxicities.

An update of this trial reported median and 5-year OS rates in patients with pancreatic head tumors of 20.5 months and 22% in those who received gemcitabine, compared with 17.2 months and 18% in those who received 5-FU. On multivariate analysis, in the subgroup of patients with pancreatic head lesions who received gemcitabine, there was a nonsignificant trend toward improved OS ($P = .08$).[85,86]

A secondary aim of RTOG-9704 was to assess the ability of post-resection CA19-9 levels to predict survival. When CA19-9 levels were analyzed in a cohort of 385 patients as a dichotomized variable (<180 IU/mL vs. ≥180 IU/mL, ≤90 IU/mL vs. >90 IU/mL), there was a significant survival difference favoring patients with CA19-9 levels of <180 IU/mL. This corresponded to a 72% reduction in the risk of death.[52] Unlike preceding randomized CRT studies, a major strength of the RTOG study was the rigorous, centralized quality control of radiation therapy techniques and delivery. A recent analysis demonstrated that patients treated per study guidelines had a significant survival advantage, indicating the importance of centralized review and treatment technique in this disease.[87]

The high rates of local failure and need for more efficacious systemic therapy, as well as controversy surrounding the role of CRT is resected patients, led to the design of the current RTOG-0848/EORTC trial. This trial randomly assigns patients with resected pancreatic head adenocarcinoma (stratified based on CA19-9 level, nodal involvement, and margin status) to receive treatment with either gemcitabine alone or gemcitabine combined with erlotinib for 5 cycles. If no progression is seen on restaging following the completion of systemic therapy, patients are further randomized either to receive an additional cycle of the previously administered chemotherapy (for a total of 6 cycles) and no further treatment or to receive CRT (50.4 Gy with concurrent capecitabine or 5-FU) using modern techniques central radiation therapy quality assurance. This trial seeks to answer two primary questions: (a) the role of the small-molecule epidermal growth factor receptor (EGFR) inhibitor, erlotinib, in the adjuvant therapy of pancreatic cancer and (b) the role of CRT in the era of modern chemotherapy, particularly in patients who do not experience early disease progression. This is the only contemporary randomized clinical trial evaluating the role of CRT in the adjuvant setting.

Single Institution Experiences

Reports of single-institution experiences with adjuvant therapy for resected pancreatic cancer have provided additional evidence to the benefit of such. A review of the Mayo Clinic experience reported the outcomes of 472 patients who underwent R0 resection between 1975 and 2005. Despite more adverse prognostic features in patients receiving CRT (higher histologic grade and greater lymph node involvement), median, 2-year and 5-year OS were significantly improved in the CRT cohort compared with patients who received no adjuvant therapy: 25.2 versus 19.2 months, 50% versus 39%, and 28% versus 17%, respectively.[88] A larger series from Johns Hopkins compared 908 patients who underwent pancreaticoduodenectomy between 1993 and 2005 and received surgery alone or CRT. Patients receiving CRT experienced a significant improvement in median, 2-year, and 5-year OS: 21.2 versus 14.4 months, 43.9% versus 31.9%, and 20.1% versus 15.4%, respectively.[89] A pooled retrospective analysis of nearly 1,100 patients from both institutions demonstrated similar results in favor of adjuvant chemoradiation.[90]

Data with the highest survival after adjuvant therapy for pancreatic cancer come from a phase II trial conducted at the Virginia Mason Clinic. Forty-three of a planned enrollment of 53 patients were treated with CRT to 50 Gy with 5-FU (200 mg/m^2/day) continuous infusion, weekly cisplatin (30 mg/m^2), and interferon-α (3 million units) subcutaneously every other day. After completion of chemoradiation, patients received further adjuvant 5-FU (200 mg/m^2/day) by continuous infusion.[91] The 2-year and 5-year OS rates were 64% and 55%, respectively. Median survival was not reached at time of initial publication. With these encouraging data came significant toxicity, as 70% of patients experienced grade 3+ toxicities and 42% required hospitalization. The American College of Surgeons Oncology Group subsequently opened a multicenter, phase II trial evaluating the Virginia Mason adjuvant regimen. Although survival outcomes were promising (median survival 25 months), the trial closed early after accrual of 89 patients due to high toxicity rates. Ninety-five percent of patients experienced grade 3+ toxicity, and 50% failed to complete the entire treatment protocol.[92]

Neoadjuvant Therapy

Even after undergoing curative resection for pancreatic cancer, 80% to 85% of patients will recur. In addition, positive margins or nodal disease increases this rate of recurrence to approximately 90%.[67,93] The use of neoadjuvant chemoradiation offers an alternative approach to improve on these figures for several reasons:

1. Approximately one-third of patients experience a significant delay or do not receive adjuvant therapy following resection.[49,94,95]
2. Twenty percent to 40% of patients will be spared the morbidity of resection as their metastatic disease becomes clinically apparent during course of neoadjuvant therapy.[96–98]
3. Preoperative therapy could theoretically be less toxic and more effective as the chemotherapy and radiation would be given without the postsurgical issues of small bowel in the radiation field, decreased oxygenation and decreased drug delivery to the remaining tumor bed.[99,100]

4. Patients with local, borderline and unresectable lesions may be able to be downstaged to allow for surgical resection and sterilization of the operative region, which potentially facilitaes R0 resection and reduces the risk of spread during surgical manipulation.

Unlike with adjuvant therapy, no phase III randomized trials of neoadjuvant CRT in resectable pancreatic lesions have been conducted, and the vast majority of data come from phase II and retrospective studies. At the MD Anderson Cancer Center, multiple trials of neoadjuvant 5-FU–based CRT have been performed. The earliest trial treated 28 patients with continuous infusion 5-FU (300 mg/m^2/day) and concurrent EBRT to 50.4 Gy over 5.5 weeks. Patients who underwent surgical resection also received intraoperative radiation therapy (IORT). Twenty-five percent of patients had evidence of metastatic disease on preoperative restaging. Fifteen percent had metastatic disease that was found on laparoscopy. For the patients who underwent surgery, median survival was 18 months, and 41% had a pathologic partial response to therapy. However, 33% of patients treated in this study required hospitalization for gastrointestinal toxicity from therapy.[101] In an effort to minimize hospitalization, this group subsequently focused on rapid fractionation EBRT. A prospective trial of 35 patients treated with EBRT to 30 Gy (3 Gy per fraction for 10 fractions) with concurrent continuous infusion 5-FU (300 mg/m^2/day) found grade 3 nausea and vomiting in only 9% of patients with no grade 4 toxicities. Twenty-seven patients were taken to surgery and 20 patients underwent resection and IORT to 10 to 15 Gy. Locoregional recurrence occurred in only 2 of 20 resected patients. Median survival for patients who underwent surgery was 25 months, with a 3-year survival rate of 23%.[102]

Trials of neoadjuvant CRT with paclitaxel as a radiosensitizer have been conducted. In radiobiologic models, paclitaxel may result in enhanced radiosensitization through synchronization of tumor cells at G_2/M, a relatively radiosensitive phase of the cell cycle, and tumor reoxygenation after apoptotic clearance of paclitaxel-damaged cells. In an MD Anderson Cancer Center study, 35 patients received weekly paclitaxel (60 mg/m^2) with concurrent EBRT to 30 Gy. Eighty percent underwent resection with 21% of pathology specimens showing >50% tumor necrosis. The 3-year survival for the patients who underwent preoperative therapy and resection was 28%. Hospitalization was required in 11% of patients for toxicity, primarily nausea and vomiting. These preliminary data show an increased toxicity without a significant improvement in histological response rate or survival.[103]

The French Fédération Francophone de Cancérologie Digestive/Société Francophone de Radiothérapie Oncologique (SFRO-FFCD) 9704 trial incorporated further radiosensitizing chemotherapy. Forty-one patients received CRT to 50 Gy with 5-FU (300 mg/m^2/day) and 2 cycles of CDDP (neoadjuvant cisplatin; 20 mg/m^2) followed by surgical resection in patients without progression. Sixty-three percent underwent curative surgery, with 80% obtaining an R0 resection and 50% of specimens showing major histologic response. In patients who underwent curative surgery, median survival was 11.7 months, with a 32% 2-year overall survival.[104]

The evolution of CRT in the neoadjuvant setting appears to parallel advances made with adjuvant therapy, with transition to gemcitabine-containing regimens. In 2008, two published phase II studies from the MD Anderson Cancer Center evaluated the use of gemcitabine as part of a neoadjuvant regimen. One trial enrolled 86 patients with radiographically resectable adenocarcinoma of the pancreatic head or uncinate. Patients received weekly gemcitabine (400 mg/m^2) with 30 Gy EBRT over 2 weeks. After restaging 4 to 6 weeks post-CRT, 73 patients (85%) underwent surgery, with 64 (74%) undergoing successful resection. Median survival in resected versus unresected patients was 34 versus 7 months, with corresponding 5-year OS rates of 36% and 0%, respectively. In patients undergoing pancreaticoduodenectomy, 11% experienced local failure, with distant failure representing the first site of failure in the majority of cases.[105]

Given the high incidence of distant disease development, a simultaneously conducted phase II trial incorporated induction CDDP and gemcitabine prior to initiation of CRT with gemcitabine. Induction chemotherapy consisted of CDDP (30 mg/m^2) and gemcitabine (750 mg/m^2) every 2 weeks for 4 cycles followed by 4 weekly infusions of gemcitabine (400 mg/m^2) with 30 Gy EBRT. Sixty-two of 90 enrolled patients (78%) underwent surgery and 52 (66%) had successful resection. The median survival for patients undergoing surgery was 31 months, compared with 10.5 months in the unresected patients.[106]

A recent review of the Surveillance, Epidemiology, and End Results (SEER) database supports the use of neoadjuvant treatment. This analysis included 3,885 patients treated for resectable pancreatic cancer: 70 patients (2%) received neoadjuvant EBRT, 1,478 (38%) received adjuvant EBRT, and 2,337 (60%) were treated with surgery alone. Given that the SEER database does not provide information on administration of chemotherapy, this variable could not be assessed. Median OS was 23 months in patients receiving neoadjuvant EBRT, 17 months with adjuvant EBRT, and 12 months in the surgery-alone cohort.[107]

Despite the potential advantages and encouraging results using a neoadjuvant CRT approach, no randomized trial results exist comparing neoadjuvant to adjuvant therapy, and its role continues to be investigational. A multicenter, randomized phase II study evaluating neoadjuvant therapy in pancreatic carcinoma has been described. This multinational study is comparing outcomes of patients with resectable disease treated with neoadjuvant gemcitabine-based CRT followed by surgery to outcomes in patients undergoing upfront surgery. Resection is followed by adjuvant gemcitabine-based chemotherapy in both arms.[108]

Therapy for Locally Advanced Carcinoma

Approximately 30% of patients present with locally advanced carcinoma of the pancreas, comprising a group of patients with an intermediate prognosis between resectable and metastatic disease. These patients have pancreatic tumors that are defined as surgically unresectable but have no evidence of distant metastases. A tumor is usually considered to be unresectable if it has one of the following features:

1. Extensive peripancreatic lymph node involvement and/or distant metastases,
2. Encasement or occlusion of the SMV or SMV/portal vein confluence that is not amenable to reconstruction, or
3. ≥180 degree involvement of the SMA; involvement of the inferior vena cava, aorta, or celiac axis.

Recent advances in surgical technique allow for resection of selected patients with tumors involving the SMV.[41,109] Treatment with radiation and chemotherapy increases median survival for patients with locally advanced cancers to approximately 8 to 14 months but rarely results in long-term survival. The therapeutic options of patients with locally advanced pancreatic cancer include chemotherapy alone, CRT, IORT, and more recently EBRT with novel chemotherapeutic and targeted agents. In evaluating the results of these various therapies, it is useful to remember that a median survival of 3 to 6 months has been reported for this subset of patients undergoing palliative gastric or biliary bypass only.[110]

Prospective Trials

Prospective trials have evaluated the role of EBRT versus CRT, variations in CRT regimens, and CRT versus chemotherapy alone. With conflicting results, there is little consensus as to the appropriate management of locally advanced patients, and all are considered reasonable options (Table 59.5). The Mayo Clinic undertook an early randomized trial in the 1960s in which 64 patients with locally unresectable, nonmetastatic stomach, large bowel, and pancreas adenocarcinoma received 35 to 40 Gy of EBRT alone or with concurrent bolus 5-FU (45 mg/kg). A significant survival advantage was seen for patients receiving EBRT with 5-FU versus EBRT only (10.4 vs. 6.3 months).[111]

The GITSG followed with a similar study comparing EBRT alone to EBRT with concurrent and maintenance 5-FU. One hundred and ninety-four eligible patients with surgically confirmed unresectable and nonmetastatic pancreatic adenocarcinoma were randomized to receive 60 Gy split course EBRT alone, 40 Gy split course EBRT with 2 to 3 cycles of concurrent bolus 5-FU chemotherapy (500 mg/m^2), or 60 Gy split course EBRT using a similar chemotherapy regimen. Patients in the latter groups received 2 years' maintenance 5-FU (500 mg/m^2) after EBRT completion. The EBRT alone arm was closed early as a result of an inferior survival rate. The 1-year survival rate in the two combined modality therapy arms was roughly 40% (with no statistical difference between CRT arms) versus 11% in the EBRT alone arm.[112]

The Eastern Oncology Group's trial ECOG-8282 randomized 114 patients to EBRT alone (59.4 Gy) with or without continuous infusion 5-FU (1,000 mg/m^2/day) on days 2 to 5 and 28 to 31 and mitomycin-C (10 mg/m^2) on day 2. There was no difference in response rates, DFS, or OS with the addition of concurrent chemotherapy. Higher rates of toxicity, primarily hematologic, where noted in the CRT group.[113]

Further studies sought to determine a more efficacious CRT regimen. A second GITSG trial randomized 157 and analyzed results for 143 eligible patients with unresectable disease to 60-Gy split course EBRT with concurrent and maintenance 5-FU (500 mg/m^2) (as in the prior GITSG trial) or 40-Gy continuous course radiation with weekly, concurrent doxorubicin chemotherapy (10 mg/m^2), followed by maintenance doxorubicin and 5-FU. A significant increase in treatment-related toxicity was seen in the doxorubicin arm, with no survival difference observed between the two groups (median survival 8.5 vs. 7.6 months). No clinical benefit was seen in substituting doxorubicin for 5-FU.[114]

As studies emerged demonstrating significant survival advantages with gemcitabine-based chemotherapy in the metastatic setting, it was incorporated into the locally advanced setting. A trial from Taipei randomized 34 patients to EBRT with concurrent 5-FU (500 mg/m^2) or gemcitabine (600 mg/m^2). Patients received 50.4 to 61.2 Gy EBRT and maintenance gemcitabine (1,000 mg/m^2) at the completion of CRT. Median OS and time to progression were prolonged in the gemcitabine arm: 14.5 months and 7.1 months (gemcitabine) versus 6.7 months and 2.7 months (5-FU). There were no observed differences in grade 3 or 4 toxicity or hospitalization days between the two arms. Study criticisms include the small number of patients and relatively poor outcomes in the 5-FU arm compared with historical controls.[115]

TABLE 59.5 PROSPECTIVE RANDOMIZED TRIALS FOR LOCALLY ADVANCED, UNRESECTABLE PANCREATIC CANCER

Series (Reference)	*Number of Patients*	*Median Survival (Month)*	*Local Failure (%)*	*1-Year (%)*	*18-Month (est %)*
EBRT Versus CRT					
Mayo Clinic (111)					
EBRT (35–40 Gy/3–4 weeks) alone	32	6.3	NA	6	6
EBRT (35–40 Gy/3–4 weeks) + 5-FU	32	10.4	NA	22	13
GITSG (112)					
EBRT (60 Gy/10 weeks) alone	25	5.3	24	10	5
EBRT (40 Gy/6 weeks) + 5-FU	83	9.7	26	35	20
EBRT (60 Gy/10 weeks) + 5-FU	86	9.3	27	46	20
ECOG (113)					
EBRT (59.4 Gy) alone	49	7.1	NA	NA	NA
EBRT (59.5 Gy) + 5-FU/MMC	55	8.4	NA	NA	NA
Variations in CRT Regimen					
GITSG (114)					
EBRT (60 Gy/10 weeks) + 5-FU	73	8.5	58 (first site)	33	15
EBRT (40 Gy/4 weeks) + doxorubicin	70	7.6	51 (first site)	27	17
Taipei (115)					
EBRT (50.4–61.2 Gy) + 5-FU	16	6.7	56	31	0 (2 year)
EBRT (50.4–61.2 Gy) + Gemcitabine	18	14.5	34	56	15 (2 year)
CRT Versus Chemotherapy					
GITSG (116,159)					
EBRT (54 Gy/6 weeks) + 5-FU and SMF	22	9.7	45 (first site)	41	18
SMF alone	21	7.4	48 (first site)	19	0
ECOG (117)					
EBRT (40 Gy/4 weeks) + 5-FU	47	8.3	32	26	11
5-FU alone	44	8.2	32	32	21
FFCD/SFRO (118)					
EBRT (60 Gy) + 5-FU/CDDP	59	8.6	NA	32	NA
Gemcitabine alone	60	13	NA	53	NA
ECOG (119)					
EBRT (50.4 Gy) + Gemcitabine	34	11.1	12 (first site)	50	29
Gemcitabine alone	37	9.2	30 (first site)	32	11

EBRT, external beam radiation therapy; CRT, chemoradiation; NA, not available; 5-FU, 5-flurouracil; CCDP, neoadjuvant cisplatin; GITSG, Gastrointestinal Tumor Study Group; ECOG, Eastern Cooperative Oncology Group; MMC, mitomycin-C; SMF, streptozocin, mitomycin-C, and 5-flurouracil; FFCD/SFRO, Fédération Francophone de Cancérologie Digestive/Société Francophone de Radiothérapie Oncologique.

A number of trials have compared CRT with chemotherapy alone. A subsequent GITSG trial compared combination streptozocin, mitomycin-C, and 5-FU (SMF) chemotherapy to chemoradiation with 5-FU. Forty-three patients were randomized to receive SMF chemotherapy or 54 Gy of EBRT with 2 cycles of concurrent bolus 5-FU chemotherapy followed by adjuvant SMF chemotherapy. The chemoradiation arm demonstrated a significant survival advantage over the chemotherapy-alone arm (1-year survival 41% vs. 19%, respectively).[116]

In contrast, the ECOG reported no benefit to chemoradiation versus chemotherapy only. In this study, 191 patients with unresectable, nonmetastatic pancreatic or gastric adenocarcinoma were randomized to receive either 5-FU chemotherapy (600 mg/m^2) alone or 40 Gy EBRT with concurrent bolus 5-FU during week 1 (600 mg/m^2) followed by maintenance chemotherapy. Patients with locally recurrent disease as well as patients undergoing surgery with residual disease were eligible for this trial. In the 91 analyzable pancreatic patients, no survival difference was observed between the two groups (median survival 8.2 vs. 8.3 months).[117]

The FFCD/SFRO trial randomized 119 patients to CRT consisting of 60 Gy EBRT with continuous infusion 5-FU (300 mg/m^2/day) on days 1 to 5 for 6 weeks and intermittent CDDP (20 mg/m^2/day) on days 1 to 5 in weeks 1 and 5 with maintenance gemcitabine (1,000 mg/m^2) versus gemcitabine alone (1,000 mg/m^2). Survival was inferior in the CRT arm at 8.6 months compared with 13 months with gemcitabine alone. Higher grade 3 or 4 toxicity rates were observed in the CRT arm during CRT (36% vs. 22%) and maintenance chemotherapy phases (32% vs. 18%). This trial closed early due to poor accrual. Many criticize the inferior survival in the CRT arm, which is similar to early GITSG trials, despite use of continuous infusion chemotherapy and modern EBRT techniques.[118]

The ECOG published results from a randomized trial of CRT (50.4 Gy with concurrent gemcitabine: 600 mg/m^2/week, weeks 1 to 5) versus gemcitabine alone (1,000 mg/m^2/week). The trial closed early due to poor accrual. Analysis of the eligible, randomized 71 patients demonstrated no difference in progression-free survival; however, a survival benefit was seen in the CRT arm: 11.1 versus 9.2 months. This benefit came at the expense of higher grade 4 or 5 toxicity rates in the CRT arm (mainly hematologic) but with no difference in quality of life.[119]

At present there is no consensus regarding the appropriate management of locally advanced patients. A meta-analysis of locally advanced patients demonstrated a survival benefit for CRT versus EBRT, but no such benefit was seen for CRT with further chemotherapy versus chemotherapy alone. Many consider upfront chemotherapy alone with subsequent response assessment and directed CRT in responders to facilitate selection of patients most likely to benefit from CRT, and is currently the topic of an ongoing phase III European study.[120] However, many patients with locally advanced disease present with local symptoms (pain, obstruction), in which case EBRT can potentially offer more prompt and durable palliation. CRT (with continuous infusion 5-FU/capecitabine or gemcitabine), gemcitabine-based chemotherapy alone or a combination of both are considered reasonable options in patients with locally advanced disease.

Borderline Resectable Disease

As surgery of the primary tumor remains the only potentially curative treatment for pancreatic cancer; neoadjuvant therapy has been evaluated to assess its ability to convert locally unresectable pancreatic cancer to resectable disease. Although the definition of borderline resectable disease is contentious, the National Comprehensive Cancer Network definition is accepted by many institutions (Table 59.2). Approximately 30% of patients with borderline resectable disease become resectable after neoadjuvant therapy.[121,122] Similarly, there appears to be higher rates of local control, R0 resection, and N0 disease in this patient subset after neoadjuvant therapy.[123–126]

A number of single institution retrospective studies have evaluated this patient subset. The earliest study from the MD Anderson Cancer Center assessed 160 patients with borderline resectable disease. Patients received 50.4 Gy in 28 fractions or 30 Gy in 10 fractions with concurrent 5-FU, paclitaxel, gemcitabine, or capecitabine at radiosensitizing doses. Forty-one percent underwent pancreatectomy with margin negative resection in 94%. Median survival in the 66 patients who completed preoperative therapy and surgery was 44 months, comparable to patients with initially resectable disease.[124]

A review from Fox Chase Cancer Center evaluated 109 patients who underwent resection of pancreatic adenocarcinoma with varying involvement of the portal vein or superior mesenteric vein as determined by CT. Patients received 5-FU or gemcitabine-based CRT. Median survival in the 74 patients who received preoperative therapy was 23 months compared with 15 months in the cohort undergoing upfront surgery. Preoperative CRT was associated with a higher rate of R0 resection and N0 disease.[125]

A smaller series from the University of Virginia reviewed the outcomes of 40 patients with borderline resectable disease. Patients received 50.4 Gy in 28 fractions or 50 Gy in 20 fractions with concurrent capecitabine. Forty-six percent of patients underwent surgery, with 75% undergoing an R0 resection. Patients undergoing surgery after neoadjuvant treatment had similar median survival rates as patients undergoing upfront surgery.[126]

The ECOG initiated a randomized phase II study of two neoadjuvant gemcitabine-containing regimens in patients with potentially resectable cancer. Patients received 50.4 Gy EBRT with weekly gemcitabine (500 mg/m^2) or induction chemotherapy with gemcitabine (175 mg/m^2), CDDP (20 mg/m^2), 5-FU (600 mg/m^2) prior to CRT with 5-FU (225 mg/m^2). All patients received adjuvant gemcitabine (1,000 mg/m^2). This trial, the only randomized trial of borderline resectable pancreatic cancer, closed early due to poor accrual with 21 patients.[127] Although the subject of ongoing study, an approach utilizing neoadjuvant chemoradiotherapy in patients with borderline resectable disease, in efforts to facilitate R0 resection, seems appropriate.

Dose Escalation

Given the limited tolerance of normal tissue in the upper abdomen (liver, kidney, spinal cord, and bowel) to EBRT, total doses of only 45 to 54 Gy in 25 to 30 Gy fractions have traditionally been administered. For an unresectable tumor, this dose of radiation is inadequate, as demonstrated by the high rates of local tumor progression and poor survival seen in both prospective and retrospective studies. Local progression as first site of failure occurred in 58% of patients treated to 60 Gy with concurrent 5-FU in the second GITSG trial.[114] Similarly, the Mayo Clinic reported a local failure rate of 72% for 122 patients with unresectable pancreatic cancer treated with an EBRT dose of 40 to 60 Gy.[128] Attempts have been made to evaluate whether increasing dose of radiation may improve outcomes through 3DCRT, IORT, IMRT, and stereotactic body radiotherapy (SBRT).

In a report from Thomas Jefferson University Hospital, 46 evaluable patients with unresectable disease by laparotomy were treated with 63 to 70 Gy EBRT with or without chemotherapy. Despite high-dose EBRT, the local failure rate was 78%.[129]

IORT is an alternative method to deliver higher radiation doses. This technique allows for administration of a single high dose of radiotherapy with the advantage of enabling healthy tissues to be displaced and shielded from radiation. IORT has been utilized postoperatively and in treatment of locally advanced disease. Institutional reports and a randomized trial have shown that surgery followed by IORT yields lower rates of locoregional recurrence; however, no significant difference in survival has been seen.[130–133] IORT has also been evaluated in patients with unresectable disease.[134,135] A study from investigators at Massachusetts General Hospital reported the results of 150 patients with unresectable pancreatic cancer treated with IORT, EBRT, and chemotherapy. Although the study spanned nearly 25 years, it demonstrated that long-term survival is possible for patients with unresectable pancreatic cancer. Furthermore, this study shows that postoperative and late treatment-related toxicity rates were acceptable.[135] A lower incidence of local failure in most series and improved median survival in some have been reported with these techniques when compared with conventional external-beam irradiation, but it is uncertain whether this is due to treatment superiority or case selection.[128]

Advances in radiation technique and delivery, such as IMRT and SBRT, also enable dose escalation and potential sparing of normal tissues. IMRT is a technique that breaks up a typical radiation treatment field into smaller beamlets. It is implemented either as dynamic IMRT (collimating leaves move in and out of the radiation beam path during treatment) or as "step-and-shoot" IMRT (leaves change field shape while the machine is off). The cumulative effect is that the prescription dose conforms around delineated target volumes, significantly reducing doses to adjacent normal tissues. This technology has increasingly been used in a number of gastrointestinal malignancies, including pancreatic cancer. Early clinical data support both the feasibility of this technique and its potential for reducing acute gastrointestinal toxicity.[136–138]

An analysis from the University of Maryland evaluated 46 patients treated with IMRT and concurrent 5-FU–based chemotherapy. Acute toxicities in these patients were compared with those in a control group enrolled in RTOG-9704 who received conventional 3D treatment. There was a statistically significant reduction in acute grade 3 or 4 gastrointestinal toxicity in the patients who received radiotherapy via IMRT compared with those who received 3D conformal radiotherapy.[138] IMRT can also result in a significant reduction of dose to normal structures, including the liver, kidneys, stomach, and small bowel.[137] This may allow alternate novel systemic agents to be administered with radiotherapy.[136]

Another radiation technique being investigated in the treatment of pancreatic cancers is SBRT, which involves the delivery of high dose-per-fraction radiation treatments over a small number of fractions (generally 1 to 5 treatments), utilizing techniques that allow very highly conformal dose delivery of external-beam radiotherapy. The postulated advantage of SBRT is potentially improving local control through the delivery of ablative doses of radiation, while minimizing associated side effects. Few institutions have published experience using this technique, and the data are largely in the setting of locally advanced disease.[139,140] Stanford University has implemented an institutional protocol for the treatment of locally advanced pancreatic cancer using a 25-Gy single fraction with systemic therapy. This single, high dose of radiation has been estimated to result in delivery of a higher biologically equivalent dose compared with a more standard, protracted course of radiation therapy, albeit at the potential for increased risk of normal tissue injury. A report from these investigators described 77 patients who were treated with SBRT and found that freedom from local progression was 91% at 6 months and 84% at 12 months. No patients experienced grade 3 acute toxicity and 9% had grade 3 or higher late toxicity.[140] Ultimately, the role of IMRT and SBRT in treatment of pancreatic cancer remains to be further defined and is currently investigational. The minimal gain with dose escalation and high rates of local and distant failures begs for improvements in both local and systemic therapies.

Chemoradiation Effects on Quality of Life

Despite the potential survival benefits for patients with locally advanced pancreatic cancer receiving therapy compared to supportive care, these gains are modest. With rare exception, all patients will ultimately succumb to their disease. In spite of this, significant palliative benefit can be achieved by chemoradiation. Pain, anorexia, fatigue, and cachexia are relatively common symptoms, which significantly impact a patient's quality of life. When using EBRT with or without chemotherapy, approximately 35% to 65% of patients will experience pain resolution as well as some improvement in cachexia and obstructive symptoms.[114,141,142] Definite but less dramatic improvements in performance status and anorexia may be observed as well.[141,142] Palliation from therapy can take many weeks for maximal effect, and alternative treatments, such as biliary and duodenal stents, may provide more rapid relief of obstructive symptoms. Given the high mortality rate associated with pancreatic cancer, quality of life should be a study end point in trials for these patients.

TARGETED THERAPIES AND FUTURE DIRECTIONS

There is much room for improvement in the diagnosis and treatment of pancreatic cancer. Screening of high-risk individuals may allow for detection of disease in earlier disease states by means of novel imaging methods or assessment of serum biomarkers.[143,144] As the biological basis of cancer is better understood, the successful use of cancer-specific targeted therapies in other cancers supports the need to identify new targets and better predictors of response to therapy in pancreatic cancer.

There is evidence of additive or synergistic effects for several targeted agents (such as antibodies against EGFR and vascular endothelial growth factor [VEGF] receptor) with both chemotherapy and radiation therapy, making these approaches promising. These targeted agents have been studied most extensively in the metastatic setting prior to evaluation in locally advanced and resectable disease. Currently, the only targeted agent that has shown a modest statistically significant survival benefit in the metastatic setting compared to chemotherapy alone is erlotinib, an anti-EGFR tyrosine kinase inhibitor. However, the survival benefit with addition of erlotinib is small, with median survival increased from 5.9 to 6.2 months and 1-year survival improvement from 17% to 24%.[145] The clinical significance of this difference has been questioned by investigators and treating physicians.

Another EGFR/*HER-1* inhibitor, cetuximab, initially showed promising phase II results in the metastatic setting. Efficacy was initially seen with the combination of cetuximab and EBRT in the treatment of locally advanced squamous cell carcinoma of the head and neck and subsequently tested in a phase III trial.[146] However, in pancreatic cancer, a phase III randomized study of gemcitabine plus cetuximab versus gemcitabine plus placebo (Southwest Oncology Group S0205) as first-line therapy in locally advanced, unresectable, or metastatic disease enrolled over 700 patients from the United States and Canada. No survival improvement was seen with the addition of cetuximab to gemcitabine (6.3 months gemcitabine plus cetuximab vs. 5.9 months gemcitabine alone). Even among patients tested for EGFR expression (90% specimens positive for expression), no benefit to cetuximab was seen in this patient subgroup.[147] An additional phase II study evaluated the efficacy and safety of multiagent chemotherapy in combination with cetuximab. Sixty-nine patients with locally advanced pancreatic cancer received cetuximab, gemcitabine, and oxaliplatin followed by cetuximab, capecitabine, and radiotherapy. Diagnostic cytology specimens were stained for Smad4 (Dpc4) expression. Median overall survival was 19.2 months, and the pattern of failure for patients with Smad4 (Dpc4) expression was primarily local, rather than distant, disease failure.[148] The addition of EGFR inhibitors in localized disease is currently being evaluated in phase I and phase II trials.

VEGF inhibitors bind to receptors involved in tumor growth via vasculogenesis and angiogenesis pathways. Preclinical data have shown that inhibition of VEGF has radiosensitizing effects. Initially promising results in the metastatic setting, however, have ultimately not shown a benefit from the addition of an anti-VEGF antibody to chemotherapy. A phase II trial of the combination of gemcitabine and bevacizumab in 52 treated patients with advanced pancreatic cancer showed a response rate of 21%, a median progression-free survival of 5.4 months, and median overall survival of 8.8 months.[149] In response to these positive results, a phase III randomized study of gemcitabine plus bevacizumab versus placebo (Cancer and Leukemia Group B CALGB-80303) was initiated. No significant difference was observed in OS or PFS.[150] Bevacizumab has also been evaluated in combination with radiotherapy. An initial phase I study of radiotherapy, capecitabine, and bevacizumab led to incorporation in the phase II setting in patients with locally advanced pancreatic cancer (RTOG-0411).[151] Eighty-two patients were treated with radiotherapy to the gross tumor, capecitabine (825 mg/m^2), and bevacizumab (5 mg/kg on days 1, 15, 29) followed by adjuvant gemcitabine (1,000 mg/m^2). The median and 1-year survival rates were 11.9 months and 47%, respectively. These results were similar to prior RTOG trials of locally advanced pancreatic cancer.[152] An additional phase II trial assessed the efficacy of full-dose gemcitabine (1000 mg/m^2), bevacizumab (10 mg/kg), and radiotherapy to 36 Gy (in 2.4 Gy fractions) with maintenance gemcitabine and bevacizumab in patients with unresected tumors with no evidence of disease progression. Median progression-free and overall survival were 9.9 and 11.8 months, respectively.[153] The incorporation of bevacizumab with radiotherapy has not led to profound improvements in treatment outcomes compared to 5-FU–based CRT.

Although improvements with targeted agents have been modest, other pathways are being evaluated. Pancreatic cells deficient in *BRCA* repair pathways are sensitive to polyadenosine diphosphate-ribose polymerase (PARP) inhibitors. PARP inhibitors have been evaluated in ovarian and breast cancer, with response rates of 40%; clinical trials of PARP inhibitors in treatment of pancreatic cancer are under way.[7] Other therapeutic agents under evaluation include hedgehog pathway inhibitors, multikinase inhibitors (sorafenib), and agents targeting v-src sarcoma, γ-secretase, stem cell factor receptor (c-kit), secreted protein acidic and rich in cysteine, mitogen-activated protein kinase, mesothelin, *RAS*, prostate stem cell antigen, tumor necrosis factor-α, Mucin-1, mammalian target of rapamycin, tumor necrosis factor superfamily member 10, and type 1 insulin-like growth factor receptor.[7,154]

SUMMARY

Treatment of pancreatic cancer remains a challenge in oncology. Despite advances in many aspects of oncologic evaluation and management, including preoperative evaluation, surgical techniques, perioperative care, systemic therapy, and radiotherapy, the 5-year OS rate for patients with resectable pancreatic cancer remains around 20%. Local tumor control has been improved by the use of specialized radiation techniques, allowing safe dose escalation. Even with these techniques, it is not clear that a survival benefit is achieved given the proclivity of metastases in this malignancy. Further advances in systemic therapies, study of the optimal sequencing of therapies, earlier detection of disease, and development of new and novel therapeutic options are urgently needed in the treatment of this formidable disease. Despite the recognized limitations of current therapy, palliation can be achieved for a high percentage of patients through combined modality treatment. Quality of life should be considered a paramount end point in the care and protocol design of clinical trials for these patients. In patients with marginal or poor performance status, gemcitabine administration alone represents a reasonable alternative to combined modality therapy. Significant improvements in long-term survival will likely be achieved through ongoing attempts at exploitation of the malignancy's basic biologic anomalies.

SELECTED REFERENCES

A full list of references for this chapter is available online.

1. American Joint Committee on Cancer. *AJCC cancer staging manual.* New York: Springer-Verlag, 2010.
2. Siegel R, Naishadham D, Jemal A. Cancer statistics, 2012. *CA Cancer J Clin* 2012; 62(1):10–29.
7. Vincent A, et al. Pancreatic cancer. *Lancet* 2011;378(9791):607–620.
13. Willett CG, et al. Locally advanced pancreatic cancer. *J Clin Oncol* 2005;23(20): 4538–4544.
14. Kinney T. Evidence-based imaging of pancreatic malignancies. *Surg Clin North Am* 2010;90(2):235–249.
15. Karmazanovsky G, et al. Pancreatic head cancer: accuracy of CT in determination of resectability. *Abdom Imaging* 2005;30(4):488–500.
19. Hariharan D, et al. The role of laparoscopy and laparoscopic ultrasound in the preoperative staging of pancreatico-biliary cancers—a meta-analysis. *Eur J Surg Oncol* 2010;36(10):941–948.
21. Bipat S, et al. Ultrasonography, computed tomography and magnetic resonance imaging for diagnosis and determining resectability of pancreatic adenocarcinoma: a meta-analysis. *J Comput Assist Tomogr* 2005;29(4):438–445.
23. Lemke AJ, et al. Retrospective digital image fusion of multidetector CT and 18F-FDG PET: clinical value in pancreatic lesions—a prospective study with 104 patients. *J Nucl Med* 2004;45(8):1279–1286.
24. Sachelarie I, et al. Integrated PET-CT: evidence-based review of oncology indications. *Oncology (Williston Park)* 2005;19(4):481–490; discussion 490–492, 495–496.
26. Grassetto G, Rubello D. Role of FDG-PET/CT in diagnosis, staging, response to treatment, and prognosis of pancreatic cancer. *Am J Clin Oncol* 2011;34(2):111–114.
30. Whipple AO, Parsons WB, Mullins CR. Treatment of carcinoma of the ampulla of Vater. *Ann Surg* 1935;102(4):763–779.
33. Cameron JL, et al. One thousand consecutive pancreaticoduodenectomies. *Ann Surg* 2006;244(1):10–15.
43. Slidell MB, et al. Impact of total lymph node count and lymph node ratio on staging and survival after pancreatectomy for pancreatic adenocarcinoma: a large, population-based analysis. *Ann Surg Oncol* 2008;15(1):165–174.
46. Farnell MB, et al. A prospective randomized trial comparing standard pancreatoduodenectomy with pancreatoduodenectomy with extended lymphadenectomy in resectable pancreatic head adenocarcinoma. *Surgery* 2005;138(4):618–630.
49. Sohn TA, et al. Resected adenocarcinoma of the pancreas—616 patients: results, outcomes, and prognostic indicators. *J Gastrointest Surg* 2000;4(6):567–579.
52. Berger AC, et al. Postresection CA19-9 predicts overall survival in patients with pancreatic cancer treated with adjuvant chemoradiation: a prospective validation by RTOG 9704. *J Clin Oncol* 2008;26(36):5918–5922.
55. Iqbal N, et al. A comparison of pancreaticoduodenectomy with pylorus preserving pancreaticoduodenectomy: a meta-analysis of 2822 patients. *Eur J Surg Oncol* 2008;34(11):1237–1245.
58. Kooby DA, Chu CK. Laparoscopic management of pancreatic malignancies. *Surg Clin North Am* 2010;90(2):427–446.
66. Allema JH, et al. Prognostic factors for survival after pancreaticoduodenectomy for patients with carcinoma of the pancreatic head region. *Cancer* 1995;75(8): 2069–2076.
67. Willett CG, et al. Resection margins in carcinoma of the head of the pancreas. Implications for radiation therapy. *Ann Surg* 1993;217(2):144–148.
68. Allema JH, et al. Results of pancreaticoduodenectomy for ampullary carcinoma and analysis of prognostic factors for survival. *Surgery* 1995;117(3):247–253.
73. Kalser MH, Ellenberg SS. Pancreatic cancer. Adjuvant combined radiation and chemotherapy following curative resection. *Arch Surg* 1985;120(8):899–903.
74. Further evidence of effective adjuvant combined radiation and chemotherapy following curative resection of pancreatic cancer. Gastrointestinal Tumor Study Group. *Cancer* 1987;59(12):2006–2010.
75. Klinkenbijl JH, et al. Adjuvant radiotherapy and 5-fluorouracil after curative resection of cancer of the pancreas and periampullary region: phase III trial of the EORTC gastrointestinal tract cancer cooperative group. *Ann Surg* 1999; 230(6):776–784.
76. Smeenk HG, et al. Long-term survival and metastatic pattern of pancreatic and periampullary cancer after adjuvant chemoradiation or observation: long-term results of EORTC trial 40891. *Ann Surg* 2007;246(5):734–740.
78. Neoptolemos JP, et al. Adjuvant chemoradiotherapy and chemotherapy in resectable pancreatic cancer: a randomised controlled trial. *Lancet* 2001;358(9293): 1576–1585.
79. Neoptolemos JP, et al. A randomized trial of chemoradiotherapy and chemotherapy after resection of pancreatic cancer. *N Engl J Med* 2004;350(12):1200–1210.
80. Oettle H, et al. Adjuvant chemotherapy with gemcitabine vs observation in patients undergoing curative-intent resection of pancreatic cancer: a randomized controlled trial. *JAMA* 2007;297(3):267–277.
81. Neuhaus P, et al. CONKO-001: final results of the randomized, prospective, multicenter phase III trial of adjuvant chemotherapy with gemcitabine versus observa-

tion in patients with resected pancreatic cancer (PC). *J Clin Oncol* 2008;26:(abstr LBA4504).
82. Ueno H, et al. A randomised phase III trial comparing gemcitabine with surgery-only in patients with resected pancreatic cancer: Japanese Study Group of Adjuvant Therapy for Pancreatic Cancer. *Br J Cancer* 2009;101(6):908–915.
83. Neoptolemos JP, et al. Adjuvant chemotherapy with fluorouracil plus folinic acid vs gemcitabine following pancreatic cancer resection: a randomized controlled trial. *JAMA* 2010;304(10):1073–1081.
84. Regine WF, et al. Fluorouracil vs gemcitabine chemotherapy before and after fluorouracil-based chemoradiation following resection of pancreatic adenocarcinoma: a randomized controlled trial. *JAMA* 2008;299(9):1019–1026.
85. Regine WF. Five-year results of the phase III intergroup trial (RTOG 97-04) of adjuvant pre- and postchemoradiation (CRT) 5-FU vs. gemcitabine (G) for resected pancreatic adenocarcinoma: implications for future international trial design. *Int J Radiat Oncol Biol Phys* 2009;75(3):S55–S56.
87. Abrams RA, et al. Failure to adhere to protocol specified radiation therapy guidelines was associated with decreased survival in RTOG 9704-A phase III trial of adjuvant chemotherapy and chemoradiotherapy for patients with resected adenocarcinoma of the pancreas. *Int J Radiat Oncol Biol Phys* 2012;82(2):809–816.
88. Corsini MM, et al. Adjuvant radiotherapy and chemotherapy for pancreatic carcinoma: the Mayo Clinic experience (1975–2005). *J Clin Oncol* 2008;26(21):3511–3516.
89. Herman JM, et al. Analysis of fluorouracil-based adjuvant chemotherapy and radiation after pancreaticoduodenectomy for ductal adenocarcinoma of the pancreas: results of a large, prospectively collected database at the Johns Hopkins Hospital. *J Clin Oncol* 2008;26(21):3503–3510.
90. Hsu CC, et al. Adjuvant chemoradiation for pancreatic adenocarcinoma: the Johns Hopkins Hospital–Mayo Clinic collaborative study. *Ann Surg Oncol* 2010; 17(4):981–990.
91. Picozzi VJ, Kozarek RA, Traverso LW. Interferon-based adjuvant chemoradiation therapy after pancreaticoduodenectomy for pancreatic adenocarcinoma. *Am J Surg* 2003;185(5):476–480.
92. Picozzi VJ, et al. Multicenter phase II trial of adjuvant therapy for resected pancreatic cancer using cisplatin, 5-fluorouracil, and interferon-alfa-2b-based chemoradiation: ACOSOG trial Z05031. *Ann Oncol* 2011;22(2):348–354.
96. Evans DB, et al. Preoperative chemoradiation strategies for localized adenocarcinoma of the pancreas. *J Hepatobiliary Pancreat Surg* 1998;5(3):242–250.
97. Raut CP, et al. Neoadjuvant therapy for resectable pancreatic cancer. *Surg Oncol Clin North Am* 2004;13(4):639–661.
98. Wayne JD, et al. Localized adenocarcinoma of the pancreas: the rationale for preoperative chemoradiation. *Oncologist* 2002;7(1):34–45.
99. White RR, Tyler DS. Neoadjuvant therapy for pancreatic cancer: the Duke experience. *Surg Oncol Clin North Am* 2004;13(4):675–684.
100. Cheng TY, et al. Effect of neoadjuvant chemoradiation on operative mortality and morbidity for pancreaticoduodenectomy. *Ann Surg Oncol* 2006;13(1):66–74.
101. Evans DB, et al. Preoperative chemoradiation and pancreaticoduodenectomy for adenocarcinoma of the pancreas. *Arch Surg* 1992;127(11):1335–1339.
102. Pisters PW, et al. Rapid-fractionation preoperative chemoradiation, pancreaticoduodenectomy, and intraoperative radiation therapy for resectable pancreatic adenocarcinoma. *J Clin Oncol* 1998;16(12):3843–3850.
103. Pisters PW, et al. Preoperative paclitaxel and concurrent rapid-fractionation radiation for resectable pancreatic adenocarcinoma: toxicities, histologic response rates, and event-free outcome. *J Clin Oncol* 2002;20(10):2537–2544.
104. Le Scodan R, et al. Preoperative chemoradiation in potentially resectable pancreatic adenocarcinoma: feasibility, treatment effect evaluation and prognostic factors, analysis of the SFRO-FFCD 9704 trial and literature review. *Ann Oncol* 2009;20(8):1387–1396.
105. Evans DB, et al. Preoperative gemcitabine-based chemoradiation for patients with resectable adenocarcinoma of the pancreatic head. *J Clin Oncol* 2008; 26(21):3496–3502.
106. Varadhachary GR, et al. Preoperative gemcitabine and cisplatin followed by gemcitabine-based chemoradiation for resectable adenocarcinoma of the pancreatic head. *J Clin Oncol* 2008;26(21):3487–3495.
107. Stessin AM, Meyer JE, Sherr DL. Neoadjuvant radiation is associated with improved survival in patients with resectable pancreatic cancer: an analysis of data from the surveillance, epidemiology, and end results (SEER) registry. *Int J Radiat Oncol Biol Phys* 2008;72(4):1128–1133.
108. Brunner TB, et al. Primary resection versus neoadjuvant chemoradiation followed by resection for locally resectable or potentially resectable pancreatic carcinoma without distant metastasis. A multi-centre prospectively randomised phase II study of the Interdisciplinary Working Group Gastrointestinal Tumours (AIO, ARO, and CAO). *BMC Cancer* 2007;7:41.
111. Moertel CG, et al. Combined 5-fluorouracil and supervoltage radiation therapy of locally unresectable gastrointestinal cancer. *Lancet* 1969;2(7626):865–867.
112. Moertel CG, et al. Therapy of locally unresectable pancreatic carcinoma: a randomized comparison of high dose (6000 rads) radiation alone, moderate dose radiation (4000 rads + 5-fluorouracil), and high dose radiation +5-fluorouracil: the Gastrointestinal Tumor Study Group. *Cancer* 1981;48(8):1705–1710.
113. Cohen SJ, et al. A randomized phase III study of radiotherapy alone or with 5-fluorouracil and mitomycin-C in patients with locally advanced adenocarcinoma of the pancreas: Eastern Cooperative Oncology Group study E8282. *Int J Radiat Oncol Biol Phys* 2005;62(5):1345–1350.
114. Radiation therapy combined with Adriamycin or 5-fluorouracil for the treatment of locally unresectable pancreatic carcinoma. Gastrointestinal Tumor Study Group. *Cancer* 1985;56(11):2563–2568.
115. Li CP, et al. Concurrent chemoradiotherapy treatment of locally advanced pancreatic cancer: gemcitabine versus 5-fluorouracil, a randomized controlled study. *Int J Radiat Oncol Biol Phys* 2003;57(1):98–104.
116. Treatment of locally unresectable carcinoma of the pancreas: comparison of combined-modality therapy (chemotherapy plus radiotherapy) to chemotherapy alone. Gastrointestinal Tumor Study Group. *J Natl Cancer Inst* 1988;80(10):751–755.
117. Klaassen DJ, et al. Treatment of locally unresectable cancer of the stomach and pancreas: a randomized comparison of 5-fluorouracil alone with radiation plus concurrent and maintenance 5-fluorouracil—an Eastern Cooperative Oncology Group study. *J Clin Oncol* 1985;3(3):373–378.
118. Chauffert B, et al. Phase III trial comparing intensive induction chemoradiotherapy (60 Gy, infusional 5-FU and intermittent cisplatin) followed by maintenance gemcitabine with gemcitabine alone for locally advanced unresectable pancreatic cancer. Definitive results of the 2000-01 FFCD/SFRO study. *Ann Oncol* 2008;19(9):1592–1599.
119. Loehrer PJ Sr, et al. Gemcitabine alone versus gemcitabine plus radiotherapy in patients with locally advanced pancreatic cancer: an eastern cooperative oncology group trial. *J Clin Oncol* 2011;29(31):4105–4112.
120. Huguet F, et al. Impact of chemoradiotherapy after disease control with chemotherapy in locally advanced pancreatic adenocarcinoma in GERCOR phase II and III studies. *J Clin Oncol* 2007;25(3):326–331.
121. Gillen S, et al. Preoperative/neoadjuvant therapy in pancreatic cancer: a systematic review and meta-analysis of response and resection percentages. *PLoS Med* 2010;7(4):e1000267.
122. Massucco P, et al. Pancreatic resections after chemoradiotherapy for locally advanced ductal adenocarcinoma: analysis of perioperative outcome and survival. *Ann Surg Oncol* 2006;13(9):1201–1208.
123. Greer SE, et al. Effect of neoadjuvant therapy on local recurrence after resection of pancreatic adenocarcinoma. *J Am Coll Surg* 2008;206(3):451–457.
124. Katz MH, et al. Borderline resectable pancreatic cancer: the importance of this emerging stage of disease. *J Am Coll Surg* 2008;206(5):833–848.
125. Chun YS, et al. Defining venous involvement in borderline resectable pancreatic cancer. *Ann Surg Oncol* 2010;17(11):2832–2838.
126. Stokes JB, et al. Preoperative capecitabine and concurrent radiation for borderline resectable pancreatic cancer. *Ann Surg Oncol* 2011;18(3):619–627.
127. Landry J, et al. Randomized phase II study of gemcitabine plus radiotherapy versus gemcitabine, 5-fluorouracil, and cisplatin followed by radiotherapy and 5-fluorouracil for patients with locally advanced, potentially resectable pancreatic adenocarcinoma. *J Surg Oncol* 2010;101(7):587–592.
128. Roldan GE, et al. External beam versus intraoperative and external beam irradiation for locally advanced pancreatic cancer. *Cancer* 1988;61(6):1110–1116.
134. Ogawa K, et al. Intraoperative radiotherapy for unresectable pancreatic cancer: a multi-institutional retrospective analysis of 144 patients. *Int J Radiat Oncol Biol Phys* 2011;80(1):111–118.
135. Willett CG, et al. Long-term results of intraoperative electron beam irradiation (IOERT) for patients with unresectable pancreatic cancer. *Ann Surg* 2005; 241(2):295–299.
136. Ben-Josef E, et al. Intensity-modulated radiotherapy (IMRT) and concurrent capecitabine for pancreatic cancer. *Int J Radiat Oncol Biol Phys* 2004;59(2): 454–459.
137. Milano MT, et al. Intensity-modulated radiotherapy in treatment of pancreatic and bile duct malignancies: toxicity and clinical outcome. *Int J Radiat Oncol Biol Phys* 2004;59(2):445–453.
138. Yovino S, et al. Intensity-modulated radiation therapy significantly improves acute gastrointestinal toxicity in pancreatic and ampullary cancers. *Int J Radiat Oncol Biol Phys* 2011;79(1):158–162.
139. Rwigema JC, et al. Stereotactic body radiotherapy in the treatment of advanced adenocarcinoma of the pancreas. *Am J Clin Oncol* 2011;34(1):63–69.
140. Chang DT, et al. Stereotactic radiotherapy for unresectable adenocarcinoma of the pancreas. *Cancer* 2009;115(3):665–672.
145. Moore MJ, et al. Erlotinib plus gemcitabine compared with gemcitabine alone in patients with advanced pancreatic cancer: a phase III trial of the National Cancer Institute of Canada Clinical Trials group. *J Clin Oncol* 2007;25(15):1960–1966.
146. Bonner JA, et al. Radiotherapy plus cetuximab for locoregionally advanced head and neck cancer: 5-year survival data from a phase 3 randomised trial, and relation between cetuximab-induced rash and survival. *Lancet Oncol* 2010;11(1): 21–28.
147. Philip PA, et al. Phase III study comparing gemcitabine plus cetuximab versus gemcitabine in patients with advanced pancreatic adenocarcinoma: Southwest Oncology Group–directed intergroup trial S0205. *J Clin Oncol* 2010;28(22): 3605–3610.
148. Crane CH, et al. Phase II trial of cetuximab, gemcitabine, and oxaliplatin followed by chemoradiation with cetuximab for locally advanced (T4) pancreatic adenocarcinoma: correlation of Smad4(Dpc4) immunostaining with pattern of disease progression. *J Clin Oncol* 2011;29(22):3037–3043.
149. Kindler HL, et al. Phase II trial of bevacizumab plus gemcitabine in patients with advanced pancreatic cancer. *J Clin Oncol* 2005;23(31):8033–8040.
150. Kindler HL, et al. Gemcitabine plus bevacizumab compared with gemcitabine plus placebo in patients with advanced pancreatic cancer: phase III trial of the Cancer and Leukemia Group B (CALGB 80303). *J Clin Oncol* 2010;28(22):3617–3622.
152. Crane CH, et al. Phase II study of bevacizumab with concurrent capecitabine and radiation followed by maintenance gemcitabine and bevacizumab for locally advanced pancreatic cancer: Radiation Therapy Oncology Group RTOG 0411. *J Clin Oncol* 2009;27(25):4096–4102.
153. Small W Jr, et al. Phase II trial of full-dose gemcitabine and bevacizumab in combination with attenuated three-dimensional conformal radiotherapy in patients with localized pancreatic cancer. *Int J Radiat Oncol Biol Phys* 2011;80(2): 476–482.
154. Hidalgo M. Pancreatic cancer. *N Engl J Med* 2010;362(17):1605–1617.
159. Phase II studies of drug combinations in advanced pancreatic carcinoma: fluorouracil plus doxorubicin plus mitomycin C and two regimens of streptozotocin plus mitomycin C plus fluorouracil. The Gastrointestinal Tumor Study Group. *J Clin Oncol* 1986;4(12):1794–1798.

Chapter 60
Cancer of the Liver and Hepatobiliary Tract

Mirrorer M. Liu, Skye H. Cheng, and Andrew T. Huang

LIVER CANCER

Hepatobiliary malignancies include hepatocellular carcinoma (HCC), gallbladder cancer, intrahepatic cholangiocarcinoma, extrahepatic cholangiocarcinoma, and rare neoplasms such as sarcoma and hepatoblastoma.[1] There were an estimated 696,000 deaths caused by liver cancer in 2008.[2] Liver cancer caused 1.2% of total death throughout the world in 2008. The male-to-female sex ratio was about 2.2 to 1.[3] People who live in eastern Asia, middle Africa, and western Africa have higher incidence of liver cancer than those who live in developed countries.[4]

Patients with liver cancer usually are asymptomatic except those symptoms related to their chronic liver disease. Clinical symptoms are associated with advanced disease; the prognosis is dismal, with a 5-year survival of 0% to 10%. Only one of five patients was amenable to curative resection in the past.[5,6] With the implementation of screening programs with α-fetoprotein (AFP) and ultrasonography, improvement of surgical technique, and liver transplantation, the resection rate can be increased to 30% to 50%.[7,8] The primary curable treatment of hepatobiliary malignancies remains surgical resection, but most patients had inoperable or unresectable disease at diagnosis. For patients with unresectable disease, modalities such as transplantation, chemoembolization, local ablation, systemic chemotherapy, and molecular target therapy were taken into consideration.

HEPATOCELLULAR CARCINOMA

Topographic Anatomy

The liver is the largest solid organ in humans. Traditionally it is divided into left and right lobes separated by the falciform ligament. The surgeon needs to understand the spatial relationship of a tumor to the hepatic vascular system preoperatively to determine resectability. Fortunately, progress in imaging techniques has made segmental division of the liver based on the anatomy of portal and hepatic veins feasible. The most common segmentation scheme proposed by Couinaud divides the liver parenchyma into right and left liver with four segments each (Fig. 60.1). The left part of the liver consists of the caudate lobe (segment I), lateral segment (segments II and III), and medial segment (segment IV). The anatomic landmark between the medial segment and lateral segment is drawn between the gallbladder and inferior vena cava (the falciform ligament). The right part of the liver comprises the anterior segments (segments V and VIII) and posterior segments (segments VI and VII). The anatomic landmark that separates the anterior from the posterior segment is the right hepatic vein; the anatomic landmark that divides the anterior segment from the left medial segment is the middle hepatic vein. No good anatomic landmarks exist that further divide the anterior and posterior segments into superior and inferior subsegments.[9]

Dynamic computerized tomography is very useful in distinctly defining segmental anatomy because the portal vein, hepatic vein, and inferior vena cava can be opacified at the same time.[10,11]

Epidemiology

HCC is the most frequent primary cancer of the liver and ranks as the fifth most common cancer in the world and the third most common cause of cancer mortality.[12] The age-standardized rate of incidence of liver cancer in 1990 worldwide was 14.7 per 100,000 men and 4.9 per 100,000 women.[13] The male-to-female ratio was 3 to 1. The highest incidence rate is seen in the male population of South Korea, China, Gambia, and Senegal (28.5 to 48.8 per 100,000 populations).[12] In low-risk areas such as Canada, Columbia, and the United Kingdom, HCC occurs in only 1 to 3 persons per 100,000.[12] But the incidence rates of primary liver cancer have a trend of decrease among Chinese population in Hong Kong, Shanghai, and Singapore.[12] In contrast, the incidence rates in some low-rate areas such as United States, United Kingdom, and Australia increased. The incidence of HCC approximately doubled between 1976 and 2000 in United States.[14] The most likely reason for this rising incidence is related to a great prevalence of hepatitis C infection.[14]

Risk Factors

HCC is clearly associated with hepatitis B (HBV) and hepatitis C (HCV) viral infections and chronic liver disease. With persistent HBV infection, the relative risk of incidence of HCC could be 223.[15] The risk of HCC is even higher in patients who are HBeAg (e antigen) positive compared with those who are HBeAg negative.[16] As high as for HBV, the relative risk of HCC among persons with chronic HCV infection and cirrhosis is also approximately 100 times the risk of uninfected persons.[17] There also exists a synergistic interaction between the two viruses to cause HCC.[18]

Other chronic liver-cell injury is also associated with the development of HCC. Chemical injury induced by ethanol, nitrites, hydrocarbons, solvents, organochlorine pesticides, primary metals, and polychlorinated biphenyls has been implicated.[19,20] Ethanol is the most common culpable chemical agent and is thought to produce HCC through the development of liver cirrhosis or to play the role of a co-carcinogen. Chronic alcohol use of greater than 80 g per day for more than 10 years increases the risk for HCC approximately fivefold. In patients with HCV, alcohol use doubles the risk of HCC.[21] Environmental toxins, including aflatoxin, contaminated drinking water, and betel nut chewing, may also be associated with the pathogenesis of HCC. Aflatoxins, well-known hepatotoxic agents, are produced by the fungi *Aspergillus flavus* and *Aspergillus parasiticus*. Aflatoxin could contaminate corn, soybeans, and peanuts. High rates of dietary aflatoxin intake have been associated with HCC.[22,23] There is a synergistic interaction on HCC between chronic HBV infection and aflatoxin exposure.[18] The risk of HCC increases dramatically when both factors are concurrently present. Patients with hereditary liver disease, such as hemochromatosis, Wilson disease, hereditary tyrosinemia, and type I glycogen storage disease, are at high risk of developing HCC.[18,24] The common mechanism of developing HCC may be related to chronic injury and inflammation of the liver.

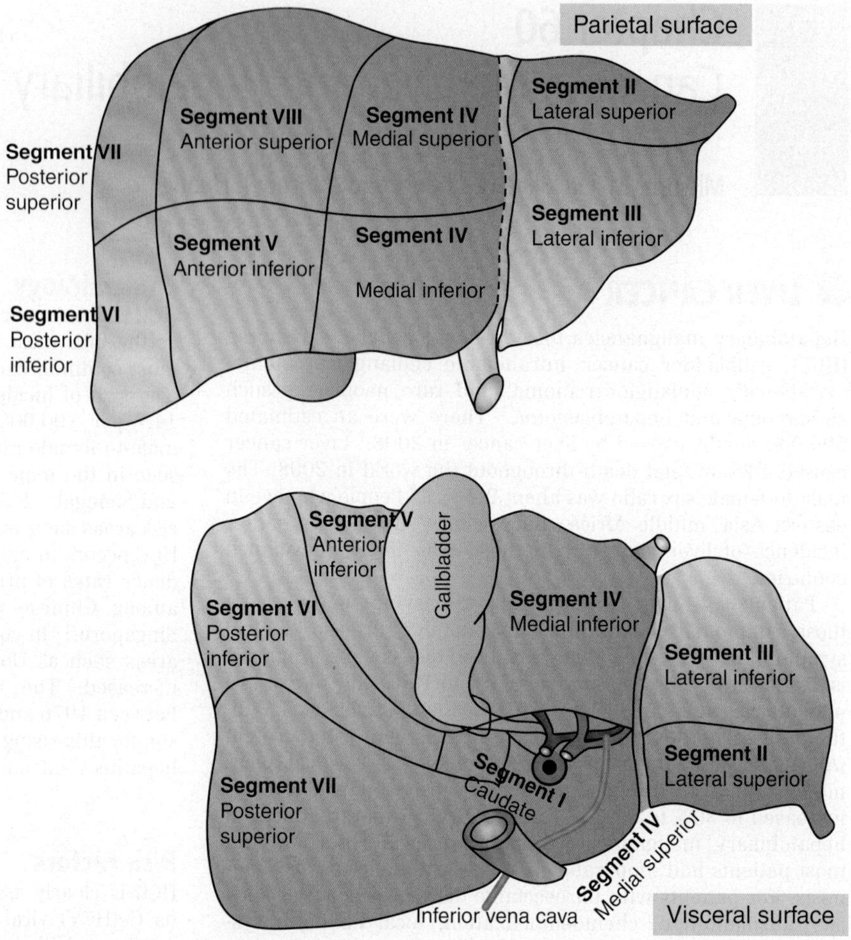

FIGURE 60.1. Segmentation schemes of the liver based on Couinaud's proposal.

Prevention

Because the development of HCC is highly related to the viral hepatitis and chemical injuries, avoidance of viral infection and chemical exposure may be helpful in prevention of HCC. The HBV vaccine has been available for decades. Universal HBV vaccination in Taiwan has showed a significant decrease of incidence of HCC (from 0.70 to 0.36 per 100,000) in children aged 6 to 14.[25] Because the development of HCV vaccination is difficult, the strategies to prevent HCV infection include blood screening, the use of disposable needles and syringes, the adoption of universal precaution for health care workers, and timely treatment of chronic HCV infection with interferon-alpha.[26] Meta-analysis suggests that long-term interferon-alfa treatment may prevent the development of HCC in HCV-infected individuals. The preventive effect is more evident among sustained responders to interferon.[27]

Surveillance

Surveillance for patients with recognized risk factors remains controversial. There is only one randomized controlled trial of surveillance versus no surveillance that has shown a survival benefit,[28] and other nonrandomized studies also showed survival benefit of surveillance in high-risk groups.[29,30] But when taking the cost into consideration, some authors questioned whether adopting a surveillance policy toward HCC should rely on the prevalence of the disease and the resources of a particular country.[30] According to the practice guideline of American Association for the Study of Liver Diseases (AASLD), surveillance is deemed cost-effective if the expected HCC risk exceeds 1.5% per year in patients with hepatitis C and 0.2% per year in patients with hepatitis B. Patients with hepatitis B virus, hepatitis C virus, and autoimmune hepatitis are candidates for surveillance. Current recommendations for surveillance according to the AASLD include:

1. Surveillance for HCC should be based on ultrasonography.
2. AFP alone should not be used for screening because of a lack of adequate sensitivity and specificity for effective surveillance and for diagnosis.
3. Patients should be screened at 6- to 12-month intervals.
4. The surveillance interval does not need to be shortened for patients at higher risk of HCC.[31,32]

Clinical Presentation

HCC in the early stage is asymptomatic; it is generally detected by elevation of AFP or ultrasonography screening or is an incidental finding in searching for other conditions such as chronic liver disease.[33] Even in the advanced stage, some patients are still asymptomatic. Patients with symptoms usually suffer from chronic hepatitis and liver cirrhosis. Clinical symptoms include general fatigue, poor appetite, ascites, jaundice, upper gastrointestinal bleeding, splenomegaly, dilated abdominal veins, palmar erythema, gynecomastia, testicular atrophy, leg edema, and weight loss. Tumor-related symptoms include palpable mass in the upper abdomen (hepatomegaly), acute onset of pain (hemorrhage from tumor rupture), and dull pain in the right upper quadrant of the abdomen, abdominal fullness, low-grade fever, obstructive jaundice, and splenomegaly.[34] Very few individuals with HCC present initially with metastatic disease involving extrahepatic organs such as lungs, bone, adrenal glands, pancreas, and neck lymph nodes.[35]

Diagnostic Workup

In a patient who is suspected of having HCC, the clinical history frequently includes a history of hepatitis, jaundice, blood transfusion, use of intravenous drugs, or exposure to aflatoxins. A family history of hepatitis or hemochromatosis is also an important indicator.[36] Details concerning alcohol abuse and job descriptions related to industrial exposure to possible carcinogenic agents are also helpful. The physical examination should include a search for signs of underlying liver disease such as jaundice, ascites, ankle edema, spider angioma on the anterior chest wall, palmar erythema, splenomegaly, increasing abdominal girth, and weight loss. Evaluation of the abdomen for liver size, existence of tumor masses, tenderness, and abdominal bruits should also be performed.

Blood tests should include serology for HBV and HCV, and AFP. If HBV or HCV serology is positive, quantitative HBV DNA or HCV RNA should be obtained.[37] Evaluation of hepatic functional reserve includes prothrombin time, activated partial thromboplastin time, and serum albumin. Platelet, red cell, and white blood cell counts also should be obtained to look for simultaneous existence of portal hypertension and hypersplenism from liver cirrhosis. Fifteen-minute retention rate of indocyanine green (ICG) before treatment is useful for determining resectability or the feasibility of radiation.[38] The diagnosis of HCC would be included in the differential diagnosis for a patient with underlying liver disease such as cirrhosis or chronic viral hepatitis. In hepatitis or cirrhotic patients, any dominant solid nodule that is not clearly a hemangioma should be considered as HCC unless proven otherwise.[39] Noninvasive criteria for diagnosing HCC suggested by the AASLD in 2005 consisted of serum AFP level >200 ng/mL or a typical enhancement pattern (arterial enhancement and portal or delayed washed out) on dynamic imaging of hepatic mass >2 cm in a cirrhotic liver.[32] The AASLD further validated the diagnostic accuracy of a single dynamic technique showing intense arterial uptake followed by "washout" of contrast in the venous-delayed phases in patients of chronic hepatitis B or cirrhosis of any etiology.[31] But histologic diagnosis of HCC is still recommended for patients who plan to have a nonsurgical therapy.[40] For surgical patients, there is a concern over the possibility of tumor seeding from biopsy or fine-needle aspiration.[40] The reported magnitude of the risk ranges from 1.6% to 5%.[41–43] In patients who have coagulopathy or significant ascites, biopsy or fine-needle aspiration may be contraindicated. At the authors' institution, fine-needle aspirations including cellblocks under ultrasound guidance are routinely performed.[44] Core biopsy of the mass is reserved for patients in whom a definitive diagnosis cannot be made by fine-needle aspirations with cellblocks. Coaxial cannula is used with fine-needle or core biopsies to reduce the chance of needle track seeding.[45] In patients who have small hepatic nodules with diagnostic possibilities ranging from well-differentiated malignancy to benign disease, ultrasonographically guided needle-core biopsy should be considered.[46] Ultrasonography, computed tomography (CT), and magnetic resonance imaging (MRI) are the most common modalities used to evaluate tumors in the liver. Ultrasound examination of the liver is commonly used as a screening tool; small tumors are often hypoechoic. As the tumor grows, the echo pattern tends to become isoechoic or hyperechoic, and HCC can be difficult to distinguish from the surrounding liver.[47] Nodules <1 cm should be followed with ultrasonography again at intervals of 3 months. Nodules >1 cm in a cirrhotic liver should be investigated further with four-phase dynamic CT

TABLE 60.1 BARCELONA CLINIC LIVER CANCER TAGING SYSTEM FOR HEPATOCELLULAR CARCINOMA

BCLC Stage	ECOG Performance Status	Tumor Features	Liver Function
0	0	Single nodule <2 cm	Child-Pugh A
A	0	Single or 3 nodules <3 cm	Child-Pugh A-B
B	0	Multinodular	Child-Pugh A-B
C	1–2	Portal invasion, N1, M1	Child-Pugh A-B
D	3–4	–	Child-Pugh C

BCLC, Barcelona Clinic Liver Cancer; ECOG, Eastern Cooperative Oncology Group; N, node classification; M, metastasis classification.

scan. If the four-phase dynamic CT scan cannot prove the diagnosis of HCC, contrast-enhanced MRI or biopsy is the next tool. The contrast-enhanced ultrasound was not recommended in the diagnosis of HCC because it may provide false-positive result in patients with cholangiocarcinoma.[31] Extrahepatic metastases are not common at presentation; they occur mainly in patients with T4 disease. The most common sites of metastases are lung, abdominal lymph nodes, and bone.[48] Routine metastatic surveys in patients with early-stage HCC are not recommended.

Staging

The prognosis in HCC patients is more complex because the underlying liver function also affects prognosis. Several factors have been identified as being important determinants of survival: the severity of underlying liver disease, the size and number of the tumor, vascular invasion, regional lymph node metastasis, and the presence of distant metastases. There is no worldwide consensus on the use of any given HCC staging system. However, most major trials of HCC therapy have chosen the Barcelona Clinic Liver Cancer Staging System (Table 60.1), making it the *de facto* reference staging system.[31] Other systems, such as the American Joint Committee on Cancer's TNM (tumor, node, metastasis) staging system,[49] Okuda staging systems,[50] and the Cancer of the Liver Italian Program scoring system,[46] are also commonly used.

Pathologic Classification

Histologic classification of malignant tumors of the liver includes HCC (conventional), HCC (fibrolamellar variant), cholangiocarcinoma (intrahepatic bile duct carcinoma), mixed hepatocellular cholangiocarcinoma, undifferentiated carcinoma, and hepatoblastoma. The fibrolamellar variant of HCC has a relatively better prognosis. It occurs more frequently in adolescents or young adults and has a more indolent clinical course than conventional HCC.[51] Hepatoblastoma occurs most commonly in young children (median age, 13 to 16 months) and usually presents in an advanced stage.[52,53]

General Management

HCC is often a multicentric disease, especially when it is associated with HCV. The incidence of multicentric disease in HCV-related HCC (53.3%) is significantly higher ($P < .05$) than in the non-HCV-related HCC (7.7%).[54] The risk of multicentric occurrence increases with the progression of chronic liver disease and cirrhosis.[55,56] Although multiple tumors occur less often in HBV-associated HCC than in HCV-associated HCC, the incidence of intrahepatic recurrence of HCC is significantly higher in patients with a sustained HBeAg-positive and high serum concentration of HBV DNA.[57] Despite these observations, the mainstay of therapy is surgical resection. The majority of patients, however, are not eligible for surgery because of the

TABLE 60.2 GRADING SYSTEM FOR CIRRHOSIS: THE CHILD-PUGH SCORE

Score	Bilirubin (mg/dL)	Albumin (g/dL)	Prothrombin Time (sec)	Hepatic Encephalopathy (grade)	Ascites
1	<2	>3.5	<4	None	None
2	2–3	2.8–3.5	4–6	1–2	Mild (detectable)
3	>3	<2.8	>6	3–4	Severe (tense)
Child-Pugh class: A, 5–6; B, 7–9; C, >9					

Modified Child-Pugh classification of the severity of liver disease according to the degree of ascites, the plasma concentrations of bilirubin and albumin, the prothrombin time, and the degree of encephalopathy.

extent of tumor involvement or underlying liver dysfunction. Several other treatment modalities are available, including liver transplantation, radiofrequency ablation (RFA), percutaneous ethanol or acetic acid ablation, transcatheter arterial chemoembolization (TACE), cryoablation, radiation therapy, and systemic chemotherapy.

Surgical Resection

Surgical resection is a reliable method to obtain long-term disease control. The main limiting factor for resection is liver function. In virus-related HCC, the extent of surgical resection of hepatic tumor depends on the functional reserve of the residual liver after surgery. Previously, the selection of patients for resection has been based on the Child-Pugh classification (Table 60.2), but this method is known to be inconsistent. Many Japanese and other Asian investigators rely on the ICG retention test.[57] In Europe and the United States, selection of optimal candidates for resection is usually based on the assessment of the presence of portal hypertension, which is assessed clinically, or by hepatic vein catheterization.[58] Clinically significant portal hypertension is suspected when the platelet count is below 100,000/mm^3, which is associated with significant splenomegaly. The goal of surgery is to remove gross tumor with a margin of 1 to 2 cm of normal liver. Today, however, the 5-year survival after resection can exceed 50%.

Liver Transplantation

Many patients are inappropriate for definitive surgery because of underlying liver dysfunction. The increasing availability of liver transplantation has made this procedure an alternative to tumor resection for selected patients. Based on the Milan study and others, liver transplantation is an effective option for HCC patients.[59] The selection criteria are solitary tumor 5 cm or up to three nodules with tumor size <3 cm. When these selection criteria are strictly applied, excellent overall 3- to 4-year actuarial (75% to 85%) and recurrence-free survival rates (83% to 92%) can be achieved.[59–61] Risk factors of recurrence after transplantation include tumor size, number of tumors, vascular invasion, and persistence of HBV infection.[61–63] A major disadvantage with orthotopic liver transplantation is the unpredictable, potentially long waiting time for donor organs.[63] Living donor transplantation can be offered for HCC if the waiting time would be so long that there is a high risk of tumor progression leading to exclusion from the waiting list.

Percutaneous Ablation

For patients with early-stage HCC who are not suitable for resection or transplantation, percutaneous ablation would be the treatment option.[64,65] Destruction of tumor cells can be achieved by the injection of chemical substances (ethanol, acetic acid) or by modifying the temperature (radiofrequency, microwave, laser, cryotherapy). Ethanol injection is highly effective for small HCC. It achieves a necrosis rate of 90% to 100% of the HCC <2 cm, but the necrosis rate could be reduced to 50% in HCC >3 cm.[66,67,68]

RFA involves the local application of radiofrequency thermal energy to the lesion. RFA is a reasonable option for patients who do not meet resectability criteria for HCC yet are candidates for a liver-directed procedure based on the presence of liver-only disease. The best outcomes are in patients with a single tumor <4 cm in diameter. The efficacy in tumors >2 cm is better than with ethanol. Randomized control trials comparing RFA and ethanol injection have shown that RFA provides better local disease control that could result in an improved survival.[69–72]

Transcatheter Arterial Chemoembolization

HCC is a highly vascular tumor supplied mostly by the hepatic or adjoining arteries and has strong neoangiogenic activity during its progression. This character provides the pathologic basis for the radiological diagnosis of disease. Its also supports arterial obstruction as a treatment option. TACE combines selectively injecting chemotherapeutic agents through the tumor artery followed by intra-arterial embolization of tumor artery with lipiodol, an iodized oily contrast agent, despite two prospectively randomized studies that failed to show significant survival benefit over conservative management in patients with unresectable HCC.[73,74] Systematic review of randomized prospective studies in more recent literature has shown TACE to have a positive impact on survival.[75] For palliative purpose, TACE has been accepted as the standard treatment for patients with unresectable HCC, and it can be used selectively for tumors of different locations and can be repeated if necessary.[1,76]

Radiotherapy

HCC is a radiosensitive tumor.[38] The major drawback of radiotherapy in treating HCC is the poor radiation tolerance of adjacent normal liver and the difficulty of tumor localization.[77,78] Recent technological and conceptual developments in the field of radiation therapy, such as intensity-modulated radiation therapy, image-guided radiation therapy, respiratory gating, and stereotactic body radiation therapy, have the potential to improve radiation treatments by conforming the delivered radiation dose distribution tightly to the tumor or target volume outline while sparing normal liver tissue from high-dose radiation.[79,80] For patients with liver-confined disease treated with conformal radiotherapy with or without TACE, local control response rates ranged from 40% to 90%, and the median survival ranged from 10 to 25 months.[81] Indications for conformal radiotherapy include large unresectable HCC, relieving portal vein thrombosis and obstructive jaundice, failure of prior TACE and as part of combined modality treatment with TACE, and percutaneous ablation therapy.[38,82,83] The combination of TACE and conformal radiotherapy in large unresectable HCC has not yet been defined in any randomized trial.

Radiation Doses

The tumor response to radiotherapy and survival of patients with HCC are related to the dose delivered.[82,84] Partial response was 18% to 23% in unresectable HCC treated with 21 Gy in 7 fractions and increased to 48% with dose around 33 Gy.[85,86] Seong et al.[87] irradiated 27 HCC patients who failed TACE and observed an objective response rate of 67% after a mean dose of 51.8 Gy ± 7.9 Gy. Dawson et al.[84] escalated radiation doses for unresectable hepatobiliary cancer and observed that patients who received radiation doses >70 Gy had better median survival (>16.4 months). It appears that the higher the radiation doses given, the higher the tumor response seen (Table 60.3).

Caution should be given in HBV-related HCC; local radiotherapy may deteriorate liver function by HBV activation, so prophylactic anti-HBV treatment should be considered.

TABLE 60.3 RADIOTHERAPY WITH AND WITHOUT CHEMOTHERAPY FOR UNRESECTABLE HEPATOCELLULAR CARCINOMA

Series (Reference)	Number of Patients	Radiation Dose (Gy)	Chemotherapy	Response Rate (%)
Stillwagon et al. (86) (RTOG)	135	21, 3 qd	Concurrent ADR, 5-FU	22
Order et al. (85) (RTOG)	105	21, 3 qd + I131 10–12 × 2 courses	Concurrent ADR and 5-FU	48
Seong et al. (87)	27	51.8 (mean), 1.8 qd	None	67
Dawson et al. (84)	25	58.5 (median), 1.5 bid	Concurrent HAI fluorodeoxy-uridine	68

RTOG, Radiation Therapy Oncology Group; qd, every day; ADR, doxorubicin; 5-FU, 5 fluorouracil; bid, twice daily; HAI, hepatic arterial infusion.

TABLE 60.4 RADIATION TREATMENT GUIDELINES FOR HEPATOCELLULAR CARCINOMA

Nontumor Part of Liver	ICG (Gy)		
	≤10%	10.1%–20%	20.1%–30%
<1/3	40 (Gy)	No RT	No RT
1/3–1/2	50 (Gy)	40 (Gy)	No RT
>1/2	60 (Gy)	50 (Gy)	40 (Gy)

ICG, indocyanine green; RT, radiation therapy.

From Cheng SH, Lin YM, Chuang VP, et al. A pilot study of three-dimensional conformal radiotherapy in unresectable hepatocellular carcinoma. *J Gastroenterol Hepatol* 1999;14:1025–1033.

Treatment Volumes

Although higher radiation doses have been shown to produce a higher response, patients with HCC usually have liver cirrhosis, which will not allow such doses. Published reports on three-dimensional conformal radiation therapy (3D-CRT) with photon energy suggest that portions of the liver can be treated with higher doses and acceptable complications. McGinn et al.[88] developed a normal tissue complication probability (NTCP) for intrahepatic malignancy. They designed a protocol in which each patient received the maximum possible dose while being subjected to a 10% risk of radiation-induced liver disease based on the NTCP model. The mean doses delivered according to this protocol were 56.6 ± 2.31 Gy (range, 40.5 to 81 Gy). They observed a complication rate of 4.8% (95% confidence interval, 0% to 23.8%), a number that did not differ significantly from the predicted 8.8% calculated on the basis of the NTCP model. This model, however, was derived using patients with relatively normal liver function, and only 4 of 21 of their study population had HCC. The NTCP model for patients with impaired liver function requires further evaluation.[89]

Multivariate analyses demonstrated that the severity of hepatic cirrhosis was the only independent predictor for radiation-induced liver disease. For cirrhotic patients with Child-Pugh grade A, the hepatic radiation tolerance was a mean dose to normal liver of 23 Gy.[90] These authors also suggested a dose–volume histogram for irradiation to normal liver so that the irradiated hepatic volume over 10 Gy, 20 Gy, 30 Gy, and 40 Gy should be less than 68%, 49%, 28%, and 20%, respectively.

ICG retention can be used to guide the treatment of HCC. In HCC patients with normal bilirubin and without ascites, if the ICG retention 15 minutes (ICG 15) is normal, the resection volume can be trisegmentectomy or bisegmentectomy; if ICG 15 is 10% to 19%, the resection volume can be left lobectomy or right monosegmentectomy; if ICG 15 is 20% to 29%, the resection can be subsegmentectomy; if ICG 15 is 30% to 39%, the resection can be done to only a limited area of the liver.[91] Therefore, the authors propose a treatment guideline using the ICG test for 3D-CRT for patients with impaired liver function (Tables 60.4 and 60.5). The authors advise no radiation treatment for patients with Child-Pugh class C liver cirrhosis or prolonged ICG retention unless only a very small portion of the liver is included in the radiation treatment fields.[38]

Stereotactic body radiotherapy (SBRT) to the intrahepatic lesion becomes the option of treatment with the improvement of planning system and linear accelerators. But the large fraction size makes a difference in normal tissue tolerance. There have been many retrospective studies but no universal consensus for hepatic tolerance of SBRT. Son et al.[96] reported that at least 800 mL of normal liver had to receive a total dose <18 Gy to reduce the risk of the deterioration of hepatic function. For lesions beside the duodenum or stomach, Mahadevan et al.[97] reported that 24 to 36 Gy (depending on the distance from the duodenum and stomach) in 3 fractions had acceptable side effects.

Design of Treatment Field

The goal of conformal radiotherapy is to precisely target the tumor(s) and to reduce damage to the surrounding normal tissue. Respiratory organ motion probably is the largest intrafractional organ motion. Aruga et al.[98] studied organ motion involving the use of CT images obtained during both the static exhalation phase and static inhalation phase for upper abdomen irradiation. They found that the tumor shifted between the two respiratory phases. The variation ranged from 2.6 to 23.7 mm: from 0.4 to 5.9 mm in the lateral direction, 2.2 to 24.5 mm in the longitudinal direction, and 0.2 to 11.7 mm in the vertical direction. Breath-gating or breath-holding irradiation may help overcome the problem of respiratory movement during irradiation.[99] In general, the radiation-field margin to the target in the lateral direction should be 6 to 9 mm, vertical direction 9 to 12 mm, superior direction 10 mm, and inferior direction 19 to 21 mm.[100,101] Controlling, gating, or tracking respiratory motion or by the use of image-guided radiation therapy, as previously mentioned, is currently under investigation.[102]

Acute and Late Complications

The dose-limiting tissue injuries in radiation treatment for HCC include the liver, stomach, duodenum, bowels, and kidneys. Acute complications include general fatigue, transient elevation of liver function test, nausea and vomiting (mainly for

TABLE 60.5 COMBINATION TRANSCATHETER ARTERIAL CHEMOEMBOLIZATION AND LOCAL RADIOTHERAPY IN UNRESECTABLE HEPATOCELLULAR CARCINOMA

Series (Reference)	Patient Number	Mean Tumor Size (cm)	Treatment	Overall Survival (3 Years) (%)	Median Survival (Months)
Guo and Yu (92)	107	10.2	TACE–RT	28	18
Cheng et al. (38)	17	8.6	TACE–RT–TACE	58 (2 yr)	>24
Yasuda et al. (93)	44	Range 3–8	TACE–RT	81	NA
Seong et al. (103)	50	8.3	TACE–RT	43%	17
Wu et al. (95)	94	10.7	TACE–RT	26	25

TACE, transcatheter arterial chemoembolization; RT, radiation therapy; NA, not available.

Clinical Radiation Oncology

tumors in the left lobe of the liver), fever, and pancytopenia.[38,87] Subacute and late complications include hepatic failure, radiation pneumonitis, and gastrointestinal bleeding (especially in tumor located in the inferior portion of the right lobe of the liver and radiation doses >50 Gy).[38,103] Hepatic failure can be avoided by an appropriate selection of patients and careful treatment planning.

Results of Combining Transcatheter Arterial Chemoembolization and Local Radiation Therapy

TACE alone rarely produces complete pathologic remission for HCC >5 cm, especially in the peripheral zone of the tumor.[104,105] Additional therapy theoretically is required to eradicate the residual disease. The combination of TACE and conformal radiotherapy shows promising results in large HCC (see Table 60.5). Guo and Yu[92] reported 107 patients with large unresectable HCC treated with TACE followed by external-beam irradiation. The greatest dimension of the tumors ranged from 5 to 18 cm. After a median follow-up interval of 24 months, the cumulative survival rates at 3 and 5 years were 28.4% and 15.8%, respectively, with a median survival of 18 months. Cheng et al.[38] reported on 17 patients with unresectable HCC treated with TACE and conformal radiotherapy. The mean tumor size was 8.6 cm (range, 3.7 to 18 cm). The overall survival rate at 2 years was 58% and local progression-free tumor control was 83%. After 24 months of median follow-up, the median survival had not been reached, and 4 of 17 patients remained progression free (Fig. 60.2).

Another study that combined TACE and local radiotherapy in 50 unresectable HCC patients reported a partial response rate of 66% and survival rates at 3 years of 43%.[103] Wu et al.[95] reported 94 patients with HCC received 3D-CRT combined with TACE. The response rate was 90.5%. The overall survival rates at 1, 2, and 3 years were 93.6%, 53.8%, and 26.0%, respectively, with the median survival of 25 months.

Patients with branch portal vein thrombosis may benefit from combined treatment. Tazawa et al.[106] reported on 19 patients with thrombus in the first branch of portal vein who received 3D-CRT with TACE. Eleven patients (58%) had an objective response, and the 1-year survival rate was 41% (eight patients). Although we do not know yet whether combined TACE and conformal radiotherapy is a superior treatment modality to TACE alone, the results of these studies suggest that in patients with large unresectable HCC, combined treatments could be a promising new treatment modality worthy of further investigation.

Chemotherapy

Systemic chemotherapy for HCC has limited value in clinical practice because only a small portion of patients obtain significant benefits at the price of remarkable toxicity.[107] In general, cytotoxic therapy should be reserved for medically appropriate patients with adequate hepatic function, preferably administered within the context of a clinical trial. The side-effect profile of any chemotherapy regimen should be considered carefully in patients with advanced liver disease and a short life-expectancy.

Several new drugs have been tested recently. One of the more promising of these drugs is gemcitabine. It has a low toxicity profile, but its antitumor activity in patients with advanced

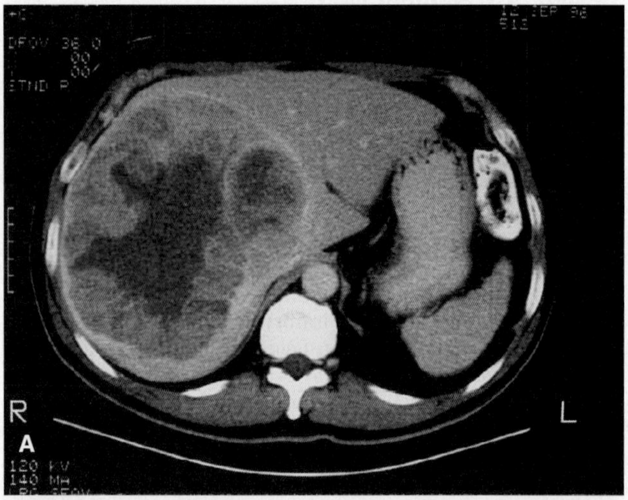

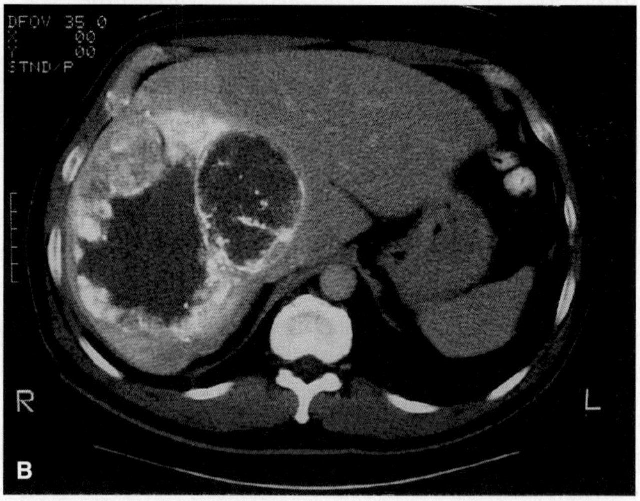

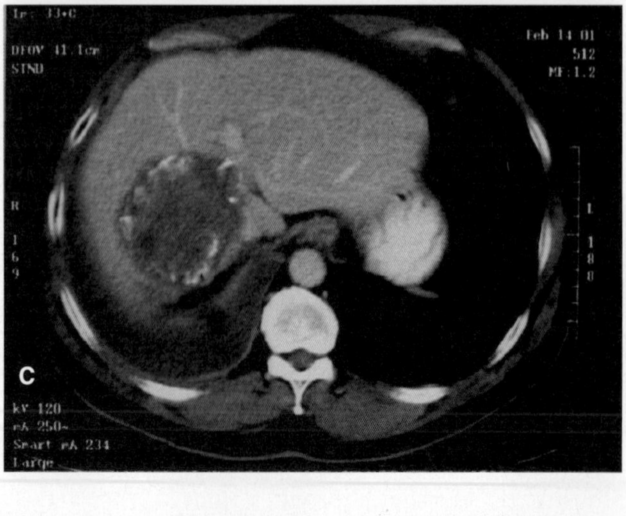

FIGURE 60.2. A: A 55-year-old man with hepatitis B virus infection developed a large hepatocellular carcinoma in right lobe of liver. The tumor measured 12 × 15 × 15 cm. Alfa-fetoprotein (AFP) was 901 ng/mL. **B:** After a first course of transcatheter arterial chemoembolization (TACE), his AFP dropped to 150 ng/mL. It rose to 440 ng/mL 3 months later. He had second TACE followed by three-dimensional conformal radiotherapy. This image was taken after the second TACE, revealing viable tumors in the peripheral zone of the main mass. **C:** Four years and 4 months after the first treatment, computed tomography revealed a non-enhancing tumor in the right lobe of the liver. His AFP remained <10 ng/mL after completion of radiotherapy.

HCC is marginal: the response rate is 18% and the response duration is 35 weeks.[108] Combination chemotherapy regimens have shown better responses. Leung et al.[109] reported on 50 patients treated with intravenous chemotherapy composed of cisplatin, doxorubicin, 5-fluorouracil (5-FU), and interferon-alfa. The partial response was 26% (13/50) and four patients achieved pathologic complete remission. Louafi et al.[110] reported 34 patients of advanced HCC treated with gemcitabine and oxaliplatin. The disease control rate was 76%. Median progression-free and overall survival times were 6.3 months and 11.5 months, respectively.

Molecular Targeted Therapy

Recent advances in molecular biology have uncovered the structures and functions of many cytokines thought to have a strong relationship with the mechanisms of the antitumor effect of biological therapies. Thalidomide, a sedative previously associated with severe fetal malformations, has limited value in the treatment of HCC.[111,112] Molecular targeted therapy to the epidermal growth factor receptor and vascular endothelial growth factor has exhibited the potential to inhibit tumor growth of HCC.[113] The randomized trial of sorafenib has showed statistic significance in median overall survival (10.7 vs. 7.9 months) and median time to radiological progression (5.5 vs. 2.8 months).[114]

Areas of Failure and Cause of Death

Survival of HCC after treatment depends on the clinical stage and liver function. Five-year survival in resectable HCC after partial hepatectomy is 50% to 73% in stage I patients, 30% to 56% in stage II patients, 10% to 29% in stage III patients, and ~10% in stage IV patients.[115,116] The 5-year survival for patients with unresectable HCC is usually <10%.[117] The major cause of failure after resection is tumor recurrence within the liver; this observation still holds true for patients who undergo TACE alone. Extrahepatic metastases in advanced-stage HCC have become more common in recent years, related to improvements in the local treatment of intrahepatic disease.[118,119]

Future Study

The overall treatment outcome in HCC is generally unsatisfactory. The main cause of failure is intrahepatic recurrence. Future efforts should be directed toward prevention of HBV and HCV infection through vaccination in hyperendemic regions and perhaps through chemoprevention for individuals who are already infected and are persistent carriers. Other approaches include early diagnosis in high-risk populations and development of effective adjuvant treatments after resection.

BILIARY TRACT CANCER

Biliary tract cancers consist of cancer of the gallbladder, the bile ducts, and the ampulla of Vater. They are highly lethal because most are locally advanced at diagnosis. Gallbladder cancer is the most common cancer of the biliary tract and accounts for two-thirds of these cancer patients, whereas bile duct cancer accounts for the remaining one-third.[120] The term *cholangiocarcinoma* was used to describe cancers arising from the epithelial cells of the bile ducts, which include intrahepatic, perihilar, and distal extrahepatic biliary tree. At present, surgical excision of all detectable biliary tract cancers is associated with improvement in long-term survival. For unresectable tumors, the purpose of treatment is to palliate symptoms such as obstructive jaundice, biliary tract infection, pain, and ascites.

CHOLANGIOCARCINOMA

Topographic Anatomy

The bile ducts originate within the liver, with the left and right hepatic ducts joining to form the common hepatic duct. At the origin of the cystic duct, it becomes the common bile duct. The cystic duct drains bile from the gallbladder into the common bile duct. The gallbladder is adjacent to the undersurface of the liver.

There is a rich lymphatic network along the submucosa of bile ducts. The primary lymphatic drainage of the biliary tract is to the lymph nodes in the pericholedochal area, periportal region, hepatoduodenal ligament, common hepatic artery, and pancreaticoduodenal groups.[80,121,122]

Epidemiology and Risk Factors

Cholangiocarcinoma is a rare tumor in developed countries; there are approximately 2,000 to 3,000 cases per year in the United States. However, it is one of the most common cancers in endemic areas of developing countries, as high as 87 per 100,000 people in northeast Thailand.[123] Cholangiocarcinoma accounts for about 15% of the primary liver cancer worldwide. But the proportion was different in different regions: 20% in Western countries, <10% in Asian nations, and as high as 90% in north Thailand.[64,124]

A number of risk factors have been identified as important in the development of cholangiocarcinoma, most of which share a history of long-standing inflammation and chronic injury of the biliary epithelium.[125] The major risk factor in Western countries is primary sclerosing cholangitis, which is closely associated with chronic inflammatory bowel disease, particularly ulcerative colitis.[126] The risk of developing cholangiocarcinoma is higher in patients with primary sclerosing cholangitis, ulcerative colitis, and colonic neoplasm than in patients with primary sclerosing cholangitis and ulcerative colitis without colonic neoplasm.[127] Studies in Japan and the United States also showed that chronic hepatitis C infection elevated the incidence of intrahepatic cholangiocarcinoma, with the odds ratio between 4 and 17.[128,129] In Asia, chronic infections of the biliary tract and infestation by certain liver flukes, such as *Clonorchis sinensis* and *Opisthorchis viverrini*, are associated with cholangiocarcinoma and hepatolithiasis.[123] Hepatolithiasis itself is also a risk factor for cholangiocarcinoma; 5% to 10% of patients with intrahepatic stones develop this complication.[130,131] Moreover, the combination of liver fluke infestation and nitrosamine exposure may explain the very high incidence of cholangiocarcinoma in northeast Thailand.[132] Other risk factors, although rare, include congenital fibropolycystic disease of the biliary system such as choledochal cysts and Caroli disease (cystic dilatation of intrahepatic bile ducts).[133] The observed incidence and mortality of intrahepatic cholangiocarcinoma has increased in the past 3 decades in Japan, the United States, and the United Kingdom.[14,134,135] In the United States, the age-adjusted mortality rate increased from 0.07 per 100,000 in 1973 to 0.69 per 100,000 in 1997; the estimated annual percentage change of mortality was 9.44%. Better case ascertainment and diagnosis because of improved diagnostic imaging, use of image-guided biopsies, or increased use of endoscopic retrograde cholangiopancreatography (ERCP) cannot fully explain this observation.[135,136]

Diagnosis

The most common presenting symptoms of biliary tract cancer are caused by obstruction of the bile duct. Those include painless jaundice, clay-colored stool, tea-colored urine, and pruritus. Other signs and symptoms include abdominal pain, fever, general malaise, abdominal distention, fullness, anorexia, and weight loss. The spectrum of cholangiocarcinoma can be classified into three broad groups: (a) intrahepatic, (b) perihilar, and (c) distal tumors. The age of onset is similar among the three groups and ranges from 60 to 65 years.[137] Patients with extrahepatic tumor usually present with jaundice and tea-colored urine. Patients with intrahepatic tumors are less likely to be jaundiced and more likely to present with abdominal symptoms.

TABLE 60.6 DIAGNOSTIC WORKUP FOR CARCINOMA OF THE BILE DUCT

General
History
Physical examination
Laboratory studies
Complete blood cell counts
Blood chemistry profile to include liver function studies
Tumor markers: CA-19-9, CEA
Radiographic studies
Standard
Computed tomography scan
Ultrasonography
Transhepatic cholangiography
Endoscopic retrograde cholangiopancreatography
Optional
Endoscopic ultrasound
Magnetic resonance cholangiopancreatography
Dynamic computed tomography scan
Arteriography

CA-19-9, carbohydrate antigen-19-9; CEA, carcinoembryonic antigen.

Modified from Gunderson LL, Willett CG. Pancreas and hepatobiliary tract. In: Perez CA, Brady LW, eds. *Principles and practice of radiation oncology*, 3rd ed. New York: Lippincott-Raven Publishers, 2010.

There are no reliable screening methods; early diagnosis is almost impossible even in patients with high-risk situations such as primary sclerosing cholangitis and hepatolithiasis.[138] Some patients are diagnosed when screening blood work demonstrates elevation of alkaline phosphatase and γ-glutamyl transferase. Ultrasonography and CT are the initial primary tools to evaluate biliary tract tumor (Table 60.6). Further tests include percutaneous transhepatic cholangiography, ERCP with brushing cytology, serum carbohydrate antigen-19-9 (CA-19-9) levels, radiologic imaging with dynamic CT scan, MRI, or both, and angiography.

A serum CA-19-9 value >100 U/mL has a sensitivity of ~75% and a specificity of ~80%.[139] The optimal cutoff value for serum CA-19-9 that best discriminates between benign or malignant biliary tract diseases is influenced by the presence of cholangitis. Thus, in patients with symptoms of acute cholangitis, serum CA-19-9 concentrations should ideally be re-evaluated after recovery. The sensitivity of serum carcinoembryonic antigen (CEA) is low and helpful in only one-third of patients.[140] Biliary CEA levels increase significantly in patients with cholangiocarcinoma and also in patients with intrahepatic cholelithiasis (average, 50.2 to 57.4 ng/mL) compared with patients with benign strictures (average, 10.1 ng/mL) and patients with sclerosing cholangitis and choledochal cysts (average, 20.0 to 21.6 ng/mL).[139] Serum AFP may increase in some cases of cholangiocarcinoma, and this would suggest a diagnosis of mixed HCC and cholangiocarcinoma.[141]

Pathology

Cholangiocarcinomas arise from the epithelium of the biliary tract; the majority of these cancers (>90%) are adenocarcinomas. Squamous cell carcinoma is the second most histologic type. Rare histologies include mucoepidermoid carcinoma, cystadenocarcinoma, and carcinoid tumor.

Adenocarcinomas are divided into three type: sclerosing, nodular, and papillary. Sclerosing tumors are characterized by an intense desmoplastic reaction. This type of tumor tends to invade the bile duct wall early and, as a result, is associated with low resectability and cure rates. Most cholangiocarcinomas are of this type.[137] The nodular cholangiocarcinomas are also highly invasive tumors. Most patients have advanced disease at diagnosis. The resection and cure rates are both very low. In contrast, papillary type tumors usually present as masses in the lumen of bile duct, causing biliary obstruction early in the course of disease. Therefore, these tumors have the most favorable prognosis.[142] Microscopically, cholangiocarcinoma are classically well differentiated to undifferentiated. Cells tend to be cuboidal or low columnar and resemble biliary epithelium; mucin is always demonstrable in the cytoplasm. Bile duct obstruction can be associated with reactive hyperplasia of subepithelial mucous glands with or without cholangiocarcinoma.[143] Cholangiocarcinomas frequently invade lymphatic, perineural, and periductal spaces and the portal tracts. Spread along the lumen of the large bile ducts can also be seen, especially in perihilar cholangiocarcinoma.[144]

The differential diagnosis of cholangiocarcinoma from HCC can be further affirmed by positive reaction with CEA, CA-19-9, and immunohistochemistry with cytokeratin-19.[145] Mutations in the *p53* tumor suppressor gene and *K-ras* proto-oncogene have been identified in cholangiocarcinoma.[146–148] *p53* overexpression and *K-ras* mutations are associated with a shortened survival.[146]

Pathways of Tumor Spread

Bile duct cancers commonly spread by direct extension through the bile duct and the abundant lymphatic network in the submucosa. These tumors also commonly involve the surrounding structures by direct invasion. Lymph node metastases in the porta hepatis and celiac axis are common. The lymph nodes in porta hepatis are more frequently involved with tumors in the intrahepatic duct and proximal extrahepatic bile duct, and the pancreaticoduodenal nodes are more often involved with tumors in the distal bile duct.[144,149]

The incidence of lymph node metastasis in intrahepatic cholangiocarcinoma ranges from 50% to 60%.[150,151] Intrahepatic cholangiocarcinomas, irrespective of their intrahepatic location, mainly spread to the nodes in the hepatoduodenal ligament, then to the para-aortic nodes, retropancreatic nodes, or common hepatic artery node group. In addition, the left peripheral type or hilar type of cholangiocarcinoma tends to spread along the left gastric nodes through the lesser curvature.[151] Lymph node metastasis in perihilar cholangiocarcinoma is common, which occurs in half of the patients, with the frequency of 43% in pericholedochal nodes, 31% in the periportal nodes, 27% in the common hepatic nodes, and 15% in the posterior pancreaticoduodenal nodes. The celiac and superior mesenteric nodes are rarely involved.[144]

Lymph node metastasis in distal duct cancer is commonly observed near the duodenopancreatic regions. Yoshida et al.[149] examined 20 consecutive patients with distal bile duct cancer who underwent pancreaticoduodenectomy with extended lymph node dissection. Histologic evidence of lymph node metastasis was seen in 55% of the patients. The areas with frequent metastases were the posterior pancreaticoduodenal lymph nodes (35%), the nodes around the hepatoduodenal ligament (35%), and those around the common hepatic artery (30%). Para-aortic lymph node involvement occurred in 25% of patients and was significantly associated with pancreatic parenchymal invasion.

Staging

The American Joint Committee on Cancer TNM classifications for intrahepatic cholangiocarcinoma are similarly to HCC. The definition of T stage were

T1: solitary tumor without vascular invasion,
T2a: solitary tumor with vascular invasion,
T2b: multiple tumors, with or without vascular invasion;
T3: tumor perforating the visceral peritoneum or involving the local extra hepatic structures by direct invasion;
T4: tumor with periductal invasion.[49]

N0 means no regional lymph node metastasis, and N1 is with regional lymph node metastasis. M0 is without distant metastasis, whereas M1 is with distant metastasis. The complete stage groups were listed on Table 60.7.

TABLE 60.7 AMERICAN JOINT COMMITTEE ON CANCER STAGE GROUPS BY TNM CLASSIFICATION

Intrahepatic Cholangiocarcinoma
Stage I: T1N0M0
Stage II: T2N0M0
Stage III: T3N0M0
Stage IVA: T4N0M0 or Any T, N1M0
Stage IVB: Any T, Any N, M1
Perihilar Cholangiocarcinoma
Stage I: T1N0M0
Stage II: T2a-bN0M0
Stage IIIA: T3N0M0
Stage IIIB: T1-3N1M0
Stage IVA: T4 Any N M0
Stage IVB: Any T, N2M0 or any T, any N, M1
Distal Cholangiocarcinoma
Stage IA: T1N0M0
Stage IB: T2N0M0
Stage IIA: T3N0M0
Stage IIB: T1-3N1M0
Stage III: T4, any N, M0
Stage IV: Any T, any N, M1

T, tumor; N, node; M, metastasis.

Used with the permission of the American Joint Committee on Cancer (AJCC), Chicago, Illinois. The original source for this material is the *AJCC Cancer Staging Manual*, 7th edition (2010) published by Springer Science and Business Media LLC, www.springer.com.

The American Joint Committee on Cancer TNM classifications for both hilar and distal cholangiocarcinoma were revised in 2010 and similar to the TNM classification of intrahepatic cholangiocarcinoma (see Table 60.7). The exception was that they added N2 disease (metastasis to periaortic, pericaval, superior mesenteric artery, or celiac artery lymph nodes) for perihilar disease. The most important prognostic factors for cholangiocarcinoma are resectability, regional lymph node metastasis, and distant metastasis.

General Management

Surgical resection provides the only possibility of cure, but the resection rates for intrahepatic, perihilar, and distal lesions were 60%, 56%, and 91%, respectively, in one large series.[137] The 5-year survival rates after resection range from 10% to 40%, depending on the location of the primary tumor.[137] Patients with unresectable cholangiocarcinoma generally have a very poor prognosis; chemotherapy and radiotherapy have been used, but the results are disappointing.[152]

Intrahepatic Cholangiocarcinoma

Intrahepatic cholangiocarcinoma accounts for 5% to 10% of all biliary tract cancers and constitutes 10% to 20% of primary liver malignancies. The resectability rate in all patients is only 30% to 50%.[153,154] The outcomes after surgery for patients with lymph node metastasis are poor regardless of the sites of nodal metastasis; the 5-year survival rate in patients with lymph node metastasis was lower than that in patients without lymph node metastasis (0% vs. 51%; $P < .0001$).[151]

Factors that affect tumor recurrence include lymph node metastasis, presence of satellite nodules, positive resection margin, tumor size, and bilobar distribution.[151,155–157] The patterns of failure after resection of intrahepatic cholangiocarcinoma are primarily in the liver (56%), regional lymph node (20%), and peritoneal seeding (24%).[158] The role of postoperative adjuvant radiotherapy with or without chemotherapy in the management of intrahepatic cholangiocarcinoma is controversial. The typical reports in the literature are retrospective, with small numbers of patients and marked variations in radiation field and dose.[159] A delineation of radiation fields based on patterns of failure analysis and lymph node spread of the disease will be necessary to rationally define the role of radiotherapy in any proposed phase III study. For unresectable cholangiocarcinoma, the purpose of treatment is palliative; however, some long-term survivals (a 4-year rate of 20%) have been observed in unresectable cholangiocarcinoma treated with conformal radiotherapy and intra-arterial infusion of fluorodeoxyuridine.[160]

Total hepatectomy with orthotopic liver transplantation also can be considered in this situation. One systemic review combining all studies that included a minimum of 10 patients reported a median survival of 11.8 months. The 1-, 3- and 5-year overall survivals were 63%, 46%, and 22%, respectively. The 1-, 3- and 5-year disease-free survivals were 58%, 22%, and 13%, respectively.[161] But orthotopic liver transplantation could not be considered as a standard treatment for localized cholangiocarcinoma at present. Such protocols should be preserved for selected patients with unresectable hilar disease only at transplantation centers.

Perihilar Cholangiocarcinoma

Perihilar cholangiocarcinoma is the most common biliary tract carcinoma and accounts for 65% to 70% of tumors of the biliary tract.[137] Perihilar tumors involving the bifurcation of the hepatic duct are also called Klatskin tumors.[162] These tumors were further classified by Bismuth et al.[163] as tumors below the confluence of the left and right hepatic ducts (type I), tumors reaching the confluence (type II), tumors occluding the common hepatic duct and the right or the left hepatic duct (types IIIa and IIIb, respectively), and tumors that are multicentric or that involve the confluence and both the right and left hepatic ducts (type IV).

Only 25% to 79% of patients are amenable for surgical resection. Definitive surgery may involve combined bile duct and liver resection with caudate lobe lobectomy.[164] The 3-year survival rate was 55% for patients without involved nodes, 32% for patients with regional node metastasis, and 12% for patients with para-aortic node metastasis.[144] In multivariate prognostic analysis, only lymph node metastases and curative resection have proven to be of independent prognostic significance.[144]

The role of postoperative radiotherapy with or without chemotherapy in patients with completely resected cholangiocarcinoma remains unproven. A retrospective analysis from Johns Hopkins suggests that postoperative adjuvant radiation therapy does not improve survival.[165] However, postoperative radiotherapy or chemoradiotherapy reduces the rate of local recurrence in patients with incomplete resection.[166,167] In addition, many retrospective series and small phase II studies suggest superior outcomes for resected patients who receive external-beam radiation therapy with or without concomitant chemotherapy.[65,168,169–170] For patients with microscopic residual disease after resection, a retrospective analysis from 63 patients with stage IV Klatskin tumor revealed that postoperative radiotherapy (with or without intraoperative radiotherapy) yielded significantly higher 5-year survival rates than in the resection alone group (33.9% vs. 13.5%).[167]

An update report from the Mayo Clinic revealed that the 5-year survival in transplant patients of unresectable hilar cholangiocarcinoma was 80% and in resection-only patients it was 21%.[171] Others also have reported similar promising results in these combined-modality treatments.[172,173]

In general, patients with inoperable perihilar cholangiocarcinoma usually have obstructive jaundice and should be treated with endoscopic or percutaneous drainage or stent placement initially. External-beam radiotherapy alone rarely controls advanced disease. Combinations of external-beam radiotherapy, chemotherapy, and intraluminal brachytherapy may relieve pain, contribute to biliary decompression, and sometimes achieve long-term survival. The most active agents include 5-FU, gemcitabine, docetaxel, and oxaliplatin.[174,175] The median survivals range from 17 to 21 months. In some cases, combined chemotherapy and radiotherapy could delay the progression of cholangiocarcinomas while patients await the chance for liver transplant.[94,168]

Distal Bile Duct Carcinoma

Primary distal bile duct adenocarcinoma, which includes carcinoma of the ampulla of Vater, accounts for 25% to 30% of biliary tract carcinomas.[137] Patients with distal duct carcinoma have the highest rate of curative resection as compared with proximal duct carcinoma. In an analysis of 171 patients who underwent surgical exploration at Mayo Clinic for extrahepatic cholangiocarcinoma from 1976 to 1985, the rate of curative resection (negative margins) by site of the primary tumor was 15% for proximal, 33% for middle, and 56% for distal duct lesions.[176] The prognosis of patients with distal duct carcinoma is also better than that of patients with proximal duct carcinoma.[127]

The role of postoperative radiotherapy is uncertain. Investigators at Thomas Jefferson University found that postoperative radiotherapy did not improve survival in distal duct carcinoma after complete resection.[177] However, studies of concurrent chemotherapy and radiotherapy show more promising results. Mehta et al.[178] from Stanford University treated 12 patients having unfavorable (mainly lymph node metastasis) ampullary carcinoma with concurrent radiotherapy and protracted venous infusion of 5-FU. Actuarial overall survival at 2 years was 89%, and median survival was 34 months. Another study conducted by the Eastern Cooperative Oncology Group revealed that unresectable pancreaticobiliary carcinoma treated with concomitant radiotherapy and protracted intravenous infusion of 5-FU achieved a 2-year survival of 19%.[170]

Systemic Chemotherapy

Although some retrospective reports showed a benefit of postoperative chemotherapy,[179,180] there was a multi-institutional randomized trial from Japan that showed only a trend toward better 5-year survival following a potential curative resection in those who received postoperative chemotherapy.[166] But it was not a statistically significant difference.

For treatment of advanced cholangiocarcinoma, a randomized trial showed a survival benefit with 5-FU–based chemotherapy compared with best supportive care alone (median survival, 6 vs. 2.5 months, respectively).[181] The most frequently used agents include 5-FU, gemcitabine, cisplatin, and oxaliplatin. Another phase III study enrolled 410 patients with locally advanced or metastatic cholangiocarcinoma, gallbladder cancer, or ampullary cancer. As compared with gemcitabine alone, cisplatin plus gemcitabine was associated with a significant survival advantage (11.7 vs. 8.1 months) without the addition of substantial toxicity. Cisplatin plus gemcitabine is an appropriate option for the treatment of patients with advanced biliary tract cancer.[182]

Radiation Therapy

The role of radiotherapy (with or without chemotherapy) in unresectable or recurrent cholangiocarcinoma is to relieve pain and biliary compression. At 1 year, 60% to 75% of patients are free of locoregional disease progression, and median survival was 7 to 12 months.[183,184] But local failure remains the first site of disease progression in 50% to 75% of patients. To enhance treatment effects, radiotherapy given with 5-FU–based chemotherapy is generally recommended.[170,178] The development of a treatment system of radiation oncology in the past few years made SBRT possible, but the experience is limited. One report included 27 patients with unresectable cholangiocarcinoma who underwent SBRT (45 Gy in 3 fractions). At a median follow-up of 5.4 months, only two patients were alive. The median progression-free and overall survival were 6.7 and 10.6 months, respectively. The local control was 84% in 1 year, but six patients had severe duodenal or pyloric ulceration and three patients developed duodenal stenosis.[185] Radiotherapy technique for intrahepatic cholangiocarcinoma is similar to treatment of HCC. The dose-limiting surrounding organs include the liver, duodenum, stomach, and spinal cord.

Treatment Volumes

The extent of the tumor within the bile duct can be defined by percutaneous cholangiography, ERCP, and magnetic resonance cholangiopancreatography. However, extraductal disease is difficult to define by any noninvasive procedure. Clip placement at the time of surgery is useful in delineating the extrahepatic portion of ductal lesions and in defining the primary tumor bed. With the incorporation of CT in radiation-treatment planning, and to reduce errors to a minimum, the authors advocate placing patients in the treatment position when performing CT, using 1 to 3 mm per slice and contrast medium to reconstruct the bile ducts and gross tumor volume (Fig. 60.3). The gross tumor volume (GTV) is defined as any visible tumor by CT or MRI. Clinical target volume (CTV) is defined as a 1.5-cm margin to the GTV, especially along the bile duct and potential lymphatic drainage areas, which include nodes along the porta hepatis, pancreaticoduodenal system, and celiac axis.[149,151,186,187] The planning target volume is defined by adding a margin of 0.5 to 1 cm to the CTV.[188]

Radiation Doses

Initial setup of radiation fields is to include GTV and CTV; the radiation fields can be coplanar or noncoplanar. The planning target volume will be treated to 45 to 50 Gy in 1.8- to 2-Gy fractions given 5 days a week, using blocks to exclude normal stomach, small intestine, kidney, and liver.[168,189] Higher radiation doses are used only to treat the GTV with the application of 3D-CRT.[84] If boost-dose irradiation is feasible with brachytherapy techniques, the GTV is carried to 45 to 50 Gy with external techniques, and 20 to 30 Gy is delivered via an intraluminal the catheter.[79] The most commonly employed brachytherapy technique for the biliary tract begins with the placement, performed by an invasive diagnostic radiologist, of a percutaneous drainage catheter through the area of tumor. The radiation oncologist then threads a catheter inside the drainage system catheter.

When a low-dose–rate system is employed, a wire with iridium-192 is then placed at the desired location inside the catheter.[190] If a remote high-dose–rate after-loading system is employed, then the appropriate dwell times and positions are selected and programmed. It is a matter of some debate as to where the brachytherapy prescription point should be placed. Some physicians select the tumor's peripheral edge, away from the catheter, as determined by CT or MRI. Other practitioners prefer a point 0.5 or 1 cm away from the catheter. It is important to be familiar with the valves used to direct bile flow in the drainage system lest, during the administration of brachytherapy, bile leaks onto the patient's skin and dressings. If the drainage system remains in place for a long period of time (i.e., a month), enteric bacterial colonization and biliary tract infection are common. The combination of external-beam irradiation and brachytherapy employed at Thomas Jefferson University resulted in 2-year and median survival rate, increasing twofold when doses were brought up to >55 Gy.[190] However, investigators at the University of Amsterdam reported no improved survival at doses >55 Gy.[191] The role of radiotherapy and its optimal dosage remain to be determined.

Acute and Late Complications

Acute complications of external-beam and intraluminal radiotherapy include nausea, vomiting, and transient elevation of transaminase. These effects are usually mild and tolerable.[35]

Late complications are associated with radiation dose to surrounding organs. The most common complications

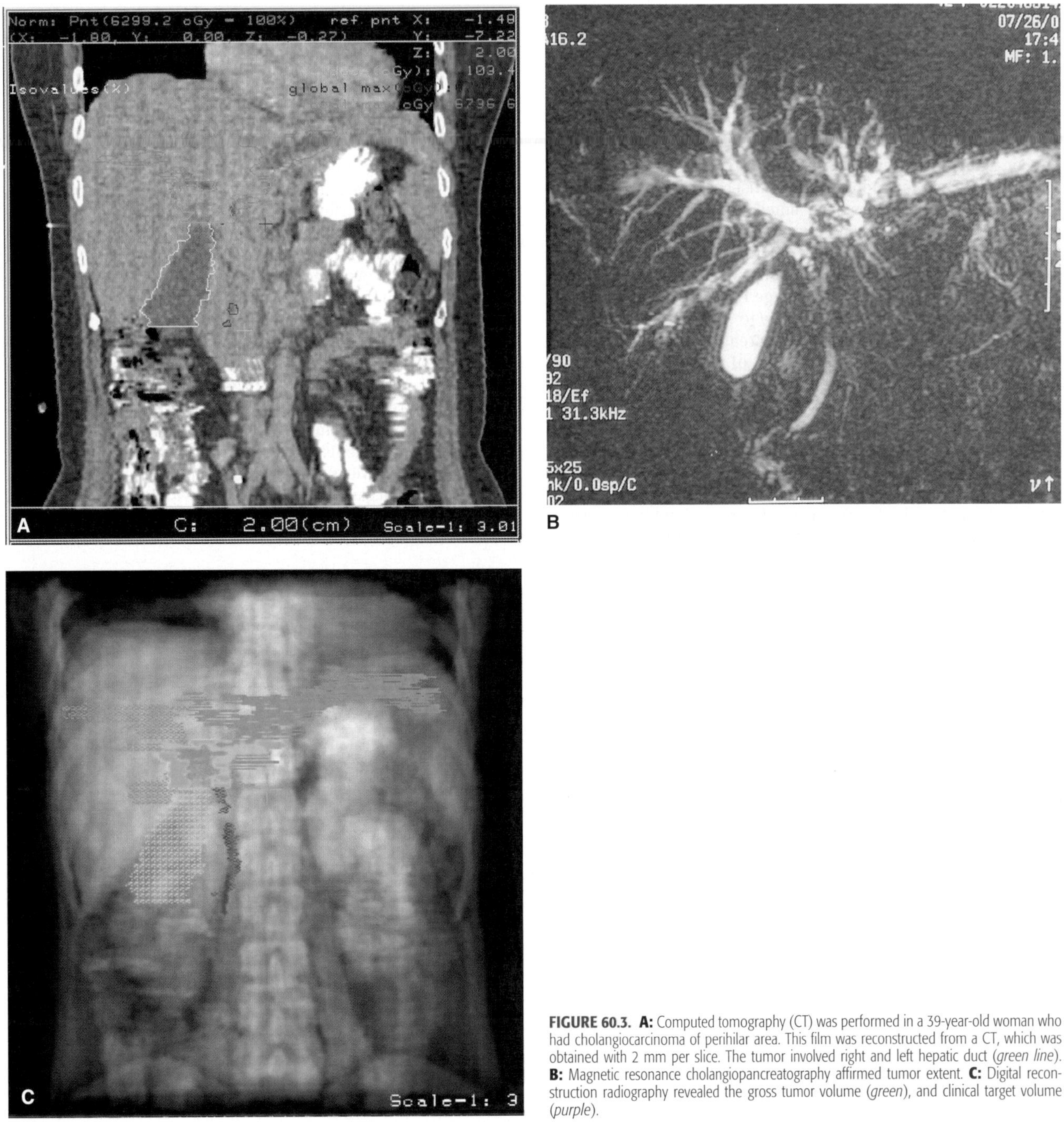

FIGURE 60.3. **A:** Computed tomography (CT) was performed in a 39-year-old woman who had cholangiocarcinoma of perihilar area. This film was reconstructed from a CT, which was obtained with 2 mm per slice. The tumor involved right and left hepatic duct (*green line*). **B:** Magnetic resonance cholangiopancreatography affirmed tumor extent. **C:** Digital reconstruction radiography revealed the gross tumor volume (*green*), and clinical target volume (*purple*).

are gastrointestinal bleeding, biliary bleeding, and duodenal stenosis.[35,190,191] With external-beam doses of <55 Gy to the duodenum or stomach, the risk of severe gastrointestinal complications varies from 5% to 10%. At doses >55 Gy, one-third of patients develop severe problems.

Future Directions

There is a paucity of phase III studies for cholangiocarcinoma, so physicians must rely on retrospective studies or prospective phase I or II trials. Further advances in treatment could potentially be made by (a) defining when to use radiation and chemotherapy for high-risk patients after curative resection, (b) investigating the use of higher doses of conformal radiotherapy and chemotherapy in unresectable cholangiocarcinoma, and (c) identifying novel chemotherapeutic agents. Patients with unresectable cholangiocarcinoma should be offered clinical trials.

ADENOCARCINOMA OF GALLBLADDER

Gallbladder carcinoma is not common; it is the fifth most common cancer of the gastrointestinal tract. The incidence indicates a large geographic variation, and it accounts for approximately 5,000 new patients per year in the United States.[192] Distinctly different from cholangiocarcinoma, the ratio of females to males is 2.5 to 1.[133] Cholelithiasis, an anomalous junction of pancreaticobiliary ducts, and porcelain gallbladder are factors that predispose to gallbladder cancer.[193] Cigarette smoking, alcohol consumption, and obesity may also increase the risk. Patients with polyps >10 mm in diameter may be at increased risk for gallbladder cancer.[194,195] Chronic infection with *Salmonella typhi* and *Helicobacter bilis* is also associated with the risk of developing carcinoma of the gallbladder.[196,197]

The most common clinical presentation is pain, followed by anorexia, nausea, or vomiting. Patients with early invasive gallbladder carcinoma are most often asymptomatic or they have nonspecific symptoms that mimic or are due to cholelithiasis or cholecystitis. In general, gallbladder carcinoma is diagnosed late, which accounts for the poor prognosis.[133] A French study of 724 patients revealed that only 4% of the patients had Tis lesions, 11% had T1 to T2 lesions, and 85% had T3 to T4 lesions.[198] Five-year survival rates according to the National Cancer Data Base were Tis disease, 60%; T1N0, 39%; T2N0, 15%; and T3N0 or node-positive disease, 5%.[199] However, improved outcomes have been noted in the past decade and attributed to more aggressive surgery and the use of postoperative adjuvant therapy.[200] Studies from Japan report a 100% 5-year survival rate in stage I patients, with stage II at 50% to 78%, stage III at 0% to 69%, and stage IV at 0% to 11%.[201,202]

Lymphatic metastasis is initially to cystic and pericholedochal nodes and then to the pancreaticoduodenal system, with later potential spread to the rest of the celiac axis or the superior mesenteric or aortic nodes.[201,203] The lymph node metastasis rate is associated with primary tumor stage: 0% to 2.5% in pT1 a disease (involvement limited to the mucosa), 15% in T1b, disease, 62% in pT2 disease, and 81% in pT3 or pT4 disease.[201,204,205]

Surgery is the only potentially curative therapy, but only 10% to 30% of patients are eligible for resection.[206] The standard surgical procedure is removal of the gallbladder, resection of various amounts of liver surrounding the gallbladder bed, resection of the extrahepatic bile duct, and dissection of the regional lymph nodes. Patients with jaundice should be considered for preoperative percutaneous transhepatic biliary drainage for relief of biliary obstruction. Overall, the curative resection rates for gallbladder carcinoma range from 10% to 30% in Western countries.[207] The prognosis is related to the possibility of curative resection, primary tumor extension, and regional lymph node metastasis.

Patients with T1 a disease often are cured after simple cholecystectomy and require no further adjuvant treatment.[205] However, for patients with ≥T2 disease, many reports support the benefit of radical resection; re-exploration is generally recommended.[200,204,208] In more advanced disease, the role of adjuvant radiotherapy is uncertain. After "curative" resection, locoregional relapse in the tumor bed or regional nodes is common. Factors predicting recurrence are positive surgical margins, lymph node metastasis, and perineural invasion.[209] Several retrospective analyses demonstrate that postoperative radiotherapy improved local control and survival.[210,211–212] Benefits are also seen in patients who have microscopic residual tumors.[212] Combination radiotherapy and chemotherapy with 5-FU also reveal similar benefits.[213–215] However, there is lack of phase III studies. Whether combination treatment is better than single modality is still unknown.

Patients with stage III and IV disease are at high risk for distant metastasis. The most frequent sites of involvement are liver, peritoneum, and lung, with less frequent spread to ovaries, spleen, bones, and other organs.[188,214] In general, patients who are locally unresectable should be referred for chemoradiotherapy. Median survival is improved in several retrospective studies.[216,217] Systemic chemotherapy has had limited success in the treatment of advanced gallbladder carcinoma. Objective response rates range from 25% to 50%. Active agents include infusion 5-FU in combination regimens, leucovorin-modulated 5-FU, capecitabine, cisplatin, oxaliplatin, gemcitabine, and docetaxel, 5-FU, and recombined interferon-alfa-2b.[218,219–220,221–223] Currently, the standard of care for systemic chemotherapy is cisplatin and gemcitabine, as mentioned above in section on cholangiocarcinoma.[182]

OTHER RARE NEOPLASMS

Primary sarcomas of the liver are extremely rare in adults and represent only 1% to 2% of primary liver cancers.[224] Leiomyosarcoma is the most common histologic type, followed by malignant fibrous histiocytoma, epithelioid hemangioendothelioma, and angiosarcoma.[93] Some patients with angiosarcoma have a history of occupational exposure to vinyl chloride monomer.[225] Histologic grade of sarcoma is the only factor significantly associated with overall patient survival. Complete resection offers a chance of long-term survival.[93]

Hemangioma is a benign lesion and generally is asymptomatic. For symptomatic hemangioma, the treatments of choice include steroids, interferon-alfa, arterial embolization, and surgery.[226] If patients fail such treatments, radiotherapy may play a role. Long symptom-free survival times have been obtained with doses as low as 13 to 30 Gy during 2.5 to 4 weeks.[227]

Hepatoblastoma is the most common malignant liver tumor of childhood. Children who have familial adenomatous polyposis are at high risk to have hepatoblastoma. The risk of hepatoblastoma in these children is 700 to 7,500 times higher than in the general population.[228,229] Surgery combined with chemotherapy has resulted in dramatic improvements in prognosis.[230] With the combination of chemotherapy and surgery, 75% to 80% of patients may be cured.[52] Preoperative chemotherapy often converts unresectable tumors to resectable and may facilitate surgery being performed with less blood loss and minimal technical complications.[231]

SELECTED REFERENCES

A full list of references for this chapter is available online.

12. El-Serag HB, Rudolph KL. Hepatocellular carcinoma: epidemiology and molecular carcinogenesis. *Gastroenterology* 2007;132:2557.
15. Beasley RP, Lin CC, Hwang LY, et al. Hepatocellular carcinoma and hepatitis B virus: a prospective study of 22,707 men in Taiwan. *Lancet* 1981;318:1129.
16. Yang HI, Lu SN, Liaw YF, et al. Hepatitis B antigen and the risk of hepatocellular carcinoma. *N Engl J Med* 2002;347:168–174.
25. Chang MH, Chen CJ, Lai MS, et al. Universal hepatitis B vaccination in Taiwan and the incidence of hepatocellular carcinoma in children. Taiwan Childhood Hepatoma Study Group. *N Engl J Med* 1997;336:1855–1859.
27. Camma C, Giunta M, Andreone P, et al. Interferon and prevention of hepatocellular carcinoma in viral cirrhosis: an evidence-based approach. *J Hepatol* 2001; 34:593–602.
31. Bruix J, Sherman M. Management of hepatocellular carcinoma: an update. *Hepatology* 2011;53:1020.
32. Bruix J, Sherman M. Management of hepatocellular carcinoma. *Hepatology* 2005; 42:1208–1236.
36. Yu MW, Chang HC, Liaw YF, et al. Familial risk of hepatocellular carcinoma among chronic hepatitis B carriers and their relatives. *J Natl Cancer Inst* 2000; 92:1159–1164.
49. Edge SB, Byrd DR, Compton CC, et al. *AJCC cancer staging manual*, 7th ed. New York: Springer, 2009.
50. Okuda K, Ohtsuki T, Obata H, et al. Natural history of hepatocellular carcinoma and prognosis in relation to treatment. Study of 850 patients. *Cancer* 1985;56: 918–928.
60. Mazzaferro V, Regalia E, Doci R, et al. Liver transplantation for the treatment of small hepatocellular carcinomas in patients with cirrhosis. *N Engl J Med* 1996; 334:693–699.
64. Chapman RW. Risk factors for biliary tract carcinogenesis. *Ann Oncol* 1999;10 (Suppl 4):308–311.
67. Lin SM, Lin CJ, Lin CC, et al. Randomised controlled trial comparing percutaneous radiofrequency thermal ablation, percutaneous ethanol injection, and percutaneous acetic acid injection to treat hepatocellular carcinoma of 3 cm or less. *Gut* 2005;54:1151–1156.
73. A comparison of lipiodol chemoembolization and conservative treatment for unresectable hepatocellular carcinoma. Groupe d'Etude et de Traitement du Carcinome Hepatocellulaire. *N Engl J Med* 1995;332:1256–1261.
75. Llovet JM, Bruix J. Systematic review of randomized trials for unresectable hepatocellular carcinoma: chemoembolization improves survival. *Hepatology* 2003;37:429–442.
81. Hawkins MA, Dawson LA. Radiation therapy for hepatocellular carcinoma: from palliation to cure. *Cancer* 2006;106:1653–1663.
82. Lin CS, Jen YM, Chiu SY, et al. Treatment of portal vein tumor thrombosis of hepatoma patients with either stereotactic radiotherapy or three-dimensional conformal radiotherapy. *Jpn J Clin Oncol* 2006;36:212–217.
90. Liang SX, Zhu XD, Xu ZY, et al. Radiation-induced liver disease in three-dimensional conformal radiation therapy for primary liver carcinoma: the risk factors and hepatic radiation tolerance. *Int J Radiat Oncol Biol Phys* 2006;65: 426–434.
92. Guo WJ, Yu EX. Evaluation of combined therapy with chemoembolization and irradiation for large hepatocellular carcinoma. *Br J Radiol* 2000;73:1091–1097.
96. Son SH, Choi BO, Ryu MR, et al. Stereotactic body radiotherapy for patients with unresectable primary hepatocellular carcinoma: dose–volume parameters predicting the hepatic complication. *Int J Radiat Oncol Biol Phys* 2010;78: 1073–1080.
97. Mahadevan A, Jain S, Goldstein M, et al. Stereotactic body radiotherapy and gemcitabine for locally advanced pancreatic cancer. *Int J Radiat Oncol Biol Phys* 2010;78:735–742.

103. Seong J, Park HC, Han KH, et al. Clinical results of 3-dimensional conformal radiotherapy combined with transarterial chemoembolization for hepatocellular carcinoma in the cirrhotic patients. *Hepatol Res* 2003;27:30–35.
106. Tazawa J, Maeda M, Sakai Y, et al. Radiation therapy in combination with transcatheter arterial chemoembolization for hepatocellular carcinoma with extensive portal vein involvement. *J Gastroenterol Hepatol* 2001;16:660.
112. Patt YZ, Hassan MM, Lozano RD, et al. Thalidomide in the treatment of patients with hepatocellular carcinoma: a phase II trial. *Cancer* 2005;103:749–755.
114. Llovet JM, Ricci S, Mazzaferro V, et al. Sorafenib in advanced hepatocellular carcinoma. *N Engl J Med* 2008; 359:378.
118. Cheng JC, Chuang VP, Cheng SH, et al. Local radiotherapy with or without transcatheter arterial chemoembolization for patients with unresectable hepatocellular carcinoma. *Int J Radiat Oncol Biol Phys* 2000;47:435–442.
122. Shirabe K, Shimada M, Harimoto N, et al. Intrahepatic cholangiocarcinoma: its mode of spreading and therapeutic modalities. *Surgery* 2002;131:S159–S164.
123. Shin HR, Oh JK, Masuyer E, et al. Epidemiology of cholangiocarcinoma: an update focusing on risk factors. *Cancer Sci* 2010;101:579.
140. Bjornsson E, Kilander A, Olsson R. CA 19-9 and CEA are unreliable markers for cholangiocarcinoma in patients with primary sclerosing cholangitis. *Liver* 1999;19:501–508.
150. Tsuji T, Hiraoka T, Kanemitsu K, et al. Lymphatic spreading pattern of intrahepatic cholangiocarcinoma. *Surgery* 2001;129:401–407.
160. Robertson JM, Lawrence TS, Andrews JC, et al. Long-term results of hepatic artery fluorodeoxyuridine and conformal radiation therapy for primary hepatobiliary cancers. *Int J Radiat Oncol Biol Phys* 1997;37:325–330.
161. Beavers KL, Bonis PAL, Lau J. Liver transplantation for patients with hepatobiliary malignancies other than hepatocellular carcinoma. Available at: https://www.cms.gov/medicare-coverage-database/.
166. Takada T, Amano H, Yasuda H, et al. Is postoperative adjuvant chemotherapy useful for gallbladder carcinoma? A phase III multicenter prospective randomized controlled trial in patients with resected pancreaticobiliary carcinoma. *Cancer* 2002;95:1685–1695.
167. Todoroki T, Ohara K, Kawamoto T, et al. Benefits of adjuvant radiotherapy after radical resection of locally advanced main hepatic duct carcinoma. *Int J Radiat Oncol Biol Phys* 2000;46:581–587.
168. Morganti AG, Trodella L, Valentini V, et al. Combined modality treatment in unresectable extrahepatic biliary carcinoma. *Int J Radiat Oncol Biol Phys* 2000;46:913–919.
171. Rea DJ, Heimbach JK, Rosen CB, et al. Liver transplantation with neoadjuvant chemoradiation is more effective than resection for hilar cholangiocarcinoma. *Ann Surg* 2005;242:451–461.
172. Heimbach JK, Gores GJ, Haddock MG, et al. Liver transplantation for unresectable perihilar cholangiocarcinoma. *Semin Liver Dis* 2004;24:201–207.
174. Alberts SR, Al-Khatib H, Mahoney MR, et al. Gemcitabine, 5-fluorouracil, and leucovorin in advanced biliary tract and gallbladder carcinoma: a North Central Cancer Treatment Group phase II trial. *Cancer* 2005;103:111–118.
175. Verderame F, Russo A, Di Leo R, et al. Gemcitabine and oxaliplatin combination chemotherapy in advanced biliary tract cancers. *Ann Oncol* 2006;17:vii68–vii72.
182. Valle J, Wasan H, Palmer DH, et al. Cisplatin plus gemcitabine versus gemcitabine for biliary tract cancer. *N Engl J Med* 2010;362:1273–1281.
184. Ben-David MA, Griffith KA, Abu-Isa E, et al. External-beam radiotherapy for localized extrahepatic cholangiocarcinoma. *Int J Radiat Oncol Biol Phys* 2006;66:772.
185. Kopek N, Holt MI, Hansen AT, et al. Stereotactic body radiotherapy for unresectable cholangiocarcinoma. *Radiothera Oncol* 2010;94:47.
187. Yamaguchi K, Chijiiwa K, Saiki S, et al. Carcinoma of the extrahepatic bile duct: mode of spread and its prognostic implications. *Hepatogastroenterology* 1997;44:1256–1261.
200. Nakeeb A, Tran KQ, Black MJ, et al. Improved survival in resected biliary malignancies. *Surgery* 2002;132:555–564.
201. Shimada H, Endo I, Togo S, et al. The role of lymph node dissection in the treatment of gallbladder carcinoma. *Cancer* 1997;79:892–899.
203. Tsukada K, Kurosaki I, Uchida K, et al. Lymph node spread from carcinoma of the gallbladder. *Cancer* 1997;80:661–667.
210. Houry S, Haccart V, Huguier M, et al. Gallbladder cancer: role of radiation therapy. *Hepatogastroenterology* 1999;46:1578–1584.
216. Czito BG, Hurwitz HI, Clough RW, et al. Adjuvant external-beam radiotherapy with concurrent chemotherapy after resection of primary gallbladder carcinoma: a 23-year experience. *Int J Radiat Oncol Biol Phys* 2005;62:1030–1034.
219. Papakostas P, Kouroussis C, Androulakis N, et al. First-line chemotherapy with docetaxel for unresectable or metastatic carcinoma of the biliary tract. A multicentre phase II study. *Eur J Cancer* 2001;37:1833–1838.
220. Patt YZ, Hassan MM, Aguayo A, et al. Oral capecitabine for the treatment of hepatocellular carcinoma, cholangiocarcinoma, and gallbladder carcinoma. *Cancer* 2004;101:578–586.

Chapter 61
Cancer of the Colon and Rectum

Manisha Palta, Christopher G. Willett, and Brian G. Czito

ANATOMY

The colorectum consists of the cecum, ascending colon, hepatic flexure, transverse colon, splenic flexure, descending colon, sigmoid colon, and rectum. Variability in the peritoneal investment, bowel mobility, and lymph node drainage of the colon and rectum presents unique therapeutic issues.[1]

The posterior and lateral surfaces of the ascending and descending colon are in direct contact with the retroperitoneum, whereas the anterior surface is draped with peritoneum.[1] These posterior attachments can prevent significant mobility, increasing the difficulty of surgical resection. In contrast, the transverse colon is completely surrounded with peritoneum and supported on a long mesentery. As the sigmoid colon evolves distally into the rectum, the peritoneal coverage recedes. The rectum, approximately 12 to 15 cm in length, extends from the rectosigmoid junction to the puborectalis ring. The upper one-third of the rectum is draped with peritoneum anteriorly and on both sides. As the middle one-third of the rectum moves deeper into the pelvis, only the anterior surface is covered with peritoneum, which forms the posterior border of the rectouterine pouch or rectovesical space. The lowest one-third of the rectum is devoid of peritoneal covering and in close proximity to adjacent structures, including the bony pelvis (Fig. 61.1). Distal rectal tumors have no serosal barrier to invasion of adjacent structures and are more difficult to resect, given the close confines of the deep pelvis.

Colonic nodal drainage consists of pericolic nodes and nodes in association with the vascular supply to the colon (i.e., mesenteric nodes). Because of the mobile and extensive nature of the colonic mesentery, complete regional lymph node coverage with external-beam radiotherapy (EBRT) is challenging but is usually well treated surgically. In contrast, the major regional groups for rectal nodal drainage can be covered within a reasonable EBRT field and include the perirectal, presacral, and internal iliac nodes.

EPIDEMIOLOGY AND RISK FACTORS

Colorectal cancer (CRC) remains a major worldwide health problem. In the United States alone, it was estimated that there would be 143,460 patients diagnosed with CRC and 51,690 deaths in 2012.[2] Worldwide, approximately 1.2 million new cases per year are diagnosed, with 600,000 deaths.[3] In the United States, incidence of CRC over the last two decades declined by 2% to 3% annually; this is largely attributed to improvements in cancer prevention, early detection, and treatment.[4]

Genetic and environmental factors can increase the likelihood of developing CRC. A number of hereditary CRC syndromes exist, including familial adenomatous polyposis (FAP), MUTYH-associated polyposis, and Lynch syndrome (hereditary nonpolyposis colorectal cancer [HNPCC]). Factors shown to increase the risk of developing CRC include the following: increasing age; male sex; family history of colorectal cancer; inflammatory bowel disease; increasing height; increasing body mass index; consumption of processed meat, refined grains, starches, and sugars; excessive alcohol intake and smoking; and low folate consumption.[5,6] Of these risk factors, only increasing age, male sex, and excessive alcohol use have been associated with rectal cancer.[7] Age is a major risk factor for the development of CRC, with median age of diagnosis in

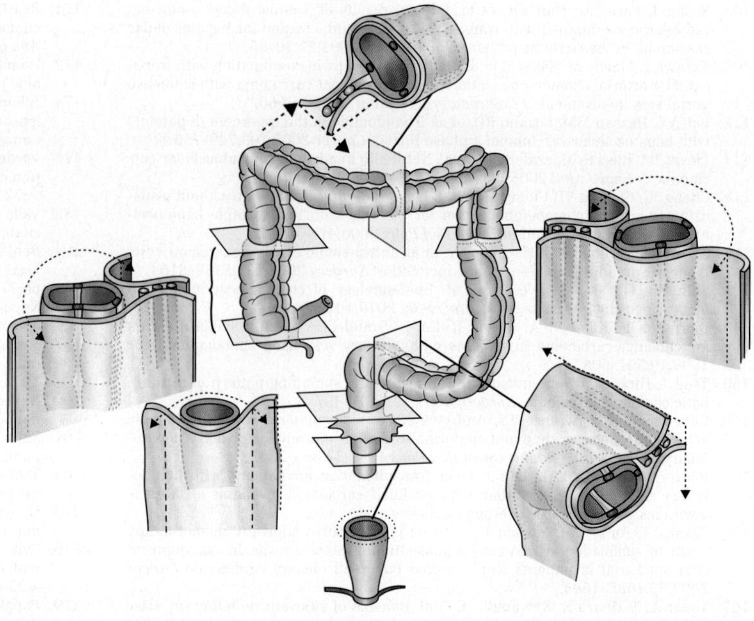

FIGURE 61.1. Idealized depiction of peritoneal relationships in the colon and rectum. The transverse and sigmoid colon are intraperitoneal, with a complete peritoneal covering (serosa) and mesentery. The ascending and descending colon are retroperitoneal, lack a true mesentery, and usually do not have a peritoneal covering posteriorly or laterally. The upper rectum begins above the peritoneal reflection and has peritoneum anteriorly and laterally. The lower one-half to two-thirds of the rectum is below the peritoneal reflection (infraperitoneal). (From Gunderson LL, O'Connell MJ. The postoperative chemotherapy/irradiation adjuvant strategy. In: Cohen AF, Winawer SJ, Friedman MA, et al., eds. *Cancer of the colon, rectum, and anus.* New York: McGraw-Hill, 1995;631–645; with permission.)

the seventh decade. Incidence rates increase dramatically between ages 40 and 50 years and each subsequent decade thereafter (data from Surveillance, Epidemiology, and End Results Program accessible online at www.seer.cancer.gov).

Although CRC may be linked to chemical carcinogens within the bowel lumen, it is not established whether these are ingested, the result of chemical activation of substances in the fecal stream, or a bacterial by-product.[8,9] The value of consumption of fruits and vegetables in the prevention of CRC remains controversial, although recent studies suggested that these associations might have been overstated.[10] Contemporary prospective and randomized data do not support a high-fiber diet in the prevention of CRC.[11] Other studies suggested that nonsteroidal anti-inflammatory drugs may serve in reducing recurrent adenomas and CRC, but long-term therapy must be weighed against potential side effects. The role of chemopreventive agents (carotenoids, aspirin, and other nonsteroidal anti-inflammatory drugs) in colorectal cancer remains an area of active investigation. A detailed discussion of the biologic and genetic pathways of development of colorectal cancer is beyond the scope of this chapter. In brief, it has been established that the development of colon cancer is a multifactorial process, involving genomic instability, mutational inactivation of tumor suppressor genes, and activation of oncogene pathways. Microsatellites are mutated short-repeat DNA sequences, usually consisting of one to five nucleotides. The majority of patients with HNPCC, as well as a minority of sporadic colorectal cancers, harbor microsatellite instability. It has been shown that this instability occurs in patients with mutations in genes encoding enzymes that repair DNA replication errors. These defects in mismatch repair lead to high-frequency microsatellite and hence genomic instability.[12] Studies suggested that patients with tumors possessing a high frequency of microsatellite instability have more-favorable outcomes and lower likelihood of developing metastatic disease.[13] CRC appears to arise through inactivation of the tumor suppressor genes adenomatous polyposis coli (APC), P53, and TGF-β, as well as activation of the RAS, BRAF, and PI3 K proto-oncogenes.[12] Further elucidation of the genetic pathways in the development of CRC remains an active area of investigation and may ultimately affect therapy of this disease.

CLINICAL PRESENTATION

CRC often produces minimal or no symptoms, emphasizing the need for screening programs in the general population. Patients with symptomatic CRC most commonly experience abdominal pain, change in bowel habits, hematochezia/melena, weakness, iron-deficiency anemia, and weight loss.[14,15] Less commonly, patients present with nausea, vomiting, or abdominal distention, which may be signs of tumor-related obstruction.

The clinical presentation of CRC is determined largely by site of the tumor. Cancers of the right colon are often exophytic and commonly associated with iron-deficiency anemia due to occult blood loss, resulting in delayed diagnosis. During the last 20 years, the incidence of cancer of the right colon appears to have increased and accounts for one-third of large-bowel cancers.[16] Cancers of the left colon and sigmoid colon are often deeply invasive, annular ("apple core lesions"), and accompanied by obstruction, rectal bleeding, and alteration in bowel habits.

SCREENING

Neoplastic polyps, including tubular adenomas, villous adenomas, and tubulovillous adenomas, are precursors of colon cancers.[8,17] Most CRC arise from pre-existing polyps. As the cumulative lifetime risk of developing CRC in the United States is about 6%, screening programs for the general population have been initiated. The goal of screening is to detect preinvasive polyps or early invasive cancer. Mounting evidence supports that screening of asymptomatic, average-risk individuals can detect CRC at early, curable stage, thereby reducing CRC mortality.[18,19–20]

Given the data in favor of screening, health organizations such as the American Cancer Society (ACS) and the United States Preventative Services Task Force recommend screening in average-risk individuals starting at age 50. The ACS advocates for tests that detect adenomatous polyps and cancer as follows:

1. Flexible sigmoidoscopy every 5 years.
2. Double contrast barium enema every 5 years.
3. Computed tomography (CT) colonography every 5 years.
4. Colonoscopy every 10 years.[19]
5. Guaiac-based fecal occult blood, fecal immunohistochemical, and stool DNA tests may be performed for CRC, but not polyp, detection.[21]

In high-risk patients (patients with adenomatous polyps, history of CRC, first-degree relative diagnosed with CRC or adenomas, inflammatory bowel disease, or high risk due to family history or genetic testing), more-intensive surveillance is recommended. Individuals with FAP initiate annual sigmoidoscopy or colonoscopy beginning at age 10 to 12 years until age 35 to 40 years if negative. Patients with HNPCC initiate annual screening at age 20 to 25 years or 10 years prior to earliest familial CRC diagnosis.[22,23] Patients with inflammatory bowel disease should initiate screening with colonoscopy 8 to 10 years after initial diagnosis.[21] The American College of Gastroenterology recommends the following for high-risk individuals based on family history[24]:

1. Colonoscopy screening.
2. If single, first-degree relative diagnosed with CRC, or advanced adenoma at age 60+ years, screening every 10 years beginning at age 50 years.
3. If single, first-degree relative diagnosed with CRC, or advanced adenoma at age <60 years or two or more first-degree relatives with CRC or advanced adenoma at any age, screening beginning at age 40 years or 10 years before the youngest relative's diagnosis. Screening should be performed every 5 years.

Although screening methods can detect colorectal cancer at an early stage, <40% of patients are diagnosed with early disease, likely reflecting low rates of disease awareness, as well as the infrequency of screening in eligible candidates.[25] Approximately 50% to 60% of adults aged 50 to 75 years underwent CRC screening in 2008.[26,27] Lower rates of screening are seen in younger patients, Hispanics, individuals of lower socioeconomic status, and individuals without insurance.[27] Although all screening tests have potential drawbacks, patients should be educated regarding relative risks and benefits of screening modalities, including potential benefits in reducing risk of CRC.

PATHOLOGY AND PATHWAYS OF SPREAD

Tumors of the colorectum arise in the mucosa and virtually all (>90%) are adenocarcinomas.[8] Other histologic types include squamous cell carcinoma, melanoma, small-cell carcinoma, carcinoid, sarcoma, and lymphoma. Most grading systems classify adenocarcinoma as well, moderately or poorly differentiated. Large-bowel tumors invade from mucosa through the bowel wall and beyond, with involvement of lymphatic channels and lymph nodes. Hematogenous spread can occur, primarily to the lung and liver. There is little propensity for colon cancer to spread longitudinally within the bowel wall, in contrast to esophageal or gastric cancers.

PATIENT EVALUATION/STAGING

Workup should include a complete history and physical exam, including digital rectal examination (DRE). On DRE, size, location, distance from the verge, mobile versus fixed, and sphincter function should be noted. Pelvic exam should be performed in women diagnosed with rectal cancer to assess for vaginal involvement where appropriate. Pretreatment evaluation should include pathologic confirmation of adenocarcinoma, colonoscopy to evaluate extent of tumor and rule out synchronous primaries (occurring in 1% to 5%), and baseline lab tests, including blood counts, liver function tests, and carcinoembryonic antigen levels.[9] India ink may be used at the time of colonoscopy to mark the proximal and distal disease extent.

Patients with CRC should undergo abdominal/pelvic CT scan and chest x-ray or chest CT to evaluate extent of local regional disease, as well as the presence or absence of distant metastases. Efforts to improve the clinical assessment of rectal cancers have been enhanced considerably with the evolution of new imaging modalities. CT appears to be more useful in identifying enlarged pelvic lymph nodes and metastasis outside the pelvis than the extent or stage of the primary tumor.[28] Standard CT does not permit the visualization of the layers of the rectal wall, and therefore its utility in the assessment of smaller primary cancers is limited.[29] The sensitivity of CT scan is reported as 50% to 80% accurate, with a 30% to 80% specificity (65% to 75% accurate for tumor staging and 55% to 65% accurate in mesorectal lymph node staging).[30] The ability of CT scans for detecting distant metastasis, including pelvic and para-aortic lymph nodes, is higher than for detecting perirectal nodal involvement (75% to 87% vs. 45%).[31,32] Any lymphadenopathy near the rectum seen on a CT scan should be considered abnormal.

For rectal malignancies, endoscopic ultrasound (EUS) or pelvic magnetic resonance imaging (MRI) can assess primary disease and, with less sensitivity, evaluate nodal extent. Transrectal EUS techniques have been more helpful in efforts to clinically stage rectal cancers. EUS is 80% to 95% accurate in tumor staging and 70% to 75% accurate in mesorectal lymph node staging.[33,34] Transrectal ultrasound is able to visualize layers of the rectal wall, including the mucosa, muscularis mucosa, submucosa, and muscularis propria.[35,36] Its use is more limited in tumors of the upper rectum or for stenosing tumors. EUS can also identify enlarged perirectal lymph nodes but is not effective outside of the perirectum.[37] One situation in which EUS can be very useful is in determining extension of disease into the anal canal, which is an area that is poorly visualized on CT but of critical importance for planning sphincter-preserving surgical procedures.[38]

More recently, MRI techniques have been found to be of high accuracy in defining the extent of rectal cancer extension into the mesorectum and in determining the location and stage of tumor.[39,40] Different approaches to MRI have been explored, including the use of body coils, endorectal MRI, and phased-array techniques. Although MRI appears to have high levels of accuracy, it requires a significant learning curve but is becoming a greater part of the standard presurgical workup for rectal cancer. Body-coil MRI, which first became available in the mid 1980s, has had an accuracy of 54% to 66% for T staging, but this has improved with the use of endorectal coil MRI, with reported accuracy rates of 80% to 95%.[16,41] A significant advantage of both endorectal and surface coil MRI is that it is less operator dependent and permits a larger field of view than EUS. It also allows assessment for proximal tumors and stenotic lesions where EUS is not possible. Another advantage of MRI is that it can detect involved lymph nodes on the basis of characteristics other than size. MRI can also be helpful in determining the extent of lateral extension of disease, which is critical in predicting the adequacy of circumferential margins for surgical excision.[17] Several studies using phased-array MRI reported accuracy rates of 80% to 97% in predicting lateral disease extent and correlated the likelihood of tumor-free resection margin by visualizing tumor involvement of the mesorectal fascia.[42]

Positron emission tomography (PET) scan, although less accurate in assessment of primary disease, is useful in evaluating patients with oligometastatic disease who may be appropriate candidates for resection of metastatic sites with curative intent.[43] Liver MRI is considered the test of choice in assessment of hepatic metastases in patients with CRC.[44] All of these imaging techniques have advantages and limitations and should be considered complementary to physical examination. They are all less accurate in predicting response after neoadjuvant therapy, with high rates of false positivity, and should be interpreted with caution in this setting.[45,46] Prognostic factors influencing survival in CRC patients include depth of tumor invasion into and beyond the bowel wall, the number of involved regional lymph nodes, and the presence or absence of distant metastases. The tumor, node, metastasis (TNM) system of the American Joint Committee on Cancer can be used as a clinical (preoperative) or postoperative staging system (Tables 61.1 and 61.2).

TREATMENT OF COLON CANCER

Surgery

Surgery is the primary treatment modality for patients with colonic tumors. Resection with curative intent is possible in approximately 75% of patients.[9] Surgery of primary colon cancer is based on the anatomy and mechanisms by which this disease spreads. Adenocarcinomas of the colon may grow by direct

TABLE 61.1 AMERICAN JOINT COMMITTEE ON CANCER 2010 TNM STAGING OF COLORECTAL CANCER

Primary Tumor (T)	
TX	Primary tumor cannot be assessed
T0	No evidence of primary tumor
Tis	Carcinoma *in situ:* intraepithelial or invasion of lamina propria
T1	Tumor invades submucosa
T2	Tumor invades muscularis propria
T3	Tumor invades through the muscularis propria into the subserosa or into pericolorectal tissues
T4a	Tumor penetrates to the surface of the visceral peritoneum[a]
T4b	Tumor directly invades or is adherent to other organs or structures[a,b]
Regional Lymph Modes (N)	
NX	Regional lymph nodes cannot be assessed
N0	No regional lymph node metastasis
N1	Metastasis in one to three regional lymph nodes
N1a	Metastasis in one regional lymph node
N1b	Metastasis in two to three lymph nodes
N1c	Tumor deposit(s) in the subserosa, mesentery, or nonperitonealized pericolorectal tissues without regional nodal metastasis
N2	Metastasis in four or more regional lymph nodes
N2a	Metastasis in four to six regional lymph nodes
N2b	Metastasis in seven or more regional lymph nodes
Distant Metastasis (M)	
MX	Distant metastasis cannot be assessed
M0	No distant metastasis
M1	Distant metastasis
M1a	Metastasis confined to one organ or site
M1b	Metastasis in more than one organ/sit or peritoneum

[a]Direct invasion in T4 includes invasion of other organs or other segments of the colorectum as a result of direct extension through the serosa, as confirmed on microscopic examination (e.g., invasion of the sigmoid colon by a carcinoma of the cecum) or, for cancers in a retroperitoneal or subperitoneal location, direct invasion of other organs or structures by virtue of extension beyond the muscularis propria (i.e., respectively, a tumor on the posterior wall of the descending colon invading the left kidney or lateral abdominal wall, or a mid or distal rectal cancer with invasion of prostate, seminal vesicles, cervix, or vagina).

[b]Tumor that is adherent to other organs or structures grossly is classified cT4b. However, if no tumor is present in the adhesion microscopically, the classification should be pT1-4a, depending on the anatomic depth of wall invasion. The V and L classifications should be used to identify the presence or absence of vascular or lymphatic invasion, whereas the PN site-specific factor should be used for perineural invasion.

Used with the permission of the American Joint Committee on Cancer (AJCC), Chicago, Illinois. The original source for this material is *AJCC Cancer Staging Handbook*, 7th ed. New York: Springer, 2010; published by Springer Science and Business Media LLC, www.springer.com.

TABLE 61.2 STAGING OF COLON AND RECTUM CANCER

	American Joint Committee on Cancer[a]				
Stage	*T*	*N*	*M*	*Dukes*[b]	*MAC*[c]
0	Tis	N0	M0	–	–
I	T1	N0	M0	A	A
	T2	N0	M0	A	B1
IIA	T3	N0	M0	B	B2
IIB	T4a	N0	M0	B	B2
IIC	T4b	N0	M0	B	B3
IIIA	T1-T2	N1/N1c	M0	C	C1
	T1	N2a	M0	C	C1
IIIB	T3-T4a	N1/N1c	M0	C	C2
	T2-T3	N2a	M0	C	C1/C2
	T1-T2	N2b	M0	C	C1
IIIC	T4a	N2a	M0	C	C2
	T3-T4a	N2b	M0	C	C2
	T4b	N1-N2	M0	C	C3
IVA	Any T	Any N	M1a	–	D
IVB	Any T	Any N	M1b		

M, metastasis; N, node; T, tumor

[a]Data from Edge SB, Byrd DR, Compton CC, eds. *AJCC Cancer Staging Handbook*, 7th ed. New York: Springer, 2010.

[b]Dukes B is a composite of better (T3 N0 M0) and worse (T4 N0 M0) prognostic groups, as is Dukes C (any TN1 M0 and Any T N2 M0).

[c]MAC, Modified Astler-Coller classification.

extension into the lymphatics of the submucosa and bowel wall. To avoid cutting across tumor intramural lymphatics, sufficient lengths of bowel must be resected proximal and distal to the primary cancer. Colon cancer often extends through the serosa into mesenteric lymphatics that run along the blood vessels draining into the portal watershed at the root of the mesentery. Resection includes removal of the major lymphatic drainage system in the mesentery. Because anatomic resections are designed to include named blood vessels and draining lymphatics, the boundaries for resecting large-bowel cancer are relatively uniform. Right hemicolectomy, transverse colectomy, left hemicolectomy, and sigmoid resection are performed by adherence to surgical oncologic principles without major sacrifice of large-bowel function. Consensus guidelines recommend that a minimum of 12 lymph nodes should be excised for appropriate staging.[47,48–49] As with other gastrointestinal and pelvic malignancies, the use of laparoscopic techniques has increased. Data suggest no difference in recurrence or survival outcomes with open versus laparoscopic resection.[50–53]

Resection results in excellent cure rates for lesions limited to the bowel wall with negative nodes (average 5-year survival, 97% for T1 N0; 85% to 90% for T2 N0). With a single high-risk feature of extension beyond the colonic wall (T3–4 N0) or involved nodes (T0–2 N+), 5-year survival with surgery falls to 65% to 75%, and adjuvant treatment is often indicated. When both high-risk features are present (T3–4 N+), 5-year survival with surgery alone drops to approximately 50% (T3 N+) and 35% (T4 N+), and adjuvant treatment is recommended.

Adjuvant Chemotherapy

The benefit of adjuvant chemotherapy has been clearly demonstrated in stage III patients, whereas benefit in stage II patients is more controversial. Prospective randomized trials have shown that the addition of 5-flourouracil (5-FU) and leucovorin (LV) improves survival for resected stage III patients.[54,55] More recently, newer agents have been investigated and have shown potential benefit. Capecitabine, an oral 5-FU prodrug, demonstrated similar overall survival (OS) and disease-free survival (DFS) rates to 5-FU/LV in patients with resected stage III colon cancer in a recent randomized trial.[56,57] Oxaliplatin has also been investigated in the adjuvant treatment of resected colon cancer. A randomized study comparing 5-FU/LV with 5-FU/LV/oxaliplatin (FOLFOX) in resected stage II or III colon cancer patients showed improved DFS and OS in patients treated with oxaliplatin-containing regimens.[58,59] These results were validated in the National Surgical Adjuvant Breast and Bowel Project (NSABP) C-07 trial, demonstrating an improvement in DFS with addition of oxaliplatin.[60,61] A Cancer and Leukemia Group B (CALGB) trial examined 5-FU/LV with and without the addition of irinotecan in resected stage III colon patients. No benefit was seen in DFS or OS.[45] These data helped to establish FOLFOX or capecitabine and oxaliplatin (XELOX) as new standard chemotherapeutic regimens in the adjuvant treatment of completely resected, high-risk colon cancer. The use of monoclonal antibodies, such as bevacizumab and cetuximab, although potentially efficacious in the metastatic setting, has not yielded similar results in the adjuvant setting.[62–65]

Adjuvant Irradiation With or Without Concurrent Chemotherapy

Given the documented efficacy of adjuvant chemotherapy, as well as the perception by many oncologists that colonic (as opposed to rectal) cancer is much more likely to relapse distantly than locally, there has been little evaluation of the efficacy of postoperative irradiation with chemotherapy. The potential indications for adjuvant radiation therapy in colon cancer are

TABLE 61.3 FIVE-YEAR ACTUARIAL LOCAL CONTROL AND RELAPSE-FREE SURVIVAL AFTER SURGERY PLUS POSTOPERATIVE RADIOTHERAPY VS. SURGERY ALONE, ACCORDING TO STAGE, FROM THE MASSACHUSETTS GENERAL HOSPITAL

	Surgery Alone			*Surgery Plus Postoperative Radiation*		
TNM Stage	*Number of Patients*	*LC (%)*	*RFS (%)*	*Number of Patients*	*LC (%)*	*RFS (%)*
T3 N0	163	90	78	23	91	72
T4 N0	83	69	63	54	93	79[a]
T3 N+	100	64	48	55	70	47
T4 N+	49	47	38	39	72	53[a]

LC, local control; RFS, relapse-free survival; TNM, tumor, node, metastasis.
[a] $p < .05$.

based on analyses of patterns of failure following resection (Table 61.3).[66,67] Advanced stage predicts for local failure in both colon and rectal cancers; however, local failure in colon cancer also depends on anatomic origin. The ascending and descending colon are considered "anatomically immobile," and their close proximity to the retroperitoneal tissues often limits wide surgical resection (Fig. 61.1). Limitations in achieving satisfactory circumferential margins increase the risk of residual disease and consequently local failure. In contrast, the mid-sigmoid and mid-transverse colon are relatively "mobile," with a wide mesentery, permitting the surgeon to obtain wide margins regardless of extent of disease invasion into the mesentery. Unless there is adjacent organ adherence/invasion by tumor, local failure at these sites is uncommon. Local failure rates for cecal, hepatic/splenic flexure, and proximal/distal sigmoid tumors are variable, depending on the amount of mesentery present, tumor extension, and the adequacy of radial margins. When colon cancers adhere to or invade adjacent structures, local failure rates exceed 30% following surgery alone. In summary, local failure occurs in patients with colonic tumors where there are anatomic constraints on radial resection margins, including tumors adherent to or invading adjacent structures.

Data evaluating the use of adjuvant radiation therapy in high-risk colon cancer patients have largely been limited to single institution retrospective analyses.[38,68–70] To summarize, these studies have suggested that operative bed failures in high-risk patients undergoing resection alone are at least 30%, and that the risk of local failure is reduced by the administration of adjuvant radiation therapy. These are discussed in detail in what follows.

A report from the Massachusetts General Hospital (MGH) evaluated outcomes in high-risk patients undergoing resection followed by adjuvant radiation therapy and compared these to a similar cohort of patients treated over the same period undergoing surgery only.[70] Irradiated patients included those with T4 N0/N+, T3 N+ disease (excluding mid-sigmoid and mid-transverse colon) and T3 N0 patients with margins of <1 cm. A total of 171 patients received postoperative radiation, with 63 patients receiving concurrent chemotherapy, usually with bolus 5-FU (500 mg/m^2 per day) for 3 consecutive days during the first and last weeks of radiation therapy. Radiation treatment was administered through parallel opposed or other multifield techniques to treat the tumor bed with an approximate 3- to 5-cm margin to a total dose of 45 Gy, followed by reduced fields to a total dose of 50.4 to 54 Gy. Draining nodes were included if they were believed to be at high risk for involvement. This cohort was compared to 395 patients with T3–4 N0/N+ tumors undergoing surgery alone during the same time period. Table 61.3 shows 5-year actuarial local control (LC) and relapse-free survival (RFS) in the adjuvant group compared to patients undergoing surgery alone. LC rates in T4 N0

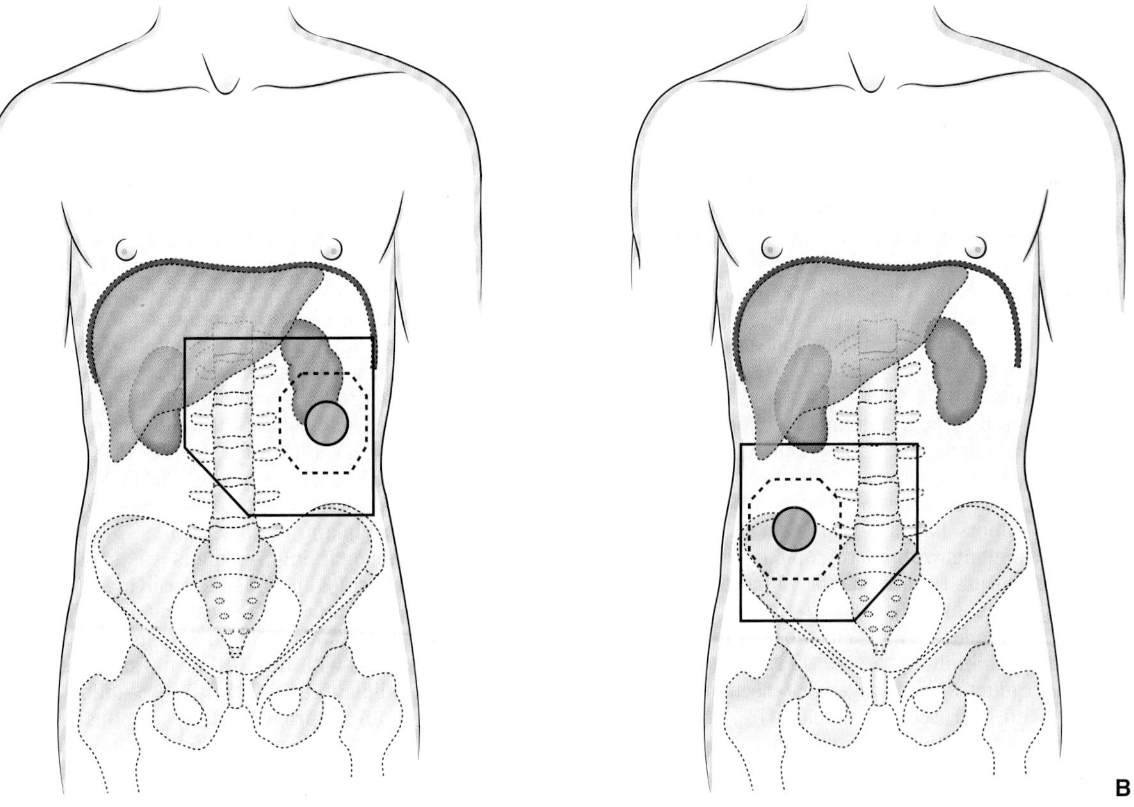
A B

FIGURE 61.2. Idealized postoperative anteroposterior–posteroanterior irradiation fields of extrapelvic colon cancer (tumor bed and nodal regions). If treated preoperatively, lateral fields could be added based on imaging with computed tomography of the abdomen and colon radiograph. **A:** Para-aortic nodes may be at risk, in addition to tumor bed, due to tumor adherence to posterior abdominal wall with descending colon cancer. **B:** External and common iliac nodes may be at risk, in addition to tumor bed, from a proximal cecal/ascending colon cancer. (From Gunderson LL, Martenson JA, Smalley SR, et al. Lower gastrointestinal cancer: rationale, results, and techniques of treatment. *Front Radiat Ther Oncol* 1994;28:140–154; with permission.)

TABLE 61.4 FIVE-YEAR ACTUARIAL LOCAL CONTROL AND RELAPSE-FREE SURVIVAL OF ADJUVANTLY IRRADIATED PATIENTS BASED ON 5-FLUOROURACIL ADMINISTRATION—MASSACHUSETTS GENERAL HOSPITAL

	Without 5-Fluorouracil			With 5-Fluorouracil		
TNM Stage	Number of Patients	LC (%)	RFS (%)	Number of Patients	LC (%)	RFS (%)
T3 N0	16	87	69	7	100	80
T4 N0	37	94	78	16	100	83
T3 N+	41	69	48	14	70	43
T4 N+	24	67	53	15	79	52

LC, local control; RFS, relapse-free survival; TNM, tumor, node, metastasis.

and T4 N+ patients treated with radiation therapy were 93% and 72%, respectively, versus 69% and 47%, respectively, in patients undergoing surgery alone. Similarly, RFS rates were 79% and 53%, respectively, in T4 N0/T4 N+ patients undergoing adjuvant radiation versus 63% and 38%, respectively, in those undergoing surgery alone. No significant outcome differences were observed in patients with T3 N0 and T3 N+ lesions; however, there may be an element of selection bias, given that most patients were referred out of concerns of adequacy of LC following surgery alone. A trend toward improved LC in patients receiving 5-FU was seen (Table 61.4). The rate of acute enteritis in patients receiving irradiation and 5-FU was 16% versus 4% in patients undergoing irradiation only. This rate of enteritis is similar to data from studies of concurrent 5-FU and radiation therapy in rectal cancer. Late bowel complication rates were not increased by concomitant 5-FU administration. The conclusion was that patients with T4 tumors, abscess/fistula formation, or margin-positive resection may benefit from postoperative radiation. In an updated analysis from MGH, 152 patients with T4 tumors received adjuvant irradiation.[38] On pathologic examination, 42 patients had tumors with positive margins. For patients with negative margins the 10-year actuarial LC in T4 N0 and T4 N+ patients was 78% and 48%, respectively. In patients with node-negative tumors, the 10-year actuarial LC and RFS rates were 87% and 58%, respectively, compared to 65% and 33%, respectively, in patients with node-positive tumors. For patients with one involved lymph node, LC and RFS rates were similar to those without nodal involvement; however, with increasing numbers of nodes involved, survival steadily decreased.

A report from the Mayo Clinic evaluated outcomes of 103 patients receiving radiation therapy following surgery for locally advanced colon cancer.[71] Microscopic and gross residual disease was present in 18 and 35 patients, respectively. Greater than 90% of patients had T4 N0/N+ disease. A median dose of 50.4 Gy was delivered through multifield techniques, and most patients received concurrent 5-FU–based chemotherapy. Eleven patients received an intraoperative radiotherapy (IORT) boost of 10 to 20 Gy. Five-year actuarial LC was 40%. Patients with margin-negative tumors had a 5-year local LC of 90%, compared to 46% for patients with microscopic residual tumor and 21% for those with gross residual tumor. In patients with residual disease, LC rates in patients undergoing intraoperative boost were 89%, compared to 18% in those undergoing external irradiation alone. Similarly, 5-year OS rates were improved in patients undergoing margin-negative resection (66%) compared to those with microscopic residual (47%) or gross residual (23%) disease. In addition, patients undergoing intraoperative boost demonstrated improved survival (76% vs. 26%).

A study from the University of Florida of patients with locally advanced but completely resected colon cancers receiving adjuvant radiation reported a LC rate of 88%, similar to the 90% reported from the Mayo Clinic series.[68] In addition, there appeared to be a dose–response relationship to LC. The 5-year rate of LC was 96% for patients receiving 50 to 55 Gy versus 76% for patients receiving <50 Gy ($p = .0095$).

These retrospective studies laid the foundation for further testing in a phase III trial. To assess whether the addition of radiation therapy to adjuvant chemotherapy would result in superior OS and LC rates in resected, high-risk colon cancer patients, the U.S. Intergroup initiated a randomized, prospective trial in 1992.[72] In this trial, patients with resected colon cancer were randomized to postoperative irradiation with 5-FU and levamisole or 5-FU and levamisole alone. Eligibility criteria included margin-negative tumors with adherence to or invasion of surrounding structures (i.e., T4 N0 or N+ disease, excluding peritoneal invasion) or tumors arising in the ascending or descending colon with metastatic regional nodes (T3 N+). Patients were randomized to receive (a) weekly 5-FU combined with levamisole for 12 months or (b) 5-FU and levamisole for 12 months with combined radiation therapy and chemotherapy beginning 1 month after the first 5-FU administration. The recommended total radiation dose was 45 Gy in 25 fractions over 5 weeks, with an optional 5.4 Gy boost.

The initial trial accrual goal was 700 patients; however, the study was closed in 1996 due to poor accrual (222 patients; 189 evaluable). Total accrual was less than one-third of the initial goal, and there was reduced statistical power to detect differences between the groups. No difference in OS or DFS was seen between the two groups. Five-year OS of patients receiving chemotherapy only was 62% versus 58% for patients randomized to chemoirradiation ($p > .50$). LR rates were identical in both arms (18 patients each). Grade III or IV hematologic toxicity was higher in patients receiving radiation therapy. Interpretation of study results was handicapped by decreased statistical power, high ineligibility rates, and lack of surgical clips or preoperative imaging to assist in the definition of appropriate radiotherapy fields in a high percentage of patients. Therefore, no definitive conclusions can be made regarding the efficacy of postoperative irradiation with 5-FU and levamisole based on this underpowered study with many flaws; however, this study provides no data supporting its routine use.

Locally Advanced Disease and Palliation

For patients with metastatic disease, 5-FU–based chemotherapy is usually administered. Prospective, randomized trials have shown that multiagent chemotherapy improves OS in patients with metastatic colorectal cancer. Saltz et al.[73] reported the results of a three-arm randomized trial comparing (a) irinotecan, 5-FU, and LV (IFL), (b) 5-FU/leucovorin, or (c) irinotecan alone. Patients receiving IFL had an improved survival (median survival 14.8 months vs. 12.6 months; $p = .04$) and response rate (39% vs. 21%; $p < .001$) compared to those treated with 5-FU and LV alone. The incidence of grade 3 or higher diarrhea was significantly higher with the three-drug regimen. A study by Goldberg et al.[74] randomized 795 patients with previously untreated, metastatic CRC patients to receive (a) irinotecan, 5-FU, and LV (FOLFIRI), (b) FOLFOX, or (c) irinotecan and oxaliplatin. Patients receiving FOLFOX had an improved median survival compared to those receiving FOLFIRI or irinotecan and oxaliplatin (19.5 vs. 15 vs. 17.4 months; $p < .05$ for oxaliplatin-containing regimens vs. irinotecan-only regimen). Response rates in patients receiving FOLFOX were significantly higher than those receiving FOLFIRI or irinotecan with oxaliplatin (45% vs. 31% vs. 35%; $p < .05$). Falcone et al.[75] reported outcomes with FOLFIRI or the same regimen with the addition of oxaliplatin (FOLFOXIRI). Evaluation of 244 patients demonstrated an improvement in response rate (41% vs. 66%), progression-free survival (6.9 vs. 9.8 months), and OS (16.7 vs. 22.6 months) at the expense of higher grade 2-3 neurotoxicity and grade 3-4 neutropenia.

A number of studies attempted to improve outcomes with the addition of biologically targeted agents. Hurwitz et al.[76] reported a randomized trial comparing FOLFIRI with or without bevacizumab, a monoclonal antibody directed against vascular endothelial growth factor. Median survival was significantly improved in the bevacizumab arm (median survival 20.3 vs. 15.6 months;

$p < .001$). In addition, response rates were improved in the bevacizumab-containing arm (45% vs. 35%; $p = .004$). Cunningham et al.[77] randomized 329 patients with metastatic colorectal cancer refractory to irinotecan-based chemotherapy regimens to receive cetuximab (a monoclonal antibody directed against the epidermal growth factor) or cetuximab with irinotecan. Response rates in patients receiving combination therapy were significantly higher (23% vs. 11%; $p = .007$), as was median time to progression (4.1 vs. 1.5 months; $p < .001$). No difference in OS was observed. Multidrug chemotherapy regimens and other novel agents remain the focus of ongoing investigation in both the metastatic and the nonmetastatic setting.

Palliative irradiation, generally in combination with 5-FU–based chemotherapy, is considered for patients with specific symptoms referable to metastatic disease—brain, bone, and other sites. The combination of radiation therapy and newer agents (irinotecan, oxaliplatin, bevacizumab, cetuximab) remains investigational.

Techniques of Irradiation

Treatment field design in colon cancer is based on patterns of failure data. As is true in the treatment of rectal carcinoma, great care must be taken in the design of postoperative treatment of adenocarcinoma of the colon. Field arrangement will vary, depending on the site of the primary disease, as well as on areas judged to be at high risk for local recurrence.[78] Patient positioning (supine, prone, decubitus) should be considered in planning. Small bowel is often a dose-limiting structure in this therapy, and it may be advantageous to position patients in the right or left decubitus position for at least a portion of their treatment, allowing displacement of the small bowel away from the treatment field. Immobilization devices may improve reproducibility. Small-bowel contrast aids in delineation of small-bowel volume within the treatment field. It may be useful to compare films in both the decubitus and supine positions to determine the actual amount of small-bowel displacement. CT-based planning may facilitate defining the tumor bed, determining beam orientation, and estimating the volume of small bowel included within the treatment fields. As in other abdominal malignancies, a portion of one kidney may be irradiated. Unilateral renal irradiation results in minimal long-term clinical sequelae, assuming that baseline function in the contralateral kidney is normal.[79]

The total radiation dose used in the adjuvant treatment of colon carcinoma depends on the amount of suspected residual disease and tolerance constraints of surrounding normal tissue. Generally, an initial dose of 45 Gy in 25 fractions at 1.8 Gy per fraction is delivered through larger fields to the primary tumor and at-risk tissues. Reduced fields may be treated to 50 Gy if only a small portion of small bowel is included. For patients with T4 tumors, the general goal is to treat the tumor bed to a total dose of 54 to 60 Gy. Surgical clips may aid in the identification of high-risk areas (i.e., positive margins) to assist in target delineation. Any treatment beyond 50 Gy generally mandates exclusion of all small bowel from the field to minimize late toxicity. Spinal cord dose should generally be limited to 45 Gy. In addition, at least two thirds of one functional kidney should receive no more than 18 to 20 Gy and at least two-thirds of the total liver volume should not receive >30 Gy. In a Mayo Clinic analysis, small-bowel obstruction rates were lower when more than two treatment fields were used, and attempts should be made to implement multifield techniques, which may be aided by CT-based planning.[80]

Generally, the primary tumor site should be covered with a 4- to 5-cm margin proximally and distally and with a 3- to 4-cm margin medially and laterally to cover areas of potential residual disease. The nodal basins in the mesentery beyond surgical margins are usually not treated, as satisfactory margin clearance is often obtained in these sites. An exception to this may be right colon tumors, for which both small bowel and right colon are supplied by ileocolic vessels, limiting the extent of resection. In some instances, treatment of the para-aortic nodes may be indicated, particularly with extensive retroperitoneal involvement by tumor. Treatment of proximal mesenteric nodes may be appropriate if nodes adjacent to the surgical or resection margin are involved. Figures 61.2 and 61.3 show idealized radiation fields for varying colonic sites, including cecum, descending, and sigmoid cancer. In many situations, it may be appropriate to exclude treatment of para-aortic nodal basins, based on operative and pathologic findings.

Conclusion

Subsets of patients with colon cancer have LR rates similar to patients with rectal cancer if surgery only is undertaken. Encouraging results from single-institution series utilizing postoperative irradiation with or without 5-FU for patients with resected high-risk colon cancers and the positive results of 5-FU and levamisole in high-risk adjuvant colon cancer prompted an Intergroup randomized trial. Patients with high risk of LR following surgery were randomized to 5-FU and levamisole or 5-FU and levamisole with tumor bed irradiation. There was no benefit in survival in patients receiving adjuvant radiation therapy; however, interpretation of these results is impaired by inadequate accrual and significant flaws, as previously discussed.

The value of adjuvant postoperative irradiation combined with systemic therapy for patients at high risk for LR is unlikely to ever be addressed in a definitive randomized trial. Treatment recommendations should be made on a case-by-case basis with existing data in the setting of an informed consent. Adjuvant tumor bed irradiation with concurrent 5-FU–based chemotherapy should be considered for patients (a) with tumors invading adjoining structures, (b) with tumors complicated by perforation or fistula, and (c) where incomplete resection is performed.

The use of IORT as a supplement to EBRT in certain T4 tumors (i.e., those with uncertain margins) may also be appropriate. For patients with tumors adherent to or invading adjacent structures, the preferred treatment sequence would be preoperative EBRT plus 5-FU–based chemotherapy, followed by resection with or without IORT and postoperative systemic therapy, based on excellent results in preliminary IORT reports from both U.S. and European institutions.[80,81,82] A similar approach would be reasonable for patients with locally recurrent cancers or with regional nodal relapse.[37,83–85]

THERAPY OF RECTAL CANCER

Management of cancer of the rectum has undergone dramatic changes in the last two decades. Surgery has been considered the primary treatment modality, but in spite of "curative" resections, historically, a significant proportion of patients developed local recurrence of disease (20% to 50%).[86,87] Local tumor recurrence is highly correlated with both the depth of penetration of the tumor and the number of regional nodes.[43] Recent results of national cooperative group studies and several European randomized trials indicate that a multimodality treatment approach, particularly neoadjuvant treatment, results in a significantly better outcome than does surgery alone.

Defining the True Rectum and Impact of Tumor Location

Rectal cancer represents a spectrum of disease stages that needs careful definition to optimize multimodality treatment strategies, and defining the true rectum is of critical importance. Traditionally, the rectum extends for 12 to 15 cm from the anal verge. The true surgical rectum begins at the anorectal ring, just proximal to the dentate line.[35] This represents the internal anal sphincteric muscle and is necessary for anal continence. It also represents the practical inferior limit for functional sphincter preservation surgery and defines the lymphatic watershed for rectal cancer spread. Tumors arising above the anorectal ring tend to metastasize along the distribution of the middle rectal vessels to the internal iliac lymph nodes, as compared to tumors that may extend into the anal canal, which may spread via nodes along the inferior rectal and external iliac pathways

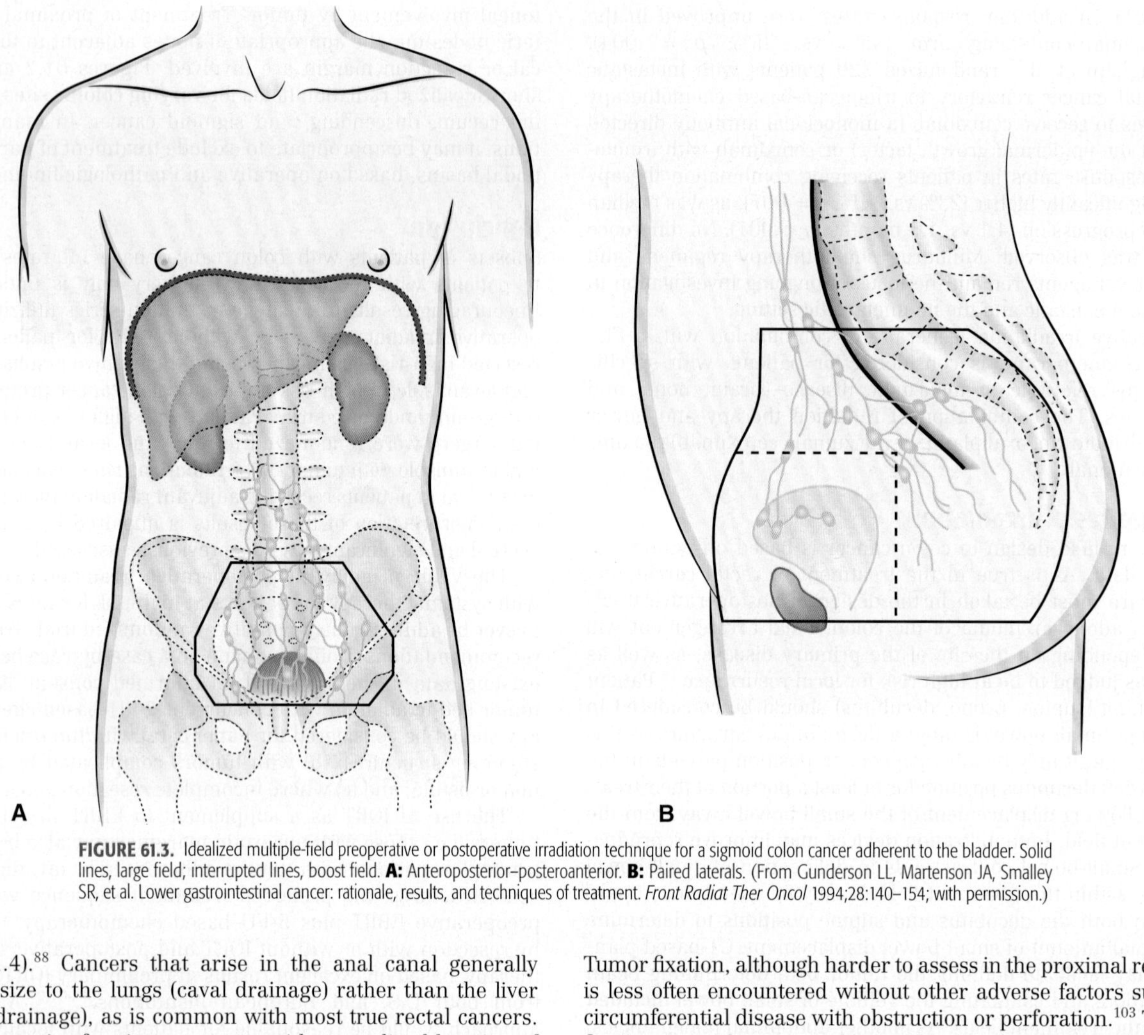

FIGURE 61.3. Idealized multiple-field preoperative or postoperative irradiation technique for a sigmoid colon cancer adherent to the bladder. Solid lines, large field; interrupted lines, boost field. **A:** Anteroposterior–posteroanterior. **B:** Paired laterals. (From Gunderson LL, Martenson JA, Smalley SR, et al. Lower gastrointestinal cancer: rationale, results, and techniques of treatment. *Front Radiat Ther Oncol* 1994;28:140–154; with permission.)

(Fig. 61.4).[88] Cancers that arise in the anal canal generally metastasize to the lungs (caval drainage) rather than the liver (portal drainage), as is common with most true rectal cancers. The prognosis of patients worsens with more distal location of cancer, and these differences persist even with the addition of adjunctive therapy.[89–91] The proximal rectum has historically been defined by the level at which the peritoneum is reflected along the anterior surface of the rectum (usually at the level of S3).[92] This is a surgical observation and difficult to define in an intact patient. The middle valve of Houston is a useful landmark that can often be identified endoscopically (usually about 6 cm from the anorectal ring) and can be used to differentiate proximal tumors from more distal lesions. Most tumors that can be digitally palpated are generally considered distal cancers.

Prognostic Factors

Several prognostic factors, in addition to tumor location, have been shown to have a significant impact on tumor behavior.[89] Tumor stage, as defined by the American Joint Committee on Cancer staging, clearly remains the dominant determinant of survival.[93,94] In some reports the presence of lymph-vascular invasion has been shown to have a negative impact on survival.[95,96] Histopathologic grade is of borderline significance; however, signet cell cancers have a particularly poor outcome.[97] Circumferential tumors or those with total or near-total obstruction (lumen, <1 cm) may respond very poorly, and tumors with deep central ulceration are associated with a high incidence of lymph node involvement.[41,95,98,99] Tumor mobility remains a key factor in both choice and outcome of treatment.[100,101] Mobile cancers have a much more favorable outcome as compared to tethered or fixed cancers. Some studies report that even among mobile cancers only 75% to 80% are completely resected with negative surgical margins.[102] Surgery for fixed cancers has proven ineffective, and these tumors are often classified as unresectable. Tumor fixation, although harder to assess in the proximal rectum, is less often encountered without other adverse factors such as circumferential disease with obstruction or perforation.[103] Tumor fixation is much more problematic in the distal rectum because the confines of the bony pelvis inhibits the surgeon's ability to achieve adequate lateral/circumferential margins. Other patient factors, such as age, gender, and ethnicity, appear to have little association with outcome but may affect choice of therapy.[104–106] As neoadjuvant therapy has emerged as the standard of care, degree of tumor regression has become an important prognostic factor.[107,108] Pathologic assessment of tumors after neoadjuvant therapy receives a special designation of ypTNM classification.

Treatment

Surgery

Surgery remains the mainstay of curative treatment for carcinoma of the rectum. Surgical management depends on the stage and location of a tumor within the rectum. Very early cancers can be manage with limited surgery (i.e., local excision) in selected situations; however, the majority of tumors tend to present as more advanced disease and require either a low anterior resection (LAR) or abdominoperineal resection (APR). The general principles of a surgical approach remain the removal of all gross and microscopic disease with negative proximal, distal, and circumferential margins. In the case of radical resection, this means removal of the adjacent mesorectal tissue (total mesorectal excision [TME]), containing the regional lymphatics and potential tumor deposits. Several studies have shown that the surgeon's experience with resection of CRC is an independent variable in the outcome of treatment.[109] The Intergroup 0114 trial found that for stage II and III rectal cancers, not only were APR rates higher in hospitals performing low-volume procedures (46% vs. 32%), but also more patients had positive resection margins.[110]

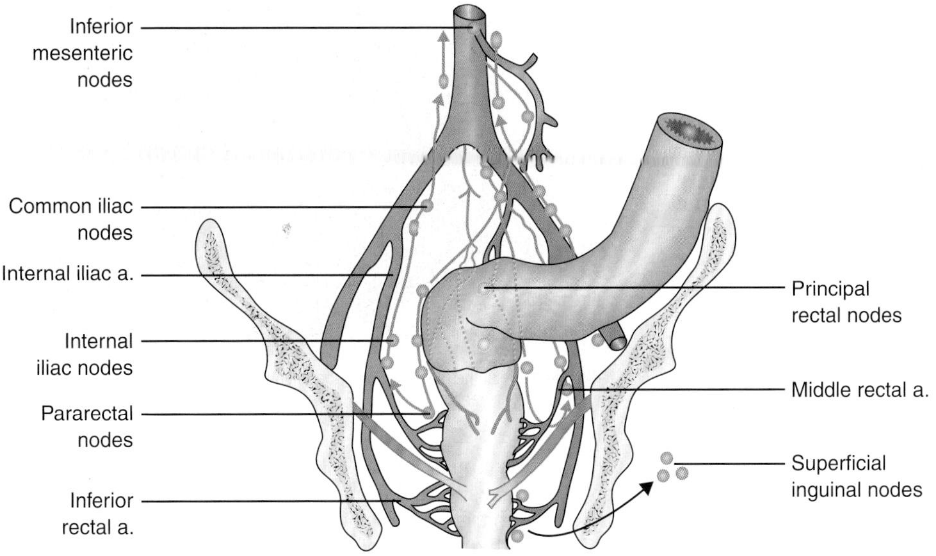

FIGURE 61.4. Lymphatics of the rectum.

Historically, the distal and proximal resection margins were considered important determinants in outcome, and a 5-cm distal margin of normal rectum was considered necessary for adequate surgical resection.[111–113] However, several retrospective studies have shown that distal intramural spread of tumor is rare beyond 1.5 cm, and, therefore, a 2-cm distal margin is currently considered acceptable, except in lesions that are poorly differentiated or widely metastatic.[114–117] The reduced requirement of 2-cm distal margin for adequate resection has led to a significant increase in the likelihood of sphincter preservation procedures in this disease.

Laparoscopic surgery has emerged offering potential advantages of reduced blood loss/perioperative morbidity and shorter hospitalizations. In the hands of an experienced surgeon outcomes from laparoscopic surgery appear no different than those from open resection in a number of randomized trials, although this remains a subject of ongoing investigation.[118–120]

Local Excision

Early rectal cancer may be resected with local excision techniques, avoiding major surgery and a colostomy, but patients should be carefully selected for these procedures. Transanal excision, transsphincteric excision (York-Mason), and a posterior parasacral approach (Kraske) permit removal of the tumor and adjoining rectum in one uninterrupted specimen. A transanal approach is usually associated with the least morbidity, but to be amenable for local excision, tumors generally need to be located <8 cm from the anal verge. An anal sphincter splitting approach can be used for tumors close to the anorectal junction, and occasionally a presacral Kraske approach can be used to access more proximal tumors, although this is now generally considered a historical procedure. An adequate resection requires full thickness (into the fat), with the tumor being removed in one uninterrupted specimen with at least a 1-cm margin so that careful pathologic assessment can be performed. A primary closure of the rectal defect may then be performed, although this is variable. The inability to sample perirectal and mesenteric lymph nodes can result in underestimation of cancer stage. Lymph node metastases have been observed in 5% to 10% of patients with T1 lesions and 20% to 35% of patients with T2 lesions.[121] Given the potential risk of lymph node spread, it is necessary to restrict local excision to patients with low-risk tumors where the risk of recurrence is <10% (i.e., very favorable T1 cancers). Properly selected T1 lesions have excellent results with local excision alone, with 5-year LC ranging from 82% to 97% and OS rates of 90% or better.[122,123] The risk of perirectal nodal metastasis and high incidence of reported local failure (LF) rates for T2 cancers following local excision alone indicate the need for further adjuvant therapy.[124]

Radiation Therapy Oncology Group (RTOG) 89-02 examined the efficacy of local excision in a study of 65 patients with distal rectal cancers. Tumors had to be grade 1 or 2, have margins ≥3 mm, no lymphovascular invasion (LVI), and no regional lymph node ≥2 cm by CT scan to be eligible for observation. T2 tumors with margins ≤3 mm received 59.4 to 65 Gy. Fourteen patients with T1 tumors were observed after surgery, whereas 13 patients with T1 tumors, 25 patients with T2 tumors, and 13 patients with T3 tumors received local excision with postoperative radiation of 50 to 65 Gy with 5-FU (1,000 mg/m^2 on days 1 to 3 and 29 to 31). None of the T1 tumors receiving postoperative treatment relapsed, compared to one distant metastasis and one local failure in the T1 observation arm. Five patients in the T2 group relapsed (2 local, 1 distant, 2 both), and 4 patients in the T3 group had recurrence (1 distant, 3 both). Therefore, 20% of T2 and 23% of T3 tumors experienced LF after local excision plus chemoradiation (CRT).[125] Therefore, although it is possible that highly selected T2 and limited T3 tumors may be treated with local excision and postoperative adjuvant therapy, the high rate of locoregional failure makes this a potentially inferior approach.

The CALGB 8984 study provides some support for postoperative CRT after local excision for T1 and T2 rectal cancers.[126] Fifty-nine patients with T1 disease were treated with local excision alone, and 51 patients with T2 disease received adjuvant therapy with 54 Gy and 5-FU (500 mg/m^2 on days 1 to 3 and 29 to 31). At 10 years, LR, DFS, and OS were 8%, 75%, and 84%, respectively, in T1 tumors. For T2 tumors LR, DFS, and OS were 18%, 64%, and 66%, respectively. Detailed information regarding salvage APR was not published in the updated study. In initial publication one of two T1 local failures and four of five T2 local failures were salvaged by APR. Of note, 25% of the clinical T1 and T2 tumors were actually pathologic T3.[127] The 20% recurrence rate and DFS of 64% for T2 cancers are considerably inferior to the results of radical surgery with TME alone or neoadjuvant therapy followed by surgery. This study supports the possibility of conservative sphincter-sparing surgery for well-selected T1 lesions, but for T2 tumors the high rate of LF despite CRT warrants caution.

Based on the available data, local excision should be limited to tumors that are small (<4 cm), clinically T1 (or favorable T2 patients in selected situations), well to moderately differentiated, and involve <40% of the circumference of the rectum. These tumors are usually mobile, polypoid, not ulcerated, and have favorable pathology, including no lymphovascular invasion.[128,129–130]

Low Anterior Resection

The availability of circular stapling devices has expanded the role of sphincter preservation surgical options in rectal cancers, and LAR is now being performed not just for cancers of the upper one-third of the rectum, but also for middle- and lower-one-third cancers.[131] Preserving adequate anorectal function becomes increasingly difficult the more distal the level of anorectal anastomosis.[132] Patients should have good anal sphincter continence prior to considering sphincter-preserving options. Patient age, pelvic anatomy, gender, and body habitus can affect suitability for sphincter preservation. A 2-cm distal margin of preserved normal rectum is considered optimal for preservation of adequate bowel function. In carefully selected patients a functional coloanal anastomosis can be achieved with significantly reduced margins for more distal cancers, particularly after neoadjuvant therapy. If LAR is planned following neoadjuvant radiation therapy, it is necessary to mobilize the splenic flexure to allow an unirradiated segment of the bowel to be used for the anastomosis. The latter can be performed with several techniques—an end-to-end, a side-to-end, or a colonic J-pouch technique to maximize preservation of sphincter function.[133,134] Several studies comparing results of LAR to APR generally reported similar outcomes for local and distant recurrence rates and survival as long as surgical margins are negative.[135,136] The absence of a colostomy, although offering a better quality of life with LAR, can be compromised with bowel urgency, frequency, or poor sphincter control.[137]

Abdominoperineal Resection

APR has been considered the gold standard for surgical resection of distal rectal cancer and requires removal of the primary tumor along with a complete proctectomy, leading to a permanent colostomy. Recent data suggest a decline in the APR rate.[36,138] APR is associated with a slightly higher morbidity and mortality than LAR and a worse quality of life related to changes in body image and depression due to the presence of a colostomy.[136,138,139] There is also a higher risk of positive margins with APR because the mesorectum is thin in the distal segment of the rectum, with margins are often restricted by the proximity of the prostate or vagina. The confines of the bony pelvis, particularly in males, can restrict surgical access.[140]

Total Mesorectal Excision

The high LR of disease following standard APR or LAR (15% to 30% or more) has been believed by some to be due to blunt dissection that violates the planes of the mesorectal circumference.[141] Lateral spread of disease has been shown to occur not only at the level of the tumor, but also distally within the mesorectum.[142] Heald et al.[143,144] recommended en bloc removal of the tumor within the envelope of the endopelvic fascia as necessary to obtain adequate lateral clearance of disease and reduced likelihood of LR. TME, as they described, has become the established standard for all radical rectal cancer resections and requires sharp dissection along the plane that separates the visceral from the parietal pelvic fascia with complete en bloc removal of the rectum so that all of the rectal mesentery remains within the envelope of the specimen.[145]

On gross pathology, an adequate TME specimen will have a bilobed, encapsulated appearance, with the surface looking smooth and unbroken, like a lipoma (Fig. 61.5). On pathologic review, an appropriate dissection should include a minimum of 12 to 15 perirectal and pelvic lymph nodes.[146–150] TME, although more difficult with APR than LAR, may be associated with a somewhat higher anastomotic leak rate, especially for low rectal lesions (15% to 17%).[102,145,151] Multiple series using TME surgery have reported low rates of LR (ranging from 5% to 10%) and an improvement in OS approaching 80% to 85% for stage II and 65% to 70% for stage III disease.[98,141,152,153–154]

Radial Margin

The National Institute of Health Consensus Conference on Rectal Cancer indicated that the principal reason for LR in resected rectal cancer appears to be related to the anatomic constraints in obtaining wide radial margins, despite adequate proximal and distal margins.[155] Using whole-mount specimens, Quirke et al. found that 27% (14 of 52) of patients showed spread to the lateral radial margin, even though the margins appeared negative with standard pathologic assessment. Eighty-six percent of those with positive radial margins developed local regional recurrence of disease, as compared to only 3% without lateral resection margin involvement.[156] In addition, pathologic assessment in a large randomized trial found that the plane of surgery—mesorectal, intramesorectal, or muscularis propria plane—predicted for LR. Three-year LR was 4% in patients undergoing complete mesorectal excision, compared with 7% and 13% in the intramesorectal and muscularis propria groups, respectively.[98] A positive radial margin is a predictor not only of LR, but also of inferior survival.[95] The mean surgical margin of resection has been shown to decrease with increasing stage of disease, ranging from 14 mm for T1 cancers to 3 mm for T4 cancers, with a corresponding increase in LR from 0% to 75%.[157]

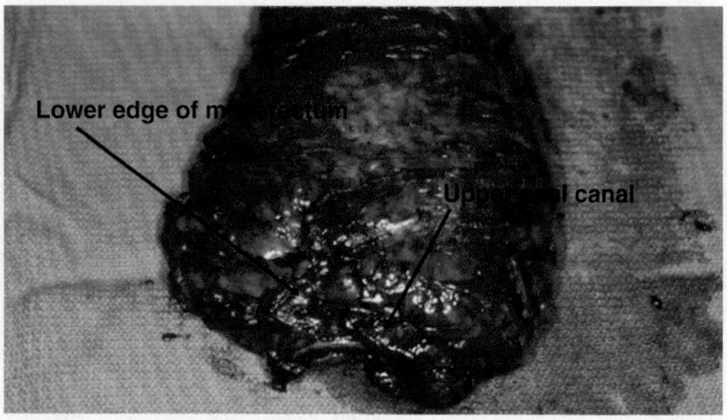

FIGURE 61.5. Total mesorectal excision specimen with designation of the lower mesorectum and upper anal canal.

Adjuvant Therapy

Postoperative

The problem of unacceptably high LR after surgery has led to many studies exploring the potential benefit of postoperative adjuvant therapy. One of the advantages of postoperative radiation is the ability to selectively treat patients at high risk of LF on the basis of pathologic criteria. Disadvantages include a potentially hypoxic postsurgical bed, making radiation and chemotherapy less effective, and potentially higher complications due to increased small bowel in the radiation field. Postoperative treatments tend to require larger treatment volumes, particularly in patients undergoing an APR where the perineal scar may need to be covered. A number of trials assessed the role of adjuvant radiotherapy compared to surgery alone. These trials showed reduced LF with radiotherapy; however, no improvement in DFS, distant metastasis (DM), or OS was seen.[158] Given this, the role of adjuvant CRT was evaluated in an effort to improve treatment outcomes. In general, surgery alone resulted in a 25% LF rate and 40% to 50% OS for T3 or T4 or node-positive patients, whereas CRT yielded a lower LF rate of 10% to 15% and higher OS of 50% to 60%.

The NSABP R-02 study enrolled 694 stage B and C patients and asked two questions in its study design: (a) Does the addition of radiation to chemotherapy improve outcome? (b) Is 5-FU, semustine, and vincristine superior to 5-FU/LV in men?[159] There were four treatment arms for male patients and two treatment arms for female patients. Five cycles of MOF were compared to six cycles of 5-FU/LV with or without radiation in male patients. For women, 5-FU/LV was compared against a similar regimen with radiation. The radiation dose was 50.4 Gy. At 5 years, the locoregional failure was 13% for the chemotherapy-only arm as compared to 8% with the addition of radiation to chemotherapy. 5-FU/LV demonstrated better RFS and DFS, but not OS, as compared to MOF chemotherapy. Although postoperative radiation treatment did not appear to improve OS, there was an improvement in LC.

Two trials of CRT demonstrating an improvement in OS were the Gastrointestinal Tumor Study Group (GITSG) and North Central Cancer Treatment Group (NCCTG) studies. The GITSG study was a four-arm trial of 227 patients with stage B2 and C rectal cancer who, after R0 resection, were randomized to (a) surgery alone, (b) postoperative chemotherapy of bolus 5-FU (500 mg/m^2 in weeks 1 and 5 and methyl-CCNU [semustine] given day 1), (c) postoperative radiation treatment of 40 to 48 Gy split course, or (d) postoperative CRT of 40 to 44 Gy plus bolus 5-FU.[34] The severe acute toxicity was 61% in the combined-modality treatment arm, as compared to 31% with chemotherapy only and 18% with radiation only. This trial was terminated early, given the significant benefit seen with CRT. In a subsequent update, postoperative CRT improved 10-year OS, 45% versus 27%, compared with observation after surgery.[160] There was a prolonged time to recurrence and a decreased recurrence rate of 33% versus 55% with CRT. LF rate was decreased to 10% versus 25% with surgery alone. Therefore, this trial concluded that there was a significant OS advantage (near doubling of survival) for patients who had CRT after surgical resection.

The Mayo–NCCTG study compared postoperative radiation therapy against postoperative CRT.[161] Two hundred four patients with T3/T4 or node-positive tumors received one cycle of 5-FU and semustine before randomization. The radiation dose was 45 to 50.4 Gy to tumor bed and adjacent lymph node regions. Bolus 5-FU (500 mg/m^2) was administered concurrently with radiotherapy. The 5-year local-regional failure was higher in the radiation-only arm, 25% versus 13%, and the 5-year OS was 40% versus 55% (in favor of CRT). Postoperative CRT reduced recurrence by 47%, LR by 46%. and DM by 37%. Cancer deaths were reduced by 36%, and overall deaths were reduced by 29%.

Given the potential benefits seen with CRT, subsequent trials attempted to refine the type and delivery of chemotherapy to maximize benefit with lower toxicity. The NCCTG 86-47-51 study compared chemotherapy regimens to be added to postoperative radiation therapy.[162] Six hundred sixty stage II or III patients were randomized 2 × 2 to systemic chemotherapy (5-FU vs. 5-FU + semustine) and the method of delivery (bolus vs. continuous infusion [CI] 5-FU). Nine weeks of chemotherapy were given, followed by the experimental chemotherapy concurrently with 50.4- to 54-Gy radiation therapy and additional chemotherapy thereafter. The bolus 5-FU dose was 500 mg/m^2 on day 1 to 5 during weeks 1 and 5, and the CI 5-FU was 225 mg/m^2 per day. With a median follow-up of 46 months, there was a 27% improvement in RFS of 63% versus 53% in favor of CI 5-FU. The 4-year OS was 70% versus 60% in favor of CI. The time to relapse and the DM rate (31% vs. 40%) were also lower. There was no difference in LR. Bolus 5-FU had a higher rate of leucopenia, whereas CI had more acute severe diarrhea, which did not persist after conclusion of CRT. Semustine was of no additional benefit beyond 5-FU chemotherapy.[163]

The Intergroup 0114 study compared different chemotherapy regimens with radiation treatment in 1,695 patients.[164] Patients were randomized to one of four arms: (a) bolus 5-FU alone, (b) 5-FU and LV, (c) 5-FU plus levamisole, and (d) 5-FU, LV, and levamisole. Levamisole was not given during the radiation treatment. The radiation treatment dose was 45 Gy with a 5.4- to 9-Gy boost to a total of 50.4 to 54 Gy. With a median follow-up of 7.4 years, there was no difference in OS or DFS among the four groups. Patients randomized to the three-drug regimen experienced greater toxicity. The addition of levamisole and/or LV did not appear to add any benefit to the 5-FU.

Favorable T3 N0

Several studies have shown that there may be a subset of tumors that might not need adjuvant therapy, given the low risk of recurrence with surgery alone. Memorial Sloan-Kettering Cancer Center evaluated 95 patients with T3 N0 rectal cancer treated by surgery alone.[165] Seventy-nine patients underwent LAR and 16 patients underwent APR, both with sharp mesorectal excision. With 53.3-month follow-up, 6% had LR, 13% had DM, and 3% had both LR and DM. Lymphovascular invasion was the only histologic factor that was important for LR. This study suggests that sharp mesorectal excision with LAR or APR for T3 N0 rectal cancers results in low LRs of <10% without the use of adjuvant therapy.

In a retrospective review of 117 patients with T3 N0 rectal cancer treated at MGH, perirectal tumor invasion ≥2 mm, LVI, and poorly differentiated histology were independent factors for increased risk of DM and worse RFS.[46] Only depth of invasion was significant for LC. Of the 25 patients with favorable histologic features (well differentiated/moderately differentiated, invading <2 mm into the perirectal fat, no LVI), the 10-year actuarial LC and RFS were 95% and 87%, respectively, as compared to 71% and 55% in the unfavorable group.

The largest series—a pooled analysis of five randomized, controlled trials—assessed survival and relapse rates by T and N stage.[94] In patients with T3 N0 disease, 5-year survival of patients undergoing surgery and adjuvant chemotherapy alone was 84% and compared favorably to the 74% to 80% survival in patients undergoing surgery and adjuvant CRT. DFS in the T3 N0 subgroup was 69%. Since many of these trials, EUS and/or pelvic MRI have become standard in staging rectal cancers. One issue for the T3 N0 subset is the concern of understaging despite these technologies. A report from Memorial Sloan-Kettering evaluated the pathologic complete response (pCR) and mesorectal lymph node involvement rate in 188 patients with either EUS or MRI staging undergoing radical resection after CRT.[166] Twenty-two percent of patients had mesorectal lymph node involvement. Although overstaging and overtreatment are possible with preoperative treatment, a larger number of patients would be understaged and require postoperative therapy. Thus, there is likely a limited subset of patients with T3 N0 rectal cancer who might have an excellent outcome with surgery alone, but there are no randomized data to support the omission of (neo) adjuvant therapy for this group of patients at the present time.

Neoadjuvant

Neoadjuvant Radiotherapy

Although both preoperative and postoperative adjuvant therapy can be effective, neoadjuvant treatment has emerged as the standard of care. Neoadjuvant therapy is associated with tumor downstaging, improved resectability and tolerance (both acute and chronic), and potential for expanded sphincter preservation options in the distal rectum. Studies from Europe have demonstrated that appropriate neoadjuvant preoperative radiation results in improvement of both LC and OS, and these results have had a significant impact on the current management of this disease.[152,167]

The Swedish Rectal Cancer Trial included 1,168 patients accrued from 1987 to 1990 with resectable, Dukes A to C rectal cancer.[168] Patients were randomized to 25 Gy in five fractions in 1 week followed by surgery 1 week later versus surgery alone. The surgery was rated as curative if margins were negative. The 5-year LR (11% vs. 27%) and OS (58% vs. 48%) were superior with preoperative radiation treatment compared to surgery alone. The LR and OS benefit persisted with long-term follow-up. At a median 13 years, LR was 9% versus 26% and OS was 38% versus 30%, both in favor of preoperative radiotherapy, with all stages benefiting.[167]

One caveat of this study is that the surgery-alone arm did not use TME, which may have resulted in an unacceptably high 5-year LF rate of 27%. Late effects suggested more bowel movement frequency, incontinence, urgency, and soiling in the preoperative radiation treatment arm, although overall quality of life was rated good.[169] A higher rate of small-bowel obstruction was also seen in the preoperative radiotherapy arm.[170] This trial set the standard of care in many European centers, but the dose of 5 Gy times five fractions may potentially contribute to late toxicity, and the short interval between radiation and surgery may not have allowed sufficient time for tumor regression (downstaging) for improved sphincter preservation.

Justification for a longer interval after preoperative radiation treatment before surgery was demonstrated in a French trial, Lyon 90–01, which delivered 39 Gy as 3 Gy per fraction (no preoperative chemotherapy).[171] Two hundred one patients were randomized to surgery within 2 weeks versus 6 to 8 weeks of radiotherapy. The LC and OS after a median follow-up of 33 months were the same in both arms of the study. However, the pCR was 7% versus 14% (p = NSS [not statistically significant]), and the pathologic downstaging was 10% versus 26% (p = .007) in favor of the longer interval before surgery.

The TME experience by Heald et al.[143] suggested that TME alone may be sufficient for achieving low LR rates. A Dutch (CKVO 95-04) multicenter, phase III study of 1,861 patients was undertaken to evaluate the role of short-course preoperative radiation with TME. Patients were randomized to TME alone versus 25 Gy in five fractions followed by TME surgery. No fixed tumors were included in the study, and approximately half of the patients had T1 or T2 disease. The 2-year OS was 82% in both arms of the study; however, the 2-year LR was 8.2% in the TME-only arm as compared to 2.4% in the preoperative arm. This highlighted the value of radiation treatment, despite use of TME. The sphincter preservation rate was the same in both arms, and there was no clear evidence of any downstaging effect. The perineal complication rate was slightly higher in the preoperative radiation arm of 26% versus 18% in the TME arm.[102,172] Ten-year follow-up indicates persistent benefit in LR of 5% (RT) vs. 11% (TME alone).[152] Updated toxicity analysis indicates a higher incidence of sexual dysfunction and slower recovery of bowel function, more fecal incontinence, and generally poorer quality of life with short-course preoperative radiation.[173,174]

Two meta-analyses of approximately 6,000 patients each were done to explore the benefit of preoperative radiation treatment. One analysis included 14 randomized, controlled trials and reported that neoadjuvant radiation treatment was associated with significantly fewer local recurrences, improved specific survival, and an overall survival benefit.[27] The second meta-analysis, provided by the Colorectal Cancer Collaborative Group, also reported on 14 randomized, controlled trials.[175] They noted a significant reduction in the risk of local recurrence and death from rectal cancer with preoperative radiotherapy.

Neoadjuvant Chemoradiation

The improvement in outcomes with CRT in the postoperative setting led to adoption of this approach in the treatment of this disease. More recently, in the United States neoadjuvant CRT has become widely accepted (see later discussion), but in other parts of the world several groups have undertaken studies to examine the potential benefit from neoadjuvant CRT compared to radiation alone.

Preoperative radiation therapy was compared with combined preoperative CRT in a French study (Fédération Francophone de la Canérologie Digestive 9203).[176] Seven hundred thirty three patients with resectable T3 and T4 tumors accessible by DRE were randomized to 45 Gy of radiation alone versus radiation with concurrent bolus 5-FU (350 mg/m^2) plus LV on days 1 to 5 during weeks 1 and 5. After surgery, four cycles of adjuvant chemotherapy were given. The primary endpoint was OS. Although there was no difference in 5-year OS between the two arms, pCR rates (11.4% vs. 3.6%) were higher and LR rates (8.1% vs. 16.5%) were lower with CRT. Grade 3/4 acute toxicity was more frequent in patients receiving CRT, at 14.6% versus 2.7%.

A similar study undertaken by the European Organization for Research and Treatment of Cancer (EORTC 22921)[177] randomized >1,000 patients to four arms (2 × 2 design): 45 Gy alone versus 45 Gy plus 5-FU (350 mg/m^2) LV followed by surgery, with patients further randomized to adjuvant therapy with 5-FU/LV or no adjuvant therapy. Results of the study were similar to those of the French study, with increased tumor downstaging (14% vs. 5.3%; p = .0001) and lower rates of LR (9% vs. 17%) but no difference in 5-year OS (65% in both arms). This information suggests that although there are lower rates of recurrence, there is no conclusive evidence that combined treatment offers a survival benefit compared to radiation alone in the neoadjuvant setting. There is, however, a higher incidence of acute toxicity associated with combined CRT.

A subsequent meta-analysis pooled four trials and compared results of preoperative radiotherapy with preoperative CRT in patients with resectable stage II or III rectal cancer.[178] The addition of chemotherapy significantly increased rates of grade 3/4 acute toxicity (odds ratio [OR], 1.68 to 10), higher rates of pCR (OR, 2.52 to 5.27) and lowered the incidence of LR (OR, 0.39 to 0.72). No difference was seen in 5-year DFS or OS. Although the aforementioned studies and meta-analysis do not show a DFS or OS benefit with the addition of chemotherapy to neoadjuvant RT, given higher pCR as well as improved LC, neoadjuvant CRT represents a reasonable standard of care.

Long Course Neoadjuvant Chemoradiotherapy vs. Short Course Neoadjuvant Radiotherapy

In parts of Europe where a hypofractionated preoperative radiotherapy regimen is preferred, a study to determine whether a short-course approach (5 Gy for five fractions) to neoadjuvant therapy is better than a protracted approach (50.4 Gy using 1.8- to 2-Gy fractions with concomitant bolus 5-FU/LV given during weeks 1 and 5) was undertaken by the Polish rectal cancer group.[180] Although a higher pCR rate was seen with CRT (16% vs. 1%) along with fewer positive radial margins (4% vs. 13%) and considerable size reduction of the tumor (by approximately 1.9 cm), no difference in the rate of sphincter preservation, LC, or OS was seen.

Results from the Australian Intergroup Trial were recently published.[179] Three hundred twenty six patients with cT3NxM0 rectal cancer within 12 cm of the anal verge were randomized to short course RT (25 Gy in 5 fractions) with surgery within 1 week or long course CRT (50.4 Gy in 28 fractions with continuous infusion 5-FU 225mg/m^2) with surgery 4-6 weeks following completion of CRT. Both regimens were followed by adjuvant 5-FU-based chemotherapy. The primary endpoint of this study was to compare LR rates at 3 years. Over 90% of patients were clinically staged with pelvic MRI or EUS. With median follow up of 5.9 years, there was no difference in 3-year LR (7.5% short course vs. 4.4% CRT), 5-year OS (74% short course vs. 70% CRT) or late toxicity. Despite tumor downstaging, there was no difference in rates of sphincter sparing surgery.

The optimal neoadjuvant approach for resectable rectal cancer is far from clear. Both short course RT (25Gy in 5 fractions) and long course CRT (50.4 Gy in 28 fractions with concurrent 5FU based chemotherapy represent reasonable therapeutic options. Many await long term data from these randomized trials to assess for differences in late toxicities which, as seen in the Swedish and Dutch experiences, can take many years to emerge.

Alternative Chemotherapy Regimens with Neoadjuvant Radiotherapy

There is considerable variability in the administration of chemotherapy in many of the trials undertaken and those that are ongoing. 5-FU has been used concurrent with radiation because of its well-established potentiating effect with radiation. However, several studies have used bolus 5-FU, whereas others have administered LV-modulated 5-FU during the first and last weeks of radiation. The results of the Intergroup study demonstrating a superiority of low-dose CI5-FU were extrapolated to the neoadjuvant setting, and it appears to be a preferred approach to treatment.[163] New drugs, including oral fluoropyrimidines (capecitabine), oxaliplatin, and irinotecan, have been shown to be effective in the treatment of metastatic colorectal cancer. Oral fluoropyrimidines, as part of a CRT regimen, are commonly replacing infusional 5-FU. The incorporation of oxaliplatin and irinotecan into the neoadjuvant regimen has been less promising.

Capecitabine is an oral fluoropyrimidine prodrug that is readily absorbed in the gastrointestinal tract and mimics the efficacy of CI 5-FU while avoiding the risk of side effects and complications due to a central line for CI 5-FU.[181] Capecitabine requires the presence of thymidine phosphorylase (TP) for conversion to the active form of 5-FU within the cells. TP is present in higher concentration in tumor cells, particularly colorectal cancer than in normal tissues, and this potentially creates a therapeutic advantage for capecitabine as compared to intravenous 5-FU.[182] Capecitabine is generally given in two divided doses twice a day during the course of radiation treatment.

Two reports from randomized control trials indicate promising results for the use of capecitabine. A German trial compared capecitabine to infusional 5-FU, initially in the adjuvant setting and then later neoadjuvantly. Initially, patients in the capecitabine group were scheduled to receive two cycles of capecitabine (2500 mg/m^2 days 1-14, repeated day 22), followed by chemoradiotherapy (50·4 Gy plus capecitabine 1650 mg/m^2 days 1-38), then three cycles of capecitabine. Patients in the fluorouracil group received two cycles of bolus fluorouracil (500 mg/m^2 days 1-5, repeated day 29), followed by chemoradiotherapy (50·4 Gy plus infusional fluorouracil 225 mg/m^2 daily), then two cycles of bolus fluorouracil. The protocol was later amended to allow a neoadjuvant cohort in which patients in the capecitabine group received chemoradiotherapy (50·4 Gy plus capecitabine 1650 mg/m^2 daily) followed by radical surgery and five cycles of capecitabine (2500 mg/m^2 per day for 14 days) and patients in the fluorouracil group received chemoradiotherapy (50·4 Gy plus infusional fluorouracil 1000 mg/m^2 days 1-5 and 29-33) followed by radical surgery and four cycles of bolus fluorouracil. 5-year overall survival in the capecitabine group was non-inferior to that in the fluorouracil group (76% [95% CI 67-2] vs 67% [58-74]; p = 0·0004; post-hoc test for superiority p = 0·05). 3-year disease-free survival was 75% (95% CI 68-81) in the capecitabine group and 67% (59-73) in the fluorouracil group (p = 0·07). Similar numbers of patients had local recurrences in each group (6% in the capecitabine group vs. 7% in the fluorouracil group, p = 0·67), but fewer patients developed distant metastases in the capecitabine group (19% vs. 28%; p = 0·04). Diarrhea was the most common adverse event in both groups (any grade: 53% patients in the capecitabine group vs. 44% in the fluorouracil group; grade 3-4: 9% vs. 2%). Patients in the capecitabine group had more hand-foot skin reaction, fatigue and proctitis than those in the fluorouracil group, whereas leukopenia was more frequent with fluorouracil arm.[183]

A second study, the NSABP R-04, compared the efficacy of four chemotherapy regimens. More than 1,600 patients were randomized to 5-FU (225 mg/m^2, 5 days/wk) or capecitabine (825 mg/m^2, twice a day, 5 days/wk) with radiation therapy with subsequent randomization to ±oxaliplatin (50 mg/m^2 per week ×5).[184] In a preliminary comparison, for patients who received 5-FU versus capecitabine, there were comparable rates of tumor downstaging, pCR, and sphincter preservation.

Several other options for neoadjuvant therapy that have been investigated include the addition of irinotecan or oxaliplatin to 5-FU–based CRT. Early data from phase I and II trials suggested that an oxaliplatin dose of 60 mg/m^2 can be combined safely with CI 5-FU and standard radiation approaches with acceptable grade 3 toxicity and promising rates of pathologic downstaging, with pCR rates of 20% to 30%.[185–188] These have not been confirmed in phase III testing, as reports from four randomized, control trials all demonstrate higher toxicity with oxaliplatin-containing regimens and no proven benefit. The STAR-01 trial randomized approximately 750 patients to CI 5-FU (225 mg/m^2 per day) ± oxaliplatin (60 mg/m^2).[189] With the addition of oxaliplatin there was no difference in pCR rate (16% in both arms), pN+ disease, or rates of positive circumferential radial margin, although higher rates of acute toxicity were seen. The ACCORD 12 study randomized approximately 600 patients with resectable T2 (low anterior) to T4 rectal cancer to CRT (45 Gy) with capecitabine (800 mg/m^2 twice daily) versus capecitabine and oxaliplatin (50 mg/m^2 weekly) delivered with 50-Gy radiation.[190] Similar to results of the STAR-01 trial, the addition of oxaliplatin increased grade 3+ acute toxicity (25% vs. 11%) and did not significantly improve pCR or sphincter preservation rates. A follow up report showed that pCR (the primary end point) was achieved in 13.9% versus 19.2% of patients, respectively (P = .09). Clinical results showed that at 3 years, there was no significant difference between the arms (cumulative incidence of local recurrence, 6.1% v 4.4%; overall survival, 87.6% v 88.3%; disease-free survival, 67.9% v 72.7%). Grade 3 to 4 toxicity was reported in four patients in the capecitabine-alone group and in two patients in the oxaliplatin-containing group. Bowel continence, erectile dysfunction, and social life disturbance were not different between groups. In multivariate analysis, the sterilization rate (Dworak score) of the operative specimen was the main significant prognostic factor (hazard ratio, 0.32; 95% CI, 0.21 to 0.50). The authors concluded that no significant difference in clinical outcome was achieved with the intensified oxaliplatin regimen and that when compared with other recent randomized trials, these results indicate that concurrent administration of oxaliplatin and RT is not recommended.[192] The preliminary results of the NSABP R-04 trial also suggest higher rates of toxicity with minimal or no improvement in outcomes. However, the German CAO/ARO/AIO-04 trial randomized patients with clinically staged T3-4 or any node-positive disease to a control group receiving standard fluorouracil-based combined modality treatment, consisting of preoperative radiotherapy of 50·4 Gy plus infusional fluorouracil (1000 mg/m^2 days 1-5 and 29-33), followed by surgery and four cycles of bolus fluorouracil (500 mg/m^2 days 1-5 and 29; fluorouracil group) versus an experimental group receiving preoperative radiotherapy of 50·4 Gy plus infusional fluorouracil (250 mg/m^2 days 1-14 and 22-35) and oxaliplatin (50 mg/m^2 days 1, 8, 22, and 29), followed by surgery and eight cycles of adjuvant chemotherapy with oxaliplatin (100 mg/m^2 days 1 and 15), leucovorin (400 mg/m^2 days 1 and 15), and infusional fluorouracil (2400 mg/m^2 days 1-2 and 15-16; fluorouracil plus oxaliplatin group). Of 1236 evaluable patients, preoperative grade 3-4 toxic effects occurred in 23% of patients who received fluorouracil and oxaliplatin during chemoradiotherapy and 20% of patients who received fluorouracil chemoradiotherapy. Grade 3-4 diarrhea was more common in those who received fluorouracil and oxaliplatin than in those who received fluorouracil (12% vs 8%), as was grade 3-4 nausea or vomiting (4% vs 1%). 85% of patients who received fluorouracil and oxaliplatin-based chemoradiotherapy had the full dose of chemotherapy, and 94% had the full dose of radiotherapy, as did 79% and 96% of patients who received fluorouracil-based chemoradiotherapy, respectively. A pathological complete response was achieved in 17% patients who underwent surgery in the fluorouracil and oxaliplatin group and in 13% of patients who underwent surgery in the fluorouracil group (odds ratio 1·40, 95% CI 1·02-1·92; p = 0·038). The authors concluded the inclusion of oxaliplatin into modified fluorouracil-based combined modality treatment was feasible and led to more patients achieving a pathological complete response than did standard treatment, with longer follow-up is needed to assess DFS, the primary endpoint.[184,192]

The addition of irinotecan to 5-FU–based chemotherapy has also been investigated. Toxicity of irinotecan with a dose of 50 mg/m^2 weekly with CI 5-FU–based CRT is somewhat higher but appears to be tolerable and also has yielded high response rates, with pCR of 25% to 30%.[193] A number of retrospective studies suggest a benefit with the addition of irinotecan to

Clinical Radiation Oncology

neoadjuvant CRT.[194–196] The RTOG conducted a randomized, phase II study of neoadjuvant CRT for distal rectal cancer.[197] One-hundred three patients with T3 or T4 distal rectal cancer (<9 cm from the dentate line) were randomized to CI 5-FU plus hyperfractionated radiation treatment of 55.2 to 60 Gy (1.2 Gy twice a day) versus CI 5-FU and irinotecan with conventional fractionation radiation of 50 to 54 Gy (1.8 Gy per fraction). The response rate between the two arms was similar, with a pCR of 28%. Other groups attempted to incorporate biologic agents into the neoadjuvant regimen. Although reports of the addition of bevacizumab and cetuximab to conventional preoperative regimens appears tolerable, the benefit remains unclear, and no phase III evaluation of these agents has been performed.[198–204]

Preoperative Versus Postoperative Therapy

A number of phase III trials have compared preoperative versus postoperative CRT treatment strategies. The first trial was an RTOG 94-01/Intergroup 0417 trial that accrued 53 patients but closed early due to poor accrual. The NSABP R-03 study was scheduled to accrue 900 patients but also closed, after accruing 267 patients.[205] In this study, individuals with operable adenocarcinoma of the rectum were randomized (and stratified based on age and sex) to surgery followed by one cycle of 5-FU/LV and then concurrent bolus (weeks 1 and 5) 5-FU/LV with radiation treatment versus 5-FU/LV for one cycle and then concurrent CRT treatment followed by surgery. All patients received adjuvant 5-FU and LV for four cycles. Although the study was underpowered, 5-year DFS was superior in the preoperative therapy group: 64.7% versus 53.4%. There was a trend, although not statistically significant, of improved 5-year OS with preoperative therapy: 74.5% vs. 65.6%. A pCR was seen in 15% of patients undergoing preoperative therapy.

A Korean trial randomized 240 patients with locally advanced (cT3/T4 or N+) rectal cancer to preoperative or postoperative CRT.[206] CRT consisted of 50 Gy in 25 fractions with concurrent capecitabine (1,650 mg/m^2 per day). Standard surgical procedure was TME. Patients received four cycles of adjuvant chemotherapy with either capecitabine (2,500 mg/m^2 per day for 14 days followed by a 1-week break) or bolus 5-FU (375 mg/m^2 per day)/LV (for 5 days every 4 weeks). The 5-year DFS, OS, and LR rates were no different between the two arms. Patients with low-lying rectal tumors (<5 cm from the anal verge) had higher rates of sphincter preservation in the preoperative arm (68% vs. 42%).

The definitive phase III study in favor of preoperative radiation therapy was the CAO/ARO/AIO-94 study performed by the German Rectal Cancer Group.[207] Eight hundred twenty-three clinically staged T3/T4 or node-positive rectal cancers were randomized to preoperative CRT followed by TME 6 weeks later or TME followed by postoperative CRT. The radiation dose was 50.4 Gy in 28 fractions in all patients, with a 5.4-Gy small-volume boost in the postoperative arm. 5-FU (1 g/m^2 per day) was administered during the weeks 1 and 5 of radiotherapy as a 120-hour CI. Both arms received four additional cycles of 5-FU (500 mg/m^2 per day for 5 days every 4 weeks). All surgeons were trained in the use of TME and were asked, prior to treatment, to evaluate the possibility of sphincter preservation. The 5-year results revealed a pelvic recurrence rate of 6% versus 13% (p = .02) in favor of the preoperative arm. The distant recurrence rate was 36% versus 38% (p = NSS), DFS was 68% versus 65% (p = NSS), and OS was 76% versus 74% (p = NSS) for preoperative radiation versus postoperative, respectively. There was significant tumor downstaging after preoperative CRT, with an 8% pCR. Nodal positivity was 25% in the preoperative versus 40% in the postoperative arm. The sphincter preservation rate in 188 patients with low-lying tumors (declared by the surgeon prior to randomization to require an APR) revealed that 39% versus 19% had a sphincter-preserving low anterior resection (p = .004) in the preoperative versus the postoperative arm. There were fewer acute (27% vs. 40%) and late toxicities (14% vs. 24%) in preoperative-treatment group. Thus, preoperative CRT resulted in half the LF and doubled the sphincter preservation rate compared to postoperative therapy. In addition, compliance rates were significantly improved in the preoperative arm. Of importance, there was no difference in OS or DFS between the two arms. An update, with a median follow up of 11 years continues to demonstrate an improvement in local control but no difference in DFS or OS with preoperative therapy.[208]

In the era of improved surgical technique, staging, and histologic assessment, the MRC CR07 trial re-evaluated the role of radiotherapy.[209] A total of 1,350 patients were randomized to preoperative radiotherapy (25 Gy in five fractions) or upfront resection with selective postoperative chemoradiotherapy (45 Gy in 25 fractions with concurrent 5-FU) in patients with a ≤1-mm circumferential resection margin. At median follow-up of 4 years the LR was significantly lower in the preoperative radiotherapy group (4.4% vs. 10.6%). Although 3-year DFS was improved in the preoperative therapy group (77.5% vs. 71.5%), there was no difference in OS. Attempts to identify patients at high risk of recurrence after resection (≤1-mm circumferential resection margin) and administration of selective CRT was inferior to upfront preoperative radiotherapy. Both the MRC CR07 and German rectal trial established preoperative therapy, either short-course (25 Gy in five fractions) or long-course chemoradiotherapy (50 Gy in 1.8-Gy fractions with concurrent 5-FU–based chemotherapy), as the current standard of care.

Locally Advanced Rectal Cancer

The definition of locally advanced rectal cancer is variable. One definition of locally advanced disease encompasses tumors that cannot be resected without high likelihood of residual gross or microscopic disease secondary to tumor fixation or adherence to adjacent structures. A preoperative therapy approach is recommended to potentially facilitate curative resections.

A number of retrospective studies have shown an advantage of CRT over radiation alone. MD Anderson Cancer Center investigators demonstrated that preoperative CRT increased OS (80% vs. 60%), LC (95% vs. 66%), and the number of sphincter-preserving procedures (35% vs. 7%) as compared to radiation alone.[210] Memorial Sloan-Kettering Cancer Center investigators reported a gross total resection rate of 97%, pCR of 25%, 4-year LC of 70%, and 4-year OS of 67% when giving preoperative chemotherapy of 5-FU and LV with 50.4 Gy of radiation followed by surgery.[211] Preoperative CRT resulted in improved resectability rates and possible improved LC and OS.

The superiority of preoperative CRT over radiotherapy alone was shown in a phase III, randomized control trial.[212] Two hundred seven patients with locally unresectable T4 primary rectal carcinoma or locally recurrent rectal cancer were randomized to CRT (50 Gy with 5-FU/LV) and further adjuvant systemic therapy for 16 weeks after surgery versus radiotherapy alone (50 Gy). Higher rates of R0 resections were seen in the CRT arm: 84% vs. 68%. Results for LC (82% vs. 67%), time to treatment failure (63% vs. 44%), and cancer-specific survival (72% vs. 55%) all favored the CRT arm. Similarly, there was a nonsignificant trend to improved OS with CRT. As would be anticipated, patients receiving concurrent chemotherapy experienced higher grade 3/4 acute toxicity with no difference in late toxicity.

Despite preoperative CRT and complete surgical resection, LR rates in this subgroup remain high. In situations in which the margin of resection is compromised, IORT offers the possibility of improved LC. The IORT experience at MGH was reviewed by Nakfoor et al.[213] Preoperative CI 5-FU plus 50.4 to 54 Gy of radiation was given, followed by a 4- to 6-week break and surgery. No IORT was given if metastases were present at surgical exploration, if there were adequate margins >1 cm, or if there was less than T4 disease. From 10 to 12.5 Gy was given for complete resection, 12.5 to 15 Gy for microscopic residual disease, and 17.5 to 20 Gy for gross residual disease. The 5-year LC was 90%, 65%, and 55%, and the disease-specific survival at 5 years was 65%, 45%, and 15%, for these three dose levels, respectively. However, the 5-year actuarial risk of complications was

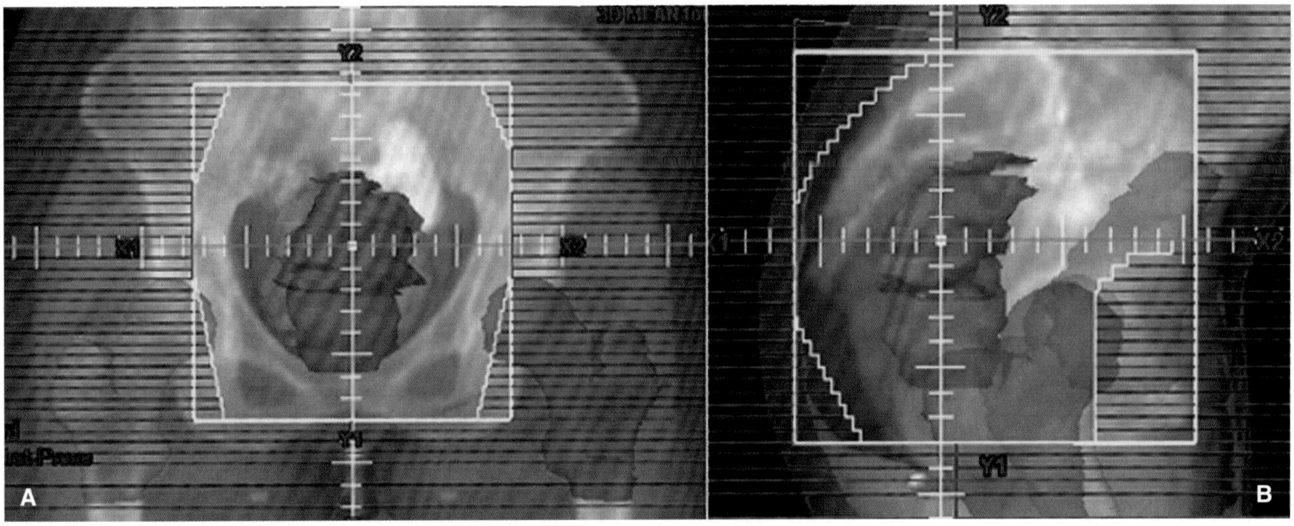

FIGURE 61.6. A: Posteroanterior treatment field of patient with T3 N1 rectal cancer. B: Lateral treatment field of a patient with T3 N1 rectal cancer. Red, gross tumor volume; brown, rectum; orange, bladder; green/blue, femoral heads.

15%. The risk of peripheral neuropathy was 20% for doses >15 Gy. IORT appeared to improve LC, especially with a gross total resection, but not OS for locally advanced rectal cancers.

A series from the Mayo clinic evaluated outcomes in 146 patients with primary locally advanced CRC.[214] Patients received conventionally fractionated EBRT (45 to 50 Gy) with chemotherapy, surgery, and IORT (10 to 20 Gy). The rates of 5-year freedom from LR and DFS were 86% and 43%, respectively. Late complications occurred in 77 patients (53%) and included peripheral neuropathy (19%), bowel obstruction (14%), and ureteral obstruction (12%). In summary, IORT is a valuable tool in an effort to improve LC in situations in which the risk of microscopic residual disease following resection remains high, albeit with potential risks for late toxicity.

Radiotherapy Treatment Technique

External-beam treatment fields for rectal carcinoma should encompass potential sites at greatest risk for harboring disease, including the presacral space, primary tumor site, and (for post-APR cases) the perineum. Other areas at risk include the internal iliac and distal common iliac nodes. Generally, the risk of disease involvement of the para-aortic region is sufficiently low, and the morbidity from treatment is sufficiently high, to exclude this region from radiation fields. The external iliac nodes may be covered for lesions involving the anterior structures, including bladder, prostate, and vagina.

In general, patients with rectal carcinoma should be treated in the prone position to reduce the volume of small bowel within the pelvis. Maneuvers to reduce the volume of small bowel include treatment with a full bladder and the use of bowel-displacement techniques such as a belly board (a device with a false tabletop to allow the upper-abdominal contents to fall anteriorly).[215] The use of shaped lateral fields reduces the dose to small bowel located in the anterior and superior aspects of the pelvis. A marker is generally placed at the anal verge and intravenous, rectal, and small-bowel contrast is often administered at the time of simulation for accurate target and normal tissue delineation.

Generally a four-field (anteroposterior/posteroanterior [AP/PA]/right/left [R/L] lateral) or three-field (PA/R/L lateral) technique is used. The superior field edge is placed at the L5/S1 interspace. The distal field edge depends on tumor location and should be roughly 3 to 5 cm below palpable tumor for patients receiving preoperative treatment. For postoperative cases the distal field edge is about 5 cm below the best estimate of the preoperative tumor bed and (if an APR has been performed) below the perineum. AP/PA fields should have at least a 1.5-cm margin on the pelvic brim.

On lateral treatment fields the superior and inferior borders remain the same as for AP/PA fields. Lateral fields should encompass the entire sacrum posteriorly to ensure adequate coverage of the presacral space. The anterior margin should be roughly 4 cm anterior to the rectum (ensuring adequate coverage of the mesorectum). If the tumor has considerable extrarectal extension, these guidelines should be modified to make certain that all disease is encompassed with appropriate margin.

The usual dose given to initial pelvic fields is 45 Gy in 25 fractions of 1.8 Gy each. An additional tumor boost may be administered, usually through opposed lateral fields, to an additional 5.4 to 9 Gy. Small bowel should be excluded from the boost volume after about 50 Gy in an effort to minimize acute and late toxicity (Fig. 61.6).

Management of Recurrent Rectal Cancer

Recurrent rectal cancer is often approached in the same way as T4 disease, often with an aggressive treatment plan of CRT, surgery, and adjuvant chemotherapy. At the time of surgery, IORT may be considered. Approximately 10% of patients with T1 and T2 N0 disease will fail locally after surgery, usually due to an inadequate lymph node/mesorectal dissection. Recurrences may occur along the pelvic sidewall or in nonpelvic sidewall areas such as the uterus, prostate, or vagina. The 5-year OS is approximately 20% for all cases. LC is roughly 40% in patients with no prior radiation and 10% to 20% in patients with prior radiotherapy.[216] Given the difficulty of surgical resection of pelvic sidewall recurrences, these tend to fare worse.

In patients with no prior history of radiation, neoadjuvant CRT followed by surgical resection is a reasonable treatment approach. In one series, 123 patients with locally recurrent CRC received a course of EBRT (45 to 54 Gy) either before or after surgical resection and IORT.[83] Five-year OS in patients undergoing gross total resection was 24%, compared to 18% in patients with gross residual disease. A second series using a similar treatment approach of neoadjuvant therapy, surgical resection, and IORT achieved 5-year LC and OS rates of 54% and 32%, respectively. The 5-year LC and OS rates in patients undergoing radical resection were 69% and 42%, respectively. A series of 35 patients with recurrent rectal cancer not amenable to upfront surgical resection was treated with a course of preoperative CRT (50.4 to 59.4 Gy with 5-FU chemotherapy).[217] Eighty percent underwent curative resection, and 60% achieved negative surgical margins. Three-year OS rate in patients with complete resection was 82%.

One randomized control trial compared outcomes of preoperative CRT or radiotherapy alone prior to surgical resection in patients with locally advanced or recurrent rectal cancer who had

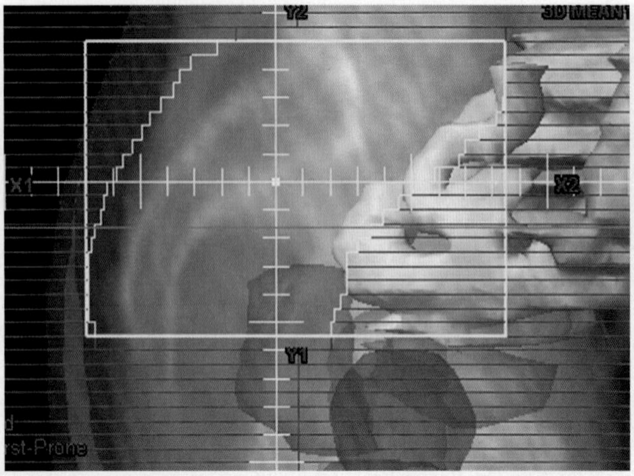

FIGURE 61.7. Lateral treatment field of patient with recurrent rectal cancer (with prior history of radiation) along presacral space. Brown, rectum; yellow, small bowel; green, bladder; orange/blue. femoral heads.

not received prior radiotherapy.[212] This series included 25 patients with recurrent disease. Higher rates of R0 resection, LC, time to treatment failure, and cancer-specific survival were seen in the chemoradiation arm (see section Locally Advanced Rectal Cancer). Five-year OS rate in patients with recurrent rectal cancer was 37%.

In patients with prior history of radiation, reirradiation is possible in carefully selected situations. Forty-seven patients in an Italian retrospective study were treated with preoperative CRT.[218] Patients who did not have prior radiation treatment received 45 Gy with CI 5-FU and mitomycin C, followed by surgery and IORT of 10 to 15 Gy. LV and 5-FU were given for six to nine cycles adjuvantly. If patients had prior radiation treatment, they received 23.4 Gy. The 5-year OS rate was 20% for all patients, 60% for resected tumors, 0% for unresected tumors, and 40% for patients treated by external beam, surgery, and IORT. The 5-year LC rate was 30% for all patients, 70% for completely resected tumors, 0% for unresectable tumors, and 80% for EBRT, surgery, and IORT. Eighty-five percent of patients had palliation of pain, with an average duration of 12 months.

Another retrospective series included 147 patients with locally recurrent rectal cancer, with the majority (127 patients) undergoing preoperative CRT.[82] Fifty-seven had received prior radiation and were reirradiated to a dose of 30.6 Gy. Preoperative treatment was followed by surgical resection and IORT. Five-year OS for the entire group was 32% and was 48% in patients with an R0 resection. Radical resection correlated significantly with improved OS, DFS, and LC rates. There was no difference in late toxicity in patients who received reirradiation.

Long-term results of reirradiation for patients with recurrent rectal carcinoma were also reported by Mohiuddin et al.[219] One-hundred three patients who developed LR after surgery with preoperative or postoperative radiation treatment (median dose, 50.4 Gy) were reirradiated with concurrent CI 5-FU. Patients were treated with opposed laterals or three-field technique (PA/L lateral/R lateral) to the presacral area and gross tumor volume with 2- to 4-cm margin. Patients received 30 Gy (1.2 Gy twice a day) or 30.6 Gy (1.8 Gy every day), followed by a boost of 6 to 20 Gy to gross tumor volume (2-cm margin). Forty-one patients were surgically explored after treatment and 34 underwent resection, with 6 patients undergoing sphincter-sparing surgery. With a median follow-up of 2 years, the 5-year OS rate was 19%. Patients who underwent resection had a higher survival rate, with tolerable acute and late toxicity. Twenty-two patients experienced late toxicity, including severe, persistent diarrhea (18 patients), small-bowel obstruction (15 patients), fistula formation (4 patients), and stricture (2 patients). Palliation of bleeding was achieved in 100% of patients.

Hyperfractionated radiotherapy may be an alternative in an effort to reduce late toxicity. A retrospective series from MD Anderson Cancer Center evaluated reirradiation outcomes in 50 patients with prior history of pelvic radiotherapy.[220] Patients were treated in 1.5-Gy fractions twice daily to total dose of 30 to 39 Gy (depending on the time interval between radiotherapy treatment courses). Concurrent chemotherapy was administered to the majority of patients. The 3-year freedom rate from local progression and OS rate in the entire cohort were 33% and 39%, respectively. Three-year OS rate was 66% in patients undergoing surgery, and the 3-year rate of grade 3/4 late toxicity was 35%.

Patients with recurrent rectal cancer and no prior history of EBRT are generally treated with a course of concurrent, preoperative CRT (50 to 54 Gy with 5-FU–based chemotherapy) followed by surgical resection (and consideration of IORT). Patients with prior history of radiotherapy may receive reirradiation to doses of 30 to 39 Gy but have the potential to experience significant late toxicity; therefore, efforts should be made to avoid small bowel within treatment fields. (Fig. 61.7).

SELECTED REFERENCES

A full list of references for this chapter is available online.

2. Siegel R, Naishadham D, Jemal A. Cancer statistics, 2012. *CA Cancer J Clin* 2012;62(1):10–29. doi:10.3322/caac.20138. Epub 2012 Jan 4.
3. Heinrich S, et al. Adjuvant gemcitabine versus NEOadjuvant gemcitabine/oxaliplatin plus adjuvant gemcitabine in resectable pancreatic cancer: a randomized multicenter phase III study (NEOPAC study). *BMC Cancer* 2011;11:346.
12. Markowitz SD, Bertagnolli MM. Molecular origins of cancer: molecular basis of colorectal cancer. *N Engl J Med* 2009;361(25):2449–2460.
13. Gryfe R, et al. Tumor microsatellite instability and clinical outcome in young patients with colorectal cancer. *N Engl J Med* 2000;342(2):69–77.
18. Screening for colorectal cancer: U.S. Preventive Services Task Force recommendation statement. *Ann Intern Med* 2008;149(9):627–637.
21. Lieberman DA. Clinical practice. Screening for colorectal cancer. *N Engl J Med* 2009;361(12):1179–1187.
34. Solomon MJ, McLeod RS. Endoluminal transrectal ultrasonography: accuracy, reliability, and validity. *Dis Colon Rectum* 1993;36:200.
37. Hildebrandt U, Feifel G. Preoperative staging of rectal cancer by intrarectal ultrasound. *Dis Colon Rectum* 1985;28:42.
38. Gualdi GF, Casciani E, Guadalaxara A, et al. Local staging of rectal cancer with transrectal ultrasound and endorectal magnetic resonance imaging: Comparison with histologic findings. *Dis Colon Rectum* 2000;43:338.
44. Nahas CS, Akhurst T, Yeung H, et al. Positron emission tomography detection of distant metastatic or synchronous disease in patients with locally advanced rectal cancer receiving preoperative chemoradiation. *Ann Surg Oncol* 2008;15(3):704–711.
45. Saltz LB, et al. Irinotecan fluorouracil plus leucovorin is not superior to fluorouracil plus leucovorin alone as adjuvant treatment for stage III colon cancer: results of CALGB 89803. *J Clin Oncol* 2007;25(23):3456–3461.
46. Freeny PC, Marks WM, Ryan JA, et al. Colorectal carcinoma evaluation with CT: Preoperative staging and detection of postoperative recurrence. *Radiology* 1986;158:347.
48. McGory ML, Shekelle PG, Ko CY. Development of quality indicators for patients undergoing colorectal cancer surgery. *J Natl Cancer Inst* 2006;98(22):1623–1633.
49. Benson AB 3rd, et al. American Society of Clinical Oncology recommendations on adjuvant chemotherapy for stage II colon cancer. *J Clin Oncol* 2004;22(16): 3408–3419.
50. The Clinical Outcomes of Surgical Therapy Study Group. A comparison of laparoscopically assisted and open colectomy for colon cancer. *N Engl J Med* 2004; 350(20):2050–2059.
51. Fleshman J, et al. Laparoscopic colectomy for cancer is not inferior to open surgery based on 5-year data from the COST Study Group trial. *Ann Surg* 2007; 246(4):655–662; discussion 662–664.
52. Bonjer HJ, et al. Laparoscopically assisted vs open colectomy for colon cancer: a meta-analysis. *Arch Surg* 2007;142(3):298–303.
53. Jackson TD, et al. Laparoscopic versus open resection for colorectal cancer: a metaanalysis of oncologic outcomes. *J Am Coll Surg* 2007;204(3):439–446.
54. Moertel CG, et al. Levamisole and fluorouracil for adjuvant therapy of resected colon carcinoma. *N Engl J Med* 1990;322(6):352–358.
55. O'Connell MJ, et al. Controlled trial of fluorouracil and low-dose leucovorin given for 6 months as postoperative adjuvant therapy for colon cancer. *J Clin Oncol* 1997;15(1):246–250.
57. Twelves C, et al. Capecitabine versus 5-fluorouracil/folinic acid as adjuvant therapy for stage III colon cancer: final results from the X-ACT trial with analysis by age and preliminary evidence of a pharmacodynamic marker of efficacy. *Ann Oncol* 2011.
58. Andre T, et al. Oxaliplatin, fluorouracil, and leucovorin as adjuvant treatment for colon cancer. *N Engl J Med* 2004;350(23):2343–2351.
59. Andre T, et al. Improved overall survival with oxaliplatin, fluorouracil, and leucovorin as adjuvant treatment in stage II or III colon cancer in the MOSAIC trial. *J Clin Oncol* 2009;27(19):3109–3116.
60. Kuebler JP, et al. Oxaliplatin combined with weekly bolus fluorouracil and leucovorin as surgical adjuvant chemotherapy for stage II and III colon cancer: results from NSABP C-07. *J Clin Oncol* 2007;25(16):2198–2204.
61. Yothers G, et al. Oxaliplatin as adjuvant therapy for colon cancer: updated results of NSABP C-07 trial, including survival and subset analyses. *J Clin Oncol* 2011;29(28):3768–3774.
62. Allegra CJ, et al. Phase III trial assessing bevacizumab in stages II and III carcinoma of the colon: results of NSABP protocol C-08. *J Clin Oncol* 2011;29(1):11–16.
63. Alberts SR Sargent DJ, Smyrk TC, et al. Adjuvant mFOLFOX6 with and without cetuximab (Cmab) in KRAS wild-type (WT) patients with resected stage III colon cancer: results from NCCTG Intergroup Phase III Trial N0147. *Clin Oncol* 2010;28:959s.
64. Goldberg RM, Sargent D, Thibodeau SN, et al. Adjuvant mFOLFOX6 plus or minus cetuximab in patients with KRAS-mutant resected stage III colon cancer: NCCTG Intergroup Phase III Trial N0147 (abstract 3508). *J Clin Oncol* 2010;28:262s.

65. De Gramont A, van Cutsem E, Tabernero J, et al. AVANT: Results from a randomized, three-arm multinational phase III study to investigate bevacizumab with either XELOX or FOLFOX4 versus FOLFOX4 alone as adjuvant treatment for colon cancer. *J Clin Oncol* 2011; 29(suppl 4):362.
66. Gunderson LL, Sosin H, Levitt S. Extrapelvic colon–areas of failure in a reoperation series: implications for adjuvant therapy. *Int J Radiat Oncol Biol Phys* 1985; 11(4):731–741.
67. Willett CG, et al. Failure patterns following curative resection of colonic carcinoma. *Ann Surg* 1984;200(6):685–690.
68. Amos EH, et al. Postoperative radiotherapy for locally advanced colon cancer. *Ann Surg Oncol* 1996;3(5):431–436.
69. Gunderson LL, et al. Locally advanced primary colorectal cancer: intraoperative electron and external beam irradiation +/- 5-FU. *Int J Radiat Oncol Biol Phys* 1997;37(3):601–614.
70. Willett CG, et al. Postoperative radiation therapy for high-risk colon carcinoma. *J Clin Oncol* 1993;11(6):1112–1117.
71. Gunderson LL, Nelson H, Martenson JA, et al. Intraoperative electron and external beam irradiation with or without 5-fluorouracil and maximum surgical resection for previously unirradiated, locally recurrent colorectal cancer. *Dis Colon Rectum.* 1996;39(12):1379–1395.
72. Martenson JA Jr, et al. Phase III study of adjuvant chemotherapy and radiation therapy compared with chemotherapy alone in the surgical adjuvant treatment of colon cancer: results of intergroup protocol 0130. *J Clin Oncol* 2004;22(16): 3277–3283.
73. Saltz LB, et al. Irinotecan plus fluorouracil and leucovorin for metastatic colorectal cancer. Irinotecan Study Group. *N Engl J Med* 2000;343(13):905–914.
74. Goldberg RM, et al. A randomized controlled trial of fluorouracil plus leucovorin, irinotecan, and oxaliplatin combinations in patients with previously untreated metastatic colorectal cancer. *J Clin Oncol* 2004;22(1):23–30.
75. Falcone A, et al. Phase III trial of infusional fluorouracil, leucovorin, oxaliplatin, and irinotecan (FOLFOXIRI) compared with infusional fluorouracil, leucovorin, and irinotecan (FOLFIRI) as first-line treatment for metastatic colorectal cancer: the Gruppo Oncologico Nord Ovest. *J Clin Oncol* 2007;25(13):1670–1676.
76. Hurwitz H, et al. Bevacizumab plus irinotecan, fluorouracil, and leucovorin for metastatic colorectal cancer. *N Engl J Med* 2004;350(23):2335–2342.
77. Cunningham D, et al. Cetuximab monotherapy and cetuximab plus irinotecan in irinotecan-refractory metastatic colorectal cancer. *N Engl J Med* 2004;351(4): 337–345.
78. Gunderson LL, et al. Lower gastrointestinal cancers: rationale, results, and techniques of treatment. *Front Radiat Ther Oncol* 1994;28:140–154.
81. Willett CG, et al. Intraoperative electron beam radiation therapy for primary locally advanced rectal and rectosigmoid carcinoma. *J Clin Oncol* 1991;9(5):843–849.
83. Gunderson LL, et al. Intraoperative electron and external beam irradiation with or without 5-fluorouracil and maximum surgical resection for previously unirradiated, locally recurrent colorectal cancer. *Dis Colon Rectum* 1996;39(12): 1379–1395.
84. Haddock MG, et al. Intraoperative electron radiotherapy as a component of salvage therapy for patients with colorectal cancer and advanced nodal metastases. *Int J Radiat Oncol Biol Phys* 2003;56(4):966–973.
85. Haddock MG, et al. Intraoperative irradiation for locally recurrent colorectal cancer in previously irradiated patients. *Int J Radiat Oncol Biol Phys* 2001;49(5): 1267–1274.
94. Gunderson LL, et al. Impact of T and N stage and treatment on survival and relapse in adjuvant rectal cancer: a pooled analysis. *J Clin Oncol* 2004;22(10): 1785–1796.
98. Quirke P, et al. Effect of the plane of surgery achieved on local recurrence in patients with operable rectal cancer: a prospective study using data from the MRC CR07 and NCIC-CTG CO16 randomised clinical trial. *Lancet* 2009;373(9666):821–828.
101. Mohiuddin M, Regine WF, Marks G. Prognostic significance of tumor fixation of rectal carcinoma. Implications for adjunctive radiation therapy. *Cancer* 1996;78(4):717–722.
102. Kapiteijn E, et al. Preoperative radiotherapy combined with total mesorectal excision for resectable rectal cancer. *N Engl J Med* 2001;345(9):638–646.
107. Rodel C, et al. Prognostic significance of tumor regression after preoperative chemoradiotherapy for rectal cancer. *J Clin Oncol* 2005;23(34):8688–8696.
110. Meyerhardt JA, et al. Impact of hospital procedure volume on surgical operation and long-term outcomes in high-risk curatively resected rectal cancer: findings from the Intergroup 0114 Study. *J Clin Oncol* 2004;22(1):166–174.
118. Kang SB, et al. Open versus laparoscopic surgery for mid or low rectal cancer after neoadjuvant chemoradiotherapy (COREAN trial): short-term outcomes of an open-label randomised controlled trial. *Lancet Oncol* 2010;11(7):637–645.
119. Lujan J, et al. Randomized clinical trial comparing laparoscopic and open surgery in patients with rectal cancer. *Br J Surg* 2009;96(9):982–989.
120. Ng SS, et al. Long-term morbidity and oncologic outcomes of laparoscopic-assisted anterior resection for upper rectal cancer: ten-year results of a prospective, randomized trial. *Dis Colon Rectum* 2009;52(4):558–566.
126. Greenberg JA, et al. Local excision of distal rectal cancer: an update of cancer and leukemia group B 8984. *Dis Colon Rectum* 2008;51(8):1185–1191; discussion 1191–1194.
127. Steele GD Jr, et al. Sphincter-sparing treatment for distal rectal adenocarcinoma. *Ann Surg Oncol* 1999;6(5):433–441.
129. You YN. Local excision: is it an adequate substitute for radical resection in T1/T2 patients? *Semin Radiat Oncol* 2011;21(3):178–184.
130. Blackstock W, et al. ACR Appropriateness Criteria: local excision in early-stage rectal cancer. *Curr Probl Cancer* 2010;34(3):193–200.
143. Heald RJ, Husband EM, Ryall RD. The mesorectum in rectal cancer surgery–the clue to pelvic recurrence? *Br J Surg* 1982;69(10):613–616.
144. Heald RJ, et al. Rectal cancer: the Basingstoke experience of total mesorectal excision, 1978-1997. *Arch Surg* 1998;133(8):894–899.
145. MacFarlane JK, Ryall RD, Heald RJ. Mesorectal excision for rectal cancer. *Lancet* 1993;341(8843):457–460.
147. Havenga K, et al. Improved survival and local control after total mesorectal excision or D3 lymphadenectomy in the treatment of primary rectal cancer: an international analysis of 1411 patients. *Eur J Surg Oncol* 1999;25(4):368–374.
148. Tepper JE, et al. Impact of number of nodes retrieved on outcome in patients with rectal cancer. *J Clin Oncol* 2001;19(1):157–163.
149. Rajput A, et al. Meeting the 12 lymph node (LN) benchmark in colon cancer. *J Surg Oncol* 2010;102(1):3–9.
152. van Gijn W, et al. Preoperative radiotherapy combined with total mesorectal excision for resectable rectal cancer: 12-year follow-up of the multicentre, randomised controlled TME trial. *Lancet Oncol* 2011;12(6):575–582.
159. Wolmark N, et al. Randomized trial of postoperative adjuvant chemotherapy with or without radiotherapy for carcinoma of the rectum: National Surgical Adjuvant Breast and Bowel Project Protocol R-02. *J Natl Cancer Inst* 2000;92(5):388–396.
160. Thomas PR, Lindblad AS. Adjuvant postoperative radiotherapy and chemotherapy in rectal carcinoma: a review of the Gastrointestinal Tumor Study Group experience. *Radiother Oncol* 1988;13(4):245–252.
161. Krook JE, et al. Effective surgical adjuvant therapy for high-risk rectal carcinoma. *N Engl J Med* 1991;324(11):709–715.
162. Miller RC, et al. Acute diarrhea during adjuvant therapy for rectal cancer: a detailed analysis from a randomized intergroup trial. *Int J Radiat Oncol Biol Phys* 2002;54(2):409–413.
163. O'Connell MJ, et al. Improving adjuvant therapy for rectal cancer by combining protracted-infusion fluorouracil with radiation therapy after curative surgery. *N Engl J Med* 1994;331(8):502–507.
164. Tepper JE, et al. Adjuvant postoperative fluorouracil-modulated chemotherapy combined with pelvic radiation therapy for rectal cancer: initial results of intergroup 0114. *J Clin Oncol* 1997;15(5):2030–2039.
166. Guillem JG, et al. cT3N0 rectal cancer: potential overtreatment with preoperative chemoradiotherapy is warranted. *J Clin Oncol* 2008;26(3):368–373.
167. Folkesson J, et al. Swedish Rectal Cancer Trial: long lasting benefits from radiotherapy on survival and local recurrence rate. *J Clin Oncol* 2005;23(24): 5644–5650.
168. Swedish Rectal Cancer Trial. Improved survival with preoperative radiotherapy in resectable rectal cancer. *N Engl J Med* 1997;336(14):980–987.
169. Birgisson H, et al. Adverse effects of preoperative radiation therapy for rectal cancer: long-term follow-up of the Swedish Rectal Cancer Trial. *J Clin Oncol* 2005;23(34):8697–8705.
170. Birgisson H, et al. Late gastrointestinal disorders after rectal cancer surgery with and without preoperative radiation therapy. *Br J Surg* 2008;95(2):206–213.
171. Francois Y, et al. Influence of the interval between preoperative radiation therapy and surgery on downstaging and on the rate of sphincter-sparing surgery for rectal cancer: the Lyon R90-01 randomized trial. *J Clin Oncol* 1999;17(8): 2396.
172. Marijnen CA, et al. Acute side effects and complications after short-term preoperative radiotherapy combined with total mesorectal excision in primary rectal cancer: report of a multicenter randomized trial. *J Clin Oncol* 2002;20(3):817–825.
173. Peeters KC, et al. Late side effects of short-course preoperative radiotherapy combined with total mesorectal excision for rectal cancer: increased bowel dysfunction in irradiated patients–a Dutch colorectal cancer group study. *J Clin Oncol* 2005;23(25):6199–6206.
174. Marijnen CA, et al. Impact of short-term preoperative radiotherapy on health-related quality of life and sexual functioning in primary rectal cancer: report of a multicenter randomized trial. *J Clin Oncol* 2005;23(9):1847–1858.
176. Gerard JP, et al. Preoperative radiotherapy with or without concurrent fluorouracil and leucovorin in T3-4 rectal cancers: results of FFCD 9203. *J Clin Oncol* 2006;24(28):4620–4625.
177. Bosset JF. Chemotherapy with preoperative radiotherapy in rectal cancer. *N Engl J Med.* 2006;355(11):1114–1123.
178. Ceelen WP, Van Nieuwenhove Y, Fierens K. Preoperative chemoradiation versus radiation alone for stage II and III resectable rectal cancer. *Cochrane Database Syst Rev* 2009(1):CD006041.
179. Ngan SY, Burmeister B, Fisher RJ, et al. Randomized trial of short-course radiotherapy versus long-course chemoradiation comparing rates of local recurrence in patients with t3 rectal cancer: trans-tasman radiation oncology group trial 01.04. *J Clin Oncol* 2012 ;30(31):3827–3833.
180. Bujko K, et al. Long-term results of a randomized trial comparing preoperative short-course radiotherapy with preoperative conventionally fractionated chemoradiation for rectal cancer. *Br J Surg* 2006;93(10):1215–1223.
183. Hofheinz ED, Wenz F, Post S, et. al. Chemoradiotherapy with capecitabine versus fl uorouracil for locally advanced rectal cancer: a randomised, multicentre, non-inferiority, phase 3 trial. *Lancet Oncol* 2012;13:579–588.
184. Roh MS, Y G, O'Connell MJ, et al. The impact of capecitabine and oxaliplatin in the preoperative multimodality treatment in patients with carcinoma of the rectum: NSABP R-04. *J Clin Oncol* 2011;29:abstract 3503.
189. Aschele C, et al. Primary tumor response to preoperative chemoradiation with or without oxaliplatin in locally advanced rectal cancer: pathologic results of the STAR-01 randomized phase III trial. *J Clin Oncol* 2011;29(20):2773–2780.
190. Gerard JP, et al. Comparison of two neoadjuvant chemoradiotherapy regimens for locally advanced rectal cancer: results of the phase III trial ACCORD 12/0405-Prodige 2. *J Clin Oncol* 2010;28(10):1638–1644.
191. Gérard JP, Azria D, Gourgou-Bourgade S, et al. Clinical Outcome of the ACCORD 12/0405 PRODIGE 2 Randomized Trial in Rectal Cancer. *J Clin Oncol.* 2012;30(36):4558–4565.
192. Rödel C, Liersch T, Becker H, et al., German Rectal Cancer Study Group. Preoperative chemoradiotherapy and postoperative chemotherapy with fluorouracil and oxaliplatin versus fluorouracil alone in locally advanced rectal cancer: initial results of the German CAO/ARO/AIO-04 randomised phase 3 trial. *Lancet Oncol.* 2012;13(7):679–687.
205. Roh MS, et al. Preoperative multimodality therapy improves disease-free survival in patients with carcinoma of the rectum: NSABP R-03. *J Clin Oncol* 2009;27(31): 5124–5130.
206. Park JH, et al. Randomized phase 3 trial comparing preoperative and postoperative chemoradiotherapy with capecitabine for locally advanced rectal cancer. *Cancer* 2011;117(16):3703–3712.
207. Sauer R, et al. Preoperative versus postoperative chemoradiotherapy for rectal cancer. *N Engl J Med* 2004;351(17):1731–1740.
209. Sebag-Montefiore D, et al. Preoperative radiotherapy versus selective postoperative chemoradiotherapy in patients with rectal cancer (MRC CR07 and NCIC-CTG C016): a multicentre, randomised trial. *Lancet* 2009;373(9666):811–820.
212. Braendengen M, et al. Randomized phase III study comparing preoperative radiotherapy with chemoradiotherapy in nonresectable rectal cancer. *J Clin Oncol* 2008;26(22):3687–3694.
214. Mathis KL, et al. Unresectable colorectal cancer can be cured with multimodality therapy. *Ann Surg* 2008;248(4):592–598.
218. Valentini V, et al. Preoperative hyperfractionated chemoradiation for locally recurrent rectal cancer in patients previously irradiated to the pelvis: A multicentric phase II study. *Int J Radiat Oncol Biol Phys* 2006;64(4):1129–1139.
219. Mohiuddin M, Marks G, Marks J. Long-term results of reirradiation for patients with recurrent rectal carcinoma. *Cancer* 2002;95(5):1144–1150.
220. Das P, et al. Hyperfractionated accelerated radiotherapy for rectal cancer in patients with prior pelvic irradiation. *Int J Radiat Oncol Biol Phys* 2010;77(1):60–65.

Chapter 62
Anal Cancer

Bernard J. Cummings and James D. Brierley

The standard treatment for primary squamous cell cancers of the anal canal is chemoradiation, using concurrent radiation therapy (RT), 5-fluorouracil (5-FU), and mitomycin-C (MMC), with surgery reserved for residual cancer. This combination, developed empirically as preoperative adjuvant therapy in the 1970s,[1] has evolved to become the standard of care. Trials of other chemotherapy agents in combination with radiation have so far not improved results. Currently, about 65% of those with cancer confined to the pelvis will survive 5 years or more and about 75% will retain anorectal function.

In this chapter, the emphasis is on the management of squamous cell cancer of the anal canal. Note is also made of the role of RT in the treatment of squamous cell cancers of the perianal skin and of adenocarcinomas of the anal region.

ANATOMY

The anal canal is 3 to 4 cm in length, the posterior wall being longer than the anterior. The canal ends superiorly at the palpable upper border of the anal sphincter and puborectalis muscle of the anorectal ring. The distal end at the anal verge is the level at which the walls of the anal canal come in contact in their normal resting state; it approximates the palpable groove between the lower edge of the internal sphincter and the subcutaneous part of the external sphincter and the junction with true skin. The American Joint Committee on Cancer Clinical Staging (AJCC)[2] and the International Union Against Cancer (UICC)[3] recommend this definition rather than a convention used by some centers under which carcinomas that are above or exactly astride the dentate line are classified as anal canal tumors and those lying mainly or entirely below that line are called anal margin tumors (Fig. 62.1). The terms *anal margin* and *perianal skin* are now generally used interchangeably. Perianal carcinomas are arbitrarily considered to be cancers arising from the skin within a 5-cm radius of the anal verge.

Four different types of epithelium are found within the anal region.[4] The perianal skin is similar to hair-bearing skin elsewhere. At the anal verge, the skin blends with a pale-colored zone, sometimes called the pecten, lined by modified squamous epithelium that lacks hair or glandular structures. This squamous zone merges just below the dentate or pectinate line, which marks the mucosal folds of the anal valves, with a transitional epithelium that incorporates features of rectal, urothelial, and squamous epithelium. The purplish red–colored transitional zone extends proximally for about 2 cm until the pinker glandular mucosa of the rectum becomes dominant.

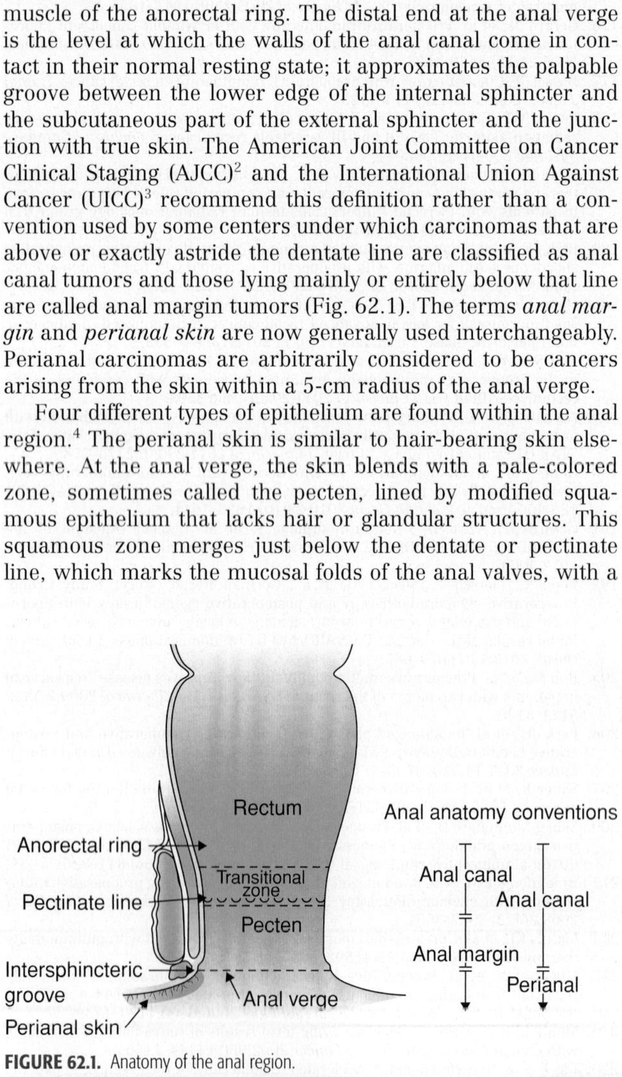

FIGURE 62.1. Anatomy of the anal region.

The major lymphatic pathways flow to three lymph node systems. The perianal skin, the anal verge, and the canal distal to the dentate line drain predominantly to the superficial inguinal nodes, with some communication to the femoral nodes and to the external iliac systems. Lymphatics from around and above the dentate line flow with those from the distal rectum to the internal pudendal, hypogastric, and obturator nodes of the internal iliac systems. The proximal canal drains to the perirectal and superior hemorrhoidal nodes of the inferior mesenteric system. There are numerous lymphatic connections between the various levels of the anal canal, and an intramural system links the lymphatics of the canal with those of the rectum.[5]

The veins of the anal canal connect with both the systemic and the portal venous systems. Venous plexuses, which lie in and surround the mucosal and muscular structures of the anal wall, anastomose around the junction of the anal verge and distal canal. The veins draining the inferior parts of these plexuses communicate with the systemic venous system via the internal pudendal and internal iliac veins, and those from the superior canal flow predominately to the inferior mesenteric vein and then to the portal system.[5]

Anorectal continence is mediated by both cerebrospinal nerves and the autonomic system. The smooth muscle of the internal sphincter is supplied by parasympathetic fibers from the second, third, and fourth sacral segments as well as sympathetic fibers from the hypogastric plexus. The upper canal has selective sensitivity for intraluminal differences in pressure, and the autonomic nerves mediate both the inhibitor and facilitator reflexes of the internal sphincter. The striated muscle of the external sphincter is under voluntary control and innervated by the internal rectal nerve, a branch of the pudendal nerve arising from the second, third, and fourth sacral nerves. The internal rectal nerve also transmits pain, touch, and other sensations from the anal lining below the dentate line and from the perianal skin.[5]

PATHOLOGIC CLASSIFICATION

The most recent revision of the World Health Organization (WHO) classification of anal tumors, published in 2000, describes intraepithelial and invasive neoplasms.[6] The term *anal intraepithelial neoplasia* (AIN) is applied to precancerous changes in the epithelium of the anal canal and perianal skin.[7]

For invasive cancers, the term *squamous cell carcinoma* is applied to all the various subtypes, squamous, large-cell keratinizing and nonkeratinizing, and basaloid, cloacogenic, and transitional, all of which were considered separate entities in the previous classification.[6] Clinicians have for some years grouped these various subtypes as epidermoid cancers because of their similar natural history; the term epidermoid is not used in the WHO classification. About 85% to 90% of primary anal canal cancers are squamous cell type. The remaining 10% to 15% are predominantly adenocarcinomas, most of which arise from anal glands or within anal fistulae. Adenocarcinomas from the rectal-type mucosa in the upper canal are classified as primary rectal cancers. The WHO system retains as separate entities rare variants such as squamous cell carcinoma with mucous microcysts, small cell, and undifferentiated cancers.

Primary cancers of the perianal skin are similar to cancers of the skin in other sites. Most are squamous cell cancers, with occasional basal cell cancers and skin adnexal adenocarcinomas.

EPIDEMIOLOGY

Anal cancers are about one-tenth as common as cancers of the rectum. Cancers arise in the canal with three to four times the frequency of perianal cancers. In North America and Europe, anal canal cancers are more common in women than in men, although this difference is decreasing[8]; perianal cancers occur with about equal frequency in both sexes. The annual age-adjusted rates per 100,000 for squamous cell cancers of the anus, anal canal, and anorectum in the U.S. Surveillance, Epidemiology, and End Results (SEER) registry for 1995 to 2004 were 0.89 for males and 1.14 for females.[8] The incidence varies widely in different parts of the world, but has been increasing in North America and Europe over the past 40 years.[8] The annual incidence of invasive and intraepithelial neoplasia almost doubled in men and rose by about half in women between the periods 1973 to 1979 and 1994 to 2000.[9] The risk of anal cancer increases with age; the median age at diagnosis is from 60 to 65 years.

RISK FACTORS

The most significant risk factors so far identified are sexually transmissible viruses, immunosuppression, and tobacco smoking. The role of sexual practices and sexually transmissible agents has been investigated intensively. Several mucosotropic types of human papilloma virus (HPV) are linked to cancer and precancerous lesions in the anogenital epithelium.[10–12] Subtypes of HPV with a high risk of association with cancer are type 16 in particular, and, to a lesser extent, types 18, 31, 33, 35, and others.[10–12] These high-risk HPV types have been found in about 85% of anal squamous cancers in many series,[10,11] more commonly in cancer of the canal than of the perianal skin.[11,13] Some geographic variation was noted in the types of high-risk HPV identified.[11,14] Case control studies suggest that a history of multiple sexual partners in homosexual or heterosexual relationships or of unprotected anal intercourse in males and in females are predictive of an increased risk of AIN and invasive anal cancer.[15] Compared to the overall annual incidence of anal cancer in white males in the United States of approximately 0.7 per 100,000 in the early 1980s, the estimated incidence in the male homosexual population, prior to the human immunodeficiency virus (HIV) epidemic, ranged from about 12 to 37 per 100,000.[16] This rate increased to about 70 per 100,000 among HIV-positive male homosexuals.[17]

Compromise of cell-mediated immunity reduces the body's ability to prevent or eliminate infection by viruses such as HPV. An increased risk of anal cancer is associated with at least two situations in which cell-mediated immunity is significantly altered: infection with HIV and iatrogenic suppression of immunity in organ transplant patients. Interactions between HPV and HIV are complex. Although anal cancer has not been designated an acquired immunodeficiency syndrome (AIDS)-defining condition, data from the U.S. AIDS Cancer Registry linkage study showed that the rate of HPV-associated cancers and precursors was increased in HIV-infected persons for all anogenital sites compared with the general population. The relative risk for anal cancers was 6.8 in women and 37.9 in men.[18] A national cohort study in Sweden of 5,931 patients who had undergone organ transplantation showed a 10-fold excess risk of developing anal cancer.[19] Whatever the cause of suppression of cell-mediated immunity, those affected have increased rates of HPV infection, higher progression rates from normal epithelium to AIN and from lower to higher grade AIN, and lower rates of clearance of HPV and regression from abnormal to normal epithelium.[20,21]

The increasing effectiveness of antiretroviral therapy has led to longer survival of HIV-infected patients and an increased number with anal cancer.[22,23] There was a 3-fold increase in incidence in the HIV-positive population from the period prior to the introduction of highly active antiretroviral therapy (HAART) in about 1996 and the later HAART era.[23] Although there was a decrease in the incidence of Kaposi's sarcoma and lymphoma by a few years after HAART became available, at the time of the review there had been no significant reduction in the incidence of less common malignancies such as anogenital cancers.[24] Early success of prophylactic vaccines against HPV in both men and women suggests that the incidence of anal cancer can be reduced in the future.[25,26]

Tobacco smoking is associated with up to a 4-fold increase in risk in several case-control studies. Current smokers are at greater risk than past smokers.[15,27] Benign conditions such as fistulae, fissures, and hemorrhoids do not appear to predispose to cancer.[28] Chronic anal inflammation due to inflammatory bowel disease has also been discounted as a risk factor.[29]

NATURAL HISTORY

Most squamous cell cancers of the anal region, especially the canal, are believed to be preceded by high-grade AIN.[7] However, it has been estimated that no more than 1% of cases with AIN develop invasive cancer per year,[30] a rate lower than that described for cervical intraepithelial neoplasia. Anal dysplasia recurs frequently despite excision, laser ablation, or topical therapies, presumably because of incomplete treatment or persistence of the HPV infection with which dysplasia is associated.[22] The natural history of AIN coexisting with anal cancers exposed to radiation, with or without chemotherapy, is unknown.

Squamous cancers of the anal canal spread most commonly by direct extension and lymphatic pathways. Hematogenous metastases are less common. Direct invasion from the anal mucosa into the sphincter muscles and perianal connective tissue spaces occurs early; in a series of 137 cases, cancers were confined to the mucosa and submucosa at diagnosis in only 12%, and to the sphincter muscles, without regional lymph node involvement, in only 34%.[31] In about half the cases, anal cancers extend into the rectum or perianal skin. Invasion of the vaginal septum and vaginal mucosa is more common than invasion of the prostate gland, but anovaginal fistulas occur in fewer than 5% of women. Extensive tumors may infiltrate the pelvic walls.

Lymphatic invasion occurs relatively early. The overall risk of regional nodal involvement at diagnosis is about 25%.[32,33] Pelvic lymph node metastases were found in as many as 30% of patients treated by abdominoperineal resection.[31,34,35] In an illustrative series, metastases were present in the superior hemorrhoidal nodes in 25% (15 of 61); in the external iliac, obturator, or hypogastric nodes in 30% (8 of 27); and in the inguinal nodes in 16% (12 of 74) of patients.[35] Inguinal metastases were detected clinically in up to approximately 20% of patients at initial diagnosis and were present subclinically in a further 10% to 20%.[31,35,36,37] Nodal metastases were associated with 30% of cancers confined to the sphincter muscles, and 60% of those that had extended through the sphincters or were more poorly differentiated.[34] Lymphatic metastases increase in frequency with progressive enlargement of the primary cancer.[34,38]

Extrapelvic metastases are identified at the time of first presentation in <10% of patients. They are found most frequently in the liver, lungs, and para-aortic nodes. Relapse after initial treatment is more common in the area of the primary tumor and the pelvic lymph nodes than in extrapelvic organs. Locoregional relapse rates of up to about 30% are common. Failure outside the pelvis occurs in up to about 20%.[31,39,40,41]

Perianal cancers tend to grow locally and may extend into the anal canal. When the site of origin is in doubt, it is conventional to classify the cancer as arising in the anal canal. The ipsilateral inguinal nodes are the most common site of metastasis and are involved in from 5% to 20% of cases. Extrapelvic metastases are uncommon except in locally advanced cancer or those with nodal metastases.

CLINICAL PRESENTATION

The symptoms of anal cancer are nonspecific, contributing to delay in presentation by the patient and in diagnosis by the physician of more than 6 months in a third of patients.[42,43] Bleeding and anal discomfort are the most common symptoms and are reported by about half the patients.[44] Less common complaints include awareness of an anal mass, pruritus, and anal discharge. Pain is uncommon but may be severe. In patients with tumors in the proximal canal, there may be an alteration in bowel habits, but this is uncommon with distal cancers.[44] Occasionally, asymptomatic tumors are found during physical examination or in the course of investigation of an enlarged inguinal node. Unsuspected microinvasive carcinoma is sometimes found in mucosa removed at hemorrhoidectomy.[45]

Small carcinomas are often nodular or plaque-like, but larger tumors are more typically ulcerated and infiltrative. Coexisting benign conditions such as anogenital warts, hemorrhoids, and anal fissures may be present. Anal sphincter tone is usually preserved and may be increased by painful spasm. Gross fecal incontinence resulting from sphincter destruction occurs in <5% of patients, although some fecal soiling is often reported. Similarly, vaginal fistulas are uncommon. Rarely, extrapelvic metastases may be the only symptomatic feature or finding.

DIAGNOSTIC WORKUP

The history and physical examination should stress features that delineate the extent of the primary tumor, including anal sphincter competence and possible invasion of adjacent organs. A biopsy of the primary tumor is necessary to establish the diagnosis and the histologic type. General anesthesia may be needed to permit detailed pelvic and anorectal examination, which should include proctoscopy. Sigmoidoscopy and colonoscopy, although often performed, infrequently disclose colonic pathology.[46] Physical examination should include detailed examination of the genital region, especially in patients who give a history of previous anogenital area dysplasia or cancer, genital warts, anal-receptive intercourse, or are HIV positive.

Only the inguinal and low perirectal lymph nodes are accessible to clinical examination. Because lymph node enlargement may be caused by reactive hyperplasia in as many as half of those with palpable inguinal nodes, clinically suspicious nodes should be assessed histologically by needle biopsy or simple excision.[44] Metastases in the internal iliac and superior hemorrhoidal node chains, about half of which are <0.5 cm in diameter,[47] cannot be identified reliably by current techniques of lymphangiography, pelvic lymphoscintigraphy, computed tomography (CT), magnetic resonance imaging (MRI), or transanorectal ultrasonography. MRI is considered the most accurate method for assessing the primary cancer and pelvic nodes.[48] Both fluorodeoxyglucose (FDG) positron emission tomography (PET) with CT and inguinal sentinel lymph node biopsy (ISLN) have been used to identify inguinal node metastases and to refine RT plans.[49–51] However, a comparison of FDG-PET-CT and ISLN biopsy in 27 patients found several false-positive PET studies (4 of 7).[52] Also, late inguinal node metastases have been reported after a previous negative ISLN biopsy.[53] Both FDG-PET-CT and ISLN biopsy are as yet of unproven value in the initial management of anal cancer.

Thoracic, abdominal, and pelvic CT and pelvic MRI identify liver or lung metastases or enlarged nodes. If the diagnosis is uncertain, image-guided biopsy should be considered. Skeletal studies are not indicated in the absence of focal symptoms.

Examination of blood and serum should include full blood count, renal and liver function tests, and, if any risk factors are present, assessment of HIV antibody status.

STAGING

The staging systems for anal canal and perianal cancers most commonly used are those proposed by the UICC[3] and the AJCC[2] (Tables 62.1 and 62.2). Most authors continue to report results by T (tumor) category or N (node) category rather than by composite TNM (tumor, node, metastasis) stages. Under the UICC and AJCC systems, the regional lymph nodes for anal canal cancer are the perirectal, internal iliac, and inguinal nodes. Spread to all other pelvic node groups, including the external iliac, common iliac, and sigmoid nodes, is classified as metastasis (M1). For perianal cancers, the only regional nodes are the ipsilateral inguinal nodes.

In a review of 19,199 patients with squamous cell carcinoma of the anal canal, diagnosed between 1985 and 2000 and recorded in the U.S. National Cancer Data Base (NCDB), the stage distribution was stage I: 25.3%, II: 51.8%, III: 17.1%, IV: 5.7%. Tumors were >5 cm in size (T3) in at least 20.6% (tumor size in T4 category not available). Nodal involvement was present in 21.8% of those for whom information on nodal status was recorded.[33]

PROGNOSTIC FACTORS

Tumor Factors

Features related to the anatomic extent of disease generally provide the most prognostic value.[54] The most adverse factor for

TABLE 62.1 ANAL CANAL TNM CLASSIFICATION

Primary Tumor (T)			
TX	Primary tumor cannot be assessed		
T0	No evidence of primary tumor		
Tis	Carcinoma *in situ*		
T1	Tumor 2 cm or less in greatest dimension		
T2	Tumor more than 2 cm but not more than 5 cm in greatest dimension		
T3	Tumor more than 5 cm in greatest dimension		
T4	Tumor of any size invades adjacent organ(s) (e.g., vagina, urethra, bladder) (involvement of the sphincter muscle(s) *alone* is not classified as T4)		
Regional Lymph Nodes (N)			
NX	Regional lymph nodes cannot be assessed		
N0	No regional lymph node metastasis		
N1	Metastasis in perirectal lymph nodes(s)		
N2	Metastasis in unilateral iliac and/or inguinal lymph node(s)		
N3	Metastasis in perirectal and inguinal lymph nodes and/or bilateral internal iliac and/or inguinal lymph nodes		
Distant Metastases (M)			
MX	Distant metastasis cannot be assessed		
M0	No distant metastasis		
M1	Distant metastasis		
Stage Grouping			
Stage 0	Tis	N0	M0
Stage I	T1	N0	M0
Stage II	T2	N0	M0
	T3	N0	M0
Stage IIIA	T1	N1	M0
	T2	N1	M0
	T3	N1	M0
	T4	N0	M0
Stage IIIB	T4	N1	M0
	Any T	N2, N3	M0
Stage IV	Any T	Any N	M1

From Sobin LH, Gospodarowicz M, Wittekind C. *TNM classification of malignant tumours*, 7th ed. New York: Wiley-Blackwell, 2009, with permission.

TABLE 62.2 PERIANAL SKIN TNM CLASSIFICATION

Primary Tumor (T)			
TX	Primary tumor (T)		
T0	No evidence of primary tumor		
Tis	Carcinoma *in situ*		
T1	Tumor 2 cm or less in greatest dimension		
T2	Tumor more than 2 cm but not more than 5 cm in greatest dimension		
T3	Tumor more than 5 cm in greatest dimension		
T4	Tumor invades deep extradermal structures (i.e., cartilage, skeletal muscle, or bone)		
Regional Lymph Nodes (N)			
NX	Regional lymph nodes cannot be assessed		
N0	No regional lymph node metastasis		
N1	Regional lymph node metastasis		
Distant Metastasis (M)			
MX	Distant metastasis cannot be assessed		
M0	No distant metastasis		
M1	Distant metastasis		
Stage Grouping			
Stage 0	Tis	N0	M0
Stage I	T1	N0	M0
Stage II	T2, T3	N0	M0
Stage III	T4	N0	M0
	Any T	N1	M0
Stage IV	Any T	Any N	M1

From Sobin LH, Gospodarowicz M, Wittekind C. *TNM classification of malignant tumours*, 7th ed. New York: Wiley-Blackwell, 2009, with permission.

survival is the presence of extrapelvic metastasis.[55,56–57] When anal cancer is confined to the pelvis, the size of the primary tumor is the most useful predictor for local control and preservation of anorectal function and survival.[39,58,59] Involvement of regional lymph nodes is an adverse factor for survival but, in most series, not for control of the primary tumor.[39,59]

Among the 19,199 patients recorded in the NCDB between 1985 and 2000, the overall 5-year survival was 58%.[33] Patients with distant metastases had a 5-year survival of 18.7% versus 59.4% for those without metastases. Patients with regional node metastases had a 5-year survival of 37.4% versus 62.9% in node-negative patients. Five-year survival rates by T category were T1: 68.5%, T2: 58.9%, T3: 43.1%, and T4: 34.3%. The survival rates by AJCC stage are shown in Figure 62.2.

In detailed analyses of data collected prospectively for Radiation Therapy Oncology Group trial RTOG-9811,[59,60] tumor diameter >5 cm correlated with an increased likelihood of colostomy (hazard ratio [HR] 1.8; $P = .008$)[59] (Table 62.3). A tumor size >5 cm and clinically positive nodes were each associated with significantly poorer 5-year disease-free and overall survival.[60] These findings were combined into prognostic groups.[60] These groups are shown in Figure 62.3, with additional data drawn from the analyses by Ajani et al.[59,60] These groupings have not been verified prospectively.

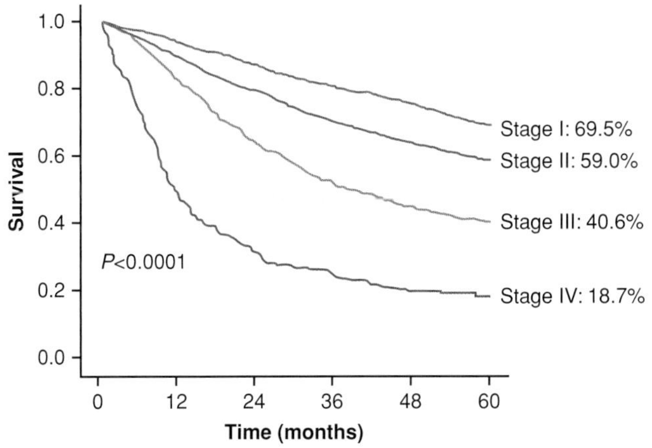

FIGURE 62.2. Five-year survival rates by American Joint Committee on Cancer Clinical Staging and the International Union Against Cancer stages, for 19,199 patients recorded in the U.S. National Cancer Data Base between 1985 and 2000. (From ref. 33, with permission.)

TABLE 62.3 PROGNOSTIC GROUPS: BASED ON DATA FROM RTOG TRIAL 9811

End Points (3 Year)	*Group 1* *T≤5 cm, N-ve (n = 365)*	*Group 2* *T>5 cm, N-ve (n = 112)*	*Group 3* *T≤5 cm, N+ve (n = 107)*	*Group 4* *T>5 cm, N+ve (n = 60)*
Disease-free survival (actuarial) (%)	74	65	48	30
Colostomy rate (crude) (%)	11	17	9	24
Overall survival (actuarial) (%)	86	75	75	63

RTOG, Radiation Therapy Oncology Group; T, primary tumor; N, any regional node.

Data from pooled trial groups treated by radiation therapy (RT), 5-fluorouracil, and mitomycin-C or RT, 5-FU and cisplatin (CDDP). Median follow-up 2.2 years. Most events occurred by 2 years.

From refs. 59 and 60.

Patient Factors

Patient-related factors are not consistent between series. Age, performance status, gender, baseline hemoglobin level, and race have all been considered prognostic in one or more series. Patients who continue to smoke tobacco may be at greater risk of local relapse.[61] In some series of HIV-positive patients, high viral load, low lymphocyte CD4-positive counts, and AIDS have been prognostic of poor local tumor control and survival, and, in some series, of impaired tolerance of RT and chemotherapy.[62–63,64]

Biochemical and Molecular Factors

A survey of nearly 50 reports on cytogenetic, flow cytometric, immunohistochemical, and other factors considered that these studies offered some insights on pathogenesis but did not help with selection of treatment or provide guidance on prognosis.[65] Recent studies suggested that biomarkers such as p53,[66] Ki-67, nuclear factor kappa B, 5HH, and Gli-1,[67] may be associated with locoregional control or disease-free survival. High levels of MCM7 protein detected in gene expression analysis were associated with improved cancer survival in one series.[68] None of these suggested markers has yet been validated in prospective studies.

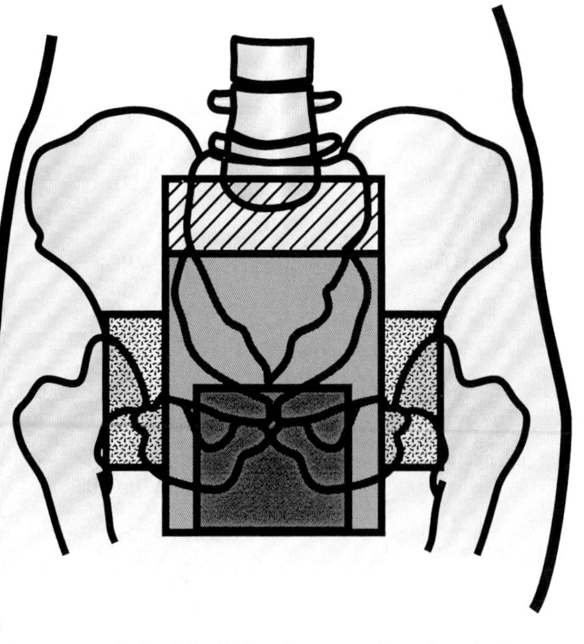

FIGURE 62.3. Example of radiation fields used to cover pelvic nodes and primary cancer. Upper border generally lowered from lumbosacral junction to lower border of sacroiliac joints part way through course. Fields are later reduced further to give higher dose to primary tumor. Separate anterior fields are applied to cover lateral inguinal nodes.

Treatment Factors

Early response, and the extent of response, to chemoradiation were correlated with survival in several multivariate analyses.[54,69,70] An association with total radiation dose or with treatment duration, while expected, has not been demonstrated consistently for either locoregional control or survival. A daily fraction size of 2.5 Gy appeared to be associated with increased acute and late toxicity, compared with 2-Gy fractions.[39]

TREATMENT OF ANAL CANCER

Although squamous cell cancer of the anal canal is a relatively uncommon malignancy, several multicenter randomized trials have been completed successfully. These have established RT, 5-FU, and MMC, with surgery reserved for failure, as the standard against which other treatments should be compared. These trials are outlined here and in Table 62.4.[41,71–78] The original references should be consulted for full details of patient eligibility, treatment regimens, outcomes, and statistical analyses. There have also been more than 100 nonrandomized studies, many of which provided hypotheses subsequently tested in the randomized studies, or information that guided the development of technical aspects of radiation treatment.[79]

It is of note that the combination of RT and chemotherapy has supplanted surgery as the preferred treatment for anal canal squamous cell cancer without formal comparison in a randomized trial. Nonrandomized comparisons of radical resection with this combination of RT, 5-FU, and MMC[32] or with radiation therapy alone[80] have shown the ability of radiation-based regimens to produce survival rates at least equal to those of surgical series, while allowing preservation of anorectal function in the majority of patients.

TABLE 62.4 SELECTED RESULTS OF PHASE III TRIALS

Trial (Reference)	*N*	*Treatment*	*Local (LF) or Locoregional (LRF) Failure (%)*	*Colostomy Rate (CR) or Colostomy-Free Survival (CFS) (%)*	*Disease-Free Survival (%)*	*Overall Survival (%)*
			3-yr LRF	3-yr CR	3 yr	3 yr
UKCCCR (ACT I) (41)	292	RT, 5-FU, MMC	39	24	np	65
	285	RT	61	40	np	58
	RR		0.54	np	np	0.86
	P		<.0001	np	np	.25
			10-yr LRF	10-yr CFS	10 yr	10 yr
Update (71)	292	RT, 5-FU, MMC	34	36	36	42
	285	RT	59	26	24	36
	HR		0.46	np	0.70	0.86
	P		<.001	sig	<.001	.12
			5-yr LRF	5-yr CFS	5 yr	5 yr
EORTC (72)	51	RT, 5-FU, MMC	32[a]	72[a]	np	58[a]
	52	RT	48[a]	40[a]	np	53[a]
	P		.02	.002	np	.17
			4-yr LF	4-yr CR	4 yr	4 yr
RTOG 8704/ECOG 1289 (73)	146	RT, 5-FU, MMC	16	9	73	76
	145	RT, 5-FU	34	22	51	67
	P		.0008	.002	.0003	.31
			5-yr LRF	3-yr CR	3 yr	3 yr
RTOG 9811 (74)	324	RT, 5-FU, MMC	25	10	60	75
	320	RT, 5-FU, CDDP	33	19	54	70
	HR		1.32	1.68	1.20	1.28
	P		.07	.02	.17	.10
			5-yr LRF	5-yr CR	5 yr	5 yr
Update (75)	325	RT, 5-FU, MMC	20	12	68	78
	324	RT, 5-FU, CDDP	27	17	58	71
	P		.089	.075	.004	.021
			3 yr	3-yr CR	3 yr[b]	3 yr[b]
UKCR (ACT II) (76)	471	RT, 5-FU, MMC	np	14	np	np
	469	RT, 5-FU, CDDP	np	11	np	np
	446	No maintenance chemo	np	np	75	85
	448	Maintenance chemo	np	np	75	84
	HR		np	11	0.89	0.79
	P			.26	.42	.19
			3-yr LF	3-yr CFS	3-yr Event-free Survival	3 yr
ACCORD-03 (77,78)	307 total	Std RT, 5-FU, CDDP	10	86	67	np
		HD RT, 5-FU, CDDP	13	80	68	np
		Ind CT + Std RTCT	20	83	70	np
		Ind CT + HD RTCT	4	85	78	np
		Ind CT arms	np	84 vs. 83		
		HD RTCT arms	np	84 vs. 83		
	P		not sig	not sig	not sig	not sig

UKCCCR, U.K. Coordination Committee for Cancer Research; EORTC, European Organisation for Research on Treatment of Cancer; RTOG, Radiation Therapy Oncology Group; ECOG, Eastern Cooperative Oncology Group; np, not published; sig, significant, not sig, not significant; RT, radiation therapy; 5-FU, 5-fluorouracil; MMC, mitomycin C; CDDP, cisplatin; Std, standard; HD RT, high dose radiation; Ind CT, induction chemotherapy; RTCT, chemoradiation.

[a]Numbers derived from curves. [b]In patients who received maintenance chemotherapy.

COMBINED RADIATION AND CHEMOTHERAPY

Radiation, 5-Fluorouracil, and Mitomycin-C Versus Radiation Alone

In both the United Kingdom and Europe in the 1970s, more so than in North America, there was already some acceptance of RT as the primary treatment for anal cancer[81]; this facilitated the development of the first multi-institutional randomized trials in which RT alone was compared with RT plus chemotherapy. The randomized trials conducted by the U.K. Coordination Committee for Cancer Research (UKCCCR)[41] and the European Organisation for Research on Treatment of Cancer (EORTC)[72] both demonstrated significant improvement in control of the primary cancer and regional nodes and in colostomy rate or colostomy-free survival in patients who received RT, 5-FU, and MMC. Overall survival rates were not improved significantly in the initial reports. However, in a later report of the UKCCCR trial after a median of 13 years' follow-up, locoregional control, colostomy-free survival, disease-free survival, and deaths due to anal cancer all significantly favored chemoradiation.[71] The absolute difference in risk of dying from all causes was 5.1% lower in the chemoradiation group at 5 years and 5.6% lower at 12 years from randomization. This difference approached statistical significance (HR 0.86; 95% confidence interval [CI], 0.70 to 1.04; $P = .12$).[71]

The UKCCCR trial included 577 patients with all stages (UICC staging system, 1987 edition) of squamous cell cancer of the anal canal (75% of patients) or anal margin (23%).[41] The radiation dose was 45 Gy in 20 to 25 fractions in 4 to 5 weeks. Those randomized to chemotherapy received 5-FU (1,000 mg/m^2/day for 4 days or 750 mg/m^2/day for 5 days) by continuous peripheral intravenous infusion in the first and final weeks of radiation treatment, plus MMC (12 mg/m^2) by bolus intravenous injection on day 1 of the first course of chemotherapy. If the primary tumor had not regressed by at least 50% by 6 weeks after treatment (as occurred in 10% in each group), surgery was recommended; otherwise, the patients received an additional 15 Gy in 6 fractions by a perineal field or 25 Gy over 2 to 3 days by iridium-192 implant. The locoregional recurrence rates at 3 years were 61% after RT and 39% after RT, 5-FU, and MMC ($P < .0001$). The overall survival rates at 3 years were 58% and 65% ($P = .25$), respectively. There were six (2%) deaths due to treatment in the combined-modality arm and two (0.7%) in the irradiation-alone arm. Acute toxicity, other than hematologic, was considered comparable in each group. In the first few years after treatment, surgery that included colostomy was necessary for management of toxicity in 10 patients (3.5%) in each group.[41] Late toxicity events (severity was not graded) after a median of 13 years' follow-up were similar in each treatment group.[71]

In the EORTC study, 103 patients with advanced cancers of the anal canal were randomized in a trial of similar design.[72] The radiation dose was 45 Gy in 25 fractions over 5 weeks. Chemotherapy included 5-FU (750 mg/m^2/day for 5 days) in weeks 1 and 5 of radiation, and a single dose of MMC (15 mg/m^2) by bolus intravenous injection on day 1 of the first course of 5-FU only. After 6 weeks, boost irradiation of 15 Gy (if complete clinical response to previous treatment had occurred) or 20 Gy (after partial response) was given by external-beam or interstitial irradiation. The 5-year locoregional recurrence rate was 48% after RT and 32% after RT, 5-FU, and MMC ($P = .02$). The difference between overall survival rates (53% and 58%, respectively) was not significant. One of 51 patients who received combined modality treatment died of toxicity. Otherwise, acute and late toxicity rates did not differ markedly. These two trials established RT, 5-FU, and MMC as the standard first-line treatment.

Radiation, 5-Fluorouracil, and Mitomycin-C Versus Radiation and 5-Fluorouracil

The RTOG and Eastern Cooperative Oncology Group (ECOG) established in a randomized trial that the combination of MMC with 5-FU and RT is more effective than 5-FU alone with RT.[73] This study was undertaken to determine whether MMC was a necessary component of the protocol and whether the hematologic toxicity of that drug could be avoided. Two hundred and ninety-one patients with cancers of the anal canal of any T and N category (RTOG staging system) who did not have evidence of extrapelvic metastases received 45 Gy to 50.4 Gy in 25 to 28 fractions over 5 weeks, plus 2 courses of 5-FU (1,000 mg/m^2/day by continuous peripheral intravenous infusion) over 4 days, with or without MMC (10 mg/m^2 by bolus intravenous injection) on the first day of each course of chemotherapy. Chemotherapy was administered in weeks 1 and 5 of radiation therapy. All patients underwent biopsy of the primary tumor site 6 weeks after treatment. Biopsies were positive in 15% of those who received 5-FU only and in 8% of those who received both MMC and 5-FU ($P = .14$). Patients with positive biopsies had the option of receiving an additional 9 Gy in 5 treatments concurrently with a 4-day infusion of 5-FU (1,000 mg/m^2/day) and a single injection of cisplatin (CDDP) (100 mg/m^2) if it was thought that anal function might still be salvaged. At 4 years, the rates of local failure (16% vs. 34%; $P = .0008$) and of colostomy (9% vs. 22%; $P = .002$), significantly favored treatment with radiation, 5-FU, and MMC. There was no significant difference in overall survival rates (76% with RT, 5-FU, and MMC vs. 67%); however, the disease-free survival rate (73% vs. 51%; $P = .0003$) was improved by the three-agent combination. Acute hematologic toxicity was more common in the patients who received MMC, but the rates of other acute and late toxic effects were similar in each treatment group. Four of 146 (2.7%) patients who received both 5-FU and MMC suffered fatal toxicity as did 1 of 145 treated with RT and 5-FU alone. On the evidence from this trial, MMC was retained in combination with RT and 5-FU.

Radiation, 5-Fluorouracil and Mitomycin-C Versus Radiation, 5-Fluorouracil, and Cisplatin

Several pilot studies suggested high tumor response rates to concurrent, induction, or induction plus concurrent 5-FU and CDDP with RT.[82–88] Cisplatin was known to be effective against squamous cell cancers in several other sites and to be associated with stronger laboratory evidence as a radiosensitizer than MMC.

The RTOG elected to evaluate a strategy of CDDP-based induction chemotherapy intended to downsize the primary tumor and nodal metastases prior to concurrent chemoradiation. This trial included a higher total radiation dose than the earlier RTOG randomized trial,[73] based on analysis of nonrandomized studies that suggested a radiation dose–control relationship,[89,90] and on pilot studies which had demonstrated that a proportion of patients could tolerate uninterrupted radiation schedules of up to 59.4 Gy over 6.5 weeks with either concurrent MMC with 5-FU[91,92] or CDDP with 5-FU.[83]

In RTOG-9811,[74] one patient group received 59 Gy in 6.5 weeks (45 Gy in 1.8-Gy fractions, followed without interruption by 14 Gy in 2-Gy fractions), together with concurrent 5-FU (1,000 mg/m^2/day) by continuous infusion on days 1 to 4 and 29 to 32 plus MMC 10 mg/m^2 intravenous bolus on days 1 and 29; the other group received 5-FU (1,000 mg/m^2/day) days 1 to 4, 29 to 32, 57 to 60, and 85 to 88 plus CDDP (75 mg/m^2 bolus injection on days 1, 29, 57, and 85) with the same 59 Gy radiation schedule (start day 57). Acute grade 3 or 4 nonhematologic toxicity rates were 75% in each arm, but hematologic toxicity was higher in the MMC group (67% vs. 47%). No treatment-related deaths were reported. The rate of severe long-term toxicity was similar in each group (11% MMC vs. 10% CDDP). The first report of this trial (after median patient follow-up of 2.5 years) described a significantly higher rate of colostomy at 3 years in those who received CDDP rather than MMC plus 5-FU and RT. There were no significant differences in disease-free or overall survival rates.

After longer follow-up, the 5-year colostomy rates and locoregional failure rates showed trends in favor of 5-FU, MMC- and RT but were not significant. However, the 5-year disease-free (68% vs. 58%; $P = .004$) and overall survival rates (78% vs. 71%; $P = .021$) significantly favored RT, 5-FU, and MMC.[75] The investigators concluded that RT, 5-FU, and MMC should remain the standard approach.

The second U.K. Anal Cancer Trial (ACT II) also has not identified a role for CDDP in addition to or in place of MMC. This trial has so far been reported in abstract only.[76] The trial incorporates a double randomization, either to 5-FU and MMC or to 5-FU and CDDP concurrently with RT; and to 2 courses of adjuvant (or maintenance) 5-FU and CDDP or to no additional chemotherapy following concurrent chemoradiation. The primary end points were improvements in complete tumor response rates and disease-free survival rates. Complete tumor response rates at 6 months were similar: 94% (MMC arm) and 95% (CDDP arm). Three-year disease-free and overall survival rates were not improved in those who received adjuvant 5-FU and CDDP. MMC-treated patients had more severe hematologic toxicity, but rates of neutropenic sepsis were similar (about 3%).

A French intergroup conducted a factorial designed four-arm trial (ACCORD 03) that evaluated the addition of induction 5-FU and CDDP and of a higher dose of boost RT (20 Gy to 25 Gy vs. standard 15 Gy). The baseline standard RT schedule was 45 Gy in 25 fractions in 5 weeks. The outcome has been reported in abstract only.[77,78] The actuarial 3-year colostomy-free survival rate (the primary study end point) ranged from 80% to 85% in the four arms, with no significant advantages for either experimental treatment. Local control, event-free survival, and overall survival rates were similar in each arm.

Other Drug–Radiation Combinations

In an effort to develop a simplified schedule, the U.K. National Cancer Research Institute Anal Subgroup conducted a phase II trial of RT (50.4 Gy in 28 fractions in 5.5 weeks), a single intravenous injection of MMC (12 mg/m^2 on day 1) and oral capecitabine (825 mg/m^2 twice daily on each RT treatment day).[93] The schedule was described as well tolerated with acceptable compliance (although only 58% received the full planned doses). The overall tumor response rate after treatment was 90% (complete in 24 of 31 and partial in 4 of 31). Although this use of oral capecitabine is promising and removes the need for continuous intravenous infusions of 5-FU, at this time, delivery of both 5-FU and MMC intravenously remains standard.

The EORTC conducted a randomized phase II trial in which RT (36 Gy + 2-week gap + 23.4 Gy) was combined with either MMC and 5-FU or MMC and CDDP. The overall response rates at 8 weeks were 92% (34 of 37) to RT, MMC, and CDDP versus 80% (31 of 39) to RT, 5-FU, and MMC, although greater compliance to the full regimen was seen with RT, 5-FU, and MMC.[94] It is not known whether this group has proceeded with a planned phase III trial.[95]

Because epidermal growth factor receptor (EGFR) is known to be overexpressed in many epithelial cancers, including squamous cell cancer of the anal canal,[96] EGFR blockers are being evaluated. The ECOG is conducting a phase II study of RT, 5-FU, CDDP, and cetuximab in HIV-negative patients.[95] The AIDS Malignancy Clinical Trials Consortium is performing a similar study in HIV-positive patients.[95] Other anti-EGFR agents under study include Nimotuzumab and panitumumab.[95] Initial laboratory studies suggest that EGFR and *K RAS* mutation analysis are not likely to be useful as a screening test for sensitivity to anti-EGFR therapy in anal canal cancer.[96]

In Sweden, bleomycin was given concurrently with RT in nonrandomized studies, but no benefit was apparent.[97–98,99] A pilot study in the United Kingdom in which all three of the major drugs investigated, 5FU, MMC, and CDDP, were combined with RT was not pursued further because of excessive toxicity.[100]

Conclusion

Much remains to be learned about the mechanisms of interaction between radiation and chemotherapy in the treatment of cancer. The synergistic interactions of various combinations of RT, 5-FU, MMC- and CDDP observed in some laboratory studies are difficult to evaluate clinically, and no trials designed to study such interactions have been performed. Also, there have not been formal comparisons of more prolonged, but less daily dose-intense, infusions of 5-FU with the 96-hour to 120-hour infusions generally favored, nor of bolus injections with continuous infusions of 5-FU or CDDP. In most series, the timing of delivery of chemotherapy each day relative to irradiation was not tightly controlled, and the importance of scheduling is not known.

The current standard chemoradiation combination is RT with two concurrent 96-hour or 120-hour continuous intravenous infusions of 5-FU and one or two bolus injections of MMC. The most effective doses have not been established. When patients are to be managed outside a clinical trial, it is suggested that a schedule used in one of the prospective randomized trials, for which there are data on efficacy and toxicity, be adopted.

RADIATION THERAPY

The use of RT alone, either brachytherapy or external beam, has been greatly reduced since the confirmation of improved outcome of combined modality therapy. Radiation alone is now recommended mainly to patients who are unable to undergo RT plus chemotherapy, or for the treatment of smaller cancers up to about 3 to 4 cm in size where the physician does not wish to add chemotherapy. As with combined RT and chemotherapy, primary tumor control is better with small tumors. Selected results, mainly from the period prior to the adoption of chemoradiation, are shown in Table 62.5.

SURGERY

For Residual and Recurrent Cancer

Random biopsies from the site of the primary tumor, or abnormal nodes, shortly after chemoradiation have been advocated by some but are not necessary. Elective biopsies at predetermined times do not appear to lead to better results than can be achieved by biopsies directed only to areas suspected clinically of harboring residual or recurrent cancer. A negative biopsy does not exclude the possibility of cancer regrowth.[105,106] Residual masses at the site of the original anal cancer may take several months to resolve fully after chemoradiation or RT alone.[39,106] Most authors now recommend biopsy only when persistent cancer is suspected clinically.

Suspected residual or recurrent cancer at the primary site or in regional nodes should be confirmed histologically if possible. Full restaging imaging is recommended. FDG-PET scans may disclose otherwise unidentified cancer.[107] Abdominoperineal resection or multivisceral pelvic resection is usually required. Survival rates are poor when R0 resection cannot be achieved.[108,109] Locoregional recurrence is common, despite apparent R0 resection.[108,110] Five-year survival rates following salvage surgery range from 30% to 50%, reflecting the varying criteria applied when selecting patients for surgery.[108,109–110,111]

Salvage for inguinal node metastases is usually by radical or selective inguinofemoral lymphadenectomy. Pelvic sidewall node metastases may not be resectable due to invasion of muscle or bone or neurovascular structures.

TABLE 62.5 SELECTED RESULTS OF RADIATION THERAPY ALONE

Author (Reference)	Radiation	Primary Tumor Control T1	T2	T3T4	Serious Complications–Colostomy	5-Year Survival
Newman et al. (101)	50 Gy/20/4 wk	8/9 (≤2 cm)	42/52 (81%) (≤5 cm)	13/20 (65%) (>5 cm or T4)	2	66%
Cummings et al. (102)	50 Gy/20/4 wk (some EB-I/I)	6/6 (≤2 cm)	19/29 (66%) (≤5 cm)	13/28 (46%) (>5 cm or T4)	6	61%
Martenson and Gunderson (103)	45–50 Gy/25–28/5–6 wk Plus boost to 55–67 Gy	9/9 (≤2 cm)	17/17 (100%) (≤5 cm)	–	2 temp	94%, actuarial
Otim-Oyet et al. (104)	60–65 Gy/30–33/6–7 wk (some with boost)	2/2 (≤2 cm)	16/22 (73%) (≤4 cm)	8/17 (47%) (>4 cm)	1	56% cause-specific
Papillon and Montbarbon (80)	42 Gy/10/2.5 wk Plus I 20 Gy at 8 wk	NS	29/39 (74%) (≤4 cm)	27/64 (42%) (>4 cm)	6	60%

EB, external beam; I, interstitial brachytherapy; NS, not stated; temp, temporary.

For Primary Cancer

Surgery is the principal treatment for anal intraepithelial neoplasia[112] but retains only a limited place in the initial management of primary invasive anal cancer. A few patients (<5% in most series) are incontinent for solid stool at presentation. This is usually due to extensive tumors that have destroyed the competence of the anal sphincters or fistulized into the vagina. Eradication of cancer by RT, with or without chemotherapy, does not restore continence in such patients, likely because the cancer is replaced by fibrous tissue rather than the specialized muscle of the anal sphincters. One approach is to perform colostomy before preoperative RT and chemotherapy using doses of 45 to 50 Gy over 5 weeks, followed by immediate or delayed resection. An alternative is initial abdominoperineal resection with postoperative RT and chemotherapy. There are insufficient data to compare the outcomes of these approaches.

Local excision, preserving anorectal function, is possible in some patients, although this is now usually restricted to small well-differentiated squamous cell cancers that have not invaded the sphincter muscles and are located distal to the dentate line.[113–115] This approach is based on the finding in surgical series that pararectal or superior hemorrhoidal system lymph node metastases were associated with <5% of well-differentiated squamous cell cancers <2 cm in size.[31,34] Local excision of small cancers of the distal canal or perianal skin is generally more expedient and associated with less morbidity than radiation-based treatments. However, if resection margins are positive or considered inadequate, and further local excision is not possible, the patient should receive chemoradiation or RT alone. There is no evidence that elective management by limited tumor excision and postoperative radiation-based protocols improves local control.[116]

The role of surgery in the management of inguinal node metastases detected at initial diagnosis has not been well defined. Although nodal metastases are generally treated successfully by the same doses of RT and chemotherapy effective against the primary cancer, there is no consensus on whether control of the nodal region involved is improved by limited node dissection prior to RT and chemotherapy and on how such an approach affects morbidity such as late limb edema.[36,38–39,40] After local excision of gross node metastases, the dose to the groin can usually be limited to 50 to 54 Gy over 5 to 6 weeks, provided imaging does not show residual metastases. The combination of local surgery and RT and chemotherapy has resulted in regional control rates in the groin of 80% or better.[38,39] However, 5-year survival rates are usually ~20% less than in those who do not present with inguinal node metastases.

Extrapelvic Metastases

Deaths from extrapelvic metastases alone are relatively infrequent. Extrapelvic metastases are identified in about 10% to 20% of patients. Among 77 patients in the UKCCCR ACT I trial who died of anal cancer after treatment with RT, 5-FU, and MMC, 38 of 77 (49% of the cancer deaths) had cancer in the pelvis only, and 21 of 77 (27%) had extrapelvic metastases only. In that trial, the overall crude rate of metastasis in those who received RT and chemotherapy was 10%, compared with 17% in those treated by RT alone.[41] In the EORTC trial, 17% of those treated by RT and chemotherapy developed metastases, as did 21% of those treated by RT only.[72] In RTOG-9811, the rates of distant metastases at 5 years were 13% in those who received RT, 5-FU, and MMC and 18% after RT, 5-FU, and CDDP.[75] In the U.K. ACT II trial, there was no suggestion in the 3-year disease-free and overall survival rates of benefit from the addition of 2 courses of adjuvant 5-FU and CDDP.[76] The rates of metastases in patients treated by chemoradiation are similar to those reported following management of the primary cancer and regional nodes by surgery or RT only. There is still considerable uncertainty regarding the effects on subclinical metastases outside the pelvis from the chemotherapy given concurrently with RT and as short-term induction or adjuvant treatment.

The median survival time after diagnosis of extrapelvic metastases ranges from 8 to about 24 months.[55,56,117] These metastases have been relatively resistant so far to all chemotherapy, RT, or combined modality protocols.[117] The most active combination is 5-FU and CDDP, although complete or durable responses are uncommon. Many recently developed drugs and molecular targeted agents have not yet been evaluated, but the possibility of new approaches is illustrated by preliminary reports of responses to cetuximab and irinotecan.[118] Radiation alone may provide useful palliation, especially for painful metastases. Stereotactic body radiation therapy or metastasectomy may be offered to selected patients, but metastases are commonly multiple.

TREATMENT OF PERIANAL CANCER

The most common histologic type of invasive cancer of the perianal skin is squamous cell carcinoma, usually keratinizing. Basal cell cancers and adenocarcinomas can also occur.

Wide local excision with a 1-cm margin is recommended for all histologic types, provided anal continence can be preserved.[115] Radiation alone or in combination with chemotherapy is also effective against squamous cell cancers.[40,69,119,120–121,122–123] Radiation-based protocols identical to those for anal canal cancer are preferred when anal continence would be impaired by surgery. In the UKCCCR ACT I trial, one of four patients had a cancer that arose in the perianal skin (anal margin). Results by site of cancer origin were not reported, but local control and cause-specific survival rates favored combined modality therapy.[41,71] The U.K. investigators also included perianal cancers in their subsequent trial.[76] In institution-based series, locoregional control rates ranged from 60% to 90%, sphincter preservation rates from 65% to 85%, and 5-year overall survival from 55% to 80%.[40,69,119,120–121,122–123] Local necrosis was seen as a complication more frequently when brachytherapy was used, although in general the rates of serious complications were <5%.

The regional nodes for the perianal skin are the ipsilateral inguinal nodes. Perirectal and pelvic node metastases are uncommon unless the cancer involves the anal canal extensively. The risk of inguinal node metastases is about 10%, principally with category T3 or T4 tumors or poorly differentiated cancers. Elective bilateral inguinal nodal irradiation may be considered when these larger tumors are treated, although some advocate elective inguinal RT for all perianal cancers.[123] The lower pelvic nodes should be included if the anal canal is invaded. The management of abnormal inguinal nodes is similar to that for anal canal cancer.

The principles of management for the uncommon basal cell and adenocarcinomas of the perianal skin are similar to those for these histological types elsewhere on the skin.

PATIENTS WITH HUMAN IMMUNODEFICIENCY VIRUS/ACQUIRED IMMUNODEFICIENCY SYNDROME

The numbers of HIV-infected patients with anal squamous cell cancer are increasing.[23] The median age at diagnosis is in the fourth decade, about 20 years earlier than in non-HIV infected patients. There is a marked preponderance of male patients.[23] HIV-infected patients were not eligible for any of the randomized trials described earlier. Anal cancers in HIV-infected patients have been treated by combined modality therapy or RT alone.[62–63,64,124,125,126,127–128] HIV-infected patients are at increased risk of toxicity, particularly in the perineal skin, anorectal mucosa, and hematologic system when treated with RT with or without chemotherapy. The mechanisms for this increased toxicity are not known.[129] Most recent reports indicate that it is not necessary to electively modify standard protocols of RT (with respect to dose, fractionation, or volume) and chemotherapy (either 5-FU and MMC, or 5-FU and CDDP), but modifications should be based on the severity of side effects in each individual patient.[62,124] Two factors may predict for heightened acute normal tissue toxicity or poor cancer control: a CD4 count $<200/\mu L$ at the start of treatment, or the presence of AIDS.[63,130] But these findings are not inevitably associated with poor tolerance. Concurrent antiretroviral therapy does not reliably reduce the severity or incidence of toxicity of RT and chemotherapy.[30]

Locoregional control rates of about 65% or better were described in some series, similar to those in HIV-negative patients. However, some investigators reported lower rates of local control and sphincter preservation in HIV-positive patients, despite earlier-stage disease and good initial tumor response.[64,128] In a study of 40 HIV-positive patients, the 5-year overall survival rate was similar to that in 81 HIV-negative patients, but the major cause of death in HIV-positive patients was anal cancer, in contradistinction to the HIV-negative patients in whom causes other than cancer predominated.[64]

ADENOCARCINOMAS

Most adenocarcinomas involving the anal canal arise from rectal-type mucosa that extends below the upper muscular boundary of the canal. They are generally treated similarly to those that arise in the rectum. The uncommon adenocarcinomas that develop from anal glands or in fistulae are more aggressive than squamous cancers and often metastasize early.[131] They have usually been managed by abdominoperineal resection. Five year survival rates following surgery alone are commonly below 50%, with local recurrence rates of about 25%.[32,115,131,132,133,134] Any advantage from adjuvant radiation and chemotherapy is unknown, although, by analogy, protocols used for primary rectal cancers are sometimes applied. A few centers have treated some anal adenocarcinomas by chemoradiation protocols developed for squamous cell cancers or rectal adenocarcinomas and have deferred surgery. Experience is limited, but anorectal function has been retained, and apparent cures have been reported, particularly in patients with smaller cancers, following treatment with RT alone or with RT and chemotherapy.[131,132,133,134–135,136–137]

SMALL CELL CARCINOMAS

Small cell carcinomas are rare cancers characterized by early metastases and have a poor prognosis.[31] The primary tumor may be managed by surgery or radiation. Systemic chemotherapy similar to that used for small cell cancers that arise elsewhere may be combined with radiation for the primary tumor and used to treat metastases, but responses are generally limited.

RADIATION THERAPY: TECHNIQUES AND DOSES

Anal Canal Cancer

Current radiation treatment strategies have been developed through better understanding of the natural history of anal cancer and correlation of sites of treatment failure with the treatment plan.[138–140] Most failures were at the site of the primary tumor, followed by the regional and other pelvic node groups.

The treatment volumes of interest are also influenced by the philosophy adopted with regard to which lymph node groups should be treated electively. Only well-differentiated squamous cell cancers ≤2 cm in size situated in the distal canal appear to have a risk of nodal metastases <5%.[31,34] The finding in surgical series of histopathologically verified metastases in the pararectal and internal iliac nodes in up to 30%, and in the inguinal nodes in up to 20%, has encouraged most radiation oncologists to irradiate these node groups electively. Retrospective and prospective studies have shown the advantages of elective nodal irradiation (ENI).[38,39] Following ENI to a total dose of 40 to 50 Gy (1.8 to 2 Gy fractions), investigators from France reported 5-year cumulative rates of inguinal recurrence of 2% in those who received ENI (n = 75) versus 16% in those who did not (n = 106). In the no-ENI group, recurrence rates were 12% from T1 to T2 and 30% from T3 to T4 tumors.[38] In a prospective study in Australasia in which patients with T1 or T2 tumors up to 4 cm in diameter did not receive inguinal ENI, inguinal node failure occurred in 9 of 40 (23%), in 5 as first site of failure.[141] Treatment of larger cancers by interstitial brachytherapy alone resulted in failure in pelvic nodes above the treated volume in 16% (14 of 88).[142] Control of most subclinical pelvic node metastases by pelvic ENI and chemotherapy can be inferred from the low failure rates reported in pelvic node sites.[138–140] The minimum effective dose for ENI is not known. Doses as low as 24 Gy in 12 fractions in 2.5 weeks appeared effective in one series,[39] but most centers give from 30.6 Gy in 17 fractions in 3.5 weeks to 50 Gy in 25 fractions in 5 weeks.[38,73,74]

The randomized trials described earlier all used radiation plans generated by two- or three-dimensional (2D or 3D) planning techniques, and, for the most part, employed predominantly anterior-posterior opposed field techniques for a substantial part of the schedule. Most radiation oncologists prefer to treat the primary tumor, the regional internal iliac, and perirectal nodes and inguinal nodes and other pelvic node groups such as the external iliac and presacral nodes in continuity. If the patient is prone, the anus can be visualized readily and bolus placed selectively over any perianal tumor extension. However, it is difficult to boost the inguinal area when the patient is prone if a 2D or 3D treatment technique is used. Alternatively, the patient may be treated supine. This facilitates boosts to the inguinal areas and reduces some of the inhomogeneities produced by the natural curvatures of the pelvic soft tissues. In that position, it is difficult to ensure that bolus placed over the anal area remains in place.

In the discussion that follows, the radiation doses described are typical of those prescribed when RT is combined with 5-FU and MMC. When an anterior-posterior opposed pair of fields is used, the upper border of the fields is placed at the lumbosacral junction if the intent is to include the common iliac, upper presacral, and lower rectosigmoid nodes, in addition to the regional nodes. This border is commonly moved down during treatment to the lower end of the sacroiliac joints (typically after 30.6 Gy in 17 fractions to 36 Gy in 20 fractions), thus encompassing in the reduced volume only the perirectal, lower presacral, and internal iliac nodes (and, if the fields are sufficiently wide, the lower external iliac nodes), in order to reduce the risk of radiation enteritis (Fig. 62.3). A further field reduction is made at 45 Gy, following which a final phase of treatment of 9 Gy in 5 fractions or 14.4 Gy in 8 fractions is delivered to the primary tumor. It is advisable to add a CTV margin of 2 to 3 cm around the primary tumor for this boost phase. If the primary tumor cannot be identified on the planning CT, the anal sphincter complex is often used as a surrogate target, adjusted for any known tumor extension beyond the anal canal. The overall total dose to the primary tumor is 54 Gy in 30 fractions in 6 weeks to 59.4 Gy in 33 fractions in 6.5 weeks when all RT is delivered by external-beam radiation. If there are metastatic nodes, these are treated by appropriate fields to the same total dose as the primary tumor. It may not be possible to deliver more than about 45 to 50.4 Gy to abnormal nodes in the pelvis if these lie adjacent to small bowel; in many cases these doses are enough to achieve control. In the absence of abnormal nodes in the lower pelvis, some consider elective treatment of radiologically normal nodes above the lower border of the sacroiliac joints unnecessary.[39,102,143]

The inferior field border is placed 3 cm distal to the lower most extension of the primary tumor, which should be indicated by a radio-opaque marker during simulation.

The position of the lateral borders depends on the philosophy adopted with respect to the desirability of treating a continuous homogeneous volume, without multiple fields and field junctions, and minimizing irradiation of the femoral head and neck. Options include anterior and posterior fields of equal size encompassing the inguinal nodes; anterior and posterior fields of equal size, but restricted to include the medial borders of the pelvis only, the inguinal nodes being treated by anterior electron beams matched to the photon fields; asymmetric photon fields, with a larger anterior field to cover the primary tumor and pelvic and inguinal nodes in continuity; and a posterior beam restricted to the primary tumor and pelvic nodes. In this latter arrangement, an anterior electron beam may be used to supplement the dose to the inguinal nodes to the desired level. The location and depth of the inguinal nodes should be obtained by axial imaging.[144] Another popular alternative, if 30.6 to 36 Gy in 3.5 to 4 weeks is felt to be sufficient dose for ENI for radiologically normal nodes, is to treat the primary and pelvic and inguinal nodes with the AP:PA fields, and then to use a three-field arrangement (posterior and two lateral fields) to encompass the primary tumor to 45 to 59.4 Gy total dose, according to the size of the primary cancer and local practice. Other field arrangements, such as oblique fields[145] and a direct perineal field coupled with a posterior partial arc beam[142] have been described. When asymmetric or matched fields are used, there is potential for both over- and underdosage.[146]

The final phase of treatment, beyond which includes both lymph nodes and primary cancer, typically delivers from 9 to 20 Gy to a reduced volume encompassing the primary tumor only. This phase may be delivered by brachytherapy. Brachytherapy is used more commonly in Europe than in North America, where external-beam treatment is favored. There are a number of reports of effective brachytherapy, including low–dose-rate (LDR),[69,147,161] pulsed–dose-rate (PDR),[148,149–150] and high–dose-rate (HDR) techniques.[151,152] Brachytherapy has usually been given 2 to 8 weeks after external-beam therapy, although one schedule introduced HDR in the interval during split-course external-beam therapy.[151] There is no agreement on whether the treatment volume should include the full extent of the initial primary cancer[69,142,149,151] or only the tumor remaining at the time of implant.[153] The brachytherapy dose depends on the composite dose of the total radiation prescription. Occasionally, significant toxicity has been encountered.

The introduction of intensity-modulated radiation therapy (IMRT) offers the possibility of further reducing the dose to normal tissues beyond that achievable with 3D conformal techniques. Several initial studies of IMRT and similar highly conformal techniques described improvements in radiation dose distributions.[139,154–157,158–159] However, it is apparent from the selected results in Table 62.6 that a wide range of severe acute toxicities was seen, and that about half the patients treated by IMRT had breaks in treatment. Comparisons of the different case series and interpretation are difficult because most studies used differing RT techniques and doses and practices for recording toxicities. There are no data as yet on long-term toxicity following IMRT for anal cancer.

Highly conformal IMRT and related techniques require considerable attention to identifying gross target volumes (GTV) and relevant elective clinical target volumes (CTV). In a trial conducted by RTOG to test the reproducibility of IMRT in multiple centers, 79% of 51 cases were found on pretreatment review to not comply with the protocol treatment volumes, particularly those for nodal regions to be irradiated electively.[158] The RTOG subsequently published an atlas of elective CTV templates developed by a consensus panel for use in planning IMRT for anal and rectal cancers.[160] When IMRT techniques

TABLE 62.6 SELECTED STUDIES OF THREE-DIMENSIONAL CONFORMAL RADIATION AND INTENSITY-MODULATED RADIATION THERAPY

Study (Reference)	RTOG 9811 MMC arm (74)	Boston (159)	RTOG 0529 (158)	Toronto (139)
No. of patients	324	43	51	58
Radiation technique	3D conformal	IMRT	IMRT	IMRT
Acute grade 3 or 4 toxicity				
Hematologic (%)	61	49	NP	38
Skin (%)	48	7	20	46
GI (%)	36	7	22 (GI/GU)	9
GU (%)	4	5	22 (GI/GU)	0
Treatment breaks	61	40	49	55
2-year results				
Locoregional control (%)	77	95 (local)	80	85
Colostomy-free survival (%)	84	94	86	87
Disease-free survival (%)	71	NP	77	75

RTOG, Radiation Therapy Oncology Group; MMC, mitomycin-C; 3D, three dimensional; IMRT, intensity-modulated radiation therapy; NP, not published; GI, gastrointestinal; GU, genitourinary.

are to be used, particular attention to patient positioning and immobilization is necessary. If possible, the accuracy of setup should be verified frequently, for example, by image-guided radiation treatment.

Although the reported results of IMRT appear similar to those achieved with 3D conformal RT, the latter is still considered the standard, as long-term clinical outcomes with IMRT have not yet been reported.

There has been increasing attention to radiation dose-time factors. Recent protocols have sought to improve local control rates, particularly for larger tumors, by intensifying RT or chemotherapy or both. Primary tumor control rates (excluding salvage treatment) in most studies of RT, 5-FU, and MMC are about 90% to 100% for tumors up to 2 cm (T1), 65% to 75% for tumors from 2 to 5 cm (T2), and 40% to 55% for those >5 cm and for most deeply invasive cancers (T3 or T4); the primary tumor control rate is about 60% overall.[39,57,106,161,162–165]

Increases in total radiation doses have been advocated. When combined with 5-FU and MMC, radiation doses of as little as 30 Gy in 15 fractions over 3 weeks have been shown to eradicate up to about 90% of cancers ≤3 cm in size. Higher doses, from 45 Gy in 25 fractions in 5 weeks to 54 Gy in 30 fractions in 6 weeks, sometimes supplemented with additional radiation after an interval of 6 to 8 weeks to a total of 60 to 65 Gy over a total time of about 12 weeks, have controlled from 65% to 75% of primary tumors >4 cm.[39,57,106,162,163–165] Recent trials in North America used up to 59 Gy in 32 fractions over 6.5 weeks for large or node-positive cancers[74,83,91,92]; the effectiveness and long-term tolerability of these increased doses has not yet been reported in detail. A recent analysis of the UKCCCR ACT I trial suggested that delivery of boost radiation of 15 to 25 Gy 6 weeks after the initial 45 Gy in 4 to 5 weeks did not improve local control but was associated with an increased risk of necrosis (8% vs. 0% if no boost was given).[166] Many centers are developing graduated dose schedules according to the size of the primary tumor and lymph node metastases.[74,138,155,159]

A potential advantage frequently proposed for IMRT is the ability to selectively increase the radiation dose to the cancer. It is not known whether this will be possible as a strategy to increase control rates for larger anal tumors because of the limited tolerances of the distal rectum, anal canal, and perianal skin.[167,168] The introduction of single-phase IMRT plans has led to the use of nonstandard dose fractionation, particularly for lymph node regions treated electively. For example, if all target volumes are to be treated to 30 fractions and the primary tumor is to receive 54 Gy at 1.8 Gy per fraction, elective treatment of uninvolved nodes to 36 Gy would be delivered at 1.2 Gy per fraction and to 45 Gy at 1.5 Gy per fraction. Some authors have also introduced biologically effective dose corrections to allow for different fractional doses or alterations in time over which the lower doses are delivered.[155,159] The long-term effectiveness of these nonstandard doses has not been determined.

In the era of 2D treatment planning, and later with 3D conformal planning, interruptions in external-beam treatment, generally of no more than 2 weeks but of up to 4 weeks in some series, were introduced into many combined modality protocols, either as elective breaks after about 3 weeks' treatment or as required by individual patients, to reduce the severity of acute anoproctitis and perineal dermatitis. Longer intervals of 6 to 8 weeks were part of some schedules to allow time for tumor regression, particularly where further RT was to be prescribed based on the extent of the clinical or histopathologic response to the first phase of treatment.[41,72,73,142] The possible adverse effects of split-course irradiation on the control of anal cancer have not been studied formally, but the limited data available on the potential tumor doubling time of anal cancer suggest that it is relatively rapid and of the order of 4 days (range 1 to 30 days; n = 26),[169] so some adverse effect may be expected from unnecessarily prolonged treatment. Recent analyses of treatment duration indicate that the overall treatment time (OTT), including time for induction chemotherapy if given and for prolonged intervals prior to boost RT, may have more influence on outcome than the duration of radiation (RTT). Review of the UKCCCR ACT I trial did not identify an association between OTT and locoregional failure.[166] Analysis of two RTOG trials[73,74] showed a trend toward an association between longer OTT and colostomy failure and a statistically significant association with local failure. RTT and OTT were not correlated with overall or colostomy-free survival rates.[170] There are many potentially confounding factors in these retrospective comparisons, and the optimum duration of overall treatment or radiation therapy is not known. The introduction of IMRT techniques does not appear to have led to a consistent reduction in interruptions in RT. The general principle recommended is to avoid, or minimize the length of, all interruptions in the delivery of radiation.

Radiation Alone

If external-beam irradiation is given without concurrent chemotherapy, it is usual, as in other cancers, to prescribe doses close to the tolerance of the normal tissues. There have been no studies to establish the optimum dose–time factors. A dose to the primary tumor of 60 to 65 Gy over 6 to 7 weeks, in 1.8- to 2-Gy fractions, is commonly prescribed, with doses to lymph nodes to be treated electively in the range of 36 Gy in 4 weeks to 50.4 Gy in 5.5 weeks. Brachytherapy may be used for part of the treatment. As with chemoradiation, interruptions in treatment should be minimized.

Perianal Cancer

If small (<4 cm) perianal cancers with low risk of regional node metastases are treated by radiation, a dose of 60 to 66 Gy in 2-Gy fractions over 6 weeks may be used. A direct perineal field is preferred as this minimizes the area of skin irradiated. Orthovoltage equipment may suffice, although electrons or low-energy megavoltage photons (with bolus) are used more commonly. Care should be taken to flatten the perineum as much as possible to avoid areas of over- or underdosage. Larger perianal cancers, or cancers invading the anal canal, are usually treated by the techniques and schedules of radiation and chemotherapy used for anal canal cancers, based on the results of the UKCCCR ACT I trial.[41] Elective nodal irradiation is given to the inguinal and lower external iliac nodes and to the lower perirectal and internal iliac nodes if the tumor extends into the anal canal. The upper border of the fields is usually placed at the lower end of the sacroiliac joints. The final phase of radiation may be given by direct perineal photon or electron therapy. Although brachytherapy may be used for the final phase, full treatment of perianal cancers by brachytherapy was associated with high rates of necrosis in some series.

SEQUELAE OF THERAPY

Surveys of published studies suggest that the delivery of chemotherapy concurrently with RT is associated more with increases in acute rather than late normal tissue toxicity, beyond that expected with RT alone. Some nonrandomized series have described higher acute and late toxicity rates from combined modality therapy than those reported in the multicenter randomized trials. This probably results from use of different criteria for recording and reporting toxicity.

In programs that combined radiation therapy, 96-hour to 120-hour infusions of 5-FU (750 to 1,000 mg/m^2/24 hours) and bolus injections of MMC (10 to 15 mg/m^2), moderate leukopenia, thrombocytopenia, anoproctitis, and perineal dermatitis were recorded in about 30% of patients after doses of 25 to 30 Gy in 2.5 to 3 weeks.[39,171] More profound proctitis and dermatitis occurred in up to 55% of those who received from 50 Gy in 4 to 5 weeks[39,106] to 59.4 Gy in 6.5 weeks.[91] When

CDDP was substituted for MMC, marrow toxicity was less, but at radiation doses of 59.4 Gy in 6.5 weeks, acute soft tissue toxicity rates were similar.[74,83] Most large studies of RT, 5-FU, and MMC or CDDP reported some mortality (<2% overall) associated with acute toxicity, usually as a result of neutropenia with sepsis. This risk can be reduced with prophylactic antibiotics[41] and aggressive supportive care.

Serious late toxicity has not been reported after doses of 30 Gy in 3 weeks with 5-FU and MMC, but significant complications, often requiring surgery, were recorded in about 5% to 10% of those receiving higher radiation doses. A review of anal cancer management in Denmark from 1995 to 2003 found 5-year cumulative incidences of tumor-related and treatment-related colostomy of 26% (95% CI, 21% to 32%) and 8% (95% CI, 5% to 12%), respectively.[172] In the randomized RTOG-9811 trial, in those who received RT, 5-FU, and MMC, only 10 of the 30 colostomy procedures performed by about 3 years were for treatment-related problems, a crude rate of about 3%.[59] It is probable that some reports, many of which were retrospective, also overlooked some treatment-related toxicity. For example, a large cohort study of 556 women aged ≥65 who developed anal cancer showed a higher risk of pelvic fracture, principally of the hip, in those who received radiation (n = 399) compared to those not irradiated (n = 157). The cumulative 5-year fracture rate was 14% versus 7.5% (P <.01).[173] One of the objectives of current 3D conformal and IMRT techniques is to reduce RT dose to the proximal femurs.

There are two additional areas of possible toxicity that need further study. Pelvic RT increases the risk of secondary malignancies,[174] and some of the chemotherapy agents used to treat anal cancer also are associated with a raised risk; these risks have not been quantified in detail for patients treated for anal cancer. Second, in the only report so far of long-term follow-up of patients in a randomized trial, it was found that there were more deaths due to causes other than cancer, particularly cardiovascular related, in the first 10 years following treatment with RT, 5-FU, and MMC.[71] This difference reached +9% at 5 years, but the effect almost disappeared by 10 years. The magnitude of this difference was less than the reduction in deaths from anal cancer. Information from other randomized trials is needed to determine whether this observation was a chance phenomenon or a risk that should be addressed by further research.

Although preservation of anorectal anatomy is an advantage of treatment by chemoradiation, late anorectal function is often abnormal. Side effects of treatment are very common and may cause patients considerable discomfort and social disability, although they are often graded as only level 1 or 2 toxicity.[175–176,177–178] These effects include changes in anorectal function such as urgency and frequency of defecation, bleeding from anorectal telangiectasia, perineal dermatitis, pelvic fibrosis, dyspareunia, and impotence. They are usually managed medically with varying success. Systematic and prospective evaluations of the function of the anorectum and of other organs potentially affected by treatment are now being reported, as are formal quality-of-life studies.[139,179] There is often dissociation between a patient's and his or her physician's assessment of anal and rectal function and continence and physiologic measurements of anorectal function. The few studies in this area have been inconclusive.[177,180] Prospective studies of pelvic organ function can be expected to assist the development of radiation treatment protocols by facilitating correlation of function with radiation–chemotherapy interactions, radiation techniques and dose distributions, and time–dose factors.

SELECTED REFERENCES

A full list of references for this chapter is available online.

1. Nigro ND, Vaitkevicius VK, Considine B. Combined therapy for cancer of the anal canal: a preliminary report. *Dis Colon Rectum* 1974;17:354–356.
2. Edge SB, Byrd DR, Compton CC, et al. eds. *AJCC cancer staging manual.* 7th ed. New York: Springer, 2010.
3. Sobin L, Gospodarowicz M, Wittekind C, eds. International Union Against Cancer (UICC). *TNM classification of malignant tumours.* 7th ed. New York: Wiley-Blackwell, 2009.
6. Fenger C, Frisch M, Marti MC, et al. Tumours of the anal canal. In: Hamilton SR, Aaltonen LA, eds. *Pathology and genetics of tumours of the digestive system.* Lyon: IARC Press, 2000:145–155.
7. Shepherd NA. Anal intraepithelial neoplasia and other neoplastic precursor lesions of the anal canal and perianal region. *Gastoenterol Clin North Am* 2007;36:969–987.
8. Cook MB, Dawsey SM, Freedman ND, et al. Sex disparities in cancer incidence by period and age. *Cancer Epidemiol Biomarkers Prev* 2009;18:1174–1182.
10. IARC Cancer Monograph Working Group. A review of human carcinogens—Part B: biologic agents. *Lancet Oncol* 2009;10:321–322.
11. Hoots BE, Palefsky JM, Pimenta JM, et al. Human papillomavirus type distribution in anal cancer and anal intraepithelial lesions. *Int J Cancer* 2009;124:2375–2383.
12. De Vuyst H, Clifford GM, Nascimento MC, et al. Prevalence and type distribution of human papillomavirus in carcinoma and intraepithelial neoplasia of the vulva, vagina, and anus: a meta-analysis. *Int J Cancer* 2009;124:1626–1636.
15. Frisch M. On the etiology of anal squamous carcinoma. *Dan Med Bull* 2002; 49:194–209.
18. Frisch M, Biggar RJ, Engels EA, et al. Association of cancer with AIDS-related immunosuppression in adults. *JAMA* 2001;285:1736–1745.
19. Adami J, Gabel H, Lindelof B, et al. Cancer risk following organ transplantation: a nationwide cohort study in Sweden. *Br J Cancer* 2003;89:1221–1227.
23. Simard EP, Pfeiffer RM, Engels EA. Spectrum of cancer risk late after AIDS onset in the United States. *Arch Intern Med* 2010;170:1337–1345.
24. International Collaboration on HIV and Cancer. Highly active antiretroviral therapy and incidence of cancer in human immunodeficiency virus-infected adults. *J Natl Cancer Inst* 2000;92:1823–1830.
28. Frisch M, Olsen JH, Bautz A, et al. Benign anal lesions and the risk of anal cancer. *N Engl J Med* 1994;331:300–302.
29. Frisch M, Johansen C. Anal carcinoma in inflammatory bowel disease. *Br J Cancer* 2000;83:89–90.
31. Boman BM, Moertel CG, O'Connell M, et al. Carcinoma of the anal canal: a clinical and pathological study of 188 cases. *Cancer* 1984;54:114–125.
32. Myerson RJ, Karnell LH, Menck HR. The National Cancer Data Base report on carcinoma of the anus. *Cancer* 1997;80:805–815.
33. Bilimoria KY, Bentrem DJ, Rock CE, et al. Outcomes and prognostic factors for squamous cell carcinoma of the anal canal: Analysis of patients from the National Cancer Data Base. *Dis Colon Rectum* 2009;52:624–631.
36. Gerard JP, Chapet O, Samiei F, et al. Management of inguinal lymph node metastases in patients with carcinoma of the anal canal. Experience in a series of 270 patients treated in Lyon and review of the literature. *Cancer* 2001;92:77–84.
38. Ortholan C, Resbeut M, Hannoun-Levi JM, et al. Anal canal cancer: management of inguinal nodes and benefit of prophylactic inguinal irradiation (CORS-03 study). *Int J Radiat Oncol Biol Phys* 2012;82(5):1988–1995.
39. Cummings BJ, Keane TJ, O'Sullivan B, et al. Epidermoid anal cancer: treatment by radiation and 5-fluorouracil with and without mitomycin C. *Int J Radiat Oncol Biol Phys* 1991;21:1115–1125.
41. UKCCCR Anal Canal Cancer Trial Working Party. Epidermoid anal cancer: results from the UKCCCR randomized trial of radiotherapy alone versus radiotherapy, 5-fluorouracil and mitomycin C. *Lancet* 1996;348:1049–1054.
52. Mistrangelo M, Pelosi E, Bello M, et al. Comparison of positron emission tomography scanning and sentinel node biopsy in the detection of inguinal node metastases in patients with anal cancer. *Int J Radiat Oncol Biol Phys* 2010;77:73–78.
53. de Jong JS, Beukema JC, Van Dam GM, et al. Limited value of staging squamous cell carcinoma of the margin and canal using the sentinel lymph node procedure: a prospective study with long-term follow-up. *Ann Surg Oncol* 2010;17:2656–2662.
54. Cummings BJ. Anal cancer. In: Gospodarowicz MK, O'Sullivan B, Sobin LH, eds. *Prognostic factors in cancer,* 3rd ed. Hoboken, NJ: Wiley, 2006:139–142.
55. Greenall MJ, Quan SHQ, Decosse JJ. Epidermoid cancer of the anus. *Br J Surg* 1985;72(Suppl):S97.
59. Ajani JA, Winter KA, Gunderson LL, et al. US Intergroup Anal Carcinoma Trial: Tumor diameter predicts for colostomy. *J Clin Oncol* 2009;27:1116–1121.
60. Ajani JA, Winter KA, Gunderson LL, et al. Prognostic factors derived from a prospective database dictate clinical biology of anal cancer. The Intergroup Trial (RTOG 98–11). *Cancer* 2010;116:4007–4013.
64. Oehler-Janne C, Huguet F, Provender S, et al. HIV-specific differences in outcome of squamous cell carcinoma of the anal canal: a multicentric cohort study of HIV-positive patients receiving highly active antiretroviral therapy. *J Clin Oncol* 2008;26:2550–2557.
65. Fenger C. Prognostic factors in anal carcinoma. *Pathology* 2002;34:573–578.
67. Ajani JA, Wang X, Izzo JG, et al. Molecular biomarkers correlate with disease-free survival in patients with anal canal carcinoma treated with chemoradiation. *Dig Dis Sci* 2010;55:1098–1105.
68. Bruland O, Fluge O, Immervoll H, et al. Gene expression reveals 2 distinct groups of anal carcinomas with clinical implications. *Br J Cancer* 2008;98:1264–1273.
69. Peiffert D, Bey P, Pernot M, et al. Conservative treatment by irradiation of epidermoid cancers of the anal canal: prognostic factors of tumoral control and complications. *Int J Radiat Oncol Biol Phys* 1997;37:313–324.
70. Chapet O, Gerard JP, Riche B, et al. Prognostic value of tumor regression evaluated after first course of radiotherapy for anal canal cancer. *Int J Radiat Oncol Biol Phys* 2005;63:1316–1324.
71. Northover J, Glynne-Jones R, Sebag-Montefiore D, et al. Chemoradiation for the treatment of epidermoid anal cancer: 13-year follow-up of the first randomized UKCCCR Anal Cancer Trial (ACT I). *Br J Cancer* 2010;102:1123–1128.
72. Bartelink H, Roelofsen F, Eschwege F, et al. Concomitant radiotherapy and chemotherapy is superior to radiotherapy alone in the treatment of locally advanced anal cancer: results of a phase III randomized trial of the European Organization for Research and Treatment of Cancer Radiotherapy and Gastrointestinal Cooperative Groups. *J Clin Oncol* 1997;15:2040–2049.
73. Flam M, John M, Pajak TF, et al. The role of mitomycin C in combination with 5-fluorouracil and radiotherapy, and of salvage chemoradiation in the definitive nonsurgical treatment of epidermoid carcinoma of the anal canal: results of a phase III randomized Intergroup study. *J Clin Oncol* 1996;14:2527–2539.
74. Ajani JA, Winter KA, Gunderson LL, et al. Fluorouracil, mitomycin, and radiotherapy vs fluorouracil, cisplatin and radiotherapy for carcinoma of the anal canal; a randomized controlled trial. *JAMA* 2008;299:1914–1921.

75. Gunderson LL, Winter KA, Ajani JA, et al. Long-term update of US GI Intergroup RTOG 98-11 phase III trial for anal carcinoma: disease-free and overall survival with RT + 5FU – mitomycin versus RT + 5FU-cisplatin. *J Clin Oncol* 2011;29(Suppl):4005.
76. James R, Wan S, Sebag-Montefiore D, et al. A randomized trial of chemoradiation using mitomycin or cisplatin, with or without maintenance cisplatin/5FU in squamous cell carcinoma of the anus (ACT II). *J Clin Oncol* 2009;27(Suppl): LBA4009.
77. Conroy T, Ducreux M, Lemanski C, et al. Treatment intensification by induction chemotherapy (ICT) and radiation dose escalation in locally advanced squamous cell anal canal carcinoma (LAAC): definitive analysis of the intergroup ACCORD 03 trial. *J Clin Oncol* 2009;27(Suppl):4033.
78. Peiffert D, Gerard JP, Ducreux M, et al. Induction chemotherapy (ICT) and dose intensification of the radiation boost in locally advanced anal canal carcinoma (LAACC): definitive analysis of the Intergroup ACCORD 03 trial (Federation Nationale des Centres de Lutte Contre le Cancer, Fondation Francaise de Cancerologie Digestive). *Radiother Oncol* 2008:88(Suppl 2):S20.
79. Lim F, Glynne-Jones R. Chemotherapy/chemoradiation in anal cancer: a systematic review. *Cancer Treat Rev* 2011;37:520–532.
80. Papillon J, Montbarbon JF. Epidermoid carcinoma of the anal canal: a series of 276 cases. *Dis Colon Rectum* 1987;30:324–333.
93. Glynne-Jones R, Meadows H, Wan S, et al. EXTRA—A multicentre phase II study using a 5-day per week oral regimen of capecitabine and intravenous mitomycin C in anal cancer. *Int J Radiat Oncol Biol Phys* 2008;72:119–126.
96. Van Damme N, Deron P, Van Roy N, et al. Epidermal growth factor receptor and K-RAS status in two cohorts of squamous cell cancers. *BMC Cancer* 2010;10:189.
99. Nilsson PJ, Svensson C, Goldman S, et al. Epidermoid anal cancer: a review of a population-based series of 308 consecutive patients treated according to prospective protocols. *Int J Radiat Oncol Biol Phys* 2005;61:92–102.
103. Martenson JA, Gunderson LL. External radiation therapy without chemotherapy in the management of anal cancer. *Cancer* 1993;71:1736–1740.
107. Schwarz JK, Siegal BA, Dehdashti F, et al. Tumor response and survival predicted by post-therapy FDG-PET/CT in anal cancer. *Int J Radiat Oncol Biol Phys* 2008;71:180–186.
109. Renehan AG, Sanders MP, Schofield PF, et al. Patterns of local disease failure and outcome after salvage surgery in patients with anal cancer. *Br J Surg* 2005;92:605–614.
110. Schiller DE, Cummings BJ, Rai S, et al. Outcomes of salvage surgery for squamous cell carcinoma of the anal canal. *Ann Surg Oncol* 2007;14:2780–2789.
116. Ortholan C, Ramaioli A, Peiffert D, et al. Anal canal carcinoma: early stage tumors ≤10 mm (T1 or Tis): therapeutic options and original pattern of local failure after radiotherapy. *Int J Radiat Oncol Biol Phys* 2005;62:479–485.
117. Eng C, Pathak P. Treatment options in metastatic squamous cell carcinoma of the anal canal. *Curr Treat Options Oncol* 2008;9:400–407.
119. Bieri S, Allal AS, Kurtz JM. Sphincter-conserving treatment of carcinomas of the anal margin. *Acta Oncol* 2001;40:29–33.
122. Papillon J, Chassard JL. Respective roles of radiotherapy and surgery in the management of epidermoid cancer of the anal margin. *Dis Colon Rectum* 1992;35:422–429.
123. Khanfir K, Ozsahin M, Bieri S, et al. Patterns of failure and outcome in patients with carcinoma of the anal margin. *Ann Surg Oncol* 2008;15:1092–1098.
125. Edelman S, Johnstone PA. Combined modality therapy for HIV-infected patients with squamous cell carcinoma of the anus: outcomes and toxicities. *Int J Radiat Oncol Biol Phys* 2006;66:206–211.
127. Hammad N, Heilbrun LK, Gupta S, et al. Squamous cell cancer of the anal canal in HIV-infected patients receiving highly active antiretroviral therapy. *Am J Clin Oncol* 2011;34:135–139.
128. Chiao EY, Giordano TP, Richardson P, et al. Human immunodeficiency virus-associated squamous cell cancer of the anus: epidemiology and outcomes in the highly active antiretroviral therapy era. *J Clin Oncol* 2008;299:1914–1921.
129. Formenti SC, Chak L, Gill P, et al. Increased radiosensitivity of normal tissue fibroblasts in patients with acquired immunodeficiency syndrome (AIDS) and with Kaposi's sarcoma. *Int J Radiat Biol* 1995;68:411–412.
132. Belkacemi Y, Berger C, Poortmans P, et al. Management of anal canal adenocarcinoma: a large retrospective study from the Rare Cancer Network. *Int J Radiat Oncol Biol Phys* 2003;56:1274–1283.
134. Chang GJ, Gonzalez RJ, Skibbar JM, et al. A twenty-year experience with adenocarcinoma of the anal canal. *Dis Colon Rectum* 2009;52:1375–1380.
135. Joon DL, Chao MW, Ngan SY, et al. Primary adenocarcinoma of the anus: a retrospective analysis. *Int J Radiat Oncol Biol Phys* 1999;45:1199–1205.
138. Wright JL, Patil SM, Temple LK, et al. Squamous cell carcinoma of the anal canal: patterns and predictors of failure and implications for intensity-modulated radiation treatment and planning. *Int J Radiat Oncol Biol Phys* 2010;78:1064–1072.
139. Han K, Craig T, Skliarenko J, et al. Prospective evaluation of IMRT for anal and perianal cancer: early patterns of failure. *Int J Radiat Oncol Biol Phys* 2011;81 (2 Suppl):S125–S126.
140. Das P, Bhatia S, Eng C, et al. Predictions and patterns of recurrence after definitive chemoradiation for anal cancer. *Int J Radiat Oncol Biol Phys* 2007;68:794–800.
142. Papillon J. *Rectal and anal cancers: conservative treatment by irradiation. an alternative to radical surgery.* Berlin: Springer-Verlag, 1982.
144. Koh WJ, Chiu M, Stelzer KJ, et al. Femoral vessel depth and the implications for groin node radiation. *Int J Radiat Oncol Biol Phys* 1993;27:969–974.
147. Papillon J, Montbarbon JF, Gerard JP, et al. Interstitial curietherapy in the conservative treatment of anal and rectal cancers. *Int J Radiat Oncol Biol Phys* 1989;17:1161–1169.
148. Gerard JP, Mauro F, Thomas L, et al. Treatment of squamous cell anal canal carcinoma with pulse dose rate brachytherapy. Feasibility study of a French Cooperative Group. *Radiother Oncol* 1999;51:129–131.
158. Kachnic L, Winter K, Myerson R, et al. RTOG 0529: A phase II evaluation of dose-painted IMRT in combination with 5-fluorouracil and mitomycin-C for reduction of acute morbidity in carcinoma of the anal canal. *Int J Radiat Oncol Biol Phys* 2009;75(Suppl):S5.
159. Kachnic LA, Tsai HK, Coen JJ, et al. Dose-painted intensity-modulated radiation therapy for anal cancer; a multi-institutional report of acute toxicity and response to therapy. *Int J Radiat Oncol Biol Phys* 2010;78(Suppl 3):S55.
160. Myerson RJ, Garofolo MC, El Naqa I, et al. Elective clinical target volumes for conformal therapy in anorectal cancer: a Radiation Therapy Oncology Group consensus panel contouring atlas. *Int J Radiat Oncol Biol Phys* 2009;74:824–830.
166. Glynne-Jones R, Sebag-Montefiore D, Adams R, et al. "Mind the gap"—the impact of variations in the duration of the treatment gap and overall treatment time in the first UK anal cancer trial (ACT I). *Int J Radiat Oncol Biol Phys* 2011;81:1488–1494.
167. Cummings BJ. Is there a limit to dose escalation for rectal cancer? *Clin Oncol* 2007;19:730–737.
168. Heemsbergen WD, Hoogeman MS, Hart GA, et al. Gastrointestinal toxicity and its relation to dose distributions in the anorectal region of prostate cancer patients treated with radiotherapy. *Int J Radiat Oncol Biol Phys* 2005;61:1101–1018.
169. Wong CS, Tsang RW, Cummings BJ, et al. Proliferation parameters in epidermoid carcinomas of the anal canal. *Radiother Oncol* 2000;56:349–353.
170. Ben-Josef E, Moughan J, Ajani JA, et al. Impact of overall treatment time on survival and local control in patients with anal cancer; a pooled data analysis of Radiation Therapy Oncology Group trials 87–04 and 98–11. *J Clin Oncol* 2010;28:5061–5066.
172. Sunesen KG, Norgaard M, Lundby L, et al. Cause-specific colostomy rates after radiotherapy for anal cancer: a Danish multicentre cohort study. *J Clin Oncol* 2011;29:3535–3540.
173. Baxter NN, Habermann EB, Tepper JE, et al. Risk of pelvic fractures in older women following pelvic irradiation. *JAMA* 2005;294:2587–2593.
174. Wright JD, St Clair CM, Deutsch I, et al. Pelvic radiotherapy and the risk of secondary leukemia and multiple myeloma. *Cancer* 2010;116:2486–2492.
177. Vordermark D, Sailer M, Flentje M, et al. Curative intent radiation therapy in anal carcinoma: quality of life and sphincter function. *Radiother Oncol* 1999;52:239–243.
178. Das P, Cantor SB, Parker CL, et al. Long-term quality of life after radiotherapy for the treatment of anal cancer. *Cancer* 2010;116:822–829.

Part H Urinary Tract

Chapter 63
Cancer of the Kidney, Renal Pelvis, and Ureter

Hiram A. Gay and Jeff M. Michalski

ANATOMY

The kidneys are retroperitoneal structures located at the level between the 11th rib and the transverse process of the 3rd lumbar vertebral body. Usually, the right kidney is inferior to the right hepatic lobe and slightly more inferior than the left kidney. The renal axis runs parallel to the lateral margin of the psoas muscle. Each kidney is approximately 11 to 12 cm in length. The kidney is encased by a fibrous capsule and surrounded by perinephric fat, which is enveloped by Gerota's fascia. At the renal hilus are the pelvis, ureter, renal artery, and vein. The organs adjacent to the right kidney include the liver superiorly, the duodenum and the vertebral bodies medially, and the transverse colon and small bowel anteriorly. On the left, the kidney abuts the spleen laterally; the stomach, pancreas, and vertebral bodies medially; and the small bowel and colon anteriorly.

The kidney consists of the cortex (glomeruli, convoluted tubules) and the medulla (Henle's loops, collecting ducts, and pyramids of converging tubules). Each papilla opens in the minor calices, which unite in the major calices and drain into the renal pelvis. The caliceal collecting systems lie on the anteromedial surface of each kidney. The ureteropelvic junction is variable in position but serves as the landmark to separate the renal pelvis and the ureter. The ureters course posteriorly and inferiorly, paralleling the lateral border of the psoas muscle until they curve anteriorly to join the bladder at the trigone. The mucosal surfaces of the renal collecting tubules, calyces, renal pelvis, ureter, bladder, and urethra all have the same embryologic origin. The renal pelvis and ureter have the following layers: epithelium, subepithelial connective tissue, and muscularis, which is continuous with a connective tissue adventitial layer.

The lymphatics of the kidney and renal pelvis drain along the renal vessels. The right kidney drains predominantly into the paracaval and interaortocaval lymph nodes, and the left kidney drains exclusively to the paraaortic lymph nodes.[1] The lymphatic drainage of the ureter is segmented and diffuse and may involve any of the renal hilar, abdominal para-aortic, paracaval, common iliac, internal iliac, or external iliac lymph nodes.

EPIDEMIOLOGY AND RISK FACTORS

The lesions discussed in this chapter are limited to adult renal cell carcinoma (RCC; e.g., hypernephroma, Grawitz's tumor) and urothelial carcinoma of the renal pelvis and ureter. Lymphomas, primary retroperitoneal sarcomas, and Wilms' tumors are discussed in Chapters 78, 83, and 85, respectively. Approximately 88% of solid renal masses are malignant, and the probability of malignancy is proportional to the size of the lesion.[2] RCCs comprise 80% to 85% of primary kidney tumors, whereas urothelial (transitional cell) carcinomas of the renal pelvis account for 7% of kidney tumors.

Renal Cell Carcinoma

Globally in 2008, the male kidney cancer incidence and mortality age-standardized rate per 100,000 (ASR) was 11.8 and 4.1 in more developed areas, and 2.5 and 1.3 in less developed areas, respectively. The estimated new kidney cancer cases in males in developed countries were 111,100, with 43,000 deaths. In contrast, the female kidney cancer incidence and mortality ASR was 5.8 and 1.7 in more developed areas, and 1.4 and 0.8 in less developed areas, respectively.[3]

In the United States in 2011, the estimated number of new cases of kidney and renal pelvis cancer was 60,920, with 13,120 deaths.[4] These figures represent approximately 4% of all new cancers and 2% of cancer-related deaths. The incidence of RCC has been increasing in the United States, whereas the size of primary RCCs has been gradually decreasing.[5] This is partly because the increased use of abdominal computed tomography (CT) and ultrasound for nonmalignant medical illnesses has increased the number of incidental RCCs.

The median age of RCC diagnosis is 65 years, and males are affected more commonly than females, with a ratio of 1.5:1. Occupations associated with a higher risk of RCC are employment in the blast-furnace, coke-oven, or iron and steel industry, as well as exposure to asbestos, cadmium, dry-cleaning solvents, gasoline, and other petroleum products.[6] In addition, several other environmental (e.g., exposure to thorium dioxide), hormonal (e.g., diethylstilbestrol), dietary (e.g., high total energy intake and fried meats increase the risk, whereas vegetables, fruits, and alcohol are protective), cellular, and genetic factors have been associated with the development of RCC.[7-9]

Long-term cigarette smoking is associated with an increased risk of developing RCC. Obesity, diabetes, hepatitis C, and hypertension are also associated with a higher relative risk for development of these tumors.[10-12] Cytotoxic chemotherapy may predispose childhood cancer survivors to translocation RCC, bearing TFE3 or TFEB gene fusions.[13]

Acquired cystic kidney disease (ACKD), which occurs in up to 50% of patients on dialysis for >3 years, is associated with a 50-fold increased risk of developing RCC.[14,15] ACKD-associated RCC is seen mostly in males, occurs approximately 20 years earlier than in the general population, and is frequently bilateral (9%) and multicentric (50%).[15]

Several inherited cancer syndromes affect the kidney: von Hippel-Lindau (VHL) disease, hereditary papillary renal cancer (HPRC), hereditary leiomyomatosis and renal cell carcinoma (HLRCC), Birt-Hogg-Dubé (BHD), and constitutional chromosome 3 translocation. VHL is autosomal dominant and is caused by germline mutations of the VHL tumor suppressor gene, located on chromosome 3p25–26. The VHL protein is involved in cell cycle regulation and angiogenesis. In patients with VHL disease, loss of the sole functioning VHL allele in somatic tissues causes a situation similar to hypoxia, with elevated levels of HIF-1alpha, despite the presence of normal oxygen tension.[16] The renal manifestations of VHL are kidney cysts and clear cell RCC. The mean age onset for VHL associated clear cell RCC is 37 years, and periodic screening with magnetic resonance imaging (MRI) should start after the age of 10 years.[17]

HPRC is autosomal dominant with high penetrance and is characterized by multiple, bilateral, late-onset papillary RCCs. HLRCC is autosomal dominant with a predisposition to papillary type 2 RCC. BHD is autosomal dominant with incomplete penetrance and is associated with multiple chromophobe and clear cell RCCs, papillary RCCs, and oncocytomas. Constitutional chromosome 3 translocation is associated with multiple, bilateral clear cell RCCs.[18] Autosomal dominant polycystic kidney disease does not appear to increase the incidence of RCC; however, the tumors are more often multicentric (28% vs. 6%), bilateral (12% vs. 1% to 5%), and sarcomatoid in type (33% vs. 1% to 5%) than in the general population.[19]

Renal Pelvis and Ureter Carcinoma

Urothelial carcinoma of the upper urinary tract accounts for 7% of all kidney tumors and 5% of all urothelial malignancies.[20] The incidence of bilateral upper urinary tract tumors is 1.5% to 2% for synchronous and 6% to 8% for asynchronous presentations.[21] Renal pelvis tumors are found two to three times more commonly in men than in women, and the peak incidence is in the fifth and sixth decades of life. Because the mucosal surfaces of the renal pelvis, ureter, and bladder have the same embryologic origin, many of the etiologic factors in renal pelvis and ureter tumors also apply to tumors of the urinary bladder. Urothelial carcinomas of the upper urinary tract tend to be multifocal owing to field cancerization, which may be caused by exposure of the urothelium to potential carcinogens. Urothelial tumors can also spread to urothelial structures that are either distal or proximal to the primary tumor and are referred to as drop metastases. About 40% to 50% of patients with upper urinary tract tumors will have a synchronous or metachronous bladder cancer.[22,23]

Cigarette smoking is the most important factor contributing to the overall incidence of urothelial cancer in Western countries. Patients with Lynch syndrome, an autosomal dominant genetic condition attributable to inherited mutations that impair DNA mismatch repair, have an increased risk of developing urinary tract cancer.[24]

Exposure to aristolochic acid has been associated with acute, near end-stage renal disease. Aristolochic acid is commonly found in the Aristolochiaceae family of plants commonly used in Chinese herbal medicine. A high incidence of cellular atypia and urothelial carcinoma of the renal pelvis, ureter, and bladder has been associated with aristolochic acid nephropathy.[25] Arsenic-contaminated water has been associated with a high incidence of upper urinary tract urothelial carcinoma in Taiwan.[26] Prolonged heavy phenacetin-containing analgesic use can lead to urothelial carcinomas of the renal pelvis, ureter, and bladder (which may be multiple and bilateral).[27]

Balkan endemic nephropathy (BEN) is a chronic tubulointerstitial disease of unknown etiology most commonly reported in southeastern Europe. A high frequency of urothelial atypia, occasionally progressing to tumors of the renal pelvis and urethra, but also involving the bladder, is associated with BEN.[27]

NATURAL HISTORY

Renal Cell Carcinoma

Primary renal cell tumors may spread by local infiltration through the renal capsule to involve the perinephric fat and Gerota's fascia. The tumor may grow directly along the venous channels to the renal vein or vena cava. Lymph node metastases occur with an incidence of 9% to 27%, and most often involve the renal hilar, para-aortic, and paracaval lymph nodes.[28,29] The renal vein is invaded by tumor in 21% of cases, and the inferior vena cava is invaded in as many as 4% of cases.[30]

Approximately 45% of patients with RCC have localized disease, 25% have regional disease, and about 30% have evidence of distant metastases at the time of diagnosis.[29,31] Of patients with metastases, about 1% to 3% have solitary lesions.[32] About half of the patients with RCC eventually develop metastatic disease.[33]

Among patients presenting with metastatic RCC, the sites of metastases include lung, bone, brain, liver, and adrenal gland. Patients with metastatic disease at diagnosis have an extremely poor prognosis, with an expected survival <5 years regardless of the site of metastasis.[29,31]

Renal Pelvis and Ureter Carcinoma

Upper urinary tract carcinoma is frequently a multifocal process. Patients with cancer at one site in the upper urinary tract are at significant risk for the development of tumors elsewhere along the urothelium. The probability of multifocal occurrence is greatest in patients with large tumors and those with carcinoma in situ. Ureteral tumors tend to occur in the distal third of the ureter.

Urothelial carcinoma of the upper urothelial tract may spread by direct extension, and by hematogenous and lymphatic metastases. Implantation of tumor cells in the bladder has been demonstrated, especially in previously traumatized areas. The incidence of lymph node metastases highly depends on the grade of the primary tumor. Low-grade tumors have a very low metastatic propensity. In a series of 94 patients, none of 43 low-grade tumors had lymph node metastases, compared with 3 of 22 grade 3 or 4 tumors.[34] Lymph node metastases were reported in 9 of 26 patients selected to receive adjuvant radiotherapy.[35]

CLINICAL PRESENTATION

Renal Cell Carcinoma

Patients with RCC may present with an occult primary tumor, or with signs and symptoms attributable to a local mass or systemic paraneoplastic syndromes. Gross hematuria, palpable flank mass, and pain describe a classic triad that occurs only in 5% to 10% of patients.[36,37] Indeed, a finding of the classic triad often suggests advanced disease with a poor prognosis. The most frequent symptom associated with RCC is hematuria, either gross or microscopic, when there is invasion of the collecting system.[38] Scrotal varicoceles, mostly left-sided, are observed in as many as 11 % of men with RCC.[39] Other symptoms include anemia, hepatic dysfunction in the absence of liver metastases (called Stauffer's syndrome and attributable to a paraneoplastic elevation in alkaline phosphatase), secondary AA amyloidosis, fever, hypercalcemia, cachexia, erythrocytosis, thrombocytosis, and a syndrome resembling polymyalgia rhumatica.[39,40,41–44,45] RCC presenting as an incidental mass on a diagnostic imaging study ordered for other purposes accounts for 61% of all diagnoses.[46]

A wide range of paraneoplastic syndromes has been associated with RCC. Parathyroidlike hormones, erythropoietin, renin, gonadotropins, placental lactogen, prolactin, enteroglucagon, insulinlike hormones, adrenocorticotropic hormone, and prostaglandins have been identified in patients with RCC.[47,48]

Renal Pelvis and Ureter Carcinoma

Gross or microscopic hematuria occurs in 70% to 95% of patients with renal pelvis or ureter tumors.[20] The other less common symptoms include pain (8% to 40%), bladder irritation (5% to 10%), or other constitutional symptoms (5%). About 10% to 20% of patients may present with a flank mass secondary to tumor or hydronephrosis.

DIAGNOSTIC WORKUP

Renal Cell Carcinoma

Renal masses are not uncommon, and most of them are benign. A central renal mass may suggest urothelial carcinoma; if so, urine cytology or ureteroscopy should be considered. Renal masses are frequently diagnosed as an incidental finding during abdominal imaging for metastatic evaluation of an unrelated malignancy or other disease.

An algorithm for the workup of renal masses has been proposed.[49] If CT or ultrasound clearly identify the mass as a cyst, no further workup is necessary. If a solid lesion is identified, then tumor removal by nephrectomy should be considered. In the case of small lesions, a follow-up CT scan to evaluate potential growth of the mass may raise the suspicion of malignancy. The diagnostic and staging workup for RCC is given in Table 63.1. The diagnosis of RCC is established clinically and radiographically in most cases. Pathologic confirmation often is made at the time of nephrectomy.

Once a radiographic diagnosis is made, a staging evaluation should be undertaken, which should include: a complete history and physical examination, complete blood count, and liver and kidney function tests. A metastatic workup should include a chest CT and an abdominal/pelvic CT (preferred) or abdominal MRI scan. Patients with symptoms suggestive of bone metastases and those with an elevated alkaline phosphatase level should undergo a bone scan. If metastatic lesions are detected, histologic confirmation should be made by biopsy of either the metastatic focus or the primary tumor. MRI can be valuable when evaluating the extent of involvement of the collecting system or inferior vena cava, or radiographic contrast cannot be administered. Renal arteriography is sometimes helpful in planning surgery.

Renal Pelvis and Ureter Carcinoma

The diagnostic workup for renal pelvis and ureter carcinoma is listed in Table 63.2. Staging includes a complete history and physical examination, complete blood count, and liver and kidney function tests. CT urography is now used to evaluate patients with renal pelvis carcinoma. CT or MRI of the abdomen and pelvis before and after contrast administration gives useful information regarding the possible extension of tumor outside the collecting system. Uteroscopic visualization of the tumor is desirable, and tissue biopsy through a uteroscope should be performed if feasible. Cystoscopy is very important because of the high incidence of multiple tumors. Urine cytology may help to determine tumor grade if tissue is not available; however, false-negative rates can be high for upper tract and low-grade tumors.

TABLE 63.1 DIAGNOSTIC WORKUP FOR RENAL CELL CARCINOMA

General
- History and physical examination

Radiographic Studies
- Abdominal/pelvic CT (preferred) or abdominal MRI with or without contrast depending on renal function. MRI is superior to CT when evaluating the inferior vena cava and right atrium for tumor involvement
- Consider CT urography, which allows imaging of both the renal parenchyma and the collecting system
- Chest CT or chest radiograph
- Bone scan, if patient has bone pain or has an elevated alkaline phosphatase
- Brain MRI, if suspecting brain metastases
- Avoid biopsy if resection is being considered. Consider needle biopsy, if clinically indicated, for small lesions to confirm diagnosis or guide surveillance, cryosurgery, or radiofrequency ablation strategies

Laboratory Studies
- Complete blood cell count
- Comprehensive metabolic panel (including lactate dehydrogenase, serum calcium, liver function tests, blood urea nitrogen, and serum creatinine)
- Urinalysis

CT, computed tomography; MRI, magnetic resonance imaging.

TABLE 63.2 DIAGNOSTIC WORKUP FOR RENAL PELVIS AND URETER CARCINOMA

General
- History and physical examination

Radiographic Studies
- CT of the abdomen and pelvic or MRI urogram
- Multidetector CT urography
- Chest CT or chest radiograph
- Bone scan, if patient has bone pain or has an elevated alkaline phosphatase
- Brain MRI, if suspecting brain metastases

Special Tests
- Cystoscopy—the entire urinary tract has to be evaluated because of the high incidence of multiple tumors
- Uteroscopic visualization of the tumor is desirable, and tissue biopsy through a uteroscope may be performed if feasible
- Urine cytology may help to determine tumor grade if tissue is not available. False negative rate can be high in upper-tract and low-grade tumors

Laboratory Studies
- Complete blood cell count
- Comprehensive metabolic panel (including liver function tests, blood urea nitrogen, and serum creatinine)
- Urinalysis

CT, computed tomography; MRI, magnetic resonance imaging.

STAGING

Renal Cell Carcinoma

The American Joint Committee on Cancer (AJCC) system is utilized to stage patients with RCC[50] (Table 63.3). T1 and T2 cancers are limited to the kidney. T3 tumors extend into major veins or perinephric tissues, although not into the ipsilateral adrenal gland, and not beyond Gerota's fascia. T4 tumors invade beyond Gerota's fascia (including contiguous extension into the ipsilateral adrenal gland). Regional lymph node metastases may involve spread to the renal hilar, paracaval, aortic, or retroperitoneal drainage sites. Metastasis in regional lymph node(s) is classified as N1. This staging system underwent significant modifications in the 2010 AJCC 7th edition of its *Cancer Staging Manual:* T2 lesions were divided into T2a (>7 cm but ≤10 cm) and T2b (>10 cm); ipsilateral adrenal involvement was reclassified as T4 if contiguous invasion and M1 if not contiguous; renal vein involvement was reclassified as T3a; and nodal involvement was simplified to N0 versus N1.

Renal Pelvis and Ureter Carcinoma

Tumors of the renal pelvis and ureter have a natural history that is not too dissimilar from that of other urothelial malignancies originating in the bladder. Their prognoses depend on tumor invasiveness and pathologic grade. The 2010 AJCC 7th edition staging classification for renal pelvis and ureter carcinoma is shown in Table 63.4.[51]

PATHOLOGIC CLASSIFICATION

Renal Cell Carcinoma

RCC is a group of malignancies arising from the epithelium of the renal tubules and comprises 90% of all malignancies in the

TABLE 63.3 AMERICAN JOINT COMMITTEE ON CANCER 2010 STAGING CLASSIFICATION FOR KIDNEY TUMORS

Primary Tumor (T)

TX	Primary tumor cannot be assessed
T0	No evidence of primary tumor
T1	Tumor 7 cm in greatest dimension, limited to the kidney
T1a	Tumor ≤4 cm in greatest dimension, limited to the kidney
T1b	Tumor >4 cm but ≤7 cm in greatest dimension, limited to the kidney
T2	Tumor >7 cm in greatest dimension, limited to the kidney
T2a	Tumor >7 cm but ≤10 cm in greatest dimension, limited to the kidney
T2b	Tumor >10 cm, limited to the kidney
T3	Tumor extends into major veins or perinephric tissues but not into the ipsilateral adrenal gland and not beyond Gerota's fascia
T3a	Tumor grossly extends into the renal vein or its segmental (muscle containing) branches, or tumor invades perirenal and/or renal sinus fat but not beyond Gerota's fascia
T3b	Tumor grossly extends into the vena cava below diaphragm
T3c	Tumor grossly extends into the vena cava above the diaphragm or invades the wall of the vena cava
T4	Tumor invades beyond Gerota's fascia (including contiguous extension into the ipsilateral adrenal gland)

Regional Lymph Nodes (N)[a]

NX	Regional lymph nodes cannot be assessed
N0	No regional lymph node metastasis
N1	Metastasis in regional lymph node(s)

Distant Metastasis (M)

MX	Presence of distant metastasis cannot be assessed
M0	No distant metastasis
M1	Distant metastasis

Stage Grouping

Stage I	T1	N0	M0
Stage II	T2	N0	M0
Stage III	T1 or T2	N1	M0
	T3	N0 or N1	M0
Stage IV	T4	Any N	M0
	Any T	Any N	M1

Histopathologic Grade

GX	Grade cannot be assessed
G1	Well differentiated
G2	Moderately differentiated
G3	Poorly differentiated
G4	Undifferentiated

[a]The regional lymph nodes are as follows: renal hilar, caval (paracaval, precaval, and retrocaval), interaortocaval, and aortic (para-aortic, preaortic, and retroaortic).

Note: Staging applies only to renal cell carcinoma (RCC), and adenomas are excluded from this classification.

TABLE 63.4 AMERICAN JOINT COMMITTEE ON CANCER 2010 STAGING CLASSIFICATION FOR RENAL PELVIS AND URETER TUMORS

Primary Tumor (T)

TX	Primary tumor cannot be assessed
T0	No evidence of primary tumor
Ta	Papillary noninvasive carcinoma
Tis	Carcinoma in situ
T1	Tumor invades subepithelial connective tissue
T2	Tumor invades muscularis
T3	(For renal pelvis only) Tumor invades beyond the muscularis into peripelvic fat or the renal parenchyma T3
	(For ureter only) Tumor invades beyond the muscularis into the periureteric fat
T4	Tumor invades adjacent organs, or through the kidney into perinephric fat

Regional Lymph Nodes (N)[a]

NX	Regional lymph nodes cannot be assessed
N0	No regional lymph node metastasis
N1	Metastasis in a single lymph node, ≤2 cm in greatest dimension
N2	Metastasis in a single lymph node, >2 cm but ≤5 cm in greatest dimension; or multiple lymph nodes, none >5 cm in greatest dimension
N3	Metastasis in a lymph node, >5 cm in greatest dimension

Distant Metastasis (M)

MX	Distant metastasis cannot be assessed
M0	No distant metastasis
M1	Distant metastasis

Stage Grouping

Stage 0a	Ta	N0	M0
Stage 0is	Tis	N0	M0
Stage I	T1	N0	M0
Stage II	T2	N0	M0
Stage III	T3	N0	M0
Stage IV	T4	N0	M0
	Any T	N1, N2, or N3	M0
	Any T	Any N	M1

Histopathologic Grade

WHO/ISUP recommended grading for urothelial histologies:

LG	Low grade
HG	High grade

If the grading system is not specified, generally the following system is used:

GX	Grade cannot be assessed
G1	Well differentiated
G2	Moderately differentiated
G3	Poorly differentiated
G4	Undifferentiated

WHO, World Health Organization; ISUP, International Society of Urologic Pathology.

[a]Laterality does not affect the N classification. The regional lymph nodes for the renal pelvis are as follows: renal, hilar, paracaval, aortic, and retroperitoneal, not otherwise specified (NOS). The regional lymph nodes for the ureter are as follows: renal hilar, iliac (common, internal [hypogastric], external), paracaval, periureteral, and pelvic, NOS.

kidney.[18] The World Health Organization (WHO) classifies renal cell tumors as clear cell RCC, multilocular clear cell RCC, papillary RCC, chromophobe RCC, carcinoma of the collecting ducts of Bellini, renal medullary carcinoma, Xp11 translocation carcinomas, carcinoma associated with neuroblastoma, mucinous tubular and spindle cell carcinoma, papillary adenoma, oncocytoma, and RCC unclassified.[18]

Clear cell RCC is the most common (80% to 90% of tumors), followed by papillary RCC (10% to 15%) and chromophobe RCC (4% to 5%). Papillary RCC can be subdivided into type 1, which tends to be low grade and have a better prognosis, and type 2, which is the opposite. Renal medullary carcinoma is a very aggressive malignancy mostly associated with young black patients with sickle cell trait and, less commonly, sickle cell disease.[52]

Renal Pelvis and Ureter Carcinoma

More than 90% of malignant tumors arising from the renal pelvis and ureter are urothelial (also called transitional cell) carcinomas. The WHO classifies urothelial tumors as infiltrating urothelial carcinoma (with squamous differentiation, glandular differentiation, trophoblastic differentiation, nested variant, microcytic variant, micropapillary variant, lymphoepitheliomalike carcinoma, lymphomalike variant, plasmacytoid variant, sarcomatoid variant, with giant cells, and undifferentiated carcinoma).[18] The most common histologic variant is squamous differentiation followed by glandular.[18] Squamous cell carcinomas account for only 7% to 8% of renal pelvis and ureter carcinomas, and are often associated with chronic calculus disease and infection. Squamous cancers of the renal pelvis and ureter are often locally advanced and associated with a high local recurrence rate.[53]

PROGNOSTIC FACTORS

Renal Cell Carcinoma

The 5-year survival rate of patients with kidney cancer has doubled over the past 50 years, from 34% in 1954 to 70.9% in 2007.[54,55] The stage at initial presentation remains the most important prognostic factor for RCC survival. Using the current 7th edition AJCC staging, the 5-year kidney cancer survival for stage I is 80.9%, 73.7% for stage II, 53.3% for stage III, and 8.2% for stage IV. Prognostic features for RCC are tumor, patient, and laboratory related. Tumor-related prognostic factors include stage, tumor size, tumor grade, histologic type, tumor necrosis, sarcomatoid transformation, and more than two sites of organ metastases. Patient-related factors include asymptomatic versus local symptoms versus systemic symptoms, weight loss, paraneoplastic syndromes, and an interval <1 year from original diagnosis to start of systemic therapy. Laboratory prognostic factors include thrombocytosis as well as elevated erythrocyte sedimentation rate (ESR) or C-reactive protein (CRP).[50,56]

For patients with metastatic RCC, the following factors were predictive of survival in a retrospective study of 670 patients: low Karnofsky performance status (KPS; <80), high lactate dehydrogenase (LDH; >1.5 times upper limit of normal), low hemoglobin (less than the lower limit of normal), high "corrected" serum calcium (>10 mg/dL or 2.5 mmol/L), and absence of prior nephrectomy.[57]

Lymph node metastases are associated with increased rates of local recurrence and distant metastasis.[36,58–59,60] Nuclear grade, sarcomatoid component, tumor size, stage, and the presence of tumor necrosis increase the likelihood of lymph node involvement.[61] The overall risk of lymph node metastases is 20%.[62,63] Patients with lymph node metastases in radical nephrectomy specimens have a local failure rate of 21%, compared with only 4% in patients without lymph node metastases ($p = .0002$).[60] A select group of patients with solitary metastases may have a 5-year survival rate of 25% to 35%.[64,65]

Nuclear grade, after stage, is the most important prognostic feature of clear cell carcinoma. Fuhrman et al.[66] developed a four-tier grading system that is based on nuclear and nucleolar size, shape, and content. Fuhrman's grade is the most widely used grading system. Grade is also an independent prognostic factor for papillary RCC and chromophobe RCC especially when using standardized criteria.[67] Worsening pathologic grade is associated with a poor 5-year disease-free survival.[31,36]

Papillary RCC has a 5-year survival rate that approaches 90% and metastasizes less frequently than clear cell RCC. The spindle cell or sarcomatoid variants of RCC are associated with statistically significant inferior 5-year survival rates, compared with pure clear, or clear and granular, histologic variants.[31,36]

Nuclear morphology is a strong predictor of tumor stage and prognosis.[66] High nuclear grade is associated with an increased incidence of advanced tumor stage, lymph node involvement, distant metastases, renal vein involvement, tumor size, and perirenal fat involvement. In a series of 190 patients reported by Bretheau et al.,[68] the 5-year actuarial survival rates of patients with grade I, II, III, and IV tumors were 76%, 72%, 51%, and 35%, respectively. Sarcomatoid differentiation carries a significantly poorer prognosis than the clear cell or granular cell subtypes. Almost half of patients with sarcomatoid RCC have bone metastases at presentation. The median survival time of patients with sarcomatoid renal cell cancer is only 6.6 months, compared with 19 months for other histologic types.[69]

Nomograms and algorithms have been described to facilitate the determination of cancer-free survival in patients with RCC. Based on 601 patients treated at Memorial Sloan-Kettering Cancer Center with radical nephrectomy, Kattan et al.[70] used variables including patient symptoms (incidental, local, or systemic), histology (chromophobe, papillary, or conventional), tumor size, and pathologic stage to predict risk of recurrence after surgery. (*Note:* Kattan et al.[70] uses the older 1997 staging and is available at the Memorial Sloan-Kettering Cancer Center website, http://nomograms.mskcc.org/Renal/PostSurgery.aspx.) Frank et al.[71] from the Mayo Clinic developed a predictive algorithm based on 1,801 patients treated with radical nephrectomy. This system combines stage, size, grade, and necrosis (SSIGN) to predict patient survival. Finally, Zisman et al.[72] from the University of California–Los Angeles (UCLA) have developed an algorithm that utilizes the AJCC TNM stage, Fuhrman's grade, and Eastern Cooperative Oncology Group (ECOG) performance status to divide patients into low-, intermediate-, and high-risk groups. This model is also known as the UISS, or the UCLA integrated staging system.

Several molecular markers are being explored for their prognostic significance, including lack of B7H1 expression,[73] immunohistochemical detection of carbonic anhydrase IX (CAIX),[74] the proliferative marker Ki67,[74] immunohistochemical expression of IMP3,[75] and others.

Renal Pelvis and Ureter Carcinoma

The major prognostic factors in patients with renal pelvis or ureter carcinoma are initial stage and grade of the tumor. There is no significant difference in prognosis between urothelial carcinomas originating in the ureter compared to those arising in the renal pelvis.[76] Using the current 7th edition AJCC staging, the 5-year renal pelvis and ureter cancer survival is as follows: stage 0a, 72.3%; stage 0is, 70.0%; stage I, 63.9%; stage II, 56.7%; stage III, 36.5%; and stage IV, 10.2%.

High-grade tumors are associated with a higher incidence of metastases and worse survival. Corrado et al.[77] reported 5-year survival rates of 83%, 75%, 52%, and 0% for grades 1 through 4, respectively. These results are comparable to those described by Heney et al.,[78] who reported 100% survival for grade 1, 81% for grade 2, and 0% for grade 3. Local recurrence was identified in 3 of 24 patients with grade 3 tumors. No survival differences were seen for patients with papillary versus solid tumors. In the series of Charbit et al.,[23] lymph node metastases were seen exclusively in patients with high-grade tumors. Of tumor-related deaths, 90% were in patients with high-grade tumors. Hall et al.[79] reported a retrospective series of 252 patients treated surgically for upper urinary tract urothelial cancers. Significant factors for recurrence included high tumor grade and advanced clinical stage. Older patients and patients treated with parenchymal-sparing surgical procedures had higher rates of recurrence. In their series of 77 patients, Akdogan et al.[80] reported from a multivariate analysis that higher recurrence rates were associated with tumor location, higher grade, and advanced T-stage. Tumors in the ureters were more likely to recur than tumors involving the renal pelvis. In a series of 86 patients, Park et al.[81] also reported a higher rate of recurrence in ureteral tumors, compared to those arising in the renal pelvis.

A prior history of bladder cancer has been reported to worsen the prognosis of patients with second urothelial cancers involving the upper tracts.[80,82] From the Memorial Sloan-Kettering Cancer Center series of 129 patients, a multivariate analysis demonstrated that patients with advanced primary tumors and a prior history of bladder cancer were associated with worse disease-free survival.[82]

Flow cytometry may aid in estimating long-term prognosis. In a multivariate analysis, Corrado et al.[77] demonstrated that although stage and grade were the most important prognostic indices, DNA pattern (diploid vs. nondiploid) and the number of lesions (unifocal vs. multifocal) identified at initial diagnosis also determined prognosis. Patients with diploid tumors had a 79% survival rate, compared with only 46% in patients with nondiploid tumors ($p = .0003$). Recent data suggest that hypermethylation of the promoter region of patients with urothelial cancers is associated with a worse prognosis. Tumors of the renal pelvis and ureters demonstrate hypermethylation in 94% of cases compared to 76% of similar-appearing tumors in the bladder (p <0.0001). Hypermethylation was also associated with higher tumor stage, tumor progression, and mortality.[83]

GENERAL MANAGEMENT

Renal Cell Carcinoma

Surgery is the therapeutic foundation for the management of kidney cancer. Radiotherapy has an important and growing role in the palliative management of RCC. Although RCC is traditionally considered to be radioresistant, it has a clear dose response to radiation.[84,85] As long as sufficient radiation dose is delivered to the tumor while respecting normal tissue dose constraints, RCC "radioresistance" can be overcome with modern techniques. At present, no effective, clinically proven, adjuvant therapy exists for RCC. The kidney cancer National Comprehensive Cancer Network (NCCN) guidelines (version 1.2013) offers the following surgical options depending on the stage[86]:

- Stage IA: Partial (preferred) or radical nephrectomy, active surveillance in selected patients, or ablative techniques for nonsurgical candidates
- Stage IB: Partial or radical nephrectomy
- Stage II and III: Radical nephrectomy
- Stage IV: Nephrectomy and surgical metastasectomy for a solitary metastasis if feasible, followed by systemic first-line therapy; cytoreductive nephrectomy if feasible when multiple metastatic sites, followed by systemic first-line therapy; or systemic first-line therapy if surgery is not feasible.

Active surveillance should be considered for patients with localized disease and short life expectancy, or significant comorbidities placing them at a surgical risk.

Surgery

A radical nephrectomy includes a perifascial resection of the kidney, perirenal fat, regional lymph nodes, and ipsilateral adrenal gland. It is the preferred treatment if the tumor extends into the inferior vena cava and usually requires the assistance of a cardiovascular surgeon if there is a caval or atrial thrombus. An experienced team should be involved in the context of a thrombus, as treatment-related mortality can reach 10%.[86] This operation is undertaken by a thoracoabdominal or transabdominal approach. Improved preoperative assessment with CT can identify patients who have no significant risk of adrenal gland involvement.[87] In 76% of cases, the adrenal gland can be spared at the time of surgery. The European Organisation for Research and Treatment of Cancer[88] (EORTC) conducted a randomized trial of radical nephrectomy with or without an elective lymph node dissection, and there was no survival advantage between the two study groups. The incidence of unsuspected lymph node metastases was low (4%).[88] Nevertheless, lymph node dissection does provide valuable prognostic information.

Radical nephrectomies should be avoided if nephron-sparing surgery is feasible for T1a and T1b renal tumors. In this setting, nephron-sparing surgery has shown equivalent outcomes to radical nephrectomy.[89,90] Radical nephrectomy–induced chronic renal insufficiency is associated with an increased risk of cardiovascular death and death from any cause.[91] For this reason, nephron-sparing surgery is preferred in T1a and T1b tumors. Nephron-sparing surgery is also preferred in patients with hereditary RCC to preserve renal function and decrease the risk of cardiovascular events.[92] In a matched pair analysis of 164 patients undergoing nephron-sparing surgery at the Mayo Clinic, the disease-free survival was 79%, which compared favorably to 77% in patients undergoing radical nephrectomy.[93] In 117 patients with renal tumors ≤4 cm undergoing partial nephrectomy at the Memorial Sloan-Kettering Cancer Center, the 5-year freedom from recurrence was 98.6% compared to 96.4% in a similar group of 173 patients undergoing radical nephrectomy. Compared to patients undergoing partial nephrectomy, those undergoing radical nephrectomy were at a higher risk of chronic renal insufficiency.[94] There is some risk that sparing of the renal parenchyma may leave microscopic residual tumor or inadequately treat multifocal cancers.[95–96,97] Bilateral RCC occurs in 2% to 3% of patients. In these patients, nephron-sparing surgery is an attractive option because bilateral radical nephrectomy sentences the patient to a lifetime of renal dialysis or the need for a renal transplant.

Following surgery, 20% to 30% of patients with localized tumors relapse, with a median time to relapse of 1 to 2 years, and most occurring within 3 years.[86] Although at present there is no role for adjuvant therapy after surgery, several recent trials are exploring the role of targeted therapy.

Patients who have local symptoms, such as hematuria, pain, hypertension, or other paraneoplastic syndromes, may benefit from palliative nephrectomy. Spontaneous regression of metastatic renal cell cancer after nephrectomy has been reported. In an extensive literature review, the incidence of regression of metastatic foci induced by nephrectomy was 0.8% (4 of 474 patients).[33] Cytoreductive surgery performed to prolong or increase the response of metastatic disease in response to systemic therapy may be beneficial.[98,99–100,101]

Thermal Ablation

Recently, the minimally invasive ablative technologies of cryoablation and radiofrequency ablation (RFA) have emerged as potential treatment options for clinically localized RCC, especially in the elderly or in patients with a solitary kidney or comorbidities impeding surgery. Long-term oncologic efficacy for these modalities remains to be established. The most favorable lesions for this approach are <4 cm and in the periphery of the kidney. Relative contraindications for RFA and cryoablation include distant metastases, tumors >5 cm, tumors in the hilum or central collecting system, and life expectancy <1 year. A meta-analysis comparing cryoablation and RFA suggested that cryoablation results in fewer re-treatments and improved local tumor control, and that cryoablation may be associated with a lower risk of metastatic progression compared with RFA.[101]

Renal Stereotactic Body Radiotherapy

Renal stereotactic body radiotherapy (SBRT) as an alternative to thermal ablation is in its infancy. Beitler et al.[102] identified nine RCC patients with primary kidney tumors who received SBRT to 8 Gy × five fractions. The tumors ranged from 1.5 to 10 cm in diameter. With a median follow up of 26.7 months, four of the nine patients were alive. One of the nine patients failed in the ipsilateral kidney, away from the initial radiation treatment volume, while the other eight patients had durable local control. One patient had a radiation injury to the stomach resulting in a 30 lb weight loss in 1 month.[102] Wersall et al.[103] reported eight patients treated with stereotactic radiotherapy to medically inoperable primary tumors using a radiation treatment schedule of 8 Gy × five fractions. Seven of the eight patients were locally controlled, and the median survival exceeded 58 months.[103] Ponsky et al.[104] also reported their initial experience on three patients treated with 4 Gy × four fractions. Two of three patients had evidence of residual disease at these low doses at the time of partial nephrectomy 8 weeks later.[104]

Svedman et al.[105] reported their SBRT experience with seven patients who were treated for metastases from a malignant kidney to its contralateral counterpart. Dose/fractionation schedules varied between 10 Gy × three fractions and 10 Gy × four fractions depending on target location and size. Local control was obtained in six of seven patients and regained after

TABLE 63.5 SURVIVAL AFTER NEPHRECTOMY OR NEOADJUVANT RADIOTHERAPY AND NEPHRECTOMY FOR RENAL CELL CARCINOMA, PROSPECTIVE RANDOMIZED TRIALS

Study (Reference)	Number of Patients	Radiation Dose/ Fraction Size (Gy)	Treatment	5-Year Survival Rate (%)	Comments
Van der Werf-Messing et al. (106,107)	85	–	N	50	No significant survival difference
	89	30–40/2	N + NART		
Juusela et al. (108)	50	–	N	63	No significant survival difference
	38	33/2.2	N + NART	47	

N, nephrectomy; NART, neoadjuvant radiotherapy.

retreatment in the one patient whose lesion progressed. Side effects were generally mild, and in five of the seven patients kidney function remained unaffected after treatment. In two patients, the creatinine levels remained moderately elevated but dialysis was not required.[105]

Neoadjuvant (Preoperative) Radiotherapy

Neoadjuvant radiotherapy is not recommended in patients with resectable RCC. Two European studies were undertaken to test the efficacy of neoadjuvant/preoperative radiotherapy in renal cell cancer (Table 63.5). A prospective randomized study of neoadjuvant radiotherapy and nephrectomy versus nephrectomy alone was conducted in Rotterdam. No advantage was demonstrated in patients receiving radiotherapy with respect to overall survival or survival free from distant metastases. In this trial, patients received a 30-Gy midplane dose to the involved kidney and regional lymph nodes, with 2 Gy daily fractions administered over a period of 3 weeks. Nephrectomy immediately followed the completion of radiotherapy. Neoadjuvant radiotherapy did appear to increase the rate of complete resectability in patients with locally advanced tumors.[106] This study was continued after the preliminary 1973 analysis. Subsequent patients received 40-Gy neoadjuvant radiotherapy. No benefit was demonstrated at the higher radiation dose.[107] In Sweden, a second prospective randomized clinical trial was also unable to demonstrate an advantage for neoadjuvant radiotherapy. In this trial, patients were randomly assigned to receive neoadjuvant radiotherapy to 33 Gy in 15 fractions administered to the flank with a betatron unit followed by nephrectomy or nephrectomy alone. Patients receiving neoadjuvant radiotherapy had a 5-year survival rate of 47%, compared with 63% for patients undergoing surgery alone.[108]

Adjuvant (Postoperative) Radiotherapy

Adjuvant radiotherapy is not recommended in RCC after complete resection. Two prospective randomized studies testing the value of adjuvant radiotherapy did not demonstrate an advantage to patients receiving radiotherapy after surgery (Table 63.6). The first study from New Castle, United Kingdom, demonstrated an inferior survival for patients receiving adjuvant radiotherapy compared with those treated by surgery alone.[109] Local recurrence rates were not affected by adjuvant radiotherapy. No stratification of patients by tumor stage or grade was made. Four patients died of fatal hepatotoxicity after radiotherapy to a right-sided nephrectomy bed. Patients in this study received 55 Gy in 2.04 Gy daily fractions.[7] A second randomized study conducted by the Copenhagen Renal Cancer Study Group compared patients with stage II or III renal cell cancer treated with nephrectomy alone with patients who received nephrectomy and adjuvant 50 Gy in 20 fractions to the kidney bed and regional ipsilateral and contralateral lymph nodes. No difference in the relapse rate was found between the two study groups. There were significant complications involving the stomach, duodenum, and liver in 44% of patients receiving adjuvant radiotherapy. In fact, 19% of deaths in the radiotherapy group were attributed to radiation-induced complications.[110]

Aref et al.[111] analyzed at the patterns of failure in 116 patients undergoing nephrectomy for RCC. They observed that locoregional failure is rare following nephrectomy and that distant metastases is the main pattern of failure. Consequently, their data did not support the role of adjuvant radiation in RCC.[111] Moreover, a retrospective study of 1,344 patients who underwent 1,390 partial nephrectomies for kidney cancer found that positive surgical margins were not associated with an increased risk of local recurrence or metastatic disease.[112] This further supports avoiding adjuvant radiotherapy for RCC.

In contrast, a meta-analysis including the two prospective randomized trials previously mentioned and five retrospective trials with a total of 735 patients observed a significant reduction in locoregional failure with adjuvant radiotherapy (p <0.0001). The patient accrual for all studies combined spanned from 1968 to 1999. There was no difference in overall survival or disease-free survival. The authors proposed a prospective randomized trial using modern radiotherapy techniques for high-risk patients with tumor size >5 cm, positive margins or gross residual disease, perinephric fat invasion, capsule invasion, renal vein/inferior vena cava invasion, positive lymph nodes, or high-grade histology.[113]

Systemic Therapy in the Treatment for Relapsed, Metastatic, or Unresectable Renal Cell Carcinoma

Until recently, systemic treatment for RCC was mostly limited to cytokine therapy. High-dose interleukin-2 (IL-2; category 2)-based immunotherapy can achieve long-lasting complete or partial remissions in a small subset of patients with predominantly clear cell carcinoma. Cytoreductive nephrectomy is recommended for patients with metastatic RCC prior to

TABLE 63.6 SURVIVAL AFTER NEPHRECTOMY OR NEPHRECTOMY AND ADJUVANT RADIOTHERAPY FOR RENAL CELL CARCINOMA, PROSPECTIVE RANDOMIZED TRIALS

Study (Reference)	Stage	Number of Patients	Radiation Dose/ Fraction Size (Gy)	Treatment	5-Year Survival Rate (%)	Local Recurrence (%)	RT-Related Mortality (%)	RT Complications (%)
Fugitt (109)	NS	48	–	N	47 (17/35)	7	18	>20
		52	55/2.04	N + ART	36 (14/39)	7		
Kjaer (64)	II, III	33	–	N	63[a]	1	19	44
		32	55/2.5	N + ART	38[a]	0		

RT, radiotherapy; NS, not stated; N, nephrectomy; ART, adjuvant radiotherapy.
[a]Interpolated from graph; number at risk not known.

Clinical Radiation Oncology

immunotherapy based on results from phase III trials from the Southwest Oncology Group (SWOG) and the EORTC. A combined analysis of these trials showed that median survival favored the surgery plus interferon (IFN)-α group (13.6 vs. 7.8 months for IFN-α alone).[99,100,114,115] Treatment with IL-2 is associated with considerable toxicity and is limited to patients with excellent performance status and normal organ function. Currently, newer targeted agents are often favored over cytokine therapy as first-line therapy owing to their efficacy and more favorable toxicity profile.

At present, seven targeted agents are U.S. Food and Drug Administration (FDA) approved in the treatment for advanced RCC: sunitinib, sorafenib, pazopanib, temsirolimus, everolimus, axitinib, and bevacizumab in combination with IFN. As first-line therapy for relapsed or medically unresectable predominantly clear cell carcinoma, the options are sunitinib (category 1), bevacizumab with IFN (category 1), pazopanib (category 1), temsirolimus (category 1 for poor-prognosis patients), sorafenib and high dose IL-2 for selected patients. Subsequent category 1 therapy following a tyrosine kinase inhibitor for predominant clear cell carcinoma includes everolimus or axitinib. Subsequent category 1 therapy following cytokine therapy for predominant clear cell carcinoma includes sorafenib, sunitinib, pazopanib, and axitinib. For non–clear cell RCC, temsirolimus is a category 1 agent.[86]

Sunitinib, an oral small-molecule multi–tyrosine kinase inhibitor, was studied in a large multinational phase III trial of 750 patients with largely good- or intermediate-prognosis metastatic clear cell RCC who had not received prior systemic therapy. Patients were randomly assigned to 6-week cycles of sunitinib (50 mg daily for 4 weeks, followed by 1 week off) or IFN-α (9 million units three times per week). The objective response rate was significantly increased with sunitinib (47% vs. 12% with IFN-α). Median progression-free survival was significantly prolonged with sunitinib (11 months vs. 5 months, hazard ratio [HR] 0.54). As well, overall survival was prolonged with sunitinib (median 26.4 months vs. 21.8 months, HR 0.82, 95% confidence interval [CI] 0.673 to 1.001, $p = .051$).[116]

Pazopanib, a multitargeted receptor tyrosine kinase inhibitor, was evaluated in a phase III trial of 435 patients who were previously untreated or had received only cytokine therapy and were randomly assigned to pazopanib or placebo. There was a significant increase in progression-free survival with pazopanib compared with placebo (median 9.2 months vs. 4.2 months, HR 0.46, 95% CI 0.34 to 0.62).[117]

Temsirolimus, a parenterally administered mTOR inhibitor, was evaluated in a phase III trial in which 626 previously untreated poor-prognosis patients with metastatic or recurrent RCC were randomly assigned to temsirolimus (25 mg intravenously per week), temsirolimus (15 mg intravenously per week) plus IFN-α (escalated up to 6 million units three times per week as tolerated), or IFN-α monotherapy (escalated up to 18 million units three times per week as tolerated). Temsirolimus as a single agent significantly prolonged the median overall survival compared to IFN-α as a single agent (10.9 months vs. 7.3 months; HR for mortality 0.73, 95% CI 0.58 to 0.92). Both overall and progression-free survival rates for the combination of temsirolimus plus IFN-α were not significantly better than with IFN-α alone.[56]

Bevacizumab, a recombinant monoclonal antibody against vascular endothelial growth factor (VEGF), was evaluated in the phase III AVOREN trial, where 649 previously untreated patients were randomly assigned to IFN-α (9 million units three times per week for 1 year) plus either bevacizumab (10 mg/kg every 2 weeks) or placebo. There was a significant prolongation of progression-free survival (10.2 months vs. 5.5 months, HR 0.63, 95% CI 0.45 to 0.72) and a significantly increased objective response rate (31% vs. 13%).[118]

Sorafenib, a small-molecule multi–tyrosine kinase and Raf inhibitor, was studied in the phase III TARGET trial, in which 903 patients with advanced RCC who had failed prior standard therapy were randomly assigned to sorafenib (400 mg orally twice daily) or placebo. The median progression-free survival was significantly longer in those receiving sorafenib compared with placebo (5.5 months vs. 2.8 months, HR 0.44, 95% CI 0.35 to 0.55). Overall survival with sorafenib was not significantly prolonged compared to placebo.[119,120]

Everolimus, an orally administered mTOR inhibitor, was studied in 410 patients with metastatic clear cell RCC whose disease had progressed on VEGF receptor–tyrosine kinase inhibitors (sunitinib, sorafenib). The median progression-free survival with everolimus was significantly prolonged compared to placebo (4.9 months vs. 1.9 months, HR 0.30, 95% CI 0.22 to 0.40). There was no statistically significant difference in overall survival.[121] Other targeted agents in development are cediranib, tivozanib, and regorafenib.

Chemotherapy has limited use in RCC because it is one of the most chemotherapy-resistant solid tumors. For patients with relapsed or medically unresectable stage IV disease with non–clear cell histology, gemcitabine in combination with doxorubicin or capecitabine has shown moderate activity in patients with sarcomatoid tumors and may be considered as first-line therapy.[86]

Metastasectomy

Patients with a solitary metastatic lesion have a 5-year survival rate of 24% (compared with 4% for those with more than one metastatic focus), and they may benefit from aggressive therapy.[122] The resection of one or a limited number of metastases in combination with nephrectomy or at relapse has been associated with a 13% to 50% 5-year survival in small series of selected patients.[123,124–125] Selected lung, bone, brain, liver, and even pancreatic metastases, among other sites, have been treated using this approach.

Whole-Brain Radiotherapy for Brain Metastases

A retrospective study of 60 patients receiving whole-brain radiotherapy (WBRT) for RCC brain metastases showed that local control at 6 months was 21% after 3 Gy × 10 fractions and 57% after higher doses of 2 Gy × 20 fractions or 3 Gy × 15 fractions ($p = .013$). The local control at 12 months was 7% and 35%, respectively. The overall survival at 6 months was 29% after 3 Gy × 10 fractions and 52% after higher doses ($p = .003$). The overall survival at 12 months was 13% and 47%, respectively. The authors[126] concluded that escalating the WBRT dose beyond 3 Gy × 10 fractions could improve the outcomes in RCC patients with brain metastases and proposed a randomized trial.

Stereotactic Radiosurgery for Brain Metastases

A retrospective study of 280 consecutive patients with metastatic brain tumors (of which 80 were RCC) treated with Gamma Knife radiosurgery (GKS) observed that to control symptomatic peritumoral edema, a higher marginal dose ≥25 Gy was necessary. The authors[127] developed an algorithm for the management of RCC metastases where lesions ≥3 cm undergo resection; lesions >2 cm with symptomatic peritumoral edema undergo resection (because 25 Gy was not considered safe for tumors >2 cm) and those without it GKS; and lesions ≤2 cm receive GKS. Another retrospective study of 46 patients and 99 RCC brain lesions treated with radiosurgery observed that the good-response group (as assessed by MRI) survived significantly longer than the poor-response group (median survival times of 18 and 9 months, respectively; $p = .025$).[128]

Kano et al.[129] reported 158 consecutive RCC patients (531 lesions) who underwent stereotactic radiosurgery (SRS). The overall survival after SRS was 60%, 38%, and 19% at 6, 12, and 24 months, respectively, with a median survival of 8.2 months. Median survival for patients with <2 brain metastases, higher KPS (>90), and no prior WBRT was 12 months after SRS. Sustained local tumor control was achieved in 92% of patients. Symptomatic adverse radiation effects occurred in 7%. Overall, 70% of patients improved or remained neurologically stable.[129]

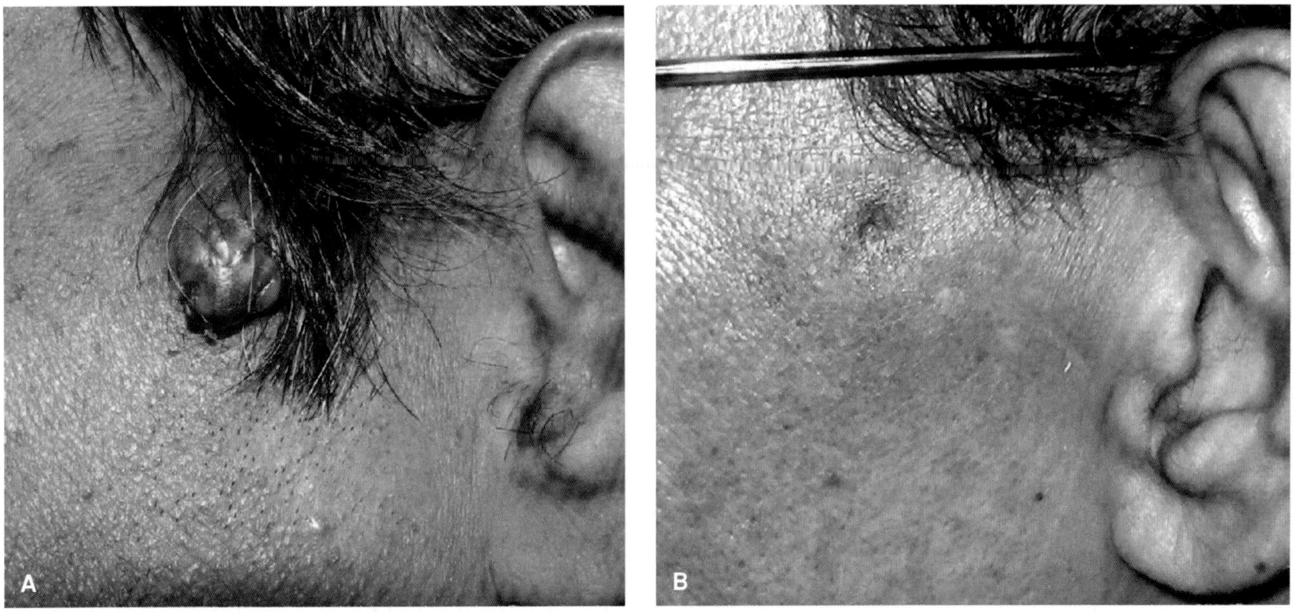

FIGURE 63.1. Patient with renal cell carcinoma (RCC) who received 375 cGy × 13 fractions over 5 weeks to a painful, fixed, and pulsatile cutaneous RCC metastasis. Appearance after 3 fractions **(A)** and complete response 6 months after the completion of treatment **(B)**. The patient had durable pain palliation without local recurrence until death. (From Gay HA, et al. Complete response in a cutaneous facial metastatic nodule from renal cell carcinoma after hypofractionated radiotherapy. *Dermatol Online J* 2007;13:6; © 2007 Dermatology Online Journal.)

Conventional Radiotherapy for Extracranial Metastases

Palliative radiotherapy is effective in relieving symptoms from metastatic RCC.[130–131,132,133] A patient with a solitary bone metastasis may have a long survival time, and a sufficient radiation dose should be administered to allow durable pain relief. If surgery is used to remove a metastatic lesion, postoperative radiotherapy is indicated to prevent its recurrence. In a prospective phase II study using validated quality-of-life questionnaires, Lee et al.[132] from the Princess Margaret Hospital demonstrated that 83% of patients treated for pain had experienced significant pain relief with 30-Gy delivered in 10 fractions. DiBiase et al.[84] observed a dose response in the palliative treatment of 107 patients with RCC. A biologically effective dose (BED) >50 Gy_{10} (α/β ratio of 10) was associated with a statistically significant increased rate of response: 59% versus 39% ($p = 0.001$).

Figure 63.1 illustrates a painful RCC cutaneous metastasis that had a complete response after 375 cGy × 13 fractions (BED = 67 Gy_{10}) over 5 weeks. The lesion was treated with electrons, a custom bolus, and a 2-cm peripheral margin.[134]

Stereotactic Body Radiation Therapy for Extracranial Metastases

In a series of 50 patients with metastatic RCC, Wersall et al.[103] reported that stereotactically delivered radiation to sites including the lung, liver, and adrenal resulted in complete regression in 30% of cases and either partial regression or stabilization of the lesions in 60%. Of 162 treated tumors, only 3 tumors recurred. Dose and fractionation ranged from 8 Gy × four fractions, 10 Gy × four fractions, and 15 Gy × three fractions all delivered in 1 week.

A retrospective study of 17 patients with metastatic melanoma (28 lesions) and 13 patients with RCC (25 lesions) to the lung, liver, and bone concluded that to achieve high rates of durable control, SBRT of at least 16 Gy × three fractions were necessary.[135] Another retrospective study of 126 extracranial metastases in 103 patients treated with single fractions observed that RCC displayed a profound dose-response effect, with an 80% local relapse-free survival at the high-dose level (23 to 24 Gy) versus 37% at low doses (≤22 Gy) ($p = .04$).[136] Further analysis of RCC patients revealed that a single 24-Gy dose had a 3-year local progression-free survival of 88%.[85]

In study of 48 patients (55 lesions) with metastatic RCC to the spine, patients received 24 Gy × one fraction, 9 Gy × three fractions, or 6 Gy × five fractions. The actuarial 1-year spine tumor progression-free survival was 82.1%. At pretreatment baseline, 23% of patients were pain free; at 1 month and 12 months post-SBRT, 44% and 52% of patients were pain free, respectively. No grade 3 or 4 neurologic toxicity was observed.[137]

A unique case report showed how a large 7-cm RCC metastasis in the parieto-occipital vertex of the skull was treated with SBRT to 7 Gy × five fractions. No significant bleeding was observed 5 weeks later at the time of tumor resection. Histologically, the tumor was largely avascular and necrotic, and the authors[138] proposed SBRT as a potential alternative to preoperative embolization.

A potential added benefit of extracranial stereotactic radiotherapy is what is called the abscopal effect, in which there is tumor response at a distance from the irradiated volume. Wersall et al.[139] observed an abscopal effect in 4 out of 28 RCC patients with treated and untreated metastatic lesions. In these 4 patients, nonirradiated metastases regressed either temporarily or seemingly permanently after treatment with SBRT of either the primary tumor or other metastatic lesions. The authors'[139] findings argued for a more active and liberal use of SBRT in metastatic RCC. They suggested that further studies were necessary to define the underlying mechanisms behind such responses or to combine SBRT with immunomodulating agents.

Ongoing Phase III Clinical Trials

There are numerous clinical trials taking place in advanced RCC. Many of these trials are employing antiangiogenesis agents, thymidine kinase inhibitors, mTOR inhibitors, and immunological therapies, alone or in combination.

Renal Pelvis and Ureter Carcinoma

Surgery is the therapeutic foundation for the management of renal pelvis and ureter carcinoma. The bladder cancer NCCN guidelines (version 1.2013) recommend the following treatment options for renal pelvis low-grade tumors: nephroureterectomy with a cuff of bladder, a nephron-sparing procedure, or endoscopic resection with or without postsurgical intrapelvic chemotherapy or bacille Calmette-Guerin (BCG).[140] High-grade renal pelvis tumors or large tumors that invade the renal parenchyma have the following management options: nephroureterectomy with a cuff of bladder and regional lymphadenectomy, with neoadjuvant chemotherapy in selected patients, extrapolating from bladder cancer series.

The management of ureter tumors depends on the location of the tumor—upper, mid, or distal—and on disease extent. Neoadjuvant chemotherapy may be considered in selected patients.[141] Tumors in the upper ureter are more commonly treated with nephroureterectomy with a cuff of bladder and regional lymphadenectomy for high-grade tumors. Low-grade tumors may be managed endoscopically.

Tumors in the mid portion of the ureter can be managed according to grade and size. Small, low-grade tumors can be treated with ureteroureterostomy, endoscopic resection, or nephroureterectomy with a cuff of bladder with or without regional lymphadenectomy. High-grade lesions are managed with nephroureterectomy with a cuff of bladder and regional lymphadenectomy with consideration of neoadjuvant chemotherapy in selected patients.

Finally, distal ureteral tumors may be managed with a distal ureterectomy and reimplantation of the ureter (ideal if feasible), endoscopic resection, or nephroureterectomy with a cuff of bladder and regional lymphadenectomy for high-grade tumors. Neoadjuvant chemotherapy may be considered in select patients.

For both renal pelvis and ureter tumors, once the pathologic staging is obtained, patients with pathologic stage pT2, pT3, pT4, or N+ should be considered for adjuvant chemotherapy with or without radiotherapy.

Surgery

Radical nephroureterectomy is the only potentially curative treatment for most patients with urothelial carcinoma of the renal pelvis or ureter. This operation includes removal of the contents of Gerota's fascia, including the ipsilateral ureter with a cuff of bladder at its distal extent. Less radical surgeries have been plagued by high local or regional recurrence rates, sometimes approaching 30%.[142] Hall et al.[79] reported an increase rate of recurrence when parenchymal-sparing procedures were performed. Conservative surgical excision should be considered only in patients with low-grade, low-stage, solitary tumors in whom radical nephrectomy is not indicated because of poor kidney function or an absent contralateral kidney.

Adjuvant Radiotherapy

There are no randomized trials on the role of postoperative radiotherapy in patients who have had a complete resection of an upper urinary tract cancer. Tumors of the renal pelvis and ureter have a significantly high local recurrence rate after nephroureterectomy, particularly in patients with high-grade tumors or deep invasion.[53] Retrospective studies suggest that adjuvant radiotherapy may diminish the likelihood of local recurrence, although it does not appear to have an impact on overall survival or reduction of future distant metastases.[34,143]

Cozad et al.[143] reported a retrospective study of 94 patients with urothelial carcinoma of the renal pelvis, of which 77 patients had resections without residual. On multivariate analysis, adjuvant radiotherapy had a significant effect on local control (p = .02). In terms of survival, the use of adjuvant radiotherapy was of borderline significance (p = .07). Of the 27 patients who were excluded from local failure and survival analysis, 19 patients had unresectable local disease, and of these, 11 patients received radiotherapy. Two long-term disease-free survivors in this group received 45 and 50.4 Gy, respectively.The authors[34] recommended consideration of adjuvant radiotherapy in patients with high grade or stage, close surgical margins, or positive lymph nodes to improve local control.

In another retrospective study of 133 patients with urothelial carcinoma of the renal pelvis, 67 patients received external-beam radiotherapy following surgery (radiotherapy group), and 66 patients received intravesical chemotherapy (nonradiotherapy group). The clinical target volume included the renal fossa, the course of the ureter to the entire bladder, and the paracaval and para-aortic lymph nodes (Fig. 63.2). The tumor bed or residual tumor was targeted in 14 patients. The median radiation dose administered was 50 Gy. There was a significant difference between the survival rates for these groups based on patients with stage T3 and T4 cancer. A significant difference was observed in the bladder tumor relapse rate between the irradiated and nonirradiated bladder groups (p = .004). The authors[144] concluded that radiotherapy may improve the overall survival for patients with T3 and T4 cancer of the renal pelvis or ureter and may delay bladder tumor recurrences.

The patterns of failure were described in 252 patients undergoing surgery at the University of Texas Southwest Medical Center for urothelial carcinoma of the upper urinary tract.[79] Local recurrence occurred only 9% of the time, whereas new invasive urothelial tumors or distant metastases occurred in 69% and 22% of cases, respectively. Isolated local recurrences were rare. Another series from the Princess Margaret Hospital confirms the high rate of distant metastases. Although local failure occurred in 35% of patients with locally advanced disease, most patients also experienced distant metastases as well.[145]

Systemic Chemotherapy

The pathologic similarity of urothelial carcinoma of the renal pelvis and ureter to bladder cancer has encouraged medical oncologists to use similar chemotherapeutic regimens in the management of upper-tract urothelial carcinomas. The MVAC regimen (methotrexate, vinblastine, doxorubicin, and cisplatin) has objective response rates of almost 70% in patients with metastatic urothelial carcinoma of the bladder, ureter, and kidney.[146,147] Gemcitabine plus cisplatin is also effective in urothelial carcinoma. Palliative chemotherapy may be considered in patients with metastatic disease.

A series of 31 patients treated with adjuvant radiotherapy for nonmetastatic urothelial cancer of the upper urinary tract was reported by Czito et al.[148] Nine patients also received chemotherapy consisting of methotrexate, cisplatin, and vinblastine prior to receiving radiation concurrent with cisplatin. The 5-year locoregional control rate was 67%. The 5-year overall and disease-specific survival appeared to be improved with the administration of concurrent chemotherapy. The overall survival for patients receiving concurrent chemotherapy and radiotherapy was 67% compared to 27% receiving postoperative radiation alone (p = .01). The disease-free survival for patients receiving concurrent chemotherapy and radiotherapy was 76% compared to 41% receiving postoperative radiation alone (p = .06).

In circumstances in which conservative resection is performed, postoperative radiotherapy should be considered. Conservative surgical options in selected cases include laparoscopic nephroureterectomy, nephrectomy and partial ureterectomy, endoscopic resection, and fulguration. The role of lymph node dissection in this disease is unclear. Patients who have the highest risk of lymph node metastases also have a high risk of systemic disease.

Ongoing Phase III Clinical Trials

Phase III Randomized Study of Gemcitabine Hydrochloride and Cisplatin with Versus without Bevacizumab in Patients with Advanced Transitional Cell Carcinoma of the Urinary Tract (NCT00942331).

RADIOTHERAPY TECHNIQUES

Normal Tissue Dose Constraints

Several organs at risk have to be taken into consideration when palliating an unresected kidney tumor or a kidney tumor bed recurrence. These organs include the spinal cord, liver, spleen, stomach, duodenum, small bowel, any normal contralateral or ipsilateral kidney, and normal adrenal gland(s).

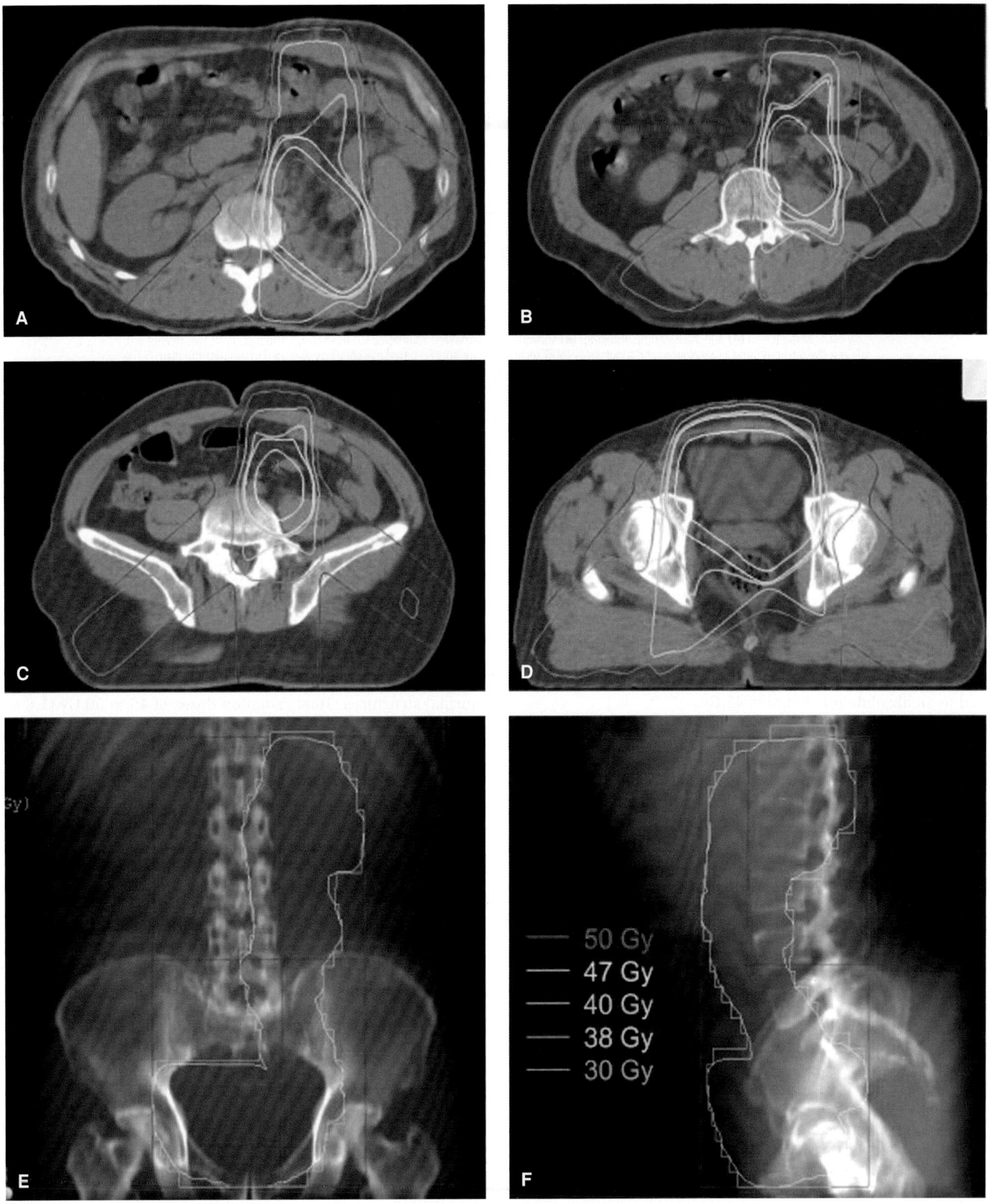

FIGURE 63.2. Dose distribution of a patient with renal pelvis cancer and beam arrangements of 0-degree, 129-degree, and 229-degree gantry. **A:** Renal fossa. **B,C:** Course of ureter. **D:** Bladder. Digitally reconstructed radiograph for views of 0-degree gantry **(E)** and 90-degree gantry **(F)**. Internal pink and yellow lines represent the clinical tumor volume $(CTV)_{50}$ and CTV_{40}, respectively. (From Chen B, et al. Radiotherapy may improve overall survival of patients with T3 and T4 transitional cell carcinoma of the renal pelvis or ureter and delay bladder tumour relapse. *BMC Cancer* 2011;11:297; © 2011 Chen et al; licensee BioMed Central Ltd.)

There are no established dose constraints for sparing the remaining kidney after nephrectomy or in the palliative setting when both kidneys are present. In the context of two normal kidneys, the Qualitative Analyses of Normal Tissue Effects in the Clinic (QUANTEC) Kidney Cancer Panel recommended a mean bilateral kidney dose <15 to 18 Gy and a bilateral kidney dose-volume histogram (DVH) with a V_{12} <55%, V_{20} <32%, V_{23} <30%, and V_{28} <20%.[149] The dose to the stomach should be kept at <45 Gy, and the small bowel V_{45} <195 cc when it is contoured as a bowel bag[150] (Fig. 63.3). The male and female

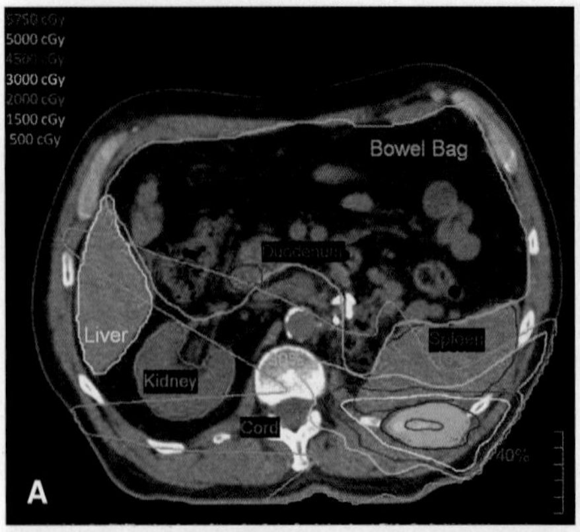

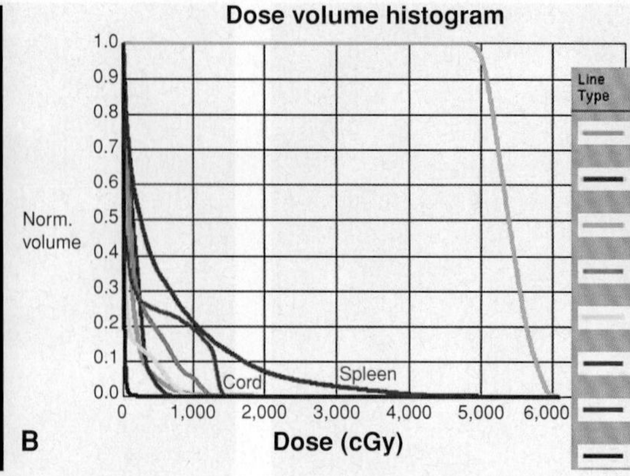

Line Type	ROI	Min.	Max.	Mean
	BOWEL_BAG	7.4	1845.3	138.1
	DUODENUM	17.9	701.8	175.4
	GTV_1000_x5	4471.5	6067.5	5404.6
	KIDNEY_R	16.5	1329.2	254.4
	LIVER	1.0	1062.8	113.5
	SPINALCORD	0.0	1477.9	302.6
	SPLEEN	6.9	4961.0	608.3
	STOMACH	7.7	200.4	22.6

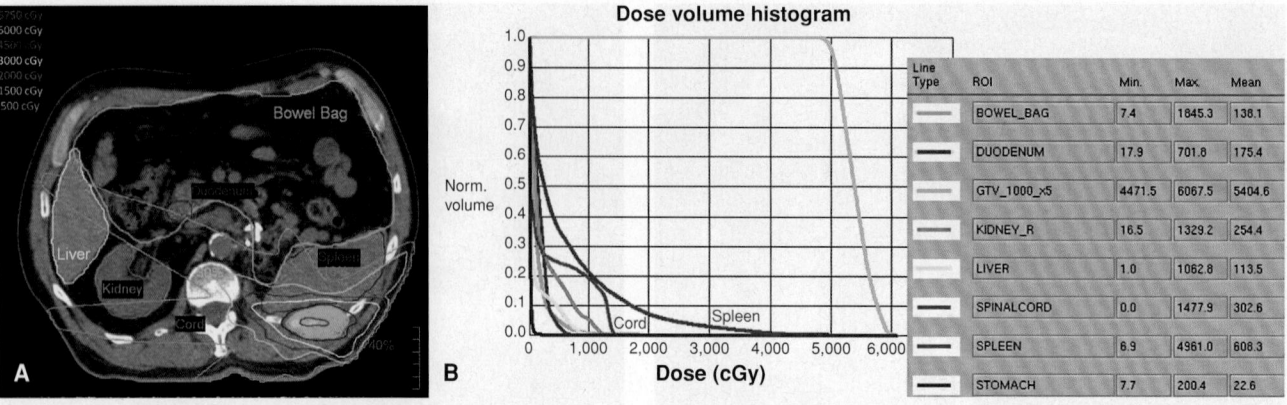

FIGURE 63.3. Patient with metastatic clear cell renal cell carcinoma (RCC) who developed a painful, destructive, 55-cc metastasis in the left 12th rib. Treatment plan **(A)** and dose-volume histogram **(B)** showing the normalized volume versus dose (cGy). The metastasis was treated with 10 Gy × five fractions using a six-field step and shoot, 6-MV IMRT technique. The isodose-based methodology was used to evaluate the plan.[158] The skin was limited to the 40% isodose (400 cGy × five fractions), the spinal cord to the 30% isodose (300 cGy × five fractions), and the spleen to the 10% isodose (100 cGy × five fractions) or less as feasible. The cyan-filled contour is the gross tumor volume (GTV). Doses to the bowel, liver, remaining kidney, and duodenum were well below tolerance. Patient was pain free one month later.

Radiation Therapy Oncology Group (RTOG) normal pelvis atlases illustrate how to contour the bowel bag (accessible at http://www.rtog.org/CoreLab/ContouringAtlases.aspx). The mean liver dose should be kept at <30 to 32 Gy, excluding patients with pre-existing liver disease or hepatocellular carcinoma who have a lower tolerance. Sparing at least 700 cc of liver from radiation is another potential strategy to avoid complications.[151] There are no recognized splenic or adrenal dose constraints. Nevertheless, based on the spleen's exquisite radiosensitivity and experience with palliative radiotherapy for myeloproliferative disorders,[152] it seems prudent to limit the spleen to a total of 5 to 10 Gy. The spinal dose should be limited to an absolute maximum of 45 Gy.

Renal Cell Carcinoma

Neoadjuvant or adjuvant radiotherapy is not routinely recommended for patients with RCC. However, there may be special cases where the clinician may consider neoadjuvant radiotherapy to improve respectability or adjuvant radiotherapy if there are clinical tumor features suggestive of a high risk of local recurrence. Careful planning is paramount because ignoring any of the critical structures surrounding the kidney or nephrectomy bed could result in serious, even fatal, patient toxicity.

Patients receiving radiotherapy to the kidney may be simulated supine, arms up, using a wing board or alpha cradle, a wire on the surgical scar, and a planning CT scan. The kidneys are mobile organs and move vertically within the retroperitoneum an average of 0.9 to 1.3 cm, and as much as 4 cm during normal respiration.[153–154,155] In going from the supine to upright position, the kidneys can shift inferiorly between 0.5 cm and 7.5 cm with an average of 3.6 cm.[156] This finding, although critical for total body irradiation treatments, further highlights the mobility of the kidneys.

The high complication rates reported in the prospective trials of postoperative radiotherapy have taught radiation oncologists an important lesson regarding radiation therapy planning, patient selection, and the tolerance of the upper abdominal viscera. Intensity-modulated radiotherapy (IMRT) may be a reasonable consideration owing to the sensitivity of adjacent surrounding structures. If IMRT is considered, a plan to manage the uncertainties in target localization such as four-dimensional (4D) CT treatment planning, image-guided radiotherapy (IGRT), abdominal immobilization devices, gating, or breathing control needs to be considered. Renal function scans may assist in the treatment planning or patient selection process, although this has not been formally studied.

In unresectable lesions, 40 to 50 Gy neoadjuvant radiotherapy (1.8 to 2 Gy per fraction) directed to the kidney tumor and regional lymphatics may improve resectability.[107] Multiple-field techniques, similar to those described for adjuvant radiotherapy, should be considered in patients receiving preoperative treatment.

CT-based treatment planning contributes to good local control with minimal morbidity. Careful definition of the target volume to encompass the nephrectomy bed, lymph node drainage sites, and surgical clips on the planning CT scan is important. Exclusive use of anterior- and posterior-field arrangements, particularly on the right side, is likely to result in irradiation of large volumes of bowel and liver beyond tolerance. The use of multiple beams is paramount for protecting the surrounding normal structures. Total radiation doses of 45 to 50 Gy (1.8 to 2 Gy per fraction) to the nephrectomy bed and regional lymph nodes with a boost to small volumes of microscopic or gross residual disease of 10 to 15 Gy (total dose 50 to 60 Gy) are appropriate. Stein et al.[157] reported two scar recurrences and recommended that the incision site be included in the target volume. If the scar cannot be covered without increasing the amount of normal tissue irradiated, an additional electron-beam field to treat the scar may be considered.

Figure 63.3 illustrates a patient with metastatic clear cell RCC, with sarcomatoid and rhabdoid differentiation, status post left radical nephrectomy, pT3aN1M1. The kidney tumor was Fuhrman nuclear grade IV and 15.5 cm in diameter. The patient was treated with temsirolimus, pazopanib, bevacizumab, and finally Adriamycin plus gemcitabine with some objective response. The patient developed a painful, destructive, 55-cc metastasis in the left 12th rib. The metastasis was treated with 10 Gy × five fractions using a six-field (RPO 210, LAO 60, LT LAT 90, LPO 120, LPO 150, PA) step and shoot, 6-MV IMRT technique. The isodose-based methodology was used to evaluate the plan and is explained in detail in Gay et al.[158] The skin was limited to the 40% isodose (400 cGy × five fractions), the spinal cord to the 30% isodose (300 cGy × five fractions), and the spleen to the 10% isodose (100 cGy × five fractions) or less as feasible. Doses to the bowel, liver, remaining kidney, and duodenum were well below tolerance (Fig. 63.3A). Daily imaging with two-dimensional (2D):2D match and cone-beam CT was used prior to the delivery of the five fractions over 3 weeks.

Because of the possibility of long survival even in the presence of distant metastases, aggressive treatment for palliation should be considered in patients who have limited metastatic disease with good performance status. Treatment fields should encompass metastatic foci with adequate (2- to 3-cm) margins. (See the following previous sections: Conventional Radiotherapy for Extracranial Metastases, Whole-Brain Radiotherapy for

Brain Metastases, and Stereotactic Radiosurgery for Brain Metastases.)

Renal Pelvis and Ureter Carcinoma

Adjuvant radiotherapy has been used in the management of renal pelvis and ureter cancers. For elective radiotherapy, the clinical target volume should include the renal fossa, the course of the ureter to the bladder, the entire bladder, and the paracaval and para-aortic lymph nodes[144] (Fig. 63.2). As in RCC, CT-based planning may facilitate dosimetric coverage of the regions at risk while minimizing dose to normal tissues. Radiation doses of 45 to 50 Gy at 1.8 to 2 Gy per day are appropriate to treat subclinical and microscopic disease. For more extensive disease (e.g., multiple positive nodes), R1 (microscopic positive margins) or R2 (macroscopic residual margins) resections, a boost of 5 to 10 Gy should be considered. For unresectable or gross residual disease, higher doses may be necessary. In this case, multiple-field arrangements including oblique and lateral fields with field reductions are important to minimize toxicity to surrounding normal structures (Fig. 63.2). CT-based simulation, three-dimensional (3D) treatment planning, and contrast-enhanced radiographs are helpful in defining the radiotherapy target volume. IMRT can be considered if organ motion is managed to avoid underdosing the planning target volume. Chemotherapy may allow a lower radiation dose for gross disease. Cozad et al.[143] reported two patients with gross residual disease who achieved local tumor control with radiation doses of 45 and 50.4 Gy. One of these patients had a pathologically proven complete response at reoperation after receiving radiotherapy and concomitant MVAC.

FOLLOW-UP

Renal Cell Carcinoma

The NCCN Kidney Cancer Panel recommends that patients be seen every 6 months for the first 2 years after surgery, then annually thereafter. Each visit should include a history and physical examination and comprehensive metabolic panel (blood urea nitrogen, serum creatinine, calcium, LDH, and liver function tests). The NCCN recommends abdominal and chest imaging 2 to 6 months after surgery and as clinically indicated thereafter.[86] The UCLA UISS (described in the Prognostic Factors section) uses the older 1997 TNM staging and also provides surveillance recommendations according to risk category.[159] The greatest risk of recurrence following surgery for RCC is in the first 3 to 5 years; however, recurrences can occur more than a decade later. Early diagnosis of metastatic disease could identify patients who may be candidates for metastasectomy and potentially result in long-term survival.

Renal Pelvis and Ureter Carcinoma

Patients with urothelial carcinoma of the upper urinary tract are at a high risk of urothelial tumors of the bladder, thus monitoring with cystoscopy at periodic intervals is necessary. For patients who have undergone a renal-sparing procedure, imaging with CT or MRI and/or ureteroscopy may be necessary. The NCCN Bladder Cancer Panel recommends a cystoscopy every 3 months for 1 year, then at increasing intervals. For endoscopic procedures, imaging (intravenous pyelogram [IVP], CT urography, retrograde pyelogram, ureteroscopy, or MRI urogram) of the upper tract collecting system at 3- to 12-month intervals is recommended. Imaging to exclude metastatic disease such as a chest radiograph, or CT scan or MRI, should be considered.

SEQUELAE OF RADIOTHERAPY

The side effects and complications from radiotherapy for cancer of the kidney, renal pelvis, and ureters are similar to those expected from irradiation of the upper abdomen and pelvis. These side effects include nausea, vomiting, diarrhea, and abdominal cramping. Patients with right-sided tumors may have significant portions of the liver irradiated, and radiation-induced liver damage is possible. The Copenhagen Renal Cancer Study Group reported that 12 (44%) of 27 patients developed significant complications: 3 patients had biochemical changes indicating radiation hepatitis, 3 patients had duodenum and small bowel stenosis, and 6 patients had duodenum and small bowel bleeding.[110] Surgery was performed on 4 of 9 patients with bowel-related radiotherapy complications, and 5 patients died of treatment-related complications. The total radiation dose in this study was 50 Gy given in 2.5-Gy fractions per day—a fractionation schedule that may account for the high rate of complications. Fugitt et al.[109] also reported four cases of "liver" failure among 52 patients who received postoperative radiotherapy.

The complication rate after radiotherapy for tumors of the kidney and upper urinary tract is related to the total dose, fraction size, and technique of irradiation. CT-based simulation and 3D treatment planning may decrease the risk of complications after elective radiotherapy in patients with upper urinary tract malignancies. In a series of 56 patients receiving 46 Gy postoperatively reported by Stein et al.,[157] significant toxicity was seen in only 3 patients (5%). These 3 patients were treated before the routine use of CT-based treatment planning. In 12 patients receiving a median dose of 45 Gy reported by Kao et al.,[160] no long-term treatment-related morbidity was identified.

ACKNOWLEDGMENTS

Thanks to Michael Watts, MS, CMD, for masterfully planning the case in Figure 63.3 and obtaining screen captures of the plan.

SELECTED REFERENCES

A full list of references for this chapter is available online.

3. Jemal A, et al. Global cancer statistics. *CA Cancer J Clin* 2011;61(2):69–90.
4. American Cancer Society. *Cancer facts and figures 2011*. Available at: http://www.cancer.org/Research/CancerFactsFigures/CancerFactsFigures/cancer-facts-figures-2011.
18. Eble JN, et al., eds. *Pathology and genetics: tumours of the urinary system and male genital organs. World Health Organization classification of tumours*. Lyon, France: IARC Press, 2004.
33. Montie JE, et al. The role of adjunctive nephrectomy in patients with metastatic renal cell carcinoma. *J Urol* 1977;117(3):272–275.
34. Cozad SC, et al. Transitional cell carcinoma of the renal pelvis or ureter: patterns of failure. *Urology* 1995;46(6):796–800.
35. Maulard-Durdux C, et al. Postoperative radiation therapy in 26 patients with invasive transitional cell carcinoma of the upper urinary tract: no impact on survival? *J Urol* 1996;155(1):115–117.
36. Skinner DG, et al. Diagnosis and management of renal cell carcinoma. A clinical and pathologic study of 309 cases. *Cancer* 1971;28(5):1165–1177.
40. Gold PJ, Fefer A, Thompson JA. Paraneoplastic manifestations of renal cell carcinoma. *Semin Urol Oncol* 1996;14(4):216–222.
45. Sidhom OA, Basalaev M, Sigal LH. Renal cell carcinoma presenting as polymyalgia rheumatica. Resolution after nephrectomy. *Arch Intern Med* 1993;153(17):2043–2045.
46. Jayson M, Sanders H. Increased incidence of serendipitously discovered renal cell carcinoma. *Urology* 1998;51(2):203–205.
49. McClennan BL. Oncologic imaging. Staging and follow-up of renal and adrenal carcinoma. *Cancer* 1991;67(4 Suppl):1199–1208.
50. Kidney. In: Edge SB, et al. *AJCC cancer staging manual*, 7th ed. New York: Springer, 2010:479–490.
51. Renal pelvis and ureter. In: Edge SB, et al. *AJCC cancer staging manual*, 7th ed. New York: Springer, 2010:491–496.
52. Bruno D, et al. Genitourinary complications of sickle cell disease. *J Urol* 2001;166(3):803–811.
54. National Cancer Institute. SEER cancer statistics review, 1975–2008, based on November 2010 SEER data submission posted to the SEER website 2011. Available at: http://seer.cancer.gov/csr/1975_2008/.
55. Pantuck AJ, Zisman A, Belldegrun AS. The changing natural history of renal cell carcinoma. *J Urol* 2001;166(5):1611–1623.
56. Hudes G, et al. Temsirolimus, interferon alfa, or both for advanced renal-cell carcinoma. *N Engl J Med* 2007;356(22):2271–2281.
57. Motzer RJ, et al. Survival and prognostic stratification of 670 patients with advanced renal cell carcinoma. *J Clin Oncol* 1999;17(8):2530–2540.
60. Rabinovitch RA, et al. Patterns of failure following surgical resection of renal cell carcinoma: implications for adjuvant local and systemic therapy. *J Clin Oncol* 1994;12(1):206–212.
61. Blute ML, et al. A protocol for performing extended lymph node dissection using primary tumor pathological features for patients treated with radical nephrectomy for clear cell renal cell carcinoma. *J Urol* 2004;172(2):465–469.

62. Pantuck AJ, et al. Renal cell carcinoma with retroperitoneal lymph nodes. Impact on survival and benefits of immunotherapy. *Cancer* 2003;97(12):2995–3002.
63. Vasselli JR, et al. Lack of retroperitoneal lymphadenopathy predicts survival of patients with metastatic renal cell carcinoma. *J Urol* 2001;166(1):68–72.
64. Kjaer M. The treatment and prognosis of patients with renal adenocarcinoma with solitary metastasis. 10 year survival results. *Int J Radiat Oncol Biol Phys* 1987;13(4):619–621.
66. Fuhrman SA, Lasky LC, Limas C. Prognostic significance of morphologic parameters in renal cell carcinoma. *Am J Surg Pathol* 1982;6(7):655–663.
67. Lohse CM, et al. Comparison of standardized and nonstandardized nuclear grade of renal cell carcinoma to predict outcome among 2,042 patients. *Am J Clin Pathol* 2002;118(6):877–886.
68. Bretheau D, et al. Prognostic value of nuclear grade of renal cell carcinoma. *Cancer* 1995;76(12):2543–2549.
70. Kattan MW, et al. A postoperative prognostic nomogram for renal cell carcinoma. *J Urol* 2001;166(1):63–67.
71. Frank I, et al. An outcome prediction model for patients with clear cell renal cell carcinoma treated with radical nephrectomy based on tumor stage, size, grade and necrosis: the SSIGN score. *J Urol* 2002;168(6):2395–2400.
72. Zisman A, et al. Improved prognostication of renal cell carcinoma using an integrated staging system. *J Clin Oncol* 2001;19(6):1649–1657.
73. Thompson RH, Kwon ED. Significance of B7-H1 overexpression in kidney cancer. *Clin Genitourin Cancer* 2006;5(3):206–211.
74. Bui MH, et al. Prognostic value of carbonic anhydrase IX and KI67 as predictors of survival for renal clear cell carcinoma. *J Urol* 2004;171(6 Pt 1):2461–2466.
75. Jiang Z, et al. Analysis of RNA-binding protein IMP3 to predict metastasis and prognosis of renal-cell carcinoma: a retrospective study. *Lancet Oncol* 2006; 7(7):556–564.
76. Raman JD, et al. Impact of tumor location on prognosis for patients with upper tract urothelial carcinoma managed by radical nephroureterectomy. *Eur Urol* 2010;57(6):1072–1079.
77. Corrado F, et al. Transitional cell carcinoma of the upper urinary tract: evaluation of prognostic factors by histopathology and flow cytometric analysis. *J Urol* 1991;145(6):1159–1163.
79. Hall MC, et al. Prognostic factors, recurrence, and survival in transitional cell carcinoma of the upper urinary tract: a 30-year experience in 252 patients. *Urology* 1998;52(4):594–601.
80. Akdogan B, et al. Prognostic significance of bladder tumor history and tumor location in upper tract transitional cell carcinoma. *J Urol* 2006;176(1):48–52.
81. Park S, et al. The impact of tumor location on prognosis of transitional cell carcinoma of the upper urinary tract. *J Urol* 2004;171(2 Pt 1):621–625.
82. Mullerad M, et al. Bladder cancer as a prognostic factor for upper tract transitional cell carcinoma. *J Urol* 2004;172(6 Pt 1):2177–2181.
83. Catto JW, et al. Promoter hypermethylation is associated with tumor location, stage, and subsequent progression in transitional cell carcinoma. *J Clin Oncol* 2005; 23(13):2903–2910. Epub 2005 Mar 7.
84. DiBiase SJ, et al. Palliative irradiation for focally symptomatic metastatic renal cell carcinoma: support for dose escalation based on a biological model. *J Urol* 1997;158(3 Pt 1):746–749.
85. Zelefsky MJ, et al. Tumor control outcomes after hypofractionated and single-dose stereotactic image-guided intensity-modulated radiotherapy for extracranial metastases from renal cell carcinoma. *Int J Radiat Oncol Biol Phys* 2012;82(5):1744–1748.
86. National Comprehensive Cancer Network. Kidney cancer. In: *NCCN clinical practice guidelines in oncology 2012,* Version 1.2013. Available at: http://www.nccn.org/professionals/physician_gls/pdf/kidney.pdf.
87. Gill IS, et al. Adrenal involvement from renal cell carcinoma: predictive value of computerized tomography. *J Urol* 1994;152(4):1082–1085.
88. Blom JH, et al. Radical nephrectomy with and without lymph-node dissection: final results of European Organization for Research and Treatment of Cancer (EORTC) randomized phase 3 trial 30881. *Eur Urol* 2009;55(1):28–34.
89. Hollingsworth JM, et al. Surgical management of low-stage renal cell carcinoma: technology does not supersede biology. *Urology* 2006;67(6):1175–1180.
90. Leibovich BC, et al. Nephron sparing surgery for appropriately selected renal cell carcinoma between 4 and 7 cm results in outcome similar to radical nephrectomy. *J Urol* 2004;171(3):1066–1070.
91. Weight CJ, et al. Nephrectomy induced chronic renal insufficiency is associated with increased risk of cardiovascular death and death from any cause in patients with localized cT1b renal masses. *J Urol* 2010;183(4):1317–1323.
92. Weight CJ, et al. Partial nephrectomy is associated with improved overall survival compared to radical nephrectomy in patients with unanticipated benign renal tumours. *Eur Urol* 2010;58(2):293–298.
93. Lau WK, et al. Matched comparison of radical nephrectomy vs nephron-sparing surgery in patients with unilateral renal cell carcinoma and a normal contralateral kidney. *Mayo Clin Proc* 2000;75(12):1236–1242.
94. McKiernan J, et al. Natural history of chronic renal insufficiency after partial and radical nephrectomy. *Urology* 2002;59(6):816–820.
97. Whang M, et al. The incidence of multifocal renal cell carcinoma in patients who are candidates for partial nephrectomy. *J Urol* 1995;154(3):968–970; discussion 970–971.
98. Bennett RT, et al. Cytoreductive surgery for stage IV renal cell carcinoma. *J Urol* 1995;154(1):32–34.
101. Kunkle DA, Uzzo RG. Cryoablation or radiofrequency ablation of the small renal mass: a meta-analysis. *Cancer* 2008;113(10):2671–2680.
102. Beitler JJ, et al. Definitive, high-dose-per-fraction, conformal, stereotactic external radiation for renal cell carcinoma. *Am J Clin Oncol* 2004;27(6):646–648.
103. Wersall PJ, et al. Extracranial stereotactic radiotherapy for primary and metastatic renal cell carcinoma. *Radiother Oncol* 2005;77(1):88–95. Epub 2005 Jun 20.
104. Ponsky LE, et al. Renal radiosurgery: initial clinical experience with histological evaluation. *Surg Innov* 2007;14(4):265–269.
105. Svedman C, et al. Stereotactic body radiotherapy of primary and metastatic renal lesions for patients with only one functioning kidney. *Acta Oncol* 2008;47(8):1578–1583.
106. Van der Werf-Messing B. Proceedings: carcinoma of the kidney. *Cancer* 1973;32(5): 1056–1061.
107. Van der Werf-Messing B, van der Heul RO, Ledeboer RC. Renal cell carcinoma trial. *Strahlentherapie [Sonderb]* 1981;76:169–715.
108. Juusela H, et al. Preoperative irradiation in the treatment of renal adenocarcinoma. *Scand J Urol Nephrol* 1977;11(3):277–281.
109. Fugitt RB, Wu GS, Martinelli LC. An evaluation of postoperative radiotherapy in hypernephroma treatment—a clinical trial. *Cancer* 1973;32(6):1332–1340.
110. Kjaer M, Frederiksen PL, Engelholm SA. Postoperative radiotherapy in stage II and III renal adenocarcinoma. A randomized trial by the Copenhagen Renal Cancer Study Group. *Int J Radiat Oncol Biol Phys* 1987;13(5):665–672.
111. Aref I, Bociek RG, Salhani D. Is post-operative radiation for renal cell carcinoma justified? *Radiother Oncol* 1997;43(2):155–157.
112. Yossepowitch O, et al. Positive surgical margins at partial nephrectomy: predictors and oncological outcomes. *J Urol* 2008;179(6):2158–2163.
113. Tunio MA, Hashmi A, Rafi M. Need for a new trial to evaluate postoperative radiotherapy in renal cell carcinoma: a meta-analysis of randomized controlled trials. *Ann Oncol* 2010;21(9):1839–1845.
114. Flanigan RC, et al. Cytoreductive nephrectomy in patients with metastatic renal cancer: a combined analysis. *J Urol* 2004;171(3):1071–1076.
115. Polcari AJ, et al. The role of cytoreductive nephrectomy in the era of molecular targeted therapy. *Int J Urol* 2009;16(3):227–233.
116. Motzer RJ, et al. Overall survival and updated results for sunitinib compared with interferon alfa in patients with metastatic renal cell carcinoma. *J Clin Oncol* 2009; 27(22):3584–3590.
117. Sternberg CN, et al. Pazopanib in locally advanced or metastatic renal cell carcinoma: results of a randomized phase III trial. *J Clin Oncol* 2010;28(6):1061–1068.
118. Escudier B, et al. Bevacizumab plus interferon alfa-2a for treatment of metastatic renal cell carcinoma: a randomised, double-blind phase III trial. *Lancet* 2007;370(9605):2103–2111.
119. Escudier B, et al. Sorafenib for treatment of renal cell carcinoma: final efficacy and safety results of the phase III treatment approaches in renal cancer global evaluation trial. *J Clin Oncol* 2009;27(20):3312–3318.
120. Escudier B, et al. Sorafenib in advanced clear-cell renal-cell carcinoma. *N Engl J Med* 2007;356(2):125–134.
121. Motzer RJ, et al. Phase 3 trial of everolimus for metastatic renal cell carcinoma: final results and analysis of prognostic factors. *Cancer* 2010;116(18):4256–4265.
124. Piltz S, et al. Long-term results after pulmonary resection of renal cell carcinoma metastases. *Ann Thorac Surg* 2002;73(4):1082–1087.
125. Zerbi A, et al. Pancreatic metastasis from renal cell carcinoma: which patients benefit from surgical resection? *Ann Surg Oncol* 2008;15(4):1161–1168.
126. Rades D, Heisterkamp C, Schild SE. Do patients receiving whole-brain radiotherapy for brain metastases from renal cell carcinoma benefit from escalation of the radiation dose? *Int J Radiat Oncol Biol Phys* 2010;78(2):398–403.
127. Shuto T, et al. Treatment strategy for metastatic brain tumors from renal cell carcinoma: selection of gamma knife surgery or craniotomy for control of growth and peritumoral edema. *J Neurooncol* 2010;98(2):169–175.
128. Kim WH, et al. Early significant tumor volume reduction after radiosurgery in brain metastases from renal cell carcinoma results in long-term survival. *Int J Radiat Oncol Biol Phys* 2012;82(5):1749–1755.
129. Kano H, et al. Outcome predictors of gamma knife radiosurgery for renal cell carcinoma metastases. *Neurosurgery* 2011;69(6):1232–1239.
132. Lee J, et al. A phase II trial of palliative radiotherapy for metastatic renal cell carcinoma. *Cancer* 2005;104(9):1894–1900.
134. Gay HA, et al. Complete response in a cutaneous facial metastatic nodule from renal cell carcinoma after hypofractionated radiotherapy. *Dermatol Online J* 2007;13(4):6.
135. Stinauer MA, et al. Stereotactic body radiation therapy for melanoma and renal cell carcinoma: impact of single fraction equivalent dose on local control. *Radiat Oncol* 2011;6(1):34.
136. Greco C, et al. Predictors of local control after single-dose stereotactic image-guided intensity-modulated radiotherapy for extracranial metastases. *Int J Radiat Oncol Biol Phys* 2011;79(4):1151–1157.
137. Nguyen Q-N, et al. Management of spinal metastases from renal cell carcinoma using stereotactic body radiotherapy. *Int J Radiat Oncol Biol Phys* 2010; 76(4):1185–1192.
138. Mitera G, et al. Preoperative stereotactic body radiotherapy to a skull renal cell metastasis: an alternative to preoperative embolization? *J Palliat Med* 2011;14(2): 157–160.
139. Wersall PJ, et al. Regression of non-irradiated metastases after extracranial stereotactic radiotherapy in metastatic renal cell carcinoma. *Acta Oncol* 2006; 45(4):493–497.
140. National Comprehensive Cancer Network. Bladder cancer. In: *NCCN clinical practice guidelines in oncology 2012,* Version 1.2013 Available at: http://www.nccn.org/professionals/physician_gls/pdf/bladder.pdf.
141. Audenet F, et al. The role of chemotherapy in the treatment of urothelial cell carcinoma of the upper urinary tract (UUT-UCC). *Urol Oncol* 2010 Sep 28. [Epub ahead of print].
143. Cozad SC, et al. Adjuvant radiotherapy in high stage transitional cell carcinoma of the renal pelvis and ureter. *Int J Radiat Oncol Biol Phys* 1992;24(4):743–745.
144. Chen B, et al. Radiotherapy may improve overall survival of patients with T3/T4 transitional cell carcinoma of the renal pelvis or ureter and delay bladder tumour relapse. *BMC Cancer* 2011;11(1):297.
145. Catton CN, et al. Transitional cell carcinoma of the renal pelvis and ureter; outcome and patterns of relapse in patients treated with postoperative radiation. *Urol Oncol* 1996;2:171–176.
148. Czito B, et al. Adjuvant radiotherapy with and without concurrent chemotherapy for locally advanced transitional cell carcinoma of the renal pelvis and ureter. *J Urol* 2004;172(4 Pt 1):1271–1275.
149. Dawson LA, et al. Radiation-associated kidney injury. *Int J Radiat Oncol Biol Phys* 2010;76(3 Suppl):S108–S115.
150. Kavanagh BD, et al. Radiation dose-volume effects in the stomach and small bowel. *Int J Radiat Oncol Biol Phys* 2010;76(3 Suppl):S101–S107.
151. Pan CC, et al. Radiation-associated liver injury. *Int J Radiat Oncol Biol Phys* 2010;76(3 Suppl):S94–S100.
155. Van Sornsen de Koste JR, et al. Renal mobility during uncoached quiet respiration: an analysis of 4DCT scans. *Int J Radiat Oncol Biol Phys* 2006;64(3):799–803.
157. Stein M, et al. The value of postoperative irradiation in renal cell cancer. *Radiother Oncol* 1992;24(1):41–44.
158. Gay HA, et al. Isodose-based methodology for minimizing the morbidity and mortality of thoracic hypofractionated radiotherapy. *Radiother Oncol* 2009; 91(3):369–378.
159. Lam JS, et al. Postoperative surveillance protocol for patients with localized and locally advanced renal cell carcinoma based on a validated prognostic nomogram and risk group stratification system. *J Urol* 2005;174(2):466–472; discussion 472; quiz 801.

Chapter 64
Bladder Cancer

Nicholas James, Richard T. Bryan, Richard Viney, Prashant Patel, and Syed A. Hussain

The basic management of bladder tumors has remained essentially unchanged for over 50 years, and in spite of its importance in terms of incidence, prognosis, and cost, bladder cancer research remains significantly underfunded.[1] Every aspect of the perceptions and management of this disease requires change; departing from the use of the term "superficial" bladder cancer is just the first step,[2] because the term is both inaccurate and implies an inappropriate lack of importance. In particular, given the very high costs to health care systems from long-term surveillance and treatment of the disease,[3] it is particularly surprising that there has not been more emphasis on the disease from health policymakers and pharmaceutical companies.

In addition, a rethinking of the view that cystectomy is the gold standard for invasive bladder cancer is long overdue. Comparisons of large surgical[4] and radiotherapy[5] series suggest very similar long-term survival rates, and population-based studies do not appear to show any survival differences linked to the mode of treatment.[6] Furthermore, most large surgical series have median ages in the mid-60s,[4,7] well below the (rising) disease population median, suggesting the results may not be applicable to many or even most patients with invasive bladder cancer. Use of bladder preservation varies worldwide from around 10% in the United States[8] to 25% in Scandinavia[9] to around 50% in the United Kingdom.[10] Moreover, there is good evidence that older or less fit patients in low-volume centers are less likely to be referred for surgery, despite the likelihood of them being fit for radiotherapy.[8,9]

In contrast, recent large randomized radiotherapy series from the United Kingdom suggest that radical radiotherapy with sensitization, either with low-dose chemotherapy[11] or with hypoxia-targeting agents,[12] is effective and well tolerated by elderly patients (median age in both studies was 72 to 73 years). Long-term functional outcomes with radiotherapy are excellent,[11–13] making it particularly suitable for less-fit patients who may struggle with major surgery or a urinary diversion.

This chapter outlines the evidence base for the current therapeutic approaches to bladder cancer and in particular will examine the proposition that bladder preservation for muscle-invasive disease is an approach that merits re-examination.

ANATOMY OF THE BLADDER

The bladder is a hollow, muscular organ situated in the pelvis when empty but able to extend up into the abdomen when full, particularly in situations where bladder emptying is impeded. At birth, the pelvis is relatively small in comparison to the abdomen, and thus the bladder has a larger abdominal component at birth and becomes more "pelvic" as growth and maturity proceed. By puberty, the bladder has migrated to the confines of the deepened true pelvis.

The bladder is described as having an apex, a superior surface, two inferolateral surfaces, a base or posterior surface, a trigone, and a neck. The apex reaches a short distance cephalad above the pubic bone and ends as a fibrous cord, the remnant of the fetal urachus, which connects the bladder to the allantois. The urachus lies anterior to the peritoneal cavity and is important as tumors can arise in the urachal remnant. The superior surface is covered by the peritoneum, again an important anatomical feature as it means that there is bowel lying superiorly to the bladder, which is potentially a critical site to consider when planning radiotherapy, particularly in men. In women it is associated with the uterus and ileum. The base of the bladder is posterior and is separated from the rectum by the vas deferens, seminal vesicles, and ureters in the male, and by the uterus and vagina in the female. The seminal vesicles form a V-shaped structure at the base of the bladder, with the vas deferens entering the middle of the "V." The ureters enter into the bladder slightly superior and lateral to the seminal vesicles, with the vas deferens coursing above and in a caudal direction to the ureters. Again these relations are critical as enlarging tumors either at the base or in the prostate can involve the ureters with consequent hydronephrosis. Inferiorly and laterally to the bladder lie the various pelvic bones and muscles: pubis, the levator ani, and obturator internus muscles. Within the pelvis, the lateral parts of the bladder are surrounded by loose connective tissue. Anteriorly the bladder is separated from the pubic bone by the retropubic space. The inferior part of the bladder is described as the neck and is in continuity with the urethra and, very importantly, the prostate gland in males. The neck of the bladder is anchored in the pelvis, and the superior portions distend and expand upward as the bladder fills.

The mucosal lining of the bladder comprises a transitional epithelium that extends from the renal pelvis to the urethra. The most common tumors arising in the urinary system are transition cell (or urothelial) carcinomas (TCC or UC). These tumors can arise from anywhere within the urothelium, so diagnosis, treatment, and surveillance protocols must take account of this important biological feature. As a distensible organ, the macroscopic appearance of the urothelium varies with distension from smooth and flat to folded when empty. A ridge called the interureteral fold lies between the ureteric orifices.

EPIDEMIOLOGY

Bladder cancer, with over 385,000 new cases reported worldwide in 2008,[14] is a major cause of cancer morbidity and mortality (Table 64.1). Median age at diagnosis is above 70 years and, as the tumor is often smoking related, many patients have significant comorbidity, posing risks for radical surgical approaches. Survival rates are poor, with around 45% of muscle-invasive cancer patients surviving 5 years irrespective of treatment modality.[4,5,7] Demographically, the industrializing nations will contribute to a significant rise in the global incidence of bladder UC,[15] with particularly large numbers likely in China given the rapid improvement in standards of living and the high prevalence of smoking. However, despite the decreasing incidence in developed nations, there remain

TABLE 64.1 2008 UROLOGICAL CANCER INCIDENCE AND MORTALITY WORLDWIDE

Cancer Site	Cases	All Cases (%)	Deaths	All Deaths (%)
Prostate	899,102	7.1	258,133	3.4
Bladder	382,660	3.0	150,282	2.0
Kidney	273,518	2.2	116,368	1.5
Testis	52,323	0.4	9,874	0.1
All cancers	12,662,554		7,564,802	

Data from GLOBOCAN http://globocan.iarc.fr.

specific challenges, mainly due to the aging population and increased life-expectancy. Within two large cohorts separated by 15 years (1991 to 1992 and 2005 to 2010), researchers have recently demonstrated an increase in the median age at presentation of 4 years, with an increase from 13% to 24% in the proportion of patients over 80 years old.[16] Overall around 75% to 80% of patients with bladder cancer are male, mostly reflecting historic trends in cigarette smoking.

There are well-known associations of squamous cell bladder carcinomas with bilharzia caused by *Schistosoma haematobium* infection in Africa, particularly in Egypt.[17] Aromatic amines, polycyclic aromatic and chlorinated hydrocarbons, arsenic-laced drinking water, aristolochic acid, cyclophosphamide exposure, and a range of industrial chemicals have been implicated in urothelial carcinogenesis. Importantly, as with most carcinogens, there are variations in individual susceptibility, and the basis of some of these polymorphisms regulating varied detoxification mechanisms has been identified.[18] With increasing awareness of these industrial associations, regulation of these processes means that these cases are becoming increasingly rare in the developed world. Their principal importance now is that those with industrially linked tumors may be entitled to compensation payments. In Egypt there have been successful public health approaches to the control of *S. haematobium* infections, leading to a substantial decline in incidence and mortality from squamous carcinomas of the bladder.[19]

Within the developed world, the overwhelming majority of bladder tumors are now TCCs, and the main known causative factor is tobacco (particularly cigarette) smoking,[20,21–22,23–25] explaining approximately half of the cases in men and one-third of the cases in women in Europe (discussed in detail below). The relation between smoking and other prognostic factors is interesting, as it could give insight into biological mechanisms of disease and, perhaps more importantly, have clinical implications by increasing our ability to identify patients at risk of more malignant disease.

NATURAL HISTORY

Non-muscle-Invasive Bladder Cancer

Most cases (70% to 80%) present with non-muscle-invasive bladder cancer (NMIBC, stage Ta, T1, and carcinoma *in situ* [Tis]), which is rarely lethal, but shows a high recurrence rate of 50% to 70% after treatment by transurethral resection of the bladder tumor (TURBT).[26] In about 10% to 20% of patients with NMIBC, the disease progresses to muscle invasion (≥T2 lesions), which can lead to metastasis and death.[26] However, the majority of patients with NMIBC will die of other causes, given the typically advanced age at presentation and the strong association with cigarette smoking,[20,21–22,23–25] although it is worth noting that up to 21% of patients with Ta tumors and 49% of patients with T1 tumors will die from bladder cancer.[27] For patients with NMIBC, it has been observed that tumor grade and stage, and also tumor number, size, presence of carcinoma *in situ* (CIS), recurrence rate, and age at diagnosis are risk factors of progression.[28–29,30] The risk of both recurrence and progression necessitates lifelong follow-up for patients with bladder tumors. However, there are factors that predict a higher risk of progression (to invasion) as opposed to recurrence in lower risk tumors, and the European Organisation for Research and Treatment of Cancer (EORTC) "bladder cancer calculator" quantifies the risk depending on the tumor characteristics imputed.[30]

Invasive Disease

Muscle-invasive bladder cancer has a poor prognosis due to a very high rate of occult metastatic disease at the time of diagnosis. Evidence for this comes from the high rate of death from metastasis after apparently successful surgery. Furthermore, reported 5-year survival rates with radiotherapy or surgery are remarkably similar at around 45% to 50%,[4,5] despite a higher rate of pelvic recurrence after radiotherapy versus surgery, suggesting that prognosis is driven by the presence or otherwise of metastases at the time of diagnosis, driven by tumor-related factors such as stage and grade.[6]

Metastatic Disease

A minority of patients (probably <10%) present with metastatic disease; most patients with metastatic disease have had prior treatment for apparently localized disease. Metastatic disease carries a poor prognosis. Overall survival from diagnosis of metastasis is difficult to ascertain as many patients receive only palliative treatment. A minority of patients are fit for systemic chemotherapy, and there are good data on outcomes with chemotherapy. In essence, extensive randomized studies, mostly carried out in the 1980s and 1990s, have demonstrated the superiority of cisplatinum-based combinations over those containing other drugs or cisplatinum alone.[31] Of the platinum-based combinations, methotrexate/vinblastine/doxorubicin (Adriamycin)/cisplatinum (MVAC)[32] and gemcitabine/cisplatinum (GC)[33] have proven to be superior to other combinations and broadly similar in efficacy to each other[34,35] (as reviewed by Hussain and James[36]). Median survival is 12 to 18 months, depending on the extent of disease and fitness of the patient. Intriguingly, however, a small minority of patients do appear to survive long term after chemotherapy for metastatic disease, but this percentage has sadly proved very hard to increase from that originally observed in the MVAC trials.

ETIOLOGY

The link between occupational exposure and an increased risk of urothelial cancer of the bladder was established more than a century ago when Rehn[37] reported on three cases of bladder cancer in a German chemical dye works in 1895.[38] During the following 40 years, similar reports appeared from around the world.[39] In 1938, Hueper et al.[39] demonstrated that when naphthylamine, an industrial arylamine used in the synthetic dye industry, was fed to dogs, it caused bladder carcinomas identical to the human disease. The link between industrial arylamines and bladder cancer was thus established and later confirmed by Case et al.[40] in 1954. These authors also identified an excess of bladder cancer in the tire industry, attributable to the use of 2-naphthylamine in the manufacture of rubber.[38,40] Around this time the "o-aminophenol hypothesis" of arylamine-induced human bladder cancer was proposed, suggesting that conjugation of aromatic amines by the liver and excretion in the urine with subsequent urinary reactions would liberate the carcinogen o-aminophenol.[41] Other workers later added to this hypothesis: arylamines are hydroxylated in the liver and conjugated with glucuronic acid, followed by excretion into urine and reliberalization of the active carcinogenic metabolite into the bladder lumen by urinary glucuronidases.[38,42,43] Slow acetylation by *N*-acetyltransferase, an enzyme involved in the metabolism of arylamines, has been shown to be a contributory risk factor for bladder carcinogenesis.[20,44,45]

Due to the widespread use of arylamines in textile dyes, hair dyes, and paint pigments, a number of high-risk occupations have been identified, including chemical, dye, textile, and rubber workers and painters and hairstylists.[21,46–48] In addition, the presence of various arylamines in tobacco smoke means that a significant proportion of bladder cancer cases can be attributed to cigarette smoking.[20,21–22,23–25] In fact, abandonment of the manufacture of many of these arylamines in the latter half of the 20th century means that smoking is currently the single most important cause of urothelial cancer.[24,25,49–51] Tobacco (particularly cigarette) smoking now explains approximately half of bladder cancer cases in men and one-third of cases in women in Europe. It has been demonstrated that an increased smoking frequency and duration and a lower age at initiation are associated with an increased risk of bladder cancer, while cessation seems to reduce the risk.[49] The relation between smoking and other prognostic factors is interesting, as it could give insight into biological mechanisms of disease and, perhaps more importantly, have clinical implications by increasing the ability to identify patients at risk of more malignant disease. Cigarette smoking also appears to be a risk factor for disease recurrence following a diagnosis of bladder UC,[49,52] although due to a lack of conclusive evidence, there is currently a low rate of physicians providing smoking cessation assistance.[49]

Studies also demonstrate a relation between *N*-acetyltransferase-2 slow acetylators and cigarette smoking, resulting in a further increase in the risk of bladder cancer, especially in those individuals with a high smoking intensity.[53–55] A similar relation has also been demonstrated with arylamine exposure.[56,57] A number of other susceptibility loci have also been identified, although such markers do not yet have sufficient discriminatory ability to be utilized for risk prediction in the general population or for prediction or prognostication in patients diagnosed with bladder cancer.[54,58,59]

CHRONIC INFLAMMATION AND BLADDER CANCER

Squamous metaplasia is considered a precursor of squamous cell carcinoma of the bladder and is a relatively common occurrence, especially on the trigone of the female bladder where a prevalence of up to 50% is reported.[60,61] Experimental evidence suggests that this does not occur by direct transformation of the superficial apical umbrella cells of the urothelium or by their dedifferentiation and redifferentiation; it is postulated that basal cells (probable stem cells) are selectively activated.[60] The normal urothelium is slowly proliferating, but urothelium undergoing squamous metaplasia becomes hyperplastic, and it may be that the hyperplasia component of urothelial squamous metaplasia is a major contributor to an enhanced risk of cancer formation.[60,61]

Squamous cell carcinoma and adenocarcinoma of the bladder often occur in the presence of chronic inflammation. In Africa and the Middle East, where these tumors are much more prevalent, the chronic inflammation occurs as a result of infestation with the parasite *S. haematobium* (bilharziasis), with a bladder carcinoma incidence of 2 to 4 per 100,000 in *S. haematobium* endemic areas.[62,63–67] This infestation can lead to malignancy through local tissue damage, mechanical irritation, bilharzial toxins, secondary bacterial infection, and the production of nitrosamines.[62,68,69] With liver involvement and subsequent liver dysfunction, tryptophan metabolism may be disturbed, resulting in excretion of carcinogenic metabolites.[62] In *S. haematobium* infected individuals, the prevalence of squamous metaplasia rises significantly during the first 10 to 15 years of life, with a plateau at roughly constant levels thereafter (30% to 40% in males and 40% to 50% in females) when the active infection may have subsided.[61] It is suggested that proliferative changes in the bladder urothelium may become independent of ongoing infection after long periods of chronic *S. haematobium*–induced inflammation.[68,69] Severe metaplasia of the bladder may represent a precancerous transformation in some individuals, but in others it may only represent a marker for the prolonged inflammation that is associated with a high cancer risk.[68,69] This sort of proliferative growth combined with the increased excretion or local formation of mutagens in the *S. haematobium*-inflamed bladder may significantly contribute to the onset of cancer formation, possibly involving mutations of the *p53* and *CDKN2* tumor-suppressor genes.[68]

In Europe and North America, the stimulus of chronic bladder inflammation is usually chronic bacterial infection, bladder calculi, or long-term indwelling catheters.[70–73] A number of metaplastic conditions (squamous metaplasia, von Brunn's nests, cystitis cystica, and cystitis glandularis) may occur prior to frank malignant change, although the premalignant nature of some of these lesions is still unclear.[70–79]

Field Cancerization and Clonality

A fundamental characteristic of neoplasia is monoclonality, in which one transformed cell gives rise to daughter cells that all exhibit the same genetic changes that provided the initial growth advantages to the originally transformed parent cell.[80] Further genetic changes accumulate in subsequent daughter cells and provide additional growth advantages.[80] However, TCC behaves as a multifocal disease, often with multiple primary tumors and frequent recurrences that can occur anywhere in the urinary tract from the renal pelvis to the urethra. These observations gave rise to the idea of a "field defect" or "field cancerization," suggesting that the whole urothelium is exposed to the same urinary carcinogens, leading to the transformation of many independent separate urothelial cells and resulting in multiple tumors developing independently in multiple sites. Such tumors are thus genetically unrelated. An alternative explanation is that the multifocality of TCC arises as a result of a single carcinogenic insult to a single cell or group of cells. The progeny or clones of these cells spread throughout the bladder, either through intraepithelial migration or through cell shedding and reimplantation, leading to multiple synchronous and metachronous tumors.[80] These tumors are thus topographically distinct but are genetically related. This is the hypothesis of clonality.

Utilizing the relatively rudimentary technique of X-inactivation,[80,81–82] the early studies in this field appeared to show that the urothelium is derived from a small number of cells (200 to 300), which subsequently develop into larger patches; each patch is clonally related and possesses different predispositions to tumorigenesis.[83] Such stem cell–derived clonal units actively replenish the urothelium during aging.[84] Multiple synchronous and metachronous TCCs in the same patient appear to be clonally related when studied by X-inactivation.[80,82,85–88] However, these studies only provide a 50% probability that one particular TCC is related to the primary TCC, although that probability improves when multiple TCCs are analyzed. Clonal patch size also needs to be taken into consideration, and because of the large patch size of the urothelium (120 mm^2), X-inactivation studies are heavily biased toward demonstrating monoclonality.[81] Ideally, these studies should have taken into account the relation of the tumors to patch boundaries.[81] In addition, DNA methylation patterns change as a natural consequence of aging.[89] Therefore, although X-inactivation studies provided an early insight into the relative importance of the processes of clonality and field cancerization, they cannot be considered as entirely accurate and reliable. Similarly, using immunohistochemistry to study specific *p53* and *pRb* mutations cannot be considered to be wholly reliable for demonstrating monoclonality.

The accuracy of these investigations has been improved by utilizing newer and more sensitive techniques such as comparative genomic hybridization, fluorescence *in situ* hybridization, and loss of heterozygosity studies. These experiments revealed both monoclonality and oligoclonality in synchronous and metachronous TCCs. More recently, research has suggested that a genetic expression profile is established early in bladder tumor development, and that this profile is stable and maintained in recurring tumors.[90–91,92] Majewski et al.[91] matched the clonal allelic losses in distinct chromosomal regions to specific phases of bladder neoplasia: these genetic changes mapped to six regions or "forerunner genes" involved in the early phases of bladder cancer development, representing critical hits driving bladder carcinogenesis. It is suggested that the clonal expansion, over vast expanses of the bladder mucosa, of urothelial cell populations containing losses of forerunner genes may represent the earliest molecular change in bladder carcinogenesis. A further wave of genetic "hits" within subregions of these clonally expanded cells leads to the first microscopically recognizable features of dysplasia, and a third and final wave is associated with the fully transformed phenotype of severe dysplasia or CIS.[91,93] The genetic changes map to six chromosomal regions that are suggested to represent the critical hits driving the development of bladder cancer.[91,93] In addition, Knowles et al.[94] have demonstrated that deletions of chromosome 9 occur in over half of bladder tumors of all grades and stages (9p, 51%; 9q, 57%). Loss of heterozygosity also occurs on 17p (32%), 11p (32%), 8p (23%), 4p (22%), and 13q (15%), and loss of heterozygosity of 5p, 8p, and 21q are significantly associated with worse grade and stage.[94] Genomic copy number alterations are also frequent in bladder TCC, with the most frequent changes involving complete or partial loss of 4q (83%) and gain of 20q (78%).[95] Other frequent losses are of 18q (65%), 8p (65%), 2q (61%), 6q (61%), 3p (56%), 13q (56%), 4p (52%), 6p (52%), 10p (52%), 10q (52%), and 5p (43%).[94]

Taken together, the studies described above show that multifocal TCCs are frequently monoclonal, whereas others show oligoclonality. The evidence for both theories is compelling (as reviewed by Duggan et al.[96]), with evidence supporting both the clonality and field cancerization theories. In reality, these theories are equally valid, with both processes seemingly often occurring simultaneously in the same patient.[86,87] In addition, many of these studies have demonstrated that deletions on chromosome 9p occur most frequently and early in transitional cell carcinogenesis with 17p13 losses (*p53* gene mutations) occurring in more advanced TCCs, shedding some light on the molecular pathology of bladder TCC.

Pathways to Muscle-Invasive and Nonmuscle-Invasive Bladder Cancer

A number of different approaches can be taken to describe the molecular alterations involved in bladder tumorigenesis (TCC). Some authors[97,98] have previously described such pathways in detail based on the six original "hallmarks of cancer" described by Hanahan and Weinberg[99] in 2000. In 2011, Hanahan and Weinberg[100] updated their original landmark review, describing genome instability and inflammation as underlying these hallmark changes and proposed "reprogramming of energy metabolism" and "evading immune destruction" as two emerging hallmarks with potential for generality. In addition, they reported that tumors exhibit another dimension of complexity by containing a repertoire of recruited, ostensibly normal cells that contribute to the acquisition of hallmark traits by creating the "tumor microenvironment."[100] The particular timing and sequence of hallmark events can vary widely between tumors of the same type and within the same tumor, but ultimately these hallmark capabilities of cancer will be reached.[99] In their 2011 update, Hanahan and Weinberg[100] also introduce the concept of "cancer stem cells," a concept that has existed for quite some time for hematopoietic malignancies.[101,102] Cancer stem cells are a subset of tumor cells that have the ability to self-renew and to generate all of the heterogeneous cells that comprise a tumor (properties that are analogous to a stem cell, the original cell of an organ, and responsible for organogenesis and organ maintenance).[101,103–106] It is proposed that these cells are responsible for tumorigenesis, tumor differentiation, tumor maintenance, tumor spread, and tumor relapse.[101,103–106] In the setting of bladder cancer, cancer stem cells appear to play a role in a subset of tumors, but their true significance has yet to be clarified.[104]

A number of other authors have also reviewed this field in detail,[107–112] and there is general consensus on a divergent pathway for the development of Ta/T1 disease and Tcis/T2+ disease, as illustrated in Figure 64.1. Significant contributions to work in this field have been made by Knowles et al.[110,113–119] (Leeds, UK); in their 2010 review, Goebell and Knowles[113] propose a third hypothetical pathway for the development of high-grade papillary tumors.

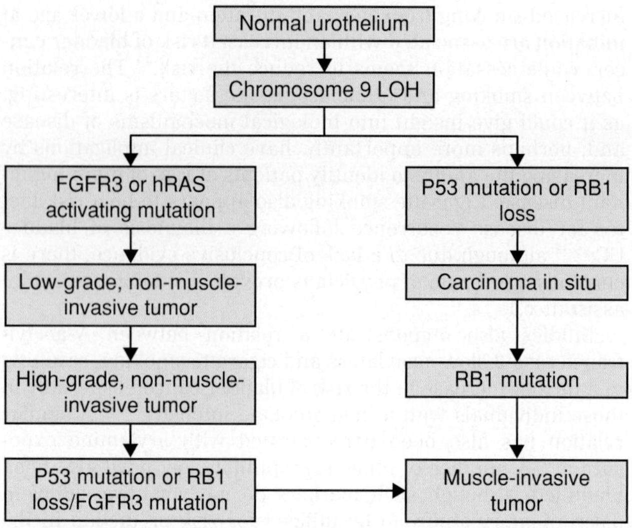

FIGURE 64.1. Pathways to development of bladder cancer. (Data from Pollard C, Smith SC, Theodorescu D. Molecular genesis of non-muscle-invasive urothelial carcinoma (NMIUC). *Expert Rev Mol Med* 2010;12:e10.)

A detailed examination of these pathways and related biomarkers is beyond the scope of this chapter. In addition, this is a rapidly changing field and new developments appear frequently with the advent of high-throughput experimental platforms, including "deep sequencing,"[120] proteomics,[121,122] and metabolomics,[123] so readers are directed to the reviews cited above or to the latest work in this field.

SYMPTOMS AND SIGNS

The typical presenting symptoms of bladder cancer include painless, visible hematuria, infection, and storage symptoms. As the first of these is typically transient and the latter two are also attributable to prostate problems, patients often go undiagnosed for considerable periods.[27] Given the intermittent nature of the hematuria associated with bladder cancer, patients presenting with a convincing episode of hematuria require urgent assessment. Similar considerations apply to male patients with a urinary tract infection. Female patients present a more difficult problem due to the higher incidence of urinary infection and the lower risk of bladder cancer. Hematuria is also more likely to be misinterpreted in women of childbearing age.

INVESTIGATION OF PATIENTS WITH BLADDER CANCER

This section is divided into the investigation of patients with suspected bladder cancer and the subsequent staging of those with an established diagnosis.

Suspected Bladder Cancer

In developed countries, most patients will be referred to some sort of rapid access hematuria or suspected bladder cancer clinic. A minority may present via other routes (e.g., gynecological clinics) or with metastatic symptoms (<10%). Hematuria clinics will generally include a clinical assessment, full blood count and biochemical profile, prostate-specific antigen (if indicated), urine cytological examination, flexible cystoscopy, and some sort of imaging of the urothelium (e.g., ultrasound, intravenous urogram, or computed tomography [CT] urogram), which will vary with local practice and facilities.[124,125] Patients identified as having a bladder tumor on flexible cystoscopy will then require further investigations to stage the disease.

Staging Bladder Cancer

The next stage for most patients will be an examination under anesthetic coupled with TURBT. The presence or absence of a mass after TURBT is also an important prognostic factor as it potentially indicates either unsuccessful clearance of tumor, extravesical extension, or both. This serves as both definitive staging of the bladder lesion as well as a substantial proportion of the initial treatment. Pathological review of the resected specimen will ascertain whether muscle invasion is present or not and whether there is CIS; these are the key determinants of further investigation and treatment. Patients with NMIBC, including CIS, do not usually require detailed further imaging, and treatment and surveillance are primarily by intravesical means. The main exception to this is patients with either extensive CIS or grade 3 lesions for whom additional cross-sectional imaging may be warranted. Patients with muscle-invasive bladder cancer (MIBC) will require detailed cross-sectional staging with CT or magnetic resonance imaging (MRI) of the chest, abdomen, and pelvis. If there are any features suggestive of bone metastasis (e.g., raised alkaline phosphatase, bone pain), an isotope bone scan will be indicated in addition.

A major confounding factor with imaging in bladder cancer is the effect of TURBT on the interpretation of the extent of the primary bladder tumor. Recent TURBT will cause perivesical changes that may be interpreted as extravesical spread. For similar reasons, enlarged pelvic nodes may be related to reactive rather than metastatic effects. On the other hand, changes such as infiltration of adjacent organs or hydronephrosis are likely to be reliable indicators of tumor stage and poor prognosis.

STAGING SYSTEM

The 2010 version of the UICC International Union Against Cancer's TNM system is the current, internationally used staging system,[126] and it is based on the size and extent of the primary tumor (T stage), presence or absence of nodal (N), and metastatic (M) spread (Table 64.2). The TNM stage must be used in conjunction with the pathological assessment of tumor removed at TURBT to decide on optimal therapy. Disappointingly, despite a substantial volume of research, no biomarkers have yet established themselves in clinical practice as either prognostic or predictive markers as has happened, for example, with estrogen-receptor or *HER2* status in breast cancer. It is hoped that the wider availability of high throughput systems such as proteomics, in-depth sequencing, and others to be developed will allow the development of such markers in the future.

PATHOLOGY

In excess of 90% of bladder cancers are transitional cell carcinomas. Of the remainder, around 5% are squamous, although it should be noted that squamous differentiation is often present in poorly differentiated TCCs, so the extent to which these are genuinely distinct is open to question. As already noted, infestation with *S. haematobium* can lead to squamous cell carcinoma, but this is rapidly decreasing due to eradication programs. Small cell carcinoma is rare but important as it is generally very chemosensitive and treatment tends to follow schedules adapted from treating small cell lung cancer. Other tumor types include melanoma, carcinosarcoma, and adenocarcinoma (particularly in the urachal remnant). Typically bladder TCCs will be graded using the standard TNM system of Gx (cannot be assessed) then G1 through to G3 (well through to poorly differentiated).[127] CIS will frequently be found in addition to a tumor mass and critically affects treatment choices.

TABLE 64.2 TNM CLASSIFICATION OF TUMORS (2009)

Tx	Primary tumor cannot be assessed		
T0	No evidence of primary tumor		
Ta	No invasive papillary carcinoma		
Tis	Carcinoma *in situ:* "Flat tumor"		
T1	Tumor invades subepithelial connective tissue		
T2	Tumor invades muscle T2a Superficial muscle (inner half) T2b Deep muscle (outer half)		
T3	Tumor invades perivesical tissue: T3a microscopically T3b macroscopically (extravesical mass)		
T4	Tumor invades any of the following: prostate stroma, seminal vesicles, uterus, vagina, pelvic wall, abdominal wall T4a Tumor invades prostate, stroma, seminal vesicles, uterus, or vagina T4b Tumor invades pelvis or abdominal wall		
N0 Regional lymph nodes	Defined as nodes of the true pelvis below the bifurcation of the common iliac arteries. Laterality does not affect the N classification.		
Nx	Nodes cannot be assessed		
N0	No lymph node metastasis		
N1	Metastasis in a single lymph node in the true pelvis (hypogastric, obturator, external iliac, or presacral)		
N2	Metastasis in multiple lymph nodes in the true pelvis (hypogastric, obturator, external iliac, or presacral)		
N3	Metastasis in a common iliac lymph node(s)		
M–Distant Metastasis			
Mx	Cannot be assessed		
M0	No distant metastasis		
M1	Distant metastasis present		
Stage Grouping			
Stage 0a	Ta	N0	M0
Stage 0is	Tis	N0	M0
Stage I	T1	N0	M0
Stage II	T2a,b	N0	M0
Stage III	T3a,b	N0	M0
	T4a	N0	M0
Stage IV	T4b	N0	M0
	Any T	N1, 2, 3	M0
	Any T	Any N	M1

From UICC International Union Against Cancer. *TNM classification of malignant tumours,* 7th ed. Hoboken, NJ: Wiley-Blackwell, 2009, with permission.

TREATMENT OF BLADDER CANCER

Non-muscle-Invasive Bladder Cancer

Around 80% of patients with bladder cancer present with non-muscle-invasive disease. These are classified as Tis, Ta, and T1 by the TMN classification system. The gold standard for diagnosis is the resection of the lesion with adequate sampling of the detrusor muscle deep to the lesion (TURBT). This will give tissue for accurate staging of the bladder lesion as well as definitive treatment for the lesion. Recurrences after TURBT are found in up to 70% of patients undergoing surveillance, and, more importantly, up to 15% of patients on surveillance will progress to muscle-invasive bladder cancer. At the time of diagnosis, the upper urinary tract also needs assessment. This can be done with intravenous urography, CT urography or ultrasound. The incidence of upper tract tumors at the time of presentation with hematuria is only 1.8%, calling into question the use of contrast imaging for the group as a whole.[128] Ultrasound is now being used more frequently, with contrast imaging modalities being used for the higher risk disease.

Prognostication and management strategy are based on accurate initial staging and grading of the disease. There can be variation in the interpretation of pathological specimens, so review of pathology is recommended (European Association of Urology [EAU] guidelines[129]). If there is uncertainty over the pathology, a further early re-resection is indicated. The risk of residual tumor can be as high as 53% in T1 tumors.[130] If the disease is defined as NMIBC, it can be characterized as low, intermediate, or high risk, and this will dictate how the disease is managed (see below). The EORTC bladder cancer calculator provides a valuable online tool for doing this and determining follow-up frequency.[131]

Following resection of the tumor, there is good evidence that a single dose of mitomycin-C administrated into the bladder for 1 hour within 24 hours of surgery will reduce the relative risk of recurrence by 24.2% but will not impact disease progression and disease survival.[132] Recurrences after TURBT are found in up to 70% of patients undergoing surveillance, and up to 15% of patients on surveillance will progress to muscle-invasive bladder cancer. Emerging endoscopic techniques employing photodynamic therapy aimed at improving diagnostic yield and thereby ultimately reducing the rates of recurrence and progression have demonstrated promising results.[133]

Low-risk tumors are single tumors that are <3 cm in diameter are graded as G1 disease and staged as Ta with no evidence of CIS. These tumors have a 15% probability of recurrence and a 0.2% risk of progression at 1 year.[30] These patients should undergo a flexible cystoscopy 3 months after the initial resection, and if this is negative, a flexible cystoscopy should be undertaken 9 months later and then annually thereafter.

Intermediate- and high-risk tumors are defined using a scoring system based on a number of clinical and pathological factors:

a. Number of tumors
b. Tumor size
c. Prior recurrence rate
d. T category
e. Presence of concurrent CIS
f. Tumor grade[131]

The high-risk tumors should be followed up with 3 monthly flexible cystoscopy for 2 years and 6 monthly for a further 5 years and then annually thereafter. Intermediate risk tumors should be followed up using a surveillance regime somewhere between that used for low- and high-risk disease, which is adapted according to personal and subjective factors. The intermediate-risk tumors have up to a 38% probability of recurrence and a 5% risk of progression at 1 year. The high-risk tumors have a 61% probability of recurrence and a 17% risk of progression at 1 year.[30]

The use of flexible cystoscopy with urine cytology is the standard of bladder surveillance. There is ongoing research into improving the sensitivity and specificity of flexible cystoscopy using variations in the wavelength of the light source used (e.g., narrow band imaging). There are a wide number of urinary biomarkers available such as NMP22, UroVysion (Abbott Laboratories, Abbott Park, Illinois), and ImmunoCyt (Scimedx, Denville, New Jersey). These agents suffer from high false-positive rates and variable sensitivity and are costly (as reviewed by Vrooman and Witjes[134]).

The presence of CIS in the bladder carries a 54% risk of disease progression without treatment.[135] Patients with high-risk tumors or CIS should be offered intravesical immunotherapy using bacille Calmette-Guérin (BCG) (EAU and American Urology Association guidelines).[129,136] There are a variety of treatment schedules in the literature, but the authors recommend an intravesical treatment once a week for 6 weeks followed by a subsequent 3 weeks as an induction treatment. If there is no cystoscopic evidence of recurrence, the patient should then be offered ongoing maintenance BCG with 6-week courses of BCG every 3 to 6 months with regular cystoscopic surveillance. In a recent meta-analysis of trials with BCG maintenance, a 32% reduction in the risk of recurrence was seen for BCG compared with mitomycin-C (P <.0001), whereas there was a 28% increase in the risk of recurrence (P = .006) for patients treated with BCG in the trials without BCG maintenance.[137] BCG is a very effective treatment, but not all patients with NMIBC should be treated with BCG due to the risk of toxicity. In a phase III study for NMIBC tumors using maintenance BCG therapy, 20.3% patients stopped BCG due to side effects, mostly local side effects; 68% who stopped due to side effects did so during the first 6 months.[138] The choice of treatment depends on the patients' risk of recurrence and progression based on EORTC subgroups. The use of BCG does not alter the natural course of tumors in the low risk of recurrence subgroup and is therefore considered to be overtreatment. In patients with tumors at high risk of progression, for whom cystectomy is not carried out, BCG including at least 1-year maintenance, is indicated. In patients at intermediate or high risk of recurrence and intermediate risk of progression, BCG with 1-year maintenance is more effective than chemotherapy for prevention of recurrence; however, it has more side effects than chemotherapy. For this reason both BCG with maintenance and intravesical chemotherapy remain options. The final choice should reflect the individual patient's risk of recurrence and progression and the efficacy and side effects of each treatment modality (EAU guidelines). In treatment refractory disease, the patient should be offered radical treatment for the bladder.

Muscle-Invasive, Nonmetastatic Disease

Relative Roles of Cystectomy and Bladder Preservation

Radiotherapy has been used as the primary treatment for muscle-invasive bladder cancer for many years, but utilization rates vary around the world from around 10% in the United States[8] to 25% in Scandinavia[139] to in excess of 50% in the United Kingdom.[10] There are no prospective randomized trials comparing surgery with radiotherapy, so the data on comparative efficacy can only be inferred indirectly. U.S. authors in particular tend to refer to surgery as the gold standard of care, with bladder preservation with radiotherapy (with or without chemotherapy) being viewed as experimental. However, this opinion seems to be based on custom and practice and not on any hard comparative data. It is thus worth examining in some detail the data that exist on this topic. There is a solitary attempt using modern techniques to compare surgery with bladder preservation combining chemotherapy and radiotherapy. The UK SPARE trial (randomized trial of Selective Bladder Preservation against Radical Excision [cystectomy] in muscle-invasive T2/T3 transitional cell carcinoma of the bladder) was a feasibility study that has now closed due to poor recruitment.[140] This phase II and III trial attempted to investigate the potential of using the response to neoadjuvant chemotherapy as a predictive tool for selecting patients for radiotherapy compared with the surgical standard. In the authors' experience, one of the problems with the trial was that the study used response to neoadjuvant chemotherapy to decide on suitability for bladder preservation. However, once this was explained to the patients in the information sheet, there were patients who had a good response but were reluctant to undergo surgery, particularly if the bladder was free of tumor at the interim cystoscopy.

Large population-based studies suggest that the main determinants of survival after diagnosis of bladder cancer are stage, grade, age, and to some extent social class. For example, Hayter et al.[6] studied patterns of care and outcomes in over 20,000 patients with bladder cancer in Ontario. They found significant variations in the use of cystectomy and radiotherapy between different districts but no evidence that these variations led to any differences in long-term outcomes. They concluded that bladder-sparing approaches were equivalent to surgery for invasive bladder cancer.

Another way to compare outcomes between surgery and radiotherapy is to look at large published series. In the United Kingdom, where both of these approaches are routinely employed, it is possible to compare the outcomes in Cancer Registry data. A recent paper from Munro et al.[10] examined outcomes in 458 patients with invasive bladder cancer treated in Yorkshire between 1993 and 1996. The ratio of cystectomy to radiotherapy was 1 to 3, reflecting UK practice at the time. Overall 10-year survival was similar between those who underwent radiotherapy (22%) versus radical cystectomy (24%). Prognostic factors for inferior outcome at 10 years were: female versus male, poor performance status, hydronephrosis and increasing T stage; treatment modality was not a factor in the prognosis.

One of the most widely quoted surgical series comes from the University of Southern California and reports the results of 1,054 patients undergoing cystectomy with overall 5- and 10 year survival rates of 60% and 43%, respectively. This series is discussed in detail below. However, this series included patients undergoing surgery for noninvasive tumors and excluded from the denominator 112 patients referred but deemed incurable at operation. If we look at the 5-year survival of those with invasive tumors, the rate drops to around 47% from the quoted 60%. A contemporary series of radiotherapy cases from Rödel et al.[5] reports 5- and 10-year survivals of 51% and 31% but included patients deemed inoperable.

Furthermore, if we look at the outcomes in the surgical control arm in the US Intergroup Neoadjuvant MVAC trial, the median survival was 38 months and the 5-year survival was 42%. Other relatively contemporary series quote similar 5-year survivals: for example, Dalbagni et al.[141] cite 45% overall and 65% disease-specific survival rates in a series of 300 patients. Furthermore, the only significant prognostic factors in this series were age, T stage, and use or nonuse of neoadjuvant chemotherapy (see the Role of Systemic Therapy section). Data also exist from single institution series with widespread use of both modalities. For example, Kotwal et al.[142] report results on 169 patients treated between March 1996 and December 2000 in Leeds, UK. There were no differences in overall, cause-specific, and distant recurrence-free survival at 5 years between the two groups, despite the radiotherapy group being older (median age, 75.3 vs. 68.2 years). There were 31 local bladder recurrences in the radiotherapy group (24 of which were solitary and hence potentially suitable for salvage surgery), but no significant difference in distant recurrence-free survival. In another more recent (2002 to 2006) cohort, the median age of radiotherapy patients but not the cystectomy patients had increased to 78.4 from 75.3 years, respectively, while the age of those undergoing surgery remained similar at 67.9 and 68.2 years for surgery, consistent with the aging trend in new bladder cancer cases. These authors concluded that although the patients undergoing radical cystectomy were significantly younger than the radiotherapy patients, treatment modality did not influence survival. They went on to state that radical radiotherapy is a viable treatment option for these patients, with the advantage of organ preservation. The data thus suggest that bladder preservation gives equivalent long-term survival to surgery when factors such as case selection are accounted for.

A proportion of patients undergoing radiotherapy will relapse within the bladder and go on to salvage cystectomy. An important consideration, therefore, is whether cystectomy after radiotherapy can be carried out safely and whether the delay compromises survival. Again, there are no randomized data on this topic. However, UK surgeons in particular have good practical experience on this topic and have commented that neither prior chemotherapy nor radiotherapy compromises surgical salvage and that long-term results appear similar to primary cystectomy series.[143,144]

Particularly intriguing in this regard is a comparison of survival rates following primary surgery or salvage surgery following failed radiotherapy from the Christie Hospital in Manchester, UK. The group examined the outcomes in 552 patients who underwent radical cystectomy between 1970 and 2005. Of these, 313 patients underwent primary radical cystectomy and 239 underwent salvage radical cystectomy following radiation failure. The median age was 62.5 years (range, 32.2 to 87.2) for the primary surgical group compared with 65.5 years for the salvage group. Overall 5-year survivals reported were 45.5% for the primary group and 42% for the salvage group, with cause-specific survivals of 51% and 50%, respectively. These differences persisted after stratification for stage, and the authors concluded that a policy of primary radiotherapy with surgical salvage did not compromise the long-term survival chances of patients.[143]

Clearly there are surgical series with much higher survival rates than this in the literature. However, there are two factors accounting for this. One is case selection, the other is that these series are, to a degree, personal, so to publish results that appear inferior to other major centers is potentially a threat to a center's (or surgeon's) reputation and will tend to have a "ratchet" effect on published results. These data also suggest that the predominant prognosis driver in bladder cancer is the presence or absence of distant micrometastasis at diagnosis of invasive disease. The (relatively modest) effect of neoadjuvant chemotherapy tends to bear this out, particularly as the biggest effect in the Medical Research Council (MRC)/EORTC trial was on metastasis-free survival rather than pelvic control rates.[145]

There is little in the way of randomized data on the efficacy of radiotherapy in either nonmuscle-invasive disease or CIS. The only randomized trial on this topic comes from the United Kingdom and compared radiotherapy with surveillance for patients with a new diagnosis of pT1G3 NXM0 transitional cell carcinoma with unifocal disease and no CIS. Patients with multifocal disease or CIS were randomized between intravesical therapy and radiotherapy. There was no evidence of benefit from radiotherapy in terms of progression-free interval (hazard ratio [HR] 1.07; 95% confidence interval [CI], 0.65 to 1.74; $P = .785$), progression-free survival (HR 1.35; 95% CI, 0.92 to 1.98; $P = .133$), or overall survival (HR 1.32; 95% CI, 0.86 to 2.04; $P = .193$).[146] There is thus no indication for radiotherapy in these groups of patients.

In truth, surgery and radiotherapy are not competing, but are complementary approaches to invasive bladder cancer. There are particular groups who appear to do poorly with primary radiotherapy, for example, those with poorly functioning bladders or extensive CIS in addition to their invasive disease. In the former case, radiotherapy is unlikely to improve bladder function; in the latter, the lack of effect of radiotherapy on CIS means that the patient remains at risk of further bladder intervention and ultimately cystectomy.[146] Similar considerations apply to patients with pT1G3 disease.[146] North American authors will also cite features such as hydronephrosis as a contraindication to radiotherapy.[147] However, hydronephrosis is also a poor prognostic factor for surgery and does not help in selecting patients one way or another.[6] On the other hand, there are many patients who may benefit from radical therapy but are poor surgical candidates, such as older patients, the obese, diabetics, poor anesthetic risk patients, or those who may struggle with whatever form of neobladder is fashioned. Although large surgical series will include patients over age 80, these will typically comprise only a few percentage of the total, whereas, with a median age at diagnosis of bladder cancer in the middle to late 70s, there are probably many more who do not make it to surgery.

Surgery

Management of Invasive Bladder Cancer

Although the majority of patients present with NMIBC, 20% to 40% will either present with or ultimately develop muscle-invasive disease. Invasive bladder cancer is a lethal malignancy; if untreated over 85% of patients will die of the disease within 2 years of diagnosis.[148] Furthermore, a certain percentage of patients with high-grade bladder tumors without involvement of the lamina propria will recur or progress or fail intravesical management, and they may be best treated with an earlier cystectomy when survival outcomes are optimal.[149] In these groups of patients, the 5-year survival rates after cystectomy exceed 80%.[150,151]

The rationale for an aggressive treatment approach employing radical cystectomy for high-grade, invasive bladder cancer is based on several important observations. First, the good long-term survival rates, coupled with the lowest local recurrences, are seen following a definitive surgical approach removing the primary bladder tumor and regional lymph nodes.[4,152,153] Although there are no randomized trials comparing radical cystectomy with bladder preserving approaches, surgery remains the preferred treatment option for many clinicians for advanced, localized invasive bladder cancer.[154] Second, the morbidity and mortality of radical cystectomy has substantially improved over the past several decades.[152,155] Third, advocates say that radical cystectomy provides accurate pathologic staging of the primary bladder tumor (p stage) and regional lymph nodes, thus, selectively determining the need for adjuvant therapy based on precise pathologic evaluation. However, it should be noted that the evidence base for adjuvant (as opposed to neoadjuvant) therapy is rather weak (see on the Role of Systemic Therapy section). For the above-mentioned reasons, radical cystectomy has become a standard form of therapy for high-grade, invasive bladder cancer. Nonetheless, many articles on cystectomy emphasize the need for careful patient selection to achieve optimal results. Although this is undoubtedly true, it begs the question of what should be done with patients who do not meet these stringent selection standards but still need to be treated. This issue is rarely, if ever, addressed in cystectomy series publications.

The evolution and improvements in lower urinary tract reconstruction, particularly orthotopic diversion, have been major components in enhancing the quality of life of patients requiring cystectomy. Currently, most men and women can safely undergo orthotopic lower urinary tract reconstruction to the native, intact urethra following cystectomy,[156] although availability varies worldwide. Orthotopic reconstruction aims to mimic the native bladder in location and function, provides a continent means to store urine, and allows volitional voiding per urethra, although patients need to do this by coordinating opening the sphincter with a Valsalva maneuver, which does require training. The orthotopic neobladder eliminates the need for a cutaneous stoma, urostomy appliance, and the need for intermittent catheterization in most cases. These efforts have improved the quality of life of patients who require removal of their bladders and have also stimulated patients and physicians to consider radical cystectomy at an earlier more curable stage for high-grade, invasive bladder cancer.[157,158]

A dedicated effort has been made to improve the surgical technique of radical cystectomy and to provide an acceptable form of urinary diversion, without compromise of a sound cancer operation.[158,159] Timing of cystectomy after the TURBT is important, and it has been demonstrated that a delay of more than 3 months undermines patient survival. This evidence forms the basis to negotiating resource needs with health care providers.[160,161] Certain technical issues regarding radical cystectomy and an appropriate lymph node dissection are critical to minimize local recurrence and positive surgical margins and to maximize cancer-specific survival.[162] Attention to surgical detail is important in optimizing the successful functional outcomes of orthotopic diversion by preserving the urinary sphincter mechanism and therefore continence. Finally, the observed associations between hospital volume and operative mortality are largely mediated by surgeon volume. Patients can often improve their chances of survival substantially, even at high-volume hospitals, by selecting surgeons who perform the operations frequently, as those centers that have adopted this strategy have demonstrated declining mortality in the past decade.[163,164]

Radical cystectomy by definition implies the *en bloc* removal of the pelvic–iliac lymph nodes along with the pelvic organs anterior to the rectum: the bladder, urachus, prostate, seminal vesicles, and visceral peritoneum in men; the bladder, urachus, ovaries, fallopian tubes, uterus, cervix, vaginal cuff, and the anterior pelvic peritoneum in women. An appropriate lymphadenectomy is an important component of radical cystectomy and is related to the clinical outcomes of patients with high-grade, invasive bladder cancer. Evidence suggests that a more extended lymphadenectomy is beneficial in both lymph node–positive and lymph node–negative patients with bladder cancer,[165,166,167] although this could be a surrogate for either case selection or surgical skill. Although the exact limits of the lymphadenectomy for patients with bladder cancer undergoing cystectomy are currently debated, the boundaries include initiation at the level of the inferior mesenteric artery (superior limits of dissection), extending laterally over the inferior vena cava or aorta to the genitofemoral nerve (lateral limits of dissection), and distally to the lymph node of Cloquet medially (on Cooper's ligament) and the circumflex iliac vein laterally. This dissection includes bilaterally all obturator, hypogastric, presciatic, and presacral lymph nodes.[168–170] Removal of more than 15 lymph nodes has been postulated to be both sufficient for the evaluation of the lymph node status as well as beneficial for overall survival in retrospective studies.[166,171–174] However, potential interindividual differences in the number of pelvic and retroperitoneal lymph nodes and difficulties in processing of the removed tissue by pathologists are issues. Furthermore, the reality is that even in today's practice the number of lymph nodes retrieved are low (<10) in a majority of patients (75%) and the chance are even lower if the patients are older, Hispanic (in the United States), and managed at low-volume, nonurban centers.[170] The true curative value of lymph node dissection and the optimal extent of dissection are both still unknown.

Technical variations from the standard cystectomy have been performed to improve patients' quality of life, including prostate-sparing cystectomy in order to preserve continence and potency. However, it carries a higher risk of missing unsuspected adenocarcinoma of the prostate. Coexistent prostate cancer and prostatic urothelial cancer are reported in 23% to 54% cases, of which 29% were clinically significant, leading to local recurrence and even metastasis.[175,176]

Radical cystectomy is an appropriate standard treatment for patients with high-grade, invasive bladder cancer. The clinical outcomes are presented in Table 64.3. These results should

TABLE 64.3 CYSTECTOMY OUTCOMES IN SELECTED SINGLE INSTITUTION SERIES

Author (Reference)	Period (Year)	Number of Patients (Male/Female)	Median Age (Year)	Median Follow-Up (Year)	Histology	30-Day Mortality (%)	Pathologic Subgroup (%) Organ Confined	Extravesical	Lymph Node Positive
Stein et al./USC (4)	1971–1997	1,054 (843/211)	66	10.2	TCC (94% high-grade)	3	56	20	24
Madersbacher et al./ Bern (153)	1985–2000	507 (400/107)	66	3.75	TCC (95% high-grade)	7	43	33	24
Hautmann et al./Ulm (155)	1986–2003	788 (652/136)	64	2.9 yrs	TCC (82% high-grade)	5	63	19	18

provide a benchmark for outcomes to which other therapies can be compared.

Both laparoscopic and robot-assisted cystectomy have been shown to be feasible and safe, but with a relatively shorter follow-up.[177,178–179] Despite an increased materials cost for a robotic-assisted cystectomy, it has been demonstrated to be cost-effective in a subgroup of patients undergoing ileal conduit when the impact of complications are considered in a single institution series.[179,180]

Morbidity and Mortality of Radical Cystectomy and Lymphadenectomy

The early clinical results and outcomes with regard to the morbidity and mortality of radical cystectomy were disappointing. Lack of universal acceptance of this procedure was attributed to the considerable complication rate and the need for improvements in urinary diversion. Prior to 1970, perioperative complication rates of radical cystectomy were approximately 35%, with a mortality rate of nearly 20%. However, with contemporary medical, surgical, and anaesthetic techniques, along with better patient selection, the mortality and morbidity from radical cystectomy have dramatically decreased (Table 64.3). Importantly, in high-volume centers, the administration of preoperative therapy (radiation or chemotherapy) and the form of urinary diversion performed (continent or incontinent) did not obviously increase the mortality rate of patients undergoing radical cystectomy.[150] The issue of the need to select patients for surgery complicates the comparison of bladder-sparing techniques, because frequently those not suitable for surgery will be the ones who appear in the radiotherapy-based series.

The early complication rate following radical cystectomy should not be underestimated in this elderly group of patients. The median age of patients undergoing cystectomy in a University of Southern California series was 66 years.[4] Of the 1,054 patients treated, 28% developed an early complication within the first 3 months of surgery. Early complications included all events related to the cystectomy, perioperative care, and urinary diversion. The administration of preoperative therapy (radiation or chemotherapy) and the form of urinary diversion did not significantly increase the early complication rate in these cystectomy patients. Most early complications following radical cystectomy are unrelated to the urinary diversion (85% diversion unrelated) and can be managed conservatively without the need for reoperation in approximately 90% of cases.[181] The most common early diversion-unrelated complication is dehydration, while the most common early diversion-related complication following radical cystectomy is prolonged urinary leakage. Overall, the most surgical complications after cystectomy are associated with urinary diversion in relation to the intestinal segments.[152,182]

Neoadjuvant chemotherapy is discussed in a later section, but it does not seem to increase the perioperative morbidity or mortality.[7,183] Preoperative radiation therapy is discussed below.

Radical cystectomy may appropriately be performed in carefully selected elderly patients,[184] however, this emphasis in the surgical literature on "careful selection" highlights as much the deficiencies as the efficacy of cystectomy as it emphasizes that the published results are not applicable to the entire population. It is emphasized that physiologic age may be more important than chronologic age when determining appropriate candidacy for radical cystectomy. Proper patient selection, strict attention to perioperative details, along with a dedicated and meticulous team-oriented surgical approach are critical components to minimize the morbidity and mortality of surgery and to ensure the best clinical outcomes in all patients following radical cystectomy.[185–187] A recommended approach from the authors' center previously pioneered by the Danish is adoption of an enhanced recovery pathway protocol (Fig. 64.2).[188]

Pathologic Stage and Subgroups

The pathologic stage of the primary bladder tumor and the presence of regional lymph node metastases are the most important survival determinants in patients undergoing cystectomy for

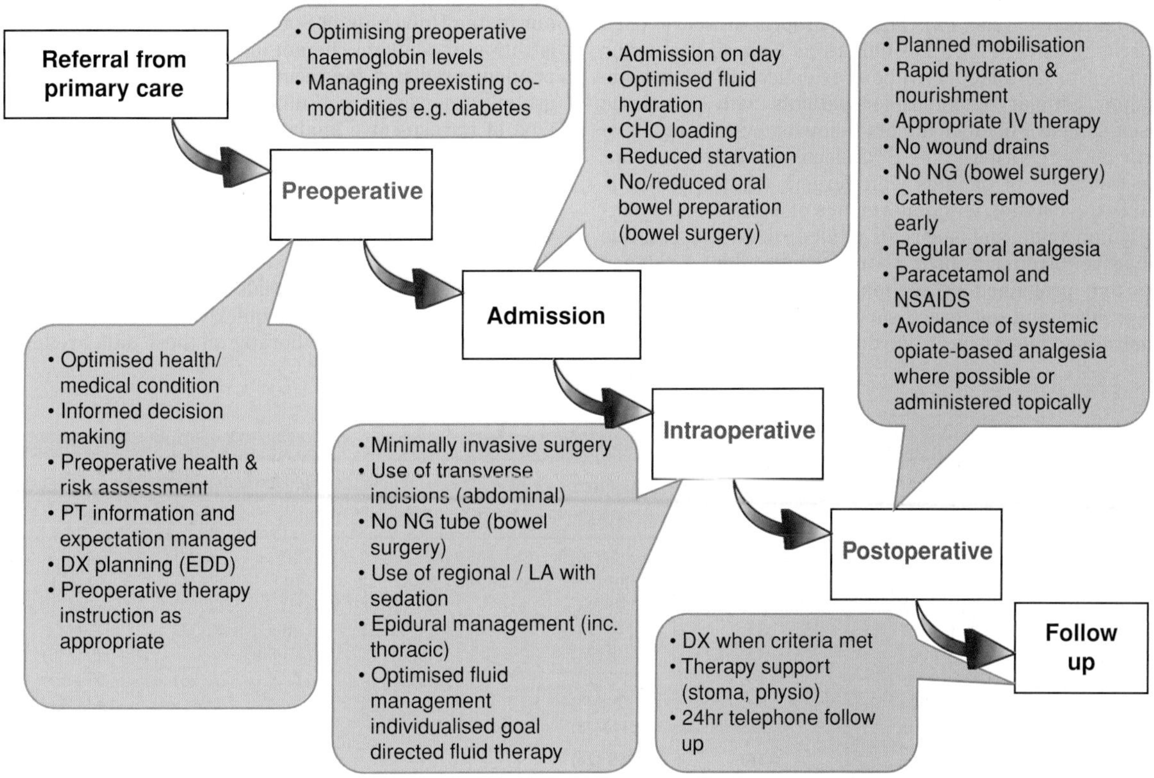

FIGURE 64.2. Schematic representation of the enhanced recovery program in patients undergoing a radical cystectomy.

TABLE 64.4 SELECTED DATA FROM THE UNIVERSITY OF SOUTHERN CALIFORNIA BLADDER CANCER STUDY OF RADICAL CYSTECTOMY

Pathologic Stage[a]	*Number of Patients*	*Probability Overall Survival (%)* 5 Years	10 Years
T2a N0	94	77	57
T2b N0	98	64	44
T3 N0	135	49	29
T4a N0	79	44	23
Extravesical N0	214	47	27
All node negative pooled	808	69	49
All node positive pooled	246	31	23

[a]From ref. 192.

bladder cancer.[4,153,155] These pathologic determinants may also be categorized into pathologic subgroups that provide risk stratification and direct the need for adjuvant therapy in the appropriately selected individual. Pathologic subgroups are defined as organ-confined, lymph node–negative tumors (P0, Pa, Pis, P1, P2a, P2b), nonorgan confined (extravesical) lymph node–negative tumors (P3, P4), and lymph node positive disease (N+); representing 56%, 20%, and 24% of patients, respectively.[155] The 5- and 10-year recurrence-free survival for the entire group of 1,054 patients in the University of Southern California series was 68% and 66%, respectively (Table 64.3). Most deaths occurred within the first 3 years following radical cystectomy and were attributed to cancer recurrence. However, with longer follow-up (>3 years), most deaths in this elderly group of patients were primarily related to comorbid diseases unrelated to bladder cancer. This underscores the effective and durable outcomes of radical cystectomy.

Organ-Confined, Lymph Node–Negative Tumors

In the University of Southern California series, 56% of patients demonstrated pathologically organ-confined, lymph node–negative tumor.[4] The outcomes in this pathologic subgroup were excellent (Table 64.4), with a 5- and 10-year recurrence-free survival of 85% and 82%, respectively. No significant survival differences were observed when comparing superficially noninvasive (Pis, Pa), lamina propria invasive (P1), and muscle-invasive (P2a, P2b) tumors as long as the tumor was confined to the bladder without evidence of lymph node involvement. Similar outcomes for patients with pathologic nonmuscle-invasive bladder tumors following cystectomy have been previously reported.[4,155,189,190] Collectively, these data support the treatment of patients with surgery when a tumor is confined to the bladder, without evidence of extravesical extension or lymph node metastasis. Treatment delays in patients with invasive bladder cancer should be avoided. Evidence suggests that prolonged delays may lead to more advanced pathologic stage and decreased survival in patients with muscle-invasive bladder cancer.[160] Furthermore, caution should be taken in delaying definitive therapy in patients with high-risk, nonmuscle-invasive bladder tumors or those with nonmuscle-invasive tumors that have not appropriately responded to conservative forms of therapy.[149]

Extravesical, Lymph Node–Negative Tumors

Nonorgan confined (extravesical), lymph node–negative tumors were found in 20% of University of Southern California series patients undergoing cystectomy (Table 64.4). No obvious survival differences between extravesical P3 and P4 (node-negative) tumors were observed. The 5- and 10-year recurrence-free survival for this pathologic subgroup was 58% and 55%, respectively. Similar outcomes were reported by Madersbacher et al.[153] and Dhar et al.,[171] who demonstrated a 56% 5-year recurrence-free survival for the same pathologic subgroup. Patients with locally advanced tumors have higher recurrence rates and decreased survival compared with those with organ-confined, lymph node–negative tumors.[191] The 1997 AJCC TNM staging system[192] used for these studies stratifies extravesical tumor involvement (previously defined as pT3b) into microscopic (pT3a) and gross (pT3b) extravesical tumor extension. No significant difference was observed in the recurrence-free and overall survival in patients when evaluating for pT3a and pT3b extravesical extension.[191] The incidence of lymph node involvement was similar (approximately 45%); however, the presence of lymph node involvement was associated with a higher risk of recurrence and worse survival compared with node-negative patients.

Lymph Node–Positive Disease

Perhaps one-fourth of patients in large cystectomy series will have positive lymph nodes (Tables 64.3 and 64.5). Although patients with lymph node tumor involvement are a high-risk group of patients, nearly one-third of these patients were alive at 5 years in the series by Stein et al.[4] It is possible that the surgical approach employing an extended lymph node dissection provides some survival advantage in selected individuals with node-positive disease.[171] The role of adjuvant therapy in these patients is difficult to assess due to the absence of adequately powered trial data (see on the Role of Systemic Therapy section). In an analysis of lymph node–positive patients carried out by the University of Southern California group, the administration of adjuvant chemotherapy was a significant and independent predictor for recurrence and overall survival in this group,[193] however, case-mix effects will be prominent in this type of retrospective analysis as patients need to survive long enough and be fit enough to even start chemotherapy to figure in the analysis. Inevitably this will bias results in favor of adjuvant chemotherapy by excluding those who died early or who never became fit enough postoperatively to receive chemotherapy. The authors own experience with attempting to recruit to adjuvant chemotherapy trials suggests that only the most fit patients are able to recover quickly enough postoperatively to undergo systemic chemotherapy, so these data are highly likely

TABLE 64.5 INCIDENCE OF LYMPH NODE METASTASIS FOLLOWING RADICAL CYSTECTOMY, CORRELATION TO PRIMARY TUMOR

Study (Reference)	*Period (Year)*	*Number of Patients*	*Lymph Node Metastasis (%)*	*Bladder Tumor Stage*[a] *(%)* P0, Pis, Pa, P1	P2a	P2b	P3	P4
Poulsen et al. (292)	1990–1997	191	50 (26)	2 (4)	4 (18)	7 (25)	33 (51)	4 (43)
Vieweg et al. (195)	1980–1990	686	193 (28)	10 (10)	12 (9)	22 (23)	97 (42)	52 (41)
Leissner et al. (166)	1999–2002	290	81 (28)	1 (3)	5 (13)	12 (22)	53 (43)	10 (50)
Stein et al. (4)	1971–1997	1,054	246 (24)	19 (5)	21 (18)	35 (27)	113 (44)	58 (42)
Vazina et al. (293)	1992–2002	176	43 (24)	1 (215)	10 (16)	–	20 (236)	12 (50)
Abdel-Latif et al. (294)	1997–1999	418	110 (26)	3 (215)	4 (7)	29 (25)	59 (48)	15 (65)
Madersbacher et al. (153)	1985–2000	507	124 (24)	2 (3)	26 (17)	–	64 (34)	32 (41)
Hautmann et al. (155)	1986–2003	788	142 (18)	2 (2)	31 (10)	–	73 (41)	36 (43)
Total		**4,110**	**989 (24)**					

[a]From ref. 192.

to be biased by underlying patient fitness. A further interesting feature of the BC2001 trial,[194] discussed in detail below, was that although no attempt was made to include pelvic nodes in the treatment field, the rate of nodal relapse was low at around 6% with radiotherapy alone, falling to 4% with chemoradiation. One possible interpretation of these data is that successful treatment of the primary, with either surgery or radiotherapy, may affect the subsequent behavior of low-volume nodal disease.

The prognosis in patients with lymph node–positive disease can be stratified by the number of lymph nodes involved (tumor burden), the stage of the primary tumor, and the presence of lymph node capsule perforation.[4,173] Patients with fewer than five positive lymph nodes among those with lymph node–positive organ-confined bladder tumors had a significantly improved recurrence-free survival rate.[4,166,195]

The number of lymph nodes involved with tumor and the extent of the lymph node dissection are both important variables for patients undergoing cystectomy for bladder cancer. Stein et al.[193] examined 246 patients with lymph node tumor involvement following radical cystectomy to evaluate other prognostic factors in this high-risk group. They used lymph node density to account for the extent of the lymph node dissection (number of lymph nodes removed) and the tumor burden (number of positive lymph nodes) following cystectomy for patients with lymph node–positive disease. Lymph node density as defined in this study was a significant and independent prognostic variable in patients with lymph node metastases. Future staging systems and the application of adjuvant therapy in clinical trials may consider applying these concepts to better stratify this high-risk group of patients.

Recurrence Following Radical Cystectomy

Recurrence following radical cystectomy for bladder cancer correlates well with the pathologic stage and subgroup.[4,153] With long-term follow-up (median, >10 years) recurrences in the University of Southern California series were classified as local (pelvic), distant, and urethral. Local recurrences were defined as those occurring within the soft tissue field of exenteration. Distant recurrences were defined as those occurring outside the pelvis, while urethral tumors were classified as a new primary tumor occurring in the retained urethra. Overall, 30% of all patients in the University of Southern California series experienced tumor recurrence.[4] The median time to any recurrence was 12 months, with 86% of all patients developing their recurrences within the first 3 years of cystectomy. Of the 311 patients who developed a recurrence, the median time to distant recurrence was 12 months, while the median time to local recurrence was 18 months. Late tumor recurrences, defined as 5 years or more after surgery, do occur and underscore the need for lifelong follow-up.

Pelvic (Local) Recurrence

Pelvic recurrence rates of 6% to 9% are reported in large series,[153,155,190] with higher rates in tumors with extravesical spread or node-positive disease at cystectomy.[4]

Metastatic (Distant) Recurrence

Recurrences following radical cystectomy are most commonly found at distant sites. This is consistent with the benefits observed in the neoadjuvant chemotherapy trials, where the maximum effect would be expected on low-volume, occult metastases rather than large-volume primary disease (discussed below). Distant recurrence rates of 20% to 35% are reported in large series (Table 64.6). However, overall death rates from bladder cancer are higher than this, so there would appear to be either underreporting of deaths in these series or the cases selected were not representative of wider experience.

Urethral Recurrence

Urethral tumor recurrence in patients with a history of bladder cancer following radical cystectomy represents a second manifestation of the multicentric defect of the primary transitional cell mucosa that led to the original bladder tumor. The term urethral recurrence is therefore somewhat misleading, suggesting a failure of definitive treatment of the bladder cancer. Most urethral tumors probably represent simply another occurrence of the transitional cell carcinoma in the remaining urothelium. Because radical cystectomy with orthotopic diversion has increasingly been performed, the fate of the retained urethra has become an increasingly important oncologic issue.

The advent of orthotopic lower urinary tract reconstruction has provided a more natural voiding pattern in patients following radical cystectomy. Approximately 85% of all patients undergoing cystectomy for TCC of the bladder at the University of Southern California research center receive an orthotopic neobladder substitute. From an oncologic perspective, only those with a positive surgical margin at the proximal urethra (distal to the apex of the prostate in men and just distal to the bladder neck in women) on intraoperative frozen section are absolutely excluded from orthotopic reconstruction. This enthusiasm to preserve the native urethra following radical cystectomy and allow for orthotopic reconstruction has rightfully increased concerns for a urethral recurrence in these patients.

Prior to the orthotopic era in women, urethral tumor recurrence was not an important oncologic issue because the entire urethra was removed at the time of cystectomy. With a better understanding of female pelvic anatomy and the innervation of the urinary sphincter and continence mechanism in women,[196] along with the identification of various pathologic risk factors for urethral tumor involvement in these patients, orthotopic diversion has now become a commonly performed form of urinary diversion in women following cystectomy.[197] Tumor involving the bladder neck is the most important risk factor for urethral tumor involvement in women.[198,199] Although bladder neck involvement is a significant risk factor for urethral tumors, not all women with tumor involving the bladder neck will have urethral tumors. Approximately 50% of female patients with tumor at the bladder neck will have an uninvolved urethra free of tumor. In this situation, the patient may potentially be considered an appropriate candidate for orthotopic diversion. Furthermore, intraoperative frozen-section analysis of the distal surgical margin is an accurate and reliable means to pathologically evaluate the proximal urethra.[199]

A growing population of male patients reconstructed to the urethra following cystectomy exists today. With longer follow-up, could this expose them to a greater risk for a urethral recurrence? The historical incidence of urethral recurrence in the retained urethra following cystectomy for bladder cancer ranges from 6% to 10%.[200,201] Specific clinical and pathologic risk factors that have been identified to provided risk assessment for urethral recurrence include multifocal tumors, CIS, tumor involvement of the prostate (particularly

TABLE 64.6 RECURRENCE-FREE SURVIVAL AND THE INCIDENCE OF RECURRENCE IN SELECTED STUDIES OF RADICAL CYSTECTOMY

Study (Reference)	Number of Patients	Median Follow-Up (Month)	Recurrence-Free Survival (%) 5 Year	Recurrence-Free Survival (%) 10 Year	Recurrence (%) Local	Recurrence (%) Distant
Stein et al./USC (4)	1,054	122	68	66	7.3	22.2
Madersbacher et al./Bern (153)	507	45	62	50	7.9	35.3
Hautmann et al./Ulm (154)	788	53	65	59	9.3	17.8
Yafi et al./Canada (190)	2,287	29	48	–	6.0	27.0

invasion of the prostatic stroma), and the form of urinary diversion (orthotopic or cutaneous) performed.[198,200,202–204]

Stein et al.[205] have evaluated urethral recurrence in a large group of male patients undergoing radical cystectomy and urinary diversion for TCC of the bladder. In this study, the clinical and pathological results of 768 consecutive male patients undergoing radical cystectomy with a median follow-up of 13 years were analyzed. Of these 768 patients, 397 men (51%) underwent an orthotopic diversion (median follow-up 10 years) and 371 men (49%) underwent a cutaneous diversion (median follow-up 19 years). Overall, 45 patients (7%) developed a urethral recurrence. The median time to a urethral recurrence was 2 years (range, 0.2 to 13.6 years). Of these 45 patients, 16 men (5%) had an orthotopic and 29 (9%) had a cutaneous form of urinary diversion. In this cohort of male patients, multiple risk factors were analyzed with regard to urethral recurrence. In a multivariate analysis, two important variables were identified that significantly increased the risk of a urethral tumor recurrence following cystectomy, including any prostate involvement and the form of urinary diversion. The estimated 5-year probability of a urethral recurrence was 5% without prostate involvement, which increased to 12% and 18% with superficial (prostatic urethra and ducts) and invasive (stroma) prostate involvement, respectively. Patients undergoing an orthotopic diversion demonstrated a statistically significantly lower risk of urethral recurrence compared with those undergoing a cutaneous form of urinary diversion.

The follow-up and management of the urethra in male patients treated for high-grade invasive bladder cancer is of importance. The indications and timing of a prophylactic urethrectomy in those undergoing cystectomy and a cutaneous diversion is debatable. It may include urethrectomy at the time of cystectomy based on preoperative clinical parameters, based on the intraoperative frozen-section analysis of the urethral margin, or a delayed urethrectomy based on final pathologic evaluation of the cystectomy specimen. These issues are best detailed with the patient preoperatively ensuring proper informed consent.

Management of the Retained Urethra Following Cystectomy

Intraoperative frozen-section analysis of the proximal urethra by an experienced pathologist is a reliable and accurate means to determine indications for orthotopic diversion in all patients. It is good practice to proceed with an orthotopic neobladder in men and women whose intraoperative frozen section of the proximal urethra is free of tumor. This approach does not appear to increase the risk of a urethral recurrence in these patients.[197,206] Male patients with known prostatic tumor involvement should not necessarily be excluded from an orthotopic substitute if the intraoperative biopsy is normal. Similarly, female patients with bladder neck involvement should not necessarily be excluded from an orthotopic neobladder if the intraoperative biopsy is also normal. All patients should be carefully counseled regarding the need for follow-up, the long-term risks of a urethral recurrence, and the possible need for urethrectomy following cystectomy.

Salvage Cystectomy

Salvage cystectomy after prior radiotherapy was discussed above in the section comparing surgical with bladder-sparing approaches.

Summary of Surgical Therapy

Surgery is an important mode of therapy for invasive bladder cancer and undoubtedly can provide durable disease control for many patients with the disease. In addition, an integrated approach with other treatment modalities such as neoadjuvant chemotherapy and radiotherapy is essential if the best results are to be achieved in the entire patient population, especially those who are borderline fit for major surgery. Radical cystectomy probably provides the best local pelvic control of the disease and provides accurate evaluation of the primary bladder tumor along with the regional lymph nodes yielding important prognostic information. This, coupled with the evolution and successful application of orthotopic lower urinary tract reconstruction in both men and women, has provided patients a more physiological and acceptable means to store and eliminate urine. However, most deaths from bladder cancer still occur due to distant metastases, presumably present at the time of original surgery, so further improvements in outcome will depend on the development of both better systemic therapies and also predictive (as opposed to prognostic) markers that will allow better selection of therapies.

Radiotherapy

External-Beam Radiotherapy

Whatever the merits or otherwise of radiotherapy as a treatment for bladder cancer, its use in the United States has declined markedly since the 1980s, and the treatment is now used mainly in certain centers such as Boston in carefully selected patients rather than as a mainstream alternative to surgery. As discussed above, patterns vary worldwide with the U.S. pattern of care predominating. Potential indications for radiotherapy are summarized in Table 64.7. Patients with radiological node-positive or metastatic disease should be managed predominantly with either chemotherapy or palliative approaches such as local radiotherapy to bulk disease (see below). Patients with radiological node-negative, muscle-invasive disease may be considered for radical radiotherapy. In North America, radiotherapy is administered as part of a package of care comprising maximal TURBT, chemotherapy, and radiotherapy, the so-called trimodality therapy (Fig. 64.3).[207,208]

The schedules used are complex but can be summarized as initial maximal TURBT followed by initial radiotherapy combined with synchronous chemotherapy, usually with cisplatinum followed by interim check cystoscopy. Patients experiencing a good response to treatment continue to consolidation chemoradiotherapy and then adjuvant polychemotherapy, usually with a cisplatinum base. Patients remain on long-term cystoscopic surveillance. Noninvasive recurrence can be managed by further TURBT and intravesical therapy. Those with isolated muscle-invasive recurrence or failure to respond (but with no systemic relapse) can undergo salvage cystectomy with or without further chemotherapy.

The optimal radiotherapy schedule has yet to be established. In North America, split schedules often used are 39 or 40 Gy in 1.8- or 2-Gy fractions with an interval cystoscopy; patients with responding disease proceed to a total dose of 64 to 66 Gy. Generally, these schedules achieve long-term survival comparable to surgical series.[209,210] A significant risk of cystectomy remains, however, with 22% undergoing immediate cystectomy, 13% delayed cystectomy for local recurrence, and 65% retaining a functioning bladder.[211]

In some countries, particularly the United Kingdom and Australia, an alternative schema is used (Fig. 64.4). As in the

TABLE 64.7 INDICATIONS FOR RADIOTHERAPY IN BLADDER CANCER

Stage	Recommendation
CIS, Ta, T1	No role for radiotherapy
T2-T4aN0M0	Potential role for radiotherapy, combined with synchronous chemotherapy if patient sufficiently fit
TanyN1–3M0 or TanyNanyM1	No role for radical radiotherapy as sole treatment for stage IV disease. It may be worth considering, however, as part of a package of "radical" palliation in concert with systemic chemotherapy. No randomized data on the use of radiotherapy in this setting beyond studies of fractionation.

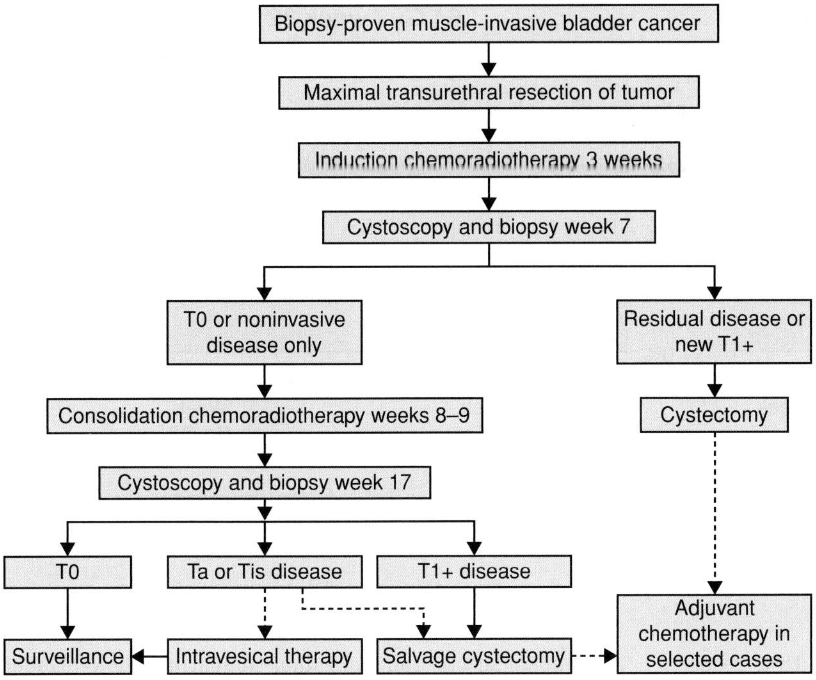

FIGURE 64.3. Trimodality therapy.

trimodality approach, patients will undergo maximal TURBT for diagnostic and staging purposes. They can then be treated either with primary surgery (as elsewhere) or alternatively with either neoadjuvant chemotherapy or primary radiotherapy. The role of cystectomy was discussed above, and the evidence and use of neoadjuvant therapy is discussed in the section Role of Systemic Therapy. In the United Kingdom, the radiotherapy itself is given as a single radical course, usually to the whole bladder, only with no attempt to treat the nodes (as discussed below). Typical dose schedules would be 64 Gy in 32 fractions or hypofractionated schedules such as 55 Gy in 20 fractions. Following radiotherapy, patients undergo cystoscopic surveillance as in the U.S. model, with salvage cystectomy for isolated local failure.

There are key differences between these two approaches. The first and most obvious is that in most disease sites radical radiotherapy is not given as a split course but as a single treatment as in the United Kingdom. To understand how this approach has arisen, it has to be understood that trimodality therapy is offered as an alternative to cystectomy in countries where the prevailing opinion is that surgery is the treatment of choice. Patients undergoing this treatment are offered what is termed "selective bladder preservation," with the multiple checkpoints allowing early exit to surgery aimed at providing reassurance to surgeons in particular that the opportunity for cure is not being lost. The median ages (mid-60s) reported in studies using this approach reflect this patient selection[147,208,212] and are similar to large surgical series.[4,141] The UK approach is completely different in this respect as there is a long tradition of using radical radiotherapy after TURBT, and the much older patient groups compared with surgical series reflect a different decision-making process in which younger, more fit patients are more likely to get surgery and older or less fit patients radiotherapy.[10,12,142,143,194] Interestingly, the long-term bladder preservation rates in older series seem similar to the rates for salvage cystectomy postradiotherapy occurring in approximately one-fourth of patients managed with radiotherapy alone at 10 years' median follow-up,[213] with around two-thirds of surviving patients retaining their bladders. The authors own more recent chemoradiotherapy series suggests a higher rate of bladder preservation with the use of synchronous chemotherapy combined with full-dose radical radiotherapy.[11]

Treatment Results

It is difficult to compare results of older series to more contemporary ones for a number of reasons. First, staging systems have changed over the years, as have imaging techniques. Patients who may have been staged as organ confined in the early or pre-CT era may now be more accurately staged as more advanced with contemporary imaging. In contrast, surgical series will report accurate pathological stage. It is well documented that more accurate staging will bring about a paradoxical improvement in reported results by stage due to upstaging of apparently early disease cases, the so-called Will Rogers phenomenon.[214] Treatment techniques in the past were obviously less refined, with little or no ability for conformal beam shaping and hence toxicity would have been higher. Nonetheless, it is clear from large series that tumor control could be attained in significant numbers of patients. For example, a study from Western General Hospital, Edinburgh, conducted between 1971 and 1982, reported treatment results from 963 patients. The reported stage mix was: T1, 20%, T2, 32%, T3, 40%, and T4, 8%, with the administered dose of 55 Gy in 20 fractions—a widely used UK schedule. The overall

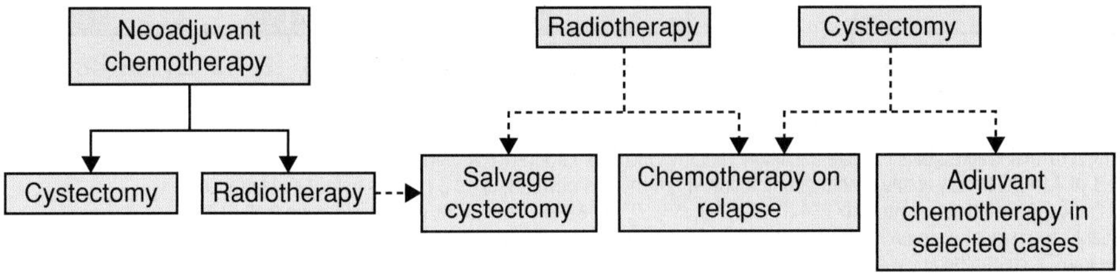

FIGURE 64.4. Integration of neoadjuvant chemotherapy, radiotherapy, and surgery in the United Kingdom.

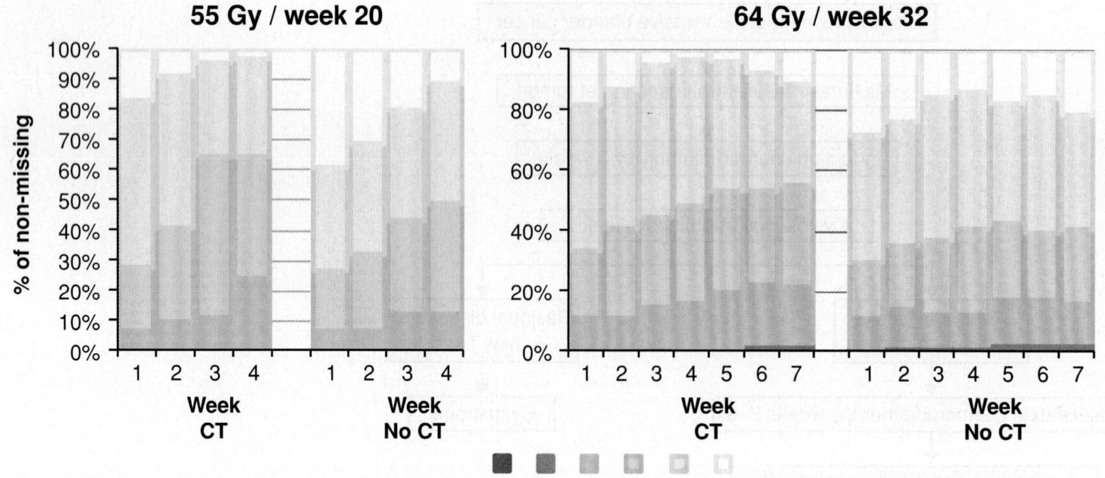

FIGURE 64.5. Acute toxicity of radiotherapy with and without synchronous chemotherapy. Graphs show worst grade of on-treatment toxicity by radiotherapy dose and week. Darkest bars indicate National Cancer Institute common terminology class grade 4; white indicates grade 0. Proportions with a grade 3 or 4 at any time on treatment: 64/178 (36.0%) chemotherapy (CT) versus 50/182 (27.5%). No CT-stratified chi-square test ($P = .07$).

5- and 10-year survival rates were 30% and 18%, respectively.[215] This study reports tumor control at cystoscopy in 46% of patients, and this seems to be a pretty typical response rate with radiotherapy alone.

Similar control rates were reported in the radiotherapy alone arm of the National Cancer Institute of Canada (NCIC) trial comparing radiotherapy with chemoradiotherapy with cisplatinum[212] and also in the radiotherapy only arms at 2 years of the UK trials BCON[12] and BC2001[194] at 2 years. The latter two trials give an accurate reflection of the results of modern radiotherapy. They ran contemporaneously between 2000 and 2009 and between them recruited more than 800 patients from around 70 UK sites, including all major UK radiotherapy centers. Both trials had similar designs, including near identical entry criteria (essentially T2–4aN0M0, with a small number of T1G3 patients entered the BCON trial), the same control arms (radical radiotherapy to bladder only to either 55 Gy in 20 fractions or 64 Gy in 32 fractions), and the same outcome measures (locoregional disease-free and overall survival). Both trials assessed both acute and late toxicity (Figs. 64.5 and 64.6). In addition, the BC2001 trial included an optional second randomization comparing whole-bladder radiotherapy with a reduced dose to uninvolved bladder of 80% of the isocenter dose. The BC2001 permitted neoadjuvant chemotherapy, which was a stratification factor. Around one-third of the chemoradiotherapy patients also received neoadjuvant chemotherapy.

The trials give a comprehensive insight into UK radiotherapy practice and great detail on outcomes. Median age in both trials was 73 to 74 years, with age range up to 90 years. Overall, around 40% of patients received 55 Gy in 20 fractions and 60% 64 Gy in 32 fractions. In both trials, over 95% of patients received at least 90% of the target dose in both arms, with no reduction associated with the two radio-sensitizing treatments. Although the protocol recommended complete debulking at TURBT, this was only achieved in one-third to one-half of the cases, probably reflecting technical factors at surgery rather than deliberate intent.

The overall 5-year survival rate was 50% for radiotherapy plus carbogen and nicotinamide compared with 39% for radiotherapy alone (48% and 35%, respectively, if T1 tumors are excluded), with the greatest effect seen in T2 tumors. For

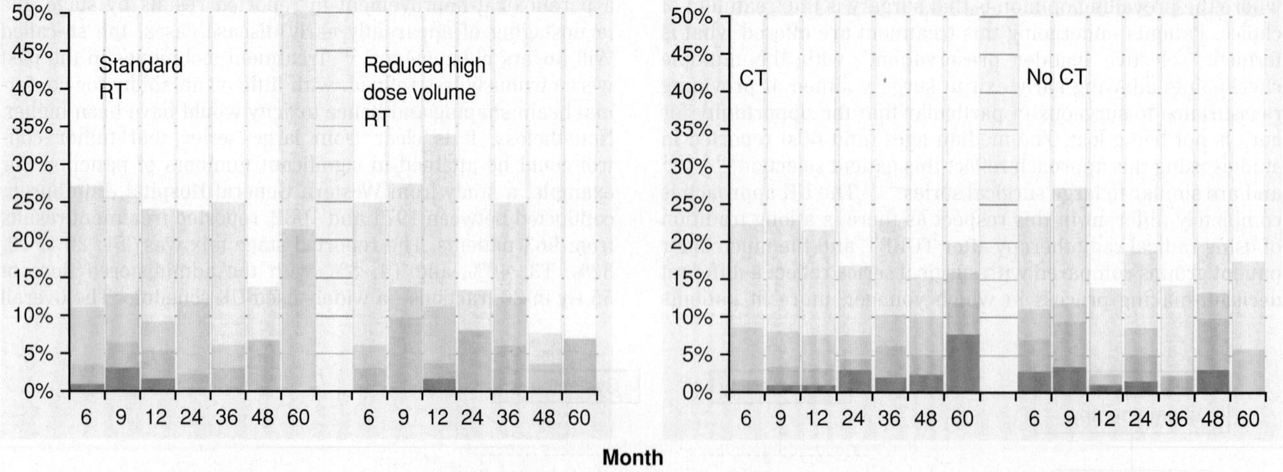

FIGURE 64.6. Late toxicity in the BC2001 trial. Darkest bars indicate Radiation Therapy Oncology Group (RTOG) grade 4; *white* indicates grade 0. Proportion of patients with grade 3 or 4 RTOG toxicity at any month during follow-up (6 months onward), up to 3 months before a recurrence: RT: 12.9% sRT vs. 17.9% RHDV; odds ratio (95% confidence interval) 1.34 (0.55, 3.24); $P = .52$; CT: 8.3% CT vs. 15.7% no CT; odds ratio 0.48 (0.21, 1.10); $P = .07$. Patients with no available assessment were excluded from analysis. RT, radiotherapy; sRT, standard volume radiotherapy; RHDV, reduced high dose volume radiotherapy; CT, chemotherapy with radiotherapy.

BC2001, the estimated 5-year survival with radiotherapy alone was very similar at 34% (95% CI, 25% to 43%).

Toxicity

The toxicity of radical radiotherapy varies with the dose and schedule used. Within BC2001 and BCON, there were two schedules: 55 Gy in 20 fractions and 64 Gy in 32 fractions. Acute toxicity is shown in Figure 64.5 for both schedules, with and without chemotherapy with 5-fluorouacil/mitomycin-C.

As can be seen, the majority of patients experience only grade 1 or 2 toxicity with very low rates of grade 4 events. Synchronous chemotherapy increased toxicity but was predominantly grade 1 or 2, with a nonstatistically significant effect on grade 3 or 4 events (27.5 vs. 36%; $P = .07$; boundary for significance set at 0.01 to reflect multiplicity of testing). The reduced volume randomization failed to demonstrate a reduction in overall toxicity. However, when the volume of bowel irradiated was calculated, this did show a significant reduction; in an exploratory analysis, volume of bowel irradiated did correlate with the risk of grade 3 or 4 toxicity. There was no increase in acute toxicity observed in BC2001 if patients had received prior neoadjuvant chemotherapy.

Treatment completion rates in both trials were very high, with an excess of 95% of patients receiving the prescribed dose. The majority of patients failing to complete did so for tumor-related reasons rather than toxicity. Late toxicity was of great interest in both trials and was analyzed somewhat differently. In BCON, the cumulative rates of grade 3 or 4 events were reported, which gives the worst-case scenario but does not reflect the overall toxicity at any given time point posttreatment. BC2001 reports the toxicity rates at prespecified time points.

There are a number of points of note here. First, late toxicity was the same with both randomizations in BC2001 (i.e., reduced-volume radiotherapy did not impact late toxicity). More significantly, the addition of synchronous chemotherapy also had no effect on reported late side effects. In addition, at any given point, 75% to 80% of patients report no late toxicity at all. This is supported by bladder capacity measurements in BC2001, which show a mean change in bladder volume at 1 and 2 years of <5 mL. Of those reported side effects, fewer than 5% report grade 4 events and fewer than 10% overall grade 3. Very similar findings pertain to the BCON trial.[12] In 2009, Efstathiou et al.[216] reported late toxicity results in 285 patients who had participated in four Radiation Therapy Oncology Group trimodality therapy trials. Overall 5.7% reported persistent late genitourinary and 1.9% gastrointestinal toxicity of grade 3 or above, consistent with the BCON and BC2001 results. The good toxicity and functional results associated with radiotherapy are borne out by surveys of quality of life and symptoms in cystectomy and radiotherapy patients carried out by Henningsohn et al.[13,217–220] Furthermore, radiotherapy and cystectomy patients report different patterns of symptoms, with sexual dysfunction being more prominent in surgical patients and bowel symptoms more prominent in radiotherapy patients. The preservation of sexual function by radiotherapy is particularly striking given that the patients were an average of around 10 years older.

Effect of Synchronous Chemotherapy

There are a large number of phase I or II trials from North America,[208,216,221–222,223,224–230,231,232–237] mainland Europe,[5,238–240] and the United Kingdom[241,242] that have examined various chemotherapy agents in combination with radiotherapy. There are, however, only a few trials reported in which radiotherapy alone is compared with radiotherapy with synchronous chemotherapy. The only randomized study using the trimodality therapy approach was carried out by the NCIC and reported in 1996.[212] This study compared radiotherapy to 40 Gy in 20 fractions with the same schedule combined with cisplatinum 100 mg/m^2 twice weekly × 3. Patients then underwent interim cystoscopy and either consolidation radiotherapy to 20 Gy in 10 fractions or cystectomy depending on response and fitness for surgery. Synchronous cisplatinum had no effect on the rate of distant metastasis, consistent with a lack of effect in neoadjuvant trials.[243] The study, however, was relatively small and could only have detected very large effects. Concurrent cisplatinum had a highly significant effect on pelvic recurrence, with 25 of 48 control patients having a pelvic recurrence, compared with 15 of 51 cisplatinum-treated patients ($P = .036$; HR 0.50; 90% CI, 0.29 to 0.86). It should be noted that a similar platinum schedule given prior to radiotherapy had no effect whatsoever on recurrences, either local or distant.[213,243]

There are two randomized trials of radio sensitization using UK schedules: the BC2001 and BCON studies, as already discussed. These two large phase III randomized control trials reported results in 2009 to 2010. These trials used radiosensitization with either concurrent chemotherapy (BC2001) or carbogen and nicotinamide (BCON). BC2001 has shown a significant improvement in locoregional disease-free survival with concurrent 5-fluorouracil and mitomycin-C of 34% (HR 0.66; 95% CI, 0.46 to 0.95) driven by a reduction of 47% in invasive locoregional recurrences (HR 0.53; $P = .007$), which is very similar to that observed in the NCIC trial with cisplatinum using the trimodality approach.[212] Figure 64.7 shows the Kaplan-Meier

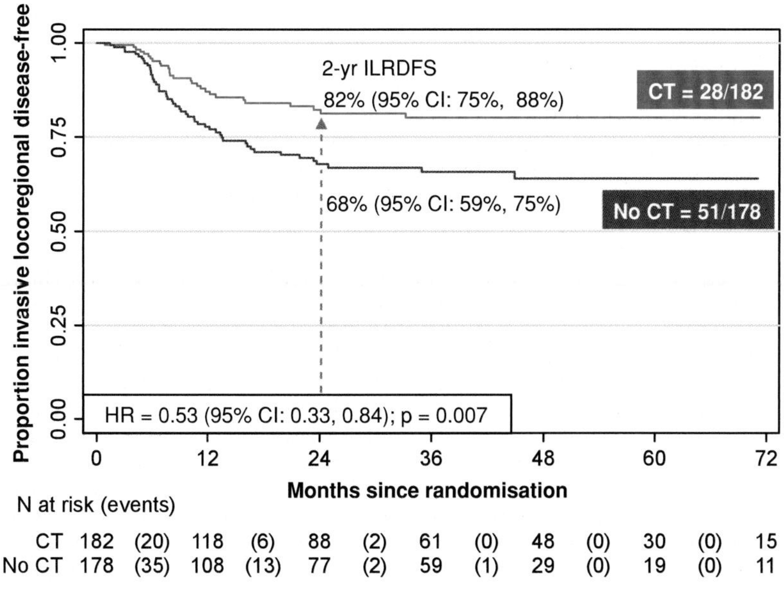

FIGURE 64.7. Invasive locoregional disease-free survival with or without chemotherapy.

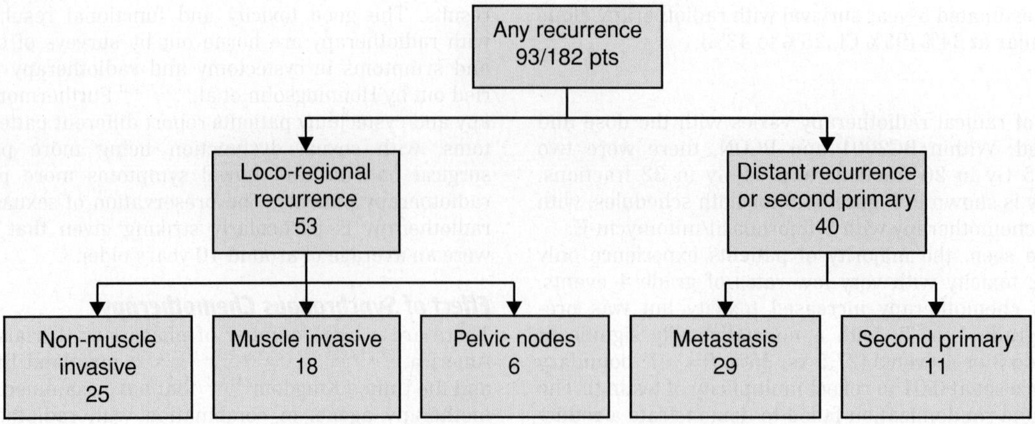

FIGURE 64.8. Patterns of failure after chemoradiotherapy in BC2001.

curves for invasive locoregional disease-free survival. Survival data show a trend toward an improvement in overall survival (HR 0.81; P = .16), although the data are immature.[194] The BCON trial[12] with synchronous carbogen and nicotinamide narrowly failed to meet its primary end point of an improvement in local relapse-free survival (HR 0.87; 63% vs. 74%; P = .1) but did report an improvement in overall survival at 3 years (46% vs. 59%; HR 0.86; 95% CI, 0.745 to 0.996; P = .04).

Taken together the trial data with chemoradiotherapy suggests good tolerability even in relatively elderly patients with excellent late toxicity profiles in the majority of patients whether treated with the North American trimodality approach[216] or the UK single treatment block.[194] The similar hazard ratios observed with cisplatinum and 5-fluorouacil/mitomycin-C suggests that a range of chemotherapy approaches can probably be used with the selection based on toxicity. It is noteworthy that comparisons of platinum and 5-fluorouacil-based chemoradiotherapy combinations have been carried out in anal cancer, with the two approaches being similarly effective.[244] The high rates of locoregional control seen make radical chemoradiotherapy a viable treatment option for many patients presenting with muscle-invasive bladder cancer.

Pattern of Failure

As already discussed above, a significant proportion of patients will experience local failure and undergo salvage surgery. The BC2001 study gives a good indication of patterns of failure using the single block approach to radical radiotherapy. A summary of relapse patterns in the chemoradiotherapy arm of the trial is shown in Figure 64.8.

There are a number of features of note here. First, the majority of locoregional failures are in the bladder, and there are more noninvasive than invasive recurrences. This underlines the need for regular surveillance postradiotherapy and the requirement for good integration of radiotherapy and surgical services if patients are to be managed by bladder conservation. In the authors' experience, the majority of noninvasive recurrences can be successfully managed conservatively without the need for cystectomy. For those with invasive recurrence, cystectomy remains an option if the patients are sufficiently fit. The low rate of nodal relapse in BC2001 is also of interest, as no attempt was made to include pelvic nodes in the field, although lower pelvic nodes would have been included in the treated volume. For improvement in the metastatic relapse rate, better systemic therapies must be found. However, the rate of second cancer is also notable and probably relates to the age of the patients and the historic high rate of tobacco consumption in the bladder cancer population.

Altered Fractionation Schedules

There are old data examining hyperfractionation in comparison to conventional treatment to 64 Gy in 32 fractions, both given as a split course. The data suggest an improvement with the hyperfractionated regimen; however, given the suboptimal nature of the control arm, it is hard to draw firm conclusions from this.[245,246] A study from the Royal Marsden Hospital compared 64 Gy in 32 fractions to 60.8 Gy in 32 fractions over 26 days in 228 patients.[247] Hypofractionated schedules are widely used in the United Kingdom and elsewhere for radical treatment and for palliation (as discussed below). There are no modern trials comparing these schedules to 64 Gy in 32 fractions.

Palliative Radiotherapy

A prospective randomized trial was conducted in 500 patients to compare the outcome in two treatment groups. Group 1 received 35 Gy in 10 fractions and group 2 received 21 Gy in 3 fractions. Five hundred patients were recruited, but data on symptomatic improvement at 3 months were only available on 272 patients. Of these, 68% achieved symptomatic improvement (71% for 35 Gy, 64% for 21 Gy), with no evidence of a difference in efficacy or toxicity between the two arms. On the basis of these results, 21 Gy in 3 fractions is widely used in the United Kingdom as a palliative schedule.[248] The data are congruent with other data on hypofractionation for palliation[249,250] as well as the growing trend for hypofractionation in other pelvic sites, in particular the prostate.

Preoperative Irradiation

Preoperative radiotherapy has been investigated in the past, but interest in the technique has waned, largely because none of the trials carried out showed any evidence of worthwhile benefit. In addition, the observed chemosensitivity of bladder cancer lead to a wave of neoadjuvant chemotherapy trials carried out in the 1980s and 1990s, effectively ending interest in the technique. Given the subsequent improvements in both radiotherapy and surgical technique, it may be appropriate to revisit the possibility of combining surgery with radiotherapy, particularly given the apparent plateau in progress with systemic therapy since the licensing of gemcitabine more than 10 years ago. Most of the studies in the literature are old, retrospective, nonrandomized comparisons and little can be concluded from them.[251]

There are few randomized trials in the literature, and those that are available are also old, for the reasons outlined above. A study from the Royal Marsden Hospital randomized patients to preoperative radiotherapy to 40 Gy in 4 weeks followed by cystectomy, against definitive radiotherapy to 60 Gy in 6 weeks. The 5-year survival in patients receiving the combined therapy was 38% versus 29% for those treated with radiotherapy alone, the difference not reaching statistical significance.[252] This trial of course did not compare radiotherapy plus surgery versus surgery alone and thus does not address the primary question in this section. However, it is noteworthy that no tumor was found in 31% of the cystectomy specimens, a similar complete response rate to that observed in the intergroup neoadjuvant MVAC study.[7] Similar response rates have been reported in other series.[253]

A second randomized study was carried out by the Memorial Sloan-Kettering Cancer Center in New York comparing radiotherapy to 40 Gy in 4 weeks followed by cystectomy 4 weeks later with a shorter 20 Gy in a 5-day course with immediate cystectomy modeled on the Swedish preoperative rectal cancer trials. Again this study is not informative on the primary issue of the utility of adding radiotherapy to surgery but does demonstrate the feasibility and safety of such an approach.[254] A retrospective review from the MD Anderson Cancer Center assessed the use of preoperative irradiation (50 Gy in 5 weeks) in patients with T3b bladder tumors.[255] The 5-year local control rate was 91% in the preoperative group (n = 92) compared with 72% for those treated with radical cystectomy alone (n = 43; P = .003).

Parsons and Million[256] reviewed the results of retrospective studies and six prospective randomized trials on the use of preoperative irradiation. They concluded that the use of the technique may improve outcomes by up to 15% to 20% at 5 years. In particular, they noted that many preoperative radiotherapy series report pathological complete response rates of around one-third, similar to that seen with neoadjuvant chemotherapy. There are no modern trials of preoperative radiotherapy, and the topic seems to be ripe for revisiting with modern techniques, particularly given the low long-term toxicity associated with chemoradiotherapy schedules, as summarized above.

Postoperative Radiotherapy

As with many areas of bladder cancer practice, there are little in the way of randomized data on the use of adjuvant radiotherapy following surgery. When used, it is mostly based on the grounds of positive surgical margins or tumor spillage at surgery, where a high local recurrence rate can be anticipated. With the use of neoadjuvant chemotherapy worldwide being at low levels, chemo-naive patients at high risk of recurrence can be offered adjuvant chemotherapy, although the evidence base for this approach is also somewhat thin. What few data there are on radiotherapy suggests that limited doses are well tolerated.[257] Given the more solid evidence base for neoadjuvant chemotherapy and the failure of adjuvant chemotherapy trials to accrue, the use of postoperative radiotherapy would also seem to be a topic well-worth revisiting with modern treatment techniques. An approach combining neoadjuvant chemotherapy, surgery, and adjuvant radiotherapy for patients at high risk of local recurrence would combine all three of the major bladder cancer treatment modalities in a novel fashion.

Electron Beam

Electron beams are really only of interest in the context of intraoperative radiotherapy. The role of intraoperative radiotherapy for carcinoma of the bladder needs to be assessed in a prospective trial and cannot at present be recommended outside of a suitable study.

Neutron Beam

There are a small number of studies examining the use of neutrons beams for bladder cancer therapy. A single randomized trial failed to show a survival advantage but did show increased morbidity.[258,259] There are currently no reasons to recommend neutron therapy for bladder cancer.

Treatment Techniques

Patient Position and Immobilization

- The patient should be planned and treated in the same position; supine with arms on their chest. Knee and ankle immobilization should be used to ensure patient positioning is reproducible.
- The rectum should be empty of flatus and feces. The use of daily microenemas may be considered.
- Patients should be asked to empty the bladder 15 minutes prior to scan.
- While breathing normally, the patient should have a CT scan performed with 3 to 5-mm slice spacing. Patients are scanned from bottom of ischial tuberosities to 3 cm above the dome of the bladder or bottom of L5 (whichever is higher). A flat top CT scanner should be used.
- Neither intravenous nor oral contrast is thought to be of benefit in this instance.
- Reference tattoos should be made at the base of the abdomen and over each hip. The location of the tattoos should be marked on the planning scan by the use of radio-opaque markers to allow cross-referencing of planning scan and setup instructions.

Volume or Field Localization

- The gross tumor volume can be difficult to define and should integrate information from the staging CT or MRI as well as the TURBT. MRI-CT fusion may be helpful, where available.
- The use of fiducial markers or contrast medium such as lipiodol at the time of TURBT has been explored and may help identify tumor for image-guided adaptive radiotherapy.
- There are few data on the optimal radiotherapy volume. A standard approach is to define the planning target volume as the whole bladder, identified by its noninvolved outer bladder wall with a 1.5-cm margin plus extravesical extent of tumor with a 2-cm margin.
- All planning and treatment should be carried out with the bladder empty to minimize the risk of geographic miss and to keep the treated volumes as small as possible. Patients with significant residual volumes post voiding should be considered for planning and treatment with a catheter *in situ,* although this is likely to increase urinary toxicity.
- There are no data to support the routine irradiation of radiologically negative lymph nodes. The nodal relapse rate in the BC2001 trial, with planning target volume and clinical target volume defined as above, was only 3% in the chemoradiotherapy arm and 6% with radiotherapy only.

Brachytherapy

There is considerable historic literature on the use of brachytherapy, particularly from the Netherlands. Reported results seem to be very good, for example, van der Werf-Messing et al.[260] report the outcomes in 328 patients treated with 3 × 3.5 Gy external irradiation followed by a radium implant. Overall 5- and 10-year survival was 56% for T2 tumors and 39% and 13%, respectively, for T3 disease. Similar results have been obtained in more recent series with iridium-192 implants and manual afterloading.[261,262] There are also descriptions in the literature of the use of high-dose rate afterloading, although one paper suggests that this may be less effective and more toxic than low-dose rate treatment.[263] The striking feature of most of these series is the very low patient numbers and long time spans reported, suggesting that these techniques are only rarely used, even in centers with the relevant expertise.

Hyperthermia

Details on hyperthermia in combination with external-beam radiation therapy or chemotherapy are beyond the scope of this chapter.

Treatment of Patients with Uncommon Bladder Tumors

Squamous cell carcinoma is uncommon in the developed world, and many reported cases may in addition reflect sampling of squamous elements within a transitional cell carcinoma. As these tumors are often excluded from systemic therapy trials, there are few data on outcomes with treatment as most papers are retrospective collections of unconnected observations.[264–265,266] It appears that local failure may be more prevalent than distant relapse, but even that observation is based on very few cases. Urachal adenocarcinomas are extremely rare. Surgical resection with a partial cystectomy and *en bloc* resection of the urachal ligament with umbilicus is the treatment of choice in the setting of localized disease. There is currently no definitive role for neoadjuvant or adjuvant chemotherapy in this tumor. Unfortunately, there are many patients who present with metastatic disease, which currently is not likely to be curable. There is no standard chemotherapy regimen for these patients. Carcinosarcoma is even more rare and appears to have a poor prognosis.[267–269] Similar considerations apply to small cell carcinoma, although the consensus seems to be that metastasis is more likely and initial response to chemotherapy is usually good. These patients generally get treated along the same lines as small cell lung carcinoma, but the benefit of prophylactic cranial irradiation is unclear.[270–275]

ROLE OF SYSTEMIC THERAPY

Up to 50% of patients will develop metastatic disease. Bladder cancer is a chemosensitive disease, with responses reported to a range of agents. Systemic combination chemotherapy can be effective and result in tumor responses and symptom control. Overall response rates may be as high as 70%,[286] with a median survival of approximately 12 to 14 months.[35] These agents were initially evaluated in the metastatic setting and subsequently in the neoadjuvant and adjuvant settings. However, despite over 30 years of research in the field, there remain many unanswered questions, including the role of adjuvant therapy and optimal second-line chemotherapy.

Neoadjuvant Chemotherapy

There are two principal rationales for neoadjuvant chemotherapy: first, to improve survival in patients with micrometastatic disease,[277] and second, to preserve the bladder by shrinking the primary tumor to facilitate radiotherapy as an alternative definitive therapy to surgery.[278] The potential disadvantage of neoadjuvant chemotherapy, and a frequent reason cited for its nonuse, is the delay in definitive treatment (cystectomy or chemoradiotherapy), because this may lead to disease progression in a proportion of nonresponding patients who may conceivably become inoperable or unsuitable for radical organ preservation treatment. However, it is equally plausible that by undergoing neoadjuvant chemotherapy these patients can be identified as those with biologically aggressive disease and therefore spared the morbidity of futile radical therapy. It should also be noted that a significant proportion, possibly up to two-thirds, of bladder cancer patients are elderly with multiple comorbidities and poor renal function and, therefore, unsuitable for neoadjuvant chemotherapy. However, in the authors' experience, a patient who is considered fit for a radical cystectomy is likely to be fit for chemotherapy as well.

There are two particularly key studies in the area of neoadjuvant chemotherapy. The South Western Oncology Group (SWOG) neoadjuvant study comparing surgery alone with 3 cycles of MVAC followed by surgery reported an estimated median survival of 6.2 years versus 3.8 years in favor of patients having neoadjuvant chemotherapy ($P = .027$).[7] Updated results from the UK MRC/EORTC neoadjuvant chemotherapy trial, which used 3 cycles of cisplatinum, methotrexate, and vinblastine (CMV) prior to surgery or radiotherapy, show a statistically significant 16% reduction in the risk of death (HR 0.84; 95% CI, 0.72 to 0.99; $P = .037$), corresponding to an increase in 10-year survival from 30% to 36% after neoadjuvant chemotherapy.[279] In total, 976 patients with high-grade T2 to T4a urothelial bladder cancer accrued over 5.5 years from 106 institutions were randomly assigned to 3 cycles of neoadjuvant CMV chemotherapy (n = 491) or no chemotherapy (n = 485), followed by the institution's choice of definitive therapy with either radical cystectomy or radiation therapy. Of patients in the chemotherapy and no chemotherapy groups, 42% and 43%, respectively, received radiation therapy alone as definitive therapy. Pathologic complete response with neoadjuvant chemotherapy was 33%. Overall survival at 3 years in the two groups was 55.5% versus 50%, respectively. The recent update, after 8 years of follow-up, showed an increase in 3-year survival from 50% to 56%, an increase in 10-year survival from 30% to 36%, and an increase in median survival time of 7 months (from 37 to 44 months) in CMV-treated patients compared with those treated with local therapy only. The SWOG study showed that of the 82% patients who underwent cystectomy, 38% had no evidence of disease pathologically. Patients who achieved pT0 status had a better prognosis than those who did not, although this difference may be accounted for by better disease biology rather than treatment effect. By definition, the SWOG study did not address organ preservation, because the mandated treatment plan was for surgery following neoadjuvant chemotherapy.

Meta-analyses show a 5% overall survival benefit at 5 years with cisplatin-containing regimens.[31] Thus, there have been two large randomized neoadjuvant studies in muscle-invasive bladder cancer, both showing significant survival advantage. Although many disciplines in cancer care would consider these data sufficient to change the standard of care, this does not seem to have taken place for the management of invasive bladder cancer.[280] The lack of widespread adoption of neoadjuvant chemotherapy may relate to the selected patients in clinical trials, not reflecting typical muscle-invasive bladder cancer patients who may be older or have impaired renal functions, which may limit the applicability of some chemotherapy regimens. GC,[33] standard,[7] or accelerated[281] MVAC are widely used with definitive radical treatment (either surgery or radiotherapy/synchronous chemoradiotherapy) 4 to 6 weeks later. It is worth noting that these trials have been restricted to patients with well-preserved renal function (typically glomerular filtration rate >60 mL/min), thus excluding a significant proportion of bladder cancer patients who are elderly or have ureteric obstruction and therefore deemed unsuitable for neoadjuvant chemotherapy. This regimen requires in-patient or prolonged hydration and therefore has a significant impact on patient quality of life and health service resources. Clinical trials investigating chemotherapy regimens that may broaden the spectrum of patients receiving cisplatin-based treatment have been conducted in palliative settings, for example, a split-dose regimen of cisplatin in combination with gemcitabine on days 1 and 8 of a 21-day schedule allowed safe treatment of patients with calculated glomerular filtration rate as low as 40 mL/min in the day-case setting.[282] This regimen could be tested within a randomized clinical trial in the neoadjuvant setting and may go far in increasing the uptake of neoadjuvant chemotherapy. It is the responsibility of urology and oncology colleagues to work together to provide state-of-art care for our patients with muscle-invasive bladder cancer, which should include neoadjuvant chemotherapy prior to surgery or organ-preservation therapy in fit patients.

Adjuvant Chemotherapy

Adjuvant chemotherapy has the potential advantage of enabling better patient selection based on the findings at surgical and pathological staging. The major disadvantages, although, are the delay in systemic therapy and the inability to assess the response to chemotherapy in the absence of measurable disease. Randomized adjuvant chemotherapy studies

TABLE 64.8 RANDOMIZED TRIALS OF ADJUVANT CHEMOTHERAPY

Author (Reference)	N	Standard Arm	Adjuvant Arm	Results
Skinner et al. (295)	91	Cystectomy	Cystectomy + CAP	Benefit, but few patients received planned therapy.
Stockle et al. (296)	49	Cystectomy	Cystectomy + MVAC	Benefit, but limited trial size, premature closure, and no therapy upon relapse.
Studer et al. (297)	77	Cystectomy	Cystectomy + cisplatinum	No benefit.
Freiha et al. (298)	55	Cystectomy	Cystectomy + CMV	Benefit limited to relapse-free survival.
Bono et al. (284)	83	Cystectomy	Cystectomy + CM	No benefit.

CAP, cyclophosphamide/Adriamycin (doxorubicin)/cisplatin; MVAC, methotrexate/vinblastine/doxorubicin (Adriamycin)/cisplatinum; CMV, cisplatinum/methotrexate/vinblastine; CM, cisplatinum/methotrexate.

(Table 64.8) have been conducted with the methodological flaws of inadequate sample size, early closure, and suboptimal choice of chemotherapy, preventing a clear interpretation of the results. A systematic review and meta-analysis of updated individual patient data from all available randomized controlled trials in the adjuvant setting has been performed. Updated data were collected, validated, and reanalyzed for 491 patients from 6 randomized controlled trials, representing 90% of all patients randomized in cisplatin-based combination chemotherapy trials and 66% of patients from all eligible trials. In view of this, the power of this meta-analysis was limited. The overall hazard ratio for survival of 0.75 (95% CI, 0.60 to 0.96; $P = .019$) suggests a 25% relative reduction in the risk of death favoring adjuvant chemotherapy. However, the impact of trials that stopped early, of patients not receiving allocated treatments, or not receiving salvage chemotherapy is less clear.[283] An Italian multicenter randomized phase III trial enrolled 194 patients (one-third of its target) with muscle-invasive TCC and assigned them to 4 cycles of GC or observation after cystectomy. The trial was stopped early due to poor accrual. After a median follow-up of 32.5 months, relapses were similar in both groups (43% vs. 45%) with no difference in disease-free survival. The 3-year overall survival was 67% for the chemotherapy arm and 48% for the observation arm and the 3-year disease-free survival was 47% and 35%, respectively, suggesting no statistically significant improvement in either survival rate with adjuvant GC in these patients.[284] A large phase III trial by EORTC (protocol 30994) evaluating observation versus adjuvant chemotherapy with one of the three chemotherapy regimens (GC, MVAC, or high-dose MVAC) in high-risk bladder cancer (pT3–4 and/or node-positive disease) was also prematurely closed due to poor accrual after enrollment of 278 of a planned 1,344 patients. This appropriately designed and sized study thus failed to conclusively address the issue of adjuvant chemotherapy following cystectomy. A possible reason for the failure of this trial was the tight window postsurgery for commencing chemotherapy. In the authors' experience, relatively few patients were able to enter the trial sufficiently soon due to slow postoperative recovery. This suggests that adjuvant chemotherapy may be less suitable than neoadjuvant chemotherapy in this patient population. The adjuvant chemotherapy question still requires international collaboration with an appropriately sized pragmatic study for a conclusive answer. In various disease sites neoadjuvant chemotherapy followed by adjuvant chemotherapy is an acceptable norm with level I evidence. With an anticipated rise in uptake of neoadjuvant chemotherapy, patients with bladder cancer should not be precluded from this strategy where neoadjuvant chemotherapy is followed by radical treatment followed by a trial of adjuvant chemotherapy versus no chemotherapy in an appropriately sized phase III trial that meets its recruitment target, thus providing a definite answer for or against this strategy. Previous failures in meeting recruitment targets can be overcome by using better-tolerated regimens in common use now and by extending the recruitment window from 12 to 16 weeks to allow full recovery postsurgery and to allow more dose-intense adjuvant chemotherapy treatment.

Choice of Chemotherapy Regimen in Metastatic Disease

Currently, systemic combination chemotherapy is the only treatment that may prolong survival in patients with metastatic disease. The chemosensitivity of bladder cancer is demonstrated by objective response rates of 12% to 73% and complete response rates of 0% to 35%.[285] Although antitumor activity has been demonstrated with several single agents, the median survival associated with single-agent therapy is short (4 to 6 months). Prior to the development of gemcitabine, a range of trials were done with doublet regimes, which typically showed median survival times of approximately 8 months.[285] The development of the four drug combination for MVAC chemotherapy extended this to over 12 months and became the established standard of care.[286]

The triplet combination CMV is also widely used but has not been compared with MVAC directly. Experimental data suggested that a combination of gemcitabine and cisplatin given using an appropriate schedule (simultaneous or close proximity exposure) can act synergistically. Synergy may be mediated either by inhibition of ribonucleotide reductase by gemcitabine, depleting the deoxynucleotide pool required for DNA replication and thereby inhibiting excision repair of cisplatin-induced DNA crosslinks, or by gemcitabine incorporation into DNA, facilitating cisplatin crosslink formation.[287,288] The combination of the two drugs proved active and tolerable[33] and was subsequently compared with MVAC in a phase III trial. Patients were randomized to GC (gemcitabine 1,000 mg/m^2 days 1, 8, and 15; cisplatin 70 mg/m^2 day 2) or standard MVAC every 28 days for a maximum of 6 cycles. Four hundred five patients were randomized (GC, n = 203; MVAC, n = 202). The groups were well balanced with respect to prognostic factors. Overall survival was similar on both arms (HR 1.04; 95% CI, 0.82 to 1.32; $P = .75$), as were time to progressive disease (HR 1.05; 95% CI, 0.85 to 1.30), time to treatment failure (HR 0.89; 95% CI, 0.72 to 1.10), and response rate (GC, 49%; MVAC, 46%). More GC patients completed 6 cycles of therapy, with fewer dose adjustments. The toxic death rate was 1% on the GC arm and 3% on the MVAC arm. More GC than MVAC patients had grade 3 or 4 anaemia (27% vs. 18%, respectively) and thrombocytopenia (57% vs. 21%, respectively). More MVAC patients, had grade 3 or 4 neutropenia (82% vs. 71%), neutropenic fever (14% vs. 2%), neutropenic sepsis (12% vs. 1%), grade 3 or 4 mucositis (22% vs. 1%), and alopecia (55% vs. 11%). Because of the higher incidence of neutropenic fever and mucositis, more hospital admissions were required for the MVAC arm (49 admissions for a total of 272 days) than for the GC group (9 admissions for a total of 33 days), resulting in considerably greater hospital resource utilization. The quality of life was maintained during treatment on both arms; however, patients on GC fared better regarding weight, performance status, and fatigue. This study thus demonstrated that GC provides a similar survival to MVAC with a better safety profile and tolerability.[34,35] Therefore, although this trial was not designed to show equivalence of the two regimens, many interpret the results as showing therapeutic noninferiority and have adopted GC as the new standard in view of the better tolerability. With the upper boundary of the confidence interval of the adjusted hazard ratio for survival close to 1.2, noninferiority can reasonably be assumed. Therefore, GC is a valuable alternative for the growing elderly patient population with metastatic bladder cancer who may derive equal benefit from this regimen as compared with MVAC but with fewer side effects.

The addition of paclitaxel to GC was evaluated in a phase III clinical trial by EORTC (protocol 30987), which enrolled 627 patients with advanced urothelial carcinoma. The regimens were well tolerated. Results showed that the GCP arm resulted in a higher rate of overall response rate (57% vs. 46%) CR (15% vs. 10%) and survival (15.7 vs. 12.8 months) compared with GC arm, but these differences were not statistically significant.[289]

Combination of docetaxel and cisplatin (DC) has been compared with MVAC in a multicenter phase III clinical trial by the Hellenic Co-operative Oncology Group.[290] Patients (n = 220) were randomly assigned to MVAC every 4 weeks versus docetaxel plus cisplatin every 3 weeks. Treatment with MVAC resulted in significantly superior response rate (54.2% vs. 37.4%), median time to progression (9.4 vs. 6.1 months), and median survival (14.2 vs. 9.3 months), suggesting that MVAC was superior to DC. Toxicity of MVAC was considerably lower than that previously reported for MVAC administered without granulocyte colony-stimulating factor. Currently GC, MVAC, and high-dose MVAC with granulocyte colony-stimulating factor support are the acceptable standard of care as first-line chemotherapy in advanced or metastatic bladder cancer setting.

Second-Line Chemotherapy Treatment

The role of salvage chemotherapy after relapse following first-line chemotherapy remains an important subject of recent clinical trials. The enrollment in such trials is challenging in view of patients' poor performance status and deranged renal functions. Although various phase I or II studies have been reported, to date there is only one completed phase III trial comparing vinflunine with best supportive care (BSC) alone. Patients (n = 370) were randomly assigned in a 2 to 1 ratio to receive vinflunine plus BSC (n = 253) or BSC alone (n = 117). Both arms were well balanced. Grade ≥3 toxicities for the vinflunine arm were neutropenia (50%), febrile neutropenia (6%), anemia (19%), fatigue (19%), and constipation (16%). A median survival advantage of 2.3 months (6.9 months for vinflunine plus BSC vs. 4.6 months for BSC) was achieved but was not statistically significant ($P = .287$). Cox multivariate analysis adjusting for prognostic factors showed a statistically significant effect of vinflunine on overall survival ($P = .036$), reducing the death risk by 23%. Objective response rate (8.6% vs. 0%), disease control (41.4% vs. 24.8%), and progression-free survival (3.0 vs. 1.5 months) were all statistically significant, favoring vinflunine. Because vinflunine was well tolerated, it is a reasonable second-line therapy option for patients with bladder cancer who have relapsed following cisplatin-based therapy.[291] Future second-line chemotherapy studies should incorporate vinflunine as the standard of care arm when testing any experimental treatment in a randomized trial.

SELECTED REFERENCES

A full list of references for this chapter is available online.

3. Riley GF, Potosky AL, Lubitz JD, et al. Medicare payments from diagnosis to death for elderly cancer patients by stage at diagnosis. *Med Care* 1995;33(8):828–841.
4. Stein JP, Lieskovsky G, Cote R, et al. Radical cystectomy in the treatment of invasive bladder cancer: long-term results in 1,054 patients. *J Clin Oncol* 2001;19(3): 666–675.
5. Rödel C, Grabenbauer GG, Kuhn R, et al. Combined-modality treatment and selective organ preservation in invasive bladder cancer: long-term results [see comment]. *J Clin Oncol* 2002;20(14):3061–3071.
6. Hayter CR, Paszat LF, Groome PA, et al. The management and outcome of bladder carcinoma in Ontario, 1982–1994. *Cancer* 2000;89(1):142–151.
8. Konety BR, Joslyn SA. Factors influencing aggressive therapy for bladder cancer: an analysis of data from the SEER program. *J Urol* 2003;170(5):1765–1771.
10. Munro NP, Sundaram SK, Weston PM, et al. A 10-year retrospective review of a nonrandomized cohort of 458 patients undergoing radical radiotherapy or cystectomy in Yorkshire, UK. *Int J Radiat Oncol Biol Phys* 2010;77(1):119–124.
11. James ND, Hussain SA, Hall E, et al. Radiotherapy with or without chemotherapy in muscle-invasive bladder cancer. *N Engl J Med* 2012;366(16):1477–1488.
12. Hoskin PJ, Rojas AM, Bentzen SM, et al. Radiotherapy with concurrent carbogen and nicotinamide in bladder carcinoma. *J Clin Oncol* 2010;28(33):4912–4918.
13. Henningsohn L, Wijkstrom H, Dickman PW, et al. Distressful symptoms after radical radiotherapy for urinary bladder cancer. *Radiother Oncol* 2002;62(2): 215–225.
21. Miller AB. The etiology of bladder cancer from the epidemiological viewpoint. *Cancer Res* 1977;37(8 Pt 2):2939–2942.
22. Hoffman D, Masuda Y, Wynder EL. Alpha-naphthylamine and beta-naphthylamine in cigarette smoke. *Nature* 1969;221(5177):255–256.
30. Sylvester RJ, van der Meijden AP, Oosterlinck W, et al. Predicting recurrence and progression in individual patients with stage Ta T1 bladder cancer using EORTC risk tables: a combined analysis of 2596 patients from seven EORTC trials. *Eur Urol* 2006;49(3):466–465.
31. Neoadjuvant chemotherapy in invasive bladder cancer: update of a systematic review and meta-analysis of individual patient data advanced bladder cancer (ABC) meta-analysis collaboration. *Eur Urol* 2005;48(2):202–205.
32. Sternberg CN, Yagoda A, Scher HI, et al. Preliminary results of M-VAC (methotrexate, vinblastine, doxorubicin and cisplatin) for transitional cell carcinoma of the urothelium. *J Urol* 1985;133(3):403–407.
33. Moore MJ, Winquist EW, Murray N, et al. Gemcitabine plus cisplatin, an active regimen in advanced urothelial cancer: a phase II trial of the National Cancer Institute of Canada Clinical Trials Group. *J Clin Oncol* 1999;17(9):2876–2881.
34. von der Maase H, Hansen SW, Roberts JT, et al. Gemcitabine and cisplatin versus methotrexate, vinblastine, doxorubicin, and cisplatin in advanced or metastatic bladder cancer: results of a large, randomized, multinational, multicenter, phase III study. *J Clin Oncol* 2000;18(17):3068–3077.
37. Rehn L. Blasengeschwultse bei Fuchsein-arbeitern. *Arch Clin Chir* 1895;50: 588–600.
38. Lower GMJ. Concepts in causality: chemically-induced human urinary bladder cancer. *Cancer* 1982;49:1056–1066.
40. Case RAM, Hosker ME, McDonald DB, et al. Tumors of the urinary bladder in workmen engaged in the manufacture and use of certain dyestuff intermediates in the British chemical industry. Role of aniline, benzidine, alpha-naphthylamine, and beta-naphthylamine. *Br J Indust Med* 1954;11:75–104.
42. King CM, Phillips B. Enzyme-catalyzed reactions of the carcinogen H-hydroxy-2-fluorenylacetamide with nucleic acid. *Science* 1968;159:1351–1353.
44. Risch A, Wallace DM, Bathers S, et al. Slow N-acetylation genotype is a susceptibility factor in occupational and smoking related bladder cancer. *Hum Mol Genet* 1995;4(2):231–236.
61. Hodder SL, Mahmoud AA, Sorenson K, et al. Predisposition to urinary tract epithelial metaplasia in *Schistosoma haematobium* infection. *Am J Trop Med Hyg* 2000;63(3–4):133–138.
62. Tawfik HN. Carcinoma of the urinary bladder associated with schistosomiasis in Egypt: the possible causal relationship. *Princess Takamatsu Symp* 1987;18: 197–209.
80. Sidransky D, Frost P, Von Eschenbach A, et al. Clonal origin bladder cancer. *N Engl J Med* 1992;326(11):737–740.
89. Jones PA, Baylin SB. The fundamental role of epigenetic events in cancer. *Nat Rev Genet* 2002;3(6):415–428.
92. Bryan RT, Zeegers MP, James ND, et al. Biomarkers in bladder cancer. *BJU Int* 2009;105(5):608–613.
94. Knowles MA, Elder PA, Williamson M, et al. Allelotype of human bladder cancer. *Cancer Res* 1994;54(2):531–538.
97. Bryan RT, Hussain SA, James ND, et al. Molecular pathways in bladder cancer: part 1. *BJU Int* 2005;95(4):485–490.
98. Bryan RT, Hussain SA, James ND, et al. Molecular pathways in bladder cancer: part 2. *BJU Int* 2005;95(4):491–496.
99. Hanahan D, Weinberg RA. The hallmarks of cancer. *Cell* 2000;100(1):57–70.
100. Hanahan D, Weinberg RA. Hallmarks of cancer: the next generation. *Cell* 2011; 144(5):646–674.
101. Reya T, Morrison SJ, Clarke MF, et al. Stem cells, cancer, and cancer stem cells. *Nature* 2001;414(6859):105–111.
110. Knowles MA. Molecular pathogenesis of bladder cancer. *Int J Clin Oncol* 2008; 13(4):287–297.
123. Hawkins RD, Hon GC, Ren B. Next-generation genomics: an integrative approach. *Nat Rev Genet* 2010;11(7):476–486.
132. Sylvester RJ, Oosterlinck W, van der Meijden AP. A single immediate postoperative instillation of chemotherapy decreases the risk of recurrence in patients with stage Ta T1 bladder cancer: a meta-analysis of published results of randomized clinical trials. *J Urol* 2004;171(6 Pt 1):2186–2190.
141. Dalbagni G, Genega E, Hashibe M, et al. Cystectomy for bladder cancer: a contemporary series. *J Urol* 2001;165(4):1111–1116.
142. Kotwal S, Choudhury A, Johnston C, et al. Similar treatment outcomes for radical cystectomy and radical radiotherapy in invasive bladder cancer treated at a United Kingdom specialist treatment center. *Int J Radiat Oncol Biol Phys* 2008; 70(2):456–463.
145. Neoadjuvant cisplatin, methotrexate, and vinblastine chemotherapy for muscle-invasive bladder cancer: a randomised controlled trial. International Collaboration of Trialists. *Lancet* 1999;354:533–540.
146. Harland SJ, Kynaston H, Grigor K, et al. A randomized trial of radical radiotherapy for the management of pT1G3 NXM0 transitional cell carcinoma of the bladder. *J Urol* 2007;178(3 Pt 1):807–813.
147. Michaelson MD, Shipley WU, Heney NM, et al. Selective bladder preservation for muscle-invasive transitional cell carcinoma of the urinary bladder. *Br J Cancer* 2004;90(3):578–581.
148. Prout GR, Marshall VF. The prognosis with untreated bladder tumors. *Cancer* 1956;9(3):551–558.
150. Shariat SF, Karakiewicz PI, Palapattu GS, et al. Outcomes of radical cystectomy for transitional cell carcinoma of the bladder: a contemporary series from the Bladder Cancer Research Consortium. *J Urol* 2006;176(6 Pt 1):2414–2422.
151. Shariat SF, Palapattu GS, Amiel GE, et al. Characteristics and outcomes of patients with carcinoma in situ only at radical cystectomy. *Urology* 2006;68(3):538–542.
152. Hautmann RE, Volkmer BG, Schumacher MC, et al. Long-term results of standard procedures in urology: the ileal neobladder. *World J Urol* 2006;24(3):305–314.

153. Madersbacher S, Hochreiter W, Burkhard F, et al. Radical cystectomy for bladder cancer today—a homogeneous series without neoadjuvant therapy. *J Clin Oncol* 2003;21(4):690–696.
155. Hautmann RE, Gschwend JE, de Petriconi RC, et al. Cystectomy for transitional cell carcinoma of the bladder: results of a surgery only series in the neobladder era. *J Urol* 2006;176(2):486–492.
159. Herr H, Lee C, Chang S, et al. Standardization of radical cystectomy and pelvic lymph node dissection for bladder cancer: a collaborative group report. *J Urol* 2004;171(5):1823–1828.
160. Sanchez-Ortiz RF, Huang WC, Mick R, et al. An interval longer than 12 weeks between the diagnosis of muscle invasion and cystectomy is associated with worse outcome in bladder carcinoma. *J Urol* 2003;169(1):110–115.
161. Lee CT, Madii R, Daignault S, et al. Cystectomy delay more than 3 months from initial bladder cancer diagnosis results in decreased disease specific and overall survival. *J Urol* 2006;175(4):1262–1267.
164. Finks JF, Osborne NH, Birkmeyer JD. Trends in hospital volume and operative mortality for high-risk surgery. *N Engl J Med* 2011;364(22):2128–2137.
166. Leissner J, Ghoneim MA, bol-Enein H, et al. Extended radical lymphadenectomy in patients with urothelial bladder cancer: results of a prospective multicenter study. *J Urol* 2004;171(1):139–144.
171. Dhar NB, Klein EA, Reuther AM, et al. Outcome after radical cystectomy with limited or extended pelvic lymph node dissection. *J Urol* 2008;179(3):873–878.
172. Herr HW, Faulkner JR, Grossman HB, et al. Surgical factors influence bladder cancer outcomes: a cooperative group report. *J Clin Oncol* 2004;22(14):2781–2789.
173. Fleischmann A, Thalmann GN, Markwalder R, et al. Extracapsular extension of pelvic lymph node metastases from urothelial carcinoma of the bladder is an independent prognostic factor. *J Clin Oncol* 2005;23(10):2358–2365.
174. Studer UE, Collette L. Morbidity from pelvic lymphadenectomy in men undergoing radical prostatectomy. *Eur Urol* 2006;50(5):887–889.
177. Challacombe BJ, Bochner BH, Dasgupta P, et al. The role of laparoscopic and robotic cystectomy in the management of muscle-invasive bladder cancer with special emphasis on cancer control and complications. *Eur Urol* 2011;60(4):767–775.
181. Stein JP, Dunn MD, Quek ML, et al. The orthotopic T pouch ileal neobladder: experience with 209 patients. *J Urol* 2004;172(2):584–587.
183. Sherif A, Holmberg L, Rintala E, et al. Neoadjuvant cisplatinum based combination chemotherapy in patients with invasive bladder cancer: a combined analysis of two Nordic studies. *Eur Urol* 2004;45(3):297–303.
190. Yafi FA, Aprikian AG, Chin JL, et al. Contemporary outcomes of 2287 patients with bladder cancer who were treated with radical cystectomy: a Canadian multicentre experience. *BJU Int* 2011;108(4):539–545.
195. Vieweg J, Gschwend JE, Herr HW, et al. Pelvic lymph node dissection can be curative in patients with node positive bladder cancer. *J Urol* 1999;161(2):449–454.
207. Zietman AL, Sacco D, Skowronski U, et al. Organ conservation in invasive bladder cancer by transurethral resection, chemotherapy and radiation: results of a urodynamic and quality of life study on long-term survivors. *J Urol* 2003;170(5):1772–1776.
208. Hagan MP, Winter KA, Kaufman DS, et al. RTOG 97–06: initial report of a phase I-II trial of selective bladder conservation using TURBT, twice-daily accelerated irradiation sensitized with cisplatin, and adjuvant MCV combination chemotherapy. *Int J Radiat Oncol Biol Phys* 2003;57(3):665–672.
209. Kaufman DS, Winter KA, Shipley WU, et al. Phase I–II RTOG study (99–06) of patients with muscle-invasive bladder cancer undergoing transurethral surgery, paclitaxel, cisplatin, and twice-daily radiotherapy followed by selective bladder preservation or radical cystectomy and adjuvant chemotherapy. *Urology* 2009;73(4):833–837.
210. Mak RH, Zietman AL, Heney NM, et al. Bladder preservation: optimizing radiotherapy and integrated treatment strategies. *BJU Int* 2008;102(9 Pt B):1345–1353.
211. Kaufman DS, Winter KA, Shipley WU, et al. The initial results in muscle-invading bladder cancer of RTOG 95–06: phase I/II trial of transurethral surgery plus radiation therapy with concurrent cisplatin and 5-fluorouracil followed by selective bladder preservation or cystectomy depending on the initial response. *Oncologist* 2000;5(6):471–476.
212. Coppin CM, Gospodarowicz MK, James K, et al. Improved local control of invasive bladder cancer by concurrent cisplatin and preoperative or definitive radiation. The National Cancer Institute of Canada Clinical Trials group. *J Clin Oncol* 1996;14(11):2901–2907.
215. Duncan W, Quilty PM. The results of a series of 963 patients with transitional cell carcinoma of the urinary bladder primarily treated by radical megavoltage X-ray therapy. *Radiother Oncol* 1986;7(4):299–310.
223. Marks LB, Kaufman SD, Prout GR Jr, et al. Invasive bladder carcinoma: preliminary report of selective bladder conservation by transurethral surgery, upfront MCV (methotrexate, cisplatin, and vinblastine) chemotherapy and pelvic irradiation plus cisplatin. *Int J Radiat Oncol Biol Phys* 1988;15(4):877–883.
231. Zietman AL, Shipley WU, Kaufman DS. The combination of cis-platin based chemotherapy and radiation in the treatment of muscle-invading transitional cell cancer of the bladder. *Int J Radiat Oncol Biol Phys* 1993;27(1):161–170.
242. Choudhury A, Swindell R, Logue JP, et al. Phase II study of conformal hypofractionated radiotherapy with concurrent gemcitabine in muscle-invasive bladder cancer. *J Clin Oncol* 2011;29(6):733–738.
243. Wallace DM, Raghavan D, Kelly KA, et al. Neo-adjuvant (pre-emptive) cisplatin therapy in invasive transitional cell carcinoma of the bladder. *Br J Urol* 1991;67(6):608–615.
247. Horwich A, Dearnaley D, Huddart R, et al. A randomised trial of accelerated radiotherapy for localised invasive bladder cancer. *Radiother Oncol* 2005;75(1):34–43.
248. Duchesne GM, Bolger JJ, Griffiths GO, et al. A randomized trial of hypofractionated schedules of palliative radiotherapy in the management of bladder carcinoma: results of medical research council trial BA09. *Int J Radiat Oncol Biol Phys* 2000;47(2):379–388.
252. Bloom HJ, Hendry WF, Wallace DM, et al. Treatment of T3 bladder cancer: controlled trial of pre-operative radiotherapy and radical cystectomy versus radical radiotherapy. *Br J Urol* 1982;54(2):136–151.
258. Duncan W, Williams JR, Kerr GR, et al. An analysis of the radiation related morbidity observed in a randomized trial of neutron therapy for bladder cancer. *Int J Radiat Oncol Biol Phys* 1986;12(12):2085–2092.
260. van der Werf-Messing BH, Menon RS, Hop WC. Carcinoma of the urinary bladder category T2, T3, NX, MO treated by interstitial radium implant. *Prog Clin Biol Res* 1988;260:511–524.
264. Kassouf W, Spiess PE, Siefker-Radtke A, et al. Outcome and patterns of recurrence of nonbilharzial pure squamous cell carcinoma of the bladder: a contemporary review of the University of Texas MD Anderson Cancer Center experience. *Cancer* 2007;110(4):764–769.
265. Kastritis E, Dimopoulos MA, Antoniou N, et al. The outcome of patients with advanced pure squamous or mixed squamous and transitional urothelial carcinomas following platinum-based chemotherapy. *Anticancer Res* 2006;26(5B):3865–3869.
276. Bajorin DF, Dodd PM, Mazumdar M, et al. Long-term survival in metastatic transitional-cell carcinoma and prognostic factors predicting outcome of therapy. *J Clin Oncol* 1999;17(10):3173–3181.
279. Griffiths G, Hall R, Sylvester R, et al. International phase III trial assessing neoadjuvant cisplatin, methotrexate, and vinblastine chemotherapy for muscle-invasive bladder cancer: long-term results of the BA06 30894 trial. *J Clin Oncol* 2011;29(16):2171–2177.
281. Sternberg CN, de Mulder PH, Schornagel JH, et al. Randomized phase III trial of high-dose-intensity methotrexate, vinblastine, doxorubicin, and cisplatin (MVAC) chemotherapy and recombinant human granulocyte colony-stimulating factor versus classic MVAC in advanced urothelial tract tumors: European Organization for Research and Treatment of Cancer Protocol no. 30924. *J Clin Oncol* 2001;19(10):2638–2646.
283. Advanced Bladder Cancer (ABC) Meta-analysis Collaboration. Adjuvant chemotherapy in invasive bladder cancer: a systematic review and meta-analysis of individual patient data Advanced Bladder Cancer (ABC) Meta-analysis Collaboration. *Eur Urol* 2005;48(2):189–199.
291. Bellmunt J, Theodore C, Demkov T, et al. Phase III trial of vinflunine plus best supportive care compared with best supportive care alone after a platinum-containing regimen in patients with advanced transitional cell carcinoma of the urothelial tract. *J Clin Oncol* 2009;27(27):4454–4461.

Part I Male Genitourinary

Chapter 65 Low-Risk Prostate Cancer

Michael J. Zelefsky, Megan E. Daly, and Richard K. Valicenti

ANATOMY

Gross Anatomy and External Architecture

The prostate gland is an ovoid-shaped structure composed of fibrous, glandular, and muscular elements. It is located in the pelvis, adjacent to the rectum, bladder, dorsal, and periprostatic venous complexes, pelvic sidewall musculature, the pelvic plexus, and cavernous nerves. Because of its shape, the prostate and the rectum curve away from each other as two convex surfaces. The prostate surrounds segments of the urethra before it passes through the genitourinary diaphragm (GUD; Fig. 65.1). The male urethra is composed of five segments: the pre-prostatic urethra adjacent to the pre-prostatic sphincter; the prostatic urethra, which is from the verumontanum to the GUD; the membranous urethra as it courses through the GUD, which is surrounded by the external sphincter; the bulbar urethra in the penile bulb; and the penile urethra as it passes through the corpus spongiosum. The paired seminal vesicles are situated posterosuperiorly to the prostate gland and secrete seminal fluid into the bilateral ductus deferens as they become the ejaculatory ducts. These ducts transverse the prostate to join the urethra at the verumontanum (Fig. 65.1, right). At this point, the urethra changes its angulation by bending 30 to 40 degrees anteriorly.

The prostate is contained within a thin, fibrous adherent capsule that is structurally continuous with the stroma of the gland. The apex of the gland rests above the GUD. The GUD surrounds the membranous sphincter and may vary in length and thickness. The puboprostatic ligaments extend anteriorly from the surface of the gland to the pubic symphysis. The prostate is separated from the rectum posteriorly by Denonvilliers' fascia (retrovesical septum), which attaches above to the peritoneum and below to the GUD. It is this portion of the prostatic fascia that restricts posterior extension of prostatic carcinoma into the rectum. The lateral margins of the prostate are usually delineated against the levator ani muscles, forming the lateral prostatic sulci.

The anterior aspect of the prostate and the lateral pelvic floor are covered with the periprostatic fascia (Fig. 65.2). The endopelvic fascia lateral to the prostate gland contains neurovascular structures, including the venous plexus of Santorini, which is the primary drainage for the penis. This venous network, also referred to as the *dorsal vein complex,* covers the anterolateral surfaces of the prostate. The primary arterial blood supply to the prostate is via branches of the internal pudendal, inferior vesical, and middle hemorrhoidal arteries. The internal pudendal arteries also provide the blood flow to the penis. The nerves originate from the pelvic plexus, containing both sympathetic

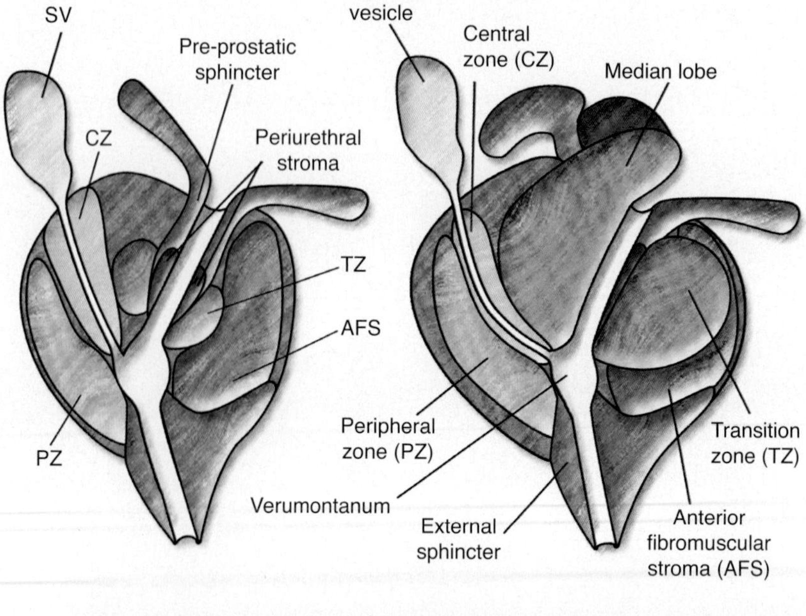

FIGURE 65.1. Zonal anatomy of the prostate. On the left, a young man with minimal transition zone (TZ) hypertrophy. Note that the preprostatic sphincter and periejaculatory duct zone (central zone of McLean) are clearly defined. On the right, an older man with TZ hypertrophy, which effaces the preprostatic sphincter and compresses the periejaculatory duct zone. AFS, anterior fibromuscular stroma; CZ, central zone; PZ, peripheral zone; SV, seminal vesicle. (From McLaughlin PW, Troyer S, Berri S, et al. Functional anatomy of the prostate: implications for treatment planning. *Int J Radiat Oncol Biol Phys* 2005;63:479–491; with permission from Elsevier.)

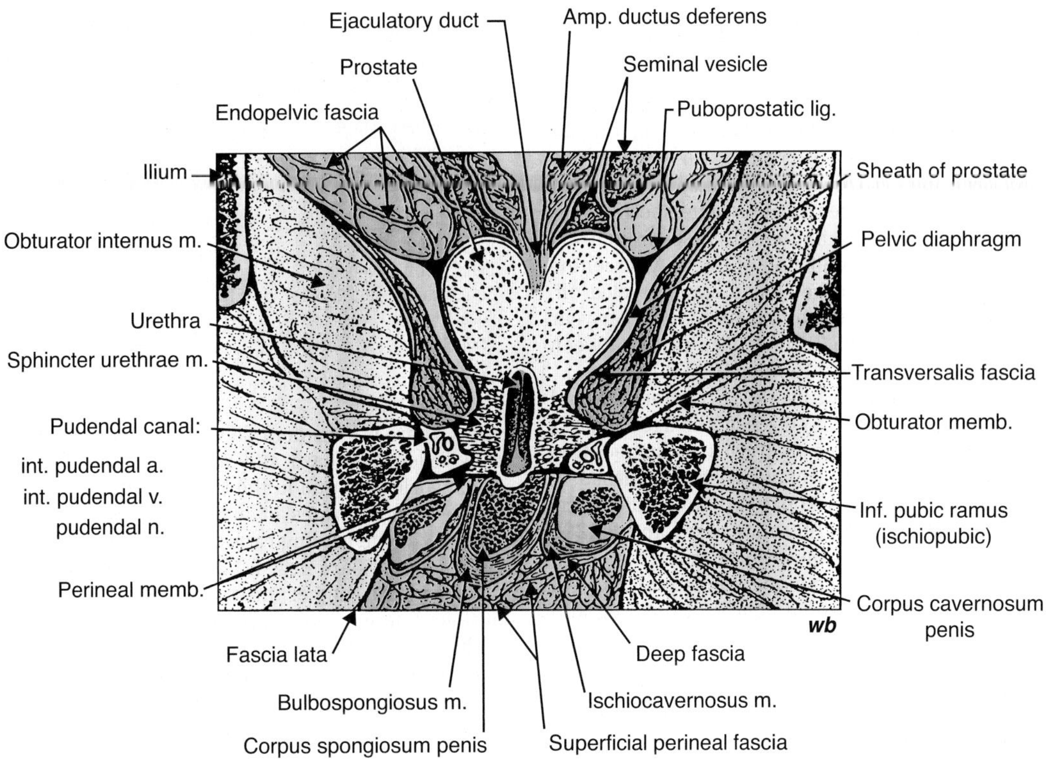

FIGURE 65.2. Frontal section of male pelvis at right angles to perineal membrane. (From Oelrich TM. The urethral sphincter muscle in the male. *Am J Anat* 1980;158:229–246;reproduced with permission of John Wiley & Sons, Inc.)

and parasympathetic fibers, and are distributed to the prostate, seminal vesicles, and the corpora cavernosa of the penis and urethra.

The prostatic apex is definable on diagnostic imaging and is important anatomically for radiation therapy treatment planning. Although the apex and the GUD, which surrounds the membranous sphincter, are easily visualized on coronal magnetic resonance imaging (MRI), it is important to recognize that the level of the GUD from the apex to the penile bulb may vary because the absence of an apical capsule contributes to the difficulty in discrimination of the gland from the GUD during computed tomography (CT)-based treatment planning. Delineation of the neurovascular bundle is also limited on CT imaging.

Prostatic Zonal Anatomy

Zonal anatomy has essentially replaced lobar anatomy of the prostate. There are four zones of the prostate (Fig. 65.1): the peripheral zone (PZ), transition zone (TZ), central zone, and anterior fibromuscular stroma zone. The central zone that surrounds the ejaculatory ducts has marked histologic differences from the PZ. It is the PZ, extending across the entire posterior surface of the gland that is palpated on rectal examination and is the location of most prostate cancers. The TZ is the location of benign prostatic hypertrophy. The anterior fibromuscular zone consists of an anterior band of fibromuscular tissue contiguous with bladder muscle and external sphincter. In young men, the PZ is the prominent zone, whereas the TZ becomes the dominant zone with age. It is important to note that there is no "median lobe" zone in this nomenclature, although such a "lobe" may be present in some prostate cancer patients and may have important implications for treatment planning and treatment selection. Histologically, the median lobe arises from the TZ or periurethral stroma, with varying proportions of fibrous, glandular, and muscle tissue.

Prostate Physiology

Histologically, the prostate consists of compound tubuloalveolar glands lined by two layers of cells. The glands are embedded in connective tissue comprising collagen and abundant smooth muscle that constitutes the prostatic stroma. This fibromuscular stroma functions both to control micturition by acting as a sphincter of the urethra and to express acidic prostatic secretions into the urethra by contracting during ejaculation.

The major function of the prostate is the production of seminal fluid that protects and nourishes the sperm after ejaculation. The prostate contributes approximately 30% to the seminal fluid, and the seminal vesicles, testicles, and bulbourethral glands provide the remaining 70%. Enzymes, including acid phosphatase and prostate-specific antigen (PSA), are secreted into the seminal fluid. PSA is a serine protease that is involved in the liquefaction of the seminal coagulum. Because PSA is produced primarily by benign and malignant prostatic epithelial cells and normally found at low concentrations in the serum, it is useful for prostate cancer screening and posttreatment monitoring of disease status.

The synthetic activity and growth of the prostate gland is regulated by androgens. The primary circulating androgen is testosterone. In the prostatic stroma, testosterone is converted to its active and more potent form, α-dihydrotestosterone, by 5-α-reductase. Secretory epithelial cells and stromal cells have intracellular androgen receptors. Dihydrotestosterone forms a complex with the dihydrotestosterone-binding domain of the androgen receptor, altering the structure of the DNA-binding domain such that it can reversibly bind DNA sequences known as *androgen response elements* in promoter or enhancer regions of androgen-regulated genes. The response includes stimulation of cell division, inhibition of apoptosis (programmed cell death), or cellular differentiation. In secretory epithelial cells, testosterone stimulation may result in the production and secretion of prostatic fluid. These mechanisms are tightly regulated at many levels, from the hypothalamus secreting luteinizing hormone–releasing hormone to maintain testosterone levels in the blood, to the local regulation of 5-α-reductase in the prostate stroma. All of these factors acting at the same time determine the balance between cellular proliferation, cell death, and differentiation of a prostatic epithelial cell.

EPIDEMIOLOGY AND RISK FACTORS

Clinical Incidence

Adenocarcinoma of the prostate is the most frequently diagnosed visceral cancer of men in the United States, accounting for 33% of non-skin cancers. The lifetime risk for American White and African American men is 18% and 21%, respectively. This corresponds to a respective lifetime risk of prostate-specific mortality of 3% and 5%.[1,2] After large annual increases from 1988 to 1992, coinciding with the introduction of the PSA screening test, prostate cancer incidence in the United States leveled off, then showed modest decreases of approximately 1.9% per year between 2000 and 2008 (Fig. 65.3). Incidence rates between 2004 and 2008 were approximately 153 per 100,000 men.[2]

Perhaps because of widespread use of PSA screening and effective early treatment for localized disease, the age-adjusted death rates have begun to decrease. It was estimated that 241,740 new cases of prostate cancer would be diagnosed in 2012, but only approximately 28,170 patients would die of the disease.[2] This compares with 189,000 new cases and 30,200 estimated deaths in 2002.[1] Despite these encouraging trends, in 2008 carcinoma of the prostate remained the second greatest cause of male cancer mortality behind cancer of the lung and bronchus.[3]

Of the known or suspected risk factors for prostate cancer, the most important is age (Table 65.1).[4] The median age at diagnosis is 68 years, and the disease incidence escalates sharply with increasing age. The incidence among men age 40 to 59 years is 1 in 38, increasing to 1 in 15 among men age 60 to 69 years and 1 in 8 among those age 70 years and older. According to autopsy data, 70% of men older than 80 years of age and 40% of men older than 50 years of age have pathologic evidence of cancer in the prostate.[5]

Although the risk for development of histologic evidence of cancer in the prostate is fairly constant across countries and races, there is considerable variability in the incidence of clinically evident disease and mortality among different populations worldwide and in the United States.[6]

The highest rates of prostate cancer are in Scandinavia, where it is the leading cause of male cancer death. The lowest recorded rates are in Asia. In the United States, incidence and mortality are higher among African Americans. A 30- to 50-fold difference in risk between African American men at the highest end of the spectrum and native Japanese at its lowest end has been reported. The mortality rates of prostate cancer in Japan dramatically increased from 1960 to 2000 in all age groups before showing modest but sustained decreases from 2000 onward.[7]

TABLE 65.1 KNOWN OR SUSPECTED RISK FACTORS FOR PROSTATE CANCER

Factor	Effect on Prostate Cancer Risk
Age	Increase
African American race	Increase
Geography	Scandinavia, high; Asia, low
Family history	Increase
Dietary fat	Increase
Agent Orange	May increase
Vasectomy	No effect
Benign prostatic conditions	No effect
Sexually transmitted diseases	No effect
Tobacco	Inconclusive data
Androgens	Inconclusive data

Risk Factors

Hormonal Influences

It is relatively well established that androgenic influences over time affect prostate carcinogenesis and disease progression.[8] Generally, androgens are required for the development of

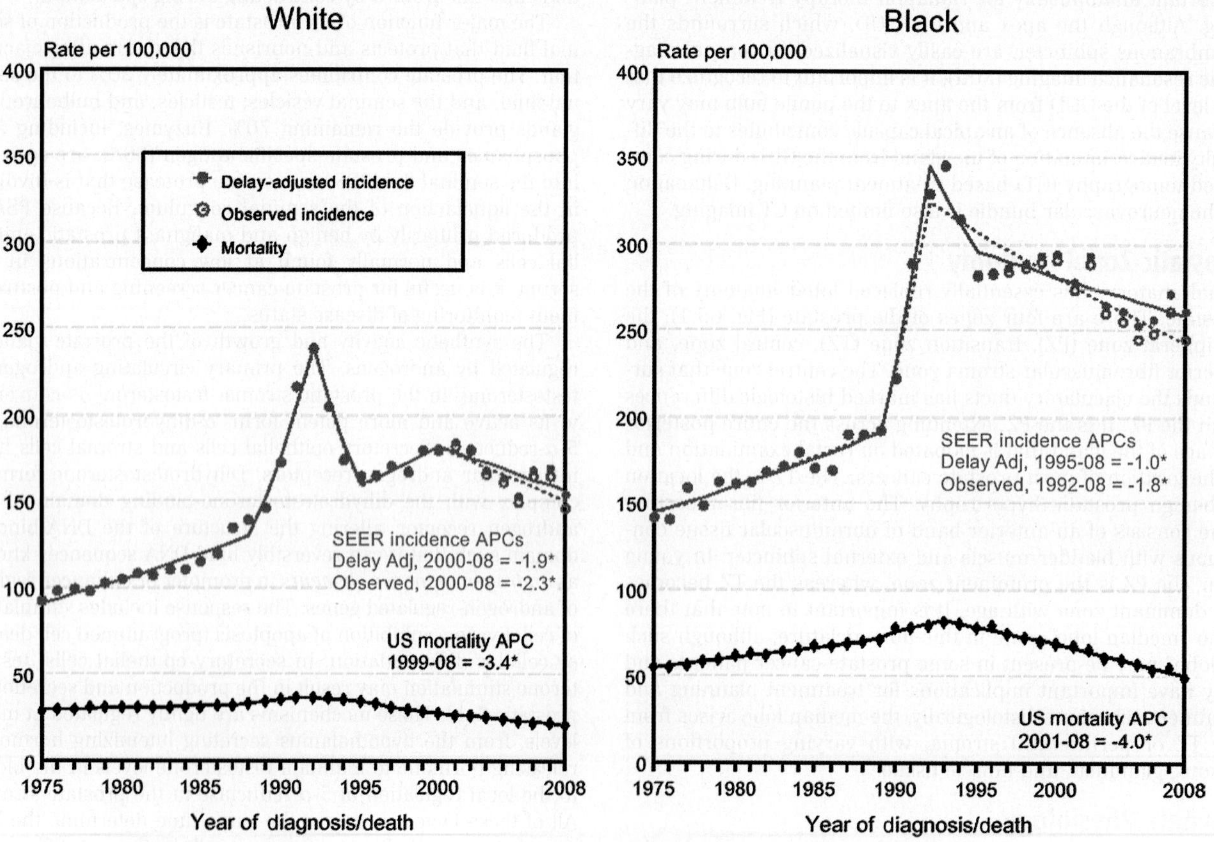

FIGURE 65.3. Surveillance, Epidemiology, and End Results (SEER) prostate cancer incidence and mortality rates by race, United States, 1975–2008. (SEER Cancer Statistics Review, 1975–2008. Available at: http://seer.cancer.gov.)

prostate cancer, and it has been noted that men deficient in 2,5α-reductase are rarely diagnosed with benign prostatic hypertrophy or prostate cancer. In a study of 1,008 men, there was a positive correlation with plasma androstenedione levels and the development of prostate cancer.[9] However, Gann et al.[10] found no clear association between individual hormone levels, including dihydrotestosterone, and the incidence of prostatic cancer. Yet, these investigators noted that high levels of testosterone in combination with low levels of the serum protein that binds testosterone, sex hormone–binding globulin, correlated with a higher risk of prostate cancer. Meikle et al.[11] observed a higher sex hormone–binding globulin level and a higher rate of testosterone synthesis in men with prostate cancer compared with control subjects.

The most conclusive evidence supporting the hormonal influence in the development of prostate cancer comes from two large, randomized trials evaluating the use of 5α-reductase inhibitors in chemoprevention. The Prostate Cancer Prevention Trial was the first large-scale, population-based trial testing the hypothesis that treatment with finasteride, which lowers intraprostatic dihydrotestosterone levels, prevents prostate cancer.[12] In this trial, a total of 18,882 men ≥55 years old and with normal digital rectal examination (DRE) and PSA level ≤3.0 ng/mL were randomized to 7 years of finasteride (5 mg/day) or placebo. This study found that the prevalence of prostate cancer was reduced by 25% in men taking finasteride compared to placebo, with the prevalence of Gleason sum 7 to 10 tumors higher in the former group. The Reduction by Dutasteride of Prostate Cancer Events (REDUCE) trial randomized 8,231 men at high risk for prostate cancer (age 50 to 60 years with a PSA of 2.5 to 10.0 or age ≥60 years with a PSA of 2.5 to 10.0 and a negative prostate biopsy within 6 months of enrollment) to dutasteride (0.5 mg daily) or placebo.[13] At 4 years, a relative risk reduction in the diagnosis or a subsequent prostate cancer of 22.8% was noted in men taking dutasteride. However, a trend toward increased Gleason 8 to 10 tumors was noted among men taking dutasteride. For both trials, it remains controversial whether this increased risk of high-Gleason tumors is real or artifactual. However, the U.S. Food and Drug Administration has declined to add chemoprevention of prostate cancer as an indication for finasteride and dutasteride.[14]

Dietary Influences

The development of prostate cancer may be attributed to both familial and environmental factors. Epidemiologic studies strongly suggest that a diet deficient in certain micronutrients is an important environmental risk factor. This has been supported through migration studies that indicate higher rates of prostate cancer in Asian men living in the United States compared with their counterparts in Japan or China.[15,16] It has been postulated that nutritional factors play a role in stimulating the progression of microscopic disease. Salient features of the "Western diet" that differ from the traditional Asian diet are high fat intake and low soy consumption. A Western diet has been associated with increased production of both androgens and estrogens and a vegetarian diet with lower levels.[17] Numerous case–control and cohort studies demonstrated an association between increased dietary fat intake and a higher risk of prostate cancer.[18] Diets high in fat content may increase the relative risk of prostate cancer by a factor of 1.6 to 1.9.[19,20] In addition, several studies showed that men with diets high in fiber and presumably lower in fat have a decreased risk of prostate cancer.[21,22]

One prospective study found that the type of fat intake was directly related to risk of prostate cancer.[23] Red meat represented the food group with the strongest positive association with advanced cancer, with a relative risk of 2.64. Fat from dairy products (with the exception of butter) or fish was unrelated to risk. When analyzed by fatty acid type, only α-linolenic acid (an omega-3 fatty acid found in red meats and butter), and not linoleic acid (omega-6 fatty acid found in fish oil), was implicated, with an increase in risk for prostate cancer of more than threefold. Conversely, a subsequent Canadian case-controlled study suggested that saturated fat consumption, not α-linolenic acid consumption, may play a role in prostate cancer progression.[24] Finally, a Swedish study of 406 men with prostate cancer and 1,208 without it (control subjects) demonstrated that body mass index and total amount of food consumed were independent risk factors.[25]

Plant-based foods and their products, such as soy, tomatoes, cruciferous vegetables, and certain nutrients, are favorably associated with prostate cancer. It is believed that these dietary factors contribute to antioxidant effects against DNA and cell damage.

Several vitamins and trace nutrients, including selenium, vitamin E, and vitamin C, have garnered attention as potential protective agents. Selenium is an essential trace nutrient that humans obtain through their diet of plants (related to soil composition; highest in Brazil nuts) and animal products (highest in seafood) and is present in nutritional supplements. Early experimental and epidemiologic data supported the anticarcinogenic effects of selenium through apoptotic, angiogenic, or antioxidative pathways.[26] The Nutrition Prevention Trial identified a 50% reduction in prostate cancer risk in men blindly and randomly assigned selenium supplements compared with placebo.[27] Promising data for vitamin E as a protective agent was reported in the Finnish Alpha-Tocopherol, Beta-Carotene Cancer (ATBC) Prevention Study, which evaluated supplementation with vitamin E and beta-carotene in male smokers for chemoprevention of lung cancer.[28] Secondary analysis suggested a 32% reduction in prostate cancer risk among men randomized to receive vitamin E. However, a large, prospective, randomized trial failed to confirm these findings for selenium or vitamin E. The Selenium and Vitamin E Cancer Prevention (SELECT) Trial randomized 35,533 men to four arms: selenium (200 μg/day), vitamin E (400 IU/day rac-α-tocopheryl acetate), both selenium and vitamin E, or placebo only.[29] With a minimum follow-up of 7 years, the study identified no reduction in risk of prostate cancer with either vitamin E or selenium supplementation but identified an increased hazard ratio for development of prostate cancer among men randomized to vitamin E alone of 1.17. Vitamin E was contemporaneously evaluated in the randomized Physicians' Health Study II, which failed to demonstrate a reduction in prostate cancer incidence by supplementation with vitamin E or C.[30]

The beneficial effects of soy are attributed to isoflavones, one of several plant pigments found in soybeans. Isoflavones are a type of phytoestrogen—compounds that have weak estrogenic, antiestrogenic, and antioxidant effects that may all be protective against progression of prostate cancer in humans. These isoflavones, most significantly genistein and daidzein, have been shown to inhibit the growth of prostate cancer cell lines in nude mice.[18] In particular, genistein has been shown to be a potent inhibitor of several steroid-metabolizing enzymes, such as aromatase, 5α-reductase, and 17β-hydroxysteroid dehydrogenase, as well as enzymes that are crucial to cellular proliferation, such as tyrosine kinase and topoisomerases I and II. Genistein is also an inhibitor of angiogenesis. It is estimated that Japanese men consume approximately 20 mg of isoflavones per day, whereas for Western men the daily consumption is <1 mg/day. This is reflected in a mean plasma concentration of genistein of 180 ng/mL in Japanese men, compared with a level of <10 ng/mL for Western men.[31]

Another protective nutrient is lycopene, prevalent in the Western diet, a carotenoid that is present in tomatoes, processed tomato products, and other fruits. It is one of the most potent antioxidants among dietary carotenoids. Although the antioxidant properties of lycopene are believed to be primarily responsible for its beneficial effects, other mechanisms may

TABLE 65.2 NUTRITIONAL RISK FACTORS FOR PROSTATE CANCER INCIDENCE, RECURRENCE, AND MORTALITY

Food or Nutrient	Direction of Association with Prostate Cancer Risk	Direction of Association with Prostate Cancer Recurrence or Mortality	Overall Quality of Evidence
Selenium	Inverse		Strong
Tomato and lycopenes	Inverse	Inverse[a]	Good
Other carotenoids	Inverse	Inverse[a]	Good[a]
Vitamin E	Inverse (seen in smokers)	Inverse[a]	Good
Vitamin D	Inverse		Good
Calcium and dairy	Null to positive		Good
Red meat	Positive		Good
Fish/omega-3	Inverse	Inverse[a]	
Soy/isoflavones	Null to inverse	Null for PSA recurrence	Fair[a]
Tea/polyphenols	Null to inverse		Fair[a]
Zinc	Positive		Fair[a]
Heterocyclic amines	Positive		Fair[a]

[a]Limited data available.

Modified from Chan JM, Gann PH, Giovannucci, EL. Role of diet in prostate cancer development and progression. *J Clin Oncol* 2005;23:8152–8160.

also be involved. In a review of 72 epidemiologic studies that investigated a link between cancer risk and consumption of tomato products, 57 linked tomato intake with a reduced risk; in 35 of those studies, the association was considered statistically significant.[32] Two large, prospective studies reported a decrease in prostate cancer risk with higher tomato product consumption.[33,34] Tomatoes were one of only four specific food items associated with significantly reduced prostate cancer risk in a prospective study of 14,000 Seventh-Day Adventist men.[34] A prospective study examined the relationship between the plasma concentration of several antioxidants and the risk for prostate cancer, using plasma samples obtained in the Physician's Health Study. Higher serum and tissue lycopene levels were found to be inversely related to the incidence of prostate cancer development.[35] In a recent meta-analysis of 21 studies, high intake of tomatoes was associated with a 10% to 20% risk reduction in prostate cancer, with lower risk due to cooked versus raw tomatoes.[36] A summary of various epidemiologic studies indicating associations of various dietary factors to prostate cancer development and morality is shown in Table 65.2.

Familial Associations

A large cohort study of the Utah Mormon population demonstrated a positive family history of prostate cancer in 6.6% of families of probands with prostate cancer and only 2.2% of families of probands without prostate cancer.[37] A subsequent study using data from the Utah State Cancer Registry reported a familial relative risk of prostate cancer of 2.2.[38] Multiple studies have confirmed these findings, including a large case–control study from Johns Hopkins.[39] Extensive cancer pedigrees were obtained from 691 prostate cancer cases and 640 spouse control subjects showing a twofold increased risk in men with a family history of prostate cancer in a single first-degree relative. There was a fivefold risk if there were two affected relatives, and the relative risk rose to 11 for three first-degree relatives with prostate cancer.

In a Canadian study, the frequency of prostate cancer detected in men who had a first-degree relative with a history of prostate cancer was 2.6 times greater than for men without such a history.[40] Aprikian et al.,[41] in a study of 2,968 patients, noted that prostate cancer was detected in 40% (1,300 patients) of men with a family history of prostate cancer, compared with 29% of 769 men without a family history ($p < .0001$). In a review of the epidemiology of prostate cancer, Giovannucci[33] reported that approximately 9% of cases may be attributed directly to a family history, although this may be as high as 43% among men younger than 55 years of age.

Despite the familial clustering of prostate cancer observed in these epidemiologic studies, causation cannot be inferred, given the shared environmental factors among family members. Segregation analyses of cancer in multiple family members have been used to examine the role of genetic factors and inheritance patterns in prostate cancer. Segregation analysis is a statistical method used to determine the best-fitting model of inheritance for a particular disease in a study population. The largest segregation analysis of prostate cancer families suggested that the familial pattern was best explained by Mendelian inheritance of a rare, autosomal dominant gene in a subset of men with early-onset prostate cancer.[42] The allele is highly penetrant, accounting for cancer by age 85 years in 88% of carriers compared with only 5% of noncarriers. Although this gene appears to be responsible for many of the early-onset cases, only 9% of all prostate cancer cases are in patients with this genetic predisposition, a percentage similar to that seen in both hereditary breast and colon cancers. Twin studies have also been used in the analysis of prostate cancer inheritance and have shown four to five times higher concordance rates for monozygotic twins.[43]

Genetic and Molecular Influences

Researchers are now focusing on the molecular level to identify genetic alterations that may be involved in the multistep process of carcinogenesis. Progress in cytogenetic studies using polymerase chain reaction (PCR)–based polymorphism analysis has facilitated the identification of regions of the genome associated with various types of cancer. Linkage analysis is used to determine whether there is an association between a particular genetic defect and clinical disease. There is ongoing investigation into the role of chromosomal deletions, oncogenes, and tumor suppressor genes in the initiation and progression of prostate cancer. Emerging data from analysis of DNA from high-risk families suggest that specific high-risk alleles exist for prostate cancer, as they do for other tumors. A major susceptibility locus for prostate cancer on the long arm of chromosome 1 (1q24-25) was identified through a genome-wide scan.[44] The gene, *HPC1* (hereditary prostate cancer 1), has been linked to families with multiple members affected with an early average age at diagnosis.[45] However, this association has not been identified in all studies. Subsequent studies have sought to identify additional susceptibility loci and germline mutations implicated in familial prostate cancer. A recent study by Ewing et al.[46] identified a recurrent mutation in HOXB13, a homeobox transcription factor gene involved in prostate development on the long arm of chromosome 17 (17q21-22) implicated in early-onset, familial prostate cancer. A number of other candidate susceptibility genes have been studied,[47] several of which are summarized in Table 65.3.

Research delving into the molecular physiology of the prostate gland has also uncovered specific DNA sequences that may be related to the occurrence and progression of prostate cancer. It is well known that prostate cancer cells, like their normal counterparts, are usually sensitive to androgens, and their growth depends on androgen-stimulated cell division. Prostate cell growth is controlled by the interaction of circulating androgens, such as testosterone and dihydrotestosterone, with the androgen receptor. The androgen receptor gene contains a polymorphic CAG repeat sequence that encodes the portion of the receptor involved in DNA transcription. The length of the CAG repeat sequence was found to be inversely proportional to the activity of the androgen receptor; therefore, shorter CAG repeat sequences may be related to prostate cancer growth.[48] Giovannucci et al.,[49] in an analysis of the activity of the androgen receptor in men with prostate cancer, found that a shorter CAG repeat sequence in the androgen receptor gene predicts higher grade and more advanced stage of prostate cancer at diagnosis, as well as metastasis and mortality from the disease. Other studies found that the prevalence of short CAG repeats is higher

TABLE 65.3 PARTIAL LIST OF PROSTATE CANCER SUSCEPTIBILITY GENES AND CANDIDATE GENES

Gene	Location	Alterations	Proposed Phenotypic Consequences
RNASEL/HPC1	1q24-25	Base substitutions Four-base deletion leading to premature truncation	Encodes endoribonuclease Early age at diagnosis
ELAC2/HPC2	17p11	Base insertion leading to premature termination Base substitutions	Unknown
MSR1	8p22-23	Base substitutions	Encodes subunit of class A macrophage-scavenger receptor
AR	Xq11-12	Polymorphic polyglutamine (CAG) and polyglycine (GGC) repeats	Encodes androgen receptor, and androgen dependent transcription factor
CYP17	10q24.3	Base substitutions in transcriptional promoter (T→C transition leading to a new Sp1 recognition site)	Encodes cytochrome P-450c17α, and enzymes that catalyzes key reactions in sex-steroid biosynthesis
SRD5A2	2p23	Base substitutions	Encodes the predominant 5-α-reductase in the prostate, converts testosterone to dihydrotestosterone
AMACR	5p13.2	Missense mutations	Unknown
BRCA2	13q12-13	Various	Possible link to higher Gleason score and stage at diagnosis
CHEK2	22q12.1	Frameshift/missense mutations	Unknown
HOXB13	17q21	Missense mutations in highly conserved functional domain	Early age at diagnosis
KFL6	10p15	DNA polymorphism	leads to alternative splicing in encoded tumor suppressor gene
MMR genes (MLH1, MSH2, HSH6, PMS2)	Various	Various	Various
NBS1	8q21	Loss of heterozygosity in carriers	Role in DNA repair
HPCX	Xq27-28	Unknown	Unknown
CAPB	1p36	Unknown	Early age at diagnosis; association with CNS malignancies

Adapted from: (1) Nelson WG, De Marzo AM, Isaacs WB. Prostate cancer. *N Engl J Med* 2003;349:366–381 (2) Langeberg WJ, Isaacs WB, Stanford JL. *Genetic Etiology of Hereditary Prostate Cancer*. Front Biosci 2007 May 1;12:4101–4110 (3) www.cancer.gov. Genetics of Prostate Cancer. Accessed December 21, 2012.

among African Americans than Whites[50] and that these sequences are longest among Chinese men.[8] These findings may partly explain the higher risk for development of prostate cancer among African Americans and the lower risk in Asian countries.

In addition to these genetic alterations identified in prostate cancer, epigenetic changes such as abnormal DNA methylation have also been observed and may play a role in upregulation or loss of expression of genes.[51] Millar et al.[52] observed that abnormal methylation of specific sites throughout the genome of prostate cancer cells leads to loss of glutathione *S*-transferase P1 (GSTP1) gene expression. The GSTP1 gene product is an enzyme that provides protection to mammalian cells against electrophilic metabolites of carcinogens and reactive oxygen species. Loss of GSTP1 may lead to a transition between proliferative inflammatory atrophy and prostatic intraepithelial neoplasia or prostate cancer.[53]

Other Risk Factors

Chronic or recurrent inflammation may have a role in the development of prostate cancer, as has been recognized in many other human cancers. Although various microbial organisms have been identified to infect prostate tissue, the specific offending pathogen causing prostatitis has not been isolated. However, the specific cause may not be necessary, as it is the host inflammatory response to an infection rather than the infectious agent itself that may lead to prostate cancer. In one large population-based study, prostate cancer risk was increased in men with a history of gonorrhea or syphilis (odds ratio, 1.6; 95% confidence interval, 1.2 to 2.1).[54] A criticism of such epidemiologic studies is the bias that men with symptomatic prostatitis compared with men without it are more likely to seek out care with urologists, have an increased serum PSA test, and have prostate biopsies.[53]

Several commonly used medications have gained attention as potential chemopreventive agents, with particular interest in 5-hydroxy-3-methylglutaryl-coenzyme A reductase inhibitors (statins). Data for the effects of statin use on subsequent risk of prostate cancer are conflicting, with some observational cohort studies and retrospective analyses suggesting a reduced risk of advanced prostate cancer,[55] reduced risk of death from prostate cancer,[56] and lower rates of relapse following radiotherapy[57] or radical prostatectomy (RP).[58] However, several large meta-analyses failed to identify a relationship between statin use and prostate cancer risk,[59,60] and no prospective, randomized studies have confirmed these observations.

Other risk factors for prostate cancer have been implicated but not corroborated. Several reports suggested an association between vasectomy and prostate cancer. In a prospective study of 10,055 vasectomized men and 37,800 nonvasectomized men, Giovannucci et al.[61] found an increased risk of 1.85 in the vasectomized men. In a retrospective study of 14,607 vasectomized or nonvasectomized men, the increased risk was 1.56.[62] A recent population-based case–control study of 923 new cases of prostate cancer among men aged 40 to 74 years from the New Zealand Cancer Registry showed no association between prostate cancer and vasectomy.[63] Although there appears to be no definite etiologic relationship, it is possible that men undergoing vasectomy are more conscious of health care and more likely to be screened for prostate cancer.[64] Circumcision has not been correlated with development of prostate cancer.[65]

Armenian et al.,[66] in a study of 296 patients with benign prostatic hyperplasia diagnosed either histologically or clinically and 299 age-matched control subjects observed from 7 to 27 years, found the incidence of prostatic cancer to be 3.7 times higher in the hyperplasia group than in the control group. This association was not observed by others.[67]

Some studies correlated smoking with increased risk of prostate cancer,[68] whereas another study did not find a significant correlation.[69] In one analysis of 359 patients,[70] a greater tumor-specific mortality rate among smokers than nonsmokers with stage A and D tumors was observed. No occupational factors have been confirmed as risks, but some evidence suggests that occupational exposure to cadmium and some aspects of farming may increase risks moderately, although these factors would account for only a small proportion of the total cases. Japanese men exposed to atomic bomb explosions in Hiroshima and Nagasaki have not had a significantly higher incidence of prostatic cancer.[71]

NATURAL HISTORY

Local Growth Patterns

The studies of prostate morphology conducted by McNeal[72] showed that almost all prostatic carcinomas (>70%) develop in the PZ of the prostate, whereas benign prostatic hyperplasia

(>90%) arises from the TZ. In addition, examination of prostatectomy specimens revealed that small tumors tend to occur in the anteromedial gland, adjacent to the fibromuscular stroma, whereas larger, more advanced T-stage tumors are often located in the posterior gland near the prostatic capsule.[73,74]

Multifocality is characteristic of prostate cancer. On DRE, there may be one nodule or many, located unilaterally or bilaterally. Histologic and molecular studies of prostatectomy specimens of patients with prostate cancer have revealed that most contain a dominant or index tumor and one or more spatially separate, often heterogeneous tumors.[75–78] Jewett[79] reported that multiple foci of disease were found throughout the prostate in 77% of prostatectomy specimens. Wise et al.[80] noted that only 17% of 486 patients treated by radical retropubic prostatectomy had one carcinoma detected by 3-mm step-section histologic examination. Of the 83% with multifocal disease, secondary cancers were mostly small; 58% were <0.5 cm^3 in volume. Qian et al.,[81] using fluorescence *in situ* hybridization to detect chromosomal abnormalities, found that an increasing incidence of chromosomal anomalies among specimens was positively correlated with progression from high-grade prostatic intraepithelial neoplasia to prostatic carcinoma. When lymph node involvement was present, there was usually evidence of one or more foci of the primary tumor sharing chromosomal anomalies with associated lymph node metastases, suggesting that just a single focus of carcinoma may give rise to metastases. This heterogeneity and multicentricity may account for the discrepancy between needle-biopsy Gleason score and the grade determined from the dominant tumor in the prostatectomy specimen.

Tumors arising from the TZ tend to demonstrate a lower frequency of extracapsular extension and may harbor large volumes of disease with relatively high PSA levels but remain confined to the prostate. Despite a high PSA value (≥10 ng/mL), these tumors should be considered to have a favorable prognosis and be managed accordingly. Noguchi et al.[82] described the histologic characteristics of 148 cases of TZ prostate cancer from RP specimens. Seventy percent were clinical stage T1c, with a preoperative serum PSA of 10 ng/mL or greater in almost two-thirds of cases. Only 63% had a positive initial prostatic biopsy. On pathologic review, 80% had organ-confined disease, and more than one-third of cases had a cancer volume >6 mL. When compared with 79 PZ cancers matched by volume, there were no differences in percentage Gleason grade 4/5, serum PSA, or prostate weight, although differences in clinical stage T1c to T2c and organ-confined cancer were highly significant. The actuarial 5-year PSA relapse–free survival rate was 71.5% among men with TZ cancer, compared with 49.2% for those with PZ cancer.

PZ cancers tend to spread along the capsular surface of the gland and may extend through the capsule of the gland, invade seminal vesicles and periprostatic tissues, and involve the bladder neck or the rectum. Clinical stage closely correlated with risk of extracapsular extension and disease progression.[83–85] The incidence of microscopic tumor extension beyond the capsule of the gland (at the time of RP) in patients with clinically organ-confined disease ranges from 8% to 57%.[86,87] Oesterling et al.,[88] in an analysis of patients with stage T1c disease treated with RP, noted that 53% had pathologically organ-confined tumors, 35% had extracapsular extension, and 9% had seminal vesicle invasion. Of the last group, 66% had positive surgical margins, an incidence comparable with that for clinical stage T2 tumors. In a similar group of patients with T1c tumors, Epstein et al.[89] found that 34% had established extracapsular extension, 6% had seminal vesicle invasion, and 17% had positive surgical margins.

Pretreatment serum PSA is also predictive of extraprostatic extension and seminal vesicle invasion. The rate of organ-confined prostate cancer ranges from 53% to 67% for men with a PSA level between 4 and 10 ng/mL and from 31% to 56% for men with a PSA level between 10 and 20 ng/mL.[90–92] D'Amico et al.,[93] in a pathologic evaluation of 347 RP specimens, reported that none of 38 patients with PSA of ≤4 ng/mL had seminal vesicle involvement, in contrast to 6% of 144 patients with PSA of 4 to 10 ng/mL, 11% of 101 with PSA of 10 to 20 ng/mL, 36% of 45 with PSA of 20 to 40 ng/mL, and 42% of 19 with PSA of >40 ng/mL. The incidence of positive surgical margins for these PSA subgroups was 11%, 20%, 33%, 56%, and 63%, respectively. The incidence of seminal vesicle involvement also is associated with the level of PSA, the Gleason score, and the clinical stage.[94,95] Seminal vesicle involvement has been observed in from 10% of patients with A2 tumors to 30% of the patients with B2 lesions.[96,97]

Roach[98] proposed formulas based on analysis of RP specimens to estimate the probability of extracapsular extension (ECE+) and seminal vesicle involvement (SV+):

$$ECE+ = 3/2\ PSA + (\text{Gleason score} - 3) \times 10$$

$$SV+ = PSA + (\text{Gleason score} - 6) \times 10$$

Regional Lymph Node Involvement

Tumor size and degree of differentiation affect the tendency of prostatic carcinoma to metastasize to regional lymphatics.[99,100] With an increasing number of patients being diagnosed in earlier stages (as a result of screening PSA), there has been a decreased incidence of lymph node metastases in patients with clinical stage T1c and T2 tumors.[101] In the low-risk prostate cancer patients, the risk of lymph node involvement is generally considered <10%.

Several groups[90,102–107] have developed models based on clinical or pathologic data that predict the risk of lymph node metastases. This information is important to decide whether a prostate cancer patient should be subjected to a staging lymphadenectomy (including laparoscopic technique) or considered for irradiation of the pelvic lymph nodes. Partin et al.[108] analyzed data from 703 patients and generated a nomogram for predicting nodal metastases based on three factors: clinical stage, preoperative PSA, and tumor biopsy grade. This model was validated in a larger multicenter study of 7,014 men and accurately predicted nodal metastases in 78% of patients.[109] The negative predictive value was 99%. Bluestein et al.[104] tested a model based on multivariate logistic regression analysis on 1,632 patients who underwent pelvic lymphadenectomy at the Mayo Clinic for staging of prostate cancer. Using this method, they determined that 29% of the patients with clinical stage T1a to T2c disease would have been spared pelvic lymphadenectomy with only a 3% rate of missed nodal metastases. Bishoff et al.[103] reported similar results demonstrating that 20% to 63% of patients with prostate cancer could be spared pelvic lymphadenectomy when accepting a 2% to 10% risk for missed nodal metastasis. These results suggest that many patients can be spared pelvic lymphadenectomy solely by analyzing preoperative PSA, Gleason grade, and clinical stage, without incurring an unacceptable risk for failing to identify regional metastasis.[110]

Stock et al.,[95] in a study of 99 patients who underwent laparoscopic lymph node dissection, correlated incidence of positive nodes with PSA, Gleason score, stage, and involvement of seminal vesicles. None of the patients with a Gleason score of 4 or lower, even those with PSA of >20 ng/mL, had positive pelvic lymph nodes, and 8% in the group with Gleason scores of 5 or 6 and PSA levels of 4 to 10 ng/mL had positive nodes. However, the incidence of positive lymph nodes increased significantly (to 24%) in patients with PSA of >20 ng/mL. These results are similar to those reported in patients treated with RP.[104,108]

In an analysis of 2,144 patients treated at two institutions, Rees et al.[111] noted that only 30 (2.2%) of 1,390 patients with a negative DRE and either PSA of 5 ng/mL or less, Gleason score of 5 or less, or a combination of PSA of <25 ng/mL and Gleason score of ≤7 had pelvic lymph node metastases.

Roach[98] suggested a formula based on pathologic findings in prostatectomy specimens to estimate the incidence of metastatic pelvic lymph nodes (Nodes+):

$$\text{Nodes+} = 2/3\ \text{PSA} + (\text{Gleason score} - 6) \times 10$$

Prognosis is closely related to the presence of regional lymph node metastases; patients with positive pelvic lymph nodes have a significantly greater probability (>85% at 10 years) for development of distant metastasis than those with negative nodes (<20%).[112] However, a single nodal metastasis is not an unfavorable prognostic sign. In a study by Cheng et al.,[113] 322 patients with positive lymph nodes after RP and bilateral pelvic lymphadenectomy were followed for a median of 6 years. Patients with prostate carcinoma who had multiple regional lymph node metastases had increased risk of death from disease, whereas patients with a single positive lymph node appeared to have a more favorable prognosis after RP and immediate adjuvant hormonal therapy. Prout et al.,[114] in 92 patients with various stages of prostatic carcinoma, noted solitary lymph node metastasis in 11 (34%) of 32 patients with positive nodes. Bilateral pelvic lymph node involvement was present in 14 (58%) of 24 patients who had more than one metastatic lymph node. Only 2 (18%) of 11 patients with a single metastasis showed tumor progression, compared with 15 (76%) of 21 with multiple lymph node involvement. Golimbu et al.[115] noted a 10-year survival rate of 50% in patients with a single positive lymph node, compared with 20% for those with multiple lymph node involvement.

The prognostic significance of multiple involved lymph nodes should be considered with the extent of lymphadenectomy. Several studies have evaluated the anatomic extent of pelvic lymph node dissection on outcome.[116,117] At Johns Hopkins University Hospital, two surgeons performed 4,000 RP with or without an extended lymph node dissection. The extended dissection removed more lymph nodes (mean 12 vs. 9; $p < .0001$) and detected more lymph node–positive prostate cancer (3.2% vs. 1.1%; $p < .0001$) than more limited procedure. If disease was found involving <15% of the extracted lymph nodes, extended lymph node dissection resulted in a more favorable 5-year PSA progression-free survival. Thus, in certain subgroups, an extended dissection may be beneficial. In another study, the number and percentage of involved lymph nodes correlated with recurrence-free and overall survival.[117] These results need additional validation in prospectively controlled studies.

CLINICAL PRESENTATION AND DIAGNOSTIC WORKUP

Screening Methods and Markers

Although DRE is still an essential element in screening and assigning clinical stage, only 25% to 50% of men with an abnormal DRE have cancer on biopsy. Moreover, because carcinoma of the prostate can be asymptomatic until attaining a significant size, if a patient presents with a palpable tumor there is a significant risk that there already may be locally advanced or metastatic disease. With the advent of PSA screening, the diagnosis of prostate cancer may precede palpable disease on DRE and the symptoms of urinary obstruction or metastatic disease by many years. DRE is associated with 70% sensitivity and 50% specificity.[118] In fact, 70% of cancers detected by PSA screening are confined to the prostate, and 40% of cancers detected by PSA are not palpable.[87]

PSA, initially identified and purified from prostatic tissue by Wang et al.[119] in 1979, is a protein with a molecular weight of 33,000. PSA is detected not only in prostatic tissue (normal tissue, benign hyperplasia, and malignant tumors) and in seminal fluid, but also in the sera of patients with prostatic cancer. It is localized in the cytoplasm of ductal epithelial cells and in secretory materials in ductal lamina.[120] PSA has been detected with immunohistochemical techniques in pancreas and salivary glands and in women; therefore, it is not absolutely specific for prostatic epithelium.[121]

Widespread use of PSA screening has come into question following publication of two landmark screening trials. The European Randomized Study of Screening for Prostate Cancer (ERSPC) randomized 162,387 men age 50 to 74 years to PSA screening an average of once every 4 years or to no such screening.[122] At a median follow-up of 9 years, PSA screening showed a modest reduction in death from prostate cancer that would require screening of 1,410 men and treatment of 48 men to prevent one death from prostate cancer. The reduction in death from prostate cancer was apparent only in men age 55 to 69 years. The contemporaneous U.S.-based Prostate, Lung, Colorectal, and Ovarian (PLCO) Cancer screening trial randomized 76,693 men age 55 to 74 years to annual PSA testing for 6 years and annual DRE for 4 years versus no such screening.[123] At a median follow-up of 7 years, no difference in mortality was noted between the arms. As of August 2008, the U.S. Preventive Services Task Force recommended against PSA screening in men age 75 years or older and concluded that current evidence is inadequate to make a PSA screening recommendation for men younger than the age of 75 years.[124] The American Urological Association continues to recommend annual DRE and PSA screening tests for men older than 40 years of age if their life expectancy is >10 years.[125]

Radioimmunoassays for prostatic acid phosphatase (PAP) have a sensitivity of approximately 10% and a specificity of about 90% for malignant tumors[118] and to a large extent have been superseded by PSA testing. Stamey et al.[126] reported PSA and PAP measurements by radioimmunoassay in 2,200 serum samples from 699 patients, 378 of whom were known to have prostatic carcinoma. PSA was elevated in 122 of 127 patients with newly diagnosed prostatic carcinoma, whereas PAP was elevated in only 57 patients with cancer and correlated less closely with tumor volume than did PSA. PSA was increased in 86% and PAP in 14% of the patients with benign prostatic hyperplasia. After RP for cancer, PSA routinely declines to undetectable levels, with an associated half-life of 2.2 days. PAP, if initially elevated, normalizes within 24 hours after surgery. Several authors concluded that PSA is more sensitive than PAP and DRE in the detection of prostatic carcinoma and that PSA would be more useful in monitoring response and recurrence after therapy.[126–128] A caveat is that both PSA and PAP may be elevated in benign prostatic hyperplasia. Hudson et al.[127] reported that only 3% of 168 men with benign prostatic hyperplasia had PSA levels of >10 ng/mL, compared with 44% of 231 patients with prostatic carcinoma.

Several investigators[129–131] reported no significant impact of DRE on the plasma levels of PSA or PAP in patients with various prostatic abnormalities in whom blood samples were collected before, immediately after, and 30 minutes after rectal examination of the prostate. Others[132–134] detected a significant increase in PSA after DRE. Ornstein et al.[134] noted an increase in both total and free PSA in 31% and 48% of men, respectively, at 1 hour after DRE. Matzkin et al.[135] found no significant change in PSA levels after inserting a urethral catheter and maintaining it for several days. Yet, significant PSA elevation has been demonstrated after prostatic massage, transrectal ultrasonography (TRUS), prostate biopsy, and transurethral resection of the prostate (TURP).[131,132,136,137] The kinetics of serum PSA elevation after DRE and needle biopsy were investigated in a Dutch study with few participants.[138] Blood samples were taken at 1 and 30 minutes and 1, 3, 6, and 12 hours and then every 24 hours until 5 days had elapsed. The peak levels were between 30 and 60 minutes after DRE and returned to baseline 24 to 72 hours after the examination. There was a threefold increase in PSA after needle biopsy, and only two of seven patients had returned to their baseline PSA at 5 days. Studies reporting the effect of ejaculation on PSA also have

TABLE 65.4A LIKELIHOOD OF DETECTING PROSTATE CANCER ON TRANSRECTAL BIOPSY FOR 2,054 MEN AGE 40 TO 80 YEARS AS A FUNCTION OF SERUM PSA LEVEL, INDEPENDENT OF DRE RESULT

	Likelihood at Given Age[a]			
PSA (ng/mL)	*<50 Year*	*51–60 Years*	*61–70 Years*	*>71 Year*
<2.5	10	14	17	23
2.6–4.0	11	15	19	24
4.1–6.0	12	16	21	26
6.1–10.0	14	18	23	29
10.1–20.0	17	23	31	37
>20.0	40	49	60	69

DRE, digital rectal examination; PSA, prostate-specific antigen. Ninety-five percent confidence intervals are within 2% to 12% for all probabilities.

[a]Recorded at time of PSA collection.

From Potter SR, Horniger W, Tinzl M, et al. Age, prostate-specific antigen, and digital rectal examination as determinants of the probability of having prostate cancer. *Urology* 2001;57:1100–1104.

TABLE 65.4B LIKELIHOOD OF DETECTING PROSTATE CANCER ON TRANSRECTAL BIOPSY FOR 2,054 MEN AGE 40 TO 80 YEARS AS A FUNCTION OF PATIENT AGE, SERUM PSA LEVEL, AND DRE FINDINGS

	Likelihood at Given Age[a]							
	<50 Year		*51–60 Years*		*61–70 Years*		*71–80 Years*	
PSA (ng/mL)	*DRE–*	*DRE+*	*DRE–*	*DRE+*	*DRE–*	*DRE+*	*DRE–*	*DRE+*
<2.5	9	37	12	39	15	42	20	44
2.6–4.0	9	41	12	42	16	44	20	47
4.1–6.0	10	41	14	44	17	47	22	48
6.1–10.0	11	–	15	48	19	50	25	42
10.1–20.0	13	55	19	54	25	58	31	60
>20.0	22	82	45	74	43	81	59	84

DRE, digital rectal examination; PSA, prostate-specific antigen. Ninety-five percent confidence intervals are within 2% to 12% for all probabilities.

[a]Recorded at time of PSA collection.

From Potter SR, Horniger W, Tinzl M, et al. Age, prostate-specific antigen, and digital rectal examination as determinants of the probability of having prostate cancer. *Urology* 2001;57:1100–1104.

contradictory results. Some authors found no effect at all,[139,140] whereas others demonstrated that ejaculation increased PSA levels in 87% of 64 men evaluated with serial determinations (at 1, 6, 24, and 48 hours).[141] A return to baseline was observed in 92% of subjects by 24 hours and in 97% by 48 hours.

Nadler et al.[142] quantified causes of elevated PSA in 148 men with PSA of >4 ng/mL (a finding suspect for cancer) and multiple negative biopsies. They were compared with 64 men who had a suspect DRE, multiple negative biopsies, and PSA of ≤4 ng/mL. Acute or chronic inflammation of the prostate was more prevalent in the high-PSA group (63% vs. 27%; $p = .0001$). Patients with elevated PSA had significantly larger prostate volumes (median, 68 cm^3) than those without PSA elevation (median, 32.5 cm^3). Simultaneous regression analysis demonstrated that prostatic size accounted for 23%, inflammation for 7%, prostatic calculi for 3%, and nonisoechoic ultrasonographic lesions for 1% of the PSA serum variances.

The positive predictive value for PSA of >4 ng/mL ranges from 31% to 54%. A greater yield is observed when elevated PSA is coupled with positive ultrasonographic and rectal examinations (Tables 65.4A and 65.4B).[143] The estimated rate of cancer detection by PSA screening ranges from 1.8% to 3.3%. The percentage of clinically localized tumors detected by PSA ranges from 81% to 97%. The percentage of pathologically localized tumors ranges from 36% to 91%, and is significantly higher when serial PSA screening is done.

An important issue is the clinical significance of small tumors detected by PSA testing. Epstein et al.[89,144] identified a subset of patients with potentially biologically insignificant tumors among men with clinical stage T1c disease who underwent RP. On multivariate analysis, the best model predicting insignificant tumor was PSA density of <0.1 ng/mL per gram and no adverse pathologic findings on needle biopsy, or PSA density of 0.1 to 0.15 ng/mL per gram, with a low- to intermediate-grade cancer <3 mm found in only one needle biopsy core specimen. The positive predictive value of the model was 95%, with a negative predictive value of 66%.[89] Dugan et al.[145] offered a definition of clinically insignificant cancer as a tumor that gives rise to no more than 20 cm^3 of cancerous tissue in the prostate by the time of expected death and a Gleason score of <4 in patients 40 years old, 5 in 50- to 59-year-old patients, 6 in 60- to 69-year-old patients, and 7 in 70- to 79-year-old patients. Using these definitions, a review of 337 prostatectomy specimens showed that, for cancer volume doubling times of 2, 3, 4, and 6 years, clinically insignificant cancer was identified in 1 (0.3%), 13 (3.9%), 25 (7.4%), and 49 (14.5%) of specimens, respectively. Humphrey et al.[146] determined that in 11% to 30% of PSA-detected prostate cancers, the tumor volumes were <0.5 mL. Therefore, by these definitions, most men treated with RP (or radiation therapy) have clinically significant cancer.

The incidence of clinically unimportant cancers has been reported to be between 4% and 16%.[89,101,147,148] Researchers at the Fred Hutchinson Cancer Center developed a computer model to estimate the rates of prostate cancer overdiagnosis because of PSA testing. Using the National Cancer Institute's Surveillance, Epidemiology, and End Results registry data as a comparison for their computer-generated incidence rates, they calculated overdiagnosis rates of 15% in Whites and 37% in Blacks. These men were predicted to have prostate cancer that would be detected only at autopsy.[149] Conversely, an epidemiologic study randomizing men from Göteborg, Sweden, to PSA screening or a control group demonstrated that screening did not lead to overdiagnosis of prostate cancer; rather, most cancers detected at PSA-guided screening would eventually develop into clinical, frequently fatal, disease.[150]

Although PSA screening–detected cancers may be smaller, they may harbor aggressive disease. Investigators from the Netherlands studied 121 RP specimens from screened patients and found that screening-detected specimens were more likely to be pathologically organ-confined tumors and to have Gleason scores of <8.[151] However, 60% of screening-detected tumors contained areas with high-grade cancer (Gleason pattern 4 or 5), and 50% had a Gleason score of 7, suggesting that most of these tumors are clinically important. Updated results from a study of expectant management of patients with nonpalpable prostate cancer believed to have small-volume disease showed a 6.5-year median survival free of intervention and a 33% intervention rate at a median of 2.2 years, with a median follow-up among the entire cohort of 2.7 years.[152] Increased PSA density and decreased percentage free PSA correlated with progression of disease. Ninety-two percent of patients had curable disease at the time of their diagnosis of progression. These investigators concluded that observation with close follow-up may be a reasonable alternative for older men with a high likelihood of harboring small-volume prostate cancer.

Refinements of the PSA screening test have been introduced to increase the sensitivity and specificity of the test. It was anticipated that such approaches would be able to more readily find curable cancers in younger men and to avoid unnecessary biopsies of benign hypertrophic disease in older men. Unfortunately, none of these modifications listed in the following sections has proven reliable enough alone on which to base a treatment decision for the individual patient.

Prostate-Specific Antigen Density

PSA density relies on the fact that cancers produce less PSA per cell than nonmalignant prostatic tissues. It is calculated by dividing the serum PSA concentration by the volume of the prostate gland measured by TRUS. A higher PSA density is associated with malignancy.

Prostate-Specific Antigen Velocity

Another method is to obtain serial PSA measurements and calculate the rate of rise in PSA, or PSA velocity. A rate of rise of >0.75 ng/mL per year has been associated with a higher frequency of cancer. Two large retrospective analyses suggested that a >2.0 ng/mL increase in PSA in the year prior to diagnosis is correlated with greater prostate cancer–specific mortality following radiotherapy[153] and RP[154] for localized prostate cancer, respectively.

Free Prostate-Specific Antigen

Serum tests for the molecular forms of PSA (free vs. complexed vs. total) have been developed to discriminate between elevated PSA levels from benign prostatic hyperplasia versus cancer. This is based on the concept that PSA exists in serum in a complexed form bound to either α_1-antichymotrypsin or α_2-macroglobulin, two extracellular protease inhibitors. Bound to α_1-antichymotrypsin or α_2-macroglobulin, the enzyme is inactive but still detectable using conventional immunoassays. In a study of free PSA, complexed PSA, and total PSA (free + complexed), the complexed-to-total ratio was higher and free PSA lower in patients with prostate cancer relative to those with benign prostatic hyperplasia.[155] Catalona et al.[156] reported on 113 patients with PSA levels between 4.1 and 10 ng/mL (63 with histologically confirmed benign prostatic hyperplasia, 30 with prostate cancer and enlarged gland, and 20 with cancer and a normal-sized gland). The median percentage of free PSA was 9.2% for men with cancer and a normal-sized gland, 15.9% for those with cancer and an enlarged gland, and 18.8% for those with benign prostatic hyperplasia ($p < .001$). Men with prostate cancer and either a normal or an enlarged gland had a significantly lower percentage of free PSA than men with benign prostatic hyperplasia only. At Washington University, a ratio of free to total PSA of ≤0.2 was most likely associated with prostate cancer and with higher percentages with benign prostatic hypertrophy. A ratio of ≤0.15 was associated with a higher Gleason score and poorer prognosis.[157]

Oesterling et al.[158] analyzed free, complexed, and total PSA in 422 healthy men aged 40 to 79 years. The respective recommended age-specific reference ranges (95th percentile) for the three forms were 0.5, 1, and 1 ng/mL for men aged 40 to 49 years; 0.7, 1.5, and 3 ng/mL for men aged 50 to 59 years; 1, 2, and 4 ng/mL for men aged 60 to 69 years; and 1.2, 3, and 5.5 ng/mL for men aged 70 to 79 years. Similar observations were made by investigators at Johns Hopkins.[159]

Reverse Transcriptase–Polymerase Chain Reaction Assay

Recent developments include using molecular biologic methods, particularly reverse transcriptase–PCR (RT-PCR), to measure markers by detecting low levels of messenger RNA (mRNA) for PSA and prostate-specific membrane antigen (PSMA) expressed by circulating metastatic prostate cancer cells.[160–164] The assay is highly specific because the only cells expressing PSA in the peripheral blood are circulating prostate cancer cells. However, there is a wide range of sensitivities of detection of PSA-expressing cells in the peripheral blood reported in the literature.[165]

Katz et al.,[166] in 94 patients on whom RT-PCR assay for PSA mRNA was performed, reported an enhanced reaction in 26 (72%) of 36 patients who had extraprostatic tumor at the time of surgery. The test was negative in 51 (88%) of 58 patients with organ-confined disease. Six months after surgery, an increased PSA level was noted in 19% and 2% of the two groups, respectively. This bioassay may have significant staging value in patients who are candidates for RP.

Cama et al.[160] noted that, in contrast to the RT-PCR assay for PSA, the assay for PSMA did not correlate with pathologic stage of prostate cancer.

Oefelein et al.,[167] using RT-PCR for PSA, identified positive cells in 20 (91%) of 22 operative field samples, and 4 (25%) of 16 had evidence of intraoperative hematogenous dissemination ($p = .046$). Their results suggest that tumor cell spillage and, less frequently, hematogenous dissemination may be associated with operative manipulation of the prostate during RP and may potentially represent the mechanism of failure after this treatment.

Israeli et al.,[168] using the PCR assay, also reported circulating prostatic tumor cells in 2 (6.7%) of 30 men. However, prostate-specific membrane primer assay demonstrated tumor cells in 19 (63%) of 30 patients. All 16 negative control subjects had negative PSA and PSMA PCR results. Using PSA mRNA as a marker for prostatic epithelial cells, Seiden et al.,[169] noted that 5 of 65 patients with clinically localized carcinoma of the prostate had PSA mRNA–detectable cells by transcription and PCR. On the other hand, 10 of 20 patients with hormone-refractory and progressive prostate cancer also demonstrated the same increased frequency of PSA mRNA–detectable cells.

Overall, most studies report a 0% PSA rate by RT-PCR in negative control cases, whereas the positive rate in the metastatic group ranges between 31% and 88%.[164] However, 25% of men with localized prostate cancer who underwent RP and had specimen-confined disease had a positive PCR PSA assay.[166] These men would be denied surgery if it was concluded that circulating prostate cancer cells are synonymous with incurable disease. A new approach is to use a combination of primers to improve the overall staging accuracy of RT-PCR. Preliminary work from the Cleveland Clinic suggests that combining RT-PCR for PSA and PSMA may improve the staging accuracy.[170] Until the significance of a positive PCR assay is determined with long-term follow-up, RT-PCR remains experimental and should not change treatment recommendations.

Staging Workup

Patients with localized prostatic carcinoma are frequently asymptomatic; the diagnosis is often made with a screening PSA test. In the pre-PSA era, asymptomatic patients were diagnosed on the basis of palpating a hard nodule on DRE. Patients with locally advanced tumors have presented with bladder outlet obstructive symptoms such as urinary hesitancy, decreased force of the urinary stream, and postvoid dribbling as the tumor impinges on the membranous urethra. Chronic obstruction and bladder distention can lead to decreased compliance of the detrusor muscle that is manifested by symptoms of urinary frequency, urgency, and nocturia. Very early–stage disease (T1a or T1b) may occasionally be diagnosed at TURP for symptoms of bladder outlet obstruction caused by benign prostatic hyperplasia. With local invasion into the urethra or ejaculatory ducts, patients may experience hematuria or hematospermia. As the disease penetrates the capsule of the prostate, there may be invasion into the neurovascular bundles that course along the lateral aspects of the prostate, leading to erectile dysfunction. Disseminated disease frequently manifests as bone pain from distant osseous metastases.

A complete clinical history and a general physical examination including DRE are mandatory. The DRE is best performed with a well-lubricated glove; the patient may be standing and bent over at the waist with his elbows resting comfortably on a firm surface or in the lateral decubitus position on the examining table. The examiner should note the size of the gland, its overall consistency, and the presence of any firm areas. A typical neoplastic nodule of prostatic carcinoma is extremely firm, often not elevated above the surface of the gland, but surrounded by compressible prostatic tissue. The examiner should determine whether the lateral sulci are involved by tumor and also the

TABLE 65.5 AMERICAN JOINT COMMITTEE ON CANCER 2010 TNM STAGING SYSTEM FOR PROSTATE CANCER

Primary Tumor (T)	
TX	Primary tumor cannot be assessed
T0	No evidence of primary tumor
T1	Clinically inapparent tumor neither palpable nor visible by imaging
T1a	Tumor incidental histologic finding in ≤5% of tissue resected
T1b	Tumor incidental histologic finding in >5% of tissue resected
T1c	Tumor identified by needle biopsy (e.g., because of elevated prostate-specific antigen)
T2	Tumor confined within prostate
T2a	Tumor involves one lobe
T2b	Tumor involves more than one-half of a lobe but not both lobes
T2c	Tumor involves both lobes
T3	Tumor extends through the prostate capsule
T3a	Extracapsular extension
T3b	Tumor invades seminal vesicle(s)
T4	Tumor is fixed or invades adjacent structures other than seminal vesicles
T4a	Tumor invades bladder neck, external sphincter, or rectum
T4b	Tumor invades levator muscles or is fixed to pelvic wall, or both
Regional Lymph Nodes (N)	
NX	Regional lymph nodes cannot be assessed
N0	No regional node metastasis
N1	Metastasis in single lymph node, ≤2 cm
N2	Metastasis in a single node, >2 cm but not >5 cm
N3	Metastasis in a node >5 cm
Distant Metastasis (M)	
MX	Presence of metastasis cannot be assessed
M0	No distant metastasis
M1	Distant metastasis
M1a	Nonregional lymph node(s)
M1b	Metastasis in bone(s)
M1c	Metastasis in other site(s)

Used with the permission of the American Joint Committee on Cancer (AJCC), Chicago, Illinois. The original source for this material is *AJCC Cancer Staging Handbook,* 7th ed. New York: Springer, 2010; published by Springer Science and Business Media LLC, www.springer.com.

degree of spread superiorly. In most patients the seminal vesicles cannot be palpated as discrete structures, and the finding of a firm area extending above the prostate suggests that the seminal vesicles are involved by malignancy. Only approximately 50% of prostatic nodules found on DRE are confirmed to be malignant on biopsy.[79] The American Joint Committee on Cancer TNM Staging System for prostate cancer is shown in Table 65.5.

An abnormal DRE result, a consistently elevated PSA, or a combination of the two warrants a biopsy to establish a pathologic diagnosis. A TRUS-guided needle biopsy is the most common method for obtaining representative samples of the prostatic tissue. Ten to 18 cores are taken, including cores from the base, mid, and apex bilaterally and additional cores from the midline and lateral peripheral zone. If clinically indicated by obstructive symptoms, a separate biopsy of the TZ is taken. The pathology report frequently includes the length of each core and the length of each core that contains tumor.

Once the tissue diagnosis of prostate cancer is ascertained, the patient should undergo a staging workup including laboratory data such as a baseline PSA, complete blood count, and testosterone level. The standard tests required in the evaluation of patients with prostatic carcinoma are listed in Table 65.6. Although a chest radiograph is recommended, a study of 236 patients undergoing RP showed abnormal findings in only 28 (11.9%), mostly related to cardiac or pulmonary problems or arterial hypertension; one primary lung cancer was found.[171] According to the American College of Radiology appropriateness criteria, a chest radiograph should be performed as part of the initial staging only with suspected metastatic disease.[172]

Imaging Studies

Diagnostic imaging studies have become an essential aspect of pretreatment evaluation and treatment selection. New techniques have allowed for more precise assessments of tumor location, volume, and extent, as well as biologic activity. As a result, clinical staging can be used more accurately as a prognostic factor for defining treatment options.

TABLE 65.6 DIAGNOSTIC WORKUP FOR CARCINOMA OF THE PROSTATE

Routine
Clinical history and clinical examination
Rectal examination
Laboratory
Complete blood cell count, blood chemistry
Serum prostate-specific antigen (total, free, percentage free)
Plasma acid phosphatases (prostatic/total)
Radiographic imaging
Magnetic resonance imaging with endorectal coil
Radioisotope bone scan (prostate-specific antigen, >20)
Computed tomography of pelvis
Chest radiograph (high risk for metastatic disease)
Transrectal ultrasonography (for biopsy guidance)
Needle biopsy of prostate (transrectal, transperineal)
Staging lymph node dissection (high risk for lymph node metastases)

Used with the permission of the American Joint Committee on Cancer (AJCC), Chicago, Illinois. The original source for this material is *AJCC Cancer Staging Handbook,* 7th ed. New York: Springer, 2010; published by Springer Science and Business Media LLC, www.springer.com.

Transrectal Ultrasonography

The normal adult prostate imaged by TRUS appears as a symmetric, triangular, relatively homogeneous structure with an echogenic capsule. TRUS is used routinely for guidance during the transrectal biopsy and during prostate brachytherapy. However, only prostate cancers located in the PZ can be reliably detected by ultrasonography. Attempts to characterize adenocarcinoma by pattern on TRUS have indicated that prostate cancers can have variable echogenicities. Rifkin et al.,[173] in 443 men undergoing TRUS of the prostate, found 130 pathologically proven cancers and 313 cases of benign prostatic disease. Cancers were hyperechoic in 69% of the cases and had poorly defined margins, whereas benign lesions were hyperechoic in only 46% of the cases. The authors concluded that there are no specific characteristics on TRUS that reliably differentiate between benign prostatic disease and malignancy.

Chodak et al.,[174] in a prospective, randomized study of TRUS in 216 men, reported a sensitivity of 86% but a specificity of only 41%; tumors <1 cm were the most difficult to detect. For staging purposes, Rifkin et al.[173] found a sensitivity of only 60% using TRUS to distinguish between T2 and T3 lesions.

Computed Tomography

The primary role of CT in prostate cancer is for size determination of the prostate gland, radiation therapy treatment planning, and assessment of pelvic nodal metastases. Roach et al.[175] compared prostate volumes defined by MRI and CT and found a 32% increase in prostate volume when defined by noncontrast CT scan. Using image fusion, they identified four areas, including the posterior aspect, the posteroinferior apical aspect of the gland, the prostatic apex, and the neurovascular bundles, which tended to be areas of discrepancy between the two imaging modalities. Kagawa et al.,[176] using CT-MRI fusion software for planning three-dimensional conformal radiation therapy (3DCRT), demonstrated that MRI was clearly superior to CT in defining the prostate apex, neurovascular bundles, and anterior rectal wall. The discrepancy in prostate location between the two imaging studies was also greatest at the apex and base of the gland.

CT lacks the soft-tissue resolution needed to detect intraprostatic disease, capsular extension, or seminal vesicle involvement. Moreover, for most patients with newly diagnosed prostate cancer, the incidence of positive lymph nodes is <5%; thus, there is little role for CT as a routine staging procedure.[177,178] CT identification of pelvic adenopathy depends on lymph node enlargement, and the correlation between nodal size and metastatic involvement is poor.[177,179,180]

Albertsen et al.[181] performed a population-based analysis to determine the positive yield of imaging studies performed on men with newly diagnosed prostate cancer. The positive yield of a CT scan was <12% for men with PSA of 4 to 20 ng/mL. More than 10% of men with PSA of >20 ng/mL and Gleason score of 6 or greater were likely to have CT scans positive for extracapsular or metastatic disease. For combinations of high Gleason scores and PSA of >50 ng/mL, the positive yield on CT scan was as high as 62%. Flanigan et al.[177] retrospectively studied 173 men who underwent preoperative CT scanning and found that none of the patients with a PSA of <25 ng/mL had an abnormality by CT scan. Of 33 patients with PSA levels of >25 ng/mL, 9 had nodal metastases, but only 3 (9%) of these 33 patients were correctly diagnosed by CT scanning. These authors concluded that routine preoperative CT scanning could not be justified in patients with a PSA of <25 ng/mL. Although the histologic incidence of positive pelvic lymph nodes is substantial when PSA levels exceed 25 ng/mL, the sensitivity of CT for detecting positive nodes is only approximately 30% to 35% even at these levels.[178]

Bone Scan

A close correlation exists between pretreatment PSA level and incidence of abnormal bone scan results.[182,183] Given the low risk of osseous metastasis in patients with early-stage prostate cancer, the yield of a bone scan is low unless the PSA is >20 ng/mL or the patient complains of bone pain. In a retrospective analysis of 589 patients with untreated carcinoma of the prostate and PSA levels of ≤20 ng/mL, Rees et al.[178] reported that only 3 (1%) of 274 patients evaluated by bone scan and 3 (1%) of 262 patients evaluated by CT scan had evidence of metastatic disease. Only 1 of 108 patients with a PSA of ≤10 ng/mL had metastatic disease, and no patient with a Gleason score of ≤5 had an abnormal bone scan or CT scan result or positive lymph nodes.

Huncharek and Muscat,[184] in an analysis of 265 patients with localized carcinoma of the prostate, noted that no patients with PSA of <4 ng/mL had a positive bone scan. In patients with PSA of 4.1 to 10 ng/mL and PSA of 10.1 to 20 ng/mL, 2.2% and 3.6%, respectively, had positive bone scans. In patients with PSA of >20 ng/mL, 6.7% had a positive bone scan.

Albertsen et al.[181] analyzed prospective data from the Prostate Cancer Outcomes Study from 1995 and found that physicians ordered bone scans for approximately two-thirds and CT for one-third of all new patients. Less than 5% of the imaging studies yielded positive results. Only 1% of bone scans were positive for metastatic disease for men with PSA of <10 ng/mL and Gleason score of ≤6. Only men with PSA of >50 ng/mL and Gleason scores of 8 to 10 had positive yields on bone scan of >10%. The guidelines established by the American College of Radiology appropriateness criteria for pretreatment staging of clinically localized prostate cancer recommend that a radionuclide bone scan be considered only for patients with PSA of ≥20 ng/ml, T3-4 disease, or Gleason score of ≥8 or for patients with skeletal symptoms.[172]

From a clinical standpoint, a baseline bone scan may be helpful before treatment with radiation therapy, especially in elderly patients or those with a history of arthritis, to document degenerative changes that may later be interpreted as metastatic osseous disease. Bone scintigraphy in routine follow-up has no value because PSA is more sensitive in detecting recurrence, and treatment of asymptomatic bone metastases (except in cases of impending pathologic fracture) cannot be justified. Periodic PSA assessment is adequate for follow-up of these patients, and bone scan should be limited to patients with rising PSA levels when clinically warranted.[185]

Endorectal Magnetic Resonance Imaging

The major development in prostate imaging has come in the field of MRI. With the maturation of MRI technology, there have been significant improvements in MR technique and performance for imaging the prostate. Some of the recent advances include the use of the endorectal coil to improve spatial resolution, analytic image correction software to eliminate artifact, fast spin-echo imaging to reduce image acquisition time and provide higher signal-to-noise ratio, and MR spectroscopy imaging (MRSI) to detect metabolic activity in the prostate.[186] Moreover, increasing reader experience has greatly improved the accuracy of MRI staging for prostate cancer. Strict MRI criteria for the diagnosis of extracapsular extension have been elucidated. Nevertheless, there is still interobserver variability, depending on the experience of the radiologist. One study demonstrated that the specificity for diagnosis of extracapsular extension was 93% for senior readers and 94% for junior readers, whereas sensitivity was only 50% for senior readers and 14% for junior readers.[187]

The appearance of the prostate and the information that can be gleaned for staging purposes depends on the MR technique used. On axial T1-weighted images, the prostate gland appears homogeneous and the zonal anatomy is not well appreciated.[188] However, there is a much larger field of view, allowing for detection of locoregional adenopathy and suspected bony lesions (Fig. 65.4A). Postbiopsy hemorrhage is evident on T1-weighted

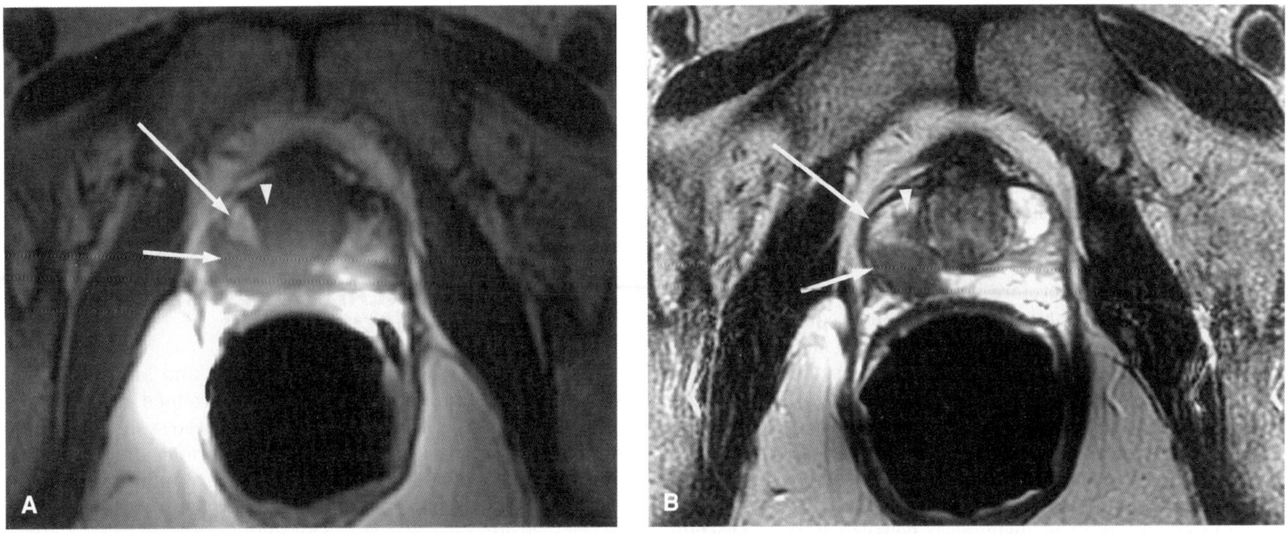

FIGURE 65.4. A: Normal T1-weighted axial magnetic resonance image. Age-related benign prostatic hyperplasia in the transition zone is evident (*long arrow*). The neurovascular bundles lie adjacent to the peripheral zone (*short arrow*). **B:** The T2-weighted axial image of the same level of the gland demonstrates areas of low signal intensity adjacent to the postbiopsy hemorrhage that are suspect for tumor (*short arrows* and *arrowheads*). This is an example of the hemorrhagic exclusion sign. (Courtesy of Steven Eberhardt, MD.)

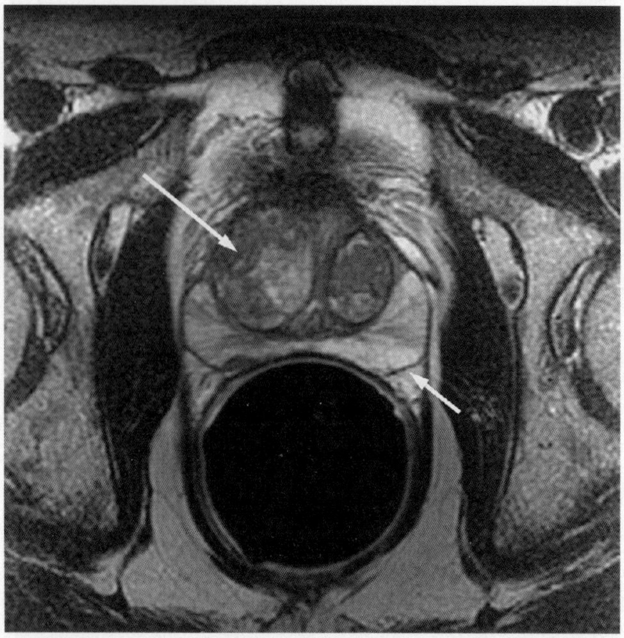

FIGURE 65.5. Normal T1-weighted axial magnetic resonance image. Age-related benign prostatic hyperplasia in the transition zone is evident (*long arrow*). The neurovascular bundles lie adjacent to the peripheral zone (*short arrow*). (Courtesy of Steven Eberhardt, MD.)

images as high T1 signal intensity (Fig. 65.4B), which may be in the prostate, seminal vesicles, or both. This is an important observation because hemorrhage may mimic tumor on T2-weighted images and because hemorrhage greatly limits the accuracy in the assessment of extracapsular extension.[189]

The zonal anatomy of the prostate is clearly depicted on axial and coronal T2-weighted images. The vas deferens and seminal vesicles are also discernible on T2-weighted axial and coronal images, whereas the neurovascular bundles can be seen best on axial images (Fig. 65.5).[188] The penile bulb is better imaged on T2-weighted coronal sections and is seen much more accurately than with CT. The PZ is normally of high signal intensity, whereas tumor appears as low signal intensity. There are many other causes of low T2 signal intensity, including hemorrhage, prostatitis, hormone treatment, and radiation therapy. An area of low signal intensity can be attributed to hemorrhage if it causes high T1 signal intensity in the corresponding region. Low T2 signal intensity due to treatment (radiation or hormonal therapy) may be suspected when the signal change is diffuse and associated with a small, featureless prostate gland. Signs of extracapsular extension are a focal, irregular capsular bulge, asymmetry or invasion of the neurovascular bundles, and obliteration of the rectoprostatic angle.[187]

Magnetic Resonance Spectroscopy Imaging

Spectroscopy is based on the principle that the electron cloud surrounding different chemical compounds shields the resonant atoms of interest to varying degrees, depending on the specific atomic structure of the compound.[190] This electron shielding causes the observed resonance frequency of the atoms to be slightly different and therefore identifiable. MRSI uses the pulse sequences from MRI, but instead of using the frequency information to provide spatial information, it uses it to identify different chemical compounds. Because MRSI uses the same clinical MRI scanner, gradients, and radiofrequency coils as MRI, it can be added to an MRI examination, and the metabolic data can then be overlaid directly on the corresponding anatomic images.[186] This modality is particularly useful in the prostate because there are metabolic compounds that localize to regions of the prostate and can be used to distinguish between normal prostate cells and malignant cells. Human prostatic glandular cells produce large amounts of citrate during cellular metabolism that are secreted into the prostatic fluid, yielding concentrations 240 to 1,300 times greater than blood plasma concentrations. High levels of citrate are found in the glandular regions of the prostate such as the PZ and lower levels in the transition and central zones. Choline is another metabolite found at intermediate levels in the normal prostate and seminal vesicles. On MRSI, regions of prostate cancer can be identified by differences in these two metabolite levels. A significant reduction in prostate citrate and a significant increase in prostate choline levels relative to the normal PZ have been observed.[186] These findings may correspond to a perturbation of cellular metabolism in malignant prostatic epithelial cells leading to less citrate production and secretion. The elevated levels of choline in prostate cancer may be attributed to the increased rate of cell proliferation, an increase in cell density in regions of cancer, and a change in the composition of the cell membrane leading to higher concentrations of choline-containing phospholipids.[186] The result of MRSI is a metabolic map of the prostate corresponding to normal and abnormal metabolic activity that can be used to pinpoint the location of prostatic tumors. This is exceptionally useful for accurate localization of prostate tumors and, in particular, when distinguishing between tumor and postbiopsy hemorrhage, which obscures MRI interpretations of prostate cancer. Moreover, there is great potential for the use of this technique for follow-up after treatment and in the development of more focused therapy.

The contribution of metabolic information gleaned from MRSI to MR anatomic imaging has improved the diagnostic accuracy of MRI both in localizing and staging prostate cancer.[190] Investigators at the University of California, San Francisco,[191] assessed the accuracy of combined MRSI and MRI for tumor detection and localization in 62 patients by comparing preoperative imaging results with histopathologic step-section examination after prostatectomy. MRI tended to have a higher sensitivity and MRSI a higher specificity for detecting definite sites of cancer. The addition of MRSI significantly improved specificity over MRI alone. Compared with step-section pathology results, the specificity for tumor location with combined MRI and MRSI reached 91%. Combined MRI/MRSI allowed localization of cancer to a sextant of the prostate with a sensitivity of up to 95% compared with MRI alone when either MRI or MRSI were positive. Moreover, a study from University of California, San Francisco,[192] found MRI and MRSI are comparable with biopsy in accurately localizing intraprostatic cancer and are more accurate than biopsy in the prostate apex.

In addition to improving prostate cancer localization, MRSI is complementary to MRI in staging and risk-stratifying patients with prostate cancer. Combined MRI/MRSI enhances the assessment of both extracapsular extension and seminal vesical invasion.[187] Furthermore, the addition of MRSI to MRI improves the accuracy of less-experienced MRI readers and reduces interobserver variability in the diagnosis of extracapsular extension.[190] Emerging data suggest that metabolic information from MRSI may also be predictive of tumor aggressiveness. Preliminary MRI/MRSI studies have shown that citrate levels are lower in poorly differentiated prostate cancers, and choline levels may be elevated in more aggressive tumors with greater membrane phospholipid synthesis.[193]

RISK STRATIFICATION SYSTEMS AND STAGING CLASSIFICATION

Based on tumor stage, pretreatment PSA, and biopsy Gleason score, PZ prostate cancer is generally grouped according to one of several risk stratification models These systems are useful to stratify disease-free survival, compare treatment results, and provide a means to appropriately recommend treatment options.[94] The most commonly used system is the prognostic risk grouping from the National Comprehensive Cancer Network (www.nccn.org), which defines low risk as PSA of ≤10 ng/mL, T1 c- T2, and Gleason score of ≤6; intermediate

TABLE 65.7 AMERICAN JOINT COMMITTEE ON CANCER 2010 ANATOMIC STAGE PROGNOSTIC GROUPS

Group	T Stage	N Stage	M Stage	Prostate-Specific Antigen	Gleason Score
I	T1a-c	N0	M0	<10	≤6
	T2a	N0	M0	≥10, <20	≤6
	T2a	N0	M0	<20	7
	T1-2a	N0	M0	X	X
IIA	T1a-c	N0	M0	<20	7
	T1a-c	N0	M0	≥10, <20	≤6
	T2a	N0	M0	<20	≤7
	T2b	N0	M0	<20	≤7
	T2b	N0	M0	X	X
IIB	T2c	N0	M0	Any	Any
	T1-2	N0	M0	≥20	Any
	T1-2	N0	M0	Any	≥8
III	T3a-b	N0	M0	Any	Any
IV	T4	N0	M0	Any	Any
	Any T	N1	M0	Any	Any
	Any T	Any N	M1	Any	Any

risk as PSA of 10 to 20 or Gleason score of 7; and high risk as PSA of >20 ng/ml, Gleason score of 8 to 10, or any T3 disease.

Traditionally, clinical and pathologic staging systems were used alone to categorize outcome, but now they are primarily used as components in risk-stratification systems. Nevertheless, it is critical to be familiar with the different updated staging systems in order to appropriately manage men with newly diagnosed prostate cancer. In 2010, the American Joint Committee on Cancer (AJCC) and International Union Against Cancer (UICC) updated the 2003 TNM classification system.[4] The TNM staging system is based on separate designations for the primary tumor, regional nodes, and distant metastases. All information that is available before first definitive treatment may be used for clinical staging, including imaging studies. The 2010 staging system maintains many of the features of the 2003 systems but reclassifies microscopic invasion of the bladder neck (previously T4) as T3 a and includes new Anatomic Stage/Prognostic Groups that incorporate both Gleason score and preoperative PSA. The 2010 AJCC/UICC staging system is summarized in Table 65.5, and the new anatomic stage/prognostic groups are outlined in Table 65.7.

PATHOLOGY

Adenocarcinoma, arising from peripheral acinar glands, is the most common tumor in the prostate. It is graded as well, moderately, or poorly differentiated according to cellular characteristics such as nuclear content, number of nuclei, pleomorphism, gland formation, and invasion of the stroma.[94]

Gleason[194,195] and Gleason and Mellinger[196] initially proposed a prognostic classification system based on the clinical stage and the degree of differentiation of primary and secondary morphologic patterns of the tumor, each graded from 1 to 5. Subsequently, only pathologic features were scored, resulting in the Gleason score that sums grades to yield nine discrete scores (range, 2 to 10). The Gleason score is one of the strongest predictors of biologic behavior in prostate cancer, including invasiveness and metastatic potential; however, it is limited by its subjectivity. There is significant interobserver and intraobserver variability reported using the Gleason grading system.[197] In addition, the treatment with hormonal therapy agents can affect the pathologist's ability to accurately identify a Gleason score.[198]

Moreover, grading errors may reflect sampling error because the needle biopsy samples a small fraction of the prostate gland, and the grade of cancer obtained on needle biopsy may not always be representative of the actual histologic subtype or degree of differentiation of the tumor. Most studies demonstrate a tendency of pathologists to undergrade biopsy specimens. Johnstone et al.[199] noted that, compared with subsequent RP specimens, the incidence of correct grading of prostatic carcinoma from needle biopsies was 71%, with 23% undergrading and 6% overgrading. In a study from Memorial Sloan-Kettering Cancer Center (MSKCC), Gleason scores from 18-gauge needle biopsies were compared with radical retropubic prostatectomy specimens in 226 consecutive patients. The biopsy score was identical to the specimen score in 31% of cases, whereas 26% were discrepant by ≥2 Gleason scores. Overall, 54% of biopsies were undergraded and 15% were overgraded.[200] University of Minnesota researchers found similar results from 466 patients.[201] The biopsy grade was the same as that of the prostatectomy specimen in 54% of the patients, with upgrading of the most common discordance in 75% of the well-differentiated tumors. When the biopsy grade was compared with the surgical pathologic stage, 49% of low-grade lesions and 82% of high-grade lesions in the biopsy had capsular penetration or locally advanced disease. A large, retrospective analysis[202] of the correlation between Gleason scores from biopsy and prostatectomy specimens and prediction of disease-free survival was carried out among 1,031 patients. Overall accuracy was 58.3%. When categorized by Gleason scores of <7, 7, and >7, patients with tumors of Gleason score <7 on prostatectomy specimens had a significant survival advantage over those with Gleason scores of <7 by biopsy, whereas disease-free survival was superior for patients with Gleason scores of >7 by biopsy than those with Gleason scores of >7 on prostatectomy specimens. The overall disease-free survival was similar among all patients with Gleason scores of 7. These data should be kept in mind when results of RP and irradiation are compared.

Predicting tumor extent and location using biopsy results was investigated by Humphrey et al.[146] in a correlative study of multiple parameters with pathologic features in 50 RP specimens. They noted that it was very difficult to predict tumor extent in the gland quadrants based on extent of tumor in the needle biopsy. There were 53 negative quadrant biopsies with carcinoma present in that quadrant in the RP specimen. Gregori et al.[203] evaluated the accuracy of sextant biopsies in predicting tumor location among 289 patients with clinically localized prostate cancer who underwent radical perineal prostatectomy. These investigators found that 33% of patients with a unilateral positive biopsy had cancer confined to one side of the gland, whereas 66% showed bilateral disease in the prostatectomy specimen.

The primary grade in the Gleason score provides additional prognostic information, particularly in Gleason score 7 prostate cancer. D'Amico et al.[204] studied pretreatment clinical and pathologic variables to predict time to postoperative PSA failure for patients with a PSA of <10 ng/mL and T1c or T2a disease. They noted that 5-year PSA failure-free survival rates were not statistically different for patients with a biopsy Gleason score of 2 to 6 versus 3 + 4 but were significantly different for patients with a biopsy Gleason score of 2 to 6 versus 4 + 3 or 2 to 6 versus 8 to 10. Five-year biochemical control rates were 79%, 81%, 62%, and 18% for patients with biopsy Gleason scores of 2 to 6 (no grade 4 or 5), 3 + 4, 4 + 3, and 8 to 10, respectively. Makarov et al.[205] at Johns Hopkins evaluated 537 patients with Gleason score 7 tumors on biopsy to determine whether Gleason score 3 + 4 = 7 and 4 + 3 = 7 cancers behave differently regardless of the number of positive cores. Five variables (3 + 4 versus 4 + 3, number of positive cores, PSA, age, and DRE) were analyzed with respect to pathologic findings after RP. Postoperative Gleason score and pathologic stage significantly correlated with preoperative PSA and preoperative Gleason scores of 4 + 3 versus 3 + 4 on biopsy.

Stamey[206] and Stamey et al.[207,208] emphasized that, with regard to natural history of prostate cancer and prognosis, it is not just the Gleason score that is important, but also how much of the tumor is present. In a study of histologic prognostic variables for PSA relapse among 372 men with prostate cancer

Clinical Radiation Oncology

followed for 3 years after retropubic prostatectomy, the most important variables predicting biochemical disease-free status for PZ cancers were percentage Gleason grade 4/5, cancer volume, serum PSA, and prostate weight.[208] Percentage Gleason grade 4/5, cancer location in the PZ, cancer volume, and lymph node involvement had prognostic value in large-volume prostate cancer. These investigators also noted that TZ cancers have a better prognosis than PZ tumors because they are separated from the neurovascular bundles and the ejaculatory ducts by the compressed surgical capsule caused by expanding benign hyperplastic nodules.[73] From the Stanford experience,[209] cancer location in the PZ and percentage Gleason grade 4/5 were the most powerful predictors of biochemical failure in men whose cancer was ≥6 cm^3 and contained in the prostatic capsule. Preoperative serum PSA was not helpful in distinguishing biochemical failure rates in large-volume cancers regardless of whether they were organ confined.

D'Amico et al.[210,211] showed that the percentage of positive prostate biopsies added clinically significant information regarding time to PSA failure among 960 men with PSA-detected or clinically palpable prostate cancer treated with RP. Investigators at the University of Michigan,[212] in an analysis of preoperative factors, including clinical stage, PSA, biopsy Gleason score, greatest percentage of a biopsy core involved by cancer, number of biopsy cores containing cancer, and perineural invasion, found that only PSA, Gleason score, and greatest percentage of a biopsy core involved by cancer were highly predictive of PSA relapse-free survival on multivariate analysis. This additional prognostic information may identify patients who are candidates for adjuvant therapy after RP. In addition, with the use of radiation therapy, histologic features from prostatectomy specimens are not available to incorporate into prognostic models, and pretreatment risk stratification is important owing to the increasing use of nonsurgical treatment options.

Prostate core biopsy histologic features have been investigated for predicting extraprostatic extension and lymph node involvement. Researchers at the Mayo Clinic[213] compared biopsy specimen Gleason scores, percentage positive cores, and percentage surface area involved in all cores with pathologic stage determined from RP specimens. Multivariate analysis using these pathologic variables, in addition to patient age, clinical disease stage, and PSA, showed that the percentage of positive cores, initial serum PSA, and Gleason score of cancer in the needle biopsy were the only parameters that jointly predicted pathologic stage (T2 versus T3 disease). Narayan et al.[106] used the combination of preoperative PSA plus biopsy Gleason score in 932 patients who had undergone pelvic lymphadenectomy to predict risk of positive pelvic lymph nodes. Patients with biopsy Gleason scores of ≤6 and preoperative PSA concentrations of ≤10 ng/mL had a <1% false-negative rate for pelvic lymph node metastases, suggesting that a staging pelvic lymphadenectomy is unnecessary.

Finally, the tumor histologic characteristics change with time and progression of disease. Cheng et al.[214] reported a trend toward histologic dedifferentiation when prostate carcinoma metastasized to regional lymph nodes. Among 242 patients treated with RP and pelvic lymphadenectomy at the Mayo Clinic, Gleason score in the lymph node metastases was higher than in the primary tumor in 45% of patients, lower in 12% of patients, and matched exactly in 43% of patients. The 5-year progression-free survival rate was significantly different between patients with histologic dedifferentiation and those without dedifferentiation.

Other Histologic Subtypes

Periurethral duct carcinoma is a separate clinicopathologic entity, usually consisting of a transitional cell type of carcinoma, although a mixture of glandular and transitional cells is also observed.[215–217] Large anaplastic tumor cells cluster in the periurethral ducts and spread into the stroma. Frequent mitoses are seen.[218] This tumor does not invade the perineural spaces as commonly as does adenocarcinoma of the prostate.

Reese et al.[219] reviewed 49 patients with *transitional cell carcinoma* of the prostate; 29 patients had stromal invasion and 20 had transitional cell carcinoma in the prostatic ducts only. Lymph node metastases were found in 14 (54%) of 26 patients with stromal invasion, compared with 4 (24%) of 17 with duct/acinar involvement. The 5-year survival rates were 80% for stromal node–negative, 45% for ductal node–negative, 55% for ductal node–positive, and 30% for stromal node–positive patients.

Ductal adenocarcinoma arises rarely from the major ducts. These tumors are usually papillary and on microscopic sections are composed of tall columnar cells with eosinophilic cytoplasm that may resemble endometrial carcinoma.[52,220–222] Originally this lesion was believed to originate in the prostatic utricle, a Müllerian remnant[223]; however, most ductal adenocarcinomas are not derived from Müllerian remnants and behave as acinar adenocarcinomas.[77]

Most reports point to aggressive behavior, with invasion of the prostatic stroma and the bladder neck and metastases to the lymph nodes, bone, and lung. In most series, the majority of patients die of the tumors within 4 years.[224,225] This tumor is moderately hormonally responsive and is sensitive to radiation therapy.[224] The treatment of choice is RP.[224,226] Kopelson et al.[216] reported a good prognosis in early stages; however, in stage C the 5-year survival rate was only 34.5%. They noted a 76% local tumor control rate and a 58% 5-year survival rate in patients treated with irradiation, in contrast to 14% local tumor control and 24% 5-year survival rates in patients not receiving this treatment. Brinker et al.[227] also observed a shortened average time to progression relative to a previous study group of men with acinar carcinoma among 58 patients treated with RP at Johns Hopkins.

Neuroendocrine tumors are a rare variant of a malignant tumor composed of small or carcinoid-like cells. Neuroendocrine cell substances found in these tumors include serotonin, neuron-specific enolase, chromogranin, calcitonin, and others. PAP and PSA are valuable to determine the prostatic origin of the tumor. Of 22 patients with stage T2 lesions, 4 died of the disease, and 3 of them had positive neuroendocrine cell findings.[228] Of 20 patients with stage T3, 5 died of the disease, and all 5 had positive neuroendocrine cell features

Mucinous carcinoma, not arising in major ducts or in the urethra, with positive histochemical stains for PAP, has been reported.[229]

Sarcomatoid carcinoma is a rare tumor and is difficult to distinguish from a true sarcoma. There is coexistence of prostatic adenocarcinoma with sarcomatoid components that have spindle cells with large pleomorphic hyperchromatic nuclei. The pattern is that of a high-grade sarcoma in most patients, similar to the malignant fibrous histiocytoma of soft tissues. Mitotic figures range from 6 to 36 per 10 high-power fields. In 12 patients reported by Shannon et al.,[230] tumor presentation was stage A or B in 4, C or D in 5, and unknown in 3 patients. Metastases data were available for 10 patients; the most common metastatic sites were bone (7 patients), lymph nodes (2 patients), lung (2 patients), liver (1 patient), and skin (1 patient). Immunostaining or electron microscopy demonstrated epithelial differentiation in the sarcomatoid areas in 6 of 11 patients on whom these studies were performed. All 9 patients for whom follow-up data were available died of disease within 3 to 48 months after diagnosis. In 3 patients, sarcomatoid elements were part of the tumor at initial diagnosis; in the other 9, the sarcomatoid component was confirmed in subsequent evaluations after initial diagnosis (2 to 89 months). Four patients were treated with radiation therapy without beneficial result. These tumors are considered a very aggressive variant of prostatic adenocarcinoma.

Endometrioid tumors occasionally arise from the verumontanum. Endometrial glands and cells with numerous mitotic figures may be seen. These tumors may have an exophytic configuration in the prostatic urethra or infiltrate the adjacent tissues.

Adenoid cystic carcinoma is a rare tumor in the prostate (representing <0.1% of all tumors of this gland). The histologic appearance is similar to that of its salivary gland counterpart.

Other epithelial tumors, such as carcinoid or small-cell carcinoma, have been reported in the prostate.[231,232] The experience with these lesions is very limited, and in most patients behavior is highly aggressive and fatal.[233] A review of the literature showed that in 130 patients reported with small-cell carcinoma of the prostate, the 2-year survival rate was 3.6%, the 3-year rate was 1.8%, and 5-year rate was <1%.[234] A subsequent Surveillance, Epidemiology, and End Results (SEER) database analysis of 241 cases of small-cell carcinoma of the prostate identified 1- and 5-year overall survival of 47.9% and 14.3%, respectively.[235] Squamous cell carcinoma originating primarily in the prostate is rare.[236] Metastatic malignant tumors from other locations to the prostate are occasionally reported.[236,237]

Sarcomas (leiomyosarcoma, rhabdomyosarcoma, or fibrosarcoma) constitute approximately 0.1% of all primary neoplasms of the prostate.[218] Leiomyosarcoma is more common in middle-aged or older men, whereas rhabdomyosarcoma is found more frequently in younger patients. Several cases of malignant schwannoma have been described.[238] These tumors tend to invade lymphatics and blood vessels, causing widespread regional lymphatic and distant metastases.

Carcinosarcoma of the prostate constitutes 0.1% of prostatic neoplasms. A mixture of adenocarcinoma invading the stroma and sarcomatous elements is seen histologically; smooth or striated muscle, fibroblasts, or other mesenchymal malignant cells may be identified.

Primary lymphoma of the prostate is rare, with <100 cases having been reported. It accounted for only 0.1% of newly diagnosed lymphomas and only 0.09% of all prostatic neoplasias at MD Anderson Cancer Center.[239]

GENERAL MANAGEMENT TRENDS IN THE UNITED STATES

The optimal management of clinically localized prostate cancer remains controversial and is often a source of great frustration and anxiety for many patients who are compelled to make a decision regarding a treatment intervention for their disease. The practitioner must be aware that the natural history of this tumor is variable and influenced by multiple prognostic factors. All of the various forms of therapy for prostate cancer can affect quality of life and sexual function in varying degrees. In the process of counseling and discussing therapeutic options, it is important to present all available data regarding the natural history of this disease, prognostic significance of the diagnosis, potential therapeutic benefit of the various modalities, and immediate as well as late treatment-related sequelae. Life expectancy and quality-of-life considerations should be carefully discussed with the patient and spouse or significant other.

Based on the available data, when comparing patients with similar prognostic features, there are no significant differences in the biochemical and disease-free survival outcomes for patients with early stages of disease treated with RP, high-dose external-beam radiation therapy (EBRT), or interstitial implantation.[240–242,243–244] In the absence of randomized trials demonstrating superiority of one treatment over another, there are wide geographic variations in the preferred therapeutic intervention for early-stage prostate cancer practiced throughout the United States.

Observations from the Cancer of the Prostate Strategic Urologic Research Endeavor (CapSURE) database—a registry of 11,000 men accrued from 36 community-based urologic practices across the United States—shed further light on practice patterns. Cooperberg et al.[245] reported that, in this cohort of patients, 50% elected to be treated with RP, 12% were treated with EBRT, 13% received brachytherapy, 4% received cryotherapy, and 14% were treated with primary ADT. In these patients it was noted that among those with higher prognostic risk features there was an increased use of primary ADT. Younger patients and especially those with low-risk disease were more often selected for prostatectomy. In addition to age playing a role in treatment selection, the presence of medical comorbidities, the socioeconomic status of the patient, and the personal practice trends of individual clinic treatment sites (irrespective of the patient's stage of disease) played important roles in treatment selection as well. There was an increasing trend observed for patients presenting at diagnosis with more favorable-risk disease in 2001–2002 (47%) compared to 1989–1990 (31%). A lower percentage of high-risk patients (defined as PSA of >20 ng/mL, Gleason 8 to 10 disease, or T3-T4 disease) was noted on initial presentation (15% compared with 41%) for 2000–2001 and 1989–1990, respectively.

A recent report[246] based on the SEER–Medicare linked database included 85,088 men with the diagnosis of prostate cancer at age 65 years and older. In this cohort of patients 42% were treated with radiotherapy, 21% were treated with RP, 17% were treated with primary ADT, and 20% were followed expectantly. The authors also noted a strong association between the type of specialist seen (urologist vs. radiation oncologist vs. medical oncologist) and the primary therapy the patient had received. For patients who were 65 to 69 years old and evaluated by a urologist, 70% underwent a prostatectomy, whereas among patients who were 70 to 74 years old, surgery was selected in 45% of patients. In addition, among men who were seen by both a urologist and a radiation oncologist, radiotherapy was the most commonly used treatment modality (83% of this cohort). These data are consistent with prior studies showing that specialists more often made treatment recommendations favoring their particular specialty.[247]

Within the practice of radiation oncology there have been new trends in radiotherapy practice and treatment delivery. Higher radiation doses and the use of adjunctive ADT with radiotherapy for various prognostic risk groups are more common than in the past. There has been a significant increase in the use of intensity-modulated radiotherapy (IMRT) for the treatment of prostate cancer and increasing use of image-guided radiotherapy with fiducial makers inserted into the prostate prior to therapy for daily target localization, as well as the use of tomotherapy and cone-beam imaging prior to the administration of the daily fraction. There is increasing interest in the use of stereotactic external-beam radiosurgery with regimens employing fraction sizes of 6.5 to 8 Gy for five treatments.

Zelefsky et al.[248] reported the results of the Quality of Research Radiation Oncology (QRRO) group, which surveyed 414 patients with clinically localized prostate cancer treated with EBRT or brachytherapy that were selected from 45 institutions in the United States. Indicators used as specific measurable clinical performance measures to represent surrogates for quality of radiotherapy delivery included established measures, such as the use of prescription doses of ≥75 Gy for intermediate- and high-risk EBRT patients and androgen-deprivation therapy (ADT) in conjunction with EBRT for patients with high-risk disease. Among favorable-risk patients, 72% were treated to ≥75 Gy. For high-risk EBRT patients, 60 (87%) were treated with ADT in conjunction with EBRT and 13% ($n = 9$) with radiotherapy alone. Among low- and intermediate-risk patients, 10% and 42%, respectively, were treated with ADT plus EBRT. For patients treated with EBRT, weekly electronic portal imaging was obtained as verification films without daily target localization in 35%, and the remaining 64% were treated with daily localization of the target, such as fiducial markers, cone-beam imaging, tomotherapy, or intrafraction localization with a ferromagnetic marker device.

For selected patients, expectant management may be a reasonable approach to offer to avoid the potential morbidity associated with any therapy. Candidates for expectant management include those patients with low PSA values with relatively slow doubling times who have low-volume disease (5% core involvement) and Gleason 6 disease based on biopsy findings. Recently, the long-term results of a phase III, randomized trial from the Scandinavian Prostate Cancer Group demonstrated a reduction in the cause-specific mortality with local therapy compared to an expectant management approach.[249] In this study, 695 men were included with early-stage T1 or T2 prostate cancer. The median follow-up was 12.8 years, the primary endpoint was death attributed to prostate cancer, and the secondary endpoint was overall survival. In the watchful-waiting group, 58% died, compared with 48% in the RP group ($p = .007$). The cumulative incidence of death directly related to prostate cancer was 14.6% in the surgery group versus 20.7% for the expectant-management cohort. The survival benefit was noted among low-risk patients, and this benefit was limited to patients who were younger than 65 years of age.

In today's health environment in the United States, it is often not considered acceptable to delay definitive therapy for many patients with localized carcinoma of the prostate, except in selected elderly patients with low Gleason scores and low-volume disease based on the biopsy findings, as well as for patients with significant medical comorbidities. Properly designed prospective clinical trials are critically needed to better define the efficacy and cost-effectiveness of various therapeutic approaches for localized carcinoma of the prostate.

Traditionally, the treatment options for patients with early-stage, clinically localized prostatic cancer (stages T1c or T2) included RP, EBRT, or permanent interstitial implantation. Surgical techniques have significantly improved with the advent of the nerve-sparing operation popularized by Walsh,[97] with a lower incidence of sexual impotence (approximately 30% to 60%, depending on the patient's age, tumor stage, and surgery extent) compared with classic RP (almost 100%), as well as improved methods available to reduce risks of post-treatment urinary incontinence. At the same time, the accuracy and safety of EBRT delivery have significantly improved with the emergence of IMRT and image-guided radiotherapy approaches. Permanent interstitial implantation using ultrasound-guided transperineal techniques and the development of intraoperative conformal optimization for prostate brachytherapy have consistently improved the dose distributions for this treatment approach, leading to improved outcomes and decreased toxicities.

Treatment Techniques

Radical Prostatectomy

RP, initially described by Young[250] in 1905 and popularized by Jewett,[79] is a therapeutic option when the tumor is confined to the prostate. In the past, according to most urologists, it had a limited role in the management of gross extracapsular disease or seminal vesicle involvement or in the presence of lymph node metastases; however, more recently there has been an increased use of surgery for locally advanced disease. Two approaches for the classic RP are used: retropubic and perineal. The procedure consists in complete removal of the prostate and its surrounding capsule together with the seminal vesicles, the ampulla, and the vas deferens. The prostate is removed completely by excision of the urethra at the prostatomembranous junction, leaving no residual prostatic tissue at the apex. The retropubic approach is preferred by many urologic surgeons; this procedure also facilitates access for performing a bilateral pelvic lymph node dissection.

In the last 5 to 10 years there has been an increasing interest and practice of laparoscopic and robotic RP approaches in both the United States and Europe. Advantages cited for the use of the laparoscopic procedure versus the open approach include improved visualization of the anatomy optical magnification, less blood loss, less postoperative pain, and more rapid resumption of normal activities. Preliminary functional and oncologic outcomes with this approach compare favorably to those achieved with open RP approaches. The Da Vinci robotic surgical system (Intuitive Surgical, Sunnyvale, CA) uses three multi-joint robotic arms, with one arm controlling the binocular endoscope and the other arms controlling small-wristed instruments. This system is controlled by the surgeon, who can be in a remote location from the patient, seated at an operative console. The stereoscopic view of the operative field provides the surgeon three-dimensional visualization with a 10-fold magnification. Fine and precise movements of the instruments can be achieved, and physiologic tremor can be eliminated. In a recent comparison of open versus laparoscopic and robot-assisted RP approaches there were no significant differences in perioperative complication rates and tumor-control outcomes among the various surgical approaches.[251] Among 239 patients evaluated with a median follow-up of 50 months, the 5-year biochemical control outcomes were 88% for open prostatectomy and 88% and 90% for laparoscopic and robotic-assisted prostatectomy, respectively. The incidence of positive margins also was similar among the different approaches. Long-term results of 184 patients treated with robot-assisted laparoscopic prostatectomy were reported by Suardi et al.[252] With a median follow-up of 67 months, the 7-year biochemical control rates for pathologic T2 and T3a and pathologic T3b disease were 85%, 84%, and 43% disease, respectively. Whether such approaches lead to significant improvements over traditional open RP outcomes is uncertain and prospective, randomized studies are required.

Radiation Therapy Techniques

Conformal and Intensity-Modulated Radiation Therapy Techniques

In the late 1980s, three-dimensional (also known as conformal) treatment techniques became increasingly available. Although these techniques vary in some aspects, they share certain common principles that offer significant advantages over conventional treatment techniques. CT-based images referenced to a reproducible patient position are used to localize the prostate and normal organs and to generate high-resolution 3D reconstructions of the patient. Treatment field directions are selected using beam's-eye-view techniques and the fields are shaped to conform to the patient's CT-defined target volume, thereby minimizing the volume of normal tissue irradiated. Conformal radiotherapy simulation, planning, and treatment incorporate various additional maneuvers to reduce treatment uncertainties and enhance setup reproducibility required during a protracted course of therapy.

IMRT is a relatively recent refinement of 3D conformal techniques that uses treatment fields with highly irregular radiation intensity patterns to deliver exquisitely conformal radiation distributions. These intensity patterns are created by using special "inverse" or "optimization" computer planning systems, the characteristics of which have been thoroughly summarized in several review articles.[253,254] Rather than define each field shape and weight as is done in conventional treatment planning, planners of IMRT treatment specify the desired dose to the target and normal tissues using mathematical descriptions referred to as "constraints" or "objectives." Sophisticated optimization methods are then used to determine the intensity pattern for each treatment field that results in a dose distribution as close to the user-defined constraints as possible.

IMRT delivery is significantly more complex than conformal delivery. Delivery of an IMRT intensity pattern requires a computer-controlled beam-shaping apparatus on the linear accelerator known as a multileaf collimator (MLC). The MLC consists of many small, individually moving leaves or fingers that can create arbitrary beam shapes. The MLC is used for IMRT delivery in either a static mode referred to as "step and shoot," which consists of multiple small, irregularly shaped fields delivered in sequence, or a dynamic mode (dynamic multileaf collimation), with the leaves moving during treatment to create the required irregular intensity patterns.[255] Since its inception, IMRT has become a common and important method for treating prostate cancer and, through its ability to tightly conform the radiation to the shape of the target, has facilitated an escalation in dose at several institutions, including MSKCC.

In the following section, the 3DCRT and IMRT techniques used at MSKCC are highlighted with reference to similar techniques developed by others.

Immobilization, Simulation, and Computed Tomography Scanning

On the evening prior to simulation, patients undergo a standard bowel preparation. Immediately before the simulation procedure and CT scan the next day, the patient is asked to void his bladder. To visualize bowel in the vicinity of the prostate and seminal vesicles, a barium sulfate suspension is administered, and the rectal lumen is visualized by inserting a rectal catheter.

Although in the past prostate cancer patients were treated in the prone position at Memorial Sloan-Kettering Cancer Center based on comparative studies[256] that demonstrated improved geometry of the normal anatomy juxtaposed to the prostate target, currently patients are routinely treated in the supine position. These changes were made based on the observation of less prostate motion observed in the supine compared to the prone position.[257] All patients undergo fiducial marker placement via transrectal ultrasound guidance 1 week prior to simulation. For immobilization, a thermoplastic mold is fabricated for simulation, CT scanning, and treatment to ensure that the patient is in the same treatment position during all procedures. The thermoplastic sheet is heated in warm water and molded to the patient's shape from the knees to mid-abdomen. Small sections of the mold are cut away to provide ports for marking and tattooing. The patient is scanned through an approximately 20- to 30-cm region around the prostate with a slice spacing and thickness of 3 mm. Before start of the CT planning study, several transverse images through the prostate and bladder are obtained to ensure that the rectal lumen is clearly visible, the bladder and rectum are not excessively filled, and the patient is properly positioned within the scan circle. With use of the CT data set, a "virtual simulation" is performed, using digitally reconstructed radiographs to localize the treatment area rather than conventional simulation films. The treatment isocenter is placed according to anatomic landmarks near the center of the prostate gland: midline, at the caudad aspect, and approximately 5 cm posterior to the symphysis pubis. The triangulation points for the isocenter are then tattooed, along with an additional alignment tattoo, along the sagittal line, approximately 10 cm superior to the isocenter. To ensure reproducible leg position, tattoos are placed on the back of the legs at the midshaft level, and the distance between the tattoos is recorded for future reference.

Target and Normal-Tissue Contouring

The clinical target volume (CTV) is defined as the prostate and seminal vesicles. The planning target volume (PTV) is defined as the CTV with a margin to account for physical uncertainties including setup reproducibility and interfractional and intrafractional organ motion. At MSKCC, a 1-cm margin is added to the CTV to form the PTV in all directions except posteriorly at the interface with the rectum, where the margin is reduced to 0.6 cm. Clinically, these margins were found to provide adequate target coverage based on a serial CT scan study evaluating organ motion during a course of 3DCRT.[258] When using image-guided approaches with daily target localization, margins are 6 mm circumferentially around the clinical target volume. Normal tissues identified on each CT slice include the inner and outer walls of the rectum and bladder, the femoral heads, and the outer skin surface. Portions of the small bowel or sigmoid colon within 1 cm of the PTV are also contoured and taken into consideration, if necessary, during planning. In addition, the central 1-cm diameter portion of the prostate encompassing the prostatic urethra is defined for dosimetric consideration and evaluation during high-dose IMRT planning.

Accurate anatomic delineation of the prostate and, in particular, the prostatic apex has been a topic of some controversy. Some have advocated urethrography at the time of simulation as a method to accurately localize the apex.[259,260] Algan et al.[259] reviewed the location of the prostatic apex in 17 patients for whom MRI scan, retrograde urethrogram, and CT of the pelvis were obtained for 3D treatment planning. The location of the prostatic apex as determined by the urethrogram alone was, on average, 5.8 mm caudad to the location on the MRI, whereas the location of the prostatic apex as determined by CT/urethrogram was 3.1 mm caudad to that on MRI. If the prostatic apex is defined as 12 mm instead of 10 mm above the urethrogram tip (junction of membranous and prostatic urethra), the difference between the urethrogram and MRI locations of the prostatic apex is removed. Milosevic et al.[260] also found differences in the position of the prostatic apex between urethrogram, CT, and MR. In an evaluation of 20 patients, the authors found relatively poor correlation between MR and CT or MR and urethrogram in determining the height of the apex above the tuberosities. In response to concerns that the position of the prostate could be altered by the urethrogram itself, Mah et al.[261] performed sagittal MR scans immediately before and after urethrogram in 13 patients. No significant systematic motion of the prostate itself or the apex was observed, leading the authors to conclude that urethrography during simulation does not introduce localization error.

The contribution of MRI to improved accuracy and reproducibility of target localization in prostate cancer has also been well studied.[175,262] Roach et al.[175] studied 10 patients with both MR and CT images of the prostate and noted that the prostate volume was 32% larger when defined by noncontrast CT than when determined by MRI. Areas of disagreement tended to occur in the posterior and posteroinferior-apical portions of the prostate, the apex (because of disagreement between urethrography and MRI), and the regions corresponding to the neurovascular bundle. Rasch et al.[263] also observed differences in CT- and MR-defined volumes. On average, the prostate and seminal vesicle volume defined on CT was 40% larger than that defined on MR. The CT-defined prostate was 8 mm larger at the base of the seminal vesicles and 6 mm larger at the prostatic apex. This difference was found to be significantly larger than interobserver variation.

Contouring Techniques

There have been several reports documenting the variability of prostate-contouring techniques among practitioners.[264,265] However, knowledge of the anatomy is essential to achieve accurate contours and should lead to less variability or discrepancies between contours drawn by different physicians. McLaughlin et al.[266] provided an excellent demonstration of common contouring errors such as overestimation of the prostatic apex and underestimation of the prostatic base. The apex and the base in particular represent regions of the target volume that can be challenging to identify on CT images and better defined with MRI imaging. Two methods recommended include the inspection of lateral view projections of the contours to detect regions of the irregularities of the target geometry and improved recognition of the GUD elements. These elements are shown in the MRI representation of the GUD in Figure 65.6 and in the CT representation in Figure 65.7.

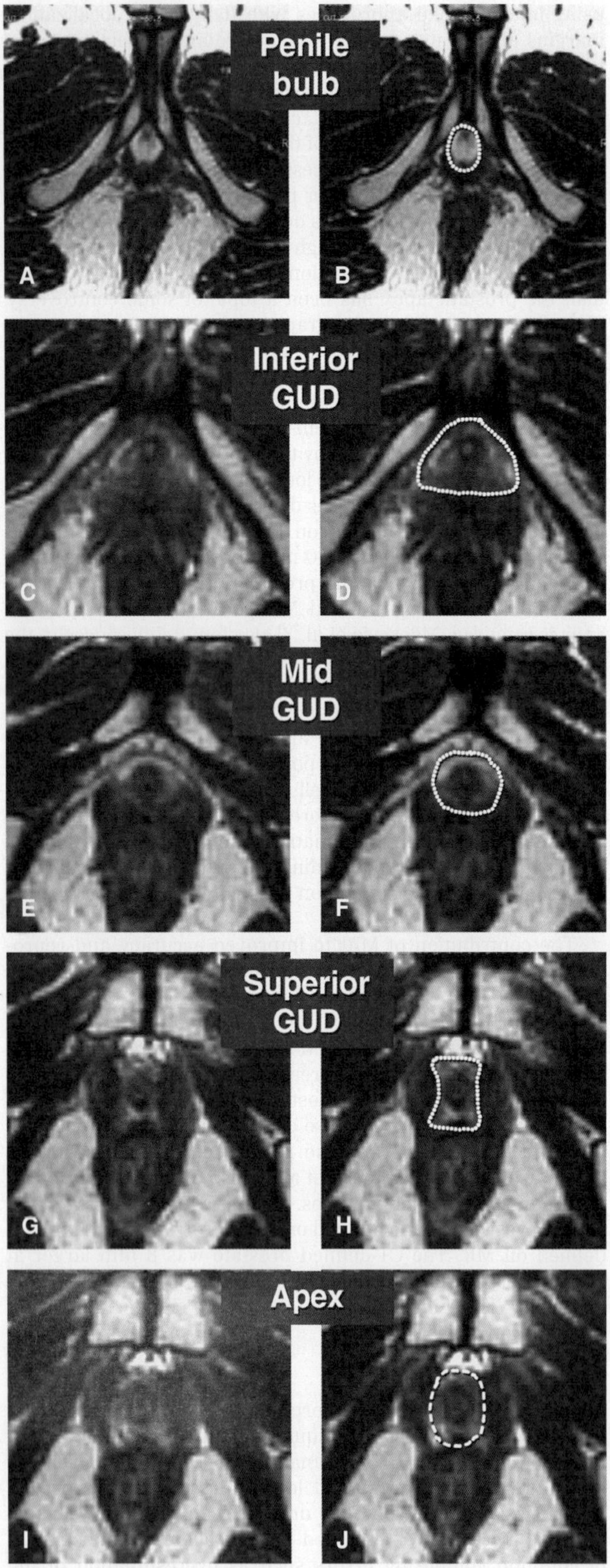

FIGURE 65.6. Representation of the genitourinary diaphragm on axial magnetic resonance imaging slices, demonstrating the anatomic configuration that can used as a guide for contouring of the clinical prostate target volume. (From McLaughlin PW, Evans C, Feng M, et al. Radiographic and anatomic basis for prostate contouring errors and methods to improve prostate contouring accuracy. *Int J Radiat Oncol Biol Phys*;76:369–378; with permission from Elsevier.)

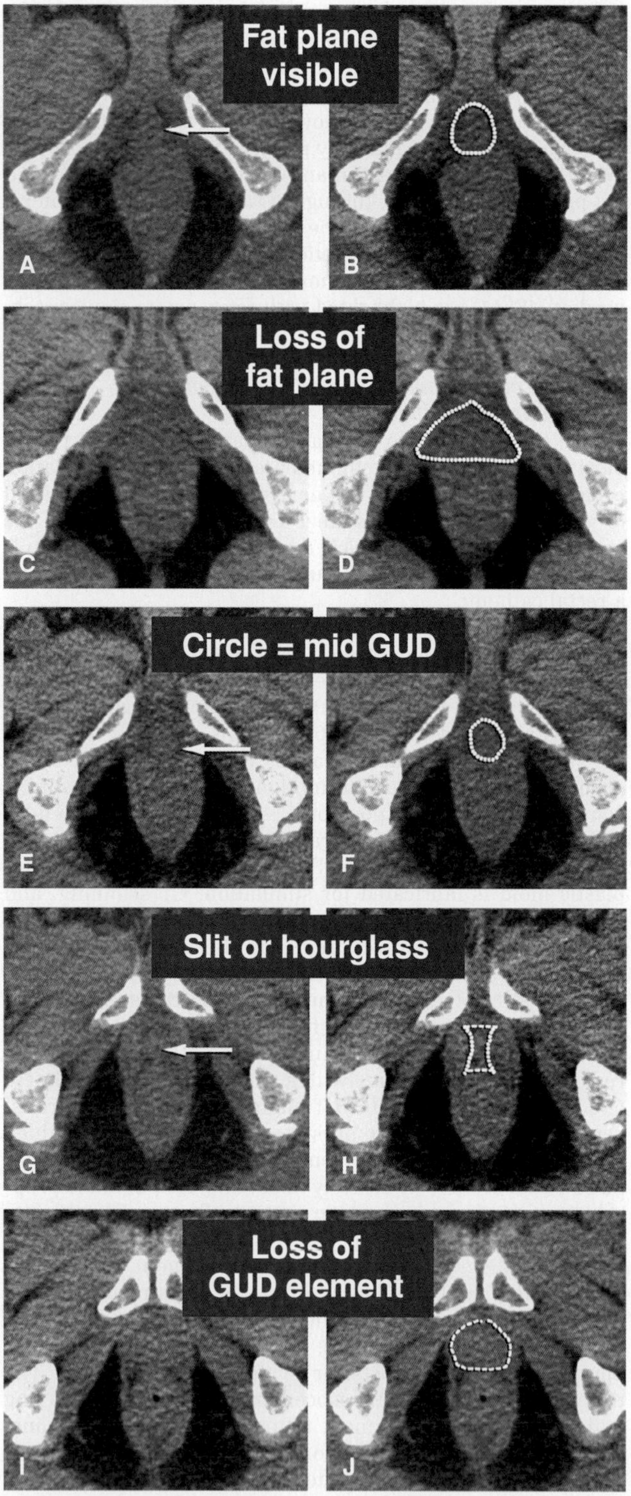

FIGURE 65.7. Representation of the genitourinary diaphragm on axial computed tomography slices, demonstrating the anatomic configuration that can used as a guide for contouring of the clinical prostate target volume. (From McLaughlin PW, Evans C, Feng M, et al. Radiographic and anatomic basis for prostate contouring errors and methods to improve prostate contouring accuracy. *Int J Radiat Oncol Biol Phys*;76:369–378; with permission from Elsevier.)

Beam Selection and Planning

3DCRT Conformal Plans. The hallmark of 3D planning is the use of a multifield beam arrangement with field apertures designed using beam's-eye-view projections that are conformal to the shape of the PTV, thereby shielding the normal tissues. At MSKCC, a standard 3D conformal beam arrangement consisted of six coplanar fields, including two lateral, two anterior, and two oblique beams. Conformal apertures were drawn around the PTV adding a margin of approximately 5 to 6 mm in the axial directions to account for beam penumbra. This margin was sufficient dosimetrically in the axial plane because of the effect of the overlapping beams, whereas in the superior and inferior directions, a margin of 1 cm was typically necessary. For the beam shaping, multileaf collimation was used, which has effectively eliminated the handling of lead–cadmium alloy blocks.

Once the treatment fields and aperture shapes were defined, the dose distribution was calculated for a few representative planes—typically transverse, coronal, and sagittal planes through the isocenter. Dose–volume histograms were generated for the PTV, femoral heads, and rectal and bladder walls. If the bowel was located near the prostate and seminal vesicles, a dose calculation for the bowel was also done. For the MSKCC six-field plan, the two lateral beams typically delivered approximately half of the dose to the isocenter, with the four oblique beams contributing the rest. The beam weights of the anterior oblique and posterior oblique beams were adjusted to obtain a uniform dose within the PTV and to place the hot spots away from the rectum. The plan was normalized so that the prescription isodose (100%) covered the PTV with a hot spot of 6% to 9% within the PTV. Although the portion of the rectal wall enclosed within the PTV was expected to receive the prescription dose or slightly higher, the rectal wall volume receiving 75.6 Gy or more did not exceed 30%. Other normal tissue dose limits for these 3DCRT plans included limiting the maximum dose to the femurs to ≤68 Gy (90%), the maximum dose to large bowel to ≤60 Gy (79%), and the maximum dose to small bowel to ≤50 Gy (66%).

Intensity-Modulated Radiation Therapy. Unlike 3DCRT treatment planning, in which the planner defines the shape, as well as the amount, of radiation to be delivered from each treatment field, planners define dose "constraints" or "objectives" for the target and normal tissues, which describe the desired dose distribution in IMRT planning. These constraints typically consist of maximum or minimum dose limits on targets and dose and dose–volume limits on normal tissues. The planner specifies as many individual constraints for a specific target or normal tissue as desired, giving each its own weight or "penalty," reflective of its clinical importance. With special computer software, these constraints are used to drive a mathematical optimization of the radiation intensities of many small "beamlets" within each treatment field. The result of this optimization is a set of intensity patterns for the treatment fields and a dose distribution with characteristics as close as possible to the constraints entered by the planner.

Because normal-tissue shielding can be accomplished by modulating the beam intensity, IMRT beam directions are often somewhat nonintuitive and can differ significantly from those typically chosen for 3DCRT. Determination of appropriate target and normal-tissue constraints can be tedious, and planners often repeat the optimization process multiple times, evaluating the dose distributions after each iteration and making small adjustments to the constraints before obtaining a final, acceptable plan. Most institutions performing IMRT planning set up templates that specify both the clinical goals of the dose distribution and initial target and normal-tissue constraints for optimization. The MSKCC template for prostate IMRT planning to 81 Gy is shown in Table 65.8. Dose and dose–volume constraints for the PTV, PTV overlap with the rectum, and rectal and bladder walls are listed. It should be noted that constraint templates vary significantly among treatment-planning systems; therefore, these constraints should be used only after a thorough evaluation on the user's system.

A variety of beam arrangements have been proposed for prostate IMRT treatment, including multifield axial or noncoplanar arrangements, in addition to intensity-modulated arc therapy.[267–269] Primarily because of concern about increased risk of secondary cancers from higher neutron doses associated with IMRT treatment at high energies,[270,271] some groups have proposed 6-MV IMRT techniques for the treatment of prostate cancer. As shown by Pirzkall et al.,[272] however, a larger number of treatment fields may be necessary to achieve a dose distribution similar to that observed with 15-MV x-rays.

The MSKCC clinical goals used to evaluate the IMRT dose distributions and dose–volume histograms for prostate patients are outlined in Table 65.8. These dosimetric guidelines defining acceptable target coverage, dose uniformity, and normal tissue doses have grown out of our 3DCRT and IMRT planning experience during the last 20 years and include several refinements resulting from retrospective outcome and toxicity analyses from our institution. Most notably, studies by Skwarchuk et al.[273] and Jackson et al.[274] retrospectively evaluating the rectal wall dose–volume histograms for patients treated to 70.2 and 75.6 Gy using 3DCRT techniques found that, on average, patients with late rectal bleeding had significantly higher rectal dose–volume histograms than patients who did not bleed. Both high- and intermediate-dose levels were found to be independently correlated with rectal bleeding. As a result of these studies, two rectal wall dose–volume histogram limits were implemented and are routinely enforced at MSKCC when treating prostate cancer: no more than 30% of the rectal wall may receive more than 75.6 Gy, and no more than 53% of the rectal wall can receive more than 47 Gy.

Typical dose distributions and dose–volume histograms for an 86.4-Gy IMRT plan are shown in Figure 65.8. The physician should carefully review the treatment plan and dose–volume histograms of the target and normal-tissue structures to select the optimal treatment plan for the patient. Target coverage should be carefully assessed, as well as the dose inhomogeneity

TABLE 65.8 OPTIMIZATION CONSTRAINT TEMPLATE AND PLANNING GOALS FOR MEMORIAL SLOAN-KETTERING CANCER CENTER 81-GY AND INTENSITY-MODULATED RADIATION THERAPY PROSTATE TREATMENT

	Optimization Constraints[a]			*Treatment Plan Goals*[b]	
Structure	*Maximum Dose (Gy)/Penalty*	*Minimum Dose (Gy)/Penalty*	*Volume (%)*	*Dose (Gy)*	*Volume (%)*
Planning target volume (excluding rectal overlap)	82.6/50	79.4/50	–	111% max	V_{95} >90
Planning target volume and rectum					
Overlap region	77.8/20	75.3/10	–	–	–
Rectal wall	77/20	–	–	75.6	30
Rectal wall	32.4/20	–	30	47	53
Bladder wall	79.4/35	–	–	–	–
Bladder wall	32.4/20	–	30	40	60

[a]Optimization constraints = initial target and normal-tissue constraints entered into the IMRT optimization planning system.

[b]Treatment plan goals = dosimetric criteria used for evaluation and acceptance of an IMRT dose distribution.

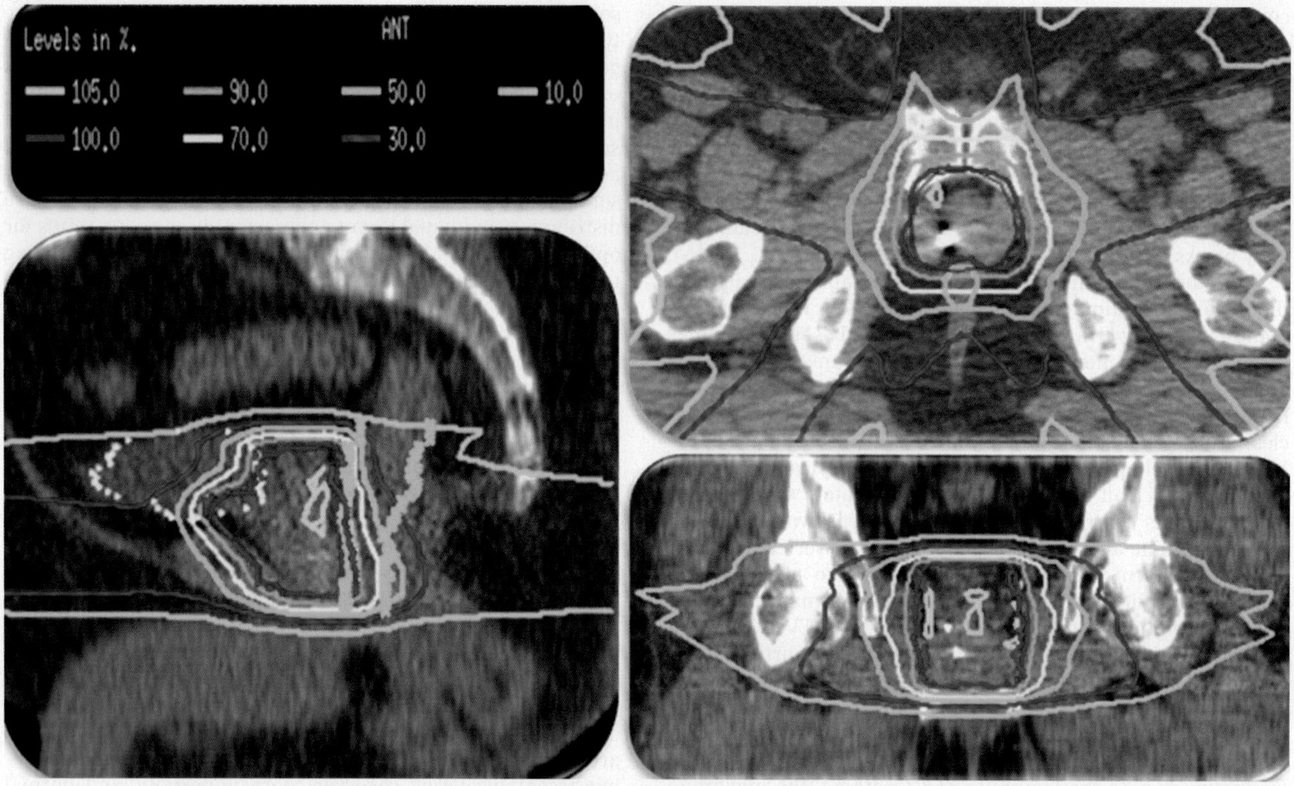

FIGURE 65.8. Dose distribution and dose–volume histogram display for a typical five-field intensity-modulated radiotherapy treatment plan whose prescription to the prostate target is 86.4 Gy. (Courtesy of Daniel Spratt MD.)

and location of hot spots. In addition, careful attention should be given to determining whether the treatment plan adequately meets acceptable dose constraints for the rectum, bladder, and bowel.

Standard Prescription Doses for 3DCRT and IMRT

At MSKCC, 81 to 86 Gy is delivered to favorable-risk patients using IMRT. Daily fractions of 1.8 to 2 Gy, five fractions per week, are routinely used; however, others have reported encouraging results with a hypofractionated scheme delivering 70 Gy with fractions of 2.5 Gy.[275,276] At MSKCC, the dose is prescribed to an isodose line that encompasses as much of the PTV as possible while still respecting the target and normal tissue goals listed in Table 65.8. Typically, at least 90% to 95% of the PTV receives the prescription dose.

Treatment Delivery and Organ-Motion Concerns

Movement of the prostate during treatment or between treatment fractions has long been a concern for prostate radiotherapy. Many studies investigating interfractional and intrafractional motion of the prostate and seminal vesicles have been reported.[277–280] Most groups have measured prostate motion relative to bony landmarks through repeated imaging of implanted radiopaque markers or serial CT studies. Although the reported magnitude of motion has varied, relatively little motion in the lateral direction and potentially significant movement in the anterior–posterior and superior–inferior directions has been consistently reported. Many studies have also observed a correlation between prostate and seminal vesicle motion and rectal or bladder filling.

Interfractional prostate motion was studied in approximately 50 patients by Crook et al.[279] Gold seeds implanted in the prostate were visualized on kilovolt radiographs taken at the simulation and approximately midway through treatment. Minimal prostate motion was observed in the lateral directions (0.1 to 0.5 cm), but inferior displacements of 0.5 and 1.0 cm or more were observed in 43% and 11% of their patients. Average displacement in the posterior direction was 0.72, 0.62, and 0.46 cm for seeds placed at the seminal vesicles, posterior aspect of the prostate, or apex of the gland, respectively; 60% of patients showed >0.5-cm posterior displacement of the prostate base, and 30% showed >1 cm.

Zelefsky et al.[258] obtained four serial CT studies for 50 patients (planning scan and three additional scans during the course of therapy). Prostate displacements in the anteroposterior and superoinferior directions were most frequently observed. The mean prostate motion in the anteroposterior, superoinferior, and left–right directions was 1.2, 0.5, and 0.6 mm, respectively. Anteroposterior movements were correlated with changes in rectal volume. Patients with large rectal volumes (>60 cm^3) and large bladder volumes (>40 cm^3) on the planning scan experienced a higher likelihood of having >3-mm systematic displacement of the prostate and seminal vesicles, leading the authors to conclude that these patients may require more generous PTV margins to ensure adequate CTV coverage. However, among patients without larger bladder and rectal volumes, a 1-cm margin around the CTV with a 6-mm margin at the prostate–rectal interface enclosed the posterior, anterior, superoinferior, and left–right aspects of the CTV within the prescription dose level with a probability of 90%, 100%, 99%, and 100%, respectively, indicating that the MSKCC margins provided adequate CTV coverage for most patients.

Intrafractional prostate motion was studied in 20 patients by Huang et al.[280] using pretreatment and posttreatment B-mode rectal ultrasound evaluations. Although the intrafractional motion was relatively insignificant in all directions, the predominant directions of motion were in the anterior and superior directions. Standard deviations of 0.4, 1.3, and 1.0 mm were observed in the lateral, anterior, and superior directions, respectively. Several methods have been developed to reduce uncertainty due to interfractional organ motion and thereby improve treatment delivery using computer-assisted transabdominal ultrasonography, radiopaque marker tracking, or CT image guidance. With the ultrasound system (BAT, Nomos Corporation, Sewickley, PA), patients are instructed to maintain a full bladder and are initially set up based on their tattoos in the supine position. The system is attached to the accelerator collimator and imports the coordinates of the isocenter, as well as to the target contours from the planning CT. Computer software facilitates 3D matching of the target contours with the prostate visualized on ultrasonography and determination of the necessary patient position modification. This system may not be reliable for patients who cannot maintain a full bladder and those with a large body habitus or other anatomic constraints because of anticipated poor image quality. It has also been noted that BAT measurements can be associated with a 2- to 3-mm error, which is sometimes in the range of the required shifts. Nevertheless, this system has been used by several investigators to verify the prostate position, and results are consistent with improved accuracy of the daily treatment delivery.[281–283] Recent technological advances have opened up the possibility of acquiring pretreatment or posttreatment megavoltage or kilovoltage CT images directly on the linear accelerator (linac) with the patient in the treatment position. One example of such a device, known as a tomotherapy unit (TomoTherapy Hi-ART, Madison, WI), consists of a 6-MV accelerator mounted within a CT-type gantry. Megavoltage CT images can be obtained prior to treatment and registered with the planning CT study, and the resulting positional corrections can then be applied prior to treatment. IMRT treatment is delivered through synchronized circular motion of the accelerator, couch translational motion, and multileaf collimation. Langen et al.[284] compared three methods of registering megavoltage CT images from a tomotherapy unit with the kilovoltage planning CT images and found that manual registration performed using implanted fiducial markers exhibited the least interobserver variability and agreed best with automatic registration computed from the center of mass of the three implanted fiducial markers.

Linac-based kilovoltage image-guidance systems are routinely used now for image-guided therapy approaches. These systems comprise a kilovoltage x-ray tube mounted 90 degrees from the accelerator head and a kilovoltage imaging plate mounted 90 degrees from the standard megavoltage imaging device. They possess capabilities for kilovoltage two-dimensional projection imaging (radiographs), fluoroscopy, and 3D cone-beam CT and are thus ideally suited for monitoring of interfractional and intrafractional motion.

Brachytherapy for Early-Stage Disease: Treatment Techniques

Preplanned Transperineal Implantation Techniques

The preplanning technique essentially attempts to map the seed-loading patterns prior to the implantation procedure, and during the procedure the brachytherapist will try to simulate the preplanned needle positions with the operative conditions and settings. The technique can be summarized as follows: TRUS imaging is obtained before the planned procedure to assess the prostate volume. A computerized plan is generated from the transverse ultrasound images, producing isodose distributions and the ideal location of seeds within the gland to deliver the prescription dose to the prostate. Several days to weeks later, the implantation procedure is performed. Needles are then placed under ultrasonographic guidance through a perineal template according to the coordinates determined by the preplan. Radioactive seeds are individually deposited in the needle with the aid of an applicator or with preloaded seeds on a semirigid strand containing the preplanned number of seeds. In the latter case, this is accomplished by stabilizing the needle obturator that holds the seed column in a fixed position while the needle is withdrawn slowly, depositing a row or series of seeds within the gland. One of the inherent advantages of a stranded-seed approach is the reduction of seed migration and embolization to the lung compared with the use of free seeds. Among patients implanted with loose seeds, usually <2% of the implanted seeds are likely to migrate. There is no evidence of any adverse effect caused by seed embolization.[285]

Careful evaluation of the preplan with attention to dose–volume histogram analyses of both the target and normal tissues is essential to ensure that the dose to the urethra and rectum are within tolerance ranges and the prescription dose is being delivered to the prostate target. In a multi-institutional analysis there remains a great deal of variability within preplans as to acceptable target volume, seed strength, dose homogeneity, treatment margins, and extracapsular seed placement, although prostate brachytherapy prescription doses are uniform.[286]

Intraoperative Planning Techniques for Prostate Brachytherapy

With the current availability of sophisticated treatment-planning programs that can rapidly generate highly conformal dose distributions in the operating room, intraoperative planning for prostate brachytherapy is an attractive method for prostate brachytherapy. Intraoperative planning takes advantage of the opportunity of using real-time measurements of the prostate during the procedure, whereas preplanning is often performed several weeks before implantation, frequently under different conditions than the actual operative procedure. Subtle changes in the position of the ultrasound probe, as well as the distortion of the prostate associated with needle placement and subsequent edema, can result in profound changes in the shape of the gland compared with the preplanned prostatic contour. Consequently, intraoperative adjustments of seed and needle placements are frequently required using a preplanned technique, and the postplan CT-based dosimetry does not always correspond to the idealized preplan. With the intraoperative real-time planning, commercially available systems track the placement of deposited seeds within the gland, which can provide feedback to the operator for the need to make adjustments to ensure target coverage and maintain constrained doses to the urethra and rectum. Yet, limitations still exist with such programs in their inability to reliably track and capture the exact coordinates of all of the deposited seeds on ultrasound because of difficulties with individual seed recognition using current ultrasound imaging techniques.

At MSKCC, intraoperative conformal optimization and planning for ultrasound-based transperineal implantation have been routinely used for well more than 10 years.[287] This technique involves a sophisticated optimization system that incorporates acceptable dose ranges allowed within the target, as well as dose constraints for the rectal wall and urethra. An ultrasound probe is positioned in the rectum, and the prostate and normal anatomies are identified. Needles are inserted through the perineal template at the periphery of the prostate. The prostate is subsequently scanned from apex to base, and these 0.5-cm images are transferred to the treatment-planning system using a PC-based video capture system. On the computer monitor, the prostate contours and the urethra are digitized on each axial image. Needle positions are identified on each image, and their coordinates are incorporated into a genetic algorithm optimization program. After the optimization program identifies the optimal seed-loading pattern and the dose calculations are completed, isodose displays are superimposed on each transverse ultrasound image and carefully evaluated. Dose–volume histograms for the target volume, rectum, and urethra are also carefully assessed. For the intraoperative plan the V100 for the prostate is set at 95% or higher, and the maximum urethral and rectal dose thresholds are set at <130% and 1-cm^3 <100% of the prescription doses, respectively. The entire planning process from the contouring of images to the generation of the seed-loading pattern requires approximately 10 minutes. Seeds are then loaded with a standard applicator.

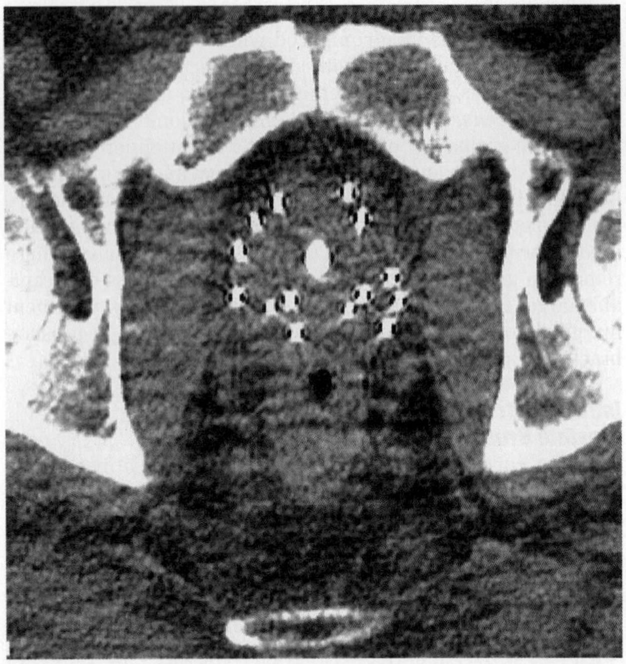

FIGURE 65.9. Postimplantation computed tomography scan after permanent transperineal ultrasound-guided seed implantation with urethral sparing.

A cone-beam CT scan from a mobile unit is routinely used to obtain postimplantation dosimetric analysis while the patient is under anesthesia before the conclusion of the procedure to ensure optimal coverage of the target volume with the prescription dose. Figure 65.9 shows a postimplantation CT image used for dosimetric evaluation.

Dose, Isotope, and Activity Considerations for Prostate Brachytherapy

At present, the commonly used dose for interstitial implantation when using ^{125}I is 144 Gy, prescribed to the isodose surface that completely encompasses the prostate as contoured from imaging studies. For ^{103}Pd, 125 Gy is the recommended prescription dose when the isotope is used as monotherapy, based on a 1999 consensus according to the National Institutes of Standards and Technology.[288] There are clear physical differences between these two isotopes. The half-life of ^{125}I is 60 days, with mean photon energy of 27 keV and an initial dose rate of 7 cGy/hour. In contrast, the half-life of ^{103}Pd is 17 days, with mean photon energy of 21 keV and an initial dose rate of 19 cGy/hour. Dosimetric analyses of treatment plans performed with either isotope have not revealed significant differences between them.[289] Most retrospective reports[290,291] failed to demonstrate any benefit in terms of local tumor control or long-term complications for either isotope. A randomized trial has been conducted comparing ^{125}I with ^{103}Pd for the treatment of early-stage prostate cancer. No differences in tumor-control outcomes have been noted between the two arms of the study. Preliminary findings from this study noted that patients treated with ^{103}Pd had more-intense radiation prostatitis in the first month after implantation but recovered from their radiation-related symptoms sooner than ^{125}I patients, consistent with palladium's shorter half-life.[292] In a retrospective analysis, Kollmeier et al.[293] reported the outcome of patients treated with ^{125}I or ^{103}Pd in conjunction with supplemental EBRT. There were no differences in toxicity or PSA relapse-free survival outcomes between patients who received the ^{103}Pd or ^{125}I boost.

Postimplantation Dosimetric Evaluation

Postimplantation dosimetric evaluation after prostate brachytherapy is recommended as the standard assessment of the quality of permanent interstitial implantation used for the treatment of prostate cancer.[294] The adequacy of the target coverage with the intended prescription doses is evaluated with surrogate parameters such as volume of the prostate treated to 100% of the prescription dose (V_{100}) and the dose delivered to 90% of the prostate target (D_{90}). These parameters have been shown by several investigators to be associated with biochemical relapse and posttreatment biopsy outcomes.[295–296,297–298] Equally important, other parameters of implant quality measure the dose exposure to the urethra and rectum. These measurements have been correlated with postimplantation urinary and rectal-related toxicities.[299,300,301,302] Commercial software is routinely available to determine the coverage of the prostate and dose to critical normal-tissue structures. Isodose curves and dose–volume histograms produce a detailed analysis of the radiation dose distribution relative to the prostate and surrounding normal tissues. Postimplantation evaluation is performed on the day of the procedure or 30 days after the procedure. Although the latter time point takes advantage of assessments when prostate edema is less significant after the implant, with potential decreased underestimate of the prostate coverage with the prescription dose, assessments made on the day of the procedure provide more rapid feedback regarding the adequacy of the dose delivered to the prostate.

A summary of published dosimetric outcomes after brachytherapy based on postimplantation CT-based dosimetric outcomes is shown in Table 65.9.

Postimplantation evaluation is considered an important quality assurance procedure for prostate brachytherapy and provides important feedback to the brachytherapist concerning the quality of the implant performed and what corrections need to be made to optimize target coverage to reduce normal tissue dosing. Postimplantation dosimetric parameters also reflect the dose delivered to the prostate and may predict the likelihood of long-term tumor control outcomes. Stock et al.[303] reported that, among patients with low-risk disease who had an optimal dose based on retrospective postimplantation dosimetry evaluation from the day-30 CT scan (D_{90} > 140 Gy; n = 49), the PSA relapse-free survival at 8 years was 94%, compared to 75% for those who received lower dose levels (p = .02). Investigators from Memorial Sloan-Kettering Cancer Center recently demonstrated that higher D_{90} values based on the postimplantation dosimetric analysis from the CT taken on day 0 (the day of the procedure) also was associated with improved long-term biochemical control outcomes.[304] In that report the 7-year PSA relapse-free survival was 99% compared to 89% for patients with D_{90} > 140 and <140 Gy, respectively (p = .005).

TABLE 65.9 POSTIMPLANT COMPUTED TOMOGRAPHY-BASED DOSIMETRIC PARAMETERS WITH PERMANENT PROSTATE BRACHYTHERAPY: TARGET COVERAGE AND NORMAL TISSUE DOSES

Institution	V_{100} (%)	D_{90} (Gy)	V_{150} (%)	Rectal Dose	Urethral Dose
BC Cancer Agency	Loose, 90	153	52.5	V_{100}, 1.29 cm^3	NS
	Stranded, 91	152	60	V_{100}, 1.5 cm^2	
Mt. Sinai Medical Center (New York)	94	175	56	D_{30}, 46 Gy	D_{30}, 209
				D_{10}, 117 Gy	D_{10}, 220
Wheeling Medical Center (West Virginia)	95	110	55	Mean, 78%	Mean, 120%
		167	68	Maximum, 115%	Maximum, 141%
Memorial Sloan-Kettering Cancer Center	96	173	67	Mean, 32%	Mean, 103%
				Maximum, 72%	Maximum, 129%

NS, Not stated.

Results of Standard Treatment Interventions for Clinically Localized Prostate Cancer

Outcome with Radical Prostatectomy

Bianco et al.[305] reported the long-term outcomes of 1,963 patients who underwent RP, all performed by one surgeon. The positive margin rate was 13%. The overall 5- and 10-year biochemical tumor-control outcomes were 82% and 77%, respectively. Among patients with pretreatment PSA levels of 4 to 10, 10 to 20, and >20 ng/mL the 10-year PSA relapse-free survival outcomes were 83%, 64%, and 47%, respectively. The overall cause-specific survival was 99% and 95%. At 24 months after surgery, 60% were potent, continent, and free of disease. Roehl et al.[306] recently reported the outcome of 3,478 men who underwent RP for clinically localized prostate cancer at Washington University. In that report, the mean follow-up was 65 months. The overall biochemical recurrence rate at 10 years was 32%, with a median time to failure of 28 months. The 10-year PSA relapse-free survival rates for patients with preoperative PSA levels of <2.6, 2.6 to 4, 4.1 to 10, and >10 ng/mL were 91%, 78%, 74%, and 49%, respectively. Multivariate analysis revealed that predictors for PSA relapse-free survival outcomes included the preoperative PSA level, clinical tumor stage, Gleason sum, pathologic stage, and treatment era. The 10-year cancer-specific and overall survival rates were 97% and 83%, respectively. The cancer-specific survival outcome was influenced by the pathologic stage ($p < .004$), Gleason sum ($p = .004$), and treatment era ($p = .04$). Of note, the 10-year biochemical relapse-free survival outcome was significantly different for those patients with pathologic Gleason 3 + 4 versus 4 + 3 (64% and 32%, respectively).

There is a relatively limited number of series reporting biochemical control outcome with median follow-up times of >10 years. A recent series was reported by the University Hospital in Hamburg, Germany, for a cohort of 432 patients with a median follow-up of 122 months.[307] During the follow-up period, 40% developed a biochemical relapse. The 10-year PSA relapse-free survival outcomes according to pathologic T stage were as follows: 87% for pT2, 53% for pT3 a, 28% for pT3b, and 6% for pT4. Patients with RP Gleason scores of 6 or less had a 90% 10-year PSA control, compared to 58% for patients with Gleason 3 + 4, 21% for patients with Gleason 4 + 3, and 11% for patients with Gleason 8 and higher. The 10-year PSA control rates for positive and negative surgical margins were 24% and 68%, respectively. Multivariate analysis demonstrated the following variables as significant for long-term biochemical tumor control: PSA level, pathologic T and nodal stage, RP Gleason score, and the surgical margin status.

Han et al.[308] reported the long-term outcome of RP from the Johns Hopkins Hospital. In that report, 2,091 men underwent RP. In this series, 79% of patients had PSA levels of <10 ng/mL, and 62% of the patients had Gleason scores of ≤6. The mean follow-up was 6.3 years. The overall 10- and 15-year PSA relapse-free survival outcomes were 85% and 79%, respectively. The 10-year PSA control rates for patients with preoperative PSA values of 0 to 4, 4 to 10, 10.1 to 20, and >20 ng/mL were 91%, 79%, 57%, and 48%, respectively.

Amling et al.[309] from the Mayo Clinic reported the outcome of 2,782 patients with clinically localized prostate cancer treated between 1987 and 1993. They noted that among patients with pathologically confirmed T2 N0 disease, 5- and 10-year PSA relapse-free survival rates were 82% and 68%, respectively. The highest risk of biochemical relapse was noted during the first 2 years after surgery, and only 6% of patients had a disease relapse after 5 years.

Outcome with Conventional External-Beam Radiation Therapy for Low-Risk Disease

Kuban et al.[310] reported the results of a large multi-institutional analysis comprising 4,839 patients with T1-T2 prostate cancer treated with EBRT between 1986 and 1995. The median follow-up was 6.3 years. In this cohort, no patient received neoadjuvant androgen-deprivation therapy. Most of the patients included (70%) were treated with conventional EBRT, and 30% were treated with 3DCRT planning techniques. Prescription doses ranged from 60 to 78 Gy. For the cohort of patients treated to dose levels of <70 Gy, the median dose was 67 Gy; among those patients who received 70 Gy or more, the median dose in this cohort was 72 Gy. PSA failure was defined according to the American Society for Therapeutic Radiology and Oncology (ASTRO) definition of three consecutive rising PSA values above the nadir value. The overall 8-year PSA control rates for patients with pretreatment PSA values of 0 to 4, 4 to 9.9, 10 to 20, and >20 to 30 ng/mL were 80%, 60%, 46%, and 34%, respectively. The overall 8-year PSA control rates for patients with posttreatment nadir PSA values of 0 to 0.49, 0.5 to 0.99, 1 to 1.99, and ≥2.0 ng/mL were 93%, 88%, 86%, and 72%, respectively. Higher prescription dose levels of ≥72 Gy were associated with a significant decrease in PSA relapse rates, and these differences were most noted among patients with intermediate- and higher-risk disease. Although there was no apparent dose response for favorable-risk patients, the number of patients with favorable-risk features who received higher doses in this study was small.

Dose Escalation for Low-Risk Disease

It has become clear that traditionally planned EBRT using conventional dose levels does not have the capacity to completely eradicate local prostatic disease in the majority of treated patients. With the increasing use of 3D conformal planning and availability of IMRT, prescription doses can be more reliably delivered to the prostate and lead to further improved outcomes. Phase III randomized trials and several single-institution trials have confirmed the advantage of high-dose CRT for patients with localized prostate cancer. These trials have shown long-term biochemical control advantages especially among patients with intermediate- and high-risk disease. More recently, however, updates of some these studies have indicated a benefit for the application of higher radiation dose levels even for patients with favorable-risk disease. The phase III trial from MD Anderson Hospital accrued 301 patients with T1 to T3 prostate cancer, of whom 150 were treated to 70 Gy (conventional EBRT) and 151 were treated to 78 Gy (conventional EBRT followed by a 3D boost). The PSA relapse-free survival rates for the 78- and 70-Gy arms were 70% and 64%, respectively ($p = .03$). In a recent update of this trial[311] a significant improvement in 8-year biochemical control was noted among low-risk patients who received 78 Gy compared to 70 Gy (88% vs. 63%; $p = .042$; Fig. 65.10).

Zietman et al.[312] reported the result of a randomized trial of 393 patients with T1-T2 prostate cancer with pretreatment PSA levels of <15 ng/mL. Patients were randomized to receive conventional EBRT to a dose level of 70.2 or 79.2 Gy. In both treatment arms, radiotherapy was delivered using a combination of photon and proton beams. The median follow-up in this study was 5.5 years. The 5-year PSA relapse-free survival rates for the low- and high-dose arms were 61% and 80%, respectively, which represented a 49% risk reduction in biochemical failure. What was most noteworthy in this trial was that a clear advantage for higher dose was observed among the subset of patients with low-risk disease, which represented the majority of patients accrued to the trial (PSA of <10 ng/mL, stage ≤T2 a, or Gleason score of <6). In this subgroup of patients, a significant advantage for higher doses was observed, with an associated 51% risk reduction in biochemical relapse (80% vs. 60% for higher vs. lower doses; $p < .001$).

The experience from MSKCC was recently reported by Zelefsky et al.[313] A total of 2,551 patients with T1-T3 prostate cancer were treated with follow-up that extended beyond 20 years. The radiation dose was systematically increased from

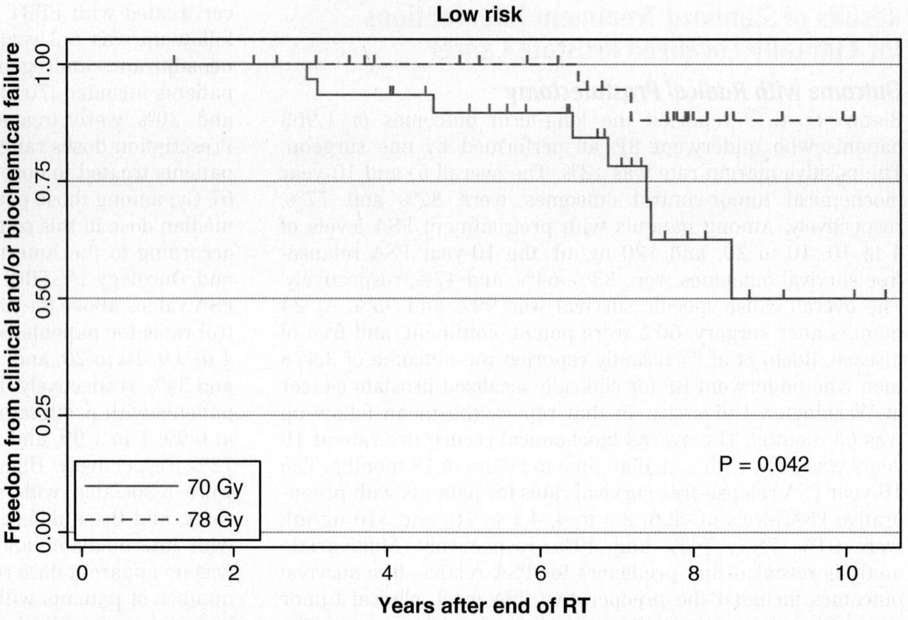

FIGURE 65.10. Freedom from biochemical failure for the subset of low-risk patients treated in the MD Anderson randomized trial with 78 versus 70 Gy. (From Kuban DA, Tucker SL, Dong L, et al. Long-term results of the M. D. Anderson randomized dose-escalation trial for prostate cancer. *Int J Radiat Oncol Biol Phys* 2008;70:67–74; with permission from Elsevier.)

64.8 to 86.4 Gy by increments of 5.4 Gy in consecutive groups of patients. This study also demonstrated an advantage for dose escalation in low-risk patients. The 10-year PSA relapse-free survival among patients with low-risk disease who received dose levels of 75.6 Gy and higher was 84%, compared to 70% for patients who received lower dose levels (*p* = .04; Fig. 65.11). In this report there were no apparent differences in long-term outcomes among patients who received 81 versus 75.5 Gy for low-risk disease. Other did not demonstrate dose-escalation advantages for low-risk disease,[314,315] but the follow-up was relatively limited in these studies. The 10-year biochemical outcomes from MSKCC patients for IMRT-treated patients have been reported.[316] The 10-year actuarial PSA relapse-free survival rates for favorable-, intermediate- and unfavorable-risk group patients were 81%, 78%, and 62%, respectively. The 10-year actuarial distant metastases–free survival outcomes for

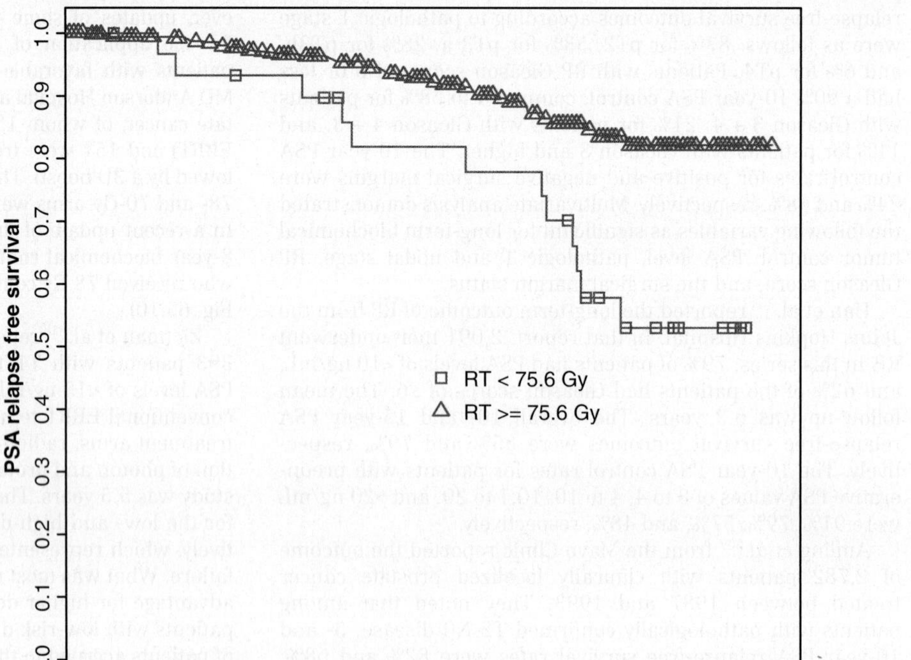

Number of subjects at risk

44	40	37	32	31	24	15	9	RT < 75.6 Gy
527	487	427	323	196	89	33	6	RT >= 75.6 Gy

FIGURE 65.11. Memorial Sloan-Kettering Cancer Center experience for prostate-specific antigen relapse-free survival outcomes for low-risk patients treated with 75.6 Gy and higher versus lower doses. (From Zelefsky MJ, Chan H, Hunt M, et al. Long-term outcome of high dose intensity modulated radiation therapy for patients with clinically localized prostate cancer. *J Urol* 2006;176:1415–1419; with permission from Elsevier.)

favorable-, intermediate-, and unfavorable-risk group were 0%, 6%, and 10%, respectively The 10-year actuarial risk of a prostate cancer–related death for favorable-, intermediate-, and unfavorable-risk group was 0%, 3%, and 14%.

Michalski et al.[317] reported the outcome of RTOG 94-06, which evaluated dose escalation using 3D conformal radiotherapy for patients with localized prostate cancer. Patients were accrued on five sequential dose levels: 68.4, 73.8, 79.2, 74, and 78 Gy. For patients with low-risk disease (n = 403), the 5-year PSA-relapse-free survival outcomes for these respective dose levels were 68%, 73%, 67%, 84%, and 80%.

Comparison of EBRT Outcomes with Surgery for Early-Stage Prostate Cancer

Kupelian et al.[316] compared the 8-year outcomes of surgery and EBRT from the Cleveland Clinic. In this report, 1,054 patients were treated with surgery and 628 were treated with EBRT. Treatments (surgery or radiotherapy) were given between 1990 and 1998, and the median follow-up was 51 months. There were significant differences in the patient groups because, in general, those treated with surgery were younger and had lower clinical stages, pretreatment PSA levels, and Gleason scores. The 8-year PSA relapse-free survival outcome for patients who underwent RP and EBRT was 72% and 70%, respectively (p = .01). Multivariate analysis demonstrated that the clinical stage, pretreatment PSA, biopsy Gleason score, use of neoadjuvant therapy, and year of treatment were all independent predictors of disease relapse, whereas the treatment modality (RT vs. surgery) did not influence likelihood of failure. These authors also noted a benefit for higher radiation doses in the favorable-risk subset of patients. Among favorable-risk patients who received 72 Gy or more, the 8-year PSA relapse-free survival outcome was similar (p = .08) to that of patients treated with RP and significantly better, in turn, than that of patients treated with RT to dose levels of <72 Gy (p < .001). Similarly, Zelefsky et al.[243] found similar distant metastases–free survival outcomes between high-dose IMRT and surgery for low-risk patients.

In the absence of randomized trials comparing surgery to RT it is difficult to definitively make claims of the superiority of one treatment over another. It has been stated frequently that, whereas the results of radiation and radical surgery are comparable up to 10 years, there is a rapid decrement in the probabilities of both disease-free and overall survival after that time point among irradiated patients. However, such conclusions are likely erroneous owing to selection bias factors favoring a younger cohort with more favorable prognostic features who are more often chosen for surgery compared with radiation therapy. In addition, because of the lack of information in most radiation therapy series of the pathologic status of the lymph nodes, patients with microscopic nodal disease will likely be included in radiation therapy reports yet routinely excluded from surgical series. An additional argument posed for surgery is that if such an approach fails, salvage radiotherapy remains a viable option, whereas for those who fail radiotherapy, salvage surgery can be associated with an increased of risk of postoperative complications. However, patients need to be informed that there are risks associated with salvage radiotherapy after a failed prostatectomy, and the likelihood of a successful outcome after well-delivered primary radiotherapy is high and comparable to surgery outcomes.

Outcome with Brachytherapy

Similar to the predictors of biochemical outcome after EBRT for prostate cancer, PSA relapse-free survival after permanent seed implantation depends on several prognostic variables, including the pretreatment PSA, biopsy Gleason score, clinical stage, and the implant dose delivered to the target volume. In general, among patients with pretreatment PSA of ≤10 ng/mL, permanent seed implantation alone is associated with excellent biochemical outcome and appears comparable with other local interventions. Fifteen-year outcomes were recently reported by Sylvester et al.[318] from 215 patients treated between 1988 and 1992. The PSA relapse-free survival outcomes were 86%, 80%, and 62% for favorable-, intermediate-, and high-risk patients, respectively. Similarly, Taira et al.[319] reported on 1,656 patients. For low-risk patients the 7-year biochemical tumor control, cause-specific survival, and overall survival outcomes were noted to be 98.6%, 99%, and 77.5%, respectively.

Eleven institutions combined data on 2,693 patients treated with permanent interstitial brachytherapy monotherapy for T1-T2 prostate cancer.[298] Of these patients, 1,831 (68%) were treated with ^{125}I (median dose, 144 Gy) and 862 (32%) were treated with ^{103}Pd (median dose, 108 Gy). The median follow-up was 63 months. The 8-year PSA relapse-free survival outcomes for favorable-, intermediate-, and unfavorable-risk patients were 82%, 70%, and 48%, respectively (p < .001) according to the ASTRO consensus definition. Among patients in whom the dose to 90% of the prostate (D_{90}) was >130 Gy, the 8-year PSA relapse-free survival outcome was 90% compared with 73% for those with D_{90} dose levels of ≤130 Gy (p < .001). The PSA nadir value at 3 years after implantation was associated with the long-term biochemical outcome. The 8-year PSA relapse-free survival outcomes were 92%, 86%, 79%, and 67%, respectively, for patients who achieved PSA nadir values of 0 to 0.49, 0.5 to 0.99, 1.0 to 1.99, and >2.0 ng/mL (p < .001). Among patients who were free of biochemical relapse at 8 years, the median nadir level was 0.1 ng/mL, and 90% of these patients achieved a nadir PSA level of <0.6 ng/mL.

Stone et al.[320] reported on 2,111 patients who underwent brachytherapy followed for a median of 6 years. In this group 56% of the patients were treated with ^{125}I, 10% were treated with ^{103}Pd, and 34% were treated with combined external-beam radiotherapy and ^{103}Pd implant. Among low-risk patients, the PSA-relapse free survival outcome at 12 years was 88%. Significant predictors of long-term biochemical tumor control included the use of androgen-deprivation therapy (p = .03), pretreatment PSA level (p = .026), and a higher biologically effective dose (p = .003). Among patients who had a posttreatment biopsy 2 years after treatment, higher biologically effective dose levels were associated with improved local tumor-control outcomes.

In an update of the outcomes of real-time intraoperative planning at MSKCC reported by Zelefsky et al.,[304] 1,466 patients with prostate cancer were treated with permanent interstitial implantation using a transrectal ultrasound-guided approach. Real-time intraoperative treatment planning, which incorporated inverse planning optimization, was used. The 5-year PSA relapse-free survival outcomes for favorable- and intermediate-risk patients were 98% and 95%, respectively. In these patients, no dosimetric parameter was identified that influenced the biochemical outcome. For this cohort of patients the use of androgen deprivation did not affect the long-term PSA relapse-free survival outcomes. Among patients treated with ^{125}I, improved biochemical control outcomes were observed for patients who had D_{90} values of >140 Gy compared to lower doses. It should be noted that this improved biochemical control outcome based on this dosimetric parameter was observed for postimplantation, CT-based assessments made on the day of the procedure (and not 30 days later).

Table 65.10 summarizes the published biochemical outcomes after low–dose-rate interstitial seed implantation according to prognostic risk groups.

ACUTE AND LATE TREATMENT-RELATED SEQUELAE OF STANDARD TREATMENT INTERVENTIONS

Sequelae of Radical Prostatectomy

Complication rates after prostatectomy vary in the literature and recently have been shown to depend on the experience

TABLE 65.10 FIVE-YEAR BIOCHEMICAL CONTROL AFTER BRACHYTHERAPY ALONE FOR CLINICALLY LOCALIZED PROSTATE CANCER ACCORDING TO PROGNOSTIC RISK-GROUP CLASSIFICATIONS

Study	Patients	Projected Results (Year)	Favorable Risk (%)
Taira et al.[319]	1,656	7	98
Sylvester et al.[318]	215	15	86
Multi-institutional[298]	2,693	8	82
Stone et al.[320]	2,111	12	88
Potters et al.[296]	1,449	12	89
Zelefsky et al.[304]	1,466	7	98

of the surgeon. Begg et al.[321] used the Medicare claim records from 11,522 patients who underwent prostatectomy between 1992 and 1996. Postoperative morbidity was found to be significantly reduced in hospitals that were considered to have high volume compared with lower-volume ones (27% vs. 32%; $p = .03$) and among surgeons with a high-volume practice compared to those with lower volumes (26% vs. 32%; $p < .001$).

Immediate intraoperative/postoperative complications include pelvic pain and transient incontinence. Although intraoperative blood loss can range from 300 to 4,000 mL, meticulous surgical technique should reduce blood loss. The operative mortality rate has been reported to be 1% to 2%, but in experienced hands the incidence is a fraction of 1%. The incidence of postoperative stress incontinence ranges from 5% to 57%.

Catalona et al.[322] reported on the complication rates in 1,870 patients who underwent RP. They reported a 2% incidence of a thromboembolic event and a 4% incidence of an anastomotic stricture. Recovery of urinary continence depended on the age of the patient. Among patients in their 50s, 60s, and 70s, the likelihood of persistent urinary incontinence was 3%, 8%, and 13%, respectively. The incidence of impotence after bilateral and unilateral nerve-sparing surgery procedures was 53% and 32%, respectively. Bilateral nerve-sparing procedure was associated with improved potency preservation among patients who were younger than 70 years of age (71% vs. 48%; $p < .001$), whereas these differences were not significant in the older age group.

Bianco et al.[305] reported continence and potency outcomes in 1,472 patients who underwent surgery since 1991 and were operated on by a single surgeon. Among 1,288 patients who were continent prior to surgery, the actuarial likelihood of maintained continence was 91% at 12 months and 95% at 24 months. Of 785 patients with potency information available, the median time to erectile function recovery was 12 months, and the 2-year likelihood of potency preservation was 70%.

A large review from the Nationwide Inpatient Sample extracted from this data set 11,889 patients who underwent robot-assisted RP (RARP) and compared the perioperative complication rates to 7,389 patients who underwent an open RP.[323] This analysis found that, among patients undergoing a RARP, significantly lower likelihoods for blood transfusions and intraoperative and postoperative complications were observed compared to the open prostatectomy procedure. In addition, a shorter duration of hospital stay was noted for the patients who underwent a RARP. However, one of the limitations of this retrospective study was the fact that these findings were not adjusted by the clinical stage of the patients and the surgeon's experience or volume, which play important roles in the frequency of surgical-related complications.

Sequelae of Conventional External-Beam Radiation Therapy

EBRT delivered with conventional techniques is fairly well tolerated, although grade 2 or higher acute rectal morbidity (discomfort, tenesmus, diarrhea) or urinary symptoms (frequency, nocturia, urgency, dysuria) requiring medication occur in approximately 60% of patients. Symptoms usually appear during the third week of treatment and resolve within days to weeks after treatment is completed. The incidence of late complications that develop ≥6 months after completion of treatment is significantly lower, whereas serious complications that require corrective surgical intervention are rare. In general the incidence of chronic urinary sequelae (i.e., cystitis, hematuria, urethral stricture, or bladder contracture) using conformal treatment delivery techniques are <5%, and the incidence of grade 3 and 4 urinary-related complications requiring major surgical interventions or hospitalization is <1%. The incidence of chronic intestinal or rectal sequelae (chronic diarrhea, proctitis, or rectal bleeding) that requires medical management ranges from 3% to 10%, and <1% of grade 3-4 complications are observed after more-targeted treatment-delivery techniques such as IMRT and image-guided radiotherapy. Fecal urgency and incontinence are documented side effects after treatment and have been reported to occur in <2% of patients, occur less than once per week, and are often associated with incontinence for flatulence.[324] Most complications attributed to radiation therapy are observed within the first 3 to 4 years after treatment, and the likelihood of complications developing after 5 years is low. The risk of complications is increased when radiation doses exceed 72 Gy. Several factors have been associated with increased bowel or rectal toxicity after EBRT,[273,324,325,326–327,328,329–330] and these include the volume of the rectum exposed to higher doses of radiation, increasing age of the patient, concomitant use of androgen-deprivation therapy, and the presence of diabetes and inflammatory bowel disease. Even patients with a prior history of inflammatory bowel disease currently in remission may have significant increases of rectal toxicity, and alternative treatments should be considered for these patients. Among patients who undergo radiotherapy and experience acute rectal side effects, a higher incidence of late rectal toxicity has been observed.[328,330]

Michalski et al.[331] reported the toxicity outcomes of various risk groups enrolled in RTOG 9406, a phase I dose-escalation study. The dose levels evaluated in this report included patients treated to the initial two dose levels of the study, 68.4 and 73.8 Gy. The median follow-up times in these subgroups ranged from 2.2 to 3.4 years. The acute grade 2 bowel/rectal toxicity rates ranged from 16% to 25%. The crude incidence of late bowel/rectal toxicities ranged from 2% to 8%. With a median follow-up of 2.5 years, the crude late grade 2 and 3 gastrointestinal toxicities for those patients treated to 78 Gy (2-Gy fractions) was 22% and 2%, respectively.

Storey et al.[332] reported late rectal toxicity among patients treated on the phase III trial form the MD Anderson Hospital. The 5-year actuarial risks of late grade 2 rectal toxicity for the 70- and 78-Gy dose level arms were 14% and 21%, respectively. In that report, the dose–volume histogram analyses of the patients treated to 78 Gy were analyzed to ascertain whether there were any predictive patterns for late rectal toxicity. These investigators reported a significant correlation for the percentage of the rectum treated to 70 Gy or higher and the likelihood of late rectal toxicity. Patients with >25% of the rectal wall treated to 70 Gy or higher had a 37% risk of grade 2 rectal toxicity, compared with 13% among patients who had <25% of the rectal wall exposed to these doses ($p = .05$). In an update of that experience, Kuban et al.[311] noted that the volume of rectum exposed to higher radiation doses was associated with the risk of rectal toxicity after external-beam radiotherapy. The incidence of grade 2 rectal toxicity was 46% when >26% of the rectal volume was exposed to >70 Gy of the prescription dose. In contrast, among patients who had lower volume of rectum exposed to these dose levels the incidence of grade 2 toxicity was significantly lower (14%).

Zelefsky et al.[333] reported the long-term tolerance of high-dose CRT at MSKCC. The 10-year actuarial rate of grade 2 or

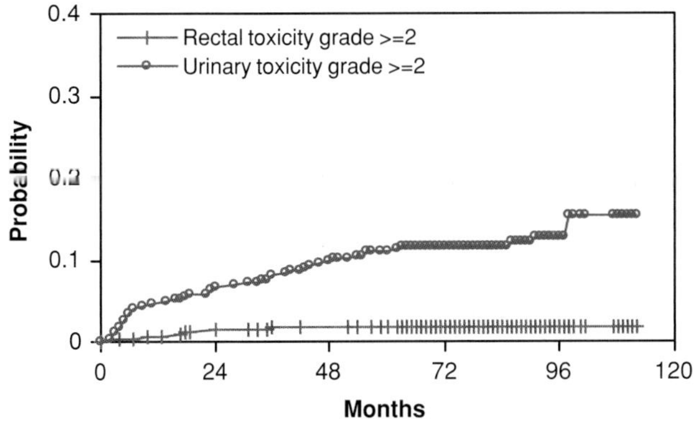

FIGURE 65.12. Actuarial likelihood of late grade 2 or greater rectal toxicities or late grade 2 or greater rectal toxicities. (From Zelefsky MJ, Chan H, Hunt M, et al. Long-term outcome of high dose intensity modulated radiation therapy for patients with clinically localized prostate cancer. *J Urol* 2006;176:1415–1419; with permission from Elsevier.)

higher rectal toxicity was 9%. The use of IMRT significantly lowered the risk of grade 2 and higher toxicities from 13% to 5% ($p < .001$). This decline in rectal toxicity was observed despite the application of higher dose levels of 81 Gy with IMRT compared to generally lower doses used with 3DCRT of 75.6 Gy (Fig. 65.12). In addition, patients who experienced acute gastrointestinal side effects during treatment were six times more likely to experience late gastrointestinal toxicities than were patients who did not experience such acute side effects (42% vs. 9%; $p < .001$). The 10-year incidence of grade 2 or higher late urinary toxicities was 15%, and the predictors for late toxicity included higher radiation doses and the presence of acute urinary symptoms during the course of EBRT. The 10-year toxicity outcomes of 81 Gy IMRT were recently updated by investigators from MSKCC.[334] The incidence of grade 2 and 3 gastrointestinal toxicities was 2% and 1%, respectively. The 10-year actuarial incidence of grade 2 and higher urinary related toxicities was 17%.

Peeters et al.[335] reported on the incidence of acute and late complications in a multicenter randomized trial comparing 68- to 78-Gy 3DCRT. The median follow-up was 31 months. The 3-year incidence of grade 2 and higher gastrointestinal and genitourinary toxicities for the 68-Gy dose arm was 23% and 28.5%, respectively. The 3-year incidence of grade 2 and higher gastrointestinal and genitourinary toxicities for the 78-Gy dose arm was 26.5% and 30%, respectively. The differences were not significant. However, the authors did note a significant increase in grade 3 rectal toxicity requiring laser cauterization for the higher-dose arm. For patients treated to 78 Gy, the incidence of grade 3 rectal bleeding at 3 years was 10%, compared to 2% for those treated to 68 Gy. The following variables were found to be predictive of late gastrointestinal toxicity: a history of abdominal surgery ($p < .001$) and the presence of pretreatment gastrointestinal symptoms ($p = .001$). The following variables were predictive of late genitourinary toxicity: pretreatment urinary symptoms ($p < .001$), the use of neoadjuvant androgen-deprivation therapy ($p < .001$), and prior transurethral resection of the prostate ($p = .006$).

Urethral strictures have been observed in 1.5% of 1,100 patients treated with 3DCRT. Grade 3 hematuria requiring fulguration was observed in <0.5% of the patients. Among patients who previously underwent a TURP, a 4% incidence of stricture development after 3DCRT was observed.[336] Other late urinary toxicities were not observed among patients with a prior history of a TURP. Lee et al.[337] observed a 2% incontinence rate among patients with a prior history of TURP who were treated with EBRT, compared with a 0.2% rate in patients without a prior TURP. At present it does not appear that the use of IMRT has significantly reduced long-term urinary symptoms compared to conventional 3DCRT.

Potency Preservation with External-Beam Radiation Therapy

The rates of erectile dysfunction after EBRT ranged from 6% to 84%.[338] The wide range of outcomes is a reflection of the varying assessment tools used and disparity in patient population, with heterogeneity of comorbidities, ages, and baseline functional status. Most studies show a progressive decline in erectile function with longer follow-ups, consistent with what is observed in an aging population with coexisting comorbidities such as hypertension, atherosclerotic heart disease, and diabetes. Investigators from the University of Chicago reported potency rates after EBRT.[339] With a median follow-up of 34 months, actuarial potency rates at 1, 20, 40, and 60 months were 96%, 75%, 59%, and 53%, respectively. In one report[340] comparing erectile function between patients who received 68 versus 78 Gy no differences were observed between the different dose levels. Overall in the studied cohort the incidence of erectile dysfunction at 1 and 2 years after therapy was 27% and 36%, respectively. Aside from erectile dysfunction, other aspects of sexual dysfunction after radiotherapy include decreased volume of ejaculate, absence of ejaculate, decreased intensity of orgasm, and decreased libido. A summary of reported potency rates after treatment is shown in Table 65.11.

Significant limitations exist with the aforementioned reported potency preservation rates because the data are derived from retrospective analyses, and information was often obtained without the use of validated questionnaires. Prospective studies suggest that when patients are assessed with validated tools, erectile dysfunction—defined as inability to achieve adequate erection sufficient for sexual intercourse—reaches 60% to 70%. What also complicates the interpretation of published incidence rates is the multifactorial nature of erectile dysfunction. The factors that impact erectile function include age, presence of medical comorbidities such as cardiac disease and diabetes, antihypertensive medications, baseline erectile function, and the use of neoadjuvant and concurrent hormonal therapy. Pinkawa et al.[341] observed that the presence of spontaneous erection in evening or morning before treatment was a strong predictor for maintained erectile function after radiotherapy.

Radiation-mediated impotence is likely multifactorial. However, it has been observed that 63% of patients evaluated for impotence after radiation therapy were diagnosed as having arteriogenic dysfunction, whereas 31% had cavernosal dysfunction. Only 3% were believed to have neurogenic impotence.[341] Sildenafil administration results in significant improvement in erectile function.[342,343] In one report, sildenafil improved erectile function in 74% of patients who underwent

TABLE 65.11 INCIDENCE OF ERECTILE DYSFUNCTION AFTER RADIATION THERAPY FOR PROSTATE CANCER

Study	*Treatment*	*Number of Patients*	*Follow-up (Month)*	*Erectile Dysfunction Incidence (%)*
Mameghan et al.	EBRT	42	55	45 at 2 yr
Roach et al.	EBRT	60	21	38
Crook et al.	EBRT	158	33	35
Mantz et al.	EBRT	68	18	25 at 2 yr
Zelefsky et al.	EBRT	544	42	39
Pilepich et al.	EBRT	230	54	72
Blasko et al.	BRT	469	38	≤70 yr of age: 15 70 yr of age: 50
Stock et al.	BRT	65	18	21
Zelefsky et al.	BRT	221	48	29
Merrick et al.	BRT	209	40	61 at 6 yr

BRT, brachytherapy; EBRT, external-beam radiation therapy.

Modified from Incrocci L, Slob AK, Levendag PC. Sexual (dys)function after radiotherapy for prostate cancer: a review. *Int J Radiat Oncol Biol Phys* 2002;52:681–693.

3DCRT (median dose, 75.6 Gy), whereas 22% of patients had no response.[343]

Low–Dose-Rate Brachytherapy: Acute and Late Toxicity

Urinary Toxicity

Acute urinary retention (AUR) is a known risk that can occur immediately after prostate brachytherapy, and the incidence varies in the literature. Roeloffzen et al.[344] recently reported the incidence and predictors of AUR in a cohort of 714 patients who were treated with ^{125}I brachytherapy. In 8% of patients, retention developed at a median of 30 days from the implantation procedure. In that report multivariate analysis revealed that patients with prostate volume >35 cm^3 experienced a higher incidence of AUR compared to patients with smaller volumes (10.4% vs. 5.4%). In addition, those with higher International Prostate Symptom Scores (IPSS) had a higher likelihood of developing urinary retention, consistent with other reports. Other reports for AUR after low–dose-rate brachytherapy range from 5% to 15%.[345,346–347] There does not seem to be any relationship between dosimetric outcomes, such as urethral dose and V_{150}, and the incidence of AUR after brachytherapy because this condition seems to be more related to acute trauma and intraprostatic inflammation and edema. Consistent with this notion is the fact that some reports demonstrated that greater number of needles placed or seeds deposited is associated with higher rates of AUR.[345,347–347] In general, almost all patients after prostate brachytherapy develop acute urinary symptoms such as urinary frequency, urgency, and occasional urge incontinence. Depending on the isotope used, these symptoms often peak at 1 to 3 months after the procedure and subsequently gradually decline over the ensuing 3 to 6 months. Most patients significantly benefit with the use of an α-blocker, which ameliorates such symptoms in 60% to 70% of patients.

Keyes et al.[348] reported on the acute and long-term urinary outcomes in 712 patients who were treated with ^{125}I permanent interstitial implantation who were followed for a median of 5 years. At 6 and 12 months after the procedure, approximately 37% and 23% experienced grade 2 acute urinary toxicities, and 4% and 2% experienced acute grade 3 urinary toxicities. Most urinary symptoms resolved within 12 months after the procedure, and significant residual toxicity was unusual. Multivariate analysis demonstrated that the use of androgen-deprivation therapy before implantation, higher baseline IPSS, and use of higher number of needles was associated with increased rates of grade 2 acute toxicity. The 5-year likelihood of developing late grade 2 and 3 urinary toxicities was 24% and 6%, respectively. Fewer than 1% of patients experienced a grade 4 urinary toxicity. In this report, predictors for increased risk of grade 2 or higher late urinary toxicity included the following variables: higher baseline IPSS, maximal postimplantation IPSS, presence of acute toxicity, and higher prostate V_{150}. The demonstration in this report that the V_{150} was an independent predictor of late urinary toxicity after brachytherapy highlights the importance of maintaining tight urethral dose constraints during the planning for brachytherapy. Urinary incontinence requiring pads was reported in <1% of treated patients. In a more recent report from MSKCC,[244] the 7-year incidence of grade 2 and 3 urinary toxicities after ^{125}I brachytherapy for low-risk patients was 15% and 2.2, respectively.

Rectal Tolerance

Zelefsky et al.[244] reported 5.1% and 1.1.% grade 2 and 3 late rectal toxicity, respectively, after prostate brachytherapy among 448 low-risk patients treated with ^{125}I implantation. Phan et al.[349] reported a 4% incidence of grade 2 rectal toxicity after permanent interstitial implantation and <1% incidence of grade 3 toxicity. In general, the incidence of grade 2 rectal toxicity after prostate brachytherapy ranges from 4% to 12%. Grade 3 or 4 rectal toxicity is unusual (<2%). Grade 2 symptoms manifest as rectal bleeding or increased mucous discharge. The onset of symptoms often peaks at 8 to 12 months and is self-limited in nature. Several reports noted that rectal bleeding is associated with the rectal dose and its volume exposed to a particular dose. Snyder et al.[301] noted that the rectal volume in cubic centimeters exposed to the prescription dose of 160 Gy correlated with the incidence of grade 2 proctitis. For patients with 0.8 cm^3 or less of rectal volume exposed to the prescription dose, no patient developed proctitis; from 0.8 to 1.8 cm^3, approximately 8% of patients developed rectal bleeding. However, among patients with >1.8 cm^3 of the rectal volume exposed to 160 Gy, 25% of patients developed rectal toxicity. The American Brachytherapy Society recommends that rectal dose constraints should be maintained to restrict the dose to 1 cm of the rectum to the prescription dose or less to reduce the risk of rectal toxicity after brachytherapy.[350]

Erectile Function

Erectile dysfunction after brachytherapy has been reported to occur in from 20% to 80% of patients. The age of the patients, baseline function, and the presence of medical comorbidities play an important role in the likelihood of maintaining durable erectile function after therapy, as described earlier after EBRT. Stone et al.[351] noted a 62% potency preservation based on a patient questionnaire among patients who underwent brachytherapy and were potent prior to treatment. The median follow-up in that cohort was 7 years. Investigators from the Princess Margaret Hospital in Toronto reported a 93% of patients with good erectile function whose baseline function was considered potential prior to therapy.[352] In that cohort, 45% of patients who were potent after therapy required a phosphodiesterase inhibitor to maintain adequate posttreatment function.

The impact of short-course androgen-deprivation therapy in conjunction with brachytherapy on long-term erectile function is unclear. Some reports suggested that ADT produces only temporary deterioration in sexual function and with testosterone recovery the function returns.[353] Data from MSKCC suggest that the use of short-course ADT for the purpose of volume reduction among patients treated with brachytherapy was not associated with a higher incidence of ED compared to patients treated with brachytherapy alone.[244]

Taira et al.[354] evaluated posttreatment erectile function after brachytherapy in 226 men with adequate preimplantation erectile function Adequate baseline function in this report was defined as an International Index of Erectile Function (IIEF-6) of >13 without pharmacologic support. The 7-year incidence of maintained erectile function was 56%. Posttreatment function depended on baseline pretreatment sexual function. Among patients with baseline IIEF scores of ≥24 and 18 to 23 the incidence of long-term erectile function preservation was 75% and 52%, respectively. Although not significant in a multivariate analysis, these investigators noted that higher doses delivered to 25% of the penile bulb created an added detrimental effect on long-term erectile function, especially among those baseline potent patients with lower IIEF scores or those who were of older age at the time of treatment. Excellent responses were observed with sildenafil citrate in the treatment of posttreatment impotence after brachytherapy, with response rates up to 85%.[355,356]

PROTON THERAPY FOR THE TREATMENT OF PROSTATE CANCER

Proton therapy, due to its known Bragg peak and physical characteristics of the beam, provides an opportunity for dose escalation and potential greater sparing of normal tissues to reduce treatment-related toxicities. In the absence of randomized trials comparing efficacy and toxicity to high-dose photon therapy, there is no cogent evidence supporting its superiority over other forms of EBRT. Investigators from Loma Linda reported the initial tumor-control outcomes and toxicity in 1,277 patients treated with early-stage disease with 74 CGE.[357] The authors noted excellent PSA relapse-free survival outcomes and low risks of late toxicity, although these findings appeared to be comparable to outcomes that are currently achieved with high-dose intensity-modulated photon therapy. It should be noted that the Proton Radiation Oncology Group 95-09 randomized trial, which randomized patients to receive 79.2 CGE of proton therapy compared to 70.2 CGE, was testing the advantage of dose escalation. This study did not attempt to compare proton to photon therapy. Such a randomized trial is essential to elucidate the role of protons in the management of localized prostate cancer and is in development in the Radiation Therapy Oncology Group.[358] Important refinements are still necessary in the further development of intensity-modulated image-guided proton therapy, which has the potential of using ultraconformal dose distributions that may pose an advantage over highly conformal IMRT using photons.[359]

STEREOTACTIC BODY RADIOTHERAPY FOR ORGAN-CONFINED PROSTATE CANCER

There has been emerging interest in the use of stereotactic body radiotherapy (SBRT) for the treatment of low- and intermediate-risk prostate cancer. Based on the use of image-guided approaches, generally five fractions of high-dose radiotherapy are used, employing tight margins to reduce the exposure of dose to normal tissues. Freeman and King[360] reported the outcomes of 41 patients who were treated with SBRT to doses of 35 to 36.25 Gy in five fractions and followed for a median of 5 years. The 5-year PSA relapse-free survival outcome was 93%. The incidence of grade 2 late rectal and urinary toxicity was 2.5% and 7%, respectively. The incidence of grade 3 rectal and urinary toxicity was 0% and 2.5%, respectively. Katz et al.[361] reported on 304 patients with a limited follow-up of 2.5 years who were treated with 35 to 36.25 Gy. Among 206 patients with a minimum follow-up of 12 months, the incidence of grade 2 urinary and rectal toxicity was 5.8% and 2.9%, respectively. One late grade 3 urinary toxicity has been observed. No information was available regarding biochemical tumor control because of the limited follow-up observations in this report.

Boike et al.[362] recently reported the preliminary outcomes of a phase I dose-escalation study for low- and intermediate-risk prostate cancer using SBRT. Cohorts of 15 patients were prospectively dose escalated from 45 to 50 Gy in 9-, 9.5-, and 10-Gy fractions. In these patients a rectal balloon was routinely used to separate the posterior and lateral walls of the rectum and reduce the volume of rectal tissue exposed to the high doses of therapy. Patients were treated every other day to further reduce toxicity, as has been demonstrated in the Stanford experience with SBRT.[363] The overall grade 2 and grade 3 rectal toxicities observed were 18% and 2%, respectively. The overall grade 2 and grade 3 urinary toxicities observed were 31% and 4%, respectively. In the 50-Gy dose cohort, two patients developed grade 3 cystitis, which developed approximately 1 year after therapy, and one patient developed a grade 4 rectal injury. At MSKCC a phase I dose-escalation study is underway in which patients with low- and intermediate-risk prostate cancer are being treated with SBRT using image-guided IMRT with margins of 5 mm around the prostate except at the prostate–rectal interface, where a 3-mm margin is used. Intrafraction tracking with a ferromagnetic marker is used for all patients, and the beam is interrupted upon organ motion exceeding 2 mm from the start position. The initial dose arm included 20 patients treated to 32.5 Gy in five fractions and subsequently to 35 Gy in five fractions. Patients are being treated to 37.5 Gy in five fractions with a final dose arm of 45 Gy in five fractions. Toxicity outcome is the primary endpoint, with a secondary endpoint of tumor control based on posttreatment biopsies performed at 2 years.

POSTIRRADIATION PROSTATE-SPECIFIC ANTIGEN

A transient increase of PSA during radiation therapy, even as soon as the first fraction, has been reported in some patients.[364,365] Because there is no prognostic significance to the PSA response during a course of radiation therapy, obtaining PSA levels during treatment is not necessary or recommended. PSA fluctuations are common in the follow-up period and have been termed *PSA bounce*. In one report,[366] 35% of patients after combined permanent interstitial implantation and EBRT experienced a transient rise in their PSA value after treatment. The median time from treatment to this bounce effect was 18 months, and 92% of the fluctuating levels were observed during the first 26 months after radiation therapy. These investigators reported fluctuations ranging from 0.11 to 15.8 ng/mL. Similar results have been reported by Cavanagh et al.[367] for patients treated with implantation alone or when combined with EBRT. Hanlon et al.[368] observed a PSA bounce effect in approximately one-third of patients treated with EBRT alone. In that series, the 5-year biochemical control rate for patients who experienced a PSA fluctuation was inferior to that in those patients who did not have a PSA bounce in their follow-up period (69% vs. 52%; p = .02). On the other hand, investigators from the MD Anderson Hospital[369] noted that, of 964 patients treated with EBRT, only 12% experienced a PSA bounce, and the 5-year PSA outcome was superior for those patients who experienced this PSA fluctuation compared with those who did not (82% vs. 58%; p = .0001).

Ciezki et al.[370] defined PSA bounce as an increased PSA level of at least 0.2 ng/mL greater than the nadir PSA with a subsequent PSA value declining back to the nadir level or lower. One hundred sixty-two patients were treated with a permanent ^{125}I implantation and followed for a minimum of 5 years. With this as the definition of a PSA bounce, almost half of the patients (46%) experienced this phenomenon. The authors observed that the patients who experienced this fluctuation were more likely to be younger and less likely to develop a biochemical relapse. The authors also noted that PSA bounces generally occurred much sooner after treatment than did a true PSA relapse. The median time to the first rise in PSA from the nadir was 15 months, compared with 30 months for an ASTRO-defined biochemical relapse or 22 months for a nadir +2 defined relapse. Other reports define PSA bounce in various ways, and for this reason the literature needs to be interpreted with caution.[371]

Although a low absolute PSA level or nadir value after radiation therapy has prognostic significance for improved disease-free survival, it is difficult to assign a specific PSA cutpoint or nadir level as a definition of biochemical relapse. Currently, the nadir + 2 definition (a rise by ≥2 ng/mL above the nadir PSA) is considered the standard definition for biochemical failure after EBRT with or without hormonal therapy. A consensus panel[372] also recommended that the date of failure be determined "at call" (not backdated). Several studies examined the significance of posttreatment PSA doubling time (PSADT). Following prostatectomy, in a single-institution experience, Pound et al.[373] noted that, for patients treated with RP, PSADT of <10 months predicted the development of metastatic disease. Zelefsky et al.[374] reported on the impact of PSADT in a cohort of patients who developed biochemical relapse after EBRT. The PSADT for favorable-, intermediate-, and unfavorable-risk patients who developed a biochemical failure was 20.0, 13.2, and 8.2 months, respectively (p < .001). The 3-year incidence of DM for patients with PSADT of 0 to 3, 3 to 6, 6 to

12, and >12 months was 49%, 41%, 20%, and 7%, respectively ($p < .001$). Patients with PSADT of 0 to 3 and 3 to 6 months demonstrated a 7.0 and 6.6 increased hazard of developing distant metastases or death, respectively, compared with patients with a doubling time of >12 months. Freedland et al.[375] noted that PSADT of <9 months correlated with prostate cancer–specific mortality but did not evaluate postprostatectomy PSADT as a surrogate for cause-specific survival. Using larger, multi-institutional databases, Albertsen et al.[181] and D'Amico et al.[376] noted that short PSADT correlated with an adverse effect on survival in patients treated with either prostatectomy or radiation therapy for prostate cancer.

Emerging data strongly correlate a rising PSA level with positive postirradiation prostate biopsies. Crook et al.[377] reported on 226 patients treated with conventional EBRT who underwent serial biopsies after treatment. At 13 months after radiation therapy, the incidence of a positive biopsy was 51%, but it decreased to 30% for biopsies obtained at 30 months. Posttreatment biopsies require an experienced pathologist to interpret because of the significant radiation effect that takes place in the prostate, which can easily be mistaken at times for residual disease. Immunohistochemical staining for high–molecular-weight keratin can often distinguish radiation atypia in benign glands from residual tumor.

SELECTED REFERENCES

A full list of references for this chapter is available online.

3. Centers for Disease Control and Prevention. Cancer among men. Available at: http://www.cdc.gov. Accessed February 2, 2012.
12. Thompson IM, Goodman PJ, Tangen CM, et al. The influence of finasteride on the development of prostate cancer. *N Engl J Med* 2003;349:215–224.
13. Andriole GL, Bostwick DG, Brawley OW, et al. Effect of dutasteride on the risk of prostate cancer. *N Engl J Med* 2010;362:1192–1202.
26. Chan JM, Gann PH, Giovannucci EL. Role of diet in prostate cancer development and progression. *J Clin Oncol* 2005;23:8152–8160.
29. Klein EA, Thompson IM Jr, Tangen CM, et al. Vitamin E and the risk of prostate cancer: the Selenium and Vitamin E Cancer Prevention Trial (SELECT). *JAMA* 2011;306:1549–1556.
30. Gaziano JM, Glynn RJ, Christen WG, et al. Vitamins E and C in the prevention of prostate and total cancer in men: the Physicians' Health Study II randomized controlled trial. *JAMA* 2009;301:52–62.
46. Ewing CM, Ray AM, Lange EM, et al. Germline mutations in HOXB13 and prostate-cancer risk. *N Engl J Med* 2012;366:141–149.
55. Platz EA, Leitzmann MF, Visvanathan K, et al. Statin drugs and risk of advanced prostate cancer. *J Natl Cancer Inst* 2006;98:1819–1825.
56. Marcella SW, David A, Ohman-Strickland PA, et al. Statin use and fatal prostate cancer: A matched case-control study. *Cancer* 2012;118:4046–4052.
57. Gutt R, Tonlaar N, Kunnavakkam R, et al. Statin use and risk of prostate cancer recurrence in men treated with radiation therapy. *J Clin Oncol* 2010;28:2653–2659.
58. Hamilton RJ, Banez LL, Aronson WJ, et al. Statin medication use and the risk of biochemical recurrence after radical prostatectomy: results from the Shared Equal Access Regional Cancer Hospital (SEARCH) Database. *Cancer* 2010;116:3389–3398.
59. Dale KM, Coleman CI, Henyan NN, et al. Statins and cancer risk: a meta-analysis. *JAMA* 2006;295:74–80.
60. Browning DR, Martin RM. Statins and risk of cancer: a systematic review and metaanalysis. *Int J Cancer* 2007;120:833–843.
109. Cagiannos I, Karakiewicz P, Eastham JA, et al. A preoperative nomogram identifying decreased risk of positive pelvic lymph nodes in patients with prostate cancer. *J Urol* 2003;170:1798–1803.
117. Daneshmand S, Quek ML, Stein JP, et al. Prognosis of patients with lymph node positive prostate cancer following radical prostatectomy: long-term results. *J Urol* 2004;172:2252–2255.
122. Schroder FH, Hugosson J, Roobol MJ, et al. Screening and prostate-cancer mortality in a randomized European study. *N Engl J Med* 2009;360:1320–1328.
123. Andriole GL, Crawford ED, Grubb RL 3rd, et al. Mortality results from a randomized prostate-cancer screening trial. *N Engl J Med* 2009;360:1310–1319.
124. Lin K, Croswell JM, Koenig H, et al. Prostate-specific antigen-based screening for prostate cancer: An evidence update for the U.S. Preventive Services Task Force. Rockville, MD: Agency for Healthcare Research and Quality (US), 2011. Available at: http://www.ncbi.nlm.nih.gov/books/NBK82303/.
125. Greene KL, Albertsen PC, Babaian RJ, et al. Prostate specific antigen best practice statement: 2009 update. *J Urol* 2009;182:2232–2241.
153. D'Amico AV, Renshaw AA, Sussman B, et al. Pretreatment PSA velocity and risk of death from prostate cancer following external beam radiation therapy. *JAMA* 2005;294:440–447.
154. D'Amico AV, Chen MH, Roehl KA, et al. Preoperative PSA velocity and the risk of death from prostate cancer after radical prostatectomy. *N Engl J Med* 2004;351:125–135.
172. Israel G, Francis I, Roach M, et al. Pretreatment staging prostate cancer. American College of Radiology Appropriateness Criteria, ACR Web Site Edition, 2009. Available at: http://www.acr.org/ac. Accessed February 2, 2012.
243. Zelefsky MJ, Eastham JA, Cronin AM, et al. Metastasis after radical prostatectomy or external beam radiotherapy for patients with clinically localized prostate cancer: a comparison of clinical cohorts adjusted for case mix. *J Clin Oncol* 2010;28:1508–1513.
244. Zelefsky MJ, Yamada Y, Pei X, et al. Comparison of tumor control and toxicity outcomes of high-dose intensity-modulated radiotherapy and brachytherapy for patients with favorable risk prostate cancer. *Urology* 2011;77:986–990.
245. Cooperberg MR, Vickers AJ, Broering JM, et al. Comparative risk-adjusted mortality outcomes after primary surgery, radiotherapy, or androgen-deprivation therapy for localized prostate cancer. *Cancer* 2010;116:5226–5234.
248. Zelefsky M, Lee W, Zietman A, et al. Evaluation of adherence to quality measures for prostate cancer radiotherapy in the United States from the Quality Research in Radiation Oncology (QRRO) survey. *Prac Radiat Oncol* 2012(14 Mar);10.1016/j.prro.2012.01.006 [Epub ahead of print].
249. Bill-Axelson A, Holmberg L, Ruutu M, et al. Radical prostatectomy versus watchful waiting in early prostate cancer. *N Engl J Med* 2011;364:1708–1717.
260. Milosevic M, Voruganti S, Blend R, et al. Magnetic resonance imaging (MRI) for localization of the prostatic apex: comparison to computed tomography (CT) and urethrography. *Radiother Oncol* 1998;47:277–284.
266. McLaughlin PW, Evans C, Feng M, et al. Radiographic and anatomic basis for prostate contouring errors and methods to improve prostate contouring accuracy. *Int J Radiat Oncol Biol Phys* 2010;76:369–378.
273. Skwarchuk MW, Jackson A, Zelefsky MJ, et al. Late rectal toxicity after conformal radiotherapy of prostate cancer (I): multivariate analysis and dose-response. *Int J Radiat Oncol Biol Phys* 2000;47:103–113.
274. Jackson A, Skwarchuk MW, Zelefsky MJ, et al. Late rectal bleeding after conformal radiotherapy of prostate cancer. II. Volume effects and dose-volume histograms. *Int J Radiat Oncol Biol Phys* 2001;49:685–698.
275. Kupelian PA, Thakkar VV, Khuntia D, et al. Hypofractionated intensity-modulated radiotherapy (70 gy at 2.5 Gy per fraction) for localized prostate cancer: long-term outcomes. *Int J Radiat Oncol Biol Phys* 2005;63:1463–1468.
276. Pollack A, Hanlon AL, Horwitz EM, et al. Dosimetry and preliminary acute toxicity in the first 100 men treated for prostate cancer on a randomized hypofractionation dose escalation trial. *Int J Radiat Oncol Biol Phys* 2006;64:518–526.
286. Merrick GS, Butler WM, Wallner KE, et al. Variability of prostate brachytherapy pre-implant dosimetry: a multi-institutional analysis. *Brachytherapy* 2005;4:241–251.
292. Herstein A, Wallner K, Merrick G, et al. I-125 versus Pd-103 for low-risk prostate cancer: long-term morbidity outcomes from a prospective randomized multicenter controlled trial. *Cancer J* 2005;11:385–389.
293. Kollmeier MA, Pei X, Algur E, et al. A comparison of the impact of isotope ((125) I vs. (103)Pd) on toxicity and biochemical outcome after interstitial brachytherapy and external beam radiation therapy for clinically localized prostate cancer. *Brachytherapy* 2012;11:271–276.
294. Nag S, Bice W, DeWyngaert K, et al. The American Brachytherapy Society recommendations for permanent prostate brachytherapy postimplant dosimetric analysis. *Int J Radiat Oncol Biol Phys* 2000;46:221–230.
297. Stone NN, Stock RG, Unger P. Intermediate term biochemical-free progression and local control following 125iodine brachytherapy for prostate cancer. *J Urol* 2005;173:803–807.
298. Zelefsky M, Kuban D, Levy L, et al. Long-term multi-institutional analysis of stage T1-T2 prostate cancer treated with permanent brachytherapy (Abstract 56). *Int J Radiat Oncol Biol Phys* 2007;67:327–333.
300. Merrick GS, Butler WM, Wallner KE, et al. The impact of radiation dose to the urethra on brachytherapy-related dysuria. *Brachytherapy* 2005;4:45–50.
302. Zelefsky MJ, Yamada Y, Marion C, et al. Improved conformality and decreased toxicity with intraoperative computer-optimized transperineal ultrasound-guided prostate brachytherapy. *Int J Radiat Oncol Biol Phys* 2003;55:956–963.
303. Stock RG, Stone NN, Dahlal M, et al. What is the optimal dose for 125I prostate implants? A dose-response analysis of biochemical control, posttreatment prostate biopsies, and long-term urinary symptoms. *Brachytherapy* 2002;1:83–89.
304. Zelefsky MJ, Chou JF, Pei X, et al. Predicting biochemical tumor control after brachytherapy for clinically localized prostate cancer: the Memorial Sloan-Kettering Cancer Center experience. *Brachytherapy* 2012;11:245–249.
305. Bianco FJ Jr, Scardino PT, Eastham JA. Radical prostatectomy: long-term cancer control and recovery of sexual and urinary function ("trifecta"). *Urology* 2005;66:83–94.
306. Roehl KA, Han M, Ramos CG, et al. Cancer progression and survival rates following anatomical radical retropubic prostatectomy in 3,478 consecutive patients: long-term results. *J Urol* 2004;172:910–914.
307. Isbarn H, Wanner M, Salomon G, et al. Long-term data on the survival of patients with prostate cancer treated with radical prostatectomy in the prostate-specific antigen era. *BJU Int* 2010;106:37–43.
308. Han M, Partin AW, Zahurak M, et al. Biochemical (prostate specific antigen) recurrence probability following radical prostatectomy for clinically localized prostate cancer. *J Urol* 2003;169:517–523.
310. Kuban DA, Thames HD, Levy LB, et al. Long-term multi-institutional analysis of stage T1-T2 prostate cancer treated with radiotherapy in the PSA era. *Int J Radiat Oncol Biol Phys* 2003;57:915–928.
311. Kuban DA, Tucker SL, Dong L, et al. Long-term results of the M. D. Anderson randomized dose-escalation trial for prostate cancer. *Int J Radiat Oncol Biol Phys* 2008;70:67–74.
312. Zietman AL, DeSilvio ML, Slater JD, et al. Comparison of conventional-dose vs high-dose conformal radiation therapy in clinically localized adenocarcinoma of the prostate: a randomized controlled trial. *JAMA* 2005;294:1233–1239.
313. Zelefsky MJ, Pei X, Chou JF, et al. Dose escalation for prostate cancer radiotherapy: predictors of long-term biochemical tumor control and distant metastases-free survival outcomes. *Eur Urol* 2011;60:1133–1139.
314. Pollack A, Hanlon AL, Horwitz EM, et al. Prostate cancer radiotherapy dose response: an update of the Fox Chase experience. *J Urol* 2004;171:1132–1136.
315. Symon Z, Griffith KA, McLaughlin PW, et al. Dose escalation for localized prostate cancer: substantial benefit observed with 3D conformal therapy. *Int J Radiat Oncol Biol Phys* 2003;57:384–390.
316. Kupelian PA, Potters L, Khuntia D, et al. Radical prostatectomy, external beam radiotherapy <72 Gy, external beam radiotherapy > or = 72 Gy, permanent seed implantation, or combined seeds/external beam radiotherapy for stage T1-T2 prostate cancer. *Int J Radiat Oncol Biol Phys* 2004;58:25–33.
317. Michalski J, Winter K, Roach M, et al. Clinical outcome of patients treated with 3D conformal radiation therapy 3D-CRT for prostate cancer on RTOG 9406. *Int J Radiat Oncol Biol Phys* 2012;83:e363–e370.

318. Sylvester JE, Grimm PD, Wong J, et al. Fifteen-year biochemical relapse-free survival, cause-specific survival, and overall survival following I(125) prostate brachytherapy in clinically localized prostate cancer: Seattle experience. *Int J Radiat Oncol Biol Phys* 2011;81:376–381.
319. Taira AV, Merrick GS, Butler WM, et al. Long-term outcome for clinically localized prostate cancer treated with permanent interstitial brachytherapy. *Int J Radiat Oncol Biol Phys* 2011;79:1336–1342.
320. Stone NN, Stone MM, Rosenstein BS, et al. Influence of pretreatment and treatment factors on intermediate to long term outcome after prostate brachytherapy. *J Urol* 2011;185:495–500.
321. Begg CB, Riedel ER, Bach PB, et al. Variations in morbidity after radical prostatectomy. *N Engl J Med* 2002;346:1138–1144.
322. Catalona WJ, Carvalhal GF, Mager DE, et al. Potency, continence and complication rates in 1,870 consecutive radical retropubic prostatectomies. *J Urol* 1999; 162:433–438.
323. Trinh Q-D, Sammona J, Sun M, et al. Perioperative outcomes of robot-assisted radical prostatectomy compared with open radical prostatectomy: results from the Nationwide Inpatient Sample. *Eur Urol* 2012;61:679–685.
324. Geinitz H, Thamm R, Keller M, et al. Longitudinal study of intestinal symptoms and fecal continence in patients with conformal radiotherapy for prostate cancer. *Int J Radiat Oncol Biol Phys* 2011;79:1373–1380.
326. Vavassori V, Fiorino C, Rancati T, et al. Predictors for rectal and intestinal acute toxicities during prostate cancer high-dose 3D-CRT: results of a prospective multicenter study. *Int J Radiat Oncol Biol Phys* 2007;67:1401–1410.
327. Huang EH, Pollack A, Levy L, et al. Late rectal toxicity: dose-volume effects of conformal radiotherapy for prostate cancer. *Int J Radiat Oncol Biol Phys* 2002; 54:1314–1321.
329. Heemsbergen WD, Peeters ST, Koper PC, et al. Acute and late gastrointestinal toxicity after radiotherapy in prostate cancer patients: consequential late damage. *Int J Radiat Oncol Biol Phys* 2006;66:3–10.
330. Zelefsky MJ, Chan H, Hunt M, et al. Long-term outcome of high dose intensity modulated radiation therapy for patients with clinically localized prostate cancer. *J Urol* 2006;176:1415–1419.
331. Michalski JM, Winter K, Purdy JA, et al. Toxicity after three-dimensional radiotherapy for prostate cancer on RTOG 9406 dose level V. *Int J Radiat Oncol Biol Phys* 2005;62:706–713.
333. Zelefsky MJ, Levin EJ, Hunt M, et al. Incidence of late rectal and urinary toxicities after three-dimensional conformal radiotherapy and intensity-modulated radiotherapy for localized prostate cancer. *Int J Radiat Oncol Biol Phys* 2008;70:1124–1129.
334. Alicikus ZA, Yamada Y, Zhang Z, et al. Ten-year outcomes of high-dose, intensity-modulated radiotherapy for localized prostate cancer. *Cancer* 2011;117: 1429–1437.
335. Peeters ST, Heemsbergen WD, van Putten WL, et al. Acute and late complications after radiotherapy for prostate cancer: results of a multicenter randomized trial comparing 68 Gy to 78 Gy. *Int J Radiat Oncol Biol Phys* 2005;61:1019–1034.
338. Incrocci L, Slob AK, Levendag PC. Sexual (dys)function after radiotherapy for prostate cancer: a review. *Int J Radiat Oncol Biol Phys* 2002;52:681–693.
339. Mantz CA, Nautiyal J, Awan A, et al. Potency preservation following conformal radiotherapy for localized prostate cancer: impact of neoadjuvant androgen blockade, treatment technique, and patient-related factors. *Cancer J Sci Am* 1999; 5:230–236.
340. van der Wielen GJ, van Putten WL, Incrocci L. Sexual function after three-dimensional conformal radiotherapy for prostate cancer: results from a dose-escalation trial. *Int J Radiat Oncol Biol Phys* 2007;68:479–484.
341. Pinkawa M, Gagel B, Piroth MD, et al. Erectile dysfunction after external beam radiotherapy for prostate cancer. *Eur Urol* 2009;55:227–234.
342. Zelefsky MJ, Eid JF. Elucidating the etiology of erectile dysfunction after definitive therapy for prostatic cancer. *Int J Radiat Oncol Biol Phys* 1998;40:129–133.
344. Roeloffzen EM, Battermann JJ, van Deursen MJ, et al. Influence of dose on risk of acute urinary retention after iodine-125 prostate brachytherapy. *Int J Radiat Oncol Biol Phys* 2011;80:1072–1079.
346. Keyes M, Schellenberg D, Moravan V, et al. Decline in urinary retention incidence in 805 patients after prostate brachytherapy: the effect of learning curve? *Int J Radiat Oncol Biol Phys* 2006;64:825–834.
347. Neill M, Studer G, Le L, et al. The nature and extent of urinary morbidity in relation to prostate brachytherapy urethral dosimetry. *Brachytherapy* 2007;6:173–179.
348. Keyes M, Miller S, Moravan V, et al. Predictive factors for acute and late urinary toxicity after permanent prostate brachytherapy: long-term outcome in 712 consecutive patients. *Int J Radiat Oncol Biol Phys* 2009;73:1023–1032.
349. Phan J, Swanson DA, Levy LB, et al. Late rectal complications after prostate brachytherapy for localized prostate cancer: incidence and management. *Cancer* 2009;115:1827–1839.
350. Davis BJ, Horwitz EM, Lee WR, et al. American Brachytherapy Society consensus guidelines for transrectal ultrasound-guided permanent prostate brachytherapy. *Brachytherapy* 2012;11:6–19.
351. Stone NN, Stock RG. Long-term urinary, sexual, and rectal morbidity in patients treated with iodine–125 prostate brachytherapy followed up for a minimum of 5 years. *Urology* 2007;69:338–342.
354. Taira AV, Merrick GS, Galbreath RW, et al. Erectile function durability following permanent prostate brachytherapy. *Int J Radiat Oncol Biol Phys* 2009;75: 639–648.
356. Raina R, Agarwal A, Goyal KK, et al. Long-term potency after iodine–125 radiotherapy for prostate cancer and role of sildenafil citrate. *Urology* 2003;62:1103–1108.
357. Slater JD, Rossi CJ Jr, Yonemoto LT, et al. Proton therapy for prostate cancer: the initial Loma Linda University experience. *Int J Radiat Oncol Biol Phys* 2004; 59:348–352.
358. Efstathiou JA, Trofimov AV, Zietman AL. Life, liberty, and the pursuit of protons: an evidence-based review of the role of particle therapy in the treatment of prostate cancer. *Cancer J* 2009;15:312–318.
359. Unkelbach J, Chan TC, Bortfeld T. Accounting for range uncertainties in the optimization of intensity modulated proton therapy. *Phys Med Biol* 2007;52: 2755–2773.
360. Freeman DE, King CR. Stereotactic body radiotherapy for low-risk prostate cancer: five-year outcomes. *Radiat Oncol* 2011;6:3.
362. Boike TP, Lotan Y, Cho LC, et al. Phase I dose-escalation study of stereotactic body radiation therapy for low- and intermediate-risk prostate cancer. *J Clin Oncol* 2011;29:2020–2026.
363. King CR, Brooks JD, Gill H, et al. Stereotactic body radiotherapy for localized prostate cancer: interim results of a prospective phase II clinical trial. *Int J Radiat Oncol Biol Phys* 2009;73:1043–1048.
369. Rosser CJ, Kuban DA, Levy LB, et al. Prostate specific antigen bounce phenomenon after external beam radiation for clinically localized prostate cancer. *J Urol* 2002;168:2001–2005.
370. Ciezki JP, Reddy CA, Garcia J, et al. PSA kinetics after prostate brachytherapy: PSA bounce phenomenon and its implications for PSA doubling time. *Int J Radiat Oncol Biol Phys* 2006;64:512–517.
371. Zelefsky MJ. PSA bounce versus biochemical failure following prostate brachytherapy. *Nat Clin Pract Urol* 2006;3:578–579.
372. Roach M 3rd, Hanks G, Thames H Jr, et al. Defining biochemical failure following radiotherapy with or without hormonal therapy in men with clinically localized prostate cancer: recommendations of the RTOG-ASTRO Phoenix Consensus Conference. *Int J Radiat Oncol Biol Phys* 2006;65:965–974.
373. Pound CR, Partin AW, Eisenberger MA, et al. Natural history of progression after PSA elevation following radical prostatectomy. *JAMA* 1999;281:1591–1597.
374. Zelefsky MJ, Ben-Porat L, Scher HI, et al. Outcome predictors for the increasing PSA state after definitive external-beam radiotherapy for prostate cancer. *J Clin Oncol* 2005;23:826–831.
375. Freedland SJ, Humphreys EB, Mangold LA, et al. Risk of prostate cancer-specific mortality following biochemical recurrence after radical prostatectomy. *JAMA* 2005;294:433–439.
376. D'Amico AV, Cote K, Loffredo M, et al. Determinants of prostate cancer-specific survival after radiation therapy for patients with clinically localized prostate cancer. *J Clin Oncol* 2002;20:4567–4573.
377. Crook JM, Perry GA, Robertson S, et al. Routine prostate biopsies following radiotherapy for prostate cancer: results for 226 patients. *Urology* 1995;45:624–631.

Chapter 66
Intermediate- and High-Risk Prostate Cancer

Hans T. Chung and Mack Roach, III

In 2010, an estimated 218,000 new cases of prostate cancer were diagnosed in the United States, representing approximately 30% of all nondermatologic cancers.[1] Prostate cancer was the second leading cause of cancer death in men, responsible for more than 30,000 deaths.[1] Most of the patients destined to die from prostate cancer initially presented with unfavorable intermediate- or high-risk disease. This chapter focuses on the management of such patients. Since the previous edition of this book, our understanding of prostate cancer has expanded substantially. With several prospective studies now demonstrating a survival advantage, hormonal therapy has become widely accepted as an integral part of treatment. Interest in adjuvant and salvage radiotherapy has been brought to the forefront with recently released prospective studies. With more mature datasets, our ability to prognosticate extends beyond merely biochemical control, but now includes distant metastases, prostate cancer-specific survival, and overall survival. High–dose-rate brachytherapy is being increasingly adopted by centers as a means to further dose escalate. Details on the management of low-risk prostate cancer and the background of prostate cancer in general can be found in Chapter 65.

EPIDEMIOLOGY

With increasing prostate-specific antigen (PSA) screening since the early 1990s, the clinical presentation of prostate cancer has changed dramatically, shifting from locally advanced or metastatic disease to clinically nonpalpable disease. Data from two national prostate cancer registries, the Cancer of the Prostate Strategic Urologic Research Endeavor (CaPSURE) and the Department of Defense Center for Prostate Disease Research (CPDR), highlight this stage migration.[2–4] According to CaPSURE, the diagnosis of high-risk disease has seen a precipitous drop from 27.4% in 1990 to 1994 to 13.7% in 2004 to 2007.[3] Similarly, the proportion of patients presenting with a pretreatment PSA >20 ng/mL has dropped from 27.0% to 8.1% in the same time periods. Conversely, clinically nonpalpable disease (stage T1) has surged from 16.9% to 49.4%, respectively. Data from CPDR mirror these findings. From 1988 to 1998, clinical stage T3 to T4 disease contracted from 19.2% to 4.4%, whereas T1c disease went from 0% to 47.8%.[4]

CLINICAL PRESENTATION

Patients with intermediate- or high-risk prostate cancer may present with locoregional symptoms, but this is not common. Lower urinary tract symptoms that may be seen include nocturia, urinary frequency, urgency, decreased flow, incomplete voiding, intermittent flow, or hesitancy. More bulky primary disease may present with difficulty in passing stool or even bloody stool. With increasing PSA and Gleason score, the risk of metastases increases. Metastatic spread is generally sequential, proceeding from the prostate to the pelvic lymph nodes then bone. Thus patients with metastatic disease may present with renal failure, lymphedema of the lower extremities, and bone pain.

PROGNOSTIC FACTORS AND RISK CLASSIFICATION SCHEMES

The traditional prognostic factors have been clinical T stage, presenting PSA, and Gleason score. To simplify treatment recommendations and prognostication, several risk classification schemes have been proposed by grouping patients with different clinical features, but similar biochemical outcomes.[5,6] The risk classification scheme proposed by D'Amico et al.[5] appears to be the most widely used, stratifies patients with clinically localized prostate cancer to three risk groups, and has since been adopted by the National Comprehensive Cancer Network (NCCN) guidelines.[7] Low risk is defined as meeting all the criteria: T1c to T2a, PSA <10 ng/mL, and Gleason score ≤6. Intermediate risk is defined as T2b or T2c, PSA 10 to 20 ng/mL, or Gleason score 7. High risk is any of the following: T3a, PSA >20 ng/mL, or Gleason score 8 to 10. Locally advanced is defined as T3b or T4 disease. It has recently been validated using a study cohort of 7,316 men from two large cancer registries (CaPSURE and CPDR) and has also been found to predict for prostate cancer–specific mortality (PCSM) after radiotherapy.[8] Of note, in the seventh edition of the American Joint Committee on Cancer (AJCC) prostate cancer staging, Gleason score and pretreatment PSA are now incorporated into the staging classification.[9]

Other pretreatment predictive factors have since been identified, including percentage of positive biopsy cores (PPC) in radiotherapy and surgery-treated patients.[10–11,12] D'Amico et al.[10] reported on the independent prognostic capabilities of PPC, calculated as the number of PPCs containing cancer divided by the total number of cores, of PSA control. Interestingly, 76% of patients with intermediate-risk disease could be reclassified into either low- or high-risk disease. Specifically, those patients with <34% PPC had similar outcomes as low-risk patients (5-year PSA control 85% vs. 91%, respectively), whereas patients with more than 50% PPC had similar outcomes as high-risk patients (5-year PSA control 30% vs. 43%, respectively). The prognostic significance of PPC has also been reported to extend to PCSM in intermediate-risk patients.[13] When stratified by ≤50% and >50% PPC, 7-year prostate cancer-specific survival was 100% versus 57% (P = .004), respectively. In patients treated with radical prostatectomy, high PPC is associated with adverse pathologic features like extracapsular extension, seminal vesicle invasion, positive surgical margins, lymphovascular invasion, perineural invasion, and pelvic lymph node involvement.[14–16]

A recent meta-analysis of four Radiation Therapy Oncology Group (RTOG) trials demonstrated that older age (>70) patients were associated with a reduced risk of PCSM and metastases, even after adjusting for the expected increased risk of non–prostate cancer–specific mortality in this subgroup.[17]

In summary, PPC (>50%) have further refined our prognostic precision in addition to the traditional predictive factors (pretreatment PSA, Gleason score, clinical T stage). At the University of California–San Francisco (UCSF), the presence of either in intermediate-risk patients, as defined by the NCCN classification, is considered as unfavorable intermediate- or high-risk disease. Single modality local therapy is likely not enough, but rather more aggressive treatment, such as hormonal therapy and pelvic irradiation, is indicated.

GENERAL MANAGEMENT

Radiation Therapy Techniques

For details on prostate only radiotherapy, please refer to Chapter 65. This section will focus on the implementation and toxicities of whole pelvic radiotherapy.

Whole-Pelvic Irradiation

Since the previous edition, intensity-modulated radiation therapy (IMRT) has been increasingly adopted by many centers in pelvic nodal irradiation. For historical purposes, with conventional technique, pelvic irradiation is usually treated with a four-field box. The target volume usually includes the prostate, seminal vesicles, obturator, and proximal internal and external iliac nodal regions. Occasionally common iliac, para-aortic, and even perirectal nodes are included in the initial target. The traditional field borders of the anteroposterior portals are as follows: superior at the L5-S1 interspace, inferior at 2 cm distal to the membranous urethra (defined by the apex of the urethrogram peak), and 1.5 to 2 cm lateral of the pelvic brim. Corner blocks are usually placed at all four corners to limit dose to the small bowel and femoral heads. In the lateral portals, the superior and inferior borders are placed at the same point as the anteroposterior portals; the anterior border is placed at the anterior most aspect of the pubic symphysis, and the posterior border is placed at the S2–3 interspace. With CT planning, the prostate, seminal vesicles, rectum, small bowel, bladder, pelvic vessels, and penile bulb may be contoured to facilitate shielding of the rectum and small bowel.

The dosimetric advantages of IMRT have led to its investigation in delivering pelvic radiotherapy. Compared to conventional technique, IMRT allows unprecedented sparing of nearby critical structures like the rectum, small bowel, bladder, and femoral heads. In a study from UCSF, Wang-Chesebro et al.[18] compared the nodal target coverage by conventional field borders with IMRT (Fig. 66.1). The nodes that were contoured included the obturator, internal or external iliac, common iliac, and presacral regions. In the conventional four-field plan, only 70.3% of the nodal target volume received the prescription dose of 45 Gy, whereas 96.2% was covered in the IMRT plan (P = .002). Even worse, conventional field placement led to 20.2% of the nodal target volume to receive <80% of the

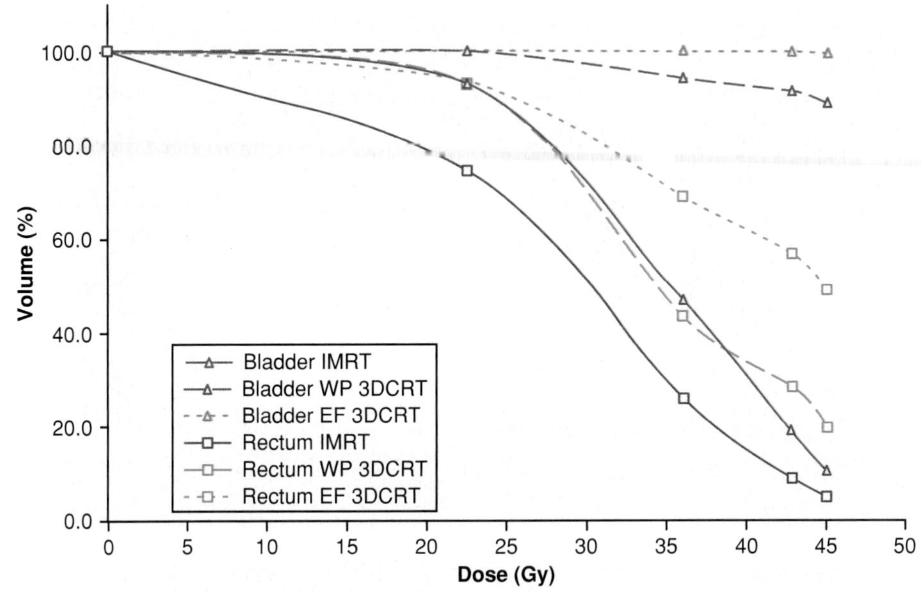

FIGURE 66.1. Comparison of dose–volume histograms for rectum and bladder for whole-pelvic only phase using intensity-modulated radiotherapy (IMRT), whole-pelvis (WP) three-dimensional conformal radiotherapy (3DCRT), and extended-field (EF) 3DCRT plans. For both bladder and rectum, IMRT significantly reduced V45, V42.75, V36, and V22.5 (P <.01 for all comparisons) compared to both WP and EF 3DCRT plans. (From Wang-Chesebro A, Xia P, Coleman J, et al. Intensity-modulated radiotherapy improves lymph node coverage and dose to critical structures compared with three-dimensional conformal radiation therapy in clinically localized prostate cancer. *Int J Radiat Oncol Biol Phys* 2006;66: 654–662, with permission from Elsevier.)

prescription dose. The rectal and bladder volume receiving 95% of the prescribed dose was significantly reduced with IMRT, with an absolute reduction of 23% and 80%, respectively.

Whereas conventional technique involved simply placing field borders based on bony anatomy, IMRT requires the delineation of a nodal target volume based on vasculature. Investigators have used lymphotropic nanoparticle-enhanced magnetic resonance imaging (MRI) and ultrasmall superparamagnetic iron oxide lymph node contrast agent, ferumoxtran-10, to develop nodal clinical target volume (CTV) models.[19,20] These MRI studies have formed the foundation for the RTOG Genitourinary Radiation Oncology Consensus on pelvic nodal CTV delineation, as shown in Figure 66.2.[21] However, the RTOG guidelines did not use sentinel lymph node imaging, which in a study by Chen et al.[22] demonstrated that the RTOG pelvic nodal CTV included all identified sentinel lymph nodes in only 30% of patients.

In the same consensus, Lawton et al.[21] recommended dose constraints to the rectum (V50 Gy ≤50%, V70 Gy ≤20%), bladder (V55 Gy ≤50%, V70 Gy ≤30%), femoral heads (V50 Gy <5%), small bowel (maximum dose <52 Gy). Based on an extensive literature search, Chan et al.[23] proposed guidelines on rectal dose constraints for patients receiving pelvic radiotherapy.

Prostate Motion

With the shift to dose escalation and IMRT and its attendant high conformality around target structures, minimization of setup errors becomes critical. The previous technique of verification of the isocenter relied on obtaining weekly port films, which only allowed comparison of bony anatomy without any consideration of the prostate and did not account for prostate motion. Questions that have since emerged are:

1. How much does the prostate move on a daily basis (i.e., interfractional) and during each treatment (i.e., intrafractional)?
2. Is the positional relationship between the prostate and bony anatomy static (i.e., can bony anatomy be used as a surrogate of the prostate location)?

The use of fiducial gold seed markers and daily electronic portal imaging (EPI) with online correction is one such strategy. In a comprehensive study from the Mayo Clinic, the inter- and intrafractional motion of the prostate and pelvic bony anatomy in 20 prostate patients, each with three or four intraprostatic gold fiducial markers, and daily pretherapy and through-treatment EPI were reported.[24] With more than 22,000 data points, Schallenkamp et al.[24] determined that the prostate moved as much as 9.1 mm (mean 2.5 mm) in the superior-inferior (SI), 16.3 mm (mean 3.7 mm) in the anterior-posterior (AP), and 15.2 mm (mean 1.9 mm) in the right-left (RL) axes, prior to any efforts to localize the fields to the fiducial markers. In recommending a margin for setup and organ motion (i.e., CTV to planning target volumes [PTV] margin), without fiducial marker localization, SI, AP, and RL margins of 5.1, 7.3, 5.0 mm, respectively, were required to cover 95% of the CTV with the prescribed dose with a 95% probability. With a daily fiducial marker localization protocol, the margins can be reduced to 2.7, 2.9, and 2.8 mm, respectively. The interfractional three-dimensional (3D) displacements of the prostate and bony anatomy were 5.6 and 4.4 mm prior to localization and 2.8 and 4.4 mm after postlocalization adjustments, respectively, suggesting that bony anatomy does not accurately reflect the position of the prostate. The average intrafractional displacements of the prostate and bony anatomy were 0.1 and –0.5, 0.4 and 0.4, and 0.1 and 0.3 mm in the AP, SI, and RL axes, respectively. Marker migration was found to be minimal, with 79% within 1 mm and 96% within 1.5 mm. The latter results have been corroborated by Kupelian et al.,[25] who demonstrated that the average absolute variation in intermarker distance was 1.01 ± 1.03 mm. Only 1% of the markers exhibited frequent movement, and it was found to be due to prostate deformation secondary to rectal filling.

Recently integrated into all contemporary linear accelerators, cone-beam computed tomography (CBCT) for online correction is gaining popularity as it allows for soft tissue matching, and does not require an invasive procedure to implant fiducial markers. Moseley et al.[26] compared kilovoltage CBCT with fiducial markers and EPI and found no significant difference as a means for image guidance.

With the development of electromagnetic transponders (Calypso Medical Technologies, Seattle WA) that can be implanted into the prostate, real-time tracking at a rate of 10 times per second is now possible. Langen et al.[27] described broadly two different types of intrafraction motions. One is by a slow, small drift, usually posteriorly and inferiorly, that is thought to be associated with pelvic muscle relaxation or the gradual movement of rectal contents away from the prostate.

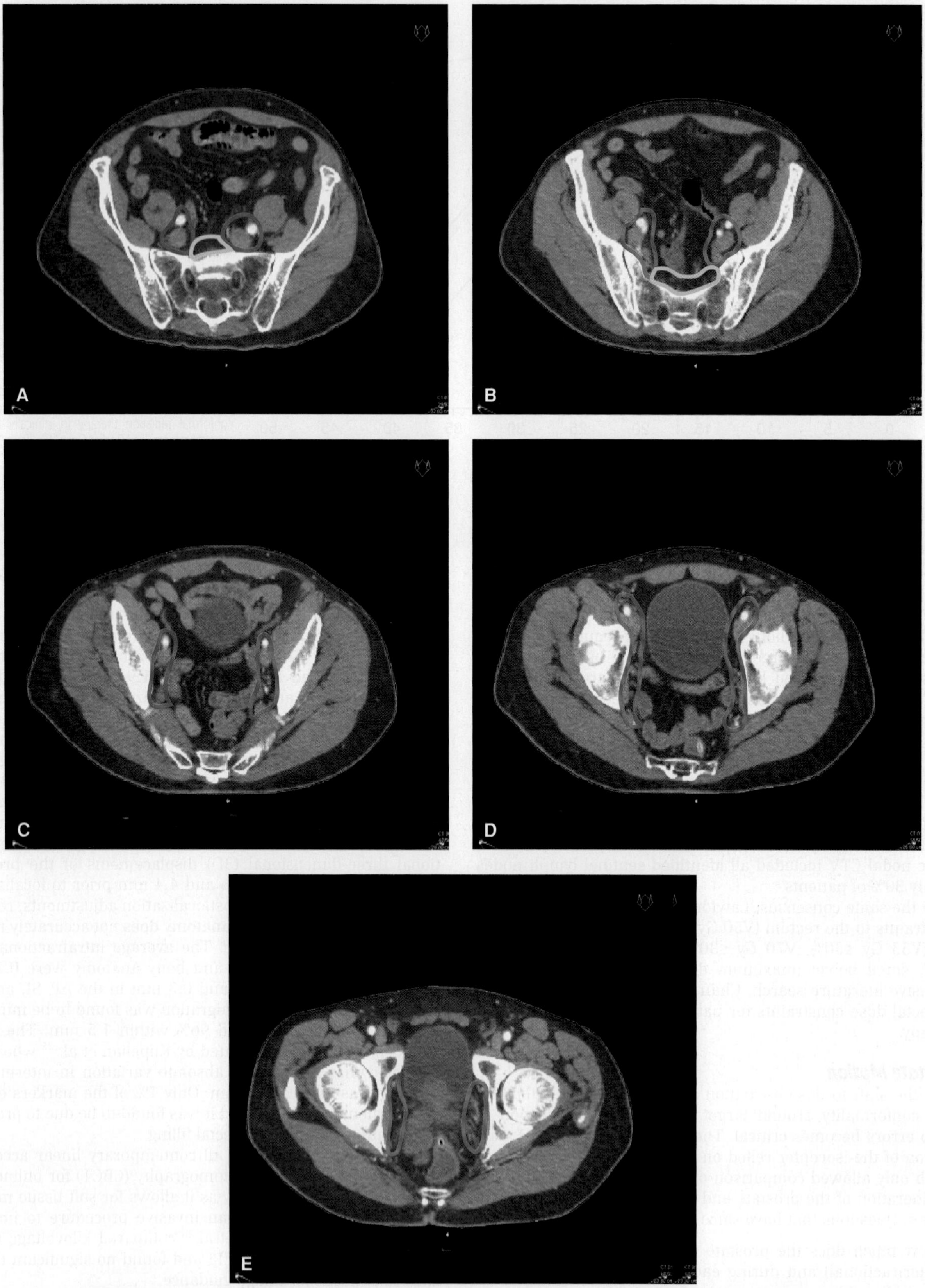

FIGURE 66.2. Representative pelvic lymph node clinical target volume contours of: **(A)** common iliac and presacral at L5-S1; **(B)** external, internal, and presacral at S1-S3; **(C)** external and internal iliac below S3; **(D)** end of external iliac at top of femoral heads (bony landmark for the inguinal ligament); **(E)** obturator at the top of the pubic symphysis. (Adapted from Lawton CA, Michalski J, El-Naga I, et al. RTOG GU radiation oncology specialists reach consensus on pelvic lymph node volumes for high-risk prostate cancer. *Int J Radiat Oncol Biol Phys* 2009;74:383–387, with permission from Elsevier.)

Second is a sudden and transient motion, usually anteriorly and superiorly, that can be significant in extent and is thought to be due to peristalsis. In the cohort of 17 patients (550 fractions), the average proportion of the total treatment time that the prostate was displaced by >3 mm and >5 mm was 13.6% and 3.3%, respectively. However, when analyzed by patient-to-patient basis, the prostate was displaced by 36.2% and 10.9%, respectively.

If the nodal target volumes are assumed to correlate with bony anatomy, pelvic IMRT that is set up to the prostate gland by intraprostatic fiducial markers could lead to significant underdosing given the lack of correlation between the prostate and bony anatomy. In a preliminary analysis of patients treated at UCSF, Chen et al.[28] demonstrated that an isocenter shift of 5 or 10 mm in the superior direction could reduce nodal target coverage by 11% and 26%, respectively, with whole pelvic IMRT. Xia et al.[29] compared multiple adaptive plans, isoshifting, and multileaf collimator (MLC) shifting and concluded that MLC shifting was the most effective in addressing the independent movement of the prostate and pelvic nodes during radiotherapy. Rossi et al.[30] performed a retrospective dosimetric review of 10 high-risk patients, who had daily onboard imaging and correction of gold intraprostatic fiducial markers, and reported that overall, there was little difference (2% to 5%) between the planned dose and the delivered dose to the pelvic nodes by IMRT. However, two patients had a significant underdosing of 9% and 29% to the pelvic nodes that was thought to be due to a difference between the planning CT simulation scan and the daily treatments rather than random prostate motion. In a study by Chung et al.,[31] patients treated with image-guided IMRT to the pelvic nodes had significantly lower dose to the rectum and bladder and fewer toxicities than those who received IMRT only.

BIOLOGIC RATIONALE FOR PROPHYLACTIC PELVIC IRRADIATION

Incidence of Occult Lymph Node Involvement

The ability of current imaging techniques to detect involved nodes is hampered by their sole reliance on size criteria. As we will see, the incidence of clinically occult disease is unexpectedly high. This observation comes from several fronts, including more sophisticated assays, different imaging agents that have increased affinity to lymph nodes, and more extensive node dissection.

From the Baylor College of Medicine, Shariat et al.[32] studied reverse-transcriptase polymerase chain reaction (RT-PCR) assay for human glandular kallikrein 2 (hK2) mRNA expression in *histopathologically* normal pelvic nodes in patients with pT3N0 prostate cancer. Of the 199 evaluable men, 20% and 40% had positive and equivocal results, respectively. In multivariate analysis, a positive RT-PCR/hK2 result was associated with PSA progression, development of distant metastases, and PCSM.

Surgical Results of Extended Pelvic Lymph Node Dissection

One of the current controversies erupting in the surgical literature is the role of an extended pelvic lymph node dissection. The traditional and most common approach is to do a limited dissection. Both procedures excise the fibrofatty and lymphatic tissues between the bifurcation of the common iliac artery superiorly to the femoral canal inferiorly and to the pelvic sidewall laterally. The critical difference between the two procedures is that in the limited dissection, the posterior extent is carried to the obturator nerve, whereas in the extended dissection, it is extended to include the obturator vessels and internal iliac vein. A second important consideration, when reviewing surgical studies, is whether only hematoxylin and eosin (H&E) staining was performed or more sensitive analyses were included, such as immunohistochemistry (IHC) or RT-PCR.

Bader et al.[33] conducted a prospective study of the anatomic extent of pelvic nodal involvement in a cohort of 365 men who underwent an extended lymph node dissection and radical prostatectomy. The median number of nodes retrieved was 21. Despite using only H&E stains to evaluate the extracted nodes, 24% of patients had node-positive disease, of which 49% of them had a PSA >20 ng/mL. The internal iliac nodes, which are not usually dissected in a limited dissection, were involved in 58% of men with node-positive disease. Of note, 19% of node-positive men had involved nodes that were exclusively found in the internal iliac region, suggesting that the lymphatic drainage of prostate cancer is variable. The rate of problematic lymphocele was only 2%.

Heidenreich et al.[34] reported on the incidence of lymph node involvement between standard and extended pelvic lymphadenectomy in 203 patients. IHC staining was performed if the H&E findings were negative. There were more dissected nodes in the extended dissection group (28 vs. 11; $P < .01$), at the expense of longer operative time (179 vs. 125 minutes; $P < .03$). There were more than twice the number of patients with positive nodes (26% and 12%; $P < .03$) in the extended dissection group, with 42% of all metastases lying outside the planes of a limited dissection. In patients deemed as high risk (Gleason score 7 to 10 and PSA ≥10.6 ng/mL) for lymph node metastasis, 60.9% of patients had histologically positive nodes. There was no difference in pelvic lymphocele or postoperative complications between the two groups.

In a large retrospective study from Johns Hopkins, the pathologic findings and biochemical outcomes were compared between two high-volume surgeons, each of whom exclusively performed either limited (n = 1,865) or extended (n = 2,135) node dissections during radical prostatectomy.[35] As expected, the extended dissection group had more lymph nodes retrieved than the limited group (11.6 vs. 8.9 nodes; $P < .0001$). Yet the proportion of patients with involved nodes was also significantly higher in the extended dissection group (3.3% vs. 1.2%; $P < .0001$). When only patients with Gleason score 7 or 8 to 10 were considered, the difference was even more striking (8.2% vs. 2.4% and 23.2% vs. 8.9%, respectively). The relative risks of detecting a patient with involved nodes were remarkably similar, varying between 2.5 to 3 when adjusted by Gleason score, organ-confined status, seminal vesicle invasion, and surgical margin status. There was a trend in favor of the extended dissection group for 5-year biochemical recurrence-free survival (34.4% vs. 16.5%; $P = .07$). Among patients with <15% positive lymph nodes, the difference was more remarkable (42.9% vs. 10%; $P = .01$), suggesting a therapeutic benefit of an extended dissection in low volume disease. Clinically significant lymphoceles occurred in only 0.3% in the extended dissection group.

Using an intraoperative gamma probe and dynamic lymphoscintigraphy, Wawroschek et al.[36] found that about a third of sentinel lymph nodes were in areas outside of a limited node dissection, such as the presacral, hypogastric, and pararectal regions. Holl et al.[37] demonstrated the feasibility of using sentinel lymph node dissection via injection of radio-labeled nanocolloid into the prostate.

On the basis of these studies, the NCCN guidelines now recommend an extended lymph node dissection for all patients who have a predicted probability of lymph node metastases of >2% for both diagnostic and potentially therapeutic reasons.[7] Although there have been numerous nomograms to predict nodal involvement, most are derived from surgical data where only limited node dissections were performed.[38,39] Recently published nomograms by Briganti et al.[39,40] help to address these limitations by using surgical data from patients who had an extended lymph node dissection to predict pelvic nodal involvement, exclusive nonobturator nodal metastases, and ideal nodal yield to accurately determine nodal involvement. Furthermore, it was recently demonstrated that the Roach et al.[41] formula still held relevance when validated with a cohort of over 3,000 patients treated with radical prostatectomy and *extended* lymph node dissections.[42] Although the accuracy of the Roach formula was found to be 80% in this cohort, Abdollah et al.[42] found that applying the recommended cutoff of ≥15% to decided on whether to treat the pelvic nodes led to missing about a third of patients with lymph node involvement, and therefore they recommended that the threshold be lowered to 6%.

Novel Imaging Techniques

The role of lymphotropic superparamagnetic nanoparticles, given with MRI, has been recently reported.[19,43] The nanoparticles are transported by lymphatic vessels, where they are filtered by lymph nodes. Lymph nodes that have been infiltrated by metastases will have distorted lymphatic flow and thus will accumulate the nanoparticles. Of the histologically involved nodes, 71.4% did not meet the MRI size criteria for malignancy.[43] The sensitivity (90.5% vs. 35.4%; $P < .001$) and specificity (97.8% vs. 90.4%; $P < .001$) of MRI with superparamagnetic nanoparticles was significantly better than conventional MRI. When only nodes that were between 5 to 10 mm in diameter on the short axis were considered, the sensitivity increased from 28.5% to 96.4% ($P < .001$). Dinniwell et al.[19] proposed a pelvic nodal modal based on nanoparticles and recommended CTV margins to the distal para-aortic (12 mm), common iliac (10 mm), external iliac (9 mm), and internal iliac (10 mm), drawn in continuity with a 12-mm expansion anterior to the sacrum and 22-mm expansion medial to the pelvic sidewall.

De Jong et al.[44] reported on C-choline positron emission tomography (PET) for preoperative nodal staging of prostate cancer. In contrast to 18-fluorine-fluorodeoxyglucose (^{18}F-FDG) PET, this radiolabeled agent does not suffer from radioactivity in the bladder, which can obscure nearby sites of metastases. The sensitivity, specificity, and accuracy were 80%, 96%, and 93%, respectively. In the 15 patients with histology-confirmed nodal disease, five patients had nodal disease in the common iliac region but otherwise had no involved nodes in the obturator region. In all five cases, ^{11}C-choline PET correctly detected them.

Implications for Radiotherapy

The surgical series suggests that an extended node dissection, not surprisingly, yields more dissected nodes. Perhaps more surprising is that more involved nodes are detected—despite negative preoperative imaging studies—suggesting that the harder one looks, the more one finds. To further put this into perspective, these nodes are often found in areas (i.e., internal iliac and presacral nodes) that are traditionally not excavated by the more common limited node dissection, meaning that a significant proportion of higher-risk patients may have residual micrometastatic disease after surgery. The location of sentinel nodes have also been shown to be remarkably variable.[36] Thus, some urologists have endorsed a more thorough node dissection in patients at higher risk of node involvement.[34,45]

The second important concept to draw from the surgical studies is that taken together, these studies suggest that minimal lymph node involvement detected by an extended lymph node dissection does not necessarily lead to inevitable relapse. It is not difficult to surmise that a patient with occult nodal disease who has been completely excised in an extended dissection would probably have a better outcome than the same patient with residual micrometastatic nodal disease after a limited dissection. Bader et al.[33,45] prospectively studied the outcomes of 92 patients with node-positive disease after radical prostatectomy and extended node dissection that was initially staged as clinically organ-confined prostate cancer. After 45 months, 39% of patients with only one positive node as compared to only 12% patients with two or more positive nodes were free of biochemical recurrence ($P = .008$). Although follow-up was short, PCSM was significantly different (8% vs. 33%, respectively; $P = .004$). In the prospective study of node-positive patients after radical prostatectomy by Messing et al.,[46] in the observation arm, 18% had no evidence of disease at a median follow-up of 7.1 years. Of note, these patients had a limited node dissection (median number of nodes retrieved was 12). The main criticism of this argument of improved outcomes with extended node dissection is that the effects of stage migration and lead time bias should not be discounted.

Collectively, these studies argue that an extended node dissection may yield a therapeutic benefit in the subgroup of patients with higher risk of nodal involvement yet have minimal nodal disease. This may in part be due to eradication of all tumor, but may also reflect the large individual variability of lymphatic drainage from the prostate gland.[36] Can we extrapolate these results to pelvic radiotherapy? Is there a volume effect for pelvic radiotherapy as seen in the extent of lymph node dissection? The results from the RTOG-9413 study would suggest so.[47]

Although RTOG-9413 affirmed the role of whole-pelvic radiotherapy and neoadjuvant androgen suppression therapy (AST) in high-risk prostate cancer, there has been some lingering reluctance among radiation oncologists to deliver whole-pelvic radiotherapy, instead opting for "minipelvic" fields or omitting the pelvic field entirely.[47] To reinforce this notion, secondary subgroup analysis of RTOG-9413 was recently presented, studying the volume dependence of outcome.[48] Because of the disparity in the time point at which the neoadjuvant and adjuvant AST arms became susceptible to relapse (i.e., end of both radiotherapy and AST), only patients (n = 649) who received neoadjuvant AST were included in this analysis. After stratifying by volume irradiated, the 7-year progression-free survival was 40%, 31%, and 27% in the groups that received whole-pelvic, minipelvic, and prostate-only radiotherapy, respectively ($P = .02$; Fig. 66.3). There was no difference in acute grade ≥3 genitourinary or gastrointestinal toxicities among the three volumes. No difference was seen in the incidence of late grade ≥3 genitourinary toxicities between the whole-pelvic, minipelvic, and prostate-only radiotherapy groups at 48 months (3.0%, 2.4%, and 0%, respectively; $P = .24$). There was a small but significant increase in the incidence of late grade ≥3 gastrointestinal toxicities with larger fields at 48 months (4.3%, 1.2%, and 0%, respectively; $P = .006$). Of note, 3D conformal radiation therapy (3DCRT), let alone IMRT, was not routinely performed in this study. It is conceivable that with either modality, late toxicities may be further decreased.

Although sentinel lymph node dissections are standard in various disease sites like breast and melanoma, its application in prostate cancer is still under study. Holl et al.[37] demonstrated that sentinel lymph node dissections using radiolabeled nanocolloid was reliable in detecting positive nodes in over 2,000 patients. Krengli et al.[49] recently reported on the application of sentinel lymph node imaging (single-photon emission computed tomography [SPECT]) in pelvic radiotherapy for prostate cancer and found that 25% of patients had nodes outside their pelvic CTV. Similarly, Chen et al.[22] reported on the feasibility of sentinel lymph node image-guided IMRT for prostate cancer and compared it to RTOG-based IMRT plans. Patients were injected with ^{99m}Tc-sulfur colloid into six prostate locations, then imaged with SPECT to generate a lymphatic drainage map. Although all patients had sentinel nodes identified in the internal or external iliac nodal basins, a startling 50% had sentinel nodes in the para-aortics, and RTOG consensus guidelines on pelvic delineation included all identified sentinel nodes in only 30% of cases. In comparative radiotherapy

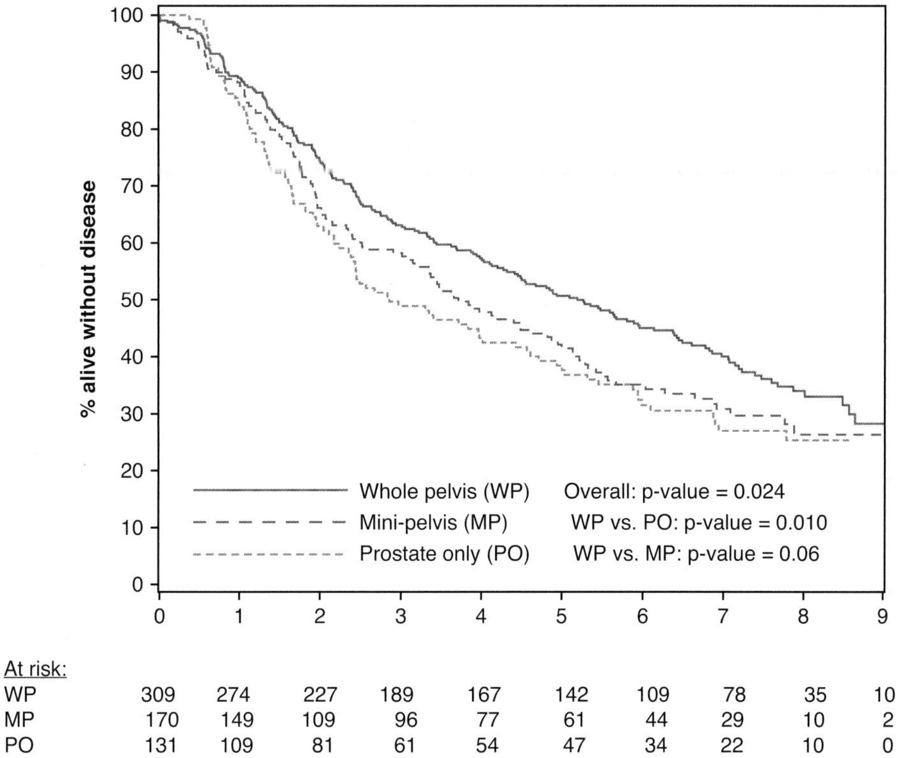

FIGURE 66.3. Progression-free survival of subgroup analysis of Radiation Therapy Oncology Group RTOG-9413 comparing whole-pelvic, minipelvic. and prostate-only radiotherapy.(From Roach M III, DeSilvio M, Valicenti R, et al. Whole pelvic, "mini-pelvic" or prostate-only external beam radiotherapy after neoadjuvant and concurrent hormonal therapy in patients treated in the Radiation Therapy Oncology Group 9413 Trial. *Int J Radiat Oncol Biol Phys* 2006;66:647–653, with permission from Elsevier.)

plans, there was no significant difference in dose to organs at risk.

Radiation Oncology Trials

RTOG-9413 is a landmark trial that featured a two-by-two factorial randomization scheme to either prostate-only radiotherapy (PORT) or whole-pelvic radiotherapy (WPRT) followed by a prostate boost, and either 4 months of neoadjuvant and concurrent hormones or 4 months of adjuvant hormones.[47] Patients with an estimated nodal risk of >15% or T2c to T4 with a Gleason score of ≥6 were eligible for the study. The 4-year progression-free survival was 54.2% and 47% in the combined WPRT arms and PORT arms (P = .02), respectively. When the four arms were analyzed separately, the neoadjuvant hormone and WPRT arm (59.6%) had a significantly better 4-year progression-free survival than the other three arms (44.3% to 49.8%; P = .008). Although there was no difference in acute (3% vs. 4%; P = .39) and late (2% vs. 2%; P = .85) grade 3 to 5 genitourinary (GU) morbidity, a trend toward increased acute (2% vs. 1%; P = .06) and late (1.7% vs. 0.6%; P = .09) grade 3 to 5 gastrointestinal (GI) morbidity was seen in the combined WPRT and prostate only arms, respectively.

Updated in 2007, there has been widespread confusion as to how to interpret the updated results, with some vocal pundits declaring that RTOG-9413 was now a "negative" study.[50,51] Contributing to this confusion was the fact that when the four arms were combined into two groups based on volume irradiated (WPRT vs. PORT), the previously significant difference in progression-free survival was no longer seen (P = .99). When the four arms were analyzed separately, there was a trend toward significance for progression-free survival in favor of the WPRT and neoadjuvant hormone arm (NHT) as compared to PORT + NHT (P = .066), WPRT and adjuvant hormonal therapy (AHT) (P = .022), but not different than PORT + AHT (P = .75). Of note, the progression-free survival end point included *death from any cause,* and therefore with longer follow-up non–prostate cancer deaths may overwhelm cancer-related events. When analyzed for biochemical failure using only the Phoenix definition (discussed below), there was a significant difference among the four arms (overall P = .047) and a significant difference in pair-wise comparisons in favor of WPRT + NHT versus PORT + NHT (P = .0098). Finally, RTOG-9413 was designed well before the results of dose-escalation trials (see Section on dose-escalation later in this chapter) that demonstrated the superiority of increased radiation doses in terms of local control and biochemical control. Indeed, its prostate dose of 70 Gy would be considered woefully inadequate in the current era. Thus, these patients would be at significant risk of local relapse, which would presumably present as later recurrences relative to distant or regional recurrences. These distinct waves of recurrences may help to explain why the initial results of RTOG-9413 were positive, but then deemed negative in the updated results.

Late toxicities were reported in the updated results of RTOG-9413.[50] Although there was no difference in grades 3 to 5 GU toxicities among the four arms (P = .16), there was a significantly greater incidence of grades 3 to 5 GI toxicities in the WPRT + NHT arm (5% vs. 1% to 2% in the other three arms; P = .002).

Preliminary results from GETUG-01 (Groupe d'Etude des Tumeurs Uro-Génitales), a French multicenter phase III trial, were recently published.[52] It randomized 444 patients with T1b-T3N0M0 prostate cancer to WPRT or PORT. Four to 8 months of neoadjuvant and concurrent hormones was not part of the protocol treatment for all patients. Instead, patients were stratified based on estimated node involvement, and only those deemed to be high risk, defined as ≥T3, Gleason score ≥7, or PSA ≥3 times normal, for nodal involvement received hormones. The total prostate dose in the study was 66 to 70 Gy. With a median follow-up of 42 months, no significant difference was seen in progression-free survival between the WPRT and PORT arms for high risk (59.8% vs. 63.4%; P = .2) and low risk (83.9% vs. 75.1%; P = .21), respectively. Yet in multivariate analyses, risk of nodal involvement was the most significant predictor of progression-free survival. WPRT slightly increased acute mild GI toxicities and late grade ≥2 GI toxicities. Although the results of GETUG-01 seem to contradict that of RTOG-9413, there are significant differences in the methodology of the two studies that warrant mention. First, more than half of the patients (~54%) had an estimated nodal risk of <15% using the Roach formula,[41] which meant that these patients had more favorable disease than those in RTOG-9413 and therefore would likely not benefit from WPRT. Second, the protocol-defined pelvic fields were smaller than those used in RTOG-9413. Specifically, the superior border was taken at the level of S1–2 interspace, rather than L5-S1 interspace, which meant that a significant portion of the presacral and common iliac nodes were not treated. Third, approximately 60% of patients received <70 Gy (RTOG-9413 mandated 70.2 Gy) to the prostate gland, which is considered suboptimal and may lead to increased risk of local recurrence.

One of the most common comments regarding RTOG-9413 is whether the beneficial finding of neoadjuvant hormones and WPRT still holds true in the dose-escalation era where doses of more than 80 Gy to the prostate alone can be given safely with IMRT. Retrospective data from Fox Chase Cancer Center were recently reported, investigating the effects of dose escalation, WPRT, and short-term hormones in the subgroup of patients who would otherwise be eligible for RTOG-9413 based on the inclusion criteria.[53] Multivariate results suggest that radiation dose (70 to 72.9 vs. 73 to 76.9 vs. ≥77 Gy), PSA, clinical T stage, and Gleason score were significant predictors of biochemical failure, whereas short-term hormones and radiation field size were not. Although provocative, there are some shortcomings of this study, as pointed out by the authors, which merit closer attention. Although the inclusion criteria was identical to RTOG-9413, 42.4% and 31.4% of patients had a PSA <10 and 10 to 20 ng/mL (median PSA 10.95 ng/mL), respectively, whereas the median PSA in RTOG-9413 was 22.6 ng/mL. In addition, only 67 patients received neoadjuvant hormones. Radiation fields were prostate only, partial pelvic, and whole-pelvis fields in 11.4%, 17.6%, and 71%, respectively. In the latter group, the whole-pelvic field extended superiorly to the inferior sacroiliac joints, which would not be considered adequate pelvic irradiation according to RTOG-9413, where a minimum unblocked field size of 16-by-16 cm was used. Total radiation doses of up to 82 Gy were given in the cohort, although the group that received at least 77 Gy had a median follow-up of only 30 months (vs. 62 and 54 months in the <73 Gy and 73 to 76.9 Gy groups, respectively). Thus, because only 16% patients received NHT and none received WPRT with the potential for selection bias (patients treated with NHT may have had worse disease than those not receiving NHT), these data do not make a compelling argument against WPRT and NHT acquired from a large phase III trial.

Vargas et al.[54] reported on the role of WPRT in a large cohort of patients treated at three institutions with external-beam radiotherapy and high–dose-rate brachytherapy. At the two German institutions, the policy was to give WPRT, whereas the American institution chose to irradiate the periprostatic area only (PORT). Of the 1,492 patients treated with this technique, 596 had an estimated nodal involvement of more than 15% based on the Roach formula,[41] and they formed the study cohort. Fifty-one percent received neoadjuvant or adjuvant hormones for ≤6 months, and 53.3% received WPRT. As opposed to the PORT group, the median PSA was higher (15.6 vs. 11.5 ng/mL), although both groups had a Gleason score of 7 and clinical T stage was slightly worse (T2b vs. T2a) in the WPRT group. Rather than show no difference, the 5-year actuarial PSA failure was significantly worse in the WPRT group (31.2% vs. 16.8%; *P* <.001) as was clinical failure (17.6% vs. 7.9%; *P* = .01), suggesting an imbalance in predictors between the two groups. In multivariate analysis, Gleason score and clinical T stage were the only predictors of clinical failure, whereas PSA, use of hormones, WPRT, and estimated risk of nodal involvement were not. Thus, the authors concluded that WPRT may not be beneficial in those with >15% risk of nodal involvement. Yet there are elements of the results and interpretation that are problematic. First, the authors chose to report only the median clinical T stage, PSA, and Gleason score (without *P* values) rather than provide a more detailed breakdown between the WPRT and PORT groups. Second, the findings of RTOG-9413 suggest a synergistic effect between neoadjuvant and concurrent hormones and WPRT. But they did not suggest that WPRT without hormones was beneficial. Rather than compare a subset of the study cohort that exclusively received WPRT and neoadjuvant hormones, this retrospective study included patients who did not receive hormones in their WPRT group. Finally, the multivariate analysis included WPRT and hormones as separate covariates.

In a retrospective study from Yale, Aizer et al.[55] analyzed the outcomes of 277 patients with an estimated nodal involvement of ≥15% who received either WPRT or PORT. The median prostate radiation dose was 75.6 Gy. Over 90% of patients in both groups received neoadjuvant and concurrent hormonal therapy. Median follow-up was only 30 months. Despite more advanced T stage, Gleason score, and pretreatment PSA, 4-year biochemical control was improved in the WPRT over the PORT group (86.3% vs. 69.4%). On multivariate analyses, WPRT was a significant predictor of biochemical control, along with Gleason score, pretreatment PSA, and the use of hormones.

Given the clinical equipoise stemming from the controversies of WPRT, in July 2011, RTOG activated its RTOG-0924 study that includes patients with unfavorable intermediate- and favorable high-risk disease, and sought to study whether the addition of WPRT could improve overall survival in patients receiving dose-escalated radiotherapy and hormones. Eschewing the simplistic NCCN risk groupings,[7] RTOG-0924 identified a subset of patients from RTOG-9413 who benefited from WPRT and incorporated the percentage of positive biopsy cores into the eligibility criteria. Patients eligible for this study should have an estimated nodal risk of at least 15% and have either:

- Gleason score 7 to 10 and T1c-T2b and PSA <50 ng/mL
- Gleason score 6 and (T2c-T4 or >50% biopsies) and PSA <50 ng/mL
- Gleason score 6 and T1c-T2b and PSA >20 ng/mL.

The phase I dose is 45 Gy in both arms and can be delivered with 3DCRT or IMRT. The phase II prostate boost can be achieved by IMRT (34.2 Gy; total dose 79.2 Gy), low–dose-rate brachytherapy (110 Gy for iodine-125 [^{125}I] and 100 Gy for palladium-103 [^{103}Pd]) or high–dose-rate brachytherapy (15 Gy in one fraction with iridium-192 [^{192}Ir]) were permitted. Patients will be stratified into 6- or 32-months of androgen suppression therapy.

Summary of University of California–San Francisco Recommendations

Whole-Pelvic Radiotherapy

At UCSF, the authors recommend prophylactic whole-pelvic IMRT to patients with an estimated nodal involvement of >15% and unfavorable intermediate- and high-risk prostate cancer. The authors recommend adherence to the RTOG GU Radiation Oncology consensus statement on pelvic nodal volumes.[21] The prostate boost is delivered with either IMRT, ^{125}I permanent seed or high–dose-rate (HDR) brachytherapy, although the authors prefer the latter approaches because of their ability to deliver maximal dose to the prostate. Brachytherapy is typically performed 1 to 2 weeks following pelvic radiotherapy. For T3 disease, the authors use an IMRT or HDR boost, which allows better coverage of extranodal disease.

Androgen Suppression Therapy

The authors give 2 months of neoadjuvant, then concurrent total androgen blockade using an luteinizing hormone-releasing hormone (LHRH) agonist and an antiandrogen. Two to

TABLE 66.1 RECOMMENDATIONS OF PELVIC RADIOTHERAPY AND HORMONES

	Low Risk	Favorable Intermediate Risk	Unfavorable Intermediate Risk	High Risk
Radiotherapy	PORT	PORT	WPRT	WPRT
Androgen suppression therapy	Not indicated	Neoadjuvant (2 mo) Concurrent	Neoadjuvant (2 mo) Concurrent ± Adjuvant (2 mo)	Neoadjuvant (2 mo) Concurrent Adjuvant (24–36 mo)

PORT, prostate-only radiotherapy; WPRT, whole-pelvic radiotherapy.

3 years of adjuvant hormones (only an LHRH agonist) is recommended for high-risk disease, but on occasion lifelong androgen deprivation is used in patients with very high-risk disease (Table 66.1).

Volumes and Setup Variation

The authors routinely place three fiducial gold seed markers into the prostate under transrectal ultrasound guidance—two in the base and one in the apex. Each marker is approximately 1.1 mm in diameter and 3 mm in length. Using an amorphous silicon flat-panel detector, the authors perform daily EPI and make any necessary adjustments prior to each treatment. As such, the authors apply a 3-mm margin around the prostate gland and seminal vesicles in defining the PTV. For patients with hip replacements, the authors use cone-beam CT for image guidance. At institutions without daily EPI to control for intra- and interfraction prostate motion, larger margins such as 0.5 to 1 cm should be considered.

Patients are instructed to empty their rectum with an enema prior to simulation. Patients are told to maintain a full bladder during simulation and treatment. A retrograde urethrogram is performed to assist in identifying the base of the prostate. Three-millimeter slice thickness is used for the CT simulation. The critical organs that are contoured include the penile bulb, small bowel, rectum, bladder, and femoral heads. The entire rectum is contoured from the anus to the rectosigmoid junction.

Intensity-Modulated Radiotherapy Treatment Planning

For patients opting for definitive external-beam radiotherapy to the pelvis and prostate, the authors use a two-phase plan. The first phase delivers 25 to 30 fractions of 1.8 Gy per fraction (total 45 to 54 Gy) to the nodes, and 2 Gy per fraction (total 54 Gy) to the seminal vesicle and prostate PTV. The second phase is a cone-down boost to the prostate PTV alone with 11 fractions of 1.8 Gy per fraction. Therefore, the minimum total dose to the prostate (prescribed to the PTV) is 73.8 Gy. The usual isodose line that the authors prescribe to is approximately 90%, meaning that the maximum dose in the prostate is approximately 82 to 84 Gy. Both phases use a seven-field isocentric technique with 18-MV photons.

For pelvic radiotherapy followed by a brachytherapy boost, the authors deliver 25 fractions of 1.8 Gy per fraction to the nodes and prostate or seminal vesicle PTV (total dose 45 Gy). In postoperative patients opting for pelvic radiotherapy, the authors prescribe 25 fractions of 1.8 Gy to the nodes (total dose 45 Gy) and 2 Gy per fraction to the tumor bed PTV (total dose 50 Gy) then 9 fractions of 1.8 Gy per fraction to the prostate bed (total minimal PTV dose 66.2 Gy, maximum dose 78 Gy).

Toxicity of Pelvic Intensity Modulated Radiotherapy

In a study from Memorial Sloan-Kettering Cancer Center, the dosimetric outcomes of pelvic radiotherapy using two-dimensional (2D), 3DCRT, and IMRT were compared in 13 patients.[56] The mean bowel dose was reduced by approximately 20% with 3DCRT and IMRT as compared to 2D planning (P = .001). Similarly, the bowel V45 was 41.7%, 22.6%, and 9.1% with 2D, 3DCRT, and IMRT. Rectal sparing was also evident with IMRT and 3DCRT. The mean dose was 40.4, 37.3, and 27.3 Gy, respectively. The V25 was significantly better with IMRT (50.5%) as compared to 2D (91.7%) and 3DCRT (86.3%). Bladder V45 was significantly better with IMRT (87.2, 56.8, and 25.6%, respectively; P <.001). Toxicity was minimal with no cases of acute grade 3 to 5 toxicities. Only one patient required medication for proctitis and none for diarrhea.

Jani et al.[57] retrospectively compared 15 patients who received pelvic IMRT versus 34 patients who received pelvic 3DCRT. The bladder (60.8% vs. 24.8%; P = .04) and rectal (65% vs. 25.1%; P = .01) V60 were significantly lower in the IMRT plans. The IMRT patients had significantly less acute GU but no difference in GI toxicities. Grade 3 (3% vs. 0%) and grade 2 GU (59% vs. 20%; P <.001) toxicities were less with IMRT.

Chung et al.[31] analyzed the dosimetry and acute toxicities of 25 high-risk patients who received pelvic radiotherapy and received either IMRT (weekly portal images) or image-guided (IG) IMRT using intraprostatic fiducial markers. Planning target volume margins differed significantly between the two groups (0.5 to 1.0 cm for IMRT vs. 0.2 to 0.3 cm for IG-IMRT). As expected, bladder and rectal doses were significantly less with IG-IMRT, which translated to significantly less RTOG grade 2 rectal (80% vs. 13%; P = .004) and bladder (60% vs. 13%; P = .014) toxicities. No grade 3 to 5 toxicities were observed.

DOSE ESCALATION

Perhaps the most polarized topic in prostate radiotherapy management is whether pelvic radiotherapy or hormonal therapy is needed in the setting of dose escalation. The crux of the argument for dose escalation in intermediate- and high-risk patients is that the relatively poor outcome observed in such patients may be due to inadequate doses of radiotherapy to the prostate itself, as suggested by postradiotherapy biopsy data, rather than occult metastatic disease. Therefore, some contend that dose escalation to the prostate obviates the need for pelvic radiation or hormonal therapy. Dose escalation can be achieved by either external-beam radiotherapy alone, or in combination with prostate brachytherapy, with the latter capable of delivering a much higher radiation dose.

External-Beam Radiotherapy Alone

To date, there have been five phase III trials comparing conventional-dose with high-dose radiotherapy. Although all have demonstrated an improvement in biochemical control, no survival advantage has been observed despite long-term follow-up. As expected, grade 3 GI toxicities appear to be worse with dose escalation.

The MD Anderson Cancer Center conducted a single-institution dose-escalation phase III trial comparing 70 with 78 Gy to the prostate.[58] Radiotherapy was conventionally planned in the 70-Gy arm and in phase I of the 78-Gy arm; a conformal boost plan was used in the 78 Gy arm. No hormonal therapy was used. With a median follow-up of 9 years, recently updated results continue to demonstrate a significant improvement with 78 Gy in 10-year PSA control of 74% versus 43% (P = .013) in patients with a presenting PSA >10 ng/mL.[59] Moreover, with longer follow-up, the high-dose arm now conferred a reduction in 10-year nodal (P = .03), distant failures (P = .016) and death from prostate cancer (3% vs. 15%; P = .03) but not overall survival. The 10-year incidence of grade ≥2 GI toxicities was 13% versus 26% (P = .013), and grade 3 GI toxicities was 1% versus 7% (P = .018) in favor of the conventional-dose arm. There was no difference in GU toxicities.[60]

The Proton Radiation Oncology Group (PROG-9509 is a phase III trial of 393 men, comparing 19.8 gray-equivalent (GyE) photon with 28.8 GyE proton boost to the prostate.[61] All patients then received 50.4 Gy using photons to the prostate and seminal vesicles with 3DCRT. In the cohort, 32% and 8% had intermediate- and high-risk disease, respectively. Updated results were recently reported with a median follow-up of 8.9 years.[62] The 10-year PSA control rates were 68% versus 82.6% for conventional- and high-dose radiotherapy, respectively (P <.001). Dose escalation clearly benefited patients with low-risk disease (hazard ratio [HR] 0.22; P <.0001) and was of borderline significance among intermediate-risk patients (HR 0.58; P = .06). The lack of dose response seen in the high-risk group may have been due to the trial limiting the accrual to a PSA <15 ng/mL and T1b to T2b stage disease. To date, there is no survival benefit from high-dose radiotherapy. Acute and late GU and GI toxicities were not significantly increased with dose escalation.

The UK Medical Research Council (MRC) recently presented the initial results of RT01, a multicenter phase III trial that randomized 843 patients to conventional-dose (64 Gy) or dose-escalated (74 Gy) 3DCRT to the prostate.[63] Both arms received neoadjuvant androgen therapy (3 to 6 months). With a median follow-up of 63 months, the 5-year biochemical control rates were superior in the dose-escalated arm.

The results of GETUG-06, a French multicenter randomized trial comparing 70 Gy with 80 Gy, were recently reported.[64] Hormonal therapy was not given. All patients received 3DCRT to the prostate and seminal vesicles (46 Gy) then a prostate-only boost to either 24 or 34 Gy. Median follow-up was 61 months. Among the 306 patients accrued, the 5-year freedom from relapse rates were 67.9% versus 76.5% (P = .09). In subgroup analyses, a significant biochemical control difference was primarily noted to be among those with an initial PSA level >15 ng/mL (HR 0.52). A trend toward increased acute rectal and urinary toxicities was seen in the 80-Gy arm. Overall, late urinary toxicities were significantly increased in the 80-Gy arm. Although there was no significant difference in overall late rectal toxicities, grade 3 toxicities were significantly >80 Gy (1.5% vs. 6.5%; P = .047).

In the Dutch multicenter CKVO96–10 study by Peeters et al.,[65] 669 men were randomized to 68 Gy versus 78 Gy to the prostate only using 3DCRT. Hormonal therapy was permitted and left to the discretion of the treating physician. Overall, 22% of patients received neoadjuvant or adjuvant hormones. Updated results were recently published after a median follow-up of 70 months.[66] The 7-year freedom from failure was significantly improved in the 78-Gy arm (45% vs. 56%; P = .03), but no survival difference was seen. Although not powered to do so, subgroup analyses suggested a significant benefit among intermediate-risk patients (odds ratio 0.6; P = .01) and borderline significance among high-risk patients, but not in the low-risk group. The 78-Gy arm had significantly higher rates of rectal bleeding, requiring laser or transfusion (3% vs. 8%; P = .01) and fecal incontinence (7% vs. 13%; P = .02) at 7-years. There was no difference seen for GU toxicities.

Zelefsky et al.[67] updated the results a single-institution phase I and II study of dose escalation from 66.0 to 86.4 Gy to the prostate alone. Of note, radiotherapy was delivered by 3DCRT or IMRT. Of a total cohort of 2,047 patients, there were 849 and 752 patients with intermediate- and high-risk disease, respectively. Approximately half of the patients received 3 months of neoadjuvant hormones with the aim of cytoreduction or for those with high-grade, unfavorable-risk disease. Median follow-up was 6.6 years. In the intermediate-risk group, doses of ≥75.6 Gy yielded significantly better PSA control rates than doses ≤70.2 Gy (P <.0001; HR 0.707). In the high-risk group, 86.4 Gy improved 5-year biochemical control as compared with 75.6 Gy (P = .05). Among the intermediate- and high-risk patients, higher doses were significant predictors of distant metastases-free survival. Postradiation biopsies taken at 2.5 years seemed to support the contention that dose escalation was efficacious, even among intermediate- and unfavorable-risk patients. Whereas only 10% and 23% of patients who received 81 and 75.6 Gy, respectively, had positive biopsies, 34% and 54% of patients who received 70.2 Gy and 64.8 Gy, respectively, had positive biopsies. The overall grade 3 late rectal toxicity was 1%. In the cohort who received 75.6 Gy or greater using 3DCRT, grade 2 late rectal toxicity was 14%. Grade 3 urethral stricture or hematuria was seen in 1.5% of patients. The 5-year rate of grade 2 late urinary toxicity was 13%.

In a separate provocative study by Zelefsky et al.[68] distant metastasis (DM)-free survival and cause-specific survival (CSS) were compared between radical prostatectomy (RP) and IMRT while controlling for differences in pretreatment characteristics by including the Kattan biochemical control nomogram[69] and NCCN risk group classification.[7] The 8-year freedom from metastatic progression was 97% for RP and 93% for IMRT (P <.001). Among intermediate- and high-risk patients, the adjusted absolute difference in DM-free survival was 3.3% and 7.8%, respectively. CSS was similarly better for RP than IMRT (P = .15). Despite euphoria from our surgical colleagues, it must be tempered by the notable limitations of this study. First, the IMRT group was severely handicapped by the lack of elective nodal irradiation, whereas extended node dissection was routinely performed in the RP arm. Second, none of the IMRT high-risk patients received adjuvant hormones, which has been shown in all phase III trials (albeit lower radiotherapy doses) to date to confer a clear survival advantage. Third, salvage therapies were given far less in the IMRT group than the RP group (43% vs. 76%) and far later (69 vs. 13 months), respectively. Salvage treatment for the IMRT group was overwhelmingly with hormones, which offers not even a glimmer of cure, whereas most in the RP group received salvage radiotherapy. Salvage brachytherapy after IMRT failure was not an option in this study. Finally, the nomogram chosen in this study found that PSA was far more predictive than clinical stage and Gleason score, whereas another nomogram specifically for the development of bone metastases[70] concluded the opposite.

Long-term toxicities of RTOG-9406, a phase I and II trial (n = 1,084) of sequential dose levels (68.4, 73.8, 79.2, 74, and 78 Gy) using 3DCRT, were recently reported. Michalski et al.[71] concluded that 79.2 Gy given in 1.8 Gy per day was the maximally well-tolerated dose. Toxicities were significantly higher with 78 Gy given in 2.0 Gy per day than the 79.2 Gy dose level. The follow-up study is RTOG-0126, a phase III multi-institutional trial that is comparing 70.2 Gy with 79.2 Gy using 3DCRT or IMRT in intermediate-risk disease, which recently completed accrual.

Of the five discussed randomized controlled trials, only the MRC RT01 and Dutch CKVO96–10 permitted hormones. In the case of the MRC study, both arms received hormones, and yet dose escalation was still beneficial. This suggests that dose escalation alone cannot replace hormones as a strategy to improve cure, and that both may be necessary in patients with intermediate- and high-risk disease. Recently, RTOG activated its RTOG-0815, which is a phase III multicenter trial evaluating the addition of 6-months of androgen blockade with dose-escalated radiotherapy, achieved by either 3DCRT or IMRT (79.2 Gy), combined low–dose-rate (110 Gy with ^{125}I or 100 Gy with ^{103}Pd) brachytherapy boost with 3DCRT or IMRT (45 Gy to the prostate and seminal vesicles), or combined high–dose-rate (2 fractions of 10.5 Gy per fractions) 3DCRT or IMRT (45 Gy to the prostate and seminal vesicles).

External-Beam Radiotherapy with Brachytherapy Boost

According to the 1999 Patterns of Care Study of radiotherapy and brachytherapy, 46% of prostate cancer patients who received brachytherapy also received supplemental external-beam radiotherapy (XRT).[72] Rather than using XRT alone, where prostate doses are limited by nearby critical organs, many have combined the advantages of dose delivery by brachytherapy with the ability to irradiate a larger volume (e.g., periprostatic or whole pelvis) with XRT that would otherwise be beyond the reach of brachytherapy. Various centers have reported using low–dose-rate (LDR) brachytherapy, whereas others have used high–dose-rate brachytherapy.

Notwithstanding the downsides that brachytherapy is an invasive procedure that requires anesthesia, additional resources, and expertise, the advantages of incorporating prostate brachytherapy as a means of boosting the dose to the prostate gland are compelling. First, the achievable biologically effective dose (BED) to the prostate far exceeds what can be achieved by IMRT, which translates into higher cure rates. Second, brachytherapy presents as a superior method of minimizing radiation to nearby critical structures, and therefore toxicities have not been significantly greater than for IMRT. Third, the overall treatment time is usually less than the usual 8 weeks of conventionally fractionated XRT and therefore more convenient for patients. Fourth, the individual unpredictable nature of prostate motion, which continues to be vexing to radiation oncologists, is not an issue with brachytherapy.

As compared to LDR brachytherapy, HDR yields the following advantages: flexibility in source positioning, accurate source positioning, immobilized target, stable geometry, adaption of dose to target and healthy organs, target volume–dose optimization, high-quality planning and dose distribution, no radiation exposition to health care personnel or public, no source preparation needed, reduced cost, and possibly more effective prostate cancer cell kill. The disadvantages of HDR are that because the dose rate is higher it is often fractionated and therefore requires more workload and careful coordination from the health care personnel.

The indications of combined XRT and brachytherapy boost are those with intermediate- or high-risk prostate cancer, in particularly patients who are relatively young and have high-volume disease. Patients not eligible for brachytherapy boost include those with a large prostate (>60 cc), prior transurethral resection of the prostate and significant urinary symptoms.

Outcomes

The Seattle Prostate Institute reported on the biochemical outcome of 232 consecutively treated patients with pelvic radiotherapy (45 Gy) followed by an ^{125}I (108 Gy) or ^{103}Pd (100 Gy) brachytherapy boost.[73] No hormones were given in this cohort. Overall, the 15-year biochemical relapse-free survival was 74%. Fifteen-year biochemical control was 86%, 80%, and 68% in the low-, intermediate-, and high-risk groups, respectively.

From McMaster University, 104 patients with T2 and T3N0 disease were randomly allocated to brachytherapy plus XRT or XRT alone.[74] The XRT-only arm received 66 Gy, whereas the brachytherapy arm received 35 Gy using ^{192}Ir seeds followed by XRT of 40 Gy (total dose 75 Gy). No adjuvant hormones were given. After a median follow-up of 8.2 years, the 5-year biochemical failure rate was significantly less in the brachytherapy arm. At 2 years, positive biopsies were significantly less in the brachytherapy arm (24% vs. 51%; P = .015). There was no difference in acute and late GI, GU, or sexual morbidity between the two arms.

Guix et al.[75] recently reported on early results of a randomized trial comparing dose-escalated external-beam radiotherapy (76 Gy) with combined external-beam radiotherapy (46 Gy) and 2 fractions (8 Gy each) of HDR brachytherapy with ^{192}Ir in patients with intermediate- or high-risk prostate cancer. After a median follow-up of 77 months, 5-year PSA relapse-free survival for intermediate- and high-risk patients in the external-beam radiotherapy only arm was 90% and 89%, respectively, whereas it was 97% and 96%, respectively, in the combined arm (P < .05). There were no grade 3 or 4 rectal or urinary toxicities observed in either arm. This study is of particular interest as it uses contemporary external-beam radiotherapy doses, unlike other studies, and is a prospective randomized trial.

In a sequential prospective study by Morton et al.,[76] HDR brachytherapy boost (10 Gy × 2 fractions, given 1 week apart) with conventional fractionation (45 Gy in 25 fractions) was compared to single-fraction HDR brachytherapy boost (15 Gy; Fig. 66.4) with hypofractionated external-beam radiotherapy (37.5 Gy in 15 fractions) in patients with intermediate-risk prostate cancer. The hypothesis was that late effects, assuming an $\alpha\beta$ ratio of 3, were equivalent between the two fractionations, and that disease control rates were comparable. With increasing reports that prostate cancer may have an $\alpha\beta$ ratio of <3, the hypofractionated arm would theoretically confer improved tumoricidal doses.[77–79] Preliminary data show no difference in 5-year PSA control rates between the single-fraction (95.1%) and two-fraction boost (97.9%; P = 0.35), although median follow-up differed at 45 versus 72 months, respectively. Two-year prostate biopsy was positive in 4% and 8%, respectively. Although acute grade 3 GU toxicity (i.e., acute urinary retention requiring catheterization) was significantly greater in the two-fraction boost group (1.6% vs. 20%; P = .0005), there was no difference in late grade 3 to 5 GU or GI toxicities as measured by the Common Terminology Criteria for Adverse Events (version 3.0), serial International Prostate Symptom Score, or Expanded Prostate Index Composite.

From UCSF, Kapréalian et al.[80] compared the outcomes of 165 patients treated with HDR brachytherapy boost using two different HDR fractionation schemes (18 Gy in 3 fractions and 19 Gy in 2 fractions). All patients received an initial 45 Gy to the prostate and seminal vesicles for those with an estimated risk of nodal involvement of ≤15% or the same dose to the pelvic nodes for those with >15% risk of nodal involvement. Patients received 4 months of neoadjuvant and concurrent hormones, except those with high-risk disease who received an additional 24 months of adjuvant hormones. There was no significant difference in overall 5-year PSA control rates between the 3- and 2-fractions HDR groups (93.5% vs. 87.3%; P = .19), despite the 2-fraction group comprising more patients with Gleason scores of 8 to 10. In the entire cohort, there were only three grade 3 GU toxicities and no grade 4 or 5 toxicities. Only one patient developed a stricture.

Hoskin et al.[81] presented preliminary results of their phase III trial comparing external-beam radiotherapy alone (55 Gy in 20 fractions) with combined external-beam radiotherapy (35.75 Gy in 13 fractions) followed by HDR prostate brachytherapy (17 Gy in 2 fractions over 24 hours) among 220 patients with clinically localized prostate cancer. With a median follow-up of 30 months, the combined arm had significantly improved PSA relapse-free survival (P = .03). There was no difference in acute GU and GI toxicity scores, except for rectal discharge, which was more frequent in the external-beam radiotherapy arm (P = .025). No difference was observed in late GU and GI grade 2+ toxicity scores.

At William Beaumont Hospital, Martinez et al.[82] published the long-term results of their phase II study of hypofractionated dose-escalated radiotherapy in 472 patients with intermediate- and high-risk disease. All patients received 46 Gy in 23 fractions to the pelvis with external-beam radiotherapy. The HDR brachytherapy procedure was delivered over 2 or 3 separate fractions during weeks 1 and 3 of the external-beam radiotherapy, for a total overall treatment time of 5 weeks. The HDR brachytherapy dose fractionation was increased in successive

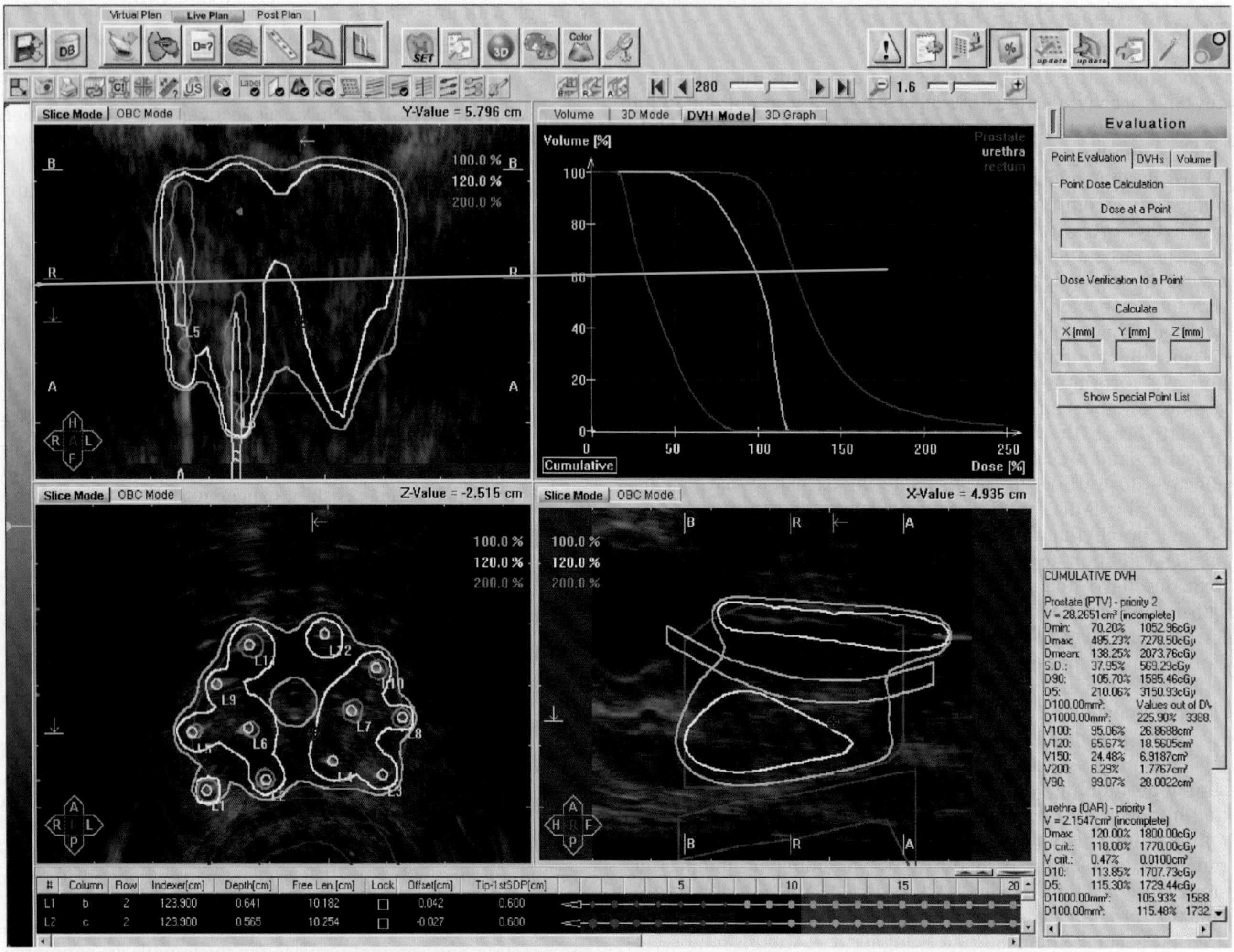

FIGURE 66.4. Isodose lines and dose–volume histogram from a representative patient treated with single-fraction 15 Gy high–dose-rate prostate brachytherapy with ultrasound-based planning. Twelve catheters were implanted. On dose–volume histogram, the prostate (*red line*), urethra (*blue line*), and rectum (*brown line*) are represented. (Courtesy of Gerard Morton, MD, Sunnybrook Odette Cancer Centre, University of Toronto.)

dose bins of 3 implants of 5.5 Gy, 6.0 Gy, and 6.5 Gy, and 2 implants of 8.25 Gy, 8.75 Gy, 9.5 Gy, 10.5 Gy, and 11.5 Gy. Assuming an $\alpha\beta$ ratio of 1.2, the HDR BED ranged from 92.13 to 243.42 Gy, and the total BED including the external-beam radiotherapy ranged from 215 to 366 Gy. For the purposes of the study, patients were separated into a low-dose-level (BED ≤268 Gy) and a high-dose-level (BED >268 Gy). The use of hormones was based on the treating physician's discretion, and in the study, 51.3% received neoadjuvant or concurrent hormones. Median follow-up was 8.2 years. At 10-years, the biochemical control rate (56.9% vs. 81.1%; P <.001) and distant metastasis-free rate (87.6% vs. 94.3%; P = .028) were superior in the high-dose-level group.

From Quebec, Bachand et al.[83] published the results of 206 patients with clinically localized prostate cancer, treated with sequential HDR dose escalation with external-beam radiotherapy (40 to 44 Gy in 2 Gy per fraction). The HDR dose fractionation increased from 3 fractions of 6 Gy and 6.5 Gy, and 2 fractions of 9 Gy, 9.5 Gy, and 10 Gy and were delivered after the external-beam radiotherapy. Half of patients received neoadjuvant or adjuvant hormones. With a median follow-up of 44 months, the 5-year PSA relapse-free survival was 95.8% in the entire cohort.

To see whether combined-modality treatment could be implemented on a nationwide scale, RTOG-P-0019, a phase II study of combined XRT with ^{125}I brachytherapy in intermediate-risk patients, was initiated.[84] The protocol mandated periprostatic XRT (45 Gy) followed by brachytherapy (108 Gy). Of 130 eligible patients, there were no grade 4 or 5 acute toxicities. All grade 3 acute toxicities were urinary (n = 10), with urinary frequency (n = 6) the most common. There were 5 and 4 late grade 3 GU and GI toxicities, respectively, and 2 cases of late grade 4 GU toxicities (bladder necrosis) but no grade 4 GI toxicities. No grade 5 late toxicities were seen. The 18- and 48-month estimates of late grade 3 GU or GI toxicities were 8% and 15%, respectively, and 4-year PSA control was 86%.

RTOG-0321 is a phase II trial designed to estimate the rates of grade 3 late GU and GI toxicities with high–dose-rate brachytherapy (19 Gy in 2 fractions) and XRT (45 Gy in 25 fractions) in intermediate- and high-risk disease.[85] Preliminary results were recently presented and showed that of 112 patients, there were only 3 acute and 4 late grade 3 GU or GI adverse events. At 18-months, the estimated late grade 3 to 5 GU or GI toxicities was only 2.56%.

Currently, there are three open RTOG studies of relevant interest. RTOG-0232 is a phase II trial comparing brachytherapy alone with combined brachytherapy and XRT in select intermediate-risk patients and is nearing completion of accrual. RTOG-0815 and RTOG-0924 are companion phase III trials that include intermediate- and favorable high-risk disease. The former trial is evaluating the addition of 6 months of neoadjuvant and concurrent hormones with dose-escalated radiotherapy, of which prostate boost is achieved by either IMRT (34.2 Gy; total dose 79.2 Gy), HDR (21 Gy in 2 fractions), or LDR (110 Gy for ^{125}I and 100 Gy for ^{103}Pd) prostate brachytherapy boost after an initial 45 Gy in 25 fractions to the prostate and seminal vesicles. RTOG-0924 is comparing WPRT with PORT in the presence of dose-escalated radiotherapy and androgen suppression therapy (6 or 32 months). Acceptable methods of dose escalation are similar to those for RTOG-0815, except for the HDR boost fractionation (15 Gy in 1 fraction), which has adopted that of Morton et al.[76]

Despite the results of RTOG-9413, there has been ongoing controversy regarding whether pelvic radiotherapy or dose escalation is more important in terms of patient outcome. At UCSF, patients with unfavorable intermediate- or high-risk disease are offered combined AST and whole-pelvic radiotherapy followed by a brachytherapy boost as a form of dose escalation or IMRT.

Technique

The external-beam radiotherapy can be delivered using a four-field box, to maintain dose homogeneity within the irradiated volume, or IMRT for better avoidance of rectum and bladder. At a minimum, the prostate, seminal vesicles, and periprostatic tissue should be irradiated. Inclusion of the first echelon lymph nodes (i.e., minipelvis) or the entire pelvic nodal contents (i.e., whole pelvis) may be considered, based on the estimated risk of involvement. The recommended external-beam radiotherapy dose is 45 to 50.4 Gy in 1.8 to 2.0 Gy per fraction.

LDR brachytherapy boost may be performed either prior to starting the external-beam radiotherapy or 2 to 4 weeks after completing external-beam radiotherapy. The technique is identical to that of LDR brachytherapy as monotherapy (see Chapter 65). The American Brachytherapy Society recommends ^{125}I and ^{103}Pd doses of 100 to 110 Gy and 80 to 90 Gy, respectively.[86] The Cesium Advisory Group recommends a boost dose of 85 Gy for cesium-131.[87]

HDR brachytherapy may be performed before, during, or after the external-beam radiotherapy. The optimal HDR dose fractionation is currently unknown, and there is significant variability across centers. Nonetheless, there is a shift toward fewer implants, fewer fractions, and higher dose per fraction because of the radiobiologic advantage of high dose per fraction in prostate cancer. Reflecting this lack of consensus, RTOG-0815 and RTOG-0924 stipulate different HDR prescription doses. In RTOG-0815, the HDR brachytherapy boost may be performed during external-beam radiotherapy or within 1 week prior to its initiation or following its completion. The prescription is 21 Gy delivered in 2 equal fractions of 10.5 Gy, separated by at least 6 hours and given within 24 hours. In RTOG-0924, the implant may be done during external-beam radiotherapy or within 2 weeks prior to its initiation or following its completion. The prescription is 15 Gy in a single fraction. In both protocols, the dose constraints to the bladder is V75 <1 cc, rectum is V75 <1 cc, and urethra is V125 <1 cc and V150 is 0%.

ANDROGEN SUPPRESSION THERAPY

AST has been increasingly used in combination with external-beam radiotherapy in the treatment of unfavorable intermediate- and high-risk adenocarcinoma of the prostate.[88–91] This practice is reflected in a recent CaPSURE report where the use of neoadjuvant hormones with radiotherapy among high-risk patients increased from 17.4% to 84.5% in 1990 to 1994 and 2004 to 2007, respectively.[2]

Biologic Basis of Combining Androgen Suppression Therapy and Radiotherapy

Animal models have provided the basis for our understanding of the mechanism behind AST and radiotherapy. In the Shionogi *in vivo* tumor system, androgen-dependent tumors, designed to mimic prostate cancer, were implanted into SCID mice.[92] The mice then received radiation or surgical orchiectomy at varying time sequences relative to each other. The results showed that androgen ablation improved the tumor response to radiation and reflected a reduction in the radiotherapy dose needed to control 50% of tumors (TCD50). More provocative was the observation that the sequence of androgen ablation and radiotherapy was also relevant. When orchiectomy was performed prior to the delivery of radiotherapy, much lower doses of radiation were required to achieve a given level of tumor control than if performed after or during radiotherapy. Thus, increased overall cell kill appears to be one of the mechanisms responsible for the combined effects of androgen deprivation and radiotherapy.

More recently, Kaminski et al.[93] studied the effects of single-fraction radiotherapy and androgen ablation sequencing in the R33270G Dunning rat prostate tumor model on tumor volume growth kinetics. There were seven groups, including a sham group, radiotherapy (RT)-alone control groups, androgen deprivation alone group, and RT before, during, and after androgen deprivation. They found that the median posttreatment doubling time was significantly longer in the group that received radiotherapy after neoadjuvant androgen ablation compared with all the other treatment groups, including the radiotherapy with concurrent or adjuvant androgen deprivation groups. Therefore, the improved outcome after combined treatment may also be explained by diminished growth velocity in the surviving prostate cancer cells after treatment.

Clinical Trials Supporting Androgen Suppression Therapy and Radiotherapy

Thus far, there have been eight phase III randomized controlled trials and a meta-analysis published in the literature that compared radiotherapy alone with radiotherapy and AST. The trials can be broadly divided based on the era (e.g., pre-PSA) when they were conducted. With greater adoption of PSA screening, a dramatic stage migration was observed in the 1990s. The CaPSURE database demonstrated that high-risk disease decreased from 36.6% of patients diagnosed in 1989 to 1992 to 16.0% in 2000 to 2002.[3] In contrast, there has been a corresponding rise in low-risk disease from 29.5% to 46.8%, respectively.[3] The pretreatment characteristics and outcome results of these seven trials are summarized in Tables 66.2 and 66.3, respectively.

High-Risk Prostate Cancer

As the first study to demonstrate a survival advantage with AST, the European Organisation of Research and Treatment of Cancer EORTC-22863 study randomized 415 men with T1 and T2 and World Health Organization grade 3 disease, or T3 or T4 disease, to either radiotherapy alone or 3 years of AST commenced on the first day of radiotherapy.[88] Ninety percent of patients had T3 or T4 disease. All patients received WPRT (50 Gy) and a prostate boost to a total dose of 70 Gy. Updated results demonstrated that after a median follow-up of 9.1 years, 10-year rates of clinical progression-free survival, prostate-cancer mortality and overall survival were significantly in favor of the AST plus radiotherapy arm.[94] AST reduced the risk of death by 40% and improved 10-year overall survival from 40% to 58% (P = .0004).

At around the same time, RTOG launched two companion trials—RTOG-8531 and RTOG-8610—which were designed to target different subsets of high-risk patients. RTOG-8531 randomized 977 men with clinical stage T1 and T2N1, T3N0–1, or pT3 after radical prostatectomy to either radiotherapy or radiotherapy with indefinite AST beginning on the last day of radiotherapy.[90] Like the EORTC trial, all patients received WPRT (44 to 46 Gy) followed by a prostate boost to a total dose of 65 to 70 Gy. In the control arm, salvage AST was offered upon failure.

TABLE 66.2 SUMMARY OF PRETREATMENT CHARACTERISTICS OF RANDOMIZED CONTROLLED TRIALS OF RADIOTHERAPY ALONE VERSUS RADIOTHERAPY WITH ANDROGEN SUPPRESSION THERAPY

				Patient Characteristics		
Study (Reference)	*Study Arms*	*Number of Patients*	*XRT Dose (Gy)*	*Clinical T Stage*	*Median PSA*	*Gleason Score*
High Risk						
EORTC-22863 (88,94)	XRT alone	208	70	T3–T4 (90%)	≤10.1 (18%)	2–6 (28%)[a]
	XRT + AST (3 yr)	207			10–20 (16%)	7–10 (33%)
					20.1–40 (24%)	Unknown (39%)
					>40 (33%)	
					Unknown (10%)	
RTOG-8531 (90,95)	XRT alone	489	65–70	NR	24[b]	2–6 (30%)[a]
	XRT + AST (indefinite)	488				7 (39%)
						8–10 (32%)
RTOG-8610 (91,96)	XRT alone	232	65–70	T3–T4 (70%)	26.3[b]	2–6 (28%)[a]
	XRT + NHT (2 mo), C-HT (2 mo)	224				7 (39%)
						8–10 (27%)
						Unknown (6%)
Quebec L-101 (101)	XRT alone	43	64			
	XRT + NHT (3 mo)	63		T2 (70%)	10.0	7–10 (27.4%)
	XRT + NHT (3 mo), C-HT (2 mo), AHT (5 mo)	55		T3 (30%)		
Granfors et al. (102,103)	XRT alone	46	65.05	T2 (65%)	NR	Grade 1 (12%)
	XRT + AST (indefinite)	45		T3–T4 (29%)		Grade 2 (70%)
						Grade 3 (18%)
TROG-96.0 (98,99)	XRT alone	276	66	T2 (60%)	15	2–6 (44%)
	XRT + NHT (2 mo), CHT (1 mo)	270		T3–T4 (40%)		7 (38%)
	XRT + NHT (5 mo), CHT (1 mo)	272				8–10 (17%)
Intermediate Risk						
BWH (89,104)	XRT alone	104	70.35	T1 (48%)	11	5–6 (27%)[a]
	XRT + NHT (2 mo), C-HT (2 mo), AHT (2 mo)	102		T2 (52%)		7 (58%)
						8–10 (15%)
RTOG-9408 (105)	XRT alone	987	66.6–68.4	T1 (49%)	<4 (11%)	2–6 (62%)
	XRT + NHT (2 mo), C-HT (2 mo)	992		T2 (51%)	4–20 (89%)	7 (28%)
						8–10 (9%)

AHT, adjuvant hormonal therapy; AST, androgen suppression therapy; BWH, Brigham and Women's Hospital; C-HT, concurrent hormonal therapy; CUOG, Canadian Urologic Oncology Group; EORTC, European Organisation of Research and Treatment of Cancer; NHT, neoadjuvant hormonal therapy; NR, not recorded; PSA, prostate-specific antigen; RTOG, Radiation Therapy Oncology Group; TROG, Trans-Tasman Radiation Oncology Group; XRT, external-beam radiotherapy; ICORG, Irish Clinical Oncology Research Group.

[a]Gleason score distribution from central review.

[b]For RTOG-8531 and RTOG-8610, pretreatment PSA was available in only 44% and 28% of patients, respectively.

In effect, this was a comparison between immediate versus delayed AST. After a median follow-up of 5.6 years, the initial published report demonstrated that immediate AST improved biochemical control but not overall survival in the entire cohort. Subgroup analyses identified a cluster of patients with centrally reviewed Gleason scores of 8 to 10 who had not undergone surgery but did have a survival advantage (66% vs. 55%; $P = .03$). The study has since been updated after a median follow-up of 7.6 years.[95] At 10 years, the overall survival advantage seen with immediate AST now extends to the entire cohort (49% vs. 39%; $P = .002$), but was preferentially in the patients with a Gleason score of 7 to 10. Ten-year PCSM (16% vs. 22%; $P = .0052$) and distant metastases failure rates (24% vs. 39%; $P < .001$) were significantly reduced in the immediate AST arm.

RTOG-8610 randomized 456 patients with bulky T2 clinical stage T2–4N0–1 or a bulky primary tumor, defined as >25 cm^2 prostate, to either radiotherapy alone or radiotherapy with 2 months of neoadjuvant and 2 months of concurrent AST (total 4 months).[91] The radiotherapy dose and technique were identical to that used in RTOG-8531. Like RTOG-8531, the initial report (median follow-up 4.5 years) showed that AST improved 5-year progression-free survival but did not impact overall survival.[91] With longer follow-up (median follow-up 11.9 to 13.2 for surviving patients years), the 10-year PCSM (23% vs. 36%; $P = .01$), and distant metastases failure (35% vs. 47%; $P = .006$) benefit from AST became more apparent, although there was no difference in overall survival (43% vs. 34%; $P = .12$).[96] In a subgroup analysis of men with Gleason score 2 to 6 tumors, there was a significant overall survival benefit with AST at 8 years (70% vs. 52%; $P = .015$).[97]

The Trans-Tasman Radiation Oncology Group TROG-96.01 study consisted of 818 men with intermediate- or high-risk prostate cancer.[98] A three-arm trial, patients were randomized to radiotherapy alone or 3 months or 6 months of neoadjuvant and concurrent hormones with radiotherapy. The protocol prescription was 66 Gy to the prostate and seminal vesicles, without WPRT. More than 80% of patients had high-risk disease. Results were recently updated with a median follow-up of 10.6 years.[99] Compared to the radiotherapy alone arm, 3-months of hormones improved the 10-year incidence of biochemical failure (73.8% vs. 60.4%; $P = .003$) and local progression (28.2% vs. 15.7%; $P = .0005$). Six months of hormones further improved the 10-year incidence of biochemical failure (73.8% vs. 52.3%; $P < .0001$), local progression (28.2% vs. 13.3%; $P = .0001$), distant progression (20.6% vs. 10.9%; $P = .001$), PCSM (22.0% vs. 11.4%; $P = .0008$), and all-cause mortality (42.5% vs. 29.2%; $P = .0008$). Compared to 3 months, 6 months of hormones significantly improved distant progression, event-free survival, PCSM and overall mortality, and nonsignificant reductions in PSA failure and local progression.

Conducted between 1991 and 1994, the Quebec L-101 study randomized 161 men with clinical stage T2 or T3

TABLE 66.3 SUMMARY OF OUTCOME RESULTS FROM RANDOMIZED CONTROLLED TRIALS OF RADIOTHERAPY ALONE VERSUS RADIOTHERAPY WITH ANDROGEN SUPPRESSION THERAPY

Study (Reference)	Median Follow-Up (Years)	Study Arms	10-Year Overall Survival	10-Year Cause-Specific Survival	10-Year Biochemical Control
High Risk					
EORTC-22863 (88,94)	9.1	XRT alone	40%	70%	23%
		XRT + AST (3 yr)	58%	90%	48%
			(*P* = .0004)	(*P* <.0001)	(*P* <.0001)
RTOG-8531 (90,95)	7.6	XRT alone	39%	78%	23%
		XRT + AST (indefinite)	49%	84%	37%
			(*P* = .002)	(*P* = .0052)	(*P* <.0001)
RTOG-8610 (91,96)	11.9–13.2[a]	XRT alone	34%	64%	20%
		XRT + NHT (2 mo), C-HT (2 mo)	43%	77%	35%
			(*P* = .12)	(*P* = .01)	(*P* <.0001)
Quebec L-101 (101)	5.0	XRT alone	NR	NR	58%
		XRT + NHT (3 mo)			76% (*P* = .009)
		XRT + NHT (3 mo), C-HT (2 mo), AHT (5 mo)			74% (*P* = .003)
Granfors et al. (102,103)	16.5[a]	XRT alone	39%	48%	28%[b]
		XRT + AST (indefinite)	58%	68%	65%
			(*P* = .03)	(*P* = .02)	(*P* = .005)
TROG-96.01 (98,99)	10.6	XRT alone	58%	78%	26%
		XRT + NHT (2 mo), C-HT (1 mo)	63% (*P* = .2)	81% (*P* = .04)	40% (*P* = .0009)
		XRT + NHT (5 mo), C-HT (1 mo)	71% (*P* = .0005)	89% (*P* = .0002)	47% (*P* <.0001)
Intermediate Risk					
BWH (89,104)	7.6	XRT alone	61%[c]	89%[c]	55%[c]
		XRT + NHT, C-HT, AHT	74%[c]	98%[c]	79%[c]
			(*P* = .01)	(*P* = .007)	(*P* <.001)
RTOG-9408 (105)	9.1	XRT alone	57%	92%	59%
		XRT + NHT (2 mo), C-HT (2 mo)	62%	96%	74%
			(*P* = .03)	(*P* = .001)	(*P* <.001)

AHT, adjuvant hormonal therapy; AST, androgen suppression therapy; BWH, Brigham and Women's Hospital; C-HT, concurrent hormonal therapy; CUOG, Canadian Urologic Oncology Group; EORTC, European Organisation of Research and Treatment of Cancer; NHT, neoadjuvant hormonal therapy; NR, not recorded; RTOG, Radiation Therapy Oncology Group; TROG, Trans-Tasman Radiation Oncology Group; XRT, external-beam radiotherapy; ICORG, Irish Clinical Oncology Research Group; NS, not significant.

[a]Value reflects surviving patients.

[b]Non-prostate-specific antigen progression-free survival.

[c]Overall survival and cause-specific survival values are at 8 years, whereas biochemical control value was at 5 years.

prostate cancer to one of three arms: radiotherapy alone, 3 months of neoadjuvant AST plus radiotherapy, or 10 months of neoadjuvant, concurrent, adjuvant AST plus radiotherapy.[100,101] The latter arm received 3 months of neoadjuvant AST and then continued for an additional 7 months during and after radiotherapy. The updated results concluded that both arms containing AST had significantly improved 7-year PSA control rates better than the control arm. There was no difference between the two experimental arms ($P = .6$). Granfors et al.[102] randomized 91 patients with T1 to T4, pN0–3 prostate cancer to radiotherapy alone or orchiectomy followed by radiotherapy. Patients were surgically staged with a pelvic lymphadenectomy. All patients received WPRT and a mean total prostate dose of 65.05 Gy. Updated results, with a mean follow-up of 16.5 years in survival, demonstrated a benefit in 10-year prostate cancer survival and overall survival in favor of the orchidectomy arm.[103] However, in subgroup analyses, only patients with positive pelvic lymph nodes benefited from orchiectomy.

In summary, the studies consistently demonstrate that combining hormones with radiotherapy can confer a PSA control and survival advantage, and as such should be recommended in the high-risk group.

Intermediate-Risk Prostate Cancer

Two studies conducted in the PSA and 3DCRT era were recently published. As expected from the PSA stage migration, the participating patients in these trials are distinctly lower risk than those in the pioneering trials and would be considered as intermediate-risk disease.

In a study from Brigham and Women's Hospital (BWH), 206 patients were randomly allocated to radiotherapy alone or 2 months each of total androgen blockade given before, during, and after radiotherapy for a total of 6 months.[104] Radiotherapy was confined to the prostate and seminal vesicles (i.e., WPRT was not performed). Nonetheless, after a median follow-up of only 4.52 years and a relatively small sample size, the AST arm had significantly improved 5-year PSA control (79% vs. 55%; $P < .001$), PCSM (0% vs. 6%; $P = .02$), and overall survival (88% vs. 78%; $P = .04$). Results were updated with a median follow-up of 7.6 years and continued to show a benefit from adding AST to radiotherapy in terms of 8-year PCSM (2% vs. 11%; $P = .007$) and overall survival (74% vs. 61%; $P = .01$). In postrandomization subgroup analysis, patients with no or minimal comorbidity had a significant overall survival benefit from AST at 8 years (90% vs. 64%; $P < .001$), whereas those with moderate or severe comorbidity did not see a significant benefit from ADT ($P = .08$).

In response to the positive findings of RTOG-8610, RTOG-9408 was designed to evaluate whether similar duration and timing of AST (2 months neoadjuvant and 2 months concurrent) could improve outcomes in patients with more favorable disease.[105] Among the 1,979 eligible patients, 54% had intermediate-risk disease and 11% had high-risk disease. All patients had prostate-only radiotherapy to 68.4 Gy, except for those with a PSA <10 ng/mL, Gleason score of 2 to 6, or negative lymph node dissection. The latter group received pelvic radiotherapy to 46.8 Gy and a total prostate dose of 66.6 Gy. With a median follow-up of 9.1 years, 10-year overall survival (57% vs. 62%; $P = .03$), PCSM (8% vs. 4%; $P = .001$), PSA failure (41% vs. 26%; $P < .001$), and distant metastases (8% vs. 6%; $P = .04$) were significantly in favor of the AST arm. In *post hoc* analyses, the benefit in overall survival and PCSM appeared to be primarily among intermediate-risk patients. Two-year positive prostate biopsy rates (39% vs. 20%; P <.001) were significantly improved with AST.

In the era of dose-escalated radiotherapy, it is unclear whether the benefit of AST, as seen in previous trials, which used much lower radiotherapy doses, was still present. Last year, RTOG-0815 was activated, which is a phase III multicenter trial evaluating the addition of 6 months of androgen blockade with dose-escalated radiotherapy in favorable intermediate-risk disease. Dose escalation is to be achieved by either 3DCRT or IMRT (79.2 Gy), combined LDR (110 Gy with ^{125}I or 100 Gy with ^{103}Pd) brachytherapy boost with 3DCRT or IMRT (45 Gy to the prostate and seminal vesicles), or combined high-dose-rate (2 fractions of 10.5 Gy per fraction) with 3DCRT or IMRT (45 Gy to the prostate and seminal vesicles).

Toxicities of Androgen Suppression

Having established that AST improves survival when combined with radiotherapy, enthusiasm has been somewhat tempered by the increasing recognition of the potentially serious complications of AST.[106,107] These include fatigue, weight gain, osteoporosis, depression, decreased cognitive function, erectile dysfunction, loss of libido, gynecomastia, anemia, decreased high-density lipoprotein, insulin resistance, and hot flashes.

In a recent study of 50,613 men with prostate cancer compiled from a linked database of Surveillance, Epidemiology, and End Results (SEER) and Medicare, the addition of AST significantly increased the risk of any fracture from 12.6% to 19.4%; fractures requiring hospitalization similarly increased from 2.37% to 5.19%.[108] Recommendations on management of osteoporosis secondary to AST have since been published.[109]

Recent studies have raised the question of whether AST, by way of increasing body fat and cholesterol levels, increases the risk of cardiovascular disease.[110] In an observational study of a population-based cohort of 73,196 patients with clinically localized prostate cancer, AST was associated with an increased risk of incident diabetes (HR 1.44; P <.001), cardiovascular disease (HR 1.16; P <.001), myocardial infarction (HR 1.11; P = .03), and sudden cardiac death (HR 1.16; P = .004). A similar study by Saigal et al.[111] of 22,816 patients accounted for ethnicity and confirmed that the use of AST was associated with a 20% increase in cardiovascular morbidity. However, data from randomized controlled trials of radiotherapy with or without AST have not shown any increased cardiovascular disease, although these studies were not powered adequately.[94,99,112,113] Nonetheless, a science advisory team from the American Health Association, American Cancer Society, and the American Urological Association was formed to review the available evidence on metabolic effects of AST and suggestions regarding management.[114]

Of note, even after cessation of AST, testosterone levels may require a year or more before recovering to noncastrate levels. During this time, men are still exposed to the potential side effects of androgen deprivation. In a study by Pickles et al.,[115] the overall median time for testosterone recovery to noncastrate levels after adjuvant AST and radiotherapy was 10 months. Testosterone recovery was dependent on the duration of the LHRH preparation, with 3- and 1-month preparations associated with a 16- and 8-month recovery time, respectively.

Sequencing of Androgen Suppression Therapy and Radiotherapy

Neoadjuvant therapy suggests delivery of the hormone prior to definitive radiation only. Yet the precise duration of androgen suppression is not so simple. One study found that the median time for testosterone recovery to noncastrate levels after cessation of AST was 10 months.[115] In effect, these definitions are artificial because patients receiving neoadjuvant AST alone are in fact receiving concurrent and short-term adjuvant AST.

Optimal Timing of Androgen Suppression Therapy

RTOG-9413 randomized 1,323 men with an estimated risk of pelvic lymph node involvement exceeding 15% in a two-by-two factorial design: WPRT followed by prostate boost radiotherapy versus PORT, and 4 months of neoadjuvant and concurrent AST (commenced 2 months prior to starting radiotherapy) versus 4 months of adjuvant AST.[41,47] Two-thirds of the study patients had T2c to T4 disease and one-third had a presenting PSA ≥30 ng/mL. Seventy-three percent had a Gleason score of 7 to 10, and approximately one-quarter had an estimated pelvic nodal involvement >35%. After a median follow-up of 59.5 months, 4-year progression-free survival was significantly improved in the arm that received WPRT and neoadjuvant AST as compared with the other three arms (60% vs. 44% to 50%; P = .008); there was no significant difference among the other three arms.[47] Because of the significant difference between the two WPRT arms, the conclusions were that the benefit was sequence dependent and that there was a favorable interaction between neoadjuvant AST and WPRT. Similarly, the lack of difference seen between the two PORT arms suggests that the benefit of AST was not sequence dependent when only the prostate was irradiated.

With the updated results in 2007, the controversies of elective pelvic nodal irradiation grew.[50] Although there remained no difference in progression-free survival between the combined neoadjuvant and adjuvant arms (P = .88 using the Phoenix definition, discussed below), the previously observed significant difference between the combined WPRT and PORT arms (P = .93) was no longer seen with longer follow-up. Furthermore, when the four arms were analyzed separately, the difference between the WPRT and NHT arm and PORT and NHT arm was now of only borderline significance (P = .066) and significantly different from the WPRT and AHT arm (P = .022). The trial investigators speculated that this loss of significance may be attributed to several factors.[51] First, the progression-free survival end point included *death from any cause* and, therefore, with longer follow-up non–prostate cancer deaths may overwhelm cancer-related events. Second, RTOG-9413 was designed well before the results of dose-escalation trials (see Section on dose-escalation above in this chapter) that demonstrated the superiority of increased radiation doses in terms of local control and biochemical control. Indeed, its prostate dose of 70 Gy would be considered woefully inadequate in the current era. Thus, these patients would be at significant risk of local relapse, which would presumably present as later recurrences relative to distant or regional recurrences. These distinct waves of recurrences may help to explain why the initial results of RTOG-9413 were positive but then deemed negative in the updated results.

Notwithstanding the controversies of the updated RTOG-9413 results, the recently activated RTOG-0924, which is evaluating the role of WPRT with dose escalation, mandates at least 2 months of neoadjuvant hormones in both arms.

Duration of Androgen Suppression Therapy

Optimal Duration of Neoadjuvant Hormonal Therapy

To date, there are three published randomized trials evaluating the optimal duration of neoadjuvant AST. The Canadian Urologic Oncology Group (CUOG) study randomized 378 patients to either 3 or 8 months of neoadjuvant AST plus radiotherapy.[116] The majority had intermediate- (43%) or high-risk (34%) disease. None received concurrent or adjuvant AST. Patients with an estimated pelvic nodal involvement of >10% to 15% received pelvic radiotherapy. Results were recently updated with a median follow-up of 6.6 years.[117] No significant difference was seen between the 3- and 6-months arms in terms of 7-year overall survival, cause-specific survival, and biochemical control. Extracted 24 to 30 months after radiotherapy, rates of positive biopsies were also not significantly different (14% vs. 9%, respectively; P = .34). Testosterone recovery was in favor of the 3-month arm (95.5% vs. 88.7%; $P = .04$).

As previously discussed, TROG-96.01 is a three-arm study with a radiotherapy-alone control group.[98,99] The other two experimental arms were 3 and 6 months of neoadjuvant AST. Although not powered to compare the two experimental arms, the 6-month arm exhibited a trend toward reduction in 10-year PSA progression (60.4% vs. 52.8%; $P = .072$) and significant reductions in distant progression (18.3% vs. 10.9%; $P = .006$), PCSM (18.9% vs. 11.4%; $P = .005$), all-cause mortality (36.7% vs. 29.2%; $P = .041$), and event-free survival (28.8% vs. 36.0%; $P = .051$). The advantage observed with 6 months of neoadjuvant AST in TROG-96.01 appear to conflict with those of CUOG. However, TROG-96.01 consisted of over 80% of patients having high-risk disease, as compared with only 34% in the CUOG trial, so perhaps the benefit of longer duration of neoadjuvant hormones may only be applicable to those more likely to have micrometastatic disease. Furthermore, subgroup analyses from CUOG demonstrated that high-risk patients benefited from longer neoadjuvant AST in terms of biochemical control.

Based on the positive results of RTOG-8610, the Irish Clinical Oncology Research Group designed a randomized study comparing 4- and 8-months of neoadjuvant AST with external-beam radiotherapy.[118] Of the 261 eligible patients, 80% were considered high or very high risk as per the NCCN definition. Despite the high-risk cohort, pelvic radiotherapy was not mandated in the protocol. The total dose was 70 Gy. Median follow-up was 8.5 years. There was no significant difference between the two arms in terms of overall survival, PCSM, or biochemical control.

In summary, there are presently three phase III trials that have reported results evaluating the optimal duration of neoadjuvant hormonal therapy. The largest study, TROG-96.01 (n = 540), showed an advantage to longer duration neoadjuvant AST, whereas the other two trials (n = 261 and n = 378) did not show any difference, although subgroup analyses in the CUOG detected a significant difference in biochemical control among high-risk patients.[99,117,118] Completed accrual, RTOG-9910 compares 8 and 28 weeks of neoadjuvant total androgen blockade in intermediate-risk patients. With over 1,500 accrued patients, the results of this study will be eagerly anticipated. Until then, the available evidence remains conflicted.

Optimal Duration of Adjuvant Hormonal Therapy

As discussed above, the Quebec L-101 trial randomized 161 intermediate-risk patients to either radiotherapy alone, 3-months of neoadjuvant AST and radiotherapy, or 10-months of neoadjuvant, concurrent, and adjuvant AST with radiotherapy.[100,101] Although the two experimental arms had superior 7-year PSA control rates over the control arm, there was no difference between the two AST arms (69% vs. 66%; $P = .6$; Table 66.4).

TABLE 66.4 SUMMARY OF OUTCOME RESULTS FROM RANDOMIZED CONTROLLED TRIALS STUDYING THE DURATION AND SEQUENCING OF ANDROGEN SUPPRESSION THERAPY

Study (Reference)	*Median Follow-Up (Years)*	*Study Arms*	*10-Year Overall Survival*	*10-Year Cause-Specific Survival*	*10-Year Biochemical Control*
Duration of Neoadjuvant Trials					
CUOG (116,117)	6.6	XRT + NHT (3 mo)	81%[a]	94%[a]	58%[a]
		XRT + NHT (8 mo)	79%[a]	93%[a]	65%[a]
			($P = .7$)	($P = .24$)	($P = .18$)
TROG-96.01 (98,99)	10.6	XRT alone	58%	78%	26%
		XRT + NHT (2 mo), C-HT (1 mo)	63% ($P = .2$)	81% ($P = .04$)	40% ($P = .0009$)
		XRT + NHT (5 mo), C-HT (1 mo)	71% ($P = .0005$)	89% ($P = .0002$)	47% ($P < .0001$)
ICORG-97-01 (118)	8.5	XRT + NHT (4 mo)	85%[b]	93%[b]	66%[b]
		XRT + NHT (8m)	77%[b]	90%[b]	63%[b]
			NS	NS	NS
Duration of Adjuvant Trials					
RTOG-9202 (121,122)	11.3	XRT + NHT (2 mo), C-HT (2 mo)	52%	84%	32%
		XRT + NHT (2 mo), C-HT (2 mo), AHT (24 mo)	54%	89%	48%
			($P = .36$)	($P = .004$)	($P < .0001$)
EORTC-22961 (123)	6.4	XRT + C-HT (2 mo), AHT (4 mo)	81%	95%	69%
		XRT + C-HT (2 mo), AHT (34 mo)	85%	97%	81%
			significant[c]	($P = .002$)	significant[c]
Quebec L-101 (101)	5	XRT alone			58%
		XRT + NHT (3 mo)			76% ($P = .009$)
		XRT + NHT (3 mo), C-HT (2 mo), AHT (5 mo)	NR	NR	74% ($P = .003$)
Quebec L-200 (101)	3.7	XRT + NHT (3 mo), C-HT (2 mo)			70%
		XRT + NHT (3 mo), C-HT (2 mo), AHT (5 mo)	NR	NR	70%
					($P = .55$)[d]
Sequencing Trials					
RTOG-9413 (50)	5	WPRT + NHT (2 mo), C-HT (2 mo)	89%	NR	69.7%
		WPRT + AHT (4 mo)	84%		63.3%
		PORT + NHT (2 mo), C-HT (2 mo)	86%		57.2%
		PORT + AHT (4 mo)	87%		63.5%
			($P = .08$)[e]		($P = .048$)[e]

AHT, adjuvant hormonal therapy; C-HT, concurrent hormonal therapy; CUOG, Canadian Urologic Oncology Group; NR, not recorded; NHT, neoadjuvant hormonal therapy; PORT, prostate-only radiotherapy; RTOG, Radiation Therapy Oncology Group; TROG, Trans-Tasman Radiation Oncology Group; WPRT, whole pelvic radiotherapy; XRT, external-beam radiotherapy; ICORG, Irish Clinical Oncology Research Group; NS, not significant.

[a]CUOG results are for 7 years.

[b]Overall survival and cause-specific survival values are at 7 years, whereas biochemical control value was at 5 years.

[c]Noninferiority test was rejected ($P = .65$) for overall survival. For clinical pregression-free survival, P value was not mentioned.

[d]L-200 biochemical control (bNED) rates are for 4 years.

[e]RTOG-9413 outcome results are 4 years. bNED rates are actuarial, whereas overall survival rates are nonactuarial.

In the subsequent confirmatory trial by Laverdiere et al.[101] (L-200 study), 296 intermediate-risk patients were randomized to either of the two experimental arms of L-101. After a median follow-up of 3.7 years, the 5-year biochemical control was identical in both arms at 70%.

Also previously discussed, in the meta-analysis of five consecutive RTOG randomized controlled prostate cancer trials (including RTOG-8531 and RTOG-8610), 2,742 men were stratified into four previously identified risk groups based on Gleason score, clinical T stage, and pelvic nodal involvement.[119,120] Risk group 1 (i.e., "low risk") did not benefit from AST. However, risk group 2 (i.e., "intermediate risk") had significantly improved 8-year disease-specific survival from 83% to 98% (P = .003) with short-term AST. Risk groups 3 and 4 (i.e., "high risk") benefited from long-term AST; 8-year overall survival increased from 28% to 44%.

After RTOG-8610 demonstrated that short-term AST was beneficial, it served as the control arm in RTOG-9202, a phase III trial that sought to determine whether the addition of 24 months of adjuvant AST could improve outcome in high-risk patients.[121] There were 1,521 eligible patients, and whole-pelvic radiotherapy (44 to 50 Gy) and a prostate dose of 65 to 70 Gy were mandated. The median pretreatment PSA was 20.4 ng/mL, 55% had clinical T3 to T4 disease, and 14% had Gleason score 8 to 10 disease on central review. Ten-year results were recently published after a median follow-up of 11.3 years.[122] Aside from overall survival, all other end points were significantly in favor of the long-term AST arm: PCSM (83.9% vs. 88.7%; P <.0001), disease-free survival (13.2% vs. 22.5%; P <.0001), and biochemical control (31.9% vs. 48.1%; P <.0001). In subgroup analysis, again patients with a Gleason score of 8 to 10 had a significant improvement in overall survival with long-term AST but not Gleason score 2 to 7. The authors speculate that the absence in overall survival difference may be due to insufficient follow-up among patients with a Gleason score of 2 to 7.

EORTC-22961 was a phase III trial that compared 6 months with 36 months of adjuvant AST in 1,113 patients with locally advanced prostate cancer.[123] Reflecting this, the overwhelming majority of patients had clinical T3 disease (73%), with the remainder having T1c-T2b (3%), T2c (19%), and T4 (4%) disease. In contrast to RTOG-9202, which included patients with node-positive disease (3.5%), 8% of patients in EORTC-22961 had clinical or pathological node-positive disease. All patients received whole-pelvic radiotherapy (50 Gy), followed by prostate boost for a total prostate dose of 70 Gy. The median follow-up was 6.4 years. Five-year overall survival (81% vs. 85%), PCSM (95% vs. 97%; P = .002), and clinical progression-free survival (69% vs. 81%) were significantly improved with long-term AST. Gleason score did not impact the difference in overall survival.

Therefore, it appears that for intermediate-risk patients, short-term AST (3 to 4 months of neoadjuvant and concurrent) appears to be sufficient, whereas for high-risk patients, the addition of long-term (≥2 years) adjuvant AST appears to confer improved outcomes.

Radiation Volume and Hormonal Therapy Considerations

There have been 14 published phase III trials studying AST and radiotherapy. All five landmark trials—four RTOG studies and EORTC-22863—mandated pelvic radiotherapy.[47,95,97,121,124] Among these studies, the pretreatment characteristics were remarkably similar—median PSA >20 ng/mL and 20% to 30% with a Gleason score of 8 to 10. Applying the Roach formula[41] to calculate the estimated occult pelvic nodal involvement, this risk is probably at least 20%. In contrast, the two contemporary studies, BWH and RTOG-9408, did not use pelvic radiotherapy.[89,98] Their pretreatment characteristics were strikingly different from the landmark trials: PSA >20 ng/mL <13%, and 9% to 15% with Gleason score 8 to 10, respectively. The estimated pelvic nodal involvement is probably <15%. Thus, it appears that omitting pelvic radiotherapy in intermediate-risk patients will not deprive them of the benefits of AST. Indeed, the recently activated RTOG-0815 is evaluating the role of 6 months of hormones in the presence of dose-escalated radiotherapy to the prostate only.

Recommendations of Androgen Suppression Therapy

On the basis of 14 published phase III trials, there is currently level 1 evidence addressing the efficacy, duration, or timing of combining AST and radiotherapy. At UCSF, the authors' practices regarding integrating pelvic radiotherapy and hormonal therapy are summarized in Table 66.1. However, it is important to consider that all 14 trials used doses <72 Gy that would be considered suboptimal by today's standard. Whether the benefit of AST remains in the current era of dose escalation is currently unclear and is the basis of the recently activated RTOG-0815 and RTOG-0924 trials.

DEFINITION OF PROSTATE-SPECIFIC ANTIGEN RELAPSE AFTER RADIOTHERAPY

Given the natural history of prostate cancer and the fact that PSA relapse precedes clinical failure by a number of years, most oncologists use PSA relapse, rightly or wrongly, as a surrogate measure of the success of treatment. In 1996, the American Society for Therapeutic Radiology and Oncology (ASTRO) developed a consensus definition of PSA relapse based on datasets of patients treated with external-beam radiotherapy alone (i.e., no hormones).[125] However, because of a lack of any other definitions, the ASTRO definition has been inappropriately applied to series using hormonal therapy as well. The ASTRO definition has also been criticized for follow-up bias, censoring artifact from backdating, and poor correlation with clinical progression.[126,127] To address these issues, RTOG-ASTRO cosponsored a conference in 2005 in Phoenix, Arizona, to develop a new definition, henceforth known as the Phoenix definition.[128] PSA relapse is defined as a rise of 2 ng/mL or more above the absolute PSA nadir. This definition is only applicable to patients treated with external-beam radiotherapy with or without short-term hormonal therapy. The date of failure is taken at the time of meeting the definition and not backdated. Any salvage therapy initiated prior to meeting the criteria should also be declared as failure. With the Phoenix definition, sensitivity and specificity is 64% and 78%, respectively.

PREDICTIVE FACTORS AFTER POSTPROSTATECTOMY BIOCHEMICAL FAILURE

Local Versus Distant Recurrence

Positive surgical margins (PSM) and extracapsular extension (ECE) are associated with increased risk of PSA recurrence and presumed local recurrence.[129,130] Rates of PSM have been reported to be 5% to 53%, with variations due to surgeon experience, surgical technique, preoperative PSA, clinical stage, and ECE.[131,132] In a multicenter study of 5,831 men treated with radical prostatectomy from eight international institutions, the 5-year biochemical control rates were 83.8% and 53.1% for men with negative and PSM, respectively (P = .0001).[133] In an analysis of patterns of treatment failure in the study by the South West Oncology Group, SWOG-8794, a randomized trial evaluating adjuvant radiotherapy in patients with adverse pathologic features (pT3a-b or PSM), the predominant site of failure was local rather than metastatic.[134] Overall, local failure was observed in 22% and 8% of patients in the observation and adjuvant radiotherapy arms, respectively. In contrast, distant metastasis was observed in 16% and 7% of patients, respectively.

Many investigators have reported on the merits of Gleason score, time to PSA relapse, postradiation PSA nadir, and PSA doubling time (PSA-DT) after PSA failure as a predictor of distant metastases versus local recurrence and PCSM. Pound et al.[135] reported that time to PSA recurrence ≤2 years after surgery, Gleason score of 8 to 10, and PSA-DT ≤10 months predicted for metastatic disease. Lee et al.[136] reported similar findings, with a PSA-DT of <12 months and an interval of <12 months from end of radiotherapy to PSA rise as significant independent predictors of distant failure. In a multi-institutional analysis of 4,839 patients treated with radiotherapy alone, PSA nadir and time to PSA nadir were significant independent predictors of biochemical and distant failure-free survival.[137] Eight-year biochemical control was 75%, 52%, 41%, and 18% and distant failure-free survival was 97%, 96%, 91%, and 73% with a PSA nadir of 0 to 0.49, 0.5 to 0.99, 1 to 1.99, and ≥2 ng/mL, respectively (P <.0001). A nomogram incorporating PSA-DT has been created to predict risk of distant metastases.[138]

On the basis of these findings, D'Amico et al.[139] demonstrated that some of these prognostic factors could be used to predict for clinically insignificant postoperative PSA rises. A preoperative PSA <10 ng/mL, <T2a, Gleason score <7, and preoperative PSA velocity ≤0.5 ng/mL per year were associated with a postoperative PSA-DT ≥12 months or no PSA failure. Conversely, patients with a Gleason score of 7 to 10 and preoperative PSA velocity >2 ng/mL per year were associated with a postoperative PSA-DT <3 months. In the first scenario, the benign rise in PSA may represent residual benign prostate tissue, and thus salvage radiotherapy may not be required. In the latter scenario, more aggressive therapies such as hormonal therapy with chemotherapy should be offered on protocol. Although provocative, these results will need to be independently validated.

Prostate Cancer-Specific Mortality

Sandler et al.[140] observed that a PSA-DT of <12 months had significantly greater PCSM than when it was >12 months. A study from Johns Hopkins found similar results, with PSA-DT, Gleason score (≤7 vs. 8 to 10), and disease-free interval (≤3 vs. >3 years) independently associated with PCSM.[141] Compiled from two multi-institutional databases with a cumulative cohort of 8,669 men treated with surgery or radiotherapy, CaPSURE and CPDR, Zhou et al.[142] showed that a PSA-DT of <3 months (P <.0001) and Gleason score of 8 to 10 (P <.0001) were significantly associated with PCSM. Zelefsky et al.[143] reported that the postradiotherapy 2-year PSA nadir of ≤1.5 ng/mL was associated with a reduced risk of developing distant metastases and PCSM.

ADJUVANT RADIOTHERAPY

The argument for adjuvant radiotherapy (ART) is that patients with PSM or ECE after radical prostatectomy are at an increased risk of local recurrence. Yet it is also known that having either ECE or PSM does not necessarily mean that local recurrence is inevitable. Epstein et al.[144] reported on 617 men with clinically confined disease treated with radical prostatectomy and found that despite ECE, the 10-year progression-free survival was 58.4% to 67.7% depending on the extent. By the same token, 10-year progression-free survival was 54.9% in men with PSM. Progression was independently predicted by Gleason score, PSM, and ECE.

How common are PSM and ECE seen? In a large series from Memorial Sloan-Kettering Cancer Center and Baylor College of Medicine, the outcomes of 4,629 men with T1 to T3 prostate cancer were analyzed.[131] Overall, PSM were seen in 20% of cases (range 0% to 48%). ECE was observed in 30.1% of cases. When only surgeons who had contributed more than 10 cases were considered, the rate of PSM ranged from 10% to 48%. Independent predictors of PSM were PSA, Gleason score, ECE, the surgeon, and surgical volume.

When one considers that data from CaPSURE show that 49% and 23% of intermediate- and high-risk patients, respectively, had a radical prostatectomy from 1999 to 2001, the number of patients who potentially have PSM or ECE is by no means trivial.[145] Yet only 8% of high-risk patients who were operated on received ART.[146] The prevalence of understaging—deemed to be clinically organ-confined disease but later found to have pathologic stage T3 to T4 or node-positive disease—of prostate cancers was reported by Grossfeld et al.[147] to be 24%. Preoperative PSA, Gleason score, and percentage of positive biopsy cores were reported to be significant predictors of understaging.

Recently, the results of three large phase III trials, which evaluated the merits of adjuvant versus expectant management in postoperative patients with PSM or pT3 disease, were reported.[148–150] EORTC-22911 consisted of 1,005 men with pT2–3N0 and at least one of the following risk factors: ECE, PSM, or seminal vesicle invasion (SVI).[148] In the ART arm, radiation was commenced at a median of 90 days postoperative. ART consisted of 50 Gy in 25 fractions to a large volume that encompassed the surgical limits and subclinical disease, followed by 10 Gy boost given over 5 fractions to a reduced margin around the prostatic bed. The protocol salvage radiotherapy dose fractionation was 70 Gy in 35 fractions. Toxicity was surprisingly mild. Radiotherapy was interrupted due to toxicities in only 3.1%, with diarrhea responsible in 8 of the 14 patients. In the ART arm, grade 3 diarrhea (5.3%) and urinary frequency (3.3%) were relatively low; the only grade 4 toxicity was urinary frequency (0.4%). There was no added risk of urinary incontinence with ART. The 5-year rates of grade 3 late toxicities was 2.6% (delayed arm) and 4.2% (ART arm; P = .0725). Five-year biochemical progression-free survival was significantly improved from 52.6% to 74.0% (P <.0001) with ART, representing a 52% reduction in PSA relapse. The treatment benefit was significant for all postoperative prognostic factors, including negative surgical margins or absence of SVI and ECE. Five-year locoregional failure was significantly lower in the ART arm (5.4% vs. 15.4%; P <.0001). Of note, in the delayed arm, 163 of 207 (79%) patients who relapsed were offered active treatment, of whom 69% (n = 113) received radiotherapy and 28% received hormonal therapy. Treatment in the delayed arm was initiated upon PSA relapse (61.3%) and locoregional progression (34.4%) and was commenced at a median time of 2.2 years.

In a separately published subgroup analysis, Van der Kwast et al.[151] reanalyzed the results of EORTC-22911 after pathology review in approximately 50% of patients. Among the cohort of patients with a postoperative PSA <0.2 ng/mL, the presence of PSM had improved outcomes with adjuvant radiotherapy. However, in contrast to the original report by Bolla et al.,[148] those with ECE, SVI, or negative surgical margins did not benefit from adjuvant radiotherapy. When analyzed by margin status and treatment arm, there was no difference in 5-year PSA progression-free survival between the negative surgical margins in the delayed (67.4%) and adjuvant (76.2%) radiotherapy arms and the arm with PSM and adjuvant radiotherapy arm (77.6%). However, the arm with PSM and delayed radiotherapy arm (48.5%) was significantly inferior. The hazard ratio for treatment benefit in the group with negative margins was 0.87 (P = .6), whereas it was 0.38 (P <.0001) in the group with PSM. When analyzed by site of PSM, there was no significant difference in treatment effect (heterogeneity, P >.1), although there was a trend for a larger benefit in patients with both positive lateral and apex margins.

SWOG-8794 randomly assigned 425 node-negative patients initially treated with radical prostatectomy but found to have either PSM or pT3 (ECE and/or SVI) disease to ART or observation.[149] Central pathology review was performed in 73% of patients, and there was a 95% concordance with the community pathologist. Ninety percent of patients had ECE or PSM. Two-thirds of patients had a postoperative PSA <0.2 ng/mL. ART consisted of 60 to 64 Gy. Median PSA relapse-free survival was significantly longer with ART (10.3 vs. 3.1 years; HR 0.43; P <.001). Updated results were recently published with a median follow-up of 12.6 years.[152] The 10-year distant metastasis-free survival (71% vs. 61%; HR 0.71; P = .016) and overall survival (74% vs. 66%; HR 0.72; P = .023) were significantly improved with ART. The median distant metastasis-free survival was prolonged from 12.9 to 14.7 years with ART, and overall survival from 13.3 to 15.2 years. On subgroup analyses, there was no interaction between the adverse pathologic features and treatment effect, and therefore the benefit in distant metastasis-free survival was seen in all subsets. Among patients in the ART arm, those with an undetectable postoperative PSA had a significantly better 10-year distant metastasis-free survival (73% vs. 65%; P = .03) than those with a PSA >0.2 ng/mL. In the observation arm, only one-third of patients eventually received salvage radiotherapy, of which the median preradiotherapy PSA was 1.0 ng/mL. Hormonal therapy was initiated later (median 12.4 vs. 9.9 years) and less frequently (39% vs. 50%) in the ART arm. Complications observed in the ART arm included proctitis (3.3% vs. 0%), urethral stricture (17.8% vs. 9.5%), and total urinary incontinence (6.5% vs. 2.8%).

From the German Cancer Society, ARO-96–02/AUO-09/95 randomized 388 patients from 22 centers with pT3 or PSM with an undetectable postoperative PSA to either ART (60 Gy in 2 Gy fractions) or observation.[150] Patients who did not achieve an undetectable postoperative PSA were categorized as having progressive disease, excluded by the protocol, and given 66.6 Gy, regardless of the original randomization. Three-dimensional CRT was directed to the prostatic fossa and region of the seminal vesicles. Of the three phase III trials, this study had the shortest median follow-up of 54 months, but it mandated central pathology review. Using intention-to-treat analysis of only patients who achieved an undetectable postoperative PSA, ART significantly improved progression-free survival (P <.0001). When analyzed according to the received treatment, 5-year progression-free survival was 72% versus 54% in favor of ART (P = .0015; HR 0.53). ART was very well tolerated, with only 3% reporting acute grade 3 bladder toxicity and none with grade 3 rectal toxicity (12% had grade 2 rectal toxicity). Late grade 2 and 3 rectal toxicity was seen in 1.4% and 0%, and bladder toxicity was observed in 2% and 0.3%, respectively. Of note, the compliance in the ART arm was surprisingly poor—23% did not proceed with radiotherapy.

A significant limitation of these three clinical trials was that they were conducted prior to the current era of ultrasensitive PSA assays, which can detect PSA levels as low as 0.01 ng/mL. For instance, the ARO trial defined undetectable PSA as those <0.1 ng/mL, of which 59% had a PSA of >0.03 to 0.1 ng/mL. In the EORTC-22911 and SWOG-8794 studies, 11% and 34% of patients, respectively, had a postoperative PSA >0.2 ng/mL. In effect, a significant proportion of patients enrolled in these trials had "measurable disease" and thus received salvage radiotherapy.[153] Although there was an initial surge in enthusiasm in embracing ART, it has given way to increasing skepticism. Given the prevalence of ultrasensitive PSA assays, it is unclear whether a strategy of active surveillance with PSA tests and the early initiation of radiotherapy only when PSA has shown an upward trend can yield equivalent or better results. The advantage of such an approach is that perhaps the 50% of patients who do not relapse after surgery will be spared from radiotherapy. The disadvantage is that biochemical control and distant metastasis-free survival (SWOG-8794) may be compromised by waiting too long to intervene with definitive treatment, which could serve as a nidus for metastatic spread. In an editorial, King[153] showed that for every 0.1 ng/mL increment in postoperative PSA, there is an estimated 4% reduction in biochemical control. Nonetheless, the EORTC-22911, SWOG-8794, and ARO-96–02 provide consistent level 1 evidence that adjuvant radiotherapy is better than expectant management in terms of biochemical control, at an acceptable toxicity. It remains to be seen whether with longer follow-up this translates into an improvement in survival. Questions also remain whether the lessons learned from the definitive radiotherapy trials, such as pelvic radiotherapy, hormonal therapy, and dose escalation, have any role in the adjuvant setting. Three important studies that will hopefully address some of these questions are the RADICALS, EORTC-220433–30041, and RTOG-0534 phase III trials. RADICALS, an MRC and National Cancer Institute of Canada led phase III trial, randomizes postoperative patients to early postoperative radiotherapy or early salvage radiotherapy. RADICALS also has a hormone duration randomization substudy in which patients are randomized to radiotherapy alone or 6 months or 2 years of adjuvant hormones. EORTC-220433–30041 is accruing postoperative patients with adverse pathologic features to adjuvant 3DCRT/IMRT radiotherapy (64 Gy) with or without 6 months of adjuvant androgen suppression therapy. RTOG-0534 is a three-arm trial evaluating the role of short-term hormones (4 to 6 months) and pelvic radiotherapy in the salvage setting.

Adjuvant Versus Salvage Radiotherapy

As discussed earlier, the findings from EORTC-22911, SWOG-8794, and ARO-96–02/AUO-09/95 strongly advocate for the use of ART. Yet none of these trials address the concept of early salvage radiotherapy given when the PSA is still low. The attraction of this strategy is that only half of the patients with adverse pathologic features will relapse.[144] Furthermore, the observed benefit from adjuvant radiotherapy as compared to salvage radiotherapy may have been augmented by some patients in the adjuvant arms who would have been cured with surgery alone.

In a multi-institutional study, Stephenson et al.[154] constructed a nomogram based on the outcomes and prognostic factors of 1,540 men who had salvage radiotherapy after a biochemical recurrence. The median follow-up after surgery and salvage radiotherapy was 90 and 53 months, respectively. In the entire cohort, the 6-year progression-free survival (PFS) was 32%, and 59% attained a PSA nadir of ≤0.1 ng/mL. Six-year PFS was clearly improved with lower preradiotherapy PSA: ≤0.5 (48%), 0.51 to 1.0 (40%), 1.01 to 1.5 (28%), >1.5 (18%). The nomogram included Gleason score, preradiotherapy PSA, surgical margins, PSA doubling time, extracapsular extension, lymph node metastasis, neoadjuvant hormones, radiotherapy dose, and SVI associated with PSA progression. On subgroup analysis, 110 patients with no adverse prognostic factors had a 6-year PFS of 69%. Interestingly, the estimated outcome of subgroups of patients with seemingly adverse features even with early salvage radiotherapy—preradiotherapy PSA ≤0.5 ng/mL—is not as futile as once thought. In the cohort with PSA doubling time of ≤10 months or Gleason score 8 to 10, the 6-year PFS was 41%. Similarly, in the group that had Gleason scores of 8 to 10 but a PSA-DT >10 months and positive surgical margins, the PFS was 50%.

In a multi-institutional matched-control analysis, Trabulsi et al.[155] demonstrated that the 5-year freedom from biochemical failure from radiotherapy was significantly improved in the adjuvant group when compared with the salvage group (73% vs. 50%; P = .0007).

As it stands, we have only retrospective data that suggest that early salvage radiotherapy is more effective than later salvage radiotherapy, and this is likely due to reduced tumor burden.[154] Whether *early* salvage radiotherapy is as good as adjuvant radiotherapy is unknown. RADICALS is a very important MRC-led phase III, two-by-three factorial design trial. It poses two questions, of which one is the timing of postoperative radiotherapy (adjuvant radiotherapy or early salvage radiotherapy) in patients with adverse pathologic features after radical prostatectomy. Early salvage radiotherapy would be mandated in the event of biochemical failure, defined as either two consecutive rises in PSA and final PSA >0.1 ng/mL or three consecutive rises in PSA. The second question posed by the trial is whether the addition of hormones to radiotherapy would improve outcomes.

Androgen Suppression Therapy and Postoperative Radiotherapy

Based on the established benefits of adding hormonal therapy to definitive radiotherapy, some investigators have extrapolated those results to the postoperative setting.[156–159,160,161–163] Selected studies are summarized in Table 66.5 and are conflicting. All were retrospective studies, except for the subgroup analysis of RTOG-8531and RTOG-9601, with varying duration of hormonal therapy, median follow-up, and PSA failure definition.[156,164] In the nomogram by Stephenson et al.,[154] the addition of neoadjuvant hormones improved PFS.

In a subset analysis of RTOG-8531, 141 postoperative patients with histologically confirmed node-positive disease were randomized to postoperative radiotherapy with immediate or delayed hormonal therapy.[156] In the immediate hormone arm, the hormones were commenced in the last week of radiotherapy and continued indefinitely. This subgroup received 60 to 65 Gy (postprostatectomy) and 65 to 70 Gy (radical treatment) with optional nodal irradiation. With a median follow-up of 6.5 years, updated results demonstrated that immediate hormones improved 5-year biochemical progression-free survival (54% vs. 10%; P <.0001).[165] On multivariate analyses, immediate hormones was associated with improved overall survival, biochemical PFS, distant metastasis-free survival.

Initial results of RTOG-9601, a phase III trial salvage radiotherapy with or without 2 years of adjuvant 150 mg daily of bicalutamide, were recently presented.[164] The protocol mandates no pelvic irradiation and a total dose of 64.8 Gy given in 1.8-Gy fractions. With a median follow-up of 7.1 years, the 7-year freedom from PSA progression was significantly in favor of the bicalutamide arm (57% vs. 40%; P <.0001). Cumulative incidence of metastatic prostate cancer at 7 years was significantly less in the bicalutamide arm (7.4% vs. 12.6%; P <.04). There did not appear to be any added radiotherapy toxicities between the two arms.

As discussed above, three phase III trials—RADICALS, EORTC-220433–30041, and RTOG-0534—are currently accruing and will determine the role of adjuvant hormones with adjuvant or salvage radiotherapy. In summary, the evidence to date suggests that the inclusion of hormonal therapy to postoperative radiotherapy may be beneficial, although the optimal type of hormones, duration, and timing remains unknown.

Postoperative Radiotherapy Dose Response

Currently, adjuvant radiotherapy doses of 60 to 64 Gy and salvage radiotherapy doses of 66 to 70 Gy appear to be the most commonly used. Valicenti et al.[166] reported on a dose–response effect in 86 patients with pT3N0 prostate cancer. None of the patients received hormonal therapy. Radiotherapy was given between 3 to 6 months after surgery in 90% of patients. The radiation dose ranged from 55 to 70.2 Gy (median dose 64.8 Gy). Among the 52 patients with an undetectable preradiotherapy PSA, 3-year PSA control was significantly better in patients who received 61.5 Gy or more than in those who received a lower dose (91% vs. 57%; P = .01). In the 21 patients with a preradiotherapy PSA of 0.2 to 2 ng/mL, a dose–response cutoff was seen with 64.8 Gy (79% vs. 33%; P = .02). These results were corroborated by Anscher et al.,[167] who found that a salvage dose of more than 65 Gy was associated with improved disease-free survival.

In a study by King and Spiotto,[168] 5-year PSA control rates (58% vs. 25%; P <.0001) were improved with salvage radiotherapy doses of 70 Gy as compared with 60 Gy. Using tumor control probabilities, King and Kapp[169] demonstrated that the dose–response relationships of salvage radiotherapy were similar to that of radical dose radiotherapy, and current adjuvant or salvage doses of 60 to 66 Gy appeared to be in the steep portion of the curve. Arguing that late toxicities remain low in the randomized adjuvant radiotherapy trials,[149,150] King and Kapp[169] contended that adjuvant and salvage radiotherapy doses may be increased further, although they cautioned that this should be explored in the context of a clinical trial.

In a retrospective study by Cozzarini et al.,[170] 334 patients with adverse pathologic features and an undetectable postoperative PSA who received adjuvant radiotherapy were analyzed for a dose response. From 1993 to 2003, the radiotherapy dose gradually increased from 55.8 to 72 Gy. When stratified by dose (<70.2 Gy [median 66.6 Gy] vs. ≥ 70.2 Gy [median 70.2 Gy]), the high-dose group had significantly better 5-year biochemical relapse-free survival (83% vs. 71%; P = .001) and disease-free survival (94% vs. 88%; P = .005).

University of California–San Francisco Recommendations of Postoperative Radiotherapy

All patients with adverse pathologic features (i.e., ECE, PSM, SVI) should be assessed by a radiation oncologist. Depending on the preoperative clinical features, such as PSA kinetics, Gleason score, percentage of positive biopsy cores, and postoperative PSA nadir, a metastatic workup may be warranted, if it has not been done already. In addition, the authors recommend a transrectal ultrasound of the tumor bed to assess

TABLE 66.5 SELECTED STUDIES COMPARING THE BIOCHEMICAL DISEASE-FREE SURVIVAL BETWEEN POSTOPERATIVE RADIOTHERAPY ALONE OR WITH HORMONAL THERAPY

Study (Reference)	Hormone Duration (Months)	Number of Patients RT/RT + HT	Biochemical Disease-Free Survival: RT Alone (%)	RT + HT (%)
Eulau et al. (158)	6	74/29	27 (5 yr)	56 (P = .004)
Lawton et al. (165)	Indefinite	75/98	33 (5 yr)	54 (P <.0001)
Song et al. (161)	4	31/30	39 (4 yr)	39 (NS)
de la Taille et al. (157)	4–6	18/34	32 (3 yr)	61 (P = .03)
Taylor et al. (163)	24	36/35	54 (5 yr)	81 (P = .03)
Katz et al. (159)	3	70/45	39 (4 yr)	59 (NS)
King et al. (160)	4	69/53	31 (5 yr)	57 (P = .0012)
RTOG-9601 (164)	24	383/387	40 (7 yr)	57
Soto et al. (162)	0.9–34	107/334	55 (3 yr)	63

HT, hormonal therapy; RT, radiotherapy; NS, not significant.

and biopsy any residual prostate tissue. Patients with a postoperative PSA nadir <0.2 are offered adjuvant radiotherapy or active surveillance. In the latter option, patients return every 3 months for history and physical examination, digital rectal examination, and PSA measurement. If there is a clear rising trend in the PSA, salvage radiotherapy is offered.

Other important considerations are the patient's postoperative urinary function and estimated life-expectancy. The authors tend to favor delaying radiotherapy in patients with significant urinary symptoms or incontinence secondary to the surgery and patients with significant comorbidities such that the estimated life-expectancy is <5 to 10 years.

the authors recommend patients to undergo implantation of two fiducial gold seed markers into the bladder neck and anastomotic site.[171] For adjuvant patients, the authors prescribe 68 Gy, whereas for salvage patients, the authors use 70.2 Gy, both of which are in 1.8-Gy fractions. Whole-pelvic radiotherapy to a dose of 45 Gy is considered depending on the extent of pelvic lymph node dissection, presence of seminal vesicle invasion, and the estimated nodal involvement. The same technique as described earlier in this chapter is used. The authors recommend adherence to the RTOG consensus guidelines on the definitions of clinical target volume in the postoperative setting. With the initial results of RTOG-9601 supporting the addition of hormonal therapy, the authors recommend including adjuvant hormones for those at high risk of metastatic spread.[71]

SELECTED REFERENCES

A full list of references for this chapter is available online.

1. Jemal A, Siegel R, Xu J, et al. Cancer statistics, 2010. *CA Cancer J Clin* 2010; 60(5):277–300.
5. D'Amico AV, Whittington R, Malkowicz SB, et al. Biochemical outcome after radical prostatectomy, external beam radiation therapy, or interstitial radiation therapy for clinically localized prostate cancer [see comments]. *JAMA* 1998;280(11):969–974.
6. Zelefsky MJ, Leibel SA, Gaudin PB, et al. Dose escalation with three-dimensional conformal radiation therapy affects the outcome in prostate cancer. *Int J Radiat Oncol Biol Phys* 1998;41(3):491–500.
7. Mohler J, Armstrong AJ, Bahnson RR, et al. NCCN clinical practice guidelines in oncology; prostate cancer, v 2.2011. 2011. Available at: www.nccn.org/professionals/physician_gls/f_guidelines.asp
9. Prostate. In: Edge SB, Byrd DR, Compton CC, et al., eds. *AJCC cancer staging manual*. 7th ed. New York: Springer, 2010:457–468.
10. D'Amico AV, Schultz D, Silver B, et al. The clinical utility of the percent of positive prostate biopsies in predicting biochemical outcome following external-beam radiation therapy for patients with clinically localized prostate cancer. *Int J Radiat Oncol Biol Phys* 2001;49(3):679–684.
11. D'Amico AV, Whittington R, Malkowicz SB, et al. Clinical utility of the percentage of positive prostate biopsies in defining biochemical outcome after radical prostatectomy for patients with clinically localized prostate cancer [see comments]. *J Clin Oncol* 2000;18(6):1164–1172.
17. Hamstra DA, Bae K, Pilepich MV, et al. Older age predicts decreased metastasis and prostate cancer-specific death for men treated with radiation therapy: meta-analysis of Radiation Therapy Oncology Group trials. *Int J Radiat Oncol Biol Phys* 2011;81(5):1293–1301.
18. Wang-Chesebro A, Xia P, Coleman J, et al. Intensity-modulated radiotherapy improves lymph node coverage and dose to critical structures compared with three-dimensional conformal radiation therapy in clinically localized prostate cancer. *Int J Radiat Oncol Biol Phys* 2006;66(3):654–662.
21. Lawton CA, Michalski J, El-Naqa I, et al. RTOG GU radiation oncology specialists reach consensus on pelvic lymph node volumes for high-risk prostate cancer. *Int J Radiat Oncol Biol Phys* 2009;74(2):383–387.
22. Chen CP, Seo Y, Shinohara K, et al. Sentinel lymph node imaging guided IMRT for prostate cancer: preliminary analysis of a prospective study at UCSF. *Int J Radiat Oncol Biol Phys* 2011;81(2):S124.
23. Chan LW, Xia P, Gottschalk AR, et al. Proposed rectal dose constraints for patients undergoing definitive whole pelvic radiotherapy for clinically localized prostate cancer. *Int J Radiat Oncol Biol Phys* 2008;72(1):69–77.
24. Schallenkamp JM, Herman MG, Kruse JJ, et al. Prostate position relative to pelvic bony anatomy based on intraprostatic gold markers and electronic portal imaging. *Int J Radiat Oncol Biol Phys* 2005;63(3):800–811.
26. Moseley DJ, White EA, Wiltshire KL, et al. Comparison of localization performance with implanted fiducial markers and cone-beam computed tomography for on-line image-guided radiotherapy of the prostate. *Int J Radiat Oncol Biol Phys* 2007;67(3):942–953.
27. Langen KM, Willoughby TR, Meeks SL, et al. Observations on real-time prostate gland motion using electromagnetic tracking. *Int J Radiat Oncol Biol Phys* 2008; 71(4):1084–1090.
29. Xia P, Qi P, Hwang A, et al. Comparison of three strategies in management of independent movement of the prostate and pelvic lymph nodes. *Med Phys* 2010;37(9):5006–5013.
30. Rossi PJ, Schreibmann E, Jani AB, et al. Boost first, eliminate systematic error, and individualize CTV to PTV margin when treating lymph nodes in high-risk prostate cancer. *Radiother Oncol* 2009;90(3):353–358.
31. Chung HT, Xia P, Chan LW, et al. Does image-guided radiotherapy improve toxicity profile in whole pelvic-treated high-risk prostate cancer? Comparison between IG-IMRT and IMRT. *Int J Radiat Oncol Biol Phys* 2009;73(1):53–60.
34. Heidenreich A, Varga Z, Von Knobloch R. Extended pelvic lymphadenectomy in patients undergoing radical prostatectomy: high incidence of lymph node metastasis. *J Urol* 2002;167(4):1681–1686.
35. Allaf ME, Palapattu GS, Trock BJ, et al. Anatomical extent of lymph node dissection: impact on men with clinically localized prostate cancer. *J Urol* 2004;172 (5 Pt 1):1840–1844.
37. Holl G, Dorn R, Wengenmair H, et al. Validation of sentinel lymph node dissection in prostate cancer: experience in more than 2,000 patients. *Eur J Nucl Med Mol Imaging* 2009;36(9):1377–1382.
38. Weckermann D, Goppelt M, Dorn R, et al. Incidence of positive pelvic lymph nodes in patients with prostate cancer, a prostate-specific antigen (PSA) level of < or = 10 ng/mL and biopsy Gleason score of < or = 6, and their influence on PSA progression-free survival after radical prostatectomy. *BJU Int* 2006;97(6): 1173–1178.
39. Briganti A, Chun FK, Salonia A, et al. Validation of a nomogram predicting the probability of lymph node invasion among patients undergoing radical prostatectomy and an extended pelvic lymphadenectomy. *Eur Urol* 2006;49(6): 1019–1027.
41. Roach M 3rd, Marquez C, Yuo HS, et al. Predicting the risk of lymph node involvement using the pre-treatment prostate specific antigen and Gleason score in men with clinically localized prostate cancer. *Int J Radiat Oncol Biol Phys* 1994;28(1):33–37.
42. Abdollah F, Cozzarini C, Suardi N, et al. The indications for pelvic nodal treatment in prostate cancer should change. Validation of the Roach formula on a large extended nodal dissection series. *Int J Radiat Oncol Biol Phys* 2012;82(2):624–629.
43. Harisinghani MG, Barentsz J, Hahn PF, et al. Noninvasive detection of clinically occult lymph-node metastases in prostate cancer. *N Engl J Med* 2003;348(25):2491–2499.
46. Messing EM, Manola J, Sarosdy M, et al. Immediate hormonal therapy compared with observation after radical prostatectomy and pelvic lymphadenectomy in men with node-positive prostate cancer. *N Engl J Med* 1999;341(24):1781–1788.
49. Krengli M, Ballare A, Cannillo B, et al. Potential advantage of studying the lymphatic drainage by sentinel node technique and SPECT-CT image fusion for pelvic irradiation of prostate cancer. *Int J Radiat Oncol Biol Phys* 2006;66(4): 1100–1104.
50. Lawton CA, DeSilvio M, Roach M 3rd, et al. An update of the phase III trial comparing whole pelvic to prostate only radiotherapy and neoadjuvant to adjuvant total androgen suppression: updated analysis of RTOG 94–13, with emphasis on unexpected hormone/radiation interactions. *Int J Radiat Oncol Biol Phys* 2007;69(3):646–655.
51. Morikawa LK, Roach M 3rd. Pelvic nodal radiotherapy in patients with unfavorable intermediate and high-risk prostate cancer: evidence, rationale, and future directions. *Int J Radiat Oncol Biol Phys* 2011;80(1):6–16.
52. Pommier P, Chabaud S, Lagrange JL, et al. Is there a role for pelvic irradiation in localized prostate adenocarcinoma? Preliminary results of GETUG-01. *J Clin Oncol* 2007;25(34):5366–5373.
58. Pollack A, Zagars GK, Starkschall G, et al. Prostate cancer radiation dose response: results of the M.D. Anderson phase III randomized trial. *Int J Radiat Oncol Biol Phys* 2002;53(5):1097–1105.
59. Kuban DA, Levy LB, Cheung MR, et al. Long-term failure patterns and survival in a randomized dose-escalation trial for prostate cancer. Who dies of disease? *Int J Radiat Oncol Biol Phys* 2011;79(5):1310–1317.
60. Kuban DA, Tucker SL, Dong L, et al. Long-term results of the M.D. Anderson randomized dose-escalation trial for prostate cancer. *Int J Radiat Oncol Biol Phys* 2008;70(1):67–74.
62. Zietman AL, Bae K, Slater JD, et al. Randomized trial comparing conventional-dose with high-dose conformal radiation therapy in early-stage adenocarcinoma of the prostate: long-term results from proton radiation oncology group/american college of radiology 95–09. *J Clin Oncol* 2010;28(7):1106–1111.
63. Dearnaley DP, Sydes MR, Graham JD, et al. Escalated-dose versus standard-dose conformal radiotherapy in prostate cancer: first results from the MRC RT01 randomised controlled trial. *Lancet Oncol* 2007;8(6):475–487.
64. Beckendorf V, Guerif S, Le Prise E, et al. 70 Gy versus 80 Gy in localized prostate cancer: 5-year results of GETUG 06 randomized trial. *Int J Radiat Oncol Biol Phys* 2011;80(4):1056–1063.
65. Peeters ST, Heemsbergen WD, Koper PC, et al. Dose-response in radiotherapy for localized prostate cancer: results of the Dutch multicenter randomized phase III trial comparing 68 Gy of radiotherapy with 78 Gy. *J Clin Oncol* 2006;24(13):1990–1996.
66. Al-Mamgani A, van Putten WL, Heemsbergen WD, et al. Update of Dutch multicenter dose-escalation trial of radiotherapy for localized prostate cancer. *Int J Radiat Oncol Biol Phys* 2008;72(4):980–988.
67. Zelefsky MJ, Yamada Y, Fuks Z, et al. Long-term results of conformal radiotherapy for prostate cancer: impact of dose escalation on biochemical tumor control and distant metastases-free survival outcomes. *Int J Radiat Oncol Biol Phys* 2008;71(4):1028–1033.
69. Stephenson AJ, Scardino PT, Eastham JA, et al. Preoperative nomogram predicting the 10-year probability of prostate cancer recurrence after radical prostatectomy. *J Natl Cancer Inst* 2006;98(10):715–717.
71. Michalski JM, Bae K, Roach M, et al. Long-term toxicity following 3D conformal radiation therapy for prostate cancer from the RTOG 9406 phase I/II dose escalation study. *Int J Radiat Oncol Biol Phys* 2010;76(1):14–22.
72. Lee WR, Moughan J, Owen JB, et al. The 1999 patterns of care study of radiotherapy in localized prostate carcinoma: a comprehensive survey of prostate brachytherapy in the United States. *Cancer* 2003;98(9):1987–1994.
73. Sylvester JE, Grimm PD, Blasko JC, et al. 15-Year biochemical relapse free survival in clinical stage T1-T3 prostate cancer following combined external beam radiotherapy and brachytherapy, Seattle experience. *Int J Radiat Oncol Biol Phys* 2007;67(1):57–64.
75. Guix B, Bartrina J, Tello J, et al. Treatment of intermediate- or high-risk prostate cancer by dose escalation with high-dose 3D-conformal radiotherapy (HD-3D-CRT) or low-dose 3D-conformal radiotherapy plus HDR brachytherapy (LD-3D-CRT+HDR-B): early results of a prospective comparative trial. *J Clin Oncol* 2010; 28(15 Suppl):4633.
76. Morton G, Loblaw A, Cheung P, et al. Is single fraction 15 Gy the preferred high dose-rate brachytherapy boost dose for prostate cancer? *Radiother Oncol* 2011;100(3):463–467.

80. Kaprealian T, Weinberg V, Speight JL, et al. High-dose-rate brachytherapy boost for prostate cancer: comparison of two different fractionation schemes. *Int J Radiat Oncol Biol Phys* 2012;82(1):222–227.
81. Hoskin PJ, Motohashi K, Bownes P, et al. High dose rate brachytherapy in combination with external beam radiotherapy in the radical treatment of prostate cancer: initial results of a randomised phase three trial. *Radiother Oncol* 2007;84(2):114–120.
82. Martinez AA, Gonzalez J, Ye H, et al. Dose escalation improves cancer-related events at 10 years for intermediate- and high-risk prostate cancer patients treated with hypofractionated high-dose-rate boost and external beam radiotherapy. *Int J Radiat Oncol Biol Phys* 2011;79(2):363–370.
85. Hsu IC, Bae K, Shinohara K, et al. Phase II trial of combined high-dose-rate brachytherapy and external beam radiotherapy for adenocarcinoma of the prostate: preliminary results of RTOG 0321. *Int J Radiat Oncol Biol Phys* 2010;78(3):751–758.
86. Nag S, Beyer D, Friedland J, et al. American Brachytherapy Society (ABS) recommendations for transperineal permanent brachytherapy of prostate cancer. *Int J Radiat Oncol Biol Phys* 1999;44(4):789–799.
88. Bolla M, Gonzalez D, Warde P, et al. Improved survival in patients with locally advanced prostate cancer treated with radiotherapy and goserelin. *N Engl J Med* 1997;337(5):295–300.
90. Pilepich MV, Caplan R, Byhardt RW, et al. Phase III trial of androgen suppression using goserelin in unfavorable-prognosis carcinoma of the prostate treated with definitive radiotherapy: report of Radiation Therapy Oncology Group protocol 85–31. *J Clin Oncol* 1997;15(3):1013–1021.
91. Pilepich MV, Krall JM, al-Sarraf M, et al. Androgen deprivation with radiation therapy compared with radiation therapy alone for locally advanced prostatic carcinoma: a randomized comparative trial of the Radiation Therapy Oncology Group. *Urology* 1995;45(4):616–623.
92. Zietman AL, Prince EA, Nakfoor BM, et al. Androgen deprivation and radiation therapy: sequencing studies using the Shionogi in vivo tumor system. *Int J Radiat Oncol Biol Phys* 1997;38(5):1067–1070.
94. Bolla M, Van Tienhoven G, Warde P, et al. External irradiation with or without long-term androgen suppression for prostate cancer with high metastatic risk: 10-year results of an EORTC randomised study. *Lancet Oncol* 2010;11(11):1066–1073.
95. Pilepich MV, Winter K, Lawton CA, et al. Androgen suppression adjuvant to definitive radiotherapy in prostate carcinoma—long-term results of phase III RTOG 85–31. *Int J Radiat Oncol Biol Phys* 2005;61(5):1285–1290.
96. Roach M 3rd, Bae K, Speight J, et al. Short-term neoadjuvant androgen deprivation therapy and external-beam radiotherapy for locally advanced prostate cancer: long-term results of RTOG 8610. *J Clin Oncol* 2008;26(4):585–591.
97. Pilepich MV, Winter K, John MJ, et al. Phase III Radiation Therapy Oncology Group (RTOG) trial 86–10 of androgen deprivation adjuvant to definitive radiotherapy in locally advanced carcinoma of the prostate. *Int J Radiat Oncol Biol Phys* 2001;50(5):1243–1252.
98. Denham JW, Steigler A, Lamb DS, et al. Short-term androgen deprivation and radiotherapy for locally advanced prostate cancer: results from the Trans-Tasman Radiation Oncology Group 96.01 randomised controlled trial. *Lancet Oncol* 2005;6(11):841–850.
99. Denham JW, Steigler A, Lamb DS, et al. Short-term neoadjuvant androgen deprivation and radiotherapy for locally advanced prostate cancer: 10-year data from the TROG 96.01 randomised trial. *Lancet Oncol* 2011;12(5):451–459.
100. Laverdiere J, Gomez JL, Cusan L, et al. Beneficial effect of combination hormonal therapy administered prior and following external beam radiation therapy in localized prostate cancer. *Int J Radiat Oncol Biol Phys* 1997;37(2):247–252.
101. Laverdiere J, Nabid A, De Bedoya LD, et al. The efficacy and sequencing of a short course of androgen suppression on freedom from biochemical failure when administered with radiation therapy for T2-T3 prostate cancer. *J Urol* 2004; 171(3):1137–1140.
103. Granfors T, Modig H, Damber JE, et al. Long-term followup of a randomized study of locally advanced prostate cancer treated with combined orchiectomy and external radiotherapy versus radiotherapy alone. *J Urol* 2006;176(2):544–547.
104. D'Amico AV, Chen MH, Renshaw AA, et al. Androgen suppression and radiation vs radiation alone for prostate cancer: a randomized trial. *JAMA* 2008; 299(3):289–295.
105. Jones CU, Hunt D, McGowan DG, et al. Radiotherapy and short-term androgen deprivation for localized prostate cancer. *N Engl J Med* 2011;365(2):107–118.
108. Shahinian VB, Kuo YF, Freeman JL, et al. Risk of fracture after androgen deprivation for prostate cancer. *N Engl J Med* 2005;352(2):154–164.
110. Keating NL, O'Malley AJ, Smith MR. Diabetes and cardiovascular disease during androgen deprivation therapy for prostate cancer. *J Clin Oncol* 2006; 24(27):4448–4456.
111. Saigal CS, Gore JL, Krupski TL, et al. Androgen deprivation therapy increases cardiovascular morbidity in men with prostate cancer. *Cancer* 2007;110(7): 1493–1500.
112. Efstathiou JA, Bae K, Shipley WU, et al. Cardiovascular mortality after androgen deprivation therapy for locally advanced prostate cancer: RTOG 85–31. *J Clin Oncol* 2009;27(1):92–99.
113. Efstathiou JA, Bae K, Shipley WU, et al. Cardiovascular mortality and duration of androgen deprivation for locally advanced prostate cancer: analysis of RTOG 92–02. *Eur Urol* 2008;54(4):816–823.
116. Crook J, Ludgate C, Malone S, et al. Report of a multicenter Canadian phase III randomized trial of 3 months vs. 8 months neoadjuvant androgen deprivation before standard-dose radiotherapy for clinically localized prostate cancer. *Int J Radiat Oncol Biol Phys* 2004;60(1):15–23.
117. Crook J, Ludgate C, Malone S, et al. Final report of multicenter Canadian phase III randomized trial of 3 versus 8 months of neoadjuvant androgen deprivation therapy before conventional-dose radiotherapy for clinically localized prostate cancer. *Int J Radiat Oncol Biol Phys* 2009;73(2):327–333.
118. Armstrong JG, Gillham CM, Dunne MT, et al. A randomized trial (Irish Clinical Oncology Research Group 97-01) comparing short versus protracted neoadjuvant hormonal therapy before radiotherapy for localized prostate cancer. *Int J Radiat Oncol Biol Phys* 2011;81(1):35–45.
119. Roach M 3rd, Lu J, Pilepich MV, et al. Predicting long-term survival, and the need for hormonal therapy: a meta-analysis of RTOG prostate cancer trials. *Int J Radiat Oncol Biol Phys* 2000;47(3):617–627.
120. Roach M 3rd, Lu J, Pilepich MV, et al. Four prognostic groups predict long-term survival from prostate cancer following radiotherapy alone on Radiation Therapy Oncology Group clinical trials. *Int J Radiat Oncol Biol Phys* 2000;47(3):609–615.
121. Hanks GE, Pajak TF, Porter A, et al. Phase III trial of long-term adjuvant androgen deprivation after neoadjuvant hormonal cytoreduction and radiotherapy in locally advanced carcinoma of the prostate: the Radiation Therapy Oncology Group protocol 92-02. *J Clin Oncol* 2003;21(21):3972–3978.
122. Horwitz EM, Bae K, Hanks GE, et al. Ten-year follow-up of Radiation Therapy Oncology Group protocol 92–02: a phase III trial of the duration of elective androgen deprivation in locally advanced prostate cancer. *J Clin Oncol* 2008; 26(15):2497–2504.
123. Bolla M, de Reijke TM, Van Tienhoven G, et al. Duration of androgen suppression in the treatment of prostate cancer. *N Engl J Med* 2009;360(24):2516–2527.
124. Bolla M, Collette L, Blank L, et al. Long-term results with immediate androgen suppression and external irradiation in patients with locally advanced prostate cancer (an EORTC study): a phase III randomised trial. *Lancet* 2002; 360(9327):103–106.
128. Roach M 3rd, Hanks G, Thames H Jr, et al. Defining biochemical failure following radiotherapy with or without hormonal therapy in men with clinically localized prostate cancer: recommendations of the RTOG-ASTRO Phoenix Consensus Conference. *Int J Radiat Oncol Biol Phys* 2006;65(4):965–974.
129. Han M, Partin AW, Pound CR, et al. Long-term biochemical disease-free and cancer-specific survival following anatomic radical retropubic prostatectomy. The 15-year Johns Hopkins experience. *Urol Clin North Am* 2001;28(3):555–565.
130. Hull GW, Rabbani F, Abbas F, et al. Cancer control with radical prostatectomy alone in 1,000 consecutive patients. *J Urol* 2002;167(2 Pt 1):528–534.
133. Karakiewicz PI, Eastham JA, Graefen M, et al. Prognostic impact of positive surgical margins in surgically treated prostate cancer: multi-institutional assessment of 5831 patients. *Urology* 2005;66(6):1245–1250.
134. Swanson GP, Hussey MA, Tangen CM, et al. Predominant treatment failure in postprostatectomy patients is local: analysis of patterns of treatment failure in SWOG 8794. *J Clin Oncol* 2007;25(16):2225–2229.
139. D'Amico AV, Chen M-H, Roehl KA, et al. Identifying patients at risk for significant versus clinically insignificant postoperative prostate-specific antigen failure. *J Clin Oncol* 2005;23(22):4975–4979.
143. Zelefsky MJ, Shi W, Yamada Y, et al. Postradiotherapy 2-year prostate-specific antigen nadir as a predictor of long-term prostate cancer mortality. *Int J Radiat Oncol Biol Phys* 2009;75(5):1350–1356.
148. Bolla M, van Poppel H, Collette L, et al. Postoperative radiotherapy after radical prostatectomy: a randomised controlled trial (EORTC trial 22911). *Lancet* 2005;366(9485):572–578.
149. Thompson IM Jr, Tangen CM, Paradelo J, et al. Adjuvant radiotherapy for pathologically advanced prostate cancer: a randomized clinical trial. *JAMA* 2006;296(19):2329–2335.
150. Wiegel T, Bottke D, Steiner U, et al. Phase III postoperative adjuvant radiotherapy after radical prostatectomy compared with radical prostatectomy alone in pT3 prostate cancer with postoperative undetectable prostate-specific antigen: ARO 96–02/AUO AP 09/95. *J Clin Oncol* 2009;27(18):2924–2930.
151. Van der Kwast TH, Bolla M, Van Poppel H, et al. Identification of patients with prostate cancer who benefit from immediate postoperative radiotherapy: EORTC 22911. *J Clin Oncol* 2007;25(27):4178–4186.
152. Thompson IM, Tangen CM, Paradelo J, et al. Adjuvant radiotherapy for pathological T3N0M0 prostate cancer significantly reduces risk of metastases and improves survival: long-term followup of a randomized clinical trial. *J Urol* 2009; 181(3):956–962.
153. King CR. Adjuvant radiotherapy after prostatectomy: does waiting for a detectable prostate-specific antigen level make sense? *Int J Radiat Oncol Biol Phys* 2011;80(1):1–3.
154. Stephenson AJ, Scardino PT, Kattan MW, et al. Predicting the outcome of salvage radiation therapy for recurrent prostate cancer after radical prostatectomy. *J Clin Oncol* 2007;25(15):2035–2041.
155. Trabulsi EJ, Valicenti RK, Hanlon AL, et al. A multi-institutional matched-control analysis of adjuvant and salvage postoperative radiation therapy for pT3–4N0 prostate cancer. *Urology* 2008;72(6):1298–1302.
160. King CR, Presti JC Jr, Gill H, et al. Radiotherapy after radical prostatectomy: does transient androgen suppression improve outcomes? *Int J Radiat Oncol Biol Phys* 2004;59(2):341–347.
164. Shipley WU, Hunt D, Lukka H, et al. Initial report of RTOG 9601: a phase III trial in prostate cancer: anti-androgen therapy (AAT) with bicalutamide during and after radiation therapy (RT) improves freedom from progression and reduces the incidence of metastatic disease in patients following radical prostatectomy (RP) with pT2–3, N0 disease, and elevated PSA levels. *Int J Radiat Oncol Biol Phys* 2010;78(3):S27.
165. Lawton CA, Winter K, Grignon D, et al. Androgen suppression plus radiation versus radiation alone for patients with stage D1/pathologic node-positive adenocarcinoma of the prostate: updated results based on national prospective randomized trial Radiation Therapy Oncology Group 85–31. *J Clin Oncol* 2005; 23(4):800–807.
169. King CR, Kapp DS. Radiotherapy after prostatectomy: is the evidence for dose escalation out there? *Int J Radiat Oncol Biol Phys* 2008;71(2):346–350.
171. Schiffner DC, Gottschalk AR, Lometti M, et al. Daily electronic portal imaging of implanted gold seed fiducials in patients undergoing radiotherapy after radical prostatectomy. *Int J Radiat Oncol Biol Phys* 2007;67(2):610–619.

Chapter 67
Testicular Cancer

Gerard C. Morton

EPIDEMIOLOGY

Testicular cancer is the most common malignancy among young men in North America and most Western European Countries. More than 95% of testicular cancers are germ cell tumors, either seminomas or nonseminomas. Seminomas are most commonly diagnosed between the ages of 30 and 34 years, whereas nonseminomas are usually diagnosed 5 to 10 years earlier. It is estimated that approximately 8,300 new cases of testicular cancer are diagnosed annually in the United States, with 350 deaths.[1]

There is marked variation in incidence worldwide. The highest incidence occurs in Northern and Western European countries (up to 9 per 100,000) and the lowest in Asian and African populations (<1 per 100,000).[2,3] In North America, incidence rates are highest among Whites and lowest among Blacks, with an overall increase in age-adjusted incidence rate in the United States of 72% between 1975 and 2004.[4,5] A similar increased incidence has been reported in Europe and Australasia.[6–8] Despite the increased incidence of both seminoma and nonseminoma, there has been a significant reduction of mortality and improvement in survival. The most dramatic reduction in mortality occurred in the 1970s with the introduction of cisplatin-based chemotherapy.[9,10] The 10-year survival for seminoma increased from 81% in 1970–1979 to 95% in 2000–2002; that for nonseminoma increased from 54% to 92%.[11]

A history of undescended testicle has long been recognized as a risk factor for the development of testicular cancer. The testes develop in the abdomen before birth and normally descend into the scrotum. In cases of testicular maldescent, normal germ cell development is impaired and the testicle is prone to malignancy. There is also an increased risk of malignancy in the normally descended contralateral testicle. The relative risk is estimated to be 6 in the undescended testicle and 2 in the contralateral testicle.[12] The mechanism of the increased risk is unclear. It is hypothesized that a common etiologic agent predisposes both to testicular maldescent and subsequent malignancy. It is also possible that the maldescended testicle is subject to a hostile and malignancy-inducing environment.

The temporal and geographic variation in incidence rates strongly suggests environmental etiologic factors. Male infertility is associated with an increased risk of testicular cancer, and infertile men with abnormal semen analyses have a 20-fold greater risk of testicular cancer than the general population.[13] The increasing incidence has paralleled decline in semen quality over the past several decades.[14,15] This has led to the hypothesis that poor semen quality, testicular cancer, cryptorchidism, and hypospadias represent a testicular dysgenesis syndrome as a result of disruption of gonadal development during embryonal development.[16] Various exogenous hormonal disruptors (e.g., exogenous estrogens) have been proposed, although with no conclusive evidence implicating one particular agent.

Approximately 2% of patients report a positive family history. Sons of cases have a 4- to 6-fold increase in risk and brothers an 8- to 10-fold increase.[17] Several candidate genes have been proposed to explain familial testicular cancer; however, it is likely that no single genetic change explains most familial cases.

In summary, germ cell tumors are thought to arise in testes predisposed to the development of malignancy owing to a combination of familial predisposition and intrauterine hormonal imbalance, later compounded by environmental factors and manifested by impaired spermatogenesis.

PATHOLOGY

More than 95% of testicular neoplasms are germ cell tumors and are divided into seminomas and nonseminomas. Nonseminomas include embryonal carcinoma, yolk sac (endodermal sinus tumour), teratoma, choriocarcinoma, and mixed germ cell tumors. Intratubular germ cell neoplasia (IGCN) is the putative precursor of most germ cell neoplasms. Sex cord–stromal tumors make up the remaining 3% to 4% of testicular neoplasms, and most are benign (Table 67.1).

CLASSIFICATION OF TESTICULAR TUMORS

Germ Cell Tumors

Intratubular Germ Cell Neoplasia

IGCN is found adjacent to invasive germ cell tumors in >95% of cases. It is also found in all clinical groups known to be at high risk for testicular cancer development: cryptorchidism (2% to 4%), infertility (1%), ambiguous genitalia (25%), and contralateral testes of patients with testicular cancer (5%).[18] IGCN is characterized by seminiferous tubules showing decreased spermatogenesis in which the normal constituents of the tubules are replaced by abnormal germ cells with the appearance of seminoma cells. These cells stain strongly for placental alkaline phosphatase (PLAP), whereas normal germ cells are negative. IGCN has a 50% risk of developing into an invasive germ cell tumor within 5 years. It is hypothesized that the cells originate from primordial germ cells early during embryogenesis, possibly owing to an excess of estrogens. They likely remain within the seminiferous tubules in a dormant stage until puberty when replication begins, possibly as a consequence of raised sex hormone levels. Transition to an invasive germ cell tumor then occurs.

TABLE 67.1 CLASSIFICATION OF TUMORS OF THE TESTIS

Germ cell tumors
Intratubular germ cell neoplasia (IGCN)
Seminoma
Classic type
Spermatocytic type
Nonseminomatous germ cell tumors
Embryonal carcinoma
Yolk sac (endodermal sinus) tumor
Teratoma
Mature
Immature
Teratoma with malignant transformation (with somatic carcinoma or sarcoma)
Choriocarcinoma
Mixed germ cell tumors
Sex Cord–Stromal Tumors
Leydig cell tumor
Sertoli cell tumor
Granulosa cell tumor
Fibroma-thecoma stromal tumor
Sex cord–stromal tumor with annular tubules
Gonadoblastoma
Sex cord–stromal tumor unclassified type

SEMINOMA

Classic Type

Seminoma accounts for >50% of all germ cell neoplasms. Serum level of human chorionic gonadotropin (HCG) is elevated in 15% to 30% of men at presentation, related to the presence of syncytiotrophoblastic cells. These may be identified in 7% of tumors on routine hematoxylin and eosin sections or by immunoperoxidase stains in 24%. Serum alpha-fetoprotein (AFP) is not elevated in pure seminoma. Grossly, seminoma is a soft tan-colored diffused multinodular mass. Focal necrosis is sometimes present. A prominent lymphocytic infiltrate is commonly seen within the fibrous stroma. More than 90% of seminomas will stain positive for PLAP.

Spermatocytic Seminoma

Spermatocytic seminoma accounts for 2% of testicular tumors. It tends to occur in an older age group at a mean age of 54 years. It is important to differentiate spermatocytic seminoma from seminoma, as the natural history and treatment is quite different. Spermatocytic seminoma is confined to the testes and is cured by orchidectomy. Metastasis is rare. The cell of origin of spermatocytic seminoma is unknown. Unlike seminoma, it does not contain glycogen and stains negative for PLAP. In fact, many authorities believe that there is little to indicate that spermatocytic seminoma is of germ cell origin.[19,20]

NONSEMINOMATOUS GERM CELL TUMORS

Nonseminomatous germ cell tumors (NSGCTs) usually contain a mixture of germ cell types (embryonal, yolk sac, teratoma, and choriocarcinoma), although tumors comprised of just one component may be found. Embryonal carcinoma is the most common component in mixed tumors and AFP- and HCG-positive cells are present in 33% and 20%, respectively. Yolk sac tumors are associated with high levels of AFP and are the most common germ cell tumors of childhood. Teratoma is not associated with elevated AFP or HCG, and both mature and immature teratomas are considered malignant with ability to metastasize. Choriocarcinoma is the least common type of pure NSGCT and is present in about 4% of mixed tumors. It is particularly aggressive, almost always metastatic at diagnosis, and associated with high levels of HCG. Seminomatous components are also common in mixed tumors. Serum markers (AFP and HCG) are elevated depending on the relative germ cell elements present.

ANATOMY AND NATURAL HISTORY

In the developing embryo, the testes originate from the genital ridge located near the second lumbar vertebra. Accompanied by their blood supply and lymphatics, they descend into the scrotum via the inguinal canal. As a result, the primary lymphatic drainage from the testis is to the retroperitoneal lymph nodes. The lymphatic vessels first drain into the collecting trunks at the hilum of the testicle. These lymphatic trunks accompany the testicular artery, vein, and spermatic cord through the internal inguinal ring and then continue proximally to the retroperitoneal lymph nodes. The retroperitoneal lymph nodes are situated anterior to the T11 to L4 vertebral bodies, concentrated at the L1-3 level. On the left, the lymphatics drain primarily into the preaortic and para-aortic lymph nodes around the left renal hilum and from there to the interaortocaval nodes (Fig. 67.1A). On the right, the first nodes involved are usually in the precaval or interaortocaval region, followed by the preaortic lymph nodes (Fig. 67.1B). Contralateral spread is mainly seen with right-sided tumors and rarely with left-sided tumors.

From the retroperitoneal nodes, the lymph drains into the cisterna chyli, thoracic duct, posterior mediastinum, and left supraclavicular fossa. The thoracic duct drains into the left subclavian vein in the left supraclavicular region. In 5% to 10% of patients, drainage into the right supraclavicular area can occur.

Aberrant lymphatic drainage may occur in the event of previous scrotal or inguinal surgery. Hernia repair alters the drainage of the testicle. The testicular lymphatic vessels anastomose with the regional lymph vessels, resulting in drainage

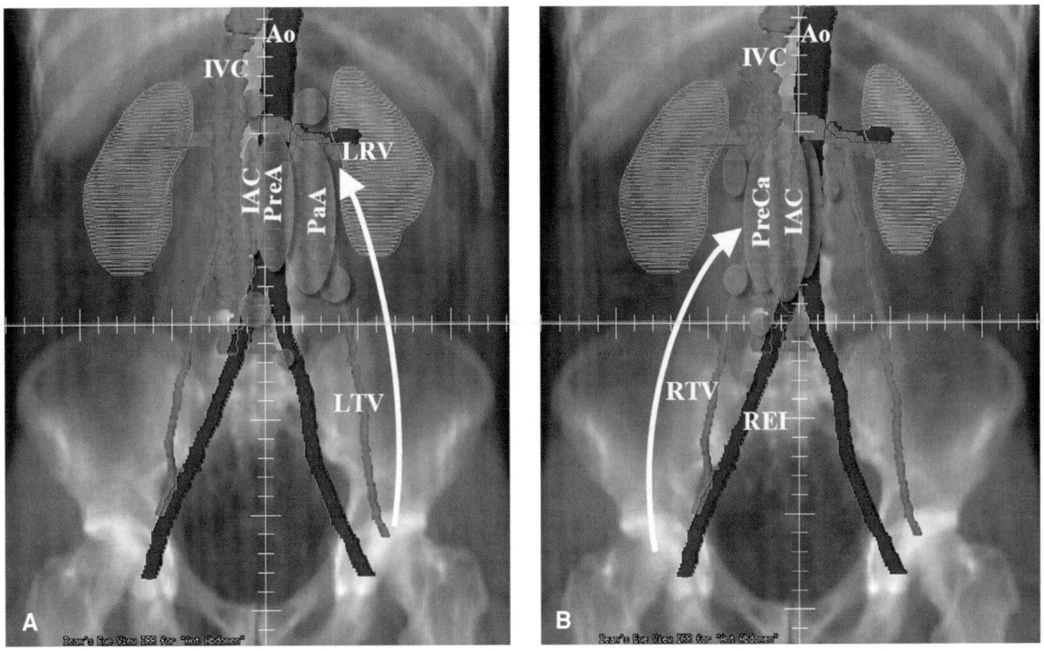

FIGURE 67.1. A: The left testis drains primarily by lymphatics along the left testicular vein (*LTV*) to lymph nodes inferior to the left renal vessels (*LRV*). Left para-aortic (*PaA*), preaortic (*PreA*), and interaortocaval (*IAC*) nodes are most commonly involved. Less commonly, nodal involvement may be found inferior to bifurcation of the aorta (*Ao*) or inferior vena cava (*IVC*), or superior to the renal vessels. **B:** Primary lymphatic drainage from the right testis (*arrow*) is along the right testicular vein (*RTV*) to precaval (*PreCa*) and then to interaortocaval and preaortic nodes. Less commonly, preaortic, right common iliac, or right external iliac (*REI*) nodes are involved.

into the ipsilateral inguinal and iliac lymph nodes. In addition, the testicular trunks may abandon the spermatic vessels at the internal inguinal ring and pass posteriorly and superiorly into the external iliac lymph nodes. The scrotum drains directly into the inguinal and external iliac lymph nodes.

Seminoma has an orderly and predictable pattern of spread. Locoregional lymphatics are the first site of metastatic disease. From the retroperitoneal lymph nodes, seminoma spreads proximally to involve the next echelon—the mediastinal lymph nodes—and then the supraclavicular lymph nodes. Very occasionally, metastases from retroperitoneal lymph nodes can drain directly via the thoracic duct to the supraclavicular fossa, resulting in supraclavicular metastases in the absence of mediastinal disease. Hematogenous metastases are rare in pure seminoma, being much more common with NSGCT. Lung is the most common site of distant disease, although bone, liver, and brain may also be involved.

CLINICAL PRESENTATION AND DIAGNOSTIC WORKUP

A testicular tumor usually presents as a painless swelling in the scrotum, although pain, heaviness, and tenderness at presentation are not uncommon. Disease in the lymph nodes of the retroperitoneum may produce back pain or abdominal swelling. Widely disseminated parenchymal disease in lungs, liver, bone, or brain is rare but, if present, may produce systemic symptoms. Gynecomastia is a rare presentation of embryonal carcinoma that may be seen in association with the very uncommon sex cord–stromal tumors. Occasionally, patients present with metastatic germ cell malignancies diagnosed by biopsy or elevated levels of serum tumor markers without evidence of a palpable mass in the testis. Occult primary disease in the testis is often detected by testicular ultrasound. If there is no evidence of a primary tumor in the testis, a diagnosis of an extratesticular germ cell tumor—usually mediastinal, retroperitoneal, or pineal—may be made.

DIAGNOSTIC WORKUP

The tests necessary to evaluate patients with testicular cancer are listed in Table 67.2. A complete history should be taken, including information about previous inguinal or scrotal surgery, cryptorchidism, retractile testes, and orchidopexy. The physical examination should pay special attention to possible sites of lymph node metastases. The contralateral testis should be examined clinically. The presence or absence of gynecomastia is an important observation. If testicular tumor is suspected, testicular ultrasound should be performed. This usually demonstrates a solid mass within the testis, often with associated testicular microlithiasis. Radical orchiectomy through an inguinal incision is diagnostic and removes the primary tumor.

TABLE 67.2 DIAGNOSTIC WORKUP FOR TUMORS OF THE TESTIS

General
History (document cryptorchidism and previous inguinal or scrotal surgery)
Physical examination
Laboratory Studies
Complete blood count
Biochemistry profile (including lactate dehydrogenase)
Serum assays
α-Fetoprotein (AFP)
β-Human chorionic gonadotropin (β-HCG)
Surgery
Radical inguinal orchiectomy
Diagnostic Radiology
Chest x-ray films, posterior/anterior and lateral views
Computed tomography (CT) scan of abdomen and pelvis
CT scan of chest for nonseminomas and stage II seminomas
Ultrasound of contralateral testis
Special Study
Semen analysis

Laboratory Studies

A routine complete blood count and chemistry screen, including renal function tests, should be done. Pulmonary or renal function tests should be performed for patients who may receive bleomycin or combination chemotherapy. NSGCTs of the testes are uniquely associated with reliable serum tumor markers: the β-subunit of human chorionic gonadotropin (β-HCG) and AFP. One or both of these serum markers are elevated in 80% to 85% of patients with disseminated nonseminomatous disease. The metabolic half-life of AFP is approximately 5 days and for β-HCG is approximately 18 to 24 hours. Although β-HCG may be modestly elevated in 15% to 30% of patients with pure seminomas, usually any elevation of AFP connotes nonseminomatous disease. Serum tumor markers may be elevated in other circumstances or conditions, such as laboratory error, cross-reactivity with luteinizing hormone, marijuana use, hepatitis, or development of antibodies to the glycoproteins. Serum lactate dehydrogenase (LDH), although nonspecific, is elevated in 80% of patients with advanced testicular cancer.

If a testicular cancer is suspected, serum tumor markers should be assayed before and after orchiectomy, and interpretation of the levels of markers should take into account their metabolic half-lives. Serum tumor markers can document persistent or recurrent cancer after surgery or chemotherapy and may predict the responsiveness of nonseminomas to treatment. The level of β-HCG should decrease by ≥90% every 21 days with each successful treatment cycle of chemotherapy. A slow decline in β-HCG after treatment may imply suboptimal response to chemotherapy, permitting early implementation of salvage therapy before the development of overt resistance to chemotherapy. The decline of AFP is less predictable.

Semen analysis and banking of sperm should be considered for patients in whom treatment is likely to compromise fertility. With newer technologies, it is possible to retrieve and bank sperm even with poorer-quality sperm.

Radiographic Studies

Investigations should routinely include chest x-ray films for all patients and computed tomography (CT) of the thorax for any patient with NSGCTs of the testis. CT scans of the abdomen and pelvis should be performed to evaluate the retroperitoneal nodal areas and assess the liver. CT of abdomen and pelvis relies on nodal size to assess the retroperitoneal nodes, with a sensitivity of 40% and a specificity of 95%.[21] There is considerable overlap between the size of normal and abnormal lymph nodes using a size limit of 10 to 20 mm. It therefore has limited ability to exclude the presence of disease, although enlarged lymph nodes in the appropriate clinical context (location, laterality, disease parameters) are very likely to be truly positive. Magnetic resonance imaging (MRI) appears equivalent to CT in determining the size and location of retroperitoneal adenopathy. Fluorodeoxyglucose positron emission tomography (FDG-PET) scan has a slightly higher sensitivity (66%) than CT with a comparable specificity (98%). It has little role in initial disease staging but may have a role where CT is questionable.[21] It is unable to detect lesions <5 mm in size or teratomas of any size owing to their very low metabolic activity. It also has an important role in evaluating residual retroperitoneal disease following chemotherapy.

Baseline ultrasonography of the remaining testis should be performed. If the contralateral testis is atrophic and the patient is <30 years of age, then there is a 30% risk of IGCN. Biopsy of the contralateral testis may be considered in this setting.

STAGING AND PROGNOSTIC FACTORS

Patients are staged according to the American Joint Committee on Cancer (AJCC) criteria as indicated in Table 67.3, which incorporates features of the primary tumor (T), node (N), metastasis (M), and level of serum tumor markers (S).[22] Approximately 80% of seminoma patients and 50% to 60% of nonseminoma patients have stage I disease at presentation. For stage I seminoma, tumor size and rete testis invasion are the most commonly reported predictors of recurrence. For nonseminomas, T-stage, extensive embryonal component, and lymphovascular invasion are prognostic. Age is an adverse prognostic factor for patients diagnosed with all stages of testicular cancer.[23]

The International Germ Cell Cancer Collaborative Group (IGCCCG) developed a widely accepted classification system for patients with metastatic germ cell malignancies, which has been incorporated into the TNM system[24] (Table 67.4). The prognostic classification is based on data collected on approximately 6,000 patients with metastatic germ cell tumor from 10 countries during the platinum era. The classification was internally validated as well as prospectively validated on a subsequent cohort of patients. The factors most strongly associated with a poor prognosis were mediastinal primary, nonpulmonary visceral metastases, or grossly elevated tumor markers (AFP >10,000 ng/mL, HCG >50,000 IU/L, or LDH >10 times normal).

TABLE 67.3 AMERICAN JOINT COMMITTEE ON CANCER 2010 STAGING FOR TESTICULAR CANCER

Primary Tumor (T) (Pathologic Classification)	
*p*Tx	Primary tumor cannot be assessed
*p*T0	No evidence of primary tumor (scar, etc.)
*p*Tis	Intratubular, noninvasive
*p*T1	Tumor limited to testis and epididymis, no vascular/lymphatic invasion
*p*T2	Tumor limited to testis and epididymis, with vascular/lymphatic invasion or involvement of the tunica vaginalis
*p*T3	Tumor invades spermatic cord
*p*T4	Tumor invades scrotum
Lymph Node (N)	
N0	No regional node metastasis
N1	Metastasis in single or multiple nodes ≤2 cm in greatest dimension
N2	Metastasis in single or multiple nodes 2–5 cm greatest dimension
N3	Metastasis in lymph nodes >5 cm in maximum diameter
Distant Metastasis (M)	
M0	No distant metastasis
M1a	Nonregional lymph node or pulmonary metastasis
M1b	Nonpulmonary visceral metastasis
Serum Tumor Markers (S)	
Sx	Serum tumor markers not performed
S0	Serum tumor markers within normal limits
S1	LDH <1.5 × N and HCG <5,000 and AFP <1,000
S2	LDH 1.5–10 × N or HCG 5,000–50,000 or AFP 1,000–10,000
S3	LDH >10 × N or HCG >50,000 or AFP >10,000
Staging Groupings	
IA	T1, N0, M0, S0
IB	T2-4, N0, M0, S0
IS	Any T, N0, M0, S1-3
IIA	Any T, N1, M0, S0/1
IIB	Any T, N2, M0, S0/1
IIC	Any T, N3, M0, S0/1
IIIA	Any T, Any N, M1a, S0/1
IIIB	Any T, Any N, M1a, S2
IIIC	Any T, Any N, M1b or S3

LDH, lactate dehydrogenase; N, node; HCG, human chorionic gonadotropin; AFP, alpha-fetoprotein.

Used with the permission of the American Joint Committee on Cancer (AJCC), Chicago, Illinois. The original source for this material is the AJCC *Cancer Staging Manual,* 7th Edition (2010) published by Springer Science and Business Media LLC, www.springer.com.

TABLE 67.4 INTERNATIONAL GERM CELL CANCER COLLABORATIVE GROUP CONSENSUS CLASSIFICATION OF METASTATIC GERM CELL CANCER[a]

Nonseminoma	*Seminoma*
Good prognosis group with all of:	
Testis/retroperitoneal primary	Any primary site
No nonpulmonary visceral metastases	No nonpulmonary visceral metastases
AFP <1,000 ng/mL	Normal AFP
HCG <5,000 IU/L	Any HCG
LDH <1.5 × normal	Any LDH
Intermediate prognosis group with all of:	
Testis/retroperitoneal primary	Any primary site
No nonpulmonary visceral metastases	Nonpulmonary visceral metastases
Intermediate markers:	
AFP >1,000 and <10,000 ng/mL *or*	Normal AFP
HCG >5,000 and <50,000 IU/L *or*	Any HCG
LDH >1.5× and <10× normal	Any LDH
Poor prognosis group with any of:	
Mediastinal primary *or*	
Nonpulmonary visceral metastases *or*	
AFP >10,000 ng/mL	
HCG >50,000 IU/L *or*	
LDH >10× normal	

AFP, alpha-fetoprotein; HCG, human chorionic gonadotropin; LDH, lactate dehydrogenase.

[a]Survival at 5 years is approximately 91%, 80%, and 50% for good, intermediate, and poor prognostic groups, respectively.

From International Germ Cell Consensus Classification: a prognostic factor-based staging system for metastatic germ cell cancers. International Germ Cell Cancer Collaborative Group. *J Clin Oncol* 1997;15(2):594–603.

Patients with NSGCT were divided into three prognostic groups (good, intermediate, and poor prognosis) and seminomas into either good or intermediate prognostic groups (Table 67.3). The good prognosis group comprised >50% of all patients with metastatic NSGCTs and 90% of seminomas and was associated with a 5-year survival >90%. The intermediate prognosis group comprised 25% to 30% of patients and had a 5-year survival of 80%. The poor prognosis group comprised 15% to 20% of patients with NSGCT and had a 5-year survival of approximately 50%.

GENERAL MANAGEMENT

The initial management of a suspected malignant germ cell tumor of the testis consists of obtaining serum AFP and β-HCG measurements and then performing a radical (inguinal) orchiectomy with division of the spermatic cord at the internal inguinal ring. Historically, it had been thought that scrotal violation (transscrotal orchiectomy, open testicular biopsy, or fine-needle aspiration) compromised prognosis. Scrotal violation is associated with a slight increase in local recurrence rate compared with inguinal orchiectomy (2.9% vs. 0.4%, respectively) but is not associated with any difference in distant recurrence rates or overall survival.[25] Orchiectomy is both diagnostic and therapeutic. Further management depends on pathologic diagnosis and the stage and extent of disease. Radiation treatment plays a significant role in the management of seminomas. Nonseminomatous tumors are generally managed by cisplatin-based combination chemotherapy and/or surgical resection.[26] A detailed discussion of the management of nonseminomatous tumors is beyond the scope of this chapter.

SEMINOMA

Stage I

Patients with stage I seminoma have a risk of relapse of approximately 20%. Either adjuvant radiotherapy or adjuvant chemotherapy with single-agent carboplatin is associated

TABLE 67.5 PATTERNS OF RECURRENCE FOR STAGE I SEMINOMA MANAGED BY SURVEILLANCE

Author (Reference)	Number	Median Follow-Up (Months)	Relapse-Free Survival (%)	Proportion Relapsing in Retroperitoneum (%)	Disease-Specific Survival (%)	Median Time to Relapse (Months)
Kollmannsberger et al. (30)	313	34	81	–	100	14
Von der Maase et al. (31)	261	48	80	94	99	14
Chung et al. (32)	203	110	82	91	99.5	17
Francis et al. (33)	120	55	82	94	100	4
Daugaard et al. (34)	394	60	83	87	100	13
Choo et al. (35)	88	145	80	76	100	14
Cummins et al. (36)	164	160	87	82	98.7	16
Aparico et al. (37)	143	52	84	84	100	11
Kamba et al. (38)	186	45	79	79	100	21
Tandstad et al. (39)	512	60	86	94	99.8	17

with a disease-free survival >95% and disease-specific survival approaching 100%.[27] Surveillance, with treatment at time of relapse, is associated with a similar survival outcome and allows 80% of patients to avoid morbidity of treatment.[28]

Surveillance

Surveillance has become the management strategy of choice for most men with stage I seminoma. A survey of Canadian radiation oncologists in 2006 revealed that 56% felt surveillance was the preferred management.[29] Kollmansberger et al.[30] document increasing use of surveillance for managing patients with stage I seminoma in a population-based cohort from British Columbia, Canada, and Oregon. Between 1999 and 2008, the proportion of patients receiving adjuvant radiotherapy decreased from 50% to 9%, and the proportion being managed by surveillance increased from 47% to 87%.

The reported series (Table 67.5) include >2,400 patients, and all report similar rates, timing, and patterns of recurrence.[30–39] When managed by surveillance, 20% of patients will relapse at a median time of around 14 months. In the series of 394 patients from Copenhagen, Denmark, median time to relapse was 13 months, with 87% occurring within the first 2 years and only 2% beyond 5 years. Choo et al.[35] reported similar results from Toronto, with a median time to relapse of 13.6 months and only 2 of 88 patients relapsing after 5 years. In the Princess Margaret Hospital (PMH) series, the risk of relapse between 5 and 10 years was 4%. Given the small event rate in the individual reports, Warde et al.[40] performed a pooled analysis from four series (PMH, Royal Marsden Hospital [RMH], Royal London Hospital, and the Danish Testicular Cancer Study Group). Individual patient data on 638 stage I seminoma patients managed by surveillance was obtained. With a median follow-up time of 7 years, the 5- and 10-year relapse-free rates were 82.3% and 78.7%, respectively. Most relapses (69%) occurred within the first 2 years of surgery, whereas 7% relapsed beyond 6 years. The 5-year cause-specific survival was 99.3%. This data is consistent with large population-based reports from Kollmansberger et al.[30] and Tandstad et al.[39]

The predominant site of relapse is in the retroperitoneum (76% to 94%). Approximately 5% to 15% of patients relapse in the mediastinum or lungs, with inguinal relapse reported in 3% to 11%, usually only after previous scrotal interference. Some variability is reported in management at time of relapse. Traditionally, most (74% to 82% of patients in the older series) were initially managed by radiation therapy, with a second relapse occurring in about 10% (6% to 16%). Second relapse almost always occurred at distant sites with a 90% to 95% rate of successfully salvage with chemotherapy. More recent series describe a greater use of chemotherapy as initial salvage treatment. In the population-based study from the Swedish Norwegian Testicular Cancer Study Group, cisplatin-based combination chemotherapy as salvage treatment was given to 89% of relapsing patients,[39] with further relapse in only 1 of 58 patients. Kollmansberger et al.[30] report the use of salvage chemotherapy in 68% of relapsing patients in the British Columbia and Oregon Testis Cancer Program database. No further relapse occurred in the 32 patients managed by chemotherapy, whereas relapse occurred in 3 of 15 patients who received salvage radiotherapy. Although salvage chemotherapy is effective, it is associated with greater toxicity than salvage radiotherapy.

In the pooled analysis,[40] tumor size, rete testis invasion, and lymphovascular invasion were predictive of relapse on univariate analysis. On multivariate analysis, tumor size (hazard ratio [HR] 2.0) and rete testis invasion (HR 1.7) remained significant. The relapse-free rate decreased from 87.8% for tumors <4 cm without rete testis invasion to 68.5% for tumors >4 cm with rete testis invasion. These risk factors, however, have not been validated on subsequent patient cohorts. Tyldesley et al.[41] also noted the importance of size >4 cm and rete testis invasion, reporting a 5-year relapse-free rate of 86%, 71% and 50% in patients with no risk factor, one risk factor, or both risk factors, respectively. Choo et al.[35] reported a reduction in 10-year relapse-free rate from 86% to 52% with rete testis invasion. However, the large population-based report from Tandstad et al.[39] failed to identify tumor size, vascular invasion, patient age, or elevated HCG as prognostic factors. Rete testis invasion was not routinely documented.

Given the varying relapse risk with time and patterns of recurrence, a reasonable surveillance policy involves four monthly assessments in the first 2 years, six monthly assessments in years 3 and 4, and annual assessments in years 5 to 10.[42] Assessment should include physical examination and CT scan of abdomen and pelvis. Although chest x-ray is also usually included, in the large series of 527 patients from PMH, all but one of the relapses was detected on abdominopelvic CT scan.[43] No relapse was detected on chest x-ray alone, and the authors suggest omitting routine chest imaging from the follow-up schedule. The use of low-dose CT[44] imaging or MRI is being investigated to further reduce long-term radiation exposure.

Surveillance is a slightly more costly approach to management than adjuvant nodal irradiation owing to the increased number of radiologic investigations.[33–45] Surveillance should be contemplated and conducted only with a compliant patient and with an understanding that because of the risk of late relapse, the patient should be monitored for at least 10 years. The survival rate of 99.5% from the large surveillance series indicates that this therapeutic option produces a result equivalent to that achieved with immediate adjuvant treatment and is a safe and effective alternative management, provided that guidelines are followed.

Adjuvant Radiotherapy

Historically, the standard postoperative management of patients with stage I seminoma has been adjuvant radiotherapy to the para-aortic and ipsilateral pelvic lymph nodes (the "dog-leg" or "hockey stick" radiation field). This is a highly effective treatment, with a reported relapse rate between 1% and 5% and a disease-specific survival of 100% in many mature series[39,46–55] (Table 67.6) and no need for ongoing abdominal imaging.[56] With the realization that most of the relapses

TABLE 67.6 RATE OF RELAPSE AND LOCATION FOR STAGE I SEMINOMA MANAGED BY ADJUVANT RADIOTHERAPY

Author (Reference)	Number	Median Follow-Up (Years)	Radiation Dose (Gy)	Fields	Number Relapsing	Para-aortic	Pelvic/Inguinal	Distant	Cause-Specific Survival (%)
Tandstad et al. (39)	481	6.1	25.2	DL	4 (0.8%)	2	0	2	100
Fossa et al. (46)	365	9.1	36–40	DL	13 (4%)	1	7	6	99
Bauman et al. (47)	169	7.5	30	DL	5 (3%)	1	0	4	100
Logue et al. (48)	431	5.2	20	PA	15 (3%)	1	9	5	99
Santoni et al. (49)	487	10	30	DL, PA	21 (4%)	4	8	9	–
Niazi et al. (50)	71	6.25	25	PA	1 (1%)	0	1	0	100%
Melchior et al. (51)	87	7.7	36	DL	3 (3%)	0	0	3	100%
Classen et al. (52)	721	5.1	26	PA	26 (4%)	6	21	5	99.6
Bruns et al. (53)	80	7.1	20	Mini PA	4 (5%)	1	3	0	100
Jones et al. (54)	313	5.1	30	PA (88%)	10 (3%)	2	6	2	100
	312		20	PA (89%)	11 (3%)	1	3	7	99.7
Oliver et al. (55)	904	6.5	20–30	PA (86%)	33 (4%)	3	11	19	99.9
Fossa et al. (57)	236	4.5	30	DL	9 (4%)	0	0	9	100
	242			PA	9 (4%)	2	4	6	99.3

DL, dog-leg; PA, para-aortic.

on surveillance occur in the para-aortic region, many have adopted smaller target volumes to reduce treatment toxicity. Series that treat just the para-aortics report a higher rate of failure in the pelvic nodes; however, the disease-free survival is minimally compromised. Classen et al.[52] reported a single-arm trial of para-aortic radiotherapy by the German Testicular Cancer Study Group, which included 721 patients with stage I seminoma. Disease-free survival at 8 years was 95%. Of 26 recurrences, 21 were within infradiaphragmatic lymph nodes beyond the treatment volume (mostly ipsilateral pelvic), with no in-field recurrences. The Medical Research Council (MRC) performed a randomized controlled trial comparing classic dog-leg irradiation to para-aortic irradiation in stage I seminoma.[57] Those with previous ipsilateral inguinal or scrotal surgery were excluded. Radiotherapy was better tolerated in the para-aortic-alone arm with a reduction in the severity and frequency of acute gastrointestinal and hematologic toxicity. At a median follow-up of 4.5 years, there was no difference in the 3-year relapse-free survival or overall survival. For those in the para-aortic radiotherapy arm, the pelvis was the most frequent site of recurrence, whereas the pelvis was a rare site of recurrence in those in the para-aortic and ipsilateral pelvic radiotherapy arm. A retrospective review showed that the median size of pelvic nodal recurrence was 7.3 cm (range, 2.8 to 13 cm) if CT scans were not included in the follow-up schedule of patients treated with para-aortic radiotherapy.[58]

Given that nearly all recurrences following para-aortic radiotherapy are in the lower common iliac or upper external iliac nodes, a common approach is to use a modified dog-leg wherein the inferior border is placed at the mid-pelvic level. This encompasses the nodal areas at risk while further reducing volume of normal tissue irradiated.

Adjuvant Chemotherapy

Adjuvant chemotherapy using single-agent carboplatin is proposed as a less toxic approach than radiotherapy for stage I seminoma. For men with advanced seminoma, carboplatin has long been known to have significant efficacy with relatively low toxicity.[59] It was logical to investigate the use of one or two cycles of carboplatin as adjuvant treatment following orchiectomy.[60–62] With a median follow-up of 75 months, Steiner et al.[63] reported a 5-year relapse-free survival of 98.1% in a population of 276 men with stage I seminoma treated with two cycles of carboplatin. Aparicio et al.[37] described a risk-adaptive strategy wherein patients with stage I seminoma deemed at low risk of recurrence were managed with surveillance and those considered at higher risk based on large tumor size or rete testis invasion received two cycles of carboplatin. With a median follow-up of 34 months, the 5-year disease-free survival following carboplatin was 96.2%. Recurrence following adjuvant carboplatin tends to be in the retroperitoneum and is readily salvaged with cisplatin-based chemotherapy, resulting in an overall disease-specific survival approaching 100%. Between 2001 and 2006, the use of single-course carboplatin following orchiectomy for stage I seminoma increased from 0% to 70% in Sweden and Norway.[39] Over the same time period, the use of adjuvant radiotherapy decreased from 40% to 5%. The relapse risk with chemotherapy was higher than that following radiotherapy (3.9% vs. 0.8%); however, overall survival was the same. In the British Columbia/Oregon database,[30] 73 patients received either one or two cycles of carboplatin, with only one relapse, yielding a relapse-free survival probability of 98% and a cause-specific survival of 100%.

The MRC has performed a randomized comparison of single-agent carboplatin and nodal irradiation in stage I seminoma.[55] Almost 1,500 patients from 14 European countries were randomized to receive either adjuvant radiotherapy or one injection of carboplatin. Radiation was limited to para-aortic fields in 87%, and the remainder also had inclusion of the ipsilateral pelvic nodes. With a median follow-up time of 6.5 years, the 5-year relapse-free survival rates were similar at 96.0% and 94.7% in the radiotherapy and carboplatin arms, respectively. In the adjuvant radiotherapy arm, the most common site of recurrence was either distant (57%) or in the pelvic nodes (31%). In the carboplatin arm, most of the relapses (74%) were in para-aortic nodes. Only one death from testicular cancer occurred in the radiotherapy group, with no cancer-related deaths in the chemotherapy group. An 80% reduction in the rate of contralateral testicular cancer was seen in the carboplatin arm (2 vs. 15 cases). Long-term toxicity (e.g., risk of leukemia) is unknown; however, the regimen is well tolerated acutely with only mild myelotoxicity. Powles et al.[64] found no increased risk of death from circulatory disease or risk of second malignancy in a cohort of 199 patients who received adjuvant carboplatin and were followed for a median of 9 years.

Mead et al.[27] analyzed mature results of three randomized noninferiority MRC clinical trials for stage I seminoma, which included nearly 2,500 patients. They concluded that either radiation therapy or carboplatin was a reasonable adjuvant therapy. It is clear that the survival of patients with stage I seminoma approaches 100%, no matter what treatment strategy is employed. The goal of management is to limit treatment morbidity without compromising chance of cure. For the compliant patient, surveillance is probably the option of choice. For patients not suitable for surveillance, adjuvant radiotherapy or adjuvant chemotherapy significantly reduces the risk of relapse. There is, however, limited data on the long-term efficacy or toxicity of adjuvant carboplatin. Furthermore, ongoing surveillance of the retroperitoneal nodes will still be required.

TABLE 67.7 RELAPSE RATE FOLLOWING INFRADIAPHRAGMATIC +/– MEDIASTINAL RADIOTHERAPY BY NODAL STAGE FOR STAGE II SEMINOMA

	Stage IIA (≤2 cm)		Stage IIB (2–5 cm)		Stage IIC (>5 cm)	
Author (Reference)	N	Relapses	N	Relapses	N	Relapses
Bauman et al. (47)	29	2	10	1	4	2
Chung et al. (65)	49	4	30	4	16	10
Classen et al. (66)	66	2	21	2	–	–
Zagars et al. (67)	6	0	38	5	25	3
Patterson et al. (68)	46	6	34	9	–	–
Whipple et al. (69)	31	2	14	3	–	–
Vallis et al. (70)	26	1	22	2	5	2
Dosmann & Zagars (71)	55	7	13	4	–	–
Mason & Kearsley (72)	–	–	25	1	24	6
Evensen et al. (73)	6	0	18	1	49	11
Total	**314**	**24 (8%)**	**225**	**32 (14%)**	**123**	**34 (28%)**

Stage II

For patients with stage II seminoma, the recommended treatment depends on the bulk of retroperitoneal nodal disease. Radiotherapy to 25 to 35 Gy is the treatment of choice for patients with stage IIA or IIB seminoma (nodal disease ≤5 cm in maximal diameter). Irradiation of the para-aortic and ipsilateral pelvic nodes is a highly effective treatment strategy with a recurrence rate <10% (Table 67.7) and a disease-specific survival rate of 97% to 100%.[47,65–73] The most common site of relapse following infradiaphragmatic radiotherapy is in the supraclavicular fossa or mediastinum. In the past, some authors[67] recommended prophylactic supraclavicular irradiation. However, the proportion of patients destined to relapse exclusively in the supraclavicular fossa is <5%, and results with infradiaphragmatic irradiation alone with chemotherapy as salvage are excellent.[74]

Patients with stage IIA/B seminoma can be cured with cisplatin-based chemotherapy, although with greater toxicity than that associated with radiotherapy alone.[75,76] Disease control rates for stage IIA/B seminoma with single-agent carboplatin appear inferior to that with radiotherapy. A phase II study by the German Testicular Cancer Study Group[77] delivered three or four cycles of carboplatin to patients with stage IIA or stage IIB seminoma, respectively. The overall failure rate was 18%, with all relapses occurring in the retroperitoneum. Although carboplatin has been combined with radiotherapy to improve outcome,[68] the reported relapse rate is within the range reported with radiotherapy alone.

Patients with stage IIC retroperitoneal disease (nodes >5 cm) are usually managed with systemic chemotherapy.[78] Radiotherapy remains a treatment option; however, the relapse rate of >30% is considered by many to be excessive. Chung et al.[65] reported recurrence in 10 of 16 patients with stage IIC disease managed with radiotherapy compared to only one relapse in a similar group of 23 patients managed by chemotherapy. The choice of modality is also influenced by the size and location of the retroperitoneal nodal mass. If the mass is centrally located and does not overlie most of one kidney or significantly overlap the liver, primary radiation therapy remains an option. If the location of the mass is such that the irradiation volume covers most of one kidney or significant volumes of the liver, then the potential morbidity of radiation therapy can be avoided by the use of primary cisplatin-containing combination chemotherapy (usually etoposide/cisplatin [EP] or bleomycin/etoposide/cisplatin [BEP]). For nodal disease >10 cm in diameter, the relapse rate is >40% with radiotherapy and such patients should be managed with systemic chemotherapy.

For the rare patient with stage III disease (i.e., supradiaphragmatic nodal disease or dissemination to parenchymal organs), or those with relapse following radiotherapy, the current standard therapy is three courses of BEP or four courses of EP chemotherapy. These patients are classified into either a good-prognosis or intermediate-prognosis group by the International Germ Cell Cancer Collaborative Group Consensus Classification, depending on the presence or absence of nonpulmonary visceral metastases, respectively. The 5-year survival is around 91% for good-prognosis patients and 80% for intermediate-prognosis patients. Despite initial favorable reports, single-agent carboplatin is not as effective as cisplatin-based combination treatment. In a pooled analysis of two randomized trials of 361 patients with metastatic seminoma, Bokemeyer et al.[79] reported an inferior progression-free (72% vs. 92%) and overall (89% vs. 94%) survival with carboplatin.

Residual Mass

For patients with stage II or III disease treated with primary chemotherapy, residual masses are present at 1 month in up to 80% of patients. Most of these then gradually regress over a period of several months. Flechon et al.[80] reported that 50% of residual masses disappeared on follow-up, and viable cancer cells were found only in masses >3 cm in size. Management strategies involve the use of consolidative radiotherapy, surgical resection, or observation. In an effort to define the role of postchemotherapy radiotherapy, the MRC Testicular Tumour Working Party conducted a retrospective review of patients with advanced seminoma managed by chemotherapy from 10 European centers.[81] Of 302 patients identified, 174 (58%) had residual masses on completion of chemotherapy, with a subsequent 3-year progression-free survival of 85%. Approximately half of these patients underwent postchemotherapy radiotherapy, with selection based predominantly on institutional preference. Radiotherapy did not significantly influence risk of progression, contributing an absolute increase in progression-free survival of only 2.3%. Instead, the most important prognostic factors for progression were the presence of prechemotherapy visceral metastases or raised LDH, or persistent visceral metastases postchemotherapy. At St. Bartholomew's Hospital, 43 of 107 patients (40%) with advanced seminoma had a residual mass postchemotherapy.[82] Positive histology was found in 3 of 19 patients (15%) who underwent surgical exploration, whereas relapse at the site of the mass occurred in 3 other patients observed. Residual disease was only found in masses >3 cm in size. Of the 107 patients, 98 patients (92%) remained alive and free from recurrence. The largest report of surgical resection following chemotherapy comes from the Memorial Sloan-Kettering Cancer Center.[83] A total of 55 patients with advanced seminoma underwent resection or biopsy of residual mass within 4 weeks of chemotherapy. Of 27 patients with a mass >3 cm, 8 patients (30%) had residual tumor. No viable tumor was found in any of the 28 patients with a residual mass <3 cm in maximal diameter.

From the reports discussed, it is clear that observation alone is adequate for a residual mass <3 cm in size. Two patterns of response to chemotherapy are evident on CT: the residual mass may be well defined with discrete borders, or the mass may have indistinct borders merging into surrounding structures and resembling a fibrous plaque. The former are more amenable to surgical resection. Furthermore, if the tumor is well defined on CT and measures >3 cm in greatest dimension, positive histology can be found in 50%. It is reasonable to resect these masses. If the mass is poorly defined, even if >3 cm, the chance of finding positive histology is <10%. Resecting such a mass is hazardous, with risk of great vessel, ureteric, and small bowel injury. These should be observed. FDG-PET scans have been shown to have a high specificity in identifying persistent disease, with a greater specificity than CT.[84] FDG-PET should be considered as a means to evaluate residual masses >3 cm as a guide to further management.[85]

Bilateral Testicular Cancer

Testicular cancer is bilateral in up to 5% of cases, with one-third being synchronous and two-thirds metachronous.[86] Although bilateral orchiectomy is an effective management strategy, the option of testis-sparing surgery and postoperative radiotherapy has emerged.[87] Partial orchiectomy should be considered for selected patients with bilateral disease or a solitary testicle. Ideally, tumors should be <2 cm in size and have negative surgical margins for invasive disease. Postoperative radiotherapy to a dose of 18 to 20 Gy is usually administered to the residual testicle to eradicate IGCN, which is found in >80% of cases.[88,89] Observation alone has also been reported.[90] In either case, some degree of hormonal dysfunction is common, and many patients may still require lifelong testosterone replacement.

RADIATION THERAPY TECHNIQUE

Target Volume and Field Borders

For stage I disease, the clinical target volume (CTV) encompasses the interaortocaval, preaortic, and para-aortic nodes (Fig. 67.1). The left renal hilar nodes are included for left-sided tumors. The ipsilateral external iliac and common iliac nodes may also be included, particularly if there is concern about aberrant drainage. Inclusion of the inguinal scar, inguinal lymph nodes, or hemiscrotum is not routinely warranted. For stage II disease, a gross tumor volume is identified from diagnostic imaging, and the CTV also usually includes the ipsilateral pelvic nodes.

The planning target volume (PTV) includes the CTV plus a margin to account for positional and setup uncertainties. To cover the known location of the retroperitoneal and iliac lymph nodes with an appropriate margin, standard anatomic field borders have been used. This is commonly referred to as the dog-leg or hockey stick field. Classically, the superior border is placed between the T9 and T10 vertebral bodies, with the inferior border at the top of the obturator foramen. A modified approach is now commonly used wherein the superior border is placed between T11 and T10 and the inferior border is placed at the superior aspect of the acetabulum (Fig. 67.2). The field is approximately 9 cm wide in the para-aortic region and usually covers the transverse processes. On the left, the lateral border is extended to include the left renal hilum, and customized shielding is positioned to reduce the amount of kidney irradiated. Field width here is typically 11 to 12 cm. At the mid-L4 level, the field is extended laterally to cover the ipsilateral external iliac nodes. Multileaf collimators are used to define the field shape. If retroperitoneal nodes alone are to be treated, the superior and lateral borders are as described previously, and the inferior border is placed at the L5/S1 disc space. Some report using a lower superior border, T10-11, and a higher inferior border, the bottom of L4.[53]

Once these borders are placed, the planning CT can be used to ensure adequate coverage of the target. Distance from the PTV to the field border is 8 to 15 mm depending on field size, energy, separation, and shielding. It should be noted that there is often a distance of several centimeters between the cranial and caudal field edges and the 95% isodose, which is related to the large field size and variability in body thickness.

In stage II disease, the PTV includes the same CTV as for stage I disease with an appropriate margin. Care must be taken to include the gross nodal disease in the CTV (Fig. 67.3). If the lymphadenopathy is >4 cm in size, a boost to gross disease is commonly used. This may be delivered either concurrently or sequentially. The advantage of a sequential approach is that it allows for reduction in disease volume and less irradiation of normal tissues. This is particularly appropriate where the initial disease is large and overlies kidney.

Simulation and Treatment Planning

A volumetric planning CT scan is acquired with the patient supine and arms at the sides. Testicular shielding (often in the form of a clamshell device) is used. Utilization of a CT-based planning technique enables visualization of the location of the lymph node regions, adjacent tissues, and critical normal structures including the kidneys and liver. In addition, the beam's eye view (BEV) allows evaluation of the coverage of the PTV, and shielding can be appropriately placed. Treatment is delivered with a linear accelerator using anterior and posterior parallel opposed fields. Depending on the separation, 6- to 18-MV photons are utilized. More elegant treatment techniques using intensity-modulated radiotherapy (IMRT) to cover the target volume with greater sparing of organs at risk are described.[91] Although IMRT enables reduction of dose to organs at risk (stomach, bowel, bone marrow), it is not clear how this is reflected in reduction of early or late side effects of treatment, including risk of second malignancy.

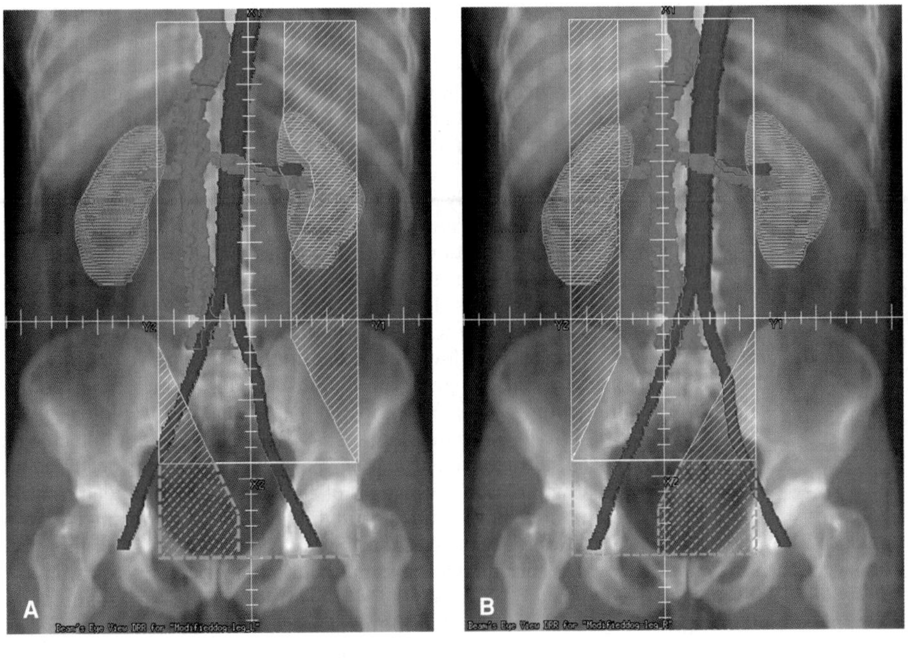

FIGURE 67.2. For stage I seminoma, a modified "dog-leg" field is used to encompass nodal regions at risk. The superior border is placed at the upper border of T10 or T11 and the inferior border at the superior aspect of the acetabulum. Traditionally, the inferior border was placed at the superior obturator foramen (indicated in *orange*) to include all external iliac nodes. These nodes are rarely involved, and using a higher border as indicated will reduce toxicity. If para-aortic fields are to be used, the inferior border is placed at the bottom of L5. The left renal hilum is included for left-sided tumors **(A)** but not for tumors on the right **(B)**.

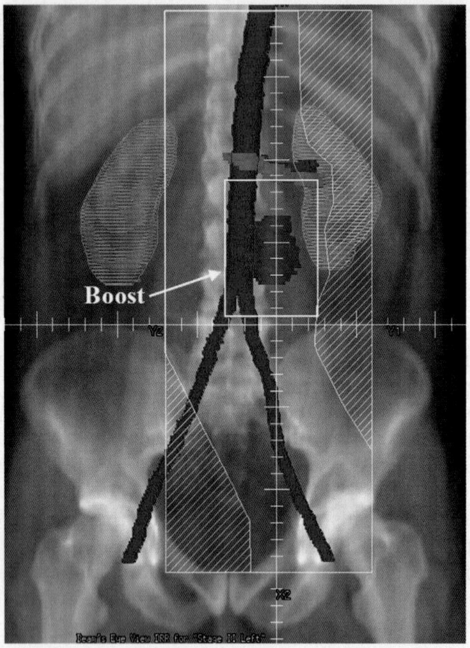

FIGURE 67.3. Stage IIA and stage IIB seminoma may be treated with a traditional or modified dog-leg to a dose of 25 Gy in 20 fractions, with a boost of 10 Gy in 5 fractions to nodes >3 cm in diameter.

Dose and Fractionation

Stage I Seminoma

Radiation dose of between 20 and 40 Gy at 1.25 to 2 Gy per fraction have been reported. A dose of 25 Gy in 20 fractions is the most commonly used dose/fractionation at North American institutions,[92] with close to 100% control of retroperitoneal disease. The United Kingdom's MRC (MRC TE18) completed a randomized controlled trial of 30 Gy in 15 fractions over 3 weeks or 20 Gy in 10 fractions over 2 weeks.[54] Relapse-free survival was similar in both groups. Acutely, there was significantly more moderate or severe lethargy and inability to carry out normal work in the group that received 30 Gy. However, by 12 weeks, there were no differences between the two groups.

Stage II Seminoma

The optimal radiation dose in stage II seminoma is yet to be determined, and several regimes are used. One regime of 25 Gy in 20 fractions is frequently used with a boost (10 Gy in 5 to 8 fractions) to the residual mass for lymphadenopathy >2 to 3 cm.[65] Alternatively, 30 Gy in 15 fractions for stage IIA and 36 Gy in 18 fractions for stage IIB seminoma have been shown to provide excellent local control.[66]

Testicular Shielding

During a fractionated course of radiotherapy to the retroperitoneal and ipsilateral iliac lymph nodes, the dose to the remaining testis ranges between 0.3 and 1.5 Gy. Dose received strongly depends on distance from the testicle to field edge. Several effective shielding devices have been described to reduce dose received by the testicle to <1% of the midplane dose.[93–95] Most departments use simple forms of gonadal shielding, such as the clamshell device, which consists of a cup that is 1 cm thick. This shields the testicle from low-energy scattered photons and effectively reduces the testicular dose by a factor of 4.

RESULTS OF THERAPY

Seminoma

The outcome of treatment with currently available therapies depends on the stage and extent of disease at presentation. Age >40 years at diagnosis is also an adverse prognostic factor.[23] For stage I disease, routine irradiation of the retroperitoneum and ipsilateral pelvic nodes results in 10-year relapse-free survival rates of 96% to 98%. Approximately 1% to 4% of patients relapse after infradiaphragmatic irradiation, usually within the first 3 years. The sites of relapse are usually evenly distributed between the mediastinum and distant sites. Occasional relapses occur as nonseminomatous germ cell malignancies, even after careful review of the initial tumor has shown a pure seminoma. Deaths from stage I seminoma are extremely rare. Most relapsing patients are salvaged with subsequent treatment, usually chemotherapy. Cause-specific survival rates in the large series are 99% to 100%.

The outcome for patients with stage II disease treated with infradiaphragmatic irradiation is shown in Table 67.6. Disease-free survival is approximately 92% and 86% for patients with stage IIA and IIB disease, respectively. Relapse most commonly occurs in the mediastinum, supraclavicular nodes, and lungs. Cisplatin-based chemotherapy is able to salvage in excess of 80% of the relapses, leading to a 5-year cause-specific survival of 96% to 100%. The relapse rate for patients with stage IIC disease managed by primary radiotherapy is >30%, and these patients are best managed with initial chemotherapy. Because of the ability to salvage patients who relapse following radiotherapy with cisplatin-based combination chemotherapy, the survival results following primary radiotherapy or chemotherapy as initial therapy even in patients with bulkier nodal disease are comparable. The potential toxicities of each approach must be evaluated for each patient, along with other factors influencing the choice of therapy.

Cisplatin-based chemotherapy (BEP × three fractions or EP × four fractions) is the standard treatment for patients with stage III seminoma, as well as for those with retroperitoneal masses >5 cm. Mencel et al.[96] reported that 93% of 142 patients with advanced seminoma achieved a favorable response to platinum-based chemotherapy, with an overall progression-free survival of 86%.

SEQUELAE OF TREATMENT

Radiation Therapy

The long-term sequelae of standard infradiaphragmatic irradiation for stages IA and IIA disease are related to the dose of radiation used. There appears to be no curative advantage for doses >25 Gy; however, there is an increase in toxicity. In the MRC randomized trial comparing 30 Gy in 15 fractions delivered to either dog-leg or para-aortic fields, 33 of 478 patients (7%) were diagnosed with a peptic ulcer during follow-up. The occurrence rate was similar in both treatment arms. Very few patients report diarrhea as a long-term consequence, and most patients report a satisfactory quality of life, with a maintained body image and few side effects.[54]

Approximately 50% of patients with testicular seminoma have some degree of impairment in spermatogenesis at the time of presentation. Exposure of the remaining testis to therapeutic irradiation may further impair fertility, and the degree of impairment is dose dependent. Available data suggest that hormonal function and spermatogenesis may be compromised at dose levels as low as 0.5 Gy and that cumulative doses >2 Gy probably lead to permanent injury.[97] Hahn et al.[98] reported the induction of aspermia in 10 of 14 patients who received >65 cGy to the remaining testis. Aspermia was not detected at doses <50 cGy. Recovery of sperm in the semen occurred in most within 30 to 80 weeks of radiotherapy. A detailed assessment of fertility and sexual function was performed in the Southwest Oncology Group Study 8711 in a series of men following orchidectomy and radiotherapy for seminoma.[99] Fourteen of 26 patients (54%) were subfertile at baseline, with a sperm count <20,000/mL. The average prescribed dose was

26 Gy in 1.6-Gy fractions, delivering a median dose of 79 cGy to the remaining testis. With a testicular dose below the median, the sperm count tended to drop to a nadir value around 6 months, with recovery of fertility by 12 months. With higher testicular dose, recovery of sperm count was further delayed. Jacobsen et al.[100] reported a 50% reduction in sperm count at 1 year in 21 men following dog-leg radiotherapy (median testis dose, 32 cGy). No change in sperm count was noted in 24 men treated with para-aortic fields (median testis dose 9 cGy). Dog-leg radiotherapy also results in an elevation of serum follicle-stimulating hormone (FSH) levels, with no change in serum testosterone. FSH levels are highest within 6 months of radiotherapy and return to normal within 3 years. With current radiation techniques, most men will have return to baseline sperm concentrations and hormone levels with minimal impact on fertility.

Patients are at increased risk of developing a second primary malignancy following treatment for testicular cancer.[101,102] Travis et al.[103] investigated the occurrence of second malignancies among >40,000 men who had undergone treatment for a testicular cancer between 1943 and 2001 from 14 population-based cancer registries in North America and Europe. The risk of developing a second solid tumor among 10-year survivors was almost twice that of the general population, with a relative risk (RR) of 1.9. The risk remained elevated for 35 years, with the highest risk for cancers of the stomach (RR 4.0), pancreas (RR 3.6), and bladder (RR 2.7). There was also an increased risk of developing cancers of the lung, esophagus, colon, and pleura. An increased risk was found for both seminomas and nonseminomas and in patients treated with radiotherapy alone (RR 2.0), chemotherapy alone (RR 1.8), and both modalities (RR 2.9). A case-control study of leukemia risk in a cohort of 18,567 patients treated for testicular cancer between 1970 and 1993 has also been reported.[104] Radiotherapy (mean dose 12.6 Gy to bone marrow) without chemotherapy was associated with a threefold elevated risk of leukemia. Risk increased with increasing dose of radiation to bone marrow, largely associated with the use of mediastinal irradiation. The cumulative dose of cisplatin was also predictive of excess leukemia risk, being 3.2 with the commonly administered dose. In absolute terms, it is estimated that 25 Gy to the retroperitoneum would result in 9 excess cases of leukemia in 10,000 patients followed for 15 years. Commonly used doses of cisplatin might result in 16 excess cases. Although treatment factors are strongly implicated in the development of second primary malignancies following treatment, an excess risk of second cancers is seen even among testicular cancer patients who have just been observed. An increased rate of spontaneous chromosomal translocations is seen in lymphocytes of patients with early-stage seminoma compared to healthy controls.[105] Following adjuvant radiotherapy, the translocation rate increases before returning to preradiotherapy levels at around 30 months.[106] It is hypothesized that this genomic instability may be a predisposing factor toward malignancy development.

Long-term survivors following radiotherapy for seminoma are also at increased risk of death related to cardiac disease, even without mediastinal irradiation,[107] with a cardiac standardized mortality ratio of 1.85 in patients followed out beyond 15 years.

Chemotherapy

Cisplatin-based chemotherapy is associated with alopecia and the potential for substantial nausea and vomiting. Modern antiemetics have improved gastrointestinal reactions. Serious short-term problems are myelosuppression, bleomycin-induced pulmonary fibrosis, and rarely cisplatin nephrotoxicity. Myelosuppression and pulmonary fibrosis are fatal in 0.5% to 4% of treated patients. A recently recognized effect of chemotherapy used in the treatment of germ cell tumors is the risk of secondary malignancy. As discussed previously, the cumulative dose of cisplatin strongly correlates with the risk of subsequent malignancy.[104] Etoposide exposure increases the risk of leukemia. Morphologically, these leukemias are usually monocytic or myelomonocytic. Characteristic chromosomal translocations are frequently but not invariably present. The onset of leukemia is ordinarily closer to chemotherapy exposure than is the typical leukemia induced by alkylating agents.

Other late toxicities reported include high-tone hearing loss, neurotoxicity, Raynaud's phenomenon, ischemic heart disease, hypertension, renal dysfunction, and pulmonary toxicity. In an observational study of 1,800 men treated with cisplatin-based chemotherapy for testicular cancer, Brydoy et al.[108] noted long-term Raynaud-like phenomena in 39%, paraesthesia in 29%, hearing impairment in 22%, and troubling tinnitus in 22%. Long-term fertility seems little impaired following chemotherapy.[109] BEP causes immediate azoospermia; however, with time, more than half of patients may recover normal or near-normal spermatogenesis.[110] The paternity rate following two to four cycles of BEP is 70% to 85%.[111,112] Symptomatic hormone dysfunction only occurs with high cumulative doses of cisplatin,[113] although subclinical endocrine abnormalities are more common.[114]

REFERENCES

1. Siegel R, Ward E, Brawley O, et al. Cancer statistics, 2011: the impact of eliminating socioeconomic and racial disparities on premature cancer deaths. *CA Cancer J Clin* 2011;61(4):212–236.
2. Chia VM, Quraishi SM, Devesa SS, et al. International trends in the incidence of testicular cancer, 1973–2002. *Cancer Epidemiol Biomarkers Prev* 2010; 19(5):1151–1159.
3. Rosen A, Jayram G, Drazer M, et al. Global trends in testicular cancer incidence and mortality. *Eur Urol* 2011;60(2):374–379.
4. Holmes LJ, Escalante C, Garrison O, et al. Testicular cancer incidence trends in the USA (1975–2004): plateau or shifting racial paradigm? *Public Health* 2008; 122(9):862–872.
5. Bray F, Ferlay J, Devesa SS, et al. Interpreting the international trends in testicular seminoma and nonseminoma incidence. *Nat Clin Pract Urol* 2006;3(10):532–543.
6. Baade P, Carriere P, Fritschi L. Trends in testicular germ cell cancer incidence in Australia. *Cancer Causes Control* 2008;19(10):1043–1049.
7. Manecksha RP, Fitzpatrick JM. Epidemiology of testicular cancer. *BJU Int* 2009; 104(9 Pt B):1329–1333.
8. Sarfati D, Shaw C, Blakely T, et al. Ethnic and socioeconomic trends in testicular cancer incidence in New Zealand. *Int J Cancer* 2011;128(7):1683–1691.
9. Bosetti C, Bertuccio P, Chatenoud L, et al. Trends in mortality from urologic cancers in Europe, 1970–2008. *Eur Urol* 2011;60(1):1–15.
10. Bertuccio P, Malvezzi M, Chatenoud L, et al. Testicular cancer mortality in the Americas, 1980–2003. *Cancer* 2007;109(4):776–779.
11. Verhoeven RH, Coebergh JW, Kiemeney LA, et al. Testicular cancer: trends in mortality are well explained by changes in treatment and survival in the southern Netherlands since 1970. *Eur J Cancer* 2007;43(17):2553–2558.
12. Akre O, Pettersson A, Richiardi L. Risk of contralateral testicular cancer among men with unilaterally undescended testis: a meta analysis. *Int J Cancer* 2009; 124(3):687–689.
13. Raman JD, Nobert CF, Goldstein M. Increased incidence of testicular cancer in men presenting with infertility and abnormal semen analysis. *J Urol* 2005; 174(5):1819–1822; discussion 1822.
14. Jorgensen N, Vierula M, Jacobsen R, et al. Recent adverse trends in semen quality and testis cancer incidence among Finnish men. *Int J Androl* 2011;34(4 Pt 2): e37–e48.
15. Jorgensen N, Asklund C, Carlsen E, et al. Coordinated European investigations of semen quality: results from studies of Scandinavian young men is a matter of concern. *Int J Androl* 2006;29(1):54–61; discussion 105–108.
16. Skakkebaek NE, Rajpert-De Meyts E, Main KM. Testicular dysgenesis syndrome: an increasingly common developmental disorder with environmental aspects. *Hum Reprod* 2001;16(5):972–978.
17. Greene MH, Kratz CP, Mai PL, et al. Familial testicular germ cell tumors in adults: 2010 summary of genetic risk factors and clinical phenotype. *Endocr Relat Cancer* 2010;17(2):R109–R121.
18. Dieckmann KP, Skakkebaek NE. Carcinoma in situ of the testis: review of biological and clinical features. *Int J Cancer* 1999;83(6):815–822.
19. Aggarwal N, Parwani AV. Spermatocytic seminoma. *Arch Pathol Lab Med* 2009; 133(12):1985–1988.
20. Looijenga LH. Spermatocytic seminoma: toward further understanding of pathogenesis. *J Pathol* 2011;224(4):431–433.
21. De Wit M, Brenner W, Hartmann M, et al. [18F]-FDG-PET in clinical stage I/II non-seminomatous germ cell tumours: results of the German multicentre trial. *Ann Oncol* 2008;19(9):1619–1623.
22. American Joint Committee on Cancer. *AJCC cancer staging manual,* 7th ed. New York: Springer, 2010.
23. Fossa SD, Cvancarova M, Chen L, et al. Adverse prognostic factors for testicular cancer-specific survival: a population-based study of 27,948 patients. *J Clin Oncol* 2011;29(8):963–970.
24. International Germ Cell Consensus Classification: a prognostic factor-based staging system for metastatic germ cell cancers. International Germ Cell Cancer Collaborative Group. *J Clin Oncol* 1997;15(2):594–603.
25. Capelouto CC, Clark PE, Ransil BJ, et al. A review of scrotal violation in testicular cancer: is adjuvant local therapy necessary? *J Urol* 1995;153(3 Pt 2):981–985.

26. Albers P, Albrecht W, Algaba F, et al. EAU guidelines on testicular cancer: 2011 update. *Eur Urol* 2011;60(2):304–319.
27. Mead GM, Fossa SD, Oliver RT, et al. Randomized trials in 2466 patients with stage I seminoma: patterns of relapse and follow-up. *J Natl Cancer Inst* 2011;103(3):241–249.
28. Chung P, Mayhew LA, Warde P, et al. Management of stage I seminomatous testicular cancer: a systematic review. *Clin Oncol (R Coll Radiol)* 2010;22(1):6–16.
29. Alomary I, Samant R, Genest P, et al. The preferred treatment for stage I seminoma: a survey of Canadian radiation oncologists. *Clin Oncol (R Coll Radiol)* 2006;18(9):696–699; discussion 693–695.
30. Kollmannsberger C, Tyldesley S, Moore C, et al. Evolution in management of testicular seminoma: population-based outcomes with selective utilization of active therapies. *Ann Oncol* 2011;22(4):808–814.
31. Von der Maase H, Specht L, Jacobsen GK, et al. Surveillance following orchidectomy for stage I seminoma of the testis. *Eur J Cancer* 1993;29A(14):1931–1934.
32. Chung P, Parker C, Panzarella T, et al. Surveillance in stage I testicular seminoma—risk of late relapse. *Can J Urol* 2002;9(5):1637–1640.
33. Francis R, Bower M, Brunstrom G, et al. Surveillance for stage I testicular germ cell tumours: results and cost benefit analysis of management options. *Eur J Cancer* 2000;36(15):1925–1932.
34. Daugaard G, Petersen PM, Rorth M. Surveillance in stage I testicular cancer. *APMIS* 2003;111(1):76–83; discussion 83–85.
35. Choo R, Thomas G, Woo T, et al. Long-term outcome of postorchiectomy surveillance for stage I testicular seminoma. *Int J Radiat Oncol Biol Phys* 2005;61(3):736–740.
36. Cummins S, Yau T, Huddart R, et al. Surveillance in stage I seminoma patients: a long-term assessment. *Eur Urol* 2010;57(4):673–678.
37. Aparicio J, Germa JR, Garcia del Muro X, et al. Risk-adapted management for patients with clinical stage I seminoma: the Second Spanish Germ Cell Cancer Cooperative Group study. *J Clin Oncol* 2005;23(34):8717–8723.
38. Kamba T, Kamoto T, Okubo K, et al. Outcome of different post-orchiectomy management for stage I seminoma: Japanese multi-institutional study including 425 patients. *Int J Urol* 2010;17(12):980–987.
39. Tandstad T, Smaaland R, Solberg A, et al. Management of seminomatous testicular cancer: a binational prospective population-based study from the Swedish Norwegian Testicular Cancer Study Group. *J Clin Oncol* 2011;29(6):719–725.
40. Warde P, Specht L, Horwich A, et al. Prognostic factors for relapse in stage I seminoma managed by surveillance: a pooled analysis. *J Clin Oncol* 2002;20(22):4448–4452.
41. Tyldesley S, Voduc D, McKenzie M, et al. Surveillance of stage I testicular seminoma: British Columbia Cancer Agency Experience 1992 to 2002. *Urology* 2006;67(3):594–598.
42. Martin JM, Panzarella T, Zwahlen DR, et al. Evidence-based guidelines for following stage 1 seminoma. *Cancer* 2007;109(11):2248–2256.
43. Tolan S, Vesprini D, Jewett MA, et al. No role for routine chest radiography in stage I seminoma surveillance. *Eur Urol* 2010;57(3):474–479.
44. O'Malley ME, Chung P, Haider M, et al. Comparison of low dose with standard dose abdominal/pelvic multidetector CT in patients with stage 1 testicular cancer under surveillance. *Eur Radiol* 2010;20(7):1624–1630.
45. Warde P, Gospodarowicz MK, Panzarella T, et al. Long term outcome and cost in the management of stage I testicular seminoma. *Can J Urol* 2000;7(2):967–972; discussion 973.
46. Fossa SD, Aass N, Kaalhus O. Radiotherapy for testicular seminoma stage I: treatment results and long-term post-irradiation morbidity in 365 patients. *Int J Radiat Oncol Biol Phys* 1989;16(2):383–388.
47. Bauman GS, Venkatesan VM, Ago CT, et al. Postoperative radiotherapy for stage I/II seminoma: results for 212 patients. *Int J Radiat Oncol Biol Phys* 1998;42(2):313–317.
48. Logue JP, Harris MA, Livsey JE, et al. Short course para-aortic radiation for stage I seminoma of the testis. *Int J Radiat Oncol Biol Phys* 2003;57(5):1304–1309.
49. Santoni R, Barbera F, Bertoni F, et al. Stage I seminoma of the testis: a bi-institutional retrospective analysis of patients treated with radiation therapy only. *BJU Int* 2003;92(1):47–52; discussion 52.
50. Niazi TM, Souhami L, Sultanem K, et al. Long-term results of para-aortic irradiation for patients with stage I seminoma of the testis. *Int J Radiat Oncol Biol Phys* 2005;61(3):741–744.
51. Melchior D, Hammer P, Fimmers R, et al. Long term results and morbidity of paraaortic compared with paraaortic and iliac adjuvant radiation in clinical stage I seminoma. *Anticancer Res* 2001;21(4B):2989–2993.
52. Classen J, Schmidberger H, Meisner C, et al. Para-aortic irradiation for stage I testicular seminoma: results of a prospective study in 675 patients. A trial of the German Testicular Cancer Study Group (GTCSG). *Br J Cancer* 2004;90(12):2305–2311.
53. Bruns F, Bremer M, Meyer A, et al. Adjuvant radiotherapy in stage I seminoma: is there a role for further reduction of treatment volume? *Acta Oncol* 2005;44(2):142–148.
54. Jones WG, Fossa SD, Mead GM, et al. Randomized trial of 30 versus 20 Gy in the adjuvant treatment of stage I testicular seminoma: a report on Medical Research Council Trial TE18, European Organisation for the Research and Treatment of Cancer Trial 30942 (ISRCTN18525328). *J Clin Oncol* 2005;23(6):1200–1208.
55. Oliver RT, Mead GM, Rustin GJ, et al. Randomized trial of carboplatin versus radiotherapy for stage I seminoma: mature results on relapse and contralateral testis cancer rates in MRC TE19/EORTC 30982 study (ISRCTN27163214). *J Clin Oncol* 2011;29(8):957–962.
56. Souchon R, Hartmann M, Krege S, et al. Interdisciplinary evidence-based recommendations for the follow-up of early stage seminomatous testicular germ cell cancer patients. *Strahlenther Onkol* 2011;187(3):158–166.
57. Fossa SD, Horwich A, Russell JM, et al. Optimal planning target volume for stage I testicular seminoma: a Medical Research Council randomized trial. Medical Research Council Testicular Tumor Working Group. *J Clin Oncol* 1999;17(4):1146.
58. Livsey JE, Taylor B, Mobarek N, et al. Patterns of relapse following radiotherapy for stage I seminoma of the testis: implications for follow-up. *Clin Oncol (R Coll Radiol)* 2001;13(4):296–300.
59. Horwich A, Dearnaley DP, Duchesne GM, et al. Simple nontoxic treatment of advanced metastatic seminoma with carboplatin. *J Clin Oncol* 1989;7(8):1150–1156.
60. Dieckmann KP, Krain J, Kuster J, et al. Adjuvant carboplatin treatment for seminoma clinical stage I. *J Cancer Res Clin Oncol* 1996;122(1):63–66.
61. Krege S, Kalund G, Otto T, et al. Phase II study: adjuvant single-agent carboplatin therapy for clinical stage I seminoma. *Eur Urol* 1997;31(4):405–407.
62. Reiter WJ, Brodowicz T, Alavi S, et al. Twelve-year experience with two courses of adjuvant single-agent carboplatin therapy for clinical stage I seminoma. *J Clin Oncol* 2001;19(1):101–104.
63. Steiner H, Scheiber K, Berger AP, et al. Retrospective multicentre study of carboplatin monotherapy for clinical stage I seminoma. *BJU Int* 2011;107(7):1074–1079.
64. Powles T, Robinson D, Shamash J, et al. The long-term risks of adjuvant carboplatin treatment for stage I seminoma of the testis. *Ann Oncol* 2008;19(3):443–447.
65. Chung PW, Gospodarowicz MK, Panzarella T, et al. Stage II testicular seminoma: patterns of recurrence and outcome of treatment. *Eur Urol* 2004;45(6):754–759; discussion 759–760.
66. Classen J, Schmidberger H, Meisner C, et al. Radiotherapy for stages IIA/B testicular seminoma: final report of a prospective multicenter clinical trial. *J Clin Oncol* 2003;21(6):1101–1106.
67. Zagars GK, Pollack A. Radiotherapy for stage II testicular seminoma. *Int J Radiat Oncol Biol Phys* 2001;51(3):643–649.
68. Patterson H, Norman AR, Mitra SS, et al. Combination carboplatin and radiotherapy in the management of stage II testicular seminoma: comparison with radiotherapy treatment alone. *Radiother Oncol* 2001;59(1):5–11.
69. Whipple GL, Sagerman RH, van Rooy EM. Long-term evaluation of postorchiectomy radiotherapy for stage II seminoma. *Am J Clin Oncol* 1997;20(2):196–201.
70. Vallis KA, Howard GC, Duncan W, et al. Radiotherapy for stages I and II testicular seminoma: results and morbidity in 238 patients. *Br J Radiol* 1995;68(808):400–405.
71. Dosmann MA, Zagars GK. Post-orchiectomy radiotherapy for stages I and II testicular seminoma. *Int J Radiat Oncol Biol Phys* 1993;26(3):381–390.
72. Mason BR, Kearsley JH. Radiotherapy for stage 2 testicular seminoma: the prognostic influence of tumor bulk. *J Clin Oncol* 1988;6(12):1856–1862.
73. Evensen JF, Fossa SD, Kjellevold K, et al. Testicular seminoma: analysis of treatment and failure for stage II disease. *Radiother Oncol* 1985;4(1):55–61.
74. Chung PW, Warde PR, Panzarella T, et al. Appropriate radiation volume for stage IIA/B testicular seminoma. *Int J Radiat Oncol Biol Phys* 2003;56(3):746–748.
75. Garcia-del-Muro X, Maroto P, Guma J, et al. Chemotherapy as an alternative to radiotherapy in the treatment of stage IIA and IIB testicular seminoma: a Spanish Germ Cell Cancer Group study. *J Clin Oncol* 2008;26(33):5416–5421.
76. Giannis M, Aristotelis B, Vassiliki K, et al. Cisplatin-based chemotherapy for advanced seminoma: report of 52 cases treated in two institutions. *J Cancer Res Clin Oncol* 2009;135(11):1495–1500.
77. Krege S, Boergermann C, Baschek R, et al. Single agent carboplatin for CS IIA/B testicular seminoma. A phase II study of the German Testicular Cancer Study Group (GTCSG). *Ann Oncol* 2006;17(2):276–280.
78. Domont J, Massard C, Patrikidou A, et al. A risk-adapted strategy of radiotherapy or cisplatin-based chemotherapy in stage II seminoma. *Urol Oncol* 2011 Jun 10. [Epub ahead of print]
79. Bokemeyer C, Kollmannsberger C, Stenning S, et al. Metastatic seminoma treated with either single agent carboplatin or cisplatin-based combination chemotherapy: a pooled analysis of two randomised trials. *Br J Cancer* 2004;91(4):683–687.
80. Flechon A, Bompas E, Biron P, et al. Management of post-chemotherapy residual masses in advanced seminoma. *J Urol* 2002;168(5):1975–1979.
81. Duchesne GM, Stenning SP, Aass N, et al. Radiotherapy after chemotherapy for metastatic seminoma—a diminishing role. MRC Testicular Tumour Working Party. *Eur J Cancer* 1997;33(6):829–835.
82. Ravi R, Ong J, Oliver RT, et al. The management of residual masses after chemotherapy in metastatic seminoma. *BJU Int* 1999;83(6):649–653.
83. Herr HW, Sheinfeld J, Puc HS, et al. Surgery for a post-chemotherapy residual mass in seminoma. *J Urol* 1997;157(3):860–862.
84. Becherer A, De Santis M, Karanikas G, et al. FDG PET is superior to CT in the prediction of viable tumour in post-chemotherapy seminoma residuals. *Eur J Radiol* 2005;54(2):284–288.
85. Becherer A. PET in testicular cancer. *Methods Mol Biol* 2011;727:225–241.
86. Klatte T, de Martino M, Arensmeier K, et al. Management and outcome of bilateral testicular germ cell tumors: a 25-year single center experience. *Int J Urol* 2008;15(9):821–826.
87. Bazzi WM, Raheem OA, Stroup SP, et al. Partial orchiectomy and testis intratubular germ cell neoplasia: world literature review. *Urol Ann* 2011;3(3):115–118.
88. Huyghe E, Soulie M, Escourrou G, et al. Conservative management of small testicular tumors relative to carcinoma in situ prevalence. *J Urol* 2005;173(3):820–823.
89. Heidenreich A, Weissbach L, Holtl W, et al. Organ sparing surgery for malignant germ cell tumor of the testis. *J Urol* 2001;166(6):2161–2165.
90. Lawrentschuk N, Zuniga A, Grabowksi AC, et al. Partial orchiectomy for presumed malignancy in patients with a solitary testis due to a prior germ cell tumor: a large North American experience. *J Urol* 2011;185(2):508–513.
91. Zilli T, Boudreau C, Doucet R, et al. Bone marrow-sparing intensity-modulated radiation therapy for stage I seminoma. *Acta Oncol* 2011;50(4):555–562.
92. Choo R, Sandler H, Warde P, et al. Survey of radiation oncologists: practice patterns of the management of stage I seminoma of testis in Canada and a selected group in the United States. *Can J Urol* 2002;9(2):1479–1485.
93. Fraass BA, Kinsella TJ, Harrington FS, et al. Peripheral dose to the testes: the design and clinical use of a practical and effective gonadal shield. *Int J Radiat Oncol Biol Phys* 1985;11(3):609–615.
94. Bieri S, Rouzaud M, Miralbell R. Seminoma of the testis: is scrotal shielding necessary when radiotherapy is limited to the para-aortic nodes? *Radiother Oncol* 1999;50(3):349–353.
95. Ravichandran R, Binukumar JP, Kannadhasan S, et al. Testicular shield for para-aortic radiotherapy and estimation of gonad doses. *J Med Phys* 2008;33(4):158–161.
96. Mencel PJ, Motzer RJ, Mazumdar M, et al. Advanced seminoma: treatment results, survival, and prognostic factors in 142 patients. *J Clin Oncol* 1994;12(1):120–126.
97. Hansen PV, Trykker H, Svennekjaer IL, et al. Long-term recovery of spermatogenesis after radiotherapy in patients with testicular cancer. *Radiother Oncol* 1990;18(2):117–125.
98. Hahn EW, Feingold SM, Simpson L, et al. Recovery from aspermia induced by low-dose radiation in seminoma patients. *Cancer* 1982;50(2):337–340.
99. Gordon WJ, Siegmund K, Stanisic TH, et al. A study of reproductive function in patients with seminoma treated with radiotherapy and orchidectomy: (SWOG-8711). Southwest Oncology Group. *Int J Radiat Oncol Biol Phys* 1997;38(1):83–94.
100. Jacobsen KD, Olsen DR, Fossa K, et al. External beam abdominal radiotherapy in patients with seminoma stage I: field type, testicular dose, and spermatogenesis. *Int J Radiat Oncol Biol Phys* 1997;38(1):95–102.

101. Fatigante L, Ducci F, Campoccia S, et al. Long-term results in patients affected by testicular seminoma treated with radiotherapy: risk of second malignancies. *Tumori* 2005;91(2):144–150.
102. Robinson D, Moller H, Horwich A. Mortality and incidence of second cancers following treatment for testicular cancer. *Br J Cancer* 2007;96(3):529–533.
103. Travis LB, Fossa SD, Schonfeld SJ, et al. Second cancers among 40,576 testicular cancer patients: focus on long-term survivors. *J Natl Cancer Inst* 2005; 97(18):1354–1365.
104. Travis LB, Andersson M, Gospodarowicz M, et al. Treatment-associated leukemia following testicular cancer. *J Natl Cancer Inst* 2000;92(14):1165–1171.
105. Schmidberger H, Virsik-Koepp P, Rave-Frank M, et al. Reciprocal translocations in patients with testicular seminoma before and after radiotherapy. *Int J Radiat Oncol Biol Phys* 2001;50(4):857–864.
106. Muller I, Geinitz H, Braselmann H, et al. Time-course of radiation-induced chromosomal aberrations in tumor patients after radiotherapy. *Int J Radiat Oncol Biol Phys* 2005;63(4):1214–1220.
107. Zagars GK, Ballo MT, Lee AK, et al. Mortality after cure of testicular seminoma. *J Clin Oncol* 2004;22(4):640–647.
108. Brydoy M, Oldenburg J, Klepp O, et al. Observational study of prevalence of long-term Raynaud like phenomena and neurological side effects in testicular cancer survivors. *J Natl Cancer Inst* 2009;101(24):1682–1695.
109. Kim C, McGlynn KA, McCorkle R, et al. Fertility among testicular cancer survivors: a case-control study in the U.S. *J Cancer Surviv* 2010;4(3):266–273.
110. Stephenson WT, Poirier SM, Rubin L, et al. Evaluation of reproductive capacity in germ cell tumor patients following treatment with cisplatin, etoposide, and bleomycin. *J Clin Oncol* 1995;13(9):2278–2280.
111. Fossa SD, Oldenburg J, Dahl AA. Short- and long-term morbidity after treatment for testicular cancer. *BJU Int* 2009;104(9 Pt B):1418–1422.
112. Brydoy M, Fossa SD, Klepp O, et al. Paternity and testicular function among testicular cancer survivors treated with two to four cycles of cisplatin-based chemotherapy. *Eur Urol* 2010;58(1):134–140.
113. Gerl A, Muhlbayer D, Hansmann G, et al. The impact of chemotherapy on Leydig cell function in long term survivors of germ cell tumors. *Cancer* 2001;91(7):1297–1303.
114. Huddart RA, Norman A, Moynihan C, et al. Fertility, gonadal and sexual function in survivors of testicular cancer. *Br J Cancer* 2005;93(2):200–207.

Chapter 68
Cancer of the Penis and Male Urethra

David B. Mansur

ANATOMY

The basic structural components of the penis include two corpora cavernosa and the corpus spongiosum. These are encased in a dense fascia (Buck's fascia), which is separated from the skin by a layer of loose connective tissue. Distally, the corpus spongiosum expands into the glans penis, which is covered by a skin fold known as the prepuce. The skin extends over and is firmly attached to the glans.

The male urethra is composed of a mucous membrane and the submucosa. It extends from the bladder neck to the external urethral meatus. The posterior urethra is subdivided into the membranous urethra, the portion passing through the urogenital diaphragm, and the prostatic urethra, which passes through the prostate. The anterior urethra passes through the corpus spongiosum and is subdivided into fossa navicularis (a widening within the glans), the penile urethra, which passes through the pendulous part of the penis, and the bulbous urethra, the dilated proximal portion of the anterior urethra. The prostatic urethra is covered by transitional epithelium only. The distal portion of the anterior urethra is covered by stratified squamous epithelium, which changes proximally to pseudostratified columnar epithelium. The columnar epithelium gradually changes into transitional epithelium in the membranous urethra.

The lymphatic channels of the prepuce and the skin of the shaft drain into the superficial inguinal nodes located above the fascia lata. The rich anastomotic network of the lymphatics within the penis and at the base of the penis means that for practical purposes lymphatic drainage may be considered bilateral. There is some disagreement as to whether the glans and the deep penile structures drain into the superficial or deep inguinal lymph nodes (those under the fascia lata). The so-called sentinel nodes located above and medial to the junction of the epigastric and saphenous veins have been identified as the primary drainage sites in carcinoma of the penis.[1] Selective biopsy of this group of nodes is of obvious importance in assessment of tumor extent, because, if they are not involved by tumor, a complete nodal dissection may not be necessary. The reliability of this procedure has not been supported by some.[2,3] Catalona[4] found that biopsy of the sentinel nodes showed false-negative results in 10% of Cabanas's[5] cases who died of carcinoma.

The lymphatics of the fossa navicularis and the penile urethra follow the lymphatics of the penis to the superficial and deep inguinal lymph nodes. The lymphatics of the bulbomembranous and prostatic urethra may follow three routes. Some pass under the pubic symphysis to the external iliac nodes, some go to the obturator and internal iliac nodes, and others end in the presacral lymph nodes. The pelvic (iliac) lymph nodes are rarely involved in the absence of inguinal lymph node involvement.[6]

EPIDEMIOLOGY

Carcinoma of the penis is rare in the United States, where an estimated 1,100 new cases will be diagnosed each year.[7] The annual incidence is estimated to be 1 in 100,000 males, accounting for less than 1% of all cancers in men.[6] There is increasing evidence that newborn circumcision has a preventive effect in the development of carcinoma of the penis.[8] This tumor is extremely rare in circumcised Jewish men;[6] circumcision performed early in life protects against carcinoma of the penis, but this is not true if the operation is done in adult life.[9] The higher incidence in some areas of South America, Africa, and Asia seems to be related to the absence of the practice of neonatal circumcision. It has been shown that male circumcision is highly effective in preventing the development of penile carcinoma in Nigeria and Uganda.[10,11] The high incidence of carcinoma of the penis in American blacks has similarly been attributed to the lower percentage of blacks undergoing neonatal circumcision. Phimosis is common in men suffering from penile carcinoma. Smegma is carcinogenic in animals, yet the component of the smegma responsible for its carcinogenic effect has not been identified.[6]

Human papilloma virus (HPV) is associated with penile carcinoma. In a systematic review of the literature, Miralles-Guri et al.[12] concluded that approximately half of all carcinomas are HPV related, with the most common serotypes being HPV-16 and HPV-18. Boon et al.[13] observed an increased incidence of cervical carcinoma and penile carcinoma in Bali in a Hindu population in whom circumcision is rare and phimosis in adult males is high. They suggested that HPV infection, estimated to be present in over 75% of Balinese patients with genital carcinoma, may be a cofactor with impeded postcoital hygiene in genital carcinogenesis. In the Netherlands, where males are usually circumcised, the male is exclusively a vector of HPV but not a victim as in Bali. Martinez[14] in Puerto Rico and Graham et al.[15] in New York also noted a significantly higher incidence of carcinoma of the cervix in the wives of males with penile carcinoma.

The quadrivalent vaccine against HPV serotypes 6, 11, 16, and 18 has been approved for females aged 9 to 26 to prevent cervical cancer. Based on the demonstrated ability to significantly decrease the incidence of penile lesions (primarily HPV-6 and HPV-11 associated genital warts) in young men, the U.S. Food and Drug Administration also approved the use of the vaccine in males aged 9 to 26. Because the incidence of penile cancer in the United States is much lower than that of genital warts, the reduction in penile cancer incidence is expected to be low. However, there is potential great benefit to vaccination in countries with much higher penile cancer rates. Perhaps the greatest benefit of vaccination of young men in the United States would be the reduced HPV infection rate in the overall population and subsequent reduced transmission to females at risk for cervical cancer.[16] Other etiologic factors, such as other viruses (herpes simplex) and venereal disease (syphilis), have been implicated,[17,18] but the evidence remains inconclusive.[5]

Carcinoma of the male urethra is also rare. There are no recognized racial or geographic predisposing factors. Although the etiology remains unknown, there seems to be some correlation between the incidence of carcinoma of the urethra and chronic irritation (infection, venereal diseases, strictures). Significant past medical history of male urethra cancer patients include venereal disease (24% to 37%), urethral stricture (35% to 54%), urethral trauma (7%), and urethral polyps (2%).[19,20] The part of the urethra covered by the transitional epithelium (prostatic and membranous urethra) may be susceptible to the same carcinogenic factors that affect the bladder and the upper urinary tract. Average age at presentation of these tumors is 58 to 60 years, although 10% occur in men younger than 40 years.[5,20]

NATURAL HISTORY

Most carcinomas of the penis start within the preputial area, arising in the glans, coronal sulcus, or the prepuce itself. Lesions arising in the skin of the shaft are rare. In most patients, carcinoma of the penis is characterized by slow locoregional progression. The penis is handled and observed daily, yet there is often significant debate as to when patient recognition and medical diagnosis should have occurred. The patient experiences fear and embarrassment, which probably contributes to delayed diagnosis. Therefore, expeditious diagnosis of all penile lesions should be the rule. Extensive primary lesions may involve the corpora cavernosa or even the abdominal wall. The inguinal lymph nodes are the most common site of metastatic spread. Pathologic evidence of nodal metastases is reported in about 35% of all patients and in approximately 50% of those with palpable lymph nodes.[5,17,21,22]

Distant metastases are uncommon (about 10%), even in patients with advanced locoregional disease, and usually occur in patients with inguinal lymph node involvement. These patients often die of septic complications, erosion of large vessels in the groin, or a combination of the two.

The natural history of carcinoma of the anterior urethra in the male is similar to that of carcinoma of the penis. Approximately 40% of tumors originate in the anterior urethra.[19] Many tumors are low grade and progress slowly at primary and regional sites rather than spread to distal areas. Tumors of the penile urethra spread to the inguinal lymph nodes first, whereas those of the bulbomembranous and prostatic urethra metastasize first to the pelvic lymph nodes. Approximately one-third of men will present with either clinically or pathologically involved lymph nodes.[19]

Urethral cancers tend to spread by direct extension to adjacent structures. Invasion into the vascular space of the corpus spongiosum in the periurethral tissues is common. Malignancies beginning in the bulbomembranous urethra often invade the deep structures of the perineum, including the urogenital diaphragm, prostate, and adjacent skin. In the majority of prostatic urethral tumors, the bulk of the prostate gland is invaded at the time of diagnosis. Hematogenous spread is uncommon except in advanced regional disease. Kaplan et al.[20] reported distant metastases in about 15% of patients; most had corpora cavernosa invasion at diagnosis.

CLINICAL PRESENTATION

Carcinoma of the penis may present as either an infiltrative-ulcerative or an exophytic papillary lesion. Figure 68.1 demonstrates the localization of penile tumors in 259 patients from 14 cancer institutes in France. The glans and the prepuce were the predominant sites of the primary lesion, whereas tumors of the shaft were rare.[23] Assessment of the primary lesion may be obscured by the presence of phimosis. Secondary infection and associated foul smell are quite common. Urethral obstruction is an unusual symptom of carcinoma of the penis. The most common presenting symptom is a mass, which occurs in over two-thirds of patients. Ulceration is also common, occurring in approximately half of patients.[22,24] In a collective series of 552 patients with penile carcinoma, the presenting symptoms were mass lesions (78%), pain or itching (12%), bleeding (7%), groin mass (7%), and urinary symptoms (4%).[25–27] Inguinal lymph nodes are palpable on presentation in 30% to 45% of patients;[5,17,21,26,28,29] however, only half contain tumor.[21,22] Enlargement of the lymph nodes is often related to inflammatory (infectious) processes. Administration of antibiotics over several weeks results in regression of inguinal lymph nodes in a substantial proportion of cases and many have advocated this practice before the status of the regional lymph nodes is definitively assessed. Conversely, between 20% and 40% of patients with clinically negative inguinal lymph nodes have occult metastases.[3,30–33]

Patients with urethral carcinoma most commonly present with obstructive symptoms (43%). Other presenting signs and symptoms include mass (28%), bleeding (20%), abscess (20%), and irritative symptoms (20%).[19] These symptoms are often attributed to urethritis or urethral stricture, which may precede the development of urethral carcinoma and may also result in delay in diagnosis. The majority of urethral carcinomas occur in the bulbomembranous (posterior) region (61%), and tumors in this location have a worse prognosis compared with those arising in the anterior urethra.[19]

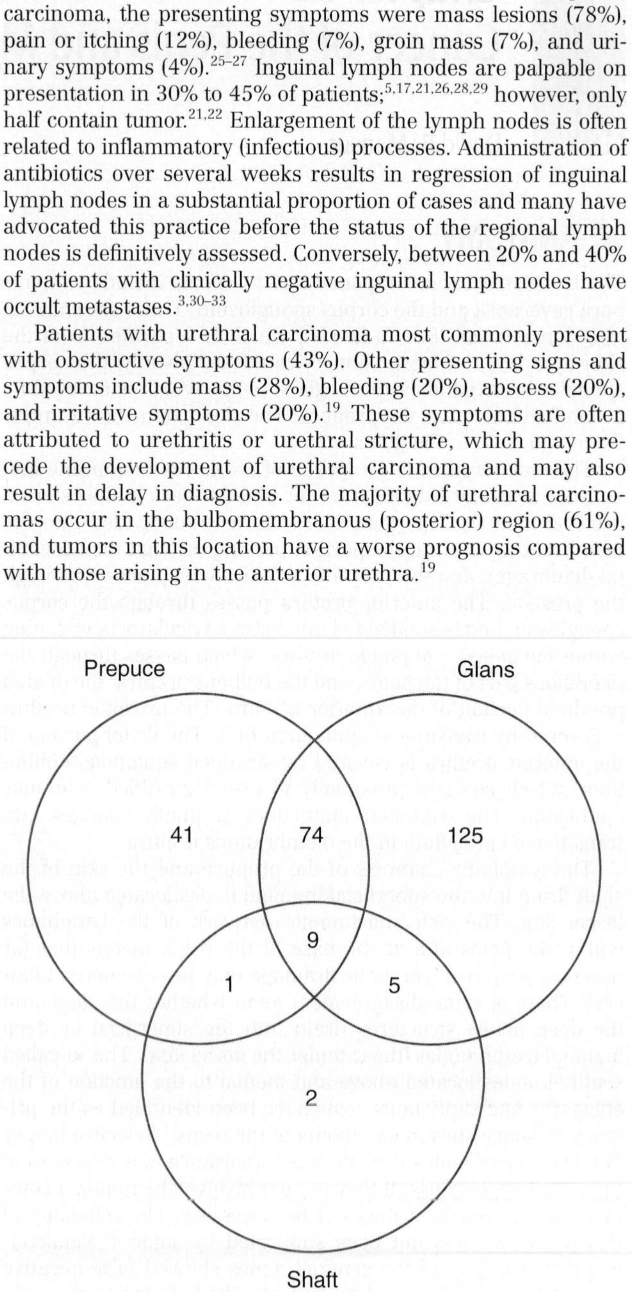

FIGURE 68.1. Localization of the primary tumor in 259 patients; each circle represents one anatomic compartment. Intersections indicate involvement of two or three compartments. Unknown: two. (From Rozan R, Albuisson E, Giraud B, et al. Interstitial brachytherapy for penile carcinoma: a multicentric survey (259 patients). *Radiother Oncol* 1995;36:83–93, copyright 1995, with permission from Elsevier.)

DIAGNOSTIC WORKUP

Diagnostic studies are required in the evaluation of patients with suspected or confirmed carcinoma of the penis and urethra. Urethroscopy and cystoscopy are essential for urethral primaries. Inguinal lymph nodes should be thoroughly evaluated. Computed tomography (CT) is useful in the identification of enlarged pelvic and periaortic lymph nodes in patients with involved inguinal lymph nodes.

Limited prospective data regarding the use of positron emission tomography (PET) with CT are available, but preliminary results show encouraging sensitivity (88%) and specificity (98%) in evaluating inguinal lymph nodes[34] and a diagnostic accuracy of 96% in evaluating pelvic lymph nodes in patients with known inguinal metastases.[35]

STAGING

The American Joint Committee on Cancer (AJCC) staging systems for carcinoma of the penis and urethra are shown in Tables 68.1 and 68.2, respectively.[36]

TABLE 68.1 AMERICAN JOINT COMMITTEE STAGING SYSTEM FOR CARCINOMA OF THE PENIS

Primary Tumor (T)			
TX	Primary tumor cannot be assessed		
T0	No evidence of primary tumor		
Tis	Carcinoma in situ		
Ta	Noninvasive verrucous carcinoma		
T1a	Tumor invades subepithelial connective tissue without lymph vascular invasion and is not poorly differentiated (i.e., grade 3–4)		
T1b	Tumor invades subepithelial connective tissue with lymph vascular invasion or is poorly differentiated		
T2	Tumor invades corpus spongiosum or cavernosum		
T3	Tumor invades urethra		
T4	Tumor invades other adjacent structures		
Regional Lymph Nodes (N)			
cNX	Regional lymph nodes cannot be assessed		
cN0	No palpable or visibly enlarged inguinal lymph nodes		
cN1	Palpable mobile unilateral lymph node		
cN2	Palpable mobile multiple or bilateral inguinal lymph nodes		
cN3	Palpable fixed inguinal nodal mass or pelvic lymphadenopathy unilateral or bilateral		
pNX	Regional lymph nodes cannot be assessed		
pN0	No regional lymph node metastasis		
pN1	Metastasis in a single inguinal lymph node		
pN2	Metastasis in multiple or bilateral inguinal lymph nodes		
pN3	Extranodal extension of lymph node metastasis or pelvic lymph node(s) unilateral or bilateral		
Distant Metastasis (M)			
M0	No distant metastasis		
M1	Distant metastasis (includes lymph node metastasis outside the true pelvis)		
Additional Descriptor	The m suffix indicates the presence of multiple primary tumors and is recorded in parentheses–e.g. pTa (m)N0M0		
Stage Grouping			
0	Tis	N0	M0
	Ta	N0	M0
I	T1a	N0	M0
II	T1b	N0	M0
	T2	N0	M0
	T3	N0	M0
IIIa	T1–3	N1	M0
IIIb	T1–3	N2	M0
IV	T4	Any N	M0
	Any T	N3	M0
	Any T	Any N	M1

Used with the permission of the American Joint Committee on Cancer (AJCC), Chicago, Illinois. The original source for this material is the *AJCC Cancer Staging Manual,* 7th Edition (2010) published by Springer Science and Business Media LLC, www.springer.com.

TABLE 68.2 AMERICAN JOINT COMMITTEE STAGING SYSTEM OF CARCINOMA OF THE URETHRA

Primary Tumor (T) (Male and Female)			
TX	Primary tumor cannot be assessed		
T0	No evidence of primary tumor		
Ta	Noninvasive papillary, polypoid, or verrucous carcinoma		
Tis	Carcinoma in situ		
T1	Tumor invades subepithelial connective tissue		
T2	Tumor invades corpus spongiosum or prostate or periurethral muscle		
T3	Tumor invades corpus cavernosum or beyond prostatic capsule or the anterior vagina or bladder neck		
T4	Tumor invades other adjacent organs		
Regional Lymph Nodes (N)			
NX	Regional lymph nodes cannot be assessed		
N0	No regional lymph node metastasis		
N1	Metastasis in a single lymph node, ≤2 cm in greatest dimension		
N2	Metastasis in a single lymph node, >2 cm in greatest dimension or metastases to multiple lymph nodes		
Distant Metastasis (M)			
MX	Presence of distant metastasis cannot be assessed		
M0	No distant metastasis		
M1	Distant metastasis		
Stage Grouping			
0a	Ta	N0	
0is	Tis	N0	
I	T1	N0	
II	T2	N0	
III	T1	N1	
	T2	N1	
	T3	N0	
	T3	N1	
IV	T4	N0	
	T4	N1	
	Any T	N2	
	Any T	Any N	M1

Used with the permission of the American Joint Committee on Cancer (AJCC), Chicago, Illinois. The original source for this material is the *AJCC Cancer Staging Manual,* 7th Edition (2010) published by Springer Science and Business Media LLC, www.springer.com.

PATHOLOGIC CLASSIFICATION

Most malignant penile tumors are well-differentiated squamous cell carcinomas.[37] Although an apparent adverse prognostic effect of anaplasia has been reported in some series,[17] others found no significant correlation between histologic grade and survival.[18,26]

Bowen disease is squamous cell carcinoma *in situ* that may involve the shaft of the penis as well as the hairy skin of the inguinal and suprapubic area. Clinically, the lesion is a solitary, dull-red plaque with areas of crusting and oozing. Approximately 25% to 50% of patients with this disease have a concomitant visceral malignancy.[6]

Erythroplasia of Queyrat is an epidermoid carcinoma *in situ* that involves the mucosal or mucocutaneous areas of the prepuce or glans.[37] It appears as a reddened, elevated, or ulcerated lesion. Graham and Helwig[38] reported that 10 of 100 patients presenting with erythroplasia of Queyrat had invasive squamous cell carcinoma at diagnosis. Mikhail[39] reported on 5 of 15 patients with the same presentation. Erythroplasia of Queyrat is not as frequently associated with internal malignancies as Bowen's disease.[40]

Basal cell carcinoma is infrequently reported, accounting for 1% to 2% of all cases of penile cancers.[41,42]

Extramammary Paget disease is a rare intraepithelial apocrine carcinoma. The most common sites are the scrotum, inguinal folds, and perineal region.[39] The lesion has a propensity to metastasize, necessitating frequent assessment of regional nodes. Radiation therapy has been recommended as palliative treatment.[39]

TABLE 68.3 PRIMARY MALIGNANCIES ASSOCIATED WITH SECONDARY CANCERS OF THE PENIS IN 219 PATIENTS

Site of Primary Malignancy	Number of Patients
Genitourinary Tract	
Bladder	65
Prostate	65
Kidney	23
Testis	10
Ureter	1
Gastrointestinal Tract	
Rectum/sigmoid	34
Colon	1
Anus	1
Liver	1
Pancreas	1
Respiratory Tract	
Lungs	8
Nasopharynx	1
Other	
Lymphosarcoma/reticulum cell sarcoma	4
Bone	2
Burkitt's lymphoma	1
Skin (malignant melanoma)	1

From Powell BL, Craig JB, Muss HB. Secondary malignancies of the penis and epididymis: a case report and review of the literature. *J Clin Oncol* 1985;3:110–116; reprinted with permission, copyright 1985 American Society of Clinical Oncology.

Soft tissue tumors are uncommon. Approximately half of the tumors are benign and may include angiomatous, neurogenous, myogenous, fibrous, and lymphoreticular tumors.[43,44] Most soft tissue tumors occur on the shaft and are malignant.

Primary lymphoma of the penis was reported in one patient with Peyronie disease, without other evidence of lymphomatous involvement. Five cases of secondary involvement of the penis by lymphoma were reported in the literature.[45]

Cancers metastatic to the penis are rare and usually represent late, advanced carcinomatosis. The most common neoplasms metastasizing to the penis are from the genitourinary organs, followed by the gastrointestinal and respiratory systems (Table 68.3). The predominant cell type is carcinoma, occurring in 202 of 219 cases.[46] Sarcomas and tumors of unknown histologic type are rare. A palpable mass, swelling, nodule, or skin change frequently occurs. Priapism as an initial presenting feature or subsequent development occurs in 40% of patients.[46]

The histological subtypes in the Memorial Sloan-Kettering Cancer Center series of urethral cancers included squamous cell carcinoma (52%), transitional cell carcinoma (33%), epidermoid carcinoma (11%), adenocarcinoma (2%), and anaplastic carcinoma (2%).[19] Primary malignant melanoma arising from the urethra has been reported.[47,48] The frequency of histologic type varies with site. Over 90% of carcinomas of the prostatic urethra are of transitional cell type. Adenocarcinomas occur only in the bulbomembranous urethra.

PROGNOSTIC FACTORS

The principal prognostic factors in carcinoma of the penis are extent of the primary lesion and status of the lymph nodes.[24,49] The incidence of nodal involvement is related to the size, location, and grade of the primary lesion. Invasion of deep-seated structures (corpora cavernosa) carries a high risk of deep inguinal node involvement.

Tumor-free regional nodes imply an excellent (80% to 90%) long-term survival or cure.[21,29,49] Patients with involvement of the inguinal nodes fare considerably worse, and only 40% to 50% survive long term.[21,29,49,50] Pelvic lymph node involvement implies a still worse prognosis; less than 20% of these patients survive.[5,21,26] Gerbaulet and Lambin[51] reported the results of 109 patients with carcinoma of penis at Institut Gustave-Roussy. The actuarial survival rates of patients with negative nodes were 82% at 5 years and 59% at 10 years. For patients with positive nodes, the survival rates were 36% and 18%, respectively. The number of positive lymph nodes has also been reported to have prognostic significance. Brkovic et al.[52] reported a 5-year survival rate of 71% in patients with solitary inguinal lymph node metastasis compared with 33% in patients with multiple positive inguinal nodes.

Tumor differentiation was shown to be an important prognostic factor by Fraley et al.[53] None of 9 patients with carcinoma *in situ,* 1 of 20 with well differentiated, 5 of 13 with moderately differentiated, and 3 of 4 with poorly differentiated lesions died of their tumors. Other investigators have confirmed the prognostic significance of tumor grade.[24,49,54,55]

Carcinoma of the penis has been reported to have greater propensity to metastasize and poorer prognosis in patients younger than 50 years of age[53] and patients older than 65 years of age.[54] Soria et al.[24] reported younger age at presentation adversely affected disease free survival, but not overall survival. Conversely, Marcial et al.[56] observed no difference in survival in relation to age.

The potential influence of HPV on prognosis was studied retrospectively in a cohort of patients treated surgically. HPV DNA was detected in paraffin-embedded specimens in 30% of patients. The presence of HPV had no prognostic significance with regard to lymph node metastasis or overall survival.[57]

Overall prognosis in males with carcinoma of the urethra varies considerably with location of the primary lesion.[19,58-63] Distal lesions generally have a prognosis similar to that of carcinoma of the penis. Lesions of the bulbomembranous urethra are usually quite extensive and are associated with a dismal prognosis. Dalbagni et al.[19] reported a 5-year overall survival of 69% in patients with anterior tumors compared with 26% in patients with posterior tumors. Other prognostic factors included lymph node status and histology (superficial vs. invasive). Tumors of the prostatic urethra show prognostic features similar to those in bladder carcinoma. Superficial lesions have a good prognosis and may be managed with transurethral resection.[61] Deeply invasive tumors have a greater tendency to develop inguinal or pelvic lymph node and distant metastases.

GENERAL MANAGEMENT

Carcinoma of the Penis

Conservative Therapies

Treatment for carcinoma *in situ* and very small penile carcinomas includes topical imiquimod and 5-fluorouracil (5-FU).[64] For larger lesions, conservative laser surgery[65] or Mohs micrographic surgery is used.[66]

Surgery

Treatment of patients with carcinoma of the penis is generally performed in two phases: initial management of the primary tumor and later treatment of the regional lymphatics. Surgical intervention at the primary site may range from local excision, including circumcision, or laser surgery[67] in a small group of highly selected patients, especially those with small lesions of the prepuce, to partial or total penectomy.[22,52,54] In very advanced proximal tumors, more aggressive resections such as total emasculation (penectomy, scrotectomy, orchiectomy) or cystoprostatectomy may be indicated.[68] Although surgical resection is a highly effective and an expedient treatment modality in most cases, it may not be acceptable to sexually active patients. Radical surgery, especially total penectomy, may be psychologically devastating to the patient. The ideal surgical procedure removes the disease with adequate margins while preserving sexual and urinary function, although this is not always possible because of the extent of disease. The high local recurrence rates described in some reports with limited surgery[69,70] illustrate the need for careful patient selection in choosing a surgical approach. Lesions confined to the prepuce may be treated with wide circumcision. Microsurgical techniques have shown local excision to be an acceptable and desirable option with small superficial lesions. A local control rate of 92% was achieved in 29 patients with a 5-year survival rate of 81% for stage I and 57% for stage II lesions.[71] Lesions on the glans penis have traditionally been treated by partial penectomy. Larger or more invasive lesions (stage III) can be treated by partial or total penectomy. Partial penectomy is the procedure of choice if surgical margins of 2 cm can be achieved. If an adequate margin cannot be achieved, total penectomy with perineal urethrotomy is warranted. Local (stump) recurrence is quite rare.[5] It is possible for some patients to remain sexually active after partial penectomy. Jensen[72] reported 45% of patients with 4 to 6 cm and 25% of patients with 2 to 4 cm of penile stump could perform sexual intercourse. D'Ancona et al.[73] evaluated the quality of life in 14 patients treated with partial penectomy. Sexual function was reported to be normal or only slightly decreased in 64% of patients. Complete loss of sexual function was reported in 14% of patients.

Surgical Treatment of Inguinal Lymph Nodes

The clinical evaluation of inguinal lymph nodes in men with cancer of the penis is unreliable. Several series have shown the sensitivity of clinical staging of the nodes to be 40% to 60% and false-negative rates to be 10% to 20%.[3,4] McDougal et al.[74] reported the correlation between clinical findings and pathologic positivity of inguinal nodes in patients with penile carcinoma. For tumors with no invasion or superficial invasion, moderately or well differentiated, only 12% of clinically enlarged inguinal nodes were pathologically positive. However, 78% to 88% of invasive or poorly differentiated tumors metastasized to inguinal nodes regardless of clinical findings. In a prospective study involving 37 patients with clinically negative groins, Solsona et al.[33] have demonstrated the predictive value of histologic grade and T stage in predicting the likelihood of occult positive lymph nodes. Three groups were identified: low, intermediate, and high risk with an incidence of occult positive nodes of 0%, 33%, and 83%, respectively (Table 68.4). Given the unreliability of clinical assessment, a rationale exists to submit all patients to the staging and therapeutic benefits of radical inguinal lymph node dissection. However, this procedure is associated with considerable morbidity. Up to one-half of patients will experience complications including wound necrosis or dehiscence, infection, lymphocele, erosion of femoral vessels, chronic lymphedema, thrombophlebitis, or pulmonary embolism.[50,68] The morbidity of radical lymphadenectomy and the relative small percentage of patients with pathologic involvement of inguinal nodes have resulted in surveillance as the initial management of regional lymph nodes in clinically negative patients at some centers.

TABLE 68.4 T STAGE AND GRADE PREDICT THE RISK OF OCCULT POSITIVE LYMPH NODES

Risk Group		Occult Positive Lymph Nodes (%)
Low	Tis, T1 grade 1	0/13 (0)
Intermediate	T1 grade 2–3 T2 grade 1	4/12 (33.3)
High	T2 grade 2 T2–3 grade 3	10/12 (83.3)

From Solsona E, Iborra I, Rubio J, et al. Prospective validation of the association of local tumor stage and grade as a predictive factor for occult lymph node micrometastasis in patients with penile carcinoma and clinically negative inguinal lymph nodes. *J Urol* 2001;165:1506, with permission.

Of concern, however, are reports describing poor salvage rates after regional failure. McDougal et al.[74] reported a 5-year disease-free survival rate of 88% for patients with clinical stage II disease who underwent immediate lymphadenectomy compared with 38% if delayed lymphadenectomy was performed. Johnson and Lo[75] reported that only one of eight patients undergoing late inguinal node dissection survived 5 years. Fraley et al.[53] noted an 88% 5-year survival rate with immediate lymphadenectomy compared with 8% with a delayed procedure. Sentinel node biopsy has been advocated as a less morbid means of evaluating inguinal nodes by some,[4] but its reliability has been questioned by others.[2,76] Catalona[4] and Colberg et al.[77] described a modified inguinal lymphadenectomy for patients with penile cancer and clinically negative groins. Long-term follow-up of nine patients reveals significantly less morbidity than the classic groin dissection designed by Daseler et al.[78] Extension of the nodal dissection into the pelvis to cover the iliac lymph nodes is justified in patients with evidence of inguinal involvement (positive biopsy of Cloquet's node). Approximately 20% of patients with pelvic lymph node involvement can be salvaged by radical pelvic lymphadenectomy.[5,79]

As demonstrated in other anatomic sites, such as the head and neck, uterine cervix, vagina, and vulva, patients with clinically negative lymph nodes who are at risk for microscopic nodal metastases (primary tumor beyond stage I or less than well-differentiated histology) can receive elective irradiation to the inguinal lymph nodes with a high probability of tumor control and low morbidity.

Radiation Therapy

The primary advantage of radiation therapy is organ preservation. In the past, radiation therapy often utilized insufficient total dose and high-dose per fraction along with poor technique, resulting in underdosage or overdosage and a high incidence of injury to normal tissues. Although historically a wide variation of techniques, doses, and fractionation schemes have been used,[17,80–84] improvement in the tumor control rate in some modern series employing adequate total doses and small daily doses is noteworthy, resulting in a decreased incidence of treatment-related sequelae. Most patients who experience local failure after radiation therapy can be salvaged surgically. Several radiation modalities are used to deliver radiation to the penis including megavoltage external-beam irradiation, iridium-192 (^{192}Ir) mold plesiotherapy, and interstitial implant using ^{192}Ir wires.[67,84–85,86,87]

Inguinal lymph node irradiation for clinically negative nodes is an integral component of successful radiotherapeutic management of this disease. Regional control has been achieved in 95% of cases. Without irradiation to the inguinal lymph nodes, as many as 20% of patients can be expected to develop positive nodes later.[17,81] For palpable nodes, groin dissection may be necessary, accepting the likelihood of postoperative morbidity. Postoperative radiation therapy to the groin adds little to the morbidity but contributes significantly to locoregional tumor control. If the inguinal lymph nodes are treated, a CT scan helps define the depth and location of the inguinal lymph node, femoral artery, and veins, which is crucial, as indicated in Chapter 74 on the vulva.

Chemotherapy

The use of systemic chemotherapy either as an adjuvant or concomitantly with radiation therapy has not been fully investigated in patients with penile cancer. Chemoradiotherapy of squamous cell carcinoma of the anus (another HPV-related carcinoma) has been used with great success, resulting in high tumor control rates and organ preservation. Similar data in penile carcinoma are lacking, however. Modern multiagent chemotherapy regimens have overall response rates ranging from 15% to 55% in patients with advanced disease (Table 68.5). The agents most commonly used include platinum, methotrexate,

TABLE 68.5 MULTIAGENT CHEMOTHERAPY IN ADVANCED PENILE CARCINOMA

Author (Reference)	*Agents*	*n*	*PR (%)*	*CR (%)*	*Median Survival (Month)*	*Life Threatening Toxicity (%)*	*Fatal Toxicity (%)*
Hass et al. (107)	Bleomycin Platinum Methotrexate	40	20	12.5	7	17	12.5
Corral et al. (108)	Bleomycin Platinum Methotrexate	29	41	14	11.5	–	3.4
Kattan et al. (109)	Varied (platinum based)	13	8	8	7.6	–	–

PR, partial response; CR, complete response.

and bleomycin. Additional clinical trials are needed to adequately define the role of chemotherapy in the management of cancer of the penis.

Carcinoma of the Male Urethra

The primary mode of therapy for carcinoma of the male urethra is surgical excision. Because of the rarity of this disease, comparison of the cure rates with radiation therapy or surgery is difficult. The principal advantage of irradiation is organ preservation. Noninvasive carcinoma of the proximal urethra can be treated with transurethral resection. In lesions of the distal urethra, results with either penectomy or radiation therapy are similar to those for carcinoma of the penis, and the 5-year survival rates are comparable (50% to 60%).[88] Involved regional lymph nodes are treated with lymphadenectomy.

Most patients, however, present with advanced invasive lesions, which are difficult to manage with either radical surgery or radiation therapy. The major problem is the high rate of local recurrence. In an attempt to improve the locoregional control rate, extended resections encompassing the inferior pubic rami, prostate, bladder, and perineum have been performed after preoperative radiation therapy. After a dose of 20 to 60 Gy, Klein et al.[60] performed an extended resection in seven patients with proximal urethral lesions. Locoregional failure was observed in two patients (29%).

Chemotherapy

Concomitant chemoradiotherapy has been investigated in only a few patients. However, these preliminary data are encouraging. Gheiler et al.[47] reported their experience with multimodality treatment of 21 patients (10 women, 11 men) with urethral carcinoma. Treatment consisted of cisplatin- and 5-FU-based chemotherapy for squamous cell carcinoma and concomitant external-beam irradiations. Patients with transitional cell carcinoma were treated with concomitant methotrexate, vinblastine, Adriamycin (doxorubicin), and cisplatin. Some patients underwent surgical resection following chemoradiation. With a median follow-up of 42 months, the overall disease-free survival rate was 62%. Of significance is the pathological complete response rate of 87.5% in eight women undergoing resection following chemoradiation.

RADIATION THERAPY TECHNIQUES

Carcinoma of the Penis

If indicated, circumcision must be performed before radiation therapy is initiated. The purpose of this procedure is to minimize radiation therapy–associated morbidity: swelling, irritation of the skin, moist desquamation, and secondary infection.

Although external-beam therapy has become prevalent in the treatment of the primary lesion in carcinoma of the penis, plastic molds or interstitial implants are still used.

External-Beam Radiation Therapy

External-beam therapy requires specially designed accessories (including bolus) necessary to achieve homogeneous dose distribution to the entire penis. Frequently, a plastic box with a central circular opening that can be fitted over the penis is used. The space between the skin and the box must be filled with tissue-equivalent material (Fig. 68.2). This box can then be treated with parallel opposed megavoltage beams. An alternative to the box technique is the use of a water-filled container to envelop the penis while the patient is in a prone position.[89]

Another more complex device consists of a Perspex tube attached to a baseplate resting on the skin.[90] This is placed as close as possible to the base of the penis, and a flexible tube is connected to a vacuum pump. The suction effect keeps the penis in a fixed position during treatment. Appropriate bolus is

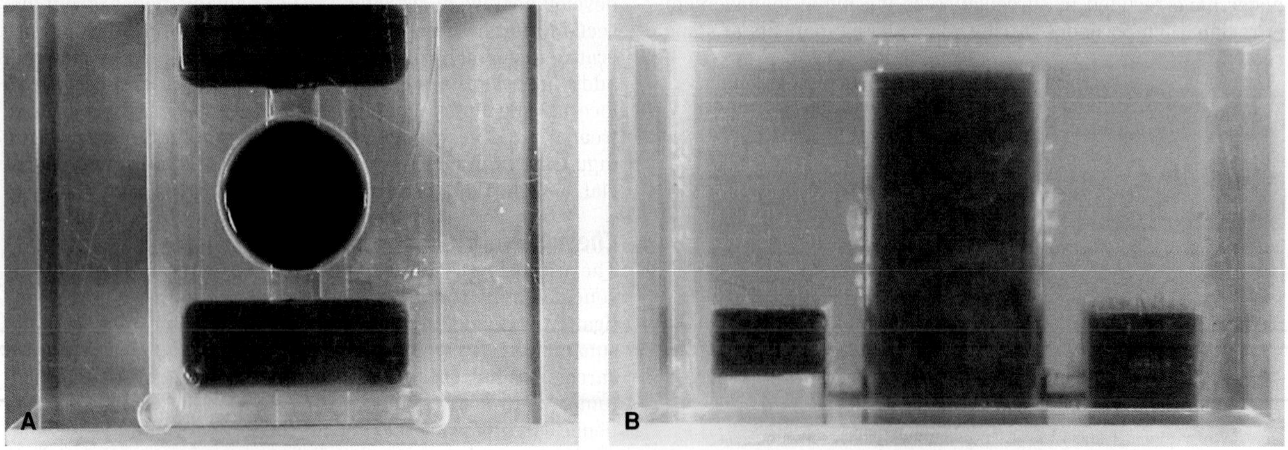

FIGURE 68.2. A: View from above of plastic box with central cylinder for external irradiation of the penis. Patient is treated in the prone position. The penis is placed in the central cylinder, and water is used to fill the surrounding volume in the box. Depth dose is calculated at the central point of box. **B:** Lateral view.

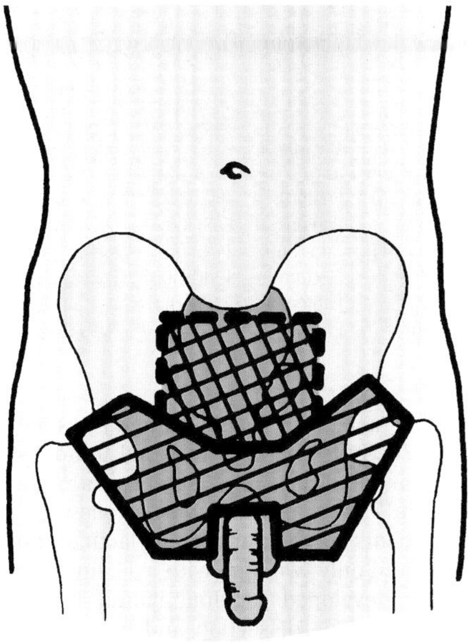

FIGURE 68.3. Portals encompassing inguinal and pelvic lymph nodes.

placed outside the tube. The patient can also be treated in the prone position, with the penis hanging through a small hole placed in the Perspex's cylinder.

Fraction size in many of the reported series has been 2.5 to 3.5 Gy (total dose of 50 to 55 Gy), although a smaller daily fraction size (1.8 to 2.0 Gy) and a higher total dose are preferable. There is a well-established association between large fraction size and late tissue damage (Chapter 1). A total of 60 to 65 Gy, with the last 5 to 10 Gy delivered to a reduced portal, should result in a reduced incidence of late fibrosis.

Regional lymphatics may be treated with external-beam megavoltage irradiation. Both groins should be irradiated. The fields should include inguinal *and* pelvic (external iliac and hypogastric) lymph nodes (Fig. 68.3). The posterior pelvis may be partially spared by anterior loading of the beams. Depending on the extent of the nodal disease and the proximity of the detectable tumor to the skin surface or the presence of skin invasion, application of a bolus to the inguinal area should be considered. If clinical and radiographic evaluation show no gross enlargement of the pelvic lymph nodes, the dose to these nodes may be limited to 50 Gy. In patients with palpable lymph nodes, doses of approximately 75 to 70 Gy over 7 to 8 weeks (1.8 to 2.0 Gy per day) with reducing fields (after 50 Gy) are advised. Alternatively, grossly involved nodes can be removed surgically either before or after inguinal radiation therapy.

Brachytherapy

A mold is usually built in the form of a box or cylinder with a central opening and channels for placement of radioactive sources (needles or wires) in the periphery of the device. The cylinder and sources should be long enough to prevent underdosage at the tip of the penis. A dose of 60 to 65 Gy at the surface and approximately 50 Gy at the center of the organ is delivered over 6 to 7 days. The mold can be applied either continuously, in which case an indwelling catheter should be in place, or intermittently. Intermittent application requires precise time record keeping. Alternatively, single- or double-plane implants can be used to deliver 60 to 70 Gy in 5 to 7 days.[87] Salaverria et al.[55] point out that molds should be reserved for stage I and II tumors. The author believes the same is true for interstitial implants. In more extensive lesions involving the shaft of the penis, it is technically difficult to obtain an adequate margin with brachytherapy procedures, similar to the problem in performing a partial penectomy.

Carcinoma of the Male Urethra

Radiation therapy for carcinoma of the anterior (distal) urethra is quite similar to that for carcinoma of the penis; lesions of the bulbomembranous urethra can be treated with a set of parallel opposed fields covering the groins and the pelvis, followed by perineal and inguinal boost. Lesions of the prostatic urethra can be treated with techniques and doses similar to those used for carcinoma of the prostate.

RESULTS

Carcinoma of the Penis

At many institutions patients with carcinoma of the penis are treated surgically. A summary of selected modern surgical series is presented in Table 68.6. Ornellas et al.[32] reported the results of 350 patients treated with surgery alone. Five-year disease-free survival was 62% for patients treated with immediate lymphadenectomy versus 8% for those treated with delayed lymphadenectomy. For all node-negative patients, 5-year disease-free survival was 87% compared with 29% for node-positive patients. Boon et al.[91] reported tumor control in 13 of 16 patients (81%) with carcinoma *in situ* or T1 and T2 tumors treated with wide local excision and lasers.

Radiation therapy has yielded comparable results at several institutions. Engelstad,[81] Cade,[93] Paterson et al.,[93] Lederman,[94] and Thurgar[95] reported 5-year survival rates ranging from 45% to 68% in groups of patients ranging from 41 to 57 years treated with various irradiation techniques (mold, interstitial, external beam). The ability of irradiation to control the tumor is closely associated with the stage of the disease.

The 20-year experience of the Institut Gustave-Rousy was reported by Soria et al.[24] One hundred and two patients with tumors <4 cm in diameter with <1 cm corpora cavernosa invasion were treated with a conservative approach consisting of limited surgery (biopsy, local excision, or therapeutic circumcision) and interstitial brachytherapy (65 to 70 Gy delivered over 5 to 7 days). Regional lymph nodes were not treated electively but were dissected in patients with clinically enlarged nodes. With a median follow-up of 111 months, local tumor recurrence rate was 25%. A regional nodal recurrence developed in 21% of patients. Disease-free survival at 5 and 10 years was 56% and 42%, respectively. Overall survival at 5 and 10 years was 63% and 50%, respectively.

Grabstald and Kelley[31] reported 90% local tumor control in 10 patients with stage I lesions treated with external-beam irradiation for 51 to 52 Gy over 6 weeks. Another series from

TABLE 68.6 SURGICAL RESULTS IN PATIENTS WITH CARCINOMA OF THE PENIS

			Local Failure (%)		
T Stage	*Author (Reference)*	*n*	*Conserving Surgery[a]*	*Partial/ Total Penile Amputation*	*5-Year Overall Survival (%)*
T1	Brkovic et al. (52)	22	56	0	77
	Horenblas et al. (70)	–	10	–	–
	Lindegaard et al. (54)	41	–	–	72
T2	Brkovic et al. (52)	23	100	18	70
	Horenblas et al. (70)	–	32	–	–
	Lindegaard et al. (54)	26	–	–	55
T3/T4	Brkovic et al. (52)	6	–	–	0
	Horenblas (70)	–	100	–	–
	Lindegaard et al. (54)	6	–	–	10
T1-T4	Lindegaard et al. (54)	63	35	5	–
	Derakhshani et al. (22)	42	–	–	78
	Zouhair et al. (110)[b]	16	–	25	–
	Lopes et al. (50)	145	–	–	54

[a]Includes wide excision, laser ablation, radical circumcision.

[b]All patients treated with postoperative radiation therapy.

the MD Anderson Cancer Center demonstrated 80% local control and retention of the phallus in early-stage disease.[25] Duncan and Jackson[96] also reported 90% local control for stage I lesions treated with a megavoltage treatment unit delivering 50 to 57 Gy over 3 weeks.

Irradiation of the involved regional lymph nodes in patients with carcinoma of the penis results in permanent control and cure in a substantial proportion of patients. In the classic series of Staubitz et al.,[18] 13 patients with proven involvement of regional lymph nodes received radiation therapy to these nodes. Five of 13 (38%) survived 5 years. Narayana et al.[26] reported 2 of 16 patients (12%) with histologically proven lymph node metastases cured with radiation therapy. No data on radiation therapy are given for either series, precluding an assessment of the doses and fields.

Jackson[97] reported a 66% 5-year survival rate and 86% tumor control rate in 58 patients with stage I carcinoma of the penis treated with irradiation compared with a 70% 5-year survival rate and 81% tumor control rate in 27 surgically treated patients. In stage II, he observed 6 of 11 patients surviving 5 years and 7 exhibiting tumor control in contrast to 6 surviving and 8 showing tumor control in 12 surgically treated patients. In stage III, four of seven irradiated patients survived 5 years with tumor control in contrast to two surviving and three with tumor control in seven treated with surgery only. Radium or cobalt molds produced the best sterilization of primary tumor; if irradiation had not controlled the primary lesion after 6 months, amputation of the penis was carried out, with a significant proportion of the patients salvaged. Two patients required amputation because of necrosis of the penis, and four developed severe phimosis, which was treated with meatotomy. Three of 37 patients (8%) initially treated surgically and 14 of 69 (20%) initially treated with irradiation developed inguinal lymph node metastases. Overall, 8% of patients treated surgically and 10% of those irradiated died of inguinal lymph node metastases and subsequent tumor spread.

Almgard and Edsmyr[80] reported tumor control in 12 of 17 patients treated with irradiation alone (superficial x-rays). Four patients underwent local radical excision for recurrence and survived from 10 to 30 years. In 17 additional patients, local irradiation was followed by amputation of the penis, and 16 had been free of recurrence for 5 to 32 years. Marcial et al.[56] noted 5-year survival in 4 of 6 patients who received irradiation alone, in 6 of 11 who were given irradiation for frank persistence after limited surgery to the penis, and in 6 of 8 to whom irradiation was administered postoperatively. Sixteen of 25 patients (64%) survived 5 years.

In a series of 145 patients reported by Knudsen and Brennhovd,[98] 99 (68%) had recurrence, as did 5 of 14 patients (36%) treated by Johnson et al.[99] and 24 of 63 patients (38%) reported by Murrell and Williams.[82] Haile and Delclos[85] reported tumor control and conservation of the penis in 16 of 20 patients (80%) treated with conservative radiation therapy methods. Whereas irradiation alone or combined with a lymph node dissection controlled lymph node metastases smaller than 2 cm in four patients, radiation therapy was successful in controlling lymph node metastases in only one of seven patients with N2 or N3 lymph nodes.

Sagerman et al.[89] reported tumor control in six of nine patients with stage I, two of three with stage II, and one of three with stage IV disease treated with irradiation alone. Two patients with stage I disease and one with stage II disease were surgically salvaged. Doses ranged from 45 Gy (15 fractions in 3 weeks) to 64 Gy (32 fractions in 6.5 weeks) with either orthovoltage x-rays or cobalt-60 and appropriate bolus. Good palliation was described in four of nine patients treated for inguinal lymph node metastases to doses ranging from 20 (5 fractions in 1 week) to 64 Gy. None of these patients survived more than 18 months.

Mazeron et al.[86] described tumor control in 8 of 9 patients with stage T1, 21 of 27 with T2, and 10 of 14 with T3 tumors treated with ^{192}Ir, using the Paris dosimetry system, to deliver doses of 60 to 70 Gy to the 85% minimal tumor isodose. The tumor-free 5-year actuarial survival rate was 63%. The penis was preserved in 75% of patients with a follow-up of 8 years. Thirty-seven patients received no prophylactic treatment to the inguinal nodes, and only two (one with a T2 and another with a T3 lesion) later developed inguinal lymph node metastases treated by inguinal node dissection and postoperative irradiation. One patient was alive with no evidence of disease at 10 years. Five patients with metastases to the lymph nodes at the time of diagnosis were treated with therapeutic nodal dissection and postoperative irradiation. Four patients had uncontrolled lymph node metastases, and all five died with distant disease.

Duncan and Jackson[96] discussed the superiority of external-beam irradiation compared with mold therapy, with 3-year tumor control rates of 90% and 47%, respectively. Salaverria et al.[55] reported a 92% 5-year survival rate in 13 stage I and II patients treated with radium-226 or ^{192}Ir molds. This compared with 10 of 13 (77%) patients who survived after partial penectomy. In stage II, four of six patients survived 5 years after ^{192}Ir mold treatment. Ten patients with stage III disease were treated with radical amputation, and eight survived 5 years. Kearsley et al.[59] described a patient with locally advanced penile carcinoma and metastatic inguinal lymph nodes who was cured with irradiation alone, a remarkable achievement because most patients with stage IV die with locoregional and disseminated disease.

Tables 68.7 and 68.8 summarize tumor control rates achieved with external-beam irradiation alone or brachytherapy

TABLE 68.7 RESULTS OF EXTERNAL-BEAM IRRADIATION FOR CARCINOMA OF THE PENIS

		Local Tumor Control		
Author (Reference)	*Modality*	*Stage I–II (%)*	*Stage III–IV (%)*	*Penis Preservation (%)*
Duncan and Jackson (96)	Photon	16/20 (80)	–	80
Haile and Delclos (85)	Photon	6/6 (100)	2/2 (100)	80
Kaushal and Harma (111)	Cobalt-60	14/16 (88)	–	93
Kelley et al. (106)	Electron	10/10 (100)	–	100
Pointon (84)	Photon	27/32 (84)	–	–
Sagerman et al. (89)	Photon	9/12 (75)	1/3 (33)	–

TABLE 68.8 RESULTS OF BRACHYTHERAPY WITH OR WITHOUT EXTERNAL-BEAM IRRADIATION FOR CARCINOMA OF THE PENIS

		Tumor Control		
Author (Reference)	*Modality*	*Stage I–II (%)*	*Stage III–IV (%)*	*Penis Preservation (%)*
Almgard and Edsmyr (80)	ISI + ERT	14/16 (88)[a]	–	–
Chaudhary et al. (105)	ISI	18/23 (78)[a]	–	–
Daly et al. (112)	ISI	21/22 (95)[a]	–	86
El-Dimry et al. (113)	Mold	17/23 (74)[a]	–	–
Gerbaulet and Lambin (51)	ISI	89/109 (82)[a]	–	–
Haile and Delclos (85)	Mold + ISI	7/7 (100)	–	–
Jackson (97)	Mold	20/45 (44)	–	44
Knudsen and Brennhovd (98)	Mold	46/145 (32)[a]	–	–
Mazeron et al. (86)	ISI	29/36 (81)[a]	10/14 (71)	74
Pierquin et al. (87)	ISI	14/14 (100)	12/31 (39)	–
Rozan et al. (23)	ISI	162/184 (88)[a]		78
Rozan et al. (23)	ISI + ERT	66/75 (88)[a]	–	64
Salaverria et al. (55)	Mold	12/13 (92)	–	77
Soria et al. (24)	ISI	26/102 (75)[a]	–	53
Suchaud et al. (114)	ISI	37/53 (70)[a]	–	58

ISI, interstitial implant; ERT, external-beam irradiation.

[a]All stages.

TABLE 68.9 LOCAL TUMOR CONTROL OF MALE URETHRAL CARCINOMA WITH RADIATION THERAPY OR *EN BLOC* RESECTION

Author (Reference)	Number of Patients	Number Controlled
Radiation Therapy		
Hopkins et al. (115)	1	1
Kaplan et al. (20)	11	9
Raghavaiah (88)	2	2
En Bloc Resection		
Anderson and McAninch (116)	2	1
Klein et al. (60)	7	5
Kaplan et al. (20)	28	25

plus external-beam irradiation. Worth mentioning are the results of a multicenter report from France.[23] With interstitial brachytherapy, no relationship was found between increasing dose and increasing local control, with doses ranging from 60 to 65 Gy. Two variables have a significant impact on tumor recurrence: the maximum diameter of the tumor and deep infiltration of the disease.

Carcinoma of the Male Urethra

Historically, men with urethral carcinoma have been treated surgically. Dalbagni et al.[19] have reported the outcome of 46 patients with carcinoma of the anterior and bulbar urethra treated at the Memorial Sloan-Kettering Cancer Center. The majority of patients were treated with definitive surgery. With a median follow-up of 125 months, the local control rate was 51%. The 5-year overall survival was 42%. Improved survival was seen in patients with anterior lesions (69%) compared with those with posterior lesions (26%).

Bracken et al.[100] described results in 11 patients with tumors at or anterior to the penoscrotal junction, 8 of which were epidermoid carcinoma, 2 transitional cell carcinoma, and 1 melanoma. Three of four patients treated with total penectomy and perineal urethrostomy had tumor control. Partial penectomy controlled the local tumor in two patients. The patient with melanoma had a local recurrence after operation. Two patients were treated with radiation therapy and a third with a combination of preoperative irradiation (45 Gy) and total penectomy. In all of these patients, tumor recurred locally. In four patients with inguinal lymph node metastases, the regional disease was controlled by bilateral lymphadenectomy. All six patients in whom local and regional tumor was controlled remain alive and disease free at 1 to 20 years. In 16 patients, the urethral tumors arose posterior to the penoscrotal junction: 13 lesions were squamous cell carcinoma, 2 transitional cell, and 1 adenocarcinoma. Penectomy was performed in five patients, all of whom had tumor control and no evidence of recurrence 5 to 29 months after therapy. Two patients treated with local excision died of disease 14 and 18 months after surgery. Irradiation was used in three patients unsuccessfully, and all died of cancer 13 to 31 months after therapy.

Kaplan et al.[20] reported on 29 patients treated at Northwestern University and reviewed the literature. In their analysis, lesions of the distal urethra carried the best prognosis and those in the bulbomembranous urethra the worst. Five-year survival rates were 22% (16 of 71 patients) with tumors in the distal urethra, 10% (10 of 99 patients) with bulbomembranous urethra lesions, and 25% (4 of 16 patients) with prostatic urethra tumors. Radiation therapy was infrequently used for these patients. Table 68.9 demonstrates equivalent local tumor control with either definitive radiation therapy or *en bloc* resection.

The combination of radiation therapy and chemotherapy using 5-FU and mitomycin-C has been reported for urethral carcinoma for organ preservation in locally advanced tumors. Reports by Baskin and Turzan,[101] Johnson et al.,[102] Licht et al.,[103] and Shah et al.[104] support the efficacy of this combination for squamous cell carcinoma of the male and female urethra. Cleveland Clinic[103] reported results of patients with locally advanced squamous cell carcinoma of the urethra treated with concomitant chemoirradiation including 5-FU (1 g/m^2 intravenous infusion on days 1 to 4 and days 29 to 32) and mitomycin-C (50 mg/m^2 bolus intravenous injection on day 1). External-beam irradiation (30 Gy in 15 fractions) to the pelvis and inguinal lymph nodes began on day 1. An additional 20-Gy tumor boost was given. Complete response was obtained in three patients, who remained disease free after 43 months of follow-up. A patient with a T2N2M0 lesion treated with 30 Gy died of myocardial infarction several months after radiation therapy. Chemotherapy was well tolerated and required no dose reduction or delay in treatment. One grade 3 acute toxicity (skin reaction) occurred that did not compromise the therapeutic plan. One patient developed urethral stricture that was managed successfully with urethral dilatation.

As previously described in this chapter, the largest chemoradiation experience for urethral carcinoma is the Wayne State experience.[47] Concomitant 5-FU and cisplatin were used for squamous cell carcinoma, while concomitant methotrexate,

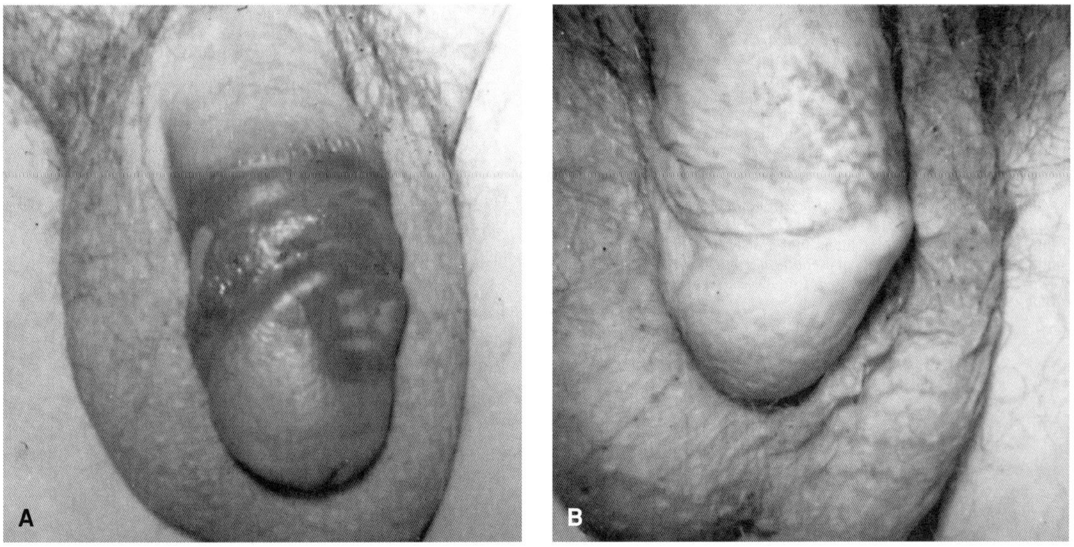

FIGURE 68.4. **A:** Squamous cell carcinoma of the balanopreputial region with extension into the glands (stage I). Patient was treated with 120 kVp x-rays, 0.3 mm Cu half-value layer, receiving 60-Gy skin dose in 5 weeks. **B:** Same patient 4 years later with no evidence of disease. Telangiectasis in present.

vinblastine, doxorubicin, and cisplatin (MVAC) were used for transitional cell carcinoma. A pathological complete response was reported in 87.5% of women undergoing resection following chemoradiation. With a median follow-up of 42 months, the overall disease-free survival rate was 62%.

SEQUELAE OF TREATMENT

Irradiation of the penis produces a brisk erythema, dry or moist desquamation, and swelling of the subcutaneous tissue of the shaft in virtually all patients. Although quite uncomfortable, these are reversible reactions that subside with conservative treatment within a few weeks. Telangiectasia is a common late consequence of radiation therapy and is usually asymptomatic (Fig. 68.4).

In the reported radiotherapy series, meatal-urethral strictures occur with a frequency of 0% to 40%.[62,83,85,104,105] This incidence compares favorably with the incidence of urethral stricture following penectomy.[22] Most strictures following radiation therapy are at the meatus.

Ulceration, necrosis of the glans, and necrosis of the skin of the shaft are rare complications in a modern series.[104] Lymphedema of the legs has been reported following inguinal and pelvic radiation therapy, but the role of irradiation in the development of this complication remains controversial. Many patients with this symptom have active disease in the lymphatics that may be responsible for lymphatic blockage.

Of all male genitourinary cancers, penile cancer poses the greatest threat to sexual function and carries the most devastating psychological impact of penectomy. Despite recent advances in treatment, sexual function is not likely to be adequately preserved in some patients. These patients and their partners need information about the physical impairments after surgical intervention and should be taught adjustment skills prior to undertaking treatment. Referral to a trained sexual consultant or therapist for help is indicated.

SELECTED REFERENCES

A full list of references for this chapter is available online.

1. Kumar S, Ananthakrishnan N, Prema V. Predicting regional lymph node metastasis in carcinoma of the penis: a comparison between fine-needle aspiration cytology, sentinel lymph node biopsy and medial inguinal lymph node biopsy. *Br J Urol* 1998;81:453–457.
2. Perinetti E, Crane DB, Catalona WJ. Unreliability of sentinel lymph node biopsy for staging penile carcinoma. *J Urol* 1980;124:734–735.
4. Catalona WJ. Modified inguinal lymphadenectomy for carcinoma of the penis with preservation of saphenous veins: technique and preliminary results. *J Urol* 1988;140:306–310.
8. Schoen EJ, Oehrli M, Colby CJ, et al. The highly protective effect of newborn circumcision against invasive penile cancer. *Pediatrics* 2000;105:E36.
9. Schrek R, Lenowitz H. Etiologic facts in carcinoma of the penis. *Cancer Res* 1947;7:180–187.
12. Miralles-Guri C, Bruni L, Cubilla AL, et al. Human papillomavirus prevalence and type distribution in penile carcinoma. *J Clin Path* 2009;62:870–878.
14. Martinez I. Relationship of squamous cell carcinoma of the cervix uteri to squamous cell carcinoma of the penis. *Cancer* 1979;24:777–780.
15. Graham S, Priore R, Graham M, et al. Genital cancer in wives of penile cancer patients. *Cancer* 1979;44:1870–1874.
16. Barroso LF, Wilkins T. Human papillomavirus vaccination in males: the state of the science. *Curr Infect Dis Rep* 2011;13:175–181.
23. Rozan R, Albuisson E, Giraud B, et al. Interstitial brachytherapy for penile carcinoma: A multicentric survey (259 patients). *Radiother Oncol* 1995;36:83–93.
31. Grabstald H, Kelley CD. Radiation therapy of penile cancer: six to ten-year follow-up. *Urology* 1980;15:575–576.
32. Ornellas AA, Seixas ALC, Marota A, et al. Surgical treatment of invasive squamous cell carcinoma of the penis: retrospective analysis of 350 cases. *J Urol* 1994;151:1244–1249.
33. Solsona E, Iborra I, Rubio J, et al. Prospective validation of the association of local tumor stage and grade as a predictive factor for occult lymph node micrometastasis in patients with penile carcinoma and clinically negative inguinal lymph nodes. *J Urol* 2001;165:1506–1509.
34. Schlenker B, Scher B, Tiling R, et al. Detection of inguinal lymph node involvement in penile squamous cell carcinoma by 18F-florodeoxyglucose PET/CT: a prospective single-center study. *Urol Oncol* 2012;30(1):55–59.
35. Graafland NM, Leijte JAP, Valdes Olmos RA, et al. Scanning with 18F-FDG-PET/CT for detection of pelvic nodal involvement in inguinal node- positive penile carcinoma. *Eur Urol* 2009;56:339–345.
43. Dehner LP, Smith BH. Soft tissue tumors of the penis: a clinicopathologic study of 46 cases. *Cancer* 1970;25:1431–1447.
47. Gheiler EL, Tefilli MV, Tiguert R, et al. Management of primary urethral cancer. *Urology* 1998;52:487–493.
48. Oliva E, Quinn TR, Amin MB, et al. Primary malignant melanoma of the urethra: a clinicopathologic analysis of 15 cases. *Am J Surg Pathol* 2000;24:785–796.
49. Villavicencio H, Rubio-Briones J, Regalado R, et al. Grade, local stage and growth pattern as prognostic factors in carcinoma of the penis. *Eur Urol* 1997;32:442–447.
50. Lopes A, Hidalgo GS, Kowalski LP, et al. Prognostic factors in carcinoma of the penis: multivariate analysis of 145 patients treated with amputation and lymphadenectomy. *J Urol* 1996;156:1637–1642.
51. Gerbaulet A, Lambin P. Radiation therapy of cancer of the penis: indications, advantages, and pitfalls. *Urol Clin North Am* 1992;19:325–332.
52. Brkovic D, Kälble T, Dörsam J, et al. Surgical treatment of invasive penile cancer—the Heidelberg experience from 1968 to 1994. *Eur Urol* 1997;31:339–342.
54. Lindegaard JC, Nielsen OS, Lundbeck FA, et al. A retrospective analysis of 82 cases of cancer of the penis. *Br J Urol* 1996;77:883–890.
57. Bezerra ALR, Lopes A, Santiago GH, et al. Human papillomavirus as a prognostic factor in carcinoma of the penis. *Cancer* 2001;91:2315–2321.
64. Shapiro D, Shasha D, Tareen M, et al. Contemporary management of localized penile cancer. *Expert Rev Anticancer Ther* 2011;11(1):29–36.
65. Solsana E, Bahl A, Brandes SB, et al. New developments in the treatment of localized penile cancer. *Urology* 2010;76(2 Suppl 1):S36–S42.
66. Salvioni R, Necchi A, Luigi P, et al. Penile cancer. *Urol Oncol* 2009;27(6):677–685.
70. Horenblas S, van Tinteren H, Delemarre JF, et al. Squamous cell carcinoma of the penis. II. Treatment of the primary tumor. *J Urol* 1992;147:1533–1538.
73. D'Ancona CAL, Botega NJ, De Moraes C, et al. Quality of life after partial penectomy for penile carcinoma. *Urology* 1997;50:593–596.
74. McDougal WS, Kirchner FK Jr, Edwards RH, et al. Treatment of carcinoma of the penis: the case for primary lymphadenectomy. *J Urol* 1986;136:38–41.
75. Johnson DE, Lo RK. Management of regional lymph nodes in penile carcinoma. *Urology* 1984;24:308–311.
76. Pettaway CA, Pisters LL, Dinney CP, et al. Sentinel lymph node dissection for penile carcinoma: the M.D. Anderson Cancer Center experience. *J Urol* 1995; 154:1999–2003.
77. Colberg JW, Andriole GL, Catalona WJ. Long-term follow-up of men undergoing modified inguinal lymphadenectomy for carcinoma of the penis. *Br J Urol* 1997;79:54–57.
86. Mazeron JJ, Langlois D, Lobo PA, et al. Interstitial radiation therapy for carcinoma of the penis using Iridium 192 wires: the Henri Mondor experience (1970–1979). *Int J Radiat Oncol Biol Phys* 1984;10:1891–1895.
88. Raghavaiah NV. Radiotherapy in the treatment of carcinoma of the male urethra. *Cancer* 1978;41:1313–1316.
89. Sagerman RH, Yu WS, Chung CT, et al. External-beam irradiation of carcinoma of the penis. *Radiology* 1984;152:183–185.
101. Baskin L, Turzan C. Carcinoma of the male urethra: management of locally advanced disease with combined chemotherapy, radiotherapy, and penile-preserving surgery. *Urology* 1992;39:21.
102. Johnson D, Kessler J, Ferrigni R, et al. Low dose combined chemotherapy/radiotherapy in the management of locally advanced urethral squamous cell carcinoma. *J Urol* 1989;141:615.
103. Licht MR, Klein EA, Bukowski R, et al. Combination radiation and chemotherapy for the treatment of squamous cell carcinoma of the male and female urethra. *J Urol* 1995;153:1918–1920.
105. Chaudhary AJ, Ghosh S, Bhalavat RL, et al. Interstitial brachytherapy in carcinoma of the penis. *Strahlenther Onkol* 1999;175:17–20.
107. Haas GP, Blumenstein BA, Gagliano RG, et al. Cisplatin, methotrexate and bleomycin for the treatment of carcinoma of the penis: a South West Oncology Group study. *J Urol* 1999;161:1823–1825.
109. Kattan J, Culine S, Droz J-P, et al. Penile cancer chemotherapy: Twelve years' experience at Institut Gustave-Roussy. *Urology* 1993;42:559–562.
110. Zouhair A, Coucke PA, Jeanneret W, et al. Radiation therapy alone or combined surgery and radiation therapy in squamous-cell carcinoma of the penis? *Eur J CA* 2001;37:198–203.
111. Kaushal V, Harma SC. Carcinoma of the penis. *Acta Oncol* 1987;26:413–417.
112. Daly N, Douchez J, Combes P. Treatment of carcinoma of the penis by iridium 192 wire implant. *Int J Radiat Oncol Biol Phys* 1982;8:1239–1243.
115. Hopkins S, Nag S, Soloway M. Primary carcinoma of the male urethra. *Urology* 1984;23:128–133.

Part J Gynecologic

Chapter 69
Uterine Cervix

Akila N. Viswanathan

ANATOMY

The uterus is a hollow, thick-walled, pear-shaped, muscular organ located in the pelvis above the vagina, behind the bladder, and in front of the rectum (Fig. 69.1). On average, it is approximately 7 to 8 cm long, 5 to 7 cm wide, and 2 to 3 cm thick. The uterus is divided into the uterine corpus superiorly and the uterine cervix inferiorly, with the most superior part of the corpus also known as the fundus and the middle portion of the corpus known as the body. The fundus is located superior to the line joining the entrance of the fallopian tubes. The body of the uterus is enclosed between layers of the broad ligament and is freely mobile. The regions of the body where the fallopian tubes enter are called the cornua. The most inferior, slightly constricted, portion of the uterus is called the isthmus or lower uterine segment (LUS). The cervix rests inferior to the LUS.

The uterus is usually bent anteriorly (anteflexed) between the cervix and the uterine body. The entire uterine-cervix structure is normally bent anteriorly (anteverted) in the pelvis. The uterus is frequently posteriorly retroverted, especially in older women who have a small uterus. The wall of the uterus has three layers: the outer serosal layer; the middle myometrium, which is approximately 12 to 15 mm of muscle through which the main blood vessels and nerves flow; and the inner coat called the endometrium.

The cervix measures approximately 3 by 3 cm and is predominantly a fibrous organ. The cervix is divided into an upper or supravaginal portion, above the ring containing the endocervical canal, and the vaginal portion, projecting in the vaginal vault. Central in the rounded vaginal region is the external os, bounded by the anterior and posterior lips of the cervix, extending inward to the internal os, the endocervical canal, and endometrial canal.

The uterus is partially covered by peritoneum in its fundal portion and posteriorly; its anterior and lateral surfaces are related to the bladder and the broad ligaments, respectively. It is attached to the surrounding structures in the pelvis by two pairs of ligaments—the broad and the round ligaments. The broad ligament is a double layer of peritoneum extending from the lateral margin of the uterus to the lateral wall of the pelvis. It contains the fallopian tubes. The two layers of peritoneum forming the broad ligament enclose the parametrium as it reaches the uterus. Inferiorly, the broad ligament follows the plane of the pelvic floor and ends medially in the upper portion of the vagina.[1]

The round ligament, a band of smooth muscle and connective tissue that contains small vessels and nerves, extends forward horizontally from its attachment in the anterolateral portion of the uterus to the lateral pelvic wall. The cord ascending from the lateral wall of the true pelvis crosses the pelvic brim and extends laterally to reach the abdominoinguinal ring, through which it leaves the abdomen to traverse the inguinal canal and terminates in the superficial fascia.

The uterosacral ligaments are paired supports for the lower uterus, extending from the uterus to the sacrum and running along the recto-uterine-peritoneal fields.[1] The cardinal ligaments, also called transverse cervical ligaments (Mackenrodt's), are thickened connective tissue and fascia arising at the upper lateral margins of the cervix and inserting into the fascial covering of the pelvic diaphragm.

The uterus including the uterine cervix has a rich lymphatic network (Fig. 69.2) that drains principally into the paracervical lymph nodes; from there it goes to the external iliac (of which the obturator nodes are the innermost component) and the hypogastric lymph nodes. The pelvic lymphatics drain into the common iliac and the para-aortic lymph nodes. Lymphatics from the fundus pass laterally across the broad ligament continuous with those of the ovary, ascending along the ovarian vessels into the para-aortic lymph nodes. Some of the fundal lymphatics also drain into the common iliac lymph nodes. The main artery supplying the uterus is the uterine artery, which originates from the anterior division of the hypogastric artery.

EPIDEMIOLOGY

Over the last 80 years, the morbidity and mortality of locally advanced invasive cervical cancer has dramatically declined in the United States and Europe due to effective screening and treatment of preinvasive lesions.[2] In the United States 50% of women who develop cervical cancer have never been screened and another 10% have not been screened within the previous 5 years. However, in the last decade, incidence rates of invasive carcinoma have remained relatively constant. The American Cancer Society estimates that approximately 12,200 new cases of invasive carcinoma of the cervix arise in the United States and about 4,200 deaths will occur per year, in addition to >60,000 cases of carcinoma *in situ.*[3]

Worldwide, cervical cancer remains the most common gynecologic cancer and the third-most-common malignancy in women, with over 500,000 women globally developing this tumor and 233,000 dying of the disease every year.[4] Unfortunately, it often affects young women, resulting in loss of the ability to bear future children. The larger societal impact from the death of young women in the prime of life and motherhood has not been measured.

In developing countries, cervical cancer is the leading cause of cancer-related death.[2] Cervical cancer is more common in areas where women have less access to screening, including

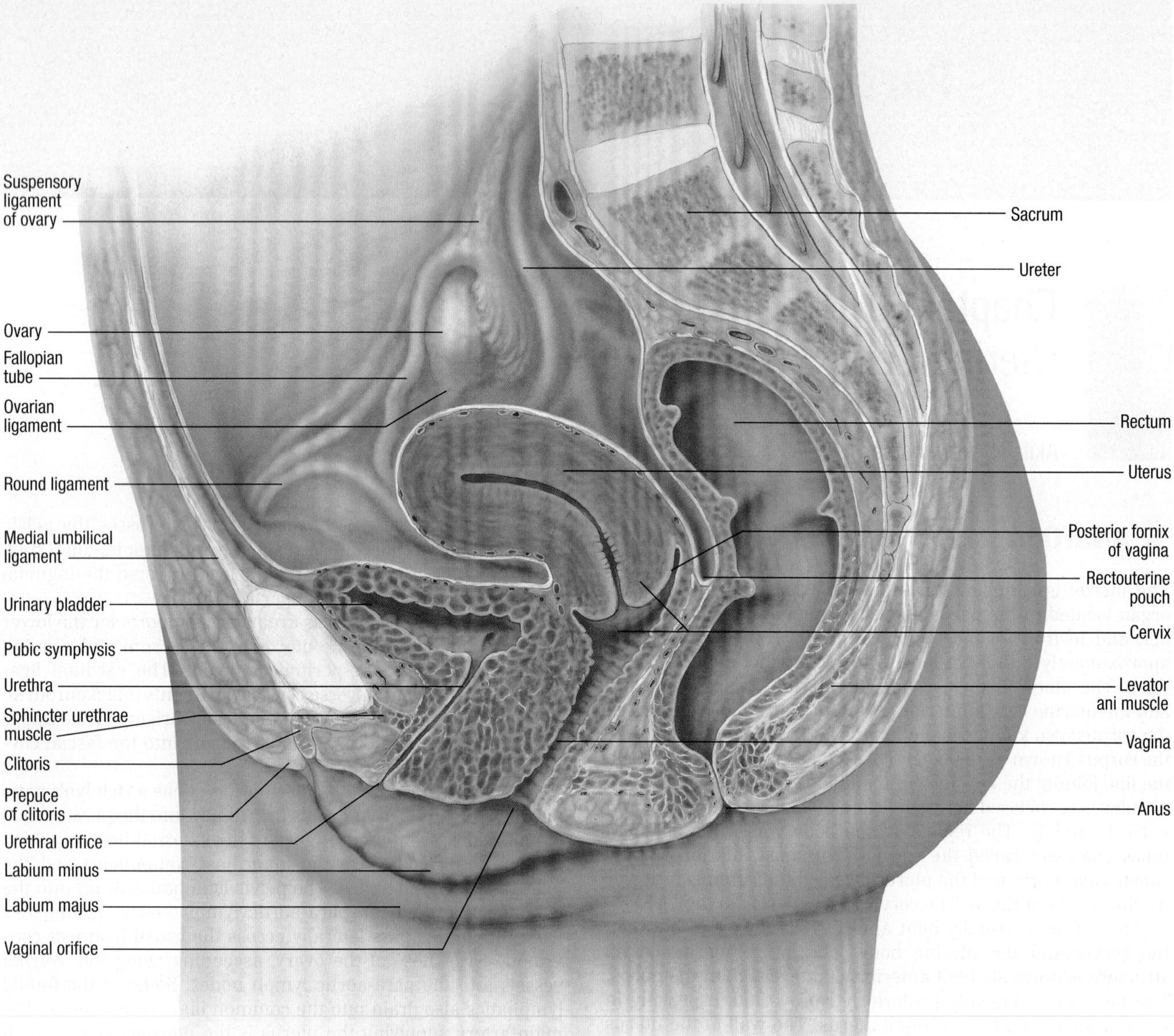

FIGURE 69.1. Anatomy of the pelvis. (Asset provided by the Anatomical Chart Company Lexington, SC.)

parts of Asia, Africa, and Central and South America. Whether regional differences in predisposition to developing cervical cancer exist is debated because it is impossible to adequately correct for unknown and known confounders, such as socioeconomic status, access to health care, parity, smoking, presence of other infections, immune status, and other factors affecting host immunity such as nutritional status.[5]

Human Papilloma Virus

Estimates indicate that >90% of cervical cancers are related to the presence of human papilloma virus (HPV) and are contracted via sexual intercourse.[6] HPV is a small, double-stranded DNA virus; HPV 16 and 18, as well as a long list of other, less frequent subtypes, including but not limited to HPV 31, 33, 35, 39, 45, 51, 52, 56, and 58, have been well characterized as causative agents for cervical cancer, with some geographic variation.[7] The HPV genome integrates into the host cell chromosomes in cervical epithelial cells and codes for six early and two late open reading frame proteins, of which three (E5, E6, and E7) alter cellular proliferation. Two viral genes, E6 and E7, are typically expressed in HPV-positive cervical-cancer cells. The E6 protein inactivates the major tumor suppressor p53; this causes chromosomal instability, inhibits apoptosis, and activates telomerase. The E7 protein affects the retinoblastoma protein (Rb), resulting in a loss of regulation of the cell's proliferation and immortalization.[8]

Although a high prevalence of HPV exists worldwide, peaking at ages 25 to 35 years, <15% of exposed women develop persistent infection that results in dysplasia,[9] whereas the majority of women clear the infection within 2 years.[10] Cervical cancer may develop 10 to 20 years after initial exposure to HPV. Social factors related to cervical cancer include those associated with HPV transmission, such as early age of first intercourse; a history of multiple sexual partners; a male partner with a history of multiple sexual partners; a large number of pregnancies;[11,12] and a history of sexually transmitted disease, including gonorrhea, chlamydia,[13] herpes simplex virus II, and/or human immunodeficiency virus (HIV).[14] A higher incidence of cervical cancer exists among women whose spouses are known or suspected to have had higher exposure to HPV[15] or whose partners have a history of penile carcinoma.[16,17] Whether circumcision may be protective to women is controversial[18] because circumcision may be a surrogate for unknown factors related to HPV transmission.[19]

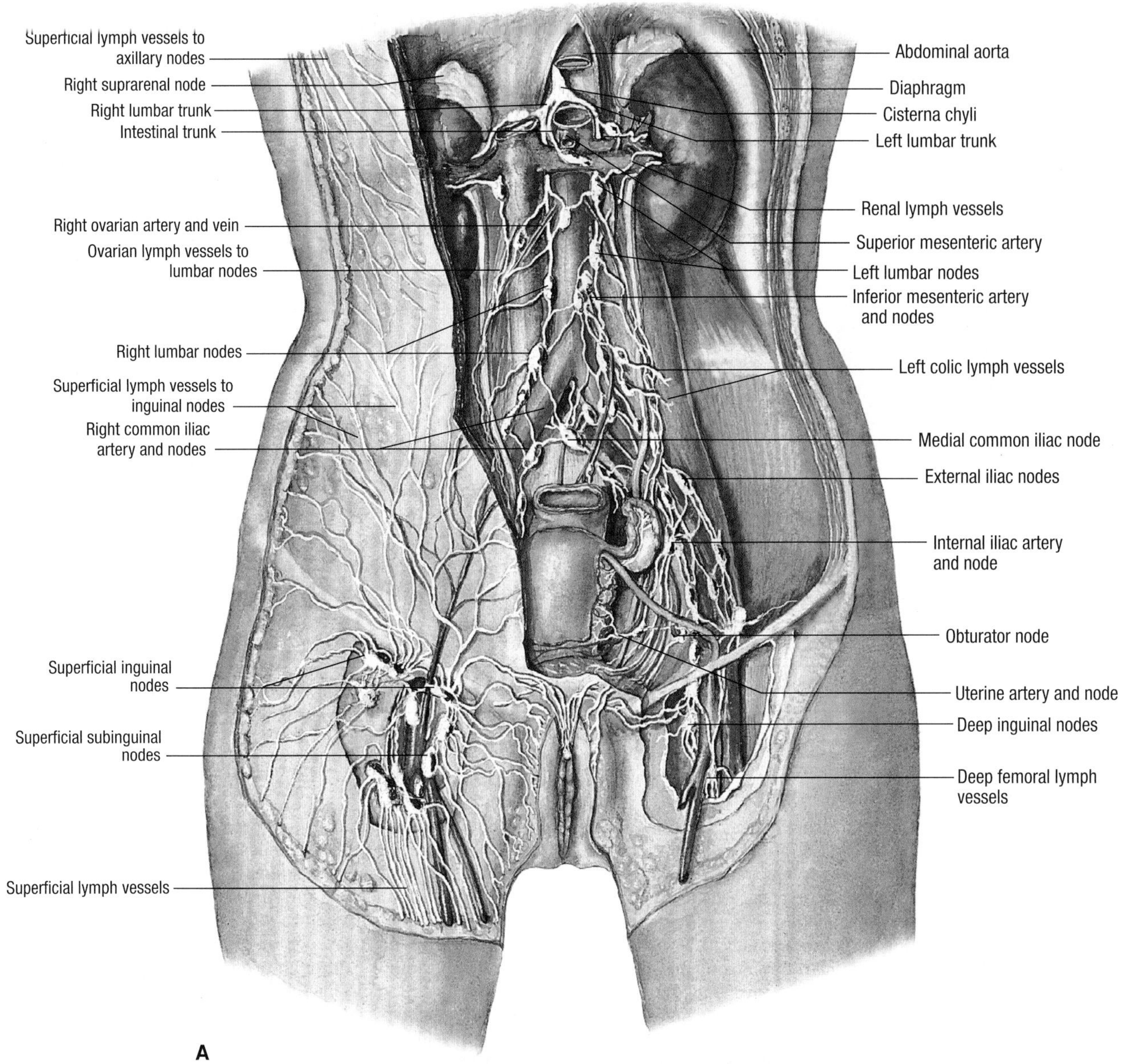

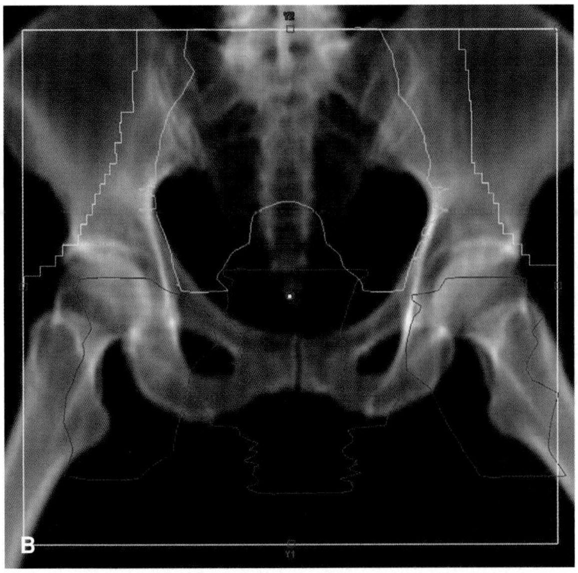

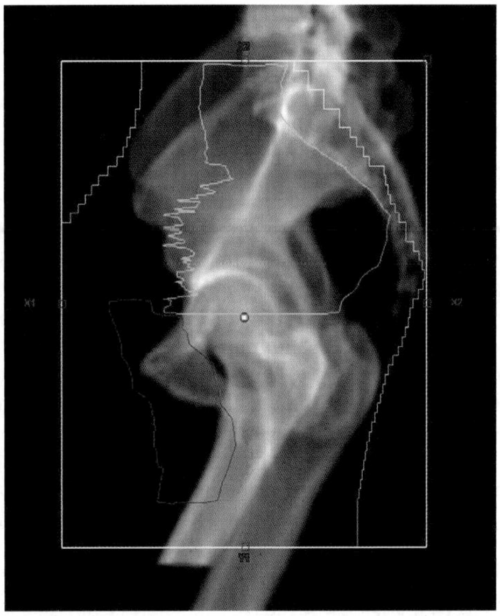

FIGURE 69.2. **A:** Lymph vessels and lymph nodes of the cervix and the body of the uterus. (Asset provided by the Anatomical Chart Company, Lexington, SC.) **B:** Three-dimensional reconstruction of location of pelvic and common iliac lymph nodes outlined on computed tomography scans in patients with carcinoma involving the distant vagina. Treatment portal is shown. **C:** The incidence of cervical cancer increased slightly in the U.S. from 2005–2010. (*continued*)

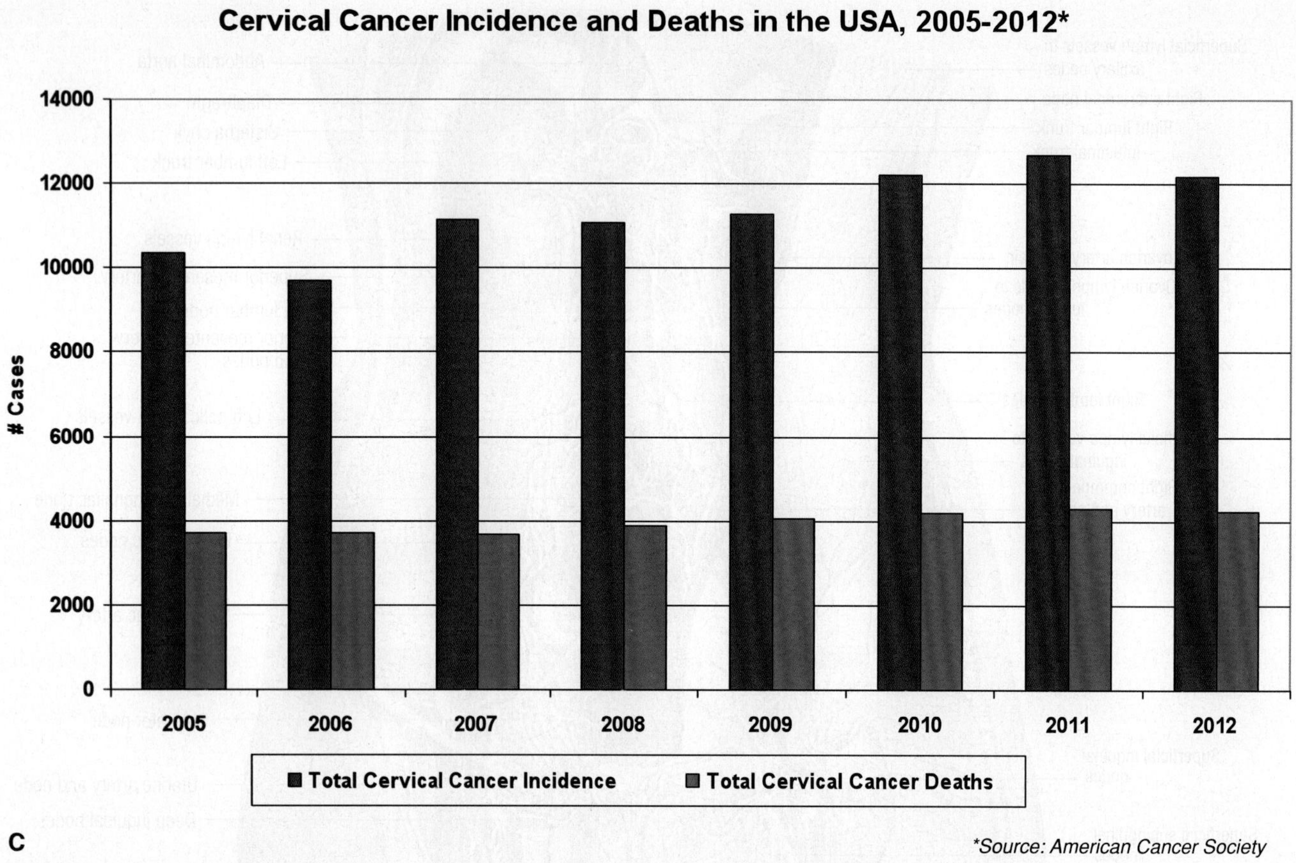

FIGURE 69.2. (*continued*)

Chemical,[20] hormonal, or other carcinogens[21] may be implicated in cervical cancer. An association between cervical carcinoma and oral contraceptive use has been reported but is considered controversial.[22] Prenatal exposure to diethylstilbestrol (DES) is linked to the development of clear-cell adenocarcinoma, although the overall incidence is small (0.14 to 1.4 per 1,000 DES-exposed women).[23–25] Cigarette smoking may increase the risk of cervical cancer.[26] However, passive smoking may not be an independent factor in the absence of active smoking.[27] A review of >50 studies considers smoking a cofactor for HPV infection and carcinogenesis,[28] although one study does not confirm this.[15] Current smoking (relative risk [RR] = 1.55) and younger age at HPV exposure (RR = 1.75) are considered risk factors among HIV-positive women.[29] Intrauterine device use may decrease cervical cancer risk, potentially through an increase in cellular immunity triggered by the device.[30]

HPV Vaccination

The quadrivalent human papillomavirus recombinant vaccine for HPV types 6, 11, 16, and 18, first approved in the United States in 2006 for girls and women ages 9 to 26 years, is now available for boys ages 9 to 26 years, with the goal of eradicating HPV-related gynecologic, penile, anal, and oropharyngeal cancers. A second vaccine with strong immunogenicity to HPV types 16 and 18, approved for girls 9 to 25 years old, is more frequently administered in Europe. Although its development is a major advance in the prevention of cancer, vaccine implementation has been hindered worldwide by cost and access. With an increase in understanding and availability, the hope is that all children will be given a vaccine covering all subtypes in the future.

NATURAL HISTORY AND PATTERNS OF SPREAD

Squamous cell carcinoma of the uterine cervix usually originates at the squamous columnar junction (transformation zone) of the endocervical canal and the portio of the cervix.

Cellular transformation follows a stepwise progression from normal to higher levels of dysplasia. Of patients diagnosed with cervical intraepithelial neoplasia (CIN) type 1, 60% have regression of the lesion, and of those with CIN2, 40% regress. Higher levels of dysplasia are more likely to progress to cancer, particularly in the presence of cofactors such as smoking or impaired immunity. Although progression typically takes 10 to 20 years,[31,32] in some instances a rapid development of carcinoma may be associated with aggressive disease.

The development of a malignant phenotype results from cells that break through the basement membrane of the epithelium and invade the cervical stroma. Invasion may result in spread to pelvic lymph nodes or other, more distant sites.[33] If the cells are detected at this stage by a Papanicolaou (Pap) or thin prepara-

TABLE 69.1 INCIDENCE OF PELVIC NODE METASTASES IN CARCINOMA OF THE UTERINE CERVIX

Authors (Reference)	Stage I (%)	Stage II (%)	Stage III (%)
No Irradiation			
Alvarez et al. (160)	12	–	–
Delgado et al. (161)	16	–	–
Piver and Chung (164)	27	–	–
Fine et al. (277)	–	23	37
Wharton et al. (278)	38	35	33
Huang et al. (878)	24	37	–
Canton-Romeo et al. (879)	11	–	–
Sentinel Node			
Gortzak-Uzan et al. (880)	17	–	–
Positron Emission Tomography/Computed Tomography			
Leblanc et al. (280)	34	16	–
Postirradiation Lymphadenectomy			
Perez et al. (406)	7	–	–

Modified from Perez CA, DiSaia PJ, Knapp RC, et al. Gynecologic tumors. In: DeVita VT Jr, Hellman S, Rosenberg SA, eds. *Cancer: Principles and Practice of Oncology,* 2nd ed. Philadelphia: JB Lippincott, 1985;1013–1041.

TABLE 69.2 METASTASES TO PARA-AORTIC LYMPH NODES IN CARCINOMA OF THE UTERINE CERVIX

Author (Reference)	*Stage IB (%)*	*Stage IIA (%)*	*Stage IIB (%)*	*Stage IIIA (%)*	*Stage IIIB (%)*	*Stage IV (%)*
Lagasse et al. (264)	8/143 (8)	4/22 (18)	19/58 (33)	0/3 (0)	19/61 (31)	1/4 (25)
Nelson et al. (390)	–	–	5/31 (16)	–	13/28 (46)	–
Piver et al. (881)	–	–	6/46 (13)	–	18/49 (37)	4/7 (57)
Wharton et al. (882)	0/21 (0)	0/10 (0)	10/47 (21)	–	14/42 (33)	–
Huang et al. (878)	7/89 (8)	–	12/48 (25)	–	–	–
Rutledge et al. (883)	9/177 (6)	–	–	–	–	–
Leblanc et al. (280)	2/43 (2)	1/9 (11)	5/46 (10)	–	3/13 (23)	3/10 (30)

Percentages are in parentheses.

Modified from Hoskins WJ, Perez CA, Young RC. Gynecologic tumors. In: DeVita VT Jr, Hellman S, Rosenberg SA, eds. *Cancer: Principles and Practice of Oncology,* 3rd ed. Philadelphia: JB Lippincott, 1989;1013–1041.

tion test, appropriate minimally invasive therapy may suffice. However, if the lesion progresses, it may present as a superficial ulceration or exophytic tumor in the ectocervix or with extensive infiltration of the endocervix. If untreated, the tumor may spread to the adjacent vaginal fornices, paracervical or parametrial tissues,[34] or adjacent organs, including the bladder, the rectum, or both. Landoni et al.[35] studied 230 patients with clinical stages IB and IIA tumors treated with radical hysterectomy with pelvic lymphadenectomy and noted that the tumor spread endocervically equally in all directions. Tumor extension into the vesicocervical ligament (anterior parametrium) was noted in 23% of cases, into the uterosacral ligaments (posterior parametrium) and the rectovaginal septum in approximately 15%, and into the parametria in 28% to 34% of cases. Paracervical extension was related to the depth of stromal invasion, tumor size, lymphatic invasion, and presence of lymph node metastasis.

Approximately 10% to 30% of patients with carcinoma of the uterine cervix have extension into the lower uterine segment and the endometrial cavity.[36] Decreased survival rates and a greater incidence of distant metastases were reported by Perez et al.[36] and Chao et al.[37] in patients with stromal endometrial invasion or replacement of normal endometrium by cervical carcinoma. Regional lymphatic or hematogenous spread may occur and increases with stage, although dissemination does not always follow an orderly sequence, and occasionally a small primary tumor may be seen infiltrating the pelvic lymph nodes, invading the bladder or rectum, or metastasizing distantly.

Both adjacent parametrial and pelvic lymph nodes may be involved. Girardi et al.[38] analyzed 359 radical hysterectomy specimens and found positive parametrial nodes in 280 patients (78%); the incidence of positive nodes was 11.4% in stage IB and 21.5% in stage IIB disease. With negative parametrial nodes, only 26% of patients had positive iliac lymph nodes, whereas 81% of patients with positive parametrial lymph nodes also had pelvic-node metastases. These data underscore the need to irradiate the parametrial tissues or carry out a complete bilateral pelvic lymphadenectomy with a radical hysterectomy in patients with invasive cervical carcinoma.

Spread of carcinoma of the cervix may progress to the obturator lymph nodes, considered a medial group of the external iliac chain, to other external iliac nodes, and to the hypogastric lymph nodes. From these, there may be tumor metastases to the common iliac or para-aortic lymph nodes.[39] The incidence of metastasis to pelvic or para-aortic lymph nodes for various stages of the disease is listed in Tables 69.1 and 69.2. In one study, pelvic lymph nodes were dissected in 225 patients with cervical carcinoma treated with radical hysterectomy; positive pelvic nodes were identified in 13 of 91 women (14.2%) with stages IB and IIA, 16 of 81 (19.8%) with stage IIB, and 11 of 40 (28%) with stage IIIB disease.[40] The most commonly involved groups were the parametrial, obturator, external iliac, and common iliac nodes (Fig. 69.3). Para-aortic lymph nodes were involved in 3 of 91 patients (3.3%) with stage IB or IIA tumors 4 cm or less and in 5 of 38 patients (13.1%) with stage IIB or III disease.

Spread through the venous plexus and the paracervical veins resulting in hematogenous dissemination, though infrequent, is relatively common with more advanced stages. In an analysis of 322 patients in whom distant metastases developed, the most frequently observed metastatic sites were the lung (21%), para-aortic lymph nodes (11%), abdominal cavity (8%), and supraclavicular lymph nodes (7%).[41] Bone metastases occurred in 16% of patients, most commonly to the lumbar and thoracic spine (Table 69.3). Spinal epidural compression from metastatic tumor, often involving lumbar segments, can occur rarely,[42] and metastasis to the brain and the heart have been reported, although it is unusual to have spread to the brain without evidence of pulmonary metastases already present,[43,44] even for small-cell carcinoma of the cervix.[45]

PAP SMEAR SCREENING

The American College of Obstetrics and Gynecology guidelines published in 2009[46] state that Pap smear screening should begin at age 21 years and continue every 2 years until age 30 years; then, if there are three normal consecutive Pap smears and no history of CIN2, CIN3, DES exposure, or HIV infection and the woman is not otherwise immunocompromised, screening should be every 3 years. Women who have had a hysterectomy for benign reasons and have no history of high-grade squamous intraepithelial lesion may discontinue testing. Co-testing of the Pap smear with an HPV DNA test is appropriate for low-risk women older than age 30 years. If negative, rescreening is not required sooner than 3 years. Women who have been treated for CIN2 or CIN3 need annual screening for at least 20 years. Those who have had a hysterectomy and a history of CIN2/CIN3 should continue to undergo screening with annual pelvic exams.

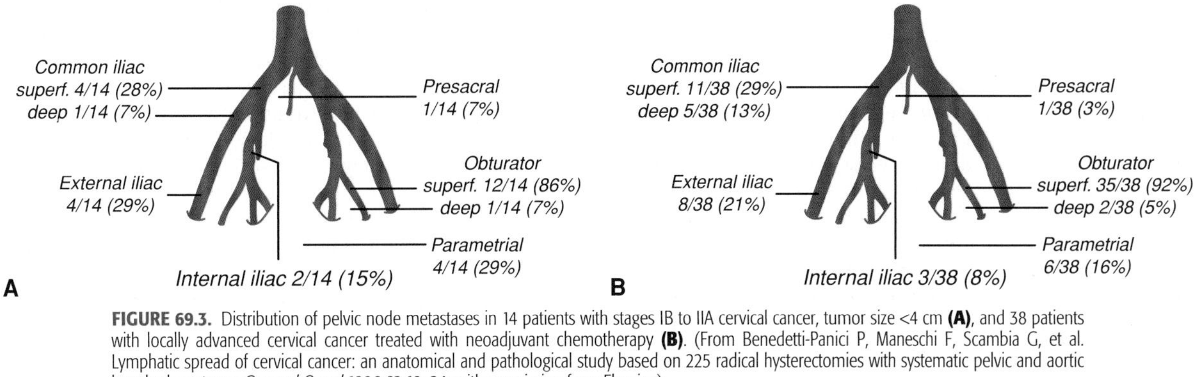

FIGURE 69.3. Distribution of pelvic node metastases in 14 patients with stages IB to IIA cervical cancer, tumor size <4 cm **(A)**, and 38 patients with locally advanced cervical cancer treated with neoadjuvant chemotherapy **(B)**. (From Benedetti-Panici P, Maneschi F, Scambia G, et al. Lymphatic spread of cervical cancer: an anatomical and pathological study based on 225 radical hysterectomies with systematic pelvic and aortic lymphadenectomy. *Gynecol Oncol* 1996;62:19–24; with permission from Elsevier.)

TABLE 69.3 CARCINOMA OF THE UTERINE CERVIX (MALLINCKRODT INSTITUTE OF RADIOLOGY 1959–1986): ANATOMIC SITE OF FIRST METASTASIS

Site	Number of Patients with Distant Metastases (n = 322)
Lung	69 (21%)
Para-aortic nodes	37 (11%)
Abdominal cavity	26 (8%)
Supraclavicular nodes	21 (7%)
Spine	21 (7%)
Gastrointestinal tract	14 (4%)
Liver	13 (4%)
Inguinal nodes	10 (3%)
Miscellaneous	111 (35%)

From Fagundes H, Perez CA, Grigsby PW, et al. Distant metastases after irradiation alone in carcinoma of the uterine cervix. *Int J Radiat Oncol Biol Phys* 1992;24:197–204; with permission from Elsevier.

When obtaining the Pap smear, special attention should be directed to not using a lubricating agent (warm water on the speculum will suffice), to obtaining good "scrapings" from the cervix and vaginal posterior fornix (without blood), and to using a small brush to obtain an endocervical sample. The patient should be instructed not to cleanse with a douche before the examination, and, if indicated, specimens should be obtained to check for trichomonas. If the cytologic smear shows atypia or mild dysplasia (class II), it should be repeated no sooner than 2 weeks after the initial test to allow representative cellular exfoliation to occur. Guidelines for reporting results of cervical and vaginal cytology were promulgated in 1988. The Bethesda system eliminated the classes of Pap cytology. The correlation between the cytologic diagnosis and subsequent histologic examination is >90%.[47] This system was modified in 1991 and in 2001.[48]

CLINICAL PRESENTATION

Cervical cancer in the United States is most frequently identified during routine gynecologic examination. Intraepithelial or early invasive carcinoma of the cervix may be detected by cytologic smears before symptoms appear; Pap smear, colposcopy and biopsies, and HPV testing have high specificity and sensitivity. Visible lesions present with an exophytic mass or a barrel-shaped cervix due to an endocervical lesion. Patients may present complaining of metrorrhagia (intermenstrual bleeding), menorrhagia (heavier menstrual flow), or postcoital bleeding. If chronic bleeding occurs, the patient may complain of fatigue or other symptoms related to anemia.

In cases with more advanced disease, bowel obstruction, renal failure, foul-smelling serosanguinous or yellowish vaginal discharge, pelvic pain, flank and/or leg pain, rectal bleeding, obstipation, dysuria, hematuria, or persistent edema of lower extremities due to lymphatic/venous blockade by pelvic sidewall disease may occur. Pain in the pelvis or hypogastrium may be caused by tumor necrosis or associated pelvic inflammatory disease. In patients with pain in the lumbosacral area, the possibility of para-aortic lymph node involvement with extension into the lumbosacral roots or hydronephrosis should be considered.

DIAGNOSTIC WORKUP

When a patient presents with an abnormal smear or if abnormal squamous cells of undetermined significance (ASCUS) are detected but HPV status is negative, follow-up in 1 year is recommended. If the second smear reveals ASCUS, regardless of HPV status, colposcopy is recommended. When both ASCUS and HPV are present or adenocarcinoma *in situ* or a squamous intraepithelial lesion is identified, directed biopsies at the time of colposcopy should be carried out. Endocervical curettage may be performed except in pregnant women. If the biopsy results are negative, the procedure should be repeated in 6 months, and, if they are positive, a conization should be performed.

TABLE 69.4 DIAGNOSTIC WORKUP FOR CARCINOMA OF THE UTERINE CERVIX

General
History
Physical examination, including bimanual pelvic and rectal examinations
Diagnostic Procedures
Cytologic smears (Papanicolaou) if not bleeding
Colposcopy
Conization (subclinical tumor)
Punch biopsies (edge of gross tumor, four quadrants)
Dilatation and curettage
Cystoscopy, rectosigmoidoscopy (stages IIB, III, and IVA)
Radiographic Studies
Standard
Chest radiography
Intravenous pyelography
Barium enema
Computed tomography
Magnetic resonance imaging
Positron emission tomography scan
Laboratory Studies
Complete blood count
Blood chemistry
Urinalysis

Patients who present with a clinically visible lesion should be jointly evaluated by the radiation and gynecologic oncologists. After obtaining a careful clinical history and performing a general physical examination, with attention to the inguinal and supraclavicular (nodal) areas, abdomen, and liver, a careful pelvic examination should be carried out with as little discomfort to the patient as possible without compromising the thoroughness of the evaluation.[49] Pelvic examination should include inspection of the external genitalia, vagina, and uterine cervix, a rectal examination, and bimanual palpation of the pelvis. Pelvic examination under anesthesia is a universally accepted component in the evaluation and clinical staging of patients in order to provide a pain-free examination that allows a clearer estimation of parametrial or sidewall tumor extension. In countries in which magnetic resonance imaging (MRI) is available, this may be used to assist with assessing tumor extension beyond the lower cervix, and in many institutions it has replaced the examination under anesthesia. Cystoscopy or rectosigmoidoscopy should be performed in all patients with symptoms consistent with presence of a fistula of the urinary or lower gastrointestinal tract, patients with clinical stage IIB, III, or IVA disease who cannot undergo an MRI, or patients with an MRI suspicious for bladder or bowel invasion. The diagnostic procedures for carcinoma of the cervix are presented in Table 69.4.

Conization/Loop Excision

Conization involves a conical removal of a large portion of the ectocervix and endocervix. Cold knife cone biopsy specimens should always be obtained with a scalpel or other appropriate instrument. At least 50% of the endocervical canal should be removed without compromising the internal sphincter. Curettage of the remaining endocervical canal should be carried out.

Conization must be performed in the following situations: no gross lesion of the cervix is noted and an endocervical tumor is suspected; the entire lesion cannot be seen with the colposcope; diagnosis of microinvasive carcinoma is made on biopsy; discrepancies are found between the cytologic and the histologic appearances of the lesion; or the patient is not reliable for all necessary follow-up. With careful selection of patients who have a negative positron emission tomography (PET) scan and an MRI with a central lesion <2 cm in width, knife conization with lymphadenectomy may be considered for fertility preservation. Laser conization and loop diathermy excision are frequently done in an office setting as an alternative to conization; loop excision is less expensive and more reliable than laser conization.

Biopsy

Multiple punch biopsies of a grossly visible lesion should be adequate to confirm the diagnosis of invasive carcinoma. Specimens should be obtained from any suspect area and from all four quadrants of the cervix and from any suspect areas in the vagina. It is important to obtain tissue from the periphery of the lesion with some adjoining normal tissue; biopsy specimens from central ulcerated or necrotic areas may not be adequate for diagnosis. Dilation and curettage is not required if the biopsy confirms a diagnosis of invasive disease.

Laboratory Studies

For invasive carcinoma, patients should have the following laboratory studies: complete peripheral blood evaluation, including hemogram, white blood cell count, differential and platelet count; blood chemistry profile, with particular attention to blood urea nitrogen and creatinine; liver function values; and urinalysis.

Imaging Studies

In countries where three-dimensional (3D) imaging is not routinely available, patients with cervical cancer should have a chest radiograph to assess for lung metastases and an intravenous pyelogram (IVP) to determine whether hydronephrosis is present. The IVP in many countries has been replaced by computed tomography (CT) scan of the pelvis and abdomen with intravenous (IV) contrast material or by PET/CT scan. In places where CT is not available, patients with stages IIB, III, and IVA disease who have symptoms in the colon and rectum may benefit from a barium enema. A skeletal survey may be performed to determine whether bone metastases are present. Historically, pedal lymphangiography was used to assess lymph node involvement in the pelvic or para-aortic nodes with mixed results.[50,51] The number of physicians trained to perform lymphangiography has declined in the United States, and instead PET scan is preferred.

Since the 1990s, the use of CT scanning has rapidly increased worldwide. A CT provides diagnostic information about the presence of metastases, enlarged lymph nodes, and the primary tumor. On a CT scan, the cervical tumor may be seen as an enlarged, irregular, hypoechoic cervix or as a mass with ill-defined margins. Parametrial regions appear dense when involved, and uterosacral involvement may be seen. Lymph nodes appear enlarged, with most >1 cm on axial dimension considered pathologic. The overall accuracy of CT scanning in staging cervical cancer ranges from 63% to 88%.[50,52] In the detection of lymph node abnormalities, the overall accuracy of conventional CT scanning is 77% to 85%, with sensitivity of 44% and specificity of 93%.[53]

In order to correlate radiographic and surgical findings, Camilien et al.[54] reported on 61 patients with carcinoma of the cervix who had both preoperative CT scans and exploratory laparotomy; results showed that 75% of the enlarged pelvic lymph nodes on CT contained metastases, and 97% of patients with negative nodes on CT scan had pathologically negative findings (specificity of 97%). However, histologically positive pelvic nodes were often missed on CT scan (sensitivity of 25%). The CT scan is more valuable in evaluation of the para-aortic lymph nodes (specificity of 100% and sensitivity of 67%).

Several studies evaluated the role of CT or PET/CT with regard to para-aortic nodal detection (Table 69.5). Heller et al.[55] conducted a prospective evaluation of 320 patients with stages IIB to IVA carcinoma of the cervix entered into a Gynecologic Oncology Group (GOG) protocol in which preoperative CT scan, lymphangiography, and ultrasonography of the aortic area were performed. Para-aortic node dissection was done in patients with negative staging studies. Lymphangiography, CT scan, and ultrasonography had false-negative frequencies for pelvic lymph node evaluation of 14.2%, 25%, and 30%, respectively. The sensitivity was 79% for lymphangiography, 34% for CT scan, and 19% for ultrasonography, and the specificity ratings were 73%, 96%, and 99%, respectively. Ultrasonography, therefore, is not reliable in preoperative detection of lymph node metastases, but it has limited value in evaluating extrauterine tumor involvement. Ultrasound has a primary role in assisting with intracavitary brachytherapy applicator insertion and may detect uterine perforation, allowing for proper positioning, which is critical for adequate dosing and affects survival.[56,57] PET has a higher sensitivity than CT and higher specificity than MR in detecting bone metastases.[58]

TABLE 69.5 COMPUTED TOMOGRAPHY AND POSITRON EMISSION TOMOGRAPHY IN THE EVALUATION OF PARA-AORTIC NODES

Author (Reference)	Number of Cases	FIGO Stage	Sensitivity (%)	Specificity (%)	Accuracy (%)
Kilcheski et al. (884)	36	I–IV	–	80	–
Camilien et al. (54)	51	IB–IIA	67	100	100
Camilien et al. (54)	10	IIB–IV	67	100	90
PET/CT					
Leblanc et al. (280)	125	IB2-IIA	33.3	94.2	–
Yildirim et al. (885)	16	IIB-IVA	50	83.3	–

FIGO, International Federation of Gynecology and Obstetrics.

Modified from Camilien L, Gordon D, Fruchter RG, et al. Predictive value of computerized tomography in the presurgical evaluation of primary carcinoma of the cervix. *Gynecol Oncol* 1988;30:209–215; with permission from Elsevier.

Magnetic Resonance Imaging

MRI is frequently used for the initial assessment of the cervical tumor and of extracervical tumor extension,[59] often in lieu of an examination under anesthesia. MRI is contraindicated in patients with pacemakers, cochlear implants, metallic prostheses, metallic fragments from prior accidents, or large vascular clips. On T2-weighted images, a cervical cancer may be seen as a mass of intermediate to high signal intensity, usually of greater intensity than the fibrocervical stroma. On T1-weighted images, tumors are usually isointense with the normal cervix and may not be seen[60] but can increase in intensity with the administration of IV contrast. Abnormal, irregular cervical margins, prominent parametrial strands, exocentric parametrial enlargement, and loss of parametrial fat planes on T1-weighted images or high signal in the parametria or cardinal/uterosacral ligaments on T2-weighted images are indicative of more extensive tumors.[52,59,61] Parametrial tumor may be identified as brighter regions on T2-weighted images when compared to the low signal intensity of the cervix and uterine ligaments.

A comparative evaluation of pretreatment tumor staging and volume as assessed by examination under anesthesia (EUA), transrectal ultrasonography (TRUS), and MRI in 60 patients with invasive carcinoma of the cervix was reported by Hawnaur et al.[62] TRUS and MRI assigned the same tumor stage in only 30% of patients, and EUA and MRI agreed on tumor stage in an additional 27%. In cases of disagreement, the MRI staging correlated better with outcome than TRUS or EUA. Sixty-two percent of patients with enlarged lymph nodes on pretreatment MRI either died or had tumor recurrence or metastases. MRI was superior to both TRUS and EUA in assessing the full extent of bulky tumors and lymph node enlargement.

Postema et al.[63] compared MRI with pelvic examination (including under general anesthesia in selected patients) and surgicopathologic findings in 103 patients with invasive cervical carcinoma. MRI was better at identifying extracervical tumor spread, but it had more false-positive results. The pelvic examination led to correct treatment decisions in 89% of patients. In a study by Hansen et al.,[64] clinical assessment (done according to International Federation of Gynecology and Obstetrics [FIGO] recommendations) was superior to low-field MRI with contrast enhancement in staging cervical cancer in 95 women who had both within 2 weeks after clinical diagnosis; the clinical staging correctly classified 57 patients (accuracy, 92%) compared with 52 for MRI (accuracy, 84%).

A prospective study by the American College of Radiology Imaging Network compared clinical examination, CT, and MRI.[53]

MRI was significantly better than clinical examination or CT for detecting uterine-body involvement or measuring tumor size,[65] but no method was accurate at evaluating the cervical stroma. MRI was significantly better[66] at detecting the tumor and parametrial involvement. MRI also somewhat increased detection of involved lymph nodes.[53]

The tumor is less likely to be as visible on MRI for adenocarcinoma cases, compared to squamous cell cancer. Haider et al.[67] evaluated 56 patients with adenocarcinoma involving the cervix using MRI and noted that 42 (75%) had a visible mass. Kodaira et al.[68] reviewed records of 84 patients with stage II cancer evaluated by MRI. The 5-year disease-free survival (DFS) rate of patients with maximal tumor size (D_{max}) of ≥50 mm was significantly lower than that for patients with $D_{max} < 50$ mm (46% vs. 88%; $p < .0001$).

Ebner et al.[69] reviewed MRI findings in 12 women with recurrent pelvic tumors and 10 with a fibrotic mass (confirmed by laparotomy or biopsy in 21 patients). They were able to differentiate between the two processes accurately in most instances. However, it is highly desirable to confirm abnormal or suspect lymph node radiographic findings with CT-guided fine-needle aspiration biopsies.

Corn et al.[70] evaluated endorectal coil MRI in 18 patients with stages IB to IIIB cervical carcinoma; in 7 patients, tumors were a higher stage by endorectal coil MRI because of proximal vaginal involvement or the combination of proximal vaginal involvement and parametrial extension. Compared with those who had a dark or intermediate signal, patients with bright signal characteristics tended to present with earlier stages, were less likely to have anemia, and were more likely to have complete response to external-beam radiation.

Radiation-induced changes detected over the course of radiation may predict local recurrence and survival. Mayr et al.[71] studied 34 patients with cervical cancer of various FIGO stages who underwent 1.5-T MRI before and after radiation therapy. Tumor volumetry (3D measurements) based on T2-weighted images quantified the tumor regression rate. Sequential tumor volumetry using MR imaging may be a very effective measure of the responsiveness of cervical cancer to irradiation. MRI dynamic contrast enhancement during the first 2 weeks of radiation therapy may provide early prediction of tumor regression rate. In 7 patients, tumor regression rates ranged from 2% to 15.2% per day and correlated positively with changes in both peak and mean tumor enhancement ($p < .01$). Hatano et al.[72] evaluated MRI in 42 patients with advanced cervical cancer treated with external-beam irradiation and high–dose-rate (HDR) brachytherapy. In biopsies performed immediately after radiation therapy (RT), no residual cancer was found in 36 patients (86%). The simultaneous MRI study demonstrated no high-signal intensity on T2-weighted images in 28 patients (75%). A high–signal-intensity area was observed in 14 patients, and this disappeared 3 months after RT in 8 patients with a negative biopsy. The sensitivity, specificity, and accuracy of MRI tumor response studies at 3 months after radiation therapy were 100%. MRI studies performed after 30 Gy of external-beam irradiation and 3 months after all radiation therapy predicted local tumor control. Similar studies were published by Gong et al.[73] and van de Bunt et al.[74] Furthermore, MRI is useful in providing accurate target volume definition in brachytherapy treatment planning (Fig. 69.4).[75]

Positron Emission Tomography

PET scanning is increasingly used in the evaluation of patients with malignant neoplasia, including invasive cervical cancer, using 2-[^{18}F]-fluoro-2-deoxy-D-glucose (FDG). Rose et al.[76] observed uptake in 91% of the primary tumors in 32 patients with locally advanced carcinoma of the cervix. Squamous cell carcinoma is more often FDG avid than is adenocarcinoma. Compared with surgical staging, PET scanning had a sensitivity of 75% and a specificity of 92% in detecting para-aortic metastasis.[77] PET-CT provides highly accurate localization of focal radiotracer uptake, which significantly improves the diagnostic accuracy compared with PET or CT alone. Diagnostic PET images may be fused with simulation CT images to ensure accurate radiation dose coverage of the target and any PET-avid lymph nodes (Fig. 69.5). Care must be taken in interpretation because physiologic FDG excretion into the urinary bladder may result in false-positive assessment of the primary tumor, and ureters may be contoured as lymph nodes; therefore, tracing the ureters and complete bladder voiding prior to imaging are recommended.

Grigsby et al.[77] compared CT and FDG-PET scanning for lymph node staging in 101 patients with carcinoma of the cervix. CT demonstrated abnormally enlarged pelvic lymph nodes in 20 patients and para-aortic lymph nodes in 7, whereas PET demonstrated abnormal FDG uptake in pelvic lymph nodes in 67, in para-aortic lymph nodes in 21, and in supraclavicular lymph nodes in 8. The 2-year progression-free survival rate, based solely on para-aortic lymph-node status, was 64% in CT-negative and PET-negative patients, 18% in CT-negative and PET-positive patients, and 14% in CT-positive and PET-positive patients ($p < .0001$). The most significant prognostic factor for progression-free survival was the presence of positive para-aortic lymph nodes on PET imaging ($p = .025$). Among 76 patients with no abnormal FDG uptake, the 2-year survival rate was 86%, with persistent abnormal uptake in 40%; there were no survivors among patients who developed new sites of abnormal uptake.[78] In a follow-up study of 152 patients, the authors reported a 5-year cause-specific survival rate of 80% in 114

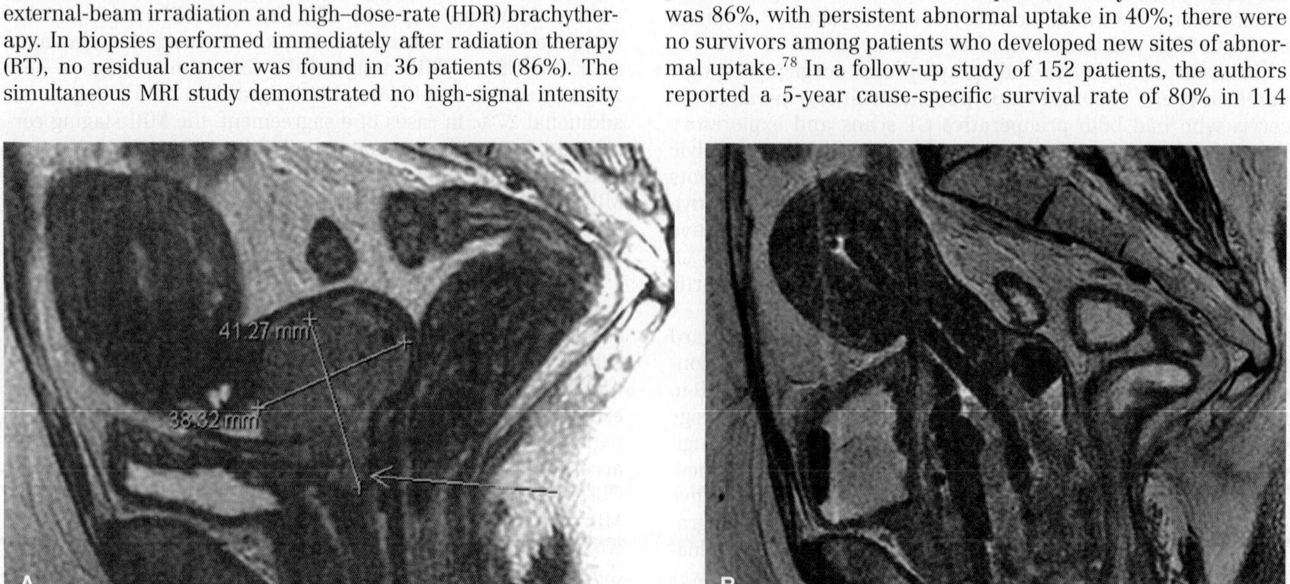

FIGURE 69.4. A: Magnetic resonance imaging (MRI) at diagnosis showing an enlarged cervical tumor. **B:** MRI with tandem and ring brachytherapy applicator in place showing dramatic shrinkage of the tumor after concurrent chemotherapy with external beam radiation.

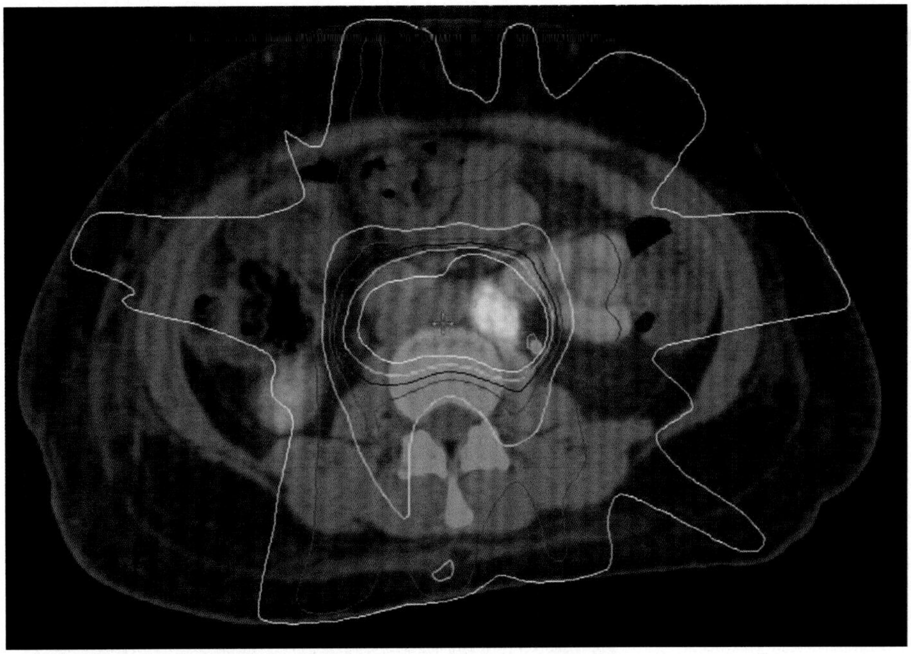

FIGURE 69.5. A fusion of a diagnostic positron emission tomography (PET) scan with simulation computed tomography delineates the hypermetabolic lymph nodes, allowing for radiation dose escalation. In this case, the entire para-aortic chain received 45 Gy, followed by a sequential boost to the PET-avid node with a 7-mm margin to approximately 65 Gy.

patients without abnormalities on posttherapy FDG-PET versus 32% in 20 patients with persistent uptake, and no survivors among 18 patients with new sites of abnormal uptake.[79] In another study, Grigsby et al.[80] noted in 208 patients a close correlation between radiation doses, number and size of positive lymph nodes and outcome (treatment failures and survival; Fig. 69.6). Hope et al.[81] performed FDG-PET scans in 58 patients with cervical carcinoma who had an endometrial biopsy or dilatation and curettage; 36 (64%) had pathologic endometrial invasion (EI). Pelvic lymph node metastasis was more commonly detected in this group than in patients without EI (70% vs. 23%; $p < .001$), as were para-aortic and supraclavicular nodal metastasis (30% vs. 0%; $p = .006$). Furthermore, 2-year survival rates were 78% versus 58%, and overall survival rates were 92% versus 65%, respectively ($p = .047$). Lin et al.,[82] using FDG-PET in 32 patients with cervical carcinoma, observed a reduction in physiologic tumor volume of 50% occurring within 20 days from the initiation of radiation therapy.

Kidd et al.[83–87] demonstrated that maximum standardized uptake value (SUV max) is an independent predictor of death from cervical cancer and is associated with persistent disease. Similarly, the SUV of the pelvic node predicts pelvic disease recurrence. Survival rates are worse with supraclavicular nodal PET positivity; para-aortic lymph node metastases portend a survival rate between those of pelvic node and supraclavicular positivity. The detection of supraclavicular metastases on FDG-PET at diagnosis and its relationship to clinical outcome for 186 cervical cancer patients was reported by Tran et al.[88] Fourteen patients (8%) had abnormal FDG uptake in left supraclavicular lymph nodes without palpable disease, confirmed on biopsy; 6 were treated with palliative intent, and 7 received definitive irradiation and concurrent chemotherapy. The median overall survival was 7.5 months; all patients developed distant metastases. After external-beam radiation is finished, an FDG-PET scan provides important information about posttreatment uptake and is prognostic with regard to outcome.[89–92]

STAGING

The FIGO staging system is based on clinical evaluation (inspection, palpation, colposcopy); roentgenographic examination of the chest, kidneys, and skeleton; and endocervical curettage and biopsies. Lymphangiograms, arteriograms, imaging findings, and laparoscopy or laparotomy findings should not be used for clinical staging. The 2009 FIGO staging system for cervical cancer has one modification from the previous version: Stage IIA has been divided into stage IIA1, with tumors invading into the upper vagina but ≤4 cm in size, and stage IIA2, with tumors >4 cm in size.[93]

Patients with hydronephrosis or a nonfunctioning kidney ascribed to extension of the tumor are classified as stage IIIB regardless of the pelvic findings. Other prognostic factors, such as endometrial extension of cervical carcinoma, stromal invasion, lymphatic/vascular permeation, and involvement of the lateral parametrium (as opposed to the medial parametrium) in

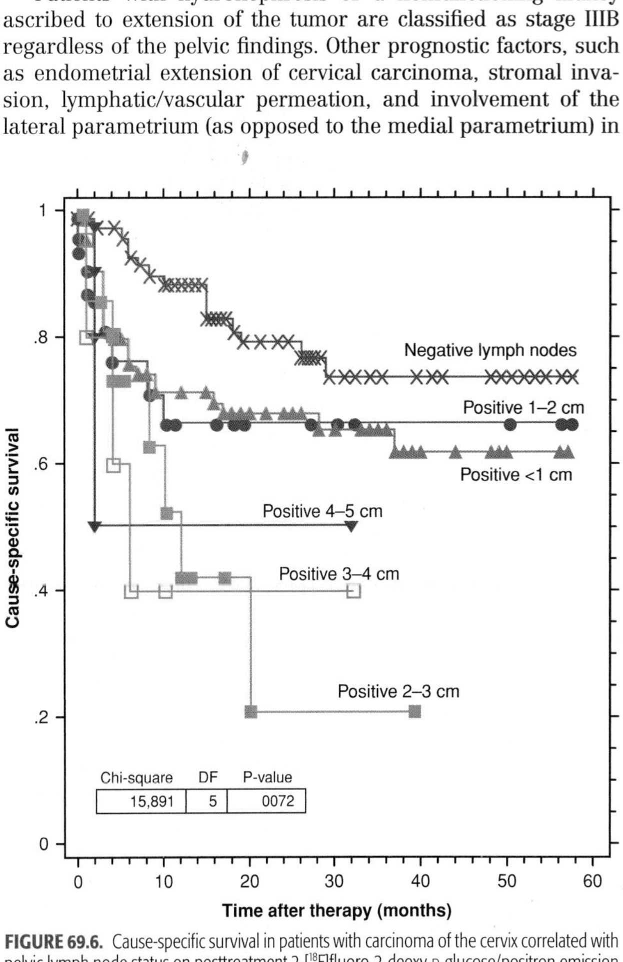

FIGURE 69.6. Cause-specific survival in patients with carcinoma of the cervix correlated with pelvic lymph node status on posttreatment 2-[^{18}F]fluoro-2-deoxy-D-glucose/positron emission tomography. (From Grigsby PW, Singh AK, Siegel BA, et al., Lymph node control in cervical cancer. *Int J Radiat Oncol Biol Phys* 2004;59:637–638; with permission from Elsevier.)

TABLE 69.6 FIGO STAGING OF CARCINOMA OF THE UTERINE CERVIX

Primary Tumor (T)	
I	Cervical carcinoma confined to uterus (extension to corpus should be disregarded)
IA	Preclinical invasive carcinoma, diagnosed by microscopy only
IA1	Minimal microscopic stromal invasion
IA2	Tumor with an invasive component ≤5 mm in depth taken from the base of the epithelium and ≤7 mm in horizontal spread
IB	Clinical lesions confined to the cervix or preclinical lesions greater than IA
IB1	Clinical lesions ≤4 cm in size
IB2	Clinical lesions ≤4 cm in size
II	Cervical carcinoma invades beyond uterus but not to the pelvic wall or to the lower one-third of vagina
IIA	Tumor in the upper two-thirds of the vagina without parametrial invasion
IIA1	Tumor in the upper two-thirds of the vagina without parametrial invasion, ≤4 cm in greatest dimension
IIA2	Tumor in the upper two-thirds of the vagina without parametrial invasion, >4 cm in greatest dimension
IIB	Tumor with parametrial invasion
III	Cervical carcinoma extends to the pelvic wall and/or involves lower one-third of vagina and/or causes hydronephrosis or nonfunctioning kidney
IIIA	Tumor involves lower one-third of the vagina, with no extension to pelvic wall
IIIB	Tumor extends to pelvic wall and/or causes hydronephrosis or nonfunctioning kidney
IVA[a]	Tumor invades mucosa of the bladder or rectum and/or extends beyond the true pelvis
IVB	Distant metastasis

FIGO, International Federation of Gynecology and Obstetrics.
[a]Presence of bullous edema is not sufficient evidence to classify a tumor as T4.

stage IIB, are not included in the staging system. Suspected invasion of the bladder or rectum should be confirmed by biopsy. Bullous edema of the bladder and swelling of the mucosa of the rectum are not accepted as definitive criteria for staging. For a lesion to be classified as stage IIIB based on tumor extension without hydronephrosis, the tumor should extend to the lateral pelvic wall, although fixation is not required.

A parallel TNM staging system is published by the American Joint Committee on Cancer;[94] however, this system requires nodal staging, which is not feasible in many settings, and radiologic nodal information is not available to most patients with cervical cancer worldwide. The FIGO system remains the standard staging system, given the lack of 3D imaging to determine nodal status in countries with the highest incidence of cervical cancer. All histologic types should be included. When there is a disagreement regarding the staging, the earlier stage should be recorded (Table 69.6 and Fig. 69.7).

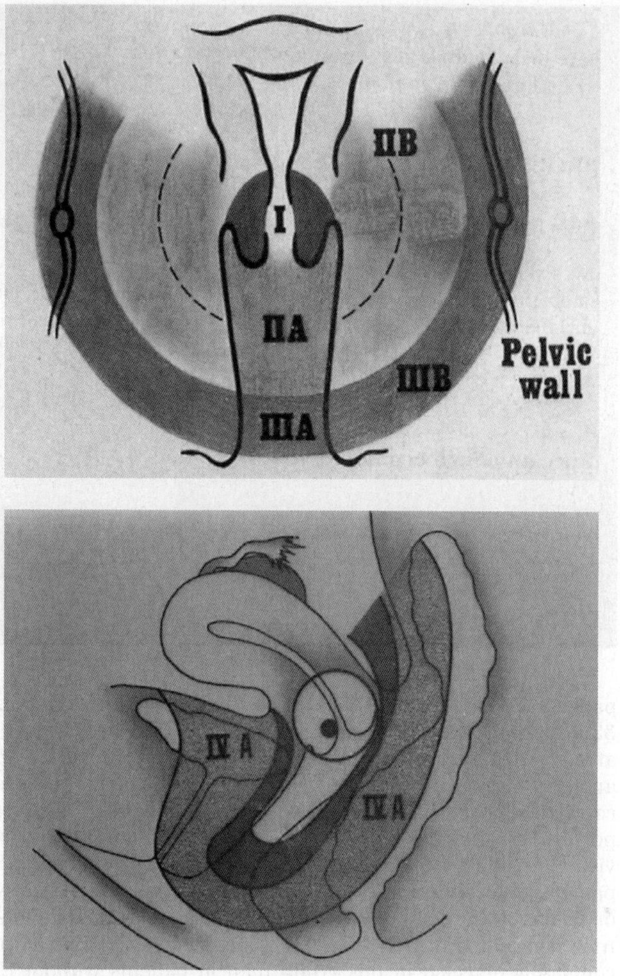

FIGURE 69.7. Diagrammatic representation of various anatomic stages of carcinoma of the uterine cervix, according to the International Federation of Gynecology and Obstetrics classification. Stage IIA has been divided into stage IIA1, with tumors invading into the upper vagina but ≤4 cm in size, and stage IIA2, with tumors >4 cm in size.

PATHOLOGIC CLASSIFICATION

More than 90% of tumors are squamous cell carcinoma. Approximately 7% to 10% are classified as adenocarcinoma, and 1% to 2% are the clear-cell mesonephric type. Squamous cell (or epidermoid) carcinoma is composed of cores and nests of epithelial cells arranged randomly; cells show central keratinization with pearls and sometimes necrosis. Nonkeratinizing tumors may be seen. Electron microscopy may show desmosomes and tonofilaments. Squamous cell carcinomas are divided into three types: large-cell keratinizing, nonkeratinizing, and small-cell carcinomas. They are subdivided according to the degree of differentiation into well, moderately, or poorly differentiated.

Verrucous carcinoma is a variant of a very well differentiated squamous cell carcinoma that characteristically has a tendency to recur locally but not to metastasize.[95] Mitotic activity is very low. It may be difficult to discriminate verrucous carcinoma from a giant condyloma with cytologic atypia or from a well-differentiated invasive squamous carcinoma. Microscopically, verrucous carcinoma is exophytic, with an undulating, hyperkeratotic surface; the deep margin is composed of large, bulbous masses that invade along a wide front in a "pushing" fashion.

Adenocarcinoma arises from the cylindrical mucosa of the endocervix or the mucus-secreting endocervical glands. Mucinous is the most common subtype of adenocarcinoma. This endocervical adenocarcinoma may form mucosal glands lined by high columnar cells and produce tubular folds oriented in many directions. In another subtype, cells resemble those of the intestines; the epithelium tends to be pseudostratified and may contain goblet cells. The third variant is the signet-ring cell adenocarcinoma, which is rare and usually mixed with the endocervical or intestinal patterns.

Endometrioid carcinoma is the most common cell type of endocervical adenocarcinoma; the cells resemble those of the endometrium, and the presence of intracytoplasmic mucin in some cells may be seen in a substantial proportion of tumors. The World Health Organization recommends that endometrioid or endocervical types of adenocarcinoma be graded according to their architecture, based on the degree of gland formation.[96]

Sometimes it is difficult to differentiate a primary endocervical adenocarcinoma from an endometrial tumor. Drescher et al.[97] described a higher incidence of involvement of the uterine corpus and the regional lymph nodes in 21 patients with adenocarcinoma compared with a similar number of patients with squamous cell carcinoma. Chao et al.[98] and Contag et al.[99] described the use of microarray analysis for gene profiling (cDNA/RNA) to understand the molecular features of these tumors, which could aid in their classification. HPV has been identified in some subtypes of adenocarcinoma of the cervix.[100]

Adenoma malignum is a rare form of cervical cancer that is difficult to diagnose, and often highly malignant and refractory to treatment.[101] Adenoma malignum is associated with Peutz-Jeghers syndrome and has an ominous natural history, with few reported cures.[102] Adenosquamous carcinoma is also relatively rare (2% to

5%) and consists of intermingled epithelial cell cores with squamous features and glandular structures. The squamous component is frequently nonkeratinizing. If the squamous component is benign metaplasia, the tumor is called adenoacanthoma.

Glassy-cell carcinoma (1% to 2%) is considered a poorly differentiated adenosquamous tumor; it is rare and highly malignant. Survival is poor after surgery or irradiation. Ulbright and Gersell,[103] in five cases of glassy-cell carcinoma evaluated by light and electron microscopy, described both glandular and squamous differentiation. Littman et al.[104] reported only 4 of 13 patients, the majority with stage II disease, surviving 5 years (6 had extrapelvic failures). Piura et al.[105] reported on 5 patients with cervical glassy-cell carcinoma, 3 with stage IB1 disease. All 3 patients were alive without disease 4, 12, and 18 months after diagnosis.

Adenoid cystic carcinoma is a rare variant of adenocarcinoma of the cervix (<1%), with an appearance similar to its counterparts in the salivary gland or the bronchial tree.[106] The tumor is composed of nests and nodules of small carcinoma cells with a few characteristic cribriform patterns. Immunohistochemical findings for type IV collagen and laminin reveal intercellular cylinders composed of basement membrane material in the solid area without a cribriform pattern. They are locally aggressive and prone to metastasize.[107]

Clear-cell carcinoma (mesonephric), not related to DES exposure, comprises approximately 2% primary cervical adenocarcinomas and is believed to arise in mesonephric remnants.[24] These tumors are submucosal, composed of clear and "hobnail" cells, and may grow in a tubular, glandular, papillary, or solid pattern. They appear at any age, with one-third occurring in women younger than 30 years of age. The clear cell is characterized by a voluminous cytoplasm filled with glycogen and the hobnail cell by single-cell apical projections into the neoplastic lumina. These tumors tend to be deeply positioned, with the bulk of the lesion on the stroma forming tubular structures, diffusely infiltrating the cervical stroma.

Cervical malignant mixed Müllerian tumors, compared with their counterparts in the corpus, are more commonly confined at presentation and may have a better prognosis. Clement et al.[108] described the clinicopathologic features with mixed Müllerian tumors of the cervix in nine patients. Gross examination revealed polypoid or pedunculated masses that invaded the cervical wall in 50% of the hysterectomy specimens. On microscopic examination, five tumors contained basaloid carcinoma or squamous cell carcinoma and four contained adenocarcinoma. In seven tumors, the sarcomatous component was homologous, usually resembling fibrosarcoma or endometrial stromal sarcoma, and two tumors contained heterologous sarcomatous elements.

Small-cell carcinoma of the cervix, according to some authors, arises from endocervical argyrophilic cells or their precursors, multipotential neuroendocrine cells; however, some small-cell tumors do not contain morphologic evidence of neuroendocrine origin. Nuclear molding, absence of nucleoli, cell necrosis, and high mitotic activity are common. One-third to one-half stain positively for neuroendocrine markers such as chromogranin, serotonin, synaptophysin, or somatostatin.[45] In the majority of patients, the cervical stroma is extensively infiltrated by single small, round cells.[109] Lymphatic and vascular invasion are significantly more common in small-cell carcinomas (noted in 58% of patients with stage IB disease; 40% of these patients had lymph-node metastases at the time of radical surgery).[110] HPV 18 has been detected in the majority of these tumors.[111]

Van Nagell et al.,[112] in an analysis of 25 patients, noted a 5-year survival rate of 54% for all stages of small-cell carcinoma, compared with 68% for matched large-cell nonkeratinizing squamous cell and 74% for keratinizing squamous cell carcinomas. Viswanathan et al.[45] studied 21 patients. All were confirmed after central pathology review to stain positively for chromogranin, synaptophysin, or CD56. The median time to first relapse from the initiation of treatment was 8.4 months. No patient had brain metastases as the sole site of first recurrence. However, 2 patients developed brain metastases concurrently with lung metastases. The overall survival rate was 29% at 5 years; none of the patients who had disease more extensive than stage IB1 or clinical evidence of lymph node metastases survived their disease.

Basaloid carcinoma or adenoid-basal carcinoma, an extremely uncommon tumor, is characterized by nests or cords of small basaloid cells, prominent peripheral palisading of cells in the tumor nests, no significant stromal reaction or capillary space invasion, and an infiltrating growth pattern. Some authors have suggested a slow growth pattern with limited local invasiveness and low probability of lymph node metastases.[113] Prognosis is excellent.[114]

Primary sarcomas of the cervix have been occasionally described (e.g., leiomyosarcoma, rhabdomyosarcoma, stromal sarcoma, carcinosarcoma).[115] Malignant lymphomas, primary or secondary in the cervix, have been sporadically reported. They should be treated like other lymphomas.[116] Melanoma of the cervix is similarly extremely rare and difficult to cure despite attempts at radical surgery. Metastasis of distant tumors to the uterine cervix is rare (about 4% of all tumors) and should be considered in the differential diagnosis. Metastases to the cervix from the breast, ovary, and kidney have been reported.[117–119]

PROGNOSTIC AND PREDICTIVE FACTORS

Patient-Related Factors

Age

According to some reports, age is not a prognostic factor in carcinoma of the cervix.[120] Other authors noted decreased survival in women younger than 35 or 40 years,[121] who have a greater frequency of poorly differentiated tumors. In contrast, two European studies showed improved outcome for younger patients.[122] This apparent contradiction may be explained by an analysis by Rutledge et al.,[123] who showed an interaction between age and stage in the relative hazard plots for 250 patients younger than 35 years of age and matched control subjects. Mitchell et al.[124] evaluated 398 patients with stage I to III cervical carcinoma treated with radiation therapy. Patients were divided into nonelderly (35 to 69 years of age; $n = 338$) and elderly (≥70 years of age; $n = 60$) groups. Comorbid conditions in the elderly resulted in diminished ability to undergo intracavitary brachytherapy. Although the 5-year actuarial disease-free and cause-specific survival (CSS) rates were comparable in the two groups, tumor recurrence and death from cervical cancer were more common beyond 5 years in the elderly group.

Race/Socioeconomic Status

Several authors noted a correlation between racial or socioeconomic characteristics of patients and outcome of therapy. Mundt et al.[125] examined factors affecting outcome in 316 African American and 94 white patients undergoing RT for cervical cancer. With a median follow-up of 72.4 months, African Americans had a trend toward poorer 8-year cause-specific survival rates (47.9% vs. 60.6%; $p = .10$) compared with white patients. Factors correlating with poor outcome, including lower hemoglobin (Hb) levels during RT ($p = .001$), lower median income ($p = .001$), and less frequent intracavitary brachytherapy ($p = .09$), were more likely to be present in the African American group. Multivariate analysis demonstrated that race was not an independent prognostic factor after controlling for differences in patient, tumor, and treatment factors. In a report on 452 white and 124 African American women with stage II or III cancer of the cervix treated with RT alone, Grigsby et al.,[126] observed 5-year CSS rates for stage II of 66% and 61% ($p = .56$) for those with stage II and of 38% and 47% ($p = 0.34$) for those with stage III disease, respectively. Overall survival rates for stage II for the two racial groups were different (60% and 51%, respectively; $p = .02$) and may be related to non–cancer-related comorbidity factors.

Brooks et al.[127] evaluated 1,009 patients with invasive carcinoma of the cervix: 606 white, 354 African American, and 5%

"other" races. African Americans were more likely to have Medicaid or to be uninsured (44% vs. 23%; $p = .001$) and were more likely to be admitted for an emergency or for a cancer-related complication ($p = .036$), to have comorbid illness ($p = .001$), to be admitted for a transfusion ($p = .01$), or to be treated with radiation rather than surgery ($p = .001$). Racial differences existed in patterns of admission, type of therapy, and severity of illness.

Moreover, in an analysis of the 1994 Patterns of Care study of 471 cases of squamous cell carcinoma treated in the United States and a randomly selected 215 additional cases from 17 institutions that admitted >40% minority patients, women who lived in low-income neighborhoods, who had only Medicaid coverage, or who were treated at large academic or minority-rich institutions tended to have a poorer initial performance status, higher-stage or bulky central tumor, and a lower pretreatment hemoglobin level.[128]

General Medical Factors

Anemia and Tumor Hypoxia

Although stage, tumor volume, histologic type of the lesion, and vascular or lymphatic invasion are known to affect the prognosis of patients with cervical carcinoma, hemoglobin levels may also contribute to patient prognosis. Many radiation oncologists routinely administer red blood cell transfusions (RBCTs) to correct anemia before treatment with radiation therapy. This may have a generally favorable effect on the patient's sense of well-being and energy level, and an impact on tumor radiosensitivity. Typically patients receive transfusion to maintain hemoglobin levels >12 to 12.5 g/dL.

Hirst[129] emphasized that in animal tumor models the opportunity to affect radiosensitivity by blood transfusion is transient. Blood transfusion is in general beneficial to the anemic patient with cancer, but it must be given as soon as possible before the first radiation dose to maximize its effects. Accounting for both the normal pulmonary and peripheral circulation and parallel flow through tumor tissue, Kavanagh et al.[130] calculated that decreasing hemoglobin–oxygen affinity should render a quantitatively greater decrease in radiobiologically hypoxic regions than what has been measured after the use of transfusions alone.[131]

Investigators have reported worse outcomes for patients whose tumors have either a median partial pressure of oxygen (Po_2) level, measured using polarographic needle electrodes for direct tumor-tissue oxygen measurements, of <10 mm Hg,[132] or a high percentage of Po_2 measurements <5 mm Hg.[133,134] Comparisons of intratumoral oxygen measurements before and after external-beam radiation therapy have usually indicated a trend toward improved oxygenation after radiation therapy,[135,136] but the significance of posttreatment measurements is unclear.[137] Hypoxic tumors are more likely to recur locoregionally than well-oxygenated tumors regardless of whether surgery or radiation therapy is the primary local treatment.[132]

Haensgen et al.[138] analyzed 70 patients with stage IIB to IVA cervical cancer treated with EBRT and brachytherapy. *In vivo* oxygenation was measured with an Eppendorf probe, and patient hemoglobin levels were recorded. Patients with a hemoglobin level of <11 g/dL had a 3-year survival rate of 27%, compared with 62% for those with a hemoglobin level of ≥11 g/dL ($p = .006$). Combining hypoxia and tp53 allowed stratification of subgroups with differing 3-year survival rates: 79% for tp53 ($n = 10$) and 47% for tp53 without hypoxia ($n = 44$).

A randomized trial reported by Bush[139] on 132 patients with stage IIB to III cervical cancer required the control arm to receive transfusions only if the hemoglobin level dropped to <10 g/dL, whereas the experimental arm had to maintain the hemoglobin level ≥12.5 g/dL. The results suggested an improved outcome for patients in the experimental arm who received transfusion; however, there was not a statistically significant difference in outcome between treatment arms when compared using an intent-to-treat analysis.[140] Second, the randomization was not stratified according to the potentially confounding influence of tumor size. Finally, the thresholds for transfusion were based on anemia during therapy, not the initial hemoglobin. Thomas[141] reviewed the Canadian experience and found that in 605 eligible patients with cervical cancer, 25% received blood transfusions, most frequently when Hb was <100 g/L. On multivariate analysis, baseline Hb was not a significant prognostic factor, but average weekly nadir during radiation therapy was significant, with those with values >120 g/L having lower incidences of local relapse and distant metastasis and a better 5-year survival rate.

Dunst et al.[142] showed that pretreatment anemia had a significant impact on 3-year relapse rates (6% in 20 patients with Hb of >13 g/dL, 15% in 47 with Hb between 11 and 13 g/dL, and 67% in 20 with Hb of <11 g/dL). The 3-year survival rate was 38% in patients with poorly oxygenated tumors, compared to 68% in patients with higher Po_2 ($p = .02$). Munstedt et al.,[143] in a study of 183 patients who received adjuvant RT after radical surgery, noted that those with Hb of <11 g/dL had lower recurrence-free and overall survival rates, primarily in a subgroup of women who had inadequate surgery.

In a retrospective review of >600 patients treated at seven different cancer centers in Canada, Grogan et al.[144] observed that the patients who maintained an average weekly hemoglobin level of >12 g/dL with or without transfusions had a significantly higher 5-year survival rate than patients with lower average weekly hemoglobin levels, regardless of the hemoglobin at presentation.

Kapp et al.[145] reported on 204 patients who received RBCT during RT when Hb level was <11 g/dL. Patients whose Hb was corrected (18.5%) had outcomes similar to those of nontransfused patients. However, nonresponders to RBCT had decreased tumor control and survival rates. Vaupel et al.,[146] in a review of published data, concluded that maximum oxygenation of tumors is expected with Hb in the range of 12 to 14 g/dL for women and that higher Hb levels may not be better.

Recombinant human erythropoietin is not routinely recommended as an alternative means of sustaining or raising hemoglobin levels during radiation therapy. Thrombotic complications[147] and the lack of any survival benefit[148] mitigate the utility of this as a therapeutic intervention.

Other Medical Factors

Jenkin and Stryker[149] observed a higher incidence of pelvic recurrences and complications in patients with arterial hypertension (diastolic pressure of >110 mm Hg). Kapp and Lawrence[150] reported on 398 patients; patients with temperatures of >101°F had a higher incidence of distant metastases and a lower survival rate. In patients with cervical cancer screened for HIV and treated with RT, Campbell et al.[151] observed a 4.2% positive HIV rate. These patients had more-advanced tumors. The duration of remission was shorter than in the HIV-negative group. RT had no effect on the HIV titers. Women who are HIV positive or have acquired immunodeficiency syndrome associated with *in situ* or invasive carcinoma of the cervix are at a higher risk for tumor recurrence after treatment and death as a consequence of the malignant process.[152,153]

Evidence continues to mount that increasing levels of plasma micronutrients are associated with a decreasing risk of cervical cancer. Increasing serum lycopene and α- and γ-tocopheral levels and higher intake of dark green and deep yellow vegetables and fruit were significantly inversely associated with cancer.[154–156] Women should be counseled to eat a well-balanced diet, particularly those at high risk for developing cervical cancer.

Tumor Factors

HPV Subtype

HPV 16 and 18 are the most frequent HPV subtypes worldwide. Studies have reported a higher risk of lymph node and other distant metastases with HPV 18 compared to HPV 16.[157,158] Wang et al.[159] studied 1,010 patients with cervical cancer after radiotherapy between 1993 and 2000. The HPV genotypes were determined by a gene chip that can detect 38 types of HPV. A total of 25 genotypes of HPV were detected in 992 specimens, of which 8 types that predominated were HPV16, 58, 18, 33, 52, 39, 31, and 45. Two high-risk HPV species were identified: α-7 (HPV18, 39, 45) and α-9 (HPV16, 31, 33, 52, 58). Risk groups determined included the high-risk group, which consisted of patients without HPV infection or those infected with the α-7 species only. The medium-risk group included patients coinfected with the α-7 and α-9 species.

Tumor Volume

There is a close correlation between depth of stromal invasion, tumor size, and incidence of parametrial and pelvic node metastases and survival in patients with cervical cancer.[160,161] In a study of women treated with radical hysterectomy, the 5-year disease-free survival rate was 90% in 181 patients with stage IB1 (≤4 cm) and 72.8% in 48 patients with stage IB2 disease (p = .02).[162]

Toita et al.,[163] in a review of 70 patients with stage IIB and IIIB carcinoma of the uterine cervix treated with RT alone, reported no significant correlation of 5-year DFS with size of the cervical tumor <60 mm (70% to 85%); however, in patients with tumor ≥60 mm, the 5-year DFS was 28.6%. Piver and Chung[164] showed a greater incidence of lymphatic and distant metastasis and lower survival rates in patients with bulky and barrel-shaped stage IB and IIA tumors treated by radical hysterectomy. In addition, a higher incidence of pelvic recurrences and distant metastases and a decreased survival rate were reported by Fletcher,[165] Eifel et al.,[166] and Perez et al.[167] in patients with larger tumors treated with irradiation. In stages IB and IIA, higher radiation doses improved local tumor control.[168,169]

Furthermore, Leveque et al.,[170] in patients with stage I to II adenocarcinoma of the cervix treated with RT alone or combined with radical surgery, noted that FIGO stage and pelvic node involvement were the most important parameters influencing overall survival. Silver et al.,[171] in 93 patients with stage I adenocarcinoma of the cervix, described patient age and tumor grade as significant prognostic variables for survival ($p < .01$ and .01, respectively); tumor size was significant ($p < .01$) for survival and progression-free survival.

In contrast, Grigsby et al.,[172] in patients with stage IB and IIA carcinoma of the cervix treated with preoperative irradiation and radical or conservative hysterectomy, observed no correlation of tumor volume with outcome. The 5-year pelvic failure rates for stage IB were 16% for tumors <3 cm and 9% for larger tumors (p = .90) and for stage IIA were 22% for tumors <3 or >3 cm (p = .75).

Several retrospective studies demonstrated decreased survival and a greater incidence of distant metastases in patients with endometrial extension of a primary cervical carcinoma (endometrial stromal invasion or replacement of the endometrium by tumor only).[36] Grimard et al.,[173] on the other hand, confirmed these findings only in patients with stage IB tumors but not in more advanced stages. Similar findings were noted by Noguchi et al.[174] Patients without uterine body invasion had a 5-year survival rate of 92.4%, compared with 53.8% in patients with invasion.

Perez et al.,[169] in an update of a previous report,[167] reviewed 1,499 patients (stages IA to IVA) treated with definitive irradiation (combination of external-beam irradiation plus two intracavitary insertions to deliver doses of 70 to 90 Gy to point A). There was a close correlation between tumor size and extent and pelvic tumor control, incidence of distant metastasis, and disease-free survival in all stages.

Margin Status After Radical Hysterectomy

In addition to the known high risk factors of positive margins, positive parametrial spread, and/or positive lymph nodes and the intermediate risk factors of depth of stromal invasion, lymphovascular invasion, and tumor size, small series have indicated the significance of close margin status.[175,176] Viswanathan et al.[177] studied 284 patients after radical hysterectomy (RH). The crude rates for any recurrence were 11%, 20%, and 38% for patients with negative (≥1 cm), close (>0 and <1 cm), and positive margins, respectively. Postoperative RT decreased the rate of local recurrence (LR) from 10% to 0% for negative, 17% to 0% for close, and 50% to 25% for positive margins. The significant predictors of decreased relapse-free survival on univariate analysis were the depth of tumor invasion (hazard ratio [HR] = 2.14/cm increase, p = .007), positive margins (HR = 3.92, p = .02), tumor size (HR = 1.3/cm increase, p = .02), lymphovascular invasion (HR = 2.19, p = .03), and margin status (HR = 0.002/increasing millimeter from cancer for those with close margins, p = .03).

Histologic Grade

Most reports have shown no significant correlation of survival or tumor behavior with the degree of differentiation of squamous cell carcinoma or adenocarcinoma of the cervix.[178–180] Alfsen et al.[178] analyzed 417 adenocarcinomas and 88 other non–squamous cell carcinomas of the cervix; on multivariate analysis, small-cell histology, corpus infiltration, vascular invasion, and positive lymph nodes were significant prognostic variables. Although Reagan and Fu[181] demonstrated prognostic value of histologic differentiation in patients treated with irradiation, Crissman et al.[182] failed to observe a correlation between histologic parameters and patient survival. In the era of chemoradiation, Monk et al.[183] showed no significant impact of histology or grade on survival in postoperative cervical cancer patients with other high-risk features.

Treatment Duration

In patients treated with radiation therapy, overall treatment time should be as short as possible, and any planned or unplanned interruptions or delays should be avoided. Timely integration of external-beam and intracavitary irradiation in patients with carcinoma of the uterine cervix is an important factor in improving pelvic tumor control (Fig. 69.8).[184] Several studies described lower pelvic tumor control and survival rates in invasive carcinoma of the uterine cervix when the overall time in a course of irradiation is prolonged.[120,185–187] Chatani et al.,[188] in 216 patients with stage IIB to III cervical carcinoma treated with a combination of external-beam and HDR brachytherapy, noted that overall treatment time was the most highly significant factor for local tumor control in multivariate analysis (p = .0005). For relapse-free survival, stage classification (p = .0001), overall treatment time (p = .0035), and hemoglobin level (p = .0174) were the three most important prognostic factors; there was no relationship between treatment time and late complications.

Fyles et al.[185] reported approximately 1% loss of tumor control per day of prolongation of treatment time beyond 30 days in 830 patients with cervical carcinoma treated with irradiation alone. Lanciano et al.,[187] in an analysis of 837 patients with squamous cell carcinoma of the cervix from the Patterns of Care Study who were treated with irradiation and received doses of 66 Gy or greater, described a 4-year actuarial in-field recurrence increase from 6% to 20% when total treatment time increased from 6 weeks or fewer to 10 weeks (p = .0001); this translated into significantly decreased survival. Girinsky et al.,[186] in 386 patients with stage IIB or III carcinoma of the cervix, also observed that the 10-year local recurrence–free survival rate decreased when overall treatment time exceeded 52 days. A 1.1% loss of pelvic tumor control per day was also observed in their regression analysis.

Perez et al.,[189] in 1,330 patients treated with definitive irradiation, noted a major impact of prolongation of treatment time on pelvic tumor control in stages IB, IIA, and IIB. In stage III, although the rate of pelvic failure was higher with prolongation of treatment time, the difference was not statistically significant. There was also a strong correlation between overall treatment time and survival. Regression analysis confirmed previous reports that prolongation of overall treatment time resulted in an increased failure rate of 0.59% per day in stage IB and IIA and 0.86% per day in stage IIB disease. Performance

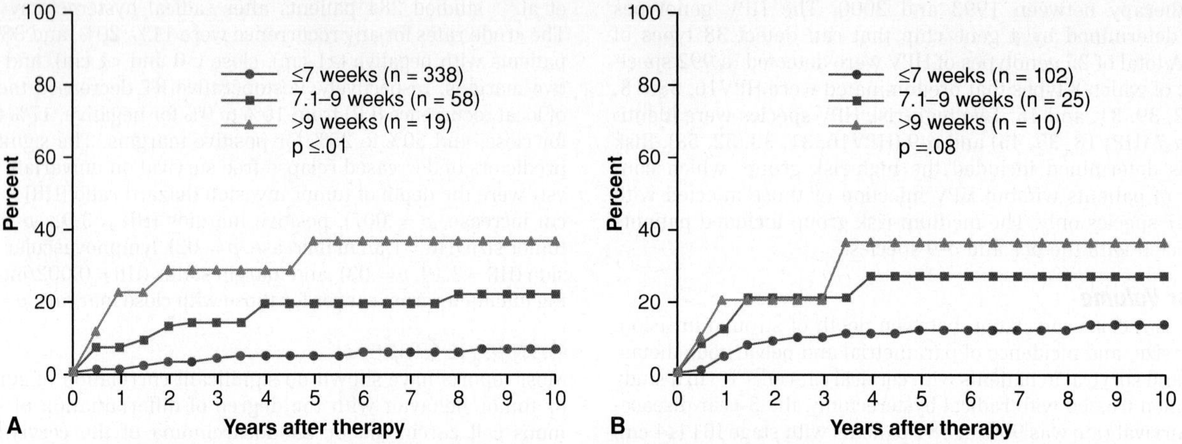

FIGURE 69.8. Pelvic failure rate correlated with length of treatment in stages IB **(A)** and IIA **(B)** carcinoma of the uterine cervix. (From Perez CA, Grigsby PW, Castro-Vita H, et al. Carcinoma of the uterine cervix: I. Impact of prolongation of treatment time and timing of brachytherapy on outcome of radiation therapy. *Int J Radiat Oncol Biol Phys* 1995;32:1275–1288; with permission from Elsevier.)

of all intracavitary insertions within 4.5 weeks from initiation of irradiation yielded lower pelvic failure rates (8.8% vs. 18% in stage IIB tumors; $p \leq .01$).

Biomarkers

Several studies assessed various biologic markers to determine whether they are prognostic; however, the majority suffered from not having multivariate analyses to determine whether these may be valid independent factors. Noordhuis et al.,[190] in a systematic review of 42 studies with 82 cell-biologic markers, reported that on univariate analysis, 34 biologic markers showed a relation with survival, 27 of which were independently associated with survival.

Angiogenesis and Hypoxia

Angiogenesis—the formation of new blood vessels—relies on the presence of proangiogenic growth factors, such as vascular endothelial growth factor (VEGF). As new blood vessels form, they deliver nutrients and oxygen to the cancerous cells. As tumors expand, the newly formed blood vessels may no longer reach the central portions of the tumor, and a hypoxic core develops. Hypoxia-inducible factor (HIF-1α) and HIF-2α regulate the response to hypoxic stress; HIF-1α but not HIF-2α has been associated with poor disease-free survival.[191-194] The HIF-2α/CD68 ratio was correlated with poor disease-free survival.[194] One study found that VEGF decreased overall survival.[195,196] Loncaster et al.,[195] in a retrospective study of 100 patients, found that VEGF expression in tumor biopsies in advanced carcinoma of the cervix was associated with a poor prognosis. Level of thymidine phosphorylase,[196] which increases hypoxic conditions, similarly was associated with poor outcomes. Nitric oxide synthase[197] and carbonic anhydrase (CA) may be prognostic for a poor outcome. In particular, CA9 is related to poor disease-free survival.[198,199] CA12, in contrast, was related to metastasis-free survival.[200]

Microvessel count is higher in patients with cervical neoplasia than in control patients and higher in patients who experience posttreatment recurrences. Obermair et al.,[201] in 166 patients with stage IB cervical cancer, observed a 5-year survival rate of 89.7% in 102 patients whose tumors had a microvessel density of 20 per field or less and 63% in 64 patients whose tumors had a microvessel density of >20 per field (log rank $p < .0001$). In a multivariate Cox model, microvessel density, lymph node involvement, tumor size, and the application of radiation therapy were independent prognostic factors for survival. Similar findings were reported by Cooper et al.[202]

Flow Cytometry Studies on DNA and Growth Fraction

Some authors noted no significant difference in recurrence rates between patients with diploid or aneuploid tumors. Kristensen et al.,[203] in a study 465 patients with invasive carcinoma of the uterine cervix on whom DNA index and S-phase fraction studies were performed, observed that neither ploidy level nor S-phase fraction had prognostic significance. Others[204] noted more relapses in tumors with an S-phase rate of 20% or greater.

Apoptosis

Whether apoptotic markers might be of importance in cervical cancer is unclear, given heterogeneity in the data. Morphologic studies have been negative, but some studies evaluating apoptotic protein expression such as that of Bcl-2 and p63 show association with poor disease-free survival.[205,206]

Ohno et al.[207] studied 20 patients before and after administration of 9 Gy and found an increase in apoptotic cell index and Bax protein. Wootipoom et al.,[205] in 174 patients with cervical cancer, noted Bax, Bcl-2, and p53 expression in 68.4%, 25.9%, and 77.6% of the cases, respectively. Bax expression was associated with better survival, whereas Bcl-2 expression was associated with poor survival. Jain et al.[208] also found that neither Bcl-2 nor p53 expression was an independent predictor of outcome in locally advanced cervical cancer.

The p53 gene controls entry into the S phase of the cell cycle. Mukherjee et al.[209] analyzed radioresistant cervical cancer cases and found that 15% had positivity for Bcl-2 and p21 proteins and 34% showed mutant p53 protein. None of the radiosensitive tumors were positive for these proteins. Seventy-five percent of the radiosensitive tumors were positive for the Bax antibody, whereas 81% of the radioresistant tumors were negative for Bax ($p < .01$). Kainz et al.,[210] in a study of 109 surgically treated patients, and Ebara et al.,[211] in 46 patients with stage IIIB squamous cell carcinoma of the cervix treated with RT alone, noted no significant difference in outcome when correlated with p53 protein expression.

Cell Cycle and Cellular Oncogenes

Cerciello et al.,[212] in 40 patients with stage IIA to IIIB cervix cancer treated with RT without chemotherapy, obtained biopsies before and after five fractions of RT. They observed significant changes in the cell cycle of cervical cancer, indicating intact G2/M checkpoint function, leading to the expectation that targeting compounds interfering with G2/M transition may enhance the effect of irradiation on cervix cancer.

In patients with carcinoma of the uterine cervix treated with irradiation, Tsang et al.,[213] observed that the most significant factors for disease-free survival were large tumor size ($p = .01$), low hemoglobin ($p = .01$), labeling index (LI) flow cytometry (disease-free survival, 67% for LI < 7%; 33% for LI ≥ 7%; $p = .03$), and potential doubling time (T_{pot}; 66% for $T_{pot} > 5$ days, 35% for $T_{pot} \leq 5$ days; $p = .04$). For small tumors (<6 cm in diameter), either a high LI (>7%) or a high apoptotic index (>1%) was associated with poorer disease-free survival. West et al.[214] evaluated the intrinsic radiosensitivity of 145 tumor biopsies from patients with cervical carcinoma (*in vitro* survival fraction at 2 Gy using a clonogenic assay). Diploid tumors tended to be more radioresistant than aneuploid tumors ($p = .07$).

The p27/Kip1 gene inhibits a variety of cyclin-dependent kinase complexes and regulates cell growth. Oka et al.[215] studied 202 biopsy specimens obtained from 77 patients with squamous cell carcinoma of the cervix before and during RT for expression of p27 and p53 proteins. A high p27 LI before radiation therapy was associated significantly with good disease-free and metastasis-free survival rates. A high p53 LI before irradiation was associated with poor overall survival.

Both specific point mutations and amplification of *ras* genes have been noted. Overexpression of the ras gene p21 product is associated with a poor prognosis and increased frequency of lymph node involvement.[216] Although loss of heterozygosity of the c-Ha-ras gene in squamous cell carcinomas was not associated with advanced-stage disease, mutations were associated with a poor prognosis. In contrast, mutations of the Ki-ras gene have been detected in a small percentage of cervical adenocarcinomas but have not been significantly associated with stage, grade, or survival.[217,218]

The c-*myc* oncogene is amplified from 3 to 30 times in approximately 20% of squamous cell carcinomas and is more frequent in high-stage compared with low-stage tumors. Overexpression of c-myc has been associated with a worse clinical outcome.[219,220]

Gadd45 belongs to the class II family of DNA damage-inducible genes, and its role in DNA repair has been proven in many experimental models. Santucci et al.,[221] in 14 patients with cervical cancer, found a correlation between the lack of gadd45 induction and a clinical response to irradiation (both local tumor control and disease-free survival) when a dose ranging from 18 to 25 Gy was delivered to the pelvis.

CD 34 is an antigen present in hemopoietic progenitor cells and is a sensitive marker for endothelial cells. In 62 patients with cervical cancer evaluated by Vieira et al.,[222] CD 34 reactivity and higher microvessel density were associated with squamous cell carcinoma. CD 109 is a cell surface protein that was found to be expressed in cervical cancer more than in endometrial adenocarcinoma.[223]

Cytokeratin Markers and the Epidermal Growth Factor Receptor Pathway

Altered expression of c-ercB-2 (HER2) protein was shown to have prognostic significance in adenocarcinoma but not in squamous cell carcinoma of the cervix.[224] HER1, as well as coexpression of epidermal growth factor receptor and HER2, has been associated with poor disease-free survival.[225] PTEN mutations have also been associated with poor prognosis.[226]

In 80 patients with carcinoma of the cervix, expression of cytokeratin 10 and 13 and involucrin was found in 24%, 64%, and 53%, respectively.[227] There was no difference in the expression of cytokeratin or involucrin between patients with positive or negative lymph nodes, although in the lymph node–positive group, survival was higher in patients lacking cytokeratin 13 expression ($p = .02$).

Squamous Cell Carcinoma Antigen and Carcinoembryonic Antigen

Tsai et al.,[228] in 117 patients with adenocarcinoma of the cervix, 28 of whom had preoperative carcinoembryonic antigen (CEA) levels of >5 ng/mL, noted a correlation with larger tumor size, deeper cervical invasion, and lymphovascular invasion ($p < .001$). A Spanish study of 96 patients with invasive carcinoma of the cervix and 7 with intraepithelial neoplasia showed elevated CEA levels in 33%, CA 19.9 in 32%, and CA 125 in 21.5% of patients.[229] Specificity for each tumor marker was 98%. Increased CEA and CA 19.9 levels were found with more advanced stages of the disease and in patients with adenocarcinoma compared with squamous cell carcinoma. At follow-up, all cases of progressive tumor or recurrence were detected by elevation of one of the three antigens. Specificity during follow-up was 92% for CEA and CA 125 and 92.6% for CA 19.9.

In a study of 272 patients with invasive carcinoma of the cervix with 1,053 samples, Bolli et al.[230] noted an elevation of squamous cell carcinoma antigen (SCC-Ag) before treatment in 53% of 103 patients, increasing with advancing tumor stage at diagnosis. In 70 patients with recurrent tumor, 81% had elevated SCC-Ag. Ngan et al.[231] also identified elevation of serum SCC-Ag in 62% of 308 women with carcinoma of the cervix. Posttreatment SCC-Ag levels were raised in 69 patients (22.4%), and this was associated with a <5% 5-year survival rate, in contrast to 87% in women with normal SCC-Ag levels.

Hong et al.,[232] in 401 patients with stage I to IV squamous cell carcinoma of the cervix treated with RT, noted that the preirradiation SCC-Ag level strongly correlated with disease stage. A persistently elevated SCC-Ag level 3 months after RT was a stronger predictor for treatment failure than residual induration by pelvic examination, and it was associated with a higher incidence of distant metastasis.

Similarly, Micke et al.,[233] in 141 patients with cervical cancer treated with RT, noted that the pretherapy serum level of SCC-Ag was elevated in 72% (>2 ng/mL). Patients with a SCC-Ag of <7.2 U/mL had better tumor response than those with higher levels. After RT, 98% of patients in complete remission and 87% of those in partial remission had a serum level below the cutoff. In recurrent tumors, 82% of patients had a significant increase in serum levels before clinical manifestation of relapse (≤0.001). Hong et al.,[234] in 1,031 patients with squamous cell cervical cancer treated with RT with or without chemotherapy, noted that independent risk factors for local relapse were advanced stage and age <45 years; 5-year local relapse-free survival was higher (90%) if squamous cell carcinoma antigen was <2. This antigen may be a useful marker in the prognosis of patients with carcinoma of the uterine cervix. Huang et al.[235,236] noted that SCC-Ag and CEA were predictive of para-aortic node failure.

Epstein-Barr Virus, Transforming Growth Factor, β-Integrin, and Other Markers

Activity of Epstein-Barr virus antigen–specific killer T cells and shedding of Epstein-Barr virus were evaluated in 55 patients with carcinoma of the cervix.[237] Activity was decreased in patients with cervical carcinoma compared with control patients; it became increasingly lower as the clinical stage of the disease advanced, and activity after treatment was clearly related to patient survival. These data may indicate an imbalance in local immunity against viral infection and impairment of T-cell immunity in patients with advanced cervical carcinoma.

In 79 patients undergoing radiation therapy for carcinoma of the cervix, pretreatment transforming growth factor-β_1 (TGF-β_1) levels were a significant prognostic factor for survival and local tumor control. There were weak significant correlations of TGF-β_1 levels with disease stage and the levels of circulating tumor markers (CA 125).[238] Hazelbag et al.[239] also assessed TGF-β_1 and plasminogen activator inhibitor (PAI-1) expression in 108 specimens of cervical carcinoma and noted that TGF was not associated with worse prognosis, whereas PAI-1 was.

Gruber et al.,[240] in biopsies of 82 patients with cervical cancer, found that β_3-integrin was expressed in 50 (61%) and correlated it with higher incidence of locoregional recurrences and decreased survival.

Cyclooxygenase-2

Gaffney et al.,[241] in 24 patients with carcinoma of the cervix treated with RT, observed that 5-year overall survival rates for tumors with low versus high COX-2 values were 75% and 35%, respectively ($p = .021$). COX-2 staining intensity was found to correlate positively with tumor size ($p = .022$).

Kim et al.[242] screened 84 patients with stage IIB squamous cell and 21 with adenocarcinoma cervical cancer and found COX-2 expression more frequently in the adenocarcinoma group (57% vs. 24%; $p = .007$). The 5-year survival rate was 83% for COX-2–negative and 57% for COX-2–positive patients, regardless of histologic subtype ($p = .001$). Pyo et al.[243] also showed that expression of COX-2 and coexpression of COX-2 and thymidine phosphorylase were correlated with high locoregional recurrence and lower survival. Moreover, Kang et al.,[244] in 84 patients with cervix adenocarcinoma, observed a higher incidence of lymph node metastasis and decreased survival with elevated expression of COX-2.

Hormonal Receptors

Suzuki et al.[245] investigated the expression of estrogen receptors and progesterone receptors (PgRs) in biopsy specimens from cervical tumors before RT in 44 patients with cervical adenocarcinoma and 22 with adenosquamous cell carcinomas. Staining for estrogen receptors or PgR was positive in 12 patients (19%). The estrogen receptor status did not correlate with the local tumor control, or disease-free, or cause-specific survival. The disease-free survival rate of PgR-positive patients was significantly higher than that of PgR-negative patients ($p = .044$), but PgR status was not statistically significant in relation to 5-year cause-specific survival or local tumor control.

TECHNIQUES USED FOR TREATMENT

Preinvasive Disease

Patients with CIN may be candidates for observation or treatment. CIN1-2 has a spontaneous regression rate in 1 to 3 years of >50%,[246] and therefore observation may be an appropriate course. For patients with persistent dysplasia, cryotherapy has a very low complication rate and is highly successful but may be less effective than laser ablation for high-grade dysplasia.[247] Cold knife conization (CKC) may be used for diagnostic and therapeutic intent, with side effects of bleeding, cellulitis, cervical stenosis, or loss of cervical competence. Loop electrosurgical excision procedure (LEEP) has become popular, although bleeding and stenosis may occur; pregnancy outcomes may be better with LEEP than with CKC.[248–250]

Invasive Disease

Surgical Techniques

Simple Conization

In patients with minimal invasion, no parametrial involvement, and small tumor size, simple conization with lymphadenectomy has been reported. Although only 36 patients were studied, after a median follow-up of 66 months, only 1 pelvic nodal relapse was observed.[251]

Radical Trachelectomy

Described in the 1960s,[252] trachelectomy entails removal of the cervix entirely. Radical trachelectomy also removes the parametrial tissue. As a means of fertility preservation in early-stage cervical-cancer patients,[253] trachelectomy should be combined with preoperative PET imaging to confirm no nodal involvement and with MRI to confirm no endocervical canal extension of tumor into the uterus.[254] A lapraroscopic lymphadenectomy should accompany the trachelectomy to confirm no nodal involvement. A nonabsorbable cerclage is placed around the uterine isthmus. Radical abdominal trachelectomy also may result in successful fertility preservation.[255] Selection criteria for a trachelectomy include those patients requesting fertility sparing surgery, age <40 years, stage IA1, IA2, or IB1 with no nodal involvement detected on MRI or PET scan, squamous cell or adenocarcinoma with a lesion <2 cm, no lymphovascular invasion on initial biopsy, and no upper endocervical involvement. The main site for recurrence is central pelvis (average 5% risk), at the cervico-uterine junction, or in the adjacent parametrial tissue.

Types of Hysterectomy

Several types of hysterectomy are used in the management of carcinoma of the uterine cervix (Table 69.7).[256]

Total (extrafascial) abdominal hysterectomy (class I) consists of removal of the cervix and adjacent tissues, as well as a small cuff of the upper vagina in a plane outside the pubocervical fascia. There is minimal disturbance of the ureters and the trigone of the bladder. This may be the surgical treatment of choice for stage IA1 cervical cancer.

The use of a radical hysterectomy for cervical cancer was first described by Wertheim in 1912.[257] In a modified radical extended hysterectomy (class II), the cervix and upper vagina are removed, including paracervical tissues, and the ureters are dissected in the paracervical tunnel to their point of entry into the bladder. Because the ureters are unsheathed and retracted laterally, parametrial and paracervical tissue can be safely removed medial to the ureter. This operation is performed with a lymphadenectomy. This is the most common surgical approach selected for stage IA2 cervical cancer.

Radical abdominal hysterectomy (class III) with bilateral pelvic lymphadenectomy consists of a wider resection of the parametrial tissues to the pelvic wall, with dissection of the ureters and mobilization of the bladder, as well as of the rectum to allow for more extensive removal of tissues. This approach was described by Meigs in 1944.[258] In addition, a vaginal cuff of at least 2 to 3 cm is always included in the procedure, as well as the uterosacral ligaments.[256] A bilateral pelvic lymphadenectomy is usually carried out. This operation is often referred to as the Wertheim or Meigs procedure. The extended radical hysterectomy (class IV) includes complete dissection of the ureter from the vesicouterine ligament, sacrifice of the superior vesicle artery, and removal of the upper three-fourths of the vagina. Due to the high rate of fistula and significant morbidity, it is rarely used.[256] In 2007, after a consensus conference in Japan, a new classification system was released based only on the lateral extent of the resection.[259] Four levels of hysterectomy are described (A to D) and four levels of lymphadenectomy (1 to 4). The levels of lymph node dissection include the internal and external iliac (level 1), common iliac and presacral (level 2), aortic inframesenteric (level 3), and

TABLE 69.7 TYPES OF ABDOMINAL HYSTERECTOMY

	Intrafascial	*Extrafascial Type I*	*Modified Radical Type II*	*Radical Type III*
Cervical fascia	Partially removed	Completely removed	———	———
Vaginal cuff removal	None	Small rim removed	Proximal 1–2 cm removed	Upper one-third to one-half removed
Bladder	Partially mobilized	———	———	Mobilized
Rectum	Not mobilized	Rectovaginal septum partially mobilized	———	Mobilized
Ureters	Not mobilized	———	Unroofed in ureteral tunnel	Completely dissected to bladder entry
Cardinal ligaments	Resected medial to ureters	———	Resected at level of ureter	Resected at pelvic sidewall
Uterosacral ligaments	Resected at level of cervix	———	Partially resected	Resected at postpelvic insertion
Uterus	Removed	———	———	———
Cervix	Partially removed	Completely removed	———	———

[a]Type IV, extended radical hysterectomy (partial removal of bladder and/or ureter), in addition to type III.

aortic infrarenal (level 4). The levels of primary tumor resection include the following:

Type A: Extrafascial hysterectomy, with minimum resection of the paracervix medial to the ureter and minimal vaginal resection <1 cm, without removal of the paracolpos.

Type B: Modified radical hysterectomy with partial resection of the vesicouterine and uterosacral ligaments, unroofing of the ureter, transection of the parametrial tissue at the ureter, and removal of at least 1 cm of the vagina. This type is divided into B1, without removal of paracervical lymph nodes, and B2, with removal of lateral paracervical nodes.

Type C: Classic radical hysterectomy, variant in which the entire uterosacral and vesicouterine ligaments are removed, 1.5 to 2 cm of vagina with paracolpos is excised, and neuronal preservation is critical.

Type D: Includes the complete radical hysterectomy and resects tissues to the pelvis sidewall, including the hypogastric (internal iliac) vessels, and exposes the sciatic nerve (type D1). Type D2 also removes the fascial and lateral muscles, called the laterally extended endopelvic resection.

Pelvic Exenteration

Pelvic exenteration has been used for en masse removal of the pelvic viscera for recurrent carcinoma of the cervix. Modern radiation therapy with concurrent chemotherapy results in high complete response rates and has made residual extensive disease a rare indication for exenteration. Patients with adjacent organ invasion are given a course of radical concurrent chemoradiation, followed by interstitial brachytherapy, with exenteration reserved for salvage.[260–262] This operation, which is not done as a palliative procedure, consists of a radical hysterectomy, pelvic lymph-node dissection, and removal of the bladder (anterior exenteration), removal of the rectosigmoid colon (posterior exenteration), or both (total exenteration). The ileum or sigmoid has been the usual means of achieving urinary diversion. Because some patients have a pelvic recurrence after radiation therapy, the bowel is used for the urinary conduit. Proof that there is no fixation to the pelvic wall and no extension of disease beyond the pelvis is mandatory. Metastases outside the pelvis, including those in para-aortic lymph nodes or any viscera, are absolute contraindications to the procedure. Bilateral ureteral obstruction secondary to tumor is also a relative contraindication.[263] Patients with sacroiliac or hip pain or leg edema rarely benefit from this procedure and should be excluded on a clinical basis.

Pretreatment Surgical Nodal Assessment

Exploratory laparotomy and nodal staging to evaluate the presence of metastases to the pelvic or para-aortic nodes may provide diagnostic information but has not had a demonstrated impact on survival (Table 69.8). In a prospective evaluation of 290 patients with carcinoma of the cervix,[264] para-aortic node metastases were found in 19 of 58 patients (32.8%) with clinical stage IIB and 19 of 61 (31.1%) with stage IIIB disease. A number of studies compared the significance of para-aortic nodal metastases with other clinical and surgical findings with regard to progression-free survival and overall survival.[265] In 626 patients treated on GOG randomized studies, the relative risk associated with positive para-aortic nodes was 11.0 for time to recurrence and 6.2 for survival time. In addition to the significant increase in risk of regional relapses, patients with para-aortic nodal metastasis are more likely to have extrapelvic failure.[266]

TABLE 69.8 CARCINOMA OF THE UTERINE CERVIX: SURVIVAL AFTER STAGING LAPAROTOMY

	Explored		*Not Explored*	
Stage	*Number of Patients*	*Percentage Surviving*	*Number of Patients*	*Percentage Surviving*
IIB	31	64.5	14	92.8
IIIA–IIIB	28	57.1	10	60.0

From Nelson JH, Macasaet MA, Lu T, et al. The incidence and significance of paraaortic lymph node metastases in late invasive carcinoma of the cervix. *Am J Obstet Gynecol* 1974;118:749–756; with permission from Elsevier.

Cosin et al.[267] reviewed 266 patients with locally advanced cervical carcinoma who underwent extraperitoneal pelvic and para-aortic lymphadenectomy before RT. Patients were divided into four groups: group A had negative lymph nodes; B, resected, microscopic lymph node metastases; C, macroscopically positive lymph nodes that were resectable at the time of surgery; and D, unresectable lymph nodes. Lymph node metastases were detected in 50% of patients. All patients received pelvic external-beam radiotherapy (EBRT; pre–intensity-modulated radiation [IMRT] era) and brachytherapy; patients with lymph-node metastases received extended-field irradiation. Five- and 10-year disease-free survival rates were similar for all patients in groups B and C. All patients in group D recurred. There was a 10.5% incidence of severe radiation-related morbidity and a 1.1% incidence of treatment-related deaths.

The potential benefit of surgical nodal debulking followed by irradiation has been studied.[268] Potish et al.[269] noted that more than half of the patients with advanced cervical cancer with grossly positive pelvic nodes that were debulked survived, compared with none with unresectable lymph nodes, findings closely paralleling those of Inoue and Morita[270]; however, these studies pre-dated the ability to implement dose escalation with IMRT to the involved nodes. Nonetheless, surgical debulking of nodes decreases the dose of radiation required to these regions. The use of high-energy photon beams and limitation of the tumor dose to extended volumes in the para-aortic region for those with completely resected but positive nodes to 45 to 50 Gy decrease the probability of complications. IMRT also enhances the sparing of adjacent abdominal normal tissues.[271,272] However, if node dissection is not feasible or would result in a treatment delay, patients may successfully be managed with IMRT with dose escalation to approximately 60 to 65 Gy to the grossly enlarged lymph nodes.[80,273,274, 275]

Complication risk may be high (Table 69.9), particularly when patients are treated with postresection RT. One study showed an 11.5% incidence of major primarily small-bowel complications with transperitoneal compared with 3.9% in the extraperitoneal lymphadenectomy group ($p = .03$).[276] Transperitoneal lymphadenectomy should be avoided.[277,278]

Due to a high rate of complications, preirradiation laparotomy was discontinued at the MD Anderson Cancer Center. The status of the lymph nodes is investigated with lymphangiography and verified when possible with percutaneous transabdominal needle biopsy. Wharton et al.[279] reported on 120 patients who had preirradiation celiotomy; 16 had fatal complications, and 32 had major intestinal complications. Most patients with positive lymph nodes died with distant metastasis. More recently, PET/CT followed by biopsy may be a useful approach. In one series of 60 patients without evidence of para-aortic lymph node involvement on preoperative CT or MRI, patients underwent a preoperative PET/CT followed by surgery. Twenty-six patients had a negative PET/CT, of whom 3 (12%) had positive nodes pathologically. Of the 27 with positive pelvic but negative para-aortic nodes on PET/CT, 6 (22%) had pathologically positive para-aortic nodes, indicating a sensitivity of 36% and a specificity of 96%. In another study, 125 patients had a PET/CT followed by para-aortic lymphadenectomy.[280] Seventeen percent had positive para-aortic metastases, 66% of whom had a negative PET/CT. The sensitivity and specificity of PET/CT were 33% and 94%, respectively. Morbidity of the surgery was 7%, and there was no delay in initiating chemoradiotherapy. A Cochrane overview of pretreatment surgical para-aortic lymph-node assessment in stage IB2-IVA cervical cancer identified one randomized trial of 61 women that favored CT or MRI over surgical staging.[281,282] Alternatively, para-aortic node sampling may

TABLE 69.9 COMPLICATION RATE FOR PRETHERAPY SURGICAL STAGING

	Transperitoneal (122/189; 64.6%)		Retroperitoneal (67/189; 35.4%)	
	Prior Laparotomy (n = 52), Group 1	No Prior Laparotomy (n = 70), Group 2	Prior Laparotomy (n = 27), Group 3	No Prior Laparotomy (n = 40), Group 4
Complications per group	32 (61.5%)	25 (37.9%)	8 (29.6%)	1 (2.5%)
Percentage of total complications (n = 66)	48.5	37.9	12.1	1.5

From Fine BA, Hempling RE, Piver MS, et al. Severe radiation morbidity in carcinoma of the cervix: impact of pretherapy surgical staging and previous surgery. *Int J Radiat Oncol Biol Phys* 1995;31:717–723; with permission from Elsevier.

be performed through a laparoscopic approach; the procedure is well tolerated, recovery is prompt, and yield is adequate.[283,284]

Aside from para-aortic nodes, supraclavicular metastases may rarely be involved. Perez-Mesa and Spratt[285] found no supraclavicular node metastasis in 73 consecutive patients with various stages of cervical carcinoma. Manetta et al.[286] also did not detect scalene node metastasis in 24 patients with recurrent carcinoma of the cervix evaluated for exploration and possible pelvic exenteration. There is no indication for removal of the supraclavicular nodes.

Sentinel Lymph Node Biopsy

Sentinel lymph node (SLN) studies show mixed results, with a 20% false-negative rate and a 50% incidence of other pelvic metastases.[287] However, the method allows for aborting surgery and pursuing RT instead. Sentinel node biopsy in patients with cervical cancer is used in several institutions; a seven-center prospective study analyzed 139 patients and detected 454 sentinel lymph nodes. Intraoperative examination did not detect micrometastasis or isolated tumor cells. Other techniques, such as molecular assays, may improve SLN assessment in the future.[288,289] The SENTICOL study[290] injected 145 stage IA1 to IB1 cervical-cancer patients with combined technetium-99 and Patent Blue. The sensitivity (92%) and lack of false-negative results were favorable, but SLN biopsy was reliable only when SLNs were detected bilaterally.

Ovarian Transposition

In premenopausal women, surgery and radiation may directly impact gonadal function. For women with early-stage cervical cancer who undergo a radical hysterectomy, ovarian function may be preserved. In patients who require postoperative radiation, transposition of ovarian tissue outside of the radiation field may help to preserve ovarian function, although even low doses to the ovaries may cause acute ovarian failure (Fig. 69.9). In women who require radical radiation to the uterus and ovarian tissue, counseling before treatment begins with a fertility expert in reproductive endocrinology may be of benefit if an intervention such as egg retrieval is desired. Care must be taken to ensure that any potential intervention does not delay the initiation of curative treatment. In addition, women with early-stage cervical cancer have an approximately 1% risk of ovarian metastasis with squamous cell carcinoma and 5% risk with adenocarcinoma. Therefore, women should be counseled on the potential risks of recurrence with ovarian preservation.[291]

In a survey of 124 patients who had undergone radical hysterectomy and lymphadenectomy with ovarian transposition, 68 responders were premenopausal at the time of surgery. Six of 30 women (20%) with ovarian preservation experienced early hormonal failure (5 had one ovary, and 1 patient had both preserved).[292] Combined-modality therapy affects ovarian function more than operation alone.[293] Anderson et al.[294] noted that only 4 of 24 patients (17%) with ovarian transposition who received postoperative pelvic irradiation had continued ovarian function. Feeney et al.[295] reported on 132 patients on whom lateral ovarian transposition was performed at the time of radical hysterectomy; 28 patients received postoperative pelvic irradiation. Fourteen of 28 patients (50%) who received pelvic irradiation had evidence of ovarian failure, in contrast to 3 of 104 patients (2.9%) on whom ovarian transposition was performed, without postoperative irradiation. Buekers et al.[296] also evaluated ovarian function in 102 patients with cervical cancer, 83 of whom underwent radical hysterectomy and 19 of whom had a staging laparotomy, all with ovarian preservation (80 included ovarian transposition); 26 patients received postoperative radiation therapy. After ovarian transposition without RT, 98% of patients retained ovarian function for a mean of 126 months, with menopause at a mean age of 45.8 years. When ovarian transposition and RT were added, 41% retained ovarian function for a mean of 43 months and experienced menopause at a mean age of 36.6 years.

Morice et al.[297] reported on 107 patients treated for cervical cancer with radical hysterectomy and lymphadenectomy, 104 of

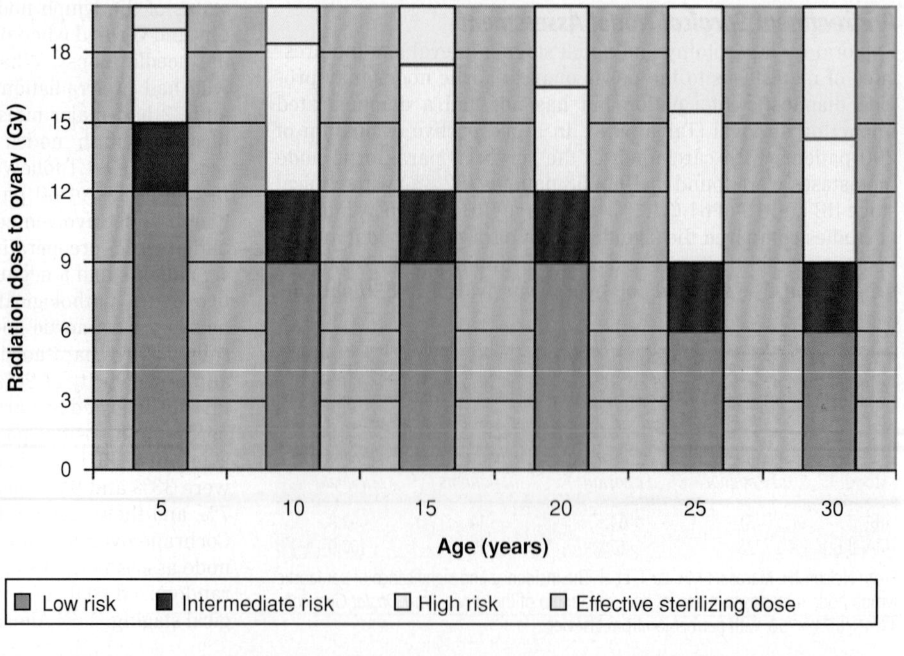

FIGURE 69.9. Risk of developing acute ovarian failure, defined as ovarian failure within 5 years, stratified by age and radiation dose to the ovary. (From Wo JY, Viswanathan AN. Impact of radiotherapy on fertility, pregnancy, and neonatal outcomes in female cancer patients. *Int J Radiat Oncol Biol Phys* 2009;73:1304–1312; with permission from Elsevier.)

whom (98%) had ovarian transposition to the paracolic gutters performed. Preservation of ovarian function was achieved in 100% for patients treated exclusively by surgery, 90% for those treated by postoperative vaginal brachytherapy, and 60% for patients treated by postoperative EBRT and vaginal brachytherapy.

Ovarian transposition or oophoropexy has been performed using laparoscopy, achieving continued hormonal function in 68% (8 of 11) and 50% (3 of 6) of the patients.[298] Mean follow-up was 8.5 years, and mean radiation absorbed dose to the displaced ovaries was 26 Gy. Stockle et al.[299] performed laparoscopic lateral ovarian transposition during staging lymphadenectomy in 11 patients with carcinoma of the cervix treated with brachytherapy (11 cases), EBRT (9 cases), and chemotherapy (2 cases). Ovarian preservation was achieved in 30% of the cases. Age was the most predictive factor for ovarian function preservation. Pahisa et al.[300] performed laparoscopic ovarian transposition on 29 FIGO stage IB1 cervical-cancer patients. After a mean follow-up of 44 months, ovarian function was preserved in 93% of the nonirradiated and 64% of the irradiated patients.

Radiation Therapy Techniques

Since the early 1900s, radiation has been used in the curative management of cervical cancer, with a combination of external-beam and brachytherapy resulting in the highest survival rates. Over the ensuing 100 years, treatment-planning techniques have evolved, as has the equipment used for treatment. Several methods have been developed to aid with conformality and normal-tissue sparing. External irradiation is used to treat the whole pelvis. Structures treated include the uterus and cervix or, in the postoperative cases, the tumor bed, the vagina, the parametrial tissue, and the pelvic lymph nodes, including the internal, external, and common iliac nodes. In selected cases the para-aortic lymph nodes may be treated. In patients with locally advanced disease, in addition to external-beam radiation, treatment of central disease (cervix, vagina, and medial parametria) relies heavily on dose given with intracavitary sources through brachytherapy. The techniques described apply, with some individualization, to most patients with locally advanced cervical carcinoma.

External-Beam Irradiation

External-beam treatments may be routinely administered to cervical cancer patients with stages IB2 to IVA in a curative fashion. Patients with stages IA to IB1 may be considered for external-beam treatment if they are deemed inoperable or prefer to avoid surgery. Patients with stage IVB disease may receive palliative radiation to the pelvis for selected indications such as to stop vaginal bleeding, relieve pain, or alleviate urethral obstruction from extrinsic compression. External-beam radiation covers the primary cervical tumor, treats any adjacent parametrial or uterosacral, uterine, or vaginal extension, and, most important, addresses microscopic disease present in pelvic lymph nodes. In treatment of invasive carcinoma of the uterine cervix, it is important to deliver adequate doses of irradiation not only to the primary tumor, but also to the pelvic lymph nodes to maximize tumor control.

The initiation of external-beam radiation typically precedes brachytherapy. Although brachytherapy may be interdigitated with external-beam treatment, based on the desire to minimize the duration of treatment, the brachytherapy dose to the normal tissues may be better optimized after maximal tumor shrinkage; therefore, many institutions prefer to wait until the completion of 45-Gy treatment before initiating brachytherapy for patients with large tumors.

Patient Positioning

Patients may be positioned in either the supine position for stability or the prone position on a belly board. The prone position aids in shifting small bowel out of the pelvis. In patients who have had a hysterectomy, small bowel may drop into the pelvic area. For those patients treated for cervical cancer with an intact cervix, the small bowel often lies superior to the uterus and above the pelvic brim, creating less need to shift the bowel out of the pelvis. For patients receiving IMRT, due to stability of the pelvis, the supine position is typically preferred with immobilization devices surrounding the pelvis to ensure minimal motion during treatment. IV contrast may be helpful to localize the pelvic vessels for contouring but is not routinely used in most centers. Oral contrast delineates the small bowel. Rectal contrast and placement of a Foley catheter for bladder contrast are not considered necessary in the majority of cases that use CT simulation because the outer wall of these normal-tissue structures can be contoured without contrast on CT.

Plain X-Ray Simulation

If CT is not available, simple plain film simulation may be performed. The standard plain radiographic simulation to the pelvis with x-rays, typically using opposed anterior–posterior:posterior–anterior (AP-PA) fields, results in comprehensive coverage of all pelvic regions. Due to the lack of visible soft-tissue detail, contrast may be placed using barium in the rectum, a vaginal tube in the vagina, and/or a wire marker over surgical scars. The superior border is set at the L4-5 interspace in order to cover the common iliac lymph nodes and the lateral borders 1.5 to 2 cm from the pelvic brim, and the inferior border covers at least the obturator foramen (Fig. 69.10). More commonly in patients with large tumors, the inferior border extends to the ischial tuberosities. When there is vaginal involvement, the entire length of this organ should be treated down to the introitus. It is very important to identify the distal extension of the tumor at the time of simulation by placing a radiopaque clip or bead on the vaginal wall or inserting a small fiducial marker in the vagina. When the tumor involves the distal half of the vagina, the portals should be modified to cover the inguinal lymph nodes because of the increased probability of metastases (see Fig. 69.2).

For the lateral field borders, in both postoperative and intact cervix settings, the posterior border must be set in such a way that the entire sacrum is covered because the uterosacral ligaments are at high risk for harboring microscopic extension. The uterosacral ligaments insert onto the sacrum, and therefore the posterior block should ensure coverage of the entire sacrum. The anterior border on the lateral field should be set at a vertical line anterior to the pubic symphysis, since the external iliac lymph nodes must be covered.

For patients with para-aortic nodal involvement, simple plain film simulation followed by AP-PA treatments to the para-aortic nodal chain may overdose the kidneys, spinal cord, and small bowel. Dose escalation to para-aortic nodes to approximately >45 Gy is not feasible with AP-PA fields, given potential bowel complications. The use of four fields, including AP-PA and two lateral fields, is implemented as an alternative to AP-PA alone as a way to reduce some of the dose to the anterior small bowel. Patients receive oral barium approximately 30 minutes before the simulation to ensure blockage of as much small bowel as feasible superiorly. The superior border covers the renal hilum, often at the T12-L1 interspace, and the inferior borders cover the obturator foramen, unless there is distal vaginal or inguinal node involvement. For the para-aortic portion of the field, the anterior border rests 2 cm in front of the vertebral body or enlarged nodes as contoured, and posteriorly the border bisects the mid-vertebral body. The pelvic portion mimics that described for the four-field pelvic setup. The use of lateral fields allows a decrease in dose to the small bowel, but care must be taken to include all structures of interest.[301–303]

Three-Dimensional Conformal Treatment Planning

CT simulation allows direct assessment of the pelvic vessels and by adjacent location the para-aortic and pelvic nodes. Oral

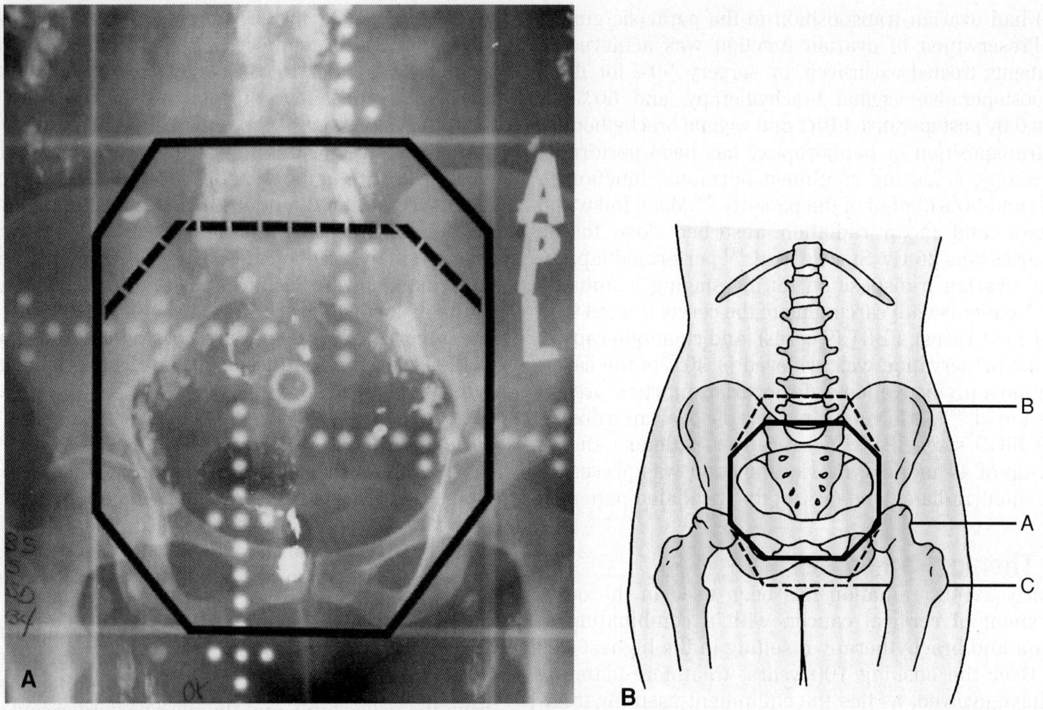

FIGURE 69.10. A: Anteroposterior simulation film of the pelvis illustrating portals used for external irradiation. The 15 by 15 cm portals at source-to-skin distance are used for stage IB (*broken line*), and 18 by 15 cm portals are used for more advanced disease (*solid line*). This allows better coverage of the common iliac lymph nodes. The distal margin is usually placed at the bottom of the obturator foramina. **B:** Diagram of pelvic portals used in external irradiation of carcinoma of uterine cervix. Standard portal for stage IB tumors is outlined (*solid line indicated as A*). When the common iliac nodes are to be covered, the upper margin is extended to the L4–5 space (*indicated in section B*). If there is vaginal tumor extension, the lower margin of the field is drawn at the introitus (*indicated in section C*).

contrast is beneficial to identify the small bowel. Cerrobend customized blocks or multileaf collimator blocking is used on each field to block the radiation to selected areas, including the skin, muscle, soft tissue, anterior small bowel, and portions of the anus and lower rectum (Fig. 69.11).

The superior border is set based on the CT-visualized bifurcation of the common iliac nodes into the external and internal iliac nodes, which may lie as high as the L3-4 interspace. If patients have positive pelvic nodes based on PET imaging, the superior border may be shifted to either the superior border of the common iliac nodes or the superior aspect of the renal hilum to treat the para-aortic nodes. In postoperative cases in which the patient has had an extensive surgical staging, the superior border may be reduced to the L5-S1 interspace. Similar to plain x-ray simulation, in patients with vaginal involvement, the inferior border is extended to cover 2 cm below the lowest extent of disease, which may lie in the vulvar tissue, and in such cases the inguinal lymph nodes are treated, resulting in a wider AP field.

On the lateral fields, the anterior border covers the front of the pubic symphysis. Bonin et al.,[304] in a review of 22 patients on whom detailed anatomic mapping of the anatomy of the pelvic lymph nodes was carried out by lymphangiography, concluded that if the criteria for adequacy of standard pelvic fields as defined in prior clinical trials were applied (anteroposterior: 1.5-cm margin on the pelvic rim; lateral field anterior edge is a vertical line anterior to the pubic symphysis and posterior border), 10 patients (45%) would have had inadequate nodal coverage in the irradiation fields. The incompletely irradiated lymph nodes were in the lowest lateral external iliac group. However, CT simulation with contouring may prevent omission of these nodes.

For the lateral borders in postoperative and intact cervix cases, posterior coverage of the entire sacral hollow is imperative. Zunino et al.[305] reviewed the appropriateness of radiation therapy box technique for cancer of the cervix in 35 sagittal MRIs and 10 lymphangiograms. If the posterior border were to be placed at the S2-3 interspace, for 50% of the patients with FIGO IB and in 67% with stage IIA disease, the posterior border of the lateral field would not adequately encompass the planning target volume (PTV). In stage IIB, the posterior border was inadequate in eight patients (42%). In patients with stage IIB and IVA disease, the PTV was not encompassed. Furthermore, Knocke et al.[306] used standard simulator planning guided by bony landmarks for pelvic irradiation in 20 patients with primary cervical carcinoma, stages I to III, using a four-field box technique. After defining the PTV with a 3D planning system, they compared the field configuration of the simulator planning with a second one based on the defined PTV. They evaluated the ability of the PTV to encompass the treatment volume (International Commission on Radiation Units and Measurements [ICRU]). Planning by simulation resulted in 1 geographic miss, and in 10 more cases the coverage of the PTV by the treatment volume was inadequate.

Finlay et al.[307] contoured pelvic blood vessels on CT scans as surrogates for lymph nodes in 43 patients and found this to be more accurate than bony landmarks for field delineation. In total, 95% of patients planned with conventional fields had inadequate coverage of some portion of lymph node coverage, whereas in 56% additional normal tissue was treated that did not require radiation. Therefore, most centers implement 3D simulation when feasible. Taylor et al.[308] used MRI to outline the pelvic lymph nodes in 20 patients and noted that with margins of 10 mm, nodal coverage was 94% and with 15 mm, 99%; with a modified 7-mm margin they ensured 99% nodal coverage with less volume of small bowel at risk.

In the postoperative setting, van den Berg et al.,[309] using 47 lymphangiograms and 15 CT scans, asked radiation oncologists ($n = 17$) to define the clinical target volume (CTV) and PTV and to delineate on simulation films the RT treatment portals to be used after a radical hysterectomy with lymph node dissection for stage IB or IIA cervical carcinoma with positive iliac lymph nodes. Large variations were observed in the portals used and

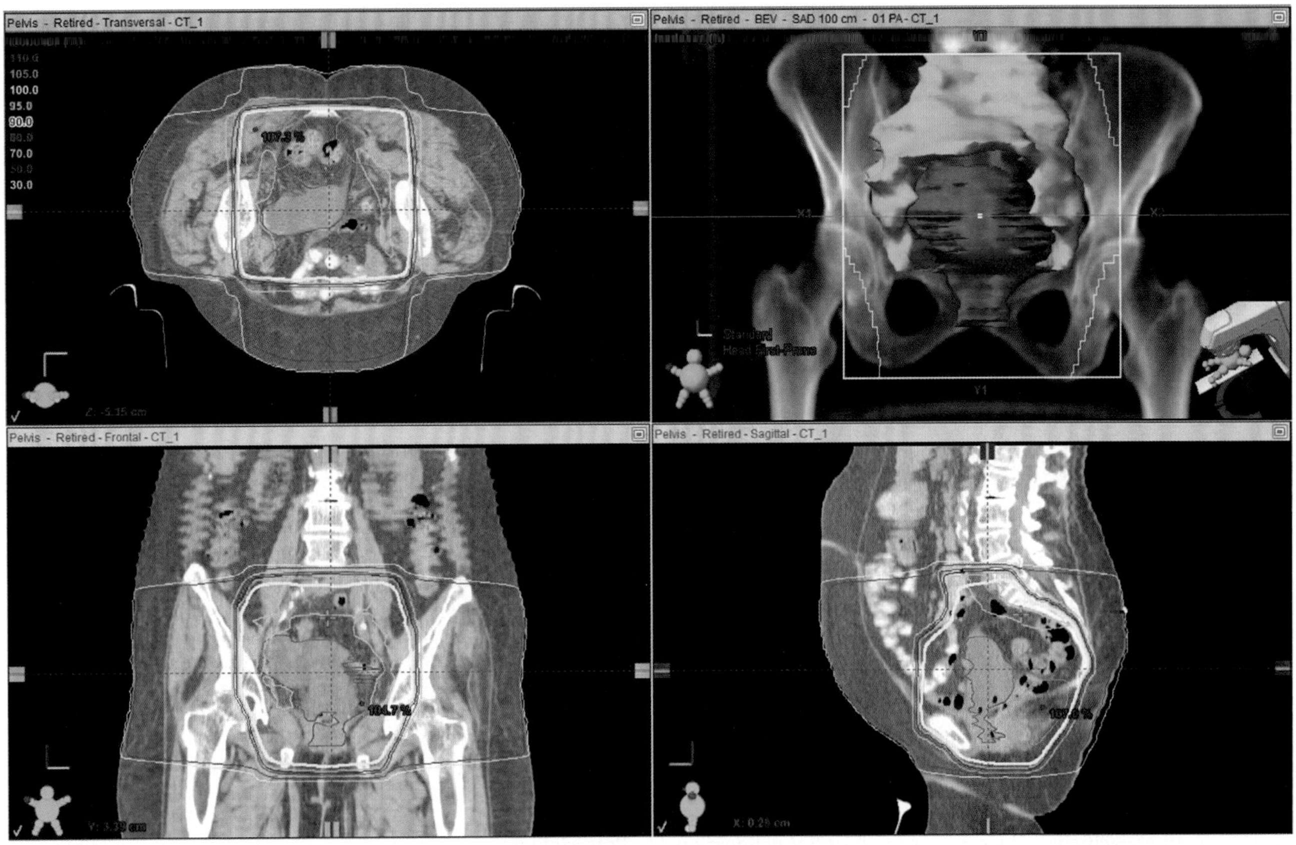

FIGURE 69.11. Anterior–posterior and lateral digitally reconstructed radiograph simulation film of the pelvis, illustrating portals used for external irradiation with the patient in the prone position on a belly board to minimize small-bowel dose. Pelvic lymph nodes are indicated in their approximate position. The uterus, cervix, and vagina are contoured to ensure adequate coverage.

in treatment techniques. From the digitized films, it appeared that in 50% of the cases the defined PTV was not covered adequately. Furthermore, 71% of the treatment plans would not cover the lateral borders of the reference PTV sufficiently. Thus, there is a need for careful adherence to standardized guidelines.

Treatment techniques may have an effect on outcome. Yamazaki et al.[310] compared 34 patients with cervical cancer treated with irregularly shaped four-field whole-pelvis radiation therapy using CT simulation and 40 patients receiving whole-pelvis EBRT with parallel-opposed fields in a nonrandomized study of postoperative radiation therapy consisting of 50 Gy in 25 fractions in 6 weeks. With a mean follow-up of 60 months, the actuarial 5-year pelvic tumor control was 94% with the two-field technique and 100% for the irregularly shaped four-field technique. The incidence of grade 2 or 3 bowel complications in the irregularly shaped–technique group (2.9%, 1 of 34) was significantly lower than that in the two-field–technique group (17.5%, 7 of 40; $p < .05$).

Burnett et al.[311] described a prosthetic silicone plastic device that is filled with saline and Renografin for x-ray visualization (capacity between 750 and 1,500 mL) to conform to the pelvis and exclude the small bowel from the irradiated volume. The device remains in place throughout the radiation therapy course and is removed through a small incision after draining the contents of the prosthesis. Seven devices had been placed to date of the report. In the postoperative period, there was one pulmonary embolism. All seven patients completed planned radiation therapy. The devices have been removed with no adhesions to the prosthesis.

Intensity-Modulated Radiation

IMRT was developed using the techniques required for inverse planning. That is, one starts with the necessary dose around the target then works backward to develop the requisite beam intensities. IMRT spatially modulates the intensity of the beam using the motion of multileaf collimators. Because of the increasing use of intensity-modulated or image-guided radiation therapy (IMRT/IGRT) in the treatment of patients with gynecologic malignancy, there is growing emphasis on imaging the pelvic anatomic structures, including lymph nodes, for treatment planning.[312] IMRT may reduce the amount of small bowel and bone marrow that receives the full dose of radiation.

The use of IMRT has been standardized in the postoperative setting but remains a topic of debate for intact cervix cases. What constitutes adequate margins in the intact cervix setting continues to be a matter of concern, given significant organ motion during treatment. Uncertainties in the definition of target volumes arise using 3D techniques. Bladder-filling and rectal-filling changes require accurate definition of margins for the PTV.[313] Beadle et al.[314] found that mean maximum changes in the center of the cervix were 2.1, 1.6, and 0.82 cm in the superior–inferior, anterior–posterior, and right–left lateral dimensions, respectively. Mean maximum changes in the perimeter of the cervix were 2.3 and 1.3 cm in the superior and inferior, 1.7 and 1.8 cm in the anterior and posterior, and 0.76 and 0.94 cm in the right and left lateral directions, respectively. Haripotepornkul et al.[315] found in 10 women with locally advanced cervical cancer that within and between radiation treatments, cervical motion averages approximately 3 mm but may be up to 18 mm in any given direction. The mean intrafractional movements in cervical seed positions in the lateral, vertical, and AP directions were 1.6 mm (standard deviation [SD] ± 2.0), 2.6 mm (SD ± 2.4), and 2.9 mm (SD ± 2.7), respectively, with a range from 0 to 15 mm for each direction. The mean interfractional movements in the lateral, vertical, and AP directions were 1.9 mm (SD ± 1.9), 4.1 mm (SD ± 3.2), and 4.2 mm (SD ± 3.5), respectively, with a range from 0 to 18 mm for each direction. Tyagi et al.[316] show that a uniform CTV planning

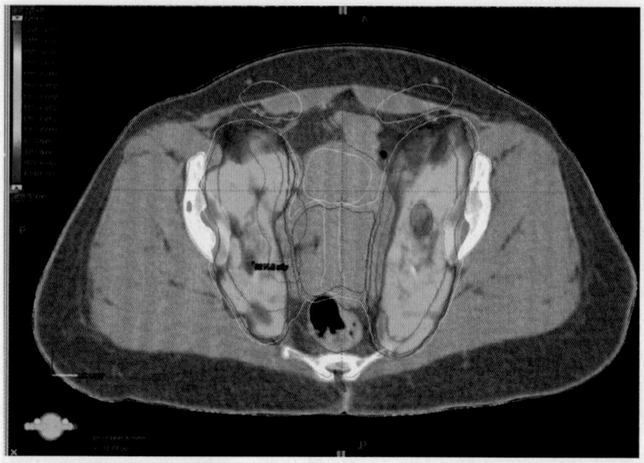

FIGURE 69.12. Intensity-modulated radiation therapy treatment plan for external irradiation of pelvic lymph nodes while sparing organs at risk.

treatment volume margin of 15 mm would not encompass the cervical CTV in 32% of fractions. With IMRT, there is a need for continual replanning (at least every other week), given rapid tumor regression and internal-organ motion.[317–319]

After a CT scan for simulation, the images are brought into a treatment-planning workstation. Contouring the gross tumor volume (GTV) may include the uterus, cervix, and/or vagina. Lim et al.[320] had 19 experts in gynecologic radiation oncology contour a case of locally advanced cervical cancer on axial magnetic resonance images of the pelvis. Substantial Simultaneous Truth and Performance Level Estimation (STAPLE) agreement sensitivity and specificity values were seen for GTV delineation (0.84 and 0.96, respectively) with a kappa statistic of 0.68 ($p < .0001$). Agreement for delineation of cervix, uterus, vagina, and parametria was moderate. The greatest variability in physician contouring was in the parametrial tissue.[320]

The CTV for the pelvic lymph nodes was based on the Radiation Therapy Oncology Group (RTOG) atlas for the female postoperative pelvis.[321] An example of dose distribution achieved with supine IMRT pelvic irradiation is illustrated in Figure 69.12. Fiducial markers may be placed in the apex of the vagina for identification on CT scan and show up to 3.5 cm of vaginal cuff motion during treatment.[322] Therefore, for postoperative patients, the vagina is contoured using a full-bladder CT scan fused to an empty-bladder CT scan to account for vaginal mobility due to differences in bladder filling.[323] This vaginal target volume has been referred to as an integrated target volume (ITV). The expansion of the CTV and/or ITV to the PTV is necessary, although given the movement of the uterus, the exact amount of margin is a matter of debate. Generous margins of approximately 2 to 3 cm are considered, particularly in the regions of the uterus and cervix or in the postoperative case around the ITV vagina. Dose constraints required for an optimal IMRT plan have not been standardized. In the RTOG postoperative clinical trial 0921 using IMRT,[324] a PTV of 7 mm around the nodal contours is recommended, and the dose is prescribed to cover 97% of the vaginal PTV and nodal PTV. A volume of 0.03 cc within any PTV should not receive >110% of the prescribed dose. No more than 0.03 cc of any PTV will receive <93% of its prescribed dose. Any contiguous volume of 0.03 cc or larger of the tissue outside the vaginal/nodal PTVs must not receive >110% of the dose prescribed to the vaginal/nodal PTV; for normal tissues the small/large bowel (30% of the entire bowel volume must not receive >40 Gy), rectum/sigmoid (60% of the rectosigmoid volume must receive ≤40 Gy), bladder (35% of the bladder volume must receive ≤45 Gy), and femoral head (15% of the femoral head volume must receive <35 Gy) constraints are being tested in RTOG 0921. Careful attention must be paid to all normal-tissue organ motion because the bladder and rectum may have 3- to 5-cm shifts due to filling changes in a short time frame.

For patients that have had a diagnostic PET or MRI before the simulation, these images may be registered to create a fused data set for contouring, particularly when a nodal boost is required. This allows the physician to visualize areas of PET enhancement or tumor volume, as seen on the MRI, onto the simulation films. Grigsby and colleagues[325] use a PET-defined target volume contoured with a metabolically active tumor specified at the 40% threshold. Normal-tissue structures, including the rectum, sigmoid, bladder, and small bowel, are routinely contoured for patients treated with IMRT who will be undergoing a nodal boost in order to limit the dose received primarily to the small bowel. Based on an overview of published data, the absolute volume of small bowel receiving ≥15 Gy should be held to <120 cc when possible to minimize severe acute toxicity if delineating the contours of bowel loops themselves. Alternatively, if the entire volume of peritoneal space in which the small bowel can move is delineated, the volume receiving >45 Gy should be <195 cc when possible.[326] For the rectum, dose–volume constraints selected as a conservative starting point that have not yet been validated for 3D treatment planning include $V_{50} < 50\%$, $V_{60} < 35\%$, $V_{65} < 25\%$, $V_{70} < 20\%$, and $V_{75} < 15\%$.[327] No dose constraint for external beam planning for the bladder could be identified, although the limits for prostate cancer may be adopted for gynecologic IMRT, including a dose constraint of no more than 15% of the volume to receive a dose >80 Gy, no more than 25% of the volume to receive a dose >75 Gy, no more than 35% of the volume to receive a dose >70 Gy, or no more than 50% of the volume to receive a dose >65 Gy.[328]

Imaging may guide more accurate definition of lymph nodes.[308] Portelance et al.[272] carried out IMRT as well as conventional planning with two- and four-field techniques in 10 patients. Prescription was 45 Gy in 25 fractions to the uterus and the pelvic and para-aortic lymph nodes. All IMRT plans were normalized to obtain a full coverage of the cervix with the 95% isodose curve (Fig. 69.13A). The volumes of small bowel receiving the prescribed dose (45 Gy) with IMRT para-aortic–only technique were, with four fields, 11%; with seven fields, 15%; and with nine fields, 13.5% (Fig. 69.13B). These dose distributions were all significantly better than with two-field or four-field conventional techniques ($p < .05$.) Ahmed et al.[329] arrived at similar conclusions in five patients with para-aortic node metastasis, and they demonstrated the feasibility of escalating the dose to 60 Gy while sparing the kidneys, spinal cord, small bowel, and bone marrow. Heron et al.,[330] in a study of 10 patients, showed that with IMRT there was a reduction of 52% in the small-bowel volume receiving >30 Gy and a decrease of 66% for the rectum and 36% for the bladder compared with 3D radiation therapy. D'Souza et al.,[331] in 10 patients, also noted a reduction of small-bowel volume (33%) with IMRT compared with four-field pelvic RT; however, small volumes of bowel received 55 to 60 Gy with the IMRT plans. Positioning the patient prone on a belly board was shown to reduce the volume of small-bowel irradiated. However, patients on a belly board may have large daily anatomic shifts that make prone IMRT unreproducible.[332]

Brixey et al.[333] and Lujan et al.[334] also used IMRT planning to spare the bone marrow of patients with gynecologic tumors. Brixey et al.,[333] in 36 patients, noted no significant difference in hematologic toxicity with IMRT or conventional RT alone; however, in patients receiving chemotherapy, less grade 2 white blood cell toxicity was observed with IMRT (31.2% vs. 60%, respectively).

Hasselle et al.[335] report on 111 patients treated with multiple different approaches, including 22 treated with postoperative IMRT, 8 with IMRT followed by intracavitary brachytherapy and adjuvant hysterectomy, and 81 with IMRT followed by planned intracavitary brachytherapy. Median follow-up time was 27 months. Acute and late grade 3 toxicity or higher was 2% (95% confidence interval [CI], 0% to 7%) and 7% (95% CI, 2% to 13%), respectively. Guerrero et al.[336] proposed using an IMRT simultaneous integrated boost (SIB) as an alternative to conventional whole-pelvis irradiation and used the linear quadratic equation to calculate equivalent

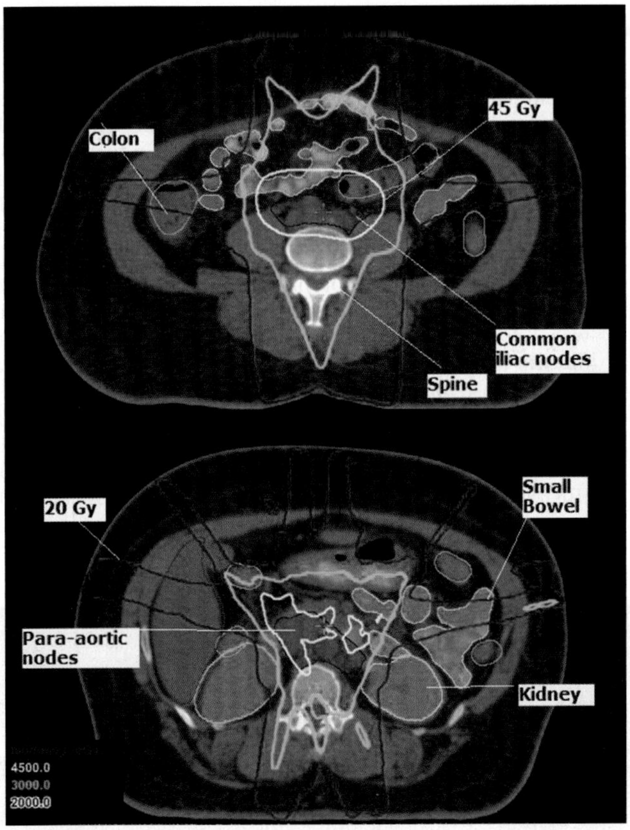

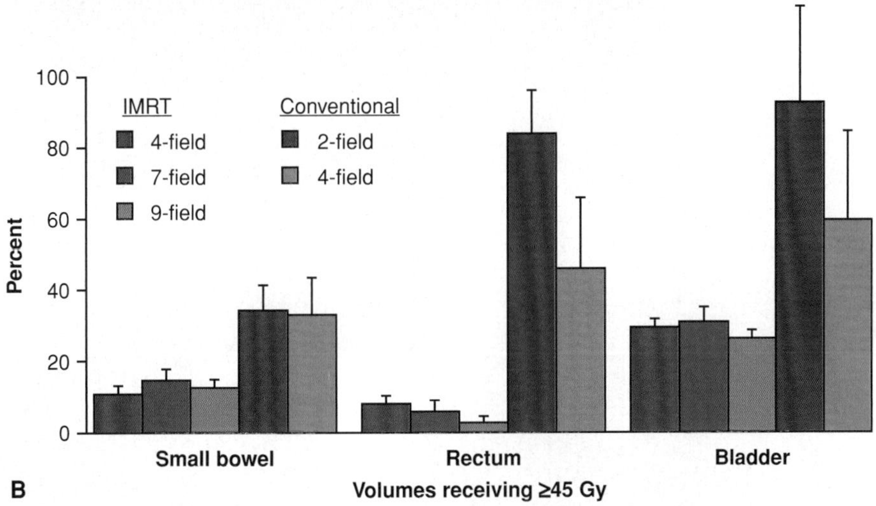

FIGURE 69.13. A: Axial views of intensity-modulated radiation therapy dose distribution. **B:** The functional volume of small bowel, rectum, and bladder receiving ≥45 Gy with intensity-modulated radiation therapy or conventional techniques when 100% of the target volume (uterus) receives ≥95% of the prescription dose (45 Gy). (From Portelance L, Chao KSCC, Grigsby PW, et al. Intensity-modulated radiation therapy [(IMRT)] reduces small bowel and bladder doses in patients with cervical cancer receiving pelvic and para-aortic irradiation. *Int J Radiat Oncol Biol Phys* 2001;51:261–266; with permission from Elsevier.)

uniform dose in multiple plans. However, a report by Kavanagh et al.[337] found that accelerated fractionation caused an unacceptably high rate of complications.

Although IMRT has dosimetric advantages over conventional RT, IMRT exposes a greater amount of normal tissues to lower irradiation levels, which has the potential to increase the incidence of radiation-induced second cancers,[338] a phenomenon already described with conventional RT techniques.[339]

Image-Guided Radiation Therapy

Although not always available, some institutions on protocol have attempted daily cone-beam CT imaging for in-room image-guided RT (IGRT).[340] Particularly in cases with a large, mobile uterus, such as is seen in young women, if an extended field is used and there is concern that the uterus may be out of the field, this may be instituted. In clinics where IMRT is used for locally advanced cervical cancer, the priority should be to treat with wide margins, so that the field mimics that of a 3D conformal (four-field) plan.[316]

Stereotactic body radiotherapy (SBRT) uses highly conformal treatments with large fraction sizes and in selected cases has been considered for a nodal boost of an isolated para-aortic node, although care must be taken to treat the entire para-aortic chain to 45 Gy with IMRT or 4 Field (4F) prior to considering an SBRT boost in order to ensure eradication of adjacent micrometastatic disease.[341] SBRT should not be used instead of brachytherapy, given the significant increase in normal-tissue doses with SBRT compared to brachytherapy.[342]

Midline Shielding in AP-PA Portals and Use of a Parametrial Boost

Depending on the institution and brachytherapy dose administered, midline shielding with rectangular or specially designed blocks has been traditionally used for a portion of the external beam dose delivered with the AP-PA ports.[302] Midline blocks may be individualized, based on the point A isodose line or a rectangular block of approximately 4-cm width. In one series, overall survival and incidence of chronic complications were not related to the type of shielding.[343] However, in the era of three-dimensional brachytherapy planning, the use of a midline block has been questioned because it may result in tumor underdosing while still contributing significant dose to the bladder, sigmoid, and rectum.[344]

Several institutions reported placing a midline block after a full course of external-beam treatment to the pelvis in order to boost the parametria or nodes for patients with persistent disease after approximately 45 to 50 Gy. When parametrial tumor persists, 50 to 60 Gy may be delivered to the parametria, with reduced anteroposterior–posteroanterior portals (8 by 12 cm for unilateral and 12 by 12 cm for bilateral parametrial coverage). However, careful estimation of dose to the small bowel, sigmoid, and rectum is needed. In the modern era, the use of highly conformal boosts with 3D planning allows an increase in normal-tissue sparing. Contours on CT of the parametrial and nodal region allow more precise tailoring of dose. For patients with enlarged nodes, when available, IMRT techniques may be best at providing conformal dose escalation to 54 to 65 Gy.

Similarly, with 3D brachytherapy and computerized optimization as available with high HDR or pulse–dose-rate (PDR) brachytherapy, the physician may cover the adjacent parametria using large enough fraction sizes that an additional external-beam boost is not needed. When one prescribes HDR brachytherapy, the per-fraction nodal dose is approximately 25% of prescription. In one study the per-fraction dose to the pelvic lymph nodes by HDR brachytherapy, when the high-risk clinical target volume (HR-CTV) received 5.5 Gy per fraction, was 1.4 Gy per fraction. Therefore, HDR brachytherapy may obviate the need for a parametrial boost, given the high per-fraction dose to the parametria and pelvic sidewall.[344]

In a comparison of three different approaches, Fenkell et al.[345] reported on parametrial boost with midline shielding in six patients with locally advanced cervical cancer (IIB to IIIB) treated with definitive chemoradiotherapy and MRI-guided brachytherapy. A three-phase plan was modeled: 45-Gy

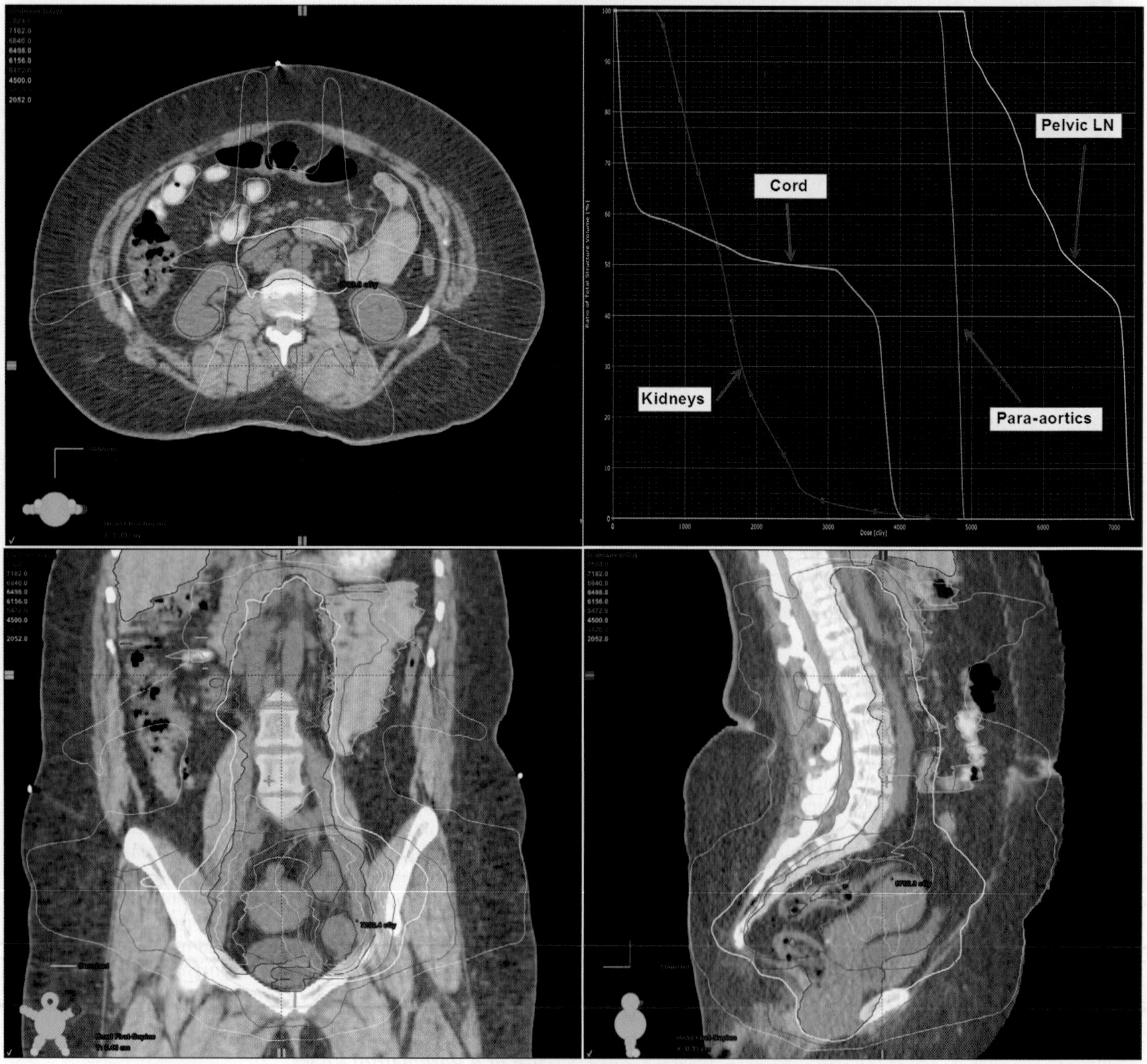

FIGURE 69.14. Extended-field intensity-modulated radiation therapy for external irradiation of uterine cervix and pelvic and para-aortic lymph nodes. Dose–volume histogram values for the spinal cord, kidneys, para-aortic nodes, and pelvic node boost are shown for a patient who had an unresectable 4-cm pelvic lymph node.

(1.8 Gy per fraction) four-field box, 9-Gy (1.8 Gy per fraction) midline-shielded anteroposterior/posteroanterior fields (MBB), and intracavitary MRI-guided brachytherapy boost of 28 Gy (7 Gy per fraction). Midline shields 3, 4, and 5 cm wide were simulated for each patient. Brachytherapy and MBB plans were volumetrically summed. After a 4-cm MBB, HR-CTV D_{90} remained <85 Gy in all cases (mean, 74 Gy; range, 64 to 82 Gy). Bladder, rectum, or sigmoid D_{2cc} increased by > 50% of the boost dose in four of six patients. The authors concluded that a midline block may not be beneficial in patients receiving 3D image-planned brachytherapy with adequate optimization of dose to the tumor and away from the normal tissues.

Para-Aortic Lymph Node Irradiation

If para-aortic node metastases are enlarged or suspected to harbor disease, patients are treated with 45 to 50 Gy to the para-aortic area plus a sequential 5- to 10-Gy boost to enlarged lymph nodes through reduced lateral or rotational portals.[275] If feasible, 3D planning with IMRT treatment is preferred to spare normal tissues, superiorly covering above the level of the renal hilum or the highest extent of disease and inferiorly covering 2 cm below the lowest extent of disease (Fig. 69.14).

The use of IMRT has allowed dose escalation to para-aortic nodes, particularly unresectable nodes. Clinical reports show excellent control of disease with dose escalation, with one report demonstrating an 85% 2-year nodal control rate after IMRT with a median dose of 63 Gy.[346] Esthappan et al.[271] described a technique using CT and FDG-PET to treat the para-aortic lymph nodes (50.4 and 59.4 Gy) with IMRT (Fig. 69.15). Acceptable dose distribution of the target volumes and sparing of the stomach, liver, and colon were achieved. Sparing of the spinal cord was dependent on the number and arrangements of the beams, as it was for the small bowel, sparing of which was limited because of overlap with the target volume. Adjusting the number of beams and prescription parameters minimally improved kidney sparing.

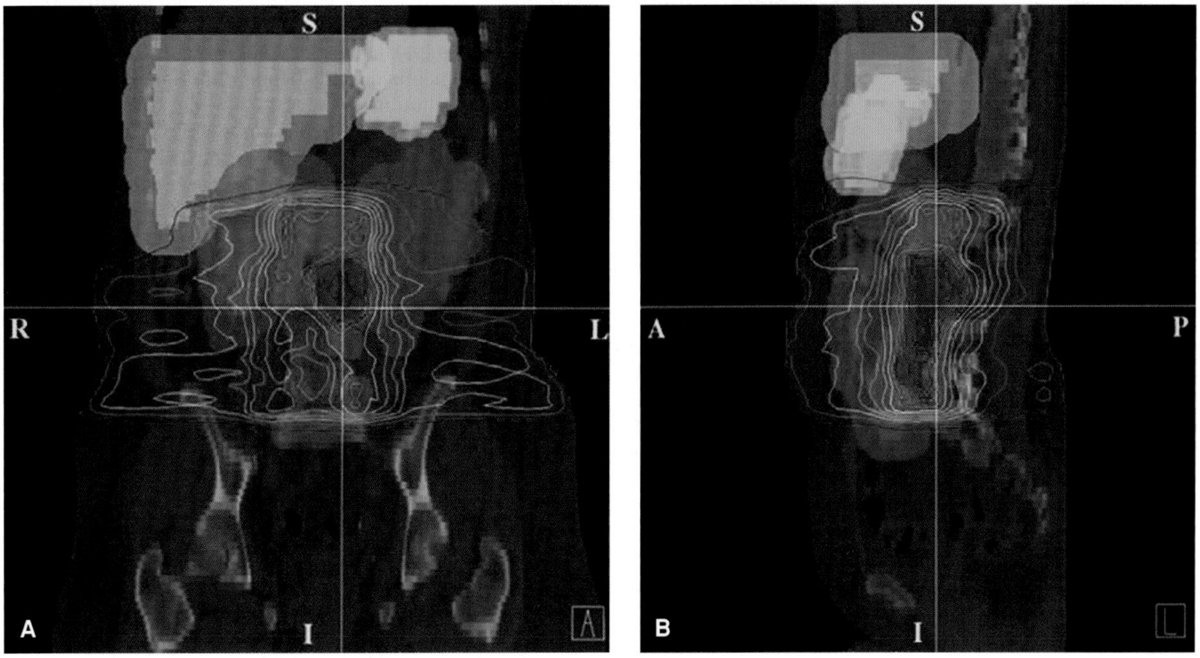

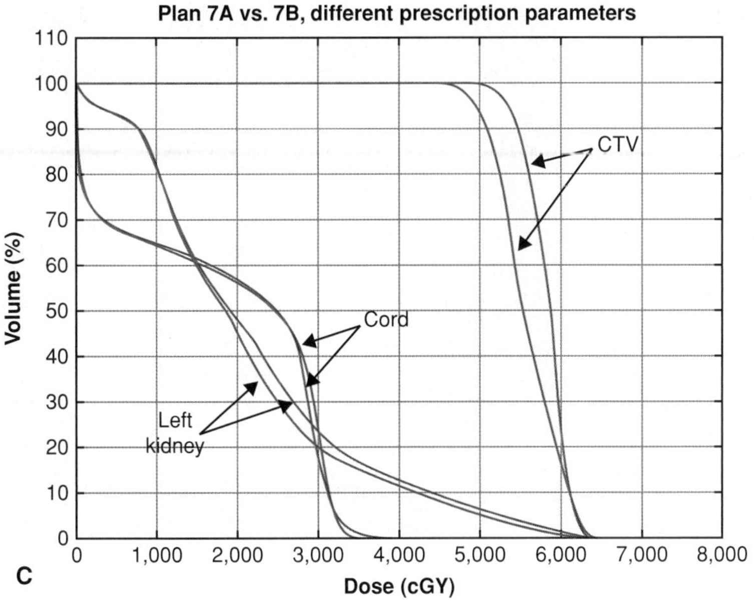

FIGURE 69.15. A, B: Example of treatment plan with intensity-modulated radiation therapy for irradiation of para-aortic lymph nodes. **C:** Dose–volume histogram illustrating sparing of left kidney and small intestine (Plan 7A, *solid line;* Plan 7B, *dashed line*). CTV, clinical target volume. (From Mutic S, Malyapa RS, Grigsby PW, et al. PET-guided IMRT for cervical carcinoma with positive para-aortic lymph nodes–a dose-escalation treatment planning study. *Int J Radiat Oncol Biol Phys* 2003;55:28–35; with permission from Elsevier.)

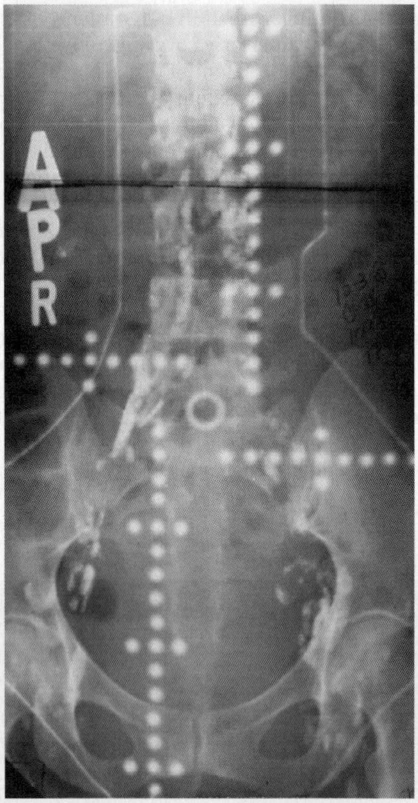

FIGURE 69.16. Extended field simulated with conventional plain films for external irradiation of pelvic and para-aortic lymph nodes.

When only conventional techniques are available, the para-aortic lymph nodes are irradiated either with an extended field, often using a four-field approach, that includes both the para-aortic nodes and the pelvis or through a separate portal (Fig. 69.16).[302,347] This may be done as one long field, or, in cases requiring extended distance, one may instead choose to separate the pelvic and para-aortic fields. This requires a "gap calculation" between the pelvic and para-aortic portals to avoid overlap and excessive dose to the small intestines. The upper margin of the field is at the T12-L1 interspace and the lower margin at L5-S1. The width of the para-aortic portals (in general, 8 to 10 cm) can be determined by CT scans, MRI, lymphangiography, FDG-PET scans, or IV pyelography outlining the ureters. The spinal cord dose (T12 to L2–3) should be kept to <45 Gy by interposing a 2-cm-wide 5–half-value-layer shield on the posterior portal (usually after 40-Gy tumor dose) or using lateral ports and limiting the kidney dose to <18 Gy. A technique using four isocentric fields weighted 2:1 anteroposterior–posteroanterior over lateral portals and 1.8-Gy fractions was described by Russell et al.[348] to deliver high-dose therapy (56 to 61 Gy). Kodaira et al.[349] evaluated a four-field para-aortic irradiation technique with 10-MV photons (mean, 50.4 Gy) in 97 patients with cervical cancer. The 5-year cause-specific survival rate was 32.2%. Grade 1 or 2 stomach and duodenum sequelae developed in 26.8%, grade 2 sequelae of small bowel in 3.1%, and grade 2 sequelae of bone in 3.1%. Rates of toxicity with IMRT may be lower.[275]

Beam Energies

For IMRT, 6-MV energy is used to provide the most homogeneous dose. However, in conventional irradiation, because of the thickness of the pelvis, high-energy photon beams (10 MV or higher) are especially suited for this treatment. They decrease the dose of radiation delivered to the peripheral normal tissues (particularly bladder and rectum) and provide a more homogeneous dose distribution in the central pelvis. With lower-energy photons (^{60}Co or 4- to 6-MV x-rays), higher maximum doses must be given, and more complicated field arrangements should be used to achieve the same midplane tumor dose (three-field or four-field pelvic box or rotational techniques) while minimizing the dose to the bladder and rectum and to avoid subcutaneous fibrosis (Fig. 69.17).[350] Biggs and Russell[351] noted that the presence of a metallic prosthesis when using lateral fields or a box pelvic irradiation technique may result in a dose decrease of approximately 2% for 25-MV x-rays and average increases of 2% for 10-MV x-rays and 5% for ^{60}Co. Allt[352] and Johns,[353] in an update of a randomized study, reported better pelvic tumor control and survival and fewer complications in 65 patients with stages IIB and III cervical carcinoma treated with 23-MV photons compared with 61 treated with external irradiation with ^{60}Co in addition to brachytherapy in both groups. In contrast, Holcomb et al.[350] compared outcome of 195 patients with stages IIB and IVA cervical carcinoma treated with ^{60}Co radiation therapy (group 1) and 53 treated with linear accelerators (group 2). There was no significant difference

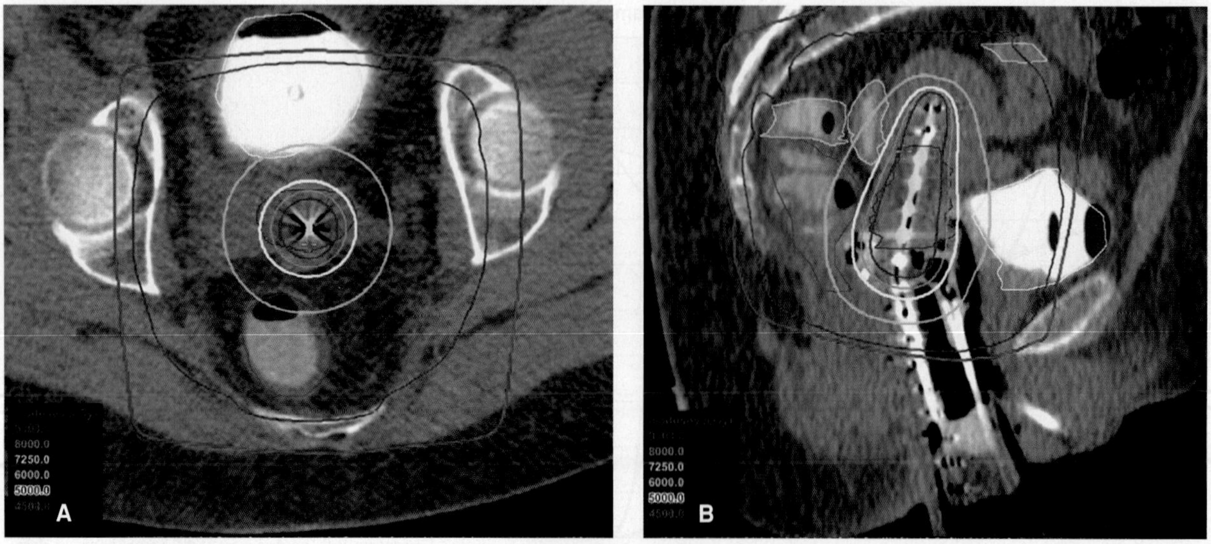

FIGURE 69.17. Example of isodose curves of 4F box irradiation of the pelvis with high-energy photons and high-dose-rate brachytherapy optimized to cover the tumor and minimize dose to the bladder and rectum.

in overall survival, although there was a trend toward increasing pelvic recurrence in the ^{60}Co group (50.8%) compared with group 2 (35.8%; p = .08). Mixed-beam external radiation with neutrons and photons resulted in unacceptably high toxicity rates and is not recommended.[354] Similarly, carbon-ion therapy was reported but resulted in major intestinal complications.[355]

Hyperfractionated or Accelerated Hyperfractionated Radiation Therapy

MacLeod et al.[356] reported on a phase II trial of 61 patients with locally advanced cervical cancer treated with accelerated hyperfractionated radiation therapy (1.25 Gy administered twice daily at least 6 hours apart to a total pelvic dose of 57.5 Gy). A boost dose was administered with either low–dose-rate (LDR) brachytherapy or EBRT to a smaller volume. Thirty patients had acute toxicity that required regular medication. One patient died of acute treatment-related toxicity. The overall 5-year survival was 27%, relapse-free survival was 36%, and actuarial local tumor control was 66%. There were eight severe late complications observed in seven patients, who required surgical intervention (actuarial rate of 27%). Five patients also required total hip replacement.

Another study reported on 30 patients with stage II or III cervical cancer randomized to receive either hyperfractionation (15 patients) or conventional fractionation (15 patients).[357] At 5 years, 2 patients in the hyperfractionation group and 8 patients in the conventional treatment group had recurrent tumor (p = .04). Delayed bowel complications (grade 2 and 3) occurred in 9 women in the hyperfractionation group and 2 patients in the conventional group (p = 0.0006).

RTOG 88-05 conducted a phase II trial of hyperfractionation (1.2 Gy to the whole pelvis twice daily at 4- to 6-hour intervals, 5 days per week) with brachytherapy in 81 patients with locally advanced carcinoma of the cervix. Total dose to the whole pelvis was 24 to 48 Gy, followed by one or two LDR intracavitary applications to deliver 85 Gy at point A and 65 Gy to the lateral pelvic nodes. Grigsby et al.[358] updated the results and noted that external irradiation was completed in 71 cases (88%). The 5-year cumulative rate of grade 3 and 4 late effects for patients with stage IB2 or IIB tumors was 7% and at 8 years was 10%, and with stage III or IVA disease, it was 12% at 5 years. The absolute survival was 48% at 8 years, and disease-free survival was 33%. Comparison with historical control patients treated on other RTOG studies showed equivalent rates of pelvic tumor control, survival, and grade 3 and 4 toxicities at 3, 5, and 8 years, respectively.

Calkins et al.[359] assessed the toxicities of multiple–daily-fractionated (twice-daily, 1.2-Gy fractions) whole-pelvis radiation plus concurrent chemotherapy for locally advanced carcinoma of the cervix. In the first study (GOG 8801), for 38 patients, hydroxyurea was given orally (80 mg/kg to a maximum of 6 g) at least 2 hours before irradiation, twice every week. In the second study (GOG 8901), for 30 patients, cisplatin and fluorouracil (5-FU) were used concomitantly with RT. Acute toxicity was primarily enteric and appeared to be dose related. The maximum tolerated dose of whole-pelvis radiation that could be delivered in a hyperfractionated setting with concomitant chemotherapy was 57.6 Gy in 48 fractions, followed by brachytherapy.

Thomas et al.[360] conducted a four-arm study in which 234 women with bulky stage IB to IVA cervical cancer were randomized to receive either standard RT (EBRT and brachytherapy to deliver 90 Gy to point A) with or without a 4-day infusion of 5-FU (1 g/m^2) on days 1 to 5 and 22 to 25, or partially hyperfractionated RT with or without the same chemotherapy regimen. The partially hyperfractionated regimen delivered two fractions, 6 hours apart, on the first 4 days of treatment, coinciding with the infusion of 5-FU. The addition of 5-FU did not improve pelvic tumor control (37% to 75% at 5 years) or overall survival. However, this study closed without reaching target patient accrual. A concomitant boost technique was reported by Kavanagh et al.[337] but had an unacceptably high rate (8 of 20 patients) of late complications.

GENERAL MANAGEMENT

Carcinoma *in Situ*

Patients with persistent high-grade carcinoma *in situ* are usually treated with a total abdominal hysterectomy with or without a small portion of the upper vagina removed. The decision to remove the ovaries depends on the age of the patient and status of the ovaries. Occasionally, when the patient wishes to have more children, carcinoma *in situ* may be treated conservatively with a therapeutic conization,[361] laser therapy, or cryotherapy.[362] This approach should be judiciously selected when the extent of tumor allows it and the patient is reliable for continued follow-up.[32] Conization microscopic margins are critical in decision making regarding a conservative approach or proceeding with a hysterectomy. A therapeutic hysterectomy can be performed 6 weeks after the conization.

Irradiation may be useful for the treatment of carcinoma *in situ,* particularly in patients with strong medical contraindications to surgery or when there is extension of the lesion to the vaginal wall or multifocal carcinoma *in situ* in both the cervix and the vagina.[302,363] In a group of 26 patients with carcinoma *in situ* treated at Washington University with intracavitary brachytherapy alone (approximately 5,000 milligram-hours [mgh], 45 Gy to point A with LDR) with tandem and ovoids, no recurrences were recorded.[364] Ogino et al.[365] used HDR brachytherapy in 14 patients with grade 3 cervical and 6 with grade 3 vaginal intraepithelial neoplasia (3 with microinvasion) and 6 with recurrent cervical intraepithelial neoplasia after hysterectomy. Seventeen patients were treated with HDR brachytherapy alone and 3 in combination with EBRT without surgery. The mean dose of HDR brachytherapy was 26.1 Gy (range, 20 to 30 Gy) prescribed at point A for intact uterus, or at 1 cm superior to the vaginal apex or 1 cm beyond vaginal mucosa for lesions of the vaginal stump. At mean follow up of 90 months, 14 patients were alive and 6 had died from intercurrent disease; none had recurrent disease. Rectal bleeding occurred in 3 patients and subsided spontaneously. Moderate and severe vaginal reactions were noted in 2 patients in whom the treatment included the entire vagina.

Invasive Disease

Based on available resources globally and the stage of disease, a debate continues among those who advocate radical surgery,[302,366,367] those who favor radiation, and those who favor chemoRT for the treatment of carcinoma of the uterine cervix. Patients should be treated with close collaboration between the gynecologic oncologist and the radiation oncologist, and an integrated team approach should be vigorously pursued. In countries with access to RT facilities and financial resources to supply chemotherapy, the use of concurrent chemoRT represents the accepted standard for patients with stage IB2 to IVA cervical cancer. For earlier-stage patients, the use of either surgery or chemoRT is recommended. The most recent survey of patterns of radiotherapy practice again documented a rise in the use of cisplatin-based concurrent chemoRT in patients with advanced stages, from 63% in 1999 to 74% in 2007.[154,368,369] Moreover, Barbera et al.[370] also reported a significant increase in the use of chemoRT in Canada after the *U.S. National Cancer Institute Bulletin* on the subject.[371]

Carcinoma of the Cervix Inadvertently Treated with a Simple Hysterectomy

Occasionally, a simple or total abdominal hysterectomy is performed and invasive carcinoma of the cervix is incidentally found in the surgical specimen. In general, extrafascial abdominal hysterectomy is not curative because the paravaginal or paracervical soft tissues and vaginal cuff are not removed. Furthermore, it may be technically difficult to perform an adequate radical opera-

TABLE 69.10 RESULTS OF POSTOPERATIVE EXTERNAL-BEAM IRRADIATION AFTER CONSERVATIVE HYSTERECTOMY IN EARLY-STAGE CARCINOMA OF THE CERVIX[a]

Author (Reference)	Number of Patients	Local Control (%)	Survival Percentage	Survival Months	Severe Complications (%)[b]
Andras et al. (372)	80[c]	89	89	60	4
Ampil et al. (42)	27[c]	89	70	60	4
Saibishkumar et al. (378)	105	72	55	60	12
Sharma et al. (886)	83	70	62	60	6

[a]Patients with postsurgery gross residual or recurrent disease before irradiation were excluded from the total number of cited cases.
[b]Remedial surgery was performed because of bowel or bladder damage in some patients in some series.
[c]All or some of the patients had additional vaginal cuff irradiation.
Modified from Ampil F, Datta R, Datta S. Elective postoperative external radiotherapy after hysterectomy in early-stage carcinoma of the cervix: is additional vaginal cuff irradiation necessary? *Cancer* 1987;60:280–288; with permission.

tion after previous simple hysterectomy. If only microinvasive carcinoma is found when a total or extrafascial hysterectomy with a wide cuff is performed, no additional therapy is necessary. For lesions with deeper stromal invasion, at most one or two vaginal intracavitary insertion(s) to deliver a 65-Gy LDR mucosal dose (or 7 Gy × six fractions prescribed at the vaginal surface, or 5 Gy at 0.5 cm × six fractions with HDR brachytherapy) to the vault are sufficient. If a less comprehensive resection was carried out, it is critical that these patients receive radiation therapy immediately with or without concurrent chemotherapy, depending on the risk factors present pathologically when their postoperative status allows it because the prognosis is worse if postoperative irradiation is not administered.

In patients with fully invasive tumor, therapy consists of approximately 40 to 45 Gy to the whole pelvis with cylinder brachytherapy to the vaginal vault for an approximately 60-Gy mucosal dose. If there is gross tumor present in the vaginal vault or parametrium, the dose to the whole pelvis should be 45 Gy with concurrent weekly cisplatin chemotherapy, followed by an additional parametrial dose of 10 to 20 Gy. An intracavitary insertion should be performed. If there is gross residual tumor, an interstitial implant should be carried out to selectively increase the dose to this volume.

Several studies have reported results of postoperative external-beam irradiation after conservative surgery (Table 69.10). Andras et al.[372] reported on 148 patients, 90 of whom were available for 10-year evaluation, who were divided into five groups, depending on tumor extent when therapy was instituted. The majority of patients were treated with 50-Gy total-pelvis irradiation (with 10-Gy parametrial boost through reduced fields), at times combined with vaginal vault intracavitary irradiation. Eight major complications were noted in 148 patients.

Ampil et al.[373] described results in 44 patients receiving postoperative irradiation after hysterectomy for stage IB and IIA carcinoma of the uterine cervix (15 patients treated with radical hysterectomy). Their 5-year results were 80% local tumor control and 63% overall survival. In 3 patients treated with intracavitary vaginal cuff irradiation only, 2 had tumor control.

Green and Morse[374] reported 9 of 30 patients (30%) surviving 5 years after definitive radiation therapy for treatment of invasive cervical carcinoma after simple hysterectomy. The same authors noted that 14 of 32 patients retreated with another surgical procedure, usually a Wertheim hysterectomy, died within 5 years. They pointed out that the 5-year cure rate was 30% in patients treated within 1 year after the hysterectomy but was only 16% in those treated after 1 year. Thus, the time at which the patient is treated and the volume of tumor are important prognostic factors.

Crane and Schneider[375] described results in 18 patients treated with RT (with or without brachytherapy) for invasive carcinoma of the cervix discovered after simple hysterectomy. The 10-year actuarial local tumor control was 88%, and the overall survival rate was 93%. Huerta Bahena et al.,[376] in 59 patients with carcinoma of the cervix incidentally found in simple hysterectomy specimens (27 with gross residual tumor) who were treated with postoperative RT, reported a 3-year survival of 59%; factors affecting prognosis included gross residual tumor, time between hysterectomy and irradiation >6 months, RT doses < 50 Gy, and histologic tumor type.

Munstedt et al.[377] reported on 119 patients who received postoperative RT after radical hysterectomy and 80 who received it after simple hysterectomy. There was a trend toward better survival in the radical hysterectomy group, but the authors concluded that postoperative RT is a good treatment in patients with invasive cervical cancer who undergo a simple hysterectomy. In another report of 105 patients with invasive cervical carcinoma found in inadequate surgery specimens treated with postoperative RT, 5-year pelvic tumor control was 72% and the survival rate was 55%. Late rectal toxicity was 19%, bladder toxicity was 4.8%, and small-bowel toxicity was 14.3%.[378]

In a series of 147 patients treated at Asan Medical Center in Korea, 48 patients with stage IA1 lesions did not receive further treatment. Another 99 patients had stage IA2 to IIA lesions incidentally identified. Of these, 26 received no further therapy, 44 had either radiation or chemoradiation, and 29 had a radical parametrectomy. For patients with stage IA1 disease who were observed, 0% relapsed, whereas 35% of patients with stage IA2 to IIA disease who were observed suffered from a recurrence.[379] Either radical parametrectomy or radiation is required for patients with stage IA2 or higher cancer after a simple hysterectomy. However, these treatments increase the risk of side effects,[380] including for those patients receiving robotic parametrectomy.[381]

Stage IA

The definition of microinvasive (stage IA) carcinoma of the cervix includes invasive carcinoma diagnosed only by microscopy. Conization is mandatory for a more accurate diagnosis. According to Kolstad,[382] lesions <1 mm in depth can be treated with conization, provided all margins are tumor free and continued careful follow-up is instituted. Raspagliesi et al.[383] used margins of 8 to 10 mm as guidelines for clearance in conization. Smaller margins or lymphovascular invasion in addition to depth of invasion were prognostic factors for recurrence.

Tumor volume in the stroma may be a more reliable criterion than depth of invasion to arrive at a definition of stage IA. Vascular space involvement does not impact stage. Depth of invasion and tumor confluence have been identified as prognostic factors that should be taken into consideration in the planning of therapy.[384]

Early invasive carcinoma of the cervix (stage IA2) is usually treated with a total abdominal or modified radical hysterectomy or in some cases with simple conization[251] or radical trachelectomy.[385] Inoperable patients may be treated with intracavitary radioactive sources alone with 6,500 to 8,000 mgh, 60 to 75 Gy to point A, in two LDR insertions, respectively, or with the equivalent dose using HDR brachytherapy, approximately 10 fractions of 5 Gy per fraction. In 47 patients with microinvasive carcinoma treated at Washington University—20 with intracavitary therapy only and 27 patients with combined external irradiation and intracavitary brachytherapy—only 1 patient had a pelvic recurrence and distant metastases 10 years later; the 5-year disease-free survival rate was 96%.[366]

When the depth of penetration of the stroma by tumor is <3 mm, the incidence of lymph node metastasis is 1% or less, and a lymph node dissection or pelvic external irradiation is not warranted.[384,385] With more extensive lesions, a Wertheim radical hysterectomy with pelvic lymphadenectomy is the preferred treatment. Tumor control with all treatment methods is >95%, with patients eventually dying of intercurrent disease. Gadducci et al.[386] treated 30 patients with conization and 82 with total and 54 with radical hysterectomy; the recurrence rates were 10%, 4.9%, and 9.3%, respectively. None of 67 patients subjected to lymphadenectomy had positive pelvic nodes. In 98 patients with adenocarcinoma of the cervix, none of 48 with depth of invasion (DOI) of ≤5 mm had involved parametria or positive nodes, in contrast to 6 of 36 (16%) with DOI of >5 mm.[387]

Vaginal trachelectomy (removal of the cervix) and laparoscopic lymphadenectomy have been used to treat young patients with microinvasive carcinoma to preserve fertility. The overall incidence of central recurrence is approximately 5%.[364] Webb et al.[388] analyzed lymph node status and survival rates of women with microinvasive cervical adenocarcinoma (FIGO stages IA1 and IA2) from the Surveillance, Epidemiology, and End Results (SEER) database between 1988 and 1997. Among reported cases, 131 had stage IA1 and 170 had stage IA2 disease. Simple hysterectomy was done in 54 women with IA1 and in 64 women with IA2 disease and radical hysterectomy in 50 and 83 women, respectively. Only 1 of 140 women who had lymphadenectomy had a single positive lymph node. There were 4 tumor-related deaths (1 with IA1 and 3 with IA2 disease). The survival rate was 98.7%.

Stages IB to IIA

The choice of definitive irradiation or radical surgery for stage IB and IIA carcinoma of the cervix remains controversial, and the preference for one procedure over another depends primarily on the impact on the patient's fertility and on the institution, the gynecologic oncologist or radiation oncologist involved, the general condition of the patient, and characteristics of the lesion. An operation has been preferred by some in young women to preserve the ovaries, attempting to prevent premature menopause. However, in some reports[294] ovarian function preservation has been observed in only 50% to 60% of surgically treated patients not receiving irradiation. Postmenopausal patients may have a survival benefit with chemoradiation and avoid the operative risks. When therapeutic results in invasive carcinoma of the cervix are evaluated, a direct comparison of surgically treated or irradiated patients is fraught with many uncertainties, including patient selection, reporting of surgical cases using staging determined by laparotomy findings, and different treatment techniques.[389] In particular, in the modern era when concurrent chemoradiation is known to be superior to radiation alone, a direct comparison of chemoradiation versus surgery in early-stage cervical cancer is needed.

Surgery provides an opportunity for a thorough pelvic and abdominal evaluation. However, surgical staging has not been shown to improve overall patient survival.[279,390] Kupets et al.[391] assessed the value of debulking large nodes and concluded that the incremental overall benefit by stage was small. Delgado et al.[161] described a GOG study in which 1,125 patients were registered before surgery; 80 were ineligible after strict pathology review, and an additional 129 patients were explored, but the hysterectomy was abandoned because of intraoperative complications in 49 patients or extent of disease beyond the uterus in 80 patients. In the era of MRI, surgeons may rely on imaging findings to screen for operability. The impact of patient selection in results of surgical series was illustrated by Whitney and Stehman,[392] who evaluated the frequency with which intended radical hysterectomy for cervical cancer is abandoned and the outcomes for those selected patients. In 1,127 patients with stage IB carcinoma of the cervix entered on GOG Protocol 49, 98 women (8.7%) were found at surgery to have extrauterine disease, and the proposed radical operation was abandoned. Subgroups of patients with extrapelvic disease[31] and pelvic extension,[387] including grossly positive pelvic nodes,[160] other pelvic implants,[393] and gross serosal extension,[163] were identified. Sixty-three (93%) patients subsequently underwent pelvic radiation therapy and brachytherapy. Para-aortic fields were added for 8 patients who were found to have positive para-aortic nodes. The disease-free survival was shorter for patients whose radical procedure was abandoned than for those patients who underwent radical hysterectomy.

The important contribution of external-beam irradiation to improve pelvic tumor control in larger lesions has been documented. Hamberger et al.,[394] in 151 patients with stage IA or IB lesions <1 cm in diameter treated with intracavitary therapy alone to high doses (8,640, 9,340, and 13,680 mgh), noted no failures in 41 patients with stage IA disease, and only 4 of 93 patients (4%) with stage IB, small-volume disease. However, 3 of 17 patients (18%) with more extensive stage IB lesions, treated with intracavitary therapy only, had regional failures. Only 3 of 151 patients (0.2%) had grade 3 complications.

Volterrani and Lombardi[395] reported 5-year survival of 82.6% in 23 patients with occult stage IB carcinoma of the cervix treated with intracavitary ^{226}Ra only (7,500 mgh), in contrast to only 64.8% with larger stage IB tumors and 50% with stage II. Unfortunately, the authors did not report the exact location of the failures. It is obvious that intracavitary therapy alone is grossly inadequate to irradiate larger primary tumors, including stage IB1.

With EBRT and brachytherapy without chemotherapy, the usual 5-year survival rate for stage IB is 86% to 92% and for stage IIA is approximately 75%.[396] Late toxicity was observed in 1% to 2% of patients. Concurrent chemotherapy significantly improves survival, including in stage IB to IIA disease. In RTOG 90-01, for the subset of 272 stage IB to IIA patients, the 8-year overall survival was 55% with RT alone versus 78% with concurrent chemoradiation ($p < .001$).[397]

Randomized Studies: Surgery Versus Radiation

Few randomized trials have compared the results of radical hysterectomy with definitive RT, and none have compared surgery to chemoradiation. Outcome between radiation alone versus surgery is comparable. Newton[398] and Roddick and Greenlaw[399] reported, in prospectively randomized studies, equivalent survival and pelvic recurrence rates in patients with stage IB and IIA carcinoma of the uterine cervix treated with a radical hysterectomy or irradiation alone. Landoni et al.[35] published results of a prospective, randomized trial of radiation therapy versus surgery; 469 women with stage IB and IIA cervical carcinoma were referred for treatment and 343 were randomized (172 to surgery and 171 to radiation therapy). Postoperative irradiation was delivered after surgery for women with surgical stage pT2b or greater, <3 mm of cervical stromal invasion and cut-through margins or positive pelvic nodes. Scheduled treatment was delivered to 169 and 158 women, respectively; 62 of 114 women with cervical diameters of <4 cm and 46 of 55 women with >4 cm received radiation therapy. After a median follow-up of 87 months (range, 57 to 120 months), 5-year overall and disease-free survival rates were nearly identical in the surgery and radiation therapy groups (83% and 74%, respectively); recurrent disease developed in 86 women: 42 (25%) in the surgery group and 44 (26%) in the radiation therapy group (Fig. 69.18). Forty-eight patients (28%) in the surgery group had severe morbidity, compared with 19 (12%) in the radiation therapy group ($p = .0004$; Table 69.11). The combination of surgery and radiation therapy had the worst morbidity, especially urologic complications.

Of note, no randomized study has compared chemoRT to radical hysterectomy, although chemoRT has a significant survival advantage over RT alone for patients with stage IB to IIA cervical cancer.[400] In a meta-analysis looking at the value of adjuvant cisplatin-based chemotherapy after radical hysterectomy, radiation therapy, or both for patients with stage IA2, IB1, or IIA cervical

Clinical Radiation Oncology

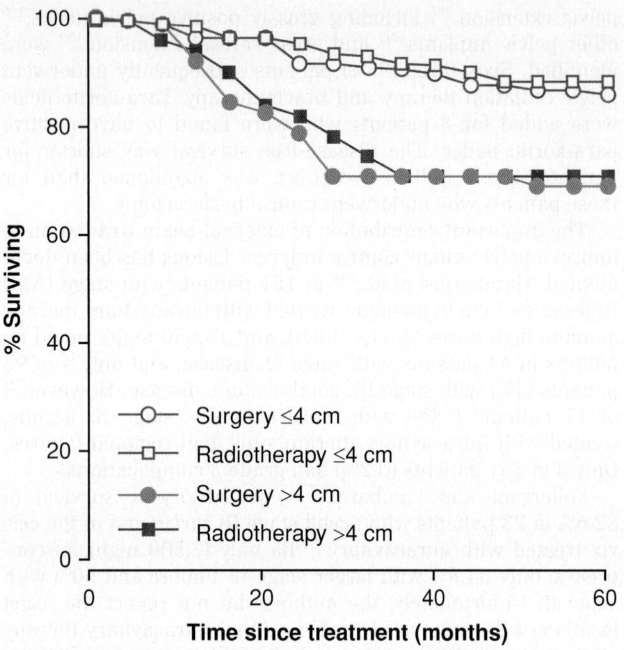

FIGURE 69.18. Overall actuarial survival of patients with carcinoma of the cervix randomized to treatment with radical surgery or radiation therapy according to treatment group and cervical diameter. (From Landoni F, Maneo A, Colombo A, et al. Randomised study of radical surgery versus radiotherapy for stage IB-IIA cervical cancer. *Lancet* 1997;350:535–540; reprinted with permission from Elsevier.)

cancer, three randomized clinical trials were evaluated.[400] Two of the three trials showed a significant benefit compared to adjuvant chemotherapy concurrent with radiation, with a reduced risk of death (HR = 0.56, 95% CI = 0.36 to 0.87). No benefit was seen when chemotherapy was given prior to radiotherapy.

Neoadjuvant chemotherapy plus surgery does not improve survival over surgery alone.[401] In a meta-analysis of six trials, although there was an improvement in progression-free survival with neoadjuvant chemotherapy (HR = 0.76, 95% CI = 0.62 to 0.94, p = .01), this did not translate into an overall survival benefit. Another meta-analysis reviewed 18 trials with locally advanced cervical-cancer patients treated with neoadjuvant chemotherapy before radiation or surgery or both and excluded concurrent chemoradiation trials; it showed significant heterogeneity and no conclusive results.[402]

Nonrandomized Studies Comparing Surgery to Radiation

Keilbinska et al.,[403] in a long-term study of 792 women treated with irradiation and 789 women treated with hysterectomy and/or irradiation for stage I cervical carcinoma, found no difference in survival, general health, incidence of recurrent carcinoma, or appearance of second primary malignancies. Piver et al.[404] treated 103 women with stage IB cervical carcinoma with either radical hysterectomy and pelvic lymphadenectomy (if tumor was <3 cm in greatest diameter) or irradiation (tumor of >3 cm or medically inoperable). The 5-year disease-free survival rate was 92.3% for the surgical group and 91.1% for the radiation therapy group. Equivalent overall 5-year survival rates were noted. Einhorn et al.,[405] in a nonrandomized study, observed a 100% 5-year survival rate in 49 patients with stage IB disease receiving combined therapy in comparison with 81% in 64 patients treated with irradiation alone. No difference was observed in 25 patients with stage IIA tumor treated with combined therapy and 40 patients treated with irradiation alone (5-year survival rate, 75%).

Perez et al.[406] reported on a prospectively randomized study of 118 patients with stage IB or IIA carcinoma of the uterine cervix in which patients were treated with RT alone or irradiation and surgery (20 Gy to the whole pelvis, one intracavitary insertion for 5,000 to 6,000 mgh, followed by a radical hysterectomy with pelvic lymphadenectomy 2 to 6 weeks later). In stage IB, the 5-year tumor-free survival was 80% and 82% (p = .23), respectively, and in stage IIA it was 56% and 79%, respectively (p = .13). The incidence of grade 2 or 3 complications for radiation alone was 13.8% and with preoperative irradiation and surgery was 11%. Subsequently, Perez et al.[407] described results in 415 patients with stage IB or limited stage IIB treated with preoperative or postoperative irradiation and surgery. The 10-year cause-specific survival rate for patients with stage IB nonbulky tumors treated with irradiation alone or irradiation combined with surgery was 84% with either modality. With bulky tumors (>5 cm), the 10-year rates were 61% and 68%, respectively (p = .5). For patients with stage IIA nonbulky tumors, the 10-year cause-specific survival rates were 66% and 71%, respectively, and with bulky tumors, 69% and 44%, respectively (p = .05). In patients with stage IIB nonbulky tumors treated with irradiation alone or combined with surgery, the 10-year cause-specific survival rates were 72% and 65%, respectively. In stage IB and IIA disease after a hysterectomy and lymphadenectomy (even combined with irradiation), patients with metastatic lymph nodes have survival rates that are approximately 50% of those of patients with negative nodes.[408]

Randomized Trials of Postoperative Radiation Therapy or Chemoradiation After Radical Hysterectomy

Patients who have undergone radical hysterectomy with no preoperative radiation therapy are considered for postoperative chemoradiation therapy if they have high-risk prognostic factors, which include positive pelvic lymph nodes, as are patients with negative nodes who have microscopic positive margins of resection or parametrial involvement.[409]

Patients with any two of deep stromal invasion, vascular/lymphatic permeation, and large tumor size are candidates for postoperative radiation.[410] These patients have an intermediate

TABLE 69.11 RANDOMIZED TRIAL OF RADICAL SURGERY OR IRRADIATION IN STAGES I TO II CERVICAL CANCER: RELAPSES AND MORBIDITY

	Surgery							
	Surgery Only		*Surgery Plus Radiation Therapy*				*Radiation Therapy Alone*	
	≤4 cm	*>4 cm*	*≤4 cm*	*>4 cm*	*Total ≤4 cm*	*>4 cm*	*≤4 cm*	*>4 cm*
Number of patients[a]	53 (52)	9 (9)	62 (62)	46 (46)	115 (114)	55 (55)	114 (105)	54 (53)
Relapses	7 (13%)	2 (22%)	15 (26%)	17 (37%)	23 (20%)	19 (34%)	21 (18%)	23 (42%)
Pelvic	4	2	7	9	11	11	12	16
Distant morbidity	3	–	9	8	12	8	9	7
Grade 2–3[b]	16 (31%)	3 (33%)	18 (29%)	11 (24%)	34 (30%)	14 (25%)	13 (12%)	6 (11%)
Short term	10 (16%)	–	22 (20%)	–	32 (19%)	–	11 (7%)	–
Long term	15 (24%)	–	31 (29%)	–	46 (27%)	–	25 (16%)	–

[a]Parentheses show number of patients who actually received this treatment instead of intention to treat.

[b]Percentage calculated for number of patients who actually received treatment.

From Landoni F, Maneo A, Colombo A, et al. Randomised study of radical surgery versus radiotherapy for stage IB–IIA cervical cancer. *Lancet* 1997;350:535–540, with permission from Elsevier.

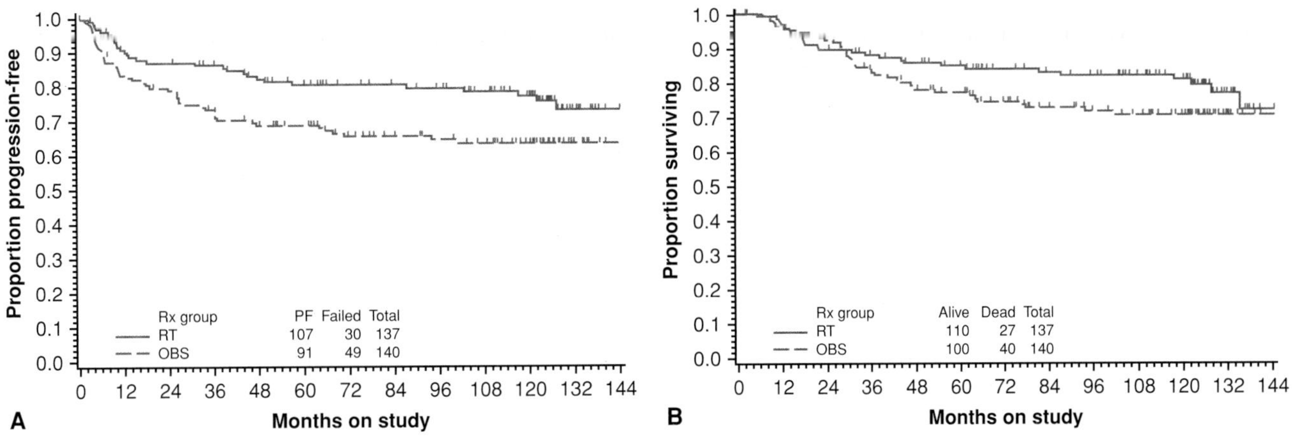

FIGURE 69.19. Recurrence-free survival **(A)** and overall survival **(B)** of patients with stage IB carcinoma of the cervix, correlated with treatment method. (From Rotman M, Sedlis A, Piedmonte MR. A phase III randomized trial of postoperative pelvic irradiation in patients with stage IB cervical carcinoma with poor prognostic features: follow up of a Gynecologic Oncology Group study. *Int J Radiat Oncol Biol Phys* 2006;65:169–176; with permission from Elsevier.)

risk of failure.[161] Whether to add concurrent chemotherapy to postoperative radiation in the intermediate risk group is being tested in an accruing randomized trial; many institutions routinely implement chemoRT for intermediate-risk patients. Song et al.[411] reported a 20-year experience in stage IB to IIA cervical-cancer patients with intermediate-risk factors (two or more of deep stromal invasion, lymphovascular invasion, and large tumor size) received postoperative RT or chemoradiation. Chemoradiation significantly decreased pelvic recurrence and distant metastases; there was no difference in acute or chronic grade 3 and 4 gastrointestinal side effects.

One randomized study showed improved recurrence-free survival with postoperative pelvic irradiation (46 to 50.4 Gy in 23 to 28 fractions) after radical surgery in the presence of positive pelvic nodes or node-negative high-risk factors in women with stage IB cervical cancer treated by radical hysterectomy and pelvic lymphadenectomy. There were 277 eligible patients with at least two of the following risk factors: greater than one-third stromal invasion, capillary lymphatic space involvement, and large clinical tumor diameter; 137 patients were randomized to pelvic radiation therapy and 140 to no further treatment. The results were updated by Rotman et al.;[412] 24 (17%) patients in the irradiation group and 43 (30.7%) in the no-further-treatment group had cancer recurrences. In the radiation therapy group 27 patients died of cancer, and in the no-further-treatment group 40 died from cancer. There was a statistically significant reduction in risk of recurrence in the irradiation group, with recurrence-free rates at 2 years of 88% versus 79% for the irradiation and no-further-treatment groups, respectively. Overall survival difference did not reach statistical difference (p = .074; Fig. 69.19). Severe or life-threatening (GOG grade 3 or 4) adverse effects occurred in 9 patients (6.6%) in the radiation therapy group and 3 (2.1%) in the observation group. A meta-analysis of trials including stage IB1 to IIA cervical cancer found that women who received postoperative radiation had a significantly lower risk of disease progression at 5 years (RR = 0.6, 95% CI = 0.4 to 0.9). The risk of serious adverse events was not significantly higher if women received radiotherapy rather than no further treatment, possibly because the rate of adverse events was low.[413]

Sundfør et al.[414] conducted a randomized study in which 122 patients with stage IIA and 20 patients with stage IIB cervix cancer were treated with intracavitary radium followed by either radical pelvic surgery including lymphadenectomy (group A, 72 patients) or EBRT (40 Gy) to the pelvis (group B, 70 patients). Postoperative RT (40 to 50 Gy) was given to patients in group A found to have node metastasis at operation. Fourteen patients in group A and 23 in group B died of recurrent cancer. The 10-year survival was 84% and 69%, respectively.

Nonrandomized Trials of Postoperative Radiation Therapy or Chemoradiation After Radical Hysterectomy

Snijders-Keilholz et al.[415] described results in 233 women who underwent radical hysterectomy for stage I or IIA cervical carcinoma; 156 were treated with surgery alone, and 77 received adjuvant radiation therapy for tumor-related high-risk prognostic factors. The most important prognostic factor for survival and disease-free survival was pelvic lymph node positivity; additional factors were depth of invasion and positive surgical margins. Twelve patients recurred after surgery alone, all in the pelvis (100%). Of the 23 recurrences after surgery and adjuvant radiation therapy, 13 were in the pelvis (56%; p = .003). Ten patients with poor prognostic factors and negative nodes received adjuvant radiation therapy, and none of these patients recurred. The incidence of severe gastrointestinal radiation-related side effects was 2%. The incidence of lymphedema of the leg was 11%, which was similar to that in the surgery-alone group.

Garipagaoglu et al.[416] investigated prognostic factors in 100 patients with stage IB or IIA cervical carcinoma treated with radical hysterectomy and postoperative irradiation. The 5-year overall survival, disease-free survival, and pelvic tumor control rates were 83.6%, 82.8%, and 91.8%, respectively. Pelvic lymph node metastasis (p = .008), interval between surgery and irradiation (p = .001), overall radiation therapy time (p = .007), and tumor size (p = .028) were significant factors for pelvic tumor control, as well as for overall survival.

Lahousen et al.[417] reported on a GOG prospectively randomized, multicenter trial in which patients with stage IB or IIB cervical cancer treated with radical hysterectomy who had pelvic lymph node metastases or vascular invasion randomly received adjuvant chemotherapy (400 mg/m^2 carboplatin and 30 mg bleomycin), external pelvic radiation therapy, or no further treatment. After a median follow-up of 4.1 years (range, 2 to 7 years), there were no statistically significant differences (p = .9539) in disease-free survival rates among the three treatment arms, suggesting that adjuvant chemotherapy or radiation does not improve survival or recurrence rates in high-risk patients with cervical cancer after radical hysterectomy.

González González et al.[418] reported that in 89 patients with stage IB or IIA cervical cancer with positive lymph nodes receiving postoperative irradiation, the 5- and 10-year survival rates were 60% and 51%, respectively. By comparison, 43 patients with negative lymph nodes had a survival rate of 85%. In the surviving patients, there were 4 gastrointestinal and 7 genitourinary severe complications requiring surgical correction. In

4 patients, asymptomatic stenosis of the ureters was detected by IV pyelography performed routinely every year.

Bianchi et al.,[419] in 60 patients receiving external irradiation for pelvic node metastasis after radical hysterectomy, observed a 65% 5-year survival rate. In contrast, in 15 patients who refused postoperative irradiation, only 3 (20%) survived 5 years.

Chatani et al.[420] reported on 128 patients with stage IB to IIB carcinoma of the cervix who underwent radical hysterectomy with bilateral pelvic lymphadenectomy and postoperative EBRT. The 5-year local and distant failure rates were, respectively, 2% and 12% for negative nodes, 23% and 25% for one positive node, and 32% and 57%, for two or more positive nodes (p = .0029 and .0051, respectively). The 5-year cause-specific survival rates were 90%, 59%, and 42%, respectively (p = .0001). The most common complication was lymphedema of the lower extremity, experienced by half of the patients (42% at 5 years and 49% at 10 years).

Uno et al.[421] evaluated results of postradical hysterectomy irradiation in 98 patients with stage IB to IIB cervical cancer; all of the patients had at least one pathologic risk factor for pelvic recurrence. The 5-year overall survival was 82%. There were pelvic recurrences in 5 cases and distant metastases in 15 cases. The 5-year overall survival rates for patients with or without pelvic lymph node metastasis were 76% and 89%, respectively (p = .018).

Kinney et al.[422] compared results of therapy in 82 patients with stage IB or IIA carcinoma of the cervix found to have pelvic lymph node metastases at Wertheim hysterectomy and bilateral lymphadenectomy without additional adjuvant therapy with 103 similar patients who received 50 Gy to the pelvis after surgery. The 5-year survival rate was 72% for the surgery-only patients and 64% for the group receiving adjuvant irradiation. The incidences of pelvic recurrence were 67% and 27%, respectively. The lack of impact on overall survival in the irradiated patients is most likely related to a higher incidence of distant metastases, which may be a reflection of shorter survival time and more high-risk patients. In 117 patients treated with radical hysterectomy and pelvic lymphadenectomy, histologically proven nodal metastatic disease was detected in 51 patients (44%; squamous cell in 35 and nonsquamous in 16). Nodal involvement was bilateral in 24 patients (47%).[423] Para-aortic lymph node dissection was performed in 14 patients, and 5 had tumor involvement. Postoperative pelvic irradiation was administered to 29 of 51 patients (51.2 Gy, two fractions). Extended fields to the para-aortic area were used in 6 patients. The 5-year survival rates were 33% for the group receiving irradiation and 50% for the nonirradiated group. Only 1 patient treated with postoperative irradiation had a pelvic failure, in contrast to 7 patients not irradiated.

Inoue and Morita[270] described results in 72 patients treated with extended-field irradiation after radical surgery for nodal metastases with stages IB (37 patients), IIA (6 patients), and IIB (29 patients) cervical cancer. The median dose to para-aortic lymph nodes was 43.5 Gy and to the pelvis was 45 Gy. The 5-year disease-free survival rates were 72% in 61 patients with squamous cell carcinoma and 27% in 11 patients with nonsquamous cell carcinoma. The 10-year disease-free survival rates were 88% for 22 patients with one positive node, 67% for 15 patients with two or three positive nodes, 64% for 16 patients with four to 17 positive nodes, and 20% for 10 patients with unresectable lymph nodes. Nineteen severe complications occurred in 17 patients; 5 were attributed to surgery, 5 to irradiation, and 9 to both modalities. Four patients (5%) died of severe complications. Another 6 patients (8%) underwent major abdominal surgery for rectovaginal and ureterovaginal fistulas.

Mitsuhashi et al.[424] described an analysis of 108 patients with carcinoma of the cervix treated with postoperative EBRT to the pelvis followed by intravaginal cone boost with electron beam to the vaginal cuff. The 5-year cause-specific survival rates were 89% for 89 patients undergoing elective radiation therapy and 56% for 19 patients undergoing salvage irradiation (p < .001). Recurrent tumors at the vaginal cuff were observed in only 2 patients in the elective irradiation group. Vesicovaginal fistula developed in 4 patients; only 1 patient had grade 2 rectal complications.

A Japanese group treated 189 stage IIB cervical cancer patients; 95 had a radical hysterectomy followed by adjuvant RT, and the other 94 patients had RT alone.[425] There was a significant increase in grade 3 to 4 late toxicities in the surgery group, 24% versus 10%, p = .048. Therefore, RT is preferable, and in the modern era, chemoRT provides a superior outcome and should be administered to all stage IIB patients. The same group reported on 55 stage IA2 to IIB patients with multiple pelvic lymph nodes positive treated either with pelvic RT and concurrent chemotherapy or extended-field RT. Overall survival significantly improved with concurrent chemotherapy (p = .03).[426]

Lee et al.[427] retrospectively compared 201 stage IB1 to IIB cervical cancer patients who had a radical hysterectomy with pelvic lymph node dissection followed by adjuvant concurrent weekly cisplatin to triweekly combination chemotherapy. With a median follow-up of 52 months, the weekly cisplatin group had the same therapeutic effect with less toxicity. The 5-year disease-free and overall survival were 82% and 81%, respectively, for patients treated with weekly cisplatin chemotherapy versus 74% and 79% for those treated with triweekly combination chemotherapy (p = NS). Leukopenia, neutropenia, thrombocytopenia, anemia, and hepatopathy were significantly more common in the triweekly combination chemotherapy group.

Postoperative External-Beam Radiation Dose

When metastatic pelvic lymph nodes are present, treatment has consisted of 45 Gy to the whole pelvis delivered with a four-field technique with concurrent weekly cisplatin. If gross residual disease is present, dose escalation to 54 to 65 Gy, depending on small-bowel dose limits (for example, D_{5cc} < 55 Gy), may be considered with a sequential IMRT nodal boost.[80] Patients with positive common iliac or para-aortic node metastases should receive 45 Gy to the entire para-aortic region with the superior border covering the renal hilum, with consideration of a boost to the tumor bed. If gross residual nodal disease is left, a nodal boost up to 65 Gy with IMRT is particularly suited to treat these patients.[271,275]

In patients for whom postoperative irradiation is indicated for deep stromal invasion in the cervix or close or positive surgical margins, an alternative is to deliver 45-Gy pelvic external irradiation in combination with an intracavitary insertion (LDR, PDR, or HDR) and LDR equivalent dose of 65 Gy to the vaginal mucosa, using colpostats or a cylinder.[428] At some institutions, external irradiation alone (50 Gy to the midplane of the pelvis) with a four-field box technique has been used. Hong et al.[176] recommended, for node-negative patients with high-risk factors, to irradiate only the low pelvis (median dose, 50 Gy), which resulted in a reduction of grade 3 small bowel morbidity (3 of 149 = 2%) in comparison with patients treated to the whole pelvis (6 of 79 = 8%). Five-year disease-specific survival was 84% and 86%, respectively.

Postoperative Intracavitary High-Dose-Rate Brachytherapy

Depending on the extent of surgical resection of the vagina, the vaginal cuff may be at risk for recurrence. There is no clear agreement on the indications for vaginal brachytherapy after radical hysterectomy, although adjuvant vaginal brachytherapy for cervical cancer is most commonly used as a boost after EBRT. Based on the American Brachytherapy Society guidelines, vaginal cuff boost should be considered in patients with a less-than-radical hysterectomy, close or positive margins, large or deeply invasive tumors, parametrial or vaginal involvement, or extensive lymphovascular invasion.[428] Consideration of postoperative vaginal intracavitary brachytherapy after external-beam therapy is recommended for patients with carcinoma at the vaginal margin of resection.[303] If parametrial margins were close or positive, defined by either surgical clips or in the region of the surgical tumor bed, an external-beam dose of at least 54 Gy for close margins and higher for positive margins is recommended.

In patients receiving postoperative irradiation, extreme care should be exercised in designing treatment techniques, including intracavitary insertions; because of the surgical extirpation of the uterus, the bladder and rectosigmoid may be closer to the radioactive sources than in the patient with an intact uterus. Furthermore, vascular supply may be affected by the surgical procedure, and adhesions can prevent mobilization of the small-bowel loops that may be fixed in the pelvis. HDR brachytherapy after surgery is particularly suited for patients with cervical cancer because it prevents the prolonged immobilization required for LDR brachytherapy. In some patients at higher risk for parametrial tumor or lymph node metastases, HDR brachytherapy is combined with external-beam pelvic irradiation.

Hart et al.[429] described results in 83 patients who received postoperative RT for early-stage cervical cancer with positive surgical margins, positive pelvic or para-aortic lymph nodes, lymphovascular space invasion, or deep stromal invasion or for disease discovered incidentally at simple hysterectomy. Twenty-eight patients were treated with LDR brachytherapy with or without EBRT and 55 with EBRT to the pelvis and HDR intracavitary. Of these 83 patients, 66 were evaluable (20 LDR and 46 HDR patients). Mean follow-up time was 101 months for the LDR group and 42 for the HDR group. The 5-year disease-free survival rates were 89% and 72%, and local tumor control rates were 90% (18 of 20) and 89% (41 of 46), respectively. Three of 20 patients (15%) receiving LDR and 4 of 46 (9%) receiving HDR experienced grade 2 or 3 late treatment-related complications. No patient in either group had grade 4 or 5 complications.

Busch et al.[430] studied the outcome of 68 patients with cervical carcinoma; 48 were treated with radical hysterectomy and, because of risk factors, with postoperative RT (group 1), and 20 patients (group 2) were pretreated with standard hysterectomy and then admitted to the hospital for postoperative radiation therapy of the whole pelvis. Postoperative pelvic RT consisted of 39.6 Gy (box technique) and 6-Gy external-beam therapy to the pelvic lymph nodes, sparing the midline, plus two HDR applications (7.5 Gy each). Survival, locoregional tumor control, and metastatic disease rates were nearly identical in both groups. Patients with positive lymph nodes had a worse prognosis (75% 3-year survival rate).

Atkovar et al.[431] described results in 126 patients treated with postoperative irradiation (median of 50 Gy in 5 weeks); 37 received vaginal cuff HDR brachytherapy (three fractions of 8 to 10 Gy at 5 mm, weekly). Overall and disease-free survival and locoregional tumor control rates were 71%, 69.9%, and 78.1%, respectively. Grade 2 and 3 complications developed in 5.5% of patients. Survival was the same in 67 patients treated with total abdominal hysterectomy and bilateral salpingo-oophorectomy and in 59 patients treated with radical hysterectomy and pelvic lymphadenectomy.

Stages IB2 to IVA: Chemoradiation

Patients with stages IB2 to IVA tumors are treated with irradiation including external beam and brachytherapy combined with concurrent chemotherapy. Numerous reports have been published on the concomitant use of irradiation and cytotoxic agents (hydroxyurea, cisplatin, and 5-FU, in some trials combined with mitomycin C) administered to obtain a radiosensitizing effect.[432–434] Cisplatin is one of the most active cytotoxic agents in squamous cell carcinoma of the uterine cervix.[435] When cisplatin and irradiation are used concomitantly, substantial enhancement of cell killing is observed. Coughlin and Richmond[433] and Douple[436] suggested two mechanisms for radiation enhancement by cisplatin: (a) in hypoxic or oxygenated cells, free radicals with altered binding of cisplatin to DNA are formed at the time of irradiation, and (b) interaction inhibits repair of sublethal damage.

It is important, however, that patients complete the full course of 45 Gy with, ideally, five to six weekly doses of cisplatin or two doses of cisplatin and 5-FU every 3 weeks. In a study of 41 patients who had weekly biopsies while receiving RT and chemotherapy for cervix cancer, increased tumor cell proliferation and accelerated repopulation was observed within 2 weeks from the initiation of therapy. Patients with a sustained yield and high S-phase fraction for 2 or more weeks were at increased risk for tumor progression.[437]

Green et al.,[438] in a search of medical databases for randomized trials of cervical cancer that compared RT with or without concurrent chemotherapy, identified 19 trials comprising 4,580 randomized patients, and they were the subjects of the meta-analysis. Concomitant chemotherapy and radiation improved tumor control and overall survival (RR = 0.71; $p < .0001$) and progression-free survival (RR = 0.61; $p < .0001$). The benefit was maximal in early-stage (I and II) disease. The absolute survival benefit was 12%. Patients receiving chemoirradiation had a higher incidence of grade 3 or 4 hematologic and gastrointestinal toxicities.

Patients with stage IVA disease (bladder and/or rectal invasion) can be treated either with higher doses of external radiation to the whole pelvis with concurrent chemotherapy followed by intracavitary or interstitial insertions (total dose to point A with LDR brachytherapy about 90 Gy) and additional parametrial irradiation, or with pelvic exenteration.[439] Niibe et al.,[440] in an analysis of 179 patients with stage IIIB adenocarcinoma, suggested that an optimal dose for large tumors was a total biological effective dose of >100 Gy.

A prospective single-arm trial, RTOG 0116, treated patients with positive para-aortic or high common iliac lymph nodes with extended-field radiation combined with cisplatin chemotherapy followed by brachytherapy.[441] IMRT was not allowed. The trial showed that this regimen is feasible, but the late grade 3 and 4 toxicity rate was 40%. There was no reduction in acute toxicity with the addition of amifostine.[442] The use of extended-field IMRT has been shown to reduce the risk of gastrointestinal toxicity in two retrospective series reports[443,275] and may be of benefit to patients with positive common or para-aortic lymph nodes requiring extended-field radiation with concurrent chemotherapy.

In countries or circumstances where a wait time exists and patients cannot immediately start on concurrent chemoradiation, induction chemotherapy may be considered. An alternative to cisplatin in this situation may be concurrent nedaplatin, which did not cause any nephrotoxicity in an analysis of 104 patients.[444]

Randomized Trials of Chemoradiation

Results from several cooperative oncology groups demonstrated that cisplatin-based chemotherapy, when given concurrently with RT, prolongs survival in women with locally advanced cervical cancers (Table 69.12), as well as in women with stage I to IIA disease who have metastatic disease in the pelvic lymph nodes, positive parametrial disease, or positive surgical margins at the time of primary surgery.[445]

The GOG conducted randomized Protocol 85, in which patients with carcinoma of the cervix, a clinical stage of IIB to IVA, and negative para-aortic nodes were treated with external pelvic irradiation (51 Gy) combined with 30 Gy to point A with LDR brachytherapy.[446] One hundred twenty- seven patients received 5-FU (IV infusion, 1 g/m^2 for 4 days) and cisplatin (50 mg/m^2 IV) on days 1, 29, and 30 to 33, and 191 patients received hydroxyurea (80 mg/kg orally twice weekly). With a median follow-up for survivors of 8.7 years, the 5-year survival rate in the cisplatin/5-FU arm was 60%, compared with 47% for women in the hydroxyurea arm.

TABLE 69.12 DETAILS OF THE TREATMENT PROTOCOLS OF THE FIVE RANDOMIZED TRIALS THAT FORMED THE BASIS OF THE NATIONAL CANCER INSTITUTE ANNOUNCEMENT

Author (Reference)	Number of Patients	Tumor Stage	Surgical Staging	Control Arm	Investigational Arm
Keys et al. (449) (GOG 123)	369	Bulky IB (≥4 cm)	Completion hysterectomy	XRT	XRT + cisplatin (40 mg/m² IV weekly × 6 wk)
Whitney et al. (446) (GOG 85)	368	IIB, III, IVA	Yes	XRT + hydroxyurea (80 mg/kg PO 2×/wk)	XRT + cisplatin (50 mg/m² IV days 1, 28) + 5-FU infusion (1 g/m² per day, days 2–5, 30–33)
Rose et al. (447) (GOG 120)	526	IIB, III, IVA	Yes	XRT + hydroxyurea (3 g/m² PO 2×/wk)	XRT + cisplatin (40 mg/m² weekly × 6 wk) versus XRT + cisplatin (50 mg/m² IV days 1, 29) + 5-FU infusion (1 g/m² per day, days 1–4, 29–33) + hydroxyurea PO (2 g/m² 2×/wk × 6 wk)
Eifel et al. (397) (RTOG 90-01)	389	IIB, III, IVA, IB, IIA + tumor ≥5 cm or positive pelvic nodes	Yes	XRT (pelvic + para-aortic)	XRT + cisplatin (75 mg/m² IV day 1) + 5-FU infusion (1 g/m² per day, days 1–5 × 3 q3 wk)
Peters et al. (409) (GOG 109)	243	IA2, IB, IIA (pathologic stage) + positive pelvic nodes and/or positive margins and/or microscopic involvement of parametria	Yes	XRT	XRT + cisplatin (70 mg/m² IV) + 5-FU infusion (1 g/m² days 1–5 × 4 q3 wk)

5-FU, 5-fluorouracil; PO, orally; XRT, pelvic external radiation therapy.

Modified from Viswanathan AN. Advances in the use of radiation for gynecologic cancers. *Hematol Oncol Clin North Am* 2012;26:157–168; with permission.

After completion of GOG 85, the group opened GOG 120[447,448] for the same patient population, which was a three-arm randomized trial comparing irradiation plus hydroxyurea versus irradiation plus weekly cisplatin versus irradiation plus hydroxyurea, cisplatin, and 5-FU. In 526 evaluable patients with a median follow-up for survivors of 106 months, the 5- and 10-year survival rates for women in both the weekly cisplatin and irradiation arm and the irradiation, 5-FU, and cisplatin arm were 60% and 53%, respectively, compared with 40% and 34% in the hydroxyurea and irradiation arm ($p \leq .01$). Overall survival was also significantly better in the two patient groups receiving cisplatin. Hematologic toxicity was greater in the group treated with the three drugs compared with cisplatin or hydroxyurea alone.

The RTOG conducted a randomized study of 389 patients with stage IB to IIA of >5 cm, proven positive pelvic lymph nodes, or stage IIB to IVA carcinoma of the cervix in which patients were treated with either pelvic and para-aortic irradiation (best arm of RTOG Protocol 79-20) or pelvic irradiation and three cycles of concomitant chemotherapy with cisplatin (75 mg/m²) and 4-day infusion of 5-FU (1,000 mg/m² per day).[449] Results were updated by Eifel et al.[397] With a median follow-up of 6.6 years for 228 survivors, the 8-year overall survival rate for women on the irradiation and cisplatin/5-FU arm was 67% versus 41% in the irradiation-only arm ($p < .0001$). Disease-free survival rates were 66% and 36%, respectively. There were no significant differences in late complications in the treatment groups.

Southwest Oncology Group 8797 was a study for women with FIGO stage IA2, IB, or IIA carcinoma of the cervix with metastatic disease in the pelvic lymph nodes, positive parametrial involvement, or positive surgical margins at the time of primary radical hysterectomy with total pelvic lymphadenectomy. Patients had confirmed negative para-aortic lymph nodes; if the para-aortic lymph nodes were not sampled, the patients had confirmed negative common iliac lymph nodes. One hundred twenty-seven patients were randomized to treatment with pelvic EBRT with 5-FU infusion and cisplatin, and 116 were treated with irradiation alone. The 3-year survival for women on the adjuvant cisplatin/5-FU and RT arm was 87%, compared with 77% for women on the pelvic irradiation arm.[409] The difference was statistically significant. An updated analysis with 5.2-year median follow-up reported 5-year overall survival of 80% versus 66%, favoring postoperative chemoradiation in high-risk patients.[183]

In GOG 123, 369 women were enrolled. One hundred eighty-three women with bulky (≥4 cm) stage IB carcinoma of the cervix with negative pelvic and para-aortic nodes radiographically or surgically determined were randomized to be treated with pelvic EBRT and brachytherapy, followed by extrafascial hysterectomy, and 186 received EBRT and brachytherapy with weekly cisplatin (40 mg/m²; total dose not to exceed 70 mg/week) followed by extrafascial hysterectomy.[450] In an updated analysis with median follow-up of 101 months[451] the 6-year progression-free survival rate for women treated with irradiation and cisplatin was 71%, compared with 60% for those treated with RT alone, after adjusting for age and tumor size ($p < .004$). The unadjusted 6-year overall survival rates were 78% and 64%, respectively ($p < .015$).

The results of randomized trials using concurrent chemoradiation are summarized in Table 69.13.[452] Curtin et al.[453] completed a small phase III trial in which 89 patients with high-risk stage IB or IIA undergoing radical hysterectomy and pelvic node dissection were randomized to be treated with postoperative cisplatin/bleomycin alone (44 patients) or combined with pelvic RT (45 patients). There were 9 and 10 recurrences, respectively, and survival was equivalent.

On the other hand, Pearcey et al.[454] reported on a Canadian randomized study in which 127 patients with stage IB to IIA of >5 cm or IIB carcinoma of the cervix were randomized to be treated with cisplatin (40 mg/m² weekly) and RT, and 126 patients were treated with RT alone (50.4 Gy to the pelvis combined with brachytherapy). With a median follow-up of 65 months, the 5-year survival rates were 59% and 56%, respectively ($p = .43$). There was a somewhat greater incidence of significant late morbidity in the RT-alone group (12% vs. 6%; $p = .08$). Possible explanations for the discrepancy in results between the five U.S. trials[371] and the Canadian study were analyzed by Lehman and Thomas.[445] Some theories include that a higher percentage of early-stage patients were accrued, who therefore had less of a difference in survival, given that the baseline survival rate for both arms was quite high; and that treatment time was short for both arms, again minimizing the difference in improving survival in the chemotherapy arm. This was the smallest of the randomized chemoradiation trials, and although the hazard ratio was reduced, given the factors equalizing the two arms, a larger number of patients would have possibly shown a significant difference.

A 2005 update of a meta-analysis of concomitant chemotherapy and radiation therapy found 24 trials and concluded that chemoradiation improves overall survival and progression-free survival, whether or not cisplatin was used, with absolute benefits of 10% and 13% respectively.[455] Similarly, a 2008 meta-analysis of the 13 trials that compared chemoradiotherapy to

TABLE 69.13 RANDOMIZED STUDIES OF CONCURRENT CHEMOIRRADIATION IN CERVICAL CARCINOMA

Author (Reference)	Drugs	Number of Patients	Median Follow-up Time (Year)	Survival: Chemoradiation Therapy (%)	Survival: Radiation Therapy (%)	p
Chemoirradiation Versus Radiation Alone						
Eifel et al. (368) (RTOG 9001)[a]	CF	389	6.6	67	41	<.0001
Keys et al. (450)/Stehman et al. (451) (GOG 123)	C	369	8.4	78	64	<.015
Peters et al. (409) (SWOG 8797)	CF	243	5.2	80	66	NR
Pearcey et al. (454) (NCIC)	C	253	6.9	62	58	.53
Comparative Trials of Chemoirradiation Regimens						
Whitney et al. (446) (GOG 85)	CF vs. H	368	8.7	55 CF	43 H	.018
Rose et al. (447) (GOG 120)	C vs. H	526	8.8	5 yr, 60; 10 yr, 53	5 yr, 40; 10 yr, 34	.002
	CHF vs. H			5 yr, 61; 10 yr, 53	5 yr, 40; 10 yr, 34	.002
Comparative Trials of Chemotherapy Regimens						
Lanciano et al. (460) (GOG 165)[b]	F vs. C	316	3.4	64	55	NR

C, cisplatin; F, 5-fluorouracil; GOG, Gynecologic Oncology Group; H, hydroxyurea; RTOG, Radiation Therapy Oncology Group; SWOG, Southwest Oncology Group.

[a]Eight-year results.

[b]Trial terminated early due to higher risk of treatment failure and higher mortality with 5-fluorouracil (HR = 1.37, 95% CI = 0.96–1.97).

Modified from Viswanathan AN. Advances in the use of radiation for gynecologic cancers. *Hematol Oncol Clin North Am* 2012;26(1): 157–168; with permission.

radiation found there was a 6% improvement in 5-year survival with concurrent chemoradiation (hazard ratio 0.81, $p < .001$). The effect was attributed to a reduction in both local and distant recurrence. Chemoradiation increased acute hematologic and gastrointestinal toxicity, but no confirmation was made about a difference in late toxicity.[456]

In the United States, weekly cisplatin has become the preferred approach, with less toxicity than an every 3-week regimen and the increased likelihood of completing the treatment on schedule. The number of completed cycles of weekly treatment was shown by Nugent et al.[457] to be predictive of survival. One hundred eighteen patients with locally advanced cervical cancer (stages IB2 to IVA) were treated with combination weekly cisplatin (40 mg/m^2) and radiation between 2003 and 2007. Thirty percent of patients completed fewer than six cycles of chemotherapy. In multivariate analyses, the number of chemotherapy cycles was independently predictive of progression-free survival (PFS) and overall survival (OS). Patients who received fewer than six cycles of cisplatin had a worse PFS (HR = 2.65; 95% CI = 1.35 to 5.17; $p = .0045$) and OS (HR = 4.47; 95% CI = 1.83 to 10.9; $p = .001$). Advanced stage, longer time to RT completion, and absence of brachytherapy were also associated with decreased OS and PFS ($p < .05$). Similar results were found when analysis was conducted using a breakpoint of at least but not less than five chemotherapy cycles. The authors concluded that aggressive supportive care to minimize missed chemotherapy treatments may improve survival after chemoradiation. A retrospective review[458] questioned whether cervical cancer patients should receive cisplatin 20 mg/m^2 × 5 days every 21 days concomitant with RT, or weekly 40 mg/m^2 weekly concomitant with RT, given that an advantage with regard to both acute toxicity and progression-free survival was seen in the 5-day regimen.

High-risk patients may benefit from adjuvant chemotherapy after chemoRT. A randomized trial of 515 cases of stages IIB to IVA cervical carcinoma treated with concurrent gemcitabine plus cisplatin followed by adjuvant gemcitabine and cisplatin compared to standard concurrent cisplatin with radiation showed a significant 3-year progression-free survival benefit 74% versus 65% ($p = .03$), as well as one in overall survival (HR = 0.68, 95% CI = 0.49 to 0.65).[459] Grades 3 and 4 toxicity was higher in the extended-chemotherapy arm, including 2 deaths. Ongoing trials comparing "outback" chemotherapy continue to accrue patients.

Alternatives to Concurrent Cisplatin-Based Chemoradiation

In GOG Protocol 165, patients with stages IIB to IVA cervical cancer received either radiation therapy and concurrent weekly cisplatin (40 mg/m^2) or radiation therapy and a protracted venous infusion (PVI) of 5-FU. Lanciano et al.[460] reported that the study was prematurely closed after an interim analysis showed a failure rate 35% higher and would not result in improved DFS with PVI 5-FU/RT compared with weekly cisplatin.

Lorvidhaya et al.[461] reported on 673 patients with predominantly stages IIB and IIIB disease randomized to receive either irradiation alone or combined with chemotherapy administered in an adjuvant, concurrent, or adjuvant and concurrent schedule. Concomitant chemotherapy consisted of mitomycin C (10 mg/m^2) given on days 1 and 30 and oral 5-FU (300 mg/m^2 per day) given on days 1 to 14 and 42 to 56. Adjuvant chemotherapy consisted of three cycles of oral 5-FU (200 mg/day) given for 4 weeks, with a 2-week rest every 6 weeks. With a median follow-up of 25 months, there was a statistically significant improvement in disease-free survival for all patients who received chemotherapy/RT, regardless of the timing of administration of the chemotherapy. However, the authors did not state the radiation dose delivered with brachytherapy, the total dose prescribed to point A, or the overall treatment time. In the absence of this information, the adequacy of the radiation therapy cannot be evaluated, and we cannot assume that the results of this study apply to all patients treated with irradiation.

In a randomized trial comparing monthly fluorouracil and cisplatin versus weekly cisplatin concurrent with pelvic radiation, Kim et al.[462] enrolled 158 stages IIB and IVA patients. With a median follow-up of 39 months, the acute grades 3 and 4 hematologic toxicity were significantly worse in the fluorouracil/cisplatin arm, 43% versus 26% ($p = .04$). The trial was not powered to detect a survival difference, and no difference in the overall or progression-free survival was noted.

Tseng et al.[463] published results of a study in which patients with advanced carcinoma of the cervix were randomly assigned to either RT alone or concurrent chemotherapy (cisplatin, vincristine, and bleomycin every 3 weeks for a total of four courses) and RT. After a median follow-up of 46.8 months, the disease-free survival and actuarial survival rates were 51.7% and 61.7% in the concurrent group and 53.2% and 64.5% in the RT group, respectively ($p = .27$). Treatment-related toxicity was higher with the combination therapy compared with irradiation alone (36.7% vs. 17.7%; $p = .02$).

Several small phase II studies have been performed showing no advantage to weekly paclitaxel over weekly cisplatin[464] and too high toxicity with concomitant cisplatin–paclitaxel.[462] Concurrent weekly carboplatin alone has been shown in many studies to be feasible,[466] including in the elderly; it is also an alternative in patients that have an elevated creatinine. Docetaxel and carboplatin concurrent with radiation was also found to be a feasible regimen.[467]

The GOG carried out a trial of irradiation with either concomitant hydroxyurea (HOU) or a placebo in patients with stage IIIB or IVA cervix cancer.[468] The study was criticized because patients were not surgically staged, half of the 190 patients were not evaluable, and radiation doses were low.[302] Piver et al.[469] published an update of a study of 130 patients (13 with para-aortic lymph node metastasis), 75 of whom were surgically staged. Of 66 patients who underwent surgical staging, 33 received hydroxyurea and 33 a placebo in combination with irradiation. Of the patients who did not have surgical staging, 27 received hydroxyurea and 37 received placebo. The 2-year survival was higher in the HOU group. Symonds et al.,[470] in a review of seven randomized trials, found no evidence to support the use of hydrea with RT in cervix cancer.

In larger randomized trial by the GOG reported by Stehman et al.,[471] 296 surgically staged patients with stage IIB to IVA disease and negative para-aortic nodes were randomized to irradiation plus either hydroxyurea (139 patients) or misonidazole (157 patients). Survival was not statistically different between the regimens, with 33.8% deaths in the hydroxyurea group and 38.9% deaths in the misonidazole group ($p = .25$). Failure limited to the pelvis occurred in 18% of patients in the hydroxyurea group and 23.6% in the misonidazole group. Of note, in a randomized RTOG trial of patients with stage III disease, Leibel et al.[472] and Overgaard et al.[473] reported lower survival in patients receiving misonidazole than in the patients treated with irradiation alone.

Grigsby et al.[474] published results of an RTOG study in which 120 patients with carcinoma of the cervix were randomized to receive irradiation alone or combined with misonidazole. The 5-year progression-free survival was 22% and 29%, respectively. These findings are similar to those reported by Overgaard et al.,[473] who, in a randomized study of 331 patients with carcinoma of the cervix treated with either misonidazole or a placebo and irradiation, found no significant difference in local tumor control (50% vs. 54%), disease-free survival (47% vs. 46%), or crude survival (39% vs. 45%).

Nonrandomized Studies of Chemotherapy and Irradiation

Numerous preliminary reports have been published on results of neoadjuvant/concomitant use of cisplatin and 5-FU, with or without mitomycin C, combined with irradiation to treat patients with locally advanced or recurrent carcinoma of the cervix.[475]

Trials with Cisplatin, 5-Fluorouracil, or Both

Perez and Grigsby[476] reported on 58 patients with locally advanced carcinoma of the cervix treated with concurrent 5-FU/cisplatin and irradiation and compared the results with 257 patients with similar stages treated with irradiation alone during the same period. Pelvic tumor control and disease-free and cause-specific survival were comparable. The incidence of rectal and bladder fistula was 7% in the chemoirradiation group and 4% with irradiation alone ($p = .61$).

Park et al.[434] described results in 113 patients with high-risk invasive cervical carcinoma treated with cisplatin and 5-FU. For adenocarcinoma, doxorubicin (45 mg/m² IV) was added. The patients subsequently received radiation therapy (not described in the publication). For patients with stage I or II tumors >4 cm, the 5-year survival rate was 78.3% with chemoirradiation and was 48% for 77 patients treated with RT alone ($p < .01$). For stages III and IV the rates were 69.1% and 57.4%, respectively. Toxicity with combined chemoirradiation was not significantly enhanced compared with irradiation alone.

Sardi et al.[477] reported results of three courses of cisplatin, vincristine, and bleomycin (days 1 to 3) at 10-day intervals combined with RT in 205 unselected patients with stage IB cervix cancer (tumors >2 cm) who were divided at random into two groups treated with surgery and RT or neoadjuvant chemotherapy, surgery, and irradiation. After 67 months, no difference in survival was seen in patients with tumors 2 to 4 cm in both groups (77% for control patients vs. 82% with neoadjuvant chemotherapy), but statistically significant differences were seen in bulky tumors (>4 cm): 61% versus 80% in favor of neoadjuvant chemotherapy.

Souhami et al.[478] treated 50 patients with bulky, locally advanced carcinoma of the cervix with a combination of weekly cisplatin (30 mg/m²) concurrent with RT. At 44 months, the actuarial survival rate was 65%, the total pelvic failure rate was 26%, and the distant metastasis rate was 24%. The incidence of late gastrointestinal toxicity was high, with 10 rectal ulcers (4 colostomies required for severe bleeding), 2 rectovaginal fistulas, and 2 small-bowel obstructions.

Park et al.[479] treated patients with stages I and II carcinoma of the cervix >4 cm with RT alone or concurrent or sequential chemoradiation with cisplatin and 5-FU. The 30-month survival rates were 100% with concurrent chemoirradiation, 89.5% with sequential treatment, and 79.5% with irradiation alone ($p < .05$).

Lee et al.[480] treated 40 women with cervix cancer using 50-Gy EBRT and brachytherapy; in 25 cases, three concurrent cycles of cisplatin/5-FU were given, and in 15 cases, six cycles of consolidation chemotherapy were given. There was no difference in 2-year survival between the two groups (98% to 100%). Grade 2 or greater hematologic toxicity was more frequent in the consolidation patients.

Grigsby et al.,[481] in a prospective study of 65 patients with cervical cancer and node negative on FDG-PET treated with RT alone (15 patients) or combined with concurrent weekly cisplatin (50 patients), noted a 5-year cause-specific survival of 78% and 74%, respectively. Severe complications included 1 rectovaginal fistula and 1 rectal stricture in the concurrent chemotherapy/RT group and 1 chemotherapy-related death.

Trials with Carboplatin

Katanyoo et al.[466] reported 148 patients with stages IIB to IVA cervical cancer treated with concurrent weekly carboplatin (100 mg/m² or area under the curve 2) for a median of six cycles and radiation. Among the 142 responders, 36 experienced recurrences: pelvic recurrences in 7 (4.7%), distant failure in 25 (16.9%), and both pelvic and distant in 4 (2.7%). The 2- and 5-year progression-free survival rates were 75.1% and 63.0%, respectively, with the corresponding 2- and 5-year overall survival rates of 81.9% and 63.5%. No grade 3 or 4 hematologic and nonhematologic toxicities were observed during treatment in any patients. Late grade 3 to 4 gastrointestinal or genitourinary toxicities were 10.1% and 0.7%, respectively.

Cetina et al.[482] looked at the use of weekly carboplatin in 59 elderly, diabetic, and/or hypertensive stage IB2 to IIIB cervical cancer patients. All patients completed radiation and 80% received five of six planned cycles, with 83% reaching a complete response. With a median follow-up of 20 months, 33% relapsed, and the 3 year overall survival rate was 63%. Although the regimen is safe and tolerable, it may have reduced efficacy compared to weekly cisplatin.

Trials with Mitomycin C or Tirapazamine

Mitomycin C acts as an alkylating agent and inhibits DNA and RNA synthesis. Activation of mitomycin C is increased in hypoxic conditions, and thus it acts as a hypoxic radiosensitizer.

Interstitial pneumonitis and pulmonary fibrosis are usually related to the dose of drug. Use of IV dexamethasone before administration of the drug may prevent pulmonary toxicity.

Christie et al.[432] described results in three groups of patients with stages IIB and III carcinoma of the cervix treated with pelvic irradiation and an intracavitary insertion combined with chemotherapy. Group A (64 patients) received 5-FU infusion during the first and last weeks of irradiation combined with mitomycin C (10 mg/m^2 IV). Group B (29 patients) received 5-FU without mitomycin C, and group C (84 patients) received irradiation alone. With median follow-up of 7.2 years, the 5-year survival rates were 56%, 32%, and 36%, and the local tumor control was 73%, 53%, and 50%, respectively. Toxicity was greater in group A (36% grade 3 and 4) compared with the 5-FU and irradiation group (14%) and the irradiation-alone group (20%).

Roberts et al.[483] reported on a trial in which 160 patients with locally advanced cervical cancer were randomized to receive RT alone (82 patients) or RT with concomitant mitomycin C (78 patients). The 4-year actuarial survival was 72% and 56%, respectively (p = .13), and the local recurrence-free survival rate was 78% and 63%, respectively (p = .11). There were no treatment-related deaths. No excess in nonhematologic toxicity has been observed with combined mitomycin C and irradiation.

Tirapazamine, a radiation sensitizer with selective cytotoxic effect on hypoxic cells, was combined with cisplatin in 56 patients with recurrent or metastatic cancer. After six cycles given every 21 days, 4 complete and 13 partial responses were noted. Overall 6-month survival was 56%. Better response was seen in patients who had not received radiosensitizing chemotherapy previously.[484]

Besides the usual hematologic and pelvic toxicity described in many of these studies with chemoradiation, Wun et al.,[485] in a retrospective analysis of 75 patients with gynecologic cancer who received erythropoietin and chemotherapy/RT, noted that 17 had upper- or lower-extremity thrombosis, in contrast to 2 of 72 who did not receive erythropoietin. Of note, Anders et al.,[486] in a review of the literature, reported that 6 of 128 patients (4.7%) treated with chemotherapy/RT without erythropoietin developed grade 4 or 5 thrombosis toxicity.

Trial with Bevacizumab Concurrent with RT

RTOG 0417 treated patients with once-weekly cisplatin (40 mg/m^2) chemotherapy and standard pelvic radiotherapy and brachytherapy. Bevacizumab was administered at 10 mg/kg intravenously every 2 weeks for three cycles. A total of 49 patients were evaluable. The median follow-up was 12.4 months (range, 4.6 to 31.4 months). There were no treatment-related serious adverse events. There were 15 (31%) protocol-specified, treatment-related adverse events within 90 days of treatment start; the most common were hematologic (12 of 15; 80%). Eighteen (37%) occurred during treatment or follow-up at any time.[487]

Trial with Epidermal Growth Factor Receptor Inhibition Concurrent with RT

Nogueira-Rodrigues et al.[488] reported a phase I study administering escalating doses of erlotinib (50/100/150 mg) combined with cisplatin (40 mg/m^2, weekly, five cycles) and radiotherapy (external beam, 4,500 cGy in 25 fractions, followed by four fractions/600 cGy weekly of brachytherapy) in squamous cell cervical carcinoma patients, stages IIB to IIIB. Fifteen patients were enrolled, 3 at dose level (DL) 50 mg, 4 at DL 100 mg, and 8 at DL 150 mg. Three patients did not complete the planned schedule. One patient at DL 100 mg withdrew informed consent due to grade 2 rash; at DL 150 mg, 1 patient presented with Raynaud's syndrome and had cisplatin interrupted, and another patient presented with grade 4 hepatotoxicity. The latter was interpreted as dose-limiting toxicity, and a new cohort of 150 mg was started. No further grade 4 toxicity occurred. Grade 3 toxicity occurred in 6 cases: diarrhea in 3 patients, rash in 2 patients, and leukopenia in 1 patient. Treatment did not lead to limiting in-field toxicity.

Intra-Arterial Chemotherapy

Intra-arterial infusion of chemotherapeutic agents in cervical carcinoma was used for some years based on the distinct arterial supply to the tumor-bearing area. Unfortunately, the responses have been uncommon and short, and the toxicity and complication rates have been significant.[489]

Onishi et al.[490] evaluated intra-arterial cisplatin through catheters inserted into both internal iliac arteries in cervix carcinoma. Patients were randomized into a concurrent intra-arterial infusion of cisplatin with RT (18 patients) or RT alone (15 patients). Five-year overall survival rates were 44.4% and 50%, respectively. In the group receiving intra-arterial infusion, grade 3 or 4 late bowel complications were seen in 44% and grade 3 or 4 myelosuppression in 33%, significantly more than in the RT group.

Neoadjuvant Chemotherapy

Thomas[491] summarized the rationale and potential limitations of neoadjuvant chemotherapy in carcinoma of the cervix. Although response rates to the chemotherapy are between 30% and 85%, none of the studies showed an advantage for pelvic tumor control or survival.[492–499] Colombo et al.,[500] in a review of the literature, concluded that the role of neoadjuvant chemotherapy followed by radiation and by concomitant chemotherapy or by surgery is controversial because no significant advantages in survival or local control have been shown, and receiving upfront chemotherapy may compromise immune status and the patient's ability to receive definitive treatment with radiation or surgery.

Souhami et al.[501] randomized 107 patients with stage IIIB carcinoma of the cervix to treatment with irradiation alone or combined with bleomycin, vincristine, mitomycin, and cisplatin. The overall 5-year survival rate for the neoadjuvant-treated patients was 23%, in contrast to 39% for those treated with irradiation alone (p = .02). Locoregional and distant failure rates were similar in both groups.

Kumar et al.[502] reported a randomized trial in which 94 patients with carcinoma of the cervix were treated with chemotherapy (two cycles of bleomycin, ifosfamide-mesna, and cisplatin) followed by RT, and 90 patients were treated with irradiation alone. In the chemotherapy/RT group, 32-month survival was 63% for stage IIB and 50% for stage III, and in the RT group, the rate was 59% for stage IIB and 27% for stage IIIB tumors (differences not statistically significant). There was no difference in radiation-induced toxicity between the two groups.

In a Swedish study,[498] 47 patients with carcinoma of the cervix were randomized to be treated with irradiation alone (64.8 Gy, 1.8-Gy fractions) and 47 with a combination of three cycles of cisplatin and 5 days of 5-FU administered every third week, followed by the same pelvic irradiation. The 5-year disease-free survival rates were 70% with chemoirradiation and 57% with irradiation alone (p = .07). The incidences of pelvic recurrence were 60% and 47%, respectively, and for distant metastasis they were 19% and 35%, respectively. Two patients in the chemoirradiation and 1 in the irradiation-alone group died as a consequence of therapy.

Response to Chemotherapy Alone for Patients with Metastatic or Recurrent Disease

Cisplatin has been combined with other cytotoxic agents. Long et al.[503] conducted a randomized study comparing methotrexate, vinblastine, doxorubicin, and cisplatin (MVAC), cisplatin/topotecan, or cisplatin alone in patients with advanced cervical cancer. The MVAC arm was closed after 4 deaths in 63 patients. In 294 patients assigned to the other arms, response rate was

27% for cisplatin/topotecan and 13% for cisplatin alone, with median survival of 9.4 and 6.5 months, respectively.

Paclitaxel, a natural product found initially in the bark of the western yew tree, produces depolymerization and irreversible bundling of tubulin in the cell. It has been shown to have a radiosensitizing effect and may also be considered for patients with metastatic disease. Rose et al.[504] reported on a phase II study of 44 patients in which the starting dose was paclitaxel (135 mg/m^2, maximum 170 mg/m^2) infused over 24 hours, followed by cisplatin (75 mg/m^2) every 21 days. Forty patients (90.9%) had received prior radiation therapy. A median of six courses of chemotherapy was given. Of the 41 assessable patients, 5 (12.2%) had a complete response and 14 (34.1%) had a partial response. Vinorelbine is a semisynthetic derivative of vinblastine. In a phase II trial in patients with prior irradiation, a 28% response rate was observed.[505] Other trials used the drug as neoadjuvant chemotherapy; in 42 patients, 2 complete and 17 partial responses (45%) were observed.[506,507]

Irinotecan and topotecan are camptothecin derivatives whose cytotoxic mechanism is believed to target topoisomerase I.[508] An international phase II trial reported a similar 21% response rate in patients predominantly with prior irradiation (1 complete and 8 partial responses among 42 patients).[509]

Gemcitabine, a nucleoside analogue, showed a 4.5% partial response and 36% stable disease in 22 patients.[510] In combination with cisplatin, it was evaluated in 32 women with previously treated cervix cancer (initial dose 800 mg/m^2 on days 1 and 8, then every 28 days); there were 7 (22%) partial responses and 12 stable disease responses.[511]

A phase II trial of docetaxel and gemcitabine showed an overall response rate of 21%. With a median survival of 7 months, 39% were alive at 1 year. Doxetaxel combined with carboplatin has been shown to have a 25% response rate.[467]

A four-arm comparison of cisplatin/paclitaxel versus cisplatin/vinorelbine, cisplatin/gemcitabine, or cisplatin/topotecan found that the standard arm of cisplatin/paclitaxel remained the best option for patients with stage IVB, recurrent or persistent cervical carcinoma.[512]

In a phase II GOG study of cetuximab 400 mg/m^2 initial dose followed by 250 mg/m^2 weekly until disease progression or prohibitive toxicity, 38 patients (15%) had no progression for at least 6 months. The median OS was 7 months. When cetuximab was combined with cisplatin, no additional benefit beyond cisplatin was identified.[513]

Ifosfamide, paclitaxel, and carboplatin as a triple regimen showed a 33% objective complete or partial response, with an overall median survival of 10 months.[514] Antiangiogenic tyrosine kinase inhibitors pazopanib and lapatinib were tested in 230 patients with stage IVB persistent/recurrent cervical carcinoma. An improvement in progression-free and overall survival was seen with pazopanib.[515]

Studies with Radiation Alone

For patients unable to tolerate concurrent chemotherapy or in countries where chemotherapy is not readily available, radiation alone may be used as an alternative to chemoradiation. Mendenhall et al.[516] analyzed 1211 patients treated with radiation alone with a minimum follow up of 3 years. In patients with Stage IB and IIA disease there was no significant correlation between doses to these points and pelvic tumor control. In Stage IIB doses of less than 6000 cGy to point A correlated with a high pelvic failure rate (8 of 12, 66.7%) in contrast to doses of 6000 to 9000 cGy (61 of 261, 23.4%) or higher than 9000 cGy (10 of 74, 13.5%) (P 0.01). In Stage III the pelvic failure rate with doses below 6000 cGy to point A was 72% (18 of 25) compared to 39% (71 of 180) for 6000 to 9000 cGy or 35% (27 of 77) with doses above 9000 cGy ($p \leq 0.01$).

Thoms et al.[517] reported on 363 patients with bulky endocervical carcinoma treated with curative intent (246 with irradiation alone and 117 with irradiation and surgery); 10-year survival was 45% and 64%, respectively. In a subset of 48 patients with similar tumors treated with irradiation alone and 45 treated with irradiation and surgery, the 10-year survival rates were comparable, and the pelvic tumor control rates were 90% and 87%, respectively.

Eifel et al.[168] evaluated 1,526 patients, of whom 371 had tumors 6 cm or greater. There were biases in treatment selection, but a statistically significantly higher 10-year survival rate was noted in patients treated with irradiation and surgery (64% vs. 45%). Tumor diameter was highly significant as a prognostic factor, and the authors concluded that only patients with lesions >8 cm in diameter benefited from adjuvant hysterectomy. In the same study, 98 patients with stages IB and IIB bulky endocervical carcinomas (≥6 cm in diameter) were treated with RT alone. Twenty-four patients received <6,000 mgh of intracavitary treatment, and 73 received higher doses. Despite having somewhat more favorably treated tumors, patients who received <6,000 mgh had a higher rate of pelvic recurrence at 5 years (33%) than those who received higher doses (16%; $p = .03$). Actuarial 5-year survival rates were 44% and 60% for low- and high-dose groups, respectively ($p = .14$).

Kim et al.[518] assessed the prognostic factors for pelvic tumor control in 40 patients with FIGO stage IB or IIA carcinoma and 25 patients with stage IIB carcinoma classified as barrel shaped (i.e., at least 5 cm in diameter) treated with curative intent. Seventy-two percent were treated with RT alone and 28% with RT and extrafascial hysterectomy. The extent of tumor regression after external-beam radiation therapy correlated with the likelihood of local tumor control ($p = .02$). For patients treated with radiation therapy alone, increased brachytherapy dose was associated with better local tumor control. The 10-year overall and cause-specific survival rates were 53% and 68%, respectively, and did not differ significantly between treatment groups.

Paley et al.[519] reported on 57 patients with barrel-shaped (mean diameter, 5 to 9 cm) cervical carcinoma treated with preoperative EBRT and BT (mean dose to point A, 79.6 Gy) followed by extrafascial hysterectomy 6 to 8 weeks later. Residual disease was present in 35 (61%) of the hysterectomy specimens; tumor sterilization correlated significantly with the mean dose to point A ($p = .016$). Ninety-five percent of the patients with negative specimens remained clinically free of disease at their last follow-up versus 31% of those with residual disease ($p < .001$).

The GOG and RTOG conducted a randomized phase III clinical trial in which 282 patients with carcinoma of the cervix measuring 4 cm or greater (exophytic or barrel shaped) were treated with either external-beam and intracavitary irradiation or a slightly lower dose of intracavitary irradiation and the same pelvic EBRT followed by an extrafascial hysterectomy.[520] The survival rates were 61.4% for irradiation alone and 64.4% for the combined irradiation and surgery group. The incidence of recurrences was 43.3% in the irradiation group compared to 34.5% with combined therapy ($p = .081$). The incidence of local recurrences was 25.8% and 14.4%, respectively. The incidence of grade 3 and 4 sequelae of therapy was 10.5% and 9.8%, respectively. Thus, the addition of hysterectomy to standard irradiation did not significantly affect survival, although there was a small reduction in the local recurrence rate. When combined therapy is used, the dose of irradiation delivered to the lymph nodes, the time of the operation, and the pathologic examination of the specimens are critical in determining the presence of postirradiation residual tumor.

Perez et al.[36] noted that in patients with primary carcinoma of the uterine cervix who had endometrial stromal invasion or tumor only in the curettings, the addition of a hysterectomy did not improve the survival rate because most of the patients failed at distant sites.

For stage IIB tumors treated with irradiation alone, the 5-year survival rate is 60% to 65%. The pelvic failure rate ranges from 18% to 39%. In an analysis of the Patterns of Care

Study in 157 patients who had stage IIB disease, Coia et al.[521] reported a better 4-year survival rate (67% and 54%) and in-field tumor control rate (78% and 68%) in patients with unilateral versus bilateral parametrial involvement, respectively. Similarly, in a review of 1,178 patients with stage IIB disease, the 5-year survival rates were 70% with medial parametrial and 58% with lateral parametrial involvement (p = .004).[522] Kim et al.,[523] in patients with stage IIB disease, found a correlation of point A dose and incidence of pelvic failures.

In stage IIIB carcinoma, the 5-year survival rates range from 25% to 48%, and pelvic failure rates range from 38% to 50%.[165,524] Hanks et al.,[525] reporting on the Patterns of Care Study, noted a 28% probability of 5-year survival in patients with stage III carcinoma of the cervix treated in a large number of facilities in the United States versus 60% survival in selected large centers (extended survey). Later, Komaki et al.[526] reported a significant increase in local pelvic tumor control (69%) in patients with stage III carcinoma of the cervix treated in 1983, compared with 37% and 49% in earlier periods (p = .03). The 5-year survival rate increased from 25% to 47% (p = .02). The improvement in pelvic tumor control may be associated with higher external-beam doses but more likely is related to the substantial increase in the percentage of patients receiving brachytherapy (96%) and more careful dosimetry and dose calculations for intracavitary therapy. They noted a decrease in major complications from 15% in the 1973 and 13% in the 1978 Patterns of Care Surveys to 7% in 1983. Montana et al.[527] reported that calculation of doses to the bladder and rectum were performed in 80% and 76% of patients, respectively, in the 1983 survey, which may also have resulted in decreased toxicity.

Arthur et al.,[528] in 89 patients with stage IIIB carcinoma of the cervix treated with external irradiation and brachytherapy, observed a locoregional tumor control rate of 22.5% and a disease-free survival rate of 15% in 16 patients treated with 78 Gy or lower doses to point A, in comparison with 53% and 47%, respectively, in 24 patients receiving higher doses.

Horiot et al.[529] reported the results of a French cooperative study of 1,383 patients with invasive carcinoma of the uterus treated with irradiation alone following the MD Anderson Hospital treatment guidelines. Survival and locoregional tumor control were similar in both groups, except in stage III, in which the pelvic and central failure rates were lower in the French patients, may be because of different tumor volumes or socioeconomic factors. Major urinary complications were noted in 2% of the patients. Grade 3 bowel complications occurred in 3% of the patients with stages I and IIA disease and in 7% of patients with stages IIB and III disease. Barillot et al.[530] updated the results in 642 patients; the analysis was divided into three periods: 1970 to 1978 (use of standard prescriptions), 1979 to 1984 (implementation of individual adjustments), and 1985 to 1994 (systematic individual adjustments). There was a significant reduction of the external radiation dose (>40 Gy in 47% of patients before 1979 vs. 36% after 1984), use of parametrial boost (55% vs. 39%), use of vaginal cylinder (28% vs. 11.5%), and combined intracavitary and external irradiation volume (842 vs. 503 cm^3 on average). The 5-year actuarial toxicity rates were as follows: grade 2, 23.5%; grade 3, 10%; and grade 4, 3%. The three main predictive factors for rectal and bladder sequelae were increased external radiation dose, higher dose rate at reference points, and whole-vagina brachytherapy.

Marcial et al.[531] described results of a randomized trial in 301 patients with stages IIB, III, and IVA carcinoma of the uterine cervix treated with split-course irradiation (10 fractions of 2.5 Gy, five weekly doses up to 25 Gy, followed by a rest period of 2 weeks, and an additional 25 Gy delivered in the same manner) or continuous irradiation (30 fractions of 1.7 Gy daily, five times per week, total dose 51 Gy) combined with LDR brachytherapy for 30 Gy to point A. There was no significant difference in tumor control, acute or late complications, or survival in the two groups.

In patients with stage IVA disease, the 5-year survival rates range from 18% to 34%, and pelvic failures from 60% to 80% after definitive irradiation.[260] Million et al.[261] reported 18 of 53 patients (34%) with bladder involvement surviving without disease after definitive irradiation, results comparable with those obtained with exenteration. Kramer et al.[260] reported on 48 patients with stage IVA carcinoma of the cervix treated with definitive RT. Patients with minimal parametrial involvement had a 5-year survival rate of 46%, compared with only 5% for those with extensive parametrial tumor. The major complication rate was 22%, consisting mostly of vesicovaginal fistula in 5 patients.

Crozier et al.[532] described equivalent 5-year survival rates after salvage pelvic exenteration (37% in 35 patients with adenocarcinoma and 39% in 70 patients with squamous cell carcinoma). In the adenocarcinoma group, 14 of 22 patients, and in the squamous cell-carcinoma group, 14 of 30 patients had distant metastases after pelvic exenteration.

Combination of Irradiation and Surgery

Preoperative Chemoirradiation

Bulky endocervical tumors and the so-called barrel-shaped cervix have a higher incidence of central recurrence, pelvic and para-aortic lymph node metastasis, and distant dissemination.[533] In the setting of plain x-ray, point-based planning for brachytherapy, because of the inability of intracavitary sources to encompass the entire tumor in a high-dose volume, larger doses of external radiation to the whole pelvis or extrafascial hysterectomy, or both, have been advocated to improve therapeutic results.[4] Alternatively, the use of 3D planning for the brachytherapy component significantly improves survival,[534] and the ability to dose escalate due to more precise dose delivery improves local control.[535] In rare cases with large residual after 45 Gy external beam, an extrafasical hysterectomy may be considered 6–12 weeks after completion of preoperative irradiation (45 Gy to the whole pelvis and one intracavitary LDR insertion for 5,500 mgh, delivering approximately 50 Gy to point A, with a total dose to point A of 70 Gy, or the equivalent dose in HDR, approximately three fractions of 6 Gy per fraction). Higher doses of irradiation alone yield equivalent pelvic tumor control and survival rates.[168,302]

Keys et al.[450] reported on 183 women with bulky (≥4 cm) stage IB carcinoma of the cervix with negative pelvic and para-aortic nodes radiographically treated with pelvic EBRT and brachytherapy, followed by extrafascial hysterectomy, or EBRT and brachytherapy (to 70 Gy) with weekly cisplatin followed by extrafascial hysterectomy. A significant survival advantage was seen with the combination of concurrent chemoradiation. However, in comparison to other trials, the survival was not significantly improved with the addition of a hysterectomy. The use of PET scanning to determine residual disease allows selection of patients who may be appropriate candidates for a hysterectomy after completion of external-beam treatment.[90] Therefore, patients should receive definitive doses of chemoradiation, with hysterectomy reserved for salvage in patients with either gross residual disease or PET-positive disease that is biopsy proven at 3 months after completion of radiation. A subsequent reanalysis including GOG 123 and GOG 71 analyzed 464 patients allocated to pelvic radiation (75 Gy, n = 291) plus hysterectomy or to pelvic radiation (75 Gy) and cisplatin (40 mg/m^2, n = 176) plus hysterectomy. A benefit to chemoradiation was seen for patients who had a poor response.[536]

Morice et al.[537] reported a randomized trial of 61 patients treated with adjuvant hysterectomy versus none after EBRT with concurrent weekly cisplatin and vaginal brachytherapy (15 Gy to intermediate-risk CTV) for stage IB2 or II cervical cancer. Hysterectomy increased the number of deaths, with an

11% nonsignificant survival advantage in the no-hysterectomy arm (86% vs. 97%). As a result of this trial, routine adjuvant hysterectomy is no longer practiced for patients who have no residual disease at 6 weeks after chemoradiation.

Motton et al.[538] retrospectively reviewed 171 patients treated with chemoradiation followed by simple extrafascial hysterectomy or extended hysterectomy. There was no difference in survival or complication rate based on type of surgery. Leguevaque et al.[539] reported on 111 patients treated with or without adjuvant hysterectomy after chemoradiation; there was no advantage to overall survival, but there was a significant difference in recurrence rates.

Touboul et al.[540] reported on toxicities for 150 patients with stages IB2 to IVA cervical cancer treated at Institut Gustave Roussy with extrafascial versus modified radical hysterectomy after chemoradiation. After a median follow-up of 3.6 years, 15% had grade 2 or greater side effects, including lymphedema, ureteral fistula, bowel fistula, iliac and vessel rupture. There were 2 postoperative deaths. Modified radical versus extrafascial hysterectomy had a higher odds ratio (OR) for complications of 2.4 ($p = .04$), as did the presence of residual disease.

Elective Para-Aortic Lymph Node Irradiation

Rotman et al.[412] updated results of an RTOG randomized study of 337 patients with stage IIB carcinoma of the uterine cervix with no clinical or radiographic evidence of para-aortic lymphadenopathy who, in addition to standard pelvic irradiation, were randomized to electively receive or not 45 Gy to the para-aortic region (1.6- to 1.8-Gy fractions). The 10-year survival rate was 55% for patients receiving elective para-aortic irradiation and 44% for those treated to the pelvis only ($p = .02$). The locoregional tumor control rate was similar (69% in the para-aortic node–irradiated group and 65% for the pelvis-irradiated group). The 10-year grade 4 or 5 (major) complication rate was 8% in the group receiving para-aortic irradiation, compared with 4% in patients treated with pelvic irradiation alone ($p = .06$).

A similar randomized study was reported by Haie et al.[541] and the European Organization for Research and Treatment of Cancer (EORTC) on 441 patients with cervical carcinoma, including stage III, who had no evidence of para-aortic lymph node involvement. In the study group, the para-aortic area either received or did not receive 45 Gy with external-beam irradiation. No statistically significant difference was found between the two treatment arms with regard to local tumor control, distant metastases, or survival. However, the incidence of para-aortic and distant metastases without pelvic failure was significantly higher in patients receiving pelvic irradiation alone. The incidence of small-bowel injury was 0.9% in the pelvic irradiation group and 2.3% in the pelvic plus para-aortic irradiation group. A severe complication rate of 9% was observed in patients receiving para-aortic irradiation, compared with 4.8% in those treated to the pelvis only.

Sood et al.[542] treated 54 patients with cervix cancer using extended fields (45 Gy) and HDR brachytherapy; 44 received concurrent cisplatin (20 mg/m^2 per day for 5 days during week 1 and 4 and once after the second HDR insertion). During a median follow-up of 28 months, 6 patients had died. The 3-year local tumor control was 100% and 85%, respectively. Late toxicity was 10% and 6%, respectively.

Huang et al.[235] assessed 758 patients and found that 38 (5%) and 42 (6%) had isolated and nonisolated para-aortic lymph node (PALN) recurrences after a median follow-up of 50 months (range, 2 to 159 months), respectively. The 3-year and 5-year overall survival rate after PALN recurrence was 35% and 28%, respectively, with those with isolated recurrences faring better than those with a nonisolated recurrence ($p < .001$). An SCC-Ag level of >40 ng/mL ($p < .001$), advanced parametrial involvement (score 4 to 6; $p = .002$), and the presence of pelvic lymphadenopathy ($p = .007$) were independent factors associated with PALN relapse on multivariate analysis. This group subsequently identified pretreatment CEA of ≥10 ng/mL as an additional risk factor of PALN relapse after definitive concurrent chemo-radiation therapy (CCRT) for SCC of the uterine cervix in patients with pretreatment SCC-Ag levels of <10 ng/mL.[236] The role of prophylactic para-aortic radiation, particularly in patients with large tumor size, parametrial involvement, or involved pelvic lymph nodes, must be carefully weighed against the potential toxicities of para-aortic radiation.

METASTASES TO PARA-AORTIC LYMPH NODES

Para-aortic lymph node metastases are frequently combined with distant dissemination but are clinically apparent in only 10% to 20% of patients who have recurrences.

Varia et al.[543] reported on GOG Protocol 125, in which 87 patients with biopsy-confirmed para-aortic lymph nodes from cervical cancer were treated with extended-field irradiation (45 Gy in 1.5-Gy fractions) and higher doses to the pelvis (approximately 80 Gy to point A) in combination with 5-FU and cisplatin. The 3-year progression-free survival rate was 33%, and the overall survival rate was 39%. Grades 3 and 4 hematologic toxicity were noted in 13 patients (15%) and chronic proctitis in 3 (3.5%), and 4 patients (4.6%) required surgery for rectal complications.

Nelson et al.[390] reported on 104 patients with stages II and III cervical carcinoma who had exploratory laparotomy and para-aortic lymph node biopsies; 12.5% of patients had stage IIA disease, 14.9% had stage IIB disease, and 38.4% had stage III disease had para-aortic lymph node metastases. They were treated with 60 Gy to the para-aortic region. Within 4 years, 50% of these patients had distant metastases, and only 1 out of 13 was alive. There was no significant increase in complications in the patients receiving para-aortic irradiation (39% and 32%). The authors concluded that the main goal of exploratory laparotomy and para-aortic lymph node biopsy is to define the extent of disease.

Lovecchio et al.[544] noted a 50% 5-year survival rate in 36 patients with stages IB and IIA cervical carcinoma who had histologically confirmed para-aortic lymph node metastases treated with RT (including 45 Gy to the para-aortic lymph nodes). Fourteen of 31 evaluable patients had pelvic recurrences (12 combined with distant metastases). Unfortunately, the authors did not specify how many patients had para-aortic recurrences, although they reported 4 abdominal failures.

Stryker and Mortel[545] determined survival after extended-field treatment of para-aortic lymph node metastasis plus brachytherapy or pelvic boost in 35 patients; 5-year survival was 41.7% for 12 patients with microscopic para-aortic lymph node metastasis and 26.1% for 23 patients with grossly enlarged lymph nodes. Three patients (8.6%) had grade 4 morbidity.

Grigsby et al.[546] reviewed 43 patients with cervical cancer and biopsy-proven positive para-aortic lymph nodes treated with external irradiation to the pelvis and para-aortic regions (45 to 50 Gy) combined with brachytherapy. The 5-year overall survival rate was 32%, and the cause-specific survival rate was 49%. Tumor recurrence occurred in 20 patients (3 in the pelvis, 9 in pelvis and distant metastasis, and 8 in distant metastasis only). Severe grade 3 complications occurred in 2 patients (1 had an enterovaginal fistula and the other had radiation myelitis).

Hacker et al.,[547] in 437 patients with invasive cervical carcinoma, 222 of whom were treated with radical hysterectomy and lymphadenectomy, identified 34 in whom resection of bulky pelvic or para-aortic lymph nodes was carried out without a complete lymphadenectomy. Thirty-three patients received pelvic external irradiation, and 28 combined pelvic and para-aortic extended-field irradiation (50.4 Gy in 1.8-Gy fractions using a four-field technique). Four cycles of cisplatin were administered to 23 patients. The 5-year survival was 80%

TABLE 69.14 RESULTS OF EXTENDED-FIELD IRRADIATION FOR PARA-AORTIC LYMPH NODE METASTASES

Author (Reference)	Number of Patients	Para-Aortic Dose (Gy)	Percentage Disease-Free Survival		Incidence of Severe Complications (%)
			2–3 Years	5 Years	
Irradiation Alone					
Piver et al. (881) (two cohorts)	21	60	9.6	61.9	–
	10	44–50	43	10.0	–
Potish (268)	81	43.5–50.75	40	2.4	–
Lovecchio et al. (544)	36	45	70	50.0	–
Podczaski et al. (347)	35	42.5–51	38	29.0	9
Kodaira et al. (349)	97	50–70	32	–	–
Irradiation and Chemotherapy					
Chou et al. (550)	26	50	19	51.0	20
Kim et al. (785)	12	–	50	–	–
Singh et al. (786)	14	–	–	–	–
Varia et al. (543)	95	45	39[a]	14.0	–
Grigsby et al. (548)	29	48 (twice a day)	49	49.0	–
Malfetano et al. (549)	13	45	62	0	–
Podczaski et al. (347)	33	42–51	37	31.0	9
Small et al. (441)	26	45–64.8	46	–	20
Kim et al. (887)	33	45–65	–	42	–
Rajasooriyar et al. (888)	39	50.4–54	–	19.4	18

[a]Only six patients treated with chemotherapy.

Modified from Goodman HM, Bowling MC, Nelson JH Jr. Cervical malignancies. In: Knapp RC, Berkowitz RS, eds. *Gynecologic Oncology.* New York: Macmillan, 1986;225–273, with permission.

in patients with pelvic and common iliac nodes and 48% in those with positive para-aortic lymph nodes. Serious long-term morbidity occurred in 6 patients (18%). Radiation enteritis was observed in 5 patients, leading to small-bowel obstruction necessitating resection.

Grigsby et al.[548] evaluated twice-daily external irradiation to the pelvis and para-aortic nodes (1.2 Gy at 4- to 6-hour intervals, 5 days/week) combined with brachytherapy and concurrent chemotherapy in 29 patients with carcinoma of the cervix and positive para-aortic lymph nodes. EBRT doses were 24 to 48 Gy to the whole pelvis, 12 to 36 Gy parametrial boost, and 48 Gy to the para-aortics, with additional boost to a total dose of 54 to 58 Gy to known metastatic para-aortic sites. One or two LDR brachytherapy applications were performed to deliver a total dose of 85 Gy to point A. Cisplatin (75 mg/m^2, days 1 and 22) and 5-FU (1,000 mg/m^2 per 24 hours for 4 days, days 1 and 22) were given for two or three cycles. Hyperfractionated external radiation therapy was completed in 86% (25 of 29). Radiation therapy toxicity was grade 2 in 34%, grade 3 in 21%, and grade 4 in 28%. An unacceptably high rate (31%, 9 of 29) of grade 4 nonhematologic toxicity was recorded. With a median follow-up of 18.9 months, at 2 years the overall survival rate was 47%, and the probability of locoregional failure was 49%.

Malfetano et al.[549] treated 67 patients with carcinoma of the cervix (44 with stage IIB and 23 with stage III disease) with cisplatin (1 mg/kg up to 60 mg weekly) and extended field radiation therapy, including the para-aortic nodes, and brachytherapy; 75% were alive without evidence of disease with a mean follow-up of 47.5 months.

Chou et al.[550] treated 19 patients with isolated para-aortic lymph node metastasis from cervix cancer, 14 of them with chemoradiation, 4 with chemotherapy, and 1 with irradiation alone. Seven of the 14 patients receiving chemoradiation survived.

Goodman et al.[551] compiled survival statistics on patients with para-aortic lymph node metastasis and found an average 5-year survival rate of approximately 40% (Table 69.14).

CARCINOMA OF THE CERVICAL STUMP

A supracervical hysterectomy, which removes the uterus and leaves the cervix behind, may be performed for benign conditions of the uterus. The use of subtotal hysterectomy has declined, given the persistent risk of cervical cancer arising in the remnant tissue and the difficulty of managing cancer of the cervical stump.

It is important to divide carcinoma of the cervical stump into true, when the first symptom occurs 3 or more years after subtotal hysterectomy, or coincidental, when the symptoms are noticed before the third postoperative year. This separation is important because the prognosis for true carcinoma of the stump is significantly better than for coincidental lesions, in which carcinoma was probably present when the hysterectomy was performed.[302]

The natural history and patterns of spread of carcinoma of the cervical stump are similar to those of the cervix in the intact uterus. The diagnostic workup, clinical staging, and basic principles of therapy are the same. Treatment also follows similar paradigms. When surgery is indicated for early stage I tumors, it may be more difficult because of the previous surgical procedures and the presence of adhesions in the pelvis. With radiation therapy, external-beam treatments are identical, although small bowel may be adherent to the superior portion of the cervix due to scar tissue, and using the prone position, as well as having the patient maintain a full bladder for treatment, may aid in attempting to move the small bowel out of the radiated field. Whole-pelvic radiation is recommended, with the superior border set at the level of the bifurcation of the common iliac nodes as determined by a CT simulation, or at the L4–5 interspace for those planned with plain film radiographs. A dose of 45 Gy in 1.8-Gy fractions over 5 weeks is the most commonly recommended dose, with concurrent weekly cisplatin at 40 mg/m^2 given for five doses. For brachytherapy, if >2 cm of the endocervical canal remain, it is best to insert a short tandem surrounded by ovoids, a ring, or, if indicated due to vaginal extension or lateral extension, interstitial catheters. For low–dose-rate insertions, as many sources as technically feasible should be inserted in the remaining cervical canal. For HDR brachytherapy, the tandem should extend from the cervical os superiorly to the full extent of the canal. When there is no opportunity to insert any sources in the cervical canal, an interstitial implant to bring the tumor dose to approximately 80 to 90 Gy for brachytherapy after completing a standard dose of 45 Gy to the whole pelvis is recommended while monitoring the radiation dose to the organs at risk (OAR). The use of external-beam radiation alone is not recommended due to the significant mobility of the cervix due to bladder motion, the low dose tolerance of the surrounding small bowel, and the high dose of radiation necessary for cure in patients with bulky disease. Total dose (external and LDR intracavitary brachytherapy) to the upper vaginal mucosa should not exceed 150 Gy, and tolerance doses to small volumes (D_{2cc}) of the bladder (90 to 100 Gy) or rectum and sigmoid (70 to 75 Gy) should be carefully monitored.

The 5-year survival rate for carcinoma of the cervical stump treated with irradiation is similar to that reported for patients with carcinoma of the intact uterus.[552,553] The anatomic sites of failure and the incidence of recurrences are similar to those of patients in whom the uterus is intact. Distant metastases also follow the same distribution. In 253 patients with carcinoma of the cervical stump treated at MD Anderson Cancer Center, median survival was 203, 140, and 32 months for stages I, II, and III, respectively.[554] Kovalic et al.[552] reported on 70 patients with carcinoma of the surgical stump treated with irradiation; 16 also underwent a surgical procedure. The 10-year disease-free survival was 79% for stage IB, 66% for stage IIB, and 39% for stage IIIB disease. The pelvic failure rates were 10%, 9%, and 50%, respectively. Major gastrointestinal complications were noted in 9% of patients and urinary complications in 3.8%. The results are comparable with those seen in patients treated for invasive carcinoma of the cervix with an intact uterus.

Hannoun-Levi et al.[555] published results in 77 patients treated for carcinoma of the cervical stump. Treatment consisted of a combination of EBRT and brachytherapy, and, in a few cases, patients underwent surgery or interstitial brachytherapy. Three-year pelvic tumor control was achieved in 59 of 77 patients (76.6%); tumor control probabilities were 77%, 73.7%, and 56% in patients with stage I, II, and III tumors, respectively. Late complications were grade 2 in 5 patients (6.5%); grade 3 in 1 patient (1.3%), and grade 4 in 2 patients (2.6%).

Hellstrom et al.[556] published a retrospective study of 145 patients treated for carcinoma of the cervical stump, representing 2.2% of all cervical cancers. Three control cases to each case were matched from the cohort of cases with cervical carcinoma with intact uterus. The dose of irradiation from the intracavitary application given to the stump cancers was lower than for comparable cases with intact uterus. Long-term prognosis for squamous cell carcinoma of the uterine stump was comparable to that of the ordinary cervical carcinomas. Stump adenocarcinomas had a worse prognosis compared with adenocarcinoma of the intact uterus ($p < .07$) and with squamous cell carcinoma stump ($p = .05$). The complication rate was higher for stump cancer cases compared with that for cervical cancers with an intact uterus.

Because of the close proximity of the bladder, rectum, and small intestine to the intracavitary sources and to the often higher doses of external-beam irradiation given to the whole pelvis, complications are somewhat more frequent than in carcinoma of the cervix with an intact uterus. Care in brachytherapy treatment planning, including the use of 3D-based treatment planning to minimize dose to the normal tissues, should be considered.

SMALL-CELL CARCINOMA OF THE CERVIX

Small-cell carcinoma of the cervix, like its counterparts in the lung and other anatomic locations, has a high proliferation rate and marked propensity for regional lymph node and distant metastases. Miller et al.[557] demonstrated that all small-cell carcinomas of the cervix are aneuploid, compared with only 30% of large-cell nonkeratinizing squamous carcinomas. The incidence of lymphatic vascular space invasion is 80% to 90%, and that of lymph node metastases has been reported to be 40% to 67%.[558] These patients must be evaluated in conjunction with a medical oncologist; the workup should include bone marrow aspiration biopsy of the iliac crest and other tests to rule out metastatic spread. Furthermore, the basic therapy should include a combination of cytotoxic agents with pelvic EBRT and intracavitary brachytherapy to doses similar to those used in squamous cell carcinoma, although some patients have been treated with radical surgery. If bleeding is present, prompt institution of radiation therapy with concurrent chemotherapy is necessary. Patients have extremely poor outcomes, with the only reported survivors having had triple-modality therapy of small tumors treated by radical hysterectomy, concurrent chemoRT, and adjuvant chemotherapy. Prophylactic cranial irradiation is not indicated because cervix cancer will most commonly spread first to lung and then to brain.

Patients with small-cell carcinoma of the cervix are treated with the same irradiation techniques as outlined for other histologic varieties of cervical carcinoma in combination with multiagent chemotherapy, including external beam radiation to 45 Gy, followed by nodal boost if PET-positive nodes are identified, followed by brachytherapy. The most frequently prescribed drugs are cisplatin and etoposide (VP-16) every 3 weeks.[559] Hoskins et al.[560] used a multimodality regimen of four cycles of cisplatin and etoposide with concurrent locoregional RT in 11 women with small-cell carcinoma of the cervix. The 3-year overall and failure-free survival rates were 28%. Four patients were alive in first remission; the remaining 7 died (2 from toxicity, 5 from cancer). Toxicity of therapy was significant, with 70% experiencing severe neutropenia; 40% were admitted to the hospital for emesis control.

Twelve patients with small-cell carcinoma of the cervix were treated with radical hysterectomy (5 received postoperative RT for lymph node metastases and 2 for close margins). With a mean follow-up of 73 months, the disease-free survival rate was 36.4%, compared with 71.6% for patients with non–small-cell carcinoma.[558] Four of five patients who received postoperative irradiation died with pelvic recurrence, and 3 also had disseminated metastases. However, only those with small lesions or those who received adjuvant irradiation were cured.

Delaloge et al.[561] reported only 2 of 10 patients with neuroendocrine small-cell carcinoma of the cervix surviving at 13 and 53 months after treatment, which included surgery, irradiation, and cisplatin/etoposide combination chemotherapy.

Boruta et al.[562] reviewed results in 11 of their and 23 other patients with early-stage neuroendocrine cervical carcinoma identified by a Medline search. Lymphovascular space invasion was present in 21 of 27 patients (78%) (7 unknown), and 15 of 29 (52%) had lymph node metastases. Fifteen patients were treated with cisplatin/etoposide (PE), 7 with vincristine/doxorubicin/cyclophosphamide (VAC), 2 with alternating cycles of VAC and PE, and 10 with other chemotherapy regimens. Twenty women were treated with radiation therapy. The presence of lymph node metastases was a poor prognostic factor ($p < .001$). PE and VAC chemotherapy were associated with increased survival ($p < .01$).

ADENOCARCINOMA OF THE CERVIX

Squamous cell carcinoma accounts for 80% of cervical cancers, adenocarcinoma for 15%, and adenosquamous carcinoma for 3% to 5%. SEER data from 1972–2002 suggest that the incidence of cervical adenocarcinoma is rising, but, based on SEER data, cause-specific mortality is not significantly different than that for SCC.[563] Adenocarcinoma has been linked to HPV 18, which has a higher rate of nodal and distant metastases than HPV 16.[159] Despite a slower regression after irradiation, reflecting cellular kinetics and slow growth, no difference in tumor control or survival has been observed in adenocarcinomas compared with squamous cell carcinomas,[564,565] although prognosis is related to clinical stage, volume of disease, and dose of irradiation.[566] Because of the predilection for endocervical involvement in adenocarcinoma, a combination of irradiation and conservative hysterectomy has been advocated by some authors,[567] although results are comparable with those obtained with irradiation alone.[564] Given a lower toxicity profile with chemoRT, this is preferable to a planned course of RT alone followed by hysterectomy upfront. Patients who have residual disease after chemoRT may be candidates for adjuvant hysterectomy.

Grigsby et al.[564] found no difference in 5-year DFS in patients with adenocarcinoma of the cervix (AC) compared with SCC treated with RT alone or combined with surgery. In contrast, Eifel et al.[568] reported that overall 5-year survival rates for patients with SCC and AC were 81% and 72%, respectively ($p < .01$). Patients with AC had a maximum cervical diameter of <4 cm more often than did those with SCC (53% vs. 47%). For 903 patients with tumors of ≥4 cm, 73% of those with SCC survived ≥5 years, compared with only 59% of those with AC ($p < .01$). Although there was no significant difference in the rate of pelvic disease recurrence for patients with AC or SCC tumors of ≥4 cm (17% vs. 13%; $p = .16$), the rate of distant metastases was greater for patients with AC (37% vs. 21%; $p < .01$). For patients with tumors of ≥4 cm, prognosis was strongly correlated with tumor size ($p < .01$) and lymphangiogram findings ($p < .01$) but not with age ($p = .58$) or tumor morphology (exophytic vs. endocervical; $p = .33$); a trend toward better survival in 165 patients who underwent adjuvant hysterectomy (78% vs. 71%) was not significant ($p = .09$). Multivariate analysis confirmed a highly significant independent association between histology and survival; patients with tumors ≥4 cm in diameter that were AC had an estimated risk of death 1.9 times that of patients with SCC ($p < .01$).

Nakano et al.[569] studied 58 patients with adenocarcinoma of the cervix treated with LDR or HDR brachytherapy and external pelvic irradiation. The 10-year survival rates for stages I, II, III, and IV were 85.7%, 60%, 27.6%, and 9.1%, respectively. The local tumor control rate with HDR treatment was 45.5%, significantly lower than with LDR (85.7%) or mixed–dose-rate treatments (72.7%). Kilgore et al.,[565] in a study of 162 patients with adenocarcinoma compared with matched patients with squamous cell carcinoma, found that clinical stage and lesion size were the most important prognostic factors. In patients with stage I tumors, no significant difference in survival was found when they were treated with radical surgery, irradiation alone, or irradiation combined with hysterectomy. In contrast, Kjorstad et al.[570] reported a worse 5-year survival rate in 102 patients with adenocarcinoma (51%) compared with that of 1,900 patients with squamous cell or other differentiated carcinomas (68%).

A Cochrane database review[571] found only one randomized trial, the Landoni study, in which a small subgroup analysis that was not powered to detect a difference showed an apparent improvement with surgery, although the majority of patients required adjuvant RT, rather than chemoradiation, which increases the rates of toxicity. Adenocarcinoma predicts worse OS on multivariate analysis (HR = 2.68, 95% CI = 1.9 to 3.8). Primary chemoradiation is considered the standard regimen for patients with locally advanced cervical adenocarcinoma.

Huang et al.[572] reported on 318 stage IB to IIB postoperative cervical cancer patients, 202 (63.5%) with SCC and 116 (36.5%) with AC/atypical squamous cells (ASC), treated by radical hysterectomy and adjuvant RT/concurrent chemo-RT (CCRT). The 5-year relapse-free survival rates for SCC and AC/ASC patients were 83.4% and 66.5%, respectively ($p < 0\ .001$). Distant metastasis was the major failure pattern in both groups. After multivariate analysis, prognostic factors for local recurrence included younger age, parametrial invasion, AC/ASC histology, and positive resection margin; for distant recurrence they included parametrial invasion, lymph node metastasis, and AC/ASC histology. Compared with SCC patients, those with AC/ASC had higher local relapse rates for the intermediate-risk group but a higher distant metastasis rate for the high-risk group. Postoperative CCRT tended to improve survival for intermediate-risk but not for high-risk AC/ASC patients.

TREATMENT OF ELDERLY PATIENTS

Oguchi et al.[573] reported on 23 patients 90 years of age or older treated for cervix carcinoma. Definitive radiation therapy was completed in 13 of the patients, and local tumor control at 6 months was attained in 9 patients. Palliative RT was completed in 7 of 11, and palliation was observed in 9 patients (81%). Seven patients were alive for 15 to 67 months. Fourteen patients died because of intercurrent disease or senility associated with active cancer and 2 because of senility without evidence of cancer. The 2-year overall and relapse-free survival rates were 30% and 21%, respectively.

CARCINOMA OF THE CERVIX AND PREGNANCY

The concurrent presence of carcinoma *in situ* or invasive carcinoma of the uterine cervix and pregnancy, although rare, poses a therapeutic dilemma to gynecologic and radiation oncologists. Reported incidence is approximately 1 to 10 per 10,000 pregnancies.[574] In the United States, the incidence has decreased. Norstrom et al.,[575] in Sweden, found that cervical cancer was diagnosed in 33 women in association with pregnancy (incidence, 11.1 cases per 100,000 deliveries and 7.5 per 100,000 pregnancies). Abnormal bleeding was the symptom that led to diagnosis in 54.5% of the women; 45.5% were asymptomatic but had an abnormal cervicovaginal cytologic test result (39.4%) or abnormal vaginal examination (6.1%) in association with pregnancy. During the follow-up, 1 of 12 women with cervix cancer in the first trimester, 4 of 12 in the third trimester, and 2 of 9 postpartum died of the disease. Primary surgery was used more frequently than radiation therapy.

For carcinoma *in situ*, if the pregnancy is allowed to reach full term, confirmation of the diagnosis by colposcopy and conservative management with monthly Pap smears constitutes the best approach. Conization has frequently been performed. Punch biopsies can be obtained, but the diagnostic accuracy is less reliable. As many as 50% of the patients have residual carcinoma *in situ* after delivery.

In patients with invasive carcinoma, the lesion is usually clinically apparent. Multiple punch biopsies are adequate to confirm the diagnosis. Management is individualized based on tumor size and stage, patient age, and desires of the patient (or couple) regarding the pregnancy. The majority of patients with cervical cancer diagnosed during pregnancy (approximately 75%) have stage I tumors.[574,576,577]

Women with tumors diagnosed early in pregnancy are often recommended to abort the fetus. Because there is a greater need to institute therapy as soon as possible, the accepted method of treatment in patients in the first 6 months of pregnancy is to carry out definitive surgery or radiation therapy, as indicated by the stage of the disease, with resultant loss of the fetus. An abortifacient may be administered before initiating radiation to ensure fetal demise and delivery of the placenta prior to initiation of treatment. The whole pelvis is irradiated (40 to 45 Gy in 4 to 5 weeks). However, in one series of 45 patients, 27% did not abort spontaneously and surgical evacuation was required;[578] alternatively, misoprostol may be administered as an alternative to surgical evacuation after failed spontaneous abortion.[579] After this dose of radiation, careful evacuation of the uterus and LDR (or equivalent-dose HDR) brachytherapy may be performed under general anesthesia. If a radical hysterectomy is performed and positive pelvic lymph nodes are found, the usual postoperative irradiation, including external beam with or without intracavitary insertion, should be carried out.

If the woman refuses abortion, serial MRI scans at 2- to 3-month intervals to ensure no growth or spread to lymph nodes is recommended. Neoadjuvant chemotherapy may be considered in selected patients.[580] Sorosky et al.[581] reported on eight pregnant women with stage I carcinoma of the cervix who had declined immediate therapy and followed until the late third trimester; a cesarean section–radical hysterectomy was performed, with delay in therapy ranging from 3 to 40 weeks during the pregnancies. There was no clinical progression of the disease with follow-up of 33 months.

When patients are diagnosed in mid-pregnancy (second trimester), consideration to keeping the pregnancy and treating with chemotherapy is given. A French series reported five cases between 2002 and 2009.[582] Three patients received neoadjuvant chemotherapy; 1 patient died of cancer. A Chinese report described treatment of two patients with neoadjuvant paclitaxel and cisplatin as feasible.[583]

Occasionally in late pregnancy (final trimester), if tumors are small and an MRI confirms no lymph node involvement, definitive therapy is postponed until after imminent delivery. In a review of the literature intentional treatment delay was associated with a recurrence rate of 4%.[362] Greer et al.[584] noted that in 600 infants without congenital abnormalities, when stage IB cervical carcinoma was diagnosed during pregnancy and fetal survival was chosen, the neonatal mortality rate decreased from 30% when the fetus was delivered at 26 to 27 weeks to 2.7% when the fetus was allowed to mature to 34 to 35 weeks. In the third trimester of pregnancy, when the fetus may be salvaged, some gynecologic oncologists prefer a postpartum cesarean section, combined with a radical hysterectomy and lymphadenectomy followed by radiation of high risk features are present. However, some authors report that vaginal delivery has no detrimental effect on the prognosis.[585]

Patients who require high doses of pelvic irradiation should be counseled regarding the permanent loss of reproductive capability, not only because of ovarian ablation (which happens with doses of 8 Gy or higher), but as a consequence of radiation effects in the uterus.[586,587]

Survival is the same regardless of the trimester of the pregnancy in which definitive treatment is instituted. Creasman et al.[585] reported on 48 patients treated by irradiation, 45 by irradiation followed by surgery, and 5 with radical hysterectomy alone. The survival was comparable with that of nonpregnant patients for similar stages. The survival rate for patients with stage I disease was comparable whether vaginal delivery was allowed or a cesarean section was performed (approximately 85% in stage I and 50% to 64% in stage II). In addition, the percentage of infants surviving (>80%) was the same in both groups.

Sood et al.[587] performed a retrospective analysis of 26 women with cervical carcinoma diagnosed during pregnancy and treated primarily with radiation therapy (mean dose, 46.7 Gy) and LDR intracavitary radiation (mean dose, 56.5 Gy to point A). These cases were matched with 26 nonpregnant control patients based on age, histology, stage, treatment, and year of treatment. There were no statistically significant differences in recurrence rates or survival between the pregnant group and the control patients. Short-term toxicity was comparable in pregnant and nonpregnant patients. Long-term complication rates were 12% in pregnant patients and 27% in control patients, but this difference was not statistically significant. Most complications were likely related to radiation techniques (particularly the predominance of ^{60}Co).

Sood et al.[588] compared the prognosis of 56 women who had cervical cancer diagnosed during pregnancy and 27 who were diagnosed within 6 months after delivery. Control patients (cervical cancer diagnosed at least 5 years since last delivery) were matched one-to-one with cases based on age, histology, stage, treatment, and time of treatment. Among the postpartum women, 11 were treated with radical hysterectomies and 14 with radiation therapy, and 2 with stage IA1 disease were treated with vaginal hysterectomies. One of 7 patients who had cesarean sections had a local and distant recurrence. In contrast, 10 of 17 (59%) patients who delivered vaginally had recurrences ($p = .04$). In multivariate analysis, vaginal delivery was the most significant predictor of recurrence, followed by high tumor stage. Survival for patients diagnosed in the postpartum period was significantly worse than for control patients and for those diagnosed during pregnancy. The authors concluded that pregnant women with cervical cancer should be delivered by cesarean section.

Jones et al.[589] published a survey by the American College of Surgeons that evaluated management of invasive cervical carcinoma in 161 pregnant patients; 86 were treated with surgery alone, 30 with radiation therapy alone, and 45 with a combination of the two modalities. Approximately one-third of patients were diagnosed in each trimester. The 5-year survival was 94.6% for patients diagnosed in the first trimester, 76.9% for the second, and 68.9% for the third. The prognosis of patients with invasive carcinoma of the cervix associated with pregnancy was similar to that of nonpregnant patients. There was no significant difference in 5-year survival between the patients delivered by cesarean section and by normal vaginal delivery.

Senekjian et al.[590] reported no difference in survival or patterns of failure in 24 women who were pregnant at the time of diagnosis of clear-cell adenocarcinoma of the cervix and vagina compared with 408 who had never been pregnant. The 5- and 10-year actuarial survival rates were 86% and 68% for the pregnant patients and 87% and 79% for the patients who had not been pregnant, respectively.

The practice popularized 30 years ago of administering a "restraining dose of radium" and deferring definitive radiation therapy until delivery is carried out should be strongly rejected. Strauss[591] reported 2 of 11 infants being born with microcephaly in addition to other complications such as alopecia, facial deformity, eye damage, and chromosomal abnormalities after this procedure.

BRACHYTHERAPY

After the discovery of radium in 1898 by the Curies, publications followed describing use of the first glass radium capsule in 1904 and a metal brachytherapy applicator for cervical cancer in 1905.[592] The incorporation of brachytherapy after external-beam treatment arose from the recognition that tumor control probability correlated with radiation dose and cancer volume.[593] Evidence confirms that brachytherapy as used for dose escalation after external-beam treatment for cervical cancer significantly improves survival.[525,594–597] Therefore, brachytherapy is a standard part of the treatment of locally advanced (stages IB2 to IVA) cervical cancer after external beam radiation; brachytherapy alone may be used as primary treatment for selected cases with early-stage (stages IA to IB1) cervical cancer.[598] The increasing complexity of brachytherapy administration, including the use of complex imaging, mandates implementation of careful quality assurance measures and a culture of open communication to ensure safe practices in the clinic.[598]

Dose Rate

The ICRU in its Report 38[599] defines brachytherapy dose rate as follows: LDR, 0.4 to 2 Gy/hr; medium dose rate (MDR) or PDR, 2 to 12 Gy/hr; and HDR, >12 Gy/hr. For LDR, the most commonly used isotope is ^{137}Cs, and for PDR and HDR it is ^{192}Ir. The use of HDR has significantly increased in the United States, from 13% in the 1996–1999 Quality Research in Radiation Oncology (formerly known as the Patterns of Care) survey to 62% in the 2007–2009 survey.[369,600] In other U.S., European, and Japanese surveys of gynecologic brachytherapy practitioners, approximately 85% state that they use HDR brachytherapy,[601–602,603] whereas in Canada the reported use is 68% HDR, 10% PDR, and 23% LDR.[604] The dose delivered per fraction for HDR and proportion of dose delivered with external beam versus brachytherapy vary substantially in different centers around the world.[602]

Most institutions in the United States have either LDR or HDR brachytherapy available. Larger centers may have LDR, PDR, and/or HDR. Overall, outcomes are similar regardless of dose rate, with the caveat that for HDR, 3D imaging should be incorporated to ensure coverage of the tumor, particularly for large-volume disease.[605] Several studies demonstrate worse survival for stage IIIB cervical cancer treated with HDR due to initiating the treatment early in the course of external beam therapy,[606] when the tumor mass was >4 cm and therefore a prescription to point A did not cover the tumor volume, or by not using 3D planning to cover large residual disease.[607]

Biology of High-Dose-Rate Brachytherapy for Cervical Carcinoma: Equivalent Dose in 2 Gy and Biologically Effective Dose

To achieve tumor control using HDR equivalent to that with LDR brachytherapy, attention to the dose/fractionation schedule and to normal tissue doses is mandatory.[608,609–610] The linear-quadratic (LQ) model provides calculation estimates of biologically equivalent dose taking into account dose rate, dose per fraction, and overall treatment time.[611,612] For comparison of LDR to HDR, the LQ model doses are normalized to an equivalent dose in 2 Gy (EQD2).[613] The α/β ratio is a critical component of the LQ model.[614] For cervix cancer, an α/β ratio of 10 Gy is used for tumor and an α/β of 3 Gy is used for normal tissues,[615] which may have inherent inaccuracies in generalizability,[616] although an α/β ratio of 3 Gy for the rectum has been correlated with late rectal complications.[617,618–619]

Spreadsheets to assist with HDR EQD2 dose conversions are available from the American Brachytherapy Society (www.americanbrachytherapy.org/guidelines). The values derived are not actual doses but biologically effective ones that take into consideration dose rate and effect of fraction size.[620]

Although use of a detailed EQD2 conversion is preferred, an approximation of these values was proposed by Orton et al.,[610] with an LDR-to-HDR reduction factor of 0.54 to 0.6 (Table 69.15), and by Patel et al.,[607] with a similar correction factor of 0.58. These conversion factors are valid when three to five HDR fractions are used, but with a higher number of fractions (six to eight), the conversion factor is closer to 0.75. Therefore, use of the EQD2 worksheet is recommended for consistency.

The importance of adopting biologically based equivalent doses when switching from LDR to HDR brachytherapy is exemplified in a report by Newman[621] on 115 patients treated with external irradiation (40 to 50 Gy) and manual afterloading cesium sources delivering 60 Gy to point A with a dose rate of 0.75 Gy/hour, or a Selectron device with 40-mCi sources, which delivered from 0.75 to 1 Gy/hour to point A. Because of the increased dose rate, the total intracavitary dose was reduced by 20%. Grade 3 genitourinary and gastrointestinal complications were observed in 3 of 87 patients (3.4%) treated with LDR, in contrast to 30 of 132 patients (22.7%) treated with the Selectron HDR sources. No significant differences in local tumor control and survival were found.

TABLE 69.15 MEAN VALUES OF THE NUMBER OF FRACTIONS, DOSE/FRACTION TO POINT A (FOR HIGH DOSE RATE) AND TREATMENT TIME, DOSE RATE FOR LOW DOSE RATE (WITH STANDARD ERRORS) AND THE RATIO OF TOTAL DOSES

	HDR		LDR		
Stage	*Fractions*	*Dose Per Fraction (Gy)*	*Treatment Time (Hour)*	*Dose Rate (Gy/Hour)*	*Ratio of Total Doses (HDR/LDR)*
I	5.3 ± 0.40	7.6 ± 0.40	75.4 ± 7.3	0.87 ± 0.14	0.60 ± 0.13
II	4.7 ± 0.30	7.4 ± 0.30	80.2 ± 7.0	0.80 ± 0.11	0.54 ± 0.10
III	4.6 ± 0.40	7.4 ± 0.40	77.3 ± 8.9	0.87 ± 0.14	0.50 ± 0.11
IV	4.7 ± 0.70	7.5 ± 0.60	79.6 ± 18.5	0.89 ± 0.27	0.50 ± 0.21
All	4.82 ± 0.21	7.45 ± 0.20	78.1 ± 4.4	0.85 ± 0.07	0.54 ± 0.06

HDR, high dose rate; LDR, low dose rate.

From Orton CG, Seyedsadr M, Somany A. Comparison of high- and low-dose rate remote afterloading for cervix cancer and the importance of fractionation. *Int J Radiat Oncol Biol Phys* 1991;21:1425–1434; with permission from Elsevier.

Figure 69.20 illustrates the late normal-tissue effect, which is proportional to log cell kill, and the relationship to the number of HDR treatment fractions.[622] Each solid curve is calculated assuming the same log cell kill. Late damage rises sharply as the number of HDR fractions is decreased. When these curves are above the dashed lines that represent the maximum late effect of 70 Gy of LDR brachytherapy given at 0.5 Gy/hour, the risk of late complications increases. Displacing the bladder and rectum away from the HDR sources for the short duration of therapy may offset the radiobiologic disadvantage of using a few brachytherapy fractions.[610]

Brachytherapy Process: Preparation and Timing

Standard procedures for pretreatment evaluation, imaging, anesthesia use, and treatment duration should follow accepted general principles in the guidelines published by the American Brachytherapy Society in 2012.[598,623,624] Planning the course of brachytherapy should begin at the time of initial presentation. An examination at diagnosis assessing disease extension and tumor size should be recorded. Periodic examinations during external beam treatment should be performed to monitor response. For patients receiving concurrent chemoradiation, rapid shrinkage should be expected because treatment may regress the tumor to 70% to 80% of the pretherapeutic volume. Therefore, a clinical gynecologic examination at the time of brachytherapy is also important.[625,626] Inserting radiopaque marker seeds ("fiducials") at the time of diagnosis that mark

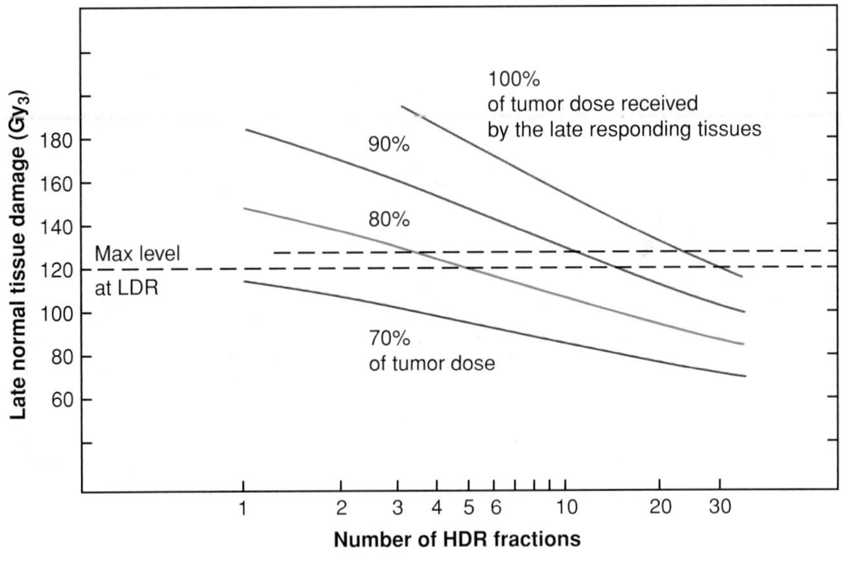

FIGURE 69.20. Relationship between number of high-dose-rate (HDR) fractions and late normal tissue effects. Solid lines show the increase in normal-tissue late effects as the number of HDR fractions used to treat cervical cancer decreases. Dotted lines indicate the maximum level of late damage calculated for conventional low-dose-rate brachytherapy of 70 Gy at 0.5 Gy/hour for 140 hours and an arbitrary level 5% above this. The intersection of the solid lines with the dotted lines indicates the number of HDR fractions needed to give equal late normal-tissue effects. In this model, the dose to late-responding tissues should be kept at 83% of the tumor dose when treating with four to six HDR fractions. (Modified from Fowler JF. The radiobiology of brachytherapy. In: Martinez AA, Orton CG, Mould RF, eds. *Brachytherapy HDR and LDR.* Leersum, Netherlands: Nucletron International BV, 1990;121–137; with permission from Elsevier.)

the inferior, lateral, and superior extension of a vaginal tumor may aid in identifying regions requiring dose escalation with brachytherapy even after complete regression during external-beam treatment.

Treatment schedules integrating external-beam irradiation and brachytherapy were initially designed with regard to the disease stage and volume.[627] For LDR, insertion of the applicator may be done after all external beam finishes, with the caveat that one or two insertions may be required, approximately 1 week apart. All treatment, including external-beam treatment and brachytherapy, should finish 8 weeks from the initiation of radiation.[184]

The optimal time–dose–fractionation scheme and the technique for remote-control afterloading intracavitary brachytherapy for cervical cancer have yet to be established through systematic clinical trials. For HDR or PDR brachytherapy, the applicator insertion and treatment may commence after external-beam treatment finishes, to ensure optimal geometry with normal tissues far from the applicator. Alternatively, the physician may choose to insert the applicator for treatment as early as during the second week of external radiation if the tumor is small enough, to minimize total treatment time. However, brachytherapy and external-beam treatments are not given on the same day.

Applicator Selection

The most frequently used applicator for locally advanced cervical cancer patients worldwide is the tandem and ovoid applicator,[602] which provides radiation dose covering the cervix, uterus, inner parametria, and approximately 1 to 2 cm of the upper vagina. The tandem and ring applicator has a slightly narrower dose distribution, but with HDR the dose distribution may be optimized and mimics that obtained with the tandem and ovoid applicator. For patients with a very narrow vagina due to stricturing, a tandem and cylinder applicator may be the only option available. However, this applicator provides insufficient dosing to the parametrial tissue and should be used with caution. For patients with large tumors with residual bulky disease after external-beam radiation or those with vaginal extension, fistulae, or pelvic sidewall invasion, a combination of tandem/ring or ovoid with interstitial applicator or tandem/interstitial applicator alone may be inserted.

Applicator Insertion

General guidelines from the American Brachytherapy Society should be followed.[598] The patient receives appropriate anesthesia for pain management. In the lithotomy position, the perineum is sterilely prepped and draped. The Foley catheter is inserted into the bladder. The catheter is clamped and the bladder filled with 150 to 200 cc of saline if ultrasound (US) is used. US with a transabdominal probe can significantly speed up the insertion process and assist with accurate placement because the uterine canal is often clearly visible after instilling fluid in the bladder (Fig. 69.21). Transabdominal US can measure uterine width and height in patients who do not have large fibroids or tumor volumes that greatly distort uterine configuration.[628] US does not define the target volume as clearly as MRI but may be used to assist with 3D-based planning when CT or MRI is unavailable.[629] Transrectal US may assist with interstitial brachytherapy when other imaging modalities are not available. For interstitial insertions, CT or MRI may be used during the insertion process iteratively using real-time guidance to ensure proper tumor coverage and no inadvertent insertions into the rectum or bladder.[630] After tandem and ovoid or tandem and ring applicator placement, vaginal packing covered with lubricant gel is placed in the vagina to separate the bladder and rectum, which also helps to maintain applicator position.

Applicator Position

An experienced brachytherapist has greater familiarity with applicator insertion and evaluation.[368] Applicator position is a critical determinant of dose specification[600,631] and pelvic control.[57,632] As Fletcher[533] emphasized, conditions for an adequate intracavitary insertion include the following:

1. The geometry of the insertion must prevent underdosing around the cervix.
2. Sufficient dose must be delivered to the paracervical areas.
3. Vaginal mucosal, bladder, and rectal tolerance doses must be respected.

For LDR Fletcher-Suit applicators, Potish et al.[633] used linear least-squares regression to show that although there was a moderately good correlation between the milligram-hours and dose to point A, it was markedly affected by the position of the colpostats and the tandem. A review of plain films of 808 LDR intracavitary applications in 396 cervical cancer patients treated at MD Anderson[634] quantified acceptable implant geometry. The median distance from the tandem to the sacrum was 4 cm, or one-third the distance from the pubis to the sacrum. The distance between the vaginal ovoids and cervical marker seeds was 7 mm, and the median distance between the tandem and the posterior edge of the ovoids was 50% of the ovoid length. In 92% of insertions, vaginal packing was posterior to or within 5 mm of a line that passed through the posterior edge of the ovoids, parallel to the tandem. The median doses to point A and

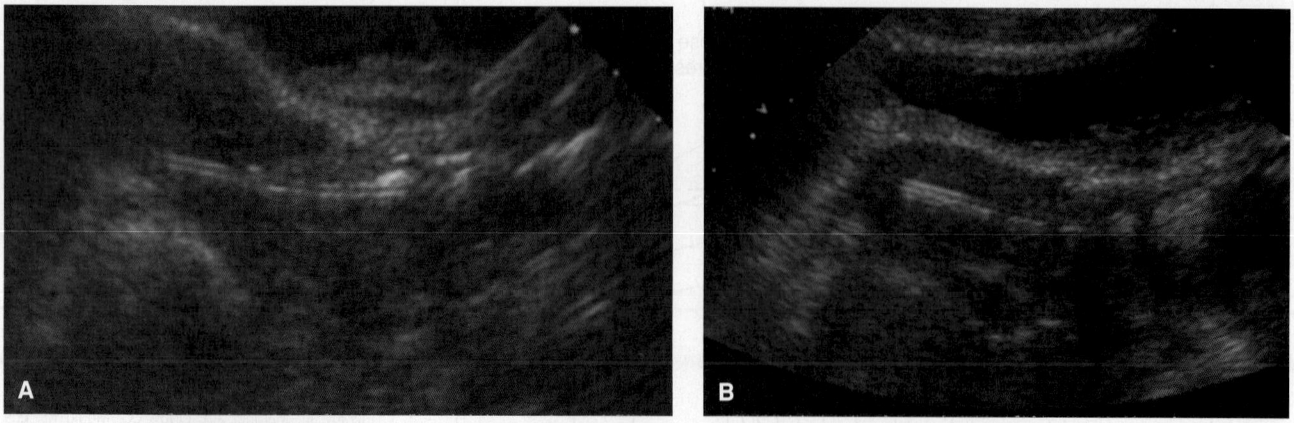

FIGURE 69.21. Ultrasound used during intrauterine tandem insertion can ensure proper placement into the intrauterine canal and shorten overall procedure time. **A:** Ultrasound depicts that the tandem is placed in the posterior myometrium. **B:** Ultrasound directs the tandem into the intrauterine canal.

rectal, bladder, and vaginal surface reference points were 87, 68, 70, and 125 Gy, respectively. Analysis of the LDR and HDR brachytherapy positions for 103 patients enrolled on RTOG trials 0116 and 0128 found that patients with unacceptable symmetry of ovoids to the tandem had a significantly higher risk of LR than patients in the acceptable group (HR = 2.67; 95% CI = 1.11 to 6.45; $p = .03$).[57] Patients with displacement of ovoids in relation to the cervical os had a significantly increased risk of LR (HR = 2.50; 95% CI = 1.05 to 5.93; $p = .04$) and a lower DFS rate (HR = 2.28; 95% CI = 1.18 to 4.41; $p = .01$). Inappropriate placement of packing resulted in a lower DFS rate (HR = 2.06; 95% CI = 1.08Y3.92; $p = .03$).

Imaging After Insertion

For LDR brachytherapy, active sources may be inserted after the films have been reviewed and the position of the applicators judged to be satisfactory.[57,634] Placing a small amount of contrast into the bladder and rectum before CT or plain film may clarify the location of these structures.

When a CT scan is obtained after applicator insertion, it also verifies proper placement (no perforation) and analyzes cervix and normal-tissue location in relationship to brachytherapy dose distribution.[601] CT provides a reasonable estimate of the location of the uterus and cervix. The CT contours of the cervix overestimate the tumor contours compared to an MRI, although the additional width contoured on a CT may not be of detriment to the patient because cervical cancer tends to spread laterally along the parametrial tissues.[635] CT depicts changes in the OAR related to tumor shrinkage, organ motion, and the location of the brachytherapy applicator in relation to the uterus. However, separating the OAR, such as the sigmoid or the small bowel from portions of the uterus or cervix, may be difficult on CT, given the lack of contrast. OAR dosimetry based on CT is similar to that based on MRI when optimized similarly.[636] CT may not provide sufficient detail of the tumor if selected dose escalation is required, such as in cases with large residual tumors. In the vast majority of cases, however, it should suffice.[637–638,639] The uterus and cervix cannot be distinguished as separate structures on a CT, whereas they can on an MRI. Therefore, CT-based contouring guidelines recommend delineating the entire cervix and uterus.[635]

In a multicenter study, MR imaging was significantly better than CT for tumor visualization and detection of parametrial involvement.[66] Other advantages of MR include multiplanar capability and excellent soft-tissue contrast resolution. The strength of a magnet in an MR scanner is expressed by a unit of measurement referred to as a tesla (T). Higher field strength produces a better overall signal-to-noise ratio and more accurate imaging.

Regardless of whether a plain film radiograph, CT, or MR is obtained after insertion to aid treatment planning, in order to properly visualize the apparatus, radiopaque markers should be inserted to identify source position to aid with dosimetric planning. For MRI, identifying the applicator using either a radiopaque marker inserted into the applicator, or, for interstitial cases undergoing MR, a special 3-T MR sequence may be used to create artifact that allows the tip of the needle to appear as a balloon on the sagittal image and as a cross on the axial images.[640]

Dose Specification

Point A

Several methods for specifying dose in brachytherapy evolved over the twentieth century.

Due to the limited availability of 3D imaging worldwide and a 100-year history of plain film radiography, the majority of institutions internationally use point-based dosimetry based on the ICRU 38 nomenclature,[599] defining point A rather than prescribing dose to a tumor volume.[601] Other institutions use a system of milligram-hours, whereas others consider the volume of the region of interest. Based on the general principles guidelines for cervical cancer brachytherapy published by the American Brachytherapy Society and the ICRU report, the point A definition was updated in 2012.[598] To determine point A, connect a line through the center of each ovoid or the lateralmost dwell position in the ring; extend this line superiorly along the radius of the ovoids (or ring), and then move an additional 2 cm superior along the tandem. From this point, extend out 2 cm on each side laterally on a line perpendicular to the tandem (Fig. 69.22). For tandem and cylinders, begin at the flange or cervical marking seed and move 2 cm superiorly along the tandem and then 2 cm laterally.

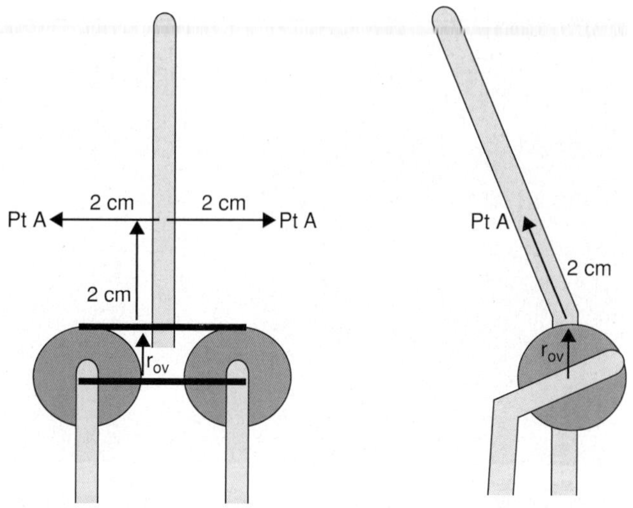

FIGURE 69.22. Definition of point A shown on a tandem and ovoid applicator based on the American Brachytherapy Society 2012 Guidelines for Cervical Cancer.

Three-dimensional image-based brachytherapy treatment planning precisely defines the tumor and aids with the precision of radiation dose delivery, which may reduce the dose to the normal tissues and reduce toxicity.[641] In the era of increasing use of HDR brachytherapy, proper applicator placement and precise estimation of the location of the normal tissue is critical. When 3D imaging is available, point-based radiographic dosimetry has limited utility for the dose adaptation required for HDR brachytherapy because point A may overestimate or underestimate the tumor dose based on 3D imaging.[642] Kim et al.[643] found that dose to point A was significantly lower than the D_{90} for HR-CTV calculated using 3D image-based optimization. With imaging, one may visualize the tumor volume and conform dose to the volume which may result in the dose to point A being lower than the prescription 100% isodose line (covering a smaller tumor volume) or a higher-than-prescription dose to point A due to a large tumor volume extending beyond the boundaries of point A. The tumor coverage relies on tumor volume at the time of brachytherapy, with larger tumors requiring greater optimization to be adequately covered by the prescribed isodose line.[642,644,645] The dose to point A should be reported to ensure consistency in terminology between centers.[646]

Accurate delineation of the tumor and OAR is critical for precise treatment planning (Fig. 69.23). Due to the rapid falloff of dose, imprecise contouring can dramatically change dosing to normal-tissue structures. Formal contouring education programs reduce the variability of interobserver contours.[647]

Computed Tomography Imaging for Brachytherapy Contouring

A CT scan can define a CTV with the lateral borders of the cervix and any parametrial extension defined based on suspicious regions seen on the scan. CT-contouring guidelines

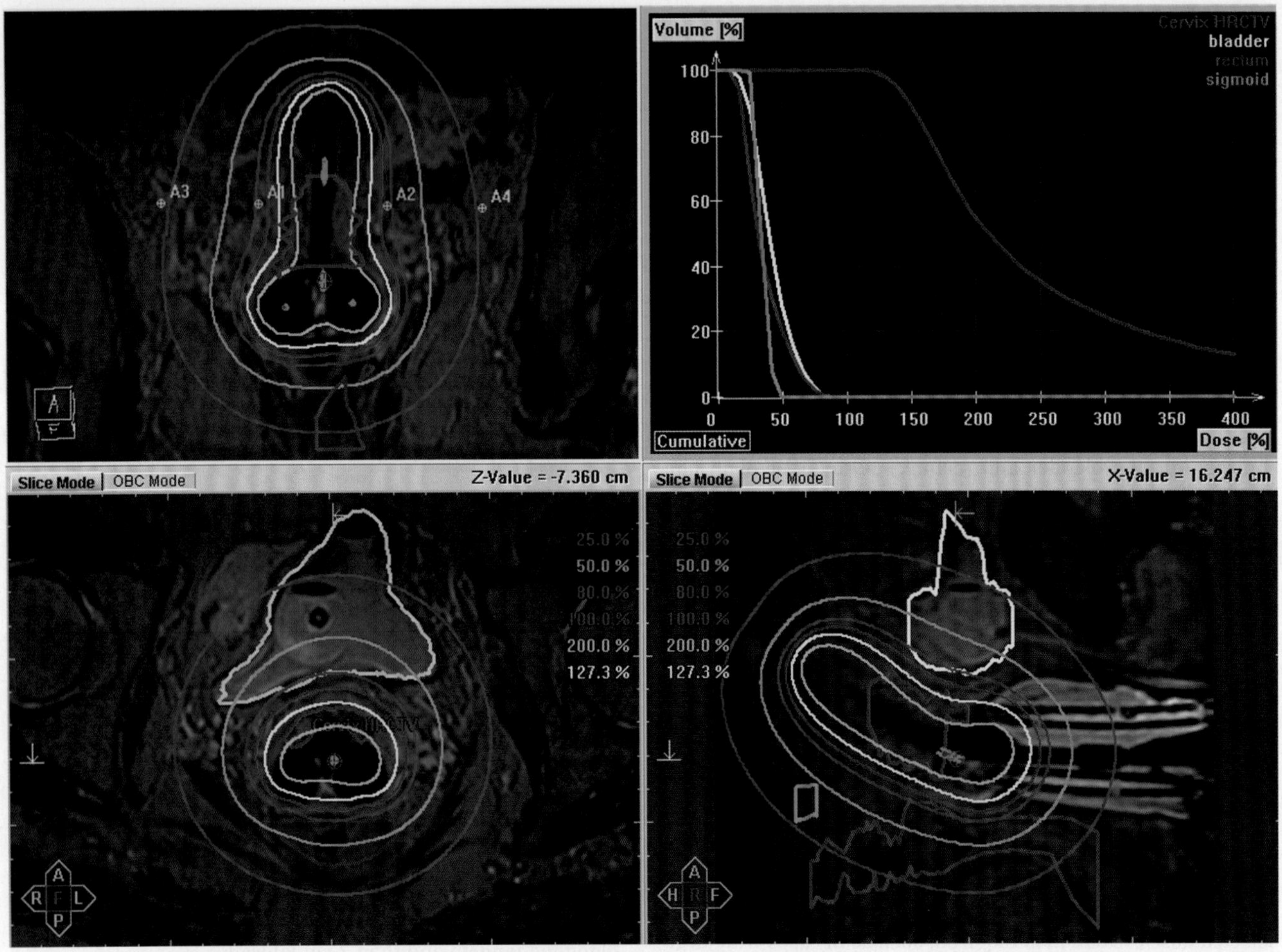

FIGURE 69.23. Tandem and ovoid implant showing the use of three-dimensional (magnetic resonance or computed tomography) imaging to adequately cover the high-risk clinical target volume (HR-CTV) while minimizing dose to the organs at risk (OAR)—the rectum, sigmoid, and bladder. Dose–volume histograms record the D_{2cc} limits to the OAR. The dose at point A is recorded but varies between patients based on optimization of the HR-CTV and OAR.

should be followed.[635] Uterosacral ligaments may be visualized on CT, and, if detected, they should be included in the CTV contours. No GTV may be identified on CT. The superior border of the cervix is not defined, but instead the entire tandem length is planned and the top dwell is optimized off the sigmoid to reduce bowel dose.

Magnetic Resonance Imaging for Brachytherapy Contouring

For MR-based contouring, the Groupe Europeen Curietherapy-European Society for Therapeutic Radiation Oncology (GEC-ESTRO) guidelines[625,626] delineate volumes for MR. The recommended volumes include the GTV, including all T2-bright areas of enhancement; the HR-CTV, which is the entire cervix, any regions of high to intermediate signal intensity in the parametria, uterus, or vagina, and any residual disease detected on clinical examination at the time of brachytherapy; and, the intermediate-risk clinical target volume (IR-CTV), which subtracts out the OARs but includes the tumor extension at the time of diagnosis, adding 1 cm to the HR-CTV volume. The IR-CTV defines regions with potential microscopic seeding of tumor cells (Fig. 69.24).[648] Lang et al.,[649] in a multicenter study, confirmed the feasibility of these recommendations, with total doses to point A from both BT and EBRT ranging from 85 to 91 Gy and to CTV from 69 to 73 cGy. Doses to organs at risk were comparable to those obtained with standard dosimetric methods, although they were more accurately determined with dose–volume histograms.

Dose–Volume Histogram Reporting

With MR-planned brachytherapy, the most common dose–volume parameters reported for target structures of the entire cervix and any residual disease at the time of brachytherapy, the HR-CTV, are D_{90}, defined as the dose received by at least 90% of the target volume, D_{100}, and V_{100}, based on the GEC-ESTRO recommendations.[650,651] The cumulative D_{90} equals the sum of D_{90} values from the individual fractions plus the dose from a homogeneous 3D conformal external-beam treatment. D_{100}, the minimum target dose, may be more sensitive to inaccuracies in contouring and dose calculation. V_{100} assesses dose coverage of the whole target volume and is 100% when the entire target is covered by the prescribed dose. V_{150} and V_{200} are often reported in interstitial brachytherapy. One may report these for CT, although the dimensions of the target will differ significantly from the absolute dimensions on MR, and the CT contour of the HR-CTV will include the cervix, residual areas in the parametria or uterosacral ligaments, and part of the uterus because the superior border of the cervix is not visible.[635] CT contours are more accurate if an MRI can be performed immediately before or with the first fraction of brachytherapy.[652] In both CT and MRI, prescribed dose is based on the physician's directive of the dose intended for the target volume, that is, the volume covered by the 100% isodose line, and point A should be recorded. Several institutions have validated the use of these guidelines with HDR, LDR, or PDR brachytherapy.[645,652,653,654,655,656]

With 3D imaging, one may define the surrounding normal tissue structures as the OAR, including the rectum, sigmoid,

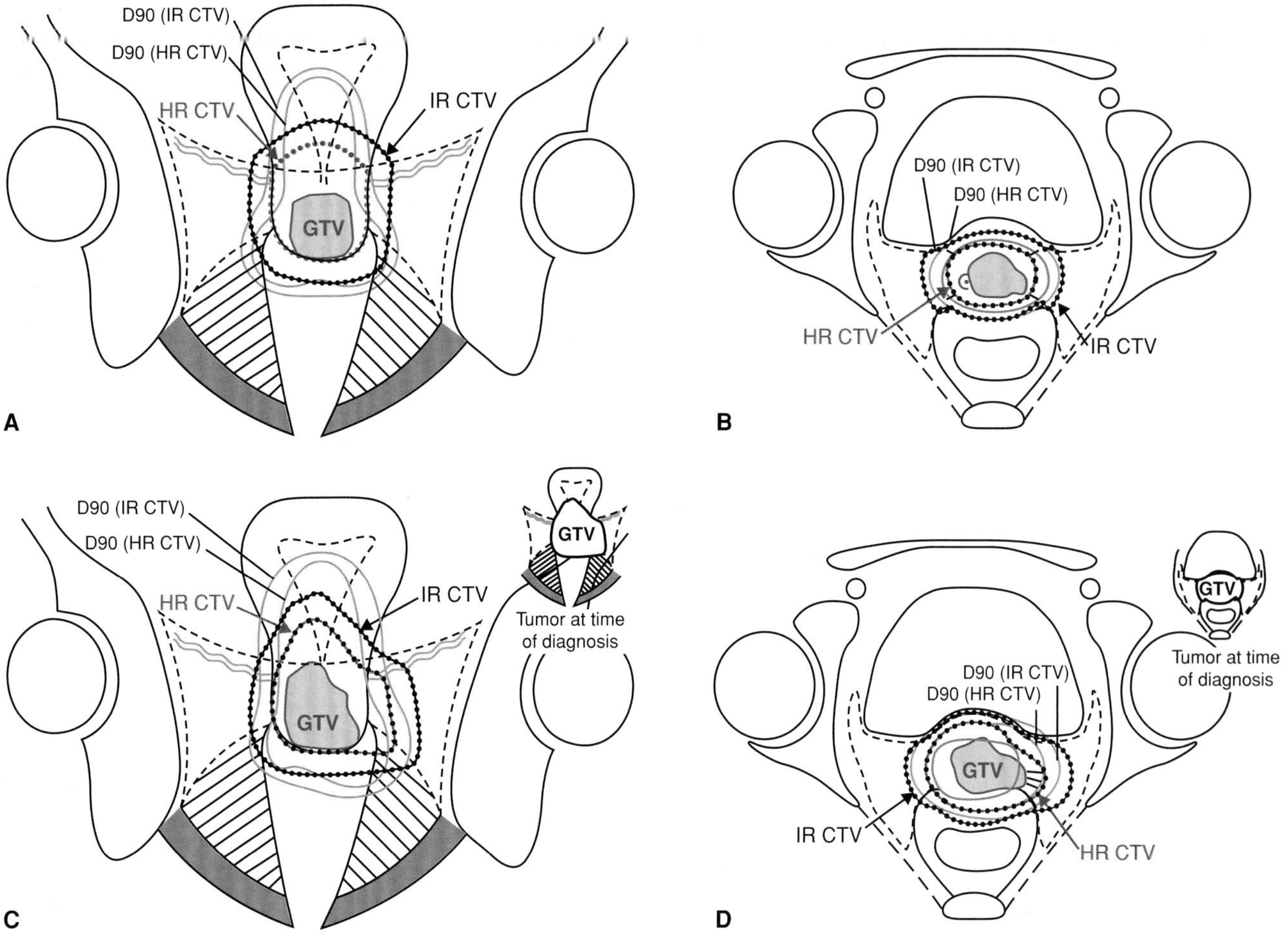

FIGURE 69.24. Diagrammatic representation of gross tumor volume (GTV) and clinical target volume (CTV) for three-dimensional treatment planning in carcinoma of uterine cervix. Coronal **(A,C)** and transverse **(B,D)** sections for limited **(A,B)** and advanced **(C,D)** disease (*gray zones in left parametrium*). (From Potter R, Haie-Meder C, Limbergen EV, et al. Recommendations from gynaecological (GYN) GEC ESTRO working group (II): Concepts and terms in 3D image-based treatment planning in cervix brachytherapy-3D dose volume parameters and aspects of 3D image-based anatomy, radiation physics, radiobiology. *Radiother Oncol* 2006;78:67–77; with permission from Elsevier.)

and bladder. With 2D imaging, the ICRU 38 report requires only reporting point estimates for the rectum and bladder because the sigmoid cannot easily be visualized.[599] However, the ICRU bladder point may underestimate maximum doses to the OAR, in particular for the bladder[657,658]; it is less likely that rectal doses will be incorrectly estimated. Numerous publications correlate the ICRU point dose and the probability of late complications for bladder and rectum.[659,660] Nevertheless, DVH metrics may provide a more reliable predictor of long-term complications.[661] In a review of 50 patients treated with LDR or HDR brachytherapy who then had a CT for treatment planning, the closest point of the sigmoid was related to sigmoid dose but varied in proximity to the tandem up to 40% between fractions, with a median distance of 1.7 cm. No sigmoid toxicity was noted after a median follow-up of 31 months.

Kapp et al.[662] analyzed 720 ^{192}Ir HDR applications in 331 patients with gynecologic tumors to evaluate the dose to normal tissues. CT-based dosimetry showed that the maximum doses to bladder and rectum were generally higher than those obtained from orthogonal films, with an average ratio of 1.44 for the bladder neck, 2.42 for the bladder base, and 1.37 for the rectum. The ratio of bladder-base dose to bladder-neck dose was 1.5 for intracervical and 1.46 for intravaginal applications. If conventional methods are used for dosimetry, the authors recommended that doses to the bladder base should be routinely calculated because single-point measurements at the bladder neck seriously underestimate the dose to the bladder. In addition, the rectal dose should be determined at several points over the length of the implant because of the wide range of anatomic variations.

Eich et al.,[663] in 11 applications of HDR brachytherapy for cervical carcinoma, calculated doses to ICRU points on orthogonal radiographs, and the doses at rectum reference points were compared with *in vivo* measurements. The *in vivo* measurements were 1.5 Gy below the doses determined for the ICRU rectum reference point (4.05 ± 0.68 vs. 6.11 ± 1.63 Gy). The advantage of *in vivo* dosimetry is the possibility to determine rectal dose during radiation. The advantages of computer-aided planning at ICRU reference points are that calculations are available before radiation and they can be taken into account for treatment planning.

Pelloski et al.[664] compared CT-based volumetric calculations and ICRU reference point radiation doses in 60 patients with cervix cancer treated with LDR brachytherapy. Of 118 insertions performed, 93 were evaluated, and the minimal doses delivered to the 2 or 3 cm of bladder or rectum (DBV2 and DRV2, respectively) were determined on a dose–volume histogram (DVH). They concluded that the ICRU dose was a reasonable surrogate for the DRV2 but not for the DBV2. Furthermore, these calculations may not be applicable to other treatment guidelines or intracavitary applicators.

Patil et al.[665] found significant correlations between ICRU point doses to the bladder and rectum and volumetric doses, particularly the D_{2cc}. However, there was significant variability, and they concluded that 3D imaging is essential to properly assess doses to the OAR.

Both CT- and MR-based OAR dosimetry report similar cumulative DVH parameters, including D_{2cc} and $D_{0.1cc}$. The D_{2cc} is the minimum dose received by the most exposed 2-cm^3 volume of the analyzed organ. For CT-based brachytherapy, contrast placed in the OAR may cause some artifact, resulting in some variation in contouring the wall of the organ. MR-based brachytherapy relies less on contrast because the organ wall may be more clearly visualized. Wachter-Gerstner et al.[666] analyzed the correlation between dose–volume histograms for bladder and rectum and found that D_{2cc} served as a good estimate for doses to the organ wall, whereas D_{5cc} was less reliable because is changed based on filling status. Rectal wall thickness did not significantly affect D_{2cc}.[667]

Based on CT-dosimetry, Koom et al.[668] showed that more-severe rectal side effects (endoscopy score >2) occurred in patients with a higher D_{2cc}. Seventy-one patients with FIGO stages IB to IIIB uterine cervical cancer had CT-based HDR intracavitary brachytherapy. The mean values of the DVH parameters and ICRU rectal point [$\alpha/\beta = 3$] were significantly greater in patients with a score of >2 than in those with a score of <2 at 12 months after brachytherapy (ICRU, 71 Gy vs. 66 Gy [$p = .02$]; $D_{0.1cc}$, 93 vs. 85 Gy [$p = .04$]; D_{1cc}, 80 vs. 73 Gy [$p = .02$]; D_{2cc}, 75 vs. 69 Gy [$p = .02$]). The probability of a score of >2 was significantly correlated with the DVH parameters and ICRU rectal point (ICRU, $p = .03$; $D_{0.1cc}$, $p = .05$; D_{1cc}, $p = .02$; D_{2cc}, $p = .02$).

For MR-based dosimetry, Georg et al.[661] tested the predictive value of dose–volume parameters for late effects of the rectum, sigmoid colon, and bladder using the D_{2cc}, D_{1cc}, and $D_{0.1cc}$ of these three OARs for 141 cervical cancer patients treated with tandem and ring HDR brachytherapy after EBRT. The mean D_{2cc} values for bladder, rectum, and sigmoid were 95 ± 22, 65 ± 12, and 62 ± 12 Gy,, respectively. This study confirmed that D_{2cc} was a predictor of late toxicity for the rectum and bladder. A rectoscopy study[669] was done in 35 patients in which EQD2 ($\alpha/\beta = 3$ Gy) of the $D_{0.1cc}$, D_{1cc}, and D_{2cc} of the rectum was recorded. After a mean follow-up time of 18 months, telangiectasia was found in 26 patients (74%), and 5 had ulceration that corresponded to the $D_{0.1cc}$ of the anterior rectal wall. The D_{2cc} was higher in patients with rectoscopy score of >3 compared to <3 (72 ± 6 vs., 62 ± 7 Gy; $p < .001$) and in symptomatic versus asymptomatic patients (72 ± 6 vs. 63 ± 8 Gy; $p < .001$). Based on these two studies, a dose limit of 70 to 75 Gy EQD2 is recommended for the rectal dose constraint.

For interstitial brachytherapy, in which a much longer portion of the anterior rectal wall is treated as part of the target volume, $D_{2cc} > 62$ Gy predicted for late toxicity.[670] The development of mucosal and clinical changes in the rectum seems to follow a clear dose effect and volume effect. For patients receiving interstitial brachytherapy who require treatment to the entire vaginal length, the dose to the rectum should be reduced as much as possible without compromising target coverage.

3D Treatment Planning for Pulse- and High–Dose-Rate Brachytherapy

Treatment planning for PDR and HDR brachytherapy can be accomplished by a variety of techniques. Treatment planning for LDR is covered in a separate chapter. For cervical cancer, customized optimization of source loading for each HDR insertion is recommended (Fig. 69.25), given significant changes in tumor and OAR dosimetry between fractions.[627,671] Himmelmann et al.[672] described individualized computer treatment optimization of source position and the dwell time for each position. Customized planning does increase the time needed for planning and requires experience on the part of the physics and dosimetry staff.[673]

CT-Based Treatment Planning

Fellner et al.[674] compared treatment planning for cervical carcinoma based on CT sections and 3D dose computations or, when these techniques were not available, dose evaluation based on orthogonal radiographs. The CT-based planning provides information on target and organ volumes and dose–volume histograms. The radiography-based planning provides dimensions and doses only at selected points. For the study, 28 patients with 35 applications receiving HDR treatment with ^{192}Ir were investigated. For a dose prescription of 7 Gy at point A, 83% (44 cm^3) of the CTV received at least 7 Gy.

Gebara et al.[675] estimated the external, internal, and common iliac dose rates using 3D CT-based dose calculations in tandem and ovoid brachytherapy in 30 patients with carcinoma of the uterine cervix treated with LDR brachytherapy using a CT-compatible Fletcher-Suit-Delclos device. Thirty-six implants were performed, and the authors concluded that the point B dose is similar to the maximum common iliac nodal dose. With HDR brachytherapy, the dose to the pelvic lymph nodes is approximately 25% of the per-fraction dose.[344]

Dewitt et al.,[676] in 15 patients with cervical cancer, defined target and organs at risk for planning of HDR brachytherapy and established guidelines for volume and dose constraint parameters using image-guided inverse treatment planning.

Careful assessment of the quality of brachytherapy and dose distributions is critical. Suyama et al.[677] analyzed the minimal radiation dose to the peripheral area of the cervix in relation to local tumor failure using CT images taken at the time of intracavitary brachytherapy in 80 patients with carcinoma of the cervix. After CT scanning, isodose curves were superimposed on the CT images. Histograms of both the minimum percentage peripheral dose and the dose to the cervical area showed significant correlation in the local tumor control and local failure groups ($p < .001$).

With HDR intracavitary applicators the use of a rectal retractor has been shown to substantially reduce the rectal dose.[610] Lee et al.,[678] in a study of 15 patients, found that this reduction was significant only in the subgroup who received >70% of the prescription dose ($p < .05$).

Wanderas et al.[679] reviewed data from 19 patients (72 fractions) retrospectively. Standard library plans were compared to individually optimized plans using a Fletcher HDR applicator. For standard treatment planning, the tolerance dose limits were exceeded in the bladder, rectum, and sigmoid in 26%, 4%, and 15% of the plans, respectively. This was observed most often for the smallest target volumes. The individualized planning of the delivered treatment gave the possibility of controlling the dose to critical organs to below certain limits. The dose was still prescribed to point A. An increase in target dose coverage was achieved when additional individual optimization was performed while keeping the dose to the OARs below predefined limits. Relatively low average target coverage was seen, however, especially for the largest volumes.

MR-Based Treatment Planning

Basic principles of MR imaging during brachytherapy have been described.[680] Several institutions have reported the dosimetric advantages of MR-based brachytherapy, with reduction in OAR doses with optimization.[645,654,681–683] Tanderup et al.[681] showed that point A dose was a poor surrogate of HR-CTV dose, and MR-based planning improved target coverage and reduced OAR dose. Starting with a standard plan is important for consistency because relative uniformity of the dose distribution should be maintained.[684]

A comparison of MR to ultrasound was reported by Van Dyk et al.[629] for 71 patients, showing comparability between the two modalities in terms of target volume and rectal point dose. Mahantshetty et al.[685] similarly confirmed the feasibility of US for institutions that do not have easy access to MR or CT.

Recommended Doses

Stage IA (microinvasive) tumors are treated with intracavitary therapy only. LDR dose is approximately 60 Gy in one insertion or 75 to 80 Gy in two insertions to point A, or with HDR an equivalent dose, with one or two fractions per week. This may be given in approximately 5 Gy per fraction for 10 fractions or other regimens based on normal-tissue exposure.

For stages IB to IVA cervical cancer in the United States, the most common EBRT dose treats the elective pelvic nodes to 45 to 50 Gy given in 1.8 Gy per fraction.[598] Some institutions instead use lower doses of whole-pelvis external irradiation (20 to 40 Gy) in addition to parametrial doses to complete 50 to 60 Gy to the involved parametrial tissues or nodal regions for more advanced stages. Brachytherapy follows, with a goal EQD2 dose of 80 to 90 Gy to point A or to the HR-CTV. For LDR, intracavitary treatment for approximately 4,000 to 5,000 mgh (36 to 50 Gy to point A at 60 cGy/hour) is given, depending on the tumor volume and stage and age of the patient. Fyles et al.[137] identified FIGO stage as the most significant prognostic factor in 965 patients with invasive carcinoma of the cervix, followed by dose of irradiation to point A and overall time of radiation therapy. The 10-year survival rate was 62% in 743 patients receiving doses to point A of 85 Gy or higher, in contrast to 53% for 222 patients receiving lower doses.

For HDR, one study found that a dose to the HR-CTV of >87 Gy resulted in a local recurrence rate of 4% compared to 20% for D_{90} < 87 Gy when the tumor was >5 cm and using an HDR tandem/ring or tandem/ring/interstitial approach. They concluded that local control rates of >95% can be achieved for patients with a poor response after EBRT if D_{90} for the HR-CTV is 87 Gy or higher.[535] The IR-CTV intended dose should be approximately 60 Gy EQD2. In the United States the most common regimen uses five fractions (5 to 6 Gy per fraction), with two fractions per week 24 to 48 hours between fractions.

DVH constraints for both PDR and HDR are 90 Gy (EQD2) for bladder and 70 to 75 Gy (EQD2) for both rectum and sigmoid as minimal doses to the most exposed D_{2cc} of the OAR.

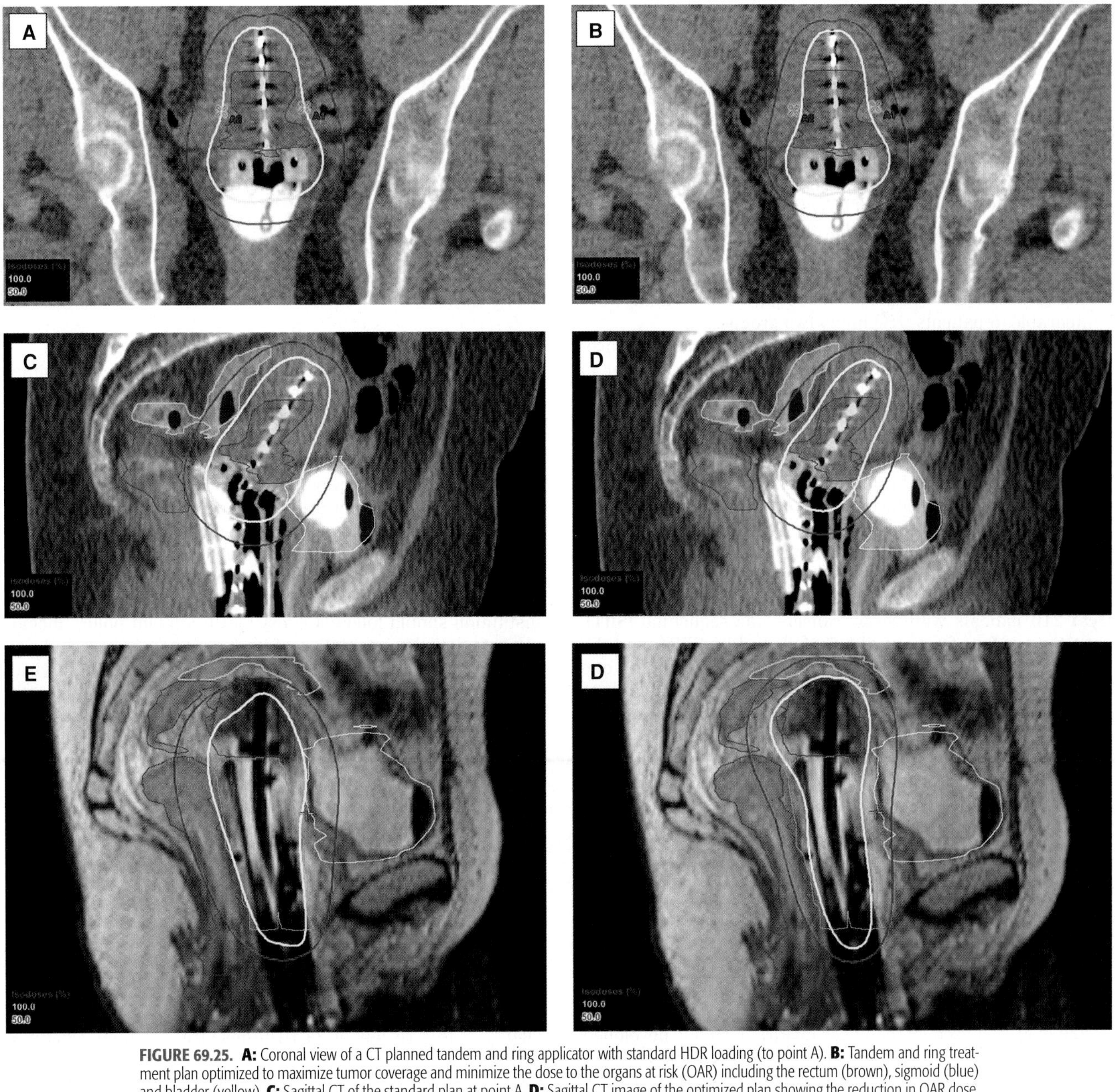

FIGURE 69.25. **A:** Coronal view of a CT planned tandem and ring applicator with standard HDR loading (to point A). **B:** Tandem and ring treatment plan optimized to maximize tumor coverage and minimize the dose to the organs at risk (OAR) including the rectum (brown), sigmoid (blue) and bladder (yellow). **C:** Sagittal CT of the standard plan at point A. **D:** Sagittal CT image of the optimized plan showing the reduction in OAR dose. **E:** Cervical stump cancer showing an MR-planned tandem and interstitial brachytherapy implant without HDR optimization. **F:** Optimized tandem and interstitial plan cover the posterior border of the cervical stump while minimizing dose to the bladder and rectum.

There are no generally accepted constraints for the 0.1-cm^3 level. Given the rapid regression of the tumor and the dramatic change in the location and size of the normal tissues, it is recommended to replan and determine the doses to the OAR with each fraction if the patient is treated on an outpatient basis.[671]

Dose Fractionation in High-Dose-Rate Brachytherapy

The relationship between dose and fractionation for HDR and LDR intracavitary irradiation of stage I and II carcinoma of the cervix was examined by Arai et al.[644] The dose rate at point A was 2 to 3 Gy/minute (120 to 180 Gy/hour) for HDR and 0.6 to 0.9 Gy/hour for LDR irradiation. Concurrent EBRT was given to the whole pelvis (23 to 30 Gy), followed by 25 to 30 Gy with central shielding, along with brachytherapy. The authors concluded that the optimal dose fractionation schedules for HDR brachytherapy were 28 ± 3 Gy in 4 to 5 fractions, 34 ± 4 Gy in 8 to 10 fractions, or 40 ± 5 Gy in 12 to 14 fractions at point A. Petereit and Pearcey,[619] based on their preliminary results and published reports in the literature, recommend doses of 45 to 50.5 Gy in a 1.8-Gy/fraction external beam followed by HDR with either 5.5 or 6 Gy per fraction in the era before the standardization of chemoradiation. Since the implementation of concurrent chemoradiation, several institutions in the United States have standardized the use of 5.5 Gy for five fractions, given some concerns about rectal toxicity with 6 Gy per fraction.[686]

Chatani et al.[687] described a study in which 165 patients with carcinoma of the cervix were randomized to a HDR brachytherapy point A dose of 6 Gy (group A) or 7.5 Gy (group B) per fraction, both combined with external irradiation. The 5-year local failure rate was 16% in both groups, and distant failure rates were 23% and 29%, respectively (p = .2955). Moderate to severe complications requiring treatment were comparable (6 patients, 7%) in the two groups.

Hama et al.[688] compared the effectiveness and safety of once- versus twice-weekly HDR brachytherapy for cervical cancer in 124 patients treated with EBRT (50 Gy); 74 patients (group A) were treated with one HDR brachytherapy insertion weekly (three fractions of 7 Gy each to point A), and 50 patients (group B) were treated twice weekly (six fractions of 4.5 Gy each to point A). Overall survival rates were 65.2% and 65.3%, respectively (p = .96). Local recurrence-free survival rates were 69% for group A and 90% for group B (p < .001). The rate of grade 2 (moderate) and grade 3 (severe) complications was significantly lower for group B (6%) versus 32% in group A (p < .001).

Mayer et al.[689] compared HDR BT in two schedules used to treat 210 patients with cervix cancer—one sequential (SRT), consisting of four fractions of 8 Gy followed by EBRT, and the other continuous (CRT), consisting of five fractions of 6 Gy one session per week integrated with EBRT (four fractions per week). Total dose to point A was 68 to 70 Gy. Progression-free survival was 71% with CRT versus 56% with SRT (p > 0.05). Late bladder and rectal morbidity were 13% in the CRT group and 25% in the SRT group (p = .037), related to the higher dose per fraction (8 Gy).

Nam and Ahn[690] compared, in a randomized study of 46 patients, two schedules of HDR BT (10 fractions of 3 Gy or five fractions of 5 Gy) followed by a small BT boost to residual tumor in combination with EBRT (30.6 Gy to whole pelvis and 14.4 Gy to parametria with midline block). Three-year pelvic tumor control was 90% in both groups, and disease-specific survival was 90.5% and 84.9% (p = .64), respectively. Late grade 2 and greater bladder or rectal morbidity was 23.8% and 9.1%, respectively (p = .24).

Liu et al.,[691] based on the linear-quadratic model, developed isoeffect tables to convert traditional LDR doses and number of fractions to point A to HDR brachytherapy; depending on dose rate, different dose values can be calculated for various fractionation schedules. They predicted that, using therapeutic gain ratio, similar results would be obtained with either brachytherapy modality with two to four fractions of LDR and four to seven fractions of HDR.

TABLE 69.16 HIGH-DOSE-RATE BRACHYTHERAPY DOSE AND FRACTIONATION REGIMENS WORLDWIDE

Percentage Respondents (Number)	Dose/Fraction	Number of Fractions	EQD2
Standard fractionation for stages IB to IIA cervical cancer			
18% (11)	6	5	40
15% (9)	6	4	32
12% (7)	7	3	29.75
8% (5)	5	6	37.5
8% (5)	7	4	39.7
5% (3)	5	5	31.25
5% (3)	5.5	5	35.52
Standard fractionation for stages IIB to IVA cervical cancer			
23% (14)	6	5	40
10% (6)	7	4	40
10% (6)	7	3	30
8% (5)	6	4	32
7% (4)	5.5	5	35.5
5% (3)	5	6	37.5
5% (3)	7	6	59.5
5% (3)	6	3	24
5% (3)	8	3	36

Gynecologic Cancer Intergroup physicians worldwide who use high-dose-rate (HDR) brachytherapy for cervical cancer were queried regarding the specific fractionation regimen that they routinely implement for stages IB to IIA and stages IIB to IVA cervical cancer patients. Results are shown for regimens reported by three or more respondents. The most common external beam dose was 45 Gy in 1.8 Gy per fraction, followed by five fractions of 5 to 6 Gy per fraction. The EQD2 formula was used to convert the HDR dose and number of fractionations and does not include the external-beam dose contribution.

Modified from Viswanathan AN, Creutzberg CL, Craighead P, et al. International brachytherapy practice patterns: a survey of the Gynecologic Cancer Intergroup (GCIG). *Int J Radiat Oncol Biol Phys* 2012;82:250–255; with permission from Elsevier.

The optimal time–dose–fractionation scheme for HDR brachytherapy for cervical cancer has yet to be established. In an international survey from the Gynecologic Cancer Intergroup, 28 different fractionation regimens were used by international cooperative group members (Table 69.16); the most common was 6 Gy for five fractions after 45 Gy.[602] The American Brachytherapy Society published recommendations for HDR brachytherapy for carcinoma of the cervix.[623] Each institution should follow a consistent treatment policy, including complete documentation of treatment parameters and correlation with clinical outcome (pelvic tumor control, survival, and complications). The goals are to treat point A to at least a total LDR equivalent of 80 to 85 Gy for early-stage disease and 85 to 90 Gy for advanced-stage disease. The pelvic sidewall dose recommendations are 50 to 55 Gy for early lesions and 55 to 65 Gy for advanced ones. As with LDR BT, every attempt should be made to keep the bladder and rectal doses to <100 Gy and 75 Gy LDR-equivalent doses, respectively. Interstitial brachytherapy should be considered when the tumor cannot be optimally encompassed by intracavitary brachytherapy. Some suggested dose and fractionation schemes for combining the external-beam radiation therapy with HDR brachytherapy for each stage of disease have been presented by the American Brachytherapy Society, although they have not been thoroughly tested. The responsibility for the medical decisions ultimately rests with the treating radiation oncologist. Petereit and Pearcy,[619] in a review of 24 HDR dose fractionation schedules published in the last three decades, found no dose relationship for either tumor control or late morbidity. Viswanathan et al.,[602] for the Gynecologic Cancer Intergroup, found significant international variation in the HDR dose/fractionation regimens

TABLE 69.17 RANDOMIZED TRIAL RESULTS OF TOXICITY AND OVERALL AND DISEASE-FREE SURVIVAL COMPARING HDR AND LDR

		Overall Survival (%)[a]		Disease-Free Survival (%)[a]		Toxicity (%)[b]	
Author (Reference)	Stage	HDR	LDR	HDR	LDR	HDR	LDR
Patel et al. (607)	Stage I, <3 cm	100	100	85	81	0.4	2.4
	Stage II, <3 cm	82	82	71	66		
	Stage I, >3 cm	87	88	75	70		
	Stage II, >3 cm	74	78	63	60		
	Stage III	71	76	43	50		
Teshima et al. (694)	Stage I	66	89[c]	85	93	7	3
	Stage II	61	73	73	78		
	Stage III	47	45	53	47		
Hareyama et al. (695)	Stage II	89	100	69	87	7.5	16.2
	Stage III	69	70	51	60		
Lertsanguansinchai et al. (696)[d]	Stage IIB	65	74	65	76	5	4
	Stage IIIB	71	63	74	59		

HDR, high dose rate; LDR, low dose rate.

[a]Five-year results unless otherwise stated. [b]Grades 3 to 5 rectal and bladder toxicity combined. [c]Statistically significant difference.

[d]Three-year results.

From Stewart AJ, Viswanathan AN. Current controversies in high-dose-rate versus low-dose-rate brachytherapy for cervical cancer. *Cancer* 2006;107:908–915; with permission.

reported, but aside from Japan, where the ratio of HDR brachytherapy dose to external beam is higher, there was consistency in converted EQD2 doses administered.

Clinical Outcomes of Brachytherapy

Randomized Studies Comparing HDR to LDR Using Plain X-Ray Dosimetry

Four randomized trials (Table 69.17) and a meta-analysis summarizing the results of these have been published comparing HDR and LDR brachytherapy for carcinoma of the cervix.[692,693] Teshima et al.[694] reported on a prospective, randomized study of 430 patients with carcinoma of the uterine cervix treated with either LDR (171 patients) or HDR (259 patients) brachytherapy combined with external irradiation. Cause-specific and overall survival rates were comparable for each clinical stage with either modality, except for stage I overall survival. The conversion factor of total intracavitary dose from LDR to HDR was 0.5 to 0.53. With HDR, four fractions usually were delivered, and with LDR, two fractions. The incidence of pelvic failures was comparable in both groups. The incidence of grade 2 and 3 morbidity was somewhat higher in the HDR group (~10%) than in the LDR group (4%; $p = .002$).

Patel et al.[607] published a randomized trial of 482 patients with invasive squamous cell carcinoma of the cervix. The overall local tumor control rate with LDR brachytherapy was 79.7%, compared with 75.8% with HDR. The 5-year survival rates were 73% with LDR and 78% with HDR in stage I, 62% and 64%, respectively, in stage II, and 50% and 43% in stage III. The only statistically significant difference was the incidence of overall rectal complications, which was 19.9% for LDR, compared with 6.4% for HDR. However, the incidences of more severe grade 3 and 4 complications were not significantly different (2.5% and 0.4%, respectively). Bladder morbidity was similar in both groups.

Hareyama et al.[695] conducted a randomized study in 132 patients with stage II or IIIB cervical carcinoma treated with LDR or HDR BT and identical pelvic EBRT. The conversion factor from LDR to HDR was 0.588. The 5-year DSS with HDR for stages II and IIIB was 69% and 51%, respectively, and with LDR it was 87% and 60%, respectively. Pelvic tumor control for stage II and III was 89% and 73% with HDR and 100% and 70% with LDR, respectively, and grade 3 or greater morbidity was 10% and 13%, respectively (differences were not statistically significant).

Lertsanguansinchai et al.[696] randomized 237 patients with cervical cancer to be treated with LDR (109 patients) or HDR (112 patients) brachytherapy and EBRT. Median follow-up was 40 and 37 months, respectively. Three-year pelvic tumor control was 89% and 86.4%, respectively, and relapse-free survival was 69% in both groups. Grade 3 or 4 morbidity was noted in 2.8% of LDR and 7.1% of HDR patients ($p = .23$).

A meta-analysis[693] including these four trials reported a pooled RR for HDR versus LDR of 0.95 (95% CI = 0.79 to 1.15), 0.93 (95% CI = 0.84 to 1.04), and 0.79 (95% CI = 0.52 to 1.20) for 3-, 5- and 10-year overall survival rates and 0.95 (95% CI = 0.84 to 1.07) and 1.02 (CI = 0.88 to 1.19) for 5- and 10-year DSS rates. For local control rates the RR was 0.95 (95% CI = 0.86 to 1.05) and 0.95 (95% CI = 0.87 to 1.05) at 3 and 5 years, respectively. For bladder, rectosigmoid, and small-bowel complications, the RR was 1.33 (95% CI = 0.53 to 3.34), 1.00 (95% CI = 0.52 to 1.91), and 3.37 (95% CI = 1.06 to 10.72), respectively, indicating no significant differences except for increased small-bowel complications with HDR ($p = .04$). Of note, none of the randomized studies used 3D imaging to optimize away from normal tissues.

The use of 3D imaging to guide brachytherapy treatment planning has allowed optimization of HDR and PDR brachytherapy, thereby reducing the high per-fraction doses to the normal tissues that might potentially cause significant side effects. A retrospective comparison of LDR and HDR with pretreatment MRI used for tumor volume determination showed a significant reduction in complications with HDR when image-based planning was implemented.[697] Similarly, the use of 3D imaging optimizes tumor coverage, which is critical with fractionated HDR therapy.

Prospective Data Using Point A Dosimetry

Haie-Meder et al.,[698] in 204 patients with cervical cancer randomized to receive one of two preoperative LDR brachytherapy procedures (0.4 or 0.8 Gy/hour), noted similar local tumor control (93%) and overall survival (85%) rates at 2 years with either dose rate. Grade 3 late complications were observed in 7% of patients treated with 0.4 Gy/hour and in 13% of patients treated with 0.8 Gy/hour. There was 1 small-bowel obstruction in the 0.4-Gy/hour group (1%), in contrast with 5 (5%) in the 0.8-Gy/hour group. Vesicovaginal fistulas were observed in 2% and 4%, respectively.

A prospective study in Japan of stage I and II cervical cancer with tumors <4 cm (by T2 MRI) and no lymphadenopathy treated 60 patients with whole-pelvis EBRT 20 Gy/10 fractions with midline block followed by 30 Gy/15 fractions and HDR 24 Gy/4 fractions (at point A).[699] The cumulative BED was 62 Gy ($\alpha/\beta = 10$) at point A, lower than that reported by any other institution worldwide. Median tumor diameter was 28 mm (range, 6 to 39 mm). Median overall treatment time was 43 days. Median follow-up was 49 months (range, 7 to 72 months). Seven patients developed recurrences: 3 patients had pelvic recurrences (2 central, 1 nodal), and 4 patients had distant metastases. The 2-year disease-free and overall survival rates were 90% (95% CI = 82% to 98%) and 95% (95% CI = 89% to 100%), respectively. The 2-year late complication rates (according to RTOG/EORTC grade ≥ 1) were 18% (95% CI = 8% to 28%)

TABLE 69.18 CLINICAL OUTCOMES WITH THREE-DIMENSIONAL PLANNED BRACHYTHERAPY

Institution (Years Reported)	*Number of Patients*	*Mode of Treatment*	*Stage*	*Imaging During BT*	*Median Follow-up (Year)*	*Local Control (%)*	*Disease-Specific Survival (%)*	*Overall Survival (%)*	*Late Grade 3–4 Toxicity (%) (Number)*
French STIC (2005–2007)[534, a]	705	–	IB–IIIB	–	2	–	–	–	–
	76	Preop LDR or PDR	–	X-ray	–	92[b]	87[b]	95[b]	14.6[b]
	89	Preop PDR	–	CT	–	100[b]	90[b]	96[b]	8.9[b]
	142	Preop ChRT/LDR or PDR	–	X-ray	–	85[b]	73[b]	85[b]	12.5[b]
	163	Preop ChRT/PDR	–	CT	–	93[b]	77[b]	86[b]	8.8[b]
	118	ChRT/LDR or PDR	–	X-ray	–	74[b]	55[b]	65[b]	22.7[b]
	117	ChRT/PDR	–	CT	–	78.5[b]	60[b]	74[b]	2.6[b]
Vienna (1993–1997)[736]	189	EB/HDR	IA–IVB	CT	2.8	78[c]	68[c]	58[c]	(3 GU), (4 GI), (31 V)[c]
Vienna (1998–2003)[742]	145	EB ± Ch[d]-HDR	IA–IVA	MR	4.3	85[c]	68[c]	58[c]	(3 GU), (4 GI), (5 V)[c]
Vienna (2001–2008)[653]	156	EB ± Ch[e]-HDR	IA–IVA	MR	3.5	95[c]	74[c]	68[c]	(3 GU), (5 GI), (2 V)[c]
UPMC (2007–2010)[652]	44	ChRT/HDR	IB–IIIB	CT + MR	0.6	88[b]	85[b]	86[b]	0
Addenbrooks (2005–2007)[737]	28	ChRT/HDR	IB1–IIIB	CT	1.9	96[c]	81[c]	–	14 (3 GI)[c]
IGR (2000–2004)[741]	39	Preop LDR	IB1–IIB	MR	4.4	9[f]	86[f]	94[f]	0
IGR (2000–2004)[655]	84	ChRT/LDR	IB2–IVB	MR	4.4	89[f]	52[f]	57[f]	(3 GU; 1 GI)[f]
IGR (2004–2006)[651]	45	ChRT/PDR	IB–IVA	MR	2.2	100[b]	73[b]	78[b]	(1 Fi)[+]
BW/DFCC (2004–2011)[738]	115	ChRT/HDR	IB–IIIB	CT	1.8	93[b]	83[b]	78[b]	–

BW/DFCC, Brigham and Women's/Dana-Farber Cancer Center; Ch, concurrent cisplatin chemotherapy; ChRT, concurrent cisplatin with external-beam radiotherapy; CT, computed tomography; EB, external beam; Fi, fistula; GI, gastrointestinal; GU, genitourinary; HDR, high–dose-rate brachytherapy; IGR, Institut Gustave Roussy; LDR, low–dose-rate brachytherapy; MR, magnetic resonance imaging; PDR, pulsed–dose-rate brachytherapy; Preop, preoperative therapy; STIC, Soutien aux Thérapeutiques Innovantes et Couteuses; UPMC, University of Pittsburgh Medical Center; V, vaginal.

[a]Prospective trial. [b]Two years. [c]Three years. [d]Ch administered to 55%. [e]Ch administered to 73%. [f]Four years.

for large intestine/rectum, 4% (95% CI = 0% to 8%) for small intestine, and 0% for bladder. No cases grade ≥3 were observed for genitourinary/gastrointestinal late complications.

The prospective French STIC trial[534] reported patients treated with x-ray simulation compared to 3D-based planning. A total of 705 patients with stages IB to IIIB cervical cancer were enrolled. Toxicity and survival were significantly improved with 3D-based treatment planning. Plain film–based 2-year local control was 74% for patients treated with chemoradiation and LDR or PDR brachytherapy. Detailed results are shown in Table 69.18.

Retrospective Data Using Point A Dosimetry for Low–Dose-Rate Brachytherapy

Fowler[700] analyzed results in 270 patients with carcinoma of the cervix treated with either 75 cGy/hour from manually loaded cesium or 150 cGy/hour by remote afterloading. There was an increase in grade 3 late complications from 4% to 22%, in spite of a reduction of 20% in dose, implying a rather large difference in biologic effect between the two systems. The effect of the increased dose rate was also described by Leborgne et al.[701] Linear-quadratic modeling was used to calculate biologically effective doses in the clinical protocols used. When the LDR was doubled, it was called MDR. The maximum ratios calculated for the biologic effective doses of 16 Gy at MDR to 20 Gy at LDR were 1.06 to 1.15, assuming $\alpha/\beta = 4$ to 2 Gy, the latter being an unlikely extreme for rectal or urinary complications. The theoretically ideal dose reduction factors, calculated using the $t_{1/2}$ values derived from the clinical data, are in the range of 24% to 29% instead of 20%.

Rodrigus et al.[702] analyzed late complications in 143 patients with cervical cancer treated with two different brachytherapy schedules and external radiation. Seventy-seven patients had two intracavitary applications with a dose rate of 0.54 Gy/hour and 66 patients with that of 1.07 Gy/hour. Because of the expected increase in complications with the higher dose rate, the latter dose per application was reduced from 25 to 20 Gy. Late intestinal and urinary complications were scored in 49 of 77 and 46 of 68 patients, respectively. Actuarial estimates at 5 years showed 42% and 54.1% late intestinal complications and 16.9% and 24.1% late urinary complications, respectively. Thus, despite the dose reduction, there was a clear dose-rate effect on late morbidity. These studies emphasize the importance of the dose rate of brachytherapy in carcinoma of the cervix.

Rotmensch et al.[703] compared the outcome in 140 patients with early-stage cervical cancer undergoing whole-pelvis radiation therapy with one versus two LDR intracavitary brachytherapy applications. The two groups had similar 5-year local tumor control ($p = .83$), disease-free ($p = .23$), and cause-specific ($p = .29$) survival. Late complications were similar in the two groups. These results support the use of a single LDR application in patients with early-stage disease undergoing definitive radiation therapy after 45-Gy external-beam pelvic irradiation.

In a retrospective analysis, Perez et al.,[169] noted that in patients with cervical cancer treated with radiation therapy alone for stage IB tumors <2 cm in diameter, the pelvic failure rate <10% with LDR doses of 70 to 80 Gy to point A, whereas for larger lesions, even doses of 85 to 90 Gy resulted in 25% to 37% pelvic failure rates. In stage IIB with LDR doses of 70 Gy to point A, the pelvic failure rate was approximately 50%, compared with 20% in nonbulky and 30% in bulky tumors with doses >80 Gy. In stage III unilateral lesions, the pelvic failure rate was approximately 50% with 70 Gy or less to point A versus 35% with higher doses, and in bilateral or bulky tumors it was 60% with doses <70 Gy and 50% with higher doses.

A study from France reported on preoperative LDR followed by radical surgery with lymph node dissection for 257 patients with stages IB1, IIA, and IIB cervical cancer of <4 cm.[704] Residual tumor was identified in 44% of patients, whereas 4.3% of patients had parametrial invasion and 17.9% of patients had lymph node involvement. Late complications of grade 2 occurred in 7.4% and of grade 3 in 2.7% of patients. Five-year actuarial overall survival and disease-free survival were 83% (CI = 78.3 to 87.5) and 80.9% (CI = 76.3 to 85.7), respectively. In multivariate analysis, lymph node involvement, parametrial involvement, and smoking factors significantly affected overall survival and disease-free survival rates.

Retrospective Results Using Point A with Pulse–Dose Rate Brachytherapy

Rogers et al.[705] treated 52 patients with cervical carcinoma, 31 of whom had staging laparotomy before radiation therapy.

Brachytherapy was interstitial in 18 patients and intracavitary in 28. The median EBRT pelvis dose was 45 Gy in 25 fractions. Median total doses were 75.8 Gy to the implant volume with interstitial and 84.1 Gy to the A points with intracavitary at a median dose rate of 0.55 Gy per pulse per hour. Six patients had laparotomy-documented para-aortic node involvement and received EBRT to this site (45 Gy in 25 fractions). Thirty patients received concomitant weekly cisplatin chemotherapy (40 mg/m^2). With a median follow-up of 25 months, the actuarial 4-year disease-free survival rates were 66% for the entire group (100% for stage IB, 69% for stage II, 68% for stage III/IVA, and 43% in patients treated for recurrences after surgery). Grade 4 complications occurred in 2 patients (4.3%). One patient (2.2%) had a grade 3 complication (frequent hematuria), and 5 (10.9%) had grade 2 complications.

Kaneyasu et al.[706] treated 419 patients with squamous cell carcinoma of the cervix from 1969 to 1999 with LDR or MDR. LDR required overnight admission, whereas MDR was given over approximately 5 hours on an outpatient basis. The 5-year overall survival rates for stages I, II, III, and IVA in the LDR group were, respectively, 78%, 72%, 55%, and 34% versus 100%, 68%, 52%, and 42% in the MDR group (not statistically different). The actuarial rates of late complications of grade 2 or greater at 5 years for the rectum, bladder, and small intestine in the LDR group were 11.1%, 5.8%, and 2.0%, respectively, whereas for the MDR group they were 11.7%, 4.2%, and 2.6%, respectively (not significantly different).

El-Baradie et al.[707] published a prospective study in which 45 patients with carcinoma of the uterine cervix were randomly allocated to either HDR or MDR. The external-beam radiation dose was the same in the two groups. The point A dose rate correction factor from LDR to HDR was 0.53, and that from LDR to MDR 0.6. The 3-year survival and locoregional tumor control rates for both modalities were equivalent (respectively 62% and 67% for HDR and 68% and 74% for MDR). The rectal and bladder complication rates were the same in both groups (29% at 3 years). Tanaka et al.[708] also compared HDR and MDR brachytherapy in 150 and 56 patients, respectively. The survival was equivalent in the two groups; grade 2 or greater late toxicity tended to be higher in the HDR group (14% vs. 6%, respectively).

Bachtiary et al.[709] reported on 109 patients treated with LDR BT and 57 who received PDR BT. The 3-year overall survival and disease-free survival rates were 70% and 57% for the LDR group and 82% and 70% for the PDR group, respectively (p = .25 and .19). The 3-year probability rate for late grade 3 or worse toxicity was 7.4% for LDR BT patients and 7.6% for PDR BT patients (p = .69) and was 6.9% and 7.6%, respectively, for concurrent chemotherapy versus none (p = .69).

Rath et al.[710] reported on 48 patients treated with PDR brachytherapy (ICRT) and pelvic irradiation. A single session delivered a dose of 27 Gy to point A by PDR (hourly pulse, 70 cGy). Ten patients had disease recurrence (5 each in stage IIB and stage IIIB). Eight patients had pelvic failure, 1 had bone metastases, and 1 had supraclavicular node metastases. Overall the grades III to IV late toxicity rate at 50 months was 6%. For the median follow-up period of 15 months, the actuarial recurrence-free survival in stages I to II was 82% and in stages III to IV was 78%.

Retrospective Results with Point A Using High–Dose Rate Brachytherapy

Many nonrandomized studies compared the results of HDR with those of historic or concurrent control patients receiving LDR at the same institution.[608,627,672,711–713] HDR in patients with stage IIIB disease or large tumors must be used cautiously because the brachytherapy prescription dose should cover the tumor volume and avoid the normal tissues as much as possible (Table 69.19). Although it is generally recommended not to give concurrent chemotherapy on the day of HDR brachytherapy,[598] several studies indicate that HDR does not increase toxicity in patients treated with chemoradiation (Table 69.20). Most studies used point A as a reference point, although the definition of point A may have differed from center to center.

A retrospective population-based cohort study of all uterine cervix cancer cases in Saskatchewan diagnosed between 1985 and 2001 had 107 LDR and 37 HDR cases with similar stage distribution. The 5-year cause-specific survival rate was 56% for HDR and 67% for LDR (p = .72). Acute toxicities were diarrhea (60%) and abdominal cramps (12.5%), and chronic toxicities were vaginal stenosis (5.5%) and small-bowel obstruction (4%).[714]

Petereit et al.[606] reported on 191 patients receiving LDR brachytherapy and 173 receiving HDR brachytherapy with equivalent external-beam radiation therapy techniques. Pelvic tumor control and survival rates were comparable with the two techniques, except in stage III; in this subgroup, outcome was better with LDR brachytherapy, but this may have been related to a lower HDR equivalent dose administered. In an analysis of 198 patients treated with LDR brachytherapy, the 3-year survival rate was 66% versus 77% for 40 patients treated with HDR brachytherapy.[715] Pelvic tumor control rates were 80% and 77%, respectively. The incidences of complications requiring hospitalization or surgery were 10% (20 of 198) and 2.5% (1 of 40), respectively.

Kapp et al.,[716] in a study of 181 patients with FIGO stages IB to IV carcinoma of the cervix, documented that prognostic factors for patients treated

TABLE 69.19 STAGE III OVERALL SURVIVAL, PELVIC CONTROL, AND TOXICITY IN RETROSPECTIVE SERIES

	Low Dose Rate				*High Dose Rate*			
	Number	*Overall Survival[a] (%)*	*Pelvic Control (%)*	*Toxicity[b] (%)*	*Number*	*Overall Survival (%)*	*Pelvic Control (%)*	*Toxicity[b] (%)*
Akine et al.[393,c,d]	212	38	61	–	37	54	64	–
Arai et al.[646,c,d]	143	46.5	–	–	508	52.2	–	–
Falkenberg et al.[718,c,e,f]	23	45	72	4.8	6	33	83	3.5
Ferrigno et al.[717,d]	69	**46**[g]	58	**4.7**[g]	56	**36**[g]	50	**0.8**[g]
Hsu et al.[724,d,h]	73	50.2	–	–	30	51.1 (6) 42.9 (4)	–	–
Kim et al.[889,d]	8	35.7	–	–	16	43.8	–	–
Kucera et al.[890,e]	212	**37.3**[g]	–	–	78	**53.8**[g]	–	9.0
Okkan et al.[891,c,d]	21	47.3	53	–	98	31.6	45	–
Orton et al.[610,d]	1464	42.6	–	–	2721	47.2	–	–
Petereit et al.[606,c,e]	50	**58**[g]	**75**[g]		50	**33**[g]	**44**[g]	
Sarkaria et al.[715,e]	57	46	63	7.0	12	58	50	2.5
Lorvidhaya et al.[730,c,d]	–	–	–	–	675	47.8	68.8	8.3
Sakata et al.[892,d]	–	–	–	–	48	–	63	–
Souhami et al.[893,c]	–	–	–	–	77	42	–	
Wong et al.[894,c,d]	–	–	–	–	51	25	63.2	–

[a]Combined grades 3 to 5 rectal and bladder late complications, reported for all stages. [b]Stage IIIB results. [c]Five-year results. [d]Three-year results. [e]Cause-specific survival reported. [f]Statistically significant differences in bold. [g]Six- and four-fraction results.

From Stewart AJ, Viswanathan AN. Current controversies in high-dose-rate versus low-dose-rate brachytherapy for cervical cancer. *Cancer* 2006;107:908–15; with permission.

TABLE 69.20 FRACTIONATION AND TOXICITY OF HIGH-DOSE-RATE AND CONCURRENT CHEMOTHERAPY

	High Dose Rate		*Toxicity (%)*[a]		*Follow-up (Month)*
	Dose (Gy)	*Number of Fractions*	*No Chemotherapy*	*Chemotherapy*	
Tseng et al.[463,b]	4.3	6	6.5 (GI) 3.2 (GU)	10 (GI) 3.3 (GU)	47
Pearcey et al.[454,b,c]	8	3	9 (GI) 7 (GU)	5 (GI) 10 (GU)	82
Sood et al.[895,d]	9	2	5 (GI)	5 (GI)	36
Saibishkumar et al.[896,d]	9	2	(GI) 1.0 (GU)	1.8 (GI) 0 (GU)	39
Sood et al.[843,d]	9	2	10	6	28
Ozsaran et al.[897,e]	8.5–9	1–2	0	0	20
Souhami et al.[478,e]	10	3		28 (GI) 6 (GU)	27
Strauss et al.[898,e]	7	5		3.7 (GI) 3.7 (GU)	19

GI, gastrointestinal; GU, genitourinary.

[a]Grades 3 to 5 late complications. [b]Prospective, randomized trial. [c]Includes high, medium, and low dose rate. [d]Retrospective comparison of patients treated with and without chemotherapy. [e]Retrospective review, all patients received chemotherapy.

From Stewart AJ, Viswanathan AN. Current controversies in high-dose-rate versus low-dose-rate brachytherapy for cervical cancer. *Cancer* 2006;107:908–915; with permission.

with HDR are similar to those in previous series with LDR brachytherapy. In multivariate analysis, tumor size was the most powerful factor for pelvic tumor control and incidence of distant metastasis.

Ferrigno et al.[717] carried out a retrospective study of 190 patients treated with LDR and 118 with HDR brachytherapy in combination with pelvic EBRT for cervical cancer. For stage I or II patients, there was no difference in outcome; however, in the stage III group local tumor control was 58% with LDR and 50% with HDR ($p = .19$), and DFS was 49% versus 37% ($p = .03$). At 5 years, rectal sequelae were 16% versus 8% ($p = .03$), bladder sequelae were 6% and 3% ($p = .13$), and small-bowel sequelae were 4.6% and 8.9% ($p = .17$).

Falkenberg et al.[718] reviewed 160 patients, 103 treated with LDR and 57 treated with HDR from 1990 to 2000. Locoregional control was 78% for LDR and 76% for HDR ($p = .96$); overall survival was 60% for LDR versus 55% for HDR ($p = .48$) at 3 years. Late complications were reported in 2 HDR patients (3.5%) and 5 LDR patients (4.8%).

Orton et al.[610] noted that dose per fraction of HDR brachytherapy significantly influenced toxicity. Morbidity rates were significantly lower for point A doses/fractions of 7 Gy or less for both severe (1.28% vs. 3.44%; $p < .0001$) and moderate plus severe injuries (7.58% vs. 19.51%; $p < .001$). The effect of dose/fractionation on cure rates was equivocal.

Kuske et al.[719] described a method to improve target coverage and locoregional tumor control with HDR tandem and ovoid applications by which HDR endocavitary and interstitial brachytherapy are applied in the same session for tumors with a lateral expansion of 25 mm or more from the axis of the cervical canal. Seventy-six combined applications were given to 41 patients. With a follow-up average of 23 months, in stage IIB tumors, 3-year DFS was 75%. No severe early or persistent late complications were observed. Combined applicators with the tandem and ring with interstitial[720] and tandem and ovoid with interstitial[656,721] are now available for HDR brachytherapy.

Forrest et al.[686] presented the results of 122 patients treated with EBRT followed by 6 Gy per fraction for five fractions of HDR. They reported a 2-year disease-free survival rate of 70% and grade 3/4 toxicity rate of 14% (13 patients). The median time to recurrence was 8 months (range, 2 to 22 months) and to toxicity was 10 months (range, 4 to 27 months). They concluded that the high toxicity of this regimen should prompt consideration of dose reduction in BT dose or use of 3D imaging to shape the dose. Several institutions in the United States now report 5.5 Gy × five fractions instead of 6 Gy per fraction for patients treated with chemoradiation.[601,602]

Anker et al.[722] treated 65 patients with HDR with 6 Gy × fractions, and 45 patients had the top dwells retracted as the tumor regressed. With a median follow-up of 24.5 months, the 3-year overall, disease-free distant metastases–free survival, and local control rates were 67%, 76%, 79%, and 97%, respectively. Acute and actuarial 3-year late grade 3 toxicity or greater occurred in 24.6% and 17% of patients, respectively.

Le Pechoux et al.[723] treated 130 patients with cervical cancer with HDR brachytherapy (for stage I, 30 Gy in six weekly sessions) in combination with EBRT (50-Gy mean dose with midline shielding). Patients with more-advanced disease received four sessions of biweekly brachytherapy for a total dose of 18 to 24 Gy and external irradiation (20 to 30 Gy to the whole pelvis, 50 to 66 Gy to parametria with midline shielding). The 5-year survival rates were 82% for patients with stage IIB and 47% with stage IIIB disease. There were 4 rectovaginal or vesicovaginal fistulas and 1 case of proctitis requiring colostomy. Survival, local tumor control, and morbidity were equivalent in 76 patients treated with 6 Gy once a week and in 54 patients receiving twice-weekly brachytherapy of 5 Gy per session.

Hsu et al.[724] dosed 92 patients with cancer of the cervix with HDR brachytherapy, six fractions of 7 Gy per fraction (42 Gy) at point A (HDR-6); 57 received four fractions of 8 Gy per fraction (32 Gy) at point A (HDR-4). A twice-daily program was used for all patients receiving HDR in two split courses. A historic control group of 259 patients was treated with LDR brachytherapy (40 Gy in two split courses). All patients received whole-pelvis external irradiation of 36 to 45 Gy (mostly 40 Gy) before brachytherapy. Five-year local tumor control rates were equivalent in the three groups (82%, 85.5% for HDR, and 89.5% for LDR). Five-year survival rates were also comparable (67.7%, 77.9%, and 74.1%, respectively). However, late complications were lower in the HDR-4 group, which received treatment more biologically equivalent to the LDR regimen, than in patients in the HDR-6 group (11% vs. 25.6%).

Selke et al.[725] published results in 187 patients with primary carcinoma of the cervix treated with whole-pelvis irradiation (46 Gy) and HDR brachytherapy with a dose rate to point A of 1.6 Gy/minute, decreasing to approximately 0.8 Gy/minute at the end of the 5-year study. Three HDR fractions (8 to 10 Gy to point A per fraction) were concurrently administered with the last 2 to 3 weeks of external irradiation. The 5-year actuarial survival rates were 72% for stage IB, 65% for IIA, 66% for IIB, 66% for IIIA, and 45% for stage IIIB. With a median follow-up of 54 months, 23 patients had 25 complications; 13 (7.6%) were grade 3 or 4. Rectal complications were significantly higher in patients who received a total rectal dose of >54 Gy ($p = .045$).

Choi et al.[726] treated 136 patients with carcinoma of the cervix with external-beam whole-pelvis irradiation (46 Gy in 23 fractions) and three weekly applications of HDR brachytherapy of 7 or 8 Gy per fraction to point A. The actuarial 5-year survival was 85% in stage IB, 64% in stage IIA, 70% in stage IIB, and 53% in stage IIIB. Grade 3 or higher complications occurred in 3% to 7% of the patients. The most significant determinants of severe rectal complications were the addition of a lower vaginal tandem ($p < .01$), uterine tandem length >5 cm, a total biologically effective dose to the rectum of >120 Gy, and stage III disease.

Kagei et al.[727] reported on 217 patients with carcinoma of the cervix (71 patients with stage II and 146 with stage III disease) who received whole-pelvis EBRT (40 Gy in 20 fractions or 39.6 Gy in 22 fractions) and an additional 10 Gy in five fractions to the parametria followed by HDR brachytherapy. Cause-specific 5-year survival rates were 77% for stage II and 50% for stage III. Pelvic failure rates were 13% and 36%, respectively. The rates of severe (grade 4) late complications were 2% for the rectum, 1% for the small intestine or sigmoid colon, and 1% for the bladder.

Takeshi et al.[728] treated 265 patients with stage III cervical carcinoma with external-beam radiation therapy (50.3 Gy) and intracavitary HDR brachytherapy (19.8 Gy). The 5-year overall survival, relapse-free survival, and locoregional event–free rates were 50.7%, 57.1%, and 71.2%, respectively. The 5-year incidence of major complications was 2.6% for bladder and 8.3% for rectum. The radiation dose in the subgroup with rectal complications was significantly greater than that in the subgroup without complications.

Wang et al.[729] reported treatment results in 173 patients with cervical carcinoma treated with HDR brachytherapy and whole-pelvis irradiation (40 to 44 Gy in 20 to 22 fractions) followed by pelvic wall boost (6 to 14 Gy in three to seven fractions with central shielding). HDR brachytherapy delivered 7.2 Gy to point A in each of three applications 1 to 2 weeks apart. Five-year pelvic tumor control rates were 94%, 87%, and 72% for stages IIA, IIB to IIIA, and IIIB to IVA, respectively. Five-year actuarial survival rates were 79%, 59%, and 41%, respectively. Sixty-six patients (38%) had rectal complications, and 19 (11%) had bladder complications. The 5-year actuarial rectal complication rates were 15%, 4%, and 3% for grades 2, 3, and 4, respectively.

Lorvidhaya et al.[730] reported the results in 1,992 patients with carcinoma of the cervix treated by external irradiation and HDR brachytherapy. There were 211 patients with stage IB, 225 with stage IIA, 902 with stage IIB, 14 with stage IIIA, 675 with stage IIIB, 16 with stage IVA, and 16 (0.8%) patients with stage IVB. With a median follow-up of 96 months, the actuarial 5-year disease-free survival rates were 70%, 59.4%, 46.1%, 32.3%, 7.8%, and 23,1%, respectively. The late complication rates (RTOG) for bowel and bladder combined were 7% for grade 3 and 1.9% for grade 4 complications.

Leborgne et al.[731] described a 4-year pelvic control rate of 93% and a disease-free survival rate of 88% for 59 patients with stage IB to IIA disease. All were treated with 18 Gy to the whole pelvis and 22 Gy to the parametria combined with six HDR fractions (14 Gy/hour to point A) of 7 Gy to point A, two in each treatment day, with 6-hour interfraction intervals. The corresponding parameters for 29 patients with stage IIB disease were 79%, 75%, and 75%. The actuarial 4-year late grade 2 and 3 complication rate was 4.7%.

In 1,148 patients with squamous cell cervical cancer treated with external RT and HDR brachytherapy with 22 years median of follow-up, the 10-year pelvic tumor control was 93% for stage IB, 82% for stage II, and 75% for stage III.[569] Cause-specific survival was 89%, 74%, and 59%, respectively. Major sequelae were 4.4% in the rectosigmoid, 0.9% in the bladder, and 3.3% in the small intestine. Nakano et al.[732] subsequently presented a study of 210 patients with stage IIIB cervical cancer from eight Asian countries treated from 1996 to 1998 with radiation and brachytherapy. Though follow-up was difficult to obtain, the reported 5-year major complication rates were 6% in the HDR group and 10% in the LDR group. The 5-year overall survival rates were 51.1% in the HDR group and 57.5% in the LDR group.

Novetsky et al.[733] presented data on 77 patients treated with external beam with concomitant cisplatin followed by two HDR brachytherapy fractions of 9 Gy each. Median follow-up was 3.5 years. The local control rate was 88% for stages IB2/II and 68% for stages III/IV. Grade 3/4 gastrointestinal acute symptoms occurred in 47%. Grade 3/4 late toxicities occurred in 5 (6%) patients. Patel et al.[734] describe 104 cervical cancer patients treated with external beam and HDR, either 9 Gy for two fractions or 6.8 Gy for three fractions, each fraction 1 week apart. Median follow-up was 31 months. The 3-year actuarial local control was 81.35% with 9 Gy versus 65.18% with 6.8 Gy ($p = .04$). The 3-year actuarial risk of developing any grade 3 or worse late toxicity was 7.47% with 9 Gy and 3.57% with 6 Gy ($p = 0.3$).

Prospective Trial with CT or MR Compared to X-Ray

The clinical outcome results from institutions using CT- or MR-based treatment planning for cervical cancer brachytherapy are listed in Table 69.18. The French STIC trial[733] collected data from 20 centers prospectively and stratified to 2D versus 3D (mainly with CT) brachytherapy. A total of 705 patients were treated with one of three arms: (a) brachytherapy followed by surgery (stage IB1, 165 patients); (b) EBRT plus chemotherapy, BT, then surgery (305 patients); or (c) EBRT plus chemotherapy and then BT (235 patients). For the 235 patients treated with concurrent chemoradiation and then brachytherapy, 2-year overall survival was 74% for 3D versus 65% for 2D ($p = .27$); disease-free survival was 60% versus 55% ($p = .09$); local regional relapse–free survival was 70% versus 61% ($p = .001$), and local-only relapse–free survival was 79% versus 74% ($p = .003$). Toxicity was reduced overall from 23% with 2D to 2.6% with 3D ($p = .002$); urinary from 9% in 2D to 1% with 3D ($p = .02$), gastrointestinal from 9% to 0% ($p = 0.17$), and gynecologic from 15% to 1% ($p = .01$).

Retrospective Comparison of CT to MR-Planned Brachytherapy

Three studies compared CT to MRI contouring for HDR tandem and ring brachytherapy. Wachter-Gerstner et al.[735] compared MR-based plans in 15 patients to those derived with either CT or orthogonal films. CT and MR enabled higher dose to the target volume with similar OAR dosing. Viswanathan et al.[635] compared CT contours to MR contours based on a standard set of guidelines; the CT contours were larger in width, but no other significant differences in DVHs were identified. A report by Eskander et al.[636] of 10 patients had an MR for the first fraction only and showed that CT volumes had a greater length on the coronal plane, whereas MR images had a greater height on the sagittal plane. No differences were found in DVH parameters after optimization.[636] Similar to the Eskander et al.[636] study, using an MR for the first fraction and CT for subsequent fractions, Beriwal et al.[652] treated 44 patients with 5- to 6-Gy per fraction HDR after EBRT. Ninety-three percent had a complete response by PET at 3 months. Of those with a CR, 2 had a local recurrence at 6 and 8 months. With a median follow up of 8 months (range, 2.5 to 38 months), 2-year local control, disease-specific, and overall survival rates were 88%, 85%, and 86%, respectively.

Retrospective Results with CT-Planned Brachytherapy

Potter et al.[736] reported results in 189 patients treated with HDR brachytherapy and EBRT (48.6 to 50 Gy). Small tumors were treated with five to six fractions of 7 Gy at point A (25 Gy in the brachytherapy volume), which is isoeffective to 76 to 86 Gy at point A. Large tumors received three to four fractions of 7 Gy after 50 Gy of EBRT, which is isoeffective to 82 to 92 Gy at point A. Three-dimensional treatment planning for brachytherapy was based on conventional x-rays and in 181 of 189 patients on CT scan. The mean brachytherapy dose was 16.2 Gy at the ICRU rectum reference point and 14.4 Gy at the

ICRU bladder point. Taking into account the dose for EBRT, the mean isoeffective dose at the ICRU rectum reference point was 69.9 Gy. After a mean follow-up of 34 months, the actuarial pelvic control rate was 78% and the late complication rate for grades 3 and 4 was 2.9% for bladder, 4% for bowel, 6.1% for rectum, and 30.6% for the vagina (shortening and obliteration).

CT-based clinical outcomes were reported by the Addenbrooks Hospital. Twenty-eight patients had HDR, 8 Gy × 3, CT-planned brachytherapy.[737] The 3-year actuarial cancer-specific survival rate in this group was 81%, with a pelvic control rate of 96%. Five of the 28 patients died of para-aortic or other distant disease, 1 of them being the only one with local recurrence presenting as a malignant vesicovaginal fistula. In 24 patients, D_{90} ≥74 Gy was achieved. The only patient with local recurrence had D_{90} = 63.8 Gy, which was a 20% improvement over historical non–image-guided controls.

At Brigham and Women's Hospital, 115 stages IB to IVA cervical cancer patients had CT-planned brachytherapy and were treated with 595 fractions of 5.5- to 6-Gy per fraction HDR brachytherapy.[738] The 2-year local relapse rate was 6.9%. The 2-year disease-specific survival was 83%, and overall survival rate was 78%.

Retrospective Results with MR-Planned LDR Brachytherapy

An initial report of MRI during intracavitary gynecologic brachytherapy was published in 1992 from the University of Michigan by Schoeppel et al.[739] Three patients had CT and MRI with their first of two intracavitary implants. A CT- and MR-compatible Fletcher applicator was used. CT could not distinguish the tumor with as much clarity as MR. Tardivon et al.[740] at Institut Gustave Roussy (IGR) treated 10 patients with MR evaluation of the tumor during intracavitary brachytherapy for cervical and vaginal cancer and found that in 7 cases MR findings were concordant with clinical examination. MR was useful to determine the tumor/applicator relationship and distinguish the adjacent OAR.

A review was published of 39 patients treated at IGR with MRI-guided LDR brachytherapy in the preoperative setting.[741] A total dose of 60 Gy to the IR-CTV was followed 6 weeks later by extrafascial hysterectomy and bilateral salpingo-oophorectomy with pelvic node dissection. Adjuvant chemoradiation was delivered to patients with pelvic lymph node involvement. After a median follow-up of 4.4 years (range, 2.6 to 6.6 years), there were no central recurrences; 1 local recurrence occurred in the lateral pelvis (2.6%). The 4-year actuarial overall and disease-free survival rates were 94% and 86%, respectively. The 2- and 4-year actuarial local relapse–free survival rates were 94% and 91%, respectively. Haie-Meder et al.[655] subsequently published a series of 84 patients treated with LDR MR-planned brachytherapy after chemoradiation. With a median follow-up of 53 months (range, 31 to 79 months), the 4-year overall survival and disease-free survival rates were 57 (95% CI = 43 to 69) and 52% (95% CI = 40 to 64), respectively. Thirty-nine late complications occurred in 28 patients (33.3%): 13 bladder, 7 rectal, 5 small bowel, 4 urethral, 3 colic, 2 vaginal, 1 pelvic fibrosis, and 4 others. Four grade 3 delayed complications were observed, and no grade 4 complication occurred.

Retrospective Results with MR-Planned PDR or HDR Brachytherapy

With a 0.2-T MRI at the Medical University of Vienna, 145 patients with stage IB to IVA cervical cancer were treated with four fractions of 7-Gy HDR from 1998 to 2003.[742] Complete remission was achieved in 138 patients (95%), with 7 patients having locally persistent or progressive disease in the central (n = 5) or noncentral (n = 2) pelvis. With a median follow-up of 40 months, the 4-year local control rate was 83%, compared to 63% for historical controls. A subsequent analysis of 156 patients treated from 2001 to 2008 with MR-based brachytherapy was reviewed.[653] Local control was 98% for tumors 2 to 5 cm and 92% for tumors >5 cm. Overall survival, however, was 72% for tumors 2 to 5 cm and 65% for tumors >5 cm, indicating that despite the increase in local control with MR-based brachytherapy, death from distant metastases remains a problem in patients with large-volume cancer.

Investigators at the IGR reported on 45 patients treated between 2004 and 2006 with a tandem and mold technique using PDR brachytherapy and MR-based contouring.[651] Until recently at IGR, surgery was often performed after brachytherapy if disease was suspected on clinical examination. A dose of ≥15 Gy (after EBRT) was prescribed to the IR-CTV. The dose to the HR-CTV was approximately 250% of the dose to the IR-CTV (i.e., 80 Gy to the HR-CTV). With a median follow-up of 26 months, the 2-year overall and disease-free survival rates were 78% and 73%, respectively. At Tata Memorial Hospital in India, 24 patients with squamous cell carcinoma were treated with MRI-based HDR. With a median follow-up of 12 months,[743] 2 patients had local failures.[616] Other European centers[645,654,656] and one Canadian center[744] reported feasibility data for MR-based cervical cancer brachytherapy, showing a reduction in the normal-tissue toxicity rate. When implementing 0.5- to 1.5-T MR-based tandem/ring or tandem/ovoid brachytherapy with MRI, specific guidelines for MR use should be followed.[680]

Toxicities

Table 69.18 lists general toxicities in series using CT- or MR-planned brachytherapy. In the Medical University of Vienna series reporting patients treated from 2001 to 2008, 73% received concurrent cisplatin chemotherapy.[653] A total of 11 grade 3 and 4 late events were recorded in 143 patients. With a median follow-up of 3.5 years, the actuarial grade 3 and 4 late morbidity at 3 and 5 years was respectively as follows: gastrointestinal, 4% and 4%; urinary, 2% and 3%; and vaginal, 1% and 3%. Two patients developed massive rectal bleeding requiring transfusions. Three patients required stoma (grade 4) for rectal wall ulceration, resulting in a fistula, a rectal perforation, and a rectovaginal fistula. Three patients developed grade 3 urinary frequency or urgency. Three patients experienced grade 3 or 4 coaptation of the vagina.

At IGR, of the 45 patients studied,[651] 23 and 2 developed acute grade 1 or 2 and grade 3 complications, respectively; 21 patients presented with delayed grade 1 or 2 complications. One other patient presented with a grade 3 vesicovaginal fistula. No grade 4 or greater complications, whether acute or delayed, were observed. In the IGR experience with LDR brachytherapy from 2000 to 2004, 39 late complications were reported; 13 bladder, 7 rectal, 5 small bowel, 4 urethral, 3 colic, 2 vaginal, 1 pelvic fibrosis, and 4 others. Grade 3 complications were 1 rectal, 2 bladder, and 1 urethral. Tan et al.[737] reported on 28 patients treated with CT-guided brachytherapy for stage IB to IIIB cervix cancer. Their overall actuarial 3-year grade 3 and 4 morbidity rate was 14%,. Two patients had grade 3 abdominal pain and 1 had a colovaginal fistula. Overall, the data indicate that a potential reduction in morbidity appears to be a benefit of image-guided brachytherapy.

Template-Based Interstitial Brachytherapy

Interstitial implants with ^{226}Ra, ^{137}Cs needles, or ^{192}Ir afterloading plastic catheters to limited tumor volumes are helpful in specific clinical situations. Indications include large residual bulky cervical tumors after external beam treatment, residual tumor with sidewall invasion, vaginal extension, presence of a fistula and/or adjacent organ invasion, or a prior supracervical hysterectomy (Fig. 69.26). Syed-Neblett[745] and Martinez[746] perineal applicators are the most commonly selected. Methods for insertion have been described.[598,747] A tandem should be inserted when a uterus is present.[748] If the os is not visible, ultrasound guidance to determine the proper placement of the

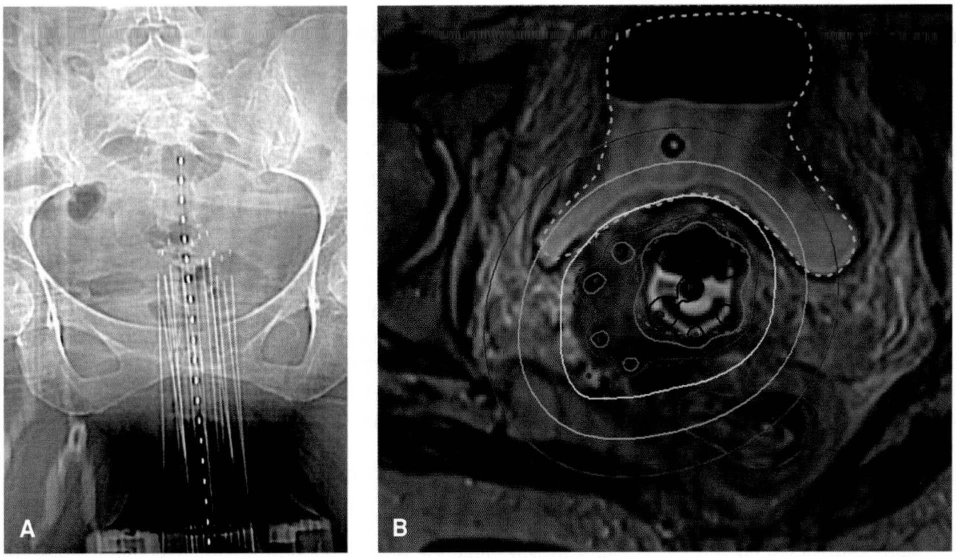

FIGURE 69.26. A: Picture of anterior scout computed tomography showing a template-based interstitial brachytherapy application. **B:** Magnetic resonance imaging during interstitial needle insertion in a patient with stage IIIB cervical cancer ensures proper placement of the catheters adjacent to the tandem. The 100% isodose line is in yellow.

tandem is advised.[749] A ring applicator modified to allow simultaneous insertion of interstitial needles[750] and ovoid application with interstitial needles have been described.[656]

Traditionally, plain x-ray films are used for brachytherapy treatment planning. Determination of normal tissue doses and optimization is not feasible, and the risk of complications is high. In these cases, consideration of laparoscopic approaches is recommended.[598] Syed et al.[751] reported on 185 locally advanced cervical cancer patients treated with LDR interstitial brachytherapy from 1977 to 1997. Patients received external-beam treatment to 50.4 Gy, followed by interstitial brachytherapy to 40 to 50 Gy. Local control was 82%; 5-year disease-free survival rates were 65%, 67%, 49%, and 17% for patients with stage IB, II, III, and IV disease, respectively. Eighteen (10%) of the 185 patients developed RTOG grade 3 or 4 late complications.

Clinical outcomes using traditional techniques have been reported by several institutions. Thirty patients with stage IIB and 37 patients with stage III carcinoma received interstitial irradiation in the parametrium to supplement the dose delivered by external-beam treatment and intracavitary brachytherapy. Despite the fact that the patients treated with interstitial implant were in a high-risk group, local tumor control was comparable to that of patients treated with standard techniques.[169] Pierquin et al.[752] described locoregional recurrences in 6% of 53 patients with T1, 11% in 47 patients with T2, and 42% of 19 patients with T3 primary tumors of the uterine cervix treated with a combination of external-beam irradiation and the Creteil method for interstitial implantation of ^{192}Ir sources in a plastic cervical-vaginal moulage and a uterine tandem. Prempree[753] reported a 96% local tumor control rate and 61% 5-year disease-free survival rate in 23 patients with stage IIIB carcinoma of the cervix treated with a combination of external irradiation and intracavitary and interstitial implants to the parametrium. Overall, major complications were noted in 8% of the patients. Martinez et al.,[746] using the Martinez Universal Perineal Interstitial applicator, treated 37 patients with advanced or recurrent carcinoma of the cervix and 26 with vaginal-urethral tumors. Doses of approximately 35 Gy were given, in addition to external irradiation (36 Gy to the whole pelvis and 14 Gy to the pelvic sidewall). They reported 6 local failures in the patients with cervical lesions and 5 in the group with vaginal-urethral tumors. The overall complication rate was 5.1%. Nag et al.[754] reported on 31 patients with carcinoma of the cervix treated with external-beam radiation therapy and fluoroscopically guided interstitial brachytherapy. With a median follow-up of 36 months, 16 patients (51%) with cervical had local tumor control. The 5-year actuarial survival rate was 34%. Only 1 patient experienced grade 3 complications (2.5%).

Recio et al.[755] used laparoscopy at the time of interstitial brachytherapy in six patients with FIGO stages IIB to IVA cervical carcinoma after completion of whole-pelvis radiation; a total of 98 needles were inserted to deliver a median interstitial brachytherapy dose of 20 Gy. Eleven perforations in the pelvic peritoneum or bladder were identified during surgery in five of the six patients, leading to immediate repositioning of needles. No acute or short-term morbidity related to the procedure was noted.

Sharma et al.[756] presented results on 42 patients treated from 2005 to 2007 in a prospective study of two weekly sessions of 10Gy, 1 week after finishing external-beam radiation. Median follow-up was 23 months. Delayed toxicity was 9%. The 3-year overall survival for all stages was 47% and the 3-year recurrence-free survival for stages IIB, IIIB, and IVA was 67%, 34%, and 20%, respectively. Sharma et al.[757] also reported on the use of transrectal ultrasound to assist with insertion of the interstitial needles.

With image-based planning including either a CT[637,638] or an MRI[630] the physician evaluates the placement of the needles and may choose either to not treat specific catheters or to lower the dose given through catheters close to normal-tissue structures. An approximate 11% rate of bowel insertion and a long-term fistula rate of 4% to 10% have been reported in studies using CT for planning after insertion.[637,638] When a physician has the facility to insert the applicator in a CT or MR suite while the patient is under anesthesia, an iterative process of image-guided needle insertion ensures proper placement of the catheters and prevents an inadvertent insertion into a surrounding normal-tissue structure, such as the rectum, sigmoid, or bladder.[630]

Dose optimization with either PDR or HDR may improve the normal-tissue doses for interstitial therapy for some patients. The University of Pittsburgh reported on 11 cervical cancer patients treated with CT-guided HDR interstitial brachytherapy (5 fractions of 3.5 Gy per fraction).[758] From 1998 to 2004 interstitial brachytherapy was chosen for cases with distorted anatomy or extensive vaginal disease. The 5-year actuarial local control rate was 63%. No patient had acute grade 3 or 4 toxicity. Grade 3 or 4 late toxicity occurred in 1 patient, with a 5-year actuarial rate of 7%. Three patients had late grade 2 rectal toxicity, and 1 patient had grade 2 small-bowel toxicity.

Dimopoulos et al.[720] reported on the use of tandem/ring with short interstitial needles and MR-planned HDR brachytherapy for 22 cervical cancer patients followed for a median of 20 months; no grade 3 or 4 toxicities were noted, and 1 patient had a local recurrence. Nomden et al.[721] described the use of tandem/ovoid application with short interstitial needles for the second insertion with MR-planned PDR brachytherapy for 20 cervical cancer patients. They compared the first insertion with just a tandem and ovoid applicator to the second insertion, which included the addition of interstitial needles. There was an average increase in dose of 4.4 Gy (SD 2.3), with better coverage of the HR-CTV with the second insertion.

Mikami et al.[759] analyzed needle applicator displacement in 10 patients treated with 30 Gy HDR in five fractions and found on daily CT scans an average of 1 to 2 mm of caudal displacement. Shifts of >3 mm were replanned. Shukla et al.[760] presented data on 20 patients with cervical cancer treated with interstitial brachytherapy who underwent every-other-fraction CT imaging. The mean needle displacement was 2.5 (range, 0 to 7.4), 17.4 (range, 0 to 27.9), 1.7 (range, 0 to 6.7), 2.1 (range, 0 to 9.5), 1.7 (range, 0 to 9.3), and 0.6 mm (range, 0 to 7.8 mm) in cranial, caudal, anterior, posterior, right, and left directions, respectively. The mean displacement in the caudal direction was higher between days 1 and 2 than that between days 2 and 3 (13.4 vs. 3.8 mm; $p = .01$). Damato et al.,[761] in a study of 10 patients treated with interstitial brachytherapy, found on average, that <1-cm displacements and deformations of the implant occurred over the course of treatment. The most significant dosimetric consequences were due to changes in organ filling rather than catheter shifts. Proper quality assurance methodologies should be in place to detect shifts that can potentially result in inadvertent insertion into normal tissue.

Brachytherapy in the Elderly

Magné et al.[762] reported on 113 patients with median age of 76 years (range, 70.7 to 94.4 years) treated by conventional LDR BT as a part of their treatment. For rectal complications, grades 1/2, 3/4, and 5 (fatal) crude incidences were 19.4% (22 of 113), 1.8% (2 of 113) and 0.9% (1 of 113), respectively. Acute toxicity death occurred in 1 patient with major diarrhea associated with a hemodynamic shock. For small-bowel complications, grades 1/2 and 3/4 crude incidences were 3.5% (4 of 113) and 0.9% (1 of 113), respectively. For urinary tract complications, grades 1/2 and 3/4 crude incidences were 11.5% (13/113) and 2.7% (3/113), respectively. With a median follow-up of 3.1 years, 10 patients developed distant metastases, and 10 others had local relapses. The 3-year specific overall survival rate was 88.6% (95% CI = 77 to 92), and the corresponding disease-free survival rate was 81% (95% CI = 72 to 88). Age did not influence the effectiveness of BT in elderly patients, and BT should be considered whenever possible, even in elderly patients presenting with a cervix cancer.

Image-Guided Brachytherapy Versus External-Beam Boost

Studies of external-beam treatment as an alternative boost instead of brachytherapy demonstrate significantly inferior survival rates compared to those that use brachytherapy. The use of ultrasound enables tandem placement in most cases, even when the os cannot be identified, and should be attempted for difficult cases. Barraclough et al.[763] reported on 44 patients with cervical cancer who did not receive brachytherapy and were treated with EBRT to 54 to 70 Gy via a three-dimensional conformal boost. After a median follow-up of 2.3 years, 48% relapsed, with 16 of 21 developing a central recurrence. The 5-year overall survival rate was 49%, which is much lower than for brachytherapy-treated patients.

The dosimetry of brachytherapy cannot be adequately mimicked by external-beam techniques. A treatment planning report compared inversely planned EBRT with photons (IMRT) and protons (IMPT) to 3D MRI-guided brachytherapy.[764] EBRT was planned to deliver the highest possible doses to the PTV while respecting D_{2cc} limits from brachytherapy, assuming the same fractionation. Volumes receiving 60 Gy (in equivalent dose in 2-Gy fractions) were approximately twice as large for IMRT compared with brachytherapy, and the high central tumor dose was lower than that seen with brachytherapy. Both IMRT and protons were inferior to 3D image-based brachytherapy.

With IMRT, there is a need for replanning due to rapid tumor regression[317–319] and an increase in integral dose, with normal tissues throughout the pelvis receiving more radiation than with brachytherapy. Given the large movement and the increased dose to the normal tissues resulting in an increase in normal-tissue toxicity, highly conformal (IMRT, IGRT, SBRT) methods for boosting the cervix are not routinely recommended. Every effort should be made to use image guidance to insert a tandem into the uterus in order to provide adequate brachytherapy doses for all cervical cancer cases receiving radiation.

External-Beam Irradiation Alone

Occasionally, brachytherapy procedures cannot be performed because of medical reasons or unusual anatomic configuration of the pelvis or the tumor (i.e., extensive lesion, inability to identify the cervical canal). These patients may be treated with higher doses of external-beam irradiation alone, although survival is significantly worse than when brachytherapy is implemented, and normal-tissue toxicity is higher due to the excessive dose to the rectum and bowel. Therefore, every attempt to treat with brachytherapy should be made because brachytherapy moves with the patient and provides high regions of dose in the central regions of the tumor. With IMRT, a significantly higher normal-tissue dose is administered, and the desired high central regions of radiation cannot safely be administered.

Coia et al.,[521] in an analysis of 565 patients with various stages of cervical carcinoma treated in the Patterns of Care Study, reported better survival (67%) and pelvic tumor control (78%) for patients treated with external irradiation and brachytherapy than for patients who had no intracavitary brachytherapy applications (36% 4-year survival rate and 47% in-field failure rate). Patients treated with two intracavitary applications had a higher 4-year survival rate (73%) and in-field tumor control rate (83%) than those receiving only one application (60% 4-year survival rate and 71% in-field tumor control rate).

Hanks et al.[525] and Montana et al.[524] reported a higher incidence of central pelvic recurrences in patients with stage III cervical carcinoma treated with external-beam therapy alone than in patients receiving brachytherapy in addition to external-beam irradiation (Table 69.21). The incidence of major complications was similar in both groups of patients.

Akine et al.[765] treated 104 patients with carcinoma of the uterine cervix with external irradiation alone (anteroposterior–posteroanterior or four-field box techniques) because of inability to perform intracavitary brachytherapy. Average doses delivered were 50 Gy to the whole pelvis, followed by additional doses with reduced portals to deliver a total of 60.8 Gy in

TABLE 69.21 CARCINOMA OF THE UTERINE CERVIX: INCIDENCE OF CENTRAL/PELVIC RECURRENCES CORRELATED WITH METHOD OF THERAPY

		Incidence of Pelvic Failures		
Author (Reference)	*Stage*	*External Beam Only*	*External Beam and Intracavitary*	*p*
Hanks et al. (525)	III	33/38 (86%)	55/109 (50%)	.0002
Montana et al. (524)	III	14/35 (40%)	12/37 (32%)	.6725
Coia et al. (521)	I,II,III	(53%)	(22%)	<.0100
Longsdon and Eifel (899)[a]	IIIB	641 (45%)	266 (24%)	<.0001

[a]Five-year disease-free survival.

Modified from Stehman FR, Perez CA, Kurman RJ, et al. Uterine cervix. In: Hoskins WJ, Perez CA, Young RC, eds. *Principles and Practice of Gynecologic Oncology,* 3rd ed. Philadelphia: Lippincott Williams & Wilkins, 2000:841–918.

6 weeks, 72.3 Gy in 7.5 weeks, or 80.5 Gy in 8 weeks, with a daily dose of 1.9 or 2 Gy. The local tumor control rate was 27% for stage II, 19% for stage III, and 15% for stage IVA disease. The 5-year survival rates were 36%, 17%, and 5%, respectively. Four patients had major complications (usually proctitis) that required surgical treatment, and 1 patient died of rectal bleeding. Eight of 23 patients treated with conformal therapy had control of the tumor and survived 5 years without major complications. Saibishkumar et al.[766] treated 146 patients with cervix cancer with EBRT alone (60 to 66 Gy) because of unsuitability for brachytherapy; 5-year pelvic tumor control was 21.9% and DFS was 11.6%.

Cost-Effectiveness of LDR Versus HDR Brachytherapy

Wright et al.[767] developed a questionnaire to elicit patient preference for two brachytherapy methods (one LDR or three HDR fractions and two HDR or five HDR fractions, assuming both methods to be isoeffective). The questionnaire was completed by 90 female staff members at their center, 18 previously treated patients, and 20 newly diagnosed patients. When both methods were assumed to be isoeffective, only 34% of the 38 patients preferred three HDR fractions to one LDR fraction. However, when HDR was assumed to be 2% more curative or 6% less toxic, 50% said they would prefer the HDR therapy. Both preference and strength of preference for LDR were significantly associated with a greater traveling distance for treatments. More studies on resource utilization[768] are needed.

Alternative Isotopes

Californium has been proposed as an alternative to iridium as the radioactive isotope. Maruyama and Muir[769] reported on 41 patients with stage IB cervix cancer treated with 40 to 50 Gy to the whole pelvis followed by a 5- to 15-Gy boost to the lateral pelvic wall and a single ^{252}Cf-neutron brachytherapy insertion in approximately 8 hours. Nearly total tumor clearance was achieved in >90% of the patients; tumor regression was more rapid in the ^{252}Cf group than in similar patients treated with ^{137}Cs and the same external-beam irradiation dose.

FOLLOW-UP

After treatment, patients should be regularly followed by both the radiation and the gynecologic oncologist. Careful history taking and a complete physical and pelvic/rectal examination usually are performed every month for the first 3 months after completion of irradiation, every 3 months for the remainder of the first year, every 4 months the second year, every 6 months during the third through the fifth year, and yearly thereafter. The use of Pap smears for cervical and vaginal cytology as a follow-up study is controversial because of postirradiation cellular morphology that renders it difficult to distinguish postirradiation changes from residual or recurrent malignant cells.[770,771] DNA analysis of postirradiation cytologic smears demonstrating atypia or dysplasia may provide ancillary information.[772]

Rintala et al.[773] evaluated the reliability of cytologic analysis and atypia after radiation therapy in 89 patients treated for cervical carcinoma. A total of 697 Pap smears were taken; during the follow-up, 44 patients had recurrent disease, which was local in 17 (39%) cases. The rate of false-positive samples was only 3%. Radiation-induced atypia was detected in 28% of the Pap smears taken during the first 4 months after radiation therapy, and its incidence decreased thereafter. In 1,000 patients treated with either surgery or radiation therapy at the MD Anderson Cancer Center for stage IB cervical cancer post-treatment, Pap smears did not detect a single asymptomatic recurrence among 133 patients with recurrent disease.[774]

The presence of apparently viable tumor cells in the cytologic smear 3 months after irradiation should be evaluated with cervical biopsies, dilation and curettage, and careful examination under anesthesia, as indicated.

Complete blood counts and chemistry profile tests are obtained as clinically indicated. Chest radiography is commonly obtained on a yearly basis, usually for the first 5 years post-treatment, although its value to detect curable lung metastasis is not proven. If radiographs are consistently negative, obtaining them every other year thereafter may be sufficient.

Other imaging studies, such as CT, MRI, PET scanning, or bone scans, are obtained when clinically warranted. When persistent or recurrent tumor is suspected, biopsies should be obtained for histologic confirmation. If a biopsy is positive, immediate treatment should be instituted, as is discussed later.

Usually, hematometra after radiation therapy for cervical carcinoma is related to recurrent disease but occasionally may be related to estrogen replacement therapy, endometrial activity, or fibrosis and obliteration of the endocervix.[775]

TREATMENT OF RECURRENT CARCINOMA OF THE CERVIX

After Previous Surgery

Radiation may salvage approximately 50% of patients with localized pelvic recurrences after surgery alone. A combination of whole-pelvis external irradiation (45 to 50 Gy) with concurrent chemotherapy followed by interstitial brachytherapy is recommended. If the tumor lies outside of an accessible region for brachytherapy, dose escalation with conformal or IMRT techniques may be attempted, depending on the location of the tumor and the need to protect bowel, with at least 65 to 70 Gy necessary for adequate control. In the setting of recurrent disease, the total mucosal dose from the external and brachytherapy can approach 140 Gy to the upper vagina and 95 Gy to the distal vagina without a high risk.[776] With interstitial brachytherapy, doses of 20 to 35 Gy are administered with single, double-plane, or volume implants, for a total tumor dose of approximately 80 Gy, depending on the extent of the tumor.

Larson et al.[777] observed 27 recurrences (11%) in 249 patients treated with radical hysterectomy and pelvic lymphadenectomy for stage IB carcinoma of the cervix; 17 (63%) had tumor recurrence in the pelvis or vulva; the other 10 patients had recurrences outside the pelvis. Eight of 15 patients (53%) treated with irradiation for an isolated recurrence in the pelvis or vulvar region were tumor free between 10 and 126 months after treatment of the recurrence (median, 48 months).

Ijaz et al.[778] reported on 50 patients treated with RT for an isolated pelvic recurrence of cervical carcinoma after radical hysterectomy; 7 patients were treated with palliative intent using hypofractionated RT. The remaining 43 patients were treated with curative intent, 33 with RT only and 10 with cisplatin-based chemoirradiation. The overall 5-year survival rate was 33% for all 50 patients, 39% for the 43 patients treated with curative intent, and 25% for patients with isolated sidewall recurrences treated with curative intent. Three patients experienced late treatment complications.

Hille et al.[779] described results in 17 patients with recurrent cervix cancer (9 had a complete microscopically incomplete resection) treated with EBRT and brachytherapy to 50 to 65 Gy. The 5-year pelvic tumor control was 48%, and relapse-free survival was 24%.

After Definitive Irradiation

Reirradiation of previously irradiated patients must be undertaken with extreme caution. It is very important to analyze the techniques used in the initial treatment (beam energy, volume, doses delivered with external or intracavitary irradiation). In addition, the period of time between the two treatments must be taken into consideration because it is postulated that some repair of the initial damage may take place in the interval. In general, external irradiation for recurrent tumor is given to limited volumes (40 to 45 Gy, 1.8-Gy tumor dose per fraction, preferentially using lateral portals). Occasionally, intracavitary or interstitial irradiation can be used to treat relatively circumscribed recurrences.

Sommers et al.[780] described the results of retreatment in 376 patients with recurrent carcinoma of the uterine cervix. Ninety-one patients received irradiation, mostly external (86.8%), occasionally combined with brachytherapy (7.7%) to control bleeding of central recurrences; brachytherapy alone was administered in 5.5% of patients. The usual dose for recurrent pelvic masses was 40 to 45 Gy, and for para-aortic lymph node metastases it was 45 to 50 Gy in 5 weeks. Other metastatic sites were treated with 35 to 40 Gy in 3 to 4 weeks. Pelvic exenteration was attempted in 23 patients, only 10 of whom were deemed to be operable (43.5%), but it was completed in only 7. The probability of 5-year survival after treatment for recurrence was 30% with combined surgery and external irradiation, 12% with surgery alone, and 4% with external irradiation alone. The 5-year survival rate for 10 patients who underwent pelvic exenteration was 16%. Only 1% of the untreated patients survived 5 years. Six of 140 patients (4.3%) experienced grade 2 or 3 complications.

Selected patients with limited pelvic recurrences not fixed to the pelvic wall and without evidence of extrapelvic metastases can be potentially salvaged by radical hysterectomy or pelvic exenteration. Coleman et al.[781] described results in 50 patients who underwent radical hysterectomy for persistent (18 patients) or recurrent (32 patients) cervical cancer after primary radiation therapy. Lymph node metastases were identified in 5 of 39 patients (13%) in whom the lymph nodes were evaluated. The 5- and 10-year survival rates were 72% and 60%, respectively.

In 65 patients on whom pelvic exenteration was carried out at Memorial Sloan-Kettering Cancer Center, the 5-year survival rate was 23%.[782] The operative mortality rate was 9.2%. The authors pointed out that the significant mortality and morbidity associated with this procedure preclude its use as palliative therapy.

Urinary diversion, either by nephrostomy or ileal bladder, may be of palliative value in patients with either recurrent carcinoma in the pelvis or complications. It must be kept in mind that diversion may prolong life but runs the risk of denying a terminally ill patient with cancer the oblivion and insensibility of uremia.

Kastritis et al.[783] treated 200 patients with stage IV or recurrent cervix cancer with cisplatin-based chemotherapy; response rate was 43.5% in 142 patients with squamous cell and 53.5% in 58 patients with nonsquamous tumors ($p = .79$). Median survival was 11.57 and 19 months, respectively. Tinker et al.[784] treated 25 women for recurrent cervical cancer with carboplatin–paclitaxel and noted a 20% cure rate and 20% progression rate, with median survival of 21 months. Brewer et al.[511] in 32 women, all of whom had previous chemotherapy and 29 of whom had previous RT, used cisplatin and gemcitabine, with a progression rate of 22% and median time to progression of 3.5 months.

Para-Aortic Lymph Node Recurrences

Isolated recurrences in the para-aortic nodes after pelvic irradiation have been described in about 3% of patients, and some may be salvaged with aggressive therapy. The advent of IMRT makes treatment easier, with less morbidity.

Kim et al.[785] treated 12 patients with isolated para-aortic lymph node metastasis with hyperfractionated RT (60 Gy in 1.2-Gy fractions twice a day) and concurrent cisplatin–paclitaxel. Fields extended from the superior plate of T12 to the lower plate of L5. Three-year survival was 19%. Grade 3 or 4 hematologic toxicity developed in two patients. Singh et al.[786] detected 14 isolated para-aortic lymph node metastases in 816 patients previously treated with RT; these women were subsequently treated with RT to the para-aortic lymph nodes combined with concurrent chemotherapy. Seven patients survived 5 years.

In a review of 1,955 patients treated with RT for cervix cancer, Jhingran et al.,[787] identified 120 patients with recurrent tumor above the pelvic fields. Initially, 10 had common iliac and 5 had para-aortic node involvement. In 104 patients, recurrences were immediately adjacent to the upper borders of the RT fields. In 15 patients treated with curative intent for the para-aortic lymph node recurrence, 5-year survival was 25%.

Intraoperative Irradiation

Intraoperative radiation therapy (IORT) has been used for treatment of locally advanced and recurrent carcinoma of the cervix, with 3-year survival rates of 8% to 21% as reported by Mahé et al.[788] and Garton et al.,[789] and a 5-year survival rate of 33% in 14 patients described by Kinney et al.[423] Patient selection may have had an impact on the different results. Abe and Shibamoto[790] noted that central recurrences, particularly in nonirradiated patients, and resection of the gross recurrent tumor in irradiated patients improve the benefit from IORT. Significant toxicity included peripheral nerve injury and ureteral stenosis (with doses >15 to 20 Gy).

IORT was used in 70 patients with pelvic recurrences in a European cooperative study.[791] Complete tumor resection was carried out in 30 patients, partial in 37, and unspecified in 3. Sixty-five patients had electron beam therapy (12 to 25 MeV), with mean doses of 18 Gy (10 to 25 Gy) after gross complete resection and 19 Gy (10 to 30 Gy) after partial resection. The 3-year overall survival rate was 8%. Grade 2 or 3 toxicity was observed in 19/70 patients (27%), with 10 complications being related to IORT.

Martinez-Monge et al.[792] reported a study of IORT in 26 patients with recurrent gynecologic tumors, some relapsing after full-dose radiation therapy (group 1) or after surgery (group 2). Cervical carcinoma was the initial tumor site of involvement in 18 patients. Treatment consisted of maximal surgical resection and IORT (10 to 25 Gy) to high-risk areas. Patients not previously irradiated also received external-beam irradiation (with or without chemotherapy) before or after surgery. There was 1 IORT-related incidence of motor neuropathy. The local tumor control rates were 33% and 77%; the 4-year actuarial survival for group 1 was 7%, and the 6-year actuarial survival rate for group 2 was 33%.

In another study, 42 patients with stages IIA to IVA cervical cancer initially received 50.4 Gy of pelvic external-beam radiation with concurrent cisplatin and 5-fluorouracil.[793] Patients then underwent radical surgery 6 to 8 weeks later with IORT. The 5-year DFS and OS were 46% and 49%, respectively, which are inferior to reported results with standard concurrent chemoradiation followed by brachytherapy without surgery or IORT. Therefore, this regimen remains of questionable value in potentially curable patients.

URGENT BLEEDING AND PALLIATIVE IRRADIATION

Frequently, the radiation oncologist is faced with the challenge of treating a patient with stage IVB or recurrent carcinoma requiring palliation of pelvic pain or bleeding. Tumors respond rapidly to radiation, and bleeding usually resolves within a few days of treatment. If vaginal bleeding is the main concern, several possibilities may be effective. In a descriptive review of eight papers that presented palliative treatment data,[794] five papers were found to report using 10 Gy per fraction, with the best resolution of bleeding and/or pain when each 10-Gy fraction was given at 3- to 4-week intervals for a total of three fractions. Alternatively, common palliative regimens used in other sites of the body, such as 4 Gy for five or six fractions or 3 Gy for 10 fractions, may be implemented. Patients who present with a new diagnosis may be treated with 3 to 4 Gy for two or three fractions, followed by standard 1.8 Gy to approximately 39.6 Gy and then brachytherapy. Alternatively, patients may receive 1 to 2 days of 1.8 Gy twice a day, switching to once-a-day treatment with 1.8 Gy per fraction after bleeding has stopped on day 2 or 3, completing treatment after 45 Gy and then commencing routine brachytherapy.

A single LDR intracavitary insertion with tandem and colpostats for approximately 6,000 mgh (55 Gy to point A) may be used for palliation. If irradiation was delivered previously, lower intracavitary doses should be prescribed (4,000 to 5,000 mgh). Grigsby et al.[795] used two fractions of HDR brachytherapy with a ring applicator (once weekly) with control of bleeding in 14 of 15 patients.

Several high-dose fractionation schedules with external-beam radiation have been used. Spanos et al.[796] reported on a phase II study of daily multifractionated split-course irradiation in 142 patients with recurrent or metastatic disease in the pelvis. Irradiation consisted of 3.7 Gy per fraction given twice daily for 2 consecutive days, repeated at 3- to 6-week intervals for a total of three courses, aiming at a total tumor dose of 44.4 Gy. Occasionally, this regimen was combined with an LDR intracavitary insertion (4,500 mgh), blocking the midline for the last 14.4-Gy external dose. Twenty-seven patients survived >1 year. There were only 2 recorded cases of grade 3 toxicity (lower gastrointestinal tract). This study was expanded to a phase III protocol randomizing 136 patients between a short (2 weeks) or a longer (4 weeks) rest period between the split courses of irradiation.[797] There was a trend toward increased acute toxicity in patients with shorter rest periods (5 of 58 vs. 0 of 68; $p = .07$). Late toxicity was not significantly different in the two groups. Pelvic tumor response was comparable in both groups (34% vs. 26%). Spanos et al.[798] reported a 6% complication rate in 290 patients treated in RTOG Protocol 85–02. No patient receiving <30 Gy experienced late toxicity. There was no significant difference in the incidence of complications for patients with a 2- or 4-week rest ($p = .47$).

IRRADIATION AND HYPERTHERMIA

Because of technical limitations in the delivery of adequate heat to large parts of the body such as the pelvis, the use of hyperthermia in the treatment of carcinoma of the uterine cervix has been rare. Hornback et al.[799] described a nonrandomized study in which the combination of microwave hyperthermia (433 MHz) and irradiation resulted in improved pelvic tumor control (72%) in a group of 79 patients with stage IIIB carcinoma compared with previously irradiated historic control patients (53%). However, 5-year survival rates were comparable in both groups (22% to 30%).

Sharma et al.[800] reported a 70% disease-free survival rate at 18 months in 20 patients with stage IIB or III carcinoma of the uterine cervix treated with a combination of irradiation and hyperthermia (13.5 MHz, 42°C to 43°C, 30 minutes before irradiation) in comparison with a 50% disease-free survival rate in 22 patients treated with irradiation alone. The grade 3 complication rate (8%) was similar in both groups.

Dinges et al.[801] treated 18 patients with advanced carcinoma of the cervix with RT plus hyperthermia (in the first and fourth weeks, two regional hyperthermia treatments were applied). The acute toxicity was low and similar to that with RT alone. The local tumor control was 48% at 2 years.

Harima et al.[802] evaluated radiation therapy or thermoirradiation (three sessions of hyperthermia) for stage IIIB cervical carcinoma; two groups of 20 patients each were randomly divided. A complete response was achieved in 50% (10 of 20) in the RT group versus 80% (16 of 20) in the thermoirradiation group ($p = .048$). The 3-year overall survival and disease-free survival rates for the patients who were treated with thermoirradiation (58.2% and 63.6%) were better than with RT (48.1% and 45%), but differences were not statistically significant. The 3-year local relapse-free survival rate of the patients who were treated with thermoirradiation (79.7%) was significantly better than that of the patients treated with irradiation alone (48.5%; $p = .048$). Thermoirradiation was well tolerated and did not add to either acute or long-term toxicity over radiation alone.

Vasanthan et al.[803] reported on 110 patients with locally advanced cervix cancer randomized to treatment with RT alone or combined with hyperthermia (minimum five sessions, 60 minutes each, once weekly). Overall 3-year pelvic tumor control was 68.5% and survival was 73.2%, with no difference in either group, although survival was lower in the patients with stage IIB treated with hyperthermia. Acute toxicity was 18% (10 of 55) in the hyperthermia patients and 4% (2 of 55) with RT alone. Late toxicity was not different in the two arms.

A Cochrane database review identified six randomized, controlled trials published between 1987 and 2009 comparing RT versus combined hyperthermia and RT. The results show 74% of patients had stage IIIB cervical cancer. A significantly higher complete response rate (RR = 0.56, 95% CI = 0.39 to 0.79) and lower local recurrence rate (HR = 0.48, 95% CI = 0.37 to 0.63) and improved overall survival (HR = 0.67, 95% CI = 0.45 to 0.99) with no difference in acute or late grade 3 to 4 toxicity were seen for patients treated with combined therapy.[804] Catheter-based ultrasound devices provide a method to deliver heat with HDR brachytherapy, but clinical results are not yet available.[805]

SIDE EFFECTS: SURGERY AND RADIATION

Descriptions of sequelae vary among institutions because toxicity-grading scales are not uniform and the scoring system for complications is not clearly stated in all reports. Surgical side effects alone depend on the extent of surgery and the amount of disease. Radical hysterectomy alone may cause long-term side effects such as urinary retention requiring chronic suprapubic catheter placement, sciatic nerve injury, postoperative seroma or hematoma formation, pelvic pain, or, when lymphadenectomy, is performed, life-long edema. Oophorectomy also may induce menopause; hysterectomy removes the ability to carry a pregnancy, and removal of a portion of the vagina may significantly change sexual function if vaginal shortening is severe.

With improved anesthesia, surgical techniques, and antibiotic therapy, the mortality rate for radical hysterectomy with pelvic lymphadenectomy has decreased to 1% or less. The most frequent sequela after radical hysterectomy is urinary dysfunction as a result of partial denervation of the detrusor muscle. Patients may have various degrees of loss of bladder sensation, inability to initiate voiding, residual urine retention, and incontinence.

In 375 patients treated with a modified radical hysterectomy for various gynecologic disorders, Magrina et al.,[806] observed some form of postoperative (within 42 days of surgery) complications in 89 patients (24%). Patients who had a pelvic lymphadenectomy experienced a greater incidence of lower-extremity lymphedema than those who did not undergo this procedure. Preoperative or postoperative pelvic irradiation was a significant predisposing factor for urinary tract infection, lymphedema, and bowel obstruction in these patients compared with those who did not receive pelvic irradiation.

Some loss of defecatory urge associated with chronic rectal dysfunction was observed by Barnes et al.[807] after radical hysterectomy. Manometric studies suggest a disruption of the spinal arcs controlling defecation.

Other complications include ureterovaginal fistula (the incidence of which has decreased to <3%), hemorrhage, infection, bowel obstruction, stricture and fibrosis of the intestine or rectosigmoid colon, and bladder and rectovaginal fistulas.

Postsurgical complications are usually more amenable to correction than are late complications after irradiation.

When postoperative radiation therapy is given to selected patients, further complications of the additional therapy are expected. The main areas of side effects due to radiation are bowel, bladder, skin, and sexual function. Because of intestinal adhesions to denuded surfaces in the pelvis, enteric complications, such as obstruction, fistula, or dysfunction, were observed in 24% of patients reported by Fiorica et al.[808] Other investigators, however, have reported no increase in the incidence of severe complications in patients treated with postoperative irradiation.[387,821]

Lower body mass index (BMI) is correlated with an increase in toxicity. A total of 404 patients with stage IB1 cervical cancer with positive lymph nodes or stage IB2 or higher were treated from 1998 to 2008. A BMI of <18.5 was associated with a decreased overall survival (HR = 2.37, $p < .01$). Grade 3 and 4 complications appeared to trend higher; overall, 17% versus 14%; specifically for fistula, 11% versus 9% ($p = .05$), for bowel obstruction, 33% versus 4% ($p < .01$), and for lymphedema, 5.6% versus. 1.2% ($p = .0$).[809]

Montz et al.[810] evaluated bowel obstruction in 98 patients undergoing radical hysterectomy for a nonadnexal gynecologic malignancy. The incidence of small-bowel obstruction was significantly higher ($p < .05$) in patients who received concomitant radiation therapy (20%). None of these patients had recurrent disease at the time of small-bowel obstruction. Findings at surgery consisted of minimal incisional adhesions but extensive matted small-bowel loops adherent to the pelvic operative sites.

When irradiation is combined with surgery, the complication rate tends to be somewhat higher, particularly because of injury to the ureter or the bladder (ureteral stricture or ureterovaginal or vesicovaginal fistula).[811] The dose of irradiation, technique, and type of surgical procedure performed are important in determining the morbidity of combined therapy. Jacobs et al.,[812] in 102 patients with invasive cervical carcinoma treated with low-dose preoperative irradiation and radical hysterectomy with lymphadenectomy or high-dose preoperative irradiation and conservative extrafascial hysterectomy, noted a major complication rate of 5%. After combined treatment, some degree of lymphedema may be observed (30% to 40%).

A significant number of complications are associated with pretherapy staging laparotomy, particularly if irradiation (>55 Gy) is given to metastatic para-aortic lymph nodes. The incidence of complications is between 5% and 20%, depending on the extent of the para-aortic lymph node dissection, use of transperitoneal or retroperitoneal approach for the operation, and dose of irradiation given.[279]

TABLE 69.22 CARCINOMA OF THE UTERINE CERVIX: GRADE 2 SEQUELAE (WASHINGTON UNIVERSITY, 1959–1989)

	Stage				
	IB	*IIA*	*IIB*	*III*	*IVA*
Total number of patients treated	415	137	391	326	23
Number of complications	51 (12%)	14 (10%)	65 (17%)	38 (12%)	3 (13%)
Rectum–Bowel	–	–	–	–	–
Rectal stricture	–	1	2	1	1
Proctitis	8	1	13	6	–
Rectal ulcer	1	–	–	2	1
Diverticulitis	–	–	1	–	–
Small-bowel obstruction	2	–	3	4	–
Malabsorption	3	–	1	1	–
Urinary	–	–	–	–	–
Chronic cystitis	–	2	12	4	–
Bladder ulcer	3	1	2	1	–
Incontinence	1	–	1	–	–
Urethral stricture	2	–	1	–	–
Extensive cystocele	–	–	–	3	–
Other					
Vaginal stenosis	21	4	7	6	1
Vault necrosis	8	2	2	5	–
Postoperative pelvic abscess	1	–	1	2	–
Lymphocyst	–	–	2	2	–
Pulmonary embolus	–	–	1	–	–
Subcutaneous fibrosis	1	–	–	–	–
Leg edema	–	–	7	3	–
Hemorrhage	–	–	1	–	–
Thrombosis of pelvic blood vessels	–	1	–	–	–
Arteriosclerosis	1	–	8	2	–
Thrombophlebitis	–	–	1	–	–
Pelvic fibrosis	–	1	–	–	–
Acute pelvic cellulitis	–	1	–	–	–
Neuritis	–	–	–	1	–

TABLE 69.23 CARCINOMA OF THE UTERINE CERVIX: GRADE 3 SEQUELAE (WASHINGTON UNIVERSITY, 1959–1989)

	Stage				
	IB	*IIA*	*IIB*	*III*	*IVA*
Total number of patients treated	415	137	391	326	23
Number of complications	26 (6%)	23 (17%)	57 (15%)	45 (14%)	2 (9%)
Rectum–Rectosigmoid					
Rectovaginal fistula	4	2	8	12	1
Rectouterine fistula	1	–	–	–	–
Colovaginal fistula	–	–	1	–	–
Rectal stricture	3	4	4	2	–
Proctitis	2	2	6	2	–
Rectal ulcer	–	–	1	–	–
Sigmoid perforation	1	–	3	1	–
Small Bowel					
Small-bowel obstruction	3	5	12	8	–
Small-bowel perforation	–	–	2	1	–
Enterocolic fistula	1	–	–	–	–
Enterocutaneous fistula	–	1	–	1	–
Enterovaginal fistula	–	–	1	–	–
Enteritis/cachexia	–	–	–	1	–
Urinary					
Vesicovaginal fistula	3	2	6	9	2
Ureterovaginal fistula	–	–	–	1	–
Cystitis	2	–	–	–	–
Bladder ulcer	–	–	–	1	–
Ureteral stricture	5	5	9	4	–
Other					
Postoperative pelvic abscess	–	–	1	1	–
Pulmonary embolus	–	–	1	–	–
Hemorrhage	–	–	1	2	–
Pelvic infection	1	–	–	–	–
Neuritis	–	1	1	–	–

Late Sequelae–Overall

The incidence of major late sequelae of radiation therapy for stages I and IIA carcinoma of the cervix ranges from 3% to 5% and for stages IIB and III between 10% and 15%. The most frequent major sequelae for the various stages are listed in Tables 69.22 and 69.23. Injury to the gastrointestinal tract usually appears within the first 2 years after radiation therapy, whereas complications of the urinary tract are seen more frequently 3 to 5 years after treatment.[570,816] Pedersen et al.,[813] in a review of morbidity of radiation therapy in 442 patients with cervical cancer stages IIB, III, and IVA, recommended that actuarial estimates rather than frequency of sequelae be reported to avoid underestimation of risks of late morbidity

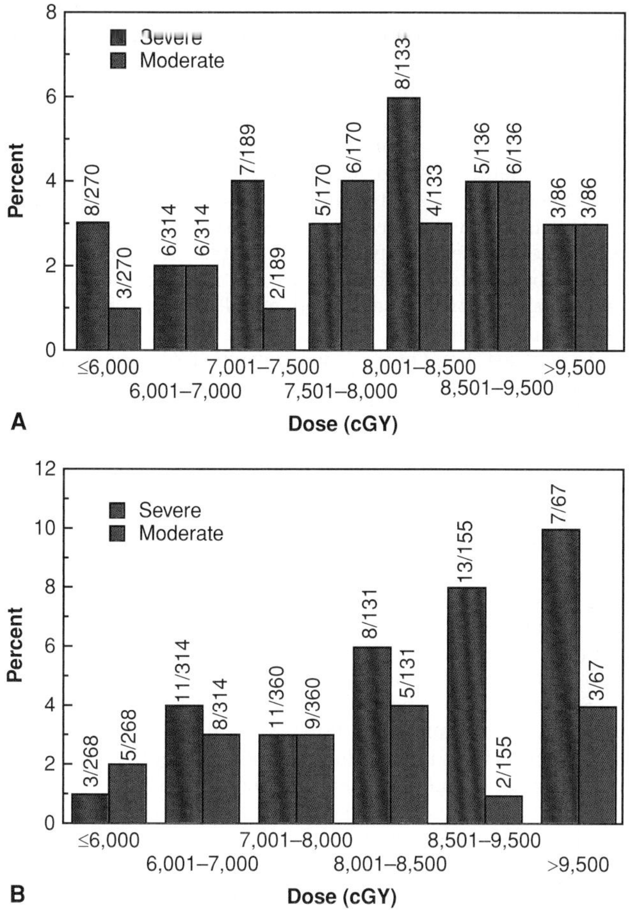

FIGURE 69.27. Incidence of moderate or severe genitourinary **(A)** or rectosigmoid **(B)** complications in patients with carcinoma of uterine cervix (all stages) treated with irradiation alone (external and brachytherapy). A greater frequency of complications is noted with maximum doses of >75 to 80 Gy to the bladder or rectum.

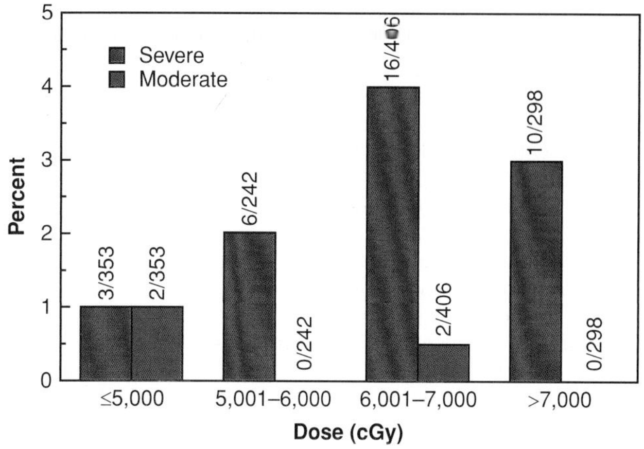

FIGURE 69.28. Incidence of moderate or severe complications in small intestine correlated with doses of irradiation.

after radiation therapy in long-term survivors. In fact, Eifel et al.,[811] in 1,784 patients with stage IB carcinoma of the cervix, noted that the greatest risk of sequelae is in the first 3 years after therapy. The risk of rectal complications declined after the first 2 years of follow-up to 0.6%/year, whereas the risk of major urinary tract complications for survivors continued at 0.3%/year, with a 20-year actuarial risk of major complications of 14.4%.

Montana et al.,[524] Perez et al.,[814] and Pourquier et al.[815] noted a greater incidence of complications with higher doses of irradiation. Perez et al.[816] and Pourquier et al.[815] reported that with doses <75 to 80 Gy delivered to limited volumes, grade 2 and 3 complications in the urinary tract and rectosigmoid were approximately 5%. However, the incidence increased to >10% with higher doses of irradiation to these organs (Fig. 69.27). Doses >60 Gy were also correlated with a greater incidence of small-bowel injury (Fig. 69.28). The same analysis showed that patients who experienced sequelae of therapy had slightly better survival rates than patients without any complications. This was related to improved tumor control with higher doses of irradiation.[816]

Perez et al.[814] quantitated the effect of total doses of irradiation, dose rate, and ratio of doses to bladder or rectum and point A on sequelae in 1,456 patients treated for cervical cancer with external-beam irradiation plus two LDR intracavitary insertions to deliver 70 to 90 Gy to point A. Median follow-up was 11 years. In stage IB, the frequency of grade 2 morbidity was 9%, and in grade 3 it was 5%; in stages IIA, IIB, III, and IVA, the frequency of grade 2 morbidity was 10% to 12% and that of grade 3 was 10%. The most frequent grade 2 urinary/rectal sequelae were cystitis and proctitis (0.7% to 3%). The most common grade 3 sequelae were vesicovaginal fistula (0.6% to 2% in patients with stage I to III tumors), rectovaginal fistula (0.8% to 3%), and intestinal obstruction (0.8% to 4%). In the bladder, doses <80 Gy correlated with a <3% incidence of morbidity, which was 5% with higher doses (p = .31). In the rectosigmoid, the incidence of significant morbidity was <4% with doses <75 Gy and increased to 9% with higher doses. For the small intestine, the incidence of morbidity was <1% with 50 Gy or less, 2% with 50 to 60 Gy, and 5% with higher doses to the lateral pelvic wall (p = .04). Multivariate analysis showed that dose to the rectal point was the only factor influencing rectosigmoid sequelae, and dose to the bladder point affected bladder morbidity.

In a review of the Patterns of Care Study, Lanciano et al.[817] observed a 5-year actuarial rate of 14% for major late complications in 1,558 patients treated with irradiation for invasive carcinoma of the cervix. Women <40 years of age or with a history of prior surgery or laparotomy for staging had a greater incidence of significant morbidity (15% to 18% vs. 8% to 9%). In addition, EBRT dose per fraction of >2 Gy, paracentral doses of 85 Gy or greater, and lateral parametrial doses >60 Gy were independently associated with a higher complication rate.

Lee et al.,[818] using 3-Gy fractions with EBRT, calculated the rectal point dose in the anterior wall at the level of the cervical os and noted that total higher BED (142.7 Gy) was associated with more frequent rectal sequelae compared with BED of <131 Gy.

Mitchell et al.[124] evaluated 398 patients with stages I to III cervical carcinoma treated with radiation therapy. Patients were divided into nonelderly (35 to 69 years of age; n = 338) and elderly (≥70 years of age; n = 60) groups. The frequency and severity of acute and chronic sequelae were equivalent in both groups.

Gastrointestinal Toxicity

When late radiation proctitis occurs, initial treatment is the same as for acute proctitis. If the symptoms and rectal bleeding persist, laser treatment of rectal telangiectasis or ulcers is frequently beneficial. Roche et al.[819] treated six patients with hemorrhagic radiation-induced proctitis using outpatient intrarectal application of formaldehyde 4%. In four cases the bleeding ceased after the first formaldehyde application; two patients continued to bleed, but another application 3 weeks later definitively controlled the hemorrhage. There were no complications, such as burns or late stenosis of the deep layers of the rectum, and this technique was well tolerated. Rubinstein et al.[820] and Seow-Choen et al.[821] also reported treatment of radiation proctitis with a similar technique. Patients are sedated, a local anesthetic block is administered, and a sponge moistened with

4% formalin is applied for 4 minutes to each bleeding area of the rectum. Care is taken to protect the perianal skin from any caustic effects of the formalin.

Occasionally, a colostomy is necessary if conservation management fails. The importance of performing colonoscopy in patients with rectal bleeding to exclude other lesions in the colon, including polyps or cancer, is emphasized. If routine screening colonoscopy is not urgent, unless there is a medical reason, the colonoscopy may be postponed until 1 year after pelvic radiation to ensure no issues with poor wound healing, bleeding, or ulceration secondary to biopsy performed at the time of colonoscopy.

Anal incontinence is occasionally observed. This sequela must be assessed in light of a report by Nelson et al.,[822] who in a survey of 6,959 nonirradiated patients, identified 153 (2.2%) who reported anal incontinence, without specific etiology. Thirty percent of incontinent subjects were >65 years of age, and 63% were women. Of those with anal incontinence, 36% were incontinent to solid feces, 54% to liquid feces, and 60% to gas.

Kim et al.[823] investigated the effects of radiation on anorectal function using manometry in 24 patients with carcinoma of the uterine cervix who had late radiation proctitis. These data were compared with those from 24 age-matched nonirradiated female volunteers. Regardless of the severity of proctitis symptoms, 75% of irradiated patients exhibited abnormal manometric parameters for sensory or motor functions. Radiation damage to nerves and to the external sphincter muscle was considered to be an important cause of motor dysfunction.

Quilty[824] noted a greater incidence of pelvic complications in patients treated with higher doses to the whole pelvis (40 to 50 Gy). The author commented that the intracavitary radium dose was not correlated with severe complications. Similar observations were made by Stryker et al.[825] who recorded a 9% incidence of fistulas and a 14% incidence of grade 2 and 3 complications in 132 patients after delivery of 50 Gy or higher to the whole pelvis (1.8-Gy daily dose) combined with intracavitary insertion. They recommended that the whole-pelvis dose should not exceed 40 to 45 Gy when doses of approximately 40 Gy are delivered to point A with LDR intracavitary insertions.

Kuske et al.,[719] reported results of therapy in 99 patients with carcinoma of the cervix on whom minicolpostats were used, noted a 15% incidence of grade 2 and 3 complications, which was higher than the 8% incidence noted in a similar group of patients treated with regular colpostats during the same period ($p = .08$).

Perez et al.[816] reported that the incidence and type of complications with interstitial therapy were approximately the same as in patients treated with intracavitary technique only. In contrast, Kasibhatla et al.[826] noted 6% small-bowel obstruction in 36 women with gynecologic cancer treated with EBRT and interstitial brachytherapy, which was aggravated by previous abdominopelvic surgery. The 3-year risk of rectovaginal fistula was 18%, and it was significantly higher in patients who received total doses of >76 Gy (100% vs. 7%; $p = .009$).

Irradiation of the para-aortic lymph nodes has been reported to cause increased morbidity, particularly if it is done after transperitoneal staging para-aortic lymphadenectomy. In a randomized study reported by Rotman et al.,[827] a somewhat higher incidence of grade 2 and 3 complications was reported in 170 patients (10 complications) given 45 Gy to the para-aortic area in addition to standard pelvic irradiation, compared with 5 complications in 167 patients treated by pelvic irradiation only. The incidence of fatal (grade 5) complications was 4 and 1, respectively. In a similar randomized study by Haie et al.[541] for the EORTC, the incidence of grade 3 small-bowel injury was 2.3% in the para-aortic irradiation group and 0.9% in the pelvic irradiation–only group. The overall incidences of severe complications were 9% and 4.8%, respectively.

Willett et al.[828] reported on 28 patients with inflammatory bowel disease (10 with Crohn's disease, 18 with ulcerative colitis) who underwent external-beam abdominal or pelvic irradiation. Patients were treated either by specialized techniques (16 patients) to minimize small- and large-bowel irradiation or by conventional approaches (12 patients). The overall incidence of severe toxicity was 46% (13 of 28 patients), and 6 patients (21%) experienced severe acute toxicity necessitating cessation of radiation therapy. Late toxicity requiring hospitalization or surgical intervention was observed in 8 of 28 patients (29%). For patients treated with conventional approaches, the 5-year actuarial rate of late toxicity was 73% versus 23% for patients treated by specialized techniques ($p = .02$). In patients with inflammatory bowel disease abdominal or pelvic irradiation, must be used judiciously.

In contrast, Song et al.,[411] in a review of 24 patients with a history of inflammatory bowel disease who received RT (median dose of 45 Gy in 1.8- to 3-Gy fractions) to fields encompassing some portion of the gastrointestinal tract, noted that 5 patients (21%) experienced acute intestinal toxicity of grade 3 or greater and 2 (8%) had grade 3 or greater late intestinal toxicity. Fifteen patients also received concurrent chemotherapy. The authors believed that the gastrointestinal toxicity in these patients was more modest than generally perceived. Tiersten and Saltz[829] noted that five patients with inflammatory bowel disease and gastrointestinal malignancy completed planned radiation therapy (30 to 54 Gy), usually with concurrent 5-FU, without difficulty.

Salama et al.[443] reported preliminary observations on acute toxicity with extended-field IMRT in 13 patients with gynecologic cancer. With median follow-up of 11 months, 2 patients treated with chemoradiation experienced grade 3 or higher morbidity and 1 (with a history of previous surgeries) developed small-bowel obstruction.

Levenback et al.[830] identified 116 of 1,784 patients (6.5%) with stage IB carcinoma of the cervix treated with irradiation in whom hemorrhagic cystitis developed, 23% grade 2 (repeated minor bleeding) and 18% grade 3 (hospitalization required for medical management). The median interval to onset of hematuria was 35.5 months. The risk of severe hematuria requiring surgical intervention was 1.4% at 10 years and 2.3% at 20 years. Minor episodes of hematuria are managed by antibiotic therapy. Cystoscopic, laser, or cautery treatment of bleeding points is indicated. Clot evacuation and continuous bladder irrigation are important elements in the acute management of patients with heavy bleeding. Occasionally, a urinary diversion is required for intractable severe hematuria.

Genitourinary Toxicity

Ureteral stricture at 20 years was observed in 2.5% of 1,784 patients with stage IB carcinoma of the cervix treated with irradiation (274 followed for up to 20 years or longer).[831] The most common presenting symptoms were flank pain and urinary tract infection. In 5 patients, ureteral stricture was complicated by a vesicovaginal fistula. Seven of 43 patients who had no evidence of cancer and had hydroureter or hydronephrosis died of radiation complications. Treatment of ureteral stenosis may consist of stenting or resection of the fibrotic segment and reimplantation of the ureter with either ureteroneocystostomy or ureteroileocystostomy. In approximately half of the patients, diversion of urinary stream and ileal conduits are necessary. Occasionally, a nephrectomy is performed for removal of a nonfunctional kidney. Buglione et al.[832] reported a 10% incidence of late urinary morbidity and 1% ureteral fibrosis, grade III or IV, in 191 patients. They postulated the role of TGF-β_1 in the activation of fibroblasts and remodeling of extracellular matrix, which may be important in the induction of these sequelae.

Patients with gynecologic malignancies, including those receiving radiation therapy, are prone to development of urinary tract infections. Prasad et al.[833] collected 216 urine samples from 36 patients receiving pelvic irradiation, 12 of whom had urinary tract infection. The most common organism isolated was

Escherichia coli, followed by *Enterococcus* species. Appropriate urine bacterial studies and cultures are indicated in patients suspected of having superimposed urinary tract infection during the course of radiation therapy.

Parkin et al.[834] reported a 26% incidence of severe urinary symptoms (urgency, incontinence, and frequency) in patients treated with irradiation alone for cervical carcinoma. They carried out urodynamic studies in 42 women and compared them with 28 women having urodynamic evaluations before and after treatment. There was no difference in the mean maximum flow rate or mean *residual* volume in the two groups. However, mean volume of full bladder sensation was significantly lower in the postirradiation group than in the pretreatment group, as was the mean maximum cystometric capacity. This same dysfunction may be noted in approximately 10% of the general female population, and the incidence increases in older women.[302]

Ureteroarterial fistula is a rare occurrence, and it is associated with a high mortality rate. When profuse urinary tract bleeding occurs in patients previously diagnosed with a gynecologic malignancy and treated with radiation therapy and extensive surgery, ureteroarterial fistula should be considered in the differential diagnoses.[835]

Neurologic Toxicity

Although extremely rare, lumbosacral plexopathy has been occasionally reported in patients treated for pelvic tumors with doses of 60 to 67.5 Gy. This syndrome was observed in 4 of 2,410 patients with cervical or endometrial carcinoma receiving 45 Gy to the para-aortic lymph nodes (without spinal cord shielding) or external pelvic irradiation (60 Gy to the parametria) and brachytherapy, with the lumbosacral plexus receiving total doses of 70 to 79 Gy.[836] Lower-extremity paralysis secondary to lumbosacral plexopathy was reported in one patient after standard radiation therapy for cervical cancer.[837]

Patients previously reported as having radiation myelopathy to the lumbar spine may have suffered a lumbar and sacral nerve plexopathy instead of or in addition to the spinal cord injury. The differential diagnosis of plexopathy with recurrent tumors is sometimes difficult. In a comparison of 20 patients with lumbosacral plexopathy after irradiation and 30 patients with plexus damage from pelvic malignancy, Thomas et al.[838] noted that indolent leg weakness occurred early in radiation-induced plexopathy (pain occurred initially in 10% of patients, although ultimately it was present in 50%), whereas pain was most frequently associated with tumor plexopathy. Muscular weakness, numbness, and paresthesia are common in both groups. Electromyography showed abnormal myokymic discharges in 57% of patients, whereas this finding was very unusual in tumor-induced plexopathy. CT is extremely helpful in the detection of pelvic masses or bone destruction caused by tumor. The authors also reported extensive retroperitoneal fibrosis of the lumbosacral plexus in 2 patients and femoral nerve fibrosis with plexopathy in 1 patient. Although cystometrograms have demonstrated bladder atonicity in some cases, several authors have failed to observe bladder or rectal sphincter disturbances. Unfortunately, as in radiation myelopathy, the neurologic deficit is irreversible, and no effective therapy other supportive care has been found.

Sexual Function

Other types of clinically significant sequelae have been described. Bruner et al.,[839] in 90 patients treated with intracavitary irradiation for either carcinoma of the cervix (42 patients) or endometrial carcinoma (48 patients), 78 of whom also received external pelvic irradiation (44.5-Gy mean dose), noted that vaginal length decreased in most patients (at 24 months, in endometrial carcinoma from 8.8 to 7.8 cm, and in cervical carcinoma from 7.6 to 6.2 cm). Pretreatment sexual activity was reported by 31% of women in comparison with 43% after treatment. However, 22% of women reported a decrease in sexual frequency and 37% a decrease in sexual satisfaction. This was correlated with increased dyspareunia, which was noted in 31% of women treated for carcinoma of the cervix and 44% of those treated for endometrial carcinoma. Grigsby et al.[840] described complex problems with sexual adjustment in women with gynecologic tumors treated with radiation therapy, with decreased frequency of sexual intercourse, desire, orgasm, and enjoyment of intercourse in 16% to 47% of patients.

Regular vaginal dilation is widely recommended to maintain vaginal health and sexual functioning; however, the compliance rate with this recommendation is not consistent. In a study to test the effectiveness of an "information-motivation-behavior skills" model, the intervention improved the use of vaginal dilation after radiotherapy, and decreased fear about sex after treatment[841] There was no evidence that the experimental intervention improved global sexual health. Jensen et al.[842] described persistent sexual dysfunction throughout 2 years after RT in 118 women; 85% had low or no sexual interest, 35% had lack of vaginal lubrication, and 55% had mild to severe dyspareunia. However, 63% of the sexually active patients before RT remained active, although with decreased frequency.

Radiation causes ovarian failure with a cessation of menses over a 6-month to 1-year period after treatment. Radiation also causes uterine fibrosis in a dose-dependent fashion. The dose required for radical cervical cancer treatment causes sufficient uterine fibrosis that even if a woman were to become pregnant through embryo donation, the pregnancy terminates as a stillbirth due to insufficient uterine distensibility.[586,843]

Bone Toxicity

Grigsby et al.,[844] in 1,313 patients with gynecologic tumors treated with radiation therapy, identified 207 who received pelvic irradiation to the inguinal areas, including the hips. Femoral neck fractures developed in 10 patients (4.8%); 4 were bilateral. The cumulative actuarial incidence of fracture was 11% at 5 years and 15% at 10 years. Most of the fractures occurred in patients receiving 45 to 63 Gy, and although radiation dose could not be correlated with the occurrence of fracture, no fractures were noted in patients receiving <42 Gy. Cigarette smoking and osteoporosis were significant prognostic factors for increased risk of fracture.

A retrospective cohort study using SEER cancer registry data linked to Medicare claims data analyzed 6,428 women of age 65 years and older diagnosed with pelvic malignancies from 1986 through 1999, and compared results for women who did (n = 2,855) with those who did not (n = 3,573) undergo radiation therapy. Results demonstrated that women who underwent radiation therapy were more likely to have a pelvic fracture than women who did not undergo radiation therapy. The cumulative 5-year fracture rate was 8.2% versus 5.9% in women with cervical cancer; the difference was statistically significant, and most fractures (90%) were hip fractures.[845] Concurrent chemoradiation may result in a higher risk than for patients treated with RT alone because the highest fracture rates were seen in patients with anal carcinoma treated with concurrent chemoradiation.

Blomlie et al.[846] reported radiation-induced insufficiency fractures of the pelvis on MRI (characterized by edema on T1-weighted images) in 16 of 18 women (9 premenopausal and 9 postmenopausal) with advanced cervical carcinoma. During the study, the fractures associated with edema subsided without treatment in 41 of 52 (79%) lesions in 15 of 16 (94%) patients. Moreno et al.[847] described eight patients with pelvic cancer who developed insufficiency fractures after pelvic irradiation, with an average onset 13.7 months after treatment. The bone and CT scan showed abnormalities in the sacroiliac joint in all cases and in the pubis in three cases. In five patients, the initial diagnosis was incorrectly labeled as bone metastases.

Huh et al.[848] reported on 463 patients treated for cervical cancer with RT alone, 1.7% of whom developed insufficiency fractures between 7 and 19 months (median, 12 months) after treatment. All had resolution of symptoms within <1 year with conservative therapy, including nonsteroidal anti-inflammatory medication and rest.

The most common complaint is persistent low back pain. Insufficiency fractures may be falsely diagnosed as metastases on PET/CT. The most common form of treatment is conservative management, followed by sacroplasty with polymethylmethacrylate. Bye et al.[849] assessed health-related quality of life (HRQOL) at 3 to 4 years after pelvic radiation therapy for carcinoma of the endometrium and cervix in 94 survivors, 79 (84%) of whom answered a survey. The treated women scored lower than the general population on role functioning (81.5 vs. 90.6; $p < .01$) and higher on diarrhea (23.8 vs. 9.5; $p < .01$). Compared with pretreatment conditions, an increase in cases with pain in the lower back, hips, and thighs was seen and was associated with deterioration in HRQOL.

Toxicities Related to Brachytherapy

Descriptions of sequelae vary among institutions because toxicity-grading scales are not uniform and the scoring system for complications is not clearly stated in all reports. It is helpful to institute preventive measures when initiating radiation; for example, Dusenbery et al.[850] reported 21 (6.4%) life-threatening complications in 327 of 462 patient implants. Lanciano et al.,[851] in 95 tandem and ovoid insertions for cervical cancer in 91 patients and for endometrial cancer in 4, observed 2 uterine perforations and a vaginal laceration in 2 patients. Twenty-four percent of implants in 16 patients were associated with temperatures >100.5°F. Five implants (5%) were removed because of presumed sepsis, pulmonary disease, arterial hypotension, change in mental status, and myocardial infarction.

Jhingran and Eifel,[852] in 4,043 patients with carcinoma of the cervix who had undergone 7,662 intracavitary procedures, observed 11 (0.3%) documented or suspected thromboembolisms, resulting in 4 deaths; the incidence of postimplant thromboembolism did not decrease significantly with the routine use of minidose heparin prophylaxis. Other life-threatening perioperative complications included myocardial infarction (1 death in 5 patients), cerebrovascular accident (2 patients), congestive heart failure (3 patients), and halothane liver toxicity (2 deaths). Intraoperative complications included uterine perforation (2.8%) and vaginal laceration (0.3%), which occurred more frequently in patients 60 years of age or older ($p < .01$).

Wollschlaeger et al.[853] reported morbidity during hospitalization in 128 patients with cervical carcinoma undergoing 110 LDR intracavitary brachytherapy insertions. Forty-two implants (24.7%) were associated with acute problems; the most common were fever/infection (14.1%) or gastrointestinal problems (5.9%).

Acute gastrointestinal side effects of pelvic irradiation include diarrhea, abdominal cramping, rectal discomfort, and occasionally rectal bleeding, which may be caused by transient enteroproctitis. Patients with hemorrhoids may experience discomfort earlier than other patients. Diarrhea and abdominal cramping can be controlled with the oral administration of diphenoxylate hydrochloride, with loperamide, atropine sulfate, or opium preparations or emollients such as kaolin and pectin. Proctitis and rectal discomfort can be alleviated by small enemas with hydrocortisone and anti-inflammatory suppositories containing bismuth, benzyl benzoate, zinc oxide, or Peruvian balsam. Some suppositories contain cortisone. Small enemas with cod liver oil are also effective. A low-residue diet with no grease or spices and increased fiber in the stool (psyllium, polycarbophil) usually helps to decrease gastrointestinal symptoms.

Genitourinary symptoms secondary to cystourethritis are dysuria, frequency, and nocturia. The urine is usually clear, although there may be microscopic or even gross hematuria. Methenamine mandelate and antispasmodics such as phenazopyridine hydrochloride or a smooth muscle antispasmodic such as flavoxate hydrochloride, hyoscyamine sulfate, oxybutynin chloride, or tolterodine tartrate can relieve symptoms. Fluid intake should be at least 2,000 to 2,500 mL daily. Urinary tract infections may occur; diagnosis should be established with appropriate urine culture studies, including sensitivity to sulfonamides and antibiotics. Therapy should be promptly instituted.

Erythema and dry or moist desquamation may develop in the perineum or intergluteal fold. Proper skin hygiene and topical application of petroleum jelly, petrolatum, or lanolin should relieve these symptoms. U.S.P. zinc oxide ointment and intensive skin care may be needed for severe cases.

Management of acute radiation vaginitis includes douching every day or at least three times weekly with a 1:5 mixture of hydrogen peroxide and water. Douching should be continued on a weekly basis until the mucositis has resolved or for 2 or 3 months as necessary. Superficial ulceration of the vagina responds to topical (intravaginal) estrogen creams, which stimulate epithelial regeneration within 3 months after irradiation. Use of vaginal dilators several times daily, started during the course of treatment, prevents vaginal stenosis. Psychoeducational intervention and motivation improve the compliance in use of dilators.[854] More-severe necrosis may require debridement on a weekly basis until healing takes place. Judicious use of biopsies is recommended to rule out persistent or recurrent cancer.

Petereit et al.[855] reported 16 acute events (9.5%) in 169 patients treated with HDR brachytherapy (128 with cervical cancer also receiving external irradiation, and 41 medically inoperable endometrial carcinomas). The overall 30-day morbidity rate for the patients with cervical cancer was 5.5%, and the 30-day mortality rate was 1.6% (2 patients; 1 died of pulmonary edema 12 days after first HDR insertion and the other had enteritis and died in a nursing home).

The complication rates for HDR and LDR techniques are usually equivalent.[608,610] Petereit et al.[606] observed a 12% 3-year actuarial overall toxicity (2.6% genitourinary and 5.6% rectum) with LDR, compared to 15% overall (3% genitourinary and 4.6% rectum) with HDR brachytherapy. However, in the series by Cikaric,[711] the rectal complication rate was significantly higher in the LDR group. Bladder complication rates reported, in general, are lower than rectal complication rates; again, except for the series by Cikaric[711] showing a higher complication rate with the LDR technique, there were no significant differences with the two techniques.

Ogino et al.,[856] in 253 patients with invasive carcinoma of the cervix treated with HDR brachytherapy, noted that grade 4 rectal complications were not observed in patients with a time–dose factor of <130 or biologic equivalent dose of <147, assuming an α/β ratio of 3 Gy for late reactions.

Spontaneous intraperitoneal rupture of the urinary bladder, an extremely rare event, was reported by Fujikawa et al.[857] after radiation therapy for cervical cancer in 6 of 148 patients treated with HDR intracavitary brachytherapy combined with EBRT. All 6 patients underwent laparotomy and repair of the perforation; however, rerupture of the bladder occurred in 3 of these patients.

Clark et al.[858] reported on 43 patients treated with pelvic EBRT (46 Gy) and three HDR intracavitary treatments given weekly combined with concomitant chemotherapy (cisplatin, 30 mg/m^2 weekly) for advanced carcinoma of the cervix. At 40 months after treatment, 9 of 13 patients who received a dose to the rectal reference point greater than the prescribed point A dose had a 46% actuarial rate of serious (grade 3 and 4) rectal complications, compared with 14% in the remainder. A strong dose response was observed, with a threshold for complications at a brachytherapy dose of 8 Gy per fraction.

Hyperbaric Oxygen

In 13 patients with hemorrhagic cystitis treated with hyperbaric oxygen, all but 1 experienced durable cessation of hematuria.[859] Lee et al.[860] also noted that, in 16 of 20 patients (80%)

with hemorrhagic radiation cystitis, significant improvement was observed after treatment with hyperbaric oxygen at 2.5 atm (44 sessions).

Several reports evaluated the efficacy of hyperbaric oxygen combined with irradiation in the treatment of a variety of human tumors, including carcinoma of the uterine cervix. Watson et al.,[861] in a randomized clinical trial of 320 patients (stages III to IVA), reported a 5-year survival rate of 33% in the oxygen-treated group in contrast to 27% in the control group treated in normal air ($p = .08$). The local recurrence rate was 33% in the 161 patients treated with oxygen and 53% in 159 patients treated in normal air ($p < .001$). Morbidity in the patients treated with oxygen was greater (20 severe and 13 moderate complications) than in those treated in normal air (6 severe and 8 moderate complications, respectively). The difference was particularly striking in the bowel (13 and 2 severe complications, respectively).

Dische et al.[862] reviewed the data in a randomized study of patients with advanced carcinoma of the cervix treated with radiation therapy and hyperbaric oxygen or air and noted that the patients treated with oxygen had improved survival at Mount Vernon and Glasgow but not at Cape Town. Data from the three centers were merged, and analysis showed that local tumor control was significantly worse in patients treated in normal air who had a prior blood transfusion, but in the oxygen group this effect was reversed. The same interaction was noted in the survival results ($p = .042$).

A trial reported by Fletcher[165] in which 233 patients with stages IIB, III, and IV carcinoma of the cervix were randomized to be treated with irradiation in normal air or with hyperbaric oxygen demonstrated no significant benefit in survival or tumor control (20 of 109 patients treated with oxygen failed in the pelvis, in contrast to 29 of 124 treated in normal air). Furthermore, morbidity was greater (26 complications) in patients treated with hyperbaric oxygen compared with the control group (15 complications).

Dische et al.[862] published results of a four-arm randomized trial of hyperbaric oxygen and radiation therapy of stages IIB and III carcinoma of the cervix in which 335 patients were randomized to treatment in 10 or 28 fractions in hyperbaric oxygen or in normal air. Data from 327 cases were analyzed. There was no advantage in tumor control with the use of hyperbaric oxygen. There was an increase in late radiation morbidity when treatment was given in hyperbaric oxygen rather than in normal air, and when using 10 fractions, a total dose of 45 Gy rather than 40 Gy was administered.

No definite conclusions can be drawn concerning the use of hyperbaric oxygen in carcinoma of the cervix. It is possible that hyperbaric oxygen administered with fewer high-dose fractions may be more efficacious than when combined with conventional dose and fractionation schemes. The trials reported have not shown an increased incidence of distant metastasis, which has been observed in a clinical study and in some animal experiments.[863]

Hormonal Replacement After Treatment of Cervical Cancer

After pelvic irradiation or bilateral salpingo-oophorectomy, usually carried out with a radical hysterectomy in patients treated for carcinoma of the uterine cervix, symptoms of menopause may occur. They can be treated with replacement hormones, although some gynecologists have expressed reservations. During the past 25 years, hormonal replacement therapy has been shown to reduce the risk of cardiovascular diseases, osteoporotic fractures, and colon carcinoma. On the other hand, there is a significant increase of the risk in breast cancer with prolonged use of estrogen plus progesterone for >5 years. Consideration may be given to progesterone alone, which does not increase the risk of endometrial cancer but has potential thromboembolic risks.[864]

Burger et al.[865] concluded that squamous cell cancers of the cervix, vulva, and vagina are unlikely to be influenced by hormonal replacement therapy. In a study of women 50 years of age or younger with ovarian cancer, estrogen replacement therapy did not have a negative influence on disease-free survival. Long-term hormonal replacement therapy in women treated for a gynecologic cancer must be based on the medical history of and discussion of risk with the individual patient (and her family when warranted). Usually, 0.625 to 1.25 mg of coagulated estrogen daily is sufficient.[866]

Second Malignancy

The risk for induction of secondary primary cancers by pelvic irradiation is low, and many potential confounders are either unknown or may not be fully accounted for, given available information.[867] Using the population-based cancer registries of Denmark, Finland, Norway, Sweden, and the United States, Chaturvedi et al.[868] found a significantly increased cancer risk in both SCC and AC survivors, with standardized incidence ratio of 1.31 (95% CI = 1.29 to 1.34) and 1.29 (95% CI = 1.22 to 1.38), respectively. The risk of smoking-related lung cancer was higher in the SCC than in the AC population, whereas second malignancies of the colon, soft tissue, melanoma, and non-Hodgkin lymphoma were higher in the AC population. Similarly, 1-year survivors of cervical cancer had an increased risk of HPV-related cancers, including pharynx, genital, and anal cancers. Higher hazard ratios for second cancer of the rectum, anus, bladder, and genital sites was seen for younger patients, with a 40-year cumulative risk of any second cancer of 22% for women diagnosed with cervical cancer before age 50 years versus 16% for those diagnosed at age >50 years.[869] In contrast, Lee et al.[870] observed no significant increase in the incidence of second malignancies in patients irradiated for carcinoma of the cervix in comparison with the Connecticut Tumor Registry prevailing rates.

Boice et al.,[339] in a review of 68,730 women with carcinoma of the cervix treated with radiation therapy, observed a second malignant tumor in 3,324, compared with 3,063 expected (4.8% increase; $p < .001$). The excess was concentrated in the lung, other genital organs, bladder, and rectum. In addition, in 10,817 women with invasive cervical cancer not treated with irradiation, 479 secondary malignant tumors were observed versus 435 expected (4.4%; $p = .02$). Thus, the incidence of secondary tumors in women treated for carcinoma of the cervix with or without irradiation is only slightly greater than in the general population. Pelvic organs receiving a high dose of irradiation appear to have a somewhat greater incidence of a second primary.

Storm,[871] in a comprehensive analysis of the Danish Cancer Registry data of 24,970 women with invasive cervical cancer and 19,470 with carcinoma *in situ* of the cervix treated between 1943 and 1982, noted a small overall excess of secondary primary cancers in the lung, stomach, pancreas, rectum, and bladder and connective tissue sarcomas, although there was a decreased incidence of breast cancer in the irradiated patients compared with nonirradiated patients (attributable to ovarian ablation by radiation therapy). In the patients irradiated for invasive carcinoma, there was an excess of 64 cases per 10,000 women per year of tumors in organs close to or at an intermediate distance from the cervix, reaching a maximum after 30 years or longer of follow-up. A high risk for development of acute nonlymphatic leukemia was observed in irradiated patients with carcinoma *in situ* but not in those with invasive lesions. This could be explained by the lower doses of irradiation delivered to the bone marrow in the *in situ* tumors treated with brachytherapy alone, with greater induction of mutations and less cell killing, which may be responsible for the leukemogenic effect. Decreased risk was noted for tumors of the brain, myeloma of the skin, and tumors of the colon other than rectal.

In a study of 117,830 women diagnosed with cervical carcinoma *in situ* and 17,556 with invasive cervical carcinoma in Sweden, treatment not specified and *in situ* lesions traditionally treated with surgery alone, there was an increased incidence (RR = 2.3 to 3) of second primary tumors in the anus, rectum, urinary bladder, pancreas, esophagus, and lung compared with the standardized incidence rate for all women.[872] The data showed consistent increases in suggested targets for HPV at tobacco-related sites. A contributing role for a depressed immune response was considered.

Werner-Wasik et al.,[873] in an analysis of 125 women with stages I and II carcinoma of the cervix treated with radiation therapy, observed 11 secondary primary tumors in 10 patients (4 breast, 2 lung, and 1 each of myeloma, non-Hodgkin lymphoma, bladder, thyroid, and vulva). All secondary primary tumors were located outside the irradiation fields. The increased relative risk of breast cancer in these patients was 2.64, higher than reported by Boice et al.[339]

In an analysis of 199,268 individuals by Wright et al.,[874] the risk of secondary leukemia increased 72% in patients who received pelvic radiotherapy, with a peak at 5 to 10 years after treatment; there was no increased risk of multiple myeloma. Mark et al.[875] identified 13 of 114 patients diagnosed with uterine sarcoma who had a prior history of pelvic irradiation (doses of 40 to 80 Gy). Criteria for radiation-induced sarcomas included a prior history of pelvic irradiation, a latent period of several years, development of sarcoma within previously irradiated field, and histologic confirmation of malignancy. Histologic types of tumor were mixed Müllerian in 6, leiomyosarcoma in 4 patients, endometrial stroma sarcoma in 1, fibrosarcoma in 1, and angiosarcoma in 1. Sarcoma developed in the uterus in 12 patients and at the vaginal cuff in 1 patient. Ten patients were treated with surgery and 2 with radiation therapy. The 5-year disease-free survival rate after salvage therapy was 17%.

In a theoretical analysis of IMRT risk in postoperative cases relative to three-dimensional conformal radiotherapy, the estimated increase in second cancer risk was 6% for 6-MV IMRT and 26% for 18 MV IMRT, with large increases in organs away from the primary beam and skin because with IMRT a much larger volume of skin was exposed.[876]

Seidman et al.[877] reviewed 15 cases of second malignancies after pelvic radiation; 5 were HPV-related vaginal primary tumors. The average latency period for development was approximately 20 years.

SELECTED REFERENCES

A full list of references for this chapter is available online.

8. zur Hausen H. Papillomaviruses causing cancer: evasion from host-cell control in early events in carcinogenesis. *J Natl Cancer Inst* 2000;92:690–698.
35. Landoni F, Maneo A, Colombo A, et al. Randomised study of radical surgery versus radiotherapy for stage Ib-IIa cervical cancer. *Lancet* 1997;350:535–540.
53. Mitchell DG, Snyder B, Coakley F, et al. Early invasive cervical cancer: MRI and CT predictors of lymphatic metastases in the ACRIN 6651/GOG 183 intergroup study. *Gynecol Oncol* 2009;112:95–103.
57. Viswanathan AN, Moughan J, Small W Jr, et al. The quality of cervical cancer brachytherapy implantation and the impact on local recurrence and disease-free survival in radiation therapy oncology group prospective trials 0116 and 0128. *Int J Gynecol Cancer* 2012;22:123–131.
71. Mayr NA, Yuh WT, Magnotta VA, et al. Tumor perfusion studies using fast magnetic resonance imaging technique in advanced cervical cancer: a new noninvasive predictive assay. *Int J Radiat Oncol Biol Phys* 1996;36:623–633.
77. Grigsby PW, Siegel BA, Dehdashti F. Lymph node staging by positron emission tomography in patients with carcinoma of the cervix. *J Clin Oncol* 2001;19:3745–3749.
91. Schwarz JK, Siegel BA, Dehdashti F, et al. Association of posttherapy positron emission tomography with tumor response and survival in cervical carcinoma. *JAMA* 2007;298:2289–2295.
161. Delgado G, Bundy BN, Fowler WC Jr, et al. A prospective surgical pathological study of stage I squamous carcinoma of the cervix: a Gynecologic Oncology Group Study. *Gynecol Oncol* 1989;35:314–320.
183. Monk BJ, Wang J, Im S, et al. Rethinking the use of radiation and chemotherapy after radical hysterectomy: a clinical-pathologic analysis of a Gynecologic Oncology Group/Southwest Oncology Group/Radiation Therapy Oncology Group trial. *Gynecol Oncol* 2005;96:721–728.
189. Perez CA, Grigsby PW, Castro-Vita H, et al. Carcinoma of the uterine cervix. I. Impact of prolongation of overall treatment time and timing of brachytherapy on outcome of radiation therapy. *Int J Radiat Oncol Biol Phys* 1995;32:1275–1288.
190. Noordhuis MG, Eijsink JJ, Roossink F, et al. Prognostic cell biological markers in cervical cancer patients primarily treated with (chemo)radiation: a systematic review. *Int J Radiat Oncol Biol Phys* 2011;79:325–334.
272. Portelance L, Chao KS, Grigsby PW, et al. Intensity-modulated radiation therapy (IMRT) reduces small bowel, rectum, and bladder doses in patients with cervical cancer receiving pelvic and para-aortic irradiation. *Int J Radiat Oncol Biol Phys* 2001;51:261–266.
274. Esthappan J, Chaudhari S, Santanam L, et al. Prospective clinical trial of positron emission tomography/computed tomography image-guided intensity-modulated radiation therapy for cervical carcinoma with positive para-aortic lymph nodes. *Int J Radiat Oncol Biol Phys* 2008;72:1134–1139.
275. Poorvu PD, Sadow CA, Townamchai K et al. Duodenal and other gastrointestinal toxicity in cervical and endometrial cancer treated with extended-field intensity modulated radiation therapy to paraaortic lymph nodes. *Int J Radiat Oncol Biol Phys* 2012; doi: 10.1016/j.ijrobp.2012.10.004. [epub ahead of print].
321. Small W Jr, Mell LK, Anderson P, et al. Consensus guidelines for delineation of clinical target volume for intensity-modulated pelvic radiotherapy in postoperative treatment of endometrial and cervical cancer. *Int J Radiat Oncol Biol Phys* 2008;71:428–434.
323. Jhingran A, Salehpour M, Sam M, et al. Vaginal motion and bladder and rectal volumes during pelvic intensity-modulated radiation therapy after hysterectomy. *Int J Radiat Oncol Biol Phys* 2012;82:256–262.
326. Kavanagh BD, Pan CC, Dawson LA, et al. Radiation dose-volume effects in the stomach and small bowel. *Int J Radiat Oncol Biol Phys* 2010;76:S101–S107.
327. Michalski JM, Gay H, Jackson A, et al. Radiation dose-volume effects in radiation-induced rectal injury. *Int J Radiat Oncol Biol Phys* 2010;76:S123–S129.
328. Viswanathan AN, Yorke ED, Marks LB, et al. Radiation dose-volume effects of the urinary bladder. *Int J Radiat Oncol Biol Phys* 2010;76:S116–S122.
329. Ahmed RS, Kim RY, Duan J, et al. IMRT dose escalation for positive para-aortic lymph nodes in patients with locally advanced cervical cancer while reducing dose to bone marrow and other organs at risk. *Int J Radiat Oncol Biol Phys* 2004;60:505–512.
369. Eifel PJ, Khalid N, Erickson B, et al. Patterns of radiotherapy practice for patients treated for intact cervical cancer in 2005–2007: a QRRO Study. *Int J Radiat Oncol Biol Phys* 2010;78:S119.
385. Abu-Rustum NR, Sonoda Y. Fertility-sparing surgery in early-stage cervical cancer: indications and applications. *J Natl Compr Canc Netw* 2010;8:1435–1438.
397. Eifel PJ, Winter K, Morris M, et al. Pelvic irradiation with concurrent chemotherapy versus pelvic and para-aortic irradiation for high-risk cervical cancer: an update of radiation therapy oncology group trial (RTOG) 90–01. *J Clin Oncol* 2004;22:872–880.
404. Piver MS, Marchetti DL, Patton T, et al. Radical hysterectomy and pelvic lymphadenectomy versus radiation therapy for small (less than or equal to 3 cm) stage IB cervical carcinoma. *Am J Clin Oncol* 1988;11:21–24.
406. Perez CA, Camel HM, Kao MS, et al. Randomized study of preoperative radiation and surgery or irradiation alone in the treatment of stage IB and IIA carcinoma of the uterine cervix: final report. *Gynecol Oncol* 1987;27:129–140.
409. Peters WA 3rd, Liu PY, Barrett RJ 2nd, et al. Concurrent chemotherapy and pelvic radiation therapy compared with pelvic radiation therapy alone as adjuvant therapy after radical surgery in high-risk early-stage cancer of the cervix. *J Clin Oncol* 2000;18:1606–1613.
410. Sedlis A, Bundy BN, Rotman MZ, et al. A randomized trial of pelvic radiation therapy versus no further therapy in selected patients with stage IB carcinoma of the cervix after radical hysterectomy and pelvic lymphadenectomy: a Gynecologic Group Study. *Gynecol Oncol* 1999;73:177–183.
412. Rotman M, Sedlis A, Piedmonte MR, et al. A phase III randomized trial of postoperative pelvic irradiation in stage IB cervical carcinoma with poor prognostic features: follow-up of a gynecologic oncology group study. *Int J Radiat Oncol Biol Phys* 2006;65:169–176.
446. Whitney CW, Sause W, Bundy BN, et al. Randomized comparison of fluorouracil plus cisplatin versus hydroxyurea as an adjunct to radiation therapy in stage IIB-IVA carcinoma of the cervix with negative para-aortic lymph nodes: a Gynecologic Oncology Group and Southwest Oncology Group study. *J Clin Oncol* 1999;17:1339–1348.
447. Rose PG, Bundy BN, Watkins EB, et al. Concurrent cisplatin-based radiotherapy and chemotherapy for locally advanced cervical cancer. *N Engl J Med* 1999;340:1144–1153.
448. Rose PG, Ali S, Watkins E, et al. Long-term follow-up of a randomized trial comparing concurrent single agent cisplatin, cisplatin-based combination chemotherapy, or hydroxyurea during pelvic irradiation for locally advanced cervical cancer: a Gynecologic Oncology Group Study. *J Clin Oncol* 2007;25:2804–2810.
450. Keys HM, Bundy BN, Stehman FB, et al. Cisplatin, radiation, and adjuvant hysterectomy compared with radiation and adjuvant hysterectomy for bulky stage IB cervical carcinoma. *N Engl J Med* 1999;340:1154–1161.
451. Stehman FB, Ali S, Keys HM, et al. Radiation therapy with or without weekly cisplatin for bulky stage 1B cervical carcinoma: follow-up of a Gynecologic Oncology Group trial. *Am J Obstet Gynecol* 2007;197:503e1–6.
454. Pearcey R, Brundage M, Drouin P, et al. Phase III trial comparing radical radiotherapy with and without cisplatin chemotherapy in patients with advanced squamous cell cancer of the cervix. *J Clin Oncol* 2002;20:966–972.
459. Duenas-Gonzalez A, Zarba JJ, Patel F, et al. Phase III, open-label, randomized study comparing concurrent gemcitabine plus cisplatin and radiation followed by adjuvant gemcitabine and cisplatin versus concurrent cisplatin and radiation in patients with stage IIB to IVA carcinoma of the cervix. *J Clin Oncol* 2011;29:1678–1685.
460. Lanciano R, Calkins A, Bundy BN, et al. Randomized comparison of weekly cisplatin or protracted venous infusion of fluorouracil in combination with pelvic radiation in advanced cervix cancer: a gynecologic oncology group study. *J Clin Oncol* 2005;23:8289–8295.
512. Monk BJ, Sill MW, McMeekin DS, et al. Phase III trial of four cisplatin-containing doublet combinations in stage IVB, recurrent, or persistent cervical carcinoma: a Gynecologic Oncology Group study. *J Clin Oncol* 2009;27:4649–4655.
524. Montana GS, Fowler WC, Varia MA, et al. Carcinoma of the cervix, stage III. Results of radiation therapy. *Cancer* 1986;57:148–154.
527. Montana GS, Hanlon AL, Brickner TJ, et al. Carcinoma of the cervix: patterns of care studies: review of 1978, 1983, and 1988–1989 surveys. *Int J Radiat Oncol Biol Phys* 1995;32:1481–1486.
534. Charra-Brunaud C, Harter V, Delannes M, et al. Impact of 3D image-based PDR brachytherapy on outcome of patients treated for cervix carcinoma in France:

results of the national STIC prospective study. *Radiother Oncol* 2012;103: 305–313.

535. Dimopoulos JC, Potter R, Lang S, et al. Dose-effect relationship for local control of cervical cancer by magnetic resonance image-guided brachytherapy. *Radiother Oncol* 2009;93:311–315.
537. Morice P, Rouanet P, Rey A, et al. Results of the GYNECO 02 Study, an FNCLCC Phase III trial comparing hysterectomy with no hysterectomy in patients with a (clinical and radiological) complete response after chemoradiation therapy for stage IB2 or II cervical cancer. *Oncologist* 2012;17:64–71.
541. Haie C, Pejovic MH, Gerbaulet A, et al. Is prophylactic para-aortic irradiation worthwhile in the treatment of advanced cervical carcinoma? Results of a controlled clinical trial of the EORTC radiotherapy group. *Radiother Oncol* 1988; 11:101–112.
543. Varia MA, Bundy BN, Deppe G, et al. Cervical carcinoma metastatic to para-aortic nodes: extended field radiation therapy with concomitant 5-fluorouracil and cisplatin chemotherapy: a Gynecologic Oncology Group study. *Int J Radiat Oncol Biol Phys* 1998;42:1015–1023.
586. Wo JY, Viswanathan AN. Impact of radiotherapy on fertility, pregnancy, and neonatal outcomes in female cancer patients. *Int J Radiat Oncol Biol Phys* 2009; 73:1304–1312.
593. Fletcher GH, Shukovsky LJ. The interplay of radiocurability and tolerance in the irradiation of human cancers. *J Radiol Electrol Med Nucl* 1975;56:383–400.
595. Lanciano RM, Martz K, Coia LR, et al. Tumor and treatment factors improving outcome in stage III-B cervix cancer. *Int J Radiat Oncol Biol Phys* 1991;20:95–100.
598. Viswanathan AN, Thomadsen B. American Brachytherapy Society consensus guidelines for locally advanced carcinoma of the cervix. Part I: General principles. *Brachytherapy* 2012;11:33–46.
600. Erickson B, Eifel P, Moughan J, et al. Patterns of brachytherapy practice for patients with carcinoma of the cervix (1996–1999): a patterns of care study. *Int J Radiat Oncol Biol Phys* 2005;63:1083–1092.
601. Viswanathan AN, Erickson BA. Three-dimensional imaging in gynecologic brachytherapy: a survey of the American Brachytherapy Society. *Int J Radiat Oncol Biol Phys* 2010;76:104–109.
602. Viswanathan AN, Creutzberg CL, Craighead P, et al. International Brachytherapy Practice Patterns: a survey of the Gynecologic Cancer Intergroup (GCIG). *Int J Radiat Oncol Biol Phys* 2012;82:250–255.
605. Stewart AJ, Viswanathan AN. Current controversies in high-dose-rate versus low-dose-rate brachytherapy for cervical cancer. *Cancer* 2006;107:908–915.
606. Petereit DG, Sarkaria JN, Potter DM, et al. High-dose-rate versus low-dose-rate brachytherapy in the treatment of cervical cancer: analysis of tumor recurrence—the University of Wisconsin experience. *Int J Radiat Oncol Biol Phys* 1999;45: 1267–1274.
607. Patel FD, Sharma SC, Negi PS, et al. Low dose rate vs. high dose rate brachytherapy in the treatment of carcinoma of the uterine cervix: a clinical trial. *Int J Radiat Oncol Biol Phys* 1994;28:335–341.
609. Hall E, Brenner D. The dose-rate effect revisited: radiobiological considerations of importance in radiotherapy. *Int J Radiat Oncol Biol Phys* 1991;21:1403–1414.
610. Orton CG, Seyedsadr M, Somnay A. Comparison of high and low dose rate remote afterloading for cervix cancer and the importance of fractionation. *Int J Radiat Oncol Biol Phys* 1991;21:1425–1434.
611. Dale RG. The application of the linear quadratic dose-effect equation to fractionated and protracted radiotherapy. *Br J Radiol* 1985;58:515–528.
615. Potter R, Haie-Meder C, Van Limbergen E, et al. Recommendations from gynaecological (GYN) GEC ESTRO working group (II): Concepts and terms in 3D image-based treatment planning in cervix cancer brachytherapy—3D dose volume parameters and aspects of 3D image-based anatomy, radiation physics, radiobiology. *Radiother Oncol* 2006;78:67–77.
618. Clark BG, Souhami L, Roman TN, et al. The prediction of late rectal complications in patients treated with high dose rate brachytherapy for carcinoma of the cervix. *Int J Radiat Oncol Biol Phys* 1997;38:989–993.
619. Petereit DG, Pearcey R. Literature analysis of high dose rate brachytherapy fractionation schedules in the treatment of cervical cancer: is there an optimal fractionation schedule? *Int J Radiat Oncol Biol Phys* 1999;43:359–366.
620. Lang S, Kirisits C, Dimopoulos J, et al. Treatment planning for MRI assisted brachytherapy of gynecologic malignancies based on total dose constraints. *Int J Radiat Oncol Biol Phys* 2007;69:619–627.
621. Viswanathan AN, Beriwal S, De Los Santos JF, et al. American Brachytherapy Society consensus guidelines for locally advanced carcinoma of the cervix. Part II: High-dose-rate brachytherapy. *Brachytherapy* 2012;11:47–52.
622. Lee LJ, Das IJ, Higgins SA, et al. American Brachytherapy Society consensus guidelines for locally advanced carcinoma of the cervix. Part III: Low-dose-rate and pulsed-dose-rate brachytherapy. *Brachytherapy* 2012;11:53–57.
623. Haie-Meder C, Potter R, Van Limbergen E, et al. Recommendations from Gynaecological (GYN) GEC-ESTRO Working Group (I): concepts and terms in 3D image based 3D treatment planning in cervix cancer brachytherapy with emphasis on MRI assessment of GTV and CTV. *Radiother Oncol* 2005;74:235–245.
628. Watkins JM, Kearney PL, Opfermann KJ, et al. Ultrasound guided tandem placement for low-dose-rate brachytherapy in advanced cervical cancer minimizes risk of intraoperative uterine perforation. *Ultrasound Obstet Gynecol* 2011;37: 241–244.
633. Potish RA, Deibel FC Jr, Khan FM. The relationship between milligram-hours and dose to point A in carcinoma of the cervix. *Radiology* 1982;145:479–483.
634. Katz A, Eifel PJ. Quantification of intracavitary brachytherapy parameters and correlation with outcome in patients with carcinoma of the cervix. *Int J Radiat Oncol Biol Phys* 2000;48:1417–1425.
635. Viswanathan AN, Dimopoulos J, Kirisits C, et al. Computed tomography versus magnetic resonance imaging-based contouring in cervical cancer brachytherapy: results of a prospective trial and preliminary guidelines for standardized contours. *Int J Radiat Oncol Biol Phys* 2007;68:491–498.
637. Eisbruch A, Johnston CM, Martel MK, et al. Customized gynecologic interstitial implants: CT-based planning, dose evaluation, and optimization aided by laparotomy. *Int J Radiat Oncol Biol Phys* 1998;40:1087–1093.
638. Erickson B, Albano K, Gillin M. CT-guided interstitial implantation of gynecologic malignancies. *Int J Radiat Oncol Biol Phys* 1996;36:699–709.
648. Potter R, Haie-Meder C, Van Limbergen E, et al. Recommendations from gynaecological (GYN) GEC ESTRO working group (II): concepts and terms in 3D image-based treatment planning in cervix cancer brachytherapy–3D dose volume parameters and aspects of 3D image-based anatomy, radiation physics, radiobiology. *Radiother Oncol* 2006;78:67–77.
650. Kirisits C, Potter R, Lang S, et al. Dose and volume parameters for MRI-based treatment planning in intracavitary brachytherapy for cervical cancer. *Int J Radiat Oncol Biol Phys* 2005;62:901–911.
651. Chargari C, Magne N, Dumas I, et al. Physics contributions and clinical outcome with 3D-MRI-based pulsed-dose-rate intracavitary brachytherapy in cervical cancer patients. *Int J Radiat Oncol Biol Phys* 2009;74:133–139.
653. Potter R, Georg P, Dimopoulos JC, et al. Clinical outcome of protocol based image (MRI) guided adaptive brachytherapy combined with 3D conformal radiotherapy with or without chemotherapy in patients with locally advanced cervical cancer. *Radiother Oncol* 2011;100:116–123.
655. Haie-Meder C, Chargari C, Rey A, et al. MRI-based low dose-rate brachytherapy experience in locally advanced cervical cancer patients initially treated by concomitant chemoradiotherapy. *Radiother Oncol* 2010;96:161–165.
661. Georg P, Lang S, Dimopoulos JC, et al. Dose-volume histogram parameters and late side effects in magnetic resonance image-guided adaptive cervical cancer brachytherapy. *Int J Radiat Oncol Biol Phys* 2011;79:356–362.
667. Olszewska AM, Saarnak AE, de Boer RW, et al. Comparison of dose-volume histograms and dose-wall histograms of the rectum of patients treated with intracavitary brachytherapy. *Radiother Oncol* 2001;61:83–85.
668. Koom WS, Sohn DK, Kim JY, et al. Computed tomography-based high-dose-rate intracavitary brachytherapy for uterine cervical cancer: preliminary demonstration of correlation between dose-volume parameters and rectal mucosal changes observed by flexible sigmoidoscopy. *Int J Radiat Oncol Biol Phys* 2007;68: 1446–1454.
669. Georg P, Kirisits C, Goldner G, et al. Correlation of dose-volume parameters, endoscopic and clinical rectal side effects in cervix cancer patients treated with definitive radiotherapy including MRI-based brachytherapy. *Radiother Oncol* 2009; 91:173–180.
670. Lee L, Viswanathan A. Predictors of toxicity following image-guided high dose rate interstitial brachytherapy for gynecologic cancer. *Int J Radiat Oncol Biol Phys* 2012;84(5):1192–1197.
680. Dimopoulos JC, Petrow P, Tanderup K, et al. Recommendations from Gynaecological (GYN) GEC-ESTRO Working Group (IV): Basic principles and parameters for MR imaging within the frame of image based adaptive cervix cancer brachytherapy. *Radiother Oncol* 2012;87:1192–1197.
698. Haie-Meder C, Kramar A, Lambin P, et al. Analysis of complications in a prospective randomized trial comparing two brachytherapy low dose rates in cervical carcinoma. *Int J Radiat Oncol Biol Phys* 1994;29:953–960.
700. Fowler JF. Dose reduction factors when increasing dose rate in LDR or MDR brachytherapy of carcinoma of the cervix. *Radiother Oncol* 1997;45:49–54.
736. Potter R, Knocke TH, Fellner C, et al. Definitive radiotherapy based on HDR brachytherapy with iridium 192 in uterine cervix carcinoma: report on the Vienna University Hospital findings (1993–1997) compared to the preceding period in the context of ICRU 38 recommendations. *Cancer Radiother* 2000;4: 159–172.
741. Haie-Meder C, Chargari C, Rey A, et al. DVH parameters and outcome for patients with early-stage cervical cancer treated with preoperative MRI-based low dose rate brachytherapy followed by surgery. *Radiother Oncol* 2009;93:316–321.
745. Syed AM, Feder BH. Technique of after-loading interstitial implants. *Radiol Clin (Basel)* 1977;46:458–475.
746. Martinez A, Edmundson GK, Cox RS, et al. Combination of external beam irradiation and multiple-site perineal applicator (MUPIT) for treatment of locally advanced or recurrent prostatic, anorectal, and gynecologic malignancies. *Int J Radiat Oncol Biol Phys* 1985;11:391–398.
747. Viswanathan AN, Erickson B, Rownd J. Image-based approaches to interstitial brachytherapy. In: Viswanathan A, Kirisits C, Erickson B, et al, eds. *Gynecologic radiation therapy: novel approaches to image-guidance and management,* 1st ed. Berlin: Springer-Verlag, 2011:247–259.
748. Viswanathan AN, Cormack R, Rawal B, et al. Increasing brachytherapy dose predicts survival for interstitial and tandem-based radiation for stage IIIB cervical cancer. *Int J Gynecol Cancer* 2009;19:1402–1406.
751. Syed AM, Puthawala AA, Abdelaziz NN, et al. Long-term results of low-dose-rate interstitial-intracavitary brachytherapy in the treatment of carcinoma of the cervix. *Int J Radiat Oncol Biol Phys* 2002;54:67–78.
766. Saibishkumar EP, Patel FD, Sharma SC, et al. Results of external-beam radiotherapy alone in invasive cancer of the uterine cervix: a retrospective analysis. *Clin Oncol (R Coll Radiol)* 2006;18:46–51.
776. Hintz BL, Kagan AR, Chan P, et al. Radiation tolerance of the vaginal mucosa. *Int J Radiat Oncol* 1980;6:711–716.
811. Eifel PJ, Levenback C, Wharton JT, et al. Time course and incidence of late complications in patients treated with radiation therapy for FIGO stage IB carcinoma of the uterine cervix. *Int J Radiat Oncol Biol Phys* 1995;32:1289–1300.
814. Perez CA, Grigsby PW, Lockett MA, et al. Radiation therapy morbidity in carcinoma of the uterine cervix: dosimetric and clinical correlation. *Int J Radiat Oncol Biol Phys* 1999;44:855–866.
827. Rotman M, Pajak TF, Choi K, et al. Prophylactic extended-field irradiation of para-aortic lymph nodes in stages IIB and bulky IB and IIA cervical carcinomas. Ten-year treatment results of RTOG 79–20. *JAMA* 1995;274:387–893.
839. Bruner DW, Lanciano R, Keegan M, et al. Vaginal stenosis and sexual function following intracavitary radiation for the treatment of cervical and endometrial carcinoma. *Int J Radiat Oncol Biol Phys* 1993;27:825–830.
845. Baxter NN, Habermann EB, Tepper JE, et al. Risk of pelvic fractures in older women following pelvic irradiation. *JAMA* 2005;294:2587–2593.
851. Lanciano R, Corn B, Martin E, et al. Perioperative morbidity of intracavitary gynecologic brachytherapy. *Int J Radiat Oncol Biol Phys* 1994;29:969–974.
852. Jhingran A, Eifel PJ. Perioperative and postoperative complications of intracavitary radiation for FIGO stage I-III carcinoma of the cervix. *Int J Radiat Oncol Biol Phys* 2000;46:1177–1183.
876. Zwahlen DR, Ruben JD, Jones P, et al. Effect of intensity-modulated pelvic radiotherapy on second cancer risk in the postoperative treatment of endometrial and cervical cancer. *Int J Radiat Oncol Biol Phys* 2009;74:539–545.
899. Logsdon MD, Eifel PJ. Figo IIIB squamous cell carcinoma of the cervix: an analysis of prognostic factors emphasizing the balance between external beam and intracavitary radiation therapy. *Int J Radiat Oncol Biol Phys* 1999;43: 763–775.

Chapter 70 Endometrial Cancer

Kaled M. Alektiar

ANATOMY

The uterus is a hollow, muscular organ located in the true pelvis between the bladder and the rectum. The average adult uterus is about 8 cm long, 5 cm wide, and 2.5 cm thick. It is divided into the fundus, body (corpus), and cervix. The junction between the body and cervix is called the isthmus. The fundus is pierced at each cornu by the fallopian tubes. The uterine surface is partially covered by peritoneum. The uterine cavity is lined by endometrium, made up of columnar cells forming many tubular glands. The thickness of the endometrium varies during the menstrual cycle, but by the end of menstruation it should be 2 to 3 mm in thickness. The wall of the uterus is composed of myometrium, consisting of smooth muscle fibers. The major supports of the uterus are the broad, round, uterosacral and cardinal ligaments. The major blood supply to the uterus is the uterine artery, which enters the uterus at the isthmus after it crosses over the ureter. The lymphatic drainage for the body of the uterus is mainly to the obturator and internal and external iliac lymph nodes. The lymphatics from the fundus accompany the ovarian artery and drain into the para-aortic lymph nodes.

EPIDEMIOLOGY AND RISK FACTORS

Endometrial cancer is the most common gynecologic cancer and the fourth most frequently diagnosed cancer in women in the United States. According to 2011 cancer statistics, the estimated number of newly diagnosed cases is 46,470, with a probability of 1 of every 39 women (2.58%) developing it during her lifetime.[1] Although it is a cancer that affects predominantly postmenopausal women, 5% to 30% of women are <50 years of age at the time of diagnosis.[2,3] The expected number of deaths from endometrial cancer in 2011 was 8,120, making it the eighth-leading cause of death from cancer in women. Prior estimates on the death rate from endometrial cancer seemed to indicate that the rate was on the rise, but the most recent data show that the death rate of 4.18 per 100,000 women did not change from the year 1990 to 2007.[1]

The age-standardized rate per 100,000 for endometrial cancer in more developed areas of the world is 12.9, with a cumulative risk of 1.6% (age 0 to 74 years), compared to 5.9 and 0.7%, respectively, in less developed areas, indicating a possible influence of environmental factors on the incidence of this disease.[4] The exact etiology of endometrial cancer remains unknown, but several risk factors have been associated with it, chiefly unopposed estrogen. It is well established that endometrial cancer risk is increased among women who have high circulating levels of bioavailable estrogens and low levels of progesterone, so that the mitogenic effect of estrogens is insufficiently counterbalanced by the opposing effect of progesterone.[5–7] The source of unopposed estrogen could be endogenous or exogenous. In a case–control study, the association between endogenous estrogen and endometrial cancer was demonstrated. In that study there was correlation between high blood concentrations of estrogens and increased risk of endometrial cancer.[7] Lifetime cumulative number of menstrual cycles, that is, menstruation span, is associated with increased risk of developing endometrial cancer. This is due to the fact that endometrial cell proliferation increases during the follicular phase, which is the longest in the menstrual cycle. Thus, *early age at menarche* (estimated relative risk [RR], 1.5 to 2) and *late age at menopause* (RR, 2 to 3), examples of increased menstruation span, are risk factors for endometrial cancer.[8,9] *Nulliparity* (RR, 3) is also associated with increased risk of endometrial cancer[8] due in part to anovulatory menstrual cycles. *Obesity* increases endometrial cancer risk (RR, 5) mainly through changes in endogenous hormone metabolism. After menopause, when ovarian production of both estrogen and progesterone ceases, the major source of estrogen is via peripheral conversion, mostly within adipose tissue, of androgens that continue being produced by the adrenal glands and ovaries. Thus with obesity there is an increase in the amount of bioavailable estrogens in the circulation and the endometrial tissue.[7,10,11] Obesity may also influence endometrial cancer risk via chronic hyperinsulinemia, which appears to be a key factor for the development of ovarian hyperandrogenism, associated with anovulation and progesterone deficiency, especially for premenopausal women.[10] *Non–insulin-dependent diabetes mellitus* and *hypertension* (RR, 1–3) also increases the risk of endometrial cancer. This is often believed to be secondary to obesity, but there are data showing that these risk factors could be independent of obesity.[12,13,14] With regard to exogenous estrogen, it is well established that the use of *estrogen-only hormone-replacement therapy* and *sequential oral contraceptives* greatly increases endometrial cancer risk (RR, 10 to 20), whereas combined preparations, that is, those that contain a progestogen as well as estrogen throughout the treatment period, have a protective effect (RR, 0.3 to 0.5).[15–16,17] The use of *tamoxifen* in patients with breast cancer has been associated with increased risk (RR, 3 to 7) of endometrial cancer.[18,19–20] The mechanism of action of tamoxifen is in competition with that of endogenous estrogen for estrogen receptors. In premenopausal women, tamoxifen has an antiestrogenic effect, but in postmenopausal women it has a weak estrogenic effect because of the upregulation of estrogen receptors. In a recent meta-analysis on adjuvant tamoxifen and endometrial cancer, for patients who were <55 years of age there was little absolute risk compared to patients in of 55 to 69 years of age, for whom the 15-year incidence was 3.8% in the tamoxifen group versus 1.1% in the control group (absolute increase 2.6% [standard error 0.6], 95% confidence interval [CI] = 1.4 to 3.8), highlighting the influence of age on the risk of endometrial cancer from tamoxifen use.[21] Initial data seemed to indicate that the majority of endometrial cancers associated with tamoxifen use were of early stage with favorable features.[22] More recent data, however, show a change in the profile of these endometrial cancers, with a rise in the rate of serous, clear-cell, carcinosarcoma, and sarcoma types.[23,24] Inherited genetic predisposition, especially in the setting of hereditary nonpolyposis colorectal cancer (HNPCC), probably accounts for <5% of all endometrial cancer cases. Mutations in one of the four mismatch repair genes *hMLH1, hMSH2, hMSH6,* or *hPMS2* have been identified in patients with Lynch syndrome. Although HNPCC is thought of primarily in terms of risk of developing colorectal cancer, it is important to note that lifetime cumulative risk of endometrial cancer for women with HNPCC is 40% to 60%, which equals or exceeds their risk of colorectal cancer.[25] There seems to be a high rate of lower uterine segment involvement in patients with HNPCC-associated endometrial cancer.[26]

CLINICAL PRESENTATION AND NATURAL HISTORY

The most common presentation for endometrial cancer is postmenopausal vaginal bleeding, which is reported by 80% to 90% of patients. The incidence of endometrial cancer in women presenting with postmenopausal bleeding is only 10% to 15%. This incidence, however, could range from 1% up to 25%, depending on patient age and the presence of other risk factors. In a recent repot of a total of 3,548 women presenting with postmenopausal vaginal bleeding, 201 (6%) had a diagnosis of endometrial carcinoma. Use of a multiple logistic regression model showed that recurrent episodes of bleeding (odds ratio [OR], 3.64), a history of diabetes (OR, 1.48), older age (1.06), and high body-mass index (OR, 1.07) increased the risk of endometrial malignancy when corrected for other characteristics.[27] Other patterns of presentations include vaginal discharge, abnormal Papanicolaou smear, or thickened endometrium on routine transvaginal ultrasound. For patients with advanced disease, they may present with urinary or rectal bleeding, constipation, pain, lower-extremity lymphedema, abdominal distension due to ascites, and cough and/or or hemoptysis.

The International Federation of Gynecology and Obstetrics (FIGO) annual report[28] showed that the 5-year survival rate for 8,110 patients with endometrial cancer treated between 1999 and 2001 was 80%. Such excellent outcome is a reflection of the fact that the majority of patients are diagnosed with early-stage disease. The tumor was limited to the corpus uteri in 71% of cases, involved the cervix in 12%, and extended beyond the uterus, but short of distant spread, in 13%. For patients with disease limited to the endometrium or with <50% myometrial invasion, the 5-year survival rate was 91%. However, the rate dropped to 66% when disease extended to adnexa/serosa/positive peritoneal cytology, to 57% with regional lymph node involvement, to 25.5% with bladder or rectal involvement, and to 20% with distant spread. For clinically staged patients, the 5-year survival rate ranged from 67% for early-stage disease down to 15% for advanced disease. Mass screening for endometrial cancer in women at average risk or increased risk due to a history of unopposed estrogen therapy, tamoxifen therapy, late menopause, nulliparity, infertility or failure to ovulate, obesity, diabetes, or hypertension is not recommended. American Cancer Society (ACS) recommends that women at average and increased risk should be informed about risks and symptoms (in particular, unexpected bleeding and spotting) of endometrial cancer at the onset of menopause and should be strongly encouraged to immediately report these symptoms to their physician. However, screening has been recommended by the ACS for women who carry, or are related to carriers of, the HNPCC mutation, starting at age 35 years, including annual transvaginal ultrasound and endometrial biopsy.[29] Prophylactic hysterectomy and bilateral salpingo-oophorectomy once childbearing is completed have been shown to effectively reduce the risk of endometrial cancer in patients with HNPCC and should be strongly considered.[30]

DIAGNOSTIC WORKUP

Endometrial tissue sampling remains the gold standard by which the diagnosis of endometrial cancer is established. This is achieved via biopsy or dilatation and curettage (D&C). *Endometrial biopsy,* which can be easily performed in the office with a Pipelle or similar device, is the preferred approach. Its sensitivity in detecting endometrial cancer in postmenopausal women is 99.6% compared to 91% in premenopausal women. Its specificity is >98% for both groups.[31] If the patient is undergoing hysterectomy, routine D&C is not necessary after an office Pipelle sampling has documented malignancy. However, if symptoms persist, the office sampling is inadequate, or the patient is being considered for conservative fertility-sparing approaches, a D&C should be performed. In addition, D&C provides more reliable assessments of final pathologic findings in hysterectomy specimens, mainly with regard to tumor grade.[32] Given that the incidence of endometrial cancer in women with postmenopausal bleeding is only 10% to 15%, it is unclear how feasible it is to perform endometrial sampling on every patient. *Transvaginal ultrasonography* (TVU) may be considered as a useful tool to assess patient's vaginal bleeding.[33] Normal endometrium looks thin and homogeneously hyperechoic, but it is thickened and heterogeneous, with hyperplasia, polyps, and cancer,[34] as shown in Figure 70.1. The consensus statement from the Society of Radiologists in Ultrasound defines an endometrial thickness of 5 mm or greater as being abnormal.[35] If the thickness of the endometrium is <5 mm, the risk of endometrial cancer is minimal; the false-negative rate is about 4%. Under such circumstances, endometrial sampling may be foregone if no further episodes of vaginal bleeding occur.[33] Recent meta-analysis seems to indicate that perhaps a cut-off of 3-mm thickness rather than <5 mm provides even better diagnostic accuracy.[36] If the TVU is abnormal but the biopsy is negative/nondiagnostic or the uterine cavity is inaccessible, then *saline-infusion sonography* or *hysteroscopy* should be considered to help exclude intracavitary lesions, especially polyps that might contain cancer.[37,38] In addition, these methods are also helpful in premenopausal women, for whom the accuracy of TVU is limited because the endometrial thickness fluctuates, depending on the level of female hormones. The potential downside to

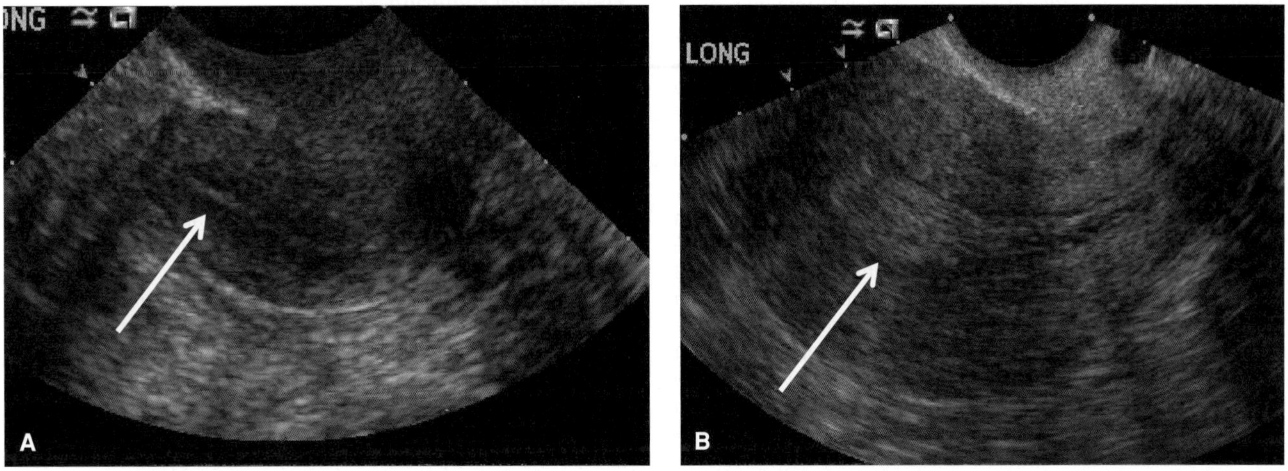

FIGURE 70.1. Sagittal view of the uterus on transvaginal ultrasound. **A:** Normal thin endometrium (*arrow*). **B:** Thickened endometrium (*arrow*).

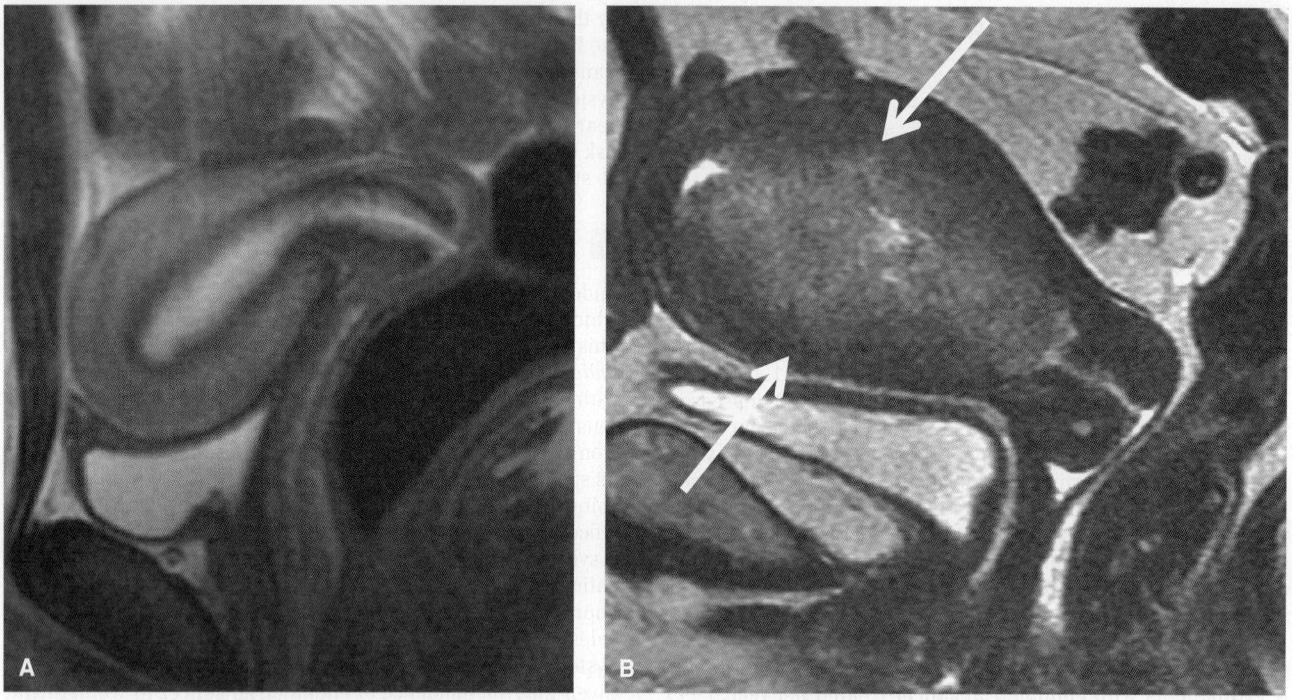

FIGURE 70.2. Sagittal magnetic resonance imaging view of the uterus. **A:** Normal uterus. **B:** Deep myometrial invasion (*arrows*).

saline infusion or hysteroscopy is that there have been reports that the insufflation of the distending medium into the canal has been associated with an increase in positive peritoneal cytology, although the prognostic implications are unclear of such positive cytology "induced" by sampling.[39] Several imaging studies are available to define the extent of disease preoperatively. Good-quality pelvic *computed tomography* (CT) scans obtained with oral and intravenous contrast can demonstrate the extent of the endometrial tumor. The endometrial carcinoma is a hypodense mass relative to the normal myometrium and may be seen as a diffuse, circumscribed vegetative or polypoidal mass within the uterine cavity. If myometrial invasion is seen, it usually implies involvement of greater than one-third to one-half of the myometrial thickness. Involvement of the cervix is seen on CT as cervical enlargement >3.5 cm in diameter with heterogeneous low-attenuation areas within the fibromuscular stroma. Parametrial or sidewall extension is seen by the loss of periureteral fat in the former and <3 mm of intervening fat between the soft tissue mass and the pelvic sidewall in the latter. Involvement of the fallopian tubes and ovaries is detected in the usual fashion, and for lymph nodes is >1 cm in diameter in the short axis.[40,41] *Magnetic resonance imaging* (MRI) is considered the most accurate imaging study to assess tumor extension in endometrial cancer, especially myometrial invasion. Dynamic contrast-enhanced MRI is the optimal MRI method for detecting myometrial invasion,[42] with an accuracy of 85% to 93%. A clear junctional zone or preservation of a sharp delineation between the tumor and the myometrium implies disease limited to the endometrium. Disease characterized by disruption of the junctional zone, increased–signal-intensity tumor in the inner half of the myometrium with preservation of the outer myometrium, or both correlate with superficial myometrial invasion. If there is extension of the high signal intensity tumor into the outer myometrium with preservation of a peripheral rim of normal, intact myometrium, then that is considered deep myometrial invasion (Fig. 70.2). MRI also helps to delineate tumor extension into the cervix. The normal cervical stroma is hypointense on T2-weighted images and is replaced by intermediate–signal-intensity tumor in cases of invasion.[34] The reported sensitivity of MRI in detecting lymph node metastasis is 27% to 66% and the specificity is 73% to 94% in surgically staged patients.[43] *Positron emission tomography/computed tomography* (PET/CT) is also being used in endometrial cancer. There seems to be little benefit in assessing the primary tumor extension. With regard to regional lymph node metastasis, the reported sensitivity is 50% to 100%, the specificity is 87% to 100%, and the accuracy is 78% to 100%. The main limitation of PET/CT is its inability to detect metastasis in lymph nodes ≤5 mm in size.[43] The FIGO staging for endometrial cancer is a surgical staging, and thus preoperative imaging studies (except chest x-rays) are not part of the staging. *Cancer antigen 125* (CA 125) serum levels could be elevated in patients with endometrial cancer. Kim et al.,[44] in a review of 413 patients, found that 23.9% of patients had >35 U/mL serum CA 125 levels. Hsieh et al.[45] found that preoperative levels of >40 U/mL correlated significantly with regional lymph nodes metastasis and suggested that such levels could be used as an indication for full pelvic and periaortic lymphadenectomy at the time of surgical staging in the absence of metastatic disease.

Pathologic Classification

Endometrial Hyperplasia

The diagnostic criterion for hyperplasia is an increase in the number and size of proliferating glands. The International Society of Gynecologic Pathologists standardized the subclassification of endometrial hyperplasia. In simple hyperplasia, there is only glandular proliferation and enlargement with increased stromal cellularity. This rarely progresses to carcinoma (<1%). Complex hyperplasia is characterized by back-to-back proliferation of glands with intraluminal papillae, epithelial pseudostratification, and few mitotic figures. If there is no cytologic atypia, the risk of malignant degeneration is again quite low, on the order of 3%. Any proliferation demonstrating cytologic abnormalities (in cellular or nuclear morphology) is classified as atypical hyperplasia. Atypical hyperplasia has a much higher risk of progression to an invasive carcinoma—8% for simple atypical hyperplasia, increasing to 29% for complex hyperplasia associated with atypia.[46] The GOG conducted a prospective trial in which all patients with atypical hyperplasia of the uterus underwent an immediate hysterectomy. The rate

TABLE 70.1 PATHOLOGIC CLASSIFICATON OF ENDOMETRIAL CANCERS

Endometrioid adenocarcinoma
Not otherwise specified
Villoglandular
Secretory adenocarcinoma
Ciliated carcinoma
Adenocarcinoma with squamous differentiation
Uterine papillary serous
Clear cell carcinoma
Mucinous carcinoma
Squamous cell carcinoma
Transitional cell carcinoma
Mixed-cell type
Undifferentiated carcinoma
Metastatic carcinoma to the endometrium

of underlying concurrent carcinoma in the uterus was 42.6% in these patients.[47] The standard recommended treatment for atypical hyperplasia of the uterus is hysterectomy if childbearing is complete and the patient has no other contraindications to surgery. In patients who desire future fertility or have an absolute contraindication to surgery, progestational therapies may be used with caution.[48]

Carcinoma of the Endometrium

Endometrioid Carcinoma

Endometrioid adenocarcinoma is the most common endometrial carcinoma, constituting 75% to 80% of all cases (Table 70.1). The classic histologic appearance is that of marked glandular proliferation with back-to-back proliferation of glands and little intervening stroma (Fig. 70.3A). The name endometrioid is derived from resemblance to proliferative-phase endometrium. Architectural grading is determined by the amount of solid mass of tumor cells compared to well-defined glands. Grade 1 is an endometrioid cancer in which <5% of the tumor growth is in solid sheets. Grade 2 is an adenocarcinoma in which 6% to 50% of the tumor is composed of solid sheets of cells. Grade 3 occurs when >50% of the tumor is made up of solid sheets. Nuclear grading is determined by the nuclear shape, size, chromatin distribution, and size of the nucleoli. The grading is primarily driven by the architectural grading, but if there is marked nuclear atypia in an otherwise grade 2 architectural grading, it should be increased to grade 3. Within endometrioid adenocarcinoma, the subtypes are endometrioid carcinoma not otherwise specified (NOS), endometrioid carcinoma with squamous differentiation, villoglandular endometrioid carcinoma, secretory carcinoma, and a ciliated cell variant.[49] Most of the endometrioid adenocarcinomas are designated NOS. Foci of squamous differentiation are often found with endometrioid adenocarcinoma. The squamous component could be benign, with the designation of adenoacanthoma, or malignant, in which case it is called adenosquamous carcinoma. Such designations have not been very useful, however, because the degree of differentiation of the squamous component parallels that of the glandular architectural grading. Therefore, most gynecologic pathologists use the term *adenocarcinoma with squamous differentiation*. Other subtypes of endometrioid adenocarcinoma include the relatively common *villoglandular carcinoma,* which grows in a papillary fashion.

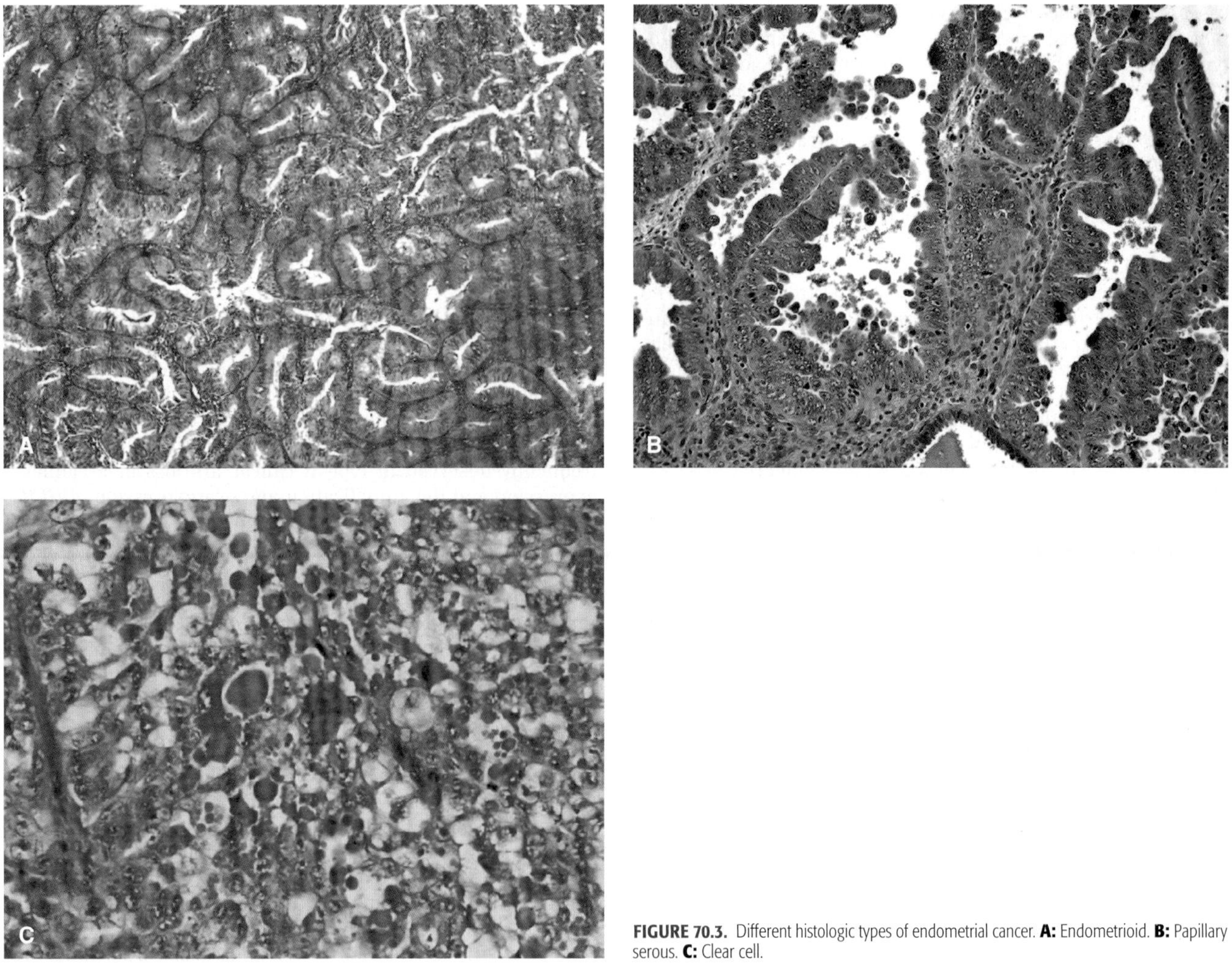

FIGURE 70.3. Different histologic types of endometrial cancer. **A:** Endometrioid. **B:** Papillary serous. **C:** Clear cell.

The prognosis of this subtype is similar to that of low-grade endometrioid cancer, and it must not be confused with serous carcinoma because of its papillary features. *Secretory carcinoma,* which represents <2% of all endometrial carcinomas, is characterized by a very well differentiated glandular pattern with much intracellular glycogen, thus resembling early secretory endometrium. Although the cells have clear cytoplasm, their histologic and cytologic features are different from those of clear-cell carcinoma. *Ciliated carcinoma* is a very rare subtype, characterized by the presence of ciliated cells comprising >75% of the tumor specimen. It is usually associated with a history of prior estrogen use, and the prognosis is quite good, since most are well differentiated.

Mucinous Carcinoma

This designation requires >50% of the tumor cells to be mucinous. These cells are carcinoembryonic antigen positive and are laden with mucin, which stains positively with mucicarmine and periodic acid–Schiff stains but is diastase resistant. Because of the resemblance to endocervical adenocarcinoma, it is essential to exclude it by endocervical curettage. Mucinous carcinomas are usually well differentiated and have the same prognosis as ordinary endometrioid carcinomas.

Serous Carcinoma

Serous carcinomas, also known as papillary serous cancers, resemble ovary cancer in terms of histology and to some extent in terms of behavior. The mere presence of papillary structure is not diagnostic because other histologic types may have papilla as well. However, the presence of marked cellular atypia in addition to papilla distinguishes serous carcinoma from others (Fig. 70.3B). Psammoma bodies are found in up to 33% of cases. The incidence of serous endometrial cancer is about 10% that of endometrial carcinomas. This is a very aggressive subtype, with a high propensity for early lymphatic and intraperitoneal dissemination, often despite little myometrial penetration.[50] In the FIGO annual report, the 5-year survival rate was 52.6% compared to 83.2% for endometrioid carcinoma.[28]

Clear-Cell Carcinoma

Clear-cell carcinoma of the endometrium resembles renal carcinoma, but its origin from Müllerian structures is now well established. Unlike vaginal and cervical clear-cell carcinoma, it is not related to intrauterine diethylstilbestrol exposure. The microscopic structure may vary from solid patterns to glandular differentiation (Fig. 70.3C). In the latter pattern, small cells resembling "hobnail" cells line spaces and glands. These are cells that extruded their cytoplasm, leaving bare nuclei that protrude into the glandular lumens. The prognosis of this cancer is somewhat similar to that of serous cancer. In the FIGO annual report, the 5-year survival rate was 62.5% compared to 83.2% for endometrioid carcinoma and 52.6% for serous carcinoma.[28]

Squamous Carcinoma

This type of cancer is extremely rare, and the diagnosis has to be made after the exclusion of cervical origin. The 5-year survival rate based on the FOGO report is 68.9% overall, but the prognosis is poor for patients with extrauterine disease or distant spread.[28]

Undifferentiated Carcinoma

The World Health Organization classification describes endometrial undifferentiated carcinomas as "malignant poorly differentiated endometrial carcinomas, lacking any evidence of differentiation" without any further characterization.[51] Undifferentiated carcinomas can also be associated with an endometrioid carcinoma component, and such tumors have been referred to as "dedifferentiated carcinomas," which is being recognized with increased frequency. Some of these tumors may belong to the spectrum of gynecologic neoplasms seen in the setting of microsatellite instability and possibly Lynch syndrome.[52]

Mixed Histology

Mixed-cell-type endometrial cancer composed of two or more pure types is not uncommon. By convention, in order to be designated as mixed, the other cell-type component has to comprise at least 10% of the tumor. Except for mixed endometrioid and serous or clear-cell carcinoma, the clinical significance of mixed cell type is questionable.

Simultaneous Tumors

Cancers of identical type may be discovered in the ovary and endometrium simultaneously. Usually, the site of the largest tumor is assigned the primary origin, but occasionally true primary endometrial and ovarian malignancies may coexist. This field effect of the Müllerian system may occur in as much as 15% to 20% of ovarian endometrioid tumors.[53] If the endometrial tumor is <5 cm in diameter, well differentiated, with no vascular invasion, limited to less than the middle one-third of the myometrium, and the ovarian lesions are bilateral, it is more likely that there are two concomitant primary tumors. Genetic profiling may represent a powerful tool in clinical practice for distinguishing between metastatic and dual primaries in patients with simultaneous ovarian/endometrial cancer and for predicting disease outcome.[54]

Molecular Biology

Several investigators pointed out that there are two distinct types of endometrial cancer.[55,56] In type I endometrial cancer there is strong correlation with prior estrogen stimulation. The cancers in this category are often indolent in nature, with minimal myometrial invasion and low-grade histology. They affect premenopausal and perimenopausal women. Type II endometrial cancer often affects postmenopausal women with no prior history of estrogen stimulation. The histology of the tumors is often high grade, such as serous or clear-cell cancers with deep invasion, and at a more advanced stage at the time of presentation. What is intriguing is the fact that at the molecular level, the existence of two distinct types of endometrial cancer seems to be validated. In a recent review by Dedes et al.,[57] the compiled data from the literature show that the most frequently altered molecular pathway in type I endometrial carcinomas is the PI3 K/PTEN/AKT pathway, which is dysregulated by oncogenic mutations, PTEN loss of function, and/or overexpression of upstream tyrosine kinase growth factor receptors, leading to uncontrolled cell proliferation and survival. On the other hand, the main pathway alterations in type II endometrial cancers involve the tumor suppressors p53 and/or p16, which cause cell cycle dysregulation and genetic instability. Other features frequently observed in type II cancer are loss of E-cadherin expression and the amplification and overexpression of *HER2*. Inactivation of the *p53* tumor suppressor gene is seen in almost 90% of cases of serous carcinoma.[58,59] Mutation in the p53 gene, however, is encountered in only 10% of endometrioid adenocarcinoma, with most occurring in grade 3 tumors. Inactivation of the cell cycle regulator *p16* is also more frequent in type II (40%) than in type I (10%). The underlying mechanism is not clear but probably involves deletion and promoter hypermethylation.[60] Reduction in the levels of the adhesion molecule *E-cadherin* is more frequent in type II (62% to 87%) than in type I (5% to 53%) tumors.[61,62] *HER2* overexpression or amplification is seen in 17% to 32% of type II compared to 3% to 10% in type I tumors.[63–64,65] In contrast, mutation in the *PTEN* tumor suppressor gene is found in 30% to 50% of type I endometrial cancer. PTEN mutations have been detected in endometrial hyperplasia with and without atypia (19% and 21%, respectively), which suggests that PTEN mutations are early events in the development of endometrial cancer.[60] Mutations in *PIK3CA* occur in 36% of type I endometrial cancer and coexist frequently with

PTEN mutations.[60] Mutation in K-ras proto-oncogene is seen in 10% to 30% of endometrial cancer patients.[59] *Microsatellite instability* (MSI), which is found in patients with HNPCC, is also seen in approximately 20% of "sporadic" endometrial cancers.[66,67] MSI, mutations in PTEN/ PIK3CA, and mutations in K-ras frequently coexist within the same tumor.[68] *B-Catenin* is important for cell differentiation, maintenance of normal tissue architecture, and signal transduction. B-Catenin mutations are seen in 25% to 40% of type I endometrial cancer. Of interest, the mutations do not usually coexist with MSI and mutations in PTEN/PIK3CA and K-ras. This suggests that type I endometrial cancers with B-catenin mutations may develop via a unique pathway.[68] Microarray analysis has further revealed distinct gene expression profiles among different histologic types of endometrial cancer.[69,70]

STAGING

Before 1988, the staging system for endometrial cancer was clinical. Stage I was tumor limited to the uterus, with IA designation if the length was ≤8 cm and IB if it was >8 cm. Stage II was for when cervix was involved, stage III when disease extension beyond uterus/cervix was limited to the true pelvis, and stage IV when it extended beyond the true pelvis or involved bladder or rectum (IVA) or distant spread (IVB). This system is applicable to the few patients who cannot have surgery and are treated with definitive radiation. Creasman et al.[71] reported a Gynecologic Oncology Group (GOG) study on 621 patients with clinically stage I endometrial cancer, that is, confined to the corpus, who underwent total abdominal hysterectomy/bilateral salpingo-oophorectomy, peritoneal cytology, and selective pelvic and para-aortic lymphadenectomy. Of the 621 patients, 144 (22%) were found to have disease outside the uterus. The rate of positive peritoneal cytology was 12%, that of adnexal involvement was 5%, and that of regional lymph node involvement was 11%. Pelvic node metastases were found in <3% of patients with grade 1 endometrium-confined disease but in >30% when grade 3 disease penetrated the outer one-third of the myometrium. Aortic nodal disease, although rare in grade 1 disease or in the absence of pelvic node metastasis, was seen in 14% and 23% of patients with deeply invasive grade 2 or 3 disease, respectively. This highlighted some of the shortcomings of the clinical staging system and led to the adoption of a surgical staging system by FIGO in 1988 in order to better estimate 5-year prognoses for patients and to better tailor adjuvant therapy to those patients most likely to benefit from it (Table 70.2).

TABLE 70.2 ENDOMETRIAL CANCER SURGICAL STAGING SYSTEM: INTERNATIONAL FEDERATION OF GYNECOLOGY AND OBSTETRICS 1988

Stages/Grades	*Definition*
Stage I	Tumor limited to the uterus
IA grades 1–3	Tumor limited to the endometrium
IB grades 1–3	Invasion to <50% of the myometrium
IC grades 1–3	Invasion to ≥50% of the myometrium
Stage II	Extension to the cervix but not beyond the uterus
IIA grades 1–3	Endocervical glandular involvement only
IIB grades 1–3	Cervical stromal invasion
Stage III	Extension outside of the uterus/cervix with/without regional metastasis
IIIA grades 1–3	Tumor invades serosa or adnexum or positive peritoneal cytology
IIIB grades 1–3	Vaginal metastasis
IIIC grades 1–3	Metastasis to pelvic and/or periaortic lymph nodes
Stage IV	
IVA grades 1–3	Tumor invades bladder and/or bowel mucosa
IVB grades 1–3	Distant metastasis including intra-abdominal and/or inguinal lymph nodes

TABLE 70.3 REVISED ENDOMETRIAL CANCER SURGICAL STAGING SYSTEM: INTERNATIONAL FEDERATION OF GYNECOLOGY AND OBSTETRICS 2009

Stage I	
IA grades 1–3	Tumor limited to the endometrium or invasion to <50% of the myometrium (includes endocervical glandular involvement)
IB grades 1–3	Invasion to ≥50% of the myometrium (includes endocervical glandular involvement)
Stage II	
II grades 1–3	Cervical stromal invasion
Stage III	
IIIA grades 1–3	Tumor invades uterine serosa or adnexae (positive cytology has to be reported separately without changing the stage)
IIIB grades 1–3	Tumor involving the vagina and/or parametria
IIIC grades 1–3	Pelvic or para-aortic lymph nodal involvement
IIIC1 grades 1–3	Pelvic nodal involvement only
IIIC2 grades 1–3	Para-aortic nodal involvement with or without pelvic nodal involvement
Stage IV	
IVA grades 1–3	Invasion of bladder, bowel mucosa, or both
IVB	Distant metastases, including intra-abdominal spread or inguinal lymph nodes

In 2009 the FIGO staging system was modified again.[72] Patients who formerly were staged as IB, that is, <50% myometrial invasion, are now considered IA. Patients with >50% myometrial invasion are designated as stage IB. Endocervical glandular involvement no longer affects staging; only patients with cervical stromal invasion are considered stage II. Having positive peritoneal cytology no longer affects staging. Parametrial extension is now considered IIIB. Patients with stage IIIC are now subdivided into IIIC1 if pelvic nodes are involved and IIIC2 if para-aortic nodes are involved (Table 70.3). The discriminating power of the new FIGO staging system is being debated. Page et al.[73] evaluated 10,839 cases from 1998 to 2006 using the Surveillance, Epidemiology, and End Results (SEER) Program. The analysis demonstrated the usefulness of two divisions rather than three for stage I in the new FIGO staging system. In contrast, a study from Memorial Sloan-Kettering Cancer Center (MSKCC) of 1,307 patients with FIGO 1988 stage I disease showed that the revised system for stage I did not improve its predictive ability over the 1988 system.[74]

Prognostic Factors

Several clinicopathologic factors have been identified in patients with endometrial carcinoma to help predict the prognosis and individualize the treatment plan. At MSKCC, a nomogram was developed for predicting overall survival of women with endometrial cancer (n = 1,735) after primary therapy.[75] Use of five prognostic factors—age, grade, histologic type, number of lymph nodes removed, and FIGO 1988 surgical stage—predicted OS with high concordance probability (Fig. 70.4).

Age

The influence of older age on worse outcome has been well established. The adverse impact of older age is often explained by pointing out that older patients tend to present with aggressive histology and more-advanced disease and are generally treated less aggressively. What is intriguing, however, is that the strongest correlation between older age and poor outcome is seen in patients with favorable characteristics. Age ≥60 years has been shown to be predictive of local-regional recurrence (hazard ratio [HR], 3.9; p = .0017) and death (HR, 2.66; p = .01) in a randomized trial limited to stage I and in which patients with deep myometrial invasion grade 3 were excluded.[76] The adverse impact of advanced age on outcome persists even when elderly patients are treated as aggressively as their younger counterparts.[77]

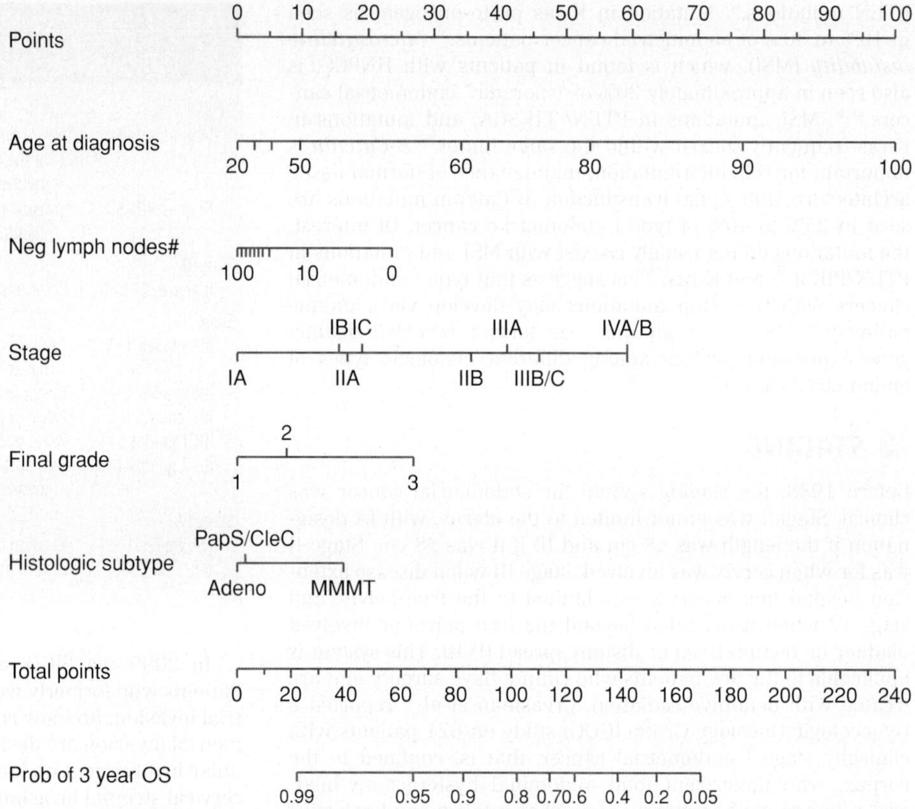

FIGURE 70.4. Nomogram for predicting overall survival in patients with endometrial cancer.

Race

White women tend to fare better than African Americans, independent of other prognostic factors.[78] It is important to note that although the prevalence of endometrial cancer is lower in African American women, the incidence of high-risk tumors in this group is higher.[79]

Histologic Subtype

According to the FIGO annual report, the 5-year survival rate was 83.2% for endometrioid adenocarcinoma, compared to 52.6% for serous cancer and 62.5% for clear-cell cancer in 8,033 surgically staged patients. Patients with endometrioid histology have surgical stage III to IV disease only in 13.8% of patients, compared to 41.7% with serous and 33% with clear-cell carcinoma, which could explain the worse outcome. However, the influence of histology was seen even in patients with surgical stage I disease ($n = 5,285$), for whom 5-year survival dropped from 90% for endometrioid histology to 79.9% with serous and 85.1% with clear-cell carcinoma.[28]

Grade

Tumor grade is one of the most sensitive indicators of prognosis. Grade directly affects the depth of myometrial penetration and the frequency of lymph node involvement. Most grade 1 tumors are limited to the endometrium or have superficial myometrial penetration, and the overall risk of pelvic and para-aortic lymph nodal metastases is 3% and 1.5%, respectively. Only 10% of grade 1 tumors have deep myometrial invasion, and pelvic and para-aortic lymph nodal involvement in these is 12% and 6%, respectively. Conversely, >50% of grade 3 tumors have >50% myometrial invasion, and these have pelvic and para-aortic nodal involvement on the order of 30% and 20%, respectively.[71] In the FIGO annual report,[28] grade 3 was an independent predictor of poor survival on multivariate analysis within each stage—stage I (HR, 2.45), II (HR, 2.14), III (HR, 2.44), and IV (HR, 2.55).

Myometrial Invasion

Regardless of grade, only 1% of tumors limited to the endometrium had lymph nodal involvement, as compared with 25% pelvic and 17% para-aortic involvement with deep penetration.[71] Before the 1988 FIGO staging system, the depth of invasion had been reported as none or inner, middle, or outer one-third of the myometrium. The 1988 FIGO staging system subdivided myometrial invasion into none or inner or outer half. Under that staging system, for patients with <50% myometrial invasion, it seems that invasion to less than versus greater than one-third is not a significant predictor of outcome.[80] In the current 2009 FIGO staging system, depth of invasion in stage I is divided into two categories: A (no or <50% myometrial invasion) and B (>50% invasion).

Lymphovascular Invasion

This is seen in about 15% of the cases of endometrial cancer. The GOG study found that lymphovascular invasion (LVI)–positive tumors were associated with a 27%, or fourfold, increase in the pelvic lymph nodal metastases, and a 19%, or sixfold, increase in para-aortic nodal metastases.[71] This translates into more frequent relapses, including vaginal recurrences,[81] and a poorer outcome.[82]

Lower Uterine Segment Involvement

The GOG study of surgical-pathologic spread patterns found a doubling of the incidence of pelvic nodal involvement from 8% to 16% and an increase in para-aortic nodal involvement from 4% to 14% when the tumor arose from or involved the isthmus.[71] There seems to be a high rate of lower uterine segment involvement in patients with HNPCC-associated endometrial cancer.[26]

Cervical Involvement

In the 1988 FIGO staging system, cervical involvement was divided into IIA when limited to endocervical glandular involvement and IIB when it involves the cervical stroma. According to the FIGO report, the 5-year survival for stage IIA was very good (89.9% for grade 1 and 83.7% for grade 2). In contrast, the corresponding figures for stage IIB were 81.2% and 76.9%, respectively.[28] This led to a change in the 2009 FIGO staging system, in which only cervical stromal invasion is considered stage II. Although the prognosis of the old stage IIA grades 1 and 2 approximated stage I rather than stage IIB, it is important to note that in the same FIGO annual report, patients with stage IIA grade 3 did not fare as well; their 5-year survival was 68.3%, which was worse than that for IC grade 3 (74.9%) and similar to that for IIB grade 3 (64.9%).

Peritoneal Cytology

Peritoneal fluid positive for malignant cells is found in 12% to 15% of all patients undergoing surgical staging. This is associated with 25% pelvic lymph node involvement and 19% para-aortic node involvement.[71] The data suggest a higher rate of positive cytology for patients undergoing laparoscopic-vaginal hysterectomy, in which there is manipulation of the uterine cavity, compared to total abdominal hysterectomy, in which there is no such manipulation.[84] The literature regarding the true impact of positive peritoneal cytology is mixed. One confounding factor, mainly in patients with no other risk factors, is whether all endometrial cancer cells that gained access to the peritoneal cavity are capable of independent growth. In a review of the literature, Wethington et al.[85] found that the overall incidence of positive washings is approximately 11%. Patients with grade 1 or 2 disease, no evidence of cervical involvement, <50% myometrial invasion, and no LVI were considered low risk. In patients with positive peritoneal cytology, the rate of recurrence for low-risk patients was 4.1% compared to 32% for those considered high risk ($p < .001$). This indicates the association of malignant cytology with other adverse prognostic factors. In the recent FIGO staging (2009), having positive peritoneal cytology is no longer considered stage IIIA.

Adnexal/Serosal Involvement

About 5% of patients with stage I and occult stage II disease have adnexal involvement.[71] This is associated with a fourfold increase in lymph node metastases; thus, pelvic lymph nodal positivity rises to 32% (as compared with 8% without adnexal spread), and para-aortic nodal involvement is seen in 20% (as opposed to only 5% in patients with no adnexal spread). The incidence of serosal involvement is less common. Jobsen et al.[86] reported on 46 patients with isolated adnexal involvement and 21 with isolated serosal involvement. There was no statistically significant difference in outcome between adnexal and serosal involvement. The 5-year disease-free survival was 76.4% versus 59.6% (p = ns), and the disease-specific survival was 76.3 % and 75.4%, respectively.

Pelvic and Para-Aortic Lymph Node Involvement

The pattern of lymphatic spread in endometrial cancer is different than that in cervical cancer. In endometrial cancer, a simultaneous spread to both pelvic and para-aortic nodes could occur, whereas in cervical cancer the spread to para-aortic nodes is almost always secondary to pelvic lymph node involvement. Overall, about 11% of patients with stage I and occult stage II endometrial cancer have pelvic nodal involvement. This increases to 25%, 30%, and 50% with deep myometrial invasion, adnexal involvement, and extrauterine spread, respectively.[71] Lymph node involvement is a major predictor of outcome; the 5-year disease-free survival rates drop to 65% to 70% in patients with pelvic lymph node involvement as their only risk factor.[87] The rate of para-aortic nodal metastases is about 5% of all patients with stage I and occult stage II disease. The biggest risk factor for para-aortic node involvement is the presence of pelvic nodal metastases; more than 30% of patients with pelvic nodal involvement have para-aortic disease. The 5-year disease-free survival rates drop to about 30% in this subpopulation.[87]

Molecular Prognostic Factors

The application of molecular biology tools to endometrial cancer has provided insights into the pathogenesis of the disease and may lead to early detection, as well as to development of novel therapeutic strategies.[88] Mutations of the tumor suppressor gene *p53* have been most extensively studied. There is a consistent observation linking the overexpression of p53 with advanced stage and poorer outcome.[89,90] Overexpression of HER-2 is also associated with more advanced disease and poor outcome.[65] PTEN mutation is associated with early-stage, nonmetastatic disease and more favorable survival outlook.[91] Data in the literature suggest a favorable survival outlook associated with microsatellite instability in endometrioid endometrial cancers.[92] As our knowledge regarding the molecular biology of endometrial cancer matures, risk stratification may soon be based on molecular alterations rather than pathologic variables.

SURGICAL MANAGEMENT

Surgery is the main treatment for endometrial cancer. It consists of simple hysterectomy, bilateral salpingo-oophorectomy (BSO), and inspection of the pelvic and abdominal cavities, with biopsy of any suspicious extrauterine lesions, accompanied in most cases by peritoneal washings. Surgical assessment of lymph nodes ranges from palpation, biopsy of suspicious nodes, to pelvic and para-aortic lymphadenectomy.

Hysterectomy

There are several approaches to simple hysterectomy, also known as extrafascial hysterectomy, but in the main it consists of removal of the entire uterine corpus and cervix without contiguous parametrial tissue. The pubocervical fascia is entered, and the ureters are not unroofed. *Total abdominal hysterectomy/BSO* (TAH/BSO) is the most prevalent and time-tested form of simple hysterectomy in endometrial cancer. It is an abdominal approach, usually via a vertical midline incision that allows thorough exploration of intra-abdominal and pelvic cavities. The main drawback of TAH/BSO is, that it is a laparotomy-based approach, in a group of patients with preexisting comorbidities such as obesity, hypertension, and diabetes. Therefore, it is not surprising that minimally invasive surgery, whether laparoscopically or robotically, has gained a great deal of acceptance in the surgical management of endometrial cancer. In *laparoscopic vaginal hysterectomy/BSO* (LAVH/BSO) the uterus is removed vaginally rather than abdominally. The benefit of using the laparoscope is to enable the surgeon to have a thorough intra-abdominal exploration and to perform BSO, which is difficult to accomplish with just a vaginal hysterectomy. The GOG completed a trial in which patients with clinical stage I to occult IIA uterine cancer were randomly assigned to laparoscopy (n = 1,696) or open laparotomy (n = 920), including hysterectomy, salpingo-oophorectomy, pelvic cytology, and pelvic and para-aortic lymphadenectomy. The main study endpoints were 6-week morbidity and mortality, hospital length of stay, conversion from laparoscopy to laparotomy, recurrence-free survival, site of recurrence, and patient-reported quality-of-life outcomes.[93] Laparoscopy had fewer moderate to severe postoperative adverse events than laparotomy (14% vs. 21%, respectively; $p < .0001$). Hospitalization of >2 days was significantly lower in laparoscopy than in laparotomy patients (52% vs. 94%, respectively; $p < .0001$). The conversion rate to laparotomy was 25.8%. With a median follow-up time of 59 months for 2,181 patients still alive, there were 309 recurrences (laparoscopy, 210, laparotomy, 99) and 350 deaths (laparoscopy, 229; laparotomy, 121). The estimated

5-year recurrence rate was 11.61% in the laparotomy arm and 13.68% for laparoscopy. The estimated 5-year overall survival rate was 89.8% for laparoscopy and 89.8% for laparotomy. The study demonstrated that surgical treatment of endometrial cancer can be performed laparoscopically with relatively small differences in recurrence rates (estimated difference at 3 years, 1.14%). These results, combined with improved quality of life and decreased complications associated with laparoscopy, are reassuring to patients and allow surgeons to reasonably suggest this method as a means to surgically treat and stage patients with presumed early-stage uterine cancers.[94] In recent years, *robotic-assisted hysterectomy*/BSO has emerged as an alternative minimally invasive surgery in endometrial cancer. It affords many advantages, including three-dimensional visualization, increased freedom of instrument movement, and enhanced ergonomics and surgeon comfort. The question of difference in cost is under debate debatable.[95] *Radical hysterectomy* is not routinely performed in endometrial cancer due to low incidence of parametrial involvement. There is no evidence to show that the cure rates are any better with such radical operations. The possible exception to this might be in patients with gross cervical involvement.[96]

Lymphadenectomy

The question of which patients need routine surgical lymph nodal staging and, if so, to what extent is a matter of great debate. The uncertainty about lymphadenectomy relates to whether the benefit from it is prognostic rather than therapeutic. Those who advocate for *no lymphadenectomy* and limit nodal assessment to inspection and removal of any enlarged/suspicious pelvic or para-aortic nodes cite the lack of documented survival advantages to lymphadenectomy. Furthermore, patients who have adverse pathologic features that increase the risk of microscopic lymph node metastasis are generally offered adjuvant pelvic radiation. Advocates for *full pelvic and para-aortic lymph node sampling* reason that surgical staging is the most accurate method to assess the extent of disease and that the sensitivity and specificity of palpation of lymph nodes are only 72% and 81%, respectively.[97] Lymphadenectomy in endometrial cancer includes removal of the fat pads surrounding the major vessels in the abdomen and pelvis without skeletonizing them. According to the GOG surgical guidelines, pelvic lymph nodes are to be removed from the distal one-half of the common iliac artery down to the circumflex iliac vein, and nodal tissue is to be removed anterior to the obturator nerve and surrounding the iliac arteries and vein. The para-aortic nodes include those overlying the vena cava, between the vena cava and aorta, and to the left of the aorta. The cephalad boundary of the para-aortic specimen is generally, but not limited to, the inferior mesenteric artery, and the distal boundary is the midpoint of the common iliac artery.[93] For the sampling to be adequate, five lymphatic stations need to be removed—para-aortic, common iliac, internal iliac, external iliac, and obturator—or total of 10 nodes. *Optional lymphadenectomy* is another approach, in which preoperative tumor grading with intraoperative assessment of depth of myometrial invasion, as well as histologic subtype, is frequently used to decide whether lymph node dissection is necessary at the time of hysterectomy. With such a policy, patients with grade 3 disease or serous or clear-cell histology and those with deep myometrial invasion on frozen section will undergo lymphadenectomy. Opponents of selective lymphadenectomy point out that depth of invasion on frozen section correlated with final pathology in only 67% of cases.[98] With regard to grade, preoperative FIGO grade 1 diagnosis correlates with final grade diagnosis in only 85% of cases of endometrial cancer.[32]

Despite the misgivings about optional or no lymphadenectomy, many surgeons have not embraced full lymphadenectomy. In a study of 27,063 women with unstaged endometrioid uterine cancer, lymphadenectomy was performed in only 30% of patients.[99] Two trials addressed the role of lymphadenectomy. The first was an Italian study[100] in which 514 eligible patients with preoperative FIGO stage I endometrial carcinoma were randomly assigned to undergo pelvic lymphadenectomy ($n = 264$) or no lymphadenectomy ($n = 250$). The median number of lymph nodes removed was 30 in the pelvic lymphadenectomy arm. Both early and late postoperative complications occurred more frequently in patients who had received pelvic systematic lymphadenectomy (81 patients in the lymphadenectomy arm and 34 patients in the no-lymphadenectomy arm; $p = .001$). Lymphadenectomy improved surgical staging, as statistically significantly more patients with lymph node metastases were found in the lymphadenectomy arm than in the no-lymphadenectomy arm (13.3% vs. 3.2%; $p < .001$). At a median follow-up of 49 months, the 5-year disease-free and overall survival rates in an intention-to-treat analysis were similar between arms (81.0% and 85.9% in the lymphadenectomy arm and 81.7% and 90.0% in the no-lymphadenectomy arm, respectively). In the second trial (Medical Research Council [MRC]/A Study in the Treatment of Endometrial Cancer [ASTEC]) patients with endometrial cancer believed preoperatively to be confined to the uterine corpus were first randomized to standard surgery consisting of hysterectomy-BSO, pelvic washing, and palpation of para-aortic nodes ($n = 704$) or to lymphadenectomy ($n = 704$). In the lymphadenectomy group patients underwent standard surgery plus systematic dissection of iliac and obturator nodes.[101] If the nodes could not be dissected, sampling of suspect nodes was recommended. Whether to dissect the para-aortic nodes was left to the discretion of the surgeon. After a median follow-up of 37 months, 191 women (88 standard surgery group, 103 lymphadenectomy group) had died, with an absolute difference in 5-year overall survival of 1% (95% CI = 4 to 6) and an absolute difference in 5-year recurrence-free survival of 6%. The conclusion from both trials was that pelvic lymphadenectomy significantly improved surgical staging, that is, it is a good prognosticator, but it did not improve disease-free or overall survival. As a trade-off between lymphadenectomy and no surgical assessment at all in patients with endometrial cancer, there has interest in adopting a sentinel lymph node approach similar to that in breast cancer (Fig. 70.5). In a recent report from MSKCC,

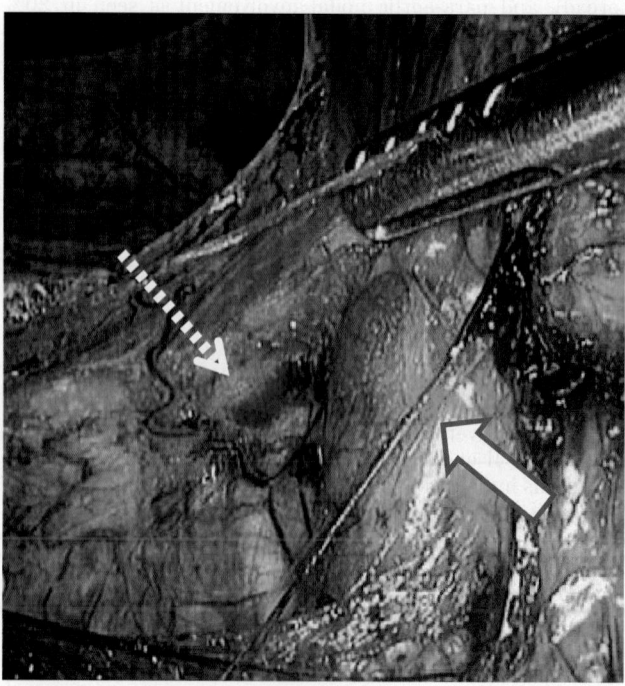

FIGURE 70.5. Sentinel lymph node. Solid arrow points to the blue dye in an external iliac node. Dashed arrow points to a lymphatic channel draining to the sentinel node.

266 patients with endometrial cancer underwent *sentinel lymph node (SLN) mapping*. At least one sentinel node was identified in 223 (84%) cases. Location of SLN was in the pelvis in 94% of cases, in the pelvis and para-aortic in 5%, and in the para-aortic in 1%. Positive nodes were diagnosed in 32 of 266 (12%) patients.[102] In a prospective trial from France, at least one SLN was detected in 111 of the 125 eligible patients. Of the 111 patients, 19 (17%) had pelvic-lymph-node metastases. Three patients had false-negative results (two had metastatic nodes in the contralateral pelvic area and one in the para-aortic area), giving a negative predictive value of 97% (95% CI = 91 to 99) and sensitivity of 84% (95% CI 62 to 95). SLN biopsy upstaged 10% of patients with low-risk and 15% of those with intermediate-risk endometrial cancer.[103] The results from these two studies suggest that SLN mapping is feasible and that adding SLN mapping to surgical staging procedures seems to increase the likelihood of detecting metastatic cancer cells in regional lymph nodes. Whether sentinel lymph node mapping will replace lymphadenectomy needs to be determined.

ROLE OF RADIATION

Radiation therapy plays a significant role in the management of endometrial cancer. It is often used as an adjuvant treatment after surgery (which will be discussed here) or as definitive treatment for patients who are medically inoperable or with local recurrence (which will be discussed later). In the past, most patients were treated with preoperative intracavitary brachytherapy with or without external-beam radiotherapy, followed by hysterectomy. This approach is not without its merit, especially in patients with gross cervical involvement. However, most patients nowadays undergo surgery first; then, depending on the prognostic features obtained from the pathology review, the need for radiotherapy is determined. In recent years there has been a plethora of data from prospective, randomized trials addressing several aspects of the management of endometrial cancer. However, unlike in cervical cancer, for which the data from the majority of the randomized trials pointed in the same direction, that is, chemoradiation is better than radiotherapy (RT) alone, the data in endometrial cancer are less conclusive. Therefore, it is important for radiation oncologists to be familiar with the methodology of these studies so that objections to the use of any form of adjuvant RT can be addressed with facts.

Role of RT in Stages I and II

Treatment options for patients with early-stage endometrial cancer after hysterectomy include observation, intravaginal RT, or pelvic RT. At MSKCC, intravaginal RT is the preferred approach for most patients because it provides the best therapeutic ratio. As the discussion will demonstrate, observation may have the best morbidity profile, but it does not provide the best therapeutic ratio because of the increased risk of local recurrence. Pelvic RT, on the other hand, although very effective in reducing recurrence, has a higher morbidity profile than intravaginal RT. The results of prospective, randomized trials will be discussed first, and then treatment recommendations based on risk factors will follow.

Results of RT Randomized Trials

There are six randomized trials regarding the role of adjuvant RT in early-stage endometrial cancer, mainly pertaining to endometrioid histology and conducted in the "modern" era.

Observation Versus Pelvic RT

Three randomized trials compared pelvic RT to observation in early-stage endometrial cancer. The first trial was the Postoperative Radiation Therapy in Endometrial Cancer (PORTEC) trial, which randomized 715 patients after total abdominal hysterectomy and bilateral salpingo-oophorectomy (TAH/BSO) to observation or pelvic RT.[104] Patients included were those with stage (FIGO 1988) IB grades 2 and 3 and those with IC grades 1 and 2. Those with IB grade 1 and those with IC grade 3 were excluded because it was felt that adjuvant RT was not indicated for the former and most physicians would not omit it for the latter. No lymph node sampling was done, and the dose of pelvic RT was 46 Gy at 2 Gy per fraction. At 5 years there was a statistically significant difference in the rates of vaginal/pelvic recurrence in favor of adjuvant pelvic RT (14% vs. 4%; $p < .001$). Overall survival, however, was not different between the two groups (81% RT vs. 85% surgery; $p = .31$), and the complications with pelvic RT were significantly higher (25% vs. 6%; $p < .0001$). In addition, many of the patients who relapsed locally after surgery alone were successfully salvaged with subsequent definitive RT. The second randomized trial was GOG 99. There were 190 patients with stage (FIGO 1988) IB to IIB (grades 1 to 3), who all underwent TAH/BSO, pelvic washing, and pelvic/para-aortic lymph node sampling and then were randomized to observation versus pelvic RT to a dose of 50.4 Gy at 1.8 Gy per fraction.[105] At 2 years there was a statistically significant difference in the rates of relapse in favor of the adjuvant pelvic RT arm (3% vs. 12%; $p = .007$). The 2-year estimated incidence of isolated vaginal/pelvic recurrence was 1.6% in the RT group and 7.4% in the surgery-alone group. There was, however, no significant difference in 4-year overall survival (92% RT vs. 86% with surgery alone; $p = .557$), but there were more complications with pelvic RT. The third trial consisted of two trials with separate randomizations consolidated into one intergroup trial. One trial was conducted by the MRC and the other by the National Cancer Institute of Canada (NCIC). Furthermore, the MRC ASTEC trial in itself consisted of two trials with separate randomizations designed to answer a surgical as well as a radiation question.[106] The surgical question was discussed earlier and regarded the need for lymphadenectomy in clinical localized endometrial cancer.[101] The radiation question was whether pelvic RT is needed. Intermediate- or high-risk early-stage patients were then randomized to observation or pelvic RT. Intermediate risk included stage (FIGO 1988) IA grade 3, IB grade 3, IC grades 1 and 2, and IIA grades 1 and 2. High risk included IC grade 3, IIA grade 3, and IA to IIA serous and clear-cell tumors. Patients who had positive pelvic nodes (stage IIIC) were allowed but not those with cervical stromal invasion (IIB). The pelvic RT was given to a total dose of 40 to 46 Gy in 20 to 25 fractions over 4- to 5 weeks. Intravaginal RT was permitted regardless of the pelvic RT randomization as long as it was the stated policy for the treating center to do so. The recommended dose was 4 Gy in two fractions prescribed to a depth of 0.5 cm treating the upper one-third of the vagina when using high dose rate and 15 Gy when using low dose rate. The NCIC had a similar design but with a few exceptions. Patients with stage IIA serous or clear-cell carcinoma were excluded, as were those with positive nodes. The dose of pelvic RT was 45 Gy in 25 fractions, and intravaginal brachytherapy was permitted in accordance with local practice.

Of the 905 patients (789 MRC and 116 NCIC) in the trial, 453 were randomized to observation and 452 to pelvic RT. The two arms were balanced except for more high-risk patients (113; 25%) in the observation arm than in the pelvic RT arm (89; 20%). There were 137 (32%) patients in the observation arm in whom nodes were removed, and 5 (4%) had positive nodes. In the pelvic RT arm, 159 (38%) had nodes removed, and 6 (4%) were positive. In the observation arm, 228 (51%) patients received intravaginal RT, 7 (2%) received pelvic and intravaginal RT, 3 (1%) received pelvic RT, and 3 (1%) were unknown. Only 212 (47%) received no form of adjuvant RT. Conversely, in the pelvic RT arm, 24 (5%) did not receive any adjuvant RT, 10 (2%) received intravaginal RT, and 2 (0.4%) were unknown. Combined intravaginal and pelvic RT was given to 232 (52%) patients, and only 184 (41%) received pelvic RT alone. The primary endpoint of this study was overall survival. With a median follow-up of 58 months, the 5-year overall survival was 84% in both arms ($p = .77$). The 5-year cumulative incidence for isolated vaginal or pelvic recurrence was 6.1% in the observation group and 3.2% in the pelvic RT group. This difference was statistically significant ($p = .2$) with a HR of 0.46 (95% CI = 0.24 to 0.89). The rate of any acute toxicity was 27% in the observation arm compared to 57% for pelvic RT. Similarly, late toxicity was more prevalent in the pelvic RT compared to observation (61% vs. 45%, respectively).

The triad of lack of overall survival advantage, increased toxicity, and high salvage rate of local recurrence for patients who are observed have led many to conclude that all forms of adjuvant RT, not simply pelvic RT, should be abandoned. The morbidity of pelvic RT and the validity of omitting adjuvant RT in favor of RT for salvage policy will discussed later in the chapter. With regard to overall survival it is considered the gold standard for primary endpoint in many randomized trials in oncology, but for early-stage endometrial cancer it is perhaps unattainable with adjuvant RT for two reasons. First, many of the patients have other, competing causes of death such as hypertension, diabetes, and obesity. In the PORTEC trial the 8-year actuarial rates of intercurrent death were 19.7% in the RT arm and 15.6% in the surgery-alone arm.[107] Endometrial cancer–related deaths in comparison were only 9.6% and 7.5%, respectively. Similarly, in the GOG 99 trial,[105] approximately half of the deaths were due to causes other than endometrial cancer or treatment (surgery alone, 19 of 36; RT, 15 of 30). This led the authors of GOG 99 to write, "With this number of intercurrent deaths in both arms, even if RT reduces the risk of endometrial cancer-related deaths, the size of this trial is not adequate to reliably detect an overall survival difference." That is why overall survival was not the primary endpoint in GOG99 but rather the disease-free interval, which was significantly different in favor of adjuvant pelvic RT over surgery alone.[105] Therefore, it is not unreasonable to conclude that neither PORTEC nor GOG 99 was large enough to conclusively show whether adjuvant pelvic RT affected overall survival. The second difficult hurdle for adjuvant RT to overcome when discussing overall survival has to do with its localized nature. In the MRC/NCIC trial, the rate of first vaginal/pelvic recurrence was reduced from 11.4% ($n = 37$ of 453) in the observation arm to 2.8% ($n = 13$ of 452) with pelvic RT. Adjuvant pelvic RT, however, did not affect distant spread; the rate of first distant spread was 8.1% ($n = 37$ of 453) in the observation compared to 9% ($n = 41$ of 452) in the pelvic RT arm.[106] One would expect adjuvant RT to make a difference in overall survival only when systemic therapy makes has an effect on the rate of distant spread. This is exactly the story learned from postoperative chest wall irradiation in breast cancer. Because pelvic RT significantly improved local control, albeit with increased toxicity, why not replace it with intravaginal RT rather than advocating observation for all early-stage endometrial cancer?

Observation Versus Intravaginal RT

In a trial reported by Sorbe et al.,[108] 645 patients with stage (FIGO 1988) IA to IB grades 1 and 2 endometrioid adenocarcinoma were randomized after surgery to observation ($n = 326$) or intravaginal RT ($n = 319$). Surgery consisted of TAH/BSO (laparoscopic surgery was allowed), pelvic washing, and removal of enlarged nodes. The dose and type of intravaginal RT varied among the six centers participating in this trial, but 347 of 645 patients were treated with high dose rate (HDR) to 18 Gy in six fractions. The proximal upper two-thirds of the vagina was treated with the dose prescribed to 0.5 cm from the surface of the cylinder. The rate of vaginal recurrence was 3.1% in the observation arm compared to 1.2% for the intravaginal RT arm ($p = .114$). The rate of pelvic recurrence was 0.9% in the observation arm and 0.3% in the treatment arm ($p = .326$). No significance difference was seen between the two arms in terms of overall survival. There was significantly more grade 1 vaginal toxicity with intravaginal RT (8.8% vs. 1.5%; $p = .00004$). There was no significant difference in gastrointestinal (GI) or genitourinary toxicity.

Pelvic RT Versus Intravaginal RT

In the PORTEC-2 trial, 427 patients were randomized to pelvic RT ($n = 214$) or intravaginal RT ($n = 213$). Patients enrolled were those with stage (FIGO 1988) IB grade 3 and >60 years old, IC grades 1 and 2 and >60 years old, and IIA grades 1 and 2 of all ages but with <50% myometrial invasion. During surgery patients underwent TAH/BSO, pelvic washing, and removal of suspicious pelvic or para-aortic lymph nodes. Routine lymphadenectomy was not performed. The dose of pelvic RT was 46 Gy given in 23 fractions. Intravaginal RT was delivered using a cylinder to treat the upper half of the vagina. The dose was prescribed to 0.5 cm from the surface of the cylinder. Three types of brachytherapy were used: HDR to 21 Gy in three fractions, low dose rate to 30 Gy at 0.5 to 0.7 Gy/hr, and medium dose rate to 28 Gy at 1 Gy/hr. With a median follow-up of 36 months, the 3-year vaginal recurrence rates were 0.9% in the intravaginal RT arm and 1.9% in the pelvic RT arm ($p = .97$). The pelvic recurrence was significantly different; the 3-year rate was 3.5% in the intravaginal RT arm compared to 0.6% in the pelvic RT arm ($p = .03$). The corresponding rates of isolated pelvic recurrence, however, were not significant: 0.6% versus 1.2%, respectively ($p = .54$). There was no significant difference in disease-free or overall survival between the two arms. The rate of grades 1 and 2 acute GI toxicity was 53% versus 12% in favor of intravaginal RT ($p < .001$). This trial showed that intravaginal RT alone is sufficient to control vaginal recurrence even in patients with intermediate- to high-risk features.[109]

In a more recent Swedish trial reported by Sorbe et al.[110] patients with stage (FIGO 1988) I endometrioid adenocarcinoma with at least one of the risk factors grade 3, ≥50% myometrial invasion, or DNA aneuploidy were randomized to adjuvant intravaginal RT (IVRT; $n = 263$) or pelvic and IVRT ($n = 264$). Lymphadenectomy was required. There was no difference in vaginal recurrence, which was 2.7% (7 of 263) in the IVRT-alone arm compared to 1.9% (5 of 264) in the combined arm ($p = .555$). Pelvic recurrence rate, however, was different: 5.3% in the IVRT arm compared to 0.4% in the pelvic plus IVRT arm ($p = .0006$). There was no significant difference in overall survival between the two arms (90% vs. 89%, respectively). The toxicity was significantly higher in the combined arm compared to IVRT alone.

Radiation Treatment Recommendations for Early-Stage Disease Based on Risk Factors

Based on the results of these trials in early-stage endometrial cancer, it is clear that pelvic RT is an excessive treatment for most of those patients. Therefore the treatment recommendations should be individualized based on risk factors. When deciding on whether to recommend observation, intravaginal RT, or pelvic RT, the risk of vaginal recurrence and pelvic recurrence should be assessed separately. With respect to vaginal recurrence, the data from randomized trials indicate that adjuvant intravaginal RT alone is sufficient to control potential microscopic disease in the vagina. The PORTEC-2 trial showed that intravaginal RT is as good as pelvic RT in controlling vaginal recurrence (0.9% vs. 1.9%, respectively; $p = .97$) despite the fact that patients included in this trial were at high risk for vaginal recurrence based on age ≥60 years old, deep myometrial invasion, or endocervical gland involvement.[109] The data from a recent Swedish randomized trial further confirmed that when it comes to vaginal control, IVRT alone is sufficient.[110] The vaginal recurrence was 2.9% in the IVRT arm compared to 1.9% ($p = .555$) in the pelvic plus intravaginal RT arm. How best to reduce pelvic recurrence is more controversial. For patients at low risk of having pelvic lymph node involvement, that is, endometrioid grade 1 or 2 with no or minimal myometrial invasion, neither lymphadenectomy nor pelvic RT is likely to be of significant benefit.[111] Those who are at higher risk of having lymph node involvement may need to have their lymph nodes surgically assessed to ensure that they are pathologically negative or receive pelvic RT to control potential microscopic disease. However, the two PORTEC trials, as well as the Swedish trial, showed that the risk of pelvic recurrence was only 2% to 6% even in the absence of lymphadenectomy.[104,109,110] This low rate of pelvic recurrence, coupled with the lack of survival advantage to lymphadenectomy and pelvic RT, raises the question of whether either approach is needed for the majority of patients with early-stage endometrial cancer. In the eyes of many, having LVI is almost indicative of nodal involvement. Cohn et al.[112] correlated LVI and the risk of positive pelvic nodes in 366 surgically staged patients. The rate of LVI was 25%, and the rate of positive pelvic nodes was 13%. Patients with LVI were significantly more likely to have nodal metastasis (35 of 92 vs. 11 of 274; $p < .001$). However, the influence of LVI on pelvic nodal metastasis was the strongest in patients with deep myometrial invasion and high grade. Data from MSKCC on 126 patients with endometrioid FIGO (1988) stages IB to IIB and LVI also showed that the mere presence of LVI should not be a trigger for giving pelvic RT, especially when patients had lymphadenectomy. Patients were divided into two groups: those from the old era, when treatment was often pelvic RT, and those from the modern era, when patients were more often treated with lymphadenectomy and intravaginal RT.[113] The rate of pelvic relapse for patients with LVI was 7% in the old era compared to 3% ($p = .3$) in the modern era.

No Myometrial Invasion, Grades 1 and 2

The risk of vaginal recurrence is almost negligible. Straughn et al.[114] reported no vaginal recurrence in 103 such patients treated with surgery alone. Pelvic lymph nodal positivity was ≤3%. The 5-year progression-free survival rate in this group was on the order of 95% to 98%. It is unlikely that postoperative pelvic or intravaginal RT would add anything to the final outcome, and therefore radiation is not routinely recommended to this group of patients.

No Myometrial Invasion, Grade 3

In GOG study 33, there were only eight patients with stage IA grade 3 disease, making it difficult to draw any meaningful conclusion.[87] There were no relapses in the three patients receiving postoperative radiation as compared with one failure in the five patients who received no postoperative therapy. Straughn et al.[114] reported on eight patients with stage IA grade 3 disease treated with surgery alone, with two of patients developing isolated vaginal recurrence. The risk of lymph node metastasis in this group of patients is not very high. At MSKCC, these patients are offered either intravaginal RT alone or observation.

Less Than 50% Myometrial Invasion, Grades 1 and 2

This group of patients constitutes the most common stage subgroup of all endometrial cancers. Straughn et al.[114] reported a 3% (9 of 296) risk of vaginal recurrence when surgery alone was done. In the surgery alone arm of the PORTEC-1 trial[115] the 5-year vaginal recurrence rate for patients with <50% myometrial invasion grade 2 was 5%. In a randomized trial reported by Sorbe et al.[108] the vaginal recurrence rate was 3.1% for those in the observation arm compared to 1.2% for those in the intravaginal RT arm ($p = .114$). The trial was designed to detect a difference of 1% versus 5% in the vaginal recurrence rate in the two groups. The data were not reported separately based on whether myometrial invasion was present or not, making it difficult to determine the true impact of intravaginal RT on the rate of vaginal recurrence in patients with myometrial invasion. Data from MSKCC on 233 patients with <50% myometrial invasion grade 1 or 2 showed a vaginal recurrence rate of only 1% using intravaginal RT alone.[116] In addition, Sorbe et al.[117] reported on 110 patients with IB grade 1 or 2 who were part of a prospective, randomized trial evaluating two different intravaginal RT doses; the rate of vaginal recurrence was 0.9%. The risk of pelvic recurrence was only 1.8%, even though lymphadenectomy was not required. This low rate of pelvic recurrence is similar to those reported by Straughn et al.[114] of 0.3% (1 of 296) and by Horowitz et al.[118] of 0% (0 of 62) in the setting of lymphadenectomy. This indicates that pelvic RT is of limited use, and therefore it seems reasonable to suggest that either observation or intravaginal RT is a reasonable option for patients with grade 1 or 2 and <50% myometrial invasion.

However, when deciding on whether adjuvant RT is needed, it is important to address two issues. First, older patients tend to have higher rates of relapse. In the study by Straughn et al.[114] 8 of the 10 vaginal/pelvic recurrences were in patients ≥60 years old. In the randomized trial by Sorbe et al.[108] comparing adjuvant intravaginal RT to observation, patients with vaginal recurrences were significantly ($p = .018$) older (mean age, 68.6 years) than patients without vaginal recurrences (mean, 62.6 years). Second, patients with LVI have a higher chance of vaginal recurrence, as demonstrated by Mariani et al.,[81] who reported on 508 patients with endometrial cancer limited to the corpus treated with surgery alone. The presence of LVI significantly increased the vaginal relapse rate from 3% to 7% ($p = .02$). The rate of vaginal relapse would have been even higher if patients without myometrial invasion (152 of 508) had been excluded because LVI is exceedingly rare in patients without myometrial invasion. At MSKCC, patients who are ≥60 years old or have LVI are recommended to have intravaginal RT.

Greater Than 50% Myometrial Invasion, Grade 3

Some advocate observation for patients with <50% myometrial invasion grade 3, yet the 5-year vaginal recurrence rate in PORTEC-1 was 14% for such patients treated with surgery alone compared to 0% for those treated with pelvic RT.[115] Perhaps a better choice for those patients is intravaginal RT. The incidence of positive pelvic lymph nodes at time of surgery in this subset of patients is not negligible. In the GOG 33 study the rate was 9% (5 of 54 of patients with inner one-third myometrial invasion), and in the study by Chi et al.[119] the rate was 7% (3 of 42) based on <50% myometrial invasion.[71] Yet the rate of pelvic recurrence, when the pelvic nodes are not surgically assessed, does not reflect these incidences. In the PORTEC-1 trial, none of the 37 patients with grade 3 disease and <50% myometrial invasion who were treated with TAH/BSO alone relapsed in the pelvis.[115] Horowitz et al.[118] ($n = 31$) and Fanning[120] ($n = 21$) reported no vaginal or pelvic recurrence in their series of patients with <50% myometrial invasion grade 3 treated with hysterectomy and lymphadenectomy followed by intravaginal RT. At MSKCC, intravaginal RT is recommended for this subset of patients irrespective of whether lymphadenectomy was performed.

Fifty Percent or Greater Myometrial Invasion, Grades 1 and 2

The risk of vaginal recurrence with surgery alone in this group of patients is not minimal. In the PORTEC-1 trial, the 5-year vaginal recurrence for patients with ≥50% myometrial invasion treated with surgery alone was 10% for those with grade 1 and 13% for grade 2. The corresponding 5-year vaginal recurrence rates for patients treated with pelvic RT were 1% and 2%, respectively.[115] Vaginal control with intravaginal RT alone in this group of patients is about 1.8% based on several series.[118,121–122,123] This highlights the fact with regard to vaginal control, pelvic RT is not superior to IVRT in patients with ≥50% myometrial invasion grade 1 or 2. With regard to pelvic control, in the PORTEC-1 trial[115] the 5-year pelvic recurrence for

TABLE 70.4 OUTCOME FOR ENDOMETRIAL CANCER WITH ≥50% MYOMETRIAL INVASION (GRADES 1 AND 2) AFTER LYMPHADENECTOMY AND INTRAVAGINAL RADIOTHERAPY ALONE

Author	Year	Number of Patients	Vaginal Recurrence	Pelvic Recurrence
Ng et al.[121]	2000	34	2.9% (1/34)	2.9% (1/34)
Horowitz et al.[118]	2002	41	2.4% (1/41)	4.8% (2/41)
Solhjem et al.[122]	2005	30	0% (0/30)	0% (0/30)
Long et al.[122]	2011	61	1.6% (1/61)	0% (0/61)
Total		**166**	**1.8% (3/166)**	**1.8% (3/166)**

TABLE 70.5 TREATMENT RECOMMENDATIONS AT MEMORIAL SLOAN-KETTERING CANCER CENTER FOR STAGE I AND II PATIENTS WITH ENDOMETRIOID ADENOCARCINOMA

Extent/Grade	1	2	3
No MI invasion	Observation	Observation	IVRT or observation[a]
<50% MI	IVRT or observation[a]	IVRT or observation[a]	IVRT
≥50% MI	IVRT	IVRT	IVRT or IMRT[b]
Endocervical gland	IVRT	IVRT	IVRT or IMRT[b]
CSI <50%	IVRT	IVRT	IVRT or IMRT[b]
CSI >50%	IMRT	IMRT	IMRT

CSI, cervical stromal invasion; IMRT, intensity-modulated radiotherapy; IVRT, intravaginal radiotherapy; MI, myometrial invasion.

[a]Observation is offered to patients <60 years old and without lymph node invasion.

[b]IMRT if high to intermediate risk.

patients with ≥50% myometrial invasion treated with surgery alone was 2% for grade 1 and 6% for grade 2. The data from the PORTEC-2 trial[109] and the Swedish trial,[110] in which patients with ≥50% myometrial invasion grade 1 or 2 were included, indicate that the omission of pelvic RT increased the risk of pelvic recurrence. In PORTEC-2 trial[109] the 3-year rate was 3.5% in the intravaginal RT arm compared to 0.6% in the pelvic RT arm ($p = .03$). In the Swedish trial[110] the pelvic recurrence rate was 5.3% in the IVRT arm compared to 0.4% in the pelvic plus intravaginal RT arm ($p = .0006$). The risk of pelvic recurrence for this subset of patients with lymphadenectomy is about 1.8% on average[118,121–122,123] from data in the literature (Table 70.4). At MSKCC, most of these patients undergo lymphadenectomy or SLN mapping, and if the nodes are pathologically negative, they undergo intravaginal RT alone.

Fifty Percent or Greater Myometrial Invasion and Grade 3

In the study by Chi et al.[119] the risk of finding positive lymph nodes in this group of patients was 28% (8 of 29). Such patients were not enrolled in the PORTEC trials because it was felt that omitting pelvic RT when lymphadenectomy was not performed could not be justified. In the registry study reported by Creutzberg et al.[115] 99 patients with ≥50% myometrial invasion grade 3 were treated with postoperative pelvic RT. The 5-year rate of vaginal recurrence was 5%, that of pelvic recurrence was 8%, and that of distant relapse was 31%. Very few investigators would recommend surgery alone for these patients. In fact an argument could be made that pelvic RT might be needed even after a negative lymphadenectomy, especially for older patients and those with LVI. In GOG 99 trial, factors associated with an increased recurrence rate (25% at 5 years) were identified using proportional hazards regression modeling of historical data from GOG 33.[105] These factors were (a) increasing age, (b) moderate to poorly differentiated tumor grade, (c) presence of lymphovascular invasion, and (d) outer one-third myometrial invasion. From the results of that analysis a subgroup of patients with high intermediate risk (HIR) was defined as follows: (a) at least 70 years of age with only one of the other risk factors, (b) at least 50 years of age with any two of the other risk factors, or (c) any age with all three of the other risk factors. Those on the RT arm demonstrated a somewhat lower overall death rate when compared to those on the observation arm (relative hazard [RH] = 0.73, 90% CI = 0.43 to 1.26) in the HIR subgroup. AT MSKCC, patients with deep myometrial invasion grade 3 who are high to intermediate risk per GOG 99 would be offered postoperative pelvic RT even in the setting of negative lymphadenectomy. If they are not HIR, then intravaginal RT could be considered, but only in the setting of adequate lymphadenectomy, that is, sampling the obturator, external iliacs, internal iliacs, common iliacs, and para-aortic lymph node stations and a minimum of 10 nodes.

Cervical Involvement

It is important to recognize the distinction between gross and occult cervical involvement. Gross involvement increases the risk of parametrial extension as well as spread to pelvic lymph nodes in a fashion similar to primary cervical cancer. Patients with gross cervical involvement from endometrial cancer could undergo radical hysterectomy and pelvic lymph node dissection or preoperative radiation including pelvic radiation and intracavitary brachytherapy followed by simple hysterectomy. For occult cervical involvement, the treatment often consists of simple hysterectomy with or without lymphadenectomy and adjuvant radiation. The type of radiation most often used is pelvic RT and intravaginal RT. Pitson et al[124] reported on 120 patients treated with such a combination. The 5-year disease-free survival rate was 68% and the rate of pelvic relapse was 5.8% (7 of 120).

There are also emerging data on the role of intravaginal RT alone in some patients with occult cervical involvement who also had surgical lymph node staging. The average rate of vaginal recurrence was 1.47% (1 of 68), and pelvic recurrence was also 1.47%. It is important to note that in these series patients treated with intravaginal RT alone were highly selected.[118,125–126,127] Patients with endocervical glandular involvement are no longer considered stage II in the new FIGO staging system. In PORTEC-2 trial patients with glandular cervical involvement were randomized to pelvic RT or intravaginal RT.[109] At MSKCC patients with endocervical glandular involvement are treated with IVRT alone, especially if there are no other adverse features or if they had lymphadenectomy. For patients with cervical stromal invasion grade 1 and 2 and the depth of cervical stromal invasion is <50%, intravaginal RT could be offered if they underwent adequate lymphadenectomy. For those with grade 3 or deep cervical stromal invasion, pelvic RT is recommended irrespective of lymphadenectomy. Table 70.5 shows overall treatment recommendations for early-stage endometrioid adenocarcinoma at MSKCC.

Role of RT in Stage III

The outcome of patients with *isolated adnexal involvement* treated with pelvic RT is reasonably good. Connell et al.[128] reported on 12 patients treated with postoperative pelvic radiation with a 5-year disease-free survival of 70.9%. The weighted average of 5-year disease-free and overall survival rates from literature review in that study was 78.6% and 67.1%, respectively. Jabson et al.[86] reported 5-year disease-free and disease specific survival of 76.4% and 76.3%, respectively, in 46 patients with isolated adnexal involvement treated with postoperative RT. The rate of local/regional recurrence was 2.2% (1 of 46) and that of distant relapse was 26.1% (12 of 46). In the same report, the outcome of patients with isolated serosal involvement ($n = 21$) was somewhat similar: the 5-year disease-free and disease-specific survival rates were 59.6% and 75.4.3%, respectively. The rate of local/regional recurrence was 14.3% (3 of 21) and that of distant relapse was 33.3% (7 of 21). If *pelvic node involvement* (IIIC) is the only major risk factor, treatment with postoperative pelvic radiotherapy can yield a 60% to 72% long-term survival rate in these patients.[87] Patients with stage IIIC disease, by virtue of *para-aortic node involvement,* represent a particularly high-risk group. After surgery, these patients are generally treated with extended-field radiation to encompass the pelvis and the para-aortic regions. With this aggressive approach, several investigators reported 30% to 40% survival rates in small patient populations.[87] The question of whether it is safe to omit radiation even after adequate surgical lymph node staging in patients with stage IIIC endometrial cancer was addressed in a study from the Mayo Clinic. Mariani et al.[129] reported on 122 patients with node-positive disease; at 5 years the risk of pelvic recurrence was 57% after inadequate lymph node dissection and/or no RT compared to 10% with adequate lymph node dissection (>10 pelvic nodes and ≥5 para-aortic nodes) and RT. This difference was statistically significant on univariate ($p < .001$) and multivariate analysis ($p = .03$) indicating the need for postoperative radiation even after adequate surgical staging.

The recognition that a significant number of patients with stage III disease fail in the abdomen has prompted a number of investigators to evaluate whole-abdomen irradiation (WAI) in these patients. The GOG did a pilot study (GOG study 94) on patients with maximally debulked stages III and IV disease using whole-abdomen radiotherapy to a total dose of 30 Gy at 1.5 Gy per fraction followed by a pelvic boost for an additional 19.8 Gy at 1.8 Gy per fraction.[130] The 3-year disease-free and overall survival rates for the 58 patients with stage III typical adenocarcinoma were both 34.5%, and for stage IV the corresponding rates were 10.4% and 21.1%, respectively.

ROLE OF SYSTEMIC THERAPY

Hormonal therapy has been used in the treatment of recurrent/advanced endometrial cancer for many years. Agents used include megestrol acetate (Megace), medroxyprogesterone acetate (Provera), and to a lesser extent tamoxifen.[131–133] The response rate rages from 9% to 33%, with an overall survival of 6 to 14 months. In GOG 107, doxorubicin was compared to doxorubicin and cisplatin.[134] The response rate was 42% vs. 25% ($p = .004$), and the progression-free interval was 5.7 versus 3.8 months ($p = .014$) in favor of combination chemotherapy. However, this did not translate into overall survival advantage (9 vs. 9.2 months). In GOG 177 trial[135] doxorubicin/cisplatin was compared doxorubicin/cisplatin/paclitaxel. The three-drug regimen was superior in terms of response rate (57% vs. 34%, $p < .01$), progression-free interval (8.3 vs. 5.3 months, $p < .01$), and survival (15.3 vs. 12.3 months, $p = .037$).

With the widespread use of chemotherapy in the recurrent/advanced setting, its use in the adjuvant setting has also started to increase and to challenge the role of adjuvant RT. There are several randomized trials addressing the role of adjuvant chemotherapy in advanced endometrial cancer.

Chemotherapy Versus RT Trials

There are three randomized trials comparing adjuvant chemotherapy to radiation. The Japanese Gynecology Oncology Group (JGOG) trial randomized 385 patients with stage (FIGO 1988) IC to III (25% with stage III) endometrial cancer to pelvic radiation (193 patients) or to chemotherapy (192 patients).[136] The surgery was hysterectomy with optional lymphadenectomy. The dose of pelvic RT was 45 to 50 Gy using open anteroposterior/posteroanterior (AP/PA) fields. Chemotherapy consisted of cyclophosphamide (333 mg/m^2), cisplatin (50 mg/m^2), and doxorubicin (40 mg/m^2) every 4 weeks for three cycles or more. There was no significant difference in progression-free ($p = .726$) or overall survival rate ($p = .462$) between the two groups. A trial from Italy had a similar design, in which 340 patients with stage (FIGO 1988) IC grade 3, stage II grade 3, and stage III (two-thirds of patients) were randomized to radiation or to chemotherapy.[137] With a median follow-up of 95.5 months, the 5-year disease-free survival rate was 63% in both arms ($p = .44$) and the 5-year overall survival rate was 69% in the radiation arm and 66% in the chemotherapy arm ($p = .77$). Again there was no significant difference in outcome despite using five cycles of Cytoxan, cisplatin, and doxorubicin. In GOG 122, 396 patients with stage (FIGO 1988) III to IV disease were randomized to whole-abdomen radiation ($n = 202$) versus doxorubicin/cisplatin ($n = 194$) for eight cycles. Progression-free survival was the primary endpoint of this study. With a median follow-up of 74 months, there was significant improvement in both progression-free (50% vs. 38%; $p = .007$) and overall survival rate (55% vs. 42%; $p = .004$), respectively, in favor of chemotherapy. However, before concluding that chemotherapy alone is the answer, a closer examination of the data is warranted. The overall absolute rate of relapse was 54% in the radiation arm compared to 50% in the chemotherapy arm, a small difference, if any, and yet the corresponding 5-year progression-free survival rates were 38% and 50% ($p = .007$), respectively. The reason for the discrepancy is that in this study, there was stage imbalance, in which there were more stage IIIA patients in the RT arm (28.2%) than in the chemotherapy arm (18%). Conversely, there were more patients with stage IIIC disease in the chemotherapy arm (51.5%) than in the RT arm (44.6%). Therefore, the 5-year disease-free survival rate for the chemotherapy arm was increased from 42% to 50%, which became significantly different than the RT arm (50 vs. 38%, $p = .007$) rather than 42% versus 38%, which is not likely to be significant. The 5-year overall survival rate in the chemotherapy arm was 55% compared to 42% for the RT arm ($p = .004$). What are we to make of the significant difference in overall survival? There were 15 deaths unrelated to endometrial cancer or protocol treatment in the radiation arm compared to only to 6 in the chemotherapy arm, raising a question about whether the two arms of the study were truly balanced, especially since no stratification was performed in that trial.[138] The results of GOG 122 have led to the adoption of adjuvant chemotherapy as the preferred treatment for stage III endometrial cancer. It is important to note, however, that GOG 122, JGOG, and the Italian study all showed no significant difference in the patterns of relapse between RT and chemotherapy. If one were to use the unadjusted progression-free survival from GOG 122, then all three randomized trials failed to show that adjuvant chemotherapy is superior to adjuvant RT.

Chemoradiation Versus RT Trials

In a trial from Finland,[139] 156 patients with stage (FIGO 1988) IA or IB grade 3 ($n = 28$) or stage IC to IIIA grade 1 to 3 ($n = 128$) were postoperatively randomized to receive radiotherapy (56 Gy) only ($n = 72$) or radiotherapy combined with three cycles of cisplatin (50 mg/m^2), epirubicin (60 mg/m^2), and cyclophosphamide (500 mg/m^2) chemotherapy ($n = 84$). The disease-specific overall 5-year survival was 84.7% in the RT arm versus 82.1% in the chemoradiation arm ($p = 0.148$). Hogberg et al.[140] reported on two trials (Mario Negri Gynecologic Oncology Group [MaNGO] and Nordic Society of Gynecological Oncology [NSGO]/European Organisation for Research and Treatment of Cancer [EORTC]) combined in one report. In the MaNGO trial there were 157 patients (two-thirds were stage III); 76 were randomized to postoperative pelvic RT (45 Gy) and 80 to chemotherapy followed by pelvic RT. The chemotherapy consisted of three cycles of doxorubicin (60 mg/m^2) and cisplatin (50 mg/m^2). The 5-year progression-free survival (PFS) was 61% in the RT group compared to 74% for the chemoradiation group, but that difference was not significant ($p = .1$). The 5-year overall survival (OS) was also not significant (73% vs. 78%, respectively; $p = .41$). In the NSGO/EORTC trial 383 patients were randomized to RT ($n = 191$) versus RT and chemotherapy ($n = 187$). The type of chemotherapy varied, and only a handful

TABLE 70.6 EFFECT OF ADJUVANT CHEMOTHERAPY ON OUTCOME IN HIGH-RISK ENDOMETRIAL CANCER

	JGOG	Italian	GOG 122	Finland	NSGO	MaNGO
Relapse	↔	↔	↔	↔	↔	↔
PFS	↔	↔	↔ Unadjusted ↑ Adjusted	↔	↑	↔
OS	↔	↔	↑, OS not primary endpoint	↔	↔	↔

The Japanese Gynecology Oncology Group (JGOG), the Italian trial, and Gynecologic Oncology Group (GOG) 122 compared chemotherapy to radiotherapy. The Finland trial, Nordic Society of Gynecological Oncology (NSGO), and Mario Negri Gynecologic Oncology Group (MaNGO) compared chemotherapy/radiotherapy to radiotherapy.
OS, overall survival; PFS, progression-free survival.
↔, chemotherapy equivalent to radiotherapy; ↑, chemotherapy better than radiotherapy.

of patients were stage III. The 5-year PFS was better for the chemoradiation arm (79% vs. 72% for RT; $p = .04$), but OS was not significantly better (83% vs. 76%, respectively; $p = .1$). Greven et al.[141] reported the results of RTOG 9708 phase II study on 44 patients with stages (FIGO 1988) I to III endometrial cancer who were treated with pelvic radiation and intravaginal RT given concurrently with cisplatin 50 mg/m^2 on days 1 and 28 of radiation followed by four cycles of cisplatin (50 mg/m^2) and Taxol (175 mg/m^2). The 4-year disease-free and overall survival rates for those with stage III disease (66% of patients) were 72% and 77%, respectively.

It is clear from the foregoing discussion that the role of adjuvant chemotherapy is gaining ground and that at least the results are equivalent to those with adjuvant RT (Table 70.6). However, adjuvant chemotherapy should not be promoted at the expense of RT, because the rate of relapse is still high even with chemotherapy.[142,143] The GOG is comparing chemoradiation (similar to RTOG 9708) to six cycles of carboplatin/paclitaxel in patients with stage III disease. PORTEC 3 is a randomized trial comparing chemoradiation to RT alone. Until the results of these trials are available, the decision on whether to give chemoradiation or chemotherapy alone should be based on risk factors.

Systemic Therapy Recommendations Based on Risk Factors

Isolated Positive Peritoneal Cytology

In the 2009 FIGO staging system, having positive peritoneal cytology is no longer considered stage IIIA. The true benefits of treatment when adverse features such as high grade or deep invasion are lacking are debatable. Eltabbakh et al.[144] reported on 29 patients with FIGO grade 1 or 2 and <50% myometrial invasion who were treated with intravaginal brachytherapy and megestrol acetate (Megace). None of the patients relapsed or died from their disease. Megace was given for 1 year, and at the end of therapy, 24 patients underwent second-look laparoscopy and peritoneal cytology. In 23 patients, the cytology was negative, and the remaining patient, with persistent positive cytology, received an additional year of Megace, after which cytology was confirmed to be negative. At MSKCC, we generally recommend intravaginal RT and Megace for such patients.

Early-Stage Serous and Clear-Cell Cancer

Serous cancer and to a lesser extent clear-cell cancer tend to spread in a fashion similar to ovarian cancer, with a high propensity for upper abdominal relapse. Therefore, it is important to perform comprehensive surgical staging because of the high rate of surgical up-staging. With such pattern of spread, it is not surprising that whole-abdomen radiation has been extensively studied in this group of patients. Lim et al.[145] reported on 78 patients with stages I to IIIA papillary serous carcinoma: 58 were treated with whole-abdomen radiation and 20 were not. The corresponding 5-year disease-specific survival rates were 74.9% and 41.3%, respectively ($p = .04$). The data from GOG 94 were less impressive.[146] The 5-year progression-free survival for stages (FIGO 1988) I and II papillary serous cancer was 38.1% and for clear-cell carcinomas was 53.9%. Alektiar et al.[147] reported on 25 patients with stages I and II serous endometrial cancer who underwent surgical staging, intravaginal RT, and six cycles of carboplatin/paclitaxel. With a median follow-up of 30 months, the 5-year progression-free and overall survival rates were 88%. None of the patients developed vaginal recurrence. In a recent update on a larger number of patients ($n = 41$) with a median follow-up time of 58 months, the 5-year disease-free and overall survival rates were 85% and 90%, respectively.[148] The 5-year actuarial recurrence rates were 9% in the pelvis, 5% in the para-aortic nodes, and 10% at distant sites. None of the patients developed vaginal recurrence. At MSKCC patients with early-stage disease who are surgically staged are being treated with intravaginal RT with concurrent carboplatin/paclitaxel.

Early-Stage High-Risk Endometrioid Adenocarcinoma

The 5-year rate of distant metastasis from the PORTEC registry study of patients with grade 3 and deep invasion was 31% despite the use of postoperative pelvic RT.[115] The rate of relapse was also 28.9% (90% distant) in a study from MSKCC despite an aggressive surgical and adjuvant RT approach.[123] Thus it is not surprising that there is an inclination toward recommending adjuvant chemotherapy in addition to RT in this group of patients. The GOG is conducting a randomized trial for patients with high to intermediate risk, as well as serous and clear-cell carcinoma, in which patients are randomized to pelvic RT versus intravaginal RT and three cycles of carboplatin/paclitaxel.

Stage IIIA

The results of postoperative external-beam RT in patients with isolated adnexal or serosal involvement are generally good. However, the rate of distant relapse is still 26% to 33%, indicating the need for adjuvant systemic therapy.[86] At MSKCC, we recommend concurrent chemoradiation followed by carboplatin/Taxol in a similar fashion to the RTOG 9708. Although the results of isolated involvement with postoperative RT are good, patients with more than one site of involvement do worse. Jobson et al.[149] reported on 141 patients with IIIA endometrioid adenocarcinoma (patients with isolated positive peritoneal cytology were excluded) treated with postoperative RT. The risk of abdominal relapse was 12.4% (11 of 89) for patients with one site of involvement compared to 36.5% (19 of 52) for more than one site ($p < .001$). Distant metastasis rate was 23.9% (21 of 89) compared to 34.6% (18 of 52), respectively. The 5-year disease-specific survival (DSS) was 70.4% for one involved site compared to 43.3% for more than one ($p = .001$). On multivariate analysis, grade 3 (HR, 2.5; $p = .045$) and more than one site involvement (HR, 2.2; $p = .012$) were independent predictors of poor DSS. In the ongoing debate on whether chemotherapy alone is better than chemoradiation in patients with stage III, it is in this group of patients with multiple sites of involvement and grade 3/aggressive histology in which chemotherapy alone might be a better choice.

Stage IIIC

The outcome of patients with isolated lymph node involvement (especially pelvic nodes), treated with postoperative pelvic RT is relatively good. At MSKCC, we recommend chemoradiation followed by carboplatin/paclitaxel to try to reduce the risk of recurrence even further. Similar to patients with IIIA, having more than one site of involvement has been shown to be a predictor of poor outcome.[150] In a recent SEER review, Garg et al.[151] showed that for patients with stage IIIC disease (n = 2,559), the 5-year disease-specific survival was 67%, which dropped to ~43% when extranodal involvement (i.e., positive washing, adnexa/serosal, and vaginal/parametrial involvement) was present ($p < .001$). Again, perhaps in this subset of patients with stage IIIC chemotherapy alone might be better.

RADIATION THERAPY TECHNIQUES

Intravaginal Radiation

The purpose of this treatment modality is to deliver the highest dose of radiation to the vaginal mucosa while limiting the dose to the surrounding normal structures such as the bladder, rectum, and small intestines. HDR brachytherapy using ^{192}Ir sources is the preferred method of delivering intravaginal RT. The type of applicator used is generally a cylinder. The treatment is given on an outpatient basis without the need for anesthesia and without the radiation exposure to medical personnel. At MSKCC, patients start their treatment 4 to 6 weeks postoperatively, depending on the vaginal cuff healing. It takes longer for the vaginal cuff to heal after LAVH/BSO and robotic hysterectomy than after TAH/BSO. The treatment is given in three fractions of 7 Gy to a total dose of 21 Gy. The interval between each fraction is 1 to 2 weeks. The dose is prescribed to 0.5-cm depth from the mucosal surface (Fig. 70.6). The treatment is usually delivered using a 3-cm-diameter cylinder to treat a 4- to 7-cm length of the vagina, depending on depth of invasion and tumor grade. For patients with grade 3, serous or clear-cell carcinoma, the length of vagina treated is generally 7 cm (assuming an average length of vagina after simple hysterectomy of about 10 cm). This is done to account for potential submucosal extension that may lead to relapse in the distal periurethral region with these aggressive histologies. For patients with grade 1 or 2 endometrioid adenocarcinoma, the treated vaginal length increases from 4 cm if myometrial invasion is <50%, to 5 cm for >50% myometrial invasion, and to 6 cm for cervical involvement. Occasionally, the dose per fraction is lowered to 6 Gy instead of 7 Gy if the diameter of the cylinder is <3 cm. This is usually done to avoid a very high dose of radiation to the vaginal mucosa. The dose per fraction is also lowered to 4 to 5 Gy when pelvic radiation is added. Intravaginal RT could be delivered with low–dose-rate ^{137}Cs sources, which requires admission to the hospital for a few days. The dose is usually 60 Gy prescribed to the vaginal mucosa or 30 to 35 Gy prescribed to a 0.5-cm depth from the vaginal mucosa.

External-Beam Radiation

Pelvic Radiation

Conventional Pelvic RT

At the time of simulation, the small bowel is opacified using oral contrast, a vaginal marker is used to define the vaginal cuff, and the rectum is opacified with barium or CT-compatible contrasts. Patients are usually placed in the prone position to displace the small intestines from the radiation field. The target volume consists of the pelvic lymph nodes, including obturator, external, internal, and lower common iliac groups, and the proximal two-thirds of the vagina. The presacral nodes are not included unless patients have gross cervical involvement. High-energy linear accelerators (15 MV) are preferred because of their sparing of the skin and subcutaneous tissue. The ideal beam arrangement with conventional radiation is the four-field pelvic-box technique to reduce the dose to the small intestines and to some extent the bladder and rectum. For AP/PA fields, the superior border is L5-S1, the inferior border is the bottom of the obturator foramina, and the lateral border is 2 cm beyond the widest point of the inlet of the true bony pelvis. For lateral fields, the anterior border is in front of the pubis symphysis and the posterior border at least at S2-3. The superior and inferior borders are the same for the AP/PA fields. All fields are treated daily to a dose of 1.8 Gy. A total dose of 50.4 Gy is generally used when pelvic radiation is used alone or 45 Gy when combined with intravaginal brachytherapy.

Intensity-Modulated RT

At MSKCC, postoperative intensity-modulated RT (IMRT) is used for most patients with endometrial cancer who need pelvic RT (Fig. 70.7). At the time of simulation patients are placed in the supine position and immobilized using Aquaplast. Oral and rectal contrasts are used to better visualize the small and large intestines. In addition, contrast is inserted in the vaginal cuff to better visualize the upper vagina. Because pelvic lymph nodes are poorly visualized by CT when normal, they should be defined by encompassing the contrast-enhanced blood vessels. Taylor et al.[152] found that a modified 7-mm margin around contrast-enhanced vessels offers a good surrogate target for pelvic lymph nodes. Small et al.[153] reported on consensus guidelines for delineation of clinical target volume for intensity-modulated pelvic radiotherapy in postoperative treatment of endometrial

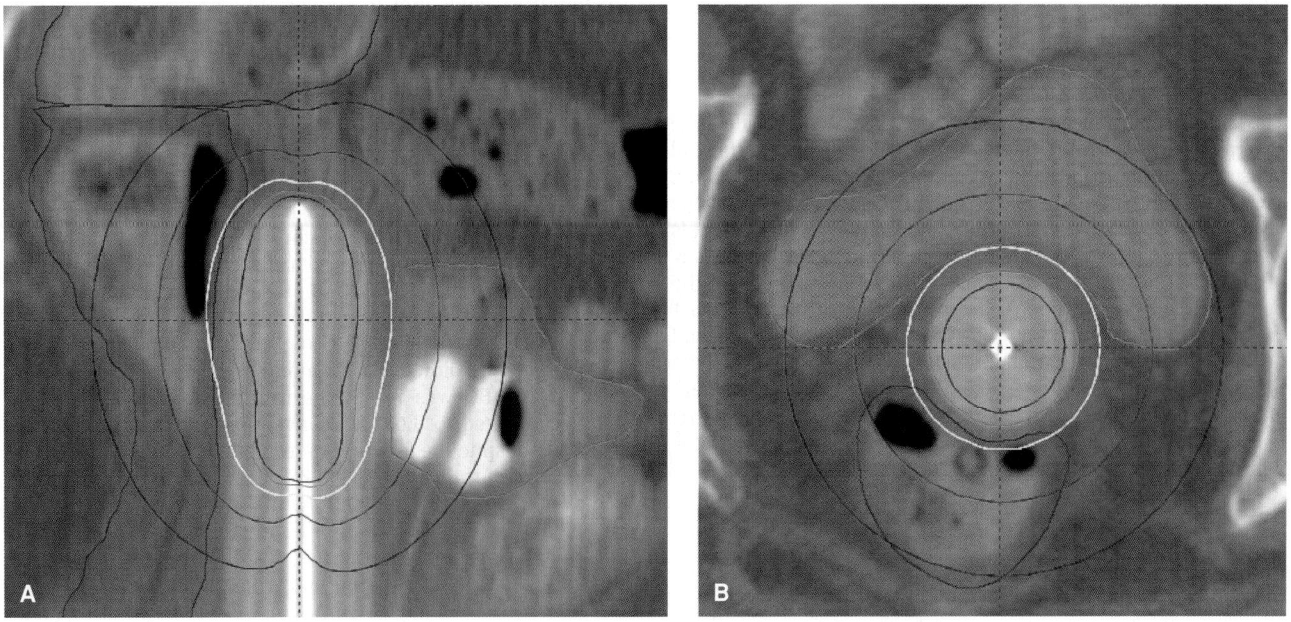

FIGURE 70.6. Dose distribution with intravaginal radiation therapy (prescription dose 7 Gy in solid yellow). **A:** Sagittal view. **B:** Axial view.

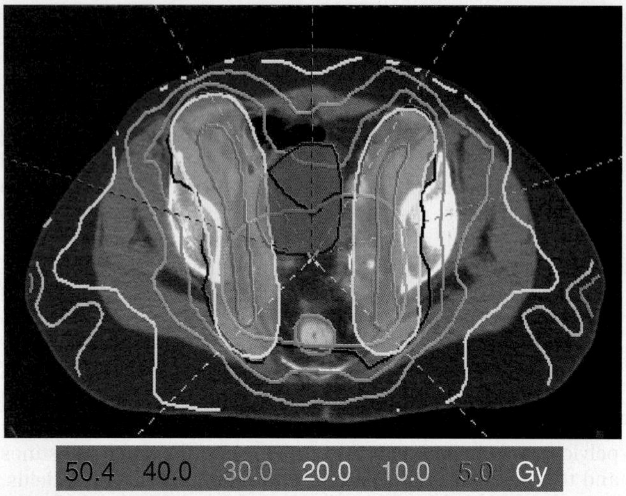

FIGURE 70.7. Pelvic intensity-modulated radiation therapy dose distribution. Outlined iliac vessels are shown in pink and nodal planning target volume in yellow.

and cervical cancer. A modified 7-mm margin (excluding bowel and muscles) is recommended around the iliac vessels to create nodal clinical target volume (CTV). To create nodal planning target volume (PTV), an additional expansion of 7 mm all around nodal CTV is generally recommended. At MSKCC vaginal PTV is created by outlining the contrast enhanced vaginal cuff and adding a 3-cm margin to account for the impact of bladder and rectal filling, as well as of vaginal motion.[154]

Extended Field

This technique is mainly used for patients with documented positive para-aortic nodes. CT simulation is crucial when treating extended fields for accurate delineation of the kidneys, small bowel, and liver in addition to nodal target. The latter should include, in addition to the pelvic nodes, the pericaval, interaortocaval and para-aortic areas, defined by contrast-enhanced blood vessels. The preferred approach is the four-field box technique rather than AP/PA in order to lower the dose to the small intestines. However, attention should be paid to the dose that the kidneys might receive with the four-field arrangement. The lower border is the same as in pelvic radiation, but the upper border is extended usually to the T12-L1 interspace. The typical dose is 45.0 Gy at 1.8 Gy or 1.5 Gy if patients develop acute gastrointestinal toxicity. At MSKCC, IMRT is also the preferred choice for extended-field radiation.

Whole-Abdomen Radiation

The target is the whole peritoneal cavity, which requires adequate coverage of the diaphragm with adequate margin during all phases of normal respiration with minimal to no liver shielding. The standard approach is AP/PA open fields with five half value layer kidney blocks placed over the PA field only (if the patient is lying supine) from the start of the treatment. The dose is usually 30.0 Gy at 1.5 Gy per fraction, followed by 19.8-Gy boost to the pelvis at 1.8 Gy per fraction. The upper border is usually placed 1 cm above the diaphragm, and the lateral borders should extend beyond the peritoneal reflections. The lower border is usually at the bottom of the obturator foramen. The para-aortic region generally receives a cone down to a total dose of 45 Gy and the pelvis to 50 Gy. IMRT may allow higher and more uniform doses to be delivered with potentially less toxicity.[155,156]

COMPLICATIONS OF TREATMENT

Surgery

In PORTEC-1 trial[104] the rate of complications in the surgery-alone arm was very low (6%). Surgical toxicity data were generally collected within 30 days of surgery, that is, before patients were enrolled in the trial. Therefore it is important to assess surgical toxicity from trials addressing a surgical question. In the GOG LAP2 trial comparing laparotomy to laproscopy[93] the rate of intraoperative complications was 8% versus 10%, respectively ($p = .106$). More important, the rate of postoperative (within 6 weeks of surgery) grade 2 or greater complications was 21% for laparotomy versus 14% for laparoscopy ($p < .001$). In the Italian randomized trial comparing hysterectomy to hysterectomy and lymphadenectomy, both early and late postoperative complications occurred significantly more frequently in the lymphadenectomy patients (81 of 264; 30.6%) than for hysterectomy alone (34 of 250, 13.6%; $p = .001$). Most of the difference in morbidity was due to lymphocysts and lymphedema, which occurred in 35 patients in the lymphadenectomy arm and 4 patients in the no-lymphadenectomy arm.[100]

Radiation

Pelvic Radiation

In the PORTEC-1 randomized trial[157] the overall (grades 1 to 4) rate of late complications was 26% in the RT group compared to 4% in the observation group ($p < .0001$). Most of the late complications in the RT group, however, were grades 1 and 2 (22%), and only 3% were grades 3 and 4. It is also important to note that many patients in this trial were treated with AP/PA fields, for which the overall rate of complications was 30%, compared to 21% for those treated with the four-field box ($p = .06$). Noute et al.[158] reported on the quality of life for patients enrolled in PORTEC-1. Patients treated with pelvic RT reported significant ($p < .01$) and clinically relevant higher rates of urinary incontinence, diarrhea, and fecal leakage, leading to more limitations in daily activities. Increased symptoms were reflected by the frequent use of incontinence materials after pelvic RT (day and night use, 42.9% vs. 15.2% for surgery alone; $p < .001$). Patients treated with pelvic RT reported lower scores on "physical functioning" ($p = .004$) and "role-physical" ($p = .003$). In GOG 99 when lymphadenectomy was performed, chronic lymphedema was seen in 2.5% of the patients randomized to surgery alone compared to 5% with postoperative pelvic RT.[105] There is an increased awareness of sacral insufficiency fractures (SIFs) as a potential complication of pelvic RT in gynecologic cancers. In a recent report from MSKCC, 13 of 223 (5.8%) patients treated with postoperative pelvic RT developed SIF (median time, 11 months after completing pelvic RT). Eight patients (62%) presented with pain, and 5 patients (38%) were diagnosed on incidental imaging. Treatment of SIF included observation in 7 patients (53%), bisphosphonate therapy in 5 patients (38%), and surgery in 1 patient (8%). On multivariate analysis, only osteoporosis was independently associated with SIF ($p = .04$), with a relative risk of 4.0 (95% CI 1.1 = 15.4). The rate of SIF was 5.5% (8 of 145) for the subset of patients with endometrial cancer.[159]

The morbidity of rate conventional pelvic radiation could be reduced by using IMRT. Mundt et al.[160,161] demonstrated significant reduction in acute and chronic gastrointestinal toxicity when IMRT was compared to conventional radiation. In a recent study from MSKCC,[162] the use of IMRT was associated with less bowel obstruction (BO) than with conventional RT. There were 223 patients; 145 (65%) had endometrial cancer. With a median follow-up of 48 months, the overall 5-year actuarial rate of BO was 7.2%. The rate in the IMRT group was 1.2%, compared to 9.6% for conventional RT ($p = .025$). This was seen despite the fact that more patients in the IMRT group had prior laparotomy (37% vs. 28%; $p = .03$), had more nodes removed (22 vs. 13 median lymph nodes; $p = .001$), and received more adjuvant chemotherapy (79% vs. 64%; $p = .016$). On multivariate analysis the use of IMRT (relative risk, 0.12, 95% CI = 0.015 to 0.987) and body mass index of >30 (relative risk, 0.12, 95% CI = 0.014 to 0.96) were associated with less bowel obstruction.

RTOG 0418 is a recently completed a phase II study on the feasibility of postoperative pelvic IMRT in cervical and endometrial cancers.[163] In the subset of evaluable patients with stages I to IIIC endometrial cancer (n = 43), with a median follow-up of 3.5 years, the 3-year DFS and OS rates were 92% and 95%, respectively. Intestinal complications were the most common; 10 patients (23%) had grade 1, 3 (7%) had grade 2, and 1 (2%) had grade 3.

Whole-Abdomen Radiation

The toxicity of whole-abdomen radiation is more pronounced than that of pelvic radiation but not as high as expected. In the radiation arm of GOG study 122, the GI toxicity did not exceed 2% for grade 4 and 11% for grade 3, whereas in the chemotherapy arm the corresponding figures were 7% and 13%. Grade 4 liver toxicity was seen in 1% of patients in the radiation arm, and the grade 4 cardiac grade toxicity was 4% in the chemotherapy arm.[138]

Intravaginal RT

The main advantage of intravaginal brachytherapy is its ability to deliver a relatively high dose of radiation to the vagina while limiting the dose to the surrounding normal structures, such as the bowels and bladder. This advantage is manifested with the low rate of severe late toxicity seen with this treatment technique, ranging from 0% to 1% in several series.[116,118,122] In the intravaginal RT arm of the Swedish trial[110] the rate of late intestinal toxicity was 2.3% for grade 1 and 0.4% for grade 2. Urinary tract toxicity was as follows: 20.2% grade 1, 2.7% grade 2, and 0.8% grade 3. Vaginal toxicity rate was 4.1% grade 1, 0.8% grade 2, and 0.8% grade 3. However, such a low rate of severe complications cannot be taken for granted because special attention needs to be paid to the depth of prescription, the dose per fraction, the length of vagina treated, and the diameter of the cylinder used. Sorbe and Smeds[164] reported a 15% late complication rate and a very high incidence of vaginal stenosis after postoperative high–dose-rate intravaginal irradiation. This was attributed to the high dose per fraction of 6 to 9 Gy; moreover, this dose was prescribed at a depth of 10 mm from the surface of the cylinder, resulting in very high vaginal mucosal, bladder, and rectal doses.

In PORTEC-2, intravaginal RT patients reported better social functioning (p = .005) and lower symptom scores for diarrhea, fecal leakage, need to stay close to a toilet, and limitation in daily activities due to bowel symptoms (p = .001) compared to pelvic RT. There were no differences in sexual functioning or symptoms between the treatment groups; however, sexual functioning was lower and sexual symptoms more frequent in both treatment groups compared to the norm population.[165]

Definitive Radiation for Inoperable Disease

Patients with medically inoperable stage I or II uterine cancer are usually treated in a fashion similar to those with cervical cancer by using intracavitary applicators with or without pelvic radiation. For patients with clinical stage I grade 1 or 2 and no evidence of myometrial invasion or lymph node metastasis on MRI, intracavitary brachytherapy alone is sufficient. Usually a Fletcher-Suit or Henschke applicator with one or two tandems (depending on uterus size) and ovoids is used to deliver 70 to 75 Gy to point A. The loading of the tandems is usually different than that in cervical cancer. This is done in order to provide wider coverage of the uterus laterally and superiorly. When pelvic radiation is added, the dose is usually 45 to 50 Gy supplemented with 30 to 35 Gy from intracavitary brachytherapy to bring the total dose to point A to 80 to 85 Gy. Rouanet et al.[166] treated 250 patients with endometrial cancer according to this approach, which yielded a 5-year disease-specific survival of 76.5%. HDR intracavitary brachytherapy is being used with increased frequency.[167,168] The American Brachytherapy Society established general guideline recommendations regarding HDR alone or in combination with external beam RT in terms of prescription point (2 cm from the central axis at the midpoint along the intrauterine sources), number of fractions, dose per fraction, combination with EBRT, and optimization.[169] Patients with stage IIIB disease (vaginal involvement), an uncommon presentation, are usually not surgical candidates and are also treated with definitive radiation, including a combination of external-beam and intracavitary/interstitial radiotherapy tailored to the extent of their disease.

Radiation Therapy for Local Recurrence

Radiation therapy can be curative in a select group of patients with small vaginal recurrences who have not received prior radiation.[170–172] The 5-year local control rate ranges from 42% to 65% and the 5-year overall survival rate from 31% to 53%. Creutzberg et al. reported on survival after relapse based on the PORTEC-1 randomized trial.[107] In patients who were initially randomized to surgery alone (n = 46 of 360), the 5-year survival after vaginal relapse was 65%. However, before adopting salvage radiation as a treatment policy for all early-stage endometrial cancer, a few aspects of this trial need to be addressed. First, the 5-year survival rate from the PORTEC trial is much higher than what is reported in the literature. Most likely, the vaginal recurrences in this trial were detected very early, unlike the situation for patients in the community. The extent and size of local recurrence in endometrial cancer are very significant predictors of outcome.[173] Second, this high rate of salvage pertains only to isolated vaginal recurrence. The rate of survival at 3 years for pelvic recurrence in the PORTEC-1 trial[107] was 0%. Third, although the trial does not mention any data on complications, it is not unrealistic to expect a higher complication rate than what is normally seen with adjuvant radiation. With salvage radiation, external-beam RT and brachytherapy are often combined, and the doses of radiation required are much higher than those used with adjuvant radiation. The study from MD Anderson Cancer Center by Jhingran et al.[170] clearly highlights these issues. They reported on 91 patients who were treated with definitive radiation for isolated vaginal recurrence. The 5-year local control and overall survival rates were 75% and 43%, respectively. The median dose of radiation was 75 Gy, which often included external radiation and brachytherapy. The rate of grade 4 complications (requiring surgery) was 9%. Thus, when talking with a patient about adjuvant radiation versus radiation reserved for salvage, these issues need to be addressed and compared to the excellent local control and low morbidity obtained with adjuvant intravaginal brachytherapy.

UTERINE SARCOMA

Uterine sarcomas are uncommon, representing about 3% to 7% of all uterine cancers.[174] The World Health Organization (WHO) classification includes endometrial stromal tumors, smooth muscle tumors, and miscellaneous mesenchymal tumors. In the mixed epithelial and mesenchymal tumors category, the WHO classification includes adenosarcoma and malignant mixed Müllerian tumors or carcinosarcoma.[51] Age-related incidences vary among the histologic types. The mean age at diagnosis for endometrial stromal sarcoma is 41 years, for leiomyosarcoma 53.5 years, for adenosarcoma 57.4 years, and for carcinosarcoma 65 years. Little is known about the risk factors for uterine sarcomas, except for history of prior radiation and carcinosarcoma.[175] Most uterine sarcomas present with vaginal bleeding, especially carcinosarcomas. Leiomyosarcomas are more commonly discovered incidentally after simple hysterectomy for presumed uterine leiomyomata.

Nodal metastases are seen in approximately 14% of carcinosarcomas at the time of surgical staging but are rarely

(<5%) seen in leiomyosarcoma unless there is obvious extrauterine disease. For stromal sarcomas, dos Santos et al.[176] reported a 19% (7 of 36) rate of nodal metastasis. The rate of occult metastasis was only 10%. The corresponding rates from the literature review were 10.1% and 8.1%, respectively.

Pathology and Staging

Endometrial stromal sarcomas are generally divided into endometrial stromal sarcomas, which are low grade by definition, and undifferentiated endometrial sarcoma, which are high grade. Tumor cells in endometrial stromal sarcoma resemble those found in the stroma of proliferative endometrial lining. In contrast, tumor cells in undifferentiated endometrial stromal sarcoma do not resemble endometrial stroma. *Leiomyosarcomas* of the uterus have a fleshy appearance, often with areas of necrosis. They display nuclear atypia, high mitotic rates, and areas of coagulative tumor necrosis. *Adenosarcomas* have two components—a benign epithelial tumor and a malignant mesenchymal component (generally low-grade sarcoma that resembles endometrial stroma). Sarcomatous overgrowth, defined as the presence of pure sarcoma, usually of high grade and without a glandular component, occupying at least 25% of the tumor, has been reported in 8% to 54% of uterine adenosarcomas.[174] Tumors containing both malignant epithelium, that is, carcinoma, and malignant soft-tissue tumors, that is, sarcomas, are called *carcinosarcomas* or *malignant mixed Müllerian tumors.* These neoplasms are often bulky, necrotic, and deeply invasive. The epithelial component is generally serous carcinoma. Homologous tumors have stroma that contains cell types normally seen in the uterus, in contrast to heterologous tumors, which may contain striated muscle cells (rhabdomyosarcoma) cartilage (chondrosarcoma), and bone (osteogenic sarcoma). Whether carcinosarcomas are epithelial tumors or sarcomas continues to be debated. Gene profiling may shed some light on that intriguing question.[177] The 2009 FIGO staging recognizes the uniqueness of each uterine sarcoma. For leiomyosarcomas and endometrial stromal sarcomas, the staging system recognizes the importance of tumor size on outcome. For adenosarcomas, the new staging system recognizes the importance of depth of myometrial invasion. For carcinosarcomas, the 2009 staging system for carcinomas of the endometrium is used, recognizing the similarity in patterns of spread.[174]

Management

The main treatment for uterine sarcoma is *surgery* in a similar fashion to endometrial adenocarcinoma. The extent of surgical staging varies, depending on the risk of lymph node involvement. Patients with carcinosarcoma should undergo comprehensive surgical staging similar to that with serous cancer. Patients with endometrial stromal sarcomas and adenosarcomas might benefit from lymph node sampling. On the other hand, for patients with leiomyosarcomas the rate of nodal involvement is too low to justify routine lymphadenectomy.[178]

A GOG clinicopathologic study of 453 patients with uterine sarcomas reported a 53% recurrence rate in carcinosarcoma and 71% in leiomyosarcoma, with the site of first recurrence being the pelvis in 21% of carcinosarcomas (19% in homologous and 24% in heterologous types) and 14% of leiomyosarcomas, respectively. Distant failure, as the first site, occurred in 14% of carcinosarcoma and 41% of leiomyosarcoma patients, respectively. Forty percent of patients with carcinosarcoma received adjuvant pelvic RT compared with 22% of leiomyosarcoma patients. The pelvic failure was 17% in patients receiving RT compared with 24% for those who did not.[179]

With regard to the role of *adjuvant radiation,* the EORTC performed a prospective, randomized trial addressing the role of postoperative pelvic RT in stages I to II uterine sarcomas. There were a total of 224 patients in the trial who underwent TAH/BSO, and 166 who had peritoneal washings. Lymphadenectomy was optional. There were 103 leiomyosarcomas (LMSs), 91 carcinosarcomas, and 28 endometrial stromal sarcomas. The 5-year cumulative incidence of locoregional recurrence was 18.8% in the pelvic RT arm compared to 35.9% in the surgery-alone arm. That difference was statistically significant ($p = .0013$). The 5-year cumulative incidence of distant relapse was 45.3% for the pelvic RT and 33.6% for surgery alone, but the difference was not statistically significant ($p = .2569$). There was no significant difference in progression-free ($p = .3254$) or overall survival ($p = .923$) between the two arms. For patients with carcinosarcoma, the rate of pelvic recurrence only was 4% in the pelvic RT arm compared to 24% for the surgery-alone arm. The corresponding rates for any local recurrence were 24% and 47%, respectively. For LMS patients, the rate of pelvic recurrence only was 2% in the pelvic RT compared to 14% in patients treated with surgery alone, and for any local recurrence it was 20% versus 24%. This seems to indicate that the pelvic control benefit is mainly seen in carcinosarcoma.[180] It is important to note that the primary endpoint of this trial was pelvic control, which it met ($p = .0013$). The study was not powered to detect a significant difference in PFS or OS. Sampath et al.[181] performed a retrospective review of uterine sarcoma patients using the National Oncology Database. The impact of adjuvant radiation was assessed in patients who presented with nonmetastatic disease and underwent definitive surgery ($n = 2,206$). In patients with carcinosarcoma, the 5-year local-regional failure-free survival was 90% for those who received adjuvant RT ($n = 490$) compared to 80% for those who received surgery alone ($n = 638$; $p <.001$). For endometrial stromal sarcoma, the rate was 97% with RT (109) versus 93% for surgery alone ($n = 252$; $p < .05$). For LMS it was 98% for RT ($n = 131$) compared to 84% with surgery alone ($n = 398$; $p < .01$).

The role of *adjuvant chemotherapy* has been evaluated mainly in carcinosarcoma. Sutton et al.[182] reported on 65 patients with completely resected stage I or II carcinosarcoma of the uterus treated with adjuvant ifosfamide and cisplatin. Overall 5-year survival was 62%. None of the patients received adjuvant RT in this GOG trial. Initial site of relapse was vaginal apex in 6 of 65 and pelvis in 4 of 64, suggesting that a combined chemoradiation approach might be ideal. GOG-150 is a phase III randomized study of WAI versus three cycles of cisplatin, ifosfamide, and Mesna (CIM). Eligible patients ($n = 206$) included those with stages I to IV uterine carcinosarcoma, no greater than 1-cm postsurgical residuum, and/or no extra-abdominal spread. Stage distribution was as follows: I, 64 (31%); II, 26 (13%); III, 92 (45%); IV, 24 (12%). The estimated crude probability of recurring within 5 years was 58% for WAI and 52% for CIM. Adjusting for stage and age, the recurrence rate was 21% lower for CIM patients than for WAI patients (RH, 0.789, 95% CI = 0.530 to 1.176; p = .245, two-tailed test). The estimated death rate was 29% lower in the CIM group (RH, 0.712, 95% CI = 0.484 to 1.048; $p = .085$, two-tailed test). The conclusion was that there was not a statistically significant advantage in recurrence rate or survival for adjuvant chemotherapy over WAI in patients with uterine carcinosarcoma. However, the observed differences favor the use of combination chemotherapy in future trials. The rate of vaginal recurrence was 4 of 105 (3.8%) in the WAI compared to 10 of 101 (9.9%). The corresponding abdominal relapse rates were 27.6% (29 of 105) and 18.8% (19 of 101). There was no difference in pelvic recurrence between the two arms. The rates of lung metastasis (14 of 105 vs. 14 of 101, respectively) or other distant sites (13 of 101 vs. 10 of 101, respectively) were similar. Analysis of the patterns of relapse from this trial also indicates the need for chemoradiation in patients with stages I to III carcinosarcoma.[183] At MSKCC, patients with surgical stages I or II carcinosarcoma are treated with intravaginal RT and chemotherapy. Stage III patients are treated with concurrent pelvic RT/cisplatin followed by carboplatin/paclitaxel.

For patients with *leiomyosarcomas* the main treatment is surgery, and the role of adjuvant treatment, whether RT or chemotherapy, is not well defined. The high rate of distant relapse in these patients overshadows any local control benefit attained with adjuvant RT. These patients should be encouraged to participate in trials assessing the role of chemotherapy and/or targeted therapy. For patients with endometrial stromal sarcomas (low grade) observation is feasible. For those with undifferentiated endometrial sarcomas adjuvant pelvic RT is reasonable. For patients with adenosarcomas, especially with sarcomatous overgrowth, adjuvant pelvic RT is also reasonable. *Carcinosarcomas* should be treated in a similar fashion to other high-risk endometrial cancers. For early-stage comprehensively staged patients, intravaginal RT and chemotherapy is recommended. Patients with stage III could be treated with concurrent pelvic RT and cisplatin followed by carboplatin/paclitaxel.

SELECTED REFERENCES

A full list of references for this chapter is available online.

4. Jemal A, Bray F, Center MM, et al. Global cancer statistics. *CA Cancer J Clin* 2011;61(2):69–90.
9. McPherson CP, Sellers TA, Potter JD, et al. Reproductive factors and risk of endometrial cancer. The Iowa Women's Health Study. *Am J Epidemiol* 1996;143:1195–1202.
10. Dossus L, Allen N, Kaaks R, et al. Reproductive risk factors and endometrial cancer: the European Prospective Investigation into Cancer and Nutrition. *Int J Cancer* 2010;127:442–451.
12. Saltzman BS, Doherty JA, Hill DA, et al. Diabetes and endometrial cancer: an evaluation of the modifying effects of other known risk factors. *Am J Epidemiol* 2008;167:607–614.
14. Friedenreich CM, Biel RK, Lau DC, et al. Case–control study of the metabolic syndrome and metabolic risk factors for endometrial cancer. *Cancer Epidemiol Biomarkers Prev* 2011;20(11):2384–2395.
17. Allen NE, Tsilidis KK, Key TJ, et al. Menopausal hormone therapy and risk of endometrial carcinoma among postmenopausal women in the European Prospective Investigation into Cancer And Nutrition. *Am J Epidemiol.* 2010; 172(12):1394–1403.
18. Pinkerton JV, Goldstein SR. Endometrial safety: a key hurdle for selective estrogen receptor modulators in development. *Menopause* 2010;17(3):642–653.
25. Meyer LA, Broaddus RR, Lu KH. Endometrial cancer and Lynch syndrome: clinical and pathologic considerations. *Cancer Control* 2009;16(1):14–22.
27. Burbos N, Musonda P, Duncan TJ, et al. Estimating the risk of endometrial cancer in symptomatic postmenopausal women: a novel clinical prediction model based on patients' characteristics. *Int J Gynecol Cancer* 2011;21(3):500–506.
28. Creasman WT, Odicino F, Maisonneuve P, et al. Carcinoma of the corpus uteri. FIGO 26th Annual Report on the Results of Treatment in Gynecological Cancer. *Int J Gynaecol Obstet* 2006;95(Suppl 1):S105–S143.
29. Smith RA, Cokkinides V, Brooks D, et al. Cancer screening in the United States, 2010: a review of current American Cancer Society guidelines and issues in cancer screening. *CA Cancer J Clin* 2010;60(2):99–119.
30. Schmeler KM, Lynch HT, Chen L, et al. prophylactic surgery to reduce the risk of gynecologic cancers in the Lynch syndrome. *N Engl J Med* 2006;354:261.
33. Smith-Bindman R, Kerlikowske K, Feldstein VA, et al. Endovaginal ultrasound to exclude endometrial cancer and other endometrial abnormalities. *JAMA* 1998; 280:1510–1517.
35. Goldstein RB, Bree RL, Benson CB, et al. Evaluation of the women with postmenopausal bleeding: Society of radiologists in ultrasound-sponsored consensus conference statement. *J Ultrasound Med* 2001;20:1025–1036.
37. de Kroon CD, Jansen FW. Saline infusion sonography in women with abnormal uterine bleeding: an update of recent findings. *Curr Opin Obstet Gynecol* 2006; 18(6):653–657.
44. Kim HS, Park CY, Lee JM, et al. Evaluation of serum CA-125 levels for preoperative counselling in endometrioid endometrial cancer: a multi-centre study. *Gynecol Oncol* 2010;118:282–288.
47. Trimble CL, Kauderer J, Zaino R, et al. Concurrent endometrial carcinoma in women with a biopsy diagnosis of atypical endometrial hyperplasia: a Gynecologic Oncology Group Study. *Cancer* 2006;106:812.
52. Tafe LJ, Garg K, Chew I, et al. Endometrial and ovarian carcinomas with undifferentiated components: clinically aggressive and frequently underrecognized neoplasms. *Mod Pathol* 2010;23(6):781–789.
54. Ramus SJ, Elmasry K, Luo Z, et al. Predicting clinical outcome in patients diagnosed with synchronous ovarian and endometrial cancer. *Clin Cancer Res* 2008;14(18):5840–5848.
57. Dedes KJ, Wetterskog D, Ashworth A, et al. Emerging therapeutic targets in endometrial cancer. *Nat Rev Clin Oncol* 2011;8(5):261–271.
58. Catasus L, Gallardo A, Cuatrecasas M, et al. Concomitant PI3 K-AKT and p53 alterations in endometrial carcinomas are associated with poor prognosis. *Mod Pathol* 2009;22, 522–529.
60. Llobet D, Pallares J, Yeramian A, et al. Molecular pathology of endometrial carcinoma: practical aspects from the diagnostic and therapeutic viewpoints. *J Clin Pathol* 2009;62(9):777–785.
63. Konecny GE, et al. HER2 gene amplification and EGFR expression in a large cohort of surgically staged patients with nonendometrioid (type II) endometrial cancer. *Br J Cancer* 2009;100:89–95.
64. Fadare O, Zheng W. Insights into endometrial serous carcinogenesis and progression. *Int J Clin Exp Pathol* 2009;2:411–432.
68. Merritt MA, Cramer DW. Molecular pathogenesis of endometrial and ovarian cancer. *Cancer Biomark* 2011;9(1–6):287–305.
70. Salvesen HB, et al. Integrated genomic profiling of endometrial carcinoma associates aggressive tumors with indicators of PI3 kinase activation. *Proc Natl Acad Sci U S A* 2009;106:4834–4839.
71. Creasman WT, Morrow CP, Bundy BN, et al. Surgical pathologic spread patterns of endometrial cancer. A Gynecologic Oncology Group Study. *Cancer* 1987; 60:2035–2041.
72. International Federation of Gynecology and Obstetrics. Revised FIGO staging for carcinoma of the vulva, cervix, and endometrium. *Int J Gynecol Obstet* 2009; 105:103.
73. Page BR, Pappas L, Cooke EW, et al. Does the FIGO 2009 endometrial cancer staging system more accurately correlate with clinical outcome in different histologies? Revised staging, endometrial cancer, histology. *Int J Gynecol Cancer* 2012;22(4):593–598.
74. Abu-Rustum NR, Zhou Q, Iasonos A, et al. The revised 2009 FIGO staging system for endometrial cancer: should the 1988 FIGO stages IA and IB be altered? *Int J Gynecol Cancer* 2011;21(3):511–516.
75. Abu-Rustum NR, Zhou Q, Gomez JD, et al. A nomogram for predicting overall survival of women with endometrial cancer following primary therapy: toward improving individualized cancer care. *Gynecol Oncol* 2010;116(3):399–403.
76. Creutzberg CL, Nout RA, Lybeert ML, et al. Fifteen-year radiotherapy outcome of the randomized PORTEC-1 Trial for endometrial carcinoma. *Int J Radiat Oncol Biol Phys* 2011;81(4):631–638.
82. Guntupalli SR, Zighelboim I, Kizer NT, et al. Lymphovascular space invasion is an independent risk factor for nodal disease and poor outcomes in endometrioid endometrial cancer. *Gynecol Oncol* 2012;124(1):31–35.
83. Kizer NT, Gao F, Guntupalli S, et al. Lower uterine segment involvement is associated with poor outcome in early-stage endometrioid endometrial carcinoma. *Ann Surg Oncol* 2011;18(5):1419–1424.
85. Wethington SL, Barrena Medel NI, Wright JD, et al. Prognostic significance and treatment implications of positive peritoneal cytology in endometrial adenocarcinoma: unraveling a mystery. *Gynecol Oncol* 2009;115(1):18–25.
86. Jobsen JJ, Naudin Ten Cate L, Lybeert ML, et al. Outcome of endometrial cancer stage IIIA with adnexa or serosal involvement only. *Obstet Gynecol Int* 2011; 2011:962518.
94. Walker JL, Piedmonte MR, Spirtos NM, et al. Recurrence and survival after random assignment to laparoscopy versus laparotomy for comprehensive surgical staging uterine cancer: Gynecology Oncology Group LAP2 study. *J Clin Oncol* 2012; 30(7):695–700.
95. Wright JD, Burke WM, Wilde ET, et al. Comparative effectiveness of robotic versus laparoscopic hysterectomy for endometrial cancer. *J Clin Oncol* 2012; 30(8):783–791.
100. Benedetti Panici P, Basile S, Maneschi F, et al. Systematic pelvic lymphadenectomy vs. no lymphadenectomy in early-stage endometrial carcinoma: randomized clinical trial. *J Natl Cancer Inst* 2008;100(23):1707–1716.
101. ASTEC Study Group. Efficacy of systematic pelvic lymphadenectomy in endometrial cancer (MRC ASTEC trial): a randomised study. *Lancet* 2009;373(9658): 125–136.
102. Khoury-Collado F, Murray MP, Hensley ML, et al. Sentinel lymph node mapping for endometrial cancer improves the detection of metastatic disease to regional lymph nodes. *Gynecol Oncol* 2011;122(2):251–254.
103. Ballester M, Dubernard G, Lécuru F, et al. Detection rate and diagnostic accuracy of sentinel-node biopsy in early stage endometrial cancer: a prospective multicentre study (SENTI-ENDO). *Lancet Oncol* 2011;12(5):469–476.
104. Creutzberg CL, van Putten WL, Koper PC, et al. Surgery and postoperative radiotherapy versus surgery alone for patients with stage-1 endometrial carcinoma: multicentre randomised trial. PORTEC Study Group. Post Operative Radiation Therapy in Endometrial Carcinoma. *Lancet* 2000;355:1404–1411.
105. Keys HM, Roberts JA, Brunetto VL, et al. A phase III trial of surgery with or without adjunctive external pelvic radiation therapy in intermediate risk endometrial adenocarcinoma: a Gynecologic Oncology Group study. *Gynecol Oncol* 2004;92(3):744–751.
106. Blake P, Swart AM, Otron J, et al. Adjuvant external beam radiotherapy in the treatment of endometrial cancer (MRC ASTEC and NCIC CTG EN.5 randomised trials): pooled trial results, systematic review, and meta-analysis. *Lancet* 2009; 373(9658):137–146.
108. Sorbe B, Nordström B, Mäenpää J, et al. Intravaginal brachytherapy in FIGO stage I low-risk endometrial cancer: a controlled randomized study. *Int J Gynecol Cancer* 2009;19(5):873–878.
109. Nout RA, Smit VT, Putter H, et al. PORTEC Study Group. Vaginal brachytherapy versus pelvic external beam radiotherapy for patients with endometrial cancer of high-intermediate risk (PORTEC-2): an open-label, non-inferiority, randomised trial. *Lancet* 2010;375(9717):816–823.
110. Sorbe B, Horvath G, Andersson H, et al. External pelvic and vaginal irradiation versus vaginal irradiation alone as postoperative therapy in medium-risk endometrial carcinoma—a prospective randomized study. *Int J Radiat Oncol Biol Phys* 2012;82(3):1249–1255.
113. Croog VJ, Abu-Rustum NR, Barakat RR, et al. Adjuvant radiation for early stage endometrial cancer with lymphovascular invasion. *Gynecol Oncol* 2008; 111(1):49–54.
115. Creutzberg CL, van Putten WL, Warlam-Rodenhuis CC, et al. Outcome of high-risk stage IC, grade 3, compared with stage I endometrial carcinoma patients: the Postoperative Radiation Therapy in Endometrial Carcinoma Trial. *J Clin Oncol* 2004;22:1234–1241.
117. Sorbe B, Straumits A, Karlsson L. Intravaginal high-dose-rate brachytherapy for stage I endometrial cancer: a randomized study of two dose-per-fraction levels. *Int J Radiat Oncol Biol Phys* 2005;62(5):1385–1389.
123. Long KC, Zhou Q, Hensley ML, et al. Patterns of recurrence in 1988 FIGO stage IC endometrioid endometrial cancer. *Gynecol Oncol* 2012;125(1):99-102.
127. Cannon GM, Geye H, Terakedis BE, et al. Outcomes following surgery and adjuvant radiation in stage II endometrial adenocarcinoma. *Gynecol Oncol* 2009; 113(2):176–180.
136. Susumu N, Sagae S, Udagawa Y, et al. Randomized phase III trial of pelvic radiotherapy versus cisplatin-based combined chemotherapy in patients with intermediate- and high-risk endometrial cancer: a Japanese Gynecologic Oncology Group study. *Gynecol Oncol* 2008;108(1):226–233.

139. Kuoppala T, Mäenpää J, Tomas E, et al. Surgically staged high-risk endometrial cancer: randomized study of adjuvant radiotherapy alone vs. sequential chemo-radiotherapy. *Gynecol Oncol* 2008;110(2):190–195.
140. Hogberg T, Signorelli M, de Oliveira CF, et al. Sequential adjuvant chemotherapy and radiotherapy in endometrial cancer—results from two randomised studies. *Eur J Cancer* 2010;46(13):2422–2431.
141. Greven K, Winter K, Underhill K, et al. Final analysis of RTOG 9708: adjuvant postoperative irradiation combined with cisplatin/paclitaxel chemotherapy following surgery for patients with high-risk endometrial cancer. *Gynecol Oncol* 2006;103(1):155–159.
143. Klopp AH, Jhingran A, Ramondetta L, et al. Node-positive adenocarcinoma of the endometrium: outcome and patterns of recurrence with and without external beam irradiation. *Gynecol Oncol* 2009;115(1):6–11.
147. Alektiar KM, Makker V, Abu-Rustum NR, et al. Concurrent carboplatin/paclitaxel and intravaginal radiation in surgical stage I-II serous endometrial cancer. *Gynecol Oncol* 2009;112(1):142–145.
148. Kiess A, Damast S, Makker V, et al. Adjuvant carboplatin/paclitaxel and intravaginal radiation for stage I-II serous endometrial cancer. *Radiother Oncol* 2012; 103:S101–S102.
149. Jobsen JJ, ten Cate LN, Lybeert ML, et al. The number of metastatic sites for stage IIIA endometrial carcinoma, endometrioid cell type, is a strong negative prognostic factor. *Gynecol Oncol* 2010;117(1):32–36.
151. Garg G, Morris RT, Solomon L, et al. Evaluating the significance of location of lymph node metastasis and extranodal disease in women with stage IIIC endometrial cancer. *Gynecol Oncol* 2011;123(2):208–213.
153. Small W Jr, Mell LK, Anderson P, et al. Consensus guidelines for delineation of clinical target volume for intensity-modulated pelvic radiotherapy in postoperative treatment of endometrial and cervical cancer. *Int J Radiat Oncol Biol Phys* 2008;71(2):428–434.
157. Creutzberg CL, van Putten WL, Koper PC, et al. The Postoperative Radiation Therapy in Endometrial Carcinoma. The morbidity of treatment for patients with stage I endometrial cancer: results from a randomized trial. *Int J Radiat Oncol Biol Phys* 2001;51(5):1246–1255.
158. Nout RA, van de Poll-Franse LV, Lybeert ML, et al. Long-term outcome and quality of life of patients with endometrial carcinoma treated with or without pelvic radiotherapy in the post operative radiation therapy in endometrial carcinoma 1 (PORTEC-1) trial. *J Clin Oncol* 2011;29(13):1692–1700.
159. Shih K, Abu-Rustum NR, Sonoda Y, et al. Sacral insufficiency fractures after postoperative pelvic radiation therapy in gynecologic malignancy. Presented at the 93rd Annual Meeting of the American Radium Society, Palm Beach, FL, 2011.
162. Shih K, Frey M, Chi D, et al. Impact of postoperative intensity-modulated radiation therapy on the rate of bowel obstruction in gynecologic malignancy. *Gynecol Oncol* 2012;125(Suppl 1):S147–S148.
163. Jhingran A, Wnter K, Portelance L, et al. Efficacy and safety of IMRT after surgery in patients with endometrial cancer: RTOG 0418 phase II study [Abstract]. *Int J Radiat Oncol Biol Phys* 2011;81(25, Suppl):S45.
165. Nout RA, Putter H, Jürgenliemk-Schulz IM, et al. Five-year quality of life of endometrial cancer patients treated in the randomised Post Operative Radiation Therapy in Endometrial Cancer (PORTEC-2) trial and comparison with norm data. *Eur J Cancer* 2012;48:1638–1648.
174. D'Angelo E, Prat J. Uterine sarcomas: a review. *Gynecol Oncol* 2010;116(1):131–139.
176. Dos Santos LA, Garg K, Diaz JP, et al. Incidence of lymph node and adnexal metastasis in endometrial stromal sarcoma. *Gynecol Oncol* 2011;121(2):319–322.
180. Reed NS, Mangioni C, Malmström H, et al. European Organisation for Research and Treatment of Cancer Gynaecological Cancer Group. Phase III randomised study to evaluate the role of adjuvant pelvic radiotherapy in the treatment of uterine sarcomas stages I and II: an European Organisation for Research and Treatment of Cancer Gynaecological Cancer Group Study (protocol 55874). *Eur J Cancer* 2008;44(6):808–818.
181. Sampath S, Schultheiss TE, Ryu JK, et al. The role of adjuvant radiation in uterine sarcomas. *Int J Radiat Oncol Biol Phys* 2010;76(3):728–734.
182. Sutton G, Kauderer J, Carson LF, et al. Gynecologic Oncology Group. Adjuvant ifosfamide and cisplatin in patients with completely resected stage I or II carcinosarcomas (mixed mesodermal tumors) of the uterus: a Gynecologic Oncology Group study. *Gynecol Oncol* 2005;96(3):630–634.

Chapter 71
Ovarian and Fallopian Tube Cancer

Larissa Lee, Ross Berkowitz, and Ursula Matulonis

Ovarian neoplasms encompass a wide array of benign and malignant tumors with diverse histologic cell types, clinical features, and survival outcomes. Primary malignant tumors of the ovary include the epithelial ovarian cancers, germ cell tumors, and sex cord tumors. Low malignant potential (LMP) tumors of the ovary are noninvasive epithelial tumors often confined to the ovary, although extraovarian tumor implants may be detected. Metastases to the ovary occur from other primary malignancies including uterine, gastrointestinal (Krukenberg tumors), and breast cancers. Primary lymphoma, sarcoma, and melanoma of the ovary are rare. Relative to its incidence, epithelial ovarian cancers have substantially high mortality because effective screening tools are lacking; only 25% are detected as stage I at diagnosis, and current therapies for advanced cancer, although improving, have reached a therapeutic plateau. Surgery is the mainstay for diagnosis, staging, and the initial treatment for ovarian cancer. Platinum-based chemotherapy is indicated for patients with high-risk or advanced disease. Novel agents, such as antiangiogenics and poly (ADP-ribose) polymerase (PARP) inhibitors, are under active investigation in the adjuvant and/or recurrent setting. The use of whole-abdomen irradiation (WAI) or intraperitoneal (IP) radioisotopes is primarily historical, and radiation therapy now has a limited role in the management of ovarian cancer. Nonetheless, palliative radiotherapy may be of significant benefit for symptomatic disease relapse or select patients with localized recurrence.

ANATOMY

In premenopausal women, the ovaries are almond-shaped, gray-pink solid organs that measure approximately 4 × 2.5 × 1 cm, with an average weight of 4 to 5 g. After menopause, the ovaries atrophy and become nonfunctional and smaller in size. When normally positioned, the ovary is attached by the meso-ovarium to the broad ligament that covers the uterus and fallopian tubes. The infundibular pelvic, or suspensory, ligament extends from the surface of the ovary to the lateral pelvic wall, forming the superior and lateral aspect of the broad ligament (Fig. 71.1). The blood supply of the ovary is derived from the ovarian arteries, which arise from the aorta immediately below the level of the renal arteries and course through the retroperitoneum and infundibular pelvic ligaments. The venous return of the ovary empties to the renal vein on the left and directly to the vena cava on the right. The primary lymphatic drainage of the ovary parallels the course of the ovarian veins, with secondary lymphatic flow passing through the inguinal canal and to the iliac nodal system.[1] Histologically, the outer cortex of the ovary is covered by a layer of pseudocolumnar or cuboidal epithelium, termed the germinal epithelium of Waldeyer or ovarian surface epithelium (OSE). The inner medulla consists of a superficial tunica albuginea and dense stromal tissue filled with blood vessels and spindled, "muscle-like" connective tissue. Within the medulla, maturing follicles are present throughout the various layers.

The fallopian tubes are positioned horizontally within the superior part of the broad ligament and extend from the superior posterior portion of the uterine fundus to the ovaries. The fallopian tubes are hollow, muscular viscera that are in direct communication with the peritoneal cavity. The ovarian artery anastomoses with the uterine artery to supply the fallopian tube, and venous drainage is through the pampiniform plexus to the ovarian vein and uterine plexus. The mucosa of the fallopian tube contains a rich network of intercommunicating

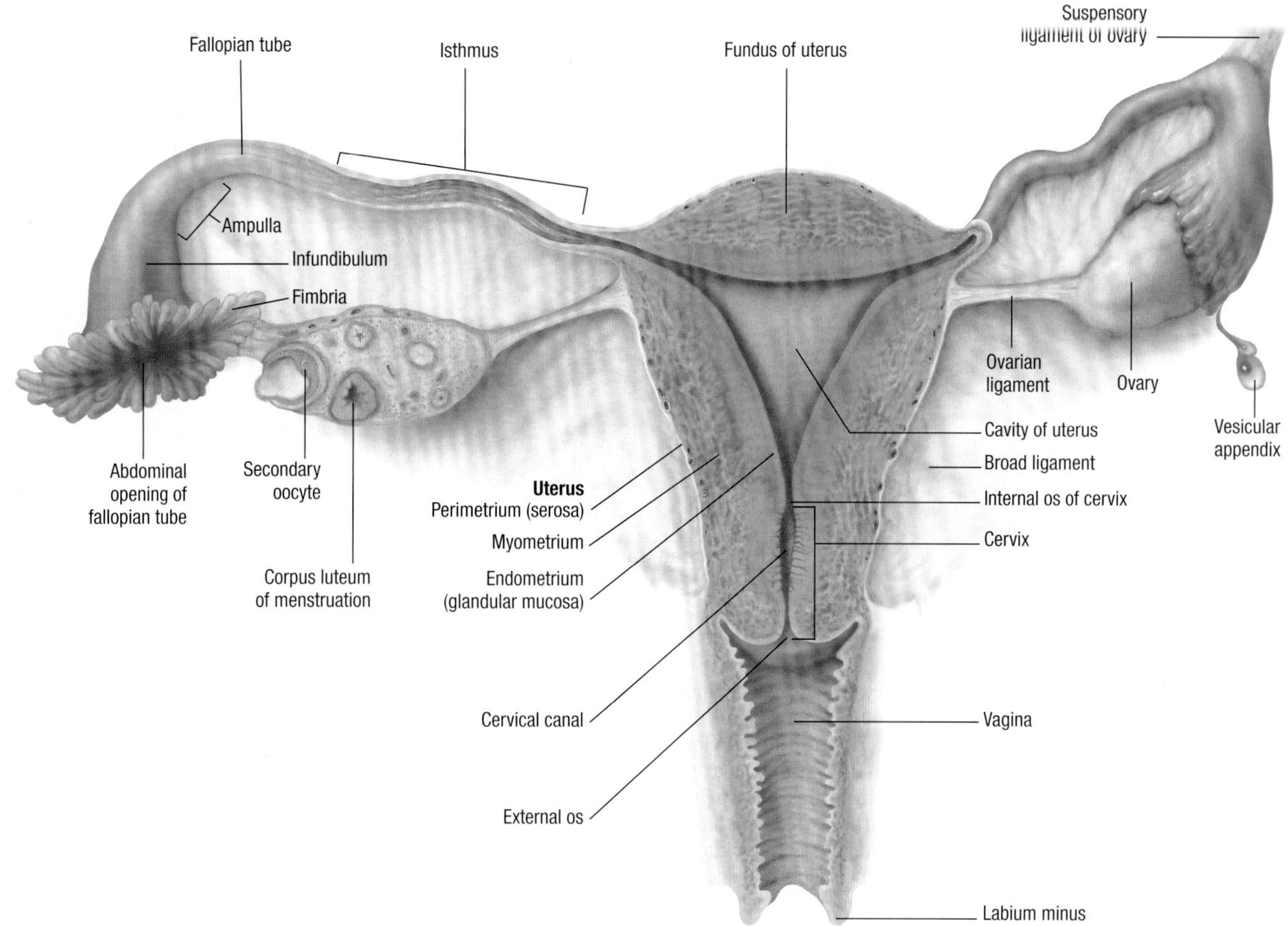

FIGURE 71.1. Anatomy of the ovary and female reproductive tract. (Asset provided by the Anatomical Chart Company.)

lymphatic sinusoids that anastomose with adjacent organs and drain into the ovarian lymphatics and para-aortic and iliac lymph nodes.[2] The fallopian tubes consist of four separate histologic layers: the mucosa, submucosa, muscularis (external longitudinal and inner circular layers), and outer serosal layer, which is continuous with the visceral peritoneum of the uterus. The mucosa is intricately folded, with the number of folds increasing from the interstitial portion to the ampulla. The epithelium is composed mainly of ciliated cells and secretory cells. Cyclic changes are evident in the tubal epithelium, similar to those of the endometrium, in response to estrogen and progesterone.

EPIDEMIOLOGY

Ovarian cancer is the second most common gynecologic malignancy in the United States after endometrial cancer. Approximately 22,280 women in the U.S. received a diagnosis of epithelial ovarian cancer in 2012, and 15,500 died of the disease[3,4] (Fig. 71.2). Ovarian cancer represents the fifth leading cause of cancer-related death in U.S. women, following lung, breast, colorectal and pancreatic cancers. The lifetime risk of ovarian cancer is approximately 1 in 72 women with a median age at diagnosis of 63 years; >80% of women are diagnosed after the age of 40 years.[5] The incidence of ovarian cancer rises with increasing age and peaks in the eighth decade of life. Differences in race and ethnicity are apparent in the age-adjusted annual incidence per 100,000 women, which in 2005 to 2009 was highest for White women (13.4), followed by Hispanic (11.3), American Indian/Alaska Native (11.2), Black (9.8), and Asian/Pacific Islanders (9.8).[5] The incidence of ovarian cancer also varies significantly by geography, with the highest rates in North America and northern Europe, which are three to seven times higher than that observed in Japan.[6] Mortality rates for ovarian cancer have been decreasing in the United States since 1975, when the 5-year survival rate reported by the Surveillance, Epidemiology, and End Results (SEER) Program was 37%. Between 2001 and 2007, 5-year survival increased to 44%, predominantly driven by survival gains among White women. Black women have disproportionately lower 5-year survival rates, estimated at 34% in the same time period.[5]

Primary cancer of the fallopian tube was once considered a rare disease, accounting for 0.2% to 0.5% of female gynecologic malignancies. However, the true incidence has likely been underestimated considering a large proportion of extrauterine high-grade serous carcinomas may actually originate in the fimbriated end of the fallopian tube.[7,8] Precursor lesions, known as tubal intraepithelial carcinomas (TICs) have been detected in the fallopian tubes of prophylactic salpingo-oophorectomy specimens from high-risk patients. The model of the fallopian tube as the primary site of origin for extrauterine high-grade serous carcinoma is supported by epidemiologic, morphologic, and genetic data, as discussed later.

PATHOGENESIS

The female reproductive tract originates from the Müllerian ducts, which are paired embryologic structures of mesodermal origin that give rise to the fallopian tubes, uterus, cervix, and upper vagina. Ovarian tissue is composed of embryonic yolk sac cells that give rise to the ova or germ cells, stromal cells

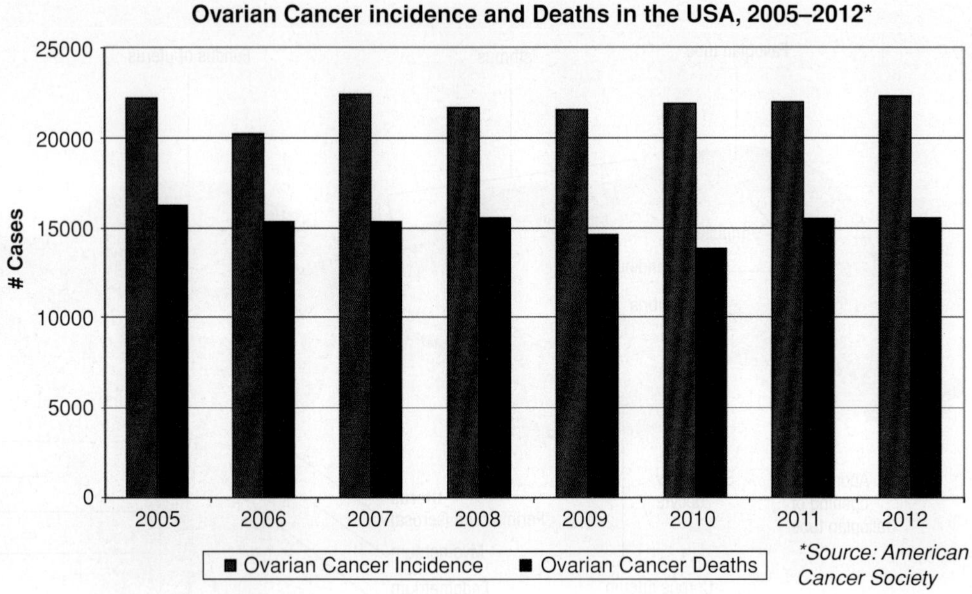

FIGURE 71.2. Ovarian cancer incidence and deaths in the United States from 2005 to 2012. (Courtesy of the American Cancer Society.)

that produce the steroid hormones, and mesothelium that provides the epithelial covering for the follicle cysts. These cell types give rise to germ cell tumors, sex cord–stromal tumors, and the epithelial tumors of the ovary, respectively. The traditional view of ovarian cancer pathogenesis is that all tumor subtypes arise from the OSE. In the "incessant ovulation hypothesis," ovarian cancer develops from an aberrant repair process as a result of repeated rupture of the surface epithelium during each ovulatory cycle, thought to produce inflammation and scarring that serves as a nidus for carcinogenesis.[9–11] A second proposed mechanism is related to hormonal and reproductive factors such as persistent exposure to gonadotropins and elevated estradiol levels that stimulate malignant transformation.[12,13] Strong evidence exists that many borderline tumors and low-grade carcinomas of the ovary arise from cortical inclusion cysts (CICs) within the ovarian parenchyma. These benign cysts are composed of Müllerian epithelium that closely resembles the fallopian tube. CICs are thought to result from invaginations of the OSE into the ovarian stroma through repeated ovulation and aging, acquiring a Müllerian phenotype through metaplasia.[8] An alternate explanation is that remnants of Müllerian-derived epithelia from the fallopian tube may adhere to the ovarian surface and become incorporated into CICs in a process known as endosalpingiosis. Nonetheless, as a result of hormone exposure, damage repair processes, and inflammation within the ovary, neoplastic transformation gives rise to a variety of Müllerian-cell type differentiations, including serous carcinomas that resemble the fallopian tube, mucinous tumors as seen in the endocervix, endometrioid tumors from the endometrium, and glycogen-rich clear cell cancers similar to secretory-phase endometrial glands.

High-grade serous ovarian carcinomas are infrequently associated with benign or borderline precursor lesions within the ovary, a contradiction of the OSE-CIC model. Furthermore, high-grade serous carcinomas of the ovary share distinct morphologic and genetic characteristics with high-grade serous carcinomas of other extrauterine sites, including serous fallopian tube carcinoma and primary peritoneal serous carcinoma. In this context, a second model of ovarian carcinogenesis has emerged with the recognition of the distal fallopian tube as the primary site of origin for many high-grade serous carcinomas. With rigorous pathologic processing, occult fallopian tube cancer has been detected in the fimbria of prophylactic salpingo-oophorectomy specimens from high-risk patients.[14,15] Furthermore, TICs have been found in a large proportion of high-grade serous carcinomas initially designated as primary ovarian cancers.[16] An adenoma-carcinoma sequence has since been described that involves a dysplastic tubal precursor lesion with loss of p53 detectable by immunohistochemical staining ("p53 signature") with progression to a TIC characterized by increased proliferation, followed by the development of frank invasive serous carcinoma.[7,17] The concept of the fallopian tube as the primary site of high-grade serous carcinoma suggests that previously undetected serous TICs may spread to the adjacent ovary or peritoneal cavity early in the disease process of serous carcinogenesis.

In the two-pathway model of ovarian carcinogenesis, type I tumors include all major histologic subtypes (serous, endometrioid, mucinous, clear cell, and transitional) with low nuclear and architectural grade that may be linked to well-defined benign precursor lesions, and type II tumors account for the bulk of high-grade serous carcinomas (Table 71.1). The type I tumors are associated with distinct molecular alterations, such as mutations in *KRAS, BRAF,* and *PTEN,* which are rarely found in type II serous tumors.[18] Mutually exclusive *KRAS* and *BRAF* mutations, both of which activate the oncogenic *MAPK* signaling pathway, are observed in 65% of serous borderline tumors but are rarely seen in high-grade serous carcinomas.[19] *KRAS* mutations also occur in Müllerian histologic subtypes, including 60% of mucinous, 5% to 16% of clear cell, and 4% to 5% of endometrioid carcinomas.[18] Mutations in *PTEN,* which lead to constitutive activation of the related PI3 kinase signaling pathway, have been detected in 20% of endometrioid carcinomas,[20] whereas activating mutations in *PIK3CA* have been

TABLE 71.1 TWO-PATHWAY MODEL OF EPITHELIAL OVARIAN CARCINOGENESIS

Type 1	*Type 2*
All Müllerian subtypes (serous, endometrioid, mucinous, clear cell, transitional)	High-grade serous carcinoma
Usually low grade	High grade
Linked to benign or borderline precursor lesions	Associated with tubal intraepithelial carcinomas (TICs)
KRAS or *BRAF* mutation (MAPK pathway)	Inactivation of *BRCA* pathway
PTEN or *PIK3CA* mutation (PI3K pathway)	
ARID1A mutation, loss of BAF250a expression	
Wild-type p53 status	High frequency of p53 mutation
Chromosomally stable	Widespread DNA copy number change
Frequently platinum insensitive	Usually platinum sensitive

Adapted from Bowtell DD. The genesis and evolution of high-grade serous ovarian cancer. *Nat Rev Cancer* 2010;10(11):803–808.

identified in 30% of clear cell cancers.[21] Somatic mutations in *ARID1A*, a novel tumor suppressor gene, were recently identified in 46% of ovarian clear cell cancers and 30% of endometrioid cancers. *ARID1A* mutation and corresponding loss of BAF250a expression, a key component in chromatin remodeling, were also seen in preneoplastic lesions and may represent an early event in the transformation of endometriosis.[22] In contrast, type II tumors exhibit a high frequency of p53 mutation and widespread DNA copy number change. Inactivation of the BRCA pathway, a critical component of DNA repair by homologous recombination, is also a hallmark of high-grade serous carcinomas.[23] Disruption of the BRCA pathway by germline or somatic mutation, epigenetic silencing, or microRNA regulation has been observed in >50% of serous cancers,[24] and functional assays show defective formation of homologous recombination repair foci following DNA damage.[25]

Angiogenesis plays an important role in normal ovarian function, as heavy vascularization occurs at the beginning of each ovulatory cycle with predictable variation in the serum levels of vascular endothelial growth factor (VEGF). Epithelial ovarian cancers frequently overexpress VEGF, fibroblast growth factor, platelet-derived growth factor (PDGF), and angiopoietin.[26] In preclinical models, expression of VEGF provides a survival advantage to transformed cells of the ovary. Other studies have found an association between preoperative serum VEGF level and clinical outcome.[27] Targeting the tumor microenvironment in ovarian cancer is an attractive treatment strategy given the inherent genomic instability of high-grade serous cancers.

RISK FACTORS

Epidemiologic studies have identified hormonal, genetic, and environmental factors that may play an important role in ovarian carcinogenesis (Table 71.2). The OSE-CIC model is consistent with well-established epidemiologic data indicating that suppression of ovulation results in substantial reduction of ovarian cancer risk. New insights into the pathogenesis of high-grade serous carcinomas have emerged through the study of high-risk populations with a genetic predisposition for the development of ovarian cancer. Nevertheless, the pathogenic mechanisms are not well understood and likely multifactorial, associated with both patient-related and environmental factors.

TABLE 71.2 FACTORS INFLUENCING THE RISK OF OVARIAN CANCER

Factor	Estimated Risk (%)	Estimated Relative Risk
Baseline lifetime risk	1.4	1
Race		
White	13.4 per 100,000	–
Hispanic or American Indian	11.3 per 100,000	–
African American	9.8 per 100,000	–
Risk factors		
Family history	9.4	5–7
BRCA1 mutation	35–46	18–29
BRCA2 mutation	13–23	16–19
Lynch II/HPNCC	3–14	6–7
Infertility	–	2–5
Obesity	–	1.1–4
Nulliparity	–	2–3
Late menopause	–	1.5–2
Early menarche	–	1–1.5
Unopposed estrogen use	–	1.2–2
Protective factors		
Multiparity	–	0.4–0.6
Oral contraceptive use	–	0.7
Hysterectomy or tubal ligation	–	0.6–0.7

HPNCC, hereditary nonpolyposis colorectal cancer.

Adapted from Holschneider CH, Berek JS. Ovarian cancer: epidemiology, biology, and prognostic factors. *Semin Surg Oncol* 2000;19(1):3–10.

Patient-Related Factors

Risk factors associated with a higher frequency of ovulatory events, such as advancing age, low parity, infertility, early menarche, and late menopause, support the proposed mechanism of incessant ovulation.[28–31] Although infertility is associated with ovarian cancer, the use of fertility drugs has not been conclusively linked.[32–34] Suppression of ovulatory events from pregnancy, breast-feeding, and oral contraceptive use may explain the observed protective benefit.[30,31,35] With oral contraceptive use for 4, 8, or 12 years, the risk of ovarian cancer is reduced by 40%, 53%, and 60%, respectively.[36] In a collaborative meta-analysis of 45 epidemiologic studies from 21 countries, the use of oral contraceptives was significantly associated with a decreased risk of ovarian cancer in ever users (hazard ratio [HR] 0.73, $p < .0001$), with larger reductions observed for longer duration of use.[37] The authors conclude that 200,000 ovarian cancers and 100,000 deaths have been prevented since the introduction of oral contraceptives 50 years ago.

Other patient-related risk factors such as polycystic ovarian disease and endometriosis may act through hormonal mechanisms attributable to elevated gonadotropins or by chronic inflammation. In a meta-analysis of eight case-control studies, women with polycystic ovarian disease had a 2.5-fold increase in ovarian cancer risk.[38] Endometriosis has been shown to be an independent risk factor for ovarian cancer with an estimated rate of malignant transformation of 2.5%.[39] Ovarian cancers that arise from endometriosis are most often low-grade tumors with endometrioid or clear cell histology and are associated with a better prognosis.[40] Altered hormonal levels such as elevated androgens may also increase risk, whereas progestins have been shown to be protective.[41] Large prospective cohort studies have demonstrated an increase in ovarian cancer risk and mortality with the use of exogenous estrogen and hormone replacement therapy.[42–44] Surgical procedures, including hysterectomy and tubal ligation, are independently associated with a 34% reduction each in ovarian cancer risk, although the protective mechanism is unknown.[29,45–47] Chronic inflammatory conditions such as pelvic inflammatory disease and tuberculous salpingitis were once believed to be causative factors in the development of fallopian tube malignancies, although this theory remains unproven.

Genetic Factors

Heredity tumors account for 10% to 15% of all ovarian cancers, and family history is the strongest risk factor after increasing age.[48,49] The risk of developing ovarian cancer in the general population is approximately 1.4%, whereas the lifetime risk for a woman with one first-degree family member with ovarian cancer is 5% and climbs to 7% with two first-degree relatives. If a hereditary syndrome is present, the lifetime risk is on the order of 25% to 50% with an age of diagnosis approximately 10 years younger than women with sporadic disease.[50]

Three distinct familial ovarian cancer syndromes have been identified by pedigree analysis with autosomal dominant patterns of inheritance.[51,52] *BRCA1* and *BRCA2* mutations are the most common genetic alterations, with up to 90% of all hereditary cases associated with a deleterious mutation of the *BRCA1* gene, located on chromosome 17q21, or the *BRCA2* gene, located on chromosome 13q22. The lifetime risk of ovarian cancer is approximately 40% in *BRCA1* mutation carriers and 18% in *BRCA2* mutation carriers.[53] BRCA-associated ovarian cancers are most frequently invasive serous adenocarcinomas and less likely borderline or mucinous tumors.[54] Mutation carriers are also more likely to present with advanced stage disease and have poorly differentiated tumors.[55] Nonetheless, *BRCA1* or *BRCA2* mutation carriers have a more favorable clinical course with a significantly longer recurrence-free and overall survival compared to noncarriers. The improved outcome appears related to a higher sensitivity to platinum chemotherapy across first and subsequent lines of treatment.[56,57,58–59,60]

The importance of the fallopian tube in the pathogenesis of extrauterine serous carcinoma was initially recognized in *BRCA1* and *BRCA2* mutation carriers. In a prospective study of 483 *BRCA1* mutation carriers, the incidence of fallopian tube cancer was reported as 120 times that of the general population.[61] High-grade serous primary peritoneal carcinomas are also frequently observed in mutation carriers.[62] Further attention was focused on the fallopian tube as the primary site of origin following reports of epithelial dysplasia and occult serous carcinomas in prophylactic salpingo-oophorectomy specimens from mutation carriers.[63–66] In contrast to the standard pathologic sampling of the ampullary region of the fallopian tube in ovarian cancer cases, more extensive complete sectioning of the tube revealed an abundance of lesions in the fimbria of the distal tube.[14,15–16] The detection of early serous carcinomas, or TICs, lent further support to the emerging concept of the fallopian tube as the primary site for extrauterine serous carcinoma. In this context, the National Comprehensive Cancer Network (NCCN) guidelines recommend that any woman with a diagnosis of ovarian, fallopian tube, or primary peritoneal carcinoma be referred to a cancer genetics professional for consideration of BRCA mutation testing.[67] BRCA screening in a population of women with non-mucinous ovarian cancer detected germline mutations in 14% of women, including 22% with high-grade serous cancer, reinforcing the importance of offering testing to all patients.[68]

Hereditary nonpolyposis colorectal syndrome, or Lynch type II cancer syndrome, is responsible for the remaining 10% of hereditary ovarian cancers.[69] In this syndrome, germline mutations of DNA mismatch repair genes lead to an increased risk of colorectal, stomach, endometrial, and ovarian cancer owing to underlying microsatellite instability. A total of seven mismatch repair genes have been identified with mutations in *MLH1* and *MSH2* accounting for 90% of the observed mutations in Lynch syndrome families.[70,71] Mutations in *MSH6* and *PMS2* have been reported in the remaining 10% of families, whereas alterations in the remaining three identified genes are uncommonly observed. Inactivating mutations in specific genes may modify the underlying cancer predisposition. Women with *MSH6* mutations are twice as likely to develop endometrial cancer compared to carriers of *MSH2* or *MLH1* gene mutations, which are the most common alterations underlying colorectal cancer risk.[72] Women with *MSH2* gene mutations have been shown to have a risk of epithelial ovarian cancer twice that of *MLH1* carriers. In contrast to *BRCA1* and *BRCA2* mutation carriers, women with Lynch syndrome may present with a variety of nonserous epithelial tumor types, including endometrioid and clear cell histologies. Ovarian cancer associated with Lynch syndrome is more often diagnosed at an earlier stage with well to moderately differentiated tumor grade. The lifetime risk of ovarian cancer in women with Lynch syndrome is estimated at 3% to 14% and is most commonly diagnosed in the fifth decade of life.[73] In women with a family or personal history suggestive of Lynch syndrome, tumor testing may be performed by microsatellite instability analysis or immunohistochemistical staining for mismatch repair genes. Direct sequencing of the mismatch repair genes is used for detection of germline mutations. Other less common germline mutations have been identified by genomic sequencing and involve the following genes: BARD1, BRIP1, CHEK2, MRE11A, NBN, PALB2, RAD50, RAD51C, and TP53.[74]

Other genetic disorders linked with nonepithelial ovarian cancers include Peutz-Jeghers syndrome, which is associated with an increased risk of sex cord–stromal tumors, and gonadal dysgenesis, associated with dysgerminomas and gonadoblastomas.

Environmental Factors

Environmental or physical causes of ovarian cancer have been investigated through numerous case-control studies. Women in developing countries have a lower incidence of ovarian cancer than those living in industrialized nations,[75] although to date, no specific chemical carcinogens have been identified. Chronic exposure to asbestos-related products, including talc products, have long been implicated in the development of ovarian cancer.[76] The Nurses' Health Study reported a modestly elevated risk of invasive serous cancers with talc use (relative risk [RR] 1.4), although no association was detected with overall ovarian cancer risk.[77] The development of mucinous ovarian cancer has been found to be associated with cigarette smoking (RR 2 to 2.2) but not other epithelial subtypes.[78,79]

Dietary and metabolic factors have also been explored in large population-based studies as possible contributors to ovarian cancer risk. To date, there have been no consistent associations of coffee or alcohol consumption with increased risk. Large epidemiologic studies also showed no relationship between consumption of animal fat and the development of ovarian cancer.[80,81] In a recent Swedish population-based cohort study of the effect of body mass index on cancer risk in >35,000 women, a 36% higher risk of cancer was observed in obese women (body mass index ≥30) relative to women with body mass index in the normal range (18.5 to 25); cancer sites most strongly related to obesity were endometrium, ovary (risk for top quartile 2.09; 95% confidence interval [CI], 1.13 to 4.13), and colon.[82] Obesity has also been associated with increased ovarian cancer mortality in a large prospective study of adults in the U.S.[83] There is no clear relationship between exercise and ovarian cancer risk.

SCREENING

In the absence of a reliable screening test, most women with ovarian cancer are diagnosed with advanced-stage disease. In contrast to women with localized disease (stage I/II) who have estimated 5-year survival rates of 70% to 90%, overall survival for women with advanced disease (stage III/IV) is poor, ranging from 20% to 45% (Table 71.3). The low sensitivity and specificity of the available screening modalities and the low prevalence of the disease in the general population have hindered the development of a robust screening test. Recent screening approaches have been associated with a low positive predictive value and unacceptable false-positive rates without impacting disease mortality in the general population or high-risk groups.

Several screening strategies have been investigated, including pelvic exam, the serum tumor marker CA-125, and transvaginal ultrasound (TVUS), either alone or in combination.[84] CA-125 values >35 U/mL are observed in 80% of patients with epithelial ovarian cancer, including 90% of women with advanced-stage disease, but only in 50% of early-stage patients.[85] CA-125 is nonspecific for ovarian cancer, as it can be elevated in benign gynecologic and nongynecologic conditions as well as nongynecologic cancers. Screening with CA-125

TABLE 71.3 EPITHELIAL OVARIAN CANCER STAGE DISTRIBUTION AND SURVIVAL BY STAGE

FIGO Stage	Patients (n = 4,825) (%)	5-Year Overall Survival (%)
IA	13	90
IB	1	86
IC	14	83
IIA	2	71
IIB	2	66
IIC	5	71
IIIA	3	47
IIIB	6	42
IIIC	42	33
IV	13	19

FIGO, International Federation of Gynecology and Obstetrics.

Adapted from Heintz APM, Odicino F, Maisonneuve P, et al. Carcinoma of the ovary. FIGO 26th Annual Report on the Results of Treatment in Gynecological Cancer. *Int J Gynaecol Obstet* 2006;95(Suppl 1):S161–S192.

alone has been found to lack specificity in an average-risk population of postmenopausal women. Ultrasound alone is able to detect early-stage disease in an average-risk population,[86–88] although the significant false-positive rate remains a concern. In a United Kingdom multimodality screening study, diagnostic surgeries were performed nine times more frequently to detect one cancer in the group screened by TVUS alone compared to multimodality screening (CA-125 and TVUS).[89]

Several large screening trials currently in progress in the United States, United Kingdom, and Japan have been designed to assess reduction in mortality with early detection of ovarian cancer. The Prostate, Lung, Colorectal, and Ovarian Cancer (PLCO) screening trial in the United States randomized 78,216 women aged 55 to 74 to annual screening with CA-125 and TVUS versus usual medical care. Following baseline screening, 570 surgical procedures, including 325 laparotomies, were performed; 29 tumors were detected, 9 of which were of LMP.[90] The positive predictive value for the detection of invasive ovarian cancer was 3.7% for an abnormal CA-125, 1.0% for an abnormal TVUS, and 23.5% for both. Publication of the mortality data with 12-year follow-up showed no difference in the stage of cancer detected by screening (90% stage III or IV) and no reduction in cause-specific or overall mortality for women who underwent screening.[91] Furthermore, diagnostic evaluation for women with false-positive screening resulted in a serious complication rate of 15%.

A second trial, the United Kingdom Collaborative Trial of Ovarian Cancer Screening (UKCTOCS), has accrued >200,000 postmenopausal women to evaluate multimodality screening with TVUS and serum CA-125. In the prevalence screen, the sensitivity, specificity, and positive predictive values of multimodality screening for invasive epithelial ovarian and tubal cancers were 89.5%, 99.8%, and 35.1%, respectively.[89] The initial results of baseline screening were more promising than the U.S. study, with 43% of invasive cancers detected as stage I or II, which may reflect differences in study design and the diagnostic algorithm. The effect of multimodality screening on mortality is awaiting further follow-up. The multicenter, randomized Japanese study utilizes a similar screening strategy with TVUS and CA-125 and has accrued >80,000 women. Unlike the U.S. and UK trials, there was a nonsignificant trend for the detection of more stage I cancers in the screened population (63% vs. 38%), although mortality rates have not yet been reported.[92]

The present data do not support routine screening for ovarian cancer in the general population. All of the North American expert groups, including the U.S. Preventive Services Task Force, the American College of Obstetricians and Gynecologists (ACOG), the Society of Gynecologic Oncologists (SGO), and the Canadian Task Force on the Periodic Health Examination, recommend against routine screening in asymptomatic women. The incidence of ovarian cancer is relatively low in the general population; thus, the concerns for false-positive screening and the associated risks of exploratory surgery are significant.[93] However, women at high risk for ovarian cancer with *BRCA1* or *BRCA2* mutations or hereditary nonpolyposis colorectal syndrome could potentially benefit from chemoprevention; screening with pelvic examinations, TVUS, and CA-125 on a biannual or annual basis; or prophylactic surgery.[94] Although the efficacy of screening has been disappointing in the high-risk population,[95] the ACOG, SGO, and NCCN guidelines recommend routine screening with pelvic exam, CA-125 and TVUS for women with hereditary ovarian cancer syndromes beginning at the age of 30 to 35, or 5 to 10 years earlier than the age of diagnosis of ovarian cancer in the family. The U.S. National Institutes of Health Consensus Development Panel recommends that prophylactic salpingo-oophorectomy be considered in women with ovarian cancer syndromes at age 35 years or after childbearing is complete, as the risk reduction with salpingo-oophorectomy is 80%.[96,97] Removal of the ovaries also reduces the risk of breast cancer in BRCA mutation carriers.[98]

HISTOLOGIC CLASSIFICATION

The World Health Organization and International Federation of Gynecology and Obstetrics (FIGO) have adopted a unified classification of the common epithelial, germ cell, sex cord, and stromal tumors[99] (Table 71.4). Most ovarian malignancies (60% to 65%) are epithelial, with germ cell tumors (20%), sex cord–stromal

TABLE 71.4 WORLD HEALTH ORGANIZATION CLASSIFICATION OF OVARIAN TUMORS

Epithelial tumors			
	Serous		
		Adenocarcinoma	
		Surface papillary carcinoma	
		Adenocarcinofibroma (malignant adenofibroma)	
	Mucinous		
		Adenocarcinoma	
		Adenocarcinofibroma (malignant adenofibroma)	
		Mucinous cystic tumor with mural nodules	
		Mucinous cystic tumor with pseudomyxoma peritonei	
	Endometrioid		
		Adenocarcinoma NOS	
		Adenocarcinofibroma (malignant adenofibroma)	
		Malignant Müllerian mixed tumor (carcinosarcoma)	
		Adenosarcoma	
		Endometrioid stromal sarcoma	
		Undifferentiated ovarian carcinoma	
	Clear cell carcinoma		
		Adenocarcinoma	
		Adenocarcinofibroma (malignant adenofibroma)	
	Transitional cell carcinoma		
	Squamous cell tumors		
	Mixed epithelial tumors		
	Undifferentiated and unclassified tumors		
Germ cell tumors			
	Dysgerminoma		
	Endodermal sinus tumor		
	Embryonal carcinoma		
	Polyembryoma		
	Choriocarcinoma		
	Teratoma		
		Immature	
		Mature	
			Solid
			Cystic
			Dermoid cyst with malignant transformation
			Monodermal
		Mixed	
Tumors composed of germ cells and sex cord–stromal derivative			
	Gonadoblastoma		
	Mixed germ cell-sex cord-stromal tumor		
Sex cord tumors			
	Granulosa-stromal cell tumors		
		Granulosa cell tumor	
		Adult type	
		Juvenile type	
	Thecoma-fibroma group		
		Thecoma	
		Fibroma-fibrosarcoma	
		Sclerosing stromal tumor	
	Sertoli-stromal cell tumors		
		Sertoli cell tumor	
		Leydig cell tumor	
		Sertoli-Leydig cell tumor	
Sex cord tumor with annular tubules			
Steroid cell tumors			
	Stromal luteoma		
	Leydig cell tumor		
	Steroid cell tumor NOS		
Unclassified			
Gynandroblastoma			

NOS, not otherwise specified.

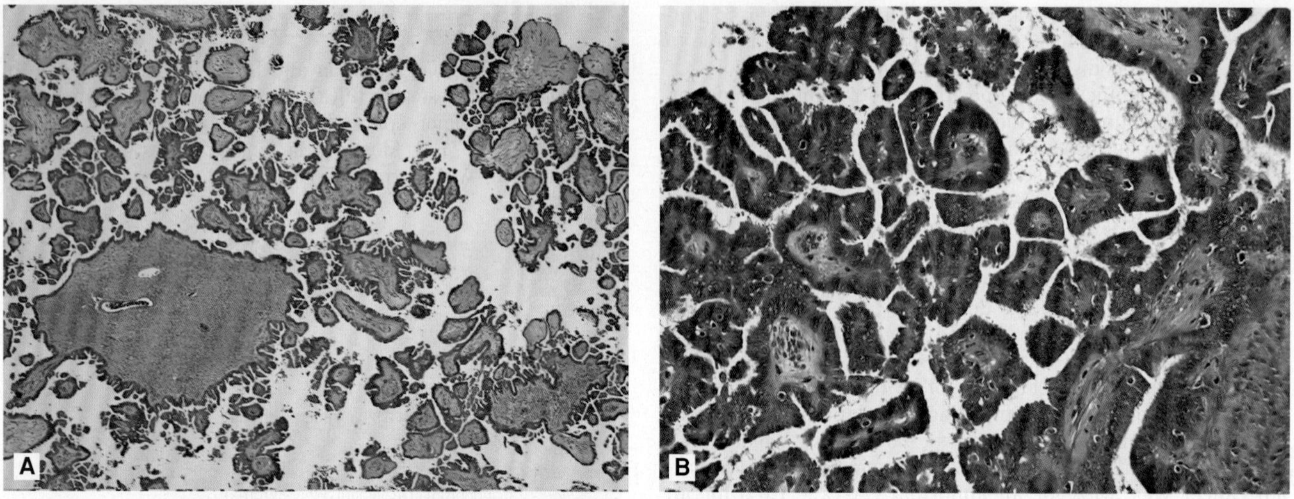

FIGURE 71.3. Serous tumor of low malignant potential of the ovary at low power **(A)** and high power **(B)**. At low power, note the progressively branching papillary fronds with fibrovascular support and detached papillary clusters; at high power, note the serous epithelium with nuclear hyperchromasia and cytologic atypia. By definition, there is no destructive stromal invasion.

tumors (5%), and metastases to the ovary (5% to 10%) accounting for the remainder.[100] Serous tumors are most common, comprising 50% to 60% of epithelial tumors. Other subtypes include mucinous carcinoma in 10%; endometrioid carcinoma, 8%; clear cell carcinoma, 3% to 5%; transitional, 3% to 5%; and undifferentiated carcinoma, 1%. Bilateral presentation occurs frequently in epithelial tumors, most commonly in serous tumors followed by endometrioid (15%) and mucinous tumors (5% to 10%).

High-grade serous carcinomas are often widely disseminated at diagnosis and account for most deaths from ovarian, tubal, and peritoneal cancers. In contrast, 5-year survival for low-grade serous carcinoma is 85%. Most serous tumors present as large ovarian masses and grossly appear nodular with multiple papillary projections and cysts filled with clear serous fluid. A two-tiered grading system separates high-grade serous carcinomas from low-grade tumors,[101,102] which have a similar prolonged natural history to noninvasive borderline tumors, or tumors of LMP.[103] As discussed previously, there is increasing evidence that high grade serous carcinomas originate in the fimbria of the fallopian tube and may spread rapidly to the adjacent ovary and peritoneal sites. Low-grade tumors appear to follow a stepwise progression from borderline tumor to invasive carcinoma and involve molecular pathways distinct from their high-grade counterparts.[104–106] Although treatment is similar for all serous tumors, low-grade tumors have been shown to be less responsive to chemotherapy.[103,107,108]

LMP or borderline tumors have nuclear abnormalities and mitotic activity intermediate between benign and malignant tumors of similar cell type but lack stromal invasion (Fig. 71.3). Borderline tumors are a subcategory of ovarian malignancies that account for 10% to 20% of all epithelial neoplasms.[109,110] The prognosis, surgical approach, and postoperative treatment recommendations are vastly different as compared with those of their invasive counterparts. The majority of LMPs (75%) present with stage I disease, which directly contrasts with the 75% advanced stages in the invasive epithelial tumors. The 5- and 10-year survival rates for women with LMP tumors are >95%. Significant heterogeneity exists in the biologic behavior of borderline tumors. Women with nonlocalized LMP tumors of the ovary have decreased survival compared to those with localized LMP tumors but are similar to that of women with localized, well-differentiated epithelial ovarian carcinoma.[111] Other pathologic features that affect prognosis include the cell type, tumor stage, implant type (invasive vs. noninvasive), the presence of micropapillary architecture, and microinvasion. Extensive sampling of all pathologic specimens is required to firmly establish the diagnosis.

Most endometrioid and clear cell carcinomas arise in foci of endometriosis and follow an adenoma to borderline tumor to carcinoma sequence. Endometrioid carcinoma of the ovary resembles its endometrial counterpart (Fig. 71.4), and synchronous primary cancers are detected in 10% of women with ovarian cancer and 5% of women with endometrial cancer.[112] Bilateral ovarian involvement, small multinodular ovaries, and surface and hilar spread suggest metastatic involvement from an endometrial primary, particularly if the endometrial tumor is high-grade, deeply invasive, and associated with lymphovascular invasion. A large, cystic, unilateral tumor of low grade arising in a focus of endometriosis likely represents a primary ovarian tumor. Endometrioid tumors appear to have a better prognosis than serous cancers regardless of tumor stage.[113] Multiple synchronous primary tumors may represent a field defect related to endometriosis, which is associated with improved survival.[114]

Mucinous tumors follow a similar progression from cystadenoma to borderline tumor prior to invasion. All subtypes are more likely to be diagnosed when confined to the ovary. Mucinous cancers may grow to a very large size, often measuring up to 20 cm in diameter and filled with large pockets of thick, necrotic, mucinous debris.[115,116] Ovarian mucinous tumors closely resemble mucin-secreting tumors originating from other sites—most commonly the gastrointestinal tract. The pathologic distinction between primary and metastatic mucinous carcinoma may be challenging, despite the use of immunohistochemical analysis. Further clinical evaluation is often required to exclude a clinically occult nonovarian primary source. Secondary involvement of the ovary may also occur in association with pseudomyxoma peritonei arising from a low-grade tumor often of appendiceal origin.[117]

Clear cell carcinoma is characterized by clear and hobnail cells with a similar histologic appearance to clear cell carcinoma of the kidney, endometrium, and vagina. Ovarian clear cell carcinoma is often seen in association with venous thromboembolism and hypercalcemia. Although more likely to be stage I than serous carcinoma, clear cell histology is associated with a lower response rate to platinum-based chemotherapy, higher recurrence rate, and worse survival.[118] The transitional cell tumors, including Brenner tumors, are benign in most cases (98%) and carry a favorable prognosis.

Ovarian germ cell tumors comprise <5% of ovarian malignancies and are classified by the World Health Organization (Table 71.4). Dysgerminomas are the most common of the germ cell tumors and occur bilaterally in 10% to 20% of cases. The other germ cell tumor types are typically unilateral. Endodermal

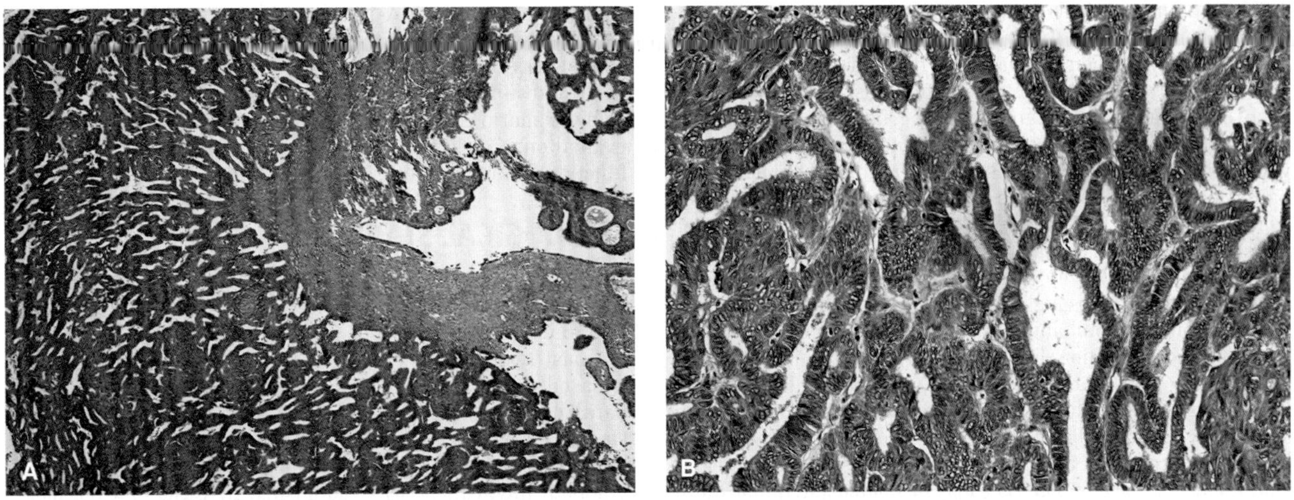

FIGURE 71.4. Endometrioid adenocarcinoma of the ovary. **A:** At low power, note the tumor composed of back-to-back endometrioid glands. **B:** At high power, note the squamous metaplasia, commonly seen in this epithelial variant. Assignment of tumor grade is based on similar criteria as for carcinomas arising in the endometrium. This tumor would qualify as well differentiated or grade 1.

sinus tumors, also known as yolk sac tumors, are characterized by Schiller-Duvall bodies. Embryonal carcinomas are rare and tend to occur in younger populations; they may be seen with nongestational choriocarcinomas as part of mixed germ cell tumors (10% of all germ cell tumors). Immature teratomas are characterized by immature elements from the germ layers. The grade, treatment recommendations, and outcome are directed by the amount of immature neural elements.

Sex cord–stromal tumors are also classified by the World Health Organization (Table 71.3), with granulosa cell tumors being the most common (70%). Histologically, the granulosa cell tumors are composed of granulosa cells that have a pale, grooved, "coffee bean" nuclei or a rosette of cells surrounding eosinophilic material, a Call-Exner body. Thecomas (hormonally active) and fibromas (hormonally inactive) are both clinically benign tumors and are most common in middle-age women.

The most common histopathology of primary fallopian tube malignancies is papillary serous adenocarcinoma. Other less common Müllerian subtypes include endometrioid, clear cell, and malignant mixed Müllerian tumors.[119,120] Rare reports of squamous cell carcinoma, immature teratoma, glassy cell tumor, and sarcoma have also been described. Benign tumors are found even less frequently than malignant neoplasms. Metastatic involvement of the fallopian tube is reported in up to 12% of women with uterine cancer and 4% with cervical cancer.[121,122]

PATTERNS OF SPREAD

The primary mode of spread for epithelial ovarian and fallopian tube cancers is transperitoneal, as malignant cells exfoliate into the peritoneal cavity. Intraperitoneal spread is favored by intestinal peristalsis and negative hydrostatic pressure below the diaphragm. The exfoliated tumor cells follow the intra-abdominal fluid stream passing along the paracolic gutters toward the diaphragm, predominately on the right side, before implantation on any peritoneal surface.[123,124] Metastatic deposits are frequently seen in the posterior cul-de-sac, paracolic gutters, diaphragmatic surfaces, liver capsule, intestinal surfaces, and omentum. Metastases may also be found in the uterus or contralateral ovary from peritoneal spread or flow through the fallopian tubes. Dense tumor "caking" can cause infiltration into the abdominal organs creating a mass effect on the omentum, ureter, bowel, liver, pancreas, spleen, or adrenals, resulting in advanced disease stage at presentation with associated ascites.

Lymphatic drainage constitutes the second most common pattern of spread. The lymphatic capillaries of the ovary converge on the hilus and follow the ovarian blood vessels in the infundibular ligament to drain to the para-aortic nodes at the level of the renal hilum. Lymphatics also drain along the broad ligament to the hypogastric and external iliac nodes in the pelvis. Less frequently, spread can occur to the inguinal nodes via the round ligament.[125] Approximately 10% to 15% of women with disease that appears confined to the ovary have para-aortic lymph node involvement,[126] which becomes increasingly common in advanced-stage disease. Because of the rich lymphatic supply of the fallopian tubes, lymph node involvement is common even in the absence of tubal musculature involvement.[127] Pelvic and para-aortic lymph node involvement has been reported in 10% to 30% of women with fallopian tube cancer at diagnosis.[128]

Transdiaphragmatic spread occurs to the pleural cavity and is the most common finding in stage IV disease. Hematogenous spread is infrequent at the time of presentation, with only 2% to 3% of patients with parenchymal liver or lung disease. Brain metastasis is also rare. However, >50% of recurrences occur both within and outside the peritoneal cavity at the time of treatment failure.

CLINICAL PRESENTATION

As ovarian cancer has insidious growth and is asymptomatic in early-stage disease, most women do not present until symptoms arise from advanced disease progression. Vague gastrointestinal complaints of dyspepsia, nausea, early satiety, bloating, constipation, or obstipation are common presenting symptoms, as are genitourinary symptoms including frequency, urgency, or incontinence. Other ill-defined symptoms include fatigue, back pain, pain with intercourse, and menstrual irregularities. These nonspecific symptoms can be present for several months but may not trigger diagnostic evaluation until after the symptoms fail to clear with other medical therapy.[129] Detection of early-stage disease may occur by palpation of an asymptomatic adnexal mass on routine examination, although most adnexal masses require moderate size for palpation. In premenopausal women, most of these masses are benign, as ovarian cancer represents <5% of adnexal neoplasms. An adnexal mass in a postmenopausal woman has a higher likelihood of malignancy, and surgical exploration is often indicated. Physical examination findings such as a fixed pelvic mass, palpable upper abdominal mass, and ascites are highly suggestive of an ovarian malignancy. According to a consensus statement on the symptoms of ovarian cancer published by the Gynecologic Cancer Foundation, SGO, and American Cancer Society, new and persistent symptoms of bloating, pelvic or abdominal pain, difficulty eating, early satiety, or urinary urgency or frequency should prompt women to seek medical evaluation.

A portion of women with fallopian tube carcinoma may present with early clinical signs and symptoms. Two triads have been described as pathognomonic for fallopian tube malignancy: (a) pelvic pain, pelvic mass, and leukorrhea and (b) vaginal bleeding, vaginal discharge, and lower abdominal pain. However, the percentage of patients presenting with either triad of symptoms has been reported as low as 11%.[130] Another classic sign—hydrops tubae profluens—is a sudden emptying of accumulated fluid in the distended fallopian tube that causes profuse, watery, serosanguineous vaginal discharge. The discharge is often accompanied by a decrease in pelvic mass size on physical examination. In a meta-analysis of 122 patients with primary fallopian tube cancer, hydrops tubae profluens was a presenting sign in only 9%.[121] In other series,[124,127] it has been specifically reported that neither a triad nor hydrops tubae profluens was present in any of the patients reviewed. When clinically apparent, the fallopian tube may be dilated and mimic more benign pathologic processes such as hydrosalpinx, pyosalpinx, or hematosalpinx.[131] In more advanced disease with tubal wall invasion, extension of a necrotic mass to involve the ovary may give the initial impression of a tubo-ovarian abscess.

Germ cell and stromal cell malignancies present at an earlier stage than epithelial ovarian or fallopian tube cancers, often related to abdominal discomfort or symptoms of excessive estrogen or androgen production. Granulosa cell tumors may lead to precocious puberty in young girls, and Sertoli-Leydig cell tumors may cause virilization.

DIAGNOSTIC WORKUP

Evaluation of a pelvic mass will be influenced by the patient's age, clinical presentation, and imaging features. An ovarian mass is more likely to be a malignant neoplasm in the pediatric, perimenopausal, and postmenopausal age groups and benign during the reproductive years. Ultrasound is often the first, noninvasive step for the evaluation of a pelvic mass. Sonographic characteristics suggestive of malignancy include irregular borders; a solid component that is not hyperechoic and often nodular or papillary; Doppler demonstration of flow in the solid component; dense multiple irregular septa (>2 to 3 mm); and the presence of ascites, peritoneal masses, enlarged nodes, or matted bowel. Computed tomography (CT) and magnetic resonance imaging (MRI) may be useful preoperatively for surgical planning to determine the extent of intra- and extra-abdominal disease. Although limited as a screening tool, an elevated CA-125 level may suggest more advanced or greater bulk of disease and high-grade serous histology but in general is a weak predictor of surgical resection.[132,133] Human chorionic gonadotropin (β-hCG), α-fetoprotein (AFP), total inhibin, and lactate dehydrogenase levels may aid in the diagnosis of and treatment for nonepithelial germ cell ovarian tumors.

Other conditions may mimic ovarian cancer in their presentation, including colon, gastric, and appendiceal carcinomas as well as metastatic breast cancer and primary lymphoma. Although ideally the primary site of disease is determined in the preoperative setting, the diagnosis often cannot be made accurately until the time of surgery, and frozen section pathologic evaluation may guide surgical approach. Primary malignancies of the fallopian tube have been difficult to diagnose prior to surgical exploration, as the clinical presentation may be similar to that of salpingitis, ovarian abscess, pelvic inflammatory disease, or even ectopic pregnancy. Occult tubal primaries may be detected only by careful pathologic processing.

Referral to a gynecologic oncologist should be considered for any woman with a suspicious pelvic mass, family history of ovarian or fallopian tube cancer, or elevated CA-125.[134] Initial evaluation should include a thorough history and full physical and pelvic examination, laboratory studies (complete blood count, chemistries, CA-125, carcinoembryonic antigen, CA 19–9), and imaging (abdominal CT/MRI, directed ultrasound, chest x-ray). Further evaluation with mammography, upper gastrointestinal endoscopy, or colonoscopy may be indicated in some scenarios. Comorbid conditions may prompt additional evaluations, including cardiac risk assessment, pulmonary function testing, and nutritional evaluation.

SURGICAL STAGING

Surgical advances in staging and the therapeutic benefit of a maximal safe tumor resection have improved the progression-free and overall survival of women with ovarian cancer over the past two decades. Traditional staging for ovarian cancer is based on the FIGO staging system shown in Table 71.5.[135] A parallel American Joint Committee on Cancer system of TNM staging also exists, with strong correlations between stage and the prognostic value of these substages. Staging of primary fallopian tube cancer was established by FIGO in 1992 based on the ovarian cancer staging system. A proposed modification was later published to permit staging of noninvasive tubal carcinomas and fimbrial carcinomas as well as the inclusion of substaging based on depth of invasion[119] (Table 71.6).

Comprehensive surgical staging is the mainstay of diagnosis and initial treatment for ovarian, fallopian tube, and peritoneal cancers.[136] In apparent early-stage cancers, surgical evaluation is required for accurate pathologic staging to guide adjuvant treatment recommendations. In patients with advanced disease, surgery represents the initial treatment by providing optimal cytoreduction. Comprehensive surgical staging begins with an exploratory laparotomy via a vertical midline incision followed by collection of peritoneal washings or any ascitic fluid for cytology. The surgeon performs a thorough inspection of all visceral and peritoneal surfaces within the abdomen and pelvis, with particular attention to the intestinal serosal surfaces, mesentery,

TABLE 71.5 FIGO STAGING FOR OVARIAN CARCINOMA

Stage I	Growth limited to the ovaries
Ia	Growth limited to 1 ovary; no ascites present containing malignant cells. No tumor on the external surface; capsule intact.
Ib	Growth limited to both ovaries; no ascites present containing malignant cells. No tumor on the external surfaces; capsules intact.
Ic	Tumor either stage Ia or Ib, but with tumor on surface of 1 or both ovaries, or with capsule ruptured, or with ascites present containing malignant cells, or with positive peritoneal washings.
Stage II	Growth involving 1 or both ovaries with pelvic extension.
IIa	Extension and/or metastases to the uterus and/or tubes.
IIb	Extension to other pelvic tissues.
IIc	Tumor either stage IIa or IIb, but with tumor on surface of 1 or both ovaries, or with ascites present containing malignant cells, or with positive peritoneal washings.
Stage III	Tumor involving 1 or both ovaries with histologically confirmed peritoneal implants outside the pelvis and/or positive retroperitoneal or inguinal nodes. Superficial liver metastases equals stage III. Tumor is limited to the true pelvis but with histologically proven malignant extension to small bowel or omentum.
IIIa	Tumor grossly limited to the true pelvis, with negative nodes, but with histologically confirmed microscopic seeding of abdominal peritoneal surfaces, or histologically proven extension to small bowel or mesentery.
IIIb	Tumor of 1 or both ovaries with histologically confirmed implants, peritoneal metastases of abdominal peritoneal surfaces with none >2 cm in diameter; nodes are negative.
IIIc	Peritoneal metastases beyond the pelvis >2 cm in diameter and/or positive retroperitoneal or inguinal nodes.
Stage IV	Growth involving 1 or both ovaries with distant metastases. If pleural effusion is present, there must be positive cytology to allot a case to stage IV. Parenchymal liver metastases equal stage IV.

FIGO, International Federation of Gynecology and Obstetrics.

Available at: http://www.igcs.org/files/TreatmentResources/FIGO_IGCS_staging.pdf. Accessed December 27, 2011.

TABLE 71.6 MODIFIED FIGO FALLOPIAN TUBE STAGING

Stage	Description
0	Carcinoma in situ (limited to tubal epithelium).
I	Growth limited to the fallopian tubes.
IA	Growth limited to 1 tube with extension into the submucosa and/or muscularis but not penetrating the serosal surface; no ascites containing malignant cells or positive peritoneal washings.
0b	Growth limited to 1 tube with no extension into lamina propria.
1b	Growth limited to 1 tube with extension into lamina propria but no extension into muscularis.
2b	Growth limited to 1 tube with extension into muscularis.
IB	Growth limited to both tubes with extension into the submucosa and/or muscularis but not penetrating the serosal sursal surface; no ascites containing malignant cells or positive peritoneal washings.
0b	Growth limited to both tubes with no extension into lamina propria.
1b	Growth limited to both tubes with extension into lamina propria but no extension into muscularis.
2b	Growth limited to both tubes with extension into muscularis.
IC	Tumor either stage IA or IB with tumor extension through or onto the tubal serosa; or with ascites present containing malignant cells or positive peritoneal washings.
I (F)	Tumor limited to fimbriated end of fallopian tube(s) without invasion of tubal wall.
II	Growth involving 1 or both fallopian tubes with pelvic extension.
IIA	Extension and/or metastasis to the uterus and/or ovaries.
IIB	Extension to other pelvic tissues.
IIC	Tumor either stage IIA or IIB with ascites present containing malignant cells or with positive peritoneal washings.
III	Tumor involves 1 or both fallopian tubes with peritoneal implants outside the pelvis and/or positive retroperitoneal or inguinal nodes. Superficial liver metastasis equals stage III. Tumor appears limited to the true pelvis but with histologically proven malignant extension to the small bowel or omentum.
IIIA	Tumor grossly limited to the true pelvis with negative nodes but with histologically confirmed microscopic seeding of abdominal peritoneal surfaces.
IIIB	Tumor involving 1 or both tubes with grossly visible histologically confirmed implants of abdominal peritoneal surfaces with none >2 cm in diameter; lymph nodes are negative.
IIIC	Abdominal implants >2 cm in diameter and/or positive retroperitoneal or inguinal nodes.
IV	Growth involving 1 or both fallopian tubes with distant metastasis. If pleural effusion is present, there must be positive cytology to be stage IV. Parenchymal liver metastases equal stage IV.

FIGO, International Federation of Gynecology and Obstetrics.

paracolic gutters, hemidiaphragms, gallbladder, and liver. Systematic biopsies of the bladder serosa, anterior and posterior cul de sac, paracolic gutters, hemidiaphragms, and any suspicious adhesions or implants should be obtained. Total hysterectomy, bilateral salpingo-oophorectomy, infracolic omentectomy, and pelvic and para-aortic lymph nodal sampling may be performed in addition to the intact removal of the adnexal mass when possible. Given the significant risk of contralateral involvement, bilateral lymph node assessment is frequently performed.[137,138] In patients with advanced disease, bowel resection, diaphragm stripping, splenectomy, nodal dissection, and radical resection of peritoneal tumor nodules are often necessary to achieve the desired surgical outcome of maximal debulking. Recently, the role of routine appendectomy has been questioned and is not recommended in the absence of visible pathology.[139]

In select cases, preservation of the contralateral unaffected ovary and the uterus can be achieved in young women wishing to retain fertility who have stage I and/or low-risk tumors (early-stage, low-grade invasive tumors, LMP lesions, or malignant stromal or germ cell tumors).[136] In the setting of unilateral salpingo-oophorectomy, comprehensive surgical staging should be performed to exclude occult disease. Exceptions to upfront surgical management include patients with significant medical comorbidities who are poor operative candidates and patients with a complex ovarian cyst where extraovarian disease has not been excluded. Neoadjuvant chemotherapy followed by interval cytoreduction may be considered in patients with bulky stage III or IV disease. Before initiation of neoadjuvant chemotherapy, the pathologic diagnosis should be confirmed by biopsy, fine-needle aspirate, or paracentesis. The NCCN guidelines recommend that patients who are evaluated for neoadjuvant chemotherapy be seen by a fellowship-trained gynecologic oncologist before being deemed a nonsurgical candidate.[136]

PROGNOSTIC FACTORS

Tumor stage, grade, histology, and optimal cytoreduction by a trained gynecologic oncologist are the most important determinants of survival for ovarian and fallopian tube cancer. Patients with FIGO stage 1A disease who have negative staging laparotomy have 5-year survival rates of 80% to 90%. If extrapelvic disease is detected at the time of surgical staging, the patient is upstaged to stage III disease with corresponding 5-year survival rates of 30% to 50%. Primary or interval cytoreductive surgery should be performed by a gynecologic oncologist based on published evidence of a 6- to 9-month median survival benefit.[140–142]

The volume of residual disease after primary surgery is also an important determinant of outcome.[143–148] Patients who have optimal cytoreduction of tumor have a 22-month improvement in median survival compared to those with suboptimal resection. A meta-analysis of >6,800 women with advanced-stage ovarian cancer treated with adjuvant platinum-based chemotherapy found a 5.5% increase in median survival for every 10% increase in maximal cytoreduction.[144] Although the definition of maximal resection varies by study, <1 mm or no visible disease has been associated with improved response to chemotherapy, less platinum resistance, and longer overall survival.[143,149,150] Preoperative CA-125 measurement is not independently prognostic, as it likely reflects disease burden. In contrast, the half-life and nadir of CA-125 during induction chemotherapy is associated with improved outcome in ovarian and fallopian tube cancers.[120,151–155]

Although a strong correlation exists between histologic grade and stage, grade has independent prognostic significance, particularly in early-stage disease. Survival rates for stage I disease with grade 1, 2, or 3 tumors are 96%, 78%, and 62%, respectively.[156] The impact of histologic subtype on survival is less robust owing to other more important clinical variables, including stage, grade, and volume of disease. Patients with mucinous and endometrioid subtypes have improved survival rates compared to serous adenocarcinoma, predominately related to the earlier stage at presentation. Clear cell carcinomas appear to be more aggressive than other epithelial malignancies. The 5-year survival rate for stage I clear cell carcinoma is 60% and for other stages is <15%.[118]

As reflected in the modified FIGO staging system, depth of tubal invasion has been found to correlate with survival in two large retrospective studies of fallopian tube carcinoma.[120,157,158] In addition to the depth of tubal invasion, the pathology report should provide information on tumor grade and the presence of lymphovascular invasion.

MANAGEMENT OF EPITHELIAL TUMORS

Treatment for ovarian and fallopian tube cancer depends largely on the stage and grade of disease at presentation. Table 71.7 presents a general schematic for treatment recommendations for women with epithelial ovarian and fallopian tube cancer. Although much less common, primary peritoneal cancers are managed in a similar manner.

Early-Stage Disease

Surgical Therapy

Comprehensive surgical staging should be performed in all women with apparent early-stage disease to confirm that the

TABLE 71.7 SCHEMATIC OF THE PRIMARY TREATMENT FOR EPITHELIAL OVARIAN CANCER

Low risk, early stage	
Stage IA/B, grade 1	Observation
Stage 1A/B, grade 2	Observation or IV taxane/carboplatin for 3–6 cycles
High risk, early stage	
Stage 1C, all grades Stage IA/B, grade 3	IV taxane/carboplatin for 3–6 cycles
Stage II	IV taxane/carboplatin for 6–8 cycles IP chemotherapy in optimally debulked patients
Advanced stage	
Optimal debulked stage III	IP chemotherapy IV taxane/carboplatin for 6–8 cycles Clinical trial
Suboptimal debulked stage III/IV	IV taxane/carboplatin for 6–8 cycles Clinical trial Interval cytoreduction if indicated by tumor response and resectability

IV, intravenous; IP, intraperitoneal.

cancer is confined to the adnexa. Fertility-sparing surgery with unilateral salpingo-oophorectomy may be considered in a small subset of women with stage IA disease if the contralateral ovary is normal in appearance.[159] In addition to abdominal exploration and full surgical staging, endometrial biopsy should be performed to sample the endometrium.

Postoperative Management

Early studies by the Gynecologic Oncology Group (GOG) and others have identified a small subgroup of patients with well- to moderately differentiated (grade 1 or 2) stage IA and 1B tumors who have a low risk of relapse and may not require adjuvant therapy.[160,161] The NCCN guidelines state that women with early-stage (FIGO 1A or 1B) grade 1 ovarian cancer may be treated with surgical resection and observation with expected 5-year survival rates on the order of 90%.[136] If observation is considered for women with early-stage grade 2 disease, full surgical staging should be performed.

Adjuvant Chemotherapy

Women with early-stage disease and a less favorable prognosis include patients with grade 3 tumors, clear cell histology, or disease extension beyond the ovarian capsule into the abdominal wall or peritoneum (stage IC or II). Various adjuvant treatment approaches have been investigated to improve clinical outcomes, although the optimal management remains controversial. Few randomized trials have been conducted in this population, and they have been limited by small sample size and lack of power to demonstrate a survival advantage.

Nonetheless, two large multi-institutional trials conducted in Europe randomized women with early-stage ovarian cancer to platinum-based chemotherapy or observation following surgery (Table 71.8). The International Collaborative Ovarian Neoplasm 1 (ICON1) trial enrolled 477 women with FIGO IA-C ovarian cancer inclusive of all tumor grades and histologic subtypes.[162] Adjuvant chemotherapy consisted of six cycles of a platinum-based regimen per institutional preference. With a median follow-up of 9.2 years, 10-year recurrence-free survival was 67% for the chemotherapy arm and 57% for observation (HR 0.7, $p = .02$).[163] Overall survival also favored the chemotherapy group (72% vs. 64%, $p = 0.06$). When stratified by histology and grade, the largest benefit for adjuvant chemotherapy was seen in patients with high-risk disease, defined as FIGO stage 1A grade 3, stages 1B or 1C grades 2 and 3, or any clear cell histology. HRs for recurrence and death for the high-risk subset were 0.52 and 0.48, respectively (both $p < .01$). The second trial, Adjuvant Chemotherapy in Ovarian Neoplasm (ACTION), assigned 448 women with early-stage ovarian cancer to four to six cycles of platinum-based adjuvant chemotherapy or observation following surgery. Women with FIGO 1A grades 2 and 3 disease, all stages IC-IIA, or any clear cell histology were eligible for the trial. Recurrence-free survival, but not overall survival, was significantly improved in the chemotherapy group (70% vs. 62% at 10 years).[164,165] The greatest benefit was seen in the subset of women with nonoptimal surgical staging. In a combined analysis of the ICON1 and ACTION trials, adjuvant chemotherapy was associated with significantly improved overall survival at 5 years (82% vs. 74%) compared to observation.[166]

The GOG conducted a randomized trial to determine the optimal duration of adjuvant chemotherapy in women with high-risk, surgical stage I disease by comparing three versus six cycles of carboplatin and Taxol chemotherapy.[167] Rates of recurrence (25% vs. 20%) and overall survival (81% vs. 83%) were similar at 5 years for three and six cycles of chemotherapy, although six cycles were associated with significantly more toxicity, including neuropathy, granulocytopenia, and anemia. However, subset analysis revealed a significantly lower risk of recurrence for women with serous tumors.[168] At 5 years, recurrence-free survival for women with serous tumors was 83% for six cycles of chemotherapy versus 60% for three cycles (HR 0.33, $p = .04$). Overall survival was also improved at 5 years (86% vs. 73%), although not statistically significant.

Adjuvant Whole-Abdomen Irradiation

WAI was an accepted standard modality in the adjuvant postoperative treatment for completely resected ovarian cancer; however, its use declined significantly after 1975. The practical advantage of WAI was the ability to treat all of the peritoneal surfaces within the abdomen and pelvis, although the

TABLE 71.8 RANDOMIZED STUDIES OF ADJUVANT CHEMOTHERAPY IN EARLY-STAGE OVARIAN CANCER

Trial	Stage	Study Design	Number of Patients	5-Year DFS%	5-Year OS%	Notes
Observation Versus Chemotherapy						
GOG (1990)	1A, IB grades 1–2	Observation	44	91	94	No survival difference; optimal staging
		Melphalan	48	98	98	
ICON1 (2003, 2007)	I/II	Observation	236	62	70	Largest benefit for high-risk group; no surgical staging
		Platinum-based	241	73[a]	79[a]	
ACTION (2003, 2010)	1A, 1B grades 2–3	Observation	224	68	78	Optimal staging in 1/3
	IC–IIA all grades	Platinum-based	224	76[a]	85	
	Clear cell					
Duration of Chemotherapy						
GOG (2006, 2010)	1A, 1B grade 3	3 cycles CT	232	75	81	No survival difference; greatest benefit for serous tumors
	1C–II all grades	6 cycles CT	225	80	83	
	Clear cell					

DFS, disease-free survival; OS, overall survival; GOG, Gynecologic Oncology Group; ICON1, International Collaborative Ovarian Neoplasm 1; ACTION, Adjuvant Chemotherapy in Ovarian Neoplasm; CT, carboplatin and paclitaxel.

[a]Statistically significant.

delivered dose was limited by the relatively low tolerance of the liver and kidneys. Interest in WAI was established following the publication from Princess Margaret Hospital of a randomized comparison of 147 patients with FIGO 1B, II, or III debulked ovarian cancer who received WAI with a pelvic boost or pelvic radiotherapy followed by chlorambucil.[169] WAI significantly improved 10-year survival rates over limited pelvic radiotherapy and chemotherapy (64% vs. 40%, respectively). The greatest magnitude of the survival benefit was observed in patients with <2 cm of residual disease (10-year survival 78% vs. 51%, respectively). No significant benefit was observed in patients with extensive residual tumor.

Subsequent randomized studies did not find a benefit for WAI compared to combined adjuvant treatment modalities. A multi-institutional trial by the National Cancer Institute of Canada (NCIC) randomized 257 high-risk stage I or optimally debulked stage II or III patients to receive melphalan, WAI, or IP ^{32}phosphorus (^{32}P).[170] All patients had previously received 22.5 Gy to the pelvis prior to study entry. The WAI arm delivered 22.5 Gy to the abdomen in 2.25-Gy fractions. Actuarial 10-year survival rates failed to demonstrate a statistically significant difference among all groups.[171] A second study from the Danish Ovarian Cancer Group (DACOVA) reported similar outcomes for women who received adjuvant WAI versus pelvic radiotherapy with cyclophosphamide or melphalan (4-year survival, 63% vs. 55%, respectively).[172]

WAI has also been shown to be comparable to single or combination chemotherapy in the adjuvant setting. A prospective study from the MD Anderson Cancer Center randomized 149 women with stage I through III ovarian cancer and <2 cm of residual disease to WAI or melphalan.[173] WAI was delivered by a moving strip technique with a pelvic boost. Overall survival at 5 years was 71% for WAI and 72% for the melphalan arm. Severe late gastrointestinal toxicity requiring surgical intervention was reported in 14% of patients who received WAI, attributed to the moving strip technique that delivered excessive pelvic dose. A second prospective trial from the Northwest Oncologic Cooperative Group of Italy randomized 70 women with early-stage high-risk disease to adjuvant WAI or six cycles of cisplatin plus cyclophosphamide. Despite protocol violations in the assigned treatment groups, there was no difference in relapse-free or overall survival when analyzed by treatment received.[174] From these studies, WAI appears equivalent to chemotherapy when delivered in patients with optimally debulked disease but is no longer used. Further dose escalation of WAI to 27.5 Gy does not appear to provide additional survival benefit.[175]

Adjuvant Intraperitoneal ^{32}Phosphorous

IP instillation of ^{32}P was extensively studied as an alternative to external-beam radiotherapy but is no longer in clinical use. In high-risk, early-stage ovarian cancer patients, randomized trials of adjuvant IP ^{32}P versus chemotherapy from the GOG and Norwegian Radium Hospital found no significant differences in disease-free or overall survival in a population with high-risk early-stage disease.[161,176,177] Given a higher incidence of bowel toxicity and limitations of delivery, ^{32}P has largely been replaced by platinum and taxane combination chemotherapy as the adjuvant treatment for early-stage and advanced disease.

Advanced-Stage Disease

Surgical Considerations

Maximal cytoreduction is one of the most important prognostic factors for survival in patients with advanced-stage ovarian cancer. Cytoreductive surgery in advanced-stage disease may improve the patient's disease-related symptoms such as abdominal pain and early satiety and allow for the ability to maintain nutritional status. Optimal debulking may also enhance chemotherapy delivery and response by removal of large hypoxic tumor masses. Bowel resection may be required to remove metastatic implants involving the bowel mesentery or serosa. Extensive upper abdominal surgery, including splenectomy, partial hepatectomy, distal pancreatectomy, and/or diaphragmatic resection, also results in prolonged palliation and improved survival.[178,179]

Second-look laparotomy (SLL) was introduced to assess the extent of residual disease following cytoreductive surgery and adjuvant chemotherapy. Up to 20% to 50% of patients may have residual disease after adjuvant therapy that was not detected on physical examination or by CA-125 levels or imaging. Although SLL demonstrated the prognostic importance of a pathologic remission, it was not found to have a therapeutic benefit in a GOG trial of 800 patients.[180] Therefore, second-look evaluations for the purposes of determining therapy, and not for interval cytoreduction, should be reserved for women enrolled in clinical trials.

Several studies have evaluated the importance of interval cytoreduction following an initial attempt at surgical debulking. In a randomized trial by the European Organisation for Research and Treatment of Cancer (EORTC), 319 women with suboptimally debulked disease (>1 cm residual) were assigned to six cycles of cisplatin/cyclophosphamide chemotherapy or interval cytoreduction after three cycles of chemotherapy, followed by an additional three cycles.[181] Progression-free and overall survival were significantly improved with interval cytoreduction (median overall survival 26 vs. 20 months, $p = .04$) without increased surgical morbidity. However, a subsequent GOG trial of 550 women failed to reproduce these results.[182] Following a suboptimal resection in the GOG trial, patients were randomized to three cycles of cisplatin and paclitaxel followed by interval debulking or chemotherapy alone for a maximum of six cycles in both arms. The absence of a survival benefit may be attributable to differences in the chemotherapy used or more aggressive initial surgical management by gynecologic oncologists in the GOG trial.

The role of neoadjuvant chemotherapy has been explored in a randomized EORTC/NCIC trial of 670 women with stage IIIC and IV ovarian, fallopian tube, or primary peritoneal cancer randomized to initial surgical debulking followed by six cycles of cisplatin-based chemotherapy or interval debulking after three cycles, followed by three additional cycles.[183] The cohort had extensive bulky disease, with >60% of patients with metastases >10 cm. Although progression-free and overall survival were similar between the two groups, interval surgery achieved optimal cytoreduction more often (81% vs. 42%) and with fewer surgical complications. A major criticism of the trial is that the median survival was significant lower than that of recently reported U.S. trials, which may be related to selection of higher-risk patients. NCCN guidelines state that more data will be necessary prior to recommending neoadjuvant chemotherapy in potentially resectable patients, and upfront debulking surgery remains the treatment of choice in the United States.[136]

Chemotherapy for Advanced-Stage Disease

Platinum agents are the most active class of compounds in the adjuvant treatment for ovarian cancer. Before 1980, alkylating-based regimens such as cyclophosphamide and doxorubicin were used with clinical response rates of 15% to 20%. GOG 47 demonstrated an improvement in clinical complete response rates (51% vs. 26%) and progression-free survival (13 months vs. 8 months) with the addition of cisplatin to cyclophosphamide and doxorubicin. Cisplatin has since been used extensively in both single-agent and multidrug studies. A meta-analysis of 49 trials from the Advanced Ovarian Cancer Trialists Group found that platinum combination chemotherapy improved survival rates over the same nonplatinum regimen (HR 0.88, 95% CI 0.79 to 0.98) and nonplatinum monotherapy (HR 0.93, 95% CI 0.83 to 1.05).[184] The women in the nonplatinum groups routinely received platinum chemotherapy at the time of relapse, likely obscuring the magnitude of the benefit.

TABLE 71.9 RANDOMIZED STUDIES OF ADJUVANT CHEMOTHERAPY IN ADVANCED-STAGE OVARIAN CANCER

Trial	Stage	Study Design	Number of Patients	Median PFS (months)	Median OS (months)	Notes
GOG 172 (2006)	III	IP/IV cisplatin/paclitaxel	415	23.6	65.6	Greater toxicity in IP/IV arm
	≤1 cm residual	IV cisplatin/paclitaxel		18.3[a]	49.7[a]	
Japanese GOG (2009)	II–IV	Dose-dense CT	631	28.0	–	More anemia with dose-dense schedule
		CT (every 21 days)		17.2[a]		
GOG 218 (2010)	III–IV	CT	1,873	10.3	39.3	Higher rates of hypertension, GI perforation, and fistula
		+ c. bevacizumab		11.2	38.7	
		+ c./m. bevacizumab		14.1[a]	39.7	
ICON7 (2010)	High risk I–II	CT	1,528	17.4	–	Greatest benefit in high-risk subset
	III–IV	+ c./m. bevacizumab		19.8[a]		

PFS, progression-free survival; OS, overall survival; IP, intraperitoneal; IV, intravenous; CT, carboplatin and paclitaxel; c., concurrent; m., maintenance; GI, gastrointestinal; ICON7, International Collaborative Ovarian Neoplasm 7.
[a]Statistically significant.

This meta-analysis also incorporated data from 11 trials that directly compared carboplatin and cisplatin, either as single agents or in combination with other drugs, which suggested no difference in efficacy between the two agents. Carboplatin clearly has fewer treatment-related side effects, including less nephrotoxicity, neurotoxicity, and emetogenic potential, and is considered standard of care. However, carboplatin does have more associated myelosuppression, primarily thrombocytopenia, which is cumulative and may be dose limiting.

In addition to platinum compounds, taxanes have become a cornerstone of the treatment schemas for women with epithelial ovarian cancer. GOG 111 was a randomized study comparing cisplatin and paclitaxel with cisplatin and cyclophosphamide in women with suboptimally debulked, large-volume ovarian cancer. The paclitaxel-containing arm demonstrated improved clinical response rates (73% vs. 60%), progression-free survival (18 months vs. 13 months), and overall survival (38 months vs. 24 months).[185] A second GOG study of 614 women with advanced disease and suboptimal resection compared single-agent cisplatin to 24-hour infusion of paclitaxel and to the combination of paclitaxel and cisplatin.[186] Cisplatin alone or in combination with paclitaxel resulted in improved clinical response rates and progression-free survival, although overall survival was similar in the three arms. Combination chemotherapy also had lower cumulative toxicity. As several trials have demonstrated the comparable efficacy of cisplatin and carboplatin, combination carboplatin and paclitaxel has become the preferred first-line chemotherapy regimen. Although the standard dosing of intravenous carboplatin and paclitaxel is every 21 days, a phase III trial from Japan demonstrated significant gains in progression-free and overall survival with a dose-dense regimen of weekly paclitaxel in combination with carboplatin given every 3 weeks[187] (Table 71.9). Grade 3 or 4 anemia was more common in the dose-dense arm, although other toxicities were similar. Dose-dense paclitaxel and carboplatin is a recommended intravenous regimen by the NCCN.[136] Carboplatin and docetaxel is also an acceptable first-line alternative and may be considered for patients at high risk for neuropathy.[188] Phase III trials have failed to show a benefit for the addition of a third agent to the carboplatin and paclitaxel regimen. GOG 182-ICON5 was a five-arm randomized trial of 4,312 women that compared the addition of gemcitabine, liposomal doxorubicin, or topotecan to carboplatin and paclitaxel. There were no improvements in progression-free or overall survival with any experimental regimen.[189]

The role of novel biologics in the first-line treatment for ovarian, fallopian tube, and primary peritoneal cancers is under active investigation. Antiangiogenics have demonstrated activity in the recurrent treatment setting, and the addition of bevacizumab to conventional first-line chemotherapy has recently been tested in two randomized trials. Bevacizumab is a humanized monoclonal antibody directed against the VEGF receptor that may inhibit tumor angiogenesis and improve chemotherapy delivery. GOG 218 reported that the addition of concurrent and maintenance bevacizumab for 15 months significantly improved progression-free survival compared to six cycles of carboplatin and paclitaxel alone (14.1 months vs. 10.3 months).[190] The benefit was not seen in the group who received concurrent bevacizumab without maintenance therapy. Rates of hypertension, gastrointestinal perforation, and fistula formation were higher with the use of bevacizumab. With a median follow up of 17.4 months, overall survival was similar between the treatment arms. The ICON7 trial also reported a progression-free but not overall survival benefit with concurrent bevacizumab and carboplatin/paclitaxel chemotherapy.[191] The greatest benefit was observed in patients at high risk for progression, defined as FIGO stage IV or >1 cm of residual disease and FIGO stage III (median progression-free survival of 16 months vs. 10.5 months). Concerns about cost and lack of an overall survival benefit have tempered the widespread adoption of bevacizumab to the first-line chemotherapy backbone. The NCCN Ovarian Cancer Panel had a major disagreement about recommending the addition of bevacizumab to upfront therapy with carboplatin/paclitaxel or as maintenance therapy, as reflected in a category 3 recommendation.[136] A phase III trial of the oral antiangiogenic nintedanib (BIBF 1120) in combination with carboplatin and paclitaxel is open to accrual for women with newly diagnosed ovarian, fallopian tube, or primary peritoneal cancer. Pazopanib, a potent multitargeted tyrosine kinase inhibitor against VEGF receptor, PDGF receptor, and c-Kit is being tested as maintenance therapy following surgical debulking and first-line chemotherapy.

Intraperitoneal Chemotherapy

Because of the unique peritoneal dissemination of epithelial ovarian and fallopian tube cancer, there has been a significant interest in evaluating IP administration of chemotherapy, which allows for a severalfold increase in drug concentration compared to systemic delivery. However, penetration into tumor tissue may be limited such that therapy is best suited for patients with minimal residual disease after surgical debulking. The National Cancer Institute published a consensus statement in 2006 stating that IP chemotherapy should be offered to every woman with optimally debulked advanced-stage ovarian cancer based on the findings of GOG 172 (Table 71.9), which showed a progression-free and overall survival benefit to IP chemotherapy when compared with intravenous therapy alone (23.6 months vs. 18.3 months and 65.6 months vs. 49.7 months, respectively).[192] Only 42% of patients completed all six cycles of IP chemotherapy owing to treatment-related toxicity and catheter-related complications, which included gastrointestinal events, abdominal pain, metabolic abnormalities, neuropathy, catheter infection, and blockage. Despite the higher incidence of toxicity, additional support for IP chemotherapy is derived from a meta-analysis of eight trials comparing IP to intravenous administration of platinum-based chemotherapy. IP delivery resulted in a 22% decrease in the risk of death, which translated into a 12-month median survival benefit.[193] NCCN guidelines state that stage II patients may also receive IP chemotherapy, although randomized evidence has not yet been published.[136] Despite the clinical advisory, IP chemotherapy has not been consistently adopted for treatment in women with optimally debulked ovarian cancer given the technical demands and increased toxicity. Patients with poor performance status, medical comorbidities, stage IV disease, or advanced age may not tolerate the IP regimen. The feasibility and effectiveness of IP carboplatin will be evaluated in a phase III GOG trial comparing a modified GOG 172 intravenous/IP cisplatin/paclitaxel regimen to IP carboplatin/weekly paclitaxel as well as intravenous carboplatin/weekly paclitaxel (dose-dense regimen). All three arms will receive concurrent and maintenance bevacizumab for 1 year.

CONSOLIDATIVE THERAPY FOR EPITHELIAL OVARIAN CANCER

Consolidative radiotherapy was introduced in hopes of eradicating subclinical residual disease in women who remain at high risk for relapse following surgical cytoreduction and adjuvant chemotherapy. Despite a negative SLL, 30% to 50% of women with confirmed clinical remission ultimately relapse, most commonly in the pelvis or upper abdomen. Consolidative WAI as well as IP radiocolloid have been evaluated in several studies, although randomized data are currently lacking. Radiotherapy is not currently used as consolidative treatment for ovarian or fallopian tube carcinomas, although it may have a role in the salvage or palliative treatment of select cases.

Consolidative Whole-Abdomen Irradiation

The efficacy of WAI has been demonstrated in early-stage patients with minimal residual disease (<2 cm) after cytoreductive surgery. A few early, prospective randomized trials have evaluated the role of consolidative WAI compared to extended chemotherapy in patients with advanced-stage disease (stage III/IV) after initial surgical cytoreduction, adjuvant chemotherapy, and SLL. In all of these trials, disease-free and overall survival rates were not found to be significantly different between WAI and chemotherapy.[194–196] A possible limitation of these trials was that women with macroscopic residual disease after SLL were eligible for enrollment.

Two recent trials have evaluated consolidative WAI in patients with complete clinical or pathologic remission following cytoreductive surgery and adjuvant chemotherapy. A randomized study from Austria demonstrated improved disease-free and overall survival for consolidative WAI, with the greatest benefit seen in stage III patients.[197] The Swedish-Norwegian Ovarian Cancer Study Group recently reported their long term results from a randomized trial of stage III patients.[198] Following primary cytoreductive surgery and four cycles of cisplatin-based chemotherapy, women with complete remission at second-look surgery were randomized to WAI, six additional cycles of chemotherapy, or observation (if pathologic remission confirmed). In the subgroup with pathologic remission, WAI improved progression-free survival compared to chemotherapy or no further therapy (56%, 36%, and 35%, respectively). Overall survival was not statistically different, although statistical power was limited because only 172 (23%) of 742 enrolled patients were randomized to consolidative treatment.

WAI does not appear to compromise the ability for patients to receive and tolerate salvage chemotherapy following relapse, as recently reported in a phase II study from Princess Margaret Hospital.[199] However, the long-term complication rate using conventional radiotherapy techniques is significant. In a multicenter retrospective study from France with a median follow up of 14 years, late symptomatic enteritis occurred in 20% of patients, of which 8% required surgical intervention for bowel obstruction, and death related to bowel complications occurred in 4%.[200] At this time, WAI is no longer included in the NCCN guidelines as an option for initial or consolidative treatment in ovarian cancer.

Consolidative Intraperitoneal ^{32}Phosphorous

Randomized data evaluating IP ^{32}P as consolidative treatment following SLL are limited. The Norwegian Radium Hospital randomized 50 patients with stage IA high-grade and IB through III disease and negative SLL to ^{32}P versus observation and found no significant difference between the arms.[176] The GOG also conducted a prospective randomized trial of 202 stage III patients with complete clinical remission and microscopically negative disease at SLL.[201] Compared with patients who received no further therapy, those who received ^{32}P (15 mCi) within 10 days of SLL did not have improved 5-year disease-free survival (36% vs. 42%, respectively) or overall survival (63% vs. 67%, respectively).

Recurrent Ovarian Cancer

Women in clinical remission following initial adjuvant treatment for ovarian cancer are followed with a combination of pelvic examination, abdominal and pelvic CT, and serial CA-125 levels. Detection of early relapse by a rising CA-125 is fairly specific, although the lead time between biochemical and clinical progression may be >6 months. Second-line chemotherapy is not curative; thus, the timing of salvage therapy is controversial. The EORTC conducted a randomized trial of early versus delayed treatment for relapsed ovarian cancer that showed no difference in overall survival between the arms.[202] However, the findings have not been widely adopted in the United States owing to criticisms regarding the study design, including lack of stratification by known prognostic factors and nonstandard second-line therapies. An SGO statement encourages physicians to discuss with their patients CA-125 monitoring and the implications regarding treatment and quality of life.

Chemotherapy

The selection of second-line chemotherapy for recurrent ovarian cancer is based on the interval to disease relapse and determination of platinum sensitivity or resistance. Patients who experience an early recurrence within 6 months of the completion of initial chemotherapy, have stable disease, or progress during initial induction chemotherapy are considered platinum-resistant with low likelihood of cure. Women who suffer an early recurrence do have treatment options, including second-line chemotherapy agents (topotecan, weekly paclitaxel, liposomal doxorubicin, gemcitabine, oral etoposide, docetaxel), hormonal therapies, targeted therapeutics, and the opportunity to participate in clinical trials. For women with a late recurrence, retreatment with a platinum-based combination is a reasonable option, and the longer the disease-free interval, the higher the response rate to the agents. With the exception of those women who have a prolonged disease-free interval, the opportunity for a meaningful second remission is low, and one needs to carefully balance quality of life, chemotherapy-related toxicity, cost, and the patient's goals of care.

Several randomized phase III studies are testing the role of antiangiogenics in the recurrent setting with combination chemotherapy. In the OCEANS trial, the addition of bevacizumab to carboplatin/paclitaxel chemotherapy resulted in improved response rates (79% vs. 57%, $p < .001$) and progression-free survival (median 12.4 months vs 8.4 months, $p < .001$) in women with platinum-sensitive recurrent disease.[203] Phase II studies of bevacizumab have demonstrated single-agent activity in patients with platinum-resistant recurrent ovarian cancer with response rates of 15% to 20%.[204,205] However, one of these studies reported a gastrointestinal perforation rate of 11% in a heavily pretreated population. A number of tyrosine kinase inhibitors have been tested in the recurrent setting as single agents with demonstrated response rates of 3% to 29%.[27,206] These agents include cediranib (targets VEGF receptor and c-Kit), sunitinib (targets VEGF receptor, c-Kit, PDGF receptor, RET, and FLT-3), sorafenib (targets VEGF receptor, c-Kit, RAF, and PDGF receptor-b), ENMD2076 (targets VEGF receptor and aurora A), pazopanib (targets VEGF receptor, PDGF receptor, and c-Kit), and cabozantinib (targets VEGF receptor and c-MET). Cabozantinib had a 29% partial response rate in patients with platinum-resistant or refractory ovarian cancer and a 40% response rate in platinum-sensitive disease.[207] A randomized phase II study of nintedanib (BIBF 1120) with activity against VEGF receptor, PDGF receptor, and fibroblast growth factor receptor demonstrated a progression-free survival benefit in the maintenance setting, and a phase III study in newly diagnosed patients is under way.

Emerging data is confirming the activity of PARP inhibitors in select patients with recurrent ovarian cancer. This new class of targeted therapy inhibits key enzymes involved in DNA repair and has been shown to be particularly active in treating cancers in BRCA mutation carriers. In the setting of BRCA deficiency, PARP inhibition results in accumulation of double-strand DNA breaks that are lethal to tumor cells through a mechanism known as synthetic lethality. A substantial number of patients with ovarian cancer have been found to have BRCA-deficient tumors related to germline or somatic mutation, epigenetic silencing, or alteration in microRNA levels. Olaparib has shown single-agent response rates ranging from 28% to 41% depending on dose and BRCA mutation status. In a recent trial of 265 women with platinum-sensitive recurrent ovarian cancer, olaparib resulted in a progression-free survival benefit of 8.4 months compared to 4.8 months with placebo (HR 0.35, 95% CI 0.25 to 0.49).[208] Further studies of PARP inhibitor agents as single agents and in combination therapy are under way in patients with platinum-sensitive and resistant disease.

Palliative Surgery

Secondary cytoreductive surgery with the intent of prolonging survival may benefit a select subset of patients with a long disease-free interval, good performance status, and single or few sites of recurrence.[209] Palliative surgery may also be considered in women who present with symptomatic tumor masses or intestinal obstruction. However, the risk of perioperative mortality and re-obstruction is significant, and the patient's medical condition, performance status, and anticipated life expectancy should be carefully considered before operative intervention. For patients who are not surgical candidates, percutaneous decompression and intravenous hydration with consideration of palliative chemotherapy and/or hospice referral may be appropriate.

Palliative Radiation Treatment

Radiation therapy may be an effective palliative treatment modality in settings where localized recurrences are causing significant symptoms that are unresponsive to systemic therapy. Symptoms such as bleeding, pain, or obstruction in the pelvis, groin, abdomen, or chest may be palliated with an abbreviated course of radiation treatment. Clinical response rates have been reported in the range of 70% to 100%, with complete clinical response rates of 30% to 70% and a median duration of 5 to 11 months.[210–213] Palliative radiotherapy is effective even in patients heavily pretreated with systemic or IP chemotherapy. Pain relief and cessation of bleeding are achieved in >80% of patients, and symptoms from bowel or ureteral obstruction in 65% to 75%.[214] Radiation therapy delivered locally to symptomatic sites appears to be of significant and durable benefit and should be considered for palliative purposes in select patients with symptomatic relapses, particularly in those who are refractory to chemotherapy.

The role of salvage radiotherapy in select patients with isolated pelvic recurrences has been suggested by several reports. In a series by Firat and Erickson,[215] 28 patients with recurrent or persistent disease involving the vagina and/or rectum received palliative radiotherapy delivered by external-beam radiotherapy, brachytherapy, or a combination of both. Bleeding was controlled in all cases, and 79% achieved a complete symptomatic response. Of the 21 patients with no evidence of liver or extra-abdominal disease, 2-year survival was 57% compared to 0% for the 7 patients with liver and extra-abdominal metastases at the time of radiotherapy. In the group of 14 patients with pelvic-confined disease, 5 patients had recurrences in the upper abdomen and 4 patients were long-term survivors >5 years after radiotherapy administration. A second study by Albuquerque et al.[216] evaluated the outcomes of 20 women treated with salvage radiotherapy for isolated extraperitoneal recurrence. Most recurrences were in the pelvis, although 3 patients had regional nodal recurrences and 1 patient had an abdominal wall recurrence. The median delivered dose to a tumor-directed volume was 50.4 Gy, and a brachytherapy boost was delivered in select cases. Local recurrence-free survival at 2 years was 89% for patients with optimal debulking prior to radiotherapy compared to 42% for patients with suboptimal debulking or gross residual disease. The corresponding disease-free survival rates at 3 years were 72% and 22%, and overall survival rates at 5 years were 50% and 19%, respectively. Given the exceptional local control rates, minimal toxicity, and long-term survival, select patients with isolated extraperitoneal recurrences may be appropriate candidates for salvage involved-field radiation treatment.

Ovarian cancer metastatic to the brain is a rare occurrence reported in <1% of patients in autopsy cases and in 2% of clinical series.[217,218] More recent series have suggested an increased incidence as chemotherapy regimens have become more effective.[218] Nonetheless, long-term prognosis is poor, as brain metastases are often a late manifestation of advanced disease, with a median survival time <12 months. In a series of 24 patients with metastatic brain disease treated with whole-brain radiotherapy, stereotactic radiosurgery (SRS), or a combination of whole-brain radiotherapy and SRS, median survival was 8.5 months. Patients with solitary metastatic lesions had significantly improved survival compared to those with multiple metastases of 17 months versus 6 months, respectively.[219] Platinum sensitivity was also recently identified as an important prognostic factor in women with metastatic brain involvement from ovarian cancer. In an analysis of 4,277 women treated at six German hospitals, 74 patients (1.7%) had clinical documentation of brain metastases, of which 61 patients received radiotherapy alone or in combination with surgical resection and chemotherapy.[220] On multivariate analysis, platinum sensitivity (HR 0.23) and good performance status (HR 0.45) were associated with improved survival, whereas multiple lesions (HR 4.4) and low tumor grade (HR 3.1) were associated with adverse outcome. Although the extent of extracranial disease was not associated with outcome in this study, it is unclear whether the prognostic importance of platinum sensitivity was related to control of intracranial or systemic disease.

RADIATION THERAPY TECHNIQUES

Whole-Abdominal Radiation Therapy

The clinical target volume for WAI includes the entire peritoneum from the diaphragm to the pelvic floor, encompassing both the visceral and parietal surfaces as well as the pelvic and para-aortic nodes. Conventionally, large anterior and posterior fields have been used. The simulation technique requires attention to the excursion of the diaphragm at the superior margin during respiration to ensure appropriate coverage. The field should encompass the pouch of Douglas inferiorly as well as the lateral extent of the peritoneal margins, which may be located outside the pelvic brim in obese patients. Fluoroscopy may be used to assess the range of quiet respiratory motion. Alternatively, image fusion of CT scans obtained at inspiration and expiration or throughout the respiratory cycle (four-dimensional [4D] CT) may be used to design the treatment fields. Extended source to skin distance may be required in some patients to ensure adequate coverage. Organs at risk that are dose limiting include the kidneys, liver, small and large bowel, and bone marrow. Kidney doses are limited to 15 Gy with customized blocking, and whole-liver tolerance is 30 Gy. The standard whole-abdomen dose is 30 Gy delivered in 1.2- to 1.5-Gy fractions. An additional boost may be delivered to the pelvis and para-aortic lymph nodes to 45 to 50 Gy, depending on the clinical requirements. Patients will need to be monitored for acute gastrointestinal and hematologic toxicity as well as nutritional support.

The use of intensity-modulated radiation therapy (IMRT) to deliver WAI has been proposed as a means to reduce the radiation dose to the bone marrow and kidneys to decrease the incidence of myelotoxicity and renal damage. Dosimetric analysis has demonstrated improved planning target volume (PTV) coverage and significant dose reductions to bones with equivalent kidney sparing using dynamic multileaf collimator IMRT when compared with conventional fields.[221] The PTV receiving 95% of the prescribed dose improved from 72% to 84%, and the volume of pelvic bones receiving >21 Gy was reduced by a relative 60% from 86% to 35%. Dose inhomogeneity, however, increased slightly, with small regions of underdosing near the kidneys. Similar improvements in PTV dose coverage were reported in a study using IMRT arc therapy.[222] It remains to be seen whether the dosimetric advantages gained from WAI-IMRT will translate to a significant and clinically relevant benefit. Furthermore, technical considerations must be considered with great care given the complex anatomy and delineation of the peritoneal cavity boundaries. Patient breathing motion and setup uncertainties will also need to be addressed.

Intraoperative Radiation for Ovarian Cancer

Several studies have suggested that intraoperative radiation therapy (IORT) as part of salvage surgery for locally recurrent gynecologic cancers, including ovarian cancer, may improve locoregional control and overall survival.[223,224–227] The largest IORT retrospective study to date that reported results of 22 ovarian cancer patients treated with IORT (median dose, 12 Gy; range, 9 to 14 Gy) suggests that the addition of IORT to cytoreductive surgery may potentially improve locoregional control and achieve palliation in highly selected patients with locally recurrent ovarian cancer.[223] Various sites were treated, most commonly the pelvic sidewall. Most patients received additional treatment after IORT, including WAI, pelvic and/or inguinal radiation, and chemotherapy. Locoregional control was achieved in 68% of patients, with a median time to recurrence of 14 months and 5-year disease-free survival of 18% and overall survival of 22%. Overall treatment-related grade 3 toxicities occurred in 41%. Bowel obstruction occurred in seven patients, all of whom received postoperative WAI and two of whom also had a component of locoregional relapse. No long-term neurologic sequelae were reported.

SEQUELAE OF TREATMENT

Acute Toxicity

Acute toxicity from WAI is common but rarely severe. The use of large radiation fields that encompass multiple abdominal organs, including the liver, kidneys, gastrointestinal tract, bladder, spleen, lungs, and pancreas, contributes to the development of predictable side effects. Gastrointestinal side effects are the most common acute and subacute toxicities encountered with WAI given the large volume of bowel within the treatment field. Up to 75% of patients treated with WAI experience mild to moderate diarrhea; severe diarrhea requiring hospitalization and intravenous hydration is seen in 10% of patients. Limiting bowel exposure through the use of shielding or appropriately timed field reductions can minimize or prevent this toxicity. Approximately 60% to 70% may also experience nausea, particularly early during treatment, although emesis occurs infrequently. Premedication with antiemetic therapy 30 to 60 minutes prior to treatment may help to mitigate this side effect. Routine intravenous hydration to prevent dehydration is also recommended. Appetite loss accompanied by weight loss is a frequent concern. It is thus essential to closely monitor and ensure proper nutrition to avoid malnourishment and dehydration that may result in hospitalization and treatment interruption.

Clinically significant liver damage is extremely rare with appropriate shielding.[228] Approximately 50% of patients will develop transiently elevated alkaline phosphatase levels; however, symptomatic hepatitis occurs in <1%.[229] Hematologic toxicity including leukopenia and thrombocytopenia occurs in 10% to 20% of patients, although significant drops in blood counts causing treatment interruption are rare. Splenic damage may occur even at low radiation doses because of the exquisite radiosensitivity of the spleen, resulting in transient reduction in platelet counts.

Urethritis and bladder spasm from pelvic irradiation may occur and should be treated symptomatically. Adequate and careful shielding of the kidneys to limit the delivered dose to <15 Gy is critical to minimize renal damage and failure. Stricture of the ureters or urethra is rare, occurring in <1% of cases and is usually not seen until 3 to 6 months postradiation. Because treatment to the entire peritoneal cavity with adequate margins requires extension of fields above the diaphragm, inclusion of the lung bases bilaterally is required. Chest radiographs may show fibrosis or bibasilar pneumonitis in 5% to 20% of patients but is generally self-limited and rarely symptomatic.

Late Toxicity

Late toxicities were more common with the moving strip technique than with the open-field technique, primarily because of the higher doses and hot spots that were generated. High radiation doses can exceed normal organ tolerances, leading to permanent organ damage and failure. Chronic gastrointestinal damage (i.e., bloating, intermittent diarrhea) occurs in <5% of treated patients. The overall incidence of bowel obstruction has been reported to be 5% to 10% at 5 years in cases in which IP ^{32}P or WAI is used independently. Approximately 50% of these patients who develop bowel obstructions will require surgical intervention (incidence, 3% to 5%); however, recent data suggest that this incidence may be higher and closer to 10% in long-term survivors at 10 years.[200] Bowel obstructions occur more frequently with doses >45 Gy and in patients with gapped or abutted split fields. In addition, adhesions in the peritoneal cavity and the combination of additional pelvic radiation to ^{32}P or WAI may double the risk of significant bowel complications up to 20% to 25%.[170,176] As with most anatomic sites, escalating doses of radiation come with an increase in rate and degree of toxicity. Major bowel complications from 10 pooled series of 1,098 patients reported an incidence of 1.4% with abdominal dose of 22.5 Gy compared with 14% with 30 Gy.[229]

MANAGEMENT OF GERM CELL TUMORS

In general, the presentation and management of nonepithelial tumors are similar to those of their epithelial counterparts, as patients usually experience vaginal bleeding, abdominal bloating, or pain and typically require surgical intervention and chemotherapy. On presentation, routine workup is identical to that for other ovarian cancers as outlined previously. Pretreatment AFP and β-hCG levels are of particular importance in diagnosis

TABLE 71.10 SERUM MARKERS FOR OVARIAN GERM CELL TUMORS

Tumor Type	AFP	hCG	LDH
Dysgerminoma	−	+/−	+
Choriocarcinoma	−	+	−
Endodermal sinus tumor	+	−	−
Immature teratoma	+/−	−	−
Mixed germ cell tumor	+/−	+/−	+/−
Embryonal carcinoma	+/−	+	−
Polyembryoma	+/−	+	−

AFP, α-fetoprotein; hCG, human chorionic gonadotrophin; LDH, lactate dehydrogenase.

and treatment. An elevated β-hCG with a normal AFP is strongly suggestive of dysgerminoma. Lactate dehydrogenase and CA-125 levels should also be drawn, as the germ cell tumors may have several tumor markers that can be followed (Table 71.10). Variations in surgical management and adjuvant chemotherapy and radiation do exist among the nonepithelial tumors, and treatments should consider the patient's desire to maintain fertility while offering the greatest chance for cure.

Most ovarian neoplasms diagnosed in children and adolescents are germ cell tumors, with approximately two-thirds of these tumors being malignant at the time of diagnosis. Germ cell tumors comprise 20% of all ovarian neoplasms and 2% to 5% of all ovarian malignancies. The most common germ cell tumor is the mature cystic teratoma (also the most common ovarian neoplasm); however, fortunately only the minority contain a malignancy or immature elements.

Dysgerminoma

Dysgerminoma is the most common of the malignant germ cell tumors and also has the highest bilaterality rate (20%), with 10% of the ovaries being grossly involved and 10% being microscopically involved. As shown in Table 71.10, dysgerminomas may secrete lactate dehydrogenase and have elevated β-hCG levels. Most women with dysgerminomas receive a diagnosis of early-stage disease, and 80% present before the age of 30 years. In many instances, young women affected by this disease wish to maintain fertility after therapy. The high rate of contralateral disease confers a greater risk with conservative surgical therapy.

Postoperative therapy for patients with dysgerminoma can be separated into those women with stage I disease and those with disease of a more advanced stage. Women with stage IA disease following careful surgical staging can be monitored closely without compromising cure. Approximately 15% to 25% of these women will experience a recurrence, although successful salvage treatment with chemotherapy results in survival rates close to 100%. For women with more advanced stage disease, chemotherapy with three to four cycles of BEP (bleomycin, etoposide, and cisplatin) is recommended.[231] In a report from MD Anderson Cancer Center, >95% of the patients with ovarian dysgerminoma were free from relapse at a median of 7 years follow-up.[230,] Of the 16 women treated with fertility-sparing surgery, 10 patients maintained menstrual function during chemotherapy and 13 patients returned to their prechemotherapy baseline. Five pregnancies were reported, and two of the women had difficulty conceiving.

Dysgerminomas are unique in that they are exquisitely radiosensitive tumors. Radiotherapy may be considered for patients who are not candidates for platinum-based chemotherapy. The appropriate radiation dose for dysgerminoma is 25 Gy in 12 to 14 fractions with a boost of 10 Gy for gross residual disease. However, radiotherapy will affect ovarian function and fertility, which must be taken into consideration when recommending adjuvant radiation therapy in a young patient.

Other Germ Cell Tumors

Nondysgerminomas are almost always unilateral. For apparent early-stage disease, unilateral salpingo-oophorectomy appears to be as effective as more extensive surgery. Patients with stage I grade 1 immature teratomas usually require no further therapy after unilateral salpingo-oophorectomy. All others, including stage I grade 2 and 3 immature teratoma, should be treated with three cycles of BEP chemotherapy. Because of the low number of diagnosed cases, large-scale studies comparing adjuvant therapy are uncommon.

Extrapolation of data regarding the efficacy of chemotherapeutic regimens in treatment for nonseminomatous testicular germ cell tumors has had a great impact on treatment in patients with nondysgerminoma ovarian germ cell tumors. Patients with less well differentiated tumors and all those with endodermal sinus tumor, embryonal carcinoma, choriocarcinoma, or mixed germ cell tumors should receive adjuvant postoperative chemotherapy. Various regimens have been used, including VAC (vincristine, dactinomycin, and cyclophosphamide), PVC (cisplatin, vincristine, and cyclophosphamide), and CVB (cyclophosphamide, vincristine, and bleomycin). The BEP regimen was prospectively evaluated by the GOG in patients with completely resected, surgically staged I, II, and III disease and resulted in a 96% disease-free survival rate.[232] NCCN guidelines recommend three to four courses of BEP as the standard treatment for well-staged patients with resected ovarian germ cell tumors. Six cycles of chemotherapy may be considered for patients with gross residual or stage IV disease.

Management of Sex Cord–Stromal Tumors

Sex cord–stromal tumors derive from the intraovarian matrix of mesenchymal and connective tissue elements that supports the germ cells. The most common sex cord–stromal tumors are the granulosa cell tumors, derived from the sex cord cells along with Sertoli cell tumors. The mesenchymal derivatives include fibromas, thecal cell tumors, and Leydig cell tumors. These tumors are responsible for <5% of all ovarian malignancies but account for 90% of all functioning ovarian neoplasms. One-third of the tumors will produce estrogen, progesterone, testosterone, or other androgens. This hormonal expression may lead to presenting signs and symptoms such as precocious puberty, postmenopausal bleeding, hirsutism, or virilization. Sex cord–stromal tumors can develop in women of any age (with the granulosa cell tumors having a bimodal age distribution) with a peak incidence in postmenopausal women around 50 years of age. These tumors typically behave in a benign fashion with LMP. Surgery remains the mainstay of treatment; however, occasionally, postoperative therapy is required, although these tumors are considered relatively insensitive.

Adult granulosa cell tumors account for 95% of all granulosa cell tumors. Most women are diagnosed after 30 years of age, with a median age of 52 years. Abdominal pain, distention, and vaginal bleeding are the most common signs and symptoms. Because of the relative state of estrogen excess produced by these tumors, 25% of women will also have concomitant endometrial pathology, such as hyperplasia or adenocarcinoma.[233] These tumors tend to be large with an average diameter of 12 cm. If a granulosa cell tumor is suspected preoperatively, inhibin A and B levels may be elevated and useful in narrowing the differential diagnosis. Ninety percent of patients present with stage I disease, and the tumors are typically unilateral in 90% of cases. Stage is the most important prognostic factor for granulosa cell tumors; other factors include tumor rupture, stage IC disease, poorly differentiated tumor, and tumor size >10 to 15 cm. The 10-year survival for women with stage I disease is approximately 90%, with 15% to 25% of stage I patients ultimately suffering a disease recurrence. The 10-year survival for women with advanced-stage disease is 26% to 49%.

Juvenile granulosa cell tumors are rare, although they account for 90% of the granulosa cell tumors that occur in prepubertal girls and women <30 years of age.[234] Similar to the adult form, the juvenile tumors may also secrete estrogen; therefore, the prepubertal girls may present with isosexual precocious puberty. This may be the most dramatic presentation, however, the most common presentation is that of an abdominal mass. As with the adult variant, the juvenile variant is rarely bilateral, with bilaterality occurring in only 5% of cases. More than 90% of cases will be stage I at the time of diagnosis, and other prognostic factors apply as with the adult variant. The 5-year survival rate is 95%, and the prognosis remains poor with advanced-stage or recurrent disease.

Most granulosa cell tumors are unilateral and can be treated with fertility-preserving therapy consisting of unilateral salpingo-oophorectomy and appropriate surgical staging. Given the rarity of pelvic and para-aortic nodal involvement, lymphadenectomy may be omitted. Endometrial sampling should be performed in all women retaining their uterus, as these tumors may be associated with concomitant hyperplasia or adenocarcinoma. In women not wishing to preserve fertility or those who are postmenopausal, complete hysterectomy with bilateral salpingo-oophorectomy is the procedure of choice. Surgery alone is typically curative. However, risk factors for relapse that should be considered in adjuvant treatment for stage 1 disease include tumor rupture, stage IC disease, poorly differentiated tumor, and tumor size >10 to 15 cm. Adjuvant treatment options for high-risk stage I and advanced-stage disease include observation, radiation therapy for localized disease, and BEP chemotherapy. Inhibin levels, if initially elevated, may be a useful tumor marker for surveillance of patients under observation.[235]

FUTURE DIRECTIONS

Ovarian cancer represents a spectrum of distinct disease processes, ranging from noninvasive borderline tumors to disseminated high-grade serous carcinomas. The cell of origin may be extraovarian in a large proportion of cases, as many high-grade serous carcinomas appear to originate in the distal fallopian tube. Clear cell, endometrioid, and mucinous cancers may arise from metaplastic transformation of the OSE, although an extraovarian origin has been proposed. Recent insights from molecular and genomic studies also support the concept of distinct biologic subtypes of ovarian cancer. Gene expression profiling has revealed greater similarity between ovarian clear cell carcinoma and renal clear cell carcinoma than other ovarian subtypes.[236] High-grade serous carcinoma shares genomic and transcriptional features with the basal subtype of breast cancer, characterized by a BRCA-deficient phenotype.[23] Driver mutations that activate the PI3 kinase signaling pathway and mutations in the tumor suppressor *ARID1A* have been identified in endometrioid and clear cell ovarian cancers, which share a strong epidemiologic link with endometriosis.

The recognition of distinct ovarian cancer subtypes has implications for prevention, early detection, clinical trial design, and the identification of new therapeutic targets, particularly for advanced stage and recurrent disease. Results from the large screening trials of postmenopausal women in the United States, United Kingdom, and Japan using CA-125 and TVUS do not at present support routine screening for ovarian and fallopian tube cancer in the general population. Future screening strategies may focus on women at greatest genetic risk by high throughput sequencing and mutation testing. Genome-wide association studies have recently identified new ovarian cancer risk loci.[237,238] Novel screening strategies will also be needed to detect precursor lesions within the fallopian tube, particularly for high-grade serous carcinomas. It is not yet known whether prophylactic salpingectomy without removal of the ovaries is an acceptable prevention strategy for premenopausal women with familial ovarian cancer syndromes. Clinical trials will soon incorporate targeted therapies with blood and imaging biomarkers to assess pathway inhibition and accurately measure disease response. Trial end points should also include robust quality-of-life tools to assess the effect of palliative chemotherapy on symptom control as well as evaluation of its toxicity. Although no longer used in the initial management of ovarian cancer, the role of radiation therapy in palliation remains of significant importance for symptomatic recurrence, particularly for women with chemotherapy-refractory disease.

SELECTED REFERENCES

A full list of references for this chapter is available online.

3. Siegel R, Naishadham D, Jemal A. Cancer statistics, 2012. *CA Cancer J Clin* 2012;62(1):10–29.
5. Howlader N, Noone AM, Krapcho M, et al. SEER cancer statistics review, 1975–2009 *(Vintage 2009 Populations)*. Available at: http://seer.cancer.gov/csr/1975_2009_pops09/.
7. Levanon K, Crum C, Drapkin R. New insights into the pathogenesis of serous ovarian cancer and its clinical impact. *J Clin Oncol* 2008;26(32):5284–5293.
8. Karst AM, Drapkin R. Ovarian cancer pathogenesis: a model in evolution. *J Oncol* 2010;2010:932371.
15. Callahan MJ, Crum CP, Medeiros F, et al. Primary fallopian tube malignancies in BRCA-positive women undergoing surgery for ovarian cancer risk reduction. *J Clin Oncol* 2007;25(25):3985–3990.
16. Kindelberger DW, Lee Y, Miron A, et al. Intraepithelial carcinoma of the fimbria and pelvic serous carcinoma: evidence for a causal relationship. *Am J Surg Pathol* 2007;31(2):161–169.
17. Lee Y, Miron A, Drapkin R, et al. A candidate precursor to serous carcinoma that originates in the distal fallopian tube. *J Pathol* 2007;211(1):26–35.
22. Wiegand KC, Shah SP, Al-Agha OM, et al. ARID1A mutations in endometriosis-associated ovarian carcinomas. *N Engl J Med* 2011;363(16):1532–1543.
23. Bowtell DD. The genesis and evolution of high-grade serous ovarian cancer. *Nat Rev* 2010;10(11):803–808.
24. Integrated genomic analyses of ovarian carcinoma. *Nature* 2011;474(7353):609–615.
25. Mukhopadhyay A, Elattar A, Cerbinskaite A, et al. Development of a functional assay for homologous recombination status in primary cultures of epithelial ovarian tumor and correlation with sensitivity to poly(ADP-ribose) polymerase inhibitors. *Clin Cancer Res* 2010;16(8):2344–2351.
26. Martin L, Schilder R. Novel approaches in advancing the treatment of epithelial ovarian cancer: the role of angiogenesis inhibition. *J Clin Oncol* 2007;25(20):2894–2901.
27. Liu J, Matulonis UA. Anti-angiogenic agents in ovarian cancer: dawn of a new era? *Curr Oncol Rep* 2011;13(6):450–458.
40. Orezzoli JP, Russell AH, Oliva E, et al. Prognostic implication of endometriosis in clear cell carcinoma of the ovary. *Gynecol Oncol* 2008;110(3):336–344.
53. Chen S, Parmigiani G. Meta-analysis of BRCA1 and BRCA2 penetrance. *J Clin Oncol* 2007;25(11):1329–1333.
56. Rubin SC, Benjamin I, Behbakht K, et al. Clinical and pathological features of ovarian cancer in women with germ-line mutations of BRCA1. *N Engl J Med* 1996;335(19):1413–1416.
58. Chetrit A, Hirsh-Yechezkel G, Ben-David Y, et al. Effect of BRCA1/2 mutations on long-term survival of patients with invasive ovarian cancer: the national Israeli study of ovarian cancer. *J Clin Oncol* 2008;26(1):20–25.
59. Cass I, Baldwin RL, Varkey T, et al. Improved survival in women with BRCA-associated ovarian carcinoma. *Cancer* 2003;97(9):2187–2195.
67. National Comprehensive Cancer Network. Genetic/familial high-risk assessment: breast and ovarian. NCCN Clinical Practice Guidelines in Oncology (NCCN Guidelines) 2012. Available at: http://www.nccn.org.
70. Pal T, Permuth-Wey J, Sellers TA. A review of the clinical relevance of mismatch-repair deficiency in ovarian cancer. *Cancer* 2008;113(4):733–742.
71. Shulman LP. Hereditary breast and ovarian cancer (HBOC): clinical features and counseling for BRCA1 and BRCA2, Lynch syndrome, Cowden syndrome, and Li-Fraumeni syndrome. *Obstet Gynecol Clin North Am* 2010;37(1):109–133.
75. Jemal A, Bray F, Center MM, et al. Global cancer statistics. *CA Cancer J Clin* 2011;61(2):69–90.
89. Menon U, Gentry-Maharaj A, Hallett R, et al. Sensitivity and specificity of multimodal and ultrasound screening for ovarian cancer, and stage distribution of detected cancers: results of the prevalence screen of the UK Collaborative Trial of Ovarian Cancer Screening (UKCTOCS). *Lancet Oncol* 2009;10(4):327–340.
90. Buys SS, Partridge E, Greene MH, et al. Ovarian cancer screening in the Prostate, Lung, Colorectal and Ovarian (PLCO) cancer screening trial: findings from the initial screen of a randomized trial. *Am J Obstet Gynecol* 2005;193(5):1630–1639.
91. Buys SS, Partridge E, Black A, et al. Effect of screening on ovarian cancer mortality: the Prostate, Lung, Colorectal and Ovarian (PLCO) Cancer Screening Randomized Controlled Trial. *JAMA* 2011;305(22):2295–2303.
92. Kobayashi H, Yamada Y, Sado T, et al. A randomized study of screening for ovarian cancer: a multicenter study in Japan. *Int J Gynecol Cancer* 2008;18(3):414–420.
96. National Institutes of Health Consensus Development Conference Statement. Ovarian cancer: screening, treatment, and follow-up. *Gynecol Oncol* 1994;55(3 Pt 2):S4–S14.
97. Finch A, Beiner M, Lubinski J, et al. Salpingo-oophorectomy and the risk of ovarian, fallopian tube, and peritoneal cancers in women with a BRCA1 or BRCA2 mutation. *JAMA* 2006;296(2):185–192.
98. Kramer JL, Velazquez IA, Chen BE, et al. Prophylactic oophorectomy reduces breast cancer penetrance during prospective, long-term follow-up of BRCA1 mutation carriers. *J Clin Oncol* 2005;23(34):8629–8635.
104. Bonome T, Lee JY, Park DC, et al. Expression profiling of serous low malignant potential, low-grade, and high-grade tumors of the ovary. *Cancer Res* 2005;65(22):10602–10612.
105. Meinhold-Heerlein I, Bauerschlag D, Hilpert F, et al. Molecular and prognostic distinction between serous ovarian carcinomas of varying grade and malignant potential. *Oncogene* 2005;24(6):1053–1065.
106. Singer G, Stohr R, Cope L, et al. Patterns of p53 mutations separate ovarian serous borderline tumors and low- and high-grade carcinomas and provide support for a new model of ovarian carcinogenesis: a mutational analysis with immunohistochemical correlation. *Am J Surg Pathol* 2005;29(2):218–224.
108. Schmeler KM, Sun CC, Bodurka DC, et al. Neoadjuvant chemotherapy for low-grade serous carcinoma of the ovary or peritoneum. *Gynecol Oncol* 2008;108(3):510–514.

111. Sherman ME, Mink PJ, Curtis R, et al. Survival among women with borderline ovarian tumors and ovarian carcinoma: a population-based analysis. *Cancer* 2004;100(5):1045–1052.
113. Storey DJ, Rush R, Stewart M, et al. Endometrioid epithelial ovarian cancer: 20 years of prospectively collected data from a single center. *Cancer* 2008; 112(10):2211–2220.
114. Zaino R, Whitney C, Brady MF, et al. Simultaneously detected endometrial and ovarian carcinomas—a prospective clinicopathologic study of 74 cases: a Gynecologic Oncology Group study. *Gynecol Oncol* 2001;83(2):355–362.
135. FIGO (International Federation of Gynecology and Obstetrics) annual report on the results of treatment in gynecological cancer. *Int J Gynaecol Obstet* 2003;83(Suppl 1):ix–xxii, 1–229.
136. National Comprehensive Cancer Network. Ovarian cancer including fallopian tube cancer and primary peritoneal cancer. NCCN Clinical Practice Guidelines in Oncology (NCCN Guidelines) 2013. Available at: http://www.nccn.org.
140. Giede KC, Kieser K, Dodge J, et al. Who should operate on patients with ovarian cancer? An evidence-based review. *Gynecol Oncol* 2005;99(2):447–461.
141. Earle CC, Schrag D, Neville BA, et al. Effect of surgeon specialty on processes of care and outcomes for ovarian cancer patients. *J Natl Cancer Inst* 2006; 98(3):172–180.
142. Du Bois A, Quinn M, Thigpen T, et al. 2004 consensus statements on the management of ovarian cancer: final document of the 3rd International Gynecologic Cancer Intergroup Ovarian Cancer Consensus Conference (GCIG OCCC 2004). *Ann Oncol* 2005;16(Suppl 8):viii7–viii12.
144. Bristow RE, Tomacruz RS, Armstrong DK, et al. Survival effect of maximal cytoreductive surgery for advanced ovarian carcinoma during the platinum era: a meta-analysis. *J Clin Oncol* 2002;20(5):1248–1259.
147. Winter WE III, Maxwell GL, Tian C, et al. Prognostic factors for stage III epithelial ovarian cancer: a Gynecologic Oncology Group study. *J Clin Oncol* 2007; 25(24):3621–3627.
149. Eisenhauer EL, Abu-Rustum NR, Sonoda Y, et al. The effect of maximal surgical cytoreduction on sensitivity to platinum-taxane chemotherapy and subsequent survival in patients with advanced ovarian cancer. *Gynecol Oncol* 2008; 108(2):276–281.
150. Winter WE III, Maxwell GL, Tian C, et al. Tumor residual after surgical cytoreduction in prediction of clinical outcome in stage IV epithelial ovarian cancer: a Gynecologic Oncology Group study. *J Clin Oncol* 2008;26(1):83–89.
154. Zorn KK, Tian C, McGuire WP, et al. The prognostic value of pretreatment CA 125 in patients with advanced ovarian carcinoma: a Gynecologic Oncology Group study. *Cancer* 2009;115(5):1028–1035.
160. Vergote I, De Brabanter J, Fyles A, et al. Prognostic importance of degree of differentiation and cyst rupture in stage I invasive epithelial ovarian carcinoma. *Lancet* 2001;357(9251):176–182.
161. Young RC, Walton LA, Ellenberg SS, et al. Adjuvant therapy in stage I and stage II epithelial ovarian cancer. Results of two prospective randomized trials. *N Engl J Med* 1990;322(15):1021–1027.
162. Colombo N, Guthrie D, Chiari S, et al. International Collaborative Ovarian Neoplasm trial 1: a randomized trial of adjuvant chemotherapy in women with early-stage ovarian cancer. *J Natl Cancer Inst* 2003;95(2):125–132.
163. Swart A. Long-term follow-up of women enrolled in a randomized trial of adjuvant chemotherapy for early stage ovarian cancer (ICON1). *J Clin Oncol* 2007; 25(Suppl 18):5509.
164. Trimbos B, Timmers P, Pecorelli S, et al. Surgical staging and treatment of early ovarian cancer: long-term analysis from a randomized trial. *J Natl Cancer Inst* 2010;102(13):982–987.
165. Trimbos JB, Vergote I, Bolis G, et al. Impact of adjuvant chemotherapy and surgical staging in early-stage ovarian carcinoma: European Organisation for Research and Treatment of Cancer-Adjuvant ChemoTherapy in Ovarian Neoplasm trial. *J Natl Cancer Inst* 2003;95(2):113–125.
166. Trimbos JB, Parmar M, Vergote I, et al. International Collaborative Ovarian Neoplasm trial 1 and Adjuvant ChemoTherapy in Ovarian Neoplasm trial: two parallel randomized phase III trials of adjuvant chemotherapy in patients with early-stage ovarian carcinoma. *J Natl Cancer Inst* 2003;95(2):105–112.
167. Bell J, Brady MF, Young RC, et al. Randomized phase III trial of three versus six cycles of adjuvant carboplatin and paclitaxel in early stage epithelial ovarian carcinoma: a Gynecologic Oncology Group study. *Gynecol Oncol* 2006;102(3):432–439.
168. Chan JK, Tian C, Fleming GF, et al. The potential benefit of 6 vs. 3 cycles of chemotherapy in subsets of women with early-stage high-risk epithelial ovarian cancer: an exploratory analysis of a Gynecologic Oncology Group study. *Gynecol Oncol* 2010;116(3):301–306.
169. Dembo AJ, Bush RS, Beale FA, et al. Ovarian carcinoma: improved survival following abdominopelvic irradiation in patients with a completed pelvic operation. *Am J Obstet Gynecol* 1979;134(7):793–800.
173. Smith JP, Rutledge FN, Delclos L. Postoperative treatment of early cancer of the ovary: a random trial between postoperative irradiation and chemotherapy. *Natl Cancer Inst Monogr* 1975;42:149–153.
174. Chiara S, Conte P, Franzone P, et al. High-risk early-stage ovarian cancer. Randomized clinical trial comparing cisplatin plus cyclophosphamide versus whole abdominal radiotherapy. *Am J Clin Oncol* 1994;17(1):72–76.
175. Fyles AW, Thomas GM, Pintilie M, et al. A randomized study of two doses of abdominopelvic radiation therapy for patients with optimally debulked stage I, II, and III ovarian cancer. *Int J Radiat Oncol Biol Phys* 1998;41(3):543–549.
180. Greer BE, Bundy BN, Ozols RF, et al. Implications of second-look laparotomy in the context of optimally resected stage III ovarian cancer: a non-randomized comparison using an explanatory analysis: a Gynecologic Oncology Group study. *Gynecol Oncol* 2005;99(1):71–79.
181. Van der Burg ME, van Lent M, Buyse M, et al. The effect of debulking surgery after induction chemotherapy on the prognosis in advanced epithelial ovarian cancer. Gynecological Cancer Cooperative Group of the European Organization for Research and Treatment of Cancer. *N Engl J Med* 1995;332(10):629–634.
182. Rose PG, Nerenstone S, Brady MF, et al. Secondary surgical cytoreduction for advanced ovarian carcinoma. *N Engl J Med* 2004;351(24):2489–2497.
183. Vergote I, Trope CG, Amant F, et al. Neoadjuvant chemotherapy or primary surgery in stage IIIC or IV ovarian cancer. *N Engl J Med* 2010;363(10):943–953.
184. Chemotherapy for advanced ovarian cancer. Advanced Ovarian Cancer Trialists Group. *Cochrane Database Syst Rev* 2000;(2):CD001418.
185. McGuire WP, Hoskins WJ, Brady MF, et al. Cyclophosphamide and cisplatin compared with paclitaxel and cisplatin in patients with stage III and stage IV ovarian cancer. *N Engl J Med* 1996;334(1):1–6.
187. Katsumata N, Yasuda M, Takahashi F, et al. Dose-dense paclitaxel once a week in combination with carboplatin every 3 weeks for advanced ovarian cancer: a phase 3, open-label, randomised controlled trial. *Lancet* 2009;374(9698):1331–1338.
188. Vasey PA, Jayson GC, Gordon A, et al. Phase III randomized trial of docetaxel-carboplatin versus paclitaxel-carboplatin as first-line chemotherapy for ovarian carcinoma. *J Natl Cancer Inst* 2004;96(22):1682–1691.
189. Bookman MA, Brady MF, McGuire WP, et al. Evaluation of new platinum-based treatment regimens in advanced-stage ovarian cancer: a phase III trial of the Gynecologic Cancer Intergroup. *J Clin Oncol* 2009;27(9):1419–1425.
190. Burger R, Brady M, Bookman M, et al. Incorporation of bevacizumab in the primary treatment of ovarian cancer. *N Engl J Med* 2011;365(26):2473–2483.
191. Perren T, Swart AM, Pfisterer J, et al. A phase 3 trial of bevacizumab in ovarian cancer. *N Engl J Med* 2011;365(26):2484–2496.
192. Armstrong DK, Bundy B, Wenzel L, et al. Intraperitoneal cisplatin and paclitaxel in ovarian cancer. *N Engl J Med* 2006;354(1):34–43.
193. Jaaback K, Johnson N. Intraperitoneal chemotherapy for the initial management of primary epithelial ovarian cancer. *Cochrane Database Syst Rev* 2006; (1):CD005340.
197. Pickel H, Lahousen M, Petru E,, et al. Consolidation radiotherapy after carboplatin-based chemotherapy in radically operated advanced ovarian cancer. *Gynecol Oncol* 1999;72(2):215–219.
198. Sorbe B. Consolidation treatment of advanced (FIGO stage III) ovarian carcinoma in complete surgical remission after induction chemotherapy: a randomized, controlled, clinical trial comparing whole abdominal radiotherapy, chemotherapy, and no further treatment. *Int J Gynecol Cancer* 2003;13(3):278–286.
199. Dinniwell R, Lock M, Pintilie M, et al. Consolidative abdominopelvic radiotherapy after surgery and carboplatin/paclitaxel chemotherapy for epithelial ovarian cancer. *Int J Radiat Oncol Biol Phys* 2005;62(1):104–110.
200. Petit T, Velten M, d'Hombres A, et al. Long-term survival of 106 stage III ovarian cancer patients with minimal residual disease after second-look laparotomy and consolidation radiotherapy. *Gynecol Oncol* 2007;104(1):104–108.
202. Rustin GJ, van der Burg ME, Griffin CL, et al. Early versus delayed treatment of relapsed ovarian cancer (MRC OV05/EORTC 55955): a randomised trial. *Lancet* 2010;376(9747):1155–1163.
203. Aghajanian C, Finkler N, Rutherford T, et al. OCEANS: a randomized, double-blinded, placebo-controlled phase III trial of chemotherapy with or without bevacizumab (BEV) in patients with platinum-sensitive recurrent epithelial ovarian (EOC), primary peritoneal (PPC), or fallopian tube cancer (FTC). *J Clin Oncol* 2011;29(Suppl):LBA5007.
206. Horowitz N, Matulonis UA. New biologic agents for the treatment of gynecologic cancers. *Hematol Oncol Clin North Am* 2012;26(1):133–156.
207. Vergote I, Sella A, Bedell C, et al. Phase II study of XL184 in a cohort of ovarian cancer patients with measurable soft tissue disease. Proceedings of the 22nd EORTC-NCI-AACR Symposium on Molecular Targets and Cancer Therapeutics conference, Berlin, Germany, November 18, 2010.
208. Ledermann J, Harter P, Gourley C, et al. Phase II randomized placebo-controlled study of olaparib (AZD2281) in patients with platinum-sensitive relapsed serous ovarian cancer. *J Clin Oncol* 2011;29(Suppl):5003.
209. Hauspy J, Covens A. Cytoreductive surgery for recurrent ovarian cancer. *Curr Opin Obstet Gynecol* 2007;19(1):15–21.
210. Gelblum D, Mychalczak B, Almadrones L, et al. Palliative benefit of external-beam radiation in the management of platinum refractory epithelial ovarian carcinoma. *Gynecol Oncol* 1998;69(1):36–41.
211. May LF, Belinson JL, Roland TA. Palliative benefit of radiation therapy in advanced ovarian cancer. *Gynecol Oncol* 1990;37(3):408–411.
212. Tinger A, Waldron T, Peluso N, et al. Effective palliative radiation therapy in advanced and recurrent ovarian carcinoma. *Int J Radiat Oncol Biol Phys* 2001; 51(5):1256–1263.
213. Corn BW, Lanciano RM, Boente M, et al. Recurrent ovarian cancer: effective radiotherapeutic palliation after chemotherapy failure. *Cancer* 1994;74(11):2979–2983.
215. Firat S, Erickson B. Selective irradiation for the treatment of recurrent ovarian carcinoma involving the vagina or rectum. *Gynecol Oncol* 2001;80(2):213–220.
218. Albuquerque KV, Singla R, Potkul RK, et al. Impact of tumor volume-directed involved field radiation therapy integrated in the management of recurrent ovarian cancer. *Gynecol Oncol* 2005;96(3):701–704.
219. Ratner ES, Toy E, O'Malley DM, et al. Brain metastases in epithelial ovarian and primary peritoneal carcinoma. *Int J Gynecol Cancer* 2009;19(5):856–859.
220. Sehouli J, Pietzner K, Harter P, et al. Prognostic role of platinum sensitivity in patients with brain metastases from ovarian cancer: results of a German multicenter study. *Ann Oncol* 2011;21(11):2201–2205.
221. Hong L, Alektiar K, Chui C, et al. IMRT of large fields: whole-abdomen irradiation. *Int J Radiat Oncol Biol Phys* 2002;54(1):278–289.
222. Duthoy W, De Gersem W, Vergote K, et al. Whole abdominopelvic radiotherapy (WAPRT) using intensity-modulated arc therapy (IMAT): first clinical experience. *Int J Radiat Oncol Biol Phys* 2003;57(4):1019–1032.
223. Yap OW, Kapp DS, Teng NN, et al. Intraoperative radiation therapy in recurrent ovarian cancer. *Int J Radiat Oncol Biol Phys* 2005;63(4):1114–1121.
229. Thomas GM, Dembo AJ. Integrating radiation therapy into the management of ovarian cancer. *Cancer* 1993;71(4 Suppl):1710–1718.
230. Brewer M, Gershenson DM, Herzog CE, et al. Outcome and reproductive function after chemotherapy for ovarian dysgerminoma. *J Clin Oncol* 1999;17(9):2670–2675.
231. Williams SD, Blessing JA, Hatch KD, et al. Chemotherapy of advanced dysgerminoma: trials of the Gynecologic Oncology Group. *J Clin Oncol* 1991;9(11):1950–1955.
232. Williams S, Blessing JA, Liao SY, et al. Adjuvant therapy of ovarian germ cell tumors with cisplatin, etoposide, and bleomycin: a trial of the Gynecologic Oncology Group. *J Clin Oncol* 1994;12(4):701–706.
236. Zorn KK, Bonome T, Gangi L, et al. Gene expression profiles of serous, endometrioid, and clear cell subtypes of ovarian and endometrial cancer. *Clin Cancer Res* 2005;11(18):6422–6430.
237. Bolton KL, Tyrer J, Song H, et al. Common variants at 19p13 are associated with susceptibility to ovarian cancer. *Nat Genet* 2010;42(10):880–884.
238. Song H, Ramus SJ, Tyrer J, et al. A genome-wide association study identifies a new ovarian cancer susceptibility locus on 9p22.2. *Nat Genet* 2009;41(9):996–1000.

Chapter 72
Vaginal Cancer

Josephine Kang and Akila N. Viswanathan

Primary vaginal cancer is a rare malignancy, constituting 1% to 2% of all gynecologic malignancies. According to the American Cancer Society estimates for 2010, there were approximately 2,300 new cases and 780 deaths from this disease.[1] The majority of malignant lesions in the vagina are metastatic from other gynecologic malignancies or involve direct extension from adjacent sites, which excludes diagnosis as a primary vaginal malignancy. According to the staging system set by the International Federation of Obstetrics and Gynecology (FIGO), a diagnosis of primary vaginal cancer excludes any tumors involving the cervix or vulva.[2] According to one study of 141 vaginal carcinoma cases, only 26% met the criteria of being a primary vaginal cancer,[3] defined as a lesion that arises in the vagina without involving the cervix or vulva.

The majority of primary vaginal malignancies are squamous cell carcinomas (SCC). According to a National Cancer Data Base (NCDB) report[4] based on 4,885 patients with primary vaginal cancer registered from 1985 to 1994, approximately 92% of patients were diagnosed with *in situ* or invasive SCC or adenocarcinomas, 4% with melanomas, 3% with sarcomas, and 1% with other or unspecified types of cancer. Sixty-six percent of all vaginal cancers were invasive, with SCC representing 79% of all invasive cases.

The peak incidence of primary vaginal cancer is in the sixth and seventh decades of life. According to data from the Surveillance, Epidemiology, and End Results (SEER) program,[1] 2,149 women in the United States were diagnosed with primary vaginal cancer from 1990 to 2004. The mean age at diagnosis was 65.7 ± 14.3 years and incidence rates increased with age. Vaginal cancer incidence is increasing in younger women, possibly due to an increase in human papilloma virus (HPV) infection or other sexually transmitted diseases. However, there has been an overall decrease in the incidence of primary vaginal tumors, possibly attributable to earlier detection and to implementation of strict exclusion criteria in the FIGO staging system. At the same time, there has been a steady increase in the diagnosis of vaginal intraepithelial neoplasia (VAIN) over the past several decades, due to expanded cytologic screening and increased awareness.[5] Due to infrequent presentation, treatment recommendations are based on results from relatively small retrospective series, the majority of which are based on heterogeneous patient populations and treatments.

ANATOMY

The vagina is a fibromuscular tube that extends from the cervix down to the vestibule, or cleft, between the labia minora (Fig. 72.1). It lies dorsal to the urethra and bladder base and ventral to the rectum. Superiorly, it joins the uterine cervix at an angle and, as a result, the posterior vaginal wall is longer than the anterior wall, with an overall average length of 7.5 cm. The upper aspect of the posterior vaginal wall is separated from the rectum by a reflection of peritoneum, the pouch of Douglas. The cervix projects into the upper lumen of the vagina, creating invaginations between the vaginal mucosa and the cervix, which are termed the anterior, posterior, and lateral fornices. Inferiorly, the vagina extends through the urogenital diaphragm and lies directly adjacent to the rectum up to where the fibromuscular perineal body tissue separates the vagina from the anal canal. Laterally, the vagina is adjacent to the pelvic fascia and levator ani muscles. At the introitus, the vagina has a perforated fold of thin connective tissue and mucous membrane known as the hymen.

The vaginal wall is composed of three layers: the mucosa, muscularis, and adventitia. The inner lining of the vagina is formed by a nonkeratinizing stratified squamous epithelium overlying a basement membrane with many papillae. The epithelium lacks glandular structures and instead receives lubrication from mucous secretions originating in the cervix. Underneath the mucosa is connective tissue composed of elastin and a thick muscularis layer composed of two layers of smooth muscle. The inner layer is arranged circularly, whereas the outer layer is arranged longitudinally. This muscular layer is covered by a thin adventitia that merges with neighboring organs. At the vaginal introitus, skeletal muscle forms a sphincter.

Proximally, the vagina is supplied by the vaginal artery, which arises from the cervical branch of the uterine artery and runs lateral to the vagina until it anastomoses with the inferior vesical and middle rectal arteries. The venous plexus runs parallel to the arteries, draining into the internal iliac vein. The vaginal vault is innervated by the lumbar plexus and pudendal nerve, with branches from sacral roots 2 to 4.[6]

The vagina has a complex, extensive network of lymphatic drainage, with vessels that course through the submucosal and muscularis layer. The uppermost portion drains primarily via cervical lymphatics. The superior anterior vagina drains along cervical channels to the interiliac and parametrial nodes, and the posterior upper vagina drains into the inferior gluteal, presacral, and anorectal nodes (Fig. 72.2). The inferior aspect of the vagina drains into the inguinal and femoral nodes and ultimately to the pelvic nodes, following drainage patterns of the vulva. Lesions in the midvagina have been shown to drain either way.[7] Lesions infiltrating the rectovaginal septum may spread to the pararectal and presacral nodes. There are multiple interconnections between lymphatic channels, and pattern of drainage cannot be reliably predicted based on location of the primary tumor. Embryologically, the vagina is believed to be of dual origin, with the upper third derived from the uterine canal, while the lower two-thirds are derived from the urogenital sinus.[8]

EPIDEMIOLOGY, PRESENTATION, AND GENERAL MANAGEMENT

Vaginal Intraepithelial Neoplasia

Epidemiology

Incidence of VAIN is estimated to be 0.2 to 0.3 cases per 100,000, with peak incidence between 40 and 60 years of age.[5,9,10] Most studies do not report differences in mean age between women with low-grade and those with high-grade VAIN,[11–15] although a few series have reported that patients with VAIN-1 or -2 were younger than patients with VAIN-3.[16–19] Incidence of *in situ* vaginal cancer is estimated to be 0.1 per

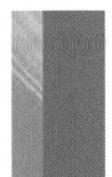

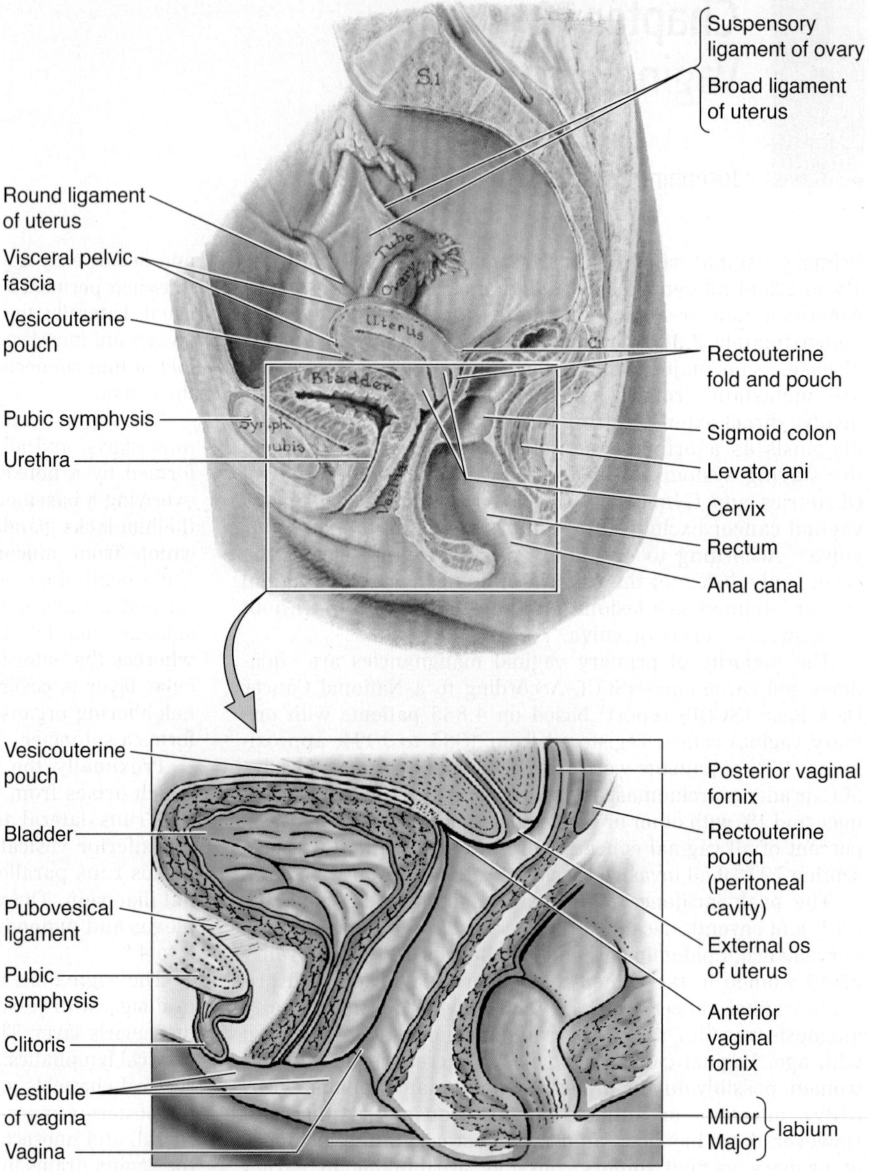

FIGURE 72.1. Median section of the female pelvis. The vagina is a fibromuscular tube situated posterior to the bladder and urethra and anterior to the rectum. The anterior and posterior fornices are formed by protrusion of the cervix into the vaginal canal. (From Moore KL. *Clinical oriented anatomy*, 4th ed. Baltimore: Lippincott Williams & Wilkins, 1999, with permission.)

100,000 women, with peak incidence between ages 70 to 79, according to data from the U.S. Centers for Disease Control and Prevention's National Program of Cancer Registries, and the National Cancer Institute's SEER program.[20] Risk factors for VAIN include low sociocultural level, history of genital warts, hysterectomy at an early age, history of cervical intraepithelial neoplasia, immunosuppression, prior pelvic radiation, smoking, exposure to diethylstilbestrol (DES), and history of sexually transmissible diseases (STDs) or HPV infection.[15,17,21,22]

The diagnosis of VAIN is associated with prior or concurrent neoplasia elsewhere in the lower genital tract. Multiple series suggest approximately 50% to 90% of patients with VAIN have concurrent or prior history of intraepithelial neoplasia or carcinoma of the cervix or vulva.[9,16,17] Immunosuppression from human immunodeficiency virus (HIV) is also a risk factor for both VAIN and HPV, although a higher incidence of invasive vaginal cancer in infected women has not been demonstrated.[23–25] The role of pelvic radiation in the development of secondary vaginal neoplasia is unclear, with conflicting data suggesting a history of ionizing radiation may predispose to VAIN or vaginal cancer after a latency period of many years.[12,26,27] *In utero* exposure to DES may double the risk of VAIN, thought to be due to transformation zone enlargement, increasing the risk of HPV infection.[28]

Natural History

Although the likelihood of VAIN progressing to invasive disease is not fully understood, several clinical series have demonstrated a significant increase in risk of invasive vaginal cancer after a diagnosis of VAIN.[12,16,29,30] Similar risk factors for VAIN and invasive vaginal cancer, as well as the younger average age at presentation of VAIN compared with invasive disease, add support to the theory that VAIN may be a precursor lesion to invasive SCC. In one series, 23 patients with VAIN, with a mean age of 41 years, were followed for at least 3 years without treatment;[16] this included multifocal lesions as well as lesions associated with cervical intraepithelial neoplasia (CIN) or vulvar dysplasia. Two cases (9%) progressed to invasive cancer; one patient had VAIN-1 and progressed to stage I vaginal carcinoma in 5 years, and the second patient had VAIN-3 and progressed to stage I vaginal carcinoma in 4 years. The overall spontaneous regression rate was 78%, with the majority (78%) occurring in patients with VAIN-1 or -2. Similarly, several additional studies have demonstrated a range of 2%

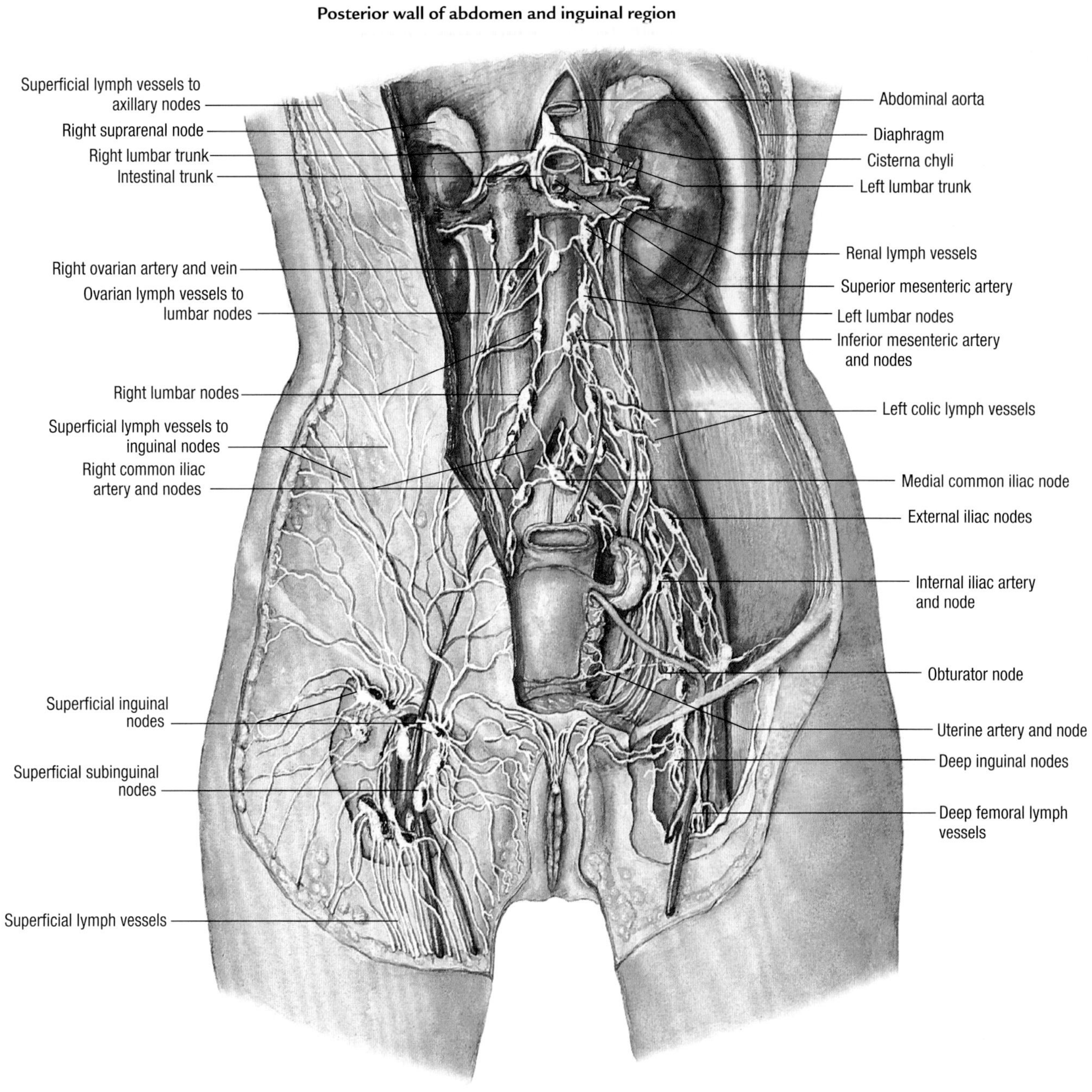

FIGURE 72.2. Lymphatic drainage of the vagina to the inguinal and pelvic lymph nodes. (Asset provided by the Anatomical Chart Company.)

to 20% of patients with VAIN progressing to invasive vaginal cancer.[12,16,29,31–33]

The rate of occult invasive disease in patients with VAIN-3 has been reported to be as high as 28%.[34] The risk of malignant transformation in VAIN-1 and -2 is less clearly elucidated; there have been reports of patients with low-grade VAIN subsequently developing invasive vaginal carcinoma.[14,15]

Pathology

VAIN is defined as the presence of squamous cell atypia without evidence of invasion (Fig. 72.3). VAIN is further classified according to depth of epithelial involvement, with involvement of the lower one-third, two-thirds, and greater than two-thirds of the epithelium classified as VAIN-1, -2 and -3, respectively. Carcinoma *in situ* encompasses the full epithelial thickness and is included under VAIN-3. Excluded from diagnosis of VAIN is the presence of glandular intraepithelial dysplasia or atypical vaginal adenosis; these entities are associated with *in utero* DES exposure and are deemed to be precursors of DES-associated clear cell adenocarcinoma.[35] VAIN is frequently multifocal and most commonly involves the upper portion of the vagina.

Histopathologically, most lesions are epidermoid and exhibit full-thickness alterations with atypical mitoses and hyperchromatism (Fig. 72.3).[36] Punctation and mosaic patterns are often noted with high-grade VAIN.[14] Most lesions are multifocal and can involve all surfaces of the vagina, although the superior one-third of the vagina is most common.[12,16]

VAIN is associated with HPV infection.[37] A review of 232 published VAIN cases documented a high prevalence of HPV using polymerase chain reaction or hybrid capture assays for detection, with 98.5% and 92.6% of VAIN-1 and VAIN-2 or -3 cases positive for HPV.[38] A series by Sugase and Matsukura[39] examining 71 biopsy specimens of VAIN found HPV in 100% of

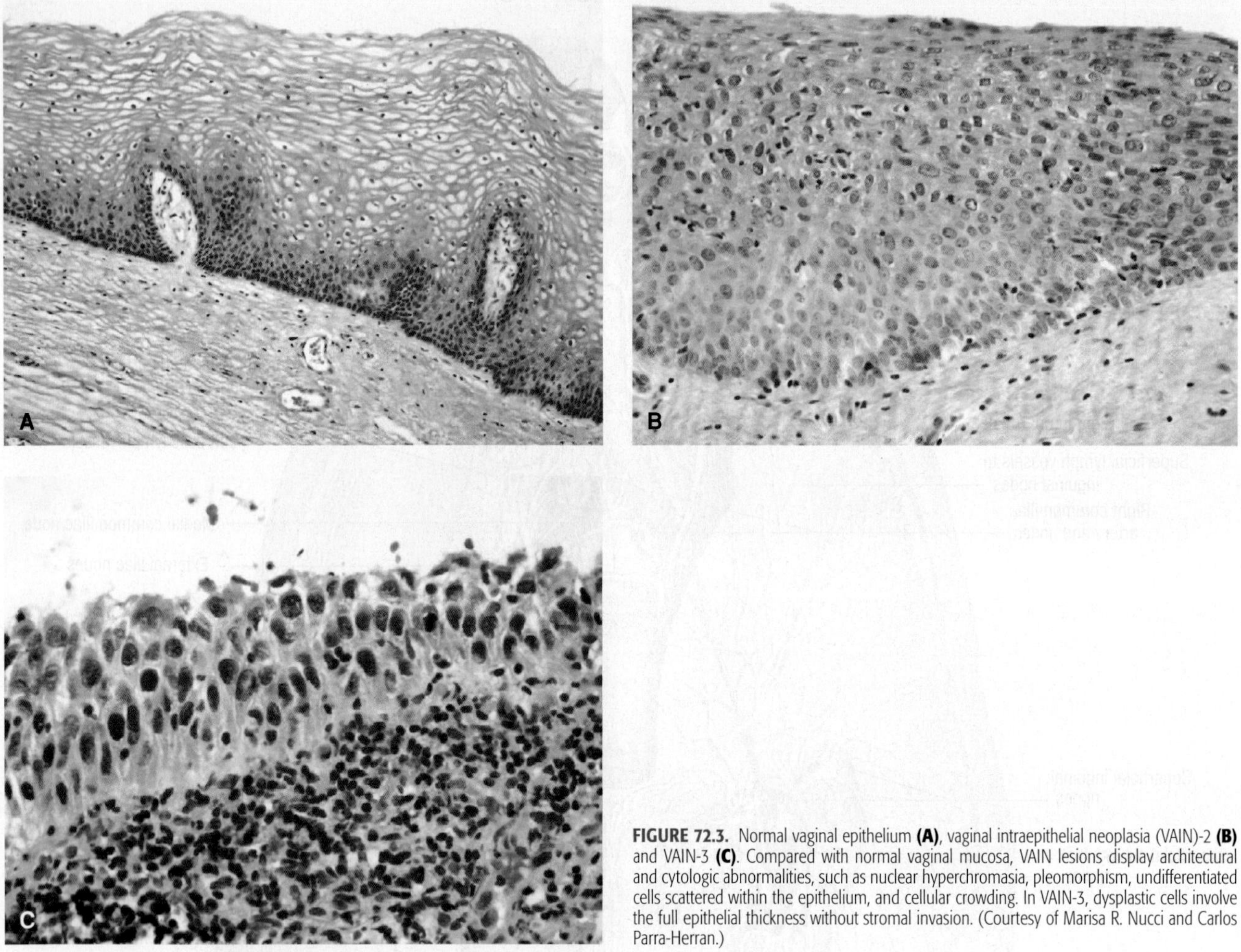

FIGURE 72.3. Normal vaginal epithelium **(A)**, vaginal intraepithelial neoplasia (VAIN)-2 **(B)** and VAIN-3 **(C)**. Compared with normal vaginal mucosa, VAIN lesions display architectural and cytologic abnormalities, such as nuclear hyperchromasia, pleomorphism, undifferentiated cells scattered within the epithelium, and cellular crowding. In VAIN-3, dysplastic cells involve the full epithelial thickness without stromal invasion. (Courtesy of Marisa R. Nucci and Carlos Parra-Herran.)

samples. Fifteen different known subtypes were identified (HPV-16, -18, -30, -31, -35, -40, -42, -43, -51, -52, -53, -54, -56, -58, -66). Types HPV-16 or -18 comprised 9%, 7%, and 67% of VAIN-1, -2, and -3 cases, respectively.

Clinical Presentation

VAIN is usually asymptomatic[12] and most commonly detected after cytologic evaluation as part of surveillance in patients with a history of CIN or invasive cervical carcinoma. According to the American Cancer Society guidelines from 2002, surveillance cytology for VAIN in posthysterectomy patients is recommended if there is a history of cervical pathology.[40] However, evidence does not support routine surveillance in patients without a history of CIN or invasive cervical cancer.

Prognostic Factors

A study by So et al.[41] on 48 women with VAIN reports a significant association between higher viral load of HPV and the likelihood of persistent disease after treatment. There is also an association between a history of pelvic radiation and development of VAIN,[33,42,43] with up to 20% of patients with prior radiation developing vaginal dysplasia. A retrospective review of 33 patients with VAIN treated at the University of Pennsylvania found patients with a history of radiation therapy to be more refractory to treatment, with a significantly higher likelihood of recurrence after surgical and ablative therapy.[31] Patients with a history of radiation had an odds ratio of 3.6 for recurrent disease (95% confidence interval, 1.5 to 9.0) compared with patients without a history of radiation.

Treatment Options

The management of VAIN is heterogeneous, with a wide variety of treatments available. There is currently no consensus on optimal treatment modality, as reported data are generally retrospective and based on decades of experience with varied treatments and patient characteristics; thus it is difficult to compare different treatment modalities (Table 72.1). Treatment approaches include local excision, partial or total vaginectomy, laser vaporization, electrocoagulation, topical 5% fluorouracil (5-FU) administration, and radiation.[14,15,17–19,47,54,64,66,67] Reported success rates for different approaches range from 48% to 100% for laser vaporization,[50,68,69] 52% to 100% for colpectomy,[34,47,51] 75% to 100% for topical 5-FU,[53,54,55,56,70,71,72,73] and 83% to 100% for radiation.[61,62,65,67,74] Given the breadth of available therapies, an individualized approach to patient management is advised, with consideration given to the patient's overall health, desire to preserve sexual function, candidacy for surgery, disease multifocality, and prior treatment failures.

Most patients with VAIN-1 are offered close surveillance. Lesions often regress spontaneously; in one study by Aho et al.,[16] 78% of patients with VAIN-1 or -2 had spontaneous regression of disease without treatment. Appropriate treatment for VAIN-2 should be determined on an individual basis, based on disease extent and associated patient factors. Therapy for

TABLE 72.1 LOCAL CONTROL OF VAGINAL INTRAEPITHELIAL NEOPLASIA BY TREATMENT MODALITY

Series (Reference)	Year	Number of Patients	Recurrence (%)	Follow-Up	Treatment Notes
Surgery					
Benedet and Sanders (44)	1984	136	25	>5 yr	WLE, PV, TV
Lenehan et al. (12)	1986	19	16	5–112 mo	PV, TV
Ireland and Monaghan (45)	1988	25	4	3 mo–11 yr	PV, TV
Hoffman et al. (34)	1992	32	17	6–73 mo	PV; 28% invasive cancer
Fanning et al. (46)	1999	15	0	1.8 yr	PV; 6.6% invasive cancer
Cheng et al. (9)	1999	35	34	1–124 mo	WLE
Dodge et al. (15)	2001	13	0	>7 mo	PV
Indermaur et al. (47)	2005	105	12	2–9 mo	PV, 12% invasive cancer
Laser Therapy					
Jobson and Homesley (48)	1983	24	17	6–27 mo	
Audet-LaPoint et al. (49)	1990	32	28	7–85 mo	3.8% invasive cancer at excision 3 of 11 w/invasive cancer at recurrence
Hoffman et al. (50)	1991	26	42	2.2 yr (mean)	
Diakomanolis et al. (51)	1996	25	32	35–82 mo	
Campagnutta et al. (52)	1999	39	23	13–90 mo	
Dodge et al. (15)	2001	42	38	>7 mo	
Topical 5-FU					
Woodruff et al. (53)	1975	9	11	3–7 yr	1%–2% 5-FU every mo
Petrilli et al. (54)	1980	15	20	2–60 mo	BID × 5 d
Kirwan and Naftalin (55)	1985	14	7	4–42 mo	Every week × 10 wk
Krebs (56)	1989	37	19	12–84 mo	Every week × 10 wk
Audet-Lapointe et al. (49)	1990	12	17	9–42 mo	Every d × 5 d
Dodge et al. (15)	2001	22	59	>7 mo	
Topical Imiquimod					
Buck and Guth (57)	2003	56	14	–	0.25 g every wk × 3 wk
Diakomonolis et al. (58)	2002	3	See note	–	3× weekly × 8 wk 3 pts with high-grade disease, therapy revealed regression to VAIN1 (n = 2) or cure (n = 1)
Radiation					
Prempree et al. (59)	1977	7	0	–	ICB 70–80 Gy
Chyle et al. (60)	1996	37	17	–	ICB or orthovoltage radiation
MacLeod et al. (61)	1997	14	14	46 mo (mean)	HDR-ICB, 34–45 Gy to vaginal surface, 4–10 fx
Ogino et al. (62)	1998	6	0	13–153 mo	HDR-ICB, mean dose 23.3 Gy
Perez et al. (63)	1999	20	6	–	ICB 60–70 Gy
Graham et al. (64)	2007	22	14	77 mo	MDR-ICB, 48 Gy to point Z
Blanchard et al. (65)	2011	28	7	79 mo (median)	LDR, 60 Gy to 5 mm below mucosa

WLE, wide local excision; PV, partial vaginectomy; TV, total vaginectomy; ICB, intracavitary brachytherapy; HDR, high-dose rate; MDR, medium-dose rate; LDR, low-dose rate.

VAIN-3 should be more aggressive, as there is a higher likelihood of progression to invasive disease, including occult invasive disease.[34,47]

Surgical and Ablative Therapies

Surgical approaches include local excision, partial vaginectomy, and, in rare cases, total vaginectomy for highly extensive disease, which provides the advantage of obtaining a complete pathologic diagnosis. Most resections can be performed through a transvaginal approach. Location of VAIN in the vaginal vault or posthysterectomy suture recesses may require partial vaginectomy for complete resection.

Local therapy is achieved through a cold-knife approach, electrosurgical loop excision, laser, or via ultrasonic surgical aspiration.[75–77] The carbon dioxide laser has been used for ablation of local tissue, with multiple treatments required in approximately one-third of patients.[49,50,52,56,69,78,79] Complications include postoperative pain, scarring, and bleeding; however, the treatment is overall fairly well tolerated, with minimum impact on sexual function.[80] Diakomanolis et al.[51] reported on 52 patients who underwent laser treatment or partial vaginectomy and found results to favor laser ablation for multifocal disease and partial vaginectomy for unifocal disease. Ultrasonic surgical aspiration is another technique that has shown efficacy similar that of to laser ablation; in one series of 110 patients, 1-year recurrence-free survival rates were 24% and 26%, respectively.[47]

Series on surgical treatment of VAIN report recurrence rates in the range of 0% to 50%, with follow-up times ranging from 3 months to 18 years.[9,12,17,34,44] Overall, series looking specifically at upper vaginectomy report control rates of 68% to 88%.[19,29,34,47,51] For example, Hoffman et al.[34] reported that 83% of patients with VAIN-3 remained free of disease with a mean follow-up time of 38 months. Of note, 28% of all patients were found to have occult invasive disease upon upper vaginectomy. A subsequent study by Indermaur et al.,[47] which retrospectively reviewed 36 patients treated with upper vaginectomy for VAIN, reported 88% to be free of recurrence with a mean follow-up time of 25 months. Thirteen patients (12%) were found to have invasive cancer; 8 of 13 had frank invasive disease, while 5 patients had microinvasive carcinoma. Complication rates of upper vaginectomy have been variably reported; in the series by Indermaur et al.,[47] there was a 9% complication rate. Potential complications from surgery depend on the extent and method of surgical resection, and they range from vaginal shortening and stenosis to standard postoperative morbidity associated with abdominal procedures. It should be noted that patients with a history of radiation treatment are at higher risk of postoperative complications, with a higher rate of fistula formation reported in one study.[9]

Topical Treatments

Topical therapies have been utilized in patients with early-stage lesions, multifocal disease, or multiple comorbidities, rendering them nonideal surgical candidates. Topical applications have also been utilized prior to surgery to reduce lesion size and improve stripping of neoplastic epithelial cells from underlying stroma.[17] Treatments include topical 5-FU and 5% imiquimod cream, with response rates in 71% to 78% of patients for imiquimod and 41% to 88% for 5-FU.[53,55,56,57,58,67,71,72,81,82] Imiquimod increases levels of interferon-alfa, interleukin-12, and tumor necrosis factor,[58] resulting in immunomodulation of the vaginal mucosa. Side effects of topical treatments include local irritation, with burning and ulceration being the most commonly reported adverse events.[53,71]

Radiation Therapy

Radiation therapy is an alternate treatment with a long history of efficacy, with several small series over the past 20 to 30 years reporting control rates ranging from 80% to 100%.[12,18,49,62,64,65,67,74,83,84] High-dose-rate (HDR), medium-dose-rate (MDR), and low-dose-rate (LDR) techniques have been reported with acceptable results, although it is difficult to compare regimens due to small patient numbers, generally short follow-up times, and overall nonuniformity among series. Generally, radiation is reserved for patients who relapse after more conservative treatments. Drawbacks to radiation include potential undertreatment of occult invasive disease, the risk of secondary malignancy, and long-term morbidity, although there are no prospective data available regarding the impact of treatment on sexual function and quality of life.

LDR treatment is most commonly delivered with an intracavitary vaginal cylinder using cesium-137. Typically, a dose of 60 Gy is prescribed to the vaginal mucosa, but a wide range of doses, depending on depth of dose prescription, as well as a variety of techniques, have been reported.[63,65,67,74,84] Chyle et al.[60] prescribed 70 to 80 Gy to the vaginal surface and reported a 17% recurrence rate at 10 years in their series of 37 patients. Perez et al.[63] treated patients to the vaginal surface with a dose of 60 to 70 Gy, and reported 1 recurrence in 20 patients. The recurrence occurred in the distal vagina and was noted to be a marginal recurrence. Blanchard et al.[65] reported on a series of 28 patients with VAIN-3 treated at Institut Gustave Roussy from 1985 to 2008. Patients were treated with LDR brachytherapy, using a vaginal mold technique, to a dose of 60 Gy prescribed 5 mm below the vaginal surface; 18 patients received treatment to the upper half of the vagina, 6 were treated to the upper two-thirds, and 4 were treated to the whole vaginal length. With a median follow-up time of 41 months, the authors report only one in-field recurrence, with a 10-year local control rate of 93%. Treatment with LDR brachytherapy is overall well tolerated; in the Blanchard et al.[65] series, there were no grade 3 or 4 late toxicities and only one grade 2 gastrointestinal toxicity noted. This is consistent with the Perez et al.[63] series, in which there was only one grade 3 urinary complication among 40 patients with VAIN-3 or stage I vaginal cancer treated with LDR. Overall, excellent local control and low toxicity have been reported for LDR brachytherapy.

Graham et al.[64] reviewed their experience using MDR intracavitary brachytherapy for VAIN-3 at the Beatson Oncology Centre in Glasgow, UK. Using a MDR Selectron (Nucletron, Holland), 48 Gy was prescribed 0.5 cm lateral to the ovoid surface (point Z) over two insertions, spaced 1 week apart. Ovoids were chosen over vaginal cylinder placement in order to adequately cover epithelium sutured into the superolateral vagina at hysterectomy. With a median follow-up duration of 77 months, recurrent or residual VAIN-3 was documented in three patients, and two of these patients subsequently developed invasive or microinvasive vaginal carcinoma. One other patient developed late progression 14 years after treatment. There were minimal acute effects during treatment; however, with longer follow-up, all patients were noted to have grade 1–2 mucosal atrophy, dryness and telangiectasia. Four patients developed grade 3 toxicity with severe vaginal stenosis, and one patient developed grade 4 toxicity, with a vaginal ulcer that presented 2 years after treatment. An additional patient developed grade 3 urinary toxicity with urethral stricture requiring intermittent self-catheterization.

HDR brachytherapy has been used for patients with VAIN-3. Ogino et al.[62] reported their experience treating six patients with VAIN-3 at Kanagawa Cancer Center from 1983 to 1993, with a mean dose of 23.3 Gy (range, 15 to 30 Gy); most treatments were delivered in 5 fractions using two ovoids, with dose calculated to a point 1 cm superior to the vaginal apex. Lesions distal to the vaginal vault had doses calculated 1 cm beyond the plane of the vaginal cylinder in order to deliver adequate dose to the entire vagina. Median follow-up was 90.5 months, and there was no evidence of disease recurrence in the treated patients. Two patients developed moderate to severe vaginal stenosis, and three patients developed rectal bleeding, which resolved. MacLeod et al.[61] reviewed their experience treating 14 patients with VAIN-3 from 1985 to 1995. Total dose was 34 to 45 Gy to the vaginal surface, in 8.5-Gy fractions delivered twice a week or 4.5-Gy fractions delivered 4 times a week. One patient developed invasive cancer, and one patient had persistent VAIN-3. There were no major acute toxicities, and two patients developed late grade 3 vaginal atrophy and stenosis. Mock et al.[83] reported treatment of six patients with HDR intracavitary brachytherapy, with 100% 5-year disease-specific survival.

Malignant Tumors of the Vagina: Squamous Cell Carcinoma

Epidemiology

A review of five series, including a total of 1,375 cases of vaginal cancer, reported a FIGO stage distribution as follows: 26% stage I, 37% stage II, 24% stage III, and 13% stage IV.[85] Consistent with these data, the NCDB review by Creasman et al.,[4] for the period of 1985 to 1994, revealed 3,244 cases of invasive primary vaginal carcinoma, with 24% of patients presenting with American Joint Committee on Cancer (AJCC) stage I disease, 20% AJCC stage II, 24% AJCC stages III an IV, and 32% unknown. Most tumors were moderately (28%) or poorly (28%) differentiated at presentation.

According to the SEER study by Shah et al.,[1] most women diagnosed with primary vaginal cancer are non-Hispanic whites (66%), followed by African Americans (14%), Hispanic whites (12%), Asian/Pacific Islanders (7%), and others (1%). Incidence rates were highest for African American women (1.24/100,000 person-years) and lowest for Asian/Pacific Islanders (0.64/100,000 person-years). The greatest proportion of women (36%) presented with stage I disease, and 65% had squamous histology, consistent with other reports.

Risk Factors

Primary vaginal SCC shares similar risk factors with VAIN and, in general, with cervical neoplasia. Potential risk factors for SCC include HPV infection, history of CIN, vulvar intraepithelial neoplasia, immunosuppression, and possibly history of pelvic radiation, although this is controversial. In a population-based case-control study of 156 women with VAIN or invasive cancer, risk factors included early onset of intercourse, increased number of lifetime sexual partners, and current smoking. HPV DNA was detectable in 80% of patients with *in situ* disease and 60% of those with invasive disease, and 30% of patients reported a history of treatment for invasive malignancy, most commonly cervix or *in situ* anogenital neoplasia.[30] A case-control study of 41 women with *in situ* disease or invasive carcinoma identified low socioeconomic status, history of genital warts, vaginal discharge or irritation, history of abnormal cytology, prior hysterectomy, and vaginal trauma as potential risk factors.[86] A larger case-control study of 36,856 women found an increased risk of vaginal cancer in alcoholic women, likely associated with a higher incidence of lifestyle factors, such as promiscuity and smoking, which are also associated with a higher incidence of HPV infection. Early hysterectomy appears to be a risk factor in some studies, if performed for malignant or premalignant disease.[30,87]

Patients with a history of cervical cancer have a significantly higher risk of developing *in situ* as well as invasive carcinoma. Studies suggest that 10% to 50% of patients with a history of VAIN or invasive carcinoma of the vagina have undergone treatment for *in situ* or invasive cervical carcinoma,[12,60,88–94] with the interval from treatment of cervical disease to development of vaginal carcinoma averaging approximately 14 years.[90,95] HIV-infected women are also at higher risk of developing vaginal carcinoma, which tends to behave more aggressively in this setting than in HIV-negative patients.[96]

The role of ionizing radiation to the pelvis in the development of vaginal carcinoma is unclear, with conflicting reports. According to one study that analyzed 1,200 patients treated over a 20-year period for carcinoma of the cervix, prior radiation therapy was not shown to result in increased secondary pelvic neoplasms.[27] A second study by Boice et al.,[26] however, reported a 14-fold increased risk of vaginal cancer in women with a history of pelvic irradiation before the age of 45, with a significant dose–response relationship.

Other proposed causes include chronic irritation of the vaginal mucosa, resulting in chronic inflammation, hyperkeratosis, thickening, and acanthosis,[96] with subsequent metaplastic and dysplastic changes. Although older studies showed that more vaginal cancers arise from the posterior vaginal wall, other studies report approximately equal distribution of invasive carcinomas on the anterior and posterior walls,[29,90,97–98,99] arguing against the theory that pooling of irritating substances in the posterior fornix contributes to development of vaginal cancers, particularly on the posterior wall. Chronic irritation from use of vaginal pessaries has also been implicated as a contributor in vaginal cancer development.[100,101]

Clinical Presentation

Vaginal tumors can spread along the vaginal walls to involve the cervix or vulva, but involvement of the cervix or vulva at the time of diagnosis excludes classification as a primary vaginal cancer. Lesions can extend radially, either into the lumen to form exophytic masses or through the vaginal wall to invade surrounding musculature and organs. Anterior wall lesions can infiltrate the vesicovaginal septum or urethra. Posterior wall lesions can infiltrate the rectovaginal septum and involve the rectal mucosa. Advanced disease can extend laterally toward the parametrium and paracolpal tissues or into the urogenital diaphragm, levator ani muscles, or pelvic fascia, and eventually to the pelvic side wall.

Grossly, SCC of the vagina can present as nodular, ulcerated, indurated, exophytic, or endophytic lesions, and it is difficult to histologically distinguish a primary vaginal SCC from recurrent cervical or vulvar carcinoma. Histologically, tumors are graded as well, moderate, or poorly differentiated and have been described as keratinizing, nonkeratinizing, basaloid, warty, or verrucous. The majority of these lesions are nonkeratinizing and moderately differentiated (Fig. 72.4).[102]

Vaginal carcinoma most frequently involves the superior one-third of the vaginal canal, with series reporting 50% to 83% of cases occurring in this region.[29,98,99,103–106] A high proportion of patients have a history of prior hysterectomy. There is approximately equal involvement of the middle and inferior thirds,[29] although some studies suggest that involvement of the lower third is more common than involvement of the middle third.[90,99] Older series report involvement of the posterior vaginal wall to be more common, although other series suggest involvement of the anterior and posterior walls occurs at equal frequencies.[90,98,99] The lateral walls are less frequently involved. Tumors may exhibit an exophytic or ulcerative, infiltrating growth pattern.

HPV has been implicated in the pathogenesis of vaginal SCC. Fuste et al.[107] examined histopathologic patterns of HPV infection and vaginal SCC. They did not find any association between the type of HPV and histology (keratinizing, basaloid, warty). Overall, 75% of specimens were positive for HPV. HPV-16 was identified in 72% of positive samples. Ferreira et al.[108] also noted a high percentage of HPV-positive tumors, with 81% of SCC specimens positive for HPV and HPV16 found in the majority of tumors.

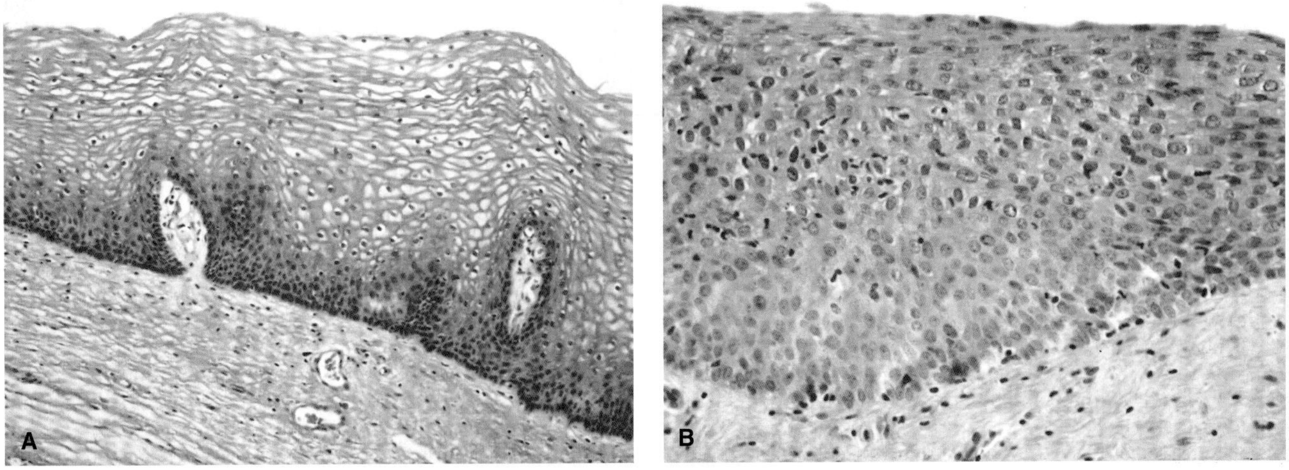

FIGURE 72.4. Invasive squamous cell carcinoma of the vagina at 10X **(A)** and 40X **(B)** magnification. (Courtesy of Marisa R. Nucci and Carlos Parra-Herran.)

Verrucous carcinoma is a distinct histologic variant of vaginal SCC that commonly presents as a well-circumscribed, soft, cauliflower-like mass that is microscopically well differentiated, with a papillary growth pattern and acanthotic epithelium.[109] There is surface maturation with parakeratosis or hyperkeratosis without koilocytosis. This variant of SCC exhibits less aggressive behavior and rarely metastasizes.[109–112] Therefore, it should be considered a distinct entity from other vaginal SCC.

Up to 65% of patients present with irregular vaginal bleeding as their primary symptom.[90,113,114] Vaginal discharge is the second most common symptom, occurring in 10% to 15% of patients. Less frequent symptoms, associated with locally advanced disease, include the presence of a mass; pain; urinary symptoms, including frequency, dysuria, or hematuria; or gastrointestinal complaints such as tenesmus, constipation, or melena. Due to the proximity of anterior wall lesions to the urethra and bladder, urinary symptoms can be seen more commonly in vaginal cancer than in cervical cancer. Up to 20% of women are asymptomatic at the time of diagnosis,[90,115] with lesions detected via cytologic screening or by speculum examination.

Patterns of Lymphatic Drainage

The lymphatic system of the vagina is complex, with many interconnections. Lymphatic channels in the mucosa run parallel to networks of channels in the submucosa and muscular layer, ultimately converging to form trunks at the vaginal wall periphery, which subsequently drain to major pelvic nodal groups. The upper vagina drains to the obturator and hypogastric nodes, similar to the cervix. The lower vagina drains to the inguinal, femoral, and external iliac nodes, and posteriorly situated lesions can drain to the inferior gluteal, presacral, or perirectal nodes. Due to considerable crossover drainage, the location of the primary tumor is not a reliable indicator of drainage site.

Frumovitz et al.[116] utilized lymphoscintigraphy to determine patterns of lymphatic drainage in 14 women diagnosed with primary vaginal cancers and found a substantial degree of anomalous drainage, resulting in a change in radiation treatment for 33% of patients. For example, among four women with lesions located in the upper third of the vagina, which is predicted to drain along the cervical lymphatic chains to the pelvis, two (50%) were found to have a sentinel node in the inguinal region. Among five women with lesions located at the vaginal introitus, a location predicted to drain along the vulvar lymphatic chains to the inguinal triangle, three (60%) were found to have a sentinel node in the pelvis.

The risk of nodal metastasis appears to increase significantly with stage, although the true incidence of positive lymph nodes is difficult to determine because most patients receive treatment with radiation therapy and do not undergo surgical lymphadenectomy. Sparse data on nodal metastases are derived from series in which exploratory laparotomies and lymphadenectomies were performed.[95] The incidence of lymph node involvement has been reported to be 0% to 14% in stage I and 21% to 32% in stage II disease.[95,117,118] The incidence of nodal involvement in stages III and IV has been reported to be as high as 78% and 83%, respectively.[99] At diagnosis, up to 20% of patients have clinically positive inguinal nodes, with reported ranges of 5.3% to 20%.[63,93] The risk of nodal failure increases significantly with local recurrence. Chyle et al.[60] reported 10-year inguinal and pelvic failure rates of 16% and 28%, respectively, in patients with local recurrence, in contrast to 2% and 4%, respectively, in patients without local recurrence.

Distant metastases can occur with advanced disease at presentation or upon recurrence after primary therapy. The most frequent site of hematogenous metastasis is the lung, with less commonly noted sites being liver and bone.[60] In a series by Perez et al.,[93] the incidence of distant metastasis was 16% for stage I, 31% for stage II, 46% for stage IIB, 62% for stage III, and 50% for stage IV. Some histologies may have a higher likelihood of distant metastases than others. Chyle et al.[60] noted a higher incidence of distant metastases in patients with adenocarcinoma (48%) than in those with SCC (10%), with correspondingly lower 10-year survival rates (20% vs. 50%). Leiomyosarcomas are also aggressive; they undergo early hematogenous dissemination, frequently occur locally,[4,119] and demonstrate frequent pulmonary metastases.[120] Vaginal melanoma and neuroendocrine small cell tumors are highly malignant, and both have a propensity for early hematogenous spread.[121,122]

Diagnostic Workup

The diagnostic workup should start with a thorough history and physical examination, with careful attention given to the pelvis. Examination under anesthesia is recommended for complete assessment of tumor extent and assessment of vaginal walls. During speculum examination, the speculum blades can obscure the anterior and posterior walls, so it is essential to rotate the speculum for visualization of all four walls from the introitus to the apex. Bimanual examination, with careful digital palpation, should be performed.

A definitive diagnosis is achieved with biopsy of suspected lesions, which can present as an exophytic mass, plaque, or ulcer. Up to 20% of vaginal malignancies are detected incidentally as a result of cytologic surveillance.[90] If a lesion is not visible in the setting of abnormal cytology, colposcopy with acetic acid, followed by Lugol's iodine stain, is conducted. Biopsies of white epithelium or atypical vascularity should be obtained after application of acetic acid. Iodine will identify Schiller-positive regions, which are nonstaining and should correspond with areas identified following application of acetic acid. Adequate biopsies should include the cervix, if present, to rule out a cervical primary. Patients can present with multiple regions of abnormality. Inguinal nodes should be palpated for disease involvement, particularly if the primary lesion is situated in the lower portion of the vagina, as 5% to 20% of patients have been reported to have involved inguinal nodes at presentation.[63,93] Suspicious nodes warrant a biopsy. Laboratory tests include a complete blood count with differential and assessment of renal and hepatic function.

FIGO staging of vaginal cancer is clinical and allows chest x-ray, intravenous pyelography (IVP), barium enema, cystoscopy, and proctosigmoidoscopy. Cystoscopy or proctosigmoidoscopy may be necessary in patients with symptoms suggestive of bladder or rectal infiltration. Computed tomographic (CT) imaging and magnetic resonance imaging (MRI) do not affect FIGO stage assignment and are commonly used. CT of the pelvis is obtained in place of IVP to assess the renal parenchyma and also to obtain information on the extent of local disease and lymph node status. MRI can provide salient treatment planning information by characterizing extent of invasion and differentiating malignant tumor, which is isointense to muscle on T1 and hyperintense on T2, from normal structures or fibrosis.[123] Advantages of MRI over other imaging modalities include superior soft tissue contrast resolution, allowing accurate assessment of tumor volume and extent of local invasion, and accurate assessment of pelvic-nodal involvement. In general, MRI is regarded as superior to CT for staging of gynecologic malignancies and should be obtained when available.

Positron emission tomography (PET) has shown efficacy in detecting the extent of primary tumor and abnormal lymph nodes in vaginal cancer with higher sensitivity than CT,[124] as is the case with cervical carcinoma. Primary vaginal carcinoma and metastatic lesions demonstrate avid uptake of 2-[fluorine-18]fluoro-2-deoxy-D-glucose (FDG). In one study, 23 patients with primary vaginal carcinoma received both PET and CT during staging. CT identified the primary tumor in only 43% of patients, whereas PET identified the tumor in 100%.

PET identified suspicious uptake in groin and pelvic nodes in 8 of 23 patients, compared with 4 of 22 with CT. Treatment planning was modified in 14% of patients due to findings from PET, and the authors concluded that PET detects primary tumor and abnormal lymph nodes more often than CT.[124] It is important that the patient have an empty bladder prior to imaging, as physiologic FDG activity in a filled bladder can potentially interfere with accurate estimation of vaginal involvement. In practice, most patients undergoing planning for radiation treatment are assessed with CT as well as MRI or PET, based on extrapolation from studies of other gynecologic malignances as well as these studies.

Staging

The AJCC[125] and FIGO[2] systems are used to stage vaginal cancer (Tables 72.2 and 72.3). FIGO is a clinical staging system that allows chest x-ray, IVP, barium enema, cystoscopy, and rectosigmoidoscopy for staging purposes. Vaginal cancer is a diagnosis of exclusion, with involvement of the cervix or vulva classified as primary cervical or vulvar cancers, respectively. Primary vaginal melanomas and lymphomas are staged according to the AJCC staging systems for melanomas and lymphomas, respectively.[125]

For patients with a prior gynecologic malignancy, a 5-year period free of disease is generally considered adequate to allow for distinction between recurrent disease and a new primary vaginal cancer. FIGO no longer recognizes carcinoma *in situ* as stage 0.

Stage I disease is defined as limited to the vaginal wall, and stage II disease involves subvaginal tissue without extension to the pelvic wall. Discriminating between stages I and II can be subjective; thin tumors <0.5 cm are generally classified as stage I, with thicker infiltrating tumors or those with paravaginal nodularity classified as stage II. Perez et al.[63] proposed a modification to the FIGO system in 1973, distinguishing tumors with paravaginal submucosal extension only (stage IIA) from tumors with parametrial infiltration (stage IIB). The study reported a 20% 5-year survival difference (55% vs. 35%) between stages IIA and IIB. This modification has not been adopted into FIGO staging; however, some investigators consider the distinction to be prognostically relevant.[59,93]

TABLE 72.2 AMERICAN JOINT COMMITTEE ON CANCER'S STAGING OF VAGINAL CANCER

Primary Tumor (T)	
Tx	Primary tumor cannot be assessed
T0	No evidence of primary tumor
Tis/0	Carcinoma *in situ*
T1/I	Tumor that is confined to the vagina
T2/II	Tumor that invades paravaginal tissues but not to the pelvic wall
T3/III	Tumor that extends to the pelvic wall[a]
T4/IVA	Tumor that invades mucosa of the bladder or rectum and/or extends beyond the pelvis (Bullous edema is not sufficient to classify a tumor as T4)
Regional Lymph Nodes (N)	
Nx	Regional lymph nodes cannot be assessed
N0	No regional lymph nodes
N1	Pelvic or inguinal lymph node metastasis
Distant Metastasis (M)	
Mx	Distant metastasis cannot be assessed
M0	No distant metastasis
M1/IVB	Distant metastasis
Stage Groupings	
Stage 0	Tis N0 M0
Stage I	T1 N0 M0
Stage II	T2 N0 M0
Stage III	T1–3 N1 M0, T3 N0 M0
Stage IVA	T4, any N, M0
Stage IVB	Any T, any N, M1

Used with the permission of the American Joint Committee on Cancer (AJCC), Chicago, Illinois. The original source for this material is the *AJCC Cancer Staging Manual,* 7th ed (2010) published by Springer Science and Business Media LLC, www.springer.com.

TABLE 72.3 INTERNATIONAL FEDERATION OF GYNECOLOGY AND OBSTETRICS STAGING SYSTEM FOR CARCINOMA OF THE VAGINA

Stage	*Description*
Stage I	Carcinoma that is limited to vaginal wall
Stage II	Carcinoma that has involved the subvaginal tissue but has not extended to the pelvic wall[a]
Stage III	Carcinoma that has extended to the pelvic wall
Stage IV	Carcinoma that has extended beyond the true pelvic or has involved the mucosa of the bladder or rectum; bullous edema as such does not permit a case to be allotted to stage IV
Stage IVA	Tumor invades bladder and/or rectal mucosa and/or direct extension beyond the true pelvis
Stage IVB	Tumor has spread to distant organs

[a]Pelvic wall is defined as muscle, fascia, neurovascular structures, or skeletal portions of the bony pelvis.

From FIGO Committee on Gynecologic Oncology. Current FIGO staging for cancer of the vagina, fallopian tube, ovary, and gestational trophoblastic neoplasia. *Int J Gynaecol Obstet* 2009;105:1, with permission.

Prognostic Factors

The most significant prognostic factor is stage at time of presentation;[1,63,91,126–129] the NCDB, the largest population-based series on vaginal cancer thus far, reports 5-year survival rates of 96% for stage 0, 73% for stage I, 58% for stage II, and 36% for stages III and IV disease.[4] The series by Shah et al.,[1] based on SEER data for women diagnosed between 1990 and 2004, also reveals the correlation between stage and outcome, with 5-year disease-specific survival rates of 84% for stage I, 75% for stage II, and 57% for stages III and IV; the adjusted hazard ratio for mortality, on multivariate analysis, was 4.67. In the Perez et al.[93] series, 165 patients with primary vaginal cancer were treated with definitive radiation therapy and had 10-year actuarial disease-free survival rates of 94% for stage 0, 75% for stage I, 55% for stage IIA, 43% for stage IIB, 32% for stage III, and 0% for stage IV. Lymph node involvement also carries an unfavorable prognosis.[130]

Size of the initial lesion is a prognostic factor that has shown significance in several series. The SEER database study,[1] which included 2,149 women with primary vaginal cancer, noted a significantly lower 5-year survival rate in women with tumors ≥4 cm than in women with tumors <4 cm (65% vs. 84%); however, size information was missing for 52% of women. After multivariate analysis, the women with the larger tumors had an adjusted hazard ratio of 1.71 for mortality. Chyle et al.,[60] in their review of 301 patients treated at the MD Anderson Cancer Center (MDACC) from 1953 to 1991, found that women with lesions >5 cm in maximum diameter had a significantly higher 10-year local recurrence rate than those with smaller lesions (40% vs. 20%). The series by Hellman et al.,[128] with 314 patients treated at the Karolinska University Hospital from 1956 to 1996, found only three factors to independently predict for poor survival on multivariate analysis: advanced age, tumor size ≥4 cm, and advanced stage. Tumors comprising two-thirds or more of the vagina and tumors growing circumferentially were associated with an extremely poor prognosis. The series by Tran et al.,[131] which reviewed records of 78 patients with SCC treated at Stanford University Medical Center from 1959 to 2005, also found size to be a prognostic factor for disease-free survival on multivariate analysis, along with stage, prior hysterectomy, and pretreatment hemoglobin level. Smaller series by Tjalma et al.[132] and Kirkbride et al.[91] also describe adverse outcomes with larger tumor size. Other series have failed to show significance, but they likely were hindered by small numbers, difficulties in accurate assessment of size, and treatment heterogeneity. Frank et al.[114] reviewed data on 193 patients treated at MDACC between 1970 and 2000 for vaginal SCC and found a nonsignificant difference in disease-specific survival rates between patients with tumors ≤4 cm in diameter and those with tumors >4 cm (82% vs. 60%, respectively). Extent of vaginal canal involvement has also been examined, as a surrogate for tumor size, in the assessment of tumor burden. In a series by Stock et al.,[98] which examined 100 cases of primary vaginal carcinoma treated at Magee Women's Hospital from 1962 to 1992, patients with involvement of one-third of the vaginal canal or less had a significantly higher 5-year disease-free survival rate (61%) than patients with more extensive involvement (25%).

There is conflicting evidence on the impact of lesion location on prognosis; it has been noted in some[60,103,133–135] but not all[93,106,136] reports. In an analysis of 110 patients by Kucera et al.,[137] 5-year survival rates were 60% for lesions of the upper third of the vagina, 37.5% for lesions of the middle third, and 37% for the lower third. Chyle et al.[60] noted a 17% rate of pelvic relapse in patients with tumors in the upper third of the vagina, 36% for patients with tumors in the middle or lower third, and 42% for patients with whole vaginal involvement. Lesions in the posterior wall were also noted to be associated with a worse prognosis than lesions involving the anterior vaginal wall,[60] with 10-year recurrence rates of 32% versus 19% on univariate analysis (<.007). The Hellman et al.[128]series found no difference in prognosis between anterior and posterior tumors.

Histologic grade has been found to be an independent significant predictor of survival in several series[91,103,135] but not others. Hellman et al.[128] evaluated the impact of tumor grade and other histopathologic variables (mitotic activity, koilocytosis, growth in vessels, lymphocytic reactions) and found no correlation with survival.

Age at diagnosis correlated significantly with poor survival in both univariate and multivariate analysis in the Hellman et al.[128] series. Age was also noted to be a significant prognostic factor in the Urbanski et al.[135] series, with 5-year survival rates of 83% for patients younger than 60 compared with 25% for those 60 years of age or older (P <.0001); other series have failed to demonstrate the statistical significance of age.[63,138]

Tran et al.[131] reviewed records of 78 patients with primary SCC of the vagina treated at Stanford University Hospital and found a hemoglobin level <12.5 g/dL prior to definitive treatment to be prognostic for worse pelvic control and disease-specific survival;[117] 5-year disease-specific survival rates were 55% for women with hemoglobin levels <12.5 g/dL and 76% for those with levels ≥12.5 g/dL. This remained significant after multivariate analysis, along with prior hysterectomy, stage, and tumor size.

Up to 62% of patients with primary vaginal cancer have had a prior hysterectomy.[139] This high rate reflects the proportion of patients with a history of cervical pathology as well as the increased hysterectomy rate in the general female population.[140] The study by Tran et al.[131] is the first to identify prior hysterectomy as a favorable prognostic factor on multivariate analysis. This may reflect more rigorous surveillance in posthysterectomy patients, resulting in tumors discovered at an earlier stage, or may be a reflection of less overall vaginal tissue as a substrate for tumorigenesis. Two studies have identified hysterectomy as a significant prognostic factor in univariate analysis.[60,128]

The prognostic role of HPV was examined by Brunner et al.[141] in their series of 35 patients with primary invasive SCC of the vagina. Using *in situ* hybridization, HPV was detected in 51.4% of cases. There was no significant influence on clinical stage, grade, or tumor size nor did prognosis differ between HPV-positive and HPV-negative tumors. However, in a subset of patients with FIGO stage III or higher disease, HPV positivity was found to correlate with improved disease-free and overall survival (P .004 and .023, respectively). In contrast, Fuste et al.[107] found a trend toward longer survival in women with HPV-positive tumors in their series of 32 patients, with median survival times of 113.9 months versus 19.7 months for women with HPV-positive and HPV-negative tumors, respectively (P = .15).

For patients treated with radiation, treatment time may be a significant factor impacting tumor control.[142,143] Lee et al.[143] found overall treatment time of ≤9 weeks to be associated with a pelvic tumor control rate of 97% as compared with 57% for treatment time >9 weeks (P <.01). Pingley et al.[142] also noted a correlation between treatment time and outcome; patients receiving brachytherapy within 4 weeks of external-beam radiation therapy (EBRT) had a 5-year disease-free survival rate of 60%, compared with a 30% rate in patients who had an interval >4 weeks.

Treatment: Surgery

For most patients with invasive vaginal cancer, radiation is the treatment of choice. Surgery is considered for highly selected patients who have early-stage lesions, when a potentially curative resection can be achieved without extensive functional morbidity. Surgery is also used for previously irradiated patients who cannot receive further radiation. A wide local excision is reserved only for carcinoma *in situ* or small, superficially invasive lesions that are well demarcated. More extensive lesions in the proximal aspect of the vaginal canal require radical hysterectomy, upper vaginectomy, and bilateral pelvic lymphadenectomy, and patients with positive margins require adjuvant radiation. Lesions that extend to the inferior vagina require a total vaginectomy with radical hysterectomy, pelvic lymphadenectomy, and possibly vulvovaginectomy and inguinofemoral lymphadenectomy.[89,90,98,99] It is not uncommon for relatively small lesions to invade the rectum or urethra early in the disease course, given the close proximity of the vagina to these structures. Older surgical series often required pelvic exenteration in 40% to 50% of cases to obtain negative margins.[95,99] Anterior exenteration removes the vagina, urethra, and bladder and is often necessary to achieve negative margins for invasive anterior wall lesions. Posterior exenteration requires resection of the vagina and rectum. Deeply invasive, circumferential lesions may require a total exenteration in order to achieve clear margins. Given the potentially devastating functional results associated with radical surgery, definitive radiation is the treatment of choice for most patients with invasive vaginal cancer and has largely replaced surgery as the primary therapeutic modality.

In select stage I patients, surgery can offer excellent results, with series reporting 5-year survival rates ranging from 56% to 100% for women with stage I disease.[4,89,95,98,132,144] The NCDB review for cancers of the vagina noted superior survival rates in patients treated with surgery,[4] although this likely reflects selection of healthier patients with good performance status for radical surgery. A more recent analysis utilizing the SEER database[1] found that women with stage I disease who underwent surgery only, had a lower risk of mortality than those treated with radiation only, combined modalities, or no treatment; however, this difference did not reach statistical significance. For stage II vaginal cancer patients, there was a similar trend toward increased mortality in women who did not have surgery alone as their primary treatment modality, but values once again did not reach statistical significance in their multivariate adjusted model.

In a review of 100 cases by Stock et al.[98] surgical treatment was noted to be a significantly favorable prognostic factor for disease-free survival, versus treatment with radiation alone, in stage II patients but not stage I patients. For stage I patients, survival rates were 56% and 80% for patients treated with surgery versus radiation, respectively. For stage II patients, survival rates were 68% and 31% after surgery and radiation, respectively, although this likely reflects selection bias, with patients with more extensive involvement offered radiation. Overall 5-year survival was 47%. Stock et al.[98] concluded that surgery that consists of radical hysterectomy, pelvic lymphadenectomy, and upper vaginectomy could be reasonable for stage I lesions and select stage II lesions, with radiation being the preferred primary modality for patients with stage IID disease. It should be noted, however, that 23 of 33 stage II patients (70%) treated with surgery required a total vaginectomy or exenterative procedure, which carries significant morbidity and functional impairment.

Other series also report excellent results with primary surgical therapy, although authors acknowledge bias resulting from selection of healthier patients with less extensive disease for primary surgery over radiation. Tjalma et al.[132] reported on 55 cases of primary vaginal SCC. Of 27 patients with stage I disease, 26 received surgery, with 4 subsequently receiving some form of adjuvant radiation. With a median follow-up time of 45 month, 5-year survival was reported to be 91%. Otton et al.,[144] in their retrospective review of 70 patients with stage I or II vaginal carcinoma treated at Queensland Centre for Gynaecological Cancer between 1982 and 1998, report that patients treated with surgery alone, or a combination of surgery and radiation, had significantly longer survival times than patients treated with radiation alone. The authors suggest that surgery may be effective in a select subset of patients with small, localized tumors that permit clear surgical margins. Peters et al.[106] reviewed records of 86 patients with vaginal carcinoma, including 68 SCC cases, treated at University of Michigan Medical Center. Twelve selected patients had surgery as primary therapy, with a 75% survival rate. Similarly, Rubin et al.[99] reported on eight patients with stage I or II disease who received surgery as primary treatment; 5-year survival was 75%, and the overall local control rate for the stage I patients was 80%, suggesting that highly selected patients can achieve excellent outcomes with surgery. Davis et al.[95] reported on 89 patients with vaginal carcinoma treated primarily at the Mayo Clinic from 1960 to 1987. A total of 52 patients were treated with surgery as primary therapy, with 5-year survival of 85% compared with 65% for patients who received radiation alone. In the stage II patients, the 5-year survival rates were 49%, 50%, and 69% for surgery, radiation, and combined treatment with surgery and radiation, respectively. However, treatment modalities cannot be effectively compared using retrospective series, which reflect strong selection biases.

Ling et al.,[145] in a small series with 4 patients who had stage I disease, report their experience using laparoscopic radical hysterectomy with vaginectomy and reconstruction of the vagina. With follow-up times ranging from 40 to 54 months, they reported all patients to be free of disease, with satisfactory sexual function. The authors suggest that laparoscopic surgery can be an option for select patients with early-stage disease, with good outcomes.

Several series report their experience using surgery for advanced stage III or IV patients, with most cases requiring pelvic exenteration.[89,90,98,99] Control rates at best were 50% in highly selected patients. In practice, given the overall poor prognosis and morbidity associated with surgery, advanced-stage patients should receive treatment with definitive radiation, typically in combination with chemotherapy.

Neoadjuvant chemotherapy followed by radical surgery has been proposed for selected patients with vaginal cancer.[146,147] Benedetti et al.[147] reported results on 11 patients with stage II SCC of the vagina, using 3 cycles of neoadjuvant paclitaxel and cisplatin. Ninety-one percent of patients obtained a partial or complete response to neoadjuvant chemotherapy; 27% achieved a complete response. All patients had disease-free resection margins after surgery, and only one patient had positive lymph nodes. At a median follow-up time of 75 months, 10 of 11 patients (91%) were alive, and of those, 8 (73%) were free of disease. Postoperative complications were mild. A case report documented the use of neoadjuvant chemotherapy, consisting of bleomycin and cisplatin, followed by radical surgery in one patient with stage II SCC of the vagina.[146] The patient was free of disease, with satisfactory sexual function, at 30 months. However, larger series of patients treated with this approach, with longer follow-up, are necessary to further evaluate the feasibility of this treatment.

Treatment: Radiation

Stage I

It is difficult to compare results for stage I and stage II disease from different series, as the distinction between them is made clinically, based on physical examination, and can be subject to variability. In general, stage I lesions are 0.5 to 1 cm in thickness. It is important to individualize radiation therapy techniques based on size, depth, and location of the lesion.

Selected patients with small, superficial tumors may be adequately treated with brachytherapy alone, with reported local control rates of 67% to 100%.[92,93,97,103,114,135,148,149] Perez et al.[63] reported pelvic tumor control of 88% in patients with stage I disease who received brachytherapy alone, using a dose of 60 to 70 Gy, prescribed 5 mm beyond the plane of the implant or vaginal mucosa, with a vaginal surface dose of 80 to 120 Gy. Frank et al.[114] reported on 21 patients with stage I disease who were treated with local radiation only, without regional node coverage. Nine received brachytherapy alone, 11 received EBRT with or without brachytherapy, and 1 received local EBRT using a transvaginal orthovoltage cone. Three of 9 patients treated with brachytherapy alone developed recurrent disease in the pelvis, resulting in a 10-year pelvic disease control rate of 67%. Patients who had received EBRT with or without brachytherapy did not have pelvic recurrences. In the series by Dancuart et al.,[148] patients treated with brachytherapy or transvaginal cone irradiation alone had a local failure rate of 18%. A pelvic relapse rate of 18% at 10 years was noted by Frank et al.,[114] with all pelvic failures occurring in patients treated with brachytherapy alone.

Typically, the entire length of the vagina is treated to a mucosal dose of 60 to 65 Gy, with an additional mucosal dose of 20 to 30 Gy delivered to the area of tumor involvement.[150] With LDR, treatment can be delivered in two applications, with the first designed to treat the entire vaginal wall and a second application to cover the tumor volume. This can be delivered with a shielded vaginal cylinder to treat the tumor with a 2-cm margin and block uninvolved mucosal surfaces. HDR can also be used to treat superficial lesions. In general, the vaginal mucosa is treated to a dose of 21 to 25 Gy, prescribed to a depth of 5 mm, in weekly fractions of 5 to 7 Gy each. An additional 21 to 25 Gy, prescribed to a depth of 5 mm, is delivered to the tumor via shielded vaginal cylinder, with weekly fractions of 5 to 7 Gy, to bring the total dose to 42 to 50 Gy. For lesions thicker than 5 mm, a combination of intracavitary and interstitial brachytherapy can be utilized. For such lesions, a vaginal cylinder typically delivers 45 Gy (LDR) or 21 to 25 Gy (HDR) to a depth of 5 mm into the vaginal mucosa. Subsequent therapy is delivered via interstitial implant, to deliver an additional dose of 25 to 35 Gy (LDR) to the tumor volume.

A combination of EBRT and brachytherapy is suggested for more extensive stage I lesions that exhibit greater infiltration or poor differentiation. Perez et al.[63] noted that tumor control in stage I vaginal carcinoma was approximately the same with brachytherapy alone as when given in combination with EBRT, consistent with observations made by some groups[137,151] but not others.[114] Given possible underestimation of submucosal disease or nodal disease, resulting in a potentially high likelihood of recurrence with brachytherapy alone, some groups recommend incorporating EBRT into treatment of all stage I patients, except for those with very small, superficial lesions.[114] Frank et al.,[114] in their series of patients with vaginal cancer treated at MDACC between 1970 and 2000, noted an increased trend toward increasing use of EBRT for stage I vaginal SCC over time.

Actuarial 5-year survival rates for stage I disease range from 60% to 85%.[1,93,114,131] Disease-specific survival rates for stage I disease, treated with definitive radiation, range from 75% to 95%.[63,60,94] The 10-year pelvic-relapse rate, comprising local, pelvic nodal, and inguinal nodal failures, was noted to be 16% by Frank et al.[114] for stage I patients. Distant metastases are uncommon and occur in about 5% of patients.[63,95,148]

Stage II

Radiation is the primary treatment for stage II disease and involves a combination of EBRT and brachytherapy. Perez et al.[63] noted a 36% pelvic tumor control rate in stage II patients treated with brachytherapy alone, compared with 67% in patients treated with a combination of EBRT and brachytherapy. The benefit of combining EBRT and brachytherapy, as opposed to using either alone, has been shown in other series as well.[60,98]

Generally, patients with stage II disease are treated with EBRT followed by interstitial or intracavitary brachytherapy. The pelvis receives 45 to 50.4 Gy in 1.8 Gy fractions, with consideration of a parametrial boost if there is extensive primary infiltration or high suspicion of nodal disease. Inguinal lymph nodes are included in a modified whole pelvic field for lesions involving the distal vaginal canal.

Chyle et al.[60] reported an 89% local-control rate in the vagina for patients treated with brachytherapy alone, although the rate of pelvic wall relapse was not reported in this cohort. Of 28 patients treated with EBRT alone, with carefully designed shrinking fields, three (11%) developed vaginal recurrences. In comparison, there were 12 recurrences (21%) in 58 patients treated with combined EBRT and brachytherapy. The authors concluded that coverage of the entire tumor volume is critical for optimal outcome.

Brachytherapy should be carefully delivered to ensure adequate coverage of tumor volume. An interstitial technique, ideally with three-dimensional (3D) imaging for treatment planning, is required for tumors >5 mm in depth.[92,152] Extensive tumors, or deeply infiltrating tumors with nondistinct margins, may be poor candidates for brachytherapy. In such cases, boosting tumors with conformal techniques or intensity-modulated radiation therapy (IMRT) may be preferred and may yield better outcomes than suboptimal brachytherapy.[114] The tumor volume should receive a minimum of 75 to 80 Gy using combined EBRT and brachytherapy. Fleming et al.[153] and Puthawala et al.[154] both report improved outcomes with higher doses of 80 to 100 Gy.

The 5-year survival rate for patients with stage II disease treated with radiation therapy alone ranges from 35% to 70% for stage IIA to 35% to 60% for stage IIB.[29,153] Pelvic relapse at 10 years has been reported to be 25% by Frank et al.,[114] consistent with recent series reporting 5-year pelvic-control rates ranging from 76% to 84%.[131] The likelihood of distant metastasis is higher for stage IIB lesions compared with stage IIA,[93,151] with overall reported rates ranging from 22% to 46%.[93,95]

Stages III and IVA

Patients with more advanced disease generally also receive EBRT to the pelvis, followed in certain cases by additional dose to the parametrium. If adequate tumor coverage can be achieved without undue toxicity, interstitial brachytherapy is employed to deliver a minimum tumor dose of 75 to 80 Gy. If brachytherapy is not feasible, due to extensive tumor infiltration of the rectovaginal septum or bladder, a shrinking-field technique or IMRT has been used to deliver additional dose to the primary lesion.[155,156] The overall cure rate for patients with stage III disease ranges from 30% to 50%. Stage IVA carries a worse prognosis. In highly selected patients with small volume stage IV disease, pelvic exenteration can yield good long-term control; however, in practice, EBRT remains the primary treatment.[1,4,63,98,99,114,135,157,158] Five-year actuarial survival rates for women with stage III disease range from 25% to 58%,[1,4,159] with local failure rates of 30% to 75%.[93,114,131] Outcomes for stage IV disease are worse, with survival rates of 0% to 40%.[60,98,160] Despite treatment with EBRT and brachytherapy, only 20% to 30% of patients with stages III and IV disease achieve local control. Pelvic recurrences occur more often than distant recurrences.[114]

Role of Chemotherapy and Radiation

There are no randomized trials that compare radiation alone with radiation plus chemotherapy in vaginal cancer, and many studies of chemoradiation for primary vaginal cancer are limited by small numbers or inclusion of other cancers, such as cervical and vulvar carcinomas. However, many clinicians incorporate the use of cisplatin for treatment of vaginal cancers, extrapolating from data demonstrating improved progression-free and overall survival in cervical cancer when cisplatin is added to radiation.[63,161–164]

Holleboom et al.[165] published a case report documenting the use of cisplatin with EBRT and brachytherapy in a patient with advanced stage SCC of the vagina. The patient was free of disease at 16 months. Evans et al.[166] reported the use of radiation with 5-FU and mitomycin-C (MMC) in seven patients with vaginal cancer. Four of seven patients were free of disease with follow-up times ranging from 19 to 39 months. Roberts et al.[167] reported results for seven patients with vaginal cancer treated with concurrent 5-FU, cisplatin, and radiation. Three patients received interstitial brachytherapy after EBRT, and two patients received intracavitary brachytherapy after EBRT. Eighty-five percent of patients achieved a complete response initially. Ultimately, 61% recurred, with a median time to recurrence of 6 months. There were three local recurrences and one distant metastasis and the 5-year overall survival rate was 22%. Kirkbride et al.[91] reported on the use of concurrent 5-FU, with or without MMC, in 26 of 153 patients with vaginal carcinoma treated at Princess Margaret Hospital. Seventy-seven percent of the patients had stage III or IV disease. Radiation was EBRT followed by interstitial or intracavitary brachytherapy to a total dose of 62 to 74 Gy. The 5-year survival rate was 50%. Dalrymple et al.[168] reported results using 5-FU-based chemotherapy in combination with radiation for treatment of primary SCC of the vagina. Thirteen of 14 patients (93%) had stage I or II disease. The median dose of radiation was 63 Gy, achieved using EBRT alone or EBRT with intracavitary brachytherapy. The 5-year survival rate was 86% for all patients, and nine patients were free of disease with a median follow-up time of 100 months, suggesting that good local control can be achieved despite the use of lower radiation doses. There was a 31% rate of severe bowel complications reported, with two deaths as a result of bowel obstruction.

A retrospective series from MDACC by Frank et al.[114] included nine patients with stage II or IVA SCC of the vagina treated with radiation therapy and concurrent cisplatin-based chemoradiation. With a mean follow-up time of 129 months, improved local control with the use of chemotherapy was noted, with 44% of patients treated with concurrent chemoradiation remaining free of disease. Samant et al.[169] published a review of 12 vaginal cancer patients, stage II to IVA, treated with concurrent weekly cisplatin at a dose of 40 mg/m^2 for 5 weeks. Patients received concurrent EBRT to a median dose of 45 Gy, with LDR interstitial or an HDR intracavitary brachytherapy boost of median dose 30 Gy. Six patients had stage II disease, four had stage III disease, and two had stage IVA. Ten of 12 (83%) patients had SCC; the other 2 had adenocarcinoma. Overall, treatment was well tolerated, with 92% of patients completing therapy as prescribed. Two of 10 patients who received interstitial brachytherapy required surgery for fistula repair. The 5-year overall survival, progression-free survival, and locoregional progression-free survival rates were 66%, 75%, and 92%, respectively, supporting use of concurrent weekly cisplatin therapy. A small series of six patients treated with chemoradiation at the University of the Ryukyus was reported by Nashiro et al.[170] All patients received EBRT to 50 Gy, followed by either a boost with shrinking fields (n = 4) or intracavitary brachytherapy (n = 2). Radiation was delivered with two to three cycles of cisplatin. Two patients had stage II, one had stage III, and three had stage IVA disease. All six achieved a complete response, and four of six patients remained free of disease at follow-up times of 18 to 55 months.

In a retrospective analysis of 71 patients with primary vaginal cancer treated at Dana-Farber Cancer Institute/Brigham and Women's Hospital from 1972 to 2009, 51 patients were treated with radiation alone and 20 were treated with chemotherapy and radiation.[170] Of patients treated with chemosensitization during radiation, 85% of patients received weekly cisplatin chemotherapy, while the remainder received either carboplatin or 5-FU. Three-year actuarial overall survival and disease-free survival was 56% for the radiation alone group, compared with 79% for the chemoradiation group (*P* = .01). Three-year disease-free survival was 43% for the radiation alone group, compared with 73% for the chemoradiation group (*P* = .01). At a median follow-up of 3 years, tumor relapse was seen in 15% of patients treated with chemoradiation compared with 45% of patients treated with radiation alone (*P* = .03).

Ghia et al.[172] published a retrospective patterns-of-care analysis using the SEER database, analyzing data from women with primary vaginal cancer treated with EBRT or brachytherapy between 1991 and 2005. Of the 326 women in the study cohort, 80.4% had SCC. It was noted that chemoradiation was used in 7.5% of patients treated before 1999 compared with 36.1% of those treated afterward (*P* <.001). Cisplatin was the most frequently utilized agent, accounting for 59% of chemoradiation treatments. Chemotherapy was significantly less likely to be used in conjunction with radiation for women over 80 years of age; otherwise, there was no difference for race, stage, grade, histologic diagnosis, comorbidities, or brachytherapy use. On multivariate analysis, chemoradiation was not found to correlate with improved cause-specific or overall survival.

Outcomes

Overall survival rates by stage, based on reports from smaller series, are shown in Table 72.4. The NCDB report by Creasman et al.,[4] which focused on 4,885 women diagnosed with vaginal

TABLE 72.4 OUTCOMES FOR VAGINAL CANCER BY TREATMENT MODALITY

Series (Reference)	Outcome	Stage I (%)	Stage II (%)	Stage III (%)	Stage IV (%)	Treatment
Dixit (1985–1989) et al. (138)	2 yr DSS	100	70	19	0	EBRT and/or BT
Fine et al. (1963–1991) (160)	5 yr OS	42	68	58	0	EBRT and/or BT
Kucera et al. (1975–1984) (137)	5 yr OS	81	44	35	32, 0[b]	EBRT and/or BT
Perez et al. (1953–1991) (63)	PC	85	66, 56[a]	65	27	EBRT and/or BT
	10 yr DFS	80	55%, 35%[a]	38	0	
de Crevoisier et al. (1970–2001) (172)	5 yr PC	79	–	62	–	EBRT and/or BT
Lee et al. (1964–1990) (143)	5 yr PC	87	88, 68[a]	80	67	EBRT and/or BT
	5 yr CSS	94	80, 39%[a]	79	62	
Frank et al. (1970–2000) (114)	5 yr PC	86	84	71	–	EBRT+BT (n = 119), EBRT (n = 63)
	5 yr DSS	85	78	58		
Chyle et al. (1953–1991) (60)	10 yr PC	84	75	60	40	EBRT+BT (n = 121), EBRT (n = 95), BT (n = 26), transvaginal cone (n = 2)
	10 yr OS	55	51	37	40	
Stryker et al. (1976–1994) (173)	5 yr DSS	78	63	33	50	EBRT+BT (n = 25), EBRT (n = 7), BT (n = 2)
Lian et al. (1986–2006) (174)	5 yr DSS	90	87	32	26	EBRT+BT (n = 28), EBRT (n = 17), BT (n = 4), S+RT (n = 6)
Tran et al. (1959–2005) (131)	5 yr PC	83	76	62	30	EBRT+BT (n = 43), EBRT (n = 22), BT (n = 10)
	5 yr DSS	92	68	44	13	
Mock et al. (1986–1999) (83)	5 yr DSS	92	57	59	0	EBRT+BT (n = 55), EBRT (n = 5), BT (n = 26)
Urbanski et al. (1965–1988) (135)	5 yr DFS	73	54	23	0	EBRT+BT (n = 77), BT (n = 11), EBRT (n = 15)
Beriwal et al. (2000–2006) (175)	2 yr crude LC	–	100	100	100	EBRT+HDR BT
Creasman et al. (1985–1994) (4)	5 yr OS	73	58	36	–	RT and/or S
Kirkbride et al. (1974–1989) (91)	5 yr DSS	72	70	53	42	RT and/or S
Rubin et al. (1958–1980) (99)	5 y OS	75	48	54	0	RT and/or S
Stock et al. (1962–1992) (98)	5 y LC	72	62	0	21	RT and/or S
	5 y DFS	67	53	0	15	
Shah et al. (1990–2004) (1)	5 yr DSS	84	75	57	–	RT and/or S
Hellman et al. (1956–1996) (176)	5 yr DSS	75	36	36	20, 0[b]	RT and/or S
Surgical Outcomes						
Ball and Berman (89)	5 yr OS	84	63	–	–	S
Creasman et al. (1985–1994) (4)	5 yr OS	90	70	–	–	S
Davis et al. (1960–1987) (95)	5 yr OS	85	49	–	–	S
Rubin et al. (1958–1980) (99)	5 yr OS	80	33	–	–	S
Tjalma et al. (132)	5 yr OS	91	–	–	–	S
Hellman et al. (1956–1996) (176)	5 yr DSS	75	36	36	20, 0[b]	RT and/or S
Chemoradiation Outcomes						
Miyamoto et al. (1972–2009) (170)	3 yr OS 79%	St I, n = 18; St II, n = 19, St III, n = 8, St IVA, n = 6				RT+cis, 5-FU or carboplatin
Dalrymple et al. (1986–1996) (168)	NED n = 9(FU 74–168 mo); DOD n = 1 (12 mo); DID n = 4 (46–109 mo)	St I, n = 1; St II, n = 10, St III, n = 1				RT+5-FU, cis/5-FU or MMC
Samant et al. (1999–2004) (169)	5 yr OS 66%	St II, n = 6; St III, n = 4; St IVA, n = 2				RT+cis
Nashiro et al. (2002–2005) (177)	DOD n = 1(25 mo); NED n = 4 (FU 19–54 mo); AWD n = 1 (FU 19 mo)	St II, n = 2; St III, n = 1; St IVA, n = 3				RT+cis or cis/5-FU

DSS, disease-specific survival; OS, overall survival; PC, pelvic control; DFS, disease-free survival; CSS, cause-specific survival; LC, local control; BT, brachytherapy; EBRT, external-beam radiation; HDR, high-dose rate; S, surgery; NED, no evidence of disease; DOD, died of disease; DID, died of intercurrent disease; St, stage; 5-FU, 5-fluorouracil; cis, cisplatin; MMC, mitomycin C; AWD, alive with disease.

[a]Outcomes for stages IIA, IIB, respectively.

[b]Outcomes for stages IVA, IVB, respectively.

cancer between 1985 and 1994, found 5-year survival rates of 96% for stage 0, 73% for stage I, 58% for stage II, and 36% for stages III and IV, with 85% of invasive cases being SCC. The more recent study by Shah et al.[1] analyzed records from the SEER database of 2,149 women diagnosed with primary vaginal cancer between 1990 and 2004. The risk of mortality is noted to have decreased over time, with a 17% decrease in the risk of death for women diagnosed after 2000 relative to those diagnosed between 1990 and 1994. The authors reported 5-year disease-specific survival rates of 84% for stage I, 75% for stage II, and 57% for stage III or IV.

Overall rates of locoregional recurrence, by stage, are shown in Table 72.4. In general, the rate of locoregional recurrence ranges from 10% to 20% for stage I and 30% to 40% for stage II. Patients with advanced disease often have persistent disease despite treatment. In a series by Dixit et al.,[138] 68% of failures in stage III patients were due to persistent disease. Most treatment failures occur within 5 years, with a median time to recurrence of 6 to 12 months,[114,178] and local recurrence is the most common pattern of treatment failure in the majority of published series. Extravaginal recurrences in the pelvic lymph nodes are less common. The reported rates of distant metastasis vary, ranging from 7% to 33%, and usually occur later in the course of disease, with approximately half of all distant metastases presenting at the time of local recurrence.[92,93,104,138]

Clear Cell Adenocarcinoma

Epidemiology

Clear cell adenocarcinoma of the vagina was first reported in 1971 by Herbst et al.[179] who documented six cases of primary vaginal clear cell carcinoma in patients 15 to 22 years of age: five of the six had been exposed to the synthetic estrogen DES *in utero* during the first trimester. This was the first report suggesting *in utero* exposure to DES, prescribed during the mid-1940s to 1960s for high-risk pregnancies, could result in an increased risk of clear cell adenocarcinoma. DES-related clear cell adenocarcinoma presents at a young age, with studies documenting median age at presentation to be within the second or third decade of life.[179,180] Studies suggest that there is a bimodal distribution for clear cell adenocarcinoma of the vagina, with the first peak among young women with a mean age of 26, most of whom were exposed to DES *in utero,* and a second peak among women with a mean age of 71 years, born prior to 1950 and thus not exposed to DES.[179,181]

The majority of patients present with stage I or II disease.[179,182] In 45% to 95% of cases, clear cell adenocarcinoma of the vagina is associated with vaginal adenosis, most commonly tuboendometrial in morphology, although three patterns of adenosis have been described: endocervical, tuboendometrial, and embryonic.[35,183,184] Grossly, clear cell adenocarcinoma has polypoid morphology and presents most commonly on the anterior vaginal wall.

Risk Factors

The risk of developing clear cell adenocarcinoma in DES-exposed women is estimated to be 1 in 1,000,[182] suggesting that there are multiple factors contributing to pathogenesis. Additional factors associated with increased risk include DES exposure prior to the 12th week of pregnancy, a maternal history of prior miscarriage, birth in autumn, and prematurity.[185]

Vaginal adenosis, defined as the abnormal presence of glandular epithelium in the vagina, is believed to be a precursor lesion to clear cell adenocarcinoma of the vagina and, therefore, is a common histologic abnormality in women who have been exposed to DES *in utero,* presenting in up to 95% of such women.[183,186] However, it is not strictly confined to this population.[187] Grossly, vaginal adenosis appears as red, velvety, grape-like clusters in the vagina. Glandular columnar epithelium of müllerian type either appears beneath the squamous epithelium or replaces it, undergoing progressive squamous metaplasia.[188]

Histology

Clear cell adenocarcinoma of the vagina is most often located in the upper third of the anterior vagina and can vary greatly in size. These cancers can also arise in the cervix. Grossly, they exhibit exophytic growth and are superficially invasive.[189] Microscopically, they are composed of vacuolated, glycogen-rich cells, hence the term clear cell carcinoma. The most common histologic pattern is tubulocystic, although solid, papillary, and mixed cell patterns have also been described.[114,190] Cells are cuboidal or columnar in shape, with large, atypical protruding nuclei, rimmed by a small amount of vacuolated cytoplasm.

Clinical Presentation

Patients with clear cell adenocarcinoma most often present with abnormal vaginal bleeding,[179] which is found in 50% to 75% of cases. Cytology is not reliable, revealing abnormality in only 33% of cases; therefore, careful assessment of the entire vaginal vault to assess for submucosal irregularity is recommended, in addition to four-quadrant cytologic assessment.[191] Abnormal discharge, urinary symptoms, and lower gastrointestinal complaints can also be noted, particularly in advanced cases. The differential diagnosis of vaginal adenocarcinoma is often challenging, because it must be distinguished from metastases from distant sites.

Prognostic Factors

For clear cell adenocarcinoma, prognostic variables associated with worse survival include advanced stage, nontubulocystic pattern of histology, size >3 cm, and depth of invasion >3 mm.[189] A study of 21 women with clear cell carcinoma of the vagina and cervix reported overexpression of wild-type p53 to be associated with a more favorable prognosis.[192] Primary adenocarcinoma of the vagina not associated with DES exposure is extremely rare. In a review of 26 such cases by Frank et al.,[193] 5-year overall survival was 34%, significantly worse than for patients with SCC.

Treatment Options

The optimal management of clear cell adenocarcinoma is unclear. There are several published series on DES-related clear cell adenocarcinomas[114,189,194–197] using conventional treatments similar to those used for squamous cell carcinoma of the vagina for stage I or II disease, including surgery with radical hysterectomy, vaginectomy, and lymphadenectomy with construction of a neovagina, or definitive radiation with consideration of radiosensitizing concurrent chemotherapy.[170,198] There has been an emphasis on preservation of ovarian and vaginal function, likely due to the earlier age at diagnosis in DES-exposed patients. According to data from the U.S. Registry for Research on Hormonal Transplacental Carcinogenesis, approximately half of all vaginal clear cell adenocarcinoma cases were treated with radical surgery alone as primary therapy.[199]

Wharton et al.[200] reported on the use of intracavitary or transvaginal irradiation for early-stage disease, with excellent tumor control and preservation of ovarian function. Herbst et al.[201] reported on 142 cases of stage I clear cell adenocarcinoma. For the 117 patients treated with radical surgery, there was an 8% risk of recurrence and 87% overall survival. For patients treated with radiation, there was a 36% risk of recurrence. The authors acknowledge that it is difficult to compare surgery to radiation, as radiation was most likely used in patients with larger lesions less amenable to resection.

A series by Senekjian et al.[195] reported on 219 cases of stage I clear cell vaginal adenocarcinoma. Forty-three patients received local therapy alone, consisting of vaginectomy, local excision, or local irradiation with or without excision, and the rest had conventional radical surgery. At 10 years, the actuarial survival rates were equivalent (88% vs. 90%) for patients who had received local therapy only and those treated conventionally, respectively. However, the actuarial recurrence rate was significantly higher (40% vs. 13%) with local excision alone. Patients who received local irradiation, with or without local excision, had decreased local recurrence compared with those treated with excision alone (P <.03).

A subsequent series by Senekjian et al.[118] reviewed 76 cases of stage II clear cell adenocarcinoma. The 10-year overall survival rate was 65%. The 5-year survival rates were 80% for patients treated with surgery, 87% for patients treated with radiation, and 85% for patients treated with both. The authors advocate treatment with combination EBRT and brachytherapy for stage II disease, with surgery reserved for smaller, more easily resectable lesions in the upper vagina. The use of pelvic exenteration for primary and recurrent lesions has been reported by Senekjian et al.[196] Survival outcomes were comparable to those of patients treated with other modalities. Thus, to minimize morbidity and preserve quality of life, exenterative approaches are advocated only for patients with disease recurrence after radiation. The 5-year survival rate after pelvic relapse is reported to be 40% by Herbst et al.[194]

Most recurrences occur within 3 years of therapy, although recurrences occurring 10 to 20 years after treatment have been reported.[202] Most recurrences are local or locoregional, with approximately one-third detected at distant sites, most commonly in the lungs or extrapelvic lymph nodes, although there have been rare cases of central nervous system metastases manifesting years after treatment.[203] The 10-year actuarial survival rate for clear cell adenocarcinoma of the vagina is 79%. For stages I and II disease, survival rates are 90% and 80%, respectively.

Other Adenocarcinomas

Most adenocarcinomas found in the vagina represent metastatic deposits from other sites. Vaginal metastases from adenocarcinoma of the breast, or other gynecological primary sites, and from renal cell carcinomas have been described.[204–206] Primary non–clear cell adenocarcinoma of the vagina is extremely rare and occurs predominantly in postmenopausal women. Histologic variants include endometrioid, mucinous, mesonephric, and papillary serous adenocarcinoma. Vaginal endometrioid adenocarcinoma is the most common non–clear cell subtype and presents most often in women with a history of endometriosis. Only a few case reports or series have been published in detail about endometrioid adenocarcinoma of the vagina.[207–217] In one series of 18 cases of primary vaginal endometrioid adenocarcinoma, 10 cases arose from the apex.[207] Fourteen of 18 cases had vaginal endometriosis, important in indicating a primary vaginal tumor rather than secondary spread from the endothelium. Median age at presentation was 57, with a range from 45 to 81 years. There have been case reports of mucinous adenocarcinoma of the vagina,[218–220] with at least one arising from a focus of endocervicosis.[221]

On gross examination, endometrioid adenocarcinomas can be polypoid, papillary, rough, granular, fungating, exophytic, or flat, and most arise from the superior aspect of the vagina. Microscopically, tumors display a predominant component of typical endometrioid carcinoma, with tubular glands lined by columnar cells that have moderate amounts of eosinophilic cytoplasm and large elongated nuclei. Only a few cases of mucinous adenocarcinoma have been described,[205,218–220] including rare cases arising in neovaginas[222] or arising from endocervicosis.[221] Mesonephric adenocarcinoma arises from the mesonephric duct remnants situated in the lateral vaginal wall.[223,224] Primary papillary serous adenocarcinoma of the vagina has rarely been reported.[225]

Melanoma

Melanomas arising from the vaginal mucosa are rare, accounting for 2.8% to 5% of all vaginal neoplasms,[226–228] with just over 100 new cases of vaginal melanoma reported each year in the United States. According to the NCDB report by Creasman et al.,[4] vaginal melanomas comprise 4% of all primary vaginal cancers. The incidence of vaginal melanoma has remained stable and is reported to be approximately 0.26 per million.[229] Most reported cases are in white women; one study of 37 women with primary melanoma of the vagina reported 84% of patients to be white and only 3% African American.[226] According to a report by Hu et al.[230] analyzing SEER data from 1992 to 2005 on 125 cases of vaginal melanoma with known race or ethnicity, there is no significant difference in the incidence rate of vaginal melanoma between whites and African American women, with a white to black ratio of 1.02 after age adjustment. In the report by Creasman et al.,[4] most patients were of advanced age at presentation, with only 23% of patients diagnosed before the age of 60; 28% were diagnosed between the ages of 60 and 69, 28% were diagnosed between the ages of 70 and 79, and 22% were diagnosed at age 80 or older.

Melanomas arising from the vaginal mucosa are thought to originate from mucosal melanocytes in regions of melanosis or from atypical melanocytic hyperplasia. Grossly, melanoma of the vagina tends to be pigmented and may present as a dark mass, plaque, or ulceration; multifocal presentation is also common. The most common appearance is polypoid-nodular.[231] The most common location at presentation is the anterior vaginal wall and lower one-third of the vagina.[226,227,232]

In a case series of 37 women with primary vaginal melanoma reported by Frumovitz et al.,[226] median tumor size at presentation was 3 cm (range, 0.4 to 5 cm), with median depth of invasion of 7 mm (range, 1 to 21 mm). Twenty-one percent of patients presented with multifocal disease; 24 patients (65%) presented with lesions in the distal third of the vagina or introitus.

Microscopically, tumors may be composed of epithelioid, spindle, or nevus-like cells and stain frequently positive for S-100 protein, HMB-45, and melan-A. When S-100 is negative or only focally positive, tyrosinase and MART-1 are useful markers. Poorly differentiated tumors may be difficult to distinguish from carcinomas or sarcomas. Tumor thickness correlates with prognosis and may be measured by the methods described by Breslow.[233]

Vaginal melanoma is a highly malignant disease with a propensity for early hematogenous spread. The most common presenting symptoms reported have been slight vaginal bleeding and vaginal discharge, which is usually blood-tinged, foul smelling, or purulent.[121] Reid et al.[234] reviewed 115 patients with primary melanoma of the vagina and found depth of invasion and lesion size >3 cm to be negative prognostic factors. Stage was not found to be prognostic for outcome, but only 42 of the 115 patients had this information available. Compared with women who have SCC, patients with vaginal melanoma have a significant 1.5-fold increased risk of mortality.[1]

Treatment Options

Primary vaginal melanoma is uncommon and, as a result, treatment outcomes for only a small number of patients have been reported[121,226,235–238] and it is difficult to make definitive treatment recommendations. Treatments used in published series include wide local excision, radical surgery, radiation and chemotherapy, or a combination of modalities. Overall prognosis is poor, with historic 5-year survival rates ranging from 5% to 30% regardless of treatment modality or extent of surgical resection.[234,235,238] There is a high rate of distant metastases, ranging from 66% to 100%.[235,239,240]

Regardless of primary treatment, outcomes have been disappointing. Some authors advocate radical surgical resection.[241–243] Geisler et al.[241] recommend primary pelvic exenteration for vaginal melanomas with >3-mm invasion, reporting a 5-year survival rate of 50% if pelvic nodes are free of disease. Morrow and DiSaia,[243] in their review of gynecologic melanoma, recommend radical surgery based on a review of the literature revealing 3 of 19 long-term survivors after exenteration with wide local excision. Chung et al.[235] reviewed 19 cases of primary vaginal melanoma treated between 1934 and 1976. All patients who received wide local excision developed recurrence. Five-year survival was only 21%. Miner et al.[244] reported on 35 patients treated at Memorial Sloan-Kettering Cancer Center from 1977 to 2001. Sixty-nine percent underwent surgery, which was either *en bloc* removal of the involved pelvic organs, wide excision, or total vaginectomy, with elective pelvic lymph node dissection in 74% of cases. Thirty-one percent of patients received definitive radiation. Primary surgical therapy was significantly associated with a longer overall survival time (25 vs. 13 months). Recurrence-free survival was not found to correlate with surgical extent.

Several series comparing radical surgery and local excision find equivalent outcomes.[121,236,245,246] In general, treatment modality does not appear to significantly affect survival. Bonner et al.[247] reported on nine cases of vaginal melanoma. Three patients were treated with wide local excision and six underwent radical surgery. All nine patients developed locoregional recurrence. As a result, these authors suggest adding pelvic radiation therapy to improve local control. The use of wide local excision followed by postoperative EBRT and brachytherapy has been proposed. A recently published review by Frumovitz et al.[226] reported that radiation after wide local excision can reduce local recurrences. However, most patients develop distant metastases, most commonly in the lungs and liver.

Given the high rates of distant metastases, chemotherapy has been used, either alone or in conjunction with radiation.[226,248] The use of systemic chemotherapy or immunotherapy has not been shown to improve patient outcomes thus far.[248] Frumovitz et al.,[226] in their review of 37 women with stage I melanoma of the vagina treated at MDACC between 1980 and 2009, report very poor prognosis even in this group of patients with localized disease, with a 5-year overall survival rate of 20%. In that study, 10% of patients received nonsurgical treatment with radiation, chemotherapy, or both. Patients treated surgically had significantly longer survival times compared with those treated nonsurgically. Radiation delivered after wide local excision reduced local recurrence and demonstrated a trend toward longer survival times, from 16.1 to 29.4 months.

Retrospective data suggest that radiation may improve local control for vaginal melanoma.[121,249] Among the few long-term survivors reported in the literature are a handful of patients who were treated with radiation. Harwood and Cummings[250] described a complete response in four patients with vaginal melanoma treated with radiation, although two subsequently relapsed. Rogo et al.,[251] in their series of 22 cases of vulvovaginal melanoma, reported comparable results for surgery and radiation, with eight patients (36%) alive 5 years after treatment. Petru et al.,[249] in their series documenting 14 patients treated for primary malignant melanoma of the vagina, noted that three of nine patients treated with radiation, either as primary treatment (n = 2) or in the postoperative setting (n = 1), survived longer than 5 years. Median overall survival for all patients was 10 months, with a 5-year disease-free survival rate of 14% and an overall survival rate of 21%. Typically, vaginal melanoma is treated similarly to vaginal carcinoma, with volumes and doses ranging from 50 Gy for subclinical disease to 75 Gy for gross tumor. Radiation is offered in the adjuvant setting based on limited data suggesting an improvement in local control.

Sarcoma

Sarcomas represent 3% of all primary vaginal cancers.[4] In a report based on data from the NCDB between 1985 and 1994,[4] there were 135 cases of primary vaginal sarcoma, with heterogeneous histologies and varying age. Twenty-two percent of patients were under 14 years of age, with a median age at presentation of approximately 50 years. In the pediatric population, embryonal rhabdomyosarcoma or sarcoma botryoides is the most common histology,[252] with 90% of cases occurring in children younger than 5 years of age.[253] Vaginal sarcoma most frequently presents as an asymptomatic vaginal mass.[119] In one series, this was the most frequent symptom, found in 35% of patients, followed by vaginal, rectal, or bladder pain (26%), bleeding or serosanguineous discharge from the vagina or rectum (18%), leucorrhea (9%), dyspareunia (7%), or difficulty in micturition (7%).

Leiomyosarcoma is the most common histology in adults, representing up to 65% of all vaginal sarcoma cases; however, overall numbers are very small, with <150 published reports in the literature.[119] Other less common histologies include malignant mixed müllerian tumor (MMT), endometrial stromal sarcoma, and angiosarcoma.[254,255] Vaginal leiomyosarcomas originate from the smooth muscle of the vaginal wall, but may also develop from smooth muscle cells in tissues adjacent to the vagina. Grossly, patients present with a palpable submucosal nodule, although advanced tumors may demonstrate palpable necrosis or exophytic polypoid tissue.[256] Criteria to distinguish between benign leiomyoma and leiomyosarcoma include more than five mitoses per 10 high-power fields, moderate or marked cytologic atypia, and infiltrating margins.[257] Due to considerable variation in smooth muscle tumors from area to area, adequate sampling is recommended to achieve an accurate diagnosis. Microscopically, leiomyosarcomas demonstrate interlacing bundles of spindle-shaped cells, with blunt-ended nuclei and fibrillar cytoplasm.[121,257] Leiomyosarcomas have a predilection for the posterior vaginal wall, with published reports suggesting approximately 43% to 45% in the posterior vagina, 17% to 21% anteriorly, and 34% to 39% laterally.[119,258]

MMT, also called carcinosarcomas, are highly aggressive, biphasic neoplasms composed of an epithelial component as well as a sarcomatous component. The epithelial component in vaginal MMT is most often SCC.[254] The sarcomatous component can be composed of fibroblasts and smooth muscle or include cartilage, striated muscle, bone, and other heterologous tissues. The metaplastic carcinoma theory suggests that there is a common cell of origin for MMT, with carcinoma giving rise to the sarcomatous component via metaplasia.[259] The most common differential diagnosis is sarcomatoid carcinoma. The spindle and carcinomatous components are positive for cytokeratin in sarcomatous carcinoma, whereas MMT demonstrates a sarcomatous component that is positive for vimentin, with the carcinomatous component positive for cytokeratin.[254]

The first case of vaginal MMT was described in 1975 by Davis and Franklin[260]; since then, only 11 cases have been reported in the literature, with age ranging from 57 to 74 years.[254,261–265] At least one case report of MMT of the vagina detected high-risk HPV in both the carcinomatous and sarcomatous components, suggesting that some vaginal MMTs may be related to HPV.[261] Fewer than 10 cases of angiosarcoma of the vagina have been reported in the literature.[266,267] A history of pelvic radiation is a risk factor for pelvic sarcomas, particularly angiosarcoma.[255]

Prognostic Factors

Review of the literature indicates that vaginal sarcomas undergo early hematogenous dissemination as well as frequent local recurrence. Pulmonary metastases are common.[119,258] Adverse prognostic factors for vaginal sarcoma include high histologic grade, stage, size >3 cm, infiltrative pushing borders, and cytologic atypia.[120]

Treatment Options

Unfortunately, most sarcomas are diagnosed at an advanced stage. Despite surgery and the use of adjuvant radiation therapy in select cases, sarcoma patients sustain poor outcomes due to a high incidence of local recurrence and distant metastasis. Locoregional control is especially important for vaginal leiomyosarcoma. A series by Peters et al.[268] reported on 17 cases comprising 10 patients with leiomyosarcoma, 4 with MMT, and 3 with other types of sarcomas. There were only three patients alive and free of disease with follow-up times of 84 to 161 months. All three of these patients had undergone pelvic exenteration. Patients who received other forms of primary therapy all died of recurrence, with the pelvis as the first site of recurrence in all cases. In 50% of cases, the pelvis was the only site of failure, stressing the importance of local treatment. Overall survival of 8 and 10 years following wide local excision have been reported.[258]

Postoperative radiation therapy has been used to manage soft tissue sarcomas in other sites to reduce locoregional recurrence rates.[269] Results from adjuvant radiation for high-grade sarcoma in other regions of the body have been extrapolated to vaginal cancer. In patients with involved margins, high doses above 62.5 Gy are generally required to achieve local control.[270] Systemic treatment with doxorubicin is standard for leiomyosarcoma.[271]

Outcomes

Five-year survival was 36% for patients with leiomyosarcoma in the Peters et al.[268] series. The survival rate for patients with MMT was even lower, at 17%. There are only a few case reports and small series detailing treatment of primary vaginal MMT. Neesham et al.[263] published a case report of a 74-year-old patient treated with wide local excision and radiation for a 5.5-cm stage I MMT. She developed distant metastases within 6 months of local therapy. Analysis of patterns of failure suggests that local therapy does not have a significant impact on survival due to early distant spread. For that reason, chemotherapy is typically administered after surgery for MMT in other sites and should be considered for primary vaginal lesions, along with adjuvant radiation as warranted. Platinum-based chemotherapy has been used for MMT occurring elsewhere in the pelvis. It has not yet been determined whether platinum agents are best administered alone or in combination with other agents. Combination regimens include a platinum agent or paclitaxel or ifosfamide.[272–275]

Lymphoma

Primary malignant lymphomas of the female genital tract account for only 1% of all primary extranodal lymphomas.[276] Of this group, lymphomas of the vagina are rare, with fewer than 30 cases reported in the literature.[277–296] In one review from the Armed Forces Institute of Pathology, only 4 of 9,500 cases of lymphoma were determined to originate from the vagina.[297] Most primary lymphomas of the vagina are of diffuse large B-cell type, although there have been reports of lymphoplasmacytic, Burkitt's, and mucosa-associated lymphoid tissue lymphomas.[284] Tumor is usually palpable on examination, with infiltrative thickening of the vaginal wall; at least one case report has described ulceration of the vaginal wall.[292] Immunohistochemical analyses are valuable techniques for confirming diagnosis, with tumors typically expressing CD20.[285,295] The most common symptom at presentation is vaginal bleeding. Leukemic infiltrates may be difficult to distinguish from lymphoma; therefore chloroacetate esterase or myeloperoxidase staining may be useful.

Although there is no established treatment protocol for primary lymphoma of the vagina, it seems reasonable to extrapolate from results for extranodal lymphomas elsewhere in the body and to use similar chemotherapeutic and response-based radiation regimens. For patients wishing to retain fertility, chemotherapy alone may be an option in select cases.

The prognosis for women with vaginal lymphoma can be excellent, particularly if diagnosed at an early stage, with 5-year survival rates ranging up to 90%. Of 10 cases reported in the literature between 1994 and 2007, all patients except one were cured of disease after treatment with chemotherapy or a combination of radiation and chemotherapy.[283,285,289,291,298–301] Follow-up periods for these 10 case reports ranged from 6 to 120 months, and one patient died from other causes. Eight patients had Ann Arbor stage IEA disease, one had IIEA, and one did not have a stage reported. The most common chemotherapy regimen was cyclophosphamide, doxorubicin, vincristine, and prednisone. Complete remission was also achieved using methotrexate, doxorubicin, cyclophosphamide, vincristine, prednisone, and bleomycin in one patient. Half of the patients did not receive radiation due to an excellent response with chemotherapy alone.

Small Cell Carcinoma and Other Histologies

Primary small cell carcinoma of the vagina is exceedingly rare, with fewer than 25 cases reported in the literature.[302] Mean age at diagnosis is 59 years, with poor outcome due to early widespread dissemination. Eighty-five percent of patients die within 1 year of diagnosis.[122,303] Microscopically, it is indistinguishable from that of the lung. Neuroendocrine differentiation is often manifested by secretory granules, argyrophilia, and expression of neuroendocrine markers,[304,305] staining positive for cytokeratin, neuron-specific enolase, chromogranin-A, and serotonin. Thyroid transcription factor-1 can also be positive and should not be used to differentiate primary from metastatic disease.[306] These tumors can occur in pure form or be associated with squamous or glandular elements.[303,304] Ectopic Cushing's syndrome has been documented to occur in primary small cell carcinoma of the vagina.[305] Treatment typically follows general principles for small cell carcinomas of the cervix, with aggressive therapy, including combination cisplatin-based chemotherapy, radiation therapy, brachytherapy, and surgery, if feasible, indicated.

Adenosquamous carcinoma of the vagina is also extremely rare. Microscopically, tumor cells are composed of glandular and squamous elements. One case report described adenosquamous carcinoma associated with small cell carcinoma of the endometrium in a 64-year-old female.[307] Treatment similarly follows general approaches for squamous cell carcinoma of the vagina, including combined consideration of combination chemoradiation for patients with gross disease.

RADIOTHERAPY TECHNIQUES

Definitive treatment of primary vaginal cancer with radiation involves EBRT, brachytherapy, or more typically a combination of the two. With advances in conformal radiation therapy, tumor dose can be escalated while the dose to surrounding normal structures, such as small bowel, rectum, bladder, urethra, and the femoral heads, can be minimized. Brachytherapy can be delivered via intracavitary or interstitial approaches, using LDR or HDR techniques. The use of 3D-based imaging to guide brachytherapy treatment planning is evolving, and recent results published for vaginal cancer show excellent short-term outcomes.[308]

External-Beam Radiotherapy

In general, when radiation is delivered as primary therapy, EBRT is prescribed prior to or, in some cases, without brachytherapy for a subset of patients with stage I and all patients with stages II to IVA disease. The treatment technique, dose prescription, and selection of the appropriate energy level must be individualized for each patient. The distal tumor margin can be identified using a radio-opaque marker at the time of simulation. CT simulation allows contouring of vessels as a surrogate for lymph node localization, allowing more precise and individualized field delineation relative to pelvic bony anatomy.[309,310] If inguinal nodes are to be treated, a "frog leg" position can be considered. Unless contraindicated, the use of oral and intravenous contrast can be helpful, allowing delineation of vascular structures and facilitating the contouring of

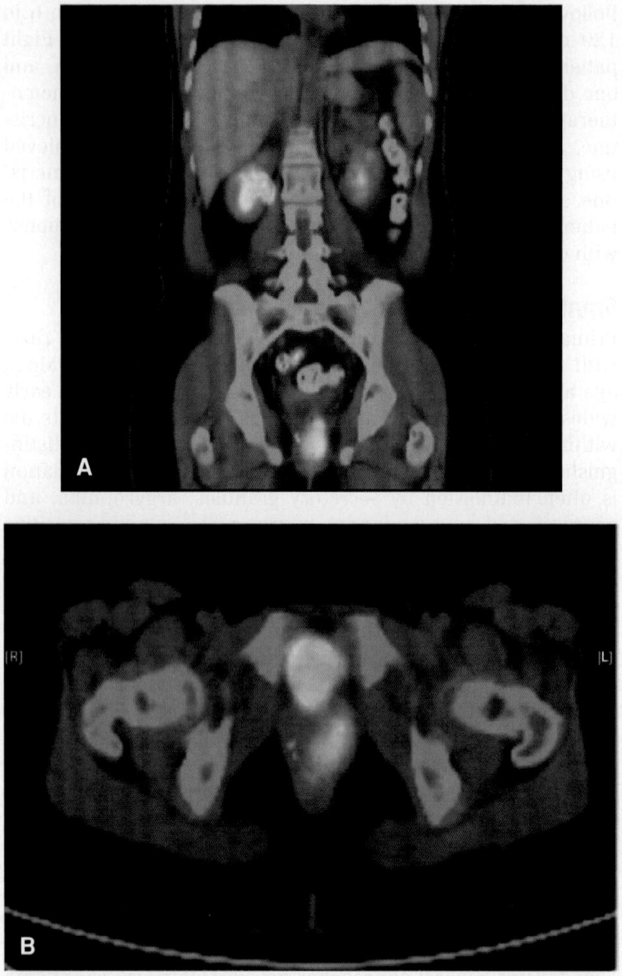

FIGURE 72.5. Computed tomography positron emission tomography fusion images of vaginal carcinoma. This localized invasive vaginal carcinoma extends into the paravaginal tissue on the left side.

bladder, small bowel, and rectum. When available, fusion of diagnostic pelvic MRI or PET-CT to the treatment planning CT can assist in defining the tumor (Fig. 72.5).

Two-Dimensional Treatment Planning

Traditionally, EBRT is delivered most commonly with opposed anterior and posterior (AP/PA) fields, although patients with extensive loops of small bowel in the treatment field may benefit from a four-field plan, with placement of small bowel blocks on lateral fields. If lateral fields are used, care must be taken to avoid shielding any potential regions of nodal involvement, including the presacral, perirectal, and anterior external iliac nodes. Selection of higher photon energy is preferred for superior dose distribution.

The target volume for EBRT is influenced by diagnostic imaging results and stage of disease. Treatment fields are designed to ensure coverage of the vagina and common iliac, external iliac, hypogastric, and obturator lymph nodes. A standard field has the L5-S1 interspace as the superior border, which ensures coverage of retroperitoneal nodes that lie caudal to the common iliac bifurcation.[311,312] However, because many initial failures occur predominantly in the vagina, paracolpos, and parametria, some authors suggest setting the superior border 1 to 2 cm superior to the inferior margin of the sacroiliac joints in patients with negative imaging of regional nodes in order to minimize treatment toxicity.[313] If there are positive pelvic lymph nodes, the superior border should be raised to the L4-5 interspace or higher in order to cover the common iliac nodes. The inferior border lies at the introitus to ensure coverage of the entire vagina, or 4 cm distal to the most caudal aspect of the vaginal tumor. Lateral borders are 1.5 to 2.0 cm lateral to the pelvic brim. Lateral fields, when utilized, should extend anteriorly to the pubic symphysis and posteriorly to the junction of the S2-3 interspace. The border should be extended accordingly to include the inguinal nodes, if warranted. The dose to the inguinal nodes should be calculated during treatment planning to ensure appropriate coverage. When designing treatment fields, the interconnectivity of vaginal lymph node drainage should be kept in mind. Unexpected nodal drainage is possible and should be considered. In a study of 14 women with vaginal cancer who received pretreatment lymphatic mapping with sentinel lymph node identification, two of four women with a lesion in the upper one-third of the vagina were found to have a sentinel lymph node in the inguinal region.[116]

Several techniques can be considered when treating the inguinal region to minimize dose to the femoral heads. An electron boost can be used to raise the inguinal dose to appropriate levels. Alternately, unequally weighted beams (2:1, AP:PA) or a combination of low- and high-energy photons (4 to 6 MV AP; 15 to 18 MV PA) can be used. Another method uses a wide AP and a narrow PA field, with a daily photon boost to the inguinal nodes delivered with asymmetric collimator jaws.[314]

Three-Dimensional Conformal Treatment

The use of 3D imaging has increased dramatically over the past decade. CT scanning is currently used in most centers for simulation; this allows treatment fields to be tailored to a patient's specific anatomy. The gross tumor volume (GTV) is defined as the extent of gross disease found on clinical examination, as well as palpable lymph nodes and suspicious lymph nodes and regions seen on CT, MRI, or PET. The GTV is expanded by 1 to 2 cm to form the clinical target volume (CTV), which also includes the entire length of the vagina, paravaginal tissue up to the pelvic sidewall, and bilateral pelvic lymph nodes. Visualization of vessels allows approximation of lymph node locations. The pelvic–nodal CTV can be defined as a 1- to 2-cm margin around blood vessels and should include the common iliac, external iliac, internal iliac, obturator, perirectal, and presacral lymph node regions. For distal vaginal involvement, inguinal lymph nodes are commonly included, with the inferior border set at the lowest aspect of the ischial tuberosity or lesser trochanter. The CTV is expanded by 1 cm to form the planning target volume (PTV). The small bowel, bladder, and rectum are contoured.

Standard dose to the pelvis is 45 to 50.4 Gy in 1.8-Gy fractions, followed in select cases by a parametrial boost ranging from 50 to 65 Gy. Elective nodal irradiation of the inguinal nodes may be delivered to 45 to 50 Gy. Gross nodal disease should receive 60 to 65 Gy, if feasible, using conformal therapy. For clinically palpable inguinal nodes, this can be achieved with reduced portals, using low-energy photons or electrons.

Radiation therapy should be tailored based on tumor location and size. After external-beam radiation to the pelvis, tumors of the vaginal apex >0.5 cm in depth can receive interstitial brachytherapy or external-beam boost; tumors <0.5 cm should receive intracavitary brachytherapy. Tumors of the midvagina, depending on location, can be treated with freehand interstitial brachytherapy or external-beam boost. In general, anterior or lateral tumors of the midvagina are better suited for interstitial brachytherapy. Tumors of the distal vagina can also either be treated with interstitial brachytherapy, especially if they are relatively confined, or external-beam boost for larger tumors. Brachytherapy follows external beam and allows dose escalation to the vaginal tumor to 70 to 80 Gy.

Intensity-Modulated Radiation Therapy

The use of IMRT must be considered with caution for any gynecologic malignancy given significant shifts in tumor position due to constant normal tissue changes and rapid tumor regression during treatment. The large degree of normal tissue and vaginal tumor movement in the pelvis results in the need to contour an integrated vaginal volume, encompassing the position of the vagina with both bladder full and bladder empty, paying close attention to rectal filling.[315] IMRT may allow dose escalation to gross disease in areas such as inguinal or pelvic lymph nodes, diffusely infiltrative disease, or sidewall tumors inaccessible to brachytherapy. Shrinking field techniques or IMRT can be used for dose escalation if brachytherapy is not feasible.[316,317] In such circumstances, a total dose of 70 to 75 Gy minimum should be delivered to gross disease. Higher doses are difficult to achieve without substantially increasing the risk of toxicity to adjacent normal tissues such as urethra, bladder, and rectum. Typical IMRT input parameters based on those used for postoperative endometrial cancer for the Radiation Therapy Oncology Group (RTOG) trial 0921 include no more than 30% of entire small and large bowel volume receiving more than 40 Gy, with a dose of 2 cc of the small bowel (D2cc) maximum of 55 Gy; at least 35% of the bladder volume must receive ≤45 Gy with a D2cc maximum of 90 Gy; at least 60% of the recto-sigmoid volume must receive ≤40 Gy, with a D2cc maximum of 70 to 75 Gy; and at least 15% of the femoral head volume must receive ≤35 Gy. The IMRT plans are optimized to minimize the volume of PTV that receives more than 110% of the prescribed dose.[318]

Brachytherapy

Patients are re-examined after EBRT to determine their suitability for intracavitary or interstitial brachytherapy. In general, patients with superficial disease that is ≤5 mm in thickness can receive intracavitary treatment, whereas thicker lesions require interstitial brachytherapy. Intracavitary brachytherapy as monotherapy is typically reserved for patients with VAIN and highly selected stage I patients with minimally invasive disease. In most cases, vaginal brachytherapy is used after EBRT to boost the cumulative dose to 70 to 80 Gy in patients with small lesions <5 mm thick.

Low-Dose-Rate Intracavitary Brachytherapy

Low-dose-rate intracavitary brachytherapy (LDR-ICB) is most commonly performed using a vaginal cylinder loaded with cesium-137 radioactive sources. A variety of vaginal applicators are available, such as those described by Declos et al, Perez et al. or Slessinger et al.[319–321] Some cylinders have lead shielding to protect regions of the vagina, bladder, and rectum. Most applicators come in different diameters, and the largest diameter cylinder that can be comfortably accommodated by the patient should be used to improve the ratio of mucosa to tumor dose. Usually, two to three cesium sources are placed along the central tandem of the cylinder. Due to the rapid decrease in dose with distance from intravaginal sources, ICB is most appropriate for lesions that are ≤5 mm thick. For LDR-ICB, the labia are typically sutured closed to secure the implant.

In cases where disease is localized to the upper vagina or vaginal fornices, an intrauterine tandem can be used to anchor the vaginal cylinder or used with vaginal colpostats. Vaginal colpostats can be used alone as well to treat the upper vagina. Some institutions report good results using custom vaginal molds.[322] It is important to avoid placing a source over the vulva, as this may increase skin toxicity. With appropriate selection of dose specification points, a uniform dose distribution can be achieved over the entire length of the vagina. Use of LDR remote control afterloading can also minimize radiation exposure to hospital personnel.

A retrospective series by Pingley et al.[142] reported their experience treating 134 women with primary vaginal cancer. Only the 75 patients who completed treatment were analyzed. Most patients received EBRT to 50 Gy, and 59 patients received subsequent brachytherapy (30 with LDR-ICB, 29 interstitial). The 5-year disease-free survival rate in patients treated with LDR-ICB was 53%; it was 30% for patients who did not receive brachytherapy. Patients who received brachytherapy within 4 weeks of EBRT had a disease-free survival rate of 60%, compared with 30% in those who did not, suggesting that a shorter interval between EBRT and brachytherapy is preferable.

High-Dose-Rate Intracavitary Brachytherapy

In order to sufficiently reduce the dose to normal tissues, 3D-treatment planning, using CT or MRI, should be performed with HDR cases. HDR-ICB delivers treatment over a span of several minutes and has the potential advantages of limiting exposure to caregivers, as well as the ability to optimize dose distribution through varying dwell times.[323,324] Compared with LDR radiation, there is less potential sublethal damage repair and thus a theoretically increased likelihood of toxicity in normal tissue. This has been best examined in cervical cancer, where several prospective and retrospective studies have failed to demonstrate any difference in local control, survival, or toxicity outcomes between HDR and LDR brachytherapy.[325]

HDR-ICB is typically performed using iridium-192, with applicators that are similar to those described for LDR. A variety of treatment regimens have been published, ranging from one to six insertions, with doses of 3 to 8 Gy per fraction.[97,308,326] There is no consensus on the optimal fractionation schedule. Single-institution studies with small numbers of patients have shown HDR to be a feasible and safe technique.[175,327]

Stock et al.[97] reported results for 49 patients treated with primary carcinoma of the vagina. Of this group, 15 patients were treated with EBRT and HDR brachytherapy for vaginal carcinoma, with dose per treatment ranging from 3 to 8 Gy. The total median dose delivered via HDR was 21 Gy, and the total median tumor dose overall was 63 Gy. No significant difference in outcome was noted between patients treated with LDR versus HDR. Five-year actuarial survival was reported to be 50% in the HDR brachytherapy group. In comparison, the 5-year survival rate for patients who received EBRT alone (n = 11) was 9% (P <.001), with a higher rate of stage IV disease in the EBRT-alone group (36%) compared with the brachytherapy group (5%).

The largest series of HDR brachytherapy for vaginal cancer is from Vienna by Mock et al.,[83] which reported on 86 patients. Patients with stage 0 to stage II disease received treatment with intracavitary HDR brachytherapy alone (n = 26). Prescribed dose per fraction ranged from 5 to 8 Gy, with a mean dose of 7 Gy, and the number of insertions ranged from two to six, with a median of five. In that series, the 5-year recurrence-free survival rates were 100%, 77%, and 50% for stages 0, I, and II, respectively. These authors noted similar local failure rates for HDR brachytherapy administered with or without EBRT, for both stages I and II disease. Treatment was well tolerated.

Nanavati et al.[326] published their experience treating 13 patients with primary vaginal cancer with EBRT to 45 Gy followed by HDR-ICB of 20 to 28 Gy, delivered in 3 to 4 fractions and calculated 0.5 cm from the surface of the applicator. All 13 patients achieved a complete response; with a median follow-up time of 2.6 years, the local control rate was 92%. No grade 3 or 4 acute or chronic intestinal or bladder toxicity was noted during this short follow-up period, but 46% of patients developed moderate to severe vaginal stenosis. All patients had stage I or II disease, and these authors concluded that EBRT plus HDR-ICB is an acceptable treatment with a high response rate, good local control and survival, and minimal toxicity.

Kucera et al.[328] described their experience with 80 patients who received treatment with HDR-ICB, with or without EBRT. Compared with a historical group of patients treated with LDR-ICB, with or without EBRT, no significant differences were noted for local and distant recurrences or rate of complications. Three-year actuarial overall and disease-specific survival rates were 51% and 61%, respectively. Three-year disease-specific survival rates for stages I and II patients were 83% and 66%, respectively.

Beriwal et al.[175] described their experience using intracavitary HDR brachytherapy in five patients with either primary or recurrent vaginal cancer treated between 2000 and 2006. The median dose for intracavitary brachytherapy was 20 Gy in 3 to 5 fractions, prescribed 0.5 cm from the surface of the applicator. One patient received intracavitary brachytherapy only, due to prior radiation therapy with EBRT and HDR brachytherapy. Interpretation is limited due to short follow-up, and the results are combined with interstitial brachytherapy patients but suggest that EBRT followed by HDR brachytherapy is efficacious in the short term as a treatment for vaginal cancer.

Interstitial Brachytherapy

Any paravaginal extension at the time of diagnosis, regardless of treatment response, merits consideration of interstitial brachytherapy, as a vaginal cylinder is unable to deliver sufficient coverage to this region. Other candidates for interstitial brachytherapy include patients with lesions thicker than 5 mm, distal vaginal extension, or those with a vagina that is unable to accommodate standard intracavitary applicators. In general, interstitial brachytherapy is delivered after completion of all EBRT.

Clinical examination provides a rough estimate of tumor thickness. MRI is superior to other imaging modalities for determination of tumor thickness, although contrast such as ultrasound gel placed to distend the vagina aids in visualization of the tumor. T1- with gadolinium and T2-weighted MRI may be obtained if possible after EBRT to assess residual disease. Use of a radio-opaque marker in the vagina placed at the time of diagnosis and after external beam will facilitate assessment of the lesion on CT imaging.

Applicator Selection

Template systems are available to secure the position of the needles in the target volumes, and include the Syed-Neblett template, the modified Syed-Neblett, and the Martinez Universal Perineal Interstitial Template.[329] These systems consist of a perineal template, a vaginal cylindrical obturator, and hollow guides for loading radionuclide sources. The vaginal obturator allows for placement of a tandem, making it possible to combine interstitial with intracavitary treatment if desired. The perineal template requires suturing to perineal skin. A freehand technique is best reserved for lower vaginal tumors, where the mass can be readily palpated and visualized.

Preoperative Assessment

Routine preoperative assessment with an anesthesiologist may occur prior to the procedure in anticipation of general, epidural, or spinal anesthesia. Patients with a history of laminectomy, significant degenerative disease, or labile blood pressure are suboptimal candidates for epidural anesthesia. Epidural anesthesia allows the patient to control the degree of pelvic anesthesia, while avoiding the systemic effects, somnolence, and potential mental-status changes that may occur with a peripheral patient-controlled anesthesia device. When feasible, a combination of general anesthesia during the insertion followed by an epidural patient-controlled anesthesia approach that continues during the entire inpatient hospitalization maximizes pain relief.

Patients on anticoagulation with medications such as warfarin should switch to low-molecular-weight (LMR) heparin approximately 1 week prior to the procedure, and LMR heparin may be discontinued 24 hours prior to insertion time and be withheld during the duration of the implant, although subcutaneous heparin for thrombosis prophylaxis may be initiated after the procedure is completed. Patients may have a gentle bowel preparation orally or an enema before the procedure.

Procedure

The patient is placed into a dorsal lithotomy position; the physician should be aware that the needles may slightly displace when the legs are lowered back to the supine position. A digital and speculum examination allows assessment of vaginal width, tumor size and location, amount and thickness of residual parametrial or paravaginal disease, and presence of a fistula. A sterile setup is used at the time of insertion. A Foley catheter is placed for bladder drainage. Radio-opaque markers can be placed to define tumor borders. For patients with an intact uterus, a central tandem may be inserted to anchor the applicator. A vaginal central plastic cylindrical is placed over the tandem and secured. The template, which contains multiple openings through which needles can be inserted, is placed onto the perineum. The tumor volume is implanted by inserting the needles through the holes of the template, with the goal of covering the GTV with a 1- to 2-cm margin, ideally using 3D imaging to confirm proper needle location. A uniform dose distribution around the tumor volume is desired.

If possible, performing implants with image guidance or under direct visualization is optimal, particularly in patients with a prior hysterectomy. To improve target localization and needle placement, there are several modalities available, including laparoscopic guidance, ultrasound, CT, and MRI. Stock et al.[330] reported the use of real-time transrectal ultrasound as guidance, allowing visualization of pelvic structures during implant placement. The ultrasound probe can be brought into close proximity to the vagina, parametria, and cervix, and the longitudinal mode of the ultrasound probe is useful in determining the optimum depth of needle insertion. Transverse imaging is also utilized during the procedure to ensure coverage of the target area and avoid entry into bladder, rectum, or small bowel. Using this technique, invasive laparotomy or laparoscopy can often be avoided.

Several investigators have used laparoscopic guidance or laparotomy to improve the accuracy and safety of interstitial implant placement.[329–334] With open laparotomy, the bladder and urethra can be visualized during needle placement. The bladder and rectum can be protected either by using slings or tissue expanders or by lysis of adhesions. Disaia and Creasman[335] described the creation of an "omental carpet," where a section of omentum is placed along the descending colon into the pelvis in order to separate the bladder and rectum from the implant and prevent small bowel adhesions. If laparotomy is performed in a two-application course of treatment, it is typically done for the first application only. There can be a significant degree of associated morbidity with the use of laparotomy, including increased operative time, longer postoperative recovery, risk of bleeding, and ileus. As an alternative to open laparotomy, laparoscopic visualization has been used. Although laparoscopy is less invasive, both laparoscopic approaches and open laparotomy are limited by an inability to visualize extraperitoneal structures, such as parts of the bladder, uterus, and cervix, as well as the vagina and paravaginal tissues. However, these techniques can be helpful, particularly in posthysterectomy patients, when CT or MRI is not available during brachytherapy, to avoid needle insertion through the small bowel and sigmoid.

The use of 3D imaging during brachytherapy has increased with the rise of CT and MR availability.[336,337] The integration of 3D treatment planning during brachytherapy allows a high dose to be delivered to the tumor volume, while sparing critical adjacent organs. Three-dimensional imaging allows determination of depth and location of insertion and enables repositioning if perforation into the bladder or rectum is detected. In cervical cancer, 3D image-based HDR brachytherapy has been shown to improve local control and decrease treatment-related toxicities.[338,339] There are fewer published reports on 3D HDR brachytherapy for primary vaginal cancer. MRI provides superior tumor delineation, whereas CT images can cause overestimation of tumor extension.[340] The use of MRI at the time of implant can be limited by lack of access, as well as the requirement for specific applicators and increased scanning time. It is not feasible at many institutions to obtain an MRI at the time of brachytherapy. A diagnostic MRI obtained after EBRT prior to brachytherapy can be used instead to assist with treatment planning. Only a few institutions have access to real time image guidance during brachytherapy[341]; most scan patients after insertion is complete, with readjustment of inappropriately placed needles after CT and MRI.

Although LDR or HDR can be used, HDR interstitial brachytherapy has the advantage of limiting exposure to caregivers and visitors and offers the ability to optimize dose distribution using 3D image-based treatment planning.[308,324,342] Permanent implants using gold-198 or iodine-125 have also been reported,[343] and they can provide long-lasting control in elderly or previously irradiated patients and are typically utilized for smaller volume disease. In general, temporary implants are preferred over permanent implants due to their relative safety or simplicity, cost-effectiveness, easy applicability, readily controlled distribution of sources, and easier modification of dose distribution. Given close proximity of the rectum and bladder, it is important to minimize treatment toxicity by avoiding overdose of critical normal structures. However, underdosing the target volume is also a serious risk, thus optimizing target localization and needle placement is critical.[344]

Vaginal cancer with gross residual disease at the time of brachytherapy is prescribed a dose of 70 to 90 Gy, with 60 Gy prescribed to the entire vaginal surface. Special care should be taken to minimize the dose to the bowel, which often lies in close proximity to gross disease. Image-based planning software, when available, allows the dose to conform to the target areas while avoiding organs at risk. As a result, optimal dose distribution can be achieved. The primary mass is contoured based on information from 3D imaging.

For HDR-ICB, different fractionation regimens are used and depend on the institution. Given the difficulty of insertion, physicians may insert the applicator once and treat patients over a several day inpatient hospitalization, with ranges of 9 to 10 fractions of 2 to 3 Gy per fraction, twice a day, or 3 to 5 fractions, ranging from 4.5 to 6.5 Gy, twice a day, with at least 6 hours between fractions. It is also feasible to perform two separate insertions with two hospitalizations required. A representative isodose distribution is depicted in Figure 72.6.[318]

For HDR patients who have 3D CT or MRI based treatment planning, the D90, D100, V100, V150, and V200 are parameters used to describe tumor volumes and the doses to those volumes. D90 and D100 are defined as the minimum dose delivered to 90% and 100% of the volume, respectively. V100, V150, and V200 are defined as the volumes receiving 100%, 150%, and 200% of the prescribed physical dose, respectively.[345] The bladder, rectum, sigmoid, urethra, and, when necessary, small bowel are contoured as volumes at risk, and the D2cc and D0.1cc calculated.[346] The high-risk CTV (HRCTV) is defined as clinically palpable disease, plus any residual disease seen on MRI, and the entire circumference of the adjacent vagina at the level of the residual tumor. The intermediate-risk CTV (IRCTV) includes the region of initial tumor extension and the remaining vagina, in order to encompass potential submucosal tumor spread. The low-risk CTV (LRCTV) is the remaining vagina. The use of MRI-guided adaptive brachytherapy in locally advanced vaginal cancer was recently reported by Dimopoulos et al.[347] with excellent outcomes. Thirteen patients with stage II to IV disease were treated, with 3-year local control and overall survival rates of 92% and 85%, respectively,

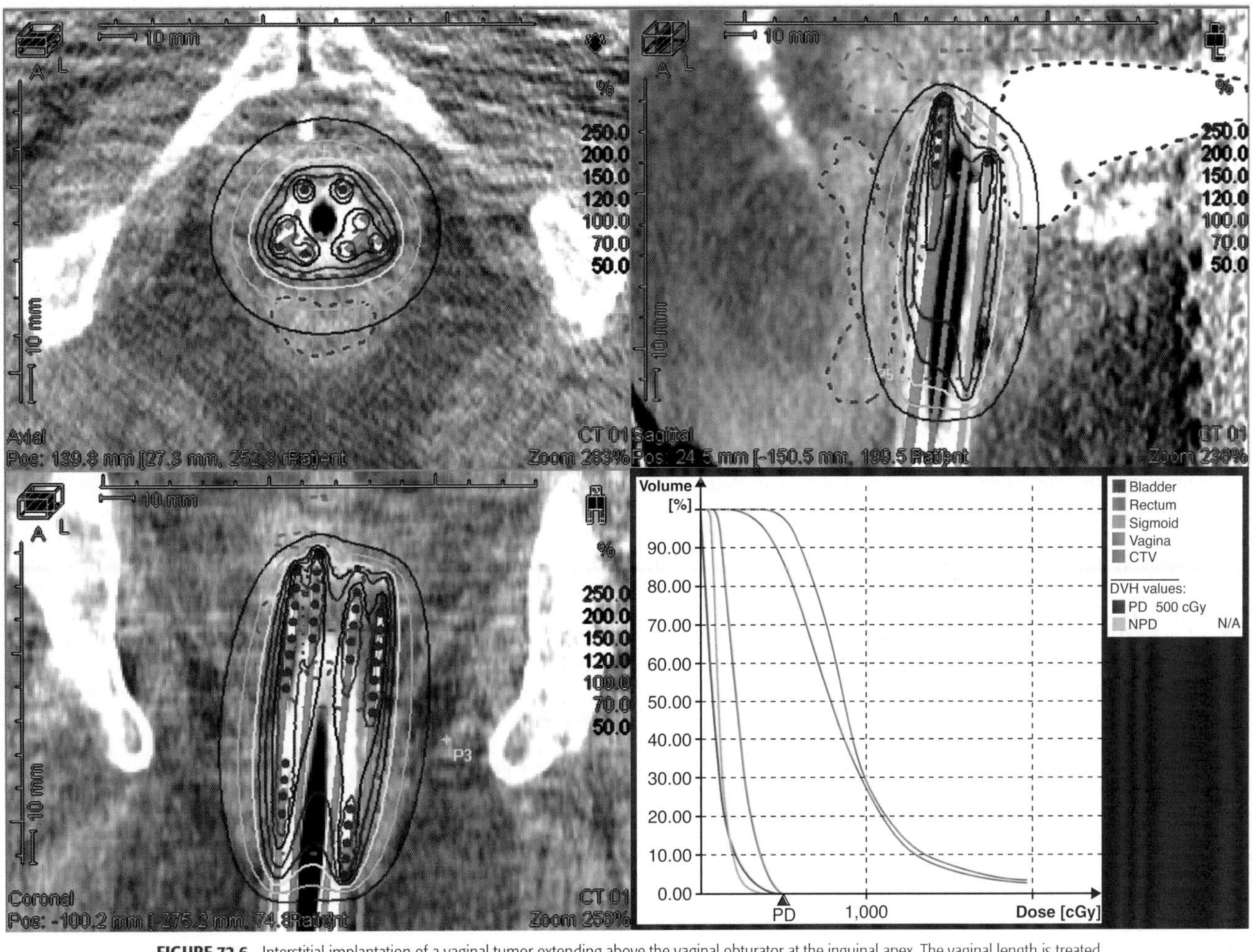

FIGURE 72.6. Interstitial implantation of a vaginal tumor extending above the vaginal obturator at the inguinal apex. The vaginal length is treated with the prescription dose in this case. Axial, sagittal, and coronal isodose distributions are depicted with a dose–volume histogram.

with a mean D90 to the HRCTV of 86 (±13) Gy. Mean D2cc doses to the bladder, urethra, rectum, and sigmoid colon were 80, 76, 70 and 60 Gy, respectively. Two patients developed fistulas and one patient had periurethral necrosis. This study supports the use of the following parameters for image-guided adaptive brachytherapy: for HRCTV, D90 of ≥85 Gy; for IRCTV, D90 ~60 Gy; and for LRCTV, D90 of ~50 Gy.

The recommended maximum equivalent dose in 2-Gy fractions (EQD2) D2cc to the rectum and sigmoid is 70 to 75 Gy and should be <70 Gy when feasible. Maximum EQD2 D2cc for the bladder should be 90 Gy. There are no dose–volume histogram parameters specific to the female urethra, but in general the D2cc should be comparable to parameters for bladder and rectum. A study from Brigham and Women's Hospital reported the grade 3 or higher complication rates in 51 women undergoing HDR 3D planned interstitial brachytherapy.[348] Median D2cc for bladder, rectum, and sigmoid were 64.6, 61.0, and 51.9 Gy, respectively. The actuarial rates of grade 3 or 4 complications at 2 years were 20% gastrointestinal, 9% vaginal, 6% skin, 3% musculoskeletal, and 2% lymphatic. The D2cc for the rectum was significantly higher in patients with grade 2 or more gastrointestinal toxicity. On univariate analysis, D2cc and D0.1cc for rectum and sigmoid, tumor size, and tumor volume at the time of brachytherapy were associated with gastrointestinal complications. This analysis validated the recommended D0.1 cc and D2cc for the rectum and sigmoid.

Precautions for Interstitial Patients

All hospitalized patients should receive subcutaneous heparin as prophylaxis against deep vein thrombosis. Patients should be checked to ensure that a decubitus ulcer has not developed prior to discharge and should be seen in follow-up 2 to 4 weeks after implant removal for a skin check, then at 3-month intervals up to a year, then every 6 months. Dilute hydrogen peroxide douching is advised for patients with tissue-necrosis development. Antibiotics with anaerobic coverage are recommended if a malodorous discharge accompanies the necrosis.

Outcomes with Interstitial Technique

Kushner et al.[349] reported outcomes of HDR brachytherapy in 19 patients with primary vaginal cancer. Two-dimensional treatment planning was performed, with interstitial brachytherapy delivered to 8 patients at a median dose of 23 Gy in 4 fractions. The 2-year overall survival rate for patients for all patients was 66.1%. Three patients (15.8%) had serious late effects, including ureteral stenosis, vaginal necrosis, and small bowel obstruction; two of these patients were treated with interstitial brachytherapy.

A series by Tewari et al.[350] reviewed long-term results using interstitial brachytherapy, with or without EBRT, in 71 patients with primary vaginal cancer. A Syed-Neblett template was used with an interstitial iridium-192 afterloading technique. Patients received a minimum of 20 Gy via implant, with a total tumor dose of approximately 80 Gy. With a median follow-up time of 66 months, 5-year disease-free survival rates were reported to be 100%, 60%, 61%, 30%, and 0% for stages I, IIA, IIB, III, and IV patients, respectively. Significant complications were noted in 13% of patients, including necrosis, fistula, and small bowel obstruction. Overall, 75% of patients achieved local control.

Beriwal et al.[308] describe results using 3D image-based HDR interstitial brachytherapy at the University of Pittsburgh Cancer Institute. A total of 30 patients with primary vaginal cancer (n = 17) or recurrent gynecologic cancer to the vagina (n = 13) were treated using the Syed-Neblett template, with CT scan done after placement of needles for confirmation and treatment planning. Of the subset of 17 patients with primary vaginal cancer, the numbers of patients with stage I, II, III, and IVA disease were 2, 9, 5, and 1, respectively. Fifty-three percent of patients received concurrent chemotherapy with weekly cisplatin at 40 mg/m^2, and apical lesions had laparoscopic guidance during needle placement. The CTV and organs at risk were contoured on CT scan for treatment planning after placement of needles. Most patients (93.3%) received EBRT to a median dose of 45 Gy, followed by HDR-ICB at 3.75 to 5 Gy per fraction in 5 fractions to a median dose of 21.3 Gy. Overall median D90 to the high-risk CTV was 74.3 Gy, and median D2cc to the bladder, rectum, and sigmoid were 58.5, 57.2, and 50 Gy, respectively, showing excellent sparing of critical organs. At a median follow-up time of 16.7 months, the 2-year locoregional control and overall survival rates were 78.8% and 70.2%, respectively, suggesting good local control. Overall, the treatment was fairly well tolerated. There were no grade 3 or higher gastrointestinal complications. One patient developed late grade 3 vaginal ulceration and another had grade 4 vaginal necrosis.

Brachytherapy Versus External-Beam Boost

Brachytherapy provides an ideal method to provide requisite radiation dose to the central regions of the tumor. Nevertheless, in special circumstances when patients are not appropriate candidates for brachytherapy, IMRT is a useful tool that can be used to boost residual gross disease. A retrospective dosimetric analysis from Princess Margaret Hospital reported data comparing IMRT boost treatment plans with conventional and four-field radiation boost plans for 12 patients with cervical (n = 8), endometrial (n = 2), or vaginal (n = 2) cancer.[351] IMRT conferred a significant improvement in dose conformity, with overall improvement in rectal and bladder dose–volume distributions, relative to conformal radiation, although inferior to brachytherapy. Overall, the use of IMRT, compared with four-field treatment, reduced the volume of rectum that received a dose >66% of prescription by 22% (P <.001) and reduced the corresponding volume of bladder by 19% (P <.001). However, when comparing an ideal photon or proton external-beam boost to brachytherapy, brachytherapy provided the best coverage and normal tissue sparing.[352]

Barraclough et al.[353] used an EBRT boost in 21 patients with cervical cancer who could not undergo intracavitary brachytherapy. A 3D-conformal boost was used to deliver a total dose of 54 to 70 Gy. With a median follow-up time of 2.3 years, 48% of patients had recurrent disease, with central recurrence in 16 of 21 patients, significantly higher than the 3% to 4% local recurrence rates reported with MRI-planned brachytherapy. These results are dramatically inferior to those reported with traditional EBRT followed by brachytherapy, suggesting that external-beam boosts should only be considered as an alternative if brachytherapy is not feasible.

Similarly, there is limited literature on the use of stereotactic body radiotherapy (SBRT) in vaginal cancer, showing inferior outcomes to standard management. A review by Higginson et al.[354] reported on two vaginal cancer patients treated with an SBRT boost instead of brachytherapy. Fiducials were placed into the paravaginal, parametrial, or cervical tissues during outpatient clinical examination. The two patients with vaginal cancer received 40 to 45 Gy EBRT followed by 25 Gy in 5 fractions of SBRT; one patient had a local recurrence at 5 months, and another developed distant disease 17 months' posttreatment. Toxicity included one acute grade 2 cystitis and one late grade 3 rectal bleeding. Therefore, SBRT is not recommended instead of brachytherapy for vaginal cancer.

PATTERNS OF FAILURE

Overall rates of locoregional recurrence, by stage, are shown in Table 72.4. In general, the rate of locoregional recurrence ranges from 10% to 20% for stage I and 30% to 40% for stage II. Patients with advanced disease often have persistent disease despite treatment. In a series by Dixit et al.,[138] 68% of failures in stage III patients were due to persistent disease. Most treatment failures occur within 5 years, with a median time to recurrence of 6 to 12 months,[114,178] and local recurrence is the most common pattern of treatment failure in the majority of published series. Extravaginal recurrences in the pelvic lymph nodes are less common. The reported rates of distant metastasis vary, ranging from 7% to 33%, and usually occur later in the course of disease, with approximately half of all distant metastases presenting at the time of local recurrence.[92,93,104,138]

GENERAL MANAGEMENT, TREATMENT OPTIONS, AND OUTCOMES: SPECIAL SCENARIOS

The Posthysterectomy Patient

According to retrospective series, approximately 60% of patients with primary vaginal cancer have had a prior hysterectomy, which likely reflects the high proportion of patients with a history of cervical neoplasia and carcinoma, as well as overall increased rates of hysterectomy in the general female population.[139,140] After hysterectomy, the small bowel tends to fall lower into the pelvis, increasing the likelihood of it being irradiated during treatment. There is also daily variation in vaginal vault position (Fig. 72.7). Finding methods to improve target positioning during EBRT becomes especially important as treatment delivery becomes increasingly more conformal, and techniques such as IMRT and image-guided brachytherapy are useful.

A study by Jhingran et al.[315] evaluated the variations in vaginal vault position and bladder and rectal volumes in posthysterectomy patients undergoing IMRT and found significant variations in the position of the vaginal vault depending on bladder and rectal filling. Patients were instructed to have a full bladder prior to radiation treatment; however, the study showed a median difference of 247 cc during IMRT treatment. It is likely that bladder movement impacts vaginal position. For patients with fiducial markers placed in the vagina, the median movement during treatment was 0.59 cm in the right-left direction, 1.46 cm in the anterior-posterior direction, and 1.2 cm in the superior-inferior direction. Thus, it is important to be mindful of target movement when delineating clinical target volumes.

To minimize underdosing the target, the authors suggest fusing planning CT scans taken with full and empty bladder in order to estimate the potential range of target volume positions during treatment. Another approach, although less practical, is to fill the bladder with a fixed volume of saline using a Foley catheter immediately prior to treatment or to use fiducial markers to adjust daily treatments. These approaches may be more useful for short treatment courses or when boosting a limited target. Alternatively, ultrasound can be used to assess bladder volume prior to treatment.

History of Prior Gynecologic Malignancy

Up to 10% to 50% of patients with VAIN or invasive carcinoma of the vagina have undergone treatment for *in situ* or invasive cervical carcinoma,[12,60,88–94] with the interval from treatment of cervical disease to development of vaginal carcinoma averaging approximately 14 years.[90,95] Ninety-five percent of recurrences after treatment of a primary carcinoma of the cervix or endometrium occur within 5 years of treatment; thus, vaginal lesions arising after 5 years are considered to be second primary lesions. Reports by Perez et al.[93] and Perez and Camel[355] on patients with primary vaginal cancer in the setting of prior gynecologic malignancy more than 5 years earlier showed survival and tumor control rates were equivalent to patients with *de novo* primary vaginal carcinoma.

For patients with a history of radiation to the pelvis, reirradiation can be considered, but it carries an increased risk of

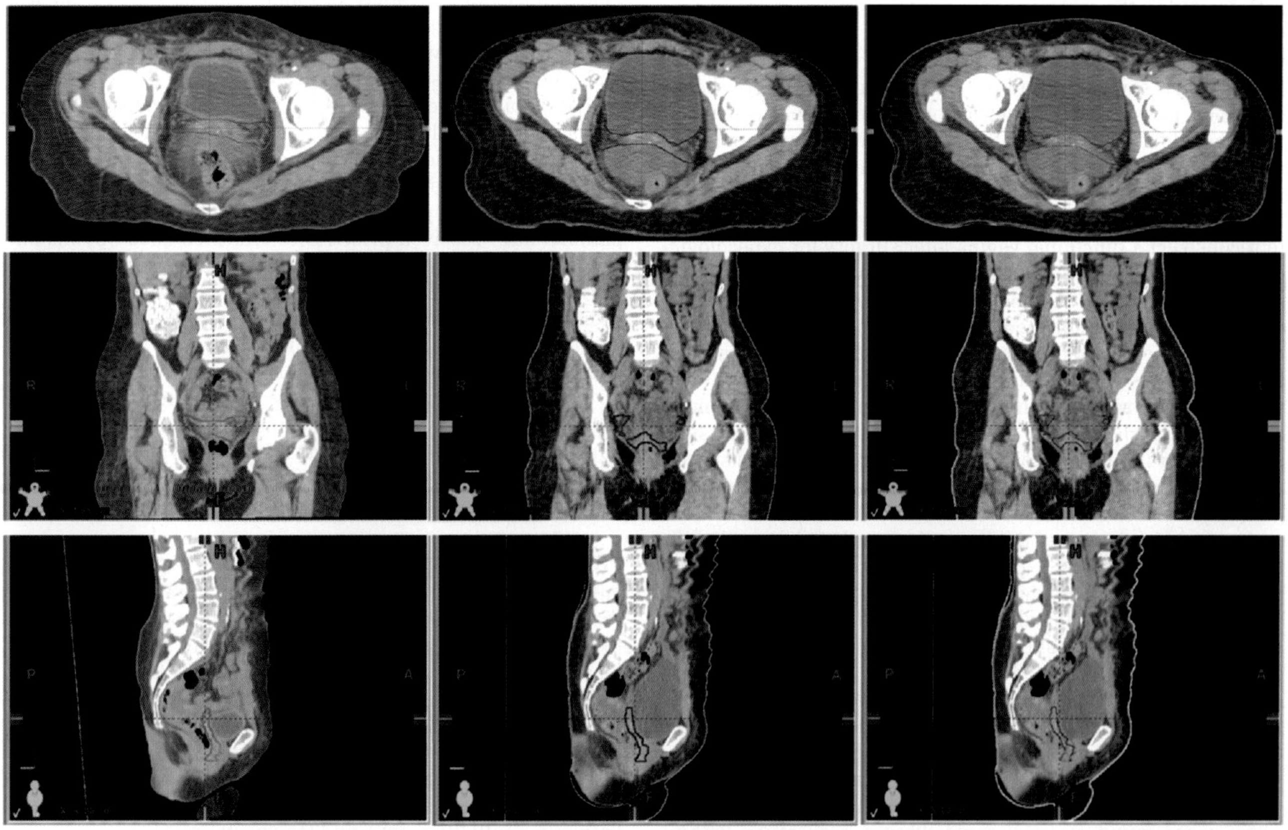

FIGURE 72.7. Displacement of the vagina with bladder filling. Axial, coronal, and sagittal images are shown for the same patient. The *left* panel shows a relatively empty bladder, with the vaginal cuff contoured in *yellow.* The *middle* panel shows a full bladder, with the vaginal cuff contoured in *blue.* The *right* panel shows a full bladder with the two vaginal contours superimposed, demonstrating the posterior deviation of the vaginal cuff that occurs with bladder filling.

toxicity. Xiang et al.[356] published a series on 73 patients with a history of radiation treatment for cervical carcinoma who received a second diagnosis of vaginal malignancy 5 to 30 years later. All patients received EBRT and brachytherapy for treatment of their initial cancer. Reirradiation for the vaginal malignancy was planned according to site and volume of the vaginal tumor and location and dose of the prior radiation. Patients received brachytherapy, using either radium delivered to the tumor base (30 to 40 Gy in 3 to 5 fractions) or HDR with cobalt-60 to the tumor base (20 to 35 Gy in 3 to 5 fractions), followed by a dose to 0.5 cm below the vaginal mucosa at 20 to 30 Gy in 4 to 6 fractions delivered using a vaginal mold. For involvement of the vulva or groin, patients additionally received EBRT to a dose of 30 to 40 Gy. Most patients received radiation alone; 11 also received chemotherapy, most typically cisplatin based. The 5-year survival rate was 40.3% and three patients survived more than 15 years. There were significant side effects with reirradiation: 18 of 73 patients developed radionecrosis. Other side effects included one (1.4%) vesicovaginal fistula and eight (11%) rectovaginal fistulas, hematuria (12.3%), and moderate to severe rectal sequelae (13.6%).

Beriwal et al.[175] reported on the use of HDR interstitial and intracavitary brachytherapy for five patients with recurrent vaginal cancer with a history of pelvic irradiation. Median time from prior radiation to recurrence was 4 years (range, 6 months to 18 years). The recurrence was within 2 cm of the prior field in two patients and within the previous field for four patients. All patients received EBRT to a median dose of 45 Gy, followed by brachytherapy. For the four patients with prior overlapping fields, the cumulative EQD2 to the vaginal mucosa ranged from 120.7 Gy to 154.54 Gy. Of these patients, one developed a rectovaginal fistula 2 years after treatment and another developed chronic vaginal ulceration with vaginal shortening to 2 cm; the EQD2 values were 142.98 and 154 Gy, respectively. There were no significant grade 3 or higher toxicities noted in the other patients.

Carcinoma of the Neovagina

In the past several decades, various methods have been described for vaginal reconstruction or neovaginal construction, including split-skin grafts, myocutaneous flaps, and formation of an artificial canal between the rectum and vagina. Such techniques have been used to construct a vaginal canal for patients with congenitally deformed or absent genitalia or to reconstruct a functional vagina after surgery for gynecologic malignancy.[357] There are very few reports of *in situ* or invasive carcinoma arising in the neovagina. A review of published literature reveals six published reports of carcinoma *in situ*.[358–363] The period of development of carcinoma *in situ* ranged from 6 months to 20 years after constructive surgery. Five patients were treated with surgical therapy. Although topical approaches such as 5-FU or laser ablation can be used, surgery offers a full pathologic evaluation. The extent of disease, patient characteristics, and treatment goals should be used to guide the choice of treatment.

Invasive carcinoma of the neovagina tends to be poorly differentiated. All reported patients have presented with large tumor masses and evidence of rapid progression.[222,364–367] Treatment options include radiation, with or without an attempt at radical resection, and, in select cases, lymph node dissection. Of 16 reported cases from a review by Steiner et al.,[357] nine received primary radiation alone, one received radiation followed by exenteration and intraoperative radiation, and four underwent exenteration. Although most cases were SCC (n = 11), there were also five cases of adenocarcinoma. Recurrence status was not documented for all patients. Three were found to have rapid disease recurrence within several months. Two patients were free of disease at 10 and 18 months, respectively. One patient had a recurrence-free interval of 3 years but died a year later from disease.

Recommendations for patients with vaginal reconstruction include regular cytologic surveillance, biopsy of suspicious granulation tissue, and avoidance of chronic irritation, which may contribute to the risk of malignancy. Although there is no optimal treatment, resection followed by consideration of adjuvant radiation is preferable to definitive radiation alone, as definitive radiation may be associated with higher recurrence rates.

Carcinoma in an Episiotomy Scar

There have been case reports documenting implantation of cervical or vulvar carcinoma in an episiotomy scar.[368–371] At presentation, the lesions have been described as nodular, or granular, ranging in size from subcentimeter to over 4 cm. Patients treated with excision and radiation do well, with no evidence of disease recurrence,[369] favoring a diagnosis of implantation over metastatic deposit. In general, patients with a history of premalignant or malignant gynecologic lesions should receive careful inspection and biopsy of any suspicious lesions in episiotomy scars during routine follow-up. Overall outcomes appear to be favorable and should be tailored to each patient given the rarity of this entity.

Salvage Therapy

For patients with recurrent or persistent disease, it is important to determine whether there is a reasonable chance of cure with salvage treatment or whether the primary goal is palliation. Thus, multiple factors, including extent of disease, site and extent of recurrence, disease-free interval, status of systemic disease, patient age, comorbidities, and overall performance status, must be considered.

Theoretically, stages I and II lesions that recur after radiation therapy can be salvaged with surgical procedures, ranging from total vaginectomy to total pelvic exenteration. A retrospective review of pelvic exenteration for recurrent gynecologic malignancies at University of California–Los Angeles Medical Center from 1956 to 2001 reported survival rates for patients with recurrent cervical and vaginal cancer to be 73% at 1 year and 54% at 5 years.[372]

Early-stage lesions that recur after limited surgical procedures can be salvaged using more extensive surgery or radiation. If radiation is used, concurrent chemotherapy with a cisplatin-based regimen may be reasonable. Recurrent disease in advanced-stage patients is more challenging to treat. Most patients have received prior EBRT and thus have options limited to radical surgery or, in patients with localized disease, reirradiation. For patients with small pelvic recurrences, reirradiation with intracavitary or interstitial brachytherapy has been reported, with control rates between 50% and 75%, and grade 3 or higher complication rates between 7% and 15%.[175,356,373–376] A recent series by Beriwal et al.[175] evaluated HDR brachytherapy for primary and recurrent vaginal malignancy. In the subset of patients with a previous malignancy, crude local control rates were 100% for patients without prior radiation and 67% for patients with a history of radiation.

Palliative Therapy

Patients with stage IVB disease have no curative options, but they can receive substantial symptomatic benefit from local radiation treatment. Advanced disease can result in vaginal bleeding, pelvic pain, lymphedema, and visceral obstruction. Although most series on palliation of gynecologic malignancies involve EBRT, brachytherapy can also be considered for effective symptom management, particularly in the case of vaginal disease. Various regimens have been used. Treatment intensity and duration must be balanced with the extent of expected palliation, potential toxicity, and life expectancy.

Vaginal bleeding is a common symptom for which radiation is prescribed. Bleeding can be minimal, due to tumor friability, or may become brisk when tumor erodes into a larger vessel.

Large fractions of radiation delivered initially during the treatment course may be useful in achieving hemostasis for such cases. Other options include embolization, infusion of vasopressin, and balloon catheterization for severe hemodynamic losses. Commonly prescribed palliative regimens, based on clinical experience from other tumor sites, are doses of 30 to 40 Gy in 10 to 20 Gy fractions, resulting in protracted treatment times. As this may not be the most appropriate regimen for patients with a limited life expectancy, shorter courses of radiation have been explored. Larger doses per fraction may increase the risk of late toxicity, but many patients may not live long enough for it to manifest these side effects.

The phase II RTOG-7905 trial explored the use of hypofractionation delivered concurrently with misonidazole, a hypoxic cell sensitizer, in patients with advanced pelvic malignancies.[377] Radiation was 10 Gy delivered every 4 weeks for a total of 3 treatments. Although the overall response rate was 41% for patients who completed all three courses, the protocol was closed early due to an unacceptably high risk of late gastrointestinal complications (45% grade 3 and 4). A follow-up study, RTOG-8502, sought to decrease toxicity with an alternative fractionation regimen of 3.7 Gy delivered twice daily, for a total of 14.8 Gy, to be repeated at 4-week intervals up to 3 times.[378] The overall tumor response rate was 32% for evaluated patients and 45% for patients who completed all 3 courses of radiation, with a substantially lower late complication rate of 7%. The phase III portion of RTOG-8502 was initiated with patients randomized to a 2- or 4-week treatment break between radiation cycles in the hope of limiting tumor repopulation by decreasing the treatment interval. However, no differences in tumor response or palliation were found. Overall, bleeding and obstruction were substantially or completely palliated in 90% of patients and 68% reported relief of pain.[379] Although there was a trend toward increased toxicity in patients with shorter rest periods, there was no significant difference in late toxicity between the two regimens.

There have been smaller series documenting use of hypofractionated regimens for palliation of gynecologic malignancies. Yan et al.[380] published a series on 51 patients with advanced gynecologic malignancies, including 10 with vaginal cancer, treated over a 10-year period at Princess Margaret Hospital. A regimen of 24 Gy delivered in 3 fractions with 7 and 14 days between subsequent fractions was used. Ninety-four percent of patients received at least 2 fractions. Overall, 92% of patients had complete or partial resolution of vaginal bleeding, and 76% reported decreased pain, comparable to other reported regimens for pelvic malignancies.

TREATMENT COMPLICATIONS AND MANAGEMENT

Radiation Toxicity

Pathologic changes in the vaginal mucosa after radiation treatment include marked mucosal atrophy with epithelial thinning and loss of the overlying stratified squamous layer. There can be hyalinization and collagenization of submucosal connective tissues, with fibrosis of the muscular layer and vasculature. Such changes result in compromised oxygenation of injured tissues, promoting ulceration and fistula formation. It is common to find cytologic abnormalities within the first 6 months after radiation, and it is important to distinguish postradiation atypia from new or recurrent malignancy during posttreatment follow-up.[381]

Clinically, vaginal stenosis and shortening can manifest several months after radiation, although presentation as late as 15 years posttreatment has been documented.[382] The reported incidence varies between series. Most of the available data are based on experience treating cervical cancer. In a retrospective review by Eifel et al.[382] of records for 1,784 patients treated with radiation for cervical cancer, the risk of severe vaginal shortening, defined as >50% of the length, was significantly higher for older patients; the 10-year incidence was 5% for those treated after the age of 50 and was 1% for younger patients. Rectovaginal and vesicovaginal fistulas form typically within 2 years of radiation therapy completion, often with preceding pelvic pain and nonhealing ulceration.[383] Symptoms include passage of vaginal stool or watery discharge. Diagnosis is made on vaginoscopy or cystoscopy, although CT or MRI with contrast can yield characteristic findings.

There are limited long-term data on late toxicity following radiation treatment of vaginal cancer. Perez et al.,[93] in their series on 205 patients treated with radiation for VAIN or vaginal carcinoma, reported a 12% crude rate of late complications in 25 patients, which included rectovaginal fistulas (n = 6), vesicovaginal fistulas (n = 3), bladder-neck contractures or urethral strictures (n = 2), rectal strictures (n = 2), and proctitis (n = 2). Other complications included rectal ulceration, vaginal necrosis, small bowel obstruction, cystitis, leg edema, neuritis, severe vaginal stenosis, and diverticulitis.

Chyle et al.,[60] in a review of 301 patients treated with radiation, reported a 19% incidence of severe complications at 20 years, including fistulas (n = 10), rectal ulceration, proctitis or stricture (n = 10), urethral stricture (n = 6), vaginal ulceration or necrosis (n = 8), and small bowel obstruction (n = 7). A subsequent series from MDACC described 193 patients with vaginal SCC treated between 1970 and 2000 with a variety of techniques.[114] The majority of patients with advanced-stage disease (66%) received radiation to a mean dose of 64 Gy. The cumulative rate of grade 3 or 4 complications was 17% at 10 years (n = 20). Nineteen of 25 total complications were gastrointestinal, with proctitis (n = 7), fistulas (n = 5), and small bowel obstruction (n = 4) being the three most frequent. Of the 11 patients with severe rectal complications, eight had tumors involving the posterior aspect of the vaginal wall. Likewise, all major genitourinary complications occurred in patients with tumor involving the anterior wall. On univariate analysis, FIGO stage and smoking status correlated significantly with the risk of late complications.

The vagina is considered to be a relatively radioresistant organ. Although the tolerance dose is not clearly defined, several studies have shown significantly increased toxicity with increased dose. Lian et al.[174] reviewed records of 68 patients treated with radiation for primary vaginal cancer at the Cross Cancer Institute in Edmonton, Canada, from 1986 to 2006. Patients were treated with EBRT, brachytherapy, or a combination of the two and total doses for the three treatment groups were 60.5 Gy, 34.5 to 60 Gy and 70.5 to 72.6 Gy, respectively. There were no reported grade 3 or 4 bowel or bladder toxicities. Six patients (10%) developed grade 3 to 4 vaginal injury, with five rectovaginal fistulas; dose >70 Gy was significantly associated with the incidence of vaginal toxicity. Beriwal et al.,[175] in a series of 18 patients treated with HDR brachytherapy, found two patients (treated to total doses of 142.98 and 154 Gy) who developed late grade 3 or 4 toxicity; one patient had a rectovaginal fistula 2 years after treatment, and the other developed a chronic vaginal ulcer with significant narrowing and shortening of the vagina.

Patient-related factors contributing to radiation injury include age at treatment, location of the primary tumor, and smoking status. Age over 50 has been shown to correlate with incidence of vaginal stenosis.[384] Several studies demonstrate an increased rate of fistula formation after treatment of vaginal cancers that invade into the bladder or rectum.[383] A retrospective review from MDACC demonstrated that current smokers had a 5-year complication risk of 25% compared with 5% for those who had never smoked.[382] There are numerous treatment-related factors that may potentially impact radiation toxicity, including fractionation pattern, size of intracavitary cylinder and resultant vaginal surface dose, use of concurrent chemotherapy, and surgery. There is no clear association between the use of chemotherapy and increased radiation sequelae; however, data are limited. Several series have shown an increased risk of fistula formation in patients who undergo surgery prior to radiation compared with patients who receive either surgery or radiation alone[382,385,386]; although these reviews were conducted on cervical cancer patients, it stands to reason that a similar association may exist in patients treated for vaginal cancer.

Symptom Management and Prevention

Acute injury to the vaginal mucosa should be managed symptomatically through hygiene, recognition and treatment of infection, and pain control. There should be a low threshold for starting antifungal medications, as candida can exacerbate vaginitis. Sitz baths and topical ointments may be useful for radiation dermatitis, and both topical and oral analgesics can be prescribed for mucositis and general discomfort during radiation.

The bladder and rectum are located in close proximity to the vagina, and it is common for patients to develop acute toxicity during treatment.[387] Increased urinary frequency, urgency, and dysuria can be managed with phenazopyridine, a urinary tract analgesic, as well as oral anticholinergic and antispasmodic medications. Antidiarrheal medications such as loperamide, and in more severe cases tincture of opium, should be prescribed for management early in the development of symptoms. Irritation of the anal mucosa can cause exacerbation of hemorrhoids and occasional hemorrhagic spotting and discomfort with defecation; topical hemorrhoidal ointments or suppositories can be used.

Regular use of a vaginal dilator to decrease stenosis and shortening should be recommended shortly after completion of radiation, as it is difficult to reverse stenosis and shortening once fibrosis has ensued. Topical estrogen, applied 3 times a week for 6 to 9 months after radiation, was shown in a randomized controlled trial published in 1975 to reduce the incidence of stenosis, dyspareunia, and cytologic changes in vaginal epithelium.[388] However, due to a small potential for systemic absorption with untoward effects on endometrial proliferation, the use of topical estrogens is not favored for all patients.

Radiation necrosis can be conservatively managed with local debridement, peroxide douches, antimicrobials, and estrogen. There is some evidence that hyperbaric oxygen can facilitate healing, with a >50% reduction in vaginal ulceration noted in one series.[389] Fistulas present more of a treatment challenge. Despite the use of interventions such as urinary or fecal diversions, additional surgical correction is often required for effective management, particularly in the case of rectovaginal fistulas.[390]

TREATMENT ALGORITHM AND CONCLUSIONS

A treatment algorithm for invasive SCC of the vagina is shown in Figure 72.8. Vaginal cancer is a rare disease with a poor prognosis. It is hoped that improvements in local control will yield superior patient outcomes. Optimizing delivery of radiation to tumor volumes while minimizing treatment toxicity remains critical for progress. The increasing use of 3D imaging, conformal external-beam treatments, and image-guided brachytherapy in gynecologic malignancies should optimize the efficacy and precision of radiation dose delivery. Given the low incidence of vaginal cancer, it is unlikely that randomized clinical trials will be undertaken; thus single-institution series will be important in guiding our understanding and management of this disease.

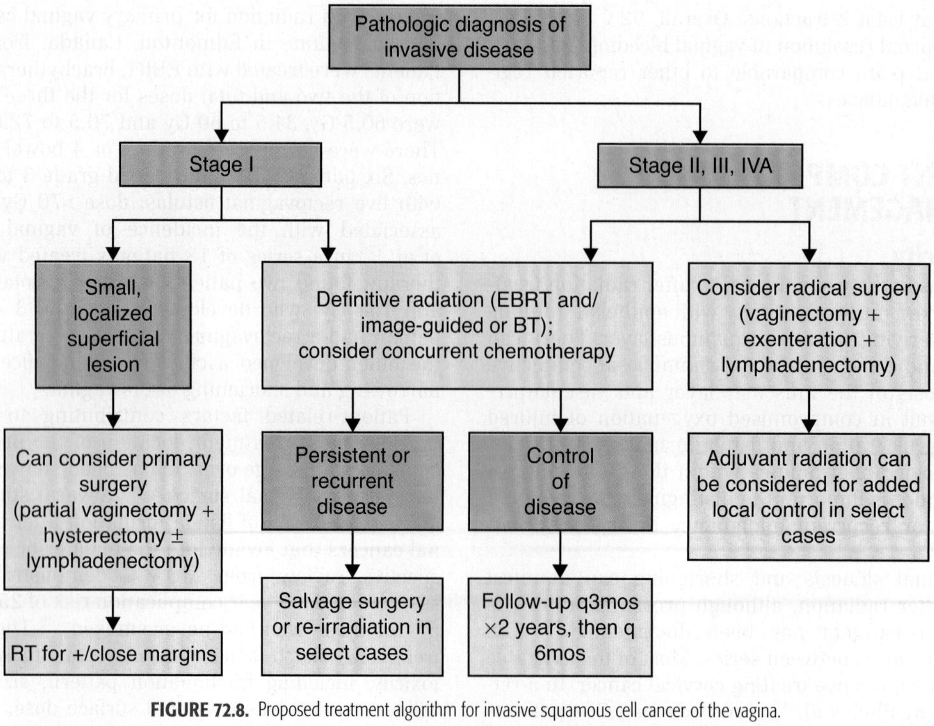

FIGURE 72.8. Proposed treatment algorithm for invasive squamous cell cancer of the vagina.

SELECTED REFERENCES

A full list of references for this chapter is available online.

1. Shah CA, et al. Factors affecting risk of mortality in women with vaginal cancer. *Obstet Gynecol* 2009;113(5):1038–1045.
47. Indermaur MD, et al. Upper vaginectomy for the treatment of vaginal intraepithelial neoplasia. *Am J Obstet Gynecol* 2005;193(2):577–580; discussion 580–581.
60. Chyle V, et al. Definitive radiotherapy for carcinoma of the vagina: outcome and prognostic factors. *Int J Radiat Oncol Biol Phys* 1996;35(5):891–905.
63. Perez CA, et al. Factors affecting long-term outcome of irradiation in carcinoma of the vagina. *Int J Radiat Oncol Biol Phys* 1999;44(1):37–45.
97. Stock RG, et al. The importance of brachytherapy technique in the management of primary carcinoma of the vagina. *Int J Radiat Oncol Biol Phys* 1992;24(4):747–753.
98. Stock RG, Chen AS, Seski J. A 30-year experience in the management of primary carcinoma of the vagina: analysis of prognostic factors and treatment modalities. *Gynecol Oncol* 1995;56(1):45–52.
114. Frank SJ, et al. Definitive radiation therapy for squamous cell carcinoma of the vagina. *Int J Radiat Oncol Biol Phys* 2005;62(1):138–147.
116. Frumovitz M, et al. Lymphatic mapping and sentinel lymph node detection in women with vaginal cancer. *Gynecol Oncol* 2008;108(3):478–481.
131. Tran PT, et al. Prognostic factors for outcomes and complications for primary squamous cell carcinoma of the vagina treated with radiation. *Gynecol Oncol* 2007;105(3):641–649.
142. Pingley S, et al. Primary carcinoma of the vagina: Tata Memorial Hospital experience. *Int J Radiat Oncol Biol Phys* 2000;46(1):101–108.
168. Dalrymple JL, et al. Chemoradiation for primary invasive squamous carcinoma of the vagina. *Int J Gynecol Cancer* 2004;14(1):110–117.
169. Samant R, et al. Primary vaginal cancer treated with concurrent chemoradiation using Cis-platinum. *Int J Radiat Oncol Biol Phys* 2007;69(3):746–750.
171. Miyamoto DT, Tanaka CK, Viswanathan AN. *Concurrent chemoradiation improves survival in patients with vaginal cancer.* San Diego, CA: Presented at the 52nd American Society for Therapeutic Radiology and Oncology Annual Meeting, 2010.
176. Beriwal S, et al. High-dose rate brachytherapy (HDRB) for primary or recurrent cancer in the vagina. *Radiat Oncol* 2008;3:7.
347. Dimopoulos JC, et al. Treatment of locally advanced vaginal cancer with radiochemotherapy and magnetic resonance image-guided adaptive brachytherapy: dose-volume parameters and first clinical results. *Int J Radiat Oncol Biol Phys* 2012;82(5):1880–1885.
348. Lee, LJ, Viswanathan, AN. Predictors of toxicity after image-guided high-dose-rate interstitial brachytherapy for gynecologic cancer. *Int J Radiat Oncol Biol Phys* 2012;84(5):1192–1197.

Chapter 73
Cancer of the Female Urethra

Tony Y. Eng

Primary urethral carcinoma is a rare tumor, accounting for <1% of all malignancies. Although previous data suggested that urethral cancer was more common in women than in men, a recent Surveillance, Epidemiology, and End Results (SEER) study reported that primary urethral cancer was more common in men.[1] The ratio of female to male predominance was approximately 1:3. Because of its rarity and lack of prospective data, optimal management of female urethral cancer is based on retrospective data and depends on the clinical stage, tumor location, extent of nodal involvement, and the patient's health status and preference.

ANATOMY

The female urethra is approximately 3 to 4 cm long and 0.6 cm in resting diameter. It is embedded in the anterior vaginal wall behind the pubis symphysis, extending inferiorly and anteriorly from the urinary bladder through the urogenital diaphragm to the vestibule, where it forms the urethral meatus. Because of the proximity of the symphysis pubis, a small curve is formed with an anterior concavity. The lower distal half of the urethra is considered the anterior urethra, and the upper proximal half is considered the posterior urethra. Figure 73.1 illustrates the urethra and adjacent organs in the female pelvis.

The wall of the urethra consists of three layers. The muscular layer is continuous with that of the bladder. At the vesicular end of the urethra, this muscular wall forms the internal sphincter. The voluntary urethral sphincter is at the plane of the urogenital diaphragm. A thin layer of erectile tissue consisting of a plexus of veins and muscle fibers forms the middle layer of the wall. The inner layer is the mucous membrane, which is continuous with the bladder proximally and with the vulva distally. This membrane consists of transitional epithelium near the bladder but distally changes to nonkeratinizing stratified squamous epithelium and pseudostratified columnar epithelium. The distal urethra also contains small mucous recesses and periurethral or Skene's glands, most of which are in the region of the meatus.

The lymphatic drainage of the distal urethra and urethral meatus parallels that of the vulva to the superficial and deep inguinal and external iliac lymph nodes. The primary drainage of the posterior or entire urethra is mainly to the obturator and internal and external iliac nodes.

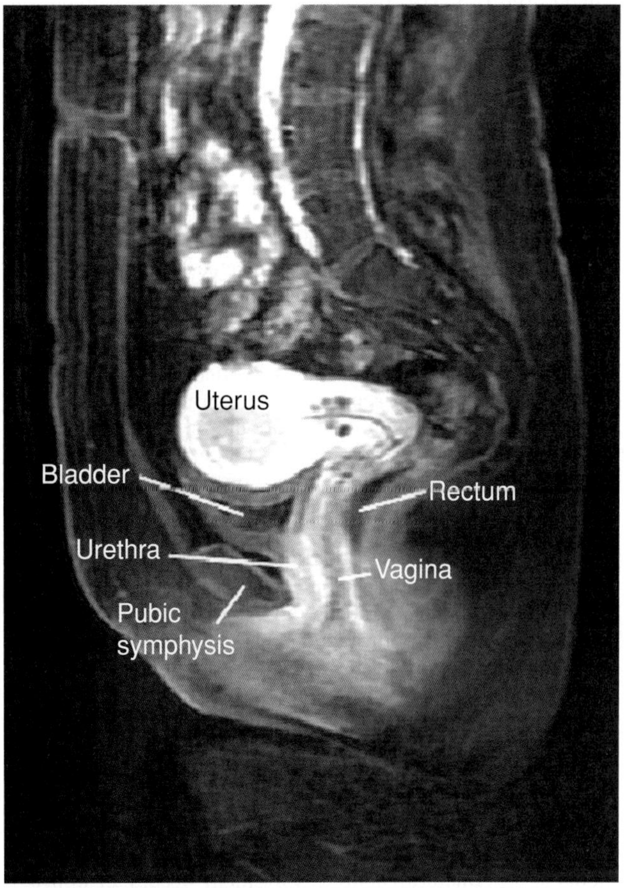

FIGURE 73.1. Magnetic resonance T1-weighted sagittal image of the female pelvis.

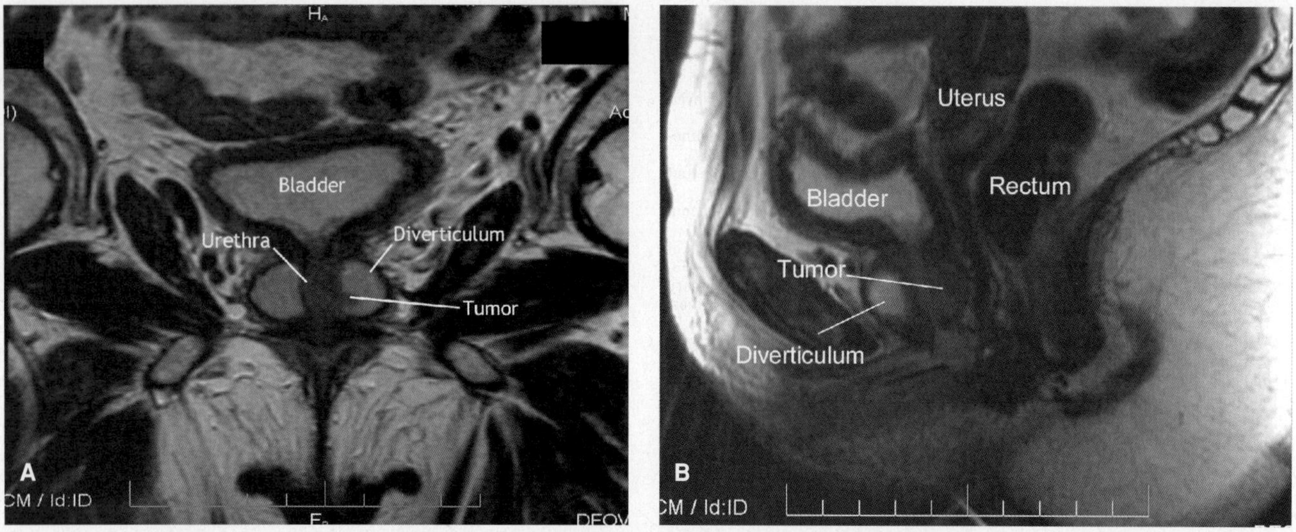

FIGURE 73.2. Coronal **(A)** and sagittal **(B)** T2-weighted magnetic resonance images demonstrate a large diverticulum surrounding the urethra with a tumor mass arising within the confines of the diverticulum posteriorly that results in an impression at the vagina.

EPIDEMIOLOGY AND ETIOLOGY

The SEER database for 1973 to 2002 identified 1,615 cases of primary urethral carcinoma, of which 540 were women.[1] The overall annual incidence was 1.5 per million for women (4.3 per million for men). Although previous observation suggested that this cancer is more common in white than in black women,[2,3] the SEER data show that the incidence is higher for African Americans and increases steadily with age. Because carcinoma of the urethra is rare in women, only a few cases are seen annually at major cancer centers.[4–7] Carcinoma of the female urethra makes up 0.02% of all cancers in women and accounts for approximately 0.1% of all gynecologic cancers.[8,9] The average patient age at the time of diagnosis is 60 years, with most patients between 50 and 80 years of age.[1,2,10–12]

Although chronic infection and local irritation have been proposed, the etiology of female urethral cancer remains obscure. Unlike other transitional cell carcinomas of the urinary tract, there is no reported correlation of cigarette smoking with urethral carcinoma. Weiner and Walther[13] analyzed archival surgical specimens of women with urethral carcinoma. Human papilloma virus (HPV) was detected in 10 of 17 patients with invasive disease. HPV type 16 was found in 8 patients. Eight women with squamous cell carcinoma and 2 with transitional cell carcinoma had HPV. Female urethral cancer may also be associated with urethral diverticula.[14–16] Figure 73.2 illustrates a carcinoma arising within a urethral diverticulum. Patients with transitional cell carcinoma of the bladder, especially the bladder neck, may have a higher risk of developing urethral cancer either synchronously or metachronously.[17,18]

NATURAL HISTORY

Most urethral cancers are clinically aggressive and historically carry a poor prognosis. During the later stages, cancers of the middle or posterior urethra tend to extend upward into the urinary bladder, downward to invade the remainder of the urethra, and posteriorly into the vaginal mucosa. Lesions involving the anterior urethra account for approximately 30% of all cases.[10,19]

Regional lymph node involvement is uncommon in early tumors (stage 0) of the urethral meatus. Advanced tumors (stages II and III) of the urethra have been associated with a 35% to 50% incidence of inguinal or pelvic lymph node involvement.[9,11,20–22] Bilateral nodal involvement occurs in approximately one-third of patients with positive nodes. Grabstald[10] confirmed nodal involvement in 24 of 25 patients with clinically palpable nodes. In his series of patients with advanced disease, 26 underwent pelvic lymph node sampling and 13 (50%) had nodal involvement.

Distant metastases are found in approximately 10% of patients at presentation, and approximately 30% to 50% ultimately die of distant disease. The most common sites of metastasis are lung, liver, bone, and brain.[10,23]

CLINICAL PRESENTATION

A majority of patients with urethral cancer present with some degree of irritative or obstructive urethral symptoms.[24] Bleeding (hematuria) or spotting is the prevailing presenting sign in 50% to 60% of patients.[2,25,26] Approximately 30% to 50% of patients experience pain or irritative symptoms, difficulty urinating, and frequent micturition. Urinary retention and overflow incontinence may occur in advanced cases. Less frequently cited signs and symptoms are a mass in the introitus (10% to 20% of patients), dyspareunia, perineal pain, and inguinal lymphadenopathy.[21,23,27] Urethrovaginal and vesicovaginal fistulas may develop in advanced, neglected cases.

Small tumors involving the urethral meatus are often mistakenly diagnosed as urethral caruncle, a benign, inflammatory lesion, or a prolapse of the mucosa through the urethral orifice. As the lesion progresses, it enlarges and eventually ulcerates.[23] Tumors may arise in a urethral diverticulum.[16,28] Larger lesions of the distal urethra are readily identified on inspection (Fig. 73.3). Tumors occupying the proximal urethra may produce a fusiform enlargement that can be palpated during pelvic examination.

DIAGNOSTIC WORKUP

An outline for the diagnostic work-up for carcinoma of the female urethra is presented in Table 73.1. A routine history and general physical examination should be performed for all patients. A detailed pelvic examination under anesthesia is necessary to fully evaluate the clinical extent of the disease. This examination can be performed at the time of urethroscopy and cystoscopy. Urine cytologic analyses have a high false-negative rate.[29] The definitive diagnosis is made by punch or incisional biopsy.

Routine radiographic evaluation should include chest radiographs, an intravenous urogram, and a computed tomography

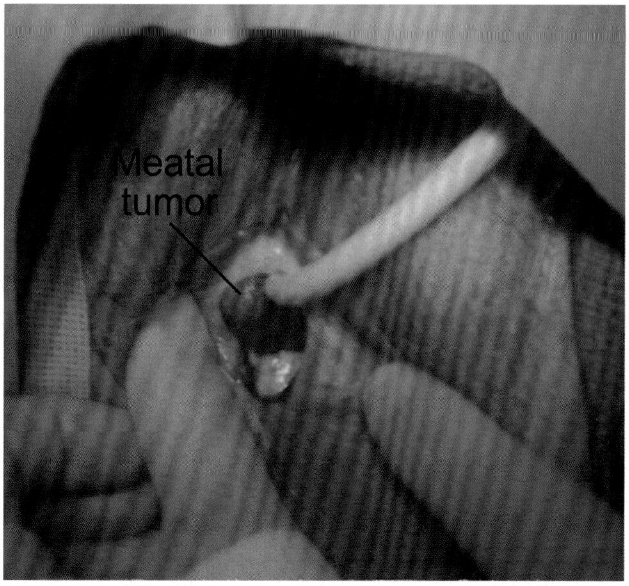

FIGURE 73.3. A meatal carcinoma of the urethra in a 68-year-old white woman presenting with hematuria.

(CT) scan of the abdomen and pelvis (Fig. 73.4).[30,31] Barium enema can be cost-effective for patients with symptoms of advanced disease. Magnetic resonance imaging of the pelvis helps delineate the tumor extent, especially when an endourethral coil is used (Fig. 73.2). It provides a discrete view of the muscular layers of the urethra.[32,33] Additional complementary studies include interactive virtual urethrography and ultrasonography, which can help detect a urethral diverticulum without contrast agent filling.[34] Multidetector CT voiding urethrography yields real-time urethral images during micturition.

Currently there are no studies to address the role of positron emission tomography (PET) with fluorodeoxyglucose (FDG) scan in urethral cancer. Perhaps some genitourinary tumors do not accumulate sufficient FDG, which may not be a useful tracer for the detection of primary genitourinary tumors because of its physiologic excretion in the urine.[35] However, PET scans may potentially be useful for identifying nodal and distant sites of disease, especially in patients with equivocal findings on conventional imaging.[36,37]

TABLE 73.1 DIAGNOSTIC WORKUP FOR CARCINOMA OF THE FEMALE URETHRA

General
History
Physical examination, including detailed pelvic examination under anesthesia
Special procedures
Punch biopsy
Urethroscopy
Cystoscopy
Rectosigmoidoscopy (advanced stages or if symptomatic)
Radiographic evaluation
Standard
Chest radiographs
Intravenous urography
Computed tomography scan (abdomen and pelvis)
Magnetic resonance imaging
Complementary
Bone scan (if symptomatic or elevated alkaline phosphatase)
Barium enema (if symptomatic or advanced stages)
Ultrasound
Urethrography
Laboratory evaluation
Complete blood count
Chemistry profile
Urinalysis

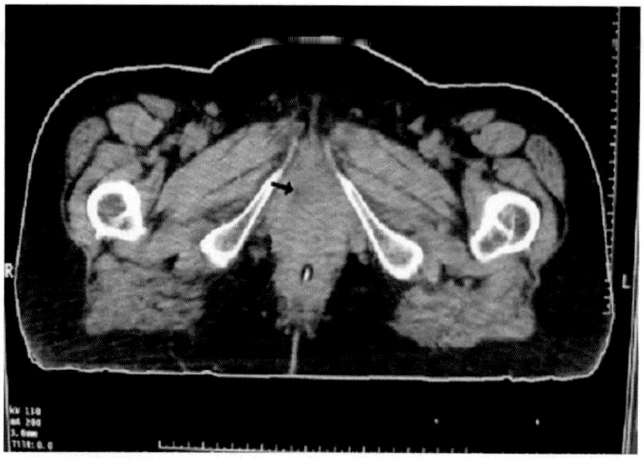

FIGURE 73.4. Transaxial computed tomography image of a patient with urethral cancer illustrating the periurethral and anterior vaginal wall expansion and deviation of the urethra (*arrow*).

STAGING SYSTEMS

Clinical staging is based on findings on physical examination, chest x-ray, and CT scan of the abdomen and pelvis. Many attempts have been made to formulate a staging system for carcinoma of the urethra. Urethral tumors can be classified in two groups: those involving the distal half of the urethra and those located in the proximal or entire urethra. Most authors have found that this classification correctly depicts the feasibility of treatment and the prognosis. A staging system based on location has been proposed by Prempree et al.[38] (Table 73.2). The current TNM staging system of the American Joint Committee on Cancer is shown in Table 73.3.[39]

PATHOLOGIC CLASSIFICATION

Because the urethra is lined by transitional cells proximally and stratified squamous cells distally, transitional cell carcinoma occurs typically in the proximal urethra, whereas squamous cell carcinoma occurs frequently in the distal urethra. The SEER data report that the most common histologic type is transitional cell carcinoma, followed by squamous cell and adenocarcinoma.[1] However, most published series suggest that squamous cell carcinoma is the most common histologic type in cancer of the female urethra, representing >50% of all cases, whereas transitional cell carcinoma and adenocarcinoma represent approximately 15% to 20% and 10% to

TABLE 73.2 PROPOSED CLINICAL STAGING SYSTEM FOR CARCINOMA OF THE FEMALE URETHRA

Tumor Stage	*Characteristics*
I	Disease limited to distal one-half of urethra
II	Disease involving entire urethra, with extension to periurethral tissues, but not involving vulva or bladder neck
III	
A	Disease involving urethra and vulva
B	Disease invading vaginal mucosa
C	Disease involving urethra and bladder neck
IV	
A	Disease invading parametrium or paracolpium
B	Metastasis
B1	Inguinal lymph nodes
B2	Pelvic lymph nodes
B3	Para-aortic nodes
B4	Distant metastasis

From Prempree T, Amornmarn R, Patanaphan V. Radiation therapy in primary carcinoma of the female urethra: II. An update on results. *Cancer* 1984;54:729–733; with permission.

TABLE 73.3 AMERICAN JOINT COMMITTEE ON CANCER STAGING OF CARCINOMA OF THE URETHRA (MALE OR FEMALE)

Primary Tumor (T)	
TX	Primary tumor cannot be assessed
T0	No evidence of primary tumor
Ta	Noninvasive papillary, polypoid, or verrucous carcinoma
Tis	Carcinoma *in situ*
T1	Tumor invades subepithelial connective tissue
T2	Tumor invades any of the following: corpus spongiosum, prostate, periurethral muscle
T3	Tumor invades any of the following: corpus cavernosum, beyond prostatic capsule, anterior vagina, bladder neck
T4	Tumor invades other adjacent organs
Regional Lymph Nodes (N)	
NX	Regional lymph nodes cannot be assessed
N0	No regional lymph node metastasis
N1	Metastasis in a single lymph node 2 cm or less in greatest dimension
N2	Metastasis in a single node more than 2 cm in greatest dimension or in multiple nodes
Distant Metastasis (M)	
M0	No distant metastasis (no pathologic M0; use clinical M to complete stage group)
M1	Distant metastasis

15%, respectively.[15,40,41] The remainder of the histologic types include adenoid cystic carcinoma, melanoma, clear-cell adenocarcinoma, anaplastic tumors, Kaposi's sarcoma, lymphomas, and metastatic lesions.[6,28,31,42–49]

PROGNOSTIC FACTORS

Conventional prognostic factors, such as grade and histology, have not been consistently predictive for recurrence or survival for female urethral cancer. In the literature, some of the most important factors in determining prognosis and survival are stage, depth of invasion, tumor size, and anatomic location.[2,15,21,50–52] Dalbagni et al.[2] showed that primary stage was one of the major independent predictors of survival in 72 female patients, with 5-year survival of 83% for low-stage tumors and 33% for high-stage tumors.

Lesions located in the meatus or distal urethra tend to be superficial, with a better prognosis; lesions in the posterior urethra are often deeply invasive and tend to have a worse prognosis.[9] Most investigators found that patients with advanced-stage disease do poorly, often irrespective of their treatment.[2,24,51,53]

Grigsby and Corn[25,54] demonstrated a worsening prognosis with increased tumor size. The 5-year progression-free survival was 81% for patients with lesions <2 cm, compared with 37% for those with lesions 2 to 4 cm and 7% for patients with lesions >4 cm ($p = .0001$). For lesions confined to the proximal urethra, local control was observed in all four patients. However, patients with tumors involving the distal urethra had a 5-year progression-free survival rate of 69%, and there was a 12% survival rate for those with involvement of the entire free urethra ($p = .0001$). Patients with meatal tumors, if diagnosed early and treated appropriately, can achieve an 80% to 90% survival rate (Figs. 73.5 and 73.6).[25] Bladder neck involvement, parametrial extension, and inguinal lymph node involvement have been identified as poor prognostic factors.

The histology of the primary lesion appears to be less important as a prognostic factor in determining response to therapy and survival. Patients with adenocarcinoma have been reported to have a good prognosis, but most studies have shown no difference in survival among patients with adenocarcinoma, squamous cell carcinoma, and transitional cell carcinoma.[10,14,38,50]

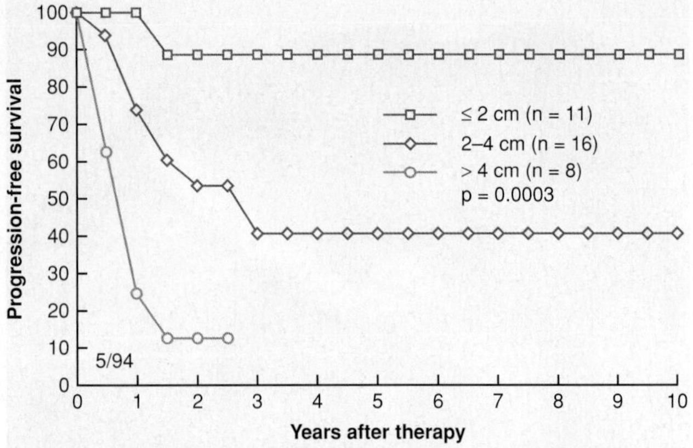

FIGURE 73.5. Progression-free survival correlated with tumor size. (From Grigsby PW, Herr HW. Urethral tumors. In: Vogelzang J, Scardino PT, Shipley WU, et al., eds. *Comprehensive textbook of genitourinary oncology.* Baltimore: Williams & Wilkins; 1996:1117–1123.)

Grigsby[25] found a worse prognosis in patients with adenocarcinoma. Primary melanoma of the urethra, although rare, has a very poor prognosis.[43,44]

GENERAL MANAGEMENT

Although various therapeutic approaches have been advocated in the management of carcinoma of the female urethra, there are no established therapeutic guidelines. The variety of treatments reflects the dimensions and locations of disease and the approaches of the treating physicians.[55] In general, surgical resection is a primary mode of treatment.[56] Radical urethral resection with urinary diversion and pelvic lymphadenectomy are commonly performed for lesions not involving the bladder neck. However, early-stage lesions of limited extent may be amenable to organ-sparing radiation therapy or conservative surgical management with or without adjuvant radiation therapy to minimize the morbidity associated with surgical intervention. Surgical approaches include neodymium:yttrium-aluminum-garnet (Nd:YAG) laser coagulation,[57] Mohs' micrographic surgery, and partial or total urethrectomy.[41] Radiation therapy may include external-beam radiation, interstitial brachytherapy, or a combination of these treatments.[58] For patients who are medically nonsurgical candidates because of potential risks of anesthesia, outpatient high–dose-rate intracavitary and intraluminal brachytherapy may be an option.[59]

For patients with locally invasive urethral carcinoma, anterior exenteration may be required. Although most available data are insufficient, in patients with more advanced disease, some

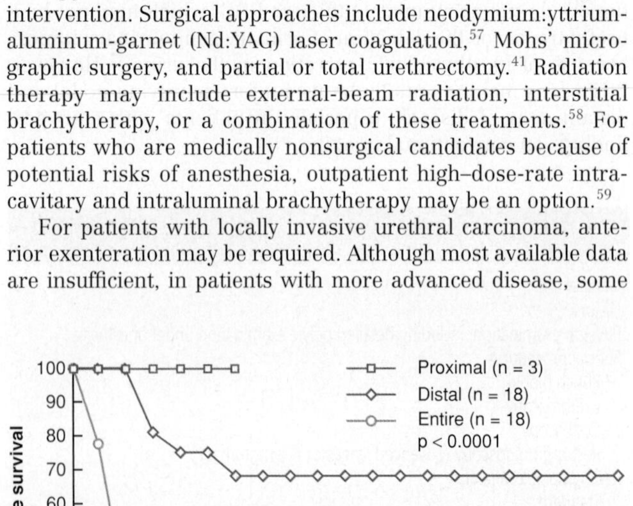

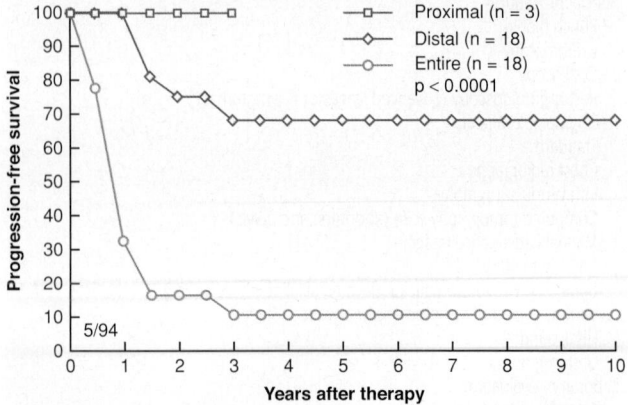

FIGURE 73.6. Progression-free survival correlated with tumor location. (From Grigsby PW, Herr HW. Urethral tumors. In: Vogelzang J, Scardino PT, Shipley WU, et al., eds. *Comprehensive textbook of genitourinary oncology.* Baltimore: Williams & Wilkins; 1996:1117–1123.)

authors have advocated adjuvant radiation therapy and/or combined irradiation and chemotherapy, including 5-fluorouracil, cisplatin, vinblastine, epirubicin, carboplatin, bleomycin, methotrexate, or mitomycin-C after surgical extirpation.[56,60–64]

Anterior (Distal) Urethral Cancer

For stage 0 and I (Ta, Tis, or small T1) lesions, open excision, electroexcision, fulguration, and laser (Nd:YAG or CO_2) coagulation are possible for tumors at the meatus or with *in situ* involvement of the distal urethra (stage 0). For larger and more invasive lesions (stage T1 and T2), surgical resection of the distal one-third of the urethra is often adequate. Alternatively, interstitial irradiation or a combination of interstitial and external-beam irradiation can be considered. For T3-T4 or recurrent anterior urethral lesions previously treated by local excision or radiation therapy, anterior exenteration and urinary diversion may be curative. Adjuvant radiation therapy may be required, depending on surgical findings.

If a limited number of inguinal nodes are involved, ipsilateral node dissection or irradiation is indicated because cure is still achievable. If no inguinal adenopathy exists, node dissection is not recommended, but prophylactic groin irradiation is recommended for patients with invasive lesions.[6,50]

Posterior (Proximal) Urethral Cancer

Cancers of the posterior or entire urethra are usually associated with invasion of the bladder, a high incidence of inguinal and pelvic lymph node metastases, and a worse prognosis. For lesions <2 cm, radical resection, definitive radiation therapy, or combined treatment may provide adequate control.[54] However, for larger lesions or locally advanced disease, the best results have been achieved with preoperative irradiation, exenterative surgery, and urinary diversion. Pelvic lymphadenectomy is performed, and inguinal node dissection may be indicated if the inguinal nodes are involved. In selected patients, it is possible to remove part of the pubic symphysis and the inferior pubic rami to maximize the surgical margin. A transpubic approach has been advocated by Golimbu et al.[65] Perineal closure and vaginal reconstruction can be accomplished with the use of myocutaneous flaps. Hedden et al.[66] advocated the use of bladder-sparing surgery with or without irradiation.

Recurrent Urethral Cancer

In most cases, locally recurrent urethral cancer after surgery alone should be considered for combination radiation therapy and wider surgical resection. Locally recurrent urethral cancer after radiation therapy should be treated by surgical excision. For patients who are not surgical candidates, local reirradiation (i.e., hyperfractionated intensity-modulated radiation therapy or brachytherapy) may be considered if radiation tolerance has not been exceeded. Patients with metastatic urethral cancer should be considered for investigational chemotherapy protocols. Palliative radiation therapy may provide good symptomatic relief.

RADIATION THERAPY TECHNIQUES

Small meatal and distal urethral lesions are curable with limited therapy. Interstitial implants have been the usual method for treating meatal carcinomas. Radioactive needles, forming a double-plane or a volume implant, have been used (Fig. 73.7). Both low–dose-rate (LDR) and high–dose-rate (HDR) afterloading implants using ^{192}Ir have replaced radium.[8,59,67] For early localized disease without involvement of adjacent organs, a volume implant composed of 8 to 12 needles arranged in an arc around the urethral orifice is used (Fig. 73.8). Radiographs may be used to verify needle placement (Fig. 73.9). Computer planning with CT-based simulation and three-dimensional treatment planning should be the standard of care to spare the

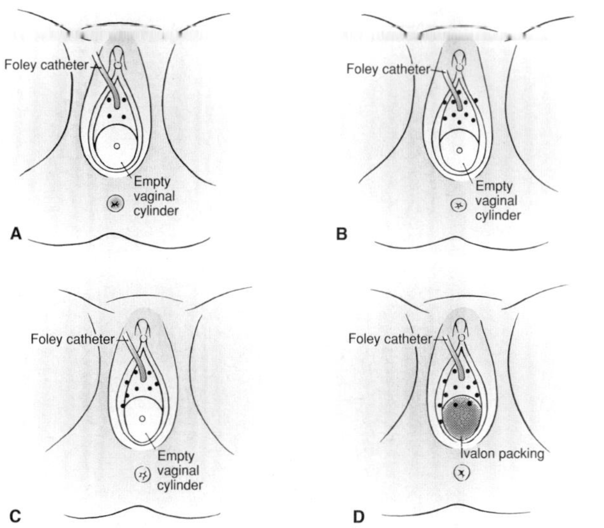

FIGURE 73.7. Diagrams of implants. **A:** Tumor limited to the urethra. **B:** Tumor extending to the periurethral tissues or originating in the periurethral glands. **C:** Tumor extending into the vagina or labia minora. **D:** Tumor involving the suburethral area. (From Delclos L. Carcinoma of the female urethra. In: Johnson DE, Boileau MA, eds. *Genitourinary tumors.* New York: Grune & Stratton, 1982:275–286, with permission; copyright Elsevier, 1892.)

adjacent normal organs. A dose of 60 to 70 Gy (LDR) should be given in 6 to 7 days (0.4 to 0.5 Gy/hr to the target volume) when an implant alone is used.

Alternatively, in patients with small, localized disease receiving radiation therapy alone, noninvasive intracavitary or intraluminal HDR brachytherapy without sedation or anesthesia after pelvic external beam radiation has been used.[51,59] Figure 73.10 illustrates an intraluminal HDR brachytherapy using a Foley catheter. The resultant conformal radiation dose covers the periurethral tissue well while sparing the surrounding normal structures. At the University of Texas Health Science Center in San Antonio, we deliver 500 to 600 cGy at twice a week, 3 days apart, to a total dose of 2,400 to 2,500 cGy with good response.

Large tumors or advance disease extending into the labia, vagina, entire urethra, or base of the bladder should not be treated with an implant alone. For these patients, a combination of external-beam irradiation and implant is recommended.[59,68,69] The external-beam portal should flash the perineum to cover the entire urethra. The conventional portal should be wide enough to cover the inguinal nodes and should

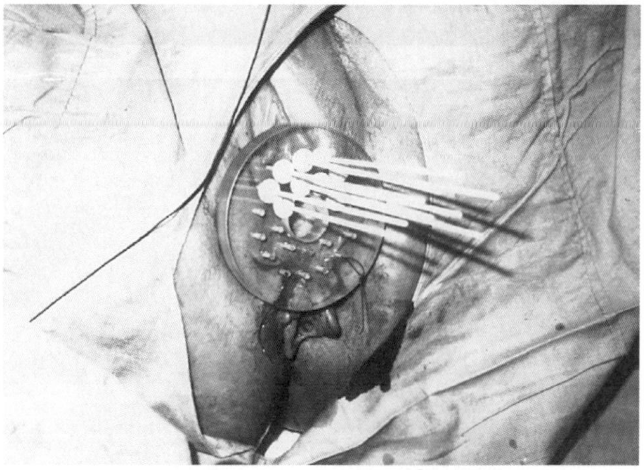

FIGURE 73.8. A template used for a curved, double-plane implant that surrounds the urethra. The closed-end flexible catheters inserted in the periurethral or vaginal tissues are glued to the template, which is sutured to the skin. The catheters are afterloaded with ^{192}Ir.

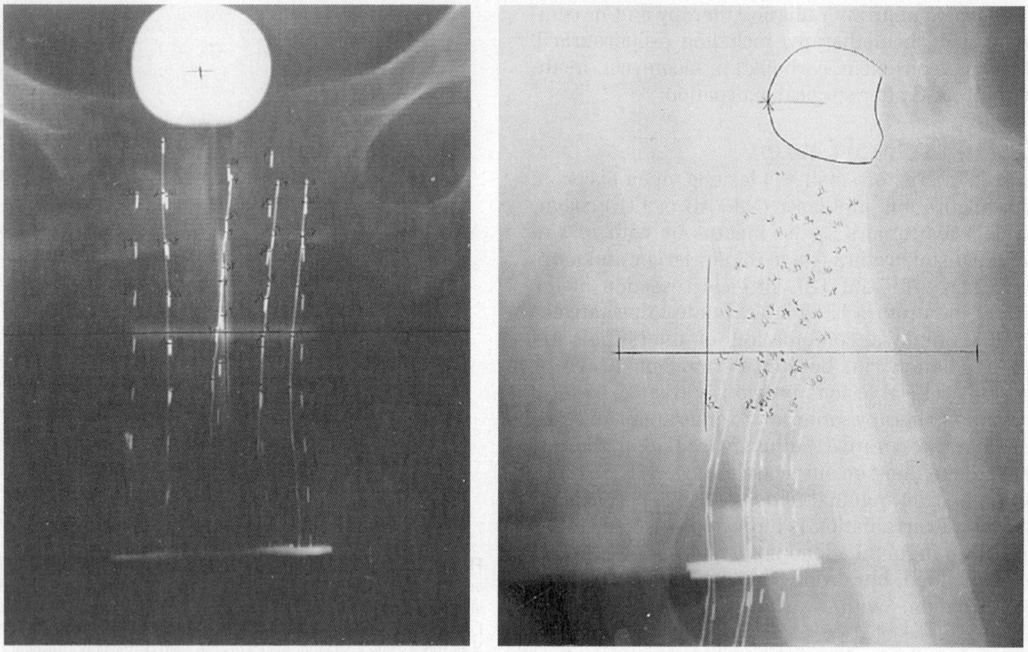

FIGURE 73.9. Anteroposterior **(A)** and lateral **(B)** simulation radiographs with dummy seeds in place. Contrast material is used to inflate the balloon of the urinary catheter, which is used to localize the bladder.

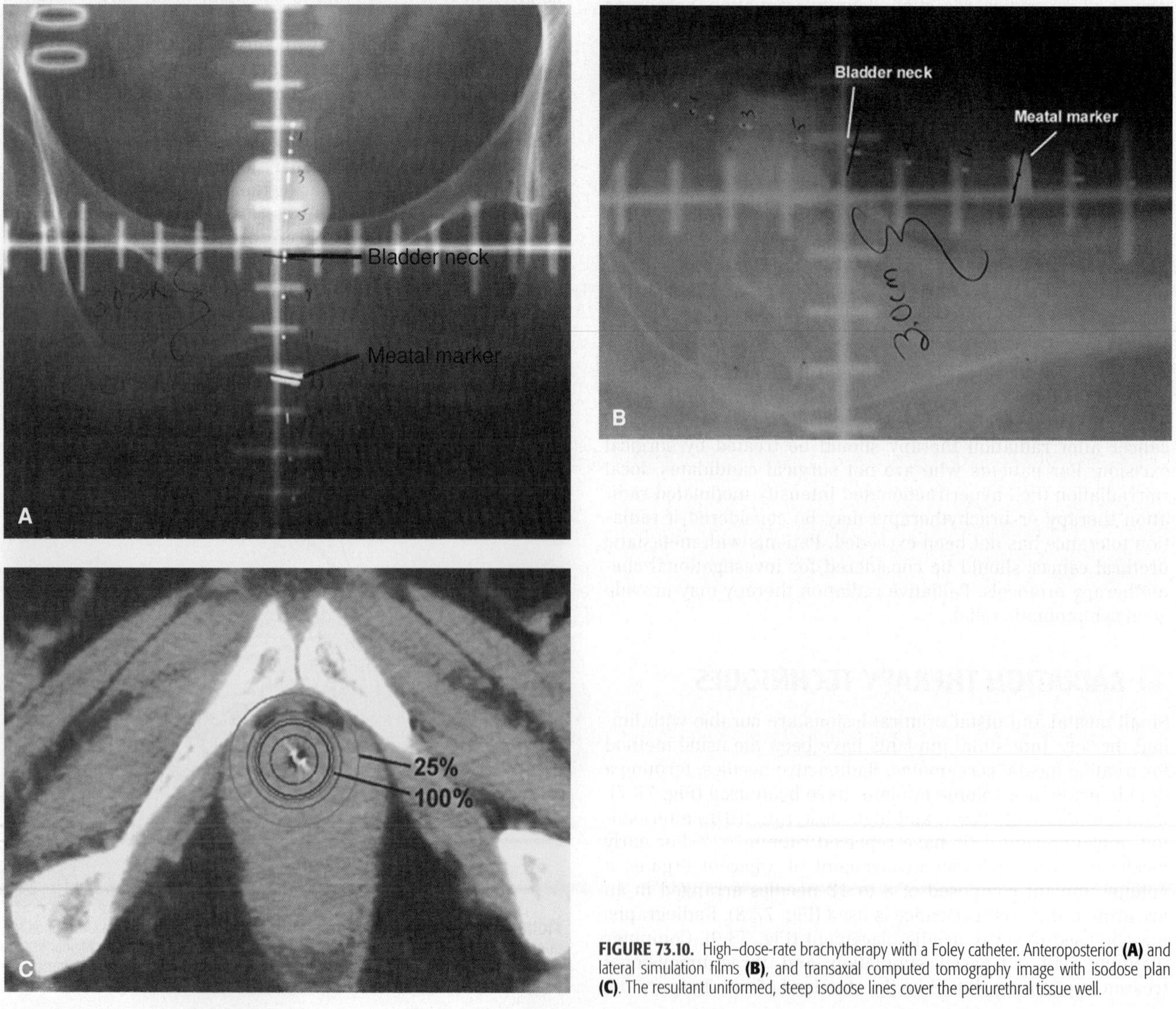

FIGURE 73.10. High-dose-rate brachytherapy with a Foley catheter. Anteroposterior **(A)** and lateral simulation films **(B)**, and transaxial computed tomography image with isodose plan **(C)**. The resultant uniformed, steep isodose lines cover the periurethral tissue well.

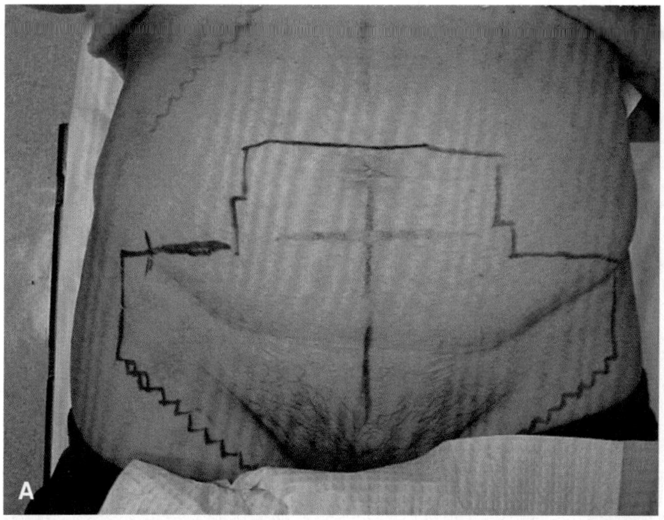

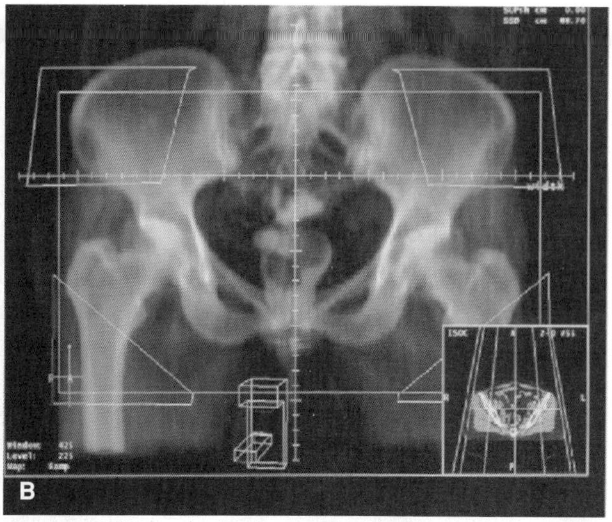

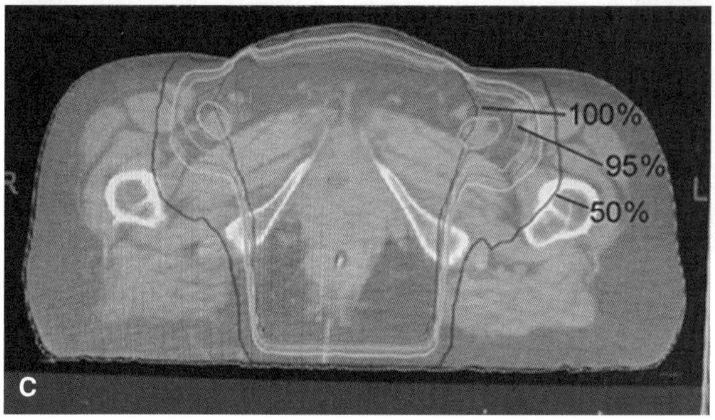

FIGURE 73.11. Whole-pelvis and inguinal field. External skin marking **(A)** and anteroposterior simulation film **(B)** of a pelvic portal showing the lateral extension to cover the inguinal lymph nodes and the isodose plan **(C)**.

extend cephalad to the L5-S1 interspace to include the pelvic nodes (Fig. 73.11).[70] A bolus, appropriate for the photon energy used, should be added to the groins when inguinal nodes are positive. This technique minimizes the hazard of groin failure due to underdosing of gross tumor. Hahn et al.[71] demonstrated the importance of treating the inguinal lymph nodes in all patients. The whole pelvis is treated to a dose of 45 to 50 Gy. A boost of 10 to 15 Gy is delivered to positive groin nodes through reduced anteroposterior fields.

After pelvic radiation therapy, the primary tumor can be treated with a vaginal cylinder to bring the dose to the entire urethra to approximately 60 Gy. An interstitial implant is administered to raise the total tumor dose to 70 to 80 Gy. For patients undergoing postoperative therapy, the tumor bed is treated after pelvic radiation therapy with an additional 10 to 15 Gy using interstitial brachytherapy.[67] Intracavitary irradiation with the vaginal cylinder and an interstitial implant are almost never used simultaneously because of the resultant high dose rate at the vaginal mucosa interface of the intracavitary and interstitial implant fields. A vaginal cylinder with partial shielding posteriorly can be used in selected patients. Gerbaulet et al.[72] demonstrated the use of a catheter or a vaginal mold applicator for intraluminal/intracavitary brachytherapy and needles or guide gutters for interstitial brachytherapy.

At the University of Texas Health Science Center in San Antonio, we commonly deliver external-beam therapy, 4,500 to 5,040 cGy, to the primary tumor and pelvic lymphatics using intensity-modulated radiation therapy technique (IMRT) with CT image-guidance (Fig. 73.12). This is followed by interstitial HDR brachytherapy, 500 to 600 cGy twice a day, 6 hours apart. A vaginal cylinder is always employed to provide spatial protection of the posterior vagina and rectum. The HDR brachytherapy is repeated in 1 week to achieve a total dose of 2,000 to 2,400 cGy (Fig. 73.13). The major advantage of interstitial HDR brachytherapy is geometric or volume optimization by changing the dwell times and dwell positions of the radioactive source along the afterloading catheters so that the target volume is well covered with good conformity while minding the surround structures and vaginal mucosal dose. Modification of dose and fractionation may be made, depending on the tumor size and response to external-beam therapy. The HDR brachytherapy is performed as an outpatient treatment procedure.

One of the limiting factors in the use of external-beam irradiation is the tolerance of the perineal and vulva skin (i.e., confluent moist desquamation). Extensive disease combined with advanced age can be a formidable obstacle to completing the irradiation course. Proper radiation therapy techniques and diligent personal hygiene and individualized skin care during and after treatment are necessary if patients are to complete the course of treatment.

Multimodality Therapy

Multimodality therapy appears to achieve similar or better overall results, even though those patients who receive combined modality tend to have more-advanced disease. Although most studies included a small number of patients, those patients who received combined therapy seem to have better disease-free survival.[15,51,53] Combination therapy often consists of either chemotherapy with radiotherapy or radiotherapy with surgery. Combined chemotherapy and radiation therapy for locally advanced urethral cancer has shown a reasonable response in several reports.[51,53,61,63,73]

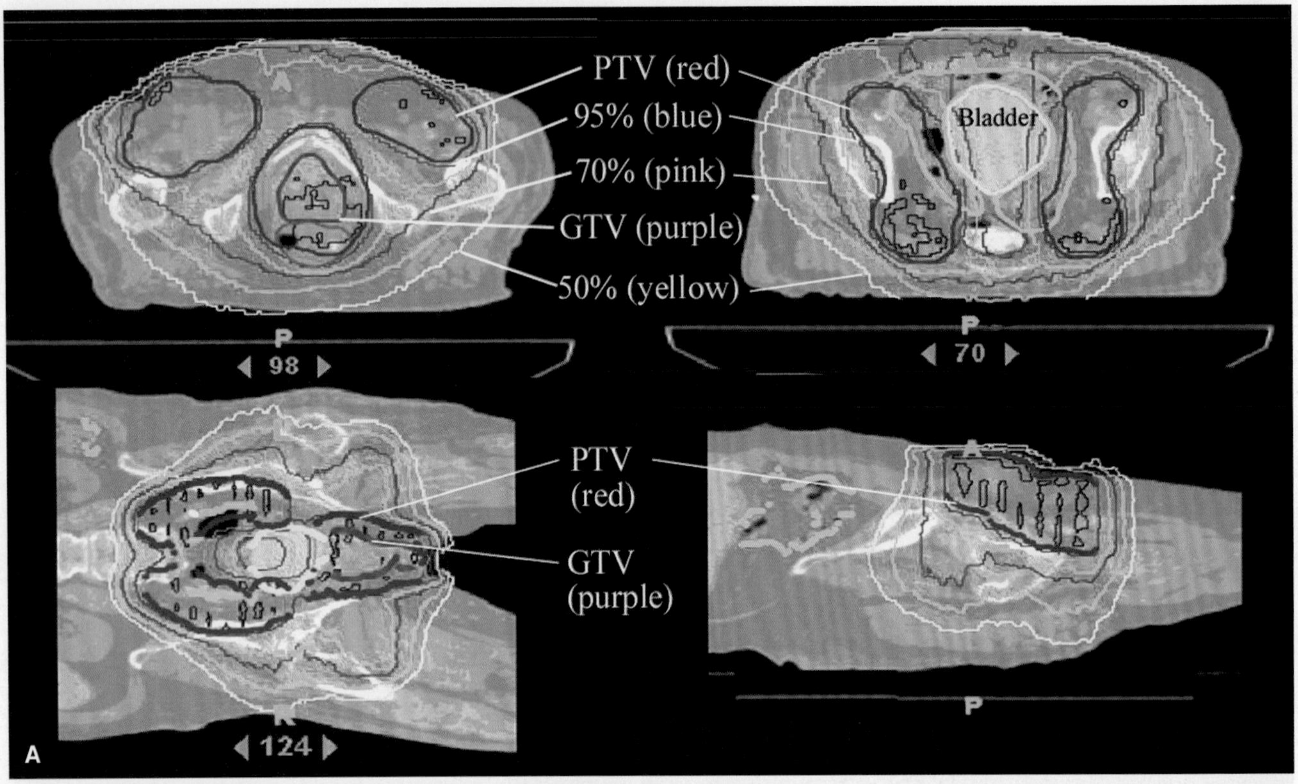

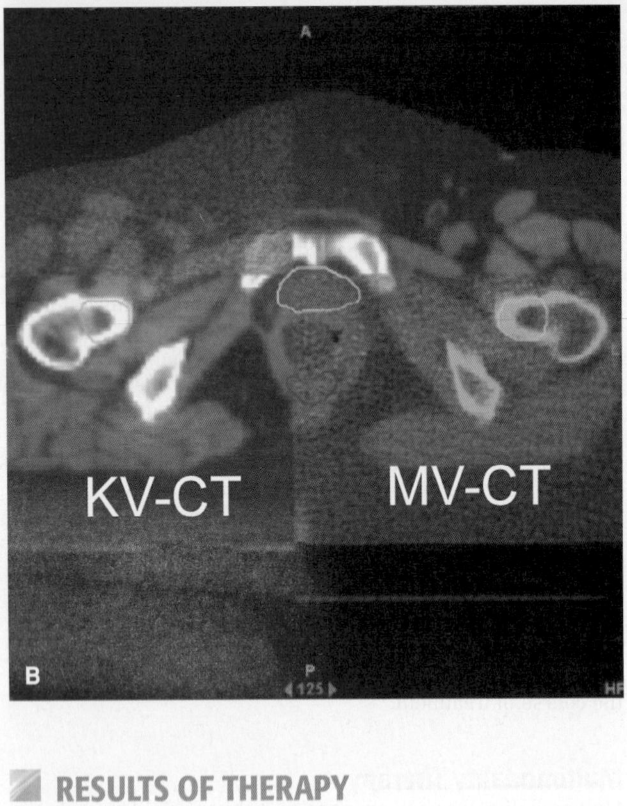

FIGURE 73.12. Pelvic intensity-modulated radiation therapy plan. **A:** Conformal dose distribution covering the lymphatics and primary target volume or the planning target volume (PTV). **B:** Daily matching of megavoltage computed tomography (CT) with the reference planning CT (kilovoltage CT) images is done prior to treatment.

RESULTS OF THERAPY

Surgery

There is a paucity of long-term outcome data. In general, female urethral cancers are clinically aggressive with high recurrence and poor survival rates.[2,10,15,22,23,53] DiMarco et al.[24] reviewed 53 female patients with primary urethral carcinoma undergoing partial urethrectomy or radical extirpation. The estimated 10-year cancer-specific survival was 60%. In a study of 72 patients treated at Memorial Sloan-Kettering Cancer Center between 1925 and 1994, the 5-year disease-specific survival was 89% for low-stage tumors and 33% for high-stage tumors.[2] The overall survival was 78% and 22%, respectively, as shown in Table 73.4.

Five of seven patients with early meatal tumors were cured of disease in the series reported by Grabstald[10] after partial urethrectomy. In the remaining two patients, both local recurrences and distant metastases developed. Bracken et al.[50] reported local control in just one of four patients treated with local excision only for distal urethral lesions. Peterson et al.[23] reported on two patients in whom squamous cell carcinomas were excised successfully. In the same series, a patient with

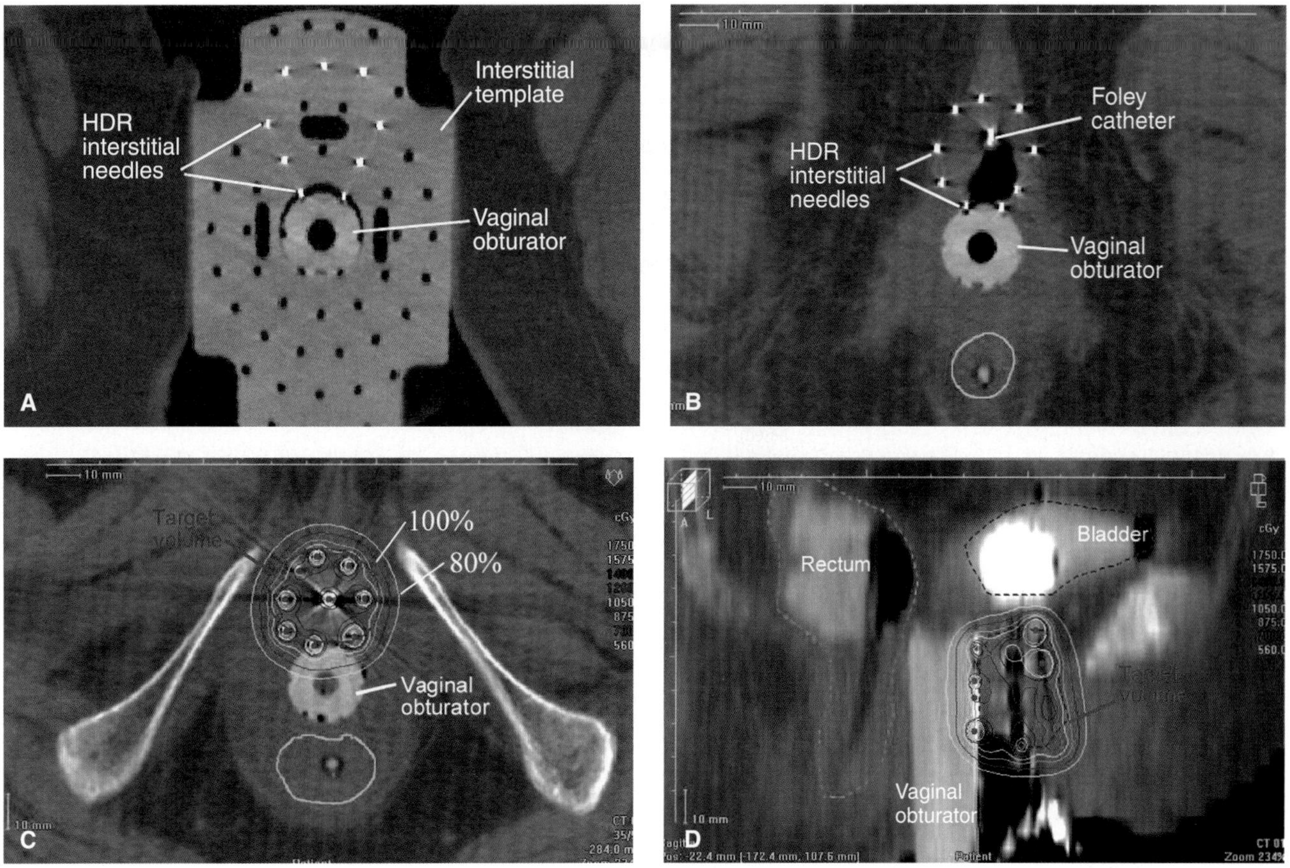

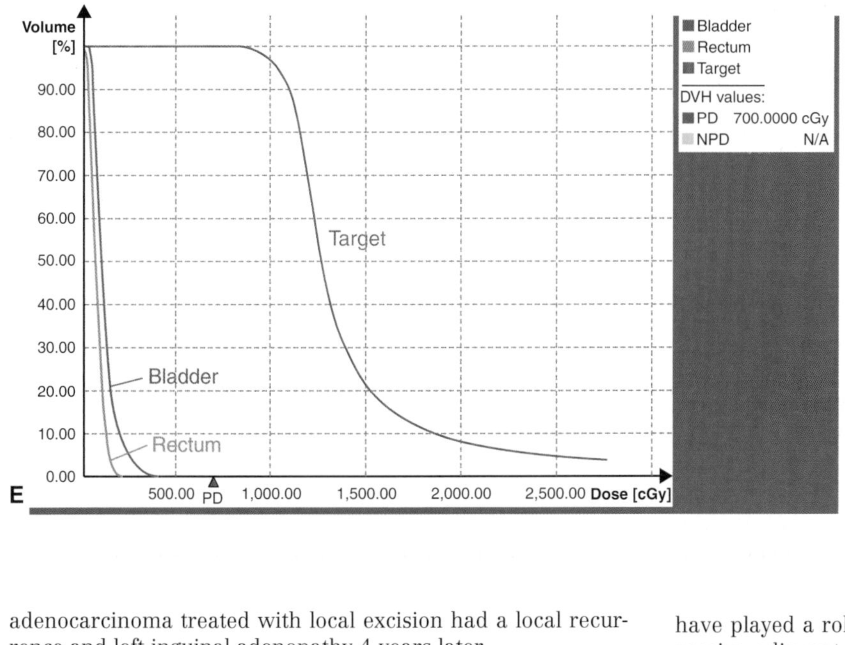

FIGURE 73.13. High-dose-rate interstitial brachytherapy. **A:** An interstitial template with a vaginal obturator is used to guide the needle placement. **B:** The needles surround the urethra at approximately 1-cm distance. **C, D:** With proper optimization, the resultant dose distribution conforms to the target volume while sparing all the surrounding organs. **E:** Dose–volume-histogram shows a large dose separation of the target from the bladder and rectum.

adenocarcinoma treated with local excision had a local recurrence and left inguinal adenopathy 4 years later.

Grabstald et al.[21] performed radical surgery on 15 patients with advanced disease; there were only 3 survivors at 5 years. Peterson et al.[23] performed radical surgery on seven patients, with three alive at 5 years. Primary radical cystectomy with anterior vaginectomy and total urethrectomy was performed on eight patients by Mayer et al.[74] Only three of these patients were free of disease at 1, 4, and 11 years.

Radiation Therapy

Although DiMarco et al.[24] found that adjuvant radiation did not improve local control or survival in the study of 53 female patients with urethral carcinoma, treatment selection bias may have played a role because the higher-stage tumors tended to receive adjuvant radiation therapy. Eng et al.[51] reported that only one of six patients with low-stage disease was referred for adjuvant radiation therapy, whereas four of five patients with advanced disease received radiation therapy. The one who did not receive radiation died 10 months after surgery. Case review of early-stage urethral cancer treated with external-beam radiotherapy, brachytherapy, or a combination of both seems to have equivalent results to surgery alone.[58,67,70,73]

Control of tumors of the urethral meatus or the distal urethra with irradiation alone is often satisfactory. Early meatal tumors have cure rates of 70% to 90%.[38] Chu[20] reported a 5-year progression-free survival rate of 64% for 11 patients with tumor involvement of the anterior urethra treated with

TABLE 73.4 FEMALE URETHRA TREATMENT SUMMARY

Authors/Site/Year	Patients	Stage	Treatment	Radiation Dose (Gy)	Follow-Up (yr)	Results	Prognostic Factors
Thyavihally et al.[52]/Tata Memorial/2005	18	T1-4, N0–N+, M0 (stages I–IV)	2 LE/RT 4 exent 4 exent/RT 4 RT 4 palliative/2 chemo	45–50 pelvis 20–25 boost	1.5–5.8	5-yr OS 33% (45%, distal vs. 16%, proximal; 50%, low vs. 0% high stage)	Stage Site (distal lesions do better)
DiMarco et al.[24]/Mayo Clinic/2004	53	pT1-3, N0–N+	26 partial urethrectomy 27 exent 20 adj RT/3 brachy 3 chemo (cis-platinum based)	20–60 (50 median)	12.8 (mean)	10-yr CSS 60% 10-yr CS 42% LR only 15 pts DM only 2 pts LR + DM 10 pts	Path stage and nodal status Partial urethrectomy (LR 22%)
Eng et al.[51]/UTHSCSA/2003	10	Tis-3, N0-2, M0-1	5 partial urethrectomy 5 RT +/– chemo	30–68 primary 50 nodes 25 brachy HDR	11 (mean)	OS 60% (4/5, low vs. 2/5, high stage)	Clinical stage
Dalbagni et al.[2]/MSKCC/1998	72	Tx-4, Nx–N+	42 exent/partial urethrectomy 25 RT/brachy 10 preop RT	No details	7.1 (median)	5-yr OS 32% (78%, low vs. 22%, high stage) 5-yr DSS 46% (89%, low vs. 33%, high stage)	Stage, nodal status, surgery type, disease site
Grigsby[25]/MIR/1998	44	T1-4, N0-2	7 surgery 25 RT 12 surgery + RT	30–73.68 (50.4 median) for adj RT 12–70 (42.59 median) + 20–95 (42.72 median) brachy for RT only	8.25 (mean)	5-yr OS 42% 5-yr DSS 40% (89%, 36%, 19% for <2, 2–4, >4 cm) LR 8 pts, LR + DM 15 pts, DM 4 pts	Size and histology
Gheiler et al.[53]/Wayne State University/1998	21 (11 males)	Ta-4, N0-2	2 urethrectomy 4 chemo + RT + exent 2 exent alone 2 chemoRT (5-FU, CDDP, MVAC)	45 pelvis 25–30 boost	3.5 (mean)	OS 62% (89%, low vs. 42%, high stage)	Clinical stage
Garden et al.[3]/MDA/1993	97	T1-4, N0–N+	86 LE + RT: (35 RT + brachy, 21 RT 30 Brachy) 11 preop RT/ cyctourethrectomy or exent	40–106 (65 median) RT 45–75 (60 median) brachy	8.75 (median)	5-yr AS 41% 10-yr AS 31% 15-yr AS 22% LC 64% (RT only)	Local extension, fixation, and involvement of entire urethra

5-FU, 5-fluorouracil; adj, adjuvant; AS, actuarial survival; brachy, brachytherapy; CDDP, cisplatin; chemo, chemotherapy; CS, crude survival; CSS, cancer-specific survival; DM, distant metastasis; DSS, disease-specific survival; exent, exenteration; HDR, high-dose-rate; LC, local control; LE, local excision; LR, local recurrence; MDA, MD Anderson Cancer Center; MIR, Mallinckrodt Institution of Radiology; MSKCC, Memorial Sloan-Kettering Cancer Center; MVAC, methotrexate, vinblastine, Adriamycin, cisplatin; OS, overall survival; preop, preoperative; pts, patients; RT, radiation therapy; UTHSCSA, University of Texas Health Science Center at San Antonio.

irradiation alone. Prempree et al.[38] treated three patients with stage I disease with interstitial irradiation alone (50 to 65 Gy) and achieved local control in all three. In the same series, two of four patients with stage II disease achieved local control and were alive 5 years after treatment. Weghaupt et al.[9] reported a 5-year survival rate of 71% for 42 patients with cancer of the anterior urethra. Their doses ranged from 55 to 70 Gy from intracavitary and external irradiation. Princess Margaret Hospital reported an 87% relapse-free survival rate in patients with stage I or II disease.[69] The majority of patients with small primary tumors received brachytherapy as a component of their treatment. Patients receiving brachytherapy and external-beam radiation therapy had a median total dose of 65 Gy.

Tumors of the proximal urethra or the entire urethra are more difficult to treat. The overall local control rate is 20% to 30%. Bracken et al.[50] treated 81 patients, and the 5-year survival rate was approximately 25% for patients with stage III and 20% for those with stage IV disease. Princess Margaret Hospital reported stage III and IV tumors to have cause-specific survival rates of 26% and 16%, respectively.[40] Weghaupt et al.[9] reported 20 patients with tumor involvement of the posterior urethra who received irradiation alone or preoperative irradiation and surgery. The 5-year survival rate for these patients was 50%. Garden et al.[3] treated 86 patients with irradiation only after excision or biopsy of the primary lesion. Radiation doses ranged from 40 to 106 Gy (median, 65 Gy). The 5-year disease-specific survival rate was 49%, and the 5-year local control rate was 64%. Preoperative irradiation combined with radical surgery is an approach used by Klein et al.[22] They treated five women in this manner and achieved a 5-year survival rate of 40%. Dalbagni et al.[67] used anterior pelvic exenteration with intraoperative tumor bed interstitial brachytherapy using ^{192}Ir, followed several weeks later by pelvic external beam radiation therapy. A variety of chemosensitizing agents were used. The median brachytherapy dose was

15 Gy, and pelvic radiation therapy given was 45 Gy. Local control was achieved in four of six women with T2 and T1 disease.

Chemotherapy and Multimodality

Gheiler et al.[53] reported a disease-free survival rate of 60% in selected patients with advanced T3 or higher disease treated with a multimodality regimen consisting of neoadjuvant chemotherapy and radiation therapy. A phase II study showed that the combination of ifosfamide, paclitaxel, and cisplatin used in 45 patients with advanced transitional carcinoma of the urothelial tract is well tolerated and results in a median survival of 20 months.[75] Similar encouraging results were reported in patients with advanced urethral cancer receiving concomitant fluorouracil, mitomycin C, and radiation therapy.[61,62,76]

SEQUELAE OF THERAPY

Complications as a result of surgery, irradiation, or combined-modality therapy vary greatly, from 0% to 42%, because of different tumor stages, the extent of surgery, and various irradiation doses.[11,20,25,50,66] In general, more aggressive treatment is expected to result in a higher complication rate. Garden et al.[3] reported that 27 of 55 patients (49%) achieving local control had complications, including urethral stenosis, fistula, necrosis, cystitis, and hemorrhage. Urethral strictures develop in some patients, necessitating dilatation or urinary diversion. Others may experience incontinence, cystitis, and vaginal stenosis. Severe complications include fistula formation, bowel obstruction, and, occasionally, operative death. In the case of advanced neoplasms, fistula formation may be unavoidable because of tumor erosion of adjacent organs and subsequent tumor necrosis. Unlike the male counterpart, the physical loss of the female urethra is not uniformly associated with sexual impotence; nevertheless, the associated treatment side effects and negative self-image may affect sexual function and quality of life.

FUTURE DIRECTIONS

Early detection and intervention provide the best chance of organ preservation and cure. Although most clinical information comes from retrospective case series accumulated over a long span of time using various treatment modalities, multimodality shows encouraging results and should always be considered, especially in patients with locally advanced or metastatic disease. Clinical trials are clearly needed to obtain prospective data. Improved knowledge of tumor and normal-tissue radiobiology and continued technological advances in external-beam radiation therapy and brachytherapy delivery will maximize organ preservation and minimize some of the treatment-related complications.

REFERENCES

1. Swartz MA, Porter MP, Lin DW, et al. Incidence of primary urethral carcinoma in the United States. *Urology* 2006;68(6):1164–1168.
2. Dalbagni G, Zhang ZF, Lacombe L, et al. Female urethral carcinoma: an analysis of treatment outcome and a plea for a standardized management strategy. *Br J Urol* 1998;82:835–841.
3. Garden AS, Zagars GK, Delclos L. Primary carcinoma of the female urethra: results of radiation therapy. *Cancer* 1993;71:3102–3108.
4. Hopkins SC, Grabstald H. Benign and malignant tumors of the male and female urethra. In: Walsh PC, Gittes RF, Perlmutter AD, et al., eds. *Campbell's urology,* 5th ed. Philadelphia: WB Saunders, 1986:1441–1462.
5. Levine RL. Urethral cancer. *Cancer* 1980;45:1965–1972.
6. Sailer SL, Shipley WU, Wang CC. Carcinoma of the female urethra: a review of results with radiation therapy. *J Urol* 1988;140:1–5.
7. Srinivas V, Khan SA. Female urethral cancer: an overview. *Int Urol Nephrol* 1987; 19:423–427.
8. Johnson DE, O'Connell JR. Primary carcinoma of the female urethra. *Urology* 1983;21:42–45.
9. Weghaupt K, Gerstner GJ, Kucera H. Radiation therapy for primary carcinoma of the female urethra: a survey over 25 years. *Gynecol Oncol* 1984;17:58–63.
10. Grabstald H. Tumors of the urethra in men and women. *Cancer* 1973;32:1236–1255.
11. Pointon RCS, Poole-Wilson DS. Primary carcinoma of the urethra. *Br J Urol* 1968; 40:682–693.
12. Turner AG, Hendry WF. Primary carcinoma of the female urethra. *Br J Urol* 1980; 52:549–554.
13. Weiner JS, Walther PJ. A high association of oncogenic human papillomaviruses with carcinomas of the female urethra: polymerase chain reaction-based analysis of multiple histological types. *J Urol* 1994;151:49–53.
14. Nakamura Y, Takahashi M, Suga A, et al. A case of adenocarcinoma arising within a urethral diverticulum diagnosed only by the surgical specimen. *Gynecol Obstet Invest* 1995;40:69–70.
15. Narayan P, Konety B. Surgical treatment of female urethral carcinoma. *Urol Clin North Am* 1992;19:373–382.
16. Rajan N, Tucci P, Mallouh C, et al. Carcinoma in female urethral diverticulum: case reports and review of management. *J Urol* 1993;150:1911–1914.
17. Chen ME, Pisters LL, Malpica A, et al. Risk of urethral, vaginal and cervical involvement in patients undergoing radical cystectomy for bladder cancer: results of a contemporary cystectomy series from M.D. Anderson Cancer Center. *J Urol* 1997; 157:2120–2123.
18. De Paepe ME, Andre R, Mahadevia P. Urethral involvement in female patients with bladder cancer. A study of 22 cystectomy specimens. *Cancer* 1990;65:1237–1241.
19. Taggart CG, Castro JR, Rutledge FN. Carcinoma of the female urethra. *AJR Am J Roentgenol* 1972;114:145–151.
20. Chu AM. Female urethral carcinoma. *Radiology* 1973;107:627–630.
21. Grabstald H, Hilaris B, Henschke U, et al. Cancer of the female urethra. *JAMA* 1966;197:835–842.
22. Klein FA, Whitmore WF, Herr HW, et al. Inferior pubic rami resection with en bloc radical excision for invasive proximal urethral carcinoma. *Cancer* 1983;51:1238–1242.
23. Peterson DT, Dockerty MB, Utz DC, et al. The peril of primary carcinoma of the urethra in women. *J Urol* 1973;110:72–75.
24. DiMarco DS, DiMarco CS, Zincke H, et al. Surgical treatment for local control of female urethral carcinoma. *Urol Oncol* 2004;22:404–409.
25. Grigsby PW. Carcinoma of the urethra in women. *Int J Radiat Oncol Biol Phys* 1998;41:535–541.
26. Moinuddin Ali M, Klein FA, et al. Primary female urethral carcinoma: a retrospective comparison of different treatment techniques. *Cancer* 1988;62:54–57.
27. Delclos L. Carcinoma of the female urethra. In: Johnson DE, Boileau MA, eds. *Genitourinary tumors.* New York: Grune & Stratton, 1982:275–286.
28. Seballos RM, Rich RR. Clear cell adenocarcinoma arising from a urethral diverticulum. *J Urol* 1995;153:1914–1915.
29. Touijer AK, Dalbagni G. Role of voided urine cytology in diagnosing primary urethral carcinoma. *Urology* 2004;63:33–35.
30. Morikawa K, Togashi K, Minami S, et al. MR and CT appearance of urethral clear cell adenocarcinoma in a woman. *J Comput Assist Tomogr* 1995;19:1001–1003.
31. Selch MT, Mark RJ, Fu YS, et al. Primary lymphoma of female urethra: Long-term control by radiation therapy. *Urology* 1993;42:343–346.
32. Fisher M, Hricak H, Reinhold C, et al. Female urethral carcinoma: MRI staging. *Am J Radiol* 1985;144:603–604.
33. Quick HH, Serfaty JM, Pannu HK, et al. Endourethral MRI. *Magn Reson Med* 2001; 45:138–146.
34. Chou CP, Levenson RB, Elsayes KM, et al. Imaging of female urethral diverticulum: an update. *Radiographics* 2008;28(7):1917–30.
35. Fanti S, Nanni C, Ambrosini V, et al. PET in genitourinary tract cancers. *Quart J Nucl Med Mol Imag* 2007;51(3):260–71.
36. Kumar R, Zhuang H, Alavi A. PET in the management of urologic malignancies. *Radiol Clin North Am* 2004;42(6):1141–53.
37. Shvarts O, Han KR, Seltzer M, et al. Positron emission tomography in urologic oncology. *Cancer Control* 2002;9(4):335–342.
38. Prempree T, Amornmarn R, Patanaphan V. Radiation therapy in primary carcinoma of the female urethra: II. An update on results. *Cancer* 1984;54:729–733.
39. Greene FL, Page DL, Fleming ID, et al., eds. *AJCC cancer staging manual,* 6th ed. Philadelphia: Lippincott-Raven, 2002.
40. Meis JM, Ayala AG, Johnson DE. Adenocarcinoma of the urethra in women: a clinicopathologic study. *Cancer* 1987;60:1038–1052.
41. Nash PA, Bihrle R, Gleason PE, et al. Mohs' micrographic surgery and distal urethrectomy with immediate urethral reconstruction for glandular carcinoma in situ with significant urethral extension. *Urology* 1996;47:108–110.
42. Ali SZ, Smilari TF, Gal D, et al. Primary adenoid cystic carcinoma of Skene's glands. *Gynecol Oncol* 1995;57:257–261.
43. Aragona F, Maio G, Piazza R, et al. Primary malignant melanoma of the female urethra: a case report. *Int Urol Nephrol* 1995;27:107–111.
44. Barbagli G, Natali A, Urso C, et al. Primary malignant melanoma of the female urethra: a case report with immunohistochemical findings. *Urol Int* 1988;43:110–112.
45. Ebisuno S, Miyai M, Nagareda T. Clear cell adenocarcinoma of the female urethra showing positive staining with antibodies to prostate-specific antigen and prostatic acid phosphatase. *Urology* 1995;45:682–685.
46. Kakizaki H, Nakada T, Sugano O, et al. Malignant lymphoma in the female urethra. *Int J Urol* 1994;1:281–282.
47. Lopez AE, Latiff GA, Ciancio G, et al. Lymphoma of urethra in patient with acquired immune deficiency syndrome. *Urology* 1993;42:596–598.
48. Millan-Rodriguez F, Montlleo-Gonzalez M, Rosales-Bordes A, et al. Kaposi's sarcoma of the urethral meatus: management by urethral dilatation. *Br J Urol* 1995;75:558.
49. Vapnek JM, Turzan CW. Primary malignant lymphoma of the female urethra: a report of a case and review of the literature. *J Urol* 1992;147:701–703.
50. Bracken RB, Johnson DE, Miller JS, et al. Primary carcinoma of the female urethra. *J Urol* 1976;116:188–192.
51. Eng TY, Naguib M, Galang T, et al. Retrospective study of the treatment of urethral cancer. *Am J Clin Oncol* 2003;26:558–562.
52. Thyavihally YB, Wuntkal R, Bakshi G, et al. Primary carcinoma of the female urethra: single center experience of 18 cases. *Jpn J Clin Oncol* 2005;35:84–87.
53. Gheiler EL, Tefilli MV, Tiguert R, et al. Management of primary urethral cancer. *Urology* 1998;52:487–493.
54. Grigsby PW, Corn B. Localized urethral tumors in women: Indications for conservative versus exenterative therapies. *J Urol* 1992;147:1516–1520.
55. Forman JD, Lichter AS. The role of radiation therapy in the management of the male and female urethra. *Urol Clin North Am* 1992;19:383–389.
56. Karnes RJ, Breau RH, Lightner DJ. Surgery for urethral cancer. *Urol Clin North Am* 2010;37(3):445–457.
57. Dann T, Schuller J, Schmeller NT, et al. Behandlung des distalen Urethrakarzinoms durch Laserkoagulation. *Urologe A* 1989;28:296.

58. Micaily B, Dzeda MF, Miyamoto CT, et al. Brachytherapy for cancer of the female urethra. *Semin Surg Oncol* 1997;13:208–214.
59. Kuettel MR, Parda DS, Harter KW, et al. Treatment of female urethral carcinoma in medically inoperable patients using external beam irradiation and high dose rate intracavitary brachytherapy. *J Urol* 1997;157:1669–1671.
60. Eisenberger MA. Chemotherapy for carcinomas of the penis and urethra. *Urol Clin North Am* 1992;19:333–338.
61. Hara I, Hikosaka S, Eto H, et al. Successful treatment for squamous cell carcinoma of the female urethra with combined radio- and chemotherapy. *Int J Urol* 2004;11:678–682.
62. Johnson DW, Kessler JF, Ferrigini RG, et al. Low dose combined chemotherapy/radiotherapy in the management of locally advanced urethral squamous cell carcinoma. *J Urol* 1989;141:615–616.
63. Licht MR, Klein EA, Bukowski R, et al. Combination radiation and chemotherapy for the treatment of squamous cell carcinoma of the male and female urethra. *J Urol* 1995;153:1918–1920.
64. Skarlos DV, Aravantinos G, Linardou E, et al. Chemotherapy with methotrexate, vinblastine, epirubicin and carboplatin (Carbo-MVE) in transitional cell urothelial cancer. A Hellenic Co-Operative Oncology Group study. *Eur Urol* 1997;31:420–427.
65. Golimbu M, Al-Askari S, Morales P. Transpubic approach for lower urinary tract surgery: a 15-year experience. *J Urol* 1990;143:72–76.
66. Hedden RJ, Husseinzadeh N, Bracken RB. Bladder sparing surgery for locally advanced female urethral cancer. *J Urol* 1993;150:1135–1137.
67. Dalbagni G, Donat SM, Eschwege P, et al. Results of high dose rate brachytherapy, anterior pelvic exenteration, and external beam radiotherapy for carcinoma of the female urethra. *J Urol* 2001;166:1759–1761.
68. Libby B, Chao D, Schneider BF. Non-surgical treatment of primary female urethral cancer. *Rare Tumor* 2010;2(3):e55.
69. Milosevic MF, Warde PR, Banerjee D, et al. Urethral carcinoma in women: results of treatment with primary radiotherapy. *Radiother Oncol* 2000;56:29–35.
70. Foens CS, Hussey DH, Staples JJ, et al. A comparison of the roles of surgery and radiation therapy in the management of carcinoma of the female urethra. *Int J Radiat Oncol Biol Phys* 1991;21:961–968.
71. Hahn P, Krepart G, Malaker K. Carcinoma of the female urethra: Manitoba experience, 1958–1987. *Urology* 1991;37:106–109.
72. Gerbaulet A, Haie-Meder C, Marsiglia H, et al. Brachytherapy in cancer of the urethra. *Ann Urol* 1994;28:312–317.
73. Koontz BF, Lee WR. Carcinoma of the urethra: radiation oncology. *Urol Clin North Am* 2010;37(3):459–466.
74. Mayer R, Fowler JE Jr, Clayton M. Localized urethral cancer in women. *Cancer* 1987;60:1548–1551.
75. Bajorin DF, McCaffrey JA, Dodd PM, et al. Ifosfamide, paclitaxel and cisplatin for patients with advanced transitional cell carcinoma of the urothelial tract: final report of a phase II trial evaluating two dose schedules. *Cancer* 2000;88:1671–1678.
76. Shah AB, Kalra JK, Silber L, et al. Squamous cell cancer of female urethra. Successful treatment with chemoradiotherapy. *Urology* 1985;25:284–286.

Chapter 74
Carcinoma of the Vulva

Junzo P. Chino, Laura J. Havrilesky, and Gustavo S. Montana

ANATOMY

Vulva

The vulva is composed of the mons pubis, clitoris, labia majora and minora, vaginal vestibule, and their supporting subcutaneous tissues. The vulva blends with the urinary meatus anteriorly and with the perineum and anus posteriorly. The mons pubis consists of prominent tissue located anteriorly to the pubic symphysis. The labia majora are two elongated skin folds that course posteriorly from the mons pubis and blend into the perineal body. The skin of the labia majora is pigmented and contains hair follicles and sebaceous glands. The labia minora are a smaller pair of skin folds located between the labia majora. Anteriorly the labia minora separates into two components that course above and below the clitoris, fusing with those of the opposite side to form the prepuce and frenulum, respectively. The skin of the labia minora contains numerous sebaceous glands but no hair follicles and has no underlying adipose tissue. The clitoris is 2 to 3 cm anterior to the urethral meatus and is supported externally by the fusion of the labia minora.

The vaginal introitus is demarcated laterally by the labia minora and posteriorly by the perineal body. Anteriorly numerous small vestibular glands are located beneath the mucosa and open onto its surface adjacent to the urethral meatus. The Bartholin's glands (or greater vestibular glands) are two small mucous-secreting glands situated within the subcutaneous tissue in the posterior aspect of the labia majora. The ducts of the Bartholin's glands open onto the posterolateral portion of the introitus. The Skene's glands (or paraurethral glands) open in the anterior aspect of the introitus but can be variable in location. The perineal body is a 3- to 4-cm band of skin that separates the vaginal introitus from the anus and forms the posterior margin of the vulva with the fusion of the labia minora, or the fourchette.

Lymphatic Drainage

The inguinofemoral nodes are located within the triangle formed by the inguinal ligament superiorly, the border of the sartorius muscle laterally, and the border of the adductor longus muscle medially. There are superficial inguinal lymph nodes that lie along the saphenous vein and its branches between Camper's fascia and the cribriform fascia overlying the femoral vessels. There are usually three to five deep nodes, the most superior of which is located under the inguinal ligament and is known as Cloquet's node. Lymph drains from these nodes into the external and common iliac pelvic lymph nodes.

Lymphatic drainage is specific to the location of a vulvar lesion. Labial lesions drain into the superficial inguinal and femoral lymph nodes, then penetrate the cribriform fascia and reach the deep femoral nodes. Lesions of the fourchette and perineum follow the lymphatics of the labia. Lymphatic drainage from the glans clitoris or perineal body enter either unilateral or bilateral superficial femoral nodes or the deep femoral and pelvic lymph nodes. Some lymphatics originating in the clitoris enter the pelvis directly, bypassing the femoral nodes to connect with the obturator and external iliac lymph nodes, though in practice, the pelvic lymph nodes are rarely involved without synchronous involvement of the inguinal nodes (Fig. 74.1).

EPIDEMIOLOGY

Vulvar cancer is a rare malignancy that represents < 1% of all the cancers diagnosed in women and <5% of all gynecologic neoplasms. In the United States, it is estimated that there were 3,900 new cases in 2010, with 920 deaths due to the disease.[1] The incidence is 2 cases per 100,000 women; however, this incidence increases to 13 per 100,000 in women of age >75 years.[2] The incidence is slightly lower in Black women (1.6 per 100,000) and Hispanics (1.5 per 100,000) compared with Whites (2.4 per 100,000), and Asians/Pacific Islanders have the lowest incidence (0.9 per 100,000).

There are two primary mechanisms believed to be involved in the carcinogenesis of this disease: human papillomavirus (HPV) and vulvar dystrophy, including lichen sclerosus and squamous hyperplasia. HPV DNA can be identified in 40% of invasive vulvar cancers, with 16, 18, and 33 being the predominant subtypes.[3,4] This is in contrast to vulvar intraepithelial neoplasia (VIN), from which HPV can be isolated in 70% to 90% of lesions.[5] Because HPV infection is related to numerous

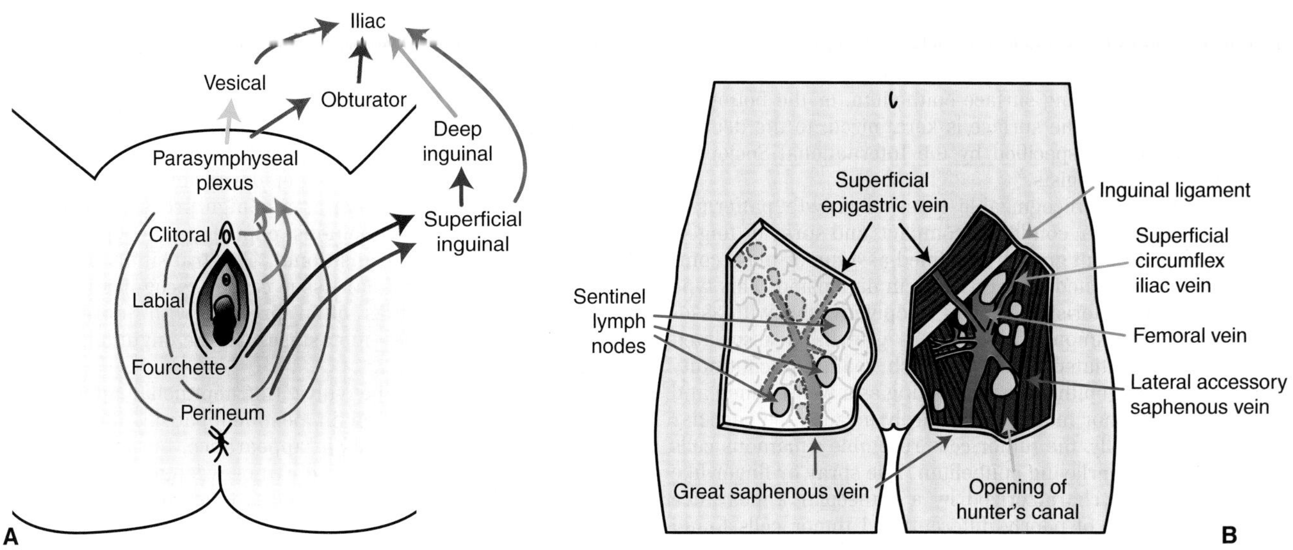

FIGURE 74.1. **A:** The lymphatic drainage of the vulva initially flows to the superficial inguinal nodes and then to the deep femoral and iliac group. Drainage from midline structures may flow directly beneath the symphysis to the pelvic nodes. (Modified from Plentl AA, Friedman EA, eds. *Lymphatic system of the female genitalia.* Philadelphia: WB Saunders, 1971.) **B:** The superficial inguinal lymph nodes comprise 8 to 10 subcutaneous nodes located between Camper's fascia and the cribriform fascia. These nodes are immediately adjacent to the saphenous vein and its branches. (Modified from DiSaia PJ, Creasman WT, Rich WM. An alternative approach to early cancer of the vulva. *Am J Obstet Gynecol* 1979;133:825.)

other cancers of the anogenital region (e.g., cervical cancer and anal canal cancer), the risk factors are similar: previous diagnosis of genital warts, multiple sexual partners, smoking history, previous abnormal Papanicolaou test, and immune suppression.[6,7] Lichen sclerosus (LS) has been found to be associated with vulvar cancer in 30% to 60% of cases in some series,[8,9] although there is no histopathologic evidence of direct transformation.[10] Women with existing LS have a 5% risk of developing invasive disease.[11] The evidence for VIN as an obligate precursor to invasive vulvar disease is much less compelling than that established between cervical intraepithelial neoplasia and cervical cancer. Only one-third of vulvar cancers have an associated VIN-3 lesion,[12] and <5% of women with an existing VIN lesion will subsequently be diagnosed with invasive disease.[13,14]

These findings have led to the hypothesis that squamous carcinoma of the vulvar can be broadly classified into two clinicopathologic entities: keratinizing squamous carcinomas (KSCs) and basaloid squamous carcinomas (BSCs).[15] KSC is more common (80% of cases), is found in older women with vulvar dystrophy, and is rarely associated with other neoplasia, HPV, or VIN.[16] p53 may or may not stain positive in KSC, because p53 mutations may play a role in pathogenesis in a subset of these neoplasms; p16 is rarely positive.[17] BSC, in contrast, is less common (20% of cases), is found in younger women, and is associated with multifocality, other anogenital neoplasia, HPV infection, and VIN. In BSC, staining for p53 is often negative, whereas p16 is often positive due to HPV infection.

PATHOLOGY

Squamous Carcinoma

Eighty-five percent of invasive disease of the vulva is squamous cell carcinoma (Fig. 74.2).[18] As noted earlier, these arise within squamous epithelium, often in or adjacent to areas of epithelial abnormalities or of premalignant conditions such as lichen sclerosus, erythroplasia of Queyrat, and Bowen's disease.[19] The depth of invasion, critical for appropriate staging

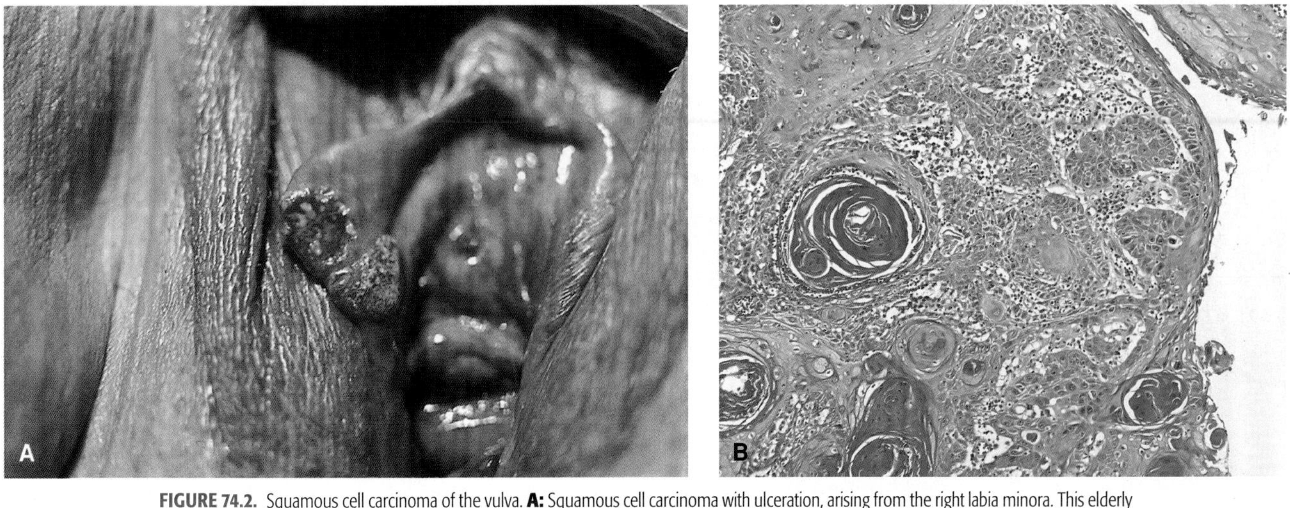

FIGURE 74.2. Squamous cell carcinoma of the vulva. **A:** Squamous cell carcinoma with ulceration, arising from the right labia minora. This elderly woman had no apparent predisposing disease. **B:** Photomicrograph of invasive keratinizing squamous cell carcinoma of the vulva. Note the keratin pearls. (Courtesy of Dr. Stanley Robboy, Duke University Medical Center, Durham, NC.)

Clinical Radiation Oncology

and management, is defined as the distance from the epithelial stromal junction of the most superficial adjacent dermal papillae to the deepest point of invasion. Tumor thickness is measured from the overlying surface epithelium, or the bottom of the granular layer if the surface is keratinized, to the deepest point of invasion as specified by the International Society of Gynecological Pathologists.[20]

There are three recognizable types of growth pattern of squamous carcinoma: confluent, compact, and spray or finger-like growth. Confluent growth is defined as a tumor mass composed of interconnected tumor >1 mm in dimension. This type of growth is characteristic for being deeply invasive with associated stromal desmoplasia. Compact growth is associated with well-differentiated tumors, which maintain continuity with the overlying epithelium, infiltrating as a well-defined and circumscribed tumor mass, which rarely invades the vascular space. Histologically, the tumor cells resemble squamous cells of adjacent and overlaying epithelium. The spray or finger-like growth pattern is characterized by a trabecular appearance with small islands of poorly differentiated tumor cells found within the dermis or submucosa, deeper than the main tumor mass. This growth pattern is often associated with desmoplastic stromal response and a lymphocytic inflammatory infiltrate. Vascular space involvement is seen more commonly with this pattern of growth than with tumors with a compact pattern of growth.[21]

Uncommon Histologic Types

Malignant melanoma of the vulva accounts for approximately 10% of all primary tumors of the vulva, occurs predominately in White women, and has a peak incidence in the sixth and seventh decades (Fig. 74.3).[22] Sometimes the tumor arises in a pre-existing pigmented lesion, and in these cases the differential diagnosis includes benign vulvar melanosis and pigmented VIN. Vulvar melanomas can be subclassified into three specific categories: superficial spreading malignant melanoma; nodular melanoma; and acral lentiginous melanoma.[23] As is the case for melanomas arising in other sites, the level of invasion and tumor thickness dictate the therapy and determine the prognosis.[24]

Adenocarcinomas of the vulva arise predominantly in the Bartholin's glands, although apocrine, eccrine, and Skene's glands can also be the site of origin. In the rare instances when adenocarcinomas arise in the absence of glandular tissue, they may be of cloacogenic origin. Carcinoma of Bartholin's gland is seen more frequently in older women and is often solid and deeply infiltrative. The overlying epidermis may remain intact, leading to misinterpretation as a benign process. Other histopathologic types are mucinous, papillary, mucoepidermoid, adenosquamous, and transitional. The transition from normal to malignant glandular tissue can be recognized in some cases. Adenocarcinomas often present with more locally advanced disease with metastases to the inguinal-femoral lymph nodes.

Paget's disease of the vulva (intraepithelial adenocarcinoma) is seen most often in postmenopausal, older White women. The disease varies in appearance, but most often it presents as an eczematoid, red can or weeping lesion, and it can be mistakenly diagnosed as eczema or contact dermatitis (Fig. 74.4). The lesion may be flat, raised, or ulcerated and may appear whitish (leukoplakia), red (erythroplastic), or hyperpigmented. This condition has a typical histologic pattern and often stains positive for carcinoembryonic antigen. Vulvar Paget's disease is associated with invasive carcinoma in 10% to 20% of the cases.[25,26,27] The invasive disease may be an underlying adenocarcinoma of the apocrine or Bartholin's glands, or it may be an adenocarcinoma arising elsewhere in the anogenital region.

Verrucous carcinomas of the vulva are uncommon, usually diagnosed in the fifth or sixth decade of life. Histologically these tumors are often well differentiated and have a low incidence of metastasis to the lymph node. In instances when the lesion is in early stage, excellent results are obtained with radical wide excision.[28] Other vulvar malignancies arising from epidermal cell types are rare. Merkel cell tumors (neuroendocrine carcinomas) of the vulva are aggressive locally, have a high incidence of distant metastasis, and carry a poor prognosis. Basal cell carcinomas, on the other hand, seldom spread to lymph nodes and are appropriately treated with wide excision alone.[29] Transitional cell carcinomas may arise from the

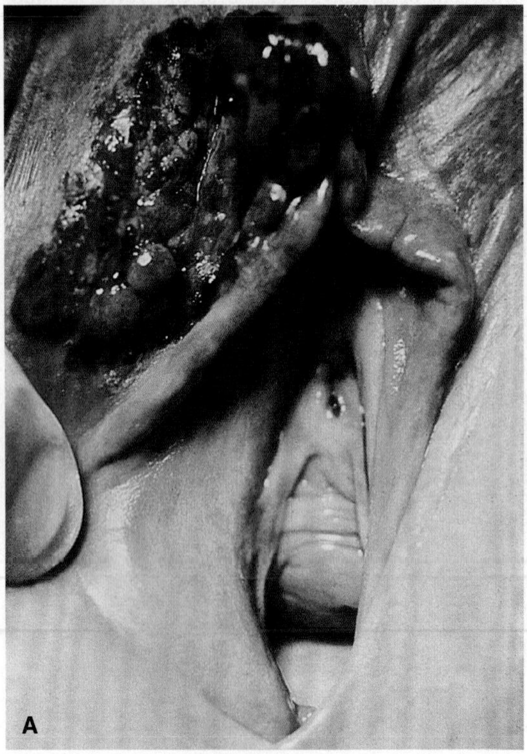

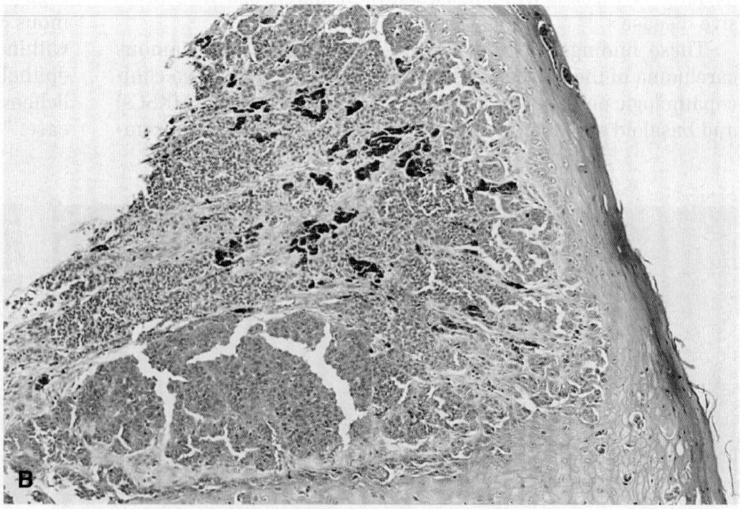

FIGURE 74.3. Melanoma of the vulva. **A:** A nodular, elevated, and darkly pigmented lesion arising from the right labia majora. **B:** Photomicrograph of invasive melanoma, with melanin apparent in portions of the tumor. (Courtesy of Dr. Stanley Robboy, Duke University Medical Center, Durham, NC.)

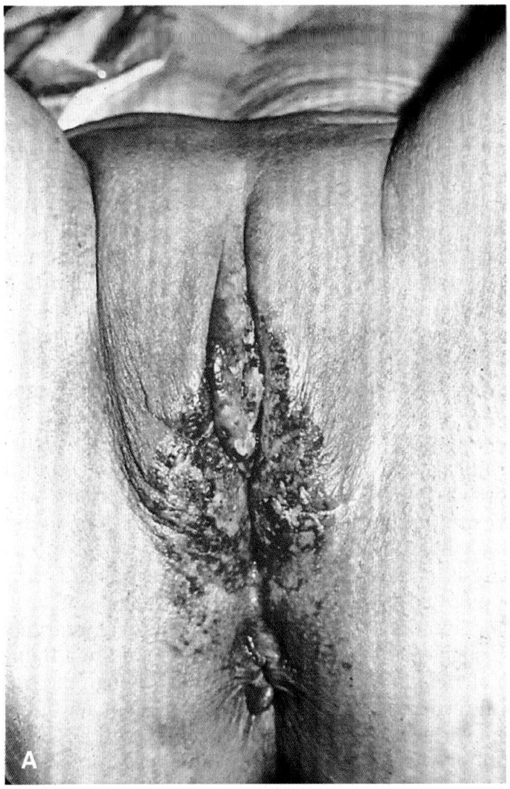

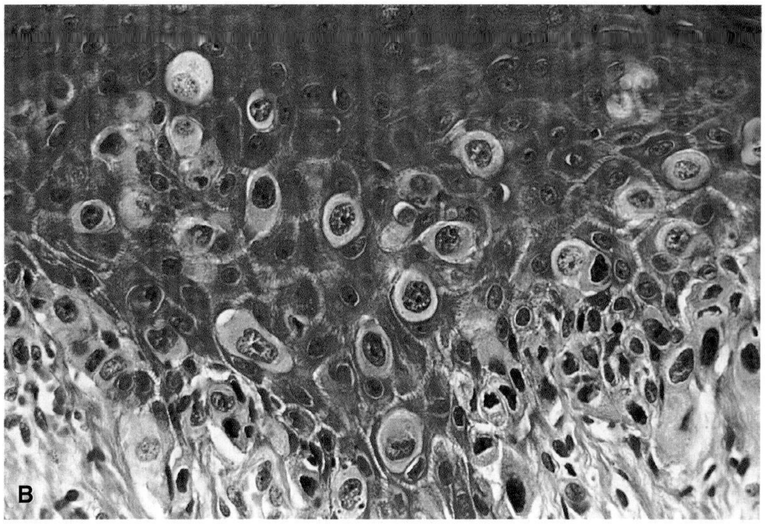

FIGURE 74.4. Paget's disease of the vulva. **A:** Photo of extensive perineal disease, extending to the perianal skin. **B:** Photomicrograph of intraepithelial Paget cells, with copious pale cytoplasm, occurring singly or in small clusters, and appearing slightly larger than neighboring squamous cells. (Courtesy of Dr. Stanley Robboy, Duke University Medical Center, Durham, NC.)

Bartholin's glands or may also represent metastasis from the bladder and/or lower urinary tract.

The most common subtypes of vulvar sarcoma are leiomyosarcomas, malignant fibrous histocytomas, epithelioid sarcomas, and rhabdomyosarcomas. Rhabdomyosarcomas of the vulva require combination therapy, chemotherapy, and radiation, as per rhabdomyosarcoma protocols of other sites. Results of treatment with other sarcomas of the vulva are unpredictable, and wide resection and/or radical radiotherapy should be considered, given the relative inactivity of chemotherapy.

CLINICAL PRESENTATION

Vulvar pruritus is the most common presenting symptom, although women may also complain of bleeding, pain, or discharge. If there is a visible lesion on physical examination, a biopsy is required to distinguish it from other vulvar lesions such as dystrophia, benign condylomata, and VIN. Unfortunately, many women have a long delay in diagnosis due to denial or minimization of symptoms and may present with a locally advanced tumor by the time of initial evaluation. These lesions may also present with symptoms related to the invasion of regional structures, including difficulty with urination or defecation. Metastatic disease is an uncommon presenting symptom because the primary lesion is usually much more problematic, although consequences of groin and distant disease may also be seen at presentation.

PATTERNS OF DISEASE AND SPREAD

Primary Site

Approximately 70% of vulvar malignancies arise in the labia majora and minora, 15% in the clitoris, 5% in the perineum and fourchette, 5% in the prepuce Bartholin's glands and urethra, and 5% are too extensive at presentation to classify.[30]

Lymphatic Spread

High-grade tumors with "spray" growth pattern and lymphatic space invasion have a proclivity to spread to the regional lymphatic nodes. The superficial inguinofemoral lymph nodes are the first echelon, followed by the deep inguinofemoral nodes. For well-lateralized lesions, metastasis to the contralateral inguinal or pelvic lymph nodes is unusual in the absence of ipsilateral inguinofemoral node involvement. Lesions of the clitoris or urethra can spread directly to pelvic lymph nodes, although this is rare without involvement of the inguinal nodes.[31,32]

The frequency of inguinal lymph node metastasis in surgically staged patients ranges from 6% to 50%, depending on tumor invasion and extent of disease (Table 74.1).[33–37] Physical examination alone is inaccurate to assess lymph node involvement: Plentl and Friedman[30] reported a 62% incidence of

TABLE 74.1 INCIDENCE OF LYMPH NODE INVOLVEMENT CORRELATED WITH PRIMARY TUMOR SIZE AND EXTENT

Primary Tumor Size and Depth of Invasion	*Number of Patients*	*Number of Patients with Positive Lymph Nodes (%)*
Depth		
<1 mm	120	0 (0)
1.1–2 mm	121	8 (6.6)
2.1–3 mm	97	8 (8.2)
3.1–4 mm	50	11 (22)
4.1–5 mm	40	10 (25)
Size		
>5 mm	32	12 (37.5)
>2 cm	168	77 (45.8)
Any size of primary tumor extending beyond the vulva	70	38 (54.2)

Adapted from Perez CA, Grigsby PW, Chao C. Vulva. In: Perez CA, Brady LW, eds. *Principles and practice of radiation oncology*, 3rd ed. Philadelphia: Lippincott-Raven, 1997.

lymph node metastases in patients with clinically palpable adenopathy and 35% involvement in patients without clinically palpable adenopathy. In a review of clinical staging, Franklin[38] noted that approximately 75% of patients with clinically suspicious lymph nodes had nodal metastasis, and 11% to 43% of patients with clinically negative nodes had metastasis to the nodes. In a Gynecologic Oncology Group (GOG) study reported by Homesley et al.[39] 23.9% of the patients with clinically negative inguinal nodes were found to have nodal metastasis on final pathology. When the lymph nodes were clinically suspicious, 76.2% of the patients had histologically positive nodes. In patients that have histologically positive inguinal nodes, the probability of having positive pelvic nodes is 30%.[39]

Multiple clinical and histologic features of the primary tumor are associated with nodal metastasis, including tumor thickness, histologic grade, capillary-like space involvement, depth of invasion, location of the tumor, and tumor size.[40,41] Rutledge et al.[42] also described the adverse effect on local control and survival of tumor size, clinical stage, positive inguinal or pelvic nodes, and positive margins at the primary site. When the tumor thickness is ≤1 mm, the probability of nodal metastasis is ≤3%, but with tumor a tumor thickness ≥5 mm, the probability increases to 33.3%. Depth of invasion of 1, 2, and 3 mm corresponds to a 4.3%, 7.8%, and 17% incidence of nodal involvement, respectively. It should be noted that in the vulva the thickness of the epithelium varies significantly from one area to another, in some areas being >0.8 mm thick, which can influence the relative value given to tumor thickness and depth of invasion. Measuring tumor thickness in superficially ulcerated tumors can be misleading and may lead to underestimating the depth of invasion. Perineural invasion correlates strongly with lymph node metastasis.[43]

In analysis of the Gynecologic Oncology Group (GOG) database on carcinoma of the vulva, several clinical and histologic tumor characteristics were identified as predictors of nodal involvement. In order of importance these are clinical node status (palpable vs. nonpalpable), grade, capillary-lymphatic space involvement, tumor thickness, and patient's age.[39,41,44] There is also a correlation between the size of the primary tumor and involvement of the lymph nodes. In Donaldson et al.'s[34] series of 66 patients, the probability of having positive inguinal nodes rose from 18.9% for patients with lesions <3 cm to 72.4% for patients with primary tumors ≥3 cm. In a GOG study of 267 patients with superficial vulvar cancer reported by Sedlis et al.,[41] the frequency of positive inguinal nodes was 18.1% for patients with lesions up to 3 cm in size and 29.3% for patients with lesions ≥3 cm. Extension of the primary tumor to the urethra, vagina, and anal area is associated with an increased incidence of nodal involvement and worsening of prognosis. The significance of this is reflected in the stage assignment of the patients.

Curry et al.[45] noted that pelvic nodes were not involved if three or fewer inguinal nodes were positive. Similar findings have been reported by Hacker et al.[46] In the GOG study reported by Homesley et al.[47] of patients with positive inguinal nodes, the incidence of pelvic node involvement was 28.3% (15 of 23). In this study, there was a correlation of pelvic node involvement with the extent of inguinal node involvement. Due to the rarity of isolated pelvic nodal metastasis, the status of the inguinal nodes determines the management of the pelvic nodes. Although deep pelvic node involvement is an ominous sign, one-fourth to one-third of the patients are still potentially curable, particularly if only a few nodes are involved.[31,33,45]

Distant Metastases

Hematogenous dissemination generally occurs late in the natural history of the disease, with the most common sites being the lungs, liver, and bones. The development of distant metastasis portends a very poor outlook.

PROGNOSTIC FACTORS

Lymph node metastasis is the most important prognostic factor in patients with vulvar cancer. The presence of inguinal node metastases is accompanied by a 50% reduction in long-term survival.[48,49] Pelvic nodal metastasis has an even more profound negative effect on survival.[31,33,45] Kurzl and Masserer[50] analyzed 124 patients with various stages of vulvar carcinoma treated with simple vulvectomy alone and local/inguinal irradiation. They found that age, disassociated growth, lymphatic spread, thickness, and ulceration of the primary tumor were important prognostic factors. In a detailed analysis of a GOG clinicopathologic study of 558 women with vulvar cancer, two significant risk factors were identified that predispose for recurrence in the vulva: tumor size >4 cm and capillary lymphatic space involvement.[44] If either of these factors was present, the risk of local recurrence after radical vulvectomy was 20.7% (30 of 184), but if neither factor was present, the risk of local recurrence was only 9.2% (37 of 404). In this study the depth of invasion did not predict for vulvar failure.

In an analysis of formalin-fixed tissue specimens, Heaps et al.[51] demonstrated a sharp rise in the incidence of local recurrence for tumors with microscopic, surgical margins <8 mm. They suggested that this would correspond to a minimum margin of 1 cm in fresh, unfixed tissue. Although the frequency of local recurrences correlates with the adequacy of the margins of the surgical resection, when dealing with larger or thicker tumors or when they involve midline structures, adequate surgical margins may be difficult to obtain.

Lymph node extracapsular tumor extension has been noted in several series and it is known to have a negative effect on prognosis. Origoni et al.[52] evaluated the significance of the size of the metastases in the lymph nodes, the number of positive lymph nodes, and extracapsular extension of the disease and found that the presence of any one of these factors worsened the prognosis. Extracapsular tumor extension as an independent adverse prognostic factor on survival was also described by van der Velden et al.[53]

INITIAL EVALUATION

A thorough examination of the genitourinary system is warranted in all women with vulvar cancer because the disease may be multifocal. Examination of the vagina, cervix, perianal skin, and anal canal is of particular importance in order to delineate the extent of disease and to identify synchronous lesions. Special attention as well is paid to the inguinofemoral basins for clinical detection of lymphatic spread.

Imaging studies may not be necessary in early lesions that may be approached with surgery as the first treatment modality. However, imaging in women with locally advanced disease or with clinically suspicious lymph nodes may aid the clinician in selecting the most appropriate treatment. Computed tomography (CT) scans may identify concerning lymphadenopathy in the inguinofemoral chains, pelvis, or para-aortic regions.[54] Contrast-enhanced magnetic resonance imaging (MRI) may also aid in the delineation of the primary lesion, as well as with the evaluation of inguinal lymph nodes, with a sensitivity of 80% and a specificity of 88%.[55] Although clinically or radiographically detected inguinal nodes may be quickly evaluated with ultrasound-guided fine-needle aspiration, a negative result does not rule out involvement.[56] Fluorodeoxyglucose-positron emission tomography has been used to evaluate the groin prior to surgical evaluation, with a sensitivity of 67% and a specificity of 95%.[57] It should be noted that the sensitivity of all imaging modalities available are insufficient to omit surgical evaluation in women with a high risk of nodal involvement.

TABLE 74.2 VULVAR CANCER: 2009 AMERICAN JOINT COMMITTEE ON CANCER (AJCC) STAGING AND CORRESPONDING INTERNATIONAL FEDERATION OF GYNECOLOGY AND OBSTETRICS (FIGO) STAGING

2009 AJCC			FIGO
Tis	Carcinoma *in situ*		–
T1a	Confined to vulva/perineum, size ≤2 cm, stromal invasion ≤1 mm	N0	IA
T1b	Confined to vulva/perineum, size >2 cm or stromal invasion >1 mm	N0	IB
T2	Adjacent spread to distal 1/3 urethra and/or vagina or anus	N0	II
T3	Extension to proximal 2/3 urethra and/or vagina, bladder/rectal mucosa, or fixation to pubic bones		IVA
N1a	1–2 lymph nodes involved, all <5 mm		IIIA
N1b	1 lymph node involved, ≥5 mm		IIIA
N2a	3 or more lymph nodes involved, all <5 mm		IIIB
N2b	2 or more lymph nodes involved, ≥5 mm		IIIB
N2c	Any lymph nodes involved with extracapsular extension		IIIC
N3	Fixed or ulcerated lymph nodes		IVA
M1	Distant metastasis (including pelvic lymph node metastasis).		IVB

According to the AJCC, femoral and inguinal nodes are considered regional spread, whereas iliac nodes are considered distant metastasis.

Used with the permission of the American Joint Committee on Cancer, Chicago, Illinois. The original source for this material is American Joint Committee on Cancer. *AJCC cancer staging handbook,* 7th ed. New York: Springer, 2010, published by Springer Science and Business Media LLC, www.springer.com.

STAGING

The staging system first adopted in 1983 was based on clinical findings. The system was modified in 1988 to give the clinical status of the nodes more importance. In 1997 the staging was revised again to create a separate category for minimally invasive lesions, stage IA, emphasizing the need for histologic assessment of the inguinal nodes in all patients presenting with primary tumors with >1 mm depth of invasion.

The most recent Federation of Gynecology and Obstetrics staging revision was performed in 2009 and contains significant changes from the 1988 framework (Table 74.2).[58,59] Stage IB now includes primary lesions >2 cm in size (previously stage II), and stage II includes lesions with involvement of adjacent perineal structures (previously stage III). Stage III is now divided into three substages, reflecting the importance of the number and size of inguinal nodes involved and the prognostic significance of extracapsular extension. Presence of pelvic nodal metastases remains stage IVB disease.

GENERAL MANAGEMENT

The treatment of carcinoma of the vulva is challenging for multiple reasons. In general patients with this disease are older and have comorbidities. The tumor, by virtue of its location, can easily involve adjacent organs such as the bladder and the rectum, and the frequency of nodal involvement is high. Because of its relatively low incidence, most published reports include rather small and heterogeneous groups of patients. Management of carcinoma of the vulva is further complicated by the major psychosexual impact that the treatment can have on patients. For the aforementioned reasons it has been difficult to study this disease and to develop treatment guidelines.

The management of vulvar carcinoma has undergone very significant changes in the last few decades. En bloc resection of the primary tumor and inguinal node dissection, which used to be the standard of care, have been replaced by multimodality therapy, with the surgery being more tailored to the extent of the disease. This change follows the recognition of the morbidity associated with radical surgery, the improved results achieved with multimodality therapy, and the recognition of the negative impact that radical surgery can have on sexual function and body image.[6,60,61] Although radical surgery retains a very important place in the management of vulvar cancer, it is no longer the mainstay of the treatment. The likelihood of controlling the primary tumor with surgery largely depends on the adequacy of the margins of resection, and it is not necessary to remove the entire vulva. A clear margin of about 1 cm in all directions is sufficient to achieve a high rate of local control of the primary tumor.[51]

There have been refinements in the surgical technique that have made the procedures more tolerable. Examples of such improvements include primary closure of the perineal wound, the use of the sartorius muscle to close the surgical defect in the inguinal area, and the use of separate incisions for the resection of the primary tumor and the inguinal nodes. These developments have resulted in a decrease in operative mortality and morbidity.

In recent decades there have been also significant advances in all aspects of radiation therapy that apply to the treatment of carcinoma of the vulva. The technical resources available now make it possible to deliver effective doses of radiation to the vulvovaginal and inguinal regions with less acute and late morbidity. With high-photon-energy units, well-collimated fields, multileaf collimators, electron beams of different energies, and intensity-modulated radiation therapy (IMRT), radiation is now delivered to the primary disease and lymph nodes with precise account of the differences in contour, tissue thickness, and extent of the disease. It is possible to tailor the treatment to the specified treatment volume while keeping the dose to the normal tissues within acceptable limits of tolerance. Brachytherapy may also be used as primary treatment in very selected cases or in combination with external beam to bring the dose higher to limited volumes.

Perhaps the most significant advance of recent decades in the management of cancer patients is the use of more than one treatment modality concurrently or sequentially. Chemotherapy, radiation, and surgery in sequence and/or in combination lessen the impact of any one modality and can achieve functional organ preservation with at least comparable or improved local tumor control and survival (Fig. 74.5).

Early Invasive Disease

Surgery

In the past even patients with early stage IB disease were considered to have diffuse disease, and a radical vulvectomy was considered the standard of care, yielding 90% survival rates but with considerable physical and emotional sequelae.[51,62] Now, small, favorable lesions, ≤2 cm in diameter and ≤5 mm in depth, are managed with wide, local excision rather than a radical vulvectomy, with very satisfactory outcomes in every respect. The local recurrence and disease survival rates are similar with either procedure, ranging from 6% to 7% and 98% to 99%, respectively.[63] However, anterior lesions close to the clitoris may not be amenable to wide local excision and may require a radical vulvectomy to obtain satisfactory margins.

Small, well-lateralized, T1 lesions with negative ipsilateral groin nodes have <1% risk of contralateral groin involvement, and treatment of the contralateral groin is not necessary.[63] Poorly differentiated tumors, with >5-mm invasion and vascular space involvement, are at higher risk for inguinal node metastasis, and both groins must be evaluated and managed as needed.[39] Centrally located lesions, within 1 cm of the introitus, are considered midline lesions and may be treated with local excision, if possible, but both groins are at risk. A deep node dissection is recommended if the superficial nodes are involved. Traditionally, primary tumors >2 cm have been treated with radical vulvectomy and bilateral groin dissection because of the high risk of nodal involvement. The indications and extent of surgery for the inguinal nodes are under re-evaluation and are the subject of further discussion later in this chapter.

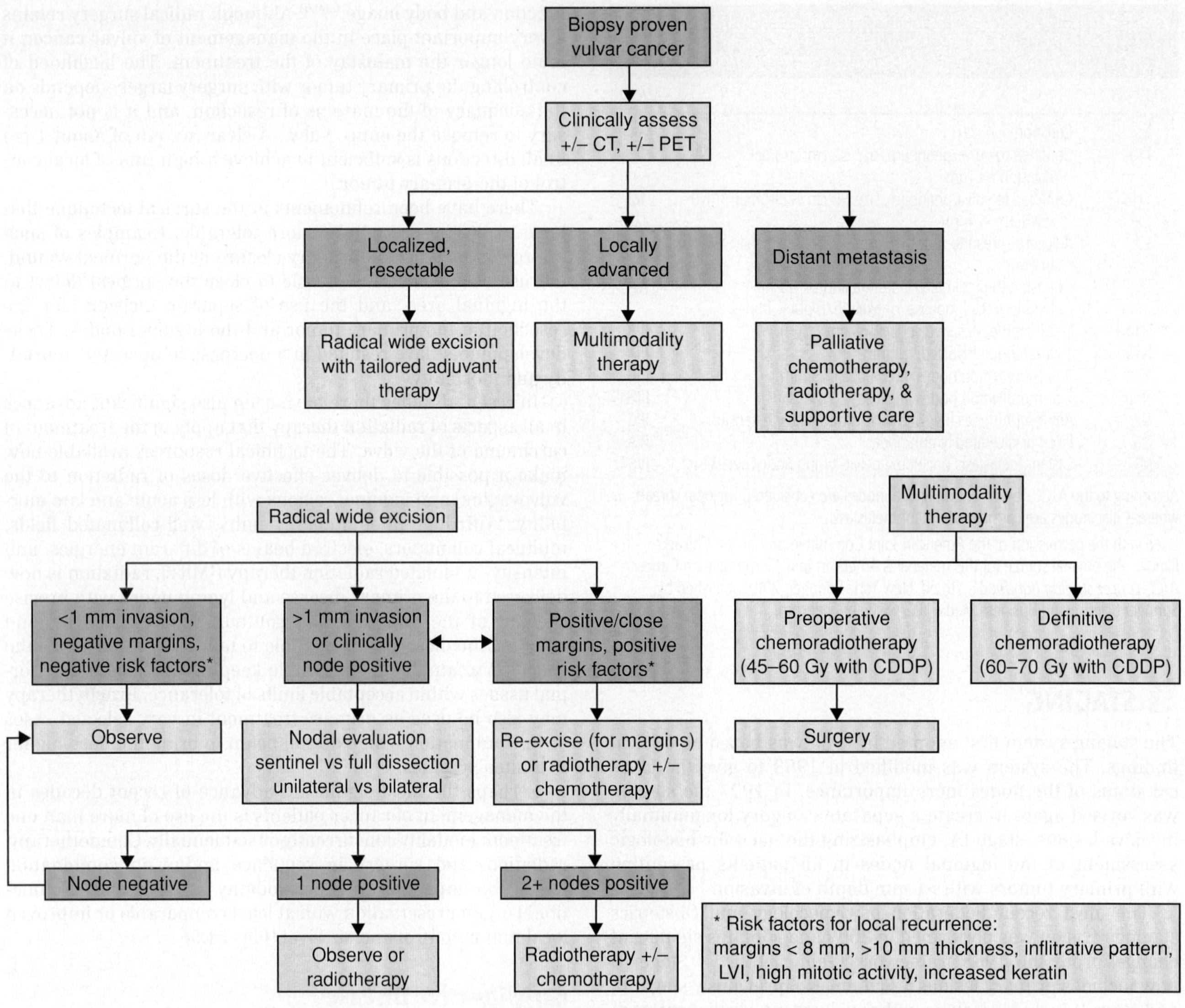

FIGURE 74.5. Treatment algorithm.

Radiation Therapy

In the setting of early invasive disease treated with wide local excision, radiation to the tumor bed may be advised to prevent local recurrence. As noted previously, pathologic features associated with higher risk of local recurrence at the primary site include lymphatic-vascular invasion (LVI), depth of invasion >5 mm, margins <8 mm, and microscopically positive margins.[51] Faul et al.[64] reported a retrospective study of 62 patients with close (≤ 8 mm) or positive surgical margins that found that local recurrence was significantly reduced from 58% with observation to 16% with postoperative radiation. Although postoperative radiation reduces the incidence of local recurrences, some recurrences may be salvaged with surgery, resulting in equivalent survival. However, in the absence of randomized trials, women with positive margins, margins <8 mm, deep invasion, and/or LVI should also be considered for adjuvant radiation. Definitive, preoperative, and postoperative radiation, with or without chemotherapy, are treatment options in patients with tumors close to the urethra, clitoris, or anal sphincter because it can be difficult to obtain an adequate margin.

The role of radiation in the management of inguinal and pelvic nodes was evaluated in a GOG trial reported in 1986.[47] In this trial patients underwent bilateral inguinal lymphadenectomy, and those with positive groin nodes were randomized to either pelvic lymphadenectomy or radiation to the pelvis and bilateral groins. The radiation group had significantly lower groin recurrence rate, 5.1% (3 of 59), compared to 23.6% (13 of 55) for the group that did not receive radiation. This translated into a 2-year significant survival benefit of 68% versus 54% ($p = .03$) in favor of the group that received postoperative radiation. Subgroup analysis of this study showed that the benefit was seen primarily in patients with more than one pathologically positive node. However, an exploratory analysis of the Surveillance, Epidemiology, and End Results data set in patients with one node positive revealed a significant survival difference in patients with <12 nodes submitted, suggesting that the benefit of radiation may be greater in patients with an insufficient nodal dissection.[65] Based on the entry criteria for the GOG study, adjuvant radiation to the pelvis and both groins should be considered for all those with nodal involvement. Patients with extracapsular extension (ECE) of tumor in the nodes or with residual disease in the inguinal areas should receive postoperative radiation to the pelvis, the groins, and the primary tumor bed area because ECE predisposes them for recurrence at the primary and the lymph node basins.[53]

Advanced Disease

Surgery alone for patients with advanced disease has yielded disappointing results, stimulating interest in multimodality treatment.[66,67] Concurrent chemoradiotherapy has been used for nearly three decades in preoperative, postoperative, and definitive settings. This multimodal approach is considered the standard of care.[68–77] Exenterations are now considered only for patients with advanced local recurrences after initial therapy and for whom there is no other alternative. In these highly selected patients, results can be acceptable in terms of the control of the disease.[78,79–80,81] However, exenterations have a very significant psychosexual impact on patients, even when measures are taken to restore some sexual function.[82]

Management of Patients with Histologic Variants

Melanoma

Melanoma is the second-most-common malignancy of the vulva. The treatment should be surgical, if possible. The prognosis is poor in general, with a 5-year overall survival of approximately 35%, and is worse in patients who have one or more of the following features: deep invasion, ulceration, nodular growth pattern, epithelioid cell type, and high mitotic rate.[83,84,85] The prognosis is also worse in older patients. The extent of the surgery needed to achieve local control depends on the size of the lesion and the depth of invasion, similar to melanomas in other parts of the body. Wide local excision is acceptable, as long as negative margins are obtained. In a study of 32 patients treated at the Royal Marsden Hospital in London, there was no difference in the outcome between patients treated with wide local excision and those treated with more radical surgical procedures.[86] Radiation may be considered for patients with positive margins or positive lymph nodes or for palliation of symptoms. As with melanomas of other sites, the prognosis is guarded due to a propensity for distant recurrence.

Bartholin's Gland Carcinoma

Carcinomas of the Bartholin's gland comprise 5% to 7% of all primary vulvar cancers. The recommended treatment consists of wide local excision and ipsilateral lymph node dissection. Contralateral groin dissection is reserved for patients with clinically suspicious nodes or for patients with involvement of the ipsilateral nodes. Similar to other types of vulvar carcinoma, pelvic node dissections are not routinely recommended. Radiation to the pelvis is advised if involvement of the pelvic nodes is suspected. The role of radiation for Bartholin's gland carcinoma has been studied by Copeland et al.[87] and Leuchter et al.[88] These two studies suggest that adjuvant radiation to the vulva and regional nodes after conservative surgery may decrease local recurrence, with 7% recurrence with radiation and 27% recurrence without it in the Copeland et al.[87] study. Five-year survival of 67% was obtained by Cardosi et al.[89] in patients who were found to have close margins and were treated with primary surgery and adjuvant radiation.

Verrucous Carcinoma

Verrucous carcinomas are locally invasive tumors that present as fungating, ulcerative masses. These lesions are usually treated by wide local excision. Inguinofemoral dissections are not recommended routinely due to the rarity of nodal metastases. The literature regarding vulvar verrucous carcinomas consists largely of case reports. with the exception of the series by Japaze et al.[90] This study was based on 24 patients, 17 of whom were treated with surgery only and 7 of whom were treated with surgery and radiation. In the surgery group only 1 patient developed recurrence and died as a result of it. In the radiation group 4 patients developed recurrence, and all died from the disease. Although it is difficult to draw definitive conclusions from this small series, there is no convincing data to recommend the routine use of radiotherapy for this disease. In addition, there is no sufficient evidence to support the notion that radiation induces anaplastic transformation.[91]

SURGERY

Primary Tumor

The surgical approach to vulvar cancer has evolved from the traditional en bloc radical vulvectomy for most patients to a more individualized and less radical procedure, alone or in combination with radiation and chemotherapy. For lesions not involving anus, vagina, or urethra, a radical local excision (also referred to as wide local excision, radical wide excision, or modified radical vulvectomy) is usually performed. At surgical resection, the depth of the excision should be to the deep perineal fascia. Excision of 2-cm margins of grossly normal-appearing tissue is recommended when possible, with a goal of obtaining at least 1-cm microscopic margins following tissue processing. If the tumor involves or abuts the clitoris, preservation of this structure may not be possible.

Radical vulvectomy is reserved for patients with large or multifocal lesions in whom preservation of normal vulvar tissue is not possible or would not serve a functional or reconstructive benefit. When the anus, vagina, or urethra are involved by malignancy, extended radical vulvectomy or pelvic exenteration is required to clear disease surgically.[78,92] Due to the high morbidity and operative mortality of extensive surgery, preoperative or primary chemoradiation should be considered for organ preservation.

Inguinofemoral Lymph Nodes

Attention to risk factors for nodal involvement is very important because inguinofemoral node dissection can lead to morbidity and sequelae. The main complications of groin surgery are wound breakdown and lower-extremity lymphedema. Although wound breakdown almost always heals successfully by secondary intention, chronic lower-extremity edema is very difficult to deal with and can lead to significant long-term disability. To reduce the frequency and the severity of these complications, an effort is made to identify patients in whom the extent of the node dissection can be decreased or eliminated altogether without compromising the likelihood of control of the disease.

Patients with small (<2-cm diameter) superficial squamous cell carcinomas with a depth of invasion 1 mm or less and no lymph vascular invasion have a very low risk of nodal involvement, and the groin dissection may be omitted.[36,93,94] For lesions with >1-mm invasion, groin node assessment should be performed in the form of superficial inguinal lymphadenectomy or sentinel node procedure. Small (<2 cm), lateralized lesions may be treated by unilateral groin dissection, whereas for midline and clitoral lesions and for those >2 cm in diameter, bilateral groins should be assessed. For patients undergoing primary surgery, palpable inguinal nodes should be removed if present.

The need to perform bilateral inguinal node dissection in patients with unilateral vulvar lesions, as well as the need to dissect the deep nodes whenever a superficial node dissection is carried out, has been re-examined in light of the additive morbidity of each procedure. When bilateral superficial and deep inguinal node dissections are performed, the potential for wound breakdown and lower-extremity lymphedema increases.[37,95] When a unilateral dissection is indicated and nodes are found to be negative, a contralateral node dissection is not required due to the low likelihood of contralateral metastasis.[96,97] The deep inguinal node dissection is usually omitted, based on the fact that if the superficial nodes are free of tumor, the deep nodes are rarely involved.[98] However, control of the disease in the lymph nodes is of utmost importance because most patients who develop groin failure will die as a result of the recurrence.[94,99]

Assessment of the groin nodes may be accomplished via full superficial inguinal dissection or alternatively via a sentinel lymph node procedure alone if performed by groups experienced in this technique. In the multicenter Groningen International Study on Sentinel Nodes in Vulvar Cancer, a sentinel node procedure using radioactive tracer and blue dye was performed in 623 groins and resulted in a 2.3% groin recurrence rate following a negative sentinel node.[100] This compares favorably to the 5% ipsilateral groin recurrence rate following negative full superficial inguinal dissection in a prospective GOG study of low-risk vulvar cancer.[99] Patients who underwent a sentinel but not a full node dissection had significantly lower groin wound breakdown (12% vs. 34%) compared to those who went on to a full inguinal dissection following the sentinel procedure. Optimal lesions for sentinel node procedures are those with small (<4 cm), unifocal lesions, and each center must have had experience with at least 10 prior sentinel procedures followed by full dissection for confirmation of proper technique.

Intraoperative diagnosis of inguinal node metastasis necessitates further diagnostic or therapeutic procedures. Because there is no established sentinel node metastasis size cutoff below which withholding further treatment of the groin can be considered safe, all women in whom a sentinel node is found to be positive should have a full ipsilateral groin dissection and/or radiotherapy to the groin.[101] In the case of non–sentinel node metastasis that is diagnosed intraoperatively, the options are to dissect the deep nodes as well as the opposite groin or to cover both groins with adjuvant radiotherapy. Standard adjuvant treatment for inguinal node metastasis consists of both inguinal and pelvic radiotherapy.[47]

Women with fixed or ulcerated inguinal nodes are rarely curable with surgery alone. These patients should have a biopsy to document the nodal involvement and should be treated with combined radiation and chemotherapy, followed by surgery for the primary and the nodes if the response to the therapy has been good and the nodes are resectable.[74,102]

Pelvic Lymph Nodes

Patients with clinically or pathologically positive groin nodes are at risk for having contralateral groin and pelvic nodal involvement. Thus, the status of the groin nodes is to be taken into consideration when determining the management of the pelvic nodes. The randomized GOG trial of pelvic node dissection versus pelvic node radiation showed that control of the disease in the pelvis could be achieved with either form of therapy.[47] Radiation to the pelvic nodes is preferred over surgery because women in need of treatment to the pelvis often also require radiation to the primary and/or inguinal nodes.

RADIATION THERAPY

The standard of care for early lesions is surgical resection; however, selected patients with small central lesions may be considered for definitive radiation, particularly when the lesions are in close proximity to the urethra, clitoris, or anus. There are few published series of radiation alone used as definitive therapy for vulvar cancer.[103–105] The reported series include patients with recurrent disease postsurgery and patients who are not medically suitable for surgery or have declined it. In Ellis's[103] series of 65 patients treated with brachytherapy and or external beam, the crude 5-year survival rate was 23% (15 of 65). Twelve of these patients were free of disease. The local control rate was 40%, and 9 patients developed necrosis. Slevin and Pointon[105] reported on the results of 58 patients treated also with brachytherapy and/or external beam, depending on the extent of the disease. The crude 5-year survival rate was 26% (15 of 58). In this series the local control rate was also 40% (23 of 58). The survival was better in the newly diagnosed group, 39% (9 of 23), compared to 17% (6 of 35) for the group of patients treated for recurrence. Nine patients developed necrosis. These series reflect the difficulty of achieving appropriate curative doses for gross disease with radiation alone without the aid of radiosensitizing chemotherapy.

Brachytherapy has been used for inoperable vulvar cancer and as a boost to the primary tumor and/or to the lymph nodes. The efficacy of this treatment is difficult to evaluate because of the variability of the clinical situation in which this type of treatment may be employed. A high rate of necrosis was reported in up to one-third of the patients.[103] A series from the Centre Alexis Vautrin Institute in France describes 34 patients, 21 with primary and 13 with recurrent disease, treated with brachytherapy only.[104] The median brachytherapy dose was 60 Gy, with a range of 53 to 88 Gy. In the group of 21 patients who underwent brachytherapy as primary treatment, 3 patients developed locoregional recurrence, for a 5-year local control rate of 80% and a disease-specific survival of 70%. In the group of 13 patients who were treated for recurrence, 8 developed local recurrence, with or without disease at other sites, for a local control rate of 19%. Of the entire group of 34, 5 patients developed necrosis. This relatively low complication rate most likely reflects that extensive experience and high quality of the brachytherapy carried out in this institution. The authors of this study advocate brachytherapy for primary vulvar cancer if the patient refuses surgery or if surgery is contraindicated. Nonetheless, due to the significant risk of necrosis, use of brachytherapy should be limited to very selected cases and performed by experienced practitioners.

In most instances radiation is used in combination with surgery and/or chemotherapy. The objective of radiation varies with the target: regions with lymphatic spread or the primary tumor in the perineum. For instance, in patients with advanced, unresectable nodes but less advanced primary tumor, complete control of the primary may be obtained with the combination of chemotherapy and radiation, obviating the need for surgery to the primary while making the nodes amenable to surgery.[74,106] Concurrent chemotherapy and radiation may also be used for definitive treatment. For patients with advanced primary tumors and limited nodal disease it is possible to render the primary resectable while sterilizing the lymph nodes. Radiation can also play a significant role for palliation of symptoms.

Treatment Volume and Technique

The radiation target volume usually encompasses the vulva, both groins and the lower pelvic nodes. Use of a midline block to spare the perineum and vagina should be avoided except for highly selected situations because this may increase the risk of local recurrence.[107] The following factors increase the risk of vulvoperineal recurrences: close or positive margins (<8 mm), primary tumor size >4 cm, lymphovascular space invasion, deep invasion (>9 mm), tumor thickness >1 cm, infiltrative growth pattern (or "spray" pattern), >25% keratin in the tumor, and high mitotic rate (>10 per 10 high-power fields).[51] All patients found to have more than one positive inguinal node should receive postoperative radiation to the inguinal and pelvic node areas because this improves overall survival.[47] The pelvis must be included in the field because patients with positive inguinal nodes have a 28% incidence of pelvic node involvement.

When planning the treatment, careful attention should be given to the location and depth at which the dose is calculated for the inguinal area. The depth of the inguinal vessels can be highly variable, ranging from 2.0 to 18.5 cm.[108] CT- or MR-based three-dimensional planning is essential to establish the location, extent, and depth of the inguinal nodes because underdosing of the nodes may easily occur, predisposing to local recurrence. Figure 74.6 demonstrates the distribution of inguinal nodes and can be used as a guideline for the design of an inguinofemoral treatment field.[109] At the time of simulation, markers should be placed on the primary, the lymph nodes, and scars from previous surgery to document the extent of the disease.

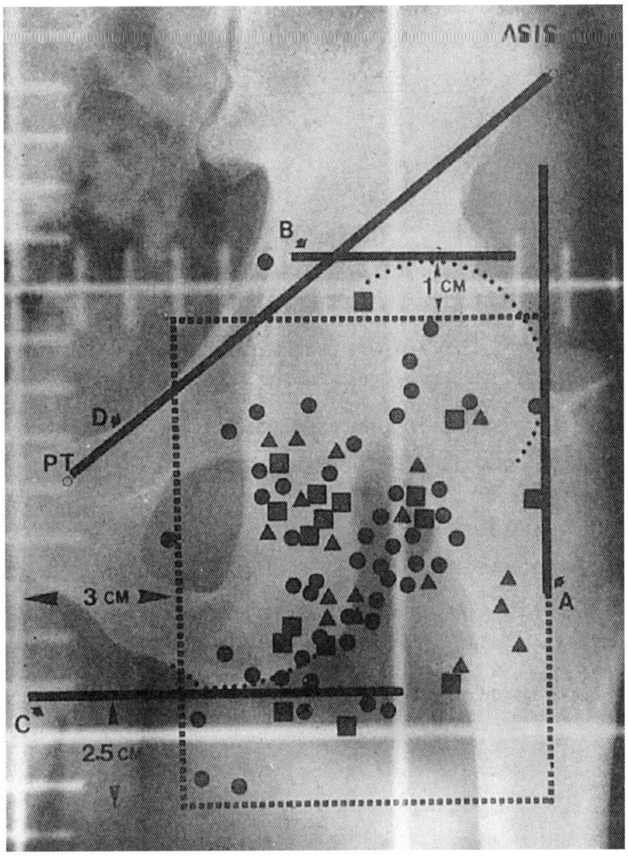

FIGURE 74.6. Topographic distribution of inguinal lymph node metastases in patients with carcinoma of the vulva–vagina–cervix (*triangles*), urethra (*squares*), or anus–low rectum (*circles*). (From Wang CJ, Chin YY, Leung SW, et al. Topographic distribution of inguinal lymph nodes metastasis: significance in determination of treatment margin for elective inguinal lymph nodes irradiation of low pelvic tumors. *Int J Radiat Oncol Biol Phys* 1996;35:133–136; copyright 1996, with permission from Elsevier.)

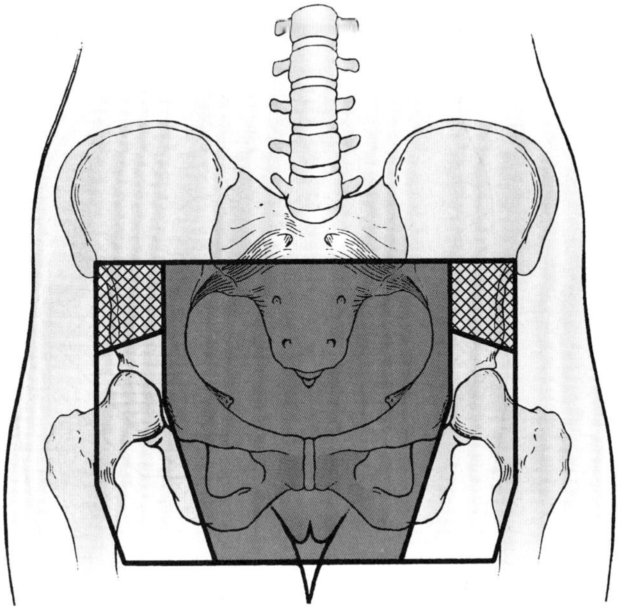

FIGURE 74.7. Treatment borders demonstrating the wide anterior field (*outer border*) and the narrow posterior field (*shaded region*).

Medium- or high-energy photon beams with anteroposterior/posteroanterior (AP/PA) fields with the patient in the supine position and with the thighs straight or in the "frog-leg" position are recommended for the delivery of external beam. The frog-leg position minimizes the bolus effect from skin folds. Documentation of the primary tumor with photos, tattoos, or fiducial markers prior to therapy may be used for objective evaluation of response to the treatment and for subsequent design of reduced fields or for brachytherapy boost. The superior border of the pelvic field should extend to the middle of the sacroiliac joints to cover the external and internal iliac nodes. If a patient has internal or external iliac node involvement, the superior border should be extended to the L3/4 interspace to cover the common iliac nodes. The inferior border should cover the entire vulva and the most superficial, inferior inguinal nodes. Laterally, the pelvic field extends 2 cm laterally to the widest point of the pelvic inlet. Although there are no data regarding scar recurrences, it is common practice to include the inguinal node dissection scars in the radiation field.

Depending on whether the inguinal/femoral lymph nodes and/or pelvic lymph nodes are to be included in the radiation volume, different field configurations may be used. To reduce the dose to the femoral heads while delivering an adequate dose to the inguinal nodes, various techniques are available. One approach is to use a wide AP field that includes the pelvic and inguinal areas, with a narrow posterior field covering only the pelvis and sparing the femoral heads. The photon fields are weighted equally, and the inguinal dose is supplemented by separate anterior electron fields matched to the pelvic field (Fig. 74.7). Bolus material should be used to ensure adequate dose to the superficial portions of the groin. An alternative method consists of using a wide AP field and narrow PA field, with a partial transmission block placed in the central portion of the AP field. The desired dose at a specified depth is delivered to the inguinal nodes through the AP field.[110] The degree of central anterior beam attenuation is calculated so that the midpoint of the pelvis receives equal doses from the AP and PA beams. This technique eliminates the dosimetric problems of photon/electron field matching, as well as the potential for daily setup variation, but the design of a precise partial transmission block is difficult. Another method consists in using matched AP/PA fields to include the primary and the pelvic nodes and treating the groins through separate anterior electron fields. This approach has the advantage of relatively easy setup, but the main drawback is ensuring an adequate dose at the match line, particularly when the match line is over gross disease. An example of an anteroposterior radiation field encompassing the inguinal/femoral and pelvic lymph nodes is shown in Figure 74.8.

Moran et al.[111] described a modified segmental boost technique using multileaf collimators with a single isocenter technique and a wide AP field to cover the vulva, pelvis, and groins and a narrow PA field to cover the vulva and pelvis. The supplemental anterior photon groin fields are angled such that the central axis is coplanar with the divergence from the PA field. The medial blocking of the groin fields is designed to match the divergence from the PA field. This technique provides a more homogeneous dose distribution and is easier to reproduce on a daily basis.

IMRT is now often used to treat the pelvis and inguinal nodes.[112,113] Beriwal et al.[112] reported 15 patients treated with IMRT using a median of seven fields. The clinical tumor volume (CTV) was defined as a 1- to 2-cm margin around bilateral external iliac, internal iliac, and inguinofemoral nodes, as well as a 1-cm margin around the entire vulvar region. Gross tumor was also expanded by 1 cm for the CTV. The planning treatment volume was defined as 1-cm margin beyond the CTV, and the prescription dose was 43 to 48 Gy for preoperative treatment and 50 Gy for postoperative treatment, delivered partly on a twice-daily schedule. This early experience yielded reasonable clinical response, with 13 of 15 patients having no evidence of disease at last follow-up. This technique also resulted in improved dose conformality and lower doses to normal structures, including rectum, bladder, small bowel, and femoral heads. A second publication by the same group expanded

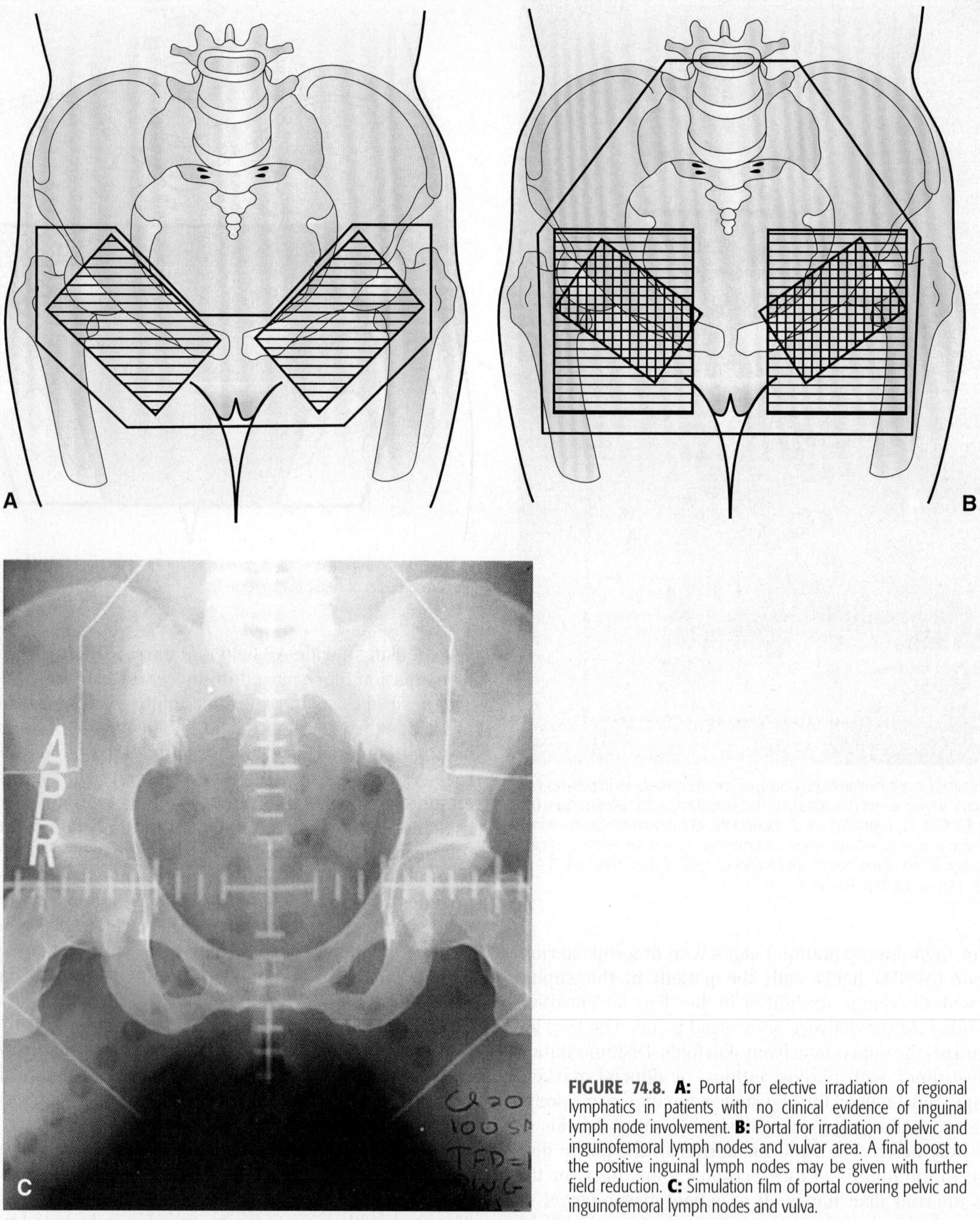

FIGURE 74.8. A: Portal for elective irradiation of regional lymphatics in patients with no clinical evidence of inguinal lymph node involvement. **B:** Portal for irradiation of pelvic and inguinofemoral lymph nodes and vulvar area. A final boost to the positive inguinal lymph nodes may be given with further field reduction. **C:** Simulation film of portal covering pelvic and inguinofemoral lymph nodes and vulva.

on the preoperative experience with 18 patients treated with concurrent cisplatin and 5-fluorouracil (5-FU), resulting in a pathologic complete response (pCR) rate of 64% and a 2-year cause-specific survival of 75%.[113] However, it must be noted that careful quality assurance is required when using IMRT. Placement of thermoluminescent dosimetry chips in the inguinal and perineum areas is recommended to document the dose given to the skin and target areas (Fig. 74.9).

Preoperative Radiation Therapy with Concurrent Chemotherapy

As the treatment for vulvar cancer has evolved with the goal of decreasing the sequelae of radical surgery and to maximize functional outcome, multimodality therapies have become the standard of care, particularly for patients with advanced stages of the disease.[74] After initial concurrent chemoradiation and healing of the reaction, the response to the therapy at the primary site and the lymph nodes is assessed. If there is complete clinical regression of the disease at the site of the primary, one option is to perform biopsies of the primary site, foregoing resection if there is a pathologic complete response.[106] In general, it is recommended to carry out the inguinal node dissection whether or not there has been complete response of the lymph nodes because residual disease is often found in the lymph nodes.[74] It also should be noted that whereas recurrences at the primary site following surgery or chemoradiation are potentially salvageable, nodal recurrences are not.

The preoperative radiation dose for the primary and the lymph nodes areas should be 45 to 55 Gy.[67,114] The most common chemotherapeutic agents used have been 5-FU, cisplatin, and mitomycin-C. Acute mucocutaneous toxicity from combined therapy is rather severe, and a preferably short treatment break during the course of the treatment is often required.[73,74,106,115] In a GOG trial for patients with advanced primary and/or nodal disease, the radiation treatment consisted

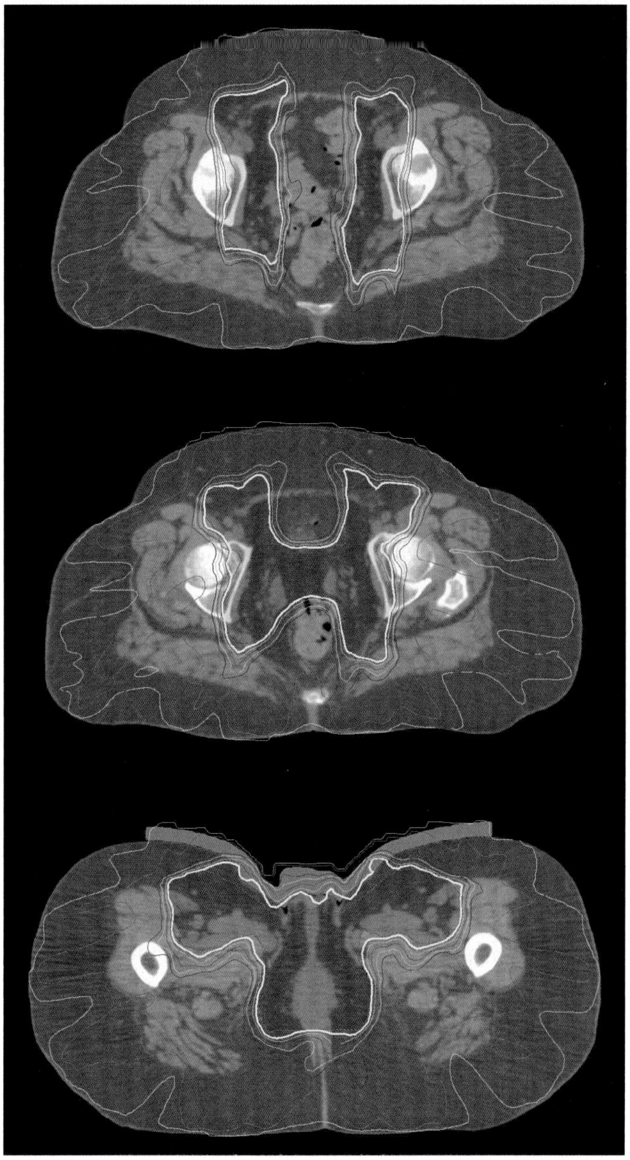

FIGURE 74.9. Intensity-modulated radiation therapy for vulvar cancer. This patient had a lesion of the posterior labia minora, involving the fourchette and the distal vagina. Three axial views are shown of the conformality of the 100% isodose line (*yellow*) and the planning treatment volume contour (*shaded red volume*). The central dose in the middle axial level is the superior margin for the vagina, added in this case due to the distal vaginal involvement.

of 170 cGy twice daily on days 1 to 4 and 170 cGy once a day on day 5 and days 8 to 12, for a dose of 2,380 cGy.[74,106] Cisplatin, 50 mg/m^2, was given on day 1, and 5-FU, 1,000 mg/m^2 by a 24-h infusion, daily on days 1 to 4. The combined cycle of chemotherapy and radiation was repeated after about a 2-week break, thus delivering a total radiation dose of 4,760 cGy. In the locally advanced cohort, the pCR rate was 34%, R0 resections were possible in 77% of the patients, and 55% were alive and without disease at last follow-up. In the group of patients with advanced nodal disease, the nodes became resectable in 83%, with a pCR rate of 40% in those who underwent surgery, with 43% of the patients being alive and disease free at last follow-up.[74]

A follow-up GOG study was recently presented by Moore et al.[102] in which T3 or T4 tumors were treated with a total dose of 5,760 cGy (180 cGy/fraction) and weekly cisplatin (40 mg/m^2). In an interim report, 40 of 58 (69%) patients were able to complete the protocol per plan, 37 of 58 (64%) achieved a complete response, and 29 of 58 (50%) had a pCR on surgical biopsy. Due to these encouraging initial results, the GOG is moving forward with radiation combined with weekly cisplatin as a potential backbone for continuing study.

Definitive Chemoradiation Therapy

Definitive chemoradiation is used for patients with advanced tumors considered unresectable at presentation or for patients who are medically inoperable (Table 74.3). This may be used when the tumor does not become resectable in the midst of preoperative intent chemoradiation or as an upfront alternative to surgically based treatment. In these patients, chemotherapy should be continued throughout the entire course of radiation for the purpose of radiosensitization of the tumor in the treatment volume and possible eradication of subclinical disease outside of the radiation field. With appropriate field reductions, the radiation dose should be brought up to 60 to 70 Gy. The total dose to certain areas is dependent upon the location and extent or bulk of the disease, the response to the therapy, and the estimated tolerance of the area requiring the high radiation dose. Often, it is the tolerance of normal tissue that limits the dose to ≤65 Gy.

Selected patients without clinically involved nodes and at very low risk of having nodal involvement may be treated to the vulvar area alone. The treatment may be delivered using electrons or low-energy photons. When the treatment is given with electrons only, a generous margin around the primary tumor should be used because the dose decreases toward the periphery of the field. Bolus material should be used also to avoid underdosing the surface of the tumor.

TABLE 74.3 STUDIES OF CONCURRENT RADIATION AND COMBINATION CHEMOTHERAPY AS PRIMARY TREATMENT FOR ADVANCED VULVAR CANCER

Authors	Number of Patients	Chemotherapy	Radiation Therapy Dose (Gy)	Number of Posttreatment Surgeries	Median and Range of Follow-up (Month)	Clinical Complete Response (%)	Clinical Outcome (%)
Moore et al.[102]	58	P	57.6	34	NS	64	NS
Mak et al.[116]	16	P	50	4	32	60	62 (2 yr DFS)
Mak et al.[116]	28	F + P/M	55	6	32	58	56 (2 yr DFS)
Tans et al.[139]	28[a]	F + M	60	NS	42	72[a]	71[a] (4 yr PFS)
Beriwal et al.[113]	18	F + P	44.6–46.4	14	22 (2–60)	72	75 (2 yr DSS)
Gerszten et al.[140]	18	F + P	44.6	14	27	72	83 (crude NED)
Montana et al.[74]	46	F + P	47.6	38	78 (56–89)	NS	54 (crude NED)
Moore et al.[106]	71	F + P	47.6	64	45	48	63 (crude NED)
Landoni et al.[141]	58[a]	F + M	54	42	(4–48)	27[a]	49[a] (crude NED)
Lupi et al.[73]	24	F + M	54	22	34 (22–73)	42	55 (5 yr OS)
Wahlen et al.[77]	19	F ± M	45–50	6	(3–67)	53	89 (5yr DSS)
Sebag-Montefiore et al.[115]	37	F + M	45	14	NS	47	37 (2 yr OS)
Koh et al.[72]	17	F ± P/M	54	10	(1–75)	53	49 (5 yr DSS)
Russell et al.[75]	18	F + P	46.8–72	1	24 (2–52)	89	75 (crude NED)

DFS, disease-free survival; DSS, disease-specific survival; F, 5-Fluorouracil; M, mitomycin-C; NS, not stated; NED, no evidence of disease; OS, overall survival; P, cisplatin; PFS, progression-free survival.

[a]Includes patients treated for recurrent disease.

There is little in the way of comparative prospective trials for chemotherapy selection with concurrent treatment; however, a recent retrospective series from Dana-Farber/Brigham and Women's Cancer Center and Massachusetts General Hospital does shed some light.[116] In this series of 44 women, 24 of whom were treated definitively without surgery, 16 received weekly platinum-based regimens and 28 received a 5-FU–based regimen every 3 to 4 weeks. The 2-year overall survival (74% platinum, 70% 5-FU), disease-free survival (62% platinum, 56% 5-FU), and locoregional recurrence (31% platinum, 33% 5-FU) were no different. The grade 3 or higher skin toxicity was higher with weekly platinum (62% platinum, 32% 5-FU), but the nonskin toxicity was higher with 5-FU (13% platinum, 46% 5-FU). Given these data and a recent GOG report of weekly platinum in preoperative treatment, weekly platinum at 40 mg/m^2 is a reasonable option for concurrent treatment.[102]

Postoperative Radiation Therapy

Adjuvant postoperative radiation can be used when limited surgery has been performed for organ conservation or when the surgical specimen reveals adverse pathologic features and local recurrence is likely to occur.[117] Local recurrence is a major cause of failure in all patients irrespective of the stage.[118] Patients with positive or close (<8 mm) margins, LVI, and depth of tumor invasion >5 mm should undergo postoperative radiation because these are factors increase the likelihood of local recurrence.[51] Patients with close margins may be considered for re-resection prior to radiation, particularly if the area in question is not in close proximity to the urethra, clitoris, or anus. Patients with more than one involved inguinal node, extracapsular extension, or gross residual nodal disease should receive adjuvant radiation to both groins and the pelvis. When the surgical margins are clear and there is no pathologic indication to treat the vulva, a midline block can be used to avoid the reaction and the sequelae of the treatment to the vulvar area, although this practice raises the probability of local recurrence.[107]

Adjuvant radiation to the primary site may be delivered with either photons or en face electrons with bolus. When treating a large area of the vulva and groins, AP/PA photon fields as described before are appropriate. If the area of involvement is small, a direct electron field can be used, and the groins are treated with separate fields. When it is indicated to treat the primary tumor bed area for possible residual microscopic disease, a dose of 50 Gy is recommended. If there is extracapsular extension of tumor in the lymph nodes, the dose to the groins should be carried to 50 to 60 Gy. If there is gross residual disease postsurgery, the dose to the area should be brought to 65 to 70 Gy.

CHEMOTHERAPY

The use of chemotherapy alone is usually reserved for patients having advanced, inoperable, or recurrent disease.

Single-Agent Chemotherapy

There is limited experience with single-agent chemotherapy for the treatment of vulvar cancer (Table 74.4). The single agents cisplatin, piperazinedione, mitoxantrone, and etoposide have all been evaluated prospectively by the GOG with disappointing results.[119–121] Paclitaxel has moderate activity, with a 14% response rate described in a phase II trial of the European Organization for Radiation Therapy and Chemotherapy (EORTC).[122] Bleomycin has been tested in older studies as a single agent in both the neoadjuvant and recurrent settings with a high initial response rate.[123,124] Limited objective responses have also been reported in a small number of patients with doxorubicin.[125]

Multiagent Regimens

Several combination chemotherapy regimens have included bleomycin, which is also associated with considerable pulmonary toxicity.[126] The Gynecological Cancer Cooperative Group of the EORTC conducted two phase II studies using a regimen of bleomycin, 5 mg intramuscularly, given on days 1 to 5, methotrexate 15 mg orally on days 1 and 4, and lomustine, 40 mg orally on days 5 to 7 in the first week, followed by bleomycin 5 mg intramuscularly and methotrexate 15 mg orally on days 1 and 4 (modified to day 1 only in the second study) for 5 additional weeks.[127,128] The overall response rate was between 55% and 65%, with a complete response rate of 8% to 11%. Unfortunately the toxicity was high. Severe mucositis was noted in up to 21% of patients, 13% had severe infections, and up to 7% developed severe pulmonary toxicity, with one death in each of the two studies possibly due to pulmonary toxicity. Other severe toxicities included nausea/vomiting and hematologic, renal, and mucocutaneous reactions. A second group prospectively evaluated cisplatin, bleomycin, and methotrexate in the neoadjuvant setting and reported a 10% response rate of the primary tumor but a 67% response rate of nodal disease after two cycles of treatment.[129]

TABLE 74.4 CHEMOTHERAPY FOR VULVAR CANCER

Authors	Number of Patients	Regimen	Partial Response (Number of Patients)	Complete Response (Number of Patients)
Geisler et al.[131]	9	FP	5	4
Geisler et al.[131]	3	P	0	0
Wagenaar et al.[128]	25	BMC	12	2
Durrant et al.[127]	31	BMC	15	3
Benedetti-Panici et al.[129]	21	PBM	Tumor, 2 Node, 3	Tumor, 0 Node, 11
Belinson et al.[142]	3	BOMP	0	0

BMC, bleomycin, methotrexate, CCNU; BOMP, bleomycin, vincristine, mitomycin-C, cisplatin; FP, 5-fluorouracil, cisplatin; P, cisplatin; PBM, cisplatin, bleomycin, methotrexate.

In other small series, combinations of cisplatin with a second agent such as vinorelbine or 5-fluorouracil showed significant activity.[130,131] In a recent small report of neoadjuvant chemotherapy with cisplatin and 5-fluorouracil, at least a partial response was observed in all 10 patients. Of interest, 3 patients were treated with cisplatin alone in the same series with no responses.[131]

Biologic Agents

Epidermal growth factor receptor (EGFR) is a tyrosine kinase that is overexpressed in many squamous cell carcinomas of the vulva.[132] Erlotinib, an EGFR inhibitor, was reported to have significant activity in a case report,[133] which resulted in development of a phase II trial of this agent for women with measurable disease in the neoadjuvant or recurrent setting. Of 19 patients on this study, 5 (26%) partial responses were reported, whereas an additional 7 (37%) had stable disease. The most common toxicities were diarrhea, fatigue, and skin changes.[134] In one other case report, the EGFR inhibitor cetuximab elicited a partial response when administered in combination with cisplatin.[135] Further studies may elucidate the role of EGRF-targeted agents and other biologics in the treatment of this disease.

In conclusion, paclitaxel and erlotinib are single agents showing activity against advanced vulvar cancer in phase II studies. Combination chemotherapy regimens, particularly those including cisplatin and 5-fluorouracil, yield improved response rates, but they are associated with significant toxicity. Bleomycin as single agent and in combination also appears to have activity but with risk of significant pulmonary toxicity. In the recurrent or metastatic setting, the choice of regimen requires consideration of single agents having modest activity but low toxicity versus combination regimens that carry both higher response rates and higher toxicity.

TREATMENT SEQUELAE

The adverse effects of treatment can be classified as acute or chronic and depend on the treatment modality or modalities used, as well as the intensity of the treatment. With early-stage disease and appropriately limited surgery to the primary site, the acute surgical complications are relatively minor and essentially consist of wound infection and hematomas. With more extensive surgery the frequency and degree of the complications can be far more significant. With single "longhorn" or "butterfly" incisions for bilateral inguinal lymphadenectomies and for resection of the primary, wound infection, necrosis, and breakdown occurred in as many as 50% to 85% of the cases. Since the use of separate incisions was adopted, the incidence of groin wound infection, necrosis, and breakdown has decreased dramatically to a low as 15%.[35,62] Other potential complications or surgery include wound infections, seromas, hemorrhage, deep vein thrombosis, pulmonary embolism, osteitis pubis, and loss of sensory perception in the anterior aspect of the thigh secondary to femoral nerve injury.

The most significant chronic surgical complication is edema of the lower extremities. Lymphedema is related to the extent of the lymphadenectomy, and it is therefore more likely to occur with a deep inguinal node dissection. The incidence of lymphedema may be as high as 69%.[62,136] Lymphedema can be progressive and very difficult to manage. Early referral for physical therapy is indicated to prevent progression and stimulate regression of symptoms. Other chronic complications reported are chronic cellulitis of the inguinal areas, stenosis of the introitus, femoral hernias, and rectovaginal or rectoperineal fistulas.

The most significant acute morbidity of radiation, alone or radiation in combination with chemotherapy, is the mucocutaneous reaction in the vulva, perineum, and inguinal folds that may develop early during the course of the treatment. The severity of the reaction depends upon the radiation fractionation schema used and the type of chemotherapy employed. Often the degree of reaction is such that a treatment interruption may be unavoidable. Topical agents, such as zinc oxide preparations, may be helpful; however, this preparation must be off the skin during radiation treatments because it can exacerbate the skin reaction. Sitz baths with sodium bicarbonate may also aid in the cleansing and soothing of the affected skin. Treatment of candidal infections with appropriate antifungal agents should be provided as required. Narcotic pain medications may also be required in the final weeks of treatment.

Acute hematologic toxicity is common and depends upon the type and intensity of the chemotherapy used. Decreased leukocytes may be managed well with colony-stimulating factors, and blood transfusions may be necessary for anemia. Chemotherapy dose adjustments or interruptions are sometimes required. Severe hematologic toxicity can lead to septicemia, with fatal consequences in some instances.[74,75]

The late complications of chemotherapy/radiation and surgery combined include telangiectasis and atrophy of the skin and mucosa of the vulva, dryness of the mucosa of the vagina and vulva, and narrowing of the vaginal introitus. Avascular necrosis of the femoral head is rare, even when AP/PA photon fields that include the inguinal nodes are used. In the GOG combined-modality study for patients with advanced disease, only one patient developed avascular necrosis of the femoral head.[74] In this study there were two instances of injury to the femoral artery. In one patient, necrosis of the femoral artery occurred immediately following surgery and was fatal. The second patient required femoral artery angioplasty.

Besides the generally recognized complications seen with surgery, radiation, and/or chemotherapy, the treatment of carcinoma of the vulva has significant psychosexual consequences. In some instances, these consequences can be far greater than expected when considering the type and extent of the therapy given. The psychosexual impact of the treatment has been studied by some investigators, but it has not received the attention that it merits, possibly because of the difficulty in its nature and impact.[82] In a study by Andersen et al.[137] of 42 patients, most of whom were treated with conservative surgery, with wide local excision in 32 patients and simple vulvectomy in 10, there was a twofold to threefold increase in the frequency of sexual dysfunction from the pretreatment level. In this study, 30% of the patients were sexually inactive at follow-up. Andersen and Hacker[82] also reported that vulvar surgery has a significant impact on sexual functioning and body image even when intercourse remains possible. As might be expected, after pelvic exenteration patients also experience significant sexual dysfunction, even when a neovagina is created.[138] The concern for the significant impact of radical surgery on patients with carcinoma of the vulva has been the principal reason for the development of multimodality therapy. Organ preservation, maintenance of function, and improved body image with reasonable control of the disease are achieved in women with this disease, particularly when the disease is early stage.

SELECTED REFERENCES

A full list of references for this chapter is available online.

3. Insinga RP, Liaw KL, Johnson LG, et al. A systematic review of the prevalence and attribution of human papillomavirus types among cervical, vaginal, and vulvar precancers and cancers in the United States. *Cancer Epidemiol Biomarkers Prev* 2008;17:1611–1622.
4. Smith JS, Backes DM, Hoots BE, et al. Human papillomavirus type-distribution in vulvar and vaginal cancers and their associated precursors. *Obstet Gynecol* 2009;113:917–924.
5. Hampl M, Sarajuuri H, Wentzensen N, et al. Effect of human papillomavirus vaccines on vulvar, vaginal, and anal intraepithelial lesions and vulvar cancer. *Obstet Gynecol* 2006;108:1361–1368.
8. Zaino RJ, Husseinzadeh N, Nahhas W, et al. Epithelial alterations in proximity to invasive squamous carcinoma of the vulva. *Int J Gynecol Pathol* 1982;1:173–184.
9. Leibowitch M, Neill S, Pelisse M, et al. The epithelial changes associated with squamous cell carcinoma of the vulva: a review of the clinical, histological and viral findings in 78 women. *Br J Obstet Gynaecol* 1990;97:1135–1139.
11. Powell JJ, Wojnarowska F. Lichen sclerosus. *Lancet* 1999;353:1777–1783.
12. Buscema J, Stern J, Woodruff JD. The significance of the histologic alterations adjacent to invasive vulvar carcinoma. *Am J Obstet Gynecol* 1980;137:902–909.
13. Hording U, Junge J, Poulsen H, et al. Vulvar intraepithelial neoplasia III: a viral disease of undetermined progressive potential. *Gynecol Oncol* 1995;56:276–279.
14. Jones RW, Rowan DM. Vulvar intraepithelial neoplasia III: a clinical study of the outcome in 113 cases with relation to the later development of invasive vulvar carcinoma. *Obstet Gynecol* 1994;84:741–745.
15. Trimble CL, Hildesheim A, Brinton LA, et al. Heterogeneous etiology of squamous carcinoma of the vulva. *Obstet Gynecol* 1996;87:59–64.
17. Santos M, Landolfi S, Olivella A, et al. p16 overexpression identifies HPV-positive vulvar squamous cell carcinomas. *Am J Surg Pathol* 2006;30:1347–1356.
18. Hunter DJ. Carcinoma of the vulva: a review of 361 patients. *Gynecol Oncol* 1975; 3:117–123.
19. Carlson JA, Ambros R, Malfetano J, et al. Vulvar lichen sclerosus and squamous cell carcinoma: a cohort, case control, and investigational study with historical perspective; implications for chronic inflammation and sclerosis in the development of neoplasia. *Hum Pathol* 1998;29:932–948.
20. Creasman WT. New gynecologic cancer staging. *Gynecol Oncol* 1995;58: 157–158.
21. Wilkinson EJ, Rico MJ, Pierson KK. Microinvasive carcinoma of the vulva. *Int J Gynecol Pathol* 1982;1:29–39.
24. Johnson TL, Kumar NB, White CD, et al. Prognostic features of vulvar melanoma: a clinicopathologic analysis. *Int J Gynecol Pathol* 1986;5:110–118.
25. Fanning J, Lambert HC, Hale TM, et al. Paget's disease of the vulva: prevalence of associated vulvar adenocarcinoma, invasive Paget's disease, and recurrence after surgical excision. *Am J Obstet Gynecol* 1999;180:24–27.
27. MacLean AB, Makwana M, Ellis PE, et al. The management of Paget's disease of the vulva. *J Obstet Gynaecol* 2004;24:124–128.
30. Plentl AA, Friedman EA. *Lymphatic system of the female genitalia: the morphologic basis of oncologic diagnosis and therapy.* Philadelphia: WB Saunders, 1971.
31. Franklin EW 3rd, Rutledge FD. Prognostic factors in epidermoid carcinoma of the vulva. *Obstet Gynecol* 1971;37:892–901.
32. Krupp PJ, Bohm JW. Lymph gland metastases in invasive squamous cell cancer of the vulva. *Am J Obstet Gynecol* 1978;130:943–952.
34. Donaldson ES, Powell DE, Hanson MB, et al. Prognostic parameters in invasive vulvar cancer. *Gynecol Oncol* 1981;11:184–190.
38. Franklin EW 3rd. Clinical staging of carcinoma of the vulva. *Obstet Gynecol* 1972;40:277–286.
39. Homesley HD, Bundy BN, Sedlis A, et al. Prognostic factors for groin node metastasis in squamous cell carcinoma of the vulva (a Gynecologic Oncology Group study). *Gynecol Oncol* 1993;49:279–283.
40. Berman ML, Soper JT, Creasman WT, et al. Conservative surgical management of superficially invasive stage I vulvar carcinoma. *Gynecol Oncol* 1989;35:352–357.
41. Sedlis A, Homesley H, Bundy BN, et al. Positive groin lymph nodes in superficial squamous cell vulvar cancer. A Gynecologic Oncology Group Study. *Am J Obstet Gynecol* 1987;156:1159–1164.
42. Rutledge FN, Mitchell MF, Munsell MF, et al. Prognostic indicators for invasive carcinoma of the vulva. *Gynecol Oncol* 1991;42:239–244.

43. Rowley KC, Gallion HH, Donaldson ES, et al. Prognostic factors in early vulvar cancer. *Gynecol Oncol* 1988;31:43–49.
44. Homesley HD, Bundy BN, Sedlis A, et al. Assessment of current International Federation of Gynecology and Obstetrics staging of vulvar carcinoma relative to prognostic factors for survival (a Gynecologic Oncology Group study). *Am J Obstet Gynecol* 1991;164:997–1003; discussion 1003–1004.
45. Curry SL, Wharton JT, Rutledge F. Positive lymph nodes in vulvar squamous carcinoma. *Gynecol Oncol* 1980;9:63–67.
46. Hacker NF, Berek JS, Lagasse LD, et al. Management of regional lymph nodes and their prognostic influence in vulvar cancer. *Obstet Gynecol* 1983;61:408–412.
47. Homesley HD, Bundy BN, Sedlis A, et al. Radiation therapy versus pelvic node resection for carcinoma of the vulva with positive groin nodes. *Obstet Gynecol* 1986;68:733–740.
49. Figge DC, Tamimi HK, Greer BE. Lymphatic spread in carcinoma of the vulva. *Am J Obstet Gynecol* 1985;152:387–394.
50. Kurzl R, Messerer D. Prognostic factors in squamous cell carcinoma of the vulva: a multivariate analysis. *Gynecol Oncol* 1989;32:143–150.
51. Heaps JM, Fu YS, Montz FJ, et al. Surgical-pathologic variables predictive of local recurrence in squamous cell carcinoma of the vulva. *Gynecol Oncol* 1990; 38:309–314.
52. Origoni M, Sideri M, Garsia S, et al. Prognostic value of pathological patterns of lymph node positivity in squamous cell carcinoma of the vulva stage III and IVA FIGO. *Gynecol Oncol* 1992;45:313–316.
53. van der Velden J, van Lindert AC, Lammes FB, et al. Extracapsular growth of lymph node metastases in squamous cell carcinoma of the vulva. The impact on recurrence and survival. *Cancer* 1995;75:2885–2890.
56. Land R, Herod J, Moskovic E, et al. Routine computerized tomography scanning, groin ultrasound with or without fine needle aspiration cytology in the surgical management of primary squamous cell carcinoma of the vulva. *Int J Gynecol Cancer* 2006;16:312–317.
57. Cohn DE, Dehdashti F, Gibb RK, et al. Prospective evaluation of positron emission tomography for the detection of groin node metastases from vulvar cancer. *Gynecol Oncol* 2002;85:179–184.
62. Podratz KC, Symmonds RE, Taylor WF, et al. Carcinoma of the vulva: analysis of treatment and survival. *Obstet Gynecol* 1983;61:63–74.
63. Hacker NF, Van der Velden J. Conservative management of early vulvar cancer. *Cancer* 1993;71:1673–1677.
64. Faul CM, Mirmow D, Huang Q, et al. Adjuvant radiation for vulvar carcinoma: improved local control. *Int J Radiat Oncol Biol Phys* 1997;38:381–389.
65. Parthasarathy A, Cheung MK, Osann K, et al. The benefit of adjuvant radiation therapy in single-node-positive squamous cell vulvar carcinoma. *Gynecol Oncol* 2006;103:1095–1099.
66. Boronow RC. Combined therapy as an alternative to exenteration for locally advanced vulvo-vaginal cancer: rationale and results. *Cancer* 1982;49:1085–1091.
67. Hacker NF, Berek JS, Juillard GJ, et al. Preoperative radiation therapy for locally advanced vulvar cancer. *Cancer* 1984;54:2056–2061.
68. Levin W, Goldberg G, Altaras M, et al. The use of concomitant chemotherapy and radiotherapy prior to surgery in advanced stage carcinoma of the vulva. *Gynecol Oncol* 1986;25:20–25.
69. Berek JS, Heaps JM, Fu YS, et al. Concurrent cisplatin and 5-fluorouracil chemotherapy and radiation therapy for advanced-stage squamous carcinoma of the vulva. *Gynecol Oncol* 1991;42:197–201.
70. Cunningham MJ, Goyer RP, Gibbons SK, et al. Primary radiation, cisplatin, and 5-fluorouracil for advanced squamous carcinoma of the vulva. *Gynecol Oncol* 1997;66:258–261.
71. Eifel PJ, Morris M, Burke TW, et al. Prolonged continuous infusion cisplatin and 5-fluorouracil with radiation for locally advanced carcinoma of the vulva. *Gynecol Oncol* 1995;59:51–56.
72. Koh WJ, Wallace HJ 3rd, Greer BE, et al. Combined radiotherapy and chemotherapy in the management of local-regionally advanced vulvar cancer. *Int J Radiat Oncol Biol Phys* 1993;26:809–816.
73. Lupi G, Raspagliesi F, Zucali R, et al. Combined preoperative chemoradiotherapy followed by radical surgery in locally advanced vulvar carcinoma. A pilot study. *Cancer* 1996;77:1472–1478.
74. Montana GS, Thomas GM, Moore DH, et al. Preoperative chemo-radiation for carcinoma of the vulva with N2/N3 nodes: a gynecologic oncology group study. *Int J Radiat Oncol Biol Phys* 2000;48:1007–1013.
75. Russell AH, Mesic JB, Scudder SA, et al. Synchronous radiation and cytotoxic chemotherapy for locally advanced or recurrent squamous cancer of the vulva. *Gynecol Oncol* 1992;47:14–20.
76. Thomas G, Dembo A, DePetrillo A, et al. Concurrent radiation and chemotherapy in vulvar carcinoma. *Gynecol Oncol* 1989;34:263–267.
77. Wahlen SA, Slater JD, Wagner RJ, et al. Concurrent radiation therapy and chemotherapy in the treatment of primary squamous cell carcinoma of the vulva. *Cancer* 1995;75:2289–2294.
79. Hopkins MP, Morley GW. Pelvic exenteration for the treatment of vulvar cancer. *Cancer* 1992;70:2835–2838.
80. Miller B, Morris M, Levenback C, et al. Pelvic exenteration for primary and recurrent vulvar cancer. *Gynecol Oncol* 1995;58:202–205.
82. Andersen BL, Hacker NF. Psychosexual adjustment after vulvar surgery. *Obstet Gynecol* 1983;62:457–462.
84. Raber G, Mempel V, Jackisch C, et al. Malignant melanoma of the vulva. Report of 89 patients. *Cancer* 1996;78:2353–2358.
87. Copeland LJ, Sneige N, Gershenson DM, et al. Bartholin gland carcinoma. *Obstet Gynecol* 1986;67:794–801.
88. Leuchter RS, Hacker NF, Voet RL, et al. Primary carcinoma of the Bartholin gland: a report of 14 cases and review of the literature. *Obstet Gynecol* 1982;60:361–368.
89. Cardosi RJ, Speights A, Fiorica JV, et al. Bartholin's gland carcinoma: a 15-year experience. *Gynecol Oncol* 2001;82:247–251.
90. Japaze H, Van Dinh T, Woodruff JD. Verrucous carcinoma of the vulva: study of 24 cases. *Obstet Gynecol* 1982;60:462–466.
93. Iversen T, Abeler V, Aalders J. Individualized treatment of stage I carcinoma of the vulva. *Obstet Gynecol* 1981;57:85–89.
95. Figge DC, Gaudenz R. Invasive carcinoma of the vulva. *Am J Obstet Gynecol* 1974; 119:382–395.
96. DeSimone CP, Van Ness JS, Cooper AL, et al. The treatment of lateral T1 and T2 squamous cell carcinomas of the vulva confined to the labium majus or minus. *Gynecol Oncol* 2007;104:390–395.
97. Gonzalez Bosquet J, Magrina JF, Magtibay PM, et al. Patterns of inguinal groin metastases in squamous cell carcinoma of the vulva. *Gynecol Oncol* 2007;105: 742–746.
98. DiSaia PJ, Creasman WT, Rich WM. An alternate approach to early cancer of the vulva. *Am J Obstet Gynecol* 1979;133:825–832.
99. Stehman FB, Bundy BN, Dvoretsky PM, et al. Early stage I carcinoma of the vulva treated with ipsilateral superficial inguinal lymphadenectomy and modified radical hemivulvectomy: a prospective study of the Gynecologic Oncology Group. *Obstet Gynecol* 1992;79:490–497.
100. Van der Zee AG, Oonk MH, De Hullu JA, et al. Sentinel node dissection is safe in the treatment of early-stage vulvar cancer. *J Clin Oncol* 2008;26:884–889.
101. Oonk MH, van Hemel BM, Hollema H, et al. Size of sentinel-node metastasis and chances of non-sentinel-node involvement and survival in early stage vulvar cancer: results from GROINSS-V, a multicentre observational study. *Lancet Oncol*;11:646–652.
102. Moore DH, Ali S, Koh WJ, et al. A phase II trial of radiotherapy and weekly cisplatin chemotherapy for the treatment of locally advanced squamous cell carcinoma of the vulva: a Gynecologic Oncology Group study. *Gynecol Oncol* 2011;120: S2–S133 (131).
103. Ellis F. Cancer of the vulva treated by radiation; an analysis of 127 cases. *Br J Radiol* 1949;22:513–520.
104. Pohar S, Hoffstetter S, Peiffert D, et al. Effectiveness of brachytherapy in treating carcinoma of the vulva. *Int J Radiat Oncol Biol Phys* 1995;32:1455–1460.
105. Slevin NJ, Pointon RC. Radical radiotherapy for carcinoma of the vulva. *Br J Radiol* 1989;62:145–147.
106. Moore DH, Thomas GM, Montana GS, et al. Preoperative chemoradiation for advanced vulvar cancer: a phase II study of the Gynecologic Oncology Group. *Int J Radiat Oncol Biol Phys* 1998;42:79–85.
107. Dusenbery KE, Carlson JW, LaPorte RM, et al. Radical vulvectomy with postoperative irradiation for vulvar cancer: therapeutic implications of a central block. *Int J Radiat Oncol Biol Phys* 1994;29:989–998.
108. Koh WJ, Chiu M, Stelzer KJ, et al. Femoral vessel depth and the implications for groin node radiation. *Int J Radiat Oncol Biol Phys* 1993;27:969–974.
109. Wang CJ, Chin YY, Leung SW, et al. Topographic distribution of inguinal lymph nodes metastasis: significance in determination of treatment margin for elective inguinal lymph nodes irradiation of low pelvic tumors. *Int J Radiat Oncol Biol Phys* 1996;35:133–136.
111. Moran M, Lund MW, Ahmad M, et al. Improved treatment of pelvis and inguinal nodes using modified segmental boost technique: dosimetric evaluation. *Int J Radiat Oncol Biol Phys* 2004;59:1523–1530.
112. Beriwal S, Heron DE, Kim H, et al. Intensity-modulated radiotherapy for the treatment of vulvar carcinoma: a comparative dosimetric study with early clinical outcome. *Int J Radiat Oncol Biol Phys* 2006;64:1395–1400.
113. Beriwal S, Coon D, Heron DE, et al. Preoperative intensity-modulated radiotherapy and chemotherapy for locally advanced vulvar carcinoma. *Gynecol Oncol* 2008; 109:291–295.
115. Sebag-Montefiore DJ, McLean C, Arnott SJ, et al. Treatment of advanced carcinoma of the vulva with chemoradiotherapy—can exenterative surgery be avoided? *Int J Gynecol Cancer* 1994;4:150–155.
116. Mak RH, Halasz LM, Tanaka CK, et al. Outcomes after radiation therapy with concurrent weekly platinum-based chemotherapy or every-3–4-week 5-fluorouracil-containing regimens for squamous cell carcinoma of the vulva. *Gynecol Oncol* 2011;120:101–107.
118. Perez CA, Grigsby PW, Chao C, et al. Irradiation in carcinoma of the vulva: factors affecting outcome. *Int J Radiat Oncol Biol Phys* 1998;42:335–344.
127. Durrant KR, Mangioni C, Lacave AJ, et al. Bleomycin, methotrexate, and CCNU in advanced inoperable squamous cell carcinoma of the vulva: a phase II study of the EORTC Gynaecological Cancer Cooperative Group (GCCG). *Gynecol Oncol* 1990;37:359–362.
128. Wagenaar HC, Colombo N, Vergote I, et al. Bleomycin, methotrexate, and CCNU in locally advanced or recurrent, inoperable, squamous-cell carcinoma of the vulva: an EORTC Gynaecological Cancer Cooperative Group Study. European Organization for Research and Treatment of Cancer. *Gynecol Oncol* 2001;81:348–354.
129. Benedetti-Panici P, Greggi S, Scambia G, et al. Cisplatin (P), bleomycin (B), and methotrexate (M) preoperative chemotherapy in locally advanced vulvar carcinoma. *Gynecol Oncol* 1993;50:49–53.
130. Cormio G, Loizzi V, Gissi F, et al. Cisplatin and vinorelbine chemotherapy in recurrent vulvar carcinoma. *Oncology* 2009;77:281–284.
131. Geisler JP, Manahan KJ, Buller RE. Neoadjuvant chemotherapy in vulvar cancer: avoiding primary exenteration. *Gynecol Oncol* 2006;100:53–57.
133. Olawaiye A, Lee LM, Krasner C, et al. Treatment of squamous cell vulvar cancer with the anti-EGFR tyrosine kinase inhibitor Tarceva. *Gynecol Oncol* 2007; 106:628–630.
134. Horowitz NS, Olawaiye A, Growdon W, et al. Phase II trial of erlotinib (Tarceva) in women with squamous cell carcinoma of the vulva. *Gynecol Oncol* 2010;116:S14.
135. Richard SD, Krivak TC, Beriwal S, et al. Recurrent metastatic vulvar carcinoma treated with cisplatin plus cetuximab. *Int J Gynecol Cancer* 2008;18:1132–1135.
136. Gould N, Kamelle S, Tillmanns T, et al. Predictors of complications after inguinal lymphadenectomy. *Gynecol Oncol* 2001;82:329–332.
137. Andersen BL, Turnquist D, LaPolla J, et al. Sexual functioning after treatment of in situ vulvar cancer: preliminary report. *Obstet Gynecol* 1988;71:15–19.
138. Andersen BL, Hacker NF. Psychosexual adjustment following pelvic exenteration. *Obstet Gynecol* 1983;61:331–338.
139. Tans L, Ansink AC, van Rooij PH, et al. The role of chemo-radiotherapy in the management of locally advanced carcinoma of the vulva: single institutional experience and review of literature. *Am J Clin Oncol* 2011;34:22–26.
140. Gerszten K, Selvaraj RN, Kelley J, et al. Preoperative chemoradiation for locally advanced carcinoma of the vulva. *Gynecol Oncol* 2005;99:640–644.
141. Landoni F, Maneo A, Zanetta G, et al. Concurrent preoperative chemotherapy with 5-fluorouracil and mitomycin C and radiotherapy (FUMIR) followed by limited surgery in locally advanced and recurrent vulvar carcinoma. *Gynecol Oncol* 1996;61:321–327.≤

Part K Retroperitoneum and Adrenal Gland

Chapter 75
Retroperitoneal Cancer

Jeffrey C. Buchsbaum, James G. Douglas, Barnali Dasgupta, and Brian D. Lawenda

Primary tumors of the retroperitoneum present in unselected series with a frequency of 0.1% to 0.2%.[1–3] They are notable for their widely disparate histologies and presentations. Morgagni published the first report of a retroperitoneal lesion in 1761 after an autopsy.[4] However, the most comprehensive work on retroperitoneal lesions was done in 1954 by Pack and Tabah.[3] They added 120 cases from the Memorial Cancer Center experience to a survey of the world's literature, which contained 750 prior reports. Recent series are histology specific (e.g., sarcomas). Older series, based on clinical presentations, are composed of a variety of tumor types and because of this continue to provide the most valuable data on presenting signs and symptoms. However, because of the tremendous variations in histologies, widely disparate therapeutic recommendations came about. Radiographic interpretation of these lesions has been aided by more recent data and ever improving technology. The focus on this chapter is on lesions that are primary to the retroperitoneum rather than metastatic to it.

ANATOMY

The retroperitoneal space is the potential space posterior to the peritoneum or abdominopelvic cavity (Fig. 75.1). The superior border of this space is the diaphragm, and its inferior border is the superior aspect of the pelvic diaphragm (the levator ani and the coccygeus muscles). In terms of vertebral levels, the retroperitoneum stretches from the 12th thoracic vertebral body to the distal coccyx. Bilaterally, the border was classically considered to be at the lateral edge of the quadratus lumborum. Pack and Tabah[3] consider the lateral extent of the 12th rib to be more valuable because this is the origin of the transversus abdominis aponeurosis as well as the mid-iliac crest. The muscles of the posterior abdominal wall, the psoas and quadratus lumborum muscles, form the posterior border of the retroperitoneum. The renal fascia forms a cone that helps to protect the pelvis from perirenal disease.[5,6]

Most of the tissue in this space consists of lymphatics and loose connective tissue. Retroperitoneal organs, either partially or fully contained, include urinary organs (adrenals, kidneys, ureters, and bladder), vascular organs (aorta and inferior vena cava), alimentary canal organs (esophagus and the upper two-thirds of the rectum), and many nerves. Organs that moved from within the peritoneum to outside of it during organogenesis include parts of the pancreas (head, neck, and body), the nonproximal duodenum, and the ascending and descending portions of the colon. The tail of the pancreas is within the splenorenal ligament and is thus intraperitoneal.

Nethercliffe et al.[7] described the surgical anatomy of the retroperitoneum in their review of retroperitoneal surgical techniques. The most common surgical approaches described include the following: (a) subcostal (below the 12th rib), (b) supracostal (above the 12th rib), (c) transcostal (removing the 11th or 12th rib), and (d) thoracoabdominal.[7]

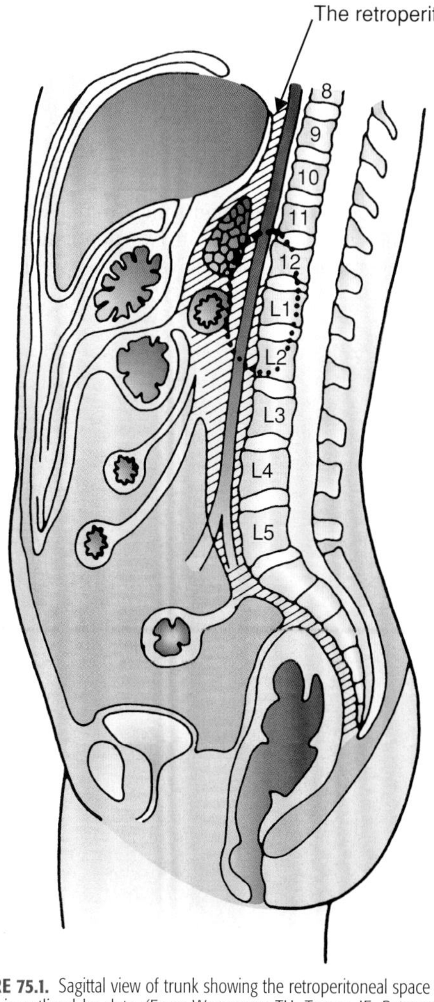

FIGURE 75.1. Sagittal view of trunk showing the retroperitoneal space (*shaded area*). The kidney is outlined by dots. (From Wasserman TH, Tepper JE. Retroperitoneum. In: Perez CA, Brady LW, eds. *Principles and practice of radiation oncology*, 3rd ed. Philadelphia, PA: Lippincott-Raven, 1997:1943–1956.)

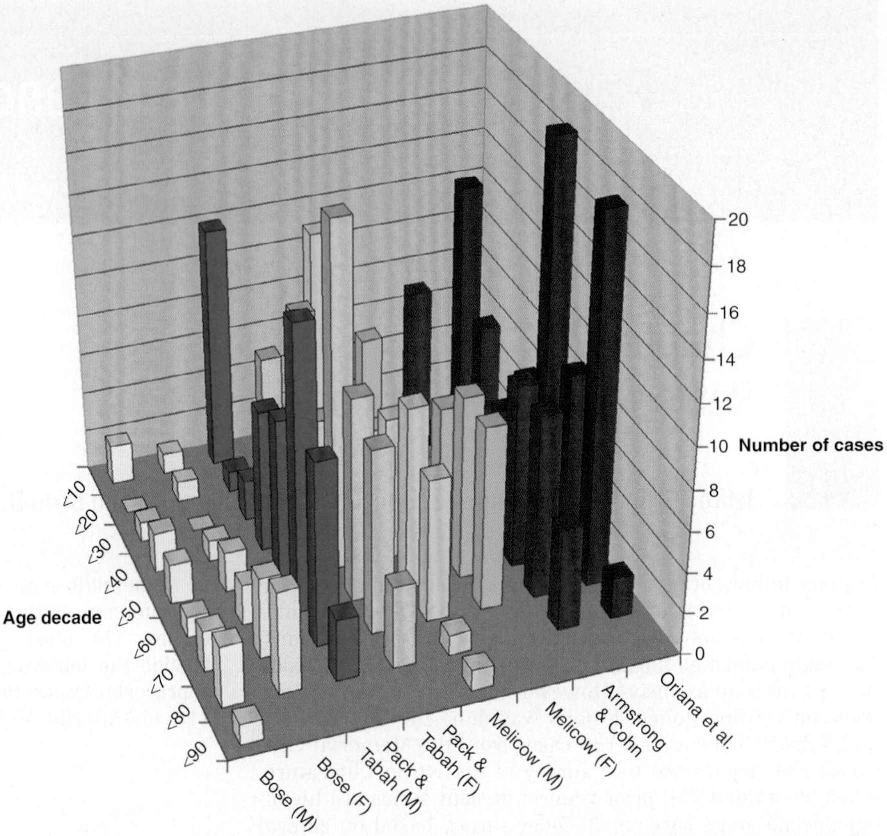

FIGURE 75.2. Age at diagnosis of malignant retroperitoneal tumors (pooled data from multiple series).

Laparoscopic and other minimally invasive techniques that cause less postoperative morbidity often defer these approaches.

EPIDEMIOLOGY

The population frequency for retroperitoneal tumors has been quoted as three per million persons in two population-based studies.[1,2] The age range of patients varied between 3 and 83 years. Fifty percent of patients are diagnosed between 60 and 80 years of age. Males and females are equally likely to develop lesions of the retroperitoneum.[2]

Figure 75.2 graphs the age at diagnosis of several large series of patients with primary retroperitoneal tumors. There are two peak age periods. The first peak occurs during the first decade and is generally caused by neuroblastoma or germ cell tumors. The second peak occurs during the sixth decade of life

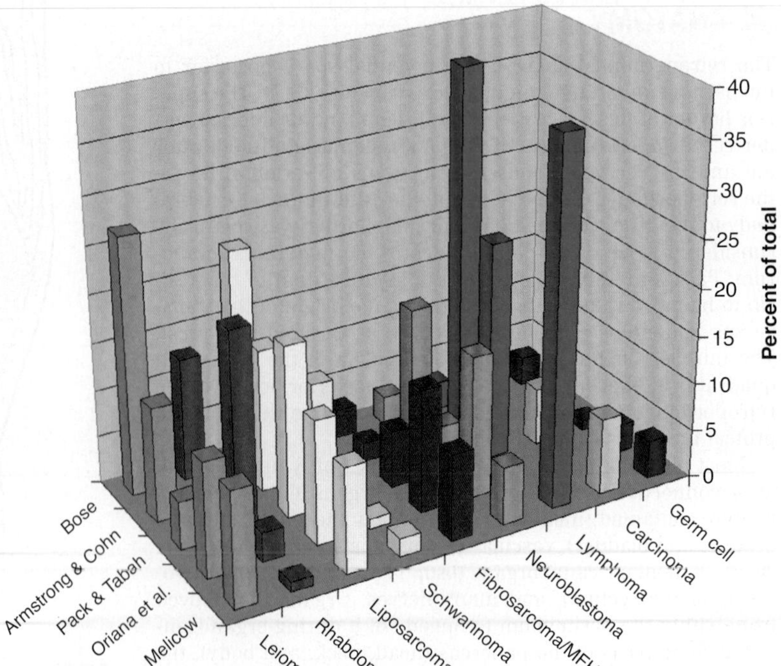

FIGURE 75.3. Percentage of retroperitoneal lesions by histology (pooled data from multiple published series).

TABLE 75.1 PRESENTING COMPLAINTS (%) OF PATIENTS WITH RETROPERITONEAL LESIONS (POOLED FROM LITERATURE SOURCES)

Sign/Symptom	Bose[2] (n = 30)	Pack and Tabah[3] (n = 120)	Oriana et al.[9] (n = 56)
Mass	83	31	42
Abdominal pain	60	51	42[a]
Back pain	20	7	NA
Weight loss	35	3	12
Anorexia	20	NS	9
Nausea/vomiting	20	20	8
Lower extremity edema	17	7	9

NS, data not stated.

[a]Indicates all patients with pain as presenting sign.

and is generally caused by mesenchymal lesions. These histologies are outlined in Figure 75.3.

NATURAL HISTORY

The natural history of these lesions varies by histology. Lesions of the peritoneum often present having achieved a substantial size owing to the anatomic properties of the region.

CLINICAL PRESENTATION

Table 75.1 shows the summary of presenting symptoms and signs of tumors in the retroperitoneum at presentation.

DIAGNOSTIC WORKUP

Melicow[8] considered the ureter to be "the 'weather vane' of the retroperitoneum" because on intravenous urography it is often displaced by tumor. Hydroureter and hydronephrosis are relative late events caused by retroperitoneal pathology given that the ureter and kidney at baseline are highly mobile. Bose[2] published that approximately 80% of these patients had such findings that were suggestive of a mass.

Two series demonstrated that the vascular bed is abnormal in patients with retroperitoneal masses. In the first of these series, which was made up of angiographic studies performed in 20 patients by Oriana et al.,[9] aberrant circulation was noted in 75% and mass effect in 85%. All patients undergoing angiography reported by Bose[2] had abnormal studies.

Neville and Herts[10] have published a comprehensive review of computed tomography (CT) appearance of primary retroperitoneal lesions. CT can differentiate between well-differentiated and dedifferentiated retroperitoneal liposarcoma. A focal nodular/water density area has been found to be a very sensitive marker of dedifferentiated tumor (sensitivity, 97.8%). CT scan can identify most dedifferentiated tumors accurately.[11] Liposarcomas frequently are large lesions with fatty components causing mass effect. Teratomas can have numerous types of tissue imaging characteristics, reflecting their capacity to be made up of differing stromal types. Nerve sheath tumors and other tumors of the nerves are commonly paraspinal. CT characteristics of retroperitoneal tumors have been used in pediatric patients as well.[12]

Magnetic resonance imaging (MRI) often demonstrates additional imaging details to further classify primary lesions of the retroperitoneum, as reported by two groups.[13,14] CT-guided needle biopsy may be performed to obtain initial tissue for histologic diagnosis when an open or laparoscopic biopsy is not possible. Positron emission tomography (PET) scans can be helpful in evaluating the extent of distant metastases during the staging workup. Fluorodeoxyglucose (FDG)-PET can complement CT and MRI for detecting high- and intermediate-grade local recurrence of retroperitoneal soft tissue sarcoma (STS).[15]

TABLE 75.2 SURVEILLANCE, EPIDEMIOLOGY, AND END RESULTS DATA: RETROPERITONEAL MALIGNANCIES, 2002[16]

Patient Data (n = 162)	Number	%
Patient sex		
Male	78	48
Female	84	52
Patient race		
White	128	79
Black	16	9.9
Other	17	10.5
Unknown	1	0.06
Histologic derivation		
Soft tissue sarcoma	126	77.8
Sympathetic nervous system	14	8.6
Epithelial	7	4.3
Germ cell	5	3
Renal	1	0.06
Other (unspecified)	9	5.6

CONTEMPORARY POPULATION-BASED DEMOGRAPHICS

A comprehensive review of the Surveillance Epidemiology and End Results (SEER) public use registry focused on retroperitoneal tumors was performed by Lawenda and Johnstone.[16] The SEER program is made up of 15 regions designed to collect information on cancer incidence, prevalence, and survival on a significant portion of the U.S. population. Table 75.2 shows the results of this review.

GENERAL MANAGEMENT OF RETROPERITONEAL SARCOMA

Gross total resection is the primary treatment for retroperitoneal sarcoma (RPS) and is attempted when possible. Aggressive surgical management is the key for long-term survival for patients with retroperitoneal STS.[17,18,19] Criteria for unresectable tumors may include spinal cord or major vessel involvement.[20] Recent series report that the rate of resectability ranges from 65% to 85%.[21–23] En bloc resection of the primary tumor has been suggested as necessary for tumor control in the retroperitoneum.[23,24]

Surgical resection is often classified by the final margin status or R status as follows:

R0—gross or macroscopically complete tumor resection with microscopically negative margins,
R1—gross or macroscopically complete tumor resection with microscopically positive margins, and
R2—incomplete or partial tumor resection with gross tumor residual.

Achieving an R1 or macroscopically negative margin is a significant prognostic factor in local control and survival; however, the significance of a microscopically positive margin is less clear.[22,25] Even with an R0 resection, the long-term outcomes of tumors of the retroperitoneum are poor: 33% to 77% (local recurrence) and 35% to 63% (5-year overall survival).[22,23,26] Local recurrence is the primary cause of death from RPS.[23,24] Local disease in the absence of metastatic disease was associated with death in 75% of patients with primary RPS in one series.[22]

No prospective data exist suggesting that postoperative radiation after surgery is superior to surgery alone for local control; multiple retrospective series support adjuvant radiation therapy.[23,26] The effect of adjuvant radiation on overall survival is less certain. Preoperative or postoperative radiation therapy can be employed. Other modalities such as hyperthermia have shown early promise and can be of use for increased local control.[20]

Postoperative radiation is felt to be more toxic than preoperative radiation therapy because the clinical target volume (CTV) may be larger and typical contains a larger amount of normal tissue. Preoperative radiation therapy may be less toxic because fields are smaller, there is less normal tissue in fields as the tumor displaces these tissues "out of the way," the tumor may be more easily resectable owing to a "rind" forming, and oxygenation may be better with an intact vasculature.

Lower dose to the region and better delineation of tumor with preoperative treatment are perhaps the most critical reasons why the trend is moving toward preoperative chemotherapy in Europe and many academic centers in North America. The role of preoperative radiation therapy was studied in the American College of Surgeons Oncology Group (ACOSOG) protocol Z9031, a phase III prospective randomized study of preoperative radiation plus surgery versus surgery alone for patients with RPS. The study, which accrued 370 patients, closed in 2006. Results have not yet been published.

Children's Oncology Group (COG) protocol ARST0332 allowed both pre- and postoperative radiation therapy as well as significant chemotherapy. It just recently closed at the time of this writing and contains significant cross sections of histologies. Most accrued cases on the study have been treated with preoperative radiation therapy and chemotherapy. It allowed enrollment for patients up to age 30 years with nonrhabdomyosarcoma STS histologies.

Completeness of resection, tumor volume, grade, and subtype are prognostic factors of RPS.[27] Preoperative radiotherapy or chemotherapy may be employed in cases of unresectable tumor as a means to attempt to shrink the tumor and make it resectable.[28] A 60% local control rate was reported in a series of unresectable RPS patients employing doses of radiation of at least 63 Gy by the Massachusetts General Hospital.[29] Patients with locally extensive tumors that are not amenable to complete resection can be offered palliative debulking surgery to help control local symptoms.[30]

Following aggressive surgery, local recurrence is a key factor determining morbidity and mortality. Local recurrence growth rate >0.9 cm per month has been associated with a poorer outcome.[31] The use of higher doses of external-beam radiation therapy (EBRT) or intraoperative radiation therapy (IORT) does not result in significant improvement in outcome in such cases.[32] Locally recurrent RPS is potentially surgically salvageable, with longer disease-free interval to recurrence being associated with better prognosis.[23] Patients who have not received prior radiation to the tumor bed should be considered for either pre- or postoperative radiation therapy. IORT has been reported to increase local control after resection in several series[33–35]; however, in a randomized prospective study at the National Institutes of Health (NIH), IORT was shown to not be significantly better than EBRT.[36]

There is no standard way to manage patients who present or recur with distant metastases. Guidelines presented by the National Comprehensive Cancer Network (NCCN) for sarcoma management (version 2.2011) suggest that the same approach used for localized sarcoma patients be employed to deal with the oligometastatic population.[37] In the case of oligometastatic disease, chemotherapy may be considered. With disease that is extensively metastatic, palliative approaches are used so as to focus on quality of life.

A histology-based system identifies RPS into three prognostic groups and can be used in both primary and recurrent RPS. Distinct risk stratification is necessary for specific assessment of prognosis and decisions regarding individualized adjuvant therapy.[38] Some authors[39] recommend the formulation of a liposarcoma-specific postoperative nomogram based on histologic subtypes, which provides more accurate survival predictions for patients with primary RPS. Well-differentiated and dedifferentiated liposarcoma differ significantly in their biologic behavior and are treated by different surgical approaches at the University of Texas MD Anderson Cancer Center.[40] Researchers at the center recommend that the American Joint Committee on Cancer (AJCC) STS staging system needs the incorporation of primary site, histologic subtype, margin status, and recurrence to shed light on prognosis.[41] Tumor size was found to have no correlation with survival.[42] Patients with dedifferentiated retroperitoneal STS carry the worst prognosis according to a small series from Italy.[43]

Assessing the response to therapy is challenging and limited to either pathologic review of biopsy or resection specimens, or to serial imaging studies (i.e., CT or MRI with contrast enhancement). Based on the findings of a recently published meta-analysis, FDG-PET imaging may not accurately reflect the response to radiation therapy.[44]

CHEMOTHERAPY

Adjuvant chemotherapy is controversial in the management of adult patients with macroscopically completely resected retroperitoneal STS. In a National Cancer Institute trial, patients with STS were randomized to chemotherapy or observation following resection; some patients had postoperative irradiation.[45] Among patients who were assigned to chemotherapy, survival was favorably affected in those with extremity tumors. However, patients with head and neck and truncal lesions (including RPS) did not benefit; the 5-year survival rate was approximately 40% in both arms. Similar findings were reported in a large meta-analysis of patients with STS.[46]

The use of neoadjuvant or adjuvant chemotherapy is not standard in the management of nonmetastatic adult retroperitoneal STS. Neoadjuvant chemotherapy has been primarily studied in the setting of high-grade extremity STS. Pisters et al.[47] demonstrated feasibility of using preoperative concurrent doxorubicin and EBRT (18 to 50.4 Gy) followed by resection and IORT (15 Gy) in patients with RPS. An R0 or R1 resection was possible in 90% of the patients who went to surgery (83%). Despite these promising results, concurrent neoadjuvant chemoradiotherapy is not recommended outside clinical protocols.[48]

RADIATION THERAPY TECHNIQUES

Three-dimensional conformal radiation therapy (3DCRT) planning is preferable to conventional planning techniques to more clearly define target and nontarget tissues and to optimize field arrangements. Intensity-modulated radiation therapy and helical tomotherapy, proton beam therapy, and IORT have reported benefits over standard 3DCRT in enhancing the delivery of higher radiation doses to the target volume while minimizing doses to normal tissues.[33–35,49–51]

We recommend preoperative radiation therapy for the reasons outlined previously. This usually requires that an initial procedure be done (CT-guided core needle biopsy, if adequate tissue can be obtained, or a small operative procedure) to obtain tissue for histologic study. Obtaining a contrast-enhanced CT scan or MRI prior to simulation will help to more clearly define tumor and normal tissues for planning purposes. The use of [F-18]FDG-PET in tumor localization has been reported and may differentiate tumor versus surrounding normal tissues.[52] Hybrid FDG-PET/CT is becoming increasingly popular for diagnosis and monitoring of treatment for RPS.[52] Most cases of RPS will require irradiating the ipsilateral kidney, except in the case of proton therapy, where some kidney may be spared on a case-by-case basis. Therefore, a renal perfusion study should be ordered as part of the initial radiation planning process to ascertain the degree of functionality of each kidney.

Target volumes are defined as follows (preoperative volumes as per ACOSOG Z9031 as an example):

1. The gross tumor volume (GTV) is the visualized GTV based on preradiotherapy imaging with CT and/or MRI. PET/CT can also be useful.

2. The CTV is defined as the tissues adjacent to the GTV that have a potential for microscopic disease and are not visible on radiographic imaging. The CTV should be contoured at least 1.5 cm outside the GTV but can be less in areas where there is minimal risk of direct invasion (i.e., peritoneum, bone, muscle).
3. The planning target volume (PTV) is an expansion volume outside the CTV that accounts for setup error and patient/organ movement.

This variable is institution dependent as well as patient dependent. A minimum of 0.5 cm expansion outside the CTV should be used. Infraction organ motion of retroperitoneal structures can be significant—that is, average movement between 11 and 19 mm (kidneys, normal breathing) and 18 and 22 mm (pancreas, normal breathing).[53] Stereotactic ultrasound-based image-guided targeting, cone-beam CT imaging, active breathing control, and respiratory gating may be useful modalities in decreasing the required PTV expansion owing to organ motion. Four-dimensional (4D) CT simulation may be of value in helping to define a GTV during the breath cycle[54] but his needs to be better evaluated on clinical trials as it has been used primarily in the lung.[55]

Critical normal structures should be contoured (i.e., liver, kidneys, spinal cord, bowel, stomach) and dose-volume histograms calculated. The spinal cord dose should be limited to 45 Gy in standard fractionation over 5 weeks. The current ACOSOG Z9031 trial limits liver doses as follows: no more than 20% of the liver volume should receive >50 Gy, and no more than 50% should receive >25 Gy. At least two-thirds of the volume of one functioning kidney should receive <20 Gy. Stomach and bowel should be limited to a maximum dose of 45 Gy. Volume expansions should be minimized in regions where tolerance doses to critical structures will be reached.

In photon-based therapy, conventional anteroposterior/posteroanterior or slightly oblique fields often provide the best target coverage with the least amount of normal tissue in the beam. The use of lateral fields can result in irradiating a substantial volume of normal tissue (i.e., liver and kidneys) and should be used sparingly.

Preoperative radiation doses of 45 to 50 Gy (in 1.8 to 2 Gy per fraction per day) are recommended. Surgical resection usually is usually delayed until 3 to 8 weeks after completion of the radiation therapy. Radiographic restaging is typically done prior to resection to assess for metastases and response to therapy.

IORT with either brachytherapy or EBRT may be used as a focal boost to deliver additional radiation to areas of concern (i.e., close or positive margins). The addition of an IORT boost has been shown to increase local control rates over resection and EBRT alone.[34,56] Although not always possible, care should be taken to avoid including critical structures from the boost (i.e., bowel, ureters, nerves). A postoperative external-beam boost can also be delivered to an area of close or positive margin. We recommend asking the surgeon to place radiopaque markers (i.e., clips, metallic seeds) at the borders of the resection cavity and in the areas where the margin may be close or positive. This will be helpful in defining these areas later if a postoperative boost is given. The boost dose is typically 10 to 15 Gy and is delivered in either a single intraoperative dose (electron beam or brachytherapy) or in a once-daily, fractionated regimen (1.8 to 2 Gy per fraction) postoperatively. Both low and high dose rate brachytherapy have similar efficacy in terms of disease control when used alone or in combination with EBRT. Brachytherapy results in fewer complications compared with combination of brachytherapy and EBRT.[57]

High dose rate intraoperative brachytherapy has been described in the treatment for primary and locally recurrent RPS. A Harrison-Anderson-Mick applicator (an array of catheters spaced 1 cm apart in a silicone rubber pad), or similar device, can be used to deliver an intraoperative dose of 12 to 15 Gy to the tumor bed, using iridium-192 (^{192}Ir) sources.[33] Adjuvant interstitial postoperative brachytherapy provides local control of tumor in both low- and high-grade STS.[58]

Postoperative radiation therapy is recommended for patients who initially present after resection. These fields frequently are more extensive than preoperative fields; thus, a larger volume of normal tissue is usually included. Normal tissues (i.e., stomach and bowel) that were previously displaced by the tumor mass will subsequently fill the resection cavity after the tumor has been removed, increasing the toxicity of the treatment and limiting the dose that can be delivered. Although not commonly employed, silicone-filled implants have been used to displace bowel and other tissues out of the radiation field.[33] Postoperative radiation fields should include the preoperative GTV (as defined on the preoperative CT or MRI) and the entire resection cavity. Defining the tumor bed can be challenging; therefore, the radiation oncologist generally needs to err on the side of treatment that affects more, rather than less, normal tissue in cases that are uncertain. Residual disease may be visible on postoperative scans; however, surgical clips placed at the time of the resection will remove much of the uncertainty of defining these areas. Boost fields can encompass areas of close margins or residual disease. Expansion volumes (CTV and PTV) should be limited in regions where the tumor did not violate fascial or peritoneal boundaries. A postoperative radiation dose of 45 Gy (1.8 Gy per fraction per day) is recommended. Limited boost fields (5.4 to 9 Gy per fraction) can be planned, although careful attention must be paid to the surrounding normal tissue tolerances. Particle therapy may be advantageous in terms of decreasing the integral dose to the abdomen and pelvis and is under study.[51,59]

RESULTS OF THERAPY

Despite poor local control rates with resection alone, complete surgical resection remains the only curative treatment modality in patients with RPS.[25] In patients with nonmetastatic, completely excised RPS, 5-year overall survival is 49% to 70%[24,25,60] (Table 75.3). Failure to achieve local control of disease is the major cause of death in patients with RPS.[21] In a large, single-institution report of RPS, patients who successfully underwent a gross total resection (n = 185) had a median survival of 103 months versus 18 months (n = 46) for those who underwent

TABLE 75.3 COMPLETE RESECTION AND SURVIVAL IN PATIENTS WITH NONMETASTATIC (M0) RETROPERITONEAL SARCOMA AND SURVIVAL

Study (Reference)	*Complete Resection (%)*	*LR (%)*	*Overall Survival (%)*	*LR with Incomplete Excision (%)*	*Overall Survival with Incomplete Excision (%)*
Ferrario & Karakousis (60)	95	Primary RPS: 41	Primary RPS: 65 (5 y), 56 (10 y)	–	–
		Recurrent: 61	Recurrent: 53 (5 y), 34 (10 y)	–	–
Stoeckle et al. (23)	65	57 (5 y)	49 (5 y)	–	–
Lewis et al. (22)	Primary RPS: 67	–	70 (5 y); median, 103 mo	–	Median, 18 mo
Catton et al. (26)	43	50 (5 y); 82 (10 y)	55 (5 y); 22 (10 y)	86 (5 y); 95 (10 y)	15 (5 y); 10 (10 y)

LR, local recurrence; RPS, retroperitoneal sarcoma.

TABLE 75.4 LOCAL RECURRENCE IN PATIENTS WITH OR WITHOUT POSTOPERATIVE RADIATION THERAPY FOLLOWING A COMPLETE RESECTION

Study (Reference)	Local Recurrence with PORT (%)	Local Recurrence without PORT (%)	p Value
Ferrario & Karakousis (60)	38 (at 41 mo)	53 (at 41 mo)	.16
Stoeckle et al. (23)	45 (5 y)	77 (5 y)	.0021
Catton et al. (26)	103 mo to LRF	30 mo to LRF	.02

PORT, postoperative radiation therapy; LRF, locoregional failure.

an incomplete resection.[21] Similarly, Stoeckle et al.[22] published actuarial 5-year overall survival rates of 62% versus 26% for patients who had a complete (n = 94) versus incomplete (n = 50) excision, respectively.

Retrospective studies demonstrate an improvement in local control with postoperative radiation therapy (Table 75.4). In the report by Stoeckle et al.,[22] patients with complete excision had a significant reduction in local recurrence risk when they received postoperative radiation therapy (median dose 50 Gy) than when they did not (relative risk [RR] 3.36; p = .0002); there was no improvement in overall survival in multivariate analysis. Catton et al.[25] found that adjuvant radiation therapy increased the time to locoregional relapse from 30 months (no radiation) to 103 months (p = .06). Similar to the trial by Stoeckle et al.,[22] radiation did not exert an effect on survival.

The optimal dose for treating RPS after resection is not known. Fein et al.[61] reported improved local control rates with adjuvant radiation doses >55 Gy (using shrinking photon fields and/or an IORT boost): 25% local failure with doses >55 Gy versus 38% local failure with doses <55 Gy. The National Cancer Institute demonstrated higher locoregional control in patients who underwent a gross total resection followed by IORT (20 Gy) and EBRT (35 to 40 Gy) compared to postoperative EBRT alone (50 to 55 Gy) of 60% versus 20%, respectively[56] (Table 75.5). Alektiar et al.[33] reported higher local control rates in patients who received IORT (12 to 15 Gy) and postoperative EBRT (45 to 50.4 Gy) compared to those who received IORT alone of 66% versus 50%, respectively.

Prospective trials have shown that intermediate- or high-grade RPS patients treated with preoperative radiotherapy and complete resection had a median survival >60 months.[62] In trials of preoperative radiation therapy, researchers from the Princess Margaret Hospital published results using preoperative EBRT (median dose 45 Gy) followed by resection and postoperative brachytherapy implant (low dose rate, median dose 25 Gy).[63] Local recurrence was 19.6% and overall survival at 2 years was 88% in the 46 patients resected with curative intent. In a Massachusetts General Hospital series, 35 patients received preoperative EBRT (45 to 50 Gy) followed by resection (79% complete resections, 11% partial resections, and 5% unresectable) and IORT (n = 20/37) using 9- to 15-MeV electrons: 10 Gy (complete resection), 12.5 to 15 Gy (microscopically involved margins), and 15 to 20 Gy for macroscopic residual disease.[34] In those patients who underwent a complete resection, there was a nonsignificant improvement for local control if they received IORT (83% vs. 61%; p = .2). Petersen et al.[35] reported the Mayo Clinic experience of primary and recurrent RPS or intrapelvic STS treated with preoperative EBRT (n = 53), postoperative EBRT (n = 12), or both (n = 12); the median EBRT dose was 47.6 Gy. IORT (median dose 15 Gy, electron beam) was also employed. Local control at 5 years for patients with gross residual disease (n = 15) was 41%; for those with microscopic residual disease (n = 56), it was 60%; and for those with complete resections (n = 16), it was 100%. The 5-year overall survival rates were 37% (in patients with gross residual disease) and 52% (in patients with microscopic and no residual disease).

TREATMENT SEQUELAE

The most common acute symptoms from EBRT of tumors in the retroperitoneum are nausea, vomiting, diarrhea, skin redness, and fatigue. Anemia, neutropenia, and thrombocytopenia may occur, especially with large radiation fields that often involve the adjacent spine. Weekly monitoring of the patient's complete blood count and daily vital signs should be performed. Reported postoperative complications include bleeding, impaired wound healing or dehiscence, infection, myocardial infarction, and death.[35,63]

TABLE 75.5 OUTCOMES WITH EXTERNAL-BEAM RADIOTHERAPY AND INTRAOPERATIVE RADIOTHERAPY BOOST FOLLOWING RESECTION OF PRIMARY AND RECURRENT RETROPERITONEAL SARCOMA

Study (Reference)	Median EBRT Dose (Gy)	Median IORT Dose (Gy)	LR (%)	OS (%)	Toxicity (%)
Petersen et al. (35)	Primary RPS: 48.6 (postop) Recurrent: 45 (postop)	Primary RPS: 12.5 Recurrent: 15	Primary RPS: 0 (CE), 8 (micro), 40 (gross); 5-y LC Recurrent: 0 (CE), 64 (micro), 33 (gross)	Primary RPS: 62 (CE), 54 (micro), 29 (gross); 5 y-OS Recurrent: 80 (CE), 44 (micro), 45 (gross)	Chronic enteritis (16), grade 3–4 GI complications (18), fistula formation (18), neuropathy (mild, 12; moderate/severe, 21)
Sindelar et al. (56)	IORT arm: 35–40 (postop) EBRT alone arm: 50–55 (postop)	20	IORT arm: time to in-field local recurrence: >127 mo EBRT alone arm: 38 mo (p <.05)	IORT arm: 45 mo EBRT alone arm: 52 (p = .39)	IORT arm: chronic enteritis (13), neuropathy (mild, 13; 47% moderate/severe, 47) EBRT alone arm: chronic enteritis (50), fistula formation (25), neuropathy (mild, 6; moderate/severe, 0)
Gieschen et al. (34)	45–50.4 (preop)	10 (CE), 12.5–15 (micro), 15–20 (gross)	*Complete excision* EBRT + IORT: 17 (5 y) EBRT alone: 39 (5 y)	*Complete excision* EBRT + IORT: 74 (5 y) EBRT alone: 30 (5 y)	Neuropathy (19), hydronephrosis (19), vaginal fistula (6), ureteral fistula (6), small bowel obstruction (6)
Alektiar et al. (33)	45–50.4 (postop)	12–15 (HDR, iridium-192)	*Complete excision* EBRT + IORT: 29 (5 y) primary RPS, 39 (5 y) recurrent, 44% (5 y) total IORT alone: NR (5 y) primary RPS, 67 (5 y) recurrent, 50% (5 y) total	Primary RPS: 75 (5 y) Recurrent: 30 (5 y)	Bowel obstruction (18), fistula (9), neuropathy (mild, 6; moderate/severe, 0), ureteral injury (3)

EBRT, external-beam radiotherapy; IORT, intraoperative radiotherapy; RPS, retroperitoneal sarcoma; LR, local recurrence; OS, overall survival; postop, postoperative; CE, complete excision; micro, microscopic residual disease; gross, gross residual disease; LC, local control; GI, gastrointestinal; preop, preoperative; HDR, high dose rate; NR, not reported.

The major long-term sequelae of surgery and radiation are small bowel enteritis, stricture, perforation, fistula, and obstruction. Development of nephritis is possible after radiation doses >30 Gy, with resultant hypertension. Late complications are associated with the number of laparotomies to which the patient has been subjected and to the radiation dose and volume.[29] A lower incidence of enteritis has been reported with the use of EBRT and an IORT boost compared with EBRT alone, as the bowel is subjected to lower radiation doses when it is able to retracted out of the field[56] (Table 75.5). One must pay careful attention to potential areas of overlap when using abutting IORT boost fields to decrease the risk of neuropathy and ureteral injury.[34,35,63] Studies of preoperative radiation therapy have demonstrated that this approach is well tolerated and appears to be less toxic than postoperative radiation therapy.[34,35,63] As mentioned previously, the role of preoperative radiation therapy is the focus of a current phase III study (ACOSOG Z9031). Proton therapy may allow decreased sequelae in that less bowel anterior to the retroperitoneum is in the treatment field.[51]

LYMPHOMAS

Lymphomas are the most frequent malignant tumors of the retroperitoneum, with non-Hodgkin lymphoma the predominant histologic variant accounting for approximately 94%. CT, MRI, and PET imaging are used in the staging workup of these tumors. CT, ultrasound, or MRI guided-needle biopsy is preferable to fine-needle aspiration for diagnostic purposes of the retroperitoneal mass if no other superficial lymph nodes are involved.[64,65] Flow cytometry and immunohistochemical stains are used to confirm the diagnosis of lymphoma. The diagnosis, staging, and management of retroperitoneal lymphoma are similar to that of other lymphoma sites and are discussed elsewhere. As with all retroperitoneal tumors, radiation doses and fields are often limited by surrounding normal tissues.

OTHER LESIONS

Neuroblastoma is the most common non–central nervous system solid tumor in children and the most common malignancy in infancy. In the United States, approximately 650 new cases are diagnosed per annum with an incidence of 0.9 per 100,000 population. Ninety-eight percent are diagnosed in children <10 years of age, with almost half (40.1%) in infants <1 year of age.[66] This tumor is extraordinarily uncommon in adults, with an estimated incidence of 0.2 per million population in those aged 30 to 39 years.[67] The paradigm for neuroblastoma treatment includes combination therapy with chemotherapy, surgery, and radiotherapy in advanced-staged disease, which is most commonly found in adults.[68,69]

Wilms tumor (WT), or nephroblastoma, is the most common intra-abdominal malignancy of childhood, with an incidence of eight per million population <16 years of age. It is the second most common extracranial solid neoplasm of childhood and the most common renal malignancy in children.[70] In contrast, it is an uncommon malignancy in patients ≥16 years of age, with an estimated incidence of 0.2 per million population.[71,72] Adults frequently present with flank pain, whereas children are more likely to present with a painless hematuria and/or abdominal distention.[66] The treatment and outcomes of patients with adult Wilms Tumor (AWT) remain controversial. Kalapurakal et al.[73] reported the outcomes of 23 adults (>16 years of age) treated on COG protocols (National Wilms Tumor Study Group; NWTS 4 and 5) and found no difference between the adults and their pediatric counterparts.[73] Similarly, the International Society of Paediatric Oncology (SIOP) published results from an SIOP retrospective review of 30 AWT patients >16 years of age, with comparable results between adults and children.[74,75] Conversely Izawa et al.[76] reported on 128 AWT patients from SIOP, as well as individual institutional reports, and concluded that the outcomes in adults were inferior to that of children. Recently, Ali et al.,[77,78] using the U.S. SEER database, concluded that the outcome in 152 AWT patients was worse than in children. Overall survival was 69% in AWT versus 88% in children (p <.001). By multivariate analysis, adult status (≥16 years), SEER stage, treatment era (before 1990), and lack of surgical staging of lymph nodes were significant prognostic factors in this cohort. A consensus statement by an international group of childhood renal experts has been recently published that recommends adoption of the pediatric paradigm for treatment for AWT patients, including surgical resection, chemotherapy agents depending on stage and histologic subtype, and local therapy with irradiation depending on the stage of disease.[79] Additionally, the current COG WT studies have revised the inclusion age criteria upward to age 30 years. The toxicities of treatment (severe acute neuropathy, grade 4 hematologic toxicity) in AWT patients may be somewhat higher than in the pediatric population[74] but are thought to be reasonable in view of the high response rates.

Retroperitoneal schwannomas are a rare tumor, accounting for approximately 4% of retroperitoneal tumors, and the most common benign tumor found is this location.[80,81] They belong in the family of peripheral nerve sheath tumors, which in addition to schwannomas includes neurofibromas, solitary circumcised neuromas, and perineuriomas.[82] Schwannomas may occur in any nerve trunk in the body, with exception of cranial nerves 1 and 2 (which are not covered by Schwann cells), and are most commonly found at peripheral nerve sites of the upper extremities and cranial nerves; only 0.3% to 3.2% of all schwannomas occur in the retroperitoneum. Benign schwannomas are associated with Von Recklinghausen's disease or neurofibromatosis 1 (NF-1) in approximately 5% to 18% of NF-1 patients, presenting most commonly between 20 and 50 years of age.[83] They are slow-growing nonaggressive tumors that displace rather than invade normal tissues[80,82] and often form large, well-circumscribed masses. They may display cystic degeneration, calcification, hemorrhage, and hyalinization on imaging studies. In several moderate to large series, there appears to be a slight female patient propensity, and the tumors often are diagnosed incidentally during radiologic examinations for unrelated symptoms.[84,85] Boney changes may occur in perispinal tumors, and invasion into nerve roots or the spinal canal may lead to neurologic symptoms including paresthesias, weakness, and pain. MRI examinations are the preferred method for imaging these soft tissue neoplasms, although CT scanning may be necessary to better visualize potential boney abnormalities, particularly in the spine. Because these tumors are frequently quite vascular, many authors do not recommend the use of CT-guided biopsies because of the risk of hemorrhage. Whenever feasible, complete surgical resection with negative margins is the treatment of choice, although adjuvant radiation therapy may be necessary for incompletely excised sacral schwannomas and malignant peripheral nerve sheath tumors (MPNST).[86] NF-1 patients have a particularly high risk of developing STS, particularly MPNST, often with an aggressive clinical presentation and poor outcome.[87]

Aggressive fibromatosis, also referred to as desmoid tumors, is a rare fibroblastic neoplasm that arises from deep musculoaponeurotic connective tissue and has an incidence of two to four cases per million population, occurring either sporadically or associated with familial adenomatous polyposis (FAP).[88–92] Ten to 30% of patients with FAP eventually develop desmoid tumors, most occurring either in the extremities or abdomen/retroperitoneum (De Carmago et al.,[93] Meazza et al.[94,95]). They occur more frequently in fertile women than in men (1.5 to 2.5:1). Although benign in nature, they are locally aggressive and may infiltrate critical structures. Complete surgical resection is the mainstay of treatment, although local recurrence is common even in the setting of a wide local resection in up to 50% of patients. Postoperative radiotherapy and/or

TABLE 75.6 THE INTERNATIONAL GERM CELL CANCER COLLABORATIVE GROUP CLASSIFICATION SYSTEM FOR ASSESSING PROGNOSIS IN NSGCT AND SGCT[103]

Tumor	*Good Prognosis*	*Intermediate Prognosis*	*Poor Prognosis*
NSGCT	• Testis/retroperitoneal primary, no nonpulmonary visceral metastases, AFP <1,000 ng/mL, β-hCG <1,000 IU/L, and LDH <1.5× upper limit of normal • 5-y PFS, 89% • 5-y survival rate, 92%	• Testis/retroperitoneal primary, no nonpulmonary visceral metastases, AFP >1,000 ng/mL and <10,000 ng/mL and/or β-hCG 5,000–50,000 IU/L and/or LDH >1.5× normal to 10× normal • 5-y PFS, 75% • 5-y survival rate, 92%	• Indicated by any of the following: mediastinal primary, nonpulmonary visceral metastases or AFP >10,000 ng/mL, β-hCG >50,000 IU/L, or LDH >10× normal • 5-y PFS, 41% • 5-y survival rate, 48%
SGCT	• Any primary site, no nonpulmonary visceral metastases, normal AFP, any β-hCG, any LDH • 5-y PFS, 92% • 5-y survival rate, 88%	• Any primary site, nonpulmonary visceral metastases, normal AFP, any β-hCG, any LDH • 5-y PFS, 67% • 5-y survival rate, 72%	• No patients classified as having poor prognosis

NSGCT, nonseminomatous germ cell tumor; SGCT, seminomatous germ cell tumor (seminoma); AFP, alpha-fetoprotein; β–hCG, beta-human chorionic gonadotropin; LDH, lactate dehydrogenase; PFS, progression-free survival.

chemotherapy may be indicated when a complete surgical resection is not achieved or not feasible or in multiply recurrent disease. The data is variable regarding the dose and treatment volumes; however, most reported series suggest that a dose of 50 to 60 Gy with margins of 5 to 7 cm is appropriate therapy. Doses >56 Gy may not be necessary to control gross disease.[96] A recent meta-analysis that included data from 22 studies suggested that local control is improved with adjuvant radiation therapy compared to surgery alone; local control after surgery alone was 72% (R0) and 41% (R1 and R2) compared to 94% (R0) and 75% (R1 and R2) after surgery and adjuvant radiation.[97] In patients with unresectable disease, radiation therapy alone is effective in providing long-term local control in up to 80% of patients.[97,98] Chemotherapy or antiestrogen therapy may also play a role in nonresectable, incompletely resected, or recurrent disease. Regimens containing anthracyclines and antiestrogens appear to be the most effective chemotherapeutic options,[93] although more recently, the tyrosine kinase inhibitor imatinib has shown activity in desmoid tumors.[99,100]

Extragonadal germ cell tumors (EGCTs) account for approximately 1% to 5% of all germ cell tumors and occur in the retroperitoneum as the second most common extragonadal site in adults after the mediastinum.[101] Primary retroperitoneal germ cell tumors account for approximately 10% of all primary malignant retroperitoneal tumors in adults and about 30% to 40% of all EGCTs. It is believed that these tumors arise from primordial germ cells, which are displaced during their migration along the urogenital ridge to the gonads.[101] When they occur in the retroperitoneum, they are considered to be metastases from an occult or "burned out" gonadal primary until proven otherwise. EGCTs are most typically found in children or young adults and mostly arise in midline locations. Most of these tumors occur in young men. In young men (in whom most of these tumors occur), histologically, seminomatous germ cell tumors (SGCTs) comprise approximately 30% to 40%, whereas the remaining tumors are nonseminomatous germ cell tumors (NSGCTs). In young women, the histologic varieties are dysgerminomas and nondysgerminomas. NSGCTs include the following histologies: teratoma, embryonal carcinoma, endodermal sinus tumor (yolk sac tumor), and choriocarcinoma, as well as mixed histologies. Any proportion of nonseminomatous components is enough to classify a tumor as an NSGCT. NSGCTs generally have a much more aggressive course than do SGCTs. Serum markers, although nonspecific, may help to categorize the histology and can be useful for following both response to therapy and the presence of recurrence. Beta human chorionic gonadotropin (β-hCG) is elevated in choriocarcinoma and embryonal carcinoma, as well as in approximately 10% to 15% of SGCTs. Serum α-fetoprotein is elevated in endodermal sinus tumors and embryonal carcinomas. These tumors often present as large masses in the retroperitoneum and frequently displace, compress, or encase abdominal vessels. There are no distinguishing features by imaging to differentiate germ cell tumors from other retroperitoneal masses; thus, biopsy by ultrasound, CT, or MRI guidance is warranted. Gonadal primaries must be ruled out using high-resolution ultrasound. A biopsy of the gonads appears to be unnecessary with a negative ultrasound. Common sites of metastases are liver, bone, brain, and lungs. The prognosis of retroperitoneal

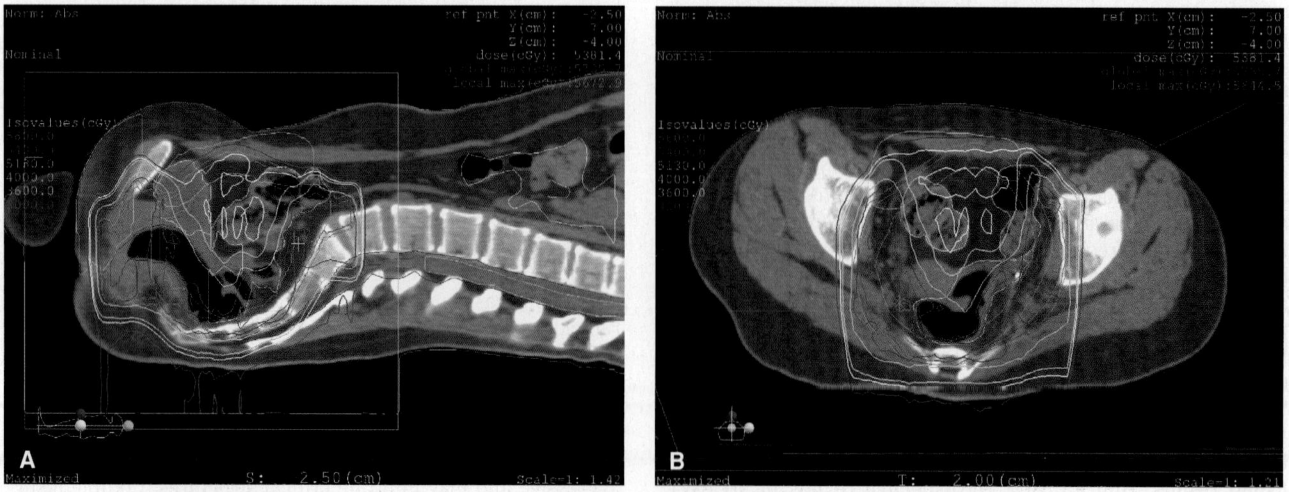

FIGURE 75.4. Proton treatment plan for retroperitoneal tumor in a young adult patient. Because of concerns specific to the case, the bowel and retroperitoneal region as shown was treated to 36 Gy. The retroperitoneal space plus a small margin was then treated to 54 Gy. Concurrent high-dose chemotherapy was employed.

SGCTs and their mediastinal counterparts are similar; however, retroperitoneal NSGCTs actually have a better prognosis than those occurring in the mediastinum.[102]

The treatment for EGCTs has evolved over the past 10 to 15 years from the use of primary radiotherapy for SGCTs to the more commonly recommended treatment using platinum-based chemotherapy regimens.[101] Treatment paradigms for early-stage SGCT and NSGCT are covered elsewhere in this book. The International Germ Cell Cancer Collaborative Group established a classification system for assessing prognosis in NSGCT and SGCT[103] (Table 75.6), which is used for treatment decisions. Some controversy remains as to the management of residual masses after three to four cycles of platinum-based chemotherapy in more advanced-stage disease or bulky retroperitoneal disease after chemotherapy or radiotherapy alone. Some authors favor surgical resection for residual masses >3 cm, particularly for NSGCT, whereas others favor observation alone. Subsequent chemotherapy is recommended for patients with viable SGCT on resection of any residual masses if radiotherapy was the sole treatment modality.[104]

CONCLUSIONS

The retroperitoneum presents the clinician with a huge variety of histologies in a complex anatomic space. Treatment is driven by the histology in general. Newer technology will play a critical role in delivering dose with fewer side effects or perhaps allowing dose escalation with the same late effects. Image-guided therapy and intensity-modulated radiotherapy are mainstays in the treatment to the retroperitoneum when normal tissue toxicity is a concern. Particle therapy can now deliver dose to large tumor volumes while sparing normal tissue via gantry systems in place in many centers, as shown in Figure 75.4. New agents will continue to come forward that will allow more individualized treatment based on histology and genetic profiling. Despite our newest radiation and chemotherapeutic technology, complete surgical resection remains the backbone of successful therapy for these lesions.[105] The rarity and poor results associated with these tumors points to a need to conduct prospective, multi-institutional trials.

REFERENCES

1. Armstrong JR, Cohn I Jr. Primary malignant tumors of the retroperitoneum. *Nebr State Med J* 1965;50(10):520–524.
2. Bose B. Primary malignant retroperitoneal tumours: analysis of 30 cases. *Can J Surg* 1979;22(3):215–220.
3. Pack GT, Tabah EJ. Primary retroperitoneal tumors: a study of 120 cases. *Int Abstr Surg* 1954;99(4):313–341.
4. Pemberton JD, Whitlock M. Large retroperitoneal lipoma. *Surg Clin North Am* 1934;14:601.
5. Raptopoulos V, et al. Why perirenal disease does not extend into the pelvis: the importance of closure of the cone of the renal fasciae. *AJR Am J Roentgenol* 1995;164(5):1179–1184.
6. Raptopoulos V, et al. Medial border of the perirenal space: CT and anatomic correlation. *Radiology* 1997;205(3):777–784.
7. Nethercliffe J, et al. Retroperitoneal and transthoracic anatomy and surgical approaches. *BJU Int* 2004;94(5):705–718.
8. Melicow MM. Primary tumors of the retroperitoneum; a clinicopathologic analysis of 162 cases; review of the literature and tables of classification. *J Int Coll Surg* 1953;19(4):401–449.
9. Oriana S, Bonardi P, Preda F. Primary retroperitoneal tumors. *Tumori* 1977;63(4):397–405.
10. Neville A, Herts BR. CT characteristics of primary retroperitoneal neoplasms. *Crit Rev Comput Tomogr* 2004;45(4):247–270.
11. Lahat G, et al. Computed tomography scan-driven selection of treatment for retroperitoneal liposarcoma histologic subtypes. *Cancer* 2009;115(5):1081–1090.
12. Xu Y, et al. CT characteristics of primary retroperitoneal neoplasms in children. *Eur J Radiol* 2010;75(3):321–328.
13. Song T, et al. Retroperitoneal liposarcoma: MR characteristics and pathological correlative analysis. *Abdom Imaging* 2007;32(5):668–674.
14. Crema MD, et al. [MR imaging of large and rare pelvic masses from non-gynecological etiology]. *J Radiol* 2008;89(7–8 Pt 1):853–861.
15. Schwarzbach MH, et al. Clinical value of [18-F] fluorodeoxyglucose positron emission tomography imaging in soft tissue sarcomas. *Ann Surg* 2000;231(3):380–386.
16. Ries LAG, Eisner MP, Kosary CL, et al., eds. *SEER cancer statistics review, 1975–2002*. Bethesda, MD: National Cancer Institute. Available at: http://seer.cancer.gov/csr/1975_2002/, based on November 2004 SEER data submission, posted to the SEER web site 2005.
17. Anaya DA, et al. Postoperative nomogram for survival of patients with retroperitoneal sarcoma treated with curative intent. *Ann Oncol* 2010;21(2):397–402.
18. Pacelli F, et al. Retroperitoneal soft tissue sarcoma: prognostic factors and therapeutic approaches. *Tumori* 2008;94(4):497–504.
19. Mendenhall WM, et al. The management of adult soft tissue sarcomas. *Am J Clin Oncol* 2009;32(4):436–442.
20. Schwarzbach MH, Hohenberger P. Current concepts in the management of retroperitoneal soft tissue sarcoma. *Recent Results Cancer Res* 2009;179:301–319.
21. Hassan I, et al. Operative management of primary retroperitoneal sarcomas: a reappraisal of an institutional experience. *Ann Surg* 2004;239(2):244–250.
22. Lewis JJ, et al. Retroperitoneal soft-tissue sarcoma: analysis of 500 patients treated and followed at a single institution. *Ann Surg* 1998;228(3):355–365.
23. Stoeckle E, et al. Prognostic factors in retroperitoneal sarcoma: a multivariate analysis of a series of 165 patients of the French Cancer Center Federation Sarcoma Group. *Cancer* 2001;92(2):359–368.
24. Gronchi A, et al. Retroperitoneal soft tissue sarcomas: patterns of recurrence in 167 patients treated at a single institution. *Cancer* 2004;100(11):2448–2455.
25. Singer S, et al. Histologic subtype and margin of resection predict pattern of recurrence and survival for retroperitoneal liposarcoma. *Ann Surg* 2003;238(3):358–370; discussion 370–371.
26. Catton CN, et al. Outcome and prognosis in retroperitoneal soft tissue sarcoma. *Int J Radiat Oncol Biol Phys* 1994;29(5):1005–1010.
27. Chen CQ, et al. Prognostic factors of retroperitoneal soft tissue sarcomas: analysis of 132 cases. *Chin Med J (Engl)* 2007;120(12):1047–1050.
28. Meric F, et al. Impact of neoadjuvant chemotherapy on postoperative morbidity in soft tissue sarcomas. *J Clin Oncol* 2000;18(19):3378–3383.
29. Kepka L, et al. Results of radiation therapy for unresected soft-tissue sarcomas. *Int J Radiat Oncol Biol Phys* 2005;63(3):852–859.
30. Shibata D, et al. Is there a role for incomplete resection in the management of retroperitoneal liposarcomas? *J Am Coll Surg* 2001;193(4):373–379.
31. Park JO, et al. Predicting outcome by growth rate of locally recurrent retroperitoneal liposarcoma: the one centimeter per month rule. *Ann Surg* 2009;250(6):977–982.
32. Ballo MT, et al. Retroperitoneal soft tissue sarcoma: an analysis of radiation and surgical treatment. *Int J Radiat Oncol Biol Phys* 2007;67(1):158–163.
33. Alektiar KM, et al. High-dose-rate intraoperative radiation therapy (HDR-IORT) for retroperitoneal sarcomas. *Int J Radiat Oncol Biol Phys* 2000;47(1):157–163.
34. Gieschen HL, et al. Long-term results of intraoperative electron beam radiotherapy for primary and recurrent retroperitoneal soft tissue sarcoma. *Int J Radiat Oncol Biol Phys* 2001;50(1):127–131.
35. Petersen IA, et al. Use of intraoperative electron beam radiotherapy in the management of retroperitoneal soft tissue sarcomas. *Int J Radiat Oncol Biol Phys* 2002;52(2):469–475.
36. Kinsella TJ, et al. Preliminary results of a randomized study of adjuvant radiation therapy in resectable adult retroperitoneal soft tissue sarcomas. *J Clin Oncol* 1988;6(1):18–25.
37. National Comprehensive Cancer Network. *NCCN practice guidelines in oncology,* Version 2.2011. Available at: http://www.nccn.org/professionals/physician_gls/pdf/sarcoma.pdf.
38. Anaya DA, et al. Establishing prognosis in retroperitoneal sarcoma: a new histology-based paradigm. *Ann Surg Oncol* 2009;16(3):667–675.
39. Dalal KM, et al. Subtype specific prognostic nomogram for patients with primary liposarcoma of the retroperitoneum, extremity, or trunk. *Ann Surg* 2006;244(3):381–391.
40. Lahat G, et al. Resectable well-differentiated versus dedifferentiated liposarcomas: two different diseases possibly requiring different treatment approaches. *Ann Surg Oncol* 2008;15(6):1585–1593.
41. Lahat G, et al. New perspectives for staging and prognosis in soft tissue sarcoma. *Ann Surg Oncol* 2008;15(10):2739–2748.
42. Nathan H, et al. Predictors of survival after resection of retroperitoneal sarcoma: a population-based analysis and critical appraisal of the AJCC staging system. *Ann Surg* 2009;250(6):970–976.
43. Mussi C, et al. The prognostic impact of dedifferentiation in retroperitoneal liposarcoma: a series of surgically treated patients at a single institution. *Cancer* 2008;113(7):1657–1665.
44. Bastiaannet E, et al. The value of FDG-PET in the detection, grading and response to therapy of soft tissue and bone sarcomas; a systematic review and meta-analysis. *Cancer Treat Rev* 2004;30(1):83–101.
45. Rosenberg SA. Prospective randomized trials demonstrating the efficacy of adjuvant chemotherapy in adult patients with soft tissue sarcomas. *Cancer Treat Rep* 1984;68(9):1067–1078.
46. Adjuvant chemotherapy for localised resectable soft-tissue sarcoma of adults: meta-analysis of individual data. Sarcoma Meta-analysis Collaboration. *Lancet* 1997;350(9092):1647–1654.
47. Pisters PW, et al. Phase I trial of preoperative concurrent doxorubicin and radiation therapy, surgical resection, and intraoperative electron-beam radiation therapy for patients with localized retroperitoneal sarcoma. *J Clin Oncol* 2003;21(16):3092–3097.
48. Adjuvant chemotherapy for localised resectable soft tissue sarcoma in adults. *Cochrane Database Syst Rev* 2000(4):CD001419.
49. DeLaney TF, et al. Advanced-technology radiation therapy in the management of bone and soft tissue sarcomas. *Cancer Control* 2005;12(1):27–35.
50. Musat E, et al. [Comparison of intensity-modulated postoperative radiotherapy with conventional postoperative conformal radiotherapy for retroperitoneal sarcoma]. *Cancer Radiother* 2004;8(4):255–261.
51. Hug EB, et al. Conformal proton radiation treatment for retroperitoneal neuroblastoma: introduction of a novel technique. *Med Pediatr Oncol* 2001;37(1):36–41.
52. Schramm N, et al. [Combined functional and morphological imaging of sarcomas: significance for diagnostics and therapy monitoring]. *Radiologe* 2010;50(4):339–348.
53. Langen KM, Jones DT. Organ motion and its management. *Int J Radiat Oncol Biol Phys* 2001;50(1):265–278.
54. Eom J, et al. Modeling respiratory motion for cancer radiation therapy based on patient-specific 4DCT data. *Med Image Comput Comput Assist Interv* 2009;12(Pt 2):348–355.
55. Liao ZX, et al. Influence of technologic advances on outcomes in patients with unresectable, locally advanced non-small-cell lung cancer receiving concomitant chemoradiotherapy. *Int J Radiat Oncol Biol Phys* 2010;76(3):775–781.
56. Sindelar WF, et al. Intraoperative radiotherapy in retroperitoneal sarcomas. Final results of a prospective, randomized, clinical trial. *Arch Surg* 1993;128(4):402–410.

57. Laskar S, et al. Perioperative interstitial brachytherapy for soft tissue sarcomas: prognostic factors and long-term results of 155 patients. *Ann Surg Oncol* 2007;14(2):560–567.
58. Mierzwa ML, et al. Interstitial brachytherapy for soft tissue sarcoma: a single institution experience. *Brachytherapy* 2007;6(4):298–303.
59. Blattmann C, et al. Non-randomized therapy trial to determine the safety and efficacy of heavy ion radiotherapy in patients with non-resectable osteosarcoma. *BMC Cancer* 2010;10:96.
60. Ferrario T, Karakousis CP. Retroperitoneal sarcomas: grade and survival. *Arch Surg* 2003;138(3):248–251.
61. Fein DA, et al. Management of retroperitoneal sarcomas: does dose escalation impact on locoregional control? *Int J Radiat Oncol Biol Phys* 1995;31(1):129–134.
62. Pawlik TM, et al. Long-term results of two prospective trials of preoperative external beam radiotherapy for localized intermediate- or high-grade retroperitoneal soft tissue sarcoma. *Ann Surg Oncol* 2006;13(4):508–517.
63. Jones JJ, et al. Initial results of a trial of preoperative external-beam radiation therapy and postoperative brachytherapy for retroperitoneal sarcoma. *Ann Surg Oncol* 2002;9(4):346–354.
64. Zangos S, et al. MR-guided biopsies of lesions in the retroperitoneal space: technique and results. *Eur Radiol* 2006;16(2):307–312.
65. Chen TC, et al. Solitary extramedullary plasmacytoma in the retroperitoneum. *Am J Hematol* 1998;58(3):235–238.
66. Pizzo P, Poplack D. *Principles and practice of pediatric oncology,* 6th ed. Philadelphia, PA: Lippincott Williams & Wilkins, 2010:1600.
67. Davis S, Rogers MA, Pendergrass TW. The incidence and epidemiologic characteristics of neuroblastoma in the United States. *Am J Epidemiol* 1987;126(6):1063–1074.
68. Ben Moualli S, et al. [Retroperitoneal neuroblastoma in the adult: case report and review of the literature]. *Ann Urol (Paris)* 2001;35(1):51–55.
69. Loeser A, Gerharz EW, Riedmiller H. Recurrent pelvic neuroblastoma in an adult patient. *Gynecol Oncol* 2007;106(1):257–258.
70. Breslow N, et al. Epidemiology of Wilms tumor. *Med Pediatr Oncol* 1993;21(3):172–181.
71. Merten DF, Yang SS, Bernstein J. Wilms' tumor in adolescence. *Cancer* 1976;37(3):1532–1538.
72. Mitry E, et al. Incidence of and survival from Wilms' tumour in adults in Europe: data from the EUROCARE study. *Eur J Cancer* 2006;42(14):2363–2368.
73. Kalapurakal JA, et al. Treatment outcomes in adults with favorable histologic type Wilms tumor—an update from the National Wilms Tumor Study Group. *Int J Radiat Oncol Biol Phys* 2004;60(5):1379–1384.
74. Reinhard H, et al. Wilms' tumor in adults: results of the Society of Pediatric Oncology (SIOP) 93-01/Society for Pediatric Oncology and Hematology (GPOH) Study. *J Clin Oncol* 2004;22(22):4500–4506.
75. Reinhard H, et al. [Wilms' tumor in adults]. *Urologe A* 2007;46(7):748–753.
76. Izawa JI, et al. Prognostic variables in adult Wilms tumour. *Can J Surg* 2008;51(4):252–256.
77. Ali AN, et al. A Surveillance, Epidemiology and End Results (SEER) program comparison of adult and pediatric Wilms' tumor. *Cancer* 2012;118(9):2541–2451.
78. Ali EM, Elnashar AT. Adult Wilms' tumor: review of literature. *J Oncol Pharm Pract* 2012;18(1):148–151.
79. Segers H, et al. Management of adults with Wilms' tumor: recommendations based on international consensus. *Expert Rev Anticancer Ther* 2011;11(7):1105–1113.
80. Theodosopoulos T, et al. Special problems encountering surgical management of large retroperitoneal schwannomas. *World J Surg Oncol* 2008;6:107.
81. Nah YW, et al. Benign retroperitoneal schwannoma: surgical consideration. *Hepatogastroenterology* 2005;52(66):1681–1684.
82. Strauss DC, et al. Management of benign retroperitoneal schwannomas: a single-center experience. *Am J Surg* 2011;202(2):194–198.
83. Antiheimo J, et al. Population based analysis of sporadic and type 2 neurofibromatosis-associated meningiomas and schwannomas. *Neurology* 2000;54:71–76.
84. Hughes MJ, et al. Imaging features of retroperitoneal and pelvic schwannomas. *Clin Radiol* 2005;60(8):886–893.
85. Li Q, et al. Analysis of 82 cases of retroperitoneal schwannoma. *ANZ J Surg* 2007;77(4):237–240.
86. Carli M, et al. Pediatric malignant peripheral nerve sheath tumor: the Italian and German soft tissue sarcoma cooperative group. *J Clin Oncol* 2005;23(33):8422–8430.
87. Ferrari A, et al. Soft-tissue sarcomas in children and adolescents with neurofibromatosis type 1. *Cancer* 2007;109(7):1406–1412.
88. Reitamo JJ, Scheinin TM, Hayry P. The desmoid syndrome. New aspects in the cause, pathogenesis and treatment of the desmoid tumor. *Am J Surg* 1986;151(2):230–237.
89. Nieuwenhuis MH, et al. A nation-wide study comparing sporadic and familial adenomatous polyposis-related desmoid-type fibromatoses. *Int J Cancer* 2011;129(1):256–261.
90. Latchford AR, et al. A 10-year review of surgery for desmoid disease associated with familial adenomatous polyposis. *Br J Surg* 2006;93(10):1258–1264.
91. Ferenc T, et al. Aggressive fibromatosis (desmoid tumors): definition, occurrence, pathology, diagnostic problems, clinical behavior, genetic background. *Pol J Pathol* 2006;57(1):5–15.
92. Lahat G, et al. Surgery for sporadic abdominal desmoid tumor: is low/no recurrence an achievable goal? *Isr Med Assoc J* 2009;11(7):398–402.
93. De Camargo VP, et al. Clinical outcomes of systemic therapy for patients with deep fibromatosis (desmoid tumor). *Cancer* 2010;116(9):2258–2265.
94. Meazza C, et al. Aggressive fibromatosis in children and adolescents: the Italian experience. *Cancer* 2010;116(1):233–240.
95. Meazza C, Alaggio R, Ferrari A. Aggressive fibromatosis in children: a changing approach. *Minerva Pediatr* 2011;63(4):305–318.
96. Ballo MT, Zagars GK, Pollack A. Radiation therapy in the management of desmoid tumors. *Int J Radiat Oncol Biol Phys* 1998;42(5):1007–1014.
97. Nuyttens JJ, et al. Surgery versus radiation therapy for patients with aggressive fibromatosis or desmoid tumors: a comparative review of 22 articles. *Cancer* 2000;88(7):1517–1523.
98. Micke O, Seegenschmiedt MH. Radiation therapy for aggressive fibromatosis (desmoid tumors): results of a national Patterns of Care Study. *Int J Radiat Oncol Biol Phys* 2005;61(3):882–891.
99. Penel N, et al. Imatinib for progressive and recurrent aggressive fibromatosis (desmoid tumors): an FNCLCC/French Sarcoma Group phase II trial with a long-term follow-up. *Ann Oncol* 2011;22(2):452–457.
100. Bhama PK, et al. Gardner's syndrome in a 40-year-old woman: successful treatment of locally aggressive desmoid tumors with cytotoxic chemotherapy. *World J Surg Oncol* 2006;4:96.
101. Bokemeyer C, et al. Extragonadal germ cell tumors of the mediastinum and retroperitoneum: results from an international analysis. *J Clin Oncol* 2002;20(7):1864–1873.
102. Jadhav AS, Pathare DB, Shingare MS. A validated stability indicating high performance reverse phase liquid chromatographic method for the determination of cilostazol in bulk drug substance. *Drug Dev Ind Pharm* 2007;33(2):173–179.
103. International Germ Cell Consensus Classification: a prognostic factor-based staging system for metastatic germ cell cancers. International Germ Cell Cancer Collaborative Group. *J Clin Oncol* 1997;15(2):594–603.
104. Lavery HJ, Bahnson RR, Sharp DS, Pohar KS. Management of the residual post-chemotherapy retroperitoneal mass in germ cell tumors. *Ther Adv Urol* 2009;1(4):199–207.
105. Mullinax JE, Zager JS, Gonzalez RJ. Current diagnosis and management of retroperitoneal sarcoma. *Cancer Control* 2011;18(3):177–187.

Chapter 76
Adrenal Cancer

Filip T. Troicki and John J. Coen

ANATOMY

The paired suprarenal (adrenal) glands are located between the superomedial aspects of the kidney and the diaphragmatic crura. They are surrounded by connective tissue containing perinephric fat. The glands are enclosed by renal fascia, but separated from the kidneys by fibrous tissue. The triangular right gland relates to the diaphragm posteriorly and the inferior vena cava and liver anteriorly. The semilunar left adrenal gland is positioned in the middle of the left crux of the diaphragm. The omental bursa separates it from the stomach. It is also related to the spleen and pancreas.[1]

The endocrine function of the adrenal glands necessitates an abundant blood supply. The superior suprarenal arteries are derived from the inferior phrenic artery, the middle suprarenal arteries from the abdominal aorta near the origin of the superior mesenteric artery, and the inferior suprarenal arteries from the renal artery. A large central vein leaves the anterior surface of the gland at the hilum. The shorter right suprarenal vein drains into the inferior vena cava and the longer left suprarenal vein drains into the left renal vein.[1]

The lymphatic drainage follows the arterial supply and is predominantly to lumbar lymph nodes. The superior lymphatic trunks end in aortocaval lymph nodes located near the origin of the celiac plexus. The inferior lymphatic trunks end in lateroaortic nodes above the renal pedicle. Some trunks may pass through the diaphragm, following the splanchnic nerves, ending in retroaortic nodes in the posterior mediastinum. On the right, some lymphatic trunks may penetrate the liver.[2]

The adrenal gland is composed of a central catecholamine-producing medulla enveloped by the steroid-secreting cortex.

Although they are in intimate contact, they represent two functionally separate organs with different embryologic origins.

EPIDEMIOLOGY

Adrenal Cortical Tumors

Adrenocortical tumors are rare. Benign tumors are more common, occurring in 1% to 8% of the general population, and the incidence of carcinoma is approximately 1 per million population in the United States.[3,4] There are approximately 75 to 115 new cases per year.[5] Adrenal cortex carcinoma deaths account for 0.2% of all yearly cancer deaths. There is a bimodal age distribution with disease peaks before the age of 5 years and in the fourth to fifth decades of life.

Overall, adrenocortical carcinoma (ACC) is slightly more common in women than men. Nonfunctional carcinomas occur in an older age population (>30 years old) and are more common in men (3:2 male-to-female ratio), although functional tumors are more common in women (7:3 female-to-male ratio) and younger patients. As they frequently present with symptoms related to hormone production, functional tumors are usually detected at an early stage.

Although most cases of ACC are sporadic, it has been described as a component of several hereditary cancer syndromes, including Li-Fraumeni syndrome (breast cancer, soft tissue and bone sarcoma, brain tumors, and ACC), Beckwith-Wiedemann syndrome (Wilms' tumor, neuroblastoma, hepatoblastoma, and ACC), multiple endocrine neoplasia type I (parathyroid, pituitary and pancreatic neuroendocrine tumors, and adrenal adenomas and carcinomas), and SBLA syndrome (sarcoma, breast, lung, ACC, and other tumors).[6–9] A role for p53 mutations in sporadic ACC is suspected.

Adrenal Medulla Tumors

Ganglioneuromas are rare, benign tumors of the adrenal medulla seen in children and young adults.[10,11] Neuroblastoma is the most common malignant tumor of the adrenal gland in children, accounting for 90% of all cases.[3,12]

Pheochromocytomas and functional ganglioneuromas (or extra-adrenal pheochromocytomas) are rare tumors that rise from chromaffin cells in the adrenal medulla and elsewhere. They secrete catecholamines and cause intermittent, episodic, or sustained hypertension. Pheochromocytomas have an estimated prevalence of 0.1% in hypertensive patients.[13] In autopsy series, there is a 0.01% to 0.1% prevalence of unsuspected pheochromocytomas. Extra-adrenal tumors are more commonly malignant.[14] Estimates of the incidence of malignancy in pheochromocytoma range from 5% to 46% in different series.[15,16] Approximately 400 new cases of malignant pheochromocytomas are expected each year in the United States.[17,18]

Pheochromocytomas may be associated with a variety of endocrine and nonendocrine inherited disorders. Bilateral pheochromocytomas are a component of multiple endocrine neoplasia type IIa (MEN-IIA) syndrome (pheochromocytoma, medullary thyroid carcinoma, and parathyroid hyperplasia) or MEN-IIB syndrome in which they are associated with marfanoid habitus, mucosal neuromas, and medullary thyroid carcinoma. Pheochromocytomas occur in 25% of patients with von Hippel-Lindau syndrome and <1% of patients with neurofibromatosis and von Recklinghausen's disease.[19,20]

NATURAL HISTORY

Fifty-nine percent of adrenal cortex tumors are functional, the left-to-right ratio is approximately 1:1, and 2.4% are bilateral.[21] Diagnosis is frequently delayed because of the rarity of disease and the deep retroperitoneal location of the adrenal glands.[22]

TABLE 76.1 TNM STAGING FOR ADRENOCORTICAL CARCINOMA

Tumor (T)
T1: Tumor ≤5 cm in size; invasion absent
T2: Tumor >5 cm in size; invasion absent
T3: Tumor outside adrenal in fat
T4: Tumor invading adjacent organs
Lymph Nodes (N)
N0: No positive lymph nodes
N1: Positive lymph nodes
Metastases (M)
M0: No distant metastases
M1: Distant metastases
Stage I–T1, N0, M0
Stage II–T2, N0, M0
Stage III–T1, N1, M0, T2, N1, M0, T3, N0, M0
Stage IV–T3, N1, M0, T4, N1, M0, Any T, any N, M1

AJCC Cancer Staging Manual, 7th ed, New York, NY: Springer-Verlag, 2010.

Nonfunctioning ACCs are typically larger tumors, >6 cm, while functioning tumors tend to be discovered at an earlier stage (for TNM staging, see Table 76.1). Incidentally discovered adrenal masses <3 cm are rarely malignant. ACC is an aggressive malignancy that frequently violates the tumor capsule and invades surrounding tissues. It metastasizes to lungs, liver, brain, and regional lymph nodes. Many patients present with widespread metastasis; most of these patients die within 6 months of diagnosis. This situation is especially common in the pediatric population. For all stages, the 5-year overall survival is only 20% to 25%.[22]

Malignant pheochromocytomas exhibit a similar pattern of spread but also metastasize to bone. They are equally common in men and women. The average age of presentation is 40 to 50 years old, but these carcinomas may also occur in children.

CLINICAL PRESENTATION

Functional adrenocortical tumors most frequently secrete cortisol and androgens, resulting in Cushing syndrome, virilization, and hypertension. Estrogen or aldosterone production is less common. Approximately 60% of ACCs are functional. In a child, virilization is the most common symptom of ACC, and Cushing syndrome is relatively uncommon. By contrast, adults usually present with either Cushing syndrome alone or mixed with virilization. Patients with nonfunctioning tumors present with nonspecific symptoms related to tumor burden, including abdominal fullness, early satiety, pain, weight loss, weakness, fever, or an abdominal mass. Nonfunctioning ACCs are more common in older patients and tend to progress more rapidly. An increasing number of adrenal tumors are incidentally discovered during abdominal imaging in the absence of any symptoms.

Pheochromocytomas arising in the setting of an inherited disorder occur in the adrenal medulla in 90% of cases, as compared with 75% of sporadic pheochromocytomas. When associated with MEN-II syndromes, 80% are bilateral. A tumor >5 cm more commonly has a malignant course than a smaller lesion. Serum catecholamines and urinary metanephrine and vanillylmandelic acid levels are elevated in 90% of pheochromocytomas. These patients present with a range of symptoms from mild labile hypertension to sudden cardiac death secondary to hypertensive crisis, myocardial infarction, or cerebrovascular accident. The classic triad of symptoms consists of episodic headaches, diaphoresis, and tachycardia.[8,23] About half of patients have paroxysmal hypertension, and others have sustained hypertension. Pheochromocytomas may also present with normal blood pressure in 5% to 15%. Other symptoms may include pallor, palpitations, panic attack symptoms, or generalized weakness. Orthostatic hypertension may occur in association with hypovolemia.

DIAGNOSTIC WORKUP AND STAGING

Patients with adrenal gland tumors should be evaluated for other primary tumors, because metastasis to the adrenal gland is common. In metastatic tumors that are not adrenal in origin, a biopsy is recommended. Prior to obtaining a biopsy, however, pheochromocytomas must be ruled out by measuring the fractionated plasma-free metanephrine, as well as the 24-hour urine fractionated metanephrines and catecholamines. Furthermore, any patient with a suspected adrenal tumor should be screened for hormonal hypersecretion, including cortisol, aldosterone, and catecholamine secretion (Table 76.2). As hypercortisolism is the most frequent abnormality, serum cortisol, a 24-hour urinary cortisol, and an overnight dexamethasone suppression test should be obtained.

Morphologic evaluation of the adrenal glands with computed tomography (CT) of the abdomen should be performed as per adrenal protocol. CT of the abdomen with thin cuts through the adrenal gland is the imaging test of choice for the evaluation of adrenal tumors. Carcinomas can mimic adenomas but are characterized by larger size, irregular margins, and heterogenous enhancement. They may also demonstrate tumor necrosis and cystic degeneration. Local invasion, tumor extension into the vena cava, as well as lymph node or other metastases are often seen in advanced ACC. Magnetic resonance imaging (MRI) is useful in the evaluation of adrenal tumors (Fig. 76.1). ACC and pheochromocytomas are hyperintense on T2-weighted images, and venous invasion is better imaged on MRI. If there is still question of vascular invasion, an angiographic study can be performed preoperatively, either selective arteriography or vena cavography. Fluorodeoxyglucose positron emission tomography may be useful in differentiating benign from malignant lesions. It may also serve as an additional staging study for patients with known ACC. A chest CT should also be performed.

The diagnosis of pheochromocytoma is confirmed by measurements of urinary and plasma fractionated metanephrines and catecholamines. Medication-induced elevation of metanephrine levels is common and should be evaluated prior to initiating further costly workup. Levels of metanephrine 4 times the normal limit are diagnostic of pheochromocytoma, and biochemical confirmation of disease is followed by imaging to locate the tumor. Other scans, including the OctreoScan (Mallinckrodt Inc., St. Luis, MO) and a bone scan, may be indicated if metastatic disease is suspected.

Levels of plasma aldosterone (high) and renin (low) activity should be assessed when suspecting primary aldosteronism (hyperaldosteronism). The ratio of aldosterone to renin above 30 is suggestive of hyperaldosteronism and should be confirmed with saline suppression or salt loading tests, and electrolytes should be measured. Although malignant hyperaldosteronism is rare, these patients require an open adrenalectomy to prevent tumor rupture. In benign cases of hyperaldosteronism, adrenal vein sampling for aldosterone is considered standard of care.

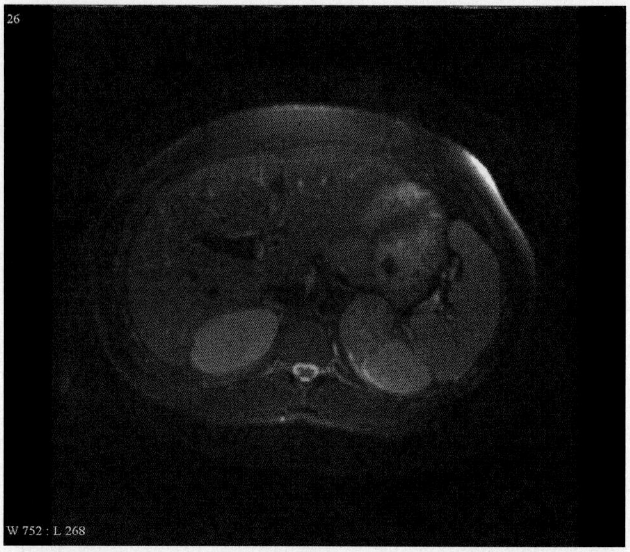

FIGURE 76.1. T2-weighted magnetic resonance image of a 35-year-old woman with a left adrenal carcinoma.

Patients with Cushing syndrome require an evaluation of serum levels of corticotropin, cortisol, as well as the sex steroid dehydroepiandrosterone sulfate (DHEA-S). If cortisol levels are elevated, a confirmatory test with dexamethasone suppression is recommended. It is important to remember that elevated corticotropin levels do not indicate adrenal origin, and further workup is necessary to look for primary causes of increased corticotropin. Benign adrenal tumors can be removed laparoscopically. Patients who present with Cushing syndrome in the presence of large (>5 cm), inhomogeneous, or invasive masses should be suspected to have malignant tumors, and imaging of the chest, abdomen, and pelvis is warranted to look for metastasis.

Pathologic Classification

Tumors <6 cm are more likely adenomas, although some smaller tumors may be malignant (Table 76.3). Hemorrhage and necrosis may be observed macroscopically in carcinomas. Numerous mitotic figures and cellular undifferentiation are common microscopic findings. Larger size, vascular invasion, or invasion of surrounding tissues and numerous mitotic figures are poor prognostic features.[24]

Pheochromocytomas have malignant features in <10% of cases. Macroscopically, they tend to be encapsulated with

TABLE 76.2 DIAGNOSTIC WORKUP FOR ADRENAL TUMORS

General
History
Physical examination
Radiology
Chest CT
Abdominal CT with thin cuts
Magnetic resonance imaging
Ultrasonography
Angiographic studies
Nuclear medicine studies
Fluorodeoxyglucose positron emission tomography
Laboratory studies
Complete blood count, blood chemistry, urinalysis
Serum and urine cortisol (adrenal cortical tumors)
Serum and urine catecholamines (pheochromocytoma)

CT, computed tomography.

TABLE 76.3 CLASSIFICATION OF ADRENAL TUMORS

Adrenal cortex
Adenoma
Functioning
Nonfunctioning
Carcinoma
Adrenal medulla
Ganglioneuroma
Pheochromocytoma
Neuroblastoma
Mixed type (ganglioneuroblastoma)
Connective tissue tumors
Myelolipomas
Lipomas
Myomas
Angiomas
Fibromas
Fibrosarcoma

areas of cystic change, hemorrhage, and necrosis. The capsule is frequently invaded, but that does not constitute malignant change. Benign and malignant pheochromocytomas may appear identical histologically. The only absolute criterion for malignancy is metastasis.[9] Histologically, cell size, nuclear size, and arrangement of cells are variable. A twisted cell cord pattern, basophilic or cytophilic staining with fine intracytoplasmic pigment granules, and periodic acid-Schiff staining of secretory droplets aid in the diagnosis.

GENERAL MANAGEMENT

Benign tumors are nonfunctioning and are most often found incidentally. After the benign nature of these tumors is confirmed, small tumors can be left untreated and can be followed up by repeat imaging 6 to 12 months after diagnosis to confirm their stability. Larger tumors (>4 cm) should be followed up with imaging in 3 to 6 months after diagnosis. A small benign mass that grows at the rate of >1 cm per year can be removed electively, but any significant growth of a larger mass should alert the clinician to a potentially malignant nature of the tumor and adrenalectomy is recommended in that case.

Nonfunctioning adrenal tumors that are >4 cm, are heterogenous, or have irregular margins are suspicious for adrenal carcinomas. Surgery with removal of adjacent lymph nodes is the primary treatment for ACC. Complete resection is the only treatment that offers long-term disease-free survival, but it is not always feasible. For patients with a macroscopically complete resection, a margin-free resection is a strong predictor for survival. Efforts to avoid tumor spillage are warranted, and the tumor capsule should remain intact. Invasion or adherence of adjacent structures often necessitates *en bloc* resection of the kidney or spleen, partial hepatectomy, or pancreatectomy. The presence of tumor thrombus in the renal vein or vena cava does not preclude resection. A lymphadenectomy is often included. The role of tumor debulking in the presence of metastatic disease is not clear. Incomplete resection of the primary tumor or metastatic disease not amenable to surgery is associated with a poor prognosis. Still, tumor debulking may help control hormonal oversecretion or relieve local symptoms in certain cases. Even with a complete resection, local recurrence and metastatic disease are common. For isolated distant metastases and locally unresectable disease, cytoreductive resection with or without radiation is recommended.

The role of radiation in the management of ACC is not well defined. It has been proposed as adjuvant therapy in high-grade adrenal carcinoma as well as after complete resection or as management of microscopic residual disease. One series reports a 10-year crude survival rate of 33% for surgical resection followed by adjuvant radiation.[25] External radiation results in good response rates and effective palliation in patients with residual macroscopic disease or bone or nodal metastasis.[18,26]

Mitotane, a chemical congener of the insecticide DDT (dichlorodiphenyltrichloroethane), is an adrenolytic compound with specific activity on the adrenal cortex. It is the chemotherapeutic agent most commonly used in the management of ACC. In patients with measurable disease, overall response rates of 14% to 36% have been reported, but most studies have reported no significant survival benefit.[27] The largest retrospective study from Italy and Germany that included 177 patients with resected ACC (stages I to III) showed improvements in disease-free survival and overall survival.[28] Unfortunately, responses are usually partial and transient, with only an occasional complete remission.[21] The role of mitotane as adjuvant therapy after complete surgical resection is questionable. Despite limited supporting data, it is frequently employed in this setting, given the high rates of locoregional and distant recurrence. Serum levels of mitotane are monitored in order to optimize therapy because objective response in the metastatic setting was associated with higher serum levels (>14 mg/L). Unfortunately, increased toxicity is also associated with higher serum levels. Side effects are predominantly gastrointestinal, particularly nausea, but anorexia and diarrhea also occur. Although less common, central nervous system toxicity can include lethargy, somnolence, ataxia, dizziness, or confusion.

Single-agent chemotherapy has proven disappointing in the management of ACC. Doxorubicin and cisplatin have both been evaluated as single-agent therapy and in combination with mitotane. Neither drug was efficacious.[29] Multiagent chemotherapy has shown more promise. A multicenter phase II study by the Italian Group for the Study of Adrenal Cancer demonstrated 49% overall response rate using a regimen of etoposide, doxorubicin, and cisplatin in combination with mitotane. The regimen was well tolerated. The most common side effects were gastrointestinal. The time to progression in responding patients was 2 years.[6] Inclusion of mitotane in a multidrug regimen is rational as ACCs are prone to multidrug resistance mediated by the multidrug resistance-1/P glycoprotein drug pump, whose mechanism is inhibited by mitotane. This multidrug regimen is worthy of further study.

Surgical resection is the definitive management of pheochromocytoma, but it is a high-risk procedure. Cardiovascular and hemodynamic parameters must be monitored closely. Preoperative medical therapy is aimed at controlling hypertension and expanding intravascular volume. Preoperative pharmacologic preparation typically includes combined α- and β-adrenergic blockade.

In patients with undiagnosed pheochromocytomas who undergo surgery for other reasons, surgical mortality rates are high because of lethal hypertensive crisis and multiorgan failure.[30] In the largest series of 147 patients undergoing surgery for pheochromocytoma, perioperative mortality and morbidity rates were 2.4% and 24%, respectively.[31] Although it results in rapid symptomatic control, surgical removal of a pheochromocytoma does not always lead to a long-time cure. In a large series of 176 patients, pheochromocytoma recurred in 16% of patients. Half of these recurrences were malignant.[32] In patients with bilateral pheochromocytomas, usually in the setting of an inherited syndrome, bilateral adrenalectomy is recommended. Hormone replacement is required in this setting. Although not curative, debulking surgery for control of symptoms is the primary therapy for malignant pheochromocytoma.

The radioisotope iodine-131 metaiodobenzylguanidine (^{131}I-MIBG) has been used as a therapeutic agent in malignant pheochromocytomas that demonstrate avid uptake of the agent. Investigators have reported partial responses, based on biochemical response as well as decreased tumor volume, ranging from 18% to 82%.[33–35] Symptomatic improvement was observed in responding patients with regard to both painful metastases and manifestations of increased catecholamine levels. Partial remissions are usually temporary, with some patients relapsing between doses of MIBG. In other patients, sustained partial remissions have been noted with durable palliation extending 2 to 3 years.[34,36] Prolonged survival has been associated with measurable responses and higher administered doses of MIBG (>500 mCi).[37] Toxicity includes bone marrow toxicity (particularly thrombocytopenia), nausea, and vomiting.

Combination chemotherapy with cyclophosphamide, vincristine, and dacarbazine has shown efficacy in a small study. In 14 treated patients, the clinical and biochemical response rates were 57% and 79%, respectively. Response was associated with objective improvement in performance status and blood pressure, and treatment was well tolerated.[38]

RADIATION THERAPY TECHNIQUES

The role of radiation in the management of ACC is controversial. Locoregional disease control remains a major problem in this disease, and some reports suggest that external radiation may reduce recurrence rates.

In the primary management of ACC, external radiation may play a role either preoperatively for unresectable tumors, postoperatively for patients with residual disease or high risk of local failure, or as definitive therapy for patients who are medically unfit for surgery. Radiation is also effective in the palliative setting for bone and nodal metastases.

For patients with macroscopic or unresectable disease, doses of 50 to 60 Gy delivered during 5 to 6 weeks should be considered. Initial fields should encompass the gross tumor with adequate margins as well as the regional lymph nodes, which should include the contralateral para-aortic lymph nodes. Dose to regional nodes can be limited to 45 Gy when they are not macroscopically involved. Care should be taken to limit dose to the spinal cord, kidneys, liver, and small bowel. For macroscopic disease for which high dose is desired, conformal techniques and intensity-modulated radiation should be considered. For patients receiving postoperative treatment for high-risk or microscopic disease, doses of 45 to 54 Gy are appropriate.

In the palliative setting, doses of 30 to 40 Gy given during the course of 2 to 3 weeks are reasonable. In patients with painful bone metastases, hypofractionated regimens should be considered for patients with poor performance status or otherwise limited life expectancy.

External-beam radiation is limited to a palliative role in the management of pheochromocytomas.

FOLLOW-UP

Patients with pheochromocytomas should have frequent follow-up that includes a thorough history and physical examination with an evaluation of vital signs and plasma markers. This should be done every 6 months for the first 3 years starting around 3 months postsurgery and annually thereafter. Advanced or persistent disease may require more frequent follow-up and symptom management.

REFERENCES

1. Moore K, Agur A. *Essential clinical anatomy.* Baltimore: Lippincott Williams & Wilkins, 2002:182–185.
2. Rouvière H. *Anatomie des lymphatiques de l'homme.* Paris: Masson, 1932.
3. Dunnick NR. Adrenal carcinoma. *Radiol Clin North Am* 1994;32:99–108.
4. McClennan BL. Oncologic imaging. Staging and follow-up of renal and adrenal carcinoma. *Cancer* 1991;67:1199–1208.
5. Shambaugh E, Ryan R. *Summary staging guide for the cancer surveillance, epidemiology and end results reporting (SEER) program.* Rockville, MD: US Dept of Health and Human Services, Public Health Service, 1977.
6. Berruti A, Terzolo M, Sperone P, et al. Etoposide, doxorubicin and cisplatin plus mitotane in the treatment of advanced adrenocortical carcinoma: a large prospective phase II trial. *Endocr Relat Cancer* 2005;12:657–666.
7. Bravo EL. Evolving concepts in the pathophysiology, diagnosis, and treatment of pheochromocytoma. *Endocr Rev* 1994;15:356–368.
8. Bravo EL. Pheochromocytoma: new concepts and future trends. *Kidney Int* 1991; 40:544–556.
9. Cotran A, Kumar V, Robbins SL. *Robbins pathologic basis of disease,* 5th ed. Philadelphia: WB Saunders, 1994:1161–1164.
10. Hubbard MM, Husami TW, Abumrad NN. Nonfunctioning adrenal tumors. Dilemmas in management. *Am Surg* 1989;55:516–522.
11. De Maria M, Barbiera F, Bonadonna F, et al. Diseases of the adrenal medulla. *Rays* 1992;17:62–86.
12. Miller RW, Fraumeni JF Jr, Hill JA. Neuroblastoma: epidemiologic approach to its origin. *Am J Dis Child* 1968;115:253–261.
13. Beard CM, Sheps SG, Kurland LT, et al. Occurrence of pheochromocytoma in Rochester, Minnesota, 1950 through 1979. *Mayo Clin Proc* 1983;58:802–804.
14. Melicow MM. One hundred cases of pheochromocytoma (107 tumors) at the Columbia-Presbyterian Medical Center, 1926–1976: a clinicopathological analysis. *Cancer* 1987;40:1987–2004.
15. Beierwaltes WH, Sisson JC, Shapiro B. Malignant potential of pheochromocytoma. *Proc Am Acad Cancer Res* 1986;27:617.
16. Cryer PE. Phaeochromocytoma. *Clin Endocrinol Metab* 1985;14:203–220.
17. Javadpour N, Woltering EA, Brennan MF. Adrenal neoplasms. *Curr Probl Surg* 1980;17:1–52.
18. Percarpio B, Knowlton AH. Radiation therapy of adrenal cortical carcinoma. *Acta Radiol Ther Phys Biol* 1976;15:288–292.
19. Loughlin KR, Gittes RF. Urological management of patients with von Hippel-Lindau's disease. *J Urol* 1986;136:789–791.
20. Nakagawara A, Ikeda K, Tsuneyoshi M, et al. Malignant pheochromocytoma with ganglioneuroblastoma elements in a patient with von Recklinghausen's disease. *Cancer* 1985;55:2794–2798.
21. Wooten MD, King DK. Adrenal cortical carcinoma. Epidemiology and treatment with mitotane and a review of the literature. *Cancer* 1993;72:3145–3155.
22. Haak HR, Hermans J, van de Velde CJ, et al. Optimal treatment of adrenocortical carcinoma with mitotane: results in a consecutive series of 96 patients. *Br J Cancer* 1994;69:947–951.
23. Stein PP, Black HR. A simplified diagnostic approach to pheochromocytoma. A review of the literature and report of one institution's experience. *Medicine* 1991;70:46–66.
24. King DR, Lack EE. Adrenal cortical carcinoma: a clinical and pathologic study of 49 cases. *Cancer* 1979;44:239–244.
25. Magee BJ, Gattamaneni HR, Pearson D. Adrenal cortical carcinoma: survival after radiotherapy. *Clin Radiol* 1987;38:587–588.
26. Markoe AM, Serber W, Micaily B, et al. Radiation therapy for adjunctive treatment of adrenal cortical carcinoma. *Am J Clin Oncol* 1991;14:170–174.
27. Pommier RF, Brennan MF. An eleven-year experience with adrenocortical carcinoma. *Surgery* 1992;112:963–971.
28. Terzolo M, Angeli A, Fassnacht M, et al. Adjuvant mitotane treatment for adrenocortical carcinoma. *N Engl J Med* 2007;356:2372–2380.
29. Ahlman H, Khorram-Manesh A, Jansson S, et al. Cytotoxic treatment of adrenocortical carcinoma. *World J Surg* 2001;25:927–933.
30. Lo CY, Lam KY, Wat MS, et al. Adrenal pheochromocytoma remains a frequently overlooked diagnosis. *Am J Surg* 2000;179:212–215.
31. Plouin PF, Duclos JM, Soppelsa F, et al. Factors associated with perioperative morbidity and mortality in patients with pheochromocytoma: analysis of 165 operations at a single center. *J Clin Endocr Metab* 2001;86:1480–1486.
32. Amar L, Servais A, Gimenez-Roqueplo AP, et al. Year of diagnosis, features at presentation, and risk of recurrence in patients with pheochromocytoma or secreting paraganglioma. *J Clin Endocr Metab* 2005;90:2110–2116.
33. Shapiro B, Gross MD, Shulkin B. Radioisotope diagnosis and therapy of malignant pheochromocytoma. *Trends Endocrinol Metab* 2001;12:469–475.
34. Shapiro B, Sisson JC, Wieland DM, et al. Radiopharmaceutical therapy of malignant pheochromocytoma with [131I]metaiodobenzylguanidine: results from ten years of experience. *J Nucl Biol Med* 1991;35:269–276.
35. Sidhu S, Sywak M, Robinson B, et al. Adrenocortical cancer: recent clinical and molecular advances. *Curr Opin Oncol* 2004;16:13–18.
36. Loh KC, Fitzgerald PA, Matthay KK, et al. The treatment of malignant pheochromocytoma with iodine-131 metaiodobenzylguanidine (131I-MIBG): a comprehensive review of 116 reported patients. *J Endocrinol Invest* 1997;20:648–658.
37. Safford SD, Coleman RE, Gockerman JP, et al. Iodine-131 metaiodobenzylguanidine is an effective treatment for malignant pheochromocytoma and paraganglioma. *Surgery* 2003;134:956–962.
38. Averbuch SD, Steakley CS, Young RC, et al. Malignant pheochromocytoma: effective treatment with a combination of cyclophosphamide, vincristine, and dacarbazine. *Ann Intern Med* 1988;109:267–273.

Part L Lymphoma and Hematologic Tumors

Chapter 77
Hodgkin Lymphoma

Richard T. Hoppe

The management of Hodgkin lymphoma (HD) continues to evolve. Since the last edition of this text, molecular imaging has taken on an expanded role as a means for "interim evaluation," that is, individualization of subsequent therapy based upon the imaging response after just a portion of treatment has been completed. Programs of combined-modality therapy have been established as the standard for early-stage disease, although challenges to the use of radiation in this setting have been raised. New, more precise techniques for radiation therapy delivery have been adopted. For the first time in more than three decades, a new systemic agent has been approved by the U.S. Food and Drug Administration (FDA) for treatment of Hodgkin lymphoma. Large prospective, randomized clinical trials have enabled us to refine treatments, and data regarding late effects continue to influence the development of management approaches.

ANATOMY

Hodgkin lymphoma almost always begins in lymph nodes. More than 80% of patients with Hodgkin lymphoma present with cervical lymph node involvement, and >50% have mediastinal disease. Isolated extralymphatic involvement in the absence of nodal disease is rare.

EPIDEMIOLOGY AND RISK FACTORS

The reported incidence of Hodgkin lymphoma is slightly less than 3 per 100,000. It accounts for 0.56% of all cancers diagnosed but only 0.23% of all cancer deaths in the United States each year, a death rate that decreased by more than one-third between 1990 and 2006 (0.85 per 100,000 to 0.56 per 100,000).[1] There is a slight male predominance (1.2:1). Hodgkin lymphoma is rare in children <10 years of age. The median age of patients at the time of diagnosis is 26 years, and the incidence has a bimodal peak as a function of age.[2] The early peak, from ages 25 to 30 years, shows an incidence of approximately 5.5 per 100,000 per year. A second peak, from age 75 to 80 years, shows a similar incidence. However, this peak in older adults may be "contaminated" by cases that were actually anaplastic large-cell or diffuse large-cell lymphoma.

Geographic clusters of patients with HD have been reported, but these are probably only coincidental.[3] A relation between HD and previous infection with Epstein-Barr virus (EBV) has been proposed.[4] Weiss et al.[5] identified components of the EBV genome in the cellular DNA of Reed–Sternberg cells in lymph nodes involved by Hodgkin lymphoma. In addition, Mueller et al.[6] identified elevated levels of immunoglobulin G and immunoglobulin A against the EBV capsid antigen and elevated levels of antibody against the EBV nuclear antigen and early antigen D in the serum of patients with Hodgkin lymphoma 3 to 156 months *before* the diagnosis of Hodgkin lymphoma.

The risk for development of Hodgkin lymphoma is 2.55 times higher among individuals who have a history of infectious mononucleosis than among noninfected control subjects.[7] Several series demonstrated an association between EBV infection and mixed-cellularity Hodgkin lymphoma, especially in children in developing countries. An international analysis based on 1,546 patients with Hodgkin lymphoma showed an increased risk for EBV-associated Hodgkin lymphoma in Hispanics (vs. Whites), those with mixed-cellularity histologic subtype (vs. nodular sclerosis), children from economically less developed (vs. more developed) regions, and young adult men (vs. women).[8] However, the ultimate relationship between EBV infection and development of Hodgkin lymphoma remains undefined. Studies attempting to link occupational exposures or other etiologic factors with the development of Hodgkin lymphoma have been inconclusive or contradictory.[3]

NATURAL HISTORY AND CLINICAL PRESENTATION

Patients with Hodgkin lymphoma usually present with painless lymphadenopathy. Some may note systemic symptoms such as unexplained fevers, drenching night sweats, weight loss, generalized pruritus, fatigue, and alcohol-induced pain in tissues involved by Hodgkin lymphoma. Still other patients are diagnosed after detection of a mediastinal mass on a routine chest radiograph.

If contiguity is assumed among the supraclavicular lymph nodes and upper para-aortic nodes/celiac axis/spleen, 90% of patients present with contiguous sites of involvement.[9,10] In addition, disease spread after treatment with limited irradiation also occurs in a contiguous fashion in most instances.[9] The theory of contiguity of spread and the development of treatment programs including presumptive treatment of uninvolved sites were important conceptual advances in the treatment of Hodgkin lymphoma in the latter half of the twentieth century.

Organ involvement by Hodgkin lymphoma may be secondary to extension from adjacent lymph nodes, such as spread from enlarged mediastinal or bronchopulmonary (pulmonary hilar) nodes directly into the pulmonary parenchyma, or it may be hematogenous, such as nodular disease in the liver or multiple bony sites. Involvement of the bones may cause blastic changes, especially in the vertebrae (creating the classic "ivory vertebra" on plain radiographs), pelvis, sternum, or ribs.

The mechanism of spread of disease to the spleen is unclear. However, the likelihood of disseminated disease, including bone marrow and liver involvement, increases as the extent of disease in the spleen increases.[11] Nearly all patients with hepatic or bone marrow involvement by Hodgkin lymphoma have extensive involvement of the spleen.[12] Hodgkin lymphoma only rarely involves the gut-associated lymphoid tissues such as Waldeyer ring and Peyer patches. It also only rarely involves the upper aerodigestive tract, central nervous system, and skin.[9]

The rapidity of Hodgkin lymphoma growth and spread is not predictable. Disease may evolve over a period of several years, demonstrated on serial radiographs or suspected by clinical history, and it is unusual to document progression during evaluation and staging.

There are three "B symptoms" included as part of the staging system for Hodgkin lymphoma (see later discussion). They are fever, drenching night sweats, and significant weight loss. One-third of patients present with one of these symptoms. Fevers may present in the classic waxing-and-waning Pel-Ebstein pattern. Night sweats may be drenching and require a change of bedclothes. The B symptoms may occur even in patients with relatively limited disease (stage II) but are uncommon in stage I disease.

Historically, children have had a particularly good prognosis compared with adults, and therefore different treatment strategies have been developed for children (see Chapter 89).[13,14–15] More recently, the results of treatment programs in adults have improved to the same level enjoyed by children. Older adults (>60 years) have a worse prognosis, which often may be secondary to intercurrent illness or the ability to tolerate standard therapies, especially bleomycin, anthracyclines, and extended-field irradiation.[16,17]

Hodgkin lymphoma may be diagnosed during pregnancy, and many women become pregnant after successful treatment. Special treatment considerations are warranted for the pregnant patient; however, no evidence exists that pregnancy *per se* has any effect on the natural history of the disease.[18,19,20] Although patients infected with human immunodeficiency virus type 1 do not appear to be at increased risk for development of Hodgkin lymphoma, the disease tends to behave differently in infected persons.[21,22,23]

DIAGNOSTIC WORKUP

Diagnostic and staging procedures commonly used for Hodgkin lymphoma are listed in Table 77.1. Patient age and the presence of intercurrent disease influence the selection of staging studies.[24–26]

Hematologic evaluation may reveal anemia, leukopenia, lymphopenia, or thrombocytosis. This is often a paraneoplastic effect, but it may be indicative of bone marrow involvement. Anemia, lymphopenia, and hypoalbuminemia are adverse prognostic factors, especially for patients with advanced disease (stage III–IV).[27] The serum alkaline phosphatase level may serve as a nonspecific marker of tumor activity or hepatic, bone marrow, or bone disease. The erythrocyte sedimentation rate (ESR) may correlate with response to treatment and subsequent disease activity and is a prognostic factor for patients with limited disease (stage I–II).[28] Other useful markers may include the lactate dehydrogenase and β_2-microglobulin levels.

Radiographic evaluation should include posteroanterior (PA) and lateral chest radiographs. Mediastinal adenopathy may be quantitated by a measurement of the maximum width of the mediastinal mass divided by the maximum intrathoracic diameter (near the level of the diaphragm) on a standing PA chest radiograph, as shown in Figure 77.1. When this ratio exceeds 1:3, the disease is defined as bulky, and this affects assignment to many clinical trials. Other definitions of bulky mediastinal adenopathy include a mass >10 cm and a ratio of mediastinal mass to the chest diameter at T5-6 exceeding 0.35 (employed in European Organization for the Treatment of Cancer [EORTC] clinical trials). Contrast-enhanced (diagnostic) computed tomographic (CT) scans of the chest, abdomen, and pelvis may reveal adenopathy or organ involvement. If irradiation to the cervical nodes is contemplated, a CT scan of the neck may be indicated in order to identify their precise location for treatment planning. Lymph nodes are usually considered to be enlarged on CT if their short axis measurement exceeds 1 cm.[29] Splenomegaly or hepatomegaly alone cannot be interpreted to represent involvement by Hodgkin lymphoma because enlarged spleens often are not involved at the time of splenectomy; however, the presence of focal nodules is usually indicative of involvement.

Positron emission tomography (PET) using 2-fluoro-2-deoxy-D-glucose (FDG), especially with fused CT images (PET-CT scan), has become an important component of initial staging in

TABLE 77.1 DIAGNOSTIC AND STAGING PROCEDURES FOR HODGKIN LYMPHOMA

History
Systemic B symptoms: unexplained fever, drenching night sweats, weight loss >10% of body weight in the last 6 mo
Other symptoms: alcohol intolerance, pruritus, respiratory problems, fatigue
Physical examination
Palpable nodes (note number, size, location, shape, consistency, mobility)
Palpable viscera
Laboratory studies
Complete blood count, differential, platelets
Erythrocyte sedimentation rate
Serum albumin, lactate dehydrogenase, liver function studies
Blood urea nitrogen, creatinine
Pregnancy test in women of childbearing age
Radiographic studies
Chest radiographs: posteroanterior and lateral
Contrast-enhanced computed tomographic (CT) scan of thorax, abdomen, and pelvis
Contrast-enhanced CT scan of neck (if neck irradiation is indicated)
Integrated positron emission tomography-CT scan
Additional biopsies, if indicated
Bone marrow, needle biopsy (if subdiaphragmatic disease or B symptoms)
Cytologic examination of effusions, if present
Percutaneous liver biopsy if abnormal liver function tests but normal CT

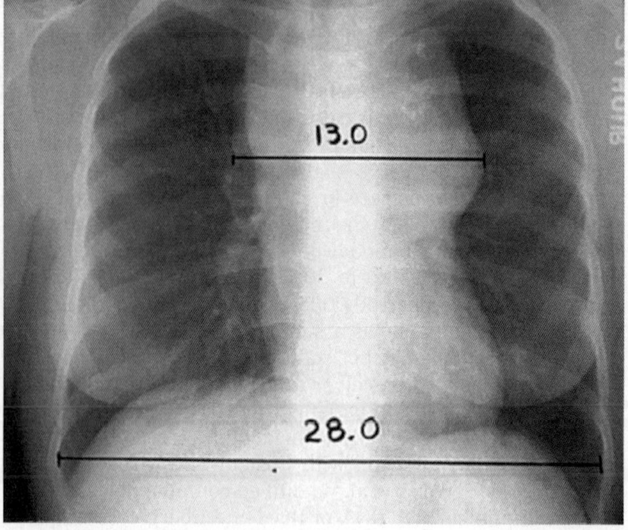

FIGURE 77.1. The mediastinal mass ratio (MMR). This ratio is defined as the maximum single horizontal mediastinal mass measurement divided by the maximum intrathoracic diameter, which is usually near the diaphragm. In this example, MMR = 13.0/28.0 = 0.46.

Hodgkin lymphoma. FDG-PET is more sensitive than CT for detecting disease.[30] It may even reveal unsuspected bone or bone marrow disease.[31] PET-CT is an essential study for response assessment, is particularly useful for the evaluation of residual masses detected by CT scanning, and may even be a useful prognostic indicator when repeated after just a portion of chemotherapy has been administered.[29,32,33]

Magnetic resonance imaging may be an alternative to chest or abdominal-pelvic CT scanning for initial staging but has not been used widely.[34] Its main value may be in the staging evaluation of women during pregnancy.[19]

A needle biopsy of the posterior iliac crest bone marrow is appropriate in selected patients. Because the yield is exceedingly low in asymptomatic patients with limited clinical disease, it should be restricted to patients with B symptoms or clinical evidence of subdiaphragmatic disease. The overall incidence of bone marrow involvement in Hodgkin lymphoma is only ~5%.

STAGING

The Ann Arbor staging system for Hodgkin lymphoma, used since 1971, is outlined in Table 77.2.[35] The lymphoid regions defined in this system are shown in Figure 77.2. The Ann Arbor system includes designation of a clinical stage, based on the results of the initial biopsy and clinical staging studies, and a pathologic stage, based on the results of any subsequent biopsies, including bone marrow biopsy and those obtained at staging laparotomy. With the exclusion of laparotomy, the generic term *stage* is now usually employed and reflects the final stage designation after completion of all appropriate staging studies. Deficiencies of the Ann Arbor system include its failure to consider bulk of disease and its lack of a more precise definition of the E-lesion (extralymphatic involvement).[36]

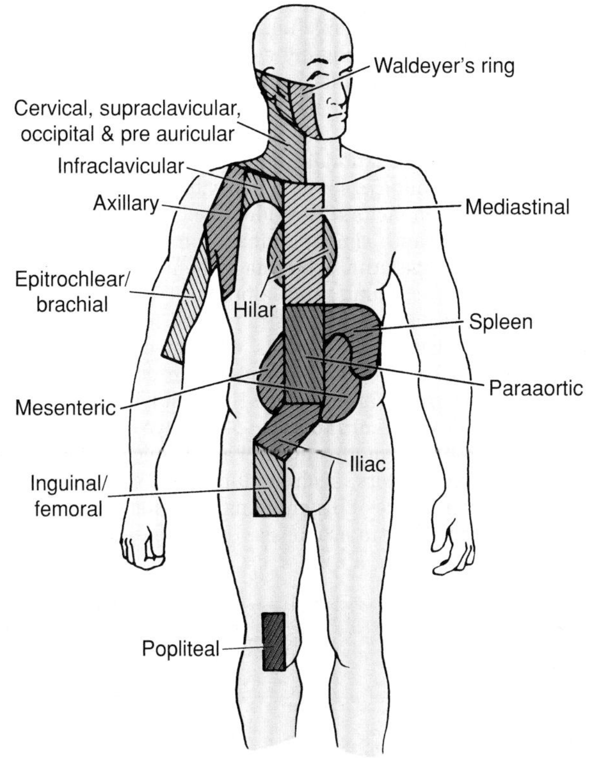

FIGURE 77.2. The lymph node regions as defined in the Ann Arbor staging system. Note that the ipsilateral supraclavicular, cervical, preauricular, and occipital nodes are defined as a single region. The mediastinum and pulmonary hila are defined as separate regions. (From Hoppe RT. The non-Hodgkin lymphomas: pathology, staging, treatment. *Curr Probl Cancer* 1987;11:363–447; with permission.)

TABLE 77.2 THE ANN ARBOR STAGING CLASSIFICATION FOR HODGKIN'S DISEASE

Stage I	Involvement of a single lymph node region
Stage II	Involvement of two or more lymph node regions on the same side of the diaphragm (II), or localized involvement of an extralymphatic organ or site and one or more lymph node regions on the same side of the diaphragm (IIE)
Stage III	Involvement of lymph node regions on both sides of the diaphragm (III), which may also be accompanied by involvement of the spleen (IIIS) or by localized involvement of an extralymphatic organ or site (IIIE) or by both (IIISE)
Stage IV	Diffuse or disseminated involvement of one or more extralymphatic organs or tissues, with or without associated lymph node involvement

The absence or presence of fever, night sweats, and/or unexplained loss of 10% or more of body weight in the 6 mo before diagnosis is denoted by the suffix letter A or B, respectively.

However, the Cotswolds modification of the Ann Arbor system employs the subscript "x" to designate large mediastinal adenopathy.[37]

PATHOLOGIC CLASSIFICATION

The neoplastic cell of classic Hodgkin lymphoma is the Reed–Sternberg cell. It is typically binucleate, with a prominent, centrally located nucleolus in each nucleus, a well-demarcated nuclear membrane, and eosinophilic cytoplasm with a perinuclear halo. However, these cells usually account for <1% of the cells in a lymph node involved by Hodgkin lymphoma. The majority are lymphoid cells, eosinophils, plasma cells, and other normal cells.[38]

Reed–Sternberg cells probably originate from B-lineage cells at various stages of development, including pre–B-cell and germinal center B-cell origin.[39,40] In most instances, the Reed–Sternberg cells stain positively with the lymphocyte activation marker CD30, PAX5, and with variable expression of the anti-granulocyte monoclonal antibody CD15. CD20, a marker of mature B cells, may be expressed on a minority of tumor cells with variable intensity in as many as 40% of cases. They stain negatively with CD45, ALK, and J chain.[41]

There are five histologic subtypes of Hodgkin lymphoma as defined by the World Health Organization modification of the Lukes and Butler system. These include nodular lymphocyte-predominant Hodgkin lymphoma and four subtypes of classic Hodgkin lymphoma: nodular sclerosis, mixed cellularity, lymphocyte-rich, and lymphocyte-depleted.[42]

Nodular lymphocyte predominant Hodgkin lymphoma (nLPHD) is characterized by an abundance of normal-appearing lymphocytes and a scarcity of abnormal cells. Unlike the other subtypes of Hodgkin lymphoma, the abnormal cells ("L and H cells" or "popcorn cells") in nLPHD are strongly reactive for CD20, CD45, CD79a, and PAX5 and negative for CD15 and CD30.[38,41] nLPHD is often diagnosed in young people. Patients frequently present with early-stage disease, usually in a solitary peripheral nodal site, and systemic symptoms are uncommon (<10%). The natural history is the most favorable of the histologic subtypes. Occasional patients demonstrate a pattern of late relapse but good survival, similar to that observed in the follicular (B-cell) lymphomas. Some investigators suggest that nLPHD would be more appropriately considered a form of non-Hodgkin B-cell lymphoma.[43,44–45] As part of its natural history, as many as 14% of patients with nLPHD may transform to an aggressive B-cell lymphoma.[46] A reactive process termed *progressive transformation of germinal centers* may be observed in conjunction with nLPHD.[47,48]

The other four histologic subtypes of Hodgkin lymphoma are variants of *classic Hodgkin lymphoma* (cHD). The Reed–Sternberg cells in these cases are CD15+, CD30+, PAX5+, and occasionally CD20+. *Nodular sclerosis classical Hodgkin lymphoma* (NSHD) is the most common histologic subtype diagnosed in developed countries. Involved nodes often have a thickened capsule and are traversed by broad bands of birefringent collagen that surround nodules of cells consisting of lymphocytes, eosinophils, plasma cells, and tissue histiocytes intermixed with a variable proportion of atypical mononuclear cells and Reed–Sternberg cells. These cells may be in empty (lacunar) spaces, which are artifacts of formalin fixation. The syncytial variant refers to cases in which there are prominent cellular aggregates of atypical cells and histiocytes. The clinical presentation includes common mediastinal involvement, and one-third of patients have B symptoms. The natural history of NSHD is less favorable than that of nLPHD.

Mixed-cellularity classic Hodgkin lymphoma (MCHD) is characterized by a diffuse effacement of lymph nodes by lymphocytes, eosinophils, plasma cells, and relatively abundant atypical mononuclear and Reed–Sternberg cells. Patients with MCHD present more commonly with advanced disease and tend to be slightly older than those with NSHD or nLPHD. The natural history of MCHD is less favorable than that of NSHD.

Lymphocyte-rich classic Hodgkin lymphoma (LRHD) is a relatively recently described entity.[49,50] It usually has a nodular growth pattern, but occasionally it has a diffuse one. Previously, many cases of LRHD may have been confused with nLPHD; however, the staining characteristics of the malignant cells in LRHD clearly are consistent with those of classic Hodgkin lymphoma. The clinical characteristics of patients affected by LRHD are similar to those of nLPHD, that is, early stage, absence of B symptoms, and excellent prognosis.

Lymphocyte-depleted classic Hodgkin lymphoma (LDHD) is variable in its microscopic appearance but is generally characterized by a paucity of normal-appearing cells and an abundance of abnormal mononuclear cells, Reed–Sternberg cells, and Reed–Sternberg variants. This subtype may be difficult to differentiate from anaplastic large-cell lymphoma.[51] It is an exceedingly uncommon subtype of Hodgkin lymphoma. It tends to occur in older patients and is more likely to be associated with advanced disease and B symptoms. It has the worst prognosis of all histologic subtypes of Hodgkin lymphoma.[52]

In addition to these major subtypes, *interfollicular Hodgkin lymphoma* is an uncommon pattern of focal involvement of a lymph node in which there is reactive hyperplasia with a small focus of Hodgkin lymphoma in the interfollicular zone. It is easy to confuse these cases with reactive lymphoid hyperplasia.[53]

Table 77.3 summarizes the characteristics of patients treated according to the major histologic subtypes of Hodgkin lymphoma at Stanford University from 1989 to 2010. These characteristics are similar to those reported from many other large centers in the United States and western Europe. However, the distribution of histologic subtypes and clinical behavior reported from South America, Asia, Africa, Eastern Europe, and even some parts of the United States indicates a greater proportion of unfavorable histologic subtypes and more aggressive clinical behavior in these developing areas.[54,55]

TABLE 77.3 MAJOR HISTOLOGIC SUBTYPES CORRELATED WITH CLINICAL CHARACTERISTICS OF 615 ADULT PATIENTS TREATED FOR HODGKIN LYMPHOMA AT STANFORD UNIVERSITY (1989–2011)

	LPHD	NSHD	MCHD
Number of patients (%)	40 (7)	468 (76)	49 (8)
Age (yr)			
Range	15–85	15–83	17–81
Median	45	30	35
Male:female ratio	23:17	228:241	32:17
Stage			
I (%)	14 (36)	30 (6)	10 (21)
II (%)	14 (36)	272 (58)	14 (29)
III (%)	11 (28)	89 (19)	12 (25)
IV (%)	0	78 (17)	12 (25)
B symptoms (%)	4 (10)	147 (31)	16 (33)

LPHD, lymphocyte-predominant Hodgkin lymphoma; MCHD, mixed-cellularity Hodgkin lymphoma; NSHD, nodular sclerosis Hodgkin lymphoma.

PROGNOSTIC FACTORS AND THERAPEUTIC IMPLICATIONS

Because most patients with Hodgkin lymphoma are cured, prognostic factors are more important for defining therapy than for predicting outcome. Historically, when treatment programs were less effectie, prognostic factors did have great importance in predicting survival.[56]

The Ann Arbor stage is likely the most important factor influencing therapy. Data generated at a time when treatment programs were more limited show a marked impact of stage on prognosis. With current management programs, this distinction has been blurred.

The bulk of disease is important, especially in the mediastinum. Bulk may be defined by absolute measurements, ratio of mass to anatomic measurements, surface area on radiographs, or volumetric determinations. In general, the risk of relapse after treatment with single-modality therapy is greater in the presence of bulky mediastinal disease than in nonbulky disease.[57] For this reason, combined-modality therapy is the established standard for patients with bulky disease.[58,59,60–63]

Other measurements of disease severity that may influence treatment selection for Hodgkin lymphoma are the presence of B symptoms, the number of sites of involvement, and the elevation of serum markers such as the ESR. Sophisticated assessments of total tumor burden correlate very well with prognosis.[64]

The histologic subtype of Hodgkin lymphoma has little impact on therapy, with the exception of identification of cases of nLPHD, for which different treatment algorithms will apply.[62] Interobserver agreement among pathologists regarding subclassification is not perfect,[65] and after the extent of disease has been determined, histologic subtype of classical Hodgkin lymphoma has little additional impact on prognosis.

Large series report a slightly worse outcome for men than for women.[1] However, gender is more important because of its influence on the choice of treatment secondary to potential reproductive complications (see Sequelae of Treatment).

An important international study evaluated a series of prognostic factors among 5,141 patients with advanced Hodgkin lymphoma.[27] Seven factors were identified, each of which had an independent and similar impact on prognosis. These included gender, age, Ann Arbor stage, hemoglobin, white cell count, lymphocyte count, and albumin (Table 77.4). This International Prognostic Score is now used for assignment of patients to clinical trials. Patients who have three or more adverse risk factors are often considered to be in an unfavorable prognostic group for advanced Hodgkin lymphoma.

Patients with stage I or II disease often have only one or two adverse factors based on this index. Large clinical trials groups have found other factors, such as number of sites of disease, age, ESR, and presence of B symptoms, to be helpful in stratifying patients according to prognosis. Unfortunately, the criteria

TABLE 77.4 INTERNATIONAL PROGNOSTIC SCORE FOR ADVANCED HODGKIN LYMPHOMA

Factor	Unfavorable Covariate
Serum albumin	<4 g/dL
Hemoglobin	<10.5 g/dL
Sex	Male
Age	≥45 yr
Stage	IV (Ann Arbor)
Leukocyte count	≥15,000/mm^3
Lymphocyte count	<600/mm^3 or <8% of white count

TABLE 77.5 DEFINITION OF "UNFAVORABLE" STAGE I TO II HODGKIN LYMPHOMA IN RECENT CLINICAL TRIALS

	EORTC	GHSG[a]	NCIC	Stanford
Age (yr)	≥50	–	≥40	–
Histology	–	–	MC/LD	–
ESR/B symptoms	≥30 mm with any B ≥50 mm without B	≥30 mm with any B ≥50 mm without B	≥50 mm or Any B sx	Any B sx
Mediastinal mass	MTR ≥0.35	MMR >0.33	MMR >0.33	10 cm or MMR >0.33
Number of nodal sites	≥4	≥3	≥4	–
E-lesion	–	Any	–	–

Patients with one or more of these factors were considered to have "unfavorable" condition.

E, extralymphatic; EORTC, European Organization for Research and Treatment of Cancer; ESR, erythrocyte sedimentation rate; GHSG, German Hodgkin Study Group; LD, lymphocyte depleted; MC, mixed cellularity; MMR, maximum mediastinal width/maximum chest width on chest x-ray; MTR, maximum mediastinal width/chest width at T5–T6 on chest x-ray; NCIC, National Cancer Institute, Canada; sx, symptoms.

[a]Patients with B symptoms and either E-lesion or large mediastinal mass treated in advanced disease clinical trials.

for defining "unfavorable" presentations of stage I–II disease vary among clinical trial groups (Table 77.5).

GENERAL MANAGEMENT

Radiation Therapy

Radiation therapy is the most effective therapeutic agent for treating Hodgkin lymphoma and has been used in its management for more than a century.[66] Optimal irradiation technique includes careful pretreatment evaluation of disease sites, precise simulation and the use of megavoltage photon beams, fields individually contoured to the patient's anatomy and tumor configuration, an adequate dose, multifield fractionated treatment, and portal film verification during therapy. Careful attention must be paid to every detail of therapy in order to maximize outcome and minimize risks.[67,68]

Chemotherapy

The initial successful drug combination for treating Hodgkin lymphoma was nitrogen mustard, vincristine, procarbazine, and prednisone (MOPP), reported by DeVita et al.[69] from the National Cancer Institute in 1970. The acute toxicities of treatment at that time were significant and included nausea, vomiting, peripheral neuropathy, constipation, leukopenia, and thrombocytopenia. Late effects of concern included sterility (especially in men) and the risk for secondary myelodysplastic syndrome or leukemia. A number of MOPP-like programs, such as chlorambucil, vinblastine, procarbazine, and prednisone (ChlVPP), achieve comparable results with similar drugs and less toxicity.[70]

With the introduction of doxorubicin (Adriamycin), completely novel drug combinations were developed. The most successful of these is ABVD, which includes doxorubicin, bleomycin, vinblastine, and dacarbazine.[71] ABVD has replaced MOPP as the gold standard of chemotherapy for Hodgkin lymphoma. This is based largely on the results of an intergroup trial that compared MOPP, ABVD, and MOPP/ABVD.[72]

More recently, in an effort to reduce toxicity, the Stanford V regimen, which almost always includes a component of radiation, was developed as an alternative to ABVD. As another approach, in an effort to enhance efficacy, the German Hodgkin Study Group (GHSG) developed the BEACOPP regimen, which may be administered in a baseline, escalated, or 14-day schedule.[73] Table 77.6 summarizes the dosages and scheduling of these drug combinations.[70]

Most recently, a completely new systemic agent has been approved by the FDA for the treatment of Hodgkin lymphoma. Brentuximab vedotin (BV) is an anti-CD30 monoclonal antibody linked to an antitubulin agent. BV has demonstrated efficacy in CD30+ lymphomas, including Hodgkin lymphoma and anaplastic large-cell lymphoma. It is approved for patients who have had disease recurrence after stem cell transplantation and is being introduced in clinical trials to define its possible use in other settings.[74]

TABLE 77.6 COMMON DRUG COMBINATIONS USED IN THE TREATMENT OF HODGKIN LYMPHOMA

Drug Combination	Agents	Dose (mg/m²)	Route	Treatment Day(s)	Cycle Duration (Days)
ABVD	Doxorubicin[a]	25	IV	1, 15	28
	Bleomycin	10	IV	1, 15	
	Vinblastine	6	IV	1, 15	
	Dacarbazine	375	IV	1, 15	
Stanford V	Doxorubicin[a]	25	IV	1, 15	28
	Vinblastine	6	IV	1, 15	
	Nitrogen mustard	6	IV	1	
	Vincristine[b]	1.4	IV	8, 22	
	Bleomycin	5	IV	8, 22	
	Etoposide	60	IV	15, 16	
	Prednisone	40	PO	Every other day	
BEACOPP	Bleomycin	10	IV	8	21
	Etoposide	100 (200)[c]	IV	1–3	
	Doxorubicin[a]	25 (35)[c]	IV	1	
	Cyclophosphamide	650 (1250)[c]	IV	1	
	Vincristine[b]	1.4	IV	8	
	Procarbazine	100	PO	1–7	
	Prednisone	40	PO	1–14	
	G-CSF		SC	8–14	

IV, intravenous; PO, oral; SC, subcutaneous.

[a]Adriamycin.

[b]Maximum, 2 mg.

[c]Higher dose is for BEACOPP escalated.

Combined-Modality Therapy

Combined-modality therapy has become the most common form of general management for patients with Hodgkin lymphoma. Important considerations include the sequence of therapy, the selection of irradiation fields, the decision to irradiate all involved sites, only initially "bulky" sites, or only sites that have not responded completely to chemotherapy, the prescription of dose, and potential overlapping toxicities. Treatment is almost always initiated with chemotherapy. This has the advantages of treating all sites of disease at the outset (especially important in stage III or IV) and reducing bulky disease to facilitate subsequent irradiation (especially in the mediastinum). The irradiation dose used in combined-modality studies in adults ranges from 20 to 36 Gy.

RADIATION THERAPY TECHNIQUES

The principal objective of radiation therapy in Hodgkin lymphoma is to treat involved nodes and regions at high risk for containing disease to a dose associated with a high likelihood

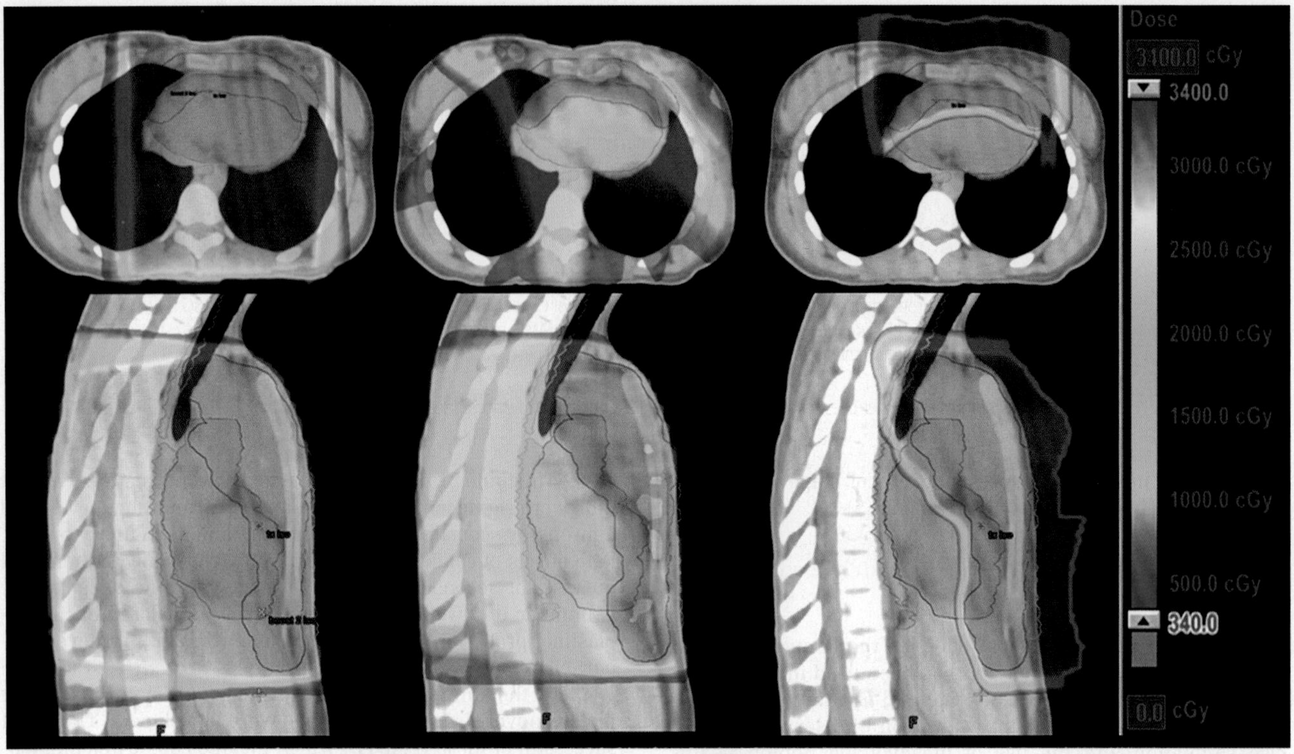

FIGURE 77.3. Color-wash dose distributions for three different plans for treating mediastinal Hodgkin lymphoma: axial sections (*top*) and sagittal sections (*bottom*) for conventional photon three-dimensional conformal anteroposterior/posteroanterior fields (*left*), intensity-modulated radiation therapy photon (*middle*), and anterior proton field (*right*). Green outline, esophagus; red outline, heart; pink outline, breasts; blue outline, clinical target volume. (Courtesy of Bradford S. Hoppe, MD, MPH.)

of tumor eradication. This requires thoughtful evaluation of all imaging studies, especially diagnostic CT and integrated PET-CT scans, a precise simulation with appropriate immobilization and consideration of organ motion, detailed treatment planning, and effective treatment delivery, including portal imaging and appropriate quality assurance measures.[67,68,75,76]

The most common techniques for field blocking include multileaf collimation, divergent Cerrobend (Cerro Metal Products, Bellefonte, PA) blocks attached to a Lucite (Lucite International, Southampton, United Kingdom) plate and mounted to the head of the machine, or a combination of both for complex-shaped fields. The use of body molds reduces body movement and rotation and may increase patient comfort.

For the majority of clinical scenarios, three-dimensional conformal treatment planning and opposed-field treatment is appropriate, but occasionally intensity-modulated radiation therapy (IMRT) may be indicated.[77] IMRT has the inherent advantage of better dose conformality, improved dose–volume histogram (DVH) criteria for the heart, coronary arteries, esophagus, and lungs, and less acute toxicity, but this is at the expense of the low-dose "bath," which may put larger volumes of normal tissue at risk for the development of secondary cancer, for example, the lungs, breasts (in women), and thyroid gland (Figs. 77.3 and 77.4). This remains a key consideration whenever the use of IMRT is contemplated. IMRT may be most useful in situations of reirradiation, when disease has relapsed in a previously treated site.

Routine three-dimensional (3D) CT simulation is required to optimize treatment field design and analyze DVHs in order to ensure adequate tumor coverage and sparing of organs at risk (OARs). When treatment includes the mediastinum, axillary, and supraclavicular areas, an arms-up position pulls the axillary nodes away from the chest wall and thereby permits more generous lung shielding but may result in an increased dose to the breasts and heart and an enhanced skin reaction in the supraclavicular area. An arms-down or akimbo position permits shielding of the humeral heads and minimizes skin reaction in the tissue folds of the supraclavicular/low neck regions and to the breasts.[78] When patients require separate treatment to adjacent regions, the calculation of field separation (gap) is exceedingly important.[79] Special additional cord blocking should be used, if possible, when adjacent fields overlie the spinal cord.

In the uncommon situations when radiation therapy alone is used for the treatment of Hodgkin lymphoma (primarily for nLPHD), the National Cancer Center Network (NCCN) guidelines recommend a dose of 30 to 36 Gy to involved and 25 to 30 Gy to uninvolved regions, fractionated at a rate of 7.5 to 10 Gy per week to involved sites.[62] Evenly weighted opposed-field treatments, all fields treated daily with fractions of 1.5 to 1.8 Gy, depending on field size and patient tolerance, are the general treatment recommendations. More commonly, radiation therapy is used in the combined-modality setting. Doses vary considerably in different trials, depending on the prognostic category of patients, bulk of disease, and type and duration of chemotherapy. The range of doses considered acceptable according to the NCCN guidelines is 20 to 30 Gy for nonbulky and 30 to 36 Gy for bulky sites of disease, 1.5 to 1.8 Gy per fraction.[62]

The classic field configurations for the treatment of Hodgkin lymphoma by radiotherapy alone included the mantle and inverted-Y. However, clinical trials have demonstrated an equivalence of "involved-field" treatment (IFRT) with "extended-field" or "subtotal-lymphoid" irradiation in the context of combined-modality therapy programs, and involved-field irradiation has been adopted as the standard for combined-modality therapy.[80–82] More recent trials are testing the application of even more restricted fields, referred to as "involved-node radiotherapy" (INRT; discussed later)[83] of "involved-region" or "involved-site" irradiation. Because these more limited fields are really portions of the classic treatment fields for Hodgkin lymphoma, an understanding of these classic fields makes the design of limited fields more logical.

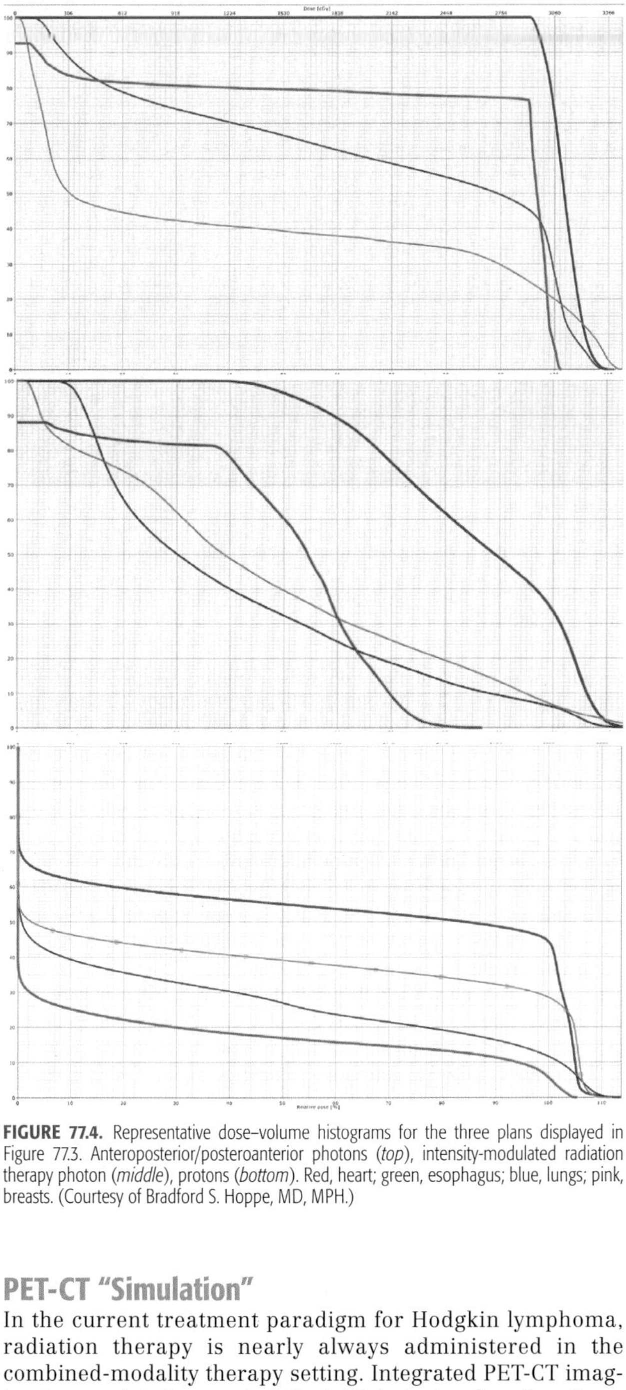

FIGURE 77.4. Representative dose–volume histograms for the three plans displayed in Figure 77.3. Anteroposterior/posteroanterior photons (*top*), intensity-modulated radiation therapy photon (*middle*), protons (*bottom*). Red, heart; green, esophagus; blue, lungs; pink, breasts. (Courtesy of Bradford S. Hoppe, MD, MPH.)

PET-CT "Simulation"

In the current treatment paradigm for Hodgkin lymphoma, radiation therapy is nearly always administered in the combined-modality therapy setting. Integrated PET-CT imaging is completed as part of the initial staging for all patients and provides accurate information regarding the initial extent of disease. However, this initial scan is not usually obtained in the treatment position or on a flat couch. After the completion of chemotherapy, the PET-CT scan is usually repeated, and generally one can expect normalization or near normalization of the PET component despite residual disease on CT.[84] After the radiation therapy simulation study has been completed (postchemotherapy), the data from the initial staging PET-CT may then be merged with it in order to localize the initial sites of disease. The accuracy of the registration will vary, depending on patient positioning for the two studies, and this needs to be accounted for in ultimate design of the treatment fields.

Supradiaphragmatic Fields

The classic mantle included all of the major lymph node regions above the diaphragm.[85] The field extended from the inferior portion of the mandible almost to the level of the insertion of the diaphragm. Individually contoured lung blocks conformed to the patient's anatomy and tumor localization. In addition to the lung blocks, blocks could be placed over the occipital region and spinal cord posteriorly, the larynx anteriorly, and the humeral heads both anteriorly and posteriorly. The use of these blocks depended on total dose planned and proximity of the adenopathy.

In the classic two-dimensional planned mantle field, the patient was set up supine, with the head fully extended. The superior margin of the field bisected the mandible and passed through the mastoid process. The lateral margins were set to flash the axillae (with humeral head blocks if the arms were at sides or akimbo). The inferior axillary margins were at the level of the inferior tips of the scapulae. The inferior mediastinal border was set at the level of the T10-11 interspace. The lung blocks were designed to provide ~1-cm margin around the mediastinal contours and also encompass the pulmonary hilar lymph nodes. The superiormost point of the lung blocks was no higher than the inferior tip of the head of the clavicle, with the tops of the lung blocks tapered laterally, often parallel to the projection of a posterior rib, in order to expose the high axillary/infraclavicular lymph nodes.

As noted previously, in contemporary management programs of combined-modality therapy, more limited fields are treated. Involved-field treatment includes just portions of the classic radiation treatment fields, and in the original definition implied treatment to the entirety of an involved lymphoid region when any portion of that region was involved. However, the definition of these regions, based on anatomic boundaries, is somewhat arbitrary. Logical considerations mandate modification of these regions in the context of individual patient management. For example, in the common scenario of supraclavicular disease (level IV) without disease any higher in the neck, the submaxillary and submandibular nodes (levels I and II) may be spared. On the other hand, the supraclavicular region is often included when the superior mediastinum is involved because a portion of the superior mediastinum actually superimposes on the lower supraclavicular area in the treatment position. The axillae are not treated unless they are involved. The two-dimensional design of these fields includes a superior border at the top or bottom of the larynx (depending on the extent of supraclavicular disease), lateral borders set at the coracoid processes of the scapulae (to include approximately two-thirds the length of the clavicle), and 0.5- to 1-cm margins beneath the clavicles. With 3D treatment planning, the initially involved lymph nodes (gross tumor volume [GTV]) and adjacent "at-risk" lymph nodes (clinical target volume [CTV]) are outlined on cross-sectional images, and field design is completed to ensure a dose range of 95% to 105% of the prescribed dose to the planning target volume (PTV). The CTV will generally extend 2 to 5 cm proximal and distal to initial PET- or CT-positive disease. The PTV expansion is then ~1 cm (Figs. 77.5A and 77.6).

In the setting of an initial large mediastinal mass, the postchemotherapy treatment fields can usually conform to the width of the residual disease only (unless there was pulmonary parenchymal extension), although the superior and inferior field margins should encompass the initial extent of disease, with margin as noted previously.[67] Although special techniques such as deep inspiration breath hold, active breathing control, and respiratory gating are infrequently used in treatment of Hodgkin lymphoma, they do demonstrate improvements in DVH criteria for the lungs and heart that would be especially useful in the setting of treatment for patients with large mediastinal masses.[86,87]

Organs at Risk

The dose range used for Hodgkin lymphoma (20 to 36 Gy) is below the threshold tolerance for many organs, including the spinal cord. However, intrathoracic structures may be affected by these doses, and careful review of dose–volume histograms is

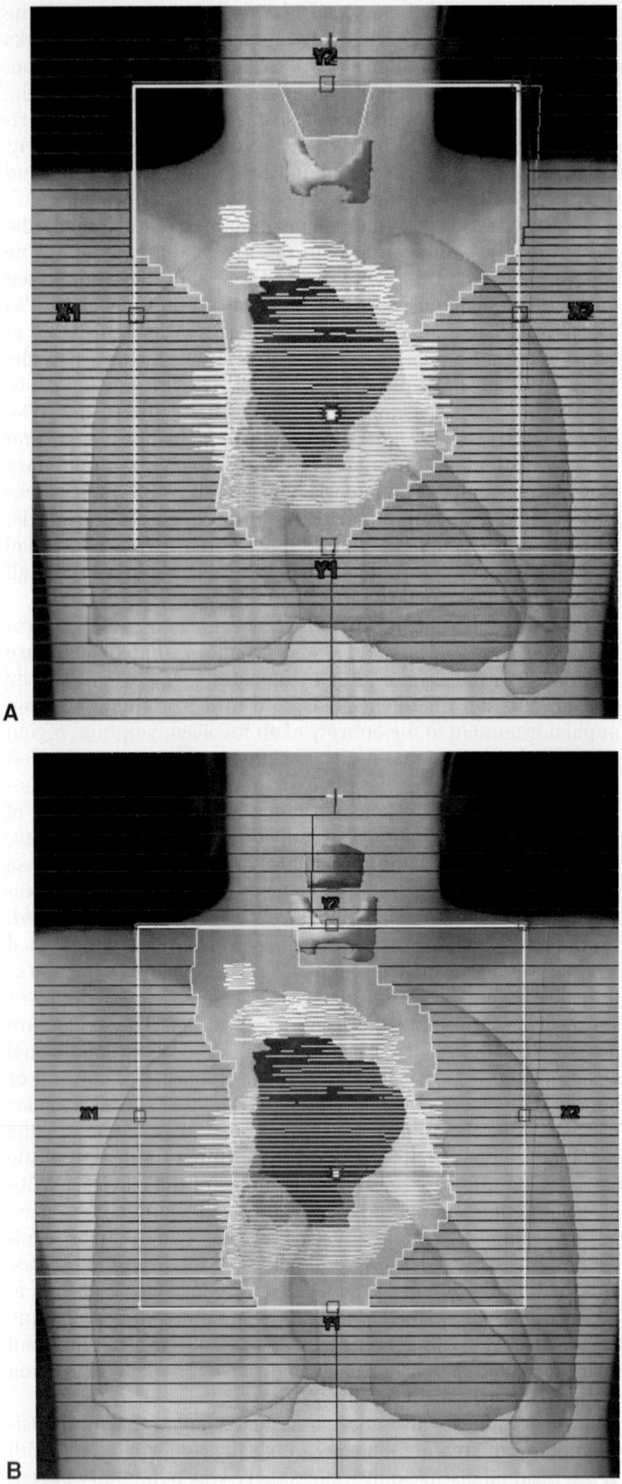

FIGURE 77.5. A 28-year-old man with massive mediastinal nodular sclerosis Hodgkin lymphoma and right supraclavicular disease, following completion of chemotherapy, with a negative positron emission tomography (PET) scan. White, pretreatment PET+ disease; black, postchemotherapy residual abnormality on computed tomography (CT). **A:** Design of a modified "involved field" to include the mediastinum, bilateral hila, and supraclavicular areas with an anterior larynx block. Note that inferiorly the field includes the entire length of the original extent of disease plus 2-cm margin. However, laterally the field encompasses only the residual disease on CT plus 2-cm margin. **B:** Design of an "involved-site" field.

warranted to minimize both acute and late effects. The risk for pneumonitis is related to volume of lung irradiated, total dose, and fraction size. The relationship between mean lung dose or V_x and pneumonitis is complex and may vary for different diseases and depend on patient age, smoking history, presence of intercurrent disease, prior chemotherapy, prior surgery, and

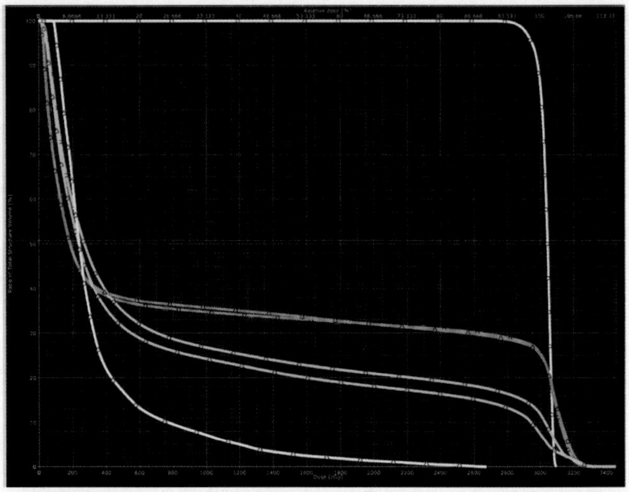

FIGURE 77.6. Representative dose–volume histograms for the fields displayed in Figure 77.5. Small triangles, involved field; small squares, involved site. Yellow, thyroid; pink, heart; blue, lungs. With this configuration of disease the most notable sparing of organs at risk is for the thyroid, with some sparing of the lungs. There is little difference in heart dose. If the disease was more superior in location, sparing of the heart using an involved region would have been more notable.

so on.[88] One study of patients with Hodgkin lymphoma identified a higher risk for Radiation Therapy Oncology Group grade 2 pneumonitis when the mean lung dose exceeded 14 Gy or the V_{20} exceeded 35%.[89] The likelihood of radiation-related pulmonary complications may be increased by the use of bleomycin,[90] and the effect that drug combinations with different doses of bleomycin may have on acceptable mean lung dose or V_{20} values is not known. A guideline followed at Stanford is not to exceed a mean lung dose of 15 Gy after treatment with ABVD or 17 Gy after treatment with Stanford V, treating with 1.5-Gy fractions. When these parameters have been followed, the risk for radiation pneumonitis has been negligible. With respect to late carcinogenesis, because data indicate that lung cancer risk may be increased after doses as low as 5 Gy, it is reasonable to define the lung V_5 and try to minimize it if multiple plans are reviewed.[91]

The criteria for cardiac dose tolerance are not well defined. Again, tolerances will be affected by comorbidities, family history, and prior treatment with cardiotoxic drugs such as doxorubicin. With respect to acute effects (pericarditis), limited data suggest keeping the mean pericardial dose to <26 to 27 Gy and the V_{30} to <46%.[92,93] Data for late cardiac events are less reliable; however, in one study of patients with Hodgkin lymphoma a threshold effect at 30 Gy was suggested for cardiac mortality.[94] A more conservative estimate, based on patients irradiated for breast cancer, is that a cardiac V_{25} of <10% is associated with a very low risk of cardiac mortality.[95] This level may be difficult to achieve in patients who present with large mediastinal adenopathy. Treatment techniques such as IMRT may succeed in reducing the cardiac dose but increase the V_5 to the lungs or V_4 to the breasts, resulting in a higher risk for secondary cancer in those organs (Figs. 77.3 and 77.4).

With respect to the breasts in women, given the excess risk of secondary breast cancer that exists for doses as low as 4 Gy, it is reasonable to track the breast V_4 and keep that volume as small as possible, especially for women <30 years of age.[96]

Subdiaphragmatic Fields

The classic subdiaphragmatic irradiation field for Hodgkin lymphoma was the inverted-Y, which included the retroperitoneal and pelvic lymph nodes and spleen. Sequential treatment to a mantle and inverted-Y field was referred to as *total lymphoid irradiation* (TLI); if the subdiaphragmatic field did not include the pelvis, the term *subtotal lymphoid irradiation* was used.

Currently, in the context of combined modality therapy, common radiation therapy fields include the spleen with or

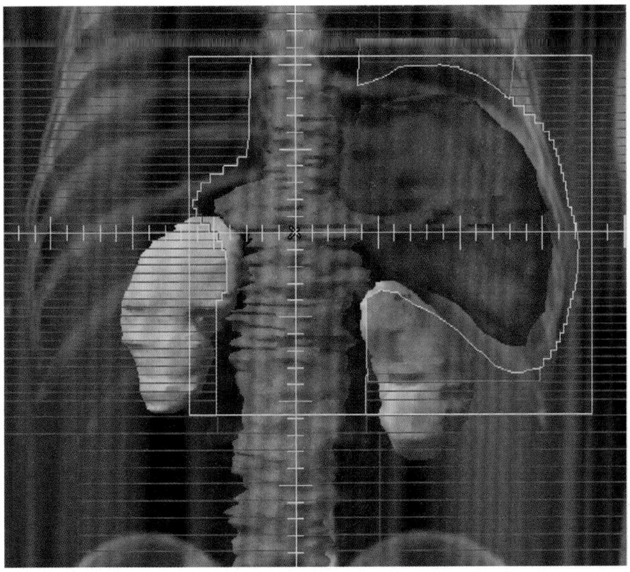

FIGURE 77.7. Example of a para-aortic–spleen field treated with respiratory gating. In this example there was a positron emission tomography+ node at the L1 level, and the inferior portion of the para-aortic field was set at the bottom of L2. The para-aortic nodes are highlighted in light red and the spleen in dark red. Due to the complex shape of this field, it is defined with a combination of multileaf collimators and Cerrobend blocks (shown in light orange) to shield the base of the left lung and the upper half of the left kidney.

without the para-aortic nodes (Fig. 77.7) and unilateral or bilateral pelvic fields (Fig. 77.8). In the two-dimensional design of a para-aortic field, the width of the field generally corresponds to the width of the transverse processes. The spleen may be treated in contiguity with this field. The design of the splenic field requires consideration of respiration and the use of generous (~2 cm) superior and inferior margins or respiratory gating. Three-dimensional planning for this field, especially if the spleen is being irradiated, is essential in order to more accurately localize the spleen and evaluate the DVH for the left kidney (Fig. 77.7). GTV, CTV, and PTV considerations for subdiaphragmatic nodal fields are similar to those for supradiaphragmatic fields, that is, GTV includes prechemotherapy disease on PET or CT, CTV includes 2 to 5 cm proximal and distal, and PTV expansion is 1 cm.

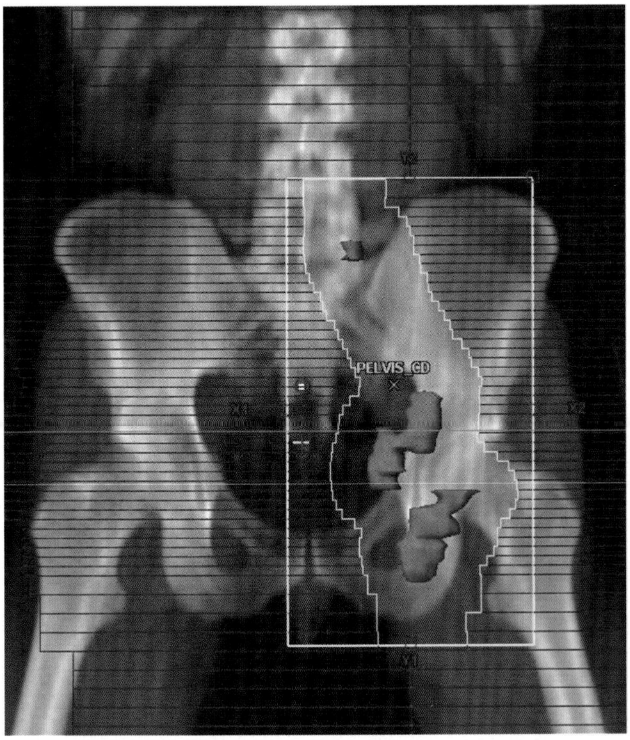

FIGURE 77.8. Typical anteroposterior/posteroanterior field for treating unilateral pelvic nodes, in this case for a 34-year-old man with stage IIA lymphocyte-predominant Hodgkin lymphoma. The initial positron emission tomography+ nodes are shown in blue. The field includes margins of at least 2 cm medial and lateral to the nodes and a field width of at least 6 cm.

Careful blocking considerations are required when the pelvic region is treated. Because the volume of marrow in the pelvis is substantial, the fields must be shaped carefully to minimize the amount of marrow treated (Fig. 77.8). With two-dimensional planning, the lateral margins are set 1.5 to 2 cm lateral to the widest point of the bony pelvis. Inferiorly, the pelvis field should extend to at least the lesser trochanters, unless there is disease that extends further inferiorly. Gonadal toxicity may also be an issue. In women, the ovaries normally overlie the iliac lymph nodes. To avoid irradiation-induced amenorrhea, an oophoropexy must be performed. This procedure is done by medial or lateral transposition of the ovaries via laparoscopy. The surgeon marks the ovaries with radiopaque sutures or clips and relocates them medially and as low as possible behind the uterine body. A double-thickness (10 half-value layers) midline block is then used; its location is guided by the position of the opacified nodes and transposed ovaries. When the ovaries are at least 2 cm from the edge of this block, the dose is decreased to 8% of that delivered to the iliac nodes.[97] Alternatively, one or both of the ovaries can be transposed laterally to a position overlying the iliac wings.

In men, if no special blocking is provided for the testes, the testicular dose may be as high as 10% of the dose delivered to the inguinal-femoral nodes. Use of a double-thickness midline block and a specially constructed testicular shield can reduce this dose to 0.75% to 3.0%, most of which results from internal scatter. The precise dose depends on the position of the testes in relation to the inferior margin of the inguinal-femoral field.

Involved-Node/Involved-Site Radiotherapy

In conjunction with the evolution of combined-modality therapy programs for all stages of Hodgkin lymphoma, the recognition that late effects may be reduced by using smaller radiation fields, and the introduction of sensitive functional imaging techniques, there has been an effort to continue to reduce radiation field size. The most recent iteration of this concept is the introduction of INRT.[83,98,99] As strictly defined by Girinsky et al.[83,98] representing the EORTC-GELA Lymphoma Group, INRT requires prechemotherapy diagnostic CT and PET-CT imaging with the patient in the treatment position, postchemotherapy contrast-enhanced CT simulation, and fusion of the prechemotherapy and postchemotherapy images. The fields are designed to treat only the initially involved nodes with modification to avoid OARs. This GTV then becomes the CTV, and a 1-cm expansion of the CTV defines the PTV.

When components of this planning process are missing, for example, the pretreatment PET-CT scan was not done in the treatment position, there is poor registration between scans, or the CT simulation scan was done without intravenous contrast, it may be risky to treat such strictly defined "involved-node" fields. However, field reduction is still possible to what one may term "involved-site" irradiation (Figs. 77.5B and 77.6).

Proton Beam Therapy

The potential dosimetric advantage of treatment with protons, as opposed to photons, is well established, and proton therapy is often employed in the management of prostate cancer and childhood tumors. There is also significant potential advantage of protons over photons (either 3D conformal radiation therapy [3DCRT] or IMRT) in the management of Hodgkin lymphoma. The use of proton beam therapy can be associated with decreased dose to the gut, bone marrow, and other organs but is especially advantageous with respect to mediastinal treatment.

Conventional 3DCRT with opposed fields minimizes lung exposure, but portions of the heart, especially the coronary arteries and valves, as well as of the esophagus, cannot be spared. IMRT plans can be quite conformal and spare those structures but at the expense of a low-dose "bath" that includes treatment to the breasts (in women) and lungs, with the potential risk for secondary cancer. With proton therapy, there can be maximal sparing of the esophagus, lungs, and cardiac subunits, thereby minimizing risk to those organs, while at the same time avoiding low-dose exposure to the breasts and lungs, minimizing potential risks and complications of therapy related to those organs (Figs. 77.3 and 77.4).[100,101–102,103] Experience is limited, but as more proton centers are established in the United States, it is likely that many patients with mediastinal Hodgkin lymphoma will be referred to these centers.

RESULTS OF THERAPY

Hodgkin lymphoma is responsive to both irradiation and chemotherapy, and a variety of programs may achieve similar survival rates. However, there may be significant differences in freedom from relapse and potential complications of therapy. The results described in the following sections emphasize treatment programs that have been identified as appropriate according to the guidelines of the NCCN.[62] The results achieved in recent clinical trials that have defined the current standards are displayed in Table 77.7.

Favorable Prognosis Stage I to IIA Classic Hodgkin Lymphoma

Favorable presentations of stage I to II include patients with stage I to II who do not have systemic symptoms or large mediastinal adenopathy. In some series from Europe and Canada, patients with an elevated ESR (>50), extralymphatic extension (E-lesion), multiple sites of disease (more than two or three), older age (>50 years), or unfavorable histology (mixed cellularity or lymphocyte-depleted) are also excluded and treated according to algorithms for intermediate prognosis (Table 77.7).[104]

Historically, patients with favorable presentations of stage I to II Hodgkin lymphoma were candidates for treatment with radiation therapy alone, with curative intent and expectations. The treatment volume generally included the mantle and para-aortic fields, as well as the spleen. Results in single-institution and cooperative group trials included 10-year survival rates of 90% and freedom from relapse rates of 80%.[57] These results are excellent, but the appearance of late risks of radiation therapy, including secondary neoplasia and cardiovascular disease, resulted in a shift of management to the use of combined-modality therapy.[105]

The current treatment of choice for these patients is abbreviated chemotherapy plus limited (IF) irradiation. The results of the HD-10 trial of the GHSG suggest that patients with very favorable presentations (no large mediastinal mass, no more than two sites of disease, no E-lesions, and ESR of <50 or <30 if B symptoms are present [see Table 77.7]) may be treated with just two cycles of ABVD, followed by 20-Gy IFRT (8-year survival [OS], 95.1%; freedom from treatment failure [FFTF], 85.9%; progression-free survival [PFS], 86.5%).[106] Other patients may be treated very effectively according to the regimen described by Bonadonna et al.[80]: ABVD times four followed by IFRT (12-year OS, 94%; freedom from progression [FFP], 94%), although the radiation dose may be reduced to 30 Gy. An alternative is to treat with 8 weeks of Stanford V chemotherapy, followed by 30-Gy IFRT (10-year OS, 96%; FFP, 94%; disease-specific survival, 99%).[107]

Important issues that have been addressed in recent clinical trials include further attenuation of the ABVD regimen by deletion of individual drugs but still incorporating IFRT (GHSG HD13 trial)[73] and trials testing the use of ABVD chemotherapy alone. The National Cancer Institute Canada HD6 trial included treatment with ABVD alone, but the comparison arms included subtotal lymphoid irradiation *alone* for the favorable patients (age, <40 years; lymphocyte predominance or nodular sclerosis histology; ESR, <50; and fewer than four involved regions) and 2 months of ABVD, followed by subtotal lymphoid irradiation for patients with any unfavorable characteristics. Although neither radiation therapy–containing arm would currently be considered appropriate management, the FFP in the two radiation-containing arms of the trial was superior to that of ABVD alone (93% vs. 87%; $p = .006$).[108] In the design of this study, patients randomized to receive ABVD alone underwent repeat CT imaging after two

TABLE 77.7 REPRESENTATIVE RESULTS FROM SELECTED CLINICAL TRIALS FOR EARLY, INTERMEDIATE, AND ADVANCED STAGES OF HODGKIN LYMPHOMA

Clinical Trial (Reference)	Treatment	Number of Patients	Percent Receiving RT	FFP % (Year)	OS % (Year)	Median Follow-Up (Month)
Early stage						
Milan (80)	ABVD x4 + IF 36–40 Gy	70	100	94 (12)	94 (12)	116
NCIC (108)	ABVD x4–6	196	0	87 (5)	96 (5)	50
EORTC H8F (82)	MOPP/ABV x3 + IF 36–40 Gy	270	100	93 (10) (EFS)	97 (10)	92
GHSG HD10 (106)	ABVD x2, 4 + 20-, 30-Gy IF	1190	100	86–90 (8) (FFTF)	94–95 (8)	90
Stanford G4 (107)	Stanford V chemo x8 wk + 30-Gy IF	87	100	94 (5)	94 (5)	120
Intermediate stage						
EORTC H7 (205)	MOPP/ABV x6 + IFRT 36–40 Gy	193	100	88 (10) (EFS)	87 (10)	NR
EORTC H8U (82)	MOPP/ABV x4, 6 + IFRT 36–40 Gy	669	100	80–82 (10) (EFS)	85–88 (10)	92
GHSG HD11 (61)	ABVD x4 + IFRT 30 Gy	356	100	81–87 (5) (FFTF)	94–95 (5)	91
ECOG E2496 (116)	ABVD x6–8 + 36-Gy RT	136	100	85 (5) (FFS)	95 (5)	66
	Stanford V + 36-Gy RT	131	100	77 (5) (FFS)	92 (5)	66
Advanced stage						
GHSG HD9 (206)	BEACOPPesc x8 ± RT 30–40 Gy	468	~66	87 (5) (FFTF)	91 (5)	48
UKNCRILGS ISRCTN64141244 (128)	ABVD x6–8 ± RT	261	53	76 (5) (PFS)	79 (5)	52
	Stanford V x12 wk + RT	259	73	74 (5) (PFS)	77 (5)	52
CALGB (207)	ABVD x6–8	115	0	54 (10) (EFS)	64 (10)	217
ECOG E2496 (127)	ABVD x6–8 + RT	404	40	73 (5) (FFS)	88 (5)	63
	Stanford V x12 wk + RT	408	73	71 (5) (FFS)	87 (5)	63
Italian (119)	ABVD x8 ± RT	166	66	73 (7)	84 (7)	NR
	BEACOPP x6 ± RT	156	67	85 (7)	89 (7)	NR

Selection criteria vary widely. See text and original papers for details.

CALGB, Cancer and Leukemia Group B; ECOG, Eastern Cooperative Oncology Group; EFS, event-free survival; EORTC, European Organization for the Research and Treatment of Cancer; FFP, freedom from progression; FFTF, freedom from treatment failure; FFS, failure-free survival; GHSG, German Hodgkin Study Group; IF, involved field; NCIC, National Cancer Institute of Canada; NR, not reported; OS, overall survival; RT, radiation therapy; UKNCRILGS, United Kingdom National Cancer Research Institute Lymphoma Group.

cycles of chemotherapy. Those patients who achieved a complete response or complete response undocumented (35% of patients) received two more cycles of ABVD and no further therapy. Of note, the 5-year FFP in this select group was ~95%.

Based on these data and consensus guidelines of the NCCN and the European Society for Medical Oncology (ESMO),[62,63] the most commonly employed treatment for favorable presentations of stage I to IIA Hodgkin lymphoma is combined-modality therapy with chemotherapy plus IFRT. The expected FFP is 90% to 95%. Selected patients may be treated with chemotherapy alone if radiation therapy is contraindicated and the increased risk for relapse is acceptable. Trials in progress (see later discussion) are testing whether interim PET imaging, done after as few as two cycles of ABVD, can help in identifying patients who are suitable for treatment with chemotherapy alone.

The use of radiation therapy alone has a long history in the successful treatment of early-stage Hodgkin lymphoma but has been abandoned for the reasons cited earlier. However, it remains a reasonable option for patients in whom there is a contraindication to chemotherapy.

Fewer than 10% of patients with stage I or II Hodgkin lymphoma present with involvement limited to subdiaphragmatic sites. For patients in whom disease is nonbulky and limited to pelvic lymph nodes with or without extension into the lower para-aortic nodes, the same general treatment principles apply to the management as for those with supradiaphragmatic presentations. In fact, many trials for stage I to II disease included such patients, and the most reasonable approach is to use combined-modality therapy, as outlined previously. In general, the outcome of treatment for these patients is equivalent to that of patients with supradiaphragmatic disease.[109,110]

Patients with bulky abdominal subdiaphragmatic presentations or those who have involvement of the spleen are generally treated according to guidelines for "unfavorable" stage I or II or else as stage III or IV disease.

Stage I to IIA Nodular Lymphocyte-Predominant Hodgkin Lymphoma

Contrary to the experience with classic Hodgkin lymphoma, it has been noted that patients with limited presentations of nLPHD may achieve long-term disease-free survival after treatment with involved-field or slightly extended field irradiation alone.[45,111,112] For example, for a high–cervical-stage IA presentation, treatment may be limited to the ipsilateral neck. For a femoral node presentation, treatment may be limited to the inguinal-femoral region with or without the ipsilateral iliac region. The usual dose is 30 to 36 Gy. There does not appear to be any benefit from the addition of chemotherapy in this setting. For example, in the retrospective review of experience with nLPHD in the GHSG, there was no significant difference in response induction, freedom from treatment failure, or overall survival for involved-field irradiation versus extended-field irradiation versus combined-modality therapy. Based upon these data and data from single-institution studies, the EORTC and GHSG adopted involved field irradiation alone, dose ~30 Gy, as the standard treatment for these patients, which also conforms with the guidelines of the ESMO and NCCN.[62,63] Lower doses have been tested, but responses have not been as durable as with conventional doses.[113]

Stage I to II Classic Hodgkin Lymphoma with Large Mediastinal Adenopathy

Patients with bulky mediastinal Hodgkin lymphoma (mediastinal mass greater than one-third of maximum intrathoracic diameter) are difficult to categorize by the Ann Arbor staging criteria and have a poor outcome when treated with single-modality therapy.[58] Early reports confirmed that these patients are best treated with combined-modality therapy.[57]

When the choice of chemotherapy is made for these patients, the potential overlapping toxicities of doxorubicin and bleomycin with irradiation (cardiac and pulmonary effects) should be considered. The recommended radiation dose in this situation varies from 20 to 36 Gy, but most data cite doses of at least 30 Gy for this cohort.[80,114] Doses in the higher part of the range may be considered when the response to chemotherapy is incomplete, PET imaging remains positive after chemotherapy, or the chemotherapy course is abbreviated.

Although ABVD remains the standard chemotherapy for this clinical presentation, both Stanford V and BEACOPP regimens have been tested in clinical trials. The GHSG HD11 trial for patients with intermediate prognosis, which included patients with large mediastinal adenopathy, elevated ESR, the presence of extranodal disease, or more than two sites of involvement, randomized the chemotherapy to BEACOPP baseline versus ABVD and the involved-field radiation therapy dose to 20 versus 30 Gy. The final analysis of that trial indicated that 20 Gy was sufficient only if BEACOPP chemotherapy was used but was inadequate in conjunction with ABVD. However, the toxicity of BEACOPP was greater, resulting in the adoption of ABVDx4 plus 30-Gy IFRT as the standard arm of the next trial of the GHSG, HD14.[61] The results for treatment with ABVDx4 plus 30 Gy included 5-year OS of 94%, PFS of 87%, and FFTF of 85%.

The Stanford V regimen has been used in the setting of patents with large mediastinal adenopathy. The 12-week chemotherapy program is followed by irradiation (30 Gy) to all sites >5 cm. In the setting of large mediastinal adenopathy this always included the mediastinum, but the bilateral hilar and supraclavicular areas were also included in the treatment fields.[115] The Eastern Cooperative Oncology Group (ECOG) compared treatment with ABVDx6–8 versus Stanford V × 12 weeks, in both cases followed by 36-Gy irradiation to mediastinum and bilateral hilar and supraclavicular areas (E2496). There were no significant differences in 5-year OS (95% and 92%) or FFS (85% and 77%).[116]

Based on consensus data, the most commonly employed treatment for stage I or II Hodgkin lymphoma in the presence of large mediastinal adenopathy is combined-modality therapy with chemotherapy plus IFRT. The expected FFP is 80% to 90%.

Stage IB or IIB Hodgkin Lymphoma

Approximately 15% to 20% of patients with stage I or II disease have B symptoms. In general, these patients are managed in a fashion analogous to those with stage III to IV disease. However, given the limited anatomic extent of disease in stage I to II, one can make a strong argument to include consolidative involved-field irradiation for these patients, as is recommended by the ESMO and NCCN.[62,63]

Stage III to IV Disease

Chemotherapy is the mainstay of treatment for patients with stage III to IV Hodgkin lymphoma.[117] With respect to the choice of chemotherapy, the landmark study was the prospective, randomized clinical trial conducted by the Cancer and Leukemia Group B. Patients with stage III_2A, IIIB, or IV Hodgkin lymphoma were randomly assigned to treatment with MOPP (six to eight cycles), MOPP/ABVD (12 months), or ABVD (six to eight cycles). The results of treatment with MOPP/ABVD and ABVD were equivalent, and both were superior to MOPP alone. Among the 115 patients treated with ABVD chemotherapy, the complete response rate was 82%, the 5-year FFS was 61%, and OS was 73%.[72] More recently, the "gold standard" of ABVD has been challenged by the GHSG, which developed the BEACOPP regimen and has demonstrated in a series of trials that results using BEACOPP escalated (often including irradiation) may be superior to those that can be achieved with ABVD. The GHSG HD9 trial compared BEACOPP escalated, BEACOPP baseline, and COPP/ABVD.[118] The outcome was best in the BEACOPP escalated arm, with 5-year FFTF of 87% and OS of 91%. However, in an Italian multi-institutional study that compared an initial treatment strategy of ABVD (four to eight cycles) with BEACOPP (four escalated plus four baseline), which took into account the possibility of autologous stem cell transplant as salvage therapy, there was no significant difference in 7-year freedom from second progression or OS (89% vs. 84%), and severe adverse events were more likely in the BEACOPP group.[119]

The use of combined-modality therapy in stage III to IV disease has a rationale because most patients who relapse after treatment with chemotherapy alone do so in sites of initial disease.[120] However, many of the early trials intended to resolve this issue were poorly designed, used chemotherapy programs that are no longer considered to be optimal, or had inadequate accruals. Nevertheless, many trials of systemic therapy for advanced disease have included the selective use of consolidative irradiation.[118,119,121]

The most definitive trial to address the question regarding effectiveness of consolidative irradiation is the EORTC–Groupe Pierre-et-Marie Curie H34 (20884) trial.[122] In this trial, patients were treated with six to eight cycles of nitrogen mustard, vincristine, procarbazine, prednisone, Adriamycin, bleomycin, and vinblastine chemotherapy, and those who achieved a complete response were randomized to no further therapy versus 25-Gy IFRT. No differences in FFTF or OS were identified. A detailed evaluation of causes of death revealed an unusually high risk for secondary myelodysplasia in the group of patients randomized to combined-modality therapy, although a similar risk was not observed in the nonrandomized patients, all of whom received irradiation to a somewhat higher dose! Those patients who achieved only a partial response (by CT criteria) received 30-Gy IFRT. The subsequent FFTF and OS for this group closely paralleled the outcome for patients who had achieved a complete response, suggesting a value to adding IFRT after only a partial response has been achieved.[123]

The GHSG HD12 trial was another effort to evaluate the impact of consolidative irradiation.[73,124] Patients were randomized to either of two different BEACOPP schedules with or without consolidative irradiation, 30 Gy to initial bulk or residual sites of disease. When analyzed "as treated," there was no significant difference in FFTF (90.4%, irradiated; 87%, nonirradiated) or OS. However, 14% of patients randomized to "no radiotherapy" were actually irradiated after a panel review of response to BEACOPP. This contamination compromises any ability to draw conclusions regarding the role of radiation therapy in advanced disease. The final conclusion of the study was that it *did not* support the omission of consolidative irradiation for patients with CT evidence of residual disease after chemotherapy.

Although the value of consolidative irradiation after complete response to conventional chemotherapy (ABVD or BEACOPP) has not been proved, there are programs of attenuated chemotherapy in which radiation therapy is an essential component. The Stanford V program includes only 12 weeks of chemotherapy, with very attenuated total doses of some of the drugs (see Table 77.7). Compared with six cycles of ABVD, there is only 50% of the cumulative dose of doxorubicin (Adriamycin) and 25% of the cumulative dose of bleomycin. Radiation therapy (30 to 36 Gy) is routinely added to initially bulky (>5 cm) sites of disease, as well as to macroscopic splenic involvement, and commences 1 to 3 weeks after completion of chemotherapy. The results of this approach have been excellent.[115,125] However, the radiation therapy component is essential, because a study that did not employ the same guidelines for radiation therapy resulted in a much worse outcome.[126] The ECOG E2496 trial compared management with ABVD versus Stanford V for patients with advanced-stage or locally advanced disease. There was no difference in 5-year FFS (73% for ABVD, 71% for Stanford V) or OS (88% for ABVD, 87% for Stanford V).[127] Lack of a difference between ABVD and Stanford V was also the result of the United Kingdom National Cancer Research Institute Lymphoma Group Study ISRCTN 64141244.[128]

A general conclusion regarding the role of combined-modality therapy compared with chemotherapy alone for patients with stage III to IV disease is that patients who achieve a complete response to a full course of conventional chemotherapy have no proven benefit from the addition of chemotherapy. Nevertheless, irradiation is often added to such programs on a selected basis, especially for bulky disease. In addition, programs of attenuated chemotherapy may realize a benefit from the addition of irradiation, and patients who achieve only a partial response to chemotherapy may have an improved outcome by the addition of irradiation. Ultimately, improved imaging and evaluation of early response to chemotherapy with FDG-PET imaging may help to identify a subset of patients who would truly benefit from consolidative irradiation (see section on Current Clinical Trials).

Pediatric Patients

Most contemporary programs for the management of pediatric Hodgkin lymphoma are based on clinical staging and use chemotherapy alone or combined-modality therapy with low-dose irradiation because higher doses of irradiation are associated with unacceptable risks for growth impairment and late effects.[13] To limit growth effects, irradiation doses should not exceed 15 to 25 Gy. Children treated with these programs, all stages combined, are reported to achieve 5-year OS rates of approximately 90% and relapse-free rates of at least 80%.[129–133]

Older Adult Patients

The treatment of Hodgkin lymphoma in older patients (>60 years) also poses a challenge.[17,134–136] They often have less favorable histology and worse performance status. They are more likely to have intercurrent disease that compromises the aggressive management programs used for younger people. Chemotherapy programs may often be modified to minimize cardiac or pulmonary toxicity, and the hematologic reserve in elderly patients more often results in dose reductions or premature discontinuation compared with younger patients.[137] Drug combinations that seem to be more tolerable for older adults include ChlVPP,[138] procarbazine, Alkeran, and vinblastine,[139] and vinblastine, bleomycin, and methotrexate (used primarily for stage I to II).[140] With respect to the radiation therapy, patients may need to be treated with slower fractionation programs and observed carefully for signs of weight loss or general decline in performance status. Extended fields are more difficult to tolerate than more limited fields.[16]

Treatment for Relapse

Treatment for relapse must be individualized. Initial disease characteristics, initial treatment and response duration, relapse sites, and general patient status must be considered in developing an effective secondary treatment program.

In general, patients who were treated initially with irradiation alone for stage I to II disease (now a relatively infrequent occurrence) should receive chemotherapy as the primary salvage treatment.[141,142] The efficacy of combination chemotherapy in this setting is similar to that achieved when chemotherapy is used in the primary management of advanced disease (rate of long-term freedom from relapse of 60% or better). The role of irradiation in combination with salvage chemotherapy has not been defined but is quite reasonable to consider if relapse is in a previously unirradiated site.[143]

More problematic is the management approach to patients who present initially with stage I to II disease and are treated with chemotherapy alone, a group for whom consensus best treatment has not been reached.[62] In these patients, relapse may be restricted to initial sites of disease and be quite limited.[144] It is possible that in this situation programs using irradiation alone, or at least emphasizing the use of radiation, may be safe and effective, especially given the success in treating some patients with initially advanced disease and limited relapse using this approach.[145,146]

For patients who present initially with stage III to IV disease and relapse after achieving a complete response to chemotherapy or combined-modality therapy, the standard salvage therapy is high-dose chemotherapy with autologous hematopoietic cell rescue.[147] The long-term PFS rate for these patients is expected to be approximately 50%.[148] Favorable prognostic factors in this group include a longer duration of response to primary therapy and absence of extranodal disease.[149,150] Allotransplantation is not used often for relapsed Hodgkin lymphoma but may be considered in situations of an unsuccessful autotransplant. Reduced-intensity conditioning regimens appear to be safer than myeloablative regimens.[151]

The Role of Radiation Therapy in Hematopoietic Cell Transplantation

Radiation therapy may be incorporated into high-dose therapy programs such as IFRT, TLI, or total-body irradiation (TBI).[147] Fractionated TBI is incorporated into a number of transplantation programs. Its value is debatable, and series that have used regimens with or without fractionated TBI report similar outcomes for both.[152] TBI is probably not the most efficacious way to use irradiation in these patients. Recurrent Hodgkin lymphoma is often a locoregional problem rather than a systemic one. In addition, data suggest that irradiation doses in the range used in TBI programs (12 to 15 Gy) are likely to eradicate disease in only about 20% of treated sites.[9] It is more logical to limit irradiation to sites of failure or those at high risk for disease, that is, initial sites of disease, especially bulky sites.

Important other issues include the timing of radiation (pretransplant or posttransplant), extent of fields, and dose. The advantages of using radiation therapy as cytoreductive treatment prior to high-dose therapy are that it can effectively reduce the tumor burden before high-dose treatment and the risk of interruption or delay of the locoregional radiation therapy is minimal. The primary disadvantages include potential delay of the high-dose therapy and the potential overlapping toxicities of the locoregional irradiation and high-dose therapy, including mucositis and pneumonitis.[153] Cytoreductive radiation treatment may include all sites of relapse, the bulky sites of relapse, sites with an incomplete response, or even more extensive treatment, such as TLI.

Many large published series of high-dose therapy for Hodgkin lymphoma included locoregional irradiation in at least selected patients. In some series, irradiation is given pretransplant, although in the majority of reports it is given after transplant.[154] The range of intervals from transplant to irradiation varies from 1 to 4 months. Often, the fields treated include sites of bulky disease (variably defined) at the time of relapse or areas of residual disease after high-dose therapy has been administered. Some included all sites involved at the time of relapse.

The range of radiation doses employed varies substantially in these series, from 18 to 40 Gy. In general, lower doses are employed in situations in which initially nonbulky disease is included in the treatment or if there has been a complete response to high-dose therapy.

The use of locoregional irradiation in high-dose therapy programs has the potential for altering the patterns of failure and perhaps reducing the risk of failure. For example, at Stanford, 49 patients with relapsed stage I to III disease who underwent high-dose therapy for relapse of Hodgkin lymphoma had IFRT as a component of their salvage treatment.[155] Their 3-year FFR, OS, and event-free survival (EFS) rates of 100%, 85%, and 85%, respectively, compared with only 67%, 60%, and 54%, respectively, for another group of patients who received high-dose chemotherapy alone. The difference in FFR was statistically significant (p = .04). A similar effect of local irradiation has been reported in cohorts of patients transplanted at several other centers.[131,156,157]

At Memorial Sloan-Kettering Cancer Center, an intensive program that incorporates pretransplant TLI has been used.[158] Patients who had not received previous irradiation were treated with IFRT to 18 Gy and TLI to 18 Gy (both with twice-daily fractionation). Patients who had prior irradiation were treated with IFRT only, if organ tolerance would not be exceeded, to a dose of 18 to 36 Gy in 5 to 10 days (twice-daily fractionation), depending on the prior doses received by the involved sites. The 10-year OS was 56%, and EFS was 56%.[159]

FOLLOW-UP

Given the effectiveness of primary therapy for Hodgkin lymphoma, the low rate of relapse, the risk for "false-positive" imaging studies, and the expense to the health care enterprise, there is debate regarding the value of routine follow-up for disease detection, beyond addressing patient symptoms.[160–162] However, there is no denying that follow-up is important to monitor for complications of therapy and late effects and to ensure health maintenance.

As a rule of thumb, all studies that initially gave abnormal results (e.g., chest radiograph, CT scan, PET scan) should be repeated at the time of completion of therapy to document the completeness of response.[26] The subsequent follow-up interval is typically every 2 to 4 months during the first 2 years, every 4 to 6 months during the third and fourth years, and annually thereafter.[62]

The most important component of follow-up is an interim history and physical examination, which leads to identification of two-thirds of relapses.[160] The frequency with which imaging studies should be repeated after the completion of therapy is not well defined. An occasional chest radiograph, especially if chest irradiation was included as a component of therapy, is justifiable. The value of more extensive imaging evaluation in the absence of symptoms or abnormalities is questionable.

The ESR, serum albumin, or other serum marker studies may be followed if these markers were abnormal at presentation. Serum thyroxine (T_4) and sensitive thyroid-stimulating hormone (TSH) levels should be obtained at least annually in patients who received irradiation to the neck, to detect subclinical hypothyroidism.

A challenging problem in follow-up evaluation in the past was the interpretation of residual mediastinal abnormality on chest radiograph or chest CT scan. However, this problem has been obviated by the introduction of FDG-PET scanning as a posttreatment assessment tool, with which concern may be limited to those patients who have residual PET activity.[32,163,164–165]

In almost every case, the first episode of relapse should be documented by biopsy. Inflammatory disease, progressive transformation of germinal centers, or the rebound growth of the thymus in young patients are other reactive processes that can be confused with recurrent Hodgkin lymphoma. All of these processes may be FDG-avid on PET scanning.

SEQUELAE OF TREATMENT

Depending on the fields treated, the acute side effects of radiation therapy may include occipital hair loss, mild skin reaction, sore throat, an altered sense of taste, dysphagia, reflux symptoms, dry cough, nausea, occasional vomiting, diarrhea, and blood count suppression. Most of these sequelae can be managed symptomatically. Complications that may arise in the early phase of the follow-up program are mild radiation pneumonitis, radiation pericarditis, hypothyroidism, herpes zoster, Lhermitte sign, and xerostomia.

Radiation pneumonitis may develop within 6 to 12 weeks after completion of mantle irradiation.[166] After classic "mantle" therapy, <5% of patients have symptomatic pneumonitis, manifested by cough, fever, pleuritic chest pain, and an infiltrate on chest radiography that usually conforms to the irradiation fields. Symptomatic management is usually sufficient; however, a small proportion of patients require treatment with corticosteroids, usually beginning with a daily dose of 40 to 60 mg of prednisone (or other corticosteroid equivalent). The initiation of corticosteroid therapy commits one to a course of at least 4 to 6 weeks, with slow, careful tapering to avoid exacerbation of symptoms.

Subclinical hypothyroidism develops in as many as half of patients who receive doses of >30 Gy to the neck.[167] It can be detected by an elevation of TSH even with a normal T_4 level. Thyroid replacement therapy with L-thyroxine is recommended, with an initial dose of up to 0.1 mg/day. The T_4 and TSH values are monitored regularly to make adjustments in the dose. Evidence suggests that thyroid replacement therapy in this setting reduces the risk for development of benign thyroid nodules.[168] It is likely that newer techniques of treatment with lower doses and better shielding of the thyroid gland will result in a decrease in this risk.

Herpes zoster can occur during treatment for Hodgkin lymphoma or within the first few years after treatment in 10% to 15% of patients.[169] The outbreak is usually limited to one or two contiguous dermatomes. Cutaneous dissemination is uncommon, and visceral involvement is extremely rare. If the cutaneous eruption is identified within 72 hours of its onset, treatment with acyclovir (800 mg five times per day for 7 to 10 days or other antiviral equivalent) can be initiated. This may limit the duration and intensity of infection and decrease the likelihood of cutaneous or visceral dissemination. Currently, zoster vaccine immunization is not recommended for patients who have been treated for lymphoma (www.cdc.gov/vaccines).

Lhermitte sign develops in approximately 10% to 15% of patients after radiation therapy that includes a significant length of the spinal cord and is more likely to occur among patients who have been treated with vinca alkaloids (vincristine and vinblastine). It is marked by paresthesias extending into the arms and legs on neck flexion and may be related to transient demyelinization of the spinal cord. Its onset is usually 1 to 2 months after completion of mantle therapy, and it generally resolves spontaneously after 2 to 6 months. This sequela is not related to the more serious problem of transverse myelitis.

Significant xerostomia may follow irradiation of the Waldeyer lymphoid region or the bilateral submandibular regions, which is rarely necessary, and permanent attention to dental care is required for these patients. Frequent dental prophylaxis and use of fluoride supplements are recommended.

An uncommon but potentially serious complication is overwhelming sepsis after splenectomy or splenic irradiation.[170,171] The most serious infections occur with Gram-positive organisms, including *Streptococcus pneumoniae,* meningococci, and *Haemophilus* strains. This risk can be minimized by immunization against these organisms. It is reasonable to immunize patients as soon as a diagnosis of Hodgkin lymphoma has been made. Recommendations for immunization of patients who have been treated previously but not immunized before therapy vary. Recent data suggest that if at least 2 years have passed since treatment, patients can develop adequate antibody titers to *H. influenzae* type b-conjugate, 4-valent meningococcal polysaccharide vaccine, and 23-valent pneumococcal polysaccharide vaccine.[172] Reimmunization is currently recommended every 5 to 7 years.

An important concern of many patients with Hodgkin lymphoma is the possible effect of treatment on reproductive potential. In men, pelvic irradiation may be followed by azoospermia if no special precautions are taken to shield the testes. However, with appropriate testicular shielding, azoospermia is usually only transient, with subsequent recovery of sperm counts to fertile levels.[173] Chemotherapy programs such as MOPP, MOPP-like combinations that include alkylating agents and procarbazine, or BEACOPP will cause sterility in most men. However, the ABVD and Stanford V regimens seem to spare male fertility.[115,174] Among women, the risk for infertility is influenced by patient age. With respect to the irradiation component, even with a proper oophoropexy and well-planned treatment fields, the scattered dose of irradiation may be sufficient to affect ovarian function and cause menopausal symptoms in women >30 years of age who receive pelvic irradiation.[175] Younger women may not have an immediate effect but may enter a premature menopause later in life. Similarly, with respect to chemotherapy that contains alkylating agents, normal menstrual function usually continues in women younger than 25 years but is altered in women older than 30 years.[175,176] Again, younger women may later experience an earlier-than-normal onset of menopause. In contrast to MOPP and BEACOPP, the ABVD and Stanford V combinations appear to spare female fertility.[115,174]

An uncommon but significant treatment complication is the "dropped-head syndrome" secondary to cervical muscle atrophy that occurs in a small proportion of patients treated with high-dose irradiation (>40 Gy) to the neck.[177] This is a late risk, not usually apparent until >10 years after therapy, and has only been reported with doses of >40 Gy. Management of this problem is challenging, with variable response to physical therapy and use of a "soft collar." Surgical intervention has been attempted in some patients.[178]

Long-term follow-up is essential to identify significant adverse late complications of treatment in all patients.[105,179,180–182] The most important long-term hazards are secondary malignancies[183] and cardiovascular disease.[184]

Secondary malignancies include leukemia, lymphoma, and solid tumors. In large series, the relative risk for development of a second malignancy after treatment for Hodgkin lymphoma is 2.3 to 2.9, and the absolute excess risk is 44.5 to 47.2 (i.e., 44.5 excess cases per 10,000 patients per year).[185,186] It is important to realize that these data are based largely on experiences with radiation therapy and chemotherapy in a different era, that is. larger fields, higher doses, and alkylating agent chemotherapy, and risks are likely much less with contemporary management programs.[102,187,188,189]

Myelodysplastic syndrome or acute myelogenous leukemia may develop after treatment that includes alkylating agents or procarbazine (e.g., MOPP or BEACOPP) after a latency of 3 to 7 years. The relative risk for this complication was 9.9 to 14.6 and the absolute excess risk 8.8 to 8.9 during the era when alkylating agent chemotherapy was commonly used.[185,186] The occurrence of leukemia after treatment with irradiation alone is unusual. It remains controversial whether the risk is greater after combined-modality therapy compared with chemotherapy alone.

Secondary lymphomas are usually of the diffuse large-cell B-cell type. The latent interval is usually >5 years. The relative risk is 5.5 to 14.0, and the absolute excess risk is 5.2 to 9.9.[185,186] The development of secondary lymphomas does not seem to be related to any specific component of therapy but may be related to underlying immunosuppression.

Secondary solid tumors are related largely to radiation therapy, although there is an increased risk from chemotherapy alone and an enhanced risk after combined-modality therapy.[185,190] Secondary solid tumors usually have a longer latency period (at least 7 to 10 years) than is seen with leukemia. The greatest risks are for lung cancer (absolute excess risk, 9.7 to 14) and female breast cancer (absolute excess risk, 3.1 to 5.1).[185,186] Other sites at increased risk reported in different studies include mouth and pharynx, esophagus, stomach, pancreas, liver, colon, bone and soft tissue, melanoma, thyroid, central nervous system, bladder, and female genital organs.

The secondary breast cancer risk has been defined more clearly recently to be greater for younger women. A recent study of >1,000 women younger than 51 years of age at the time of treatment for Hodgkin lymphoma reported a 5.6-fold increased risk for developing invasive breast cancer compared with the general population of women (absolute excess risk, 57 cases per 10,000 persons per year).[188] The increased risk was primarily among women who were younger than 40 years at the time they were treated, and the risk was greater for women treated to a full mantle field compared with mediastinal irradiation only. The risk may also be related to radiation dose. Travis et al.[96] reported that doses exceeding 4 Gy were associated with an increased risk for developing a secondary cancer. This escalated risk for breast cancer mandates that women should begin mammographic screening as soon as 5 to 7 years after completion of mantle irradiation.[62]

The lung cancer risk after irradiation exposure is also dose related, with an increased risk for lung cancer following doses as low as 5 Gy.[91] In addition, it has been clearly demonstrated that the lung cancer risk is extraordinarily high among irradiated patients who continue to smoke after treatment.[191] Because of this inordinately high risk for lung cancer, patients who continue to smoke after treatment should be urged to stop and encouraged to enter into smoking-cessation programs.

Cardiac complications following treatment for Hodgkin lymphoma include pericarditis (which may occur during therapy), valvular dysfunction, conduction abnormalities, coronary artery disease, and ventricular dysfunction.[184] Radiation pericarditis is a potential risk if the majority of the cardiac silhouette is treated, an uncommon scenario with current management programs. It presents as an acute febrile syndrome associated with chest pain and friction rub, an asymptomatic pericardial effusion diagnosed by chest radiograph or echocardiogram, or constrictive pericarditis or tamponade. Mild manifestations may be managed with conservative medical treatment including analgesics and nonsteroidal anti-inflammatory agents; it usually clears within a few weeks. The syndrome of tamponade or constrictive pericarditis is the most serious. It is seen only rarely in this era and may require surgical intervention.

Long-term cardiovascular sequelae result in increased morbidity and mortality.[192,193] Compared with the general population, the risk for cardiac morbidity requiring hospitalization is 2.77 fold for patients treated with both mediastinal irradiation and Adriamycin and 1.82 fold for mediastinal irradiation alone. The relative risk of death from cardiac disease is 3.1 among patients treated for Hodgkin lymphoma.[194] Screening studies have shown a significant risk of asymptomatic coronary artery disease, although optimal screening guidelines for patients after mediastinal irradiation have not yet been defined.[195] Aggressive management of hypertension, diabetes, and serum lipid abnormalities is recommended for all patients.[62,196]

Another group of sequelae involves psychosocial problems, fatigue, marital difficulties, and employment issues.[197–200] Identification of these problems may promote the development of rehabilitation programs to anticipate and deal with these issues early in the course of treatment.

CURRENT CLINICAL TRIALS

Interim PET Imaging

As noted earlier, the results of PET-CT imaging performed after as few as two cycles of chemotherapy are very predictive of outcome.[33] This strategy has been adopted in a number of clinical trials in which treatment is either escalated to more aggressive therapy for patients with positive interim scans or de-escalated for patients with negative studies.

For early-stage lymphoma, several clinical trials groups are testing the deletion of radiation therapy for patients who have negative interim PET scans. In the UK RAPID trial, a PET scan is obtained after ABVDx3, and, if it is negative, patients are randomized to IFRT or no further therapy. In the GHSG HD16 trial, a PET scan is obtained after only two cycles of ABVD, and, if it is negative, patients are randomized to IFRT or no further therapy. In the GHSG HD17 trial (unfavorable stage I or II), patients who have a negative interim PET after BEACOPP escalatedx2 plus ABVDx2 are randomized to IFRT or no further therapy, whereas those with a positive PET are randomized to IFRT or INRT. In the EORTC/GELA/IIT H10 trial, a PET scan was obtained after ABVDx2, and, if it is negative, patients were treated with 1 more month of ABVD (2 more months in H10U) plus INRT (control arm) or two more cycles of ABVD (four more in H10U). Before the study reached its accrual goal, the protocol monitoring committee identified an excess number of events for ABVD alone both in the H10F and H10U, and all subsequent patients went on to receive INRT. The Cancer and Leukemia Group B recently activated studies 50604 and 50801, with virtually identical design as the closed EORTC trials.

In advanced disease, PET is being used to attempt to define the group of patients who may benefit from the addition of irradiation. In the GHSG HD15 trial, patients who have residual masses >2.5 cm at the completion of chemotherapy undergo PET imaging. If the PET scan is positive, they receive IFRT, and if it is negative, they are simply followed.

Systemic Therapy

Because nLPHD marks as a B-cell lymphoma and is CD20+, there has been interest and experience using rituximab, an anti-CD20 monoclonal antibody, in its management. Response rates are high (94% to 97%), with complete response rates of 38% to 41%. This has resulted in the incorporation of rituximab into systemic treatment programs for nLPHD.[201,202] In addition, because the Reed–Sternberg cells of cHD sometimes express CD20 and there are benign reactive B cells in the milieu of the lymph nodes affected by cHD, rituximab has been incorporated as a systemic therapy in some trials for cHD.[203] Recently, the FDA approved the use of brentuximab vedotin for patients with Hodgkin lymphoma who had relapse after hematopoietic cell transplant. The pivotal trial for this agent reported an overall response rate of 75%, with one-third of patients achieving a complete response.[204] This remarkable response rate has led to the rapid incorporation of this agent into trials for advanced or relapsed disease.

SELECTED REFERENCES

A full list of references for this chapter is available online.

9. Kaplan H. *Hodgkin disease.* Cambridge, MA: Harvard University Press, 1980.
12. Hoppe RT, Cox RS, Rosenberg SA, et al. Prognostic factors in pathologic stage III Hodgkin's disease. *Cancer Treat Rep* 1982;66(4):743–749.
13. Hudson M, Korholz D, Donaldson SS. Pediatric Hodgkin lymphoma. In: Hoppe R, Armitage J, Diehl V, eds. *Hodgkin lymphoma.* Philadelphia: Lippincott Williams & Wilkins, 2007:293–318.
17. Evens AM, Sweetenham JW, Horning SJ. Hodgkin lymphoma in older patients: an uncommon disease in need of study. *Oncology.* 2008;22(12):1369–1379.
19. Portlock CS, Yahalom J. The management of Hodgkin lymphoma during pregnancy. In: Hoppe R, Armitage J, Diehl V, eds. *Hodgkin lymphoma.* Philadelphia: Lippincott Williams & Wilkins, 2007:419–426.
22. Tirelli U, Carbone A, Straus DJ. HIV-related Hodgkin disease. In: Mauch P, Armitage J, Diehl V, eds. *Hodgkin disease.* Philadelphia: Lippincott Williams & Wilkins, 1999:701–712.
24. Gossmann A. Anatomic imaging in Hodgkin Lymphoma. In: Hoppe R, Armitage J, Diehl V, eds. *Hodgkin lymphoma.* Philadelphia: Lippincott Williams & Wilkins, 2007:133–142.
25. Erturk SM, Ng AK, van den Abbeele AK. Functional imaging in Hodgkin lymphoma. In: Hoppe R, Armitage J, Diehl V, eds. *Hodgkin lymphoma.* Philadelphia: Lippincott Williams & Wilkins, 2007:143–156.
26. Hodgson D, Gospodarowicz M. Clinical evaluation and staging of Hodgkin lymphoma. In: Hoppe R, Armitage J, Diehl V, eds. *Hodgkin lymphoma.* Philadelphia: Lippincott Williams & Wilkins, 2007:123–132.
27. Hasenclever D, Diehl V. A prognostic score for advanced Hodgkin's disease. International Prognostic Factors Project on Advanced Hodgkin's Disease. *N Engl J Med* 1998;339(21):1506–1514.
29. Cheson BD, Pfistner B, Juweid ME, et al. Revised response criteria for malignant lymphoma. *J Clin Oncol* 2007;25(5):579–586.
33. Gallamini A, Hutchings M, Rigacci L, et al. Early interim 2-[18F]fluoro-2-deoxy-D-glucose positron emission tomography is prognostically superior to international prognostic score in advanced-stage Hodgkin's lymphoma: a report from a joint Italian-Danish study. *J Clin Oncol* 2007;25(24):3746–3752.
35. Carbone PP, Kaplan HS, Musshoff K, et al. Report of the Committee on Hodgkin's Disease Staging Classification. *Cancer Res* 1971;31(11):1860–1861.

37. Lister TA, Crowther D, Sutcliffe SB, et al. Report of a committee convened to discuss the evaluation and staging of patients with Hodgkin's disease: Cotswolds meeting. *J Clin Oncol* 1989;7:1630–1636.
42. Swerdlow S, Campo E, Harris N, et al. *WHO Classification of tumours of haematopoietic and lymphoid tissues*. Lyon, France: IARC, 2008.
44. Nogová L, Reineke T, Brillant C, et al. Lymphocyte-predominant and classical Hodgkin's lymphoma: a comprehensive analysis from the German Hodgkin Study Group. *J Clin Oncol* 2008;26(3):434.
45. Chen RC, Chin MS, Ng AK, et al. Early-stage, lymphocyte-predominant Hodgkin's lymphoma: patient outcomes from a large, single-institution series with long follow-up. *J Clin Oncol* 2010;28(1):136.
46. Al-Mansour M, Connors JM, Gascoyne RD, et al. Transformation to aggressive lymphoma in nodular lymphocyte-predominant Hodgkin's lymphoma. *J Clin Oncol* 2010;28(5):793.
49. Shimabukuro-Vornhagen A, Haverkamp H, Engert A, et al. Lymphocyte-rich classical Hodgkin's lymphoma: clinical presentation and treatment outcome in 100 patients treated within German Hodgkin's Study Group trials. *J Clin Oncol* 2005;23(24):5739.
52. Klimm B, Franklin J, Stein H, et al. Lymphocyte-depleted classical Hodgkin's lymphoma: a comprehensive analysis from the German Hodgkin study group. *J Clin Oncol* Oct 10 2011;29(29):3914–3920.
56. Specht L, Hasenclever D. Prognostic factors in Hodgkin lymphoma. In: Hoppe R, Armitage J, Diehl V, eds. *Hodgkin lymphoma*. Philadelphia: Lippincott Williams & Wilkins, 2007:157–176.
57. Hoppe RT, Coleman CN, Cox RS, et al. The management of stage I–II Hodgkin's disease with irradiation alone or combined modality therapy: the Stanford experience. *Blood* 1982;59(3):455–465.
58. Hoppe R, Engert A, Noordijk EM. Treatment of unfavorable prognosis, stage I-II Hodgkin's disease. In: Mauch P, Armitage JO, Diehl V, et al., eds. *Hodgkin's disease*. Philadelphia: Lippincott Williams & Wilkins, 2007.
60. Eghbali H, Raemaekers J, Carde P. The EORTC strategy in the treatment of Hodgkin's lymphoma. *Eur J Haematol Suppl* 2005(66):135–140.
61. Eich HT, Diehl V, Görgen H, et al. Intensified chemotherapy and dose-reduced involved-field radiotherapy in patients with early unfavorable Hodgkin's lymphoma: final analysis of the German Hodgkin Study Group HD11 trial. *J Clin Oncol* 2010;28(27):4199–4206.
62. Hoppe RT, Advani RH, Ai WZ, et al. Hodgkin lymphoma. *J Natl Compr Canc Netw* 2011;9(9):1020–1058.
63. Eichenaur D, Engert A, Dreyling M. Hodgkin's lymphoma: ESMO Clinical Practice Guidelines for diagnosis, treatment and follow-up. *Ann Oncol* 2011;22(Suppl 6):vi55–vi58.
67. Yahalom J, Hoppe RT, Mauch P. Principles and techniques of radiation therapy for Hodgkin lymphoma. In: Hoppe R, Armitage J, Diehl V, eds. *Hodgkin lymphoma*. Philadelphia: Lippincott Williams & Wilkins, 2007:177–188.
70. Hough R, Hancock BW. Principles of chemotherapy in Hodgkin lymphoma. In: Hoppe R, Armitage J, Diehl V, eds. *Hodgkin lymphoma*. Philadelphia: Lippincott Williams & Wilkins, 2007:189–204.
72. Canellos GP, Anderson JR, Propert KJ, et al. Chemotherapy of advanced Hodgkin's disease with MOPP, ABVD, or MOPP alternating with ABVD. *N Engl J Med* 1992;327(21):1478–1484.
73. Diehl V, Fuchs M. Early, intermediate and advanced Hodgkin's lymphoma: modern treatment strategies. *Ann Oncol* 2007;18(Suppl 9):ix71–ix79.
74. Younes A. CD30-targeted antibody therapy. *Curr Opin Oncol* 2011;23(6):587.
76. Hoppe RT, Hanlon AL, Hanks GE, et al. Progress in the treatment of Hodgkin's disease in the United States, 1973 versus 1983. The Patterns of Care Study. *Cancer* 1994;74(12):3198–3203.
77. Girinsky T, Pichenot C, Beaudre A, et al. Is intensity-modulated radiotherapy better than conventional radiation treatment and three-dimensional conformal radiotherapy for mediastinal masses in patients with Hodgkin's disease, and is there a role for beam orientation optimization and dose constraints assigned to virtual volumes? *Int J Radiat Oncol Biol Phys* 2006;64:218–226.
80. Bonadonna G, Bonfante V, Viviani S, et al. ABVD plus subtotal nodal versus involved-field radiotherapy in early-stage Hodgkin's disease: long-term results. *J Clin Oncol* 2004;22(14):2835–2841.
81. Engert A, Schiller P, Josting A, et al. Involved-field radiotherapy is equally effective and less toxic compared with extended-field radiotherapy after four cycles of chemotherapy in patients with early-stage unfavorable Hodgkin's lymphoma: results of the HD8 trial of the German Hodgkin's Lymphoma Study Group. *J Clin Oncol* 2003;21(19):3601–3608.
82. Ferme C, Eghbali H, Meerwaldt JH, et al. Chemotherapy plus involved-field radiation in early-stage Hodgkin's disease. *N Engl J Med* 2007;357(19):1916–1927.
83. Girinsky T, van der Maazen R, Specht L, et al. Involved-node radiotherapy (INRT) in patients with early Hodgkin lymphoma: concepts and guidelines. *Radiother Oncol* 2006;79:270–277.
85. Kaplan HS. The radical radiotherapy of regionally localized Hodgkin's disease. *Radiology* 1962;78:553–561.
86. Claude L, Malet C, Pommier P, et al. Active breathing control for Hodgkin's disease in childhood and adolescence: feasibility, advantages, and limits. *Int J Radiat Oncol Biol Phys* 2007;67(5):1470–1475.
89. Koh E-S, Sun A, Tran TH, et al. Clinical dose-volume histogram analysis in predicting radiation pneumonitis in Hodgkin's lymphoma. *Int J Radiat Oncol Biol Phys* 2006;66:223–228.
91. Travis LB, Gospodarowicz M, Curtis RE, et al. Lung cancer following chemotherapy and radiotherapy for Hodgkin's disease. *J Natl Cancer Inst* 2002;94(3):182–192.
92. Martel MK, Sahijdak WM, Ten Haken RK, et al. Fraction size and dose parameters related to the incidence of pericardial effusions. *Int J Radiat Oncol Biol Phys* 1998;40(1):155–161.
94. Hancock SL, Tucker MA, Hoppe RT. Factors affecting late mortality from heart disease after treatment of Hodgkin's disease. *JAMA* 1993;270(16):1949–1955.
95. Gagliardi G, Constine LS, Moiseenko V, et al. Radiation dose-volume effects in the heart. *Int J Radiat Oncol Biol Phys* 2010;76(3 Suppl):S77–S85.
96. Travis LB, Hill DA, Dores GM, et al. Breast cancer following radiotherapy and chemotherapy among young women with Hodgkin disease. *JAMA* 2003;290:465–475.
98. Girinsky T, Ghalibafian M, Bonniaud G, et al. Is FDG-PET scan in patients with early stage Hodgkin lymphoma of any value in the implementation of the involved-node radiotherapy concept and dose painting? *Radiother Oncol* 2007; 85(2):178–186.
100. Hoppe BS, Flampouri S, Su Z, et al. Consolidative involved-node proton therapy for stage IA-IIIB mediastinal Hodgkin lymphoma: preliminary dosimetric outcomes from a phase ii study. *Int J Radiat Oncol Biol Phys* 2012;83(1):260–267.
103. Hoppe B, Slopsema R, Specht L. Proton therapy for Hodgkin lymphoma. In: Specht L, Yahalom J, eds. *Radiotherapy for Hodgkin lymphoma*. Berlin: Springer, 2011:197–204.
104. Mauch P. Treatment of favorable prognosis stage I-II Hodgkin lymphoma. In: Hoppe R, Armitage J, Diehl V, eds. *Hodgkin lymphoma*. Philadelphia: Lippincott Williams & Wilkins, 2007.
105. Hoppe RT. Hodgkin's disease: complications of therapy and excess mortality. *Ann Oncol* 1997;8(Suppl 1):115–118.
106. Engert A, Plütschow A, Eich HT, et al. Reduced treatment intensity in patients with early-stage Hodgkin's lymphoma. *N Engl J Med* 2010;363(7):640–652.
107. Advani RH, Hoppe R, Baer D, et al. Efficacy of abbreviated Stanford V chemotherapy and involved field radiotherapy in early stage Hodgkin lymphoma: mature results of the G4 trial. *Ann Oncol* 2012.doi:10.1093/annonc/mds542.
108. Meyer RM, Gospodarowicz MK, Connors JM, et al. Randomized comparison of ABVD chemotherapy with a strategy that includes radiation therapy in patients with limited-stage Hodgkin's lymphoma: National Cancer Institute of Canada Clinical Trials Group and the Eastern Cooperative Oncology Group. *J Clin Oncol* 2005;23(21):4634–4642.
111. Wirth A, Yuen K, Barton M, et al. Long-term outcome after radiotherapy alone for lymphocyte-predominant Hodgkin lymphoma: a retrospective multicenter study of the Australasian Radiation Oncology Lymphoma Group. *Cancer* 2005; 104(6):1221–1229.
112. Nogova L, Reineke T, Eich HT, et al. Extended field radiotherapy, combined modality treatment or involved field radiotherapy for patients with stage IA lymphocyte-predominant Hodgkin's lymphoma: a retrospective analysis from the German Hodgkin Study Group (GHSG). *Ann Oncol* 2005;16(10):1683–1687.
114. Horning SJ, Williams J, Bartlett NL, et al. Assessment of the stanford V regimen and consolidative radiotherapy for bulky and advanced Hodgkin's disease: Eastern Cooperative Oncology Group pilot study E1492. *J Clin Oncol* 2000;18:972–980.
115. Horning SJ, Hoppe RT, Breslin S, et al. Stanford V and radiotherapy for locally extensive and advanced Hodgkin's disease: mature results of a prospective clinical trial. *J Clin Oncol* 2002;20(3):630–637.
116. Advani R, Hong F, Fisher R. Randomized phase III trial comparing ABVD +radiotherapy and the Stanford V regimen in patients with stage I/II bulky mediastinal Hodgkin lymphoma: a subset analysis of the US Intergroup trial E2496. *Blood* 2010;116(21):4–7.
117. Diehl V, Behringer K, Raemaekers J. Treatment of stage III–IV Hodgkin lymphoma. In: Hoppe R, Armitage J, Diehl V, eds. *Hodgkin lymphoma*. Philadelphia: Lippincott Williams & Wilkins, 2007:253–270.
121. Johnson PWM, Sydes MR, Hancock BW, et al. Consolidation radiotherapy in patients with advanced Hodgkin's lymphoma: survival data from the UKLG LY09 randomized controlled trial (ISRCTN97144519). *J Clin Oncol* 2010;28(20):3352.
122. Aleman BM, Raemaekers JM, Tirelli U, et al. Involved-field radiotherapy for advanced Hodgkin's lymphoma. *N Engl J Med* 2003;348(24):2396–2406.
123. Aleman BM, Raemaekers JM, Tomisic R, et al. Involved-field radiotherapy for patients in partial remission after chemotherapy for advanced Hodgkin's lymphoma. *Int J Radiat Oncol Biol Phys* 2007;67(1):19–30.
124. Borchmann P, Haverkamp H, Diehl V, et al. Eight cycles of escalated-dose BEACOPP compared with four cycles of escalated-dose BEACOPP followed by four cycles of baseline-dose BEACOPP with or without radiotherapy in patients with advanced-stage Hodgkin's lymphoma: final analysis of the HD12 Trial of the German Hodgkin Study Group. *J Clin Oncol* 2011;29:4234–4242.
125. Edwards-Bennett SM, Jacks LM, Moskowitz CH, et al. Stanford V program for locally extensive and advanced Hodgkin lymphoma: the Memorial Sloan-Kettering Cancer Center experience. *Ann Oncol* 2010;21(3):574–581.
126. Chisei T, Bellei M, Luminari S, et al. Long-term follow-up analysis of HD9601 Trial comparing ABVD versus Stanford V versus MOPP/EBV/CAD in patients with newly diagnosed advanced-stage Hodgkin's lymphoma: a study from the Intergruppo Italiano Linfomi. *J Clin Oncol* 2011;29(36):4227–4233.
127. Gordon LI, Hong F, Fisher RI, et al. A randomized phase III trial of ABVD vs. Stanford V+/- radiation therapy in locally extensive and advanced stage Hodgkin's lymphoma: an Intergroup study coordinated by the Eastern Cooperative Oncology Group (E2496) [Abstract]. *Blood* 2010;116(21):415.
128. Hoskin PJ, Lowry L, Horwich A, et al. Randomized comparison of the Stanford V regimen and ABVD in the treatment of advanced Hodgkin's Lymphoma: United Kingdom National Cancer Research Institute Lymphoma Group Study ISRCTN 64141244. *J Clin Oncol* 2009;27(32):5390–5396.
137. Engert A, Ballova V, Haverkamp H, et al. Hodgkin's lymphoma in elderly patients: a comprehensive retrospective analysis from the German Hodgkin's Study Group. *J Clin Oncol* 2005;23(22):5052–5060.
139. Horning SJ, Ang PT, Hoppe RT, et al. The Stanford experience with combined procarbazine, Alkeran and vinblastine (PAVe) and radiotherapy for locally extensive and advanced stage Hodgkin's disease. *Ann Oncol* 1992;3:747–754.
141. Canellos G, Josting A. Management of recurrent Hodgkin lymphoma. In: Hoppe R, Armitage J, Diehl V, eds. *Hodgkin lymphoma*. Philadelphia: Lippincott Williams & Wilkins, 2007.
144. Shahidi M, Kamangari N, Ashley S, et al. Site of relapse after chemotherapy alone for stage I and II Hodgkin's disease. *Radiother Oncol* 2006;78(1):1–5.
146. Rueda A, Olmos D, Viciana R, Alba E. Treatment for relapse in stage I/II Hodgkin's lymphoma after initial single-modality treatment. *Clin Lymphoma Myeloma* 2006;6(5):389–392.
147. Armitage J, Carella A, Schnitz N. Role of hematopoietic stem-cell transplantation in Hodgkin lymphoma. In: Hoppe R, Armitage J, Diehl V, eds. *Hodgkin lymphoma*. Philadelphia: Lippincott Williams & Wilkins, 2007:281–292.
148. Lavoie JC, Connors JM, Phillips GL, et al. High-dose chemotherapy and autologous stem cell transplantation for primary refractory or relapsed Hodgkin lymphoma: long-term outcome in the first 100 patients treated in Vancouver. *Blood* 2005;106:1473–1478.
153. Tsang RW, Gospodarowicz MK, Sutcliffe SB, et al. Thoracic radiation therapy before autologous bone marrow transplantation in relapsed or refractory Hodgkin's disease. PMH Lymphoma Group, and the Toronto Autologous BMT Group. *Eur J Cancer* 1999;35:73–78.
154. Fermé C, Mounier N, Diviné M, et al. Intensive salvage therapy with high-dose chemotherapy for patients with Advanced hodgkin's disease in relapse or failure after initial chemotherapy: results of the Groupe d'Études des Lymphomes de l'Adulte H89 Trial. *J Clin Oncol* 2002;20(2):467–475.
155. Poen JC, Hoppe RT, Horning SJ. High-dose therapy and autologous bone marrow transplantation for relapsed/refractory Hodgkin's disease: the impact of involved field radiotherapy on patterns of failure and survival. *Int J Radiat Oncol Biol Phys* 1996;36(1):3–12.

157. Kahn S, Flowers C, Xu Z, et al. Does the addition of involved field radiotherapy to high-dose chemotherapy and stem cell transplantation improve outcomes for patients with relapsed/refractory Hodgkin lymphoma? *Int J Radiat Oncol Biol Phys* 2011;81(1):175–180.
159. Yahalom J, Rimner A, Tsang R. Salvage therapy for relapsed adn refractory Hodgkin Lymphoma. In: Specht L, Yahalom J, eds. *Radiotherapy for Hodgkin lymphoma*. Berlin: Springer, 2011:31–44.
161. Thompson CA, Charlson ME, Schenkein E, et al. Surveillance CT scans are a source of anxiety and fear of recurrence in long-term lymphoma survivors. *Ann Oncol* 2010;21(11):2262–2266.
163. Advani R, Maeda L, Lavori P, et al. Impact of positive positron emission tomography on prediction of freedom from progression after Stanford V chemotherapy in Hodgkin's disease. *J Clin Oncol* 2007;25:3902–3907.
166. Vose JM, Constine LS, Sutcliffe SB. Other complications of the treatment of Hodgkin Lymphoma. In: Hoppe R, Armitage J, Diehl V, eds. *Hodgkin lymphoma*. Philadelphia: Lippincott Williams & Wilkins, 2007:383–392.
167. Hancock SL, Cox RS, McDougall IR. Thyroid diseases after treatment of Hodgkin's disease. *N Engl J Med* 1991;325(9):599–605.
173. Pedrick TJ, Hoppe RT. Recovery of spermatogenesis following pelvic irradiation for Hodgkin's disease. *Int J Radiat Oncol Biol Phys* 1986;12:117–121.
174. Viviani S, Santoro A, Ragni G, et al. Gonadal toxicity after combination chemotherapy for Hodgkin's disease. Comparative results of MOPP vs ABVD. *Eur J Cancer Clin Oncol* 1985;21:601–605.
175. Horning SJ, Hoppe RT, Hancock SL, et al. Vinblastine, bleomycin, and methotrexate: an effective adjuvant in favorable Hodgkin's disease. *J Clin Oncol* 1988;6:1822–1831.
176. Behringer K, Breuer K, Reineke T, et al. Secondary amenorrhea after Hodgkin's lymphoma is influenced by age at treatment, stage of disease, chemotherapy regimen, and the use of oral contraceptives during therapy: a report from the German Hodgkin's Lymphoma Study Group. *J Clin Oncol* 2005;23:7555–7564.
177. van Leeuwen-Segarceanu EM, Dorresteijn LD, Pillen S, et al. Progressive muscle atrophy and weakness after treatment by mantle field radiotherapy in Hodgkin lymphoma survivors. *Int J Radiat Oncol Biol Phys* 2012;82(2):612–618.
179. Ng AK, Mauch P, Hoppe R. Life expectancy in Hodgkin lymphoma. In: Hoppe R, Armitage J, Diehl V, eds. *Hodgkin lymphoma*. Philadelphia: Lippincott Williams & Wilkins, 2007.
183. van leeuwen FA, Swerdlow AJ, Travis LB. Second cancers after treatment of Hodgkin lymphoma. In: Hoppe R, Armitage J, Diehl V, eds. *Hodgkin lymphoma*. Philadelphia: Lippincott Williams & Wilkins, 2007:347–370.
184. Hancock S. Cardiovascular late effects after treatment of Hodgkin lymphoma. In: Hoppe R, Armitage J, Diehl V, eds. *Hodgkin lymphoma*. Philadelphia: Lippincott Williams & Wilkins, 2007:371–382.
185. Swerdlow A, Higgins C, Smith P, et al. Second cancer risk after chemotherapy for Hodgkin's lymphoma: a collaborative British cohort study. *J Clin Oncol* 2011; 29:4096–4104.
188. De Bruin ML, Sparidans J, van't Veer MB, et al. Breast cancer risk in female survivors of Hodgkin's lymphoma: lower risk after smaller radiation volumes. *J Clin Oncol* 2009;27(26):4239–4246.
191. Travis LB, Gilbert E. Lung cancer after Hodgkin lymphoma: the roles of chemotherapy, radiotherapy and tobacco use. *Radiat Res* 2005;163:695–696.
194. Hancock SL, Hoppe RT. Long-term complications of treatment and causes of mortality after Hodgkin's Disease. *Semin Radiat Oncol* 1996;6:225–242.
195. Heidenreich PA, Schnittger I, Strauss HW, et al. Screening for coronary artery disease after mediastinal irradiation for Hodgkin's disease. *J Clin Oncol* 2007; 25:43–49.
198. Fobair P, Hoppe RT, Bloom J, et al. Psychosocial problems among survivors of Hodgkin's disease. *J Clin Oncol* 1986;4:805–814.
201. Ekstrand BC, Lucas JB, Horwitz SM, et al. Rituximab in lymphocyte-predominant Hodgkin disease: results of a phase 2 trial. *Blood* 2003;101(11):4285–4289.
204. Katz J, Janik JE, Younes A. Brentuximab Vedotin (SGN-35). *Clin Cancer Res* 2011; 17(20):6428–6436.
205. Noordijk EM, Carde P, Dupouy N, et al. Combined-modality therapy for clinical stage I or II Hodgkin's lymphoma: long-term results of the European Organisation for Research and Treatment of Cancer H7 randomized controlled trials. *J Clin Oncol* 2006;24(19):3128–3135.

Chapter 78
Non-Hodgkin Lymphomas

Leonard R. Prosnitz, Manisha Palta, and Christopher R. Kelsey

Non-Hodgkin lymphomas (NHL) are a heterogeneous group of malignancies of the lymphoid system characterized by an abnormal clonal proliferation of B cells, T cells, or both. Scientific knowledge regarding NHL has increased dramatically in the past two decades, resulting in specific advances in the spheres of molecular biology and immunobiology and leading to new histopathologic classifications and therapies.

EPIDEMIOLOGY

The U.S. age-adjusted incidence rate for NHL was 19.8 per 100,000 between 2004 and 2008, according to the Surveillance, Epidemiology, and End Results (SEER) program of the National Cancer Institute.[1] In 2010, the estimated number of new NHL cases in the United States was 65,500; deaths from NHL were 21,000.[2] In 2008, worldwide estimated incidence was 356,000 new cases and 191,000 deaths. International NHL incidence rates vary, with the highest incidence rates in North America, Europe, and Australia/New Zealand. The lowest rates have been reported in Asia and the Caribbean.[3] NHL is primarily a disease of older populations, with a median age of 65 at diagnosis.[4]

There has been a striking increase in NHL incidence rates over the past four decades, with a doubling between 1970 and 1990. The rate of increase has slowed since 1990, with a modest increase in incidence from 18.5 per 100,000 to 20.5 per 100,000 between 1990 and 2005.[5] Incidence rates have remained at approximately 20 to 21 per 100,000 over the past decade. The mortality rate for NHL has risen steadily, peaking in the late 1990s, with more recent decline over the past decade. The U.S. mortality rate rose from 5.6 per 100,000 to 8.2 per 100,000 between 1975 and 2000. Since a peak of 8.9 per 100,000 in 1997, the mortality rate has steadily declined with most recent SEER data reports of 6.5 per 100,000 deaths in 2007.[6] Similar increases have been noted in international cancer registries.[7]

The increased incidence of NHL has been partly attributed to advances in molecular diagnostic techniques, aging of the population, immunosuppression from human immunodeficiency virus (HIV), infectious agents, and occupational or environmental exposures.[8] There are likely other contributing factors that remain unknown at present.

ETIOLOGY

Several genetic diseases, environmental agents, and infectious agents have been associated with the development of lymphoma. Familial clustering of NHL has been described. However, it is not clear whether the familial aggregations are due to hereditary factors or shared environmental exposures.[9]

Immunodeficiency

The frequency of NHL is greatly increased in immunocompromised patients. The two most common clinical circumstances are among HIV-infected patients and solid organ transplant recipients, both associated with prolonged immunosuppression.[10,11] In HIV patients, NHL is the second most common malignancy, with a rate of 1.2% per year.[12] The introduction of highly active antiretroviral therapy (HAART), however, has resulted in a decline with subsequent stabilization in the incidence. Treatment outcomes of NHL in this population have improved as well.[13,14]

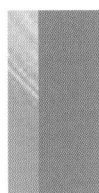

Patients with autoimmune and chronic inflammatory disorders, including Sjögren syndrome, Hashimoto's thyroiditis, systemic lupus erythematosus, and less commonly, celiac sprue also have an increased risk of NHL.[15,16] Several rare inherited disorders are associated with up to a 25% lifetime risk for development of lymphoma.[17] These include severe combined immunodeficiency, hypogammaglobulinemia, common variable immunodeficiency, Wiskott-Aldrich syndrome, Chediak-Higashi syndrome, and ataxia-telangiectasia. Lymphomas associated with these disorders are often Epstein-Barr virus (EBV) related and usually highly aggressive in their behavior.

Infectious Agents

A number of viral infectious agents are implicated in the pathogenesis of NHL. EBV is associated with Burkitt's lymphoma, posttransplant lymphoproliferative disorders (PTLD), acquired immunodeficiency syndrome (AIDS)-associated primary central nervous system lymphoma (PCNSL), congenital immunodeficiency associated lymphomas, and natural killer (NK) T-cell lymphomas.[18] The human T-cell lymphotropic virus type 1 (HTLV-1) is an RNA virus responsible for adult T-cell leukemia/lymphoma (ATL).[19] In endemic areas, more than 50% of all NHL cases are ATL, although the risk for development of disease is only approximately 5% in infected patients. Human herpes virus 8 (HHV-8), the causative agent for Kaposi's sarcoma, is also associated with several rare lymphoproliferative diseases, including primary effusion lymphoma.[20] The hepatitis C virus (HCV) is linked with several NHL subtypes, including splenic marginal zone lymphoma.[21,22]

The strongest association between infectious agents and NHL is in marginal zone lymphomas (MZL). The bacterium *Helicobacter pylori* has been linked to gastric mucosa-associated lymphoid tissue (MALT) lymphomas.[23,24] It has been suggested that several other bacteria, including *Borrelia burgdorferi, Campylobacter jejuni,* and *Chlamydia psittaci,* may also play a role in the pathogenesis of MZL of other sites.[21,25,26]

Environmental and Occupational Exposures

Occupations associated with a higher risk of developing NHL include farmers, teachers, dry cleaners, butchers, printers, wood workers, mechanics, and agricultural workers.[27,28] Several studies have shown an increased risk of NHL in relation to pesticide exposure, particularly phenoxyl herbicides and organochlorines.[29,30] The development of NHL has also been linked to hair dyes, organic solvents, high levels of nitrates in drinking water, arsenic, pesticides, fungicides, lead, vinyl chloride, and asbestos.[29] Radiation has been suggested as a causative agent with increased lymphoma incidence in survivors of nuclear explosions or atomic reactor accidents.[31] NHL is also observed as a late effect of prior radiation therapy or chemotherapy.[32] Dietary factors and tobacco and alcohol use may affect the risk of developing NHL.[33]

PATHOLOGY AND IMMUNOBIOLOGY

NHL is a group of many different disease entities, often difficult to diagnosis, with a correspondingly complex histopathologic classification that has changed relatively frequently over the years. The changing classifications reflect new knowledge gained as well as difficulties with older systems that were recognized with the passage of time, such as interobserver variability, difficulties with reproducibility, and a somewhat confusing picture with respect to clinical–pathologic correlates. The predecessor to the currently utilized World Health Organization (WHO) classification was the Working Formulation.[34] It subdivided NHL by biologic behavior; low grade, intermediate grade, and high grade; and indolent or aggressive behavior groups. This staging characterization has been abandoned in the new WHO classification. Such groupings were convenient and appeared clinically useful, but represented an oversimplification and did not account for several distinct clinical–pathologic entities.

The WHO 2008 classification divides NHL into B-cell and T-cell neoplasms, with over 40 different lymphomas delineated, as shown in Table 78.1.[35] These specific entities are distinguished on the basis of reproducibly identifiable morphologic, immunologic, and genetic characteristics. The specific diseases

TABLE 78.1 WORLD HEALTH ORGANIZATION 2008 CLASSIFICATION OF MATURE

B-Cell, T-Cell, and NK-Cell Lymphoid Neoplasms
B-Cell Neoplasms
Chronic lymphocytic leukemia/small lymphocytic lymphoma
B-cell prolymphocytic leukemia
Splenic marginal zone lymphoma
Hairy cell leukemia
Splenic B-cell lymphoma/leukemia, unclassifiable
Splenic diffuse red pulp small B-cell lymphoma
Hairy cell leukemia-variant
Lymphoplasmacytic lymphoma
Heavy chain diseases
Gamma heavy chain disease
Mu heavy chain disease
Alpha heavy chain disease
Plasma cell neoplasms
Monoclonal gammopathy of undetermined significance (MGUS)
Plasma cell myeloma
Solitary plasmacytoma of bone
Extraosseous plasmacytoma
Monoclonal immunoglobulin deposition diseases
Extranodal marginal zone lymphoma of mucosa-associated lymphoid tissue (MALT lymphoma)
Nodal marginal zone lymphoma
Follicular lymphoma
Primary cutaneous follicle center lymphoma
Mantle cell lymphoma
Diffuse large B-cell lymphoma (DLBCL)
T-cell/histiocyte-rich large B-cell lymphoma
Primary DLBCL of the CNS
Primary cutaneous DLBCL, leg type
EBV positive DLBCL of the elderly
DLBCL associated with chronic inflammation
Lymphomatoid granulomatosis
Primary mediastinal large B-cell lymphoma
Intravascular large B-cell lymphoma
ALK positive large B-cell lymphoma
Plasmablastic lymphoma
Large B-cell lymphoma arising in HHV-8 associated multicentric Castleman disease
Primary effusion lymphoma
Burkitt lymphoma
B-cell lymphoma, unclassifiable, with features intermediate between DLBCL and Burkitt lymphoma
B-cell lymphoma, unclassifiable, with features intermediate between DLBCL and classical Hodgkin lymphoma
T-Cell and NK-Cell Neoplasms
T-cell prolymphocytic leukemia
T-cell large granular lymphocytic leukemia
Chronic lymphoproliferative disorder of NK cells
Aggressive NK cell leukemia
Epstein-Barr virus (EBV) positive T-cell lymphoproliferative diseases of childhood
Systemic EBV+ T-cell lymphoproliferative disease of childhood
Hydroa vacciniforme-like lymphoma
Adult T-cell lymphoma/leukemia (human T-cell leukemia virus type 1 positive)
Extranodal NK/T-cell lymphoma, nasal type
Enteropathy-associated T-cell lymphoma
Hepatosplenic T-cell lymphoma
Subcutaneous panniculitis-like T-cell lymphoma
Mycosis fungoides
Sézary syndrome
Primary cutaneous CD30 positive T-cell lymphoproliferative disorders
Primary cutaneous peripheral T-cell lymphomas, rare subtypes
Primary cutaneous gamma-delta T cell lymphoma
Primary cutaneous CD8 positive aggressive epidermotropic cytotoxic T-cell lymphoma
Primary cutaneous CD4 positive small/medium T-cell lymphoma
Peripheral T cell lymphoma, not otherwise specified (NOS)
Angioimmunoblastic T-cell lymphoma
Anaplastic large cell lymphoma, ALK positive
Anaplastic large cell lymphoma, ALK negative

Adapted from Swerdlow SH, Campo E, Harris NL, et al., eds. *WHO classification of tumours of haematopoietic and lymphoid tissues*. 4th ed. Lyon, France: International Agency for Research on Cancer, 2008.

described may be either indolent or aggressive in behavior. Within a given disease there may be a range of behaviors (e.g., anaplastic large cell lymphoma [ALCL]). Similarly, the histologic grade and the biologic behavior may vary within a specific disease entity (e.g., follicular lymphoma [FL]). In addition, the WHO classification describes new disease categories not clearly recognized in the Working Formulation, notably marginal zone lymphoma (MZL), mantle cell lymphoma (MCL), peripheral T-cell lymphomas (PTCL), ALCL, and primary mediastinal large B-cell lymphoma.

A description of all the varieties of NHL is not practical and beyond the scope of this chapter. This chapter will focus on the most common entities in order of decreasing frequency, namely, diffuse large B-cell lymphoma (DLBCL), FL, MZL, MCL, PTCL, and chronic lymphocytic leukemia (CLL) or small lymphocytic lymphoma (SLL), although other less common entities are also discussed. Incidence data are derived largely from the NHL Classification Project,[36] which evaluated 1,403 cases of NHL at nine study sites around the world, establishing the frequency of the subtypes, geographic variation in incidence, and clinical correlates.

It must be emphasized that lymphoma pathology is complex with a long history of interobserver disagreement. National Comprehensive Cancer Network (NCCN) guidelines describe as "essential" specialized hematopathology review of all slides and adequate immunophenotyping to establish the diagnosis.[37] Fine-needle aspiration alone is rarely acceptable for the initial diagnosis of lymphoma due to lack of nodal architecture.[38]

Diffuse Large B-Cell Lymphoma

DLBCL is a neoplasm of large, transformed B cells with a diffuse growth pattern and a high (>40%) proliferation fraction. The cells may resemble centroblasts, immunoblasts, multilobated cells, or anaplastic large cells. It is the most common type of NHL (31% of all cases, 33% if primary DLBCL of the mediastinum is included).[36] DLBCL is a heterogeneous group of neoplasms with multiple distinct variants described in the current WHO classification.[35] In addition, DNA microarrays (oligonucleotides or cDNA probes) show that three different subgroups of DLBCL with unique molecular abnormalities can be identified.[39] These include the germinal center B-cell subtype and the activated B-cell subtype. Primary mediastinal DLBCL also has a unique molecular signature that closely resembles classical Hodgkin lymphoma (HL).[40] Models predictive of clinical outcome using gene-expression data have also been developed.[41–42,43] Treatment tailored to molecular subclassification of this disease is premature at present but may become part of future routine clinical practice.

DLBCL express one or more pan B-cell markers (CD19, CD20, CD22, and CD79a), as well as CD45, and often surface immunoglobulin.[44] Twenty-five percent to 80% in various studies express BCL-2 protein.[45] Approximately 70% express BCL-6 protein, consistent with a germinal center origin.[45,46] Most cases of DLBCL have somatic mutations in the immunoglobulin variable region genes, suggesting they have progressed through the germinal center where immunoglobulin affinity maturation occurs. The *BCL-2* gene is rearranged in 15% to 30% of cases, the *C-MYC* gene is rearranged in 5% to 15%, and the *BCL-6* gene is rearranged in 20% to 40% of cases.[45]

Follicular Lymphoma

The next most common type of NHL is FL (22% of all cases). In the Working Formulation, it was described as low grade or indolent. It has also been referred to as follicle center cell lymphoma.[36] In North America, the frequency is somewhat higher at 31% versus 14% at other geographic sites.[47] Thus, in North America FL and DLBCL are approximately equal in frequency.

FL is a tumor of follicle center B cells (centrocytes and centroblasts) with a follicular (nodular) pattern that morphologically is similar to normal germinal centers.[48] The neoplastic follicles may be present in the entire tumor, or the lymphoma may contain a diffuse component as well. FL is graded based on morphology. There is either a predominance of small cleaved cells (grade 1), a mixture of small cleaved and large cells (grade 2), or predominantly large cells (grade 3). In the WHO classification, the number of large cells per high-power field (0 to 5, 5 to 15, >15) is used to assign grades (1 to 3, respectively). However, if there are diffuse areas comprised predominantly of blastic cells, a diagnosis of DLBCL is also made.

Clinically, grades 1 and 2 are closely related with no apparent differences in biologic behavior or response to therapy. FL grade 3 tends to have a somewhat higher relapse rate with an outlook favorably influenced by anthracycline-containing chemotherapy. Although grade 3 FL is not the same as DLBCL, it may contain areas of the latter, which further suggests the need for more aggressive therapy.

The tumor cells of FL are usually surface immunoglobulin positive, express pan-B-cell–associated antigens (CD19, CD20), CD21, CD10 (60% of the time), but lack CD5. Most cases are *BCL-2* positive; nuclear *BCL-6* is expressed by at least some of the neoplastic cells. T(14;18) and *BCL-2* gene rearrangement are present in the majority of the cases (85%). BCL-2 protein is expressed in most cases, ranging from 100% in grade 1 to 75% in grade 3 FL.[49]

Marginal Zone Lymphomas

MZL is now recognized as a distinctive subtype of NHL in the WHO classification, accounting for approximately 10% of all cases of NHL. MZL entities include nodal MZL, splenic MZL, and extranodal MZL of MALT. MALT as a distinct clinical pathologic type of lymphoma was first described in 1983.[50]

Extranodal MZL is characterized by a polymorphous infiltrate of small lymphocytes, marginal zone (centrocyte-like) B cells, monocytoid B cells, and plasma cells, as well as rare large basophilic blast cells (centroblast- or immunoblast-like). In epithelial tissues, the marginal zone B cells typically infiltrate the epithelium, forming lymphoepithelial lesions defined by invasion and partial obstruction of mucosal glands by tumor cells.[51] Although transformed large cells are typically present, they are in the minority. If present in large numbers, a diagnosis of DLBCL is warranted.

The tumor cells express surface immunoglobulin and lack immunoglobulin D. Forty percent to 60% have monotypic cytoplasmic immunoglobulin, indicating plasmacytoid differentiation. They express pan B-cell–associated antigens (CD19, CD20, CD22, CD79a) but are generally negative for CD5 and CD10. There is no specific marker for MZL at present. Immunophenotyping studies are useful in confirming malignancy (light chain restriction) and in excluding B-cell chronic lymphocytic leukemia (B-CLL; CD5+), mantle cell (CD5+), and follicular lymphomas (CD10+).[52]

Immunoglobulin genes are rearranged; the variable region has a high degree of somatic mutation, as well as intraclonal diversity consistent with a postgerminal center stage of B-cell development.[53] The most common reported cytogenetic abnormalities are trisomy 3, seen in 60%, and t(11;18), seen in 25% to 40% of patients.[52,54] These changes are characteristically found in extranodal but not nodal MZL.

The most common site of MALT is the stomach. Lymphoid tissue is not normally present in the stomach, but in response to an antigenic stimulus brought about by *H. pylori,* normally present T cells in the gastric mucosa attract a B-cell population, giving rise to lymphoid follicles and, after prolonged antigenic stimulation, lymphomas.[55]

Peripheral T-Cell Lymphomas

PTCLs are the group most confusing to clinicians. They were not a separate entity in the Working Formulation but were frequently classified as either diffuse poorly differentiated lymphocytic lymphoma or diffuse mixed lymphocytic-histiocytic lymphoma. The term *peripheral T-cell lymphoma* is often misinterpreted. It refers not to the anatomic distribution of the lymphomas but to their origin from so-called peripheral or mature T cells outside the thymus, as opposed to thymic (precursor) T lymphocytes. The T-cell lymphomas collectively make up approximately 10% of all NHL.[56] They are a diverse group that includes 14 different entities (Table 78.1).

PTCLs constitute the most frequently occurring variety of T-cell lymphoma. In the International Lymphoma Study Group (ILSG) report, PTCLs comprised 7% of the total cases, making them approximately equal in frequency to MZL, SLL, and MCL.[56] Their frequency is quite different, however, by geographic locale. ILSG data showed a roughly 3% incidence of PTCL in North America compared with 9% in South Africa, Hong Kong, and London.[47] EBV may be associated with T-cell lymphomas originating in the nasal cavity.[57]

PTCLs typically contain a mixture of small and large atypical cells. The architectural pattern is diffuse. T-cell–associated antigens (CD2, CD3, CD4) are variably expressed, with some tumors expressing CD8. Sometimes the T-cell antigens CD5 and CD7 are lost. B-cell–associated antigens are lacking. The T-cell receptor genes (*TCR*) are usually, but not always, rearranged. No specific cytogenetic or oncogene abnormality has been reported.

ALCL is a special variant of PTCL.[58,59] In the ILSG project, ALCL comprised 2% of all NHL.[36] The tumor is usually composed of large cells with round, pleomorphic, or horseshoe-shaped nuclei with single or multiple prominent nucleoli and abundant cytoplasm, giving the cells an epithelial or histiocyte-like appearance. The cells express CD30 (Ki-1) and usually express CD25 and either T-cell or null lineage–specific antigens.[58] CD30 was originally recognized on HL cells. In some cases, there may be confusion between ALCL and HL, but distinction between the two on the basis of immunophenotyping and morphology is usually possible.

The overexpression of a novel tyrosine kinase gene on chromosome 2 known as anaplastic lymphoma kinase (ALK) is a characteristic feature of ALCL.[59] Approximately 60% of cases overexpress the ALK protein; such cases have a better prognosis than ALK-negative cases, except for skin cases. ALCL in children or young adults is usually ALK positive.[59]

Small Lymphocytic Lymphoma

SLL is the nodal equivalent of B-CLL.[48] In the WHO classification these are considered a single entity (CLL/SLL). It is a neoplasm composed predominantly of small lymphocytes with condensed chromatin and round nuclei. Larger lymphoid cells (prolymphocytes and paraimmunoblasts) with more prominent nucleoli and dispersed chromatin are always present, usually clustered in pseudofollicles. SLL comprises approximately 7% of all NHL.

The tumor cells of SLL express human leukocyte antigen (HLA)-DR, B-cell–associated antigens (CD19, CD20, CD22, CD79a), and both CD5 and CD23 and have faint surface immunoglobulin. CD23 is particularly useful in distinguishing CLL/SLL from MCL.

Approximately 50% of cases have abnormal karyotypes.[60] Trisomy 12 is reported in one-third of cases with cytogenetic abnormalities and correlates with atypical histology and an aggressive clinical course.[60] Abnormalities of 13q are reported in no more than 25% of the cases and are associated with long survival. CLL/SLL can transform to DLBCL (Richter syndrome).[61]

Mantle Cell Lymphoma

MCL was first distinguished in the 1980s by Weisenburger et al.,[62] who described a type of FL in which there were wide mantles of malignant cells around apparently benign germinal centers. The term *mantle zone lymphoma* was proposed, subsequently modified to *mantle cell.* It was thought to represent a variant of FL and was classified under the Working Formulation as a low-grade lymphoma. Its behavior, however, is more characteristic of aggressive disease. MCL represents about 7% of all NHL.[36]

Since the original description by Weisenburger et al.,[62] additional features of this disease have been recognized. It is a neoplasm of small to medium-sized B cells with irregular nuclei that resemble the cleaved cells (centrocytes) of germinal centers. The morphologic pattern may be diffuse, nodular, a mantle zone, or some combination thereof. Tumor cells are typically CD5 positive, CD23 negative, CD20 positive, and CD10 negative. A characteristic cytogenetic abnormality is t(11;14) involving the *BCL-1* gene and resulting in the overexpression of cyclin D1. The product of the cyclin D1 gene can be detected in paraffin-embedded tissue sections with the immunoperoxidase technique and is useful in distinguishing MCL from other lymphoma variants.[63,64]

CLINICAL FEATURES: GENERAL

Nodal Versus Extranodal Disease

NHL is primarily a disease of older adults (in contrast to HL), with a median age at presentation from 55 to 65 years.[65–67] There is a slight male over female preponderance (55% to 60% male). NHL may involve lymph nodes in almost any area of the body but may also present in extranodal sites, presumably arising from lymphoid tissue widely distributed throughout the body. Approximately two-thirds of NHL is nodal at presentation and one-third extranodal, again in contrast to HL, where extranodal presentation is rare.[65,68]

Patients with primarily nodal disease usually present with an asymptomatic lump in the neck or inguinal area; B symptoms (fevers, night sweats, weight loss) may be present in 20% to 30% of patients. There is often a history of some spontaneous regression and then regrowth of the nodes.

The most frequent sites of nodal involvement are the neck in approximately 70% of patients, the groin in approximately 60%, and the axilla in approximately half.[66,67] Although patients with nodal presentations may appear to have localized disease initially, full staging evaluation results in assignment to a more advanced stage in two-thirds.[69]

Patients presenting with extranodal lymphoma, on the other hand, usually have localized disease. Indeed, some authorities conclude that the definition of primary extranodal disease should be restricted to those with stage I or II disease.[70] The symptoms relate to the site of involvement. The gastrointestinal (GI) tract is the most common (25% to 35% of extranodal disease), followed closely by Waldeyer's ring and other head and neck sites (18% to 28%) and skin.[68,71] Epigastric discomfort, abdominal pain or bleeding, and sore throat or difficulty swallowing are among the usual symptoms for these locations.

The histologic picture of most primary extranodal lymphomas is that of DLBCL, although depending on anatomic site, other histologies are commonly seen (e.g., MALT lymphoma of the stomach). Nodal presentations, conversely, are more commonly FL. Nodal and extranodal disease of similar histologic type, stage, and other prognostic variables are treated in an equivalent fashion and have a similar outcome.[72,73] For example, DLBCL, stage IA in the neck, treated with combination chemotherapy and radiotherapy, would have the same outcome as stage IA DLBCL in the stomach treated similarly. These characteristics are summarized in Table 78.2. There are notable exceptions, however. For example, localized disease in the central nervous system (CNS) has a much worse prognosis as does primary testicular disease and perhaps lymphoma in the breast (to be discussed subsequently).[74,75,76]

TABLE 78.2 CHARACTERISTICS OF NODAL VERSUS EXTRANODAL NON-HODGKIN LYMPHOMA

	Nodal	*EN*
Histology	FL, MCL, SLL	DLBCL, MZL
Stage	III, IV	I, II
Location	Neck, groin	GI, head and neck, skin
Outcome: Equivalent by stage and histology		

EN, extranodal; FL, follicular lymphoma; MCL, mantle cell lymphoma; SLL, small lymphocytic lymphoma; DLBCL, diffuse large B-cell lymphoma; MZL, marginal zone lymphomas; GI, gastrointestinal.

Evaluation and Staging

A careful history and physical examination are required. The history should record presence or absence of B symptoms (fever, night sweats, weight loss), performance status, duration of lymph node enlargement and growth history, and any specific symptoms suggestive of extranodal involvement. All peripheral nodal areas should be examined clinically, enlarged nodes measured with suitable calipers and two-dimensional measurements recorded, and inspection of the skin, oral cavity, and tonsils performed. Patients with suspected or established head and neck lymphoma or GI tract involvement should undergo direct fiberoptic laryngoscopy or endoscopy.[77] Staging procedures are summarized in Table 78.3.

The use of functional imaging, initially with gallium, now largely with positron emission tomography (PET) using ^{18}F-fluorodeoxyglucose (FDG) has increased dramatically in the past decade.[78,79,80,81,82] PET has largely replaced gallium because of greater accuracy, particularly in the abdomen, convenience, and the ability to perform at one examination an integrated PET and computed tomography (CT) scan.[79,83] The fused images obtainable from an integrated PET-CT increase the accuracy of diagnosis by more precisely localizing anatomically areas of increased isotope uptake (Fig. 78.1). The fused images are also very helpful to the radiation oncologist in planning radiation fields. A number of authors in relatively small series have suggested that PET imaging is the most sensitive indicator of disease present initially, surpassing CT scans in this regard with a sensitivity exceeding 90%, compared with 60% to 70% for conventional imaging.[80,81]

TABLE 78.3 CLINICAL, LABORATORY, AND RADIOLOGIC EVALUATION OF PATIENTS WITH NON-HODGKIN LYMPHOMA

History and physical examination
Blood studies
Complete blood count
Lactate dehydrogenase
Liver function studies and blood chemistries
Pregnancy test (if appropriate)
Hepatitis serologies and human immunodeficiency virus testing when appropriate
Bone marrow aspirate and biopsy
Imaging studies
Chest radiograph
Computed tomography scan of chest, abdomen, pelvis, head and neck where indicated
Positron emission tomography/gallium scanning
Positron emission tomography/computed tomography (if available, can replace separate studies)
Appropriate endoscopic studies
Upper gastrointestinal series/small bowel where indicated

Some authors have suggested PET imaging at diagnosis is unnecessary in the presence of obvious generalized disease and should be omitted to conserve resources and reduce costs.[84] Because PET is so often now performed to evaluate response (however, see below), a pretreatment scan is quite useful for comparison if resources permit. Further, PET-CT scanning (contrast-enhanced CT) eliminates the need for a separate CT.

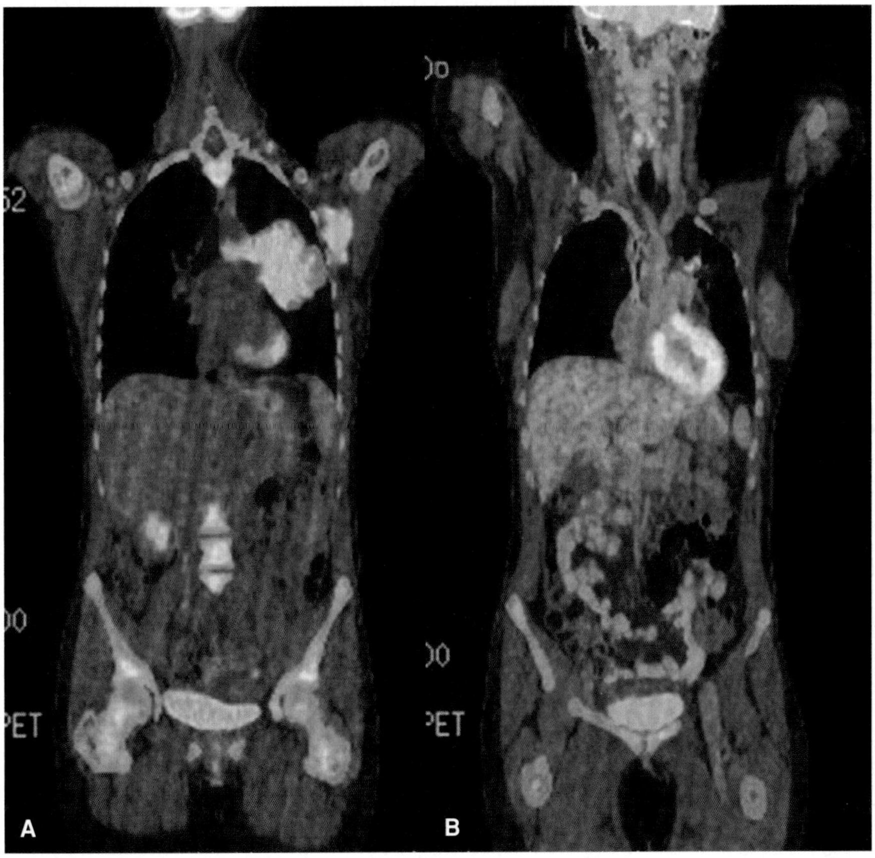

FIGURE 78.1. Fused coronal positron emission tomography (PET) computed tomography images of a patient with diffuse large B-cell lymphoma before **(A)** and after **(B)** chemotherapy. The postchemotherapy PET was scored as positive in the mediastinum. Biopsy confirmed persistent disease.

PET with gallium scanning is particularly useful after therapy, where residual anatomic abnormalities on CT scan are common.[85,86,87–88] Positive functional imaging studies after therapy are a poor prognostic sign, predicting for early relapse and suggesting that minimal cell kill has been accomplished by the therapy, because enough viable cells remain to take up the isotope in question. In contrast, patients with residual anatomic abnormalities as imaged on CT who have negative PET or gallium studies enjoy an outlook comparable with PET negative or gallium-negative patients without residual static abnormalities. A positive PET scan following salvage chemotherapy for relapsed DLBCL (in preparation for high-dose chemotherapy) has also been reported as a poor prognostic sign and a relative contraindication to proceeding with transplant.[89,90]

Other important staging studies include bilateral bone marrow aspirate and biopsy and routine blood studies, particularly lactate dehydrogenase (LDH), because this is an important prognostic factor. Patients should be evaluated for the presence of hepatitis B antigen because of concerns of reactivation of this virus with chemotherapy and particularly if rituximab is administered.[91]

Other staging studies will be indicated for suspected primary extranodal disease depending on the site of involvement. For example, lymphoma arising in the head and neck region may require magnetic resonance imaging (MRI) for precise anatomic delineation or lumbar puncture for CNS evaluation in the case of testicular or sinus lymphoma (see specific lymphoma sections for additional details).

The most widely used staging system is the anatomically based Ann Arbor system (Table 78.4), originally devised at a conference in Rye, New York, in 1965[92] and modified at Ann Arbor, Michigan, in 1970[93] and again at the Cotswolds conference in England in 1988.[94] The principal changes introduced at Cotswolds were the use of the subscript "x" to designate "bulky" disease (i.e., a mass of ≥10 cm in maximum diameter), and the definition of criteria for liver or spleen involvement as evidence of focal defects with two or more imaging modalities. Abnormal liver function study results were to be ignored for staging purposes.

The Cotswolds conference and a subsequent workshop[95] also discussed categories of response to treatment.[96] It has been long recognized that many patients had good clinical responses with improvement but not complete disappearance of disease on follow-up static imaging such as CT scans. Although the Cotswolds conference did not consider functional imaging in the assessment of response, it has been incorporated by the International Working Group.[96] A complete response has now been redefined to include residual masses on CT scan that have become PET negative.

TABLE 78.4 THE ANN ARBOR/COTSWOLDS STAGING CLASSIFICATION FOR HODGKIN LYMPHOMA AND NON-HODGKIN LYMPHOMA

Stage I	Involvement of a single lymph node region (1) or single extralymphatic organ or site (I_E)
Stage II	Involvement of two or more lymph node regions on the same side of the diaphragm (II) or localized involvement of an extralymphatic organ or site (II_E) and one lymph node region on the same side of the diaphragm. The number of anatomic regions involved is indicated by a subscript (e.g., II_3).
Stage III	Involvement of lymph node regions on both sides of the diaphragm (III), which may also be accompanied by involvement of the spleen (III_S) or by localized contiguous involvement of only one extranodal organ site (III_E), or both (III_{SE}).
Stage III_1	With or without involvement of splenic, hilar, celiac, or portal nodes
Stage III_2	With involvement of para-aortic, iliac, and mesenteric nodes
Stage IV	Diffuse or disseminated involvement of one or more extranodal organs or tissues, with or without associated lymph node involvement
Designations Applicable to any Disease State	
A	No symptoms
B	Fever (temperature >38°C), drenching night sweats, unexplained loss of >10% body weight within the preceding 6 months
X	Bulky disease (a widening of the mediastinum by more than one-third or the presence of a nodal mass with a maximal dimension >10 cm)
E	Involvement of a single extranodal site that is contiguous or proximal to the known nodal site
CS	Clinical stage
PS	Pathologic stage (as determined by a laparotomy)

From Lister TA, Crowther D, Sutcliffe SB, et al. Report of a committee convened to discuss the evaluation and staging of patients with Hodgkin's disease: Cotswolds meeting. *J Clin Oncol* 1989;7:1630–1636, with permission.

Prognostic Factors

Anatomic stage of disease, tumor mass, and systemic symptoms are important prognostic indicators. Other prognostic variables investigated have included patient age, performance status, histologic type of lymphoma, tumor size, number of nodal or extranodal sites, tumor phenotype (B or T cell), LDH, β_2-microglobulin levels, serum albumin, hemoglobin, and proliferation indices.[97,98] Many of these variables were shown to be significant in univariate and multivariate analyses but in small series from individual institutions.

In an attempt to develop a better prognostic model, the International Non-Hodgkin Lymphoma Prognostic Factors project examined data on 2,031 patients, all with aggressive-histology NHL.[99,100] Two indices were developed, the International Prognostic Index (IPI) and the Age Adjusted International Prognostic Index, because age was found to be a highly significant prognostic variable (>60 years vs. ≤60 years). For both indices, four risk groups were identified—low, low intermediate, high intermediate, and high—depending on the number of risk factors present in a given patient. Five prognostic variables were found to be significant: age, performance status, stage (I/II vs. III/IV), number of extranodal sites, and LDH (Table 78.5). When patients were divided by age, three factors remained independently significant: performance status, stage, and LDH.

With the widespread utilization of rituximab therapy and improved outcome for patients with DLBCL, some authors have suggested revisions to the IPI to allow for more separation of prognostic groups.[101] Essentially these authors regrouped the IPI into three rather than four groups, with the best outlook for those with zero adverse factors (94% survival), a good outcome for those with one or two adverse factors (80%), and a poor outcome (55% survival) for those with three or more adverse factors. The German High-Grade Non-Hodgkin Lymphoma Study Group has found, however, the IPI to still be a valid predictor in the rituximab era.[102] Others have suggested an elderly prognostic index (for patients older than 70).[103] At present, IPI remains the standard with no consensus on modifications.

The IPI was developed primarily for patients with DLBCL. It has also been successfully applied with some modifications to patients with PTCL.[104,105,106] There were initial attempts to apply the IPI to FL, but here it was less useful because most patients fell into a favorable prognostic category. A recent international effort has addressed this problem, however.[107]

TABLE 78.5 INTERNATIONAL PROGNOSTIC INDEX FOR DIFFUSE LARGE B-CELL LYMPHOMA

Adverse Factors	*Risk Groups*	*5-Year Survival (%)*
Age >60	Low (0–1 factor)	73
Performance status 2–4	Low Intermediate (2 factors)	51
Stage III–IV	High Intermediate (3 factors)	43
LDH >1 X normal	High (4–5 factors)	26
>1 involved EN site		

LDH, lactate dehydrogenase; EN, extranodal.
From ref. 99.

TABLE 78.6 FOLLICULAR LYMPHOMA INTERNATIONAL PROGNOSTIC INDEX

Adverse Factors	Risk Groups	10-Year Survival (%)
Age ≥ 60 y	Low (0–1 factor)	70.7
>4 nodal sites	Intermediate (2 factors)	50.9
LDH >1X normal	High (≥3 factors)	35.5
Stage III–IV		
Hemoglobin < 120 g/L		

LDH, lactate dehydrogenase.
From ref. 107.

Patient characteristics were collected from 4,167 patients with FL diagnosed between 1985 and 1992. Five adverse prognostic factors were identified on multivariate analysis, including age (>60 years vs. <60 years), stage (I/II vs. III/IV), hemoglobin level (<120 g/L vs. ≥120 g/L), number of nodal areas (>4 vs. ≤4), and serum LDH. Three risk groups were identified: low risk (zero to one adverse factor), intermediate risk (two factors), and poor risk (three or more adverse factors). Patients were approximately equally divided among the three groups. There was good separation between the groups in terms of survival (Table 78.6). The resulting index is known as the follicular lymphoma international prognostic index (FLIPI).

The FLIPI has subsequently been revised to predict for progression-free survival (PFS) in the rituximab era.[108] The significance of FLIPI-2 remains to be determined with additional follow-up studies. In the original FLIPI study, neither tumor size nor histologic grade was considered. Other groups have suggested these are important variables.[109]

The molecular features of DLBCL have been examined using gene-expression profiling as assessed by DNA microarrays or polymerase chain reaction (PCR). These studies have involved patients receiving chemotherapy for DLBCL who had been classified according to the IPI risk categories.[43] One study used 13 key genes, another 17 to divide patients into two or four groups, respectively, with markedly different survival rates, accounting for IPI risk categories.[42,43] In general, the outcome for patients with germinal center B-cell–like DLBCL differs from that of activated B-cell–like DLBCL, the latter being considerably worse.[108]

Gene-expression profiling has also been investigated in FL,[110,111] with two reports differing significantly, in that one examined the molecular features of tumor infiltrating cells and the other the actual lymphoma cells. Dave et al.[110] were able to group the patients into four quartiles with widely disparate median lengths of survival depending on two gene-expression signatures. This trial controlled for clinical features as determined by the IPI but not by the FLIPI. Similarly, the study by Glas et al.[111] used gene-expression profiling to predicate clinical behavior. Again, the IPI was the clinical classification utilized rather than the FLIPI. Further investigation is needed to determine the value of gene-expression profiling in FL if patients are subdivided according to the FLIPI rather than the IPI. Additionally, it remains to be determined whether the tumor-infiltrating immune cells are the appropriate targets for gene-expression profiling or the tumor itself. In general, gene-expression profiling is not widely available clinically and must still be considered investigational.

A number of other biomarkers have been investigated for their influence on outcome in DLBCL, FL, and other histologic variants of lymphoma. Results, however, have been inconsistent so that clinical indices remain the standard prognostic evaluation tool at this time.[45,112]

CLINICAL–HISTOPATHOLOGIC CORRELATES

The pathology and immunobiology of the most frequently encountered varieties of NHL have already been discussed. This section examines the clinical features of the most commonly encountered NHLs. Data from the NHL classification project are invaluable in this regard.[36,113]

Diffuse Large B-Cell Lymphoma

Patients most often present with an enlarging peripheral nodal mass or with symptoms related to a primary extranodal site of involvement, such as abdominal or epigastric pain. DLBCL is primarily a disease of older adults, with a median age of 64 years and a slight preponderance of men (55%). B symptoms are present in approximately one-third of patients. Just over half the patients (55%) have localized disease (stages I or II) at onset. Just over half the patients with stage I or II disease have extranodal presentations. When subdivided according to IPI score, one-third of patients have a score of 0 or 1, one-half a score of 2 or 3, and the remainder a score of 4 or 5.[36,113] Lymphomas that present extranodally are most commonly DLBCL.[72]

The WHO recognizes several distinct variants of DLBCL. The most notable include primary mediastinal DLBCL, T-cell/histiocyte-rich large B-cell lymphoma, and primary DLBCL of the CNS (discussed later).

Primary mediastinal DLBCL is believed to arise from thymic medullary B cells. Microarray studies have revealed a unique molecular signature for primary mediastinal DLBCL with a resemblance to nodular sclerosis HL.[114] There are characteristic genetic changes, notably absence of *BCL2* and *BCL6* rearrangements, as well as consistent increases in chromosome 9P and 2P, the former being rather specific for primary mediastinal DLBCL and observed in up to 75% of cases.

Primary mediastinal DLBCL comprises about 2.4% of all NHL, about 7% of all DLBCL. The disease affects primarily young women (median age 37) and is generally confined to the anterior mediastinum, sometimes with supraclavicular or cervical adenopathy. Relapses tend to be extranodal, however. When grouped according to the IPI, the prognosis is similar to that of DLBCL generally, perhaps a bit more favorable,[114,115] with a plateau observed in the PFS curve after 18 to 24 months. Rituximab appears to improve outcomes to the same extent as other subtypes of DLBCL.[116] The role of consolidation radiation therapy (RT) has been questioned, given the more favorable prognosis. However, omitting consolidation RT for early-stage primary mediastinal DLBCL has not been formally studied.[115]

T-cell/histiocyte-rich B-cell lymphoma consists of large malignant B cells with a florid background of inflammatory T cells, with or without histiocytes. Clinically, it occurs in a younger population compared with DLBCL, generally with a male predominance.[117,118] This entity is also more likely to present with B symptoms and involve the spleen, liver, and bone marrow. Treatment recommendations are similar to DLBCL, not otherwise specified.

Follicular Lymphoma

FL affects primarily older adults (median age, 59 years). There is a slight female preponderance. In contrast to DLBCL, approximately 70% of patients present with generalized disease, most with stage IV disease. The bone marrow is the principal extranodal organ involved. Localized extranodal presentation is uncommon, reported in only 6% of the ILSG series, again in contrast to DLBCL.[113] FL, in general, has a favorable outcome in the intermediate term, with 5- to 8-year survival rates from 70% to 80%. The failure-free survival (FFS) rate is considerably less, however, at approximately 40%.[119–121] Furthermore, there is little evidence of flattening of the survival curves with time, suggesting that relapse occurs continually over the course of many years. An exception may be the small percentage of patients who present with localized disease and are treated definitively with radiotherapy, a significant number of whom may be cured with that treatment.[122,123] Despite being considered an indolent disease, the leading cause of death is lymphoma, often after histologic transformation to DLBCL.

Marginal Zone Lymphoma

MZL includes both nodal and extranodal varieties and the unique entity of splenic MZL.[124] The more familiar name for extranodal MZL is MALT lymphoma. Approximately 70% of MZL is extranodal, with the remainder divided about equally between splenic and nodal MZL. Two-thirds to three-fourths of patients have stage I or II disease, the former more common than the latter. The prognosis is generally excellent with 85% to 90% 5-year survival irrespective of stage, although FFS is less.[74,125–127] In the MD Anderson Cancer Center series, splenic MZL had the best survival (93% at 5 years), although the disease was invariably stage IV at diagnosis, confirming the indolent nature of these diseases.[128]

Extranodal MALT lymphoma occurs primarily in the stomach, but a number of other anatomic sites are commonly seen, including the thyroid, parotid glands, orbit, and skin. Recently, an association with bacterial infection for MALT at sites other than the stomach has been described.[21] *C. psittaci* has been found in many cases of ocular adnexal lymphoma; antibiotic treatment has been shown to result in lymphoma regression in some series but not in others.[129,130] Additionally, *B. burgdorferi* and *C. jejuni* have been associated with MZL arising in the skin and small intestine.[21,131] Unlike gastric MALT, the standard initial treatment for these conditions, however, remains local radiotherapy, with very high rates of complete response and local control in excess of 90%, similar to what has been reported for gastric MALT.[127,132]

Splenic MZL patients usually present with splenomegaly.[126,133,134] Almost all have stage IV disease, principally because of bone marrow involvement. The disease is relatively indolent, with three-quarters of patients alive at 5 years, but a more aggressive subset does exist. The most effective therapy appears to be splenectomy. Indeed, the diagnosis is usually not clearly established until this time. Radiotherapy to the spleen has infrequently been used.

Peripheral T-Cell Lymphoma

The International Peripheral T-Cell Lymphoma Project recognized 12 varieties of PTCL, accounting for 5% to 10% of NHL in Western countries but 5% to 20% of NHL in Asia where NK/T-cell lymphoma and adult T-cell leukemia/lymphoma are far more common.[135,136] This section will discuss only the more common variants.

Most common in the West is PTCL, not otherwise specified (NOS), accounting for about one-third of cases (vs. 20% in Asia). This is a disease of older adults, with a median age of 61 years.[56,113,137–139] Slightly more than half of the affected patients are male. Most patients present with nodal disease in a similar fashion to B-cell lymphoma. In contrast to DLBCL, however, the great majority of patients (70%) have stage III or IV disease at diagnosis.[137,139] Approximately half of the patients have B symptomatology. The IPI also tends to be more advanced, with 52% of patients having a score of 2 or 3 and 31% with a score of 4 or 5. Many patients have some preceding disorder of the immune system (27% in the U.S. combined series) such as angioimmunoblastic lymphadenopathy, mononucleosis, lymphomatoid granulomatosis, or papulosis.[137]

Extranodal NK/T-cell lymphoma is a T-cell lymphoma of special interest. This lymphoma has a variety of names in the older literature, including angiocentric lymphoma, midline malignant reticulosis, polymorphic reticulosis, and lethal midline granuloma.[140–143] It is much more frequent in Asia (about 22% of T-cell lymphomas) than in the United States and is often associated with EBV.[144] In contrast to most lymphomas, tissue destruction of the nasal or facial area is common. The response to chemotherapy and radiotherapy is variable and slow, in contrast to the usual rapid response observed in most other lymphomas.[145]

ALCL is another T-cell lymphoma. Two forms may be distinguished: a systemic illness with widespread involvement of lymph nodes and extranodal sites and a type primarily limited to the skin.[59,146,147–150] The systemic type may in turn be separated into those patients who are ALK positive and those who do not overexpress this protein. The clinical features and prognosis differ widely among these two categories. Patients with ALK-positive ALCL are predominantly young men and, despite advanced-stage disease, respond well to combination chemotherapy, with survival rates in the range of 75% to 90%. Patients who are ALK negative, in contrast, tend to be older with a more nearly equal male to female ratio. Their response to chemotherapy is much worse, with survival rates reported in the 20% range.

Cutaneous ALCL constitutes a special situation.[146] It is almost invariably ALK negative but carries an excellent prognosis. It is often difficult to distinguish from benign lymphomatoid papulosis (LyP). The latter may spontaneously remit and tends to run a benign clinical course over many years. ALCL of the skin is quite responsive to localized radiotherapy (see the section on lymphomas of the skin).[151]

Overall ALCL has one of the best survival rates of any lymphoma, approximately 75% at 5 years in the ILSG study, despite its aggressive appearance under the microscope. The heterogeneity and complexity of this particular variant of NHL well illustrates past difficulties of attempting to group lymphomas into categories of low grade, intermediate grade, and high grade, indolent or aggressive, favorable or unfavorable, on the basis of histologic appearance alone.

Small Lymphocytic Lymphoma

SLL is morphologically and immunotypically identical to CLL; the two are classified as one entity by the WHO. Of combined cases, about 85% are CLL and 15% SLL. Clinically, SLL is distinguished from CLL by the absence of peripheral blood involvement and <30% infiltration of the bone marrow. SLL is generally manifest by widespread nodal involvement with or without hepatosplenomegaly.[152] In those uncommon instances where it is localized, however, radiotherapy may make it curable. The median age is 65 years, the oldest for any lymphoma. The male to female ratio is approximately even. Ninety percent of cases are generalized (i.e., stages III or IV), with 90% of those being stage IV (or 80% of the total). This is truly an indolent lymphoma. Survival may be prolonged even in the absence of therapy. In the ILSG project, the overall survival (OS) rate was approximately 50% at 5 years; the FFS rate was considerably less, however, at 25%.

Mantle Cell Lymphoma

MCL has a 74% male preponderance and a median age of 63 years.[113,153] Eighty percent of patients have stage III or IV disease at onset. IPI scores are high, with 23% of patients with a score of 4 or 5, 54% with a score of 2 or 3, and only 23% with a score of 0 or 1. In common with FL, the organ most likely to be involved is the bone marrow, which is positive in two-thirds of patients at the time of diagnosis. GI tract involvement is frequent as well.

Although originally classified among the low-grade/indolent tumors in the Rappaport system, the clinical course for MCL is unfavorable in the great majority of patients. The 5-year survival rate in the ILSG project was only 27%, with an FFS rate of 11%.[113] This FFS rate is, in fact, among the worst for virtually any type of lymphoma. The poor overall 5-year survival rate is matched only by PTCL and lymphoblastic lymphoma. The shape of the survival curve is continually negative, with no plateau to suggest cure in any significant percentage of patients. The situation is somewhat analogous to FL, but the latter usually has a much more prolonged natural history.

PRINCIPLES OF TREATMENT

Surgery

Before modern radiotherapy and chemotherapy, surgical resection constituted the only potentially curative treatment for NHL. It was commonly used for extranodal sites such as the stomach or head and neck and was curative in a significant percentage of patients when the disease was truly localized. Similarly, patients with nodal presentations and localized disease were managed by radical surgical procedures. The surgical approach subsided rapidly with the development of radiotherapy and chemotherapy and the recognition of the unique radiosensitivity and chemotherapy responsiveness of lymphomas.

Surgery, however, is still widely used to establish a diagnosis by biopsy. That may involve a major surgical operation, such as exploratory laparotomy for the diagnosis of stomach, intestinal, retroperitoneal, or mesenteric lymphoma. This is becoming much less common, however, with the use of endoscopic and laparoscopic techniques. With an established diagnosis of lymphoma, surgical resection as primary treatment should be a rare event, with radiotherapy and chemotherapy forming the mainstays of treatment. For example, lymphoma of the stomach should almost never be primarily resected, as the results are equal or better with radiotherapy with or without chemotherapy.

Radiation Therapy

Dose of Radiation Therapy When Used Alone

Malignant lymphomas are, in general, uniquely sensitive to ionizing radiation. For the great majority of anatomic locations, the sensitivity of the tumor is greater than that of the corresponding normal tissue, usually by a considerable amount, a luxury not available when treating most solid tumors. As a consequence, radiation fields can often be somewhat larger to cover potential microscopic areas of spread. Three-dimensional treatment planning and intensity-modulated RT may be less important for lymphomas than for solid tumors because of the lower doses generally used but have a definite role in many situations.

Dose–response data for RT of NHL are sparse. Most data come from phase II retrospective analyses; almost all of these analyses were carried out years ago, well before the latest WHO pathologic classification. The diseases most often studied were what we now know as DLBCL and FL, with a reasonable amount of information also available for MALT lymphomas. On the other hand, diseases such as PTCL, MCL, and ALCL have never been analyzed separately, so one is forced to extrapolate from the data for DLBCL and FL.

The classic articles in this regard are from Stanford University and Princess Margaret Hospital. Fuks and Kaplan[154] in 1973 reported that doses in the range of 44 Gy achieved local control of FL in >95% of instances. For diffuse histiocytic lymphoma (corresponding roughly to DLBCL), local failure rates, however, were in the range of 20% to 30%, regardless of the dose of RT delivered (Fig. 78.1). These data have been widely misinterpreted as suggesting or justifying a dose of 50 Gy for DLBCL. In fact, they suggest a subset of resistant disease in the range of 20%, regardless of the dose of RT delivered.

A series of articles from Princess Margaret Hospital also addressed this issue.[155–157] Dose–response curves were constructed for both diffuse histiocytic lymphoma (mostly DLBCL) and FL. For DLBCL patients with medium- or large-bulk disease, defined as 2.5 to 5 cm in size and >5 cm, respectively, an approximately 50% local control rate was achieved with a dose of 20 Gy, rising to 70% at 30 Gy and 80% at 40 Gy with a plateau thereafter, and no apparent improvement with additional dose (Fig. 78.2). For patients with small volume (<2.5 cm) DLBCL, a local control rate >90% was achieved regardless of dose. For patients with nodular (follicular) disease, doses in the range of 25 to 35 Gy produced a local control rate >90%.[158]

Similar data were reported in a more contemporary series from the University of Florida.[159] For patients with low-grade lymphomas treated with RT alone (mostly FL), doses of 30 Gy achieved local control in >90% of patients. For those with intermediate- or high-grade disease, doses of 30 to 50 Gy also achieved local control in >95% of instances.

There was a suggestion that tumor bulk appeared to influence the outcome. Patients with tumor size >6 cm were treated with combined modality therapy (CMT). It was suggested that doses of at least 40 Gy were necessary in these circumstances for optimal local control, although the data demonstrate local failure in 1 of 51 patients treated with >40 Gy as part of a CMT program versus 4 of 70 patients treated with doses of 30 to 40 Gy.

For MZL, particularly MALT of the stomach, high local control rates are achieved with doses of approximately 30 Gy. Data from Princess Margaret Hospital demonstrate a 96% complete response (CR) with 4% partial response (PR) and an overall local control rate of 95%.[132,160,161] In a smaller series of patients from Memorial Sloan-Kettering Cancer Center, the response and local control rates were 100% with similar doses (30 Gy).[162] One hundred percent local control with 30 Gy was also achieved in a Harvard series.[127] Similar data, although in smaller numbers, are available for MZL at sites other than the stomach.

It is unclear if tumor size affects the dose required for local control in FL and MZL. Smaller tumors may do well with <30 Gy.

Recently a phase III dose–response trial was carried out by the British National Lymphoma Investigation (BNLI) group.[163] This multicenter trial randomized 1,001 patients between 1997 and 2005, 361 with indolent lymphomas, predominantly FL and to a lesser extent MZL, and 640 with aggressive lymphomas, predominantly DLBCL, between two different radiation schedules: 24 Gy versus 40 to 45 Gy for indolent disease and 30 Gy versus 40 to 45 Gy for aggressive disease. About 20% of indolent disease patients had received chemotherapy, but 80% of aggressive histology patients did. Thus, this is primarily a trial of the dose of RT alone for indolent disease and the dose of RT in a combined modality program for aggressive disease. Tumor bulk was not considered in the randomization process.

For indolent disease the outcomes (survival, PFS, and local control) were virtually identical regardless of dose. The latter approximated 70% at 10 years (Fig. 78.2). From these data and the phase II data cited above, there is no justification for RT doses exceeding 30 Gy for indolent disease when RT is used as a single modality.

Dose of Radiation Therapy in a Combined Modality Therapy Program

For DLCBL, almost all patients, including those with localized disease, are treated with CMT, now typically R-CHOP (rituximab, cyclophosphamide, doxorubicin, vincristine, prednisone) chemotherapy followed by RT. Thus, a more relevant question than the dose of RT required for local control in patients treated with RT alone is the required dose in a CMT program.

There are many phase II reports in the literature of CMT for DLBCL with rather widely varying doses of RT used. The Vancouver group reported 308 patients with stage I and II DLBCL treated with CHOP (and related combinations) followed by involved field radiotherapy (IFRT) to doses of 30 to 35 Gy (2 to 3 Gy per fraction).[164] The 10-year cause-specific survival rate was 82%. In-field local failures occurred in 3% of patients.

Investigators at the MD Anderson Cancer Center reviewed 469 patients with DLBCL treated between 2001 and 2007 with R-CHOP (6 to 8 cycles) with or without RT. Forty percent had stage I or II disease and 60% had stage III or IV. Overall, 30% had consolidation IFRT following CR to chemotherapy with doses of 30 to 39 Gy. Local control was achieved in 100% of patients with all relapses outside the RT field.[165]

Krol et al.[166] at the Daniel den Hoed Cancer Center in Rotterdam looked at 26 versus 40 Gy for patients with stage I DLBCL who had experienced a CR to CHOP. There was no difference in outcome for the two doses in this retrospective analysis.

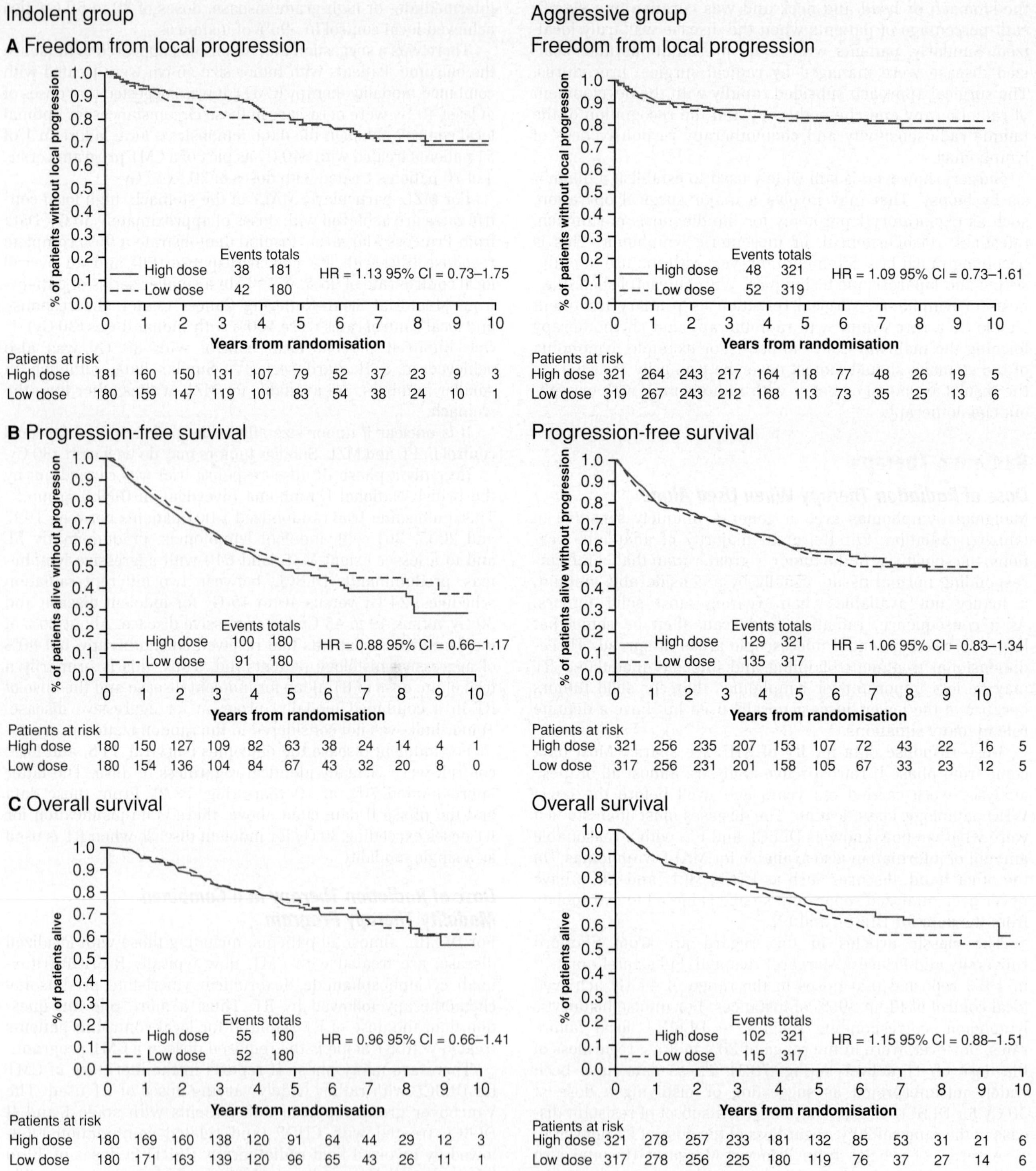

FIGURE 78.2. Freedom from local progression **(A)**, progression-free survival **(B)**, and overall survival **(C)** for indolent and aggressive non-Hodgkin lymphomas according to radiation dose. (From Lowry L, Smith P, Qian W, et al. Reduced dose radiotherapy for local control in non-Hodgkin lymphoma: a randomised phase III trial. *Radiol Oncol* 2011;100:86–92, with permission.)

At Duke University, the authors examined 45 patients with stage I and II DLBCL treated with CHOP who experienced a CR, defined by anatomic imaging and the presence of a negative gallium scan at the completion of therapy. Doses of RT ranged from 10 to 50 Gy but were clustered largely around 30 Gy. Durable local control was achieved in 92% of patients.

The phase III data from the BNLI again demonstrate virtually superimposable curves for local control, PFS, and OS for 30 versus 40 to 45 Gy.[163] Again, there is no mention of bulk disease in the BNLI study nor was functional imaging commonly employed to determine CR.

The issue of the dose of RT for FL or MZL in CMT programs has usually not been considered because of the lack of efficacy of chemotherapy group for localized FL or MZL. Thus, the optimal RT dose in CMT programs (for aggressive histology patients achieving CR with chemotherapy) appears to be 30 Gy, on the basis of the phase II and III data cited above. Even smaller doses may suffice and are under investigation at Duke University. There is no convincing evidence that so-called bulk disease requires more, particularly if PET negative after systemic therapy. For patients who respond to chemotherapy but have persistent PET-positive disease (Fig. 78.1), higher doses of consolidation RT may be required to achieve optimal local control (~40 Gy).[167]

An unresolved and controversial question is what to do with the patient who is PET positive after chemotherapy. This section will address only the dose of RT to be used if RT alone is selected for treatment. The BNLI study found no difference in outcome between 30 and 40 to 45 Gy for the small number of aggressive histology patients treated with RT without chemotherapy, but no details are given. Nonetheless, in view of the phase II data above, the authors favor a dose 40 Gy under these circumstances.

Field Size and Treatment Volume

The optimal treatment volume or field size for RT of localized NHL is also a matter of some controversy, because definitive phase III trials to resolve the issues are not available. Many of the conclusions regarding appropriate field size are extrapolated from information regarding patterns of failure.

For DLBCL, the pattern of failure after CMT is usually disseminated disease, with a small percentage with local failure.[168] After chemotherapy alone, more local failure occurs.[168,169] Failure in nodal areas adjacent to the original disease is uncommon.

The question frequently arises as to the appropriate treatment volume or field size when the patient with DLBCL has experienced CR to chemotherapy. Should one treat the original prechemotherapy tumor volume, the postchemotherapy tumor volume, or the original volume plus adjacent nodal areas? What kind of margin should be employed? The policy at Vancouver, for example, was to cover the nodal or extranodal area in question with a margin of about 5 cm, without, however, specifying whether to treat the prechemotherapy or postchemotherapy volume.[164]

In view of the patterns of failure data cited above, treatment of the original volume plus adjacent nodal areas has pretty much been abandoned. Thus, IFRT seems most appropriate. Whether the involved field is the pre- or postchemotherapy tumor volume depends a lot on where the original tumor was and the tolerance of surrounding normal tissues. With DLBCL of the stomach, for example, the entire organ would be treated regardless of the response to chemotherapy. For patients presenting with nodal disease in the neck unilaterally, the entire neck on that side would generally receive RT after chemotherapy. It would not be necessary or desirable to "prophylactically" treat Waldeyer's ring for neck presentations of DLBCL.

For tonsil, base of tongue, or nasopharynx presentations of DLBCL, after a CR to chemotherapy, the specific primary site should be radiated with appropriate three-dimensional planning at a minimum or IMRT (Fig. 78.3). One would usually not irradiate all of Waldeyer's ring but only the specific primary site. In the absence of clinical involvement of the neck at diagnosis, it would not be necessary to "prophylactically" treat the neck. Indeed, omission of neck radiation in these instances would facilitate parotid-sparing treatment plans. Mouth dryness seems to be a real problem for these patients, despite a relatively modest dose of radiation.

Conversely, for a large mediastinal mass, concerns about excessive pulmonary toxicity usually lead to treatment of the reduced tumor mass in the lateral dimensions or the normal mediastinal and hilar structures in the event of a CR to chemotherapy, not the original tumor volume.[170]

For FL, a number of authors have reported on patterns of failure and appropriate field sizes for patients with stage I or II disease.[158,171] For patients presenting with nodal disease, most studies have suggested that FFS is improved with the use of total lymphoid irradiation (TLI), as opposed to IFRT.[123,157,159,172] None of these studies has shown an improvement in OS, however, leading most centers to conclude that the morbidity and expense of TLI are not justified.[170]

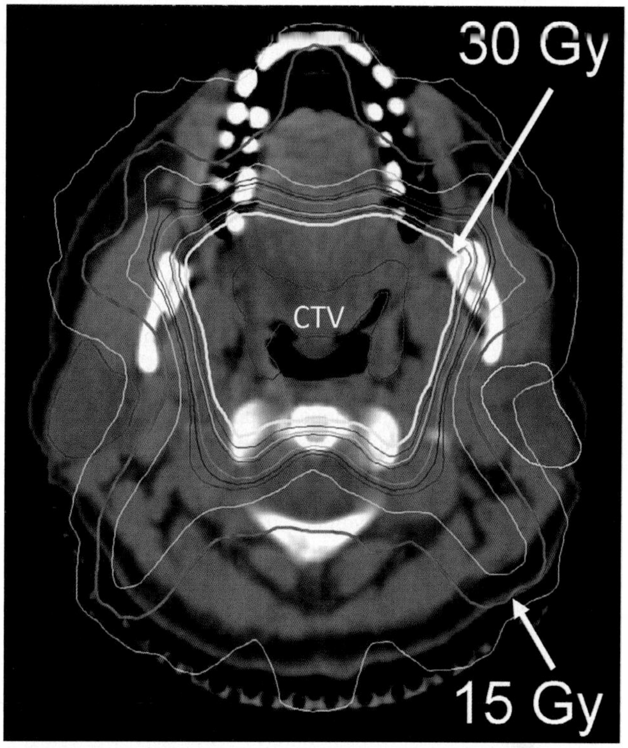

FIGURE 78.3. Axial image from planning computer tomography scan of patients with marginal zone lymphoma of Waldeyer's ring (base of tongue and bilateral tonsils). The clinical target volume (CTV) is labeled. The planning target volume was a 1-cm expansion around the CTV. The 15 Gy (*pink*) and 30 Gy (*yellow*) isodose lines are marked with *white arrows*. Note sparing of the parotid glands.

Recently the Vancouver group has explored the use of involved nodal RT compared with IFRT, the former defined as covering just the involved nodal group with a margin of up to 5 cm and the latter defined as the involved nodal group and one or more immediately adjacent uninvolved nodal groups.[109] This retrospective study was done in 237 FL patients. There were no significant outcome differences.

RT may be used alone to treat stage IIIA FL, although seldom done currently.[173] In this instance, TLI would be required. The techniques of TLI (i.e., the mantle, para-aortic nodes, spleen, and pelvis) are discussed in Chapter 77.

Two additional specialized techniques may be applicable to NHL. Total body irradiation (TBI) was used years ago for palliation of advanced FL but has largely been supplanted in this regard by a variety of newer systemic agents. It is still used, however, as part of various regimens of high-dose chemotherapy (HDC) in conjunction with stem cell transplantation.[174] When used in the setting of a myeloablative conditioning regimen, TBI is typically administered in a dose of 12 to 15 Gy, 1.2 to 2.0 Gy per fraction, once or twice daily, all depending on institutional preference. One randomized trial of single-dose (10 Gy) TBI (dose rate 0.125 Gy/min) versus 14.85 Gy in 11 fractions over 5 days (dose rate 0.25 Gy/min) revealed similar therapeutic efficacy but a lesser degree of veno-occlusive disease in the fractionated group.[175] Both groups had the lungs shielded after 8 to 9 Gy. In the setting of a nonmyeloablative conditioning regimen, 2 Gy TBI is often utilized.

Patients are treated at an extended source to skin distance, the exact arrangement depending on the geometry of the treatment room. At Duke University, patients typically sit on a stretcher with the knees drawn up. Treatment is administered utilizing lateral fields. Unlike TBI for acute leukemia, a testicular boost is not used. The arms are crossed over the chest to provide some self-shielding of the lungs. Dose to the lungs is usually in the neighborhood of 8 to 10 Gy for a 13.5 Gy overall dose, to reduce the risk of pneumonitis. Most, but not all, institutions use some type of lung shielding to reduce the lung dose to approximately 8 to 10 Gy. Other toxicities of TBI include nausea, vomiting, diarrhea, and suppression of the blood counts. This dose would also be expected to cause permanent ovarian ablation in the majority of premenopausal women, sterility in men, and the long-term risk of cataract formation.[176,177] In contrast, the acute and late toxicity of 2 Gy TBI in nonmyeloablative regimens are expected to be much less.

Whole-abdomen irradiation (WAI) may also be undertaken more frequently in NHL compared with HL. Mesenteric lymph nodes are commonly involved in NHL, unlike HL. If treating with CMT in a patient with stage II disease and widespread abdominal involvement, the radiation oncologist might wish to use WAI or a modified version excluding the pelvis or liver. The usual Duke University technique is opposed anterior and posterior fields from the diaphragm to the superior portion of the pelvis or the inferior portion of the obturator foramen with partial shielding of the iliac bones and femoral heads. Unless there is known liver involvement, the right lobe of the liver is also shielded. If doses <18 Gy are being used, kidney blocks are not used. If higher doses are desired, either kidney blocks need to be used or different field arrangements made. This depends on the exact location of the disease to be treated. If treating only mesenteric nodes, cross-table lateral fields may be appropriate. Three-dimensional planning is done in most patients. The kidneys are easily localized with CT simulation or with intravenous contrast on a conventional simulator. Modified WAI may also be undertaken as single-treatment modality for FL of the mesentery.

Radiation Therapy for Palliation

RT is a very effective palliative agent and should be considered more often in patients not responding to multiple courses of drug treatment.[170] Often relatively small doses of radiation in brief courses can be quite effective. A Dutch trial described 304 sites treated in 109 patients with indolent lymphomas (mostly FL).[178] Patients received 4 Gy, either in 1 or 2 fractions, to the symptomatic areas. The overall response rate was 92% with a CR in 61% of patients and a PR in 31%. A French trial had similar results.[179] The median time to local progression was 25 months. In this study the number of prior chemotherapy regimens did not influence the response rate. Patients with FL that is behaving in an indolent fashion may sometimes be managed with judicious palliative irradiation for many years without systemic therapy.[122,143] For critical local problems occurring in the palliative setting, such as spinal cord compression, RT is the treatment of choice. In this setting, where the goal is to maximize the chances of long-term freedom from local progression, doses of 30 Gy (2 Gy per day) would achieve that objective in 90% to 95% of instances.

For the more aggressive NHL histologies, responses to such low doses would not be predicted, but, in fact, response rates of 50% to 80% have been reported with a dose of 2 Gy × 2 and a median time to progression of about 1 year.[180,181] Certainly effective palliation can be accomplished with doses well below 30 to 40 Gy.

Chemotherapy

Chemotherapy forms the mainstay of treatment for the great majority of patients with NHL, because these diseases are most often generalized. As with radiation, malignant lymphomas are, in general, very responsive to chemotherapy. This responsiveness, unfortunately, does not translate to cure of the patient in most instances. Of all the pathologic variants of NHL in the WHO classification, consistent curability with advanced disease is seen only in patients with DLBCL and to a lesser extent in some patients with PTCL and ALCL. Some of the more "indolent" lymphomas such as FL do not appear curable with conventional chemotherapy. A few patients with advanced indolent disease may be curable with an allogeneic transplant.

A large variety of drugs are available for the treatment of malignant lymphomas, including alkylating agents such as cyclophosphamide, corticosteroids, vinca alkaloids, purine analogs, and anthracyclines. They are typically used in combination in order to circumvent problems of drug resistance. The most widely used combination for the treatment of DLBCL has been CHOP.[182] For patients with advanced DLBCL, this combination produces an approximate 50% to 60% CR rate, just over half of which are durable responses, for an overall cure rate of approximately 30% to 40%. Results are significantly improved by the addition of the anti-CD20 antibody rituximab, so that R-CHOP has rapidly become the new standard.[183,184]

Similarly, R-CHOP is probably the most widely used combination in the United States for the treatment of FL,[185] although its superiority to other less aggressive combinations has not been established in phase III studies. These data are discussed in greater detail in the sections on the specific types of NHL.

Stem Cell Transplantation and High-Dose Chemotherapy

There has been a great interest in the application of HDC with stem cell rescue in the treatment of malignant lymphomas, both for relapsed disease following initial treatment and for those patients deemed to be at high risk for relapse at diagnosis. The underlying concept is that larger doses of conventional chemotherapy will result in greater tumor cell kill and increased cure rates. The doses involved are so large that they would be lethal because of hematopoietic toxicity without a rescue strategy. Accordingly, hematopoietic progenitor cells are harvested from the patient before the HDC, either from the bone marrow itself or more often mobilized from the patient's peripheral blood and then reinfused to re-establish marrow function (autologous stem cell transplantation [ASCT]). The high frequency of bone marrow involvement in certain types of NHL limits this strategy, as well as chemotherapy resistance.

Alternatively, an allogeneic transplant may be carried out in individuals with a suitable matched donor in which the stem cells are harvested from the donor. In this procedure, it is hoped that the infused donor stem cells will additionally mount an immunologic attack on the tumor. Allogeneic transplantation may be preceded by full-dose (myeloablative) chemotherapy designed to have not only an antitumor effect, but also to condition the patient for the infusion of the donor cells, or it may be preceded by a nonmyeloablative or reduced intensity conditioning (RIC) program designed primarily to enable the recipient to accept the donor stem cells. In this latter situation the major antitumor effect is postulated to derive from the infused donor stem cells. RIC allogeneic transplants are associated with a much lower treatment-related mortality (10% to 20%) compared with myeloablative allogeneic transplants (40% to 50%).[186,187] TBI is often a component of the conditioning program, with doses varying quite widely from 2 to 13.5 Gy (see the section Principles of Treatment: Radiation Therapy).

Studies of ASCT have been carried out in many varieties of NHL but primarily in DLBCL. Numerous phase I, II, and III trials have been reported. An expert committee of the American Society for Blood and Marrow Transplantation has recently comprehensively reviewed all published trials and issued recommendations.[188]

In general, ASCT has been investigated in three types of situations: (a) patients who have been treated with conventional chemotherapy and then relapsed; (b) patients who fail conventional chemotherapy from the onset (so-called primary refractory disease); and (c) patients who have responded well to primary chemotherapy but are considered at high risk for relapse. The most widely accepted use is for the treatment of patients with DLBCL who have relapsed following initial CHOP or R-CHOP chemotherapy. In a phase III trial from the Parma group, patients with DLBCL who had relapsed following initial CHOP chemotherapy and who were responsive to a salvage program (dexamethasone, cisplatin, cytarabine [DHAP]) were then randomly assigned to receive either four additional cycles of DHAP or a high-dose chemotherapy program.[189] Those receiving the HDC program had a markedly improved FFS and OS compared with those getting conventional chemotherapy (46% FFS vs. 12%, 53% OS vs. 32%). Note that in both arms of this trial, IFRT to original bulky sites of disease (≥5 cm) was utilized, with a dose of 35 Gy in 20 fractions in the conventional chemotherapy arm and 26 Gy in 1.3 Gy fractions twice a day in the HDC arm. All patients in the Parma trial were <60 years of age. Patients with a favorable IPI score of 0 did not benefit.[190] Those with a short remission after initial chemotherapy had a worse outcome.[191]

The Parma trial and associated phase II studies have led to the adaptation of ASCT as standard of care for patients <60 years of age with DLBCL relapsing after initial chemotherapy, although the Parma trial is the only phase III investigation of relapsed DLBCL patients ever done. It is also important to note that in this as well as almost all other trials, patients who do not respond to the initial salvage program do poorly with subsequent HDC and are not considered good candidates. PET scanning has also been utilized to define response; those with a persistently positive PET after a salvage program do poorly with HDC.[89]

A number of groups have explored the incorporation of HDC programs into initial therapy for patients with aggressive histology lymphomas considered at high risk for relapse. Between 1999 and 2010, two meta-analyses and nine prospective randomized trials have examined this issue and are described by the American Society for Blood and Marrow Transplantation expert committee. Rituximab was not included in any of these trials. The committee concluded the evidence was insufficient to recommend HDC/ASCT for any patient group.[188]

The final issue addressed by ASCT studies is the role of this procedure in patients with primary refractory DLBCL (i.e., those who are chemotherapy-induction failures). This group, in general, has a very poor prognosis. Several studies have attempted to assess the role of HDC, none of them in phase III. An initial report from the University of Nebraska indicated no patients with primary refractory disease were disease free beyond 1 year after HDC.[192,193] These patients were not sensitive, however, to second-line chemotherapy. Other trials suggested better results could be obtained in patients responsive to second-line salvage programs.[194–197] More recently, however, a large international phase III trial looking at salvage regimens demonstrated a 10% 3-year event-free survival in patients who had relapsed <12 months after induction therapy.[198] The expert committee recommended against the use of HDC ASCT for newly diagnosed aggressive lymphoma patients with a partial response to induction chemotherapy without specifically addressing the issue of those patients who are nonresponders.

HDC and ASCT have generally not been successful in improving survival and curing patients with indolent disease (e.g., FL). These data have also been comprehensively reviewed recently.[199] In brief, OS for indolent lymphomas does not appear to be improved with HDC/ASCT for relapsed disease. Late consequences, particularly the development of myelodysplasia or acute leukemia, are a real concern. The data on the use of allogeneic SCT are all from phase II trials, and, while promising, this procedure is still inhibited by the substantial treatment-related mortality, about 20% at 3 years for RIC transplants and 40% for myeloablative transplants. Thus, allogeneic SCT remains investigational.

The role of radiotherapy in patients undergoing HDC with SCT, either autologous or allogeneic, is undefined. The authors have recently reviewed this issue.[200] The rationale for RT lies in the observation that most treatment failures after HDC SCT occur at sites of initial involvement. As mentioned above, consolidation RT was employed in the landmark Parma trial. It is also commonly used at a number of institutions, usually directed at bulk disease sites present before the start of salvage chemotherapy, but with considerable interinstitutional variation and without a clear definition of what constitutes bulk disease. There are a number of phase II trials but no phase III trials addressing this issue. The majority of phase II trials do suggest benefit. The authors recommend doses of 20 to 30 Gy for those patients who have not received prior RT, depending on clinical circumstances and also dependent on whether or not TBI is planned as part of the conditioning regimen. Generally, it is preferable to irradiate prior to reinfusion of stem cells.

Immunotherapy

Perhaps the most promising new approach to the treatment of NHL has been the recent development of effective immunotherapy. The malignant lymphomas express a variety of surface antigens, most notably the B-cell antigen CD20. The ubiquitous presence of the CD20 antigen in many varieties of B-cell lymphomas led to the genetic engineering of a human chimeric anti-CD20 antibody rituximab. In contrast to prior murine derived monoclonal antibodies, rituximab is quite well tolerated in humans. Rituximab was the first antibody of any type to receive U.S. Food and Drug Administration (FDA) approval (1997) for the treatment of any human malignancy.

Numerous trials of rituximab have been carried out in virtually all B-cell lymphomas.[201–207] Responses as a single agent are seen frequently in FL, CLL, MCL, and MZL. Although responses are infrequent in DLBCL, the addition of rituximab to the standard CHOP program significantly improves outcomes.[183,184] Indeed, the addition of rituximab to chemotherapy for DLBCL represents *the* major advance of the past several decades in the systemic treatment of DLBCL. The effect is so substantial as to force a re-evaluation of prognostic factors as well as other adjuvant therapies (such as stem cell transplantation or radiotherapy) in the rituximab era.

Rituximab is also employed frequently in combination with chemotherapy for FL, both in the induction phase as well as for maintenance, and significantly improves both response rate and duration of response. Its effect on survival for FL is less clear. It has been combined with chemotherapy for MCL as well.[204,208,209,210–211]

In parallel with the development of rituximab, efforts were undertaken to link radioactive isotopes to anti-CD20 antibodies, in view of the known radiosensitivity of lymphomas. Currently two such radiolabeled anti-CD20 antibodies have been successfully developed: iodine-131 [^{131}I] tositumomab (Bexxar) and yttrium-90 [^{90}Y] ibritumomab tiuxetan (Zevalin). Both of these agents were FDA approved in 2002 and 2003, respectively. Both demonstrate significant antilymphoma activity, either alone or in combination with other chemotherapeutic regimens.[212,213] They demonstrate efficacy in patients resistant to both chemotherapy and rituximab.[214]

Most of the experience has been gained with FL. The overall response rates are in the range of 80% with approximately one-third of patients achieving CR. In relapsed large cell lymphoma patients, response rates are somewhat lower (approximately 40%). In one trial of untreated FL patients very high response rates of 95% overall with 75% CR were achieved.[215] In a phase III Canadian trial for advanced FL, consolidation ^{90}Y-ibritumomab tiuxetan significantly improved CR rates (53% vs. 87%) as well as the median PFS (13.3 vs. 36.5 months).[216] There is additional evidence to suggest efficacy of radioimmunotherapy as consolidation for aggressive histologies.[217] The optimal timing of radioimmunotherapy, selection of appropriate patients, and integration into other available therapeutic modalities has not been established. These data have recently been reviewed by the Seattle group.[218]

TREATMENT OF SPECIFIC LYMPHOMAS

Diffuse Large B-Cell Lymphoma, Stage I or II

Historically in the prechemotherapy era, early-stage DLBCL was treated with RT alone.[155,159,171,219–222] Ten-year FFS and OS in these series ranged from 30% to 60%, depending on the mix of patients and prognostic variables. The doses of RT varied widely from 30 to 60 Gy. The CR rate was high, usually >80%. Field sizes and arrangements also varied widely but, in general, IFRT was used.

The pattern of failure in these series was primarily distal, either organ involvement or nodal sites remote from the primary site. Patients with both nodal and extranodal disease were included in these series and appear to have equivalent prognoses. Stage II patients had a long-term FFS and OS in the range of 25%, in contrast to patients with stage I disease where the FFS and OS were in the 50% to 60% range.

In the late 1970s and early 1980s, efforts to improve on these results by the addition of combination chemotherapy were begun. The phase III trials in many instances antedated the phase II trials, but the former were typically carried out with older combinations such as CVP (cyclophosphamide, vincristine, prednisone) with results not as good as the more modern phase II studies incorporating CHOP.[223,224] These latter trials demonstrated a substantial improvement in both FFS and OS with CMT compared with RT alone. CR rates of approximately 90% are reported with FFS and OS in the range of 70% to 85%.[164,225]

These studies differed widely in their design. The number of cycles of chemotherapy varied between 2 and 8. The radiation dose ranged from 20 to 60 Gy, with the larger doses of radiation generally for patients not experiencing a CR. None of the trials used rituximab as part of the therapy (now standard) nor was functional imaging employed for assessment of response. Radiotherapy fields were generally IFRT only, although the latter was vaguely, if at all, defined in most reports. Usually they covered the original site of disease before chemotherapy with a margin.

After improved outcomes were seen with the addition of chemotherapy, the question was raised whether RT was still necessary. Five randomized studies were subsequently conducted comparing chemotherapy with a combined modality program (Table 78.7).[168,226–230] Again, none of these studies used rituximab as part of the treatment regimen nor was functional imaging utilized for response assessment. Interpretation of the trials can be challenging, given their individual peculiarities, requiring a brief overview of each.[231]

The South West Oncology Group (SWOG) study demonstrated that brief CHOP chemotherapy (3 cycles) plus RT was superior to a more extended CHOP regimen (8 cycles).[168] Both PFS and OS were improved in the combined modality arm with less toxicity (Fig. 78.4). However, it has been reported that more late systemic relapses occurred in the combined modality arm with longer follow-up, suggesting that 3 cycles of chemotherapy may be inadequate to control systemic disease long term in some early-stage patients.[229]

The Eastern Cooperative Oncology Group study demonstrated that consolidation RT reduced the risk of relapse even with extended chemotherapy (8 cycles of CHOP in this case).[227] Disease-free survival at 6 years was 73% with consolidation RT versus 56% with observation ($P = .05$) (Fig. 78.5).

The Groupe d'Etude des Lymphomes de l'Adulte study GELA-93-4 enrolled older patients (>60 years) with early-stage disease without adverse risk factors.[226] Crude rates of local failure were less with RT (18% vs. 7%). However, neither PFS nor OS was improved with consolidation RT after 4 cycles of chemotherapy. Thus, older patients, especially those with favorable prognostic factors or medical comorbidities, may derive less benefit from consolidation RT.

GELA-93-1 demonstrated that an aggressive chemotherapy regimen was superior to CHOP plus RT, at the expense of increased toxicity.[230] Quality control issues have been raised, however, regarding the RT in this trial. Despite the apparent advantage of the aggressive chemotherapy program, this regimen has not been generally adopted due to its toxicity profile.

Finally, International Extranodal Lymphoma Study Group (IELSG) enrolled a small number of patients with gastric DLBCL to CHOP versus CHOP plus RT. PFS was improved with the combined approach.[228] These trials have led to a general acceptance of treatment with CMT therapy for early-stage DLBCL. The advantage of CMT has also been confirmed using SEER data.[232]

These results must be interpreted in the light of rituximab not having been used. A recent large retrospective analysis demonstrated an advantage of RT even with R-CHOP.[165] However, no phase III trials comparing R-CHOP with or without RT for stage I or II DLBCL are in progress to the authors' knowledge. Similarly, functional imaging was not utilized in any of the randomized studies, and how to incorporate interim and posttreatment PET response into a treatment algorithm remains an area of investigation.

Although a range of RT doses were utilized in the randomized trials, 30 Gy appears adequate in the setting of a CR after chemotherapy.[163,227] The original extent of disease should be treated, if not an entire involved field, depending on the circumstances. It is generally appropriate to restrict treatment to the postchemotherapy volume in situations where excessive

TABLE 78.7 RANDOMIZED TRIALS EVALUATING CONSOLIDATION RADIATION THERAPY IN EARLY-STAGE DIFFUSE LARGE B-CELL LYMPHOMA

Study (Reference)	n	Disease Characteristics	Randomization	Progression-Free Survival[a]	Comments
SWOG (168)	401	I	CHOP × 8	64%	More late systemic relapses
		II (nonbulky)	CHOP × 3 + RT	77% (P =.03)	reported in arm 2(228)
ECOG (227)	172	I (high-risk)	CHOP × 8	56%	Only patients in CR randomized
		II	CHOP × 8 + RT	73%[b] (P =.05)	
GELA-93-4 (226)	576	I–II without risk factors	CHOP × 4	61%	Only patients ≥60 yr old
			CHOP × 4 + RT	64% (P = .6)	
GELA-93-1 (230)	647	I–II without risk factors	ACVBP × 3[c]	82%	Only patients ≤61 yr old
			CHOP × 3 + RT	74% (P < 01)	
IELSG (228)	44	I–II gastric DLBCL	CHOP[d]	82%	Closed early due to poor accrual
			CHOP[d] + RT	100% (P =.04)	

RT, radiation therapy; DLBCL, diffuse large B-cell lymphoma; SWOG, South West Oncology Group; CHOP, cyclophosphamide, doxorubicin, vincristine, prednisone; ECOG, Eastern Cooperative Oncology Group; GELA, Groupe d'Étude des Lymphomas de l'Adulte; ACVBP, doxorubicin, cyclophosphamide, vindesine, bleomycin, and prednisone; IELSG, International Extranodal Lymphoma Study Group.

[a]Five-year unless otherwise noted. [b]Six year.

[c]Plus consolidation chemotherapy with methotrexate, etoposide, ifosfamide, and cytarabine. [d]CHOP or CHOP-like chemotherapy.

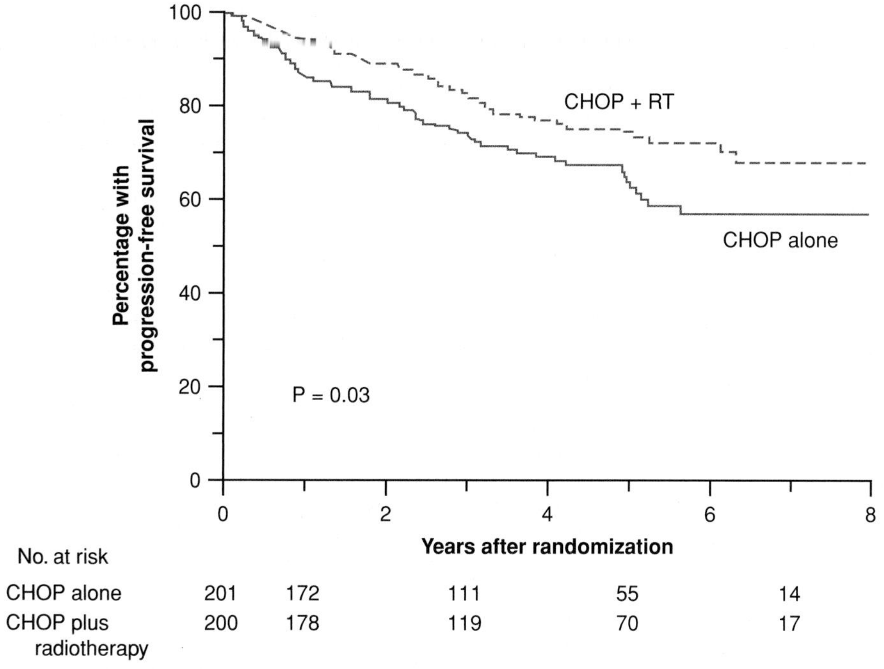

FIGURE 78.4. Progression-free survival for patients randomized to CHOP (cyclophosphamide, doxorubicin, vincristine, prednisone) × 8 versus CHOP × 3 plus consolidation radiotherapy in the South West Oncology Group randomized trial. (From Miller TP, Dahlberg S, Cassady JR, et al. Chemotherapy alone compared with chemotherapy plus radiotherapy for localized intermediate- and high-grade non-Hodgkin lymphoma. *N Engl J Med* 1998;339:21–26, with permission; copyright Massachusetts Medical Society.)

dose to normal tissue might result, such as with DLBCL of the mediastinum or abdomen. For these sites, the field reduction would typically be in the lateral dimensions to spare normal lung and kidney, but superior inferior margins may be more generous.

Diffuse Large B-Cell Lymphoma, Stage III or IV

The mainstay of treatment of disseminated DLBCL is clearly systemic chemotherapy. RT has been thought to play little, if any, role.[233] A re-examination, however, may be in order, given some trials that do suggest benefit.[234,235–236] The standard chemotherapeutic combination has been CHOP, first introduced in the late 1970s.[237] With this combination, CR in the range of 60% to 70% were reported with most of these (approximately 60%) being durable, for a long-term cure rate of 35% to 40%.[182,238]

Although these results were better than those in the past, they were far from optimal. Over the next several decades, there were numerous attempts to improve on the CHOP program with promising phase II trials of new combinations, but unfortunately, that promise was unsupported by follow-up phase III studies. The best known of the latter was the Intergroup/SWOG trial comparing CHOP, M-BACOD, Pro-MACE-CYTABOM (prednisone, methotrexate, doxorubicin, cyclophosphamide, etoposide, cytarabine, bleomycin, and vincristine) and MACOP-B (CHOP plus methotrexate and bleomycin).[182] This trial analyzed approximately 900 patients. Three-year survival rates were 50% with 3-year FFS rates of 41% with no differences between the four-drug combinations. The least toxic combination, CHOP, thus became the standard treatment.

A recently published overview of chemotherapy for "aggressive" NHL histologic type reviewed 111 scientific reports including 35 randomized trials with a total of approximately 22,000 patients. The overview concluded that in unselected patients with advanced-stage disease, CHOP was curative in approximately one-third.[239]

A major improvement in the outcome for patients with DLBCL has come with the introduction of rituximab. Several phase III trials have now demonstrated the value of adding rituximab to standard CHOP. The GELA study compared CHOP alone with rituximab and CHOP in 399 patients >60 years

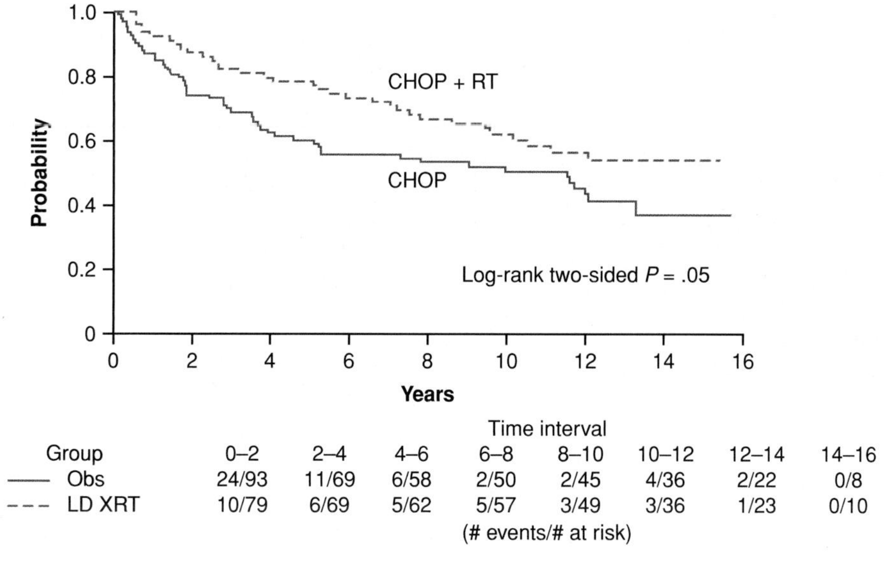

FIGURE 78.5. Disease-free survival for complete remission patients in the Eastern Cooperative Oncology Group randomized trial. Observation (*solid line*) and consolidation radiotherapy (*dotted line*) are shown. (From Horning SJ, Weller E, Kim K, et al. Chemotherapy with or without radiotherapy in limited-stage diffuse aggressive non-Hodgkin lymphoma: Eastern Cooperative Oncology Group study 1484. *J Clin Oncol* 2004;22:3032–3038, with permission.)

old.[183] FFS improved from 30% to 54% and 5-year OS from 45% to 58%.

Similarly, a European cooperative trial compared R-CHOP and CHOP in 824 patients aged 18 to 60 with stages II to IV DLBCL.[184] Three-year FFS was 79% in the R-CHOP group compared with 59% in the CHOP group. Three-year OS was 93% and 84%, respectively. In this trial, unlike the GELA trial, RT was given to select patients with bulky disease or extranodal disease. These studies have led to the rapid adaptation of R-CHOP as standard initial therapy of DLBCL for all stages of disease.

There have also been attempts to improve on the CHOP combination by the introduction of HDC and ASCT for patients with a poor prognosis in first remission, as mentioned above. Thus far, no proven benefit has been demonstrated.[240] The use of HDC/ASCT for DLBCL patients in first remission has not been explored in patients treated with R-CHOP.

A comparatively unexplored approach is the use of consolidation RT in combination with chemotherapy for advanced DLBCL. One rationale for the use of such RT is the tendency of patients with advanced lymphoma to relapse at sites of disease present at diagnosis and, in particular, sites of bulky disease present at diagnosis.[241–243] This observation is somewhat controversial.[233] In view of the efficacy of CMT in localized disease, the exploration of its value in more advanced disease appears worthwhile.

There have been a few reports regarding its use. Aviles et al.[236,244] performed a phase III trial in which patients with DLBCL who experienced a CR with CHOP and who had preexisting bulky disease were randomized to receive RT (40 to 50 Gy) to prior sites of bulky disease or not. The FFS rate was 72% in those receiving CMT compared with 35% in those treated with chemotherapy alone. Corresponding OS was 81% and 55%, respectively, all differences being statistically significant.

A retrospective analysis at MD Anderson Cancer Center compared a group of patients with stage III or IV DLBCL treated with chemotherapy only with a similar group treated with CMT.[234] RT dramatically improved local control (89% vs. 52%) and freedom from progression (5-year rates of 85% vs. 51%), but not OS (87% vs. 81%).

A similar analysis from Milan examined 94 patients with stage III or IV DLBCL and bulky disease (tumor mass ≥6 cm).[245] Forty patients received consolidation RT, whereas 54 did not. Doses and field sizes varied between 30 and 46 Gy. Improvements were noted in OS as well as FFS. These reports raise the issue of additional phase III trials to evaluate further this concept.[234]

Follicular Lymphoma, Stages I and II

The treatment historically for stage I or II FL has been RT alone. Representative series are shown in Table 78.8.[123,155,159,171,172,221,246–249] The largest experiences are from the Princess Margaret Hospital,[155] BNLI,[221] and Stanford University.[172] The reported series were accumulated over a long period, with patients staged in different ways and treated with differing doses and fields of radiation. Although these series are grouped as FL, most of them included patients with other histologic types classified as low-grade lymphoma in older pathologic classifications.

Despite the heterogeneity of the patient population and the lack of uniformity in data reporting, certain conclusions may be drawn:

1. Five- and 10-year OS is high, in the range of 75% to 90%, particularly if cause-specific survival is the quantity measured. Early deaths from lymphoma in this group are quite uncommon.
2. The FFS rate is less, with wide variability from 40% to 80%. Most series report much better FFS rates for patients with stage I versus stage II disease. Most series also suggest few relapses beyond 10 years.
3. Although radiation doses varied widely, local control was >90% in almost all instances with doses of ≥30 Gy, with no dose–response demonstrated above 30 Gy. A recent randomized trial confirmed that doses as low as 24 Gy are adequate for low-grade lymphomas.[163]
4. Radiation field sizes varied widely as well, with no evidence for improved survival with increasing field size. Prophylactic coverage of uninvolved adjacent lymph node regions does not decrease overall recurrence risk.[109]
5. Although a long median survival is observed, the leading cause of death is relapsed lymphoma.[250]

There have been a few attempts to improve on these results with the use of CMT. Two phase III trials published in the early 1980s that showed positive results for the effects of CMT, compared with RT alone for DLBCL, showed no benefit for the use of CMT in FL.[223,224] Very small numbers of patients were included, however, so the studies were grossly underpowered to detect meaningful differences. Two additional phase III trials were published in the 1990s.[251,252] The Memorial Sloan-Kettering Cancer Center trial similarly contained very small numbers of patients with FL. The BNLI had by far the largest number of patients. Single-agent chlorambucil was the chemotherapy; the trial was negative.

This lack of enthusiasm for CMT for stage I or II disease no doubt mirrors the general attitude toward advanced disease, where, to date, combination chemotherapy has not shown curative potential.[119,253,254] As with DLBCL, all these series antedate rituximab, which has a profound effect on FL. Additionally, they antedate the introduction of the FLIPI, so whether certain prognostic groups might benefit from CMT is unknown.

The predominant pattern of failure for patients with stage I or II disease treated with RT alone is distant. Local failure of

TABLE 78.8 RADIATION THERAPY OF STAGE I/II FOLLICULAR LYMPHOMA SELECTED PHASE II TRIALS

Study (Reference)	*Year*	*Number of Patients*	*Stage*	*Radiation Dose (Gy)*	*Complete Response Rate*	*Failure-Free Survival (%)*	*Survival Years (%)*
Bush and Gospodarowicz (155)	1982	130	I/IIA	25–40	–	53	72 (10)
Chen et al. (171)	1979	25	I/IIA	35–40	–	83	100 (5)
Kamath et al. (159)	1999	72	I/II	30–50	–	59	46 (10)
Krol et al. (246)	1998	56	I	–	87	75	73 (5)
MacManus and Hoppe. (172)	1996	177	I/II	35–50		43	65 (10)
McLaughlin et al. (247)	1986	50	I/II	30–40	–	35	72 (5)
Pendlebury et al. (248)	1995	40	I	30–54	–	43	82 (10)
		18	II			42	76 (10)
Reddy et al. (249)	1989	14	I	–	–	82	90 (10)
		24	II	–	–	46	54 (10)
Vaughan Hudson et al. (221)	1994	208	I	~35	98	49	71 (64)
Wilder et al. (123)	2001	33	I	26–50		66	87 (15)

any type, either alone or combined with distant failure, occurs in <10% of patients. Nodal extension is an uncommon pattern of failure, seen in perhaps 20% of patients.

The question frequently arises as to whether patients with localized FL who respond well to RT and experience a prolonged disease-free survival are truly cured of their disease. Although the OS and FFS curves appear to flatten beyond 10 years, concern has been raised by reports of persistent molecular abnormalities in such patients. In particular, circulating t(14:18)-positive cells were noted in one-third of patients with FL in prolonged remission in one report.[255] On the other hand, such cells were also found in 23% of normal individuals.[256] Thus, the issue of molecular cure remains unsettled. Additionally, one Stanford University study suggests an equivalent outcome with a watch-and-wait policy for early-stage disease.[257] Majority opinion, however, would support involved field RT for patients with early-stage FL. Nonetheless, the view that FL is an indolent process leads to underutilization of RT for localized disease. Recent studies have shown that only ~30% of patients with early-stage FL receive RT, despite national and international guideline recommendations.[258,259] A SEER analysis suggested a possible detriment in long-term survival when RT is not given.[259]

Follicular Lymphoma, Stages III and IV

The treatment of advanced-stage FL is a special challenge. The disease has a long natural history.[120,253,254,260] Median survivals ranging from 6 to 11 years have been described with or without treatment. FL is quite responsive to a variety of systemic agents, including alkylating agents, anthracyclines, purine analogs, vinca alkaloids, corticosteroids, and monoclonal antibodies. Examination of published survival curves after a variety of therapeutic approaches, however, demonstrates a continuing pattern of relapse and death, albeit over a long period, with no evidence for flattening of the survival curve, the pattern usually associated with cure. There is also no clear evidence for the superiority of any one drug or combinations of drugs in the treatment of this disease. Studied agents have ranged from single-agent chlorambucil or cyclophosphamide to aggressive combinations such as ProMACE/MOPP (prednisone, methotrexate, doxorubicin, cyclophosphamide, etoposide, Mustargen, vincristine, procarbazine). As would be expected, the CHOP combination has been extensively studied in FL. Although superior to less aggressive therapies for DLBCL, CHOP has no proven advantage in FL. An extensive review of multiple SWOG trials involving doxorubicin-containing combinations for the treatment of FL showed no benefit for this drug combination compared with less aggressive combinations.[261]

Accordingly, there remains interest in deferral of therapy for this disease. In selected patients with low tumor burden followed expectantly, OS was 73% at 10 years.[120] Of interest, spontaneous regressions were noted in approximately 25% of patients. Histologic transformation to a higher-grade lymphoma occurred both before and after therapy with a frequency similar to that seen in patients treated at initial diagnosis. This study was nonrandomized, but similar findings have been observed in the randomized trial by Groupe d'Etude des Lymphomes Folliculaires.[262]

The lack of evidence that the natural history of FL is greatly altered by conventional chemotherapy has stimulated the search for new agents and new treatment strategies. Some of these approaches are as follows:

Immunotherapy: Rituximab produces responses in about 50% of relapsed FL patients as a single agent. As first-line therapy, the response rate is about 70%. More often, however, rituximab has been combined with chemotherapy. Numerous phase III trials have been conducted utilizing a variety of drug combinations with rituximab.[208,211,263–265,266–267] These studies have consistently shown an improvement in OS when rituximab is added to a combination chemotherapy regimen. To which chemotherapy program one should add rituximab, however, is not clear. In the United States, the most popular combination has been R-CHOP.[185]

Of primary interest currently is the issue of immunotherapy in the maintenance setting. Multiple phase III trials, using various induction regimens, have demonstrated an improvement in PFS with rituximab maintenance,[268–269,270] with a meta-analysis demonstrating an OS benefit.[268] However, the largest trial conducted to date, which used R-CHOP induction, did not show an advantage in overall survival, possibly due to more effective induction therapy, rituximab use at relapse, or simply inadequate follow-up.[270] The optimal schedule and duration of maintenance rituximab has not been formally studied. The primary risk is infections.

Radioimmunotherapy: This has also been extensively investigated in FL, both for the treatment of relapsed disease as well as an initial therapy. The two agents in wide use are ^{90}Y ibritumomab tiuxetan and ^{131}I-tositumomab, the former a pure β-emitter, the latter a γ- and β-emitter. Both agents demonstrate comparable activity with response rates of 60% to 80% in relapsed FL patients.[271–273] In a select group of previously untreated patients, a 95% response rate was obtained with ^{131}I-tositumomab (75% CR) with half of the patients in continuous CR at 4 years.[215] These radiolabeled antibodies have been cautiously combined with chemotherapy, because their primary toxicity is myelosuppression.

In a SWOG phase II trial of CHOP followed by ^{131}I-tositumomab, 5-year FFS was 67% and OS was 87%.[213] A phase III trial randomized patients with stage III or IV FL in CR or PR after a variety of induction regimens to observation or consolidation with ^{90}Y ibritumomab.[216] PFS was increased from 13.3 to 36.5 months (P <.0001) with manageable toxicity. This has not been widely adopted given the lack of rituximab in the control arm. The SWOG recently completed a randomized study comparing R-CHOP with CHOP and consolidation ^{131}I-tositumomab. Final results have not yet been reported. There are no studies to the authors' knowledge combining radioimmunoconjugates with external-beam radiotherapy.

Interferon: A large number of trials have been conducted examining the effect of this agent, both as a part of induction therapy and as maintenance after chemotherapy. A recent meta-analysis concluded that when given in the context of relatively intensive initial chemotherapy interferon-alfa prolongs both remission duration and survival.[274] Nonetheless, its toxicity has inhibited widespread use, and further, all those trials preceded the rituximab era.

Stem cell transplantation: A number of studies have examined the role of autologous and allogeneic transplantation in FL, for both relapsed disease and FL in first remission following induction chemotherapy.[275–282] Although a number of phase II trials looked promising, most phase III trials using ASCT have not shown an improvement in OS, although most have shown an improvement in PFS.

Allogeneic SCT has been used less frequently, particularly with myeloablative conditioning, given high rates of treatment-related mortality in the range of 30% to 40%. More recent studies have used RIC regimens, which are associated with less but still significant nonrelapse mortality.[276,278,282] The curative potential of allogeneic SCT is evident, although many questions remain including optimal conditioning regimen, appropriate donor sources, graft versus host disease prophylaxis, and posttransplant interventions such as donor lymphocyte infusions.

Role of Radiation Therapy in Advanced Follicular Lymphoma

The curative potential of RT for localized FL together with the early HL experience led to the initiation of trials of TLI for patients with stage III FL, primarily by the Stanford University group.[173] Sixty-six patients with stage III FL were treated either with TLI (61 patients) or TBI (5 patients). The FFS rate was 35% at 15 years, the cause-specific survival was 58%, and the OS was 35%, reflecting additional mortality from nonlymphoma causes. A small cohort of eight patients with a lower tumor burden, so-called limited stage III disease, defined as fewer than five disease sites and no tumor mass >10 cm, had an FFS of 88% and cause-specific survival of 100% at 15 years. Doses of RT used were 40 to 48 Gy, much larger than would be considered optimal currently. There were few relapses occurring beyond the 10th year. Similar data have been reported from the University of Florida, the Medical College of Wisconsin, and the MD Anderson Cancer Center.[283–285]

RT has also been advocated as consolidation therapy after chemotherapy in patients with advanced stage FL. A phase III trial by Aviles et al.[286] randomized 118 untreated patients with stage III or IV FL to receive CVP chemotherapy alone or the same chemotherapy followed by IFRT to initially involved nodal sites, at doses of 35 to 45 Gy. The 7-year FFS was 33% in the group treated by chemotherapy alone and 66% in those receiving CMT. The 7-year OS was also doubled from approximately 40% to 80%. The improvement in FFS was highly significant, and the survival showed improvement of borderline statistical significance (P = .06). There have been no additional studies attempting to replicate these results.

Follicular Lymphoma, Grade 3

Grade 3 FL comprises cases where there are >15 centroblasts per high-power field. In the current WHO classification, patients with FL who have diffuse areas in the pathological specimen comprised predominantly or entirely of large blastic cells are also reported to have DLBCL.[35] FL grade 3 is an uncommon variety of FL, comprising approximately 15% of all cases of FL.[287–290] The biologic behavior of this specific type of lymphoma is somewhat controversial because of its infrequency and the relatively small number of patients reported in various retrospective series in the literature.

Initial reports suggested an unfavorable outlook; a median survival >10 years was reported in the Stanford University series, but only 22% of patients were disease free at that time.[289] The advent of anthracycline-based chemotherapy appears to have resulted in some improvement in that prognosis and perhaps a plateauing of the FFS curve. The University of Nebraska group reported 3-year survival rates of 76% and 61% for patients with stage I or II disease and III or IV disease, respectively, but FFS rates of only 61% and 34%, respectively, results not that different from those seen with other FLs.[287] On the other hand, the MD Anderson Cancer Center group reported 5-year survival rates of 72% in a series of 100 patients with stage I to IV disease and an FFS rate of 67%, with a "possible plateau in the FFS curve for patients with stage I–III disease."[290] In both series, patients received anthracycline-containing combination chemotherapy, with the patients with earlier-stage disease receiving IFRT as well in varying dosages. The aforementioned as well as other series have led to a consensus that patients with FL grade 3 should be treated similarly to patients with DLBCL in terms of chemotherapy.[288,291] The prognosis, in general, is better than for DLBCL but median survivals are shorter than for FL.

Data regarding dose–response information for RT are lacking. Because virtually all patients are receiving chemotherapy, however, the authors consolidate patients with early-stage disease with 30 Gy IFRT in a fashion similar to that for early-stage DLBCL.

Marginal Zone Lymphomas

Extranodal MZL or MALT lymphomas are the most common variant, the most common location being the stomach. The treatment of MALT lymphoma of the stomach is discussed in the section on primary extranodal lymphomas. Other commonly involved extranodal sites include skin, salivary glands, and orbit (in descending order of frequency).[128] MALT lymphoma involving sites other than the stomach and GI tract behaves similarly, but there is no association with *H. pylori.* The disease is very responsive to RT. Doses of approximately 30 Gy produce long-term control in more than 90% of patients. In one large series combining MALT of all sites, the overall local control rate was 97%, the OS was 96%, and FFS at 5 years was 76%.[132,161] When MALT lymphoma relapses, it tends to have a prolonged clinical course.

Occasional patients with MALT lymphoma present with isolated organ involvement that is, however, bilateral (e.g., involvement of the salivary glands or conjunctivae). This behavior, referred to as *lymphocyte homing,* is not well understood. Such patients may be treated with local RT to both paired sites with apparent long-term FFS observed.[292]

MALT lymphoma is responsive to chemotherapy in a high percentage of patients. With single-agent chlorambucil, a 75% CR rate was observed in one series.[293] A large SWOG analysis, however, indicated that FFS and OS rates were similar to those observed in FL, with no plateauing of the survival curve.[294] Thus, chemotherapy is palliative and reserved for patients with generalized disease who are symptomatic. MALT lymphomas also respond well to rituximab, but either alone or in combination with chemotherapy this agent is not curative either.[74] Asymptomatic individuals with generalized disease should be considered for observation, similar to patients with generalized FL because the course is so often indolent. Patients with generalized disease with symptoms due to a localized tumor mass may be easily palliated with modest doses of radiation to the mass in question. That approach is often superior to systemic chemotherapy.

Nodal and splenic MZL have been discussed previously in the section on clinical–histopathologic correlates. Both are most often generalized and managed similarly to advanced FL.

Peripheral T-Cell Lymphomas

PTCL of the nodal type, not otherwise specified, resembles DLBCL in its clinical characteristics and presentation.[36,56,113,138,295–298] Overall, there is a worse outlook. PTCL is more often generalized, the IPI tends to be worse, and approximately half of patients have B symptomatology. Response to treatment is generally unsatisfactory. The International T-Cell Lymphoma Project reported 10-year survivals in the range of 20%.[136] There was no clear benefit for the addition of anthracyclines to a chemotherapy program and no standardized regimen has emerged. CHOP is probably the most commonly employed regimen in the United States. Because this is a T-cell lymphoma, there is no role for rituximab. Patients who present with localized PTCL should be treated with chemotherapy (type and duration uncertain) and IFRT. Doses and field sizes of RT are probably comparable with those used for DLBCL. PTCL patients were included in the BNLI trial but constituted only 5% of aggressive histologies.[163] Given these uncertainties and considering that PTCL is less responsive to chemotherapy then DLBCL, a dose of approximately 40 Gy in 2 Gy fractions is recommended. Few data exist regarding the role of RT for advanced disease. As for DLBCL, the concept may warrant further exploration.

In contrast to most patients with PTCL, those with ALCL have a much better prognosis, among the best of any of the lymphoma categories and certainly the best of the ostensibly "aggressive" histologic types. The presence of the anaplastic lymphoma kinase (*ALK*) translocation, with subsequent expression of the ALK protein, distinguishes prognostic groups. ALK-positive patients have a good prognosis when treated with CHOP. OS is around 70% at 10 years.[299,300] ALK-negative patients have a considerably worse outlook, with OS from 14% to 40% following CHOP therapy. ALCL of the skin is discussed in the section on primary extranodal lymphomas.

Small Lymphocytic Lymphoma

SLL is a rare disease, histologically and phenotypically identical to CLL and subsumed into one category by the WHO classification. SLL is most often generalized. The distinction between SLL and CLL is somewhat arbitrary and depends on the absence of leukemic cells in the blood in the former ($<5 \times 10^9$/L monoclonal lymphocytes in the peripheral blood). Treatment is essentially that of CLL except when localized. The purine analogs appear to be the most active agents.[301,302] The disease is also responsive to alkylating agent chemotherapy such as chlorambucil or combination chemotherapy, with CHOP, for example. Rituximab also plays a major role. As with FL and MZL, there is neither evidence for a plateauing of the survival curve nor definite benefit from combination chemotherapy, as opposed to single-agent treatment.[303,304]

In that rare situation where the disease is localized (i.e., stage I or II nodal only), one would predict RT might achieve long-term FFS for some patients with doses and field sizes similar to those used for FL, namely, approximately 30 Gy in 3 weeks' time to a generous involved field. Accordingly, RT has been recommended as the treatment of choice in this situation.[152]

Mantle Cell Lymphoma

The treatment of MCL is unsatisfactory. This recently designated disease is distinguished by one of the worst outlooks for any lymphoma. Another way of describing the survival pattern of MCL is that it resembles FL in its response to therapy and FFS (i.e., no plateauing of the FFS curve and thus no indication of cure), but DLBCL in its overall survival (i.e., much shorter than FL).[305–308]

The therapy of MCL has been explored in a number of retrospective analyses as well as prospective phase II and limited phase III trials using a variety of chemotherapy programs.[153,306,308] Chemotherapy programs can be generally grouped as CHOP-like, now usually including rituximab, which does have activity in MCL, purine analog containing programs (e.g., R-FCM [fludarabine, cyclophosphamide, mitoxantrone]) or more intensive programs such as hyperCVAD (cyclophosphamide, vincristine, doxorubicin, dexamethasone, cytarabine, and methotrexate). High response rates are seen (80% to 90%), but relapse usually occurs with no plateauing of FFS. There is no clear evidence for superiority of one regimen over another. The addition of rituximab to chemotherapy does seem beneficial.[309]

HDC and SCT have also been employed, both autologous as well as allogeneic, both in first remission and for rela pse.[153,310,311] One phase III trial did demonstrate improved FFS for SCT in first remission, but no survival benefit as yet.[312] Thus, SCT must still be considered unproven. It has been suggested that apparent improvements in survival with programs such as HDC and SCT may be attributed to better supportive care, patient selection, and failure to account for prognostic factors.[307,313] NCCN guidelines indicate no standard therapy for MCL.[314] Entry into clinical trial is recommended.

Patients with localized MCL (stage I or II) are seldom encountered. One small series from British Columbia has been reported, however.[315] Seventeen patients treated with RT (30 to 35 Gy) with or without chemotherapy had a 5-year FFS of 68% and OS of 71%. Adjuvant chemotherapy did not seem to influence the outcome. Thus, RT appears to have an important role for those few patients with limited stage MCL. RT is also very effective palliation for patients with advanced disease.[316] Clinically the disease is quite sensitive to radiation, and low doses (<20 Gy) may suffice.[316]

Finally, there may be a group of patients with MCL with favorable prognostic factors in whom observation is a reasonable strategy. In a small series from New York Hospital, survival was not compromised by an initial period of observation prior to initiation of therapy when and if disease progression occurred.[307]

PRIMARY EXTRANODAL LYMPHOMAS

Thus far this chapter has considered NHL primarily from the standpoint of the histopathologic classification. NHL may also be clinically divided, however, on the basis of origin from nodal or extranodal tissue; the latter may be further subdivided as to site of origin. The frequency of extranodal lymphoma (ENL) and certain characteristic clinical entities associated with lymphoma in various extranodal sites makes the discussion of ENL as such appropriate.

It is important to re-emphasize certain principles that recur in this section: localized disease, whether presenting nodally or extranodally, seems to have the same prognosis (Fig. 78.5). The management strategy for localized nodal lymphoma of a given histologic type usually applies as well to that same histologic type when presenting extranodally.

Extranodal disease accounts for approximately 35% to 40% of all patients with NHL and approximately half of those with stage I and II NHL.[71,72,317] The most common sites of involvement are the GI tract, accounting for approximately 25% to 35% of all ENL, the head and neck region, which accounts for approximately 20% to 30% (including Waldeyer's ring and other head and neck sites, but excluding brain), and skin, with a variety of miscellaneous sites accounting for the rest. PCNSL, which accounts for approximately 10% of all ENL, is discussed separately.

Histopathologically, ENLs are classified in much the same fashion as nodal lymphomas. The extranodal location may cause difficulties in histopathologic diagnosis. Immunophenotyping as well as cellular morphology may be helpful in this respect. Establishing the diagnosis of ENL on the basis of fine-needle aspirate or similarly sized biopsy, however, is an unwise practice. Accurate histopathologic classification is essential for proper management and almost always requires at least a core of tissue.[38]

Gastrointestinal Lymphoma

The stomach is the most common site of involvement (50% to 80% of all cases of GI lymphoma).[72,318–320] The remaining GI lymphomas occur in the small and large intestines, primarily ileum, followed by colon and rectum, but lymphomas may arise in any of the GI tissues. Histopathologically, 90% to 95% of gastric lymphomas are MALT or DLBCL, the two being approximately equal in frequency.[320–322]

Patients with gastric lymphoma usually present with symptoms of abdominal pain (~80%).[320] Other common complaints are loss of appetite (~50%), weight loss (25%), and bleeding (20%). B symptomatology is uncommon (10% of patients). In this regard, only fever and night sweats are significant because weight loss is so often a function of direct effects on the stomach. Perforation as an initial symptom is very uncommon, occurring in <2% of patients. Many cases of gastric MZL are detected incidentally during endoscopic examinations.

The diagnosis of gastric lymphoma is usually established endoscopically, although in past years laparotomy was often necessary.[323] Surgical resection has traditionally been the cornerstone of treatment, followed by adjuvant RT or chemotherapy. This approach at the Princess Margaret Hospital, for example, resulted in an FFS of 81% and cause-specific survival of 88% in 149 patients treated between 1967 and 1996.[324] Other surgical series have been extensively reviewed by Bozzetti et al.[325] and Thirlby,[326] with OS of 60% to 100% in stage I patients and 40% to 80% for stage II disease.

Beginning in the 1980s, however, some authors began to question the necessity for surgery in a disease that is usually quite responsive to RT or chemotherapy. Subsequently a number of reports showed equivalent outcomes when patients were treated with RT and chemotherapy without surgery.[320,327–328,329,330] A large series of gastric lymphomas reported by the German GI

Tumor Study Group is representative.[330,331] They reported on 398 stage I and II patients with primary gastric lymphoma about equally divided between MALT and DLBCL. Three hundred thirty-five were managed conservatively without surgical resection; 63 had subtotal gastrectomy. Outcomes were essentially identical with an 80% 5-year survival.

Gastric Diffuse Large B-Cell Lymphoma

The historical experience with the treatment of localized DLBCL of the stomach without systemic therapy demonstrated an OS in the range of 25% to 50%, as with DLBCL generally. The use of systemic chemotherapy has resulted in considerable improvement. Multiple centers now report 5-year OS in the range of 70% to 80% for patients with localized disease treated with chemotherapy with or without RT.[320,332–334] Although some authors have suggested that chemotherapy alone is adequate treatment,[332,334] most studies have used CMT.

A multicenter randomized trial from the IELSG formally evaluated the role of RT in patients with high-grade NHL (principally DLBCL) of the stomach.[228] Patients with a CR after 4 cycles of a CHOP-like regimen were randomized to consolidation RT (minimum of 30 Gy) or 2 additional cycles of chemotherapy. Patients with a PR after 4 cycles received an additional 2 cycles of chemotherapy, and if they obtained a CR, were then randomized to radiation versus observation. Due to poor accrual, the study was closed after enrolling 55 of a planned 125 patients. Four patients (three local failures and one distant failure) recurred in the chemotherapy alone arm, while there were no recurrences after consolidation RT, resulting in a disease-free survival of 100% with RT versus 82% without (P = .04).

Although most studies of gastric DLBCL have utilized CHOP, treatment should be initiated with R-CHOP in view of the results cited above. The risk of chemotherapy-induced gastric perforation is very low, 1% to 2%. The number of cycles is not well defined; 3 to 6 cycles have been most often used, with the precise number depending on the rapidity of response, initial volume of disease, and investigator preference, as with stage I and II disease in general.[164,168] The response to chemotherapy should be assessed with appropriate imaging studies, usually a repetition of those studies that were positive before the onset of chemotherapy. Repeat endoscopic evaluation and biopsy are particularly useful for assessing the completeness of response.

Radiation doses and field sizes to be used for gastric DLBCL are not well defined. Excellent results have been reported in patients treated with 25 Gy after surgical resection.[335] For patients treated without resection, a wide variety of radiation doses have been reported, ranging from 30 to 50 Gy, similar to what has been described for the treatment of nodal DLBCL. Treatment fields have also varied considerably from whole abdomen to IF. There is no apparent correlation between field size or dose and outcome. Local control in almost all the reported series has been high, in the range of 90%. FFS and OS for patients with stage I and II disease have also ranged from 70% to 80%.[292,321,324,329,330,333,336]

The radiation field should probably encompass the entire stomach and perigastric lymph nodes along the greater and lesser curvature of the stomach as well as any other involved nodal areas with an appropriate margin. Patients should be fasting for several hours prior to simulation and treatment. CT-based planning is preferred. Respiratory-induced motion should be assessed and accounted for using fluoroscopy or four-dimensional CT. The typical field arrangement is parallel-opposed anterior and posterior fields. More complex field arrangements may be necessary depending on the position of the kidneys in relation to the target volume. In the event the patient has responded completely to chemotherapy by negative endoscopic examination and biopsy, a dose of 30 Gy is appropriate, similar to what would be done for nodal disease (see the section Principles of Treatment). If there is persistent biopsy-documented disease after chemotherapy, other systemic therapy should be considered or higher doses of radiation must be used, in the range of 40 Gy.

Gastric Lymphoma, Mucosa-Associated Lymphoid Tissue Type

MALT lymphoma is a distinct clinical-pathologic entity first described by Isaacson and Wright[50] and occurring most often in the stomach. A unique feature of gastric MALT is the association with *H. pylori* infection, initially reported by Isaacson's group.[23,337] *H. pylori* can be identified in up to 92% of patients.[23]

Accordingly, first-line treatment for patients who are *H. pylori* positive is appropriate antibiotics. A frequently recommended combination is omeprazole, metronidazole, and clarithromycin.[338] Numerous studies have confirmed the efficacy of antibiotics for gastric MALT. The complete remission rate is approximately 75%. Approximately two-thirds of complete responders remain in remission at 5 years,[339,340,341] for an overall 5-year FFS of about 50%. The 5-year OS is much higher at 90% with most deaths due to causes other than lymphoma.[341] Response of *H. pylori*-negative cases to antibiotics has also been reported.[342]

Several factors have been associated with resistance to antibiotics, including deep invasion of the gastric wall[343,344] and the (11:18) translocation.[345] Additionally, some patients in CR will have persistent B cell monoclonality on PCR analysis and are at higher risk of relapse.[341]

These results appear inferior to those achieved with RT where the CR rate exceeds 95% and the relapse rate is <10% with doses of 30 Gy,[132] although no direct comparison has even been done. Nonetheless, national and international guidelines call for initial therapy with antibiotics and close follow-up because of the simplicity of this approach and the slow growth of MALT lymphomas.[24,314] RT is reserved for patients who are *H. pylori* negative or who fail antibiotic therapy. The same techniques utilized for gastric DLBCL apply. Doses of 25 to 30 Gy are adequate. Interestingly, the initial clone can be detected by PCR in the majority of patients after RT, despite durable clinical remissions.[346]

There is no apparent role for adjuvant chemotherapy in localized gastric MALT lymphoma. Rituximab has been used in patients not suitable for RT with promising but very short-term results.[347] For patients with advanced disease, chemotherapy is not a curative modality and observation may be warranted if the patient is asymptomatic. In general, management of advanced MALT is similar to advanced FL.

Intestinal Lymphomas

Small intestinal lymphomas may comprise 20% to 30% of all GI lymphomas.[318,320,336,348] The majority are B-cell lymphomas, predominantly DLBCL.[318,349,350] DLBCL of the intestine is seen primarily in Western countries and resembles primary DLBCL of the stomach. The clinical presentation is usually with abdominal pain, anorexia, and weight loss. However, ileus or perforation is much more common than in gastric lymphoma, occurring in approximately 40% of the patients in the German series.[320] Most patients have localized disease at onset, but the usual staging workup is appropriate. PET-CT should be performed, primarily for delineation of disease outside the intestinal tract and determination of the size of mass lesions in the intestinal tract. Intraluminal disease is probably better visualized with conventional barium studies.

Because of the frequent presentation with obstructive signs and symptoms, along with the complexity of establishing a diagnosis endoscopically, surgery is more commonly used, both for diagnosis and for therapy, than it is for gastric lymphoma. For surgically resected, localized intestinal lymphoma of the DLBCL type, anthracycline-based chemotherapy with rituximab should be given after surgery, as for localized DLBCL of other sites. For completely resected disease, adjuvant RT is probably not necessary. In the case of localized disease incompletely resected, some authorities recommend the addition of WAI,[324] although more conformal fields may be used if the target region can be appropriately demarcated.

From 20% to 30% of patients with B-cell lymphomas of the intestine present with histologies other than DLBCL, primarily MALT, although Burkitt's, mantle cell, and FL have all been observed.[330,349,350–351] Mantle cell lymphoma has a propensity to present with multicentric involvement.[350] Primary FL of the duodenum is a rare presentation of FL and may have a more favorable prognosis compared with nodal FL. Complete and durable remissions after RT have been reported and would be the standard treatment for a localized FL.[351] Even with no treatment, distant dissemination is rare.

MALT intestinal lymphomas are not thought to be *H. pylori* related. They are managed primarily with RT. The role of chemotherapy is limited. Crump et al.[324] recommend WAI for intestinal MALT after surgical resection with a dose of 20 to 25 Gy in 1- to 1.25-Gy fractions. Depending on the segment of intestine involved and the extent, less than WAI may also be used to similar doses (25 to 30 Gy). CT-based planning with field arrangements that limit dose to the kidneys and liver is critical. The technique of cross-table laterals for treatment of mesenteric adenopathy may be applicable. Precise data as to the prognosis of localized intestinal B-cell lymphoma are lacking. Underlying histology affects prognosis. MZL appears to have the best prognosis, as would be expected, while the prognosis for mantle cell lymphoma is poor. Lymphomas of the ileocecal region are more likely to present with obstruction, leading to surgical resection. This may lead to a better prognosis.[350]

T-cell lymphomas account for approximately 10% to 20% of all intestinal lymphomas, and multiple subtypes have been known to arise in the bowel, including extranodal NK/T-cell lymphoma, anaplastic large cell lymphoma, and $\gamma\delta$ T-cell lymphoma. A distinct intestinal lymphoma entity in the WHO classification is *enteropathy-associated T-cell lymphoma,* which occurs primarily in the presence of celiac disease. This has also been described as malignant histiocytosis of the intestine, but it is now known to represent a T-cell lymphoma.[352] Patients with celiac disease have an approximately 200-fold increased risk for development of intestinal T-cell lymphoma.[72]

The clinical presentation is similar to that described for B-cell intestinal lymphomas. Diarrhea is prominent, reported in approximately 40% of patients. Presentation with perforation or obstruction occurs in approximately 40% of patients.[353] There is a greater tendency for these patients to have widespread bowel involvement. The diagnosis is usually established with laparotomy. After surgical resection, treatment has usually consisted of anthracycline-based chemotherapy. The outcome, however, has been poor, with 5-year survivals of 20% to 25%.[349,353] These patients usually have a worse performance status and tolerate chemotherapy poorly. Intestinal perforation after chemotherapy is not unusual.

There are no reported results for RT. For patients with residual disease after surgery, it is possible that a protracted course of RT with small fractions followed by chemotherapy might reduce the frequency of intestinal perforation reported after conventional doses of CHOP. Field sizes and arrangements would be similar to those described for intestinal MALT. More dose is presumably required (30 to 40 Gy) but would be difficult to administer because of tolerance problems.

Immunoproliferative small intestinal disease (IPSID), also referred to as *Mediterranean lymphoma,* occurs mainly in young adults in the Middle East and North Africa.[354] In Western series it is quite uncommon. IPSID is a B-cell lymphoma, believed to arise from the clonal proliferation of B lymphocytes that produce immunoglobulin-A (IgA heavy chain). *C. jejuni* has recently been shown to have an etiologic role. In its early stages, the disease responds to antibiotic therapy. The disease frequently affects the entire small intestine. Symptoms of malabsorption predominate. Treatment has usually consisted of chemotherapy.[354,355] The prognosis has been poor, with survival rates not exceeding 20%. WAI has been reported to be useful in selected patients.[354]

Head and Neck Lymphomas

Head and neck lymphomas are the second most frequent variant of ENL after those of the GI tract, representing approximately 20% of all ENL.[68,71,72,317,356,357] They occur in a variety of sites, including Waldeyer's ring, the thyroid, salivary glands, nasal cavity, paranasal sinuses, and orbit, with differing histologic types and clinical characteristics depending on the site of origin. Most appear to be of B-cell origin and most of those are DLBCL. MZL is less common but constitutes a majority of salivary gland lymphomas. A special entity is that of nasal NK/T-cell lymphoma.[140–142,358,359] This disease for a number of years was of uncertain cause but is now believed to represent a T-cell lymphoma. It went by many names in the past, including angiocentric lymphoma, lethal midline granuloma, midline malignant reticulosis, and polymorphic reticulosis, reflecting its uncertain etiology. The preferred terminology, however, is NK/T-cell lymphoma.

Lymphomas presenting in Waldeyer's ring typically involve the tonsil, base of tongue, or nasopharynx. The clinical symptoms are those associated with epithelial tumors in those sites, such as dysphagia, sore throat, nasal congestion, and eustachian tube blockage. The lesions are frequently clinically apparent on thorough head and neck examination. Neck adenopathy is common.

The usual lymphoma staging studies are appropriate, including CT or PET-CT scans of head and neck, chest, and abdomen and bone marrow examination. MRI may be necessary for precise anatomic delineation. There is a predilection for Waldeyer's ring lymphomas to have GI tract involvement as well, so direct imaging (i.e., upper GI series or endoscopy) is indicated. Most cases are stage I or II after full staging evaluation.

The pathologic type is usually DLBCL. The treatment guidelines are those for nodal stage I and II DLBCL. Older series report results of RT alone: 50% survival rates in patients with stage I disease and 25% to 50% in stage II, but more often the former number, results clearly suboptimal.[356,360] Consequently, almost all centers now report the use of CMT, 3 to 6 cycles of CHOP followed by IFRT. Again R-CHOP would now be the preferred combination. Retrospective analyses show an improvement in survival rates to approximately 80% for patients with stage I disease and 50% for those with stage II disease after CMT.[356,361] Even better results would be expected today with the use of R-CHOP.

The one phase III study is that of Aviles et al.,[362] who randomized 316 patients to RT alone, CMT, or chemotherapy alone. Although a CR was achieved in over 90% of patients in all three groups, relapses were frequent for the single-modality arms. The 5-year survival rate was approximately 90% in the CMT arm versus approximately 50% for the chemotherapy and RT alone arms.

Paranasal sinus and nasal cavity lymphomas are often grouped together but in reality appear to have a different prognosis and should be discussed separately. Most paranasal sinus tumors are B cell in origin and usually present in men in the sixth or seventh decade. The outlook when treated with RT alone seems to be particularly poor for both stage I and II disease, with 12% long-term survival in the Stanford University series and approximately 30% in an MD Anderson Cancer Center report.[363,364] Some authors have described a predilection for CNS spread;[363] others have not found this to be the case.[142,364] In any event, the outlook improves markedly when patients are treated with CMT. In the MD Anderson Cancer Center report, FFS approximately doubled from 34% to 63% at 10 years with the addition of chemotherapy to RT.[364] With CMT, survival rates in the range of 70% to 80% are expected, similar to those seen in other sites. CNS prophylaxis for these patients is controversial. In the MD Anderson Cancer Center series, only 1 of 70 patients relapsed in the CNS.[364]

Nasal cavity lymphomas, on the other hand, appear to be of predominantly T-cell origin and fall into the category of NK/T-cell lymphomas. They are seen more commonly in Asia and Central and South America. The disease affects primarily men, mostly in the fifth decade. It often presents as a destructive necrotizing process. Because of this, histologic diagnosis may be difficult. The disease appears to progress primarily locally with only a small predilection for regional or systemic failure.[141] Treatment approaches have consisted of RT alone, chemotherapy alone, and the two combined. With RT alone, approximately two-thirds of patients achieved CR,[141,142,358] but half of those relapsed. The prognosis appears somewhat worse for stage II than stage I.[142]

The contribution of chemotherapy to the management of NK/T-cell lymphoma is unclear. When treated initially with chemotherapy, CR occurs in only a minority of patients,[142,143,145,365] in contrast to the results seen with most other head and neck lymphomas. Recently, Japanese and Korean investigators have reported the use of concurrent chemotherapy and radiation with encouraging results.[366,367] The Japanese series used concurrent dexamethasone, etoposide, carboplatin, and ifosfamide with a dose of 50 Gy. The CR rate was 77% and the 2-year survival rate was 78% compared with historical controls of 45%.[366] The Korean series employed concurrent cisplatin and radiation, with the dose of the latter 40 to 50 Gy, followed by 3 cycles of cisplatin, dexamethasone, ifosfamide, and etoposide. The CR rate was 83% and the 3-year survival rate was 86%.[367] In both series, the number of patients is small (33 and 30 patients, respectively), but the results are quite promising and worthy of further study. The large experience with concurrent cisplatin and radiation in head and neck carcinomas argues for the feasibility of this approach in nasal type NK/T-cell lymphomas.

In contrast to most other head and neck lymphomas, salivary gland lymphomas are frequently of a more indolent histologic type (i.e., MZL).[368] In Asian countries, the percentage of MZL may be lower. These patients usually present with painless enlargement of the parotid gland. There is an association with Sjögren syndrome.[357] Treatment usually consists of RT alone. The prognosis is excellent, with survival >90%.[357,368] One small randomized trial explored the use of chemotherapy in addition to RT.[369] In this trial, 5-year survival rates of 90% were achieved with RT alone or with CMT. These data are consistent with the lack of improvement shown for the addition of chemotherapy to RT for MZL in other sites, as well as the lack of benefit for chemotherapy in addition to RT in localized FL.

There are occasional patients with salivary gland lymphomas presenting with bilateral paired organ involvement (e.g., both parotid glands). When the histologic type is MZL, such patients, although not stage II in the conventional sense, appear to do quite well with localized RT directed to both parotids.

The appropriate radiation dose for head and neck lymphomas may be derived from the general principles of lymphoma treatment. For DLBCL, which in almost all instances will be treated initially with R-CHOP or similar combinations, patients achieving CR should receive 30 Gy consolidation (2 Gy per fraction). Less information is available for those not achieving CR. Doses from 30 to 40 Gy are reasonable. For NK/T-cell tumors, few data are available. The authors recommend a dose of 40 to 50 Gy in combination with chemotherapy. The NCCN guidelines recommend a dose of at least 50 Gy. Indolent histologies involving the head and neck should be treated with RT alone to a maximum of 30 Gy.

The field size is involved region with a generous margin without prophylactic nodal radiation. IMRT should be utilized in most patients to maximize parotid sparing as well as shielding to the minor salivary glands. Lymphoma patients may have unusual susceptibility to xerostomia.[370]

Cutaneous Lymphomas

The term primary cutaneous lymphoma (PCL) is used to define those lymphomas that present in and are confined to the skin without evidence of extracutaneous disease. Including mycosis fungoides (discussed in Chapter 79), PCL is the third most common ENL, closely following GI and head and neck lymphomas. PCL is a relatively unique type of lymphoma whose clinical behavior seems to be governed more by presentation in the skin than by its histologic appearance, in contrast with most other lymphomas, where the histopathologic appearance predicts the clinical behavior. Further, where in the skin the disease originates may have a significant bearing on outcome. DLBCL originating on the legs has a much worse outlook than that originating on skin surfaces elsewhere.[146,371] The biologic explanation for this phenomenon is unknown.

PCL is an uncommon entity with an overall incidence of 1 to 1.5 per 100,000. Separate pathologic classifications were devised by the European Organisation for Research and Treatment of Cancer (EORTC)[372] and WHO[48] but have recently been reconciled (Table 78.9).[373] About 75% of all PCL is of T-cell origin and 25% of B-cell origin. Most cutaneous T-cell lymphomas are mycosis fungoides.

Most other cutaneous T-cell lymphomas consist of the closely related categories of LyP and primary cutaneous ALCL. LyP and cutaneous ALCL have overlapping clinical, histologic, and immunophenotypical characteristics. They are characteristically referred to as CD30-positive lymphoproliferative disorders. The largest reported experience is from the Dutch Cutaneous Lymphoma Group.[146] These authors described 219 patients in the period 1983 through 1998, approximately equally divided between LyP and cutaneous ALCL. The distinction between the two was often difficult, but both had an excellent prognosis. The disease is almost invariably confined to the skin. Only 2% of patients with LyP and 4% of those with cutaneous ALCL died of lymphoma. This has implications for initial staging, where some authorities discourage imaging studies looking for systemic disease.[374] LyP is often generalized (in the skin), and spontaneous remissions are a characteristic feature and an important clue as to diagnosis. Cutaneous ALCL, on the other hand, is localized or regional in approximately 80% of cases.

The treatment of choice for cutaneous ALCL is local radiotherapy. A dose of 40 Gy is generally recommended.[146] About 40% of patients will relapse elsewhere in the skin but may often still be sufficiently localized so they can be treated again with radiation. As stated above, death from lymphoma is infrequent. LyP, if it can be distinguished from cutaneous ALCL, should be left untreated as spontaneous regression is a characteristic feature. There is generally no role for chemotherapy for cutaneous ALCL, although a variety of agents have been tried for LyP that is sufficiently symptomatic to require treatment. The natural history of LyP and its tendency for spontaneous regression makes evaluation of various chemotherapeutic agents quite problematic.[374]

TABLE 78.9 WORLD HEALTH ORGANIZATION–EUROPEAN ORGANISATION FOR RESEARCH AND TREATMENT OF CANCER CLASSIFICATION OF CUTANEOUS LYMPHOMAS

Type	*Frequency (%)*	*5-Year Cause-Specific Survival (%)*
Cutaneous T Cell		
Mycosis fungoides	44	88
Lymphomatoid papulosis	12	100
Anaplastic large cell lymphoma	8	95
Cutaneous B Cell		
Marginal zone lymphomas	7	99
Follicle center	11	95
Diffuse large B-cell lymphoma, leg-type	4	55

From ref. 373.

As mentioned previously, there is a difference between cutaneous ALCL arising in the skin and ALCL that originates elsewhere. The latter has a highly variable course depending on whether the ALK protein is overexpressed. ALK-negative patients have a worse outlook. ALCL in the skin, however, is ALK negative, with the determining factor in biologic behavior the site of origin.

Cutaneous B-cell lymphoma comprises about 25% of skin lymphomas. In the new WHO-EORTC classification, it is divided into primary cutaneous follicle center lymphoma (PCFCL), primary cutaneous marginal zone lymphoma (PCMZL), and primary cutaneous large cell lymphoma, leg type (PCLBCL-LT).[373,375] The term diffuse large B-cell lymphoma of the skin is no longer used; these patients are now included in the PCFCL group, which also contains follicular lymphoma of the skin. An unusual feature of a minority of cases of PCMZL is the association with *B. burgdorferi* infection, in which case the disease may respond to antibiotics.[21]

Both PCFCL and PCMZL have an excellent prognosis. The treatment of choice is RT, with the dose of 40 Gy for the former and 30 Gy for the latter, as for MZL elsewhere. The 5-year disease-specific survival for both conditions exceeds 95%.[371,373,375] Adjuvant chemotherapy is not recommended.

PCLBCL-LT, however, has a much worse prognosis with a cause-specific survival of about 50% at 5 years. In addition to local radiation, chemotherapy with R-CHOP is usually recommended, although it is not clear if this favorably influences outcome.[371,376]

Orbital Lymphomas

Lymphomas of the eye may involve either the extraocular orbital tissues such as the conjunctiva, retrobulbar region, or lacrimal gland, or may involve the globe itself. The latter condition is referred to as primary intraocular lymphoma and is, in essence, a subset of PCNSL in which lymphoma cells are initially present only in the eyes, without evidence of disease in the brain or other CNS tissues.[377] Its management is essentially that of PCNSL, which is discussed later.

Orbital lymphomas comprise approximately 4% of all ENL. They typically arise in superficial tissues such as conjunctiva and eyelids and are most commonly seen in an older population, with a median age of approximately 60 years.[72] Histopathologically, approximately two-thirds of these tumors are MZL. Most of the remainder are DLBCL.

Patients typically present with mass lesions in the conjunctivae or lids, described in the literature as "salmon pink" in color. Tumors of the retrobulbar region may present with swelling and proptosis and associated disturbances in function of the extraocular muscles. Bilaterality is not unusual, occurring in 10% to 15% of cases. Similar to salivary gland and skin tumors, this does not adversely affect prognosis.

The usual staging studies for systemic disease should be performed. MRI of the orbit should be done to delineate precisely the anatomic extent of disease for RT planning purposes.

The treatment principles for lymphomas generally apply. MZL is treated with RT alone. No more than 30 Gy is required for local control. Doses of 20 to 30 Gy have been reported as equally effective.[378,379–381] The BNLI study provides support for doses at the lower end of this range.[163] Local control exceeds 95% as does 5-year cause-specific survival. Most series report about 20% of patients relapsing, almost always at distant sites. There is, however, no established role for adjuvant chemotherapy or rituximab.

Field arrangements are somewhat controversial. Some authors suggest the entire orbit be treated to avoid marginal misses.[378,380] This may be done with a single anterior field or a wedged pair. Three-dimensional planning and IMRT may be helpful. A lens shield is often used to prevent cataracts, but this may increase marginal misses. With whole-orbital doses of 20 to 30 Gy, cataract formation is the principal risk, occurring in 20% to 30% of patients.[380] Some dryness may result from inclusion in the field of a portion of the lacrimal gland and meibomian glands. As mentioned, orbital MZL may involve both eyes at presentation. Under these circumstances, RT alone remains the treatment of choice, with careful attention to treatment planning and prescribed dose to minimize eye complications.

Orbital MZL has recently joined the group of MZL's associated with infectious agents, in this instance *C. psittaci*.[25] A trial of antibiotic therapy has been suggested for patients in whom this organism is identified,[382] but a meta-analysis has shown highly variable results of antibiotic therapy, with an overall incidence of *C. psittaci* of 23%.[130] It has also been suggested that observation only is a reasonable strategy. In a Japanese series of 36 patients, 70% did not require treatment with a median follow-up of 7 years.[383] However, radiotherapy remains the standard of care.

A much smaller percentage of patients (10% to 30%) presents with orbital disease that is DLBCL. The prognosis in the literature in the past has been poor—a 33% survival rate in Florida, and 50% at the Royal Marsden Hospital with RT alone.[384,385] The treatment of choice is CMT, R-CHOP followed by IFRT. After CR to chemotherapy, the appropriate dose of RT is no more than 30 Gy. It is particularly important to minimize dose to the eye to avoid late complications. With this program, cure rates of 80% would be expected and have been reported.[386]

Extranodal Lymphomas of Other Sites

In addition to the areas previously described, NHL may arise in almost any organ or tissue of the body, including but not limited to bone, testis, ovary, kidney, bladder, female genital tract, breasts, and lung. Lymphoma in any of these sites is quite uncommon. General principles of evaluation and management apply. Accurate histopathologic diagnosis is essential, followed by full staging workup with treatment decisions governed by stage and histopathologic diagnosis.

A few brief comments regarding the special features of testicular, bone, breast, and lung lymphomas are appropriate. Testicular lymphoma is rare, accounting for approximately 2% to 3% of all ENL and <1% of all NHL.[387,388,389] It presents typically in elderly men in their seventh and eighth decades. Most patients have stage I or II disease. The histologic type is typically DLBCL. Approximately one-fourth of patients have stage IV disease at presentation, with a predilection for unusual sites of involvement such as CNS, skin, and lung. In most reported series, patients have been treated in a variety of ways because of the rarity of the disease and the long period over which cases are collected from any one institution.

The disease is typically diagnosed by orchiectomy. In the past that was frequently followed by RT to pelvic and para-aortic nodes in a fashion similar to that for testicular carcinoma. Such treatment programs were notably unsuccessful, with probably <20% OS.[389] The introduction of CHOP combined with RT and surgery did not improved matters much. Treatment programs of surgery, CHOP, and RT have still resulted in only an approximately 30% long-term survival.[390,391] There is a high predilection for both contralateral testis relapse as well as CNS relapse, with some 30% to 40% of patients failing in these sites as well as other generalized sites.[389,392,393]

Accordingly, more recent treatment programs have advocated the use of CNS prophylaxis coupled with prophylactic RT to the contralateral testis and sometimes pelvic and para-aortic nodes. The IELSG recently reported a multi-institutional series of 53 stage I or II patients treated with R-CHOP, 6 to 8 cycles, prophylactic intrathecal methotrexate, and radiotherapy to the contralateral testis and para-aortic and pelvic nodes in the case of stage II patients.[76] Five-year survival and PFS were 85% and 74%, respectively. In a previous IELSG study, both survival and PFS were about 50% at 5 years and declined further at the 10-year mark.[393] The rarity of testicular lymphoma most likely precludes phase III trials.

ENL of bone is another uncommon entity, representing <5% of all ENL.[394–396] Patients tend to be somewhat younger, with a median age in the fifth decade. The long bones are primarily affected. The presenting signs and symptoms are usually local bone pain, with or without soft tissue swelling, and occasionally a palpable mass lesion or a pathologic fracture. Approximately two-thirds to three-fourths of patients have stage I and II disease at presentation, with the remainder having stage IV disease. A recent large series from British Columbia showed 50% of patients with stage IV disease and equal involvement of long bones and spine.[397] Histopathologically, 70% to 90% of patients have DLBCL.[394] Staging studies should include the usual workup for systemic disease. MRI to determine the extent of disease in the bone in limited stage patients should be performed as well.

The disease is managed similarly to stage I or II NHL of other sites. Thus, for DLBCL therapy is initiated with R-CHOP followed by involved field RT. Although a dose of 30 Gy is appropriate for patients achieving CR, that determination may be difficult in bone disease. The normal reparative processes may cloud the imaging determination of a CR. Therefore, the authors often use 40 Gy consolidative RT but try and avoid this dose to entire joints because of the risk of avascular necrosis. Treatment volume should include the original tumor volume as determined by MRI with a margin of several centimeters. Radiation of the entire bone is probably unnecessary. FFS and OS are high, 85% to 95% in a recent series.[396]

Another quite uncommon variety of ENL is that arising in the lung.[398,399] Although secondary involvement in the lung in NHL is common, primary involvement in the lung represents approximately 1% of all ENL presentations. The prognosis of primary lung lymphoma is good, because these are primarily MZL. They are known as BALT tumors because they arise from bronchus-associated lymphoid tissue. Five-year survival rates in the range of 90% have been reported from the Mayo Clinic and a large French series.[398,400]

Patients usually present with an asymptomatic abnormality on chest radiograph. It is difficult to obtain sufficient tissue at bronchoscopy with bronchial washings or with fine-needle aspirate to establish the diagnosis. An open procedure, either thoracoscopy or thoracotomy, is usually required. Most of the reported patients in the literature have been treated with surgical resection, sometimes followed by chemotherapy. There are very few patients reported treated with radiation, either alone or in combination with surgery and chemotherapy. Excellent local tumor control would be predicted for RT, however, in modest doses typical for MZL. It is therefore the treatment of choice in unresectable BALT lymphoma or where the extent of pulmonary resection would significantly compromise lung function. If only a small amount of lung needs to be surgically removed to encompass the tumor, surgical resection may carry less morbidity than RT.

The role of chemotherapy in BALT lymphoma is not well studied but would be predicted to be quite similar to that in MALT or FL—that is, the disease is chemotherapy responsive, with no data to suggest that the natural history is altered or survival prolonged by initiation of chemotherapy at diagnosis.

A small percentage of pulmonary lymphomas are DLBCL. These should be managed in accordance with the accepted principles of management of DLBCL, namely, R-CHOP. If the disease has been completely resected to establish the diagnosis, no additional RT appears necessary. If resection has not been accomplished, R-CHOP should be followed by RT, with the dose chosen reflecting the adequacy of response to R-CHOP. The treatment volume is problematic. A balance should be struck between treatment of the original tumor volume, which could conceivably involve a large amount of normal lung, and treatment of the postchemotherapy tumor volume, where the disease may all have disappeared.[399]

Breast is another quite uncommon primary site for lymphoma but with some unusual characteristics. Most cases are DLBCL, but FL and MZL have been reported as well. Most data are derived from two retrospective IELSG series reporting on DLBCL and indolent lymphomas involving the breast, respectively.[74,401] For the DLBCL group treated largely with CHOP and radiation without rituximab, 5-year survival was 63%. Although some have reported a tendency for CNS relapse, which was not seen in the IELSG series, and CNS prophylaxis was not done. There was a tendency for opposite breast relapse as well as systemic failure. Appropriate treatment presently would consist of R-CHOP and radiotherapy to the whole breast, with a dose of 30 Gy for patients in CR. Mastectomy is unnecessary. For patients with indolent histologies, radiotherapy alone, with a dose of 26 to 30 Gy, is indicated without systemic therapy and without mastectomy.

Primary Central Nervous System Lymphoma

PCNSL is a rare form of extranodal NHL but with increasing incidence. From 1973 to 1992, the estimated frequency of brain lymphoma increased more than 10-fold, from 2.5 to 30 cases per 10 million population.[402] This increase is, only partially, attributable to HIV-associated cases, with a significant rise in immunocompetent patients. The median age at presentation is 55 years for immunocompetent patients and 31 years for patients with AIDS. Neurologic symptoms are usually of brief duration, 3 months or less. Specific neurologic deficits depend on tumor location. Generalized symptomatology such as altered mental status, seizures, and symptoms of increased intracranial pressure such as headache, nausea, and vomiting may occur. Immunocompetent patients are more likely to have localized neurological deficits in contrast to patients with AIDS who more often have diffuse disease with generalized symptomatology.[403,404]

Radiologic imaging often suggests a diagnosis. PCNSL is usually isodense or hyperdense on nonenhanced CT scans, in contradistinction to other primary brain tumors or metastatic lesions. The preferred imaging modality for PCNSL is MRI, which can detect up to 10% of lesions missed by CT. Lesions appear isointense to hypointense on T1-weighted images and approximately 50% are hyperintense on T2-weighted imaging. Homogeneous contrast enhancement is commonly seen in immunocompetent patients.[405] Despite the appearance of a focal mass on CT or MRI, diffuse parenchymal infiltration is underestimated by imaging. The location of the lesion may also suggest the diagnosis as the majority of PCNSLs occur in a periventricular distribution, involving the corpus callosum, thalamus, or basal ganglia. In patients with HIV infection, disease is often multifocal in the brain and may be difficult to distinguish from CNS infections.[403]

At diagnosis, although most patients with PCNSL have a solitary brain lesion, the presence of leptomeningeal and ocular involvement is seen in approximately one-third and 20% of cases, respectively. Evaluation of these areas is indicated, including lumbar puncture (if the intracranial pressure is not increased and it can be done safely) and full ophthalmologic evaluation of the eye. Staging to evaluate for extracranial disease is often done, although additional disease outside the CNS is rarely found.[403,406] In the absence of specific signs or symptoms suggesting presence of extracranial disease, staging is of limited value.

The role of surgery in the management of PCNSL is limited to establishing the diagnosis, preferably by stereotactic biopsy. Corticosteroids, commonly used to alleviate symptoms including intracranial pressure, have a direct antitumor effect.[406] Tumor regression may lead to difficulties in establishing diagnosis. Accordingly, steroids should be withheld, if possible, until after biopsy, if the diagnosis of lymphoma is suspected. PCNSL is usually not amenable to surgical resection due to deep location and involvement of critical structures. Occasionally, surgical decompression and shunt placement is necessary for relief of increased intracranial pressure. Cerebrospinal fluid (CSF) analysis, including immunoglobulin gene rearrangement studies, can identify clonal populations to establish the diagnosis of PCNSL.[407]

The histologic appearance of PCNSL in an immunocompetent patient is typically that of DLBCL. Further, immunophenotyping suggests the tumor is the same as DLBCL occurring outside the nervous system, raising the question as to why it responds so differently to therapy, a question that remains unanswered.[408] In HIV-positive patients, aggressive or high-grade histopathologic pictures are common. In addition, the tumor is virtually always associated with EBV.[409] EBV is rare in immunocompetent patients with PCNSL.

Almost all studies reveal age and performance status to be important independent prognostic factors. Patients <60 years had a 42% survival in the Princess Margaret series compared with 9% for those >60 years. A prognostic model developed at Memorial Sloan-Kettering Cancer Center from 338 patients with PCNSL incorporates age and Karnofsky performance status, dividing patients into three prognostic classes.[410] The IELSG has also reported elevated LDH, increased CSF protein, and tumor location within the deep regions of the brain as significant prognostic variables.[410–411,412]

The management of PCNSL has evolved over recent years. Historically, the treatment was whole-brain radiotherapy (WBRT) alone to address the disease's multifocal nature. Results were poor, however, despite the known radiosensitivity of NHL outside the CNS. Two representative series from the Radiation Therapy Oncology Group (RTOG) and Princess Margaret Hospital report median survivals of 12.2 months and 17 months, respectively, and 5-year survivals of 10% to 20%.[413,414] Although the tumor initially responds to RT, regrowth is common and uncontrolled disease in the brain is the primary cause of death. Attempts at dose escalation beyond 50 Gy resulted in high toxicity rates without survival improvement in RTOG-8315, and a dose of 40 to 50 Gy was recommended.[414]

Given the poor results achieved with RT alone and the chemoresponsiveness of lymphomas generally, evaluation of systemic chemotherapy for PCNSL was soon undertaken. Initial programs consisted of CHOP and variations on that combination. Despite the efficacy of this combination in NHL outside the CNS, the results in PCNSL have been quite disappointing. A randomized trial by the Medical Research Council showed no benefit for CHOP added to RT.[415] Other studies have come to similar conclusions. This lack of efficacy may be due to the failure of many drugs to penetrate the blood–brain barrier (BBB).

Methotrexate (MTX), particularly in high doses, is known to penetrate the BBB. It was first used for treatment of PCNSL in 1980, with subsequent use becoming widespread.[403] There has been much variability in dosage, scheduling, and combinations with intrathecal MTX and other cytotoxics such as cytarabine, vincristine, or thiotepa. MTX appears to represent an important advance. The phase II RTOG-9310 study treated patients with combination chemotherapy, including high-dose MTX, and WBRT. The 5-year OS was 32% and the FFS 25%, results better than historically obtained with RT alone.[416]

A recent phase III noninferiority trial from Germany treated 550 patients with high-dose MTX and subsequent randomization to WBRT or no further therapy. WBRT was delivered to a dose of 45 Gy in 1.5-Gy daily fractions. There was no significant difference in median overall survival in the treatment arms, 32 months in MTX plus WBRT arm and 37 months in the chemotherapy-alone arm (estimated 5-year OS was 25% to 30%). However, 2-year PFS was 43.5% in the WBRT group and 30.7% in the group not receiving WBRT; this may represent a clinically significant advantage in selected populations. Neurotoxicity data were collected from a subset of patients in the WBRT arm. Forty-nine percent of patients in the WBRT arm experienced clinically defined neurotoxicity after a median of 20 months and 71% had evidence of delayed neurotoxicity as assessed by CT or MRI at a median of 50 months. The potential advantage in PFS must be balanced against the higher rates of neurotoxicity in the WBRT arm by clinical and radiographic assessment.[417] Criticisms of this trial include poor protocol adherence, randomization caveats, low statistical power, and prolonged accrual time, leaving the question of consolidation WBRT unanswered.[418] In addition, the inferior survival in the WBRT arm may be a function of neurotoxicity-associated death due, in part, to high radiation doses.

The Memorial Sloan-Kettering Cancer Center group evaluated 57 patients treated with MTX-based chemotherapy followed by selective WBRT to 45 Gy. Of the entire cohort, 30% of patients developed treatment-related neurotoxicity. Thirty-five patients received WBRT as salvage or initial therapy and 16 (46%) developed treatment-related neurotoxicity.[419] In a series of 226 patient with PCNSL (162 received WBRT), a 26% rate of severe neurotoxicity was seen at 6 years.[420]

Neurologic complications can arise as early as 3 months posttreatment with symptoms of attention deficit, memory impairment, ataxia, and urinary incontinence and could ultimately lead to dementia.[421] It is difficult to determine the precise incidence, because actuarial complication rates are seldom reported.

An additional multi-institutional retrospective series reported a 30% 5-year actuarial rate of neurotoxicity overall, while patients >60 years had a 58% risk of neurotoxicity at 7 years.[422] Given higher neurologic toxicity rates in the elderly, many institutions treat this subset of patients with chemotherapy alone.[423,424]

In an effort to reduce neurologic complications, radiation dose reduction has been investigated. Bessell et al.[425] reduced RT dose to 30 Gy in 26 patients who had achieved CR to chemotherapy. The 3-year overall survival was 92% versus 60% for a retrospective comparison group receiving 45 Gy plus a 10 Gy boost. This series, however, utilized eight drugs with a MTX dose of 1.5 g/m^2 and delivered the 30.6 Gy of RT over 5 weeks.

Recently the Memorial Sloan-Kettering Cancer Center group has reduced the dose to 23.4 Gy for patients achieving CR to rituximab and MTX-based chemotherapy with promising short-term results. Two-year OS and PFS were 67% and 57%, respectively. With a median follow-up of 37 months, no treatment-related neurotoxicity was observed.[426]

In a recent phase II Italian trial, patients <60 years old received high-dose MTX and were randomized to cytarabine or no further chemotherapy. Patients who developed a CR were consolidated with WBRT to a dose of 36 Gy in both arms.[427] The addition of cytarabine appeared to improve clinical outcomes.

Future areas of research include additional chemotherapeutic drugs in combination with high-dose MTX. Regimens including cytarabine and rituximab have been reported in the literature.[426,427] Rituximab appears to be a reasonable addition to the chemotherapy regimen, given its efficacy in systemic DLBCL.

HDC with ASCT has also been evaluated. Soussain et al.[428] reported a 96% CR after HDC and ASCT. Two-year OS was 45% among the entire cohort and 69% among the 27 patients undergoing HDC and ASCT. Additional studies have evaluated the use of HDC and ASCT, many in combination with WBRT, in newly diagnosed PCNSL.[429–434] Currently, a randomized trial for patients <60 years old comparing WBRT or HDC-ASCT as consolidation after high-dose MTX is ongoing.[421]

Thus, the treatment of PCNSL remains unsettled with few phase III trials. High-dose MTX, >3 g/m^2 every 2 to 4 weeks, is the cornerstone of therapy. Whether doses >3 g/m^2 are helpful is unresolved. The addition of other drugs and the role of stem cell transplant remain controversial. The role of WBRT after high-dose MTX is especially controversial, particularly in patients achieving a CR and in those >60 years old. It seems clear that 45 Gy WBRT results in unacceptable toxicity in older patients and perhaps in younger ones as well. Given the overall unsatisfactory results of therapy, the addition of low-dose RT (24 Gy) to chemotherapy for patients achieving a CR is a promising approach.

CONCLUSION

Radiation therapy continues to play an important role in the management of NHL. Participation by radiation oncologists in the multi-disciplinary management of patients with these disorders is vital. This requires a sound understanding of the natural history and optimal treatment approach for each of the many NHL subtypes.

SELECTED REFERENCES

A full list of references for this chapter is available online.

7. Muller AM, Ihorst G, Mertelsmann R, et al. Epidemiology of non-Hodgkin's lymphoma (NHL): trends, geographic distribution, and etiology. *Ann Hematol* 2005;84:1–12.
10. Behler CM, Kaplan LD. Advances in the management of HIV-related non-Hodgkin lymphoma. *Curr Opin Oncol* 2006;18:437–443.
11. Gottschalk S, Rooney CM, Heslop HE. Post-transplant lymphoproliferative disorders. *Annu Rev Med* 2005;56:29–44.
23. Wotherspoon AC, Ortiz-Hidalgo C, Falzon MR, et al. Helicobacter pylori-associated gastritis and primary B-cell gastric lymphoma. *Lancet* 1991;338:1175–1176.
24. Zucca E, Dreyling M. Gastric marginal zone lymphoma of MALT type: ESMO clinical practice guidelines for diagnosis, treatment and follow-up. *Ann Oncol* 2010;21(Suppl 5):v175–v176.
32. Rueffer U, Josting A, Franklin J, et al. Non-Hodgkin's lymphoma after primary Hodgkin's disease in the German Hodgkin's Lymphoma Study Group: incidence, treatment, and prognosis. *J Clin Oncol* 2001;19:2026–2032.
35. Swerdlow SH, Campo E, Harris NL, et al, eds. *WHO classification of tumours of haematopoietic and lymphoid tissues.* 4th ed. Lyon, France: International Agency for Research on Cancer, 2008.
39. Alizadeh AA, Eisen MB, Davis RE, et al. Distinct types of diffuse large B-cell lymphoma identified by gene expression profiling. *Nature* 2000;403:503–511.
41. Lossos IS, Czerwinski DK, Alizadeh AA, et al. Prediction of survival in diffuse large-B-cell lymphoma based on the expression of six genes. *N Engl J Med* 2004;350:1828–1837.
42. Rosenwald A, Wright G, Chan WC, et al. The use of molecular profiling to predict survival after chemotherapy for diffuse large-B-cell lymphoma. *N Engl J Med* 2002;346:1937–1947.
46. Winter JN, Weller EA, Horning SJ, et al. Prognostic significance of Bcl-6 protein expression in DLBCL treated with CHOP or R-CHOP: a prospective correlative study. *Blood* 2006;107:4207–4213.
47. Anderson JR, Armitage JO, Weisenburger DD. Epidemiology of the non-Hodgkin's lymphomas: distributions of the major subtypes differ by geographic locations. Non-Hodgkin's Lymphoma Classification Project. *Ann Oncol* 1998;9:717–720.
52. Farinha P, Gascoyne RD. Molecular pathogenesis of mucosa-associated lymphoid tissue lymphoma. *J Clin Oncol* 2005;23:6370–6378.
56. Rudiger T, Weisenburger DD, Anderson JR, et al. Peripheral T-cell lymphoma (excluding anaplastic large cell lymphoma): results from the Non-Hodgkin's Lymphoma Classification Project. *Ann Oncol* 2002;13:140–149.
58. Kutok JL, Aster JC. Molecular biology of anaplastic lymphoma kinase-positive anaplastic large-cell lymphoma. *J Clin Oncol* 2002;20:3691–3702.
74. Ryan G, Martinelli G, Kuper-Hommel M, et al. Primary diffuse large B-cell lymphoma of the breast: prognostic factors and outcomes of a study by the International Extranodal Lymphoma Study Group. *Ann Oncol* 2008;19:233–241.
76. Vitolo U, Chiappella A, Ferreri AJ, et al. First-line treatment for primary testicular diffuse large B-cell lymphoma with rituximab-CHOP, CNS prophylaxis, and contralateral testis irradiation: final results of an international phase II trial. *J Clin Oncol* 2011;29:2766–2772.
79. Kostakoglu L, Leonard JP, Kuji I, et al. Comparison of fluorine-18 fluorodeoxyglucose positron emission tomography and G1–67 scintigraphy in evaluation of lymphoma. *Cancer* 2002;94:879–888.
81. Juweid ME, Cheson BD. Role of positron emission tomography in lymphoma. *J Clin Oncol* 2005;23:4577–4580.
83. Cheson B. Role of functional imaging in the management of lymphoma. *J Clin Oncol* 2011;29:1844–1854.
86. Juweid ME, Wiseman GA, Vose JM, et al. Response assessment of aggressive non-Hodgkin's lymphoma by integrated International Workshop Criteria and fluorine-18-fluorodeoxyglucose positron emission tomography. *J Clin Oncol* 2005;23:4652–4661.
89. Spaepen K, Stroobants S, Dupont P, et al. Prognostic value of pretransplantation positron emission tomography using fluorine 18-fluorodeoxyglucose in patients with aggressive lymphoma treated with high-dose chemotherapy and stem cell transplantation. *Blood* 2003;102:53–59.
90. Hoppe BS, Moskowitz CH, Zhang Z, et al. The role of FDG-PET imaging and involved field radiotherapy in relapsed or refractory diffuse large B-cell lymphoma. *Bone Marrow Transplant* 2009;43:941–948.
96. Cheson BD, Pfistner B, Juweid ME, et al. Revised response criteria for malignant lymphoma. *J Clin Oncol* 2007;25:579–586.
99. A predictive model for aggressive non-Hodgkin's lymphoma. The International Non-Hodgkin's Lymphoma Prognostic Factors Project. *N Engl J Med* 1993; 329:987–994.
101. Sehn LH, Berry B, Chhanabhai M, et al. The revised International Prognostic Index (R-IPI) is a better predictor of outcome than the standard IPI for patients with diffuse large B-cell lymphoma treated with R-CHOP. *Blood* 2007;109:1857–1861.
102. Ziepert M, Hasenclever D, Kuhnt E, et al. Standard International Prognostic Index remains a valid predictor of outcome for patients with aggressive CD20+ B-cell lymphoma in the rituximab era. *J Clin Oncol* 2010;28:2373–2380.
103. Advani RH, Chen H, Habermann TM, et al. Comparison of conventional prognostic indices in patients older than 60 years with diffuse large B-cell lymphoma treated with R-CHOP in the US Intergroup Study (ECOG 4494, CALGB 9793): consideration of age greater than 70 years in an elderly prognostic index (E-IPI). *Br J Haematol* 2010;151:143–151.
105. Sonnen R, Schmidt WP, Muller-Hermelink HK, et al. The International Prognostic Index determines the outcome of patients with nodal mature T-cell lymphomas. *Br J Haematol* 2005;129:366–372.
107. Solal-Celigny P, Roy P, Colombat P, et al. Follicular lymphoma international prognostic index. *Blood* 2004;104:1258–1265.
109. Campbell BA, Voss N, Woods R, et al. Long-term outcomes for patients with limited stage follicular lymphoma: involved regional radiotherapy versus involved node radiotherapy. *Cancer* 2010;116:3797–3806.
110. Dave SS, Wright G, Tan B, et al. Prediction of survival in follicular lymphoma based on molecular features of tumor-infiltrating immune cells. *N Engl J Med* 2004;351:2159–2169.
112. Relander T, Johnson NA, Farinha P, et al. Prognostic factors in follicular lymphoma. *J Clin Oncol* 2010;28:2902–2913.
113. A clinical evaluation of the International Lymphoma Study Group classification of non-Hodgkin's lymphoma. The Non-Hodgkin's Lymphoma Classification Project. *Blood* 1997;89:3909–3918.
114. Savage KJ, Monti S, Kutok JL, et al. The molecular signature of mediastinal large B-cell lymphoma differs from that of other diffuse large B-cell lymphomas and shares features with classical Hodgkin lymphoma. *Blood* 2003;102:3871–3879.
115. Savage KJ, Al-Rajhi N, Voss N, et al. Favorable outcome of primary mediastinal large B-cell lymphoma in a single institution: the British Columbia experience. *Ann Oncol* 2006;17:123–130.
116. Rieger M, Osterborg A, Pettengell R, et al. Primary mediastinal B-cell lymphoma treated with CHOP-like chemotherapy with or without rituximab: results of the Mabthera International Trial Group study. *Ann Oncol* 2011;22:664–670.
132. Tsang RW, Gospodarowicz MK, Pintilie M, et al. Localized mucosa-associated lymphoid tissue lymphoma treated with radiation therapy has excellent clinical outcome. *J Clin Oncol* 2003;21:4157–4164.
146. Bekkenk MW, Geelen FA, van Voorst Vader PC, et al. Primary and secondary cutaneous CD30(+) lymphoproliferative disorders: a report from the Dutch Cutaneous Lymphoma Group on the long-term follow-up data of 219 patients and guidelines for diagnosis and treatment. *Blood* 2000;95:3653–3661.
163. Lowry L, Smith P, Qian W, et al. Reduced dose radiotherapy for local control in non-Hodgkin lymphoma: a randomised phase III trial. *Radiother Oncol* 2011;100:86–92.
164. Shenkier TN, Voss N, Fairey R, et al. Brief chemotherapy and involved-region irradiation for limited-stage diffuse large-cell lymphoma: an 18-year experience from the British Columbia Cancer Agency. *J Clin Oncol* 2002;20:197–204.
165. Phan J, Mazloom A, Medeiros J, et al. Benefit of consolidative radiation therapy in patients with diffuse large B-cell lymphoma treated with R-CHOP chemotherapy. *J Clin Oncol* 2010; 28:4170–4176.
167. Dorth JA, Chino JP, Prosnitz LR, et al. The impact of radiation therapy in patients with diffuse large B-cell lymphoma with positive post-chemotherapy FDG-PET or gallium-67 scans. *Ann Oncol* 2011;22:405–410.
168. Miller TP, Dahlberg S, Cassady JR, et al. Chemotherapy alone compared with chemotherapy plus radiotherapy for localized intermediate- and high-grade non-Hodgkin's lymphoma. *N Engl J Med* 1998;339:21–26.
178. Haas RL, Poortmans P, de Jong D, et al. High response rates and lasting remissions after low-dose involved field radiotherapy in indolent lymphomas. *J Clin Oncol* 2003;21:2474–2480.
180. Haas RL, Poortmans P, de Jong D, et al. Effective palliation by low dose local radiotherapy for recurrent and/or chemotherapy refractory non-follicular lymphoma patients. *Eur J Cancer* 2005;41:1724–1730.
182. Fisher RI, Gaynor ER, Dahlberg S, et al. Comparison of a standard regimen (CHOP) with three intensive chemotherapy regimens for advanced non-Hodgkin's lymphoma. *N Engl J Med* 1993;328:1002–1006.
184. Pfreundschuh M, Trumper L, Osterborg A, et al. CHOP-like chemotherapy plus rituximab versus CHOP-like chemotherapy alone in young patients with good-prognosis diffuse large-B-cell lymphoma: a randomised controlled trial by the MabThera International Trial (MInT) Group. *Lancet Oncol* 2006;7:379–391.
192. Philip T, Armitage JO, Spitzer G, et al. High-dose therapy and autologous bone marrow transplantation after failure of conventional chemotherapy in adults with intermediate-grade or high-grade non-Hodgkin's lymphoma. *N Engl J Med* 1987;316:1493–1498.
209. Lenz G, Dreyling M, Hoster E, et al. Immunochemotherapy with rituximab and cyclophosphamide, doxorubicin, vincristine, and prednisone significantly improves response and time to treatment failure, but not long-term outcome in patients with previously untreated mantle cell lymphoma: results of a prospective randomized trial of the German Low Grade Lymphoma Study Group (GLSG). *J Clin Oncol* 2005;23:1984–1992.
213. Press OW, Unger JM, Braziel RM, et al. Phase II trial of CHOP chemotherapy followed by tositumomab/iodine I-131 tositumomab for previously untreated follicular non-Hodgkin's lymphoma: five-year follow-up of Southwest Oncology Group Protocol S9911. *J Clin Oncol* 2006;24:4143–4149.
216. Morschhauser F, Radford J, Van Hoof A, et al. Phase III trial of consolidation therapy with yttrium-90-ibritumomab tiuxetan compared with no additional therapy after first remission in advanced follicular lymphoma. *J Clin Oncol* 2008;26:5156–5164.
226. Bonnot C, Fillot G, Mounier N, et al. CHOP alone compared with CHOP plus radiotherapy for localized aggressive lymphoma in elderly patients: a study by the Groupe d'Etude des Lymphomes de l'Adulte. *J Clin Oncol* 2007;25:787–792.
227. Horning SJ, Weller E, Kim K, et al. Chemotherapy with or without radiotherapy in limited-stage diffuse aggressive non-Hodgkin's lymphoma: Eastern Cooperative Oncology Group study 1484. *J Clin Oncol* 2004;22:3032–3038.
228. Martinelli G, Gigli F, Calabrese L, et al. Early stage gastric diffuse large B-cell lymphomas: results of a randomized trial comparing chemotherapy alone ver-

sus chemotherapy + involved field radiotherapy (IELSG 4) [corrected]. *Leuk Lymphoma* 2009;50:925–931.
229. Miller TP, LeBlanc M, Spier C. CHOP alone compared to CHOP plus radiotherapy for early stage aggressive non-Hodgkin's lymphomas: update of the Southwest Oncology Group (SWOG) randomized trial. *Blood* 2001;98:724a.
230. Reyes F, Lepage E, Ganem G, et al. ACVBP versus CHOP plus radiotherapy for localized aggressive lymphoma. *N Engl J Med* 2005;352:1197–1205.
232. Ballonoff A, Rusthoven KE, Schwer A, et al. Outcomes and effect of radiotherapy in patients with stage I or II diffuse large B-cell lymphoma: a surveillance, epidemiology, and end results analysis. *Int J Radiat Oncol Biol Phys* 2008;72:1465–1471.
235. Aviles A, Delgado S, Fernandez R, et al. Combined therapy in advanced stages (III and IV) of follicular lymphoma increases the possibility of cure: results of a large controlled clinical trial. *Eur J Haematol* 2002;68:144–149.
236. Aviles A, Fernandezb R, Perez F, et al. Adjuvant radiotherapy in stage IV diffuse large cell lymphoma improves outcome. *Leuk Lymphoma* 2004;45:1385–1389.
244. Aviles A, Delgado S, Nambo MJ, et al. Adjuvant radiotherapy to sites of previous bulky disease in patients stage IV diffuse large cell lymphoma. *Int J Radiat Oncol Biol Phys* 1994;30:799–803.
251. Kelsey SM, Newland AC, Hudson GV, et al. A British National Lymphoma Investigation randomised trial of single agent chlorambucil plus radiotherapy versus radiotherapy alone in low grade, localised non-Hodgkins lymphoma. *Med Oncol* 1994;11:19–25.
259. Pugh TJ, Ballonoff A, Newman F, et al. Improved survival in patients with early stage low-grade follicular lymphoma treated with radiation: a Surveillance, Epidemiology, and End Results database analysis. *Cancer* 2010;116:3843–3851.
266. Marcus R, Imrie K, Solal-Celigny P, et al. Phase III study of R-CVP compared with cyclophosphamide, vincristine, and prednisone alone in patients with previously untreated advanced follicular lymphoma. *J Clin Oncol* 2008;26:4579–4586.
267. Herold M, Haas A, Srock S, et al. Rituximab added to first-line mitoxantrone, chlorambucil, and prednisolone chemotherapy followed by interferon maintenance prolongs survival in patients with advanced follicular lymphoma: an East German Study Group Hematology and Oncology Study. *J Clin Oncol* 2007; 25:1986–1992.
270. Salles G, Seymour JF, Offner F, et al. Rituximab maintenance for 2 years in patients with high tumour burden follicular lymphoma responding to rituximab plus chemotherapy (PRIMA): a phase 3, randomised controlled trial. *Lancet* 2011;377:42–51.
286. Aviles A, Diaz-Maqueo JC, Sanchez E, et al. Long-term results in patients with low-grade nodular non-Hodgkin's lymphoma. A randomized trial comparing chemotherapy plus radiotherapy with chemotherapy alone. *Acta Oncol* 1991; 30:329–333.
300. Gascoyne RD, Aoun P, Wu D, et al. Prognostic significance of anaplastic lymphoma kinase (ALK) protein expression in adults with anaplastic large cell lymphoma. *Blood* 1999;93:3913–3921.
301. Coiffier B, Neidhardt-Berard EM, Tilly H, et al. Fludarabine alone compared to CHVP plus interferon in elderly patients with follicular lymphoma and adverse prognostic parameters: a GELA study. Groupe d'Etudes des Lymphomes de l'Adulte. *Ann Oncol* 1999;10:1191–1197.
312. Dreyling M, Lenz G, Hoster E, et al. Early consolidation by myeloablative radiochemotherapy followed by autologous stem cell transplantation in first remission significantly prolongs progression-free survival in mantle-cell lymphoma: results of a prospective randomized trial of the European MCL Network. *Blood* 2005;105:2677–2684.
314. NCCN. Non-Hodgkin's lymphoma clinical practice guidelines in oncology. National Comprehensive Cancer Network. 2011. Available at: http://www.nccn.org.
315. Leitch HA, Gascoyne RD, Chhanabhai M, et al. Limited-stage mantle-cell lymphoma. *Ann Oncol* 2003;14:1555–1561.
329. Ibrahim EM, Ezzat AA, Raja MA, et al. Primary gastric non-Hodgkin's lymphoma: clinical features, management, and prognosis of 185 patients with diffuse large B-cell lymphoma. *Ann Oncol* 1999;10:1441–1449.
337. Wotherspoon AC, Doglioni C, Diss TC, et al. Regression of primary low-grade B-cell gastric lymphoma of mucosa-associated lymphoid tissue type after eradication of *Helicobacter pylori*. *Lancet* 1993;342:575–577.
339. Chen LT, Lin JT, Tai JJ, et al. Long-term results of anti-Helicobacter pylori therapy in early-stage gastric high-grade transformed MALT lymphoma. *J Natl Cancer Inst* 2005;97:1345–1353.
341. Wundisch T, Thiede C, Morgner A, et al. Long-term follow-up of gastric MALT lymphoma after *Helicobacter pylori* eradication. *J Clin Oncol* 2005;23:8018–8024.
346. Noy A, Yahalom J, Zaretsky L, et al. Gastric mucosa-associated lymphoid tissue lymphoma detected by clonotypic polymorase chain reaction despite continuous pathologic remission induced by involved-field radiotherapy. *J Clin Oncol* 2005;23:3768–3772.
350. Kim SJ, Choi CW, Mun YC, et al. Multicenter retrospective analysis of 581 patients with primary intestinal non-hodgkin lymphoma from the Consortium for Improving Survival of Lymphoma (CISL). *BMC Cancer* 2011;11:321.
351. Schmatz AI, Streubel B, Kretschmer-Chott E, et al. Primary follicular lymphoma of the duodenum is a distinct mucosal/submucosal variant of follicular lymphoma: a retrospective study of 63 cases. *J Clin Oncol* 2011;29:1445–1451.
362. Aviles A, Delgado S, Ruiz H, et al. Treatment of non-Hodgkin's lymphoma of Waldeyer's ring: radiotherapy versus chemotherapy versus combined therapy. *Eur J Cancer B Oral Oncol* 1996;32B:19–23.
365. Li YX, Yao B, Jin J, et al. Radiotherapy as primary treatment for stage IE and IIE nasal natural killer/T-cell lymphoma. *J Clin Oncol* 2006;24:181–189.
366. Yamaguchi M, Tobinai K, Oguchi M, et al. Phase I/II study of concurrent chemoradiotherapy for localized nasal natural killer/T-cell lymphoma: Japan Clinical Oncology Group Study JCOG0211. *J Clin Oncol* 2009;27:5594–5600.
367. Kim SJ, Kim K, Kim BS, et al. Phase II trial of concurrent radiation and weekly cisplatin followed by VIPD chemotherapy in newly diagnosed, stage IE to IIE, nasal, extranodal NK/T-Cell Lymphoma: Consortium for Improving Survival of Lymphoma study. *J Clin Oncol* 2009;27:6027–6032.
369. Aviles A, Delgado S, Huerta-Guzman J. Marginal zone B cell lymphoma of the parotid glands: results of a randomised trial comparing radiotherapy to combined therapy. *Eur J Cancer B Oral Oncol* 1996;32B:420–422.
371. Grange F, Bekkenk MW, Wechsler J, et al. Prognostic factors in primary cutaneous large B-cell lymphomas: a European multicenter study. *J Clin Oncol* 2001;19:3602–3610.
373. Willemze R, Jaffe ES, Burg G, et al. WHO-EORTC classification for cutaneous lymphomas. *Blood* 2005;105:3768–3785.
374. Querfeld C, Kuzel TM, Guitart J, et al. Primary cutaneous CD30 +lymphoproliferative disorders: new insights into biology and therapy. *Oncology* 2007;21:689–696; discussion 699–700.
375. Senff NJ, Hoefnagel JJ, Jansen PM, et al. Reclassification of 300 primary cutaneous B-Cell lymphomas according to the new WHO-EORTC classification for cutaneous lymphomas: comparison with previous classifications and identification of prognostic markers. *J Clin Oncol* 2007;25:1581–1587.
378. Pfeffer MR, Rabin T, Tsvang L, et al. Orbital lymphoma: is it necessary to treat the entire orbit? *Int J Radiat Oncol Biol Phys* 2004;60:527–530.
388. Moller MB, d'Amore F, Christensen BE. Testicular lymphoma: a population-based study of incidence, clinicopathological correlations and prognosis. The Danish Lymphoma Study Group, LYFO. *Eur J Cancer* 1994;30A:1760–1764.
393. Zucca E, Conconi A, Mughal TI, et al. Patterns of outcome and prognostic factors in primary large-cell lymphoma of the testis in a survey by the International Extranodal Lymphoma Study Group. *J Clin Oncol* 2003;21:20–27.
403. Batchelor T, Loeffler JS. Primary CNS lymphoma. *J Clin Oncol* 2006;24:1281–1288.
410. Abrey LE, Ben-Porat L, Panageas KS, et al. Primary central nervous system lymphoma: the Memorial Sloan-Kettering Cancer Center prognostic model. *J Clin Oncol* 2006;24:5711–5715.
411. Ferreri AJ, Abrey LE, Blay JY, et al. Summary statement on primary central nervous system lymphomas from the Eighth International Conference on Malignant Lymphoma, Lugano, Switzerland, June 12 to 15, 2002. *J Clin Oncol* 2003;21:2407–2414.
415. Mead GM, Bleehen NM, Gregor A, et al. A medical research council randomized trial in patients with primary cerebral non-Hodgkin lymphoma: cerebral radiotherapy with and without cyclophosphamide, doxorubicin, vincristine, and prednisone chemotherapy. *Cancer* 2000;89:1359–1370.
417. Thiel E, Korfel A, Martus P, et al. High-dose methotrexate with or without whole brain radiotherapy for primary CNS lymphoma (G-PCNSL-SG-1): a phase 3, randomised, non-inferiority trial. *Lancet Oncol*;11:1036–1047.
419. Gavrilovic IT, Hormigo A, Yahalom J, et al. Long-term follow-up of high-dose methotrexate-based therapy with and without whole brain irradiation for newly diagnosed primary CNS lymphoma. *J Clin Oncol* 2006;24:4570–4574.
420. Blay JY, Conroy T, Chevreau C, et al. High-dose methotrexate for the treatment of primary cerebral lymphomas: analysis of survival and late neurologic toxicity in a retrospective series. *J Clin Oncol* 1998;16:864–871.
425. Bessell EM, Lopez-Guillermo A, Villa S, et al. Importance of radiotherapy in the outcome of patients with primary CNS lymphoma: an analysis of the CHOD/BVAM regimen followed by two different radiotherapy treatments. *J Clin Oncol* 2002;20:231–236.
426. Shah GD, Yahalom J, Correa DD, et al. Combined immunochemotherapy with reduced whole-brain radiotherapy for newly diagnosed primary CNS lymphoma. *J Clin Oncol* 2007;25:4730–4735.

Chapter 79
Primary Cutaneous Lymphomas

James E. Hansen, Youn H. Kim, Richard T. Hoppe, and Lynn D. Wilson

Primary cutaneous lymphoma is defined by an accumulation of malignant lymphoid cells in the skin without evidence of extracutaneous disease at the time of diagnosis. The distinction between a primary cutaneous lymphoma and a nodal lymphoma with secondary cutaneous involvement is important and markedly impacts evaluation, staging, prognosis, and therapeutic management. The term *primary cutaneous lymphoma* encompasses a heterogeneous group of extranodal non-Hodgkin lymphomas, and in 2005 the World Health Organization (WHO) and European Organisation for Research and Treatment of Cancer (EORTC) endorsed a consensus classification system that defines three categories of primary cutaneous lymphomas: cutaneous T-cell and NK-cell lymphomas, cutaneous B-cell lymphomas, and precursor

TABLE 79.1 WHO-EORTC CLASSIFICATION[1]

Cutaneous T-Cell and NK-/T-Cell Lymphomas
Mycosis fungoides and variants (folliculotropic mycosis fungoides, pagetoid reticulosis, and granulomatous slack skin)
Sézary syndrome
CD30+ lymphoproliferative disorders (primary cutaneous anaplastic large cell lymphoma and lymphomatoid papulosis)
Extranodal NK-/T-cell lymphoma, nasal type
Subcutaneous panniculitis-like T-cell lymphoma
Primary cutaneous peripheral T-cell lymphoma, unspecified
Primary cutaneous aggressive epidermotropic CD8+ T-cell lymphoma (provisional)
Primary cutaneous γ/δ T-cell lymphoma (provisional)
Primary cutaneous CD4+ small/medium-sized pleomorphic T-cell lymphoma (provisional)
Cutaneous B-Cell Lymphomas
Primary cutaneous marginal zone lymphoma
Primary cutaneous follicle center lymphoma
Primary cutaneous diffuse large B-cell lymphoma, leg type
Primary cutaneous diffuse large B-cell lymphoma, other
Precursor Hematologic Neoplasm
CD4+/CD56+ hematodermic neoplasm (blastic NK-cell lymphoma)

WHO, World Health Organization; EORTC, European Organisation for Research and Treatment of Cancer.

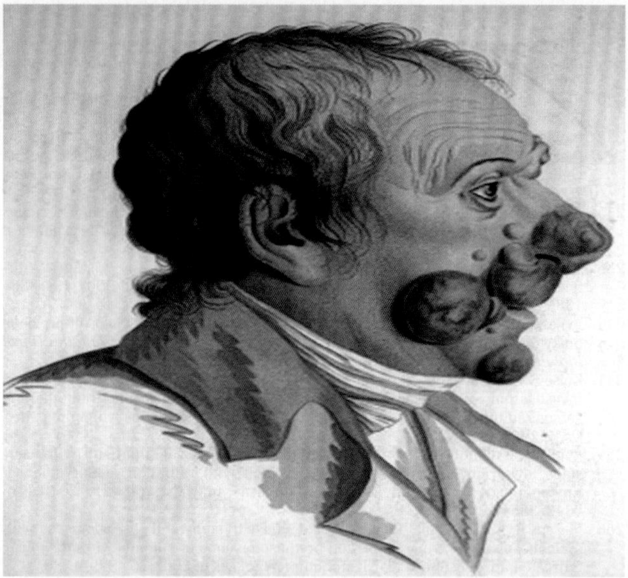

FIGURE 79.1. Pian fungoide, from Jean-Louis-Marc Alibert's atlas of dermatoses, *Descriptions des Maladies de la Peau.*

hematologic neoplasms/immature hematologic malignancies (Table 79.1).[1] This chapter will review the primary cutaneous lymphomas in the context of this consensus system. A slightly modified classification system was released by the WHO in 2008.[2]

CUTANEOUS T-CELL AND NK-CELL LYMPHOMAS

Cutaneous T-cell lymphoma (CTCL) is the most common primary cutaneous lymphoma. In the United States, 71% of the 3,884 cases of primary cutaneous lymphoma diagnosed during 2001–2005 were CTCL.[3] Similarly, 78% of primary cutaneous lymphoma diagnoses recorded in the Dutch and Austrian Cutaneous Lymphoma Group registry over 1986–2002[1] and 85% of diagnoses in the Central Cutaneous Lymphoma Registry of the German Society of Dermatology over 1999–2004 were CTCL.[4]

CTCL subtypes include mycosis fungoides (MF); CD30+ lymphoproliferative disorders; extranodal NK-/T-cell lymphoma, nasal type; subcutaneous panniculitis-like T-cell lymphoma; adult T-cell leukemia/lymphoma; and primary cutaneous peripheral T-cell lymphomas. MF is the most common CTCL, responsible for 54% of CTCL diagnoses in the United States over 2001–2005.[3] CD30+ T-cell lymphoproliferative disorders and cutaneous peripheral T-cell lymphomas represent the majority of the remaining cases of CTCL. The remaining CTCL subtypes are extremely rare and represent <1% of primary cutaneous lymphomas.

Mycosis Fungoides

MF is the archetype cutaneous lymphoma. The first case of MF was reported in 1806 by the French dermatologist Jean-Louis-Marc Alibert in his atlas of dermatoses, *Descriptions des maladies de la peau* (Fig. 79.1). After Alibert released his depiction of MF, approximately 300 similar cases were reported over the next decade, and in modern times approximately 1,500 new cases of MF were diagnosed during 2001–2005.[3] MF is a disease of skin-homing CD4+ T-helper cells[5] and is most commonly diagnosed in men (male:female ratio of 1.6–2.0:1) with a median age at diagnosis of 55 to 60.[1] Significant advances in MF therapy have been made over the past 200 years, but the precise etiology responsible for the development of MF remains elusive.

Cutaneous Disease

Pruritus, either diffuse or localized to areas of involved skin, is the most common symptom associated with MF. Ulcerated lesions may also cause patients significant pain. Cutaneous lesions in classic (or Alibert-Bazin) MF follow a predictable evolutionary course, and a consensus statement from the International Society for Cutaneous Lymphomas (ISCL), U.S. Cutaneous Lymphoma Consortium (USCLC), and EORTC defines the lesions found in distinct phases of MF.[6] In the *premycotic phase* a small number of red, scaled, macular or patchlike lesions develop in sun-shielded areas of the skin such as the trunk, pelvis, and extremities. These early lesions are unstable and usually regress, followed by development of new lesions. Biopsies of premycotic lesions are rarely diagnostic due to a paucity of malignant lymphocytes in the lesion. With increased deposition of malignant T cells in the skin, the lesions become increasingly durable, and persistent cutaneous patches are characteristic of the *patch phase.* The ISCL/USCLC/EORTC consensus definition of an MF patch is "any size lesion without induration or significant elevation above the surrounding uninvolved skin: poikiloderma may be present".[6] As the lesions become more densely infiltrated by both malignant and reactive lymphocytes, they evolve into plaques with thickened and raised borders in the *plaque phase* of classic MF. Plaques are defined by the ISCL/USCLC/EORTC as "any size lesion that is elevated or indurated: crusting or poikiloderma may be present".[6] Plaques may evolve into cutaneous tumors, which the ISCL/USCLC/EORTC defines as "any solid or nodular lesion ≥1 cm in diameter with evidence of deep infiltration in the skin and/or vertical growth".[6] The presence of cutaneous tumors designates the tumor phase of MF. MF may also progress to or present with erythroderma, in which a diffuse erythema involves >80% of the skin surface area.[6] Representative images of patches, plaques, tumors, and erythroderma are shown in Figure 79.2.

Leukemic CTCL and the Sézary Syndrome

In rare CTCL cases circulating malignant T cells are identified in the peripheral blood. This phenomenon, sometimes referred to as leukemic CTCL or the Sézary syndrome (SS), most commonly occurs in association with erythroderma but may occur in patients with minimal cutaneous disease.[1] The circulating malignant T cells (also called Sézary cells) are atypical T cells with hyperconvoluted nuclei seen at analysis of peripheral buffy coat smear. The circulating cells most commonly possess a CD4+/CD7− or CD4+/CD26− immunophenotype, and flow

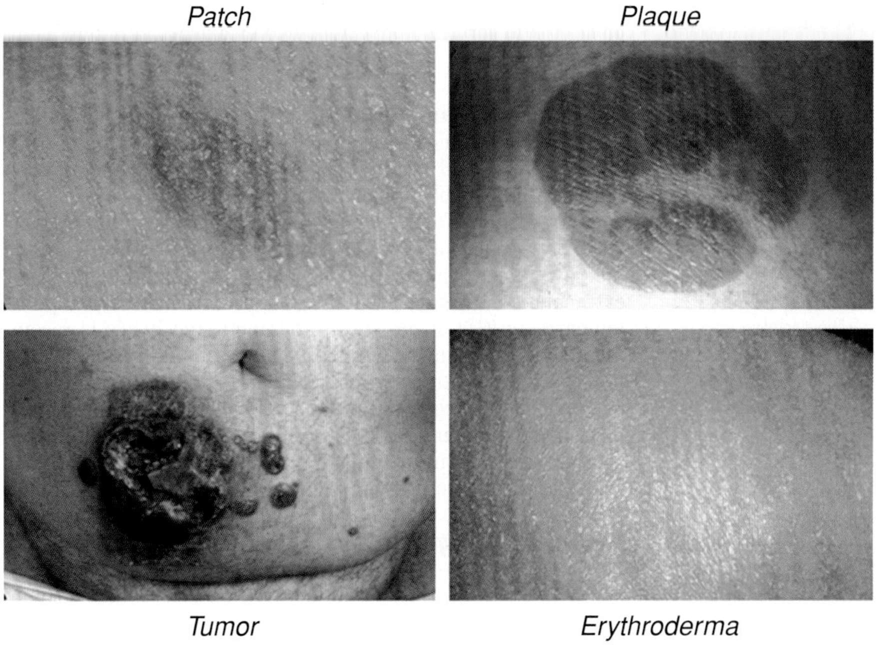

FIGURE 79.2. Representative images of cutaneous lesions in mycosis fungoides. (From Smith BD, Wilson LD. Management of mycosis fungoides. Part 1. Diagnosis, staging, and prognosis. *Oncology* 2003;17:1419–1428, with permission.)

cytometry allows for quantification of the proportion of circulating malignant T cells. In addition, presence of a dominant circulating malignant clone may be demonstrated by evaluation of the T-cell receptor (TCR) by polymerase chain reaction (PCR) or Southern blotting. The degree of tumor burden in the peripheral blood is denoted as B0 (≤5% atypical or Sézary cells seen on examination of buffy coat smear), B1 (>5% of cells on buffy coat analysis are atypical, but further criteria meeting B2 disease are not met), or B2 (combination of presence of a dominant T-cell clone in the peripheral blood identified by PCR or Southern blot and either ≥1,000 Sézary cells/mm^3, an increased amount of CD3+ or CD4+ T cells with CD4:CD8 ratios >10, or increased quantities of abnormal T cells defined as loss of CD7 in >40% of cells or CD26 in >30% of cells).[6] If peripheral blood is evaluated for a circulating clone by PCR or Southern blot, B0 or B1 disease may be stratified into B0a or B1a (absence of circulating clone) or B0b or B1b (presence of circulating clone). The mechanism responsible for the development of leukemic disease in MF is unknown and in some cases may simply reflect disease progression. In other cases erythroderma and circulating disease develop simultaneously, which has historically been referred to as SS. The distinction between SS and erythrodermic MF with leukemic involvement (or SS syndrome preceded by MF) has been a point of controversy, and it remains unclear whether the two diseases are distinct or merely variants of one another. At present, SS is specifically defined as the combination of erythroderma with B2 disease.[6]

Extracutaneous Disease

In advanced stages of disease MF may progress to involve regional or distant lymph nodes or extracutaneous organ systems (most commonly the lungs, oral cavity, pharynx, or central nervous system), and these sites may cause patients significant pain or functional impairment.[7] Of note, in advanced cases of MF the extent of cutaneous or extracutaneous disease may vary significantly in patients of the same clinical stage. Clinical trials that report results by stage alone may therefore be difficult to interpret. The ISCL/USCLC/EORTC consensus statement on clinical end points and response criteria should facilitate improved communication of the degree of disease and response to treatment in future clinical trials.[6]

Molecular and Cellular Pathophysiology

Examination of early phase MF lesions by hematoxylin and eosin staining commonly reveals epidermotropism, a profound infiltration of lymphocytes into the epidermis. As the lesions progress and become thickened, epidermotropism is gradually lost as the lymphocytes begin to localize more diffusely in the skin. Only a fraction of the skin-homing lymphocytes in MF are malignant, and the malignant T cells may be identified by visualization of their small to medium-sized hyperconvoluted (or cerebriform) nuclei and surrounding lacunae, which give them the impression of being surrounded by a halo. A Pautrier's microabscess (Langerhans cell surrounded by atypical T cells in the epidermis) is a less common but pathognomonic histologic finding associated with MF.[1,5] The malignant cells in MF are CD4+ T-helper cells, which most commonly express a CD3+, CD4+, CD45RO+, CLA+, CCR4+ immunophenotype. Evaluation of the TCR profile of malignant T cells in MF reveals a predominant TCR rearrangement indicative of clonal dominance in a majority of cases.

The specific stimuli and molecular events responsible for activation and development of clonal dominance of a specific T cell are unknown. Genetic profiling studies have identified a number of chromosomal deletions and duplications associated with MF/SS, and microRNA profiling is beginning to reveal distinct molecular profiles associated with different phases of MF. In addition to the molecular aberrations intrinsic to the malignant T cells, the cutaneous microenvironment is also likely to play a key role in the development and maintenance of disease.[5,8–11]

Diagnosis and Evaluation

Evaluation of a patient with suspected or recently diagnosed MF should include a comprehensive history/physical examination, biopsy of cutaneous lesion(s) and suspicious lymph nodes, and appropriate laboratory and imaging studies. The ISCL has designed a diagnostic algorithm for early-stage MF (not applicable to MF variants) (Table 79.2),[12] and specific recommendations for patient evaluation have been released by the ISCL/EORTC.[13]

History and Physical Examination. The duration of symptoms, evolutionary course of cutaneous disease, and presence or absence of B symptoms should be determined. The percentage of body surface area involved by disease and

TABLE 79.2 DIAGNOSTIC CRITERIA FOR EARLY STAGE MYCOSIS FUNGOIDES[a,12]

Clinical	*Immunopathologic*
Persistent and/or progressive patches and plaques plus: 1. Non-sun-exposed location 2. Size/shape variation 3. Poikiloderma *Scoring:* Two points if two or more criteria met. One point if only one criterion met.	1. CD2, 3, 5 <50% of T cells 2. CD7 <10% of T cells 3. Epidermal discordance from expression of CD2, 3, 5, or 7 on dermal T cells *Scoring:* One point if any criterion met.
Molecular/Biologic	*Histopathologic*
1. Clonal TCR gene rearrangement *Scoring:* One point if present.	1. Epidermotropism without spongiosis 2. Lymphoid atypia *Scoring:* One point for each.

TCR, T-cell receptor.

[a]Not applicable to mycosis fungoides variants. Diagnosis made with 4 points or more.

presence or absence of cutaneous tumors should be documented, and a thorough evaluation of the lymphatic system should be performed. Appropriate images of cutaneous lesions should be recorded so that disease progression or response to therapy may be monitored.

Skin Biopsy. Biopsies should be taken from a minimum of two distinct sites of disease. Lesions of the greatest induration will be most likely to yield a diagnosis due to greater numbers of malignant cells. However, scaled lesions are more likely to show epidermotropism. Tissue should be evaluated with hematoxylin and eosin staining, immunostaining for surface marker expression profiles (including CD2, CD3, CD4, CD5, CD7, CD8, CD20, CD30, CD26, CD56, TIA1, granzyme B, βF1), and PCR for clonal TCR rearrangement. Slides should be reviewed by a dermatopathologist.

Excisional biopsies of enlarged or otherwise suspicious lymph nodes (fixed or matted lymph nodes, or lymph nodes ≥1.5 cm or ≥1 cm in the head and neck) should be evaluated as described previously. When multiple suspicious lymph nodes are encountered, the choice of lymph node to be excised should be based on size, fluorodeoxyglucose (FDG) avidity, and location, with priority given to the largest lymph node draining an affected area of skin or the lymph node with the highest standardized uptake value (SUV) on positron emission tomography (PET) scan. If all other factors are equal, priority should be given first to cervical nodes, followed by axillary and then inguinal nodes.[13]

Laboratory and Imaging Studies. Laboratory studies should include a complete blood count, chemistry panel, liver function tests, and lactate dehydrogenase (LDH). Examination of the peripheral blood for circulating disease by PCR and flow cytometry should also be considered, particularly for patients with erythroderma, nodal, or extracutaneous disease. Bone marrow biopsy should be considered if peripheral blood or extracutaneous organs are found to harbor disease.[13] Computed tomography (CT) of the chest, abdomen, and pelvis is recommended in the evaluation of all patients with MF with the exception of patients with patch/plaque disease limited to 10% or less of the body surface area. In these cases a chest x-ray or nodal ultrasound may suffice. PET scanning was shown to be more sensitive than CT in identifying involved lymph nodes, and the role of PET in MF continues to evolve.[14]

Staging and Prognosis

MF is presently staged using the modified TNMB system proposed by the ISCL/EORTC (Table 79.3).[13] Based on a review of 525 patients with MF (staged using the previous 1979 TNMB system), the majority of patients present with early stage disease (30% IA, 25% IB, 11% IIA, 16% IIB, 3% IIIA, 8% IIIB, 6% IVA, and 1% IVB). Only 7% of patients presented with peripheral blood involvement. The correlation of clinical stage to overall and disease-specific survival is presented in Figure 79.3.[7] Similar results were obtained in a validation study of the current staging system.[15] Of note, stage IA MF is not associated with any increase in mortality risk in comparison to an age- and ethnicity-matched control population, and is associated with only a 16% rate of disease progression at 20 years of follow-up.[7]

Skin-Directed Therapy

MF is not generally considered to be curable, although extended periods of disease-free survival after treatment have been reported. Efforts to treat MF are primarily focused on preventing progression and ameliorating symptoms. In early-stage disease a number of skin-directed treatments are effective and should be considered as first-line therapy. Topical therapies include corticosteroids (complete response [CR] rates of 63% for T1 and 25% for T2 disease),[16] nitrogen mustard (CR

TABLE 79.3 ISCL/EORTC REVISIONS TO MYCOSIS FUNGOIDES STAGING[13]

T Stage	*N Stage*
T1: Limited patches, papules, and/or plaques covering <10% of the skin surface. May further stratify into T1a (patch only) vs. T1b (plaque/patch) T2: Patches, papules, or plaques covering ≥10% of the skin surface. May further stratify into T2a (patch only) vs. T2b (plaque/patch). T3: One or more tumors (≥1-cm diameter) T4: Confluence of erythema covering >80% body surface area	N0: No clinically abnormal peripheral lymph nodes; biopsy not required N1: Clinically abnormal peripheral lymph nodes; histopathology Dutch grade 1 or NCI LN0–2 (N1a: clone negative, N1b: clone positive N2: Clinically abnormal peripheral lymph nodes; histopathology Dutch grade 2 or NCI LN3 N3: Clinically abnormal peripheral lymph nodes; histopathology Dutch grades 3 or 4 or NCI LN4; clone positive or negative NX: Clinically abnormal peripheral lymph nodes; no histologic confirmation
B Stage	*M Stage*
B0: Absence of significant blood involvement: <5% of peripheral blood lymphocytes are atypical (Sézary) cells B1: Low blood tumor burden: >5% of peripheral blood lymphocytes are atypical (Sézary) cells but does not meet B2 criteria B2: High blood tumor burden: ≥1,000/μL Sézary cells with positive clone	M0: No visceral organ involvement M1: Visceral involvement (must have pathology confirmation and organ involved should be specified)
Staging Groups	
IA: T1 N0 M0 B0–1 IB: T2 N0 M0 B0–1 IIA: T1–2 N1–2 M0 B0 IIB: T3 N0–2 M0 B0–1	IIIA: T4 N0–2 M0 B0 IIIB: T4 N0–2 M0 B1 IVA1: T1–4 N0–2 M0 B0–2 IVA2: T1–4 N3 M0 B0–2 IVB: T1–4 N0–3 M1 B0–2

ISCL, International Society for Cutaneous Lymphomas; EORTC, European Organisation for Research and Treatment of Cancer; NCI, National Cancer Institute.

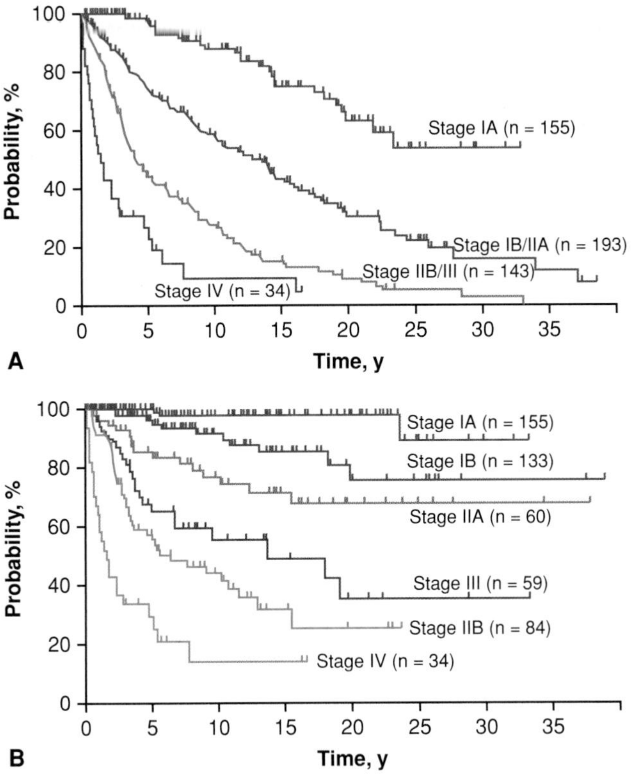

FIGURE 79.3. Overall **(A)** and disease-specific **(B)** survival in mycosis fungoides by stage. (Reprinted with permission from Kim YH, Liu HL, Mraz-Gernhard S, et al. Long-term outcome of 525 patients with mycosis fungoides and Sezary syndrome. *Arch Dermatol* 2003;139: 857–866; copyright © 2003 American Medical Association. All rights reserved.)

rates of 76% to 80% for stage IA and 35% to 68% for stage IB),[17] carmustine (CR rates of 86% for T1 and 47% for T2 disease),[18] and bexarotene gel (CR rate of 21% in early-stage MF).[19] Phototherapy with narrow-band ultraviolet B (NB-UVB) (54% CR in stages IA or IB)[20] or psoralen + UVA (PUVA) (CR rate of 65%)[21] is also frequently used. However, the most effective skin-directed therapy for MF is ionizing radiation.

Ionizing radiation is well suited to the treatment of cutaneous lymphoma. Lymphocytes are highly radiosensitive, and radiation doses may be effectively limited to the epidermis and dermis by appropriate selection of photon or electron energies. Options for irradiation include local superficial irradiation or irradiation of the entirety of the skin via total skin electron beam therapy (TSEBT).

Local Superficial Irradiation

A small portion (~5%) of patients with stage IA MF present with "minimal" disease, defined as a solitary lesion or two to three MF lesions clustered sufficiently close to one another that they are amenable to treatment with a single or abutting radiation fields.[22] For these patients, treatment with local superficial irradiation may be considered. Treatment fields should be designed to encompass the entirety of the lesion (determined by visual inspection, palpation, and/or appropriate imaging) with a 1- to 2-cm margin, with use of a lead or Cerrobend cutout to conform field borders to the anatomy of the cutaneous lesion. Treatment is most commonly provided with electrons, with energies (usually 6 to 16 MeV) carefully selected to optimize dose penetration. The EORTC recommends that the 80% isodose line is set at the deep border of the dermis,[23] which is commonly at a depth of approximately 4.5 mm.

Local superficial radiation is very effective in generating a CR for patients with "minimal" stage IA MF. In a review of 21 patients with "minimal" stage IA MF treated with local superficial radiation (superficial or orthovoltage x-rays or megavoltage electrons) to doses ranging from 20 to 40 Gy in four to five or 10 to 15 fractions, Wilson et al.[22] found a CR rate of 97%. Importantly, review of the recurrence rates associated with different total doses of local superficial radiation revealed a 25% local recurrence rate (two of eight fields) with treatment to 20 Gy and an 8% local recurrence rate (two of 25 fields) with treatment to 20 to 40 Gy. Similarly, Cotter et al.[24] reported a local recurrence rate of 42% for fields treated to 10 Gy or less, but 0% for fields treated to >30 Gy. More recently, treatment to 8 Gy in 4-Gy fractions has been shown to yield a CR rate of 92%.[25] Based on these studies, it is recommended that "minimal" stage IA (i.e., unilesional or up to three closely approximated sites) MF lesions are treated to a dose of 30 to 36 Gy, and treatment as low as 8 Gy in two fractions may be considered as a palliative treatment. Side effects of local superficial radiation are usually limited to mild dermatitis, local alopecia, and pigmentation changes.

Total Skin Electron Beam Therapy

Technique. Total skin electron beam therapy (TSEBT) is technically challenging and should only be attempted in centers with special expertise in its provision, including skilled physics support. EORTC recommendations regarding the technical aspects of TSEBT are presented in Table 79.4. Modern TSEBT is usually accomplished with 6- to 9-MeV electrons generated by a medical linear accelerator directed at a patient standing behind a polycarbonate screen ~3.8 meters from the linear accelerator head. The polycarbonate screen scatters the incident electron beam and contributes to an improved surface dose. Treatment is provided in "cycles," with one cycle composed of treatment of the patient in six different positions (Fig. 79.4A) over 2 days (three positions each day). Typically, a dose of 2 Gy is provided to the entirety of the skin during one cycle, and two cycles are usually administered per week. Treatment in six positions optimizes dose distribution at the skin surface (Fig. 79.4B). At Yale and Stanford, the anterior, right posterior oblique, and left posterior oblique positions are treated on cycle day 1, and the posterior, right anterior oblique, and left anterior oblique positions on cycle day 2.[26,27] When the patient stands in a treatment position, a dual-field technique is used to deliver treatment to a superior and inferior field by angling the gantry 16 to 17.5 degrees above and below horizontal, respectively, the specific angle dependent upon individual machine characteristics (Fig. 79.5). Treatment to the six positions using the dual-field technique, which is in use at Yale and Stanford, delivers maximum dose to a depth of 1 mm, 80% dose to 6 to 7 mm, and 20% dose to 12.5 mm.[26,27]

TABLE 79.4 EORTC TECHNICAL RECOMMENDATIONS FOR TSEBT[23]
The primary target in TSEBT is the epidermis, adnexal structures, and dermis.
The goal of treatment (either by primary or supplemental treatments) is to deliver a dose of 26 to 28 Gy to a depth of 4 mm below the skin surface, which usually translates to a truncal dose of 31 to 36 Gy.
Treatment should be provided in 30 to 36 fractions (1 to 1.2 Gy/fraction) over 6 to 10 weeks. Fraction sizes should not exceed 2 to 2.5 Gy due to increased acute and late side effects.
The 80% isodose line should extend to 4 mm below the skin surface, the dose 20 mm deep to the skin must be <20% of the maximum dose at skin, and the dose at curved skin sites must not exceed 120% of the prescribed skin dose.
Patient positioning is critical, and patients must be positioned in a manner to maximize unfolding of the skin. A minimum of six treatment positions is recommended.
The optimal source-to-patient distance is 3 to 8 meters, and dose should be homogenous to within 10% across the entire vertical and lateral dimensions of the beam at the patient's surface.
The globe of the eye must be limited to <15% of the maximum skin dose, and photon contamination at the bone marrow must be limited to <0.7 Gy.

EORTC, European Organisation for Research and Treatment of Cancer; TSEBT, total skin electron beam therapy.

Clinical Radiation Oncology

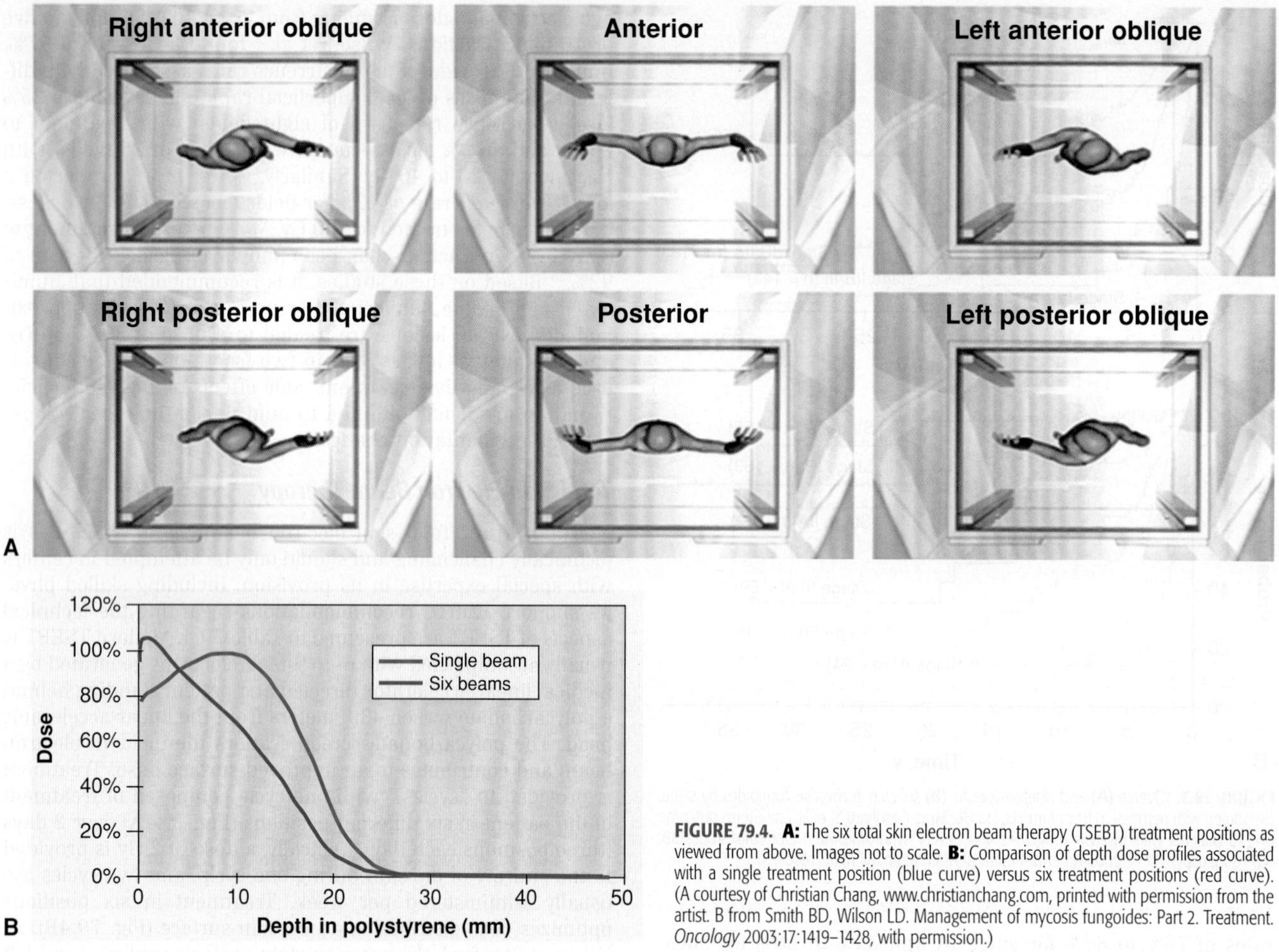

FIGURE 79.4. **A:** The six total skin electron beam therapy (TSEBT) treatment positions as viewed from above. Images not to scale. **B:** Comparison of depth dose profiles associated with a single treatment position (blue curve) versus six treatment positions (red curve). (A courtesy of Christian Chang, www.christianchang.com, printed with permission from the artist. B from Smith BD, Wilson LD. Management of mycosis fungoides: Part 2. Treatment. *Oncology* 2003;17:1419–1428, with permission.)

Dose and Fractionation. Sublethal damage repair does not appear to be a major factor in determining the response of MF to ionizing radiation,[28] and modern TSEBT is provided with a relatively protracted course of two cycles per week for 9 weeks, which provides a total dose of 36 Gy to the skin surface. The total radiation dose appears to be directly associated with complete response rates, with 18% CR with treatment to <10 Gy, 55% CR with treatment to 10 to 20 Gy, 66% CR with treatment to 20 to 25 Gy, 75% CR with treatment to 25 to 30 Gy, and 94% CR with treatment to 30 to 36 Gy.[29] However, lower doses yield impressive rates of overall response (defined as a >50% reduction in cutaneous disease), overall survival, progression-free survival, and relapse-free survival rates. Relapse rates are relatively high even in patients in which a CR is obtained, and the absolute benefit of a CR relative to the increased side effects at higher doses of TSEBT is unclear. The application of reduced-dose TSEBT (10 to 20 Gy) in combination with additional therapies may be a viable alternative to the current standard of 36 Gy,[30] but additional studies are necessary before any conclusions may be made in this regard.

Supplemental Treatments. The six treatment positions in TSEBT maximize unfolding of the skin and exposure of the skin surface to the incident electron beam, but areas such as the soles of the feet, perineum, and scalp remain obscured and require supplemental doses to ensure that a minimum of 20 to 28 Gy is administered to a depth of approximately 4 mm. Supplemental treatment to these areas may be accomplished by the use of 120-kV superficial photons with half-value layer (HVL) 4.2-mm Al or low-energy (~6 MeV) electrons with 1-cm bolus to treat the soles of the feet (1 Gy per fraction) and the perineum (1 Gy per fraction). In some setups, the scalp is treated by placing an angled electron reflector above the patient,[26] but supplemental boosting is an alternative approach that is incorporated in some centers. Additional areas that may need supplemental dose include thick cutaneous tumors and skin folds secondary to body habitus, and the need for supplemental dose to such areas is based on the judgement of the radiation oncologist.[26,27]

Side Effects. In a review of perceptions of MF therapy, patients overall considered TSEBT to be a more difficult treatment to endure as compared to other treatments,[31] and it is important that patients are advised that symptoms such as pruritus and cutaneous erythema may be exacerbated during therapy. Additional acute side effects that commonly occur include xerosis, dry desquamation, extremity edema, blister/bullae formation over the lower extremities, alopecia (including hair of the scalp, eyebrows, eyelashes, and body), and nail changes (nails may ultimately be lost but usually regrow). Hypohydrosis secondary to damage to sweat glands may occur. Similarly, dryness and irritation of the nasal mucosa may result in nose bleeds. Gynecomastia is a rare occurrence. Late/chronic side effects are minimal and include cataract formation, chronic xerosis, persistent alopecia, dystrophic nails, telangiectasia, and secondary skin cancers including squamous and basal cell carcinomas and melanomas.[23,32–35]

In an effort to minimize side effects, areas that are most susceptible to TSEBT such as the eyes, lips, hands, fingernails, feet, and testes are blocked during certain cycles of treatment. Shielding of the eye and lens may be accomplished by a combination of internal/external shields, selected based upon the

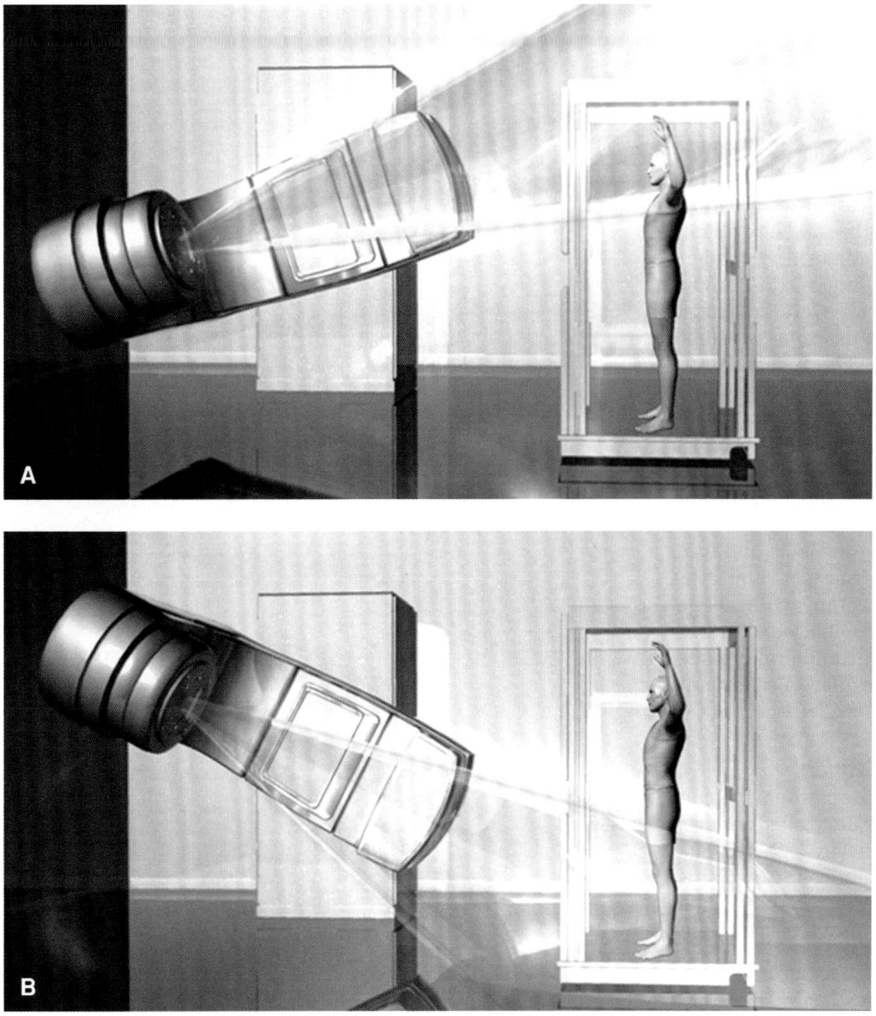

FIGURE 79.5. Dual-field technique for total skin electron beam therapy (TSEBT). **A:** Treatment of superior field. **B:** Treatment of inferior field. Images not to scale. (Courtesy of Christian Chang, www.christianchang.com, printed with permission from the artist.)

proximity of clinical disease. Usually, if internal eyeshields are used, they are used for only a portion of the therapy (7 to 20 Gy). The lips, hands, and fingernails may be blocked by lead mitts or fingernail shields as clinical circumstances warrant. The feet may be blocked by footboards for a portion of the treatment. A testicular shield may be used during perineal boost treatments.[26]

Clinical Efficacy. TSEBT is very effective, particularly for early-stage disease. TSEBT yields a complete response rate of >90% with a 15-year relapse-free survival of 40% in patients with T1 disease, although it is no longer recommended for such limited disease.[29] Of note, patients with recurrent disease after a course of TSEBT most commonly have disease restricted to <5% of the skin surface area, and these recurrences are therefore amenable to local salvage therapy with topical therapy or limited superficial radiation. When successful salvage of such limited recurrences is taken into account, relapse-free survival improves to 70% at 15 years.[36–38]

In T2 disease TSEBT is similarly effective, with a complete response rate of 76% to 90% and a 50% relapse-free survival rate at 5 years and 10% at 10 years. Relapse-free survival is significantly improved by addition of adjuvant PUVA or nitrogen mustard. Specifically, adjuvant PUVA improves 5-year relapse-free survival to 85%, and nitrogen mustard improves 10-year relapse-free survival to 40%.[23,38–40]

When cutaneous tumors are present (T3 disease), TSEBT is less effective but still yields an impressive complete response rate of 44% to 54% of patients, much greater than any other single modality. Adjuvant treatment should be considered, and retrospective studies suggest that nitrogen mustard may increase the durability of response. Alternatively, a combination of nitrogen mustard and local superficial radiation may be considered for tumors localized to a small percentage of the skin surface.[38,40,41] Supplemental boosts should be considered for patients with tumors, and such boost treatment should be provided concomitantly with the initiation of TSEBT or prior to its initiation. The purpose of the boost is to diminish the thickness of the lesion so that electrons from TSEBT can effectively penetrate the entire lesion.

In erythrodermic MF (T4 disease), TSEBT yields a 70% to 100% response rate (for patients with T4N0 disease) and 5-year progression-free survival of 25% to 69%. When disease involves the peripheral circulation or extracutaneous sites, TSEBT is less effective and response and progression-free survival rates decrease to 74% and 36%, respectively. TSEBT appears to be synergistic with extracorporeal photopheresis (ECP), and the combination of TSEBT and ECP is associated with improved disease-specific survival and decreased levels of circulating malignant cells.[42–45]

Palliative Radiotherapy

Symptomatic nodal or visceral disease may be effectively palliated by a brief course of localized radiotherapy, usually to a total dose of 12 to 30 Gy. If this treatment is given in conjunction with a course of TSEBT, a similar dose may be used. In the subset of patients that develop extensive recurrence of cutaneous disease after a previous course of TSEBT, additional courses of TSEBT to lower total doses can be considered and have proven effective in studies at Yale and Stanford.[46,47]

Systemic Therapy

Skin-directed therapy should be attempted first for patients with early-stage disease, but in patients with advanced or refractory disease systemic therapy may be considered. Options for systemic therapy include oral bexarotene (response rate up to 54% in refractory CTCL at a dose of 300 mg/m^2, and bexarotene may be used in combination with other therapies),[48,49] denileukin diftitox (a fusion protein consisting of interleukin-2 and a portion of the diphtheria toxin that yields an overall response rate of 30% in refractory CTCL),[50] histone deacetylase inhibitors (such as vorinostat and romidepsin, ~30% response rate in refractory CTCL),[51,52] alemtuzumab (a monoclonal antibody targeted against the CD52 surface marker with a 38% overall response rate in relapsed or refractory CTCL and 86% response rate in SS),[53,54] interferon-α2a (IFN-α) (a biologic modifier with a response rate of 40% to 80% in CTCL as a single agent and with synergistic activity with other MF therapies),[55–61] ECP (associated with improvement in peripheral blood and skin involvement, especially in those with T4 disease),[62] and cytotoxic chemotherapy (single-agent chemotherapy with agents such as purine or nucleoside analogs, liposomal doxorubicin, and antifolate agents, including methotrexate and pralatrexate, is preferred because no distinct advantages have been identified with the use of multiagent regimens).[63–69]

Autologous or Allogeneic Stem Cell Transplant

Patients with MF/SS refractory to other therapies may be considered for stem cell transplant. Although autologous stem cell transplants have not proven to be overly effective, greater success has been achieved with allogeneic stem cell transplants. Additional studies are necessary to fully define the role of stem cell transplant in MF. This approach may prove to be a valuable option for patients with refractory disease.[70–74]

Treatment Recommendations by Stage

Treatment recommendations for MF/SS are presented by stage in Table 79.5.[71] The National Comprehensive Cancer Network (NCCN) has also published treatment guidelines for MF/SS.[75]

TABLE 79.5 RECOMMENDATIONS FOR TREATMENT OF MF BY STAGE

Stage	First-Line Therapies	Options for Refractory or Relapsed Disease
"Minimal" IA	Local superficial irradiation	Consider standard stage IA first-line therapies
IA, IB, IIA	Expectant observation (for stage IA) Topical therapies (corticosteroids, nitrogen mustard, BCNU, bexarotene) Phototherapy (PUVA, NB-UVB) TSEBT (consider adjuvant PUVA or nitrogen mustard)	Second course TSEBT Oral bexarotene IFN-α Low-dose MTX Vorinostat Denileukin diftitox Clinical trials NOTE: Chemotherapy is not recommended
IIB	TSEBT (consider boosts to cutaneous tumors and adjuvant PUVA or nitrogen mustard) IFN-α PUVA	Second course TSEBT Oral bexarotene Vorinostat Denileukin diftitox Clinical trials Chemotherapy
IIIA, IIIB, leukemic CTCL or SS	TSEBT + ECP ECP alone IFN-α PUVA + IFN-α MTX	Second course TSEBT Oral bexarotene Vorinostat Denileukin diftitox Alemtuzumab Clinical trials Chemotherapy Allogeneic stem cell transplant
IVA(1–2), IVB	Chemotherapy TSEBT for palliation Oral bexarotene Denileukin diftitox IFN-α Vorinostat Romidepsin Low-dose MTX Clinical trials	Allogeneic stem cell transplant

BCNU, bis-chloroethylnitrosourea; PUVA, psoralen plus ultraviolet A; NB-UVB, narrow-band ultraviolet B; TSEBT, total skin electron beam therapy; IFN-α, interferon-alpha; MTX, methotrexate; CTCL, cutaneous T-cell lymphoma; SS, Sézary syndrome; ECP, extracorporeal photopheresis.

Transformed Disease

In some cases, large cell transformation of MF may occur, which is identified on biopsy by >25% large cells in the sample. Large cell transformation may be associated with decreased survival rates and occurs in 8% to 39% of cases. Patients with advanced stage or high levels of β_2-microglobulin or LDH are at the greatest risk of large cell transformation. Treatment options include systemic chemotherapy, stem cell transplant, and consolidative or local radiation for localized disease.[71]

Variants of Mycosis Fungoides

Variant forms of MF that share histologic and clinical features with classic MF but exhibit distinct clinical behavior have been recognized and include folliculotropic MF, Woringer-Kolopp disease, granulomatous slack skin, and hypopigmented MF.

Folliculotropic MF is characterized by a folliculotropic pattern of cutaneous infiltration of malignant T cells. Folliculotropic MF lesions present as patches, plaques, or tumors or may manifest in an acneiform pattern. Lesions primarily develop over the head and neck and are rarely found over the trunk. Localized alopecia secondary to the folliculotropic pattern is common. Folliculotropic MF is associated with a 15-year survival of 41% for early-stage disease. Early-stage disease may be treated with PUVA combined with bexarotene or IFN-α. Local radiation therapy may be advantageous because it can effectively treat to deeper depths of involvement seen in this variant. Advanced-stage disease is minimally responsive to cytotoxic chemotherapy, and alternate options such as irradiation or allogeneic stem cell transplant should be considered.[1,76]

Woringer-Kolopp disease (pagetoid reticulosis) is characterized by a solitary erythematous and scaling cutaneous patch on an extremity. Biopsy results are similar to classic MF, and the malignant T cells commonly carry a CD3+/CD4+/CD8– or CD3+/CD4–/CD8+ immunophenotype. If CD8+ disease is identified, it is important to consider the alternative diagnosis of CD8+ aggressive peripheral cutaneous T-cell lymphoma, and the distinction between these diagnoses is made by the aggressiveness of disease. Specifically, as compared to CD8+ aggressive peripheral cutaneous T-cell lymphoma, Woringer-Kolopp disease is very slowly progressive and carries an excellent prognosis. Treatment options include skin-directed therapies such as corticosteroids, nitrogen mustard, resection, or local irradiation. Local radiation may be very successful in achieving long-term local control even in locally very advanced disease. In rare cases of diffuse or refractory disease, irradiation is also recommended.[1,77]

Granulomatous slack skin (GSS) is an extremely rare variant of MF, with <100 cases reported in the literature. It is characterized by cutaneous infiltration of a clonal population of malignant T cells coupled with a granulomatous infiltration. The granulomatous infiltrate ultimately causes destruction of local elastin fibers and impairs the structural integrity and elasticity of the skin, which results in loose or "slack" skin. This loosening of the skin is most commonly observed in the axilla, groin, neck, and breast. Although GSS is itself an indolent disease, it is

TABLE 79.6 ISCL/EORTC TNM CLASSIFICATION OF CUTANEOUS LYMPHOMA OTHER THAN MF/SS[81]

T Stage	N Stage	M Stage
T1: Solitary skin involvement T1a: A solitary lesion <5 cm in diameter T1b: A solitary lesion >5 cm in diameter T2: Regional skin involvement: multiple lesions limited to 1 body region or 2 contiguous body regions T2a: All-disease-encompassing in a <15-cm-diameter circular area T2b: All-disease-encompassing in a >15- and <30-cm-diameter circular area T2c: All-disease-encompassing in a >30-cm-diameter circular area T3: Generalized skin involvement T3a: Multiple lesions involving 2 noncontiguous body regions T3b: Multiple lesions involving & ≥3 body regions	N0: No clinical or pathologic lymph node involvement N1: Involvement of 1 peripheral lymph node region that drains an area of current or prior skin involvement N2: Involvement of 2 or more peripheral lymph node regions or involvement of any lymph node region that does not drain an area of current or prior skin involvement N3: Involvement of central lymph nodes	M0: No evidence of extracutaneous non–lymph node disease M1: Extracutaneous non–lymph node disease present

ISCL, International Society for Cutaneous Lymphomas; EORTC, European Organisation for Research and Treatment of Cancer; MF, mycosis fungoides; SS, Sézary syndrome.

associated with an increased incidence of secondary lymphomas, most commonly Hodgkin lymphoma or MF. Given the rarity of this disease, it is difficult to make definitive recommendations regarding therapy, but surgical resection or local superficial radiation may be effective.[1,78]

Hypopigmented MF presents at an earlier age (childhood or adolescence) than classic MF and is characterized by development of hypopigmented patches frequently over the trunk or extremities. In contrast to classic MF, the malignant T cells are often CD8+. Treatment and disease course are otherwise similar to classic MF.[79,80]

Non–Mycosis Fungoides CTCL

Staging

In 2007 the ISCL and EORTC presented a new TNM staging system for non-MF/SS cutaneous lymphomas (Table 79.6).[81]

CD30+ Lymphoproliferative Disorders

A review of the SEER registry identified 268 cases of primary cutaneous CD30+ lymphoproliferative disorders recorded between 1974 and 2004 (58% male and 42% female patients). The median age of diagnosis was 61, and population-matched 3-year relative survival was 87%, with 5-year disease-specific survival 92%. Localization of disease in the head and neck appears to be a negative prognostic factor.[82] The primary cutaneous CD30+ lymphoproliferative disorders recognized by the WHO/EORTC are primary cutaneous anaplastic large cell lymphoma and lymphomatoid papulosis.[1] These cannot be differentiated histologically. It is essential to take a careful clinical history to document the distribution of lesions and their clinical course (e.g., history of spontaneous regression). The diagnosis is a clinical-pathologic one. Recently the EORTC, ISCL, and USCLC released consensus recommendations regarding the evaluation and treatment of primary cutaneous CD30+ lymphoproliferative disorders.[83]

Primary cutaneous anaplastic large cell lymphoma (C-ALCL) is characterized by development of cutaneous plaques, nodules, or tumors that are usually solitary or clustered into a localized area. Multifocal disease is uncommon (occurring in only 20% of patients), and lymph nodes are involved in only 10% of cases. Extracutaneous disease is rarely found. C-ALCL is most commonly diagnosed in males, with a male:female ratio of 2–3:1. When disease is localized to the skin and regional lymph nodes, prognoses are excellent, with anticipated 5-year overall survival and 10-year disease-specific survival rates of 90%. Progression to extracutaneous disease is associated with overall survival, and extensive limb disease (defined as "initial presentation or progression to multiple skin tumors in 1 limb or contiguous body regions"[84]) is associated with disease-specific survival. Biopsies of C-ALCL lesions reveal a diffuse infiltration of large anaplastic CD4+ T cells, and at least 75% of these anaplastic T cells express CD30. Similar to MF, clonal dominance is frequently detected by PCR evaluation for TCR rearrangement.[1]

Limited resection or local superficial irradiation is very effective in controlling localized cutaneous disease, and low-dose methotrexate may be considered when widespread cutaneous disease precludes simple resection or irradiation. Local superficial radiation to a dose of 34 to 44 Gy was associated with a 100% CR rate,[85] and treatment to 36 to 40 Gy in 2-Gy fractions is recommended. In rare cases in which extracutaneous disease is found, doxorubicin-based chemotherapy should be considered.

Of note, prior to initiating therapy, it is critically important to verify that C-ALCL has been correctly distinguished from the more common systemic ALCL. Molecular studies to evaluate the presence of the (2:5)(p23;q35) chromosomal translocation and expression of anaplastic lymphoma kinase (ALK) or epithelial membrane antigen (EMA) are useful in making this distinction, because the (2:5) translocation and expression of ALK and EMA are found in systemic ALCL but rarely found in C-ALCL.[1,86]

Lymphomatoid papulosis (LyP) carries an excellent prognosis, with a 5-year overall survival rate of 100%. However, 15% to 20% of patients with LyP will develop MF, C-ALCL, or a Hodgkin lymphoma. LyP is characterized by development of violaceous papular or papulonodular lesions over the trunk or extremities, which typically regress after 3 to 12 weeks, often leaving a residual scar. Biopsy of LyP cutaneous lesions reveals epidermotropic atypical CD3+/CD4+/CD8– lymphocytes, and clonal TCR rearrangement is identified in 60% to 70% of cases. Three distinct histologic subtypes are recognized: LyP A, B, and C. LyP A (characterized by large multinucleated CD30+ cells intermixed with an inflammatory infiltrate) and C (characterized by large CD30+ cells with minimal inflammatory infiltrate) represent 90% of cases. In contrast to types A and C, atypical lymphocytes in LyP B are CD3+/CD4+/CD30–, reminiscent of MF.[1]

Aggressive therapies such as chemotherapy or radiation should be avoided in LyP. In the rare patient with a large cutaneous burden of disease, skin-directed therapy with PUVA or a topical chemotherapy agent may be considered. In addition, low-dose oral methotrexate may be effective in suppressing the development of new lesions and should be considered if previous LyP lesions caused significant scarring.[1]

Extranodal NK-/T-Cell Lymphoma, Nasal Type

Extranodal NK-/T-cell lymphoma, nasal type most commonly arises in the nasal cavity and nasopharynx but in select cases may present with cutaneous plaques or tumors over the extremities and trunk and is therefore included in the WHO/EORTC classification of cutaneous lymphomas. Biopsy of a cutaneous lesion reveals a dense lymphoid infiltrate, which may exhibit an epidermotropic component. The malignant cells are most commonly NK in origin with a CD3–/CD2+/CD56+ immunophenotype, but on occasion the malignant cells are derived from cytotoxic T cells. Epstein Barr virus (EBV) is directly associated with disease development, and cutaneous lesions are nearly always EBV+. Consistent with an EBV-mediated pathophysiology, the disease occurs more commonly in geographic distributions in which EBV is endemic (Central America, South America, South Asia). The TCR usually remains in germline configuration when the malignant cells are of NK-cell origin, but clonal TCR rearrangement may be observed in cases in which the malignant cells are derived from cytotoxic T cells. Optimal treatment regimens for cutaneous extranodal NK-/T-cell lymphoma, nasal type have not yet been determined. Treatment with extended field radiotherapy to a median dose of 50 Gy yields a CR rate of 95.4% in early-stage disease, but local or distant recurrences are common and adjuvant therapy with L-asparaginase and other regimens should be considered. Advanced-stage disease is treated primarily with chemotherapy.[1,87–89]

Subcutaneous Panniculitis-Like T-Cell Lymphoma

Subcutaneous panniculitis-like T-cell lymphoma presents with subcutaneous nodules and/or plaques, which are commonly localized over the legs or trunk. Biopsy reveals a lymphoid infiltrate composed primarily of malignant cytotoxic CD8+ T cells. Prior to the establishment of the WHO/EORTC classification system, α/β and γ/δ T-cell forms of disease were each recognized as subcutaneous panniculitis-like T-cell lymphoma. However, γ/δ T-cell lymphoma is now recognized as a distinct, more aggressive disease and is categorized as a primary cutaneous peripheral T-cell lymphoma. The 5-year survival of the less aggressive α/β disease approaches 80%, and treatment involves combinations of corticosteroids and radiation, and potentially chemotherapy for refractory disease.[1] Notably, presence of the hemophagocytic syndrome predicts a worse prognosis.

Adult T-Cell Leukemia/Lymphoma

Infection with the human T-lymphotropic virus 1 (HTLV-1) may result in adult T-cell leukemia/lymphoma in approximately 1% to 5% individuals, and patients may develop associated cutaneous disease characterized by papules, plaques, and tumors. In smoldering disease, cutaneous lesions may be the only sign of pathology. Chemotherapy is the primary therapy for acute adult T-cell leukemia/lymphoma, while smoldering cases may be treated with skin-directed therapies.[1]

Primary Cutaneous Peripheral T-Cell Lymphoma

Additional CTCLs that do not fit into the previously discussed categories are grouped as "primary cutaneous peripheral T-cell lymphomas," and provisional subsets of this category described by the WHO/EORTC include primary cutaneous aggressive epidermotropic CD8+ cytotoxic T-cell lymphoma (characterized by cutaneous papules/plaques, nodules, and tumors with ulceration and a propensity for extracutaneous spread of disease), cutaneous γ/δ T-cell lymphoma (most commonly characterized by subcutaneous plaques or tumors in the extremities), primary cutaneous CD4+ small/medium-sized pleomorphic T-cell lymphoma (usually presents as a single cutaneous plaque or tumor on the head and neck or upper trunk and has an indolent clinical behavior), and primary cutaneous peripheral T-cell lymphoma, unspecified (most commonly presents as solitary or generalized nodules). The primary cutaneous peripheral T-cell lymphomas are primarily treated with chemotherapy, with the exception of primary cutaneous CD4+ small/medium-sized pleomorphic T-cell lymphoma, which may be treated with local resection or radiation.[1]

CUTANEOUS B-CELL LYMPHOMAS

Primary cutaneous B-cell lymphoma (PCBCL) was first recognized as a distinct clinical entity in 1981 and accounts for only 29% of the 3,884 cases of primary cutaneous lymphoma diagnosed in the United States during 2001–2005.[3] The WHO/EORTC classification system recognizes three primary categories of CBCL: primary cutaneous marginal zone B-cell lymphoma (PCMZL), primary cutaneous follicle center B-cell lymphoma (PCFCL), and primary cutaneous diffuse large B-cell lymphoma, leg type (PCLBCL-LT).[1] Of the CBCL cases diagnosed in the United States in 2001–2005, the most common subtype was primary cutaneous DLBCL (40%, of which only 23% were of leg type), followed closely by cutaneous follicle center lymphoma (30%) and cutaneous marginal zone B-cell lymphoma (25%).[3] However, it should be noted that the histopathologic criteria for PLCBCL changed upon adoption of the WHO/EORTC consensus system, and it is likely that most of the PLCBCL cases diagnosed during 2001–2005 would now be reclassified as PCFCL. In a recent review 65% of CBCL cases classified as DLBCL using the older WHO criteria were found to be PCFCL under the current WHO/EORTC classification.[90]

Primary Cutaneous Marginal Zone B-Cell Lymphoma

PCMZL commonly presents with isolated or multifocal red or violaceous papules, plaques, and/or nodules on the trunk or extremities. The malignant cells are marginal zone B cells with a CD20+/CD79a+/CD5–/CD10– immunophenotype. Biopsies reveal an infiltrate composed of numerous lymphoid cells including marginal zone B cells, lymphoplasmacytoid cells, plasma cells, centroblastlike and immunoblastlike cells, reactive T cells, and reactive germinal centers. The prognosis for patients with PCMZL is excellent, and extracutaneous disease is rarely seen. Five-year overall survival rates of approximately 99% are expected, and cutaneous disease is very responsive to therapy. Cutaneous relapses are common but do not predict decreased survival.[1]

Primary Cutaneous Follicle Center Lymphoma

In contrast to PCMZL, PCFCL frequently presents with solitary or clustered plaques and tumors on the scalp, forehead, and trunk. Biopsy reveals a nodular or diffuse lymphoid infiltrate containing varying proportions of centrocytes, centroblasts, and reactive T cells growing in patterns ranging from follicular to diffuse. Similar to PCMZL, the malignant cells in PCFCL are of a CD20+/CD79a+ immunophenotype. Clonal rearrangement of immunoglobulin genes is usually observed. Importantly, the chromosomal translocation t(14:18) is infrequently seen in PCFCL, and therefore detection of this translocation should prompt consideration of a nodal or systemic follicular lymphoma. Similar to PCMZL, cutaneous lesions respond well to treatment, but rates of cutaneous relapse are relatively high at 20% overall. Extracutaneous disease is detected in 5% to 10% of patients, and bone marrow biopsy is an important component of evaluation. The 5-year overall survival rate for PCFCL is estimated at 95%.[1]

Primary Cutaneous Diffuse Large B-Cell Lymphoma, Leg Type

PCLBCL, leg type most commonly presents with violaceous cutaneous tumors over the lower extremities. Despite the nomenclature, anatomic restriction to the legs is not a requirement and in rare cases PCLBCL, leg type may be found in other cutaneous sites than the leg. The disease is characterized by diffuse lymphoid infiltrates with a predominance of centroblasts and immunoblasts, with absence of any significant numbers of centrocytes being a key distinguishing feature from PCFCL. A CD20+, CD79a+, Bcl-6+/–, CD10–, Bcl-2+, MUM-1+, FOXP1+ immunophenotype is usually observed. In contrast to PCMZL and PCFCL, both cutaneous relapses and development of extracutaneous disease are common, and the 5-year overall survival is decreased to 50%. A very small subset of PCLBCL (such as intravascular PCLBCL or anaplastic or plasmablastic PCLBCL) is categorized as "PCLBCL, other."[1]

TABLE 79.7 CUTANEOUS B-CELL LYMPHOMA PROGNOSTIC INDEX

CBCL-PI Group[93]	Histology	Site	% 5-Year OS	% Relative 5-Year OS
IA	Any indolent	Any	81	94
IB	Diffuse large B cell	Favorable	72	96
II	Diffuse large B cell	Unfavorable	48	60
	Immunoblastic diffuse large B cell	Favorable		
III	Immunoblastic diffuse large B cell	Unfavorable	27	34

CBCL-PI, cutaneous B-cell lymphoma prognostic index; OS, overall survival.

Diagnosis and Evaluation

Evaluation of patients with suspected PCBCL should follow the basic protocol recommended by ISCL/USCLC/EORTC previously discussed.[13] In addition, a bone marrow biopsy is needed for PCBCL-LT and should be strongly considered in PCFCL (rate of bone marrow involvement may be as high as 11%). In other cases the need for bone marrow biopsy is left to the discretion of the treating physician. A further component to evaluation of PCBCL in European nations includes evaluation for *Borrelia burgdorferi* infection.[1,91] The *Borrelia* subspecies *B. afzelii* that appears to be the causative organism is not found in the United States.[92]

Staging and Prognosis

PCBCLs should be staged in accordance with the ISCL/EORTC staging system for non-MF/SS cutaneous lymphomas (Table 79.6). A cutaneous B-cell lymphoma prognostic index (CBCL-PI) was developed by correlating outcome data from the Surveillance, Epidemiology, and End Results (SEER) database with PCBCL histology and anatomic location (Table 79.7).[93] Four prognostic groups (IA, IB, II, III) were defined by the CBCL-PI based on specific combinations of histology and anatomic location. However, as described earlier, the histologic criteria in use during the years on which the CBCL-PI is based (1973–2001) were changed with the 2005 release of the WHO/EORTC consensus classification system,[1] and the CBCL-PI should be used with caution when modern histopathologic classification criteria are used.

In 2011, the International Extranodal Lymphoma Study Group (IELSG) released the cutaneous lymphoma international prognostic index (CLIPI) for indolent CBCL. Independent prognostic factors associated with progression-free survival included serum LDH, morphology (nodule vs. other), and number of distinct cutaneous sites of disease (greater than two). One point is scored for each factor, and patients are grouped into low risk (score 0), intermediate risk (score 1), and high risk (score 2 or 3) with associated 5-year progression-free survival rates of 91%, 64%, and 48%, respectively.[94] The clinical utility of this prognostic system in determining risk-adapted therapy remains unclear.

Treatment

No prospective randomized clinical trial data are available to help guide treatment decisions, but the ISCL/EORTC recently performed an extensive survey of the literature pertaining to treatment of the PCBCLs and published consensus recommendations.[95] The NCCN has also published treatment guidelines for PCBCLs.[96]

PCMZL and PCFCL

PCMZL and PCFCL are not expected to be associated with decreased survival relative to control populations (although PCFCL arising in the leg may have a worsened prognosis under the WHO/EORTC classification), and therefore side effects of proposed treatments should be carefully considered. Treatment options include local superficial irradiation, surgical excision, intralesional IFN-α, local and systemic rituximab, antibiotics (where *B. burgdorferi* is endemic), and chemotherapy.

Local Superficial Irradiation. In the ISCL/EORTC literature review, 132 patients with PCMZL treated with local superficial irradiation were identified, and a 99% complete response rate was observed. Doses ranged from 30 to 45 Gy, and field margins ranged from 1 to 5 cm. Although cutaneous relapse of disease occurred in 46% of patients, extracutaneous progression occurred in only 2% of patients. For PCFCL, 460 patients treated with radiation were reviewed, and the complete response rate was 99% with a 30% relapse rate. Doses ranged from 20 to 54 Gy and margins were 0.5 to 5+ cm. Recently, local superficial irradiation to 4 Gy in two fractions was shown to yield a 72% complete response rate for PCMZL and PCFCL and is recommended as a palliative dose.[25,95]

Surgery. Excision is associated with a 99% CR rate and 43% cutaneous relapse rate in PCMZL and a 98% CR rate and 40% cutaneous relapse rate in PCFCL.[95]

IFN-α. Intralesional IFN-α yields a 100% CR rate and 25% local relapse rate for PCMZL and a 100% CR rate and 29% local relapse rate for PCFCL.[95]

Rituximab. Systemic rituximab (monoclonal antibody targeted against CD20) has proven effective as a treatment for non-Hodgkin lymphomas and has been applied to the treatment of PCBCL. In a review of five patients with PCMZL treated with systemic rituximab, the overall response rate was 60%, and in 10 patients with PCFCL treated with systemic rituximab a 100% overall response rate and 80% complete response rate was observed. Intralesional rituximab may also be effective, with a reported complete response rate of 89% in nine patients with PCMZL, but with a high relapse rate of 62%. Twelve patients with PCFCL treated with intralesional rituximab had a complete response rate of 83% with 40% relapse.[97]

Chemotherapy. Single-agent treatment with chlorambucil was evaluated in 14 patients with PCMZL, and a complete response rate of 64% with 33% relapse rate was observed. Multiagent chemotherapy with cyclophosphamide, doxorubicin, vincristine, and prednisone (CHOP) was also evaluated in 33 patients with PCMZL, and an 85% complete response rate with 57% relapse rate was observed. In 104 patients with PCFCL treated with CHOP or CHOP-like regimens, an 85% complete response rate with 48% relapse rate was reported.[95]

ISCL/EORTC Recommendations. For patients who have only one or a few lesions clustered in one region, radiation (30 Gy or more) using a margin of 1 to 1.5 cm is highly effective. Patients presenting with a single small lesion may be treated with resection alone. Scattered lesions that cannot easily be encompassed in one or a few radiation fields may be carefully observed, with treatment reserved for only the most concerning or symptomatic sites. In the setting of diffuse disease, systemic rituximab should be considered. Of note, cutaneous relapses are common, and relapsed disease often responds to retreatment and does not predict for worsened overall survival rate.[95]

PCLBCL, Leg Type (PCBCL-LT)

PCLBCL-LT is a significantly more aggressive entity in comparison to PCMZL and PCFCL. The primary treatment options that are used in therapy for PCBCL-LT are radiation, rituximab, and multiagent chemotherapy.

Local Superficial Irradiation. The ISCL/EORTC literature review found 101 patients with PCLBCL-LT treated with radiation. In contrast to the more indolent lymphomas in which CR rates were close to 100%, the CR rate for PCLBCL-LT was lower at 88%. The rate of cutaneous relapse rate was high

(58%), and even more concerning, 30% of patients were found to have extracutaneous progression of disease.

Rituximab. Systemic rituximab in PCLBCL-LT has been investigated (dose 375 mg/m^2 weekly for 4 to 8 weeks) and yielded a CR rate of 38%. Relapse rates are as yet unknown, and additional follow-up is necessary.[95]

Chemotherapy. Multiagent chemotherapy regimens have been tested in PCLBCL-LT, and in 32 patients treated with CHOP or CHOP-like regimens, an 81% complete response rate has been observed. However, despite aggressive therapy, relapse rates remain high at 54%.[95]

ISCL/EORTC Recommendations. Based on the aggressive nature of PCLBCL-LT and its propensity to develop extracutaneous disease, recommended treatment in patients able to tolerate multiagent chemotherapy is R-CHOP, with the possible addition of local superficial radiation to distinct cutaneous lesions. In the subset of patients unable to tolerate a multiagent course of chemotherapy, systemic rituximab may be considered. Alternatively, an aggressive course of radiation to all cutaneous sites of disease may be considered, but relapse is expected.[95]

PRECURSOR HEMATOLOGIC NEOPLASMS

The third category of cutaneous lymphomas in the WHO/EORTC system is precursor hematologic neoplasms/immature hematologic malignancies. At present this category primarily references CD4+/CD56+ hematodermic neoplasm (also referred to as blastic NK-cell lymphoma or blastic plasmacytoid dendritic cell neoplasm), which is characterized by development of red or violaceous cutaneous nodules. Biopsy reveals cutaneous infiltration of abnormal cells with an appearance reminiscent of lymphoblasts and myeloblasts. The origin of the tumor cells in CD4+/CD56+ hematodermic neoplasm is unclear. Immunohistochemistry indicates that the tumor cells lack CD3 and CD8 and express both CD4 and CD56. The expression of CD56 initially led investigators to believe these cells were of NK origin. However, the concomitant expression of CD4 and CD56 is unusual, and further exploration led to the identification of expression of CD123 and TCL1 in these tumor cells, which suggests a possible origin in plasmacytoid dendritic cells. Examination of TCR status in these cells indicates it remains in germline configuration, providing further support for the notion that these cells are not derived from a B- or T-cell lineage. CD4+/CD56+ hematodermic neoplasm is an aggressive malignancy, and it is common for patients to harbor nodal or systemic disease at diagnosis. Due to the propensity for systemic spread of disease, skin-directed therapies are usually unlikely to control disease and chemotherapy is often necessary. Although chemotherapy may induce remission of disease, the duration of remission is typically relatively brief and median survival is only 14 months.[1]

SUMMARY

The primary cutaneous lymphomas are a diverse group of extranodal non-Hodgkin lymphomas, each with distinct biologic activity. A correct histopathologic diagnosis is therefore critical to the determination of appropriate management. Although significant advances in therapy have been made since the recognition of MF in 1806, numerous questions remain unanswered regarding the pathophysiology and optimal treatment of the cutaneous lymphomas. Recent efforts to develop uniform criteria for classification of disease and response to treatment should facilitate international collaborations. Due to the rarity of these diseases, such international collaborations are critical to the advancement of our understanding of the primary cutaneous lymphomas.

REFERENCES

1. Willemze R, Jaffe ES, Burg G, et al. WHO-EORTC classification for cutaneous lymphomas. *Blood* 2005;105:3768–3785.
2. *WHO classification of tumours of haematopoeitic and lymphoid tissues,* 4th ed. Lyon, France: IARC, 2008.
3. Bradford PT, Devesa SS, Anderson WS, et al. Cutaneous lymphoma incidence patterns in the United States: a population-based study of 3884 cases. *Blood* 2009;113(21):5064–5073.
4. Assaf C, Gellrich S, Steinhoff M, et al. Cutaneous lymphomas in Germany: an analysis of the Central Cutaneous Lymphoma Registry of the German Society of Dermatology (DDG). *J Dtsch Dermatol Ges* 2007;5(8):662–668.
5. Girardi M, Heald PW, Wilson LD. The pathogenesis of mycosis fungoides. *N Engl J Med* 2004;350:1978–1988.
6. Olsen EA, Whittaker S, Kim YH, et al. Clinical end points and response criteria in mycosis fungoides and Sezary syndrome: a consensus statement of the International Society for Cutaneous Lymphomas, the United States Cutaneous Lymphoma Consortium, and the Cutaneous Lymphoma Task Force of the European Organisation for Research and Treatment of Cancer. *J Clin Oncol* 2011; 29(18):2598–2607.
7. Kim YH, Liu HL, Mraz-Gernhard S, et al. Long-term outcome of 525 patients with mycosis fungoides and Sezary syndrome. *Arch Dermatol* 2003;139:857–866.
8. Salgado R, Servitje O, Gallardo F, et al. Oligonucleotide array-CGH identifies genomic subgroups and prognostic markers for tumor stage mycosis fungoides. *J Invest Dermatol* 2010;130(4):1126–1135.
9. Van Doorn R, van Kester MS, Dijkman R, et al. Oncogenomic analysis of mycosis fungoides reveals major differences with Sezary syndrome. *Blood* 2009;113(1): 127–136.
10. Ballabio E, Mitchell T, van Kester MS, et al. MicroRNA expression in Sezary syndrome: identification, function, and diagnostic potential. *Blood* 2010;116(7): 1105–1113.
11. van Kester MS, Ballabio E, Benner MF, et al. miRNA expression profiling of mycosis fungoides. *Mol Oncol* 2011;5(3):273–280.
12. Pimpinelli N, Olsen EA, Santucci M, et al. Defining early mycosis fungoides. *J Am Acad Dermatol* 2005;53(6):1053–1063.
13. Olsen E, Vonderheid E, Pimpinelli N, et al. Revisions to the staging and classification of mycosis fungoides and Sezary syndrome: a proposal of the International Society for Cutaneous Lymphomas (ISCL) and the Cutaneous Lymphoma Task Force of the European Organization of Research and Treatment of Cancer (EORTC). *Blood* 2007;110(6):1713–1722.
14. Tsai EY, Taur A, Espinosa L, et al. Staging accuracy in mycosis fungoides and Sezary syndrome using integrated positron emission tomography and computed tomography. *Arch Dermatol* 2006;142(5):577–584.
15. Agar NS, Wedgeworth E, Crichton S, et al. Survival outcomes and prognostic factors in mycosis fungoides/Sezary syndrome: validation of the revised International Society for Cutaneous Lymphomas/European Organisation for Research and Treatment of Cancer staging proposal. *J Clin Oncol* 2010;28: 4730–4739.
16. Zackheim HS, Kashani-Sabet M, Amin S. Topical corticosteroids for mycosis fungoides. Experience in 79 patients. *Arch Dermatol* 1998;134(8):949–954.
17. Kim YH. Management with topical nitrogen mustard in mycosis fungoides. *Dermatol Ther* 2003;16:288–298.
18. Zackheim HS. Topical carmustine (BCNU) in the treatment of mycosis fungoides. *Dermatol Ther* 2003;16(4):299–302.
19. Breneman D, Duvic M, Kuzel T, et al. Phase 1 and 2 trial of bexarotene gel for skin-directed treatment of patients with cutaneous T-cell lymphoma. *Arch Dermatol* 2002;138(3):325–332.
20. Gathers RC, Scherschun L, Malick F, et al. Narrowband UVB phototherapy for early-stage mycosis fungoides. *J Am Acad Dermatol* 2002;47(2):191–197.
21. Hermann JJ, Roenigk HH Jr, Hurria A, et al. Treatment of mycosis fungoides with photochemotherapy (PUVA): long-term follow-up. *J Am Acad Dermatol* 1995;33(2 Pt 1):234–242.
22. Wilson LD, Kacinski BM, Jones GW. Local superficial radiotherapy in the management of minimal stage IA cutaneous T-cell lymphoma (mycosis fungoides). *Int J Radiat Oncol Biol Phys* 1998;40(1):109–115.
23. Jones GW, Kacinski BM, Wilson LD, et al. Total skin electron radiation in the management of mycosis fungoides: consensus of the European Organization for Research and Treatment of Cancer (EORTC) Cutaneous Lymphoma Project Group. *J Am Acad Dermatol* 2002;47(3):364–370.
24. Cotter GW, Baglan RJ, Wasserman TH, et al. Palliative radiation treatment of cutaneous mycosis fungoides–a dose response. *Int J Radiat Oncol Biol Phys* 1983; 9(10):1477–1480.
25. Neelis KJ, Schimmel EC, Vermeer MH, et al. Low dose palliative radiotherapy for cutaneous B- and T-cell lymphomas. *Int J Radiat Oncol Biol Phys* 2009;74(1): 154–158.
26. Chen Z, Agostinelli AG, Wilson LD, et al. Matching the dosimetry characteristics of a dual-field Stanford technique to a customized single-field Stanford technique for total skin electron therapy. *Int J Radiat Oncol Biol Phys* 2004;59(3):872–885.
27. Hoppe RT, Fuks Z, Bagshaw MA. Radiation therapy in the management of cutaneous T-cell lymphomas. *Cancer Treat Rep* 1979;63:625–632.
28. Kim JH, Nisce LZ, D'Anglo GJ. Dose-time fractionation study in patients with mycosis fungoides and lymphoma cutis. *Radiology* 1976;119(2):439–442.
29. Hoppe RT, Fuks Z, Bagshaw MA. The rationale for curative radiotherapy in mycosis fungoides. *Int J Radiat Oncol Biol Phys* 1977;2:843–851.
30. Harrison C, Young J, Navi D, et al. Revisiting low dose total skin electron beam therapy in mycosis fungoides. *Int J Radiat Oncol Biol Phys* 2011;81(4):e651–e657.
31. Yu JB, Khan AM, Jones AW, et al. Patient perspectives regarding the value of total skin electron beam therapy for cutaneous T-cell lymphoma/mycosis fungoides: a pilot study. *Am J Clin Oncol* 2009;32(2):142–144.
32. Price NM. Electron beam therapy. Its effect on eccrine gland function in mycosis fungoides patients. *Arch Dermatol* 1979;115:1068–1070.
33. Price NM. Radiation dermatitis following electron beam therapy. An evaluation of patients ten years after total skin irradiation for mycosis fungoides. *Arch Dermatol* 1978;114:63–66.
34. Licata AG, Wilson LD, Braverman IM, et al. Malignant melanoma and other second cutaneous malignancies in cutaneous T-cell lymphoma. The influence of additional therapy after total skin electron beam radiation. *Arch Dermatol* 1995;131:432–435.

35. Desai KR, Pezner RD, Lipsett JA, et al. Total skin electron irradiation for mycosis fungoides. Relationship between acute toxicities and measured dose at different anatomic sites. *Int J Radiat Oncol Biol Phys* 1988;15:641–645.
36. Jones GW, Hoppe RT, Glatstein E, et al. Electron beam treatment for cutaneous T-cell lymphoma. *Hematol Oncol Clin North Am* 1995;9:1057–1076.
37. Kim YH, Jensen RA, Watanabe GL, et al. Clinical stage IA (limited patch and plaque) mycosis fungoides. A long-term outcome analysis. *Arch Dermatol* 1996; 132:1309–1313.
38. Jones G, Wilson LD, Fox-Goguen L. Total skin electron beam radiotherapy for patients who have mycosis fungoides. *Hematol Oncol Clin North Am* 2003;17: 1421–1434.
39. Quiros PA, Jones GW, Kacinski BM, et al. Total skin electron beam therapy followed by adjuvant psoralen/ultraviolet-A light in the management of patients with T1 and T2 cutaneous T-cell lymphoma (mycosis fungoides). *Int J Radiat Oncol Biol Phys* 1997;38:1027–1035.
40. Chinn DM, Chow S, Kim YH, et al. Total skin electron beam therapy with or without adjuvant topical nitrogen mustard or nitrogen mustard alone as initial treatment of T2 and T3 mycosis fungoides. *Int J Radiat Oncol Biol Phys* 1999;43: 951–958.
41. Wilson LD, Licata AL, Braverman IM, et al. Systemic chemotherapy and extracorporeal photochemotherapy for T3 and T4 cutaneous T-cell lymphoma patients who have achieved a complete response to total skin electron beam therapy. *Int J Radiat Oncol Biol Phys* 1995;32:987–995.
42. Jones GW, Rosenthal D, Wilson LD. Total skin electron radiation for patients with erythrodermic cutaneous T-cell lymphoma (mycosis fungoides and the Sezary syndrome). *Cancer* 1999;85:1985–1995.
43. Wilson LD, Jones GW, Kim D, et al. Experience with total skin electron beam therapy in combination with extracorporeal photopheresis in the management of patients with erythrodermic (T4) mycosis fungoides. *J Am Acad Dermatol* 2000;43:54–60.
44. Introcaso CE, Micaily B, Richardson SK, et al. Total skin electron beam therapy may be associated with improvement of peripheral blood disease in Sezary syndrome. *J Am Acad Dermatol* 2008;58:592–595.
45. Hansen JE, Wilson LD, Carlson K, et al. Addition of TSEBT to ECP reduces circulating malignant cells in leukemic cutaneous T-cell lymphoma. *Int J Radiat Oncol Biol Phys* 2009;75(3 Suppl):S480–S481.
46. Wilson LD, Quiros PA, Kolenik SA, et al. Additional courses of total skin electron beam therapy in the treatment of patients with recurrent cutaneous T-cell lymphoma. *J Am Acad Dermatol* 1996;35:69–73.
47. Becker M, Hoppe RT, Knox SJ. Multiple courses of high-dose total skin electron beam therapy in the management of mycosis fungoides. *Int J Radiat Oncol Biol Phys* 1995;32:1445–1449.
48. Duvic M, Martin AG, Kim Y, et al. Phase 2 and 3 clinical trial of oral bexarotene (Targretin capsules) for the treatment of refractory or persistent early-stage cutaneous T-cell lymphoma. *Arch Dermatol* 2001;137(5):581–593.
49. Duvic M, Hymes K, Heald P, et al. Bexarotene is effective and safe for treatment of refractory advanced- stage cutaneous T-cell lymphoma. Multinational phase II-III trial results. *J Clin Oncol* 2001;19:2456–2471.
50. Olsen E, Duvic M, Frankel A, et al. Pivotal phase III trial of two dose levels of denileukin diftitox for the treatment of cutaneous T-cell lymphoma. *J Clin Oncol* 2001;19:376–388.
51. Olsen EA, Kim YH, Kuzel TM, et al. Phase IIb multicenter trial of vorinostat in patients with persistent, progressive, or treatment refractory cutaneous T-cell lymphoma. *J Clin Oncol* 2007;25:3109–3115.
52. Whittaker SJ, Demierre MF, Kim EJ, et al. Final results from a multicenter, international, pivotal study of romidepsin in refractory cutaneous T-cell lymphoma. *J Clin Oncol* 2010;28(29):4485–4491.
53. Kennedy GA, Seymour JF, Wolf M, et al. Treatment of patients with advanced mycosis fungoides and Sézary syndrome with alemtuzumab. *Eur J Haematol* 2003; 71(4):250–256.
54. Bernengo MG, Martin AG, Kim Y, et al. Low-dose intermittent alemtuzumab in the treatment of Sézary syndrome: clinical and immunologic findings in 14 patients. *Haematologica* 2007;92(6):784–794.
55. Ross C, Tingsgaard P, Jorgensen H, et al. Interferon treatment of cutaneous T-cell lymphoma. *Eur J Haematol* 1993;51:63–72.
56. Jumbou O, N'Guyen JM, Tessier MH, et al. Long-term follow-up in 51 patients with mycosis fungoides and Sezary syndrome treated by interferon-alpha. *Br J Dermatol* 1999;140:427–431.
57. Roenigk HH Jr, Kuzel TM, Skoutelis AP, et al. Photochemotherapy alone or combined with interferon alpha-2a in the treatment of cutaneous T-cell lymphoma. *J Invest Dermatol* 1990;95:198S–205S.
58. Kuzel TM, Roenigk HH Jr, Samuelson E, et al. Effectiveness of interferon-alpha-2a combined with phototherapy for mycosis fungoides and the Sezary syndrome. *J Clin Oncol* 1995;13:257–263.
59. Chiarion-Sileni V, Bononi A, Fornasa CV, et al. Phase II trial of interferon-alpha-2a plus psolaren with ultraviolet light A in patients with cutaneous T-cell lymphoma. *Cancer* 2002;95:569–575.
60. Wollina U, Looks A, Meyer J, et al. Treatment of stage II cutaneous T-cell lymphoma with interferon alfa-2a and extracorporeal photochemotherapy: a prospective controlled trial. *J Am Acad Dermatol* 2001;44:253–260.
61. Stadler R, Otte HG, Luger T, et al. Prospective randomized multicenter clinical trial on the use of interferon -2a plus acitretin versus interferon-2a plus PUVA in patients with cutaneous T-cell lymphoma stages I and II. *Blood* 1998;92: 3578–3581.
62. Lim HW, Edelson RL. Photopheresis for the treatment of cutaneous T-cell lymphoma. *Hematol Oncol Clin North Am* 1995;9:1117–1126.
63. Koizumi K, Sawada K, Nishio M, et al. Effective high-dose chemotherapy followed by autologous peripheral blood stem cell transplantation in a patient with the aggressive form of cytophagic histiocytic panniculitis. *Bone Marrow Transplant* 1997; 20:171.
64. Foss FM, Ihde DC, Breneman DL, et al. Phase II study of pentostatin and intermittent high-dose recombinant interferon alfa-2a in advanced mycosis fungoides/Sezary syndrome. *J Clin Oncol* 1992;10:1907.
65. Foss FM, Ihde DC, Linnoila IR, et al. Phase II trial of fludarabine phosphate and interferon alfa-2a in advanced mycosis fungoides/Sezary syndrome. *J Clin Oncol* 1994;12:2051.
66. Duvic M, Talpur R, Wen S, et al. Phase II evaluation of gemcitabine monotherapy for cutaneous T-cell lymphoma. *Clin Lymphoma Myeloma* 2006;7:51.
67. Duvic M, Forero-Torres A, Foss F, et al. Oral forodesine is clinically active in refractory cutaneous T-cell lymphoma: results of a phase I/II Study. *Blood* 2006;108: 2467.
68. Wollina U, Dummer R, Brockmeyer NH, et al. Multicenter study of pegylated liposomal doxorubicin in patients with cutaneous T-cell lymphoma. *Cancer* 2003; 98(5):993–1001.
69. Foss FM. Evaluation of the pharmacokinetics, preclinical and clinical efficacy of pralatrexate for the treatment of T-cell lymphoma. *Expert Opin Drug Metab Toxicol* 2011;7(9):1141–1152.
70. Molina A, Zain J, Arber DA, et al. Durable clinical, cytogenetic, and molecular remissions after allogeneic hematopoietic cell transplantation for refractory Sezary syndrome and mycosis fungoides. *J Clin Oncol* 2005;23:6163.
71. Prince HM, Whittaker S, Hoppe RT. How I treat mycosis fungoides and Sezary syndrome. *Blood* 2009;114(20):4337–4353.
72. Wu PA, Kim YH, Lavori PW, et al. A meta-analysis of patients receiving allogeneic or autologous hematopoietic stem cell transplant in mycosis fungoides and Sézary syndrome. *Biol Blood Marrow Transplant* 2009;15(8):982–990.
73. Jacobsen ED, Kim HT, Ho VT, et al. A large single-center experience with allogeneic stem cell transplantation for peripheral T-cell non-Hodgkin lymphoma and advanced mycosis fungoides/Sezary syndrome. *Ann Oncol* 2011;22(7):1608–1613.
74. Duvic M, Donato M, Dabaja B, et al. Total skin electron beam and non-myeloablative allogeneic hematopoietic stem-cell transplantation in advanced mycosis fungoides and Sezary syndrome. *J Clin Oncol* 2010;28(14):2365–2372.
75. National Comprehensive Cancer Network Guidelines Version 4.2011, Mycosis fungoides/Sezary syndrome.
76. Gerami P, Rosen S, Kuzel T, et al. Folliculotropic mycosis fungoides: an aggressive variant of cutaneous T-cell lymphoma. *Arch Dermatol* 2008;144(6):738–746.
77. Lee J, Viakhireva N, Cesca C, et al. Clinicopathologic features and treatment outcomes in Woringer-Kolopp disease. *J Am Acad Dermatol* 2008;59(4):706–712.
78. Kempf W, Ostheeren-Michaelis S, Paulli M, et al. Granulomatous mycosis fungoides and granulomatous slack skin: a multicenter study of the Cutaneous Lymphoma Histopathology Task Force Group of the European Organization For Research and Treatment of Cancer (EORTC). *Arch Dermatol* 2008;144(12):1609–1617.
79. Neuhaus IM, Ramos-Caro FA, Hassanein AM. Hypopigmented mycosis fungoides in childhood and adolescence. *Pediatr Dermatol* 2000;17(5):403–406.
80. El-Shabrawi-Caelen L, Cerroni L, Medeiros LJ, et al. Hypopigmented mycosis fungoides: frequent expression of a CD8+ T-cell phenotype. *Am J Surg Pathol* 2002;26(4):450–457.
81. Kim YH, Willemze R, Pimpinelli N, et al. TNM classification system for primary cutaneous lymphomas other than mycosis fungoides and Sezary syndrome: a proposal of the International Society for Cutaneous Lymphomas (ISCL) and the Cutaneous Lymphoma Task Force of the European Organization of Research and Treatment of Cancer (EORTC). *Blood* 2007;110(2):479–484.
82. Yu JB, Blitzblau RC, Decker RH, et al. Analysis of primary CD30+ cutaneous lymphoproliferative disease and survival from the Surveillance, Epidemiology, and End Results database. *J Clin Oncol* 2008;26(9):1483–1488.
83. Kempf W, Pfaltz K, Vermeer MH, et al. European Organization for Research and Treatment of Cancer (EORTC), International Society of Cutaneous Lymphoma (ISCL) and United States Cutaneous Lymphoma Consortium (USCLC) consensus recommendations for the treatment of primary cutaneous CD30-positive lymphoproliferative disorders: lymphomatoid papulosis and primary cutaneous anaplastic large-cell lymphoma. *Blood* 2011;118(15):4024–4035.
84. Woo DK, Jones CR, Vanoli-Storz MN, et al. Prognostic factors in primary cutaneous anaplastic large cell lymphoma: characterization of clinical subset with worse outcome. *Arch Dermatol* 2009;145(6):667–674.
85. Yu JB, McNiff JM, Lund MW, et al. Treatment of primary cutaneous CD30+ anaplastic large-cell lymphoma with radiation therapy. *Int J Radiat Oncol Biol Phys* 2008;70(5):1542–1545.
86. Liu HL, Hoppe RT, Kohler S, et al. CD30+ cutaneous lymphoproliferative disorders. The Stanford experience in lymphomatoid papulosis and primary cutaneous anaplastic large cell lymphoma. *J Am Acad Dermatol* 2003;49:1049–1058.
87. Li YX, Wang H, Jin J, et al. Radiotherapy alone with curative intent in patients with stage I extranodal nasal-type NK/T-cell lymphoma. *Int J Radiat Oncol Biol Phys* 2012;82(5):1809–1815.
88. Jaccard A, Hermine O. Extranodal/natural killer T-cell lymphoma: advances in the management. *Curr Opin Oncol* 2011;23(5):429–435.
89. Mraz-Gernhard S, Natkunam Y, Hoppe RT, et al. Natural killer/natural killer-like T-cell lymphoma, CD56+, presenting in the skin: an increasingly recognized entity with an aggressive course. *J Clin Oncol* 2001;19:2179–2188.
90. Senff NJ, Hoefnagel JJ, Jansen PM, et al. Reclassification of 300 primary cutaneous B-cell lymphomas according to the new WHO-EORTC classification for cutaneous lymphomas: comparison with previous classifications and identification of prognostic markers. *J Clin Oncol* 2007;25(12):1581–1587.
91. Kutting B, Bonsmann G, Metze D, et al. Borrelia burgdorferi-associated primary cutaneous B cell lymphoma: complete clearing of skin lesions after antibiotic pulse therapy or intralesional injection of interferon alpha-2a. *J Am Acad Dermatol* 1997;36(2 Pt 2):311–314.
92. Aberer E, Fingerle V, Wutte N, et al. Within European margins. *Lancet* 2011; 377(9760):178.
93. Smith BD, Smith GL, Cooper DL, et al. The cutaneous B-cell lymphoma prognostic index: a novel prognostic index derived from a population-based registry. *J Clin Oncol* 2005;23(15):3390–3395.
94. Mian M, Marcheselli L, Luminari S, et al. CLIPI: a new prognostic index for indolent cutaneous B cell lymphoma proposed by the International Extranodal Lymphoma Study Group (IELSG 11). *Ann Hematol* 2011;90(4):401–408.
95. Senff NJ, Noordijk EM, Kim YH, et al. European Organization for Research and Treatment of Cancer and International Society for Cutaneous Lymphoma consensus recommendations for the management of cutaneous B-cell lymphomas. *Blood* 2008;112(5):1600–1609.
96. National Comprehensive Cancer Network Guidelines Version 4.2011, Primary cutaneous B-cell lymphoma.
97. Morales AV, Advani R, Horwitz SM, et al. Indolent primary cutaneous B-cell lymphoma: experience using systemic rituximab. *J Am Acad Dermatol* 2008; 59(6):953–957.

Chapter 80
Leukemia

Kenneth B. Roberts, Stuart Seropian, and Peter W. Marks

The leukemias are a group of neoplastic disorders of the hematopoietic system, characterized by aberrant or arrested differentiation. The role of radiotherapy (RT) in conventional curative treatment is largely to deliver central nervous system (CNS) treatment in combination with systemic therapy for patients with acute lymphocytic leukemia (ALL). While the role of CNS prophylaxis has declined over the last 15 years because of toxicity concerns, it remains an important component of therapy for high-risk patients. Radiation oncologists must also be familiar with certain palliative situations unique to the leukemias as well as total body irradiation (discussed elsewhere), as the latter is often part of a stem cell transplant program.

Childhood ALL can now be cured in 80% to 89% of cases, with initial remissions generally occurring in about 90%.[1–3] In adults, initial remission rates are generally equally high, but cure rates are only in the 30% to 45% range.[4] In contrast to the situation in pediatric ALL, pediatric acute myeloid leukemia (AML) generally fairs less well, with 60% cure rates, although this represents a marked improvement since the 1970s when cure rates were roughly 20%.[2] Adult AML cures are less frequent in the overall population, in large part a reflection that this disease principally afflicts older individuals. In the United States, the estimated annual incidence and mortality from AML are 12,330 cases and 8,950 deaths.[2] Allogeneic stem cell transplantation has specifically targeted refractory/recurrent ALL and AML. Reduced-intensity transplants are being investigated to address the needs of high-risk or elderly patients with acute leukemia.

Chronic myelogenous leukemia (CML) and chronic lymphocytic leukemia (CLL) are primarily diseases of adults and have natural histories measured in years to decades. Both have the ability to transform to more aggressive diseases, though CML, in particular, reliably progresses to a more acute disease or blast crisis in its terminal phase. Allogeneic stem cell transplantation is associated with a high cure rate for patients with CML if conducted early in the chronic phase of the disease. However, due to the widespread use of the ABL tyrosine kinase inhibitors, the use of allogenic transplant for CML has declined dramatically over the past decade.[5]

ANATOMIC CONSIDERATIONS

The radiation oncologist must be knowledgeable about the anatomy of the CNS, particularly the meninges (dura mater, arachnoid, and pia mater) and subarachnoid space for the proper design of CNS-directed radiation treatments. The epidural space lies between periosteum and the dura, whereas the potential space between the dura and arachnoid is called the *subdural space*. The pia and arachnoid are often described as a combined membrane called the *leptomeninges*. Between the arachnoid and pia is the subarachnoid space, which is filled with cerebrospinal fluid (CSF). The pia hugs the surface of the brain extending into sulci, fissures, and the internal cavities or ventricles while the bulk of the arachnoid follows along the dura except for the fine trabeculations and into some of the major fissures of the brain. Arachnoid sheathes both nerves and blood vessels penetrating the pia and exiting the CNS, creating relatively short segments of subarachnoid space, which is of particular anatomical importance in the vertebral column.

In the design of the inferior aspect of craniospinal radiation fields, the subarachnoid space extends laterally to the spinal ganglia, which are located within the intervertebral foramina.[6,7] Thus, coverage of the entire sacroiliac joints in such spinal field design is excessive. The caudad extent of the subarachnoid space is variable within the sacrum.[8] Clinically, the end of the thecal sac is now routinely determined on magnetic resonance image scanning. Pathologically, CNS leukemia originates as a perivascular infiltrate along the subpial blood vessels. As this progresses, the leukemia infiltrates preferentially into the subarachnoid space as well as into the brain parenchyma.[9]

Base of skull anatomy is also of importance to the radiation oncologist in the design of lateral cranial fields. The middle cranial fossa and temporal lobe project over the sphenoid sinuses on lateral radiographs. The cribriform plate projects along the roof of the orbit along an imaginary line that connects to the inferior aspect of the frontal sinuses. Several radiologic-anatomic studies have pointed out how the eye's lens in this "beam's-eye view" is <1 cm away from the cribriform plate, having implications in field design. Insuring coverage of the entire subarachnoid space should supersede the concerns of radiation-induced cataracts.[10,11] Moreover, because subarachnoid space extends as a sheath along the optic nerve, it is standard to include the posterior half of the eye globes within cranial radiation fields by using the anterolateral aspect of the bony orbit as an anatomic landmark, as it typically lies along a line that roughly bisects the eye[11] (Figs. 80.1 and 80.2).

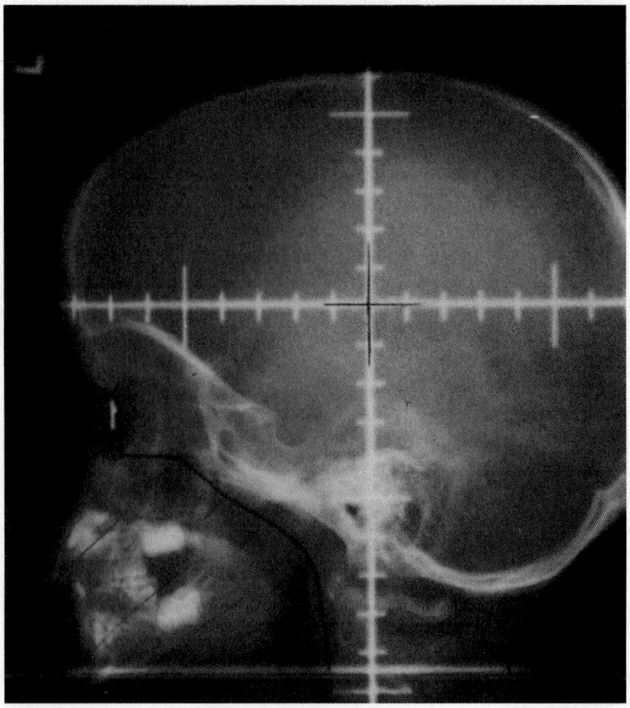

FIGURE 80.1. Cranial irradiation field outlining treatment that encompasses the entire cranial subarachnoid space. The radio-opaque markers outline the anterior aspect of the bony orbit so as to demarcate inclusion of the posterior aspect of the eye within the treatment fields.

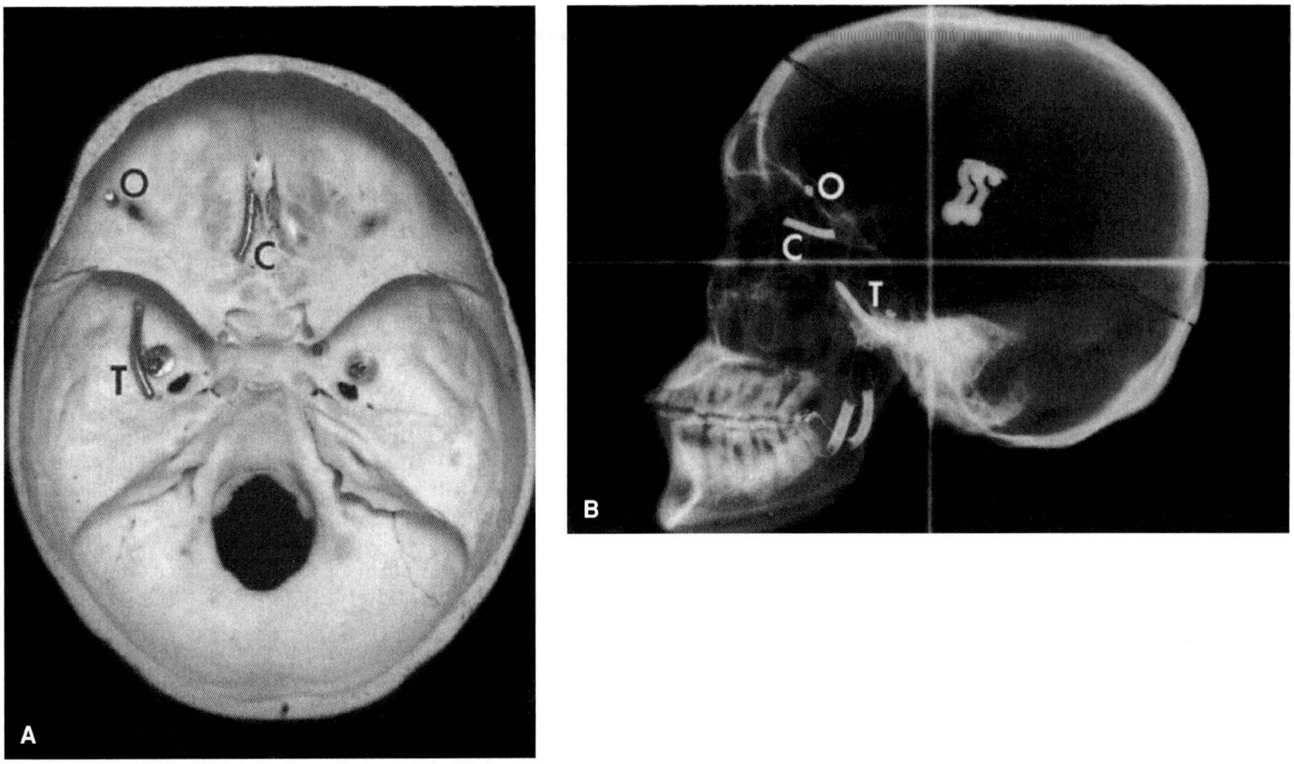

FIGURE 80.2. Skull views outlining anatomic limits of the base of skull for inclusion of the cranial subarachnoid space. **A:** Radio-opaque markers have been placed at the cribriform plate (C), roof of the orbit (O), and the temporal fossa (T). **B:** Plain lateral radiograph shows the projection of the cribriform plate, orbital roof, and temporal fossa.

To compensate for the blood–brain barrier, certain drugs are administered directly into the subarachnoid space either via lumbar puncture or via an intraventricular reservoir (e.g., an Ommaya reservoir). Intrathecal (IT) drugs distribute unevenly, however, throughout the subarachnoid space.[12,13] This is not surprising given the knowledge of brain anatomy and CSF circulation. CSF is mainly formed in the brain ventricles by the choroid plexuses, which are specialized capillary-rich tufted structures. This fluid then flows through the intraventricular foramina and the cerebral aqueduct of the midbrain into the fourth ventricle, from where it communicates with the rest of the subarachnoid space. CSF is resorbed principally in the dural sinuses via buttonlike projections called *arachnoid villi.* Thus, IT therapy theoretically undertreats the ventricular spaces and cerebral/cerebellar sulci as well as any gross disease extending into the brain substance. This concern has led to the concept of combining cranial RT with IT chemotherapy; the latter to cover the spinal subarachnoid space. Similarly, when craniospinal irradiation (CSI) is needed to treat a higher burden of CNS leukemia, IT therapy allows the spine to be treated to a lower dose than the brain.

ACUTE LEUKEMIAS

Classification Systems, Pathology, and Risk Stratification

Acute leukemias have traditionally been classified using the French-American-British (FAB) morphologic criteria. AML and its subtypes can most often be identified microscopically by the presence of Auer rods, staining for myeloperoxidase or monocyte-associated esterases, and other cytologic features of differentiation. Certain chromosome translocations are common to each AML subtype (Table 80.1). AML with minimal or no myeloid differentiation (M1 and M0 subtypes) can be confused with ALL but for flow cytometric identification of early myeloid antigens. The more differentiated AML subtypes M2-M6 are usually recognizable by morphology and cytochemistry.

The FAB assignment of subtypes is increasingly being replaced by the World Health Organization (WHO) classification scheme for myeloid neoplasms.[14] The WHO classification creates four key subgroups: AML with recurrent genetic abnormalities (including t(8;21), inv(16), t(15;17), t(9;11) among others), AML with myelodysplasia-related changes, therapy-related neoplasms, and AML not otherwise specified. The new subgroups are meant to highlight meaningful biologic and genetic differences between disease entities with differing prognoses and clinical behavior. In addition, in the WHO scheme, the number of blasts in the blood or bone marrow required to confirm a diagnosis of AML is 20%, instead of the 30% specified by the older FAB criteria.

The FAB classification for ALL specified three subtypes based on morphology, which is largely of historical interest. L1 is the predominant type in 85% of childhood ALL. It is characterized by small cells with scanty cytoplasm and inconspicuous nucleoli. L2 is common in ALL of adults and is identified morphologically by blasts that show prominent nucleoli, abundant cytoplasm,

TABLE 80.1 CORRELATION OF FRENCH-AMERICAN-BRITISH (FAB) CLASSIFICATION OF ACUTE MYELOGENOUS LEUKEMIA (AML) WITH COMMON CYTOGENETIC ABNORMALITIES

FAB Type	*Cytogenetic Finding*
M0, M1 (Undifferentiated AML)	trisomy 11, t(10;11)
M2 (Acute myeloid leukemia)	t(8;21)
M3 (Acute promyelocytic leukemia)	t(15;17), t(11;17), t(5;17)
M4Eo (Acute myelomonocytic leukemia with eosinophilia)	inv(16)
M5 (Acute monocytic leukemia)	t(11;23)
M6 (Acute erythroleukemia)	t(3;5)
M7 (Acute megakaryocytic leukemia)	t(3;3), t(3;12)

and more variability in size. L3 lymphoblasts are large cells with cytoplasmic basophilia and vacuolization, similar to Burkitt's lymphoma cells. The common ALL antigen (CALLA) is expressed in about 85% of ALL cases. At least with childhood ALL, this FAB system has not proved to be terribly useful with high interobserver variability and a lack of correlation with the more prognostically important immunologic and genetic features for ALL.[15] In the WHO classification, most of these entities, with the exception of Burkitt's, fall under the category of precursor lymphoid neoplasms. These are subcategorized into B-cell lymphoblastic leukemia/lymphoma, not otherwise specified; B-cell leukemia/lymphoma with recurrent genetic abnormalities; and T-lymphoblastic leukemia/lymphoma.[16]

As may be apparent from the above discussion of the transition from the FAB to the WHO criteria for categorization, immunophenotyping and molecular markers have become very important in the classification of leukemia. Flow cytometry using specific monoclonal antibodies can be used to assay for a panel of antigens, often known as *cluster of differentiation (CD) molecules,* that define leukocyte maturation. For instance, CD19 and cytoplasmic CD79a define B-cell lineage, whereas CD7 and CD3 define T-cell lineage. Myeloid cells are correlated with positivity for CD13, CD33, and cytoplasmic myeloperoxidase. With other markers defining different degrees of differentiation and maturation, ALL is now conventionally divided into T-cell and B-cell lineage. B-cell leukemia has four distinct subclasses: early pre-B, pre-B, transitional pre-B, and the more mature B-cell. The transitional pre-B subclass is relatively new and is associated with a relatively good prognosis in children.[17]

Cytogenetic or chromosomal abnormalities occur in up to 90% of ALL cases. Of these, roughly two-thirds are nonrandom, falling into distinct patterns. Some of these have distinct prognostic and therapeutic implications. Adult and childhood forms of ALL have distinctly different patterns of genetic abnormalities as well as immunophenotyping (Table 80.2). This may partially explain the poorer prognosis in older patients. For example, the Philadelphia chromosome or *bcr-abl* gene fusion/t(9;22) translocation in precursor B-cell ALL is associated with a poorer prognosis. It occurs in 4% of childhood ALL cases compared to about 25% in adults, but it now represents an important therapeutic target with the development of tyrosine kinase inhibitors. Abnormal DNA ploidy is extremely common, but two patterns seem to be clinically important. Hyperdiploidy with >51 chromosomes per cell (or DNA index >1.6) occurs in 25% of children with ALL. Although there is some association with favorable clinical factors (age >10 years and low presenting leukocyte counts), hyperdiploidy is an independent favorable factor; however, in adults with ALL, outcomes are poor even in presence of hyperdiploidy. In childhood ALL, trisomies 4, 10, and 17 are associated with a good prognosis. Similarly, *TEL/AML1* fusion gene expression (cryptic t(12;21) translocation, is a common translocation, occurring in 15% of pediatric ALL patients, in which an in utero event juxtaposes the *RUNX1* gene on chromosome 21 with the *ETV6* gene on chromosome 12. The resulting chimeric protein impairs normal hematopoietic differentiation, increasing the self-renewal capacity of early progenitor cells. Distinct poor molecular prognostic factors in pediatric ALL include not only the aforementioned Philadelphia chromosome but also MLL-AF4 or t(4;11), which primarily occurs in infants as well as hypodiploidy (<44 paired chromosomes).

The aforementioned laboratory assessment and clinical disease features have led to distinct risk stratification categories, at least as far as childhood ALL is concerned. Clinical prognostic features of B-cell leukemias have been commonly used to place patients into risk groups. Using the National Cancer Institute's (NCI) risk classification scheme, standard risk includes patients (two thirds of pediatric B-cell ALL patients) whose age at diagnosis is between 1 and 10 years as well as a presenting leukocyte count of <50,000/μL, in the absence of CNS involvement, was historically associated with an 80% 4-year disease-free survival.[18] High-risk patients—defined as a high white blood cell (WBC) count, age below 1 year or above 10 years, or CNS involvement at diagnosis—had a corresponding 65% 4-year disease-free survival. T-cell phenotype occurs in 12% to 15% of pediatric ALL cases and was once thought to convey a relatively poorer prognosis. This prejudice has been due to numerous unfavorable clinical correlations, including older age, male sex, elevated WBC count, extensive extramedullary disease including mediastinal and peripheral adenopathy or hepatosplenomegaly, and a higher tendency for relapse in the CNS and testes in males.[19] Current clinical practice is for T-cell leukemias to be treated on different protocols than B-lineage ALL. Nevertheless, when one factors out unfavorable clinical features, the prognostic difference between T- and B-cell ALL is difficult to discern. In regards to B-cell ALL, current protocols assign patients to low, standard, and high risk. Low-risk patients are operationally defined by standard risk features along with a rapid early response to induction chemotherapy.[20] Age is also an important prognostic factor. Apart from this, the intensity of the treatment program is of importance as shown by the fact that adolescents treated on pediatric leukemia regimens have had better outcomes than those treated on adult programs.[21]

The response to induction chemotherapy has also been proven to be an extremely important prognostic category. In pediatric ALL, the concept of minimal residual disease (MRD) detected by flow cytometry of postinduction peripheral blood or marrow aspirates has led to critical prognostic stratification. A contemporary analysis of MRD in a pediatric cooperative group trial showed that even up to 0.01% blasts from day 8 postinduction mononuclear peripheral blood cells conferred a poorer prognosis.[22] Moreover, day 29 and end of consolidation bone marrow MRD was able to further segregate unfavorable patient subgroups taking into account other prognostic factors such as *TEL/AML1,* trisomies 4 and 10, and NCI risk class. From the assessment of MRD, the concept of risk-adapted therapy has allowed for improved outcomes with the intensification of therapy in those patients who continue to have detectable lymphoblasts after initial chemotherapy.

Assessment of CNS involvement at diagnosis in acute leukemia is critical as to risk stratification, which is of course of particular importance to the radiation oncologist. Unfortunately, a traumatic lumbar puncture has been noted to be associated with a worse prognosis.[23] Regardless, CNS involvement has been unequivocally defined by a CSF leukocyte count of ≥5 WBC/μL along with either blast cells on cytospin or the presence of cranial nerve palsy. By convention, this is now classified as CNS-3. CNS-1 is defined as no blast cells on CSF

TABLE 80.2 FREQUENCY AND DISEASE CONTROL ASSOCIATED WITH IMMUNOPHENOTYPES AND CYTOGENETIC ABNORMALITIES AND SURVIVAL IN ACUTE LYMPHOBLASTIC LEUKEMIAIN CHILDREN (AGES 1–18) VERSUS ADULTS (AGES 18 AND OLDER)

	Frequency (%)		*5-Year Disease-Free Survival (%)*	
Pattern	*Children*	*Adults*	*Children*	*Adults*
Pre B cell	80–85	75–80	80	30–40
B cell	2	3–5	45–85	45–65
T cell	15	20 25	65 75	40 60
TEL/AML1 t(12;21)	20–25	1–3	90	rare
MLL/AF4 t(4;11)	2	5–7	20	20
BCR/ABL t(9;22)	5	25–30	20–40	<10
Hyperdiploid	25	5	80–90	10–40
Normal karyotype	9–37	30	70–87	40

Adapted from DeAngelo DJ. The treatment of adolescents and young adults with acute lymphoblastic leukemia. *Hematology* 2005;1:123–130.

cytology, whereas CNS-2 is <5 WBC/μL with blast cells present. Clinical data is conflicting as to the prognostic importance of CNS-2, reflecting the fact that CNS involvement is not simply a distinction of being present or absent, but that it has also been associated with improved control with more intensive systemic and IT therapies.[24,25] Patients with CNS-3 disease who have more intensive IT chemotherapy along with cranial radiation within the first year of therapy have similar event-free survival as CNS-2 patients. For patients in remission who undergo surveillance lumbar punctures, there is even controversy regarding the prognostic importance of finding low numbers of blast or atypical cells in the CSF.[26,27]

Radiotherapeutic Emergencies

The radiation oncologist will be called on to assist with certain emergencies when the patient first presents with leukemia or at the time of relapse. Mediastinal adenopathy causing airway compression or spinal cord compression from epidural disease are clear indications for emergent RT. Generally, only one to three 1.5- to 2.0-Gy fractions are required while the diagnosis is being established and systemic therapy is being initiated (Fig. 80.3). Glucocorticoids are an important adjunct to CNS RT but can produce rapid lysis of some lymphoblastic lymphomas/leukemias, which may hamper diagnostic evaluation. In the presence of cranial nerve palsies at diagnosis, some radiation oncologists recommend 10 to 15 Gy to the base of skull early in the treatment course to try and reverse the neurologic deficits.[28,29] Extreme leukocytosis with blast counts over 75,000 to 100,000/μL is a concern with myeloid leukemia, as leukostasis may occur, particularly in the vessels of the brain or lung. Lymphoid blasts are less adhesive to vessel walls and blast counts of up to 400,000/μL or more are often well tolerated. In decades past, RT directed at the whole brain was employed using low doses on the order of 6 to 10 Gy in various fractionations. However, the role of RT in this setting has been questioned,[15,30,31] but may be considered when leukophoresis or exchange transfusion is contraindicated or unavailable.

Treatment of Acute Myeloid Leukemias

Classical induction therapy for AML is an anthracycline on days 1 to 3 with cytarabine (cytosine arabinoside, ara-C) for 7 days. Acute promyelocytic leukemia (M3 AML, APL) represents an exception to this rule. In many cases, the disseminated intravascular coagulation and associated PML-RAR fusion in APL are best managed with a combination of anthracycline and all-*trans*-retinoic acid or single-agent arsenic trioxide.[32] For the remainder of the AML subtypes, daunorubicin and idarubicin are the anthracyclines most commonly used in induction chemotherapy regimens. Although a meta-analysis of multiple trials suggested that idarubicin has a higher complete response (CR) rate and survival over daunomycin,[33] more recent data from dose escalation trials using daunorubicin as part of the induction regimen suggest that when equivalently dosed, responses are similar.[34] Remission rates vary from 50% to 80% dependant on patient age, karyotype, and subtype of AML. Patients younger than age 60 have CR rates of 70% to 80%, whereas older patients tend to have lower CR rates of 50% to 60%. Patients who develop secondary AML following chemotherapy for other cancers have CR rates in the 40% to 60% range. Some induction regimens in children have added other drugs such as etoposide. Adding other chemotherapy drugs to anthracycline and cytarabine has yet to be shown to produce a convincing survival benefit for AML induction in adults.[35] Adults older than 60 years of age with AML and intermediate or unfavorable cytogenetics who are not candidates for hematopoietic stem cell transplantation are generally considered suitable for treatment with low-intensity palliative therapies such as low-dose subcutaneous cytarabine, azacitidine, or decitabine.[36] Alternatively, such patients may be referred for clinical trials of novel agents.

Once remission is achieved, the need for additional therapy has been well documented in large randomized trials. Current data suggests that optimal postremission consolidative therapy begins with high-dose ara-C for up to four cycles.[37] Alternatively, additional cycles of anthracycline for 2 days along with conventional-dose cytarabine for 5 days has been used in both

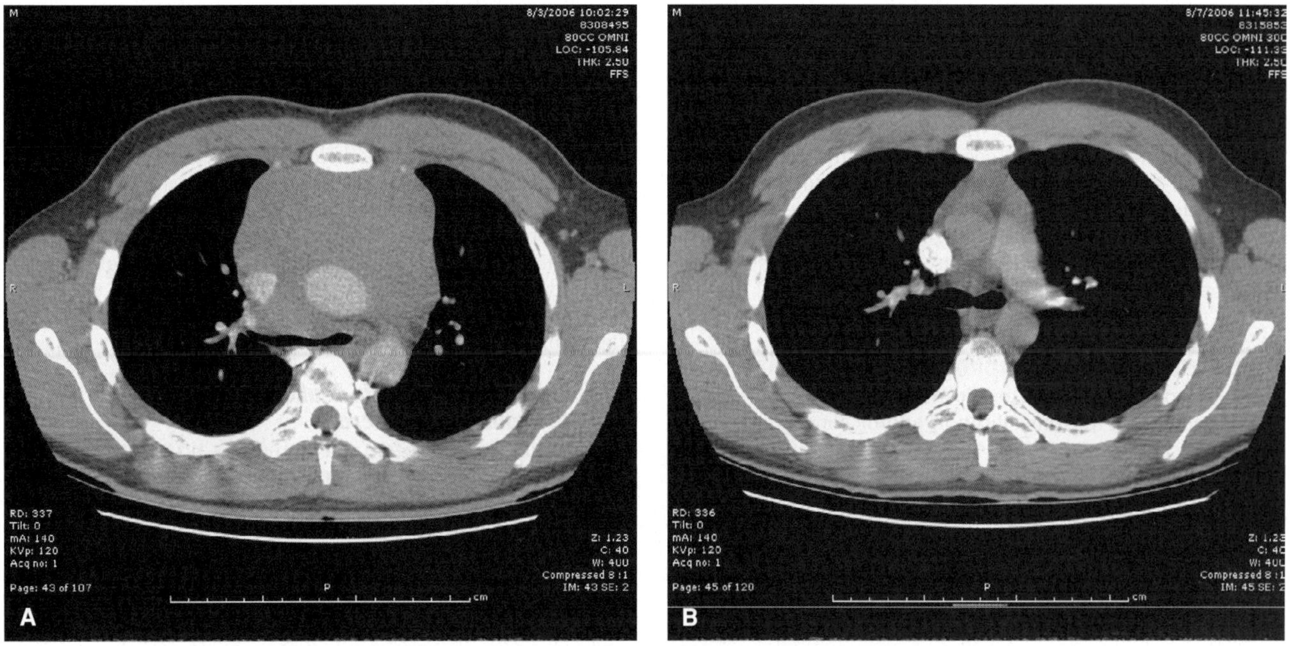

FIGURE 80.3. Computed tomography scans of chest before **(A)** and after **(B)** palliative radiotherapy (RT) for mediastinal mass associated with T-cell acute lymphocytic leukemia. A 16-year-old boy presented with dyspnea and chest pain. A chest x-ray showed a mediastinal mass while blood counts revealed a lymphocytosis. Diagnosis was established by flow cytometry of blood. Initial treatment with steroids, doxorubicin, vincristine, and methotrexate failed to produce immediate response. Megavoltage RT with anterior and posterior opposed beams for 6 Gy in three fractions was administered, subsequently relieving acute symptoms and allowing for general anesthesia to take place without risk for complete airway obstruction in order for central line placement and lumbar puncture to be performed.

younger and older individuals with AML. Lumping all types of AML together as one group, the roughly 10% to 20% of patients who then remain in remission for 3 years have a high likelihood of being cured. High-dose ara-C has considerable CNS toxicity in elderly patients and has also been avoided in pediatric protocols. Other drugs used for consolidative treatment or for second-line induction therapy include etoposide, 6-mercaptopurine, amsacrine, 5-azacytidine, and methotrexate (MTX), but no one regimen is clearly advantageous.

The role of CNS prophylaxis is not well defined for AML, particularly because CNS relapse rates are relatively infrequent (at roughly 5% to 10%). Some studies show no difference in relapse rates with cranial radiation. Nevertheless, many pediatric regimens employ IT drugs such as ara-C. Patients with a high WBC count at diagnosis or monocytic variants of AML are believed to have a higher risk for CNS relapse, which may justify both IT chemotherapy and cranial radiation in this setting. At least one study of childhood AML demonstrated a lower systemic relapse rate after cranial radiation.[38]

Leukemia-free survival rates vary widely from 15% to 80% in AML and are dependent on risk stratification. Younger patients with standard risk M2 AML or with favorable cytogenetic abnormalities have relatively better prognoses, whereas those with older age, induction failure, adverse cytogenetic abnormalities, or other FAB subtypes of AML do worse.[39,40] An exception is acute promyelocytic leukemia, which is among the most curable types of AML thanks to the efficacy of all-*trans*-retinoic acid (ATRA) in the management of this leukemic subtype. Postremission therapy for AML patients with adverse features may include transplantation with autologous or allogeneic stem cells.

The radiation oncologist may be called on to treat myeloid or granulocytic sarcoma, which may predate a diagnosis of leukemia or be a harbinger of systemic relapse, and are typically associated with AML, but may also be seen with myeloproliferative disorders.[41,42] Also called a *chloroma,* these solid masses of leukemic infiltrates are responsive to modest doses of RT. The name chloroma derives from the fact that myeloid cells contain myeloperoxidase, which manifests a greenish color on gross inspection. These may occur in all varieties of extramedullary sites including periosteum, skin, soft tissues, gastrointestinal tract, the spine, and in epidural spaces or meninges.[43–46] Pathologic misclassifications are common, as this is a rare clinicopathologic disorder. Based on various case reports in the literature, symptomatic problems from chloromas may be readily relieved with doses of 10 to 20 Gy. The fractionation and total dose needs to take into consideration any normal tissue toxicities and the potential for future total body irradiation (TBI) should the patient be a potential candidate for an allotransplant. Although overall survival may be better than AML in many chloromas, long-term disease control usually requires systemic therapy used for AML.[41,47–48,49,50]

Treatment of Acute Lymphoblastic Leukemia

The four components of specific ALL therapy are (i) induction of remission, (ii) intensification and/or consolidation, (iii) maintenance therapy, and (iv) CNS prophylaxis. In the 1960s, the problem of CNS recurrence was addressed with CNS radiation and IT chemotherapy. Subsequent improvements in ALL cure rates over the last 2 to 3 decades has resulted from improved risk stratification of patients with more effective, tailored multidrug regimens. As discussed in the following text, the late sequela of 24-Gy cranial irradiation were recognized in the 1980s and 1990s, leading to the elimination of cranial RT in favor of intermediate- or high-dose MTX in all but high-risk patients or those with CNS-3 disease. While not a standard worldwide, investigators at St. Jude Children's Research Hospital (SJCRH) have completely eliminated the use of upfront cranial RT in their protocols of pediatric ALL, accepting a small incidence of CNS relapse in their high-risk patients.[51] In addition, with the improvements in systemic therapy, testicular relapse in males has become a rare event.[52] Testicular irradiation is rarely necessary except in the setting of testicular relapse or bone marrow transplantation.

Induction therapy for ALL as a minimum typically includes a glucocorticoid, vincristine, and L-asparaginase. Higher-risk patients often receive additional drugs such as an anthracycline, especially for adult ALL. Other four or greater multidrug regimens have been used, all of which has resulted in initial remission rates of 95% to 99% in children and 75% to 90% in adults. Dexamethasone is now the preferred systemic steroid treatment as suggested in two clinical reports comparing it to prednisone, with dexamethasone reducing both CNS and systemic relapse in pediatric ALL.[53,54] This may be related to dexamethasone's better penetration into the CSF and longer half-life, providing enhanced protection against CNS relapse.[55]

Following induction and achieving CR, patients then receive intensification therapies that have been developed by cooperative groups in the United States and Europe.[56,57] This may consist of high doses of antimetabolites such as MTX, ara-C, or L-asparaginase. Additional anthracycline therapy is beneficial in high-risk patients.[58] It is believed that high-dose MTX helps control CNS disease, which has allowed for less use of cranial radiation in some pediatric programs.

Following intensification therapy, patients undergo a phase of maintenance treatment. In all but mature B-cell ALL, maintenance therapy over 2 to 3 years with agents such as weekly low-dose MTX and mercaptopurine appears to be quite important, albeit for unclear reasons. In high-risk patients, cooperative group studies have demonstrated a benefit to an additional "delayed" intensification after a period of maintenance therapy.[56,59]

For ALL in adults, particularly those with the L3 subtype, patients have experienced improved remission rates with multiagent induction regimens that include high-dose MTX, cyclophosphamide, and sometimes ara-C. These drugs in combination with vincristine, steroids, L-asparaginase, and sometimes doxorubicin have been associated with 68% to 85% CR rates.

For relapsed ALL, a second induction generally consists of multiple drugs including vincristine, prednisone, L-asparaginase, an anthracycline with or without MTX, VP-16 or teniposide, and ara-C. If the CNS is involved, IT treatment is given along with RT.[60] If testicular relapse occurs, bilateral testicular irradiation is administered. When isolated CNS or testicular relapse develops, systemic therapy is indicated along with local RT.[61]

If a second remission develops, as occurs in 70% to 90% of cases, subsequent treatment includes either allogeneic transplantation or consolidative chemotherapy.[61,62] There are no randomized trials to indicate which is better, but comparative analysis suggests that survival is improved with allogeneic transplantation, particularly in ALL patients who had brief initial remissions.[62,63]

CNS Prophylaxis of Acute Leukemia and the Role of Cranial Radiotherapy

Historically, as multiagent chemotherapy proved to be highly effective in producing remissions in childhood ALL, numerous investigators noted a significant increase in CNS relapses. The CNS was recognized as a sanctuary site, protected from chemotherapy by the blood–brain barrier. In addition, CNS recurrences invariably led to systemic recurrence suggesting that CNS disease was capable of reseeding the blood and marrow.

This observation led to a long series of CNS preventative therapy trials, which initially utilized craniospinal irradiation (CSI). For instance, studies V and VI in 1962–1967 from SJCRH established that CSI to 24 Gy in 15 to 16 fractions reduced the isolated CNS relapse rate from 67% to 4%.[64,65] CSI doses of 12 Gy did not appear to be effective with the early chemotherapy regimens from this time.[66] Concerns that full spinal RT would be associated with more acute myelosuppression, late musculoskeletal hypoplasia, as well as the technical difficulties of CSI, led SJCRH investigators to compare CSI with cranial radiation plus IT MTX in study VII.[67] Here, the two CNS preventative regimens were found to be equivalent with roughly an 8% risk of CNS relapse.

In SJCRH study VIII (1972–1975), all patients received 24-Gy cranial radiation plus IT MTX. Patients were randomized to one of four maintenance regimens: (i) weekly intravenous (IV) MTX begun during cranial radiation, (ii) oral MTX and 6-mercaptopurine, (iii) oral MTX, mercaptopurine, and cyclophosphamide, and (iv) same three drugs plus ara-C.[68] The incidence of CNS relapse was 5.0%, 1.5%, 20%, and 11.4%, respectively. More troublesome, however, was the development in some patients of leukoencephalopathy, a disabling syndrome of lethargy, seizures, spasticity, paresis, and ataxia. The incidence of leukoencephalopathy in the four randomization groups was 55%, 0%, 7.1%, and 1.4%, respectively. Thus, standard maintenance with oral MTX and mercaptopurine following CNS treatment with cranial radiation along with IT MTX to treat the spinal subarachnoid space was found to have the lowest CNS relapse rate and the least toxicity. The major lesson learned was that IV MTX and cranial radiation in close temporal proximity should be avoided.

In the 1970s and 1980s, additional phase III trials further defined appropriate preventative CNS therapy for childhood ALL. The Children's Cancer Study Group (CCSG) trial #101 compared: (i) 24-Gy CSI plus extended field RT encompassing the liver, spleen, and gonads; (ii) 24-Gy CSI alone; (iii) 24-Gy cranial RT plus IT MTX; and (iv) IT MTX alone. Overall, the different radiation regimens were comparable in preventing CNS relapse while statistically superior to IT chemotherapy alone.[69] This finding was further confirmed in a cross-study comparison[70] as well as a Cancer and Leukemia Group B trial.[52] The CCSG further compared cranial RT plus IT MTX with CSI in high-risk patients, defined by a WBC at diagnosis of >50,000/μL; cranial irradiation and IT MTX proved to be significantly superior with respect to both CNS and systemic relapse rates.

Further cooperative group trials have refined the efficacy of CNS-directed therapies within patient groups stratified by risk. Several trials have compared cranial RT with intermediate- or high-dose IV MTX along with IT chemotherapy (some with the addition of IT hydrocortisone and ara-C to MTX know as "triple" IT therapy).[52,71,72] The essential findings have been that in patients with low- or standard-risk ALL (e.g., age 3 to 6 years and WBC count <10,000/μL) who are managed without cranial radiation by substituting IT MTX throughout induction, consolidation, and maintenance therapy, CNS relapse rates have remained at a low level of 5% or less.[73–75] Additionally, with triple IT chemotherapy, there was a trend toward fewer systemic failures as well as excellent CNS control when given throughout consolidation and maintenance therapy. This may be at the expense of increased neurotoxicity, however, when given in conjunction with intermediate-dose IV MTX.[75]

Moreover, a meta-analysis of 65 randomized trials of pediatric ALL worldwide initiated prior to 1993 that evaluated the role cranial RT concluded that in the vast majority of patients, cranial RT may be avoided with the use of extended IT therapy.[76] IV MTX was particularly advantageous in reducing systemic relapse. One notable exception to the conclusions of aggregated trials of this meta-analysis was the CCG-105 trial of intermediate-risk ALL. In CCG-105, 1,388 patients (with a complex matrix of adverse risk factors defined by patient age, presenting WBC count, and FAB subtype) were randomly assigned to receive either IT MTX alone or cranial radiation for CNS treatment.[77] A secondary complex randomization scheme allocated patients to standard or intensive chemotherapy. Intensive chemotherapy included either more drugs for induction or the addition of a delayed intensification chemotherapy phase after consolidative and CNS therapies. CNS recurrence rates were comparable in all groups at roughly 5% to 7% except in those patients receiving standard chemotherapy without cranial radiation, where the CNS recurrence was 20%. Thus, more intensive systemic therapy can lower CNS recurrence rates, abrogating any benefit to cranial irradiation. Finally, one interesting subanalysis of this systematic review of cranial RT for ALL looked at 809 patients across seven trials[78,79–82] that compared different doses of radiation (generally 18 to 21 Gy versus 24 Gy). There were no differences in CNS or non-CNS relapse rates that could be discerned.

Regarding present-day use of prophylactic cranial RT, investigators have been focusing on patients who are at the highest risk for CNS relapse. At one extreme is the St. Jude's group, which has become particularly concerned about the late effects of 24 Gy to the brain in terms of neurocognitive disabilities, hypothalamic/pituitary dysfunction, and secondary malignancies. With risk-adapted intensification of chemotherapy, Pui et al.[51] have reported favorable results with the complete elimination of cranial RT in all newly diagnosed ALL patients.[51] In their St. Jude Total XV trial, 498 patients were treated without cranial RT yielding an 86.6% 5-year event-free survival, which was comparable to their prior studies that had included cranial RT. CNS-directed therapy used five cycles of high-dose MTX including, as part of induction therapy, dexamethasone, and extended IT chemotherapy. High-risk ALL patients received up to 16 to 25 IT chemotherapy sessions, whereas low-risk patients received 13 to 18 doses of IT chemotherapy. Patients who were at increased risk of CNS relapse were those who had positive CSF cytology (CNS-2 or -3) or T-cell ALL. Moreover, a relatively high 7% of patients in first remission went on to undergo an allogeneic stem cell transplant correlating with high-risk features of MRD and adverse cytogenetic markers.

Elsewhere worldwide, the philosophy on the use of cranial RT in pediatric ALL has been to use it judiciously in high-risk patients while at the same time also reducing radiation doses to address the concerns about late effects, which includes learning disabilities and other cognitive defects, growth retardation, hypopituitarism, secondary malignancies, and the aforementioned leukoencephalopathy. The European BFM-ALL trials since 1990 have reduced the cranial radiation dose to 12 Gy with their risk-adapted intensification schemes, although those with CNS-3 disease received 24 Gy in their BFM-90 trial and 18 Gy in the more recent BFM-95 trial. Currently, the Children's Oncology Group (COG) has followed suit with a reduction in cranial radiation doses in its current ALL trials.

High-risk B-cell ALL patients who continue to receive cranial radiation are generally defined by age and high presenting WBC counts per NCI criteria, by adverse cytogenetics (e.g., *bcr-abl*, MLL, and hypodiploidy), and by MRD after induction chemotherapy. Most T-cell ALL patients are at increased risk for CNS relapse due to accompanying risk factors and, therefore, continue to receive cranial irradiation. An analysis of T-cell ALL patients (generally with other poor-risk features) treated within several Pediatric Oncology Group (POG) protocols suggested that omitting cranial radiation had an adverse impact on CNS relapse rates.[83] Specifically, the 3-year CNS relapse rate was 18% for those who did not receive RT compared to 7% who did. On the other hand, a European report looking at a subgroup of favorable T-cell ALL patients, generally those with young age and low WBCs, suggests that it may be safe to omit cranial radiation in this subgroup.[73] However, as most T-cell ALL patients present with high WBC counts, Conter et al.[73] published a relevant comparison of the AIEOP-91 trial with the BFM-90 trial in which similar backbone chemotherapy is used. The AIEOP-91 trial omits cranial RT albeit with more IT chemotherapy, leading to a significantly higher CNS relapse along with a 3-year event-free survival of 62% compared to 88% for the BFM-90 patients who received cranial RT. Multivariate analysis showed that age younger than 10 years and WBC >100,000 in particular defined a group of T-cell ALL patients who should receive cranial RT.

To reduce the toxicity of prophylactic cranial radiation, several investigations have explored a reduction in radiation dose. The use of 18 Gy in 9 or 10 fractions along with IT MTX yields comparable disease control rates as 24 Gy.[84] Although there were some initial reports of reduced cognitive dysfunction even with such a dose reduction,[85] this issue is by no means completely settled.[86–88] Nevertheless, a dose of 18 Gy for prophylactic cranial irradiation had become more or less standard for pediatric ALL being treated off-protocol. As noted in the following text, however, patients being treated with BFM-type chemotherapy programs may be treated with lower cranial RT doses of 12 Gy. For adults with ALL, various protocols have used 24 Gy, whereas others employ 18 Gy.[87,89] Some programs such as HyperCVAD omit the use of cranial RT in the face of high-dose MTX and ara-C, which effectively penetrate the blood–brain barrier. The Dana Farber Cancer Institute ALL Consortium has studied the role of hyperfractionated cranial radiation (0.9 Gy twice daily) compared to standard daily fractionated treatments (1.8 Gy daily) to 18 Gy in high-risk patients.[90,91] Results from Dana Farber ALL 87–04 show excellent CNS control rates with both the standard or hyperfractionated treatments. Late neurocognitive sequela has been similar in which systemic therapy emphasizes L-asparaginase and omits high-dose MTX. A follow-up Dana Farber ALL trial 95-01, compared hyperfractionated 18 Gy cranial RT to extended IT chemotherapy without cranial RT. The interesting finding here is that quantitative measurements of neurocognitive function were similar in both groups.[92]

The German-Austrian-Swiss ALL-BFM ("Berlin-Frankfurt-Munich") Study Group has further reduced the radiation dose to 12 Gy, initially in a selected group of standard-risk pediatric patients.[74] With modern chemotherapy regimens as opposed to the older SJCRH experience, this further reduction in radiation dose was associated with excellent CNS control. Moreover, the ALL-BFM 90 protocol stopped using cranial RT in low- or standard-risk patients, but both the medium- and high-risk patients received 12-Gy prophylactic cranial radiation resulting in CNS recurrence rates well below 5%.[58] For the ALL-BFM 95 trial, cranial RT was deleted for the intermediate-risk B-cell ALL patients. This has resulted in a small increased risk for CNS relapse, which is considered clinically acceptable in order to avoid the late effects of such RT.[93] Specifically comparing intermediate-risk BFM 90 to BFM 95 patients, the isolated CNS relapse rate at 6 years is 0.5% versus 1.9%, $p < 0.01$. The 6-year "any-CNS" relapse rate was also statistically different at 2.2% versus 4.4%. Further follow-up and additional experience within the COG with this lower cranial radiation dose will be of interest in the years to come, hopefully seeing a reduction in late toxicity without compromising efficacy as cranial RT continues as used in a subset of high-risk pediatric ALL patients.

Meningeal Leukemia at Diagnosis

At the time of diagnosis of ALL, approximately 3% to 5% of patients will present with clinically detectable CNS involvement (i.e., CNS-3 disease). Meningeal leukemia at diagnosis is typically managed as high-risk leukemia with cranial RT. The St. Jude investigators may disagree with the use of RT even here, but their latest results of their Total XV protocol included nine patients with CNS-3 disease whose 5-year event-free survival was only 43%.[51] These high-risk patients receive chemotherapy programs that include dose intensive therapy with agents that penetrate the blood–brain barrier as well as IT therapy. Cranial radiation doses may vary from 18 to 25 Gy. Historically, CSI has been used, but modern practice has dispensed with the spine fields as the IT and systemic chemotherapy programs appear to be effective in assisting with CNS control. In children with ALL, meningeal involvement no longer carries a dire prognosis, as 5-year disease-free survival rates approaching 70% are commonly seen.[94]

Within the older Children's Cancer Study Group (CCG) clinical trials for ALL, CSI has been consistently used in the management of CNS-3 disease. Until 1983, the cranial and spinal doses were 24 Gy and 12 Gy, respectively. Subsequent trials through 1989, utilized more intensive consolidation chemotherapy with a decrease in spinal radiation doses to 6 Gy. This allowed for a nonrandomized comparison of 6- and 12-Gy doses to the spine (in 2-Gy fractions). Interestingly, the patients who received a reduced spinal dose did just as well as those who received 12 Gy with less intensive chemotherapy. The 5-year event-free survival rate for patients with CNS-3 disease was 69%, compared to 67% for patients enrolled in all CCG ALL protocols in 1983–1989 who were without CNS-3 disease.[94]

Delay in RT up to 12 months has been found to be safe as long as intensive chemotherapy is being given first.[95,96] This avoids the marrow compromise that could potentially occur with early spine irradiation. In addition, with doses <16 Gy to the spine, myelosuppression has not been a major problem. Musculoskeletal hypoplasia would not be expected to be a significant problem for long-term survivors. The sequencing of RT *after* rather than *before* potentially neurotoxic drug therapy such as MTX may theoretically result in a lower incidence of cognitive dysfunction or encephalopathy. Some pediatric protocols will also tailor the dose to the brain based on patient age. For instance, the ALL-BFM 90 protocol, which utilizes cranial rather than CSI, avoids any RT for those younger than 1 year of age, 18 Gy for ages 1 to 2 years, and 24 Gy for older patients. In this large multicenter trial, 54 patients presented with CNS-3 disease and achieved a 48% 6-year event-free survival.[58] Arguably, this is inferior to protocols that use CSI, such as those reported by the CCG.[94] However, in the ALL-BFM 95, there were 64 patients with CNS-3 disease who had a 6-year event-free survival of 57.7% in which therapy included cranial radiation to 18 Gy without irradiation of the spine.

Summary of Cranial RT for Initial ALL Management

In summary, cranial RT may be used to prevent CNS relapse of leukemia. From a historical perspective that considered the brain as a sanctuary site, cranial RT has been well documented to improve outcomes for selected patients with pediatric ALL. With concerns about late sequela and improvements in systemic therapy including agents that can better penetrate the blood–brain barrier, cranial RT is used much less frequently in the upfront management of ALL. Overall, only 15% to 20% of pediatric ALL patients who have high-risk features require cranial RT currently. In current practice, cranial radiation is employed selectively in high-risk ALL patients. Although the definition of high risk has been shifting, one needs to take into account the intensity and specifics of risk-adapted chemotherapy. Nevertheless, ALL patients who benefit from cranial RT include older age (e.g., older than 10 years of age, and probably increasing benefit at ages older than 13 years); T-cell phenotype, especially in older patients with high presenting WBC over 100.000; and risk groups CNS-2 or -3 by CSF findings. Additionally, among B-cell patients, those with MRD and adverse cytogenetics should be strongly considered for cranial RT. All adults with ALL may be considered to be at high risk for CNS relapse, but there are no standard recommendations on cranial RT. Patients with AML, except for specific subtypes such as monocytic variants, are not generally treated with prophylactic cranial radiation at the present as the risk for CNS relapse is <5%. Unless otherwise indicated, in a specific treatment protocol, the radiation prescription for prophylactic cranial radiation to prevent ALL relapse is 18 Gy in 9 or 10 fractions. When BFM-type chemotherapy programs are used, the radiation dose has been reduced to 12 Gy with favorable outcomes. The spinal region is specifically treated by IT chemotherapy rather than RT, although an open question is whether there would be an incremental benefit to low radiation doses to the spine with meningeal leukemia at diagnosis.

Therapeutic CNS Irradiation for Meningeal Relapse

With modern chemotherapy programs incorporating CNS-directed treatment, CNS relapse rates are typically <10%. As in overt CNS leukemia at diagnosis, RT has a central role. Formally, CNS relapse was thought to have a poor prognosis. Studies in the 1970s and 1980s describe disease control rates of 25% to 50%.[97–103] More recent trials, however, utilizing more intensive chemotherapy as well as RT, have reported ALL 5-year survivals of 50% to 70%.[95,104–107] Almost all trials have employed RT; the debate has been between cranial RT alone or CSI. Doses used have generally been approximately 24 Gy to the brain and 10 to 15 Gy to the spine. Most comparisons have not been randomized, but superior outcomes seem to be achieved with CSI.[58,95,104–105,106,107] One small phase III trial did show superiority for CSI compared to cranial RT.[104]

Although CNS relapse may ostensibly occur without over systemic disease, the latter is viewed as inevitable without additional systemic therapy. Therefore, intensive chemotherapy is an essential component of the treatment of meningeal relapse.[108]

Several prognostic factors have been found to be of importance in the setting of CNS relapse.[109–111] Patients who were originally deemed at diagnosis to be at low risk for CNS relapse by virtue of a low initial leukocyte count (<20,000/μL), who originally did not receive cranial irradiation, or whose CNS relapse occurred at a relatively long period after the original diagnosis have a better prognosis after CNS recurrence. An isolated CNS relapse has generally been more prognostically favorable compared to combined CNS and systemic relapse. After completing chemotherapy, those children with CNS relapse have better outcomes with longer disease-free intervals. For instance, experience within the Pediatric Oncology Group (POG) with isolated CNS relapse of ALL in which RT used a cranial dose of 24 Gy and a spine dose of 15 Gy. The 4-year event-free survival was 71%. Those patients who presented with greater than an 18-month disease-free interval prior to CNS relapse had a 4-year event-free survival of 83% compared to 46% for those with shorter initial remission durations.[95] This has led subsequent POG trials that omit RT to the spine if there is a long disease-free interval, but if the disease-free interval is <18 months, 24 Gy is given to brain while 15 Gy is delivered to the spine. Whether the omission of spinal RT in this favorable subgroup is detrimental is unclear. However, high-dose Ara-C has generally been added to the management of CNS relapse of ALL. With this agent, Mora et al.[112] reported a favorable 63% complete response rate. These concepts have been maintained with current COG trials for CNS relapse of ALL, but with intensification of systemic therapy, spinal RT has been proposed to be dropped even for short disease-free intervals, while the brain is treated to 18 Gy. As for adults with CNS leukemia, most of the published experience and commentary from medical oncologists has been opposed to the use of CSI mainly for fear of excessive myelosuppression.[87] Cranial irradiation is relatively standard, however. Quite possibly, the avoidance in treating the entire CNS is detrimental, although admittedly this is not a settled issue.

Selected high-risk patients with CNS relapse may be candidates for allogeneic transplants. TBI is often a component of the preparative regimen. One function of the TBI is to specifically treat the CNS burden of disease. Because doses on the order of 12 to 15 Gy are employed here, it makes sense to boost the head prior to TBI to bring total doses to the cranium to 18 to 25 Gy.

Testicular Relapse

In boys with ALL, particularly those with T-cell subtype, testicular involvement was once a common problem. Overt testicular involvement by leukemia at diagnosis occurs in approximately 2% of males with ALL, and is a particularly poor prognostic situation. Microscopic burden in the testes is estimated to be higher at 5% to 15% based on biopsy data and the historic risk for testicular relapse. With modern chemotherapy, especially the use of intermediate- to high-dose MTX, this is now rare. Similar to the experience with CNS relapse, there once was speculation as to whether the testes acted as a sanctuary site due to a physiologic blood–testes barrier. In 1980, a trial of prophylactic testicular irradiation significantly reduced the risk of testicular relapse but did not improve survival.[113]

In cases of testicular relapse, systemic and/or CNS relapse usually follows.[114] Both intensive systemic therapy and local RT are indicated. Doses <12 Gy are generally thought to be suboptimal, whereas doses of 24 to 26 Gy over 2.5 to 3.5 weeks are considered standard. Case reports of local recurrences despite adequate RT have led some to suggest higher doses. When only one testes is clinically involved, imaging or biopsy of the contralateral testes frequently reveals bilateral disease. Similarly, unilateral irradiation or orchiectomy as local management is felt to be associated with a significant risk of contralateral testicular relapse, justifying treatment directed at both testes for leukemia management, despite the expectation of infertility from RT. Data from CCG and POG studies suggests that local irradiation and intensive systemic therapy results in prolonged event-free survival in roughly 50% to 65% of patients.[61,115] Where allogeneic transplantation is indicated, TBI is often part of the conditioning regimen. One retrospective series from the Memorial Sloan-Kettering Cancer Center suggests that for TBI/cyclophosphamide preparative regimens, the risk of testicular relapse is significantly reduced with a local boost to the scrotum of 4 Gy to bring the total testicular dose to 16 to 20 Gy.[116] Regardless, there is not universal agreement about the need for a testicular boost in this setting.

THE CHRONIC LEUKEMIAS

Chronic Myelogenous Leukemia

CML is a chronic myeloproliferative disorder arising from clonal expansion of the primitive hematopoietic stem cell. It involves myeloid, erythroid, megakaryocytic, and sometimes lymphoid elements. It is the first neoplastic process to be characterized by a specific cytogenetic marker, the Philadelphia chromosome (Ph+), t(9;22) described in 1960.[117] This is detectable by cytogenetics in 90% to 95% of patients and by molecular analysis in most other patients.[118] This translocation results in a fusion protein that has tyrosine kinase activity critical for leukemic transformation.

Clinically, the disease manifests several phases: an initial chronic indolent phase of 3 to 4 years with progression to an accelerated phase and finally an acute transformation to blast phase, which occurs in 75% to 85% of patients, with a survival of 3 to 6 months. As the disease advances, the accelerated phase is characterized by increasing difficulty in controlling the peripheral WBC count, increasing splenomegaly, increasing blasts in the peripheral blood and bone marrow, and increasing basophilia and eosinophilia. The blast crisis resembles acute leukemia with >30% blasts in blood or bone marrow with symptoms such as bone pain, sweats, fever, anorexia, or weight loss. Anemia, thrombopenia, and extramedullary disease involving bones, skin, CNS, and lymph nodes are common. In about 20% of cases, blasts are lymphoid by phenotype.

Prognostic factors have been identified in CML and include age, splenic size, platelet count, percent of basophils in blood, and marrow. Poor prognosis factors are age >60 years, spleen >l0 cm below the costal margin, blasts >3% in blood or marrow, basophilia >7% in blood or marrow, and platelets >700,000/μL.[119,120] A poor response to therapy and a short duration of remission also are considered unfavorable, as well as failure to achieve significant cytogenetic remission.[121]

Therapy of CML

The first effective therapy for chronic leukemias was RT to the spleen and sometimes the liver, initiated in 1902 by Pusey[122] and assessed in 1924 by Minot et al.[123] Today, RT is primarily used in a palliative setting to relieve painful splenomegaly or other extramedullary sites when indicated. In some centers, TBI plays an important role in allogeneic transplantation.

There is a long history of treating CML in chronic phase with alkylating agents, hydroxyurea, cytarabine,and interferon alpha, which is beyond the scope of this chapter. Over the past decade, such therapies, as well as hematopoietic stem cell transplant, have largely been relegated to the salvage setting through the introduction of ABL tyrosine kinase inhibitors effective in inducing and maintaining long-term remissions in CML.[124] Imatinib is a relatively nontoxic oral medication that has been shown to be effective in CML in both chronic and accelerated phases.[125,126] This agent has been a paradigm for molecularly targeted therapies and is now used as upfront therapy for CML along with two other more recently introduced agents dasatinib and nilotinib.[127] For those who do not respond adequately to the tyrosine kinase inhibitors or who lose response, allogeneic transplantation remains an important option.[128,129] About 70% of good-risk patients achieve long-term disease-free survival.[130] Allotransplantation and total body irradiation are further discussed in Chapter 15.

Palliative RT may be of benefit in those patients with massive splenomegaly with responses seen with doses in the 10- to 20-Gy range or lower. The radiation oncologist is well advised to understand the extreme radiosensitivity of the malignant stem cells in CML and in other hematopoietic disorders causing splenomegaly with the admonition to use very low doses per fraction (25 to 100 cGy) once or twice a week with close monitoring of blood counts (see below).

Chronic Lymphocytic Leukemia

CLL is a chronic leukemia of B-cell origin. The course of the disease demonstrates marked variability. Many patients live a normal lifespan, never require therapy, and die of unrelated causes. Others progress within a few years despite treatment. The usual course is characterized by gradual progression from no significant physical findings to lymphadenopathy, gradual increase in peripheral blood lymphocyte count, and increasing splenomegaly, sometimes massive in size. Nonlymphoid organ involvement may occur with advanced stage of disease. As disease progression occurs, anemia and thrombocytopenia occur.

An occasional patient with CLL demonstrates transformation to an aggressive large B-cell lymphoma referred to as *Richter's syndrome*.[131] Its incidence ranges from 3% to 5% of CLL cases.[132] It may arise in the setting of active disease or during a CR. It is characterized by an abrupt onset of asymmetric adenopathy, fever, and elevated LDH. Other transformations include evolution to prolymphocytic leukemia with development of progressive refractory disease and a majority of prolymphocytes in the blood. Rarely, ALL or myeloma develop in the course of CLL.[133,134]

The clinical diagnosis is based upon the blood lymphocyte count, which must be at least $5 \times 10^3/\mu L$ in an adult. The malignant B cells have a distinct immunophenotype with expression of surface markers CD5 and CD23 in addition to immunoglobulin light chain restriction.[135] Healthy individuals may harbor monoclonal B-cells of this phenotype and are classified as monoclonal B-cell lymphocytosis provided there are $<5 \times 10^3/\mu L$ and no other evidence of disease is present. Patients with lymphadenopathy or other tissue morphology and similar phenotype without leukemic involvement are diagnosed with small lymphocytic lymphoma. There have been many staging systems proposed, but the most widely used are those modified by Rai et al.[136] and Binet et al.,[137] the former used in the United States and the latter in Europe (Table 80.3). Clinical stage is the most important predictor of survival in patients with CLL. Numerous other factors have been reported to have an impact on survival and include age, sex, lymphocyte doubling time, pattern of marrow involvement, β-2 microglobulin levels, and immunophenotype of malignant cells.[138] Cytogenetic and molecular abnormalities have more recently emerged as powerful predictors of outcome and may impact treatment decisions.[139] For example, deletion of chromosome 17p or p53 mutation confer both an inferior overall survival as well as resistance to purine analog and alkylator-based therapy.

TABLE 80.3 CHRONIC LYMPHOCYTIC LEUKEMIA STAGING SYSTEMS

Staging System	Clinical Features	Median Survival (Year)
Rai staging		
Low risk		>10
0	Lymphocytosis of blood and marrow	
Intermediate risk		7
I	Lymphadenopathy	
II	Splenomegaly	
High risk		2–4
III	Anemia, Hgb <10 g/dL (unrelated to hemolysis)	
IV	Thrombocytopenia <100,000 platelets/μL	
Binet staging		
A	<3 Areas of lymphadenopathy	12
B	≥3 Involved nodal areas	7
C	Anemia and/or thrombocytopenia	2

Hgb, hemoglobin.

Asymptomatic early-stage patients may be followed without therapy. About 20% of such patients will have an indolent course indefinitely. Of the remaining patients, the decision to intervene therapeutically is often challenging. The NCI has established guidelines for the initiation of treatment which include constitutional symptoms due to CLL, symptomatic lymphadenopathy and/or hepatosplenomegaly, lymphocyte doubling time <6 months, anemia (hemoglobin <10 g/dL), thrombocytopenia (platelets <100,000/μL), and refractory autoimmune disease.[140] The absolute lymphocyte count should not be used as an indication for treatment, as symptoms associated with marked lymphocytoses due to leukocyte aggregation do not typically occur in patients with CLL.

For many years, the standard treatment for CLL included single-agent chlorambucil with or without prednisone.[141] The newer purine analogs, 2-deoxycoformycin, fludarabine, and 2-chloro-2′-deoxy-β-D-adenosine (cladribine or 2-CDA) have been tested in CLL and, of these, fludarabine has shown a high response rate.[142] In a phase III trial comparing fludarabine to chlorambucil, the complete response rate with chlorambucil was 4% and with fludarabine 20%.[143,144] Overall response rates were 37% with chlorambucil and 63% with fludarabine. The median survival was 66 months (fludarabine) versus 56 months. For these reasons, fludarabine is now accepted as a standard therapy for CLL. More recently, a combination of fludarabine, cyclophosphamide, and the anti-CD20 antibody, rituximab, has resulted in a very high complete remission rate of 70% in patients with CLL, with a median time to progression of 80 months.[145]

Allogeneic transplantation has been employed with increasing frequency in the past decade with the recognition of graft-versus-leukemia effects and the advent of reduced-intensity conditioning. Earlier studies of allografting showed promising results in young patients with regard to disease control at the expense of significant treatment related toxicity.[146–148] Several groups have reported favorable disease control and survival in high-risk patients with reduced-intensity conditioning regimens that are fludarabine or low-dose TBI based. Of note, patients with chromosome 17p deletion appear to respond as well to allografting as those without 17p deletion.[149,150] Indications for consideration of allografting have been proposed by the European Group for Blood and Marrow Transplantation and include early relapse following chemoimmunotherapy, resistance to fludarabine, chromosome 17p deletion, and Richter's transformation.[150] It is not clear whether a survival advantage will occur with stem cell transplantation because there are no controlled trials. Newer approaches to the treatment of CLL involve vaccines, cell cycle inhibitors, antiapoptotic agents, immunomodulatory agents, and monoclonal antibodies.[151] The anti-CD52 antibody, alemtuzumab, has established single-agent activity in patients refractory to fludarabine and appears effective in patients harboring chromosome 17p deletions. The additive benefit of alemtuzumab in combination with other agents, such as fludarabine, has been tempered by increased infectious toxicity. Recently approved agents with documented efficacy include the novel alkylating agent bendamustine and a new humanized anti-CD20 monoclonal antibody, ofatumumab. The immunomodulatory drug, lenalidomide has also shown clinical efficacy and is under active study in combination with other agents.[152]

RT, once the initial effective therapy for CLL, is now used in the management of painful splenomegaly or occasionally for cytopenias associated with splenomegaly when splenectomy is not an option. It is also indicated in instances of unresponsive disease to alleviate symptomatic adenopathy or nonlymphoid organ involvement. Historically, low-dose TBI without stem cell support was used to control CLL. Remarkably low doses on the order of several Gray can be effective for palliation, though fractionated doses up to 20 Gy are also reasonable.

IRRADIATION TECHNIQUES

Cranial Radiation

The volume of treatment must include the subarachnoid space within the cranial vault. The inferior margin has by convention extended to the bottom of either the first or second cervical vertebra and includes the whole vertebral body. This may facilitate matching of potential future treatment fields to the spine. Other field boundaries typically involve "flashing" over the scalp. With regard to blocking the anterior facial structures, attention must be given to the base of skull anatomy to adequately cover the cribriform plate and the middle cranial fossa. The cribriform plate is somewhat variable as a function of the age of the patient but is generally in line with the bottom of the frontal sinuses extending posteriorly for several centimeters. The middle cranial or temporal fossa projects on lateral radiographs over the sphenoid sinuses. Figure 80.3 shows plain radiographs of an adult skull with radio-opaque markers at various anatomic landmarks. The posterior globe of the eye is typically included given concerns of leukemic relapse in the posterior retina near where there is subarachnoid space extending alone the optic nerves. Radio-opaque markers on the anterior aspect of the bony orbit are generally a good anatomic landmark that bifurcates the globe.

Figure 80.1 shows an example of lateral fields used to treat a patient with ALL. Head immobilization with Aquaplast or similar thermoplastic material facilitates a high degree of treatment position reproducibility. Accounting for setup variation and beam penumbra leads to field design that clearly must encroach on the eye. With forward gaze of the eyes, this would imply that the superior half of the lens is within the dose build-up region of the treatment fields. With the exception of very young children who cannot cooperate, voluntary rotation of the eye downward ("looking toward one's toes") would theoretically reduce the risk of cataracts. Another important caveat in treatment technique to minimize dose to the anterior portion of the eyes is the alignment of the anterior beam edge divergence. Figure 80.4 depicts this concept of angling the gantry 3 to 5 degrees to achieve a parallel anterior beam margin behind the lens, bisecting the eye producing a relatively tight radiation dose gradient. The simple trigonometric equation to determine the proper gantry rotation is:

$$\tan A = D/SAD,$$

where A is the desired rotation angle, D is the anterior-posterior distance between the central axis (i.e., isocenter) and the projection of the anterior aspect of the bony orbit at midplane, and SAD is the source to axis (or isocenter) distance (which is generally 100 cm for most linear accelerator geometries. Since $\tan A \cong A$ (in radians) for small angles and the conversion factor for radians to degrees is approximately 57 (i.e., 180 degrees per π radians), this further simplifies to:

$$A = (D)(0.57) \text{ for a source to axis/isocenter distance of } 100 \text{ cm}.$$

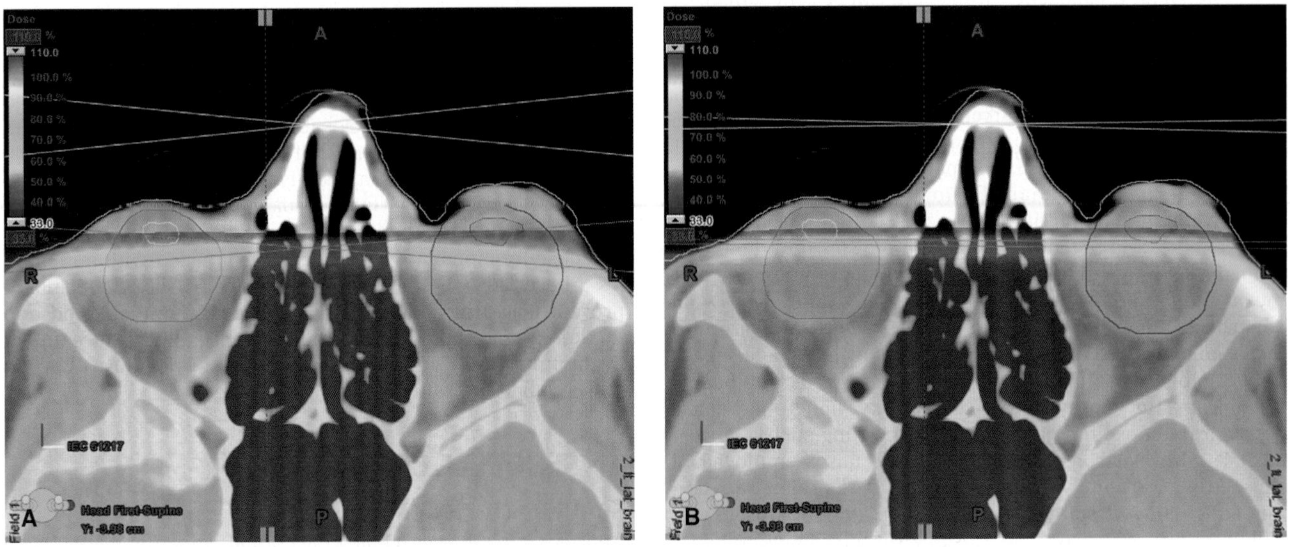

FIGURE 80.4. An 8-year-old boy with T-cell acute lymphoblastic leukemia, CNS-3 at diagnosis, requiring cranial RT to 18 Gy in 12 fractions after remission from systemic therapy. Alignment of anterior divergence of lateral cranial fields showing beam edge and color wash of radiation dose superimposed on axial CT scan at level of eyes. **A:** Parallel opposed fields result in widened dose gradient within anterior aspect of eyes. **B:** Gantry angle of 3 to 5 degrees results in alignment of anterior margin beam divergence from lateral fields and tighter dose gradient.

Some radiation oncologists prefer to simply place the isocenter of the treatment beam just posterior to the lens so that the anterior eye is protected by a modified "half-beam block." This is a fine technique for linear accelerators equipped with independent primary collimators so that block trays are not excessively heavy. With the advent of CT simulators, alignment of beam divergence can be performed graphically without the need for trigonometric calculations. The standard radiation dose for prophylactic cranial radiation in pediatric ALL is 18 Gy in 9 to 10 fractions, but increasing use of 12 Gy in 8 fractions is based on evolving experience with selected patients being treated with BFM-type ALL programs. Although this is a reasonable dose for adults, some protocols still continue to utilize 24 Gy in 12 fractions. Photon energies >6 MV should not be used so that the dose build-up region at initial depths is superficial to the meninges.

Craniospinal Radiation and Therapeutic Cranial Radiation for CNS Leukemia

The techniques of cranial spinal radiation involve precise matching of beam divergence between a PA spine field and lateral parallel opposed cranial fields. This topic is discussed in detail in the chapter on medulloblastoma (see Chapter 84). It is recommended that there be minimal or no gap between the spine and cranial fields. The field junction may be shifted or "feathered" by 1 to 2 cm once or twice to avoid any excessive overlap of dose over the cervical spine. Some physicians prefer to place the beam isocenter at the inferior or caudad border of the initial craniocervical field so as to avoid the complexity of a couch rotation in the treatment setup. A gantry rotation to align the anterior beam divergence near the eye may still be performed. Other physicians place the isocenter near the eye to avoid divergence into the anterior globe, which can be done in conjunction with an appropriate couch rotation to match divergence with the posteroanterior spine field.

Maximum beam energy of 6 MV is recommended. Radiation doses for overt CNS leukemia are 18 to 30 Gy to the cranium in 1.5- to 1.8-Gy fractions. The authors recognize that it is increasingly rare that overt CNS leukemia for children or adults be treated with craniospinal fields, but there can be clinical circumstances where this may still be rationale. In such cases, along with the administration of IT chemotherapy, the spine may be treated to lower doses than the brain to total doses of 6 to 15 Gy depending on individual circumstances. Plans for possible TBI must be taken into account. This part of the preparative regimen for an allogeneic transplant can be conceptualized as being in part CNS therapy.

Testicular Irradiation

For the management of leukemic infiltration of the testes, both gonads and the scrotum can be irradiated with either electrons or photons. With the patient in a "frog-leg" position and the penile shaft taped onto the abdomen, an anterior inferior oblique photon field works well. Attention to the cremaster reflex and potential ascent of the testes into the inguinal canal is important so as to avoid a geographic miss. For megavoltage photon beams, bolus may be required to avoid superficial underdosing. In young boys where the scrotum/testes thickness is under 2 cm, 250-kV orthovoltage x-rays may also be used. Alternatively, direct en face electron beams of appropriate energy work adequately. Though there are considerable dose inhomogeneities in treating such a curved surface with electrons, the relatively low doses employed in this setting translates into relatively low risks related to skin and subcutaneous soft tissue reactions. Radiation doses typically used are 24 to 26 Gy in 1.5- to 2.0-Gy fractions. When a testicular boost is given in conjunction with TBI for a hematopoietic stem cell transplant, the dose is either 4 Gy × 1 fraction or 2 Gy × 2 fractions.

Splenic Irradiation

Massive splenomegaly may be seen with CML, CLL, hairy cell leukemia, and splenic marginal zone lymphomas where the spleen can extend into the pelvis. Significant splenomegaly may also occur with prolymphocytic leukemia, myeloproliferative disorders such as polycythemia vera or essential thrombocytosis, or myelofibrosis. One type of myelofibrosis called *agnogenic myeloid metaplasia* is characterized by progressive bone marrow failure, splenomegaly, and extramedullary hematopoiesis. It is therapeutically important to recognize which conditions of splenomegaly are due to extramedullary hematopoiesis rather than leukemic infiltration as whole spleen RT with modest radiation doses can result in severe, long-lasting pancytopenia when the spleen is the primary hematopoiesis site.[153] Splenic hematopoiesis can also occur with late stages of CML, myeloproliferative disorders, and hairy cell leukemia. Extreme care is required to proceed slowly with RT in these circumstances.

Historically, splenic RT was commonly employed for palliation, but it is now uncommon, as more effective systemic treatments have been developed. Nevertheless, the radiation oncologist is called on to assist with the management of symptomatic splenomegaly from these hematologic disorders from time to time, often with excellent results.[154] Symptomatic problems include pain, early satiety, diaphragmatic irritation, and bleeding risk related to sequestration of platelets. Leukemic infiltration of the spleen responds to relatively low doses of radiation.[155] Particularly in an elderly patient with other comorbidities, palliative splenic RT can offer significantly less risk than splenectomy.[156] Splenic irradiation has been reviewed by Weinmann et al.[157]

Anterior and posterior opposed portals for photon treatments are generally employed. In cases of leukemic infiltration, standard practice is to treat the whole spleen in 0.25- to 1.0-Gy fractions either daily or two to three times a week with doses titrated to response and hematologic tolerance.[158] As the spleen responds, one may progressively shrink the treatment fields accordingly. Generally, it is prudent to start treatment very conservatively. Blood counts may need to be monitored several times a week. Total radiation dose delivered is determined clinically by when palliation is achieved. Total doses are typically in the range of 4 to 10 Gy with usually no more than 20 Gy required. Occasionally, a large spleen that is extensively fibrotic will not response to RT. CLL and prolymphocytic leukemia are particularly radiosensitive, with occasional abscopal effects seen with splenic irradiation.

In patients with extramedullary hematopoiesis, the potential for severe neutropenia or thrombocytopenia is very high with even modest radiation doses. Dose per fraction may need to be as low as 0.1 to 0.5 Gy treating several times a week to avoid severe and protracted myelosuppression. Another strategy in this situation is to treat only half of the spleen. For myelodysplastic conditions or extramedullary/intrasplenic hematopoiesis, total doses of 1 to 9 Gy are usually adequate.

With splenic irradiation, nausea is uncommon with these low-dose fractions but can be readily managed with antiemetics if necessary. As there can be rapid cell lysis, allopurinol to prevent uric acid nephropathy is advised. Cumulative dose to the left kidney should be monitored, especially as retreatment in the future may be required, but it is rare for doses beyond 20 Gy to be required.

SEQUELAE OF THERAPY

Somnolence Syndrome

Approximately 1 month following cranial radiation, up to 40% to 50% of patients may develop lethargy, irritability, anorexia, and even fevers. This has been termed *somnolence syndrome.* It has been associated with electroencephalographic abnormalities and CSF pleocytosis.[159,160] This syndrome is self-limited and typically reverses within 1 to 3 weeks. Glucocorticoids in acute management may be helpful. Two reports suggest that the incidence of this syndrome is reduced if patients receive steroids during cranial RT.[161,162]

Pituitary Dysfunction

Hypothalamic-pituitary irradiation can impact endocrine function in a dose and age dependant manner. For the doses used in leukemia management, growth hormone (GH) deficiency is the most common abnormality observed. Age younger than 5 years at the time of RT is associated with particular susceptibility to the development of GH deficiency. Higher radiation doses as well as younger age correlate with an increased incidence of GH deficiency and a shorter time period for its clinical manifestations.[163] It is more common after 24 Gy than 18 Gy.[164,165] Up to 22% of adult survivors of pediatric ALL who have received cranial RT may have diminished GH responses to provocative testing.[166] Precocious puberty has been reported with radiation doses to the hypothalamic-pituitary region as low as 18 Gy, although it seems to be more prevalent in females who receive doses of 24 Gy or higher.[167] Doses <35 to 40 Gy are rarely associated with other pituitary hormone deficiencies or abnormalities. Thus, patients receiving cranial RT for leukemia, particularly in childhood, require regular follow-up of their linear growth and sexual development. Abnormalities should then lead to appropriate endocrinologic evaluation so as to determine the need for therapy with either GH replacement or gonadotropin-releasing hormone agonists.

Cognitive Dysfunction

Intellectual and psychological impairments from the treatment of leukemia have received wide attention. Evidence that RT is to blame has been a major impetus in investigations aimed at lowering the dose delivered to the brain or eliminating it completely. Increasingly, however, there is evidence that chemotherapy may also be causing similar detriments. Objective measures of cognitive function and social functioning are inherently difficult. Nevertheless, a variety of assessment tools, intelligence quotients, or scales have been verified as useful measures of language, reasoning, and performance skills. Other descriptive measures of lowered school achievement have also been reported. Cognitive dysfunction is thought to be the result of white matter injury causing deficits in the speed of information processing.[168] These effects are most pronounced in children younger than age 5 years and probably most pronounced in those younger than 3 years of age when the brain is still undergoing growth and development especially with myelinization.

Some reports have suggested a gender difference in susceptibility to radiation injury, with females more likely than males to develop intellectual impairments, although this has not been consistently reported.[169,170] The Dana Farber group has suggested that the reduction in IQ seen in girls was the result of an interaction between high-dose MTX and cranial radiation.[171] Moreover, an impairment in verbal memory observed in both boys and girls was independent of cranial radiation, suggesting toxicity from systemic therapy.[171]

A reduction in radiation dose from 24 Gy to 18 Gy has not consistently reported to result in a lower cognitive difficulties.[85,86,88] Further reduction to 12 Gy is under study. Overall, for these radiation doses, the cognitive deficits have been arguably small with average full-scale IQ measures decreasing by no more than 10%, while other studies fail to show measurable changes. Perhaps a more important statistic is the proportion of patients with significant reductions, say >15 points in IQ scales; the SJCRH group has reported that up to 22% to 30% of children have such deficits after 18 Gy, 24 Gy, or no cranial RT.[170] One hypothesis is that a component of cognitive difficulties is related to chemotherapy rather than RT. Regardless, a recent report from the Dana Farber group suggests that in high-risk ALL patients receiving 18-Gy cranial radiation, neurocognitive function many years after therapy is not significantly different from that of the general population.[90] Importantly, this was a group of patients who experienced a favorable 5-year disease-free survival of 75% with a 1% CNS relapse rate. The Dana Farber group has been investigating hyperfractionated cranial radiation for CNS prophylaxis (0.9 Gy twice daily versus 1.8 Gy daily to a total dose of 18 Gy). There are no obvious differences between standard or hyperfractionated RT in terms of late neurotoxicity reported thus far, although there are numerous methodological problems inherent in such a comparison.[90,91,92] An emerging experience suggests that stimulants such as methylphenidate may be of help in managing treatment-related cognitive problems, particularly some attentional or social deficits.[172]

Leukoencephalopathy

Some early prophylactic cranial radiation studies for childhood ALL showed an significant incidence of profound encephalopathy occurring months after irradiation.[108,173] The highest incidence was seen when cranial radiation with doses as low as 24 Gy were combined with IV MTX. Leukoencephalopathy is thought to represent a demyelinating condition that may be initiated by endothelial damage and a subsequent cytokine cascade with ischemic microinfarcts.[174] While concomitant IV MTX seems to be a significant synergistic factor, leukoencephalopathy has been observed at low incidence rates with RT alone at doses >30 to 35 Gy, with IT MTX, or in conjunction with other chemotherapy agents. High-dose chemotherapy alone is becoming increasingly recognized as causing similar dementialike syndromes. One should also remember that after cranial RT, the blood–brain barrier is thought to be more permeable, which may contribute to chemotherapy effects on cognitive function.[175] Regardless, the risk of leukoencephalopathy is decidedly rare after doses of <20 Gy.

Secondary Malignancies

One of the larger single institution series of pediatric ALL with extended follow-up of 2,169 patients from SJCRH treated between 1962 and 1998 reported that the cumulative incidence of secondary cancers were 4.2% and 10.9% at 15 and 30 years, respectively.[176] The incidence does not appear to plateau, although second malignancies occurring after 20 years tend to be lower-grade malignancies that include meningiomas and basal cell skin cancers. The Childhood Cancer Survivor Study (CCSG) has also documented an elevated risk for nonmelanoma skin cancers in pediatric ALL survivors, with a cumulative incidence of 10% at 30 years.[177] Cranial MRI surveillance imaging may also increase the detection of asymptomatic radiation associated meningiomas, estimated to have an incidence of 15% at 20 years and which may sometimes be multifocal.[178] Other secondary cancers attributable to RT include gliomas, parotid gland tumors, thyroid cancers, and sarcomas (bone and soft tissue).[176,179,180,181] The types of secondary brain tumors from RT tend to be evenly split between meningiomas and high-grade gliomas.[176] In an earlier report from the CCSG of 9,720 patients treated for ALL, 43 secondary cancers were observed after a mean follow-up of 6 years.[182] Of these, 24 were CNS tumors in patients who had previously received 24-Gy cranial RT. All but one of these patients with CNS tumors had been younger than 5 years of age at diagnosis of their acute leukemia, suggesting an age-related susceptibility. Additional data from the CCSG suggests that the risk of gliomas and meningiomas both have a linear radiation dose response relationship.[181,182] While there is hope that a reduction in cranial radiation doses to as low as 12 Gy may reduce the incidence of secondary tumors, the German BFM group has observed in the long-term follow-up of their ALL-BFM 90 trial a 3.4% actuarial incidence of secondary brain tumors at 16 years of follow-up.[93] In comparison, for those children with ALL not receiving cranial RT, the incidence of subsequent brain tumors was 1.2% at 15 years.[179] In a review of 3,182 children treated by an allogeneic bone marrow transplant, 25 solid tumors were observed compared to an expected incidence of one case.[183] A majority of these cancers originated in the CNS or thyroid gland. Moreover, most of these patients had received TBI as part of their preparative regimen before transplant.

Testicular Effects from RT

Gonadal dysfunction is quite rare from cranial RT for leukemia management unless patients undergo re-treatment that results in high cumulative doses. Direct effects from testicular irradiation, however, are very common. Doses as low as 1 Gy, even from scattered dose from adjacent external-beam fields, will cause transient oligospermia or azoospermia. Higher doses, particularly those used in TBI or therapeutic testicular radiation, would be expected to cause permanent infertility. Leydig cell function, on the other hand, is more radioresistent.[184] Low serum testosterone levels or delayed puberty are unusual with doses <29 Gy to the testes. One report of 60 male survivors of ALL showed significant germ cell dysfunction as manifested by increased FSH levels and testicular atrophy in 55% of patients treated with testicular RT and in 17% treated with craniospinal RT. The incidence of Leydig cell dysfunction was very low.[184]

SELECTED REFERENCES

A full list of references for this chapter is available online.

6. Halperin EC. Concerning the inferior portion of the spinal radiotherapy field for malignancies that disseminate via the cerebrospinal fluid. *Int J Radiat Oncol Biol Phys* 1993;26(2):357–362.
8. Dunbar SF, Barnes PD, Tarbell NJ. Radiologic determination of the caudal border of the spinal field in cranial spinal irradiation. *Int J Radiat Oncol Biol Phys* 1993;26(4):669–673.
11. Weiss E, Krebeck M, Kohler B, et al. Does the standardized helmet technique lead to adequate coverage of the cribriform plate? An analysis of current practice with respect to the ICRU 50 report. *Int J Radiat Oncol Biol Phys* 2001;49(5):1475–1480.
15. Pui CH. Childhood leukemias. *N Engl J Med* 1995;332(24):1618–1630.
16. Campo E, Swerdlow SH, Harris NL, et al. The 2008 WHO classification of lymphoid neoplasms and beyond: evolving concepts and practical applications. *Blood* 2011;117(19):5019–5032.
22. Borowitz MJ, Devidas M, Hunger SP, et al. Clinical significance of minimal residual disease in childhood acute lymphoblastic leukemia and its relationship to other prognostic factors: a Children's Oncology Group study. *Blood* 2008; 111(12):5477–5485.
32. Sanz MA, Lo-Coco F. Modern approaches to treating acute promyelocytic leukemia. *J Clin Oncol* 2011;29(5):495–503.
35. Fernandez HF. New trends in the standard of care for initial therapy of acute myeloid leukemia. *Hematology Am Soc Hematol Educ Program* 2010;2010:56–61.
36. Pollyea DA, Kohrt HE, Medeiros BC. Acute myeloid leukaemia in the elderly: a review. *Br J Haematol* 2011;152(5):524–542.
45. Paydas S, Zorludemir S, Ergin M. Granulocytic sarcoma: 32 cases and review of the literature. *Leuk Lymphoma* 2006;47(12):2527–2541.
49. Tsimberidou AM, Kantarjian HM, Wen S, et al. Myeloid sarcoma is associated with superior event-free survival and overall survival compared with acute myeloid leukemia. *Cancer* 2008;113(6):1370–1378.
51. Pui CH, Campana D, Pei D, et al. Treating childhood acute lymphoblastic leukemia without cranial irradiation. *N Engl J Med* 2009;360(26):2730–2741.
56. Schorin MA, Blattner S, Gelber RD, et al. Treatment of childhood acute lymphoblastic leukemia: results of Dana-Farber Cancer Institute/Children's Hospital Acute Lymphoblastic Leukemia Consortium Protocol 85-01. *J Clin Oncol* 1994;12(4): 740–747.
57. Reiter A, Schrappe M, Ludwig WD, et al. Chemotherapy in 998 unselected childhood acute lymphoblastic leukemia patients. Results and conclusions of the multicenter trial ALL-BFM 86. *Blood* 1994;84(9):3122–3133.
58. Schrappe M, Reiter A, Ludwig WD, et al. Improved outcome in childhood acute lymphoblastic leukemia despite reduced use of anthracyclines and cranial radiotherapy: results of trial ALL-BFM 90. German-Austrian-Swiss ALL-BFM Study Group. *Blood* 2000;95(11):3310–3322.
74. Buhrer C, Henze G, Hofmann J, et al. Central nervous system relapse prevention in 1165 standard-risk children with acute lymphoblastic leukemia in five BFM trials. *Hamatol Bluttransfus* 1990;33:500–503.
76. Clarke M, Gaynon P, Hann I, et al. CNS-directed therapy for childhood acute lymphoblastic leukemia: Childhood ALL Collaborative Group overview of 43 randomized trials. *J Clin Oncol* 2003;21(9):1798–1809.
78. Schrappe M, Reiter A, Henze G, et al. Prevention of CNS recurrence in childhood ALL: results with reduced radiotherapy combined with CNS-directed chemotherapy in four consecutive ALL-BFM trials. *Klin Padiatr* 1998;210(4):192–199.
83. Laver JH, Barredo JC, Amylon M, et al. Effects of cranial radiation in children with high risk T cell acute lymphoblastic leukemia: a Pediatric Oncology Group report. *Leukemia* 2000;14(3):369–373.
84. Nesbit ME Jr, Sather HN, Robison LL, et al. Presymptomatic central nervous system therapy in previously untreated childhood acute lymphoblastic leukaemia: comparison of 1800 rad and 2400 rad. A report for Children's Cancer Study Group. *Lancet* 1981;1(8218):461–466.
89. Larson RA, Dodge RK, Burns CP, et al. A five-drug remission induction regimen with intensive consolidation for adults with acute lymphoblastic leukemia: cancer and leukemia group B study 8811. *Blood* 1995;85(8):2025–2037.
90. Waber DP, Shapiro BL, Carpentieri SC, et al. Excellent therapeutic efficacy and minimal late neurotoxicity in children treated with 18 grays of cranial radiation therapy for high-risk acute lymphoblastic leukemia: a 7-year follow-up study of the Dana-Farber Cancer Institute Consortium Protocol 87-01. *Cancer* 2001;92(1):15–22.
92. Waber DP, Turek J, Catania L, et al. Neuropsychological Outcomes From a Randomized Trial of Triple Intrathecal Chemotherapy Compared With 18 Gy Cranial Radiation As CNS Treatment in Acute Lymphoblastic Leukemia: Findings From Dana-Farber Cancer Institute ALL Consortium Protocol 95-01. *J Clin Oncol* 2007;25(31):4914–4921.
93. Möricke A, Reiter A, Zimmermann M, et al. Risk-adjusted therapy of acute lymphoblastic leukemia can decrease treatment burden and improve survival: Treatment results of 2169 unselected pediatric and adolescent patients enrolled in the trial ALL-BFM 95. *Blood* 2008;111(9):4477–4489.
94. Cherlow JM, Sather H, Steinherz P, et al. Craniospinal irradiation for acute lymphoblastic leukemia with central nervous system disease at diagnosis: a report from the Children's Cancer Group. *Int J Radiat Oncol Biol Phys* 1996;36(1):19–27.
106. Ribeiro RC, Rivera GK, Hudson M, et al. An intensive re-treatment protocol for children with an isolated CNS relapse of acute lymphoblastic leukemia. *J Clin Oncol* 1995;13(2):333–338.
124. O'Brien SG, Guilhot F, Larson RA, et al. Imatinib compared with interferon and low-dose cytarabine for newly diagnosed chronic-phase chronic myeloid leukemia. *N Engl J Med* 2003;348(11):994–1004.
125. Druker BJ, Talpaz M, Resta DJ, et al. Efficacy and safety of a specific inhibitor of the BCR-ABL tyrosine kinase in chronic myeloid leukemia. *N Engl J Med* 2001; 344(14):1031–1037.
126. Druker BJ, Sawyers CL, Kantarjian H, et al. Activity of a specific inhibitor of the BCR-ABL tyrosine kinase in the blast crisis of chronic myeloid leukemia and acute lymphoblastic leukemia with the Philadelphia chromosome. *N Engl J Med* 2001;344(14):1038–1042.
138. Furman RR. Prognostic markers and stratification of chronic lymphocytic leukemia. *Hematology Am Soc Hematol Educ Program* 2010;2010:77–81.
140. Cheson BD, Bennett JM, Grever M, et al. National Cancer Institute-sponsored Working Group guidelines for chronic lymphocytic leukemia: revised guidelines for diagnosis and treatment. *Blood* 1996;87(12):4990–4997.
144. Rai KR, Peterson BL, Applebaum FR, et al. Long-term survival analysis of the North American Intergroup Study C9011 comparing fludarabine and chlorambucil in previously untreated patients with chronic lymphocytic leukemia (CLL). *Blood* 2009;114:224.
145. Tam CS, O'Brien S, Wierda W, et al. Long-term results of the fludarabine, cyclophosphamide, and rituximab regimen as initial therapy of chronic lymphocytic leukemia. *Blood* 2008;112(4):975–980.
149. Sorror ML, Storer BE, Sandmaier BM, et al. Five-year follow-up of patients with advanced chronic lymphocytic leukemia treated with allogeneic hematopoietic cell transplantation after nonmyeloablative conditioning. *J Clin Oncol* 2008; 26(30):4912–4920.
150. Dreger P, Corradini P, Kimby E, et al. Indications for allogeneic stem cell transplantation in chronic lymphocytic leukemia: the EBMT transplant consensus. *Leukemia* 2007;21(1):12–17.
151. Hallek M. State-of-the-art treatment of chronic lymphocytic leukemia. *Hematology Am Soc Hematol Educ Program* 2009;2009(1):440–449.
154. Kriz J, Micke O, Bruns F, et al. Radiotherapy of splenomegaly : a palliative treatment option for a benign phenomenon in malignant diseases. *Strahlenther Onkol* 2011;187(4):221–224.
157. Weinmann M, Becker G, Einsele H, et al. Clinical indications and biological mechanisms of splenic irradiation in chronic leukaemias and myeloproliferative disorders. *Radiother Oncol* 2001;58(3):235–246.
165. Stubberfield TG, Byrne GC, Jones TW. Growth and growth hormone secretion after treatment for acute lymphoblastic leukemia in childhood. 18-Gy versus 24-Gy cranial irradiation. *J Pediatr Hematol Oncol* 1995;17(2):167–171.
170. Mulhern RK, Fairclough D, Ochs J. A prospective comparison of neuropsychologic performance of children surviving leukemia who received 18-Gy, 24-Gy, or no cranial irradiation. *J Clin Oncol* 1991;9(8):1348–1356.
171. Waber DP, Tarbell NJ, Fairclough D, et al. Cognitive sequelae of treatment in childhood acute lymphoblastic leukemia: cranial radiation requires an accomplice. *J Clin Oncol* 1995;13(10):2490–2496.
176. Hijiya N, Hudson MM, Lensing S, et al. Cumulative incidence of secondary neoplasms as a first event after childhood acute lymphoblastic leukemia. *JAMA* 2007;297(11):1207–1215.
177. Friedman DL, Whitton J, Leisenring W, et al. Subsequent neoplasms in 5-year survivors of childhood cancer: the Childhood Cancer Survivor Study. *J Natl Cancer Inst* 2010;102(14):1083–1095.
178. Goshen Y, Stark B, Kornreich L, et al. High incidence of meningioma in cranial irradiated survivors of childhood acute lymphoblastic leukemia. *Pediatr Blood Cancer* 2007;49(3):294–297.
180. Mody R, Li S, Dover DC, et al. Twenty-five-year follow-up among survivors of childhood acute lymphoblastic leukemia: a report from the Childhood Cancer Survivor Study. *Blood* 2008;111(12):5515–5523.

Chapter 81
Plasma Cell Myeloma and Plasmacytoma

David C. Hodgson, Joseph Mikhael, and Richard W. Tsang

EPIDEMIOLOGY AND ETIOLOGY

Plasma cell neoplasms account for 22% of all mature B-cell neoplasms in the Surveillance, Epidemiology, and End Results (SEER) program of the United States.[1] The majority of plasma cell neoplasms are multiple myeloma, with solitary plasmacytoma accounting for ≤6% of cases, and plasma cell leukemia rarely. Although the incidence of multiple myeloma gradually increased in the 1970s through 1990s, recently there has been a plateau in the U.S. incidence from 1992 to 2008.[2] Data from SEER indicate an incidence in the United States of 7.2 per 100,000 men per year and 4.6 per 100,000 women during the period 2004 to 2008,[2] and for 2011, it is estimated that there will be 20,520 new cases and 10,610 deaths due to multiple myeloma in the United States.[3] The incidence exceeds that of Hodgkin lymphoma and is about one-quarter that of non-Hodgkin lymphoma. The incidence rises with advancing age, with a median age at diagnosis of 70 years,[4] and <1% of cases are diagnosed in those younger than 35. Nonregistry studies usually report a lower median age ranging from 60 to 66 years.[5,6] There is a slight male predominance, and for black Americans, the incidence and mortality rates are approximately double that for whites. The 5-year relative survival rates have increased, from 26% in 1975 to 40% in 2003.[2]

Little is known about the cause of multiple myeloma. There are studies reporting association with prior exposure to radiation (e.g., atomic bomb survivors in Hiroshima)[7] and certain chemicals such as petroleum products.[8,9] It is now thought that all cases of myeloma are preceded by monoclonal gammopathy of unknown significance (MGUS).[10,11,12]

PATHOPHYSIOLOGY

Multiple myeloma arises from malignant transformation of a late-state B cell. Although the full cascade of genetic abnormalities has yet to be defined, one of the earliest genetic events is the illegitimate switch recombination of partner oncogenes into the immunoglobulin heavy chain (IgH).[13] Other events may occur such as cytogenetic hyperploidy and up-regulation of cell cycle control genes. The result of these genetic abnormalities is the development and propagation of a clonal population of B cells within the bone marrow; this, however, is common and can be seen in up to 5% of the general population over the age of 70 (MGUS).[14] Most of these will not go on to develop myeloma, so there must be additional events to create the malignant phenotype of multiple myeloma. These secondary events may include mutations of kinases, deletions of chromosomes, and up-regulation of enzymes such as c-myc.[15] Having sustained a secondary event, the malignant plasma cells begin to proliferate in the bone marrow microenvironment, producing monoclonal proteins and causing osteolytic bone disease. The slow accumulation of these malignant cells gradually results in the characteristic clinical features of myeloma: anemia, bone resorption, hypercalcemia, renal failure, and immunodeficiency. Established myeloma is sustained by a number of microenvironment features, including the bone marrow stroma itself and the cytokines interleukin-6 and insulin-like growth factor-1.[16] The bone disease that arises in myeloma appears to be mediated in part by Rank ligand/osteprotegrin and the Wnt signaling antagonist Dickkopf1.[17]

CLINICAL PRESENTATION

Multiple myeloma has a wide clinical spectrum, ranging from the preclinical condition of MGUS to the most aggressive form, plasma cell leukemia (Table 81.1). In all cases, a plasma cell clone exists, and the secretion of a monoclonal protein by these plasma cells, along with their interaction with the bone marrow environment, is the source of organ damage in patients with this illness.[16] These concepts have become particularly important as the molecular mechanisms by which the disease progresses through these "stages" provide essential information that may help us to better understand the disease and its potential therapies.

Monoclonal Gammopathy of Unknown Significance

MGUS has traditionally been considered a benign or a premalignant condition, in which only a small proportion of patients will progress to multiple myeloma or related diseases (Table 81.1). In MGUS, the monoclonal protein is <3 g/dL and the bone marrow clonal plasma cells are <10% with no related organ damage. This condition is likely much more common than initially thought, as it has been documented in 3% of the population and 5% in those over the age of 70.[14] The risk of transformation to myeloma and related diseases (such as amyloidosis or Waldenstrom's macroglobulinemia) has been estimated at 1% per year, based on a 30-year follow-up of 1,384 patients at the Mayo Clinic.[10]

Asymptomatic Multiple Myeloma (Smoldering Myeloma)

This category of myeloma represents an intermediate form of myeloma whereby patients do meet serological monoclonal protein and bone marrow criteria for the diagnosis of myeloma

TABLE 81.1 THE SPECTRUM OF MYELOMA

	MGUS	Asymptomatic Multiple Myeloma	Symptomatic Multiple Myeloma	Plasma Cell Leukemia
Clinical	No organ damage	No organ damage	Organ damage[a]	Organ damage
Marrow disease	<10% plasma cells	>10% plasmacytosis	>10% plasmacytosis	Plasma cells in peripheral blood
Management	Monitor	Close follow-up	Chemotherapy	High-dose chemotherapy
Transformation rate	1% per year	20% per year	–	–

MGUS, monoclonal gammopathy of unknown significance.

[a]Organ damage definition: hypercalcemia (corrected calcium >2.75 mmol/L); renal insufficiency attributable to myeloma; anemia (hemoglobin <10 g/dL); bone lesions (lytic lesions or osteoporosis with compression fractures (from ref. 27).

Clinical Radiation Oncology

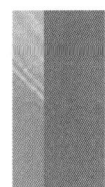

(in excess of 10% clonal plasmacytosis) but have yet to develop evidence of end organ damage (Table 81.1). These patients are not significantly anemic, do not have renal insufficiency, and do not have bony disease. Although the risk of transformation to multiple myeloma is much higher than in MGUS (20% per year), some patients' disease may remain asymptomatic without significant progression for many years. These patients generally do not require therapy but should be followed closely to monitor for progression.

Solitary Plasmacytomas

The median age at diagnosis of solitary plasmacytoma (SP) is 55 to 65 years, on average about 10 years younger than patients with multiple myeloma.[18,19–20] Males are affected predominately (male-to-female ratio 2:1).[18] A diagnosis of SP is made if all the following criteria are satisfied at presentation: a histologically confirmed single lesion with negative skeletal imaging outside the primary site, normal bone marrow biopsy (<10% monoclonal plasma cells), and no myeloma-related organ dysfunction.[21] A monoclonal protein is present in 30% to 75% of cases (particularly for an osseous presentation), and the level is usually minimally elevated (IgG <3.5 g/dL, IgA <2.0 g/dL, and urine monoclonal κ or λ <1.0 g/24 hours).[21,22]

The disease more commonly presents in bone (80%). Such cases are considered stage I multiple myeloma according to the Durie Salmon staging system.[23] The most common location is the vertebra.[18] Patients with bone involvement often present with pain, neurologic compromise, and occasionally pathologic fracture. A lytic lesion is typical, with or without adjacent soft tissue mass. Less commonly, SP presents in an extramedullary site (20%), usually as a mass in the upper aerorespiratory passages, and produces local compressive symptoms.[18,19,24,25] The histologic diagnosis of extramedullary plasmacytoma (EMP) can be difficult, with the main differential diagnosis being extranodal marginal zone lymphoma (mucosa-associated lymphoid tissue type), where there can be extensive infiltration by plasmacytoid cells.[24,26]

Multiple Myeloma

By definition, myeloma involves end organ damage, described by the mnemonic CRAB (*C*alcium elevation, *R*enal insufficiency, *A*nemia, and *B*one disease).[27] Bone pain and symptoms due to anemia, such as easy fatigability, are the most common.[5] Because of the myriad effects of the disease, other insidious symptoms can result from a combination of hypercalcemia, renal impairment, infection, neurologic compression, and occasionally, hyperviscosity. Bone disease manifesting as generalized osteopenia and multiple lytic bone lesions can frequently lead to pathologic fractures. In the vertebral column, this often results in a diminished height. Sclerotic lesions at presentation are rare.

Laboratory evaluation generally confirms anemia, high erythrocyte sedimentation rate, and a variable degree of granulocytopenia and thrombocytopenia. An abnormal monoclonal immunoglobulin (M protein) in the blood or urine is characteristic,[5] most commonly IgG or IgA. Biclonal disease is also recognized, and rarely, nonsecretory disease. In up to 10% of cases, only monoclonal light chains are detected. It is important to assess for hypercalcemia, renal dysfunction, and integrity of the skeleton because these complications require appropriate management. A constellation of polyneuropathy, organomegaly, endocrinopathy, M protein, and skin changes characterize a rare plasma cell dyscrasia known as POEMS syndrome.[28]

Plasma Cell Leukemia

This is a very rare variant of multiple myeloma, where the proliferation of plasma cells is not confined to the bone marrow but may be detected in the peripheral blood. It carries a very poor prognosis, with median survival <1 year and shortest when occurring as secondary plasma cell leukemia.[29,30] There is currently no standard therapy for this condition, but patients are usually treated with high-dose, multiagent chemotherapeutic regimens or with experimental therapies.

TABLE 81.2 DIAGNOSTIC WORKUP FOR PLASMA CELL NEOPLASMS

General
History and physical examination
Complete blood count and blood smear, chemistry panel including calcium and creatinine

Standard Laboratory Tests
Bone marrow aspirate and trephine biopsy, or biopsy of mass if solitary lesion (clonality, immunophenotype and cytogenetic studies (both conventional cytogenetics and fluorescence *in situ* hybridization), plasma cell labeling index)
Serum β_2 microglobulin, albumin, C-reactive protein, and lactate dehydrogenase
M-component measurement:

- serum protein electrophoresis, and immunofixation for quantification of immunoglobulins
- Urine protein electrophoresis
- Free light chain measurements if conventional M-component is negative or equivocal (serum and urine)

Imaging Studies
Skeletal survey
Computed tomography and magnetic resonance imaging where indicated (e.g., to visualize soft tissue tumor, detailed assessment of local disease extent and bulk, assessing vertebral column osteopenia and compression fractures, and spinal cord compression)
Fluorine-18 fluorodeoxyglucose positron emission tomography or magnetic resonance imaging may be ordered to detect occult disease if clinically indicated

DIAGNOSTIC WORKUP AND STAGING

The recommended tests for the diagnosis of plasma cell neoplasms are outlined in Table 81.2. The most important components relate to the measurement and quantification of the M protein, bone marrow examination with ancillary studies, serum β_2 microglobulin and albumin, and diagnostic imaging. The M protein should be measured with serum protein electrophoresis. Quantification of the monoclonal Ig with immunofixation techniques is also acceptable and especially useful if the M component is at a low level. If no M protein is detectable, assays for free light chains should be performed in the serum and in the urine (Bence-Jones proteinuria). The standard imaging is the skeletal survey, as radionuclide bone scan usually does not detect lytic disease and has limited value.[21] For localized areas of concern, both computed tomography (CT) or magnetic resonance imaging (MRI) should be liberally utilized. MRI is preferred to assess the extent of vertebral disease and the presence of spinal cord or nerve root compression. With advances in diagnostic imaging, it is likely that "stage migration" has occurred.[31] It has been documented that some patients with presumed solitary plasmacytoma of bone will be upstaged following the detection of multiple vertebral lesions or bone marrow disease by MRI or by 18-fluorine (^{18}F) fluorodeoxyglucose positron emission tomography (FDG-PET).[32,33–34] The optimal role of PET in myeloma is yet to be determined but will likely evolve rapidly, and it will likely be of most benefit in nonsecretory disease.[35,36–37] The staging criteria for the historical Durie Salmon staging system are detailed in Table 81.3.[23] The newer International Myeloma Staging System (ISS) is simple, validated, and of importance particularly for present and future clinical trials (Table 81.3).[6] Criteria for the diagnosis of MGUS and asymptomatic (smoldering) myeloma are also well established.[21,30]

PROGNOSTIC FACTORS

Solitary Plasmacytoma

With respect to local control, tumor bulk appears to be an important unfavorable factor. Tumors <5 cm achieved a high

TABLE 81.3 STAGING OF MULTIPLE MYELOMA (DURIE SALMON AND THE NEW INTERNATIONAL STAGING SYSTEM)

Clinical Stage	Durie and Salmon Staging System (from Ref. 23)	
Stage I	All of the following: • Hemoglobin >10 g/dL • Serum calcium normal • Normal bone structure or solitary plasmacytoma only • Low M-component (IgG <5 g/dL, IgA <3 g/dL, urine light chains <4 g/24 hours)[a]	
Stage II	Fitting neither stage I nor stage III	
Stage III	One or more of the following: • Hemoglobin <8.5 g/dL • Serum calcium >12 mg/dL • Advanced lytic bone lesions • High M-component (IgG >7 g/dL, IgA >3 g/dL, urine light chains >12 g/24 hours)	
Subclassified:		
A	Relatively normal renal function (serum creatinine <2 mg/dL)	
B	Abnormal renal function (serum creatinine ≥2 mg/dL)	
	International Staging System (ISS; from Ref. 6)	*Median Survival*
Stage I	Serum β_2 microglobulin <3.5 mg/L, and Serum albumin >35 g/L	62 months
Stage II	Neither I nor III i.e., β_2 microglobulin <3.5 mg/L, with albumin <35 g/L, or β_2 microglobulin 3.5 to 5.5 mg/L	44 months
Stage III	Serum β_2 microglobulin >5.5 mg/L	29 months

Ig, immunoglobulin.

[a]For solitary plasmacytoma, current recommendations are IgG <3.5 g/dL, IgA <2 g/dL.

level of local control with 35 Gy, whereas those ≥5 cm had a local failure rate of 58% (7 of 12 patients, total dose range 25 to 50 Gy).[20] The importance of tumor bulk is also supported by other studies.[18,39,40]

Age is a factor that affects the risk of progression to myeloma in some series[20,41,42–43] but not in others.[18,39,40,44,45] A bony presentation has been consistently demonstrated to have a significantly higher risk of subsequent development of myeloma with a 10-year rate of 76%, compared with an extramedullary presentation where the 10-year rate was 36% (Fig. 81.1).[18] Subclinical bone disease, either detected as generalized osteopenia[46] or abnormal MRI scan of the spine,[33,34,47] predicts for rapid progression to symptomatic multiple myeloma. A suppression of the normal immunoglobulin classes has been shown to correlate with a higher risk of progressing to myeloma.[46,48] Where there was an elevation of M protein pretreatment, persistence of the M protein following radiation therapy (RT) predicts for progression to myeloma.[22,32] Many of these factors reflect the presence of occult myeloma. Therefore, it is not surprising that generalized disease becomes manifest once the local disease is controlled. Pathologic factors have been examined in some studies, with the finding that anaplastic plasmacytomas (those with a higher histologic grade)[49] and those tumors expressing a high level of angiogenesis are associated with a poor outcome.[50] Anaplastic plasmacytomas share some common pathologic and clinical features with aggressive B-cell lymphomas (plasmablastic type) and can arise in the context of immunosuppression and Epstein-Barr virus infection.[51,52]

Multiple Myeloma

Analysis of over 1,000 patients evaluated at the Mayo Clinic revealed the following adverse prognostic risk factors: Eastern Cooperative Oncology Group performance status 3 or 4, serum albumin <3 g/dL, serum creatinine ≥2 mg/dL, platelet count <150,000/μL, age ≥70 years, β_2 microglobulin >4 mg/L, plasma cell labeling index ≥1%, serum calcium ≥11 mg/dL, hemoglobin <10 g/dL, and bone marrow plasma cell percentage ≥50%.[5] The ISS has been validated to assist in prognostication.[6] Over 10,000 patients were evaluated, and the three-stage system was developed based on two variables: serum albumin and β_2 microglobulin (Table 81.3). In addition to stage, cytogenetic abnormalities affect prognosis. Some abnormalities demonstrated to carry a poorer prognosis include: deletion of chromosome 13,[53] presence of the t(4;14) translocation,[54] and p53 deletion.[55] Risk stratification by means of conventional cytogenetics and fluorescence *in situ* hybridization not only influences prognosis but now also affects therapeutic choices.[56]

MANAGEMENT OF SOLITARY PLASMACYTOMA

RT is the standard treatment for solitary plasmacytoma. Surgery should be considered for structural instability of bone or rapidly progressive neurologic compromise such as spinal cord compression.[21,57,58] For patients treated with gross tumor excision, RT is still indicated due to a high likelihood of microscopic residual disease. Surgery alone without RT leads to an unacceptably high local recurrence rate.[18] A review of the literature for solitary bone plasmacytoma (Table 81.4) indicates a high local control rate with RT (79% to 95%), yet a modest overall survival of approximately 50% at 10 years. This is due to

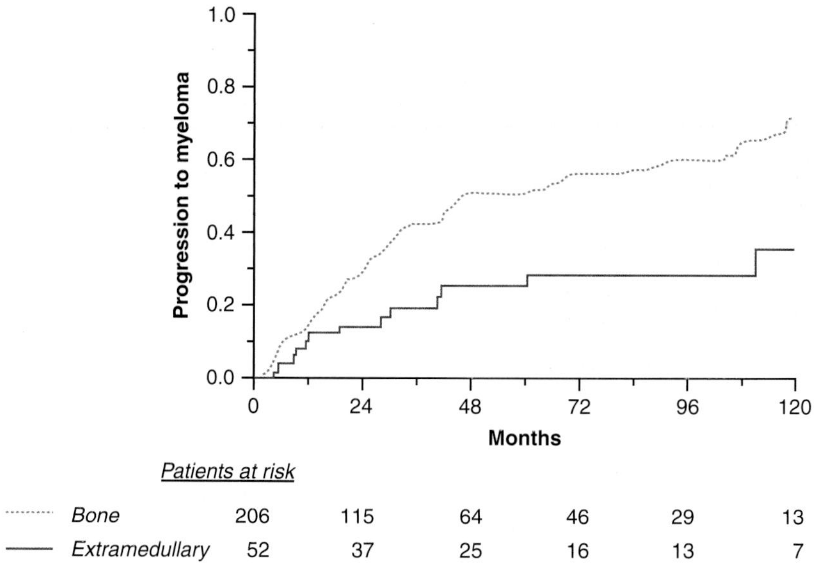

FIGURE 81.1. Probability of progression to multiple myeloma according to bone (*dotted line*) versus extramedullary (*solid line*) solitary plasmacytoma in 258 patients (*P* = .0009). (From Ozsahin M, Tsang RW, Poortmans P, et al. Outcomes and patterns of failure in solitary plasmacytoma: a multicenter Rare Cancer Network study of 258 patients. *Int J Radiat Oncol Biol Phys* 2006;64(1):210–217, copyright 2006, with permission from Elsevier.)

TABLE 81.4 SOLITARY PLASMACYTOMA OF BONE: REPRESENTATIVE TREATMENT RESULTS (SERIES INCLUDING MORE THAN 30 PATIENTS)

Study (Reference)	*Institution*	*Number of Patients (Median f/u)*	*Local Control (%)*	*Progression to Myeloma (10-Year Rate %)*	*Overall Survival (10-Year Rate %)*
Bataille and Sany 1981 (41)	Hospital St. Eloi, France	114 (>10 year)	88	58	68[a]
Chak et al. 1987 (42)	Stanford[b]	65[b] (87 months)	95	77	52
Frassica et al. 1989 (59)	Mayo Clinic	46 (90 months)	89	54[a]	45
Jackson and Scarffe 1990 (48)	Christie Hospital	32 (101 months)	97[a]	~76	~45
Holland et al. 1992 (40)	Mallinckrodt	32 (66 months)	94	53[a]	–
Galieni et al. 1995 (46,68)	Siena, Italy[b]	32[b] (69 months)	91[a]	~68	49
Tsang et al. 2001 (20)	Princess Margaret Hospital	32 (95 months)	87	64 (8-year rate)	65 (8-year rate)
Wilder et al. 2002 (22)	MD Anderson Cancer Center	60 (94 months)	90	62	59
Ozsahin et al. 2006 (18)	RARE Cancer Network[b]	206[b] (56 months)	79 (10-year rate)	72	52

[a]Crude rate.
[b]Multiple institutions.

a high rate of progression to multiple myeloma in the bone plasmacytomas, a finding consistently reported from all series.[18,20,22,40–41,42,46,48,59,60] As shown in Table 81.4, over 60% of patients with solitary bone tumor progressed to myeloma, at a median of 2 to 3 years after treatment. When actuarial methods were not used, the progression rate is slightly lower (crude rates ranges, 53% to 54%).[40,59] Therefore, solitary plasmacytoma of bone appears to be an early form of multiple myeloma. Studies have documented about 29% to 50% of patients with apparent solitary plasmacytoma will have multiple asymptomatic lesions detected in the spine on MRI.[33,34,61] Provided that all the other diagnostic criteria for solitary plasmacytoma are satisfied, it is still appropriate to treat with local RT to the presenting site.[57] For these patients the risk of developing symptomatic myeloma in a short time is high.[33,34,47,62] Chemotherapy can be started at the time of symptomatic progression. The presence of low level M protein preradiation is extremely common and is not associated with a higher risk of progression to multiple myeloma. However, its persistence following radiation is highly predictive of subsequent systemic failure,[22,32,46,63] attesting to the importance of monitoring this as part of posttreatment follow-up. It has been observed that some patients recur with plasmacytoma(s) of bone or soft tissues, without bone marrow involvement.[40,41,64] This is infrequent and the subsequent development of multiple myeloma is high, 75% in one series.[41]

The addition of adjuvant chemotherapy is theoretically attractive, both in enhancing local control and eradicating subclinical disease to prevent the development of myeloma. One randomized trial suggested a benefit with adjuvant melphalan and prednisone given for 3 years after RT.[65] With a median follow-up of 8.9 years, those treated with chemotherapy had a myeloma progression rate of 12%, whereas with RT alone it was 54%. However, this was a small study, and the risk of diminishing stem cell reserve or inducing leukemia makes the prolonged use of alkylating agents an undesirable treatment option for most patients.

In the management of EMP, while complete surgical excision may be curative for small lesions, most patients with larger lesions or with tumor location not amenable to complete excision should receive local RT. Postoperative RT is indicated for incompletely excised lesions. In contrast to bone plasmacytoma, EMPs are frequently controlled with local radiation (Table 81.5), with a lower rate of progression to myeloma, ranging from 8% to 44%,[18,19,25,49,64,66,67–68,69–73] indicating a significant proportion of patients are cured of their disease. Although the 10-year survival varies widely in the reported literature (range, 31% to 90%), the two largest series report 10-year survival rates of 72%[18] and 78%.[68] The issue of dose will be discussed later.

Initial Treatment of Symptomatic Multiple Myeloma

Patients who have symptomatic multiple myeloma require treatment of the malignant plasma cell clone. Once the decision

TABLE 81.5 SOLITARY EXTRAMEDULLARY PLASMACYTOMA: REPRESENTATIVE TREATMENT RESULTS (SERIES INCLUDING MORE THAN 15 PATIENTS)

Study (Reference)	*Number of Patients (Median f/u)*	*Local Control (%)*	*Progression to Myeloma (10-Year Rate %)*	*Overall Survival (10-Year Rate %)*
Kapadia et al. 1982 (70)	17 (62 mo)	85	31[a]	31[a] (5-yr)
Knowling et al. 1983 (64)	25 (71 mo)	88	28	43
Brinch et al. 1990 (66)	18	–	–	90
Soeson et al. 1992 (71)	25 (44 mo)	88	–	~50
Susnerwala et al. 1997 (49)	25 (73 mo)	79	8[a]	59 (5-yr)
Liebross et al. 1999 (67)	22	95	44 (5-yr)	50
Galieni et al. 2000 (68)	46[b] (118 mo)	92	15[a]	78 (15-yr)
Strojan et al. 2002 (19)	26 (61 mo)	87	8	61
Chao et al. 2005 (69)	16 (66 mo)	100	31	54
Ozsahin et al. 2006 (18)	52[b] (56 mo)	74 (10-yr)	36	72
Tournier-Rangeard et al. 2006 (25)	17 (80.5 mo)	73 (10-yr)	36	63
Bachar et al. 2008 (73)	56 (96 mo)	88 (10-yr)	28 (10-yr)	56 (10-yr)

[a]Crude rate.
[b]Multiple institutions.

is made to treat, however, the first step is to determine candidacy for autologous stem cell transplantation (ASCT). As this modality has become the standard of care for eligible patients, it is necessary to stratify patients initially so that the ability to collect stem cells is not compromised by induction therapy.[74]

Patients Eligible for Autologous Stem Cell Transplantation

In patients who are candidates for ASCT, various regimens can be used to induce response prior to stem cell collection. Historically, most regimens were steroid based, either with high-dose dexamethasone alone[75] or with vincristine, Adriamycin (doxorubicin), and dexamethasone (VAD).[76] Newer agents that have been validated in the relapse setting are now being used as initial therapy with superior results, including bortezomib and lenalidomide. Both have recently been established into initial treatment or for relapsed disease.

Bortezomib

Bortezomib was the first proteasome inhibitor to be used in clinical trials and has demonstrated efficacy and safety in frontline therapy when used in combination. Indeed, response rates have dramatically improved when compared with VAD or dexamethasone alone. A randomized comparison of bortezomib plus dexamethasone (BD) versus VAD as induction therapy before ASCT showed that BD produced superior complete response or near complete response: 14.8% versus 6.4%, at least very good partial response: 37.7% versus 15.1%, and overall response (78.5% vs. 62.8%) than VAD. Median progression-free survival was 36.0 months (BD) versus 29.7 months (VAD; $P = .064$).[77] Even as a single agent, with dexamethasone or with doxorubicin, bortezomib has remarkable efficacy and safety in initial therapy.[78,79] It is often the preferred agent in patients with renal insufficiency and high-risk disease. Its greatest challenge, however, remains neuropathy, occurring in 13% to 15% of patients at ≥grade 3; this may be reduced, however, with weekly use[80] or when given subcutaneously.[81]

Lenalidomide

Lenalidomide is an immunomodulatory drug derived from thalidomide that has also been shown to be effective, both as upfront therapy and in relapsed disease. It is most commonly used in combination with low-dose dexamethasone.[82] A phase III trial of lenalidomide with low-dose dexamethasone versus lenalidomide with high-dose dexamethasone found that despite a higher rate of complete or partial response with high-dose therapy, overall 1-year survival was 87% in the high-dose group versus 96% in the low-dose group ($P = .0002$), largely due to the significant toxicity of the former. As a result, the trial was stopped and patients on high-dose therapy were crossed over to low-dose therapy. Three-year overall survival rates now exceed 85%. This has resulted in the extensive use of this combination in upfront myeloma.[82]

Lenalidomide has also been used in combination with conventional chemotherapy and most recently with bortezomib.[83] This has resulted in even higher response rates and complete remission rates of >50%.

Thalidomide

An alternative to VAD induction is the combination of thalidomide and dexamethasone (TD). Early reports indicate that this combination yields a response rate of 64% (similar to VAD), without compromising the ability to collect stem cells, but with a rate of deep vein thrombosis of 12%.[84] The Medical Research Council Myeloma IX trial compared cyclophosphamide-thalidomide-dexamethasone (CTD) with cyclophosphamide-VAD as induction before ASCT. In a preliminary analysis, the complete response rate was 20.3% after CTD and 11.7% after cyclophosphamide-VAD.[85]

In a randomized trial of 480 patients, Cavo et al.[86] reported that the addition of bortezomib to TD prior to tandem autologous stem cell transplant increased the complete or near-complete response rate to 31% versus 11% without bortezomib.

In summary, preferred initial regimens include bortezomib or lenalidomide, but alternatives include thalidomide or doxorubicin prior to ASCT.

Patients Not Eligible for Autologous Stem Cell Transplantation

In patients who will not be undergoing a transplant, there are various options available for initial therapy. Historically, most transplant-ineligible patients received melphalan and prednisone (MP), which produced partial remissions in approximately 55% of patients, with the occasional complete response.[87] San Miguel et al.[88] reported the results of a randomized trial of 682 patients randomized to receive either 9 6-week cycles of MP or the same chemotherapy with bortezomib. The addition of bortezomib increased the proportion of patients achieving and complete response (30% and 4%;, $P < .001$) and improved median duration of response (19.9 vs. 13.1 months), time to progression (24.0 vs.16.6 months; $P < .001$), and the risk of death (hazard ratio 0.61 for the bortezomib group; $P = .008$).

The addition of thalidomide to melphalan and prednisone (MPT) also improves outcome compared with MP alone. For patients aged 60 to 85, Palumbo et al.[89] demonstrated a 76% response rate with MPT, superior to the 48% among patients treated with MP; however, thromboses were more common with thalidomide with an incidence of 12% (vs. 2% in the MP group).

In an updated analysis with median follow-up of 38.1 months, the median progression-free survival was 21.8 months for MPT and 14.5 months for MP ($P = .004$). The median overall survival was not significantly improved with MPT (45.0 vs. 47.6 months for MP, $P = .79$).[90]

In a randomized trial of 292 patients aged 75 years or older, Hulin et al.[91] found that the addition of thalidomide to MP increased overall survival compared with MP alone (median survival 44.0 vs. 29.1 months; $P = .028$). Another randomized comparison of MPT versus MP among 357 elderly patients found that the addition of thalidomide increased the rate of good partial response or better (23% vs. 7%; $P < .001$) but did not improve progression-free or overall survival.[92]

A recent meta-analysis of MP versus MPT concluded that MPT increases response rates and overall survival, but with increased toxicity such as thrombosis and somnolence.[93]

These results provide several options for the initial therapy of patients who will not proceed to ASCT, including all three novel agents, thalidomide, bortezomib, and lenalidomide, with or without melphalan.

Autologous Stem Cell Transplantation

ASCT has become the standard of care for eligible patients, as it has been demonstrated in multiple trials to improve the likelihood of complete response, prolong disease-free survival, and extend overall survival.[94–96] Treatment-related mortality rates are now <2%, and often the transplant can be performed entirely as an outpatient. Melphalan 200 mg/m^2 is the most commonly used conditioning regimen, although it may be reduced in elderly patients or patients with renal insufficiency.

Tandem Transplantation

Tandem or double transplantation refers to a planned second ASCT after the patient has recovered from the first. A phase III trial in France evaluated tandem transplant versus single ASCT and demonstrated superior overall survival in the tandem group[97]; however, when further analyzed, the patients who benefited most from the second transplant were those who did not achieve a 90% reduction in their disease after the first ASCT. Therefore, it may be more prudent to consider tandem transplantation only in patients whose response to the first ASCT is suboptimal.

Allogeneic Stem Cell Transplantation

Myeloablative stem cell transplant is perhaps the only current potential cure for patients with myeloma, as the graft is not contaminated with tumor cells and may produce a profound graft versus myeloma effect.[98] However, its use is very limited due to the lack of donors, age restriction, high treatment-related mortality, and graft versus host disease. Reduced intensity nonmyeloablative allogeneic transplant following ASCT has also been investigated as a means of inducing a graft versus myeloma effect. In one study of 102 patients undergoing nonmyeloablative transplant, 5-year overall survival and progression-free survival were 64% and 36%, respectively, although the 5-year rate of nonmyeloma mortality was 18%.[99]

Maintenance Therapy

Much investigation of late has been directed at the use of maintenance therapy post-ASCT to prolong remission and survival. Two large randomized trials are being conducted using maintenance lenalidomide versus placebo, with publication pending.[100,101] In both trials progression-free survival was prolonged by approximately 20 months, although overall survival data are pending. The use of maintenance therapy post-ASCT remains controversial, and most guidelines do not recommend its use unless the patient is at high risk of rapid recurrence.

Relapse After Autologous Stem Cell Transplantation

The general approach to myeloma is to provide sequential therapies to patients, knowing each will not be curative but will prolong the period of disease control. The goal is to convert the disease into a chronic illness. Whereas there used to be very limited treatment options, the armamentarium available has grown considerably over the past few years. This has contributed to a prolongation of the median survival of patients with myeloma. Patients will relapse after a median of 2 years after the first ASCT,[102] and several options may be pursued for treatment (Table 81.6). The most commonly used agents are again the three key drugs in myeloma: thalidomide, bortezomib, and lenalidomide. All three have been validated extensively in relapsed disease. Even with retreatment, these agents can confer prolonged progression-free and overall survival.

The most promising agents that will likely be added to this list are carfilzomib and pomalidomide. Carfilzomib is a irreversible proteasome inhibitor with significant activity in relapsed myeloma.[103,104] It is currently under U.S. Food and Drug Administration review for approval. Pomalidomide is a novel immunomodulatory drug, in the family of thalidomide and lenalidomide, that has also demonstrated efficacy in relapsed myeloma, even in patients refractory to both bortezomib and lenlidomide.[105]

TABLE 81.6 TREATMENT OPTIONS FOR RELAPSED MULTIPLE MYELOMA

Conventional Therapy
Repeated courses of alkylator based therapy (melphalan)
Cyclophosphamide (IV or PO) and steroids
Transplantation
Second autologous stem cell transplant
High-Dose Chemotherapy
DTPACE
High-dose cyclophosphamide
Novel Agents
Thalidomide
Bortezomib
Lenalidomide
Combination Conventional and Novel Agent
CyBorD (cyclophosphamide, bortezomib, dexamethasone)
CRD (cyclophosphamide, lenalidomide, dexamethasone)
Vel-Doxil (bortezomib, liposomal doxorubicin)

IV, intravenous; PO, by mouth; DTPACE, dexamethasone, thalidomide, cisplatin, doxorubicin, cyclophosphamide, and etoposide.

Supportive Care

A description of therapy of myeloma would not be complete without addressing the need to treat not only the disease itself but also the complications of this disease. Erythropoietic agents assist in the management of chemotherapy induced anemia, leading to reduction and transfusions. Bisphosphonates are critical to the optimal therapy of bone disease and may even have an effect on overall survival in certain patients.[85,106–109]

Local RT for bony disease remains valuable in pain control and debulking disease. Patients often present with bony disease and anemia; both of these complications are treatable, allowing an improved quality of life and local RT for bony disease. Newer surgical techniques such as vertebroplasty and kyphoplasty are also being used to improve back pain and spinal symptoms.

RADIATION THERAPY OF MULTIPLE MYELOMA

Total Body Irradiation

Some high-dose chemotherapy protocols for multiple myeloma incorporate total body irradiation (TBI) into the conditioning regimen. Because of toxicity concerns (mucosal and hematologic) with TBI, many programs use chemotherapy alone, most commonly melphalan. A phase III French study (IFM [Intergroupe Francophone du Mye'lome] trial 9502) examined melphalan, 200 mg/m^2 alone (M200) versus melphalan 140 mg/m^2 with TBI, 8 Gy in 4 fractions (M140/TBI),[110] and found that patients in the TBI-containing arm suffered more grade 3 or 4 mucosal toxicity, heavier transfusion requirement, and longer hospitalization stay. There was a higher toxic death rate in the M140/TBI arm (3.6% vs. 0% for the M200 arm). The event-free survival was no different between the two treatments, but the 45-month overall survival favored the M200 arm (M200: 65.8%; M140/TBI: 45.5%; $P = .05$).

Similarly, another IFM protocol tested TBI in the tandem transplant setting by intensifying the conditioning regimen for the second transplant to melphalan 200 mg/m^2 without TBI, and comparing this with the standard tandem regimen (M140 for the first, M140/TBI for the second). There was no benefit with TBI, and increased toxicity was again observed. Therefore, all subsequent IFM trials abandoned the use of TBI.[111] Similar findings have been reported by others.[112,113] In an effort to facilitate donor marrow engraftment without increasing toxicity, some investigators have used reduced-dose TBI (2 Gy in a single fraction) as part of allogeneic bone marrow transplant following ASCT.[99,114]

Hemibody Radiation

Diffuse bone pain involving wide areas of the skeleton can be effectively palliated by half-body radiation with single doses of 5 to 8 Gy,[115–117] although this is rarely used now. The bone marrow in the unirradiated half-body serves as a stem cell reserve and will slowly repopulate the irradiated marrow after treatment. The dose for upper half-body should not exceed 8 Gy due to lung tolerance.[118] The main toxicity is myelosuppression. The use of hemibody radiation must be carefully considered in patients heavily pretreated with chemotherapy. Growth factor support may be helpful, while transfusions of blood products should be given as needed. The sequential hemibody radiation technique has been used in phase II[119,120] and phase III trials as "systemic" treatment to control myeloma, in patients with or without skeletal pain. A phase III trial by the South West Oncology Group included newly diagnosed patients treated initially with chemotherapy, with complete responders randomized to sequential hemibody radiation (7.5 Gy in 5 fractions, upper hemibody, followed 6 weeks later by lower hemibody) or further chemotherapy.[121] Survival in this trial was significantly poorer with radiation compared with chemotherapy. At present, there is no standard role for sequential hemibody radiation as systemic treatment for myeloma outside of a clinical trial, although it may remain useful for palliation of advanced disease in chemotherapy-refractory patients.

Local External Beam for Palliation

The most common use of RT in the management of plasma cell tumors is for palliative treatment of bony disease[117,122,123] and relief of compression of spinal cord,[124–126] cranial nerves, or peripheral nerves. It has been estimated that approximately 40% of patients with multiple myeloma will require palliative radiation therapy for bone pain at some time during the course of their disease.[127] In practice the actual proportion is lower than estimated, varying from 24% to 34%, leading investigators in Australia to suggest that this potentially useful modality of treatment has been underutilized, even taking into account the beneficial effect of bisphosphonates, particularly for the elderly.[127] Palliative RT to the spine reduces the incidence of future vertebral fractures or the appearance of new lesions.[128] However, the role of RT in preventing impending pathologic fracture is unclear. In general, lesions at high risk for pathologic fracture should be referred for surgical stabilization, and RT can be administered after surgery for control of residual disease at the local site.

When RT is given for pain due to disease involving a long bone, a local field suffices. It is unnecessary to treat the entire bone.[129] Doses of 10 to 20 Gy (in 5 to 10 fractions) are effective, although the pain relief is often partial.[130] Leigh et al.[123] found a symptomatic response rate of 97% (complete pain relief in 26%, and partial relief in 71%) after an average dose of 25 Gy given to 306 sites in 101 patients. There was no dose–response relationship above 10 Gy. Recurrence of symptoms requiring further treatment was seen in 6% of sites after a median of 16 months.

It is not clear if pain relief is better if RT is given concurrently with chemotherapy. A study by Adamietz et al.[122] reported complete pain relief in 80% of patients receiving RT with chemotherapy, compared with 40% among those receiving RT alone. In contrast, Leigh et al.[123] found no significant difference in pain relief when RT was given with or without concurrent chemotherapy.

For spinal cord compression, motor improvement is expected in approximately 50% of irradiated patients. A multicenter study suggested that a longer fractionated regimen (30 Gy in 10 fractions or higher) was associated with better neurologic recovery than 20 Gy in 5 fractions or a single 8 Gy.[126] With the availability of newer drugs, the advantage of radiation sensitizing efforts with drug–radiation combinations requires continued investigation, both in terms of enhancing local control[131] and possible toxicity. Bortezomib and spinal radiation given concurrently was reported to result in severe enteritis.[132] The use of bisphosphonates (e.g., pamidronate) has been shown to reduce skeletal complications and pain,[106–109] with a reduction of the use of RT from 50% to 34% in one study.[108]

Radioimmunotherapy Approaches

Bone seeking radiopharmaceuticals targeting the bone marrow have been studied as an alternative to TBI. Typically a β-emitting isotope is conjugated to a phosphonate complex, such as samarium-153-ethylene diamine tetramethylene phosphonate (^{153}Sm-EDTMP, or Quadramet™). The isotope also emits a γ-ray, permitting scanning to locate areas of uptake. This agent has been used for palliation of bone metastasis.[133,134] The feasibility of this approach in a small number of myeloma patients has been reported for stem cell transplantation both in the autologous[135,136] and allogeneic settings.[137] Another bone seeking pharmaceutical is holmium-166-DOTMP (^{166}Ho-1,4,7,10-tetraazacyclododecane-1,4,7,10-tetramethylene-phosphonic acid), with a higher energy β emission (maximum energy 1.85 MeV) than ^{153}Sm and a shorter $T_{1/2}$ of 26.8 hours. It also has a γ emission (81 KeV) suitable for imaging. A phase I and II study incorporating ^{166}Ho-DOTMP into a transplant regimen has been performed at the MD Anderson Cancer Center with encouraging results.[138] With the ability to deliver much higher doses to the bone marrow than TBI, in the range of 30 to 60 Gy, yet sparing the dose-limiting normal tissues such as lung, mucosa, and kidneys, the concept of targeted radiation therapy is tantalizing. However, there remains a problem of heterogeneity of uptake in the skeleton, and the dosimetric variation may be even larger at a microscopic level due to the limited range of the β particle. Whether this approach will have a more favorable therapeutic ratio than standard conditioning regimens in the transplant setting awaits larger scale phase II and phase III trials.

RADIATION THERAPY TECHNIQUES

Radical Radiation Therapy for Local Control of Solitary Plasmacytoma

Accurate evaluation of tumor extent is an important feature of radical RT for solitary plasmacytoma. MRI is useful to evaluate the extent of disease both within and beyond bone. This is particularly true for the paranasal sinuses, where inflammatory changes may be difficult to distinguish from tumor on CT imaging. Currently, the accuracy of FDG-PET in the evaluation of tumor extent is uncertain.

There are few data to support specific guidelines regarding RT treatment volumes. CT and MRI imaging should be used to determine gross tumor volumes. Clinical target volumes (CTV) should encompass probable routes of microscopic spread, recognizing that barriers to the extension of local disease will vary according to anatomic location, as will the morbidity of treating adjacent normal tissues (Fig. 81.2). For the spine, inclusion of two vertebral bodies above and below the grossly involved vertebra(e) is a common practice. As this is based on relapse patterns seen following RT for spinal metastases for solid tumors, it may not be directly applicable to solitary plasmacytoma.

For RT of long bone lesions, while coverage of the entire involved bone has been recommended by some authors, a study of palliative RT to only the symptomatic area for multiple myeloma found that recurrence in the untreated portion of the involved bone was rare,[129] and similarly, no marginal recurrences were seen among 30 patients with solitary plasmacytoma treated with RT that encompassed only the tumor with a margin.[139] Prophylactic regional nodal coverage is not necessary in solitary plasmacytoma of bone as multiple studies have found a very low risk of regional nodal failure after involved-field radiation without intentional coverage of adjacent nodes (i.e., 0% to 4%).[20,49,67,139] For extramedullary plasmacytoma, nodal involvement at presentation is observed in 10% to 20%, and occasional nodal failure in the literature led to a common practice of extending the RT coverage to the draining lymph node region.[20,57,110] Some authors specifically recommend this practice if the primary disease involves a lymphatic structure (e.g., lymph nodes or Waldeyer's ring).[39,64,140] However, this is controversial as some series reported a low incidence of regional nodal failure without routine prophylactic nodal irradiation,[39,64,140] leading to variation in practices between centers.[19] After reviewing their own series of 26 patients with EMP and contrasting the results with the literature, Strojan et al.[19] concluded that prophylactic nodal radiation is probably unnecessary.

Planning target volumes (PTV) should account for day-to-day setup variation and will typically add 5 to 10 mm around CTV volumes depending on the immobilization technique employed (Fig. 81.2). Overall, RT field edges are typically 2 to 3 cm from gross tumor seen on imaging. Although parallel-opposed fields

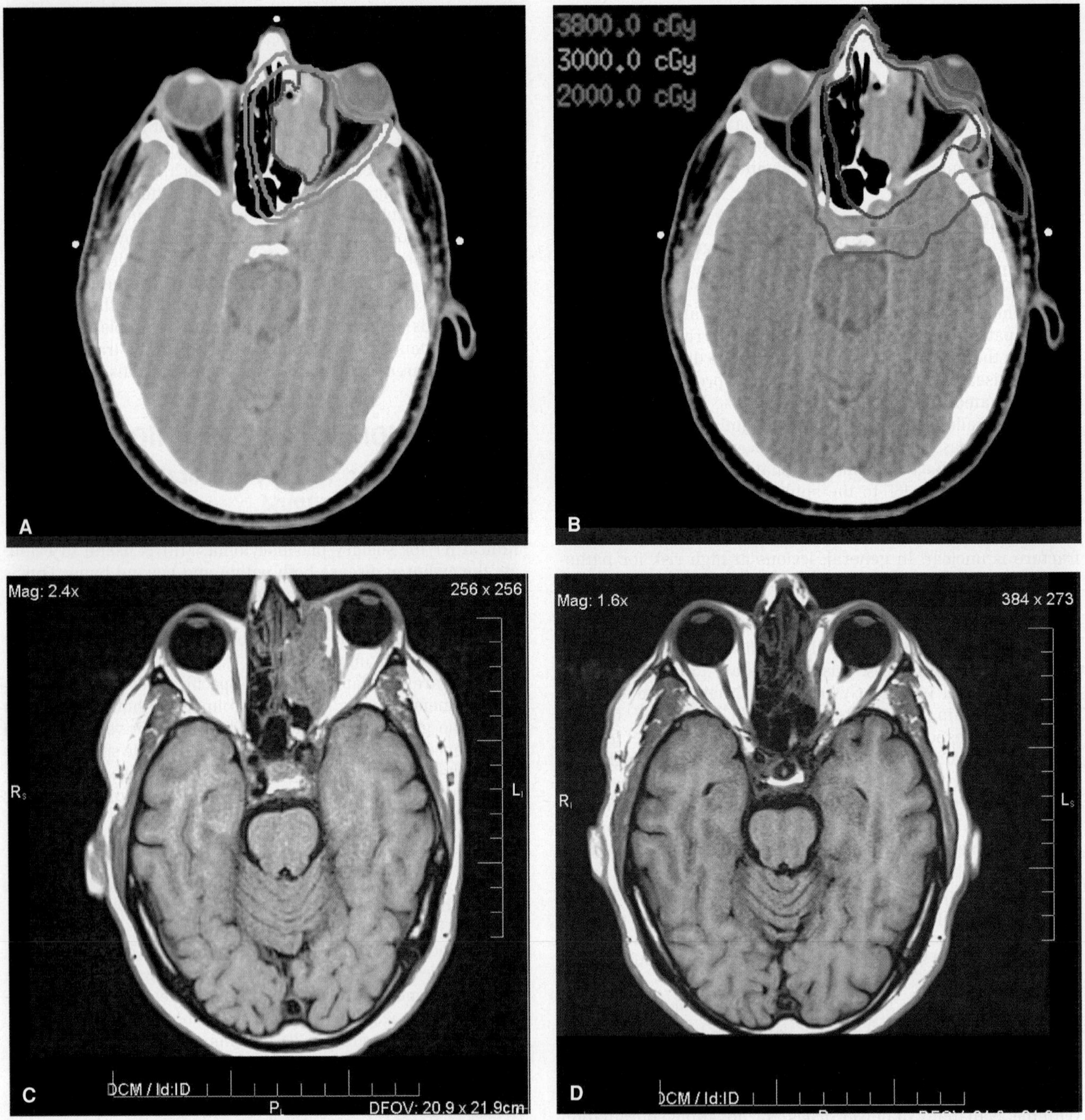

FIGURE 81.2. Radiation treatment plan for a solitary plasmacytoma of the left orbit **(A)**. The entire orbit was contoured as the clinical target volume and received 36 Gy; the gross tumor volume received a subsequent boost to a total of 40Gy **(B)**. The initial mass on magnetic resonance imaging resolved 6 months after treatment **(C,D)**.

are commonly adequate to encompass disease without significant irradiation of normal tissues, CT-based planning and the use of conformal techniques, including intensity-modulated radiation therapy, should be employed when needed to treat the PTV adjacent to critical structures. This can be particularly important in extramedullary disease involving the paranasal sinuses, where avoidance of the optic structures and salivary glands is desirable.

Radiation Therapy Dose

Studies evaluating RT dose response in plasmacytoma have produced differing results. Most studies have found response rates >85% among patients treated with ≥ 35Gy; some investigators have found better local control following doses ≥45 Gy,[25,59] while others have found no indication of improved outcome with higher doses.[18,139] Based on a dose–response analysis of 81 patients by Mendenhall et al.[141] reported in 1980, a minimum dose of 40 Gy was recommended, including osseous and extramedullary lesions. A total dose of 40 Gy and above resulted in a local failure rate of 6% versus 31% for lower doses. Therefore, the usual practice is to administer a dose of 40 to 45 Gy or even higher for bulky tumors. However, in the largest of these studies (n = 258), there was no evidence of improved local control with RT doses ranging from 30 to 50 Gy, including a subset of patients with tumors >4 cm.[18] In fact there was a worse local control rate for the group receiving total dose ≥50 Gy, although not statistically significant.[18] It should be noted, however, that retrospective studies of dose response are typically confounded by selection bias, as higher doses are prescribed to larger tumors with worse prognosis. Several studies have demonstrated durable local control in >85% of tumors <5 cm with 35 to 40 Gy, and there is little evidence that higher doses are necessary for small tumors, regardless of bone or EMP locations. In contrast, plasmacytomas >5 cm have worse local control,[18,20] and doses of 45 to 50 Gy are recommended in these bulkier tumors, which also tend to be EMPs. However, one should be aware that the quality of evidence supporting the use of higher RT doses is limited, and local failures are occasionally observed even after doses exceeding 50 Gy.[18,20]

Assessment of Response and Follow-Up

Reimaging is of greatest value in the response assessment of extramedullary plasmacytoma. Repeat imaging, preferably with MRI, should be done approximately 6 to 8 weeks following completion of treatment. It is rare to have symptoms suggestive of local progression that necessitate reimaging prior to this. It is common for a residual soft tissue abnormality to persist on follow-up imaging, and periodic reimaging may be required every 4 to 6 months until any residual mass disappears or remains stable on consecutive scans. It is generally not beneficial to continue to reimage a stable abnormality.

Bone destruction caused by tumor can produce persistent abnormalities on imaging following RT for painful bone metastases or isolated plasmacytoma of bone. Consequently, repeat imaging is of less value in establishing response in such cases.

With a high risk of recurrence of disease as multiple myeloma, the occurrence of new bone pain requires further investigations, including imaging as appropriate. Repeat measurement of the M protein often detects the onset of systemic disease prior to the development of symptoms and can be used as an indicator of disease burden.[22,142] Complete blood counts should be taken periodically to evaluate bone marrow function. A team of international investigators have recently developed recommendations for uniform response criteria for assessing the treatment of multiple myeloma.[143]

The RT doses used for myeloma are rarely associated with significant delayed side effects. Treatment of significant volumes of the parotid or submandibular glands may result in prolonged xerostomia and should be avoided. As noted previously, TBI has been associated with significant toxicity and is not widely used. Evaluation of renal function should be undertaken prior to initiating RT, which may include the kidneys, and blood counts should be evaluated prior to treating a large volume of bone marrow in the spine or pelvis. Reirradiation of vertebral metastases is possible, but careful evaluation of all prior RT records is required to ensure that the tolerance of the spinal cord is not exceeded.

SELECTED REFERENCES

A full list of references for this chapter is available online.

6. Greipp PR, San Miguel J, Durie BG, et al. International staging system for multiple myeloma. *J Clin Oncol* 2005;23(15):3412–3420.
10. Kyle RA, Therneau TM, Rajkumar SV, et al. A long-term study of prognosis in monoclonal gammopathy of undetermined significance. *N Engl J Med* 2002;346(8):564–569.
12. Weiss BM, Abadie J, Verma P, et al. A monoclonal gammopathy precedes multiple myeloma in most patients. *Blood* 2009;113(22):5418–5422.
13. Kuehl WM, Bergsagel PL. Multiple myeloma: evolving genetic events and host interactions. *Nat Rev Cancer* 2002;2(3):175–187.
16. Hideshima T, Bergsagel PL, Kuehl WM, et al. Advances in biology of multiple myeloma: clinical applications. *Blood* 2004;104(3):607–618.
17. Tian E, Zhan F, Walker R, et al. The role of the Wnt-signaling antagonist DKK1 in the development of osteolytic lesions in multiple myeloma. *N Engl J Med* 2003;349(26):2483–2494.
18. Ozsahin M, Tsang RW, Poortmans P, et al. Outcomes and patterns of failure in solitary plasmacytoma: a multicenter Rare Cancer Network study of 258 patients. *Int J Radiat Oncol Biol Phys* 2006;64(1):210–217.
21. Durie BG, Kyle RA, Belch A, et al. Myeloma management guidelines: a consensus report from the scientific advisors of the International Myeloma Foundation. *Hematol J* 2003;4(6):379–398.
22. Wilder RB, Ha CS, Cox JD, et al. Persistence of myeloma protein for more than one year after radiotherapy is an adverse prognostic factor in solitary plasmacytoma of bone. *Cancer* 2002;94(5):1532–1537.
23. Durie BG, Salmon SE. A clinical staging system for multiple myeloma. Correlation of measured myeloma cell mass with presenting clinical features, response to treatment, and survival. *Cancer* 1975;36(3):842–854.
27. Criteria for the classification of monoclonal gammopathies, multiple myeloma and related disorders: a report of the International Myeloma Working Group. *Br J Haematol* 2003;121(5):749–757.
29. Tiedemann RE, Gonzalez-Paz N, Kyle RA, et al. Genetic aberrations and survival in plasma cell leukemia. *Leukemia* 2008;22(5):1044–1052.
33. Mariette X, Zagdanski AM, Guermazi A, et al. Prognostic value of vertebral lesions detected by magnetic resonance imaging in patients with stage I multiple myeloma. *Br J Haematol* 1999;104(4):723–729.
34. Van de Berg BC, Lecouvet FE, Michaux L, et al. Stage I multiple myeloma: value of MR imaging of the bone marrow in the determination of prognosis. *Radiology* 1996;201(1):243–246.
36. Schirrmeister H, Buck AK, Bergmann L, et al. Positron emission tomography (PET) for staging of solitary plasmacytoma. *Cancer Biother Radiopharm* 2003;18(5):841–845.
37. Kim PJ, Hicks RJ, Wirth A, et al. Impact of 18F-fluorodeoxyglucose positron emission tomography before and after definitive radiation therapy in patients with apparently solitary plasmacytoma. *Int J Radiat Oncol Biol Phys* 2009;74(3):740–746.
38. Group TIMW. Criteria for the classification of monoclonal gammopathies, multiple myeloma and related disorders: a report of the International Myeloma Working Group. *Br J Haematol* 2003;121(5):749–757.
42. Chak LY, Cox RS, Bostwick DG, et al. Solitary plasmacytoma of bone: treatment, progression, and survival. *J Clin Oncol* 1987;5(11):1811–1815.
43. Reed V, Shah J, Medeiros LJ, et al. Solitary plasmacytomas: outcome and prognostic factors after definitive radiation therapy. *Cancer* 2011;117(19):4468–4474.
47. Moulopoulos LA, Dimopoulos MA, Smith TL, et al. Prognostic significance of magnetic resonance imaging in patients with asymptomatic multiple myeloma. *J Clin Oncol* 1995;13(1):251–256.
49. Susnerwala SS, Shanks JH, Banerjee SS, et al. Extramedullary plasmacytoma of the head and neck region: clinicopathological correlation in 25 cases. *Br J Cancer* 1997;75(6):921–927.
54. Chang H, Sloan S, Li D, et al. The t(4;14) is associated with poor prognosis in myeloma patients undergoing autologous stem cell transplant. *Br J Haematol* 2004;125(1):64–68.
57. Soutar R, Lucraft H, Jackson G, et al. Guidelines on the diagnosis and management of solitary plasmacytoma of bone and solitary extramedullary plasmacytoma. *Clin Oncol (R Coll Radiol)* 2004;16(6):405–413.
60. Knobel D, Zouhair A, Tsang RW, et al. Prognostic factors in solitary plasmacytoma of the bone: a multicenter Rare Cancer Network study. *BMC Cancer* 2006;6(1):118.
61. Moulopoulos LA, Dimopoulos MA, Weber D, et al. Magnetic resonance imaging in the staging of solitary plasmacytoma of bone. *J Clin Oncol* 1993;11(7):1311–1315.
62. Sasaki R, Yasuda K, Abe E, et al. Multi-institutional analysis of solitary extramedullary plasmacytoma of the head and neck treated with curative radiotherapy. *Int J Radiat Oncol Biol Phys* 2012;82(2):626–634.
63. Dimopoulos MA, Goldstein J, Fuller L, et al. Curability of solitary bone plasmacytoma. *J Clin Oncol* 1992;10(4):587–590.
64. Knowling MA, Harwood AR, Bergsagel DE. Comparison of extramedullary plasmacytomas with solitary and multiple plasma cell tumors of bone. *J Clin Oncol* 1983;1(4):255–262.
67. Liebross RH, Ha CS, Cox JD, et al. Clinical course of solitary extramedullary plasmacytoma. *Radiother Oncol* 1999;52(3):245–249.
68. Galieni P, Cavo M, Pulsoni A, et al. Clinical outcome of extramedullary plasmacytoma. *Haematologica* 2000;85(1):47–51.
76. Samson D, Gaminara E, Newland A, et al. Infusion of vincristine and doxorubicin with oral dexamethasone as first-line therapy for multiple myeloma. *Lancet* 1989;2(8668):882–885.
77. Harousseau JL, Attal M, Avet-Loiseau H, et al. Bortezomib plus dexamethasone is superior to vincristine plus doxorubicin plus dexamethasone as induction treatment prior to autologous stem-cell transplantation in newly diagnosed multiple myeloma: results of the IFM 2005-01 phase III trial. *J Clin Oncol* 2010;28(30):4621–4629.
78. Jagannath S, Durie BG, Wolf J, et al. Bortezomib therapy alone and in combination with dexamethasone for previously untreated symptomatic multiple myeloma. *Br J Haematol* 2005;129(6):776–783.
79. Richardson P, Jagannath S, Hussein M, et al. Safety and efficacy of single-agent lenalidomide in patients with relapsed and refractory multiple myeloma. *Blood* 2009;114(4):772–778.
80. Reeder CB, Reece DE, Kukreti V, et al. Once- versus twice-weekly bortezomib induction therapy with CyBorD in newly diagnosed multiple myeloma. *Blood* 2010;115(16):3416–3417.
81. Moreau P, Pylypenko H, Grosicki S, et al. Subcutaneous versus intravenous administration of bortezomib in patients with relapsed multiple myeloma: a randomised, phase 3, non-inferiority study. *Lancet Oncol* 2011;12(5):431–440.
82. Rajkumar SV, Jacobus S, Callander NS, et al. Lenalidomide plus high-dose dexamethasone versus lenalidomide plus low-dose dexamethasone as initial therapy for newly diagnosed multiple myeloma: an open-label randomised controlled trial [Erratum appears in *Lancet Oncol* 2010;11(1):14]. *Lancet Oncol* 2010;11(1):29–37.
83. Richardson PG, Weller E, Lonial S, et al. Lenalidomide, bortezomib, and dexamethasone combination therapy in patients with newly diagnosed multiple myeloma. *Blood* 2010;116(5):679–686.
84. Rajkumar SV, Hayman S, Gertz MA, et al. Combination therapy with thalidomide plus dexamethasone for newly diagnosed myeloma. *J Clin Oncol* 2002;20(21):4319–4323.
85. Morgan GJ, Davies FE, Gregory WM, et al. First-line treatment with zoledronic acid as compared with clodronic acid in multiple myeloma (MRC Myeloma IX): a randomised controlled trial. *Lancet* 2010;376(9757):1989–1999.
86. Cavo M, Tacchetti P, Patriarca F, et al. Bortezomib with thalidomide plus dexamethasone compared with thalidomide plus dexamethasone as induction therapy before, and consolidation therapy after, double autologous stem-cell transplantation in newly diagnosed multiple myeloma: a randomised phase 3 study. *Lancet* 2010;376(9758):2075–2085.
88. San Miguel JF, Schlag R, Khuageva NK, et al. Bortezomib plus melphalan and prednisone for initial treatment of multiple myeloma. *N Engl J Med* 2008;359(9):906–917.
89. Palumbo A, Bringhen S, Caravita T, et al. Oral melphalan and prednisone chemotherapy plus thalidomide compared with melphalan and prednisone alone in elderly patients with multiple myeloma: randomised controlled trial. *Lancet* 2006;367(9513):825–831.

90. Palumbo A, Bringhen S, Liberati AM, et al. Oral melphalan, prednisone, and thalidomide in elderly patients with multiple myeloma: updated results of a randomized controlled trial. *Blood* 2008;112(8):3107–3114.
91. Hulin C, Facon T, Rodon P, et al. Efficacy of melphalan and prednisone plus thalidomide in patients older than 75 years with newly diagnosed multiple myeloma: IFM 01/01 trial. *J Clin Oncol* 2009;27(22):3664–3670.
92. Waage A, Gimsing P, Fayers P, et al. Melphalan and prednisone plus thalidomide or placebo in elderly patients with multiple myeloma. *Blood* 2010;116(9):1405–1412.
93. Fayers PM, Palumbo A, Hulin C, et al. Thalidomide for previously untreated elderly patients with multiple myeloma: meta-analysis of 1685 individual patient data from 6 randomized clinical trials. *Blood* 2011;118(5):1239–1247.
94. Attal M, Harousseau JL, Stoppa AM, et al. A prospective, randomized trial of autologous bone marrow transplantation and chemotherapy in multiple myeloma. *N Engl J Med* 1996;335(2):91–97.
95. Kumar A, Loughran T, Alsina M, et al. Management of multiple myeloma: a systematic review and critical appraisal of published studies. *Lancet Oncol* 2003; 4(5):293–304.
96. Blade J, Vesole DH, Gertz M. High-dose therapy in multiple myeloma. *Blood* 2003;102(10):3469–3470.
97. Attal M, Harousseau JL, Facon T, et al. Single versus double autologous stem-cell transplantation for multiple myeloma. *N Engl J Med* 2003;349(26):2495–2502.
99. Rotta M, Storer BE, Sahebi F, et al. Long-term outcome of patients with multiple myeloma after autologous hematopoietic cell transplantation and nonmyeloablative allografting. *Blood* 2009;113(14):3383–3391.
101. McCarthy PL, Owzar K, Anderson KC, et al. Phase III intergroup study of lenalidomide versus placebo maintenance therapy following single autologous hematopoietic stem cell transplantation (AHSCT) for multiple myeloma: CALGB 100104. ASH Annual Meeting Abstracts. *Blood*2010;116:(abstr 37).
102. Mikhael J, Samiee S, Stewart AK, et al. Second autologous stem cell transplantation as salvage therapy in patients with relapsed multiple myeloma: improved outcomes in patients with longer disease free interval after first autologous stem cell transplantation. *Biol Blood Marrow Transplant* 2006;12(2 Suppl 1):117.
104. Khan ML, Stewart AK. Carfilzomib: a novel second-generation proteasome inhibitor. *Future Oncol* 2011;7(5):607–612.
106. Djulbegovic B, Wheatley K, Ross J, et al. Bisphosphonates in multiple myeloma. *Cochrane Database Syst Rev* 2002;3:CD003188.
107. Berenson JR, Lichtenstein A, Porter L, et al. Efficacy of pamidronate in reducing skeletal events in patients with advanced multiple myeloma. Myeloma Aredia Study Group. *N Engl J Med* 1996;334(8):488–493.
108. Berenson JR, Lichtenstein A, Porter L, et al. Long-term pamidronate treatment of advanced multiple myeloma patients reduces skeletal events. Myeloma Aredia Study Group. *J Clin Oncol* 1998;16(2):593–602.
109. Berenson JR, Hillner BE, Kyle RA, et al. American Society of Clinical Oncology clinical practice guidelines: the role of bisphosphonates in multiple myeloma. *J Clin Oncol* 2002;20(17):3719–3736.
110. Moreau P, Facon T, Attal M, et al. Comparison of 200 mg/m(2) melphalan and 8 Gy total body irradiation plus 140 mg/m(2) melphalan as conditioning regimens for peripheral blood stem cell transplantation in patients with newly diagnosed multiple myeloma: final analysis of the Intergroupe Francophone du Myelome 9502 randomized trial. *Blood* 2002;99(3):731–735.
113. Abraham R, Chen C, Tsang R, et al. Intensification of the stem cell transplant induction regimen results in increased treatment-related mortality without improved outcome in multiple myeloma. *Bone Marrow Transplant* 1999;24(12): 1291–1297.
121. Salmon SE, Tesh D, Crowley J, et al. Chemotherapy is superior to sequential hemibody irradiation for remission consolidation in multiple myeloma: a Southwest Oncology Group study. *J Clin Oncol* 1990;8(9):1575–1584.
124. Ampil FL, Chin HW. Radiotherapy alone for extradural compression by spinal myeloma. *Radiat Med* 1995;13(3):129–131.
125. Wallington M, Mendis S, Premawardhana U, et al. Local control and survival in spinal cord compression from lymphoma and myeloma. *Radiother Oncol* 1997; 42(1):43–47.
126. Rades D, Stalpers LJ, Veninga T, et al. Evaluation of five radiation schedules and prognostic factors for metastatic spinal cord compression. *J Clin Oncol* 2005; 23(15):3366–3375.
128. Lecouvet F, Richard F, Vande Berg B, et al. Long-term effects of localized spinal radiation therapy on vertebral fractures and focal lesions appearance in patients with multiple myeloma. *Br J Haematol* 1997;96(4):743–745.
130. Mill WB, Griffith R. The role of radiation therapy in the management of plasma cell tumors. *Cancer* 1980;45(4):647–652.
132. Mohiuddin MM, Harmon DC, Delaney TF. Severe acute enteritis in a multiple myeloma patient receiving bortezomib and spinal radiotherapy: case report. *J Chemother* 2005;17(3):343–346.
133. Anderson PM, Wiseman GA, Dispenzieri A, et al. High-dose samarium-153 ethylene diamine tetramethylene phosphonate: low toxicity of skeletal irradiation in patients with osteosarcoma and bone metastases. *J Clin Oncol* 2002;20(1): 189–196.
139. Jyothirmayi R, Gangadharan VP, Nair MK, Rajan B. Radiotherapy in the treatment of solitary plasmacytoma. *Br J Radiol* 1997;70(833):511–516.
141. Mendenhall CM, Thar TL, Million RR. Solitary plasmacytoma of bone and soft tissue. *Int J Radiat Oncol Biol Phys* 1980;6(11):1497–1501.
143. Durie BG, Harousseau JL, Miguel JS, et al. International uniform response criteria for multiple myeloma. *Leukemia* 2006;20(9):1467–1473.

Part M Bone and Soft Tissue

Chapter 82
Osteosarcoma and Other Primary Tumors of Bone

Jaroslaw T. Hepel and Timothy J. Kinsella

Primary malignant tumors of bone are rare neoplasms accounting for <0.2% of all cancers. In 2010, an estimated 2,650 new cases and 1,460 related deaths were expected.[1] Osteosarcoma, chondrosarcoma, and Ewing sarcoma are the most common, comprising 35%, 30%, and 16% of cases, respectively. Other rare entities include malignant fibrous histiocytoma, fibrosarcoma, and chordoma. Ewing sarcoma is discussed in detail in Chapter 88. Osteosarcoma and the other malignant bone tumors will be discussed here.

OSTEOSARCOMA

Epidemiology

Osteosarcoma is a rare primary malignant tumor of bone, accounting for approximately 750 to 900 new cases in the United States annually. Despite its rarity, osteosarcoma is the fifth-most-common malignancy and the most common malignant bone tumor in children and adolescents.[2,3] It has a bimodal age distribution, with peak incidence in early adolescence and another smaller peak in adults older than 65 years of age.[4] In childhood, osteosarcoma typically occurs sporadically, whereas in adulthood it is more commonly associated with sarcomatous degeneration of Paget's disease or other benign bone lesions. There is a slight male predilection, with a ratio of 1.2:1.[2]

Pathogenesis and Risk Factors

The etiology of osteosarcoma is unknown, but there is a suggestion of a relationship with rapid bone growth. The peak incidence of osteosarcoma occurs during the adolescent growth spurt; this peak is earlier in girls corresponding to their earlier bone development. The most frequent sites of involvement correspond to the areas of greatest increase in bone length the metaphysis of the distal femur, proximal tibia, and proximal humerus. It has been suggested that an aberration in the natural process of bone growth leads to osteosarcoma, but the specific etiology has not been elucidated. Unlike other pediatric tumors, no characteristic translocation or genetic abnormality has been defined for osteosarcoma.

Several risk factors have been associated with osteosarcoma. Development of osteosarcoma after radiation therapy exposure in childhood has been reported. The mean latency period is generally >10 years.[5–7] Similarly, chemotherapy, especially alkylating agents, has been implicated with secondary osteosarcoma.[7] Benign bone lesions, particularly Paget's disease, have also been associated with osteosarcoma. Paget's disease of bone is a focal skeletal disorder characterized by accelerated bone turnover. Sarcomatous transformation is usually seen in long-standing Paget's and occurs in only 0.7% to 1% of cases.[8] Other benign bone lesions have also been associated with risk of osteosarcoma, including chronic osteomyelitis, multiple hereditary exostoses, fibrous dysplasia, osteochondromas, enchondromas, sites of bone infarcts, and sites of metallic implants.[9] Several genetic conditions have been linked to an increase risk of osteosarcoma. Retinoblastoma is associated with an increased risk of secondary tumors, more than half of which are soft-tissue sarcomas and osteosarcomas.[10] Li–Fraumeni syndrome is associated with a spectrum of malignancies, including breast, adrenocortical, brain, leukemia, and sarcomas, including osteosarcoma. Li–Fraumeni syndrome involves a germline inactivation of p53, a key cell cycle regulatory gene.[11] Rothmund–Thomson, Bloom, and Werner syndromes have also been associated with osteosarcoma.[12]

Clinical Presentation

Most patients present with localized pain in the affected bone. Pain is usually of several months duration and may wax and wane. There may be associated soft-tissue swelling or a palpable mass. Some patients present with pathologic fracture. Osteosarcoma has a predilection for involvement of the metaphysis of long bones. The most common site of involvement is the knee (distal femur or proximal tibia), followed by the proximal humerus, mid and proximal femur, and then other bones.[13] Although most patients have micrometastatic disease at the time of presentation, only 10% to 20% of patients present with clinical evident macrometastases. The lung is the most common site of metastatic involvement, followed by bone.[14]

Diagnostic Evaluation

Plain x-ray of the affected bone classically demonstrates destruction of the normal trabecular bone with lytic and/or sclerotic lesions, osteoid formation under the periosteum (Codman's triangle), and variable ossification of the associated soft tissue mass (Fig. 82.1). Magnetic resonance imaging (MRI) of the affected bone is essential to fully delineate the extent of the lesion, evaluate any soft-tissue component, and evaluate for involvement of joint, nerves, and vasculature (Fig. 82.2). The entire affected bone should be imaged to evaluate for the presence of skip lesions. Skip metastases are well recognized in osteosarcoma but occur infrequently, with <5% incidence.[15,16] Systemic staging should include a computed tomography (CT) scan of the chest and radionuclide bone scan to evaluate for pulmonary and bone metastases, respectively. Positron emission tomography (PET) scan can be used as an alternative for systemic staging but may have less sensitivity than CT and bone scan.[17,18] PET scan has also been used to assess response to preoperative chemotherapy.[19]

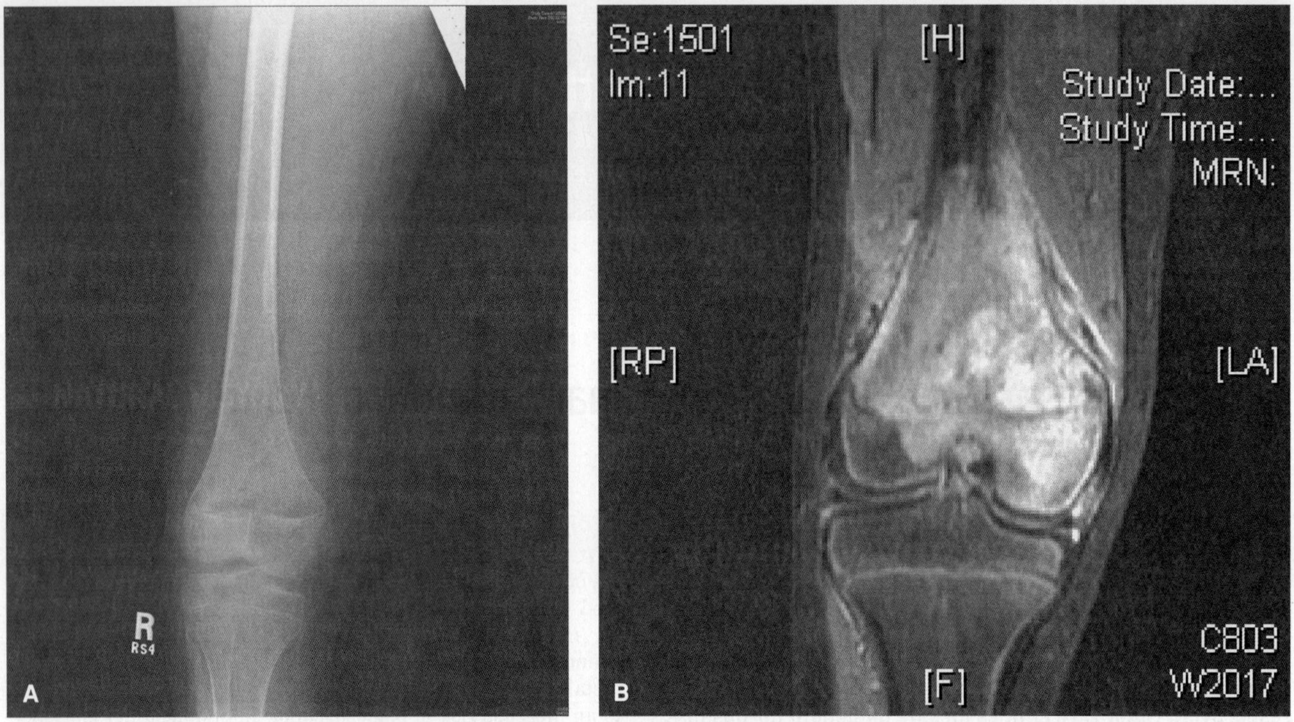

FIGURE 82.1. **A:** Plain radiograph of a distal femur osteosarcoma showing a lytic region and Codman's triangle in the medial distal femur. **B:** Magnetic resonance image scan of the same lesion.

Biopsy of the tumor should be performed to confirm the diagnosis and to differentiate from other bone lesions. Similar to soft-tissue sarcomas, the biopsy should be performed at a center with expertise in bone tumors and should be carried out by or in conjunction with the orthopedic surgeon who will be performing future definitive surgery in order to not jeopardize subsequent treatment, particularly a limb-preserving procedure.

Staging Systems

There are two staging systems commonly used for osteosarcoma (Table 82.1). The Musculoskeletal Tumor Society (MSTS) staging system is a surgical staging system stratifying tumors by grade and subdividing by local extent.[20] The American Joint Committee on Cancer system is less often used.[21]

Pathology

Osteosarcoma is characterized by the presence of malignant sarcomatous stroma with associated osteoid (immature bone) production.[22] Osteosarcoma is believed to arise from mesenchymal stem cells with the capacity to have fibrous tissue, cartilage, and bone differentiation. Thus, osteosarcoma shares many features with chondrosarcomas and fibrosarcomas. However, only osteosarcoma produces woven bone matrix, a key element for diagnosis.

Osteosarcoma is classified into two main categories: conventional (intramedullary) and surface.[23] The conventional type accounts for 90% of osteosarcomas and is associated with the typical presentation in adolescence. The majority of conventional osteosarcomas are high-grade tumors. Conventional

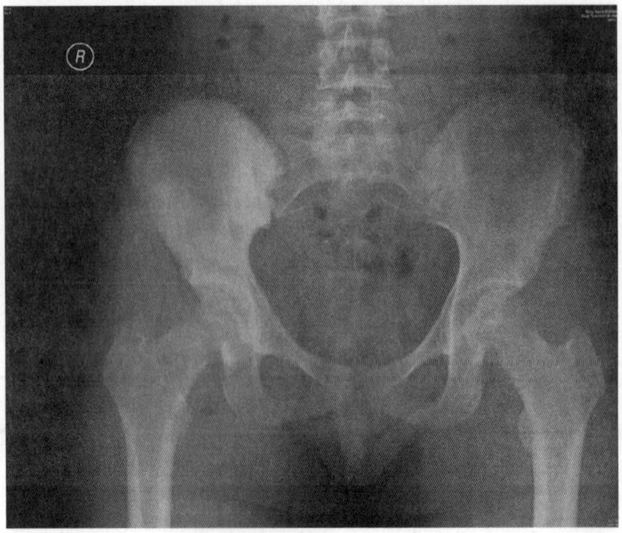

FIGURE 82.2. Plain radiograph of a sclerotic pelvic osteosarcoma.

TABLE 82.1 STAGING OF OSTEOSARCOMA

Stage	*Grade*	*Site*	*Metastases*
Enneking Staging System			
IA	Low	Intracompartmental	None
IB	Low	Extracompartmental	None
IIA	High	Intracompartmental	None
IIB	High	Extracompartmental	None
III	Any	Any	Present
Stage	*Grade*	*Local Extent (cm)*	*Metastases*
AJCC Staging System[a]			
IA	Low	≤8	None
IB	Low	>8 or discontinuous	None
IIA	High	≤8	None
IIB	High	>8	None
III	High	discontinuous	None
IVA	Any	Any	Pulmonary metastases
IVB	Any	Any	Other metastases

[a]Used with the permission of the American Joint Committee on Cancer, Chicago, Illinois. The original source for this material is *AJCC cancer staging handbook,* 7th ed. New York: Springer, 2010; published by Springer Science and Business Media LLC, www.springer.com.

osteosarcoma is further subdivided into osteoblastic, chondroblastic, fibroblastic, and mixed subtypes. Other, less common histologic variants of conventional osteosarcoma include small cell, telangiectatic, malignant fibrous histiocytoma, and multifocal. Multifocal osteosarcoma typically carries a worse prognosis.

Surface osteosarcoma is subdivided into parosteal, periosteal, and high-grade surface.[24,25] Parosteal variant is considered to be a low-grade tumor with a low metastatic potential. Periosteal variant is intermediate in grade, with an intermediate rate of developing metastases, between parosteal and conventional osteosarcoma, about 20%. A rare variant, extraosseous osteosarcoma, arises in soft tissues and is generally associated with prior radiation exposure.[26]

Treatment

Chemotherapy plays a critical role in the management of most patients with osteosarcoma. Although only 10% to 20% of patients present with overt metastatic disease, the vast majority of patients harbor subclinical metastatic disease at the time of presentation. Before effective chemotherapy, 80% to 90% of patients subsequently developed distant metastases and died of their disease despite achieving local disease control.[27] The typical treatment sequence for intermediate- and high-grade osteosarcoma is neoadjuvant chemotherapy, followed by surgery with a limb-sparing procedure if possible, and then followed by further adjuvant chemotherapy. With this approach, 60% to 70% of patients without overt metastases at diagnosis are expected to be long-term survivors.[28] Those with isolated lung metastases have an overall survival of 35% to 40%, whereas those with more extensive metastatic disease at diagnosis have <20% likelihood of long-term survival. For the less common low-grade tumors such as parosteal osteosarcoma, treatment with surgery alone is appropriate because the risk of developing metastases is low. These patients have an 80% to 90% likelihood of long-term survival.[29]

Surgery

The mainstay of surgical management is the complete *en bloc* resection of tumor. The extent and functional implications of surgery have dramatically evolved over time, with an emphasis on more conservative, limb-sparing resections with maintenance of function rather than amputation. Neoadjuvant chemotherapy has played an important role in this evolution.

For extremity lesions, limb preservation is preferred and can be accomplished in the majority of cases. Retrospective studies have shown equivalent results of limb-sparing surgery and amputation as long as adequate margins can be achieved.[30–32] Contraindications to limb-sparing surgery include nerve or vascular encasement, presence of large, biopsy-related hematoma, and pathologic fracture. Some data suggest that pathologic fracture does not increase the risk of local recurrence after limb-sparing surgery as previously believed.[33,34] Reconstructive options include use of allografts, endoprostheses, and occasionally rotationplasty.

Axial tumors, although much less common, pose a particular challenge because achieving complete surgical resection can be difficult. As a result, these lesions have a worse prognosis compared to extremity tumors. Pelvic tumors typically require a hemipelvectomy for *en bloc* resection. Some patients can undergo resection of the hemipelvis with preservation of the extremity (internal hemipelvectomy). This has a better functional outcome compared to an external hemipelvectomy, also referred to as a hindquarter amputation. Adjuvant radiation has been used to improve outcomes in patients with incomplete resections of pelvic tumors. Spinal tumors are also particularly difficult to resect with negative margins. Typically, an *en bloc* resection with vertebrectomy is performed, combined with mechanical stabilization. Postoperative radiation therapy can be used when negative margins cannot be obtained, particularly when there is microscopic dural involvement.

Chemotherapy

In the absence of chemotherapy, 80% to 90% of patients will subsequently develop distant metastases.[27] Chemotherapy thus plays an important role for all patients with intermediate- and high-grade tumors. Level I evidence for the benefit of chemotherapy was established by two randomized trials in the 1980s. Eilber et al.[35] reported on 59 patients with nonmetastatic osteosarcoma randomized to surgery followed by observation versus adjuvant chemotherapy. Disease-free survival at 2 years was 55% with chemotherapy and 20% with observation ($p < .01$). Overall survival was also superior at 2 years: 80% versus 48% with and without chemotherapy, respectively ($p < .01$). Link et al.[36] reported similar results in a group of 36 patients with nonmetastatic, high-grade osteosarcoma randomized to observation versus adjuvant chemotherapy after primary surgery. Disease-free survival at 2 years was 66% with chemotherapy and 17% with observation ($p < .001$).

The concept of neoadjuvant chemotherapy arose in conjunction with evolving surgical techniques striving for limb-preserving procedures and improved functional outcomes. This led to a randomized clinical trial by the Pediatric Oncology Group (POG).[37] POG 8651 randomized patients with nonmetastatic, high-grade osteosarcoma to neoadjuvant chemotherapy followed by surgery or surgery followed by the same chemotherapy. The 5-year relapse-free survival was not statistically different between the two groups (65% vs. 61%, respectively), nor was the rate of limb salvage (55% vs. 50%, respectively). Although this trial did not show improved outcomes with neoadjuvant chemotherapy, it did show equivalence and established a benchmark for comparison with future trials. Neoadjuvant chemotherapy is favored by most centers, with the belief that the likelihood of limb-sparing surgery and, ultimately, functional outcome can be improved with this approach. Furthermore, the response to neoadjuvant chemotherapy has been shown to be prognostic.[38] This allows for the stratification of patients for more intensive postoperative treatment.

The optimal choice of chemotherapy and administration schedule remains a subject of active research. The Memorial Sloan-Kettering Cancer Center T10 regimen is frequently used for nonprotocol patients and consists of high-dose methotrexate, doxorubicin, bleomycin, cyclophosphamide, and actinomycin D.[39] Patients are being accrued to EURAMOS I (AOST 0331), an international collaborative group trial sponsored by European and American Osteosarcoma Study Group, as well as by other groups, including the Children's Oncology Group.[40] This trial is evaluating the benefit of additional chemotherapy after preoperative and postoperative chemotherapy consisting of methotrexate, doxorubicin, and cisplatin. Patients with a poor response to preoperative chemotherapy are randomized to the addition of ifosfamide and etoposide, whereas those with a good response to preoperative chemotherapy are randomized to the addition of interferon.

Radiation

Historically, radiation has been used for the treatment of osteosarcoma; however, high local failure rates with the use of radiation alone, improved surgical techniques, allowing for limb preservation, and effective use of chemotherapy limits the use of radiation therapy for osteosarcoma today. With a combined approach of chemotherapy and surgery with negative margins, local control rates of 90% to 98% have been reported.[30–32,41]

Patients who have tumor resection with inadequate or positive margins or who have unresectable tumors, however, have high rates of local recurrence. The Cooperative Osteosarcoma Study Group (COSS) performed a multivariate analysis of 1,702 patients and found that poor response to neoadjuvant chemotherapy and incomplete surgical resection predicted negatively for overall survival.[42] Picci et al.[43] also reported that local recurrence was higher for limb-salvage surgery if wide, negative margins were not achieved. Furthermore, high recurrence rates have been reported in locations where complete surgery is usually not possible, including a recurrence rate of 70% in the pelvis, 68% in the spine, and 50% in the skull regions.[44–46] Radiation can potentially improve local control in these patients. Therefore, indications for integration of radiation therapy with other treatment modalities currently include incompletely resected tumors with positive margins and unresectable tumors or for palliation of symptoms.

Radiation Therapy Techniques

As with other sarcomas, proper patient position at the time of simulation and treatment is essential to achieve optimal tumor coverage and normal-tissue sparing. Customized immobilization devices may need to be constructed to achieve optimal positioning that is reproducible on a daily basis. Three-dimensional treatment planning with the aid of presurgical and postsurgical imaging is used to define gross tumor volumes and areas of subclinical disease. Typically, a 2-cm margin is used for axial tumors, which can be extended to 4 to 5 cm for extremity tumors. These margins can be restricted at natural tissue and fascial boundaries. The radiation technique used, either three-dimensional conformal or intensity-modulated radiation therapy, should be tailored to the individual patient. Dose to uninvolved organs should be minimized to prevent late organ dysfunction, as should the integral dose to minimize risk of secondary malignancy.

A prescription dose of 60 Gy in 2-Gy fractions is typically used for microscopically involved margins, whereas 66 Gy is used for macroscopic residual disease and 70 Gy is used for inoperable tumors. Chemotherapy should not be interrupted to deliver local radiation therapy. Radiation can be given concurrently but is usually delivered after chemotherapy due to increased acute toxicity with concurrent administration.

Intraoperative radiation therapy has been used to deliver dose directly to close or involved surgical margins.[47,48] Proton particle therapy has been used in an attempt to escalate radiation dose, particularly in unresectable tumors.[49,50] Radionuclide therapy with rhenium,[51] strontium,[52] and samarium[53] has been used for palliation of extensive bone metastases with good effects.

Results of Radiation Therapy

In the prechemotherapy era, Cade[54] pioneered a technique of radiotherapy with delayed amputation in patients who did not develop distant metastases. The primary tumor was controlled in some patients who refused amputation. However, the overall results were poor, with most patients dying of metastatic disease. The incorporation of chemotherapy with optimal surgery has resulted in significantly improved outcomes, obviating the need for radiation therapy for most patients. Dincbas et al.[55] evaluated the addition of preoperative radiation therapy to chemotherapy followed by limb-sparing surgery. They reported on a series of 46 patients, most of whom received 35 Gy in 10 fractions. Local control and overall survival rates at 5 years were 97.5% and 48.4%, respectively. Although the results were excellent, it is not clear whether preoperative radiation therapy improved outcomes, given that the rate of local control with chemotherapy follow by surgery in the absence of adjuvant radiation is high, as previously summarized.

For patients who have incomplete tumor resection or unresectable tumors, the risk of local recurrence/progression is high. These patients, therefore, can potentially benefit from radiation therapy. Machak et al.[56] reported on a series of 187 patients with nonmetastatic osteosarcoma treated with induction chemotherapy. Of these, 31 patients refused surgery and were treated with radiation to a mean dose of 60 Gy. Local control was related to response to induction chemotherapy. There were no local recurrences in 11 patients who had a good response to chemotherapy. However, local progression-free survival was 31% at 3 years and 0% at 5 years for nonresponders. Schwarz et al.[57] reported on an analysis of 100 patients treated with radiation therapy in the COSS registry. Local control and overall survival for the whole group were 30% and 36%, respectively, at 5 years. Local control was significantly better when surgery was combined with radiation compared to radiation alone: 48% vs. 22%, respectively ($p = .002$). Local control was also higher for primary tumors compared with recurrent tumors: 40% vs. 17%, respectively. DeLaney et al.[50] reported on the Massachusetts General Hospital (MGH) experience. Forty-one patients with osteosarcoma underwent radiation for close or positive margins or for unresectable disease. Anatomic sites included 17 skull, 8 extremity, 8 spine, 7 pelvis, and 1 trunk. Patients received a median dose of 66 Gy (10–80 Gy), with about half of patients receiving a portion of their treatment with protons. The overall local control rate was 68% at 5 years. Local control was similar between patients who underwent a gross total resection or subtotal resection but was significantly better than for those who underwent biopsy only: 78% versus 78% versus 40% at 5 years, respectively ($p < .01$).

Overall, it appears that radiation is most effective when the tumor burden is small, with the best results achieved in patients who have a good response to chemotherapy or are able to undergo gross total or subtotal tumor resection. Total dose may also be an important factor. Gaitán-Yanguas[58] showed a dose–response relationship for osteosarcoma, with no lesions controlled at doses ≤30 Gy and all lesions controlled at doses of >90 Gy. The best clinical results were reported in the MGH series.[50] A median dose of 66 Gy was used, and half of the patients received proton therapy as part of their treatment. The unique dose–depth properties of proton radiation therapy allows for dose escalation while maintaining normal-tissue sparing. This approach may explain the improved outcomes reported. However, this study did fail to show a dose–response relationship.

Whole-Lung Irradiation

Whole-lung irradiation has been shown to be beneficial in several other pediatric tumors with a propensity for lung metastases. This led to the rationale that this treatment may improve outcomes in osteosarcoma, which has a high propensity for metastases and for which the lung is the most common site of spread. Two initial small randomized trials in the prechemotherapy era showed a trend for improved disease-free and overall survival for whole-lung irradiation.[59,60] This led to the EORTC-20781/SIOP-03 phase III trial, which randomized 240 patients to three arms: chemotherapy, whole-lung irradiation, or both.[61] The whole-lung dose was 20 Gy. The 4-year disease-free survival and overall survival were 43% and 24%, respectively, with no difference between the arms. Therefore, with the recognition of the other advantages of systemic therapy, whole-lung irradiation has fallen out of favor.[62]

Surveillance and Sequelae of Treatment

Surveillance for recurrence should include imaging of the primary site with CT or MRI and chest imaging. Late complications are largely related to chemotherapy and surgical interventions. Limb functional outcomes are related to location of tumor and type of resection and reconstruction performed. Complications related to radiation therapy include joint fibrosis with decreased range of motion, bone weakening and fracture, loss of allograft, and secondary malignancy.[50] Careful consideration of radiation technique and physical rehabilitative therapy are essential to minimizing late functional impairment.

CHONDROSARCOMA

Epidemiology

Chondrosarcoma is characterized by a neoplastic process with associated cartilage matrix production that is devoid of osteoid, a characteristic of osteosarcoma. It is the second-most-common primary bone tumor, accounting for approximately 30% of cases.[63] Chondrosarcoma may arise at any age but typically occurs in middle-aged and older adults.[64]

Pathogenesis and Risk Factors

The etiology of chondrosarcoma is not fully understood. It is usually sporadic but can also develop from malignant transformation of benign cartilaginous lesions—osteochondromas and enchondromas. Osteochondroma is a cartilage-capped bony projection arising on the external surface of bones. It is usually located on long bones, particularly around the knee. Multiple osteochondromas are associated with hereditary multiple exostoses, an autosomal dominant syndrome. Malignant transformation occurs in 5% of patients with either solitary or multiple osteochondromas.[65,66] Enchondroma is a benign cartilaginous tumor developing in the marrow cavity of bone. Multiple enchondromas, or enchondromatosis, are usually associated with congenital disorders such as Ollier disease or Maffucci syndrome. Malignant transformation of solitary enchondromas is extremely rare, but the risk with enchondromatosis is as high as 25% to 30%.[66,67]

Clinical Presentation and Diagnostic Evaluation

Patients typically present with localized pain in the affected bone with or without associated soft-tissue swelling or a palpable mass. Plain radiograph is obtained for initial evaluation, but CT and MRI are essential to characterize the lesion(s) and determine the full extent of disease.

Tissue biopsy of the tumor is necessary to confirm the diagnosis and to differentiate it from other malignant bone tumors. Biopsy should be aimed at the most aggressive portion as determined by imaging. This can help avoid biopsy a portion of a benign precursor lesion. It also helps avoid less aggressive surgical approaches used for low-grade lesions if a high-grade component is present.[68]

The rate of metastatic disease for chondrosarcoma is very dependent on tumor grade. Low-grade lesions have a <10% risk of metastases, intermediate-grade lesions have a 10% to 50% risk, and high-grade lesion have a 50% to 70% risk.[69,70] The lungs are the main site of metastases. Staging evaluation thus should include a chest CT for intermediate- and high-grade lesions.

Staging Systems

As with osteosarcoma, both the MSTS staging system and the American Joint Committee on Cancer staging system can be used (Table 82.1). MSTS is used more often.[20,21]

Pathology

Chondrosarcoma pathologically is divided into conventional, which comprises 85% to 90% of cases, and other, uncommon variants. Conventional chondrosarcoma is further subdivided into central, peripheral, and periosteal.[71,72] Central chondrosarcoma is the most common type, accounting for 75% of all chondrosarcomas. Most are sporadic, but as many as 40% may arise for underlying enchondromas. Most commonly the proximal femur, pelvis, and proximal humerus are involved.[73] Peripheral chondrosarcoma by definition arises from a pre-existing osteochondroma. The long bones, pelvis, and shoulder girdle are most commonly affected.[66] Periosteal chondrosarcoma arises from the surface of bone and is rare. It usually affects adults at a younger age, in their 20s and 30s, and tends to have a good prognosis.[74] Nonconventional chondrosarcoma variants include clear cell, dedifferentiated, myxoid, and mesenchymal. Clinical behavior of chondrosarcoma is highly dependent on histologic grade.[69,75,76]

Treatment

Histologic grade and tumor location are important determinates of treatment approach. Surgical excision is the primary treatment modality for chondrosarcoma. For low-grade tumors, which constitute the vast majority of chondrosarcomas, surgical resection alone is sufficient to achieve a high rate of disease control. For low-grade central tumors, intralesional excision or curettage is the preferred method of resection. This can be combined with local adjuvant chemical treatment or cryotherapy. These approaches result in good local control rates and minimize the morbidity of more extensive surgical resection.[77–80] The best outcomes are obtained with small tumors located in the extremities. Larger tumors, tumors with intra-articular or soft-tissue involvement, and axial or pelvic tumors have higher local recurrence rates with these more conservative treatments and are better treated with wide excision.[81,82] For the less common intermediate- and high-grade tumors, wide *en bloc* excision is the optimal surgical approach.[76] Radiation therapy is indicated for incompletely resected high-grade or locally recurrent tumors and tumors that are unresectable. Chemotherapy is generally not very effective for chondrosarcoma, especially for the most prevalent conventional type. There is no established adjuvant chemotherapy regime for these patients. There is some suggestion that dedifferentiated and mesenchymal chondrosarcomas may potentially benefit from chemotherapy, but phase III randomized data are lacking in these rare tumors.[83–85]

Radiation

As with osteosarcoma, no level 1 evidence exists for radiation therapy in chondrosarcoma. Based on first principles and results of published case series, radiation therapy is indicated to improve on high local failure rates after incomplete resection of high-risk tumors. These indications include intermediate- to high-grade tumors, locally recurrent tumors, and tumors in locations where surgical resection is challenging or limited. Definitive radiation can also be used for unresectable tumors. Doses of 50 Gy preoperatively and 60 to 66 Gy postoperatively for close or positive margins are typically used. Doses of ≥70 Gy are needed for definitive treatment.

Results of Radiation Therapy

Although chondrosarcoma was traditionally considered to be a "radioresistant" tumor, modern series have shown good outcomes with radiation therapy. Goda et al.[86] presented the Princess Margaret Hospital experience of combined surgery and radiation therapy for high-risk extracranial chondrosarcoma. They reported on 60 patients with a median follow-up of 75 months and showed local control rates of 100%, 94%, and 42% for R0, R1, and R2 resected patients, respectively. Ten-year overall survival was 86%. Definitive radiation therapy has also been used for locations where complete surgical resection is difficult to achieve, that is, the spine and base of skull.[87–90] In these locations, *en bloc* resection is generally not possible, and even piecemeal resection is often not complete. Proton radiation therapy has been used in this setting. The unique depth–dose properties of protons allows for dose escalation while sparing neighboring critical structures. A large series was reported from Massachusetts General Hospital consisting of 200 patients with base-of-skull chondrosarcoma treated using a combination of photon and proton radiation therapy.[91] With median dose of 72 cobalt-gray-equivalent (CGE), they reported a 10-year local control rate of 98%. Similar local control rates have been reported by other institutions using various conformal radiation methods to achieve a high tumor dose, including

TABLE 82.2 SELECTED STUDIES OF BASE-OF-SKULL CHORDOMA AND CHONDROSARCOMA

Institution/Study	Number of Patients	Radiation Modality	Median Dose (Range)	Median Follow-Up (Month)	Local Control	Overall Survival
MGH Terahara et al.[96]	132 chordoma	Mixed photon/proton	68.9 CGE (66.6–79.2 CGE)	41	5 yr 59% 10 yr 44%	NR
MGH Rosenberg et al.[91]	200 chondrosarcoma	Mixed photon/proton	72.1 CGE (64.2–79.6 CGE)	63	5 yr 99% 10 yr 98%	5 yr 99% DSS 10 yr 99% DSS
Institut Curie Noël et al.[97]	100 chordoma	Mixed photon/proton	67 CGE	31	2 yr 86% 4 yr 54%	2 yr 94% 5 yr 81%
Paul Scherrer Institute Ares et al.[92]	64 total: 42 chordoma 22 chondrosarcoma	Mixed photon/proton	Chordoma 73.5 CGE Chondrosarcoma 68.4 CGE	38	Chordoma 5 yr 81% Chondrosarcoma 5 yr 94%	Chordoma 5 yr 62% Chondrosarcoma 5 yr 91%
Loma Linda University Hug et al.[93]	58 total: 33 chordoma 25 chondrosarcoma	Proton	70.7 CGE (64.8–79.2 CGE)	33	Chordoma 5 yr 76% Chondrosarcoma 5 yr 92%	Chordoma 5 yr 79% Chondrosarcoma 5 yr 100%
University of Heidelberg Schulz-Ertner et al.[98]	96 chordoma	Carbon ions	60 CGE (60–70 CGE)	31	3 yr 81% 5 yr 70%	3 yr 92% 5 yr 89%
University of Heidelberg Schulz-Ertner et al.[94]	54 chondrosarcoma	Carbon ions	60 CGE	33	4 yr 90%	5 yr 98%
North American Gamma Knife Consortium Kano et al.[99]	71 chordoma	SRS-Gamma knife	15 Gy (9–25 Gy)	60	5 yr 66%	5 yr 80%
University of Heidelberg Debus et al.[95]	45 total: 37 chordoma 8 chondrosarcoma	F-SRT-photon	Chordoma 66.6 Gy Chondrosarcoma 64.9 Gy	27	Chordoma 2 yr 82% 5 yr 50% Chondrosarcoma 5 yr 100%	2 yr 97% 5 yr 82%

CGE, cobalt gray equivalents; F-SRT; fractionated stereotactic radiation therapy; MGH, Massachusetts General Hospital; NR, not reported; SRS, stereotactic radiosurgery.

protons, fractionated stereotactic photon, and carbon ions.[92–95] Tables 82.2 and 82.3 summarize the results of selected studies of radiation therapy for chondrosarcoma involving the base of skull and the spine, respectively.

Surveillance and Sequelae of Treatment

Functional assessment, rehabilitation, and physical therapy are important to minimize the long-term morbidity of surgery and/or radiation therapy. Surveillance for recurrence should include history and physical exam, CT or MRI imaging of the primary area, and chest imaging on a periodic basis. Follow-up should continue for a minimum of 10 years because late recurrences are more commonly observed with chondrosarcoma than with other sarcomas.[105]

CHORDOMA

Epidemiology

Chordoma is a rare, malignant neoplasm arising from the remnant of the primitive notochord. Chordoma accounts for 1% to 4% of primary bone tumors, with an annual incidence in the United States of 0.08 cases per 100,000.[106] Median age at presentation is 60 years, but base-of-skull location typically present at a younger age, usually in the third to fourth decade of life.

Pathogenesis

In normal embryologic development, the notochord regresses as the embryo matures. Remnants can be found anywhere along the tract of the notochord from the base of skull to the sacrum. The largest foci remain at the cranial and caudal ends. This corresponds well with the anatomic distribution of chordoma, with half arising in the sacrococcygeal region and one-third at the base of skull, typically the clivus.[106] The rest occur in the vertebral bodies of the spine. Chordomas in other locations are exceedingly rare.[107]

Clinical Presentation and Diagnostic Evaluation

Chordomas are slow-growing but locally destructive tumors. They typically present with pain at the affected area that may be of long-standing duration. Neurologic symptoms based on location are frequent. Base-of-skull tumors can present with cranial nerve deficits, particularly cranial nerve 3 or 6 palsies

TABLE 82.3 SELECTED STUDIES OF SACRAL/SPINE CHORDOMA AND CHONDROSARCOMA

Institution/Study	Number of Patients	Radiation Modality	Median Dose (Range)	Median Follow-Up (Month)	Local Control	Overall Survival
MGH DeLaney et al.[100]	29 chordoma 14 chondrosarcoma 7 other	Mixed photon/proton	76.6 CGE (59.4–77.4 CGE)	78	5 yr 78% Chordoma 90% Chondrosarcoma 57%	5 yr 87%
Paul Scherrer Institute Rutz et al.[101]	26 chordoma	Mixed photon/proton	72 CGE (59.4–74.4 CGE)	35	3 yr 86%	3 yr 84%
University of Heidelberg Zabel-du Bois et al.[102]	34 chordoma	IMRT-photons	66 Gy (54–72 Gy)	54	2 yr 55% 5 yr 27%	2 yr 91% 5 yr 70%
Chiba RCH Imai et al.[103]	38 chordoma	Carbon ions	70.4 CGE (52.8–73.6 CGE)	80	5 yr 89%	5 yr 86%
Berkeley Schoenthaler et al.[104]	14 chordoma	Helium/neon ions	75.6 CGE	60	5 yr 55%	5 yr 85%

CGE, cobalt Gray equivalents; IMRT, intensity-modulated radiation therapy; MGH, Massachusetts General Hospital; RCH, Research Center Hospital.

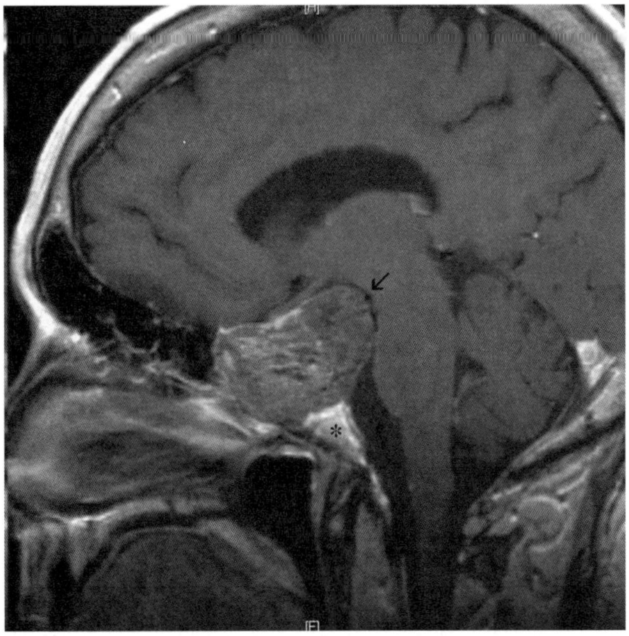

FIGURE 82.3. Base-of-skull chordoma. Fifty-year-old patient who presented with several months of headaches and visual field deficits. T1-weighted, postgadolinium sagittal magnetic resonance imaging of the head depicts a chordoma (*arrow*) arising from the clivus (*asterisk*) with mass effect and posterior displacement of the brainstem.

(Fig. 82.3). Hydrocephalus and sensorimotor deficits can also occur. In the sacral region, sacral nerve roots can be affected, resulting in bowel or bladder dysfunction. Diagnostic evaluation includes CT and MRI to characterize the extent of the primary tumor and involvement or neighboring neural structures (Fig. 82.4). Biopsy should be performed to establish the pathologic diagnosis.

Chordomas have a low metastatic potential, but metastases may occur in as many as 10% to 40% of patients.[108–112] These typically occur late in the disease course and can involve lung, bone, liver, lymph nodes, or soft tissues. Metastatic deposits

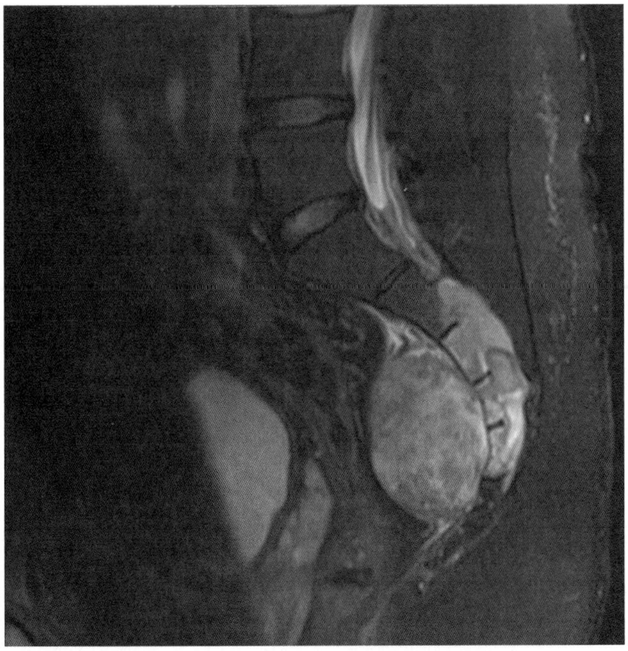

FIGURE 82.4. Sacral chordoma. Forty-five-year-old patient who presented with 1 year of low back pain radiating to the coccyx. T2-weighted sagittal magnetic resonance imaging of the pelvis depicts a 5-cm chordoma involving the inferior sacrum up to the level of S2.

tend to be slow growing, and control of local disease progression remains the major therapeutic challenge in most patients.[113]

Pathology

Chordomas are classified histologically into conventional (classic), chondroid, and dedifferentiated. The majority are conventional. Chondroid chordoma accounts for 5% to 15% and tends to have a better prognosis. Dedifferentiated chordoma account for <5% of chordomas but are more aggressive, faster growing, and more likely to metastasize.[113] Chordoma can be histologically difficult to differentiate from low-grade chondrosarcoma. The latter has a better prognosis, so the distinction is prognostically important. A careful pathologic review by a pathologist experienced in these tumors is recommended.[114]

Treatment

Although chordoma has the potential to metastasize, the dominant failure pattern is local recurrence, and this typically dictates morbidity and mortality for these patients. Salvage after local recurrence can achieve disease control for a period of time, but the ultimate outcomes tends to be poor. Thus, aggressive upfront treatment affords the best potential for cure.

Surgery has been the primary approach for these tumors. Complete *en bloc* resection with negative margins has been reported to achieve local control in 70% to 80% of patients.[115] However, when negative margins cannot be achieved, the failure rate is >70%.[115,116] Unfortunately, less than half of sacral tumors and even fewer base-of-skull tumors are amenable to complete resection. Aggressive surgery can also result in significant morbidity. Base-of-skull resection can result in cranial nerve deficits.[117] Resection of sacral chordomas can result in bowel and bladder dysfunction when S2 or S3 nerve roots are injured or sacrificed.[118,119]

Chordomas are considered relatively "radioresistant" tumors, and so doses of >66 Gy are required. These doses have traditionally been difficult to achieve with conventional external beam techniques, given the location of these tumors abutting sensitive neural structures. Given the advantages of the physical dose properties of the Bragg peak of charged particles, these tumors were treated early in the advent of this technology. Thus far, the best results in the treatment of chordomas have been achieved with a combination of surgery and high-dose proton radiation therapy. Local control rates of 54% to 90% have been reported.[92,93,96,97,100,101]

Chemotherapy has long been known to be inactive in chordoma, and thus chemotherapy has not played a role in the definitive management of these patients. Recently, expression of Platelet-derived growth factor and epidermal growth factor receptors on these tumors and antitumor activity of targeted therapies against these receptors have been described, renewing interest in systemic treatment.[120,121] Imatinib, cetuximab, and gefitinib have been used, but clinical experience is limited.[122,123]

Results of Radiation therapy

For base-of-skull chordomas, one of the largest experiences has been reported from Massachusetts General Hospital.[112] A crude local control of 69% was achieved in 204 patients treated using proton radiation therapy to a dose of 66.6 to 79.2 CGE. Reports of using heavier charged particle have shown similar outcomes.[98] With improvement in technology, dose escalation using conventional photons has also been achieved using intensity-modulated radiation therapy, fractionated stereotactic radiation therapy, and stereotactic radiosurgery techniques.[92–94,97–99] The outcomes with these approaches have been comparable to those reported for proton techniques. Table 82.2 summarizes the results of selected published studies for base-of-skull chordomas.

For sacral chordomas, the published literature is less robust but has shown similar results. DeLaney et al.[100] reported local control in 90% of 29 patients with sacral chordoma at a median follow-up of 4 years. Five-year actuarial local control was 100% for primary treatment versus 56% for salvage. There was no statistical difference based on extent of resection. Table 82.3 summarizes the results of published studies for spine sarcomas, including chordoma.

Sequelae of Radiation Therapy

Due to the high dose required for treatment of chordomas and the proximity of sensitive structures, late complications are not infrequent, and patients need to be followed and monitored closely. For base-of-skull chordoma, hypopituitarism, memory impairment, cranial nerve injury, sensory neural hearing loss, and central nervous system necrosis have been reported.[88,92,110] For sacral chordoma, sacral nerve root injury, erectile dysfunction, rectal bleeding, and sacral insufficiency factures have been reported.[100]

RARE MALIGNANT BONE TUMORS

Fibrosarcoma of bone is a very rare tumor, accounting for <5% of all primary bone tumors.[124] It is a malignant neoplasm of mesenchymal origin characterized by predominance of fibroblasts without tumor osteoid or cartilage production. It has a predilection for long bones and has a high metastatic potential. It is treated with complete surgical resection and often with adjuvant or neoadjuvant chemotherapy. Radiation therapy can be used for incompletely resected or unresectable tumors.

Malignant fibrous histiocytoma of bone also accounts for <5% of bone tumors.[124] It is characterized by a mixture of spindle-shaped fibroblastic cells in a storiform pattern and admixed with mononuclear cells with histiocytic morphology and anaplastic giant cells without tumor osteoid or cartilage production. The mainstay of treatment is complete surgical resection. Like osteosarcoma, it has a high rate of metastases. Malignant fibrous histiocytoma of bone is typically treated similarly to osteosarcoma and has been shown to benefit from chemotherapy.[125]

SELECTED REFERENCES

A full list of references for this chapter is available online.

5. Hawkins MM, Wilson LM, Burton HS, et al. Radiotherapy, alkylating agents, and risk of bone cancer after childhood cancer. *J Natl Cancer Inst* 1996;88(5):270.
6. Le Vu B, de Vathaire F, Shamsaldin A, et al. Radiation dose, chemotherapy and risk of osteosarcoma after solid tumours during childhood. *Int J Cancer* 1998;77(3): 370.
7. Tucker MA, D'Angio GJ, Boice JD Jr, et al. Bone sarcomas linked to radiotherapy and chemotherapy in children. *N Engl J Med* 1987;317(10):588.
20. Enneking WF, Spanie SS, Goodman MA. A system for the surgical staging of musculoskeletal sarcoma. *Clin Orthop Rel Res* 2003;415:4–18.
21. American Joint Committee on Cancer. *Cancer staging manual*, 7th ed. New York: Springer-Verlag, 2010.
34. Bacci G, Ferrari S, Lari S, et al. Osteosarcoma of the limb. Amputation or limb salvage in patients treated by neoadjuvant chemotherapy. *J Bone Joint Surg Br* 2002;84(1):88.
35. Eilber F, Giuliano A, Eckardt J, et al. Adjuvant chemotherapy for osteosarcoma: a randomized prospective trial. *J Clin Oncol* 1987;5:21–26.
36. Link MP, Goorin AM, Miser AW, et al. The effect of adjuvant chemotherapy on relapse-free survival in patients with osteosarcoma of the extremity. *N Engl J Med* 1986;314(25):1600.
37. Goorin AM, Schwartzentruber DJ, Devidas M, et al. Presurgical chemotherapy compared with immediate surgery and adjuvant chemotherapy for nonmetastatic osteosarcoma: Pediatric Oncology Group POG-8651. *J Clin Oncol* 2003;21: 1574–1580.
38. Bielack SS, Kempf-Bielack B, Delling G, et al. Prognostic factors in high-grade osteosarcoma of the extremities or trunk: an analysis of 1,702 patients treated on neoadjuvant cooperative osteosarcoma study group protocols. *J Clin Oncol* 2002; 20(3):776.
39. Rosen G, Caparros B, Huvos AG, et al. Preoperative chemotherapy for osteogenic sarcoma: selection of postoperative adjuvant chemotherapy based on the response of the primary tumor to preoperative chemotherapy. *Cancer* 1982;49(6): 1221.
40. European and American Osteosarcoma Study Group. Available at: http://www.ctu.mrc.ac.uk/euramos. Accessed August 8, 2011.
41. Bacci G, Ferrari S, Bertoni F, et al. Long-term outcome for patients with nonmetastatic osteosarcoma of the extremity treated at the Istituto Ortopedico Rizzoli according to the Istituto Ortopedico Rizzoli/Osteosarcoma-2 Protocol: an updated report. *J Clin Oncol* 2000;18(24):4016–4027.
42. Bielack SS, Kempf-Bielack B, Delling G, et al. Prognostic factors in high-grade osteosarcoma of the extremities or trunk: an analysis of 1,702 patients treated on neoadjuvant cooperative osteosarcoma study group protocols. *J Clin Oncol* 2002;20(3):776–790.
43. Picci P, Sangiorgi L, Bahamonde L, et al. Risk factors for local recurrences after limb-salvage surgery for high-grade osteosarcoma of the extremities. *Ann Oncol* 1997;8(9):899–903.
44. Ozaki T, Flege S, Kevric M, et al. Osteosarcoma of the pelvis: experience of the Cooperative Osteosarcoma Study Group. *J Clin Oncol* 2003;21(2):334–341.
45. Ozaki T, Flege S, Liljenqvist U, et al. Osteosarcoma of the spine: experience of the Cooperative Osteosarcoma Study Group. *Cancer.* 2002;94(4):1069–1077.
46. Kassir RR, Rassekh CH, Kinsella JB, et al. Osteosarcoma of the head and neck: meta-analysis of nonrandomized studies. *Laryngoscope* 1997;107(1):56–61.
47. Oya N, Kobubo M, Mizowaki T, et al. Definitive intraoperative very high dose radiotherapy for localized osteosarcoma in the extremities. *Int J Radiat Oncol Biol Phys* 2001;51:878–893.
48. Tsuboyama T, Toguchida J, Kotoura Y, et al. Intra-operative radiation therapy for osteosarcoma in the extremities. *Int Orthop* 2000;24:202–207.
49. Hug EB, Fitzek MM, Liebsch NJ, et al. Locally challenging osteo- and chondrogenic tumors of the axial skeleton: results of combined proton and photon radiation therapy using three dimensional treatment planning. *Int J Radiat Oncol Biol Phys* 1995;31:467–476.
50. DeLaney TF, Park L, Goldberg S, et al. Radiotherapy for local control of osteosarcoma. *Int J Radiat Oncol Biol Phys* 2005;61:492–498.
51. Sawyer EJ, Cassoni AM, Waddington W, et al. Rhenium-186 HEDP as a boost to external beam irradiation in osteosarcoma. *Br J Radiol* 1999;72:1225–1229.
52. Gompakis N, Sidi B, Salem N, et al. Strontium-89 for palliation of bone pain. *Med Pediatr Oncol* 2003;40:136.
53. Bruland OS, Skretting A, Solheim OP, et al. Targeted radiotherapy of osteosarcoma using 153Sm-EDTMP. *Acta Oncol* 1996;35:381–384.
54. Cade S. Osteogenic sarcoma. A study based on 133 patients. *Clin Orthop Rel Res* 1991;264:4–9.
55. Dincbas FO, Koca S, Mandel NM, et al. The role of preoperative radiotherapy in nonmetastatic high-grade osteosarcoma of the extremities for limb-sparing surgery. *Int J Radiat Oncol Biol Phys* 2005;62:820–828.
56. Machak GN, Tkachev SI, Solovyev YN, et al. Neoadjuvant chemotherapy and local radiotherapy for high-grade osteosarcoma of the extremities. *Mayo Clin Proc* 2003;78:147–155.
57. Schwarz R, Bruland O, Cassoni A, et al. The role of radiotherapy in osteosarcoma. *Cancer Treat Res* 2009;152:147–64.
58. Gaitán-Yanguas M. A study of the response of osteogenic sarcoma and adjacent normal tissues to radiation. *Int J Radiat Oncol Biol Phys* 1981;7(5):593–595.
59. Breur K, Cohen P, Schweisguh O, et al. Irradiation of the lungs of an adjuvant therapy in the treatment of osteosarcoma of the limbs. An EORTC randomized study. *Eur J Cancer* 1978;14:461–471.
60. Rab GT, Ivins JC, Childs DS, et al. Elective whole lung irradiation in the treatment of osteogenic sarcoma. *Cancer* 1976;38:939–942.
61. Burgers JM, van Glabbeke M, Busson A, et al. Osteosarcoma of the limbs. Report of the EORTC-SIOP o3 trial 20781 investigating the value of adjuvant therapy with chemotherapy and/or prophylactic lung irradiation.*Cancer* 1988;61:1024–1031.
62. Whelan JS, Burcombe RJ, Janinis J, et al. A systematic review of the role of pulmonary irradiation in the management of primary bone tumors. *Ann Oncol* 2002; 13:23–30.
69. Evans HL, Ayala AG, Romsdahl MM. Prognostic factors in chondrosarcoma of bone: a clinicopathologic analysis with emphasis on histologic grading. *Cancer* 1977; 40:818.
70. Björnsson J, McLeod RA, Unni KK, et al. Primary chondrosarcoma of long bones and limb girdles. *Cancer* 1998;83(10):2105.
75. Giuffrida AY, Burgueno JE, Koniaris LG, et al. Chondrosarcoma in the United States (1973 to 2003): an analysis of 2890 cases from the SEER database. *J Bone Joint Surg Am* 2009;91(5):1063.
76. Fiorenza F, Abudu A, Grimer RJ, et al. Risk factors for survival and local control in chondrosarcoma of bone. *J Bone Joint Surg Br* 2002;84(1):93.
77. Veth R, Schreuder B, van Beem H, et al. Cryosurgery in aggressive, benign, and low-grade malignant bone tumours. *Lancet Oncol* 2005;6(1):25.
78. Leerapun T, Hugate RR, Inwards CY, et al. Surgical management of conventional grade I chondrosarcoma of long bones. *Clin Orthop Relat Res* 2007;463:166.
79. van der Geest IC, de Valk MH, de Rooy JW, et al. Oncological and functional results of cryosurgical therapy of enchondromas and chondrosarcomas grade 1. *J Surg Oncol* 2008;98(6):421.
80. Marcove RC. A 17-year review of cryosurgery in the treatment of bone tumors. *Clin Orthop Relat Res* 1982;(163):231–234.
81. Streitbürger A, Ahrens H, Balke M, et al. Grade I chondrosarcoma of bone: the Münster experience. *J Cancer Res Clin Oncol* 2009;135(4):543.
82. Wirbel RJ, Schulte M, Maier B, et al. Chondrosarcoma of the pelvis: oncologic and functional outcome. *Sarcoma* 2000;4(4):161.
83. Mitchell AD, Ayoub K, Mangham DC, et al. Experience in the treatment of dedifferentiated chondrosarcoma. *J Bone Joint Surg Br* 2000;82(1):55–61.
84. Cesari M, Bertoni F, Bacchini P, et al. Mesenchymal chondrosarcoma. An analysis of patients treated at a single institution. *Tumori* 2007;93(5):423–427.
85. Dantonello TM, Int-Veen C, Leuschner I, et al. Mesenchymal chondrosarcoma of soft tissues and bone in children, adolescents, and young adults: experiences of the CWS and COSS study groups. *Cancer* 2008 Jun;112(11):2424–31.
86. Goda JS, Ferguson PC, O'Sullivan B, et al. High-risk extracranial chondrosarcoma: Long-term results of surgery and radiation therapy. *Cancer* 2011;117: 2513– 2519.
87. York JE, Berk RH, Fuller GN, et al. Chondrosarcoma of the spine: 1954 to 1997. *J Neurosurg* 1999;90(1 Suppl):73–78.
88. Noël G, Habrand JL, Jauffret E, et al. Radiation therapy for chordoma and chondrosarcoma of the skull base and the cervical spine. Prognostic factors and patterns of failure. *Strahlenther Onkol* 2003;179(4):241–248.
89. Austin-Seymour M, Munzenrider J, Goitein M, et al. Fractionated proton radiation therapy of chordoma and low-grade chondrosarcoma of the base of the skull. *J Neurosurg* 1989;70(1):13–17.
90. Hug EB, Loredo LN, Slater JD, et al. Proton radiation therapy for chordomas and chondrosarcomas of the skull base. *J Neurosurg* 1999;91(3):432–439.
91. Rosenberg AE, Nielsen GP, Keel SB, et al. Chondrosarcoma of the base of the skull: a clinicopathologic study of 200 cases with emphasis on its distinction from chordoma. *Am J Surg Pathol* 1999;23(11):1370–1378.
92. Ares C, Hug EB, Lomax AJ, et al. Effectiveness and safety of spot scanning proton radiation therapy for chordomas and chondrosarcomas of the skull base: first long-term report. *Int J Radiat Oncol Biol Phys* 2009;75(4):1111–1118.

93. Hug EB, Loredo LN, Slater JD, et al. Proton radiation therapy for chordomas and chondrosarcomas of the skull base. *J Neurosurg* 1999;91(3):432–439.
94. Schulz-Ertner D, Nikoghosyan A, Hof H, et al. Carbon ion radiotherapy of skull base chondrosarcomas. *Int J Radiat Oncol Biol Phys* 2007;67(1):171–177.
95. Debus J, Schulz-Ertner D, Schad L, et al. Stereotactic fractionated radiotherapy for chordomas and chondrosarcomas of the skull base. *Int J Radiat Oncol Biol Phys* 2000 1;47(3):591–596.
96. Terahara A, Niemierko A, Goitein M, et al. Analysis of the relationship between tumor dose inhomogeneity and local control in patients with skull base chordoma. *Int J Radiat Oncol Biol Phys* 1999;45(2):351–358.
97. Noël G, Feuvret L, Calugaru V, et al. Chordomas of the base of the skull and upper cervical spine. One hundred patients irradiated by a 3D conformal technique combining photon and proton beams. *Acta Oncol*2005;44(7):700–708.
98. Schulz-Ertner D, Karger CP, Feuerhake A, et al. Effectiveness of carbon ion radiotherapy in the treatment of skull-base chordomas. *Int J Radiat Oncol Biol Phys* 2007;68(2):449–457.
99. Kano H, Iqbal FO, Sheehan J, et al. Stereotactic radiosurgery for chordoma: a report from the North American Gamma Knife Consortium. *Neurosurgery* 2011;68(2):379–389.
100. DeLaney TF, Liebsch NJ, Pedlow FX, et al. Phase II study of high-dose photon/proton radiotherapy in the management of spine sarcomas. *Int J Radiat Oncol Biol Phys* 2009;74(3):732–9.
101. Rutz HP, Weber DC, Sugahara S, et al. Extracranial chordoma: outcome in patients treated with function-preserving surgery followed by spot-scanning proton beam irradiation. *Int J Radiat Oncol Biol Phys* 2007;67(2):512–520.
102. Zabel-du Bois A, Nikoghosyan A, Schwahofer A, et al. Intensity modulated radiotherapy in the management of sacral chordoma in primary versus recurrent disease. *Radiother Oncol* 2010;97(3):408–412.
103. Imai R, Kamada T, Tsuji H, et al, Working Group for Bone and Soft Tissue Sarcomas. Effect of carbon ion radiotherapy for sacral chordoma: results of phase I-II and phase II clinical trials. *Int J Radiat Oncol Biol Phys* 2010;77(5):1470–1476.
104. Schoenthaler R, Castro JR, Petti PL, et al. Charged particle irradiation of sacral chordomas. *Int J Radiat Oncol Biol Phys* 1993;26(2):291–298.
105. Lee FY, Mankin HJ, Fondren G, et al. Chondrosarcoma of bone: an assessment of outcome. *J Bone Joint Surg Am* 1999;81(3):326–338.
106. McMaster ML, Goldstein AM, Bromley CM, et al. Chordoma: incidence and survival patterns in the United States, 1973–1995. *Cancer Causes Control* 2001;12(1):1–11.
107. Tirabosco R, Mangham DC, Rosenberg AE, et al. Brachyury expression in extra-axial skeletal and soft tissue chordomas: a marker that distinguishes chordoma from mixed tumor/myoepithelioma/parachordoma in soft tissue. *Am J Surg Pathol* 2008;32(4):572–580.
108. Rich TA, Schiller A, Suit HD, et al. Clinical and pathologic review of 48 cases of chordoma. *Cancer* 1985;56(1):182–187.
109. Higinbotham NL, Phillips RF, Farr HW, et al. Chordoma: thirty-five-year study at Memorial Hospital. *Cancer* 1967;20(11):1841–1850.
110. Catton C, O'Sullivan B, Bell R, et al. Chordoma: long-term follow-up after radical photon irradiation. *Radiother Oncol* 1996;41(1):67–72.
111. Chambers PW, Schwinn CP. Chordoma. A clinicopathologic study of metastasis. *Am J Clin Pathol* 1979;72(5):765–776.
112. Fagundes MA, Hug EB, Liebsch NJ, et al. Radiation therapy for chordomas of the base of skull and cervical spine: patterns of failure and outcome after relapse. *Int J Radiat Oncol Biol Phys* 1995;33(3):579–584.
113. Chugh R, Tawbi H, Lucas DR, et al. Chordoma: the nonsarcoma primary bone tumor. *Oncologist* 2007;12(11):1344–1350.
114. Rosenberg AE, Nielsen GP, Keel SB, et al. Chondrosarcoma of the base of the skull: a clinicopathologic study of 200 cases with emphasis on its distinction from chordoma. *Am J Surg Pathol* 1999;23(11):1370–1378.
115. Boriani S, Bandiera S, Biagini R, et al. Chordoma of the mobile spine: fifty years of experience. Spine (Phila Pa 1976) 2006;31(4):493–503.
116. Tzortzidis F, Elahi F, Wright D, et al. Patient outcome at long-term follow-up after aggressive microsurgical resection of cranial base chordomas. *Neurosurgery* 2006;59(2):230–237.
117. Gay E, Sekhar LN, Rubinstein E, et al. Chordomas and chondrosarcomas of the cranial base: results and follow-up of 60 patients. *Neurosurgery* 1995;36(5):887–896.
118. Devin C, Chong PY, Holt GE, et al. Level-adjusted perioperative risk of sacral amputations. *J Surg Oncol* 2006;94(3):203–211.
119. Cheng EY, Ozerdemoglu RA, Transfeldt EE, et al. Lumbosacral chordoma. Prognostic factors and treatment. Spine (Phila Pa 1976) 1999;24(16):1639–1645.
120. Tamborini E, Miselli F, Negri T, et al. Molecular and biochemical analyses of platelet-derived growth factor receptor (PDGFR) B, PDGFRA, and KIT receptors in chordomas. *Clin Cancer Res* 2006;12(23):6920–6928.
121. Weinberger PM, Yu Z, Kowalski D, et al. Differential expression of epidermal growth factor receptor, c-Met, and HER2/neu in chordoma compared with 17 other malignancies. *Arch Otolaryngol Head Neck Surg* 2005;131(8):707–711.
122. Casali PG, Messina A, Stacchiotti S, et al. Imatinib mesylate in chordoma. *Cancer* 2004;101(9):2086–2097.
123. Hof H, Welzel T, Debus J. Effectiveness of cetuximab/gefitinib in the therapy of a sacral chordoma. *Onkologie* 2006;29(12):572–574.
124. Dorfman HD, Czerniak B. Bone cancers. *Cancer* 1995;75(1 Suppl):203–210.
125. Bramwell VH, Steward WP, Nooij M, et al. Neoadjuvant chemotherapy with doxorubicin and cisplatin in malignant fibrous histiocytoma of bone: a European Osteosarcoma Intergroup study. *J Clin Oncol* 1999;17(10):3260–3269.Chapter 83 Auther Query

Chapter 83
Soft Tissue Sarcoma (Excluding Retroperitoneum)

Elizabeth H. Baldini

INCIDENCE

Soft tissue sarcomas (STS) comprise a heterogeneous group of rare malignancies that vary extensively by anatomic location, histology, and biologic behavior. They arise from connective tissues and can occur at any anatomic site. Annually, there are almost 11,000 expected new cases of STS in the United States, and this accounts for approximately 0.7% of all new cancer diagnoses.[1] The median age at diagnosis for all STS is 65 years, but incidence varies by histologic subtype.[2] For example, embryonal rhabdomyosarcoma is common in children; synovial sarcoma occurs mostly in young adults; and pleomorphic high-grade sarcoma, liposarcoma, and leiomyosarcoma are seen mostly in the elderly.

ETIOLOGY AND GENETICS

For the great majority of STS, there is no known etiology. A minority of cases can be attributed to environmental or genetic factors.[2,3] Associated environmental factors include radiation exposure; chemical exposures, such as vinyl chloride, dioxin, arsenical pesticides, and phenoxyherbicides; immunosuppression; lymphedema (Stewart-Treves syndrome); and viruses (human immunodeficiency virus, human herpes virus type 8). Certain clinical syndromes are associated with a genetic predisposition for the development of sarcoma. A few examples include Li-Fraumeni syndrome and Werner syndrome, which are associated with the development of STS as well as other malignancies; neurofibromatosis type 1, which is associated with the development of malignant peripheral nerve sheath tumors; and familial adenomatous polyposis (Gardner syndrome), which is associated with the development of abdominal desmoid tumors.

HISTOLOGIC CLASSIFICATION

The World Health Organization divides soft tissue tumors into four categories: benign; intermediate, locally aggressive (e.g., desmoid fibromatosis); intermediate, rarely metastasizing (e.g., plexiform fibrohistiocytic tumor); and malignant.[2] Further, there are more than 50 histologic subtypes of STS. The most common subtypes include high-grade pleomorphic sarcoma, liposarcoma, leiomyosarcoma, synovial sarcoma, and malignant peripheral nerve sheath tumor. Together, these account for about 75% of STS cases.[2] Histologic diagnosis is determined largely by tumor cell morphology. Immunohistochemical staining helps refine the diagnosis in many cases, and several of the histologic subtypes have characteristic translocations. Some of these characteristic translocations include: Ewing's tumor, t(11,22); synovial sarcoma, t(X,18); myxoid liposarcoma, t(12,16); and clear cell sarcoma, t(12,22).[2] There are several grading systems. The two most widely used are the U.S. National Cancer Institute (NCI) and the French Federation Nationale des Centres de Lutte Contre le Cancer grading systems, both of which employ a three-tiered system of low, intermediate, and high grade.[4] Furthermore, there are certain STS subtypes for which grading is not applicable.[2]

Given the rarity of STS as well as the numerous histologic subtypes, it is not surprising that diagnoses vary even among STS specialists. Several reports have examined concordance rates for histologic diagnosis or grade among pathologists. Agreement rates between nonspecialists and specialists range from 24% to 68%[5–9] Even among sarcoma specialists, concordance rates can vary from 60% to 90%.[10,11] For this reason, it is very important to submit diagnostic slides for review by an experienced sarcoma pathologist prior to embarking on definitive treatment.

NATURAL HISTORY

STS can occur anywhere in the body. The most common site of presentation is an extremity, specifically the thigh. The approximate distribution of STS sites at presentation is extremity, 60% (lower extremity, 45%, upper extremity, 15%); trunk, 15% to 20%; retroperitoneum, 10% to 15%; and head and neck, 8%.[12–14,15] Interestingly, certain histologic subtypes have predilections for specific sites. For example, angiosarcoma commonly occurs in the head and neck, desmoid tumors frequently occur in the abdomen associated with Gardner syndrome, and epithelioid carcinoma often involves the hand or forearm.[16–18]

In the classic reports by Simon and Enneking[19] and Enneking et al.,[20] the local behavior of STS is well described. STS tends to invade longitudinally along musculoaponeurotic planes. These tumors rarely transgress fascial boundaries or invade bone. As the sarcoma grows, it compresses surrounding normal tissue to form a pseudocapsule, which contains a compression zone and a reactive zone. The latter comprises edema, inflammatory cells, and tumor cells. Furthermore, Simon and Enneking[19] have shown that microscopic tumor cells perforate through and extend beyond the pseudocapsule.

Unlike most solid tumors, STS rarely spread to lymph nodes. Three series, each with more than 1,000 consecutive patients with STS, cited only 1.8% to 3.7% of lymph node involvement at the time of initial presentation.[21–23] However, there are a few histologic subtypes for which lymph node involvement is more common. Notable lymph node involvement rates have been demonstrated for epithelioid sarcoma (20% to 35%), clear cell sarcoma (10% to 18%), rhabdomyosarcoma (20% to 25%), and cutaneous angiosarcoma (10% to 15%).[18,22–26]

The American College of Surgeons Patterns of Care Study for adult STS showed that during the years of that study, 23% of patients had metastatic disease at presentation.[15] The single most common site of distant metastasis (34%) was the lung; other metastatic sites included bone (24%), liver (16%), brain (3%), and "other" (24%). Two additional studies that examined patterns of distant recurrence (primarily in high-grade STS) also showed the lung to be the most common site for distant spread, reporting 38% to 52% of first recurrences in the lung.[13,27] Furthermore, as was the case for lymph node spread, certain histologic subtypes exhibit distinct patterns of recurrence. For example, myxoid liposarcoma has a predilection for spread to the retroperitoneum as well as other extrapulmonary sites. Among reported recurrences, 48% to 71% occur in the retroperitoneum, 20% in extrapulmonary soft tissue, and 15% to 17% in bone.[28,29–30] For retroperitoneal STS, the most common site of recurrence is locally in the retroperitoneum.[31–34] These tumors also have a predilection for spread to the liver as well as the lung.[32–34] Lastly, myxofibrosarcoma exhibits higher local recurrences rates than other STS, sometimes with multiple local recurrences necessitating amputation; conversely, the rate of distant recurrence to the lung for this histology is lower than for other STS types.[35–37]

INITIAL EVALUATION

Most STS cases present as a painless mass. When taking a history, one should ask how long the mass has been present, if it has changed in size and at what rate, and if there are any associated local or systemic symptoms. It is also important to ask about potential risk factors for STS, including a history of radiation exposure or a family history of malignancies including STS. On physical examination, one should assess the mass for characteristics such as size, depth, fixation to underlying structures, the presence of overlying skin changes, and potential evidence of neurovascular compromise. On the general examination, one should also note if there are any stigmata of neurofibromatosis, such as neurofibromas or café au lait spots (as there is an association between neurofibromatosis type I and malignant peripheral nerve sheath tumors).[3]

Imaging workup should include evaluation of the primary site as well as sites of potential metastatic spread. For STS of the extremity, trunk, or head and neck, evaluation of the primary tumor with a magnetic resonance imaging (MRI) scan is generally preferred to computed tomography (CT) scanning.[38–39,40] The T1-weighted images of the MRI scan provide excellent definition of the anatomic relation between the tumor and adjacent structures. T2-weighted images demonstrate the tumor and associated edema. As peritumoral edema can contain malignant cells, it is crucial to identify this for both radiation and surgical planning.[41] Demas et al.[39] compared MRI and CT for STS lesions in the extremity and reported that for 23% of cases, the MRI scans showed tumor involvement in muscles

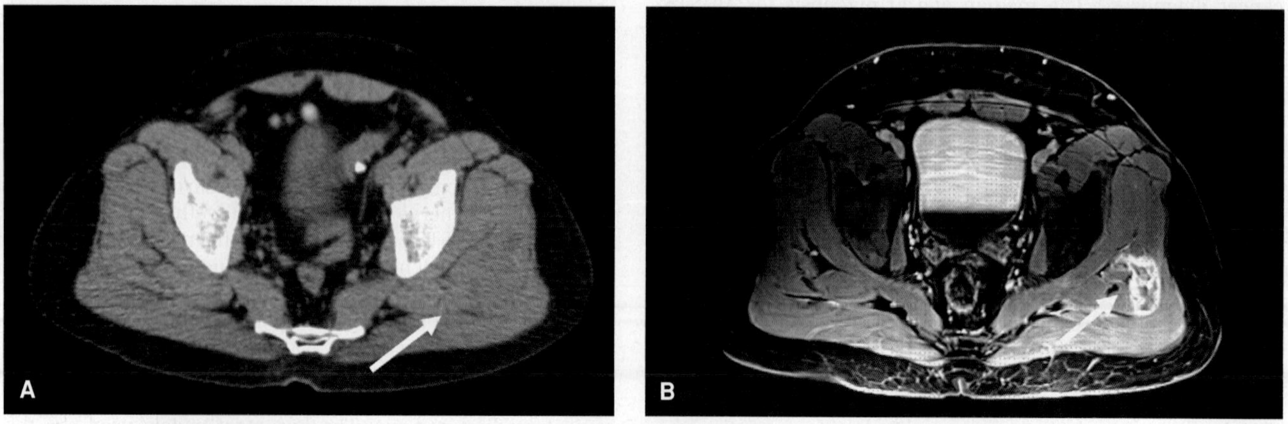

FIGURE 83.1. Comparison of computed tomography (CT) and magnetic resonance imaging (MRI) axial slices for a synovial sarcoma of the left gluteus medius muscle in a 56-year-old man. **A:** The CT axial slice shows a vaguely defined soft tissue mass in the left gluteus medius muscle. **B:** The anatomic definition of the soft tissue sarcoma is seen much more clearly on the corresponding T1 postgadolinium axial slice of the MRI.

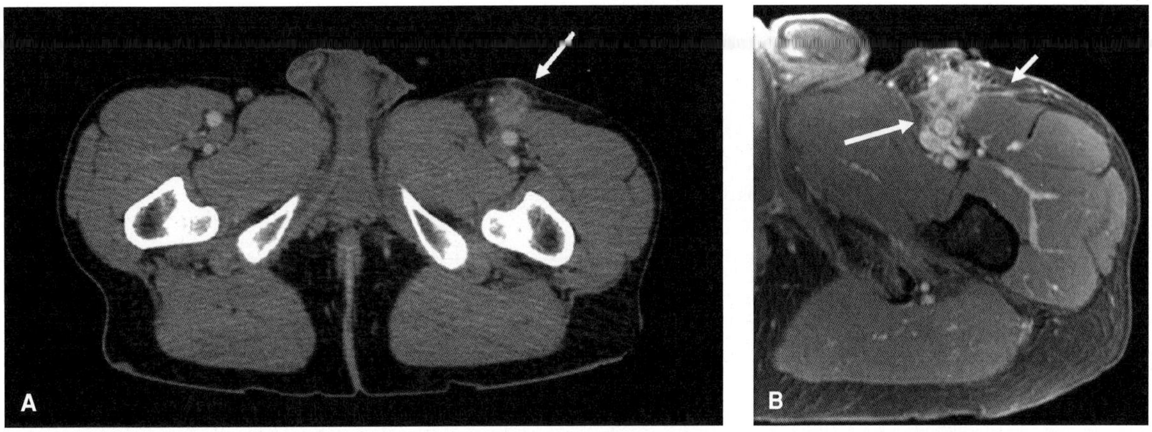

FIGURE 83.2. Comparison of computed tomography (CT) and magnetic resonance imaging (MRI) axial slices for a high-grade leiomyosarcoma of the proximal anterior thigh in a 53-year-old man. **A:** The CT axial slice shows a soft tissue mass in the left anterior upper thigh anterior to the superficial femoral artery and vein. **B:** The T1 postgadolinium image of the MRI at the same level provides superior resolution compared to the CT. It shows a loss of fat plane between the mass and the superficial femoral artery suggestive of arterial invasion (*long arrow*), linear fascial enhancement overlying the vastus medialis muscle (*short arrow*), and tumor spiculations into adjacent subcutaneous fat and to the skin along the biopsy tract.

that appeared normal on CT scan. On the other hand, a prospective study showed no significant difference between the two imaging modalities when performed for preoperative evaluation.[42] Nonetheless, most practitioners believe that MRI is superior to CT for evaluation of soft tissue tumors of the extremity, trunk, and head and neck. Figure 83.1 depicts a case of synovial sarcoma of the left gluteus medius muscle. The mass is difficult to discern on CT imaging (Fig. 83.1A) but very clearly delineated on MRI (Fig. 83.1B). Figure 83.2 is a second comparative example of CT and MRI and shows a leiomyosarcoma of the proximal anterior thigh. Although, the differences between the imaging modalities are not as pronounced as in Figure 83.1, the MRI again provides superior information compared to the CT scan. The MRI demonstrates probable arterial wall invasion, fascial enhancement of the vastus medialis muscle, and definition of tumor spiculations into the adjacent fat and along the biopsy tract. Chest CT scan is recommended to rule out pulmonary metastases for all cases except low-grade tumors or small (<5 cm) high-grade lesions, and even in these latter cases, the author often obtains a baseline chest CT at her institution. Currently, there is no clearly defined role for positron emission tomography (PET) as part of the diagnostic evaluation. However, PET scanning may have potential utility to help distinguish malignant peripheral nerve sheath tumors from benign neurofibromas in patients with neurofibromatosis.[43] Lastly, given that myxoid liposarcoma has a predilection for spread to the retroperitoneum, CT of the abdomen and pelvis is recommended as part of the initial evaluation for patients with this histologic subtype.[28,29–30]

Incisional biopsy or CT-guided core biopsy are the desired diagnostic approaches, and they are preferred to fine-needle aspiration (FNA).[44,45] Each of these procedures typically provides enough tissue for adequate pathologic assessment of both histologic subtype and tumor grade. FNA can confirm malignancy for recurrent disease, but typically does not yield enough tissue to establish an initial diagnosis. The diagnostic biopsy should be performed carefully with the subsequent definitive resection in mind.[38,46] Tumor cells can potentially seed a biopsy tract or incision, thereby necessitating removal of tracts and skin incisions at the time of surgical resection. It is important that the biopsy approach does not transgress an uninvolved compartment or joint as this would create a situation where a much more radical resection would need to be performed. Consequences of inappropriately placed biopsies can be significant and include the need to perform more complex operations, including amputation, with the potential for subsequent loss of function, local recurrence, and death.[46]

STAGING

The American Joint Committee on Cancer (AJCC) published the seventh edition of the TNM (tumor, node, metastasis) staging manual in 2010.[47] The significant factors related to staging of STS include grade (1 to 3), tumor size (≤5 cm vs. >5 cm), location superficial or deep to fascia, and presence of lymph node or distant organ involvement. Stage groupings are shown in Table 83.1. The AJCC staging system for STS does not account for histologic subtype or tumor site, nor does it stratify for tumor size >5 cm. This is unfortunate, given that all of these factors are predictive of survival, but understandable given the complexities of staging systems.

PROGNOSTIC FACTORS FOR SURVIVAL AND LOCAL RECURRENCE

Many reports have evaluated patient and tumor characteristics to determine prognostic factors for disease-free survival (DFS) or overall survival (OS) and local recurrence (LR). The most powerful predictor for DFS and OS is the AJCC TNM stage of the tumor. Five-year DFS rates for stages I, II, and III STS are 86%, 72%, and 52%, respectively.[47] The staging system incorporates several variables, the two most important of which are grade and tumor size. It is also valuable to consider predictive factors individually. Results of multivariate analyses for DFS from several large studies are shown in Table 83.2. Although

TABLE 83.1 AMERICAN JOINT COMMITTEE ON CANCER TNM STAGE GROUPINGS FOR SOFT TISSUE SARCOMAS

Stage IA	G1,X	T1a,b	N0	M0	Low grade, small
Stage IB	G1,X	T2a,b	N0	M0	Low grade, large
Stage IIA	G2,3	T1a,b	N0	M0	Moderate/high grade, small
Stage IIB	G2	T2a,b	N0	M0	Moderate grade, large
Stage III	G3 Any Grade	T2a,b	N0	M0	High grade, large or
		Any T	N1	M0	Node positive
Stage IV	Any Grade	Any T	Any N	M1	Metastatic

GX, grade cannot be assessed; G, grade; T1, tumor ≤5 cm; T2, tumor >5 cm; a, superficial to fascia; b, deep to fascia; NX, regional lymph nodes (LN) cannot be assessed; N0, no regional LN metastasis; N1, regional LN metastasis; M0, No distant metastasis; M1, distant metastasis.

TABLE 83.2 SIGNIFICANT ADVERSE PROGNOSTIC FACTORS FOR DISEASE SPECIFIC SURVIVAL OR OVERALL SURVIVAL ON MULTIVARIATE ANALYSES FROM SEVERAL LARGE PATIENT SERIES

Study	High Grade	Size >5 cm	Deep to Fascia	Tumor Site	Recurrent Disease at Presentation	Positive Margin	Old Age	Histologic Subtype	Bone or Neurovascular Invasion	Gender	Race
Pisters[48] MSKCC N = 1,041 (Extremity)	+	+ (>5 cm, >10 cm)	+	+ Proximal LE	+	+	– (>50)	+ LMS, MPNST	–	–	NA
Zagars[49] MDACC N = 1,225 (All sites)	+	+	NA	+ H+N, RP	–	+	+ (>64)	+ Epithelioid, RMS, clear cell	NA	–	NA
Coindre[50] FFCC N = 1,240 (All sites)	+	+ (>5 cm, >10 cm)	+	–	NA	NA	– (≥50)	–	+	–	NA
Parsons[51] SEER N = 6,215 (Extremity)	+	+	NA	NA	NA	NA	+	+ MFH	NA	+ Male	+ African American
Sampath[54] NODB N = 821 (All sites)	–	+	NA	+ H+N	NA	–	+	+ Spindle cell, synovial, LMS	NA	+ Female	NA
LeVay[52] PMH N = 389 (All except RP)	+	+	NA	+ H+N, trunk	–	–	–	NA	+ (or invasion of skin, and adjacent organs)	NA	NA
Gutierrez[55] FCDS N = 8,249 (All sites)	–	–	NA	+ Trunk, RP	NA	NA	+ (>50, >70)	+ MFH, LMS, GIST	NA	+ Male	+ Non-Caucasian

MSKCC, Memorial Sloan-Kettering Cancer Center; MDACC, MD Anderson Cancer Center; FFCC, French Federation of Cancer Centers; NODB, National Oncology Database; PMH, Princess Margaret Hospital; FCDS, Florida Center Data System; NA, not assessed; LE, lower extremity; H+N, head and neck; RP, retroperitoneum; LMS, leiomyosarcoma; MPNST, malignant peripheral nerve sheath tumor; RMS, rhabdomyosarcoma; MFH, malignant fibrous histiocytoma; GIST, gastrointestinal stromal tumor.

Note: + denotes that factor is statistically significant; – denotes that it is not significant.

there are differences among series, several independent prognostic factors are consistently demonstrated. The single most important individual prognostic factor for lower survival rates is high grade.[48–53] Five-year DFS rates range from 44% to 67% for high-grade tumors compared to 90% to 100% for low-grade tumors.[48–50,53] Other significant predictors for DFS include tumor size, depth, and site. Tumors >5 cm are associated with 5-year DFS rates of about 55% to 70% compared to rates of about 78% to 100% for tumors <5 cm.[48,50,53] DFS rates for tumors >10 cm are even lower and range from 33% to 60%.[48,50] Five-year DFS rates for tumors that are deep to the fascia range from 58% to 70%, whereas those for tumors superficial to fascia are 81% to 92%.[48,50] Furthermore, patients with tumors located in the head and neck or retroperitoneum have lower survival rates than those with tumors located in the extremity or superficial trunk.[49,52,54,55] Reports vary regarding the impact of histologic subtype on DFS, but several cite leiomyosarcoma and malignant peripheral nerve sheath tumor as adverse prognostic factors.[48,54–56] Older age at presentation, positive resection margins, bone or neurovascular invasion, gender, and race all show mixed results regarding their predictive value for DFS (Table 83.2). As stated earlier, lymph node involvement for STS is rare; but if present, it is an adverse prognostic factor.[21–23]

Consistently demonstrated significant predictors for LR include positive margins of resection, presentation with locally recurrent disease, older age, and head and neck or retroperitoneal location. Rates of LR for tumors resected with positive margins range from 28% to 56% compared to 0% to 20% for those with negative margins.[48,49,57–63] Patients who present with locally recurrent disease are at higher risk for LR (25% to 47%) than those who present with primary disease (11% to 21%).[48,58,61] Age has been analyzed with varying cutoff values including >50 years, >64 years, and as a continuous variable. Repeatedly, older age has been associated with higher LR rates.[48,49,52,54]

MANAGEMENT AND OUTCOME FOR SOFT TISSUE SARCOMAS OF EXTREMITY AND TRUNK

Because of the rarity of STS and the numerous forms in which it can present with respect to tumor histology, site, and size, there are many nuances related to optimal management. Furthermore, delivery of treatment requires a multimodality team that includes experienced pathologists; radiologists; surgeons from the disciplines of surgical oncology, orthopedics, and reconstructive surgery; radiation oncologists; medical oncologists; nurses; physical therapists; and social workers. Treatment goals include complete eradication of tumor with optimal function preservation and minimal treatment-related toxicities. Execution of these goals is complex, and, for this reason, STS is best treated by an experienced team at a specialized sarcoma center. Reports from Sweden, the United Kingdom, and the United States have shown inferior quality of treatment delivery and outcome for STS treated outside of specialized centers.[64–66]

Surgery

In almost all cases, appropriate surgical resection is a prerequisite for curative treatment of STS. A range of surgical procedures has been employed for the treatment of STS with varying levels of success. These procedures include marginal resection or excisional biopsy, wide resection, and radical resection or amputation. A marginal resection refers to simple removal of the tumor with its pseudocapsule. This is also often described as a "shell-out," and this is the procedure commonly performed when the diagnosis of STS is not suspected. LR rates after marginal resection range from 42% to 93%.[12,20,67–70] This is not surprising as it is known that microscopic tumor cells can extend beyond the pseudocapsule and up to several centimeters beyond palpable gross tumor.[19,41] Marginal resection is not an appropriate treatment.

At the other end of the spectrum is radical resection, which involves removal of all of the muscles and neurovascular structures within the compartment where the tumor resides or amputation. Reported LR rates after radical resection are much lower and range from 0% to 18%.[12,20,59,67–69] These LR rates are acceptable, but the cost of loss of limb (or loss of an entire compartment) is high. Amputation was a common procedure for STS of the extremities up to the 1970s. The intermediate procedure is a wide resection. Wide resection is also described as conservative surgery (CS), limb-sparing surgery, or function-sparing surgery. It involves *en bloc* removal of tumor with a rim of normal tissue varying in width from about 1 cm to several centimeters depending on anatomic constraints. This procedure preserves good function (limb salvage) but as a treatment by itself is usually associated with moderately high LR rates, ranging from 25% to 60%.[12,20,67–69] Wide resection/CS combined with pre- or postoperative radiation therapy (RT) is the current standard of care for most high-grade STS.

Surgeons should attempt to attain negative margins at the time of definitive resection. As previously stated, the presence of positive margins is consistently associated with increased LR rates even when RT is used.[48,49,52,57–63,71] Because STS is so rare in comparison to benign soft tissue lesions, the initial procedure performed for a STS is often an unplanned excision (shell-out) with resulting positive margins. It is important to perform a definitive re-excision in these situations, if possible, as the likelihood of finding significant residual disease is on the order of 24% to 63%.[8,72,73–75,76–79] As part of the re-resection, incisions, biopsy tracts, drain sites, and any tissues contaminated by the first surgery need to be removed *en bloc* along with tumor-bed margins. Unfortunately, this often results in a greater scope of surgery and increased functional deficit than if an initial planned excision had been performed by an experienced oncologic surgeon.[46] Lastly, although the goal of resection is to attain negative margins, if this would require debilitating surgery, such as resection of a nerve, vessel, or bone, a function-sparing approach with a planned positive margin is sometimes accepted. These decisions are best handled by experienced sarcoma surgeons. Gerrand et al.[60] compared LR rates resulting from procedures with planned positive margins (abutting critical structures) to those of procedures with unplanned (unexpected) positive margins. They found a 4% LR rate for the former compared with a 32% to 38% LR rate for the latter.

Conservative Surgery and Radiation Therapy

Three sentinel randomized trials have been performed and have established RT combined with CS as the standard management for most (high-grade) STS of the extremities and trunk (Table 83.3). The first of these trials was conducted by Rosenberg et al.[59] at the NCI. Patients with high-grade STS of the extremity were randomized to amputation or to CS and postoperative external beam RT (60 to 70 Gy). Patients in both treatment arms received postoperative doxorubicin, cyclophosphamide, and methotrexate; in the RT arm, chemotherapy was started 3 days prior to RT and continued concurrently with RT. LR rates were 0% (0 of 16) and 15% (4 of 27) for patients treated with amputation and with CS and RT, respectively (P = .06). There was no significant difference in survival

TABLE 83.3 RANDOMIZED CONTROLLED TRIALS INCLUDING RADIATION THERAPY FOR SOFT TISSUE SARCOMAS OF THE EXTREMITIES AND TRUNK

Study	Treatment Arms	Local Recurrence	OS or DFS
Rosenberg[59] NCI 1982 N = 43 (Extremity)	Amputation vs. CS + EBRT (60–70 Gy) (both arms received doxorubicin, cyclophosphamide, methotrexate)	0% (0/16) 15% (4/27) P = .06	88% 83% P = .99 (5-yr OS)
Pisters[71] MSKCC 1996 N = 164 (Extremity + trunk)	High grade (n = 119) CS vs. CS + BRT (42–45 Gy) Low grade (n = 45) CS vs. CS + BRT (42–45 Gy)	30% (19/63) 9% (5/56) P = .0025 26% (6/23) 36% (8/22) P = .49	All patients 81% 84% P = .65 (5-yr DFS)
Yang[82] NCI 1998 N = 141 (Extremity)	High grade (n = 91) CS vs. CS + EBRT (63 Gy) (both arms received doxorubicin, cyclophosphamide) Low grade (n = 50) CS vs. CS + EBRT (63 Gy)	19% (9/47) 0% (0/44) P = .003 33% (8/24) 4% (1/26) P = .016	74% 75% P = .71 (10-yr OS) 92% (22/24) 92% (24/26) (no. alive)
O'Sullivan[86,109] CSG 2004 N = 190 (Extremity)	Preop RT (50 Gy) + CS CS + postop RT (66 Gy)	7% 8% P = NS (5-yr LR)	73% 67% P = .48 (5-yr OS)

NCI, National Cancer Institute; MSKCC, Memorial Sloan-Kettering Cancer Center; CSG, Canadian Sarcoma Group; CS, conservative (limb-sparing) surgery; EBRT, external-beam radiation therapy; BRT, brachytherapy; preop, preoperative; postop, postoperative; OS, overall survival; DFS, disease-free survival.

rates. This trial was instrumental in setting a new standard for limb-sparing local management of STS. Amputations are now performed sparingly and in <15% of cases.[80,81]

The next question posed was whether adjuvant RT is necessary. Two more hallmark trials randomized patients between CS alone and CS plus RT.[71,82] Both of these trials showed improved local control with the addition of RT. At the NCI, patients with high-grade STS of the extremity were randomized to treatment with CS and postoperative chemotherapy (doxorubicin and cyclophosphamide) with or without concurrent external-beam RT (63 Gy). Patients with low-grade tumors were randomized to CS with or without postoperative external-beam RT (63 Gy). LR rates for the high-grade tumors were 20% (9 of 44) for CS and chemotherapy compared to 0% (0 of 47) for CS, chemotherapy, and RT (P = .003). For the low-grade tumors, LR rates were 33% (8 of 24) for CS alone and 4% (1 of 26) for CS and RT (P = .016). There were no significant differences in survival rates between the two groups. At Memorial Sloan-Kettering Cancer Center (MSKCC), patients with STS of the extremity and trunk were randomized to treatment with CS alone or CS plus adjuvant brachytherapy (BRT).[71] BRT catheters were sewn into the tumor bed in a parallel array with 1-cm spacing between catheters and extension of catheters 1.5 to 2.0 cm beyond the tumor bed. Iridium-192 was loaded into the catheters and a dose of 42 to 45 Gy was delivered over 4 to 6 days. LR rates for high-grade tumors were 30% (19 of 63) for CS alone compared with 9% (5 of 56) for CS plus BRT (P = .0025). No difference in LR rates by treatment was seen for low-grade tumors; rates were 26% (6 of 23) and 36% (8 of 22) for patients treated with CS alone and CS plus BRT, respectively. As in the two prior trials, there were no significant differences in survival outcomes. Given that BRT did not improve local control for low-grade tumors in this trial, BRT is not recommended for low-grade STS. Furthermore, for high-grade tumors treated with BRT, LR rates are higher in the setting of positive margins.[83] Therefore, BRT as monotherapy is only recommended for high-grade tumors resected with negative margins.[84] (In the setting of positive resection margins, a combination of external-beam RT and BRT or external-beam RT alone is preferred.) These two randomized trials have established the role for RT combined with CS for the management of high-grade (and, in select cases, low-grade) STS. In modern series, local control following CS and RT is excellent, with most reported LR rates being <15%.[53,58,63,85–91]

It is important to note that the current treatment recommendation for most low-grade STS of the extremity and trunk is wide excision alone.[92] As long as negative margins are obtained, LR rates are expected to be well under 20%. Relative indications for RT in the setting of low-grade tumors include situations of positive resection margins, locally recurrent disease following initial wide excision, and tumor location that would not be amenable to subsequent salvage surgery.

Radiation Therapy

Positioning the Patient

The first step of RT planning is to determine the appropriate positioning of the patient. This can be challenging, and sometimes simulation needs to be performed in a few different positions to ascertain the optimal arrangement. A limb should be positioned to allow treatment with as many potential beam angles as possible. In general, this requires that the limb is positioned as far away from the trunk (for upper extremities) or from the opposite limb (for lower extremities) as possible. Suitable positions for upper extremity lesions often include abduction of the arm away from the body with supination or pronation of the arm determined by the location of the tumor. Another good approach for upper extremity lesions is the "swimmer position," whereby the patient is prone with the arm extended above the head (Fig. 83.3A). This position enables an almost 360-degree approach for all but proximal lesions close to the head. For lower extremity lesions, there are several potential positions. Tumors in the medial compartments are often treated with the majority of the beams in an anterior-posterior/posterior-anterior–like orientation and therefore positioning the patient supine with the legs spread apart often suffices. For proximal thigh lesions, one or both legs are often abducted and flexed in the "frog-leg position" to enable reduction of skin folds in the inguinal region, optimal sparing of the perineum and genitalia, and maximal separation from the contralateral leg. Tumors in the true anterior or posterior compartments are often the most challenging. Sometimes the supine position and oblique fields will be feasible, but, for most of these cases, the author's approach is to place the patient in a decubitus position (Fig. 83.3B). The author places the patient in the right-sided decubitus position for right-sided tumors (and vice versa), as she finds it is more stable to have the treated leg directly on the table. The untreated leg is flexed at the knee and placed either posterior or anterior to the treated leg, and the legs are separated as much as possible. For men with proximal thigh lesions, the author typically places the genitalia in netting, which is pulled to the contralateral side. Most of time, the genitalia can be positioned such that they will be out of the path of any beams, but the dose delivered from internal scatter cannot be avoided. For this reason, the author counsels all men with treatment fields close to the genitalia to consider sperm banking if they wish to preserve fertility. Similarly, the author recommends fertility consultation for women with treatment fields close to the ovaries. The author also typically calculates and documents doses delivered to the testicles or ovaries in appropriate situations. Patients with an extremity STS that is to be treated with intensity-modulated RT (IMRT) are often positioned in a more neutral supine posture.[93] This is possible because of the multiple beam angles used in IMRT planning. Once the position is determined, the patient is immobilized in a reproducible fashion. A custom cast is highly recommended for almost all scenarios.

Target Volumes and Treatment Fields

Preoperative Radiation Therapy

Definitions of appropriate treatment volumes for STS of the extremities and trunk have not been formally tested. Historically, large longitudinal margins of at least 5 cm and sometimes >10 cm have been used with good success. The Radiation Therapy Oncology Group (RTOG) Sarcoma Working Group reported a consensus for appropriate target volumes for preoperative RT and this is described as follows.[94] The gross tumor volume (GTV) is defined as the gross tumor delineated by the T1 postgadolinium MRI. Fusion of the diagnostic MRI and planning CT for optimal target definition is strongly encouraged. Clinical target volume (CTV) is defined as the GTV plus 3-cm margins in the longitudinal directions and 1.5-cm margins radially. These margins can be truncated if they extend beyond the compartment or into an intact fascial barrier, bone, or skin. Peritumoral edema on T2 MRI will often be included within the CTV as defined above. If the edema is more extensive and appears suspicious, the CTV can be enlarged to include it at the discretion of the radiation oncologist. Of

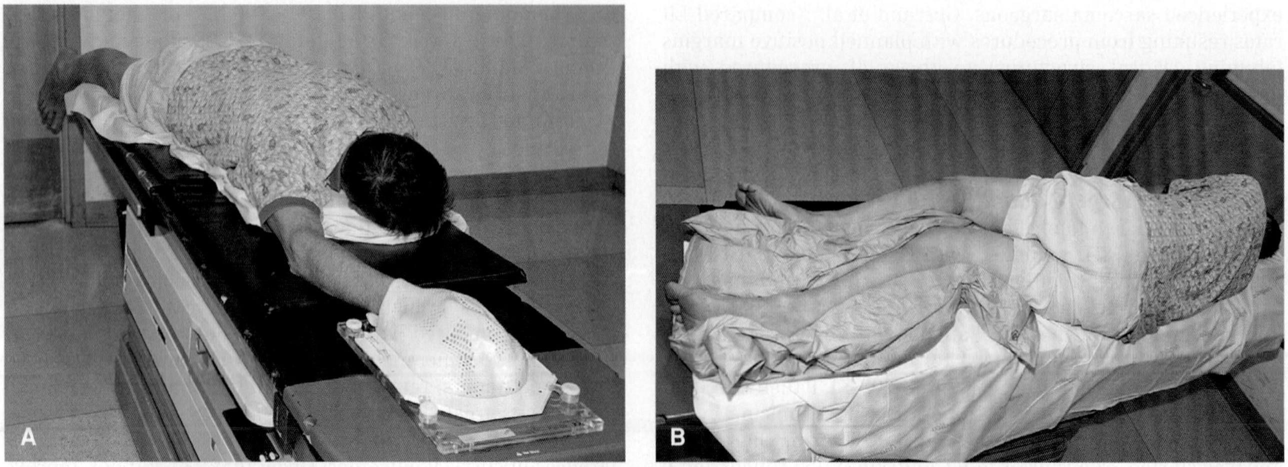

FIGURE 83.3. Examples of patient positions for treatment of upper and lower extremity soft tissue sarcoma (STS). Patients are immobilized in custom casts. **A:** The "swimmer position" is often an ideal position for treating STS of the hand, forearm, or distal upper arm. **B:** This is a right decubitus position to treat a STS in the right posterior or anterior distal thigh or lower leg. The right leg is placed directly on the table. The left leg is flexed at the knee, positioned anterior to the right leg, and the legs are separated as much as possible.

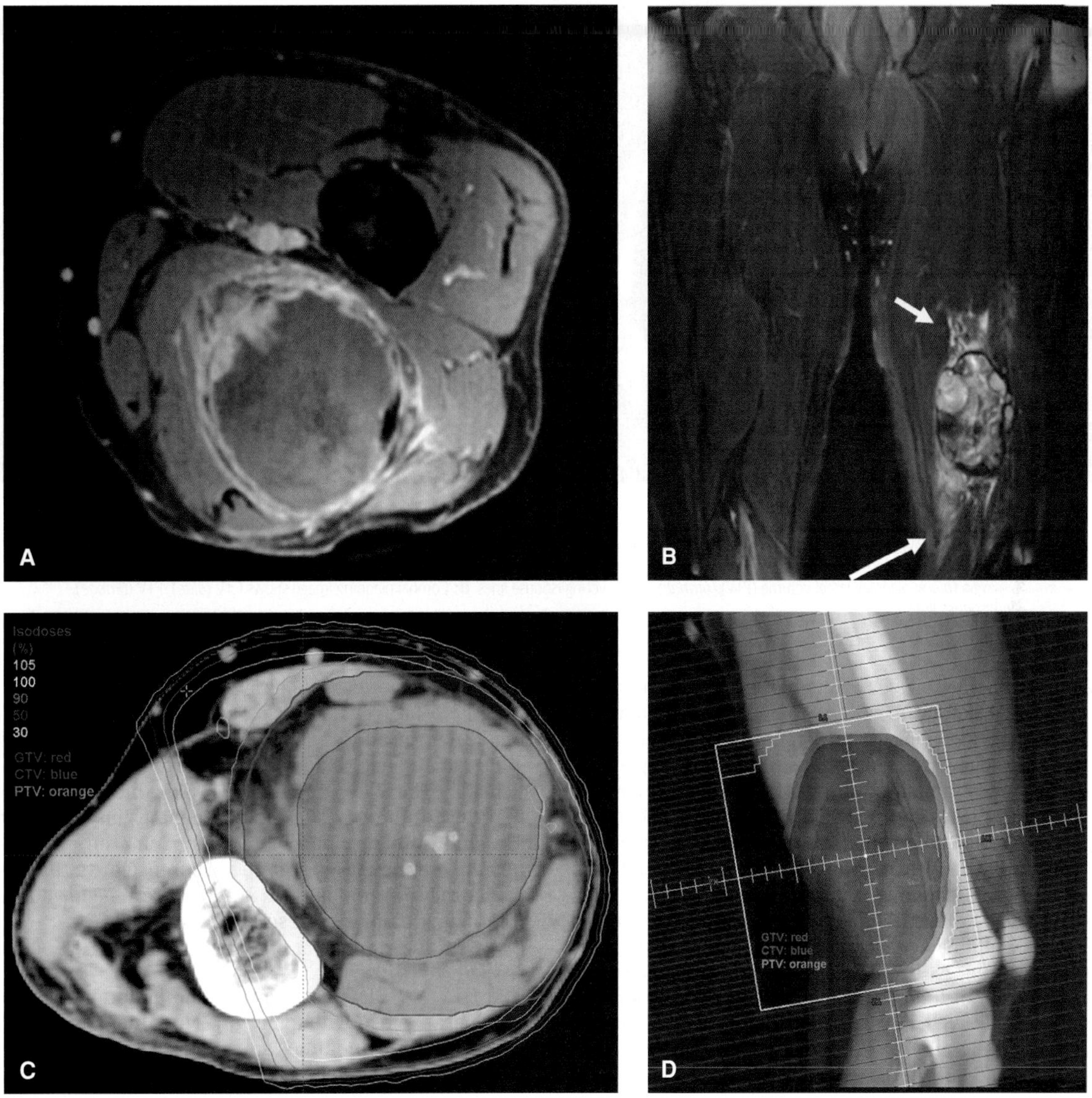

FIGURE 83.4. An unclassified pleomorphic high-grade sarcoma of the posterior left thigh in a 61-year-old man that was treated with preoperative three-dimensional-conformal radiation therapy (50 Gy) using opposed oblique fields. **A:** T1 postgadolinium image of the magnetic resonance imaging (MRI) scan. **B:** T2 image of the MRI scan showing peritumoral edema (*arrows*). **C:** Axial slice of the graphic plan showing the gross tumor volume (*red*), clinical target volume (*blue*), planning target volume (*orange*), and covering isodose lines. **D:** Digital reconstructed radiograph showing the treatment field and target volumes.

note, more clarity is needed to determine in which situations peritumoral edema should be included in the CTV. One report showed the presence of sarcoma cells beyond the gross tumor in 10 of 15 patients. The location of the cells varied from 1 to 4 cm beyond the tumor but did not correlate with the location or extent of peritumoral edema on MRI.[41] It is reasonable to try to include the edema in the CTV, but if this would require a significant increase in the treatment field beyond the RTOG consensus guidelines, it becomes a judgment call. The planning target volume (PTV) definition is not specified in the consensus statement, but typically it is defined as the CTV plus 5 to 10 mm. Application of the GTV and CTV definitions of the RTOG consensus group results in treatment planning fields very similar to the historical standard of 5-cm margins and 2.5- to 3-cm margins from GTV to the field edge in the longitudinal and radial dimensions, respectively. Figure 83.4 depicts MRI, dosimetry, and treatment field images for a STS of the left posterior thigh that was treated with three-dimensional (3D) conformal preoperative RT.

Several series using treatment volumes similar to those described above have reported excellent local control rates. Kim et al.[88] reported a series of 56 patients treated using target volume definitions very similar to the consensus recommendations and described a local control rate of 88.5%. The Canadian Sarcoma Group's randomized trial of preoperative versus postoperative RT also employed similar preoperative treatment fields (except that the CTV expansion in the longitudinal direction was typically 4 cm rather than 3 cm) and reported a 5-year actuarial local control rate of 93%.[86] Lastly, a review of 768 patients treated with preoperative and postoperative RT at Princess Margaret Hospital between 1990 and 2006 demonstrated a local control rate of 92%. Among the 60 recurrences, 82% occurred within the treatment fields.[87] As a group, these three publications provide firm support that the current guidelines produce treatment fields that are sufficiently large.

Postoperative Radiation Therapy

For postoperative treatment, the nomenclature for GTV and CTV is variably described and partly a matter of semantics given that there is actually no "gross tumor." It can be helpful to draw a GTV in the location where the gross tumor was

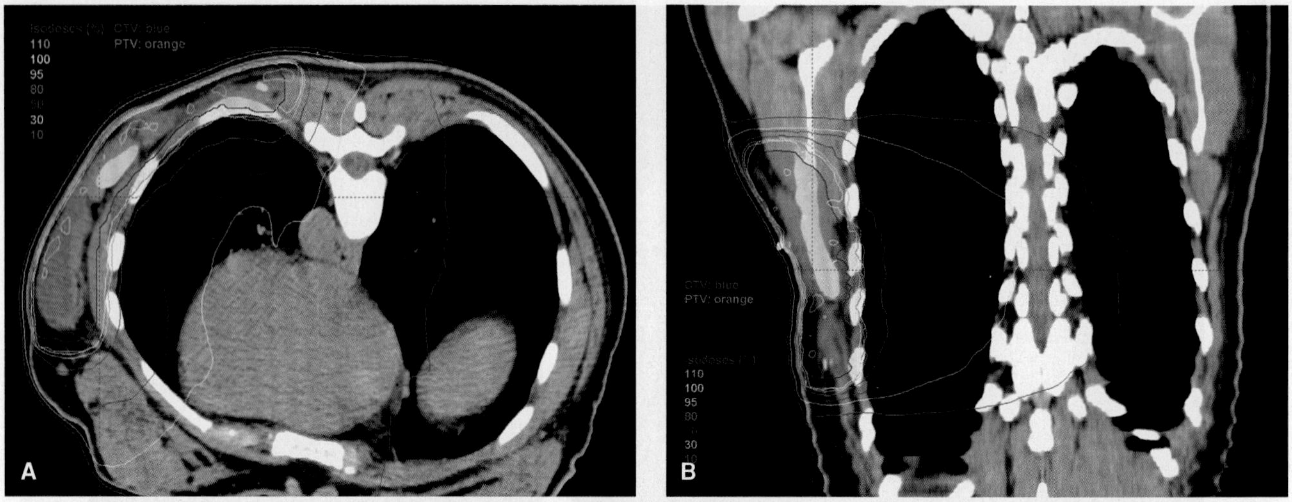

FIGURE 83.5. A malignant solitary fibrous tumor of the left upper back in a 45-year-old woman who underwent marginal excision of a 3.5 cm tumor with multiple positive margins. Radical re-excision showed residual microscopic tumor and negative margins. Postoperative radiation therapy was delivered using intensity-modulated radiation therapy (50.4 Gy) for the first course and opposed oblique fields for the second course (12.6 Gy) to a total dose of 63 Gy. **A:** Axial slice of a planning image shows the clinical target volume (CTV), which includes the operative bed with a margin (*blue*), planning target volume (PTV) (*orange*), and covering isodose lines. **B:** Coronal planning image shows CTV (*blue*), PTV (*orange*), and isodose lines.

preoperatively, as sometimes this volume is used for cone-down volumes. The CTV should encompass all the tissues handled during the surgery including the incision and any drain sites. (Postoperative changes seen on MRI help define the operative bed.) An additional longitudinal margin of 2 to 4 cm and a radial margin of 1.5 to 2 cm is generally added to the operative bed to form the CTV. The same principles apply as listed above in terms of using the T1 postgadolinium images for GTV definition, fusing the planning CT and MRI when possible, and editing the CTV to exclude bone, an intact fascial plane, skin, or extension beyond an uncontaminated compartment. The PTV is typically CTV plus 5 to 10 mm. As is the case in the preoperative guidelines, the end result of these GTV and CTV definitions is a distance from the operative bed to the field edge of about 2 to 5 cm in the longitudinal direction, which matches the historical standard. A second (and sometimes third) course field reduction is typically used in the postoperative setting. CTV margins for the reduced field(s) vary and can include about 2 cm on the operative bed or on the initial GTV.[95,96] These postoperative treatment field definitions are associated with excellent local control rates and are the current standard of care.[86,87,93,97,98] Figure 83.5 shows dosimetry images for a malignant solitary fibrous tumor of the left upper back that was treated with postoperative RT using IMRT.

The excellent local control rates resulting from the use of standard preoperative and postoperative treatment fields establish that these fields are adequately large, but they do not address the question of whether these field sizes could be reduced. As such, the necessity of such large treatment fields has been called into question. Initial development of these large fields predated the CT and MRI era, when imaging modalities to define STS were suboptimal. Moreover, the BRT experience at MSKCC produced excellent local control rates using treatment volumes that extended only 1.5 to 2 cm beyond the tumor bed.[71] Lastly, several single-institution series of treatment with surgery alone have been associated with very good local control rates ranging from 0% to 20% (see the Surgery Alone section).[99,100–106] Specifically, Baldini et al.[102] found no recurrences in 36 patients with resection margins ≥1 cm compared to an actuarial 10-year LR rate of 13% (4 of 38) for those with margins <1 cm. Based on these observations, it is reasonable to query whether treatment field sizes can be reduced. Two ongoing studies ask this question. The first is a trial, in which patients receiving postoperative RT were randomized to standard fields with 5-cm margins or to tailored fields.[107] The CTV for the tailored fields was defined as GTV plus 2 cm in all directions. The second study is RTOG-0630, which is a phase II study using image-guided RT and reduced fields.[108] The CTV is defined as GTV plus 2-cm longitudinal margins for tumors <8 cm and 3-cm margins for tumors >8 cm. The CTV also includes suspicious edema on MRI T2 images. Results of these trials will be very informative, but until more evidence is available, the author recommends the standard treatment volumes as described above.

Brachytherapy

The CTV for BRT treatment as monotherapy should include the operative bed with a margin. The American Brachytherapy Society recommendations state that there is no clear consensus for the appropriate size of the margin.[84] The MSKCC randomized trial used margins of 1.5 to 2 cm beyond the tumor bed.[71] A more detailed description of BRT modalities, techniques, and indications is beyond the scope of this chapter. The American Brachytherapy Society published detailed recommendations in 2001 and those are a good reference.[84]

Doses

The standard dose for preoperative external-beam RT is 50 Gy delivered in 2-Gy fractions.[49,53,89,109] In the situation of positive margins, a postoperative external-beam RT boost of 16 to 20 Gy (delivered in 1.8- to 2-Gy fractions) is sometimes delivered. The efficacy of this boost dose has not been proven and, as it may be associated with increased toxicity, its use has been called into question.[110] Other techniques to deliver an additional boost dose include BRT (both low-dose rate and high-dose rate) and intraoperative electron therapy. Due to variabilities in patient selection for these procedures, it is difficult to determine the relative benefit of the additional dose delivered by these modalities.[95,111,112–115] For postoperative external-beam RT, treatment usually commences about 4 to 6 weeks following surgery and once the wound is fully healed. Recommended total doses are 60 to 66 Gy (delivered in 1.8- or 2-Gy fractions) for the case of negative margins and 66 to 68 Gy for positive margins.[49,63,97,98,116,117] The first course of treatment is typically treated to a dose of 45 to 50 Gy and the balance of the dose is either given in one reduced field or split about evenly between two reduced fields. The standard dose for low–dose-rate BRT is 45 Gy.[71,84] For treatment combining external-beam RT with BRT as a boost, doses are typically 45 to 50 Gy for external beam and 15 to 25 Gy for the BRT component, for a total of approximately 65 Gy.[84,111]

Principles of Treatment Planning

As for any other malignancy, the basic principles of RT planning are to achieve good coverage of the PTV with maximal sparing of adjacent normal structures. For extremity lesions, the important normal structures are the limb itself, soft tissues, bones, and joints. For proximal thigh lesions, the perineum and genitals are also relevant. For STS of the trunk, adjacent normal structures can include small bowel, kidneys, spinal cord, stomach, liver, and lung. Basic tenets for treating the extremity are to "spare a strip" of the limb circumference (to prevent subsequent lymphedema and pain), to avoid treating the whole thickness of bone to high doses (to diminish risk of fracture), and to avoid treating an entire joint to high doses (to decrease joint stiffness). It is not always possible to preserve fertility (and in any borderline situation, one should offer sperm banking or fertility consultation). Every effort should be made to place the testicles as far out of the field as possible to avoid direct treatment and to minimize the contribution from internal scatter.

Specific dosing guidelines for structures of the extremity are as follows. Spare as much as possible of the limb circumference from receiving any dose, and try to spare a 1-cm thickness at a minimum. With 3D-conformal techniques, part of the limb can usually be excluded entirely from the treatment fields (Fig. 83.4C,D). With IMRT, in order to achieve more dose conformality, the tradeoff is that the volume of tissue that receives a low dose is increased; for some of these cases, the entire circumference of the limb may receive some low dose. The acceptable low dose that can be delivered to the entire limb has not been well established and will most likely vary with factors such as the total dose delivered, total volume of tissue treated, and the location in the limb. However, as a guideline, it is helpful to contour a strip of limb circumference to use as an avoidance structure in order to keep part of the treated limb dose to a minimum. The whole-joint dose should be <40 to 45 Gy. Higher doses can be delivered to part of the joint if needed. Full thickness bone irradiation should be avoided if possible, and the mean and maximum doses to the whole bone should also be kept to a minimum. Dickie et al.[118] performed a detailed analysis of dosimetric predictors for bone fracture using a matched pair analysis and found that radiation-related bone fractures were reduced if the following parameters were met: volume of bone receiving ≥40 Gy (V40) <64%, mean dose to bone <37 Gy, and maximum dose to bone <59 Gy. Normal-tissue complication probabilities for organs that may be affected by treatment of a truncal STS are listed in the Quantitative Analysis of Normal Tissue Effects in the Clinic document.[119] If RT treatment of a trunk lesion may potentially ablate ipsilateral kidney function, a renal scan should be performed to ensure adequate function of the contralateral kidney. To achieve sufficient coverage of superficial target volumes (in either the preoperative or postoperative setting), tissue-equivalent bolus material is often applied to intact skin as well as to incision sites. In the preoperative setting, if one reviews the case with the surgeon and determines that an appropriately sized paddle of skin will be removed along with a superficial tumor, one can consider omitting bolus.

Three-dimensional-conformal RT (3D-CRT) and IMRT are both acceptable external-beam treatment techniques. The principal dosimetric differences between these two techniques are that, compared with 3D-CRT, IMRT typically achieves comparable full target coverage, improved conformality of the dose distribution around the target volume, reduced volumes of high doses to normal tissues, greater volumes of low doses to normal tissues, and greater total body exposure due to increased monitor units.[120,121] Three-dimensional-CRT has a longer track record for STS treatment with well-established outcomes and toxicity end points. Fewer long-term data are available for IMRT, and optimal dose–volume histogram metrics for normal structures, such as limb circumference, are yet to be defined. The data for IMRT that do exist, however, are encouraging. Alektiar et al.[93] reported a series of 41 patients with STS of the lower extremity treated with IMRT. With a median follow-up time of 3 years, local control was excellent (94%) and the toxicity profile was comparable to that of 3D-CRT series. Alektiar et al.[122] performed a second analysis comparing outcomes for patients with high-grade STS of the extremity treated with either BRT or IMRT at MSKCC. The authors acknowledged the limitations of this retrospective comparison, but reported superior local control for IMRT compared to BRT with 5-year local control rates of 92% and 81%, respectively ($P = .04$). On the other hand, Hall[120] raised a caveat that IMRT may be associated with a higher rate of radiation-associated second cancers compared to 3D-CRT, resulting from the use of more monitor units with a greater total body exposure from leakage, and from a larger volume of normal tissue exposure to low doses of RT, resulting from the greater number of treatment fields. He estimated a potential doubling of second cancers in older patients from a rate of approximately 1.5% to 3% at 10 years. (These rates could be higher for children.) Larger patient numbers and longer follow-up are still needed to confirm the favorable findings reported for IMRT thus far.

There are several other exciting technological advances for treatment, which include IMRT dose painting, image-guided radiation therapy (IGRT), adaptive RT, particle-beam radiotherapy (protons, carbon ions), and stereotactic body RT (SBRT). *Dose painting* is an advanced application of IMRT in which differential doses are delivered to different areas of the target volume simultaneously. The idea is to deliver higher doses to areas of the tumor that are believed to be more radioresistant (such as hypoxic regions), areas that may contain a higher burden of disease, or areas where the surgeon may have more difficulty with resection. This technique has been used in the setting of retroperitoneal sarcoma and is appealing.[123] *Image-guided radiation therapy* refers to serial imaging of patient setup prior to treatment so that appropriate positional adjustments can be made beforehand. Because of the increased certainty of treatment accuracy, in many cases the added margins for "setup error" can be reduced, which allows for smaller treatment fields and potential dose escalation without undue normal tissue toxicity. For example, although spinal cord tolerance is 50 Gy, Hansen et al.[124] described the ability to treat paraspinal sarcomas to 59.4 Gy using IGRT with CT imaging to better assess patient position prior to treatment. IGRT and reduced treatment fields were also used in the phase II RTOG-0630 trial; patient accrual is complete and the results are awaited.[108] Another benefit of IGRT is that if imaging during a course of treatment demonstrates changes in patient anatomy (e.g., due to weight loss) or changes in tumor shape, a second radiation plan can be developed to adapt to these new data. This is referred to as *adaptive radiation therapy* and might be relevant for sarcomas that respond dramatically to radiation, such as myxoid liposarcoma.[125,126]

Particle beams such as protons and heavier ions (carbon ions) have more favorable physical and biologic characteristics than photons, which make them appealing for clinical use. Specifically, because of the Bragg peak dose distribution property, treatment plans can be created with steep dose falloff at field borders.[127] This allows for ideal sparing of adjacent critical normal structures as well as opportunities for safe dose escalation. Proton-beam treatment for malignancies has been in use at a few centers for several decades. There are published data for treatment of chordomas and chondrosarcomas of the skull base as well as for paraspinal and sacral bone tumors. There have been no randomized studies comparing photons and protons, but there are several single-institution

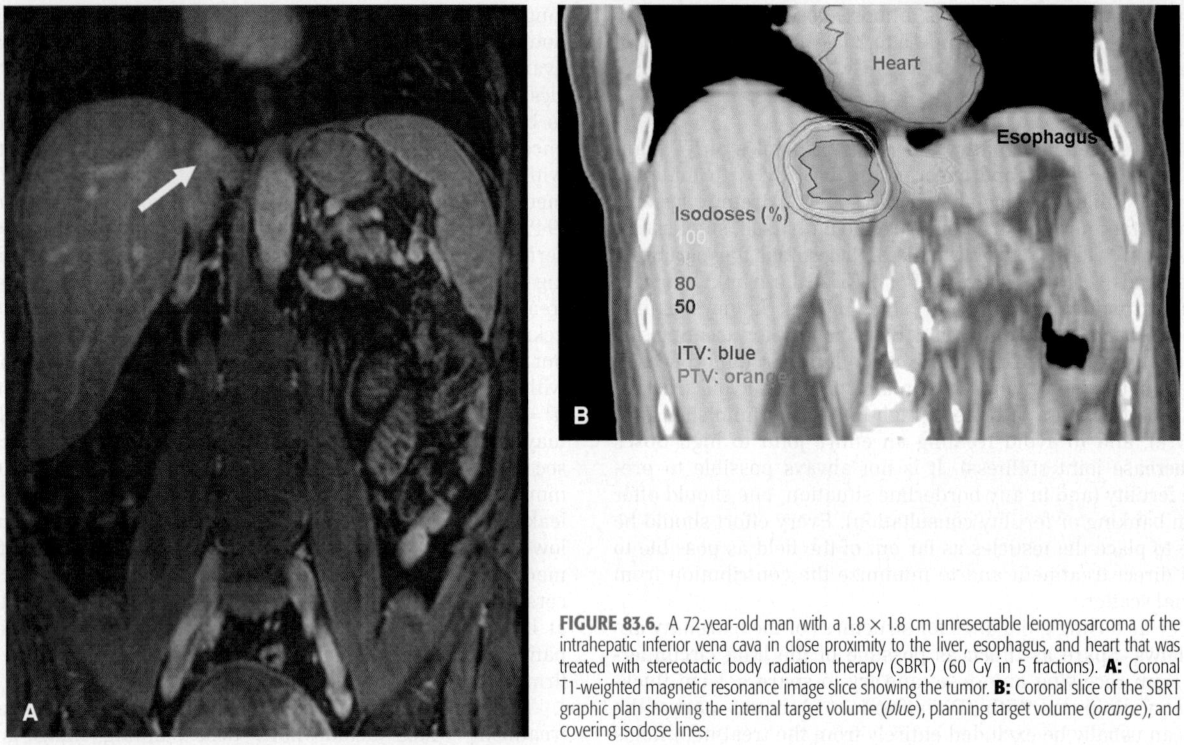

FIGURE 83.6. A 72-year-old man with a 1.8 × 1.8 cm unresectable leiomyosarcoma of the intrahepatic inferior vena cava in close proximity to the liver, esophagus, and heart that was treated with stereotactic body radiation therapy (SBRT) (60 Gy in 5 fractions). **A:** Coronal T1-weighted magnetic resonance image slice showing the tumor. **B:** Coronal slice of the SBRT graphic plan showing the internal target volume (*blue*), planning target volume (*orange*), and covering isodose lines.

reports for protons that show very good results. Local control rates for skull-base chordomas treated with protons range from 46% to 90% and for skull-base chondrosarcomas range from 75% to 100%.[128,129,130–132,133,134–135] Carbon ions have been used for clinical treatment only since the 1990s. Schulz-Ertner et al.[136,137] reported a 74% 4-year local control rate for skull-base chordomas treated with carbon ions and a 90% local-control rate for skull-base chondrosarcomas. The group from Chiba, Japan, reported a 73% local-control rate for unresectable bone and STS and a 96% local-control rate for sacral chordomas.[138,139] These early results are impressive, but confirmatory long-term follow-up data are needed.

Stereotactic body radiation therapy is a technique that delivers highly focused photon radiation doses to extracranial lesions. Typically the dose schedules are hypofractionated, with large ablative fraction sizes ranging from 6 to 30 Gy per fraction, for a course of 1 to 5 treatments. With respect to sarcoma, SBRT may have a role in the treatment of oligometastatic disease. Excellent local control rates, ranging from 73% to 96%, have been reported for treatment of metastases to the lung as well as other sites for a mix of tumors including sarcoma.[140,141,142] There are less data regarding the role of SBRT for definitive treatment of primary sarcomas, but there may be a role in select patients with tumors located in or adjacent to sensitive normal structures. For example, a study of SBRT for 14 patients with primary sarcoma of the spine reported local control for 5 of 7 patients treated with SBRT alone and for 5 of 7 patients treated with SBRT and surgery.[143] Figure 83.6 shows an MRI and dosimetry for a case of an unresectable leiomyosarcoma of the inferior vena cava that was treated with definitive SBRT at Brigham and Women's Hospital.

IMRT with or without dose painting, IGRT, adaptive RT, particle beams, and SBRT all show potential dosimetric and biological advantages compared to conventional 3D-CRT photon treatment. Promising data are available for all of these approaches, but they are limited. There will likely be appropriate places for all of these technologies in the armamentarium for sarcoma treatment, but further careful study is needed to define the optimal role of each technology and to ensure that toxicities are acceptable.

Radiation Therapy Toxicities

Acute Radiation Therapy Toxicities

Acute toxicities following RT treatment of the extremities include skin erythema and possible desquamation in high-dose areas, problems with wound healing, localized alopecia, and fatigue. Moist desquamation can be quite uncomfortable, but this heals typically quickly after completion of RT. Depending on tumor location, treatment of STS of the superficial trunk can be associated with additional toxicities such as nausea, bowel irritability, or esophagitis.

The most significant of these acute sequelae is problems with wound healing. Several retrospective single-institution series have reported wound complication rates following preoperative RT of 25% to 46%.[89–91,95,144,145–147,148] Rates following postoperative RT are lower and range from 6% to 29%.[90,91,144,146] The most definitive data pertaining to wound complications are provided by the landmark randomized trial performed by the Canadian Sarcoma Group, in which the study end point was major wound complications within 120 days of surgery.[109] Major wound complications were defined as those requiring a second operation for wound repair or wound management requiring an invasive procedure, readmission, or persistent deep packing for 120 days or longer. This trial randomized 190 patients to preoperative RT (50 Gy ± 16 to 20 Gy postoperative boost) or postoperative RT (66 to 70 Gy). With a median follow-up time of 3.3 years, the study met early stopping rules and closed. Wound complication rates were 35% for patients treated with preoperative RT compared to 17% for those treated with postoperative RT ($P = .01$). Further, lower extremity site and tumor size >10 cm were independent predictors for wound complications on multivariate analysis. Others have also found large tumor size and lower extremity site to be risk factors for wound complications.[89,145,146] Baldini et al.[89] reviewed the experience at Brigham and Women's Hospital and Dana-Farber Cancer Institute for 103 patients with STS of the trunk or extremity treated with preoperative RT. On multivariate analysis, significant independent predictors for wound complications were tumor size >10 cm, tumor proximity to skin surface <3 mm, vascularized flap closure, and diabetes mellitus. In an attempt to decrease wound complications following preoperative RT, Dickie et al.[149] conducted a phase II trial for 59 patients with lower-extremity sarcoma. Together with the surgeon, the radiation oncologist contoured the area of the subsequent surgical flaps and designated it as an avoidance structure for IMRT planning. The resulting rate of wound complications was 30.5%, which was not statistically different from the value reported in the randomized trial. Interestingly, for patients who developed wound complications, there was a trend for higher mean and maximum doses to the flaps. It may be that higher doses to the flaps were a necessary planning outcome for patients with tumors in close proximity to the skin surface, which would be consistent with the Baldini report showing increased complications for tumors within 3 mm of the skin surface. Efforts continue to minimize postoperative wound complications.

Chronic Radiation Therapy Toxicities

The most significant chronic toxicities following RT to the extremities include edema, subcutaneous fibrosis, decreased muscle strength, decreased range of motion, pain, and, less commonly, bone fracture and peripheral nerve damage. Published rates of these toxicities vary significantly, as series have different patient inclusion criteria (with respect to tumor site and treatment) and some report only moderate or severe complications, while others report any degree of complication. Nonetheless, reported rates for edema are 10% to 20%, for fibrosis they are 30% to 60%, and for bone fracture they are 0.07% to 7%.[97,150–152,153,154–156] Stinson et al.[150] reviewed 145 patients treated at the NCI with surgery and RT and reported the following complication rates: fibrosis 57%, moderate to severe decreased range of motion 32%, moderate to severe decreased muscle strength 20%, contracture 20%, ≥ grade 2 edema 19%, pain requiring narcotics 7%, and bone fracture 6%. Furthermore, several studies have correlated higher complication rates with higher doses and larger field sizes. Doses >60 or 63 Gy have been associated with higher rates of fibrosis, edema, bone fracture, pain, decreased muscle strength, and decreased range of motion.[97,118,150,151,154,157] Large RT field sizes have also been associated with more edema, fibrosis, and joint stiffness.[150,151]

Radiation Timing: Preoperative Versus Postoperative

External-beam RT can be delivered either prior to or following definitive resection. Reported local recurrence rates with each approach are similar and range from 3% to 27% for preoperative RT and 8% to 28% for postoperative RT.[53,86–88,90,91,158,159,160] The randomized trial of preoperative versus postoperative RT conducted by the Canadian Sarcoma Group showed local control rates of 93% and 92% for the preoperative and postoperative groups, respectively.[86] Similarly, there is no clear difference in DFS or OS associated with either approach. The Canadian randomized trial initially showed improved survival for the preoperative RT treatment arm, but updated 7-year results showed no differences in any recurrence or survival outcomes.[86,109] One retrospective report that assessed 821 patients using the National Oncology Database showed improved DFS rates for patients treated with preoperative RT.[54] However, these results should be considered with caution given the retrospective nature of the report and associated potential selection biases.

Although the efficacy of these approaches seems to be similar, the toxicity profiles are clearly different. Preoperative RT is associated with a well-established increased risk of acute wound complications. Several retrospective reports have described wound complication rates on the order of 25% to 46%.[89,90,95,145–147] As described in detail above (see the Acute Radiation Therapy Toxicities section), the definitive data for wound complication rates come from the Canadian randomized trial in which the primary end point was wound complications. In that trial, wound complication rates were 35% for patients treated with preoperative RT compared to 17% for those treated with postoperative RT (P = .01).[109] Although wound complications adversely affected functional outcome for patients in the early postoperative period (6 weeks after surgery), this toxicity was largely reversible, as evidenced by the fact that function was equivalent between the treatment arms 1 year after resection.

On the other hand, patients treated with postoperative RT have a higher rate of chronic and generally irreversible toxicities, which include subcutaneous fibrosis, joint stiffness, edema, and bone fractures. These late toxicities have been reported in retrospective series but, again, good data come from the Canadian randomized trial.[150,151,154,157,161] Davis et al.[151] reported that grade 2 or higher late toxicity rates were higher for the postoperative RT group than the preoperative group. Specifically, for the postoperative and preoperative groups, respectively, rates of grade 2+ complications were as follows: subcutaneous fibrosis, 48% versus 31.5%; joint stiffness, 23% versus 18%; and edema, 23% versus 15.5%. These differences were not statistically significant, but the study was not powered to detect these differences. Statistically significant associations were seen between larger field size and rates of fibrosis, joint stiffness, and edema. Additionally, in a retrospective series, Holt et al.[154] reported increased rates of bone fracture for patients treated postoperatively (60 to 66 Gy) compared to those treated preoperatively (50 Gy). The rates were 7% and 0.6%, respectively (P = .007).

It is helpful to summarize the relative advantages and disadvantages for preoperative versus postoperative RT. For preoperative RT, the advantages include the ability to treat with smaller RT fields and lower doses, both of which are associated with reduced long-term toxicities. Lower RT doses are also associated with reduced treatment time, lower costs, and a hypothetical possibility of lower second-malignancy risks. Other potential advantages of preoperative RT include the ability to render unresectable or marginally resectable tumors resectable, the potential to prevent tumor seeding of the operative bed or systemic circulation, and an increased efficacy of RT from good oxygenation of tissues due to unperturbed tumor vasculature. Furthermore, in most cases, defining the tumor volume for RT planning is relatively straightforward given that it is *in situ*. The main disadvantage of preoperative RT is the higher risk of major wound complications and its concomitant increased morbidity and cost. However, most major wound complications are treatable and, therefore, this toxicity is generally considered reversible. Another disadvantage of preoperative RT is that the resected specimen is potentially less informative on pathology review due to the prior treatment.

Postoperative RT has the advantage that the complete tumor specimen is available for pathology review for determination of histology and margin status. Another important advantage is the lower risk of major wound complications. A disadvantage of postoperative RT is the necessity for larger treatment volumes and higher doses, which are associated with higher chronic long-term toxicities such as subcutaneous fibrosis, joint stiffness, edema, pain, and bone fractures. For the most part, these toxicities are irreversible. In theory, the interrupted vasculature related to surgery may create a hypoxic environment, rendering RT less effective (this is a potential explanation for the need for higher doses compared to the preoperative setting). Lastly, determining an RT target definition is often more complex in the postoperative setting, as it requires reconstruction of where the tumor resided as well as definition of the entire operative field.

In conclusion, pre- and postoperative RT are associated with equivalent efficacies but different toxicity profiles, the most salient of which are increased (reversible) wound complications for preoperative RT and increased (irreversible) long-term toxicities of fibrosis, edema, and joint stiffness for postoperative RT. The topic is controversial, but preoperative RT is generally the author's preferred approach for STS of the extremities or trunk. Even when a patient is at high risk of developing a wound complication, the author often prefers preoperative RT, as most wound problems are highly treatable with eventual recovery of good function.

Surgery Alone

As stated previously, conservative surgery and RT is the standard treatment for high-grade STS of the extremity and trunk. However, there are also several reports that demonstrate excellent outcomes following treatment with surgery alone (Table 83.4). It is important to acknowledge that these are all single-institution series, all but one are retrospective, and patients were highly selected for treatment. These factors render the results less generalizable, so caution is recommended when considering this approach. Nonetheless, crude and actuarial LR rates in these select studies range from 0% to 20% and most are 10% or lower.[99,100–106,162] What the appropriate selection criteria for this approach are remains unclear, but potential factors can be inferred by close analysis of these reports. Excellent local control appears to be associated with wide resection performed for tumors in a subcutaneous location. Rydholm et al.[103] described only 4 local recurrences (5%) among 73 subcutaneous tumors treated with wide excision. In addition, Gibbs et al.[105] reported no local recurrences among 35 patients with subcutaneous STS treated with wide excision alone. Among these tumors, 47% were high grade and 32% were >5 cm.

Pisters et al.[104] described a prospective series of patients with tumors <5 cm who had negative resection margins and were treated with surgery alone. The overall crude LR rate was 8%, and among the subcutaneous tumors, the rate was only 5%. Furthermore, surgical technique and margin status are important. In the series reported by Rydholm et al.,[100] a large proportion of the cases were resected without an initial biopsy and, thus, without the potential for tumor seeding of intervening tissues.

Several of the reports also describe a meticulous surgical approach to wide resection with removal of a cuff of normal tissue as well as intact fascia.[100,103,105] In the prospective trial of Pisters et al.,[104] negative resection margins were a required criterion for treatment by resection alone. The report by Baldini et al.[102] quantified surgical resection margins. In that series, 74 patients were treated with surgery alone and the overall 10-year actuarial LR rate was 7%. Interestingly, there were no recurrences seen for 36 patients with resection margins ≥1 cm compared to a 10-year actuarial LR rate of 13% (4 of 38) for those with margins <1 cm.

Conversely, the authors of a retrospective study from the Institut Gustave Roussy also quantified margin status.[163] They reported a 10-year actuarial LR rate of 35% for patients treated with surgery alone who had resection margins ≥1 cm. Further, they found the addition of RT for patients with these characteristics was not associated with a significant local control benefit. As the local recurrence rate in that series is high, it is difficult to draw meaningful conclusions except to reinforce the concept that treatment with surgery alone should be done with care.

Cahlon et al.[162] assessed 200 patients who were treated with surgery alone at MSKCC following re-resection showing no evidence of disease. Although the overall 5-year actuarial LR rate was only 9%, on multivariate analysis, age >50 and stage III disease were both predictors for higher LR rates. If both of these factors were present, the LR rate was 31%. The LR rates for low-grade tumors treated with surgery alone in these series were all very low and range from 0% to 5%.[100,102–105,164] In fact, the standard treatment recommendation for low-grade STS is wide resection alone. With this approach and negative margins, LR rates are typically <20%.[92] (Indications for adjuvant RT for low-grade tumors include positive resection margins, locally recurrent disease following initial treatment with surgery alone, or a tumor location that would not be amenable to subsequent salvage surgery.)

In sum, there is most certainly a subset of patients with STS of the extremity and trunk for whom wide excision alone is appropriate treatment. The selection criteria for this strategy remain undefined but will perhaps include, but not be limited to, some of the following: subcutaneous tumors; tumors resected with wide negative margins >1 cm or an intact fascia; low-grade tumors; tumors representing primary presentation of disease (e.g., not locally recurrent); tumor locations amenable to limb-sparing salvage surgery for recurrence; and patient willingness to comply with follow-up. Before surgery alone can become standard of care for select patients with STS, the eligibility criteria need to be elucidated and tested in a prospective multi-institutional trial. Other than for low-grade tumors resected with negative margins, treatment with surgery alone should be employed cautiously.

TABLE 83.4 RESULTS OF SELECT SINGLE-INSTITUTION SERIES OF SOFT TISSUE SARCOMAS TREATED WITH SURGERY ALONE

Study	*Crude LR Rate*	*Comments and Crude LR Rates*
Rydholm[100] University Hospital, Lund Sweden 1991 N = 56	7% (4/56)	Subcutaneous & intramuscular tumors; All had "wide margins"
Rydholm[103] University Hospital, Lund Sweden 1991 N = 73	5% (4/73)	All subcutaneous; All had "wide margins" Low grade: 0% (0/14) High grade: 7% (4/49)
Karakousis[101] Roswell Park 1995 N = 116	10% (12/116)	Wide or radical resection (including 9 amputations) Low grade: 0% (0/19) High grade 12% (12/97)
Gibbs[105] University of Chicago 1997 N = 35	0% (0/35)	All subcutaneous All had "wide resection"
Baldini[102] Brigham & Women's Hospital and Dana-Farber Cancer Institute 1999 N = 74	5% (4/74)	Margin <1 cm: 11% (4/38) Margin >1 cm: 0% (0/36) Low grade: 2.5% (1/40) High grade: 9% (3/24)
Fabrizio[164] Mayo Clinic 2000 N = 34	15% (5/34)	Low grade: 0% (0/18) High grade: 31% (5/16)
Alektiar[106] MSKCC 2002 N = 116	18% (21/116)	All were high grade, size <5 cm and resection margin negative
Pisters[104] MDACC 2007 N = 74	8% (6/74)	Only prospective trial All resection margins negative All tumors <5 cm For subcutaneous tumors, LR: 5%
Cahlon[162] MSKCC 2008 N = 200	10% (20/200)	All had negative re-resection; Age ≤50: 5% (6/123) Age >50: 18% (14/77) Stage I/II: 7% (13/178) Stage III: 32% (7/22)

LR, local recurrence; MSKCC, Memorial Sloan-Kettering Cancer Center; MDACC, MD Anderson Cancer Center.

Neoadjuvant, Concurrent, or Adjuvant Chemotherapy

Locally advanced (stage III) STS of the extremities and trunk has a significant risk of distant recurrence, and for this reason, the addition of systemic therapy to treatment algorithms is appealing. There is an established role for chemotherapy as part of the treatment for rhabdomyosarcoma and Ewing's sarcoma in children and in adults treated per pediatric protocols, many of which include adults up to age 50.[165,166] For other histologies of adult STS, no clear role for chemotherapy has been defined, and this group is the subject of the discussion below. The two most standardly used drugs in the management of STS are doxorubicin and ifosfamide, with gemcitabine-based regimens increasingly used, particularly in patients with leiomyosarcoma.[167,168]

There are several potential benefits to a neoadjuvant chemotherapy approach. These include the potential to treat micrometastatic disease early in the treatment course; the potential to decrease the scope of the resection if sufficient response is achieved; the ability to ascertain the chemotherapy response or lack thereof for an individual patient, which could guide the use of additional (postoperative) chemotherapy; and enhanced drug delivery to the tumor with corresponding increased efficacy, given that the tumor vasculature has not been disrupted in the neoadjuvant setting. Few reports address the role of neoadjuvant chemotherapy for high-risk STS of the extremities and trunk. A prospective randomized phase II trial conducted by the European Organisation for Research and Treatment of Cancer included 137 patients who were randomized to receive or not receive 3 cycles of doxorubicin and ifosphamide prior to resection with selective use of postoperative RT.[169] Unfortunately, the study was closed due to poor accrual and therefore lacks sufficient power for one to draw definitive conclusions. The results showed no statistically significant differences between treatment arms for DFS or OS. Specifically, the 5-year DFS rate for the chemotherapy group was 56% compared with 52% for the observation group; the corresponding 5-year OS rates were 65% and 64%, respectively. Two other retrospective reports on the use of neoadjuvant chemotherapy showed mixed results.[170,171]

Similarly, informative data are scarce regarding the use of concurrent preoperative chemotherapy and radiotherapy. Several trials have shown that treatment with RT and concurrent doxorubicin, ifosphamide, gemcitabine, or temozolomide is both feasible and safe.[172–176] There are also two reports of an interdigitated chemotherapy and RT approach. The first was a pilot trial conducted at the Massachusetts General Hospital, which enrolled 48 patients. Treatment involved an interdigitated approach of chemotherapy (mesna, doxorubicin, ifosphamide, and dacarbazine) and 44 Gy given as a split course.[177] Results were very good and associated with improved survival compared with historical controls. The RTOG subsequently enrolled 66 patients in a phase II trial with a very similar treatment approach.[178] Efficacy was somewhat comparable to that of the pilot study, but toxicities were greater, with 5% treatment-related deaths and 83% grade 4 toxicities reported.

The most data available pertain to the use of chemotherapy in the adjuvant setting. A meta-analysis reported by the Sarcoma Meta-Analysis Collaboration (SMAC) included 1,568 patients treated in 14 randomized trials using adjuvant doxorubicin-based chemotherapy. It showed that chemotherapy was associated with statistically higher rates of LR-free survival and DFS at 10 years.[179] Ten-year LR-free survival rates were 81% and 75%, respectively, for the chemotherapy and observation groups (P = .02); the corresponding values for 10-year DFS were 55% and 45% (P = .001). For 10-year OS, there was no clear benefit, with rates of 54% for the chemotherapy group and 50% for the observation group (P = .12). However, exploratory analysis showed a significant 7% survival benefit for the subset of patients with STS of the extremities. Subsequent to this meta-analysis, several more randomized trials of adjuvant chemotherapy were performed using anthracycline or ifosphamide-based chemotherapy; many of these showed trends for survival benefits with chemotherapy, but none were statistically significant.[180–184] (One study from Italy initially reported a significant survival benefit due to chemotherapy at 4 years, but the survival benefit did not hold up with 7.5-year follow-up.[180,181]) SMAC updated their meta-analysis in 2008 with the inclusion of four additional trials (three adjuvant and one neoadjuvant).[169,180,182,183,185] The new analysis included 18 randomized trials with 1,953 patients and reported statistically significant absolute reductions of 4% for LR and 9% for distant recurrence and an absolute improvement of 6% for survival attributable to chemotherapy.[185] However, the fact that this update did not include the largest negative trial renders the results less conclusive.[184]

All of the above studies included a mix of STS histologic subtypes, which is probably not appropriate as we learn more about the varied biologic behaviors of individual STS entities. For example, several trials have shown that synovial sarcoma and round cell liposarcoma are particularly sensitive to chemotherapy.[186–189] It may be that a small survival benefit does indeed exist for select subsets of patients (such as those with synovial sarcoma or round cell liposarcoma), but the available studies are underpowered and hindered by the inclusion of a mix of histologic subtypes and tumor sites. Going forward, trials should include centralized pathology review and stratification by histology.

In totality, although there are hints of efficacy for certain subgroups, the available data do not support the routine use of chemotherapy for locally advanced STS. However, for select high-risk patients with high-grade and large tumors (>8 to 10 cm), it is reasonable to address the pros and cons of neoadjuvant, concurrent or interdigitated, or adjuvant chemotherapy on an individual patient basis. As toxicity can be significant, concurrent approaches are best undertaken at experienced centers.

Isolated Limb Perfusion, Isolated Limb Infusion, and Chemotherapy with Regional Hyperthermia

Isolated limb perfusion (ILP) is a complicated technique that has been used in Europe for the treatment of locally advanced STS that would otherwise require amputation. This procedure involves isolating the arterial and venous circulation of the limb by connecting it to an extracorporeal circulation, where it is oxygenated and instilled with systemic agents, most commonly, melphalan and tumor necrosis factor. A tourniquet is applied to the limb to prevent leakage into the systemic circulation and the limb is often treated with hyperthermia as well. The treatment can have significant morbidity, but reported limb salvage success rates are quite high.[190–193] *Isolated limb infusion* (ILI) employs low-flow isolated limb perfusion without oxygenation and has been developed as a simpler alternative to ILP. Available data suggest comparable efficacy and less toxicity for ILI compared to ILP.[194,195] Lastly, chemotherapy with regional hyperthermia (delivered via an external electromagnetic field) is another approach for locally advanced disease. A randomized trial of doxorubicin, ifosphamide, and etoposide, with or without regional hyperthermia delivered before and after local therapy, has shown superior DFS and progression-free survival rates for the regional hyperthermia group.[196] All of these techniques are complicated to deliver and associated with significant potential toxicities. However, they represent valuable potential alternatives to amputation in such settings as in transit metastases of epithelioid or clear cell sarcoma or extensive local recurrences after prior surgery and RT.

FUTURE DIRECTIONS

In summary, success rates for the treatment of stages I and II STS of the extremities and trunk are currently high, with local control rates of ≥85% and 5-year survival rates of 90% and 81%, respectively.[47] For these patients, we should continue to explore ways to reduce treatment-related morbidity related to surgery and RT. These strategies should include development of innovative techniques to reduce postoperative wound complications, efforts to reduce RT field sizes and to deliver more conformal therapy, and definition of patient subsets that can be effectively treated with surgery alone. For situations in which it is difficult to achieve local control, more aggressive local treatment is needed; this could include the use of RT dose escalation using IGRT, IMRT with dose painting, heavy particles, SBRT, or concurrent chemoradiation strategies. Lastly, patients with stage III disease have a high rate of distant relapse and death. For these patients, novel systemic therapies are needed. The discovery of the targeted agent imatinib mesylate for the treatment of gastrointestinal stromal tumors has been associated with great success, and similar discoveries for other histologies are anticipated.[197] As the field of STS continues to move forward, it is likely that treatment algorithms for the various histologic subtypes will be developed.

ACKNOWLEDGMENT

I would like to acknowledge the editorial assistance of Susanna Hilfer and Barbara Silver.

SELECTED REFERENCES

A full list of references for this chapter is available online.

2. Fletcher CDM, Unni KK, Mertens F, eds. *World Health Orgnization classification of tumours: pathology and genetics of tumours of soft tissue and bone.* Lyon: IARC Press, 2002.
15. Lawrence W Jr, Donegan WL, Natarajan N, et al. Adult soft tissue sarcomas. A pattern of care survey of the American College of Surgeons. *Ann Surg* 1987;205(4):349–359.
19. Simon MA, Enneking WF. The management of soft-tissue sarcomas of the extremities. *J Bone Joint Surg Am* 1976;58(3):317–327.
20. Enneking WF, Spanier SS, Malawer MM. The effect of the Anatomic setting on the results of surgical procedures for soft parts sarcoma of the thigh. *Cancer* 1981;47(5):1005–1022.
28. Guadagnolo BA, Zagars GK, Ballo MT, et al. Excellent local control rates and distinctive patterns of failure in myxoid liposarcoma treated with conservation surgery and radiotherapy. *Int J Radiat Oncol Biol Phys* 2008;70(3):760–765.
35. Haglund KE, Raut CP, Nascimento AF, et al. Recurrence patterns and survival for patients with intermediate- and high-grade myxofibrosarcoma. *Int J Radiat Oncol Biol Phys* 2012;82(1):361–367.
36. Mutter RW, Singer S, Zhang Z, et al. The enigma of myxofibrosarcoma of the extremity. *Cancer* 2012;118(2):518–527.
37. Sanfilippo R, Miceli R, Grosso F, et al. Myxofibrosarcoma: prognostic factors and survival in a series of patients treated at a single institution. *Ann Surg Oncol* 2011;18(3):720–725.
38. Toomayan GA, Robertson F, Major NM. Lower extremity compartmental anatomy: clinical relevance to radiologists. *Skeletal Radiol* 2005;34(6):307–313.
39. Demas BE, Heelan RT, Lane J, et al. Soft-tissue sarcomas of the extremities: comparison of MR and CT in determining the extent of disease. *AJR Am J Roentgenol* 1988;150(3):615–620.
41. White LM, Wunder JS, Bell RS, et al. Histologic assessment of peritumoral edema in soft tissue sarcoma. *Int J Radiat Oncol Biol Phys* 2005;61(5):1439–1445.
42. Panicek DM, Gatsonis C, Rosenthal DI, et al. CT and MR imaging in the local staging of primary malignant musculoskeletal neoplasms: report of the Radiology Diagnostic Oncology Group. *Radiology* 1997;202(1):237–246.
46. Mankin HJ, Mankin CJ, Simon MA. The hazards of the biopsy, revisited. Members of the Musculoskeletal Tumor Society. *J Bone Joint Surg Am* 1996;78(5):656–663.
47. Edge SB, Byrd DR, Compton CC, et al., eds. *AJCC cancer staging manual.* 7th ed. New York: Springer, 2010.
48. Pisters PW, Leung DH, Woodruff J, et al. Analysis of prognostic factors in 1,041 patients with localized soft tissue sarcomas of the extremities. *J Clin Oncol* 1996;14(5):1679–1689.
49. Zagars GK, Ballo MT, Pisters PW, et al. Prognostic factors for patients with localized soft-tissue sarcoma treated with conservation surgery and radiation therapy: an analysis of 1225 patients. *Cancer* 2003;97(10):2530–2543.
50. Coindre JM, Terrier P, Guillou L, et al. Predictive value of grade for metastasis development in the main histologic types of adult soft tissue sarcomas: a study of 1240 patients from the French Federation of Cancer Centers Sarcoma Group. *Cancer* 2001;91(10):1914–1926.
51. Parsons HM, Habermann EB, Tuttle TM, et al. Conditional survival of extremity soft-tissue sarcoma: results beyond the staging system. *Cancer* 2011;117(5):1055–1060.
52. LeVay J, O'Sullivan B, Catton C, et al. Outcome and prognostic factors in soft tissue sarcoma in the adult. *Int J Radiat Oncol Biol Phys* 1993;27(5):1091–1099.
53. Suit HD, Mankin HJ, Wood WC, et al. Treatment of the patient with stage M0 soft tissue sarcoma. *J Clin Oncol* 1988;6(5):854–862.
54. Sampath S, Schultheiss TE, Hitchcock YJ, et al. Preoperative versus postoperative radiotherapy in soft-tissue sarcoma: multi-institutional analysis of 821 patients. *Int J Radiat Oncol Biol Phys* 2011;81(2):498–505.
55. Gutierrez JC, Perez EA, Franceschi D, et al. Outcomes for soft-tissue sarcoma in 8249 cases from a large state cancer registry. *J Surg Res* 2007;141(1):105–114.
56. Cantor RJ, Beal E, Borys D, et al. Interaction of histologic subtype and histologic grade in predicting survival for soft-tissue sarcomas. *J Am Coll Surg* 2010,210(2).191–198.
57. Trovik CS, Bauer HC, Alvegard TA, et al. Surgical margins, local recurrence and metastasis in soft tissue sarcomas: 559 surgically-treated patients from the Scandinavian Sarcoma Group Register. *Eur J Cancer* 2000;36(6):710–716.
58. Gronchi A, Casali PG, Mariani L, et al. Status of surgical margins and prognosis in adult soft tissue sarcomas of the extremities: a series of patients treated at a single institution. *J Clin Oncol* 2005;23(1):96–104.
59. Rosenberg SA, Tepper J, Glatstein E, et al. The treatment of soft-tissue sarcomas of the extremities: prospective randomized evaluations of (1) limb-sparing surgery plus radiation therapy compared with amputation and (2) the role of adjuvant chemotherapy. *Ann Surg* 1982;196(3):305–315.
60. Gerrand CH, Wunder JS, Kandel RA, et al. Classification of positive margins after resection of soft-tissue sarcoma of the limb predicts the risk of local recurrence. *J Bone Joint Surg Br* 2001;83(8):1149–1155.
61. Singer S, Corson JM, Gonin R, et al. Prognostic factors predictive of survival and local recurrence for extremity soft tissue sarcoma. *Ann Surg* 1994;219(2):165–173.
62. Stefanovski PD, Bidoli E, De Paoli A, et al. Prognostic factors in soft tissue sarcomas: a study of 395 patients. *Eur J Surg Oncol* 2002;28(2):153–164.
63. Fein DA, Lee WR, Lanciano RM, et al. Management of extremity soft tissue sarcomas with limb-sparing surgery and postoperative irradiation: do total dose, overall treatment time, and the surgery-radiotherapy interval impact on local control? *Int J Radiat Oncol Biol Phys* 1995;32(4):969–976.
64. Gustafson P, Dreinhofer KE, Rydholm A. Soft tissue sarcoma should be treated at a tumor center. A comparison of quality of surgery in 375 patients. *Acta Orthop Scand* 1994;65(1):47–50.
65. Clasby R, Tilling K, Smith MA, et al. Variable management of soft tissue sarcoma: regional audit with implications for specialist care. *Br J Surg* 1997;84(12):1692–1696.
66. Guadagnolo BA, Xu Y, Zagars GK, et al. A population-based study of the quality of care in the diagnosis of large (≥5 cm) soft tissue sarcomas. *Am J Clin Oncol* 2011 (in press).
71. Pisters PW, Harrison LB, Leung DH, et al. Long-term results of a prospective randomized trial of adjuvant brachytherapy in soft tissue sarcoma. *J Clin Oncol* 1996;14(3):859–868.
72. Fiore M, Casali PG, Miceli R, et al. Prognostic effect of re-excision in adult soft tissue sarcoma of the extremity. *Ann Surg Oncol* 2006;13(1):110–117.
76. Zagars GK, Ballo MT, Pisters PW, et al. Surgical margins and reresection in the management of patients with soft tissue sarcoma using conservative surgery and radiation therapy. *Cancer* 2003;97(10):2544–2553.
77. Lewis JJ, Leung D, Espat J, et al. Effect of reresection in extremity soft tissue sarcoma. *Ann Surg* 2000;231(5):655–663.
78. Davis AM, Kandel RA, Wunder JS, et al. The impact of residual disease on local recurrence in patients treated by initial unplanned resection for soft tissue sarcoma of the extremity. *J Surg Oncol* 1997;66(2):81–87.
79. Giuliano AE, Eilber FR. The rationale for planned reoperation after unplanned total excision of soft-tissue sarcomas. *J Clin Oncol* 1985;3(10):1344–1348.
80. Williard WC, Hajdu SI, Casper ES, et al. Comparison of amputation with limb-sparing operations for adult soft tissue sarcoma of the extremity. *Ann Surg* 1992;215(3):269–275.
82. Yang JC, Chang AE, Baker AR, et al. Randomized prospective study of the benefit of adjuvant radiation therapy in the treatment of soft tissue sarcomas of the extremity. *J Clin Oncol* 1998;16(1):197–203.
83. Alektiar KM, Leung D, Zelefsky MJ, et al. Adjuvant brachytherapy for primary high-grade soft tissue sarcoma of the extremity. *Ann Surg Oncol* 2002;9(1):48–56.
84. Nag S, Shasha D, Janjan N, et al. The American Brachytherapy Society recommendations for brachytherapy of soft tissue sarcomas. *Int J Radiat Oncol Biol Phys* 2001;49(4):1033–1043.
85. Lewis JJ, Leung D, Heslin M, et al. Association of local recurrence with subsequent survival in extremity soft tissue sarcoma. *J Clin Oncol* 1997;15(2):646–652.
86. O'Sullivan B, Davis A, Turcotte R, et al. Five-year results of a randomized phase III trial of pre-operative vs post-operative radiotherapy in extremity soft tissue sarcoma. ASCO Annual Meeting Proceedings 2004. *J Clin Oncol* 2004;22(14 Suppl): (abstr 9007).
87. Dickie CI, Griffin AM, Parent AL, et al. The relationship between local recurrence and radiotherapy treatment volume for soft tissue sarcomas treated with external beam radiotherapy and function preservation surgery. *Int J Radiat Oncol Biol Phys* 2012;82(4):1528–1534.
88. Kim B, Chen YL, Kirsch DG, et al. An effective preoperative three-dimensional radiotherapy target volume for extremity soft tissue sarcoma and the effect of margin width on local control. *Int J Radiat Oncol Biol Phys* 2010;77(3):843–850.
89. Baldini EH, Lapidus MR, Wang Q, et al. Predictors for major wound complications following pre-operative radiotherapy and surgery for soft tissue sarcoma of the extremity and trunk: importance of tumor proximity to skin surface. *Ann Surg Oncol* 2011 (in press).
90. Cheng EY, Dusenbery KE, Winters MR, et al. Soft tissue sarcomas: preoperative versus postoperative radiotherapy. *J Surg Oncol* 1996;61(2):90–99.
91. Kuklo TR, Temple HT, Owens BD, et al. Preoperative versus postoperative radiation therapy for soft-tissue sarcomas. *Am J Orthop (Belle Mead NJ)* 2005;34(2):75–80.
92. Mendenhall WM, Indelicato DJ, Scarborough MT, et al. The management of adult soft tissue sarcomas. *Am J Clin Oncol* 2009;32(4):436–442.
93. Alektiar KM, Brennan MF, Healey JH, et al. Impact of intensity-modulated radiation therapy on local control in primary soft-tissue sarcoma of the extremity. *J Clin Oncol* 2008;26(20):3440–3444.
94. Wang D, Bosch W, Roberge D, et al. RTOG sarcoma radiation oncologists reach consensus on gross tumor volume and clinical target volume on computed tomographic images for preoperative radiotherapy of primary soft tissue sarcoma of extremity in Radiation Therapy Oncology Group studies. *Int J Radiat Oncol Biol Phys* 2011;81(4):e528.
95. Devisetty K, Kobayashi W, Suit HD, et al. Low-dose neoadjuvant external beam radiation therapy for soft tissue sarcoma. *Int J Radiat Oncol Biol Phys* 2011;80(3):779–786.
96. O'Sullivan B, Wunder J, Pisters PWT. Target description for radiotherapy of soft tissue sarcoma. In: Gregoire V, Scalliet P, Ang KK, eds. *Clinical target volumes in conformal and intensity modulated radiation therapy: a clinical guide to cancer treatment.* New York: Springer-Verlag, 2004:205–227.
97. Mundt AJ, Awan A, Sibley GS, et al. Conservative surgery and adjuvant radiation therapy in the management of adult soft tissue sarcoma of the extremities: clinical and radiobiological results. *Int J Radiat Oncol Biol Phys* 1995;32(4):977–985.
100. Rydholm A, Gustafson P, Rooser B, et al. Limb-sparing surgery without radiotherapy based on anatomic location of soft tissue sarcoma. *J Clin Oncol* 1991;9(10):1757–1765.
101. Karakousis CP, Proimakis C, Walsh DL. Primary soft tissue sarcoma of the extremities in adults. *Br J Surg* 1995;82(9):1208–1212.
102. Baldini EH, Goldberg J, Jenner C, et al. Long-term outcomes after function-sparing surgery without radiotherapy for soft tissue sarcoma of the extremities and trunk. *J Clin Oncol* 1999;17(10):3252–3259.
103. Rydholm A, Gustafson P, Rooser B, et al. Subcutaneous sarcoma. A population-based study of 129 patients. *J Bone Joint Surg Br* 1991;73(4):662–667.
104. Pisters PW, Pollock RE, Lewis VO, et al. Long-term results of prospective trial of surgery alone with selective use of radiation for patients with T1 extremity and trunk soft tissue sarcomas. *Ann Surg* 2007;246(4):675–681; discussion 81–82.

105. Gibbs CP, Peabody TD, Mundt AJ, et al. Oncological outcomes of operative treatment of subcutaneous soft-tissue sarcomas of the extremities. *J Bone Joint Surg Am* 1997;79(6):888–897.
106. Alektiar KM, Leung D, Zelefsky MJ, et al. Adjuvant radiation for stage II-B soft tissue sarcoma of the extremity. *J Clin Oncol* 2002;20(6):1643–1650.
108. O'Sullivan B, Davis AM, Turcotte R, et al. Preoperative versus postoperative radiotherapy in soft-tissue sarcoma of the limbs: a randomised trial. *Lancet* 2002;359(9325):2235–2241.
109. Al Yami A, Griffin AM, Ferguson PC, et al. Positive surgical margins in soft tissue sarcoma treated with preoperative radiation: is a postoperative boost necessary? *Int J Radiat Oncol Biol Phys* 2010;77(4):1191–1197.
111. Alektiar KM, Velasco J, Zelefsky MJ, et al. Adjuvant radiotherapy for margin-positive high-grade soft tissue sarcoma of the extremity. *Int J Radiat Oncol Biol Phys* 2000;48(4):1051–1058.
116. Delaney TF, Kepka L, Goldberg SI, et al. Radiation therapy for control of soft-tissue sarcomas resected with positive margins. *Int J Radiat Oncol Biol Phys* 2007;67(5):1460–1469.
117. Ballo MT, Zagars GK, Cormier JN, et al. Interval between surgery and radiotherapy: effect on local control of soft tissue sarcoma. *Int J Radiat Oncol Biol Phys* 2004;58(5):1461–1467.
118. Dickie CI, Parent AL, Griffin AM, et al. Bone fractures following external beam radiotherapy and limb-preservation surgery for lower extremity soft tissue sarcoma: relationship to irradiated bone length, volume, tumor location and dose. *Int J Radiat Oncol Biol Phys* 2009;75(4):1119–1124.
119. Marks LB, Yorke ED, Jackson A, et al. Use of normal tissue complication probability models in the clinic. *Int J Radiat Oncol Biol Phys* 2010;76(3 Suppl):S10–S19.
120. Hall EJ. Intensity-modulated radiation therapy, protons, and the risk of second cancers. *Int J Radiat Oncol Biol Phys* 2006;65(1):1–7.
121. Hong L, Alektiar KM, Hunt M, et al. Intensity-modulated radiotherapy for soft tissue sarcoma of the thigh. *Int J Radiat Oncol Biol Phys* 2004;59(3):752–759.
122. Alektiar KM, Brennan MF, Singer S. Local control comparison of adjuvant brachytherapy to intensity-modulated radiotherapy in primary high-grade sarcoma of the extremity. *Cancer* 2011;117(14):3229–3234.
123. Koshy M, Landry JC, Lawson JD, et al. Intensity modulated radiation therapy for retroperitoneal sarcoma: a case for dose escalation and organ at risk toxicity reduction. *Sarcoma* 2003;7(3–4):137–148.
124. Hansen EK, Larson DA, Aubin M, et al. Image-guided radiotherapy using megavoltage cone-beam computed tomography for treatment of paraspinous tumors in the presence of orthopedic hardware. *Int J Radiat Oncol Biol Phys* 2006;66(2):323–326.
125. Pitson G, Robinson P, Wilke D, et al. Radiation response: an additional unique signature of myxoid liposarcoma. *Int J Radiat Oncol Biol Phys* 2004;60(2):522–526.
129. Terahara A, Niemierko A, Goitein M, et al. Analysis of the relationship between tumor dose inhomogeneity and local control in patients with skull base chordoma. *Int J Radiat Oncol Biol Phys* 1999;45(2):351–358.
133. Weber DC, Rutz HP, Pedroni ES, et al. Results of spot-scanning proton radiation therapy for chordoma and chondrosarcoma of the skull base: the Paul Scherrer Institut experience. *Int J Radiat Oncol Biol Phys* 2005;63(2):401–409.
137. Schulz-Ertner D, Nikoghosyan A, Hof H, et al. Carbon ion radiotherapy of skull base chondrosarcomas. *Int J Radiat Oncol Biol Phys* 2007;67(1):171–177.
138. Kamada T, Tsujii H, Tsuji H, et al. Efficacy and safety of carbon ion radiotherapy in bone and soft tissue sarcomas. *J Clin Oncol* 2002;20(22):4466–4471.
141. Milano MT, Katz AW, Schell MC, et al. Descriptive analysis of oligometastatic lesions treated with curative-intent stereotactic body radiotherapy. *Int J Radiat Oncol Biol Phys* 2008;72(5):1516–1522.
143. Levine AM, Coleman C, Horasek S. Stereotactic radiosurgery for the treatment of primary sarcomas and sarcoma metastases of the spine. *Neurosurgery* 2009;64(2 Suppl):A54–A59.
144. Pollack A, Zagars GK, Goswitz MS, et al. Preoperative vs. postoperative radiotherapy in the treatment of soft tissue sarcomas: a matter of presentation. *Int J Radiat Oncol Biol Phys* 1998;42(3):563–572.
148. Curtis KK, Ashman JB, Beauchamp CP, et al. Neoadjuvant chemoradiation compared to neoadjuvant radiation alone and surgery alone for stage II and III soft tissue sarcoma of the extremities. *Radiat Oncol* 2011;6(1):91.
149. Dickie CI, Griffin A, Parent A, et al. Phase II study of preoperative intensity modulated radiation therapy for lower limb soft tissue sarcoma. *Int J Radiat Oncol Biol Phys* 2010;78(3 Suppl):S84–S85 (abstr 181).
150. Stinson SF, DeLaney TF, Greenberg J, et al. Acute and long-term effects on limb function of combined modality limb sparing therapy for extremity soft tissue sarcoma. *Int J Radiat Oncol Biol Phys* 1991;21(6):1493–1499.
151. Davis AM, O'Sullivan B, Turcotte R, et al. Late radiation morbidity following randomization to preoperative versus postoperative radiotherapy in extremity soft tissue sarcoma. *Radiother Oncol* 2005;75(1):48–53.
152. Rimner A, Brennan MF, Zhang Z, et al. Influence of compartmental involvement on the patterns of morbidity in soft tissue sarcoma of the thigh. *Cancer* 2009;115(1):149–157.
154. Holt GE, Griffin AM, Pintilie M, et al. Fractures following radiotherapy and limb-salvage surgery for lower extremity soft-tissue sarcomas. A comparison of high-dose and low-dose radiotherapy. *J Bone Joint Surg Am* 2005;87(2):315–319.
155. Helmstedter CS, Goebel M, Zlotecki R, et al. Pathologic fractures after surgery and radiation for soft tissue tumors. *Clin Orthop Relat Res* 2001(389):165–172.
156. Alektiar KM, Zelefsky MJ, Brennan MF. Morbidity of adjuvant brachytherapy in soft tissue sarcoma of the extremity and superficial trunk. *Int J Radiat Oncol Biol Phys* 2000;47(5):1273–1279.
158. Zagars GK, Ballo MT, Pisters PW, et al. Preoperative vs. postoperative radiation therapy for soft tissue sarcoma: a retrospective comparative evaluation of disease outcome. *Int J Radiat Oncol Biol Phys* 2003;56(2):482–488.
160. Al-Absi E, Farrokhyar F, Sharma R, et al. A systematic review and meta-analysis of oncologic outcomes of pre- versus postoperative radiation in localized resectable soft-tissue sarcoma. *Ann Surg Oncol* 2010;17(5):1367–1374.
162. Cahlon O, Spierer M, Brennan MF, et al. Long-term outcomes in extremity soft tissue sarcoma after a pathologically negative re-resection and without radiotherapy. *Cancer* 2008;112(12):2774–2779.
164. Fabrizio PL, Stafford SL, Pritchard DJ. Extremity soft-tissue sarcomas selectively treated with surgery alone. *Int J Radiat Oncol Biol Phys* 2000;48(1):227–232.
177. DeLaney TF, Spiro IJ, Suit HD, et al. Neoadjuvant chemotherapy and radiotherapy for large extremity soft-tissue sarcomas. *Int J Radiat Oncol Biol Phys* 2003;56(4):1117–1127.
178. Kraybill WG, Harris J, Spiro IJ, et al. Phase II study of neoadjuvant chemotherapy and radiation therapy in the management of high-risk, high-grade, soft tissue sarcomas of the extremities and body wall: Radiation Therapy Oncology Group Trial 9514. *J Clin Oncol* 2006;24(4):619–625.
179. Adjuvant chemotherapy for localised resectable soft-tissue sarcoma of adults: meta-analysis of individual data. Sarcoma Meta-analysis Collaboration. *Lancet* 1997;350(9092):1647–1654.
185. Pervaiz N, Colterjohn N, Farrokhyar F, et al. A systematic meta-analysis of randomized controlled trials of adjuvant chemotherapy for localized resectable soft-tissue sarcoma. *Cancer* 2008;113(3):573–581.
197. Demetri GD, von Mehren M, Blanke CD, et al. Efficacy and safety of imatinib mesylate in advanced gastrointestinal stromal tumors. *N Engl J Med* 2002;347(7):472–480.

Part N Pediatric

Chapter 84
Central Nervous System Tumors in Children

Carolyn R. Freeman, Jean-Pierre Farmer, and Roger E. Taylor

Central nervous system (CNS) tumors account for 20% to 25% of all malignancies that occur in childhood. According to the North American Association of Central Cancer Registries (NAACCR), the age-standardized incidence rate was 48.47 per million in the 0- to 19-year age group for the period 2004–2007.[1] The incidence was highest among children 1 to 4 years of age and lowest among 10- to 14-year-olds.

The etiology of pediatric CNS tumors remains largely unknown. Only 2% to 5% can be ascribed to a known genetic predisposition. Included in this category are those seen in patients with neurofibromatosis types 1 (NF-1) and 2 (NF-2), tuberous sclerosis, nevoid basal cell (Gorlin's) syndrome, familial adenomatous polyposis, and Li-Fraumeni syndrome. An even smaller percentage can be attributed to ionizing radiation used for diagnostic or therapeutic purposes. For the majority of patients, no predisposing factors can be identified.

The management of children with CNS tumors has changed substantially over the past three decades. Routine use of magnetic resonance imaging (MRI), and now frequently also functional imaging, and improved neuropathologic examination and molecular diagnostics have contributed to better characterization of the different tumor types. Improved neurosurgical techniques and perioperative care permit greater degrees of surgical resection even for tumors previously considered inoperable because of their location in eloquent areas of the brain. All of these, as well as improved radiotherapy techniques, newer chemotherapy agents and regimens, and national and international clinical trials, have contributed to improved outcomes for children and adolescents with CNS tumors. According to the NAACCR, 5-year survival has increased from 62.9% for patients diagnosed in 1980–1989 to 75.3% for those diagnosed in 2000–2006.[1]

RADIOTHERAPY FOR PEDIATRIC CNS TUMORS: GENERAL ISSUES

Radiotherapy is an essential component of treatment for many children with CNS tumors. However, survivors are at significant risk for the development of long-term sequelae,[2,3] many of which, while usually multifactorial, are in large part due to radiotherapy; many of the strategies used in the management of children with CNS tumors over the past three decades have been designed to reduce the risks associated with treatment. Recent developments in radiotherapy including improved targeting and new technologies and techniques for treatment, as well as new treatment modalities such as protons, all offer important opportunities for therapeutic gain that will be discussed below and in each section of this chapter.

Long-Term Effects of Radiotherapy

The quality of survival of children with brain tumors may be compromised by long-term sequelae. While some patients (e.g., patients with NF-1) may be at particular risk and while some sequelae (e.g., neurologic deficits) are more often due to the tumor and/or surgery, it is clear that radiotherapy is directly, alone or modulated by other factors, responsible for many late effects. A review by Kortmann et al.[4] gives an excellent account of radiation-related sequelae in children treated for low-grade glioma including effects on brain parenchyma, neurologic deficits, neurocognitive and behavioral effects, endocrine dysfunction, vasculopathy, and the development of second tumors.

The neurocognitive sequelae of radiotherapy have become much better characterized over recent years. It is now known that myelinization and functional maturation of the CNS continue until well into adolescence and even into young adulthood. Through its effect on the microvasculature as well as on the oligodendrocyte precursor cells that produce myelin, radiotherapy causes disrupted neurogenesis and cortical atrophy. Patients fail to acquire new knowledge and skills at an age-appropriate rate and show a progressive decline in IQ over time.[5] The magnitude of the deficit depends most importantly on age at treatment, but many other host (e.g., NF-1 or not), tumor (e.g., location, hydrocephalus or not), and treatment factors (e.g., radiotherapy volume and dose,[6–8] use of chemotherapy[9,10]) play a role. Moreover, the development of other deficits such as behavioral difficulties related to the location of the tumor and/or surgery or hearing impairment due to cisplatinum may have a modulating effect. The end result for many patients is impaired school and social performance that deteriorates over time. There is increasing evidence that intervention using cognitive or behavioral therapy or pharmacotherapy and even exercise may be useful and that this should start soon after treatment for best results.[5,11,12]

Endocrine deficits are very common after radiotherapy.[13] Even though a substantial proportion of patients may have had deficits prior to radiotherapy due to the tumor or to surgery,[14,15] and even though there may be modulating factors such as chemotherapy that affect the frequency of deficits, radiotherapy is primarily responsible for the growth hormone deficiency that correlates with the dose of radiotherapy to the hypothalamic–pituitary axis[16,17–18] and the primary hypothyroidism seen after craniospinal radiotherapy. There may be direct and indirect effects on musculoskeletal development. Osteopenia is a rather common finding that may put patients, particularly those with residual neurologic deficits, at significant risk for fracture.

Radiotherapy has been implicated as well in the development of cardiovascular complications including cerebrovascular events and coronary heart disease.[15,19] Although again the etiology is likely multifactorial, it is important to be cognizant of the risks and to minimize the dose to vascular structures and the heart.

Strategies that have been used to avoid or minimize the long-term effects of treatment for pediatric brain tumors include the following:

- Avoidance of radiotherapy altogether (e.g., in patients with low-grade astrocytoma for whom surgery alone may be a good option)
- Delay of radiotherapy for young children (i.e., those younger than age 3 to 8) by the use of chemotherapy
- Use of daily anesthesia, improved immobilization techniques (e.g., rigid casts or a stereotactic frame), and/or daily pretreatment image verification, all of which allow the use of reduced safety margins
- Use of image-based treatment planning using computed tomography (CT)–MRI or CT–MRI–functional imaging coregistration and better treatment-planning and delivery techniques that result in greater sparing of normal brain and organs at risk
- Use of new radiation modalities (e.g., proton therapy that provides even greater sparing of the surrounding normal brain and organs at risk)
- Use of reduced radiotherapy target volumes when it is shown safe to do so (e.g., tumor bed rather than whole posterior fossa for the boost in standard-risk medulloblastoma)
- Reduction of radiotherapy dose (e.g., in young patients with standard-risk medulloblastoma for whom in the North American studies the dose for craniospinal irradiation has been reduced progressively from 35 to 36 Gy to 23.4 Gy and, in current studies, to 18 Gy for children younger than 8)
- Use of smaller fraction sizes where appropriate (e.g., 1.5 Gy/day for patients with radiosensitive tumors such as germinoma)
- Use of hyperfractionated radiotherapy (HFRT) (e.g., as in the current European studies for standard-risk medulloblastoma)

These will be discussed later in each relevant clinical situation.

Preparation for Radiotherapy

The planning and delivery of radiotherapy for children with CNS tumors are technically challenging and labor intensive for the entire interprofessional team. The expertise of specialist personnel such as pediatric nurses and play therapists can be pivotal in encouraging a young child to lie still for the making of an immobilization device, for radiotherapy-planning procedures, and for treatment itself. For children younger than age 4 or 5 years, daily anesthesia will almost always be necessary, and this will require a skilled pediatric anesthetist because anesthesia will be administered in an environment without all of the support available in an operating room.

Radiotherapy Target Volumes and Treatment Techniques

Focal, Tumor or Tumor Bed Radiotherapy

For most tumor types, target volume definition is best accomplished using CT simulation with CT–MRI image coregistration. For patients who have undergone cerebrospinal fluid (CSF) diversion or surgical resection or in whom tumor shrinkage has occurred with chemotherapy, it will be important to take into account any anatomic shifts that may have taken place. This will be more of an issue for tumors arising in some areas than others and often adds significantly to the time required for contouring. The clinical target volume (CTV) will be tumor type specific, while the planning target volume (PTV) will be technique specific, ranging from 1 to 5 mm depending on the type of immobilization device used and whether daily pretreatment image verification is to be performed.

Modern radiotherapy treatment-planning and delivery techniques make it easier to achieve conformity of the treated volume to the target and sparing of uninvolved normal structures than in the past. The choice of technique in an individual patient will require careful analysis of the dosimetry in the context of the available options. A recent article by Beltran et al.[20] provides an excellent example of the issues to be considered now when weighing alternatives.

Other options for focal treatment include brachytherapy and intracystic injection of radioactive colloids. These will be discussed in the context of the relevant clinical situation.

Whole-Ventricle Radiotherapy

Whole-ventricular irradiation is used most frequently in patients with CNS germ cell tumors. Because subependymal spread is common, the target volume logically would include the lateral, third, and fourth ventricles with a margin of 1 to 1.5 cm. If lateral opposed fields are used, the volume of brain spared will be small. Better sparing can be achieved using intensity-modulated image-guided radiotherapy.[21–23]

Craniospinal Radiotherapy

The CTV for craniospinal radiotherapy has an irregular shape that consists of the whole brain and spinal cord and their overlying meninges. In standard techniques, the lower borders of lateral whole-brain fields are matched to the cephalad border of a posterior spine field, usually with a moving junction between the brain and spine fields to minimize the risk of underdose or overdose in the cervical spinal cord. Compensators may be needed to achieve dose homogeneity throughout the target volume.

Patient Positioning and Immobilization

Patients have traditionally received craniospinal irradiation (CSI) in the prone position, but modern technology allows safe treatment in the supine position that in general is more comfortable and, if anesthesia is required, allows better control of the airway. In either case, immobilization is essential and involves the use of a head shell or full-body immobilization. Careful attention to positioning at the time of simulation is critical to minimize or even eliminate the risk of certain long-term effects. For example, using neck extension together with careful selection of the level for the junction of the brain and spine fields, it is possible to avoid including the dentition in the exit from the superior aspect of the spinal field and thus damage to developing teeth.

Target Volume Definition

CT simulation is necessary to ensure adequate coverage of the CTV in the subfrontal region at the cribriform plate. Traditionally, blocks have been used in the lateral fields to shield not only the facial structures but also the lenses. However, in most children it is impossible to adequately irradiate the cribriform plate and shield the lenses (Fig. 84.1), and adequate PTV coverage should take precedence.

CT simulation is helpful, too, in identifying the lateral aspect of CTV for the spine field that includes the extensions of the meninges along the nerve roots to the lateral aspects of the spinal ganglia (Fig. 84.2). The field will be narrower in the dorsal region to avoid unnecessary irradiation of the heart and lungs and wider in the lumbar region, although here it is important to avoid an excessively wide field that will result in unnecessary irradiation of the bone marrow and gonads. The lower limit of the CTV for the spine field is best determined by MRI. Traditionally, the lower border of the spine field was placed at the lower border of the second sacral foramen, but it is well documented that the lower border of the thecal sac can be as high as L5 or as low as S3. In the interest of both CTV

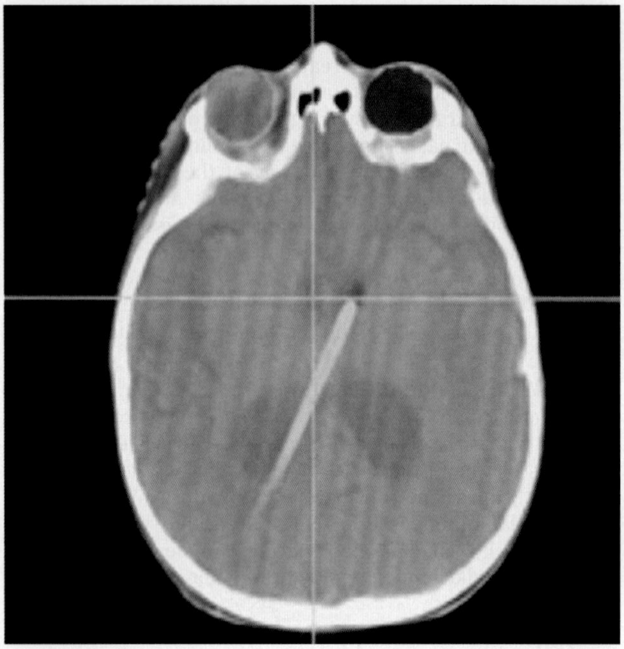

FIGURE 84.1. The use of computed tomography simulation is superior to conventional radiographs for determination of the clinical target volume for craniospinal irradiation and ensures coverage of the meninges in the subfrontal region. In most children adequate coverage of the planning target volume precludes significant sparing of the lens.

coverage and normal tissue sparing, it is important that the lower border be individualized according to the MRI findings.

Treatment Planning and Delivery

There are many issues that need to be addressed in designing a CSI technique (Table 84.1). Many of the different solutions[24] add further complexity. Using modern tools for treatment planning and delivery, it is possible to greatly simplify the technique and substantially reduce planning and delivery times. One such technique is shown in Figure 84.3.[25] In general, photons in the 6- to 10-MV range provide satisfactory coverage of the PTV. A variation of dose along the spinal axis of >10% will require the use of dose compensation that can be achieved using multileaf collimation.

TABLE 84.1 TECHNICAL CONSIDERATIONS FOR CRANIOSPINAL IRRADIATION

Problem	*Possible Solutions*
Target volume definition may be difficult using conventional simulation	Use CT simulation with CT-MRI coregistration
Prone position	Supine position preferred
Uncomfortable	
Difficult to monitor airway	
Field matching over cervical spine/risk of over- or underdosage	Angle brain fields
	Use half-beam block for brain fields
	Use couch rotation or match line wedge
Choice of extended SSD or second field for treatment of spinal axis	Two fields preferred
Inhomogeneity along spinal axis	Use compensator, MLC
Irradiation of normal tissues	
Mandible/teeth	Neck extension
Thyroid	Care with level of junction
Heart	Use lower junction
	Care with width of spine field
GI tract	Use electrons, IMRT, protons
Gonads	Use electrons, IMRT, protons
	Care with lower limit and width of spine field

CT, computed tomography; MRI, magnetic resonance imaging; SSD, source-to-surface distance; MLC, multileaf collimator; IMRT, intensity-modulated radiation therapy; GI, gastrointestinal.

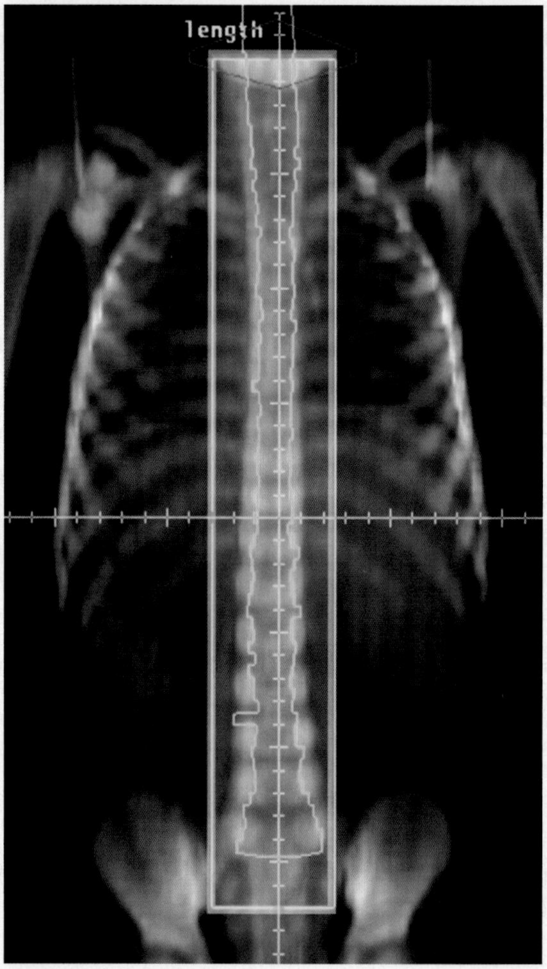

FIGURE 84.2. The use of computed tomography simulation with contouring of the cord and overlying meninges that extend laterally to the lateral aspect of the spinal ganglia results in a field width that is narrower than one based on bony anatomy. The addition of shielding further reduces the volume of normal tissues included in the treated volume.

Electrons are used in some centers to treat the spinal axis and in fact may be of greater interest now than in the past because of improved dose calculation algorithms and even electron dose modulation techniques. However, at the same time newer treatment-planning and delivery methods such as intensity-modulated radiation therapy (IMRT) together with daily image verification allow for improved dosimetry with photons with clinically relevant dose reductions to structures anterior to the target volume such as the heart, gastrointestinal (GI) tract, and gonads.[26] The use of IMRT and smaller PTV margins raises new issues that are not as relevant when lateral opposed fields are used, such as the need to ensure adequate coverage of all CSF extensions including those along the optic nerves and into the internal auditory canals (Fig. 84.4).

New Treatment Modalities for CSI

Protons provide a dose distribution for CSI that cannot be achieved by even the most sophisticated photon beam treatment planning, with significant reduction in low-dose exposure outside the target volume.[27] For now, however, access to proton therapy is limited and the cost prohibitive.

Radiation Dose and Dose-Fractionation Regimens

The conventional daily fraction size for the treatment of most pediatric CNS tumors is 1.8 Gy and the total dose typically on the order of 54 to 55.8 Gy. When treating a primary tumor of the spinal cord, it is conventional to use a lower total dose (e.g., 50.4 Gy). It is also usual to use lower doses for children

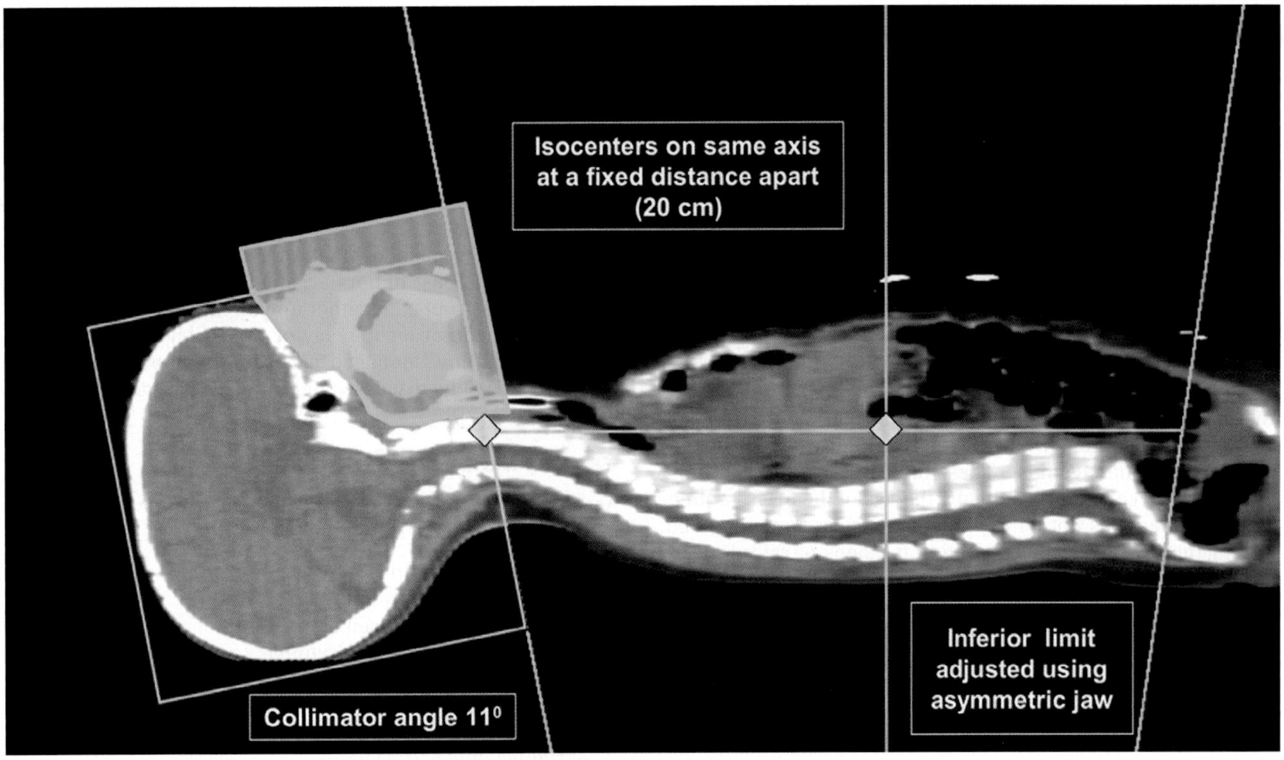

FIGURE 84.3. To cover the clinical target volume for craniospinal irradiation, lateral opposed fields are used to treat the brain and a direct posterior field is used to cover the spinal axis. Magnetic resonance imaging is used to identify the caudal extent of the thecal sac. The field junction over the cervical cord should be at a level that avoids the inclusion of the teeth in the exit of the spinal field and usually is moved weekly ("feathered") to avoid over- or underdosage. The supine position is more comfortable for the patient and safer if sedation or anesthesia is required. In the technique shown, fixed field parameters are used, which greatly facilitates treatment planning and delivery. (From Parker WA, Freeman CR. A simple technique for craniospinal radiotherapy in the supine position. *Radiother Oncol* 2006;78[2]:217–222.)

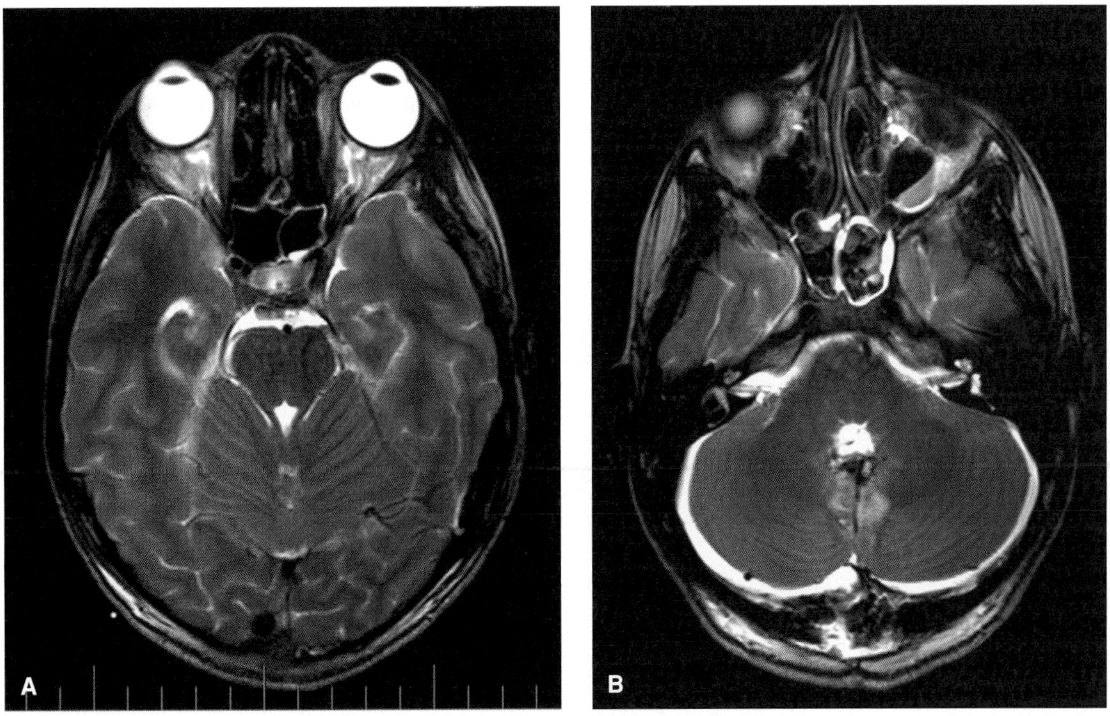

FIGURE 84.4. Postoperative axial T2-weighted magnetic resonance imaging for a patient receiving craniospinal irradiation (CSI) for medulloblastoma showing extension of cerebrospinal fluid along the optic nerves to the lamina cribrosa **(A)** and into the internal auditory canals **(B)**. Care is necessary to identify all such extensions when using intensity-modulated radiation therapy for CSI given that the margins are much tighter than when using conventional lateral opposed fields.

younger than age 3 years to reduce the risk of neurocognitive deficits. When treating radiosensitive tumors such as intracranial germinoma, radiotherapy may be delivered using a lower dose per fraction (e.g., 1.5 Gy) and lower total doses of 30 to 45 Gy.

Many pediatric brain tumors exhibit a dose–response relationship for tumor control and in some cases local progression is not prevented by the use of a conventional "CNS tolerance" radiation dose. When the target contains only a small volume of normal brain tissue, dose escalation may be possible using newer treatment-planning and delivery techniques. HFRT may be a useful strategy in situations where dose escalation cannot be achieved safely using conventional fractionation.

Follow-Up During and After Radiotherapy

An excellent review by Donahue[28] describes the acute reactions seen during treatment with radiotherapy and provides guidelines for their management. These days nausea and vomiting almost always can be prevented by the use of the 5HT-3 antagonists. Headache is not an expected side effect and should be investigated by physical examination for signs of raised intracranial pressure and by imaging as appropriate. Steroids, if used, usually can be tapered by the second or third week of treatment. Fatigue is a rather common symptom and is cumulative. The neurologic status of the patient, especially coordination and gait, may appear to worsen during the last weeks of treatment because of this. Children usually recover relatively quickly and often can get back to their usual routine quite soon after completion of treatment.

Predictable effects of treatment include hormonal deficits, especially primary hypothyroidism when CSI is delivered using photons and growth hormone deficit secondary to inclusion of the hypothalamic–pituitary axis. Patients should be monitored closely in follow-up and treatment instituted as appropriate. Many will also need regular follow-up in ophthalmology and audiology.

Extra pedagogic support may be necessary. Patients should have ready access to a neuropsychologist for evaluation of any special needs and in the longer term to vocational assessment and counseling.

RADIOTHERAPY FOR SPECIFIC TUMOR TYPES

The World Health Organization (WHO) classification of tumors of the nervous system[29] is given in Table 84.2 and the distribution by tumor type and location in Figure 84.5. There are important differences between tumors seen in childhood and those occurring in adults. In children, almost half of all tumors arise in the infratentorial compartment. Low-grade astrocytic tumors as a group account for approximately one-third to half of all CNS tumors, but medulloblastoma is the most common distinct entity. High-grade gliomas, which account for the majority of primary brain tumors seen in adults, are much less common in children.

This chapter will follow the order of the WHO classification. Although in the past tumors arising in infants and very young children were grouped together and all managed similarly with chemotherapy in order to delay or if possible avoid radiotherapy, they are now managed according to the specific tumor type and so will be discussed here in each relevant section.

TABLE 84.2 WORLD HEALTH ORGANIZATION CLASSIFICATION OF TUMORS OF THE CENTRAL NERVOUS SYSTEM

Tumors of neuroepithelial tissue
Astrocytic tumors[a]
Oligodendroglial tumors
Mixed gliomas
Ependymal tumors[a]
Choroid plexus tumors[a]
Glial tumors of uncertain origin
Neuronal and mixed neuronal-glial tumors[a]
Neuroblastic tumors
Pineal parenchymal tumors[a]
Embryonal tumors[a]
Tumors of the meninges
Lymphomas and hematopoietic neoplasms
Germ cell tumors[a]
Tumors of the sellar region[a]
Metastatic tumors

[a]Topics addressed in this chapter; the remainder are uncommon in the pediatric population and generally speaking will be managed as in adult populations.

From Louis DN, International Agency for Research on Cancer. *WHO classification of tumours of the central nervous system*. Lyon, France: International Agency for Research on Cancer, 2007.

ASTROCYTIC TUMORS

According to the WHO classification, astrocytic tumors comprise the following clinicopathologic entities:

- Pilocytic astrocytoma (WHO grade I)
  –Pilomyxoid astrocytoma
- Subependymal giant cell astrocytoma
- Pleomorphic xanthoastrocytoma
- Diffuse astrocytoma (WHO grade II)
  –Fibrillary astrocytoma
  –Gemistocytic astrocytoma
  –Protoplasmic astrocytoma
- Anaplastic astrocytoma (WHO grade III)
- Glioblastoma multiforme (WHO grade IV)
  –Giant cell glioblastoma
  –Gliosarcoma
- Gliomatosis cerebri

These tumors are heterogeneous with respect to clinical presentation (age, gender, location in the CNS, imaging findings) as well as to growth potential and rate of progression. Two, pleomorphic xanthoastrocytoma and subependymal giant cell astrocytoma, are rare tumors. Their clinical presentation and imaging findings are quite characteristic and surgery is usually curative. They will not be discussed further here.

Low-Grade Astrocytoma (WHO Grades I and II)

So-called benign or low-grade astrocytomas (LGAs) comprise a heterogeneous group of tumors with behavior patterns that are fairly typical according to location and pathologic type. In general, in children, they follow an indolent clinical course with overall survival rates at 10 and 15 years as high as 80% to 100%. LGAs can be grouped according to their anatomic location:

- Cerebellar astrocytomas (15% to 20% of all CNS tumors)
- Hemispheric astrocytomas (10% to 15% of all CNS tumors)
- Midline supratentorial tumors, including the corpus callosum, lateral and third ventricles, and hypothalamus and thalamus (10% to 15% of all CNS tumors)
- Optic pathway tumors (approximately 5% of all CNS tumors)
- Brainstem LGAs (brainstem tumors account for 10% to 15% of all CNS tumors; 20% to 30% of these are LGAs)
- LGAs of the spinal cord (spinal cord tumors account for 3% to 6% of all CNS tumors; approximately 60% of these are LGAs)

Pilocytic astrocytomas are the most common type in the pediatric age group, accounting for almost all of the LGAs at certain sites (e.g., the cerebellum and the anterior optic pathway). They account for a smaller proportion of LGAs arising in the deep midline structures and in the cerebral hemispheres. Macroscopically, pilocytic astrocytomas appear well circumscribed and frequently have an associated cystic component. Pilocytic astrocytomas are characterized histologically by a

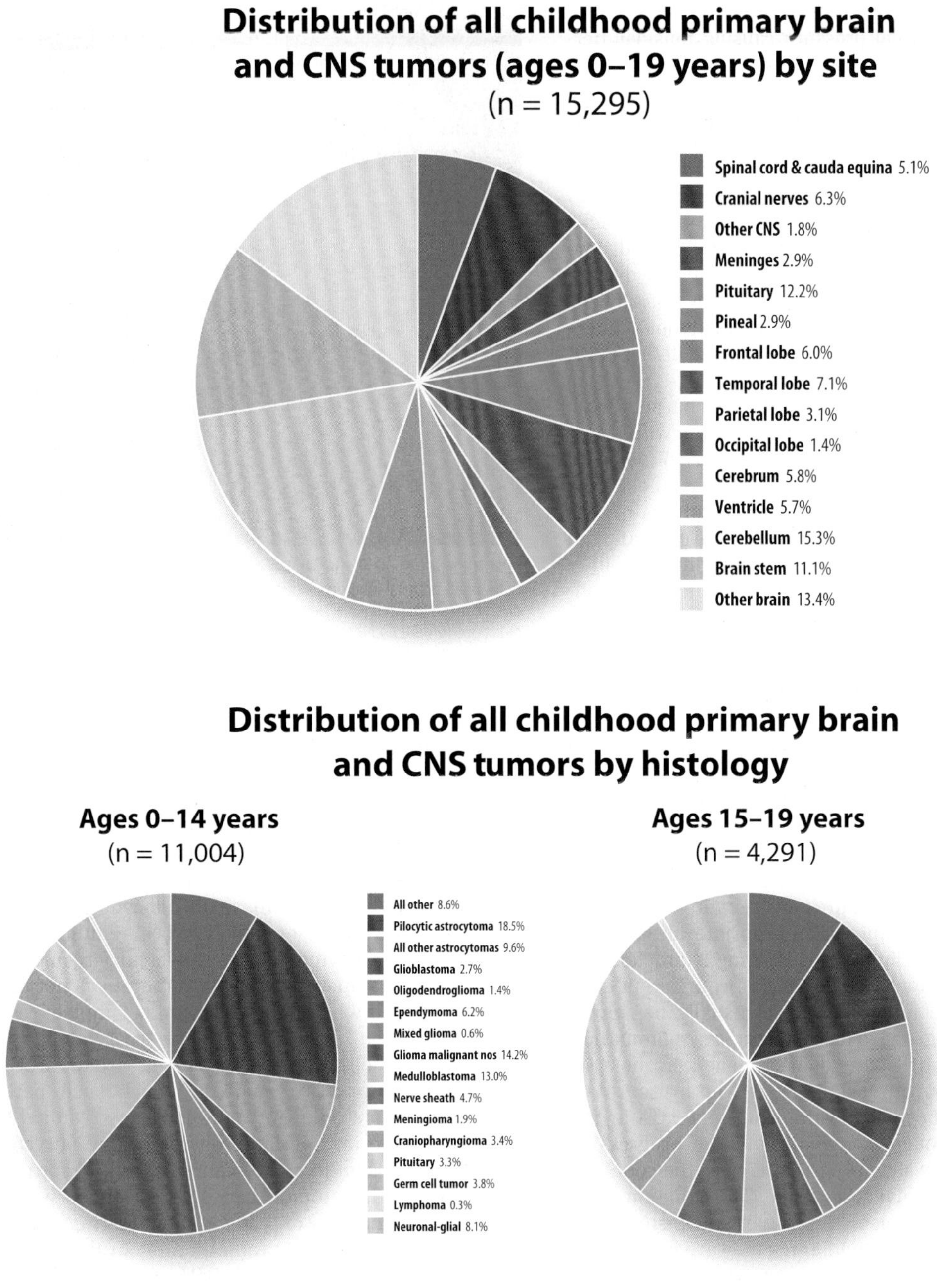

FIGURE 84.5. Distribution of central nervous system tumors by site **(A)** and histology **(B)** for the years 2004–2007. Data from the Central Brain Tumor Registry of the United States (www.cbtrus.org).

biphasic pattern with a varying proportion of compacted bipolar cells with Rosenthal fibers and loose-textured multipolar cells with microcysts and granular bodies. Rare mitoses, occasional hyperchromatic nuclei, microvascular proliferation, and even infiltration of the meninges are compatible with a diagnosis of pilocytic astrocytoma and not a sign of malignancy. A variant, pilomyxoid astrocytoma, first described in infants and young children with chiasmatic/hypothalamic tumors, appears to be associated with more aggressive behavior that may include leptomeningeal seeding.[30]

Diffuse astrocytomas account for only approximately 10% to 15% of all LGAs in children but for a relatively higher proportion of those seen in infants and adolescents. Most intrinsic pontine tumors and a large proportion of astrocytomas arising in the cerebral hemispheres are diffuse astrocytomas. Diffuse astrocytomas grow by infiltration rather than destruction of anatomic structures and usually are not well circumscribed. Microscopically, they are composed of well-differentiated fibrillary or gemistocytic neoplastic astrocytes on a background of loosely structured, often microcystic, tumor matrix. Cellularity is moderately increased. The presence of nuclear atypia is a diagnostic criterion, but mitotic activity, necrosis, and microvascular proliferation are absent. The growth fraction as determined by Ki-67 and MIB-1 labeling indices is usually low. Diffuse astrocytomas may undergo malignant progression, although this is not common in the pediatric age group with the notable exception of tumors arising in the pons.

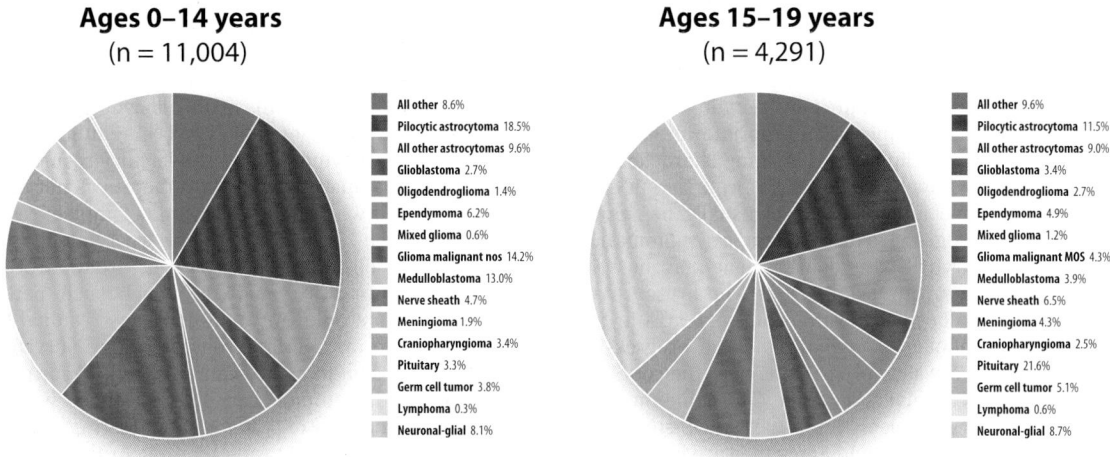

Patients with LGAs typically present with a long history of nonspecific and nonlocalizing symptoms. Symptoms and signs of raised intracranial pressure may be seen in patients with midline and cerebellar tumors. Patients with posterior fossa tumors may present with neck stiffness and a head tilt as a manifestation of raised intracranial pressure causing tonsillar herniation, altitudinal diplopia, or spinal accessory nerve irritation. Seizures are present in as many as three-quarters of patients with hemispheric lesions. Other symptoms relatively less frequent and usually of more recent onset relate to the location of the tumor. These may include, for example, focal motor deficits with hemispheric tumors, visual field deficits with tumors compressing or involving the optic pathway, neuroendocrine deficits with hypothalamic tumors, and the diencephalic syndrome (consisting of emaciation with loss of subcutaneous fat despite normal or increased appetite, alert appearance, increased vigor and euphoria, pallor without anemia, and nystagmoid movements of the eyes) in young children with chiasmatic/hypothalamic tumors.

Neuroimaging findings are usually quite characteristic. Pilocytic astrocytomas are well circumscribed, often with a cystic component that may be large relative to the size of the solid component. There is usually little edema or mass effect. The solid component enhances brightly and uniformly with contrast material. Diffuse or fibrillary astrocytomas are usually not well seen on nonenhanced CT or MRI and usually show little enhancement with contrast material. T2-weighted or fluid-attenuated inversion recovery (FLAIR) MRI sequences usually best demonstrate the extent of disease.

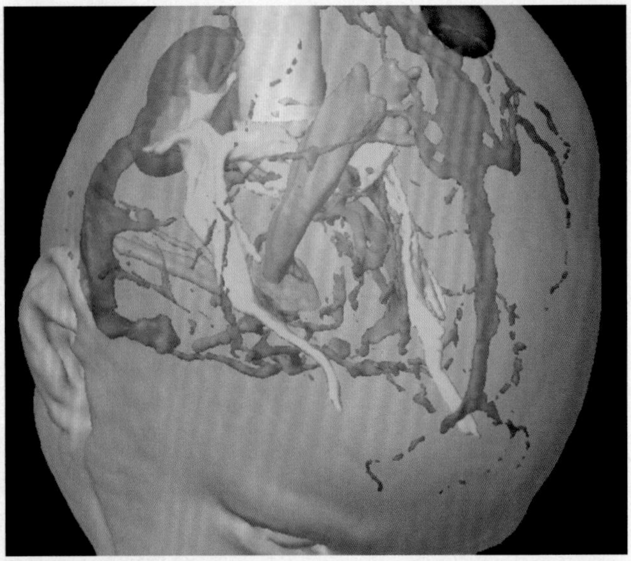

FIGURE 84.6. Surgical planning for a dysembryoplastic neuroepithelial tumor (*light blue*) in the right occipital lobe presenting with seizures. Functional magnetic resonance imaging data are used to identify the 1-degree visual cortex (*purple*). Fiber tracking identifies the optic radiations (*green*) and the corticospinal tract (*darker blue*). These data are then used to plan the trajectory (*yellow*). By identifying regions to be selectively avoided, similar information could be helpful in radiotherapy treatment planning.

Management of Low-Grade Astrocytomas: General Principles

Some children with LGAs may not require any tumor-specific treatment. These include, for example, patients with NF-1, as many as 15% of whom have optic pathway tumors.[31] NF-1 patients also may have astrocytic tumors in other parts of the CNS as well as hamartomatous lesions, typically in the brainstem. These lesions may be detected on routine imaging, but even tumors that are symptomatic may remain stable over long periods so that surveillance is appropriate initial management.[32–34] A number of clinical and imaging characteristics have been correlated with a more aggressive course, but even for these patients active intervention will usually be undertaken only at time of progressive disease that is symptomatic.

Progression-free survival without treatment may be very good as well for patients with tectal lesions who present with hydrocephalus without localizing brainstem signs. LGA in this region may be very indolent, showing either no progression (the majority) or only very slow progression over the course of many years following CSF diversion alone. The common characteristics of these very indolent tumors are their small size (<1.5 or 2 cm) and the fact that on imaging they are hypodense/hypointense and nonenhancing. Follow-up with MRI is essential to identify patients with progressive lesions as manifested by increasing size and/or enhancement with gadolinium. Treatment (usually radiotherapy but sometimes now surgery) at time of progression is associated with a high probability of long-term tumor control.

These special situations underscore the need for careful evaluation and individualization of management of patients with LGAs depending on the specific clinical situation and tumor type. If in doubt, a period of surveillance generally will be an acceptable initial approach.

Surgery is the mainstay of treatment for LGAs. Complete resection is more likely to be accomplished in patients with smaller tumors and those arising in noneloquent parts of the brain as well as in patients with the generally well-circumscribed pilocytic tumors. Modern surgical techniques that include, for example, computer-assisted resections ("neuronavigation") aided by preoperative functional MRI, MR tractography, and intraoperative mapping of eloquent areas (Fig. 84.6) together with intraoperative MRI permit greater degrees of resection in larger proportions of patients, including many who in the past would have been considered to have inoperable lesions. Complete resection is now achieved in >80% of cerebral, cerebellar, and spinal cord tumors and about 50% of diencephalic tumors.

Children with LGAs who undergo complete resection fare very well, with long-term disease-free and overall survival rates of 80% to 100%.[35–39,40] In most series, results are better (close to 100%) for patients with pilocytic astrocytomas than for those with diffuse or fibrillary LGAs, although some have disputed this, showing equally satisfactory results for both. In either type, postoperative adjuvant therapy is not indicated.

For children who undergo less than complete resection, the progression-free survival rate after surgery alone is less satisfactory. In a joint Children's Cancer Group (CCG)–Pediatric Oncology Group (POG) study in which such patients were observed without adjuvant treatment, any residual tumor was associated with an inferior progression-free survival rate: the 8-year progression-free survival rate was 56% for patients with <1.5 cm^3 residual tumor and 45% for those with >1.5 cm^3. However, the majority of patients can be salvaged with a second surgical resection and/or radiotherapy. In the CCG–POG study, overall survival at 8 years was 95% and 90%, respectively.[41]

The role of postoperative radiotherapy following less than complete resection remains unclear. In most series, the use of radiotherapy in this situation results in improved disease-free survival without any benefit in terms of overall survival. Because only approximately half of all patients will develop progressive disease, the usual recommendation for a patient who is neurologically stable will be surveillance, with MRI performed at least every 6 months for the first 3 years, the period during which risk of progression is greatest.[42] A second surgical procedure would usually be considered at time of progression, and other treatment, either radiotherapy or chemotherapy, reserved for patients with progressive, inoperable disease (Fig. 84.7).

In the past, patients with deep midline and other tumors considered surgically inaccessible were treated with radiotherapy, often even without histologic confirmation of diagnosis. However, using modern neurosurgical techniques, it is feasible to resect surgically about half of these lesions (Fig. 84.8), and the overall strategy for these patients should now be as for patients with LGAs at other locations, albeit with the understanding that outcome is not as satisfactory. The 8-year progression-free and overall survival rates in the CCG–POG study

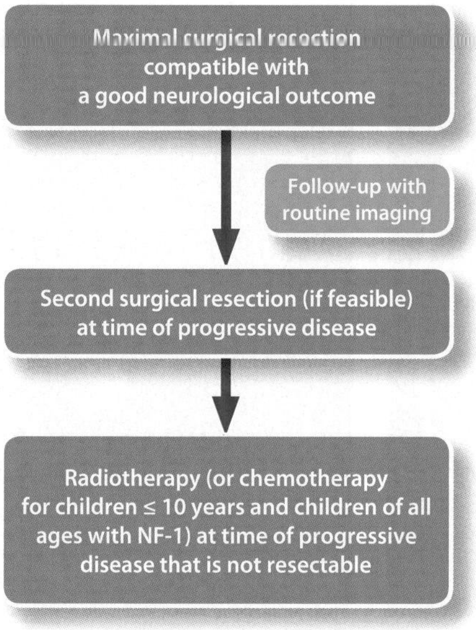

FIGURE 84.7. An algorithm for the management of patients with low-grade astrocytoma.

for patients with midline chiasmatic tumors were 25% and 84%, respectively.[41]

When adjuvant therapy is indicated, the options include chemotherapy, particularly for infants and young children and for patients of all ages with NF-1 who are at greatest risk of developing neurocognitive, vaso-occlusive, and neuroendocrine sequelae of treatment. Complete responses to chemotherapy are not common, but overall response rates that include stable disease range from 70% to 100% and the use of chemotherapy has been shown to permit delay of radiotherapy by 2 to as many as 4+ years.[43–46] The age limit below which chemotherapy should be used is controversial. It is likely that delaying radiotherapy for 2 to 3 years will be of benefit for a child younger than age 5 to 8. However, the benefit from a similar delay for an older child is less clear, particularly when any benefit may be offset by neurologic compromise from further tumor progression as well as the need for a larger radiotherapy target volume. Moreover, recent advances in radiotherapy practice that have the potential to reduce the risks of radiotherapy have led to a reassessment of the role of radiotherapy in LGAs and better acceptance of its earlier use even in very young children.

Radiotherapy in LGAs

Due largely to improvements in surgery and to a lesser extent to successful treatment of younger children with chemotherapy, there has been a substantial decrease in the use of radiotherapy over recent years. Currently only approximately 10% of all children with LGAs receive radiotherapy.

Indications for Radiotherapy

- Radiotherapy is not indicated after complete resection
- Radiotherapy may be indicated following incomplete resection in situations when tumor progression would compromise neurologic function (e.g., "threat to vision")
- The clearest indication for radiotherapy is in patients with progressive and/or symptomatic disease that is unresectable

Radiotherapy Target Volume

The radiotherapy target volume (the gross tumor volume or GTV) consists of all disease seen on MRI performed just prior to treatment (Fig. 84.9). The resulting treatment volume usually will be considerably smaller than one based on preoperative imaging, which until recently would have constituted standard

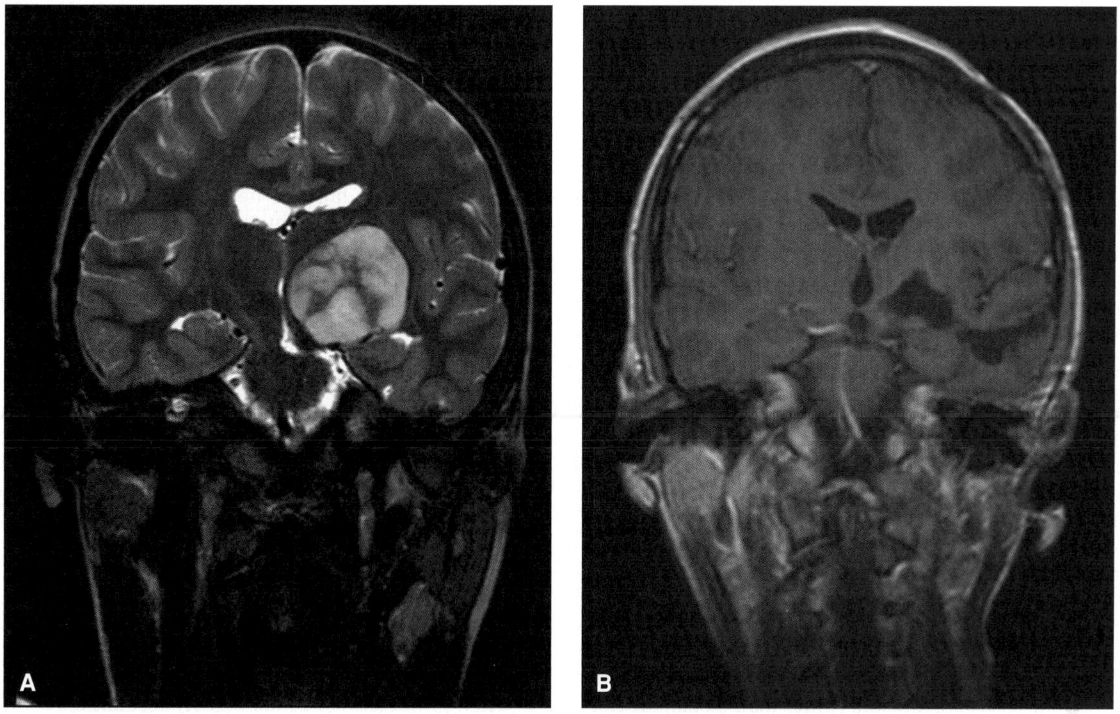

FIGURE 84.8. A 12-year-old boy referred to the radiation oncology department 3 years after diagnosis of a biopsy-proven JPA of the left thalamus at another institution. He had been deemed inoperable at diagnosis and had received chemotherapy first with vincristine and carboplatin and then with weekly vinblastine. **A:** At the time of referral he was having more frequent choreoathetotic movements of his right hand and there was evidence of progressive disease on magnetic resonance imaging (MRI). **B:** He underwent complete resection without complications and has no evidence of residual disease on his most recent MRI. This was a far better approach than radiotherapy, avoiding the neurocognitive, endocrine, and vascular complications associated with radiotherapy for tumors in this region, and with a greater probability of long-term tumor control.

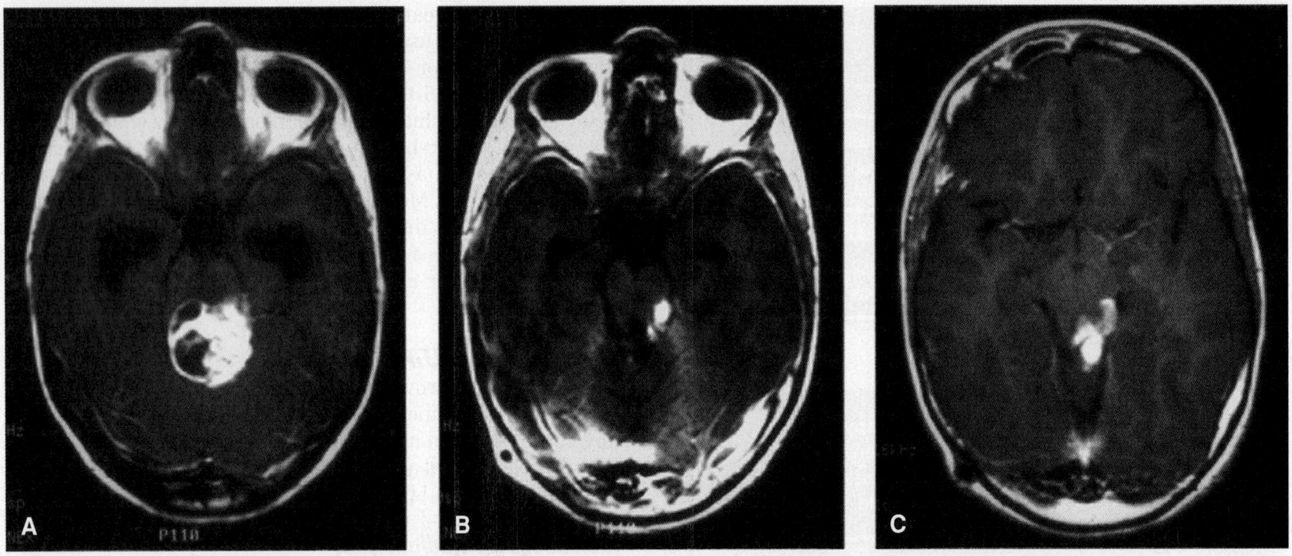

FIGURE 84.9. This patient underwent subtotal resection of a low-grade astrocytoma of the left cerebellar peduncle at age 8 (**A:** preoperative, **B:** postoperative). **C:** Three years later routine imaging showed evidence of progressive disease. The gross tumor volume for radiotherapy consists of the tumor as seen on magnetic resonance imaging at the time of treatment.

practice. Similarly, margins that were considered standard (and still are in adult practice) are unnecessary, particularly for the well-circumscribed pilocytic tumor for which a CTV margin of 1 cm[40] or even 0 cm (i.e., CTV = GTV)[47] around the GTV as seen on T1-weighted gadolinium-enhanced images has been shown to result in excellent local control. More generous margins of 1 to 1.5 cm around the GTV as seen on T2-weighted or FLAIR images may be more appropriate for the more infiltrative diffuse fibrillary tumors.

Radiotherapy Dose

Evidence for a dose–response correlation in LGAs in children is scant. Although the European and North American studies that randomized adult patients with LGAs between low-dose (45 and 50.4 Gy, respectively) and high-dose (59.4 and 64.8 Gy, respectively) radiotherapy failed to demonstrate any advantage for the higher dose, it may be unwise to extrapolate that in children doses of 45 to 50 Gy are as effective as the higher doses of 54 to 55 Gy that until now have constituted standard practice. There are biologic differences between LGAs in children and in adults. As well, children who have progressed on chemotherapy may have tumors that are less sensitive. For now, the recommendation for children with LGAs would be a "standard" dose of 50 to 54 Gy depending on the age of the child and the location of the tumor and its relationship to critical normal structures such as the optic chiasm.

Radiotherapy Technique

External-beam radiotherapy using a conventional dose-fractionation schedule should be considered the standard of care in LGAs and the technique to be used that which provides homogeneous irradiation of the CTV and best spares surrounding normal tissues.

Other approaches that have been used in LGAs include radiosurgery using the Gamma knife or linear accelerator–based techniques.[48] While the use of a single fraction, typically of 10 to 20 Gy, to the periphery of the lesion or a small number of large fractions may not be optimal for diffuse or fibrillary LGAs with tumor cells embedded in rather than displacing normal brain, such treatment may be of interest for part or even all of the treatment for the less invasive pilocytic astrocytomas that are often small at time of progression.

Another option for treatment is brachytherapy, which has been used with some success particularly in European centers.[49–53] As for radiosurgery, the principal limitation with respect to the use of brachytherapy is the size of the target volume. Brachytherapy series necessarily select for smaller tumors, and there is no evidence that brachytherapy is a better treatment option than external-beam radiotherapy. Radioactive solutions such as ^{32}P, ^{90}Y, ^{198}Au, and ^{186}Re may be useful in cystic LGAs, particularly for patients with recurrent disease after radiotherapy in whom symptoms not infrequently relate more to the cyst than to the solid component of tumor. Simple aspiration with or without placement of an internal shunt usually will alleviate symptoms for protracted periods, but in some cases, particularly those in which the cyst wall enhances and is felt to be biologically active, control of the cyst may be difficult, and the use of radioactive solutions could be considered. However, this is not a procedure without risks and care has to be taken to avoid leakage.

Follow-Up After Radiotherapy

Tumor regression after radiotherapy typically is slow and patients and their families need to be warned that the tumor may remain stable or sometimes even increase in size in the first months after completion of treatment. It is important not to assume that changes seen on MRI represent progressive disease. Close follow-up with early repeat imaging usually will be the best approach in this situation.

High-Grade Astrocytoma (WHO Grades III and IV)

Anaplastic astrocytoma (AA) is a diffusely infiltrating malignant astrocytoma characterized by nuclear atypia, increased cellularity, and significant proliferative activity. Glioblastoma multiforme (GBM) is the most malignant astrocytic tumor. Histopathologic features include nuclear atypia, cellular pleomorphism, mitotic activity, vascular thrombosis, microvascular proliferation, and necrosis. Both AA and GBM may develop from WHO grade II astrocytomas. However, with the exception of tumors that arise in the pons, they arise almost always in the pediatric age group *de novo* without evidence of a less malignant precursor lesion.

High-grade astrocytomas (HGAs) account for 5% of all CNS tumors in the pediatric age group. They are the most common tumor type in older adolescents. Two-thirds of HGAs are located in the cerebral hemispheres and the remainder approximately equally divided between the deep midline structures (thalamus and basal ganglia) and cerebellum. Patients with HGAs usually present with symptoms of short duration that relate to the location of the lesion.

Surgery is an important component of treatment. Because most studies show a survival advantage for patients who have undergone complete resection,[54–58] maximal surgical resection compatible with a good neurologic outcome should be the goal for all patients and a second surgical procedure should be considered if there is significant residual tumor after the first. Postoperative radiotherapy always is indicated. Although leptomeningeal seeding is seen in a substantial minority (10% to 30%) of patients, the predominant failure pattern is local and the radiotherapy target volume is local, with a GTV that consists of the tumor bed and any residual enhancing or nonenhancing residual tumor plus any abnormality seen on T2-weighted MRI with a margin for the CTV of 1.5 cm. Because these are often large tumors and doses beyond tolerance levels for structures such as the optic chiasm are required, it is usual to consider a volume reduction at 50 to 54 Gy to a CTV that consists of the tumor bed and any residual tumor plus a reduced margin of 1 cm. The dose to the CTV should be at least 54 Gy given over 6 weeks, but a dose of 59 to 60 Gy is more usual if feasible. There is no evidence that higher doses delivered using radiosurgery or stereotactic boosts, boosts with brachytherapy, or HFRT result in improved outcome, but IMRT delivering accelerated treatment to a component of the target volume (such as the GTV) may be of interest, if only to decrease the overall treatment duration.

The role of chemotherapy remains to be defined. Although responses are seen to many different agents and regimens, results have often been difficult to interpret because of small patient numbers, inconsistent inclusion criteria with respect to pathology, and confounding variables such as tumor location and extent of surgical resection. The cooperative groups in North America and Europe are investigating a number of approaches that include newer chemotherapeutic and biologic agents, some of which have radiosensitizing properties. Whenever possible, patients should be treated on such protocols. Off study it may be difficult to make a recommendation with respect to adjuvant chemotherapy, although the poor prognosis, particularly for patients with macroscopic residual disease following surgery, usually is given as an argument for the use of the "current best" regimen, most often now temozolomide as in adults.

The prognosis for children with HGAs is poor, with a median time to progression of 10 to 11 months and an overall survival at 5 years of only approximately 20%. Several factors correlate with outcome. Patients with lesions in the cerebral hemispheres fare better than those with tumors in other locations, apparently independent of extent of surgical resection. The prognosis for children with thalamic lesions appears to be particularly poor.[59] Age also may be an important factor. In contrast to most other tumor types, children younger than age 3 with HGAs fare better than older children, with overall survival at 3 to 5 years in the 33% to 50% range in the North American and United Kingdom Children's Cancer Study Group/International Paediatric Oncology Society (UKCCSG/SIOP) baby studies.[60–63] The prognosis may be even better for children younger than age 1.[64] Histologic grade (AA vs. GBM) has not been shown consistently to affect outcome, but p53 overexpression and a high MIB-1 labeling index appear to identify patients with a particularly adverse prognosis.[65]

Management of Astrocytic Tumors in Specific Locations

Optic Pathway Gliomas

Optic pathway gliomas collectively account for approximately 5% of all CNS tumors in the pediatric age group. These are tumors of young children: the peak age incidence is between 2 and 6 years and 75% of all patients are younger than 10. One-third of patients have NF-1. They may be divided into three clinicopathologic entities: tumors confined to the optic nerve(s), tumors of the optic chiasm with or without optic nerve involvement (collectively "anterior" tumors), and tumors that involve the hypothalamus or adjacent structures ("chiasmatic/hypothalamic" or "posterior" tumors). Management of patients with optic pathway gliomas is often said to be controversial but is really not when differences in behavior between the different tumor types and between patients with and without NF-1 are taken into consideration.

Optic nerve gliomas may involve one or both optic nerves. Bilateral involvement is pathognomonic of NF-1. In a substantial proportion of cases, the optic nerve tumors are incidental findings on routine imaging and patients may remain asymptomatic with nonprogressive lesions over long periods; even spontaneous regression is well documented. The frequency of progression is difficult to establish, ranging from lows of <10% among patients followed in NF-1 clinics to 40% to 50% in series reported by oncology centers. Even in patients with symptomatic tumors, the course can be quite variable: only 30% to 60% of such patients will develop progressive disease that requires treatment.[34,66] Thus, management of patients with optic nerve tumors will usually consist initially of close follow-up with regular ophthalmologic examinations and MRI, with active intervention, usually chemotherapy, reserved for patients with clear evidence of progression that is symptomatic.[66–68]

Patients with unilateral optic nerve involvement may not have NF-1. They present most frequently with proptosis that may be relatively long-standing. Findings on examination may include optic atrophy and impaired visual acuity. On MRI, optic nerve tumors are usually relatively small and well circumscribed, with bright enhancement typical for pilocytic astrocytoma. Biopsy is not necessary to make a diagnosis. Treatment usually, although not always, will be necessary and the approach will depend on whether there is useful vision. If not, then surgical resection will be the treatment of choice. If useful vision is preserved, chemotherapy would be the preferred option for infants and very young children up to age 5 and for patients of all ages with NF-1. Radiotherapy could be considered for older children. Overall, the prognosis is very good. Visual acuity remains stable or improves in the majority of cases following chemotherapy or radiotherapy. Long-term tumor control approaches 100% with either modality.[69]

Chiasmatic gliomas are tumors that involve the optic chiasm and sometimes one or both optic nerves as well. Patients typically present with loss of visual acuity and temporal field defects. On imaging, the tumors are usually relatively small and well circumscribed and enhance uniformly and brightly with contrast material, suggestive of pilocytic histology. Biopsy is usually not necessary.

A period of surveillance is appropriate initial management, particularly for patients with NF-1. For patients without NF-1, especially those who present before age 5, there is a high probability of early progression and the majority of patients will require treatment within a few months following diagnosis. Surgery is rarely an option for tumors in this location. As for optic nerve tumors, chemotherapy usually will be the treatment of choice for infants and young children and for patients with NF-1. Radiotherapy is reserved for salvage after chemotherapy and for definitive treatment of older children without NF-1, providing a reasonable expectation that vision will not deteriorate further and a probability of long-term progression-free survival in the 60% to 90% range.[68,70–73] Overall survival for patients with chiasmatic tumors is in the 90% to 100% range.

Posterior, or chiasmatic/hypothalamic, gliomas account for approximately 70% of all optic pathway gliomas in children. They are typically rather large lesions that probably arise in the optic chiasm and extend to involve the hypothalamus. They may extend posteriorly along the optic tracts as well. They often fill the third ventricle, eventually causing hydrocephalus. Early findings consist of nystagmus, impaired visual acuity, and visual field deficits; only later do patients present increasing head circumference and/or symptoms and signs of raised intracranial pressure.

Treatment consists of CSF diversion, if necessary, and surgical resection, particularly if tumor is growing exophytically into the basal cistern because this may provide rapid relief of symptoms. In most patients, however, resection will be incomplete. As for LGAs at other locations, a period of surveillance following surgery is reasonable, although most patients will require adjuvant therapy.[44,69] The treatment of choice for children younger than 5 and those with NF-1 usually will be chemotherapy. Progression-free survival at 3 to 5 years is rather low at 20% to at best 60%.[44–46,74] However, some patients will never need further treatment, and for those who do, the use of chemotherapy allows radiotherapy to be deferred by a median of 2 to 4+ years without jeopardizing overall survival.

The indications for radiotherapy are (a) progressive disease on chemotherapy for children younger than 10 and (b) progressive disease at diagnosis or after surgery for older patients. Radiotherapy in this situation, given to local fields to a dose of 45 to 50 Gy for younger children and of 50 to 54 Gy for those older than 5, results in local tumor control in 70% to 80% of cases.[44,69,73,75,76] Overall, however, outcomes are less satisfactory for this group of patients than for those with anterior tumors. Long-term survival is in the 50% to 80% range, and many patients will be left with significant neuroendocrine and neuropsychologic sequelae. Patients with NF-1 are particularly at risk. They may have subnormal IQ even without chemotherapy and/or radiotherapy.[77] They are also at greater risk for moyamoya syndrome, a progressive vaso-occlusive process involving the circle of Willis. This may be seen without radiotherapy, but when radiotherapy is used in patients with NF-1 it is important to include MR angiography as part of the regular follow-up imaging protocol and intervene surgically if necessary to avoid a cerebrovascular accident.

Brainstem Gliomas

Tumors arising in the midbrain, pons, and medulla oblongata account for 10% to 15% of all CNS tumors in the pediatric age group. They are of several distinct types that can be broadly grouped as the more favorable low-grade focal, dorsal exophytic, and cervicomedullary tumors and the much more aggressive diffuse intrinsic pontine tumors.[78,79,80]

Focal tumors by definition are tumors of limited size (<2 cm) that on MRI are well circumscribed, without evidence of infiltration, and without edema. They may be cystic, and, as with cystic tumors at other sites, the cystic component may be large relative to the solid, biologically active, component. Focal tumors may occur at any level in the brainstem but most frequently are seen in the midbrain and medulla. They usually present with a long history of localizing findings such as an isolated cranial nerve deficit and a contralateral hemiparesis. Signs and symptoms of raised intracranial pressure are uncommon except in patients with tumors arising in the tectal region that may cause aqueduct stenosis while still small.

The management depends on the location of the tumor in the brainstem and the specific imaging characteristics of the tumor. As noted previously, patients with nonenhancing focal tumors in the tectal region who present with only hydrocephalus may do well without any treatment other than CSF diversionary procedures, usually endoscopic third ventriculostomy. Active intervention, including biopsy, is reserved for patients with clinical and radiologic evidence of progressive tumor. This is important because surgery for tumors in this location is associated with a substantial risk of morbidity even with modern techniques.

Surgery is the treatment of choice for focal tumors at other locations that are surgically accessible (meaning that they extend either toward the surface of the brainstem laterally or at the floor of the fourth ventricle) and have imaging characteristics suggestive of low-grade histology. In this regard, uniform bright enhancement with contrast material, which correlates with pilocytic histology, and the absence of peritumoral hypodensity are of particular importance. In experienced hands, the risk of morbidity for well-selected patients is low and, as with completely or subtotally resected LGAs at other sites, results may be excellent with freedom from progression in a majority of cases.[81,82] Outcomes are less satisfactory for patients with bulky tumors and for patients with tumors in the medulla with lower cranial nerve deficits who are at risk of developing postoperative feeding and/or breathing difficulties.

There are several treatment options for patients with surgically inaccessible focal lesions. By extrapolation from series reporting results of treatment using conventional radiotherapy in brainstem tumors in which outcome correlates with location (pons vs. other), imaging appearance (tumor volume, density on CT, enhancement pattern), and histology (malignant vs. benign), it is reasonable to assume that 50% to 70% of focal lesions may be permanently controlled with such treatment. Similar results have been obtained in small numbers of patients treated with HFRT and with interstitial irradiation using ^{125}I.[49,51,53] There is also some experience with the use of radiosurgery. However, standard treatment is as for LGAs at other locations, that is, external-beam radiotherapy using a margin for the CTV of 0.5 cm, to a total dose on the order of 54 Gy given over 6 weeks. The risks of HFRT, radiosurgery, or stereotactic irradiation with large fraction sizes, or interstitial irradiation in inexperienced hands cannot be justified in the absence of any established superiority.

Dorsal exophytic tumors arise from the floor of the fourth ventricle. They are usually large, filling the fourth ventricle, but do not invade the brainstem to any significant extent. They present insidiously with failure to thrive in younger children and symptoms and signs of raised intracranial pressure in older patients. Cranial nerve deficits are seen in about half of the patients. On MRI, they are sharply delineated from surrounding structures. They are hypointense on T1-weighted images, are hyperintense on T2-weighted images, and enhance uniformly and brightly after gadolinium injection. Most are pilocytic astrocytomas.

Surgery is the treatment of choice for dorsal exophytic tumors. Intraoperative image guidance is essential to achieve a maximal degree of tumor resection. However, because there is usually no definite tumor–brainstem interface, even an optimal resection will leave a thin layer of tumor on the floor of the fourth ventricle. Nonetheless, the majority of children do well following surgery and routine postoperative adjuvant therapy is not indicated. Radiotherapy should be considered for the rare patient who is found to have a high-grade lesion or for patients with low-grade tumors who develop progressive disease in the early (<9 months) postoperative period. For patients whose tumors recur later, further surgery should be considered and radiotherapy reserved for those with inoperable disease. The radiotherapy volume and dose should be similar to those used for LGAs in other locations. The literature suggests that salvage is possible in the majority of cases and overall the prognosis for patients with dorsal exophytic tumors is excellent.[83–85]

Cervicomedullary tumors arise in the upper cervical cord and grow rostrally beyond the foramen magnum. Most are low-grade lesions whose axial growth is limited by the pyramidal decussations located ventrally at the junction of the cervical cord and medulla. At this point, the tumor grows posteriorly, causing a bulge in the dorsal aspect of the medulla, toward the fourth ventricle.[78] These tumors typically present with lower cranial nerve deficits, sleep apnea and feeding difficulties in younger children, long tract signs, and sometimes torticollis. Hydrocephalus is unusual.

Surgery is the treatment of choice. Gross total resection may be achieved in 70% to 80% of cases and subtotal removal in most of the remainder. The probability of long-term tumor control after such treatment appears to be excellent for the typical low-grade lesion. There is, therefore, no indication for routine postoperative radiotherapy for these patients.

Diffuse intrinsic pontine tumors (DIPGs) account for 70% to 80% of all brainstem tumors. They arise in the pons and cause diffuse enlargement of the brainstem. Extension to the midbrain and medulla and/or exophytic growth is seen in at least two-thirds of cases. In contrast to the other types of brainstem tumors, the majority of DIPGs are fibrillary astrocytomas with a propensity for malignant change and a very poor prognosis.

DIPGs typically present with a short duration of symptoms consisting of multiple, bilateral, cranial nerve deficits (especially VI and VII) as well as long tract signs and ataxia. About 10% of patients have hydrocephalus at diagnosis. On CT, DIPGs are isodense or hypodense, with little enhancement after contrast injection, similar to diffuse fibrillary astrocytomas at other sites. They are best seen on T2-weighted or FLAIR MRI. The presence of ring enhancement is suggestive of high-grade histology.

Surgery has no role in the management of patients with DIPGs. Outside a clinical trial, even biopsy, a relatively nonmorbid procedure now, is considered unnecessary because in the context of a typical clinical presentation, the MRI findings are characteristic and histology does not influence treatment.[86,87] Treated with conventional radiotherapy, the majority (70% or more) of patients with DIPGs will improve clinically. However, the progression-free interval is short (median <6 months) and survival is poor, with a median survival of <1 year and survival rates at 2 years <20%.

So far all attempts to improve the outcome for children with DIPGs have proved futile. HFRT was tested in a series of phase I/II studies using doses ranging from 64.8 to 78 Gy. Time to progression and overall survival were not improved in comparison with conventional radiotherapy.[88,89] Moreover, at the higher doses of HFRT of 75.6 Gy and 78 Gy, morbidity was considerable. This included steroid dependency, vascular events, and white matter changes outside the radiation field, as well as hearing loss, hormone deficiencies, and late-developing seizure disorders in the small number of long-term survivors.[88,90–92] Accelerated and hypofractionated radiotherapy regimens have also been tested in single-institution studies using, respectively, a total dose of 50.4 Gy given in 28 twice-daily fractions of 1.8 Gy over 3 weeks[93] and 39 Gy in 13 daily fractions and 45 Gy in 15 daily fractions.[94,95] Progression-free and overall survival rates were similar to those seen in the HFRT studies.

Alternative approaches that use chemotherapy in combination with radiotherapy also have been disappointing. None of the many single-agent and multiagent regimens that have been tested in this patient population have been shown to provide a survival advantage compared with radiotherapy alone. New agents and novel chemotherapy–radiotherapy combinations are under investigation by the pediatric cooperative groups in North America and Europe.

Currently, standard treatment for DIPGs consists of radiotherapy given to the GTV as usually best demonstrated on T2-weighted or FLAIR MRI with a margin for the CTV of 1 to 1.5 cm to a dose of 54 Gy given in 30 daily fractions over 6 weeks that because of the initial rapid progression of neurologic deficit treatment often needs to be started on a semi-urgent basis. Because no unexpected toxicity was seen with the hypofractionated regimens, these in some cases could be considered an alternative to conventional radiotherapy that reduces the burden of treatment for the child and family.

Improvement in clinical status is usually evident as early as 2 to 3 weeks into treatment and steroids, if used, usually can be discontinued at that point. This improvement is often impressive and well appreciated by the family, despite being of only short duration. Treatment at time of progression may include experimental chemotherapy regimens or supportive care, or even retreatment with radiotherapy in selected cases.[96,97]

Astrocytoma of the Spinal Cord

Intramedullary spinal cord tumors account for 3% to 6% of all CNS tumors in the pediatric age group. About 60% are astrocytomas, the majority of which are LGAs; 30% are ependymomas; and the remainder, gangliogliomas and developmental tumors such as teratomas, lipomas, and dermoid and epidermoid cysts.

Patients typically present with pain and motor deficits, often of long duration. Rapid progression of symptoms and signs is suggestive of high-grade histology. On imaging, astrocytomas most often are seen to comprise a solid component and one or more cysts that may be intratumoral and/or extend rostrally and caudally beyond the solid component. Most enhance heterogeneously with the use of contrast material. Ependymomas, in contrast, only rarely harbor intratumoral cysts (although they may have an associated syrinx) and usually enhance homogeneously.

The management of spinal cord tumors has changed over recent years.[98] In the past, patients typically were treated with biopsy followed by radiotherapy, and there is evidence to suggest that this is effective treatment in more than half of children with LGAs.[99] However, improvements in surgery and the routine use of surgical adjuncts such as ultrasonic aspiration and support systems such as intraoperative ultrasonography and sensory and more recently motor evoked potential monitoring improve the safety and completeness of resection so that complete or subtotal resection is now possible in approximately 80% of children with pilocytic astrocytoma (the majority), especially those with a syrinx. Resection is more difficult and less likely to be complete in patients with grade II astrocytoma because of the more infiltrative nature of these tumors and the absence of a clear interface.[98] Because outcome following complete or subtotal resection for LGAs is very good, with long-term progression-free survival in the 70% to 90% range,[100–102] routine postoperative adjuvant therapy is not indicated. For children in whom complete or subtotal resection is not possible, the options will be as for patients with LGAs in other locations, that is, early second surgery if feasible, or close follow-up with second surgery and/or radiotherapy at the time of progression. As for LGAs in other locations, chemotherapy may be an alternative to radiotherapy for young children.[103,104] The benefit of surgical resection in HGAs is less clear and the more usual approach is biopsy followed by postoperative radiotherapy.[105]

The radiotherapy target volume for LGAs consists of the solid portion of the tumor (including intratumoral cysts) with a margin for the CTV of 1 to 1.5 cm. The usual dose is 50.4 Gy given in 28 daily fractions over approximately 6 weeks. The CTV should be larger for patients with HGAs for whom a margin beyond the entire lesion of at least 1.5 cm (or one vertebral body) would be more appropriate. The dose usually will be as for LGA because of the substantial risk of morbidity at higher doses but often chemotherapy will be given as well. While older studies[99,100] and data from the Surveillance, Epidemiology, and End Results (SEER) registry[106] and from the German cooperative group[107] all suggest that 20% to 35% of children with high-grade gliomas will survive following such treatment, a recent study from St. Jude Children's Research Hospital presents an even bleaker picture with a very high rate of both local progression and leptomeningeal spread and no long-term survivors among patients with GBM.[105]

EPENDYMAL TUMORS

The following types are seen in children:

- Myxopapillary ependymoma (WHO grade I)
- Ependymoma (WHO grade II)
- Anaplastic ependymoma (WHO grade III)

Myxopapillary Ependymoma

Myxopapillary ependymomas are slowly growing lesions almost always located in the conus filum terminale region of the spinal cord. They are the most common spinal cord tumor in this location. They usually present with back pain. On imaging, myxopapillary ependymomas are well circumscribed and usually enhance brightly after contrast injection. Despite their low-grade histology, leptomeningeal spread is not uncommon even at diagnosis and all patients should have an MRI of the whole spine and brain as part of their initial workup.

Surgical resection is the treatment of choice. If the tumor is contained within the filum, complete resection may be possible after mobilization of the filum. Whether postoperative radiotherapy is necessary after complete resection is unclear. A significant proportion of tumors recur locally and/or with leptomeningeal metastases, but salvage with further surgery and/or with radiotherapy seems to be possible in most.[108–110] If the tumor is in continuity with the conus, resection is more difficult and more likely to result in significant sequelae so that there frequently will be residual tumor. If the tumor is not resected en bloc or if there is macroscopic residual tumor, the risk of recurrence is high. Postoperative radiotherapy in this situation results in improved local control.[101,111–113] The radiotherapy target volume is local (macroscopic disease plus a margin cephalad and caudad of 1.5 cm [or one vertebral body]) for the CTV and the dose, 50.4 Gy.[113] Patients with leptomeningeal seeding at diagnosis or at relapse after surgery alone should be treated with curative intent with CSI followed by a boost to the primary site with a reasonable expectation of long-term tumor control.[101,109,112,114]

Ependymoma

Ependymoma is the third most common CNS tumor in children. About half of all cases arise in children younger than 5. Ependymoma can occur at any site in the ventricular system or in the spinal canal, but in children approximately two-thirds arise in the ependymal lining of the fourth ventricle. Tumors in this location typically present with symptoms and signs of raised intracranial pressure. On imaging the tumor is usually large but relatively well circumscribed, with displacement rather than invasion of adjacent structures. Extension through the foramen magnum into the upper cervical region is not uncommon (Fig. 84.10). Tumors that arise in the supratentorial compartment, some of which arise outside the ventricular system, present with focal neurologic deficits. Intramedullary ependymomas, which account for approximately 30% of all spinal cord tumors arising in childhood, usually present initially with dysesthesia and sensory deficits due to their central location in the cord and only later with pain and motor deficits.

Spread of ependymoma is primarily local. However, 5% to 10% of patients have leptomeningeal seeding at diagnosis, and gadolinium-enhanced MRI of the whole CNS and CSF cytology are essential components of the workup for all patients.

Management of Ependymoma

The completeness of the surgical resection is the factor that has the greatest impact on the outcome of patients with ependymoma.[115–123,124] Currently, it is estimated that complete resection is achieved in 70% to 90% of supratentorial ependymomas and in a similar percentage of spinal ependymomas. Complete resection is less frequently possible in patients with infratentorial ependymomas. Most commonly, residual tumor is left behind on the floor of the fourth ventricle or laterally at the cerebellopontine angle where tumor protruding through the foramen of Luschka encircles lower cranial nerves and vessels. "Second-look" surgery may be considered, if feasible, either after the realignment of structures that takes place following resection of an initially bulky tumor in an often unstable young child or after chemotherapy.

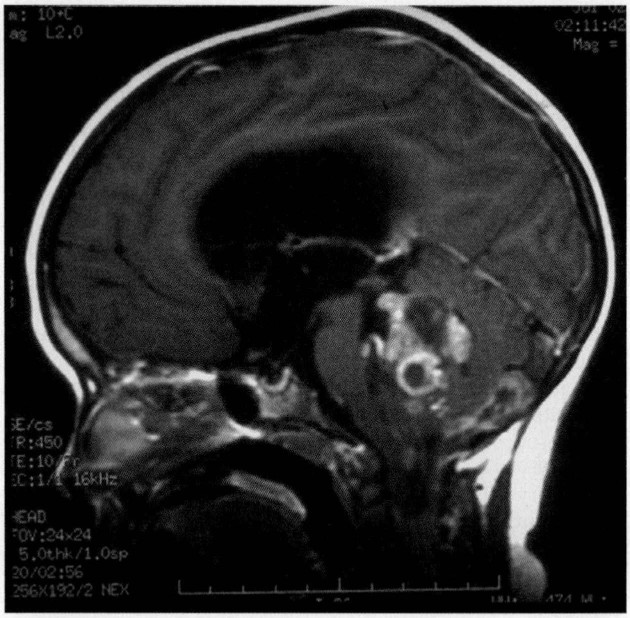

FIGURE 84.10. Typical appearance of an ependymoma that fills the fourth ventricle causing hydrocephalus and extends inferiorly below the foramen magnum over the dorsal aspect of the spinal cord to the level of C4.

Postoperative radiotherapy is the standard of care for all children with ependymoma. Some have questioned the need for such treatment for patients who have undergone complete resection.[121,125,126] However, a number of studies including studies in young children in which the goal was to delay or avoid altogether radiotherapy suggest that such a strategy results in worse disease-free and overall survival and in the long term greater morbidity[122,127–130] and therefore can be considered acceptable only for (a) patients with ependymoma of the spinal cord who have undergone complete resection for whom disease-free survival in contemporary series approaches 100%[131–134] and (b) selected patients with supratentorial ependymoma, such as those with intraventricular tumors or with extraventricular tumors that are solid and located in noneloquent areas and can be resected with a wider margin.[126]

Radiotherapy Target Volume

In the past, CSI was recommended for treatment of infratentorial ependymoma. However, there is no evidence that the use of CSI affects outcome, and local radiotherapy is now accepted as the standard of care.[135,136] The GTV is a composite of the tumor bed, including any extension caudal to the foramen magnum and taking into account any anatomic shifts due to surgery plus any residual tumor. In the St. Jude prospective study of conformal radiotherapy that included both ependymoma and anaplastic ependymoma, the margin for the CTV was 1 cm.[124] In the subset of 107 patients in that study that received immediate postoperative radiotherapy, local control was excellent (cumulative incidence of local failure 7.8%) for patients who had undergone gross total resection, while patients who had undergone near-total or subtotal resection fared less well. All failures were reported to be within the 95% isodose. The current Children's Oncology Group (COG) study uses an even smaller margin for the CTV of 0.5 cm.

Radiotherapy Dose

There is evidence for a dose–response in ependymoma, with improved tumor control with doses >45 to 50 and even 54 Gy.[135] Although the lower doses may be the maximum possible for spinal ependymomas, the current standard is a dose of at least 54 Gy for children older than 18 months with infra- or supratentorial tumors. Moreover, because failure most often

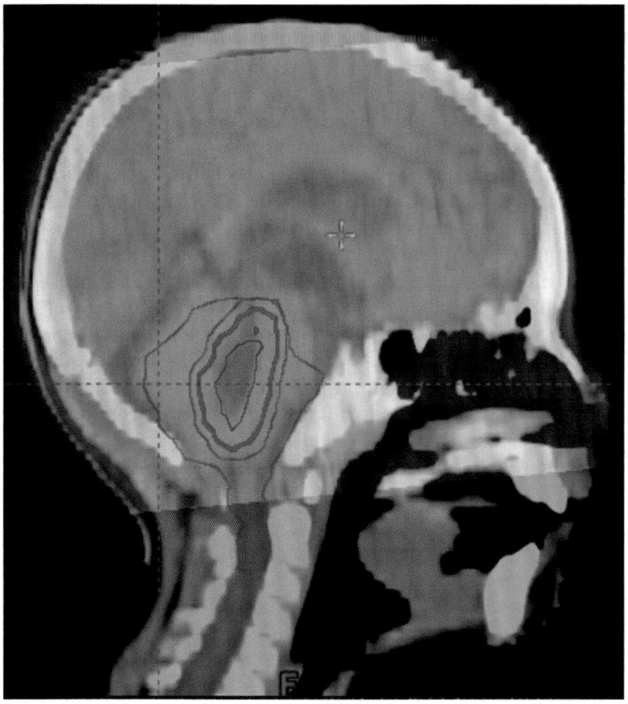

FIGURE 84.11. Care is necessary to ensure that the inferior extent of disease is included in the radiotherapy target volume. Volume reduction at 54 Gy is necessary to respect the tolerance of the spinal cord.

occurs at the site of macroscopic residual disease, even higher doses may be desirable and most would reduce the CTV at 54 Gy to respect the tolerance of the spinal cord and/or other structures and continue to a total dose of 59.4 Gy (Fig. 84.11).

HFRT has been explored in ependymoma as a strategy to more safely deliver these higher radiotherapy doses. Studies from the Children's Hospital of Philadelphia in which the majority of patients received HFRT to a mean dose of 70.7 Gy,[137] from the Italian pediatric oncology group that used a dose of 70.4 Gy,[138] and from the French pediatric oncology group that used a lower total dose of 60 Gy in 60 fractions[139] all reported HFRT to be feasible. However, in none of these studies was there any clear evidence of benefit, particularly in the context of improved surgery and modern radiotherapy.

The role of chemotherapy in ependymoma remains to be defined. There is some evidence of efficacy, but even in the more recent infant studies in which chemotherapy was used because of the desire to delay or even avoid altogether radiotherapy, more than half of the patients progressed on chemotherapy,[63,128,130,140,141] and in the COG baby study, prolonged use of chemotherapy and a delay to radiotherapy of more than 1 year was associated with a worse survival.[127] Consequently, most would now use radiotherapy for all children older than 12 months following complete resection. In patients with residual disease, chemotherapy has been justified because of the poor prognosis. As well, it may facilitate complete resection of residual disease at second-look surgery, and current North American and European trials are testing chemotherapy in this setting.

Reirradiation for Ependymoma

For patients who fail standard treatment with either local recurrence or, less frequently, leptomeningeal dissemination, retreatment with radiotherapy is an option that may result in durable control in a proportion of patients.[142,143]

Anaplastic Ependymoma

By definition, an anaplastic ependymoma is a malignant glioma of ependymal differentiation that is characterized by high mitotic activity, often accompanied by microvascular proliferation and pseudopalisading necrosis. There are no histopathologic features that can reliably differentiate anaplastic ependymomas from the more slowly growing and more favorable ependymomas, which probably explains the controversy in the literature with respect to the prognostic significance of tumor grade. Proliferation markers may be more useful in this regard, but several groups also are investigating genetic and expression profiles based on preliminary data that suggest that a molecular classification system can be built that will prove useful for risk stratification.

Management of anaplastic ependymoma begins with maximum surgical resection consistent with a good neurologic outcome and a workup consisting of a gadolinium-enhanced MRI of the spinal axis and CSF cytology to rule out leptomeningeal seeding, which is only slightly more frequent than in ependymoma. Postoperatively all patients receive radiotherapy. As for ependymoma, the role of chemotherapy remains to be defined but may be an option in very young children to delay the use of radiotherapy.

CSI was previously the standard of care for anaplastic ependymoma, but several institutional studies, a careful retrospective review, and prospective studies by the POG all suggest that there is no survival advantage for CSI.[116,144–148] Thus, a target volume consisting of the tumor bed and any macroscopic residual disease with a margin for the CTV of 1 cm is used for patients with localized disease and only patients with leptomeningeal seeding at diagnosis receive CSI. As for ependymoma, the dose should be at least 54 to 55 Gy and, if feasible, 59 to 60 Gy.

In contemporary series, disease-free survival for patients with anaplastic ependymoma is typically still only in the 30% to 45% range at 3 to 5 years,[138,148] although results were better in the St. Jude series, with event-free survival at 7 years of 61.3% and overall survival, 71.8%.[124] This may be in part at least due to the high rate of gross total resection in that series because, as others have shown, the prognosis is better for patients in whom complete resection has been achieved than for those with residual disease.[147,148] Patients with leptomeningeal dissemination at diagnosis fare poorly despite intensive treatment that includes CSI and chemotherapy.

CHOROID PLEXUS TUMORS

Choroid plexus tumors arise from the epithelium of the choroid plexus of the cerebral ventricles. They include:

- Choroid plexus papilloma (WHO grade I)
- Atypical choroid plexus papilloma (WHO grade II)
- Choroid plexus carcinoma (WHO grade III)

Choroid plexus tumors account for only 2% to 4% of all brain tumors that occur in children but as many as 10% to 20% of those seen in the first year of life. Choroid plexus papillomas (CPPs), which account for more than half of choroid plexus tumors in children, are composed of delicate fibrovascular connective tissue fronds covered by a single layer of uniform cuboidal columnar epithelial cells with round or oval basally situated monomorphic nuclei. Mitotic activity is low and increased mitotic activity in a CPP defines an atypical choroid plexus papilloma. In contrast to both, choroid plexus carcinomas (CPCs) are solid tumors that tend to transgress the ventricular wall and invade the brain. Histologically CPCs show frank evidence of malignancy including frequent mitoses (>5%/10 HPF), increased cellular density, nuclear pleomorphism, blurring of the papillary pattern with poorly structured sheets of tumor cells, and necrotic areas.

In children, most choroid plexus tumors arise in the lateral ventricles causing obstruction to CSF flow. Infants commonly present with increasing head circumference and older children with symptoms and signs of raised intracranial pressure. On neuroimaging, choroid plexus tumors are usually hyperdense, contrast-enhancing masses. Even papillomas seed into the CSF space and workup for both benign and malignant lesions should include a gadolinium-enhanced MRI of the spinal axis and CSF cytology.

Management of Choroid Plexus Tumors

Surgery is the treatment of choice for CPPs both for the primary lesion and for metastatic deposits, if feasible. Complete resection is achieved in a high percentage of cases now and outcome in this situation is excellent. Less than 10% of tumors recur and overall survival is close to 100%.[149–152] The role of radiotherapy following incomplete resection is unclear, but because not all patients will progress, follow-up without adjuvant treatment would be the usual strategy, with consideration of further surgery, if feasible, and/or radiotherapy only at the time of progression.

Results are less satisfactory for patients with CPCs. Surgery is an important component of treatment but often difficult. Blood loss may be considerable and staged procedures may be necessary to obtain maximal resection. In most series, results are better for patients who have undergone complete resection[149,153–161,162] and the need for adjuvant therapy in this situation is not clearly established. In one series of pooled data, survival was significantly better when radiotherapy had been given postoperatively despite a probable bias toward the use of radiotherapy in patients considered to have more unfavorable disease.[156,159] Others have reported excellent results following complete resection, in some cases with chemotherapy but without radiotherapy.[153,154,157,158] In contrast, patients who have residual disease fare very poorly. Postoperative radiotherapy appears to be useful,[162] but the desire to avoid radiotherapy in infants and very young children may mean that chemotherapy is used instead despite less convincing evidence of efficacy. When both are used, radiotherapy is usually delivered early (following two cycles of chemotherapy) with the exception of infants and very young children in whom radiotherapy is delayed until age 3 years. Genetic and genomic analyses may in the future help guide therapy. A substantial percentage of patients with CPCs have TP53 mutations, and patients without such mutations are reported to have a more favorable prognosis and be successfully treated without radiotherapy.[163]

The radiotherapy target volume is also controversial. CSI was traditionally used in patients with CPCs, and a recent literature review showed that the use of CSI was associated with improved progression-free survival as compared with radiotherapy to the whole brain or tumor bed only.[162] Importantly, more than half of all failures occurred outside the treatment field. This is problematic given the young age of the patients, and a pragmatic approach in which local fields are used for patients with CPPs with postoperative residual (including metastatic sites) as well as for patients with atypical CPPs or CPCs without evidence of leptomeningeal seeding and only patients with atypical CPPs or CPCs with leptomeningeal seeding receive CSI would seem reasonable for now.

NEURONAL AND MIXED NEURONAL-GLIAL TUMORS

These are uncommon tumors that are characterized by the presence of both neuronal and glial elements in variable amounts. They include entities such as desmoplastic infantile astrocytoma and dysembryoplastic neuroepithelial tumor. Most will be cured by surgery, but radiotherapy may be indicated in two tumor types:

- Ganglioglioma and anaplastic ganglioglioma
- Central neurocytoma

Ganglioglioma and Anaplastic Ganglioglioma

Gangliogliomas are well-differentiated slowly growing tumors composed of mature ganglion cells in combination with neoplastic glial cells (WHO grade I or II). Tumors in which the glial component shows anaplastic features (WHO grade III) are called anaplastic gangliogliomas.

Although these tumors can arise anywhere within the CNS, most in children arise in the temporal region and typically present with seizures. Surgery is the treatment of choice. When resection is complete, the probability of long-term tumor control in patients with ganglioglioma is excellent.[164–166] The indications for radiotherapy are as for patients with LGAs, that is, for patients with progressive or recurrent disease that is not resectable, and the radiotherapy target volume and dose likewise. The significance of a high proliferation index or of the presence of anaplasia in patients with ganglioglioma is controversial. Although it seems clear that the risk of recurrence is higher in patients with these features,[164,165,167] the indications for postoperative radiotherapy remain undefined except for patients with anaplastic gangliogliomas who have undergone less than complete resection in whom the use of radiotherapy has been shown to result in improved progression-free survival.[166,168]

Central Neurocytoma

This is a neoplasm composed of uniform round cells with neuronal differentiation that arises in the lateral or third ventricles, typically the former, that is seen predominantly in adolescents and young adults. Patients usually present with symptoms and signs of raised intracranial pressure. Surgery is the treatment of choice, and when complete resection is achieved long-term tumor control is excellent without adjuvant treatment.[169] Patients in whom complete resection cannot be achieved as well as those with tumors with atypical histology or a high mitotic rate fare less well,[169,170] and postoperative radiotherapy should be considered in these situations. While a dose of 50 Gy appears adequate for patients with typical neurocytomas,[171] there is evidence of improved tumor control at doses of at least 54 Gy in patients with atypical neurocytoma.[172]

PINEAL PARENCHYMAL TUMORS

Pineal region tumors account for 2% to 8% of intracranial tumors in children. Approximately half are germ cell tumors, one-fourth to one-third are pineal parenchymal tumors, and most of the remainder are astrocytic tumors. Pineal parenchymal tumors are derived from pineocytoma, which are cells with photosensory and neuroendocrine functions, or their embryonal precursors. According to the WHO classification, the following entities can be distinguished:

- Pineocytoma (WHO grade I)
- Pineal parenchymal tumor of intermediate differentiation
- Pineoblastoma (WHO grade IV)

Pineocytoma

Pineocytoma is a slow-growing tumor composed of small uniform mature cells resembling pineocytes, with occasional large pineocytomatous rosettes, that accounts for approximately half of pineal parenchymal tumors and in childhood most commonly occurs in the teenage years. Patients typically present with symptoms and signs of raised intracranial pressure. Some will have symptoms of upper mesencephalic tegmental dysfunction (Parinaud's syndrome), consisting of limitation of upward gaze, lid retraction, retraction nystagmus, and pupils that react more poorly to light than to accommodation. On MRI, pineocytomas are usually spherical, well-circumscribed masses, hypointense on T1 and hyperintense on T2 weighted images, with homogeneous contrast enhancement. Leptomeningeal spread has been described in pineocytoma,[173] but it is probable that the explanation for this lies in sampling error. With better imaging and more extensive surgery with more complete histologic evaluation of the tumor, it seems that leptomeningeal spread can be considered to be an uncommon event.[174]

Treatment consists of surgical resection via an occipital transtentorial or an infratentorial supracerebellar approach using modern operative adjuncts such as functional MRI and MR tractography in relation to the location of the primary visual cortex and deep MR venography. If complete or subtotal resection is accomplished, progression-free survival is in the 90% to 100% range.[175,176] Patients who undergo lesser degrees of resection or only biopsy fare less well and, although some have questioned its usefulness based on the results of a systematic review,[176] postoperative radiotherapy usually is recommended.[177] The target volume is local, consisting of macroscopic residual disease with a margin for the CTV of 1 cm, and the dose, 50 to 55 Gy over 6 weeks.

Pineal Parenchymal Tumor of Intermediate Differentiation

Pineal parenchymal tumors of intermediate differentiation are composed of diffuse sheets or large lobules of uniform cells with mild to moderate nuclear atypia and low to moderate mitotic activity. They are rare tumors, accounting for only 10% of pineal parenchymal tumors, and optimal management remains to be defined. In one series, three patients treated with surgery alone survived free of disease.[175] At the other extreme, another group considers these to be tumors "with seeding potential" and recommends postoperative treatment with CSI as for pineoblastoma.[174]

Pineoblastoma

Pineoblastoma is a highly malignant tumor composed of patternless sheets of densely packed small cells with round to irregular nuclei and scant cytoplasm.

Pineoblastomas most frequently affect infants and very young children, who typically present with an enlarged head circumference or symptoms and signs of short duration of raised intracranial pressure. On MRI, pineoblastomas are usually multilobulated and often enhance heterogeneously, with areas of necrosis and/or hemorrhage. Infiltration of surrounding structures is common. Leptomeningeal spread is seen in as many as 50% of patients at diagnosis.

Surgery for lesions in the pineal region is difficult and complete resection is often not possible. Postoperatively, children older than 3 are treated with CSI and chemotherapy, as for high-risk medulloblastoma and supratentorial PNETs (see later). Five-year survival in this age group is in the 50% to 70% range.[174,178,179] However, infants treated with chemotherapy without radiotherapy fare extremely poorly: in prospective studies of the POG and CCG, all tumors recurred within the first 11 months (POG) and 1.2 years (CCG) and all patients died of disease.[180,181] Thus, more aggressive treatment that includes chemotherapy dose intensification is necessary. Patients with familial bilateral retinoblastoma with pineoblastoma ("trilateral retinoblastoma") also have an extremely poor prognosis, most dying within a year following diagnosis.

EMBRYONAL TUMORS

Embryonal tumors as a group are the second most common type of CNS tumor in the pediatric age group. They include:

- Medulloblastoma
  - –Desmoplastic/nodular medulloblastoma
  - –Medulloblastoma with extensive nodularity
  - –Anaplastic medulloblastoma
  - –Large cell medulloblastoma
- Supratentorial PNET
  - –CNS neuroblastoma
  - –Medulloepithelioma
  - –Ependymoblastoma
- Atypical teratoid/rhabdoid tumor

Medulloblastoma

Medulloblastoma accounts for 15% to 20% of all CNS tumors in children with a median age at presentation of 6 years. It is a malignant invasive embryonal tumor of the cerebellum with predominantly neuronal differentiation and an inherent tendency to metastasize via CSF pathways. In the majority of cases the tumor arises in the cerebellar vermis and projects into the fourth ventricle. Patients typically present with symptoms and signs of raised intracranial pressure (i.e., headache and morning vomiting). On MRI medulloblastomas appear as solid masses that enhance usually fairly homogeneously with contrast material (Fig. 84.12). The frequency of leptomeningeal

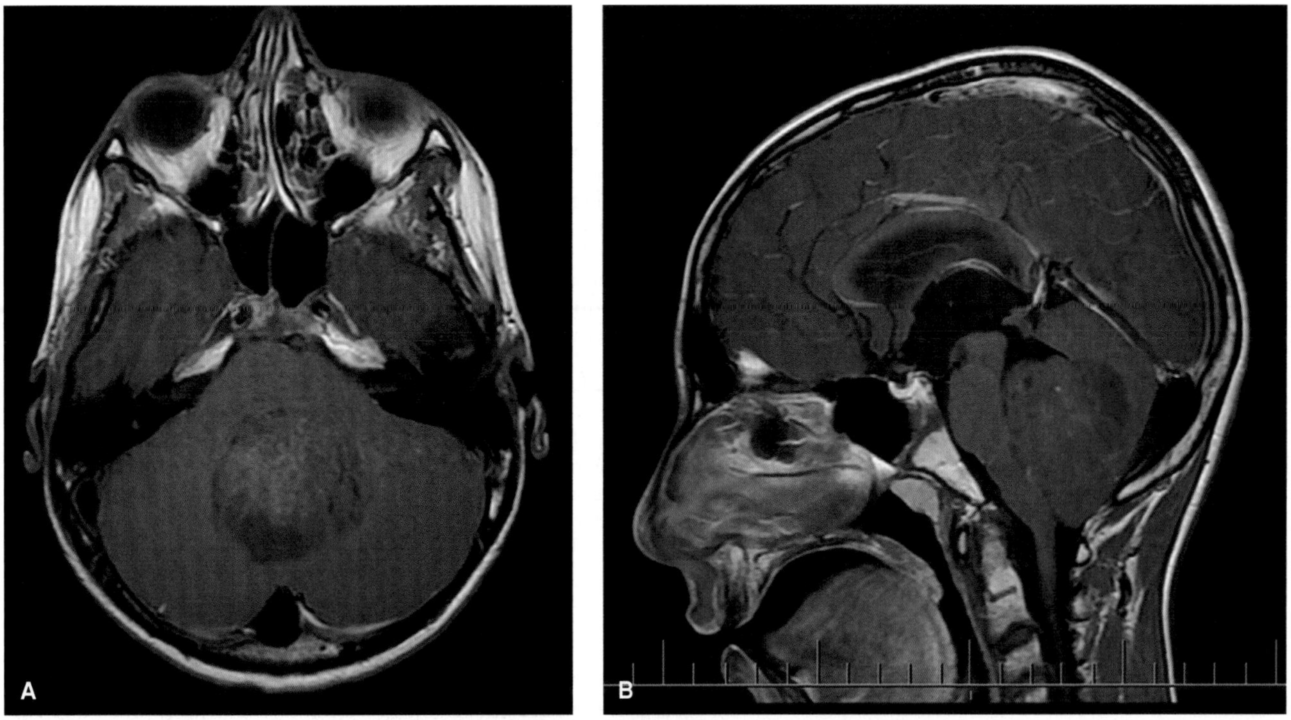

FIGURE 84.12. T1 axial **(A)** and T1 gadolinium-enhanced sagittal **(B)** magnetic resonance images of a medulloblastoma in an 11-year-old boy. Note the typical midline location of the tumor that is causing ventricular outlet obstruction with dilatation of the third and lateral ventricles.

seeding at diagnosis is approximately 30% to 35% and investigation at diagnosis must include a gadolinium-enhanced MRI of the spinal axis and CSF cytology. The former should be obtained whenever possible preoperatively or else at least 2 weeks postoperatively because of the artifactual changes that may be seen in the early postoperative period. CSF cytology, which should be obtained by lumbar puncture, usually cannot be obtained safely preoperatively because of the presence of raised intracranial pressure and more commonly is obtained at least 2 weeks postoperatively to avoid false positives that may be seen in the early postoperative period. Medulloblastoma is one of the few CNS tumors to spread outside the CNS (to lymph nodes, bone), but this is a very uncommon event at diagnosis and other studies such as a bone scan or bone marrow aspiration or biopsy are not justified as a routine.

Factors that correlate with outcome include age at diagnosis, the presence or absence of leptomeningeal spread at diagnosis, and the completeness of the surgical resection. Patients are allocated to one of two risk categories: standard and high risk. Those who have undergone complete or subtotal resection with <1.5 cm^2 of residual tumor on postoperative MRI performed within 48 to 72 hours of surgery and no evidence of CSF dissemination (M0) are considered to have standard-risk disease, whereas patients who have larger-volume residual tumor and those with evidence of CSF dissemination at diagnosis are characterized as high risk. With contemporary neurosurgical techniques, complete or near-total resection is accomplished in approximately 80% of cases. Overall, approximately two-thirds of patients will be standard risk and one-third will be high risk.

Management of Standard-Risk Medulloblastoma

Until the 1990s, the standard of care for patients older than 3 years with standard-risk disease consisted of postoperative radiotherapy to the craniospinal axis to a dose of 35 to 36 Gy followed by a boost to the whole posterior fossa to a total dose of 54 to 55.8 Gy. In multi-institution studies, such treatment results in long-term event-free survival in 60% to 65% of patients.[10,182,183] Sequelae of treatment include hormonal deficits, decreased bone growth, and neurocognitive deficits that correlate with the age of the child and the radiation dose.[7]

Several treatment strategies designed to reduce the morbidity associated with the use of radiotherapy have been tested. An attempt by the French Cooperative Group (SFOP) to reduce the radiotherapy target volume to avoid supratentorial radiation produced disastrous results,[184] and CSI remains the standard of care. The use of reduced-dose CSI (23.4 Gy) alone (without chemotherapy) in the North American intergroup study (CCG-923/POG#8631) resulted in a significantly increased risk of isolated neuraxis failure and an event-free survival at 5 and 8 years of only 52%.[183] HFRT may be a more promising strategy. In an SFOP pilot study that tested HFRT to a CSI dose of 36 Gy without chemotherapy, early toxicity was reduced and progression-free survival at 3 years was 81%.[185] The results of the European SIOP PNET-4 study in which patients were randomized to HFRT or conventional radiotherapy are pending.

An alternative strategy consists of reduced-dose CSI followed by a boost to the posterior fossa to a total dose of 55.8 Gy in combination with systemic chemotherapy. Progression-free survival was 79% at 5 years in a CCG pilot study that used CSI to a dose of 23.4 Gy in combination with weekly vincristine followed by adjuvant systemic chemotherapy consisting of vincristine 1.5 mg/m^2, CCNU 75 mg/m^2, and cisplatinum 75 mg/m^2.[186] In the joint CCG/POG phase III randomized study (A9961) that followed, this regimen was compared to a regimen in which the CCNU was replaced by cyclophosphamide. Event-free survival at 4 years was approximately 85% in both arms,[187] and such an approach is now considered to be the standard of care for children with standard-risk medulloblastoma in North America. The current COG study is testing the safety of an even lower dose of CSI (18 Gy) in children aged 3 to 8 years and of a reduced-volume posterior fossa boost in children of all ages.

In the next generation of studies in medulloblastoma, risk stratification will be based on biologic parameters in addition to clinical and pathologic features. Already, patients with anaplastic large cell histology are no longer included in the standard-risk group given their poorer outcome. As well, evidence now suggests that β-catenin nucleo-positivity is associated with a better prognosis and MYC gene amplification with a worse one, opening up the possibility of reduced-intensity treatment, even perhaps elimination of radiotherapy, in the former group, while maintaining or even increasing the intensity of treatment in the latter.[188]

Management of High-Risk Medulloblastoma

Patients with residual disease >1.5 cm^2 and/or those with leptomeningeal seeding are considered to have high-risk disease. This is the group of patients in which the use of chemotherapy was shown in the prospective randomized phase III studies conducted in the 1970s to result in significant improvement in disease-free survival. Research since then has largely focused on the chemotherapy regimens, including changes in scheduling in relation to radiotherapy and in doses and routes of delivery of chemotherapy. Some have used higher-dose CSI or altered radiotherapy fractionation schedules. An overview of studies performed by the North American and European cooperative groups up until the early 2000s is given in Freeman et al.[189]

It is important to note that the definition of risk factors has evolved considerably over the past two decades, making comparison of published data quite problematic. Better postoperative imaging and more complete staging as well as identification of unfavorable pathologic features (e.g., large cell and anaplastic histology) have led to transfer of patients from the standard-risk to the high-risk category, which may partly explain the improving results for both standard-risk and high-risk disease. The category of high-risk disease is heterogeneous and includes more favorable subsets such as patients with postoperative residual disease without leptomeningeal spread, and even those with M1 (cytology-positive) disease, for whom it may be appropriate to consider a treatment approach different from that for patients with M2/3 disease with nodular seeding. For example, for patients with residual disease, M0, it would be logical to consider using a boost to residual disease in the posterior fossa to a dose higher than the standard 55.8 Gy. Management of patients with M1 disease remains controversial, but the weight of evidence suggests that they should be treated similarly to those with M2/3 disease.[190] Results for patients with M2/3 disease remain quite poor, although an impressive 81% 4-year overall survival was reported for patients treated on a COG pilot study using carboplatin daily during radiotherapy as a radiosensitizer. This forms the backbone of the current COG study for high-risk medulloblastoma, while the standard of care in many centers in Europe is now a hyperfractionated accelerated radiotherapy (HART) regimen given in combination with pre- and postradiotherapy chemotherapy.[191]

Management of Medulloblastoma in Infants

Medulloblastoma accounts for 20% to 40% of all CNS tumors in infants. While up to half of infants have more favorable histologic types (desmoplastic/nodular or medulloblastoma with extensive nodularity), the prognosis overall is worse than in older children. The explanation for this is likely multifactorial. In addition to biology, the rate of complete resection is lower in this age group and the frequency of leptomeningeal seeding at diagnosis higher (as much as 50%), but also, many patients do not receive optimal treatment.[192] Because of the significant risks with respect to neurocognitive function associated with the use of radiotherapy in infants and very young children, chemotherapy has been used in an attempt to either delay or avoid radiotherapy altogether. Infants with M0 disease who have undergone total resection may do well with chemotherapy alone, with a 5-year overall survival of 69% in the first POG infant study[193] and of 93% in the German study,[194] although it is noteworthy that treatment in the latter included intraventricular methotrexate for which there are also concerns about the risk of neurocognitive sequelae. In other studies results were less satisfactory, in some because of the need for aggressive salvage regimens that were associated with significant long-term sequelae.[195] In fact, with the possible exception of very young children with desmoplastic/nodular medulloblastoma without residual disease, evidence suggests that radiotherapy is an important component of treatment,[62] and because recurrences are generally early (6 to 12 months) and local,[62,193,196] the recently completed North American study used early radiotherapy to a limited treatment volume consisting of the tumor bed plus an anatomically confined margin for the CTV of 1 cm for patients without leptomeningeal seeding. Infants with M2/3 disease generally are treated with intensive chemotherapy regimens. While patients with desmoplastic/nodular histology may do quite well, with an overall survival at 5 years of 52.9% in the UKCCSG/SIOP baby study, for example,[63] the prognosis for those with other subtypes is much less satisfactory. Despite this, the goal of treatment generally will still be to avoid radiotherapy (especially CSI) and the decision to use it highly individualized based on the clinical situation and the wishes of the parents.

Radiotherapy for Medulloblastoma

CSI is the standard of care, and careful attention to coverage of the entire target volume that includes the meninges overlying the brain and spine including extensions along nerve roots is critical. In the SFOP M-7 protocol, 50% of relapses could be correlated with targeting deviations. In the subsequent studies (MSFOP-93 and MSFOP-98) the relapse rate was 17% in patients who had inadequate coverage of only one part of the CTV (a typical example being the cribriform plate), 28% for patients who had inadequate coverage at two sites, and 67% for patients who had inadequate coverage at three or more sites.[197,198] In an SFOP pilot study that tested reduced-dose CSI for standard-risk disease, overall survival at 5 years was significantly worse for patients with inadequate coverage at two or more sites as compared with no or only one major deviation (54.4% vs. 79.3%).[199]

CSI is followed by a boost to the posterior fossa. Traditionally, the entire posterior fossa has been treated to a total dose of 54 to 55.8 Gy. Using conformal treatment techniques, it is possible to reduce the dose to the inner ear, which is important in children who will also be receiving chemotherapy with cisplatinum, but there will be little sparing of other structures such as, and most especially, supratentorial brain. Better sparing of the cochlea,[200] pituitary and hypothalamus, and the temporal lobes can be achieved using a reduced target volume for the boost (Fig. 84.13). Fukunaga-Johnson et al.[201] found a low risk of isolated failure outside the tumor bed in the posterior fossa in a cohort of 114 patients, and data from several other centers as well as an SFOP pilot study that used a conformal boost limited to the tumor bed similarly support such an approach.[185,202–205] The optimal CTV for a reduced-volume posterior fossa boost remains to be defined, although an anatomically confined expansion of 1.5 cm around the GTV (any macroscopic residual tumor and the surgical bed) seems to be reasonable and this is the volume under investigation in the current COG study for standard-risk disease.

Delay to radiotherapy may be associated with poorer outcomes, and CSI should ideally start within 28 to 30 days following surgery. There is evidence, too, that it is important to deliver radiotherapy in a timely fashion, avoiding unnecessary gaps in treatment resulting from machine servicing, holidays, and the like. In the SIOP PNET-3 study event-free and overall survival were significantly worse when the duration of treatment exceeded 50 days as compared with the results for children treated as planned over 45 to 47 days.[206] When CSI has to be interrupted, for example, because of hematologic toxicity, treatment should continue to the posterior fossa boost volume while waiting for the blood counts to recover. Granulocyte colony-stimulating factor may be used to hasten recovery of the counts.

Supratentorial Primitive Neuroectodermal Tumor

By definition, supratentorial primitive neuroectodermal tumor (stPNET) is an embryonal tumor composed of undifferentiated or poorly differentiated neuroepithelial cells. Tumors with only neuronal differentiation are termed cerebral neuroblastoma or ganglioneuroblastoma. Tumors that re-create features of neural tube formation are called medulloepithelioma. Tumors with ependymoblastic rosettes are called ependymoblastoma. All are highly malignant tumors that show aggressive clinical behavior.

stPNETs account for <5% of all CNS tumors in the pediatric age group. Patients are typically young, with a median age at presentation of 3 years, and usually present with symptoms and signs of raised intracranial pressure. Tumors arising in the cerebral hemispheres in particular may be very large. On imaging they are often quite heterogeneous, with cystic or necrotic areas and areas of hemorrhage. Leptomeningeal seeding is present at diagnosis in up to 40% of patients and MRI of the spinal axis and lumbar puncture for CSF cytology are mandatory prior to treatment.

Over the past two decades, patients with stPNETs have been treated using an approach similar to that used for patients with high-risk medulloblastoma, that is, with postoperative radiotherapy (standard-dose CSI plus a boost) and chemotherapy. Overall survival is at best only 30% to 50%. Factors that have been associated with a better outcome include smaller size (<5 cm),[207] location in the pineal region, and complete resection,[193,208–210] while younger patients[62,63,193,211] and patients M+ at diagnosis[179,207,209,212–214] fare significantly worse, with survival in the 0% to 30% range. Radiotherapy appears to be an important component of treatment that is associated with improved progression-free and overall survival.[179,210,211] However, the benefit of chemotherapy remains rather unclear despite its widespread use and the high risk of recurrence despite chemotherapy and the short time to progression, together with poor salvage rates, has led to recommendations for early radiotherapy particularly in patients with macroscopic residual tumor.[210]

Radiotherapy treatment factors including timing of radiotherapy (i.e., its use immediately postoperatively rather than following completion of chemotherapy[212]), the use of CSI rather than reduced (whole-brain or local) volumes,[212,214,215] and dose (CSI dose >35 Gy and dose to the primary site >54 Gy)[212] have all been shown to be associated with improved outcomes. Even in contemporary series, however, failure at both the primary site and in the leptomeninges is a significant problem: local failure was seen in 42% of patients with M0 disease treated on the CCG 921 protocol, and failure in the leptomeninges as a first site of failure was seen in 43% of M+ patients.[213] Both HFRT and HART have been tested as a means to more safely deliver the higher radiotherapy doses that seem to be needed in patients with stPNETs. Of five patients treated with HFRT at Duke University, four survived without evidence of disease 4.3 to 8 years following diagnosis.[216] Preliminary results from the Italian cooperative group using HART were interpreted as promising, with progression-free survival at 3 years of 54%.[217]

For now, the usual approach for a child older than 3 with a stPNET without leptomeningeal spread consists of maximal surgical resection followed by postoperative radiotherapy (CSI followed by a boost) and chemotherapy. Experimental regimens such as high-dose chemotherapy with stem cell rescue are used in infants and young children and in patients with M+ disease. The use in more favorable patients of a lower CSI dose or even local radiotherapy rather than CSI, while certainly of interest as a strategy to reduce the risk of long-term sequelae

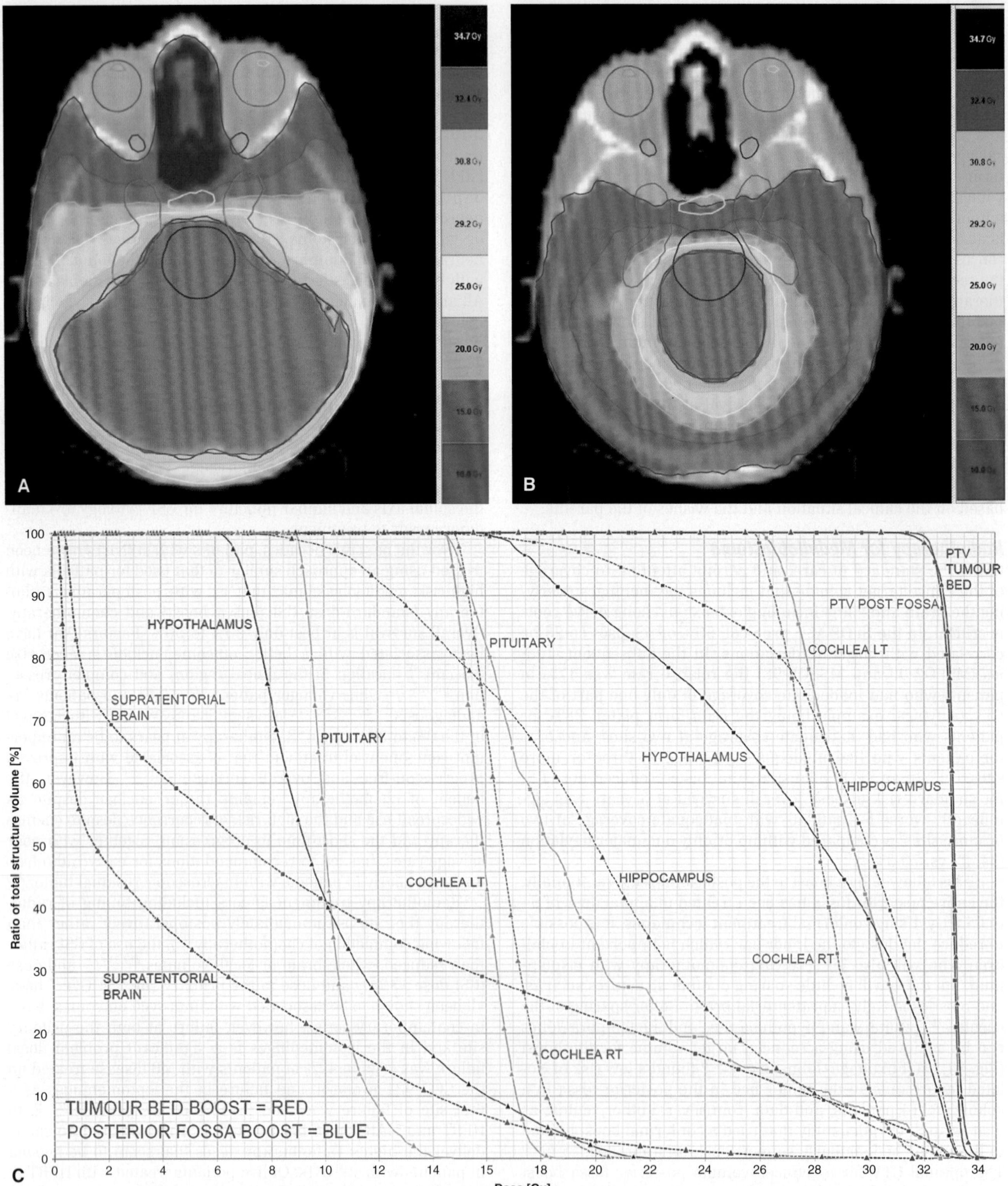

FIGURE 84.13. Axial images of an intensity-modulated radiation therapy/image-guide radiation therapy plan for a whole posterior fossa **(A)** and a reduced-volume posterior fossa boost **(B)** for a patient with medulloblastoma. **C:** Dose–volume histograms show significant sparing of organs at risk with the reduced-volume boost.

of treatment, should be considered experimental for lack of evidence to support such an approach at this time.

Atypical Teratoid/Rhabdoid Tumor

Atypical teratoid/rhabdoid tumor (ATRT) is a highly malignant embryonal tumor seen in very young children with a peak incidence in the birth to 2-year age group, at which age in one population-based study ATRT was as common as PNET and medulloblastoma.[218] Composed of rhabdoid cells with or without fields resembling a classical PNET, ATRT is diagnosed on the basis of the characteristic molecular findings, namely, deletion and/or mutation of the INI1 locus on chromosome 22. ATRT can arise at any location within the CNS, including the spine. Leptomeningeal seeding is seen at diagnosis in a quarter to a third of patients.

Since recognition of ATRT as a separate entity with a high frequency of early relapse and a very poor prognosis, patients have been treated with increasingly intensive chemotherapy regimens. Radiotherapy appears to be an important component of treatment.[219–222,223,224,225] In a series of 37 patients treated at St. Jude, early use of radiotherapy and the use of CSI were found to be associated with improved outcomes,[223] and it has been suggested that the worse survival reported for children younger than age 3 may be due in part to the less frequent use of radiotherapy and, when used, to the use of local radiotherapy rather than CSI in this age group. However, in a recent update limited to patients who received age- and risk-stratified radiotherapy, delay to radiotherapy was found to be the important factor.[226] In the current COG study, the treatment plan calls for early radiotherapy (after completion of two cycles of induction chemotherapy), although in practice the use and timing of radiotherapy depend on the age of the child, the location (infra- or supratentorial), and the extent of disease at diagnosis (M0 or M+). Thus, children younger than 6 months at completion of chemotherapy with an infratentorial tumor and those younger than 12 months with a supratentorial tumor receive radiotherapy later, upon completion of both induction and consolidation chemotherapy. The radiotherapy target volume is local (tumor bed and any macroscopic residual disease plus a margin for the CTV of 1 cm) for children with localized disease and CSI followed by a boost for those with leptomeningeal spread. Doses are age dependent for both local radiotherapy and CSI (50.4 Gy vs. 54 Gy and 23.4 Gy vs. 36 Gy for children younger and older than 3 years, respectively). In Europe, patients with nonmetastatic ATRT receive doxorubicin-based chemotherapy and local radiotherapy to a dose of 54 Gy, while those with metastatic disease receive CSI. An ATRT registry (EURHAB) has been established to collect multi-institutional and multinational data on patient management and outcome.

GERM CELL TUMORS

Germ cell tumors of the CNS constitute a group of rare tumors that are morphologic homologs of germinal neoplasms arising in the gonads and at other extragonadal sites. They include the following entities although in many cases more than one tumor type is present:

- Germinoma
- Embryonal carcinoma
- Yolk-sac tumor (endodermal sinus tumor)
- Choriocarcinoma
- Teratoma
  - –Mature
  - –Immature
  - –Teratoma with malignant transformation
- Mixed germ cell tumor

A teratoma is a tumor composed of an admixture of different tissue types representative of ectoderm, endoderm, and mesoderm. A mature teratoma is composed exclusively of fully differentiated tissues, sometimes arranged in such a manner as to resemble normal tissue relationships. Mitoses are absent or rare. An immature teratoma is composed of incompletely differentiated tissues resembling those of the fetus. Mitoses typically are present.

In the West, CNS germ cell tumors are relatively rare, accounting for 3% to 5% of all CNS tumors in the pediatric age group. They are more common in Asia, where they account for as many as 15% to 18% of all CNS tumors occurring in childhood. The peak age incidence is 10 to 12 years. Boys are affected more frequently than girls, with a ratio of approximately 3:1. CNS germ cell tumors arise from primordial germ cells in structures about the third ventricle, with the region of the pineal gland being the most common site of origin followed by the suprasellar region. Nongerminomatous germ cell tumors (NGGCTs) are the most common tumor type in the former area and germinomas in the latter.

The presenting symptoms and signs depend on the tumor type and the location of the tumor. Tumors in the pineal region cause obstruction to CSF flow at the aqueduct of Sylvius resulting in hydrocephalus, and most patients with tumors in this region present with a relatively short history with symptoms and signs of raised intracranial pressure. Another characteristic presentation of tumors in this region is Parinaud's syndrome as a result of dorsal midbrain compression. In contrast, patients with tumors in the suprasellar region usually present with a longer history initially of neuroendocrine deficits, especially diabetes insipidus, growth failure, and precocious puberty, and only later of visual field deficits and, later still, of symptoms and signs of raised intracranial pressure. On imaging, most germ cell tumors appear as solid masses. Teratomas are more heterogeneous with cysts, areas of calcification, and sometimes fat, whereas choriocarcinomas often contain areas of hemorrhage. Bi- or multifocal disease around the third ventricle is seen in approximately 10% of patients with germinomas. Gadolinium-enhanced MRI of the spinal axis is an essential part of the workup to exclude leptomeningeal dissemination, which is found at diagnosis in approximately 10% of patients with germinomas and 10% to 15% of patients with NGGCTs. Measurement of serum and CSF tumor markers is another essential part of the initial workup. Modest elevation of β-human chorionic gonadotropin (β-hCG) (<100 IU/mL) may be seen with pure germinomas that may contain syncytiotrophoblastic cells. Higher levels of β-hCG are more suggestive of a choriocarcinoma. An elevated α-fetoprotein (α-FP) is diagnostic of a yolk-sac tumor.

In the past, many lesions arising in or about the third ventricle were treated without histologic confirmation of diagnosis. This is no longer considered acceptable practice because the differential diagnosis includes many disparate entities (such as Langerhans cell histiocytosis, astrocytoma, and ependymoma) and all patients should undergo biopsy unless CSF and/or serum markers confirm the presence of an NGGCT (elevated α-FP and/or β-hCG >100 IU/mL) or unless a histologic diagnosis is made by other means (e.g., CSF cytology). For tumors in the pineal region with hydrocephalus, the usual surgical approach is an endoscopic third ventriculostomy, which allows access to the lesion for biopsy purposes. Intraventricular lesions have to be biopsied with care because hemorrhage, which is not infrequent, may be difficult to manage endoscopically. A stereotactic approach is also possible, but this may be quite challenging because of the proximity of deep cerebral veins and, moreover, may be suboptimal for diagnosis because of the potential for sampling error. Occasionally complete resection will be possible; this would be a reasonable strategy for patients with NGGCTs if it can be accomplished without major morbidity because it would ensure complete characterization of the pathology and may even obviate the need for further therapy.

Germinoma

In the past, standard treatment for patients with germinoma, whether localized or disseminated, was radiotherapy alone. Results of treatment using CSI followed by a boost to the primary site are excellent, with long-term disease-free survival rates of 100% in some series.[227–231] For patients with unifocal disease without leptomeningeal spread, radiotherapy alone to limited volumes, that is, whole brain[232,233] or whole ventricle,[227,229,234] results in a high probability of local control and a low (0% to 5%) risk of failure in the spinal axis. Experience with local radiotherapy (tumor plus a margin) alone generally has been less satisfactory,[232–233,234,235,236] although some have reported excellent results.[237] To reduce the risk of morbidity associated with radiotherapy, chemotherapy has been considered another option, either alone or in combination with reduced-volume and/or reduced-dose radiotherapy. Several studies have shown clearly that the former, that is, the use of chemotherapy alone, is not acceptable: only 40% to 50% of patients remain disease free, and although salvage using further chemotherapy together with radiotherapy is possible in most cases and overall survival is high, this is achieved at the cost of considerable toxicity.[238–241]

In contrast, a combined approach using platinum-based chemotherapy followed by reduced-volume, reduced-dose radiotherapy is an attractive option that results in disease-free survival rates in the 90% to 96% range.[239,242–244] The optimal radiotherapy target volume using such an approach remains to be defined. Local failures were seen in 10 of 60 patients treated in the SFOP TGM-TC-90 study with chemotherapy followed by local radiotherapy[245] and with even greater frequency in some single-institution studies, which, although with a patient population with a median age in adolescence, included adult patients.[236,246] Local failure appears to be less frequent after whole ventricular radiotherapy[246] and this is becoming generally accepted as the appropriate volume in this context (Fig. 84.14), but prospective data are lacking for now.

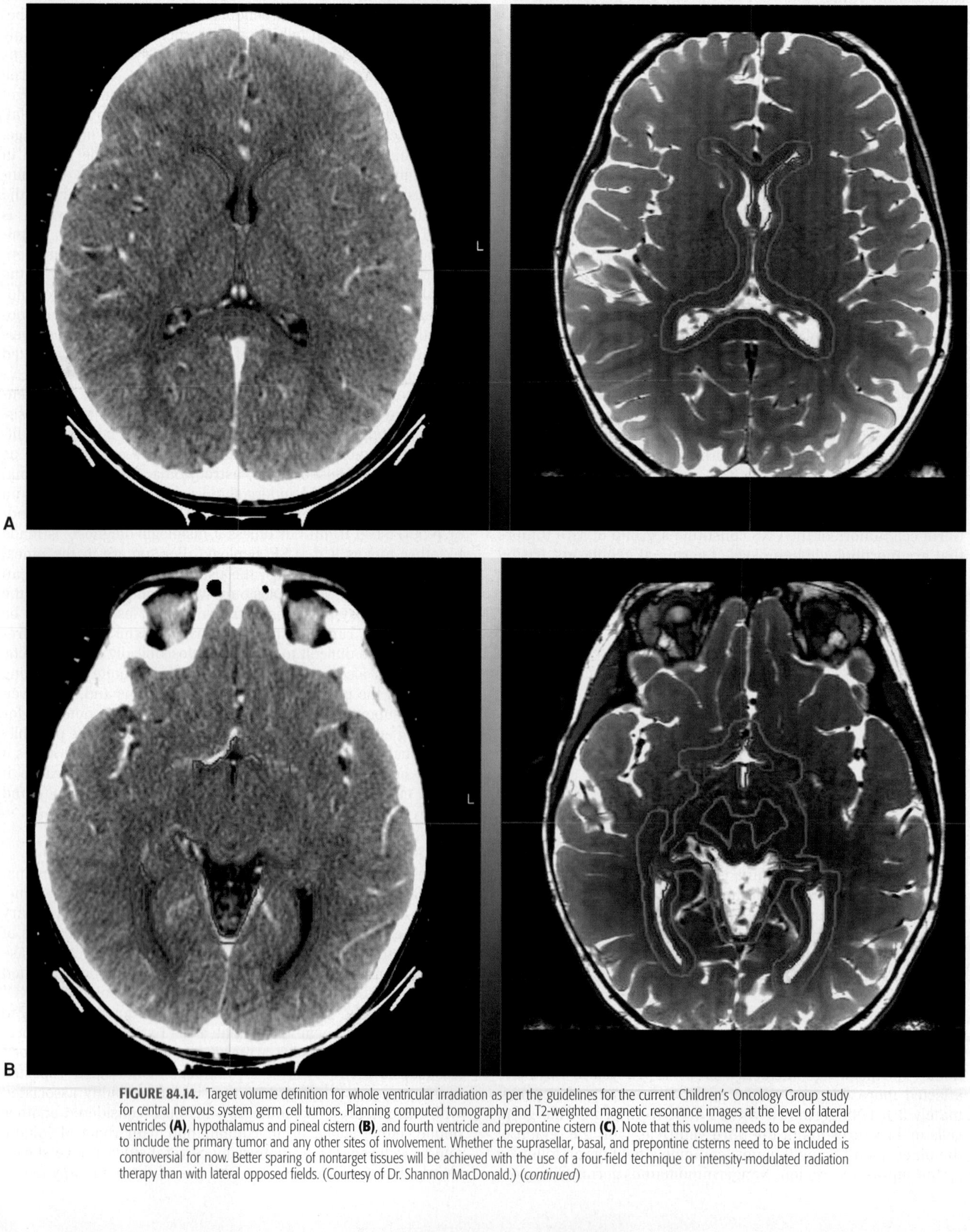

FIGURE 84.14. Target volume definition for whole ventricular irradiation as per the guidelines for the current Children's Oncology Group study for central nervous system germ cell tumors. Planning computed tomography and T2-weighted magnetic resonance images at the level of lateral ventricles **(A)**, hypothalamus and pineal cistern **(B)**, and fourth ventricle and prepontine cistern **(C)**. Note that this volume needs to be expanded to include the primary tumor and any other sites of involvement. Whether the suprasellar, basal, and prepontine cisterns need to be included is controversial for now. Better sparing of nontarget tissues will be achieved with the use of a four-field technique or intensity-modulated radiation therapy than with lateral opposed fields. (Courtesy of Dr. Shannon MacDonald.) *(continued)*

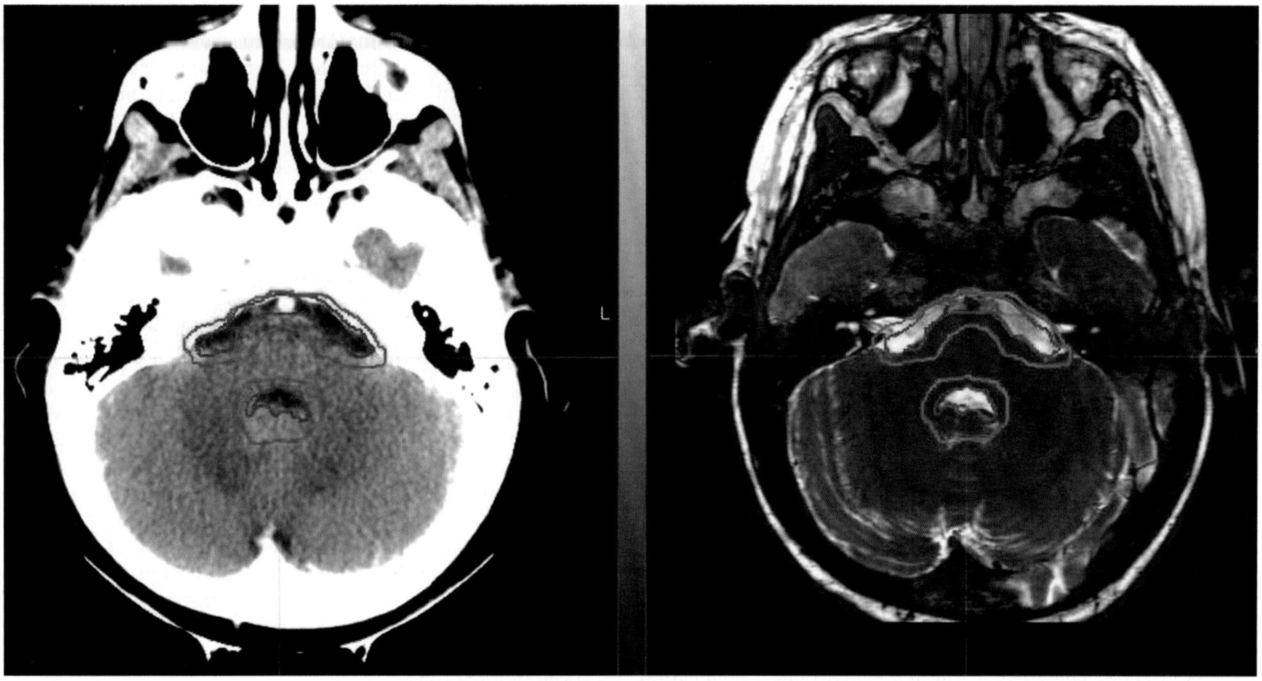

FIGURE 84.14. (Continued)

For patients with leptomeningeal spread at diagnosis, radiotherapy alone using CSI with boosts to macroscopic disease is certainly an option, although in North America chemotherapy followed by CSI followed by a boost to all sites of involvement would be the more usual approach. Management of patients with bi- or multifocal midline tumors is controversial. In the past these patients were treated as having disseminated disease, but at least some, that is, those with bifocal disease by imaging or by inference (e.g., in a patient with a pineal region primary who has diabetes insipidus), are now more usually treated with chemotherapy and whole ventricular radiotherapy.

There is less controversy now with regard to the radiotherapy dose and dose-fractionation schedule for germinoma. Results are excellent with a CSI dose as low as 21 Gy even in patients with leptomeningeal spread. The total dose to the primary site has typically been 40 to 45 Gy but probably can be safely reduced to 30 Gy or even to 24 Gy[239,244] in patients treated with a combined chemotherapy–radiotherapy regimen who have had a complete response to chemotherapy. Finally, because germinoma is a very radiosensitive tumor, a fraction size of 1.5 Gy can be used, which, in theory, further reduces the risk of injury to normal structures.

Nongerminomatous Germ Cell Tumors

For NGGCTs the diagnosis can be made in as many as one-third of all patients on the basis of imaging findings (location and appearance) plus tumor markers. NGGCTs are of several different histopathologic types that carry different prognoses (Table 84.3). Patients with mature teratomas without any associated malignant elements can be managed with surgery alone, while those with mature teratoma with germinomatous elements will be treated as germinomas. All other patients with intermediate- and poor-prognosis tumor types[247] require more aggressive treatment. The results of treatment using radiotherapy alone are very poor, with overall survival in the 10% to 30% range. Results are better with chemotherapy alone, although 40% to 60% of patients relapse following chemotherapy and will be subjected to aggressive salvage regimens.[238,248,249] A multimodality approach that includes both chemotherapy and radiotherapy appears to be associated with the best outcome. Event-free survival was 81% in the German/Italian pilot study that led to the most recent SIOP CNS GCT study.[250] The current standard of care therefore consists of platinum-based chemotherapy followed by radiotherapy.

There is controversy with respect to the radiotherapy target volume for NGGCT. Although good results have been reported by some groups using chemotherapy followed by local radiotherapy,[177] others show a high rate of failure outside the primary site.[249,251–255] Thus, as for germinoma, a whole-ventricle volume may be a better option for more favorable patients (e.g., the intermediate-risk group, α-FP <1,000 ng/mL), while CSI would be used for those with less favorable or disseminated disease. The usual dose to the whole-ventricle volume or CSI is 30 to 36 Gy and to the primary site, 54 Gy.

Patients who have less than a complete response to chemotherapy fare poorly. Second-look surgery may be useful to both exclude the possibility that the residual imaging abnormality represents mature teratoma and/or resect residual viable tumor. This would be followed by CSI and more intensive chemotherapy such as high-dose chemotherapy with stem cell rescue.

TABLE 84.3 CLASSIFICATION OF NONGERMINOMATOUS GERM CELL TUMORS

Good Prognosis
Mature teratoma
Intermediate Prognosis
Immature teratoma
Mixed germ cell tumors consisting of germinoma with either mature or immature teratoma
Poor Prognosis
Teratoma with malignant transformation
Embryonal carcinoma
Yolk-sac tumor
Choriocarcinoma
Mixed germ cell tumors including a component of embryonal carcinoma, yolk-sac tumor, choriocarcinoma, or teratoma with malignant transformation

Adapted from Sawamura Y, Ikeda J, Shirato H, et al. Germ cell tumours of the central nervous system: treatment consideration based on 111 cases and their long-term clinical outcomes. *Eur J Cancer* 1998;34:104–110.

TUMORS OF THE SELLAR REGION

Tumors arising in the sellar region in children include the following:

- Craniopharyngioma
  –Adamantinomatous
  –Papillary
- Pituitary adenomas

Craniopharyngioma

By definition, craniopharyngiomas are benign partly cystic epithelial tumors that arise in the sellar region from remnants of Rathke's pouch. In children, almost all are of the adamantinomatous type. They account for approximately 5% of intracranial tumors in the pediatric age group with a peak incidence between the ages of 5 and 14 years.

In the majority of patients, craniopharyngiomas have both suprasellar and intrasellar components. Children typically present with neuroendocrine deficits, especially diabetes insipidus and growth failure. Visual field deficits often go unnoticed initially. Cognitive and behavioral changes are not uncommon. Compression of or tumor growth within the third ventricle may lead to hydrocephalus and symptoms and signs of raised intracranial pressure. On neuroimaging, the findings are very typical, with solid and cystic areas in varying proportions. Calcification is seen in the majority of cases. The solid portion(s) and the cyst capsule usually enhance with the use of contrast material.

Treatment of craniopharyngiomas, although long considered a controversial issue,[256] in practice depends on the characteristics of the tumor and the availability of the surgical expertise required. The argument for surgical resection is based on single-institution (mostly specialist center) reports of long-term tumor control after complete resection as confirmed on postoperative imaging in 85% to 100% of patients.[257] However, in a three-nation prospective study event-free survival at 3 years was only 64%.[258] Moreover, while visual deficits, if present, improve after surgery in the majority of cases, new neuroendocrine deficits are very common and hypothalamic damage is a major concern particularly in patients with tumors that have grown retro-chiasmatically into the floor of the third ventricle.[259–261] Devastating sequelae that include rage, aggressivity, and hyperphagia permanently compromise the quality of life of the patient and his or her family. The transsphenoidal approach that has been used more frequently in recent years, even in younger children and even in patients with tumors with a supradiaphragmatic component, is associated with fewer complications. In general, therefore, tumors that are smaller and/or subdiaphragmatic in location and without hypothalamic involvement would be managed surgically. Patients who have residual tumor following surgery are at high risk for progressive disease within the first 2 to 3 years following surgery,[258,262–265] mandating close follow-up with MRI performed at 3-month intervals during that time period. Patients at greater risk for complications secondary to surgery would be managed with biopsy, cyst decompression, if necessary, and radiotherapy.[266–271]

Radiotherapy may, therefore, be given as the sole therapy after biopsy, after incomplete surgery, or at time of progression/recurrence after surgery, and the heterogeneity of tumor types and situations means that one of several approaches may be used. For example, a lesion with a small solid component and a simple cyst may be well treated with intracavitary injection of liquid radioactive material. Most contemporary experience is with β emitters such as ^{32}P and ^{90}Y delivering a high dose (i.e., 200 Gy) to the cyst wall. Intracavitary injection of radioactive material is not always easy.[272] Sometimes the cyst fluid is very thick in consistency and there may be little or no communication between multiple cysts. It is essential to use contrast material to ensure that the catheter is well placed in the cavity and that there is no leakage of material outside the cyst before injecting radioactive material. This could be combined with radiosurgery or fractionated stereotactic irradiation to the associated solid component, although it may be reasonable to do so only later and only if there is evidence of progressive disease. Special care is needed if, as is usually the case, the tumor is in close proximity to the optic chiasm or optic nerves.[273] Tumor control rates using this approach are good for carefully selected patients.[274] However, conventionally fractionated external-beam radiotherapy may be a better option for all except very small tumors, with a lower risk of morbidity.[256,275]

The target volume for external-beam radiotherapy consists of the entire lesion (i.e., both the solid and cystic components) as demonstrated on MRI performed just prior to treatment. While some have used a margin for the CTV of 1 cm,[276] a smaller margin of 0.5 cm or even 0 cm (i.e., CTV = GTV) can be justified on the basis of excellent tumor control using such margins.[277–279] A dose of 54 to 55 Gy given in 30 daily fractions over 6 weeks appears to be necessary to achieve a high probability of tumor control. Cyst enlargement during treatment or within the first 2 to 3 months after completion of radiotherapy is not uncommon. Early recognition and appropriate management consisting usually of cyst decompression is essential to avoid further neurologic compromise or even death.[280] The long-term prognosis is good, with event-free survival of 80% to 100% in most series.[258,276,279,281,282]

Pituitary Adenomas

Pituitary adenomas are rare in childhood. Almost all cases arise in adolescence. Most are functioning adenomas that present with endocrine dysfunction, most often menstrual irregularities and galactorrhea in girls and delayed puberty in boys. They may be quite large, with extrasellar extension, and appear to be more invasive than those seen in adults.[283–285] Visual loss, when present, may be more severe and more likely to be associated with optic atrophy.[284]

Management will, in general, parallel that for adult patients. Prolactin- and growth hormone–secreting adenomas are managed medically as in adults. When surgery is necessary, a transsphenoidal approach using neuronavigation appears to be feasible and safe in children, even in those with poor pneumatization of the sphenoid sinus.[283,285] Radiotherapy is indicated if surgical resection is not possible or if hormone levels remain elevated following surgery. Highly conformal treatment with a margin for the CTV of 0.5 cm beyond macroscopic disease is appropriate in most cases, the technique used being that which optimally spares adjacent critical structures including major vessels. The usual dose, as in adults, will be 45 to 50 Gy over 5 to 6 weeks. Close follow-up by an endocrinologist is essential to ensure appropriate management of hormone deficits.

SELECTED REFERENCES

A full list of references for this chapter is available online.

2. Armstrong GT, Liu Q, Yasui Y, et al. Long-term outcomes among adult survivors of childhood central nervous system malignancies in the Childhood Cancer Survivor Study. *J Natl Cancer Inst* 2009;101(13):946–958.
3. Vinchon M, Baroncini M, Leblond P, et al. Morbidity and tumor-related mortality among adult survivors of pediatric brain tumors: a review. *Childs Nerv Syst* 2011;27(5):697–704.
4. Kortmann RD, Timmermann B, Taylor RE, et al. Current and future strategies in radiotherapy of childhood low-grade glioma of the brain. Part II: treatment-related late toxicity. *Strahlenther Onkol* 2003;179(9):585–597.
5. Mulhern RK, Merchant TE, Gajjar A, et al. Late neurocognitive sequelae in survivors of brain tumours in childhood. *Lancet Oncol* 2004;5(7):399–408.
13. Meacham L. Endocrine late effects of childhood cancer therapy. *Curr Probl Pediatr Adolesc Health Care* 2003;33(7):217–242.
16. Sklar CA, Constine LS. Chronic neuroendocrinological sequelae of radiation therapy. *Int J Radiat Oncol Biol Phys* 1995;31(5):1113–1121.
20. Beltran C, Naik M, Merchant TE. Dosimetric effect of setup motion and target volume margin reduction in pediatric ependymoma. *Radiother Oncol* 2010;96(2): 216–222.
24. Urie M, FitzGerald TJ, Followill D, et al. Current calibration, treatment, and treatment planning techniques among institutions participating in the Children's Oncology Group. *Int J Radiat Oncol Biol Phys* 2003;55(1):245–260.

25. Parker WA, Freeman CR. A simple technique for craniospinal radiotherapy in the supine position. *Radiother Oncol* 2006;78(2):217–222.
26. Parker W, Filion E, Roberge D, et al. Intensity-modulated radiotherapy for craniospinal irradiation: target volume considerations, dose constraints, and competing risks. *Int J Radiat Oncol Biol Phys* 2007;69(1):251–257.
28. Donahue B. Short- and long-term complications of radiation therapy for pediatric brain tumors. *Pediatr Neurosurg* 1992;18(4):207–217.
29. Louis DN, International Agency for Research on Cancer. *WHO classification of tumours of the central nervous system.* Lyon, France: International Agency for Research on Cancer, 2007.
40. Merchant TE, Kun LE, Wu S, et al. Phase II trial of conformal radiation therapy for pediatric low-grade glioma. *J Clin Oncol* 2009;27(22):3598–3604.
41. Wisoff JH, Sanford RA, Heier LA, et al. Primary neurosurgery for pediatric low-grade gliomas: a prospective multi-institutional study from the Children's Oncology Group. *Neurosurgery* 2011;68(6):1548–1554; discussion 54–55.
79. Freeman CR, Farmer JP. Pediatric brain stem gliomas: a review. *Int J Radiat Oncol Biol Phys* 1998;40(2):265–271.
124. Merchant TE, Li C, Xiong X, et al. Conformal radiotherapy after surgery for paediatric ependymoma: a prospective study. *Lancet Oncol* 2009;10(3):258–266.
136. Merchant TE, Fouladi M. Ependymoma: new therapeutic approaches including radiation and chemotherapy. *J Neurooncol* 2005;75(3):287–299.
162. Mazloom A, Wolff JE, Paulino AC. The impact of radiotherapy fields in the treatment of patients with choroid plexus carcinoma. *Int J Radiat Oncol Biol Phys* 2010; 78(1):79–84.
183. Thomas PR, Deutsch M, Kepner JL, et al. Low-stage medulloblastoma: final analysis of trial comparing standard-dose with reduced-dose neuraxis irradiation. *J Clin Oncol* 2000;18(16):3004–3011.
185. Carrie C, Muracciole X, Gomez F, et al. Conformal radiotherapy, reduced boost volume, hyperfractionated radiotherapy, and online quality control in standard-risk medulloblastoma without chemotherapy: results of the French M-SFOP 98 protocol. *Int J Radiat Oncol Biol Phys* 2005;63(3):711–716.
187. Packer RJ, Gajjar A, Vezina G, et al. Phase III study of craniospinal radiation therapy followed by adjuvant chemotherapy for newly diagnosed average-risk medulloblastoma. *J Clin Oncol* 2006;24(25):4202–4208.
188. Ellison DW, Kocak M, Dalton J, et al. Definition of disease-risk stratification groups in childhood medulloblastoma using combined clinical, pathologic, and molecular variables. *J Clin Oncol* 2011;29(11):1400–1407.
189. Freeman CR, Taylor RE, Kortmann RD, et al. Radiotherapy for medulloblastoma in children: a perspective on current international clinical research efforts. *Med Pediatr Oncol* 2002;39(2):99–108.
191. Gandola L, Massimino M, Cefalo G, et al. Hyperfractionated accelerated radiotherapy in the Milan strategy for metastatic medulloblastoma. *J Clin Oncol* 2009; 27(4):566–571.
197. Carrie C, Alapetite C, Mere P, et al. Quality control of radiotherapeutic treatment of medulloblastoma in a multicentric study: the contribution of radiotherapy technique to tumour relapse. The French Medulloblastoma Group. *Radiother Oncol* 1992;24(2):77–81.
198. Carrie C, Hoffstetter S, Gomez F, et al. Impact of targeting deviations on outcome in medulloblastoma: study of the French Society of Pediatric Oncology (SFOP). *Int J Radiat Oncol Biol Phys* 1999;45(2):435–439.
206. Taylor RE, Bailey CC, Robinson KJ, et al. Impact of radiotherapy parameters on outcome in the International Society of Paediatric Oncology/United Kingdom Children's Cancer Study Group PNET-3 study of preradiotherapy chemotherapy for M0-M1 medulloblastoma. *Int J Radiat Oncol Biol Phys* 2004;58(4): 1184–1193.
207. Pizer BL, Weston CL, Robinson KJ, et al. Analysis of patients with supratentorial primitive neuro-ectodermal tumours entered into the SIOP/UKCCSG PNET 3 study. *Eur J Cancer* 2006;42(8):1120–1128.
217. Massimino M, Gandola L, Spreafico F, et al. Supratentorial primitive neuroectodermal tumors (S-PNET) in children: a prospective experience with adjuvant intensive chemotherapy and hyperfractionated accelerated radiotherapy. *Int J Radiat Oncol Biol Phys* 2006;64(4):1031–1037.
223. Tekautz TM, Fuller CE, Blaney S, et al. Atypical teratoid/rhabdoid tumors (ATRT): improved survival in children 3 years of age and older with radiation therapy and high-dose alkylator-based chemotherapy. *J Clin Oncol* 2005;23(7):1491–1499.
225. Athale UH, Duckworth J, Odame I, et al. Childhood atypical teratoid rhabdoid tumor of the central nervous system: a meta-analysis of observational studies. *J Pediatr Hematol Oncol* 2009;31(9):651–663.
226. Pai Panandiker AS, Merchant TE, Beltran C, et al. Sequencing of local therapy affects the pattern of treatment failure and survival in children with atypical teratoid rhabdoid tumors of the central nervous system. *Int J Radiat Oncol Biol Phys* 2012;82(5):1756–1763.
234. Shirato H, Aoyama H, Ikeda J, et al. Impact of margin for target volume in low-dose involved field radiotherapy after induction chemotherapy for intracranial germinoma. *Int J Radiat Oncol Biol Phys* 2004;60(1):214–217.
236. Jensen AW, Laack NN, Buckner JC, et al. Long-term follow-up of dose-adapted and reduced-field radiotherapy with or without chemotherapy for central nervous system germinoma. *Int J Radiat Oncol Biol Phys* 2010;77(5):1449–1456.
237. Shibamoto Y, Sasai K, Oya N, et al. Intracranial germinoma: radiation therapy with tumor volume-based dose selection. *Radiology* 2001;218(2):452–456.
245. Alapetite C, Brisse H, Patte C, et al. Pattern of relapse and outcome of non-metastatic germinoma patients treated with chemotherapy and limited field radiation: the SFOP experience. *Neuro Oncol* 2010;12(12):1318–1325.
247. Sawamura Y, Ikeda J, Shirato H, et al. Germ cell tumours of the central nervous system: treatment consideration based on 111 cases and their long-term clinical outcomes. *Eur J Cancer* 1998;34(1):104–110.
258. Muller HL, Gebhardt U, Schroder S, et al. Analyses of treatment variables for patients with childhood craniopharyngioma–results of the multicenter prospective trial KRANIOPHARYNGEOM 2000 after three years of follow-up. *Horm Res Paediatr* 2010;73(3):175–180.

Chapter 85
Wilms Tumor

John A. Kalapurakal and Patrick R.M. Thomas

Wilms tumor (WT, nephroblastoma) is a highly curable childhood neoplasm. The prognosis of children with WT has improved considerably from a very high mortality rate at the beginning of the 20th century to the current cure rate of >90%.[1] The management of WT is a paradigm for successful interdisciplinary treatment of solid tumors of childhood to maximize cure rates and minimize treatment-related complications.

EPIDEMIOLOGY

WT is the most common malignant renal tumor of childhood. It occurs with an annual incidence of 7 cases per million children <15 years of age. Approximately 500 new cases are diagnosed each year in North America. The peak incidence is between 3 and 4 years of age. WT may arise as sporadic or hereditary tumors or in the setting of specific genetic disorders.[2] Most WTs are solitary lesions, multifocal within a single kidney in 12% and bilateral in 7%.[3] The clinical syndromes associated with WT include WAGR syndrome (*W*T, *A*niridia, *G*enitourinary malformations, mental *R*etardation), Denys-Drash syndrome (pseudohermaphroditism, mesangial sclerosis, renal failure, and WT), and overgrowth syndromes like Beckwith-Wiedemann syndrome (somatic gigantism, omphalocele, macroglossia, genitourinary abnormalities, ear creases, hypoglycemia, hemihypertrophy, and a predisposition to WT and other malignancies) and Simpson-Golabi-Behmel syndrome.[4,5]

BIOLOGY

Among the various genetic changes implicated in the development of WT, the most widely studied involves *WT1,* which is a tumor suppressor gene at chromosome 11p13 that was isolated from a child with WAGR syndrome.[6] *WT1* is likely to play a specific role in glomerular and gonadal development.[7] *WT1* can also act as a dominant negative oncogene resulting in abnormal cell growth such as in Denys-Drash syndrome.[8] Germline *WT1* mutations are observed in approximately 82% of WT patients who have genitourinary anomalies or renal failure. The frequency of *WT1* mutations in sporadic and familial WT is much lower at ~20% and ~4%, respectively.[9] Beckwith-Wiedemann syndrome maps to chromosome 11p15.5; this locus is also referred to as *WT2*.[10]

Patients with loss of heterozygosity (LOH) at 16q and 1p have higher relapse and mortality rates.[11] The National Wilms Tumor Study-5 (NWTS-5) prospectively evaluated the prognostic significance of LOH on 16q and 1p. Analysis of these data revealed that the relative risks (RR) for relapse for patients with stages I to IV favorable histology (FH) tumors with LOH stratified by stage were 1.8 for LOH 1p ($P < .01$) and 1.4 for LOH 16q ($P = .05$). When the effects of LOH for both 1p and 16q were considered jointly, the RR for relapse in stages I and II FH disease was 2.9 (P = .001) and for stages III and IV FH disease was 2.4 (P = .01). The RR for death for patients with stages I and II FH disease with LOH for both regions was 4.3 (P = .01) and for stages III and IV was 2.7 (P = .04). Based on these results, it was proposed that in future WT trials, the therapy for children with LOH at both 1p and 16q be augmented by the addition of doxorubicin to regimen EE4A (discussed below) for early-stage (stages I and II) tumors and cyclophosphamide/etoposide to regimen DD4A (discussed below) for advanced-stage tumors (stages III and IV).[12]

A novel Wilms tumor suppressor gene on the X chromosome, *WTX*, was recently discovered. This gene is inactivated in approximately one-third of sporadic WT cases.[13] Anaplastic tumors have shown changes on 17p consistent with *TP53* deletion and specific genomic loss or underexpression on 4q and 14q and focal gain of *MYCN*.[14] Rhabdoid tumors are characterized by the genetic loss of the *SMARCB1/hSNF5/INI-1* gene located at chromosome 22q11. Global gene expression studies have shown that loss of *SMARCB1* results in repression of neural crest development and loss of cyclin-dependent kinase inhibition.[15] In children with very low-risk WT treated with just surgery alone, the presence of *WT1* mutation and 11p15 loss have been prospectively validated to be an important predictor of relapse. These biomarkers may be used to stratify patients to receive reduced chemotherapy in the future.[16]

PATHOLOGIC CLASSIFICATION

Although histopathologists had attempted to relate appearance to prognosis, no generally acceptable classification was available until the report of Beckwith and Palmer[17] from the National Wilms Tumor Study-1 (NWTS-1). The NWTS classifies all tumors as having either FH or unfavorable histology (UH). The UH tumors include anaplastic tumors, clear cell sarcoma, and rhabdoid tumor of kidney. Of 1,465 patients randomly assigned on NWTS-3, 163 (11.1%) had UH.[18] WTs are usually sharply demarcated, spherical masses with a "pushing" border and a surrounding distinct intrarenal pseudocapsule. Histologically, WT reflects the development of the normal kidney, consisting of three components: blastemal, epithelial (tubules), and stromal elements, in varying proportions.[17] The proportion of the different components has prognostic significance.[19] Nephrogenic rests consist of embryonal nephroblastic tissue and are found in 35% of kidneys with unilateral WT and in nearly 100% of kidneys with bilateral WT.[20] Nephrogenic rests may be intralobar or perilobar based on their location within the kidney.[21] Most nephrogenic rests undergo spontaneous regression and only a small proportion (1% to 5%) transform into WT.[22] The histologic feature of greatest clinical significance in WT is anaplasia.[23] Anaplasia may be focal (FA) or diffuse (DA). The definitions of FA and DA have been revised to reflect the distribution of anaplastic cells in the tumor rather than their quantitative density. These revised definitions are of prognostic significance. The 4-year survival rates for patients with stages II, III, and IV FA were 90%, 100%, and 100%, compared with 55%, 45%, and 4%, respectively, for patients with similar stage DA WT.[24]

Clear cell sarcoma of kidney (CCSK) and malignant rhabdoid tumor of kidney (RTK) are no longer considered true WT, but they have been included in NWTS protocols.[17] CCSK has a propensity to metastasize to bone, and a skeletal survey and bone scan should be performed. RTK is the most lethal renal neoplasm in children. Primitive neuroepithelial tumors of the cerebellum or pineal region may be seen in 10% to 15% of patients with RTK.[25]

CLINICAL PRESENTATION

The classic presentation for WT is that of a healthy child in whom abdominal swelling is discovered by the child's mother or by a physician during a routine physical examination. A smooth, firm, nontender mass on one side of the abdomen is felt. Gross hematuria occurs in as many as 25% of these cases.[26] The child may be hypertensive or have nonspecific symptoms such as malaise or fever.[27] Only rarely does a patient present with symptomatic metastases.

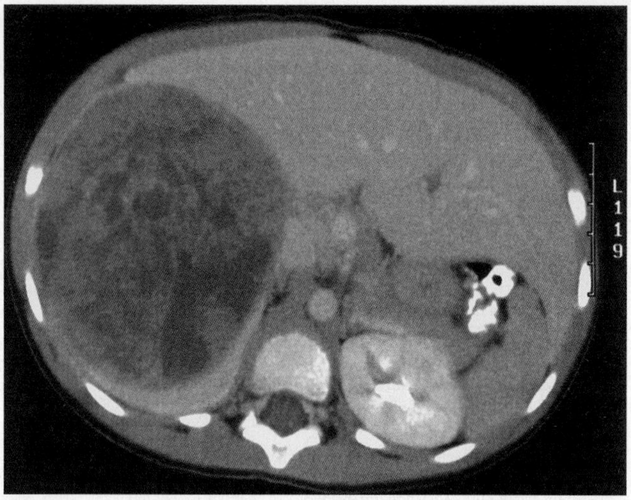

FIGURE 85.1. Computed tomography scan of a 4-year-old girl with a large right-sided Wilms' tumor measuring 10.5 × 8.4 × 13.5 cm. The left kidney did not show any lesions. At laparotomy, the tumor was found to invade the diaphragm. She underwent a right radical nephrectomy. Surgical margins of resection were positive and she had metastases in the para-aortic lymph nodes. The tumor was classified as stage III favorable histology and received 10.8 Gy to the right flank and chemotherapy with vincristine, dactinomycin, and doxorubicin.

DIAGNOSTIC WORK-UP

The differential diagnosis of WT includes other malignant childhood lesions of the kidney, neuroblastoma, and benign conditions such as hydronephrosis, polycystic disease, and splenomegaly in left-sided tumors. Plain films of the abdomen may demonstrate calcifications, which occur in 60% to 70% of neuroblastomas but in only 5% to 10% of WT. Excretory urography (intravenous pyelography) was once the mainstay of imaging in WT and now has largely been replaced by ultrasonography and computed tomography (CT) scanning. Ultrasonography is very useful because it is readily available and is cost-effective.[28] A specific advantage of ultrasonography is its ability to assess vessels for flow and tumor thrombus with duplex and color Doppler.[29] Routine use of Doppler sonography after abdominal CT scans was not found to be useful in detecting cavoatrial thrombus in a Children's Oncology Group (COG) study.[30] Abdominal CT scans can demonstrate gross extrarenal spread, lymph node involvement, liver metastases, and the status of the opposite kidney (Fig. 85.1).[31] Magnetic resonance imaging (MRI) has several advantages over CT scans, especially in identifying renal origin and vascular extension of the tumor.[32] CT and MRI are useful in the detection and follow-up of patients with nephrogenic rests.[33] Clinical and imaging impressions do not, however, obviate the need for inspection at laparotomy.[34] Plain chest radiography and chest CT are also essential because asymptomatic pulmonary metastases are common.[35] A complete blood cell count and urinalysis should be performed. Patients with WT can be anemic from hematuria. Serum blood urea nitrogen and creatinine levels and liver function tests are routine. If neuroblastoma is not ruled out, a test for urinary catecholamines should be performed. Table 85.1 outlines the pretreatment investigations recommended by the COG.

NATURAL HISTORY

The disease is often localized at diagnosis, as evidenced by the fact that surgery and radiation therapy is curative in almost

TABLE 85.1 PRETREATMENT WORK-UP

History	Record pre-existing conditions, family history of cancer, or congenital defects
Physical examination	Blood pressure, weight, height, presence of abdominal masses, congenital anomalies particularly genitourinary, hemihypertrophy, and aniridia
Laboratory	Hemoglobin, white cell, and differential counts, platelets, urinalysis, serum blood urea nitrogen, creatinine, protein, alanine, and aspartate aminotransferases, alkaline phosphatase, bilirubin
Radiology	CT or MRI scan of the abdomen and pelvis, abdominal ultrasonography, chest CT scan, chest x-ray
	Bone scan and MRI of the brain (CCSK, RTK, and renal cell carcinoma)

CT, computed tomography; MRI, magnetic resonance imaging; CCSK, clear cell sarcoma of kidney; RTK, rhabdoid tumor of kidney.

50% of cases.[36] The first signs of local tumor spread beyond the pseudocapsule are invasion into the renal sinus or the intrarenal blood and lymphatic vessels. Spread throughout the peritoneal cavity may also occur, especially if there has been preoperative rupture or the disease has been spilled at surgery.[37,38] The most common sites of metastases of WT are in the lungs, lymph nodes, and liver. Among patients with stage IV disease, lungs were the only metastatic site in approximately 80% and 15% have liver metastases.[39] The NWTS-2 study demonstrated the prognostic importance of lymph node involvement. The 2-year relapse-free survival (RFS) with and without lymph node involvement was 54% and 82%, respectively.[37]

STAGING

Tumor staging is performed after examining the radiologic, operative, and histopathologic findings.[38,39] In NWTS-1 and NWTS-2, a tumor grouping system was used for staging and treatment stratification. After analyzing the prognostic significance of several clinicopathologic factors in NWTS-1 and NWTS-2, a new staging system was adopted in NWTS-3. The presence of lymph node involvement was upstaged to stage III instead of group II, and local tumor spill was downstaged from group III to stage II.[38] In NWTS-5, the most significant change was the distinction between stages I and II. The criteria for stage I was revised to accommodate an important subset of WT that is being managed by nephrectomy alone. Before NWTS-5, the distinction between stages I and II in the renal sinus was established by the hilar plane, which was an imaginary plane connecting the most medial aspects of the upper and lower poles of the kidney. This criterion was difficult to apply because of tumor distortion, and thus the hilar plane criterion has been replaced with renal sinus vascular or lymphatic invasion. This definition includes not only the involvement of vessels within the hilar soft tissue, but also the vessels located in the radial extensions of the renal sinus into the renal parenchyma.[40,41] The COG staging guidelines for WT are shown in Table 85.2. The major change from NWTS-5 is that children with tumor spillage are upstaged from stage II to stage III because of the higher risk for relapse with two-drug chemotherapy alone.[42] The COG risk group classification for treatment assignment in the new generation of WT protocols is shown in Table 85.3. In addition to tumor stage, this classification will also consider

TABLE 85.2 CHILDREN'S ONCOLOGY GROUP STAGING OF WILMS' TUMOR, RHABDOID TUMOR, AND CLEAR CELL SARCOMA OF THE KIDNEY

Stage I: Tumor limited to kidney, completely resected. The renal capsule is intact. The tumor was not ruptured or biopsied prior to removal. The vessels of the renal sinus are not involved. There is no evidence of tumor at or beyond the margins of resection. *Note:* For a tumor to qualify for certain therapeutic protocols as stage I, regional lymph nodes must be examined microscopically.

Stage II: The tumor is completely resected and there is no evidence of tumor at or beyond the margins of resection. The tumor extends beyond kidney, as is evidenced by any one of the following criteria[a]:
- There is regional extension of the tumor (i.e., penetration of the renal capsule or extensive invasion of the soft tissue of the renal sinus)
- Blood vessels within the nephrectomy specimen outside the renal parenchyma, including those of the renal sinus, contain tumor.

Stage III: Residual nonhematogenous tumor present following surgery and confined to abdomen. Any one of the following may occur:
- Lymph nodes within the abdomen or pelvis are involved by tumor. (Lymph node involvement in the thorax or other extra-abdominal sites is a criterion for stage IV.)
- The tumor has penetrated through the peritoneal surface
- Tumor implants are found on the peritoneal surface
- Gross or microscopic tumor remains postoperatively (e.g., tumor cells are found at the margin of surgical resection on microscopic examination)
- The tumor is not completely resectable because of local infiltration into vital structures
- Tumor spillage occurring either before or during surgery
- The tumor was biopsied (whether tru-cut, open, or fine-needle aspiration) before removal
- Tumor is removed in more than one piece (e.g., tumor cells are found in a separately excised adrenal gland; a tumor thrombus within the renal vein is removed separately from the nephrectomy specimen)

Stage IV: Hematogenous metastases (i.e., lung, liver, bone, brain) or lymph node metastases outside the abdominopelvic region are present. (The presence of tumor within the adrenal gland is not interpreted as metastasis and staging depends on all other staging parameters present.)

Stage V: Bilateral renal involvement by tumor is present at diagnosis. An attempt should be made to stage each side according to the criteria here on the basis of the extent of disease.

[a]Rupture or spillage confined to the flank, including biopsy of the tumor, is no longer included in stage II and is now included in stage III.

TABLE 85.3 CHILDREN'S ONCOLOGY GROUP RISK GROUP CLASSIFICATION FOR FAVORABLE HISTOLOGY WILMS' TUMORS

Age	Tumor Weight	Stage	LOH	Rapid Response	Risk Group	COG Study	Treatment
<2 yr	<550 g	I	Any	N/A	Very Low	AREN0532	Surgery only
Any	≥550 g	I	None	N/A	Low	AREN0532	EE4A
≥2 yr	Any	I	None	N/A	Low	AREN0532	EE4A
Any	Any	II	None	N/A	Low	AREN0532	EE4A
≥2 yr	Any	I	Yes	N/A	Standard	AREN0532	DD4A
Any	≥550 g	I	Yes	N/A	Standard	AREN0532	DD4A
Any	Any	II	Yes	N/A	Standard	AREN0532	DD4A
Any	Any	III	None	Any	Standard	AREN0532	DD4A
Any	Any	III	Yes	Any	Higher	AREN0533	M
Any	Any	IV	Yes	Any	Higher	AREN0533	M
Any	Any	IV	None	Yes	Standard	AREN0533	DD4A
Any	Any	IV	None	No	Higher	AREN0533	M

LOH, loss of heterozygosity at both 1p and 16q; N/A, not applicable; DD4A (V [vincristine] A [dactinomycin], D [doxorubicin]); M (VAD/Cy [cyclophosphamide], E [etoposide]); EE4A (VA).

the patient's age, tumor weight, presence or absence of LOH at 1p and 16q, and response to chemotherapy in children with FH tumors and lung metastases.

GENERAL MANAGEMENT

The diagnosis of WT is usually made before surgery and confirmed at surgery. A transverse transabdominal, transperitoneal incision is recommended for adequate exposure and thorough abdominal exploration.[43] The surgeon must excise all tumors without spillage, if possible. Lymph node sampling from the para-aortic, celiac, and iliac areas must be performed. The use of titanium clips to identify residual tumor and margins of resection is also recommended. Routine exploration of the contralateral kidney was mandated in the past, but it is no longer recommended due to better imaging of the contralateral kidney with CT and MRI scans.

The chemotherapy and radiation therapy (RT) regimens for WT in the COG protocols are outlined in Tables 85.4 and 85.5.

RADIATION THERAPY TECHNIQUES

RT guidelines used for primary and recurrent WT in the COG protocols are shown in Table 85.5.

Timing of Radiation Therapy

The NWTS has shown that although RT does not need to be given immediately after surgery,[36] a delay of ≥10 days after surgery was associated with a significantly higher abdominal relapse rate, particularly among patients with UH tumors.[44–47]

TABLE 85.4 OUTLINE OF CHILDREN'S ONCOLOGY GROUP RENAL TUMOR STUDY

Tumor Risk Classification	*Multimodality Treatment*
Very Low-Risk FH Wilms Tumor	
<2 yr, stage I, tumor weight <550 g	Nephrectomy without adjuvant therapy, if node sampling and central pathology review has been performed.
Low-Risk FH Wilms Tumor	
≥2 yr, stage I, tumor weight ≥550 g, stage II without LOH	Nephrectomy, no RT, regimen EE4A
Standard-Risk FH Wilms Tumor	
Stage I and II with LOH	Nephrectomy, no RT, regimen DD4A
Stage III without LOH	Nephrectomy, RT, regimen DD4A
Stage IV FH: rapid responders of lung metastases at week 6 with regimen DD4A, without LOH	Nephrectomy, RT, regimen DD4A; no WLI
Higher-Risk FH Wilms Tumor	
Stage III with LOH	Nephrectomy, RT, regimen M
Stage IV slow responders (lung) and nonpulmonary metastases, with LOH	Nephrectomy, RT, regimen M, WLI and RT to metastases
High-Risk UH Renal Tumors	
Stages I–IV focal anaplasia	Nephrectomy, RT, regimen DD 4A
Stage I diffuse anaplasia	Nephrectomy, RT, regimen DD 4A
Stage I–III CCSK	Nephrectomy, RT, regimen I
Stage II–IV diffuse anaplasia	Nephrectomy, RT, regimen UH1, RT to all metastatic sites
Stage IV CCSK	Nephrectomy, RT, regimen UH1, RT to all metastatic sites
Stage I–IV RTK	Nephrectomy, RT, regimen UH1, RT to all metastatic sites

FH, favorable histology; LOH, loss of heterozygosity at 1p and 16q; RT, flank or abdominal irradiation; regimen EE4A (VA); regimen DD 4A (V [vincristine], A [dactinomycin], D [doxorubicin]); WLI, whole-lung irradiation; regimen M (VAD/Cy [cyclophosphamide], E [etoposide]); UH, unfavorable histology; CCSK, clear cell sarcoma of kidney; RTK, rhabdoid tumor of kidney; regimen I (alternating VDCy/CyE); regimen UH1 (alternating VDCy/CyC [carboplatin] E).

TABLE 85.5 CHILDREN'S ONCOLOGY GROUP RENAL TUMOR PROTOCOL RADIATION THERAPY GUIDELINES

Abdominal Tumor Stage and Histology	*RT Dose/RT Field[a]*
Stage I and II FH Wilms tumor	None
Stage III FH, stage I–III focal anaplasia	10.8 Gy to the flank[b]
Stage I–II DA, stage I–III CCSK[c]	10.8 Gy to the flank[b]
Stage III DA, stage I–III RTK	19.8 Gy flank[b] RT, infants ≤12 months 10.8 Gy
Recurrent abdominal Wilms tumor	12.6–18 Gy (<12 months)[b] 21.6 Gy (older children, previous RT ≤10.8 Gy) Boost dose of 9 Gy to gross residual tumor
Lung metastases (favorable histology)	12 Gy WLI in 8 fractions[d]
Lung metastases (unfavorable histology)	12 Gy WLI in 8 fractions
Brain metastases	30.6 Gy whole brain in 17 fractions, or 21.6 Gy whole brain + 10.8 Gy IMRT or stereotactic boost
Liver metastases	19.8 Gy whole liver in 11 fractions
Bone metastases	25.2 Gy to the lesion plus 3-cm margin
Unresected lymph node metastases	19.8 Gy

RT, radiation therapy; FH, favorable histology; CCSK, clear cell sarcoma of the kidney; RTK, rhabdoid tumor of kidney; DA, diffuse anaplasia; WLI, whole-lung irradiation; IMRT, intensity-modulated RT.

[a]Timing of RT (RT delay): RT should begin as close to the beginning of chemotherapy as possible, preferably by day 9 (surgery is day 0), but no later than day 14, unless medically contraindicated or when there is a delay in central pathology review.

[b]Whole-abdomen irradiation (WAI) is indicated when there is diffuse tumor spillage, preoperative or intraperitoneal tumor rupture, peritoneal tumor seeding, or hemorrhagic or cytology positive ascites. When WAI dose is >10 Gy, renal shielding is required to limit the dose to the remaining kidney to <14.4 Gy. Gross residual disease after surgery should receive a boost of 10 Gy. WAI dose is not to exceed 10 Gy in infants ≤12 months.

[c]COG protocol (AREN0321) is studying the possibility of eliminating RT in children with stage I CCSK tumors who have lymph node sampling and central pathology review.

[d]COG protocol (AREN0533) is studying the possibility of eliminating WLI in children with lung metastases who are rapid responders (completer response of lung metastasis after three-drug chemotherapy on central review of computed tomography [CT] scans at week 6). Tumor size, number of lesions, and CT or x-ray detectability are not considered indications for WLI in FH tumors.

Because the pathologist cannot always rule out UH quickly, all patients with WT should be scheduled to start RT no later than day 9, the day of surgery being day 0. Although most patients may not be irradiated, it is easier to cancel than to make arrangements to start RT for a small child on short notice. The influence of RT delay on abdominal tumor recurrence in patients with FH tumors treated on NWTS-3 and NWTS-4 has been reported. The mean RT delay was 10.9 days. Although univariate and multivariate analysis did not reveal RT delay of ≥10 days to adversely influence flank and abdominal recurrence, it is important to note that in 59% of children the RT delay ranged from 8 to 12 days.[48] For the COG protocols, it is recommended that RT be given preferably by day 9 but no later than day 14 after surgery.

Radiation Therapy Dose

In NWTS-1 and NWTS-2 RT dosages to the operative bed were given according to the age of the patient, however, no significant dose–response association was detected.[45,47] In NWTS-3, there was a randomization for patients with FH tumors that resulted in elimination of RT for stage II FH, and a reduction of dose to 10 Gy for stage III patients.[46] NWTS-3 and NWTS-4 data showed no RT dose response for CCSK and anaplastic tumors.[49] Therefore, it was decided to treat all abdominal disease with 10 Gy. In the COG protocols, the dose is 10 Gy for most indications except for stage III DA and stages I to III RTK, where a higher dose of 19.8 Gy is recommended (Table 85.5).[50,51]

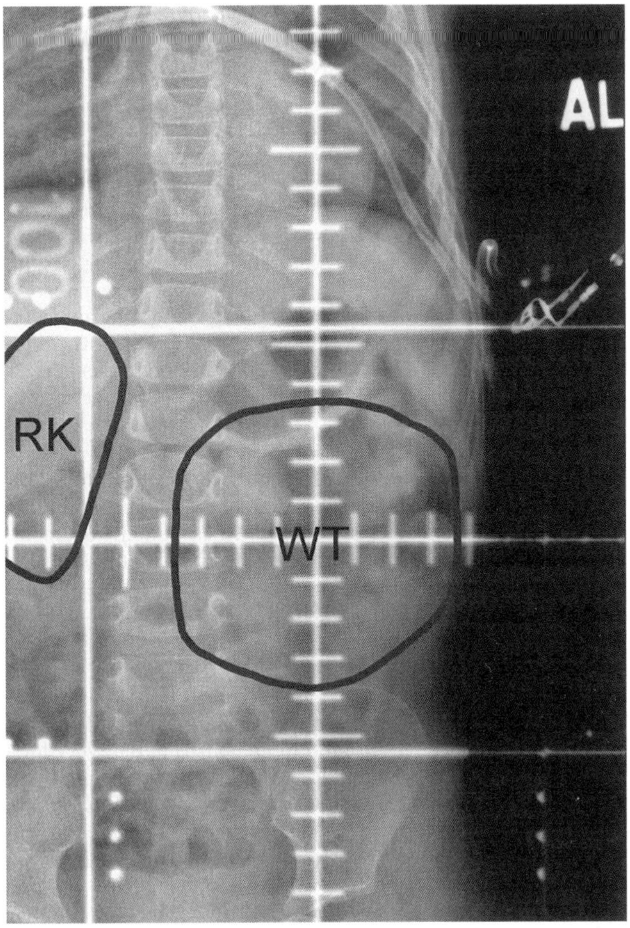

FIGURE 85.2. Anteroposterior flank irradiation portal in a 2-year-old child with a left-sided stage III favorable histology Wilms tumor (WT), showing inclusion of the entire width of the vertebral body in the irradiated volume. The outline of the right kidney (RK) and the WT from the preoperative computed tomography scan is shown.

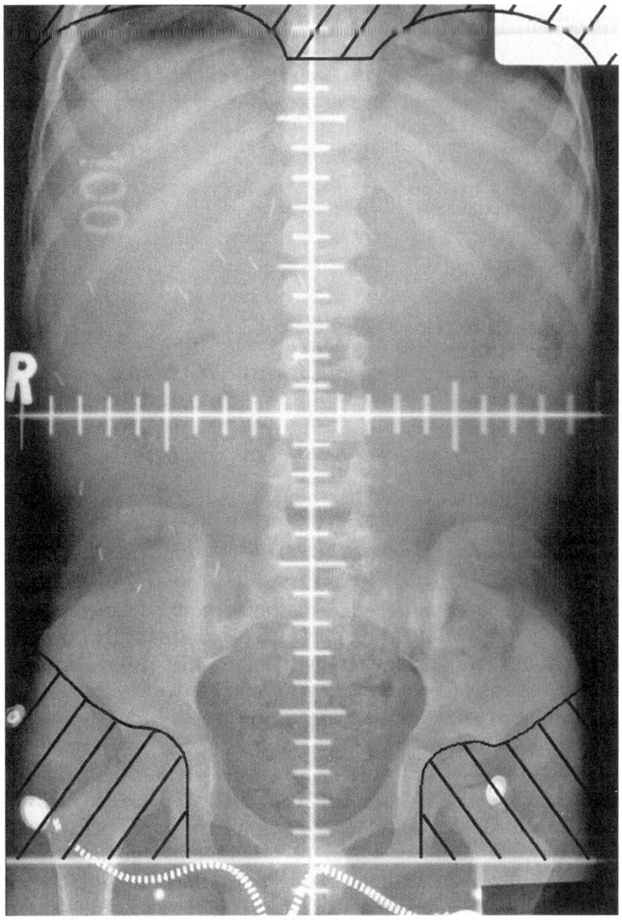

FIGURE 85.3. Anteroposterior whole-abdomen irradiation portal in a patient with stage III Wilms tumor and diffuse peritoneal tumor spillage. The upper margin of the abdominal field must include the diaphragm. The acetabulum and femoral head should be excluded from the irradiated volume to decrease the probability of slipped femoral capital epiphysis. The pants zipper can be seen low on the hips. In general, it is advisable to remove the trousers completely to ensure a reproducible setup.

Radiation Therapy Volume

Parallel-opposed fields using 4 or 6 MV photons are preferred. The flank RT field is determined by the CT or MRI scan performed at diagnosis before any chemotherapy is administered. The planning target volume is the tumor bed (outline of the kidney and associated tumor on the initial CT or MRI) with a 1-cm margin. The medial border must cross the midline to include the entire width of the vertebrae so as to minimize growth disturbances. An example of a flank RT portal is shown in Figure 85.2.[44] When whole-abdomen RT is administered, the femoral heads and acetabulum must be shielded (Fig. 85.3). Whole-lung Irradiation (WLI) portals are shown in Figure 85.4. If the lungs and either the flank or whole abdomen have to be treated simultaneously, it is preferable to include them in one treatment portal.

SUMMARY OF CLINICAL TRIALS

No tumor has been studied by clinical trials as thoroughly and effectively as WT. The NWTS has been active in North America since 1969. There have also been successful studies run by the International Society for Pediatric Oncology (SIOP). The long-term results of NWTS-3 and NWTS-4 are shown in Table 85.6.

First National Wilms Tumor Study (1969–1974)

NWTS-1 showed that postoperative RT was not necessary for children younger than 2 years of age with group I tumors, and that combined dactinomycin and vincristine for irradiated patients with group II and III tumors was better than therapy with either agent alone. The RFS with and without RT among

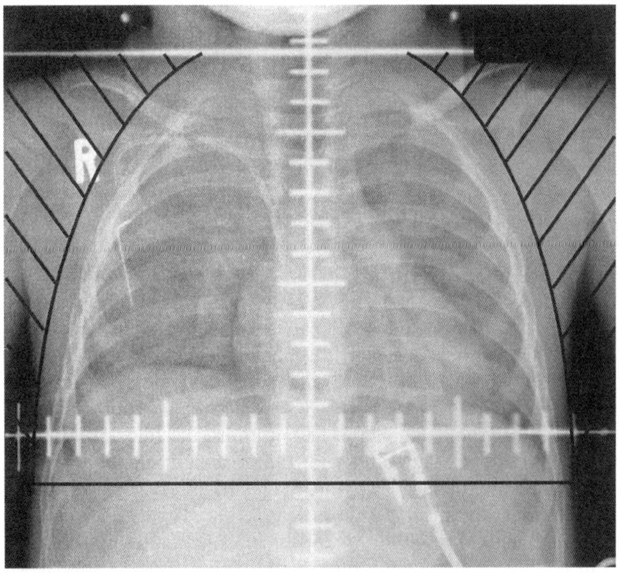

FIGURE 85.4. Anteroposterior whole-lung irradiation portal in a patient with stage IV favorable histology Wilms tumor. The axial, coronal, and sagittal chest computed tomography simulation scans should be carefully reviewed to ascertain inclusion of the anterior and posterior costophrenic angles at the inferior edge of the treatment volume with a 1-cm margin.

Clinical Radiation Oncology

TABLE 85.6 LONG-TERM RESULTS OF NATIONAL WILMS TUMOR STUDIES 3 AND 4[a]

Category	Number of Patients	10-Year RFS (%)	10-Year OS (%)
Stage I FH	1,582	91.4	96.6
Stage II FH	1,006	85.5	93.4
Stage III FH	1,038	84.2	89.5
Stage IV FH	592	75.2	80.7
Stage V FH	344	65.1	77.9
All FH	4,562	84.4	90.8
Clear cell sarcoma	170	67.1	77.1
Stage II–III anaplasia	128	43.0	49.2
Stage IV anaplasia	55	18.2	18.2
Rhabdoid tumor	88	27.3	28.4

FH, favorable histology; RFS, relapse-free survival; OS, overall survival.
[a]National Wilms' Tumor Study unpublished data.

patients with group I tumors younger than 2 years of age was 90% and 88%, respectively.[44]

Second National Wilms Tumor Study (1974–1979)

NWTS-2 showed that in patients with group I tumors there was no survival difference between 6 months or 15 months of dactinomycin plus vincristine. Patients with groups II to IV tumors had a superior 2-year RFS of 77% with doxorubicin, dactinomycin, and vincristine compared with 63% with dactinomycin and vincristine alone.[37]

Third National Wilms Tumor Study (1979–1985)

The overall objective of NWTS-3 was to reduce therapy for low-risk patients (stages I to III FH) and to intensify treatment by adding a fourth drug, cyclophosphamide, for stage IV tumors with FH and all UH tumors. The results of this study demonstrated that RT and doxorubicin could be eliminated in children with stage II FH tumors. Patients with stage III FH tumors who received doxorubicin or 20 Gy had fewer abdominal relapses than those receiving 10 Gy without doxorubicin.[46] The addition of cyclophosphamide in high-risk patients did not improve outcomes.[49]

Fourth National Wilms Tumor Study (1986–1994)

By the conclusion of NWTS-3, it was clear that the treatment of WT had been refined for the majority of patients; 62% of patients with WT have stage I or II FH disease and therefore require neither flank RT nor the potentially cardiotoxic doxorubicin. NWTS-4 was designed with cost containment in mind. The results proved that the survival was similar among patients who received standard-course (5 days) or single-dose, pulse-intensive dactinomycin chemotherapy. Further, pulse-intensive therapy was associated with less hematologic toxicity and marked reduction of treatment costs.[52,53]

Fifth National Wilms Tumor Study (1995–2001)

One of the major goals of the NWTS-5 trial was to prospectively analyze the prognostic significance of LOH at chromosomes 1p and 16q. These results have been discussed elsewhere.[12] Patients with stage I FH and anaplastic histology and stage II FH tumors were treated with 18 weeks of dactinomycin and vincristine without RT. Stage I FH tumors in children younger than 24 months of age and with tumor weight less than 550 g were treated with surgery alone. Stages III and IV FH and stages II to IV focal anaplastic tumors were treated with 24 weeks of dactinomycin, vincristine, doxorubicin, and irradiation. Stages II to IV diffuse anaplastic tumors and stages I to IV CCSK were treated with cyclophosphamide, vincristine, doxorubicin, and etoposide along with irradiation. Stages I to IV RTK were treated with carboplatin, etoposide, cyclophosphamide, and irradiation. The RT guidelines in NWTS-5 were similar to those used in NWTS-4 except for anaplastic tumors, where a dose of 10.8 Gy to the flank and abdomen was recommended compared to an age-adjusted schedule used in NWTS-1 to NWTS-4.

Children's Oncology Group Studies (2002–)

The COG renal tumors committee is the successor of the NWTS. The COG staging and risk-group classification for treatment assignment in the new generation of WT protocols are shown in Tables 85.2 and 85.3. This classification will, in addition to tumor stage, also consider the patient's age, tumor weight, presence or absence of LOH at 1p and 16q, and response to chemotherapy in children with FH tumors and lung metastases. The main objectives of the first generation of COG protocols are listed below. The COG chemotherapy regimens and RT guidelines are outlined in Tables 85.4 and 85.5, respectively.

AREN0321

This is a study for children with high-risk renal tumors. This study will determine whether a regimen of cyclophosphamide/carboplatin/etoposide alternating with vincristine/doxorubicin/cyclophosphamide improves the survival of patients with DA and RTK. This study will also determine whether the excellent event-free survival in stage I CCSK can be maintained without the use of abdominal RT.

AREN0532

This is a study for children with very low and standard risk FH WT. The main objectives are: (a) to demonstrate that very low-risk patients treated by nephrectomy and observation alone will have a 4-year RFS of ≥85% and overall survival (OS) of ≥95%; (b) to document continued excellent outcome for patients with stage III WT without LOH of 1p and 16q treated with vincristine, dactinomycin, doxorubicin, and RT (regimen DD4A); (c) to improve the current 4-year RFS for patients with stages I and II WT with LOH of 1p and 16q by adding doxorubicin but not RT to the standard dactinomycin and vincristine regimen.

AREN0533

This is a study for higher risk FH WT. The main objectives are: (a) to demonstrate that patients with stage IV tumors with pulmonary metastases only, who have complete resolution of the pulmonary lesions after 6 weeks of regimen DD4A chemotherapy (rapid complete responders) will have a 4-year RFS of 85% with additional chemotherapy (regimen DD4A) and without WLI; (b) to demonstrate that stage IV patients who do not have resolution of pulmonary metastases by week 6 (slow incomplete responders) will have a 4-year RFS of 85% with the addition of cyclophosphamide and etoposide to a modified regimen DD4A (regimen M) and WLI; (c) to improve the 4-year RFS to 75% for patients with stage III or IV FH WT with LOH of chromosomes 1p and 16q.

AREN0534

This is a study for patients with bilateral, multicentric, or bilaterally predisposed unilateral WT. The main objectives are: (a) to improve 4-year RFS to 73% for patients with bilateral Wilms tumor (BWT); (b) to prevent complete removal of at least one kidney in 50% of patients with BWT by using prenephrectomy three-drug chemotherapy induction with vincristine, dactinomycin, and doxorubicin; (c) to have 75% of children with BWT undergo definitive surgical treatment by 12 weeks after initiation of chemotherapy.

Outcomes of Children with Wilms Tumor

Lung Metastases

Patients with stage IV FH with lung metastases had a 4-year survival of 80% on NWTS-3, whereas survival for those with stage IV UH was 55%.[18,39,49] In a United Kingdom Children's

Cancer Study Group (UKCCSG) trial, patients with stage IV FH were spared WLI if they had complete resolution of pulmonary metastases after chemotherapy. The 6-year RFS and OS were 50% and 65%, respectively.[54] These results appear to be somewhat worse than the 4-year survival rate of 82% on NWTS-3 and 75% in the second UKCCSG Wilms tumor study due to the greater use of WLI.[18,55] In children with FH tumors enrolled in NWTS-3 and NWTS-4 who had negative chest radiographs and CT scans positive for pulmonary metastases, the 4-year RFS with and without WLI was similar at 89% and 80%, respectively.[56] In a report from NWTS-4 and NWTS-5, among children with lung metastases detected only by CT scans, the 5-year RFS after three drugs with or without WLI was significantly higher than those receiving two drugs (80% vs. 56%). There was no difference seen in 5-year OS between the three-drug and two-drug subsets (87% vs. 86%). There were no significant differences in RFS (82% vs. 72%) or OS (91% vs. 83%) based on whether these patients did or did not receive WLI. This report concluded that in patients with CT-only lung lesions, the addition of doxorubicin may improve RFS but not OS, and there was no added benefit from WLI.[57] In COG protocol AREN0533, chemotherapy response at week 6 will be used to determine whether WLI is delivered or not. Patients with FH tumors and lung metastasis who achieve a complete radiologic response to three-drug chemotherapy at week 6 will not receive WLI, all others will receive WLI. All patients with UH WT and lung metastases will receive WLI, regardless of response to chemotherapy (Tables 85.4 and 85.5).

Liver Metastases

Patients with liver metastasis undergo hepatic RT if the metastatic lesions are not completely resected at the time of initial diagnosis before any chemotherapy is delivered. Whole-liver RT is given for diffuse disease, with supplementary boosts to gross disease as indicated. When possible, however, more limited RT fields are used if the disease is more localized in the liver. In a report from NWTS-4 and NWTS-5, the RFS for patients with FH WT and liver metastases was 76%, and this was similar to the RFS in patients with lung metastases (76%), liver and lung metastases (70%), and metastases to other sites (64%).[58]

Bilateral Wilms Tumor

The goals of treatment in BWT are to maximize cure rates and to preserve functional renal parenchyma; thus, the role of radical nephrectomy and RT has been restricted. Initial surgical resections should be performed only if more than two-thirds of each kidney can be preserved.[59] The initial surgery should confirm histologic diagnosis, assess extent of disease in the kidney, and perform a lymph node biopsy. Systemic chemotherapy is then delivered, after which second-look surgery is done in order to perform tumor resection with maximal preservation of renal function. Unpublished 10-year data from the NWTS-3 and NWTS-4 showed that BWT patients, compared with those who have stages I to IV unilateral FH tumors, had lower RFS (65% and 86%) and OS (78% and 92%). In NWTS-4, the 8-year RFS and OS were 74% and 89%, respectively, for FH and 40% and 45%, respectively, for UH BWT. The incidence of end-stage renal disease was 12% among stage V patients.[60] In NWTS-5, BWT patients had a 4-year RFS and OS of only 61% and 80%, respectively. The factors that might have contributed to these poor outcomes were understaging or undertreatment, delay in definitive surgical resection, and increased incidence of anaplasia.[61,62] The current COG protocol (AREN0534) recommends earlier biopsies or resection of nonresponsive tumors so that ineffective therapies for patients with DA could be avoided. This study will intensify chemotherapy upfront (three drugs), require second-look surgery at 6 weeks and definitive surgery at 12 weeks, and recommends chemotherapy based on histologic response after definitive surgery. Radiation therapy is indicated for stage III FH tumors, stages I to III UH tumors, or when chemotherapy and several surgeries do not result in complete tumor resection with negative margins. Unlike in unilateral WT, the performance of a tumor biopsy or the use of chemotherapy before definitive surgery is not an indication for flank RT in BWT.

Effect of Tumor Spillage on Outcome in Patients with Stages II and III Disease

Operative tumor spillage was identified in 24% of patients in NWTS-3 and NWTS-4, and 22% of the spills were classified as diffuse.[42,63,64] An analysis was undertaken to determine the influence of RT and chemotherapy on abdominal tumor recurrence caused by spilled cells in abdominal stages II and III FH WT. The odds ratio for the risk of recurrence relative to no RT was 0.35 for 10 Gy ($P = .01$) and 0.08 for 20 Gy ($P = .01$). Thus, RT (10 or 20 Gy) significantly reduced abdominal tumor recurrence rates following tumor spillage. After adjusting for RT, the effect of doxorubicin on tumor recurrence was not significant. For stage II patients (NWTS-4), the 8-year RFS and OS with and without spillage were 74% and 85% ($P = .02$) and 90% and 94% ($P = .4$), respectively. The higher relapse rate among stage II children with spillage was the reason for upstaging patients with tumor spillage to stage III in the new COG staging system (Table 85.2). These patients will now receive three drugs and flank RT.[42]

Nephrectomy Only for Patients with Stage I Favorable Histology Wilms Tumor

In NWTS-5, a single-arm study was conducted to evaluate the efficacy of nephrectomy alone in children younger than 24 months of age with small (<550 g) stage I FH WT. A total of 75 children were enrolled and the 2-year RFS and OS were 87% and 100%, respectively. This study was ended because of stringent stopping rules.[65] In a recent update, the 5-year RFS and OS for these children treated with just surgery alone were 85% and 98%, respectively. These outcomes were similar after treatment with surgery and two-drug chemotherapy (regimen EE4A).[66]

The COG will again examine the possibility of avoiding any chemotherapy or irradiation in these children. However, only those children (<24 months, tumors <550 g) who have stage I FH tumors after central pathology review, lymph nodes sampling, and CT scan staging will be eligible for the surgery-only therapy.

Wilms Tumor with Peritoneal Implants

The outcome of 57 patients with FH WT and peritoneal implants at the time of nephrectomy in NWTS-4 and NWTS-5 were analyzed. All children received multimodality therapy with three-drug chemotherapy and RT. Forty-seven patients (82%) received whole-abdominal RT to a dose of 10.5 Gy. The overall abdominal and systemic tumor control rates were 97% and 93%, respectively. The detection of peritoneal implants was not associated with inferior survival. The 5-year RFS with and without peritoneal implants was 90% and 83%, respectively.[67]

Clear Cell Sarcoma

In the NWTS-1 through NWTS-4 experience for 351 patients with CCSK, the OS rate was 69%. Multivariate analysis revealed four independent prognostic factors for survival: treatment with doxorubicin, tumor stage, age at diagnosis, and tumor necrosis.[68] In NWTS-4, there was no significant difference among those patients initially randomized to pulse-intensive (PI) or standard chemotherapy with vincristine, dactinomycin, and doxorubicin. The 8-year RFS and OS were 72% and 87% for PI and 70% and 84% for standard chemotherapy, respectively. The second randomization to short-duration and long-duration chemotherapy also did not show any significant difference in survival between the two arms. The survival in NWTS-4 was significantly superior to that of NWTS-3 (83% vs. 67%). The PI chemotherapy administration of dactinomycin and doxorubicin in NWTS-4 was presumed to be one of the reasons for the improvement in outcomes.[69]

Rhabdoid Tumor of Kidney

A total of 142 children with RTK were enrolled in the NWTS-1 through NWTS-5 trials. The OS at 4 years was 23%. The survival rate for children with stages I or II tumors (42%) was significantly higher than for those with stages II or III tumors (16%; $P = .014$). The survival rate in infants <6 months of age was 9% compared with 41% in children >2 years of age ($P < .001$). Children who received a higher dose of RT (>25 Gy) had a significantly better outcome. However, the dose of RT was not an independent predictor of survival.[51]

Anaplastic Wilms Tumor

In NWTS-5, among 2,596 patients who were enrolled, 281 (11%) had anaplastic WT. The 4-year RFS and OS for patients with stage I anaplasia treated with vincristine and dactinomycin without RT were 70% and 83%, respectively. The 4-year RFS for anaplastic tumor patients who underwent immediate nephrectomy and regimen-I chemotherapy was 83%, 65%, and 33% for stages II, III and IV tumors, respectively. The 4-year RFS and OS for stage V tumors were 44% and 55%, respectively. Based on these results, the therapy for stages I, III, IV, and V tumors will be augmented in the new COG protocols (Tables 85.4 and 85.5).[50]

Recurrent Wilms Tumor

Children with relapsed FH WT have a variable prognosis depending on the site of relapse, the time from initial diagnosis to relapse, and their previous therapy. The favorable prognostic factors include no previous treatment with doxorubicin; relapse more than 12 months after diagnosis; and intra-abdominal relapse in a patient not previously treated with abdominal RT.[70] In NWTS-5 relapse protocol, patients who relapsed after initial treatment with vincristine and dactinomycin only without RT were treated on stratum "B" with regimen "I" chemotherapy, surgery, and RT. The 4-year RFS and OS were 71% and 81% for all patients, 68% and 81% for those who relapsed in the lung only, and 78% and 83% for those who relapsed in the operative bed with or without lung metastasis.[71] Patients who relapsed after treatment with vincristine, dactinomycin, doxorubicin, and RT were treated on stratum "C" of NWTS-5 protocol, with alternating courses of drug pairs; cyclophosphamide/etoposide and carboplatin/etoposide, surgery, and RT. The 4-year RFS and OS were 42% and 48% for all patients, and 49% and 53% for those who relapsed in the lung only.[72] The COG protocol (Table 85.5) recommends postoperative RT for all children with abdominal relapse because these tumors are generally large and infiltrative, and surgical resection with negative margins is unlikely.

Wilms Tumor in Older Patients

WT is rarely seen in patients ≥16 years of age. Their survival is similar to that of children and they should be treated similarly.[73,74]

International Society of Pediatric Oncology Trials

The SIOP studies have primarily used preoperative therapy. The goals of administering preoperative therapy are to facilitate surgical removal of the tumor without rupture, to allow for early treatment of micrometastases, and to stratify patients for postoperative therapy based on pathologic tumor response at the time of surgery. The first SIOP trial found that preoperative RT reduced the incidence of tumor spillage but did not increase survival.[75] SIOP-5, reported in 1983, showed that preoperative chemotherapy with vincristine and dactinomycin was as effective as preoperative RT plus dactinomycin in preventing tumor rupture.[76] In SIOP-6, patients with stage I disease were randomly assigned to either 17 or 38 weeks of vincristine and dactinomycin and showed no difference in survival. Among patients with stage II disease and negative lymph nodes (SIOP staging is not identical to NWTS staging) who were randomly assigned to not receive RT, there was a higher recurrence rate.[77] In SIOP-9, there was a randomization of the duration of prenephrectomy therapy with vincristine and dactinomycin (4 weeks vs. 8 weeks). No advantage was noted for 8 weeks of therapy. Among patients with stage II disease with negative lymph nodes, the rate of abdominal relapse was reduced to 7% by the addition of epirubicin.[78] SIOP-93–01 further stratified treatment according to the pathologic response to preoperative chemotherapy. The recommended dose of RT in SIOP-9 and SIOP-93-01 was 15 Gy in patients with low- and intermediate-risk stage III disease and 30 Gy in high-risk patients.[79] SIOP-93-01 showed that the amount of postoperative chemotherapy of stage I patients with either intermediate-risk histology or anaplasia could be reduced to four doses of vincristine and one course of dactinomycin with 5-year RFS and OS rates of 87% and 95%, respectively.[80]

United Kingdom Children's Cancer Study Group

The first UKCCSG Wilms tumor study (UKW1) showed that vincristine could be used alone in patients with stage I FH disease. Among patients with lung metastases, the 6-year survival rate of 65% was significantly worse than the 4-year survival rate of 82% on NWTS-3, probably because of the inclusion of routine WLI in the NWTS.[54] In the second UKCCSG WT study (UKW2), stage I FH patients had similar survival rates as NWTS stage I patients after 10 weekly doses of vincristine. The 4-year survival rate in patients with stage IV disease was higher than in UKW1, at 75%, probably due to the greater use of WLI. The flank RT doses used for stage III FH and UH tumors are 20 Gy and 30 Gy, respectively.[55] The UKW3 trial conducted a randomized comparison of a primary nephrectomy followed by adjuvant therapy based on surgical stage (NWTS approach) and a preoperative chemotherapy followed by nephrectomy and adjuvant therapy (SIOP approach). The 4-year RFS and OS were equivalent in the primary nephrectomy arm (80% and 85%) and in the preoperative chemotherapy arm (79% and 95%), respectively. The UKCCSG has now joined the current SIOP clinical study.[81]

LATE EFFECTS OF TREATMENT

The study of late effects is of paramount importance to prevent survivors of childhood cancer from becoming chronically sick adults.

Scoliosis

A series from Washington University showed a high incidence of scoliosis in 54% of patients who were treated with a median dose of 30 Gy. However, there was minimal functional disability.[82] In another report, the incidence of scoliosis after 10 to 12 Gy, 12.1 to 23.9 Gy, and 24 to 40 Gy was 8%, 46%, and 63%, respectively.[83] Thus, at present, with the use of megavoltage x-rays, lower doses and coverage of the entire width of the vertebra, the incidence of scoliosis should be low.

Congestive Heart Failure

The cumulative frequency of congestive heart failure among patients on NWTS-1 through NWTS-4 was 4.4% at 20 years among patients treated initially with doxorubicin and 17.4% among patients treated with doxorubicin for their first or subsequent relapse. The factors that were significantly associated with the incidence of heart failure were female sex, cumulative doxorubicin dose, WLI, and left abdominal RT.[84]

Pregnancy Outcome in Wilms Tumor Survivors

The NWTS Long-Term Follow-Up Study analyzed pregnancy outcomes among WT survivors. Malposition of the fetus and premature labor were significantly more frequent among previously irradiated women. The offspring of female patients who received flank RT were more likely to be of low birth weight (<2,500 g), premature (<36 weeks of gestation), and to have congenital malformations. A flank RT dose response was identified with higher complication rates at doses >25 Gy. A number of radiation-induced side effects involving the spine, uterus, and ovaries may all have been responsible.[85–87] The pregnancy outcomes in survivors who received abdominal RT on NWTS protocols were also analyzed. Fertility could be preserved in children with upper abdominal RT that did not include the pelvis. In rare instances, fertility could be preserved after whole-abdominal RT to 10.5 Gy. However, higher doses to the abdomen and pelvis resulted in miscarriages and fetal deaths.[88]

END-STAGE RENAL DISEASE

The 20-year cumulative incidence of end-stage renal disease among WT survivors after unilateral nephrectomy on NWTS protocols was 74% for children with Denys-Drash syndrome, 36% for children with WAGR syndrome, 7% for children with genitourinary anomalies, and 0.6% for patients with none of these conditions. The importance of long-term screening for high-risk children to facilitate early detection and treatment of impaired renal function was emphasized.[89]

Second Malignant Neoplasm

Among NWTS patients, the 15-year cumulative risk of second malignant neoplasm (SMN) was 1.6%. The risk of developing a lymphoma or leukemia was 0.4% at 8 years, after which no cases occurred. However, the risk of developing a solid tumor continued to rise sharply with time. Approximately 73% of solid tumors arose within a previous RT field. Higher doses of abdominal RT, doxorubicin use, and treatment for relapse were the significant factors correlated with the development of second tumors.[90] In another NWTS report, the standardized mortality ratio was 24.3 within 5 years of diagnosis, 12.6 for the next 5 years, and >3.0 thereafter. The main cause of mortality within the first 5 years was the original disease (91%). However, beyond 5 years the two important causes of mortality were the original disease (40%) and late effects of treatment (39%). The three common treatment-related late effects that contributed to mortality were SMNs, congestive heart failure, and end-stage renal disease. The risk of death, particularly from treatment-related late effects, remained elevated even 20 years after diagnosis.[91] Similar results have been shown recently by the Childhood Cancer Survivor Study after a follow-up of 25 years.[92] In the British Cancer Survivor Study, the cumulative incidence of a second primary neoplasm at 30, 40, and 50 years of age was 2%, 7%, and 12%, respectively.[93]

FUTURE DIRECTIONS

The first generation of WT protocols conducted by the COG is expected to close in 2013. Study proposals are presently being considered for the second generation of COG protocols. All of these proposals are aimed at further refining the treatment of low-risk patients to decrease treatment-related toxicity and intensify treatment of high-risk tumors to improve outcomes. The following are some of the proposals under consideration: to include tumor molecular signatures as part of the COG risk stratification system to further refine the definition of very low-risk and low-risk WT that will be treated either by surgery alone or surgery followed by two-drug chemotherapy; to use cardiac-sparing intensity-modulated radiation therapy (IMRT) in children receiving WLI to reduce cardiac toxicity[94]; to use IMRT to reduce renal toxicity in children receiving whole-liver irradiation[95]; to re-evaluate the necessity of irradiating all children who receive chemotherapy before nephrectomy; to re-evaluate the current recommendation for using whole-abdomen RT in children with localized preoperative tumor rupture limited to the flank without any ascites or peritoneal implants; to add new biologic agents to the currently used chemotherapy regimens in children with diffuse anaplastic WT and rhabdoid tumors; and to intensify therapy for children with FH WT and lymph node metastases who have a higher risk of tumor relapse. The biologic samples banks of COG will continue to be a valuable source of tissue for studies aimed at identifying new biologic markers that may be of prognostic significance.

REFERENCES

1. Coppes MJ, Ritchey ML, D'Angio GJ. Preface: the path to progress in medical science: a Wilms' tumor conspectus. *Hematol Oncol Clin North Am* 1995;9:xiii–xviii.
2. Birch JM, Breslow N. Epidemiologic features of Wilms' tumor. *Hematol Oncol Clin North Am* 1995;9:1157–1178.
3. Breslow N, Beckwith JB, Ciol M, et al. Age distribution of Wilms' tumor: report from the National Wilms' Tumor Study. *Cancer Res* 1988;48:1653–1657.
4. Breslow NE, Olshan A, Beckwith JB, et al. Epidemiology of Wilms' tumor. *Med Pediatr Oncol* 1983;21:172–181.
5. Coppes MJ, Egeler RM. Genetics of Wilms' tumor. *Semin Urol Oncol* 1999;17:2–10.
6. Call KM, Glaser T, Ito CY, et al. Isolation and characterization of a zinc finger polypeptide gene at the human chromosome 11 Wilms' tumor locus. *Cell* 1990; 60:509–520.
7. Pritchard-Jones K, Fleming S, Davidson D, et al. The candidate Wilms' tumor gene is involved in genitourinary development. *Nature* 1990;346:194–197.
8. Pelletier J, Bruening W, Kashtan CE, et al. Germline mutations in the Wilms' tumor suppressor gene are associated with abnormal urogenital development in Denys-Drash syndrome. *Cell* 1991;67:437–447.
9. Huff V. Wilms' tumor genetics. *Am J Hum Genet* 1998;79:260–267.
10. Koufos A, Grundy P, Morgan K, et al. Familial Wiedemann-Beckwith syndrome and a second Wilms' tumor locus both map to 11p15.5. *Am J Hum Genet* 1989; 44:711–719.
11. Grundy PE, Telzerow PE, Breslow N, et al. Loss of heterozygosity for chromosomes 16q and 1p in Wilms' tumors predicts an adverse outcome. *Cancer Res* 1994;54: 2331–2333.
12. Grundy PE, Breslow NE, Li S, et al. Loss of heterozygosity for chromosomes 1p and 16q is an adverse prognostic factor in favorable histology Wilms tumor: a report from the National Wilms Tumor Study Group. *J Clin Oncol* 2005;23:7312–7321.
13. Rivera MN, Kim WJ, Wells J, et al. An X chromosome gene, WTX, is commonly inactivated in Wilms tumor. *Science* 2007;315:642–645.
14. Williams RD, Al-Saadi R, Natrajan R, et al. Molecular profiling reveals frequent gain of *MYCN* and anaplasia-specific loss of 4q and 14q in Wilms' tumor. *Genes Chromosomes Cancer* 2011;50:982–995.
15. Gadd S, Sredni ST, Huang CC, et al. Rhabdoid tumor: gene expression clues to pathogenesis and potential therapeutic targets. *Lab Invest* 2010;90:724–738.
16. Perlman EJ, Grundy PE, Anderson JR, et al. *WT1* mutation and 11p15 loss predict relapse in very low-risk Wilms' tumor treated with surgery alone: a Children's Oncology Group Study. *J Clin Oncol* 2010;26:698–703.
17. Beckwith JB, Palmer NJ. Histopathology and prognosis of Wilms' tumor: results from the first National Wilms' Tumor Study. *Cancer* 1978;41:1937–1948.
18. D'Angio GJ, Breslow N, Beckwith JB, et al. The treatment of Wilms' tumor: results of the Third National Wilms' Tumor Study. *Cancer* 1989;64:349–360.
19. Beckwith JB, Zuppan CE, Browning NG, et al. Histological analysis of aggressiveness and responsiveness in Wilms' tumor. *Med Pediatr Oncol* 1996;27:422–428.
20. Beckwith JB. Precursor lesions of Wilms' tumor: clinical and biological implications. *Med Pediatr Oncol* 1993;21:158–168.
21. Beckwith JB. Nephrogenic rests and the pathogenesis of Wilms' tumor: developmental and clinical considerations. *Am J Med Genet* 1998;79:268–273.
22. Coppes MJ, Arnold M, Beckwith JB, et al. Factors affecting the risk of contralateral Wilms' tumor development: a report from the National Wilms' Tumor Study Group. *Cancer* 1999;85:1616–1625.
23. Bonadio JF, Storer B, Norkool P, et al. Anaplastic Wilms' tumor: clinical and pathologic studies. *J Clin Oncol* 1985;3:513–520.
24. Faria P, Beckwith JB, Mishra K, et al. Focal versus diffuse anaplasia in Wilms' tumor: new definitions with prognostic significance. A report from the National Wilms' Tumor Study Group. *Am J Surg Pathol* 1996;20:909–920.
25. Schmidt D, Beckwith JB. Histopathology of childhood renal tumors. *Hematol Oncol Clin North Am* 1995;9:1179–1200.
26. Ledlie EM, Mynors LS, Draper GJ, et al. Natural history and treatment of Wilms' tumor: an analysis of 335 cases occurring in England and Wales 1962–1966. *BMJ* 1970;4:195–200.
27. Sukarochana K, Tolentino W, Kiesewetter WB. Wilms' tumor and hypertension. *J Pediatr Surg* 1972;7:573–576.
28. Hartman DS, Sanders RC. Wilms' tumor versus neuroblastoma: usefulness of ultrasound in differentiation. *J Ultrasound Med* 1982;1:117–122.
29. Ramos IM, Taylor KJW, Kier R, et al. Tumor vascular signals in renal masses: detection with Doppler US. *Radiology* 1988;168:633.
30. Khanna G, Rosen N, Anderson JR, et al. Evaluation of diagnostic performance of CT for detection of tumor thrombus in children with Wilms tumor: a report from the Children's Oncology Group. *Pediatr Blood Cancer* 2012;58(4):551–555.
31. Reiman TAH, Siegel MJ, Shackelford GD. Wilms' tumor in children: abdominal CT and US evaluation. *Radiology* 1986;160:501–505.
32. Belt TG, Cohen MD, Smith JA, et al. MRI of Wilms' tumor: promise as the primary imaging modality. *AJR Am J Roentgenol* 1986;146:955–961.
33. Gylys-Morin V, Hoffer FA, Kozakewich H, et al. Wilms' tumor and nephroblastomatosis: imaging characteristics at gadolinium-enhanced MR imaging. *Radiology* 1993;188:517–521.

34. Ritchey ML, Green DM, Breslow NB, et al. Accuracy of current imaging modalities in the diagnosis of synchronous bilateral Wilms' tumor: a report from the National Wilms' Tumor Study Group. *Cancer* 1995;75:600–604.
35. Cohen MD. Current controversy: is computed tomography scan of the chest needed in patients with Wilms' tumor? *Am J Pediatr Hematol Oncol* 1994;16:191–193.
36. Gross RE, Neuhauser EBD. Treatment of mixed tumors of the kidney in childhood. *Pediatrics* 1950;6:843.
37. D'Angio GJ, Evans AE, Breslow NE, et al. The treatment of Wilms' tumor: results of the Second National Wilms' Tumor Study. *Cancer* 1981;47:2302–2311.
38. Farewell VT, D'Angio GJ, Breslow N, et al. Retrospective validation of a new staging system for Wilms' tumor. *Cancer Clin Trials* 1981;4:167–171.
39. Breslow N, Churchill G, Nesmith B, et al. Clinicopathologic features and prognosis for Wilms' tumor patients with metastases at diagnosis. *Cancer* 1986;58:2501–2511.
40. Beckwith JB. National Wilms' Tumor Study: an update for pathologists. *Pediatr Dev Pathol* 1998;1:79–84.
41. Weeks DA, Beckwith JB, Luckey DW. Relapse-associated variables in stage I favorable histology Wilms' tumor: a report of the National Wilms' Tumor Study. *Cancer* 1987;60:1204–1212.
42. Kalapurakal JA, Li SM, Breslow NE, et al. Intraoperative spillage of favorable histology Wilms tumor cells: influence of irradiation and chemotherapy regimens on abdominal recurrence: a report from the National Wilms Tumor Study. *Int J Radiat Oncol Biol Phys* 2010;76:201–206.
43. Leape LL, Breslow NE, Bishop HC. The surgical treatment of Wilms' tumor: results of the National Wilms' Tumor Study. *Ann Surg* 1978;187:351–356.
44. D'Angio GJ, Evans AE, Breslow NE, et al. The treatment of Wilms' tumor: results of the National Wilms' Tumor Study. *Cancer* 1976;38:633–646.
45. D'Angio GJ, Tefft M, Breslow NE, et al. Radiation therapy of Wilms' tumor: results according to dose, field, postoperative timing and histology. *Int J Radiat Oncol Biol Phys* 1978;4:769–780.
46. Thomas PRM, Tefft M, Compaan PJ, et al. Results of two radiotherapy randomizations in the third National Wilms' Tumor Study (NWTS-3). *Cancer* 1991;68: 1703–1707.
47. Thomas PRM, Tefft M, Farewell VT, et al. Abdominal relapses in the Second National Wilms' Tumor Study patients. *J Clin Oncol* 1984;2:1098–1101.
48. Kalapurakal JA, Li SM, Breslow NE, et al. Influence of radiation therapy delay on abdominal tumor recurrence in patients with favorable histology Wilms tumor treated on NWTS-3 and -4: a report from the National Wilms Tumor Study Group. *Int J Radiat Oncol Biol Phys* 2003;57:495–499.
49. Green DM, Beckwith JB, Breslow NE, et al. The treatment of children with stages II–IV anaplastic Wilms' tumor: a report from the National Wilms' Tumor Study Group. *J Clin Oncol* 1994;12:2126–2131.
50. Dome JS, Cotton CA, Perlman EJ, et al. Treatment of anaplastic histology Wilms tumor: results from the fifth National Wilms Tumor Study. *J Clin Oncol* 2006;24: 2352–2358.
51. Tomlinson GE, Breslow NE, Dome J, et al. Rhabdoid tumor of the kidney in the National Wilms Tumor Study: age at diagnosis as a prognostic factor. *J Clin Oncol* 2005;23:7641–7645.
52. Green DM, Breslow NE, Beckwith JB, et al. Comparison between single-dose and divided-dose administration of dactinomycin and doxorubicin for patients with Wilms' tumor: a report from the National Wilms' Tumor Study Group. *J Clin Oncol* 1998;16:237–245.
53. Green DM, Breslow NE, Evans I, et al. The effect of chemotherapy dose intensity on the hematological toxicity of the treatment for Wilms' tumor: a report from the National Wilms' Tumor Study. *Am J Pediatr Hematol Oncol* 1994;16:207–212.
54. Pritchard J, Imeson J, Barnes J, et al. Results of the United Kingdom Children's Cancer Study Group First Wilms' Tumor Study. *J Clin Oncol* 1995;13:124–133.
55. Mitchell C, Jones PM, Kelsey A, et al. The treatment of Wilms' tumor: results of the United Kingdom Children's Cancer Study Group (UKCCSG) second Wilms' tumor study. *Br J Cancer* 2000;83:602–608.
56. Meisel JA, Guthrie KA, Breslow NE, et al. Significance and management of computed tomography detected pulmonary nodules: a report from the National Wilms' Tumor Study Group. *Int J Radiat Oncol Biol Phys* 1999;44:579–585.
57. Grundy P, Li SM, Green DM, et al. Event free but not overall survival is improved for Wilms tumour patients with pulmonary lesions detectable only by computed tomography by the addition of doxorubicin but not from pulmonary irradiation: results of National Wilms Tumour Studies 4 and 5. *Pediatr Blood Cancer* 2012;59(4):631–635.
58. Ehrlich PF, Ferrerar F, Ritchey M, et al. Hepatic metastasis at diagnosis in favorable histology Wilms tumor is not an independent adverse prognostic factor. A report from the National Wilms Tumor Study Group. *Ann Surg* 2009;250:642–648.
59. Blute ML, Kelalis PP, Offord KP, et al. Bilateral Wilms' tumor. *J Urol* 1987;138: 968–973.
60. Hamilton TE, Ritchey ML, Haase GL, et al. The management of synchronous bilateral Wilms tumor: a report from the National Wilms Tumor Study Group. *Ann Surg* 2011;253:1004–1010.
61. Shamberger RC, Haase GC, Argani P, et al. Bilateral Wilms tumors with progressive or nonresponsive disease. *J Pediatr Surg* 2006;41:652–657.
62. Hamilton TE, Green DM, Perlman EJ, et al. Bilateral Wilms tumor with anaplasia: lessons from the National Wilms Tumor Study. *J Pediatr Surg* 2006;41:1641–1644.
63. Breslow NE, Beckwith JB, Haase GM, et al. Radiation therapy for favorable histology Wilms' tumor: prevention of flank recurrence did not improve survival on National Wilms Tumor Studies 3 and 4. *Int J Radiat Oncol Biol Phys* 2006;65:203–209.
64. Shamberger RC, Guthrie KA, Ritchey ML, et al. Surgery-related factors and local recurrence of Wilms' tumor in National Wilms' Tumor Study 4. *Ann Surg* 1999; 229:292–297.
65. Green DM, Breslow NE, Beckwith JB, et al. Treatment with nephrectomy only for small, stage I/favorable histology Wilms' tumor: a report from the National Wilms' Tumor Study Group. *J Clin Oncol* 2001;19:3719–3724.
66. Shamberger RC, Anderson JR, Breslow NE, et al. Long term outcomes of infants with very low risk Wilms tumor treated with surgery alone on National Wilms Tumor Study-5. *Ann Surg* 2010;251:555–558.
67. Kalapurakal JA, Green DM, Haase G, et al. Outcomes of children with favorable histology Wilms 'tumor and peritoneal implants treated on National Wilms' Tumor Studies-4 and -5. *Int J Radiat Oncol Biol Phys* 2010;77:554–558.
68. Argani P, Perlman EJ, Breslow NE, et al. Clear cell sarcoma of the kidney: a review of 351 cases from the National Wilms' Tumor Study Group Pathology Center. *Am J Surg Pathol* 2000;24:4–18.
69. Seibel N, Li S, Breslow NE, et al. Effect of duration of treatment on treatment outcome for patients with clear-cell sarcoma of the kidney: a report from the National Wilms' Tumor Study Group. *J Clin Oncol* 2004;22:468–473.
70. Grundy P, Breslow NE, Green DM, et al. Prognostic factors of children with recurrent Wilms' tumor: results from the second and third National Wilms' Tumor Study. *J Clin Oncol* 1989;7:638–647.
71. Green DM, Cotton CA, Malogolowkin M, et al. Treatment of Wilms tumor relapsing after initial therapy with vincristine and actinomycin D. A report from the National Wilms Tumor Study Group. *Pediatr Blood Cancer* 2007;48:493–499.
72. Malogolowkin M, Cotton CA, Green DM, et al. Treatment of Wilms tumor relapsing after initial treatment with vincristine, actinomycin D and doxorubicin. A report from the National Wilms tumor Study Group. *Pediatr Blood Cancer* 2008;50: 236–241.
73. Kalapurakal JA, Nan B, Norkool P, et al. Treatment outcomes in adults with favorable histologic type Wilms tumor: an update from the National Wilms Tumor Study Group. *Int J Radiat Oncol Biol Phys* 2004;60:1379–1384.
74. Segers H, van den Heuvel-Eibrink MM, Pritchard-Jones K, et al Management of adults with Wilms' tumor: recommendations based on international consensus. *Expert Rev Anticancer Ther* 2011;11:1105–1113.
75. Lemerle J, Vote PA, Tournade MF, et al. Preoperative versus postoperative radiotherapy, single versus multiple courses of actinomycin D in the treatment of Wilms' tumor. *Cancer* 1976;38:647–654.
76. Lemerle J, Vote PA, Tournade MF, et al. Effectiveness of preoperative chemotherapy in Wilms' tumor: results of an International Society of Pediatric Oncology (SIOP) trial. *J Clin Oncol* 1983;1:604–609.
77. Jereb B, Burgers MV, Tournade M-F, et al. Radiotherapy in the SIOP (International Society of Paediatric Oncology) nephroblastoma studies: a review. *Med Pediatr Oncol* 1994;22:221–227.
78. DeKraker J, Weitzman S, Vote PA. Preoperative strategies in the management of Wilms' tumor. *Hematol Oncol Clin North Am* 1995;9:1275–1285.
79. Graf N, Tournade MF, de Kraker J. The role of preoperative chemotherapy in the management of Wilms' tumor. The SIOP studies. *Urol Clin North Am* 2000;27: 443–454.
80. De Kraker J, Graf N, van Tinteren H, et al. Reduction of postoperative chemotherapy in children with stage I intermediate-risk and anaplastic Wilms tumor (SIOP-93–01): a randomized trial. *Lancet* 2004;364:1229–1235.
81. Mitchell C, Shannon R, Vujanic GM, et al. The treatment of Wilms tumor: results of the United Kingdom Children's Cancer Study group Third Wilms Tumor Study. *Med Pediatr Oncol* 2003;41:289.
82. Thomas PRM, Griffith KD, Fineberg BB, et al. Late effects of treatment for Wilms' tumor. *Int J Radiat Oncol Biol Phys* 1983;9:651–657.
83. Paulino AC, Wen BC, Brown CK, et al. Late effects in children treated with radiation therapy for Wilms' tumor. *Int J Radiat Oncol Biol Phys* 2000;46:1239–1246.
84. Green DM, Grigoriev YA, Nan B, et al. Congestive heart failure after treatment for Wilms' tumor: a report from the National Wilms' Tumor Study Group. *J Clin Oncol* 2001;19:1926–1934.
85. Critchley HOD. Factors of importance for implantation and problems after treatment for childhood cancer. *Med Pediatr Oncol* 1999;33:9–14.
86. Green DM, Peabody EM, Nan B, et al. Pregnancy outcome after treatment for Wilms' tumor. *J Clin Oncol* 2002;20:2506–2513.
87. Green DM, Lange JM, Peabody EM, et al Pregnancy outcome after treatment for Wilms tumor: a report from the national Wilms tumor long-term follow-up study. *J Clin Oncol* 2010;28:2824–2830.
88. Kalapurakal JA, Peterson S, Peabody EM, et al. Pregnancy outcomes after abdominal irradiation that included or excluded the pelvis in childhood Wilms tumor survivors: a report of the National Wilms Tumor Study. *Int J Radiat Oncol Biol Phys* 2004;58:1364–1368.
89. Breslow NE, Collins AJ, Ritchey ML, et al. End stage renal disease in patients with Wilms tumor: results from the National Wilms Tumor Study Group and the United States renal data system. *J Urol* 2005;174:1972–1975.
90. Breslow NE, Takashima JR, Whitton JA, et al. Second malignant neoplasms following treatment for Wilms' tumor: a report from the National Wilms' Tumor Study Group. *J Clin Oncol* 1995;13:1851–1859.
91. Cotton CA, Peterson S, Norkool PA, et al. Early and late mortality after diagnosis of Wilms tumor. *J Clin Oncol* 2009;27:1304–1309.
92. Termhuhlen AM, Tersak JM, Liu Q, et al. Twenty-five year follow up of childhood Wilms tumor. A report from the Childhood Cancer Survivor Study. *Pediatr Blood Cancer* 2011;57:1210–1216.
93. Taylor AJ, Winter DL, Pritchard-Jones K, et al. Second primary neoplasms in survivors of Wilms tumor: a population-based cohort study from the British Cancer Survivor Study. *Int J Cancer* 2008;122:2085–2093.
94. Kalapurakal JA, Gopalakrishnan M, Zhang Y, et al. Advantages of cardiac-sparing whole lung IMRT in children with lung metastases from Wilms' tumor, rhabdomyosarcoma or Ewing Sarcoma: a dosimetry study based on 4-D gated chest CT scans. *Int J Radiat Oncol Biol Phys* 2011;18(2):S662.
95. Kalapurakal JA, Zhang Y, Sathiaseelan V, et al. Advantages of whole liver IMRT compared to standard AP-PA technique in children with liver metastasis from right or left sided unilateral Wilms' tumor: a 3–4D CT dosimetry study *Int J Radiat Oncol Biol Phys* 2011;18(2):S663.

Chapter 86
Neuroblastoma

David B. Mansur and Jeff M. Michalski

Neuroblastoma is an enigmatic malignant neoplasm. In its early stages it can be readily cured with surgery or, in some circumstances, can even spontaneously regress or mature to a benign ganglioneuroma. In the more common advanced stages, the disease is often fatal. The unique biology of neuroblastoma has attracted the interest of many prominent scientists and is one of the first malignancies in which molecular biologic assays have influenced treatment and prognosis.

EPIDEMIOLOGY

After brain tumors and leukemia, neuroblastoma is the third-most-common malignancy diagnosed in children, with an annual incidence of 9 new cases per 1 million children in the United States. It is the most common cancer diagnosed before the age of 12 months, accounting for almost half of all cancers in infants. The median age at diagnosis is 2 years. The relatively good prognosis of infants diagnosed with early-stage neuroblastoma prompted the initiation of infant-screening studies.[1]

Screening of infants for neuroblastoma has been studied systematically in large clinical trials conducted in Japan, North America, and Europe.[2–5] Excretion of catecholamine metabolites in the urine of children with neuroblastoma has served as the basis of these screening tests. Urine samples were collected and dried on filter paper and returned to screening centers to be tested qualitatively for vanillylmandelic acid (VMA) levels or quantitatively for VMA and homovanillic acid (HVA) measured by high-performance liquid chromatography and normalized to urinary creatinine levels. Children with elevated levels of these metabolites subsequently were referred for further diagnostic evaluation. The incidences of the diagnosis and death rates from neuroblastoma in the screened populations were compared to control populations in the same country or continent. The study populations generally were chosen because of access to an existing screening infrastructure that could readily be adapted to neuroblastoma. The Japanese study screened children at 6 months of age. The Quebec study screened children at 3 weeks and 6 months of age. The German study tested children at their first year's birthday.

The results and conclusions of these three large screening trials on three continents are remarkably similar. In Japan, 1,142,519 children were screened using a qualitative test, and another 550,331 were screened with the quantitative test; they all were compared to 713,025 children in a control population. The incidence rates per 100,000 were 1.12 in the control group compared to 5.69 in the qualitative group and 17.81 in the quantitative group. Despite this increased incidence in the screened group, the neuroblastoma mortality rates were unchanged by the screening.[5] In Germany, 1,475,773 children were screened between 1994 and 1999. Screening detected neuroblastoma in 149 children, 3 of whom died. Despite the screening at 12 months, another 55 children subsequently developed neuroblastoma, 14 of whom died. Compared to the control group, the incidence of stage 4 neuroblastoma was similar. The death rate from neuroblastoma was unaffected by the screening.[3] In Quebec, a total of 425,838 children were enrolled in the neuroblastoma screening trial (89% of births during a 5-year study period from 1989 to 1994). The standardized incidence ratios of neuroblastoma death in the Quebec cohort were nearly identical to those in control groups in Ontario, Minnesota, Florida, and the Greater Delaware Valley.[4] In summary, each of these trials demonstrates that screening does not affect the mortality rate of neuroblastoma. Furthermore, the overdiagnosis of clinically insignificant disease may lead to significant financial, emotional, and physical burdens on the children and their families. This tumor has a high frequency of spontaneous regression in infancy. The mass screening programs have led to the diagnosis of biologically favorable and clinically insignificant tumors.[6,7]

NATURAL HISTORY

Neuroblastoma, along with ganglioneuroma and ganglioneuroblastoma, may arise from any site in the sympathetic nervous system. The most common sites of origin are the adrenal medulla (30% to 40%) and paraspinal ganglia in the abdomen or pelvis (25%). Thoracic (15%) and head and neck primary tumors (5%) are slightly more common in infants than in older children. More than 70% of patients have metastatic disease at presentation. The most frequent metastatic sites are lymph nodes, bone, bone marrow, skin (or subcutaneous tissues), and liver.[8] The lung and central nervous system are rare sites of involvement.

Neuroblastoma has the highest spontaneous remission rate of any human neoplasm, usually by maturation to ganglioneuroma.[9] Microscopic neuroblastomas have been found in the autopsy material of the adrenal glands of young infants at >40 times the expected rate. It has been suggested that most potential neuroblastomas are never clinically manifested, because of spontaneous regression.[10] Despite these peculiarities, clinically obvious neuroblastoma is frequently a progressive and relentless disease.

CLINICAL PRESENTATION

Pain is the most common presenting symptom. This frequently is caused by bone, liver, or bone marrow metastases or local visceral invasion by the primary tumor. Other constitutional symptoms may include weight loss, anorexia, malaise, and fever. Respiratory distress may accompany massive hepatomegaly, especially in infants with stage IV-S disease.[8] Horner's syndrome can accompany a primary tumor originating in the neck. Spinal cord compression with paralysis of the lower extremities can accompany the so-called dumbbell-shaped tumor that extends from its origin along the sympathetic ganglia through the adjacent neural foramina. Orbital metastases are not uncommon and can cause proptosis and ecchymosis. Skin metastases may have a bluish tinge, giving the classic "blueberry muffin" sign. When pressed, the release of catecholamine into the tissue causes transient blanching of the adjacent skin. An unusual presentation of localized neuroblastoma is the opsoclonus–myoclonus syndrome, manifested by truncal ataxia and cerebellar encephalopathy. This syndrome typically indicates a favorable prognosis from the tumor, but patients may have persistent neurologic sequelae after successful tumor therapy.[11,12]

DIAGNOSTIC WORKUP

As in the case of any suspected malignant neoplasm in children, the diagnosis of neuroblastoma must be established by pathologic evaluation. Tumor tissue may be obtained from the suspected primary tumor site or from involved lymph nodes by excision (if the tumor is resectable) or incisional biopsy. Bone marrow aspirate and biopsy frequently show metastatic tumor deposits that can establish the diagnosis. Pathologic evaluation of bone marrow is also a requirement for staging of neuroblastoma. Characteristically, neuroblastoma in bone marrow appears in clumps and pseudorosettes. The absence of pseudorosettes does not eliminate the possibility of neuroblastoma.

Laboratory studies should include measurement of urinary catecholamines and their metabolites. Either HVA or VMA, metabolites of dopa/norepinephrine and epinephrine, respectively, is elevated in >90% of patients with stage IV neuroblastoma. A ratio of VMA to HVA of >1.5 is associated with a favorable prognosis in patients with metastatic neuroblastoma. An assay for urinary VMA is the basis for screening studies of infants in Japan, Europe, and North America. Anemia secondary to bone marrow involvement with tumor can be evaluated with a complete blood cell count. Serum ferritin, lactate dehydrogenase (LDH), and other liver function indicators should be assayed routinely.

Appropriate use of imaging studies assists in staging and in planning an approach to therapy. X-ray studies demonstrate intrinsic speckled calcifications in 85% of neuroblastomas. Computed tomography (CT) of the abdomen with intravenous contrast is more sensitive than intravenous pyelography and provides more information about lymph-node or hepatic metastases as well as tumor resectability.[13] Increasingly, high-quality magnetic resonance imaging (MRI) scans are replacing the routine use of CT in evaluation of suspicious thoracic or abdominal masses in children. Although MRI cannot demonstrate intratumoral calcifications, it allows better evaluation of blood vessel encasement, intraspinal extension (dumbbell tumors), diffuse hepatic replacement, and bone marrow involvement (Fig. 86.1). Each of these findings improves staging accuracy and facilitates

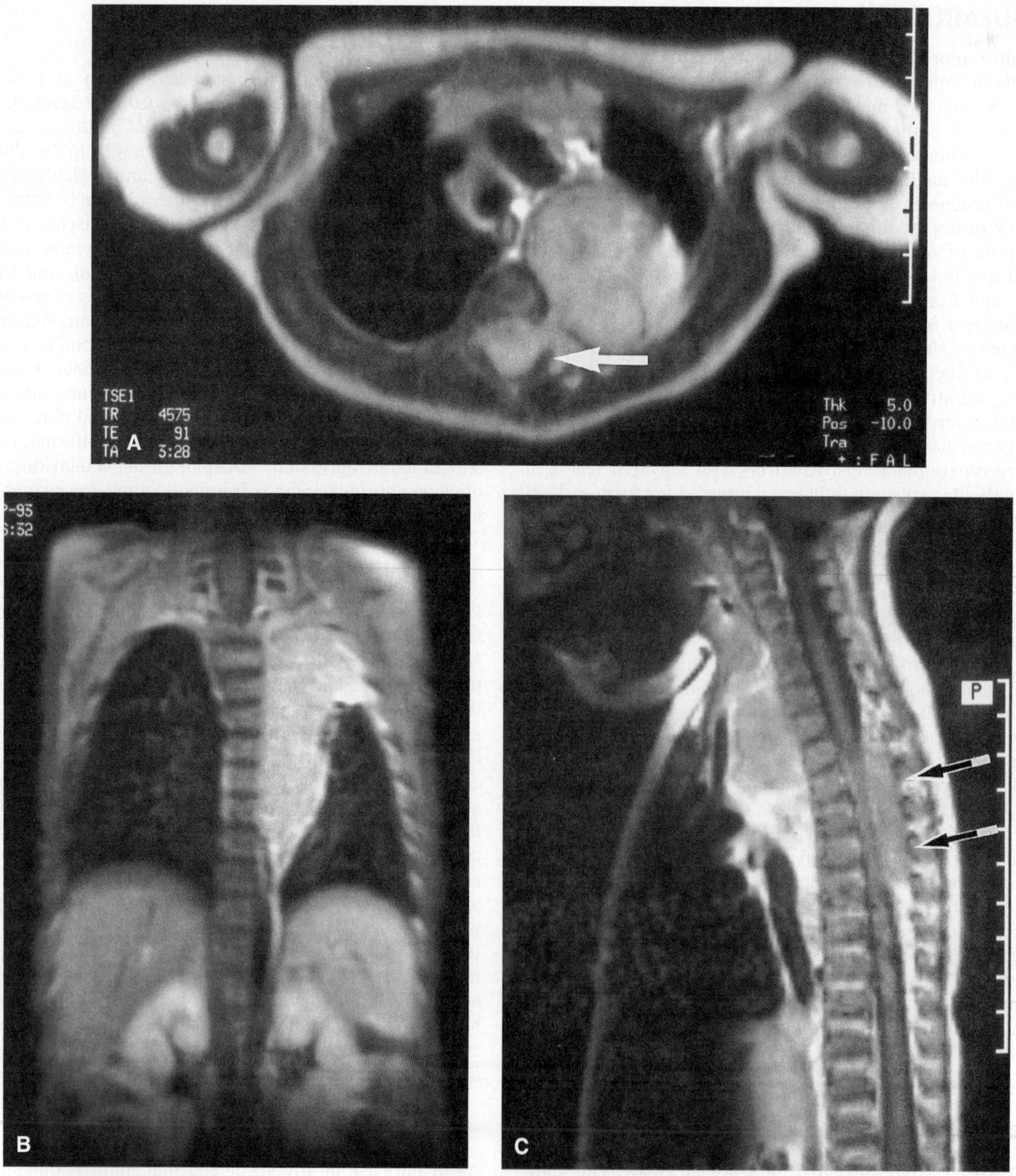

FIGURE 86.1. Magnetic resonance imaging scans of a 4-month-old child with a thoracic neuroblastoma. The dumbbell shape of the paraspinal mass can be appreciated on axial **(A)**, coronal **(B)**, and sagittal **(C)** images. The intraspinal component is indicated by arrows. The three views of this child's tumor are helpful in radiation-therapy field design.

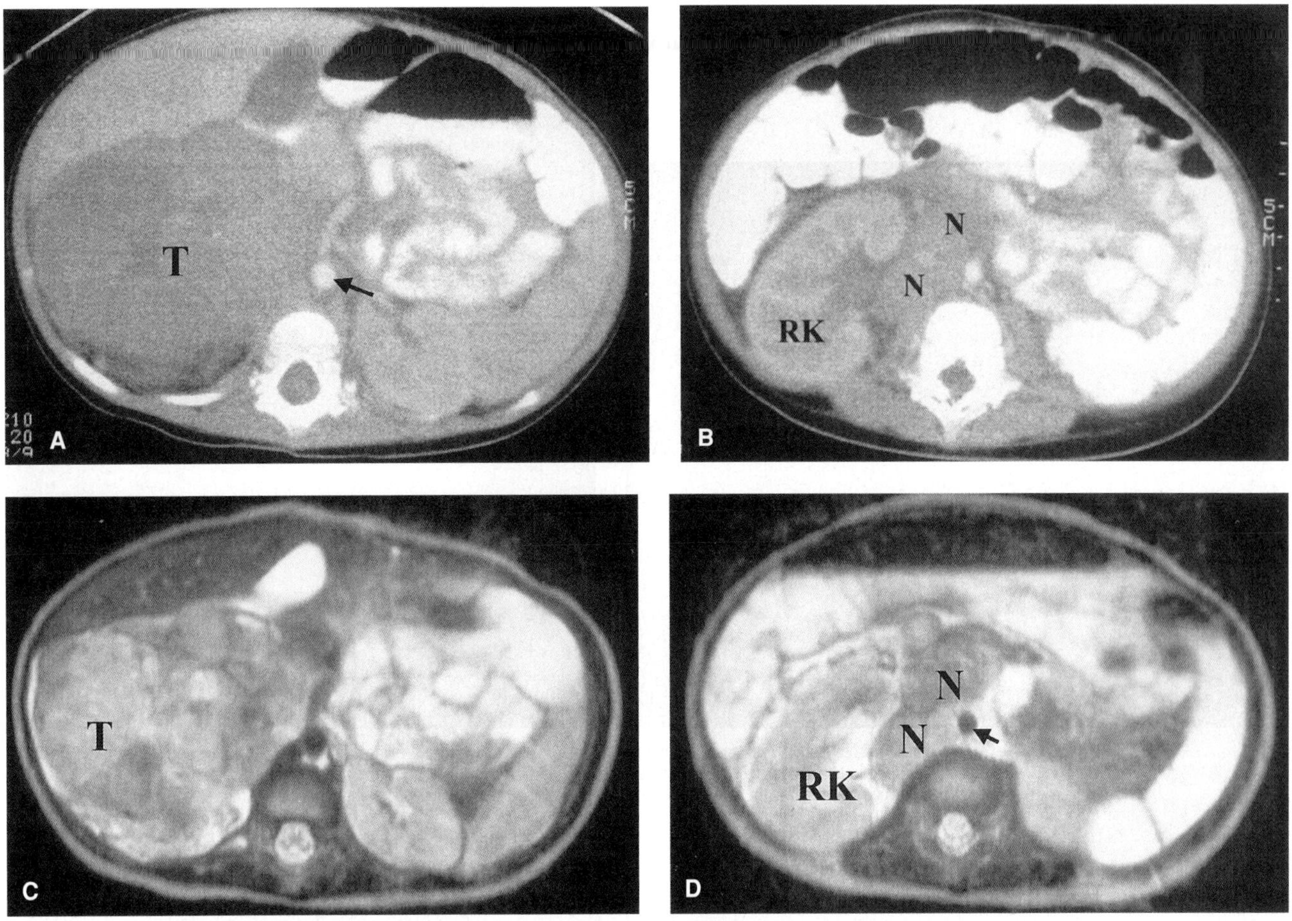

FIGURE 86.2. Neuroblastoma with nodal involvement in a 3-year-old boy. **A:** Computed tomography (CT) through the upper abdomen shows a large soft-tissue mass (*T*) arising in the right adrenal gland and extending to the midline (aorta, *arrow*). **B:** A CT scan several centimeters lower shows several small nodes (*N*) in the right pararenal area. **C:** T_2-weighted axial image shows a high–signal intensity tumor (*T*) in the right suprarenal area. **D:** T_2-weighted image at a lower level shows enlarged, mildly enhancing paracaval lymph nodes (*N*). (R, right kidney; arrow, aorta). (Courtesy of Dr. Marilyn Siegel, Mallinckrodt Institute of Radiology, St. Louis, MO.)

the decision-making process regarding appropriate surgical interventions.[14–17]

Nuclear medicine scans are helpful in determining the extent of metastatic disease. Because neuroblastoma has a predilection for bony metastases, a radionuclide bone scan is a mandatory investigation. It is more sensitive than a skeletal survey in detecting bone metastases[18] *Meta*-iodobenzylguanidine (MIBG) is concentrated by neurosecretory granules of both normal and neoplastic tissues of neural crest origin and can be used to image primary and metastatic sites of neuroblastoma. MIBG labeled with either ^{131}I or ^{123}I has a sensitivity of 85% to 90% and a specificity of almost 95% in the detection of metastatic neuroblastoma.[19] Poor scintigraphic response on ^{123}I-MIBG scans after induction chemotherapy has been shown to predict for a poor event-free survival in patients undergoing high-dose chemotherapy with stem cell rescue.[20] Like other neural crest–derived neoplasms, neuroblastoma can express somatostatin receptors. The long-acting somatostatin analog octreotide labeled with ^{123}I has been used to image neuroblastoma with a sensitivity comparable to that of ^{131}I-MIBG.[21] The expression of somatostatin receptors by neuroblastoma tissues is a favorable prognostic factor.[22]

The Radiology Diagnostic Oncology Group enrolled 96 children with newly diagnosed neuroblastoma in a multicenter prospective cohort study prior to surgery. CT, MRI, and bone scintigraphy were used to evaluate tumor stage. The results show that MRI is more accurate than CT for detection of stage IV disease (sensitivities 0.83 and 0.43, respectively). When combined with bone scintigraphy, both imaging tests have high accuracy for the detection of metastases. Figures 86.2 to 86.4 illustrate the value of CT and MRI in staging patients with metastatic disease. The prevalence of determinants of local disease was relatively low in this study because patients who had extensive disease at time of entry underwent delayed surgery after induction chemotherapy. Although the numbers are small, the data suggest the following: (a) in stage I tumor, abdominal extent was more likely to be staged correctly with CT than with MRI, which often overstaged tumor; (b) for stage II and III tumors, both CT and MRI were more likely to understage than overstage tumor; and (c) for stage II tumor, understaging was more likely with CT than MRI.

STAGING

The most commonly used staging system is the International Neuroblastoma Staging System (INSS). It is based on clinical, radiographic, and surgical findings.[23] The INSS integrates many of the concepts of previous staging systems promoted by the Children's Cancer Group (CCG) and Pediatric Oncology Group (POG)[24,25] and unifies them into a single system. Each of these systems is summarized in Table 86.1.

PATHOLOGIC CLASSIFICATION

Neuroblastomas are derived from primitive neural crest cells arising from within sympathetic ganglia. Three types of tumors, representing different degrees of differentiation, are recognized. *Ganglioneuroma* consists of mature ganglion cells,

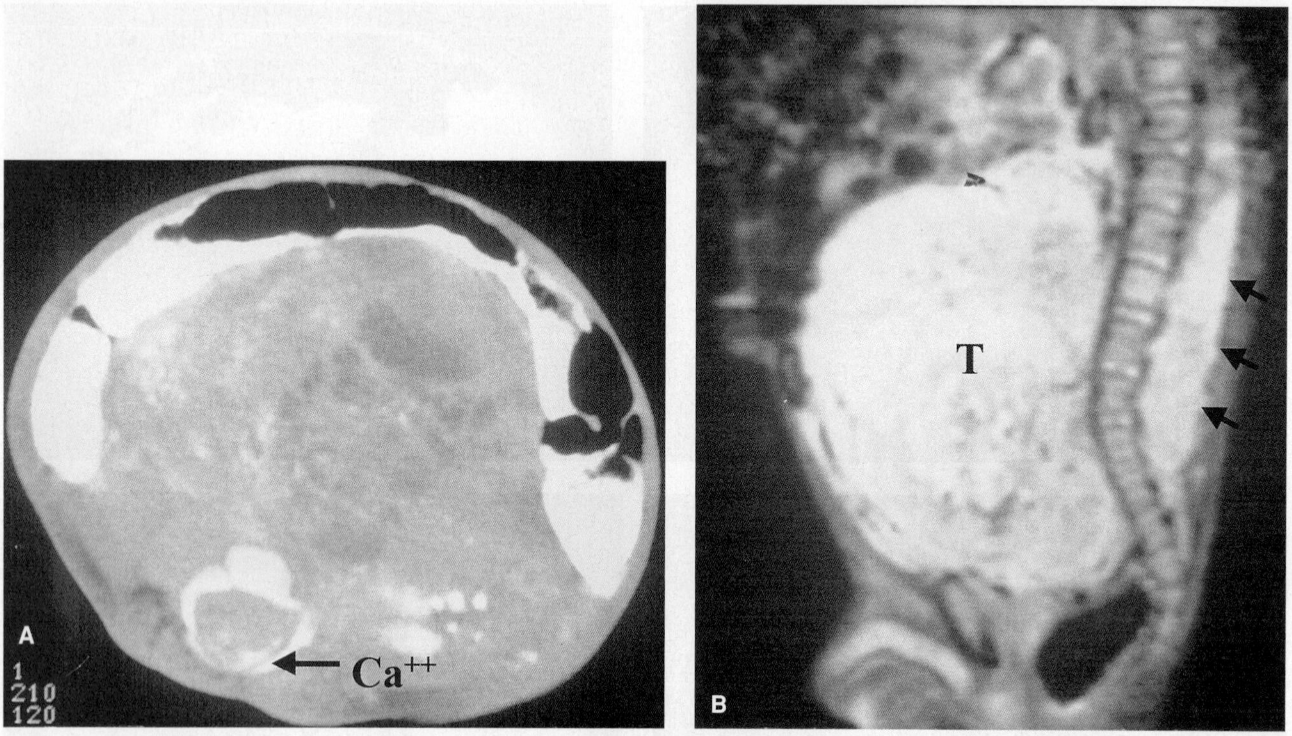

FIGURE 86.3. A 1-year-old child with constipation and a palpable mass, also noted to have lower leg weakness. **A:** Computed tomography shows a large soft-tissue mass with calcifications and necrosis filling the retroperitoneum. Tumor calcification (*arrow*) is noted in the spinal cord. **B:** Sagittal, short-tau inversion recovery image shows the large prevertebral mass displacing bowel loops superiorly. Intraspinal tumor extends from the lower thoracic level through the lumbar level. The patient underwent emergent resection of the intraspinal tumor (*arrows*). (Courtesy of Dr. Marilyn Siegel, Mallinckrodt Institute of Radiology, St. Louis, MO.)

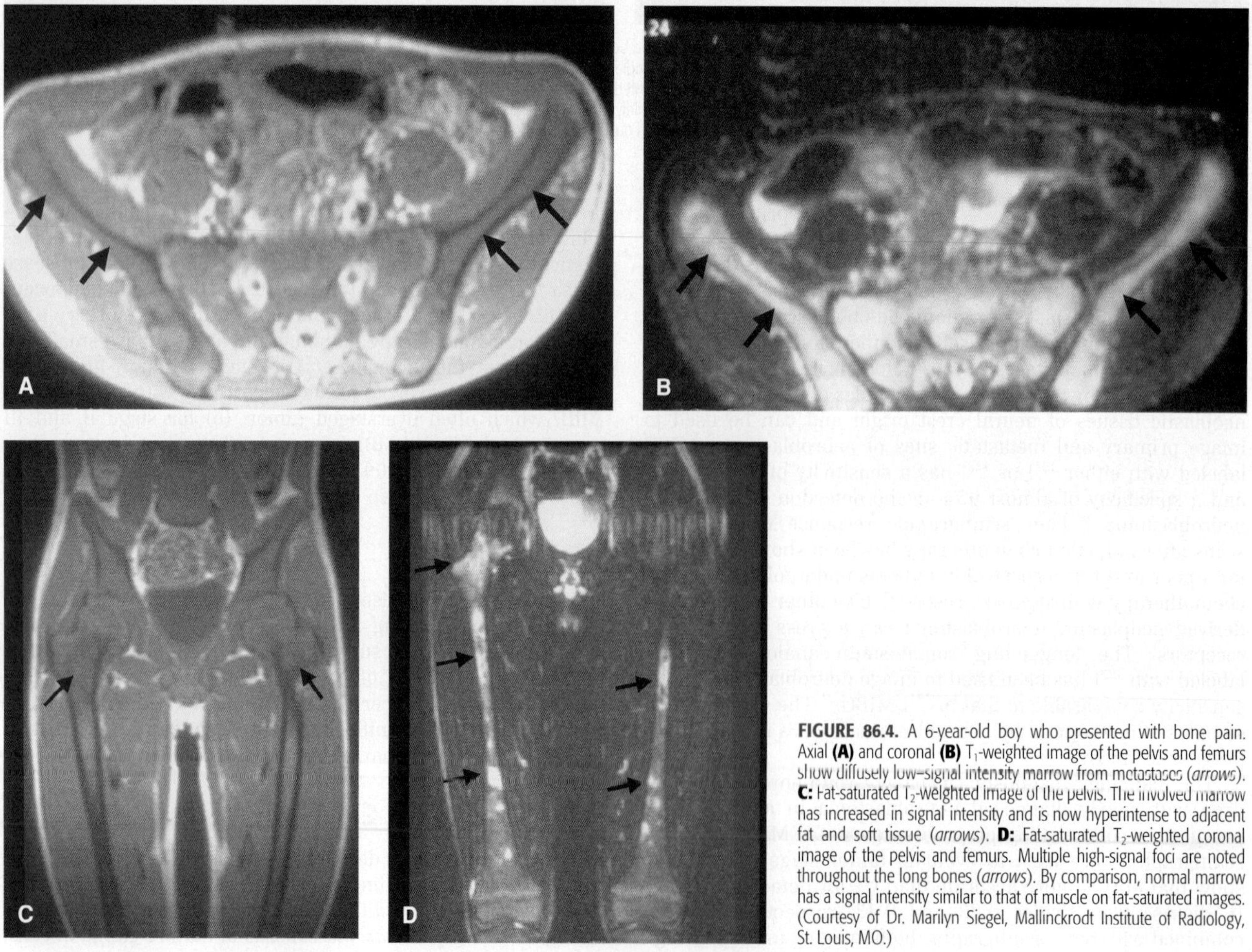

FIGURE 86.4. A 6-year-old boy who presented with bone pain. Axial **(A)** and coronal **(B)** T_1-weighted image of the pelvis and femurs show diffusely low–signal intensity marrow from metastases (*arrows*). **C:** Fat-saturated T_2-weighted image of the pelvis. The involved marrow has increased in signal intensity and is now hyperintense to adjacent fat and soft tissue (*arrows*). **D:** Fat-saturated T_2-weighted coronal image of the pelvis and femurs. Multiple high-signal foci are noted throughout the long bones (*arrows*). By comparison, normal marrow has a signal intensity similar to that of muscle on fat-saturated images. (Courtesy of Dr. Marilyn Siegel, Mallinckrodt Institute of Radiology, St. Louis, MO.)

TABLE 86.1 NEUROBLASTOMA STAGING SYSTEMS

Evans and D'Angio	Pediatric Oncology Group	International Staging System
Stage I Tumor confined to the organ or structure of origin	**Stage A** Complete gross resection of primary tumor, with or without microscopic residual; intracavitary lymph nodes, not adhered to and removed with primary (nodes adhered to or within tumor resection may be positive for tumor without upstaging patient to stage C), histologically free of tumor; if primary in abdomen or pelvis, liver histologically free of tumor	**Stage 1** Localized tumor with complete gross excision, without microscopic residual disease; representative ipsilateral lymph nodes negative for tumor microscopically (nodes attached to and removed with the primary tumor may be positive)
Stage II Tumor extending in continuity beyond the organ midline; regional lymph nodes on the ipsilateral side may be involved	**Stage B** Grossly unresected primary tumor; nodes and liver same as stage A	**Stage 2A** Localized tumor with incomplete gross excision; representative ipsilateral nonadherent lymph nodes negative for tumor microscopically
Stage III Tumor extending in continuity beyond the midline; regional lymph nodes may be involved bilaterally	**Stage C** Complete or incomplete resection of primary, intracavitary nodes not adhered to primary histologically positive for tumor; liver as in stage A	**Stage 2B** Localized tumor with or without complete gross excision, with ipsilateral nonadherent lymph nodes positive for tumor; enlarged contralateral lymph nodes must be negative microscopically
Stage IV Remote disease involving skeleton, bone marrow, soft tissue, distant lymph-node groups, etc. (see stage IV-S)	**Stage D** Any dissemination of disease beyond intracavitary nodes (i.e., extracavitary nodes, liver, skin, bone marrow, bone)	**Stage 3** Unresectable unilateral tumor infiltrating across the midline,[a] with or without regional lymph-node involvement; or localized unilateral tumor with contralateral regional lymph-node involvement; or midline tumor with bilateral extension by infiltration (unresectable) or by lymph-node involvement
Stage IV-S Patients who would otherwise be stage I or II but who have remote disease confined to liver, skin, or bone marrow (without radiographic evidence of bone metastases on complete skeletal survey)	**Stage DS** Infants <1 yr of age with stage IV-S disease (see Evans and D'Angio)	**Stage 4** Any primary tumor with dissemination to distant lymph nodes, bone, bone marrow, liver, skin, and/or other organs (except as defined for stage 4S)
		Stage 4S Localized primary tumor as defined for stage 1, 2A, or 2B with dissemination limited to skin, liver, and/or bone marrow[b] (limited to infants <1 yr of age)

Multifocal primary tumors (e.g., bilateral adrenal primary tumors) should be staged according to the greatest extent of disease, as defined in the table, and followed by a subscript letter M (e.g., 3_M).

[a]The midline is defined as the vertebral column. Tumors originating on one side and crossing the midline must infiltrate to or beyond the opposite side of the vertebral column.

[b]Marrow involvement in stage 4S should be minimal, i.e., <10% of total nucleated cells identified as malignant on bone marrow biopsy or on marrow aspirate. More extensive marrow involvement would be considered to be stage 4. The *meta*-iodobenzylguanidine scan (if performed) should be negative in the marrow.

Modified from Halperin EC, Constine LS, Tarbell NJ, et al., eds. *Pediatric radiation oncology*. New York: Raven Press, 1994:171–214.

Schwann cells, and nerve bundles and is benign in appearance and nature. It frequently is calcified and may represent a matured neuroblastoma.[26] Cases of maturation of proven neuroblastomas to ganglioneuromas, either spontaneously or after therapy, have been reported.[9] *Ganglioneuroblastoma* is the intermediate form between ganglioneuroma and neuroblastoma. Both mature ganglion cells and undifferentiated neuroblasts are evident.

Neuroblastoma is at the undifferentiated end of the spectrum of neural crest tumors. It is a small, round, blue cell tumor composed of dense nests of hyperchromatic cells. Homer Wright rosettes with a central fibrillary core can be present. Areas of necrosis, hemorrhage, and calcium are frequently present. Immunohistochemical stains may help distinguish neuroblastoma from other undifferentiated malignant neoplasms of childhood. Neuroblastoma characteristically stains positive for neurofilaments, neuron-specific enolase (NSE), synaptophysin, and chromogranin A and negative for muscle and leukocyte common antigens. The use of electron microscopy to demonstrate neurosecretory granules is required infrequently to establish the diagnosis.

A grading system has been proposed by Shimada et al.,[27] and its significance has been confirmed by the CCG.[28,29] This clinicopathologic staging system evaluates tumor specimens for stromal development (i.e., stromal-rich and stromal-poor tumors), neuroblastic differentiation, and mitosis-karyorrhexis index of neuroblastic cells. These three histologic features and the patient's age at diagnosis divide children into favorable and unfavorable prognostic groups. The stroma-rich tumors are characterized by an extensive Schwann cell stroma. The well-differentiated stroma-rich tumors may correspond to ganglioneuroma, and the "intermixed" stroma-rich tumors may correspond to the ganglioneuroblastomas. To be reliable, the Shimada classification requires pretreatment evaluation of the entire primary tumor specimen. However, primary tumors often are not completely resectable, or the presence of widespread metastases makes thorough tumor resection inappropriate before introduction of initial systemic therapy, thereby limiting the usefulness of this system.

PROGNOSTIC FACTORS

Patient age and stage at initial presentation remain the two most important factors that influence outcome (Table 86.2). In general >75% of infants and children <2 years old survive, as do 90% to 100% of children with INSS stages 1 and 2.[30–40] The presence of tumor in regional lymph nodes is a poor prognostic factor and was recognized as such by the POG in their staging system.[41] Infants <12 months old with metastatic disease confined to the liver, bone marrow (not bone), or skin (stage IV-S) have a remarkably good prognosis; <75% of these children survive with little or no treatment.[8,42] Treatment should be directed at relief of the acute presenting event (often respiratory distress secondary to hepatomegaly), and the temptation to aggressively treat these patients in the absence of other bad prognostic factors should be avoided.

Patients with more-differentiated tumors (e.g., ganglioneuroma, ganglioneuroblastoma) fare better than children with

TABLE 86.2 PROGNOSTIC VARIABLES IN NEUROBLASTOMA

Prognostic Factor	Favorable	Unfavorable	Survival (%) Favorable	Survival (%) Unfavorable
Age	<2 yr	>2 yr	77	38
Stage	I, II, IV-S	III, IV	90–100	50, 30
Pathology (Shimada)	Favorable	Unfavorable	90	23
Ferritin	<143 ng/mL	>143 ng/mL	83	19
Neuron-specific enolase	<100	>100	79	10
Chromogranin	<190 ng/mL	>190 ng/mL	69	30
GD2 ganglioside	<103 pmol/mL	>568 pmol/mL	70	24
Urine VMA/HVA	<1	>1	84	44
gp 140TRK-A	High expression	Low expression	78	14
N-*myc*	Single copy	Amplified	70	5
DNA index	>1.1	1	100	10
1p deletion	No 1p deletion	1p deletion	90	10

HVA, homovanillic acid; VMA, vanillylmandelic acid.

Modified from Matthay KK Neuroblastoma. A clinical challenge and biologic puzzle. *CA Cancer J Clin* 1995; 45:179–192.

TABLE 86.3 NEUROBLASTOMA RISK ASSESSMENT

Risk	Stage	Age	MYCN	Ploidy	Histology	Other
Low	1	Any	Any	Any	Any	
Low	2a/2b	Any	Non amp	Any	Any	Resection ≥50%
Inter	2a/2b	Any	Non amp	Any	Any	Resection <50%
Inter	2a/2b	Any	Non amp	Any	Any	Biopsy only
	2a/2b	Any	Amp	Any	Any	Any degree of resection
Inter	3	<547 d	Non amp	Any	Any	
Inter	3	≥547 d	Non amp	Any	FH	
High	3	Any	Amp	Any	Any	
High	3	≥547 d	Non amp	Any	UH	
High	4	<365 d	Amp	Any	Any	
Inter	4	<365d	Non amp	Any	Any	
High	4	365 to <547 d	Amp	Any	Any	
High	4	365 to <547 d	Any	DI = 1	Any	
High	4	365 to <547 d	Any	Any	UH	
Inter	4	365 to <547 d	Non amp	DI > 1	FH	
High	4	>547 d	Any	Any	Any	
Low	4s	<365 d	Non amp	DI > 1	FH	Asymptomatic
Inter	4s	<365 d	Non amp	DI = 1	Any	Asymptomatic or symptomatic
Inter	4s	<365 d	Missing	Missing	Missing	Too sick for biopsy
Inter	4s	<365 d	Non amp	Any	Any	Symptomatic
Inter	4s	<365 d	Non amp	Any	UH	Asymptomatic or symptomatic
High	4s	<365 d	Amp	Any	Any	Asymptomatic or symptomatic

amp, amplified; DI, DNA index; FH, favorable Shimada histology; UH, unfavorable Shimada histology.

poorly differentiated or undifferentiated neuroblastomas. A favorable Shimada stage is associated with 90% survival, compared with 22% with unfavorable Shimada stages. Elevated serum ferritin (>142 ng/mL), NSE (>100 ng/mL), and LDH (>1,500 IU) are all associated with advanced disease and a poor prognosis.[32,43–45]

MYCN (N-*myc*) is a proto-oncogene that resides on the short arm of chromosome 2. An increased number of *MYCN* gene copies is associated with an extremely poor prognosis (5% survival).[46,47] *MYCN* amplification has been associated with the multidrug-resistance gene and may account for this tumor's notorious resistance to therapy.[48] A tumor with a DNA index of 1 (diploid or near-diploid) paradoxically gives a worse prognosis than tumors that are aneuploid.[49] Hyperdiploid tumors occur more often in lower stages and are associated with better chemotherapy responsiveness. Allelic loss of the short arm of chromosome 1 represents a loss of heterozygosity of a tumor suppressor gene and is also associated with a poor prognosis independent of age and stage. It reliably identifies patients with stage I, II, or IV-S disease who have a high risk of relapse and require aggressive therapy.[50]

GENERAL MANAGEMENT

Because of the biologic heterogeneity of neuroblastoma, the following treatment recommendations should be considered as guidelines. The prognostic implications of a tumor's biologic indices, such as *MYCN* amplification and DNA index, may warrant more aggressive therapy in young patients with otherwise a favorable stage (Table 86.3).

Low-Risk Disease

Low-stage, resectable tumors (INSS stage 1, 2, or 3 with negative nodes) have an excellent prognosis after complete gross surgical excision. Adjuvant chemotherapy or irradiation has not improved the outcome in children with completely resected tumors with favorable biologic features.[38,51–54] Positive surgical margins or microscopic residual disease does not uniformly require more aggressive therapy. Patients with *MYCN* amplification or low DNA index may require adjuvant therapy and should be enrolled in clinical trials.[49]

Unresectable tumors that are otherwise of low stage (INSS stages 1 to 3 with negative lymph nodes) may require preoperative chemotherapy and occasionally radiation therapy to convert them into a resectable status. Second-look surgery is performed to remove a previously unresectable primary tumor and achieve a complete remission after induction chemotherapy. Complete resection can be achieved in almost two-thirds of previously unresectable stage III to IV primary tumors.[55] The CCG reported that eventual complete resection of the primary tumor in advanced disease may have a favorable impact on outcome.[55] The benefit to complete resection in patients with advanced disease has not been uniformly established. Patients with biologically favorable tumors may be more amenable to surgery after chemotherapy, and the apparent benefit of complete resection may be a result of patient selection.[56] POG-8104 enrolled patients with INSS stage 1 (POG stage A) disease. In that trial, *MYCN* amplification and DNA index were not evaluated uniformly. Treatment was surgery only. Regardless of the presence of residual microscopic disease, the 2-year disease-free survival rate was 89%.[25] In the CCG experience (CCG trial 3881) with stage 1 disease, the 4-year event-free and overall survival rates for children treated initially with surgery alone were 93% and 99%, respectively. For patients with stage 2 disease, the event-free and overall survival rates were 81% and 98%, respectively. In that trial, only 13% of patients with stage 2 disease received any chemotherapy or radiotherapy, despite the fact that 104 patients had INSS stage 2b disease. The authors ascribe the favorable results to improved surgical management and better staging with MIBG scanning.[57]

Intermediate-Risk Disease

Locally advanced and regionally metastatic tumors (INSS stage 2b to 3 with positive lymph nodes) require more intensive therapy. Infants <1 year of age should undergo complete resection of the primary tumor and receive adjuvant chemotherapy.[56,58–60] In unresectable cases, chemotherapy may be administered initially, and surgery can be performed after response to systemic treatment. In older children with lymph-node metastases, adjuvant radiation therapy to the primary and regional lymph nodes has improved the disease-free and overall survival rates. A prospective, randomized trial of postoperative chemotherapy or chemotherapy plus regional irradiation demonstrated 31% disease-free survival in children treated with chemotherapy, compared with 58% in those who also received radiation therapy.[61] However, the value of radiation therapy in intermediate-risk patients is not universally accepted. De Bernardi et al.[62] failed to demonstrate a benefit from the addition of radiotherapy in 29 children >1 year of age with postoperative residual tumor or positive regional lymph nodes. Children in that randomized study received two cycles of peptichemio with or without radiation. Progression-free survival was 64% in the radiotherapy arm and 73% in the arm without radiotherapy.[62] Coupled with the risk of late effects from even moderate radiotherapy doses, this small trial provided an argument that systematic radiation therapy, even for POG stage C patients, may not be necessary. Current COG trials reflect this bias because the use of radiation therapy is decreasing.

Patients with intraspinal extension of neuroblastoma pose a unique problem. They frequently have severe neurologic compromise resulting from spinal cord compression. Historically, these patients were treated with laminectomy and surgical debulking with or without radiation therapy and chemotherapy.[63] Because the morbidity of this approach is significant, with a high rate of spinal growth deformity, a number of investigators have proceeded with treatment of these patients using primary chemotherapy.[55] A prospective series of 42 patients treated with primary chemotherapy demonstrated a 92% improvement in neurologic deficits, allowing children to avoid neurosurgical decompression in >60% of cases when receiving courses of carboplatin and etoposide alternating with cyclophosphamide, vincristine, and doxorubicin.

The POG experience (POG trials 8742 and 9244) with stages 2b to 3 disease demonstrates an 85% event-free survival with completely resected tumors at diagnosis, compared to 70% with incomplete resection at diagnosis (p = .259). In both of these studies, patients underwent maximum safe tumor resection followed by five courses of induction chemotherapy. In POG-8742 they received cisplatinum and etoposide alternating with cyclophosphamide and doxorubicin. In POG-9244 they received alternating cycles of vincristine, cisplatinum, etoposide, and cyclophosphamide (OPEC) and vincristine, carboplatin, etoposide, and cyclophosphamide. After second-look surgery the same chemotherapy was given as maintenance. Radiotherapy was given to patients with viable residual tumor discovered at the time of the second-look operation. Children age 12 to 24 months at the time of radiation therapy received 24 Gy in 1.5-Gy fractions to the primary tumor site. Older children received 30 Gy in 1.5-Gy fractions. Of the 37 patients on these two protocols who survived "event free," 11 (30%) received radiotherapy. Patients with favorable Shimada histology tumors had a 92% event-free survival, compared with 58% with unfavorable tumors (p = .009). Patients with *MYCN* amplification did poorly, with outcomes comparable to those for stage D patients.[27]

Based on CCG and POG data, patients with intermediate-risk neuroblastoma have an estimated 3-year survival of between 75% and 98%. Cyclophosphamide, doxorubicin, carboplatin, and etoposide are the four most active agents.[64–66] The COG now is evaluating the role of chemotherapy dose intensity and duration for children based on tumor biology.

Surgery plays a critical role in the primary management of neuroblastoma. The goals of surgery are to establish a diagnosis; provide tissue for evaluation of prognostic biologic markers; stage the disease according to INSS criteria; and attempt to totally excise the primary, if feasible. The extent of surgery has an important impact on outcome. O'Neill et al.[67] reported that 55 of 59 patients with a complete or near-complete resection were alive and free of disease 2 years after surgery, compared to only 13 of 24 cases with a subtotal resection. Just as Haase had reported, Grosfield and Baehner[34] found evidence for improved outcome in stage 4 patients attaining complete resection of primary tumor at delayed second-look procedures.

High-Risk Disease

The majority of patients with neuroblastoma present with metastatic disease. With the exception of infants with favorable biologic disease confined to the skin, bone marrow, or liver, the outcome is poor. Extremely aggressive treatment regimens have been used in these patients to prolong survival and achieve cure. Intensive high-dose chemotherapy regimens appear to be superior to less intensive regimens. Active drugs in advanced neuroblastoma include cyclophosphamide, cisplatin, doxorubicin, etoposide, and teniposide.[68]

Many recent clinical trials have sought to intensify treatment of metastatic neuroblastoma through the use of high-dose myeloablative chemotherapy with stem cell rescue or bone marrow transplantation (BMT). The French Lyon-Marseille-Curie East group reported a 40% progression-free survival at 2 years and 20% at 5 years in 62 patients proceeding to autologous bone marrow transplant (ABMT).[69] The CCG reported a 43% 2-year event-free survival in 43 children undergoing consolidation melphalan, cisplatin, teniposide, doxorubicin, and total-body irradiation (TBI) to 1,000 cGy in three fractions of 330 cGy/day. The toxic death rate was 22%.[70] Australian investigators tested a less intense preparative regimen with a TBI regimen consisting of 12 Gy in six twice-daily fractions.[71] Of 28 patients registered, 19 achieved complete remission after induction chemotherapy. Seventeen of these 19 patients underwent ABMT and 15 (87%) remained free of disease at 5 years from ABMT. Of the 28 patients registered, 50% have survived 5 years.

Uncertain that ABMT could be studied successfully in a cooperative group, the CCG conducted two pilot studies for children with stage 4 disease. In CCG-321, patients received induction chemotherapy consisting of cisplatin, etoposide, doxorubicin, and cyclophosphamide. Of 207 patients, 159 remained disease free during induction chemotherapy. Of these patients, 67 received myeloablative chemotherapy and ABMT, whereas 74 continued conventional chemotherapy for a total of 13 cycles. The patients receiving the ABMT had a higher event-free survival than patients continuing standard chemotherapy (40% vs. 19%, p = .019).[72] Because they are not randomized trials, these studies potentially may have allowed a biased allocation of patients to one arm based on clinical concerns or prognostic risk factors. The POG failed to show a benefit to BMT in high-risk metastatic neuroblastoma (POG 8340).[45]

The European Neuroblastoma Study Group studied the role of consolidative ABMT with high-dose melphalan versus no further treatment following induction chemotherapy with the OPEC regimen in patients with stage 3 and 4 disease.[73,74] With a median follow-up of 14.3 years for surviving children, they report an improvement in event-free survival (38% vs. 27%) and overall survival (47% and 30%) for the high-dose melphalan arm, but these differences did not reach statistical significance. The subset of patients with stage IV disease who were >1 year of age, however, did show statistically significant improvement in event-free survival (33% vs. 17%, p = .01) and overall survival (46% vs. 21%, p = .03).

The CCG conducted a randomized trial comparing continued chemotherapy with myeloablative therapy (including 10 Gy TBI in 3 daily fractions) and autologous bone marrow transplantation in children with high risk neuroblastoma. All patients received radiation therapy to the primary site and select metastatic sites. A second randomization following cytotoxic therapy included 6 cycles of 13-*cis*-retinoic acid or no further therapy. Initial results demonstrated an event-free survival advantage to both bone marrow transplantation and 13-*cis*-retinoic acid therapy, but no overall survival advantage.[75] However, after a median follow-up of more than 7 years, a statistically significant advantage to overall survival was demonstrated for the cohort treated with both myeloablative therapy and 13-*cis*-retinoic acid therapy.[76]

Berthold et al.[77] in Germany reported results of a prospective, randomized trial in children with high-risk neuroblastoma comparing myeloablative therapy with melphalan, etoposide, and carboplatin and autologous stem cell rescue with maintenance chemotherapy with cyclophosphamide. When analyzed as-treated, statistically significantly improved 3-year event-free survival (53% vs. 30%) and overall survival (68% vs. 53%) were seen with myeloablative therapy.

Local control of the primary tumor in stage 4 neuroblastoma is an important element of patient management. The role of surgical resection in metastatic disease remains controversial. Many authors have reported more favorable outcome in patients undergoing complete resection.[78,79] There is a strong association between chemotherapy dose intensity and surgical respectability, which reduces the significance of aggressive resection as an independent favorable factor. It can be assumed that tumors that are amenable to resection may have an inherently less aggressive biology.

In the CCG-321-P3 pilot there was a 33% rate of local relapse in patients not undergoing a complete resection at their initial surgery, irrespective of their ultimate surgical resection status, including second-look operations.[80] This high local failure rate suggests that there is a role for local radiation therapy. In that pilot study, patients received radiotherapy if they had gross residual disease after second-look surgery. Although the local control in patients receiving radiotherapy was the same as in unirradiated patients, it should be noted that only patients with gross residual disease received this local treatment, suggesting that the radiotherapy (RT) was beneficial.

In a reanalysis of CCG-3891, Hass-Kogan et al.[81] compared locoregional control rates in patients on the non-ABMT arm who received 10 to 20 Gy to gross residual disease after induction therapy to patients in the ABMT arm who received similar RT to residual disease but also received 10-Gy TBI in 3.33-Gy daily fractions in their conditioning regimens The patients in the ABMT arm had a lower locoregional recurrence rate (33% vs. 51%, $p = .004$). Although this affect may be due to the higher dose of RT delivered in this group of patients, it is not possible to separate the RT effect from that of the more intense systemic therapy also given to these patients in the ABMT arm.

Laprie et al.[82] analyzed locoregional control in MYCN-amplified INSS stage 2 and 3 patients treated with different regimens over different eras. Their approach varied from conventional chemotherapy and RT only to gross residual disease after surgery in patients >1 year of age, to high-dose chemotherapy with ABMT, to local radiation therapy to all patients. They noted an improvement in event-free survival with ABMT and RT (83% vs. 25%, $p = .001$). Again, conclusions regarding the effect of RT independent of the intensified systemic therapy are difficult to make because this was not a randomized comparison.

Local therapy to the primary tumor and metastatic sites may be beneficial in the curative therapy of children with disseminated disease. Surgical resection of the primary tumor has been associated with improved survival and local control after aggressive systemic therapy.[55,80] There is a predilection for recurrence in previous sites of disease, and it is conceivable that additional local therapy with irradiation to the primary tumor site and distant metastases may enhance tumor control and cure rates.[80,83]

The POG reported that patients with persistent disease at primary or metastatic sites received boost irradiation of 12 Gy prior to TBI for BMT. Only 2 of 27 patients relapsed at irradiated sites. Six of 10 first-remission patients given local radiation remained in remission, compared to only 13 of 40 who were not irradiated, despite the fact that irradiated patients had residual disease.[84]

Radiation therapy plays an extremely important role in the palliative management of patients with end-stage symptomatic neuroblastoma. Pain from bone or other visceral metastases often can be relieved with external-beam radiation therapy. Mass effect from a rapidly enlarging tumor can respond dramatically to radiation therapy. In a series of 10 patients treated at Duke University Medical Center, Halperin[85] reported 7 complete responses to radiation therapy, either alone or in conjunction with chemotherapy. Radiation doses ranged from 4 to 24.4 Gy at a rate of 1 to 1.5 Gy/fraction. The 7 patients with complete response survived without recurrence.

Systemic radionuclide therapy with ^{131}I-MIBG has been tested in several European and U.S. centers with early encouraging results. This radioactive agent produced objective responses in previously treated and chemoresistant stage 4 neuroblastoma.[86,87] These early positive results prompted some investigators to test this agent in previously untreated metastatic neuroblastoma. DeKraker et al.[88] reported that a combination of ^{131}I-MIBG and second-look surgery produced response rates comparable to those of multidrug chemotherapy. Preliminary research on the combination of ^{131}I-MIBG with systemic chemotherapy and/or TBI with BMT demonstrated that this is a safe treatment and worthy of more investigation.[89–91]

The current approach by the Children's Oncology Group for patients with high-risk disease is to combine induction chemotherapy, surgical resection, autologous stem cell rescue, radiation therapy to the primary site and select metastatic sites, and 13-*cis*-retinoic acid in an attempt to improve outcome in these patients. The current protocol explores further intensification of therapy by randomizing patients to either one myeloablative transplant or two myeloablative transplants. It will also include a higher radiation total dose of 36 Gy for patients with gross residual disease at their primary sites.

RADIATION-THERAPY TECHNIQUES: TREATMENT PLANNING AND FIELD DESIGN

Significant reductions in irradiation-associated morbidity have accompanied technological advances. The transition from orthovoltage to megavoltage x-rays has decreased the risk of severe growth-related skeletal defects.[92] CT-assisted simulation and three-dimensional radiation-therapy treatment planning have the potential to decrease the volume of normal tissues irradiated and thereby decrease the incidence of late effects (Fig. 86.5). As in Wilms' tumor, the radiation oncologist must be aware of the increased risk of spinal deformity or other skeletal anomalies if symmetric irradiation of the bone is not administered. The clinician needs to balance the treatment of disease and normal tissues to maximize tumor coverage while not sacrificing the growing tissues.

Radiation therapy portals to a primary tumor site should treat the gross residual tumor remaining after chemotherapy with at least a 2-cm margin from the tumor to the block edge. This mar-

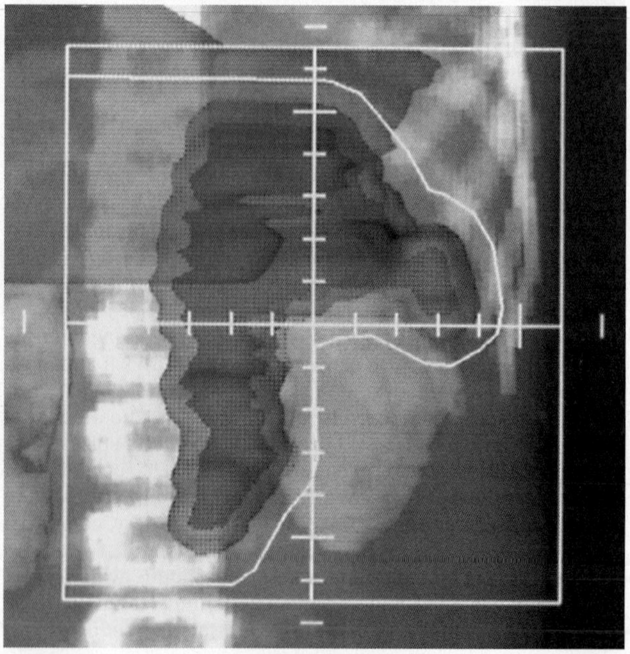

FIGURE 86.5. Radiation therapy treatment field for a child with a left adrenal primary neuroblastoma and para-aortic lymph-node metastases. The beam's-eye-view display with a digital reconstructed radiograph allows for adequate coverage of the target volume and lymph-node region with sparing of the ipsilateral kidney and liver while homogeneously irradiating the adjacent spine.

gin usually ensures adequate dosimetric coverage of the residual tumor, taking into account treatment-related positional uncertainties and beam penumbra. Children who are not sedated may require more margin if they tend to shift or move on the treatment table. Regional lymph-node sites should be covered if nodes were radiographically or pathologically involved at any time during the disease course. The POG study that demonstrated an advantage to radiation therapy for POG stage C disease included extended-field radiation therapy to adjacent lymph-node sites (i.e., elective mediastinal irradiation for abdominal primary tumors).[61] It is not clear that this extended-field treatment contributed to the beneficial effect of radiation therapy, and current POG trials do not include it. Halperin[93] reviewed the patterns of failure in 13 children with stage C neuroblastoma treated with systemic therapy and radiation therapy directed to the primary tumor and without "prophylactic" irradiation of contiguous lymph-node regions. Of the 7 patients who failed, 2 of them developed a recurrence in contiguous lymph-node regions. In both these circumstances these regional failures were accompanied by local or distant failure. Considering the morbidity associated with the additional radiation volume and its impact on the tolerance to subsequent chemotherapy, he recommended against this prophylactic regional irradiation.

CT or MRI scans should be used to define the full extent of disease when a radiation therapy portal is designed. In many instances, parallel opposed anterior and posterior portals may suffice for tumor coverage. They have the added advantage of allowing homogeneous irradiation of the spine in paraspinal tumors.

Radiation therapy of metastatic sites should include generous margins. Bony metastases often are more extensive than a plain radiograph may suggest. Orbital metastases may require treatment of the entire orbit. Hepatic metastases do not require whole-liver irradiation, but adequate margins must be used to account for respiratory motion during treatment. The patient's life expectancy should influence the selection of radiation-therapy portals, field shaping, and dose fractionation. Children who have end-stage disease with tumors that are resistant to most chemotherapy drugs should be treated with wide fields and a rapid fractionation schedule. Complex field design and prolonged fractionation schedules may prevent the terminal child from spending quality time off therapy. The exception is infants with stage 4S disease. These children frequently have a very good prognosis, and sparing of normal tissues is an important goal.

Low-dose TBI has been used with variable success in the curative management of children with metastatic neuroblastoma.[94,95] More important has been the use of TBI as part of the preparative regimen for patients undergoing BMT for high-risk metastatic disease. It is not clear if TBI is essential in the preoperative program for a transplant. Patterns of failure after BMT are predominately in sites of prior disease, including the original primary tumor and previously documented metastatic sites.[80,83] These data suggest that involved-field boost irradiation, before or after BMT with TBI, may be beneficial.

The appropriate radiation dose is debatable. Laboratory data suggest that neuroblastoma is very radiosensitive and that neuroblasts exhibit very little repair capacity between fractions.[96] This makes hyperfractionated radiation therapy an attractive option because comparable tumoricidal doses can be achieved with minimization of the risk of late effects.[97,98] However, despite irradiation doses that approach normal-tissue tolerance in the young, local recurrences after radiation therapy still occur. The irradiation dose required to control gross disease may be age dependent.[29,39,99] In infants <1 year of age, a dose of 12 Gy appears sufficient for durable local control.[29,99] Tumors in children aged 12 to 48 months may require doses of at least 25 Gy. Children >4 years of age frequently develop local failures even with doses of > 25 Gy. Local control of the primary tumor site in patients with high-risk disease may be improved with the use of local radiation to the primary site and regional lymph nodes. Kushner et al.[52] updated the experience from Memorial Sloan-Kettering Cancer Center, reporting that 21 Gy of hyperfractionated radiation therapy resulted in 90% primary-site local control at 5 years. Radiation was delivered after all chemotherapy with a minimum interval of 4 hours between fractions. No TBI was administered in this group of patients. If patients had a gross total resection, the local control was 100%, whereas in seven patients with gross disease, three had recurrence.[52,100] In Kushner et al.'s series, 92% of metastatic sites were controlled with 21 Gy of hyperfractionated radiation therapy at 36 months.

Haas-Kogan[101] described the results of intraoperative radiation therapy (IORT) in patients with high-risk disease. A single fraction of 7 to 16 Gy (median 10 Gy) to the primary tumor bed was associated with a local control rate of 100% in patients who had gross total resection, whereas IORT was unable to control any patients with gross residual disease.

Children treated palliatively for symptomatic metastatic disease should receive adequate irradiation doses for durable tumor control if they have a reasonable expectation of long survival. Total dose and fractionation regimens similar to those used for curative therapy should be considered. Low-dose, short-fractionation schedules are appropriate if the child is not expected to live beyond 6 to 12 months. In these instances, minimizing a child's visits to the radiation-therapy facility while rapidly relieving symptoms is a worthwhile goal. If the likelihood of long survival is small, 5 to 20 Gy in one to five daily fractions can allow rapid palliation.

RESULTS OF THERAPY

Low-Risk Disease

Survival rates after surgery alone of 85% to 90% or better can be expected.[25,51,54,57,102] Additional therapy usually is not indicated unless unfavorable biologic features are present.

Intermediate-Risk Disease

Children with large, initially unresectable tumors often respond to primary chemotherapy with combinations of drugs, including cyclophosphamide, vincristine, cisplatin, etoposide, doxorubicin, or teniposide. Children with unresponsive, unresectable gross residual disease may require external-beam irradiation. Frequently, these children can undergo resection of the tumor at a second-look operation[55] and achieve a survival rate of 60% to 90%.[54,102]

The presence of lymph-node metastases, even with a localized primary tumor, negatively affects prognosis. These children have a 50% to 75% survival rate even with aggressive systemic therapy and adjuvant radiation therapy.[61,102] Infants with lymph node–positive disease have a more favorable outcome, with a 3-year disease-free survival rate of 93% after treatment with cyclophosphamide and doxorubicin and complete resection without irradiation.[59]

High-Risk Disease

Children >1 year of age with metastatic neuroblastoma continue to have a poor prognosis, with expected 3- or 4-year survival rates of <10% to 30%. The addition of cisplatin and teniposide to the chemotherapy armamentarium improved the expected 4-year survival rate from 7% to 28% in a series of trials conducted from 1962 to 1988 at St. Jude Children's Research Hospital.[58] The CCG reported that ABMT can improve outcome in selected patients with metastatic neuroblastoma. With this aggressive therapy, the 3-year event-free survival was 34%. The addition of *cis*-retinoic acid was associated with a 47% event-free survival.[75] The COG is investigating even more intensive systemic therapy with tandem stem cell transplant.

Infants with metastatic disease have a uniquely favorable outcome. In stage 4S, survival rates can be as high as 75% to 90%.[103,104] In these patients, the goal of therapy should be limited to the relief of acute presenting symptoms. Local-field, fractionated low-dose irradiation (<12 Gy), minimal chemotherapy, or supportive care may be sufficient to achieve high survival rates. Infants with metastases to other sites (brain, bone, or lung) or who have tumors with poor biologic features (DNA index of 1, *MYCN* amplification) should be managed with more aggressive regimens.[49,105] Halperin[85] reported 7 complete responses to hepatic radiation in 10 infants with symptomatic liver metastases. All 7 of these children survived.

SEQUELAE OF TREATMENT

Early Complications

Acute side effects of radiation therapy depend on tumor site and fields of treatment. The short-term effects are those that can be expected for any patient receiving radiation therapy. Acute effects, especially skin reactions and mucositis, may be enhanced if concurrent chemotherapy or a hyperfractionated irradiation schedule is used.

Late Effects

Long-term effects depend on the site irradiated and the total dose of both radiation and chemotherapy agents used. Age at the time of treatment may influence the risk and severity of skeletal anomalies,[106] which may include spinal deformities such as kyphosis, scoliosis, or limb shortening. Generally, younger children are more prone to late radiation injury than older children. Fortunately, in neuroblastoma, the youngest children require radiation therapy infrequently or at lower total doses. Table 86.4 lists the late sequelae associated with radiation therapy in the management of neuroblastoma at Washington University.[107] Chemotherapy may increase the risk of irradiation sequelae, and the expected tolerance may be reduced.[108]

Neve et al.[109] reported a high rate of pulmonary function impairment in children receiving TBI as part of their conditioning regimen for ABMT. The impairment was most severe in younger children or patients requiring more chemotherapy. TBI was fractionated: a total of 12 Gy was given in six fractions over 3 days, with a dose rate of 50 cGy/minute with lung shielding at 10 Gy. TBI also has been associated with poor growth in survivors of neuroblastoma treated with ABMT. Hovi et al.[110] described a series of 31 children, 15 of whom were treated with high-dose chemotherapy and no TBI and 16 of whom received TBI of 10 to 12 Gy in five or six fractions over 3 days. After 10 years of follow-up, the height standard deviation score of the TBI group was –2.0 compared to –0.7 to –0.9 for the nonirradiated group. This loss of height may have been related to growth-hormone deficiency. The majority of patients in both groups responded to growth hormone deficiency with a mean increase in their height standard deviation score of 0.8 at 3 years.

TABLE 86.4 WASHINGTON UNIVERSITY NEUROBLASTOMA STUDY OF LONG-TERM SEQUELAE RELATED TO RADIATION THERAPY

Complication	Number of Patients	Dose (Gy)
Scoliosis (mild)	6	8–30
Scoliosis (severe)	6	16–37
Muscle hypoplasia	3	28–30
Bone hypoplasia	4	28–30
Breast hypoplasia	5	28–30
Kidney hypoplasia	2	30–33
Pulmonary hypoplasia	3	28–30
Lung fibrosis	1	48 (possibly fatal)
Liver fibrosis	1	39.5 (fatal)
Rib necrosis	1	48
Thyroid adenocarcinoma	1	20
Chondrosarcoma	1	20
Cataracts	1	20
Hypopituitarism	1	20
Urinary tract infection	1	20
Thyroid adenoma	1	18
Total	**38**	

REFERENCES

1. Woods WG, Tuchman M, Bernstein ML, et al. Screening for neuroblastoma in North America: 2-year results from the Quebec Project. *Am J Pediatr Hematol Oncol* 1992;14(4):312–319.
2. Schilling FH, Berthold F, Erttmann R, et al. Population-based and controlled study to evaluate neuroblastoma screening at one year of age in Germany: interim results. *Med Pediatr Oncol* 2000;35(6):701–704.
3. Schilling FH, Spix C, Berthold F, et al. Neuroblastoma screening at one year of age. *N Engl J Med* 2002;346(14):1047–1053.
4. Woods WG, Gao RN, Shuster JJ, et al. Screening of infants and mortality due to neuroblastoma. *N Engl J Med* 2002;346(14):1041–1046.
5. Yamamoto K, Ohta S, Ito E, et al. Marginal decrease in mortality and marked increase in incidence as a result of neuroblastoma screening at 6 months of age: cohort study in seven prefectures in Japan. *J Clin Oncol* 2002;20(5):1209–1214.
6. Murphy SB, Cohn SL, Craft AW, et al. Do children benefit from mass screening for neuroblastoma: consensus statement from the American Cancer Society Workshop on Neuroblastoma Screening. *Lancet* 1991;337(8737):344–346.
7. Yamamoto K, Hayaski Y, Hanada R, et al. Mass screening and age-specific incidence of neuroblastoma in Suitama Prefecture Japan. *J Clin Oncol* 1995;13(8):2033–2038.
8. Evans AE, Chatten J, D'Angio GJ, et al. A review of 17-IV-S neuroblastoma patients at the Children's Hospital of Philadelphia. *Cancer* 1980;45(4):833–839.
9. Everson EC, Cole WH. *Spontaneous regression of cancer.* Philadelphia: WB Saunders, 1966:88–163.
10. Beckwith JB, Perrin EV. *In situ* neuroblastomas: a contribution to the natural history of neural crest tumors. *Am J Pathol* 1963;43:1089–1104.
11. Bray PF, Ziter FA, Lahey ME, et al. The coincidence of neuroblastoma and acute cerebellar encephalopathy. *J Pediatr* 1969;75(6):983–990.
12. Pranzatelli MR The neurobiology of the opsoclonus-myoclonus syndrome. *Clin Neuropharmacol* 1992;19(1):1–47.
13. Boechat MI, Ortega J, Hoffman AD, et al. Computed tomography in stage III neuroblastoma. *AJR Am J Roentgenol* 1985;145:1283–1287.
14. Couanet D, Geoffray A, Hartmann O, et al. Bone marrow metastases in children's neuroblastoma studies by magnetic resonance imaging. *Prog Clin Biol Res* 1988;271:547–555.
15. Fletcher BD, Kopiwoda SY, Strandjord SE, et al. Abdominal neuroblastoma: magnetic resonance imaging and tissue characterization. *Radiology* 1985;155(3):699–703.
16. Petrus LV, Hall TR, Boechat MI, et al. The pediatric patient with suspected adrenal neoplasm: which radiological test to use? *Med Pediatr Oncol* 1992;20(1):53–57.
17. Siegel M, Jamroz GA, Glazer HS, et al. MR imaging of intraspinal extension of neuroblastoma. *J Comput Assist Tomogr* 1986;10(4):593–595.
18. Turba E, Fagioli G, Mancini AF, et al. Evaluation of stage 4 neuroblastoma patients by means of MIBG and 99mTc-MDP scintigraphy. *J Nucl Biol Med* 1993;37(3):107–114.
19. Shapiro B. Imaging of catecholamine-secreting tumors: uses of MIBG in diagnosis and treatment. *Ballieres Clin Endocrinol Metab* 1993;7(2):491–507.
20. Katzenstein HM, Cohn SL, Shore RM, et al. Scintigraphic response by 123I-metaiodobenzylguanidine scan correlates with event-free survival in high-risk neuroblastoma. *J Clin Oncol* 2004;22(19):3909–3915.
21. O'dorisio MS, Hauger M, Cecalupo AJ. Somatostatin receptors in neuroblastoma: diagnosis and therapeutic implications. *Semin Oncol* 1994;21(5, Suppl 13):33–37.
22. Moertel CL, Reubi JC, Scheithaur BS. Expression of somatostatin receptors in childhood neuroblastoma. *Am J Clin Pathol* 1994;102(6):752–756.
23. Brodeur GM, Seeger RC, Barrett A, et al. International criteria for diagnosis staging and response to treatment in patients with neuroblastoma. *J Clin Oncol* 1988;6(12):1874–1881.
24. Evans AE, D'Angio GJ, Randolph J. A proposed staging for children with neuroblastoma. Children's cancer study group A. *Cancer* 1971;27(2):374–378.
25. Nitschke R, Smith EI, Shochat S, et al. Localized neuroblastoma treated by surgery: a Pediatric Oncology Group study. *J Clin Oncol* 1988;6(8):1271–1279.
26. Willis RA. *The pathology of tumors in children.* Springfield IL: Charles C Thomas, 1962:7–17.
27. Shimada H, Chatten J, Newton WA, et al. Histopathologic prognostic factors in neuroblastic tumors: definition of subtypes of ganglioneuroblastoma and an age-linked classification of neuroblastomas. *J Natl Cancer Inst* 1984;73(7):405–416.
28. Chatten J, Shimada H, Sather HN, et al. Prognostic value of histopathology in advanced neuroblastoma: a report from the Children's Cancer Study Group. *Hum Pathol* 1988;19(10):1187–1198.
29. Jacobson GM, Sause WT, O'Brien RT. Dose response analysis of pediatric neuroblastoma to megavoltage radiation. *Am J Clin Oncol* 1984;7(6):693–697.
30. Carlsen NL, Christensen IJ, Schroeder H, et al. Prognostic factors in neuroblastoma treated in Denmark from 1943 to 1980: a statistical estimate of prognosis based on 253 cases. *Cancer* 1986;58(12):2726–2735.
31. Coldman AJ, Fryer CJH, Elwood JM, et al. Neuroblastoma: influence of age at diagnosis stage tumor site and sex on prognosis. *Cancer* 1980;46(8):1896–1901.
32. Evans AE, D'Angio GJ, Propert K, et al. Prognostic factors in neuroblastoma. *Cancer* 1987;59(11):1853–1859.
33. Evans AE, D'Angio GJ, Sather HN, et al. A comparison of four staging systems for localized and regional neuroblastoma: a report from the Children's Cancer Study Group. *J Clin Oncol* 1990;8(4):678–688.
34. Grosfeld JL, Baehner RL. Neuroblastoma: an analysis of 160 cases. *World J Surg* 1980;4(1):29–37.
35. Halperin EC, Cox EB. Radiation therapy in the management of neuroblastoma: the Duke University Medical Center experience 1967–1984. *Int J Radiat Oncol Biol Phys* 1986;12(10):1829–1837.
36. Hayes FA, Green AA. Neuroblastoma. *Pediatr Ann* 1983;12(5):366–367.
37. Hayes FA, Thompson EI, Huizdala E, et al. Chemotherapy as an alternative to laminectomy and radiation in the management of epidural tumor. *J Pediatr* 1984;104(2):221–224.
38. Ninane J, Wese FX. Treatment of localized neuroblastoma. *Am J Pediatr Hematol Oncol* 1986;8(3):248–252.
39. Rosen EM, Cassady JR, Frantz CN, et al. Neuroblastoma: the Joint Center for Radiation Therapy/Dana Farber Cancer Institute/Children's Hospital experience. *J Clin Oncol* 1984;2(7):719–732.
40. Simone JV. The treatment of neuroblastoma. *J Clin Oncol* 1984;2(7):717–718.
41. Hayes FA, Green AA, Hustu HO, et al. Surgicopathologic staging of neuroblastoma: prognostic significance of regional lymph node metastases. *J Pediatr* 1983;102:59.
42. Evans AE, Baum E, Chard R. Do infants with stage IV-S neuroblastoma need treatment? *Arch Dis Child* 1981;56(4):271–274.

43. Berthold F, Trechow R, Utsch S, et al. Prognostic factors in metastatic neuroblastoma: a multivariate analysis of 182 cases. *Am J Pediatr Hematol Oncol* 1992;14:207–215.
44. Brodeur G, Castleberry R. Neuroblastoma. In: Pizzo P, Poplack D, eds. *Principles and practice of pediatric oncology.* Philadelphia: Lippincott Williams & Wilkins, 1993:739–767.
45. Shuster J, McWilliams N, Castleberry R, et al. Serum lactate dehydrogenase in childhood neuroblastoma: a Pediatric Oncology Group recursive partitioning study. *Am J Clin Oncol* 1992;15(4):295–303.
46. Brodeur GM, Seeger RC, Schwab M, et al. Amplification of N-myc in untreated human neuroblastomas correlates with advanced disease stage. *Science* 1984;224(4653):1121–1124.
47. Seeger RC, Brodeur GM, Sather H, et al. Association of multiple copies of the N-myc oncogene with rapid progression of neuroblastomas. *N Engl J Med* 1985;313(18):1111–1116.
48. Norris MD, Bordow SB, Marshall GM, et al. Expression of the gene for multidrug-resistance-associated protein and outcome in patients with neuroblastoma. *N Engl J Med* 1996;334(4):231–238.
49. Look A, Hayes FA, Shuster J, et al. Clinical relevance of tumor cell ploidy and N-myc gene amplification in childhood neuroblastoma: a Pediatric Oncology Group Study. *J Clin Oncol* 1991;9(4):581–591.
50. Caron H, van Sluis P, De Kraker J, et al. Allelic loss of chromosome 1p as a predictor of unfavorable outcome in patients with neuroblastoma. *N Engl J Med* 1996;334(4):225–230.
51. Evans AE, Brand W, de Lorimier A, et al. Results in children with local and regional neuroblastoma managed with and without vincristine cyclophosphamide and imidazole carboxamide: a report from the Children's Cancer Study Group. *Am J Clin Oncol* 1984;6:3.
52. Kushner BH, Cheung N-K, LaQuaglia MP, et al. International neuroblastoma staging system stage 1 neuroblastoma: a prospective study and literature review. *J Clin Oncol* 1996;14(7):2174–2180.
53. Matthay KK, Sather HN, Seeger RC, et al. Excellent outcome of stage II neuroblastoma is independent of residual disease and radiation therapy. *J Clin Oncol* 1989;7(2):236–244.
54. Nitschke R, Smith EI, Altshuler G, et al. Postoperative treatment of nonmetastatic visible residual neuroblastoma: a Pediatric Oncology Group study. *J Clin Oncol* 1991;9(7):1181–1188.
55. Haase GM, O'Leary MC, Ramsay NKC, et al. Aggressive surgery combined with intensive chemotherapy improves survival in poor-risk neuroblastoma. *J Pediatr Surg* 1991;26(9):11119–1123.
56. Shorter NA, Davidoff AM, Evans AE, et al. The role of surgery in the management of stage IV neuroblastoma: a single institution study. *Med Pediatr Oncol* 1995;24(5):287–291.
57. Perez CA, Matthay KK, Atkinson JB, et al. Biologic variables in the outcome of stages I and II neuroblastoma treated with surgery as primary therapy: a Children's Cancer Group study. *J Clin Oncol* 2000;18(1):18–26.
58. Bowman LC, Hancock ML, Santana VM, et al. Impact of intensified therapy on clinical outcome in infants and children with neuroblastoma: the St. Jude Children's Research Hospital experience 1962–1988. *J Clin Oncol* 1991;9:1599–1608.
59. Castleberry RP, Shuster JJ, Altshuler G, et al. Infants with neuroblastoma and regional lymph node metastases have a favorable outlook after limited post-operative chemotherapy: a Pediatric Oncology Group study. *J Clin Oncol* 1992; 10(8):1299–1304.
60. Guglielmi M, DeBernardi B, Rizzo A, et al. Resection of primary tumor at diagnosis in stage IV-S neuroblastoma: does it affect the clinical course? *J Clin Oncol* 1996;14(5):1537–1544.
61. Castleberry RP, Kun LE, Shuster JJ, et al. Radiotherapy improves the outlook for patients older than 1 year with Pediatric Oncology Group stage C neuroblastoma. *J Clin Oncol* 1991;9(5):789–795.
62. de Bernardi B, Rogers D, Carli M, et al. Localized neuroblastoma: surgical and pathologic staging. *Cancer* 1987;60:1066–1072.
63. Plantaz D, Rubie H, Michon J, et al. The treatment of neuroblastoma with intraspinal extension with chemotherapy followed by surgical removal of residual disease. *Cancer* 1996;78(2):311–319.
64. Castleberry RP, Cantor AB, Green AA, et al. Phase II investigational window using carboplatin iproplatin ifosfamide and epirubicin in children with untreated disseminated neuroblastoma: a Pediatric Oncology Group study. *J Clin Oncol* 1994;12(8):1616–1620.
65. Ettinger LJ, Gaynon PS, Krailo MD, et al. A phase II study of carboplatin in children with recurrent or progressive solid tumors: a report from the Childrens Cancer Group. *Cancer* 1994;73(4):1297–1301.
66. Philip T, Gentet JC, Carrie C, et al. Phase II studies of combinations of drugs with high dose carboplatin in neuroblastoma (800 mg/m^2 to 1 g $250/m^2$): a report from the LMCE group. *Prog Clin Biol Res* 1988;271:573–582.
67. O'Neill JA, Littman P, Blitzer P, et al. The role of surgery in localized neuroblastoma. *J Pediatr Surg* 1985;20(6):708–712.
68. Cheung NV, Heller G. Chemotherapy dose intensity correlates strongly with response median survival and median progression-free survival in metastatic neuroblastoma (Review). *J Clin Oncol* 1991;9(6):1050–1058.
69. Philip T, Zucker JM, Bernard JL, et al. Improved survival at 2 and 5 years in the LMCE1 unselected group of 72 children with stage IV neuroblastoma older than 1 year of age at diagnosis: is cure possible in a small subgroup? *J Clin Oncol* 1991;9(6):1037–1044.
70. Seeger RC, Villablanca JG, Matthay KK, et al. Intensive chemoradiotherapy and autologous bone marrow transplantation for poor prognosis neuroblastoma. *Prog Clin Biol Res* 1991;366:527–533.
71. McCowage GB, Vowels MR, Shaw PJ, et al. Autologous bone marrow transplantation for advanced neuroblastoma using teniposide doxorubicin melphalan cisplatin and total body irradiation. *J Clin Oncol* 1995;13(11):2789–2795.
72. Stram DO, Matthay KK, O'Leary M, et al. Consolidation chemoradiotherapy and autologous bone marrow transplantation versus continued chemotherapy for metastatic neuroblastoma: a report of two concurrent Children's Cancer Group studies. *J Clin Oncol* 1996;14(9):2417–2426.
73. Pinkerton CR. ENSG 1-randomized study of high-dose melphalan in neuroblastoma. *Bone Marrow Transplant* 1991;7(Suppl 3):112–113.
74. Pritchard J, Cotterill SJ, Germond SM, et al. High dose melphalan in the treatment of advanced neuroblastoma: results of a randomised trial (ENSG-1) by the European Neuroblastoma Study Group. *Pediatr Blood Cancer* 2005;44(4):348–357.
75. Matthay KK, Villablanca JG, Seeger RC, et al. Treatment of high-risk neuroblastoma with intensive chemotherapy radiotherapy autologous bone marrow transplantation and 13-cis-retinoic acid. Children's Cancer Group. *New Engl J Med* 1999;341(16):1165–1173
76. Matthay KK, et al. Long-term results for children with high-risk neuroblastoma treated on randomized trial of myeloblative therapy followed by 13-cis-retinoic acid: a Children's Oncology Group Study. *J Clin Oncol* 2009;27(7):1007–1013.
77. Berthold F, Boos J, Burdach S, et al. Myeloablative megatherapy with autologous stem-cell rescue versus oral maintenance chemotherapy as consolidation treatment in patients with high-risk neuroblastoma: a randomised controlled trial. *Lancet Oncol* 2005;6(9):649–658.
78. Cecchetto G, Luzzatto C, Carli M, et al. The role of surgery in non-localized neuroblastoma. Analysis of 59 cases. *Tumori* 1983;69(4):327–329.
79. La Quaglia MP, Kushner BH, Heller G, et al. Stage 4 neuroblastoma diagnosed at more than 1 year of age: gross total resection and clinical outcome. *J Pediatr Surg* 1994;29(8):1162–1165.
80. Matthay KK, Atkinson JB, Stram DO, et al. Patterns of relapse after autologous purged bone marrow transplantation for neuroblastoma: a Children's Cancer Group pilot study. *J Clin Oncol* 1993;11(11):2226–2233.
81. Haas-Kogan DA, Swift PS, Selch M, et al. Impact of radiotherapy for high-risk neuroblastoma: a Children's Cancer Group study. *Int J Radiat Oncol Biol Phys* 2003;56(1):28–39.
82. Laprie A, Michon J, Hartmann O, et al. High-dose chemotherapy followed by locoregional irradiation improves the outcome of patients with international neuroblastoma staging system stage II and III neuroblastoma with MYCN amplification. *Cancer* 2004;101(5):1081–1089.
83. Sibley GS, Mundt AJ, Goldman S, et al. Patterns of failure following total body irradiation and bone marrow transplantation with or without a radiotherapy boost for advanced neuroblastoma. *Int J Radiat Oncol Biol Phys* 1995; 32(4):1127–1135.
84. Graham-Pole J, Casper J, Elfenbein G, et al. High-dose chemoradiotherapy supported by marrow infusions for advanced neuroblastoma: a Pediatric Oncology Group study. *J Clin Oncol* 1991;9:152.
85. Halperin EC. Hepatic metastasis from neuroblastoma. *South Med J* 1987;80(11): 1370–1373.
86. Hutchinson RJ, Sisson JC, Shapiro B, et al. 131-I-metaiodobenzylguanidine treatment in patients with refractory advanced neuroblastoma. *Am J Clin Oncol* 1992;15(3):226–232.
87. Lashford LS, Lewis IJ, Fielding SL, et al. Phase I/II study of iodine 131 metaiodobenzylguanidine in chemoresistant neuroblastoma: a United Kingdom Children's Cancer Study Group investigation. *J Clin Oncol* 1992;10(12):1889–1896.
88. DeKraker J, Hoefnagel CA, Caron H, et al. First line targeted radiotherapy: a new concept in the treatment of advanced stage neuroblastoma. *Eur J Cancer* 1995;31A(4):600–602.
89. Gaze MN, Wheldon TE, O'Donoghue JA, et al. Multi-modality megatherapy with [131I]meta-iodobenzylguanidine high dose melphalan and total body irradiation with bone marrow rescue: feasibility study of a new strategy for advanced neuroblastoma. *Eur J Cancer* 1995;31A(2):252–256.
90. Mastrangelo R, Tornesello A, Riccardi R, et al. A new approach in the treatment of stage IV neuroblastoma using a combination of [131I]meta-iodobenzylguanidine (MIBG) and cisplatin. *Eur J Cancer* 1995;31A(4):606–611.
91. Yanik GA, Levine JE, Matthay KK, et al. Pilot study of iodine-131-metaiodobenzylguanidine in combination with myeloablative chemotherapy and autologous stem-cell support for the treatment of neuroblastoma. *J Clin Oncol* 2002; 20(8):2142–2149.
92. Thomas PR, Griffith KD, Fineberg BB, et al. Late effects of treatment for Wilms' Tumor. *Int J Radiat Oncol Biol Phys* 1983;9(5):651–657.
93. Halperin EC Long-term results of therapy for stage C neuroblastoma. *J Surg Oncol Suppl* 1996;63(3):172–178.
94. D'Angio GJ, Evans A. Cyclic low-dose total body irradiation for metastatic neuroblastoma. *Int J Radiat Oncol Biol Phys* 1983;9:1961.
95. Kun LE, Casper JT, Kline RW, et al. Fractionated total body irradiation for metastatic neuroblastoma. *Int J Radiat Oncol Biol Phys* 1981;7(11):1599–1602.
96. Wheldon TE, Wilson L, Livingstone A, et al. Radiation studies on multicellular tumor spheroids derived from human neuroblastoma: absence of sparing effect of dose fractionation. *Eur J Cancer Clin Oncol* 1986;22(5):563–566.
97. Eifel PJ. Decreased bone growth arrest in weanling rats with multiple radiation fractions per day. *Int J Radiat Oncol Biol Phys* 1988;15(1):141–145.
98. Eifel PJ, Sampson CM, Tucker SL. Radiation fractionation sensitivity of epiphyseal cartilage in a weanling rat model. *Int J Radiat Oncol Biol Phys* 1990;19(3):661–664.
99. Michalski JM, Ratheesan K, Grigsby PW. Neuroblastoma: treatment and patient factors influencing local tumor control by radiotherapy. In: *Proceedings of the American Radium Society 87th Annual Meeting,* Paris, 1995.
100. Wolden SL, Gollamudi SV, Kushner BH, et al. Local control with multimodality therapy for stage 4 neuroblastoma. *Int J Radiat Oncol Biol Phys* 2000;46(4):969–974.
101. Haas-Kogan DA. *Int J Radiat Oncol Biol Phys* 2000;47(4):985–992.
102. Haase GM, Atkinson JB, Stram DO, et al. Surgical management and outcome of locoregional neuroblastoma: comparison of the Children's Cancer Group and the International Staging Systems. *J Pediatr Surg* 1995;30(2):289–294.
103. Nickerson HJ, Nesbit ME, Grosfeld JL, et al. Comparison of stage IV and IV-S neuroblastoma in the first year of life. *Med Pediatr Oncol* 1985;13(5):261–268.
104. Strother D, Shuster JJ, McWilliams N, et al. Results of Pediatric Oncology Group 8104 for infants with stages D and DS neuroblastoma. *J Pediatr Hematol Oncol* 1995;17(3):254–259.
105. Paul SR, Tarbell NJ, Korf B, et al. Stage IV neuroblastoma in infants: long-term survival. *Cancer* 1991;67(6):1493–1497.
106. Wallace WH, Shalet SM. Chemotherapy with actinomycin D influences the growth of the spine following abdominal irradiation. *Med Pediatr Oncol* 1992;20(2):177.
107. Thomas PRM, Lee JY, Fineberg BB, et al. An analysis of neuroblastoma at a single institution. *Cancer* 1984;53(10):2079–2082.
108. Wallace WHB, Shalet SM, Morris-Jones PH, et al. Effect of abdominal irradiation on growth in boys treated for a Wilms' tumor. *Med Pediatr Oncol* 1990;18(6):441–446.
109. Neve V, Foot AB, Michon J, et al. Longitudinal clinical and functional pulmonary follow-up after megatherapy fractionated total body irradiation and autologous bone marrow transplantation for metastatic neuroblastoma. *Med Pediatr Oncol* 1999;32(3):170–176.
110. Hovi L, Saarinen-Pihkala UM, Vettenranta K, et al. Growth in children with poor-risk neuroblastoma after regimens with or without total body irradiation in preparation for autologous bone marrow transplantation. *Bone Marrow Transplant* 1999;24(10):1131–1136.

Chapter 87 Rhabdomyosarcoma

John C. Breneman and Sarah S. Donaldson

ANATOMY

Rhabdomyosarcoma (RMS) is a highly malignant soft tissue sarcoma that arises from unsegmented, undifferentiated mesoderm or myotome-derived skeletal muscle. It may occur at any site in the body, but the most frequently involved sites are the orbit, 9%; head and neck (excluding parameningeal tumors), 7%; parameningeal, 25%; genitourinary 31%; extremity, 13%; trunk, 5%; retroperitoneum, 7%, and other sites 3%.[1]

Epidemiology and Risk Factors

RMS is the most common of the childhood soft tissue sarcomas, with an annual incidence of 4.4 per 1 million whites and 1.3 per 1 million blacks. The male-to-female ratio is ~1.5 to 1.0, and males may have slightly better overall survival.[2]

The great majority of patients are <10 years of age at the time of diagnosis, and approximately 5% are <1 year of age. There are two peak age frequencies, at ages 2 to 6 and in adolescence. Tumors in the younger age group are likely to be of embryonal histology (or one of its subtypes). About 25% of patients are ≥10 years at diagnosis and their tumors are more commonly of alveolar histology. Age has been identified as an independent predictor of prognosis, with children <1 year and >10 years having inferior survival.[3] Adults with RMS have been reported to have poor outcomes, although there is evidence that when treated aggressively using pediatric-type protocols, the prognosis may be similar to that of younger patients.[4,5]

The cause of RMS is unknown; however, it is associated with several environmental exposures including paternal cigarette use, prenatal x-ray exposure, and maternal recreational drug use.[2] RMS is also associated with disorders in development, including central nervous system, genitourinary, gastrointestinal, and cardiovascular anomalies, and with congenital disorders including congenital pulmonary cysts, Gorlin basal cell nevus syndrome, and neurofibromatosis. In addition, RMS is the most frequently occurring childhood cancer in families with Li-Fraumeni syndrome, and its incidence is increased in children with neurofibromatosis type 1, Beckwith-Wiedemann syndrome, and Costello syndrome.

Recent developments in cytogenetics and molecular genetics now provide a more comprehensive understanding of the origin and biologic behavior of RMS. These are discussed in more detail later.

NATURAL HISTORY AND PATTERNS OF SPREAD

There are unexplained associations of site of primary tumor with age at diagnosis and tumor histology. For example, tumors arising in the urinary bladder and vagina occur primarily in infants and often are of the embryonal or botryoid histologic type. Tumors arising in the trunk and extremity occur in adolescents and are often alveolar or undifferentiated type. Tumors of the head and neck area occur throughout childhood and are commonly of the embryonal type.

RMS, a locally invasive tumor often with a pseudocapsule, has the potential for local spread along fascial or muscle planes, lymphatic extension, and hematogenous dissemination. The overall risk of regional lymphatic spread is approximately 15%, but varies with the site of the primary lesion. Lymph node metastases are rare in orbital tumors, but they occur in approximately 15% of tumors at other head and neck sites, most commonly the nasopharynx. Accounting for staging inaccuracies, regional lymph node extension occurs in approximately 25% of children with paratesticular, extremity, and truncal tumors.[6] The risk for lymph node involvement also correlates with primary tumor invasiveness and large tumor size.

Hematogenous metastases are detected at the time of presentation in approximately 15% of patients, particularly those with truncal and extremity primary tumors. The most common sites of hematogenous dissemination are lungs, bone marrow, and bone. Malignant pleural and peritoneal effusions may also accompany tumors primary to the chest and abdomen or pelvis, respectively.[7]

CLINICAL PRESENTATION

Because RMS occurs in multiple primary sites, there are many site-specific clinical signs and symptoms. It usually presents, however, as an asymptomatic mass. When symptoms are present, they relate to mass effect on associated organs and tissues. Tumors of the orbit may cause proptosis and ophthalmoplegia. Patients with parameningeal tumors often present with nasal, aural, or sinus obstruction, cranial nerve palsy, and headache. Genitourinary tumors may cause hematuria, urinary obstruction, or constipation.

DIAGNOSTIC WORKUP

Determination of tumor extent is best done with a multidisciplinary approach by a radiation oncologist, pediatric oncologist, and appropriate subspecialty surgeon. An expeditious local and systemic workup is essential because these tumors have the potential to grow rapidly. The initial assessment by all members of the team permits accurate staging and the formation of a uniform treatment plan. Table 87.1 provides recommendation for diagnostic workup at various sites. Early experience with combined positron emission tomography (PET) and computed tomography (CT) scanning indicates this modality may be a valuable component of staging[8] and may in fact provide more accurate staging than conventional imaging.[9] PET-CT may be especially valuable in assessing response to therapy, as conventional imaging has not shown a good correlation of tumor response to long-term clinical outcome.[10,11] Some children whose tumors exhibit characteristic fusion transcripts can be shown to have micrometastatic disease using reverse-transcriptase polymerase chain reaction techniques, even when there is no evidence of metastases from routine diagnostic procedures. The clinical significance of this is, however, unknown.[12]

STAGING SYSTEMS

The clinical grouping classification used extensively by the Intergroup Rhabdomyosarcoma Study Group (now known as the Children's Oncology Group Soft Tissue Sarcoma [COG

TABLE 87.1 RECOMMENDED WORKUP FOR TUMORS AT VARIOUS SITES

All Patients	Optional
All sites	
History	
Physical examination by several observers (including a pediatric oncologist, surgical oncologist and radiation oncologist)	Examination under anesthesia for infants and youngsters
Laboratory studies	Plain films of bones abnormal on scans
Complete blood count	Abdomen-pelvis CT, MRI, or ultrasound
Liver function tests	
Renal function tests	
Urinalysis	
Imaging studies	
PET-CT (this study can likely replace chest/abdomen/pelvis CT and bone scan studies)	
MRI or CT of primary tumor	
Bone marrow biopsy and aspirate	
Head and neck	
MRI or CT of primary tumor (with contrast)	Plain films of area
Lumbar puncture with cytologic examination of fluid (in parameningeal primary tumors)	Dental evaluation and x-rays
	Paranasal sinus and skull films
	MRI of spine if cerebrospinal fluid is positive or patient is symptomatic
Genitourinary	
CT of MRI of abdomen-pelvis (with contrast)	Ultrasound of pelvis
Pelvic examination under anesthesia	Cystoscopy
Extremity and truncal lesions	
MRI or CT of primary lesion (with contrast)	Plain films of primary site
	Ultrasound
	Barium gastrointestinal contrast studies

CT, computed tomography; MRI, magnetic resonance imaging; PET, positron emission tomography.

STS] committee) investigators is somewhat of a misnomer because it actually requires surgical pathologic evaluation (Table 87.2). It is not a staging system and does not accurately reflect the biology of the disease, rather it reflects the surgical procedure selected for an individual patient. It is, however, useful for guiding decisions for radiotherapy, based on the amount of residual tumor after the initial surgical procedure. A more valid pretreatment staging system uses a TNM (tumor, node, metastasis) approach, which emphasizes characteristics of the primary tumor, size and invasiveness, nodal status, and systemic spread. Noninvasiveness, small size, and an absence of metastases have been shown to influence prognosis.[13] The site of primary tumor also has a significant impact on survival.[14,15] The Intergroup Rhabdomyosarcoma Study IV (IRS-IV) has prospectively demonstrated the validity

TABLE 87.2 INTERGROUP RHABDOMYOSARCOMA STUDY CLINICAL GROUPING CLASSIFICATION

Group I	Localized disease, completely resected
A	Confined to organ or muscle of origin
B	Infiltration outside organ or muscle of origin; regional nodes not involved
Group II	Compromised or regional resection
A	Grossly resected tumor with microscopic residual disease
B	Regional disease, completely resected, in which nodes may be involved or extension of tumor into adjacent organ may exist
C	Regional disease with involved nodes, grossly resected, but with evidence of microscopic residual disease
Group III	Incomplete resection or biopsy with gross residual disease
Group IV	Distant metastases at diagnosis

Adapted from Mauer HM. The Intergroup Rhabdomyosarcoma Study: objectives and clinical staging classification. *J Pediatr Surg* 1980;15:371–372.

TABLE 87.3 INTERGROUP RHABDOMYOSARCOMA STUDY PRETREATMENT STAGING SYSTEM

Stage	Site[a]	Invasiveness	Size	Nodal Status	Metastases
I	Favorable	T1 or T2	a or b	N0 or N1	M0
II	Unfavorable	T1 or T2	a	N0	M0
III	Unfavorable	T1 or T2	b	N0	M0
			a or b	N1	M0
IV	Any site		T1 or T2	N0 or N1	M1

T1, tumor confined to site or organ of origin; T2, regional extension beyond the site or organ of origin; a, ≤5 cm; b, >5 cm; N0, no evidence of regional node involvement; N1, evidence of regional node involvement (enlargement of nodes on radiographic imaging is considered evidence of involvement, although histologic confirmation is recommended when possible); M0, no distant metastasis; M1, evidence of distant metastasis.

[a]Favorable sites: orbit, head and neck (nonparameningeal), genitourinary (non–bladder-prostate); unfavorable sites: genitourinary (bladder-prostate), extremity, parameningeal, other.

of a staging system incorporating TNM classification along with primary tumor site (Table 87.3). Three-year failure-free survival was 86% for stage 1 tumors, 80% for stage 2, 68% for stage 3, and 25% for stage 4.[1,7] Of note, the clinical grouping did not correlate as well with survival. In fact, failure-free survival for clinical group II patients in the IRS-IV study was superior to clinical group I patients (86% vs. 83%), probably reflecting the routine use of radiotherapy for group II patients.

PATHOLOGIC CLASSIFICATION

The histogenesis of RMS can be traced from mesoderm to mesenchyme and ultimately to striated muscle tissue. The classification of RMS initially used by the IRS investigators consisted of four histologic subtypes: embryonal, botryoid subtype of embryonal, alveolar, and pleomorphic. Embryonal histologies comprise approximately two-thirds of all cases, with most of the rest having alveolar histology.[16] Other variants including a "solid" alveolar pattern, considered a subtype of alveolar RMS, a spindle cell subtype of embryonal RMS, and a diffuse anaplastic variant have also been described.[17]

To improve reproducibility of pathologic subtyping and prognostic utility, pediatric pathologists developed an updated classification system: the International Classification of Rhabdomyosarcoma. This system is based on a review of IRS-II data and it groups pathologic subtypes into distinct prognostic groups (Table 87.4). The International Classification of Rhabdomyosarcoma system appears to be predictive of outcome and has been reproduced by several reference pediatric pathologists.[17,18] The superior prognosis group, comprising of two subsets (botryoid and spindle cell), carries a projected 5-year survival rate of 88% to 95%.[18] The botryoid subtype, a polypoid variant of embryonal RMS, has a grapelike appearance. The stroma consists of loose cellular tissue with a myxoid appearance. Under the superficial stroma is a hypercellular

TABLE 87.4 INTERNATIONAL CLASSIFICATION OF RHABDOMYOSARCOMA

I. Superior prognosis
  a. Botryoid rhabdomyosarcoma
  b. Spindle cell rhabdomyosarcoma
II. Intermediate prognosis
  a. Embryonal rhabdomyosarcoma
III. Poor prognosis
  a. Alveolar rhabdomyosarcoma
  b. Undifferentiated sarcoma
  c. Anaplastic rhabdomyosarcoma
IV. Subtypes whose prognosis is not presently evaluable
  a. Rhabdomyosarcoma with rhabdoid features

zone of tumor cells called the cambium layer of Nicholson. Botryoid tumors are usually noninvasive and localized and occur in mucosal-lined organs such as the vagina, urinary bladder, middle ear, biliary tree, and nasopharynx. The spindle cell subtype of embryonal RMS has a spindled appearance, often with a storiform pattern. It is frequently found in paratesticular sites.

Patients with embryonal RMS have an intermediate prognosis, with an 83% failure-free survival at 3 years.[14] The embryonal type consists of blastemal mesenchymal cells that tend to differentiate into cross-striated muscle cells. There is often a considerable variation in degree of cytoplasmic development, ranging from primitive mesenchymal to highly differentiated muscle tumor cells. Most of the tumor cells have eosinophilic cytoplasm, which is positive by periodic acid Schiff staining. Immunohistochemistry may demonstrate actin- or desmin-positive reactions. Ultrastructural studies exhibit evidence of myogenesis with the presence of thick and thin cytoplasmic intermediate filaments or Z-band material. Ribbon or strap-shaped cells and tadpole cells are characteristic. The presence of cross-striations confirms the diagnosis. The embryonal form may be distinguished from the other subtypes by specific structural abnormalities. A consistent loss of heterozygosity at the chromosome 11p15.5 locus suggests that this site is specific for the embryonal subtype,[19] although, unlike alveolar histology, no characteristic translocation has been identified. Immunohistochemical presence of epidermal growth factor receptor and fibrillin-2 appears to be highly specific for embryonal histology and is predictive of a favorable outcome.[20,21] Dysregulation of the RAS pathway has also been found in some patients and may be involved in the pathogenesis of this subtype.[22] The embryonal histology is found most commonly in the orbit, head and neck, and genitourinary sites.

The group with poor prognosis includes alveolar, diffuse anaplastic, and undifferentiated sarcomas. With routine use of immunohistochemistry and molecular genetic analysis, about one-third of RMSs are now classified as alveolar; it is most commonly found in adolescents with truncal, retroperitoneal, and extremity tumors. The alveolar subtype is characterized by a pseudoalveolar pattern of connective tissue trabeculae, lined by large rhabdomyoblasts and multinucleated giant cells. The "solid" variant of alveolar RMS grows as solid nests of closely aggregated tumor cells with less alveolar pattern. Alveolar histology is strongly associated with hyperdiploid content.[23] Approximately 75% of children with alveolar RMS exhibit a characteristic translocation involving chromosomes 2 and 13, t(2;13)(q35;q14) and occasionally a 1;13 translocation.[19,24] These translocations correspond to abnormal fusion genes involving *PAX3-FKHR* and *PAX7-FKHR*, respectively, and are probably the initial oncogenic events in these tumors.[25,26] Immunohistochemical presence of AP2-β and P-cadherin is also highly specific for alveolar histology.[20,21] The projected 3-year failure-free survival for children with the alveolar subtype is 66%.[1] Recent data suggest that fusion-negative alveolar RMS is more similar to embryonal histology, both clinically and molecularly, and may be more appropriately managed with those treatment algorithms.[27]

Undifferentiated sarcoma is largely a diagnosis of exclusion; it consists of a diffuse cell population of primitive, noncommitted mesenchymal cells. The 3-year failure-free survival rate of patients with undifferentiated sarcoma is 55%.[1] Today, sarcomas that lack characteristics of differentiation are most appropriately managed as non-RMS soft tissue sarcomas.

The pleomorphic type is extremely rare; many cases formerly classified as pleomorphic RMS are currently considered to be malignant fibrous histiocytoma. Previously, tumors classified as extraosseous Ewing's sarcoma were treated using guidelines for RMS. These are more appropriately considered in the Ewing family of tumors and are managed as such.

PROGNOSTIC FACTORS AND THERAPEUTIC CONSIDERATIONS

Because RMS is protean in presentation, factors such as age, site, stage, extent of disease, and pathologic characteristics of the tumor influence therapeutic decisions. These prognostic factors are interrelated and are best discussed as a function of the specific site (Fig. 87.1). Although most treatment failures occur within 3 years of diagnosis, about 10% of children who are free of disease at 5 years will subsequently experience disease recurrence.[28]

Orbit

The orbit has long been recognized as a favorable prognostic site. In addition to prompt recognition of the tumor, the paucity of lymphatics in this area means that lymphatic extension is rare. Most tumors in this site have embryonal histology, and hematogenous metastasis at the time of diagnosis is uncommon. Approximately 10% are alveolar histology, however, and the prognosis for these children is more guarded.[29]

When treatment for orbital tumors is individualized, it is generally agreed that no surgical procedure should be used that may compromise vision. In most patients, this means that biopsy only should be performed to provide the diagnosis. Primary treatment typically consists of vincristine, actinomycin-D, and cyclophosphamide (VAC) or vincristine and actinomycin-D (VA) chemotherapy with local radiotherapy beginning between the 3rd and 12th week of treatment. Radiation doses of approximately 50 Gy are often used, although results from the IRS-V study suggest that 45 Gy may be sufficient when given with a cyclophosphamide-containing chemotherapy combination.[30,31] Using this approach, cure rates of >90% can be achieved.[14] Chemotherapy without irradiation has resulted in local relapse and inferior event-free survival.[32] Although salvage radiotherapy for these patients can still be curative, functional vision in this setting is often poor.[33] Orbital exenteration should be reserved for salvage treatment and enucleation for management of posttreatment ocular complications.

With a combined-modality approach, radiotherapy can be directed to the tumor plus a margin without necessarily irradiating the entire orbit. Technique is very important for minimizing corneal and lacrimal gland dose and for preserving useful vision, ocular function, and appearance. Photon irradiation with the eyelid open can minimize the corneal dose when an anterior field is used and may be associated with improved long-term functional outcome.[34] Three-dimensional conformal or intensity-modulated radiotherapy technique is optimal for treating the target volume and sparing normal structures, and proton radiation has also been used successfully.[35]

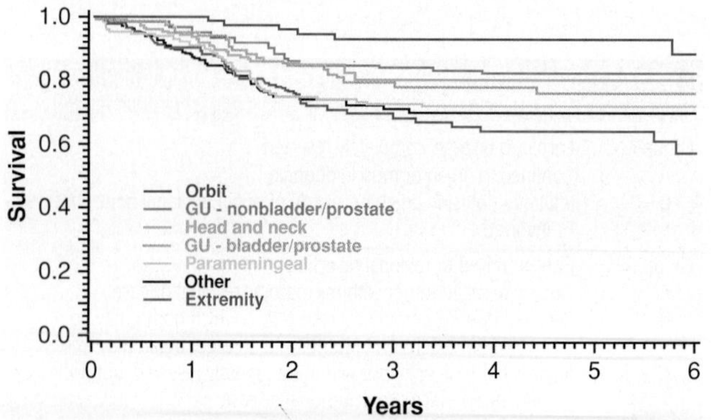

FIGURE 87.1. Survival curves for 883 children with nonmetastatic disease entered onto the fourth Intergroup Rhabdomyosarcoma Study are shown by anatomic site of the primary tumor. GU, genitourinary; B/P, bladder-prostate. (Adapted from Crist WM, Anderson JR, Meza JL, et al. The Intergroup Rhabdomyosarcoma Study-IV: results for patients with nonmetastatic disease. *J Clin Oncol* 2001;19:3091–3102.)

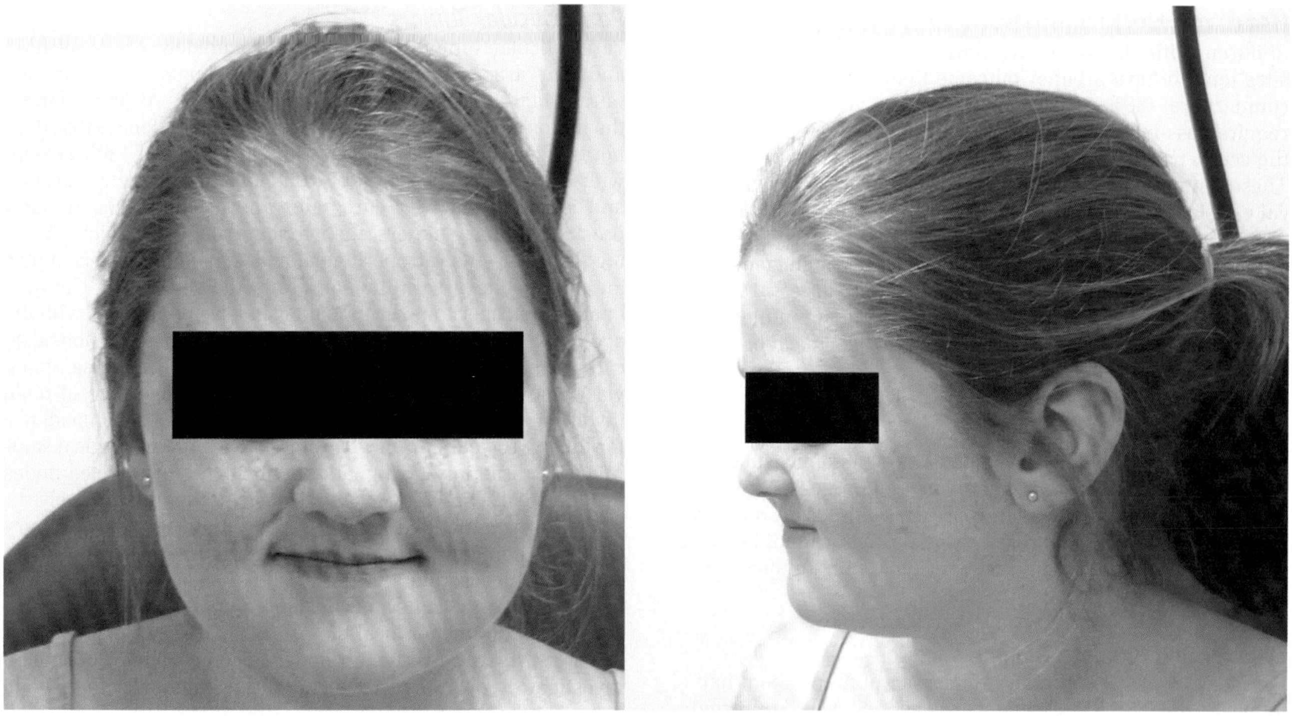

FIGURE 87.2. This 12-year-old girl was treated at age 3 years for an embryonal rhabdomyosarcoma of the nasal cavity. Her treatment consisted of excisional biopsy, followed by VAC (vincristine, actinomycin-D, and cyclophosphamide) chemotherapy and 41.4 Gy radiotherapy. Slight hypoplasia of the midface is evident, but overall cosmesis is excellent.

Head and Neck: Parameningeal Sites

Nonorbital RMS of the head and neck is grouped into parameningeal sites (nasopharynx, nasal cavity, paranasal sinuses, middle ear, pterygopalatine fossa, and infratemporal fossa) and nonparameningeal sites based on differences in natural history, treatment, and prognosis. Parameningeal RMS represent the majority of nonorbital head and neck RMS, and radiotherapy is essential for maximizing the chance of cure.[14,36] These tumors have a propensity for invading the base of the skull, creating a potential for cranial nerve palsy and direct extension into the central nervous system, a pattern of spread that is seen in as many as 41% of these patients.[37] Historically, as many as 35% of children with tumor arising in a parameningeal site would later have meningeal extension, and previous irradiation regimens called for whole-brain irradiation as part of central nervous system prophylaxis.[38] However, the prognosis of these patients is markedly improved with appropriate imaging, multiagent chemotherapy, and adequate irradiation of the primary tumor and adjacent meninges, and studies demonstrate that whole-brain irradiation is not necessary, even in the presence of direct intracranial tumor extension.[39] Patients with known meningeal dissemination should receive craniospinal irradiation. A radiation dose of 50.4 Gy in 28 fractions to the primary site is commonly used. Data from the IRS studies show improved local control in patients with intracranial tumor extension when radiotherapy is started within 2 weeks of diagnosis,[37] although other reports show no disadvantage with delayed radiotherapy.[40]

Aggressive surgery is rarely indicated because complete resection usually is not possible, does not obviate the need for high-dose radiation therapy, and often results in a delay of systemic chemotherapy because of postoperative complications. Surgical approaches to these tumors have been described by proponents of multispecialty skull-base surgery, but the efficacy of these approaches has not been firmly established.[41] Delayed surgical resection has been proposed as beneficial for children with residual tumor after completing chemotherapy and radiotherapy but is not considered standard of care.[42,43] The role of postradiation surgical resection is being investigated in select intermediate-risk patients enrolled onto IRS-V.

Five-year survival for patients with parameningeal RMS is approximately 75% with adequate radiotherapy.[44] For the subset of parameningeal tumors arising in the nasopharynx or nasal cavity, middle ear, and parapharyngeal locations, survival may be even higher,[39] and functional and cosmetic outcome can by good in spite of an aggressive treatment regimen (Figs. 87.2 and 87.3).

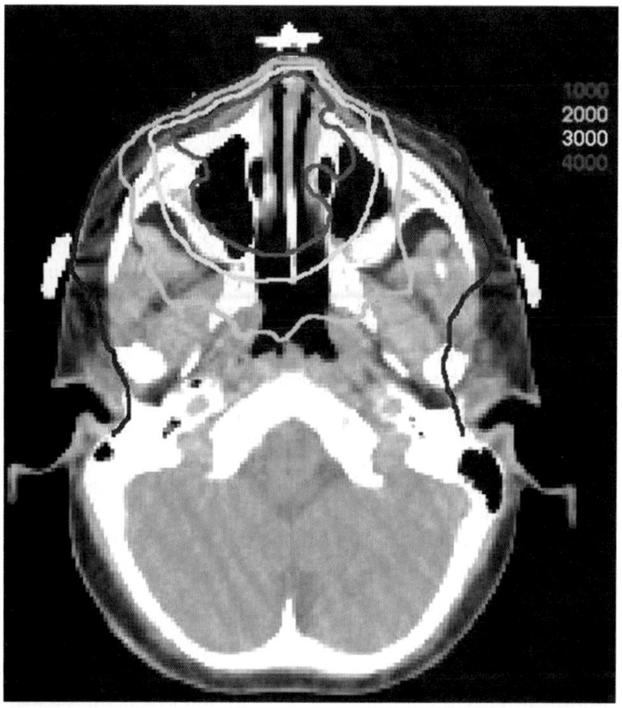

FIGURE 87.3. Isodose distribution from the treatment of the child in Figure 87.2 (doses in cGy).

Head and Neck: Nonparameningeal Sites

Children with tumors in nonparameningeal head and neck sites tend to have a better outcome than their parameningeal counterparts (80% 5-year failure-free survival in IRS-IV) and require less-intensive chemotherapy.[1,14] These sites include the scalp, parotid, oral cavity, larynx, oropharynx, and cheek. These tumors may be more amenable to complete gross surgical excision compared with their parameningeal counterparts. Approximately 15% of these patients present with regional lymph node metastases. Radiotherapeutic management is based on the amount of residual tumor after surgery. Draining regional lymph nodes are not routinely irradiated unless they are considered to be involved with tumor by clinical or pathologic assessment.

Pelvis

Pelvic tumors usually are divided into anatomic subgroups because the natural history, treatment, and prognosis are different for each site. Some children present with locally advanced pelvic tumors for which an exact site of origin cannot be determined. These large tumors are associated with an unfavorable prognosis.

Bladder and Prostate Tumors

Bladder and prostate primary tumors account for about half of all pelvic RMS[36]; 75% of patients are age <5 years at presentation, and more than 90% of these tumors are of the embryonal histologic subtype, with approximately one-third having a botryoid morphology. In boys, it is often difficult to differentiate a tumor of prostatic origin from one of bladder origin because disease usually involves both structures. However, patients with tumors arising in the prostate have significantly inferior survival compared with those with tumor confined to the bladder.[45]

Historically, anterior pelvic exenteration (or partial cystectomy for small tumors arising from the dome of the bladder) combined with chemotherapy and irradiation for microscopic or gross residual disease has been associated with a survival rate of approximately 70%.[15] More recently, emphasis has been on limited surgery to preserve bladder function. The IRS-II study treated these patients primarily with chemotherapy followed by delayed surgery or radiation therapy when there was residual or recurrent disease. This approach resulted in an inferior 3-year disease-free survival rate of 52%, compared with 80% for a primary radical surgical approach and only 22% of patients survived with intact bladders.[46] Subsequently, IRS-III intensified the therapy with systematic use of planned irradiation 6 weeks after the start of treatment and added cisplatin and doxorubicin (Adriamycin) chemotherapy.[47] The 5-year survival rate for patients with locoregional disease was 82%, with 64% of surviving patients retaining functional bladders, demonstrating the necessity of routine radiation therapy early in treatment.[48] Survival of patients with locoregional bladder or prostate tumors treated on IRS-IV was similar, with 40% of all enrolled patients reporting normal bladder function at follow-up.[49] A more recent analysis showed maintenance of continence in 69% treated with conservative surgery in a multimodality treatment program.[50]

The German Cooperative Weichteilsarkom Studiengruppe CWS-96 protocol treated children with bladder or prostate RMS using multiagent chemotherapy followed by response-adapted radiotherapy and surgery. Children with complete resection did not have radiotherapy, while others received 32 to 44.8 Gy using 1.6 Gy twice a day, depending on the tumor's IRS group and response to chemotherapy. Five-year event-free survival was 70%.[51]

A pooled analysis of patients treated prospectively on several cooperative group trials from North America and Europe showed improved local control for those who received radiotherapy as part of their initial treatment, but this did not translate into improvement in overall survival.[52]

Paratesticular Tumors

Paratesticular tumors represent approximately 7% of all RMS and may arise anywhere along the spermatic cord, from the intrascrotal area through the inguinal canal.[53] At presentation, the tumor usually is a painless scrotal or inguinal mass that does not transilluminate. Most boys with paratesticular RMS present with early-stage disease that is amenable to complete resection and is associated with cure rates approaching 90%. As with prostatic primary tumors, the lymphatic network is rich, draining directly to the retroperitoneal nodes along the external iliac and spermatic vessels, the aorta, and the vena cava. The incidence of retroperitoneal lymph node involvement varies with the age of the patient and method of staging (surgical vs. nonsurgical). In the IRS-III study, retroperitoneal lymph node sampling was done in most patients, showing a 14% incidence of node involvement for children <10 years of age and a 47% incidence for those ≥10 years. In IRS-IV, thin-cut CT without surgical sampling was used for staging, and the incidence of detected nodes dropped to 4% and 13% for the two age groups, respectively.[53]

The recommended surgical procedure for the primary tumor is inguinal orchiectomy. If there is no evidence of invasion into the scrotum and the proximal spermatic cord is free of tumor, this procedure is considered equivalent to an amputation, and no further local therapy is necessary. Surgical staging of retroperitoneal lymph nodes is controversial. European investigators do not recommend retroperitoneal lymph node sampling for these patients, preferring to treat with intensified chemotherapy in high-risk patients and salvage radiotherapy, if necessary.[54,55] In the IRS, the high risk of nodal involvement in certain subsets of these patients has led to the recommendation for ipsilateral retroperitoneal nerve-sparing node dissection for staging of all children ≥10 years of age.[53] In the absence of histologic documentation, enlargement of retroperitoneal lymph nodes on thin-section CT imaging is considered evidence of tumor involvement.

Patients with nodal disease have a 5-year survival rate of 69%, compared with 96% for those without regional nodal disease (P <.001). Regional lymph node irradiation to the periaortic and ipsilateral iliac nodes is recommended when there is nodal involvement.[56] Surgical violation of the scrotum or tumor extension to the structure is an indication for hemiscrotectomy or, less commonly, scrotal irradiation. If scrotal irradiation is used, orchiopexy should be considered prior to treatment to protect the remaining testes. Treatment programs must be planned to reduce morbidity, particularly among this group with high likelihood of cure.

Gynecologic Tumors

Tumors arising in the vulva, vagina, cervix, and uterus are about one-third as common as bladder and prostate primary tumors and account for 4% of all RMS.[57] Within this group, the vagina is the most common site of origin.

Patients with vaginal tumors are often much younger than those with other pelvic RMS, with most girls diagnosed before the age of 3 years. Most present with a vaginal mass or discharge; botryoid morphology is common. Initial surgery is used primarily for diagnosis, although gross tumor resection is occasionally possible without cosmetic or functional deformity. These tumors are often quite sensitive to chemotherapy, and treatment regimens have previously used a strategy of chemotherapy only, reserving surgery and radiotherapy for persistent or recurrent tumor.[57–59] However, analysis of data from the IRS-IV and IRS-V studies have revealed high rates of local failure for vaginal tumors when local control with surgery or radiotherapy is omitted.[31,60] Current guidelines from the COG STS committee call for radiotherapy in all patients with post-surgical microscopic or macroscopic tumor.

Uterine, cervical, and vulvar tumors receive chemotherapy and radiotherapy based on the amount of tumor present after initial surgery. Intracavitary and interstitial brachytherapy are useful irradiation techniques in some of these patients.[61] Data are limited, but with proper patient selection, disease control is excellent and late normal tissue effects may be significantly less with brachytherapy than is seen with external-beam techniques.[62] Permanent implants with iodine-125, temporary low–dose-rate, and high–dose-rate brachytherapy have all been used, and there are no clear differences among these techniques in terms of disease control or late effects. When temporary implants are used, high–dose-rate brachytherapy has the practical advantage of minimizing radiation exposure to the family and medical personnel caring for the child.

Survival after treatment is excellent. Children ages 1 to 9 years have a 98% 5-year survival. Survival for infants and adolescents approaches 90%, although these patients may require more intensive systemic therapy for cure.[57]

Other Pelvic Sites

These tumors include perianal, perirectal, and perineal primary sites. Regional lymph node involvement is relatively common. The location of these primary tumors creates surgical and irradiation challenges. Combined chemotherapy and radiation therapy programs are favored over primary surgical procedures if excision requires exenteration with urinary and fecal diversion procedures or is associated with organ or sphincter dysfunction.

Extremity

Tumors arising in the extremity are often of the alveolar or undifferentiated subtypes, large, deeply invasive, and associated with a high probability of lymphatic and hematogenous metastasis.[63] Complete surgical resection is difficult to achieve, usually requires extensive dissection, and is associated with a high risk of residual disease. Because radiation therapy and multiagent chemotherapy have been shown to provide excellent local control, it is advisable to avoid disfiguring and mutilating surgical procedures, with their attendant functional disabilities, and to recommend limb-salvage procedures including irradiation and chemotherapy.

Regional lymph node involvement is present in approximately 24% of patients and confers a more guarded prognosis.[63] Aggressive surgical staging of draining lymph node basins is important to define extent of involvement, although if lymph node dissection is performed, it is for the purpose of staging, not for treatment. Sentinel lymph node mapping and biopsy are being investigated for their diagnostic and prognostic value.[64,65] Radiotherapy of involved regional lymphatics is mandatory, and aggressive treatment of in-transit nodal sites may improve overall local control.[66]

Radiation therapy for extremity primary tumors requires careful immobilization techniques, sparing of nonirradiated skin for lymphatic drainage, and use of shrinking fields. Routine physical therapy during and after radiation therapy is important for obtaining an optimal functional result. Overall survival at 3 years for these patients is about 70%, although failure-free survival is only 55%.[67]

Other Sites

Patients with tumors arising in sites such as a paraspinal, retroperitoneal, or intrathoracic location have a poor outcome compared with other patients.[14] Most patients with tumors in these locations are unable to undergo complete resection of the tumor. Both local and distant relapse are common. These patients should be treated aggressively with high-dose radiation therapy and multiagent chemotherapy.

Metastatic Disease

Hematogenous or distant lymph node metastasis at the time of diagnosis is an ominous finding, although not all these children do poorly. The subset of patients who are <10 years of age and have only one or two sites of metastatic disease may have long-term survival chances of >50%.[7] Intensive multiagent chemotherapy plays a major role in the treatment of these patients, although marrow ablative techniques have not improved efficacy compared with conventional chemotherapy approaches.[68,69] Local control of the primary tumor is site specific, as previously described. Metastatic sites should be treated with radiotherapy when feasible.

GENERAL MANAGEMENT

A multidisciplinary approach using surgery, irradiation, and chemotherapy is important in the management of RMS; however, the optimal sequence and specific application of each modality continue to be investigated. Although the primary goal remains long-term cure, improvement in therapeutic results necessitates considerations of quality of life, with particular attention to maximization of functional and cosmetic results.

Surgery

Before the era of multidisciplinary therapy, surgical ablation resulted in a long-term survival rate of approximately 20% of those patients able to undergo resection.[70] Certain primary sites represented exceptions to these data; for example, approximately 50% of those with localized disease of the orbit survived after orbital exenteration.[71] However, with the introduction of effective adjunctive treatment, preservation of function and appearance became major goals. The concept of reasonable surgery has evolved. It involves removal of the bulk of tumor with maximal conservation of anatomic structures, including preservation of bladder, bowel, and sexual function in patients with tumors of genitourinary origin; limb function in patients with extremity tumors; and vision, voice, deglutition, and appearance in patients with head and neck tumors.

Resection of RMS from normal surrounding tissues is often technically challenging. Only 20% of tumors are located in sites where complete excision can readily be accomplished without an undesirable loss of function or cosmesis.[14] An additional 20% of patients have compromised surgical procedures, leaving microscopic residual disease. Sixty percent of patients have tumors amenable to biopsy only or present with metastatic disease and are not candidates for primary resection. When the IRS surgical grouping system is used, patients with tumor amenable to complete excision fare better than those who have subtotal resection or biopsy alone. However, the tumors that are most accessible to surgical excision are small and noninvasive and are confined to the organ or structure of origin. Assessment using a TNM system demonstrates that prognosis is dictated by tumor size and invasiveness rather than by the initial surgical approach.[72] Furthermore, combined-modality therapy provides good local control of the primary tumor, even after subtotal excision.[73] For these reasons, the trend has been toward less-aggressive surgical resection, with more reliance on radiation therapy and chemotherapy to provide local control.[14]

In cases of suspected RMS, the initial surgical procedure should be an incisional biopsy. Surgical excision is indicated if it can be done without compromise of function or cosmesis. Normal tissue margins of at least 5 mm around the tumor are usually required to consider the resection complete (IRS group I), although this is sometimes not feasible in some anatomic sites and smaller margins may suffice. If microscopic disease remains after initial resection, a primary re-excision can be considered prior to beginning chemotherapy. Those children who can be rendered microscopically free of disease by this procedure have an improved outcome, compared with children who remain in clinical group II following initial surgery.[74,75] Amputation of an extremity, orbital exenteration, mutilating surgery of the head and neck area, therapeutic lymphadenectomy, and radical neck dissection are procedures reserved in case initial therapy fails.

Second-look operations (also termed delayed primary excisions) may be useful for converting partial responses after chemotherapy into complete responses, and there is evidence that these procedures may improve survival.[43] However, data regarding efficacy of second-look operations are mixed, with some finding no benefit with this procedure.[10] To investigate if second-look surgery might allow a reduction in the amount of radiotherapy that is necessary to provide local tumor control, the IRS-V study evaluated this approach; preliminary results suggest that only select primary sites are appropriate for this approach, and final results are currently pending. Some investigators have used second-look operations in an attempt to eliminate radiotherapy, although this approach has resulted in inferior local control and survival.[76] Second-look operations may be used to evaluate therapeutic response after chemotherapy or radiation therapy. In the IRS-III study, 28% of patients categorized as having clinical partial response and 43% of those scored as having no response to induction chemotherapy were reclassified as having pathologic complete response after second-look operation.[77] These children enjoyed a survival rate similar to that of children who were able to undergo complete surgical excision at the time of initial diagnosis. Therefore, a clinical or radiographic evaluation indicating residual tumor after initial therapy may be misleading.

Chemotherapy

Chemotherapy is necessary in all cases. Several drugs have demonstrated single-agent activity measured as a percentage response rate, including vincristine (59%), dactinomycin (24%), cyclophosphamide (54%), cisplatin (15% to 21%), dacarbazine (11%), mitomycin-C (36%), etoposide (15% to 21%), ifosfamide (86%), irinotecan (23%), and topotecan (46%).[78–80] Agents with known activity against central nervous system tumors, such as the nitrosoureas and methotrexate, have not shown activity against RMS.

The most extensive experience in combination chemotherapy is with VAC or VAC plus doxorubicin (VACA). Some studies have suggested that patients with embryonal histology tumors in favorable sites who have no gross residual disease or lymph node involvement after the initial surgical resection may be adequately treated with VA for 1 year, provided that irradiation is given for microscopic residual disease.[14] However, data from the recently completed IRS-V study suggest that local control may be compromised when alkylating agents are omitted.[30,31] Patients with unresectable pelvic tumors may benefit from the addition of doxorubicin and cisplatin to VAC, but tumors in other sites do not seem to benefit from the addition of these drugs compared with an intensive regimen of VAC alone.

Some subsets of patients, such as those with tumors of unfavorable histology or unfavorable site and those with extensive tumor burden, continue to fare poorly. Some of these patients with embryonal histology may benefit from intensification of the cyclophosphamide or ifosfamide component of their chemotherapy, although there are conflicting data regarding this.[81,82] Patients with metastatic RMS benefit from the addition of ifosfamide and etoposide to the standard VAC regimen.[83] High-dose chemotherapy with total-body irradiation and autologous bone marrow transplantation has not improved the outcome in these high-risk patients.[68,69]

Initial intensive chemotherapy has been used as a means of pharmacologic debulking, potentially allowing for a more conservative surgical approach or less-aggressive radiation therapy.[46,84,85] However, response to induction chemotherapy—whether complete, partial, or no response—does not predict ultimate outcome.[86] When chemotherapy alone is used for tumors in sites such as the head and neck or pelvis, most children require radiation therapy with or without a follow-up surgical procedure because of incomplete response or local recurrence.[15,32,87,88] Omission of radiotherapy in these patients may result in inferior survival.[76,89] Even patients with only microscopic disease after initial resection (group II) require radiotherapy to achieve optimal local control.[90] In patients with group II disease who routinely receive radiotherapy, local control is 92%.[91] The approach of initial chemotherapy followed by limited irradiation or less radical surgery may be appropriate in the management of infants and very young children, in whom late effects of aggressive surgery or high-dose, large-volume irradiation are particularly severe, although this may lead to inferior local control and survival.

Radiation Therapy

Adequate irradiation implies careful attention to volume and dose. It is essential to evaluate the soft tissue extent of the primary lesion by CT scan or magnetic resonance imaging. Because RMS tends to infiltrate tissue planes widely, tumors often extend beyond a fascial compartment and beyond the obvious visible margins. Careful examination by a radiation oncologist at the time of initial diagnosis, even if the treatment plan calls for neoadjuvant chemotherapy, is essential to establish the appropriate tumor volume.

Treatment portals are designed to encompass the involved region at the time of presentation (before chemotherapy) with margins that encompass surgical sites and biopsy tracts. A biopsy should be performed of clinically suspicious lymph nodes, or they should be included in the radiation therapy portal. Prophylactic lymph node irradiation is not necessary in children with clinically negative findings who will be receiving combination chemotherapy. The gross tumor volume is defined as the tumor as seen at the time of initial diagnosis. A clinical target volume of 1 cm is added and can be modified to account for anatomic barriers to tumor spread (such as the bony orbit in primary orbital tumors) or to account for regression of "pushing" the tumor border after chemotherapy, such as may occur in large pelvic tumors that initially displace contents of the peritoneal cavity. The planning target volume adds a patient-specific margin, which is typically about 5 mm. Many current treatment protocols use a cone-down boost or simultaneous integrated boost to any gross posttreatment tumor volume after a microscopic tumor dose has been delivered. Patients with tumors at parameningeal sites (middle ear, paranasal sinuses, nasopharynx, nasal cavity, infratemporal fossa, and parapharyngeal area) have developed meningeal extension of tumor when inadequate irradiation portals were used.[39] Radiation therapy portals that cover the adjacent meninges in these patients can prevent meningeal relapse.[14,37]

Three-dimensional conformal and intensity-modulated radiotherapy treatment planning techniques are valuable for ensuring adequate treatment of the tumor volume and minimizing acute and chronic toxicity from the irradiation of uninvolved, adjacent structures.[37,92–94] Proton-beam radiotherapy is being increasingly utilized as access to this form of therapy increases,[35] and dosimetric studies consistently demonstrate decreases of integral dose to normal structures compared to photon-based techniques for many children with RMS (Fig. 87.4).[95] The long-term clinical significance of these differences in integral dose has not been studied, but as the number of proton centers increases, many clinicians are recommending proton radiotherapy for most affected children. Others, however, express concern regarding the increased neutron dose associated with many current proton delivery technologies and urge caution before adopting protons as standard of care for RMS.[96] Immobilization techniques that ensure reproducible portals are essential. Sedation or anesthesia may be necessary to ensure adequate implementation of the treatment plan. These complex programs are best conducted in regional centers by an experienced team of physicians, including a pediatric surgeon, pediatric anesthesiologist, pediatric oncologist, and radiation oncologist.

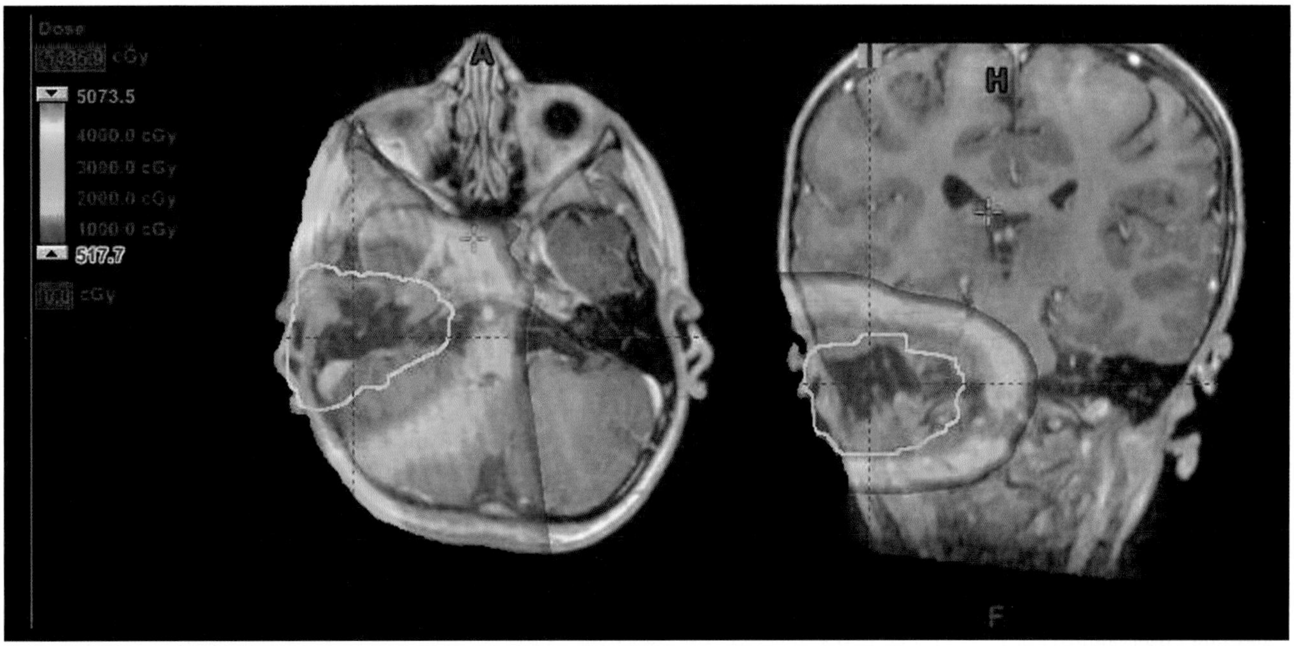

FIGURE 87.4. Isodose distribution in the axial and coronal planes for treatment of a middle ear RMS using protons. The physical properties of protons permit complete sparing of the contralateral structures and ipsilateral eye. (Courtesy of Danny Indelicato, MD.)

Radiation is necessary to ensure local tumor control in patients who are unable to undergo complete surgical resection. Local control of gross disease in most anatomic sites requires doses of 50 to 55 Gy. Data from the IRS-V D9602 study support a somewhat lesser dose of 45 Gy for gross tumor at orbital sites, especially if cyclophosphamide is included in the systemic therapy regimen.[30,31] In the IRS-IV study, investigators studied the efficacy of a higher radiation dose, 59.4 Gy, given in 1.1-Gy fractions twice daily at 6-hour intervals for children with gross residual disease.[97] This hyperfractionated regimen was compared in a prospective, randomized fashion to a standard radiotherapy regimen consisting of 50.4 Gy given as 1.8 Gy once daily. There was no difference in locoregional disease control, failure-free survival, or overall survival between the two groups. Therefore, the standard of care for group III RMS continues to be conventionally fractionated radiation with chemotherapy.

Ninety percent of patients with microscopic residual tumor achieve local control with 41.4 Gy, and the D9602 study results suggest that 36 Gy may be adequate for microscopically positive margins that are not associated with lymph node involvement. Investigators have been unable to generate a strict dose–response curve but have observed an association with age that suggests that lower doses, often given to infants and youngsters, are associated with higher relapse rates.[98] They also suggest that local tumor control is greater for tumors <5 cm in diameter than for larger lesions, supporting the adult experience with soft tissue sarcomas.[99,100]

Results of the IRS-I study had indicated that radiotherapy was not needed for patients whose tumors were completely resected at diagnosis (group I). Subsequently, a reanalysis of data from the IRS-I to IRS-III studies suggested that the subset of group I patients with alveolar or undifferentiated histology had improved overall and failure-free survival when radiotherapy was given to the primary tumor site.[101] A more recent analysis using data from IRS-IV did not, however, show a significant advantage for radiotherapy in group I alveolar tumors, and this practice is currently under review for the next generation of RMS protocols.[102]

Interstitial radiation therapy may play a role as primary treatment or as a boost after external-beam therapy for selected sites.[41,62] The advantages of precise shaping of the dose distribution, sharp falloff of radiation dose, and shortening of overall treatment time are especially attractive in dealing with infants and young children. Some investigators report a decrease in late normal tissue effects when compared with external-beam techniques.[103] There are no data regarding comparative efficacy or toxicity between high–dose-rate and low–dose-rate techniques. However, high–dose-rate remote brachytherapy may be particularly attractive in this patient population for logistical reasons. These children often require extensive care from family members and medical personnel during their treatment, and high–dose-rate techniques can eliminate radiation exposure to these caregivers.

The timing of radiation therapy must be carefully coordinated with planned surgical intervention and combination chemotherapy scheduling to optimize local control and ensure optimization of drug doses and unimpaired postoperative healing. Although radiation therapy is often delayed for several weeks to allow administration of neoadjuvant chemotherapy, some data suggest that earlier irradiation, particularly in high-risk patients, may provide better local tumor control and survival.[37,104,105] Interaction between radiation and some of the commonly used chemotherapeutic drugs can produce undesirable early and late effects. This is particularly true of dactinomycin and doxorubicin. Radiation therapy given concurrently with these agents is usually avoided. In contrast, systemic treatment with drugs such as vincristine and cyclophosphamide can usually be continued concurrently with the administration of irradiation.

Salvage Therapy

Salvage after recurrence of RMS is difficult, which probably accounts for the inferior survival seen with treatment approaches that do not maximize therapy at the time of initial diagnosis.[89,106] Because local recurrence is the most common pattern of failure, surgery and radiotherapy play especially important roles in the treatment of these children. Aggressive treatment programs utilizing radical resection and brachytherapy have had success in selected patients.[41] There is evidence that salvage is more successful if radiotherapy was not used in the initially treatment and can be maximized for salvage therapy. Care must be taken when evaluating patients for local recurrence. Residual masses can be seen in as many as 40% of children who are shown to be pathologically free of tumor.[107]

RESULTS OF THERAPY: SUMMARY OF CLINICAL TRIALS

Because of the low incidence of RMS, much of what has been learned about its treatment has come from cooperative group trials performed in North America and Europe. Various cooperative groups have used different philosophies of treatment. In general, the North American IRS studies have emphasized the role of local control measures and European studies have focused more on chemotherapeutic approaches.

Intergroup Rhabdomyosarcoma Studies

The IRS began intergroup clinical trials for RMS in 1972 and has enrolled several thousand children with this disease since then. A primary goal has been to test the efficacy of chemotherapy and radiation therapy as a function of surgical stage. In the first IRS study (IRS-I), radiation therapy was given initially for patients with group I and II disease and was delayed until week 6 for those with group III and IV disease. All patients received multiagent chemotherapy for 2 years. This study made several important observations[108]:

1. For localized tumors amenable to complete resection (IRS group I), postoperative radiation therapy is unnecessary if the patient is given 2 years of VAC. For these patients, the relapse-free survival rate in IRS-I at 5 years was 80%, and the 5-year survival rate was 81% to 93%. Subsequent analysis has shown a benefit to postoperative radiation therapy for patients with group I tumors of alveolar or undifferentiated histology.[101]
2. VAC failed to improve results obtained with intensive VA for patients with group II disease if postoperative radiation therapy was given. For these patients, the relapse-free survival rate at 5 years was 65% to 72%, and the overall 5-year survival rate was 72%.
3. VACA provided no advantage over VAC for patients with group III disease (gross residual) or group IV disease (metastasis) if routine radiation therapy was used in addition. The complete remission rate for group III patients was 69%, and for group IV patients it was 50%. Those who achieved complete remission had a 60% chance of staying in remission for 5 years in group III and a 30% chance in group IV. The survival rate at 5 years was 52% for group III and 20% for group IV patients.
4. The 5-year survival rate for the entire group was 55%.
5. Survival after relapse was poor—32% at 1 year and 17% at 2 years.
6. The risk of distant metastasis was much greater than the risk of local recurrence.
7. Primary tumors of the orbit and genitourinary tract carried the best prognoses, and tumors of the retroperitoneum had the worst.
8. The alveolar histologic subset had a poor prognosis, especially in extremity lesions.

A second IRS study (IRS-II) was built on the findings of IRS-I.[36] The results from this study include:

1. The 5-year survival rate for the IRS-II group was 62%, a 7% improvement over the IRS-I rate.
2. Patients in group I (excluding alveolar extremity patients) had better disease-free status with VAC (82%) than those who received only VA (68%), but they had similar survival rates (82% and 88%) at 5 years. Cyclophosphamide could not be withdrawn safely from the standard VAC regimen if irradiation was omitted from patients with group I disease.
3. Intensive (cyclic-sequential) VA therapy was as effective as repetitive pulse VAC therapy for patients with group II disease, if all patients received postoperative irradiation. At 5 years, 68% to 75% remained disease free and 77% to 90% were alive, with no differences between the two therapy groups.
4. Repetitive pulse chemotherapy for 2 years increased survival in children with group III disease but not in those with group IV disease; doxorubicin and dactinomycin had comparable efficacy in the pulse regimens used. The complete remission rates were 72%. At 5 years, 70% remained in complete remission and 64% were surviving.
5. In IRS-I, patients having tumors in parameningeal sites with high-risk factors (cranial nerve palsy, erosion of the base of the skull, or intracranial extension) had a high incidence of central nervous system relapse. In IRS-II, whole-brain radiotherapy irradiation, with or without intrathecal chemotherapy, was introduced. This prevented meningeal recurrence and increased survival in these patients with high-risk parameningeal primary tumors.
6. Primary repetitive pulse VAC for patients with special pelvic primary tumors (i.e., bladder, prostate, uterus, vagina) did not reduce the frequency of total cystectomy or produce durable bladder salvage, although survival was not compromised.
7. Survival after relapse was only 17% at 5 years.

The third IRS study (IRS-III) covered the period 1984 to 1991. This study revealed the following[14]:

1. The 5-year survival rate for the IRS-III group was 71%, an 8% improvement over the IRS-II rate. The 5-year progression-free survival rate was 65%, a 10% improvement over IRS-II.
2. Patients with group I favorable-histology tumors fared as well on a 1-year regimen of VA as did a comparable group treated with VA plus cyclophosphamide. The 5-year progression-free survival rates were 83% and 76%, respectively ($P = .18$).
3. Results for patients with group II favorable-histology tumors, excluding orbit, head, and paratesticular sites, were not improved with the addition of doxorubicin over VA chemotherapy × 1 year and radiation therapy.
4. Patients with group III tumors, excluding those in special pelvic, orbit, and other selected head sites (scalp, parotid, oral cavity, larynx, oropharynx, and cheek), fared better on the more intensive regimens of IRS-III than on pulsed VAC or VAC vincristine and doxorubicin (VADR) in IRS-II; the 5-year progression-free survival rates were 62% and 52%, respectively. The intensive regimen from IRS-III included multiple agents (VAC + doxorubicin + cisplatin + etoposide) plus radiation therapy plus second-look surgery. There were no differences in outcome among the three chemotherapy programs on IRS-III.
5. Patients with group IV tumors did not benefit from the aggressive therapy of IRS-III.
6. Patients with tumors in the bladder, vagina, and central pelvis in clinical group III had significantly improved outcome as compared with IRS-II patients, primarily because of the routine administration of early radiation therapy, which improved the bladder salvage rate from 25% in IRS-II to 60% in IRS-III.
7. Patients with unfavorable histology, in clinical groups I and II, who received VADR-VAC + cisplatin and radiation therapy had improved outcome over patients in IRS-II receiving VA or VAC and irradiation.
8. Patients with favorable-histology group II paratesticular tumors and those with favorable-histology orbit and head tumors in groups II and III do not require cyclophosphamide when VA × 1 year plus radiation therapy is used.
9. Whole-brain radiotherapy was omitted for patients with parameningeal primary tumors and cranial nerve palsy or base of skull erosion (although patients with intracranial extension of tumor still received this treatment). Risk

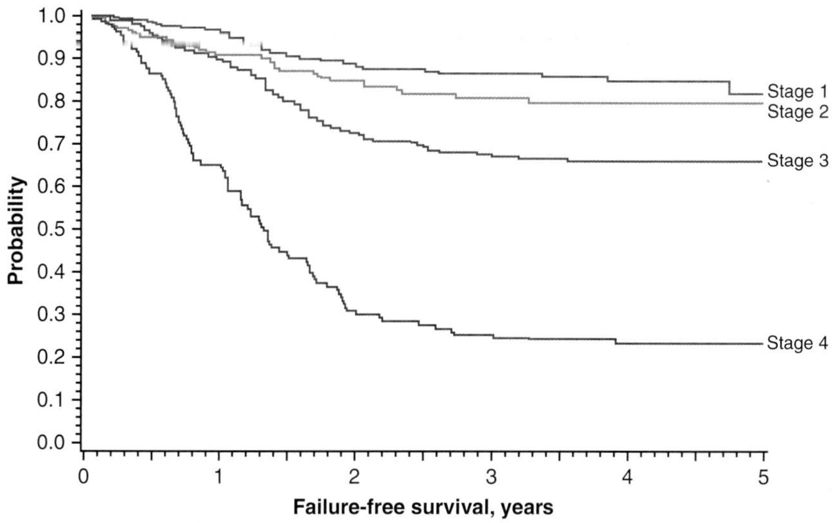

FIGURE 87.5. Survival curves of 1,010 children with rhabdomyosarcoma entered into the fourth Intergroup Rhabdomyosarcoma Study are shown by stage. (Adapted from Breneman JC, Lyden E, Pappo AS, et al. Prognostic factors and outcome in children with metastatic rhabdomyosarcoma: a report from the Intergroup Rhabdomyosarcoma Study IV. *J Clin Oncol* 2003;21:78–84; and from Crist WM, Anderson JR, Meza JL, et al. The Intergroup Rhabdomyosarcoma Study-IV: results for patients with nonmetastatic disease. *J Clin Oncol* 2001;19:3091–3102.)

of central nervous system relapse and survival were not compromised by this change if adequate local fields were used.

The fourth IRS study (IRS-IV) was conducted from 1991 to 1997 (Fig. 87.5).[1] Results from this study are as follows:

1. For patients with group III tumors, hyperfractionated radiotherapy was no more effective than conventional radiotherapy for tumor control and survival.
2. There was no difference in survival between VAC versus vincristine/actinomycin/ifosfamide versus vincristine/ifosfamide/etoposide in children with nonmetastatic disease.
3. Failure-free survival at 3 years for patients with embryonal histology was superior to results seen in IRS-III (83% vs. 74%), but no difference was seen for alveolar or undifferentiated subtypes.
4. Survival for patients with group I or II orbit or eyelid tumors was excellent when treated with VA and radiotherapy for group II disease.
5. Prognostic subsets of patients based on histologic subtype, stage, and group could be identified as follows: low-risk patients had embryonal histology and were stage 1 (all groups), or stage 2 or 3 and group I or II. All other patients with locoregional disease were intermediate risk.
6. Survival for patients with metastatic disease was superior with the drug pair ifosfamide/etoposide when compared with vincristine/melphalan.[83]
7. Whole-brain radiotherapy was omitted for all patients with parameningeal primary tumors except when there was cytologic evidence of cerebrospinal fluid involvement. Survival was not compromised by this approach.

The fifth IRS studies (IRS-V) were conducted from 1997 to 2005. They studied a number of questions that included:

1. Can a subset of the most favorable patients be treated without alkylating agents?
2. Can radiation dose be reduced to 36 Gy for microscopic disease and 45 Gy for gross tumor in the subset of patients with orbital primaries?
3. Can radiation dose be reduced for group III patients after induction chemotherapy and second-look operation?
4. What is the activity of topotecan and irinotecan in the treatment of RMS?

Results from some of these studies are now available and show that failure-free survival for low-risk patients (treated without cyclophosphamide and given decreased radiation doses as described above) was similar to results seen in IRS-III, which also did not use cyclophosphamide, but was inferior to results from IRS-IV where cyclophosphamide or ifosfamide was given. The conclusion of this study was that reduced radiotherapy doses did not appear to compromise local control, but the inclusion of an alkylating chemotherapy agent in the treatment regimen may be important for maximizing outcomes in these patients. These same reduced radiotherapy doses continue to be studied for low-risk patients in the current COG STS studies.[30,31] For patients with intermediate-risk disease, the addition of topotecan to the standard VAC regimen did not improve failure-free survival.[109]

Societe Internationale D'oncologie Pediatrique Studies

SIOP (the French acronym for the International Society of Pediatric Oncology) began multi-institutional trials for RMS in 1975 and has reported results from three studies to date.[87,110,111] The focus of these studies has been to minimize local therapy by using risk-adapted intensification of chemotherapy, with attempted salvage of patients who fail locally.

The first SIOP study (RMS-75) used VAC chemotherapy plus doxorubicin. Group III patients were randomized to early local therapy versus response-based delayed local therapy (surgery preferred over radiotherapy) after maximal chemotherapy response. No survival difference was seen between these arms, although overall survival was only 40%.

The second SIOP study, MMT-84 (malignant mesenchymal tumor), used a similar strategy of limited radiotherapy only when there was residual tumor after chemotherapy and surgery. Overall survival at 5 years was 68%, although event-free survival was only 53%, and 29% of patients had isolated local relapse.

The third SIOP study, MMT-89, concluded that alkylating agents can be omitted for patients with the most favorable prognosis. The use of radiotherapy was again limited, resulting in a local failure rate of 34%.

The SIOP and IRS studies differ significantly in their use of local therapy, with IRS studies emphasizing early introduction of radiotherapy for patients with residual tumor after surgery, and SIOP studies avoiding radiotherapy except for proven residual tumor after chemotherapy and surgery. A comparison of the results of the two studies has been performed, and although it is clear that some children can be cured without radiotherapy, the routine use of radiotherapy for residual tumor after initial surgery as used in the IRS studies results in higher survival rates for most subsets of patients.[89]

Cooperative Weichteilsarkom Studiengruppe Studies

The German-based CWS studies have taken an approach to local control that is intermediate between that of the IRS and SIOP trials. The CWS-81 trial used response-adapted radiotherapy after chemotherapy and second-look surgery with children receiving no radiotherapy, 40 or 50 Gy depending on tumor status. Results of this study showed that children who have a complete response to chemotherapy have a prognosis equal to those who have an initial complete resection of their tumor. However, those patients who do not have a complete response to chemotherapy by week 9 should have early surgery or radiotherapy. Overall disease-free survival after 5 years was 68% for children with nonmetastatic disease.[84,112] Local recurrence was the most common cause of failure.

The CWS-86 study used ifosfamide for all patients, with an abbreviated course of chemotherapy for favorable patients with early-stage disease, and altered the way radiotherapy was given.[113] Patients who had an early complete response to chemotherapy did not receive radiotherapy. Most received hyperfractionated accelerated radiotherapy of 1.6 Gy twice daily concurrent with ifosfamide and doxorubicin containing chemotherapy, using 32 Gy after a good response and 54.4 Gy after a poor response. Conclusions from this study were:

1. Duration of chemotherapy can be reduced to as little as 16 weeks for the most favorable patients.
2. Ifosfamide gives improved response rates compared with cyclophosphamide.
3. Hyperfractionated accelerated radiotherapy concurrent with chemotherapy as used in the study is tolerable and provided acceptable local control.

Like CWS-81, the majority of failures in this study were local, with an especially high local recurrence rate in those group II and III patients who did not receive radiotherapy.

The CWS-91 study continued the strategy of risk-adapted therapy.[114] Patients were initially stratified for treatment according to IRS group, tumor site, and histologic subtype. After induction chemotherapy, second-look surgery was encouraged, and those with a complete resection and no high-risk features did not receive radiotherapy. Others received 32 or 48 Gy (1.6 Gy twice daily) depending on risk factors and response to initial chemotherapy. Outcomes were compared to historical controls from the CWS-86 study. Major findings were:

1. Local control and event-free survival were improved in those patients who received radiotherapy when compared to those who did not receive radiotherapy, in spite of more unfavorable risk factors in the former group.
2. Results for patients receiving 32 or 48 Gy on CWS-91 were similar to results in similar patients treated with higher radiation doses on the CWS-86 study.
3. Patients with group I and group II tumors and favorable risk factors had equivalent outcomes with decreased intensity chemotherapy compared with similar patients treated in CWS-86.

SEQUELAE OF TREATMENT

Acute Effects

Acute side effects from surgery are primarily postoperative complications that are usually reversible and not serious. The acute toxicity from chemotherapy includes nausea, vomiting, mucositis, alopecia, and hematopoietic suppression. Drug-induced granulocytopenia significantly increases the risk of fever and infection, although the routine use of granulocyte colony-stimulating factor has lessened these risks. Newer protocols using more aggressive therapy, including topoisomerase inhibitors, ifosfamide, etoposide, and other agents, have other acute side effects, including renal and electrolyte imbalance, which demand close monitoring.

Acute radiation toxicity is related to the regions irradiated and the dose administered. It can be especially pronounced for tumors of the head and neck, abdomen, and pelvis. The synergistic effect of chemotherapeutic drugs such as dactinomycin and doxorubicin can be severe and may require modification of the treatment plan. Both dactinomycin and doxorubicin are known to accentuate a "recall" of radiation injury if given during or immediately after the course of radiation therapy.

Prompt attention to skin care is important. Moisturizers and steroid creams are effective symptomatic treatments for erythema and dry desquamation. Moist desquamation may be treated with aluminum acetate soaks or hydrocolloid dressings. Occasionally, a delay in radiation therapy is necessary to permit healing.

After orbital irradiation, an acute inflammatory reaction of the cornea and conjunctiva may be seen within weeks of completion of treatment. This can result in pain and photophobia. Topical steroids should be administered under the direction of an ophthalmologist for these symptoms.

Acute otitis externa or media with hyperemia and swelling of the membranes of the eustachian tube is common during or soon after treatment of head and neck areas. Decongestants are helpful in reducing the swelling. Erythematous mucositis, leading to a patchy, fibrinous exudate, is seen after head and neck irradiation, after drug therapy, and almost universally if the two are used simultaneously. Mouthwashes such as baking soda, 1% hydrogen peroxide, or combinations of diphenhydramine elixir, hydrocortisone, and antibiotics partially alleviate the reaction. Bacterial or fungal superinfection requires specific drug management. Pretreatment evaluation by a dentist is important to correct pre-existing problems and help guide preventive therapy such as dental hygiene and fluoride applications.

Acute gastrointestinal sequelae, such as vomiting and diarrhea, are usually managed by supportive care. Parenteral nutritional support may be necessary to prevent protein or calorie malnutrition.

Late Effects

Life-threatening late events occur in approximately 9% of survivors after treatment.[28] A higher percentage experience lesser degrees of late morbidity, with the risks dependent on factors such as primary tumor site, disease stage, and the treatment modalities employed.

Long-term sequelae related to specific chemotherapy drugs are usually site specific, and the morbidity may be accentuated by radiation therapy. Cyclophosphamide may induce hemorrhagic cystitis, and doxorubicin is implicated in late myocardiopathies.[115] Cisplatin carries a high incidence of hearing impairment. Alkylating agents and topoisomerase inhibitors are associated with the development of secondary neoplasms, particularly acute myeloid leukemia.[116,117]

Late radiation effects are related to the irradiated site, the dose of radiation, and the age of the child at the time of treatment. Effects include bone and soft tissue growth disturbances, dental abnormalities, cataract, hypopituitarism, gonadal dysfunction, induction of second malignant tumors (particularly bone sarcomas), and chronic organ dysfunction.[50,116,118–120] Long-term follow-up and treatment are important to minimize the impact of these, particularly for endocrine and dental complications.[121] Combined-modality treatment programs are significantly implicated in many of these complications.

Late surgical complications depend mainly on the choice of surgical procedure for primary treatment of the tumor. They include disfigurement and loss of function. Serious late effects of surgical treatment include the consequences of fecal and urinary diversion as well as ejaculatory impotence after retroperitoneal lymph node dissection.

FUTURE DIRECTIONS AND RESEARCH

Advances in molecular biology are providing a more comprehensive understanding of the biologic behavior of RMS and direct new research initiatives.

Chromosome aberrations are common in RMS. A consistent loss of heterozygosity at 11p15.5 is seen in embryonal RMS. Cytogenetic studies of alveolar RMS often demonstrate a translocation involving chromosomes 2 and 13, which affects the *PAX3* gene in band 2q35 and the *FKHR* gene in band 13q14.[122,123] The reciprocal translocation t(2;13) fuses *PAX3* to the *FKHR* gene, resulting in a chimeric structure that functions as an oncoprotein, resulting in dysregulation of cell growth and transformation.[124] Similarly, t(1;13) juxtaposes the *PAX7* gene on chromosome 1p36 with the *FKHR* gene on chromosome 13q14, again producing a chimeric transcript. These findings suggest that there may be a set of target genes involved in the pathogenesis of RMS, and work is currently under way to engineer vaccines against the resulting fusion proteins.[26] The identification of genes in alveolar RMS has permitted the development of molecular diagnostic assays, including reverse-transcriptase polymerase chain reaction and fluorescence *in situ* hybridization, for improved detection of alveolar RMS cells.[125]

Proto-oncogene research has focused on nuclear transcription factors. Embryonal RMS does not reveal amplification of either N-*myc* or c-*myc;* however, the majority of alveolar cases do have N-*myc* amplification. Survival among N-*myc*–amplified patients is poor.[126] Recent investigations link N-*myc* regulation to the *PAX3-FKHR* fusion gene present in many patients with alveolar RMS and may suggest targets for biologic manipulations.[127] Overexpression of the histone H3 lysine 9 (H3K9) methyltransferase KMT1A has been shown to block differentiation of alveolar RMS by repressing a myogenic gene expression program and is a potential target for novel therapies.[128]

The hedgehog pathway has been found to be activated in a subset of patients with embryonal and fusion-negative alveolar RMS.[129] These children have a significantly worse outlook than those with similar phenotypes without hedgehog activation. Inhibitors of the hedgehog pathway may offer therapeutic options in this group of patients. STAT3 is also an important signaling pathway in the oncogenesis of RMS, and targeting of this cascade is also being explored.[130]

Increased expression of the insulinlike growth factor 1 receptor (IGF1R) has been demonstrated in several RMS cell lines, and IGF1R inhibitors have shown significant preclinical antitumor activity.[131] Future studies will examine the efficacy of these drugs in the clinical setting.[132] Antibodies to the death receptor DR-5, present on many RMS cells, have also shown significant preclinical activity.[133]

Alteration of tumor suppressor genes is described in RMS, although their significance is unclear. Investigators have reported that >50% of both alveolar and embryonal RMS in established cell lines contain a mutant *p53* tumor suppressor gene.[134] However, more recent data indicate that the actual incidence of mutant *p53* in tissue derived directly from patient biopsies is much lower, and data regarding its predictive value for survival are mixed.[135,136] Studies of multiple-drug resistance genes, which encode P-glycoprotein, suggest that in RMS, high levels of P-glycoprotein lead to tumor resistance. In these tumors, there appears to be a correlation between P-glycoprotein positivity and poor outcome.[137]

The current generation of COG STS studies tests a number a clinical hypothesis. These include testing the ability to reduce the duration of chemotherapy for favorable prognosis tumors, studying the effect of delivering radiotherapy early in the course of treatment (week 4) concurrently with irinotecan for intermediate-risk patients, and evaluating the prognostic value of early treatment response as assessed by PET imaging.

Future directions and research in RMS are being driven by many exciting molecular biologic and technologic advances. Such new findings provide hope for more refined risk-based therapy in RMS and potentially for gene therapy to be added to the therapeutic armamentarium.

SELECTED REFERENCES

A full list of references for this chapter is available online.

1. Crist WM, Anderson JR, Meza JL, et al. Intergroup rhabdomyosarcoma study-IV: results for patients with nonmetastatic disease. *J Clin Oncol* 2001;19:3091–3102.
2. Ognjanovic S, Linabery AM, Charbonneau B, et al. Trends in childhood rhabdomyosarcoma incidence and survival in the United States, 1975–2005. *Cancer* 2009; 115:4218–4226.
3. Joshi D, Anderson JR, Paidas C, et al. Age is an independent prognostic factor in rhabdomyosarcoma: a report from the Soft Tissue Sarcoma Committee of the Children's Oncology Group. *Pediatr Blood Cancer* 2004;42:64–73.
4. Ferrari A, Dileo P, Casanova M, et al. Rhabdomyosarcoma in adults. A retrospective analysis of 171 patients treated at a single institution. *Cancer* 2003;98:571–580.
5. Ogilvie CM, Crawford EA, Slotcavage RL, et al. Treatment of adult rhabdomyosarcoma. *Am J Clin Oncol* 2010;33:128–131.
6. La TH, Wolden SL, Rodeberg DA, et al. Regional nodal involvement and patterns of spread along in-transit pathways in children with rhabdomyosarcoma of the extremity: a report from the Children's Oncology Group. *Int J Radiat Oncol Biol Phys* 2011;80:1151–1157.
7. Breneman JC, Lyden E, Pappo AS, et al. Prognostic factors and clinical outcomes in children and adolescents with metastatic rhabdomyosarcoma—a report from the Intergroup Rhabdomyosarcoma Study IV. *J Clin Oncol* 2003;21:78–84.
8. McCarville MB, Christie R, Daw NC, et al. PET/CT in the evaluation of childhood sarcomas. *AJR Am J Roentgenol* 2005;184:1293–1304.
9. Tateishi U, Hosono A, Makimoto A, et al. Comparative study of FDG PET/CT and conventional imaging in the staging of rhabdomyosarcoma. *Ann Nucl Med* 2009;23:155–161.
10. Rodeberg DA, Stoner JA, Hayes-Jordan A, et al. Prognostic significance of tumor response at the end of therapy in group III rhabdomyosarcoma: a report from the Children's Oncology Group. *J Clin Oncol* 2009;27:3705–3711.
11. Burke M, Anderson JR, Kao SC, et al. Assessment of response to induction therapy and its influence on 5-year failure-free survival in group III rhabdomyosarcoma: the Intergroup Rhabdomyosarcoma Study-IV experience—a report from the Soft Tissue Sarcoma Committee of the Children's Oncology Group. *J Clin Oncol* 2007;25:4909–4913.
14. Crist W, Gehan EA, Ragab AH, et al. The third Intergroup Rhabdomyosarcoma Study. *J Clin Oncol* 1995;13:610–630.
15. Rodary C, Gehan EA, Flamant F, et al. Prognostic factors in 951 nonmetastatic rhabdomyosarcoma in children: a report from the International Rhabdomyosarcoma Workshop. *Med Pediatr Oncol* 1991;19:89–95.
17. Qualman SJ, Coffin CM, Newton WA, et al. Intergroup Rhabdomyosarcoma Study: update for pathologists. *Pediatr Dev Pathol* 1998;1:550–561.
20. Wachtel M, Runge T, Leuschner I, et al. Subtype and prognostic classification of rhabdomyosarcoma by immunohistochemistry. *J Clin Oncol* 2006;24:816–822.
21. Grass B, Wachtel M, Behnke S, et al. Immunohistochemical detection of EGFR, fibrillin-2, P-cadherin and AP2beta as biomarkers for rhabdomyosarcoma diagnostics. *Histopathology* 2009;54:873–879.
22. Martinelli S, McDowell HP, Vigne SD, et al. RAS signaling dysregulation in human embryonal rhabdomyosarcoma. *Genes Chromosomes Cancer* 2009;48:975–982.
26. van den Broeke LT, Pendleton CD, Mackall C, et al. Identification and epitope enhancement of a PAX-FKHR fusion protein breakpoint epitope in alveolar rhabdomyosarcoma cells created by a tumorigenic chromosomal translocation inducing CTL capable of lysing human tumors. *Cancer Res* 2006;66:1818–1823.
27. Williamson D, Missiaglia E, de Reynies A, et al. Fusion gene-negative alveolar rhabdomyosarcoma is clinically and molecularly indistinguishable from embryonal rhabdomyosarcoma. *J Clin Oncol* 2010;28:2151–2158.
28. Sung L, Anderson JR, Donaldson SS, et al. Late events occurring five years or more after successful therapy for childhood rhabdomyosarcoma: a report from the Soft Tissue Sarcoma Committee of the Children's Oncology Group. *Eur J Cancer* 2004;40:1878–1885.
30. Raney R, Walterhouse DO, Meza JL, et al. Results of the Intergroup Rhabdomyosarcoma Study Group D9602 protocol, using vincristine and dactinomycin with or without cyclophosphamide and radiation therapy, for newly diagnosed patients with low-risk embryonal rhabdomyosarcoma: a report from the Soft Tissue Sarcoma Committee of the Children's Oncology Group. *J Clin Oncol* 2011; 29:1312–1318.
31. Breneman J, Meza J, Donaldson S, et al. Local control with reduced dose radiotherapy for low risk rhabdomyosarcoma: a report from the Children's Oncology Group D9602 study. *Int J Radiat Oncol Biol Phys* 2012;83(2):720–726.
32. Rousseau P, Flamant F, Quintana E, et al. Primary chemotherapy in rhabdomyosarcomas and other malignant mesenchymal tumors of the orbit: results of the International Society of Pediatric Oncology MMT 84 Study. *J Clin Oncol* 1994; 12:516–521.
35. Yock T, Schneider R, Friedmann A, et al. Proton radiotherapy for orbital rhabdomyosarcoma: clinical outcome and a dosimetric comparison with photons. *Int J Radiat Oncol Biol Phys* 2005;63:1161–1168.
36. Maurer HM, Gehan EA, Beltangady M, et al. The Intergroup Rhabdomyosarcoma Study-II. *Cancer* 1993;71:1904–1922.
37. Michalski JM, Meza J, Breneman JC, et al. Influence of radiation therapy parameters on outcome in children treated with radiation therapy for localized parameningeal rhabdomyosarcoma in Intergroup Rhabdomyosarcoma Study Group trials II through IV. *Int J Radiat Oncol Biol Phys* 2004;59:1027–1038.
40. Douglas JG, Arndt CA, Hawkins DS. Delayed radiotherapy following dose intensive chemotherapy for parameningeal rhabdomyosarcoma (PM-RMS) of childhood. *Eur J Cancer* 2007;43:1045–1050.
46. Raney RB Jr, Gehan EA, Hays DM, et al. Primary chemotherapy with or without radiation therapy and/or surgery for children with localized sarcoma of the bladder, prostate, vagina, uterus, and cervix. A comparison of the results in Intergroup Rhabdomyosarcoma Studies I and II. *Cancer* 1990;66:2072–2081.
49. Arndt C, Rodeberg D, Breitfeld PP, et al. Does bladder preservation (as a surgical principle) lead to retaining bladder function in bladder/prostate

rhabdomyosarcoma? Results from Intergroup Rhabdomyosarcoma Study IV. *J Urol* 2004;171:2396–403.
50. Raney B, Anderson J, Jenney M, et al. Late effects in 164 patients with rhabdomyosarcoma of the bladder/prostate region: a report from the international workshop. *J Urol* 2006;176:2190–2194; discussion 4–5.
51. Seitz G, Dantonello TM, Int-Veen C, et al. Treatment efficiency, outcome and surgical treatment problems in patients suffering from localized embryonal bladder/prostate rhabdomyosarcoma: a report from the cooperative soft tissue sarcoma trial CWS-96. *Pediatr Blood Cancer* 2011;56(5):718–724.
52. Rodeberg DA, Anderson JR, Arndt CA, et al. Comparison of outcomes based on treatment algorithms for rhabdomyosarcoma of the bladder/prostate: combined results from the Children's Oncology Group, German Cooperative Soft Tissue Sarcoma Study, Italian Cooperative Group, and International Society of Pediatric Oncology Malignant Mesenchymal Tumors Committee. *Int J Cancer* 2011;128:1232–1239.
53. Wiener ES, Anderson JR, Ojimba JI, et al. Controversies in the management of paratesticular rhabdomyosarcoma: is staging retroperitoneal lymph node dissection necessary for adolescents with resected paratesticular rhabdomyosarcoma? *Semin Pediatr Surg* 2001;10:146–152.
56. Wiener ES, Lawrence W, Hays D, et al. Retroperitoneal node biopsy in paratesticular rhabdomyosarcoma. *J Pediatr Surg* 1994;29:171–177; discussion 8.
60. Walterhouse DO, Meza JL, Breneman JC, et al. Local control and outcome in children with localized vaginal rhabdomyosarcoma: a report from the Soft Tissue Sarcoma Committee of the Children's Oncology Group. *Pediatr Blood Cancer* 2011;57(1):76–83.
61. Magne N, Oberlin O, Martelli H, et al. Vulval and vaginal rhabdomyosarcoma in children: update and reappraisal of Institut Gustave Roussy brachytherapy experience. *Int J Radiat Oncol Biol Phys* 2008;72:878–883.
64. McMulkin HM, Yanchar NL, Fernandez CV, et al. Sentinel lymph node mapping and biopsy: a potentially valuable tool in the management of childhood extremity rhabdomyosarcoma. *Pediatr Surg Int* 2003;19:453–456.
65. Weiss BD, Dasgupta R, Gelfand MJ, et al. Use of sentinel node biopsy for staging parameningeal rhabdomyosarcoma. *Pediatr Blood Cancer* 2011;57:520–523.
66. La TH, Wolden SL, Rodeberg DA, et al. Regional nodal involvement and patterns of spread along in-transit pathways in children with rhabdomyosarcoma of the extremity: a report from the Children's Oncology Group. *Int J Radiat Oncol Biol Phys* 2010;80:1151–1157.
69. McDowell HP, Foot AB, Ellershaw C, et al. Outcomes in paediatric metastatic rhabdomyosarcoma: results of The International Society of Paediatric Oncology (SIOP) study MMT-98. *Eur J Cancer* 2010;46:1588–1595.
72. Pedrick TJ, Donaldson SS, Cox RS. Rhabdomyosarcoma: the Stanford experience using a TNM staging system. *J Clin Oncol* 1986;4:370–378.
74. Cecchetto G, Carli M, Sotti G, et al. Importance of local treatment in pediatric soft tissue sarcomas with microscopic residual after primary surgery: results of the Italian Cooperative Study RMS-88. *Med Pediatr Oncol* 2000;34:97–101.
76. Cecchetto G, Carretto E, Bisogno G, et al. Complete second look operation and radiotherapy in locally advanced non-alveolar rhabdomyosarcoma in children: a report from the AIEOP Soft Tissue Sarcoma Committee. *Pediatr Blood Cancer* 2008;51:593–597.
79. Pappo AS, Lyden E, Breneman J, et al. Up-front window trial of topotecan in previously untreated children and adolescents with metastatic rhabdomyosarcoma: an Intergroup Rhabdomyosarcoma Study. *J Clin Oncol* 2001;19:213–219.
81. Baker KS, Anderson JR, Link MP, et al. Benefit of intensified therapy for patients with local or regional embryonal rhabdomyosarcoma: results from the Intergroup Rhabdomyosarcoma Study IV. *J Clin Oncol* 2000;18:2427–2434.
83. Breitfeld PP, Lyden E, Raney RB, et al. Ifosfamide and etoposide are superior to vincristine and melphalan for pediatric metastatic rhabdomyosarcoma when administered with irradiation and combination chemotherapy: a report from the Intergroup Rhabdomyosarcoma Study Group. *J Pediatr Hematol Oncol* 2001; 23:225–233.
84. Koscielniak E, Jurgens H, Winkler K, et al. Treatment of soft tissue sarcoma in childhood and adolescence. A report of the German Cooperative Soft Tissue Sarcoma Study. *Cancer* 1992;70:2557–2567.
87. Stevens MC, Rey A, Bouvet N, et al. Treatment of nonmetastatic rhabdomyosarcoma in childhood and adolescence: third study of the International Society of Paediatric Oncology—SIOP Malignant Mesenchymal Tumor 89. *J Clin Oncol* 2005;23:2618–2628.
89. Donaldson SS, Anderson JR. Rhabdomyosarcoma: many similarities, a few philosophical differences. *J Clin Oncol* 2005;23:2586–2587.
90. Schuck A, Mattke AC, Schmidt B, et al. Group II rhabdomyosarcoma and rhabdomyosarcomalike tumors: is radiotherapy necessary? *J Clin Oncol* 2004;22:143–149.
95. Cotter SE, Herrup DA, Friedmann A, et al. Proton radiotherapy for pediatric bladder/prostate rhabdomyosarcoma: clinical outcomes and dosimetry compared to intensity-modulated radiation therapy. *Int J Radiat Oncol Biol Phys* 2011;81(5):1367–1373.
97. Donaldson SS, Meza J, Breneman JC, et al. Results from the IRS-IV randomized trial of hyperfractionated radiotherapy in children with rhabdomyosarcoma—a report from the IRSG. *Int J Radiat Oncol Biol Phys* 2001;51:718–728.
98. Malempati S, Rodeberg DA, Donaldson SS, et al. Rhabdomyosarcoma in infants younger than 1 year: a report from the Children's Oncology Group. *Cancer* 2011;117(15):3493–3501.
99. Wharam MD, Hanfelt JJ, Tefft MC, et al. Radiation therapy for rhabdomyosarcoma: local failure risk for clinical group III patients on Intergroup Rhabdomyosarcoma Study II. *Int J Radiat Oncol Biol Phys* 1997;38:797–804.
100. Wharam MD, Meza J, Anderson J, et al. Failure pattern and factors predictive of local failure in rhabdomyosarcoma: a report of group III patients on the third Intergroup Rhabdomyosarcoma Study. *J Clin Oncol* 2004;22:1902–1908.
101. Wolden SL, Anderson JR, Crist WM, et al. Indications for radiotherapy and chemotherapy after complete resection in rhabdomyosarcoma: a report from the Intergroup Rhabdomyosarcoma studies I to III. *J Clin Oncol* 1999;17:3468–3475.
102. Raney RB, Anderson JR, Brown KL, et al. Treatment results for patients with localized, completely resected (group I) alveolar rhabdomyosarcoma on Intergroup Rhabdomyosarcoma Study Group (IRSG) protocols III and IV, 1984–1997: a report from the Children's Oncology Group. *Pediatr Blood Cancer* 2010;55:612–616.
108. Maurer HM, Beltangady M, Gehan EA, et al. The Intergroup Rhabdomyosarcoma Study-I. A final report. *Cancer* 1988;61:209–220.
109. Arndt CA, Stoner JA, Hawkins DS, et al. Vincristine, actinomycin, and cyclophosphamide compared with vincristine, actinomycin, and cyclophosphamide alternating with vincristine, topotecan, and cyclophosphamide for intermediate-risk rhabdomyosarcoma: Children's Oncology Group Study D9803. *J Clin Oncol* 2009;27:5182–5188.
110. Flamant F, Rodary C, Rey A, et al. Treatment of non-metastatic rhabdomyosarcomas in childhood and adolescence. Results of the second study of the International Society of Paediatric Oncology: MMT84. *Eur J Cancer* 1998;34:1050–1062.
112. Treuner J, Kuhl J, Beck J, et al. New aspects in the treatment of childhood rhabdomyosarcoma: results of the German Cooperative Soft-Tissue Sarcoma Study (CWS-81). *Prog Pediatr Surg* 1989;22:162–173.
113. Koscielniak E, Harms D, Henze G, et al. Results of treatment for soft tissue sarcoma in childhood and adolescence: a final report of the German Cooperative Soft Tissue Sarcoma Study CWS-86. *J Clin Oncol* 1999;17:3706–3719.
114. Dantonello TM, Int-Veen C, Harms D, et al. Cooperative trial CWS-91 for localized soft tissue sarcoma in children, adolescents, and young adults. *J Clin Oncol* 2009;27:1446–1455.
115. Punyko JA, Mertens AC, Gurney JG, et al. Long-term medical effects of childhood and adolescent rhabdomyosarcoma: a report from the childhood cancer survivor study. *Pediatr Blood Cancer* 2005;44:643–653.
127. Mercado GE, Xia SJ, Zhang C, et al. Identification of PAX3-FKHR-regulated genes differentially expressed between alveolar and embryonal rhabdomyosarcoma: focus on MYCN as a biologically relevant target. *Genes Chromosomes Cancer* 2008;47:510–520.
128. Lee MH, Jothi M, Gudkov AV, et al. Histone methyltransferase KMT1A restrains entry of alveolar rhabdomyosarcoma cells into a myogenic differentiated state. *Cancer Res* 2011;71(11):3921–3931.
129. Zibat A, Missiaglia E, Rosenberger A, et al. Activation of the hedgehog pathway confers a poor prognosis in embryonal and fusion gene-negative alveolar rhabdomyosarcoma. *Oncogene* 2010;29:6323–6330.
130. Reed S, Li H, Li C, et al. Celecoxib inhibits STAT3 phosphorylation and suppresses cell migration and colony forming ability in rhabdomyosarcoma cells. *Biochem Biophys Res Commun* 2011;407:450–455.
131. Mayeenuddin LH, Yu Y, Kang Z, et al. Insulin-like growth factor 1 receptor antibody induces rhabdomyosarcoma cell death via a process involving AKT and Bcl-x(L). *Oncogene* 2010;29:6367–6377.
132. Kolb EA, Gorlick R, Lock R, et al. Initial testing (stage 1) of the IGF-1 receptor inhibitor BMS-754807 by the pediatric preclinical testing program. *Pediatr Blood Cancer* 2011;56:595–603.
133. Kang Z, Chen J, Yu Y, et al. Drozitumab, a human antibody to death receptor 5, has potent anti-tumor activity against rhabdomyosarcoma with the expression of caspase-8 predictive of response. *Clin Cancer Res* 2011;17(10):3181–3192.

Chapter 88
Ewing Tumor

Robert B. Marcus, Jr.

EPIDEMIOLOGY

Ewing sarcoma family tumor (ESFT) is the second most common primary tumor of bone in childhood, and also arises in soft tissues. ESFT is uncommon before 8 years of age and after 25 years of age.[1] In the European Intergroup Cooperative Ewing Sarcoma Study group (EICESS), the median age was 14 years, with 57% of the patients male and 43% female, although a majority of the patients below 10 years of age were female.[1] The malignancy is rare in African Americans.[2] In the EICESS, 24.7% of lesions are located in the pelvis, 16.4% in the femur, 16.7% below the knee, 12.1% in the ribs, 8.0% in the spine, and 4.8% in the humerus.[1]

PATHOLOGY AND CYTOGENETICS

Light microscopy shows a tumor of small, round blue cells that lack markers for lymphoma, neuroblastoma, or rhabdomyosarcoma. Cytogenetics has shown that Ewing tumors of bone and soft tissue are the most undifferentiated members of a tumor family that shares a common neuroectodermal precursor cell, arrested at different stages of differentiation.[3,4] Approximately 95% of ESFTs have a translocation between the EWS gene on chromosome 22 and the FLI1 gene on chromosome 11 (t[11;22][q24;q12]) or the ERG gene on chromosome 21 (t[21;22][q22;q12]),[5,6] although in an analysis of 222 consecutive tumors at the Rizzoli Institute in Italy with a presumptive diagnosis of Ewing tumor, an occasional other translocation was noted.[7] The translocations are present only in tumor cells and occur in bone and soft-tissue Ewing tumors, primitive neuroectodermal tumors of bone and soft tissue, peripheral primitive neuroectodermal tumors, Askin tumors, some esthesioneuroblastomas in children, and some central nervous system (CNS) tumors.[8] Intra-abdominal desmoplastic small round cell tumor appears to have a different translocation at t(11;22)(p13;q12), indicating it is not one of these neoplasms.[9] The proto-oncogene c-myc, not seen in neuroblastoma, is expressed in the ESFT, whereas n-myc is not amplified.[9]

CLINICAL PRESENTATION

The most frequent presenting symptoms are pain and swelling. Pain can wax and wane as the tumor progresses. Symptoms of systemic disease occur at times, including low-grade fevers, malaise, and weakness. ESFT patients exhibit a mean lag time of 146 days between the onset of symptoms and diagnosis, the longest lag time of any pediatric solid tumor.[10] Both patients and physicians contribute to this delay. Overall, patients with the EWS-FLI1 fusion have a similar clinical presentation and prognosis to those with the less common EWS-ERG fusion.[11]

DIAGNOSTIC WORKUP

In Ewing tumor of bone, plain films usually reveal a mottled or moth-eaten lesion. Lytic and blastic areas may be present; lytic areas are more commonly seen. Subperiosteal reactive new bone may be present, producing an "onion skin" appearance. Like an osteosarcoma, Ewing tumors may produce spicules radiating from the cortex of the involved bone, or expansion of the bone may produce a cystic-appearing tumor. Occasionally, the tumor may appear to arise on the surface of the bone, producing a saucerlike indentation of the surface.[12] A magnetic resonance imaging (MRI) scan of the primary lesion will show the extent of bone marrow involvement and soft-tissue invasion, whereas bone destruction is best seen using computed tomography (CT). The radiographic differential includes osteosarcoma, osteomyelitis, eosinophilic granuloma, primary lymphoma of the bone, and even an occasional metastatic malignancy.

The systemic workup should include blood studies, a chest roentgenogram, a CT scan of the chest, a bone scan, and a bone marrow biopsy. Fluorodeoxyglucose (FDG)-positron emission tomography (PET) scans have been shown to detect considerably more bone metastases than traditional bone scans, both at diagnosis and recurrence. Whole-body MRI has also been reported to be superior to bone scan in detecting bone metastases in patients with Ewing tumors, particularly diffusion-weighted images or short-time inversion recovery (STIR) images, but some lesions are found on bone scans that are not seen on MRI.[13,14] MRI has also been reported as better than FDG-PET.[15] Because few lesions <8 mm are detectable using PET imaging, CT scans are still more accurate for the screening of lung metastases.[16] Nevertheless, routine CT scans of the abdomen and pelvis rarely pick up metastatic disease not shown on other studies, either in the initial workup or during follow-up.[17]

In a large cooperative group study, approximately 20% of patients presented with metastatic disease. Of these patients, 44% presented with lung metastases only, 51% with bone or bone marrow involvement (with or without lung metastases), and 5% with metastases in other organs.[1] However, three times as many bone lesions are diagnosed in studies utilizing whole-body MRI scans,[13,14] so it is quite possible that the standard workup using only bone scans underestimates the incidence of bone metastases. Because of the specific cytogenetic identity of ESFTs, cytogenetic analyses have been shown to occasionally diagnose a Ewing tumor in the setting of an unknown primary tumor.[18]

PROGNOSTIC FEATURES

Metastases at diagnosis, a large or pelvic or truncal primary tumor, the presence of a large soft-tissue mass, an older age at diagnosis, a poor response to induction chemotherapy, not using surgery as part of the treatment of the primary lesion, and a filigree histologic pattern have all been proposed as poor prognostic factors.[1,19,20,21,22,23,24,25,26,27] These factors are interrelated; 90% of tumors in the pelvis and femur are usually large, have a large soft-tissue mass, and occur more often in older adolescents and adults.[28] The presence of necrosis on pretreatment MRI scans has been linked to an increased risk of metastases at diagnosis.[29]

There are differing opinions regarding the prognosis of skeletal versus nonskeletal primary lesions. Some reports show an advantage for skeletal primary sites,[30] but if size, site, and other tumor characteristics are stratified, the prognosis may be identical.[31]

The radiologic or histologic response of the soft-tissue mass to induction chemotherapy is an extremely good prognostic indicator[1,24,27,32]; the PET scan response is different from osteosarcoma and not as useful.[33]

Ewing tumors with p53, p16/p14ARF alterations or the presence of vascular endothelial growth factor respond poorly to chemotherapy and have a poor prognosis.[34,35,36] The matricellular protein CCN3, which plays an important role in bone formation, has been reported to be associated with a worse prognosis if fully expressed.[36]

Although in the past the type 1 fusion abnormality, which is the EWS-FLI1 transcript created as a result of fusion between exons 7 of *EWS* and 6 of *FLI1,* has been reported to have a favorable prognosis, more recent analyses do not confirm this. A re-examination of this association in a prospective cohort of patients with ESFT treated according to current Children's Oncology Group (COG) protocols using more intensive chemotherapy show no advantage.[37] In a report from the Euro-Ewing 99 trial, no type of translocation impacted disease progression or relapse.[38]

The EWS-FLI1 transcript can sometimes be detected in the peripheral blood or bone marrow, where it may indicate residual occult disease.[39]

GENERAL MANAGEMENT

Effective local *and* systemic therapy is necessary for the cure of ESFTs. Most chemotherapy regimens combine cyclophosphamide, doxorubicin HCl (Adriamycin), vincristine, dactinomycin, ifosfamide, and etoposide.[21,23,27,40,41,42,43,44] Induction chemotherapy is preferred over starting the systemic therapy and local therapy concomitantly. There are several advantages to this approach:

1. Administering the chemotherapy first allows an evaluation of the effectiveness of the regimen for each patient;
2. Shrinkage of the soft-tissue mass may help the surgeon or radiation oncologist decrease the volume of the local therapy;
3. Shrinkage of the soft-tissue mass may allow the surgeon to achieve better margins; and
4. Some bone healing takes place during the chemotherapy, which may diminish the risk of pathologic fracture if radiation therapy is used to treat the primary lesion.

Response rates to induction chemotherapy are high, with radiologic complete response and partial response rates of up to 90% reported.[32,45,46] For institutions that use surgery for the treatment of the primary lesion, excellent necrosis rates have been reported in many patients.[19,27] Almost all patients whose lesions show a poor response either radiologically or histologically die.[19,24,27,32]

The biopsy should be performed at the same institution where the treatment will be performed, and the biopsy specimen should only be taken from the soft-tissue component, if present. Enough tissue should be collected for light and electron microscopy as well as cytogenetics. In experienced hands, a large-needle biopsy may be sufficient, although usually a larger sample is preferred, particularly because cytogenetics is becoming increasingly important.

For definitive therapy, limb-salvage surgery is preferable over amputation, but amputation may be an option for younger patients with lesions of the fibula, tibia, and foot. In older patients, lesions of the proximal fibula, ribs, scapula, clavicle, and wing of the ilium are easier to resect than other sites. Lesions of the bones of the hands and feet may be resectable with a ray resection. Other sites may be resectable with major reconstructive procedures and significant morbidity.[47]

RADIOTHERAPY TECHNIQUES

For gross disease, standard treatment is a total dose of 55.8 Gy at 1.8 Gy per day, with a field reduction at 45 Gy, although 36 Gy may be adequate for the initial field.[48,49,50,51] Local control rates of 53% to 93% have been reported with these doses (Table 88.1). Local control at doses <40 Gy is significantly worse, even for small lesions.[57]

Twice-a-day irradiation has been used in several trials. To treat ESFTs, radiation oncologists at the University of Florida used 1.2 Gy twice a day to a total dose of 50.4 Gy, 55.2 Gy, or 60 Gy, depending on the tumor response to induction chemotherapy, and showed that late effects could be decreased while maintaining good local control, even for large primary tumors.[48,51] In CESS 86, doses of 1.6 Gy twice a day to a total of 60 Gy were given, although not in a continuous course. The Italian SE-91 trial also used 1.6 Gy twice a day to a total of 60.8 Gy, but in a continuous course. The CESS 86 trial showed no advantage for the accelerated hyperfractionated approach, but the early results of SE-91 are promising with regard to local control.[52,56] Both of the latter regimens would be theoretically expected to increase late effects.

The Pediatric Oncology Group trial (POG 8346) showed, in a randomized fashion, that the traditional approach of irradiating the entire marrow cavity was not necessary.[58] Although "tailored" fields are the standard of care today, attention to the requisite volume is critical to obtaining maximal control rates; geographic miss has been a frequent source of failure in cooperative group studies.[26,58] Three-dimensional treatment planning is essential. In the present open COG trial, the initial clinical target volume 1 includes the prechemotherapy tumor volume with a 1-cm margin, with at least a 0.5-cm addition for planned target volume 1. The boost is to the residual tumor volume at the time of radiotherapy plus a 1-cm margin, with or without a 0.5-cm planned target volume 2. PET-CT may be helpful for planning. Any initial bone or bone marrow abnormalities in the primary bone should be included in gross tumor volume 2. These margins are much tighter than in previous studies, and only additional follow-up will show whether they will be adequate.

Extremity lesions require sparing at least a 1- to 2-cm strip of tissue to prevent lymphedema, which can be very difficult at times, particularly in arm lesions, although the arm is less likely to develop lymphedema than the leg. It may be necessary to consider surgery as an alternative if a strip of tissue cannot be spared. It is more important to cover the tumor adequately than to spare adjacent growth plates and joints.

With the high doses of cyclophosphamide or ifosfamide given in chemotherapy regimens for Ewing tumor, it is important to minimize the dose to the bladder. Radiation cystitis can be a significant risk even at doses as low as 20 Gy. Because pelvic lesions rarely infiltrate into the tissues around the bladder, but instead tend to push aside those structures, neoadjuvant chemotherapy allows additional bladder to be spared if good shrinkage is obtained. A 1-cm medial margin on the residual disease at the time of treatment is adequate from the beginning of radiation therapy.

Rib lesions should be treated conformally with a minimum of lung and heart in the high-dose field. However, rib primary tumors often present with pleural effusions, and in the EICESS and COG trials hemithorax irradiation was used, even for surgically resected lesions. A dose of 15 Gy for patients younger than 14 years and 20 Gy for older patients was given, corrected for lung transmission. In the EICESS 92 trial, the 7-year rate of event-free survival (EFS) was 63% with hemithorax irradiation versus 46% without.[59] Another option is ^{32}P colloid, which has been used in addition to standard radiation, but not hemithorax, in high-risk but localized chest wall tumors in an attempt to decrease chest or pleural recurrence, with no relapses in the patients receiving it.[60]

In the United States, the standard dose for vertebral lesions is 45 Gy; it is not clear whether this decreases local control and survival rates. The average dose used in the CESS 81, CESS 86, and EICESS 92 trials was 49.6 Gy, although sometimes spinal shielding was used.[61,62] In these trials, neurologic late effects were seen in one of 47 patients irradiated, occurring at a dose of 44.8 Gy at 1.6 Gy twice a day. Sacral lesions should be treated to the full dose.

Doxorubicin and dactinomycin given during the course of radiation therapy will often cause moist desquamation, particularly with beams of 6 MV or

TABLE 88.1 SURVIVAL AND LOCAL CONTROL BY METHOD OF TREATMENT TO PRIMARY LESIONS IN MAJOR COOPERATIVE GROUP TRIALS (LOCALIZED LESIONS ONLY)

		Local Control (%)			*5-Year Survival (%)*			
Trial	*Years Open*	*RT*	*Surgery*	*Both*	*RT*	*Surgery*	*Both*	*Overall*
IESS-I[44]	1973–1978	–	–	–	–	–	–	50[a]
IESS-II[40]	1978–1982	–	–	–	–	–	–	70[a]
IESS-II (pelvic)[41]	1978–1982	85	91	100	59	73	62	63
CESS 81[26]	1981–1985	53	91	80	44	55	67	50
CESS 86[52]	1986–1991	86	100	95	70	66	74	70
UKCCSG ET-2[53]	1987–1993	82	71	100	–	–	–	62
CCG/POG Intergroup I[54]	1988–1992	–	–	–	–	–	–	66[a]
CESS 81, CESS 86, EICESS 92[b, 55]	1981–1999	74	96	92	–	–	–	–
SE 91-CNR[c, 56]	1991–1997	93	93	94	75[a]	77[a]	87[a]	–
CCG/POG Intergroup II[42]	1995–1998	–	–	–	–	–	–	79
CCG/POG Intergroup II[d, 4]	1995–1998	75	75	89.5	52	41.7	47.4	49

RT, radiotherapy; IESS, Intergroup Ewing's Sarcoma Study; CESS, Cooperative Ewing's Sarcoma Study; UKCCSG, United Kingdom Children's Cancer Study Group; ET, Ewing tumor; SE 91-CNR, Italian Cooperative Study of Ewing Sarcoma; EICESS, European Intergroup Cooperative Ewing Sarcoma Study; CCG/POG, Children's Cancer Group and Pediatric Oncology Group.

[a]Estimated from results of individual arms.

[b]Combined; data for EICESS 92 alone not available.

[c]Only 3-year survival available.

[d]Pelvic primaries only.

TABLE 88.2 RECOMMENDATIONS FOR RADIATION THERAPY FIELDS AND DOSES

Clinical Situation	Total Dose (%)		Dose Per Fraction (%)	Volume	Margin (cm)
Gross disease (after biopsy only or intralesional resection)					
Treatment once a day	Initial field	36–45	1.8 qd	Original bone and soft-tissue mass	1
	Boost field	10.8–18[a]	1.8 qd	Original bone and *residual* soft-tissue mass	1
Treatment twice a day	Initial field	36	1.2 bid	Original bone and soft-tissue mass	1
	Boost field	19.2	1.2 bid	Original bone and *residual* soft-tissue mass	1
After marginal resection or poor histologic response at surgery		41.4–45	1.8 qd	Original bone and soft-tissue mass plus surgical scars and drains if feasible	1
Preoperative radiotherapy: consider for patients with poor clinical response (<50% shrinkage of soft-tissue mass) to induction chemotherapy		36 (doses as low as 35 have been successful)	1.8 qd	Original bone and soft-tissue mass	1

qd, once a day; bid, twice a day.
[a]Depending on initial dose.

less, tangential irradiation, or skin folds. These drugs may also cause a "recall" phenomenon of the dry or moist desquamation when given after the end of radiation therapy.

The indications for adjuvant radiotherapy with surgery are not completely defined. Jereb et al.[63] found that the local recurrence rate after conservative surgery was high without irradiation. Ozaki et al.[64] also reported a slight advantage for adding postoperative irradiation for patients with inadequate margins. Dunst and Schuck[65] reported that patients with a wide resection alone but a poor histologic response had a local failure rate of 12%, in comparison with 6% for similar patients who received postoperative radiotherapy. With present data, postoperative radiotherapy should probably be given to all patients with marginal margins and all patients with a poor histologic response. Intralesional surgery is not indicated as the EICESS trials showed no improvement in local control in patients with intralesional surgery plus radiotherapy versus radiotherapy alone.[65]

In the COG trials, a dose of 50.4 Gy at 1.8 Gy once a day is given if postoperative radiotherapy is indicated. Doses in the range of 30 to 44.8 Gy at 1.8 Gy a day have also been reported to be effective for subclinical disease.[64,66] Intralesional resections should be treated to the same dose as in patients receiving radiotherapy alone. Table 88.2 lists the recommended doses and fields for different clinical situations.

In a review of 153 patients treated with surgery followed by postoperative radiotherapy from CESS 86 and EICESS 92, Schuck et al.[67] showed that the interval between surgery and radiotherapy did not influence survival, although there was a slight trend for improved local control in patients receiving radiotherapy <90 days postoperatively.

Good results have also been reported with preoperative radiotherapy for patients with a poor response (<50% reduction of the evaluable soft-tissue mass) after two cycles of chemotherapy.[61,64] Doses of 36 to 63 Gy have been used.[64]

Radiation therapy doses and margins are shown in Table 88.2.

RESULTS OF THERAPY

The majority of studies reported in the literature reflect the results of therapy only for Ewing tumor of bone, because before 1991 soft-tissue Ewing tumors were treated on Intergroup Rhabdomyosarcoma Study (IRS) Group protocols. The addition of chemotherapy to local therapy increased the survival for Ewing tumor of bone from <10% to >40% at 5 years for patients with localized disease at diagnosis.[68] Modern protocols show better results and Surveillance, Epidemiology and End Results (SEER) data confirm this gradual improvement in survival rates over time. Five-year survival improved from 36% for patients treated from 1973 to 1977 to 59% for patients treated from 1993 to 1997.[69] However, late recurrences and deaths from complications continue to occur for years, yielding 10- and 15-year survival rates 10% to 15% lower than 5-year rates.[32,70]

Local control and survival rates are shown in Table 88.1 for patients treated with different local control strategies in cooperative group trials that reported appropriate data. Surgery has become the treatment of choice for the primary lesion at most centers, and many series report superior local control for patients receiving surgery as a component of their local treatment, particularly if radiotherapy compliance was poor.[26,58] The influence of different local control strategies on survival is less certain. In CESS 86, with good radiotherapy compliance, survival rates were not influenced by the method of therapy to the primary tumor.[52] Nor was there an advantage for surgery in pelvic primary lesions treated in Intergroup 0091.[4] Other trials show an advantage for surgery or a combination of surgery and radiotherapy. With no randomized studies addressing this question and considerable selection going into the choice of local treatment, conclusions regarding the relative influence of different local therapies on survival are based more on opinion than fact.[26]

However, systemic therapy does influence the rate of detectable local relapse. The first Intergroup Ewing's Sarcoma Study (IESS-I) reported that the addition of doxorubicin improved local control.[6] The first Children's Cancer Group/Pediatric Oncology Group (CCG/POG) intergroup study showed an improvement in survival in the intensified arm for patients with localized disease and large primary or pelvic tumors. The improvement with the more intensive regimen resulted from a decrease in the rate of local relapse; the rate of distant metastases was similar in both arms.[42] The time interval between initiation of chemotherapy and start of radiotherapy has also been reported to influence survival (local control was not evaluated), with early radiotherapy preferable to late radiotherapy.[65]

RESULTS OF CLINICAL TRIALS FOR PATIENTS WITH LOCALIZED DISEASE AT DIAGNOSIS

IESS-I showed that VACA chemotherapy (vincristine, dactinomycin, cyclophosphamide, and doxorubicin) produced superior 5-year relapse-free survival rates over a VAC (vincristine, dactinomycin, and cyclophosphamide) regimen alone. The third arm combined bilateral whole-lung irradiation (WLI) with VAC and produced survival rates better than VAC alone, but less than VACA, indicating that bilateral WLI is an effective adjuvant, although it has not been studied in any subsequent trial except in patients with lung metastases at diagnosis.[44] IESS-I also showed poorer survival rates in all arms for patients with pelvic tumors; intensifying systemic therapy in IESS-II improved the results for pelvic tumors. IESS-II also showed that induction chemotherapy was a viable option.[41] A trial at St. Jude Children's Research Hospital (Memphis, TN) confirmed this approach, and it has since been the standard of care.[45]

Based on data from previous trials,[25] both the University of Florida and the German Cooperative Ewing Sarcoma Study stratified ESFTs by tumor size and intensified treatment for large localized tumors. Although neither approach was randomized, both the University of Florida studies and CESS 86 found that intensifying treatment improved survival closer to the level as achieved with smaller primary lesions and less-aggressive chemotherapy.[32,51,71]

In the first CCG/POG intergroup study starting in 1988, a randomization between VACA chemotherapy alone versus VACA alternating with etoposide and ifosfamide showed that adding etoposide–ifosfamide improved the survival rates, particularly for patients with primary tumors of the pelvis.[42] The United Kingdom Children's Cancer Study Group trials ET-1 and ET-2 showed a better survival rate in the ET-2 trial if ifosfamide was substituted for most of the cyclophosphamide used in ET-1; however, the dose intensity in ET-2 was also higher.[53]

The second POG and CCG intergroup trial, accruing 483 eligible patients between 1995 and 1998, built on the previous intergroup protocol. The 48-week vincristine, doxorubicin, cyclophosphamide, ifosfamide, and etoposide regimen was used as the standard arm, compared with the same drugs given in fewer cycles but with higher drug doses per cycle. There was no significant difference in survival rates in the two arms, with a 5-year EFS of 71% and an overall survival of 79%.[54]

The first COG trial used the more standard doses but decreased the interval of chemotherapy to 2 weeks if there was blood count recovery. The 3-year EFS was 76% for the interval compression arm versus only 63% for the more standard arm.[72] Because of the results of the interval compression study, the five-drug standard of vincristine, cyclophosphamide, doxorubicin, ifosfamide, and etoposide with interval compression is now considered the standard Ewing sarcoma regimen in North American institutions. The present phase III COG study is evaluating the addition of the regimen vincristine, topotecan, and cyclophosphamide to the five-drug intensive regimen.

The EICESS 92 trial showed that for standard-risk patients (<100 mL and no metastases at diagnosis), a regimen substituting cyclophosphamide (VACA) for ifosfamide (VAIA) was equivalent.[73] In high-risk patients (metastases at diagnosis or primary lesions >100 mL), the addition of etoposide provided superior survival results than VAIA alone.[5]

Raney et al.[74] reported the results of treating extraosseous Ewing tumors on the IRS until 1991. Long-term survival of these patients was probably better than for patients with bony primaries, with 10-year survival of 62%, 61%, and 77% for IRS-I, IRS-II, and IRS-III therapeutic protocols, respectively. Survival rates were better for patients with primary lesions of the head and neck, extremities, and trunk and for those with gross tumor removal. Extraosseous primary lesions are now treated on the same protocol as osseous lesions.

RESULTS OF CLINICAL TRIALS FOR PATIENTS WITH METASTATIC DISEASE AT DIAGNOSIS

Patients with metastatic disease at diagnosis have a poor prognosis. In a report from the EICESS, the 5-year relapse-free survival for patients with lung metastases only was 29%; for patients with bone and bone marrow metastases, it was 19%; and for patients with both lung and bone metastases at diagnosis, it was only 8%.[1] Although there was an improvement in survival rates in patients with localized disease treated in the first intergroup CCG/POG trial, adding ifosfamide–etoposide did not improve survival for patients with metastatic disease at diagnosis.[75]

WLI improved survival in the CESS 81, CESS 86, and EICESS 92 trials for patients with lung metastases as the only site of metastatic disease at diagnosis.[76] The CESS 81 and 86 studies also showed increasing survival rates with an increasing radiation dose to the lung fields, particularly with a dose of >18 Gy (corrected for lung transmission) at either 1.5 Gy once a day or 1.25 Gy twice a day. Individual residual lesions were boosted.[3] Some institutions only use WLI in patients with lung metastases who respond poorly to chemotherapy.[77]

In patients with disseminated disease, results are better with adequate treatment of the primary as well as all the metastases. EURO-EWING 99 showed that the 3-year EFS was better (47%) for patients receiving both surgery and radiation to the primary lesion versus either surgery alone (25%) or radiation therapy alone (23%). Without local therapy, the EFS was 13%.[78] Obviously, selection bias cannot be excluded. At Memorial Sloan-Kettering Cancer Center (New York, NY), local control was worse for patients with metastatic disease (61%) than those with localized disease (84%),[79] although in a large series from St. Jude Children's Hospital, the local control in the two groups was equal.[80]

Recent evidence shows improved survival in patients with disseminated bone metastases if all the lesions are treated. Of 120 patients enrolled on arm R3 of EURO-EWING, which suggested but did not mandate local therapy (radiation, surgery, or both) to all sites of disease, 40% received local therapy (either surgery or radiation) or both to all sites of metastatic disease, and 60% received no local therapy. Three-year EFS was 35% in those patients who received radiation therapy to metastatic sites compared to 16% in those who received no local therapy.[78] Paulino et al.[81] show similar results with local therapy to all sites of metastatic disease. It is acceptable to delay the radiotherapy until close to the end of chemotherapy if a significant amount of bone marrow would be treated.

HIGH-DOSE THERAPY WITH STEM CELL RESCUE

Many institutions have investigated end-intensification with megatherapy and stem cell rescue using high-dose chemotherapy with and without total-body irradiation. Patients with metastatic disease treated on EICESS studies between 1990 and 1995 had a superior 4-year EFS when megatherapy was added to the end of therapy, but CCG-7951 showed no improvement with this approach over a matched cohort from other Ewing tumor studies for patients with bone or bone marrow metastases.[76,82] Some institutional pilot studies without strict selection criteria show promising but not conclusive results.[32,43,83,84] The use of two sequential transplants (tandem transplants) has produced promising early results.[5] Total-body irradiation has been reported to add to toxicity but not improve EFS.[5,85]

A few institutions have used a single transplant to treat high-risk patients (large primary tumors or tumors of the pelvis or trunk) with localized disease. Five-year survival rates of 48% to 71% have been reported.[5,32,43,86] Although the results are clearly better than standard treatment for similar high-risk groups treated historically, recent intensified regimens without end-intensification appear to give similar results,[19,32,42,54] showing that intensifying systemic therapy for patients with high-risk localized disease has improved survival rates, whether the intensification is with an ablative approach or more intensive conventional chemotherapy.

However, high-dose therapy has become increasingly accepted for patients with metastatic disease or recurrence, particularly in Europe. TBI has been largely abandoned as part of the conditioning regimen. Many different regimens have been used, most a combination of melphalan with etoposide, busulfan, carboplatin, and thiotepa.[87] The results of high-risk localized disease are usually lumped together with multifocal disease in the high-dose therapy reports, but the survival of patients with bone metastases at diagnosis appears much better than with standard therapy in some reports. EFS rates as high as 43% have been reported.[88] The use of whole-body MRI to detect bone metastases followed by compartmental irradiation to doses up to 54 Gy and high-dose chemotherapy and stem cell rescue has also been reported to produce a 5-year survival rate of 45%.[89] Although it was a small series, over half the patients had lung metastases and multiple bone metastases.

TREATMENT AFTER RELAPSE

The prognosis after relapse is poor, with a 5-year overall survival of only 13% for patients recurring after treatment in the CESS 81, CESS 86, and EICESS 92 studies. Patients experiencing either late (>2 years) or strictly localized relapses fared slightly better.[1,90] Relapse occurring only at the local site warrants aggressive attempts at salvage.[91] Patients who relapse only with lung metastases can sometimes be salvaged with additional chemotherapy and lung irradiation. Resecting the lung metastases, if there are fewer than four lesions, may also be beneficial.[92] Patients with late pulmonary relapses fare better than those with early relapses.[53] Patients who relapse with bone metastases, however, are essentially incurable with standard therapy.

SEQUELAE OF TREATMENT

Ewing tumor has been reported to have an actuarial complication rate of 70% at 35 years.[93] Paulino et al.[35] reported that 10 (53%) of 19 patients receiving radiotherapy alone, four (25%) of 16 receiving surgery alone, and two (40%) of five undergoing combined surgery and radiation therapy had significant late effects.[35] Neither study included loss of function related to planned surgical resection as a complication.

The most common skeletal complication of radiotherapy is abnormal growth and development of the irradiated tissues. Radiation can cause premature closure of active epiphyses, producing growth deficits and limb-length discrepancies. The degree of discrepancy depends on the radiation dose, patient's age, and epiphysis radiated. Because 65% of leg growth is from the distal femoral (37%) and proximal tibial (28%) epiphyses, typical radiotherapy doses to the knee in boys younger than 14 years of age and girls younger than 12 years of age will usually cause a severe enough leg-length discrepancy to require intervention.[94] Deficits of 2 to 6 cm can usually be managed by a shoe lift; larger deficits require surgical treatment.[95]

Approximately 15% of long-bone lesions develop pathologic fractures at some time in their course, 5% at diagnosis and 10% after radiation therapy, although approximately one-third of the latter are caused by tumor recurrence or occasionally a secondary malignancy.[96] Whether the fracture is disease or treatment related, the most common site is the femur, particularly the proximal femur. Radiotherapy-related fractures usually occur within 24 months after treatment, but can be much later. Doses below 40 Gy using once-a-day doses of 1.8 to 2.0 Gy appear to have a very low risk, as does a hyperfractionated approach using 1.2 Gy twice a day from 50.4 to 55.2 Gy.[48,96]

Extremity weakness, decreased range of motion secondary to fibrosis, pain in the extremity (particularly in the early morning), discoloration of the skin, and lymphedema can also occur after radiotherapy, even with careful planning and sparing of an adequate strip of tissue.

The risk of secondary neoplasia at the site of the primary lesion is related to radiation therapy dose, with an increased risk at doses >60 Gy.[5] Sarcomas, often osteosarcoma, are the most common second tumor, and the risk for megavoltage treatment has been reported as 1% to 4% at 20 years.[44,97,98] With more intensive chemotherapy regimens and the increased use of etoposide, the risk of secondary leukemia is about 2%.[54]

FUTURE CONSIDERATIONS

Although the 5-year survival rate of patients with ESFT appears to have improved since 1970, almost half of all patients diagnosed with Ewing tumor die of it within 10 years.[69] Intensifying systemic treatment appears to improve survival as the recently completed (in 2005) COG trial evaluating the role of interval compression chemotherapy shows. High-dose chemotherapy and stem cell rescue may also produce better results, particularly for patients with metastatic disease at diagnosis, but the limits of intensification have probably been reached with the presently available drugs. Other drugs are being tested and newer approaches are also promising. The Ewing family of tumors is characterized by the t(11;22)(q24;q12) translocation that generates the EWS-FLI1 fusion transcription factor producing the malignant EWS cell. Because continued expression of EWS-FLI1 is believed to be critical for ESFT cell survival, clinically effective small-molecule inhibitors have been sought.

Mithramycin has been reported to inhibit expression of EWS-FLI1 downstream targets at the messenger RNA and protein levels.[99] YK-4-279, a small molecule found by researchers at Georgetown University (Washington, DC) in a library of small molecules supplied by the National Cancer Institute, stops EWS-FLI1's fusion protein from sticking to RNA helicase A, inducing apoptosis in ESFT cells, and reduces the growth of tumor cells.[100] Other approaches are also being studied.[101]

These findings provide proof of principle that inhibiting the interaction of mutant cancer-specific transcription factors with the normal cellular binding partners required for their oncogenic activity provides a promising strategy for the development of uniquely effective, tumor-specific anticancer agents.

With regard to local therapy, the focus should be on improving function and decreasing the incidence of long-term sequelae. The use of image-guided intensity-modulated radiation therapy and proton therapy, as well as smaller margins, should spare significantly more normal tissues than older techniques, probably decreasing late effects. However, it is unlikely that refinements in local therapy with radiotherapy or surgery will significantly improve the cure rate for patients with apparent localized disease, although treating all metastases with radiation or surgery appears to be promising for high-risk patients.

REFERENCES

1. Cotterill SJ, Ahrens S, Paulussen M, et al. Prognostic factors in Ewing's tumor of bone: analysis of 975 patients from the European Intergroup Cooperative Ewing's Sarcoma Study Group. *J Clin Oncol* 2000;18:3108–3114.
2. Kissane JM, Askin FB, Foulkes M, et al. Ewing's sarcoma of bone: clinicopathologic aspects of 303 cases from the Intergroup Ewing's Sarcoma Study. *Hum Pathol* 1983;14:773–779.
3. Dunst J, Paulussen M, Jurgens H. Lung irradiation for Ewing's sarcoma with pulmonary metastases at diagnosis: results of the CESS-studies. *Strahlenther Onkol* 1993;169:621–623.
4. Yock TI, Krailo M, Fryer CJ, et al. Local control in pelvic Ewing sarcoma: analysis from INT-0091–a report from the Children's Oncology Group. *J Clin Oncol* 2006;24:3838–3843.
5. Ladenstein R, Hartmann O, Pinkerton R, et al. A multivariate and matched pair analysis on high-risk Ewing tumor (ET) patients treated by megatherapy (MGT) and stem cell reinfusion (SCR) in Europe (Meeting abstract). 1999 ASCO Annual Meeting, Vol 18. Atlanta, Georgia, 1999:555.
6. Perez CA, Tefft M, Nesbit ME Jr, et al. Radiation therapy in the multimodal management of Ewing's sarcoma of bone: report of the Intergroup Ewing's Sarcoma Study. *Natl Cancer Inst Monogr* 1981:263–271.
7. Gamberi G, Cocchi S, Benini S, et al. Molecular diagnosis in Ewing family tumors: the Rizzoli experience–222 consecutive cases in four years. *J Mol Diagn* 2011;13:313–324.
8. Hadfield MG, Quezado MM, Williams RL, et al. Ewing's family of tumors involving structures related to the central nervous system: a review. *Pediatr Dev Pathol* 2000;3:203–210.
9. Sandberg AA, Bridge JA. Updates on cytogenetics and molecular genetics of bone and soft tissue tumors: Ewing sarcoma and peripheral primitive neuroectodermal tumors. *Cancer Genet Cytogenet* 2000;123:1–26.
10. Pollock BH, Krischer JP, Vietti TJ. Interval between symptom onset and diagnosis of pediatric solid tumors. *J Pediatr* 1991;119:725–732.

11. Ginsberg JP, de Alava E, Ladanyi M, et al. EWS-FLI1 and EWS-ERG gene fusions are associated with similar clinical phenotypes in Ewing's sarcoma. *J Clin Oncol* 1999;17:1809–1814.
12. Edeiken J, Karasick D. Imaging in bone cancer. *CA Cancer J Clin* 1987;37: 239–245.
13. Mentzel HJ, Kentouche K, Sauner D, et al. Comparison of whole-body STIR-MRI and 99mTc-methylene-diphosphonate scintigraphy in children with suspected multifocal bone lesions. *Eur Radiol* 2004;14:2297–2302.
14. Nakanishi K, Kobayashi M, Nakaguchi K, et al. Whole-body MRI for detecting metastatic bone tumor: diagnostic value of diffusion-weighted images. *Magn Reson Med Sci* 2007;6:147–155.
15. Daldrup-Link HE, Franzius C, Link TM, et al. Whole-body MR imaging for detection of bone metastases in children and young adults: comparison with skeletal scintigraphy and FDG PET. *AJR Am J Roentgenol* 2001;177:229–236.
16. Gyorke T, Zajic T, Lange A, et al. Impact of FDG PET for staging of Ewing sarcomas and primitive neuroectodermal tumours. *Nucl Med Commun* 2006;27:17–24.
17. Dobbs MD, Lowas SR, Hernanz-Schulman M, et al. Impact of abdominopelvic CT on Ewing sarcoma management. *Acad Radiol* 2010;17:1288–1291.
18. Pantou D, Tsarouha H, Papadopoulou A, et al. Cytogenetic profile of unknown primary tumors: clues for their pathogenesis and clinical management. *Neoplasia* 2003;5:23–31.
19. Ahrens S, Hoffmann C, Jabar S, et al. Evaluation of prognostic factors in a tumor volume-adapted treatment strategy for localized Ewing sarcoma of bone: the CESS 86 experience. Cooperative Ewing Sarcoma Study. *Med Pediatr Oncol* 1999;32: 186–195.
20. Aparicio J, Munarriz B, Pastor M, et al. Long-term follow-up and prognostic factors in Ewing's sarcoma. A multivariate analysis of 116 patients from a single institution. *Oncology* 1998;55:20–26.
21. Bacci G, Picci P, Mercuri M, et al. Predictive factors of histological response to primary chemotherapy in Ewing's sarcoma. *Acta Oncol* 1998;37:671–676.
22. Barbieri E, Emiliani E, Zini G, et al. Combined therapy of localized Ewing's sarcoma of bone: analysis of results in 100 patients. *Int J Radiat Oncol Biol Phys* 1990;19:1165–1170.
23. Fizazi K, Dohollou N, Blay JY, et al. Ewing's family of tumors in adults: multivariate analysis of survival and long-term results of multimodality therapy in 182 patients. *J Clin Oncol* 1998;16:3736–3743.
24. Lee JA, Kim DH, Cho J, et al. Treatment outcome of Korean patients with localized Ewing sarcoma family of tumors: a single institution experience. *Jpn J Clin Oncol* 2011;41:776–782.
25. Marcus RB, Million RR. The effect of primary tumor size on the prognosis of Ewing's sarcoma. *Int J Radiat Oncol Biol Phys* 1984;10(Suppl 2).
26. Sauer R, Jurgens H, Burgers JM, et al. Prognostic factors in the treatment of Ewing's sarcoma. The Ewing's Sarcoma Study Group of the German Society of Paediatric Oncology CESS 81. *Radiother Oncol* 1987;10:101–110.
27. Wunder JS, Paulian G, Huvos AG, et al. The histological response to chemotherapy as a predictor of the oncological outcome of operative treatment of Ewing sarcoma. *J Bone Joint Surg Am* 1998;80:1020–1033.
28. Hense HW, Ahrens S, Paulussen M, et al. Factors associated with tumor volume and primary metastases in Ewing tumors: results from the (EI)CESS studies. *Ann Oncol* 1999;10:1073–1077.
29. Dunst J, Ahrens S, Paulussen M, et al. Prognostic impact of tumor perfusion in MR-imaging studies in Ewing tumors. *Strahlenther Onkol* 2001;177:153–159.
30. Applebaum MA, Worch J, Matthay KK, et al. Clinical features and outcomes in patients with extraskeletal Ewing sarcoma. *Cancer* 2011;117:3027–3032.
31. Pradhan A, Grimer RJ, Spooner D, et al. Oncological outcomes of patients with Ewing's sarcoma: is there a difference between skeletal and extra-skeletal Ewing's sarcoma? *J Bone Joint Surg Br* 2011;93:531–536.
32. Marcus RB Jr, Berrey BH, Graham-Pole J, et al. The treatment of Ewing's sarcoma of bone at the University of Florida: 1969 to 1998. *Clin Orthop Relat Res* 2002:290–297.
33. Gaston LL, Di Bella C, Slavin J, et al. 18F-FDG PET response to neoadjuvant chemotherapy for Ewing sarcoma and osteosarcoma are different. *Skeletal Radiol* 2011;40:1007–1015.
34. Fuchs B, Inwards CY, Janknecht R. Vascular endothelial growth factor expression is up-regulated by EWS-ETS oncoproteins and Sp1 and may represent an independent predictor of survival in Ewing's sarcoma. *Clin Cancer Res* 2004; 10:1344–1353.
35. Paulino AC, Nguyen TX, Mai WY. An analysis of primary site control and late effects according to local control modality in non-metastatic Ewing sarcoma. *Pediatr Blood Cancer* 2007;48:423–429.
36. Perbal B, Lazar N, Zambelli D, et al. Prognostic relevance of CCN3 in Ewing sarcoma. *Hum Pathol* 2009;40:1479–1486.
37. van Doorninck JA, Ji L, Schaub B, et al. Current treatment protocols have eliminated the prognostic advantage of type 1 fusions in Ewing sarcoma: a report from the Children's Oncology Group. *J Clin Oncol* 2010;28:1989–1994.
38. Le Deley MC, Delattre O, Schaefer KL, et al. Impact of EWS-ETS fusion type on disease progression in Ewing's sarcoma/peripheral primitive neuroectodermal tumor: prospective results from the cooperative Euro-E.W.I.N.G. 99 trial. *J Clin Oncol* 2010;28:1982–1988.
39. Avigad S, Cohen IJ, Zilberstein J, et al. The predictive potential of molecular detection in the nonmetastatic Ewing family of tumors. *Cancer* 2004;100: 1053–1058.
40. Burgert EO Jr, Nesbit ME, Garnsey LA, et al. Multimodal therapy for the management of nonpelvic, localized Ewing's sarcoma of bone: intergroup study IESS-II. *J Clin Oncol* 1990;8:1514–1524.
41. Evans RG, Nesbit ME, Gehan EA, et al. Multimodal therapy for the management of localized Ewing's sarcoma of pelvic and sacral bones: a report from the second intergroup study. *J Clin Oncol* 1991;9:1173–1180.
42. Grier HE, Krailo MD, Tarbell NJ, et al. Addition of ifosfamide and etoposide to standard chemotherapy for Ewing's sarcoma and primitive neuroectodermal tumor of bone. *N Engl J Med* 2003;348:694–701.
43. Horowitz ME, Kinsella TJ, Wexler LH, et al. Total-body irradiation and autologous bone marrow transplant in the treatment of high-risk Ewing's sarcoma and rhabdomyosarcoma. *J Clin Oncol* 1993;11:1911–1918.
44. Nesbit ME Jr, Gehan EA, Burgert EO Jr, et al. Multimodal therapy for the management of primary, nonmetastatic Ewing's sarcoma of bone: a long-term follow-up of the First Intergroup study. *J Clin Oncol* 1990;8:1664–1674.
45. Hayes FA, Thompson EI, Meyer WH, et al. Therapy for localized Ewing's sarcoma of bone. *J Clin Oncol* 1989;7:208–213.
46. Oberlin O, Patte C, Demeocq F, et al. The response to initial chemotherapy as a prognostic factor in localized Ewing's sarcoma. *Eur J Cancer Clin Oncol* 1985; 21:463–467.
47. Scully SP, Temple HT, O'Keefe RJ, et al. Role of surgical resection in pelvic Ewing's sarcoma. *J Clin Oncol* 1995;13:2336–2341.
48. Bolek TW, Marcus RB Jr, Mendenhall NP, et al. Local control and functional results after twice-daily radiotherapy for Ewing's sarcoma of the extremities. *Int J Radiat Oncol Biol Phys* 1996;35:687–692.
49. Donaldson SS. Ewing sarcoma: radiation dose and target volume. *Pediatr Blood Cancer* 2004;42:471–476.
50. Korah MP, Esiashvili N, Mazewski CM, et al. Incidence, risks, and sequelae of posterior fossa syndrome in pediatric medulloblastoma. *Int J Radiat Oncol Biol Phys* 2010;77:106–112.
51. Marcus RB Jr, Cantor A, Heare TC, et al. Local control and function after twice-a-day radiotherapy for Ewing's sarcoma of bone. *Int J Radiat Oncol Biol Phys* 1991;21:1509–1515.
52. Dunst J, Jurgens H, Sauer R, et al. Radiation therapy in Ewing's sarcoma: an update of the CESS 86 trial. *Int J Radiat Oncol Biol Phys* 1995;32:919–930.
53. Craft A, Cotterill S, Malcolm A, et al. Ifosfamide-containing chemotherapy in Ewing's sarcoma: the Second United Kingdom Children's Cancer Study Group and the Medical Research Council Ewing's Tumor Study. *J Clin Oncol* 1998;16: 3628–3633.
54. Granowetter L. COG Public Report, 8/29/01. Available from: COG Statistical Center, 440 E Huntington Drive, Suite 300, Arcadia, CA 91006.
55. Schuck A, Ahrens S, Paulussen M, et al. Local therapy in localized Ewing tumors: results of 1058 patients treated in the CESS 81, CESS 86, and EICESS 92 trials. *Int J Radiat Oncol Biol Phys* 2003;55:168–177.
56. Rosito P, Mancini AF, Rondelli R, et al. Italian Cooperative Study for the treatment of children and young adults with localized Ewing sarcoma of bone: a preliminary report of 6 years of experience. *Cancer* 1999;86:421–428.
57. Krasin MJ, Rodriguez-Galindo C, Billups CA, et al. Definitive irradiation in multidisciplinary management of localized Ewing sarcoma family of tumors in pediatric patients: outcome and prognostic factors. *Int J Radiat Oncol Biol Phys* 2004;60:830–838.
58. Donaldson SS, Torrey M, Link MP, et al. A multidisciplinary study investigating radiotherapy in Ewing's sarcoma: end results of POG #8346. Pediatric Oncology Group. *Int J Radiat Oncol Biol Phys* 1998;42:125–135.
59. Schuck A, Ahrens S, Konarzewska A, et al. Hemithorax irradiation for Ewing tumors of the chest wall. *Int J Radiat Oncol Biol Phys* 2002;54:830–838.
60. Shamberger RC, Grier HE, Weinstein HJ, et al. Chest wall tumors in infancy and childhood. *Cancer* 1989;63:774–785.
61. Schuck A, Ahrens S, von Schorlemer I, et al. Radiotherapy in Ewing tumors of the vertebrae: treatment results and local relapse analysis of the CESS 81/86 and EICESS 92 trials. *Int J Radiat Oncol Biol Phys* 2005;63:1562–1567.
62. Venkateswaran L, Rodriguez-Galindo C, Merchant TE, et al. Primary Ewing tumor of the vertebrae: clinical characteristics, prognostic factors, and outcome. *Med Pediatr Oncol* 2001;37:30–35.
63. Jereb B, Ong RL, Mohan M, et al. Redefined role of radiation in combined treatment of Ewing's sarcoma. *Pediatr Hematol Oncol* 1986;3:111–118.
64. Ozaki T, Hillmann A, Hoffmann C, et al. Significance of surgical margin on the prognosis of patients with Ewing's sarcoma. A report from the Cooperative Ewing's Sarcoma Study. *Cancer* 1996;78:892–900.
65. Dunst J, Schuck A. Role of radiotherapy in Ewing tumors. *Pediatr Blood Cancer* 2004;42:465–470.
66. Merchant TE, Kushner BH, Sheldon JM, et al. Effect of low-dose radiation therapy when combined with surgical resection for Ewing sarcoma. *Med Pediatr Oncol* 1999;33:65–70.
67. Schuck A, Rube C, Konemann S, et al. Postoperative radiotherapy in the treatment of Ewing tumors: influence of the interval between surgery and radiotherapy. *Strahlenther Onkol* 2002;178:25–31.
68. Chan RC, Sutow WW, Lindberg RD, et al. Management and results of localized Ewing's sarcoma. *Cancer* 1979;43:1001–1006.
69. Esiashvili N, Goodman M, Marcus RB. Incidence and survival of patients with Ewing sarcoma of bone over the past three decades based on surveillance epidemiology and end results data. 38th Annual Congress of International Society of Pediatric Oncology (SIOP), Geneva, Switzerland, 2006.
70. Gasparini M, Lombardi F, Ballerini E, et al. Long-term outcome of patients with monostotic Ewing's sarcoma treated with combined modality. *Med Pediatr Oncol* 1994;23:406–412.
71. Paulussen M, Ahrens S, Dunst J, et al. Localized Ewing tumor of bone: final results of the cooperative Ewing's Sarcoma Study CESS 86. *J Clin Oncol* 2001;19: 1818–1829.
72. Womer RB, West DC, Krailo MD, et al. Randomized comparison of every-two-week v. every-three-week chemotherapy in Ewing sarcoma family tumors (ESFT). *J Clin Oncol* 2008;26:abstr 10504.
73. Paulussen M, Craft AW, Lewis I, et al. Results of the EICESS-92 Study: two randomized trials of Ewing's sarcoma treatment–cyclophosphamide compared with ifosfamide in standard-risk patients and assessment of benefit of etoposide added to standard treatment in high-risk patients. *J Clin Oncol* 2008;26: 4385–4393.
74. Raney RB, Asmar L, Newton WA Jr, et al. Ewing's sarcoma of soft tissues in childhood: a report from the Intergroup Rhabdomyosarcoma Study, 1972 to 1991. *J Clin Oncol* 1997;15:574–582.
75. Miser JS, Krailo MD, Tarbell NJ, et al. Treatment of metastatic Ewing's sarcoma or primitive neuroectodermal tumor of bone: evaluation of combination ifosfamide and etoposide–a Children's Cancer Group and Pediatric Oncology Group study. *J Clin Oncol* 2004;22:2873–2876.
76. Paulussen M, Ahrens S, Craft AW, et al. Ewing's tumors with primary lung metastases: survival analysis of 114 (European Intergroup) Cooperative Ewing's Sarcoma Studies patients. *J Clin Oncol* 1998;16:3044–3052.
77. Spunt SL, McCarville MB, Kun LE, et al. Selective use of whole-lung irradiation for patients with Ewing sarcoma family tumors and pulmonary metastases at the time of diagnosis. *J Pediatr Hematol Oncol* 2001;23:93–98.
78. Haeusler J, Ranft A, Boelling T, et al. The value of local treatment in patients with primary, disseminated, multifocal Ewing sarcoma (PDMES). *Cancer* 2010; 116:443–450.
79. La TH, Meyers PA, Wexler LH, et al. Radiation therapy for Ewing's sarcoma: results from Memorial Sloan-Kettering in the modern era. *Int J Radiat Oncol Biol Phys* 2006;64:544–550.

80. Rodriguez-Galindo C, Navid F, Liu T, et al. Prognostic factors for local and distant control in Ewing sarcoma family of tumors. *Ann Oncol* 2008;19:814–820.
81. Paulino AC, Mai WY, Teh BS. Radiotherapy in metastatic Ewing sarcoma. *Am J Clin Oncol* 2012012 [Epub ahead of print].
82. Meyers PA, Krailo MD, Ladanyi M, et al. High-dose melphalan, etoposide, total-body irradiation, and autologous stem-cell reconstitution as consolidation therapy for high-risk Ewing's sarcoma does not improve prognosis. *J Clin Oncol* 2001;19:2812–2820.
83. Kushner BH, Meyers PA. How effective is dose-intensive/myeloablative therapy against Ewing's sarcoma/primitive neuroectodermal tumor metastatic to bone or bone marrow? The Memorial Sloan-Kettering experience and a literature review. *J Clin Oncol* 2001;19:870–880.
84. Pinkerton CR, Bataillard A, Guillo S, et al. Treatment strategies for metastatic Ewing's sarcoma. *Eur J Cancer* 2001;37:1338–1344.
85. Burdach S, Meyer-Bahlburg A, Laws HJ, et al. High-dose therapy for patients with primary multifocal and early relapsed Ewing's tumors: results of two consecutive regimens assessing the role of total-body irradiation. *J Clin Oncol* 2003; 21:3072–3078.
86. Madero L, Munoz A, Sanchez de Toledo J, et al. Megatherapy in children with high-risk Ewing's sarcoma in first complete remission. *Bone Marrow Transplant* 1998;21:795–799.
87. Rosenthal J, Pawlowska AB. High-dose chemotherapy and stem cell rescue for high-risk Ewing's family of tumors. *Expert Rev Anticancer Ther* 2011;11:251–262.
88. Oberlin O, Rey A, Desfachelles AS, et al. Impact of high-dose busulfan plus melphalan as consolidation in metastatic Ewing tumors: a study by the Societe Francaise des Cancers de l'Enfant. *J Clin Oncol* 2006;24:3997–4002.
89. Burdach S, Thiel U, Schoniger M, et al. Total body MRI-governed involved compartment irradiation combined with high-dose chemotherapy and stem cell rescue improves long-term survival in Ewing tumor patients with multiple primary bone metastases. *Bone Marrow Transplant* 2010;45:483–489.
90. Stahl M, Ranft A, Paulussen M, et al. Risk of recurrence and survival after relapse in patients with Ewing sarcoma. *Pediatr Blood Cancer* 2011;57:549–553.
91. Hayes FA, Thompson EI, Kumar M, et al. Long-term survival in patients with Ewing's sarcoma relapsing after completing therapy. *Med Pediatr Oncol* 1987;15: 254–256.
92. Lanza LA, Miser JS, Pass HI, et al. The role of resection in the treatment of pulmonary metastases from Ewing's sarcoma. *J Thorac Cardiovasc Surg* 1987;94: 181–187.
93. Fuchs B, Valenzuela RG, Inwards C, et al. Complications in long-term survivors of Ewing sarcoma. *Cancer* 2003;98:2687–2692.
94. Anderson M, Green WT, Messner MB. Growth and predictions of growth in the lower extremities. *J Bone Joint Surg Am* 1963;45-A:1–14.
95. Moseley CF. Leg-length discrepancy. In: RT M, ed. *Lovell and Winter's pediatric orthopaedics,* vol 2, 3rd ed. Philadelphia: Lippincott Williams & Wilkins, 1990: 767–813.
96. Wagner LM, Neel MD, Pappo AS, et al. Fractures in pediatric Ewing sarcoma. *J Pediatr Hematol Oncol* 2001;23:568–571.
97. Kuttesch JF Jr, Wexler LH, Marcus RB, et al. Second malignancies after Ewing's sarcoma: radiation dose-dependency of secondary sarcomas. *J Clin Oncol* 1996;14: 2818–2825.
98. Tucker MA, D'Angio GJ, Boice JD Jr, et al. Bone sarcomas linked to radiotherapy and chemotherapy in children. *N Engl J Med* 1987;317:588–593.
99. Grohar PJ, Woldemichael GM, Griffin LB, et al. Identification of an inhibitor of the EWS-FLI1 oncogenic transcription factor by high-throughput screening. *J Natl Cancer Inst* 2011;103:962–978.
100. Erkizan HV, Kong Y, Merchant M, et al. A small molecule blocking oncogenic protein EWS-FLI1 interaction with RNA helicase A inhibits growth of Ewing's sarcoma. *Nat Med* 2009;15:750–756.
101. Subbiah V, Anderson P. Targeted therapy of Ewing's sarcoma. *Sarcoma* 2011;2011: 686985.

Chapter 89
Lymphomas in Children

Monika L. Metzger, Hiroto Inaba, Stephanie Terezakis, and Louis S. Constine

Childhood lymphomas are gratifying to treat because of their curability. Central to this progress has been single and multi-institutional clinical trials that, in turn, have benefited from advances in our understanding of the normal immune system, through diagnostic imaging and pathology. The primary focus of pediatric trials in the past decade has been stratification of patients into risk groups to refine treatment as follows: (a) less morbid therapy in children with a favorable prognosis, and (b) intensification of therapy in children with an unfavorable prognosis. Furthermore, early response to therapy has been recognized as a very important tool in identifying patients with more sensitive disease in whom therapy can be reduced or patients with more aggressive disease that may benefit from therapy escalation.

Commensurate with the increasingly effective use of chemotherapy has been a more restrictive role for radiotherapy. Our recognition of the long-term sequelae of therapy has played a prominent role in the development of effective treatment strategies.

HODGKIN LYMPHOMA

Historically, irradiation techniques and doses used successfully in adults caused substantial morbidities (primarily musculoskeletal growth inhibition) in children.[1,2] Contemporary treatment programs use a risk-adapted approach in which patients receive varying intensities of multiagent chemotherapy and low-dose involved field irradiation.[3–6,7–9,10–11,12,13,14,15,16,17,18,19–20,21–24,25–27] It is now clear that the vast majority of children with Hodgkin lymphoma (HL) can be cured, prompting increased attention to devising nonmorbid therapy for these patients. Considering the excellent outcome for the majority of children and adolescents diagnosed with HL, the identification of biologic factors predicting very good or very poor outcome is critical to direct future refinements in therapy.

EPIDEMIOLOGY

Lymphomas are the third most common form of childhood cancer, comprising 15% of cancer diagnoses in individuals younger than age 20 years. Overall, pediatric HL is more common than non-Hodgkin lymphoma (NHL), with an annual incidence rate of 12.8 per 1 million children (≤19 years old).[28]

Childhood HL has unique epidemiologic presentations that vary geographically:

- The childhood form occurs in patients age 14 years or younger. It is rare in children <4 years of age, usually occurring in children >10 years. The childhood form of HL is associated with increasing family size and decreasing socioeconomic status. Early and intense exposure to an infectious agent has been speculated to increase the risk for the childhood form of HL.[29,30]
- The young adult form affects patients aged 15 to 34 years and has a roughly equal incidence between older adolescent males and females. In contrast to childhood HL, young adult HL is associated with a higher socioeconomic status, as found in high-income countries. The risk for young adult HL also decreases significantly with increased sibship size and later birth order.[31] Delayed exposure to an infectious agent has been proposed as a risk factor for the development of young adult HL because its epidemiologic features are similar to those seen with paralytic poliomyelitis.[30] However, Chang et al.[29] demonstrated that early exposure to other children at nursery school and day care seems to decrease the risk of young adult HL, most likely by facilitating childhood exposure to common infections and promoting maturation of cellular immunity.

Biology

HL is unique among the lymphomas because the malignant Hodgkin and Reed-Sternberg (HRS) cells, lymphocytic and histiocytic (L&H) cells, and their variants account for <1% of the tumor cell population. Identical immunologic gene rearrangements in HRS and L&H cells support their origin from a single transformed B cell that subsequently undergoes monoclonal expansion.[32,33,34] Two distinct immunophenotypes of HL exist. The first immunophenotype, characteristic of L&H cells, consistently expresses CD20 and J chain and does not express CD30 and CD15.[34,35] The second immunophenotype, characteristic of HRS cells, consistently expresses CD30, frequently expresses CD15, and does not express J chain. These immunophenotypes differentiate lymphocyte-predominant HL from classical HL, as outlined in the World Health Organization's (WHO) classification.[36,37] Substantial data exist to support a strong association between HL and the Epstein-Barr virus (EBV).[38,39] The incidence of EBV-associated HL varies by age, gender, ethnicity, histologic subtype, and regional economic level.[39] EBV-positive tumor genomes are more frequent in children <10 years of age and in those who live in low-income countries (see Chapter 77). HL is also associated with congenital (e.g., ataxia telangiectasia) and acquired (e.g., human immunodeficiency virus [HIV]) immunodeficiency states.[40] Familial cases of HL suggest a genetic predisposition to the disease or a common environmental exposure. Concordance of HL has been observed in first-degree relatives (particularly of the same gender) and in parent–child pairs.[41]

Pathologic Classification

The WHO classification categorizes HL into two major groups of HL—classical HL and lymphocyte predominant (LP) HL—according to their biological and clinical features.[36,37] Classical HL is further subclassified into nodular sclerosing (NS), mixed cellularity (MC), lymphocyte-rich (LR), and lymphocyte-depleted (LD) histologies based on their unique morphology. The pathologic characteristics are the same as in adults and are described in Chapter 77. The relative distribution of the subtypes differs in younger children compared with adolescents and adults. LP is relatively more common (13%) in children younger than age 10, whereas LD is exceedingly rare. Although NS is the most common subtype in all age groups, it is more frequent in adolescents (77%) and adults (72%) than in younger children (44%). Conversely, MC is more common in younger children (33%) than in adolescents (11%) or adults (17%).[42]

Clinical Presentation

Most children (80%) present with cervical lymphadenopathy. The lymph nodes are often fixed, firm, rubbery, and painless. Mediastinal involvement is present in 76% of adolescents but only in 33% of children aged 1 to 10 years.[43] Occasionally patients are diagnosed after the onset of respiratory distress, although isolated mediastinal disease is rare as is isolated infradiaphragmatic HL, both occurring in <5% of patients. One-third of patients have one or more of the so-called B symptoms at diagnosis (unexplained fever >38°C with recurrent episodes during the previous month, drenching night sweats recurrent during the previous month, or weight loss of more than 10% in the 6 months preceding diagnosis).[43,44] Cytokine production induced by the HRS cells are responsible for these manifestations as well as a variety of other clinical and pathologic features of HL, including anorexia, pruritus, fibrosis, eosinophilia, thrombocytosis, plasmacytosis, and immunodeficiency.[45]

Diagnostic Work-Up

The diagnosis of HL is made by lymph node biopsy and is confirmed pathologically by the presence of HRS cells and their mononuclear variants. The diagnosis is facilitated through an excisional lymph node biopsy, which enables evaluation of the malignant HRS cells within the characteristic architectural changes associated with the specific histologic subtypes. The recommended procedures for pretreatment evaluation of the child with HL are similar to those for the adult. Because bone marrow involvement at initial presentation is uncommon and rarely occurs as an isolated site of extranodal disease, bone marrow biopsy can be restricted to patients with B symptoms or stage III or IV disease.

Imaging studies of the thorax include a chest radiograph and a computed tomography (CT) scan, which alters treatment decisions in at least 10% of patients through delineation of radiographically inapparent disease involving subcarinal, hilar, or cardiophrenic angle nodes, and in extranodal sites (pleura, chest wall, or pericardium). Using the ratio of the measurement of the mediastinal mass to the maximum diameter of the intrathoracic cavity on an upright chest radiograph is a standard method to assess mediastinal bulk (mediastinal to thoracic ratio of ≥33%). Infradiaphragmatic disease is best assessed by CT scan or magnetic resonance imaging (MRI). The optimal CT evaluation requires oral and intravenous contrast agents to distinguish lymphadenopathy from other infradiaphragmatic structures. CT evaluation of abdominopelvic disease may be compromised in suboptimally contrasted studies and in children who lack retroperitoneal fat. In these cases, MRI may provide better assessment of disease involvement in the retroperitoneal lymph nodes.[46] Nuclear imaging studies such as positron emission tomography (PET) scanning are helpful in staging and monitoring treatment response, particularly in cases with persistent radiographic abnormalities or "rebound" thymic growth after completion of therapy.[47] Splenic and hepatic involvement by HL is suggested by the presence of enlarged organs with areas of abnormal density on CT or MRI scans, as well as increased fluorodeoxyglucose (FDG) uptake on PET scan.

Staging Systems

As for adults, children with HL are staged according to the system devised at the Ann Arbor Staging Conference in 1970 and revised at the Cotswolds meeting. Refer to Chapter 77 for complete staging information.

Prognostic Factors

As the treatment of HL has improved, the factors that influence outcome have diminished in importance. However, several factors continue to influence the choice and success of therapy. These factors are interrelated in that disease stage, bulk, and biologic aggressiveness are frequently codependent.[48,49] A further complication in the determination of prognostic factors is that relevant variables often depend on staging evaluation and treatment. Similarly, patients with early stage disease have different prognosticators than patients with advanced stage disease.[48] Illustrating the complexity of this subject are data from a multi-institutional study that specifically address prognostic factors in 320 children with clinical stage I to IV disease. On univariate analysis stage IV, NS HL, B symptoms, white blood cell count (WBC) of ≥11,500/mm³, hemoglobin ≤11.0 g/dL, bulky mediastinal disease, extranodal disease, and erythrocyte sedimentation rate (ESR) ≥50 mm per hour were significant for inferior disease-free survival (DFS) and overall survival (OS). By multivariate analysis, male gender; stage IIB, IIIB, or IV disease; WBC ≥11,500/mm³; and hemoglobin ≤11.0 g/dL were significant for inferior DFS and OS. Prognosis was associated with the number of adverse factors.[50]

The following are some generalizations regarding prognostic variables derived from both adult and pediatric data:

- *Stage of disease* is the most significant prognosticator of treatment outcome. Stage IV disease with multiple organ involvement confers an exceptionally poor prognosis when managed with conventional therapy.[50,51]
- *Bulk of disease* is reflected in the disease stage but more specifically is determined by the volume of distinct areas of involvement and the number of disease sites. Large mediastinal adenopathy, defined as a mass of more than one-third

of the intrathoracic diameter, is associated with an increased risk of disease recurrence, particularly when managed with radiation therapy alone.[43,52–55] However, overall survival remains high because of the effectiveness of salvage chemotherapy.[52,53,55] Patients with multiple sites of involvement (usually defined as three or more sites) have an inferior freedom from relapse and survival in some but not all reports.[54–57]

- *Presence of systemic symptoms* (B disease), which result from cytokine secretion, reflects biologic aggressiveness and correlates with an increased risk of relapse compared with the absence of such symptoms (A disease).[44,50]
- *Abnormally high levels of certain serum markers* have been reported to be prognosticators of a negative outcome.[58] Whether these elevated levels are caused by more malignant biology of disease or by increased tumor volume is unclear. In most reports, independent prognostic significance for serum markers is unproven except in select clinical scenarios.[48,50]
- *Histologic subtype* may correlate with prognosis. LD histology confers a worse outcome than do the other subtypes, but it is exceedingly rare.[55] Patients with LP histology are more commonly early stage[59] and have an excellent outcome. Most modern combined modality trials do not show any histology survival difference.[21,50] Recently, the Children's Oncology Group (COG) reported a survival advantage for patients with mixed cellularity HL treated in their low-risk study AHOD0431.[60]
- Finally, *patient age* appears to be a determinant of patient outcome.[42,61] Children <10 years of age have been observed to fare better than older patients, possibly because they are more likely to have early stage or A disease.[42,62]

The use of these prognostic factors is reflected in the risk grouping that various pediatric trials employ for assignment of therapy. Such stratification is discussed below in the "Combination Chemotherapy, Combined Modality Therapy, and Risk-Adapted Therapy" section and is reflected in the summary treatment recommendations.

General Management

Although HL is one of the few pediatric malignancies that has an adult counterpart with similar natural history and biology, determination of the optimal therapeutic approach for children with this disease is complicated by their longevity and increased risk for adverse treatment-related side effects over time. In particular, radiation therapy doses and fields used in adults can produce significant musculoskeletal growth retardation and cardiovascular and pulmonary effects, as described later in this chapter.[1,2,63] Consequently, the various successful approaches to treatment of HL in children (Tables 89.1, 89.2, and 89.3) must be considered in terms of efficacy and morbidity, and this is influenced by the developmental status of the patient.

Radiation Therapy

Radiation therapy (RT) to extended fields to a curative dose range of 30 to 40 Gy produced the first cures in patients with HL, and similar treatment paradigms were used for adults and children. Five-year DFS rates following extended-field radiation therapy in surgically staged children with early stage disease ranged from 60% to 80%.[4,5,9,64,65] However, it became apparent that the late effects of RT posed significant risks in terms of morbidity and mortality in pediatric HL survivors.[1,52,63,83–88,89,90–92]

Combined-modality treatment programs evolved in an effort to reduce therapy-related toxicities; reduced radiation dose was combined with non–cross-resistant chemotherapy in pediatric patients. These regimens reduced the dose-related toxicity of both chemotherapeutic agents and RT and improved DFS in advanced stage patients.[1,8,10,11,26,27,93] Advances in radiation technology and diagnostic imaging led to a reduction in RT field size, permitting involved-field radiotherapy (IFRT) treatment

TABLE 89.1 TREATMENT RESULTS OF COMBINED-MODALITY TRIALS OF PEDIATRIC HODGKIN LYMPHOMA

				Percentage Outcome (Year)			
Chemotherapy/Study (Reference)	*Radiation Therapy*	*Stage*	*Number of Patients*	*EFS*	*DFS*	*RFS/FFP*	*Survival*
Stanford							
3 MOPP/3 ABVD (11)	15–25.5 Gy, IF	CS/PS I–IV	57	96 (10)	–	–	93 (10)
6 MOPP (1)	15–25.5 Gy, IF	PS I–IV	55	–	–	90 (15)	89 (15)
St. Jude							
4–5 COP(P)/3–4 ABVD (10)	20 Gy, IF	CS II–IV	85	–	93 (5)	–	93 (5)
St. Jude/Stanford/Dana Farber Consortium							
VAMP (64,65)	15–25.5 Gy, IF	CS I–II	110	89 (10)	–	–	96 (10)
Toronto							
6 MOPP (12)	20–30 Gy, EF	CS IIA–IV	57	–	–	80 (10)	85 (10)
Children's Cancer Group							
6 ABVD (66)	21 Gy, EF	PS III–IV	54	87 (4)	–	–	90 (4)
12 ABVD (8)	21 Gy, R	PS III–IV	64	87 (3)	–	–	89 (3)
4 COPP/ABV (67)	21 Gy, IF	CS IA/IB,IIA	294	100	–	–	100
6 COPP/ABV (67)	± 21 Gy, IF	CS I/II adverse, CS IIB, III	394	88 (IF)	–	–	95 (IF)
COPP/ABV, CHOP, Ara-C/VP-16 (67)	± 21 Gy, IF	CS IV	141	91 (IF)	–	–	100 (IF)
Pediatric Oncology Group							
4 MOPP/4 ABVD (26)	21 Gy, EF	CS/PS IIB, IIIA2, IIIB–IV	80	80 (5)	–	–	87 (5)
4 MOPP/4 ABVD (27)	21 Gy, TLI	CS/PS IIB, IIIA2, IIIB, IV	62	77 (3)	–	–	91 (3)
DBVE (68)	25.5 Gy, IF	CS/PS I/II/IIIA	51	91	–	–	98
P9425 (69)			216	84 (5)	–	–	95 (5)
RER: 3 × ABVE-PC	21 Gy, IF	IB, II, III, IV		86 (5)	–	–	–
SER: 5 × ABVE-PC	21 Gy, IF	IB, II, III, IV		83 (5)	–	–	–
Children's Oncology Group							
C5943 (70)			98	94 (5)	–	–	97 (5)
RER: 4 × esc BEACOPP							
Females: + 4 × COPP/ABV	–	IIB, IIIB, IV	38	–	–	–	–
Males: + 2 ABVD	21 Gy, IF	IIB, IIIB, IV	34	–	–	–	–
SER: 8 × esc BEACOPP	21 Gy, IF	IIB, IIIB, IV	15	–	–	–	–

(continued)

TABLE 89.1 (CONTINUED)

Chemotherapy/Study (Reference)	*Radiation Therapy*	*Stage*	*Number of Patients*	*Percentage Outcome (Year)*			
				EFS	*DFS*	*RFS/FFP*	*Survival*
Intergroup Hodgkin's							
6 MOPP (9)	35 Gy, IF	PS I–II	97	–	–	95 (5)	90 (5)
Gustave-Roussy (15)							
			60	–	–	86 (5)	93 (5)
3 MOPP	40 Gy, IF	All stages	40	–	–	–	–
6 MOPP	40 Gy, IF	–	20	–	–	–	–
SFOP MDH-82 (71)							
			238	–	86 (6)	–	92 (6)
4 ABVD	20–40 Gy, IF	CS I–IIA	79	–	89 (6)	90 (6)	–
2 MOPP/2 ABVD	20–40 Gy, IF	CS I–IIA	67	–	89 (6)	87 (6)	–
3 MOPP/3 ABVD	20–40 Gy, EF	CS IB–IIB	31	–	89 (6)	–	–
3 MOPP/3 ABVD	20–40 Gy, EF	CS III	40	–	82 (6)	–	–
3 MOPP/3 ABVD	20–40 Gy, EF	CS IV	21	–	62 (6)	–	–
SFOP MDH-90 (13)							
	–	–	202	91 (5)	–	–	98 (5)
4 VBVP, good responders	20 Gy, IF	I–II	171	91 (5)	–	–	–
4 VBVP + 1–2 OPPA, poor responders	20 Gy, IF	I–II	27	78 (5)	–	–	–
AEIOP-MH-83 (25)							
			215	–	–	82 (7)	86 (7)
Group A			83	–	–	95 (7)	–
3 ABVD	20–40 Gy, IF	IA	–	–	–	–	–
3 ABVD	20–40 Gy, R	IIA (M/T <0.33)	–	–	–	–	–
Group B			83			81 (7)	
3 MOPP/3 ABVD	20–40 Gy, R	IIA (M/T = 0.33)	–	–	–	–	–
3 MOPP/3 ABVD	20–40 Gy, EF	IIIA	–	–	–	–	–
Group C							
5 MOPP/5 ABVD	20–40 Gy, EF	IIIB–IV	49	–	–	60	–
Germany-Austria							
HD-82 (72)							
2 OPPA	35 Gy, IF	IA/IB–IIA	100	98 (9)	–	–	100 (9)
2 OPPA/2 COPP	30 Gy, IF	IIB–IIIA	53	94 (9)	–	–	96 (9)
2 OPPA/4 COPP	25 Gy, IF	IIIB–IV	50	86 (9)	–	–	85 (9)
HD-85 (72)							
2 OPA	35 Gy, IF	IA/IB–IIA	53	85 (6)	–	–	98 (6)
2 OPA/2 COMP	30 Gy, IF	IIB–IIIA	21	55 (6)	–	–	95
2 OPA/4 COMP	25 Gy, IF	IIIB–IV	24	49 (6)	–	–	100
HD-90 (73)							
2 OEPA/OPPA	25 Gy, IF	IA/IB–IIA	275	94/95 (5)	–	–	99 (5)
2 OEPA/OPPA + 2 COPP	25 Gy, IF	IIB–IIIA	124	90/96 (5)	–	–	97 (5)
2 OEPA/OPPA + 4 COPP	20 Gy, IF	IIIB–IV	179	84/89 (5)	–	–	94 (5)
GPOH-HD95 (74,75)							
			830	90 (3)			97 (3)
	CR no RT	TG1, TG2, or TG3	185	–	–	89 (3)	–
	20–35 Gy, IF for PR	–	611	–	–	93 (3)	–
2 OEPA/OPPA	IA/B, IIA	–	326	94 (3)	–	–	–
2 OPEA/OPPA + 2 COPP	IIEA, IIB, IIIA	–	224	91 (3)	–	–	–
2 OEPA/OPPA + 4 COPP	IIEB, IIIEA/B, IIIB, IVA/B	–	280	84 (3)	–	–	–
GPOH-HD-2002 (76)							
2 O(E/P)A	CR no RT	IA/IB–IIA	62	93 (5)	–	–	100 (5)
	20 Gy, IF		133	92 (5)	–	–	
2 O(E/P)A + 2 COP(P/DAC)	20 Gy, IF	IIB–IIIA	139	88 (5)	–	–	99 (5)
2 O(E/P)A + 4 COP(P/DAC)	20 Gy, IF	IIIB–IV (21)	239	87 (5)	–	–	95 (5)
United Kingdom Children's Cancer Study Group							
6–10 ChlVPP	35 Gy, IF	II	125	–	–	85 (10)	92 (10)
6–10 ChlVPP	35 Gy, IF	III	80	–	–	73 (10)	84 (10)
6–10 ChlVPP	35 Gy, IF	IV	27	–	–	38 (10)	71 (10)
Argentina (GATLA) (18)			64	–	–	–	81 (5)
Intermediate[a]							
6 CVPP	30–40 Gy, IF	I–IV	43	–	–	87 (5)	–
6 AOPE	30–40 Gy, IF	I–IV	21	–	–	67 (5)	–
Unfavorable[a]							
CCOPP/CAPTe	30–40 Gy, IF	I–IV	24	–	–	83 (5)	–

EFS, event-free survival; DFS, disease-free survival; RFS, relapse-free survival; FFP, freedom from progression; MOPP, Mustargen, Oncovin, procarbazine, prednisone; ABVD, Adriamycin, bleomycin, vinblastine, dacarbazine; IF, involved field; CS, clinical stage; PS, pathologic stage; COPP, cyclophosphamide, Oncovin, Procarbazine, prednisone; EF, extended field; R, regional; TLI, total lymphoid Irradiation; VBVP, vinblastine bleomycin etoposide (VP16) prednisone; M/T, mediastinal mass/thoracic ration; OPPA, Oncovin, prednisone, procarbazine, Adriamycin; OPA, Oncovin, prednisone, Adriamycin; COMP, cyclophosphamide, Oncovin, methotrexate, prednisone; OEPA, Oncovin, etoposide, prednisone, Adriamycin; PR, partial response; ChiVPP, chlorambucil, vinblastine, procarbazine, prednisone; GATLA, The Grupo Argentino de Tratamiento de Leucemia Aguda; CVPP, cyclophosphamide, vincristine, prednisone, procarbazine; AOPE, Adriamycin, Oncovin, prednisone, etoposide; CCOPP/CAPTe, CCNU, vincristine, procarbazine, prednisone/cyclophosphamide, Adriamycin, prednisone, teniposide.

[a]Intermediate and unfavorable prognostic group determined on the basis of age, symptoms, stage, and number of nodal regions.

TABLE 89.2 TREATMENT RESULTS OF CHEMOTHERAPY ALONE IN PEDIATRIC HODGKIN LYMPHOMA TRIALS

			Percentage Outcome (Year)			
Chemotherapy/Study (Reference)	Stage	Number of Patients	EFS	DFS	RFS/FFP	Survival
Children's Cancer Group (66)						
		111	82 (4)	–	–	87 (4)
6 MOPP/6 ABVD	PS III/IV	57	77 (4)	–	–	84 (4)
Pediatric Oncology Group						
6 MOPP-ABVD (77)	I, IIA, IIIA1	78	83 (8)	–	–	94 (8)
8 MOPP-ABVD (27)	CS IIB, IIIA2, IIIB, IV	81	79 (5)	–	–	96 (5)
Australia/New Zealand						
5–6 VEEP (7)	All stages	53	59 (3)	78 (5)	–	92 (5)
3 EVAP/ABV (78)	CS IA–IVA	25	–	–	79 (3)	100 (3)
6–8 MOPP or 6 ChlVPP (78)	CS I–IV	38	–	–	98 (4)	94 (4)
Costa Rica (14)						
6 CVPP	CS I–IIIA	52	–	–	90 (5)	100 (5)
6 CVPP/EBO	CS IIIB/IV	24	–	–	60 (5)	81 (5)
Argentina (GATLA) (18)						
3 CVPP	CS IA, IIA	10	86 (6.7)	–	–	–
6 CVPP	CS IB, IIB	16	87 (6.7)	–	–	–
Nicaragua (3)						
6 COPP	CS I, IIA	14	100 (3)	–	–	100 (3)
8–10 COPP-ABV	CS IIB, III, IV	34	75 (3)	–	–	–
Madras, India						
6 COPP/ABV (22)	CS I–IIA	10	89 (5)	–	–	–
6 COPP/ABV (22)	CS IIB–IVB	43	90 (5)	–	–	–
4 COPP/4 ABVD (79)	CS I–IV	133	88 (5)	–	–	92 (5)
The Netherlands (24)						
6 MOPP (24)	CS I–IV (lymph nodes <4 cm)	21	91 (10)	–	–	100 (10)
6 ABVD (24)	CS I–IV (lymph nodes <4 cm)	17	70 (10)	–	–	94 (10)
6 ABVD/MOPP (24)	CS I–IV	21	91 (10)	–	–	91 (10)
Rotterdam-HD-84 (80)		46	91 (10)	–	–	95 (10)
6 EBVD	I–IIA	23	96 (10)	–	–	100 (10)
3–5 EBVD/MOPP	IIB–IV	23	87 (10)	–	–	91 (10)
Uganda (16)						
6 MOPP	CS I–IIIA	38	–	–	–	75 (5)
6 MOPP	CS IIIB–IV	10	–	–	–	60 (5)

ABVD, doxorubicin, bleomycin, vinblastine, dacarbazine; ChlVPP, vinblastine, procarbazine, prednisone; COPP, cyclophosphamide, Vincristine, procarbazine, prednisone; CS, clinical stage; CVPP, cyclophosphamide, vincristine, procarbazine, prednisone; DFS, disease-free survival; EBO, epirubicin, bleomycin, Vincristine; EFS, event-free survival; EVAP, etoposide, vinblastine, cytosine arabinoside, cisplatinum; FFP, freedom from progression; GATLA, Grupo Argentino de Tratamiento de Leucemia Aguda; MOPP, Mustargen, Vincristine, procarbazine, prednisone; PS, pathologic stage; RFS, relapse-free survival; VEEP, vincristine, etoposide, epirubicin, prednisone.

approaches that more effectively shield normal tissues. Although radiation alone has been largely abandoned as a treatment strategy in children, risk-adapted treatment strategies still integrate low-dose (15 to 25.5 Gy) IFRT as a critical component of combined-modality regimens and as salvage therapy for patients with refractory or relapsed disease.

TABLE 89.3 TREATMENT RESULTS IN CHILDREN WITH HODGKIN LYMPHOMA WITH RADIATION THERAPY ALONE

Group/Institution and Study (Reference)	Number of Patients (Dose and Field)	Stage	Percentage Survival (Year)	
			Overall	Relapse-Free
Joint Center/Harvard (2,81)	50	PS I, IIA	97 (5)	82 (5)
St. Bartholomew's Great Ormond St. (82)	28	CS I, II	95.5 (10)	79 (10)
Stanford University (82)	48	PS I, II	86 (10)	82 (10)
Intergroup Hodgkin's Study (9)	39 (IF)	PS I, II	95 (5)	41 (5)
	58 (EF)	PS I, II	96 (5)	67 (5)
University of Toronto (12)	8 (EF) 23 (IF)	CS, PS I	95	87
	42 (EF)	PS IIA, IIIA	85	45
Gustave-Roussy (5)	33 (EF)	PS I	80 (5)	33 (5)
Royal Marsden Hospital (21)	99 (IF)	CS I	92 (10)	70 (10)

PS, pathologic stage; CS, clinical stage; EF, extended field; IF, involved field.

Combination Chemotherapy, Combined Modality Therapy, and Risk-Adapted Therapy

The development of non–cross-resistant chemotherapy combinations provided the first effective therapy for advanced HL and formed the cornerstone for contemporary risk-adapted therapy. The specific chemotherapeutic combinations have changed as their morbidities have become better understood, but most treatment regimens include MOPP (mechlorethamine, vincristine, procarbazine, and prednisone), ABVD (doxorubicin, bleomycin, vinblastine, and dacarbazine), or therapies derived from one of the combinations (Table 89.2).

Despite the excellent disease control with ABVD,[6,85,93,94] bleomycin and doxorubicin cause pulmonary and cardiovascular damage, respectively. To reduce the treatment-related toxicities associated with 6 cycles of either MOPP or ABVD, strategies alternating the two regimens, and using fewer cycles of each, have been developed. The combined ABVD and MOPP regimens used for children have produced excellent disease control with apparent diminished toxicity.[10,11,27]

Contemporary therapy for pediatric HL using chemotherapy alone or combined-modality therapy produces long-term DFS in 85% to 100% of patients with localized disease and 70% to 90% of patients with advanced disease.[3,6,7–8,10,11,13,14,15,16,17,18,20,22–24,25–27,67,71,73,74,77,78,83,94,95] Single-modality chemotherapy treatment usually involves more cycles of chemotherapy, whereas combined-modality therapies prescribe low-dose, involved-field radiation in lieu of several chemotherapy cycles. Although early treatment results appear comparable with results of more mature trials of combined-modality therapy, the long-term efficacy and treatment toxicities associated with chemotherapy alone have not been reported. Earlier randomized pediatric trials prospectively comparing outcomes in patients treated with chemotherapy alone with those treated with combined-modality therapy have not definitively established the superiority of one treatment approach over the other.[26,93] However, other trials suggest a better outcome in patients with intermediate or advanced disease treated with combined-modality therapy.[26,74] Children's Cancer Group (CCG) investigators closed enrollment into a randomized controlled trial comparing outcomes in patients treated with contemporary risk-adapted combined-modality therapy with COPP/ABV (cyclophosphamide, vincristine, prednisone, procarbazine/doxorubicin, bleomycin, vinblastine) hybrid chemotherapy and low-dose, involved-field radiation to those treated with COPP/ABV chemotherapy alone based on a significantly higher 3-year event-free survival (EFS) in patients randomized to also receive radiotherapy.[67] However, early follow-up did not demonstrate a significant difference in OS among the groups due to the successful retrieval of relapsed patients following salvage therapy. Similarly, the German HL-DAL-90 protocol treated intermediate- and high-risk patients with 2 cycles of OPPA (vincristine, prednisone, procarbazine, doxorubicin) or OEPA (vincristine, etoposide, prednisone, doxorubicin) (females and males, respectively), followed by 2 to 4 cycles of COPP. All patients received 20 to 35 Gy IFRT. Five-year EFS in the intermediate- and high-risk groups was 93% and 86%, respectively, which was comparable to that seen in the low-risk group. OS (5-year) for all three risk groups was ≥94%.[17,20,74,75] In the subsequent HL-95 trial, which employed the same chemotherapy but omitted IFRT in complete responders, the EFS for intermediate- and high-risk patients combined who did not receive radiotherapy dropped to 79% compared with 91% for those who did get radiotherapy.[74]

Currently, consensus regarding the optimal therapy for children and adolescents with HL has not been established. Treatment with chemotherapy alone is preferred by many investigators desiring to avoid long-term sequelae of radiation, including musculoskeletal growth impairment, cardiovascular dysfunction, and solid tumor carcinogenesis. However, single modality chemotherapy protocols typically use higher cumulative doses of chemotherapeutic agents with dose-related toxicity, especially alkylating agents. Moreover, low-dose involved-field radiation therapy has substantially reduced many of the undesirable radiation-associated sequelae. Therefore, current investigations aim to selectively combine chemotherapy and radiation in an effort to improve the therapeutic ratio.

Ongoing risk-adapted trials aim to identify patients who require radiation to optimize DFS and patients who can be cured by limited chemotherapy alone (Table 89.4).

TABLE 89.4 INVOLVED FIELD RADIATION GUIDELINES

Involved Node(s)	*Radiation Field*
Unilateral neck	Unilateral neck[a] + ipsilateral supraclavicular
Supraclavicular	Supraclavicular + mid/low neck + infraclavicular
Axilla	Axilla ± infraclavicular/supraclavicular
Mediastinum	Mediastinum + hila + infraclavicular/supraclavicular[b]
Hila	Hila ± mediastinum
Spleen	Spleen ± adjacent para-aortics
Para-aortics	Para-aortics ± spleen
Iliac	Iliacs + inguinal/femoral

[a]Upper neck region not treated if supraclavicular involvement is extension of the mediastinal disease.

[b]Clinical target volume encompasses postchemotherapy mediastinal width laterally and prechemotherapy extent in superior-inferior direction.

Favorable Risk

In the 1990s, pediatric HL investigators evaluated risk-adapted therapies using fewer cycles of combination chemotherapy and lower radiation doses and treatment volumes in clinically staged patients with favorable disease presentations. Favorable disease presentations were characterized by localized nodal involvement in the absence of B symptoms and bulky mediastinal lymphadenopathy. The number of involved nodal regions, the presence of extranodal extension, hilar lymphadenopathy, and peripheral nodal bulk comprised the other risk factors considered in some of these studies. Most treatment regimens prescribed 2 to 4 cycles of novel chemotherapy combinations that limited or omitted alkylating agent and anthracycline chemotherapy and bleomycin. The results of these trials demonstrated that excellent treatment outcomes could be maintained in patients with favorable presentations of localized HL using minimal therapy.[13,17,19,20,25,65,67,68,71,74,96] Ongoing trials are testing the feasibility of omitting chemotherapy in patients with excellent response to chemotherapy.

Intermediate and Unfavorable Risks

In most clinical trials, intermediate risk consists of stage I, II, and IIIA patients with unfavorable disease features such as more than three nodal sites, presence of bulky mediastinal lymphadenopathy (mediastinal ratio ≥33%, peripheral nodal mass ≥6 to 10 cm), or extranodal extension. High-risk HL patients are those with stage IIIB and any with stage IV. Patients with stage IIB disease are sometimes considered intermediate and sometimes high risk according to the study group. Two treatment approaches are used for intermediate and high-risk patients, both of which include chemotherapy regimens derived from the original MOPP and ABVD combinations. MOPP has largely been replaced by COPP because cyclophosphamide is less myelosuppressive and leukemogenic than mechlorethamine.[97]

In the conventional treatment approach, combination chemotherapy is administered on a twice monthly schedule for 6 to 8 months.[8,10,11,17,19,20,26,27,67,72,74,93] More recent trials are evaluating the second treatment approach, which has been used successfully in adults with HL. These protocols prescribe dose-intensive, multiagent chemotherapy in an abbreviated schedule over a period of 3 to 5 months. Prototypes of the dose-intensive therapy include the MOPP/ABV hybrid, Stanford V, or BEACOPP (bleomycin, etoposide, doxorubicin, cyclophosphamide, vincristine, procarbazine, prednisone) regimens.[67,70,98,99,100] These treatments alternate myelosuppressive and nonmyelosuppressive chemotherapy combinations in a weekly schedule with the aim of reducing the development of resistant disease. Growth factor support is required to facilitate bone marrow recovery and maintain the compacted treatment schedule. Low-dose, involved-field radiation therapy generally is used to consolidate remission after completion of chemotherapy. In ongoing pediatric trials, the response to chemotherapy influences the ultimate amount of therapy. For example, in the Stanford/St. Jude/Dana Farber protocols, rapid early responders to chemotherapy, defined by complete response after 2 cycles of chemotherapy, are being targeted for reduced treatment (less or no radiation therapy, depending on the risk group). In the last COG trial for high-risk patients, rapidity of response was evaluated after 4 cycles of BEACOPP. Rapid responders received consolidation therapy according to gender in order to avoid or minimize sex-specific long-term toxicities of therapy. Females received 4 cycles of COPP/ABV without IFRT to avoid secondary breast cancers, while males received 2 cycles of ABVD with IFRT. Slow responders received 4 more cycles of BEACOPP followed by IFRT. OS was 97%, with significant acute hematologic toxicity and two patients developing secondary leukemia.[70] The current European trial, based on the long-standing German experience, is also testing a gender-based approach in which a procarbazine-free OEPA/COPDAC (cyclophosphamide, vincristine, prednisone, dacarbazine) is given to boys and OEPA/COPP to girls, in order to reduce the alkylator exposure in boys and maintain fertility.[76]

The last COG intermediate risk HL study treated patients with stage IA or IIA bulky, IB, IIB, IIIA, or IVA disease with 2 cycles of ABVE-PC (doxorubicin, bleomycin, vincristine, etoposide, prednisone, cyclophosphamide) prior to response evaluation. Those with a rapid early response to therapy (>60% reduction in the tumor dimension) and those who achieve complete recovery after an additional 2 cycles of the same chemotherapy were randomized to 21 Gy IFRT or no additional treatment. Patients with slow early response after 2 cycles of chemotherapy were randomized to either standard therapy (an additional 2 cycles of ABVE-PC + 21 Gy IFRT) or intensified therapy (2 cycles of ABVE-PC, 2 cycles of DECA [dexamethasone, etoposide, cisplatin, cytarabine] + 21 Gy IFRT). Early results show an improved outcome for rapid early responders of 87% compared with 78% for slow early responders ($P = .0001$), while radiotherapy did not improve outcome in the rapid early responders ($P = .07$).[101]

Sequence of Therapy

The most effective sequence of therapy in the setting of combined chemotherapy and irradiation is not unequivocally established. However, chemotherapy is usually the first modality. This allows assessment of drug response, maximization of the amount of drug treatment, and shrinkage of disease and more limited fields of irradiation. Rarely, focal irradiation prior to chemotherapy is necessary due to significant symptomatic compromise such as airway obstruction.

Refractory or Relapsed Disease

Treatment failures in pediatric HL patients typically develop within the first 3 years, although late relapses have been reported, particularly in patients with lymphocyte-predominant HL. The most common site of relapse following risk-adapted therapies remains the primary site of disease.[102] Because of the excellent outcome for the majority of children and adolescents with HL, investigations regarding salvage strategy have been limited. Prognosis following relapse is dependent on the primary therapy given and the timing of relapse. Standard multiagent chemotherapy and radiation therapy may salvage 40% to 50% of patients who relapse 1 or more years after primary therapy, but treatment complications such as second malignancies may reduce long-term survival. More aggressive salvage chemotherapy without stem cell transplant has been shown to provide satisfactory outcome for patients with late relapses.[103] Patients with primary refractory disease (i.e., those unresponsive to initial therapy or who relapse within 1 year of primary therapy) have a very poor prognosis. Intensive cytoreductive chemotherapy followed by myeloablation and autologous hematopoietic stem cell transplantation is reported to salvage 30% to 60% of these patients, but relapses after 5 years have been observed, and long-term treatment complications may predispose to early mortality.[104,105–107]

Historically, because of higher treatment-related mortality, allogeneic transplantation did not provide a survival advantage compared with autologous stem cell transplantation. However, allogeneic bone marrow transplantation has been shown to be a useful treatment in healthy patients who have failed or cannot have an autologous transplant.[108]

Techniques of Radiation Therapy

As discussed above, most children with HL will be treated with combined chemotherapy and low-dose IFRT using a risk-adapted approach. The use of radiation therapy alone has been largely abandoned due to concerns for late effects, including cardiac complications and secondary malignancies. The Patterns of Care studies demonstrated the relation between radiation technique and outcome.[57] The results of patients treated with RT alone were improved in institutions that treated a large number of HL patients. The HD-DAL 90 trial (German-Austrian pediatric multicenter trial) showed that upfront centralized review of patients entered into the study altered the treatment approach for a large number of children.[109] Because technique is discussed in Chapter 77, only select points applicable to children will be discussed here.

Using risk-adapted strategies, most children with HL are treated with combined chemotherapy and low-dose IFRT. The definition of involved fields depends on the anatomy of the region in terms of lymph node distribution and patterns of disease extension into regional areas. Involved fields typically should include not just the identifiably abnormal lymph nodes but also the entire lymph node region containing the involved nodes (Table 89.5). Historically, consideration has been given to radiating the treatment area bilaterally (e.g., both sides of the neck) in young children in an effort to avoid growth asymmetry. However, current combined modality treatment strategies use low radiation doses of 15 to 25 Gy and, therefore, unilateral radiation fields are appropriate if the disease is confined to one side of the neck. However, field definitions often are protocol specific.

Strong consideration must be given to excluding normal tissues in an effort to reduce the risk of acute and late effects,

TABLE 89.5 GUIDELINES FOR TREATMENT SELECTION IN PEDIATRIC HODGKIN LYMPHOMA

Stage	*Clinical Presentation*	*Therapy Considerations*
IA, IIA	*Favorable risk* Without bulk No extranodal extension 3 or less involved nodal regions	*Recommended therapy* 2–4 cycles non–cross-resistant chemotherapy (OEPA, VAMP, COPP-ABV, AV-PC). Response-based low-dose, involved-field radiation (15 Gy to 25.5 Gy). **Other considerations: Consider use of IFRT based on early response to chemotherapy** If CR after 2 OEPA no need for RT
IA, IIA, IIIA Selected IIB	*Intermediate risk* Bulky lymphadenopathy Mediastinal ratio ≥33% Peripheral nodes ≥6–10 cm More than 3 involved nodal regions	*Recommended therapy* 3–6 cycles compacted, dose-intensive, non-cross-resistant chemotherapy (OEPA/COPP, ABVE-PC) plus low-dose, involved-field radiation (15 Gy to 25.5 Gy). **Other considerations: Early response to therapy may be considered in determining need for radiation in those achieving CR.**
IIB, IIIB, IVA/B	*High risk*	*Recommended therapy* 4–6 compacted, dose-intensive cycles of non–cross-resistant chemotherapy (OEPA/COPP, ABVE-PC) plus low-dose, involved-field radiation (15 Gy to 25.5 Gy). **Other considerations:** 8 cycles non–cross-resistant chemotherapy alone (BEACOPP).

CR, complete remission; RT, radiation therapy; OEPA, Oncovin, etoposide, prednisone, Adriamycin; COPP, cyclophosphamide, Vincristine, procarbazine, prednisone; VAMP, vinblastine, doxorubicin, methotrexate, prednisone; ABVE-PC, Adriamycin, bleomycin, vincristine, etoposide, prednisone, cyclophosphamide; BEACOPP, bleomycin, etoposide, doxorubicin, cyclophosphamide, vincristine, procarbazine, prednisone.

including secondary malignancies and cardiac complications. Every effort should be made to exclude breast tissue, and potentially the thyroid gland, in patients with isolated mediastinal disease with no evidence of axillary or neck involvement. Clearly, careful planning and judgment are necessary. With the use of CT-based treatment planning, normal structures can be identified and doses minimized.[89,110,111–115] The treatment of involved supradiaphragmatic fields or a mantle field can pose a clinical challenge to treat precisely the lymph node regions that are involved while still protecting critical adjacent normal tissues. These fields can be simulated with the arms up over the head or down with hands on the hips. The former pulls the axillary lymph nodes away from the lungs, allowing greater lung shielding. However, the axillary lymph nodes then move into the vicinity of the humeral heads, which should be blocked in growing children. Thus, the position chosen involves weighing concerns regarding lymph nodes, lung, and humeral heads. Attempts should be made to exclude or position breast tissue under the lung–axillary blocking.

In risk-adapted strategies using combined modality therapy, radiation dose is dependent on the choice of systemic therapy that is variously defined and often protocol specific. In general, doses of 15 to 25 Gy are used, with modifications based on patient age, treatment response, the presence of bulk or residual (postchemotherapy) disease, and normal tissue concerns. In some situations, a boost of 5 Gy is appropriate. Although IFRT remains the standard when patients are treated with combined-modality therapy, response-adapted RT, which is limited to areas of initial bulk disease (generally defined as ≥5 or 6 cm at the time of disease presentation) or postchemotherapy residual disease (generally defined as ≥2 cm, or residual PET avidity), is under investigation.

An approach studied in Europe by the European Organisation for Research and Treatment Center–Groupe d'Etudes des Lymphomes de l'Adulte is the use of involved node RT (INRT), which restricts RT to the initially involved lymph node.[116] This is based on the premise that chemotherapy can effectively eliminate microscopic disease that may exist within adjacent but clinically uninvolved nodes. This concept is supported by the observation that among patients treated with chemotherapy alone, initially involved lymph nodes are the most common site of recurrence.[117] INRT uses all available clinical information including pre- and postchemotherapy imaging with CT and FDG-PET scan to define the treatment field according to the prechemotherapy extent of disease.[118,119] However, uninvolved lymph node regions are not necessarily included within the clinical target volume (CTV). For example, in contrast to conventional IFRT, uninvolved hila are not included in the CTV for mediastinal presentations, and the length of the treated volume is not routinely extended beyond 1 cm for the planning target volume (Fig. 89.1). However, the margins for INRT are defined differently depending on the protocol and cooperative group.[112,120,121] Regardless, successive reduction in treatment volume may reduce the toxicity of therapy.

Steep radiation dose gradients, using modern radiation techniques such as three-dimensional conformal radiation (3D-CRT) and intensity-modulated radiotherapy (IMRT), are achieved to spare normal structures, particularly for patients who are at risk for treatment complications. For example, 3D-CRT of an anterior mediastinal mass could avoid radiation to normal structures, such as the spine, breast, heart, or lung tissue located behind the mass. IMRT utilizes multiple beams to create concavities and avoid dose to surrounding tissues.[110,111–114,122] Although conformality is improved, the radiation dose is spread over a larger volume of tissue, and additional monitoring units are required to deliver treatment compared to conventional methods. As a result, integral dose is increased, which has limited the use of IMRT in the pediatrics population, particularly because low doses are required for treatment of HL. IMRT remains controversial in the treatment of children as a result of the concerns that increased integral dose, and increased radiation scatter within the smaller body habitus of a child could lead to an increase in the development of secondary malignancies.[123,124] However, IMRT may still provide dosimetric advantages in particular cases, such as patients who have received prior radiation or in patients with bulky mediastinal disease.

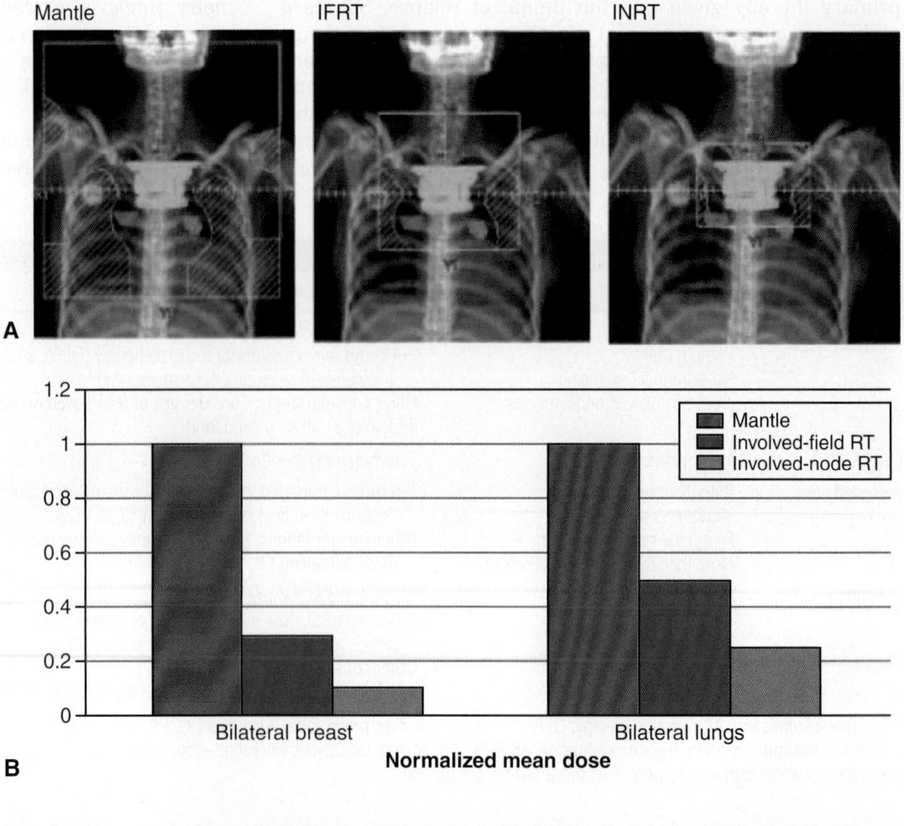

FIGURE 89.1. A: Digitally reconstructed radiographs demonstrating typical radiation therapy (RT) fields for historic mantle RT, contemporary involved-field RT (IFRT), and involved node RT (INRT) for a female patient with stage I disease involving the upper mediastinum. The postchemotherapy volume of initially involved mediastinal nodes is shown in *green*. Hila are shown in *blue* and *violet*. **B:** Reduction in dose to breast and lung for the same patient. For each volume the prescribed dose to the CTV is the same. The resulting mean dose to breast and lung tissue with mantle RT is a set value equal to 1. The proportional reduction in normal tissue dose occurs as a result of the reduction in treated volume with IFRT and INRT. (From Hodgson DC, Hudson MM, Constine LS. Pediatric Hodgkin lymphoma: maximizing efficacy and minimizing toxicity. *Semin Radiat Oncol* 2007;17:230–242; copyright 2007, with permission from Elsevier.)

Proton therapy for pediatric HL is also an area under current active investigation. In particular, the steep dose gradient offered by protons may improve the dose distribution in specific clinical scenarios, such as in patients with superior mediastinal masses in whom the dose to breast and lung may be reduced.[125,126]

Ultimately, each clinical scenario must be considered independently to determine the optimum RT technique, taking into account the characteristics of the tumor, patient's age, normal structures at risk, and comorbidities.

Complications of Radiation Therapy

Acute Effects

The acute side effects of radiation therapy are related to the involved site treated. Due to the lower doses used in pediatrics, the most common toxicities include temporary loss or change in taste, xerostomia, esophagitis, low posterior scalp epilation, skin erythema, and occasionally dyspepsia, nausea, and vomiting. Acute effects of para-aortic irradiation include early onset nausea and vomiting, which usually abates after the second or third treatment without antiemetic therapy. Patients who receive larger fields may be subject to bone marrow suppression, the severity of which may be influenced by the systemic regimen preceding radiation.

Long-Term Effects

Musculoskeletal

Height reduction is a potential long-term consequence of irradiation, most frequently with doses >20 Gy and most severe in prepubertal children. Growth arrest or delay is modest with the low doses currently used in modern pediatric HL treatment strategies (Fig. 89.2).[2,127,128] Interclavicular shortening and hypoplasia of the neck muscles may occur in children irradiated before puberty, which is particularly dependent on dose delivered; the severity of these complications is more pronounced in children <5 years of age at the time of irradiation. Slipped capital femoral epiphysis occurs in ≤50% of young children whose femoral heads have been irradiated. Avascular necrosis of the femoral or humeral heads is rare if appropriate shielding is provided. Radiation doses of 20 to 40 Gy to the mandible may result in dental abnormalities, such as stunted tooth development, incomplete calcification, premature apical closure or eruption, and root tapering with apical constriction if the tooth germ tissue is in the irradiated field.[129]

Cardiovascular

Radiation-associated pericardial and myocardial disease are related to dose (including fraction size) and volume and are complicated by the use of anthracyclines. Cardiac sequelae, including pericarditis and effusion, valvular thickening, biventricular dysfunction, and coronary artery disease, all are observed with irradiation to the heart.[1,63,68,85,130] Increase in mortality risk, due to premature coronary artery disease and acute myocardial infarction, has been demonstrated in patients who received mediastinal radiation in doses >30 Gy before 20 years of age.[83] Conversely, modern treatment approaches based on tailored low-dose radiation and less cardiotoxic chemotherapy, sometimes including cardioprotectants, will optimistically reduce such effects. Radiation doses of <30 Gy and techniques that use adequate cardiac shielding and avoid anterior weighting of the treatment fields appear to reduce the risk of cardiac complications, particularly pericarditis and myocarditis.[63,85] Although the proximal coronary arteries are not shielded by a central cardiac block, the 45-fold excess mortality risk from acute myocardial infarction associated with higher radiation doses has diminished substantially with current approaches.[131] Also, dose to the heart can now be calculated using advanced radiation techniques and dose can be constrained using conformal techniques in order to keep the risk of long-term development of cardiac injury to a minimum. Unfortunately, the impact of low-dose RT to the heart may not become apparent until larger cohorts of survivors treated with modern combined modality regimens have longer follow-up.

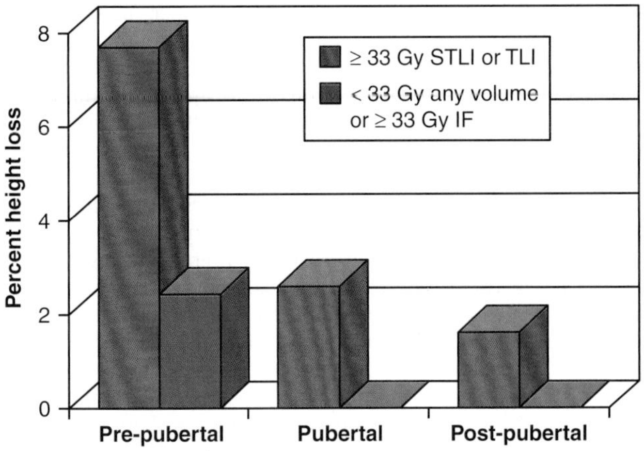

FIGURE 89.2. Relative height impairment for different age and treatment groups in pediatric Hodgkin lymphoma. (From Willman K, Cox K, Donaldson S. Radiation induced height impairment in pediatric Hodgkin's disease. *Int J Radiat Oncol Biol Phys* 1994;28:85–92; copyright 1997, with permission from Elsevier.)

Pulmonary

With doses of 25 Gy,[132] the incidence of pulmonary complications, including pneumonitis or fibrosis, is low. Use of bleomycin can increase the risk of acute pulmonary pneumonitis and late pulmonary fibrosis in patients receiving pulmonary RT. In a report from the CCG, 9% of children treated with ABVD and 21 Gy of mantle irradiation exhibited clinically significant pulmonary damage.[8] These results were confirmed recently in a study evaluating pediatric patients with any chest radiation who developed radiation pneumonitis. The incidence was found to be low and most often related to therapies including bleomycin.[133]

Thyroid

Thyroid dysfunction may result from neck or upper mediastinal irradiation and most often is manifested by an elevated serum concentration of thyroid-stimulating hormone (TSH). The incidence of hypothyroidism varies, but it appears to be directly related to irradiation dose. Constine et al.[134] noted an increased serum TSH in 4 of 24 (17%) children who received mantle irradiation of ≤26 Gy and in 74 of 95 (78%) who received >26 Gy. Approximately one-fourth of these children had a concomitant low thyroxine level. In this series, 36% of children experienced spontaneous improvement in thyroid function.

In a Childhood Cancer Survivor Study, thyroid abnormalities were self-reported by 34% of patients surveyed. Hypothyroidism was the most common thyroid disturbance, with a relative risk of 17.1 (P <.0001) compared with sibling controls. Risk factors for hypothyroidism include increased dose of radiation, older age at diagnosis of HL, female sex, and white race.[135] The estimated actuarial risk of hypothyroidism for survivors treated with ≥45 Gy was 50% at 20 years from diagnosis. Other thyroid abnormalities identified in excess from sibling controls included hyperthyroidism (eightfold excess risk), thyroid nodules (27-fold excess risk), and thyroid cancer (18-fold excess risk).[136]

Pelvic Late Effects

Gonadal injuries, including infertility and impaired secretion of sex hormones, are potential complications of pelvic irradiation.[137] In women, irradiation of the pelvis can affect the ovaries, resulting in premature menopause or fertility impairment.[137] In a report of female HL survivors by the Late Effects Study Group, 42% of women treated with alkylating agent chemotherapy and subdiaphragmatic radiation had experienced menopause by age 31 years, compared with 5% of control subjects.[138] In childhood cancer survivors who continued to have spontaneous menses more than 5 years after their cancer diagnosis, the cumulative incidence of nonsurgical menopause was 8% by age 40 years, representing a 13-fold higher risk compared with a sibling control group. Risk factors for premature menopause include attained age, exposure to increasing doses of ovarian radiation, increasing alkylating agent score (based on number of agents and cumulative dose), and diagnosis of HL.[136] Normal pregnancies, without increased risk of fetal wastage, spontaneous abortion, or birth defects, have been reported after pelvic irradiation.[137] In an effort to preserve ovarian function, it is recommended that the ovaries are transposed via oophoropexy to a shielded area laterally or inferomedially near the uterine cervix prior to the initiation of radiation.

In boys irradiated to the pelvis, oligospermia is common, but it is reversible (usually by 18 to 24 months) in most cases if the radiation dose scattered to the shielded testes is small.[2,139,140] Permanent oligospermia may occur, however, after full-dose pelvic irradiation.[140] Several investigations have demonstrated that fertility is compromised in boys treated with gonadotoxic combinations like COPP, even when cycles of alkylating agent chemotherapy are limited.[141,142] Anthracycline-based regimens such as ABVD (or similar hybrid) are associated with recovery of spermatogenesis after a temporary period of azoospermia.[143,144] In the modern treatment era, risk-adapted strategies seek to reduce or eliminate gonadotoxic treatments, resulting in excellent prospects to preserve fertility in boys.[141]

Second Malignant Neoplasm

The 15-year actuarial risk of second malignant neoplasms ranges from 8% to 15%.[83,131,145–146,147,148–155] Patients are at risk for developing secondary malignancies including leukemias (e.g., acute myeloblastic leukemia) and solid tumors, most commonly breast, thyroid, bone, and soft tissues. The risk of leukemia, which exhibits a peak frequency in the first 5 to 10 years after treatment, is associated primarily with the use of alkylating agents.[145,147] In contrast to secondary hematopoietic malignancies, the risk of developing a second solid tumor increases with time after therapy, with a latency usually exceeding 10 years from diagnosis.

Several studies reveal an increased ratio of observed to expected risk of second tumors for girls compared with boys, with median follow-up of 10 to 16 years.[81,145,156] A portion of this risk results from breast cancer, which is the most common solid second malignant neoplasm following the treatment of children. The increased risk of breast cancer is a significant concern for women treated for HL at a younger age. This increase in risk of breast cancer is related to the patient's age at the time of RT and has also been shown to decrease with a decrease in radiation dose.[157,158] Travis et al.[158] reported a large case-control study that included 105 women who developed breast cancer within a cohort of more than 3,800 female survivors diagnosed with HL at age ≤30. This cohort also included patients who had received either very low-dose RT (<4 Gy) or no radiation to the breast area where breast cancer developed. For all patients who received RT alone (>4 Gy), the relative risk of breast cancer was 3.2 and increased to 8.0 in the highest radiation dose group. This study demonstrated a dose–response relation between RT and the risk of breast cancer development.

Multiple studies have now demonstrated that lower RT dose and smaller treatment fields should translate into a reduction in late effects when used judiciously.[89,91,159,160] Historical extended field treatments included a substantial amount of breast tissue in the field design, which were then exposed to full-dose RT. Interestingly, breast tissue exposure was most significant when the axillae was irradiated in a typical mantle field as opposed to the mediastinal and hilar region. The practice of prophylactically irradiating the axillae is no longer performed, and, thus, the volume of breast tissue exposed to RT using involved field or involved node radiotherapy approaches is substantially less.[89] Using CT-based planning, the breast tissue can also be contoured as an avoidance structure and thereby shielded appropriately when designing RT fields in the region, a practice that was not used 30 years ago.

Current recommendations for the screening of late effects of therapy after childhood cancer can be found in the long-term follow-up guidelines developed by the COG, which are constantly updated (http://www.survivorshipguidelines.org).

Future Investigations

Analyzing patterns of disease recurrence should enhance our understanding of directions for therapeutic intensification. Most patients will relapse in areas of initial disease involvement, even in this era of combined-modality therapy.[161,162] Preventing these recurrences will require ingenuity if additional toxicity is to be avoided. Some generalizations regarding ongoing efforts in clinical trials for pediatric HL are as follows:

- Identification of prognostic biologic markers that correlate with tumor response for a more accurate risk stratification.
- Patients with early stage disease have an excellent prognosis, and, therefore, therapeutic aims focus on reducing the intensity of therapy.
- Patients with disease of an intermediate stage or prognosis are studied appropriately with questions that are intended to increase efficacy without increasing toxicity. Usually this entails modification of existing chemoradiation programs. The rapidity of response to therapy may offer a means to risk adapt subsequent treatment and is under investigation.
- Patients with advanced-stage disease require more effective treatment regimens. This may be attained by increasing the dose intensity or the rate of drug delivery; however, more attractive approaches under discussion are the incorporation of some of the new agents found to be effective in heavily pretreated patients (like brentuximab vedotin) into existing regimens. The role of radiation therapy in such trials will continue to be important.
- Identification of genetic host predisposition to treatment toxicity to better guide risk-adapted therapy.

Targeted therapy for HL focuses either on monoclonal antibodies directed against receptors and antigens expressed on the surface of HRS or on small molecules that target the well-defined signaling pathways that promote HRS survival and are triggered by these receptors.[163] Brentuximab vedotin, an anti-CD30 antibody conjugated to a synthetic antimicrotubule agent, monomethyl auristatin E, recently approved by the U.S. Food and Drug Administration for the treatment of relapsed or refractory HL, has shown excellent response in refractory HL.[164] Previous trials with naked anti-CD30 antibodies were disappointing.[165,166] Histone deacetylase (HDAC) inhibitors are small molecules that affect gene transcription by inhibiting posttranscriptional histone modification. Although there are a variety of enzymes that play a role in this process, the most studied drugs are vorinostat[167] and panobinostat,[168] both inhibit class I and II (pan-HDAC inhibitors). Everolimus, an inhibitor of mammalian target of rapamycin, a frequently activated pathway in HRS, has produced encouraging clinical responses in relapsed HL.[169] Other compounds under investigation directly or indirectly inhibit NF-κB, a nuclear transcription factor that regulates the expression of a variety of genes that play a crucial role in viral replication, tumorigenesis, apoptosis, various autoimmune diseases, and inflammation.[170]

Identifying the most promising agents and moving them into frontline therapy in order to spare further toxicity escalation while improving outcome will be the goal of upcoming trials. Adoptive immunotherapy with EBV-specific cytotoxic T-lymphocytes and other tumor-specific T cells are other attractive strategies under investigation for the therapy of relapsed or refractory HL.[171–173]

NON-HODGKIN LYMPHOMA

Childhood NHLs are a heterogeneous group of malignancies with variable histopathology, site of origin, and clinical manifestations. Childhood NHLs are diffuse, high grade, and poorly differentiated; extranodal involvement is common, and dissemination occurs early and often.[174] This is in striking contrast to adult NHL, in which low- and intermediate-grade nodal disease predominate.[174,175] These differences in pathology and clinical behavior observed between children and adults explain the markedly different presentations, staging practices, and treatment strategies for these age groups.

Epidemiology

In the United States, NHL is diagnosed in approximately 800 children and adolescents younger than 20 years of age, each year. According to the Surveillance, Epidemiology, and End Results program of the National Cancer Institute, NHL accounts for about 8% of all cases of childhood cancer.[28] The incidence increases with age, being rare in the child <3 years old; incidence is higher in males than in females (ratio of 3 to 1), and higher in whites than in African Americans (ratio of 1.5 to 1). In younger children, NHL is more frequent than HL, whereas the reverse is true for adolescents.

Although NHL is related to several genetic and environmental factors, its cause and pathogenesis remain unclear.[174,176] A small proportion of cases are seen in association with inherited immunodeficiencies (e.g., Wiskott-Aldrich syndrome, X-linked lymphoproliferative disease, ataxia-telangiectasia),[177,178] or acquired immunodeficiencies (e.g., HIV infection or immunosuppressive therapy in patients receiving solid organ or bone marrow transplants).[179,180] Evidence of EBV infection has been demonstrated in the majority of endemic (mainly in equatorial Africa) Burkitt tumors and in about 15% of sporadic cases (outside of Africa), suggesting a significant role for this virus in lymphomagenesis through unknown mechanisms.[181,182–183] EBV infection has also been associated with the development of posttransplant lymphoproliferative disease (PTLD), a B-cell lymphoproliferative disorder seen in patients after solid organ or hematopoietic stem cell transplantation.[184,185]

Pathologic Classification

The classification of NHL by the WHO was updated in 2008 (Table 89.6). Pediatric NHL cases are divided into four major histopathologic subtypes based on morphology and immunophenotype in the order of frequency: (a) Burkitt lymphoma (BL), (b) lymphoblastic lymphoma (LL), (c) diffuse large B-cell lymphoma (DLBCL), and (d) anaplastic large cell lymphoma (ALCL).[28,37,176] Identification of large numbers of monoclonal antibodies directed against surface antigens has allowed subclassification of the NHLs according to immunophenotype (see Chapter 78).[186] Thorough and efficient evaluation of histology and immunophenotype is a key to the determination of diagnosis, prognosis, and appropriate course of treatment because pediatric NHLs are usually aggressive. Cytogenetic analysis and identification of molecular markers provide a more precise means of characterization of these tumors and will likely contribute to the understanding of pathogenesis as well as the development of novel therapeutic approaches.[187–189]

TABLE 89.7 CLINICAL CHARACTERISTICS OF CHILDHOOD NON-HODGKIN LYMPHOMA

Histologic Subtype	Proportion of Cases (%)	Most Common Sites of Presentation
Burkitt lymphoma	35–40	Abdomen or head and neck
Lymphoblastic lymphoma		
T	15–20	Mediastinum with adenopathy
B	3	Cutaneous masses, isolated nodes, and bone
Diffuse large B-cell lymphoma	15–20	Nodes, abdomen, and bone
Mediastinal large B-cell lymphoma	1–2	Mediastinum
Anaplastic large cell lymphoma	15–20	Skin, nodes, and bone

Modified from Sandlund JT. Childhood Lymphoma. In: Abeloff MD, Armitage JO, Lichter AS, et al., eds. *Clinical oncology*, 2nd ed. New York: Churchill Livingstone, 2000:2438.

Clinical Presentation

The signs and symptoms in children with NHL correlate with the histologic subtype, disease site(s), and extent of involvement (Table 89.7). Clinical presentation is different between endemic and sporadic BL. Abdomen is the most common site of disease in sporadic BL, which presents with abdominal pain, distension, mass, nausea, vomiting, and gastrointestinal bleeding, followed by head and neck region involvement. Bone marrow involvement is seen in about 20% of sporadic disease and can present as BL.[190] However, in endemic BL, jaw involvement is the most common, and bone marrow involvement is rare.[191]

The majority (50% to 70%) of children with precursor T-cell LL present with rapidly enlarging neck and mediastinal lymphadenopathy.[176,188] Mediastinal masses can cause respiratory symptoms (e.g., cough, wheezing, shortness of breath, and orthopnea) by compressing airways or cause neck, face, and upper extremity swelling due to obstruction of the superior vena cava (SVC). Hemodynamic compromise due to pericardial effusions may also occur. However, children and adolescents with precursor B-cell LL tend to have limited disease in sites including skin, bone, and peripheral lymph nodes.[192,193]

DLBCL usually presents with nodal disease, especially in the abdomen, although bone (single or multiple sites) is also a

TABLE 89.6 BIOLOGIC CHARACTERISTICS OF THE FOUR MAJOR SUBTYPES OF CHILDHOOD NON-HODGKIN LYMPHOMA AS DEFINED BY HISTOLOGY AND IMMUNOPHENOTYPE

Histology	Immunology	Cytogenetics[a]	Molecular Genetics
Burkitt lymphoma	B-cell (sIg+)	t(8;14)(q24;q32)	IgH/c-myc
		t(2;8)(p11;q24)	Igκ/c-myc
		t(8;22)(q24;q11)	Igλ/c-myc
Lymphoblastic lymphoma	Immature T cell (80%)	t(1;14)(p32;q11)	TCRad/TAL1
		t(11;14)(p13;q11)	TCRad/RHOMB2
		t(11;14)(p15;q11)	TCRad/RHOMB1
		t(10;14)(q24;q11)	TCRad/HOX11
		t(7;19)(q35;p13)	TCRb/LYL1
		and others	
	Precursor B cell (20%)	Hyperdiploid	Ig gene rearrangement
Diffuse large B-cell lymphoma	B cell (of germinal center or postgerminal center)		Ig gene rearrangement
(Mediastinal large B cell)	(B cells of medullary thymus)		
Anaplastic large cell lymphoma	T cell (mostly), null cell, or natural killer cell	t(2;5)(p23;q25)	NPM/ALK

[a]Not all tumors in each category contain one of the translocations or molecular lesions described.

Modified from Shad A, Magrath I. Non-Hodgkin's lymphoma. *Pediatr Clin North Am* 1997;44(4):863–890, and Gross TG, Perkins SL: Malignant non-hodgkin lymphomas in children. In: Pizzo PA, Poplack DG, eds. *Principles and practice of pediatric oncology*, 6th ed. Philadelphia: Lippincott Williams & Wilkins, 2011:663–682.

relatively common site.[194,195] Primary mediastinal large B-cell lymphoma can be locally invasive and may present with SVC syndrome.[196]

The most frequent sites of involvement in systemic ALCL are peripheral nodes, mediastinal lymph nodes, and extranodal sites such as skin, soft tissue, and bone.[197,198] Spontaneous regression or waxing and waning of disease has been observed.

Diagnostic Evaluation

Tissue diagnosis and investigation to determine the clinical extent of disease should be completed expeditiously. It is important that appropriate therapy be initiated promptly because of the extremely rapid growth rate of pediatric NHL.[174] Although histology and immunophenotype remain the primary means of establishing the definitive diagnosis, karyotype and molecular studies will be vital for implementation of an optimal treatment plan. Thus, it is critical that an adequate amount of tissue be obtained at biopsy by performing either open biopsy or core-needle biopsy. If the patient's condition does not permit an open biopsy (e.g., a large mediastinal mass is causing airway obstruction or compression of SVC), then use of a less invasive means of sampling tumor cells with as minimal anesthesia as possible, such as percutaneous fine-needle aspiration or examination of pleural fluid, ascites, peripheral blood, or bone marrow (Table 89.8), is warranted.[199,200] The use of irradiation or steroids before biopsy for respiratory distress may result in rapid shrinkage of the mediastinal mass but may jeopardize the ability to establish a tissue diagnosis.[201,202]

Bilateral bone marrow biopsies are superior to a single aspirate or biopsy for identifying bone marrow involvement, which is often patchy in distribution in NHL.[176] Omitting this procedure may result in understaging. FDG-PET scan combined with CT is now widely available and preferred to gallium scans as part of the assessment of the extent of disease at diagnosis, speed of response to therapy, and posttherapy remission status.[203,204] Data in adults with HL and NHL and children with HL suggest that PET scanning to assess the rapidity of response may be prognostic.[205,206] However, further confirmation is needed to determine whether PET scanning has predictive value for detecting recurrence of pediatric NHL.

TABLE 89.8 INVESTIGATIONS REQUIRED FOR ACCURATE STAGING AND DIAGNOSIS OF CHILDHOOD LYMPHOMAS

History and physical examination
Complete blood count
Chemistry panel
Serum electrolytes with calcium, phosphorus, and magnesium
Liver enzymes with bilirubin
BUN, serum creatinine, LDH, and uric acid
Imaging studies
Chest radiograph
Neck, chest, abdominal and pelvis CT scan
Fluorine-18 FDG-PET imaging
Tissue biopsy (specimen type)
Morphology (fixed)
Immunophenotypic analysis (fresh or fixed)
Cytogenetics (fresh)
Molecular analysis (fresh or fixed)
FISH for specific translocation (fresh or fixed)
Immunoglobulin gene rearrangements (fresh or fixed)
Bone-marrow examination (bilateral aspirates and biopsies)
Cerebrospinal fluid examination (cell counts and cytology)

BUN, blood urea nitrogen; CT, computed tomography; FDG-PET, fluorodeoxyglucose positron emission tomography; FISH, fluorescence *in situ* hybridization; LDH, lactate dehydrogenase.

Adapted from Shad A, Magrath I. Non-Hodgkin's lymphoma. *Pediatr Clin North Am* 1997;44(4):863–890, and Gross TG, Perkins SL. Malignant non-Hodgkin lymphomas in Children. In: Pizzo PA, Poplack DG, eds. *Principles and practice of pediatric oncology*, 6th ed. Philadelphia: Lippincott Williams & Wilkins, 2011:663–682.

TABLE 89.9 STAGING AND GROUPING SYSTEM FOR CHILDHOOD NON-HODGKIN LYMPHOMA

Stage/Group	Description
St. Jude Staging System	
I	A single tumor (extranodal) or single anatomic area (nodal), excluding the mediastinum or abdomen
II	A single tumor (extranodal) with regional lymph node involvement on same side of the diaphragm:
	(a) Two or more nodal areas
	(b) Two single (extranodal) tumors with or without regional node involvement
	A primary gastrointestinal tract tumor (usually ileocecal) with or without associated mesenteric node involvement, grossly completely resected
III	On both sides of the diaphragm:
	(a) Two single tumors (extranodal)
	(b) Two or more nodal areas
	All primary intrathoracic tumors (mediastinal, pleural, thymic)
	All extensive primary intra-abdominal disease; unresectable
	All primary paraspinal or epidural tumors regardless of other sites
IV	Any of the above with initial central nervous system or bone marrow involvement (<25% blasts)
Group Classification in the B-Cell Lymphomas	
A	Completely resected stage I or completely resected abdominal stage II lesions.
B	All cases not eligible for group A or group C. (Murphy stage III and non-CNS stage IV)
C	Any CNS involvement and/or bone marrow involvement ≥25% blasts. For CNS involvement one or more of the following applies:
	(1) Any L3 blasts in CSF
	(2) Cranial nerve palsy (if not explained by extracranial tumor)
	(3) Clinical spinal cord compression
	(4) Isolated intracerebral mass
	(5) Parameningeal extension: cranial and/or spinal

CNS, central nervous system; CSF, cerebrospinal fluid

Data from Murphy SB. Classification, staging and end results of treatment of childhood non-Hodgkin's lymphomas: dissimilarities from lymphomas in adults. *Semin Oncol* 1980;7:332–339; and Patte C, et al. The Societe Francaise d'Oncologie Pediatrique LMB89 protocol: highly effective multiagent chemotherapy tailored to the tumor burden and initial response in 561 unselected children with B-cell lymphomas and L3 leukemia. *Blood* 2001;97:3370–3379.

Laparotomy is not performed routinely for staging purposes because combination chemotherapy is part of the primary treatment. Still, laparotomy may be necessary in selected cases for diagnostic purposes, but aggressive debulking procedures are not advised. MRI may be helpful in detecting disease at specific sites, particularly the nervous system, but it is not routinely used.

Staging Systems

The Ann Arbor staging system (commonly used in adult NHL) has proved to be of limited use in pediatric NHL because of the unique clinical presentation and course of the disease in children. These special features of childhood NHL include the preponderance of extranodal presentations, the noncontiguous pattern of disease spread, and a tendency to evolve into leukemia and to involve the central nervous system (CNS). To address the uniqueness of childhood NHL, staging systems specific for pediatric NHL have been developed. The St. Jude Children's Research Hospital staging system is used most widely (Table 89.9).[175]

The distinction between lymphoma and leukemia lies in the percentage of malignant cells in a bone marrow aspirate. Patients with more than 25% blasts in bone marrow are considered to have acute leukemia, and those with between 5% and 25% marrow involvement are considered to have stage IV NHL. However, any identifiable tumor cell in the cerebrospinal fluid constitutes CNS disease and therefore stage IV disease.

Of interest, several of the clinical cooperative groups have adopted the designation of limited disease (including stages I and II) versus advanced disease (stages III and IV) for the purpose of determining appropriate treatment strategies. European investigators have developed a clinical grouping system of the B cell lymphomas (i.e., BL and DLBCL) that is based on extent of disease, modified St. Jude staging criteria, and relative risk of relapse.[207] Treatment intensity is based on the designation of group A, B, or C disease, which correlates to low-, intermediate-, or high-risk disease, respectively (Table 89.9). This strategy has also proven very effective in recent treatment trials.[208–210]

Prognostic Factors

The most important factor in determining prognosis in childhood NHL is stage, which takes into account other known prognostic variables such as tumor burden, site, and extent of involvement[211] as well as response to therapy.[210] The fact that most cases of pediatric NHL are of the diffuse, high-grade, and aggressive subtypes may have obscured the prognostic value of histology; few reports support its role as a prognostic factor.[212]

More sensitive techniques such as flow cytometry to detect lymphoma-specific immunophenotype and RT polymerase chain reaction to evaluate chromosomal translocations or immunoglobulin rearrangements have shown that bone marrow and blood involvement are much more frequent than would be predicted by morphologic examination.[213,214,215–216] Higher detected amounts of minimal disseminated disease at diagnosis are associated with worse prognosis in all the major subtypes of pediatric NHL.

With genetic analyses of mature B-cell NHL in children and adolescents, it was shown that deletions of 13q and gains of 7q in addition to c-myc translocations have a significant, negative effect on prognosis.[217,218]

In pediatric CD30-positive ALCL, there almost always is an anaplastic lymphoma kinase (ALK) rearrangement with translocation t(2;5)(p23;q35), which is associated with a favorable prognosis. This is in contrast with adult cases of ALCL, in which ALK rearrangements are less common and are associated with poor prognosis. In addition, ALK autoantibodies were detected frequently in pediatric patients. High antibody titers correlated with significantly lower amounts of circulating tumor cells and cumulative incidence of relapses, suggesting that a robust pre-existing immune response to an oncoantigen from an oncogenic chromosomal translocation inhibits lymphoma dissemination and relapse.[219]

Treatment and Results

The overall survival of children with NHL was poor before the advent of multiagent chemotherapy in the mid-1970s.[211] Even in cases in which the disease apparently was localized, cure rates as low as 20% were reported. Failure, in most cases, was caused by early systemic dissemination of disease. In modern regimens, chemotherapy is the primary therapeutic modality for all histologies and stages of childhood NHL. The dramatic improvement in the overall rate of survival of those with childhood NHL can be attributed not only to the development of highly effective, multiagent chemotherapy regimens but also to the systematic evaluation of these diseases and their treatment by pediatric cooperative group clinical trials. Cure rates of 85% to 95% in patients with limited disease and 70% to 90% in those with extensive involvement have been reported (Tables 89.10 and 89.11).

Surgery is indicated only for diagnostic purposes or in the case of an abdominal emergency, such as intussusception or acute appendicitis due to abdominal mass effect at presentation. Patients with extensive NHL may present with a number of life-threatening complications that require urgent intervention, including respiratory distress from airway obstruction, SVC syndrome, spinal cord compression, intestinal obstruction, hydronephrosis, renal insufficiency, or tumor lysis syndrome. The priority in these situations is to maximize supportive care and initiate specific chemotherapy as soon as a diagnosis has been established.

TABLE 89.10 TREATMENT OUTCOMES FOR LIMITED STAGE NON-HODGKIN LYMPHOMA

Protocol (Reference)	Stage/ Group	Number of Patients	Event-Free Survival
POG 1983–1991 (220)	I/II	138/202	5 yr = 89%, 86%, 88% for 3 treatment groups
Small non-cleaved cell (SNCC)	I/II	185	5 yr = 89%
Lymphoblastic lymphoma	I/II	50	5 yr = 63%
Large cell lymphoma (LCL)	I/II	81	5 yr = 88%
SFOP LMB 89[a] (207)	I/II	119	5 yr = 98%
NHL-BFM 90[a] (221)	I/II	164	6 yr = 98%
CCG[a]-COMP (nonlymphoblastic) (222)	I/II	104	5 yr >95%
CCG–lymphoblastic lymphoma (222)	I/II	15	5 yr = 67%
FAB/LMB 96 (Burkitt/diffuse large B-cell lymphoma (209)	A	132	4 yr = 98%

[a]Includes B-cell lymphomas with SNCC, Burkitt, and LCL subtypes.

POG, Pediatric Oncology Group; SFOP, societe francaise d'oncologie pediatrique; LMB, protocol for mature B-cell lymphomas; NHL, non-Hodgkin lymphomas; BFM, Berlin-Frankfurt-Muenster Study Group; CCG, Childhood Cancer Group; COMP, cyclophosphamide, vincristine, methotrexate, and prednisone; FAB, French-American-British Study Group.

Systemic Chemotherapy

The importance of tailoring therapy to address the inherent biologic differences of the various histologic subtypes became evident early in the evolution of NHL therapy (Tables 89.10 and 89.11). The CCG performed an important randomized clinical trial to compare the cyclophosphamide-based four-drug regimen COMP (cyclophosphamide, vincristine, methotrexate [MTX], and prednisone) and the 10-drug LSA_2L_2 regimen (cyclophosphamide, vincristine, prednisone, daunomycin, MTX, cytarabine, thioguanine, asparaginase, carmustine [BCNU], and hydroxyurea).[223,244,245] COMP was a lymphoma-targeted regimen and LSA_2L_2 was designed for acute lymphoblastic leukemia (ALL) therapy. For localized NHL, no difference was seen between the two treatment regimens, regardless of histology (Fig. 89.3A). However, outcomes of patients with stage 3 or 4 disease were significantly related to treatment arm and histology. The LSA_2L_2 regimen (ALL approach) was superior to COMP for lymphoblastic lymphoma (Fig. 89.3B; 5-year EFS 64% vs. 35%), whereas the COMP regimen was superior to LSA_2L_2 for BL (Fig. 89.3C; 5-year EFS 50% vs. 29%).

Based on these results, further refinements were performed for BL and DLBCL. The St. Jude Total B regimen incorporated sequential high-dose (HD) MTX and escalating continuous infusion of cytarabine.[190] This regimen resulted in an excellent outcome for patients with stage III disease; however, those with stage IV disease had only a 20% long-term EFS rate. The Pediatric Oncology Group (POG), POG-8617 protocol, derived from the Total B regimen, which incorporated early administration of high-dose pulse cytarabine, resulted in improved outcomes for patients with stage IV disease.[246] During this same time period, a study from the National Cancer Institute (NCI-77–04) showed an equally improved result for patients with advanced stage disease using a cyclophosphamide, doxorubicin, vincristine, and prednisone (CHOP) and HD-MTX regimen.[247] Further improvement in treatment outcome has been reported by Patte et al.[248] and Reiter et al.[249] These regimens incorporated the above mentioned agents (COMP, HD-MTX, and high-dose cytarabine) and etoposide (VP-16) and/or ifosfamide. Patte et al.[210] have reported excellent results for children with mature B-cell lymphomas using the Lymphoma Malignancy B (LMB) LMB-89 regimen, with approximately 87% of patients with stage IV disease or B-ALL experiencing long-term EFS. For patients with CNS disease, a group with a poorer prognosis, they reported a 79% long-term EFS rate. Burkitt lymphoma/leukemia is a rapidly growing tumor and is often associated

TABLE 89.11 TREATMENT OUTCOMES FOR ADVANCED STAGE NON-HODGKIN LYMPHOMA BASED ON HISTOLOGIC SUBTYPE

Protocol (Reference)	Stage/Group	Number of Patients	Event-Free Survival
Burkitt and Burkitt-Like Lymphoma			
CCG 551–LSA_2L_2	III/IV/B-ALL	44	5 yr = 29%
vs. COMP (223)	III/IV/B-ALL	93	5 yr = 50%
POG 8616–Comparison 8106	III	65	2 yr = 64%
vs. SJCRH Total B (224)	III	58	2 yr = 79%
SFOP LMB 89[a] (207)	I–II	119	5 yr = 98%
	III	278	5 yr = 91%
	IV	62	5 yr = 87%
	B-ALL	102	5 yr = 87%
	Burkitt	420	5 yr = 92%
	DLBCL	63	5 yr = 89%
FAB/LMB 96 (208,210)	B	762	4 yr = 90%
	C (full intensity)	96	4 yr = 90%
	C (reduced intensity)	94	4 yr = 80%
NHL-BFM 90[a] (221)	I, II,	164	6 yr = 98%
	III	169	6 yr = 88%
	IV	24	6 yr = 73%
	B-ALL	56	6 yr = 74%
NHL-BFM 95[a] (225)	All	505	3 yr = 89%
	I/II	172	3 yr = 98%
	III	221	3 yr = 87%
	IV	33	3 yr = 81%
	B-ALL	79	3 yr = 77%
Burkitt	All	283	3 yr = 93%
CCG 5911–Orange/French (226)	III/IV/B-ALL	46	4 yr = 80%
vs. 552 (CHOP-AraC/VP/MTX)	III/IV/B-ALL	52	4 yr = 58%
vs. 503 (COMP, D-COMP)	III/IV/B-ALL	241	4 yr = 60%
Lymphoblastic Lymphoma			
CCG 551-LSA_2L_2	III/IV	124	5 yr = 64%
vs. COMP (223)	III/IV	40	5 yr = 35%
MSKCC–LSA_2L_2 (modified)	III	41	5 yr = 85%
(227)	IV/ALL	19/27	5 yr = 73%/70%
BFM 86 (228)	III/IV	73	7 yr = 82%
BFM 90 (229)	III/IV/T-ALL	101	5 yr = 90%
BFM 95[b] (230)	III/IV	156	5 yr = 82%
DFCI 81, 85, 87, 91-01 (231)	III/IV	15	5 yr = 87%
	T-ALL	125	5 yr = 75%
POG 8704–with ASP intensi-	III/IV	84	4 yr (CCR) = 78%
fication (232)	T-ALL	160	4 yr (CCR) = 68%
POG 9404 (233) –with	III/IV	71	5 yr = 82%
HD-MTX		66	5 yr = 88%
–without HD-MTX			
–with HD-MTX	T-ALL	148	5 yr = 80%
–without HD-MTX		151	5 yr = 68%
CCG 5941 (234)	III/IV	85	5 yr = 78%
Large Cell Lymphoma			
CCG 551 - LSA_2L_2	III/IV	18	5 yr = 43%
vs. COMP (223)	III/IV	42	5 yr = 52%
MSKCC–LSA_2L_2, LSA_4 (227)	III/IV	19	5 yr = 56% (OS 84%)
SJCRH 1975–1990 (198)	I/II	4	5 yr = 75%
	III/IV	14	5 yr = 57%
BFM 83, 86, 90 (235)	I/II	4/16	5 yr = 75%/68%
	III/IV	35/7	5 yr = 86%/86%
CCG 503–COMP vs. D-COMP (236)	I–III	106	10 yr = 48%
	IV	14	10 yr = 39%
SFOP HM-89, HM-91 (237)	I/II	23	3 yr = 94%
	III/IV	59	3 yr = 55%
CCG 5911 Orange (CCG	III/IV	12	5 yr = 92%
hybrid) (238)	III/IV	27[c]	5 yr = 70%
CCG 5911 (Orange/French) (194)	Disseminated	18	5 yr = 65%
vs. pre-5911 (1983–1990)	Disseminated	173	5 yr = 49%
POG 8615–APO vs.	III	93	8 yr = 68%
ACOP+[a] (239)	IV	27	8 yr = 59%
POG 9315–APO vs. IDM/HiDAC (240)	III/IV	85/90	4 yr = 67% (all)
Anaplastic LCL	III/IV	86	4 yr = 72%
Diffuse B-cell LCL	III/IV	71	4 yr = 64%
NHL-BFM 90	All	56	3 events
Diffuse B-cell LCL (221)			
Anaplastic LCL (241)	All	89	5 yr = 76%
NHL-BFM 95	All	81	3 yr = 93%
Diffuse B-cell LCL (225)			
Primary mediastinal B cell LCL	III	15	3 yr = 53%
EICNHL (anaplastic LCL) (242)			
HD-MTX (1g) + IT vs.	All	175	2 yr = 74%
HD-MTX (3g)	All	177	2 yr = 75%
ALCL99 (anaplastic LCL) (243)			
NHL-BFM90 + vinblastine vs.	All	110	2 yr = 73%
NHL-BFM90	All	107	2 yr = 70%

ALL, acute lymphoblastic leukemia; LCL, large cell lymphoma; DLBCL, diffuse large B-cell lymphoma; CCR, complete clinical remission; OS, overall survival.

[a]Includes patients with B-cell large cell non-Hodgkin lymphoma.

[b]Excludes patients with central nervous system positive disease and those who had insufficient response on day 33.

[c]Median observation time 4.3 years.

CCG, Childhood Cancer Group; LSA_2L_2, cyclophosphamide, vincristine, prenisone, daunomycin, methotrexate, cytarabine, thioguanine, asparaginase, carmustine, and hydroxyurea; POG, Pediatric Oncology Group; SFOP, societe francaise d'oncologie pediatrique; LMB, protocol for mature B-cell lymphomas; FAB, French-American-British Study Group; NHL, non-Hodgkin lymphomas; BFM, Berlin-Frankfurt-Muenster Study Group; CHOP, cyclophosphamide, doxorubicin, vincristine, prednisone; COMP, cyclophosphamide, vincristine, methotrexate, and prednisone; MSKCC, Memorial Sloan Kettering Cancer Center; DFCI, Dana Farber Cancer Institute; HD-MTX, high dose methotrexate.

with tumor lysis syndrome (including hyperuricemia). Careful attention to the control of metabolic abnormalities during induction greatly reduced early mortality associated with initial treatment. The international LMB-96 study (CCG, Societe Francaise d'Oncologie Pediatrique [SFOP], and United Kingdom Children's Cancer Study Group [UKCCG]) randomized patients with group B and C disease to receive standard LMB doses versus stepwise-reduced doses. Efficacy data show that the 4-year EFS of group B patients was >90% in all arms of the study.[210] Thus, in Group B patients, nonescalation of cyclophosphamide in the second course of COPADM3 (cyclophosphamide, Oncovin [vincristine], prednisone, Adriamycin [doxorubicin], HD-MTX 3 g/m^2) and deletion of the maintenance sequence did not compromise the excellent outcome. In contrast, dose reduction for group C patients was associated with a poorer outcome: 4-year EFS was 90% for the full-dose arm versus only 80% for the dose-reduced arm.[208] Finally, group C patients with CNS involvement had an inferior outcome, with 3-year EFS rates of 71% (vs. 87% for group C patients without CNS involvement). Patients with mediastinal large B-cell lymphoma were also associated with a poorer treatment outcome. In the LMB-96 study, the 4-year EFS for these patients was 72%, a finding consistent with those of other studies. It appears, therefore, that these patients require either novel or more intensive therapy.[210]

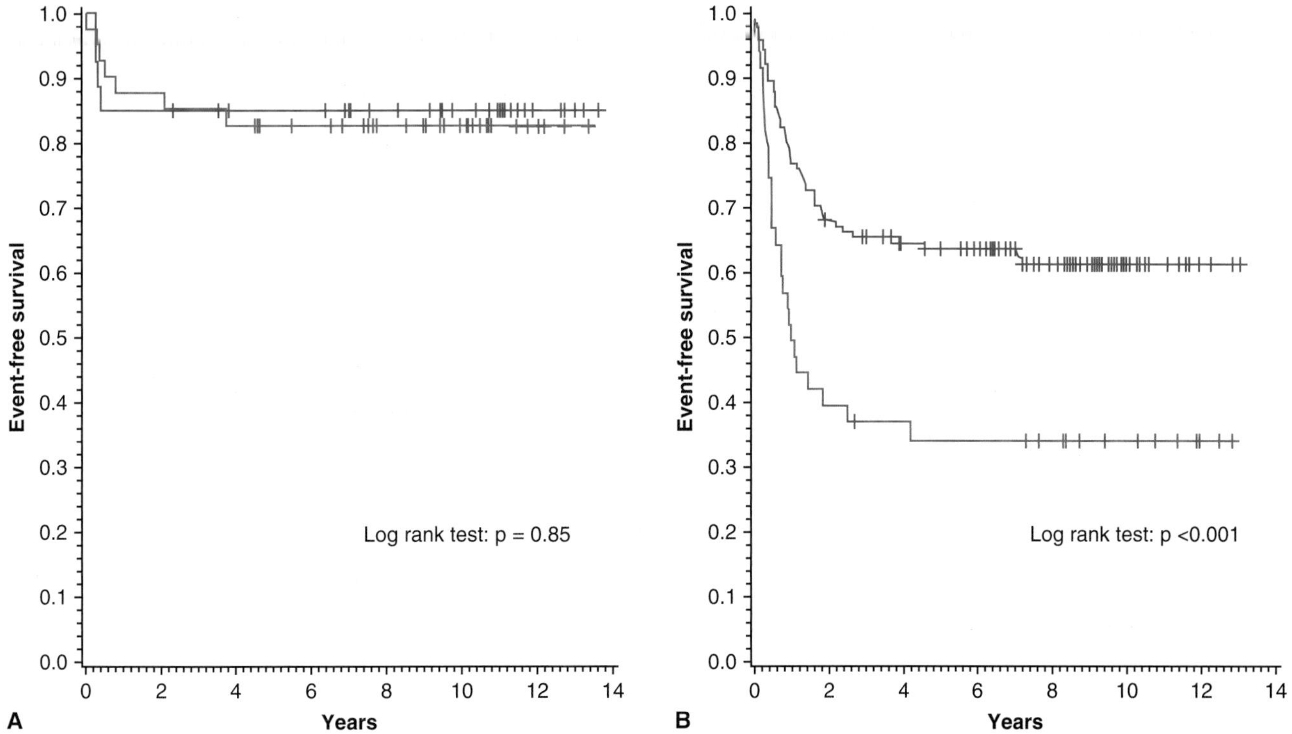

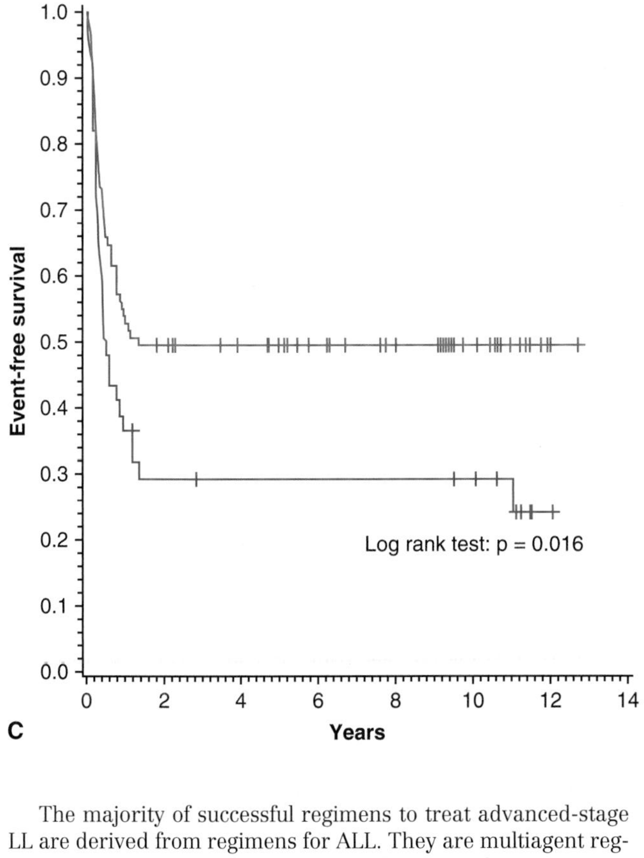

FIGURE 89.3. **A:** Event-free survival of 68 non-Hodgkin lymphoma patients with localized disease by treatment group. *Solid line,* COMP (41 patients); *dotted line,* LSA_2L_2 (27 patients). **B:** Event-free survival of patients with disseminated lymphoblastic lymphoma by treatment group. *Solid line,* COMP (40 patients); *dotted line,* LSA_2L_2 (124 patients). **C:** Event-free survival of patients with disseminated undifferentiated lymphoma by treatment group. *Solid line,* COMP (93 patients); *dotted line,* LSA_2L_2 (44 patients). COMP, cyclophosphamide, vincristine, methotrexate, and prednisone; LSA, cyclophosphamide, vincristine, prednisone, daunomycin, methotrexate, cytarabine, thioguanine, asparaginase, carmustine [BCNU], and hydroxyurea. (From Anderson JR, Jenkin RDT, Wilson JF, et al. Long-term follow-up of patients treated with COMP or LSA_2L_2 therapy for childhood non-Hodgkin's lymphoma: a report of CCG-551 from the Children's Cancer Group. *J Clin Oncol* 1993;11:1024–1032; reprinted with permission. © 1993, American Society of Clinical Oncology.)

The majority of successful regimens to treat advanced-stage LL are derived from regimens for ALL. They are multiagent regimens comprising induction, consolidation, and maintenance phases delivered over 18 to 30 months. The early St. Jude study, Total X-High Risk, demonstrated the survival efficacy of the addition of cytarabine and teniposide to an otherwise standard antimetabolite-based ALL regimen.[250] Epipodophyllotoxins have also been used in other protocols[232,234] but have been omitted from recent regimens because of the risk of secondary leukemia. Controversy still exists about the role of HD-MTX in the management of advanced-stage LL. Excellent results were achieved with the LMT81 regimen of the SFOP when multiple courses of HD-MTX (3 g/m^2 per course) were added to an LSA_2L_2 backbone.[251] The BFM (Berlin-Frankfurt-Munster) -90 regimen included 4 courses of HD-MTX (5 g/m^2 per dose) as a consolidation phase and produced one of the best outcomes to date (5-year EFS for stage III 90% and stage IV 95%).[229] The POG-9404 regimen, which examined the role of HD-MTX in a backbone of intensive doxorubicin and weekly l-asparaginase, was terminated early because of an inferior outcome for children with T-ALL in the arm without HD-MTX.[233] Although the POG study was not powered to examine the effect of HD-MTX in advanced-stage precursor T-LL, the 5-year EFS rate of patients not receiving HD-MTX (87.8%) was higher than that of those receiving it (81.7%) ($P = .38$). Asparaginase is thought to be an important component of effective LL therapy. The POG-8704 study demonstrated a survival advantage for patients who received an additional 20 weekly doses of l-asparaginase after consolidation therapy.[232] Anthracyclines are also thought to be important in the treatment of precursor T-cell ALL and LL[231]; and the use of anthracyclines in reinduction (delayed intensification) phases, a strategy used in the BFM regimens, COG-A5971, and St. Jude Total studies, may also improve outcome.[229,252]

Advanced systemic ALCL has been treated with short-pulse chemotherapy, proven effective in B-cell lymphomas, or with modifications of high-risk ALL protocols.[240,241,242] In the BFM B-NHL studies, children with stage II unresected and stage III ALCL received 6 courses of chemotherapy, and patients with stage IV or multifocal bone disease received 6 intensified courses, which included moderate or HD-MTX, dexamethasone, ifosfamide, cyclophosphamide, VP-16, cytarabine, doxorubicin, and intrathecal chemotherapy. The EFS rate was about 75% for patients with stages II, III, and IV disease.[241] A follow-up study using this backbone of chemotherapy demonstrated that intrathecal chemotherapy can be eliminated if HD-MTX is given.[242] However, adding vinblastine during induction and as maintenance for a total treatment duration of 1 year in the ALCL-99 study significantly delayed the occurrence of relapses but did not reduce the risk of failure.[243] Importantly, the failure rate for incompletely resected stage I disease was similar to that for stage II and stage III or IV disease in this study.[253] The POG study used the APO (doxorubicin, prednisone, vincristine) regimen for children with large cell lymphoma, which included systemic ALCL.[240] Randomized study with or without the addition of consolidation cycles of intermediate-dose MTX and HD-cytarabine did not show a benefit of such regimens, and the EFS rate was approximately 70% for patients with stages III and IV ALCL.

Role of Radiation Therapy

With the development of effective multiagent chemotherapy regimens, radiation therapy for local control of primary disease (exclusive of bone) or for CNS prophylaxis has been virtually eliminated. Radiation is reserved for emergency treatment of mediastinal disease or symptomatic neurologic compromise such as spinal cord compression, palliation of pain, consolidation before bone marrow transplantation in patients with recurrent disease, and treatment of overt symptomatic CNS lymphoma at diagnosis or relapse.

Primary Site and Involved-Field Irradiation (Exclusive of Primary Bone Lesions)

To reduce the potential acute and late effects associated with radiation therapy, protocols have reduced treatment-field size and radiation dose to approximately 20 Gy.[222,254] Results of these limited trials showed that lower doses and smaller treatment fields can induce local control and survival rates similar to those achieved with extended fields in early-stage NHL. In a randomized trial, POG observed no difference in results between induction therapy with CHOP alone and CHOP plus 27 Gy IFRT.[255] Most investigators have abandoned the use of IFRT in localized early-stage pediatric NHL.

The role of RT in advanced-stage disease is limited. In the one published randomized trial that studied the use of chemotherapy with or without irradiation, the 2-year EFS rate in both treatment arms was only 38%, a value so low that the potential contribution of RT may have been masked by ineffective systemic control.[175] Nonetheless, because of concern for the potential of RT to compromise the delivery of chemotherapy and cause late effects in the pediatric population, IFRT has been eliminated from the design of advanced-stage pediatric NHL trials. Recent results of chemotherapy-alone trials tend to support this practice.[256]

RT can be considered for treatment of localized residual disease after induction chemotherapy or at the time of relapse. The RT dose prescribed is dependent on histologic subtype and involved site of disease, but frequently a dose range of 30 to 40 Gy is used (e.g., 30 Gy is often used for small-cell lymphocyte/LL, but higher doses may be used for large-cell subtypes). The data for the dose–response relation by histology in adult NHL are reviewed in detail in Chapter 78. For palliation, RT at total doses as low as 4 Gy in 2-Gy fractions can result in rapid relief from symptoms associated with such conditions as SVC syndrome, acute respiratory distress, spinal cord compression, and orbital proptosis.[257] Local radiotherapy delivered at a dose range of 20 to 30 Gy may be more appropriate for palliation of cranial nerve deficits.[258]

Primary Non-Hodgkin Lymphoma of Bone

Primary NHL of bone (PBL) is a heterogeneous type of NHL that comprises approximately 2% of NHL in children and adolescents. It has a high rate of systemic spread, even in patients with clinically apparent early-stage presentation. Localized RT to the involved bone was included as part of standard management in early chemotherapy trials. Total doses used for PBL (45 to 55 Gy) have historically been higher than those used for nodal disease. Studies attempting to reduce the risk of late morbidity by eliminating irradiation have been successful because of the increased incidence of second primary bone tumors observed after combined-modality therapy and the potential for growth delay or arrest in young children.[259]

Prophylaxis and Overt Central Nervous System Disease

CNS involvement was diagnosed in 141 of 2,381 (5.9%) patients and was associated with an advanced stage of NHL in BFM studies.[260] The percentage of patients with CNS involvement was as follows: Burkitt lymphoma/leukemia (8.8%), precursor B–lymphoblastic lymphoma (5.4%), anaplastic large-cell lymphoma (3.3%), T-cell–lymphoblastic lymphoma (3.2%), diffuse large B-cell lymphoma (2.6%), and primary mediastinal large B-cell lymphoma (0%).

In the only published randomized trial of CNS presymptomatic therapy in pediatric NHL, 1 of 18 (6%) children randomly assigned to cranial irradiation and intrathecal MTX experienced an isolated CNS relapse, whereas 4 of 16 (25%) of those who did not receive any specific form of CNS prophylactic therapy experienced CNS relapse.[175]

Concern for increased neurotoxicity with the use of cranial irradiation in children prompted investigators to test the efficacy of intrathecal chemotherapy alone for CNS prophylaxis. Prophylactic cranial irradiation was not used in BFM-95 for patients with LL, but the outcome of these patients was not inferior to that of patients on BFM-90 or BFM-86 therapies.[230] St. Jude NHL-13 included intensive intrathecal (IT) chemotherapy for CNS therapy and excluded prophylactic cranial radiation.[261]

Indications for cranial irradiation are currently limited to patients with overt symptomatic CNS lymphoma at diagnosis, particularly when unresponsive to initiation of chemotherapy or dexamethasone or when there is CNS relapse.[262] Due to the relative efficacy of intrathecal MTX and cranial irradiation compared with that of chemotherapy alone, CNS-directed RT is often integrated at the time of CNS relapse. Importantly, St. Jude TOTXV[252] and the Dutch Childhood Oncology Group ALL-9[263] studies showed that cranial irradiation can be safely eliminated from ALL treatment if effective risk-directed chemotherapy and IT therapy are given. The 5-year cumulative risk of isolated CNS relapse in patients in these studies was 2.7% and 2.6%, respectively, which is within the range (1.5% to 4.5%) of risk of CNS relapse observed in clinical ALL trials using prophylactic cranial irradiation. Careful follow-up of patients after CNS therapy to assess disease status and treatment-related complications is crucial, regardless of whether cranial irradiation is used. Current recommendations for the screening of late effects of therapy after childhood cancer can be found in the long-term follow-up guidelines developed by the COG, which are constantly updated.

Testicular Lymphoma

Testicular involvement at diagnosis is uncommon (about 5% of children with disseminated BL and Burkitt-like NHL).[264] Testicular disease does not seem to confer a poor prognosis, and it is curable with intensive combination chemotherapy alone. Local treatment (i.e., surgery or radiation) is avoidable; therefore, gonadal function can be preserved.

Posttransplant Lymphoproliferative Disorder

PTLD encompasses a spectrum of abnormal B-cell lymphoid proliferation that occurs following transplant (mostly within 2 years) in the setting of compromised T-cell immunity, antirejection immunosuppressive therapy and is almost always associated with EBV infection.[184,265]

As knowledge of the risk factors for PTLD increases, attention has turned to prevention of disease. Limiting the amount of immunosuppression by adjusting the type, combination, and doses of drugs after transplant is important. Although their efficacy is not proven, antiviral agents such as acyclovir and ganciclovir, along with high doses of intravenous immunoglobulin, are commonly used as prophylaxis of PTLD.[184,266] EBV-associated PTLD is usually preceded by an increase in the number of latently infected B cells. It is generally accepted practice to perform serial peripheral quantitative blood EBV-PCR monitoring, with a planned decrease or change in immunosuppressive drugs in the event of rising EBV load.[184] Historically, withdrawal of immune suppression has been the mainstay of therapy, but the reported success varies greatly, from 20% to 80%. Patients with localized or polymorphic disease are more likely to respond than those with disseminated or monomorphic PTLD.[185] However, even if patients are responsive to reduction of immunosuppression, there is an increased risk of rejection, which may threaten the viability of the allograft.[267] The use of rituximab, a humanized anti-CD20 monoclonal antibody, was associated with better survival in those with PTLD.[268] However, the significant effect of rituximab causing B-cell lymphocytopenia and hypogammaglobulinemia must be monitored. Chemotherapy is considered for patients for whom reduction of immunosuppression and rituximab have failed.[184,185] To avoid toxicity, regimens with lower doses of chemotherapy (e.g., cyclophosphamide, prednisone) than those used to treat B-cell NHL in children have been used. Other strategies include cytokine therapy (e.g., alfa-interferon) and cellular immunotherapy (e.g., EBV-specific T cells).

Future Investigations

In children with localized disease (stages I and II), the excellent survival rates achieved with reduced therapy support the practice of minimizing treatment to reduce the incidence and severity of adverse late effects. For the small number of children who do suffer a relapse, secondary treatment with salvage chemotherapy regimens is highly successful. In children with advanced stage NHL (stages III and IV), future trials are aimed at developing more effective therapeutic regimens that include new types of active chemical agents, monoclonal antibodies, and molecularly targeting agents. Nelarabine, a pro-drug of the deoxyguanosine analog ara-G, has been evaluated in pediatric T-cell malignancies.[269] The use of monoclonal antibodies directed to B-cell antigens, particularly CD20, in addition to CHOP therapy, improves the initial response rates and durations of remission for adults with B-cell lymphoma.[270] Similar approaches are being explored in the pediatric B-cell lymphomas. Similarly, antibodies to the CD30 antigen on ALCL cells, as well as small-molecule inhibitors, such as ALK inhibitors, are in early-phase trials.[271] New diagnostic strategies such as PET scan with FDG or scans with newer radioisotopes may contribute to improved outcomes through more accurate staging and response monitoring, thus allowing early intervention when primary treatments fail. Detection of minimal disseminated or minimal residual disease, which has proven to be an effective end point of therapeutic efficacy in children with leukemia, is being evaluated in childhood NHL. The challenges lie in using new technologies to investigate the cytogenetic and molecular subtypes of pediatric NHL, understand the key events in lymphomagenesis, identify critical genes that can be used for targeted therapy, develop techniques to assess minimal disseminated or residual disease, and develop therapeutic strategies that are more effective but less toxic.

SELECTED REFERENCES

A full list of references for this chapter is available online.

1. Donaldson SS, Hancock SL, Hoppe RT. The Janeway lecture. Hodgkin's disease—finding the balance between cure and late effects. *Cancer J Sci Am* 1999;5(6):325–333.
3. Baez F, Ocampo E, Conter V, et al. Treatment of childhood Hodgkin's disease with COPP or COPP-ABV (hybrid) without radiotherapy in Nicaragua. *Ann Oncol* 1997;8(3):247–250.
4. Barrett A, Crennan E, Barnes J, et al. Treatment of clinical stage I Hodgkin's disease by local radiation therapy alone. A United Kingdom Childrens Cancer Study Group study. *Cancer* 1990;66(4):670–674.
5. Bayle-Weisgerber C, Lemercier N, Teillet F, et al. Hodgkin's disease in children. Results of therapy in a mixed group of 178 clinical and pathologically staged patients over 13 years. *Cancer* 1984;54(2):215–222.
6. Behrendt H, Brinkhuis M, Van Leeuwen EF. Treatment of childhood Hodgkin's disease with ABVD without radiotherapy. *Med Pediatr Oncol* 1996;26(4):244–248.
10. Hudson MM, Poquette CA, Lee J, et al. Increased mortality after successful treatment for Hodgkin's disease. *J Clin Oncol* 1998;16(11):3592–3600.
11. Hunger SP, Link MP, Donaldson SS. ABVD/MOPP and low-dose involved-field radiotherapy in pediatric Hodgkin's disease: the Stanford experience. *J Clin Oncol* 1994;12(10):2160–2166.
13. Landman-Parker J, Pacquement H, Leblanc T, et al. Localized childhood Hodgkin's disease: response-adapted chemotherapy with etoposide, bleomycin, vinblastine, and prednisone before low-dose radiation therapy-results of the French Society of Pediatric Oncology Study MDH90. *J Clin Oncol* 2000;18(7):1500–1507.
15. Oberlin O, Boilletot A, Leverger G. Clinical staging, primary chemotherapy and involved field radiotherapy in childhood Hodgkin's disease. *Eur Paediatr Haematol Oncol* 1985;2:65.
17. Ruhl U, Albrecht M, Dieckmann K, et al. Response-adapted radiotherapy in the treatment of pediatric Hodgkin's disease: an interim report at 5 years of the German GPOH-HD 95 trial. *Int J Radiat Oncol Biol Phys* 2001;51(5):1209–1218.
19. Schellong G. The balance between cure and late effects in childhood Hodgkin's lymphoma: the experience of the German-Austrian Study-Group since 1978. German-Austrian Pediatric Hodgkin's Disease Study Group. *Ann Oncol* 1996;7(Suppl 4):67–72.
20. Schellong G, Dorffel W, Claviez A, et al. Salvage therapy of progressive and recurrent Hodgkin's disease: results from a multicenter study of the pediatric DAL/GPOH-HD study group. *J Clin Oncol* 2005;23(25):6181–6189.
25. Vecchi V, Pileri S, Burnelli R, et al. Treatment of pediatric Hodgkin disease tailored to stage, mediastinal mass, and age. An Italian (AIEOP) multicenter study on 215 patients. *Cancer* 1993;72(6):2049–2057.
26. Weiner MA, Leventhal BG, Marcus R, et al. Intensive chemotherapy and low-dose radiotherapy for the treatment of advanced-stage Hodgkin's disease in pediatric patients: a Pediatric Oncology Group study. *J Clin Oncol* 1991;9(9):1591–1598.
27. Weiner MA, Leventhal B, Brecher ML, et al. Randomized study of intensive MOPP-ABVD with or without low-dose total-nodal radiation therapy in the treatment of stages IIB, IIIA2, IIIB, and IV Hodgkin's disease in pediatric patients: a Pediatric Oncology Group study. *J Clin Oncol* 1997;15(8):2769–2779.
33. Kuppers R, Rajewsky K. The origin of Hodgkin and Reed/Sternberg cells in Hodgkin's disease. *Annu Rev Immunol* 1998;16:471–493.
50. Smith RS, Chen Q, Hudson MM, et al. Prognostic factors for children with Hodgkin's disease treated with combined-modality therapy. *J Clin Oncol* 2003;21(10):2026–2033.
59. Bodis S, Kraus MD, Pinkus G, et al. Clinical presentation and outcome in lymphocyte-predominant Hodgkin's disease. *J Clin Oncol* 1997;15(9):3060–3066.
65. Donaldson SS, Link MP, Weinstein HJ, et al. Final results of a prospective clinical trial with VAMP and low-dose involved-field radiation for children with low-risk Hodgkin's disease. *J Clin Oncol* 2007;25(3):332–337.
66. Hutchinson RJ, Fryer CJ, Davis PC, et al. MOPP or radiation in addition to ABVD in the treatment of pathologically staged advanced Hodgkin's disease in children: results of the Children's Cancer Group phase III trial. *J Clin Oncol* 1998;16(3):897–906.
67. Nachman JB, Sposto R, Herzog P, et al. Randomized comparison of low-dose involved-field radiotherapy and no radiotherapy for children with Hodgkin's disease who achieve a complete response to chemotherapy. *J Clin Oncol* 2002;20(18):3765–3771.
68. Tebbi CK, Mendenhall N, London WB, et al. Treatment of stage I, IIA, IIIA(1) pediatric Hodgkin disease with doxorubicin, bleomycin, vincristine and etoposide (DBVE) and radiation: a Pediatric Oncology Group (POG) study. *Pediatr Blood Cancer* 2006;46(2):198–202.
69. Schwartz CL, Constine LS, Villaluna D, et al. A risk-adapted, response-based approach using ABVE-PC for children and adolescents with intermediate- and high-risk Hodgkin lymphoma: the results of P9425. *Blood* 2009;114(10):2051–2059.
70. Kelly KM, Sposto R, Hutchinson R, et al. BEACOPP chemotherapy is a highly effective regimen in children and adolescents with high-risk Hodgkin lymphoma: a report from the Children's Oncology Group. *Blood* 2011;117(9):2596–2603.

71. Oberlin O, Leverger G, Pacquement H, et al. Low-dose radiation therapy and reduced chemotherapy in childhood Hodgkin's disease: the experience of the French Society of Pediatric Oncology. *J Clin Oncol* 1992;10(10):1602–1608.
74. Dorffel W, Luders H, Ruhl U, et al. Preliminary results of the multicenter trial GPOH-HD 95 for the treatment of Hodgkin's disease in children and adolescents: analysis and outlook. *Klin Padiatr* 2003;215(3):139–145.
75. Ruhl U, Albrecht M. The German multinational GPOH-HD 95 trial: treatment results and analysis of failures in pediatric Hodgkin's disease using combination chemotherapy with and without radiation. *Int J Radiat Oncol Biol Phys* 2004; 60(1):S31.
76. Mauz-Korholz C, Hasenclever D, Dorffel W, et al. Procarbazine-free OEPA-COPDAC chemotherapy in boys and standard OPPA-COPP in girls have comparable effectiveness in pediatric Hodgkin's lymphoma: the GPOH-HD-2002 study. *J Clin Oncol* 2010;28(23):3680–3686.
77. Kung FH, Schwartz CL, Ferree CR, et al. POG 8625: a randomized trial comparing chemotherapy with chemoradiotherapy for children and adolescents with stages I, IIA, IIIA1 Hodgkin disease: a report from the Children's Oncology Group. *J Pediatr Hematol Oncol* 2006;28(6):362–368.
89. Hodgson DC, Hudson MM, Constine LS. Pediatric Hodgkin lymphoma: maximizing efficacy and minimizing toxicity. *Semin Radiat Oncol* 2007;17(3):230–242.
97. Schellong G, Potter R, Bramswig J, et al. High cure rates and reduced long-term toxicity in pediatric Hodgkin's disease: the German-Austrian multicenter trial DAL-HD-90. The German-Austrian Pediatric Hodgkin's Disease Study Group. *J Clin Oncol* 1999;17(12):3736–3744.
98. Diehl V, Franklin J, Hasenclever D, et al. BEACOPP, a new dose-escalated and accelerated regimen, is at least as effective as COPP/ABVD in patients with advanced-stage Hodgkin's lymphoma: interim report from a trial of the German Hodgkin's Lymphoma Study Group. *J Clin Oncol* 1998;16(12):3810–3821.
100. Horning SJ, Hoppe RT, Breslin S, et al. Stanford V and radiotherapy for locally extensive and advanced Hodgkin's disease: mature results of a prospective clinical trial. *J Clin Oncol* 2002;20(3):630–637.
103. Schellong G, Dorffel W, Claviez A, et al. Salvage therapy of progressive and recurrent Hodgkin's disease: results from a multicenter study of the pediatric DAL/GPOH-HD study group. *J Clin Oncol* 2005;23(25):6181–6189.
104. Claviez A, Sureda A, Schmitz N. Haematopoietic SCT for children and adolescents with relapsed and refractory Hodgkin's lymphoma. *Bone Marrow Transplant* 2008;42(Suppl 2):S16–S24.
108. Claviez A, Canals C, Dierickx D, et al. Allogeneic hematopoietic stem cell transplantation in children and adolescents with recurrent and refractory Hodgkin's lymphoma: an analysis of the European Group for Blood and Marrow Transplantation. *Blood* 2009;114(10):2060–2067.
110. Cella L, Liuzzi R, Magliulo M, et al. Radiotherapy of large target volumes in Hodgkin's lymphoma: normal tissue sparing capability of forward IMRT versus conventional techniques. *Radiat Oncol* 2010;5:33.
116. Girinsky T, Van Der MR, Specht L, et al. Involved-node radiotherapy (INRT) in patients with early Hodgkin lymphoma: concepts and guidelines. *Radiother Oncol* 2006;79(3):270–277.
119. Girinsky T, Specht L, Ghalibafian M, et al. The conundrum of Hodgkin lymphoma nodes: to be or not to be included in the involved node radiation fields. The EORTC-GELA lymphoma group guidelines. *Radiother Oncol* 2008;88(2):202–210.
127. Donaldson SS. Effects of irradiation on skeletal growth and development. In: Green DM, D'Angio GJ, eds. *Late effects of treatment for childhood cancer.* New York: Wiley-Liss, 1992.
130. King V, Constine LS, Clark D, et al. Symptomatic coronary artery disease after mantle irradiation for Hodgkin's disease. *Int J Radiat Oncol Biol Phys* 1996; 36(4):881–889.
136. Sklar CA, Mertens AC, Mitby P, et al. Premature menopause in survivors of childhood cancer: a report from the childhood cancer survivor study. *J Natl Cancer Inst* 2006;98(13):890–896.
147. Bhatia S, Yasui Y, Robison LL, et al. High risk of subsequent neoplasms continues with extended follow-up of childhood Hodgkin's disease: report from the Late Effects Study Group. *J Clin Oncol* 2003;21(23):4386–4394.
164. Younes A, Bartlett NL, Leonard JP, et al. Brentuximab vedotin (SGN-35) for relapsed CD30-positive lymphomas. *N Engl J Med* 2010;363(19):1812–1821.
174. Gross T, Perkins S. Malignant non-Hodgkin lymphomas in children. In: Pizzo PA, Poplack DG, eds. *Principles and practice of pediatric oncology,* 6th ed. Philadelphia: Lippincott Williams & Wilkins, 2011:663–682.
175. Murphy SB. Classification, staging and end results of treatment of childhood non-Hodgkin's lymphomas: dissimilarities from lymphomas in adults. *Semin Oncol* 1980;7(3):332–339.
181. Burkitt D. Determining the climatic limitations of a children's cancer common in Africa. *Br Med J* 1962;2(5311):1019–1023.
184. Gross TG, Savoldo B, Punnett A. Posttransplant lymphoproliferative diseases. *Pediatr Clin North Am* 2010;57(2):481–503.
186. Jaffe ES. The role of immunophenotypic markers in the classification of non-Hodgkin's lymphomas. *Semin Oncol* 1990;17(1):11–19.
191. Magrath IT. African Burkitt's lymphoma. History, biology, clinical features, and treatment. *Am J Pediatr Hematol Oncol* 1991;13(2):222–246.
196. Seidemann K, Tiemann M, Lauterbach I, et al. Primary mediastinal large B-cell lymphoma with sclerosis in pediatric and adolescent patients: treatment and results from three therapeutic studies of the Berlin-Frankfurt-Munster Group. *J Clin Oncol* 2003;21(9):1782–1789.
208. Cairo MS, Gerrard M, Sposto R, et al. Results of a randomized international study of high-risk central nervous system B non-Hodgkin lymphoma and B acute lymphoblastic leukemia in children and adolescents. *Blood* 2007;109(7):2736–2743.
209. Gerrard M, Cairo MS, Weston C, et al. Excellent survival following two courses of COPAD chemotherapy in children and adolescents with resected localized B-cell non-Hodgkin's lymphoma: results of the FAB/LMB 96 international study. *Br J Haematol* 2008;141(6):840–847.
210. Patte C, Auperin A, Gerrard M, et al. Results of the randomized international FAB/LMB96 trial for intermediate risk B-cell non-Hodgkin lymphoma in children and adolescents: it is possible to reduce treatment for the early responding patients. *Blood* 2007;109(7):2773–2780.
213. Coustan-Smith E, Sandlund JT, Perkins SL, et al. Minimal disseminated disease in childhood T-cell lymphoblastic lymphoma: a report from the Children's Oncology Group. *J Clin Oncol* 2009;27(21):3533–3539.
215. Mussolin L, Pillon M, d'Amore ES, et al. Minimal disseminated disease in high-risk Burkitt's lymphoma identifies patients with different prognosis. *J Clin Oncol* 2011;29(13):1779–1784.
216. Shiramizu B, Goldman S, Kusao I, et al. Minimal disease assessment in the treatment of children and adolescents with intermediate-risk (stage III/IV) B-cell non-Hodgkin lymphoma: a Children's Oncology Group report. *Br J Haematol* 2011; 153(6):758–763.
218. Poirel HA, Cairo MS, Heerema NA, et al. Specific cytogenetic abnormalities are associated with a significantly inferior outcome in children and adolescents with mature B-cell non-Hodgkin's lymphoma: results of the FAB/LMB 96 international study. *Leukemia* 2009;23(2):323–331.
220. Link MP, Shuster JJ, Donaldson SS, et al. Treatment of children and young adults with early-stage non-Hodgkin's lymphoma. *N Engl J Med* 1997;337(18):1259–1266.
221. Reiter A, Schrappe M, Tiemann M, et al. Improved treatment results in childhood B-cell neoplasms with tailored intensification of therapy: a report of the Berlin-Frankfurt-Munster Group trial NHL-BFM 90. *Blood* 1999;94(10):3294–3306.
225. Woessmann W, Seidemann K, Mann G, et al. The impact of the methotrexate administration schedule and dose in the treatment of children and adolescents with B-cell neoplasms: a report of the BFM Group study NHL-BFM95. *Blood* 2005; 105(3):948–958.
227. Mora J, Filippa DA, Qin J, Wollner N. Lymphoblastic lymphoma of childhood and the LSA2-L2 protocol: the 30-year experience at Memorial Sloan-Kettering Cancer Center. *Cancer* 2003;98(6):1283–1291.
228. Reiter A, Schrappe M, Parwaresch R, et al. Non-Hodgkin's lymphomas of childhood and adolescence: results of a treatment stratified for biologic subtypes and stage—a report of the Berlin-Frankfurt-Munster Group. *J Clin Oncol* 1995; 13(2):359–372.
229. Reiter A, Schrappe M, Ludwig WD, et al. Intensive ALL-type therapy without local radiotherapy provides a 90% event-free survival for children with T-cell lymphoblastic lymphoma: a BFM group report. *Blood* 2000;95(2):416–421.
230. Burkhardt B, Woessmann W, Zimmermann M, et al. Impact of cranial radiotherapy on central nervous system prophylaxis in children and adolescents with central nervous system-negative stage III or IV lymphoblastic lymphoma. *J Clin Oncol* 2006;24(3):491–499.
232. Amylon MD, Shuster J, Pullen J, et al. Intensive high-dose asparaginase consolidation improves survival for pediatric patients with T cell acute lymphoblastic leukemia and advanced stage lymphoblastic lymphoma: a Pediatric Oncology Group study. *Leukemia* 1999;13(3):335–342.
233. Asselin BL, Devidas M, Wang C, et al. Effectiveness of high-dose methotrexate in T-cell lymphoblastic leukemia and advanced-stage lymphoblastic lymphoma: a randomized study by the Children's Oncology Group (POG 9404). *Blood* 2011; 118(4):874–883.
234. Abromowitch M, Sposto R, Perkins S, et al. Shortened intensified multi-agent chemotherapy and non-cross resistant maintenance therapy for advanced lymphoblastic lymphoma in children and adolescents: report from the Children's Oncology Group. *Br J Haematol* 2008;143(2):261–267.
235. Reiter A, Schrappe M, Tiemann M, et al. Successful treatment strategy for Ki-1 anaplastic large-cell lymphoma of childhood: a prospective analysis of 62 patients enrolled in three consecutive Berlin-Frankfurt-Munster Group studies. *J Clin Oncol* 1994;12(5):899–908.
237. Brugieres L, Deley MC, Pacquement H, et al. CD30(+) anaplastic large-cell lymphoma in children: analysis of 82 patients enrolled in two consecutive studies of the French Society of Pediatric Oncology. *Blood* 1998;92(10):3591–3598.
238. Cairo MS, Krailo MD, Morse M, et al. Long-term follow-up of short intensive multiagent chemotherapy without high-dose methotrexate ('Orange') in children with advanced non-lymphoblastic non-Hodgkin's lymphoma: a children's cancer group report. *Leukemia* 2002;16(4):594–600.
239. Laver JH, Mahmoud H, Pick TE, et al. Results of a randomized phase III trial in children and adolescents with advanced stage diffuse large cell non-Hodgkin's lymphoma: a Pediatric Oncology Group study. *Leuk Lymphoma* 2002;43:105–109.
240. Laver JH, Kraveka JM, Hutchison RE, et al. Advanced-stage large-cell lymphoma in children and adolescents: results of a randomized trial incorporating intermediate-dose methotrexate and high-dose cytarabine in the maintenance phase of the APO regimen: a Pediatric Oncology Group phase III trial. *J Clin Oncol* 2005; 23(3):541–547.
241. Seidemann K, Tiemann M, Schrappe M, et al. Short-pulse B-non-Hodgkin lymphoma-type chemotherapy is efficacious treatment for pediatric anaplastic large cell lymphoma: a report of the Berlin-Frankfurt-Munster Group Trial NHL-BFM 90. *Blood* 2001;97(12):3699–3706.
242. Brugieres L, Le Deley MC, Rosolen A, et al. Impact of the methotrexate administration dose on the need for intrathecal treatment in children and adolescents with anaplastic large-cell lymphoma: results of a randomized trial of the EICNHL Group. *J Clin Oncol* 2009;27(6):897–903.
243. Le Deley MC, Rosolen A, Williams DM, et al. Vinblastine in children and adolescents with high-risk anaplastic large-cell lymphoma: results of the randomized ALCL99-vinblastine trial. *J Clin Oncol* 2010;28(25):3987–3993.
253. Attarbaschi A, Mann G, Rosolen A, et al. Limited stage I disease is not necessarily indicative of an excellent prognosis in childhood anaplastic large cell lymphoma. *Blood* 2011;117(21):5616–5619.
255. Link MP, Donaldson SS, Berard CW, et al. Results of treatment of childhood localized non-Hodgkin's lymphoma with combination chemotherapy with or without radiotherapy. *N Engl J Med* 1990;322(17):1169–1174.
260. Salzburg J, Burkhardt B, Zimmermann M, et al. Prevalence, clinical pattern, and outcome of CNS involvement in childhood and adolescent non-Hodgkin's lymphoma differ by non-Hodgkin's lymphoma subtype: a Berlin-Frankfurt-Munster Group report. *J Clin Oncol* 2007;25(25):3915–3922.
261. Sandlund JT, Pui CH, Zhou Y, et al. Effective treatment of advanced-stage childhood lymphoblastic lymphoma without prophylactic cranial irradiation: results of St. Jude NHL13 study. *Leukemia* 2009;23(6):1127–1130.
262. Barredo JC, Devidas M, Lauer SJ, et al. Isolated CNS relapse of acute lymphoblastic leukemia treated with intensive systemic chemotherapy and delayed CNS radiation: a Pediatric Oncology Group study. *J Clin Oncol* 2006;24(19):3142–3149.
263. Veerman AJ, Kamps WA, Van Den BH, et al. Dexamethasone-based therapy for childhood acute lymphoblastic leukaemia: results of the prospective Dutch Childhood Oncology Group (DCOG) protocol ALL-9 (1997–2004). *Lancet Oncol* 2009;10(10):957–966.
266. Gross TG, Steinbuch M, DeFor T, et al. B cell lymphoproliferative disorders following hematopoietic stem cell transplantation: risk factors, treatment and outcome. *Bone Marrow Transplant* 1999;23(3):251–258.
271. Merkel O, Hamacher F, Sifft E, et al. Novel therapeutic options in anaplastic large cell lymphoma: molecular targets and immunological tools. *Mol Cancer Ther* 2011;10(7):1127–1136.

Chapter 90
Unusual Tumors in Children

Christian Carrie and Abraham Kuten

Some unusual and rare childhood tumors are comparable to those that occur in the adult population and require the same therapeutic strategy, with particular attention given to late sequelae. Some of these tumors are more characteristic of children and require specific radiotherapeutic strategies.

NASOPHARYNGEAL CARCINOMA IN CHILDHOOD

Nasopharyngeal carcinoma (NPC) is a rare malignant tumor in childhood and adolescence (<1% of pediatric malignancies). The frequency differs greatly by geographic area: 1 case per 100,000 in Europe, the United States, and Australia; 10 per 100,000 in North Africa; and 80 per 100,000 in South China, Malaysia, and Greenland. According to the World Health Organization, there are three distinct classification groups: type I, keratinizing squamous cell carcinoma; type II, nonkeratinizing carcinoma; and type III, undifferentiated carcinoma. Most pediatric NPC cases are type III.[1] As in older patients, Epstein–Barr virus is associated with this type of NPC. The virus is found in the tumoral cells and not in the surrounding lymphocytes. Antibody and antigen titers are useful for both diagnosis and follow-up (Table 90.1).[2] The association between dietary factors and NPC has been suspected in China and seems to be confirmed in the last case–control study published by Jia et al.[3]

Clinical Presentation

The mean age at presentation is 14 years; boys are more often affected than girls.[4] The tumor usually originates in the fossa of Rosenmuller, followed early on by locoregional extension, including extensive pharyngeal involvement and often bone, lung, and cervical lymph node metastases. The most frequent clinical symptoms are nasal obstruction, epistaxis, otitis, and neck and facial pain.

On clinical examination, bilateral lymphadenopathy and cranial nerve palsies are found; a nasopharyngeal mass can be seen by direct or indirect nasopharyngoscopy, and sometimes a protruding mass can be seen in the oral cavity.

The diagnostic workup must include a cranial and neck computed tomography (CT) scan and magnetic resonance imaging (MRI), a thorax CT scan, and bone scintigraphy. Pathologic confirmation is obtained by biopsy. Commonly used staging systems are the TNM/American Joint Committee on Cancer (AJC), Kyoto, and Ho classifications. The Ho and Kyoto systems are based on topographic extension; the more commonly used TNM/AJC classification is based on tumor volume and CT information.[5]

TABLE 90.1 ANTIGEN AND ANTIBODY EPSTEIN–BARR VIRUS TITERS

	IgG VCA	Ig EA	IgM VCA	IgA VCA	IgA EA	EBNA
Naive patient	0	0	0	0	0	0
Immune patient	Mild	0	0	0	0	Mild
Burkitt lymphoma	Raised	Raised	0	0	0	Raised
AIDS	Very raised	Raised	0	0	0	0
NC	Very raised	Very raised	Mild	Raised	Raised	Very raised

AIDS, acquired immunodeficiency syndrome; Ig, immunoglobulin; EA, early antigen (active disease); EBNA, EBV-associated nuclear antigen (cellular immunity); NC, nasopharynx carcinoma; VCA, vision capsid antigen (immune status).

Treatment

In adult NPC, concomitant radiotherapy and chemotherapy (cisplatin and 5-fluorouracil) is the standard of care.[6,7] Because of the scarcity of pediatric NPC cases, it is not feasible to perform randomized studies in this age group. Based on adult trials, multimodality treatment is generally accepted as standard of care for children. Usually two courses of 5-fluorouracil/*cis*-diamminedichloroplatinum II (cisplatin) are given on weeks 1 and 5 of radiotherapy.[8] Others have used neoadjuvant cisplatin-based chemotherapy, followed by radiation.[9]

Radiation Therapy

A dose–response relationship for local control with a threshold at 60 Gy has been reported in a number of series.[4,8,10] However, more recently Habrand et al.[11] reported interesting results with lower doses of radiation therapy (50 Gy) in patients with good response to chemotherapy. These results are in accordance with the reports of Polychronopoulou et al.[12] and Orbach et al.[13] In this series, 70% of children achieved local control with doses of <60 Gy (50% received only 52 Gy). A recent study from St. Jude also reported a better outcome for patients receiving cisplatin and dose of radiotherapy >50 Gy.[14] Techniques include CT for dosimetric purposes, three-dimensional (3D) dosimetry, customized blocking, and, if possible, MRI/CT scan image fusion for intensity-modulated radiotherapy (IMRT). Proton beam therapy is appropriate where available.

The target volume encompasses the tumor site and the neck (even in N0 disease) due to the severity of late sequelae after standard techniques. The standard of care for radiotherapy is IMRT, if available.[15] High–dose-rate, pulsed low–dose-rate, or conventional low–dose-rate intraluminal brachytherapy is used for the boost at some institutions. For some physicians, hyperfractionated radiotherapy is believed to be standard of care. A recent publication concerning hyperfractionated radiotherapy shows an increased rate of neurologic complication.[16] The overall survival for T1-T2 disease is 70% to 90%. The survival for T3-T4 disease using combined modality is 50% to 60%. For advanced stage, innovative targeted therapies are in the development process. These include induction of the lytic viral cycle with ganciclovir, gene therapy, or antitumor vaccination against the viral protein LMP2.[17,18]

Late Effects

Xerostomia is the main side effect of treatment, followed by dental caries, trismus, muscular atrophy, nerve palsies, and endocrine dysfunction resulting from pituitary irradiation. Significant auditory late toxicity and sporadic cases of visual morbidity, secondary to radiotherapy with or without cisplatin-based chemotherapy have been reported.[19] The St. Jude retrospective analysis reported a rate of 8.5% of subsequent malignancies 8.6 to 27 years after treatment.[14]

New techniques such as IMRT or radioprotective drugs such as amifostine may be able to decrease late sequelae.

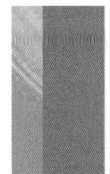

OTHER HEAD AND NECK TUMORS

Carcinoma of the Oropharynx and Salivary Glands

Schwaab et al.[20] reported the largest pediatric series, with only 2% squamous cell carcinoma among 380 head and neck tumors. The more frequent sites of disease are the tongue, lip, tonsil palate, and salivary glands. Cigarette smoking or use of smokeless tobacco have been shown to be the etiologic factors for adolescent tongue carcinoma.[21] For other sites, passive smoking, poor oral hygiene, or genetic predispositions (xeroderma pigmentosum or retinoblastoma) have been suggested.

Special attention must be paid to larynx carcinoma because some of the cases may develop from juvenile papillomatisis, a benign condition of the aerodigestive tract that may undergo malignant degeneration. Guidelines for surgery and radiation therapy are the same as those for adults. Combined chemotherapy and radiation can be attempted for organ conservation.[22] The node area to treat does not differ from adults and must follow the Gregoire definition.[23]

Psychological support and rehabilitation programs are an essential part of the comprehensive treatment for children who undergo major surgical resection.

Esthesioneuroblastoma

Esthesioneuroblastoma is a malignant tumor arising from the olfactory nerve in the upper nasal cavity. Intracranial extension is common at the time of diagnosis. Esthesioneuroblastoma is mostly seen in patients in their 20s or 60s. Positive S-100 and neuron-specific enolase stains combined with negative epithelial markers strongly suggest a neurogenic origin.[24] The clinical presentation includes nasal obstruction, loss of smell, epistaxis, and, sometimes, enlarged cervical lymph nodes. Bony structures are often involved, as well as the ethmoid and maxillary sinuses. The most commonly used staging/grouping system is by Kadish et al.[24] and is based on degree of local tumor extension.

Standard treatment has not yet been defined. Localized tumors are often treated by surgery alone, but local relapse is very frequent. Therefore, postoperative radiotherapy is often proposed. In patients treated by combined surgery and irradiation, local control can be obtained in >75% of cases.[25] Eich et al.[26] and Broich et al.[27] recommend combined surgery and radiotherapy in all stages. Demiroz et al.[28] reviewed 26 patients treated between 1995 and 2007. The relapse rate for patients treated with surgery alone was 29% versus 0% for those treated by surgery and postoperative radiotherapy. The recommended dose is 50 to 60 Gy. Elective neck irradiation or dissection is not advocated because <10% of early-stage cases exhibit nodal involvement. However, node metastases are frequent if the tumor extends beyond the paranasal sinuses. In this case, lymph node dissection or prophylactic irradiation should be considered. Chemotherapy has not yet been accepted as part of routine first-line treatment, although responses to chemotherapy have been reported.[29] Chemotherapy can be employed to reduce tumor volume prior to surgery or radiotherapy, as well as for palliative purposes in advanced cases. Promising results with cyclophosphamide, doxorubicin, vincristine, *cis*-platinum, and etoposide, combined with radiotherapy and stem cell support, have been reported recently by Mishima et al.[30] They obtained 8 complete responses in 12 Kadish stage C and D patients. Neoadjuvant concurrent chemoradiotherapy as preoperative treatment for locally advanced esthesioneuroblastoma has been reported by Sohrabi et al.[31] with very promising results.

Juvenile Nasopharyngeal Angiofibroma

Juvenile nasopharyngeal angiofibroma (JNA) is a malignant vascular tumor most often arising from the posterior lateral wall of the nasopharynx. The lesion tends to extend into the nasal cavities, maxillary and sphenoid sinuses, orbit, and infratemporal fossa. Several classifications have been proposed, but the classification of Radkowski et al.[32] appears to be the most appropriate, at least for the surgical purposes (Table 90.2). Common symptoms are epistaxis, cheek swelling, a visible orbital tumor, and cranial nerve palsies. JNA is more frequent in familial adenomatous polyposis patients. A mutation in the cluster region of the APC gene was reported in several studies, suggesting that JNA is perhaps a familial adenomatous polyposis tumor.[33,34]

TABLE 90.2 STAGING CLASSIFICATION FOR JUVENILE NASOPHARYNGEAL ANGIOFIBROMA

Stage	Description
Ia	Limited to the nose and/or nasopharynx
Ib	Same as Ia, but with extension into one or more paranasal sinuses
IIa	Minimal extension through the sphenopalatine foramen, into and including a minimal part of the medialmost part of pterygomaxillary fossa
IIb	Full occupation of the pterygomaxillary fossa, displacing the posterior wall of the maxillary antrum forward; lateral and/or anterior displacement of branches of the maxillary artery; superior extension may occur, eroding orbital bones
IIc	Extension through the pterygomaxillary fossa into the cheek and temporal fossa or posterior to the pterygoid plates
IIIa	Erosion of the skull base with minimal intracranial extension
IIIb	Erosion of the skull base with extensive intracranial extension with or without cavernous sinus invasion

Based on the classification of Radkowski et al.[32]

Treatment consists of surgery for small lesions, often with preoperative embolization or hormone therapy. Surgery carries a risk of significant operative blood loss. For localized JNA, the cure rate obtained by surgery alone can be as high as 90%. Resection with negative margins is required because inadequate margins will result in a high local failure rate.[35] Minimally invasive endoscopic resection has recently been proposed for early-stage JNA. Lesions limited to the nasal cavity and/or nasopharynx or lesions with minimal extension through the sphenopalatine foramen are suitable for this procedure. A craniofacial approach is recommended for lesions extending into the pterygoid plates.[36,37] Radiation therapy is used either as adjuvant treatment or as sole treatment in locally advanced lesions. Modern techniques such as IMRT have been successfully applied in unresectable and recurrent tumors.[38] A wide range of doses have been used, but there is no proof that doses of >36 Gy are advantageous. Chakraborty et al.[39] treated eight patients with intensity-modulated radiotherapy with a median dose of 39 Gy. The local control rate was 87% with a mean of follow-up of 2 years. There is no role for cytotoxic chemotherapy in JNA. The role of antiangiogenesis agents is speculative.

LUNG CANCER

Bronchogenic Carcinoma

Pediatric bronchogenic carcinoma is extremely rare, and its management does not differ from that of adults. Most of the tumors occur during adolescence. Histology is more frequently undifferentiated adenocarcinoma or carcinoid tumors rather than squamous cell carcinoma.[40]

Of 230 cases of primary pulmonary neoplasms of childhood reviewed by Hartman and Shochat,[41] <25% were bronchogenic carcinoma. The survival rate was very similar to that of adults, stage for stage.

Pleuropulmonary Blastoma

Fewer than 100 cases of pleuropulmonary blastoma (PPB) have been reported. This tumor can occur from the neonatal period up to 12 years of age.[42] PPB was often mixed with pulmonary blastoma until it was accepted that PPB is purely a pediatric tumor. The main histologic difference between pulmonary

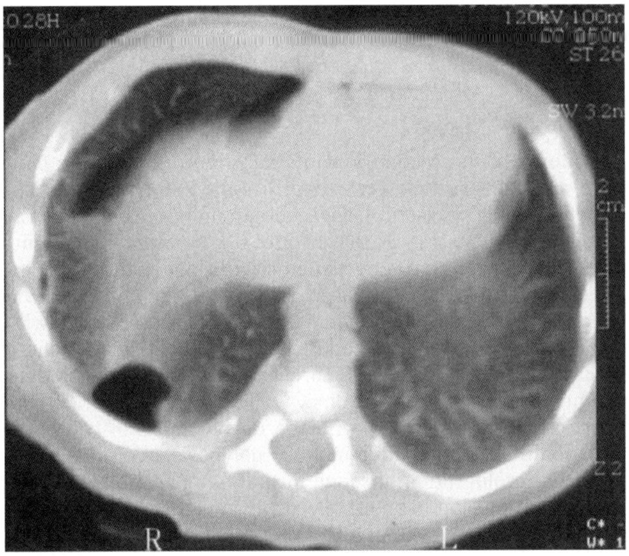

FIGURE 90.1. Pleuropneumoblastoma in a 1-year-old girl.

blastoma and PPB is the absence of epithelial carcinomatous components in PPB; PPB consists of mesenchymal stroma only. The tumor usually begins in pulmonary tissue, but it can also originate in the pleura or mediastinum.[43] According to the Dehner et al.[44] classification, three pathologic features can occur: cystic, mixed, and solid. However, it seems that this subdivision has neither prognostic nor therapeutic value.[45,46] Some reports also described PPB associated with pre-existing pulmonary cyst.[47] It is unclear whether PPB arises in pre-existing malformation or whether PPB induces cystic lesion formation. The report from the International Pleuropulmonary Blastoma Registry showed that great vessel or cardiac extension is present at diagnosis in 3% of cases.[48]

Clinically, PPB exhibits no specific symptoms. The usual presentation is cough, thoracic pain, and fever. Respiratory impairment is unusual. Radiologic findings depend on the extent of the cystic component (Fig. 90.1). The standard treatment is surgery, which can be curative in early-stage disease, but the prognosis is often poor even after complete excision, especially if the size of tumor exceeds 5 cm.[49]

Priest et al.[42] reported only 8% survival rate at 5 years among 50 patients.[50] Postoperative radiation therapy can be offered for a positive margin resection or in recurrent disease. The recommended dose is 50 Gy to the tumor bed and, because most of the relapses are local or metastatic, it is our opinion that lymphatic irradiation is not necessary. The value of chemotherapy is controversial. There are, however, long-term survivals reported with multiagent combinations such as actinomycin D, cyclophosphamide, cisplatin, etoposide, Adriamycin, and vincristine.[43,51–53,54] Multimodal therapy with surgery followed by chemotherapy and radiotherapy (10.5 Gy) has been reported with good results at 3 years,[55] and recommendations have been published by the International PPB Registry.[48]

BREAST TUMORS

Malignant breast tumors account for <1% of all childhood cancers and <0.1% of all breast cancers.[56–59]

A review of adolescents seen at the MD Anderson Cancer Center during a 40-year period identified breast cancer in 16 patients <20 years of age. Ten patients had primary adenocarcinoma of the breast, 4 had cystosarcoma phylloides, and 2 had breast metastases from other primary tumors. Four of the 16 patients had a family history of breast disease.[60] Roisman et al.[61] reported seven female patients, ages 14 to 17 years, who were treated in various hospitals in Israel for malignancy of the breast during 1967 to 1989. There were two cases of undifferentiated carcinoma with positive axillary lymph nodes, two cases of cystosarcoma phylloides, one case of rhabdomyosarcoma, and two cases of malignant lymphoma, one of them Burkitt's type. Umanah et al.[62] reported 1 case (1.2%) of an invasive ductal carcinoma among 84 breast tumor materials from patients aged 10 to 19 years in a Nigerian city.

Breast self-examination is recommended for girls who carry the BRCA1 or BRCA2 gene, beginning at age 18 to 21 years.[63,64] Ultrasonography is the most appropriate initial investigation in any adolescent patient with a breast mass because dense breast tissue adversely affects the quality of mammography.[65] MRI is recommended for diagnosing breast cancer when conventional imaging is complex and indeterminate, especially in young patients with dense mammographies.

Juvenile secretory carcinoma of the breast is rare and was first described by McDivitt and Stewart[66] in 1966 in seven girls ages 3 to 15 years, all of whom had a benign clinical course. The tumor cells are characterized by abundant mucin- and mucopolysaccharide-containing materials.[67] Hormonal receptors are generally negative.[68] Local tumor excision alone may be adequate therapy, although simple and radical mastectomies have also been used.[68–70]

The histology and patterns of spread of adenocarcinoma of the breast in children and adolescents are similar to those in adults. Because most publications refer to isolated cases, neither a consensus of opinion nor specific guidelines exist with regard to treatment. In general, principles of clinical management established for adults should be adopted. Because recurrences were found in 25% of patients treated with excisional biopsy alone, this seems inadequate, and a simple mastectomy with axillary lymph node dissection should probably be performed.[71] Sentinel lymph node biopsy offers an approach to stage the axillary lymphatic drainage with a lower complication rate than formal dissection.[72] On the other hand, McDivitt and Stewart[66] believed that the disease tends to run a relatively favorable course and that radical therapy is therefore unnecessary. Hartman and Magrish[73] considered it important to avoid radiotherapy in young children, and instead they recommended radical mastectomy.

Inflammatory carcinoma of the breast is extremely rare in children.[74,75]

There have been case reports of primary lymphoma, rhabdomyosarcoma, adenoid cystic carcinoma, radiation-induced sarcoma, and cystosarcoma phylloides of the breast in children.[76–81]

Cystosarcoma phylloides appears as a large breast mass; in 25% of cases it is bilateral. Norris and Taylor[80] were the first to separate benign from malignant lesions in this disorder. The distinction is based on tumor size, stromal invasion, cellular atypia, degree of mitotic activity, focal calcification, and/or patterns of infiltration. Metastases occur in the lungs and bones. Lymph node metastases are extremely rare. Simple or wide local excision or simple mastectomy, with rare local recurrences, may adequately treat histologically benign lesions. In malignant cystosarcoma phylloides some authors recommend radical mastectomy with or without axillary lymph node dissection, and others are in favor of simple mastectomy.[82–86] The use of radiotherapy and postoperative chemotherapy in cystosarcoma phylloides is controversial. These modalities should be reserved for locally advanced, palliative, and disseminated cases.

Rhabdomyosarcoma of the breast, either primary or metastatic, is rare. Billroth[87] reported the first case of primary rhabdomyosarcoma in a 16-year-old girl in 1860. In a series of 108 patients <20 years of age with this malignancy, Howarth et al.[88] reported 7 patients who had metastatic tumors to the breast with primary rhabdomyosarcoma located on an extremity or buttock. Six of the 7 patients had alveolar histology. Rhabdomyosarcoma of the breast and other sarcomas of the breast are treated primarily by surgery followed, in most cases, by adjuvant radiation and chemotherapy.

Breast metastases in the pediatric age group include hepatocarcinoma, non-Hodgkin lymphoma, rhabdomyosarcoma Hodgkin disease, neuroblastoma, and adenocarcinoma.[89]

GASTROINTESTINAL TUMORS OF CHILDHOOD

Gastrointestinal tract malignant tumors are relatively rare in children. Carcinoid and hepatobiliary tumors are the most common.[90] Others are adenocarcinoma, lymphoma, and leiomyosarcoma. More common are benign tumors such as hamartoma, leiomyoma, neurofibroma, and hemangioma.

Esophagus

In most cases, an esophageal tumor is of epithelial origin, either squamous cell carcinoma or adenocarcinoma. Rarely, sarcomas may develop in the esophagus (leiomyosarcoma, carcinosarcoma, malignant schwannoma). Malignization of a chemical injury to the esophagus has been described.[91] Carcinoma of the esophagus may develop in association with Barrett's esophagus and Cornelia de Lange syndrome.[92,93] The most common benign tumor of the esophagus in the pediatric age group is leiomyoma; desmoid and teratoma may also occur.[94–96] The management of esophageal cancer in the pediatric age group follows the same guidelines of treatment as in adults.[97]

Stomach

Non-Hodgkin lymphoma is the most frequent gastric malignancy in the pediatric age group, followed by leiomyosarcoma and leiomyoblastoma.[98] Adenocarcinoma is extremely rare; it may arise in association with Peutz–Jeghers syndrome.[99] The management of non-Hodgkin lymphoma follows the treatment guidelines of non-Hodgkin lymphoma in adults.

Leiomyosarcoma of the stomach is treated primarily with surgery. Postoperative irradiation is given to patients with high risk of local recurrence (such as positive surgical margins or extension into the retroperitoneum).

As in the adult age group, subtotal gastrectomy with resection of associated lymph nodes is the treatment of choice for children with gastric carcinoma. No data are available on adjuvant radiation–chemotherapy in the pediatric age group. However, based on the results of a randomized study in adult patients with locoregionally advanced gastric carcinoma,[100] one could assume that the use of combined irradiation and chemotherapy (5-fluorouracil and leucovorin) after surgery is beneficial.

Radiotherapy guidelines are similar to those for the adult age group. At the time of radiotherapy planning, attention should be given to vital structures such as spinal cord, kidneys, small bowel, and liver. During treatment, acute side effects may occur, such as nausea, weight loss, and fatigue.

Several combination chemotherapy regimens have been used in the adjuvant setting and for locally advanced or metastatic gastric carcinoma. Numerous phase II and phase III studies were reported in the adult age group.[101] More than 20% of gastric cancers and up to 33% of gastroesophageal junction tumors show HER2 overexpression.[102] This gives new therapeutic options, adding trastuzumab to chemotherapy.[103]

Small Bowel

According to the Surveillance, Epidemiology, and End Results (SEER) data, the incidence of malignant small intestine tumors is low in patients <30 years of age.[104] The most common malignancy of the small intestine in children is non-Hodgkin lymphoma.[105] Sarcomas of the small bowel and carcinoids may also develop in children. Small intestine adenocarcinoma may develop spontaneously or in association with Peutz–Jeghers syndrome.[106]

Treatment guidelines are similar to those of the adult age group. Adjuvant irradiation can be given after surgery for duodenal sarcomas or adenocarcinomas arising in the segment fixed to the retroperitoneum or for palliative purposes such as for pain or bleeding.

Colorectal Cancer

Carcinoma of the rectum and the large bowel is rare in children and adolescents. According to the SEER data, approximately 145,000 cases of colorectal carcinoma occur annually in the United States. Of these, only 0.1% occurs in patients <20 years of age.[107] Young patients with long-standing ulcerative colitis have an increased risk of developing colorectal cancer.[108] Several genetic conditions may be associated with colorectal carcinoma in childhood and adolescence. These include familial polyposis, Turcot syndrome, Oldfield syndrome, and Gardner syndrome.[100,101,102–103,104–108,109,110–112] The genetic events associated with the development of colorectal carcinoma in familial adenomatous polyposis syndrome, from epithelial proliferation, through formation of adenomas, to the sequential development of colorectal malignancy, have been described by Vogelstein et al.[113]

Similar to the adult age group, signs and symptoms of colorectal cancer are related to the segment of the large bowel where the tumor is located. Because of its rarity in the pediatric and adolescent age groups, diagnosis of colorectal carcinoma is often delayed, and patients usually present with acute symptoms that necessitate urgent laparotomy. Colorectal cancer in the young is usually diagnosed at an advanced stage with metastases involving the omentum, peritoneum, mesenteric lymph nodes, liver, ovaries, and sometimes lungs, brain, and bones, and therefore it carries a poor prognosis.[114]

Colorectal carcinoma is diagnosed by direct fiberoptic colonoscopy. Radiographic studies include barium enema with air contrast, CT scan, and radioisotope studies (fluorodeoxyglucose-positron emission tomography [FDG-PET]) to determine metastatic spread. Preoperative carcinoembryonic antigen (CEA) level is important both as a prognosticator and for follow-up purposes. CA19-9 essay has been less valuable, although some tumors produce CA19-9 without CEA production.

Adenocarcinoma of the colorectum may be well, moderately, or poorly differentiated. The mucinous variety and signet cell types are associated with extremely poor prognosis. Mucinous adenocarcinoma is the most common histotype in the pediatric age group.[115] Unlike adult patients, in whom 60% of colonic cancers are located within 25 cm of the anus and in whom the rectum and sigmoid are also common sites for mucinous adenocarcinoma, tumors in children are probably more evenly distributed in all parts of the colon.[95,116,117] In a series reported by Andersson and Bergdahl,[118] the most common area was the transverse colon (39%). In a series of 20 patients reported by Karnak et al.[119] from Turkey, the rectosigmoid area was the most frequent site of location of the primary tumor (65%, the same as in adults).

Surgery is the primary and most effective treatment for colorectal carcinoma. Because of late diagnosis, the rate of complete resection has been less than optimal in children. In the series of Karnak et al.,[119] complete resection was possible in only 6 of 20 patients. The surgical guidelines are similar to those of adult patients. Similarly, the use of chemotherapy and radiotherapy follows the guidelines of the adult age group. Special attention should be given to radiochemotherapy sequelae on the reproductive system.

Appendix

The most frequent malignant tumors of the appendix in the pediatric age group are carcinoids. These tumors are usually diagnosed incidentally during surgery for acute appendicitis or during other abdominal surgery. Complete surgical removal is the treatment of choice.[120,121]

Pancreas

Pancreatic tumors are rare in children. The most important types are the functional tumors, pancreatoblastomas, and solid papillary epithelial neoplasms.[122,123] The adult form of pancreatic adenocarcinoma rarely occurs in children.

Functional islet cell tumors are characterized by their hormonal activity. The diagnostic procedures and management follow the same guidelines set for adults.

The pediatric type of carcinoma of the pancreas, pancreatoblastoma, is a rare tumor; <100 cases have been reported in the literature. The European Cooperative Study Group for pediatric rare tumors analyzed 20 patients diagnosed between 2000 and 2009.[124] The tumor is characterized by adenocarcinomatous tissue with ductal cells, acinar cells, squamoid corpuscles and sometimes islet cell differentiation. These tumors stain positively by periodic acid-Schiff, α-trypsin, and α-keratin, and in many cases can be associated with increased levels of α-fetoprotein (AFP).[125–127]

In most cases the tumor is located in the head of the pancreas. In patients with a solitary noninfiltrative tumor, complete local resection without radical pancreatoduodenectomy is recommended. Unlike patients with local disease, in whom local resection can be curative, in many other cases the tumor is clearly malignant, with invasion, local recurrences, and nodal and disseminated metastases. The prognosis for these patients is very poor.[128,129]

Radiation therapy is used in the postoperative setting, in locoregional recurrences, and in the neoadjuvant setting. A dose of 40 to 50 Gy is recommended.[127,130] Technical guidelines of radiotherapy planning are similar to those of the adults. Intraoperative radiotherapy for recurrent disease has also been used.

Chemotherapy has been used for unresectable tumors, to treat metastatic disease, or in the adjuvant setting. 5-Fluorouracil, cyclophosphamide, actinomycin D, vincristine, vinblastine, mitomycin c, bleomycin, ifosfamide, etoposide, cisplatin, doxorubicin, and gemcitabine, alone or in combination, have been used with very modest results.[131,132] Because the disease is so rare, it is impossible to set firm guidelines and treatment policies for chemotherapy in pediatric pancreatoblastoma.

Papillary cystic tumors of the pancreas, also known as Frantz tumors, are usually encapsulated lesions that can develop throughout the pancreas. They are characterized by cystic or pseudocystic spaces surrounded by residual solid tissue. Only 15% of these tumors are malignant, and they usually occur in female patients at a mean age of 24 years at diagnosis.[133]

These tumors usually present as an upper abdominal mass. Unlike other malignant pancreatic tumors, their prognosis is excellent after complete surgical excision.[134]

The adult type of pancreatic adenocarcinoma is extremely rare in the pediatric and adolescent age groups. Signs and symptoms are similar to those of adult carcinoma of the pancreas.[130] These tumors are managed according to guidelines of treatment set for adult patients.

Hepatobiliary Tumors

Hepatobiliary tumors are the most common neoplasms of the gastrointestinal tract to occur in children. They constitute 0.5% to 2% of pediatric cancer in Europe and in the United States. Hepatocellular carcinoma (HCC) occurs more frequently in Saharan Africa and the Asia.[62,135–139] This geographic clustering may be explained by the high rates of hepatitis B infection and hepatitis B serum antigen positivity.[140]

Benign hepatic tumors are more frequent than malignant tumors in young children. In older children, malignant tumors become more common. Benign tumors are classified according to the cell of origin: mesenchymal (hemangioma, hemangioendothelioma, hamartoma, peliosis hepatis) or epithelial (cysts, focal nodal hyperplasia, adenoma).[141] On rare occasions, radiation therapy may be used for the treatment of hemangiomas.

Malignant tumors of the liver are classified according to the tissue of origin, with hepatocellular tumors (hepatoblastoma [HBL] and HCC) most common, constituting 75% to 90% of primary hepatic malignant tumors of childhood. Other tumors include malignant mesenchymoma, undifferentiated embryonal sarcoma, primary hepatic malignant tumors with rhabdoid features, leiomyosarcoma, angiosarcoma, hepatic sinusoid tumors, carcinoid, and non-Hodgkin lymphoma.

Bile duct adenocarcinoma (cholangiocarcinoma) is extremely rare before the age of 30 years. This tumor has been associated with certain rare congenital biliary anomalies, ulcerated colitis, cystic fibrosis, and sclerosing cholangitis.[141,142] The liver is also a common site for metastatic disease.

Of the malignant tumors of the liver in childhood, HBL is the most common. HBL occurs almost exclusively in small infants, although isolated instances in older children and in young adolescents have been reported. These tumors occur more frequently among males.

HBL is associated with Beckwith–Wiedemann syndrome, familial adenomatous polyposis, and congenital anomalies like hemihypertrophy and cleft palate, Wilms tumor, and glycogen storage diseases.[143–146] Although the association between HBL and Beckwith–Wiedemann syndrome indicates abnormalities on chromosome 11 and loss of heterozygosity on chromosome 11p, increased incidence of HBL in families with familial adenomatous polyposis indicates a possible significance for abnormalities of chromosome 5q.[145,147]

The presenting signs and symptoms are distention of the abdomen, anorexia, vomiting, anemia, fever, and jaundice. Isosexual precocity secondary to human chorionic gonadotropin (HCG) secretion by the tumor can be seen in some cases.[146]

Serum AFP produced by the embryonal endoderm is increased in 84% to 90% of patients with HBL.[148] HCG and cystathionase may also serve as tumor markers.[149] Histologically, hepatoblastomas (Fig. 90.2) are classified into five subtypes (Table 90.3). These subtypes can occur together in varying properties, but present definitions do not take this into account, which makes it difficult to relate a specific histologic subtype with prognosis. Pure fetal histology has a better outcome, but the definition of "pure fetal" is not clear. The prognosis of the rare (3%) small-cell undifferentiated subtype is poor. In long-term survivors of HBL, the most common histologic variant is the conventional type with predominantly fetal cell patterns. A trial performed by the Pediatric Oncology Group (POG) and the Children's Cancer Study Group (CCSG) demonstrated the importance of the distinction between fetal hepatoblastoma and the other histologic subtypes in stage I disease.[150] A German study (HB 89–94)[151] identified several poor prognostic factors in HBL: metastatic disease, AFP >1,000,000 ng/mL, extrahepatic and intrahepatic vascular invasion, multifocal disease, involvement of both liver lobes, stage (TNM), and poorly differentiated epithelial histology.

HCC is the second-most-common primary malignant liver tumor in the pediatric age group and accounts for about one-fourth to one-third of hepatic malignancies. Although reported in children as young as 21 months, most reports indicate that

TABLE 90.3 HISTOLOGIC CLASSIFICATION OF HEPATOBLASTOMA

Epithelial type (56%)	Mixed epithelial and mesenchymal type (44%)
Fetal pattern (31%)	Without teratoid features (34%)
Embryonal and fetal pattern (19%)	With teratoid features (10%)
Macrotrabecular pattern (3%)	
Small-cell undifferentiated pattern (3%)	

Modified from Stocker.[350]

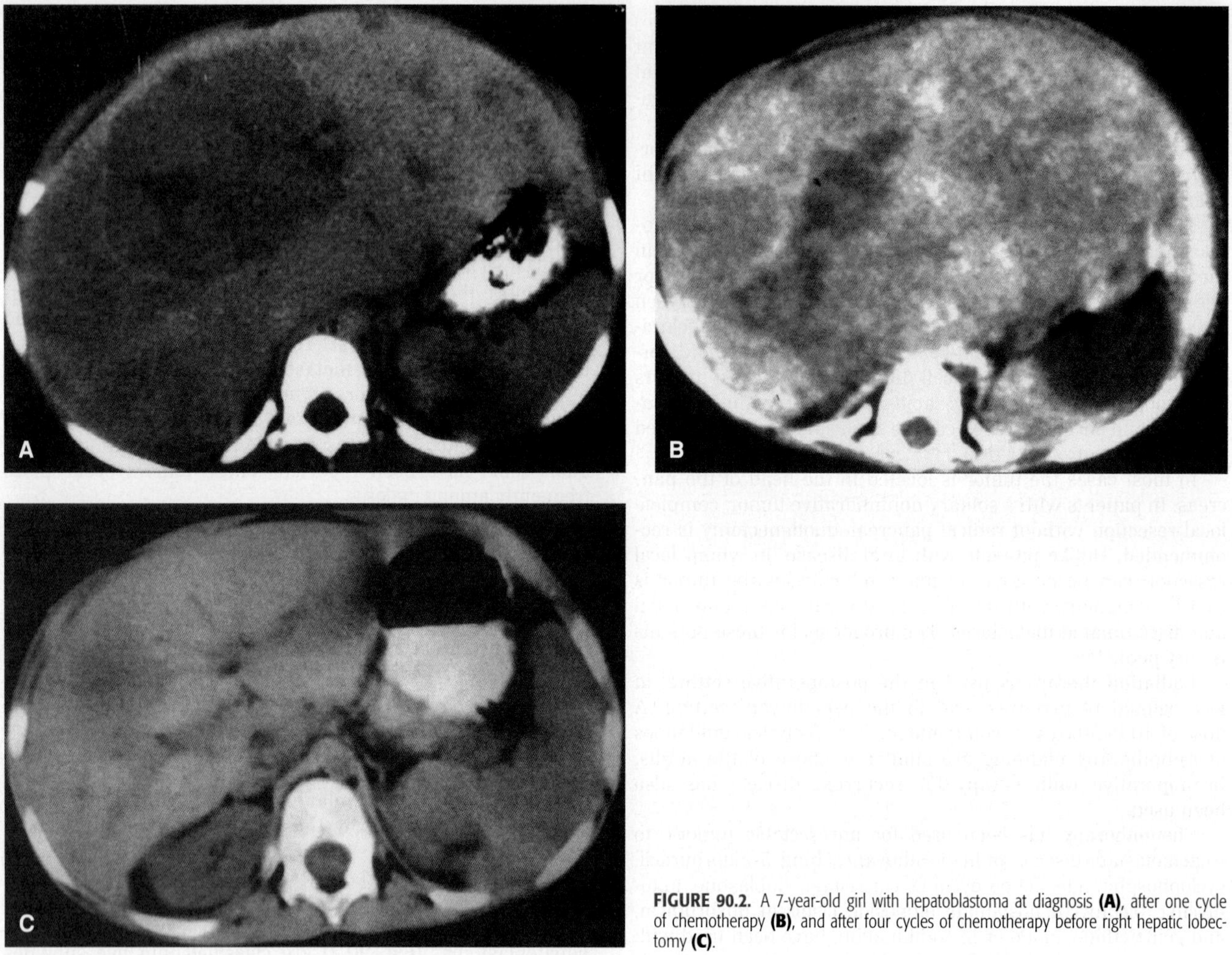

FIGURE 90.2. A 7-year-old girl with hepatoblastoma at diagnosis **(A)**, after one cycle of chemotherapy **(B)**, and after four cycles of chemotherapy before right hepatic lobectomy **(C)**.

HCC usually develops in early adolescence.[152,153] This is in contrast to HBL, which occurs primarily in infancy and is seldom seen in children older than 3 years. Similar to HBL, HCC occurs mainly in males.[154,155] The fibrolamellar carcinoma variant of HCC occurs mainly in young adults around the age of 20 years but has also been reported in childhood.[156,157]

Approximately 25% of HCC cases in childhood are associated with cirrhosis secondary to biliary atresia, Fanconi anemia, glucose-6-phosphatase deficiency, and hereditary tyrosinemia.[158] The most important known etiologic factor for HCC is the high incidence of maternal transmission of the hepatitis B surface antigen in Africa and Asia.[159,160] Other etiologic factors include exposure to aflatoxins, hepatic fibrosis, anabolic steroids, inherited disorders of metabolism, membranous obstruction of the inferior vena cava, and possibly ethanol abuse.[139,155,161] However, these etiologic factors apply mostly to HCC in the adult age group. In adult Black South African patients, deletions of alleles on chromosome 17p and P53 (codon 249) have been identified[162,163]; the exact molecular mechanisms responsible for the development of HCC are not known.

Similar to HBL, two-thirds of children with HCC have an elevated AFP.[164] AFP levels are high in the healthy newborn and drop rapidly by the age of 1 month and should not be detectable by age 2 years.[165] Initial AFP level is a significant prognostic factor: In a study performed by the Radiation Therapy Oncology Group,[166] the mortality in HCC was 1.8 times higher in patients with strongly positive AFP. AFP is an indicator of tumor growth and can serve as a valuable marker of response to therapy. After complete tumor resection, AFP level should return to normal within 2 months.[167] Increasing levels of AFP during the follow-up period after surgery indicate local recurrence or metastatic disease.[164]

The CCSG intergroup and POG staging systems for primary malignant liver tumors are based on resectability and on the histologic subtype (Tables 90.4[168,169] and 90.5[170]).

Successful therapy of localized HBL or HCC depends mainly on the feasibility of complete surgical excision.[151] Up to two-thirds of HBL patients have resectable tumors at presentation

TABLE 90.4 CHILDREN'S CANCER STUDY GROUP STAGING SYSTEM FOR PRIMARY MALIGNANT LIVER TUMORS

Stage	*Description*
I	Complete excision
A	Favorable histology (fetal HBL)
B	Unfavorable histology (embryonal HBL, HCC)
II	Microscopic residual disease
A	In liver
B	Extrahepatic
III	Gross residual disease ± node involvement ± spilled tumor
A	Tumor completely removed; tumor spilled, residual gross disease in nodes, or both
B	Gross tumor not completely removed ± positive nodes ± spill
IV	Metastatic disease
A	Primary tumor completely excised
B	Primary tumor not completely excised

HBL, hepatoblastoma; HCC, hepatocellular carcinoma.

Data derived from Cohen et al.[168] and Perilongo et al.[169]

TABLE 90.5 PEDIATRIC ONCOLOGY GROUP STAGING SYSTEM FOR PRIMARY MALIGNANT LIVER TUMORS

Stage	Description
I	Complete resection achieved
II	Microscopic residual tumor remaining
III	Gross residual tumor remaining
IV	Metastatic disease present at diagnosis

Modified from Bowman LC, Riely CA. Management of pediatric liver tumors. *Surg Oncol Clin North Am* 1996;5:451–459.

because these tumors are usually unifocal and encapsulated. Cure can be achieved in one-third of the successfully operated patients, typically those with fetal HBL.[143,150,171] In contrast, only 30% of the cases of HCC are suitable for complete resection at the time of diagnosis because of the multifocal involvement or size. From 50% to 75% of the fibrolamellar variant of HCC is amenable to complete resection at the time of presentation.[172,173] In principle, tumor resectability is determined by the tumor size, the existence of bilobar involvement necessitating the resection of more than three liver segments, vascular invasion, or metastatic spread. Patients with advanced disease who are not suitable for primary surgery may be considered for neoadjuvant preoperative cytoreductive chemotherapy. In these cases, the diagnosis can either be based on clinical presentation, on imaging findings, including FDG-PET scan[174] and tumor markers, or on tissue diagnosis obtained via open biopsy or CT/ultrasound-guided needle biopsy, although there are some concerns that a needle biopsy may cause a significant hemorrhage. Preoperative cytoreductive chemotherapy can reduce the size of the tumor in the majority of HBL patients and in a significant percentage of HCC patients, rendering them resectable. Chemotherapy regimens include combinations of cisplatin, vincristine, and 5-fluorouracil[175]; ifosfamide, cisplatin, and doxorubicin[176]; vincristine, doxorubicin, cyclophosphamide or vincristine, cyclophosphamide, cisplatin-carboplatin-based combinations[172,177]; the camptothecin analogues topotecan and irinotecan; a novel platinum derivative, oxaliplatin; and liposomal doxorubicin (Doxil).[151] Recently, surafemib, a multiphase inhibitor, was introduced as first-line treatment of HCC, and bevacizumab has shown a survival benefit in a phase II trial.[178,179] If resectability cannot be achieved using chemotherapy, there is still a chance to render unresectable tumors resectable by radiotherapy.[172] The perioperative mortality of hepatic lobectomy is in the order of 5% to 10% in specialized centers applying improved surgical techniques, modern methods of anesthesia, and state-of-the-art postoperative intensive care.[180]

Surgical resection of pulmonary metastases can be attempted if they persist after chemotherapy and if the primary tumor can be completely resected. Patients who are successfully operated on for stage I disease and later develop a solitary lung metastasis are also suitable for metastasectomy.

Total hepatectomy and liver transplantation can be attempted in unresectable HBL (about 10% after chemotherapy) and HCC (>50% are unresectable at diagnosis) with tumor confined to the liver without penetration of the capsule and in the absence of lymph node and distant metastases. The overall survival is between 50% and 83%, with a minimum follow-up of 2 years. The best outcome was achieved in patients with a good response to chemotherapy who had a "first-line transplant" (i.e., not after an unsuccessful attempt at resection).[151,181–183]

Although it has been used preoperatively and postoperatively in children with HBL and HCC, radiation therapy has a limited role in curative management.

Preoperative radiation was given to children who remained unresectable after initial chemotherapy.[172,184,185] In the postoperative setting, it has been shown that patients with residual disease after surgery may benefit from postoperative irradiation. In a combined POG-CCSG protocol,[150] patients with microscopic residual disease after surgery received postoperative chemotherapy and limited field irradiation, 45 Gy to the tumor bed. Their 3-year progression-free survival was 60%. Patients who were unable to undergo complete resection after preoperative chemotherapy received whole-liver irradiation, 30 Gy. Their 3-year progression-free survival was 22%.

According to the Institut Gustave Roussy protocol,[172] children were treated with preoperative chemotherapy followed by surgery. If there was evidence for microscopic or gross persistent tumor at surgery, more chemotherapy was given and limited field irradiation was administered to the site of residual tumor, 25 to 45 Gy. Fifteen patients were reported by Habrand et al.,[172] 11 with HBL, 2 with HCC, and 2 without tissue diagnosis. Nine patients who underwent surgical resection of the primary tumor received either preoperative or postoperative chemotherapy consisting of vincristine, doxorubicin, and cyclophosphamide, alternating with vincristine, cyclophosphamide, and *cis*-platinum. Radiotherapy with a median dose of 40 Gy was given to 8 incompletely resected patients. Six of 8 patients were alive at a median of 45 months from the time of diagnosis. One inoperable patient was rendered operable by whole-liver irradiation (24 Gy) and concurrent 5-fluorouracil and *cis*-platinum. This patient was alive at 68 months after radiation therapy. Of 4 unresectable primaries, 1 was controlled by radiotherapy. Two children received whole-lung irradiation, 18 to 20 Gy, for pulmonary metastases; neither of them was controlled. One of these 2 patients underwent pulmonary metastasectomy and was alive without evidence of disease 41 months after surgery.

When radiotherapy is given to children with HBL or HCC, careful assessment of the tumor volume is essential to reduce the amount of normal liver tissue irradiated. Parallel opposed high-energy beams or multiple-field techniques, using 3D treatment-planning systems or IMRT, should be employed. When limited irradiation volume is administered, a dose of 35 to 45 Gy is appropriate for bulky disease and 25 to 45 Gy for microscopic residual disease. For children treated with a palliative intent, whole-liver irradiation, 20 to 25 Gy in 2 to 2.5 weeks, is adequate.

The results of whole-lung irradiation for macroscopic pulmonary metastases are discouraging. A total dose of 12- to 13-Gy whole-lung irradiation might be considered in patients with microscopic residual pulmonary metastatic disease after chemotherapy or surgery and chemotherapy.

A number of multicenter trials have been performed by cooperative study groups to test the value of preoperative and postoperative combination chemotherapy in HBL and HCC. In some of the studies, radiotherapy was included as part of the treatment protocol. It has been demonstrated that a significant number of initially unresected tumors could be surgically removed after chemotherapy and that complete resection followed by adjuvant chemotherapy was superior to surgery alone.

In CCG trial 831,[186] patients with residual disease in one lobe after surgery received actinomycin D, vincristine, and cyclophosphamide combination chemotherapy and involved-field irradiation. Patients with disseminated tumors received chemotherapy alone. Of 40 children entered into the study, there were only 7 long-term survivors: those with either stage I disease or minor residual tumor who received irradiation.

In CCG trial 881,[186] doxorubicin and 5-fluorouracil were added to the actinomycin D, vincristine, and cyclophosphamide combination used in CCG 831. A response rate of 44% was observed in patients with measurable disease, and 83% of patients receiving the drug combination as an adjuvant treatment were disease-free at 30 months.

In CCG trial 823F,[186] patients with HBL (33 children) or HCC (14 children) confined to the liver received doxorubicin and cisplatin prior to definitive surgery. Although only 2 of 14 HCC patients survived, 78% of 25 HBL patients who completed chemotherapy and were eligible for surgery were alive without evidence of disease. In 16 patients, complete resection was performed, and no viable tumor was found in 9 of them at the time of surgery. Fifteen of these patients were alive and disease free. It was found that, for children with unresectable or metastatic HBL entered into this study, early changes in AFP levels were a reliable predictor of outcome and could identify poor responders to therapy. The authors suggested that if the AFP level failed to decrease by two logs prior to surgery, a surgical approach should probably not be attempted.[187]

In a trial performed by the Pediatric Hepatoma Study Intergroup (CCG 8881/POG 8945),[188] patients were allocated to receive either cisplatin, vincristine, and 5-fluorouracil or cisplatin and doxorubicin. Both chemotherapy regimens were equally effective in terms of overall and disease-free survival; however, the cisplatin plus doxorubicin combination was significantly more toxic.

POG study 8679[189] enrolled children with stage I to IV HBL. Children with stage I favorable histology received surgery alone. Children with stage I unfavorable histology or stage II disease received surgery and adjuvant cisplatin, vincristine, and 5-fluorouracil. Children with stage III or IV disease received five cycles of chemotherapy, after which they were evaluated for surgery. Unresectable patients received limited field irradiation, 33 to 39 Gy, and additional chemotherapy. The 3-year disease-free survival for stage I unfavorable histology and stage II patients was 91, for stage III it was 67, and for stage IV patients it was 13. Three of five irradiated patients underwent complete resection and were free of disease.

The International Society of Pediatric Oncology (SIOP) designed a series of clinical trials based on a risk-adapted treatment approach philosophy. In the SIOPEL I trial patients underwent a preoperative cisplatin-doxorubicin (PLADO) regimen.[190] The investigators concluded that the extent of pretreatment hepatic disease and the presence of pulmonary metastases were significant prognosticators of 5-year event-free survival. Survival for HCC patients was significantly inferior to that of children with HBL, and complete tumor excision remained the only realistic chance of cure. A novel staging system was developed, called *PRETEXT* (pretreatment extent of disease), and two risk clusters for treatment failure were identified: a "standard-risk" group, comprising patients with disease confined to the liver and involving up to three hepatic sectors, and a "high-risk" group, with disease extending to all four hepatic sectors or with extrahepatic spread. It was suggested that PLADO chemotherapy followed by delayed surgery and a short course of postoperative chemotherapy used in the SIOPEL I trial should be regarded as best treatment for children with HBL and that future treatment programs should be measured against this standard.[191,192]

In the SIOPEL II trial, patients were stratified according to standard- and high-risk groups. For high-risk HBL patients, treatment was intensified by adding carboplatin to the cisplatin/doxorubicin regimen used in the SIOPEL I trial, in a rapidly alternating sequence of administration.

For standard-risk HBL patients, 3-year overall and progression-free survivals were 91% and 89%, and for the high-risk HBL group, they were 53% and 48%, respectively. Despite chemotherapy intensification, only half of the high risk HBL patients were long-term survivors.[193] For standard-risk HBL patients, the efficacy of cisplatin monotherapy and cisplatin/doxorubicin combination are being compared in a prospective SIOPEL III randomized trial.[151]

Investigators from the United States analyzed the effectiveness of intrahepatic chemotherapy[194] and intrahepatic chemoembolization.[195] They concluded that these treatment modalities can halt the progression and possibly downstage advanced hepatic malignancies.

Japanese investigators used transarterial chemoembolization with lipiodol and cisplatin/etoposide, concluding that this treatment modality was particularly useful in potentiating the cytoreductive effect of antitumor drugs and also useful in reducing toxicities.[196]

Other Japanese investigators analyzed the survival outcome for patients with HBL treated by preoperative and/or postoperative chemotherapy using a combination of cisplatin and tetrahydropyranyl–Adriamycin.[197] They concluded that preoperative chemotherapy resulted in an improved resectability of the tumor, whereas postoperative chemotherapy played an important role in the increased cure rate of patients with an incomplete tumor resection or metastasis.

In the prospective, multicenter, single-arm German Liver Tumor Study HB94, children undergoing primary surgery received ifosfamide, cisplatin, and Adriamycin (IPA) chemotherapy and or etoposide and carboplatin. Treatment was risk stratified according to stage: stage I patients receive IPA ×2; stage II patients receive IPA ×2 to 3; and stage III or IV patients receive carboplatin/etoposide plus IPA. Growth pattern of the liver tumor, vascular tumor invasion, occurrence of distant metastases, initial AFP level, and surgical radicality were found to be pretreatment prognostic factors.[198]

In an interim analysis of the German Liver Tumor Study HB 99, it was shown that adding high-dose carboplatin and etoposide to the regimen for high-risk HBL patients was highly efficient and induced a remission in the majority of patients with advanced and metastasized high-risk HBL.[199]

Innovative radiotherapeutic approaches include intraoperative irradiation, intra-arterial yttrium-90 microspheres,[200,201–202] and intraluminal iridium-192 with or without regional hyperthermia.[203–205]

LANGERHANS CELL HISTIOCYTOSIS

Pathology

Histiocytosis results from dysregulation of the mononuclear cell line. Usually, after maturation in the bone marrow, monocytes migrate to the liver (Kupffer cells), bone marrow (macrophages), or connective tissue and skin (histiocytes). The Langerhans cell is characterized by the presence of the intracytoplasmic Birbeck granule of unknown origin but which develops only after an antigenic stimulation. Langerhans cell histiocytosis (LCH) is a proliferative disorder in which infiltration by Langerhans cells leads to tissue damage. The pathogenesis is not completely understood, but excessive production of interleukin 1, interleukin 17a prostaglandin, and metalloproteases MMP9 and MMP12,[206] as well as of prostaglandin E_2, has been demonstrated in affected bone. These factors can play a major role in osteoclast activation.

In the past, three subentities of LCH were recognized. In 1893, Hand[207] was the first to describe the *craniohypophysis xanthomatoses*. This was followed by reports by Christian and Schuller. Hand–Schuller–Christian disease is characterized by skull lesions, exophthalmos, and diabetes insipidus and occurs in children older than age 2 years.

Twenty years later, Letterer and Siwe described an entity in children younger than age 2 years, with splenomegaly, hepatomegaly, anemia, and hemorrhagic diathesis.

Twenty years after this, Otani and Erblich described the solitary eosinophilic granuloma in children older than 2 years with a characteristic bony site.[90,167,208] Lichtenstein[209] merged the variants into one entity, which he called *histiocytosis X*. It should be emphasized that it is not yet clear whether LCH is a malignant disorder. The finding of monoclonality has been described, but is not sufficient to establish the existence of malignancy. Moreover, Langerhans cells are not aneuploid, and LCH has been reported with Hodgkin disease.

Clinical Presentation

The annual incidence of LCH is 0.5 to 2 cases per 100,000 children.[210] The clinical presentation is age related. In children <2 years old, the disseminated form (Letterer–Siwe) is more frequent, with wasting, hepatosplenomegaly, and pancytopenia and sometimes with massive seborrheic dermatitis on the groin and scalp. The infant is often irritable and fails to thrive.[211,212]

In children older than 2 years, the disease is less aggressive, with widespread bone granulomas causing pain, otitis, diabetes insipidus (42%), and exophthalmos. Eosinophilic granuloma is characterized by bone involvement only and with symptoms related to the location of the granuloma.

Central nervous system involvement is possible; most frequently, meningeal and pituitary lesions occur, but intraparenchymal lesions, especially hypothalamic and cerebellar, can also be encountered.

Whatever the clinical presentation, the definitive diagnosis is made by biopsy confirming the presence of the Birbeck granule in a Langerhans cell. Staging procedures include a skeletal survey (rather than isotopic bone scan). Many prognostic scores have been proposed, all based on the extent of disease, age at diagnosis, and demonstrable organ dysfunction.[210] As suggested by Halperin et al.,[210] patients are classified into three groups:

1. Very favorable, with unifocal lesion requiring minimal therapy.
2. Very unfavorable, with organ dysfunction necessitating intensive therapy.
3. All others, not well defined, for which treatment by surgery, steroids, chemotherapy and/or radiotherapy may be required.

Treatment

Many cases of LCH are indolent or resolve spontaneously. Aggressive treatment therefore should not be given if there is no organ dysfunction.

Surgery

The POG 8047 study demonstrated that a similar control rate can be achieved (70% to 90%) with biopsy, curettage, or tumor excision.[213] Wide excision is recommended for expendable bones (clavicle, ribs) and biopsy for other sites. Curettage is not indicated if there is a risk of instability (cervical vertebra, femoral neck) or if a poor cosmetic or orthopedic outcome is likely.

Radiation Therapy

Radiation therapy was widely used in the 1960s but is no longer indicated in the large majority of cases. Radiation therapy could be discussed in a case of resistant cerebral location. The international study LCH2 compared vinblastine and etoposide, with no benefit seen for the latter. Thus, due to the risk of etoposide-induced leukemia, the drug should not be used as first-line therapy.[214]

Medical Treatment

In Situ Injection of Steroids

The procedure is performed under general anesthesia and fluoroscopic guidance. Methylprednisolone is injected directly into the granuloma.[215] It has not been proven whether the steroid or the local trauma is responsible for the effects.

Chemotherapy

The exact point in the course of the disease at which chemotherapy should be considered is controversial. There is little agreement on the factors that should be considered as bad prognostic signs. Only organ dysfunction and/or multiorgan disease have been generally accepted as indications for chemotherapy. Initially, high-dose steroids are used and followed, when necessary, by vinblastine. The LCH3 protocol failed also to find any advantage for methotrexate.[216] There is no proof that a multidrug regimen is more effective than single-agent chemotherapy as first-line therapy. Furthermore, it is unknown whether early treatment prevents the development of diabetes insipidus at a later stage.[217,218] Recently, promising results were reported using thalidomide for treatment of disseminated LCH.[219]

For resistant disease (especially in infants), a more aggressive approach, including cyclosporine, liver transplantation, bone marrow transplantation, and/or monoclonal antibody therapy, is under investigation.[220,221] Pamidronate has been shown to be effective in reducing bone pain secondary to skeletal involvement by LCH.[222]

ENDOCRINE TUMORS

Adrenocortical Carcinoma

Adrenocortical carcinoma (ACC) accounts for 0.2% of childhood cancer and in 75% of the cases occurs in children younger than 5 years, more commonly in females.[223–229] ACC is sometimes associated with Beckwith–Wiedemann syndrome and hemihypertrophy.[230]

Children with ACC may present with abdominal pain and a palpable mass. More than 75% of the tumors are functional, secreting one or more hormones: androgens, cortisol, aldosterone, or estrogens. The most common presenting sign is virilization, with deepening of the voice, hirsutism, premature pubic hair, clitoromegaly, phallomegaly, excessive muscular development, and advanced bone age. Pure Cushing syndrome (moon face, plethora, hypertension, striae, weight gain, acne, and "buffalo hump") is rare in children. Feminization or aldosterone-secreting tumors are also rare.[228]

Urinary 17-ketocorticosteroids and 17-hydroxycorticosteroids are usually elevated, with steroid production not influenced by adrenocorticotropic hormone suppression.

Diagnostic imaging studies include CT and/or MRI. It is sometimes difficult to separate ACC from adenoma. However, at presentation, most carcinomas are >6 cm and calcified, whereas benign adenomas are small and nonfunctional. A characteristic echogenic star pattern can be seen on ultrasonography, and CT scan shows an inhomogeneous tumor with irregular contrast material. Recently, the use of 18-FDG-PET has been shown to be effective in discriminating between benign and malignant adrenal lesions.[231,232] Because both benign adenomas and ACC may exhibit abnormal mitoses and cellular and nuclear pleomorphism, malignancy is determined by the finding of capsular penetration, invasion of the inferior vena cava up to the right atrium, lymph node, and distant metastases.[223]

Generally, the prognosis of ACC is poor.[233–235] Small, well-encapsulated, and easily excised tumors can be cured by surgery alone. In locally advanced cases, there is a significant risk of locoregional and metastatic relapse.[228,229] Repeat complete resection of local recurrences and discrete metastatic lesions can improve survival.[236]

The literature on adjuvant radiation therapy after resection of ACC is scarce and relatively old and consists of small series or case reports. Postoperative whole-abdominal irradiation (15 to 30 Gy) was administered by Stewart et al.[237] Three of four irradiated patients were long-term survivors. Percarpio and Knowlton[238] used preoperative irradiation, 45 to 50 Gy, to treat two patients and postoperative irradiation to treat four patients with unresectable tumors or spillage at the time of surgery. One patient who was treated preoperatively was rendered operable; three of four postoperatively treated patients relapsed in the field of radiation and one outside the field.

Magee et al.[239] reported a series of 15 patients with ACC, 9 of whom received postoperative irradiation. Three of the irradiated patients were girls under the age of 2 years, who received

Clinical Radiation Oncology

30 Gy in 4 weeks. Two of these girls died as the result of a second malignancy arising in the irradiated volume.

Based on these results and the results of similar small retrospective series,[224,240–241,242] it is difficult to make any firm recommendations on the role of radiotherapy in ACC. Investigators from the United Kingdom reported a relatively high frequency of second, fatal, primary tumors, especially if radiotherapy was part of the treatment protocol.[243]

Mitotane (o,p-DDD) is the most frequently used chemotherapeutic agent for recurrent or metastatic ACC, with a response rate of approximately 20%. Other agents include suramin, doxorubicin, 5-fluorouracil, streptozotocin, cisplatin, and etoposide, alone or in combination, with response rates of 20% to 30%.[244] The administration of adjuvant chemotherapy is controversial. Some investigators advocate the use of adjuvant mitotane after surgery[240]; however, the administration of this drug is associated with significant gastrointestinal, neuromuscular, and skin toxicity, as well as with abnormal platelet aggregation and prolongation of bleeding time. There is also a significant decrease in urinary 17-hydroxysteroids and 17-ketosteroids. The response rates to mitotane are highly dependent on obtaining adequate serum levels (>10 to 14 mcg/mL), and the therapeutic window between toxicity and efficacy is quite narrow. Hence, most authorities agree that in the absence of solid data based on randomized, well-controlled clinical trials, it is difficult to justify the administration of radiation or chemotherapy in the adjuvant setting.[154,243,245]

PHEOCHROMOCYTOMA AND PARAGANGLIOMA

Pheochromocytoma and paraganglioma are rare tumors of childhood and adolescence.[246–251] Pediatric pheochromocytoma occurs usually between 8 and 14 years of age, more frequently in males. More than 90% of all pheochromocytomas in adults, and 70% of pheochromocytomas in children, originate in the adrenal gland, but the tumor can occur at any site in the sympathetic chain, most commonly below the diaphragm. The most common sites of occurrence of extra-adrenal pheochromocytoma are the superior para-aortic region, between the diaphragm and the lower renal poles, in the paraganglia, the organs of Zuckerkandl, and the bladder. Extra-abdominal tumors may develop in the brain, thorax, and the bladder.[246,250,252,253] Approximately 10% of all patients with pheochromocytoma are children, but several characteristics distinguish them from their adult counterparts. Unlike pheochromocytomas of the adult age group, children with pheochromocytoma have a higher incidence of bilaterality, a higher association with the multiple endocrine neoplasia (MEN) syndromes, and a lower incidence of malignant neoplasms.[246,252,254–256]

Familial pheochromocytoma is associated with other endocrine tumors in the MEN IIa and IIb syndromes.[252,257,258–259]

In addition to the familial syndrome of isolated pheochromocytomas, pheochromocytomas in the pediatric age group can be associated with other inherited diseases, such as von Hippel–Lindau disease (retinocerebral angiomatosis), tuberous sclerosis, and von Recklinghausen neurofibromatosis.

Malignant pheochromocytomas occur in 10% of the pediatric cases of pheochromocytoma. The definition of malignancy is based on biologic and clinical behavior and not on histologic features alone.

Pheochromocytoma is responsible for 1% of cases of childhood hypertension, which, unlike the situation in adults, is sustained and not paroxysmal. Other signs and symptoms include diaphoresis, flushing, fatigue, headache, and convulsions.[260]

Adrenal pheochromocytomas produce epinephrine and norepinephrine, but most extra-adrenal pheochromocytomas produce only norepinephrine.

Urinary epinephrine, norepinephrine, metanephrine, and vanillylmandelic acid values remain the gold standard for biochemical screening of pheochromocytoma. On some occasions, urinary catecholamine levels may be normal while serum levels are elevated. Imaging studies include ultrasonography, CT scan, and/or MRI. Iodine-131 metaiodobenzylguanidine (MIBG) scan provides the most accurate and direct method of diagnosing adrenal, extra-adrenal, or metastatic pheochromocytoma because MIBG, which has a molecular structure similar to that of norepinephrine, is actively concentrated and stored in catecholamine storage vesicles of pheochromocytoma cells.[246,252,261–263]

Surgery is the definitive therapy. The most significant reduction in preoperative and postoperative mortality has come from the control of perioperative hypertension using alpha and beta blockers.[25,264]

External-beam irradiation is used for palliation of lymph node, bone, brain, and spinal cord metastases. High-dose iodine-131 MIBG has been used with modest results in metastatic disease. Streptozotocin or cyclophosphamide, vincristine, and dacarbazine may produce modest decreases in catecholamine secretion in patients with malignant pheochromocytoma.[244] Patients with malignant pheochromocytoma require chronic medical control of their elevated blood pressure by alpha and beta blockade or inhibition of catecholamine synthesis with α-methyl-para-tyrosine.[265–267]

THYROID CARCINOMA

Thyroid carcinoma accounts for 1% to 1.5% of all cases of cancer in the pediatric and adolescent age groups, with between 0.4 and 1.5 cases per million, two to three times as frequent in girls as in boys.[268,269] After the April 26, 1986, Chernobyl nuclear reactor accident, a remarkable increase of incidence was observed in children exposed to radioactive iodine (RAI) fallout.[270,271] The incidence of thyroid cancer in Belarus and Ukraine began to rise sharply in 1989 to 1990: in adults, the number of new cases increased twofold to threefold, and in children <20 years of age, and particularly during the first 5 years of life, the number of new cases increased 20- to 30-fold.[270,272] Almost all new pediatric cases were papillary tumors (94% to 98%), with a relatively high incidence of lymph node (65%) and lung (5%) metastases at presentation (Table 90.6).[272]

Follicular carcinoma is characterized by vascular invasion and accounts for 16% to 20% of cases.

Medullary carcinomas are rare. These tumors develop from the neural crest parafollicular or C cells and tend to be more aggressive than the differentiated carcinomas and can be fatal. They are associated with the immunoreactive thyrocalcitonin

TABLE 90.6 HISTOLOGIC TYPES OF CHILDHOOD THYROID CANCER

Type	Frequency (%)	Characteristics
1. Differentiated carcinoma		
A. Papillary carcinoma	70–80	Infiltrative and multicentric; lymph node metastases in 70%–90% of cases; hematogenous spread (mainly lung) in 5%–10% of cases
B. Follicular carcinoma	16–20	Vascular invasion
2. Medullary carcinoma	Rare	Occurs in isolation, but more frequently associated with one of the multiple endocrine neoplasia syndromes; usually aggressive and can be fatal
3. Undifferentiated carcinoma	Rare	Aggressive, usually fatal within 6 months of diagnosis
4. Insular carcinoma	Very rare	A variant of the poorly differentiated carcinoma; aggressive, poor prognosis

marker. Because of the aggressive clinical course, experts advocate genetic testing to identify affected individuals with specific mutations in the ret oncogene that predict for MEN syndromes. Those individuals could be candidates for prophylactic thyroidectomy at an earlier age than if the increase in serum calcitonin was used to identify C-cell hyperplasia or early carcinoma. At present, genetic testing should be performed at birth in children suspected of having the MEN IIa syndrome and no later than 1 year of age for those with possible MEN IIb.[273–275]

Children with thyroid cancer are commonly euthyroid and usually present with a thyroid nodule or palpable cervical lymph node. Conventional radiographs may show calcifications in the region of the thyroid gland (psammoma bodies). Iodine radionuclide scan may show a cold nodule.

Paradoxically, despite the fact that 70% to 80% of patients present with regional lymph node involvement and approximately 20% have distant metastases at diagnosis, the prognosis of differentiated thyroid cancer in children and adolescents is excellent.[1,275,276,277] In the Mayo Clinic series, survival rates for children did not differ significantly from those of matched controls at 20 to 30 years.[278] In the Royal Marsden series,[279] the median overall survival was 53 years, and the median survival for patients who developed recurrence was 30 years. The only presenting feature predictive of poorer survival was the presence of metastases at diagnosis. According to a study reported by the Surgical Discipline Committee of the Children's Cancer Group, the overall survival for children presenting with distant metastases was 100% at 10 years. The progression-free survival rate was 76% at 5 years and 66% at 10 years. In a series of 14 children with papillary thyroid cancer and pulmonary metastases treated at the Mayo Clinic[280] by various surgical procedures, RAI, external-beam irradiation (one patient), and suppressive hormone therapy, at a mean follow-up time of 19.3 years 50% were alive completely free of disease and 50% were alive and asymptomatic with residual pulmonary disease.

Thyroid carcinoma is treated primarily by surgery. The extent of surgery for the primary tumor (subtotal lobectomy, lobectomy, total thyroidectomy) and involved lymph nodes (node picking, modified or radical neck dissection) is controversial.[281]

The arguments in favor of total thyroidectomy include the multifocality of the tumor, decrease in neck recurrences, the ability to use serum thyroglobulin as a tumor marker after radical surgery, and the ability to detect pulmonary metastases by radioactive iodine scan earlier. The arguments for more limited surgery are mainly the increased complication rate of radical surgery, with apparently no clear survival advantage.[1,274–275,276,279,282–284,285,286]

The use of RAI for routine ablation of remaining thyroid tissue after surgery in patients without any known metastatic disease is another area of controversy. Because the mortality rate of pediatric thyroid cancer is extremely low and recurrences can develop many years after surgery, it is impossible to perform randomized trials to answer therapeutic questions. However, most authorities support the administration of RAI in this setting because of the high incidence of nodal and systemic metastases of thyroid cancer in the young.[272,287]

RAI is indicated in patients with cervical lymph node involvement or distant metastases. The radiopharmaceutical is taken up by 50% to 80% of well-differentiated tumors and is able to deliver high focal doses of irradiation to any remaining thyroid tissue.

Side effects of RAI include nausea, glossalgia, hypogeusia, thyroiditis, and gastrointestinal discomfort. Potential and rare long-term complications include myelosuppression, leukemia, bladder cancer, salivary cancer, gastric cancer, breast cancer, and infertility. These complications were mainly reported in the past, when high, repetitive doses of RAI were used and should not occur, or occur rarely, with today's treatment policies and dosages.[272,287]

RAI concentrates in the salivary glands and is secreted into the saliva. Following the administration of high dose RAI, salivary gland swelling and pain, usually involving the parotid gland, can be seen in conjunction with radiation sialadenitis. Secondary complications reported include xerostomia, taste alterations, increases in caries, stomatitis, and candidiasis.[288,289]

Exogenous thyroid hormone is given to suppress thyroid-stimulating hormone production and to decrease the probability of tumor recurrence. Exogenous thyroid hormone is also given as replacement therapy to keep the patients euthyroid despite thyroidectomy.[45,279,280]

External-beam irradiation in children with differentiated thyroid cancer is indicated for unresectable primary tumor or cervical or mediastinal lymph nodes that do not take up RAI. It also has a role in advanced locoregional disease, with extensive extrathyroid extension, or where there is gross residual tumor after attempted surgical excision or when definitive resection has not been possible. Although external-beam irradiation is useful for palliative therapy of advanced or metastatic disease, the lack of randomized controlled studies makes its role as part of initial adjuvant treatment controversial, and it is rarely indicated for microscopic residual disease. Radiotherapy, with or without chemotherapy, can be administered in children with anaplastic thyroid carcinoma.[277]

External-beam irradiation for thyroid cancer requires careful and meticulous treatment planning in order to minimize acute toxicity and avoid serious long-term complications. The volume of irradiation is adjusted according to operative and pathologic findings and can range from whole-neck and upper mediastinal irradiation to just treating the thyroid gland or thyroid bed.

The anatomy of the area causes significant technical difficulties, especially because the treatment volume curves around the vertebral bodies. CT-based planning, three-dimensional treatment planning, or IMRT is advocated to allow the administration of curative doses (in the range of 55 to 65 Gy) to the target volume without compromising spinal cord tolerance. This can be achieved by a variety of techniques.[290]

GERM CELL TUMORS

Gonadal or extragonadal germ cell tumors (GCTs) represent <2% of pediatric cancer. Their cure rate is high and strongly correlated with adherence to strict treatment guidelines.

Pathology

The tumor is the result of neoplastic transformation of primitive germ cells or totipotent embryonal cells (Fig. 90.3).[291] The site of the tumor depends on the site of arrest of the neoplastic cell during migration from the brain to the sacrococcygeal region in the fetal period. The most common sites are testis, ovary, sacrococcygeal region, retroperitoneum, and mediastinum. Aberrant migration can occur, which explains unusual tumor sites.[292] The Children's Oncology Group evaluated the link between a family history of cancer and pediatric GCT in a case–control study of 274 cases. The risk of GCT decreased among female cases with a family history with onset before 40 years but increased for boys, especially for those with a family history of melanoma.[293] The most frequent cytogenetic abnormality is the isochromosome 12p for both gonadal and extragonadal GCT, except for children <3 years of age at diagnosis. Klinefelter syndrome can be associated with GCT in boys.[270] Intracranial germ cell tumors are discussed in Chapter 84.

Clinical Presentation

Abdominal pain, abdominal distention, and sacrococcygeal or buttock swelling are the frequent presenting signs.[294] Staging includes imaging both of the primary tumor and most frequent sites of metastatic dissemination (lungs, liver, brain, and bone).

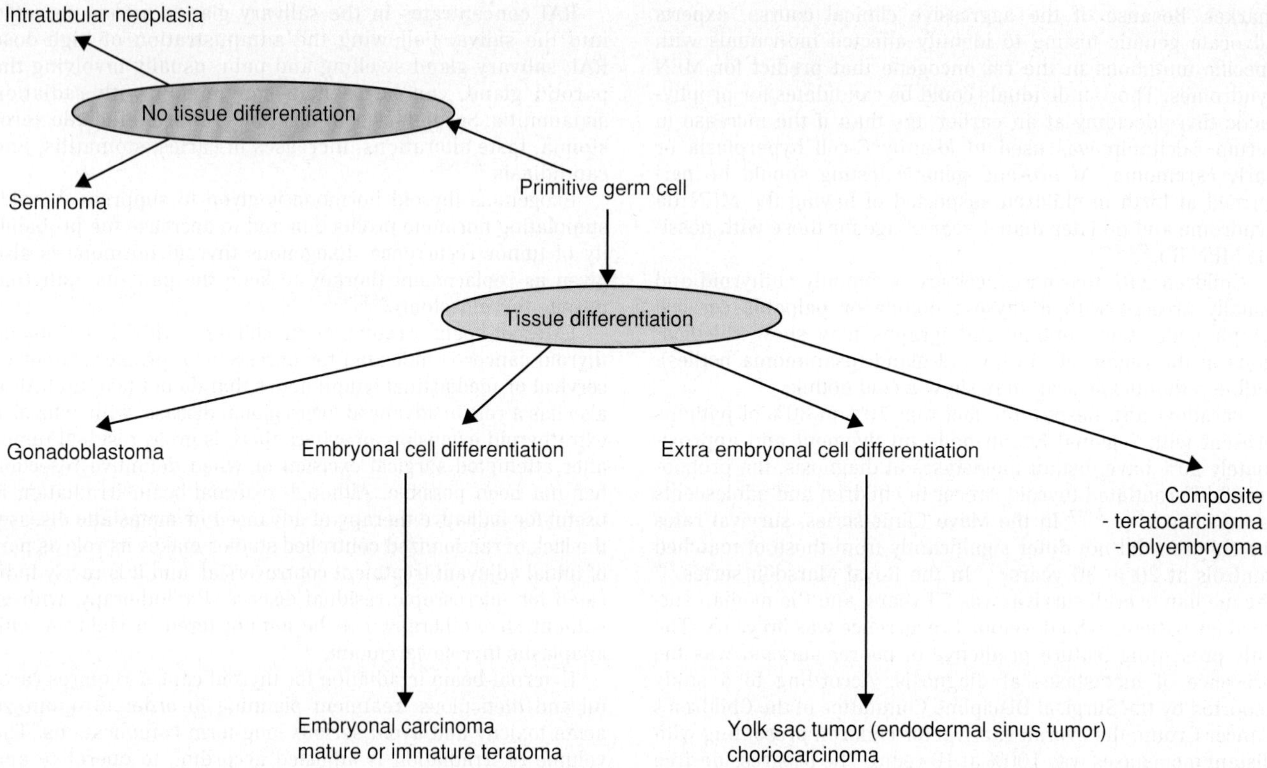

FIGURE 90.3. Classification of germ cell tumors.

Serum AFP, β-HCG, lactate dehydrogenase, CEA, and placental alkaline phosphatase levels are mandatory prior to the initiation of any treatment. Serum AFP level must be interpreted according to patient age (level >1,000 mg/mL is normal until the age of 1 month). Clinical markers are strongly correlated with some histologic features (Table 90.7); however, high AFP levels can be detected in infectious diseases of the liver, and increased β-HCG level can be associated with malignancies other than choriocarcinoma. The half-life time of AFP is 5 to 7 days and that of β-HCG is 24 to 36 hours. Both are very useful tools for predicting and monitoring treatment response, progression of disease, and relapse.[295]

Treatment

Surgery is the standard treatment for mature teratomas and sacrococcygeal tumors (with complete removal of the tumor and the coccyx), but it may be combined with chemotherapy to limit the extent of irradiation. Surgery is often the first treatment for malignant gonadal GCT: orchiectomy with high inguinal ligation or ovariectomy with careful peritoneal cavity exploration. Lymph node dissection is not recommended in early-stage GCT, especially in germinomas. Second-look surgery can be indicated in cases of residual disease (clinical or biochemical) after chemotherapy.

TABLE 90.7 GERM CELL TUMOR AND CLINICAL MARKERS

Tumor Type	β-HCG	AFP	LDH	CEA	PLAP
Embryonal carcinoma	+	+		+	
Mature teratoma					
Immature teratoma	+	+	+	+	
Yolk sac tumor		+++	+	+	
Choriocarcinoma	+++		+		
Germinoma	+		+	+	+++

AFP, α-fetoprotein; β-HCG, human chorionic gonadotropin; CEA, carcinoembryonic antigen; LDH, lactate dehydrogenase; PLAP, placental alkaline phosphatase.

Since the introduction of cisplatin-based chemotherapy, the survival rate of GCT has risen from 60% to 90%,[296] and regimens used are similar to those used in the adult age group. There is now a trend to use carboplatin in order to reduce late toxicities.[297] The value of rate of decline of serum tumor markers has been proven to be of prognostic significance and must be used in the management of poor-risk patients.[191] Radiotherapy is rarely indicated except for some cases of early-stage ovarian germinoma in adolescents (dose, 20 to 25 Gy). The use of radiotherapy for ovarian germinoma in the young, however, must be compared with salvage chemotherapy after surgery alone. In advanced cases of ovarian dysgerminoma, careful surgical staging followed by conservative resection and chemotherapy without radiotherapy results in an overall survival rate as high as 85% without compromising the possibility of future pregnancy.[50] There is no indication for radiotherapy after complete response in extragonadal GCT. For stage IA ovarian dysgerminoma, conservative surgery is the gold standard, even in a case of incomplete staging, and chemotherapy is given only in the event of relapse, according to the last Italian group report.[298]

HEMANGIOMAS AND LYMPHANGIOMA

Hemangiomas

Hemangiomas constitute a very common vascular abnormality of infancy. In some cases their development can be associated with adverse cosmetic effects, unacceptable symptoms, and organ compression that in certain cases could be life-threatening. Such cases require therapy. There are two distinct types of hemangiomas[299]: dynamic lesions, which include cellular hemangiomas, capillary hemangiomas, and cavernous hemangiomas; and adynamic lesions, which include port wine stains, telangiectasias, and venous lakes. Radiation therapy is very rarely used in the treatment of hemangiomas. It is generally considered only for lesions that are not likely to spontaneously regress and when other therapies have been tried and

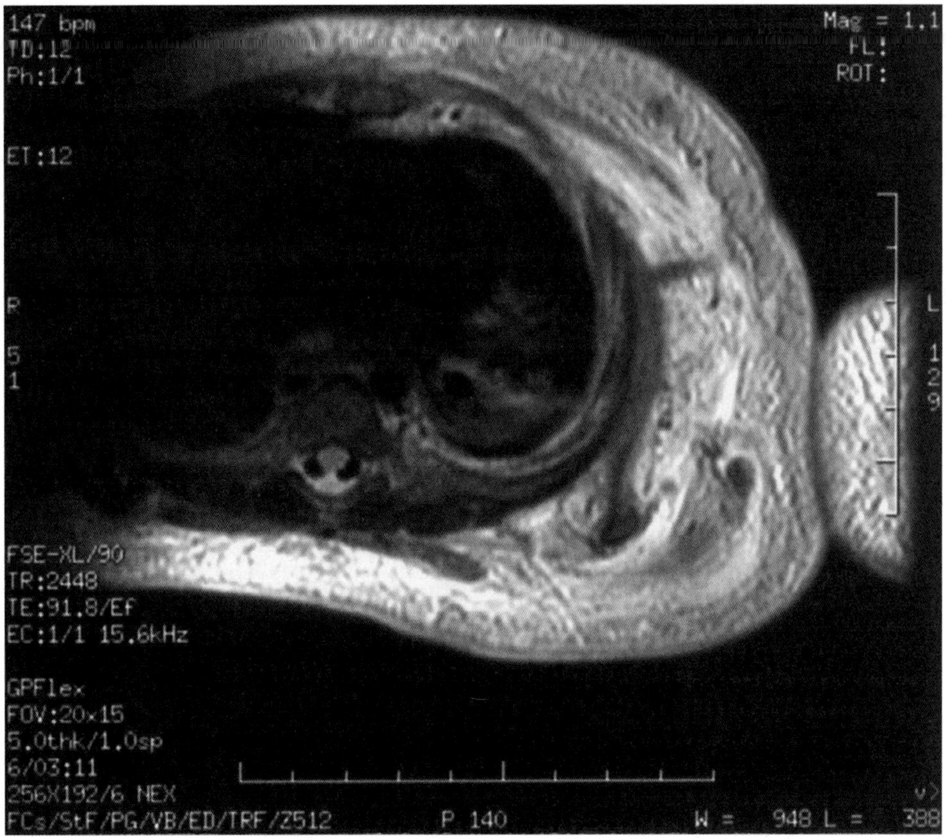

FIGURE 90.4. Kasabach–Merritt syndrome. Massive left hemithorax infiltration and involvement of the left arm.

failed. Second malignant neoplasms have been described in long-term survivors of radiotherapy for hemangioma. Steroids or interferon are considered first-line therapy. Only cavernous and capillary hemangiomas are suitable for radiotherapy. In infants, a total dose of 7.5 Gy in three fractions is often sufficient for capillary hemangioma. Higher doses (30 to 40 Gy) are used in older patients for large and progressive lesions. Special attention must be given to the Kasabach–Merritt syndrome (KMS) (Fig. 90.4), which is defined as combination of cutaneous vascular abnormalities with or without visceral involvement and thrombopenia due to intravascular coagulopathy. KMS is associated only with Kaposi-like hemangioendothelioma or tufted angioma. Kaposi-like hemangioendothelioma must be distinguished from infantile hemangioma, which disappears spontaneously.[300,301] There are alarming hemangiomas with life-threatening lesions (mediastinum, lower extremities, abdomen) either due to compression or secondary to a thrombocytic coagulopathy or high-output cardiac failure. A dose of 10 Gy in 10 fractions can be given; it is not mandatory to encompass the whole hemangioma in the target volume.[302,303]

Cavernous hemangiomas can be located in the epidural space and cause spinal cord compression. Surgical resection is the standard treatment.[304]

Gamma-knife radiosurgery has been employed successfully for circumscribed choroidal hemangioma.[305]

Lymphangiomas

Histologically, lymphangiomas are a benign proliferation of lymph vessels. Four types are recognized: (a) capillary lymphangiomas, (b) cavernous lymphangiomas, (c) cystic hygromas, and (d) lymphangeal hemangiomas. Surgery is the treatment of choice.

Special attention must be given to the Gorham syndrome, also known as the bone-vanishing syndrome or massive osteolysis of bone.[306] Gorham syndrome is a bone hamartoma with various percentages of lymphangioma and hemangioma, characterized by well-margined osteolytic scattered lesions that progressively affect the cortex, with no respect for joint boundaries (Fig. 90.5). All bones can be affected (vertebrae, ribs, scapula). Progression is unpredictable, from spontaneous remission to bone absorption and sometimes even death. The prognosis is very poor when pleural or visceral involvement develops. Some encouraging results have been reported using antiresorptive therapy such as calcitonin or biphosphonates.[307] Although radiotherapy is the last resort for the patient, encouraging results have been reported for patients with chylothorax and with patients with rib, thorax, and vertebral body involvement. The usual dose is ~18 Gy to the hemithorax and ~40 Gy to the affected bone.[308] An encouraging response has been reported for base-of-skull lesions with doses of 40 Gy.[309,310]

DESMOPLASTIC SMALL ROUND-CELL TUMOR

Desmoplastic small round-cell tumor (DSRCT) was first described in 1989.[311] It is a rare aggressive neoplasm with typical clinical, histologic, karyotypic, and biologic characteristics. DSRCT mainly affects male adolescents and young adults, but it sometimes occurs in young females. Clinically, patients present with a bulky abdominal or pelvic mass, but intracranial, testicular, renal soft tissue, and bone DSRCTs have also been described.[312,313,314–315]

The tumor is characterized by a desmoplastic stroma with circumscribed tumor cells and encased nests of primitive undifferentiated cells. The tumoral cells express epithelial (keratin, EMA), conjunctival (vimentin), muscular (desmin), and neuroendocrinal markers.

Reciprocal translocation (11:22) (p13:q12) has been described, which results from a fusion between the terminal part of the Ewing sarcoma gene (EWS) and the carboxy terminus part of the Wilms tumor gene (WT1).[316]

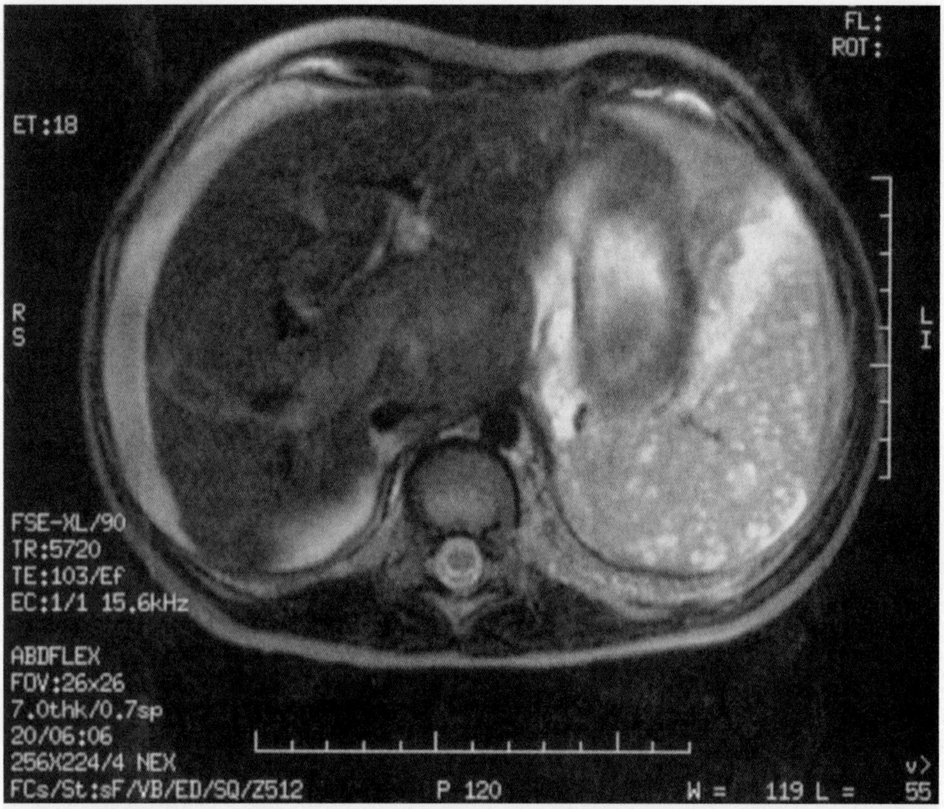

FIGURE 90.5. Gorham disease in a 3-year-old girl. Diffuse lymphangiomatosis affecting pelvic bones, ribs, spleen, and liver.

The DSRCTs are highly chemosensitive, but the prognosis is still poor. Kretschmar et al.,[317] reviewed 101 cases of DSRCT: after 2 years, only 2 patients were still alive, and the median survival was 17 months.

More recently, investigators from the Memorial Sloan-Kettering Cancer Center reported a series of 66 patients treated with high-dose alkylating agents–based chemotherapy with autologous bone marrow transplantation, surgical debulking, and whole-abdominopelvic radiotherapy. The dose to the whole abdomen was 30 Gy (1.5 Gy twice daily), and patients with gross residual disease received a boost of 6 to 15 Gy. The 3-year overall survival was 48%, but the progression-free survival was only 35% in the first report.[317] In a more recent publication, a slightly better survival rate at 3 years (55%) was reported.[318] Survival at 3 years was only 27% when the three modalities were not used, with only 10 patients surviving without evidence of disease at a median follow-up of 2.4 years.

MD Anderson Cancer Center published an outpatient and home chemotherapy program, including neoadjuvant chemotherapy, continuous hyperthermic peritoneal perfusion with cisplatin, and abdominal radiation (30 Gy) with simultaneous temozolomide with an overall survival at 3 years of 71% among eight patients.[319,320]

SKIN CANCER

Basal and squamous cell carcinomas are rare in children and adolescents. When they occur in the pediatric and adolescent age groups, there is usually an underlying predisposing genetic disorder, such as basal cell nevus syndrome (BCNS) or Gorlin–Goltz syndrome and xeroderma pigmentosum. Basal and squamous carcinomas have also been reported to arise in nevus sebaceous[321] and after radiation for benign or malignant conditions.[322,323]

BCNS or Gorlin–Goltz syndrome[208,324–326] is an autosomal dominant disorder with variable penetration characterized by a "coarse face" with hypertelorism and frontal bossing, multiple basal cell carcinomas presenting at a young age, pits on the palms and soles, skeletal abnormalities (e.g., bifid ribs, hemivertebrae, fusion of vertebral bodies), jaw cysts, epidermic cysts and hamartomas, oculoneurologic abnormalities, and ectopic calcification of the falx cerebri and other structures. Skin lesions located in the head and neck tend to invade the deep structures. Several patients with BCNS were reported to have developed medulloblastoma at early childhood and ovarian fibromas.[134,208,327–332]

Mutation of the human homologue of *Drosophila* Patched (PTC) gene is considered to be the molecular defect in BCNS.[332,333] The Gorlin–Goltz syndrome is a unique example of the genetic–environmental interaction for the production of malignancies: children treated for medulloblastoma by craniospinal irradiation developed multiple skin cancers in the irradiated area, an unusual and special illustration of multihit mutagenesis, suggesting that radiotherapy should probably be omitted or limited in children with BCNS.[332]

Xeroderma pigmentosum (XP) is an extremely rare, autosomal-recessive inherited disease characterized by abnormal pigmentation and >1,000-fold increase in nonmelanoma skin cancer (basal cell carcinoma and squamous cell carcinoma) on sun-exposed skin. XP patients are also at a significant risk to develop melanoma.[334,335] Neurologic abnormalities such as areflexia and mental retardation are sometimes associated with XP.

The genetic abnormality underlying XP leads to defects in nucleotide excision repair of ultraviolet-induced DNA damage.[334,336,337]

Skin cancer in affected children is treated by standard techniques (such as surgery, cryosurgery, chemosurgery). There should not be any contraindication to using radiotherapy to treat skin cancer or any other malignancy in XP patients because ionizing radiation damage is normally repaired in these patients.[338]

MALIGNANT MELANOMA

Childhood melanoma can sometimes be associated with large congenital nevocytic nevi, dysplastic nevus syndrome, immunosuppression, transplacental malignant melanoma, and xeroderma pigmentosum.[339–345] Pediatric malignant melanoma should be distinguished from the juvenile melanoma or Spitz nevus characterized by a relatively benign course and long-term survival.[346–348]

The management of childhood melanoma follows the guidelines set for adult patients.[349] The prognosis is related to the Breslow's or Clark's thickness of the primary lesion and nodal status. Radiotherapy has a role mainly for palliation of metastatic disease or in locally advanced lesions.

SELECTED REFERENCES

A full list of references for this chapter is available online.

6. Al Sarraf M, LeBlanc M, Giri PG, et al. Chemoradiotherapy versus radiotherapy in patients with advanced nasopharyngeal cancer: phase III randomized Intergroup study 0099. *J Clin Oncol* 1998;16:1310–1317.
7. Cheng SH, Jian JJ, Tsai SY, et al. Long-term survival of nasopharyngeal carcinoma following concomitant radiotherapy and chemotherapy. *Int J Radiat Oncol Biol Phys* 2000;48:1323–1330
8. Wolden SL, Steinherz PG, Kraus DH, et al. Improved long-term survival with combined modality therapy for pediatric nasopharynx cancer. *Int J Radiat Oncol Biol Phys* 2000;46:859–864.
10. Uzel O, Yoruk SO, Sahinler I, et al. Nasopharyngeal carcinoma in childhood: long-term results of 32 patients. *Radiother Oncol* 2001;58:137–141.
13. Orbach D, Brisse H, Helfre S, et al. Radiation and chemotherapy combination for nasopharyngeal carcinoma in children: radiotherapy dose adaptation after chemotherapy response to minimize late effects. *Pediatr Blood Cancer* 2008;50: 849–853.
14. Cheuk DK, Billups CA, Martin MG, et al. Prognostic factors and long-term outcomes of childhood nasopharyngeal carcinoma. *Cancer* 2011;117:197–206.
15. Lai SZ, Li WF, Chen L, et al. How does intensity-modulated radiotherapy versus conventional two-dimensional radiotherapy influence the treatment results in nasopharyngeal carcinoma patients? *Int J Radiat Oncol Biol Phys* 2011;80: 661–668.
19. Rosenblatt E, Brook OR, Erlich N, et al. Late visual and auditory toxicity of radiotherapy for nasopharyngeal carcinoma. *Tumori* 2003;89:68–74.
23. Gregoire V, Levendag P, Ang KK, et al. CT-based delineation of lymph node levels and related CTVs in the node-negative neck: DAHANCA, EORTC, GORTEC, NCIC, RTOG consensus guidelines. *Radiother Oncol* 2003;69: 227–236.
26. Eich HT, Staar S, Micke O, et al. Radiotherapy of esthesioneuroblastoma. *Int J Radiat Oncol Biol Phys* 2001;49:155–160.
27. Broich G, Pagliari A, Ottaviani F. Esthesioneuroblastoma: a general review of the cases published since the discovery of the tumour in 1924. *Anticancer Res* 1997;17:2683–2706.
28. Demiroz C, Gutfeld O, Aboziada M, et al. Esthesioneuroblastoma: is there a need for elective neck treatment? *Int J Radiat Oncol Biol Phys* 2011;81:255–261.
30. Mishima Y, Nagasaki E, Terui Y, et al. Combination chemotherapy (cyclophosphamide, doxorubicin, and vincristine with continuous-infusion cisplatin and etoposide) and radiotherapy with stem cell support can be beneficial for adolescents and adults with estheisoneuroblastoma. *Cancer* 2004;101:1437–1444.
31. Sohrabi S, Drabick JJ, Crist H, et al. Neoadjuvant concurrent chemoradiation for advanced esthesioneuroblastoma: a case series and review of the literature. *J Clin Oncol* 2011;29:358–361.
34. Valanzano R, Curia MC, Aceto G, et al. Genetic evidence that juvenile nasopharyngeal angiofibroma is an integral FAP tumour. *Gut* 2005;54:1046–1047.
36. Enepekides DJ. Recent advances in the treatment of juvenile angiofibroma. *Curr Opin Otolaryngol Head Neck Surg* 2004;12:495–499.
37. Wormald PJ, Van Hasselt A. Endoscopic removal of juvenile angiofibromas. *Otolaryngol Head Neck Surg* 2003;129:684–691.
39. Chakraborty S, Ghoshal S, Patil VM, et al. Conformal radiotherapy in the treatment of advanced juvenile nasopharyngeal angiofibroma with intracranial extension: an institutional experience. *Int J Radiat Oncol Biol Phys* 2011;80: 1398–1404.
47. Dosios T, Stinios J, Nicolaides P, et al. Pleuropulmonary blastoma in childhood. A malignant degeneration of pulmonary cysts. *Pediatr Surg Int* 2004;20: 863–865.
48. Priest JR, Andic D, Arbuckle S, Gonzalez-Gomez I, Hill DA, Williams G. Great vessel/cardiac extension and tumor embolism in pleuropulmonary blastoma: a report from the International Pleuropulmonary Blastoma Registry. *Pediatr Blood Cancer* 2011;56:604–609.
50. Ayhan A, Bildirici I, Gunalp S, et al. Pure dysgerminoma of the ovary: a review of 45 well staged cases. *Eur J Gynaecol Oncol* 2000;21:98–101.
54. Parsons SK, Fishman SJ, Hoorntie LE, et al. Aggressive multimodal treatment of pleuropulmonary blastoma. *Ann Thorac Surg* 2001;72:939–942.
55. Pinarli FG, Oguz A, Ceyda K, et al. Type II pleuropulmonary blastoma responsive to multimodal therapy. *Pediatr Hematol Oncol* 2005;22:71–76.
62. Umanah IN, Akhiwu W, Ojo OS. Breast tumors of adolescents in an African population. *Afr J Paediatr Surg* 2010;7:78–80.
72. Bond SJ, Buchino JJ, Nagaraj HS, et al. Sentinel lymph node biopsy in juvenile secretory carcinoma. *J Pediatr Surg* 2004;39:120–121.
97. Brenner B, Ilson DH, Minsky BD. Treatment of localized esophageal cancer. *Semin Oncol* 2004;31:554–65.
98. Jaeger HJ, Schmitz-Stolbrink A, Albrecht M, et al. Gastric leiomyosarcoma in a child. *Eur J Radiol* 1996;23:111–114.
99. Harting MT, Blakely ML, Herzog CE, et al. Treatment issues in pediatric gastric adenocarcinoma. *J Pediatr Surg* 2004;39:8–10.
100. Macdonald JS, Smalley S, Bendedetti J, et al. Postoperative combined radiation and chemotherapy improves disease-free survival (DFS) and overall survival (OS) in resected adenocarcinoma of the stomach and G.E. junction. *N Engl J Med* 2001;345:725–730.
102. Albarello L, Pecciarini L, Doglioni C. HER2 testing in gastric cancer. *Adv Anat Pathol* 2011;18:53–59.
103. Yiang Y, Ajani JA. Multidisciplinary management of gastric cancer. *Curr Opin Gastroenterol* 2010;26:640–646.
109. Church JM, McGannon E, Burke C, et al. Teenagers with familial adenomatous polyposis: what is their risk for colorectal cancer. *Dis Colon Rectum* 2002;45: 887–889.
114. Hill DA, Furman WL, Billups CA, et al. Colorectal carcinoma in childhood and adolescence: a clinicopathologic review. *J Clin Oncol* 2007;25:5808–5814.
115. Kravarusic D, Feigin E, Dlugy E, et al. Colorectal carcinoma in childhood: a retrospective multicenter study. *J Pediatr Gastroenterol Nutr* 2007;44:209–211.
121. Moertel CG, Weiland LH, Nagorney DM, et al. Carcinoid tumor of the appendix: treatment and prognosis. *N Engl J Med* 1987;317:1699–1701.
123. Shorter NA, Glick RD, Klimstra DS, et al. Malignant pancreatic tumors in childhood and adolescence: the Memorial Sloan-Kettering experience, 1967 to present. *J Pediatr Surg* 2002;37:887–892.
124. Bien E, Godzinski J, Dall'igna P, et al. Pancreatoblastoma: a report from the European cooperative study group for paediatric rare tumors (EXPeRT). *Eur J Cancer* 2011;47:2347–2352.
131. Defachelles AS, Martin De Lassalle E, Boutard P, et al. Pancreatoblastoma in childhood: clinical course and therapeutic management of seven patients. *Med Pediatr Oncol* 2001;37:47–52.
172. Habrand J-L, Nehme D, Kalifa C, et al. Is there a place for radiation therapy in the management of hepatoblastoma and hepatocellular carcinomas in children. *Int J Radiat Oncol Biol Phys* 1992;23:525–531.
174. Mody RJ, Pohlen JA, Malde S, et al. FDG PET for the study of primary hepatic malignancies in children. *Pediatr Blood Cancer* 2006;47:51–55.
177. Casanova M, Massimino M, Ferrari A, et al. Etoposide, cisplatin, epirubicin chemotherapy in the treatment of pediatric liver tumors. *Pediatr Hematol Oncol* 2005; 22:189–198.
178. Cheng AL, Kang YK, Chen Z, et al. Efficacy and safety of soratenib in the Asia-Pacific region with advanced hepatocellular carcinoma: a phase III randomized, double blind, placebo-controlled trial. *Lancet Oncol* 2009;10:25–34.
190. Czauderna P, Mackinlay G, Perilongo G, et al. Liver Tumors Study Group of the International Society of Pediatric Oncology. Hepatocellular carcinoma in children: results of the first prospective study of the International Society of Pediatric Oncology group. *J Clin Oncol* 2002;15;20:2798–2804.
192. Pritchard J, Brown J, Shafford E, et al. Doxorubicin and delayed surgery for childhood hepatoblastoma: a successful approach—results of the first prospective study of the International Society of Pediatric Oncology. *J Clin Oncol* 2000;18: 3819–3828.
193. Perilongo G, Shafford E, Maibach R, et al. Risk-adapted treatment for childhood hepatoblastoma. Final report of the second study of the International Society of Paediatric Oncology-SIOPEL 2. *Eur J Cancer* 2004;40:411–421.
195. Arcement CM, Towbin RB, Meza MP, et al. Intrahepatic chemoembolization in unresectable pediatric liver malignancies. *Pediatr Radiol* 2000;30:779–85.
197. Suita S, Tajiri T, Takamatsu H, et al; Committee for Pediatric Solid Malignant Tumors in the Kyushu Area, Japan. Improved survival outcome for hepatoblastoma based on an optimal chemotherapeutic regimen—a report from the study group for pediatric solid malignant tumors in the Kyushu area. *J Pediatr Surg* 2004;39: 195–198.
198. Fuchs J, Rydzynski J, Von Schweinitz D, et al. Study Committee of the Cooperative Pediatric Liver Tumor Study Hb 94 for the German Society for Pediatric Oncology and Hematology. Pretreatment prognostic factors and treatment results in children with hepatoblastoma: a report from the German Cooperative Pediatric Liver Tumor Study HB 94. *Cancer* 2002;95:172–182.
199. Haberle B, Bode U, von Schweinitz D. Differentiated treatment protocols for high- and standard-risk hepatoblastoma—an interim report of the German Liver Tumor Study HB99 [in German]. *Klin Padiatr* 2003;215:159–165.
200. Goin JE, Salem R, Carr BI, et al. Treatment of unresectable hepatocellular carcinoma with intrahepatic yttrium 90 microspheres: a risk-stratification analysis. *J Vasc Interv Radiol* 2005;16:195–203
214. Gadner H, Grois N, Arico M, et al. A randomized trial of treatment for multisystem Langerhans' cell histiocytosis. *J Pediatr* 2001;138:728–734.
216. Gadner H, Grois N, Potschger U, et al. Improved outcome in multisystem Langerhans cell histiocytosis is associated with therapy intensification. *Blood* 2008;111:2556–2562.
220. Akkari V, Donadieu J, Piguet C, et al. French Langerhans Cell Study Group. Hematopoietic stem cell transplantation in patients with severe Langerhans cell histiocytosis and hematological dysfunction: experience of the French Langerhans Cell Study Group. *Bone Marrow Transplant* 2003;31:1097–1103.
231. Tenenbaum F, Groussin L, Foehrenbach H, et al. 18F-fluorodeoxyglucose positron emission tomography as a diagnostic tool for malignancy of adrenocortical tumours. Preliminary results in 13 consecutive patients. *Eur J Endocrinol* 2004; 150:789–792.
232. Zettinig G, Mitterhauser M, Wadsak W, et al. Positron emission tomography imaging of adrenal masses: (18)F-fluorodeoxyglucose and the 11beta-hydroxylase tracer (11)C-metomidate. *Eur J Nucl Ed Mol Imaging* 2004;31:1224–1230.
242. Zografos GC, Driscoll DL, Karakousis CP, et al. Adrenal adenocarcinoma: a review of 53 cases. *J Surg Oncol* 1994;56:160–164.
244. Norton JA. Adrenal tumors. In: DeVita V, Hellman S, Rosenberg S, eds. *Cancer principles and practice,* 7th ed. Philadelphia: Lippincott Williams & Wilkins, 2005:1528–1539.
257. Fassbender WJ, Krohn-Grimberghe B, Gortz B, et al. Multiple endocrine neoplasia (MEN): an overview and case report. Patient with sporadic bilateral pheochromocytoma, hyperparathyroidism and marfanoid habitus. *Anticancer Res* 2000; 20:4877–4887.
276. Vassilopoulou-Sellin R, Goepfert H, Raney B, et al. Differentiated thyroid cancer in children and adolescents: clinical outcome and mortality after long-term follow-up. *Head Neck* 1998;20:549–555.
278. Zimmerman D, Hay ID, Gough IR, et al. Papillary thyroid carcinoma in children and adults: long term follow-up of 1039 patients conservatively treated at one institution during three decades. *Surgery* 1988;104:1157–1166.

280. Brink JS, van Heerden JA, McIver B, et al. Papillary thyroid cancer with pulmonary metasteses in children: long term prognosis. *Surgery* 2000;128:881–887.
285. Ontai S, Straehley CJ. The surgical treatment of well-differentiated carcinoma of the thyroid. *Am Surg* 1985;51:653–657.
294. Powles TB, Bhardwa J, Shamash J, et al. The changing presentation of germ cell tumours of the testis between 1983 and 2002. *BJU Int* 2005;95:1197–1200.
296. Einhorn LH, Williams SD, Loehrer PJ, et al. Evaluation of optimal duration of chemotherapy in favorable-prognosis disseminated germ cell tumors: a Southeastern Cancer Study Group protocol. *J Clin Oncol* 1989;7:387–391.
297. Pinkerton CR, Broadbent V, Horwich A, et al. 'JEB'—a carboplatin based regimen for malignant germ cell tumours in children. *Br J Cancer* 1990;62:257–262.
298. Mangili G, Sigismondi C, Lorusso D, et al. Is surgical restaging indicated in apparent stage IA pure ovarian dysgerminoma? The MITO group retrospective experience. *Gynecol Oncol* 2011;121:280–284.
304. Minh NH. Cervicothoracic spinal epidural cavernous hemangioma: case report and review of the literature. *Surg Neurol* 2005;64:83–85.
306. Moller G, Priemel M, Amling M, et al. The Gorham-Stout syndrome (Gorham's massive osteolysis). A report of six cases with histopathological findings. *J Bone Joint Surg Br* 1999;81:501–506.
314. Goodman KA, Wolden SL, La Quaglia MP, et al. Whole abdominopelvic radiotherapy for desmoplastic small round-cell tumor. *Int J Radiat Oncol Biol Phys* 2002; 54:170–176.
315. Su MC, Jeng YM, Chu YC. Desmoplastic small round cell tumor of the kidney. *Am J Surg Pathol* 2004;28:1379–1383.
316. Gerald WL, Ladanyi M, de Alava E, et al. Clinical, pathologic, and molecular spectrum of tumors associated with t(11;22)(p13;q12): desmoplastic small round-cell tumor and its variants. *J Clin Oncol* 1998;16:3028–3036.
318. Lal DR, Su WT, Wolden SL, et al. Results of multimodal treatment for desmoplastic small round cell tumors. *J Pediatr Surg* 2005;40:251–255.
319. Aguilera D, Hayes-Jordan A, Anderson P, et al. Outpatient and home chemotherapy with novel local control strategies in desmoplastic small round cell tumor. *Sarcoma* 2008;2008:261589.
320. Hayes-Jordan A, Anderson PM. The diagnosis and management of desmoplastic small round cell tumor: a review. *Curr Opin Oncol* 2011;23: 385–389.
336. Berneburg M, Lehmann AR. Xeroderma pigmentosum and related disorders: defects in DNA repair and transcription. *Adv Genet* 2001;43:71–102.
340. Handerfield-Jones SE, Smith NP. Malignant melanoma in childhood. *Br J Dematol* 1996;134:607–616.

Part O Benign Diseases

Chapter 91
Nonmalignant Diseases

Karen M. Winkfield, Jose G. Bazan, Iris C. Gibbs, Tony Y. Eng, and Charles R. Thomas

Benign diseases generally include a class of localized tumors or growths that have a low potential for progression and do not invade surrounding tissue or metastasize to distant sites. Pathologically, they are composed of well-differentiated cells that are considered nonmalignant and usually do not require any treatment. However, clinically, not all benign diseases have benign consequences. Some untreated benign diseases can produce bothersome mass or secretory effects. Others can be locally aggressive and cause secondary debilitating symptoms. For example, Graves ophthalmopathy can lead to local pain and visual impairment without therapeutic intervention[1]; a hormonally active pituitary adenoma may cause growth abnormality in addition to blindness[2]; desmoid tumors, can be locally persistent even after surgical resection and some are therefore managed aggressively, similar to their malignant counterparts and may require adjuvant radiation therapy after radical resection.[3]

Documented empirical use of radiation in imaging and the treatment of benign diseases or conditions occurred soon after the discovery of x-rays by Wilhelm Röntgen in 1895.[4] An estimate of over 1 million Americans, mostly young adults and children, received x-ray treatments to the head and neck region for benign conditions between 1920 and 1960.[5,6] The painless x-ray treatment and its visible efficacy led to many benign conditions being treated with radiation, such as acne, body hair, scalp ringworm, enlarged tonsils, enlarged thymus, enlarged lymph neck nodes, whooping cough, and others. Radiation therapy was used in some instances due to a lack of effective alternative therapies.[7]

Over the past decades, advances in medical and surgical therapies have provided new treatment options for many diseases. With improved awareness of late radiation sequelae on normal tissue, particularly radiation carcinogenesis, there has been a gradual decline in the use of radiation therapy for treatment of benign conditions. However, with modern radiation therapy techniques and better understanding of radiobiology, judicial use of radiation still provides good local control in and relief of associated symptoms from a variety of benign diseases.

RADIOBIOLOGICAL EFFECTS ON BENIGN DISEASES

The precise radiobiological mechanisms of radiation effects on benign diseases are not well defined. Radiation is believed to work through a complex of multicellular interactions that affect different cell types in our body system.[8] Specific cellular and functional mechanisms depend on the specific disease and site. Although most benign lesions have no known stimuli or causes, some benign lesions may be triggered by trauma as seen in keloid formation after body piercing or heterotopic bone formation after surgery. In conditions that arise following trauma, local inflammation and repair occur, which is often characterized by stimulation of growth factors and accelerated cellular proliferation. For example, in the development of keloids, fibroblast proliferation is responsible for most of the hyperproliferative process. Even with the lower doses commonly used in benign diseases, radiotherapy is clinically effective in inhibiting cell proliferation and suppressing cell differentiation without inducing cell death, as is typically seen with tumoricidal doses of radiation. Yet, radiation can induce apoptosis in selected target cells by influencing the expression of cytokines in macrophages, leukocytes, endothelial, and other cells and thereby modulating the inflammatory cascade.

Among the major sites of radiation effects are the blood vessels; vascular endothelial cells respond rapidly to radiation damage by up-regulating the cytokine-mediated cellular reactions responsible for inflammatory tissue response. Low-dose irradiation (<12 Gy) exerts anti-inflammatory effects on the endothelial cells of capillaries and mononuclear cells of the immune system.[9]

Cell adhesion molecules, selectins, are mobilized to the cell membrane and change the capillary permeability, allowing the inflammatory cells (lymphocytes, macrophages, monocytes) to migrate into interstitial space. The anti-inflammatory effect is attributed to the modulation of cytokine and adhesion molecule expression on the activated endothelial cells and leukocytes. These cells are known to be radiosensitive. They express proinflammatory cytokines (e.g., interleukin-1, interleukin-6) or necrosis factors (e.g., tumor necrosis factor-α), which influence the complement cascade and enzymes of inflammatory reaction. Interleukin-1 stimulates the production and release of proinflammatory prostaglandins, leading to a change in synthesis of inducible nitric oxide synthetase.

The radiation-induced modulation of nitric oxide production and oxidative burst in activated macrophages and native granulocytes lead to modification of the immune response and inflammatory process as well as clinical analgesic effects. Although endothelial cells possess a high proliferative potential and are sensitive to radiation damage at high doses, they are not prone to rapid mitotic radiation death at low doses.

Chronic inflammatory processes are triggered by antigen–antibody reactions and mediated by mononuclear peripheral blood cells in the immune system. Ionizing radiation helps suppress some of these cell populations, such as T-lymphocytes, in the inflammation process or modulate their effects. Although low doses of radiation can exert an anti-inflammatory response, high doses of radiation as used in malignant tumors can elicit proinflammatory effects and fibrotic change in normal tissue.[10] At higher single or total doses, endothelial cell damage can lead to sclerosis and obliteration of blood vessels. In vascular disorders such as hemangiomas or arteriovenous malformations, high radiation doses may induce occlusion of pathologic vessels. In addition to inhibition of cell proliferation, cell killing may play a part in the management of benign meningiomas, pituitary adenomas, or neuromas where higher, tumoricidal doses of radiation may be required.

RISK OF SECOND MALIGNANCIES

The induction of cancer or genetic defects by radiation exposure is attributed to stochastic effects where there is no threshold level of radiation exposure below which cancer induction or genetic effects will not occur. Increasing the radiation dose or the volume of exposure will increase the probability that a cancer or genetic effect will occur. Sometimes, the radiation effects are difficult to separate from inherent genetic effects. For example, in patients with retinoblastoma, the *Rb1* gene plays an important role in the development of radiation-induced sarcomas.[11,12] In a study of 384 retinoblastoma patients treated with radiation, the actuarial risk for developing a sarcoma in the treatment field 18 years after treatment was 6.6%.[11] In another study of 693 patients, the cumulative risk for any sarcoma 50 years after radiotherapy was 13.1%.[12] Although most sarcomas were within the irradiated fields, 18 of 69 sarcomas developed outside the treatment fields. *Rb1* mutations appear to confer a genetic predisposition to developing sarcomas, especially after radiation exposure.

The risk of the induction of secondary tumors was overestimated in the past.[13] Trott and Kamprad[14] used the epidemiologic data from long-term follow-up studies on patients treated with radiotherapy for benign diseases to estimate the risk of cancer induction. Taking all known modifying and organ-specific factors into account, including doses of radiation and volume irradiated, the estimated absolute lifetime risk for sarcoma induction was <0.0001% for 1 Gy and a 100-cm^2 field. Table 91.1 lists the absolute lifetime risk for other malignancies.

Jansen et al.[15] applied the effective dose concept and estimated the carcinogenic risk in patients after radiotherapy of benign diseases (heterotopic ossification, omarthritis, gonarthrosis, heel spurs, and hidradenitis suppurativa). Special risk modifying factors, including age at exposure and gender, were taken into account. For an average-aged population, the estimated number of radiation-induced fatal tumors was between 0.5 and 40 persons per 1,000 patients treated. The range of effective doses was also found to be large (5 to 400 mSv). In addition to age and gender, the individual risk also depends on individual inherent sensitivity, anatomic site, type of disease, and treatment technique, such as dose and fractionation.

TABLE 91.1 THE ESTIMATED ABSOLUTE LIFETIME RISK FOR MALIGNANCIES AFTER RADIATION THERAPY FOR BENIGN DISEASES

Types	Absolute Lifetime Risk
Skin (basal cell carcinoma)	0.1% for 100-cm^2 field
Osteosarcoma	<0.0001% for 1 Gy and a 100-cm^2 field
Leukemia	1% for 1 Gy TBI
Brain tumor	0.2% after 20 Gy for endocrine orbitopathy
Thyroid carcinoma	1% per Gy for children <10 years
Breast carcinoma	5% for one breast, 1 Gy, age <35 (<3% for age 35–45)
Lung carcinoma	1% within 25 years after a mean lung dose of 1 Gy

INDICATION FOR RADIOTHERAPY

The majority of benign diseases can be classified as inflammatory, degenerative, hyperproliferative, or functional. Therefore, therapeutic approaches vary widely and are regionally customized, in part because of geographic traditions and differences in clinical training. Radiation treatment of benign diseases is less commonly used in the United States than in other parts of the world where variation in indications and treatment schedules are institutionally based.[16] Within Germany, a pattern of care study revealed significant geographic and institutional differences.[17] Although most radiation treatments for benign disease are delivered in the low-dose range (<10 to 15 Gy), the prescribed dose varied widely and inconsistently within geographic regions and among institutions.

Degenerative processes in tendons, ligaments, and joints can cause pain by chronic inflammation and trigger secondary functional impairment of the involved musculoskeletal system. Although radiation does not halt the degenerative process, it may reduce the inflammation and provide partial or complete pain relief. This clinical effect is well established in reports of osteoarthritis, synovitis, and bursitis, where low-dose radiation therapy has improved the function of affected joints.[17,18]

Benign diseases may have a significant effect on self-image and self-esteem because of cosmetic appearance (e.g., facial keloids, juvenile angiofibroma) or have a lasting impact on quality of life because of chronic pain or other secondary symptoms (e.g., heterotopic bone, macular degeneration). When benign diseases become locally invasive with aggressive growth, therapeutic intervention can prevent or limit functional loss of organs. In rare cases of large hemangioma with associated thrombocytopenia and consumption coagulopathy (Kasabach-Merritt syndrome), potentially fatal complications can occur, and timely therapeutic intervention can be life-saving.[19]

Although there is a lack of international consensus, the German Working Group on Radiotherapy of Benign Diseases published their consensus guidelines for radiation therapy of nonmalignant diseases. The guidelines were to serve as a starting point for quality assessment, prospective clinical trials, and outcomes research.[18] In brief, treatment is indicated when benign diseases are symptomatic or potentially symptomatic. When other methods are unavailable or have failed, radiation therapy should be considered. As medical professionals, we remain mindful of therapeutic gain and potential treatment side effects and complications. A thorough risk–benefit analysis is always pertinent. Organ-specific acute and chronic toxicities, including potential effects on fertility and induction of secondary tumors in the future, must be explained to and discussed with patients, especially those who are young and have a long life-expectancy. Informed consent, which is required for all medical interventions, is certainly required for treatment of benign diseases and should be obtained prior to the delivery of radiation therapy.

This chapter covers some of the more common benign conditions that are still encountered in the practice of radiation oncology. Details on the therapeutic approaches and data on radiation dose regimens for different benign diseases are summarized in the individual corresponding sections.

BENIGN NEOPLASMS OF THE BRAIN, HEAD, AND NECK

Nonmalignant tumors of the central nervous system (CNS) and neck can lead to severe, life-threatening symptoms due to pressure and mass effect on critical structures from tumor growth. However, depending on tumor growth rate and location, the surrounding tissue may adapt, leading to a delay in the clinical diagnosis.

Meningioma

Background and Clinical Aspects

Meningiomas are the most common benign tumors of the CNS. The incidence peaks in the seventh decade of life with a 2 to 1 female-to-male predominance. The majority (>90%) of meningiomas are benign and classified by the World Health Organization (WHO) as grade I tumors.[20] WHO grade II meningiomas (atypical, clear cell, or chordoid) have a higher tendency for local recurrence, and WHO grade III malignant meningiomas (anaplastic, rhabdoid, papillary) are exceedingly rare.

The most common presenting symptom is headache, but patients may present with other localizing symptoms depending on the tumor location. The radiographic diagnosis of meningioma is often made on computed tomography (CT) or magnetic resonance imaging (MRI) based on the appearance of a homogeneously and intensely enhancing extra-axial mass with or without the presence of a dural tail.

Surgical Management

Surgical resection is the treatment of choice for the majority of patients, as this will relieve symptoms and also provide a pathologic diagnosis. The primary goal of surgery is to remove as much tumor burden as possible while minimizing the risk of neurologic deficits (maximal safe resection). Gross total resection (GTR) is generally attempted for patients with tumors in locations such as the convexity and olfactory groove.[21,22] After GTR, the relapse rate is as low as 10%, but this depends on the Simpson classification, which grades tumors according to extent of resection and degree of dural involvement (Table 91.2).[23] Local recurrence rates are as high as 40% for patients with incomplete resection,[23] although these rates can be substantially reduced with the use of adjuvant radiotherapy.

Meningiomas tend to be highly vascularized tumors. In select patients, preoperative embolization is used to decrease blood loss and improve the extent of resection.[24,25]

Active Surveillance

Asymptomatic patients with small meningiomas may be observed clinically. At the time of tumor growth or the development of symptoms, patients can be treated with surgery or radiation therapy. The safety and reasoning for this approach was established in a large retrospective series from Japan that demonstrated that the majority of patients do not require intervention in the short term.[26]

Systemic Therapy

Interest in the use of medical therapy to treat meningiomas stems from the observation that up to 67% of meningiomas express the progesterone receptor or androgen receptor, and approximately 10% express the estrogen receptor.[17] However, response rates to antihormonal agents are low. Overall, studies that have investigated the role of chemotherapy, such as hydroxyurea, in the management of recurrent disease have demonstrated little efficacy.[27]

TABLE 91.2 SIMPSON GRADING SYSTEM FOR POSTOPERATIVE MENINGIOMAS WITH ASSOCIATED RATES OF RECURRENCE

Simpson Grade	Description	Recurrence Rate
I	Complete macroscopic tumor removal with adherent dura as well as the possibly affected part of the cranial calotte	8.9% (8/90 patients)
II	Complete macroscopic tumor removal with adherent dura via diathermia	15.8% (18/114 patients)
III	Complete macroscopic tumor removal without adherent dura or possibly additional extradural parts	29.2% (7/24 patients)
IV	Partial macroscopic tumor removal while leaving intradural tumor parts	39.2% (20/51 patients)
V	Simple decompressive and bioptic removal of tumor	88.9% (8/9 patients)

Adapted from Simpson D. The recurrence of intracranial meningiomas after surgical treatment. *J Neurol Neurosurg Psychiatry* 1957;20:22–39.

Radiotherapy

Primary radiotherapy (RT) is indicated for tumors in locations in which complete resection is not feasible (i.e., optic nerve, cavernous sinus, major venous sinus) or for patients who are poor surgical candidates. Adjuvant RT is indicated for patients with subtotal resection (STR), recurrent disease, or for WHO grade II or III tumors. RT techniques include conventionally fractionated three-dimensional conformal radiotherapy (3D-CRT), conventionally fractionated intensity-modulated radiation therapy (IMRT), frame-based or linear accelerator–based fractionated stereotactic radiotherapy (FSRT), stereotactic radiosurgery (SRS), or protons and heavy ions.

The MRI sequences that best delineate the gross tumor volume (GTV) should be coregistered with the treatment-planning CT scan for optimal treatment planning and delivery. Particularly for patients receiving FSRT or SRS, it is important that a neuroradiologist and neurosurgeon be involved in assisting with GTV delineation, as enhancement from residual tumor versus postoperative change is often difficult to ascertain.

For 3D-CRT or IMRT treatments, the clinical target volume (CTV) is constructed by adding a 1- or 2-cm symmetric margin around the GTV, respecting normal tissue boundaries. An additional 3 to 5 mm is added for the final planning target volume (PTV). These margins may be modified based on institutional policy and other considerations, such as the availability of daily image guidance (i.e., kilovolt imaging or cone-beam CT).

For benign meningiomas, the typical dose prescription to the PTV is 50 to 54 Gy given in 1.8- to 2-Gy daily fractions. Retrospective data suggest that local control is inferior for patients treated with doses of <52 Gy.[28] For patients with more aggressive histology (WHO grade II or III tumors), the GTV is expanded by at least 2 cm, with a higher dose prescription in the range of 59.4 to 63 Gy. Several modern series of radiotherapy show 5-year local control rates ranging from 89% to 98%, with three-dimensional conformal therapy demonstrating local control rates >95% (Table 91.2).[28–30,31–32]

Because meningiomas are frequently noninvasive and well-circumscribed tumors, SRS and FSRT are increasingly being used in their treatment. The decision to fractionate depends largely on tumor size and proximity to critical structures, such as the optic apparatus or brainstem. Typical dose prescriptions for frame-based SRS range from 12 to 16 Gy prescribed to the 50% isodose line (IDL) and 14 to 18 Gy prescribed to the 80% IDL for a frameless robotic radiosurgery platform. In patients with tumors that require fractionated treatment, dose prescriptions vary and are dependent on the individual case. For example, at Stanford University, primary or residual meningiomas of the convexity and skull base are treated with 15 to 18 Gy in 1 or 2 fractions. Additionally, a select group of perioptic tumors, including meningiomas, have been treated with a prescription of 24 to 30 Gy in 3 to 5 fractions (to the 80% IDL) with high rates of tumor control and visual preservation (Fig. 91.1).[33] Recent nonrandomized, prospective evidence indicates that FSRT should be the treatment of choice for optic nerve sheath meningiomas due to the high rate of preservation of visual acuity.[34]

Reported results with SRS are excellent, with 5-year local control rates as high as 98% to 100% (Table 91.3).[35–41,42,43,44] DiBiase et al.[45] demonstrated that male gender, conformality index <1.4, and size >10 mL predict for worse outcome after SRS. That article also showed improved disease-free survival in patients in which the dural tail was covered as part of the target volume. The benefit of including the dural tail has to be

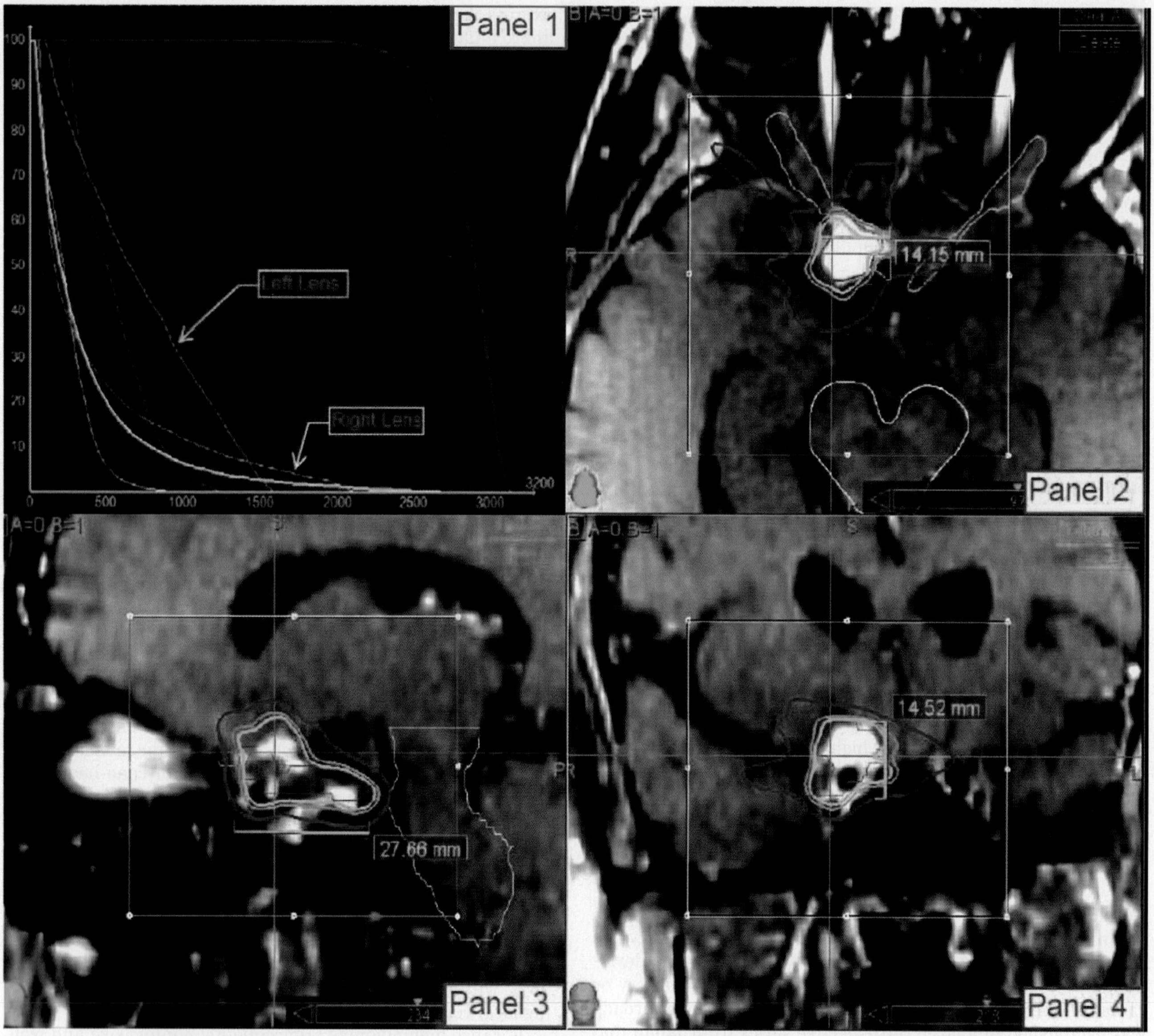

FIGURE 91.1. Radiosurgery treatment plan of a patient with a right optic nerve sheath meningioma treated to a dose of 24 Gy in 3 fractions. The lesion is intensely enhancing on the postcontrast stereotactic magnetic resonance imaging sequences. *Panel 1* demonstrates the dose–volume histogram for the patient. The maximum dose to the ipsilateral optic nerve was 22.3 Gy. *Panels 2–4* demonstrate the isodose curves for the treatment in the axial, sagittal, and coronal planes, respectively. The 100% (24 Gy) isodose line is *green,* the 88% (21 Gy) isodose line is *orange,* and the 50% (12 Gy) isodose line is *blue.*

weighed against the risk of toxicity from increasing the target volume for each individual case.

Due to their physical properties, protons and heavy ions (i.e., carbon) are attractive choices for the treatment of meningiomas, particularly for those located near critical structures. Several studies have shown excellent local control rates with the combination of protons and photons or protons alone.[46–49] In the study by Weber et al.,[48] patients were treated to a median dose of 56 cobalt gray equivalents (GyE) given in 1.8 to 2.0 GyE per day.

Pituitary Adenoma

Background and Clinical Aspects

Pituitary adenomas comprise 10% to 15% of all intracranial tumors. Approximately 75% of these tumors are functional (secretory), thereby producing increased amounts of hormones. Prolactinomas and growth-hormone (GH)–secreting adenomas are the most frequently encountered. Functional adenomas are more common in women, while nonfunctioning and GH-secreting adenomas are more common in men.

Adenomas are often classified by size, with a picoadenoma <0.3 cm, microadenoma <1 cm, and macroadenoma >1cm. Macroadenomas may exert mass effect upon the optic chiasm, leading to the classic sign of bitemporal hemianopsia. Headaches are seen in approximately 20% of patients. If the adenoma extends to the cavernous sinus, cranial nerve deficits may be present. Involvement of the hypothalamus by the adenoma results in hypopituitarism.

Patients with functional adenomas present with signs and symptoms that correspond to the excess hormone: galactorrhea, amenorrhea, diminished libido, and infertility in patients with prolactinomas; acromegaly or gigantism in patients with GH-secreting adenomas, Cushing disease in adrenocorticotropic hormone (ACTH)–secreting adenomas; hyperthyroidism in patients with thyroid-stimulating hormone (TSH)–secreting adenomas. In patients who have had bilateral adrenalectomy, up to 40% will develop Nelson syndrome, which is characterized by an ACTH-secreting adenoma and increased skin pigmentation secondary to increased release of α-melanocyte–stimulating hormone.

TABLE 91.3 CLINICAL OUTCOMES OF STEREOTACTIC RADIOSURGERY OR EXTERNAL-BEAM RADIOTHERAPY (WITH OR WITHOUT SURGERY) FOR MENINGIOMAS IN MODERN SERIES

Study (Reference)	Number of Patients	Radiation	S + R/R (%)	Dose (Median or Mean, Gy)	Local Control (%)
Ganz et al. (2009) (37)	97	SRS	NA	12	100 (2 yr)
Takanisha et al. (2009) (43)	101	SRS	24/76	13.2	97 (1 yr)
Han et al. (2008) (38)	98	SRS	36/64	12.7	90 (5 yr)
Iwai et al. (2008) (40)	108	SRS	NA	12	93 (5 yr) 83 (10 yr)
Kondziolka et al. (2008) (42)	972	SRS	49/51	14	87 (10 yr)
Davidson et al. (2007) (35)	36	SRS	100/0	16	100 (5 yr) 95 (10 yr)
Feigl et al. (2007) (36)	214	SRS	43/57	13.6	86.3 (4 yr)
Hasegawa et al. (2007) (39)	115	SRS	57/43	13 Gy	87 (5 yr) 73 (10 yr)
Kollova et al. (2007) (41)	368	SRS	30/70	12.5	98 (5 yr)
Zachenhofe et al. (2006) (44)	36	SRS	70/30	17	94 (9 yr)
Goldsmith et al. (1994) (28)	117	EBRT	100/0	54	89 (5 yr) 77 (10 yr)
Mendenhall et al. (2003) (29)	101	EBRT	35/65	54	95 (5 yr) 92 (10 yr)
Nutting et al. (1999) (31)	82	EBRT	100%/0%	55–60	92 (5 yr) 83 (10 yr)
Vendrely et al. (1999) (32)	156	EBRT	51/49	50	79 (5 yr)

S, surgery; R, radiation; SRS, stereotactic radiosurgery; EBRT, external-beam radiotherapy; NA, not available.

Adapted from Minniti G, Amichetti M, Enrici RM. Radiotherapy and radiosurgery for benign skull base meningiomas. *Radiat Oncol 2009*;4:42.

In addition to history and detailed physical examination (H&P), workup of a pituitary tumor includes laboratory analysis of pituitary hormone levels, contrast enhanced MRI with thin slices through the pituitary (Fig. 91.2A,B), and tissue diagnosis to rule out other causes of pituitary masses, including craniopharyngioma, meningioma, suprasellar germ cell tumor, metastatic disease, or a benign lesion (i.e., cyst).

Surgical Management

Surgery is generally the treatment of choice for pituitary adenomas. Surgery provides immediate relief of compressive symptoms and helps to decrease hormone secretion. The most common surgical technique is through a transsphenoidal approach. In some cases, a more aggressive surgery (i.e., frontal craniotomy) may be indicated for patients with extensive intracranial and skull-based involvement. Overall, local control rates range from 50% to 80% after surgery alone for both functioning and nonfunctioning adenomas.[50] In patients who continue to have abnormally elevated hormones after surgical resection, adjuvant treatment with pharmacotherapy or radiation therapy is pursued.

Pharmacotherapy

Pharmacotherapy, such as bromocriptine and cabergoline for prolactinomas, octreotide for GH adenomas and TSH adenomas, and ketoconazole for ACTH adenomas, is often used as an adjunct to surgery for patients with functioning adenomas. With the exception of prolactinomas, the use of these drugs as monotherapy is generally not curative. Prolactinomas can often be managed with pharmacotherapy alone, but a high proportion of patients are unable to tolerate bromocriptine for long periods of time due to nausea, headache, and fatigue.

Radiotherapy

Except for medically inoperable patients in which RT is used in the primary setting, the role of RT is generally in the adjuvant setting with the following indications: recurrent tumor after surgery; persistence of hormone elevation after surgery; residual disease after STR or debulking procedure. Tumor growth control is excellent, particularly for patients with nonfunctioning adenomas.[51,52–53] Endocrine control after treatment of functioning adenomas, as demonstrated by normalization of pituitary hormone levels, takes years to develop. At a median of 2 years after RT, growth hormone levels stabilize quickest; normalization is slowest for TSH-secreting adenomas.[54] Pharmacologic therapy should be discontinued 1 to 2 months prior to the initiation of RT based on evidence demonstrating lower RT sensitivity with concurrent medical treatment.[55]

RT techniques include 3D-CRT, IMRT, single-fraction SRS, and FSRT. Delineation of the GTV (or preoperative GTV in the case of GTR) should be performed by coregistration of the postoperative MRI to the treatment planning CT scan.

For 3D-CRT and IMRT, the CTV is constructed by adding 1 to 1.5 cm to the GTV; an additional 3 to 5 mm is added to the CTV to create the PTV. These margins may be modified based on institutional policy and other considerations, such as the availability of daily image guidance. Nonfunctional adenomas are typically prescribed a dose of 45 to 50.4 Gy given in 1.8- to 2.0-Gy daily fractions (Fig. 91.2C–E). Higher doses in the range of 50.4 to 54 Gy are recommended for secretory adenomas.

SRS remains an attractive option for the treatment of pituitary adenomas. General principles apply in that FSRT is used over SRS for large lesions (>3 cm) or lesions near critical structures (<1 or 2 mm from the chiasm). Similar to 3D-CRT or IMRT, higher doses are needed for functional adenomas compared with nonfunctional adenomas. Numerous retrospective studies have demonstrated excellent local control rates of 92% to 100% for nonfunctional adenomas, using doses of 14 to 25 Gy (at the edge of the tumor) in a single fraction.[56] Commonly used prescriptions are 16 to 20 Gy in a single fraction for nonfunctional adenomas and 20 to 25 Gy in a single fraction for functional adenomas using a frameless robotic radiosurgery platform.

Craniopharyngioma

Background and Clinical Aspects

Craniopharyngiomas comprise 6% to 10% of pediatric CNS tumors, or approximately 300 to 350 cases per year in the United States. The median age of diagnosis is 5 to 10 years, with a second peak in patients >40 years old.

These benign tumors are epithelial, arising from remnants of Rathke's pouch (hypophyseal-pharyngeal duct), and are most commonly located in the suprasellar region, although they may be found in the sella proper. Craniopharyngiomas generally abut the hypothalamus and third ventricle. Histologically, they are divided into the adamantinomatous and squamous subtypes. The adamantinomatous subtype is characterized by a

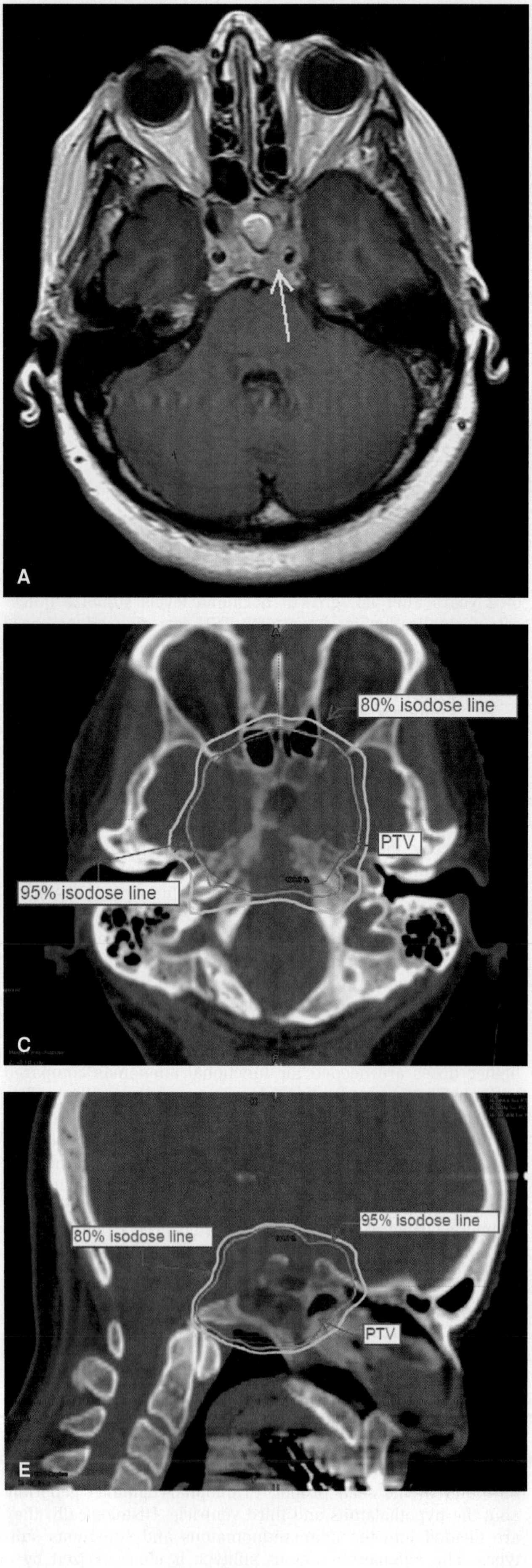

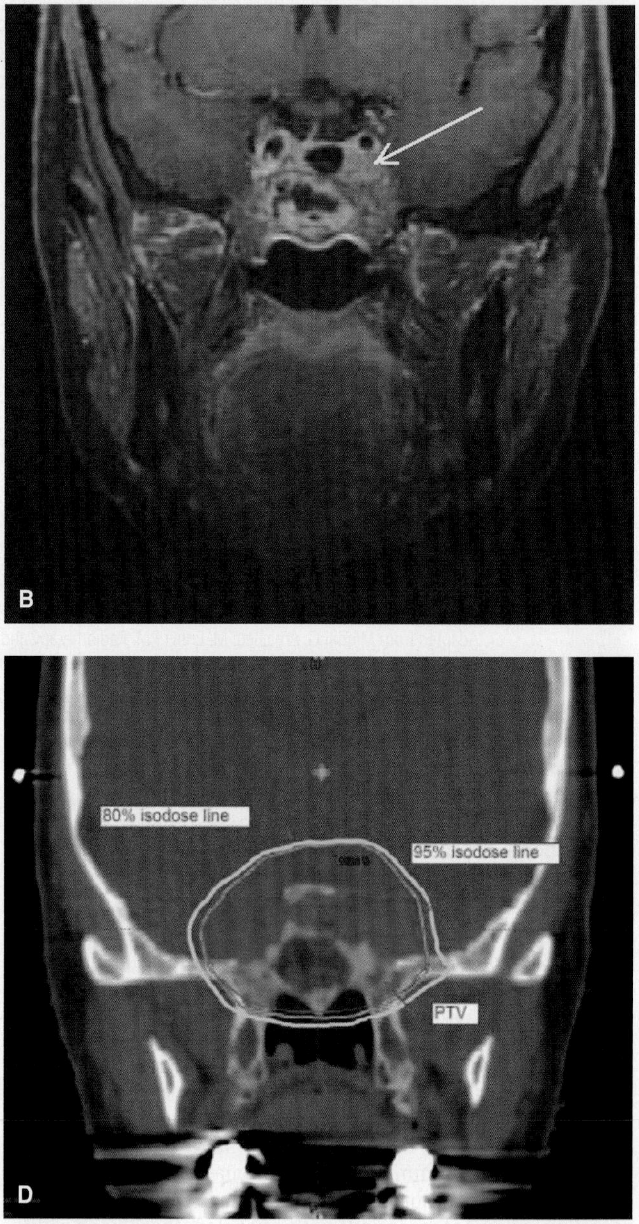

FIGURE 91.2. A recurrent nonfunctioning pituitary adenoma 7 years after surgical resection in the axial **(A)** and coronal **(B)** planes. The *yellow arrows* denote invasion into the left cavernous sinus. Rapid arc intensity-modulated radiotherapy treatment plan for the same patient in the axial **(C)**, coronal **(D)**, and sagittal **(E)** planes. The planning target volume (*purple shaded area*) was prescribed at 50.4 Gy in 28 fractions.

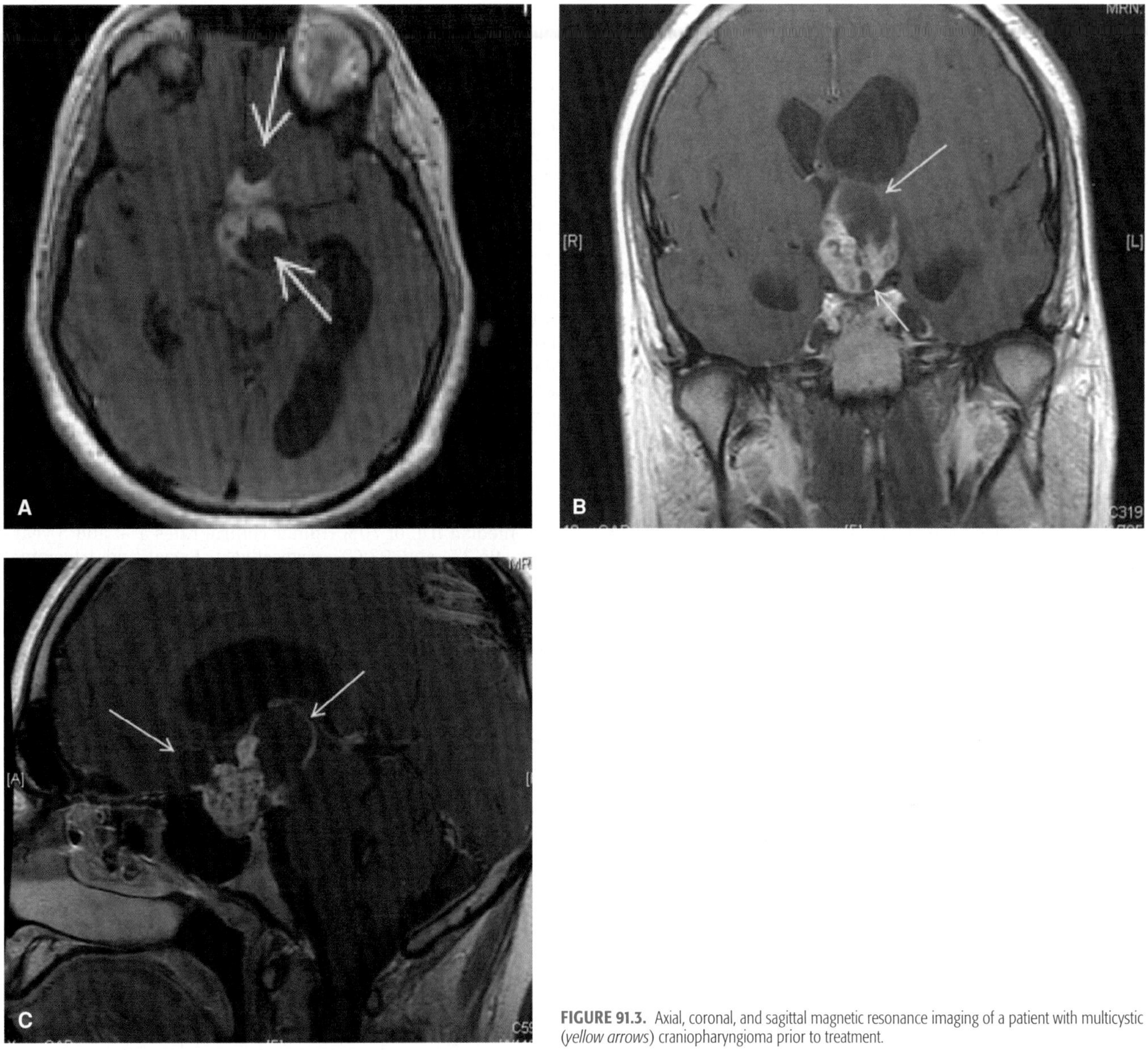

FIGURE 91.3. Axial, coronal, and sagittal magnetic resonance imaging of a patient with multicystic (*yellow arrows*) craniopharyngioma prior to treatment.

solid and cystic pattern with the well-known description of "machine oil-like" cystic fluid.

Presenting signs and symptoms include headache, nausea and vomiting, bitemporal hemianopsia, and endocrine dysfunction (diabetes insipidus, dwarfism, fat tissue disturbance, adrenal cortical insufficiency). The most common hormone deficiency is lack of GH. The workup is similar to that of pituitary adenoma and includes H&P, pituitary hormone levels, and brain MRI with thin slices through the sella (Fig. 91.3).

Surgery

The primary goal of surgery is complete resection. However, GTR may be associated with high rates of neurologic sequelae, including visual impairment and panhypopituitarism. In order to minimize morbidity, most patients are treated with maximal safe resection followed by adjuvant RT. In some cases, intralesional bleomycin may be directly injected into the cyst to decrease the rate of cyst recurrence.

Radiotherapy

Radiation therapy is often used in the adjuvant setting. In select patients (i.e., <3 years old), observation following STR may be an option as local control rates are similar with RT at the time of relapse ("salvage" RT) compared with adjuvant RT with no compromise in overall survival.[57]

RT techniques include 3D-CRT, IMRT, FSRT, proton therapy, and intralesional RT with β-emitting isotopes (yttrium-90, phosphorous-32). The GTV is the postoperative residual tumor volume, including the cyst wall, if present. The postoperative MRI should be fused with the treatment planning CT scan for optimal target delineation. A margin of 1 to 1.5 cm is added to the GTV to create the PTV. Dose prescriptions for 3D-CRT and IMRT are typically 54 Gy given in 1.8-Gy daily fractions.

Fractionated proton radiotherapy has demonstrated excellent results. The Loma Linda series treated 15 patients to a total dose of 50.4 to 59.4 GyE given in 1.8-GyE daily fractions.[58] Local control was achieved in 14 of 15 patients, with few long-term complications. In a series from the Massachusetts General Hospital (MGH), no failures were seen in 24 patients who received fractionated proton radiotherapy to a total dose of 52.2 to 54 GyE in 1.8 GyE per fraction.[59]

It has been well established that cysts may regrow during the several weeks of fractionated treatment. The MGH proton study recommends that reimaging (CT, or MRI if the cyst is not well visualized on CT) be performed within 2 weeks of the treatment planning scan and every 2 weeks thereafter; for large cysts or those that demonstrate growth during RT, weekly reimaging is recommended.[59] The emergence of image-guided radiotherapy techniques now allows for the convenient monitoring of cyst regrowth with cone-beam CT scans while patients are on the treatment table.

SRS and FSRT have been used with success in the treatment of craniopharyngioma. In one series from Stanford University using a frameless robotic platform,[60] 16 patients were treated postoperatively with doses of 18 to 38 Gy given over 3 to 10 fractions prescribed to mean IDL of 75%. Local control was 91% in this cohort of patients with no visual or neuroendocrine complications. Similar results have been demonstrated with use of a frame-based platform.[61–64]

Cystic craniopharyngiomas may also be managed by the use of intralesional radioactive isotope injection using a β-emitter. Typical prescriptions range from 200 to 250 Gy prescribed to the cyst wall. Optimal results are seen in patients whose tumors have one cyst and lack a large solid component.[65,66]

Acoustic Neuroma (Vestibular Schwannoma)

Background and Clinical Aspects

Acoustic neuromas (AN) represent 5% to 8% of primary CNS brain tumors. They are derived from Schwann cells of the neurilemma of the vestibulocochlear nerve (CN VIII). The vast majority of cases (90%) are unilateral and sporadic. Bilateral AN occur in about 10% of cases and are associated with the autosomal dominant disorder neurofibromatosis type II.

Symptoms include sensorineural hearing loss, tinnitus, and vertigo. Hearing loss is correlated more with tumor location (intracanalicular) rather than tumor size. In a minority of patients (5%), facial nerve symptoms may be present. As the AN grows, it may affect the trigeminal nerve (CN V) and brainstem.

During the initial workup, physical examination should include the Rinne test (air conduction greater than bone conduction on the affected side) and Weber test (vibratory sound louder on the unaffected side) to test for sensorineural hearing loss, as well as detailed examination of CN V and CN VII. All patients should undergo audiometry when the diagnosis of AN is suspected; this will often reveal asymmetric hearing loss more prominent at high frequencies as well as impairments in speech discrimination score. Imaging should include a contrast-enhanced MRI with thin slices through the internal auditory canal. The entire neuraxis should be imaged in patients with neurofibromatosis type II.

Surgery

For many years, the standard treatment for patients with AN was microsurgical resection, either via a translabyrinthine approach or middle cranial fossa approach. Surgery remains the preferred treatment for patients with large, symptomatic lesions. Hearing preservation is approximately 50% to 60% after surgery, and facial nerve preservation ranges from 80% to 90%.[67,68]

Active Surveillance

Observation is appropriate management for asymptomatic patients with small tumors. Serial MRI and audiometry (at least once per year) should be performed in this patient cohort for surveillance. Treatment is initiated when the lesion demonstrates rapid and significant growth or when the patient becomes symptomatic.

Radiotherapy

RT in the form of SRS or FSRT is an option for the primary treatment of AN, often with higher rates of hearing preservation and facial nerve presentation compared with surgery. Proton therapy has also been used to treat AN.

SRS doses using frame-based platforms are generally 12 to 13 Gy prescribed to the 50% IDL. Although earlier studies demonstrated lower hearing preservation rates with higher SRS doses,[69] current results are significantly improved. Flickinger et al.[70] demonstrated a local control rate of 98.6%, hearing preservation rate of 70.3%, trigeminal neuropathy rate of 4.4%, and no incidence of facial nerve dysfunction. Using a frameless robotic radiosurgery platform to treat 383 AN to a dose of 18 to 21 Gy given in 3 fractions, Stanford University researchers demonstrated a 98% local control, 76% hearing preservation, 2% incidence of trigeminal nerve dysfunction (transient in four of the eight affected patients), and no facial nerve dysfunction.[71]

Common dose prescriptions employing FSRT include 25 Gy in 5 fractions, 30 Gy in 10 fractions, and 50 to 55 Gy in 25 to 30 fractions. A nonrandomized prospective trial compared SRS (10 to 12.5 Gy) to FSRT (20 to 25 Gy in 5 fractions). This study demonstrated comparable rates of local control, hearing preservation, and CN V and CN VII preservation between the two groups.[72]

Proton beam SRS has also been used to treat AN, although with low rates of hearing preservation compared with other RT techniques. In a series from MGH, 88 patients were treated to a median dose of 12 GyE given in a single fraction prescribed to a median IDL of 70%. Tumor control rates at 2 and 5 years were 95.3% and 93.6%, respectively. Facial and trigeminal nerve preservation rates were 90%. Only 33% of patients retained serviceable hearing.[73] In a study of FSRT using a proton beam, local control was excellent but the hearing preservation rate was poor at 42%.[74]

Chordoma

Background and Clinical Aspects

Chordomas are rare, slowly growing midline tumors originating from the embryonal notochord rests in the skull base (35%), vertebral column (15%), or sacral regions (50%). The most common sites of skull-based tumors include the clivus, dorsum sella, and nasopharynx.

Patients typically present with signs and symptoms attributable to the primary site of the tumor. Workup includes MRI with contrast enhancement. CT may complement MRI to assess for local bony destruction. A biopsy is necessary primarily to distinguish chordoma from chondrosarcoma, which has a better prognosis, and other malignancies. In children, biopsy is essential to distinguish chordoma from rhabdomyosarcoma, which can frequently present in the same location.

Surgery

Complete surgical resection is the mainstay of treatment. However, due to location, GTR is often not possible. Relapse rates are as high as 50% even after surgical resection with negative margins.[75] Poor prognostic factors include large tumors, recurrent tumors, older age, and presence of necrosis on biopsy.[76–77,78]

Systemic Therapy

Approximately 25% of chordomas metastasize to the lungs, liver, or bone. In these patients, or in patients with recurrent disease after surgical resection and radiation therapy, molecularly targeted agents may be considered. Several small studies have demonstrated some benefit to the use of imatinib or the combination of imatinib and sirolimus in this situation.[79–81]

Radiotherapy

Adjuvant radiation therapy is indicated to reduce recurrence rates for skull-based chordomas. Retrospective data suggest that salvage RT is inferior to adjuvant RT with 5- and 10-year overall survival rates of 50% and 0%, respectively, for those treated with salvage RT compared with 80% and 65%, respectively, for patients treated with adjuvant RT.[82] RT techniques for treatment of skull-based chordomas include conventionally fractionated 3D-CRT or IMRT, fractionated charged particle therapy (protons, carbon ions), and FSRT.

Determination of the GTV should be made by coregistration of the preoperative and/or postoperative MRI to the treatment planning CT scan. Particularly for pediatric cases in which IMRT will be used with tight margins, a neuroradiologist should be available at the time of treatment planning to assist in creating the GTV. Margins for CTV should be 1 to 2 cm with an additional 3 to 5 mm for the PTV. Dose prescriptions to the PTV for patients receiving photon-based treatment should be at least 60 Gy given in 1.8- to 2.0-Gy daily fractions.

Proton-based therapy can achieve higher doses with good results. In a series of 195 chordomas treated at the MGH, 5-year progression-free survival was 70% with doses of 63 to 79.2 GyE given in 1.8- to 2.0-GyE daily fractions.[83] Research at Loma Linda examined 33 cases of chordomas treated with a median of 70 GyE and found a 76% 5-year local control and 79% 5-year overall survival.[78]

In a report of 96 chordomas treated using carbon ion therapy at the University of Heidelberg, with median total dose of 60 GyE (range 60 to 70 GyE) delivered in 20 fractions within 3 weeks, good local control rates of 81% at 3 years and 70% at 5 years were observed.[84] There was a trend to improved local control in patients who received >60 GyE.

FSRT and SRS are less well established than charged-particle therapy. The North American Gamma Knife Consortium published the experience of 71 patients who underwent Gamma Knife (Elekta Corp, Stockholm) SRS as primary, adjuvant, or salvage therapy for skull-base chordomas.[85] The median dose to the tumor margin was 15 Gy (range 9 to 25 Gy). Five-year local control was 66% for the entire cohort (69% for the no prior RT group and 62% for the prior RT group). Debus et al.[86] reported on 37 patients with chordomas treated with FSRT to a median dose of 66.6 Gy given in 1.8-Gy daily fractions; the target volume was encompassed by 90% of the dose. Local control was 82% at 2 years and 50% at 5 years.

Glomus Tumor, Chemodectoma, and Paraganglioma

Background and Clinical Aspects

Glomus tumors are rare, benign tumors that occur at and along the carotid artery near the bifurcation (carotid body tumor), the jugular bulb (glomus jugulare), or the middle ear (globus tympanicum). The peak age is in the fifth decade of life. Bilateral or multiple tumors occur in 10% to 20% of affected patients.

Symptoms include headache, cranial nerve dysfunction, dysphagia, pulsatile tinnitus, vertigo, and large, pulsating masses in the neck. In rare cases, patients present with episodic hypertension, which may be related to the secretion of vasoactive substances by the tumor. In this situation, urine and serum metanephrines should be measured. The clinical presentation coupled with imaging (high-resolution CT, MRI, or angiography) often establish the diagnosis. In patients in which multiple tumors are suspected, imaging with metaiodobenzylguanidine may be useful.

Surgery

In the carotid region, primary tumor resection after previous embolization is the therapy of choice. At the skull base or tympanum, neurosurgical intervention is often deferred due to the high rates of complications, including stroke and cranial nerve injury.[87]

Radiotherapy

RT is indicated for patients with tumors in unsuitable locations (i.e., skull base), as adjuvant therapy after STR, or as salvage therapy at the time of relapse after surgery. RT techniques include conventionally fractionated 3D-CRT or IMRT, SRS, and FSRT.

The diagnostic MRI should be coregistered with the treatment planning CT scan. The GTV is delineated and 1 to 1.5 cm is added for clinical and setup margin. With conventional techniques, doses are often 45 to 55 Gy given in 1.8- to 2.0-Gy daily fractions with local control rates near or >90% in several series.[88–91]

Results with SRS have been comparable to that of conventionally fractionated RT. Using a frame-based platform, reported tumor margin doses range from 12.5 to 20 Gy prescribed to the 50% IDL[92,93–94] and 15 to 25 Gy for linac-based SRS.[87] Local control rates in these series range from 90% to 100%. A recent meta-analysis of SRS published by the Johns Hopkins Hospital reviewed 335 patients treated with SRS across 19 different studies.[95] In the eight studies with median follow-up >3 years, clinical control was 95% and tumor control was 96%. The control rates were equal among patients treated with linac-based platforms and frame-based platforms. Complications were rare and often transient in each of the studies examined. On the basis of these findings, the authors advocate for the use of SRS as primary treatment of glomus jugulare tumors.[95]

Juvenile Nasopharyngeal Angiofibroma

Background and Clinical Aspects

Juvenile nasopharyngeal angiofibroma (JNA) is a rare, benign, vascularized tumor in the head and neck, affecting mostly male adolescents. JNAs develop from the sphenoethmoidal suture and spread from the nasal cavity to the sphenopalatine foramen and pterygopalatine fossa. Other routes of local spread include the paranasal sinuses, infratemporal fossa, orbital space, and middle cranial fossa.

Symptoms initially include recurrent epistaxis and impaired nose breathing. As local extension occurs, patients may develop facial swelling, orbital symptoms (blindness), cranial nerve deficits, and headaches from intracranial extension.

Diagnosis is often made with the clinical presentation and CT or MRI-based imaging. Biopsy may cause massive bleeding. Numerous staging systems are used to categorize the tumors based on extent of local extension, including the Chandler et al.,[96] Fisch,[97] and Radkowski et al.[98] systems (Table 91.4).

Surgery

Surgery combined with embolization is the preferred treatment. Through surgery, most JNAs without intracranial extension (i.e., Chandler stage I to III) have local control rates of near 100%. In patients with intracranial extension, complete resection is often not possible.

Radiotherapy

Tumors with intracranial extension or tumors in patients who are medically inoperable are generally treated with RT as the primary modality. Indications for postoperative RT include relapse after surgery. Fractionated IMRT is currently the RT technique of choice to limit collateral radiation to critical structures near the target volume.

The PTV is generally treated to 30 to 50 Gy given in fraction sizes of 2 to 3 Gy per day. In modern series, local control rates

TABLE 91.4 CHANDLER STAGING SYSTEM FOR JUVENILE NASOPHARYNGEAL ANGIOFIBROMA[a]

Stage	Description
I	Confined to nasopharynx
II	Extension into nasal cavity and/or sphenoid sinus
III	Extension into ≥1 of the following: cheeks, infratemporal fossa, pterygomaxillary fossa, ethmoid sinus, maxillary antrum
IV	Intracranial extension

Adapted from Chandler JR, Goulding R, Moskowitz L, et al. Nasopharyngeal angiofibromas: staging and management. *Ann Otol Rhinol Laryngol* 1984;93(4 Pt 1):322–329.

[a]See refs. 97 and 98 for the Fisch and Radkowski staging, respectively.

TABLE 91.5 CLINICAL RESULTS OF RADIOTHERAPY IN JUVENILE NASOPHARYNGEAL ANGIOFIBROMA

Study (Reference)	Number of Patients	Study Period	Dose (Gy)	Local Control (%)	Side Effects
Chakraborty et al. (2011) (99)	9	2006–2009	30–46	87.5 (2 yr)	No late toxicity
McAfee et al. (2006) (101)	22	1975–2003	30–36	90 (10 yr)	Cataracts (6), transient CNS syndrome (2), "in field" BCC (2)
Lee et al. (2002) (100)	27	1960–2000	30–55	85 (5 yr)	15% late toxicity (growth retardation, panhypopituitarism, TLN, cataracts)
Reddy et al. (2001) (102)	15	1980–1991	30–35	85 (5 yr)	Cataracts (3), CNS syndrome (1), BCC (1)

CNS, central nervous system; BCC, basal cell carcinoma; TLN, temporal lobe necrosis.

range from 85% to 100% (Table 91.5).[99,100,101,102] After RT, JNA remission is slow, and late recurrences may occur.

Langerhans Cell Histiocytosis (Histiocytosis-X)

Background and Clinical Aspects

Langerhans cell histiocytosis (LCH) is a rare disorder that affects approximately 300 individuals with a higher incidence in children (3 to 5 per million) than adults (1 to 2 per million). Age is an important prognostic factor, with children having better outcomes than adults. In the past, it was felt that children younger than 2 years old were felt to have a poor prognosis, but recent data from the LCH-II study now refute that point.[103]

The disease is due to an accumulation or proliferation of cells that phenotypically resemble the Langerhans skin cell and can cause tissue damage by production of cytokines and infiltration. The actual Langerhans cell is a myeloid dendritic cell that expresses the same antigens (CD1a and CD207) as the Langerhans skin cell.[104] On electron microscopy, Birbeck granules are the classic finding.

LCH can affect a variety of organ systems. Patients are typically stratified into groups based on the extent of disease: single-system disease at a single site, single-system disease involving multiple sites, or multisystem disease. The clinical presentation is dependent on the sites of disease. Involvement of the skeletal system is the most common site for children and may manifests as pain, palpable mass, motion deficit, or chronic otitis in the case of mastoid or middle ear involvement. Bony lesions from LCH are predominantly lytic in appearance, and the skull is the most frequently involved bony structure.

Cutaneous involvement affects primarily the skin of the scalp and groin and resembles a seborrheic dermatitis. Patients with cranial involvement (posterior pituitary or hypothalamus) may present with diabetes insipidus (DI). The disease may also involve the cervical lymph nodes. Pulmonary involvement is more typically seen in adults. Hepatomegaly, splenomegaly, bone marrow infiltration, and involvement of the gastrointestinal tract are further potential sites of disease.

Evaluation of the patient with suspected LCH should include complete H&P. Routine laboratory work should include white cell blood count with differential. Patients who have symptoms of DI should also undergo a water restriction test. A skeletal survey with or without bone scan should be performed to assess for potential lytic lesions. Further imaging with CT of the head should be performed in patients with skull, orbital, or mastoid involvement. MRI of the head is indicated for patients with DI and those suspected of having brain parenchymal disease involvement. CT of the chest is performed to evaluate patients with pulmonary involvement. An MRI of the abdomen should be performed for patients with palpable hepatomegaly or splenomegaly.

Management Principles

Treatment of LCH depends on the site and extent of disease. Asymptomatic lesions may be observed. For patients with involvement of only the skeletal system, treatment options include curettage, excision, or intralesional steroid injection. Response rates with curettage or excision alone range from 70% to 90%.[105] Single system multifocal bone disease may be effectively treated with corticosteroids or chemotherapy, such as vinblastine. For skin-only disease, topical nitrogen mustard and methotrexate are considered effective treatments.

In patients with multisystem disease with symptoms (fever, pain, failure to thrive) or organ dysfunction, treatment with systemic therapy is indicated. In LCH-II, all patients received initial treatment with prednisone and vinblastine and were randomized to intensification with or without etoposide.[103,106] The patients treated with intensification demonstrated superior rapid response rates and decreased mortality rates compared with the standard arm.[106] Exogenous antidiuretic hormone (ADH; vasopressin) is used to treat children with DI.

Radiotherapy

Due to the excellent response rates to nonradiotherapeutic measures, the role of RT in the treatment of LCH bony lesions has decreased. Indications for radiation therapy to bony sites include relapse after surgery, no signs of clinical healing after other interventions, pain relief, potential compromise of critical structures from an expansile lesion (i.e., cord compression), or if the bony site is not amenable to other local therapies. Collapsed vertebral lesions should not be irradiated unless they are painful. DI is another recognized potential indication for treatment with RT. When the decision is made to treat, 3D-CRT should be the technique of choice.

The target volume for patients with bony disease should encompass the abnormality seen on imaging with a small margin. For children, low doses on the order of 5 to 10 Gy given in 1.5- to 2.0-Gy daily fractions should be sufficient to control most bony lesions. Higher doses can be used in adults. In an early study by Smith et al.,[107] 92% of patients received total doses in the range of 4.5 to 10.0 Gy with an 87% local control rate. A study at the University of California–Los Angeles found local control rates of 88% with doses in the range of 6 to 15 Gy for previously untreated lesions and 8 to 15 Gy for recurrent lesions.[108]

The target volume for patients receiving treatment for DI should encompass the hypothalamus and pituitary gland. The recommended prescribed dose is 15 Gy in 1.5-Gy daily fractions. In a report from the Mayo Clinic, 36% of 28 evaluable patients responded to radiotherapy.[109] The response rates were 60% (3 of 5 patients) in those treated with >15 Gy compared with 30% (7 of 23 patients) treated with doses of <15 Gy. Six patients had a complete response to therapy, five of whom received treatment within 14 days from diagnosis of DI.

Controversy still remains regarding the role of RT in the management of DI. In a retrospective series from MGH, 14 of 17 patients with DI received irradiation to the hypothalamic–pituitary axis.[110] Only two of these patients had a complete response (cessation of ADH therapy), and no patients had a partial response. The others argue that treatment of DI from LCH is "no longer justified."[110]

VASCULAR DISORDERS

Vascular disorders are broadly categorized into vascular tumors, most commonly benign hemangiomas, and vascular malformations, including arteriovenous malformations (AVMs) and cavernous hemangiomas. Radiosurgery has emerged as an important and common treatment option for AVMs. Although radiation was used commonly in the past to treat hemangiomas in children, the recognition of late effects associated with radiotherapy, especially secondary malignancies, has rendered this practice less common.

Arteriovenous Malformations

Background and Clinical Aspects

Intracranial AVMs are congenital vessel abnormalities consisting of widened arteries connected to the normal capillary bed. The nidus of an AVM is made up of tangled arteries and veins that are connected by one or more fistulas. The overall prevalence is low, affecting approximately 18 in 100,000 individuals, with age at presentation typically between 20 and 40 years old.

Clinical concern comes from the high risk of bleeding, estimated to be 2% to 4% per year. Approximately 50% of patients present with hemorrhage and 50% present with nonfocal (headache, nausea) symptoms or incidentally found focal neurologic deficits. The risk of death per bleed is up to 10%, and approximately 30% have serious morbidity associated with each bleed.

Diagnostic imaging includes angiography, which is invasive but allows for full grading of the AVM according to the Spetzler-Martin scale. MRI, MR angiography, and CT angiography are noninvasive and complementary studies that may be used to visualize the AVM.

Surgery

The goal of any therapy for AVM is to completely obliterate the nidus. Partial obliteration of the nidus does not decrease the bleeding risk. Complete surgical excision provides immediate cure but carries a risk of intraoperative bleeding, ischemic cerebrovascular accident, infection, and death. Surgery is particularly indicated for AVMs in superficial, noneloquent regions of the brain. Endovascular therapy (embolization) is not curative but may be used to decrease the risk of intraoperative bleeding or to decrease the size of the nidus before planned radiotherapy.

TABLE 91.6 FLICKINGER'S PREDICTED RATES OF IN-FIELD ARTERIOVENOUS MALFORMATIONS OBLITERATION BASED ON THE MINIMUM DOSE WITHIN THE TARGET VOLUME

Minimum Dose to Target (Gy)	*Predicted AVM Obliteration Rate (%)*
27	99
25	98
22	95
20	90
17	80
16	70
13	50

AVM, arteriovenous malformations.

Adapted from Flickinger JC, Pollock BE, Kondziolka D, et al. A dose-response analysis of arteriovenous malformation obliteration after radiosurgery. *Int J Radiat Oncol Biol Phys* 1996;36:873–879.

Radiotherapy

SRS is the radiation modality of choice for the treatment of AVMs. SRS is indicated mostly for lesions in deep or eloquent regions of the brain and is particularly safe and successful for lesions that are <3 cm. Unlike surgery, the time to obliteration ranges from 1 to 4 years after SRS, so the patient remains at a continued bleeding risk. Even with time, Maruyama et al.[111] demonstrated that the bleeding risk is not completely eliminated but reduced by approximately 88%.

Based on the Flickinger et al.[112] dose–response data, typical prescriptions for treatment of AVM are 21 to 22 Gy prescribed to the 50% IDL for frame-based radiosurgery (Table 91.6). The prescription should be lowered for AVMs near the brainstem or larger lesions (>3 cm). For linac-based SRS, prescriptions generally range from 16 to 24 Gy in a single fraction to 20 to 22 Gy in 2 fractions for spinal AVMs (Fig. 91.4).[113]

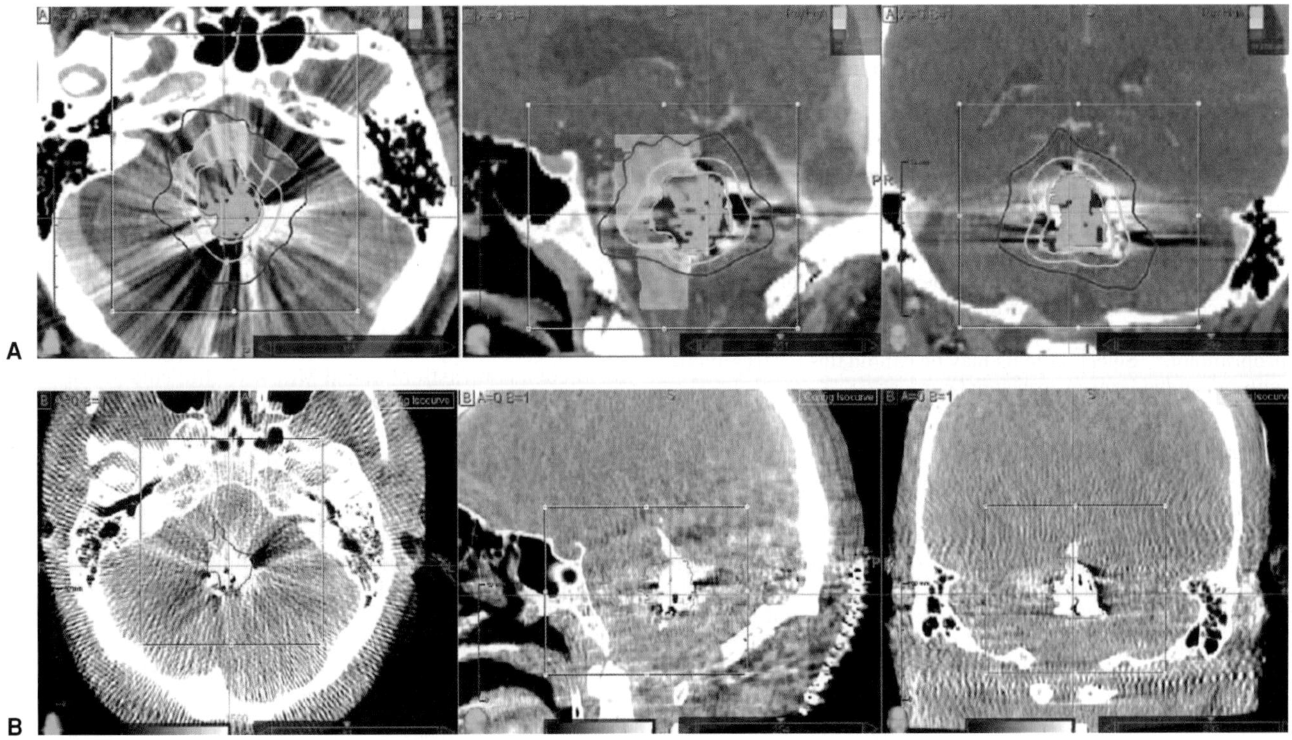

FIGURE 91.4. A: Stereotactic radiosurgery plan for an arteriovenous malformations (AVM) (*red*) in the dorsal pons treated with 22 Gy in 2 fractions. The prominent streak artifacts are present due to embolization 1 year prior to treatment. **B:** Computed tomography angiogram of the same patient used to assist in defining the AVM nidus (*red contour*).

Hemangioma and Kasabach-Merritt Syndrome

Background and Clinical Aspects

Hemangiomas are dynamic vascular tumors characterized by a proliferative phase followed by an involution phase. Approximately 20% of hemangiomas are present at birth, while the remaining 80% usually form within the first few weeks of life. Most hemangiomas present no problems to the patient and require no treatment. The spontaneous involution rate is approximately 10% per year.[114] However, potential complications that may require treatment include obstruction of vision (eyelid hemangioma), ulceration and infection, cosmetic deformity from a facial hemangioma, and high-output cardiac failure.

Previously, it was felt that extremely large hemangiomas predisposed patients to Kasabach-Merritt syndrome (KMS). This syndrome consists of platelet trapping and destruction within the vascular tumor with a resultant consumptive coagulopathy (disseminated intravascular coagulation) that can be life-threatening. It is now recognized that this phenomenon is associated with a type of vascular tumor known as the kaposiform hemangioendothelioma, and not the classical infantile hemangioma.[115]

Systemic Therapy

Treatment options for hemangiomas include local and systemic pharmacotherapy, laser therapy, and surgery. Glucocorticoids have been the mainstay of systemic treatment for patients with hemangiomas. However, long-term use of steroids in children leads to many complications, including growth retardation, metabolic disorders, cushingoid facies, personality changes, and increased risk of infections. Recently, propranolol has been recognized as a potential therapeutic agent for hemangiomas. The first report of its use was published in the *New England Journal of Medicine* in 2008 when two patients with hemangiomas with resultant heart failure were treated with propranolol and were noted to have softening, change in color, and ultimately regression of the lesions.[116] Both of these children were able to sustain a clinical response, even after being weaned off of steroids. Additional studies of propranolol have shown promising results, with most children exhibiting significant regression of their lesions and the ability to wean off of steroids without a rebound effect.[117]

For patients with KMS, vincristine and interferon-alfa have been used, particularly in situations in which a quick clinical response is needed or when the disease has become refractory to steroids and propranolol. Patients with KMS should also be managed with supportive measures, such as blood or platelet transfusions, as needed.

Patients with small lesions may be candidates for local therapy, such as intralesional or topical steroids. Topical timolol is also being investigated, given the promising results seen with propranolol.[118] Select patients may be candidates for treatment with pulse-dye laser or excisional surgery.

Radiotherapy

Radiotherapy is indicated only in patients who have exhausted all other treatment options. When RT is used, responses are often quick and dramatic. With low-dose RT (<10 Gy), scarring should be minimal, but patients must be followed closely for secondary malignancies.

The CTV should include the clinically visible and palpable lesion with a margin. Imaging of the affected area with MRI is useful to delineate the depth and full extent of disease. Although there are no prospective trials to guide total dose and daily dose, most reports have used fractionation schedules of 1 to 3 Gy per day to a total dose of ≤10 Gy.[19,119] When patients have not responded to low-dose RT, higher doses may be used to achieve a response.

FUNCTIONAL DISORDERS

SRS is widely used for the treatment of benign tumors. However, a significant number of patients benefit from the use of SRS to treat functional disorders such as trigeminal neuralgia, tremors, and epilepsy. Over the past several years, there have been increasing reports of the use of SRS for the treatment of refractory psychiatric disorders including obsessive-compulsive disorder and major depressive disorder.

Trigeminal Neuralgia (Tic Douloureux)

Background and Clinical Aspects

Trigeminal neuralgia (TN) is a common problem that affects approximately 15,000 patients each year in the United States. There is a slight female predominance (1.5 to 1). The disorder is currently classified into type I TN and type II TN, which is based on pain characteristics, as opposed to the traditional classification system, which divided patients into idiopathic TN versus secondary TN.[120–121,122] Patients with type I TN describe pain as being predominantly (>50%) sharp, lancinating, and shock-like with pain-free intervals. Patients with type II TN predominantly experience burning, aching, or throbbing pain. This system also carries prognostic significance, with type I TN patients more likely to be pain free and have longer disease control than patients with type II TN after decompression.[120]

The classic clinical feature is recurrent episodes of sudden, brief, severe, stabbing, or lancinating pain in the area of the trigeminal nerve sensory distribution. It is most commonly unilateral, but some cases are bilateral. Common triggers for attacks include talking, chewing, brushing teeth, and cold air. The diagnosis is often suspected on the basis of the above clinical symptoms, but an MRI of the brain should be performed to rule out structural abnormalities that may be causing secondary TN.

Medical Therapy

TN is first treated with pharmacotherapy, with carbamazepine being the most common and extensively studied agent. Oxcarbazepine is an option for patients who are unable to tolerate carbamazepine. Numerous other agents have been used to treat carbamazepine-refractory patients including lamotrigine, gabapentin, pimozide, tizanidine, and topiramate.

Surgery

In patients who have medically refractory disease, microvascular decompression is the treatment of choice for immediate relief of symptoms. Other options include rhizotomy with either radiofrequency ablation, glycerol injection, or balloon compression.

Radiotherapy

SRS has emerged as a successful and minimally invasive procedure to treat classical TN. Treatment planning involves fusion of a contrast-enhanced MRI with thin cuts to the treatment planning CT scan. The target for SRS varies from the root entry zone of the trigeminal nerve as it enters the pons to the semilunar ganglion.[123–129] Typical doses using a frame-based radiosurgery platform are 70 to 90 Gy, prescribed to the 50% IDL. This dose range is largely based on a trial that prospectively assigned patients to low-dose (60 to 65 Gy) or high-dose (70 to 90 Gy) SRS and demonstrated higher rates of pain relief in the high-dose arm (72% vs. 9% for patients treated with >70 Gy vs. <70 Gy), with a median time to pain relief of 1 month.[125]

The main concern with treating larger segments of the nerve with higher doses of radiation is the delayed onset of facial numbness. This is based on a prospective study by Flickinger et al.[130] who randomized patients to 75 Gy targeted to a shorter (1 isocenter) or longer (2 isocenters) segment of the trigeminal nerve. The rates of pain relief were surprisingly identical between the two groups. There was a trend toward a higher incidence of numbness or paresthesias in the 2 isocenter patients, and overall, the nerve length irradiated was significantly correlated with the development of numbness and paresthesias. However, in a report by Adler et al.,[131] 46 patients received treatment with a frameless robotic radiosurgery platform to a 6-mm segment of the trigeminal nerve with a mean marginal prescription dose of 58.3 Gy and mean maximal dose of 73.5 Gy. In this cohort of patients, 85% experienced a complete response and, at a mean follow-up of 15 months, 96% reported excellent or good outcomes. Only 15% of patients experienced ipsilateral facial numbness.

Epilepsy

Background and Clinical Aspects

Epilepsy is a disorder characterized by recurring seizures. It affects 0.5% to 1% of the population, and its etiology is unknown in the vast majority of cases. The clinical presentation of patients with seizures is broad, depending on the type of seizure and the area of the brain involved. Seizures are generally classified into simple versus complex (loss of consciousness) and generalized versus partial (affecting only one focus in the brain).

Nonradiotherapeutic Treatment

Antiepileptic drugs are the treatment of choice for patients with epilepsy. Surgery is an option for patients who develop medically refractory disease, particularly for temporal lobe epilepsy.[132]

Radiotherapy

SRS may be an alternative to surgery in medically refractory epilepsy for patients who are not surgical candidates. In a multi-intuitional study, Regis et al.[133] treated 20 patients with SRS for intractable mesial temporal lobe epilepsy. The mesial temporal lobe was treated to a dose of 24 to 25 Gy in a single fraction with Gamma Knife. At a follow-up of 2 years, 65% of the patients were seizure free. However, there was a 1-year lag between treatment and maximal effect, and there was a transient increase in seizures before the seizures started to diminish. In a study by Barbaro et al.,[134] 30 patients were randomized to low-dose (20 Gy) or high-dose (24 Gy) radiosurgery targeting the amygdala, hippocampus, and parahippocampal gyrus. At 3 years, the seizure-free rate was 67% among all patients with a trend toward a higher response rate (77% vs. 59%) and earlier responses in the high-dose compared with the low-dose group of patients. No serious toxicity was reported in the study.

In general, the use of SRS to treat epilepsy is not routine, and nonradiosurgical options should be employed first. Further study is needed to establish the long-term safety and efficacy of SRS in the treatment of epilepsy.

Parkinson Disease

Background and Clinical Aspects

Parkinson disease (PD) results from the loss of dopaminergic neurons in the substantia nigra. It is a debilitating and progressive neurodegenerative disorder that affects approximately 1 million people in the United States. The hallmark clinical symptoms include masked facies, resting tremor, slow movements, shuffling gait, and muscle rigidity. Some patients also develop dementia as part of the disorder.

Nonradiotherapeutic Treatment

Pharmacotherapy with dopamine agonists and other compounds is the treatment of choice for patients with PD. Once refractory to medical therapy, surgery (thalamotomy or pallidotomy) may be used to remove the overactive brain nuclei. Deep brain stimulation is another invasive procedure done under stereotactic guidance that can be used in medically refractory PD.

Radiotherapy

Patients who are poor candidates for surgery may receive SRS for the treatment of medically refractory PD. To relieve tremor, the target is the ventralis medialis nucleus with a dose in the range of 120 to 180 Gy. Young et al.[135,136] reported a long-term success rate of 80% to 90% in relieving symptoms from PD tremor with a very low rate of permanent complications.

Mixed results have been found with regard to the treatment of PD-related akinesia, dyskinesia, and rigidity. Treatment entails targeting the globus pallidus internus (pallidotomy) with doses in the range of 120 to 180 Gy. Rand et al.[137] reported that four of eight patients received relief in rigidity with no serious complications. However, Friedman et al.[138] achieved a response in only one of four patients, while causing dementia and psychosis in the only patient responder. Young et al.[139] treated 29 patients with SRS pallidotomy with an 80% success rate at mean follow-up of 2 years and only one (3.4%) complication at 9 months (homonymous hemianopia).

Psychiatric Disorders

Background and Clinical Aspects

Psychiatric disorders such as obsessive-compulsive disorder (OCD), bipolar disorder, and major depressive disorder are debilitating illnesses. Radiosurgery has been used for the treatment of some of these psychiatric illnesses, with the majority of the experience in patients with OCD. OCD is characterized by intrusive thoughts (obsessions) that lead to repetitive behaviors (compulsions).

Nonradiotherapeutic Treatment

The combination of pharmacotherapy (i.e., selective serotonin reuptake inhibitors) and behavior therapy are the treatments of choice for patients with mood disorders and OCD. Surgical management and deep brain stimulation are used for extreme and severe cases.

Radiotherapy

Patient selection for the use of SRS to treat psychiatric disorders is complex. Friehs et al.[140] recommend that such patients must be enrolled on an institutional protocol after carefully being evaluated by a multidisciplinary team. Similar strict criteria were used by Kondziolka et al.[141]

The treatment of OCD involves targeting the bilateral anterior capsules to a total dose of 120 to 140 Gy (Fig. 91.5). Kondziolka et al.[141] delivered a maximum dose of 140 to 150 Gy to the anterior limb of the internal capsule in three patients. At a minimum follow-up of 28 months, all patients noted significant functional improvements with no treatment-related complications. In a pilot study by Lopes et al.,[142] five patients were treated with SRS to a maximum dose of 180 Gy to the anterior limb of the internal capsule. At 3 years, three patients had a complete response to treatment, and one patient had a partial response based on changes in scores on an OCD assessment tool. Based on these findings, the group has opened a double-blind, randomized controlled study on the use of SRS to treat refractory OCD.

Summary

SRS is a well-established, safe, and effective treatment modality for TN. Its use in the treatment of PD, epilepsy, and psychiatric disorders remains an active area of investigation with limited data to support the widespread use of SRS in these situations.

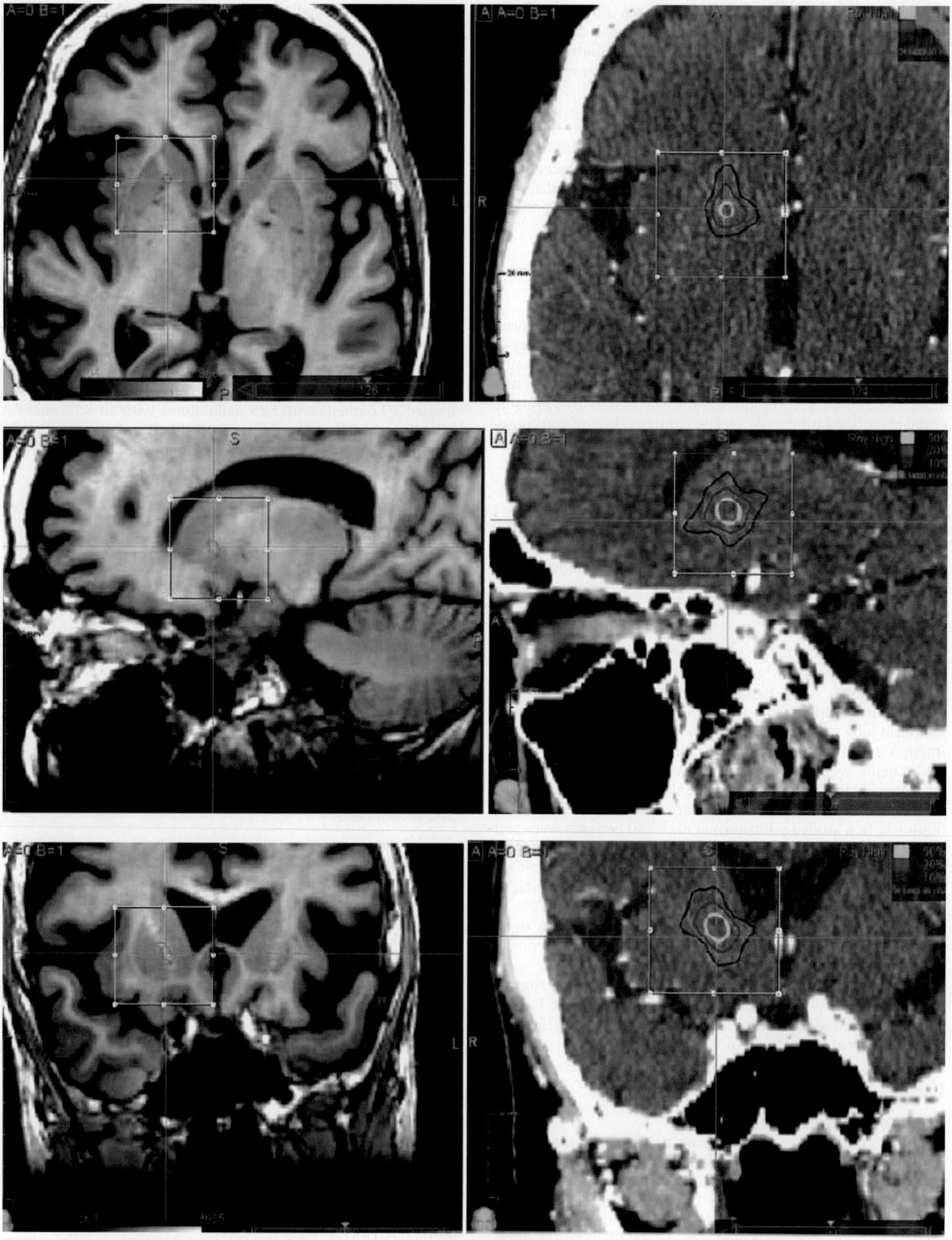

FIGURE 91.5. Stereotactic magnetic resonance imaging sequences (*left side*) demonstrating the contoured anterior limbs of the internal capsule bilaterally and the corresponding treatment plan for the right internal capsule (*right side*) for a patient with refractory obsessive-compulsive disorder. The right internal capsule was prescribed at 70 Gy to the 50% isodose line (140 Gy maximum dose) in a single fraction.

In particular, patients with psychiatric disorders should only be treated with SRS as part of a strict institutional protocol.

DISEASES OF THE EYE AND ORBIT

Pterygium

Background and Clinical Aspects

Pterygium is a chronic fibrovascular and degenerative process that arises from the conjunctival–corneal border that extends from the nasal corner of the eye to the cornea. Its name ("pterygium") refers to the shape of the tissue, which is wing-like. The exact prevalence of this problem is unknown, but it is well established that the frequency is higher in tropical regions. Most patients are asymptomatic and present for medical attention on the basis of cosmetic concerns, but symptoms may include redness and irritation of the eye. Pterygium may impair vision by producing an irregular astigmatism as it grows onto the cornea.

Surgery

Treatment is indicated when vision is threatened and less commonly to improve cosmesis. The treatment of choice for pterygium is surgical excision with an adjunct to help improve local control rates (i.e., sliding conjunctival flap; rotational conjunctival autograft; free conjunctival or limbal autograft). Intraoperative or postoperative mitomycin-C has also been used to improve local control rates, although this leads to increased risk of scleral ulceration, secondary glaucoma, iritis, and cataracts.

Radiotherapy

Local radiation therapy with strontium-90 plays an important role as an adjunct to surgery to prevent relapse. Outcomes with radiotherapy have been excellent at decreasing relapse rates.

The first prospective randomized study comparing postoperative radiation to observation after surgery was performed by de Keizer.[143] In this study, 19 pterygia were treated with bare scleral excision with a recurrence rate of 68% at 4 months compared with no recurrences in the 18 pterygia treated with postoperative fractionated irradiation (3 × 10 Gy, once a week). Numerous retrospective studies have also demonstrated the efficacy of postoperative radiation in preventing recurrence of pterygium, including a large series of 1,300 pterygia by Van de Brenk[144] and 825 pterygia by Paryani et al.,[145] both of which showed a low recurrence rate of 1.7% using fractionated radiotherapy.

In 2004, a European randomized trial compared single-dose (as opposed to fractionated) postoperative radiotherapy (25 Gy) compared with sham RT.[146] Patients who received radiotherapy had a local control rate of 93.2% compared with 33.3% in the placebo arm, indicating that single-dose radiotherapy is effective. In another randomized study, Viani et al.[147] compared low fractionation dose (2 Gy in 10 fractions) to high fractionation dose (5 Gy in 7 fractions) β-radiotherapy in the postoperative setting. Control rates were similar between the two groups (93.8% vs. 92.3%), with a significantly lower incidence of poorer cosmesis, photophobia, eye irritation, and scleromalacia in the low fractionation dose arm.

Choroidal Hemangioma

Background and Clinical Aspects

Choroidal hemangiomas (CH) are rare vascular tumors that arise from the choroid. CH can be classified as circumscribed, which occur in older patients, or diffuse, which are associated with the Sturge-Weber syndrome.[148]

Clinically, these lesions are often asymptomatic, but patients may present with a visual disturbance by several mechanisms, including retinal detachment, macular edema, and retinal pigment changes.[149] Lesions are detected on funduscopic examination. Further workup includes ultrasonography, angiography with fluorescent dyes, and CT or MRI.

Surgery

Among the surgical treatment options available, CH that are not near the central visual structures (macula and papilla) are often treated with photodynamic therapy with a low rate of complications.[148] Other treatment modalities include laser photocoagulation and transpupillary thermotherapy. In general, radiation therapy is preferred over photodynamic therapy for the treatment of diffuse CH, although several small studies have reported encouraging results with the use of photodynamic therapy.[148]

Radiation Therapy

RT is indicated to treat lesions near the macula and papilla and in cases that did not respond to other therapeutic maneuvers. RT techniques to treat CH include conventional 3D-CRT, proton-beam therapy, and brachytherapy.

Typical dose prescriptions for 3D-CRT are 18 to 20 Gy for circumscribed CH and 30 Gy for diffuse CH given in 1.8- to 2.0-Gy daily fractions. Schilling et al.[150] irradiated 36 circumscribed CH with 20 Gy in 10 fractions. Retinal reattachment occurred in 64% of the cases with improved vision in 50% and stable vision in 50%.

Fractionated proton radiotherapy doses range from 16.4 to 30 Gy in 4 fractions.[151–153] In the study by Zografos et al.,[153] all 54 cases experienced retinal reattachment, and visual acuity was improved in 70%. A recent study from Paris also demonstrated a 100% rate of retinal reattachment and substantial improvement in visual acuity using proton-beam therapy.[154]

Plaque brachytherapy using cobalt-60, iodine-125, or ruthenium-106 has been used to treat circumscribed lesions.[149,153,155,156] Typical doses prescribed to the apex of the lesion range from 25 to 50 Gy. Each isotope has advantages and disadvantages depending on the physical properties (i.e., energy, half-life), and there is no evidence to support the use of one over the other.

Age-Related Macular Degeneration

Age-related macular degeneration (AMD) is the leading causes of blindness in the developed world.[157] The development of AMD is dependent on age, with a prevalence of up to 35% in the eighth decade of life. External-beam radiotherapy with photons or protons and brachytherapy have been used in the past to treat macular degeneration. Overall, results of radiotherapy in the management of this disease have been mixed. A Cochrane meta-analysis in 2010 analyzed 14 randomized trials utilizing RT as a treatment for AMD and concluded that the review "does not provide convincing evidence that radiotherapy is an effective treatment for neovascular AMD."[158] Given that there is no clear benefit or indication for RT, its use should be limited for the treatment of AMD.

Graves Ophthalmopathy

Background and Clinical Aspects

Graves ophthalmopathy (GO), also referred to as Graves orbitopathy or thyroid eye disease, is an autoimmune disorder affecting the musculature of the orbits. The presence of activated T-lymphocytes leads to an inflammatory reaction secondary to the release of cytokines. It is estimated that up to 50% of patients with Graves disease will develop orbitopathy, but 10% of patients are euthyroid and some are hypothyroid at presentation.[1] Smoking is the greatest risk factor for the development of GO and also predicts for a poorer response to therapy.[1]

A multidisciplinary team, including an ophthalmologist, endocrinologist, and radiation oncologist, should be involved in the evaluation of the patient with GO. Clinical features of patients with GO include proptosis (measured by the Hertel exophthalmometer on physical examination), photophobia,

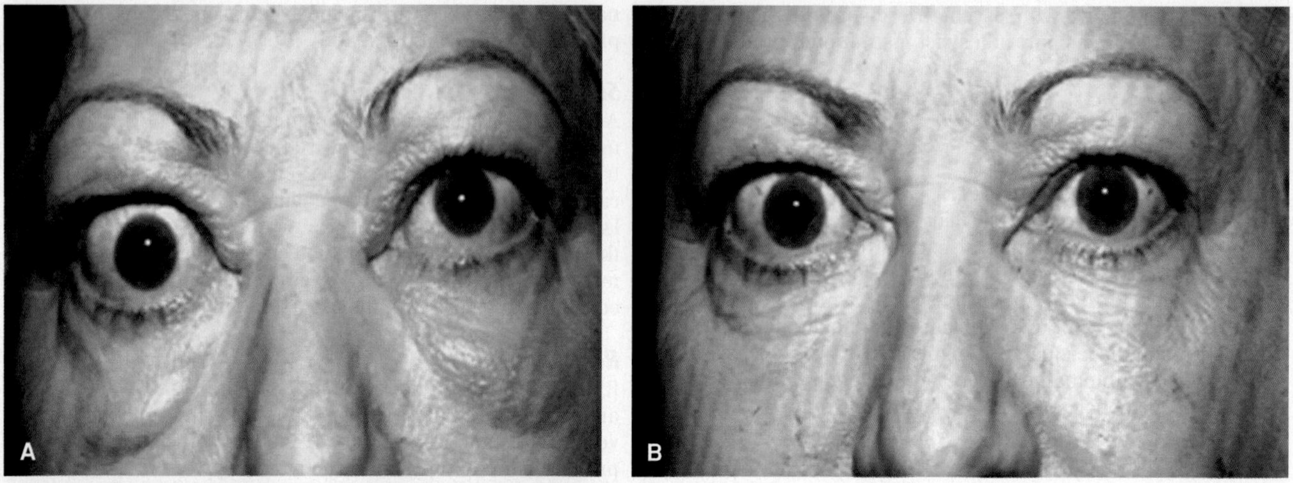

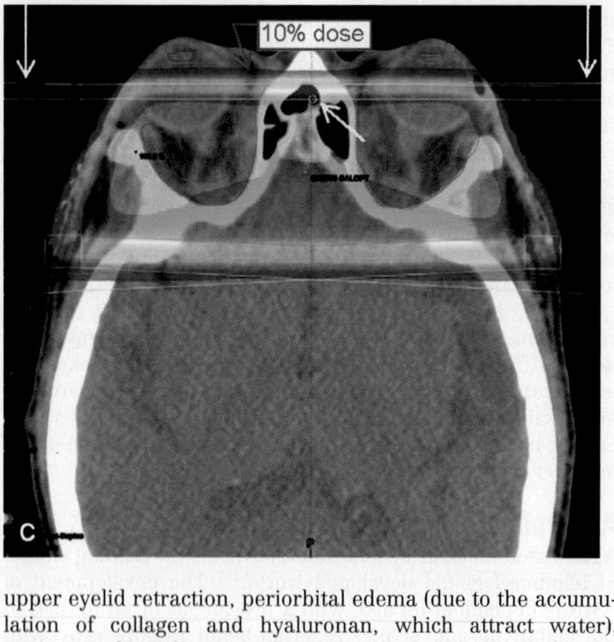

FIGURE 91.6. A 50-year-old woman with Graves ophthalmopathy before **(A)** and after **(B)** treatment with corticosteroids and radiotherapy for prominent eyelid edema and strabismus. **C:** Three-dimensional conformal radiotherapy treatment plan for a patient with Graves ophthalmopathy. The isocenter (*yellow arrow*) is placed a few millimeters posterior to the lenses (*magenta*), and the opposing fields are beam split anteriorly (*white arrows*). The extraocular muscles are contoured in *red.* The color wash display demonstrates that <10% of the dose reaches the lens.

upper eyelid retraction, periorbital edema (due to the accumulation of collagen and hyaluronan, which attract water), conjunctival erythema and tearing, and visual impairment (Fig. 91.6A,B). Patients may complain of a "gritty" sensation in their eyes. Several classification systems are available to document the extent of disease, although the one favored at Stanford University is the SPECS Ophthalmic Index (Table 91.7), which assigns a score of 1 to 3 on the basis of six categories: *S*oft tissue involvement, *P*roptosis, *E*xtraocular movements, *C*orneal involvement, and *S*ight (visual acuity).

Imaging studies, such as CT or MRI, will demonstrate abnormalities, including enlargement of the extraocular muscles and fatty infiltration, in 70% to 80% of cases.[1] The most commonly involved muscles include the inferior and medial rectus muscles.[159]

Management Overview

Treatment options for GO include glucocorticoids, orbital radiotherapy, and surgery (orbital decompression, eye muscle surgery, eyelid surgery). Smokers should be encouraged to quit. Prior to the initiation of treatment, the patient's thyroid function should be normalized, as this may help improve the GO.[160] Radioiodine therapy, but not antithyroid drugs, may cause worsening of GO.[161,162] Once thyroid function is stabilized, the treatment of GO depends on the severity of the disease.

Medical Management (Glucocorticoids)

Glucocorticoids (GCs) are a mainstay of treatment for GO. Immediate treatment with high-dose steroids (intravenous or oral) is required for patients whose vision is threatened by

TABLE 91.7 SPECS CLASSIFICATION SYSTEM FOR GRAVES OPHTHALMOPATHY

Clinical Feature	*Grade 1 (1 Point)*	*Grade 2 (2 Points)*	*Grade 3 (3 Points)*
S (soft tissue involvement)	Minimal objective symptoms: redness, chemosis, slight periorbital edema	Moderate objective symptoms: redness, chemosis; moderate periorbital edema	Severe objective symptoms: conjunctival exposition, prominent periorbital edema
P (proptosis)	>20–23 mm	24–27 mm	>27 mm
E (eye muscle dysfunction)	Rare diplopia; none in primary position	Frequent diplopia; moderate mobility impairment	Severe constant muscular dysfunction
C (corneal involvement)	Slight corneal changes and no symptoms	Prominent corneal changes and moderate symptoms	Keratitis or other severe eye symptoms
S (sight loss)	20/25–20/40	20/45–20/100	>20/100

Adapted from Marquez SD, Lum BL, McDougall IR, et al. Long-term results of irradiation for patients with progressive Graves' ophthalmopathy. *Int J Radiat Oncol Biol Phys* 2001;51(3):766–774.

TABLE 91.8 CLINICAL GUIDELINES FOR USE OF RADIOTHERAPY IN GRAVES OPHTHALMOPATHY

Radiotherapy Goal	Precondition/Indications	Contraindications
Induce clinical regression	*Pretherapeutic diagnostics:* evidence of autoimmune thyroid disease; CT/MRI	Stable GO without clinical progression
Reduce/eliminate functional deficits	*Ophthalmologic diagnostics:* documented progressive disease	Lack of euthyrosis
Improve cosmetics/esthetics	*Subjective/objective findings:* evidence of functional deficits and disorders	"Cosmetic" indication alone without functional impairment
Avoid/decrease undesired effects of other measures	*Exclusion of risk factors:* no other eye disease (i.e., diabetic retinopathy)	No consent to planned therapy

GO, Graves ophthalmopathy; CT, computed tomography; MRI, magnetic resonance imaging.
Adapted from Donaldson SS. *Radiotherapy of intraocular and orbital tumors*. Berlin: Springer, 2002.

optic neuropathy.[163] GCs may also be used to treat patients with moderate to severe active ophthalmopathy.[163]

Surgery

In the event that GCs fail to improve optic neuropathy, urgent orbital decompression is necessary.[164,165] Another indication for urgent orbital decompression is when exposure keratopathy is not relieved by topical therapies.[164] In order to improve extraocular muscle function and cosmesis, other procedures such as strabismus surgery and lid surgery may be performed. It is recommended that the GO be inactive for at least 6 months before pursuing these procedures.[164]

Radiotherapy

Indications for RT in the management of GO have been outlined by Donaldson[166] and include inducing clinical regression, improving functional deficits, improving cosmesis, and avoiding side effects of other treatments (Table 91.8).

RT is generally administered with 3D-CRT. Both orbits, including the entire length of the extraocular muscles, are treated to a total dose of 20 Gy in 2-Gy fractions using opposed lateral fields with the isocenter placed a few millimeters posterior to the lenses using a beam-split technique (Fig. 91.6C).

In a double-blind, placebo-controlled study, untreated euthyroid patients with GO were randomized to oral steroids or 20 Gy orbital irradiation.[167] Both groups experienced response rates of 50%, with greater improvements in eye motility and fewer side effects in the radiation arm. Two prospective studies have demonstrated a benefit of the combination of steroids and radiation compared with single modality treatment.[168,169]

For patients with progressive GO, retrospective data suggest that orbital RT is an effective treatment modality. Marquez et al.[170] reviewed the records of 197 patients treated at Stanford University, all of whom received 20 to 30 Gy to the bilateral retrobulbar region. Outcomes assessed included SPECS score and patient satisfaction. There was a 96% overall response rate and 98% patient satisfaction rate, with the largest improvements in soft tissue findings (89%), extraocular muscle dysfunction (85%), and corneal abnormalities (96%).

Reactive Lymphoid Hyperplasia and Orbital Pseudotumor

Background and Clinical Presentation

Disease of the lymphoid tissue in the orbit is rare and may include orbital pseudotumor (OP) or malignant lymphomas. OP is an inflammatory condition of unclear etiology that affects the soft tissue of the orbits, most often unilaterally.[159] Most patients present between the fifth and sixth decades of life.[171]

Clinical features of OP include periorbital edema, retrobulbar pain, extraocular muscle dysfunction, palpable mass, and exophthalmos.[159] Symptoms usually develop acutely. Imaging with CT or MRI of the orbits should be obtained for further evaluation. Imaging findings include enlarged extraocular muscles, optic nerve thickening, and infiltrates in the retrobulbar adipose tissue with enhancement after administration of iodinated contrast or gadolinium.[159] Biopsy should be obtained to establish the diagnosis, especially for lesions that are easily accessible.

Medical Therapy

Corticosteroids are the treatment of choice for the majority of patients. Response rates for optic neuropathy are as high as 92% with an overall response rate of 78%.[159] However, only 33% of patients experience long-term control with a single course of steroids.[172]

Surgery

Surgical excision may be used for easily accessible lesions. Relapses are common after surgery.

Radiation Therapy

Indications for RT include recurrent lesions after surgery, steroid-refractory lesions, and lesions not amenable to other treatments. The RT technique of choice is 3D-CRT.

A planning CT should be obtained and coregistered with the diagnostic MRI or diagnostic CT to delineate the target volume when visible. Unilateral treatment is typically performed with a single lateral field or with an anterior and lateral field, weighted more heavily laterally. Bilateral orbital involvement is treated in a manner similar to GO. Occasionally, superficial lesions may be treated with electrons. Typically, the prescription dose is 20 Gy given in 10 fractions.[159]

In a modern retrospective series from the University of Oklahoma, 20 orbits in 16 patients were treated with RT for OP.[173] With a mean dose of 20 Gy in 10 fractions, 87.5% of the patients experienced a response (clinical improvement or tapering of corticosteroid dose). Corticosteroid use was stopped or reduced in 81% of the patients. No significant late effects were reported.

BENIGN DISEASES OF SOFT TISSUE AND BONES

General Overview of Inflammatory Conditions of Joints and Tendons

The role of radiation therapy in the treatment of benign inflammatory conditions involving the joints or tendons is controversial. Osteoarthritis (OA), tendonitis, bursitis, rotator's cuff syndrome, and tennis elbow are examples of inflammatory conditions for which radiation therapy has been used in the past. These soft tissue syndromes may result from repetitive activities that cause overuse or injury to the joint areas, incorrect posture, stress on the soft tissues due to an abnormal or poor positioned joint or bone, or other diseases, such as autoimmune diseases or infection.

Although the cause of each disorder may be different, the clinical presentation and general treatment plan are frequently similar. Symptoms include pain, swelling, or inflammation in the tissues and structures around a joint, such as the tendons,

TABLE 91.9 RADIATION THERAPY MECHANISM OF ACTION DOSE CONCEPTS

Mechanisms of Action	Single Dose (Gy)	Total Dose (Gy)
Cellular gene and protein expression (e.g., eczemas)	<2.0	<2
Inhibition of inflammation in lymphocytes (e.g., in pseudotumor orbitae)	0.3–1.0	2–6
Inhibition of fibroblast proliferation (e.g., in keloids)	1.5–3.0	8–12
Inhibition of proliferation in benign tumors (e.g., in desmoids)	1.8–3.0	45–60

ligaments, bursae, and muscles. Treatment generally involves a combination of exercise, lifestyle modification, and analgesics. If pain becomes debilitating, joint replacement surgery may be used to improve the quality of life. In rare instances, low-dose radiation therapy (<10 to 15 Gy) can be employed. The low dose required to improve symptoms suggests the possible mechanism of action for radiation therapy (Table 91.9).

Osteoarthritis

OA is the most common joint disorder. It presents with pain associated with cartilage destruction, bone modification, and structural changes of capsule and synovia. Symptoms are caused by reactive inflammation of joint surface and joint capsule lining (synovia). Although in many instances the cause of OA is unknown, age is a major risk factor. Other risk factors include obesity, bone fracture or joint injury, whether by an accident or overuse from work or sports, and other medical conditions.

Nonradiotherapeutic Treatment

Hunter and Lo[174] provide a general overview of the diagnosis, investigation, and treatment of OA. The treatment of early OA is intended to reduce the primary symptoms of joint pain and stiffness with the goal of maintaining and improving the functional capacity of the affected joint(s).[175] Exercise, weight reduction, and joint braces, among other measures, have shown some success at unloading damaged joints and improving symptoms.[176,177] For osteoarthritis of the hip and knee, exercises that strengthen muscles and improve aerobic condition are most effective.[178]

Oral analgesics are the mainstay of treatment for OA. Although acetaminophen is frequently offered due to its relative safety and effectiveness, a nonsteroidal anti-inflammatory drug (NSAID) may be added or substituted.[179] NSAIDs can be used in patients with symptomatic OA of the hand, hip, or knee. The goal is to administer the lowest effective dose for the shortest duration. The use of stronger analgesics, such as weak opioids and narcotics, may be considered when other methods have been ineffective or if certain drugs are contraindicated.[176] Glucosamine and chondroitin sulfate are over-the-counter remedies that are frequently used to reduce pain, but their efficacy has not been proven.[180] Corticosteroids and other analgesics may be injected directly into the joint; injections may temporarily reduce swelling and pain. Acupuncture and other complementary and alternative treatment modalities have been used, but their efficacy has yet to be proven.[181]

Surgery is reserved for patients with severe OA and those who have not responded to noninvasive therapies. Total or partial joint replacement is most commonly used for OA involving the knee, hip, and shoulder and is considered when structural damage is visible on x-rays. However, there are modern surgical procedures that can obviate or delay the need for joint replacement, including osteotomies and joint resurfacing.[182] Joint fusion or arthrodesis may be used to treat arthritis of the spine, ankles, hands, and feet. Arthroscopy, or arthroscopic surgery, is a minimally invasive surgical procedure that can be used to examine and treat the interior surface of a damaged joint. Arthroscopic procedures can help relieve pain for a short time and allow the joints to move better. Although arthroscopy may delay the need for joint replacement surgery, it does not improve the arthritis itself.[183]

Radiotherapeutic Options

In nonsurgical candidates, low-dose RT may be considered if pharmacotherapy has failed. RT can lead to primary freedom from pain and secondary to improved joint function.[184] Several single-institution studies have been published that report long-term pain relief and functional gain in 50% to 75% of patients. In Germany from 2006 to 2008, a pattern of care study investigated the use of RT for the treatment of OA of the knee (gonarthrosis).[185] Almost 80% of institutions in Germany have used RT to treat OA in the 2-year period analyzed. Treatment of 4,544 patients was performed annually at 188 institutions. The median total dose was 6 Gy (range 3 to 12 Gy), with a median single dose of 1 Gy (0.25 to 3 Gy). Long-term clinical outcomes were available in 5,069 cases. The majority of patients experienced pain reduction for at least 3 months, but pain management for up to 12 months was reported. In 30% of patients, a second course of RT was used for inadequate pain response or early pain recurrence.

As with arthroscopy, radiation may reduce pain and pain-related dysfunction, but it does not improve the arthritis itself. Due to its efficacy and relative safety, RT may provide an alternative to conventional conservative treatment for patients who are not surgical candidates.

DISEASES OF CONNECTIVE TISSUE AND SKIN

Desmoid Tumors

Background and Clinical Aspects

Desmoid tumors (also called aggressive fibromatosis or deep musculoaponeurotic fibromatosis) are benign tumors of connective tissue tumors that arise from muscle fascias, aponeuroses, tendons, and scar tissue. They are slightly more predominant in females and tend to occur during the third and fourth decades of life, although children and the elderly can be affected. In the general population, desmoids are rare; the estimated incidence is 2 to 4 per million per year. Genetic factors, trauma, or surgery predispose the development of desmoids. Most desmoids arise sporadically; however, approximately 2% are associated with familial adenomatous polyposis (FAP). Desmoid tumors affect between 10% to 20% of patients with FAP. The development of desmoid tumors in patients with FAP is called Gardner syndrome.

Tumors can develop anywhere in the body, but most commonly involve the trunk or extremity, abdominal wall, and intra-abdominal sites, including the bowel and mesentery. Approximately 30% of patients with desmoid tumors have a history of prior trauma at the tumor site.[186,187] Sporadic cases commonly involve the extremities, the shoulder girdle, and the buttock.[187] In patients with FAP, intra-abdominal desmoids predominate and tend to be associated with surgical sites and anastomoses following colectomy.[188] Desmoid tumors in women can occur during or after pregnancy and therefore may be associated with high estrogen states. Women who have been pregnant are more likely to have abdominal desmoid tumors that develop within 10 years of the last pregnancy.[189]

Although desmoids have no known potential for metastasis or dedifferentiation, they are locally aggressive and commonly have a high rate of recurrence even after complete resection. Diagnostics workup with MRI helps to estimate size and infiltration into other organs and should be obtained prior to incisional biopsy obtained to confirm diagnosis.

Nonradiotherapeutic Treatment

Observation is a viable option for stable, asymptomatic desmoids. Treatment is indicated for symptomatic patients, if there is risk to adjacent structures, or to improve cosmesis. Complete resection of the tumor with negative microscopic margins is the treatment of choice for most desmoid tumors. Due to the size and infiltrative nature of extra-abdominal desmoids, resection may require skin grafting or flap reconstruction. Desmoid tumors have a high rate of recurrence following even complete surgical removal, and the contribution of incomplete resection to local recurrence rates is unclear.[190] Furthermore, resection does not appear to affect survival, which is not surprising in view of the histologically benign nature of desmoids. Given these issues, the overall surgical strategy should be an attempt at complete removal using function-preserving surgical approaches to minimize major morbidity (functional or cosmetic).[191]

Although extra-abdominal desmoid tumors can generally be treated effectively with local therapy, surgical intervention tends to be counterproductive in intra-abdominal variants, especially the ones associated with FAP. In some instances, systemic therapy may achieve significant and durable cytoreduction, obviating the need for resection. Patients with desmoid tumors have been treated with NSAIDs. The most widely used NSAID for treatment of desmoid tumors is sulindac. Hormonal agents such as tamoxifen, raloxifene, and progesterone have been used, often in combination with NSAIDs. Tamoxifen has been used most widely and is typically prescribed at doses similar to those used for breast cancer (10 mg daily). Much higher doses (120 mg daily) have been recommended,[192] but high-dose tamoxifen is difficult to tolerate and there is no evidence to suggest that higher doses of tamoxifen are better than lower doses.

A variety of palliative chemotherapeutic regimens have been used.[193–194,195–196] With the waxing and waning natural history of desmoids, it is difficult to say whether systemic therapy provides much benefit over observation. In one series, 142 patients presented with either a primary (n = 74) or recurrent (n = 68) desmoid tumor. Eighty-three patients were treated with observation alone, and 59 received either hormone therapy or chemotherapy. There was no statistically significant difference in progression-free survival between the two groups.

Desmoid tumors also respond to the tyrosine kinase inhibitor imatinib.[197,198] The response is thought to be due to expression of one of Gleevec's molecular targets, platelet-derived growth factor receptor, on desmoid tumors.[199] In a phase II clinical trial to assess the efficacy of imatinib (400 mg per day for 1 year) in the treatment of progressive and recurrent aggressive fibromatosis, the 2-year progression-free and overall survival rates after the use of imatinib were 55% and 95%, respectively.[198]

Intralesional injections[200] and radiofrequency ablation[201] have also been used. Although the techniques led to some tumor shrinkage, the experience to date is limited and the long-term results are not yet known.

Radiotherapeutic Options

Radiation therapy is a viable option for inoperable patients and may also be used in combination with surgery or chemotherapy. Spear et al.[202] retrospectively compared the efficacy of surgery alone, radiation alone, and combined modality therapy (radiation and surgery) in the treatment of desmoid tumors. Five-year local control rates among surgery, radiation therapy, and combined modality groups were 69%, 93%, and 72%, respectively. The study recommended radiation doses of 60 to 65 Gy for inoperable or recurrent desmoids. However, long-term results at another institution show increased posttreatment toxicity in patients who receive RT doses >56 Gy.[191,203]

Young age (≤30 years) was also associated with increased late toxicity. In a retrospective study of 30 patients under the age of 30, younger age (<18 years) is associated with inferior local-regional control following RT. Although actuarial control rates were better with RT doses of ≥55 Gy, almost 50% of patients experienced grade 3 or 4 complications, including pathologic fractures, impaired range of motion, pain, and in-field skin cancers.[204] Because long-term results suggest that unresectable tumors respond to 56 Gy with a 75% expectation of local control, the lower dose may be more appropriate.

When an R0 resection is not possible, doses of 50 Gy postoperatively should be given to improve local control. RT is often not considered for intra-abdominal tumors because the dose and increased field size required increase risk of bowel injury. Due to the complexities involved in managing the disease, a multidisciplinary approach must be taken.[205]

Peyronie Disease

Background and Clinical Aspects

Peyronie disease (also known as Induratio penis plastica) is a chronic inflammatory connective tissue disorder involving the penile tunica albuginea that results in tissue proliferation and the development of hard plaques, most commonly on the dorsal surface of the penis, which may cause a curvature and changes in the length or circumference of the penis while erect. Symptoms may lead to difficult intercourse, penile pain, and erectile dysfunction.

Peyronie disease affects up to 10% of men, although a recent population-based study suggests the condition may be underreported in the United States.[206] Although Peyronie disease can affect teenagers, peak incidence is between 40 to 60 years of age. The cause is unknown, but diabetes mellitus and arterial and venous vascular disease are risk factors, along with an assumed genetic predisposition. The disorder results in pain, abnormal curvature, erectile dysfunction, indentation, loss of girth, and shortening. Slow progression over several months is typical, but spontaneous remission may occasionally occur.

Nonradiotherapeutic Treatment

Results of nonsurgical treatment of Peyronie disease are mixed and are controversial.[207,208] Some success has been reported with vitamin E supplementation, but results have not been confirmed in larger studies.[209] A combination of vitamin E and colchicine may delay disease progression.[210] Other agents that specifically target inflammatory pathways have also shown mixed benefit, including, tumor growth factor-β1 inhibitors,[211] coenzyme Q10,[212] and sildenafil, among others.[213] Topical therapies have largely been ineffective, but penile injection with verapamil or collagenase, intended to break up scar tissue formed by the inflammation, have shown some efficacy.[214] Physical therapy and extracorporeal shock treatments have also had limited benefit.

Surgical options for Peyronie disease are complex procedures that should only be performed by experienced urologists and are reserved for patients not responding to other therapies.[215] Although the nonsurgical treatments discussed may not reliably treat the disease, they can be used to stabilize the scarring process and may result in some reduction of deformity. A combination of nonsurgical techniques may have even more efficacy.[216]

Radiotherapeutic Options

The largest experience with the use of RT in the treatment of Peyronie disease has been in Europe. Retrospective studies showed symptom improvement with the use of RT. Although some studies suggested improvement in curvature,[217] the majority of studies suggest that radiation therapy primarily provides relief of pain associated with Peyronie disease. These data suggest that the benefit of RT might best be in the treatment of early stages of disease, when radio-responsive inflammatory cells and fibroblasts are still active in the disease. There may be little improvement in penile contracture once the plaques have fully formed.

As with radiation therapy for other rare benign conditions, the treatment regimens for Peyronie disease vary among institutions.[17] A survey of European practices show that most practices give a total dose of approximately 20 Gy (3 to 30 Gy) in 2-Gy fractions (range 0.5 to 8.0 Gy). Most of the institutions used electrons (n = 44), however, orthovoltage was still used at a number of practices (n = 32). One retrospective study from the Netherlands indicated that low-dose RT, either 13.5 Gy (9 × 1.5 Gy, 3 fractions per week) or 12 Gy (6 × 2 Gy, daily fractions) resulted in pain relief in the majority of the 179 patients evaluated.[217] Sexual dysfunction was a reported side effect, although this is confounded by the underlying disease.

As experimental models improve our understanding of the pathogenesis of the Peyronie disease, the use of radiation therapy may further decline, as concern regarding radiation induction of fibrosis surface and new more effective therapies to emerge.[218,219]

Dupuytren's Contracture

Background and Clinical Aspects

Dupuytren's contracture, also known as Morbus Dupuytren (MD) and Morbus Ledderhose (ML), depending on involvement of the hands or feet, respectively, is a connective tissue disorder that affects the palmar or plantar fascia. Incidence increases after the age of 40, and the condition affects men more often than women. Although there is a familial disposition, alcohol abuse, diabetes mellitus, epilepsy, and other conditions are associated. Initially, there is an inflammatory proliferative phase with fibroblast activity.

In the early stage, subcutaneous nodules appear, which may be fixed to the overlying skin. As the disease progresses, cords develop and become visibly predominant. With further progression, the cords reach the periosteum of the bones and lead to the characteristic appearance of palmar or plantar contraction. The fourth or fifth phalanges of the hand (MD) or the first or second toes of the foot (ML) are the most commonly affected digits (Fig. 91.7). With increased thickening of the fascia and progressive contracture, the fingers and toes begin to curl, resulting in impaired function. Flexion contractures in the metacarpal or proximal interphalangeal joints lead to difficulty grabbing (MD) or walking (ML).

Nonradiotherapeutic Treatment

Excision of diseased cords and fascia via limited or selective fasciectomy is widely considered the gold standard treatment for Dupuytren's contracture.[220,221] A 20-year review of open surgery for Dupuytren's contracture showed that major complications occurred in 15.7% of cases and wound complications were seen in 22% of cases.[222] Even with excellent surgical resection, relapse is common, with 30% to 50% recurrence rate at 3 years.

Modern minimally invasive techniques have substantially reduced the complication rates. Percutaneous needle fasciotomy is a technique where cords are weakened through the insertion and manipulation of a small 25-gauge needle mounted on a 10 mL syringe.[223] The procedure is performed under local anesthesia and patients may return to full usage of the affected limb within 24 hours. Because the cords and nodules are not fully excised, minimally invasive surgery has an even higher recurrence rate than surgical excision. A randomized study comparing percutaneous needle fasciotomy with limited fasciectomy showed an 85% recurrence rate after 5 years with the minimally invasive procedure.[224]

During the early stage of Dupuytren's, medication (steroids, allopurinol, nonsteroidals, vitamin E) may provide benefit, but the effects are temporary. Injectable collagenase extracted from *Clostridium histolyticum* has been approved for the treatment of Dupuytren's contracture. Injection of small amounts of the enzyme collagenase weaken cords by breaking the peptide bonds in collagen.[225] Treatments should only be applied by an experienced provider, as the amount of enzyme injected varies depending on the affected joint and also has a very high recurrence rate.[226,227]

Radiotherapeutic Options

Several clinical trials support the concept of prophylactic radiation therapy in the treatment of Dupuytren's contracture.[228–229,230,231] Radiotherapy is effective for prevention of disease progression in early stages of disease when only small lumps or cords are present and only moderate extension deficits (≤10 degrees) are present. Treatment can be administered with either electrons or orthovoltage radiation, and a variety of dose levels have been used. Because the target cells are proliferating and radiosensitive fibroblasts and inflammatory cells, low-dose radiation therapy can be applied.[228,230]

In a recent prospective trial involving 129 patients, two different dose regimens were compared for safety and efficacy. In group A, 63 patients received 10 × 3 Gy (30 Gy) via a split course (5 × 3 Gy) separated by 8 weeks; in group B, 66 patients

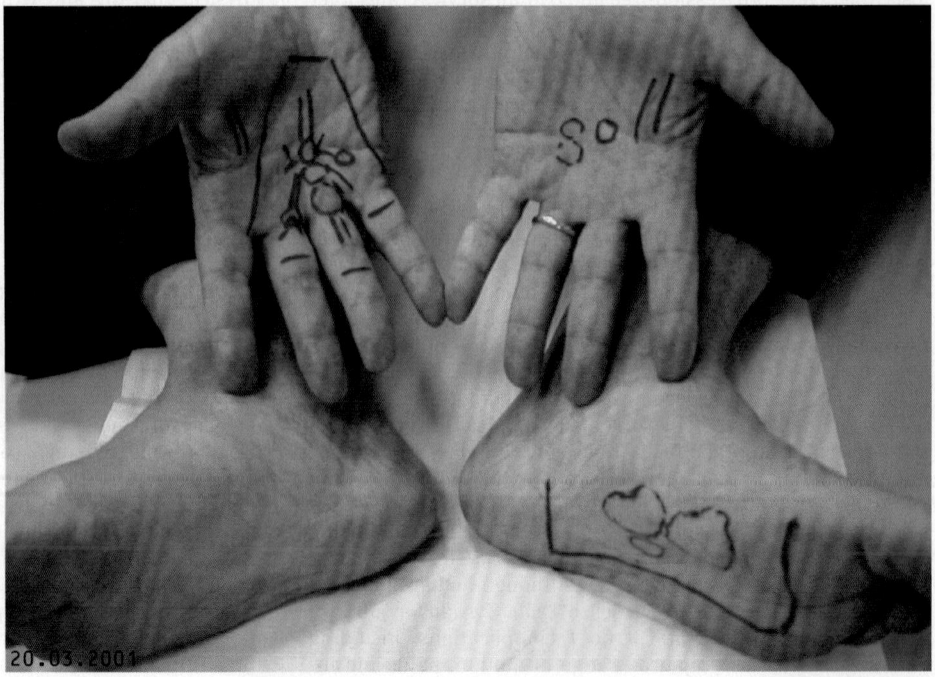

FIGURE 91.7. Dupuytren's contracture of both hands and the left foot.

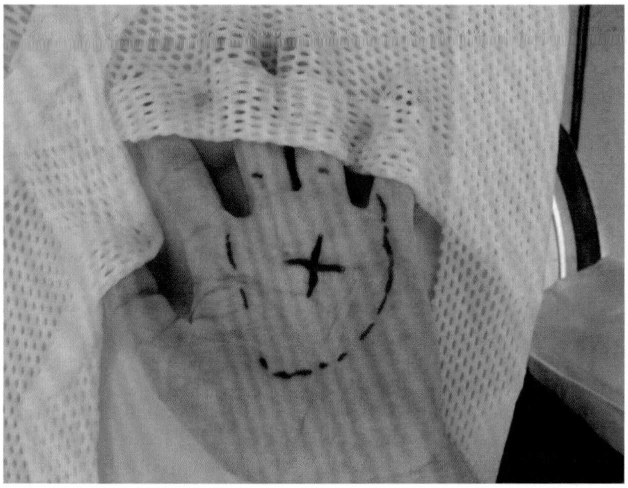

FIGURE 91.8. Immobilization for treatment of Dupuytren's contracture with electrons.

were treated with 7 × 3 Gy (21 Gy) delivered over 2 weeks. There was no difference in treatment outcomes between the two groups. Regardless of dose regimen, approximately 90% of patients had stable or improved disease. Overall and mean number of nodules, cords, and skin changes decreased at 3 and 12 months. There was an 8% treatment failure rate at 1 year. Acute toxicity was more pronounced in group B, but long-term toxicity was comparable and included dryness, desquamation, skin atrophy, and altered sensation. Although long-term results of this study are pending, prior retrospective data indicated that prophylactic RT is well tolerated by patients and is effective at preventing disease progression. Irrespective of dose regimen, appropriate immobilization and shielding of unaffected joints is required (Fig. 91.8).

Keloids and Hypertrophic Scars

Background and Clinical Aspects

Keloids are an excessive tissue proliferation around scars after skin injury from surgery, heat, chemical burns, inflammation (e.g., acne), or even spontaneous proliferation. They differ from hypertrophic scars by their typical infiltrative growth pattern, causing local pain and inflammatory reactions, and sometimes long-term progression; hypertrophic scars show thickening without surrounding reaction and can flatten spontaneously. Keloids appear mostly in the upper body and in regions with high skin tension (e.g., sternum, earlobes). The cause is still unknown, although there is a genetic and race-specific predisposition that is already noted during adolescence. Keloids at the earlobe after piercing are typical. In some patients, the resulting lesions are severely disfiguring and painful (Fig. 91.9). Recurrence is common after treatment.

Nonradiotherapeutic Treatment

Silicone bandages, pressure dressings, and cryosurgery have all been used to treat keloids, with varying efficacy.[232–234] Intralesional injections remain the first-line therapy for most keloids. Corticosteroids, 5-fluorouacil, and verapamil have all been directly injected into keloid lesions with symptom improvement. Up to 70% of patients respond to intralesional corticosteroid injection with flattening of keloids, although the recurrence rate is high in some studies (up to 50% at 5 years).[235]

Surgical excision may be indicated if injection therapy alone does not result in improvement. In patients treated with excision alone, recurrence rates range from 45% to 100%,[236] therefore, excision is typically combined with perioperative or postoperative injections of either triamcinolone or interferon.[235]

Radiotherapeutic Options

Radiotherapy should be considered in cases of repeat recurrences postoperatively or where there is a high-risk of recurrence (e.g., marginal resection, large lesion, unfavorable location). Primary RT can be considered in instances where resection would result in functional impairment and in actively proliferating disorders within about 6 months after the triggering trauma. Because proliferating fibroblasts and mesenchymal and inflammatory cells are the target cells for RT, fully matured keloids have minimal response to RT alone. Prophylactic RT immediately following excision is most effective and reduces the risk of recurrence to 20% or 25% in most series.

RT is initiated 24 hours after surgery. The target volume is limited to the scar plus a 1-cm margin; lead shielding can be constructed to protect normal tissue. An analysis of multicenter data on the use of postoperative RT for earlobe keloids shows that higher dose per fraction and use of deeper penetrating electrons are preferable to standard 2-Gy fractionation schemes or use of brachytherapy techniques that have rapid dose falloff.[237] Radiation dose is typically 12 to 20 Gy, delivered in 3 or 4 fractions within 1 week.[238] Single-fraction RT with 7.5 to 10 Gy is also effective.[239] Clinical end points are long-term control, low relapse rate, and good cosmesis.

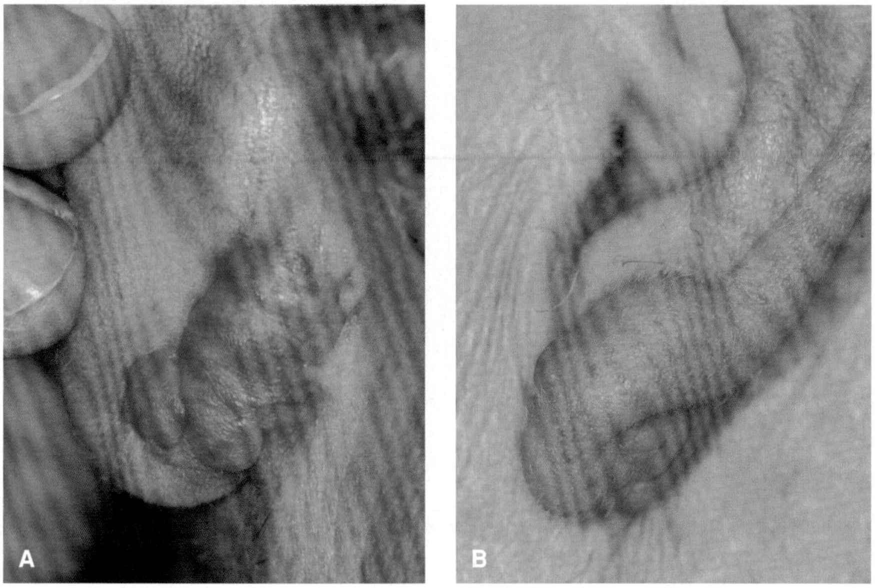

FIGURE 91.9. A: Keloid behind left earlobe. **B:** Status of keloid following resection plus 4 × 4 Gy radiotherapy.

Diseases of Bone

Gorham-Stout Syndrome

Gorham-Stout syndrome, also known as disappearing bone disease or essential osteolysis, is a rare bone disorder of unknown etiology. It is characterized by painless bone destruction due to progressive proliferation of small blood or lymph vessels. There may also be significant osteoclast activation. The symptoms are nonspecific but include muscular weakness, limb tenderness, and pathologic fracture occurring after minimal trauma. Involvement of the cervical spine or skull base could be fatal. Case reports indicate limited efficacy of systemic therapies such as zoledronic acid and interferon-alfa.[240,241] Radiation therapy has also been used.[242,243] Heyd et al.[244] completed a national patterns-of-care study and literature review that summarizes the scant data available for this rare disorder. The 38 articles listed therein provide evidence from treatment of 44 patients that indicate conventionally fractionated external-beam RT (total dose of 36 to 45 Gy) may prevent disease progression in 77% to 80% of cases.

Pigmented Villonodular Synovitis

Pigmented villonodular synovitis or tenosynovial giant cell tumor is a rare proliferative disorder of synovial tissue. Symptoms include sudden onset, unexplained joint swelling, and pain that frequently involves a single joint. The knee and foot are most commonly affected, but there are reports of shoulder, hand, and hip involvement.[245] Decreased motion, joint stiffness, and increased pain occur as the disorder progresses. Surgical resection with either synovectomy or joint replacement is the treatment of choice.[246,247]

Radiation therapy is indicated in cases of diffuse disease, bulky disease resulting in bone destruction, or in the rare instance of multiple recurrences after resection. Although intrasynovial injection of radioactive isotopes postoperatively has been used in the past for high-risk patients,[248] most institutions use external-beam radiation therapy. RT to a dose of 35 to 50 Gy has been effective.[249,250] MRI is essential for delineating disease pre- and postoperatively. Final dose of RT should be tailored to amount of residual disease.[251]

Vertebral Hemangiomas

Hemangiomas are benign proliferations of blood vessels that can affect any tissue and are typically asymptomatic. About 50% of hemangiomas involving the vertebral body are associated with pain and therefore may require treatment. Treatment options include surgical resection or more conservative interventions such as vertebroplasty or intralesional injections.[252] Radiation therapy either alone or postoperatively has been successful in reducing pain caused by vertebral hemangiomas.[253] In this study, a total of 84 patients with 96 symptomatic lesions were irradiated for a symptomatic vertebral hemangioma. At a median 68 months' follow-up, 90% of patients had either complete or partial pain relief. Radiation doses ≥34 Gy resulted in significantly improved pain relief. A total radiation dose of 36 to 40 Gy delivered in 2 Gy per fraction has been recommended.[254]

Heterotopic Ossification

Background and Clinical Aspects

Heterotopic ossification (HO) is a common complication of total hip arthroplasty, hip trauma, or acetabular fracture. HO occurs when the soft tissues around the hip become ossified. Following trauma, primitive mesenchymal cells in the surrounding soft tissues are transformed into osteoblastic tissue that then forms mature bone. The hip is the most common joint affected; HO typically occurs around the femoral neck and adjacent to the greater trochanter. The risk factors for development of HO are unknown, but the incidence is greater in men and occurs in more than 80% in patients who have a history of ipsilateral or contralateral HO. It is also more common in patients with a known history of osteoarthritis, ankylosing spondylitis, and diffuse and Paget disease.[255] Hip stiffness is the primary symptom, and the diagnosis is made radiographically. Pain is typically not associated with HO.

Nonradiotherapeutic Treatment

The treatment for HO is surgical excision followed by some form of HO prophylaxis. Prophylaxis is only applied to patients at high risk for developing HO. A meta-analysis showed that NSAIDs are effective in reducing the risk of postoperative HO.[256] Indomethacin is the most commonly used NSAID for HO prophylaxis. Indomethacin is a prostaglandin synthase inhibitor that also suppresses mesenchymal cells. The limited data available have not shown a clear benefit to the use of selective cyclo-oxygenase-2 inhibitors in HO prophylaxis.[257,258] Bisphosphonates have been used for prophylaxis because they delay mineralization of osteoid and appear to have some efficacy in preventing HO if used at the appropriate time. In one

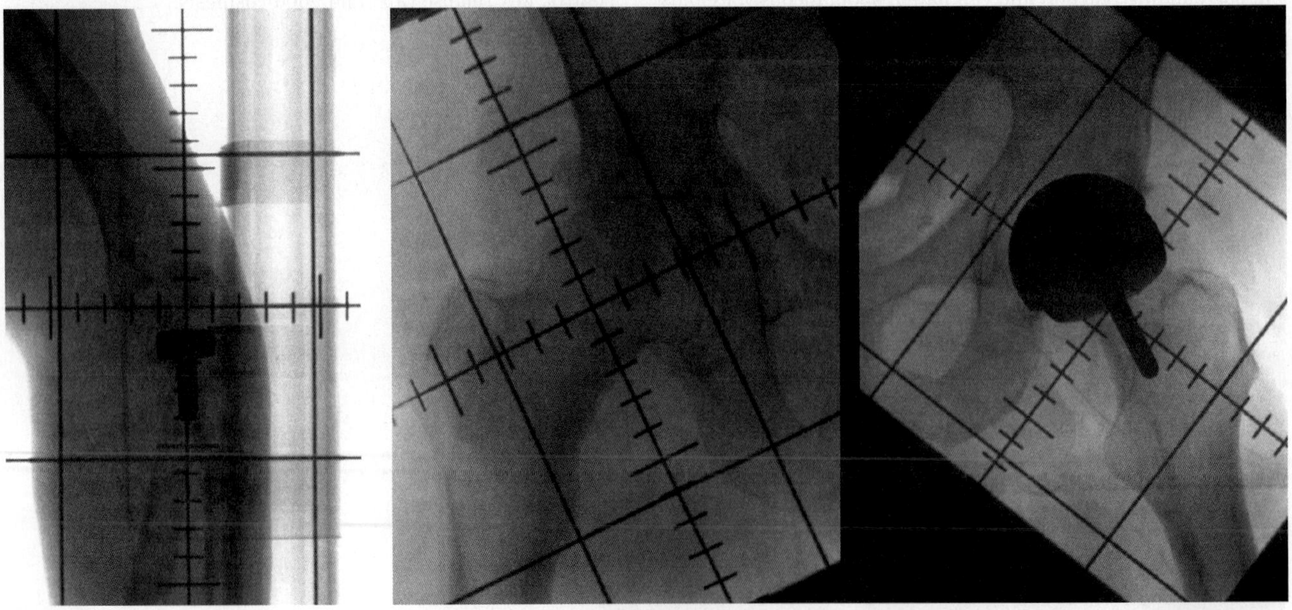

FIGURE 91.10. Typical treatment field for heterotopic ossification.

study, the cost of bisphosphonate was prohibitive for routine use when compared with indomethacin.[259]

Radiotherapeutic Options

External-beam radiation is an effective method for prevention of HO after total hip arthroplasty. Prophylactic radiation therapy for the prevention of HO has been used since the 1970s. A single fraction of 7 or 8 Gy to the at-risk region (Fig. 91.10) is recommended and should be delivered in the perioperative period, either preoperatively (within 24 hours) or postoperatively (within 72 hours).[260,261,262] When comparing radiation therapy and NSAIDs, there is no clear benefit for use of one modality over another. A prospective, randomized study demonstrated that radiation therapy and indomethacin are both effective in the prevention of postoperative HO.[263] Although one meta-analysis of seven randomized studies concluded that radiotherapy is more effective than NSAIDs for HO prophylaxis,[264] a more recent analysis of nine studies involving 1,295 patients found no statistically significant difference between the two.[265] An economic analysis using the same nine studies and the meta-analysis suggests that radiation therapy is not cost-effective when compared with use of NSAIDs.[266] This analysis has yet to be validated.

CONCLUSION

This chapter has reviewed the therapeutic approaches and supporting data for a variety of benign diseases and disorders. For some conditions, the use of radiation therapy has been well-established and the literature provides sufficient data regarding the radiation techniques, dose regimens, and outcomes. In instances where there are not yet sufficient data to make recommendations, the radiation therapy should be used cautiously, and preferably, in the context of a clinical trial.

Radiation therapy is a powerful tool and must always be used safely and judiciously. While radiation oncologists are trained to be mindful of acute toxicities, disease outcomes, and long-term treatment sequelae, special care must be taken when radiation is used for the treatment of benign disorders. When other therapeutic options exist, a thoughtful multidisciplinary approach should be considered to ascertain which modality is in a patient's best interest.

SELECTED REFERENCES

A full list of references for this chapter is available online.

8. Trott KR, Kamprad F. Radiobiological mechanisms of anti-inflammatory radiotherapy. *Radiother Oncol* 1999;51(3):197–203.
9. Rodel F, Keilholz L, Herrmann M, et al. Radiobiological mechanisms in inflammatory diseases of low-dose radiation therapy. *Int J Radiat Biol* 2007;83(6):357–366.
13. Leer JW, van Houtte P, Seegenschmiedt H. Radiotherapy of non-malignant disorders: where do we stand? *Radiother Oncol* 2007;83(2):175–177.
14. Trott KR, Kamprad F. Estimation of cancer risks from radiotherapy of benign diseases. *Strahlenther Onkol* 2006;182(8):431–436.
18. Micke O, Seegenschmiedt MH. Consensus guidelines for radiation therapy of benign diseases: a multicenter approach in Germany. *Int J Radiat Oncol Biol Phys* 2002;52(2):496–513.
20. Louis DN OH, Wiestler OD, et al. *WHO classification of tumours of the nervous system.* Lyon: IARC Press, 2007.
23. Simpson D. The recurrence of intracranial meningiomas after surgical treatment. *J Neurol Neurosurg Psychiatry* 1957;20(1):22–39.
26. Yano S, Kuratsu J. Indications for surgery in patients with asymptomatic meningiomas based on an extensive experience. *J Neurosurg* 2006;105(4):538–543.
28. Goldsmith BJ, Wara WM, Wilson CB, et al. Postoperative irradiation for subtotally resected meningiomas. A retrospective analysis of 140 patients treated from 1967 to 1990. *J Neurosurg* 1994;80(2):195–201.
29. Mendenhall WM, Morris CG, Amdur RJ, et al. Radiotherapy alone or after subtotal resection for benign skull base meningiomas. *Cancer* 2003;98(7):1473–1482.
30. Minniti G, Amichetti M, Enrici RM. Radiotherapy and radiosurgery for benign skull base meningiomas. *Radiat Oncol* 2009;4:42.
33. Adler JR Jr, Gibbs IC, Puataweepong P, et al. Visual field preservation after multisession cyberknife radiosurgery for perioptic lesions. *Neurosurgery* 2008;62(Suppl 2):733–743.
34. Paulsen F, Doerr S, Wilhelm H, et al. Fractionated stereotactic radiotherapy in patients with optic nerve sheath meningioma. *Int J Radiat Oncol Biol Phys* 2012;82(2):773–778.
42. Kondziolka D, Mathieu D, Lunsford LD, et al. Radiosurgery as definitive management of intracranial meningiomas. *Neurosurgery* 2008;62(1):53–60.
44. Zachenhofer I, Wolfsberger S, Aichholzer M, et al. Gamma-Knife radiosurgery for cranial base meningiomas: experience of tumor control, clinical course, and morbidity in a follow-up of more than 8 years. *Neurosurgery* 2006;58(1):28–36.
45. DiBiase SJ, Kwok Y, Yovino S, et al. Factors predicting local tumor control after Gamma Knife stereotactic radiosurgery for benign intracranial meningiomas. *Int J Radiat Oncol Biol Phys* 2004;60(5):1515–1519.
50. Laws ER, Sheehan JP, Sheehan JM, et al. Stereotactic radiosurgery for pituitary adenomas: a review of the literature. *J Neurooncol* 2004;69(1–3):257–272.
51. Brada M, Rajan B, Traish D, et al. The long-term efficacy of conservative surgery and radiotherapy in the control of pituitary adenomas. *Clin Endocrinol (Oxf)* 1993;38(6):571–578.
54. Littley MD, Shalet SM, Beardwell CG, et al. Hypopituitarism following external radiotherapy for pituitary tumours in adults. *Q J Med* 1989;70(262):145–160.
55. Landolt AM, Haller D, Lomax N, et al. Octreotide may act as a radioprotective agent in acromegaly. *J Clin Endocrinol Metab* 2000;85(3):1287–1289.
57. Stripp DC, Maity A, Janss AJ, et al. Surgery with or without radiation therapy in the management of craniopharyngiomas in children and young adults. *Int J Radiat Oncol Biol Phys* 2004;58(3):714–720.
59. Winkfield KM, Linsenmeier C, Yock TI, et al. Surveillance of craniopharyngioma cyst growth in children treated with proton radiotherapy. *Int J Radiat Oncol Biol Phys* 2009;73(3):716–721.
60. Lee M, Kalani MY, Cheshier S, et al. Radiation therapy and CyberKnife radiosurgery in the management of craniopharyngiomas. *Neurosurg Focus* 2008;24(5):E4.
62. Kobayashi T, Kida Y, Mori Y, et al. Long-term results of gamma knife surgery for the treatment of craniopharyngioma in 98 consecutive cases. *J Neurosurg* 2005;103(6 Suppl):482–488.
69. Kondziolka D, Lunsford LD, McLaughlin MR, et al. Long-term outcomes after radiosurgery for acoustic neuromas. *N Engl J Med* 1998;339(20):1426–1433.
70. Flickinger JC, Kondziolka D, Niranjan A, et al. Acoustic neuroma radiosurgery with marginal tumor doses of 12 to 13 Gy. *Int J Radiat Oncol Biol Phys* 2004;60(1):225–230.
71. Hansasuta A, Choi CY, Gibbs IC, et al. Multi-session stereotactic radiosurgery for vestibular schwannomas: single institution experience with 383 cases. *Neurosurgery* 2011;69(6):1200–1209.
73. Weber DC, Chan AW, Bussiere MR, et al. Proton beam radiosurgery for vestibular schwannoma: tumor control and cranial nerve toxicity. *Neurosurgery* 2003;53(3):577–588.
74. Vernimmen FJ, Mohamed Z, Slabbert JP, et al. Long-term results of stereotactic proton beam radiotherapy for acoustic neuromas. *Radiother Oncol* 2009;90(2):208–212.
78. Hug EB, Loredo LN, Slater JD, et al. Proton radiation therapy for chordomas and chondrosarcomas of the skull base. *J Neurosurg* 1999;91(3):432–439.
82. Carpentier A, Polivka M, Blanquet A, et al. Suboccipital and cervical chordomas: the value of aggressive treatment at first presentation of the disease. *J Neurosurg* 2002;97(5):1070–1077.
84. Schulz-Ertner D, Karger CP, Feuerhake A, et al. Effectiveness of carbon ion radiotherapy in the treatment of skull-base chordomas. *Int J Radiat Oncol Biol Phys* 2007;68(2):449–457.
85. Kano H, Iqbal FO, Sheehan J, et al. Stereotactic radiosurgery for chordoma: a report from the North American Gamma Knife Consortium. *Neurosurgery* 2011;68(2):379–389.
87. Li G, Chang S, Adler JR Jr, et al. Irradiation of glomus jugulare tumors: a historical perspective. *Neurosurg Focus* 2007;23(6):E13.
89. Hinerman RW, Amdur RJ, Morris CG, et al. Definitive radiotherapy in the management of paragangliomas arising in the head and neck: a 35-year experience. *Head Neck* 2008;30(11):1431–1438.
92. Foote RL, Pollock BE, Gorman DA, et al. Glomus jugulare tumor: tumor control and complications after stereotactic radiosurgery. *Head Neck* 2002;24(4):332–339.
95. Guss ZD, Batra S, Limb CJ, et al. Radiosurgery of glomus jugulare tumors: a meta-analysis. *Int J Radiat Oncol Biol Phys* 2011;81(4):e497–e502.
96. Chandler JR, Goulding R, Moskowitz L, et al. Nasopharyngeal angiofibromas: staging and management. *Ann Otol Rhinol Laryngol* 1984;93(4 Pt 1):322–329.
99. Chakraborty S, Ghoshal S, Patil VM, et al. Conformal radiotherapy in the treatment of advanced juvenile nasopharyngeal angiofibroma with intracranial extension: an institutional experience. *Int J Radiat Oncol Biol Phys* 2011;80(5):1398–1404.
101. McAfee WJ, Morris CG, Amdur RJ, et al. Definitive radiotherapy for juvenile nasopharyngeal angiofibroma. *Am J Clin Oncol* 2006;29(2):168–170.
103. Gadner H, Grois N, Arico M, et al. A randomized trial of treatment for multisystem Langerhans' cell histiocytosis. *J Pediatr* 2001;138(5):728–734.
107. Smith DG, Nesbit ME Jr, D'Angio GJ, et al. Histiocytosis X: role of radiation therapy in management with special reference to dose levels employed. *Radiology* 1973;106(2):419–422.
108. Selch MT, Parker RG. Radiation therapy in the management of Langerhans cell histiocytosis. *Med Pediatr Oncol* 1990;18(2):97–102.
109. Minehan KJ, Chen MG, Zimmerman D, et al. Radiation therapy for diabetes insipidus caused by Langerhans cell histiocytosis. *Int J Radiat Oncol Biol Phys* 1992;23(3):519–524.
110. Rosenzweig KE, Arceci RJ, Tarbell NJ. Diabetes insipidus secondary to Langerhans' cell histiocytosis: is radiation therapy indicated? *Med Pediatr Oncol* 1997;29(1):36–40.
111. Maruyama K, Kawahara N, Shin M, et al. The risk of hemorrhage after radiosurgery for cerebral arteriovenous malformations. *N Engl J Med* 2005;352(2):146–153.
112. Flickinger JC, Pollock BE, Kondziolka D, et al. A dose–response analysis of arteriovenous malformation obliteration after radiosurgery. *Int J Radiat Oncol Biol Phys* 1996;36(4):873–879.
117. Sans V, de la Roque ED, Berge J, et al. Propranolol for severe infantile hemangiomas: follow-up report. *Pediatrics* 2009;124(3):e423–e431.
119. Ogino I, Torikai K, Kobayasi S, et al. Radiation therapy for life- or function-threatening infant hemangioma. *Radiology* 2001;218(3):834–839.
122. Miller JP, Acar F, Burchiel KJ. Classification of trigeminal neuralgia: clinical, therapeutic, and prognostic implications in a series of 144 patients undergoing microvascular decompression. *J Neurosurg* 2009;111(6):1231–1234.
130. Flickinger JC, Pollock BE, Kondziolka D, et al. Does increased nerve length within the treatment volume improve trigeminal neuralgia radiosurgery? A prospective double-blind, randomized study. *Int J Radiat Oncol Biol Phys* 2001;51(2):449–454.
131. Adler JR Jr, Bower R, Gupta G, et al. Nonisocentric radiosurgical rhizotomy for trigeminal neuralgia. *Neurosurgery* 2009;64(2 Suppl):A84–A90.

132. Wiebe S, Blume WT, Girvin JP, et al. A randomized, controlled trial of surgery for temporal-lobe epilepsy. *N Engl J Med* 2001;345(5):311–318.
134. Barbaro NM, Quigg M, Broshek DK, et al. A multicenter, prospective pilot study of Gamma Knife radiosurgery for mesial temporal lobe epilepsy: seizure response, adverse events, and verbal memory. *Ann Neurol* 2009;65(2):167–175.
139. Young RF, Vermeulen S, Posewitz A, et al. Pallidotomy with the Gamma Knife: a positive experience. *Stereotact Funct Neurosurg* 1998;70(Suppl 1):218–228.
140. Friehs GM, Park MC, Goldman MA, et al. Stereotactic radiosurgery for functional disorders. *Neurosurg Focus* 2007;23(6):E3.
142. Lopes AC, Greenberg BD, Noren G, et al. Treatment of resistant obsessive-compulsive disorder with ventral capsular/ventral striatal gamma capsulotomy: a pilot prospective study. *J Neuropsychiatry Clin Neurosci* 2009;21(4):381–392.
143. de Keizer RJ. Pterygium excision with or without postoperative irradiation, a double-blind study. *Doc Ophthalmol* 29 1982;52(3–4):309–315.
147. Viani GA, De Fendi LI, Fonseca EC, et al. Low or high fractionation dose beta-radiotherapy for pterygium? A randomized clinical trial. *Int J Radiat Oncol Biol Phys* 2012;82(2):e181–e185.
149. Lopez-Caballero C, Saornil MA, De Frutos J, et al. High-dose iodine-125 episcleral brachytherapy for circumscribed choroidal haemangioma. *Br J Ophthalmol* 2010; 94(4):470–473.
154. Levy-Gabriel C, Rouic LL, Plancher C, et al. Long-term results of low-dose proton beam therapy for circumscribed choroidal hemangiomas. *Retina* 2009;29(2): 170–175.
156. Shields CL, Honavar SG, Shields JA, et al. Circumscribed choroidal hemangioma: clinical manifestations and factors predictive of visual outcome in 200 consecutive cases. *Ophthalmology* 2001;108(12):2237–2248.
158. Evans JR, Sivagnanavel V, Chong V. Radiotherapy for neovascular age-related macular degeneration. *Cochrane Database Syst Rev* 2010;5:CD004004.
159. Smitt MC, Donaldson SS. Radiation therapy for benign disease of the orbit. *Semin Radiat Oncol* 1999;9(2):179–189.
161. Bartalena L, Marcocci C, Bogazzi F, et al. Relation between therapy for hyperthyroidism and the course of Graves' ophthalmopathy. *N Engl J Med* 1998;338(2): 73–78.
164. Bartalena L, Baldeschi L, Dickinson AJ, et al. Consensus statement of the European Group on Graves' Orbitopathy (EUGOGO) on management of Graves' orbitopathy. *Thyroid* 2008;18(3):333–346.
165. Wakelkamp IM, Baldeschi L, Saeed P, et al. Surgical or medical decompression as a first-line treatment of optic neuropathy in Graves' ophthalmopathy? A randomized controlled trial. *Clin Endocrinol (Oxf)* 2005;63(3):323–328.
173. Matthiesen C, Bogardus C Jr, Thompson JS, et al. The efficacy of radiotherapy in the treatment of orbital pseudotumor. *Int J Radiat Oncol Biol Phys* 2011;79(5): 1496–1502.
174. Hunter DJ, Lo GH. The management of osteoarthritis: an overview and call to appropriate conservative treatment. *Med Clin North Am* 2009;93(1):127–143.
176. Zhang W, Nuki G, Moskowitz RW, et al. OARSI recommendations for the management of hip and knee osteoarthritis: part III: Changes in evidence following systematic cumulative update of research published through January 2009. *Osteoarthritis Cartilage* 2010;18(4):476–499.
182. Ronn K, Reischl N, Gautier E, et al. Current surgical treatment of knee osteoarthritis. *Arthritis* 2011;2011:454873.
185. Mucke R, Seegenschmiedt MH, Heyd R, et al. [Radiotherapy in painful gonarthrosis. *Results of a national patterns-of-care study*]. *Strahlenther Onkol* 2010;186(1): 7–17.
191. Ballo MT, Zagars GK, Pollack A, et al. Desmoid tumor: prognostic factors and outcome after surgery, radiation therapy, or combined surgery and radiation therapy. *J Clin Oncol* 1999;17(1):158–167.
192. Hansmann A, Adolph C, Vogel T, et al. High-dose tamoxifen and sulindac as first-line treatment for desmoid tumors. *Cancer* 2004;100(3):612–620.
193. Gega M, Yanagi H, Yoshikawa R, et al. Successful chemotherapeutic modality of doxorubicin plus dacarbazine for the treatment of desmoid tumors in association with familial adenomatous polyposis. *J Clin Oncol* 2006;24(1):102–105.
194. Garbay D, Le Cesne A, Penel N, et al. Chemotherapy in patients with desmoid tumors: a study from the French Sarcoma Group (FSG). *Ann Oncol* 2012;23(1): 182–186.
198. Penel N, Le Cesne A, Bui BN, et al. Imatinib for progressive and recurrent aggressive fibromatosis (desmoid tumors): an FNCLCC/French Sarcoma Group phase II trial with a long-term follow-up. *Ann Oncol* 2011;22(2):452–457.
203. Guadagnolo BA, Zagars GK, Ballo MT. Long-term outcomes for desmoid tumors treated with radiation therapy. *Int J Radiat Oncol Biol Phys* 2008;71(2):441–447.
205. Lev D, Kotilingam D, Wei C, et al. Optimizing treatment of desmoid tumors. *J Clin Oncol* 2007;25(13):1785–1791.
206. Dibenedetti DB, Nguyen D, Zografos L, et al. A population-based study of Peyronie's disease: prevalence and treatment patterns in the United States. *Adv Urol* 2011;2011:282503.
208. Hauck EW, Diemer T, Schmelz HU, et al. A critical analysis of nonsurgical treatment of Peyronie's disease. *Eur Urol* 2006;49(6):987–997.
213. Trost LW, Gur S, Hellstrom WJ. Pharmacological management of Peyronie's disease. *Drugs* 2007;67(4):527–545.
214. Kuehhas FE, Weibl P, Georgi T, et al. Peyronie's disease: nonsurgical therapy options. *Rev Urol* 2011;13(3):139–146.
224. van Rijssen AL, Ter Linden H, Werker PM. 5-year results of randomized clinical trial on treatment in Dupuytren's disease: percutaneous needle fasciotomy versus limited fasciectomy. *Plast Reconstr Surg* 2012;129(2):469–477.
226. Thomas A, Bayat A. The emerging role of *Clostridium histolyticum* collagenase in the treatment of Dupuytren disease. *Ther Clin Risk Manag* 2010;6:557–572.
230. Betz N, Ott OJ, Adamietz B, et al. Radiotherapy in early-stage Dupuytren's contracture. Long-term results after 13 years. *Strahlenther Onkol* 2010;186(2):82–90.
237. Flickinger JC. A radiobiological analysis of multicenter data for postoperative keloid radiotherapy. *Int J Radiat Oncol Biol Phys* 2011;79(4):1164–1170.
239. Ragoowansi R, Cornes PG, Moss AL, et al. Treatment of keloids by surgical excision and immediate postoperative single-fraction radiotherapy. *Plast Reconstr Surg* 2003;111(6):1853–1859.
241. Kuriyama DK, McElligott SC, Glaser DW, et a;. Treatment of Gorham-Stout disease with zoledronic acid and interferon-alpha: a case report and literature review. *J Pediatr Hematol Oncol* 2010;32(8):579–584.
244. Heyd R, Micke O, Surholt C, et al. Radiation therapy for Gorham-Stout syndrome: results of a national patterns-of-care study and literature review. *Int J Radiat Oncol Biol Phys* 2011;81(3):e179–e185.
253. Heyd R, Seegenschmiedt MH, Rades D, et al. Radiotherapy for symptomatic vertebral hemangiomas: results of a multicenter study and literature review. *Int J Radiat Oncol Biol Phys* 2010;77(1):217–225.
260. Healy WL, Lo TC, DeSimone AA, et al. Single-dose irradiation for the prevention of heterotopic ossification after total hip arthroplasty. A comparison of doses of five hundred and fifty and seven hundred centigray. *J Bone Joint Surg Am* 1995; 77(4):590–595.
262. Gregoritch SJ, Chadha M, Pelligrini VD, et al. Randomized trial comparing preoperative versus postoperative irradiation for prevention of heterotopic ossification following prosthetic total hip replacement: preliminary results. *Int J Radiat Oncol Biol Phys* 1994;30(1):55–62.
264. Pakos EE, Ioannidis JP. Radiotherapy vs. nonsteroidal anti-inflammatory drugs for the prevention of heterotopic ossification after major hip procedures: a meta-analysis of randomized trials. *Int J Radiat Oncol Biol Phys* 2004;60(3):888–895.

Chapter 92
Endovascular Brachytherapy

Ray Lin and Prabhakar Tripuraneni

Vascular brachytherapy (VBT) continues to have a role in the treatment of coronary in-stent restenosis and has a promising role in the treatment of restenosis following intervention of the peripheral arterial system. With the introduction of drug-eluting stents (DESs) midway through the last decade, the incidence of coronary in-stent restenosis has declined following percutaneous coronary intervention.[1] The future of VBT in the treatment of coronary in-stent restenosis at one point seemed uncertain. However, after several years of declining use of VBT for in-stent restenosis, some centers including Scripps Green/Scripps Clinic (La Jolla, CA) have recently seen a gradual rise in the number of patients needing VBT for coronary in-stent restenosis as some patients have developed in-stent restenosis following multiple DESs.

Patients with small vessel disease and diabetes are particularly prone to develop coronary in-stent restenosis, with rates as high as 10% or more.[2] Repeated percutaneous coronary interventions and surgical revascularization procedures are also associated with high rates of restenosis, with rates as high as 14% being reported.[3] DESs can reduce recurrences of in-stent restenosis by 50% to 70%.[4] Nonetheless, restenosis still can occur following DESs at rates between 2% and 10%.[5]

There are more than 1.5 million coronary interventions performed worldwide each year for coronary stenosis.[6] Coronary stenting with metallic stents has become a standard of care in treating patients with coronary stenosis. Restenosis has been the major complication of percutaneous transluminal coronary angioplasty since the introduction of balloon angioplasty by Gruentzig in the mid-1970s.[7–9] This process has been thought to consist of three separate mechanisms: vascular recoil, neointimal hyperplasia, and negative remodeling.

VBT has been shown in several double-blinded randomized trials to demonstrate its efficacy in reducing rates of in-stent restenosis. The potential usefulness of vascular radiation therapy to prevent restenosis emerged rapidly, from positive preclinical studies carried out in animals in the late 1980s and early 1990s, to a large number of feasibility trials and randomized clinical trials in the mid- to late 1990s, to U.S. Food and Drug Administration (FDA) approval of the first commercial devices in the last quarter of 2000. Although initial preclinical studies have included evaluation of both teletherapy and brachytherapy approaches, only vascular systems have been tested extensively in human coronary vessels.

Of the 1 million angioplasties expected in the United States annually, approximately 80% to 90% of these patients will undergo stenting. In-stent restenosis will develop in approximately 15% of these patients, and these patients present a considerable management problem to the interventional cardiologist. Restenosis rates approaching 80% for long, diffuse lesions in small vessels have been reported.

Studies on DESs have now matured. Interventional cardiologists have implanted several million DESs worldwide.[10] DESs using antiproliferative agents such as paclitaxel[11] and immunosuppressive agents such as sirolimus[12–15] have been shown to be effective in treating in-stent restenosis. Published randomized trials show DESs to be superior to VBT in treating in-stent restenosis.[16–18] DESs have replaced VBT as first-line therapy for coronary in-stent restenosis. Additionally, interventional cardiologists may simply prefer DESs over VBT in order to avoid the logistics and expense of having radiation oncology involved in the catheterization laboratory.[12,14] However, adverse events such as acute stent thrombosis, aneurysm, and incomplete apposition do occur with DESs, although some randomized trials have not shown a difference in the incidence of stent thrombosis between patients with DESs or bare-metal stents (BMSs).[19]

VBT has found a niche in treatment of patients who fail DESs. The Checkmate system (Cordis Corporation, Miami Lakes, FL) and the Galileo system (Guidant Corporation, Indianapolis, IN) are no longer commercially available. The Novoste Beta-Cath 3.5F System (Novoste Corporation, Norcross, GA) using ^{90}Sr is the only system clinically available for use in coronary artery in-stent restenosis following repeat intervention.

Approximately 400,000 peripheral vascular procedures are done each year in United States. The risk of restenosis after angioplasty and stent placement varies considerably in different parts of the peripheral arterial tree. Initial clinical trials of VBT in superficial femoral arteries and renal artery in-stent restenosis[20,21] show similar results as observed in the coronary system. VBT appears to be safe and effective in certain patients with restenosis in the peripheral vascular system.

HISTORICAL PERSPECTIVE

VBT was empirically tried in Frankfurt, Germany, by Liermann and colleagues on restenosed femoral popliteal arteries starting in 1990. A small cohort of patients has been followed for 10 years, and no long-term adverse events have been reported.[22] The first coronary brachytherapy procedure was performed in Caracas, Venezuela, by Condado et al.[23] in 1994, and the results of their initial feasibility trial were reported in 1997. At 5-year follow-up, the data from this landmark study are durable and demonstrate the feasibility of brachytherapy for preventing coronary artery restenosis. The first randomized trial of VBT was carried out by investigators at the Scripps Clinic in 1995, and the positive results from this trial were subsequently published in the *New England Journal of Medicine*.[24] That led to GAMMA I, the first multi-institutional, double-blind, randomized pivotal trial using ^{192}Ir, which led to the approval of the Checkmate system (Cordis Corporation, Miami Lakes, FL) for native coronary in-stent restenosis.[25]

In the mid-1990s, a Geneva group and a second group at Emory University began testing the feasibility of intracoronary brachytherapy using β-emitting sources.[26,27] The Beta-Cath System (developed by Novoste Corporation, now owned by Best Vascular, Inc., Norcross, GA), which was piloted at Emory, became the focus of the START trial, the second pivotal trial. In November 2000, it was approved, along with the Checkmate system, for in-stent restenosis.[28] The INHIBIT trial testing the Galileo system represents the third pivotal trial of VBT for in-stent restenosis and led to the approval of this device in November 2001.[29] The only randomized trial comparing VBT for *de novo* lesions in native coronary vessels to stents used the Beta-Cath System and was reported as a negative trial.[30]

The approval of VBT is unique in radiation oncology in a number of ways. It is the first time that level I evidence supported by multi-institutional, randomized trials was required by FDA mandate before VBT became available in the routine clinical setting. Likewise, under FDA and Nuclear Regulatory Commission mandate, it was the first time that all specialists, including radiation oncologists (therapeutic radiologists and oncologists), interventional cardiologists, and medical physicists, were required to be part of the team delivering VBT. Since 1995, more than 6,000 patients have been enrolled in approximately 50 protocols testing the efficacy of VBT.[31]

CORONARY ANATOMY

(This section is modified with permission from Windecker S, Meier B. Basics of interventional cardiology. In: Tripuraneni P, Jani S, Minar E, et al., eds. *Intravascular brachytherapy: from theory to practice.* London: Remedica, 2001:83–86.) The coronary arteries originate as the only branches of the ascending aorta from the aortic root.[32] Coronary arteries usually have an epicardial course and terminate as arterioles in the capillary network. The left and right coronary arteries surround the epicardial surface as a ring-loop system in two orthogonal planes defined by the fibrous skeleton of the heart. Thus, the right coronary artery (RCA) and the left circumflex coronary artery (LCX) run around the atrioventricular groove and form a circle between the atria and ventricles at the base of the heart. Perpendicular to this plane, the left anterior descending coronary artery (LAD) and the posterior descending RCA constitute a semicircle around the interventricular groove and encircle the left ventricular apex.

Left Coronary Artery

The left coronary artery usually originates from a single ostium in the middle portion of the left sinus of Valsalva (Fig. 92.1). The vessel originating from the left ostium is termed the *left main coronary artery* (LM) if it subsequently gives rise to both the LAD and the LCX. The LM measures 3 to 10 mm in diameter and is usually <40 mm long. The LM has no side branches and divides into the LAD and the LCX, although in 20% to 40% of cases a trifurcation with an intermediate branch between the LAD and LCX can be seen.

The LAD leads, in direct continuation of the LM, to the anterior interventricular groove toward the apex and supplies 40% to 60% of the left ventricular myocardium.

The LAD gives rise to septal branches, diagonal branches, and branches to the free right ventricular wall. The LCX originates at an almost vertical angle from the LM and courses posteriorly at variable length along the left atrioventricular groove, beneath the left atrial appendage and toward the crux of the heart. The LCX gives off one to three obtuse marginal branches, which supply the free lateral left ventricular wall and have the same course as the diagonal branches of the LAD.

Right Coronary Artery

Usually the RCA arises from the right sinus of Valsalva and runs in the right atrioventricular groove toward the crux of the heart. The segment from the ostium to the right-angled turn into the vertical part of the RCA is called the *proximal RCA*, the mid-RCA is defined as the vertical segment, and the distal RCA extends from the right-angled turn at the distal end of the vertical segment to the bifurcation into the posterior descending coronary artery and posterolateral branches.

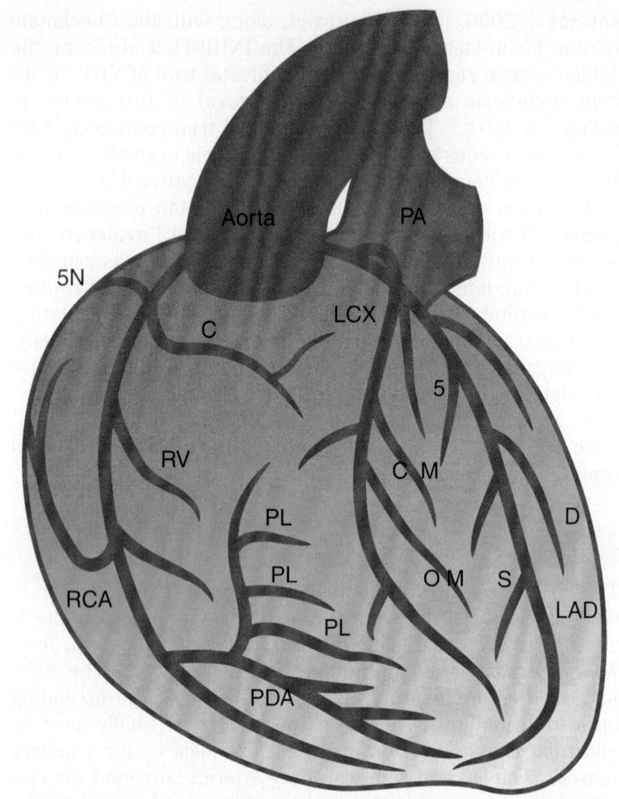

FIGURE 92.1. Schematic representation of the major epicardial coronary arteries as seen in an anteroposterior projection. The left coronary artery originates left and posterior from the cusp of the aortic root as the left main (LM) coronary artery. The LM coronary artery divides after a variable length into the left anterior descending (LAD) artery and the left circumflex (LCX) artery. The LAD runs as a direct continuation of the LM anteriorly along the interventricular groove to the ventricular apex. The LAD gives rise to the septal branches, which take off at a vertical angle and immediately become intramural in the interventricular septum. The LAD also gives rise to the diagonal branches, which course epicardially over the anterolateral free wall. The LCX originates at a nearly vertical angle from the LM and courses posteriorly along the left atrioventricular groove. It gives rise to the obtuse marginal branches, which course epicardially and supply the free lateral wall. The right coronary artery (RCA) takes off anteriorly from the right coronary cusp and follows the right atrioventricular groove. The first branch of the RCA is the conal or infundibular artery, followed by the sinus node artery as the second branch. In the vertical portion of the atrioventricular groove, the RCA gives rise to the right ventricular marginal branches, which supply the right ventricular free wall. The RCA then courses posteriorly and divides at the crux of the heart base into the posterior descending artery (PDA) and a variable number of posterolateral branches. The PDA courses along the posterior interventricular groove toward the left ventricular apex. It closes a loop with the LAD along with the interventricular groove, whereas the posterolateral branches of RCA close a second perpendicular loop of blood supply with the LCX along with the atrioventricular groove. C, conus branch; D, diagonal branch; OM, obtuse marginal branch; PA, pulmonary artery; PL, posterolateral branch; RV, right ventricular branch; S, septal branch; SN, sinus node artery.

PERCUTANEOUS CORONARY INTERVENTION

(This section is modified with permission from Windecker S, Meier B. Basics of interventional cardiology. In: Tripuraneni P, Jani S, Minar E, et al., eds. *Intravascular brachytherapy: from theory to practice.* London: Remedica, 2001:88–100.) The indications for percutaneous coronary intervention (PCI) have expanded during the past two decades, and there is currently no absolute contraindication to this technique. Arterial access is usually gained through an anterior wall stick of the right femoral artery using the Seldinger technique. The coronary guidewire is advanced by the coronary guiding catheter into the coronary artery and is cautiously navigated through the narrowing (stenosis) into the periphery of the vessel to be treated. It secures access to the coronary artery during the intervention and allows for the rapid exchange of balloons, stents, and other devices (Fig. 92.2).

The balloon catheter not only is central to balloon angioplasty but also serves as a complementary instrument for other intracoronary interventions, such as delivery of stents, local drugs, or radiation sources. Balloon catheters consist of a shaft providing support when pushing the catheter through vessels, a central lumen for the coronary guidewire, and an inflation channel for balloon expansion.

During conventional balloon angioplasty (percutaneous transluminal coronary angioplasty), a balloon catheter is advanced over the previously inserted coronary guidewire into the target stenosis and subsequently inflated until the balloon is fully expanded. The chief limitations to event-free survival after balloon angioplasty have been abrupt vessel closure (a short-term complication) and restenosis (a long-term complication).[6] Abrupt vessel closure, defined as the sudden occlusion of the target vessel during or after angioplasty, has been reported in 4% to 8% of cases. Restenosis, defined as stenosis >50% diameter at follow-up angiography, has been the most important long-term limitation of balloon angioplasty, with an incidence of 30% to 50% and with 20% to 30% of patients requiring target vessel revascularization. Most restenoses occur during the first 4 months after balloon angioplasty.

The therapeutic effect of arterial vessel enlargement through PCI is accompanied by various degrees of arterial injury with exposure of thrombogenic components. This may result in intracoronary thrombus formation with its subsequent ischemic sequelae. Therefore, inhibition of platelets and the coagulation system has always been a central focus of interventional investigations. In patients undergoing PCI, aspirin is recommended at a low dose (75 to 325 mg/day), ideally administered at least 1 day before the procedure and continued indefinitely thereafter. Ticlopidine and clopidogrel are typically administered with a loading dose before or after the procedure. Additionally, they are prescribed for ≥6 months after VBT if a new stent was not placed and ≥12 months if a new stent was placed under the discretion of the interventional cardiologist.[18]

EXTERNAL-BEAM IRRADIATION STUDIES

Results using external-beam irradiation have been mixed.[33–38] Studies of external-beam irradiation in the pig coronary balloon angioplasty model, done at Emory University, revealed that when 14 Gy was administered immediately before or after or 2 days after balloon injury, there was reduced neointima formation compared with controls, but the lumens were smaller owing to negative remodeling (contracture) of the vessel. Results from studies using 21 Gy after either angioplasty or stenting indicate a profound and consistent suppression of neointima formation.[38,39] The lack of benefit seen with a 14-Gy external beam compared with 14 Gy delivered by VBT at a 2-mm radius from the source suggests that the minimum dose delivered to the vessel wall is not the only factor in determining outcome. Studies of 14- and 21-Gy external radiation treatment have shown focal myocardial necrosis, an effect never seen with endovascular irradiation at any dose. This suggests that sophisticated treatment techniques, limiting the dose to normal tissues, will be essential for external-beam therapy to be adopted.

ENDOVASCULAR IRRADIATION STUDIES

In contrast to the disparate results from studies using external radiation, numerous studies have consistently demonstrated remarkable suppression of neointima formation using radiation from a variety of isotopes delivered by an endoluminal approach. At least three groups have documented similar results in the pig coronary artery model of restenosis after balloon angioplasty, using the γ emitter ^{192}Ir at roughly comparable doses.[40–42]

VBT typically reduces the neointima formation and maintains the patency of the lumen. Scanning electron microscopy of arteries irradiated to 14 Gy showed no morphologic differences from controls at 2 weeks; a confluent layer of endothelial or endothelial-like cells was present throughout the region of

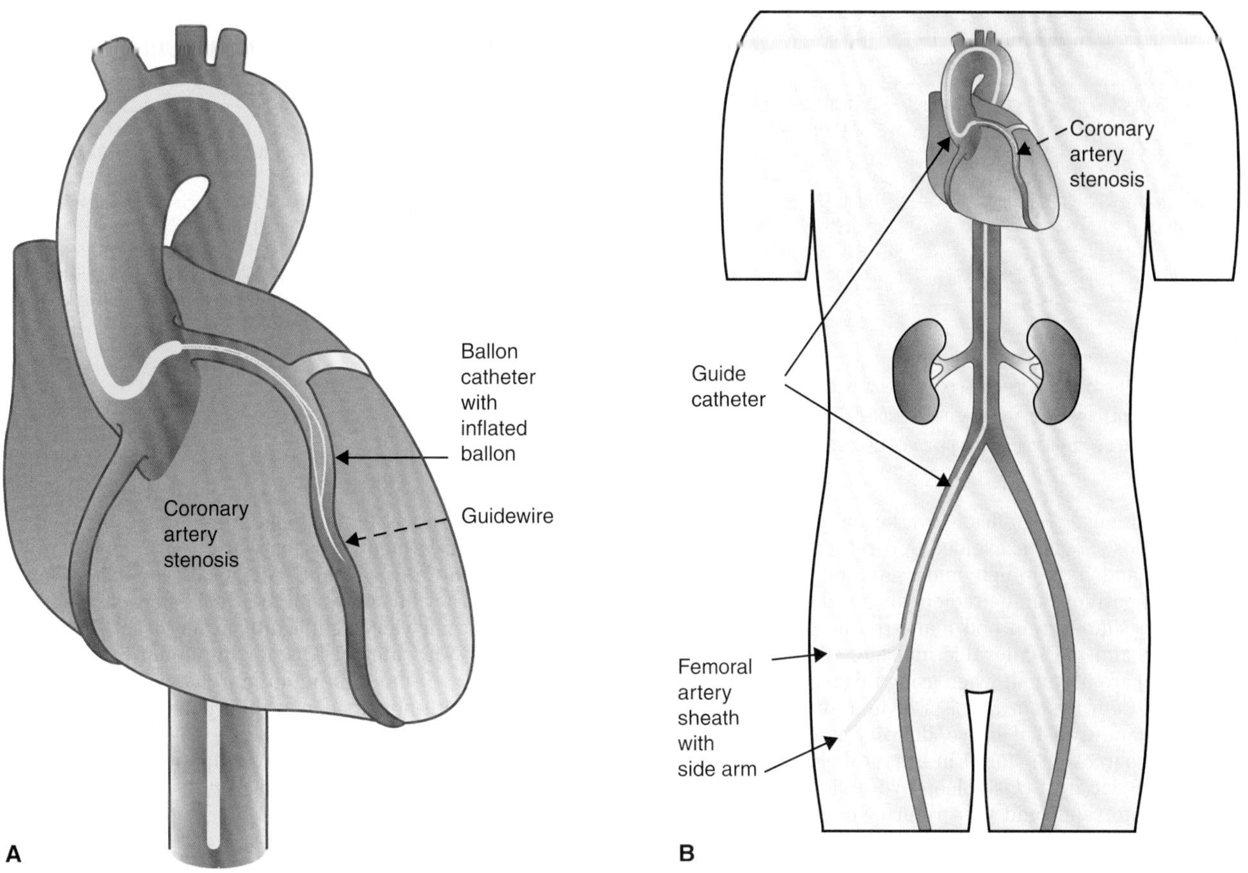

FIGURE 92.2. Schematic diagram of access to the coronary arteries during percutaneous coronary interventions. **A:** An introducer sheath with side arm is placed in the artery chosen for vascular access. A guiding catheter is introduced through the vascular access sheath and advanced to the coronary artery ostium chosen for the intervention. **B:** A guidewire is advanced through the guiding catheter into the coronary artery, navigated through the artery, and placed distal to the stenosis to be treated. A balloon catheter is then placed in the coronary stenosis for dilatation.

the angioplasty injury. However, at 28 and 56 Gy, neointima formation was nearly eradicated and endothelial coverage was incomplete. Inadequate endothelial recovery of an irradiated artery after angioplasty might render its luminal surface prothrombotic. In the setting of an appropriate physiologic stimulus, this can result in thrombotic occlusion. The problem of late thrombosis observed in clinical trials certainly is compatible with the delayed healing observed in the animal studies.

With stents playing an increasingly important role in the management of coronary stenosis, it became important to test whether radiation might prove a useful adjunct to coronary stenting. Studies carried out with β and γ emitters have demonstrated conclusively that the excess intimal hyperplasia occurring in a stent can be effectively eliminated by radiation delivered either before or after stenting.[43]

VASCULAR BRACHYTHERAPY PHYSICS AND DEVICES

The initial evaluation of radiation therapy in animal models of restenosis focused on testing the effect of radiation with commercially available radiation sources. Testing has included both teletherapy and brachytherapy. Although occasional positive results have been reported with teletherapy in experimental models of restenosis, consistently positive results emerged from a variety of brachytherapy approaches. These approaches have included both temporary (VBT) and permanent implants (radioactive stents). Although many isotopes have been proposed for VBT, only approximately half a dozen have been used in human clinical trials, and of those, only three have seen widespread use. The three isotopes, which have been used for well over 95% of all clinical trials of catheter-based systems, are ^{192}Ir, ^{90}Sr/Y, and ^{32}P (Table 92.1).

BETA-CATH SYSTEM FOR CORONARY IN-STENT RESTENOSIS

The Beta-Cath System is the only system currently manufactured that is offered for in-stent restenosis. ^{90}Sr is a pure β emitter with a 28.8-year half-life (10,519.25 days) and 546-KeV maximum β energy. The daughter isotope ^{90}Y is also a pure β emitter with a 64-hour half-life and 2.27-MeV maximum β energy. It is primarily the ^{90}Y β emissions that are used for therapy because the ^{90}Sr β particles are mostly absorbed by the stainless steel encapsulation and the surrounding catheter. The Beta-Cath System contains sources that are 0.38 mm in diameter and 2.5 mm in length confined within a flexible steel coil between radiopaque end plug markers that are maximum 0.495 mm in diameter and 2.5 mm in length. Source trains of 12, 16, and 24 sources (30-, 40-, and 60-mm active lengths, respectively) are commercially available. The nonradioactive marker plugs are located both proximally and distally to the radioactive sources in the jacketed train (Fig. 92.3). The markers permit fluoroscopic verification of the source train arriving at the end of the delivery catheter for treatment. For lesions plus margins longer than the available source train, a "pullback technique" is used in which the most distal portion of the lesion is treated first, and then the catheter is carefully pulled back to treat the more proximal lesion. At Scripps Clinic, we have the 60-mm source train available. A 60-mm source train can be used with a pullback technique to cover a distance of 120 mm. This technique could also be used for treatment of lesions at

TABLE 92.1 SUMMARY OF CATHETER-BASED SYSTEMS

System	Isotope/Half-Life	Delivery Method/Length of Source	Centering System	Approved Injury Length/Diameter/Dosimetry
Checkmate (Cordis/Best)[a]	^{192}Ir gamma/74 days	Manual (hand-delivered) 6, 10, and 14 seeds (23, 39, and 55 mm long)	Noncentered (3.7-Fr delivery catheter)	≤45 mm/2.75–4 mm/intravascular ultrasonography based; 8 Gy at farthest junction of media and adventitia and <30 Gy to the closest
Beta-Cath (Novoste)[b]	^{90}Sr/Y beta/28.8 years	Manual (hydraulic) 12, 16, and 24 seeds (30, 40, and 60-mm length jacketed trains)	Noncentered (3.5-Fr delivery catheter)	≤60 mm/2.7–4 mm/fixed length dose for in-stent restenosis; 18.4 Gy @ 2 mm for 2.7–3.35 mm RVD, or 23 Gy @ 2 mm for > 3.35–4 mm RVD
Galileo (Guidant)[c]	^{32}P beta/14 days	Computerized source delivery 27-mm wire (manual tandem stepping to 54 mm long)	Centering catheter, 2.5, 3.0, and 3.5 mm diameter, allowing distal, side branch flow	≤47 mm/2.4–3.7 mm/fixed dosimetry of 20 Gy at 1.0 mm into vessel wall from balloon surface

RVD, reference vessel diameter.

[a]18 and 22 seeds (71 and 87 mm long, respectively) and fixed dosimetry in clinical trials in the United States. No longer manufactured.

[b]30-, 40-, and 60-mm source train currently manufactured.

[c]A 20-mm-long source with automated computerized stepping. No longer manufactured.

vessel bifurcations.[44] Significant overlap or gaps between the treatment fields should be avoided. A careful review of the cine angiograms and a thorough understanding of the quantity, spacing, and positions of the radiopaque markers in the system (i.e., the two source train end markers, the delivery catheter stop marker, and the removable indicator of the source train marker wire) are pertinent when using this technique.

The Beta-Cath System consists of four main components: the source train, transfer device, delivery catheter, and accessories. The sources are stored in a hand-held transfer device and are advanced by a closed-loop hydraulic system that uses sterile water to send (and then return) the source train. The advantage of the Beta-Cath System is the relatively short treatment times (3 to 5 minutes) and the absence of radiation exposure to catheterization laboratory staff. The long half-life of the isotope permits a total shelf life of 12 months divided into two 6-month use periods, which allows for a decay correction of a few seconds in the second 6-month dwell times. A potential disadvantage of this system is the inferior depth–dose gradient compared with the γ source, attenuation by calcifications or stents, and lack of utility in larger vessels (Fig. 92.4).

A dose of 18.4 Gy is recommended at a 2-mm radius from the centerline of the source train axis for vessels with a reference diameter between 2.7 and 3.35 mm. For reference diameters between 3.35 and 4 mm and for most saphenous vein grafts, a dose of 23 Gy is recommended. The gross target volume is the stenotic area itself. The clinical target volume is the dilated part of the vessel. The planning target includes at least 5 mm proximal and distal to the clinical target volume[45–47] for the 30-mm source train and at least 10 mm for the 40-mm and 60-mm source trains. Although both minimum 5-mm and minimum 10-mm treatment margins were proven safe and effective in the Beta-Cath System START trials, a cumulative comparison of efficacy outcomes out to 5 years suggests that longer treatment margins yield significantly lower target vessel revascularization (TVR) rates of 51% for minimum 5-mm margins versus 19% for 10-mm minimum margins versus 55% for the placebo, and with nonsignificant differences in major adverse coronary event (MACE) rates of 63% with minimum 5-mm margins versus 67% for minimum 10-mm margins versus 68% for the placebo (User's Manual, Novoste Beta-Cath System).

Roles and Responsibilities

(This text is modified and printed with permission from Tripuraneni P. In: Tripuraneni P, Jani S, Minar E, et al., eds. *Intravascular brachytherapy: from theory to practice.* London: Remedica, 2001:272–274.) The FDA has mandated that VBT be carried out by a team consisting of an interventional cardiologist/radiologist, a radiation oncologist/therapeutic radiologist and oncologist, and a medical physicist. The roles and responsibilities of these specialists are listed in the following sections.[31]

Interventional Cardiologist/Radiologist

1. Perform preprocedure evaluation and communicate patient's status (risk factors, interventions) with radiation oncologist.
2. Perform angioplasty with or without stenting as necessary.
3. Define the anatomic location of diseased vessel amenable to intervention, length/volume of intervention, angioplasty and stenting, and reference vessel diameter (including

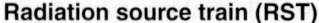

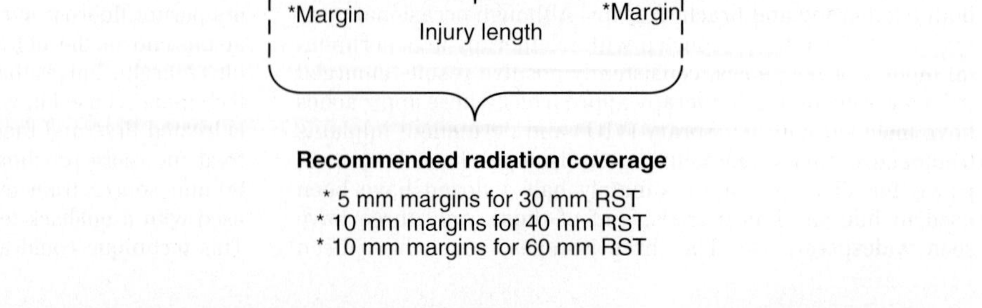

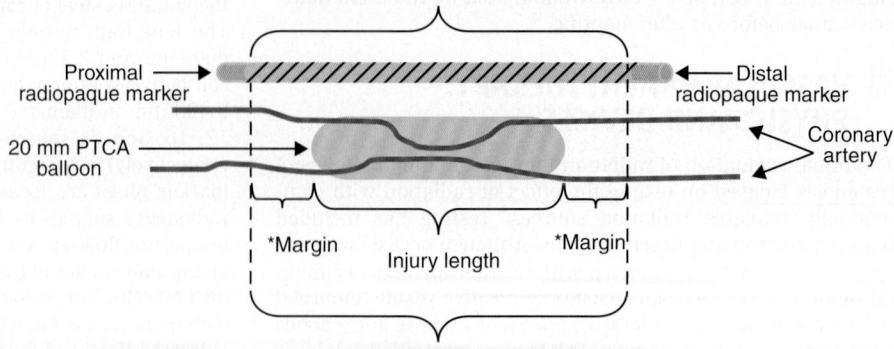

FIGURE 92.3. Radiation source train with proximal and distal radiopaque markers noted. (Courtesy of Novoste Corporation, Norcross, GA.)

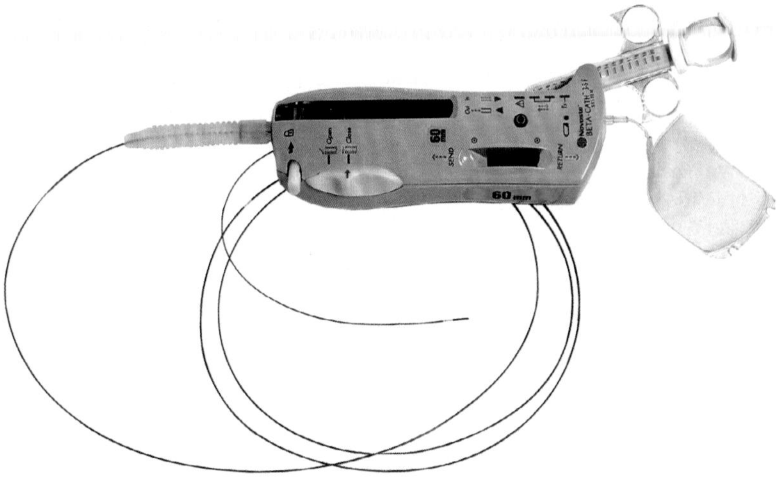

FIGURE 92.4. The Beta-Cath system is a hydraulic delivery system with a noncentered, 5-Fr, closed, over-the-wire delivery catheter. ^{90}Sr seeds 24 source train (60 mm in length) is available. The delivery unit is shown. (Courtesy of Novoste Corporation, Norcross, GA.)

preintervention and postintervention vessel segment diameters), and communicate with radiation oncologist.
4. Determine the target volumes, jointly with the radiation oncologist and medical physicist.
5. Place delivery catheter and make final adjustment, in consultation with the radiation oncologist.
6. Advise the radiation oncologist of any changes in the delivery catheter position during the delivery of radiation.
7. Assist the radiation oncologist with any procedural details.
8. Assist the radiation oncologist in source removal as needed. In cases of medical or radiation emergencies, have procedures in place to ensure that radiation treatments are preplanned and nothing is left to chance.

Therapeutic Radiologist/Oncologist (Authorized User)

1. Review preprocedure evaluation, including patient's status (including risk factors and interventions), with interventional cardiologist for the advisability of using intravascular radiation.
2. Review the anatomic location of diseased vessels amenable to intervention, length/volume of intervention, angioplasty, and stenting, and reference vessel diameter (including preintervention and postintervention vessel segment) with the interventional cardiologist.
3. Determine the target volumes together with the interventional cardiologist.
4. Obtain proper informed consent for VBT after discussions with the patient.
5. Review the final placement of the delivery catheter and any adjustments as needed.
6. Prescribe radiation dose and sign prescription.
7. Calculate treatment times, along with the medical physicist.
8. Insert radiation source.
9. Provide appropriate delivery of radiation.
10. Remove radiation source.
11. Supervise overall radiation delivery.
12. Participate in decisions and implementation of emergency source removal in case of medical or radiation emergencies.

Medical Physicist

1. Survey catheterization laboratory or radiation source delivery room and make appropriate preparations and modifications as needed.
2. Order radiation sources, under the direction of the radiation oncologist.
3. Calibrate sources upon arrival.
4. Ensure safe-keeping of radiation sources.
5. Prepare sources for clinical use.
6. Calculate treatment delivery times.
7. Conduct radiation survey of patient before and during treatment.
8. Assist radiation oncologist and interventional cardiologist in source removal in cases of radiation or medical emergencies.
9. Conduct radiation survey of patient after source removal.
10. In case of radiation or medical mishaps, inform appropriate regulatory authorities.
11. Participate in preparation of license application for medical use of VBT sources.
12. Develop and oversee quality assurance and improvement programs for efficacious and safe use of VBT sources in consultation with the radiation oncologist and interventional cardiologist as appropriate.

CLINICAL TRIALS OF CORONARY BRACHYTHERAPY

Nearly 5,000 patients have participated in clinical trials to determine the safety and efficacy of VBT.[25,48,49] There have been seven double-blind randomized trials investigating the use of VBT on patients with in-stent restenosis.[24,25,48,50–55] These trials led to the approval of one γ system using ^{192}Ir and two β systems using ^{32}P and ^{90}Sr/Y isotopes.[25,56,57]

Of note, Rha et al.[58] have reported that results from commercially available VBT are superior to the results obtained during investigational VBT trials as MACEs were lower with commercial radiation. This is likely from the lessons learned through clinical trials as dosimetry was optimized (higher doses, wider margins) and prolonged antiplatelet therapy was administered to reduce late thrombotic events. More recently, a rhenium-188–filled balloon source has also been shown to be effective for in-stent restenosis and improving long-term outcomes.[59]

γ-Radiation In-Stent Coronary Artery Restenosis Trials

The SCRIPPS I trial was the first double-blind, randomized radiation trial for coronary in-stent restenosis and restenosis without stents.[24,43,52,60–62] It was a single-institution trial with off-site analysis involving the treatment of 55 patients during a 9-month period. Twenty-six patients were randomized to ^{192}Ir and 29 to placebo. At 5-year follow-up, the target lesion revascularization (TLR) was significantly lower in the ^{192}Ir group (23.1% vs. 48.3%; p = .05). There were two TLRs between years 3 and 5 in the treated patients, but none in the patients receiving placebo. The event-free survival rate (freedom from death, myocardial infarction, or TLR) was significantly lower in ^{192}Ir-treated patients (34.5% vs. 61.5%; p = .028).

A second single-institution, randomized study of radiation for in-stent restenosis was carried out at the Washington

TABLE 92.2 SUMMARY OF PUBLISHED OR PRESENTED TRIAL RESULTS FOR CORONARY IN-STENT RESTENOSIS[a]

Study/System	Lesion Length (mm)/Dose (Gy)	Percentage Target Lesion Revascularization (Radiation vs. Placebo)	Percentage Angiographic In-Stent Restenosis (Radiation vs. Placebo)
SCRIPPS I/Checkmate	≤30/<8 farthest EEM, <30 closest EEM	15 vs. 48	33 vs. 64
WRIST/Checkmate	≤47/15 at 2 or 2.4 mm	14 vs. 63	19 vs. 58
GAMMA I/Checkmate	≤45/<8 farthest EEM, <30 closest EEM	24 vs. 45	22 vs. 51
GAMMA II Registry/Checkmate	≤45/14 at 2 mm	23	25
Long WRIST/Checkmate	36–80/15 at 2 mm	30 vs. 60	32 vs. 71
Long WRIST HD Registry/Checkmate	36–80/18 at 2 mm	17	24
SVG WRIST/Checkmate[b]	≤80/15 at 2 or 2.4 mm	10 vs. 48	10 vs. 48
START/Beta-Cath	≤20/18.4 or 23 at 2 mm (5-mm minimum margins)	13.6 vs. 22.4 5-year TVR reduced 51 vs. 59	14 vs. 41
START 40/20 Registry/Beta-Cath	≤20/18 or 23 at 2 mm (10-mm minimum margins)	12 vs. 24.4 5-year TVR reduced 19 vs. 59	15.4 vs. 41.2 @ 240 days
INHIBIT/Galileo	<47/20 at 1 mm	11 vs. 29	16 vs. 49
BETA WRIST Registry/Schneider	≤47/20.6 at 1 mm	16	22

EEM, external elastic lamina; TVR, target vessel revascularization.

[a]Some of the above results have not been published yet. The results may not be directly comparable because the enrollment and reporting criteria are sometimes different. All of the above trials are statistically significantly positive in favor of radiation.

[b]Saphenous vein graft.

Hospital Center in Washington, DC, and is known as the WRIST trial.[55,63] The WRIST trial randomized 130 patients to either ^{192}Ir or placebo. Fixed dosimetry was used, prescribing 15 Gy at either 2 or 2.4 mm depending on lumen diameter for lesions ≤47 mm. Six-month follow-up confirmed a statistically significant reduction in TLR from 63% to 14% and in angiographic restenosis from 58% to 19% in favor of radiation over placebo.

The GAMMA I trial was the first multi-institutional, randomized radiation trial for in-stent restenosis.[25] A total of 252 patients at 12 centers were enrolled, and radiation therapy was delivered using intravascular ultrasound (IVUS)-based dosimetry (similar to the SCRIPPS trial dosimetry) for lesions ≤45 mm. A dose of 8 Gy was delivered to the farthest junction of the media and adventitia as long as the dose to the closest junction was <30 Gy, using IVUS. There were significant reductions in the rates of both TLR, from 45% to 24% at 9-month follow-up, and angiographic restenosis, from 50.5% to 21.6% at 6-month follow-up, in favor of radiation over placebo.

The GAMMA II registry included 125 patients at 12 centers and used fixed dosimetry for lesions ≤45 mm (same entry criteria as GAMMA I trial), with 14 Gy prescribed at a 2-mm radius for all patients.[64] There was a TLR rate of 23% at the 9-month follow-up and an angiographic restenosis rate of 25% at the 6-month follow-up. This registry showed that the results with ^{192}Ir were reproducible and similar to those in the GAMMA I trial with simplified dosimetry.[65]

The LONG WRIST trial was a two-institution, 120-patient randomized trial that used fixed dosimetry of 15 Gy at a 2- or 2.4-mm radius, for longer lesions of 36 to 80 mm. There was a statistically significant decrease in the 6-month angiographic restenosis rate (32% vs. 71%; p = .0002) in favor of radiation.[66] The PLAVIX WRIST trial was a registry of 120 patients who received 6 months of clopidogrel. Six-month follow-up has demonstrated that extended antiplatelet therapy is able to eliminate the problem of late thrombosis observed in the WRIST and GAMMA studies[67] (Table 92.2).

β-Radiation In-Stent Coronary Artery Restenosis Trials

The START trial (Beta-Cath system) was a 50-center multi-institutional, double-blind, randomized trial of 476 patients with in-stent restenosis.[68] A 30-mm-long ^{90}Sr/Y source was used to treat lesions ≤20 mm; the dose prescribed was 18.4 Gy at a 2-mm radius for vessels ≥2.7 and ≤3.35 mm in diameter, and 23 Gy at a 2-mm radius for vessels ≥3.35 and ≤4 mm in diameter. At 8-month follow-up, the TLR rate was statistically decreased from 22% to 13% (p <.008), and the angiographic in-stent restenosis rate was also significantly decreased from 41% to 14% in favor of radiation over placebo.

The START 40/20 trial was a registry of 207 patients with the same entry criteria as START, except the source train was 40 mm long.[69] The 8-month binary angiographic in-stent restenosis rate was 16%. The frequency of geographic misses with the longer source train in the START 40/20 trial was 6% compared with 15% in the START 30 trial.

The PREVENT trial (Galileo system) was a six-institution feasibility study involving 105 patients, 70% of whom had *de novo* lesions and 61% of whom were stented.[51] The patients were randomized to placebo or 16, 20, or 24 Gy at 1 mm from the balloon surface for lesions ≤25 mm. The TLR rate was statistically decreased with ^{32}P versus placebo from 24% to 10%, and the in-stent angiographic restenosis rate was decreased from 39% to 8%. The INHIBIT trial (Galileo system), a multi-institutional, double-blind, randomized study, enrolled 332 patients with in-stent restenosis at 27 centers. Fixed dosimetry was used to prescribe 20 Gy at 1 mm from the balloon surface for lesions with an injury length of ≤47 mm.[29,49] Because the source is only 27 mm in length, manual repositioning of the balloon catheter was used to treat the longer lesions. At 9-month follow-up, the rate of MACEs was decreased from 31% to 15% (p = .0006), and the rate of angiographic in-stent restenosis was also significantly decreased from 49% to 16% (p <.0001) in favor of radiation over placebo. Sixty-four patients in the radiation group and 76 patients from the placebo group were treated with the pullback technique for lesions longer than 20 mm. No safety issues were identified in patients in whom there had been a significant overlap of active sources at the junction.

The Beta WRIST trial was a registry of 50 patients with in-stent restenosis treated with the Boston Scientific/Schneider system at the Washington Hospital Center using the same entry criteria as the WRIST trial.[55] An angiographic restenosis rate of 22% and a TLR rate of 16% at 6 months were noted, which were similar to the results obtained in the radiation arm of the WRIST study (Tables 92.3 and 92.4).

Trials on Drug-Eluting Stents for Coronary In-Stent Restenosis

The role of VBT in coronary in-stent restenosis has clearly changed with the introduction of effective DESs. The first trial using DESs was a Brazilian study involving 31 patients. There was no incidence of restenosis reported on initial evaluation of patients at 4 months. No clinical events were reported at

TABLE 92.3 SUMMARY OF THE PIVOTAL MULTI-INSTITUTION RANDOMIZED TRIALS AND REGISTRIES FOR CORONARY IN-STENT RESTENOSIS

Trial	Isotope	Patients/Centers	Randomization	Centering Balloon	Lesion Maximum Length/Diameter (mm)	Dose (Gy)
GAMMA I	^{192}Ir	252/12	Yes	No	45/2.75–4.0	Intravascular ultrasonography-based 8–30
GAMMA II	^{192}Ir	125/12	No	No	45/2.75–4.0	14 at 2-mm radius
START	Sr/^{90}Y	476/50	Yes	No	20/2.7–4.0	18.4–23 at 2-mm radius
START 40/20	Sr/^{90}Y	207/22	No	No	20/2.7–4.0	18.4–23 at 2-mm radius
INHIBIT	^{32}P	332/27	Yes	Yes	47/2.4–3.7	20 at 1-mm radius from balloon surface

From Tripuraneni P, Teirstein P. Radiation therapy in coronary arteries: catheter based trials. In: Tripuraneni P, Janis P, Minar E, et al., eds. *Intravascular brachytherapy: from theory to practice*. London: Remedica, 2001:210.

8 months.[15] There are also data showing that DESs can be safely and effectively delivered after VBT.[70]

The RAVEL (Randomized Study with Sirolimus-eluting Velocity Balloon-Expandable Stent) involved 238 patients randomized to either DESs or BMSs.[13] At 3 years, event-free survival rates for target lesion revascularization were 93.7% in the DES arm versus 75% for the control group (p <.001).[71]

Paclitaxel-eluting stents have been investigated in the series of TAXUS trials I through IV.[11,72–74] TAXUS I evaluated 61 patients randomized to 15-mm TAXUS NIRx paclitaxel-eluting stent (Boston Scientific, Natick, MA) or similar drug-free stent. At 6 months, there were no incidences of in-stent restenosis in the DES arm and three patients developed restenosis in the BMS arm (p = .112).[11] TAXUS II investigated two different drug formulations and compared them to BMSs. No differences were noted between the two drug arms, but a statistical advantage was noted in the DES arms compared with BMSs.[72] TAXUS IV randomized 1,314 patients to EXPRESS BMSs or EXPRESS DESs. Nine-month angiographic results were available in 559 patients. A relative risk of restenosis was reduced by 70% in the DES arm (p <.001).[73] The TAXUS V and VI trials evaluated the EXPRESS DESs in patients with more complex diseases.

The two major trials comparing DESs to VBT have now been completed.[75] The TAXUS V trial is a multicenter randomized trial with 396 patients enrolled. This study demonstrated that paclitaxel-eluting stents when compared to VBT significantly reduced the ischemic target lesion revascularization rate by 40% at 9 months: 6.3% for DESs versus 13.9% for VBT. Relative reductions in total target lesion (61%) and target vessel (49%) revascularization events were higher in patients treated with paclitaxel-eluting stents rather than those receiving VBT when considering only ischemic-related events. Additionally, the 9-month rate of major adverse coronary events was reduced by 43% in the DES arm versus the VBT arm.[17] The SISR trial is a prospective, multicenter randomized trial with 384 patients enrolled. Patients were randomized to sirolimus-eluting stents versus VBT for restenosis following BMS implantation. At 6 months, the DES arm had superior clinical and angiographic outcomes when compared with VBT. At 3-year follow-up, patients treated with DESs had improved survival-free TLR and TVR compared to VBT. MACEs and stent thrombosis did not reach a statistical difference between the two groups.[18]

Nonetheless, there have been some reports of DES-associated arteriopathy with late stent malapposition, aneurysm formation, hypersensitivity reactions, and DES-induced spasms. The more recent VBT trials have seen very few of these complications.[76,77] Still, short-term results of DESs compare favorable with VBT and long-term results will hopefully address these concerns.

Vascular Brachytherapy for In-Stent Restenosis Following DESs

VBT following DES failure has been shown to be effective and safe. Up to 10% of patients develop restenosis following DESs. The optimal treatment remains unclear for patients who fail DESs. Options include balloon angioplasty, additional DESs with either the same or a different drug, or VBT.

The RESCUE Registry is a multicenter international electronic registry for patients who receive VBT for recurrent restenosis following DESs. The purpose of the registry is to evaluate the safety and efficacy of VBT following DESs and to compare it to repeat DESs following in-stenosis of DESs.

Sixty-one patients received VBT following DESs and were compared with 50 patients who received additional DESs (Taxus or Cypher stents) after DES restenosis. The patient's demographic and angiographic characteristics were similar in both groups. Torguson et al.[78] presented the data at the 2005 American Heart Association Scientific Sessions. VBT appeared to be safe. At 6 months, target vessel revascularization rates were 3.3% versus 16% (p = .04) in favor of VBT. TLR rates were 3.3% versus 8% (p = .24) in favor of VBT as well. At 8 months, VBT was associated with fewer MACEs compared with repeat DESs (9.8% vs. 24%; p = 0.044).[79]

At Scripps Clinic, the clinical experience on the first 41 patients treated with VBT following DESs has been reviewed. Median follow-up is 8 months. TLR rates are 22% and TVR (target vessel failure) rates are 2%.

TABLE 92.4 RESULTS OF PIVOTAL TRIALS AND REGISTRIES FOR CORONARY IN-STENT RESTENOSIS[a]

Trial	Percentage Target Lesion Revascularization	Percentage Major Adverse Cardiac Events	Percentage In-Stent Restenosis	Percentage Analysis Restenosis	In-Stent Late Loss (mm)
GAMMA I	42 vs. 24	46 vs. 29	52 vs. 22	56 vs. 33[b]	1.14 vs. 073
GAMMA II	23	30	25	34[b]	0.61
START	22 vs. 13 5-year TVR 59 vs. 51	26 vs. 18 5-year MACE 68 vs. 63 (ns)	41 vs. 14	45 vs. 29	0.67 vs. 0.21
START 40/20	24 vs. 12 5-year TVR 59 vs. 19 (p <.0000)	28 vs. 20 5-year MACE 68 vs. 67 (ns)	16	22	0.20
INHIBIT	29 vs. 11	33 vs. 22	49 vs. 16	52 vs. 26	

TVR, target vessel revascularization; MACE, major adverse coronary event.

[a]The results may not be directly comparable because the reporting criteria and enrollment criteria are sometimes different. GAMMA II and START 40/20 are single-arm registries with the same entry criteria as GAMMA I and START, respectively. Results are placebo versus radiation.

[b]In-lesion.

From Tripuraneni P, Teirstein P. Radiation therapy in coronary arteries: catheter based trials. In: Tripuraneni P, Janis P, Minar E, et al., eds. *Intravascular brachytherapy: from theory to practice*. London: Remedica, 2001:210.

Saphenous Vein Graft In-Stent Restenosis Clinical Trials

Saphenous vein grafts often are larger vessels with luminal diameters of >4 mm. Allowances must be made to deliver adequate doses when using IVUS-based or fixed dosimetry. All SCRIPPS trials included patients with saphenous vein grafts. However, the number of patients enrolled into SCRIPPS I was too small to reach any conclusions. Thirty of 130 patients in the WRIST trial were treated for in-stent restenosis of saphenous vein grafts. Subgroup analysis of WRIST suggests that radiation was as effective in saphenous vein grafts as in native coronary vessels. The more definitive study, SVG WRIST, a multi-institutional, randomized trial testing the efficacy of the Checkmate system with ^{192}Ir, enrolled 120 patients with lesions <47 mm in length.[80] A dose of 15 Gy at a 2-mm radius for vessels of 2.5- to 4-mm radius and 18 Gy at a 2-mm radius for vessels of 4- to 5-mm radius was delivered. A statistically significant reduction in the rate of in-stent restenosis of 43% versus 15% ($p = .004$), in favor of radiation over placebo, was observed. Likewise, the TLR rate at 6 months was statistically significantly decreased (10% vs. 48%; $p < .01$) in favor of radiation over placebo. At 36-month follow-up, TLR rate was still in favor of the radiation arm (43% vs. 66%; $p = .02$).[81] With appropriate doses, the in-stent rate of saphenous vein grafts can be reduced with adjuvant brachytherapy after appropriate recanalization.

In summary, there are numerous multi-institutional, randomized trials confirming the efficacy of radiation in decreasing in-stent restenosis. The three pivotal trials, GAMMA I, START, and INHIBIT, led to the approval of VBT for use in native coronary in-stent restenosis after recanalization. The Beta-Cath system, the only commercial system that is currently available, was approved based on the START trial. The system has been used successfully and has a registry confirming that longer margins decrease edge restenosis. This system was initially approved for 20-mm-long injured length with 2-mm radius prescription dosimetry. Doses would need to be adjusted for vessels with larger diameters between 3 and 5 mm.[82]

De Novo Coronary Artery Stenosis Clinical Trials

There are limited data supporting the use of routine radiation therapy to prevent restenosis for *de novo* coronary artery stenosis after recanalization. However, data in the Beta-Cath trial indicate that radiation may indeed decrease the rate of restenosis in patients. This trial was a multi-institution, double-blind randomized study with 1,456 patients.[30] After balloon angioplasty, patients received either radiation doses of 14 or 18 Gy depending on vessel diameter or no adjuvant radiation. The 8-month angiographic analysis showed a statistically significant decrease in restenosis in favor of radiation (34.3% vs. 21.4%; $p = .003$). However, with edge failures, this did not translate into a clinical benefit. Likewise, the GENEVA dose-finding trial[83,84] confirmed the dose response with increasing doses, with the effect being more profound in the patients receiving angioplasty only without stenting. Nevertheless, with emerging data from the DES trials, it seems unlikely that VBT will be used routinely in *de novo* coronary artery stenosis. However, for special situations of high-risk *de novo* stenosis in which stents may not be optimal, such as small-diameter vessels, longer lesions, or branch vessels, VBT may possibly find a niche role.

RADIOACTIVE STENTS

Currently, the majority of patients undergoing PCI receive coronary stents. Coupling the radiation delivery to the stent appears attractive in that it simplifies the delivery of treatment. Most clinical investigations have been undertaken with the ^{32}P β-emitting stent.[85] Stents have been tested with activities ranging from 0.5 to 20 μCi. These stents are of extremely low activity and can be handled with the aid of a 1-cm acrylic shield. Unfortunately, clinical trials using the ^{32}P stent demonstrated restenosis rates of approximately 50%, largely owing to intimal proliferation at the stent edges. These are often called *candy wrapper* edge failures. These clinical failures have inspired recent investigation of variations of the ^{32}P-coated stent with "cold" ends, "hot" ends, low-pressure balloon deployment systems, and so forth; ^{103}Pd (a γ-emitting isotope)-emitting stents; and ^{198}Au-emitting stents. Because studies to date indicate a lack of efficacy, currently there are no clinical trials evaluating the efficacy of radioactive-coated stents.

PERIPHERAL VASCULAR BRACHYTHERAPY TRIALS

Peripheral vascular disease involves more organs than coronary artery disease (CAD), and hence there are more diverse clinical situations, manifestations, and end points.[86] It is challenging to define measurable clinical end points for a diverse group of "host" organs (e.g., extremities, kidney, liver) that differ not only anatomically but also in function. Unlike coronary vessels, most peripheral vessels have a diameter >3 mm and, in fact, are typically approximately 7 to 10 mm. Peripheral vascular lesions tend to be much longer and are more likely to be multifocal. Because of the larger vessel diameter and increased thickness of the vessel wall, VBT in peripheral arteries is likely to require the use of either a more penetrating γ source (^{192}Ir) or a β source that is in direct contact with the vessel wall.

Most trials in peripheral vessels have used an high–dose-rate (HDR) afterloader and treatment of the superficial femoral or popliteal artery. After successful percutaneous transluminal angioplasty (PTA) of these arteries, the restenotic rate at 6 months varies from 25% to 77%.[87,88] In a Veterans Administration study, the actuarial restenosis rate was 41% at 36 months.[89]

The feasibility of VBT for peripheral vascular systems in humans was first documented in a study from Frankfurt, Germany.[22] In this study, 30 patients with in-stent restenotic lesions in femoropopliteal arteries were treated with repeat PTA, stent implant, and VBT. A dose of 12 Gy at 3 mm was administered with a ^{192}Ir HDR afterloader through a 5-Fr, non-centered catheter. At last follow-up, the median follow-up time was 32.9 months for 28 patients (range, 7 to 84 months). There were no adverse effects from the brachytherapy. The 5-year vessel patency rate was 82% (23 of 28 patients) based on Doppler ultrasonography. Stenosis developed in the treated vessel in three of 28 patients (11%); two (7%) had complete occlusion of the vessel due to thrombosis after 16 and 37 months.

Investigators in Vienna, Austria, have mounted a series of trials exploring the use of VBT in similar patients.[90,91] The Vienna II trial enrolled 107 patients with symptomatic *de novo* or restenotic femoropopliteal lesions treated with angioplasty and then randomly assigned patients to either additional radiation therapy or no further treatment. A fixed dose of 12 Gy at a 3-mm radius from the source center and a margin of 1 cm at each end of the injured segment were delivered with a ^{192}Ir HDR afterloading system. At 6 months, the angiographic restenosis rate was significantly lower in the radiation group compared with the control group (28% vs. 54%; $p < .05$). The cumulative patency rate at 12 months was significantly higher in the radiation group than in the control group (64% vs. 35%; $p < .005$). Subgroup analysis demonstrated that restenotic lesions, occlusions, and long lesions benefit the most from VBT. Despite radiation, the recurrence rate in the radiation arm was 28%. It is postulated that this may be due to the relatively modest radiation dose and the absence of a centering catheter. At 5-year follow-up, the stenosis recurrence rate was similar in each group, 72.5% each arm, ($p > .99$).[92] This showed that the radiation resulted in a delay but not an inhibition in restenosis.

The Vienna III trial enrolled 134 patients. This double-blind study randomized patients following angioplasty to brachytherapy or placebo irradiation. Patients had either *de novo* lesions ≥5 cm or restenosis following femoropopliteal angioplasty. A dose of 18 Gy (γ-irradiation) was prescribed 2 mm from the surface of the centering balloons. At 24 months, patency rates based on intention-to-treat analysis was 54% in the brachytherapy arm and 27% in the placebo arm (p <.005). VBT, however, reduced the restenosis rates for recurrent lesions only and not for *de novo* lesions.

The Vienna V trial studied 88 patients with femoropopliteal lesions at high risk for restenosis (mean treatment length, 16.8 ± 7.3 cm). This double-blind study randomized patients to receive either brachytherapy with ^{192}Ir (14 Gy to 2 mm into arterial wall) or with nonradioactive seeds. In this trial, brachytherapy did not improve 6-month patency after femoropopliteal stent in high-risk patients mainly because of a high incidence of early and late thrombotic events.[93]

The Peripheral Artery Radiation Investigational Study (PARIS) is the pivotal multi-institutional, randomized trial of VBT in superficial femoropopliteal arteries using the Nucletron HDR afterloader (Nucleotron, The Netherlands). This study consists of two phases: an initial lead-in phase of 40 patients, followed by a second phase in which 300 patients were randomized to receive or not receive radiation after PTA. In the initial phase, 35 of 40 patients were successfully irradiated with no procedural complications.[55] The angiographic restenosis rate at 6 months was 17.2%, which is very promising. The second phase started in early 1998 as the first multicenter, multinational, prospective, double-blind, randomized trial. Although initial results were promising at 6 months, the restenosis rates were similar in both groups (27.5% placebo and 28.6% brachytherapy) at 12 months (Table 92.5).

Krueger et al.[94] reported on 30 patients who underwent PTA for *de novo* femoropopliteal stenosis. Patients received either 14-Gy centered VBT or no radiation. Rates of restenosis were statistically significantly lower in the radiated group at 6 (p = .006) and 12 (p = .042) months.

Compared with the femoropopliteal arteries, the tibioperoneal arteries are smaller; hence, post-PTA restenosis tends to occur more frequently. Long-term success is limited mostly by neointimal hyperplasia. In a study of 55 PTA lesions in 40 patients, 44% remained patent at an average follow-up of 25.8 months.[95] There are no clinical data reported on the use of radiation therapy for the tibial-peroneal vessels, but this remains a potentially fertile site for further investigation.

There are two types of stenosis in renal arteries: ostial (at the origin of the renal artery from the aorta) and nonostial (beyond the ostium). Ostial stenoses are more difficult to treat and tend to recur; hence, they are often treated with stenting. The restenosis rates as determined by angiography are somewhat lower, at 23%, for nonostial regions compared with 30% for both ostial and nonostial lesions together.[96,97] Renal artery stenosis also lends itself to exploration with VBT. In certain clinical subgroups, the prevalence of serious renal artery disease is as high as 43%, especially in the growing population of patients older than 50 years of age with multiple manifestations of atherosclerosis.[98] Renal artery disease may account for up to 15% of patients with renal failure in the dialysis population older than 50 years of age. The morbidity and mortality among these patients are very high; hence, any potential benefit of VBT in the treatment of renal artery disease deserves investigation. In recent years, there have been some limited and selected cases published in the literature demonstrating the efficacy and safety of VBT for the treatment of renal artery in-stent restenosis.[99–102]

There are more than 120,000 patients with end-stage renal disease in the United States who require vascular access for hemodialysis. The most common forms of vascular access are arteriovenous (AV) grafts and central venous canalization. AV grafts typically fail within 14 to 19 months, with a reported primary occlusion rate of 15% to 50% at 1 year.[103] The most common cause of failure is stenosis at the anastomosis. The most common causes are thrombosis and intimal hyperplasia. Development of intimal hyperplasia at the site of venous anastomosis is due to several factors, including high-flow turbulence, compliance mismatch, vessel vibration, and platelet activation The restenosis rates for AV dialysis grafts after PTA are 9% at 3 months, 29% at 6 months, and 61% at 12 months; the restenosis rate for the subclavian vein after PTA alone is 71% at 6 months.[104] The restenosis rate after PTA and stenting for the subclavian vein is 30% to 53% at 1 year. An FDA-approved pilot study at New York Hospital used external-beam radiation (8 to 12 Gy, given in two equal fractions 48 hours apart) in a total of 10 patients to prevent restenosis. Unfortunately, all patients had restenosis by 18 months, suggesting no benefit from the therapy.[90] A feasibility study involving a series of eight patients with restenosis of AV fistula in hemodialysis patients has been recently published.[105] Although it appeared that radiation with ^{192}Ir after PTA of fistula stenosis appeared as a safe and feasible method in these patients, the radiation did not seem to decrease the incidence of restenosis. Different fractionation schemes are currently under investigation.

Compared with trials in CAD, peripheral vascular disease clinical trials testing the efficacy of VBT in reducing restenosis are in earlier stages with mixed results. VBT has now been tried in numerous sites outside the coronary arteries, including vein grafts, renal artery in-stent restenosis, femoropopliteal arteries, and even the carotid arteries.[106] The Vienna II and III trials, single-institution randomized trials, initially supported its efficacy in peripheral vascular disease. However, 5-year results were disappointing in the Vienna II trial. Certainly, there are opportunities to explore the role of VBT in peripheral arterial disease.

TABLE 92.5 DETAILS OF FEMORAL POPLITEAL ARTERY BRACHYTHERAPY TRIALS[a]

Trial	*Number of Patients*	*Randomization*	*Centering Catheter*	*Dose (Gy)*	*Dose (mm)*	*Patency*
Frankfurt	40	No	No	12	3	82%
Vienna I	10	No	No	12	3	60%
Vienna II[b]	113	Yes	No	12	3	72% p <.004
Vienna III	200	Yes	Yes	18	R +2	–
Vienna IV		Yes	Yes	14	R +2	–
Vienna V	88	Yes	Yes	14	R +2	–
Swiss	320	Yes	No	14	R +2	–
Paris[c]	300	Yes	Yes	14	R +2	–

R, radius of the vessel.

[a]The general trend of more recent trials of peripheral artery brachytherapy is the use of a high–dose-rate remote afterloader with ^{192}Ir gamma source and centering catheter.

[b]Single-institution randomized trial for high-risk *de novo* and in-stent restenosis lesions. Statistically significant improvement in patency at 12 months.

[c]Multi-institution randomized trial for high-risk *de novo* stenosis. Feasibility phase results encouraging. Completed enrollment of randomized phase and results expected in late 2002.

ADDITIONAL CLINICAL CONSIDERATIONS

Edge Restenosis

When restenosis occurs after VBT, the renarrowing is found at the treatment edges in one-third to one-half of patients. The etiology of edge failure is likely to be multifactorial but most likely results from inadequate radiation dose delivered to injured lesion margins. Many factors can lead to higher-than-expected rates of edge failure. These include geographic miss, which arises from misalignment of the radioactive source in the injured segment of the vessel.[107,108] In several studies using catheter-based radiation, careful, quantitative coronary angiographic measurements have documented a surprisingly high incidence of inadequate coverage of the injured region by the radioactive source. The balloon catheters used initially to open the stenotic segment can slip forward or backward ("watermelon seeding"), causing unintended injury to the lesion margins. Also, barotrauma from both angioplasty and stent deployment contributes to arterial wall injury beyond the nominal lengths of the balloons or stents.[109] Longitudinal seed displacement may also contribute to higher-than-expected restenotic rates at lesion margins owing to the movement of the radioactive seeds relative to the coronary vessel during the cardiac cycle. In a seed movement analysis of 19 cineangiograms, proximal movement of 0 to 2 mm and distal movement of 1 to 5 mm were observed.[110] In addition to more movement in the distal portion of arteries, the movement also varies with the particular artery (possibly more in the circumflex, for example). Uncertainty in target localization can arise because of the difficulty in visual estimation of proximal and distal lesion ends. This uncertainty is compounded by different magnifications and obliquity of various projections during fluoroscopy and cineangiography and the relative lack of reference points available (branch vessels are commonly used as reference points for targeting). Last, the dose falloff and penumbra effect of the particular isotope used can contribute to marginal failure.[111]

VBT cannot be effective in regions injured by angioplasty or atherectomy where radiation is not delivered. Although the causes of edge failure are still unclear and most likely multifactorial, several strategies have been used to decrease edge failures. First, careful cineangiographic documentation of injury to the vessel should be carried out at every balloon angioplasty or stent placement (discouraged to minimize late thrombosis). Second, the most proximal and distal extents of the injury to the vessel should be carefully determined, ideally with a side-branch reference point. Finally, a very wide margin (i.e., 5 to 10 mm) of the radiation source should be provided on either side of the injured vessel region. These measures will not eliminate edge failure but will probably considerably reduce its occurrence.[57]

TERMINOLOGY

Based on the International Commission on Radiation Units and Measurements Report 50, terminology for VBT volumes was proposed that takes into consideration both radial and longitudinal dimensions.[111] This terminology will help to define the target volume with attention to appropriate margins to decrease edge failures. The gross target volume (GTV) is the length of stenotic segment with an appropriate radius that may vary along the length. The clinical target volume (CTV) is the interventional length, which is delineated by the most proximal and distal extents of injury, and is always larger than GTV. The planning target volume (PTV) is the CTV plus a margin to account for both heart and catheter movements and inaccuracies in the visual delineation of the ends of the CTV. The uncertainty or magnitude of the margin depends on the location of the target in the vessel, the delivery system (centered or noncentered), and the cardiac cycle. The target volume is the volume irradiated based on the PTV and the penumbra of the isotope's effect, which depends on the isotope, source design, and prescription distance. In practice, it is necessary to give at least a 4- to 8-mm margin to the longest injured length of the vessel (Table 92.6).

TABLE 92.6 VASCULAR BRACHYTHERAPY TREATMENT TERMINOLOGY[a]

Target Volume Definition	*Description*
Gross target volume (GTV)	Stenotic or restenotic lesion
Clinical target volume (CTV)	Intervened or injured (angioplasty, stent, stent deployment, atherectomy) length
Planning target volume (PTV)	CTV + uncertainty for heart/catheter movement + uncertainty in target localization
Treatment volume (TV)	PTV + penumbra effect

[a]Volume includes the length and radius of the vessel. The target radius varies depending on the vessel, plaque in the vessel wall, and location of the delivery catheter in the lumen of the vessel. Intravascular ultrasonography may be helpful in determining target radius but is not widely available and not widely used. It is common practice to accept a 2-mm radius for noncentered systems and 1 mm into the vessel wall for centered systems as the target radius.

Modified from Tripuraneni P, Parikh S, Giap H, et al. How long is enough? Defining the treatment length in endovascular brachytherapy. *Cathet Cardiovasc Intervent* 2000;51:147–153.

SUBACUTE THROMBOSIS

Similar to the first attempts at stent implantation, initial enthusiasm for VBT was dampened by reports of target thrombosis, particularly thrombosis occurring late (>30 days) after treatment. In early trials, late thrombosis after VBT was observed in 3% to 10% of patients independent of the isotope and delivery system tested.[67,112] The thrombotic episode usually manifested itself as a sudden target vessel occlusion resulting in myocardial infarction 1 to 9 months after radiation treatment. There is no uniform definition or criteria for subacute thrombosis. Total occlusions can be subdivided into two groups: (a) symptomatic late thrombosis, occurring more than 30 days after the index procedure and resulting in myocardial infarction, and confirmed by angiography; and (b) silent late occlusions, occurring more than 30 days after the index procedure. These total occlusions are seen on the protocol-required follow-up angiogram without clinical symptoms of myocardial infarction.[113]

The emergence of this complication seriously jeopardized radiation as a viable treatment modality for CAD. Careful study, however, yielded two helpful clues that led to a dramatic reduction in radiation-associated late thrombosis: (a) the overwhelming majority of patients sustaining a late thrombosis had a new stent implanted at the time of the radiation procedure, and (b) almost all patients sustaining late thrombosis had discontinued antiplatelet therapy. Two strategies to prevent late thrombosis were initiated. First, the implantation of new stents during or immediately after treatment with brachytherapy was strongly discouraged. Second, antiplatelet therapy was extended for 6 to 12 months after the radiation therapy procedure. This strategy has now been tested with apparent success in several large series. In more recent trials using the aforementioned strategies, the incidence of late thrombosis was similar to that in the placebo arm, in the range of 1% to 3%. In the SCRIPPS III trial, the late thrombosis rate is zero.[114]

Stent placement at time of radiation delivery can cause both increased late thrombosis and possibly decreased efficacy of the brachytherapy itself. Pooled retrospective data from the SCRIPPS I, WRIST, and GAMMA I trials for patients with in-stent restenosis show an even more pronounced effect of brachytherapy in patients without new stent placement than in patients with stent placement. The Geneva dose-finding study of *de novo* stenosis confirmed these results, with decreased restenosis rates with radiation after angioplasty only compared with angioplasty and stenting.

SUMMARY

VBT is the first proven, clinically effective therapy in the management of in-stent restenosis. The Beta-Cath system using $^{90}Sr/Y$ is currently the only available system used in the treatment of coronary in-stent restenosis.

Results of DES trials have decreased the need for VBT in coronary in-stent restenosis. The TAXUS V study and the SISR randomized trials demonstrate that DESs may be superior to VBT in treating coronary in-stent restenosis.[74] However, VBT can't be entirely eliminated as there are still concerns with long-term complications with DESs. Long-term result studies of DESs are starting to address these concerns.

Outcomes from the RESCUE Registry have shown VBT to be safe and effective following in-stent restenosis of DESs. Overall MACEs were lower in the VBT group when compared to retreatment with DESs. Additionally, there are cost issues as well with multiple stents as there are concerns for stent thrombosis, increased DES failures, and additional interventional procedures. Also, it may be difficult to implant additional DESs in small vessel disease.

VBT is finding a niche role in the treatment of coronary artery disease. Although DESs may become even more efficacious as the next generation of DESs are released, VBT should be considered for earlier use in patients with DES failure, diffuse long lesions, small vessels, vein grafts, bifurcation lesions, possibly *de novo* lesions, and diabetic lesions. Although the initial cost for treatments with VBT may be high, cost-effective analysis performed from GAMMA I and INHIBIT studies show that these costs are offset in the long run due to reduced need for additional bypass surgeries and coronary interventions.

VBT may have an increased role in the treatment of vein graft in-stent restenosis and for peripheral vascular disease. The role of VBT for peripheral vascular disease will mainly be defined based on results of current clinical trials. The dose and volume to be treated will need to be refined to improve efficacy further. VBT has certainly come a long way, becoming more user-friendly and cost-effective.

REFERENCES

1. Babapulle NM, Joseph L, Belisle P, et al. A hierarchical Bayesian meta-analysis of randomized clinical trials of drug-eluting stents. *Lancet* 2004;364:583–591.
2. Lemos PA, Arampatzis CA, Saia F, et al. Treatment of very early vessels with 2.25mm diameter sirolimus-eluting stents. *Am J Cardiol* 2004;93:633–636.
3. Williams DO, Holubkov R, Yeh W, et al. Percutaneous coronary intervention in the current era compared with 1985–1986: the National Heart, Lung, and Blood Institute Registries. *Circulation* 2001;102:2945–2951.
4. Moses JW, Leon MB, Popma JJ, et al. Sirolimus-eluting stents versus standard stents in patients with stenosis in native coronary artery. *N Eng J Med* 2003;349:1315–1323.
5. Dobesh PP, Stacy ZA, Ansara AJ, et al. Drug-eluting stents: a mechanical & pharmacologic approach to coronary artery disease. *Pharmacotherapy* 2004;24: 1554–1577.
6. Landau C, Lange RA, Hillis LD. Percutaneous transluminal coronary angioplasty. *N Engl J Med* 1994;330:981–983.
7. Hillegass WB, Ohman EM, Califf RM. Restenosis: the clinical issues. In: Topol EJ, ed. *Textbook of interventional cardiology*, vol 1, 2nd ed. Philadelphia: WB Saunders, 1994:415–435.
8. Klein LW, Rosenblum J. Restenosis after successful percutaneous transluminal coronary angioplasty. *Prog Cardiovasc Dis* 1990;32:365–382.
9. Ludbrook PA. Coronary restenosis: its mechanisms and modification—overview. *Coron Artery Dis* 1993;4:225–228.
10. Raja SG, Berg GA. Safety of drug eluting stents: current concerns and controversies. *Curr Drug Saf* 2007;2:212–219.
11. Grube E, Silber S, Hauptamann KE, et al. TAXUS I: six- and twelve-month results form a randomized double-blind trial on the slow release paclitaxel-eluting stent for de novo coronary lesions. *Circulation* 2003;107:38–42.
12. Degertekin M, Regar E, Tanabe K, et al. Sirolimus-eluting stent for treatment of complex in-stent restenosis: the first clinical experience. *J Am Coll Cardiol* 2003;41:184–189.
13. Morice MC, Serruys PW, Sousa JE, et al. A randomized comparison of a sirolimus-eluting stent with a standard stent for coronary revascularization. *N Engl J Med* 2002;346:1315–1323.
14. Saia F, Lemos PA, Sianos G, et al. Effectiveness of sirolimus-eluting stent implantation for recurrent in-stent restenosis after brachytherapy. *Am J Cardiol* 2003;41: 184–189.
15. Sousa JE, Costa MA, Abizaid A, et al. Lack of neointimal proliferation after implantation of sirolimus-coated stents in human coronary arteries: a quantitative coronary angiography and three-dimensional intravascular ultrasound study. *Circulation* 2001;103:192–195.
16. Holmes DR, Teirstein P, Satler L, et al. Sirolimus-eluting stents vs. vascular brachytherapy for in-stent restenosis within bare-metal stents. *JAMA* 2006;295: 1264–1273.
17. Stone GW, Ellis SC, O'Shaughnessy CD, et al. Paclitaxel-eluting stents versus vascular brachytherapy for in-stent restenosis within bare metal stents: the TAXUS V ISR randomized trial. *JAMA* 2006;295:1253–1263.
18. Holmes DR, Teirstein P, Satler L, et al. 3-year follow-up of the SISR (sirolimus-eluting stents versus vascular brachytherapy for in-stent restenosis) trial. *J A Coll Crdiol Intv* 2008;1:439–448.
19. Mauri L, Hsieh WH, Massaro JM, et al. Stent thrombosis in randomized clinical trials of drug-eluting stents. *N Engl J Med* 2007;356:1020–1029.
20. Jahraus, CD, St Clair W, Gurley J, et al. Endovascular brachytherapy for the treatment of renal artery in-stent restenosis using a beta-emitting source: a report of five patients. *South Med J* 2003;96:1165–1168.
21. Waksman, R. an update on peripheral brachytherapy. *Endovasc Today* 2004; October:43–52.
22. Schopohl B, Leirmann D, Pohlit LH, et al. ^{192}Ir endovascular brachytherapy for avoidance of intimal hyperplasia after percutaneous transluminal angioplasty and stent implantation in peripheral vessels: 6 years of experience. *Int J Radiat Oncol Biol Phys* 1996;36:835–840.
23. Condado JA, Waksman R, Gurdiel O. Long-term angiographic and clinical outcome after percutaneous transluminal coronary angioplasty and intracoronary radiation therapy in humans. *Circulation* 1997;96:727–732.
24. Teirstein PS, Masullo V, Jani S, et al. Catheter-based radiotherapy to inhibit restenosis after coronary stenting. *N Engl J Med* 1997;336:1697–1703.
25. Leon MB, Teirstein PS, Moses JW, et al. Localized intracoronary gamma-radiation therapy to inhibit the recurrence of restenosis after stenting. *N Engl J Med* 2001;344:250–256.
26. King SB, Williams DO, Prakash C, et al. Endovascular beta-radiation to reduce restenosis after coronary balloon angioplasty: results of the Beta Energy Restenosis Trial (BERT). *Circulation* 1998;97:2025–2030.
27. Verin V, Urban P, Popowski Y, et al. Feasibility of intracoronary β-irradiation to reduce restenosis after balloon angioplasty. *Circulation* 1997;95:1138–1144.
28. Lansky A, Desai K, Costantino C, et al. Predictors of stent and stent-edge restenosis after Sr-90 radiation in the START trial. *J Am Coll Cardiol* 2001;37:54A.
29. Waksman R, Raizner A, Chiu K, et al. Beta radiation to inhibit recurrence of in-stent restenosis: clinical and angiographic results of the multicenter, randomized double blind study. *Circulation Online* 2000;102:e9046.
30. Kuntz RE, Speiser B, Joyal M, et al. Acute and midterm clinical outcomes after use of $^{90}Sr/^{90}Y$ beta radiation for the treatment of native coronary artery obstructions: acute results from the Novoste™ Beta-Cath™ System trial. Presented at the American College of Cardiology, 49th Annual Scientific Session, Anaheim, CA, March 12–16;2000.
31. Tripuraneni P, Berger B. Summary and future of vascular brachytherapy in 2000. In: Meyer JL, ed. *Radiation therapy for benign diseases: current indications and techniques*. Basel: Karger, 2001:211–215.
32. Windecker S, Meier B. Basics of interventional cardiology. In: Tripuraneni P, Jani S, Minar E, et al., eds. *Intravascular brachytherapy: from theory to practice.* London: Remedica, 2001:83–100.
33. Abbas MA, Afshari NA, Stadius ML, et al. External beam irradiation inhibits neointimal hyperplasia following balloon angioplasty. *Int J Cardiol* 1994;44:191–202.
34. Marijianowski M, Crocker I, Styles T, et al. Fibrocellular tissue responses to endovascular and external beam irradiation in the porcine model of restenosis. *Int J Radiat Oncol Biol Phys* 1999;44:633–641.
35. Schwartz RS, Koval TM, Edwards WD, et al. Effect of external beam irradiation on neointimal hyperplasia after experimental coronary artery injury. *J Am Coll Cardiol* 1992;19:1106–1113.
36. Shimatokahara S, Mayberg MR. Gamma irradiation inhibits neointimal hyperplasia in rats after arterial injury. *Stroke* 1994;25:424–428.
37. Styles T, Marijianowski MMH, Robinson KA, et al. Effects of external irradiation of the heart on the coronary artery response to balloon angioplasty injury in pigs. *Proceedings from Advances in Cardiovascular Radiation Therapy* 1997;11.
38. Verheye S, Salame M, Cui J, et al. High-dose external beam irradiation prevents lumen loss and inhibits neointima formation in stented pig coronary arteries. *Int J Radiat Oncol Biol Phys* 2001;51:820–827.
39. Robinson KA, Verheye S, Salame MY, et al. External radiation for restenosis. *J Intervent Cardiol* 1999;12:235–241.
40. Waksman R, Robinson KA, Crocker IR, et al. Endovascular low dose irradiation inhibits neointima formation after coronary artery balloon injury in swine: a possible role for radiation therapy in restenosis prevention. *Circulation* 1955; 91:1553–1539.
41. Wiedermann JG, Marboe C, Amols H, et al. Intracoronary irradiation markedly reduces neointimal proliferation after ballon angioplasty in swine: persistent benefit at 6-month follow-up. *J Am Coll Cardiol* 1995;25:1451–1456.
42. Wiedermann JG, Marboe C, Schwartz A, et al. Intracoronary irradiation reduces restenosis after balloon angioplasty in a porcine model. *J Am Coll Cardiol* 1994; 23:1491–1498.
43. Massullo VM, Teirstein PS, Jani SK, et al. Endovascular brachytherapy to inhibit coronary artery restenosis: an introduction to the Scripps Coronary Radiation to inhibit proliferation post stenting trial. *Int J Radiat Oncol Biol Phys* 1996;36:973–975.
44. Costa R, Joyal M, Harel F, et al. Treatment of bifurcation in-stent restenotic lesions with beta radiation using strontium 90 and sequential positioning pullback technique: procedural details and clinical outcomes. *J Invasive Cardiol* 2003;15: 469–473.
45. Giap H, Massullo V, Teirstein P, et al. Theoretical assessment of late cardiac complication from endovascular brachytherapy for restenosis prevention. *Cardiovasc Radiat Med* 1999;1:233–238.
46. Giap H, Tripuraneni P, Teirstein P, et al. Theoretical assessment of dose-rate effect in endovascular brachytherapy. *Cardiovasc Radiat Med* 1999;1:227–232.
47. Tripuraneni P. Coronary artery radiation therapy for the prevention of restenosis after percutaneous coronary angioplasty, II: outcomes of clinical trials. *Semin Radiat Oncol* 2002;12:17–30.
48. Popma J, Suntharanlingam M, Lansky AJ, et al. Randomized trial of 90Sr/90Y b-radiation versus placebo control for treatment of in-stent restenosis. *Circulation* 2002;106:1090–1096.
49. Waksman R, Ajani A, White RL, et al. Two year follow up after beta and gamma intracoronary radiation therapy for patients with diffuse in-stent restenosis. *Am J Cardiol* 2001;88:425–428.
50. Grise MA, Massullo V, Jani S, et al. Five-year clinical follow-up after intracoronary radiation: results of a randomized clinical trial. *Circulation* 2002;105:2737–2740.

51. Raizner AE, Oesterle SN, Waksman R, et al. Inhibition of restenosis with beta-emitting radiotherapy: report of the proliferation reduction with vascular energy trial. *Circulation* 2000;102:951–958.
52. Teirstein PS, Masullo V, Jani S, et al. Three-year clinical and angiographic follow-up after coronary radiation: results of a randomized clinical trial. *Circulation* 2000;101:360–365.
53. Waksman R, Ajani AE, White RL, et al. Intravascular gamma radiation for in-stent restenosis in saphenous-vein bypass grafts. *N Engl J Med* 2002;346:1194–1199.
54. Waksman R, Raizer AE, Yeung AC, et al. Use of localized intracoronary β radiation in treatment of in-stent restenosis: the INHIBIT randomized controlled trial. *Lancet* 2002;350:551–557.
55. Waksman R, White L, Chan RC, et al., for the Washington Radiation for In-Stent Restenosis Trial (WRIST) Investigators. Intracoronary γ-radiation therapy after angioplasty inhibits recurrence in patients with in-Stent restenosis. *Circulation* 2000;101:2165–2171.
56. Silber S, Popma JJ, Suntharalingam M, et al. Two-year clinical follow-up of 90 Sr/90 Y beta-radiation versus placebo control for the treatment of in-stent restenosis. *Am Heart J* 2005;149:689–694.
57. Urban P, Serruys P, Baumgart D, et al. A multicentre European registry of intraluminal coronary beta brachytherapy. *Eur Heart J* 2003;24:604–612.
58. Rha SW, Kuchulakanti P, Pakala R, et al. Real-world clinical practice of intracoronary radiation therapy as compared to investigational trials. *Catheter Cardiovasc Interv* 2005;64:61–66.
59. Hang CL, Hsieh BT, Wu CJ, et al. Six-year clinical follow-up after treatment of diffuse in-stent restenosis with cutting balloon angioplasty followed by intracoronary brachytherapy with liquid rhenium-188-filled balloon via transradial approach. *Circ J* 2011;75:113–120.
60. Teirstein PS, Massullo V, Jani S. Radiation therapy to inhibit restenosis: early clinical results. *Mt Sinai J Med* 2001;68:192–196.
61. Teirstein PS, Masullo V, Jani S, et al. A subgroup analysis of the Scripps Coronary Radiation to Inhibit Proliferation Poststenting Trial. *Int J Radiat Oncol Biol Phys* 1998;42:1097–1104.
62. Teirstein PS, Masullo V, Jani S, et al. Two-year follow-up after catheter based radiotherapy to inhibit coronary restenosis. *Circulation* 1999;99:243–247.
63. Waksman R, Bhargava B, White LR, et al. Intracoronary beta radiation therapy inhibits recurrence of in-stent restenosis. *Circulation* 2000;101:1895–1898.
64. Tripuraneni P, Leon MB, Teirstein PS, et al. Gamma II, a prospective multicenter registry, with fixed dosing regimen compared to the gamma I trial, using Ir-192 in the treatment of coronary treatment of coronary in-stent restenosis. *Int J Radiat Oncol Biol Phys* 2000;48(Suppl 3):183–184.
65. Sanfilippo NJ, Tripuraneni P. Intravascular brachytherapy trials for coronary heart disease using gamma sources. *Front Radiat Ther Oncol* 2001;35: 202–210.
66. Mehran R, Lansky A, Waksman R. Gamma radiation vs placebo in focal vs. diffuse in-stent restenosis: the length makes the difference. *J Am Coll Cardiol* 2001;35:82A.
67. Waksman R, Ajani AE, White RL, et al. Prolonged antiplatelet therapy to prevent late thrombosis after intracoronary gamma-radiation in patients with in-stent restenosis: Washington Radiation for In-Stent Restenosis Trial Plus 6 Months of Clopidogrel (WRIST PLUS). *Circulation* 2001;103:2332–2335.
68. Popma J, Heuser R, Suntharalingam M, et al., for the START Investigators. Late clinical and angiographic outcomes after use of ^{90}Sr/Y beta radiation for the treatment of in-stent restenosis. *J Am Coll Cardiol* 2000;36:311–312.
69. Suntharalingam M, Laskey W, Lansky W, et al. Analysis of clinical outcomes from the START and START 40 trials:the efficacy of Sr-90 radiation in the treatment of long lesion in-stent restenosis. *Int J Radiat Oncol Biol Phys* 2001;51(Suppl 3): 142.
70. Zahn R, Hamm CW, Zeymer U, et al. Coronary stenting with the sirolimus-eluting stent in patients with restenosis after intracoronary brachytherapy: results from the prospective multicentre German Cypher Stent Registry. *Clin Res Cardiol* 2010; 99:99–106.
71. Fajadet J, Morice MC, Bode C, et al. Maintenance of long-term clinical benefit with sirolimus-eluting coronary stents: three-year results of the RAVEL trail. *Circulation* 2005;111:958–960.
72. Colombo A, Drzewiecki J, Banning A, et al. Randomized study to assess the effectiveness of slow- and moderate-release polymer-based paclitaxel-eluting stent for coronary artery lesions. *Circulation* 2003;108:788–794.
73. Stone GW, Ellis SG, Cox DA, et al. A polymer-based, paclitaxel-eluting stent in patients with coronary artery disease. *N Engl J Med* 2004;350:221–231.
74. Tanabe K, Serruys PW, Grube E, et al. TAXUS III: in-stent restenosis treated with stent-based delivery of paclitaxel incorporated in a slow-release polymer formation. *Circulation* 2003;107:559–564.
75. Tripuraneni P. The future of CART in the era of drug-eluting stents: "It's not over until it's over." counterpoint. *Brachytherapy* 2003;2:74–76.
76. Park S-W, Lee S-W, Koo BK, et al. Treatment of diffuse intent restenosis with drug-eluting stents vs. intracoronary beta-radiation therapy: INDEED study. *Int J Cardiol* 2008;31:70–77.
77. Ellis SG, O'Shaughnessy CD, Martin SL, et al. Two-year clinical outcomes after paclitaxel-eluting stent or brachytherapy treatment for bare metal stent restenosis: the TAXUS V ISR trial. *Eur Heart J* 2008;29:1625–1634.
78. Torguson R, Sabate M, Okubagzi P, et al. Intravascular brachytherapy for the treatment of patients with drug-eluting stent restenosis: the RESCUE Registry. *Presented at Annual Meeting of the American Heart Association, November 13–16,* 2005, Dallas, Texas.
79. Xiong-Jie L, Rha SW, Wani SP, et al. Vascular brachytherapy revisited for in-stent restenosis in the drug-eluting stent era: current status and future perspective. *Chin Med J* 2009;122(18):2174–2179.
80. Castagna M, Mintz G, Weissman N, et al. Intravascular ultrasound analysis of the impact of gamma radiation on the treatment of saphenous vein graft in stent restenosis. *Am J Cardiol* 2002;90(12):1378–1381.
81. Rha SW, Kuchulakanti P, Ajani AE, et al. Three-year follow up after intravascular gamma radiation for in-stent restenosis in saphenous vein grafts. *Catheter Cardiovasc Interv* 2005;65:257–262.
82. Schiele TM, Regar E, Silber S, et al. Clinical and angiographic acute and follow up results of intracoronary beta brachytherapy in saphenous vein bypass grafts: a subgroup analysis of multicentric European registry of intraluminal coronary beta brachytherapy (RENO). *Heart* 2003;89:640–644.
83. Erbel R, Verin V, Popowski Y, et al. Intracoronary beta-irradiation to reduce restenosis after balloon angioplasty: results of a multicenter European dose-finding study (abstr). *Circulation* 1999;100:1–154.
84. Verin V, Popowski Y, de Bruyne B. Endoluminal beta-radiation therapy for the prevention of coronary restenosis after balloon angioplasty: the Dose-Finding Study Group. *N Engl J Med* 2001;344:243–249.
85. Albiero R, Colombo A. Radiation therapy in coronary arteries: radioactive stent trials. In: Tripuraneni P, Jani S, Minar E, et al., eds. *Intravascular brachytherapy: from theory to practice.* London: Remedica, 2001:215–224.
86. Tripuraneni P, Giap H, Jani S. Endovascular brachytherapy for peripheral vascular disease. *Semin Radiat Oncol* 1999;9:190–202.
87. Johnsons KW. Femoral and popliteal arteries: reanalysis of results of angioplasty. *Radiology* 1992;183:767–771.
88. Murray RRJ, Hewes RC, White RIJ, et al. Long-segment femoro-popliteal stenoses: is angioplasty a boon or a bust. *Radiology* 1987;162:473–476.
89. Wilson SE, Wolf GL, Cross AP. Percutaneous transluminal angioplasty versus operation for peripheral arteriosclerosis: report of a prospective randomized trial in a selected group of patients. *J Vasc Surg* 1989;9:1–9.
90. Minar E, Parikh S. Peripheral trials of radiation therapy for prophylaxis of restenosis. In: Tripuraneni P, Jani S, Minar E, et al., eds. *Intravascular brachytherapy: from theory topractice.* London:Remedica, 2001:225–242.
91. Pokrajac B, Potter R, Maca T, et al. Intra arterial high dose rate brachytherapy for prophylaxis of restenosis after femoropopliteal percutaneous transluminal angioplasty: the prospective randomized Vienna 2 trial radiotherapy parameters and risk factor analysis. *Int J Radiat Oncol Biol Phys* 2000;48:923–931.
92. Wolfram RM, Budinsky AC, Pokrajac B, et al. Endovascular brachytherapy for prophylaxis of restenosis after femoropopliteal angioplasty: five-year follow-up-prospective randomized study. *Radiology* 2006;240(3):878–884.
93. Wolfram RM, Budinsky AC, Pokrajac B, et al. Endovascular brachytherapy: restenosis in de novo versus recurrent lesions of femoropopliteal artery-the Vienna experience. *Radiology* 2005;236:338–342.
94. Krueger K, Zaehringer M, Bendel M, et al. De novo femoropopliteal stenoses: endovascular gamma irradiation following angioplasty—angiographic and clinical follow-up in a prospective randomized controlled trial. *Radiology* 2004;231:546–551.
95. Brown KT, Moore ED, Getrajdman GI, et al. Infrapopliteal angioplasty: long-term follow up. *J Vasc Intervent Radiol* 1993;4:139–144.
96. Martin LG, Rees CR, O'Bryant T. Percutaneous angioplasty of the renal arteries. In: Strandness DE, vanBreda A, eds. *Vascular diseases: surgical and interventional therapy.* New York. :Churchill Livingstone, 1994:721–742.
97. Schwarten DE. Percutaneous transluminal angioplasty of the renal arteries: intravenous digital subtraction angiography for follow-up. *Radiology* 1984;150:369–373.
98. Holley KE, Hunt JC, Brown AL, et al. Renal artery stenosis: clinical pathologic study. *Am J Med* 1964;37:14–22.
99. Aslam MS, Balasubramanian J, Greenspahn BR. Brachytherapy for renal artery in-stent restenosis. *Catheter Cardiovasc Interv* 2003;58:151–154.
100. Chrysant GS, Goldstein JA, Casserly IP, et al. Endovascular brachytherapy for treatment of bilateral renal artery in-stent restenosis. *Catheter Cardiovasc Interv* 2003;59:251–254.
101. Ellis K, Murtagh B, Loghin C, et al. The use of brachytherapy to treat renal artery in-stent restenosis. *J Interv Cardiol* 2005;18:49–54.
102. Jahraus CD, Meigooni AS. Vascular brachytherapy: a new approach to renal artery in-stent restenosis. *J Invasive Cardiol* 2004;16:224–227.
103. Palder SR, Kirkman RL, Whittermore AD, et al. Vascular access for hemodialysis: patency rates and results of revision. *Ann Surg* 1995;202:235–239.
104. Beathard GA. Percutaneous transvenous angioplasty in the treatment of vascular access stenosis. *Kidney Int* 1992;42:1390–1397.
105. Krueger K, Bendel M, Zaehringer M, et al. Centered endovascular irradiation to prevent postangioplasty restenosis of arteriovenous fistula in hemodialysis patients; results of a feasibility study. *Cardiovasc Radiat Med* 2004;5:1–8.
106. Chan AW, Roffi M, Mukherjee D, et al. Carotid brachytherapy for in-stent restenosis. *Catheter Cardiovasc Interv* 2003;58:86–92.
107. Kim HS, Waksman R, Kollum M. Edge stenosis after intracoronary radiotherapy: angiographic, intravascular, and histological findings. *Circulation* 2001;103:2219–2220.
108. Sabate M, Costa MA, Kozuma K, et al. Geographic miss: a cause of treatment failure in radio-oncology applied to intracoronary radiation therapy. *Circulation* 2000;101:2467–2471.
109. Giap H, Teirstein P, Massullo V, et al. Barotrauma due to stent deployment in endovascular brachytherapy for restenosis prevention. *Int J Radiat Oncol Biol Phys* 2000;47:1021–1024.
110. Giap HB, Bendre DD, Huppe GB, et al. Source displacement during the cardiac cycle in coronary endovascular brachytherapy. *Int J Radiat Oncol Biol Phys* 2001;49:273–277.
111. Tripuraneni P, Parikh S, Giap H, et al. How long is enough? Defining the treatment length in endovascular brachytherapy. *Cathet Cardiovasc Intervent* 2000;51: 147–153.
112. Waksman R, Bhargava B, Leon MB. Late thrombosis following intracoronary brachytherapy. *Cathet Cardiovasc Intervent* 2000;49:344–347.
113. Waksman R, Bhargava B, Mintz GS, et al. Late total occlusion after intracoronary brachytherapy for patients with in-stent restenosis. *J Am Coll Cardiol* 2000; 36:65–68.
114. Teirstein PS, Moses JW, Casterella PJ, et al. Late thrombosis after coronary radiation may be eliminated by longer antiplatelet therapy and reduced stenting: the Scripps III results. *J Am Coll Cardiol* 2001;37(Suppl A):60 A.

SECTION IV PALLIATIVE AND SUPPORTIVE CARE

Chapter 93
Palliation of Brain and Spinal Cord Metastases

Elizabeth M. Nichols, Roy A. Patchell, William F. Regine, and Young Kwok

BRAIN METASTASIS

Brain metastasis is very common, with an annual incidence of approximately 170,000 to 200,000. The rising incidence of brain metastasis is most likely from a combination of increasing survival from recent advances in systemic therapy and a greater availability and use of magnetic resonance imaging (MRI). The most common primary site is the lung followed by breast. Metastatic brain tumors outnumber primary brain tumors by a factor of 10 to 1, with autopsy series demonstrating a 10% to 30% incidence rate for all patients with a diagnosis of cancer (Table 93.1).[1,2]

Clinical Presentation, Diagnosis, and Prognosis

The majority of patients present with neurologic signs and symptoms (Table 93.2).[3] Although differential diagnoses such as an abscess or a stroke must be considered, new-onset neurologic symptoms in a known cancer patient should always be presumed to be from brain metastasis until proven otherwise.

Given its ability to image in multiple orientations and sequences, including superior resolution and accuracy compared to computed tomography (CT), MRI has become the standard of care for imaging of the central nervous system (CNS) in cancer patients.[4] MRI will frequently pick up smaller lesions not seen on CT scans, which can have a significant effect on the patient's prognosis and treatment course. Full systemic workup (e.g., positron emission tomography [PET] and CT) should be promptly initiated if brain metastasis is the presenting event. The incidence of unknown primaries may subsequently decrease with the increasing popularity of integrated PET-CT scans.

Performance status and extracranial disease status have consistently been shown to impact prognosis. Gaspar et al.[5] reported on the Radiation Oncology Therapy Group (RTOG) experience of 1,200 patients. This analysis revealed three recursive partitioning analysis (RPA) classes, with the RPA class I (Karnofsky performance score [KPS] ≥70, controlled primary, age <65 years, brain metastasis only), II (not meeting requirements of classes I or III), and III (KPS <70) having median survivals of 7.1 months, 4.2 months, and 2.3 months, respectively.

Corticosteroids

The initial therapy should promptly start with corticosteroids (e.g., dexamethasone or methylprednisolone), which effectively improve edema and neurologic deficits in approximately two-thirds of patients.[6] The only randomized trial evaluating dosage was reported by Vecht et al.[7] This trial included two successive groups of patients. The first group (n = 47) evaluated 8 mg per day versus 16 mg per day initial dexamethasone doses, with tapering schedules over 4 weeks. The second group (n = 49) evaluated 4 mg per day versus 16 mg per day of initial dexamethasone, with continuation of these doses for 28 days before tapering. The patients were scheduled for whole-brain radiotherapy (WBRT) and concurrent ranitidine. All arms had similar KPS improvements at 7 days (54% to 70%) and 28 days (50% to 81%). The study concludes that 4 mg per day of dexamethasone (with a taper over 4 weeks) is the preferable regimen. One should be cautious, however, in interpreting the results of this study. Patients in the 4 mg per day arm had to have the medication be reinstituted at a higher rate than the patients in the 8 or 16 mg per day arms. Furthermore, the arm with the greatest improvement in the KPS was the 16 mg per day arm when this was tapered over 4 weeks, compared with any of the other arms. It can be argued that higher KPS improvement arose from the maximal anti-inflammatory effects of the initial higher doses, with the 4-week taper minimizing the late toxicity associated with corticosteroids.

A reasonable corticosteroid regimen in patients with brain metastases is a 10 mg intravenous (IV) or oral bolus, followed by a 4 to 6 mg every 6 to 8 hours of dexamethasone equivalent dose (with a concurrent proton-pump inhibitor [PPI]), before this is tapered in a clinically cautious manner. In asymptomatic patients with little peritumoral edema or mass effect, initial corticosteroids may be reserved until the first sign of neurologic symptoms.

Whole-Brain Radiotherapy

WBRT continues to be the standard of care in patients with brain metastasis. In general, WBRT should be given soon after the diagnosis of brain metastasis. There has never been any evidence to suggest that delaying systemic chemotherapy for WBRT compromises overall survival, especially when one considers that progression in the brain frequently leads directly to the death of the patient.

There is still no agreement on the dose and fractionation schedule for WBRT, despite numerous studies designed to determine the optimal delivery. Table 93.3 summarizes selected randomized fractionation studies.[8–12] Typically, the radiographic and clinical response rates range from 50% to 75%. Most of these studies have been negative, and the overall survival has

TABLE 93.1 EPIDEMIOLOGY OF BRAIN METASTASIS

Primary Site	
Lung	50%
Breast	15%–20%
Other known primary	10%–15%
Unknown primary	10%–15%
Melanoma	10%
Colon	5%
Relevant Facts	
Median survival	<1 yr
Mean age	60 yr
Annual U.S. incidence	>170,000
Autopsy incidence	10%–30%
Clinical incidence	15%–30%
Metastatic/primary ratio	10:1

From refs. 1 and 2.

TABLE 93.2 CLINICAL PRESENTATION OF BRAIN METASTASIS

Symptom	*Percentage of Patients*	*Sign*	*Percentage of Patients*
Headache	49	Hemiparesis	59
Mental problems	32	Cognitive deficits	58
Focal weakness	30	Sensory deficits	21
Ataxia	21	Papilledema	20
Seizures	18	Ataxia	19
Speech problems	12	Apraxia	18

Data from Posner JB. Brain metastases: 1995. A brief review. *J Neurooncol* 1996;27:287–293.

TABLE 93.3 SELECTED RANDOMIZED TRIALS EXAMINING VARIOUS FRACTIONATION SCHEDULES FOR BRAIN METASTASIS

Author/Study Group (Reference)	Dose/ Fractions	N	Median Survival	P
Borgelt et al./RTOG (8)				
1st study (1971–1973)	30 Gy/10	233	21 wk	NS
	30 Gy/15	217	18 wk	
	40 Gy/15	233	18 wk	
	40 Gy/20	227	16 wk	
2nd study (1973–1976)	20 Gy/5	447	15 wk	NS
	30 Gy/10	228	15 wk	
	40 Gy/15	227	18 wk	
Haie-Meder et al./French (10)	25 Gy/10	110	4.2 mo	NS
(1986–1989)	36 Gy/6[a]	106	5.3 mo	
Priestman et al./Royal College (12)	30 Gy/10	263	84 day	.04
of Radiology (1990–1993)	12 Gy/2	270	77 day	
Murray et al./RTOG-91-04 (11)	30 Gy/10	213	4.5 mo	NS
(1991–1995)	54.4 Gy/34[b]	216	4.5 mo	
Graham et al./Australia (9)	40 Gy/20[c]	57	6.1 mo	NS
(1996–2006)	20 Gy/4	56	6.6 mo	

NS, not significant; RTOG, Radiation Therapy Oncology Group.

[a]18 Gy/3 split course with another 18 Gy/3 within 1 month.

[b]54.4 Gy in 1.6 Gy twice a day hyperfractionation for the entire course of therapy.

[c]40 Gy in 1.0 Gy twice a day hyperfractionation for the entire course of therapy.

TABLE 93.4 RANDOMIZED TRIALS OF SURGICAL RESECTION OF SINGLE BRAIN METASTASIS

Author/Study Group (Reference)	Surgery + RT	RT Alone	P
Patchell et al./University of Kentucky (n = 48) (16)			
Primary end point	(36 Gy/12 fx)		
Overall survival	40 wk	15 wk	<.01
Secondary end points			
Local control			
Local failure	20%	52%	<.02
Time to local failure	>59 wk	21 wk	<.0001
Time to neurologic death	62 wk	26 wk	<.0009
KPS ≥70 maintenance	38 wk	8 wk	<.005
Noordijk et al./Dutch (n = 63) (15)			
Primary end points	(40 Gy/20 fx)[a]		
Overall survival	10 mo	6 mo	.04
FIS[1b]	7.5 mo	3.5 mo	.06
Mintz et al./Canadian (n = 84) (14)			
Primary end point	(30 Gy/10 fx)		
Overall survival	5.6 mo	6.3 mo	NS
Secondary end points			
FIS (proportion of days, mean)[2b]	32%	32%	NS
Quality of life (Spitzer score)			
1–3 months (mean)	6.38	5.36	NS
4–6 months (mean)	6.32	6.15	NS

RT, whole-brain radiotherapy; KPS, Karnofsky performance score; fx, fraction number, WHO, World Health Organization.

[a]40 Gy total in 2 Gy twice a day hyperfractionation for the entire course of therapy.

[b]Functionally independent survival as defined by:

[1]WHO performance status ≤1 and neurologic condition ≤1.

[2]KPS ≥70.

not improved appreciably over the past 25 to 30 years. A total of 30 Gy in 10 fractions continues to be the standard for a vast majority of patients. In chemotherapy refractory RPA class III patients, a shorter fractionation scheme (e.g., 20 Gy in 5 fractions) should be considered. However, short fractionation schemes should be avoided in chemotherapy-naive patients with brain metastasis as the presenting event in the cancer diagnosis. The natural disease course of such patients can be frequently unpredictable, so they may live sufficiently long enough to experience late radiation toxicity posed by such short fractionation schedules.[13]

Surgical Resection

Surgical resection can provide immediate relief of the tumor mass effect (Fig. 93.1). On the other hand, radiation typically takes several days to work. Radiobiologically, 30 Gy in 10 fractions to a solid tumor (excluding radiosensitive tumors) is not adequate to achieve long-term tumor control. This issue is especially germane because historically up to one-half of all patients died from neurologic causes after being treated with WBRT alone.

There have now been three phase III trials testing the hypothesis that surgical resection to single brain metastasis is potentially beneficial. All three trials were on patients with a single lesion, which is defined as the presence of only one lesion in the brain regardless of the extracranial disease status, while a solitary lesion is defined as the presence of the CNS metastasis as the only site of the metastatic disease burden. Table 93.4 summarizes the three trials.[14–16] The studies by Patchell et al.[16] (KPS ≥70) and Noordijk et al.[15] (World Health Organization grade ≤2) included better performance status patients compared with the Mintz et al.[14] study (KPS ≥50), which mainly contributed to the differences in the survival outcomes between the studies. The results of these studies suggest that surgical resection should be reserved for lesions causing life-threatening complications or for those patients with good performance status (i.e., KPS ≥70).

Radiosurgery Boost Trials

Radiosurgery provides a substitute or alternative to conventional surgery. The three randomized trials of surgical resection were performed before the widespread availability of stereotactic radiosurgery (SRS). Although no randomized trials have been performed comparing surgery with SRS, SRS appears to provide similar local control rates (in the order of 80% to 90% only when combined with WBRT). Unless the tumor causes significant edema and mass effect, with consequent hydrocephalus or herniation requiring urgent surgical intervention, SRS can serve as a noninvasive alternative. Frequently, a patient may not be a craniotomy candidate because of tumor location in eloquent areas or existing medical contraindications. Although two of the three conventional surgery trials have shown a survival benefit in single brain metastasis, there have been no randomized trials addressing multiple lesions, and the retrospective data available are contradictory. For SRS there have been three randomized trials assessing the efficacy of SRS in the treatment of multiple metastases (Table 93.5).

The first randomized trial was reported by Kondziolka et al.[17] from the University of Pittsburgh. This small study was stopped early at a planned interim analysis of 60% patient accrual because the authors reported having found a large difference in the primary end point of local control in favor of SRS (92% vs. 0%; P = .0016). Unfortunately, the study used nonstandard end points to measure recurrence, defining it as *any* increase in the lesion size on MRI. Furthermore, no attempt was made to control for steroid use, radiation changes, or other factors that might produce small fluctuations in the lesion size on MRI. Therefore, this study is difficult to interpret.

Chougule et al.[18] from Brown University reported the second trial, although this is published only in abstract form. This trial had three treatment arms and randomized patients to treatment with SRS alone with Gamma Knife (Elekta Corp, Stockholm), SRS plus WBRT, or WBRT alone. This trial suffers from several methodological problems. Although the authors conclude that the survival times among the treatment arms were similar and that patients treated with SRS experienced superior local control and fewer brain metastases, no probability values are given. Furthermore, 51 of the patients had surgical resection for at least one symptomatic brain metastasis prior to entry into the study, and no attempt was made to stratify for previous surgery. The inclusion of the surgically resected patients effectively

Palliative and Supportive Care

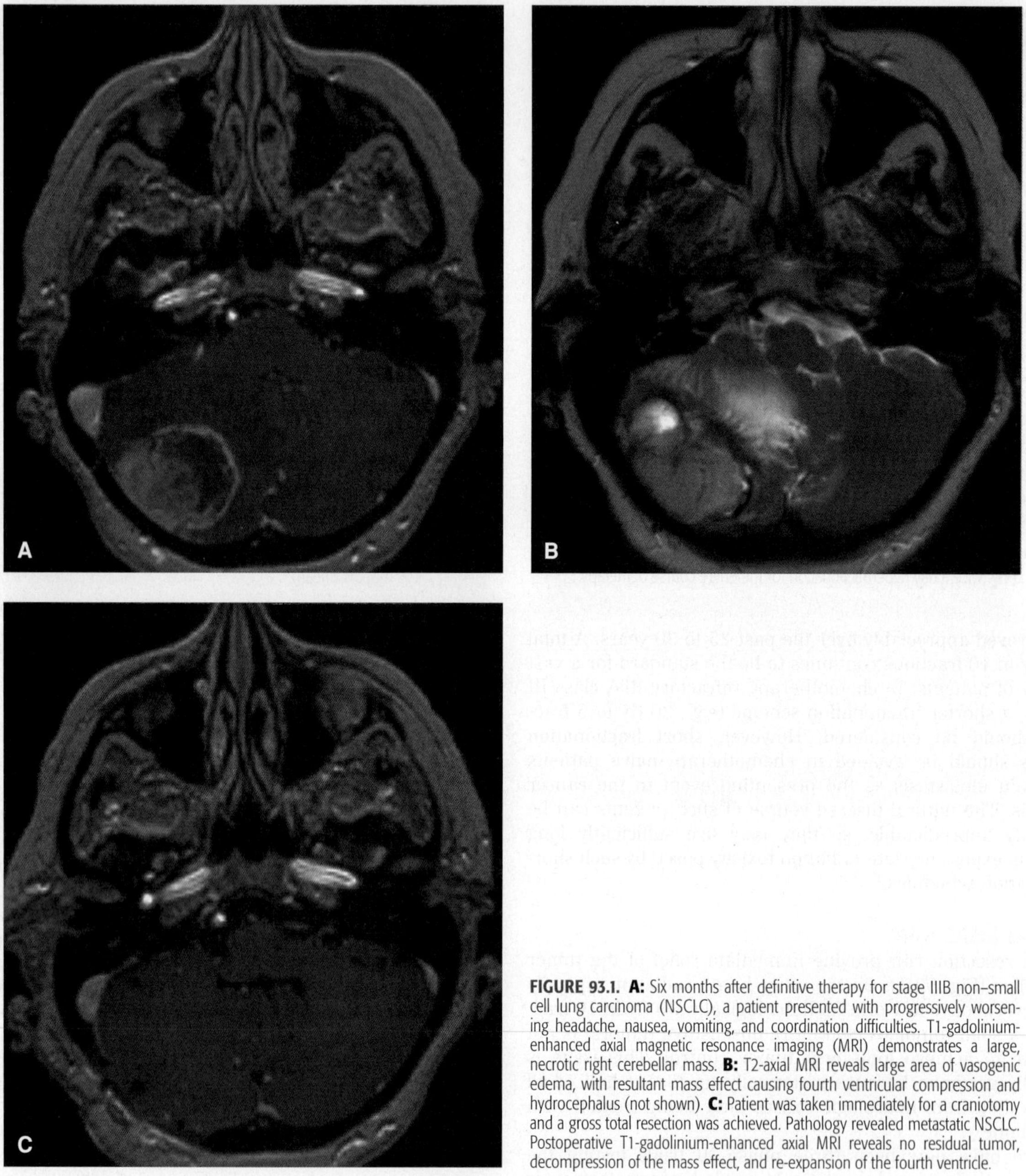

FIGURE 93.1. A: Six months after definitive therapy for stage IIIB non–small cell lung carcinoma (NSCLC), a patient presented with progressively worsening headache, nausea, vomiting, and coordination difficulties. T1-gadolinium-enhanced axial magnetic resonance imaging (MRI) demonstrates a large, necrotic right cerebellar mass. B: T2-axial MRI reveals large area of vasogenic edema, with resultant mass effect causing fourth ventricular compression and hydrocephalus (not shown). C: Patient was taken immediately for a craniotomy and a gross total resection was achieved. Pathology revealed metastatic NSCLC. Postoperative T1-gadolinium-enhanced axial MRI reveals no residual tumor, decompression of the mass effect, and re-expansion of the fourth ventricle.

made this a six-arm trial and, therefore, the size of this trial was not large enough to support a meaningful analysis. Finally, the radiation doses used in the SRS arms cannot be considered conventional because the peripheral dose was not individualized based on the tumor size or volume.

In the third study, RTOG-95-08, the primary end point was overall survival, which was not statistically different between the WBRT plus SRS and WBRT alone arms (6.5 months and 5.7 months, respectively; $P = .1356$), although the SRS boost improved the survival in the subgroup (planned analysis) of patients with single metastasis.[19] For secondary end points, the local control and performance measures, were higher in the SRS boost arm, but this did not translate into a lower death rate from neurologic progression. Multiple, unplanned subgroup analyses were made, and an overall survival benefit with the SRS boost was found in several subgroups that included patients with RPA class 1, tumor size ≥2 cm, and non–small cell lung cancer or metastatic squamous histology from any site. Unfortunately, these subset analyses were not planned or prespecified, and the probability values needed for significance should have been adjusted for inflation of the type I error. When this was done, none of these subgroup analyses showed a positive benefit for SRS.[20] On the other hand, this trial did demonstrate that SRS is associated with lower edema and corticosteroid use, countering a commonly held notion that SRS actually increases the edema risk. However, regarding the major end points for multiple metastases, this study should be considered a negative trial.

Although SRS boost is indicated (from RTOG-95-08 and from the extrapolation of surgical resection data) in patients with a single metastasis, it is difficult to justify its routine use in patients with multiple metastases in light of the equivocal phase III SRS boost trials.

Postoperative or Postradiosurgery Whole-Brain Radiotherapy

A controversy in the treatment of brain metastasis is the routine use of postoperative or post-SRS WBRT. In a multi-institutional retrospective SRS study, Sneed et al.[21] argue for the

TABLE 93.5 RANDOMIZED TRIALS OF STEREOTACTIC RADIOSURGERY BOOST IN BRAIN METASTASES

Author/Study Group (Reference)	*RT + SRS*	*RT Alone*	*SRS Alone*	*P*
Andrews/RTOG 95-08 (n = 333; 1–3 lesions) (19)				
Primary end point (overall survival)	(37.5 Gy/10 fx)			
1–3 lesions	5.7 mo	6.5 mo		NS
Single brain metastasis (planned subgroup analysis)	6.5 mo	4.9 mo		.04
Secondary end points				
Local control (1 year)	82%	71%		.01
Neurologic death rate	28%	31%		NS
Performance outcome				
KPS stable/improve				
at 3 mo	50%	33%		.02
at 6 mo	43%	27%		.03
Mental status				NS
Unplanned subgroup analysis (overall survival)				
Largest tumor >2 cm	6.5 mo	5.3 mo		.04
RPA class I	11.6 mo	9.6 mo		.05
Squamous/NSCLC	5.9 mo	3.9 mo		.05
Other outcomes				
Response rate (3 mo)				
Tumor	73%	62%		.04
Edema	70%	47%		.002
Kondziolka et al./University of Pittsburgh (n = 27; 2–4 lesions) (17)				
Primary end point (30 Gy/12 fx)				
Local control (1 yr)	92%	0%		.0016
Time to local failure	36 mo	6 mo		.005
Time to any brain failure	34 mo	5 mo		.002
Secondary end points				
Overall survival	11 mo	7.5 mo		NS
Treatment morbidity	0	0		
Progression-free survival	not reported			
Need for retreatment	not reported			
Chougule et al./Brown University (n = 109; 1–3 lesions) (18)				
Endpoints (abstract only)	(30 Gy + 20 Gy SRS)	(30 Gy/10 fx)	(30 Gy SRS)	
Overall survival	5 mo	9 mo	7 mo	not reported
Local control	91%	62%	87%	not reported
New brain lesions	19%	23%	43%	not reported

RT, whole-brain radiotherapy; SRS, stereotactic radiosurgery; RPA, recursive partitioning analysis; NSCLC, non–small cell lung cancer; NS, not significant; KPS, Karnofsky performance score; fx, fraction number.

omission of upfront WBRT because this does not compromise overall survival. Unfortunately, only an overall survival analysis was performed, and no local control or retreatment data were given. In an earlier study by Sneed et al.[22] on the University of California–San Francisco SRS experience, patients who were initially treated with SRS alone without WBRT experienced worse freedom from new brain metastasis and overall brain freedom from progression despite the imbalance of the prognostic factors that favored the SRS alone group, although the overall survival was not different. Because of the equivalency of overall survival, many have advocated withholding upfront WBRT. They often use repeat SRS for the failures, which can be very expensive. Furthermore, brain failure can lead to unacceptable consequences. Many incorrectly assume that with close follow-up, recurrences can be diagnosed early before symptoms. For example, Regine et al.[23] reported on 36 patients with planned observation after initial SRS alone. Even with close follow-up with examinations and high-resolution MRIs, 47% of patients experienced brain failure, with 71% and 59% experiencing symptomatic relapse and neurologic deficits, respectively.

The omission of upfront WBRT may have even more serious consequences for patients with more radioresistant tumors such as renal-cell carcinoma (RCC). The SRS dose given is typically limited by tumor size and volume, not by whether the patient received additional dose with WBRT. Therefore, a patient treated with WBRT plus SRS receives much higher tumor dose than SRS alone. It is then not a surprise that the Eastern Cooperative Oncology Group protocol E6397 demonstrates very disappointing results.[24] In this phase II trial that evaluated SRS alone in radioresistant tumors (RCC, melanoma, sarcoma), Manon et al.[24] reported a 6-month total brain failure rate of 48.3%. The authors correctly conclude that routine avoidance of WBRT should be approached judiciously.

Fortunately, there have been five phase III trials that have assessed the use of postoperative or postradiosurgery WBRT (Table 93.6). Patchell et al.[25] demonstrated that surgical resection without WBRT led to a failure rate at the original site and the entire brain of 46% and 70%, respectively. More importantly, 44% of the patients in the surgery alone arm died as a result of neurologic sequelae from brain failure. The results of this study have been frequently misinterpreted in the literature. Some have justified the withholding of upfront WBRT based on the fact that this study demonstrated equivalent survivals. In fact this study was designed with brain tumor recurrence rate as the primary end point and not overall survival. To show an overall survival difference, this trial needed to enroll over 2,000 patients. This study met its primary end point and confirmed the importance of postoperative WBRT in preventing brain failure and death from neurologic causes.

In the Japanese Radiation Oncology Study Group JROSG-99-1 phase III trial of one to four lesions, the SRS-only arm experienced worse 1-year total brain recurrence rate ($P < .001$) and more frequently required salvage therapy ($P < .001$).[26] Furthermore, the average time until Mini-Mental State Examination (MMSE) deterioration was significantly longer for the combined arm (16.5 vs. 7.6 months; $P = .05$).[27] The main drawback of this study was the designation of overall survival as the primary end point. There is very little evidence that adjuvant WBRT after surgery is likely to improve overall survival. However, this study did demonstrate the importance of WBRT in decreasing brain failure, corroborating the findings of the Patchell et al.[25] study.

Muacevic et al.[28] randomized single brain metastasis patients (KPS ≥70, size ≤3 cm, stable systemic disease) to SRS alone versus resection plus WBRT. Those randomized to SRS alone experienced worse local ($P = .06$) and distant ($P = .04$) recurrences, but there were no differences in neurologic death rates or overall survival.

The results of EORTC-22952-26001 have been reported with the primary end point of evaluating duration of functional independence.[29] In this study, patients with one to three brain metastases underwent local therapy with either surgery or SRS and were then randomized to the addition of WBRT versus observation. WBRT did not improve duration of functional independence or overall survival but was associated

Palliative and Supportive Care

TABLE 93.6 RANDOMIZED TRIALS OF POSTOPERATIVE/POSTRADIOSURGERY WHOLE-BRAIN RADIOTHERAPY

Study (Reference)	*Surgery + RT*	*Surgery Only*	*P*
Patchell et al./University of Kentucky (n = 95; single lesion) (25)			
Primary end point (50.4 Gy/28 fx) craniotomy			
Brain tumor recurrence			
Total brain recurrence	18%	70%	<.001
Original site only	4%	33%	
Distant site only	8%	24%	
Original and distant	6%	13%	
Distant site total	14%	37%	<.01
Original site total	10%	46%	<.001
Secondary end points			
Cause of death			
Neurologic	14%	44%	.003
Systemic	84%	46%	<.001
Functional independence[a]	37 wk	35 wk	NS
Overall survival	48 wk	43 wk	NS
Aoyama et al./Japanese JROSG-99-1 (n = 132; 1–4 lesions) (26)			
Primary end point (30 Gy/10 fx) SRS			
Overall survival			
1 year[b]	39%	28%	NS
Median	7.5 mo	8.0 mo	NS
Secondary Endpoints			
Brain recurrence (total)[b]	47%	76%	<.001
Functional preservation[a,b]	34%	27%	NS
Neurologic death	23%	19%	NS
Need for salvage therapy	10 patients	29 patients	<.001
Radiation morbidity			
Acute	4 patients	8 patients	NS
Late	7 patients	3 patients	NS
Muacevic et al./German (n = 70; 1 lesion) (28)			
Primary end point (40 Gy/20 fx)	SRS or craniotomy[c]		
Overall survival	9.5 ms	10.3 ms	NS
Secondary end point			
Brain recurrence			
Local (1 yr)	3.4%	18%	.06
Distant (1 yr)	3%	25.8%	.04
Kocher et al./EORTC-22952-26001 (n = 359; 1–3 lesions) (29)			
Primary end point (30 Gy/10 fx) SRS or craniotomy			
Functional independence	9.5 mo	10 mo	NS
Secondary end points			
Brain tumor recurrence			
Original site: SRS	31%	19%	.040
Distant site: SRS	48%	33%	.023
Original site: S	59%	27%	<.001
Distant site: S	42%	23%	.008
Progression-free survival	4.6 mo	3.4 mo	NS
Overall survival	10.7 mo	10.9 mo	NS
Chang et al./MDACC (n = 58; 1–3 lesions) (30)			
Primary end point (30 Gy/12 fx) SRS			
Neurocognitive function (HVLT-R drop)	52%	24%	Significant
Secondary end points			
Local control (1 yr)	100%	67%	.012
Distant brain control (1 yr)	73%	45%	.02
Overall survival	5.7 mo	15.2 mo	.003

fx, fraction number; NS, not significant; KPS, Karnofsky performance score; RT, whole-brain radiotherapy; S, surgery; SRS, stereotactic radiosurgery; HVLT-R, Hopkins Verbal Learning Test-Revised; JROSG, Japanese Radiation Oncology Study Group.

[a]As defined by KPS ≥70 maintenance.

[b]One-year actuarial rates.

[c]SRS alone versus craniotomy plus WBRT.

with a decreased 2-year local and distant brain relapse rate of roughly 30%, resulting in a 16% decrease in neurologic death. Although there was no difference in duration of functional independence between the two arms, the authors conclude that this is likely due to a variety of factors, including the subjective grading of the performance status, the routine MRI imaging rendering the majority of recurrences as asymptomatic, and the potential impact of systemic agents on performance status.

Recently, Chang et al.[30] reported on a series of 58 patients with one to three brain metastases randomized to WBRT with or without SRS. The primary end point of the study was neurocognitive function, which was assessed using the Hopkins Verbal Learning Test-Revised at 4 months after therapy. They found that patients receiving combined therapy were more likely to have a decline in learning and memory function at 4 months compared with patients who did not receive WBRT. The median survival was 15.2 months for the SRS alone group and 5.7 months for the WBRT/SRS group (P = .003). However, the local (67% vs. 45%; P = .012) and distant (100% vs. 73%; P = .02) brain control were worse in the SRS alone group compared with the WBRT/SRS group. There are multiple criticisms of this study worth noting.[31] First, because the primary end point was neurocognitive function, the authors did not stratify by baseline neurocognitive function or other factors known to impact neurocognition. Second, the authors chose a single test at a single time point. Ideally, a whole battery of tests should be performed at multiple time points to adequately assess the trend of something as complex as neurocognition. Most importantly, the combined arm inexplicably had a shorter survival, contrary to the four previously mentioned trials that demonstrated equivalent survivals. The median survival of 5.7 months was within 2 months of the primary end point mark, which classically falls within the time point of progressively worsening cognition seen in terminally ill patients.[32,33] The superior survival in spite of inferior local and distant brain control is unprecedented and can possibly be explained by an improper randomization, which is possible in a small study.

In summary, four of the five phase III local with or without WBRT trials unequivocally show a meaningful benefit of WBRT in terms of preventing neurologic deaths or brain failure. It is difficult to ignore the level I evidence provided by these phase III trials. Adjuvant WBRT, therefore, should be considered the standard of care after local therapy with surgical resection or SRS.

Repeat Whole-Brain Radiotherapy

Occasionally, patients will fail in the brain with multiple lesions after initial WBRT. Repeat WBRT should strongly be considered. Wong et al.[34] reported on a series of 86 patients who underwent repeat WBRT. The median dose for the first course was 30 Gy, while the median dose for the second course was 20 Gy. A total of 70% experienced neurologic improvement, with 27% experiencing complete neurologic resolution while 43% had partial improvement after repeat WBRT. A retreatment dose of >20 Gy was associated with a significantly longer survival. Only one patient experienced dementia thought to be caused by radiation.

Son et al.[35] similarly reported on a series of 17 patients who underwent whole brain reirradiation. The median RT dose for the first course of treatment was 35 Gy and for the second course 21.6 Gy. The median survival time for all patients after retreatment was 5.2 months. In patients with stable extracranial disease, the median survival time after retreatment was 19.8 months compared with 2.5 months in patients with progressive extracranial disease. Eighty percent of patients experienced improved symptomatology, but acute mild to moderate adverse reactions were seen in 70.5% of patients.

Repeat WBRT is relatively safe because a vast majority of patients have limited survival with recurrent or progressive brain metastases after initial WBRT. A minimum of 20 Gy in 1.8 to 2 Gy fractions should be given.

Concurrent Radiosensitizers

Although a majority of patients with brain metastases ultimately succumb to systemic progression, a significant percentage will die from neurologic progression. Multiple randomized trials of concomitant radiosensitizers have been performed in an attempt to optimize brain control (Table 93.7).[25,36–43] No trial has demonstrated a survival advantage, although a few have demonstrated an increased response rate. The two trials with temozolomide show promise. Temozolomide is an oral alkylating agent with excellent CNS penetration. However, the findings of these two relatively small trials need to be confirmed in a larger trial. Concurrent temozolomide with WBRT should be considered in a patient with bulky brain metastases burden who is unlikely to become a SRS candidate. Otherwise, a patient should be treated with a concomitant radiosensitizer only on a prospective trial.

TABLE 93.7 SELECTED RANDOMIZED TRIALS OF RADIOSENSITIZERS IN BRAIN METASTASIS

Author/Study Group (Reference)	*Arms*	*Response Rate (%)*	*P*	*Median Survival*	*P*
Komarnicky et al./ RTOG 79-16 (39) (n = 859)	RT (30 Gy/10 fx)	45[a]	NS	4.5 mo	NS
	RT+misonidazole	42[a]	NS	3.9 mo	NS
	RT (30 Gy/6 fx)	42[a]		4.1 mo	
	RT+misonidazole	45[a]		3.1 mo	
Ushio et al./ Japan (42)[b] (n = 88)	RT (40 Gy/20 fx)	36	<.05	27 wk	NS
	RT+nitrosurea	69		31 wk	
	RT+nitrosurea+tegafur	74		29 wk	
Phillips et al./ RTOG-89-05 (86) (n = 72)	RT (37.5 Gy /15 fx)	50	NS	6.1 mo	NS
	RT+BrdUrd	63		4.3 mo	
Guerrieri et al./ Australia (37)[b] (n = 42)	RT (20 Gy/5 fx)	10	NS	4.4 mo	NS
	RT+carboplatin	29		3.7 mo	
Antonadou et al./ Greece (36) (n = 52)	RT (40 Gy/20 fx)	67	.017	7.0 mo	NS
	RT+temozolomide	96		8.6 mo	
Verger et al./ Spain (43) (n = 82)	RT (30 Gy/10 fx)	54[c]	.03	3.1 mo	NS
	RT+temozolomide	72[c]		4.5 mo	
Mehta et al./ SMART Trial (40) (n = 401)	RT (30 Gy/10 fx)	51	NS	4.9 mo	NS
	RT+MGd	46		5.2 mo	
Suh et al./REACH Trial (41) (n = 515)	RT (30 Gy/10 fx)	38	NS	4.4 mo	NS
	RT+efaproxiral	46		5.4 mo	
Knisely et al./ RTOG-01-18 (38) (n = 175)	RT (37.5 Gy/15 fx)			3.9 mo	NS
	RT+thalidomide			3.9 mo	

SWOG, South West Oncology Group; RTOG, Radiation Therapy and Oncology Group; RT, whole-brain radiotherapy; NS, not significant; fx, fractions; BrdUrd, bromodeoxyuridine; MGd, motexafin gadolinium; KPS, Karnofsky performance score.

[a]Percentage of survival time in KPS 90–100 range.

[b]Only lung cancer patients.

[c]Ninety-day freedom from brain metastasis.

Causes of Neurocognitive Decline in Brain Tumor Patients

Historically, brain radiation has been frequently cited as the major cause of neurocognitive decline in cancer patients. One of the most misinterpreted studies on this subject is the Memorial Sloan-Kettering Cancer Center experience reported by DeAngelis et al.[13] An 11% risk of radiation-induced dementia is reported in patients undergoing WBRT for brain metastasis. The 11% figure is very misleading. Of the 47 patients who survived 1 year after WBRT, 5 patients (11%) developed severe dementia. When these five patients were examined, all were treated in a fashion that would significantly increase the risk of late radiation toxicity (i.e., large daily fractions and concurrent radiosensitizer). Three patients received 5 Gy and 6 Gy daily fractions, while a fourth patient received 6 Gy fractions with concurrent Adriamycin. Only one patient received what is considered a standard radiation fractionation scheme (i.e., 30 Gy in 10 fractions), but this patient received a concurrent radiosensitizer (lonidamine). *No* patient who received the standard 30 Gy in 10 fractions WBRT alone experienced dementia.

The accuracy of the 11% dementia rate is further questioned by the nature of the statistical interpretation utilized. Although the study included 232 patients in the initial analysis, it only examined the 47 patients who survived at least 1 year. The principles of conditional probability dictate that the 11% risk is accurate only if a patient survives 1 year, which is significantly longer than most reported series. Therefore, a radiation-induced dementia risk of 2% (5 of 232) would reflect the true probability *ab initio* for patients presenting with brain metastasis. Indeed, in a separate study of a larger cohort, DeAngelis et al.[44] estimated the risk of radiation-induced dementia to be 1.9% to 5.2% for all patients presenting with brain metastasis. In the authors' opinion, this risk of dementia is not high enough to warrant withholding quality-of-life–prolonging WBRT.

Many have argued that the increased local control with adjuvant WBRT does not translate into a survival benefit, and that performing repeat SRS or deferring WBRT for recurrences is a reasonable approach. However, WBRT may actually improve neurocognition in a significant number of patients, and brain recurrence or progression is associated with a decrease in neurocognitive function.[45] In a neurocognitive analysis of RTOG-91-04, Regine et al.[46] demonstrated that approximately one-third of patients treated with WBRT experienced improvement in their MMSE; most importantly, those who had uncontrolled brain metastases had an average decrement of 6 points on the MMSE.

The DeAngelis et al.[13] experience, as well as other studies that employed MMSE, did not utilize sophisticated neurocognitive testing. It is possible that subtle neurocognitive dysfunction may indeed result from WBRT. Recent studies that have used sophisticated neurocognitive testing clearly demonstrated that the brain tumor (presence, recurrence, and progression) has the greatest effect on neurocognitive decline. In the large phase III motexafin gadolinium study, the neurocognitive battery examined memory recall, memory recognition, memory delayed recall, verbal fluency, pegboard hand coordinate, and executive function.[47] This study demonstrated that 21.0% to 65.1% of patients had impaired functioning *at baseline* before treatment with WBRT. Furthermore, patients who progressed in the brain after treatment experienced significantly worse scores in all of these individual tests.

There are now strong data that other factors, such as anticonvulsants, benzodiazepines, opioids, chemotherapy, craniotomy, and, most importantly, the brain tumor contribute significantly to the neurocognitive decline of patients with brain tumor.[48–52]

Anticonvulsants

Patients frequently present to the radiation oncologist already started on prophylactic anticonvulsants. This represents one of the most preventable causes of neurocognitive decline in brain tumor patients. Anticonvulsants are clearly known to impact negatively on quality of life and neurocognition. In a study of 156 patients with low-grade glioma (85% experiencing a seizure), Klein et al.[50] correlated seizure burden with quality of life and neurocognitive function. This study convincingly demonstrates the significant correlation between the increase in the number anticonvulsants (even with lack of seizures) with the decrease in quality of life and neurocognitive function.

Based on four negative randomized trials, the American Academy of Neurology recommends that prophylactic anticonvulsants not be initiated in newly diagnosed brain tumor patients who have not experienced a seizure.[53] It is safe to taper a patient off of anticonvulsants provided the patient has not experienced a seizure.

SPINAL CORD COMPRESSION

In the United States, more than 20,000 cases of metastatic spinal cord compression (MSCC) are diagnosed annually, and it is estimated to develop in approximately 5% to 14% of all cancer patients.[54,55] MSCC is a devastating complication of cancer. It is considered a true medical emergency, and immediate intervention is required. Even with aggressive therapy, results can often be unsatisfactory. Although most patients with MSCC have limited survival, up to one-third will survive beyond 1 year.[56] Therefore, aggressive therapy should always be considered to preserve or improve the quality of life.

Pathophysiology

MSCC develops primarily in one of three ways: (a) continued growth and expansion of vertebral bone metastasis into the epidural space; (b) neural foramina extension by a paraspinal mass; or (c) destruction of vertebral cortical bone, causing vertebral body collapse with displacement of bony fragments into the epidural space. Although complex, the most significant damage caused by MSCC appears to be vascular in nature. Epidural tumor extension causes epidural venous plexus compression, which leads to edema of the spinal cord. This increase in vascular permeability and edema cause increased pressure on the small arterioles. Capillary blood flow diminishes as the disease progresses, leading to white matter ischemia. Prolonged ischemia eventually results in white matter infarction and permanent cord damage.[57]

Clinical Presentation, Diagnosis, and Prognosis

The vast majority of patients with MSCC have a cancer diagnosis history. In a review by Fuller et al.,[58] of more than 1,000 patients with MSCC, the most common tumor types are breast cancer (29%), lung cancer (17%), and prostate cancer (14%). This reflects the high natural incidence of these tumors. New-onset back pain in cancer patients needs to be taken seriously and worked up. Even without a prior cancer diagnosis, MSCC should be suspected in anyone who presents with progressively worsening back pain, incontinence, or paraplegia, especially in the high-risk population such as longtime smokers. The most common level of the MSCC involvement is in the thoracic spine (59% to 78%), followed by lumbar (16% to 33%) and cervical spine (4% to 15%), while multiple levels are involved in up to half of the patients.[58–60] Back pain is the most common presenting symptom (88% to 96%), followed by weakness (76% to 86%), sensory deficits (51% to 80%), and autonomic dysfunction (40% to 64%).[59,61–65]

MRI is the standard modality for spine imaging. It has a very high sensitivity (93%), specificity (97%), and accuracy (95%) in diagnosing MSCC.[66,67] Because patients can have synchronous, multifocal MSCC, an MRI of the entire spine with and without contrast should be promptly performed in anyone suspected of having MSCC.[68] High-resolution CT scan or CT myelogram of the spine should be performed for those with contraindications to MRI.

Prognostic factors predicting survival are generally similar to patients with brain metastasis, as discussed above. In terms of predicting ambulatory outcome, one of the most important factors is the rapidity of symptom onset. Other important prognostic factors include radiosensitive histology (e.g., multiple myeloma, germ cell tumors, small cell carcinoma) and pretherapy ambulatory function. In a prospective study of 98 patients with MSCC reported by Rades et al.,[69] the single strongest predictor for ambulatory status after therapy on multivariate analysis was time to development of motor deficits before radiation ($P < .001$) from the start of any symptoms. This cohort was separated into three groups according to the time to motor deficits before radiation therapy: 1 to 7 days (group A), 8 to 14 days (group B), and >14 days (group C). The ambulatory rates after therapy for groups A, B, and C were 35%, 55%, and 86% ($P < .001$), respectively. The symptom improvement rates for groups A, B, and C were 10%, 29%, and 86% ($P = .026$), respectively. The other factor significant on the multivariate analysis for posttherapy ambulatory status was favorable histology ($P = .005$), and there was a trend regarding pretherapy ambulatory status ($P = .076$). Acute, rapid deterioration is predictive of irreversible spinal cord infarction. Only 10% of the patients in group A had symptom improvement; therefore, prompt diagnosis and treatment of MSCC are essential.

Corticosteroids

Corticosteroids must be started as soon as possible in anyone suspected of having MSCC, even before radiographic diagnosis, because this can be rapidly discontinued with a negative diagnosis. Corticosteroids effectively decrease cord edema and serve as an effective bridge to definitive treatment. Although multiple retrospective studies have demonstrated their clinical efficacy, Sorensen et al.[70] reported the only randomized controlled study (n = 57) on the utility of high-dose corticosteroids before definitive radiotherapy in MSCC from solid tumors. The treatment arm consisted of 96 mg of IV bolus of dexamethasone followed by 96 mg oral per day for 3 days and a 10-day taper versus no corticosteroid therapy. This study demonstrated 3-month and 6-month ambulatory rates of 81% versus 63% and 59% versus 33% ($P < .05$), respectively, in favor of high-dose dexamethasone.

The optimal maintenance dose of corticosteroids is unknown. Vecht et al.[71] reported the only randomized study (n = 37) comparing corticosteroid doses in patients with MSCC, but this study only evaluated the IV loading dose. It compared IV loading doses of 10 mg versus 100 mg, followed in both arms by the same oral regimen of 16 mg per day. Both arms demonstrated significant reductions in pain from baseline ($P < .001$); however, there was no difference between the two arms with respect to pain reduction, ambulation, or bladder function.

Very high doses of corticosteroids are associated with significant side effects. The Sorensen et al.[70] phase III study reported an 11% incidence of serious side effects for patients in the treatment arm, while Heimdal et al.[72] reported a 14.3% incidence of serious gastrointestinal (GI) side effects in 28 consecutive patients treated with 96 mg of IV dexamethasone per day. The toxicities in the Heimdal et al.[77] report included one fatal ulcer hemorrhage, one rectal bleeding, and two bowel perforations. Subsequently, the dexamethasone dose was decreased to 16 mg per day for the next 38 consecutive patients, and there were no incidences of serious side effects ($P <.05$). Most importantly, the ambulatory rates were not different between the two dexamethasone doses.

Based on these data, a loading disc of 10 mg of IV dexamethasone followed by a maintenance dose of 4 to 6 mg every 6 to 8 hours should be sufficient before being tapered. Patients can be safely switched to a oral regimen after 24 to 48 hours because there is good oral bioavailability of corticosteroids. Furthermore, patients should be started on a PPI for GI prophylaxis. Although here has been no randomized trial utilizing PPIs in patients receiving corticosteroids, there have been multiple phase III studies demonstrating the protective effects of PPIs against peptic ulcers in patients receiving chronic nonsteroidal anti-inflammatory drugs (NSAIDs).[73] NSAIDs and corticosteroids both cause GI mucosal injury by decreasing mucosal-protective prostaglandin levels. Therefore, it is not an unreasonable extrapolation to assume that PPIs provide a similar mucosal protective effect with corticosteroids, especially considering that the morbidity of GI toxicity can be life-threatening. Chronic use of oral antacids should be avoided because the short half-life of these agents requires a large amount to be ingested per day. Increased popularity of over-the-counter antacids as a means of calcium supplementation has been recognized as an important cause of the recent increase in milk-alkali syndrome and resultant hypercalcemia.[74,75]

TABLE 93.8 KEY FINDINGS OF A PHASE III STUDY (77) OF PATIENTS WITH METASTATIC SPINAL CORD COMPRESSION

	Surgery + Radiation Median (n = 50)	*Radiation Alone Median (n = 51)*	*P*
Primary end point			
<Ability to walk			
Rate	84% (42/50)	57% (29/51)	.001
Time	122 days	13 days	.003
Secondary end points			
Maintenance of continence	156 days	17 days	.016
Maintenance of ASIA score[a]	566 days	72 days	.001
Maintenance of Frankel score[a]	566 days	72 days	.0006
Overall survival	126 days	100 days	.033
Other end points			
Mean daily morphine[b]	0.4 mg	4.8 mg	.002
Mean daily dexamethasone[b]	1.6 mg	4.2 mg	.0093
In patients ambulatory at study entry			
Ability to walk (maintaining)			
Rate	94% (32/34)	74% (26/34)	.024
Time	153 days	54 days	.024
In patients nonambulatory at study entry			
Ability to walk (regaining)			
Rate	62% (10/16)	19% (3/16)	.012
Time	59 days	0 days	.04

ASIA, American Spinal Injury Association.
[a]Measures of spinal function after injury.
[b]Converted into equivalent doses.

Surgery

Radiation for nonradiosensitive tumors typically takes several days to have an effect and does not stabilize the spine, while surgery allows for immediate cord decompression and provides an opportunity to stabilize the spine intraoperatively. At some institutions, surgery was used infrequently because several retrospective studies and one small randomized study showed no benefit to surgery plus radiation over radiation alone. Young et al.[76] randomized 29 patients with MSCC to decompressive laminectomy followed by radiation versus radiation alone. Although this trial showed no benefit to surgery in terms of pain relief, ambulation, or sphincter function, it is difficult to draw any conclusion because of the small sample size. All of these studies used posterior laminectomy in conjunction with radiotherapy; however, most of the lesions in MSCC involve the anterior portion of the vertebral body.[54] Therefore, a laminectomy does not effectively relieve the compression and may actually worsen the stability of the spine.

Recently, several authors have advocated the use of direct surgical decompression, tumor debulking, and spinal stabilization via instrumentation to improve on the results from radiation alone. Patchell et al.[77] reported the first phase III randomized trial testing the efficacy of direct decompressive surgery in patients with MSCC (Table 93.8). The study compared radiation alone (standard 30 Gy in 10 fractions) versus decompressive and stabilization surgery within 24 hours of diagnosis followed by the same radiotherapy (within 2 weeks of surgery). The trial was terminated early when early-stopping rules were met regarding the primary end point of ambulation after treatment. This trial definitively demonstrated an advantage to surgery for every end point at statistically significant levels. For nonambulatory patients, the combined treatment patients had a significantly higher chance of regaining the ability to walk after therapy. Maintenance of continence, maintenance of American Spinal Cord Injury (ASIA) and Frankel scores (measures of spinal function after injury), median overall survival, and median mean daily dexamethasone and morphine equivalent doses all favored the surgery arm.

If operable, patients should undergo surgical decompression and stabilization followed by radiotherapy. Even for radiosensitive tumors, surgery can often stabilize the spine. Therefore, all patients with MSCC should be evaluated by a surgeon. Effective multidisciplinary teamwork is critical to the rapid evaluation and management of patients with MSCC.

Radiotherapy

Palliative radiotherapy has been the standard of care in the treatment of patients with MSCC. Although a total of 30 Gy in 10 fractions is the most frequently employed fractionation schedule, multiple fractionation schemes have been reported, which undoubtedly reflects the heterogeneity in the patient population and tumor histology.[66] In one of the largest studies to date, Rades et al.[78] reported a retrospective series of 1,304 patients with MSCC. The patients were separated into five schedules: 8 Gy × 1 in 1 day (n = 261, group 1), 4 Gy × 5 in 1 week (n = 279, group 2), 3 Gy × 10 in 2 weeks (n = 274, group 3), 2.5 Gy × 15 in 3 weeks (n = 233, group 4), and 2 Gy × 20 in 4 weeks (n = 257, group 5). All of the groups had similar posttreatment ambulatory rates (63% to 74%) and motor function improvements (26% to 31%). However, in-field recurrence rates were much lower for the protracted schedules. The 2-year in-field recurrence rates for groups 1, 2, 3, 4, and 5 were 24%, 26%, 14%, 9%, and 7% ($P <.001$), respectively. They recommend that a single fraction of 8 Gy should be used in MSCC patients with limited survival expectations, and that 30 Gy in 10 fractions should be used for all other patients.

Maranzano et al.[56,79] have reported the only randomized trials on radiation schedule for patients with MSCC. In the first trial, they compared two hypofractionation schemes, a short course (8 Gy × 1 → 6-day break → 8 Gy × 1; 16 Gy total in 1 week) versus a split course (5 Gy × 3 → 4-day break → 3 Gy × 5; 30 Gy total in 2 weeks). The study concludes that the treatment with short versus split courses of RT resulted in similar back pain relief (56% vs. 59%), ambulatory maintenance (68% vs. 71%), and good bladder function (90% vs. 89%) rates. Therefore, they recommend that an 8 Gy × 2 regimen should be used for patients with MSCC. But physicians should be cautious before implementing this recommendation. When one limits the definition of response to regaining motor function and sphincter control, the rates of success decrease to 29% and

14%, respectively. Confounding variables included having patients with favorable histology, excellent performance status, and the use of nonstandard, large fraction sizes in both arms.[80] It is conceivable that the 5% who progressed to paraplegia without in-field recurrence may have suffered from late radiation-induced toxicity, even if it was not scored by the authors. Based on these results, the authors then performed another randomized trial in patients with an estimated life expectancy of ≤6 months, comparing 8 Gy × 1 versus 8 Gy × 1 → 6-day break → 8 Gy × 1; 16 Gy total in 1 week. These results showed equivalence in terms of median duration of response and overall survival. From this study the authors conclude that an 8 Gy × 1 regimen can be used to effectively palliate patients with MSCC with minimal toxicity and inconvenience.[79] The same cautions should be applied to this recommendation, especially in those who are treatment naive or patients with favorable features. Furthermore, neither study compared the short schedules with the standard 30 Gy in 10 fractions.

For patients receiving radiotherapy for MSCC from solid tumors, 30 Gy in 10 fractions is considered the standard of care. Shorter fractionation schedules, such as 8 Gy × 1 or 4 Gy × 5, should only be reserved for those with clear evidence of progressive disease, refractory to systemic therapy. Furthermore, these short schedules should be avoided in newly diagnosed, chemotherapy naive patients because the clinical course can be quite variable and unpredictable. Chemotherapy may be considered in select, newly diagnosed patients with excellent neurologic functional status and very chemosensitive tumors (e.g., lymphoma, multiple myeloma, germ cell tumors), but this is still considered outside the accepted standard. If the patient is found to have unresectable or inoperable tumor but otherwise has good performance status, oligometastatic disease, and controlled primary disease, then consideration should be made to escalate the total dose beyond 30 Gy because this will not be sufficient to achieve long-term gross tumor control. Special techniques such as intensity-modulated radiation therapy (IMRT) or fractionated stereotactic body radiation therapy (SBRT) should be considered to safely escalate the total dose (Fig. 93.2). However, the routine use of IMRT or SBRT cannot be recommended because the technology is expensive, and it has yet to show definite benefit over conventional delivery of radiation in a patient population who has a median survival of 6 months or less.

Caution Against Short, Hypofractionated Radiotherapy

A common mistake made by those who advocate a short hypofractionated regimen (e.g., 8 Gy × 2 or 4 Gy × 5) for MSCC is equat-

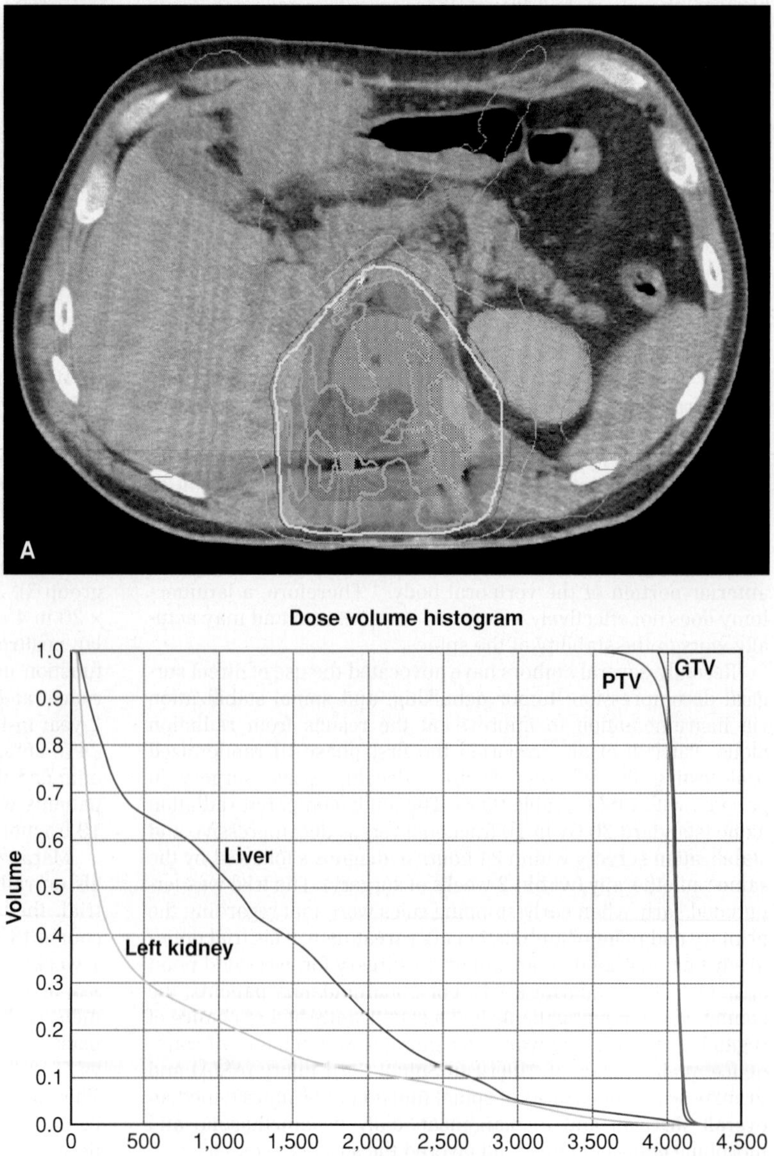

FIGURE 93.2. A: Five years after undergoing a right nephrectomy for a stage I renal call carcinoma (RCC), patient presented with progressively worsening midback pain. Magnetic resonance image of the spine revealed a T11–12 right-sided paraspinal mass invading the right lateral T12 vertebral body and neural foramina causing T12 spinal cord compression. Patient underwent a gross total resection and instrumentation to stabilize the spine. A full metastatic workup revealed the vertebral disease as the solitary site of recurrent RCC. Chemistries revealed a mild chronic renal insufficiency, with a creatinine level of 2.1 mg/dL. Intensity-modulated radiation therapy (IMRT) was used to minimize the dose to the left kidney. The figure shows an axial computed tomography image of the IMRT plan generated, with the *red* and *blue* color washes representing gross tumor volume (GTV) and planning target volume (PTV), respectively. **B:** The dose–volume histogram of the IMRT plan is shown. A total of 40 Gy in 20 fractions was delivered to the PTV (GTV + 1 cm). The PTV was modified so the margin was decreased to 8 mm along the left lateral edge of the vertebral body next to the left kidney.

ing the safety and equivalency of these abbreviated schedules in bone and lung metastases trials as a justification for the safety of such regimens in MSCC. The consequence of progression of a bone metastasis despite prior radiotherapy (i.e., 8 Gy × 1) is an increase in pain, which leads to an increased need for pain medications and usually reirradiation. By contrast, the consequences of MSCC progression despite prior radiotherapy are an increase in pain, paralysis, and incontinence, which usually contribute significantly to the direct demise of the patient. Because some studies, but not all, suggest that single fraction radiotherapy for bone metastasis is associated with a higher retreatment rate than fractionated therapy, a note of caution is appropriate for single fraction radiotherapy for MSCC.[81]

The predominant mechanism of cord injury by both MSCC and radiation-induced myelopathy (RIM) is vascular damage leading to ischemia.[82] There are many studies that have established the vascular effects of high fraction dose. Dose response to single dose of SRS for arteriovenous malformation obliteration starts at doses as low as 8 Gy and as soon as 6 months or earlier.[83] It is possible that a compressed cord has a lower threshold for RIM when a short, hypofractionated schedule of radiation therapy is used. Chow et al.[84] demonstrated that oncologists are not accurate in predicting survival times. As systemic therapy improves for patients with metastatic disease, the ability to predict survival will undoubtedly become less accurate. Therefore, these abbreviated schedules should be routinely avoided unless the patient is chemotherapy refractory and has convincing evidence of progressive systemic disease with limited expected survival.

Pediatric Spinal Cord Compression

MSCC in the pediatric population differs from adult MSCC. Histologic subtypes commonly encountered in children (e.g., neuroblastoma, Wilms' tumor, and Ewing sarcoma) rarely occur in adults. In adults, most cases of MSCC are caused by direct invasion into the epidural space by metastatic vertebral body tumors, although, in children, most are caused by direct neural foraminal invasion, causing the characteristic "dumbbell" tumor. Chemotherapy plays a central role in the treatment of pediatric MSCC.[85]

Neuroblastoma is the most common histology of pediatric MSCC.[86] Hayes et al.[87] (nine cases of neuroblastoma and five cases of Ewing sarcoma) and Sanderson et al.[88] (four cases of neuroblastoma) demonstrated that chemotherapy alone allowed complete recovery of spinal cord function in all cases. The French Society of Pediatric Oncology protocol NBL-90 included 42 nonmetastatic neuroblastoma patients with intraspinal extension and consequent MSCC.[89] All were treated with initial chemotherapy, and this resulted in intraspinal tumor shrinkage, avoidance of surgery, and neurologic deficit improvement in 58%, 60%, and 92% of the patients, respectively. Severe neurologic sequelae occurred in only six patients (15%).

Emergent surgery should be offered to any pediatric patient with rapid neurologic progression at initial presentation or while on chemotherapy. In most circumstances, this should be followed by definitive chemotherapy. In stable or mildly symptomatic patients, chemotherapy can obviate the need for surgery, which is often associated with long-term skeletal deformities. Radiation should be reserved only for those who require palliation for progressive disease after failure of multiple systemic regimens, those who progress neurologically despite the initial treatment with chemotherapy or surgery, and those who present with primary vertebral tumors (e.g., primary vertebral Ewing sarcoma) in which definitive surgery is rarely feasible.

Intramedullary Spinal Cord Metastasis

Intramedullary spinal cord metastasis (ISCM) is rare, representing only 1% of all intramedullary tumors. According to a review by Kalayci et al.,[90] ISCM is most commonly secondary to a lung primary (54%), followed by breast cancer (11%), in contrast to patients with MSCC. Although back pain is common in >90% of MSCC patients, back or neck pain was seen in only 38% with ISCM. However, high sensory deficits (79%), sphincter dysfunction (60%), and weakness (91%) are more common in ISCM. The most striking difference between ISCM and MSCC is the high incidence of synchronous brain metastasis (41%) in patients presenting with ISCM. This is not surprising when one considers the route of spread and the high incidence of lung primaries in patients with ISCM. An MRI of the brain should be obtained.

The treatment of ISCM should be approached very similarly to MSCC, save for the role of surgery. Most surgeons are reluctant to operate in ISCM because surgery carries a high morbidity rate. Only 32 cases of surgery in ISCM have ever been reported.[90] Corticosteroids as well as radiation therapy should be promptly initiated.

Leptomeningeal Carcinomatosis

Leptomeningeal carcinomatosis (LCM) is a rare complication of multiple cancers that portends a poor prognosis. The most frequent cancers associated with LCM are lung (22% to 36%) and breast (27% to 50%). In breast cancer it is often seen in patients who have *HER2-neu* overexpression. It occurs in approximately 1% to 6% of patients with lung cancer, and it is most commonly involved by adenocarcinoma (50% to 56%), followed by squamous cell carcinoma (26% to 36%) and small cell carcinoma (13% to 14%).[91–95]

The majority of patients present with signs and symptoms. According to the review by Gleissner and Chamberlain,[93] spinal symptoms (>60%) are the most common, followed by cerebral (50%) and cranial nerve symptoms (40%). Contrast-enhanced MRI is the radiographic modality of choice. The entire neuraxis must be imaged if LCM is clinically suspected in a patient with a known malignancy. In most patients, the MRI will reveal leptomeningeal enhancement that is frequently associated with cranial nerve enhancement and gross tumor deposits. Although Collie et al.[96] found that all 25 patients with solid tumors exhibited abnormal gadolinium-enhanced MRI, Straathof et al.[97] found MRI to have a diagnostic sensitivity and specificity of LCM of 76% and 77%, respectively.

If MRI is equivocal, then cerebrospinal fluid (CSF) should be obtained if safe. Multiple samples may need to be obtained because the initial yield of a lumbar tap may be only 50%.[93] Neurosurgery must be consulted to evaluate the need for (a) shunting if hydrocephalus is suspected, and (b) placement of Rickham or Ommaya reservoirs for possible intrathecal (IT) chemotherapy. Chamberlain[92] and Gleissner and Chamberlain[93] argue that CSF flow studies should be performed with indium-111 or technetium-99, because up to one-half of patients have abnormal CSF flow from gross tumor deposits that may disrupt adequate IT chemotherapy delivery. However, flow studies are not performed by many centers because gross tumor nodules, most likely to cause flow disruption and not effectively treated by IT chemotherapy, are treated with radiation anyway. Thus, CSF flow studies typically do not change the overall management of patients with LCM who require treatment decisions to be made in an expedient manner.

There is no consensus on the optimal management of patients with LCM. This is mainly because of the lack of large published experiences, limited number of randomized trials, nonuniform treatment regimens in single institution experiences, and inclusion of various primary tumor histologies in the clinical trials. However, most would agree that an aggressive treatment with radiation (either WBRT or focal spinal radiation to symptomatic sites) and IT chemotherapy are indicated in patients with good performance status.[98] The optimal dose and fractionation schedule of radiation therapy delivered in the setting of LCM remains unknown; however, similar to WBRT and MSCC, 30 Gy in 10 fractions is the most typical scheduled used. In patients with poor performance

TABLE 93.9 RANDOMIZED TRIALS OF SOLID TUMOR PATIENTS WITH LEPTOMENINGEAL CARCINOMATOSIS

Study (Ref.)	N	Histology	Arms[a]	RR[b] (%)	Median Survival	Survival P
Hitchins et al. (1987) (104)	44	Solid tumors	IT MTX 15 mg	61	12 wk	.08
			IT MTX + Ara-C 50 mg/m^2	45	7 wk	
			Concurrent RT (not randomized)	75		
			No concurrent RT	35		<.05
Grossman et al. (1993) (103)	52	Nonleukemic[c]	IT MTX 10 mg	0	16 wk	NS
			IT thiotepa 10 mg	0	14 wk	
Glantz et al. (1999) (102)	61	Solid tumors	IT MTX 10 mg	20	11 wk	.15
			IT DepoCyt 50 mg	26	15 wk	
Kim et al. (2003) (105)	55	Solid tumors	IT MTX 15 mg	14	10 wk	.03
			IT MTX + Ara-C 30 mg/m^2 + Hydrocortisone 15 mg/m^2	39	19 wk	
			Concurrent RT (not randomized)	82		
			No concurrent RT	50		.014
Boogerd et al. (2004) (101)	35	Breast	IT chemotherapy[d]	41	18 wk	.32
			Non-IT chemotherapy	39	30 wk	

IT, intrathecal; MTX, methotrexate; Ara-C, cytarabine; DepoCyt, sustained-release cytarabine; RR, response rate; NS, not significant.
[a]All studies allowed palliative radiation when necessary.
[b]RR determination by neurologic and CSF improvements as predefined by each study.
[c]Fourteen patients (19%) had lymphoma, the rest had solid tumors.
[d]All patients started with MTX and switched to Ara-C if no response.

status, larger fractions may be more advantageous because these patients will rarely live long enough to experience late radiation toxicity and larger fractions may result in a faster symptomatic response. In the largest published experience to date on LCM from small cell lung cancer (n = 36), the dismal median survival of 1.3 months is a direct result of only 14 patients being offered some kind of therapy (n = 9 for radiation, n = 5 for chemotherapy).[99] In contrast, Chamberlain and Kormanik,[100] in the largest series of patients with LCM from non–small cell lung cancer (n = 32), treated all patients prospectively with radiotherapy followed by IT chemotherapy. The median survival for the entire cohort was 5 months, while patients with normal CSF flow had a significantly longer median survival compared with patients with interrupted CSF flow (6 vs. 4 months; P <.05). This suggests that an aggressive multimodality approach can produce survival times that are comparable to patients with multiple brain parenchymal metastases.

All of the randomized clinical trials on patients with LCM from solid tumors have included IT methotrexate (MTX)-based regimens (Table 93.9).[101–105] The only trial that compared IT versus non-IT (i.e., systemic) chemotherapy was reported by Boogerd et al.[101] However, this negative trial only included patients with breast primaries. Glantz et al.[102] reported that IT DepoCyt (cytarabine liposome injection) led to a greater median time to neurologic progression (8 vs. 4 weeks; P = .007), although the overall survival was not statistically different. The only positive trial reported to date has been by Kim et al.[105] from Seoul National University. Patients randomized to IT MTX, Ara-C (arabinofuranosyl cytidine), and hydrocortisone had a significantly longer survival than those randomized to IT MTX alone (18.2 vs. 10.4 weeks; P = .029). Patients with adenocarcinoma of the lung in the multiagent arm had a significant, longer survival (23.9 vs. 10.4 weeks; P = .038). Multiple other agents have been studied, but none have demonstrated significant responses.

There is ample evidence that focal radiation, such as WBRT or spinal radiation, provides added benefit to IT chemotherapy. This is particularly true in patients with bulky meningeal disease because IT chemotherapy only penetrates 2 to 3 mm. In the randomized IT chemotherapy trial reported by Hitchins et al.,[104] patients who received concurrent CNS radiation had a higher response rate compared with those who did not (73% vs. 35% P <.05). Likewise, in the randomized trial reported by Kim et al.,[105] those who received concurrent CNS radiation had a significant higher neurologic response rate (81.5% vs. 50.0% P = .014).

There is a concern that concurrent radiation and IT chemotherapy could potentially increase toxicity. However, the vast majority of patients do not survive long enough to see the late neurologic toxicity manifest.

CONCLUSION

A significant percentage of cancer patients will require palliative radiation therapy at some point during their natural history. On the basis of randomized data, patients with a limited number of brain metastases should be treated with a combination of local therapy such as surgery or SRS and whole-brain irradiation while those with numerous brain metastases should be treated with whole-brain irradiation alone. In patients with spinal cord compression, surgical decompression should be strongly considered in patients with single-level disease and good performance status followed by radiation therapy. Radiation therapy alone can also be considered for all patients with spinal cord compression with the most common fractionation scheme being 30 Gy in 10 fractions. Leptomeningeal carcinomatosis continues to have an unfavorable prognosis and the use of radiation therapy should based on the palliation of individual signs and symptoms.

REFERENCES

1. Li KC, Poon PY. Sensitivity and specificity of MRI in detecting malignant spinal cord compression and in distinguishing malignant from benign compression fractures of vertebrae. *Magn Reson Imaging* 1988;6:547–556.
2. Wen PY, McLaren Black P, Loeffler JS. Treatment of metastatic cancer. In: DeVita VT, Hellman S, Rosenberg SA, eds. *Cancer: principles and practice of oncology.* Philadelphia, PA: Lippincott Williams & Wilkins, 2001:2655–2670.
3. Posner JB. Brain metastases: 1995. A brief review. *J Neurooncol* 1996;27:287–293.
4. Davis PC, Hudgins PA, Peterman SB, et al. Diagnosis of cerebral metastases: double-dose delayed CT vs contrast-enhanced MR imaging. *AJNR Am J Neuroradiol* 1991;12:293–300.
5. Gaspar L, Scott C, Rotman M, et al. Recursive partitioning analysis (RPA) of prognostic factors in three Radiation Therapy Oncology Group (RTOG) brain metastases trials. *Int J Radiat Oncol Biol Phys* 1997;37:745–751.
6. Ruderman NB, Hall TC. Use of glucocorticoids in the palliative treatment of metastatic brain tumors. *Cancer* 1965;18:298–306.
7. Vecht CJ, Hovestadt A, Verbiest HB, et al. Dose-effect relationship of dexamethasone on Karnofsky performance in metastatic brain tumors: a randomized study of doses of 4, 8, and 16 mg per day. *Neurology* 1994;44:675–680.
8. Borgelt B, Gelber R, Kramer S, et al. The palliation of brain metastases: final results of the first two studies by the Radiation Therapy Oncology Group. *Int J Radiat Oncol Biol Phys* 1980;6(1):1–9.
9. Graham PH, Bucci J, Browne L. Randomized comparison of whole brain radiotherapy, 20 Gy in four daily fractions versus 40 Gy in 20 twice-daily fractions, for brain metastases. *Int J Radiat Oncol Biol Phys* 2010:77(3):648–654.
10. Haie-Meder C, Pellae-Cosset B, Laplanche A, et al. Results of a randomized clinical trial comparing two radiation schedules in the palliative treatment of brain metastases. *Radiother Oncol* 1993;26:111–116.
11. Murray KJ, Scott C, Greenberg HM, et al. A randomized phase III study of accelerated hyperfractionation versus standard in patients with unresected brain metastases: a report of the Radiation Therapy Oncology Group (RTOG) 9104. *Int J Radiat Oncol Biol Phys* 1997;39:571–574.
12. Priestman TJ, Dunn J, Brada M, et al. Final results of the Royal College of Radiologists' trial comparing two different radiotherapy schedules in the treatment of cerebral metastases. *Clin Oncol (R Coll Radiol)* 1996;8:308–315.
13. DeAngelis LM, Delattre JV, Posner JB. Radiation induced dementia in patients cured of brain metastases. *Neurology* 1989;39:789–796.
14. Mintz AH, Kestle J, Rathbone MP, et al. A randomized trial to assess the efficacy of surgery in addition to radiotherapy in patients with a single cerebral metastasis. *Cancer* 1996;78:1470–1476.
15. Noordijk EM, Vecht CJ, Haaxma-Reiche H, et al. The choice of treatment of single brain metastasis should be based on extracranial tumor activity and age. *Int J Radiat Oncol Biol Phys* 1994;29:711–717.
16. Patchell RA, Tibbs PA, Walsh JW, et al. A randomized trial of surgery in the treatment of single metastases to the brain. *N Engl J Med* 1990;322:494–500.

17. Kondziolka D, Patel A, Lunsford LD, et al. Stereotactic radiosurgery plus whole brain radiotherapy versus radiotherapy alone for patients with multiple brain metastases. *Int J Radiat Oncol Biol Phys* 1999;45:427–434.
18. Chougule PB, Burton-Williams M, Saris S, et al. Randomized treatment of brain metastases with gamma knife radiosurgery, whole brain radiotherapy or both. *Int J Radiat Oncol Biol Phys* 2000;48:114.
19. Andrews DW, Scott CB, Sperduto PW, et al. Whole brain radiation therapy with and without stereotactic radiosurgery boost for patients with one to three brain metastases: phase III results of the RTOG 9508 randomized trial. *Lancet* 2004;363:1665–1672.
20. Elveen T, Andrews DW. Summary of RTOG 95–01 phase III randomized trial of whole brain radiation with and without stereotactic radiosurgery boost, including presentation of a clinical case study. *Am J Oncol Rev* 2004;3:592–600.
21. Sneed PK, Suh JH, Goetsch SJ, et al. A multi-institutional review of radiosurgery alone vs. radiosurgery with whole brain radiotherapy as the initial management of brain metastases. *Int J Radiat Oncol Biol Phys* 2002;53:519–526.
22. Sneed PK, Lamborn KR, Forstner JM, et al. Radiosurgery for brain metastases: is whole brain radiotherapy necessary? *Int J Radiat Oncol Biol Phys* 1999;43: 549–558.
23. Regine WF, Huhn JL, Patchell RA, et al. Risk of symptomatic brain tumor recurrence and neurologic deficit after radiosurgery alone in patients with newly diagnosed brain metastases: results and implications [Erratum in: *Int J Radiat Oncol Biol Phys* 2002;53:259.] *Int J Radiat Oncol Biol Phys* 2002;52:333–338.
24. Manon R, O'Neill A, Knisely J, et al. Phase II trial of radiosurgery for one to three newly diagnosed brain metastases from renal cell carcinoma, melanoma, and sarcoma: an Eastern Cooperative Oncology Group study (E 6397). *J Clin Oncol* 2005;23:8870–8876.
25. Patchell RA, Tibbs PA, Regine WF, et al. Postoperative radiotherapy in the treatment of single metastases to the brain: a randomized trial. *JAMA* 1998;280: 1485–1489.
26. Aoyama H, Shirato H, Tago MK, et al. Stereotactic radiosurgery plus whole-brain radiation therapy vs stereotactic radiosurgery alone for treatment of brain metastases. *JAMA* 2006:295:2483–2491.
27. Aoyama H, Tago M, Kato N, et al. Neurocognitive function in patients with brain metastasis who received either who whole brain radiotherapy plus stereotactic radiosurgery or radiosurgery alone. *Int J Radiat Oncol Biol Phys* 2007;68: 1388–1395.
28. Muacevic A, Wowra B, Siefert A, et al. Microsurgery plus whole brain irradiation versus Gamma Knife surgery alone for treatment of single metastases to the brain: a randomized controlled multicentre phase III trial. *J Neurooncol* 2008;87:299–307.
29. Kocher M, Soffietti R, Abacioglu U, et al. Adjuvant whole-brain radiotherapy versus observation after radiosurgery or surgical resection of one to three cerebral metastases: results of the EORTC 22952–26001 study. *J Clin Oncol* 2011:29(2):134–141.
30. Chang EL, Wefel JS, Hess KR, et al. Neurocognition in patients with brain metastases treated with radiosurgery or radiosurgery plus whole-brain irradiation: a randomized controlled trial. *Lancet Oncol* 2009:10(11):1037–1044.
31. Mahmood U, Kwok Y, Regine WF, et al. Whole-brain irradiation for patients with brain metastases: still the standard of care. *Lancet Oncol* 2010;11:221–222.
32. Lawlor PG, Gagnon B, Mancini IL, et al. Occurrence, causes, and outcome of delirium in patients with advanced cancer. *Arch Intern Med* 2000;160:786–794.
33. Pereira J, Hanson J, Bruera E. The frequency and clinical course of cognitive impairment in patients with terminal cancer. *Cancer* 1997;79(4):835–842.
34. Wong WW, Schild SE, Sawyer TE, et al. Analysis of outcome in patients reirradiated for brain metastases. *Int J Radiat Oncol Biol Phys* 1996;34:585–590.
35. Son CH, Jimenez R, Niemierko A, et al. Outcomes after whole brain re-irradiation in patients with brain metastases. *Int J Radiat Oncol Biol Phys* 2012;82(2): e167–e172.
36. Antonadou D, Paraskevaidis M, Sarris G, et al. Phase II randomized trial of temozolomide and concurrent radiotherapy in patients with brain metastases. *J Clin Oncol* 2002;20:3644–3650.
37. Guerrieri M, Wong K, Ryan G, et al. A randomised phase III study of palliative radiation with concomitant carboplatin for brain metastases from non-small cell carcinoma of the lung. *Cancer* 2004;46:107–111.
38. Knisely JPS, Berkey B, Chakravarti A, et al. A phase III study of conventional radiation therapy plus thalidomide versus conventional radiation therapy for multiple brain metastases (RTOG 0118). *Int J Radiation Oncology Biol Phys* 2008: 71(1):79–86.
39. Komarnicky LT, Phillips TL, Martz K, et al. A randomized phase III protocol for the evaluation of misonidazole combined with radiation in the treatment of patients with brain metastases (RTOG-7916). *Int J Radiat Oncol Biol Phys* 1991;20:53–58.
40. Mehta MP, Rodrigus P, Terhaard CH, et al. Survival and neurologic outcomes in a randomized trial of motexafin gadolinium and whole-brain radiation therapy in brain metastases. *J Clin Oncol* 2003;21:2529–2536.
41. Suh JH, Stea B, Nabid A, et al. Phase III study of efaproxiral as an adjunct to whole-brain radiation therapy for brain metastases. *J Clin Oncol* 2006;24:106–114.
42. Ushio Y, Arita N, Hayakawa T, et al. Chemotherapy of brain metastases from lung carcinoma: a controlled randomized study. *Neurosurgery* 1991;28:201–205.
43. Verger E, Gil M, Yaya R, et al. Temozolomide and concomitant whole brain radiotherapy in patients with brain metastases: a phase II randomized trial. *Int J Radiat Oncol Biol Phys* 2005;61:185–191.
44. DeAngelis LM, Mandell LR, Thaler T, et al. The role of postoperative radiotherapy after resection of single brain metastases. *Neurosurgery* 1989;24:798–805.
45. Taylor BV, Buckner JC, Cascino TL, et al. Effects of radiation and chemotherapy on cognitive function in patients with high-grade glioma. *J Clin Oncol* 1998;16: 2195–2201.
46. Regine WF, Scott C, Murray K, et al. Neurocognitive outcome in brain metastases patients treated with accelerated-fractionation vs. accelerated-hyperfractionated radiotherapy: an analysis from Radiation Therapy Oncology Group Study 91–04. *Int J Radiat Oncol Biol Phys* 2001;51:711–717.
47. Meyers CA, Smith JA, Bezjak A, et al. Neurocognitive function and progression in patients with brain metastases treated with whole-brain radiation and motexafin gadolinium: results of a randomized phase III trial. *J Clin Oncol* 2004;22:157–165.
48. Brezden CB, Phillips KA, Abdolell M, et al. Cognitive function in breast cancer patients receiving adjuvant chemotherapy. *J Clin Oncol* 2000;18:2695–2701.
49. Klein M, Engelberts NH, van der Ploeg HM, et al. Epilepsy in low-grade gliomas: the impact on cognitive function and quality of life. *Ann Neurol* 2003;54:514–520.
50. Klein M, Heimans JJ, Aaronson NK, et al. Effect of radiotherapy and other treatment-related factors on mid-term to long-term cognitive sequelae in low-grade gliomas: a comparative study. *Lancet* 2002;360(9343):1361–1368.
51. Sonderkaer S, Schmiegelow M, Carstensen H, et al. Long-term neurological outcome of childhood brain tumors treated by surgery only. *J Clin Oncol* 2003;21: 1347–1351.
52. Zacny JP, Gutierrez S. Characterizing the subjective, psychomotor, and physiological effects of oral oxycodone in non-drug-abusing volunteers. *Psychopharmacology (Berl)* 2003;170:242–254.
53. Glantz MJ, Cole BF, Forsyth PA, et al. Practice parameter: anticonvulsant prophylaxis in patients with newly diagnosed brain tumors: report of the Quality Standards Subcommittee of the American Academy of Neurology. *Neurology* 2000; 54:1886–1893.
54. Byrne TN. Spinal cord compression from epidural metastases. *N Engl J Med* 1992;327:614–619.
55. Quinn JA, DeAngelis LM. Neurologic emergencies in the cancer patient. *Semin Oncol* 2000;27:311–321.
56. Maranzano E, Bellavita R, Rossi R, et al. Short-course versus split-course radiotherapy in metastatic spinal cord compression: results of a phase III, randomized, multicenter trial. *J Clin Oncol* 2005;23:3358–3365.
57. Kato A, Ushio Y, Hayakawa T, et al. Circulatory disturbance of the spinal cord with epidural neoplasm in rats. *J Neurosurg* 1985;63:260–265.
58. Fuller BG, Heiss JD, Oldfield EH. Spinal cord compression. In: DeVita VT, Hellman S, Rosenberg SA, eds. *Cancer: principles and practice of oncology.* Philadelphia, PA: Lippincott Williams & Wilkins, 2001:2617–2633.
59. Heldmann U, Myschetzky PS, Thomsen HS. Frequency of unexpected multifocal metastasis in patients with acute spinal cord compression. Evaluation by low-field MR imaging in cancer patients. *Acta Radiol* 1997;38:372–375.
60. Schiff D, O'Neill BP, Wang CH, et al. Neuroimaging and treatment implications of patients with multiple epidural spinal metastases. *Cancer* 1998;83:1593–1601.
61. Gilbert RW, Kim JH, Posner JB. Epidural spinal cord compression from metastatic tumor: diagnosis and treatment. *Ann Neurol* 1978;3:40–51.
62. Maranzano E, Latini P, Checcaglini F, et al. Radiation therapy in metastatic spinal cord compression: a prospective analysis of 105 consecutive patients. *Cancer* 1991;67:1311–1317.
63. Martenson JA, Evans RG, Lie MR, et al. Treatment outcome and complications in patients treated for malignant epidural spinal cord compression (SCC). *J Neurooncol* 1985;3:77–84.
64. Torma T. Malignant tumors of the spine and spinal epidural space: a study based on 250 histologically verified cases. *Acta Chir Scand* 1957;225:1–176.
65. Helweg-Larsen S, Sorensen PS. Symptoms and sings in metastatic spinal cord compression: a study of progression from first symptom until diagnosis in 153 patients. *Eur J Cancer* 1994;30A:396.
66. Larson DA, Rubenstein JL, McDermott MW. Treatment of metastatic cancer. In: DeVita VT, Hellman S, Rosenberg SA, eds. *Cancer: principles and practice of oncology.* Philadelphia, PA: Lippincott Williams & Wilkins, 2005:2323–2336.
67. Loughrey GJ, Collins CD, Todd SM, et al. Magnetic resonance imaging in the management of suspected spinal canal disease in patients with known malignancy. *Clin Radiol* 2000;55:849–855.
68. Loblaw DA, Laperriere NJ. Emergency treatment of malignant extradural spinal cord compression: an evidence-based guideline. *J Clin Oncol* 1998;16:1613–1624.
69. Rades D, Heidenreich F, Karstens JH. Final results of a prospective study of the prognostic value of the time to develop motor deficits before irradiation in metastatic spinal cord compression. *Int J Radiat Oncol Biol Phys* 2002;53:975–979.
70. Sorensen S, Helweg-Larsen S, Mouridsen H, et al. Effect of high-dose dexamethasone in carcinomatous metastatic spinal cord compression treated with radiotherapy: a randomised trial. *Eur J Cancer* 1994;30A:22–27.
71. Vecht CJ, Haaxma-Reiche H, van Putten WL, et al. Initial bolus of conventional versus high-dose dexamethasone in metastatic spinal cord compression. *Neurology* 1989;39:1255–1257.
72. Heimdal K, Hirschberg H, Slettebo H, et al. High incidence of serious side effects of high-dose dexamethasone treatment in patients with epidural spinal cord compression. *J Neurooncol* 1992;12:141–144.
73. Lai KC, Lam SK, Chu KM, et al. Lansoprazole for the prevention of recurrences of ulcer complications from long-term low-dose aspirin use. *N Engl J Med* 2002; 346:2033–2038.
74. Scofield RH. Milk-alkali syndrome. Available at: http://www.emedicine.com/med/topic1477.htm.
75. Ziegler R. Hypercalcemic crisis. *J Am Soc Nephrol* 2001;12:S3–S9.
76. Young RF, Post EM, King GA. Treatment of spinal epidural metastases: randomized prospective comparison of laminectomy and radiotherapy. *J Neurosurg* 1980; 53:741–748.
77. Patchell RA, Tibbs PA, Regine WF, et al. Direct decompressive surgical resection in the treatment of spinal cord compression caused by metastatic cancer: a randomised trial. *Lancet* 2005;366:643–648.
78. Rades D, Stalpers LJ, Veninga T, et al. Evaluation of five radiation schedules and prognostic factors for metastatic spinal cord compression. *J Clin Oncol* 2005;23: 3366–3375.
79. Maranzano E, Trippa F, Casale M, et al. 8 Gy single-dose radiotherapy is effective in metastatic spinal cord compression: results of a phase III randomized multicentre Italian trial. *Radiother Oncol* 2009:93:174–179.
80. Kwok Y, Regine WF, Patchell RA. Radiation therapy alone for spinal cord compression: time to improve upon a relatively ineffective status quo. *J Clin Oncol* 2005;23:3308–3310.
81. Wu JS, Wong R, Johnston M, et al. Meta-analysis of dose-fractionation radiotherapy trials for the palliation of painful bone metastases. *Int J Radiat Oncol Biol Phys* 2003;55:594–605.
82. St Clair WH, Arnold SM, Sloan AE, et al. Spinal cord and peripheral nerve injury: current management and investigations. *Semin Radiat Oncol* 2003;13:322–332.
83. Flickinger JC, Pollock BE, Kondziolka D, et al. A dose-response analysis of arteriovenous malformation obliteration after radiosurgery. *Int J Radiat Oncol Biol Phys* 1996;36:873–879.
84. Chow E, Davis L, Panzarella T, et al. Accuracy of survival prediction by palliative radiation oncologists. *Int J Radiat Oncol Biol Phys* 2005;61:870–873.
85. Klein SL, Sanford SA, Muhlbauer MS. Pediatric spinal epidural metastases. *J Neurosurg* 1991;74:70–75.
86. Phillips TL, Scott CB, Leibel SA, et al. Results of a randomized comparison of radiotherapy and bromodeoxyuridine with radiotherapy alone for brain metastases: report of RTOG trial 89–05. *Int J Radiat Oncol Biol Phys* 1995;33:339–348.
87. Hayes FA, Thompson EI, Hvizdala E. Chemotherapy as an alternative to laminectomy and radiation in the management of epidural tumor. *J Pediatr* 1984;104: 221–224

88. Sanderson IR, Pritchard J, Marsh HT. Chemotherapy as the initial treatment of spinal cord compression due to disseminated neuroblastoma. *J Neurosurg* 1989; 70:688–690.
89. Plantaz D, Rubie H, Michon J, et al. The treatment of neuroblastoma with intraspinal extension with chemotherapy followed by surgical removal of residual disease. A prospective study of 42 patients—results of the NBL 90 Study of the French Society of Pediatric Oncology. *Cancer* 1996;78:311–319.
90. Kalayci M, Cagavi F, Gul S, et al. Intramedullary spinal cord metastases: diagnosis and treatment—an illustrated review. *Acta Neurochir (Wien)* 2004;146:1347–1354.
91. Boogerd W, Hart AAM, van der Sande JJ, et al. Meningeal carcinomatosis in breast cancer. *Cancer* 1991;67:1685–1695.
92. Chamberlain MC. Neoplastic meningitis. *J Clin Oncol* 2005;23(15):3605–3613.
93. Gleissner B, Chamberlain MC. Neoplastic meningitis. *Lancet Neurol* 2006;5:443–452.
94. Kaplan JG, DeSouza TG, Farkash A, et al. Leptomeningeal metastases: Comparison of clinical features and laboratory data of solid tumors, lymphomas and leukemias. *J Neurooncol* 1990;9:225–229.
95. Wasserstrom WR, Glass JP, Posner JB. Diagnosis and treatment of leptomeningeal metastases from solid tumors: experience with 90 patients. *Cancer* 1982; 49:759–772.
96. Collie DA, Brush JP, Lammie GA, et al. Imaging features of leptomeningeal metastases. *Clin Radiol* 1999;54(11):765–771.
97. Straathof CA, de Bruin HG, Dippel DW, et al. The diagnostic accuracy of magnetic resonance imaging and cerebrospinal fluid cytology in leptomeningeal metastasis. *J Neurol* 1999;246(9):810–814.
98. Central nervous system cancers. NCCN Clinical Practice Guidelines in Oncology. V.2. 2011. Available at: www.nccn.org/professionals/physician_gls/PDF/cns.pdf.
99. Seute T, Leffers P, ten Velde GPM, et al. Leptomeningeal metastases from small cell lung carcinoma. *Cancer* 2005;104:1700–1705.
100. Chamberlain MC, Kormanik P. Carcinoma meningitis secondary to non-small cell lung cancer. *Arch Neurol* 1998;55:506–512.
101. Boogerd W, van den Bent MJ, Koehler PJ, et al. The relevance of intraventricular chemotherapy for leptomeningeal metastasis in breast cancer: a randomised study. *Eur J Cancer* 2004;40:2726–2733.
102. Glantz MJ, Jaeckle KA, Chamberlain MC, et al. A randomized controlled trial comparing intrathecal sustained-release cytarabine (DepoCyt) to intrathecal methotrexate in patients with neoplastic meningitis from solid tumors. *Clin Cancer Res* 1999;5:3394–3402.
103. Grossman SA, Finkelstein DM, Ruckdeschel JC, et al. Randomized prospective comparison of intraventricular methotrexate and thiotepa in patients with previously untreated neoplastic meningitis. *J Clin Oncol* 1993;11:561–569.
104. Hitchins RN, Bell DR, Woods RL, et al. A prospective randomized trial of single-agent versus combination chemotherapy in meningeal carcinomatosis. *J Clin Oncol* 1987;5(10):1655–1662.
105. Kim DY, Lee KW, Yun T, et al. Comparison of intrathecal chemotherapy for leptomeningeal carcinomatosis of a solid tumor: methotrexate alone versus methotrexate in combination with cytosine arabinoside and hydrocortisone. *Jpn J Clin Oncol* 2003;33:608–612.

Chapter 94
Palliation of Bone Metastases

William F. Hartsell and Santosh Yajnik

BACKGROUND AND INCIDENCE

Metastatic disease to the bone is a common cause of pain and other significant symptoms that are detrimental to quality of life. The exact incidence of bone metastases is difficult to determine, but estimates are that >100,000 people in the United States will develop osseous metastatic disease annually.[1,2] The incidence of bone metastases varies significantly, depending on the primary site, with breast and prostate cancer accounting for up to 70% of patients with metastatic disease.[3] Bone metastases may be found in up to 85% of patients dying from breast, prostate, or lung cancer. Other primary sites with a propensity for bone metastases include thyroid, melanoma, and kidney. On the other hand, gastrointestinal sites of primary malignancy give rise to bone metastasis in only 3% to 15% of patients with metastatic disease.[4] Some hematologic malignancies, including myeloma and lymphoma, can also cause significant pain and bone destruction.

The ultimate prognosis for patients with bone metastases is poor, with median survival typically measured in months rather than years. Overall survival depends on the primary site and the presence or absence of visceral metastases. Patients with bone metastases from lung cancer have short median survival durations of 6 months. However, patients with bone metastases from breast or prostate primary sites may have significantly longer survival times. In patients with bone-only metastatic prostate or breast cancer, median survivals of 2 to 4 years have been reported.[3,5,6] Whether the survival time is only a few months or extends to multiple years, these patients will often require active treatment because of pain, difficulty with ambulation and immobility, hypercalcemia, pathologic fractures, neurologic deficits, anxiety, depression, spinal cord or nerve root compression, fatigue, insomnia or sleep disturbances, and general deterioration of quality of life.[4,7,8]

The axial skeleton is the most common site of bone metastasis, with metastasis most frequently occurring in the spine, pelvis, and ribs. The lumbar spine is the most frequent site of bone metastasis.[9–12] In the appendicular skeleton, the proximal femurs are the most common site of metastatic disease, and humeral lesions also occur frequently. The acral sites (feet and hands) are rarely involved. Certain skeletal sites are associated with specific areas of bone metastases. For example, scapular metastases are seen more frequently from renal primaries.[13] Involvement of the skull is more common with breast primaries. The distal appendicular skeleton (tibia, fibula) and acral sites (especially the hands) are more common with lung primaries, and involvement of the toes is seen more commonly with genitourinary primaries (Fig. 94.1).

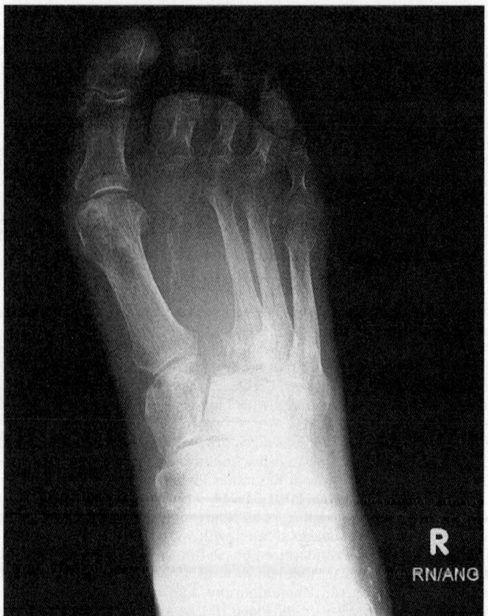

FIGURE 94.1. Radiograph of right foot of a patient with metastatic transitional cell carcinoma of the bladder. Note the destruction of the second metatarsal.

The most common symptom of bone metastases is slowly progressive, insidious pain that is fairly well localized. The pain may be worse at night. Pain from the femur or acetabulum may worsen with weight bearing or ambulation. In contrast, pain from the inferior ischium or sacrum may be worse with sitting but less bothersome with ambulation. Although the pain is frequently localized, pain may radiate to other areas. This is most frequently seen with pain in the lower back, pelvis, or hips that may radiate down the legs. Pain that radiates does not necessarily indicate nerve impingement because radicular pain can also be caused by spasm of muscles that originate or insert near the area of disease (e.g., pain in the hip radiating to the knee).

PATHOPHYSIOLOGY

There are primarily three types of cells within mature bone: osteocytes, osteoblasts, and osteoclasts. Osteoblasts originate from osteogenic cells, found in the periosteum or endosteum. The osteogenic cells differentiate into osteoblasts when there is a mechanical or chemical stimulus for remodeling or repair. The osteoblasts build bone by depositing collagen type I into the extracellular space. An inorganic complex of calcium and phosphate (hydroxyapatite) is laid down within this organic matrix to provide the strength and density of the bone. The osteoblasts then mature into osteocytes, which maintain the bone structure. Osteoclasts are multinucleated giant cells that originate from pluripotent hematopoietic bone marrow cells and are adherent to the bone surface.[14] These cells create an acidophilic environment that causes dissolution of the hydroxyapatite crystals and proteolysis of the bone matrix.

The differentiation and activation of osteoclasts occurs because of the effects of a group of proteins that are related to tumor necrosis factor, including osteoprotegerin, receptor activator of nuclear factor-κB (RANK), and the RANK ligand (RANKL). Osteoblasts and stromal cells express RANKL, and activated T cells may also release RANKL. The RANKL binds to the RANK receptor on osteoclast precursors, which then induces the formation of mature osteoclasts. Osteoprotegerin is a decoy receptor for RANKL and inhibits the differentiation and activation of osteoclasts.[14] The destruction of bone by osteolytic metastases is mediated by the osteoclasts, not by the tumor cells. However, the factors that activate the osteoclasts are likely produced by the tumor cells, including RANKL, interleukin-1, interleukin-6, and macrophage inflammatory protein 1α. The mechanisms for osteoblastic activation are not clearly delineated, but it appears that bone resorption occurs first even in osteoblastic metastases from prostate cancer.[15]

Normal bone is constantly being remodeled in a cycle lasting about 120 to 200 days (3 to 6 months). For the first 20 to 40 days of the cycle, the bone is resorbed by osteoclasts. The bone is then rebuilt by osteoblasts during the next 100 to 150 days.[16]

The structure of the bone changes during growth and development. All bones are immature, woven bone at the time of birth. Woven bone is more cellular, with no organized orientation to the collagen fibers of the bone. As the woven bone is absorbed, it is replaced by lamellar bone. The lamellar bone is organized circumferentially around neurovascular canals. This cylindrical structure provides much more strength than the haphazard orientation of woven bone. Most adult bone is lamellar.

The strength of bone is provided primarily by cortical bone, which is the dense, compact bone found in the diaphysis of long bones and along the exterior surfaces of cuboidal bones. Cortical bone comprises most of the mass of the skeletal system and provides most of the strength of the skeleton. Trabecular bone is the spongy, cancellous bone found in the center of cuboidal bones and in the center of the metaphysis and diaphysis of long bones. There is much more rapid remodeling of trabecular bone, with replacement of 25% of trabecular bone per year, compared with 3% of cortical bone.[17]

Long bones consist of the epiphysis, metaphysis, and diaphysis. The diaphysis is the long shaft of the bone. The epiphyses are at the ends of the bone. These are composed of hyaline cartilage initially, which becomes ossified during puberty. The metaphysis is the area between the epiphysis and diaphysis. The metaphysis is an area of rapidly growing trabecular bone.

Metastases to the bone most often occur in the red marrow, which is found in highest concentration in the axial skeleton. This most often occurs by hematogenous spread but may occur by direct extension as well. Involvement of adjacent bone by direct extension (e.g., mandibular involvement from an oral cavity cancer) does not necessarily imply that there is a higher likelihood of distant bone metastases, and its management is very different from that of bone metastases from hematogenous spread. The predilection of certain tumor sites to metastasize to bone may be related to local growth factors in the bone such as transforming growth factor-β, insulin-like growth factors I and II, fibroblastic growth factors, or platelet-derived growth factors, preferential adherence to endothelial surfaces in certain bones by cell adhesion molecules, or chemotactic attraction from bone cells by osteocalcin or type I collagen.[4,14,18] The relatively high proportion of hematogenous metastasis to bone compared with other sites in the body cannot simply be explained by blood flow, which is >30 times greater in lung than in red bone marrow.[19]

Bone metastases are often described as either osteolytic or osteoblastic, but these are different representations of abnormalities in the normal bone-remodeling process. Breast and lung cancers more commonly cause osteolytic-appearing lesions, and lesions caused by prostate and thyroid cancers more often have an osteoblastic appearance. However, only myeloma is associated with purely osteolytic lesions.[14] Most other tumors have a combination of osteolytic and osteoblastic components. Even in osteoblastic-appearing prostate cancer metastases, increased bone resorption does occur.

The mechanism of pain from bone metastases is not clearly understood. Possible mechanisms include mechanical instability, irritation of periosteal stretch receptors, tumor-directed osteoclast-mediated osteolysis, tumor cells themselves, or tumor-induced nerve injury, production of nerve growth factor, or stimulation of other cytokine receptors.[2,3,20,21] Because the mechanisms of pain may be multifactorial, a combination of therapies may be superior to any one therapy alone.[20]

EVALUATION

The physical examination is an important step in evaluating a patient with bone metastases. The physical examination may help make decisions regarding appropriate subsequent imaging studies. Firm palpation will often elicit the specific area of pain, with "point tenderness" often pointing directly to the affected area in the bone. It is important to carefully evaluate the entire skeletal system with examination because intense pain at one site often masks subjective reports of pain at other sites. A careful physical examination may reveal hidden pain in other locations. A thorough neurologic examination is also important, especially in patients with spinal metastases, to carefully evaluate for the possibility of spinal cord, cauda equina, or nerve root compression.

For symptomatic patients with point tenderness, plain radiographs are typically the most appropriate first imaging study. Such radiographs are easy to obtain and inexpensive. The appearance of bone metastases on x-rays varies depending on the primary site and histology. Most bone metastases from lung cancer and breast cancer appear osteolytic, whereas most from prostate cancer appear osteoblastic (Fig. 94.2). However, nearly all bone metastases have components of both osteolytic and osteoblastic processes. The primary disadvantage of plain radiographs is that small lesions are rarely seen. Approximately 30% to 50% of the bone mineral content must be lost before the lesion will be apparent on x-rays.

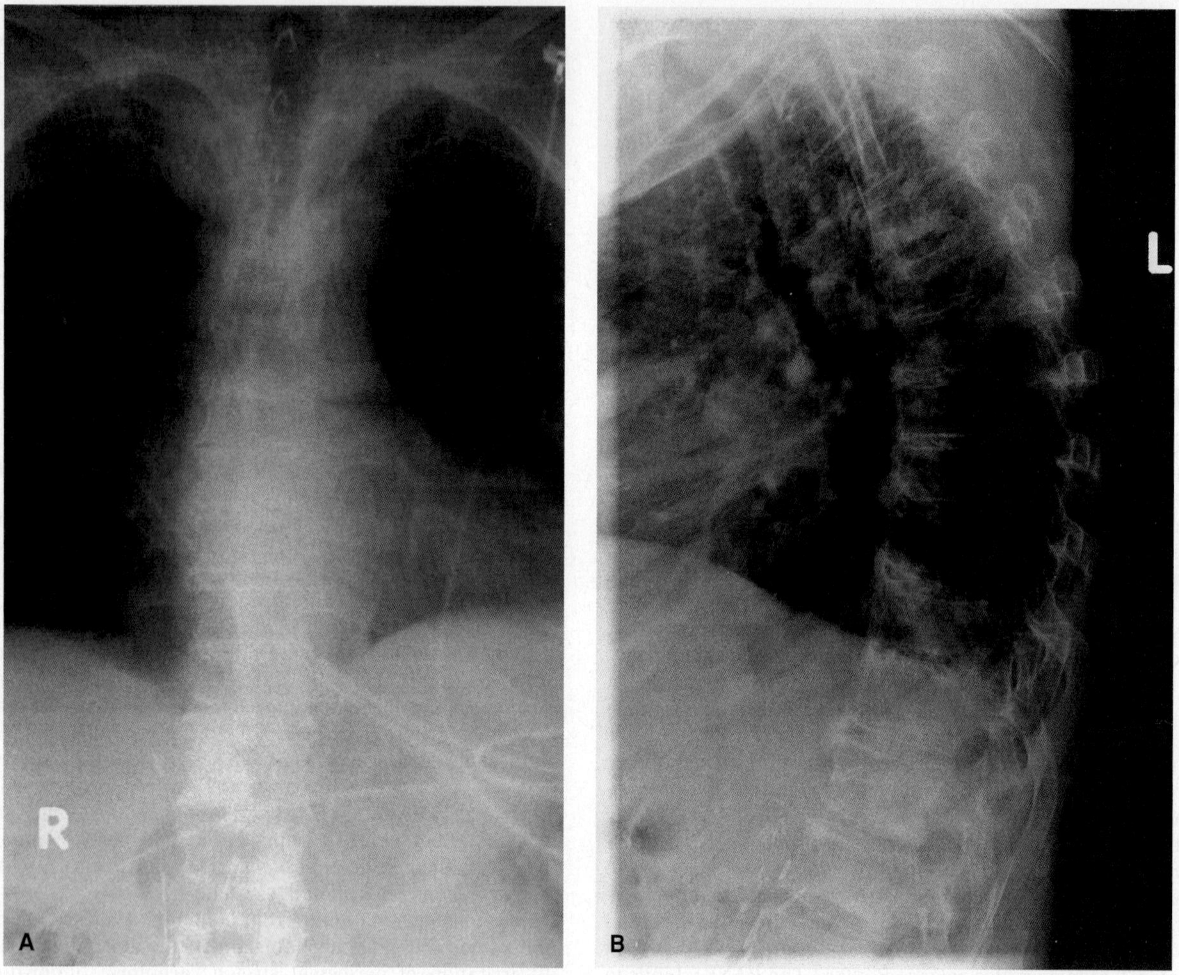

FIGURE 94.2. Anteroposterior **(A)** and lateral **(B)** spine radiographs from a patient with metastatic prostate cancer. There are osteoblastic lesions seen in T12 and L1.

Technetium-99m bone scintigraphy (nuclear medicine bone scan) is the best method for screening patients at risk for bone metastasis and is useful to evaluate the extent of metastatic disease in the bone. Bone scintigraphy is an indicator of osteoblastic activity. Because multiple myeloma is frequently purely osteolytic, bone scans are less useful for evaluating extent of disease in myeloma. Bone scintigraphy is not specific for metastatic disease, and positive findings must often be confirmed using other imaging studies. A confirmatory study is especially important in a weight-bearing bone such as the proximal femur. False-positive readings may be seen in areas of arthritis, trauma, or Paget's disease. In addition, the osteoblastic activity in healing bone after treatment may give the appearance of progressive disease. False-negative readings may occur in fast-growing, highly aggressive tumors, especially if these are mainly osteolytic.

Computed tomography (CT) scans are more sensitive than plain radiographs and may be better able to localize the lesion within the bone. However, CT scans are more expensive, more time-consuming, and may not be useful as a screening tool for skeletal metastasis. The CT may be useful in defining the extent of cortical destruction and helping to assess the risk of a pathologic fracture.[22] In addition, the CT scan may be used to guide needle biopsies to obtain a tissue diagnosis. CT scans have limited usefulness in detecting marrow involvement but are much better than plain radiographs at evaluating soft tissue extension of disease.

Magnetic resonance imaging (MRI) is better than plain radiography or nuclear medicine bone scintigraphy at assessing the involvement of trabecular bone (red marrow), especially in the vertebral bodies. The findings are typically best seen on T1 contrast-enhanced images and short-tau inversion recovery (STIR) images. Metastatic prostate cancer is visible as high-intensity lesions on the STIR images and is visible prior to its appearance on bone scintigraphy.[23] In addition, MRI scans are useful in determining the involvement of neurovascular structures. MRI scans are not useful as a screening tool for bone metastases. However, MRI scans may be more sensitive than bone scintigraphy in the vertebral body region (Fig. 94.3). The sensitivity of MRI scanning has been reported as 91% to 100%, compared with 62% to 85% for bone scintigraphy.[23,24] In addition, MRI images can help distinguish whether a vertebral body compression fracture is from malignancy or from osteoporosis.

Positron emission tomography (PET) scanning evaluates areas of increased metabolic activity, most commonly using the 18-fluorodeoxyglucose (FDG) isotope. These scans are useful in detecting osteolytic bone metastases but are less sensitive for osteoblastic metastases. In addition, precise determination of the location of lesions is difficult with PET scans, but the use of simultaneous CT scans allows for much better localization of the abnormal FDG uptake.[25] PET scans may be useful as a whole-body screening tool.[25,26] Comparative studies have shown PET scans to be more sensitive than Tc-99m scintigraphy or whole-body MRI scans in detecting bone metastases.[27,28] There may be limitations in the sensitivity of PET scanning in certain areas such as the skull, where the intense physiologic uptake from the adjacent brain parenchyma may obscure small skull metastases.

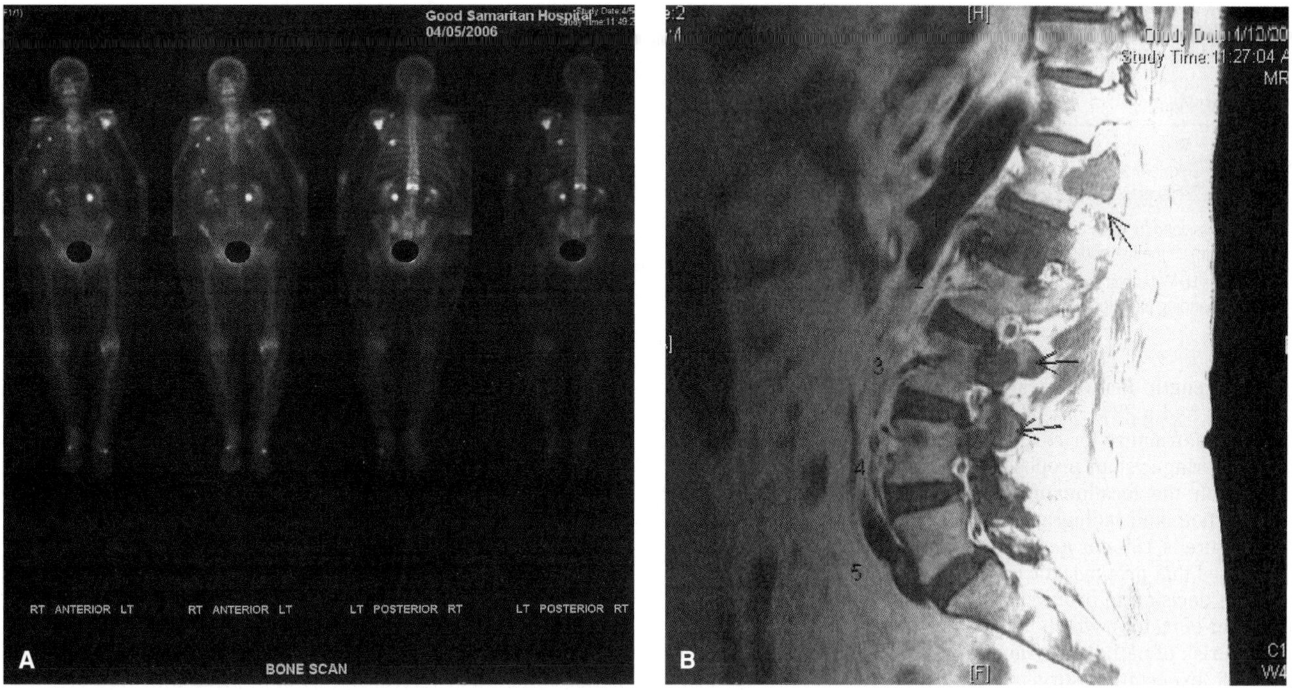

FIGURE 94.3. Nuclear medicine bone scan **(A)** and sagittal T1 magnetic resonance image (MRI) scan **(B)** from a woman with metastatic breast cancer. The bone scan shows the abnormality at L1, but the MR shows lesions at multiple levels, including the pedicles of T12, L3, and L4 (*arrows*).

PAIN MANAGEMENT

The majority of patients with bone metastases will experience pain during their disease course, and pain control can significantly improve their quality of life. Pain management may be achieved either by debulking disease using cytotoxic therapy or by symptomatic control with pharmacologic interventions.

Despite increasing understanding about the effective treatment of pain, patients with pain from bone metastases frequently have inadequate pain management. Barriers to pain treatment include physician underestimation of the patient's pain and reluctance by the patient to report pain.[29] There is a significant discrepancy between the physician estimate of pain and the pain level reported by the patient.[30] The use of a validated pain scale, such as the Brief Pain Inventory, gives the patient an opportunity to describe the severity of pain and the interference of pain with function in a manner that can be understood both by the patient and the physician.[29] This also allows for comparisons of pain levels over time, to better assess the effectiveness of treatments.

Pain control can be achieved in the majority of patients using the World Health Organization analgesic ladder. Step I uses nonopioid analgesics such as acetaminophen or nonsteroidal anti-inflammatory drugs; step II uses weak opioids such as codeine; step III uses strong opioids such as morphine. These medications are increased as necessary until the patient is free of pain. Typically, the medications are given on a routine schedule ("by the clock") rather than waiting until a certain level of pain is reached ("on demand"). Using this schedule, 70% to 76% of patients will have good pain relief.[31,32] Adjuvant medications such as gabapentin, pregabalin, or amitriptyline may be added for neuropathic pain. Antianxiety or antidepressant medications may also be of benefit in selected patients.

The opioid-based pain medications frequently cause constipation and may cause nausea. Patients using opioid medications should routinely be administered a fiber medication with or without a stool softener to minimize constipation. Other side effects of the opioid analgesics may include sedation, mental status changes, and mood changes.

SURGICAL MANAGEMENT

Surgical management of bone metastases is performed primarily to prevent or treat pathologic fractures. The goals of surgical intervention are to prevent or relieve pain, improve motor function, and improve overall quality of life. Treatment techniques are simpler and more effective when the procedure is performed prophylactically for an impending fracture rather than after the occurrence of a pathologic fracture. The risk of pathologic fracture depends on multiple factors, including location and extent of the lesion; whether the lesion is osteolytic, osteoblastic, or mixed; and the primary cancer site.

Fractures of the weight-bearing bones are the most likely to cause significant functional deficits. The proximal femur may have a higher propensity for fracture than other sites, but some authors have suggested that the fracture risk in upper limbs is similar to the risk in the femur. Whether or not there is a difference in the risk of fracture, the peritrochanteric femur is the site most likely to cause serious morbidity, and therefore the threshold for prophylactic intervention should be relatively low. The femur accounts for 65% of pathologic fractures requiring surgical intervention.[33] The humerus and vertebral bodies are also sites that require special attention because of the potential functional deficits from pathologic fractures.

The size of the bone metastasis is an important predictor of risk of fracture, especially with regard to the extent of cortical destruction. Various models have been used to predict the risk of pathologic fracture based on the size of the lesion. In series using plain radiographs, lesions ≥2.5 cm in the cortex of the femur were significantly more likely to fracture.[34] The proportion of cortical destruction is important as well. The risk of pathologic fracture of the femur begins to significantly increase when there is destruction of >50% of the cortex; the risk of fracture is 80% when >75% of the cortex is destroyed.[35] The location within the bone is important as well. An experimental model has shown that the greatest reduction in strength of the femur occurs with lesions in the inferior and medial aspect of the femoral neck, and posterior lesions have the least impact.[36] The use of CT scans may offer more accurate assessment of the

TABLE 94.1 MIRELS' SCORING SYSTEM OF PREDICTION OF PATHOLOGIC FRACTURE RISK

Score	*Pain*	*Location*	*Cortical Destruction*	*Radiographic Appearance*
1	Mild	Upper limb	<1/3	Blastic
2	Moderate	Lower limb	1/3–2/3	Mixed
3	Severe	Peritrochanteric	>2/3	Lytic

A score is assigned for each of the four categories, and the sum of those scores is used to estimate the risk of pathologic fracture.

From Mirels H. Metastatic disease in long bones: a proposed scoring system for diagnosing impending pathologic fractures. *Clin Orthop Relat Res* 1989;249:256–264.

bone strength. Femoral lesions with axial cortical destruction >30 mm had a 23% risk of pathologic fracture, compared with 3% risk of fracture for cortical destruction ≤30 mm.[37]

A scoring system proposed by Mirels[38] has a 12-point scale based on the location of the lesion, pain, extent of cortical destruction, and radiographic appearance (Table 94.1). The risk of fracture is 15% for a score of 8 and 33% for a score of 9. He proposed that prophylactic fixation is indicated for a score of ≥9.

The decision to proceed with surgery should be based on a number of factors, which include but are not limited to the estimated risk of pathologic fracture. For patients with a very limited life expectancy, surgery may not be indicated even if the risk of pathologic fracture is relatively high.[33] Clinical prediction of survival may be more accurate than relying on specific parameters such as diagnosis (primary site), performance status, number of bone metastases, presence of visceral metastases, and hemoglobin level.[39]

Fractures of the femoral neck can be managed either by total hip arthroplasty (which replaces both the femoral head and acetabulum) or a proximal femoral endoprosthesis alone.[33] Fractures of the intertrochanteric area may be managed by open reduction and internal fixation without the use of a prosthesis. This may allow for better long-term gait because of preservation of the hip flexor and adductor strength.[33] Lytic disease that extends below the intertrochanteric area is treated with a long intramedullary rod that provides stability throughout the length of the femur (Fig. 94.4). If there is significant destruction of the greater trochanter and femoral neck or head in addition to subtrochanteric involvement, a prosthetic replacement would be more appropriate than a reconstruction nail.[40] Fractures of the distal femur may be managed either with a plate and compression screw or with an intracondylar nail and screws augmented by intramedullary methylmethacrylate cement. The latter method may reduce the risk of late failure of the repair, especially in patients receiving postoperative radiation therapy.[33]

Repair of pathologic fractures of the humerus may be more problematic because of the small intramedullary canal and because of the proximity of the radial nerve, which may require extensive dissection.[33] Pathologic fractures of the proximal humerus will frequently require prosthetic replacement.[33] Fractures in the diaphysis may be repaired with a compression plate and screws. An alternative is to use a segmental diaphyseal replacement prosthetic device, which involves a prosthetic device than can be cemented into an allograft.[40] Supracondylar fractures are difficult to manage because the shape of the bone is not conducive to a plate and screws; these lesions may require intramedullary rods inserted in a retrograde manner through both the medial and lateral condyles, supplemented by intramedullary cement.[33]

Most pathologic fractures of the pelvis do not require surgical intervention, except for those involving the acetabulum.[33] Repair of acetabular fractures may involve the use of a total hip acetabular prosthesis, but more extensive lesions may require reconstruction that transfers the load-bearing stresses into more structurally intact bone in the iliac bone or sacroiliac joint.[33]

INTERVENTIONAL TECHNIQUES

Vertebroplasty is an effective method of palliating pain from vertebral body metastases, even in patients who have received prior radiotherapy.[41] Most patients experience pain relief within 48 hours. The procedure involves percutaneous injection of methylmethacrylate under CT or fluoroscopic guidance. Retropulsion of bone, epidural tumor, or collapse of the bone to less than one-third of its original height are relative contraindications to percutaneous vertebroplasty because of the risk of extrusion of the cement into the spinal canal, potentially causing neurologic complications. In some patients with epidural tumor, percutaneous vertebroplasty can be performed safely and effectively with a relatively low risk of serious complications.[42,43] However, the procedure should be considered with some caution; in a systematic review of 987 patients, there were 5 deaths and 19 other serious complications.[44]

Kyphoplasty involves percutaneous placement of a balloon-like device into a symptomatic spinal metastasis (most commonly into a fractured or compressed vertebral body).[45] The balloon is then inflated to restore the height of the vertebral body, and methylmethacrylate is subsequently injected into this cavity. This procedure may provide significant relief of pain and improve overall functioning, especially in patients with mechanical instability of the vertebral body.[46,47] Kyphoplasty may be a better option than vertebroplasty in patients with vertebral wall deficiency.[46]

An ablative procedure is frequently coupled with vertebroplasty or kyphoplasty.[48] Radiofrequency ablation (RFA) may be used to ablate the tumor but is most effective for tumors that are osteolytic or mixed osteolytic and blastic. The RFA may not be as effective in tumors that are primarily sclerotic. Cryoablation may be used for larger lesions or those that are sclerotic. For both of these procedures, special attention to cord and nerve temperatures is required to minimize the risk of complications.

SYSTEMIC TREATMENT

The rationale for using systemic therapy in the management of bone metastasis is compelling. The pathophysiology of bone metastasis involves hematogenous dissemination, and most patients with bone metastasis suffer from multiple synchronous sites of disease. In theory, administering systemic cytotoxic therapy should deliver palliative benefit by simultaneously addressing all sites of bone metastasis. A localized therapy such as external-beam radiation may be most appropriate for palliation if symptoms are localized. On the other hand, systemic chemotherapy may offer palliative benefit if symptoms are diffuse or constitutional and disease is widespread.

Measurement of response to systemic therapy has generally been with the same criteria used for solid metastatic tumors: a measurable radiographic change. This works well for lung and liver metastasis but not as well for bone metastasis. For bone metastases, the definition of a complete response is complete disappearance of all lesions on radiographs for at least 4 weeks. This is unlikely to occur even if all tumor cells are eradicated. A partial response requires some recalcification of lytic lesions, which may not be evident for 6 months or more.[49] PET scans may be more accurate at assessing response in a timely manner but are too expensive to be used as a routine follow-up evaluation for bone metastases. Markers of bone resorption may be a good way to detect response to therapy but are not clinically available at this time. Response to therapy for other modalities (i.e., radiotherapy, bisphosphonates) is measured in terms of pain relief and quality-of-life measures. Unfortunately, there is not much literature on accurate and reliable response criteria to palliative systemic therapy for bone metastasis. Most of the studies of chemotherapy for metastatic disease involve patients with visceral as well as osseous metastases. The responses in terms of pain are typically reported for all patients, not just

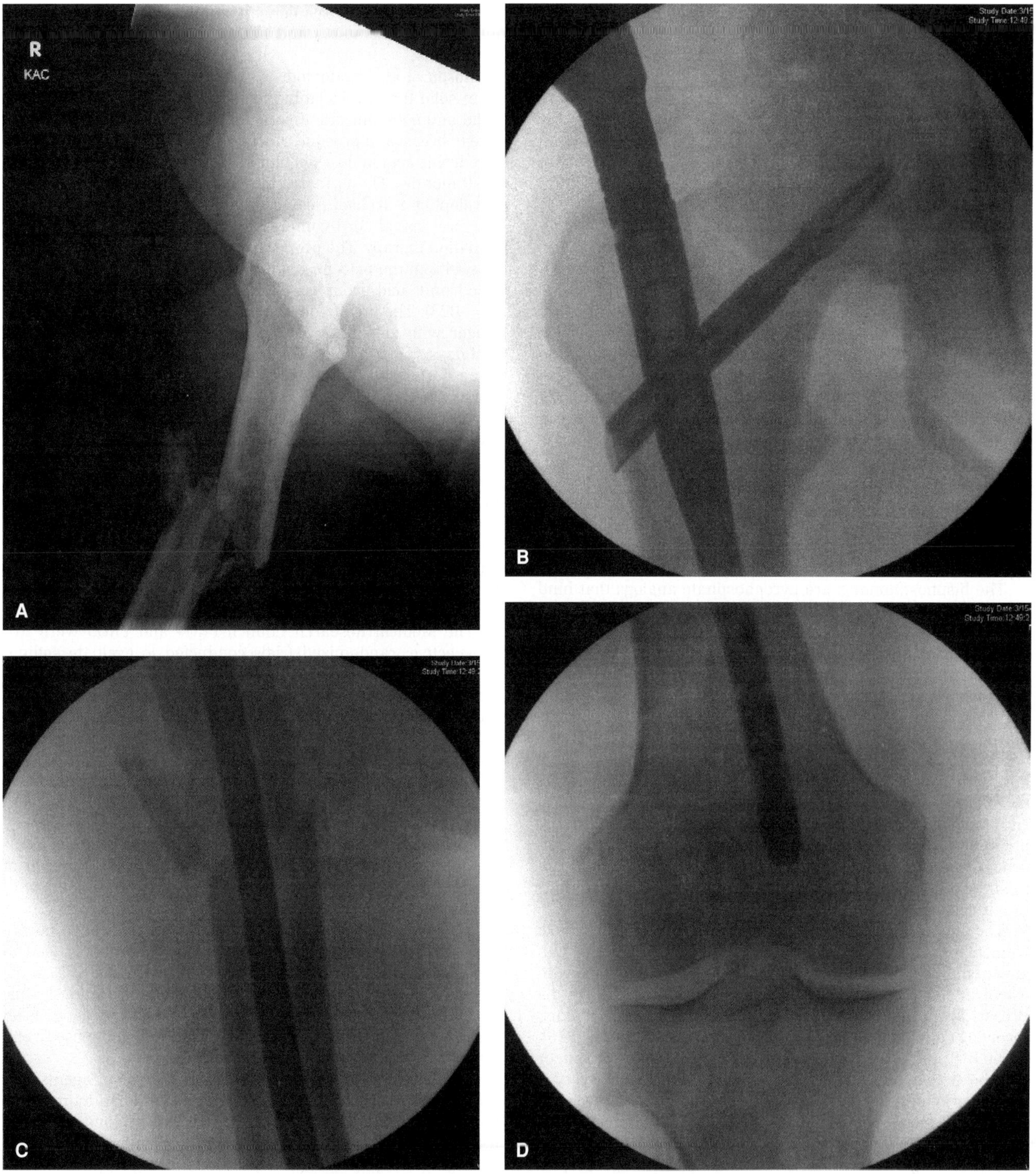

FIGURE 94.4. Anteroposterior radiograph **(A)** of a diaphyseal fracture of the femur in a patient with diffuse large-cell lymphoma. Intraoperative fluoroscopic views of the proximal **(B)**, mid-shaft **(C)**, and distal **(D)** femur after internal fixation with a trochanter fixation nail (TFN) nail.

those with bone metastases. There is more information regarding response to chemotherapy for patients with metastatic prostate cancer because this more frequently involves bone-only metastatic disease. The chemotherapy drugs are frequently given with bisphosphonates or corticosteroids, which may affect the response rates.

Tannock et al.[50] recommended using more relevant endpoints of palliation. They performed a randomized trial of mitoxantrone plus prednisone versus prednisone alone for patients with hormone-refractory prostate cancer and pain. Improvement in pain was seen in 29% of patients receiving the chemotherapy, compared with 12% of those who received prednisone alone. In a subsequent study, they compared mitoxantrone and prednisone plus or minus clodronate for a similar group of patients. Most had mild pain at study entry (160 of 209; 77%), and the remainder had moderate pain scores. The patients with moderate pain who received chemotherapy and clodronate had a 58% response rate (≥2-point improvement in pain score) compared with 26% for those who received chemotherapy alone. The median duration of pain response was 6 months. The TAX327 phase III trial was conducted in 1,006 men with hormone-resistant metastatic prostate cancer and randomized patients to receive prednisone combined with either docetaxel or mitoxantrone. The docetaxel arm showed an improvement in overall survival, lower cancer-induced bone pain, and better objective tumor response.[51]

In patients with bone metastasis, there is seldom reason to combine chemotherapy with concurrent radiation therapy because of the potential for increased toxicity when both modalities are delivered concurrently.

A number of hormonal therapies are available in the management of metastatic prostate and breast cancer. In properly selected patients, hormonal therapy has the potential for providing excellent palliation of metastatic disease with limited morbidity. In 1984, the Medical Research Council started a prospective, randomized trial in which 938 patients who either had asymptomatic metastatic prostate cancer or were not medical candidates for definitive therapy were randomized to immediate versus delayed hormone ablation therapy. Hormone ablation was achieved using either a leutinizing hormone–releasing hormone agonist or by orchiectomy. This study showed that immediate versus delayed initiation of hormone ablation therapy in the subset of patients with metastatic prostate cancer helped to prevent serious complications from metastatic disease. Serious complications including pathologic fracture, spinal cord compression, development of extraskeletal metastases, and ureteral obstruction were twofold more frequent in patients whose hormonal therapy was deferred compared with patients who received immediate hormone ablation therapy.[52]

The bisphosphonates are pyrophosphate analogs that bind to calcium phosphate with high affinity and are potent agents affecting bone resorption.[53] There is emerging evidence that the bisphosphonates also induce apoptosis in cancer cells.[54] Clodronate is a first-generation, non–nitrogen-containing bisphosphonate. Clodronate has a high affinity for bone mineral and is subsequently taken up into activated osteoclasts during bone resorption, thereby ensuring high concentrations within osteoclasts.[55] The nitrogen-containing bisphosphonates inhibit the key enzyme farnesyl diphosphonate synthase in the mevalonate pathway.[56] This prevents the action of several additional enzymes required for bone resorption. The bisphosphonates include pamidronate, alendronate, ibandronate, risedronate, and zoledronic acid. Zoledronate is much more potent than the other bisphosphonates, in part because it also inhibits tumor cell adhesion to the extracellular matrix.

The initial studies of bisphosphonate usage were primarily in women with metastatic breast cancer. Pamidronate was evaluated in multiple randomized, prospective studies of women with osteolytic bone metastases from breast cancer. The Aredia Breast Cancer Study Group Protocols 18 and 19 enrolled women receiving either chemotherapy (P19) or hormonal therapy (P18). In the P18 study, 372 women were randomized to receive either placebo or pamidronate 90 mg as a 2-hour infusion every 4 weeks for 24 cycles.[57] The primary endpoint was the prevention of "skeletal-related complications" (pathologic fractures, spinal cord compression, hypercalcemia, or the requirement for surgery or radiation therapy on bone). There were fewer skeletal-related complications in the pamidronate arm (475 events vs. 648 in the placebo group), but the benefit in reducing pathologic fractures and hypercalcemia was not significant until 18 to 24 months of treatment. The primary difference was that twice as many placebo patients required radiation therapy for palliation of pain, most often in the first 6 to 12 months. There was no difference in survival, although pain levels and serum markers of bone resorption were significantly lower in the group receiving pamidronate.

In the P19 study, women with stage IV breast cancer who were receiving chemotherapy and had lytic bone metastasis were given placebo or pamidronate for 12 monthly cycles.[58] Patients in the pamidronate arm suffered fewer overall skeletal complications and had a greater median time to first skeletal complication when compared with patients in the placebo arm of the study. Women treated with pamidronate maintained better performance status and had less bone pain secondary to metastasis.

Rosen et al.[59] evaluated 773 patients with bone metastases from solid tumors, including lung cancer, renal cell carcinoma, head and neck cancers, thyroid, and other primary sites (exclusive of breast and prostate cancer). They compared placebo with zoledronic acid in doses of either 4 or 8 mg given every 3 weeks for 9 months. The primary endpoint was proportion of patients developing a skeletal-related event (SRE), including pathologic fracture, spinal cord compression, or the need for surgery or radiation therapy. The proportion of patients developing an SRE was 44% in the placebo group compared with 38% in the 4-mg zoledronic acid group ($p = .127$) and 35% in the 8-mg group ($p = .023$). The time to development of an SRE was significantly longer with zoledronic acid compared with placebo (230 vs. 163 days; $p = .017$). The dose of the 8-mg group was reduced to 4 mg during the latter part of the study because of safety concerns, and thus 25% of patients in the 8-mg treatment arm actually received only 4 mg per dose. In addition, only 25% of patients received the full 9-month course of treatment because of death (27%), adverse events (21%), patient decision to discontinue (15%), or "insufficient efficacy" (7%). There was no improvement in two specific events—surgery to bone and spinal cord compression—in the patients receiving zoledronic acid compared with placebo. In addition, the need for analgesics gradually increased and functional capacity decreased from baseline to month 9 in all groups, with no differences between zoledronic acid and placebo.

The Medical Research Council PRO4 and PRO5 were two prospective, randomized trials conducted to evaluate sodium clodronate in men with prostate cancer. Long-term data showed that sodium clodronate improved overall survival in men with metastatic prostate cancer who were starting hormone therapy, but there was no improvement in overall survival for men with nonmetastatic disease.[60]

Complications of supportive therapy with bisphosphonates include osteoradionecrosis (particularly of the jaw) and renal insufficiency.[61] The mechanism of bisphosphonate-induced osteoradionecrosis is not known. Risk factors include the intravenous use of pamidronate and zoledronic acid, duration of treatment of 36 months or longer, older age in patients with multiple myeloma, and need for periodontal procedures.[62]

Bisphosphonates are not metabolized by the body and are excreted by the kidneys. Bisphosphonate therapy can lead to renal toxicity. The incidence of renal toxicity is 9% to 15% in trials when 4 mg of zoledronic acid is delivered intravenously during 15 minutes.[61] Moreover, the rate of renal toxicity depends on underlying renal disease, dose of bisphosphonate used, and duration of the infusion.

Another form of systemic therapy is the use of agents that target the RANK pathway. Denosumab is a human monoclonal antibody specific for the RANK ligand. The antibody binds to RANKL and thus inhibits the formation, activation, maturation, and survival of osteoclasts.[63] In randomized, prospective comparisons of denosumab with zoledronic acid in patients with metastatic breast or prostate cancer, denosumab was superior to zoledronic acid in delaying or preventing the time to skeletal-related events.[64,65]

RADIATION THERAPY

Radiation therapy has been reported to be effective in palliating painful bone metastases, with partial pain relief seen in 80% to 90% of patients and complete pain relief in 50% of patients (Fig. 94.5). These data are primarily from studies using physician evaluation of pain. When patient evaluation of pain is used, pain improvement is seen in 60% to 80% of patients and complete pain relief is seen in 15% to 40% of patients.[66] The response to treatment depends on a large number of factors,

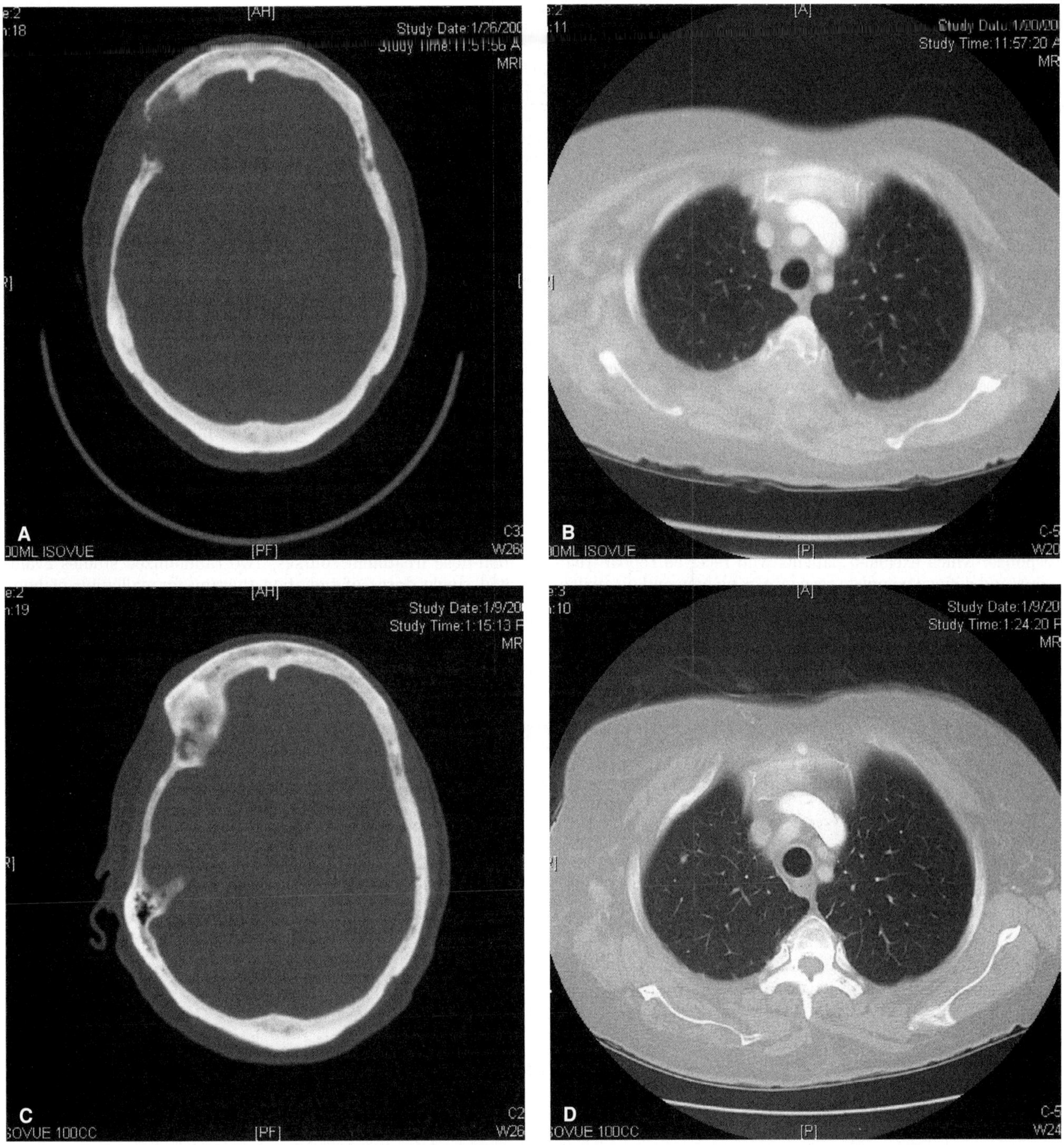

FIGURE 94.5. Axial computed tomography scans from a patient with metastatic breast cancer. Images through the frontal skull **(A)** and thoracic spine **(B)** show large, destructive, osseous lesions. Images 1 year later **(C, D)**, after palliative external-beam radiation, show significant healing of the bone.

including sex, primary site and histology, performance status, type of lesion (osteolytic vs. osteoblastic), location of the metastases, weight-bearing vs. non–weight-bearing site, extent of disease, number of painful sites, marital status, and level of pain prior to treatment. The effectiveness of the treatment also depends on the goal: palliation of pain, prevention of pathologic fracture, avoidance of future treatments, or local control of the disease. The doses required and volumes treated may be quite different for each of these goals. In addition to pain relief, other symptoms may be relieved by radiotherapy. Patients who have improvement in pain after radiotherapy may also have improvement in emotional functioning, decreased insomnia and decreased constipation, and overall improvement in quality-of-life scores.[67] Radiation therapy should be an integral part of palliative treatment for bone metastases for treatment of pain and prevention of other symptoms.[68]

Local-field external-beam radiation therapy is typically used for palliation of a few discrete areas of painful metastases. The first large randomized study evaluating different dose and fractionation schemes was the Radiation Therapy Oncology Group (RTOG) 74-02 trial.[69] Patients with solitary bone metastases were randomized to 40.5 Gy in 15 fractions versus 20 Gy in 5 fractions. Patients with multiple painful metastases were allocated to one of four treatment schedules: 30 Gy in 10 fractions, 15 Gy in 5 fractions, 20 Gy in 5 fractions, or 25 Gy in 5 fractions. The initial analysis by Tong et al.[69] in 1982 showed no

TABLE 94.2 RANDOMIZED TRIALS WITH ≥100 EVALUABLE PATIENTS COMPARING MULTIPLE-FRACTION TREATMENTS FOR PALLIATION OF BONE METASTASES

Study	*Number of Patients (Number of Evaluable)*	*Dose (Gy)/Number of Fractions*	*Complete Response[a] (%)*	*Overall Response[a] (%)*	*Pathologic Fractures (%)*
Tong et al.,[69] 1982, U.S.	266 (146)	20/5	53	82	4
(solitary treatment site)		40/15	61	85	18
Tong et al.,[69] 1982, U.S.	750 (613)	15/5	49	87	5
(multiple sites)		20/5	56	85	7
		25/5	49	83	9
		30/10	57	78	8
Hirokawa et al.,[75] 1988,	128 (128)	25/5	NA	75	NA
Japan		30/10		75	
Rasmusson et al.,[82] 1995,	217 (127)	15/3	NA	69	NA
Denmark		30/10		66	
Niewald et al.,[81] 1996,	100 (100)	20/5	33	77	8
Germany		30/15	31	86	13

Number of patients entered on study and number of patients evaluable for response; dosage schedule; complete and overall responses; and proportion of patients with pathologic fractures after treatment. NA, not available from published report.
[a]Response rates listed are for pain relief.

statistically significant difference in response rates between any of the treatment arms, with complete responses in 49% to 61% of patients. These results were questioned by Blitzer,[70] who reanalyzed the data using different criteria for complete response, which excluded patients who received repeat treatment, and defined complete response as no pain and no analgesic usage. With this adjustment in response definition, there was a significant difference in response favoring the longer treatment courses: 40.5 Gy in 15 fractions for the solitary metastases and 30 Gy in 10 fractions for multiple metastases. This was offered as evidence that higher doses were necessary for optimal palliation, even though one of the highest biologic doses for multiple fractions (25 Gy in 5 fractions) had one of the lower response rates. This reanalysis highlighted the importance of retreatment in this group of patients, especially in those given lower total doses during the initial course of radiation therapy.

There have been multiple randomized, prospective trials evaluating different dose and fractionation schemes.[69,71–83] Most of the earlier studies evaluated different multifraction treatment regimens (Table 94.2). No significant difference was seen between longer-course treatments and the shorter-duration, lower-total-dose treatment courses. Two randomized studies evaluated single doses of radiation therapy for palliation of bone metastases. Hoskin et al.[84] randomized patients to 4 versus 8 Gy, and Jeremic et al.[85] randomized patients to one of three dose levels, 4 versus 6 versus 8 Gy. In both of these studies, the

TABLE 94.3 RANDOMIZED TRIALS OF SINGLE VERSUS MULTIPLE FRACTIONS WITH ≥100 EVALUABLE PATIENTS: DEMOGRAPHICS AND STUDY DESIGN

Study	*Number of Patients (Number Evaluable)*	*Primary Endpoint*	*Secondary Endpoint(s)*	*Primary Site*	*Treatment Site*	*Response Evaluation Time[a]*	*Percentage Severe Pain Pretreatment[b]*
Foro Arnalot et al.,[72] 2008, Spain	160	Pain relief and analgesics	–	Breast, 27% Lung, 26% Prostate, 25%	Pelvis, 39% Spine, 36% Long bones, 14%	–	50 (median pain score of 7)
Kaasa et al.,[76] 2006, Norway/Sweden	376	Pain relief	Fatigue, quality of life	Prostate, 38% Breast, 30% Lung, 11%	Spine, 38% Pelvis, 35% Extremities, 20%	–	35–41
Hartsell et al.,[74] 2005, U.S./Canada	949 (898)	Pain relief	Analgesic use, toxicity, path fracture rate, retreatment rate	Breast, 50% Prostate, 50%	C spine, 5% T spine, 19% L spine, 27%	3 mo	72–73
Kirkbride et al.,[77] 2000, Canada	398 (287)	Pain relief and analgesics	–	Breast, 40% Lung, 26% Prostate, 23%	Spine, 30% Pelvis, 29%	3 mo	–
Steenland et al.,[83] 1999, Netherlands	1,171 (1,073)	Pain relief	Quality of life	Breast, 39% Lung, 25% Prostate, 23%	TL spine, 30% Pelvis, 36% Femur, 10% Ribs, 8% Humerus, 6%	During first year	Mean pain score 6.3 (moderate)
Bone Pain Working Group,[71] 1999, U.K./New Zealand	765	Pain relief	Nausea and vomiting	Breast, 36% Prostate, 34% Lung, 12%	Pelvis/hip, 28% L spine, 20% Ribs, 11% T spine, 9% Femur, 6%	–	22–23
Koswig and Budach,[78] 1999, Germany	107	Pain relief	Recalcification	Breast, 58% Lung, 24% Prostate, 10% Kidney, 7%	Spine, 81% Extremities, 13%	6 wk	–
Nielsen et al.,[80] 1998, Denmark	241 (239)	Pain relief	Quality of life, analgesic use	Breast, 39% Prostate, 34% Lung, 13%	TL spine, 42% Pelvis, 21% Hips/femur, 18% Other, 19%	12 wk	–
Gaze et al.,[73] 1997, U.K.	265 (240)	Pain relief	Side effects, quality of life	Any epithelial tumor	–	–	–

C, cervical; L, lumbar; T, thoracic. NA, not available from published report.
[a]Time from study entry to assessment of response.
[b]Proportion of patients with severe pain scores at the time of study entry.

TABLE 94.4 RANDOMIZED TRIALS OF SINGLE VERSUS MULTIPLE FRACTIONS: RESULTS

Study	Number of Patients (Number Evaluable)	Dose (Gy)/ Fractions	Median Survival (mo)	Complete Response[a]	Overall Response[a]	Retreatment Rate (%)	Pathologic Fractures[b] (%)	Toxicity
Foro Arnalot et al.,[72] 2008,	160	8/1 vs. 30/10	6.5	15	75	2	NA	12%
Spain			7.6	13	86	28		18%
Kaasa et al.,[76] 2006,	376	8/1 vs.	9.6	NA	No difference	16	4	NA
Norway/Sweden		30/10	7.9			4	11	
Hartsell et al.,[74] 2005, U.S./	949 (898)	8/1 vs.	9.1	15	65	18	5	10% grade 2–4
Canada		30/10	9.3	18	66	9	4	17% $p = .002$
Kirkbride et al.,[77] 2000,	398 (287)	8/1 vs.	NA	22	51	NA	NA	NA
Canada		20/5		29	48			
Steenland et al.,[83] 1999,	1171 (1073)	8/1 vs.	7	37	72	25	4	No difference
Netherlands		20/5		33	69	7	2	
Bone Pain Working Party,[71]	761 (681)	8/1 vs.	NA	57	78	23	2	No difference
1999, U.K./New Zealand		20/5[c]		58	78	10	<1	
Koswig and Budach,[78]	107 (107)	8/1 vs.	NA	33	81	NA	NA	NA
1999, Germany		30/10		31	78			
Nielsen et al.,[80] 1998,	241 (239)	8/1 vs.	NA	15	73	21	NA	No difference
Denmark		20/5		15	76	12		
Gaze et al.,[73] 1997, U.K.	265 (240)	10/1 vs.	NA	37	81	NA	NA	21% p = NS
		22.5/5		47	76			26% emesis

NA, not available from published report; NS, not statistically significant.

[a]Proportion of patients with pathologic fractures after treatment.

[b]Response rates listed are for pain relief.

[c]A regimen of 30 Gy/10 was also allowed; 98% of patients received 20 Gy/5.

Palliative and Supportive Care

8-Gy arm was superior to 4 Gy, indicating that there is a threshold dose necessary to achieve adequate palliation. Most of the randomized trials during the last 15 years used a multiple fraction treatment scheme as the control arm and a single dose of 8 to 10 Gy as the study arm (Tables 94.3 and 94.4).

Two recent large studies compared single-dose treatment to longer courses of radiation therapy. The Dutch trial evaluated patients with bone metastases from solid tumors, primarily breast (39%), prostate (23%), and lung (25%); metastatic melanoma and renal cell carcinomas were excluded.[83] The primary endpoint was patient-assessed pain relief, evaluated on an 11-point scale (0 = no pain, 10 = worst imaginable pain). A total of 1,171 patients were randomized to either 8 Gy in a single fraction or 24 Gy in six fractions. The painful areas had to be included in a single treatment volume. The spine (36%) and pelvis (30%) were the two most common sites of treatment. The median pain score was 6.3, with a minimum score of 2. About half of the patient were receiving narcotic pain medications prior to randomization, and slightly more than half (53%) were receiving systemic therapy. The median survival after treatment was 30 weeks, with no difference between the two treatment groups. There was no difference in overall or complete response rates between the single-dose versus longer-course treatment arms. Overall, 71% of patients achieved a response to therapy during follow-up, with 35% achieving a complete response. Most of the responses occurred within the first 4 to 6 weeks after treatment. Complete response rates were higher for patients with breast and prostate primaries than with lung or other primary sites (44% and 41% vs. 21% and 16%, respectively).

There were two significant differences between the two treatment groups: retreatment rates and pathologic fracture rates. The rate of pathologic fracture in the treated area was 4% for the 8-Gy single-treatment arm compared with 2% for the 24 Gy/six fraction group. The median time to fracture was similar for the two groups at 21 and 17 weeks. Although there was a significant difference in pathologic fracture between the two groups, these rates are still relatively low. There was also a significant difference in retreatment rates between the two arms of the study, with a much higher likelihood of a second course of treatment in the single-treatment group. The group of patients receiving 24 Gy in six fractions initially was given a second course of treatment 7% of the time, whereas 25% of the 8-Gy single-fraction group was given retreatment. Retreatment occurred more commonly with lung/other tumors than with breast/prostate primaries. In addition, the retreatment was given at a lower pain score (median 6.8 for 8-Gy single-fraction compared with 7.5 for the multiple fraction group) and at an earlier time (14 weeks after initial treatment compared with 23 weeks). This may indicate a greater willingness to reirradiate after a single dose of 8 Gy or more reluctance to give retreatment after a higher initial dose of radiation therapy.

The second large study of single-dose versus longer-course treatment for palliation of bone metastases was RTOG study 9714, which was conducted in the United States and Canada.[74] This was limited to patients with painful bone metastases from breast or prostate primaries, with up to three painful sites allowed. Pain was evaluated using the Brief Pain Inventory, an 11-point scale. At the time of randomization, the patient was required to have a minimum pain score of 5 or a high narcotic pain medication requirement of the equivalent of >60 mg of morphine per day. More than 70% of the patients had severe pain at study entry (pain scores of 7 to 10). Patients were randomized to 8 Gy in a single fraction versus 30 Gy in 10 treatments. The median survival was 9.3 months. Overall toxicity rates were low, with fewer patients in the 8-Gy treatment group experiencing acute toxicity. There were no significant differences in complete (17%) and partial pain response rates (49%) between the two treatment groups. Complete pain and narcotic response (0 pain score and no narcotic pain medication use) was seen in 11%; these responses were all determined at the 3-month posttreatment evaluation. As in the Dutch trial, the rate of retreatment was higher in the 8-Gy treatment group, with 18% in that group receiving retreatment compared with 9% in the 30-Gy group. This disparity in the rate of retreatment occurred despite nearly identical rates of stable (26% vs. 24%) or progressive pain scores (9% vs. 10%) and similar rates of narcotic use between the two groups.

In contrast to the Dutch trial, there was no difference in the rate of pathologic fractures between the two groups (5% for 8 Gy vs. 4% for 30 Gy). Further analysis of this study has shown that certain subgroups may benefit from the longer course of palliative radiation therapy. Konski et al.[86] showed that although married men and single and married women were more likely to receive retreatment after receiving 8 versus 30 Gy of palliative radiation therapy, there was no difference in retreatment rates among single men. The authors suggest that social support factors may significantly affect the ability of some patients to access repeat therapies for painful bone metastasis, especially as their health declines. Such subgroups of patients may benefit from the longer 10-fraction course of therapy.

These two large prospective, randomized trials comparing single-fraction to multiple-fraction palliative radiation therapy have similar results and help to clarify the role of palliative radiotherapy for bone metastases. The assessment of pain was performed by the patients rather than by physicians or other health care providers. The studies with the highest response rates generally used physician assessment of pain response (e.g., the RTOG 7402 study). Even with patient assessment of response, the single-fraction treatment yields similar response rates to the longer-course treatment. The patients in the Dutch trial were treated when their pain was in the moderate range, with only half on narcotic pain medications, compared with severe pain and high-dose narcotic pain medication for most of the patients entered on the RTOG trial. This may account for the higher rates of complete response on the Dutch trial. In the RTOG trial, the group of patients with a single area of pain or with moderate pain scores at the time of study entry had higher complete response rates. Thus, it appears that the outcome is much better if patients are treated with palliative radiotherapy earlier in the course of their bone metastases rather than waiting until pain is severe or narcotic pain medication requirements are significant. There was no difference in pain response whether the treated bone metastases were in the spine or in extremity sites. The rates of pathologic fracture after treatment are relatively low, but it is not clear whether higher doses provide greater protection from fractures. The rates of retreatment are significantly higher with the single-dose schedules, but there may be some physician bias partially accounting for this difference because the retreatment tends to be offered at an earlier time and at lower levels of pain following the single-dose treatment.

There have been multiple randomized, prospective trials in the last 30 years comparing shorter-course, lower–total-dose treatment to the more "standard" longer-course, higher–dose treatment. Several conclusions are clear from these studies:

1. Single-dose treatments of 8 Gy provide similar pain relief to longer-treatment regimens (30 Gy in 10 fractions or 20 to 24 Gy in five to eight treatments).
2. The retreatment rates are higher after short-course treatment by a factor of two to three.
3. Response rates are lower when scored by the patient instead of by the treating physician.
4. Response rates are better when the initial pain scores are lower, that is, when the patients are treated for moderate pain rather than severe pain.
5. There is no consistent dose–response relationship for palliation of bone metastases.

The lack of a dose–response relationship suggests that the mechanism of initial pain relief is not a reduction in tumor burden but more likely a change in the local environment that has caused activation of bone resorption by osteoclasts.[2] This helps to explain the seeming paradox of similar pain improvement with single-dose treatment compared with higher–total-dose, longer-course treatment. The treatment paradigm for bone metastases may be more analogous to treatments for certain benign conditions such as prevention of heterotopic ossification or keloid formation. In those conditions, a single or few treatments are given to diminish the activation of osteoblasts or fibroblasts.

This mechanism of pain relief may also help to explain the higher rates of retreatment after single-dose 8-Gy treatment because there will be less cell kill with this dose compared with 30 Gy in 10 fractions. Thus, for patients with a longer lifespan, there is a greater opportunity for regrowth of the tumor, which may again affect the local milieu, causing osteoclast activation.

For patients with a poor performance status, difficulty making multiple trips for treatment, extensive nonosseous metastases, and/or a short life expectancy, the most appropriate treatment is a single fraction of 8 Gy. Even with a limited expectancy (<3 months), the majority of patients experience pain relief, and palliative radiotherapy should still be considered for those patients.[87,88] For patients with a longer life expectancy, bone-only metastases, and good performance status, a longer course of treatment (30 Gy in 10 fractions) may be more appropriate to minimize the risk of retreatment. For selected patients with a solitary bone metastasis ("oligometastasis"), an even higher dose of treatment may be indicated, although this must be tempered by potential weakening of surrounding normal bone.

The single large-fraction treatment may be more likely to cause a "flare" reaction, with a temporary increase in pain at the site of the metastases.[89] The risk of this side effect may be diminished by the use of anti-inflammatory medications, either corticosteroids or nonsteroidal anti-inflammatory medications. Although the risk of significant acute toxicity has been low in the randomized trials, another potential concern is the risk of nausea or emesis if a significant portion of the stomach is within the treatment field (e.g., with a field covering the lower thoracic spine). It may be beneficial to give prophylactic antiemetics 1 to 2 hours before the treatment to minimize the possibility of this side effect.

Stereotactic radiosurgery has also been evaluated for the treatment of bone metastasis, particularly in the spinal region. The Radiation Therapy Oncology Group (RTOG) 0631 is a phase II/III study evaluating the role of stereotactic radiosurgery for patients with spine metastasis. Patients on this trial are randomized to either single-fraction external-beam radiation to 8 Gy or to single-fraction image-guided stereotactic radiosurgery to 16 Gy. The primary endpoint of this study is assessment of pain control at the treated site(s), and results of this study are pending.

A prospective, nonrandomized cohort study conducted at the University of Pittsburgh in 500 cases of spinal metastasis treated with single-fraction radiosurgery to a maximum intratumor dose of 12.5 to 25 Gy demonstrated long-term pain level improvement in 86% of cases. Long-term tumor control was demonstrated in 90% of cases when radiosurgery was used as the primary treatment modality.[90]

The use of bisphosphonates with external-beam radiotherapy may further improve the outcome in terms of both pain and bone healing. A prospective trial by Vassiliou et al.[91] evaluated 45 patients who received both external-beam irradiation and monthly ibandronate for painful bone metastases from solid tumors. All of the patients had improvement in pain, with 57% complete responses and 43% partial responses when using the same response criteria as RTOG 9714. The average pain score decreased from 6.3 to 0.8, and opioid pain medication use decreased from 84% of the patients before treatment to 24% after treatment. Bone density in the area of the metastases increased by 73% by 10 months after treatment. A similar study using pamidronate and 30 Gy of external-beam radiotherapy in women with painful bone metastases from breast cancer found that 88% of patients had complete radiographic response by International Union Against Cancer criteria.[92]

The majority of patients with osseous metastases have multiple lesions. Although radiation therapy is effective at palliating pain in a few sites, it cannot be used to treat widespread disease. Two techniques that have been used to treat more-diffuse metastases are hemibody irradiation and intravenous radiopharmaceuticals.

Hemibody Radiation Therapy

Hemibody irradiation (HBI), or wide-field radiation therapy, refers to the technique of treating a large portion of the body with external-beam irradiation. Although the term *hemibody irradiation* is used, typically the field does not cover half of the body, but more accurately treats about one-third of the body. The treatment has been used for palliation of symptoms and as an adjuvant to prevent the development of new bone metastases. The treatment for palliation of pain is most useful in patients who have diffuse, widespread bone metastases.

The treatment volumes have been divided into upper, middle, and lower HBI. The fields for upper HBI cover the thorax and abdomen from the neck to the top of the iliac crests. For midbody HBI, the fields include the abdomen and pelvis from the diaphragm to the ischial tuberosities, and for lower HBI treatment, the field borders are from the top of the pelvis to the inferior portion of the femurs. The toxicities from each of the fields depend on the critical structures included. The most problematic of these is the risk of radiation pneumonitis with upper HBI. This is the dose-limiting toxicity for upper HBI, and dose-inhomogeneity corrections for the lung are necessary to minimize the risk of fatal pneumonitis. A lower total dose can be given to the upper hemibody fields compared with the middle or lower hemibody areas.

RTOG 78-10 was a dose-searching prospective protocol evaluating the maximum tolerated dose (MTD) for single-dose HBI.[93] The MTD for middle and lower hemibody treatment was 8 Gy. The MTD for the upper HBI was 6 Gy if the lung dose was uncorrected and 7 Gy if lung corrections were used. Improvement in pain was noted in 80% of patients with breast cancer and 90% of patients with prostate cancer. Overall, the response rate in terms of pain relief was 73%, with complete relief of symptoms seen in 19%. Pain relief was seen relatively rapidly, with 50% of responses occurring within 2 days and 95% of responses within 2 weeks. The subsequent study RTOG 82-06 evaluated the use of HBI in addition to local radiotherapy to determine whether the HBI would prevent the development of new sites of disease.[94] All of the patients received involved-field irradiation to one or more painful sites, and half of the patients were randomly assigned to receive single-dose HBI as well. The median time to progression was 6.3 months in the local-treatment-only group compared with 12.6 months for those receiving HBI. Fewer patients receiving HBI required additional treatment. The incidence of severe hematologic toxicity was low and transitory but was seen only in the group receiving HBI.

Both the RTOG and the International Atomic Energy Agency performed trials evaluating multifraction courses of HBI.[95,96] The doses per fraction ranged from 2.5 to 4 Gy to a total of 8 to 20 Gy. The maximum tolerated dose on the RTOG 88–08 study was 17.5 Gy in seven fractions. On the International Atomic Energy Agency study, 3 Gy twice daily for 2 days (12 Gy total) or 3 Gy daily for 5 days (15 Gy total) was more effective than 4 Gy daily for 2 days. The primary toxicities were hematologic and gastrointestinal. The rationale for these doses was to decrease the acute toxicity. However, each of these regimens requires multiple treatments during several days, and the acute toxicities are not appreciably different than the single-dose treatment. With the use of appropriate antiemetic premedications and with cytokines to aid in hematologic recovery, there does not appear to be any appreciable benefit to the fractionated HBI compared with the single dose.

Premedication with antiemetics and anti-inflammatory medications significantly reduce the acute side effects of treatment. Before the development of the 5-HT3 receptor antagonists, nausea was a significant side effect of treatment, even with pretreatment and posttreatment use of steroids, prochlorperazine, and intravenous hydration. With the use of ondansetron, granisetron, or other 5-HT3 receptor antagonists, the incidence of acute nausea and emesis has been minimized and HBI is well tolerated.[97] A typical premedication regimen consists of dexamethasone, 8 to 16 mg, and ondansetron, 8 to 16 mg, 1 hour before treatment with HBI.[98]

Radiopharmaceuticals

The concept of radiopharmaceutical treatment is compelling.[99] Calcium (and to a lesser extent phosphorous) analogs will preferentially accumulate in bone, especially in areas of active bone turnover. A radioactive isotope that is a β-emitter or low-energy γ-source will allow localized treatment in the areas in which the radiopharmaceutical accumulates, thus minimizing side effects and giving an excellent therapeutic ratio. The radiopharmaceuticals are given in a single injection that is easily administered. The treatment can be combined with other modalities, including chemotherapy or external-beam radiation therapy.

The first radiopharmaceutical used for treatment of bone metastases was phosphorous-32 (P-32). Treatment with P-32 for diffuse bone metastases was successful in giving subjective pain relief but with unacceptable bone marrow toxicity. Other radioisotopes have been used for the palliation of diffuse osseous metastases with a better therapeutic ratio than P-32. Strontium-89 (Sr-89) is chemically similar to calcium and is deposited in the bone matrix, preferentially in sites of active osteogenesis. Sr-89 is a pure β-emitter with an energy of 1.4 MeV and a half-life of 50.6 days.[100] Samarium-153 (Sm-153) is primarily a β-emitter but also has a component of gamma emission, which is useful for imaging purposes. The Sm-153 ethylenediaminetetra methylenephosphoric acid (EDTMP) is concentrated in areas of high bone turnover, accumulating in areas of hydroxyapatite. The physical half-life of Sr-153 is 46.3 hours, but the biologic half-life is much shorter because about half of the compound is excreted in the urine within 8 hours of injection.[101] These two isotopes have been evaluated in multiple prospective trials. There are other, newer isotopes that are being evaluated, including rhenium-186, rhenium-188, and tin-117m. All of these isotopes accumulate in areas of osteoblastic activity, especially in areas of increased uptake on bone scintigraphy; for this reason, most of the patients entered on prospective trials have metastatic prostate cancer.

Strontium-89

The first study of Sr-89 with substantial numbers of patients was a randomized, prospective trial of Sr-89 versus placebo in 126 men with metastatic prostate cancer, reported by Porter and McEwan[102] in 1993. The patients were randomized after involved-field radiation therapy in a double-blind fashion to 400 MBq of Sr-89 versus placebo. Although there was no statistically significant difference in the primary endpoint of pain relief, there were several secondary endpoints that were improved with the Sr-89. More patients were able to discontinue pain medications (17% vs. 2%), and there were fewer sites of new pain requiring additional radiotherapy in the patients who received Sr-89. Smeland et al.[103] reported on a similar study of Sr-89 versus placebo after involved-field radiation therapy, which showed no difference in outcome between the two groups. In this study, the dose of Sr-89 was only 150 MBq.

There have been two randomized trials of Sr-89 versus external-beam radiation therapy. A study by Quilty et al.[104] from the United Kingdom evaluated Sr-89 given in a dose of 200 MBq compared with external-beam radiotherapy. For patients with a few bone metastases, the randomization was Sr-89 versus local-field radiation therapy. Patients with more widespread metastases were randomized to Sr-89 versus HBI of 8 Gy to the lower hemibody or 6 Gy to the upper hemibody. There was no difference in pain relief, toxicity, or median survival between the groups. In the patients with diffuse disease, there were fewer new pain sites after Sr-89 than HBI. The trial by Oosterhof et al.[105] evaluated 203 patients with hormone-refractory metastatic prostate cancer, randomly assigning patients to receive local-field radiation therapy or 150 MBq of intravenous Sr-89. There was no difference in pain relief or toxicity between the two treatment arms.

Sr-89 can be given concomitantly with chemotherapy. Two randomized, prospective trials evaluated concomitant chemotherapy with Sr-89 for patients with hormone-refractory metastatic prostate cancer. In the trial by Sciuto et al.,[106] 70 patients received 148 MBq of Sr-89 on day 0. They were randomly assigned to receive cisplatin, 18 mg/m^2 intravenously on day 0 and 16 mg/m^2 on days 10 and 11, or placebo on the same days. The group that received cisplatin and Sr-89 had significantly more patients with pain relief (91% vs. 63%), longer duration of pain palliation (120 vs. 60 days), longer median survival (9 vs. 6 months), and a significantly greater proportion of patients with improvement in performance status (66% vs. 26%), with no significant difference in toxicity. Tu et al.[107] performed a phase II randomized study of doxorubicin, 20 mg/m^2 per week given intravenously, with randomization between 2.035 MBq/kg of intravenous Sr-89 versus placebo. Neutropenia and anemia were common in the combined Sr-89 plus doxorubicin group compared with doxorubicin alone, but the median survival was also significantly better (28 vs. 17 months).

An economic evaluation of the Trans-Canada randomized study found Sr-89 treatment to be cost-effective.[108] The patients who received the Sr-89 had significantly lower subsequent costs for palliative medications, hormonal therapy, and subsequent radiation therapy. However, Oosterhof et al.[105] found that Sr-89 was associated with higher costs than external-beam radiotherapy.

Samarium-153

Samarium-153 is chelated with ethylenediaminetetra-methylenephosphoric acid to form Sm-153 EDTMP, a compound that is preferentially taken up in newly formed bone. The unbound remainder of the drug is rapidly cleared via urinary excretion. Phase I/II studies showed that doses of >2.5 mCi/kg are associated with neutropenia. In a dose-escalation study, Collins et al.[109] evaluated doses from 0.5 to 3.0 mCi/kg. There was no significant difference in clinical response between 1.0 and 2.5 mCi. There have been at least five randomized, prospective evaluations of Sm-153 for metastatic cancers (primarily for prostate cancers).[101,110–113] Two of these studies used a placebo arm in comparison to 1.0 mCi/kg[112] or 0.5 and 1.0 mCi/kg.[101] In both of these studies, the 1.0-mCi/kg dose gave significant improvement in pain relief compared to placebo. The average opioid dose decreased for the patients receiving Sm-153, compared to an increase in the patients receiving placebo. Transient marrow suppression was seen, with a nadir at 4 to 6 weeks and recovery by 8 weeks; this was primarily manifest as grade ≥3 neutropenia (14% compared with 0% for placebo).

The other phase III study evaluated three dose levels of Sm-153 (0.5, 1.0, and 1.5 mCi/kg). Olea et al.[110] reported no difference in response rates among the different dose levels, with an overall pain relief response rate of 73%. Two randomized phase II studies compared doses of 0.5 with 1.0 mCi/kg, with no placebo arm.[111,113] In these two studies, there was no significant difference between the two dose levels for response or toxicity. There was no difference in response by primary site, although the numbers of patients were small for each primary site. The study by Tian et al.[113] is the only one in which metastatic prostate cancer patients did not comprise the majority of patients included.

Patient Selection

Radiopharmaceuticals, specifically Sr-89 and Sm-153, are effective in providing pain relief for patients with diffuse osseous metastases. This is primarily true for metastases that have an osteoblastic component. In general, if a Tc-99m nuclear medicine bone scan shows localized areas of increased uptake, then radiopharmaceutical treatment is likely to be of benefit. An advantage of radioisotope treatment is that it can be combined with other modalities, such as external-beam radiation therapy or chemotherapy. Because the targets of treatment are similar, treatment with bisphosphonates should not be given simultaneously with radioisotopes because this may reduce the efficacy of both medications. Relative contraindications to therapy would be impaired renal or hepatic function or inadequate hematologic reserve.

Radiopharmaceuticals: Summary

The primary advantages of Sm-153 compared with Sr-89 are reduced radiation safety issues (because of the much shorter half-life) and the ability to image the distribution of the Sm-153. Although there has not been a randomized comparison of Sr-89 and Sm-153, there does not appear to be a significant difference in the incidence, severity, onset, or duration of hematologic toxicity, despite the short half-life of the Sm-153. Both radiopharmaceuticals appear equally effective at palliating pain from bone metastasis. These radiopharmaceuticals add to the growing armamentarium of therapies designed to palliate pain and improve the quality of life of patients with bone metastasis from cancer.

CONCLUSION

Palliative radiation therapy is of significant benefit to patients after painful bone metastasis, with most patients experiencing relief in the magnitude of pain following treatment. Response rates to palliative radiation therapy for localized sites of pain are consistently higher than response rates from palliative systemic therapy, and palliative external-beam radiation therapy remains the mainstay of treatment for clinically localized painful bone metastasis. Providing shorter, single-fraction palliative treatment schedules (i.e., 800 cGy × one fraction) for properly selected patients with bone metastasis can help better integrate palliative radiation therapy into the multidisciplinary management of patients with metastatic cancer and offer equivalent palliation compared with longer courses of palliative radiation therapy. Systemic targeted therapies including Sm-153 and Sr-89 offer yet another means to target painful sites of blastic bone metastasis without limiting the ability to use localized external-beam radiation therapy and systemic chemotherapy.

REFERENCES

1. Ratanatharathorn V, Powers WE, Moss WT, et al. Bone metastasis: review and critical analysis of random allocation trials of local field treatment. *Int J Radiat Oncol Biol Phys* 1999;44:1–18.
2. Smith HS. Painful osseous metastases. *Pain physician* 2011;14:E373–E405.
3. Coleman RE. Skeletal complications of malignancy. *Cancer* 1997;80(Suppl 8): 1588–1594.
4. Nielsen OS, Munro AJ, Tannock IF. Bone metastases: pathophysiology and management policy. *J Clin Oncol* 1991;9:509–524.
5. Coleman RE, Rubens RD. The clinical course of bone metastases from breast cancer. *Br J Cancer* 1987;55:61–66.
6. Singh D, Yi WS, Brasacchio RA, et al. Is there a favorable subset of patients with prostate cancer who develop oligometeastases? *Int J Radiat Oncol Biol Phys* 2004;58:3–10.
7. Khan L, Uy C, Nguyen L, et al. Self-reported rates of sleep disturbance in patients with symptomatic bone metastases attending an outpatient radiotherapy clinic. *J Palliat Med* 2011;14:708–714.
8. Nguyen J, Cramarossa G, Bruner D, et al. A literature review of symptom clusters in patients with breast cancer. *Expert Rev Pharmacoecon Outcomes Res* 2011; 11:533–539.
9. Asdourian PL, Weidenbaum M, DeWald RL, et al. The pattern of vertebral involvement in metastatic vertebral breast cancer. *Clin Orthop Relat Res* 1990; 250:164–170.
10. Hitchins RN, Philip PA, Wignall B, et al. Bone disease in testicular and extragonadal germ cell tumours. *Br J Cancer* 1988;58:793–796.
11. Matsuyama T, Tsukamoto N, Imachi M, et al. Bone metastasis from cervix cancer. *Gynecol Oncol* 1989;32:72–75.
12. Steinmetz MP, Mekhail A, Benzel EC. Management of metastatic tumors of the spine: strategies and operative indications. *Neurosurg Focus* 2001;11:e2.
13. Gurney H, Larcos G, McKay M, et al. Bone metastases in hypernephroma. Frequency of scapular involvement. *Cancer* 1989;64:1429–1431.
14. Roodman GD. Mechanisms of bone metastases. *N Engl J Med* 2004;350:1655–1664.
15. Roodman GD. Biology of osteoclast activation in cancer. *J Clin Oncol* 2001;19: 3562–3571.
16. Eriksen EF. Cellular mechanisms of bone remodeling. *Rev Endocr Metab Disord* 2010;11:219–227.
17. Manolagas SC, Jilka RL. Bone marrow, cytokines and bone remodeling. Emerging insights into the pathophysiology of osteoporosis. *N Engl J Med* 1995;332: 305–311.

18. Ratanatharathorn V, Powers WE, Temple HT. In: Perez CA, Brady LW, Halperin EC, et al., eds. *Principles and practice of radiation oncology*, 4th ed. Philadelphia: JB Lippincott, 2003:2383–2404.
19. Zetter BR. The cellular basis of site-specific tumor metastasis. *N Engl J Med* 1990;322:605–612.
20. Goblirsch MJ, Zwolak PP, Clohisy DR. Biology of bone cancer pain. *Clin Cancer Res* 2006;12:6231s–6235s.
21. Hoskin PJ, Stratford MRL, Folkes LK, et al. Effect of local radiotherapy for bone pain on urinary markers of osteoclast activity. *Lancet* 2000;355:1428–1429.
22. Schmidt GP, Schoenberg SO, Reiser MF, et al. Whole-body MR imaging of bone marrow. *Eur J Radiol* 2005;55:33–40.
23. Flickinger FW, Sanal SM. Bone marrow MRI: techniques and accuracy for detecting breast cancer metastases. *Magn Reson Imaging* 1994;12:829–835.
24. Hamaoka T, Madewell JE, Podoloff DA, et al. Bone imaging in metastatic breast cancer. *J Clin Oncol* 2004;22:2942–2953.
25. Evan-Sapr E, Mester U, Mishani E, et al. The detection of bone metastases in patients with high-risk prostate cancer: 99mTc-MDP Planar bone scintigraphy, single- and multi-field-of-view SPECT, 18F-fluoride PET, and 18F-fluoride PET/CT. *J Nucl Med* 2006;47:287–297.
26. Fujimoto R, Higashi T, Nakamoto Y, et al. Diagnostic accuracy of bone metastases detection in cancer patients: comparison between bone scintigraphy and whole-body FDG-PET. *Ann Nucl Med* 2006;20:399–408.
27. Daldrup-Link HE, Franzius C, Link TM. Whole-body MR imaging for detection of bone metastases in children and young adults: comparison with skeletal scintigraphy and FDG PET. *Am J Roentgenol* 2001;177:229–236.
28. Ohta M, Tokuda Y, Suzuki Y, et al. Whole body PET for the evaluation of bony metastases in patients with breast cancer: comparison with 99Tcm-MDP bone scintigraphy. *Nucl Med Commun* 2001;22:875–879.
29. Cleeland CS. The measurement of pain from metastatic bone disease: capturing the patient's experience. *Clin Cancer Res* 2006;12:6236s–6242s.
30. Cleeland CS, Gonin R, Hatfield AK, et al. Pain and its treatment in outpatients with metastatic cancer. *N Engl J Med* 1994;330:592–596.
31. Meuser T, Pietruck C, Radbruch L, et al. Symptoms during cancer pain treatment following WHO-guidelines: a longitudinal follow-up study of symptom prevalence, severity and etiology. *Pain* 2001;93:247–257.
32. Zech DF, Grond S, Lynch J, et al. Validation of World Health Organization guidelines for cancer pain relief: a 10-year prospective study. *Pain* 1995;63:65–76.
33. Harrington KD. Orthopaedic management of extremity and pelvic lesions. *Clin Orthop Relat Res* 1995;312:136–147.
34. Beals RK, Lawton GD, Snell WE. Prophylactic internal fixation of the femur in metastatic breast cancer. *Cancer* 1971;28:1350–1354.
35. Fidler M. Incidence of fracture through metastases in long bones. *Acta Orthop Scand* 1981;52:623–627.
36. Cheal EJ, Hipp JA, Hayes WC. Evaluation of finite element analysis for prediction of the strength reduction due to metastatic lesions in the femoral neck. *J Biomech* 1993;26:251–264.
37. Van der Linden Y, Dijkstra PD, Kroon HM, et al. Comparative analysis of risk factors for pathological fracture with femoral metastases. *J Bone Joint Surg Br* 2004;86:566–573.
38. Mirels H. Metastatic disease in long bones: a proposed scoring system for diagnosing impending pathologic fractures. *Clin Orthop Relat Res* 1989;249:256–264.
39. Nathan SS, Healey JH, Mellano D, et al. Survival in patients operated on for pathologic fractures: implication for end-of-life orthopedic care. *J Clin Oncol* 2005;23:6072–6082.
40. Sim FH, Frassica FJ, Chao EYS. Orthopaedic management using new devices and prostheses. *Clin Orthop Rel Res* 1995;312:160–172.
41. Chow E, Holden L, Danjoux C, et al. Successful salvage using percutaneous vertebroplasty in cancer patients with painful spinal metastases or osteoporotic compression fractures. *Radiother Oncol* 2004;70:265–267.
42. Hentschel SJ, Burton AW, Fourney DR, et al. Percutaneous vertebroplasty and kyphoplasty performed at a cancer center: refuting proposed contraindications. *J Neurosurg Spine* 2005;2:436–440.
43. Shimony JS, Gilula LA, Zeller AJ, et al. Percutaneous vertebroplasty for malignant compression fractures with epidural involvement. *Radiology* 2004;232:846–853.
44. Chew C, Craig L, Edwards R, et al. Safety and efficacy of percutaneous vertebroplasty in malignancy: a systematic review. *Clin Radiol* 2011;66:63–72.
45. Kassamali RH, Ganeshan A, Hoey ET, et al. Pain management in spinal metastases: the role of percutaneous vertebral augmentation. *Ann Oncol* 2011;22:782–6.
46. Qian Z, Sun Z, Gu Y, et al. Kyphoplasty for the treatment of malignant vertebral compression fractures caused by metastasis. *J Clin Neurosci* 2011;18:763–767.
47. Tancioni F, Lorenzetti MA, Navarria P, et al. Percutaneous vertebral augmentation in metastatic disease: state of the art. *J Support Oncol* 2011;9:4–10.
48. Callstrom MR, Charboneau JW. Image guided palliation of painful metastases using percutaneous ablation. *Tech Vasc Interv Radiol* 2007;10:120–131.
49. Houston SJ, Rubens RD. The systemic treatment of bone metastases. *Clin Orthop Relat Res* 1995;312:95–104.
50. Tannock IF, Osoba D, Stockler MR, et al. Chemotherapy with mitoxantrone plus prednisone or prednisone alone for symptomatic hormone-resistant prostate cancer: a Canadian randomized trial with palliative end points. *J Clin Oncol* 1996;14:1756–1764.
51. Berthold, DR, Pond, GR, Soban, F, et al. Docetaxel plus prednisone or mitoxantrone and prednisone for advanced refractory prostate cancer: updated survival in the TAX327 study. *J Clin Oncol* 2008;26:242–245.
52. Medical Research Council Prostate Cancer Working Party Investigators Group. Immediate versus deferred treatment for advanced prostatic cancer: initial results of the MRC trial. *Br J Urol* 1997;79:235–246.
53. Michaelson MD, Smith MR. Bisphosphonates for treatment and prevention of bone metastases. *J Clin Oncol* 2005;23:8219–8224.
54. Senaratne SG, Pirianov G, Mansi JL, et al. Bisphosphonates induce apoptosis in human breast cancer cell lines. *Br J Cancer* 2000;82:1459–1468.
55. Green JR. Bisphosphonates: preclinical review. *Oncologist* 2004;9(Suppl):3–13.
56. Russell RG, Rogers MJ, Frith JC, et al. The pharmacology of bisphosphonates and new insights into their mechanisms of action. *J Bone Miner Res* 1999;14(Suppl 2):53–65.
57. Theriault RL, Lipton A, Hortobagyi GN, et al. Pamidronate reduces skeletal morbidity in women with advanced breast cancer and lytic bone lesions: a randomized, placebo-controlled trial. Protocol 18 Aredia Breast Cancer Study Group. *J Clin Oncol* 1999;17:8464–8454.
58. Hortobagyi GN, Theriault RL, Porter L. Efficacy of pamidronate in reducing skeletal complications in patients with breast cancer and lytic bone metastases. Protocol 19 Aredia Breast Cancer Study Group. *N Engl J Med* 1996;335:1785–1791.
59. Rosen LS, Gordon L, Tchekmedyian NS, et al. Long-term efficacy and safety of zoledronic acid in the treatment of skeletal metastases in patients with nonsmall cell lung carcinoma and other solid tumors: a randomized, phase III, double-blind, placebo-controlled trial. *Cancer* 2004;100:2613–2621.
60. Dearnaley DP, Mason, MD, Parmar, MK, et al. Adjuvant therapy with oral sodium clodronate in locally advanced and metastatic prostate cancer: long-term overall survival results from the MRC PRO4 and PRO5 randomized controlled trials. *Lancet Oncol* 2009;10:872–876.
61. Mehrotra B, Ruggiero S. Bisphosphonate complications including osteonecrosis of the jaw. *Hematology* 2006;1:356–360.
62. Migliorati CA, Siegel MA, Elting LS. Bisphosphonate-associated osteonecrosis: a long-term complication of bisphosphonate treatment. *Lancet Oncol* 2006;7:508–514.
63. Lipton A, Goessl C. Clinical development of anti-RANKL therapies for treatment and prevention of bone metastases. *Bone* 2011;48:96–99.
64. Fizazi K, Carducci M, Smith M, et al. Denusomab compared with zoledronic acid for treatment of bone metastases in men with castration-resistant prostate cancer: a randomized, double-blind study. *Lancet* 2011;377:813–822.
65. Stopeck AT, Lipton A, Body JJ, et al. Denusomab compared with zoledronic acid for the treatment of bone metastases in patients with advanced breast cancer: a randomized, double-blind study. *J Clin Oncol* 2010;28:5132–5139.
66. Wu JS, Wong R, Johnston M, et al. Meta-analysis of dose-fractionation radiotherapy trials for the palliation of painful bone metastases. *Int J Radiat Oncol Biol Phys* 2003;55:594–605.
67. Caissie A, Zeng L, Nguyen J, et al. Assessment of health-related quality of life with European Organization for Research and Treatment of Cancer QLQ-C15-PAL after palliative radiotherapy of bone metastases. *Clin Oncol (R Coll Radiol)* 2012;24:125–133.
68. Lutz S, Berk L, Chang E, et al. Palliative radiotherapy for bone metastases: an ASTRO evidence-based guideline. *Int J Radiat Oncol Biol Phys* 2011;79:965–976.
69. Tong D, Gillick L, Hendrickson FR. The palliation of symptomatic osseous metastases: final results of the study by the Radiation Therapy Oncology Group. *Cancer* 1982;50:893–899.
70. Blitzer P. Reanalysis of the RTOG study of the palliation of symptomatic osseous metastasis. *Cancer* 1985;55:1468–1472.
71. Bone Pain Trial Working Party. 8 Gy single fraction radiotherapy for the treatment of metastatic skeletal pain: randomised comparison with a multifraction schedule over 12 months of patient follow-up. *Radiother Oncol* 1999;52:111–121.
72. Foro Arnalot P, Fontanals AV, Galcerán JC. Randomized clinical trial with two palliative radiotherapy regimens in painful bone metastases: 30 Gy in 10 fractions compared to 8 Gy in single fraction. *Radiother Oncol* 2008;89:150–155.
73. Gaze MN, Kelly CG, Kerr GR, et al. Pain relief and quality of life following radiotherapy for bone metastases: a randomized trial of two fractionation schedules. *Radiother Oncol* 1997;45:109–116.
74. Hartsell WF, Scott CB, Bruner DW, et al. Randomized trial of short-versus long-course radiotherapy for palliation of painful bone metastases. *J Natl Cancer Inst* 2005;97:798–804.
75. Hirokawa Y, Wadasaki K, Kashiwado K, et al. A multiinstitutional prospective randomized study of radiation therapy of bone metastases [in Japanese]. *Nippon Igaku Hoshasen Gakkai Zasshi* 1988;48:1425–1431.
76. Kaasa S, Brenne E, Lund JA, et al. Prospective randomized multicenter trial on single fraction radiotherapy (8 Gy × 1) versus multiple fractions (3 Gy × 10) in the treatment of painful bone metastases. *Radiother Oncol* 2006;79:278–284.
77. Kirkbride P, Warde RR, Panzarella T, et al. A randomized trial comparing the efficacy of a single radiation fraction with fractionated radiation therapy in the palliation of skeletal metastases. *Int J Radiat Oncol Biol Phys* 2000;48(Suppl 1]):185.
78. Koswig S, Budach V. Remineralization and pain relief in bone metastases after different radiotherapy fractions (10 time 3 Gy vs 1 time 8 Gy). A prospective study. *Strahlenther Onkol* 1999;175:500–508.
79. Madsen EL. Painful bone metastasis: Efficacy of radiotherapy assessed by the patients—a randomized trial comparing 4 Gy × 6 versus 10 Gy × 2. *Int J Radiat Oncol Biol Phys* 1983;9:1775–1779.
80. Nielsen OS, Bentzen SM, Sandberg E, et al. Randomized trial of single dose versus fractionated palliative radiotherapy of bone metastases. *Radiother Oncol* 1998;47:233–240.
81. Niewald M, Tkocz HJ, Abel U, et al. Rapid course radiation therapy vs. more standard treatment: a randomized trial for bone metastases. *Int J Radiat Oncol Biol Phys* 1996;36:1085–1089.
82. Rasmusson B, Vejborg I, Jensen AB, et al. Irradiation of bone metastases in breast cancer patients: a randomized study with 1 year follow-up. *Radiother Oncol* 1995;34:179–184.
83. Steenland E, Leer JW, van Houwelingen H, et al. The effect of a single fraction compared to multiple fractions on painful bone metastases: a global analysis of the Dutch Bone Metastases Study. *Radiother Oncol* 1999;52:101–109.
84. Hoskin PJ, Price P, Easton D, et al. A prospective randomized trial of 4 Gy or 8 Gy single doses in the treatment of metastatic bone pain. *Radiother Oncol* 1992;23:74–78.
85. Jeremic B, Shibamoto Y, Acimovic L, et al. A randomized trial of three single-dose radiation therapy regimens in the treatment of metastatic bone pain. *Int J Radiat Oncol Biol Phys* 1998;42:161–167.
86. Konski A, DeSilvio M, Hartsell W, et al. Continuing evidence for poorer treatment outcomes for single male patients: retreatment data from RTOG 97 14. *Int J Radiat Oncol Biol Phys* 2006;66:229–233.
87. Dennis K, Wong K, Zhang L, et al. Palliative radiotherapy for bone metastases in the last 3 months of life: worthwhile or futile? *Clin Oncol (R Coll Radiol)* 2011;23:709–715.
88. Meeuse JJ, van der Linden YM, van Tienhoven G, et al. Efficacy of radiotherapy for painful bone metastases during the last 12 weeks of life: results from the Dutch Bone Metastasis Study. *Cancer* 2010;116:2716–2725.
89. Loblaw DA, Wu JS, Kirkbride P, et al. Pain flare in patients with bone metastases after palliative radiotherapy—a nested randomized control trial. *Support Care Cancer* 2007;15:451–455.
90. Gerszten PC, Burton SA, Ozhasoglu C, et al. Radiosurgery for spinal metastases: clinical experience of 500 cases from a single institution. *Spine* 2007;15:193–199.

91. Vassiliou V, Kalogeropoulou G, Christopoulos C, et al. Combination ibandronate and radiotherapy for the treatment of bone metastases: clinical evaluation and radiographic assessment. *Int J Radiat Oncol Biol Phys* 2007;67:264–272.
92. Kouloulias V, Matsopoulos G, Kouvaris J, et al. Radiotherapy in conjunction with intravenous infusion of 180 mg of disodium pamidronate in management of osteolytic metastases from breast cancer: clinical evaluation, biochemical markers, quality of life, and monitoring of recalcification using assessments of gray-level histogram in plain radiographs. *Int J Radiat Oncol Biol Phys* 2003;57:143–157.
93. Salazar OM, Rubin P, Hendrickson F, et al. Single dose half-body irradiation for palliation of multiple bone metastases from solid tumors: final Radiation Therapy Oncology Group Report. *Cancer* 1986;58:29–36.
94. Poulter C, Cosmatos D, Rubin P, et al. A report of RTOG 82-06: a phase III study of whether the addition of single dose hemibody irradiation is more effective than local field irradiation alone in the treatment of symptomatic osseous metastases. *Int Radiat Oncol Biol Phys* 1992;23:207–214.
95. Salazar OM, Sandhu T, da Motta NW, et al. Fractionated half-body irradiation (HBI) for the rapid palliation of widespread, symptomatic, metastatic bone disease: a randomized phase III trial of the International Atomic Energy Agency (IAEA). *Int J Radiat Oncol Biol Phys* 2001;50:765–775.
96. Scarantino CW, Caplan R, Rotman M, et al. A phase I/II study to evaluate the effect of fractionated hemibody irradiation in the treatment of osseous metastases—RTOG 88-22. *Int J Radiat Oncol Biol Phys* 1996;36:37–48.
97. Scarantino C, Omitz, RD, Hoffman LG, et al. On the mechanism of radiation induced emesis: the role of serotonin. *Int J Radiat Oncol Biol Phys* 1994;30: 825–830.
98. Sarin R, Budrukkar A. Efficacy, toxicity and cost-effectiveness of single-dose versus fractionated hemibody irradiation (HBI) [Letter]. *Int J Radiat Oncol Biol Phys* 2002;52:1146.
99. Bauman G, Charette M, Reid R, et al. Radiopharmaceuticals for the palliation of painful bone metastasis—a systemic review. *Radiother Oncol* 2005;75:258–270.
100. Siegel HJ, Luck JV Jr, Siegel ME. Advances in radionuclide therapeutics in orthopaedics. *J Am Acad Orthop Surg* 2004;12:55–64.
101. Serafini AN, Houston SJ, Resche I, et al. Palliation of pain associated with metastatic bone cancer using samarium-153 lexidronam: a double-blind placebo controlled clinical trial. *J Clin Oncol* 1998;16:1574–1581.
102. Porter AT, McEwan AJ. Strontium-89 as an adjuvant to external beam radiation improves pain relief and delays disease progression in advanced prostate cancer: results of a randomized controlled trial. *Semin Oncol* 1993;20: 38–43.
103. Smeland S, Erikstein B, Aas M, et al. Role of strontium-89 as adjuvant to palliative external beam radiotherapy is questionable: results of a double-blind randomized study. *Int J Radiat Oncol Biol Phys* 2003;56:1397–1404.
104. Quilty PM, Kirk D, Bolger JJ, et al. A comparison of the palliative effects of strontium-89 and external beam radiotherapy in metastatic prostate cancer. *Radiother Oncol* 1994;31:33–40.
105. Oosterhof GON, Roberts JT, De Reijke T, et al. Strontium89 chloride versus palliative local field radiotherapy in patients with hormonal escaped prostate cancer: a phase III study of the European organisation for research and treatment of cancer genitourinary group. *Eur Urol* 2003;44:519–526.
106. Sciuto R, Festa A, Rea S, et al. Effects of low-dose cisplatin on 89Sr therapy for painful bone metastases from prostate cancer: a randomized clinical trial. *J Nucl Med* 2002;43:79–86.
107. Tu S-M, Delpassand ES, Jones D, et al. Strontium-89 combined with doxorubicin in the treatment of patients with androgen independent prostate cancer. *Urol Oncol* 1996;2:191–197.
108. McEwan AJ, Amyotte GA, McGowan DG, et al. A retrospective analysis of the cost effectiveness of treatment with Metastron (89Sr-chloride) in patients with prostate cancer metastatic to bone. *Nucl Med Commun* 1994;15:499–504.
109. Collins C, Eary JF, Donaldson G, et al. Samarium-153-EDTMP in bone metastases of hormone refractory prostate carcinoma: a phase I/II trial. *J Nucl Med* 1993; 34:1839–1844.
110. Olea E, Riccabona G, Tian J, et al. Efficacy and toxicity of 153Sm EDTMP in the palliative treatment of painful skeleton metastases: results of an IAEA international multicenter study [Abstract]. *J Nucl Med* 2000;51:146P.
111. Resche I, Chatal JF, Pecking A, et al. A dose-controlled study of 153Sm-ethylenediaminetetramethylenephosphonate (EDTMP) in the treatment of patients with painful bone metastases. *Eur J Cancer* 1997;33:1583–1591.
112. Sartor O, Quick D, Reid R, et al. A double blind placebo controlled study of 153samarium-EDTMP for palliation of bone pain in patients with hormone-refractory prostate cancer [Abstract]. *J Urol* 1997;157:321.
113. Tian JH, Zhang JM, Hou QT, et al. Multicentre trial on the efficacy and toxicity of single-dose samarium-153-ethylene diamine tetramethylene phosphonate as a palliative treatment for painful skeletal metastases in China. *Eur J Nucl Med* 1999;26:2–7.

Chapter 95

Palliation of Visceral Recurrences and Metastases and Treatment of Oligometastatic Disease

Ramji R. Rajendran, Siavash Jabbari, and William F. Hartsell

The 5-year survival and overall cure rates for many cancers have significantly improved over the past 40 years. Unfortunately, there is still a substantial minority of patients who develop recurrent or metastatic disease. The most common sites of metastatic disease are bones, brain, lungs, and liver. In addition, there are other visceral sites of recurrence or metastatic disease that may cause significant symptoms. Palliative radiation therapy for treatment of bone and brain metastases is well established, with multiple randomized prospective trials evaluating best treatment practices. However, there is less information on treatment of visceral metastases, although radiation oncologists recognize that radiation therapy is frequently effective at palliating symptoms from visceral metastases.

The specific goals of treatment will depend on the symptoms, treatment site, functional status of the patient, and other patient-specific factors. The indications for treatment may include pain, visceral obstruction, bleeding, or other symptoms that negatively impact the quality of life. In general, this treatment is given with the goal of improving the quality of life, not the quantity of life. For some disease sites, this can be done with a very short course, low-dose treatment. For other sites, this will require higher doses given to control the local disease.

Some visceral metastases will cause pain. For example, liver or adrenal metastases may cause significant pain. Splenic metastases from hematologic metastases may cause abdominal pain, early satiety, and abdominal distention. In contrast, pulmonary metastases rarely cause pain. These lesions may cause airway obstruction or hemoptysis. Metastatic lesions in the gastrointestinal system may cause bleeding or obstructive symptoms (esophageal obstruction, gastric outlet obstruction, gastric bleeding, biliary obstruction, rectal obstruction). In addition to rectal obstruction, pelvic masses may cause bleeding (vaginal, bladder, or rectal), ureteral obstruction, or pain from involvement of the sacrum or sacral nerves.

There has been a revolution in the understanding of the metastatic process in the past decade. Traditionally in solid tumor biology, cancer cells are thought to undergo some genetic change that potentiates them to grow into tumors and cause daughter cells to spread through the lymphatic or circulatory system to lymph nodes and distant sites. However, recent understanding of the epithelial–mesenchymal transition demonstrates that cancer cells develop embryonic stem cell–like properties that allow them to disseminate to distant sites. The microenvironment surrounding the primary tumor and metastatic sites can regulate the metastatic process. In addition, metastasis occurs much earlier than clinical detection of lymphadenopathy and radiographic or symptomatic evidence of the development of distant visceral disease.[1] Treatment of visceral metastases in the oligometastatic setting may allow for improved palliation and may also improve the overall survival in carefully selected patients.

MALIGNANT LOWER AIRWAY OBSTRUCTION

The lower airway is generally defined as being below the first tracheal ring. Upper airway obstructions can be emergently treated with a tracheostomy. The lower airway can become compromised from either primary or metastatic malignancy. Patients may have intrinsic compression caused by an endobronchial tumor or extrinsic airway compression by a tumor

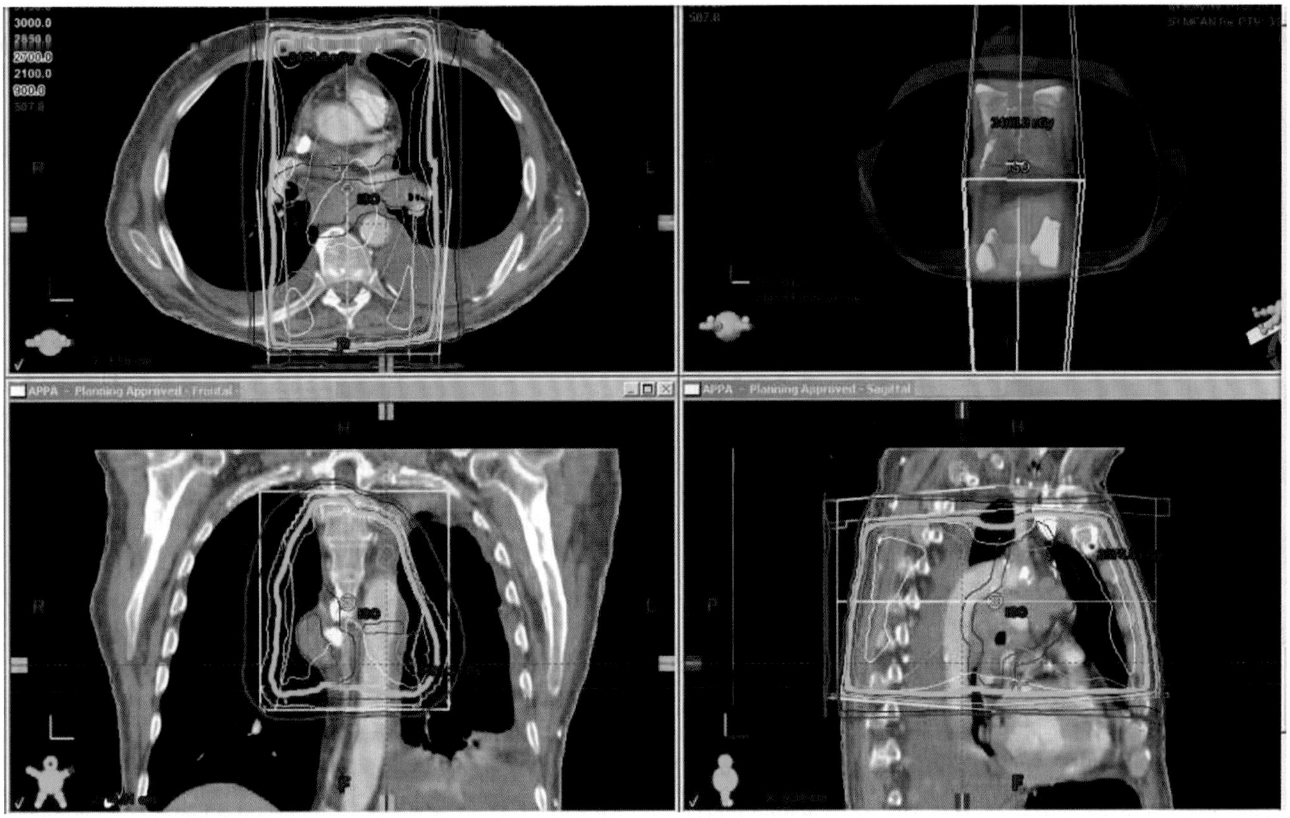

FIGURE 95.1. Digitally reconstructed images from computed tomography simulation, showing axial, sagittal, coronal, and three-dimensional representations of a palliative lung treatment field. This treatment field is in a patient with hemoptysis from central airway involvement as well as superior vena caval compression.

mass in the lung parenchyma or bulky lymphadenopathy during the course of their illness. Clinical symptoms, bronchoscopy, and radiographic imaging are used to determine the extent of luminal obstruction. It is important to determine whether the airway obstruction is endobronchial or from external compression of the airway in order to select the most appropriate treatment. For intrinsic compression of a tumor mass growing inside the bronchial lumen, interventional bronchoscopy techniques offer immediate benefit in many patients. These interventional techniques can result in relief of dyspnea, decreased risk of postobstructive pneumonia, and improved functional status.[2–4] Either laser resection of tumor or endobronchial stent placement, along with radiation therapy, is effective in maintaining the patency of the lower airway.[5,6] The additional treatment of the airway can be given with either external-beam radiation therapy, endobronchial brachytherapy, or photodynamic therapy. Brachytherapy is typically the best option in patients who have recurred after prior external-beam radiation therapy. For endobronchial therapy, the recommended doses are 7.5 Gy × 3 or 10 Gy × 2.[7]

External-beam radiation therapy is typically used for treatment of airway compromise caused by extrinsic compression of a bronchus. Endobronchial brachytherapy typically does not improve symptoms when there is external compression of the airways.[8,9] The highest doses from brachytherapy will be given to the (relatively) normal mucosa of the airway, with a much lower dose to the extrinsic tumor that is causing the compression.

There is no standard fractionation scheme or total dose for palliative external-beam treatment for lung cancer. A review by Fairchild et al.[10] found the best results, in terms of palliation of symptoms, with relatively high doses of radiation therapy: 3 Gy per fraction to a total of 30 to 45 Gy, or 2 Gy per fraction to 50 to 60 Gy. The trade-off is that there is a higher rate of acute esophagitis with these higher doses. The American Society for Radiation Oncology clinical practice guideline consensus statement recommends doses equivalent to 30 Gy in 10 fractions or greater.[11] For patients with a poor performance status or who have difficulty traveling for multiple treatments, shorter fractionation schemes such as 20 Gy in 5 fractions can be used. Very short regimens (17 Gy in 2 fractions or 10 Gy in 1 fraction) may be useful in certain situations; however, there are reports of radiation myelopathy with these regimens (17 Gy in 2 fractions).[11] Figure 95.1 demonstrates an example of a digitally reconstructed radiograph of a palliative lung treatment field. The major acute side effect from this treatment is dysphagia, but careful attention should be made to limit normal lung tissue.

In most patients who receive radiation therapy for palliation of pulmonary symptoms, there is no benefit to the addition of chemotherapy. Combined chemotherapy and radiation therapy may improve response rates slightly, but with significantly greater acute toxicity.[11]

LIVER METASTASES

The liver is a common metastatic site. It is the most frequent site of distant metastatic disease from gastrointestinal tumors, especially colorectal, but also including esophageal, stomach, and pancreatic cancers. The liver is also a frequent site of metastases from lung cancer, breast cancer, and melanoma. A patient with liver metastases may have symptoms of anorexia or early satiety, weight loss, nausea, right upper quadrant or epigastric pain, jaundice, and fever.

For patients with few metastatic lesions in the liver and no evidence of extrahepatic metastases, 12% to 36% may be cured with surgical resection.[12] The risk factors associated with the best outcome are clear resection margins, low levels of carcinoembryonic antigen, a single metastatic deposit, metachronous presentation of the liver metastasis, and node-negative disease (with the original primary).[12] There are multiple other treatments that can be used for patients with one or a few hepatic metastases, including radiofrequency ablation, microwave coagulation therapy, transarterial chemoembolization, and stereotactic body radiotherapy.[13]

Most patients with liver metastases are found to have multiple lesions, extrahepatic disease, or other risk factors that make them unsuitable for these surgical or interventional procedures. It is common for these patients to undergo multiple courses of systemic therapy prior to being seen and evaluated by a radiation oncologist. For many years, the only viable chemotherapy option for metastatic gastrointestinal tumors was 5-fluorouracil, often given in combination with leucovorin. More recently, multiple drug regimens including oxaliplatin or irinotecan have significantly improved the response rates and increased the median duration of survival. Targeted agents such as cetuximab or bevacizumab may improve the response rates even further. These new combinations have changed the goal of treatment from palliation to prolonging survival; with this new paradigm, the multiple drug regimens are given as neoadjuvant therapy with the goal of downsizing tumor bulk in order to facilitate a resection.[14] Hepatic arterial infusion of chemotherapy gives higher local concentrations of the chemotherapy agents and also gives higher response rates. A meta-analysis of hepatic arterial infusion chemotherapy for liver metastases demonstrated a significantly higher response rate but showed no improvement in survival duration.[15]

The group of patients who are referred to a radiation oncologist for palliation of liver metastases tend to be the patients who have more medical comorbidities, a greater tumor burden, and who have been previously treated with multiple other therapies. Despite these poor prognostic factors, radiation therapy can be effective in palliating symptoms (Fig. 95.2).[16]

Palliative treatment of the liver is limited by radiation-induced liver toxicity (RILD). This toxicity becomes apparent 1 week to 3 months after treatment and may result in liver failure and death.[17] Both dose and volume of liver irradiated are important in avoiding RILD. For treatment of the whole liver, the threshold for RILD is approximately 30 Gy in 2 Gy fractions or 33 Gy in 1.5 Gy twice daily fractions.[18,19] The Radiation Therapy Oncology Group's trial RTOG-7605 evaluated multiple regimens in patients with multiple liver metastases: 30 Gy in 15 fractions, 25.6 Gy in 16 fractions, 20 Gy in 10 fractions, and 21 Gy in 7 fractions.[20] Improvement in symptoms was seen in 55% of the patients, with no difference among the four treatment regimens. A subsequent RTOG trial evaluated whole-liver radiation therapy with a dose of 21 Gy in 7 fractions; patients were randomized to receive the radiation alone or with the addition of misonidazole to the radiation.[21] There was minimal toxicity and a rapid symptomatic response in the majority of patients. Complete pain relief was reported in 54% of the patients, and 80% of the patients noted an improvement in pain following treatment. Overall, there was no significant benefit with the addition of misonidazole. The best response rates were seen in patients with colorectal primaries. Bydder et al.[22] reported on a series of 28 patients treated with a hypofractionated regimen of 10 Gy in 2 fractions to the whole liver. The overall response rate was 54%, with two patients experiencing grade 3 toxicity (emesis and diarrhea).

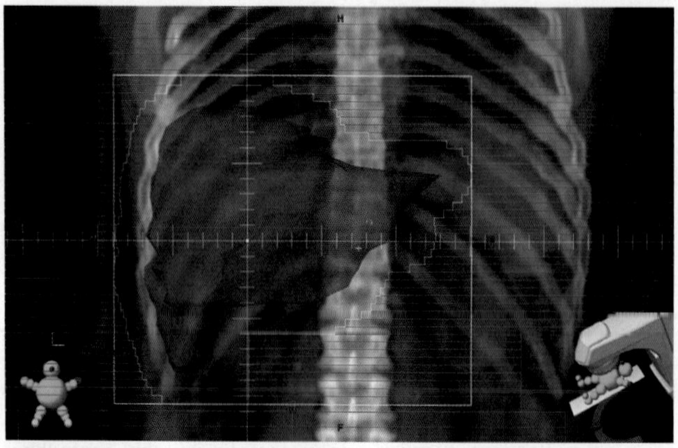

FIGURE 95.2. Digitally reconstructed image from computed tomography simulation. The field covers the whole liver volume in a patient with multiple liver metastases from a metastatic rectal cancer.

Selective internal radiation therapy (SIRT) is another option for patients with diffuse liver metastases. This technique involves the use yttrium-90 (^{90}Y) glass or resin microspheres that are given through intra-arterial infusions into the liver. A phase III trial of patients with liver metastases from colorectal cancer evaluated intra-arterial floxuridine alone compared to intra-arterial floxuridine plus SIRT with ^{90}Y resin microspheres.[23] The patients who received SIRT had a significantly better overall response rate, time-to-tumor progression, and overall survival. The addition of SIRT did not increase grade 3 or 4 toxicity.

In summary, patients with multiple symptomatic liver metastases may be palliated by whole-liver radiation therapy. Relatively low doses of 21 Gy in 7 fractions or 30 Gy in 15 fractions are generally well tolerated and provide symptomatic relief for the majority of patients.[16,21]

BILIARY OBSTRUCTION

Malignant biliary obstruction may be caused either by a tumor mass causing extrinsic compression or intrinsic compression from tumor progression within the bile duct lumen. This obstruction can lead to hyperbilirubinemia and jaundice, which can cause pruritus, anorexia, and weight loss. The biliary obstruction may be a life-threatening emergency. Emergent drainage of the bile duct is achieved initially by external stent. These stents are later converted to internal endoprostheses; however, these catheters typically only remain patent for 4 to 8 months.[24] The patency of these stents can be extended with the use of intraluminal brachytherapy, photodynamic therapy, or external-beam radiation therapy. Intraluminal brachytherapy extends stent patency and lengthens survival duration in patients with inoperable cholangiocarcinoma.[25,26] Although there are few data specifically for the use of external-beam radiation therapy for palliative treatment of metastatic biliary obstruction, it may be of benefit especially for treatment of extrinsic bile duct compression by a tumor mass.

PAINFUL ADRENAL METASTASES

The adrenal glands are a common site of metastatic disease from many types of cancer, primarily due to the rich blood supply of the adrenal gland. Lung cancer is the most common source of adrenal metastases. These metastases are frequently asymptomatic, but occasionally may cause pain. For patients with a good performance status and few sites of metastatic disease, surgical management may be appropriate. Radiation therapy is also appropriate for palliative treatment.

Palliative radiotherapy typically has been given with conventional external-beam techniques. Soffen et al.[27] reported the results in 16 patients with painful adrenal metastases treated with palliative radiation therapy. The majority of the patients received 30 Gy in 10 to 12 treatments. A response was seen in 12 of 16 patients (75%), with 6 of those patients having complete response for the duration of their survival. Nearly half of the patients (44%) experienced nausea, which may have been related to the technique of treatment with anterior and posterior fields. No late toxicity was seen, but the median survival was only 3 months. There are multiple recent reports evaluating the use of intensity-modulated radiation therapy techniques or stereotactic body radiation therapy techniques for treatment of adrenal metastases. Most of these patients were treated for

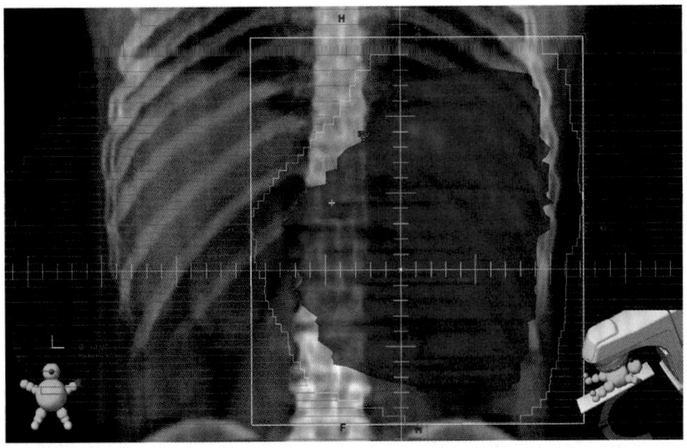

FIGURE 95.3. Digitally reconstructed rendering of an anterior-posterior treatment field of the spleen. Splenomegaly may respond rapidly to low doses of radiation therapy. The fields should be checked clinically on a frequent basis to determine if the blocks or multileaf collimators need to be adjusted.

asymptomatic adrenal metastases, rather than for palliation of symptoms. These treatments appear to provide a high rate of local control, and may be appropriate for patients with limited volume disease (oligometastases). In the palliative setting, there is a benefit with a dose of 30 Gy in 10 to 12 treatments using conventional techniques.

SPLENIC METASTASES

It is relatively uncommon for solid tumors to metastasize to the spleen. Splenomegaly is more often associated with hematologic malignancies and disorders such as leukemia or myeloproliferative diseases. The spleen can become massively enlarged, causing pain, early satiety, nausea, or emesis. These symptoms may also occur when the spleen is enlarged because of extramedullary hematopoiesis due to marrow failure.[28]

Treatment with radiation therapy can be very effective at reducing the size of the spleen and palliating the other symptoms associated with splenomegaly. The doses required for palliation of symptoms are much lower than the doses typically used for palliation of other visceral metastases. The response may be quite rapid as well, which necessitates evaluation of the field sizes on a frequent basis (Fig. 95.3). The regimens frequently used include doses of 0.25 to 1 Gy given 2 to 3 times per week. It is important to evaluate blood counts on a frequent basis, since anemia and thrombocytopenia may occur rapidly with precipitous drops in the counts over a very short period. A typical regimen is the one reported by McFarland et al.[29] Their patients were treated twice-weekly beginning at 0.5 Gy per fraction the first week, increasing to 0.75 Gy per fraction in the second week and 1 Gy per fraction on the third week. A complete blood count was obtained prior to each treatment. The total dose was typically <5 Gy. Even with these low doses, 14 of 16 patients had subjective improvement in their symptoms, and 12 of 16 patients had objective decrease in the splenomegaly. Treatment of the spleen may cause an abscopal effect as well, with decrease in size of involved lymph nodes distant to the treated spleen.[29]

VAGINAL BLEEDING OR DISCHARGE

Vaginal bleeding is a common symptom at diagnosis in several gynecologic tumors, especially cervical, uterine, and vaginal tumors.[30] The initial treatment should be with vaginal packing.[31] Radiation therapy is also effective at controlling this type vaginal bleeding. A hypofractionated treatment course is typically used, usually with 2.5 to 4 Gy per fraction. A typical course of treatment would be 30 Gy in 10 fractions.[30] Often, the bleeding will slow or stop after 3 to 5 treatments. The treatment can be continued to definitive doses at that point, using more standard fractionation of 1.8 to 2.0 Gy per fraction (Fig. 95.4) An alternative method of palliating bleeding and vaginal discharge is to use a single large fraction of 10 Gy.[32–34] This will result in a high likelihood of reducing or stopping the bleeding, often within 24 to 48 hours of the first dose. This dose of 10 Gy can be repeated at 1-month intervals. The risk of complications increases when this dose is repeated a third or fourth time, so this should be limited to one to two fractions.[35]

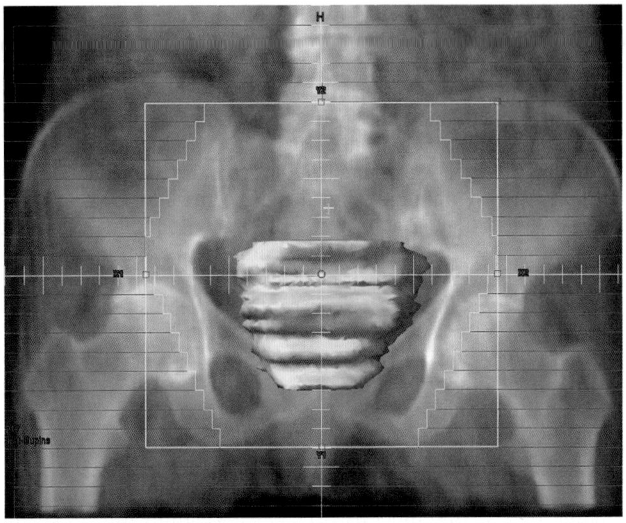

FIGURE 95.4. Digitally reconstructed anterior-posterior radiograph of a palliative pelvic field. This palliative field arrangement would be appropriate to treat a patient with hemorrhage from a cervical or bladder cancer.

PELVIC RECURRENCE

Recurrent pelvic malignancies may cause significant symptoms, including pain, bleeding, or obstruction. The choice of the appropriate palliative treatment depends on multiple factors, including the type and amount of prior treatment. In contrast to palliative treatment of other sites of recurrent disease, aggressive combined modality treatment may provide the best chance of palliation of symptoms for recurrent pelvic malignancies.

Recurrent colorectal cancer may cause life-threatening problems from bowel obstruction. For most patients in this circumstance, surgical intervention is the most appropriate treatment. This may involve complete surgical removal of the disease, if possible, or a diverting colostomy to alleviate the symptoms of obstruction.[36] There is a high risk of perioperative complications in this group of patients, primarily because it is frequently difficult to perform an adequate bowel preparation prior to surgery.

Hydronephrosis and severe pain may be signs of a more advanced tumor and are relative contraindications to surgical resection.[37] The majority of patients with recurrent rectal cancers have posterior or posterolateral involvement of the pelvis, which makes surgery more difficult.[38] The presence of severe pain may indicate invasion of the sacrum or sacral nerve roots. Tumors that invade these structures are more difficult to resect completely. Melton et al.[39] and Wells et al.[40] reported that patients who underwent an aggressive surgical resection of locally recurrent rectal cancers had a high risk of significant complications. Patients who had sacral resection as part of the surgical treatment had a 42% risk of significant complications.[40]

Patients with bulky pelvic recurrences who have not previously received radiation therapy are appropriate candidates for combined chemotherapy and radiation therapy. A prospective randomized Danish trial evaluated radiation therapy alone (50 Gy in 25 fractions, with a boost of 10 to 20 Gy in 5 to 10 fractions) compared with the same radiation therapy with concomitant weekly bolus dose of 5-fluorouracil.[41] This treatment was given to patients with locally recurrent or inoperable rectal cancers. There was no improvement in survival with the addition of chemotherapy, but there was a higher rate of acute complications (33% with chemotherapy vs. 13% with radiation alone). In several retrospective studies, the addition of chemotherapy was beneficial. Ito et al.[42] reported on 30 patients with symptomatic intrapelvic recurrent rectal cancers. They noted a higher pain relief rate in the patients receiving chemotherapy (100% vs. 77% for radiation alone) and a near doubling of the median survival time (7.8 vs. 4 months). For these patients with locally recurrent rectal cancers, combined modality therapy is usually recommended to improve the likelihood of local control.

Relatively high doses of radiation therapy are required for palliation of symptoms. A review by Wong et al.[43] showed that total dose was important in achieving a response, with the highest responses seen in patients receiving ≥50 Gy. In their series, the patients with the best prognostic factors received higher doses, but the dose–response relationship was still predictive of local control and survival in a multi-variate analysis. Bae et al.[44] also found improvement in the rate and duration of symptom control in patients who received higher doses. They recommended a biologic effective dose >40 Gy_{10} when possible.

Patients who have received prior irradiation and subsequently develop locally recurrent rectal cancer are frequently treated with surgery, chemotherapy, or a combination of the two. However, there are circumstances in which additional radiation therapy may be beneficial. The radiation therapy may be given as hyperfractionated external-beam radiation, intraoperative radiation therapy (IORT), or brachytherapy. Lingareddy et al.[45] utilized hyperfractionation with 1.2 Gy twice a day to a median dose of 30.6 Gy for reirradiation of patients with locally recurrent rectal cancer; these patients had received full-dose pelvic radiation therapy as part of their initial treatment. They used limited fields for the reirradiation, excluding the bladder and small bowels. Most of the patients (90%) received concurrent 5-fluorouracil chemotherapy. There was improvement in pain in 65% of these patients and cessation of bleeding in 100%. The late toxicity of treatment was significantly lower in patients who received hyperfractionated treatment compared to single daily treatments (18% vs. 47%). The most frequent late toxicities were small bowel obstruction (17%) and fistula formation (8%). An Italian prospective study evaluated patients with recurrent rectal cancer who had previously received radiation therapy.[46] Patients with biopsy-proven recurrent disease were given preoperative combined modality treatment, with hyperfractionated radiation therapy (30.6 Gy using 1.2 Gy twice a day, followed by a 10.8 Gy boost also with 1.2 Gy twice a day) and continuous infusion 5-fluorouracil. The patients were then evaluated for resection, and surgery was performed at 4 to 6 weeks following the chemoradiotherapy, when feasible. Fifty-one (86%) of the patients completed the preoperative treatment as planned, and 30 (50.8%) underwent resection. The overall median survival was 42 months, and the 5-year survival was 39%. Seven patients had late grade 3 toxicity, and there were no grade 4 toxicities.

Intraoperative radiation therapy may be useful in some patients with locally recurrent rectal cancer. The patients who may benefit from this treatment are those with locally advanced recurrent rectal cancer who have no evidence of metastatic disease. Haddock et al.[47] reported on a series of 51 previously irradiated patients with recurrent rectal cancer who underwent maximal resection followed by intraoperative radiation therapy using electrons. The dose given was 10 to 30 Gy, with a median of 20 Gy. Thirty-seven patients received additional external-beam radiation therapy (median 25.2 Gy) following the surgery and IORT. The 2-year survival rate was 48%, but the 5-year survival rate was only 12%. The local control rate was 60% at 2 years, with a trend toward better local control in patients who received ≥30 Gy external-beam treatment in addition to the IORT (81% local control vs. 54% for those who received no external-beam treatment or doses <30 Gy). The toxicity included peripheral neuropathy in 32% of patients and ureteral narrowing or obstruction in 14%.

Brachytherapy is another alternative method to deliver radiation dose to a relatively limited volume. Alektiar et al.[48] reported on 74 patients with locally recurrent colorectal cancers. The patients underwent surgical resection of the recurrence, followed by high-dose-rate intraoperative brachytherapy, with doses of 10 to 18 Gy. The 5-year overall survival rate was 23% with a 5-year local control rate of 39%. The primary toxicity was peripheral neuropathy, which occurred in 16% of the patients. Patients with negative margins of resection had a higher likelihood of local control compared to those who had positive margins (43% vs. 28%). Kolotas et al.[49] evaluated palliative interstitial high-dose-rate brachytherapy in a group of 38 patients. Only four of the patients had the catheters implanted intraoperatively; most were placed using computed tomography guidance, with the catheters implanted through the perineum or sacrum. This group of patients had bulky disease at the time of implant. The median survival was 15 months following brachytherapy, with most deaths caused by distant metastases. There was stable disease in 28 of 38 patients, with pain relief in 89.5% of patients.

In summary, palliative radiation therapy is effective in reducing pain or bleeding from recurrent pelvic malignancies. Because of the location and nature of pelvic recurrences, combined modality treatment with chemotherapy, radiation therapy, and surgery may be needed. Relatively high doses of radiation may also be needed to provide the palliative benefits of treatment.

RADIATION THERAPY IN THE SETTING OF OLIGOMETASTATIC DISEASE

As reviewed in the preceding sections, the radiotherapeutic management of metastatic disease has historically been limited to palliation, typically utilizing relatively low overall doses and abbreviated treatment schedules. The goal of this approach has been to provide short- to moderate-term palliation, while limiting treatment-related toxicity and minimizing duration of therapy. Until recently, this paradigm has been generalized to nearly all patients staged as metastatic, with an essentially uniform treatment strategy applied to a widely heterogenous group of patients, presentations, and disease biology. The paradigm shift of "curative" local therapy, including radiation therapy for select presentations of "oligometastatic" disease, was first proposed by Weichselbaum and Hellman[50] in a 1995 editorial. According to this concept, select patients with controlled locoregional disease and a limited number of metastatic sites may theoretically be cured with definitive local therapy, especially in the setting of effective systemic therapy. During the era of Weichselbaum and Hellman's writing, limitations in radiotherapy technique precluded effective ablation of most sites of oligometastatic disease without significant toxicity. Furthermore, available systemic therapy was largely ineffective in eliminating microscopic systemic disease. However, interval advances in highly conformal image-guided radiotherapy and the increased efficacy of systemic and molecular therapies have allowed for the translation of this theoretical concept into clinical investigation and practice.

Early investigations of definitive radiation therapy for metastatic disease included isolated metastatic liver disease.[51] Investigators at the University of Michigan first pioneered the

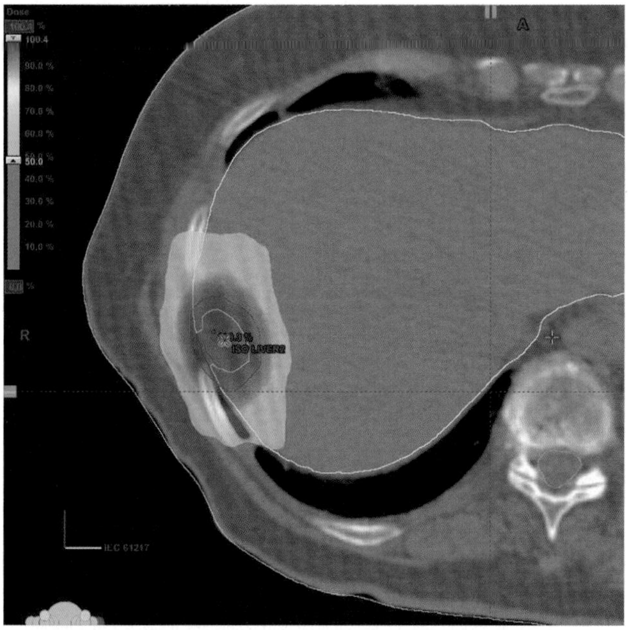

FIGURE 95.5. Axial computed tomography images showing the dose distribution from stereotactic body radiotherapy treatment of a liver metastasis.

paradigm of high-dose three-dimensional conformal radiation therapy in a cohort of patients that included both primary hepatocellular carcinoma and hepatic metastasis, achieving acceptable local control and toxicity (Fig. 95.5). With the advent of image-guided stereotactic body radiotherapy (SBRT), the definitive treatment of isolated hepatic metastasis has been the focus of intense clinical investigation and practice.[52] A multi-institutional phase I and II trial of 47 patients with one to three liver lesions (each <6 cm in size) tested dose-escalated SBRT of 36 to 60 Gy in 3 fractions, reporting a 2-year local control of 92% for all lesions. Local control rates of 100% for lesions ≤3 cm and 77% for lesions >3 cm were also achieved in the 60-Gy cohort. With a median follow-up of 16 months, an overall survival of 20.5 months was reported, with no documented radiation-induced liver disease and grade ≥3 toxicity of 2%.[53] A recent pooled analysis of 65 patients from three institutions has also demonstrated an excellent efficacy and toxicity profile for SBRT in the definitive treatment of colorectal liver metastasis, recommending a prescription dose of at least 48 Gy for a 3-fraction regiment for optimal local control.[54]

With rapid advances in SBRT technique and experience in the definitive treatment of primary lung malignancies, the definitive SBRT treatment of oligometastatic disease involving the lung has also been the subject of numerous clinical reports.[55,56] A recent multi-institutional phase I and II trial of SBRT for lung metastasis dose-escalated 38 patients with one to three lesions and cumulative maximal tumor diameters of <7 cm from 48 to 60 Gy in 3 fractions. A median survival of 19 months and local control rate of 96% at 2 years were achieved, while symptomatic radiation pneumonitis was uncommon (2.6%) and grade ≥3 toxicity was reported as 8%.[57]

The curative treatment of oligometastatic sites in addition to lung and liver has also shown promise in published clinical reports. In most series, the oligometastatic state has been defined as one to five sites of metastatic disease, with inconsistent application of primary disease status, overall disease volume, or maximal lesion size as constraints for oligometastatic disease. Investigators from the University of Chicago have reported a dose-escalation trial of 29 patients with one to five sites of metastatic disease, concluding no to minimal toxicity and potential clinical benefit from this approach.[58] Another prospective study of 121 curative-intent SBRT with five or fewer oligometastatic lesions yielded 4-year survival rates of 28%, progression-free survival of 20%, and local control of 60%.[59] Twenty-nine patients were alive and with no evidence of disease at last follow-up, leading the authors to conclude that "oligometastatic disease is a potentially curable state of distant cancer spread."

Other investigators have also examined the curative role of oligometastatic disease for specific primary sites of disease. Milano et al.[60] examined the role of curative SBRT for 51 metastatic breast cancer patients, concluding prolonged survival and possible cure for select patients with limited metastatic disease, as well as the utility of palliative-intent SBRT for symptomatic or potentially symptomatic sites. Recent international guideline statements have also addressed the management of select oligometastatic breast cancer patients in consensus recommendations, stating "a small but very important subset of metastatic breast cancer patients, for example those with a solitary metastatic lesion, can achieve complete remission and a long survival."[61] Early reports have also documented the potential utility of curative SBRT for oligometastatic disease from gynecological and non–small cell lung primary sites, as well as involved oligometastatic sites such abdominal nodal metastases and adrenal gland metastasis.[62–67]

In summary, SBRT may be beneficial in selected patients with a small number of metastatic sites; these patients should be treated on prospective trials in order to obtain a better understanding of the appropriate use of this technology.

REFERENCES

1. Hendrix MJC. Charting a course to a distant site. *Nat Rev Cancer* 2009;9:237.
2. Ferrell B, Koczywas M, Grannis F, et al. Palliative care in lung cancer. *Surg Clin North Am* 2011;91:403–417.
3. Jung B, Murgu S, Colt H. Rigid bronchoscopy for malignant central airway obstruction from small cell lung cancer complicated by SVC syndrome. *Ann Thorac Cardiovasc Surg* 2011;17:53–57.
4. Ranu H, Madden BP. Endobronchial stenting in the management of large airway pathology. *Postgrad Med J* 2009;85:682–687.
5. Canak V, Zarić B, Milivancev A, et al. Combination of interventional pulmonology techniques (Nd:YAG laser resection and brachytherapy) with external beam radiotherapy in the treatment of lung cancer patients with Karnofsky index ≤50. *J BUON* 2006;11:447–456.
6. Zarić B, Canak V, Milivancev A, et al. The effect of Nd:YAG laser resection on symptom control, time to progression and survival in lung cancer patients. *J BUON* 2007;12:361–368.
7. Nag S, Kelly JF, Horton JL, et al. Brachytherapy for carcinoma of the lung. *Oncology* 2001;15:371–381.
8. Suh J, Dass KK, Pagliaccio L, et al. Endobronchial radiation therapy with or without neodymium yttrium aluminum garnet laser resection for managing malignant airway obstruction. *Cancer* 1994;73:2583–2588.
9. Allen MD, Baldwin JC, Fish VJ, et al. Combined laser therapy and endobronchial radiotherapy for unresectable lung carcinoma with bronchial obstruction. *Am J Surg* 1985;150:71–77.
10. Fairchild A, Harris K, Barnes E, et al. Palliative thoracic radiotherapy for lung cancer: a systematic review. *J Clin Oncol* 2008;26:4001–4011.
11. Rodrigues G, Videtic GMM, Sur R, et al. Palliative thoracic radiotherapy in lung cancer: an American Society for Radiation Oncology evidence-based clinical practice guideline. *Pract Radiat Oncol* 2011;1:60–71.
12. Abbas S, Lam V, Hollands M. Ten-year survival after liver resection for colorectal metastases: systematic review and meta-analysis. *ISRN Oncol* 2011;2011:763245.
13. Qian J. Interventional therapies of unresectable liver metastases. *J Cancer Res Clin Oncol* 2011;137:1763–1772.
14. Alberts SR, Wagman LD. Chemotherapy for colorectal liver metastases. *Oncologist* 2008;13:1063–1073.
15. Mocellin S, Pilati P, Lise M, et al. Hepatic arterial infusion (HAI) compared to systemic chemotherapy for the treatment of unresectable liver metastases from colorectal carcinoma: a systematic review and meta-analysis of randomized controlled trials. *J Clin Oncol* 2007;25:5649–5654.
16. Malik U, Mohiuddin M. External-beam radiotherapy in the management of liver metastases. *Semin Oncol* 2002;29:196–201.
17. Lawrence TS, Robertson JM, Anscher MS, et al. Hepatic toxicity from cancer treatment. *Int J Radiat Oncol Biol Phys* 1995;31:1237–1248.
18. Ingold JA, Reed GB, Kaplan HS, et al. Radiation hepatitis. *Am J Roentgenol Radium Ther Nucl Med* 1965;93:200–208.
19. Russell AH, Clyde C, Wasserman TH, et al. Accelerated hyperfractionated hepatic irradiation in the management of patients with liver metastases: results of the RTOG dose escalating protocol. *Int J Radiat Oncol Biol Phys* 1993;27:117–123.
20. Borgelt BB, Gelber R, Brady LW, et al. The palliation of hepatic metastases: results of the Radiation Therapy Oncology Group pilot study. *Int J Radiat Biol Phys* 1981;7:587–591.

21. Leibel SA, Pajak TF, Massullo V, et al. A comparison of misonidazole sensitized radiation therapy to radiation therapy alone for the palliation of hepatic metastases: results of a Radiation Therapy Oncology Group randomized prospective protocol. *Int J Radiat Oncol Biol Phys* 1987;13:1057–1064.
22. Bydder S, Spry NA, Christie DR, et al. A prospective trial of short-fractionation for the palliation of liver metastases. *Australas Radiol* 2003;47:284–288.
23. Gray B, Van Hazel G, Hope M, et al. Randomised trial of SIR-spheres plus chemotherapy vs. chemotherapy alone for treating patients with liver metastases from primary large bowel cancer. *Ann Oncol* 2001;12:1711–1720.
24. Shapiro MJ. Management of malignant biliary obstruction: nonoperative and palliative techniques. *Oncology* 1995;9:493–496.
25. Shinohara ET, Mitra N, Guo M, et al. Radiotherapy is associated with improved survival in adjuvant and palliative treatment of extrahepatic cholangiocarcinomas. *Int J Radiat Oncol Biol Phys* 2009;74:1191–1198.
26. Eschelman DJ, Shapiro MJ, Bonn J, et al. Malignant biliary duct obstruction: long-term experience with Gianturco stents and combined-modality radiation therapy. *Radiology* 1996;200:717–724.
27. Soffen EM, Solin LJ, Rubenstein JH, et al. Palliative radiotherapy for symptomatic adrenal metastases. *Cancer* 1990;65:1318–1320.
28. Barosi G, Rosti V, Vannucchi AM. Therapeutic approaches in myelofibrosis. *Expert Opin Pharmacother* 2011;12:1597–1611.
29. McFarland JT, Kuzma C, Millard FE, et al. Palliative irradiation of the spleen. *Am J Clin Oncol* 2003;26:178–183.
30. Mishra SK, Laskar S, Muckaden MA, et al. Monthly palliative pelvic radiotherapy in advanced carcinoma of uterine cervix. *J Cancer Res Ther* 2005;1:208–212.
31. Smith SC, Koh WJ. Palliative radiation therapy for gynaecological malignancies. *Best Pract Res Clin Obstet Gynaecol* 2001;15:265–278.
32. Adelson MD, Wharton JT, Delclos L, et al. Palliative radiotherapy for ovarian cancer. *Int J Radiat Oncol Biol Phys* 1987;13:17–21.
33. Onsrud M, Hagen B, Strickert T. 10-Gy single-fraction pelvic irradiation for palliation and life prolongation in patients with cancer of the cervix and corpus uteri. *Gynecol Oncol* 2001;82:167–171.
34. Tinger A, Waldron T, Peluso N, et al. Effective palliative radiation therapy in advanced and recurrent ovarian carcinoma. *Int J Radiat Oncol Biol Phys* 2001;51:1256–1263.
35. Konski A, Feigenberg S, Chow E. Palliative radiation therapy. *Semin Oncol* 2005;32:156–164.
36. Hahnloser D, Nelson H, Gunderson LL, et al. Curative potential of multimodality therapy for locally recurrent rectal cancer. *Ann Surg* 2003;237:502–508.
37. deWilt JHW, Vermaas M, Ferenschild FTJ, et al. Management of locally advanced primary and recurrent rectal cancer. *Clin Colon Rectal Surg* 2007;20:255–263.
38. Moriya Y. Treatment strategy for locally recurrent rectal cancer. *Jpn J Clin Oncol* 2006;36:127–131.
39. Melton GB, Paty PB, Boland PJ, et al. Sacral resection for recurrent rectal cancer: analysis of morbidity and treatment results. *Dis Colon Rectum* 2006;49:1099–1107.
40. Wells BJ, Stotland P, Ko MA, et al. Results of an aggressive approach to resection of locally recurrent rectal cancer. *Ann Surg Oncol* 2007;14:390–395.
41. Overgaard M, Bertelsen K, Dalmark M, et al. A randomized feasibility study evaluating the effect of radiotherapy alone or combined with 5-fluorouracil in the treatment of locally recurrent or inoperable colorectal carcinoma. *Acta Oncol* 1993;32:547–553.
42. Ito Y, Ohtsu A, Ishikura S, et al. Efficacy of chemoradiotherapy on pain relief in patients with intrapelvic recurrence of rectal cancer. *Jpn J Clin Oncol* 2003;33:180–185.
43. Wong R, Thomas G, Cummings B, et al. In search of a dose-response relationship with radiotherapy in the management of recurrent rectal carcinoma in the pelvis: a systematic review. *Int J Radiat Oncol Biol Phys* 1998; 40:437–446.
44. Bae SH, Park W, Choi DH, et al. Palliative radiotherapy in patients with a symptomatic pelvic mass of metastatic colorectal cancer. *Radiat Oncol* 2011;6:52.
45. Lingareddy V, Ahmad NR, Mohiuddin M. Palliative reirradiation for recurrent rectal cancer. *Int J Radiat Oncol Biol Phys* 1997;38:785–790.
46. Valentini V, Morganti AG, Gambacorta MA, et al. Preoperative hyperfractionated chemoradiation for locally recurrent rectal cancer in patients previously irradiated to the pelvis: a multicentric phase II study. *Int J Radiat Oncol Biol Phys* 2006;64:1129–1139.
47. Haddock MG, Gunderson LL, Nelson H, et al. Intraoperative irradiation for locally recurrent colorectal cancer in previously irradiated patients. *Int J Radiat Oncol Biol Phys* 2001;49:1267–1274.
48. Alektiar KM, Zelefsky MJ, Paty PB, et al. High-dose-rate intraoperative brachytherapy for recurrent colorectal cancer. *Int J Radiat Oncol Biol Phys* 2000;48:219–226.
49. Kolotas C, Röddiger S, Strassmann G, et al. Palliative interstitial HDR brachytherapy for recurrent rectal cancer. Implantation techniques and results. *Strahlenther Onkol* 2003;179:458–463.
50. Hellman S, Weichselbaum RR. Oligometastases. *J Clin Oncol* 1995;13:8–10.
51. Dawson LA, McGinn CJ, Normolle D, et al. Escalated focal liver radiation and concurrent hepatic artery fluorodeoxyuridine for unresectable intrahepatic malignancies. *J Clin Oncol* 2000;18:2210–2218.
52. Sawrie SM, Fiveash JB, Caudell JJ. Stereotactic body radiation therapy for liver metastases and primary hepatocellular carcinoma: normal tissue tolerances and toxicity. *Cancer Control* 2010;17:111–119.
53. Rusthoven KE, Kavanagh BD, Cardenes H, et al. Multi-institutional phase I/II trial of stereotactic body radiation therapy for liver metastases. *J Clin Oncol* 2009;27:1572–1578.
54. Chang DT, Swaminath A, Kozak M, et al. Stereotactic body radiotherapy for colorectal liver metastases: a pooled analysis. *Cancer* 2011;117:4060–4069.
55. Norihisa Y, Nagata Y, Takayama K, et al. Stereotactic body radiotherapy for oligometastatic lung tumors. *Int J Radiat Oncol Biol Phys* 2008;72:398–403.
56. Siva S, MacManus M, Ball D. Stereotactic radiotherapy for pulmonary oligometastases: a systematic review. *J Thorac Oncol* 2010;5:1091–1099.
57. Rusthoven KE, Kavanagh BD, Burri SH, et al. Multi-institutional phase I/II trial of stereotactic body radiation therapy for lung metastases. *J Clin Oncol* 2009;27:1579–1584.
58. Salama JK, Chmura SJ, Mehta N, et al. An initial report of a radiation dose-escalation trial in patients with one to five sites of metastatic disease. *Clin Cancer Res* 2008;14:5255–5259.
59. Milano MT, Katz AW, Muhs AG, et al. A prospective pilot study of curative-intent stereotactic body radiation therapy in patients with 5 or fewer oligometastatic lesions. *Cancer* 2008;112:650–658.
60. Milano MT, Zhang H, Metcalfe SK, et al. Oligometastatic breast cancer treated with curative-intent stereotactic body radiation therapy. *Breast Cancer Res Treat* 2009;115:601–608.
61. Cardoso F, Winer EP, Fallowfield LJ. Metastatic breast cancer. Recommendations proposal from the European School of Oncology (ESO)-MBC Task Force. *Breast* 2007;16:9–10.
62. Higginson DS, Morris DE, Jones EL, et al. Stereotactic body radiotherapy (SBRT): technological innovation and application in gynecologic oncology. *Gynecol Oncol* 2011;120:404–412.
63. Yano T, Haro A, Yoshida T, et al. Prognostic impact of local treatment against postoperative oligometastases in non-small cell lung cancer. *J Surg Oncol* 2010;102:852–855.
64. Khan AJ, Mehta PS, Zusag TW, et al. Long term disease-free survival resulting from combined modality management of patients presenting with oligometastatic, non-small cell lung carcinoma (NSCLC). *Radiother Oncol* 2006;81:163–167.
65. Bignardi M, Navarria P, Mancosu P, et al. Clinical outcome of hypofractionated stereotactic radiotherapy for abdominal lymph node metastases. *Int J Radiat Oncol Biol Phys* 2010;81:831–838.
66. Casamassima F, Livi L, Masciullo S, et al. Stereotactic radiotherapy for adrenal gland metastases: University of Florence experience. *Int J Radiat Oncol Biol Phys* 2012;82:919–923.
67. Scorsetti M, Bignardi M, Alongi F, et al. Stereotactic body radiation therapy for abdominal targets using volumetric intensity modulated arc therapy with RapidArc: feasibility and clinical preliminary results. *Acta Oncol* 2011;50:528–538.

Chapter 96
Pain Management

Gary Deng, Amitabh Gulati, and Barrie R. Cassileth

Pain can significantly decrease patients' quality of life during and after radiotherapy, but appropriate and adequate pain management remains imperfect. More than half of patients who undergo radiotherapy experience pain,[1] and the majority of patients and physicians feel that patients' pain is inadequately controlled.[2]

Pain may result from tissue damage caused by the tumor, such as bone destruction by a metastasis from prostate cancer or invasion of the celiac plexus by pancreatic cancer, or from the delivery of radiotherapy and subsequent complications. Irradiation of normal tissues, especially those with a rapid growth turnover rate, causes cell death and triggers a cascade of proinflammatory cytokines and thrombotic and growth factors, propagating local painful reactions.[3,4] Radiation oncologists must be knowledgeable about pain management during and after radiotherapy. In this chapter we discuss the pathophysiology of pain, treatment options, and practice guidelines for developing a stepwise, integrated treatment plan.

Radiotherapy is also a valuable modality in the treatment of cancer pain. It is commonly used in the palliative setting when a radiosensitive cancer invades bone, soft tissue, or nerves.[5] Radiotherapy for the palliation of pain caused by various types of cancer is covered in their respective chapters elsewhere in this book.

TYPES OF PAIN

Pain generally can be defined as either nociceptive or nonnociceptive. Nociceptive pain refers to the nervous system response that is proportionate to the tissue damage initiating the response. Nociceptive pain is divided into somatic pain and visceral pain, depending on the location and symptoms of the painful stimulus. Typically, somatic pain presents as a well-localized sharp, stabbing (knifelike), and achy pain as a response to skin, muscle, and connective tissue damage. Conversely, patients typically find it difficult to localize visceral pain, which also may have a somatic referral pattern, often complaining of cramping or a dull ache.[6]

Nonnociceptive pain encompasses both neuropathic and psychogenic (or idiopathic) pain syndromes. In these cases, nervous system responses are not what would be expected from the damage causing the response. In fact, responses may occur without tissue damage. Neuropathic pain involves abnormal pain processing by the peripheral or central nervous system. Patients may complain of burning, shooting, tingling, or numbness, which generally occurs along a nerve distribution.[7] Patients also may experience pain that is out of proportion to physical injury. Psychogenic causes such as depression and anxiety may exacerbate the perception of painful stimuli.

Understanding a patient's symptoms allows the physician to determine the pathophysiology of the pain syndrome. Each type of pain syndrome is amenable to treatment with different modalities. For example, somatic pain, localized sharp pain, may be better treated with opioid medications, whereas anticonvulsants or antidepressants may be more effective against neuropathic pain. Other modalities, such as acupuncture, have been shown to help either type of pain.[8]

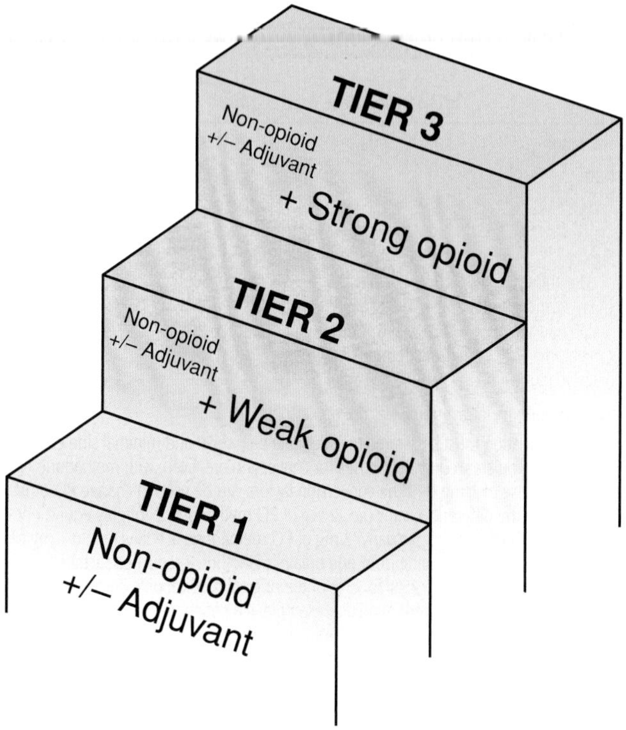

FIGURE 96.1. World Health Organization (WHO) guidelines for initial medical treatment for cancer pain. A three-tiered system broadly indicating the use of opiate medications for continued pain control is shown. As pain symptoms worsen, a physician may enter a higher tier of medications for pain control. (Adapted from World Health Organization. *WHO guidelines cancer pain relief*, 2nd ed. Geneva: World Health Organization, 1996.)

MEDICAL MANAGEMENT

Many national and international organizations have developed guidelines for pain management. Despite variations in the details, the principles and approaches are consistent across guidelines. The World Health Organization (WHO), American Pain Society (APS), and National Comprehensive Cancer Network (NCCN) guidelines are discussed here.

WHO Pain Ladder

The WHO guidelines for analgesic management of cancer pain, first described in the early 1980s,[9,10] consist of a three-step approach that has been validated in recent trials.[11] Despite some debate on its effectiveness,[12] it establishes a widely practiced, stepwise approach in the treatment of various levels of pain severity.

The first tier involves the use of nonopiate medications, primarily nonsteroidal anti-inflammatory drugs (NSAIDs) (Table 96.1). These medications include acetaminophen, nonspecific cyclo-oxygenase inhibitors (including ibuprofen, diclofenac, aspirin), and cyclo-oxygenase-2 inhibitors (celecoxib).[13] NSAIDs are considered the first group of medications to administer. If the patient's pain persists or worsens, the second tier adds a weak opioid in addition to the nonopiate. Finally, continued treatment for worsening pain includes the addition of a strong opioid to replace the weak opiate, the third tier (Fig. 96.1).

Five simple principles are recommended to make the pharmacologic treatments effective: (a) oral administration of analgesics should be used whenever possible; (b) analgesics should be given at regular intervals; (c) analgesics should be prescribed according to pain intensity as evaluated with a pain scale; (d) dosing of analgesics should be adapted to the individual; and (e) analgesics should be prescribed with a constant concern for detail.[14]

Physicians using the WHO guidelines may find it difficult to select among opioids or other medications to start with and to determine dosages to use when changing medications (Table 96.2). Often a patient may not respond to a weak opioid but may respond well to a strong opioid. When pain control becomes inadequate, the physician can climb a higher tier for guidance for better pain control.[14] In light of advances in pharmacogenomics, it is increasingly clear that genetics plays a role in each individual's sensitivity to an analgesic.[15,16] If a patient does not respond or develops tolerance to a particular agent, the current medical regimen should be increased to the maximum tolerated dose or the patient rotated to a different agent.

Over time, adaptations of the WHO ladder have been proposed. In refractory pain or crises of chronic pain, a fourth step may be considered, which includes invasive techniques such as nerve blocks, neurolysis, or surgical or other interventions.[9,17] Adjuvant medications including steroids, anxiolytics, antidepressants, hypnotics, anticonvulsants, antiepileptic-like gabapentinoids (gabapentin and pregabalin), membrane stabilizers, sodium channel blockers, *N*-methyl-D-aspartate receptor antagonists, and cannabinoids may be used in the treatment of neuropathic pain.[18,19]

TABLE 96.1 GUIDE TO COMMON NONOPIATE MEDICATIONS AND STARTING DOSES FOR ADULTS

Medication	*Starting Dose (Maximum Daily Dose in mg)*
Acetaminophen	500, 3–4 × day (4,000)
Nonsteroidal anti-inflammatory drugs	
Aspirin	325, 3–4 × day (4,000)
Ibuprofen	200, 3 × day (2,400)
Naproxen	250, 2 × day (1,250)
Ketorolac	IV 15–30 up to 4 doses
Diclofenac	50, 3 × day (150 mg)
Specific COX-2 inhibitors	
Celecoxib	100, 2 × day (400–800)

IV, intravenous; COX-2, cyclo-oxygenase 2.

Palliative and Supportive Care

TABLE 96.2 GUIDE TO COMMON WEAK AND STRONG OPIOID MEDICATIONS AND POTENTIAL STARTING DOSES[a]

Opioid	*PO Starting Dose (mg)*	*PO Conversion (mg)*	*IV Conversion (mg)*
Tramadol	50, 2–3 × day	–	–
Weak			
Codeine	30, 4–6 × day	–	–
Hydrocodone	5, 4–6 × day	–	–
Strong			
Morphine	15, 4–6 × day	30	10
Hydromorphone	2–4, 4–6 × day	8	2
Methadone	2.5–5, 2–3 × day	2	1
Fentanyl	Transdermal 25 μg/day	NA	0.2
Oxycodone	5–15, 4–6 × day	20	NA

PO, by mouth; IV, intravenous; NA, not applicable.

[a]Opiate medication must be titrated for adequate pain relief and minimal side effects. For the strong opiates, equivalent doses for conversion are given, with methadone IV as the base dose of 1 mg.[73–75] The conversion factors can be used to change PO or IV doses among the different opiates (i.e., 2 mg of PO methadone is roughly equivalent to 30 mg of PO morphine). Similarly, 2 mg of PO methadone is equivalent to 1 mg of IV methadone. When changing from one opiate to another, a reduction factor is sometimes applied (usually 25% to 75% of the original medication's dose) because of less tolerance to the new medication. For example, if a patient is using 60 mg of PO morphine every 4 hours, an equivalent oxycodone dose may be 40 mg × a 50% reduction, leading to 20 mg every 4 hours.

APS and NCCN Guidelines

As the understanding of pain physiology and treatments expands, so does the management strategy. Although the WHO guidelines are a good initial step in pain management, other organizations have modified and expanded these strategies to improve treatment for cancer pain. These guides provide initial medication dosages, the addition of adjuvant medications, and information on appropriate dose increases, allowing the radiation oncologist to further develop pain management skills.

The 2005 APS *Guideline for the Management of Cancer Pain in Adults and Children* contains detailed discussions of cancer pain management algorithms, pharmacologic strategies, coanalgesics, psychological strategies, supportive therapy, integration of nonpharmacologic and pharmacologic treatments, physical strategies, nerve blocks, surgical strategies, radiation therapy, chemotherapy, and pain management in special populations. It also discusses patient education and the importance of patients' adherence to the pain management plan, as well as how to improve quality of care in pain management.[4]

The latest (2010) NCCN guidelines for adult cancer pain contain the following required components: (a) pain intensity must be quantified by the patient (whenever possible); (b) a formal comprehensive pain assessment must be performed; (c) reassessment of pain intensity must be performed at specified intervals to ensure that the therapy selected is having the desired effect; (d) psychosocial support must be available; and (e) specific educational material must be provided to the patient. The guidelines also acknowledge the range of complex decisions faced in caring for these patients. They provide specific suggestions for dosing of NSAIDs, opioids, and coanalgesics; titrating and rotating of opioids; escalation of opioid dosage; management of opioid adverse effects; and when and how to proceed to other techniques/interventions for the management of cancer pain.[20]

Universal screening of pain should take place for cancer patients, followed by comprehensive assessment of the characteristics, underlying pathophysiology and etiology, psychosocial issues, and risk factors for undertreatment of pain. Patients' goals and expectations should be sought for any patient whose pain score is not zero (on a visual analog or a numerical rating scale). Patients are then stratified based on the urgency and severity of the pain and treated with escalating aggressiveness. Repeat reassessments are done frequently to adjust treatment plans until patients' goals and expectations in comfort and function are met. It is preferable to convert short-acting opioids to long-acting ones when the dose required to provide adequate pain control is determined. Rescue dosing with short-acting agents should be provided for breakthrough pain during maintenance therapy.

Opiate Side Effects

Patients taking opioids also should be provided with a bowel regimen. Side effects may limit the maximal tolerable dose of opioid analgesics. Treating a patient's pain is a balance of maximizing analgesic effects and minimizing side effects.[21] Common opioid side effects include gastrointestinal (constipation, nausea, and emesis), respiratory (decreased respiratory rate), dermatologic (pruritus and dry mouth), and central nervous system (sedation, hallucinations, and seizures) effects. Many strategies are implemented in balancing analgesic effects and side effects.[22,23] Although no consensus exists, physicians can manage side effects with the following strategies:

1. Pharmacologic treatment of the side effects (e.g., high water intake, dietary fiber, stool softeners, laxatives, or the peripherally acting opioid antagonist methylnaltrexone for constipation);
2. Reduction of opiate dose;
3. Addition of adjuvant medications for pain management (see following discussion), and opioid rotation.

Opioid rotation refers to drug-switching within a group, for example, changing hydrocodone to codeine because of nausea.[24] Medications should be changed every 2 to 3 months so that the patient does not become tolerant to an agent.

Adjuvant Therapy

Using the WHO ladder, pain related to cancer can be managed with oral medications in 70% to 85% of patients.[11,25] At any point on the WHO analgesic ladder, adjuvant therapy can be initiated to supplement NSAIDs and opioid treatment. Benefits of adjuvant therapy include use of medications tailored to specific causes of nociceptive responses (i.e., neuropathic pain) and reduction of opiate side effects.

Because neuropathic pain generally is not responsive to opioid medications unless high doses are applied, other classes of medications often are prescribed.[26] Anticonvulsants, such as gabapentin, carbamazepine, and pregabalin, are effective in managing neuropathic symptoms.[7] Both gabapentin and pregabalin are renally excreted and have minimal drug–drug interactions, which renders these medications effective first-line treatments for neuropathic pain.[7]

Like anticonvulsants, antidepressants are a broad category of medications that stabilize neurons involved in neuropathic pain. Tricyclic antidepressants in low doses, such as amitriptyline, have been well studied for pain relief.[27] Serotonin reuptake inhibitors and newer classes of antidepressants, including selective serotonin and norepinephrine reuptake inhibitors (milnacipran, duloxetine, and venlafaxine), are less well studied but often prescribed for neuropathic pain. Because many patients with neuropathic pain experience depression or anxiety, antidepressants may play a dual treatment role, resulting in improved efficacy in pain control.[27]

When faced with a patient with neuropathic pain, the radiation oncologist may prescribe an anticonvulsant, such as gabapentin, at low doses and titrate the medication to improve analgesia while monitoring side effects. Some physicians may initiate antidepressant treatment, especially if patients also exhibit signs of depression or anxiety, and then add the anticonvulsant as a secondary medication. In any case, both medications can be used synergistically to improve analgesia for neuropathic pain.

TABLE 96.3 COMMON ADJUVANT MEDICATIONS WITH STARTING DOSAGES AND COMMON SIDE EFFECTS

Medication	Starting Dose (PO unless Otherwise Specified; mg)	Significant Side Effects
Antidepressants		
Amitriptyline	10–25 at night	Cardiac, CNS
Nortriptyline	10–25 at night	Cardiac, CNS
Venlafaxine	37.5 every day	CNS
Duloxetine	60 every day	Nausea, somnolence
Anticonvulsants		
Gabapentin	100, 3 × day	CNS, sedation
Carbamazepine	100, 2 × day	Bone marrow, liver, CNS
Pregabalin	75, 2 × day	CNS, sedation
Topicals		
Lidocaine 5%	1–3 patches for 12 hours	CNS, cardiac
Capsaicin	0.025% Cream	Burning
Muscle relaxants		
Baclofen	5, 3 × day	CNS
Cyclobenzaprine	5, 3 × day	Drowsiness, dry mouth
Tizanidine	2 every night (4 mg tid)	Weakness, dry mouth
N-methyl-D-aspartate antagonist		
Ketamine	Intravenous infusion	Hallucinations, CNS

PO, by mouth; tid, three times a day.

The NMDA (*N*-methyl-D-aspartate) receptor has received much attention for its role in modulating pain signals throughout the nervous system. Methadone is a long-acting opioid receptor antagonist, which may act also as an NMDA receptor antagonist, preventing morphine tolerance and NMDA hyperalgesia effects.[28] Pain management specialists have also used ketamine, a specific NMDA receptor antagonist, to relieve cancer and neuropathic pain, especially refractory pain.[29]

Other adjuvant analgesic drug classes used in cancer therapy include local anesthetics, steroids, muscle relaxants, benzodiazepines, α-adrenergic agonists, and bisphosphonates.[29] In recent years there has been a resurgence in clinical trials of cannabis extracts and analogs in the treatment of refractory cancer pain.[30] Many of these medications are used in specific pain syndromes, which may be useful for the radiation oncologist (Table 96.3).

Nonoral Routes of Administration

Chemotherapy, surgery, and radiotherapy often produce significant side effects. Pain medications given by mouth may not be the most appropriate mode of delivery. When changing from oral to another delivery mode, care must be taken to give equipotent analgesic doses. Conversion charts for opioids are readily available in the literature.[22]

Some pain medications come in formulations that can be delivered rectally, intramuscularly, intravenously, or topically. NSAIDs and opioids are commercially available in suppository form. Intramuscular delivery of morphine and other medications shows variable efficacy and is not recommended.[31] Patient-controlled analgesia allows patients to regularly administer intravenous medications without nursing assistance, especially in the inpatient setting. Both fentanyl and lidocaine are available in a transdermal patch.[32] Capsaicin cream and a newer transdermal patch are effective for the local treatment of neuropathic pain.[33,34]

INTERVENTIONAL MANAGEMENT

Although most cancer pain can be managed medically, some patients require interventional procedures to achieve pain relief. Such interventions include peripheral nerve blocks, neuroablation, and neuroaxial and implantable techniques.

During Radiotherapy Procedure

Most patients tolerate the radiotherapy procedure, but occasional individuals may not tolerate proper positioning secondary to pain. Most patients can be managed with oral or intravenous pain medications, primarily with opioids such as morphine or fentanyl. When these methods fail, the radiation oncologist may need the assistance of an anesthesiologist.

If the region of radiotherapy is an extremity, the specific nerves to an extremity may be anesthetized with local anesthetic or peripheral nerve block.[35] For multiple-day procedures, a peripheral nerve catheter may be placed for delivery of continuous anesthetic.[36] Patients with abdominal or thoracic pain may benefit with local anesthetic delivered through an epidural catheter.[37] If these methods are contraindicated, general anesthesia may be the only option.

Neuroablative Techniques

Although most pain symptoms can be managed with oral and intravenous medications, the regimen may become insufficient (e.g., due to medication tolerance), or side effects may become intolerable. Interventional pain management specialists offer a myriad of neurolytic procedures that reduce pain medication requirements.

Peripheral nerves, once leaving the spinal cord, can be visualized with magnetic resonance imaging or ultrasound and are amenable to various neurolytic procedures. Common nerves targeted include intercostal nerves for thoracic chest wall or abdominal wall pain, maxillary and mandibular nerves for facial pain, and median branch nerves for facet arthropathy.[38] Cryoanalgesia techniques apply subzero temperatures to induce wallerian degeneration of neurons, while allowing normal regrowth of axons. Radiofrequency techniques use heat to cause nerve damage. Chemical neurolysis can be achieved with phenol or alcohol preparations.

Pain signals initiating from the perineal, pelvic, and abdominal regions may be transmitted via visceral afferents following the sympathetic nervous system. Along with these fibers, the sympathetic nerves coalesce at specific ganglia (impar, superior and inferior hypogastric, and celiac plexus). At these sites, image-guided neurolytic procedures can be performed.[39] When pain fibers are destroyed in this process, the associated region also is sympathetically denervated.

Not all cancer patient pain is caused by tumors and somatic in nature. Sympathetically mediated pain, complex regional pain syndromes (CRPSs) I and II, may present in an extremity with symptoms of swelling, redness, and temperature change. These typically result from nerve injury and consequent dysautomania of the sympathetic system. Chronic skin changes, hair loss, and muscle atrophy and disuse may follow.[40] Along with pharmacologic treatment, neuroablative techniques targeting sympathetic fibers to the upper extremity (stellate ganglion) and lower extremity (lumbar sympathetics) can be used to treat these syndromes.[41]

Neuroaxial Techniques

Neuroaxial procedures involving drug delivery systems are indicated when oral opioid doses are escalated without significant pain relief or when side effects are intolerable.[42] Either semipermanent epidural systems or permanent intrathecal delivery systems can be used to deliver local anesthetic and opiate medications in low concentrations to appropriate spinal cord root levels.[43] The benefits of these methods include the use of local anesthetics in concentrations that are not toxic but can provide analgesia at the spinal cord level and the use of adjuvants (such as clonidine, baclofen, and ziconotide). These should not be given at equivalent oral doses because of side effects.[44]

Electrostimulation techniques also may be applied to disrupt the flow of pain signals in the spinal cord. Transcutaneous electrical nerve stimulation, spinal cord stimulation at thoracic and lumbar regions, and deep-brain stimulation at the thalamus or motor cortex can interfere with the conduction of pain signals.[23] The stimulation of large motor fibers inhibits the conduction of pain signals by small nerve fibers and has shown efficacy for various pain syndromes.[45]

Neurosurgical techniques are generally reserved for refractory pain and specific indications. Plexus root avulsions may be responsive to dorsal root entry zone lesioning, but the indications and success rates are limited.[46] More specific lesions at the spinal cord and central nervous system (e.g., thalamotomy and deep-brain stimulation) have also been used with variable success and significant side effects.[47] Finally, various chemoneurolytic medications can be delivered intrathecally for destruction of specific nerve roots or parts of the spinal cord for the treatment of refractory cancer pain.[48]

COMPLEMENTARY THERAPIES

Conventional medical regimens may not satisfactorily treat cancer-related pain syndromes. Several complementary modalities such as hypnosis, biofeedback, massage, music therapy, mind–body exercises, and dietary supplementation have been shown to reduce anxiety and chronic pain,[49] yet more multi-institutional, randomized, controlled trials are needed to confirm their effectiveness in this setting.[50]

Acupuncture is perhaps the most extensively studied method for pain control.[51] Acupuncture relieves both acute pain (e.g., postoperative dental pain) and chronic pain (e.g., headache, osteoarthritis).[52–54] Acupuncture appears effective against cancer-related pain. A randomized, placebo-controlled trial tested auricular acupuncture for patients with cancer pain despite stable medication. Pain intensity decreased by 36% at 2 months from baseline in the treatment group, a statistically significant difference compared with the two control groups for whom little pain reduction was seen.[8] Most patients in this study had neuropathic pain, which is often refractory to conventional treatment.

Neurophysiologic studies show that acupuncture-induced analgesia appears to be mediated by endogenous opioids and other neurotransmitters.[55] Functional brain imaging studies suggest that acupuncture also modulates the affective-cognitive aspect of pain perception.[56] Correlations between functional magnetic resonance imaging signal intensities and analgesic effects induced by acupuncture have been reported.[57]

SPECIFIC SCENARIOS

The following section identifies common pain syndromes that radiation oncologists may face.

Muscle Spasm

Muscle fibers, once thought to be radioresistant, may undergo significant change, especially months after radiation exposure.[58] One-time muscle exposures to 10 to 20 Gy or fractionated doses >55 Gy are associated with myokymia, pain, and decreased muscle strength and range of motion.[58] Specific cancer locations susceptible to muscle complications include head and neck cancers and soft-tissue cancers (e.g., Ewing sarcoma).[58] Treatment regimen includes early physical therapy and orthopedic exercises and pharmacologic therapy such as muscle relaxants (e.g., baclofen). Novel treatments involve the use of botulinum toxin injected in small doses (15 to 25 units) into the muscle to relieve contracture or spasm.[59,60]

Plexopathy

Similar to muscle fibers, nerve bundles exposed to a one-time dose of 28 Gy, or fractionated doses totaling 60 Gy, undergo significant decreases in large nerve fiber density.[61] Significant pain may ensue months to years after radiotherapy, especially in the brachial plexus distribution.[62] Rates of radiation-induced plexopathy range from 1% to 5%, with 10% of this population having complicated pain syndromes such as CRPSs, dysesthesias, and numbness.[63] Treatments involve early physical and occupational therapy, multimodality pain regimens (opioid and neuropathic pain medications as previously discussed), neurolytic procedures (e.g., stellate ganglion), and electrical stimulation (transcutaneous electrical nerve stimulation or spinal cord stimulators).[64]

Mucositis and Proctitis

Pain associated with mucositis (up to 75% of patients treated with radiation) is debilitating and may result in dose limitations of radiotherapy.[65] Pain control strategies include NSAIDs and oral opioids, with intravenous patient-controlled analgesia providing good management of pain when patients are hospitalized. Topical analgesics, such as viscous lidocaine, ice chips, capsaicin, benzydamine (Gelclair, Sinclair Pharma Ltd., United Kingdom), and diphenhydramine, may provide relief prior to ingestion of food.[66] Some helpful interventions include good oral hygiene, honey, hydrolytic enzymes, zinc, laser therapy, Gelclair, and povidone.[67,68]

Similar to oral mucosa, the rectum is susceptible to late radiation damage and proctitis, with patients presenting with tenesmus and rectal pain. Medical treatments involve reducing inflammation with NSAIDs and steroids, such as hydrocortisone cream, and the use of sucralfate.[69] Novel therapies, including hyperbaric oxygen and heat therapy (laser therapy), have also been used successfully to heal rectal mucosa and reduce tenesmus.[70–72]

SUMMARY

Pain is a common problem in patients with advanced cancer. Radiotherapy can be used to treat pain caused by the underlying cancer (e.g., pain from bone metastasis and pain due to treatment side effects). A multimodal management approach should be applied, starting with oral analgesics administered according to clinical practice guidelines, and also confounding factors such as psychological issues should be addressed. For patients who experience refractory pain despite medical management, interventional procedures may be necessary. Complementary therapies may be helpful in some patients, although their efficacy has not been definitively established.

REFERENCES

1. Pignon T, et al. Impact of radiation oncology practice on pain: a cross-sectional survey. *Int J Radiat Oncol Biol Phys* 2004;60(4):1204–1210.
2. Cleeland CS, et al. Cancer pain management by radiotherapists: a survey of radiation therapy oncology group physicians. *Int J Radiat Oncol Biol Phys* 2000; 47(1):203–208.
3. Cherny N, et al. Strategies to manage the adverse effects of oral morphine: an evidence-based report. *J Clin Oncol* 2001;19(9):2542–2554.
4. Gordon DB, et al. American pain society recommendations for improving the quality of acute and cancer pain management: American Pain Society Quality of Care Task Force. *Arch Intern Med* 2005;165(14):1574–1580.
5. Friedland J. Local and systemic radiation for palliation of metastatic disease. *Urol Clin North Am* 1999;26(2):391–402.
6. Besson JM, Chaouch A. Peripheral and spinal mechanisms of nociception. *Physiol Rev* 1987;67(1):67–186.
7. Irving GA. Contemporary assessment and management of neuropathic pain. *Neurology* 2005;64(12 Suppl 3):S21–S27.
8. Alimi D, et al. Analgesic effect of auricular acupuncture for cancer pain: a randomized, blinded, controlled trial. *J Clin Oncol* 2003;21(22):4120–4126.
9. Jadad AR, Browman GP. The WHO analgesic ladder for cancer pain management. Stepping up the quality of its evaluation. *JAMA* 1995;274(23):1870–1873.
10. Ventafridda V, et al. WHO guidelines for the use of analgesics in cancer pain. *Int J Tissue React* 1985;7(1):93–96.
11. Zech DF, et al. Validation of World Health Organization Guidelines for cancer pain relief: a 10-year prospective study. *Pain* 1995;63(1):65–76.
12. Azevedo Sao Leao Ferreira K, Kimura M, Jacobsen Teixeira M. The WHO analgesic ladder for cancer pain control, twenty years of use. How much pain relief does one get from using it? *Support Care Cancer* 2006;14(11):1086–1093.
13. Bruera E. Mechanism of action of nonsteroidal anti-inflammatory drugs. *Cancer Invest* 1998;16(7):538–539.
14. World Health Organization. *WHO guidelines cancer pain relief*, 2nd ed. Geneva: World Health Organization, 1996.
15. Palmer SN, et al. Pharmacogenetics of anesthetic and analgesic agents. *Anesthesiology* 2005;102(3):663–671.
16. Stamer UM, Bayerer B, Stuber F. Genetics and variability in opioid response. *Eur J Pain* 2005;9(2):101–104.

17. Cahana A, et al. Do minimally invasive procedures have a place in the treatment of chronic low back pain? *Expert Rev Neurother* 2004;4(3):479–490.
18. Moulin DE, et al. Pharmacological management of chronic neuropathic pain - consensus statement and guidelines from the Canadian Pain Society. *Pain Res Manag* 2007; 12(1):13–21.
19. Dworkin RH, et al. Pharmacologic management of neuropathic pain: evidence-based recommendations. *Pain* 2007;132(3):237–251.
20. Swarm R, et al. Adult cancer pain. *J Natl Compr Canc Netw* 2010;8(9):1046–1086.
21. Cherny NI. The management of cancer pain. *CA Cancer J Clin* 2000;50(2):70–116; quiz 117–120.
22. Cherny NI, Portenoy RK. Cancer pain management. Current strategy. *Cancer* 1993; 72(11 Suppl):3393–3415.
23. McNicol E, et al. Management of opioid side effects in cancer-related and chronic noncancer pain: a systematic review. *J Pain* 2003;4(5):231–256.
24. Quigley C. Opioid switching to improve pain relief and drug tolerability. *Cochrane Database Syst Rev* 2004;(3):CD004847.
25. Ventafridda V, et al. A validation study of the WHO method for cancer pain relief. *Cancer* 1987;59(4):850–856.
26. Milch RA. Neuropathic pain: implications for the surgeon. *Surg Clin North Am* 2005;85(2):225–236.
27. Hainline B. Chronic pain: physiological, diagnostic, and management considerations. *Psychiatr Clin North Am* 2005;28(3):713–735.
28. Inturrisi CE. Pharmacology of methadone and its isomers. *Minerva Anestesiol* 2005;71(7–8):435–437.
29. Lussier D, Huskey AG, Portenoy RK. Adjuvant analgesics in cancer pain management. *Oncologist* 2004;9(5):571–591.
30. Farquhar-Smith WP. Do cannabinoids have a role in cancer pain management? *Curr Opin Support Palliat Care* 2009;3(1):7–13.
31. McQuay HJ, Carroll D, Moore RA. Injected morphine in postoperative pain: a quantitative systematic review. *J Pain Symptom Manage* 1999;17(3):164–174.
32. Priano L, Gasco MR, Mauro A. Transdermal treatment options for neurological disorders: impact on the elderly. *Drugs Aging* 2006;23(5):357–375.
33. Sawynok J. Topical analgesics in neuropathic pain. *Curr Pharm Des* 2005; 11(23):2995–3004.
34. Jones VM, Moore KA, Peterson DM. Capsaicin 8% topical patch (Qutenza)–a review of the evidence. *J Pain Palliat Care Pharmacother* 2011;25(1):32–41.
35. Marhofer P, Greher M, Kapral S. Ultrasound guidance in regional anaesthesia. *Br J Anaesth* 2005;94(1):7–17.
36. Grossi P, Allegri M. Continuous peripheral nerve blocks: state of the art. *Curr Opin Anaesthesiol* 2005;18(5):522–526.
37. Waurick R, Van Aken H. Update in thoracic epidural anaesthesia. *Best Pract Res Clin Anaesthesiol* 2005;19(2):201–213.
38. Trescot AM. Cryoanalgesia in interventional pain management. *Pain Physician* 2003;6(3):345–360.
39. de Leon-Casasola OA. Critical evaluation of chemical neurolysis of the sympathetic axis for cancer pain. *Cancer Control* 2000;7(2):142–148.
40. Aprile AE. Complex regional pain syndrome. *AANA J* 1997;65(6):557–560.
41. Mekhail N, Kapural L. Complex regional pain syndrome type I in cancer patients. *Curr Rev Pain* 2000;4(3):227–233.
42. Mercadante S. Neuraxial techniques for cancer pain: an opinion about unresolved therapeutic dilemmas. *Reg Anesth Pain Med* 1999;24(1):74–83.
43. Lordon SP. Interventional approach to cancer pain. *Curr Pain Headache Rep* 2002; 6(3):202–206.
44. Deer TR, et al. Comprehensive consensus based guidelines on intrathecal drug delivery systems in the treatment of pain caused by cancer pain. *Pain Physician* 2011;14(3): E283–E312.
45. Rushton DN. Electrical stimulation in the treatment of pain. *Disabil Rehabil* 2002; 24(8):407–415.
46. Sindou M, Mertens P. Neurosurgical management of neuropathic pain. *Stereotact Funct Neurosurg* 2000;75(2–3):76–80.
47. Slavik E, Ivanovic S. Cancer pain (neurosurgical management). *Acta Chir Iugosl* 2004;51(4):15–23.
48. Candido K, Stevens RA. Intrathecal neurolytic blocks for the relief of cancer pain. *Best Pract Res Clin Anaesthesiol* 2003;17(3):407–428.
49. Deng G, Cassileth BR. Integrative oncology: complementary therapies for pain, anxiety, and mood disturbance. *CA Cancer J Clin* 2005;55(2):109–116.
50. Bardia A, et al. Efficacy of complementary and alternative medicine therapies in relieving cancer pain: a systematic review. *J Clin Oncol* 2006;24(34):5457–5464.
51. Park J, et al. The status and future of acupuncture clinical research. *J Altern Complement Med* 2008;14(7):871–881.
52. Berman BM, et al. Effectiveness of acupuncture as adjunctive therapy in osteoarthritis of the knee: a randomized, controlled trial. *Ann Intern Med* 2004;141(12): 901–910.
53. NIH Consensus Conference. Acupuncture. *JAMA* 1998;280(17):1518–1524.
54. Melchart D, et al. Acupuncture for recurrent headaches: a systematic review of randomized controlled trials. *Cephalalgia* 1999;19(9):779–786; discussion 765.
55. Han JS. Acupuncture and endorphins. *Neurosci Lett* 2004;361(1–3):258–261.
56. Wu MT, et al. Central nervous pathway for acupuncture stimulation: localization of processing with functional MR imaging of the brain–preliminary experience. *Radiology* 1999;212(1):133–141.
57. Zhang WT, et al. Relations between brain network activation and analgesic effect induced by low vs. high frequency electrical acupoint stimulation in different subjects: a functional magnetic resonance imaging study. *Brain Res* 2003;982(2): 168–178.
58. Gillette EL, et al. Late radiation injury to muscle and peripheral nerves. *Int J Radiat Oncol Biol Phys* 1995;31(5):1309–1318.
59. Lou JS, Pleninger P, Kurlan R. Botulinum toxin A is effective in treating trismus associated with postradiation myokymia and muscle spasm. *Mov Disord* 1995; 10(5):680–681.
60. Van Daele DJ, et al. Head and neck muscle spasm after radiotherapy: management with botulinum toxin A injection. *Arch Otolaryngol Head Neck Surg* 2002; 128(8):956–959.
61. Vujaskovic Z, et al. Ultrastructural morphometric analysis of peripheral nerves after intraoperative irradiation. *Int J Radiat Biol* 1995;68(1):71–76.
62. Galecki J, et al. Radiation-induced brachial plexopathy and hypofractionated regimens in adjuvant irradiation of patients with breast cancer–a review. *Acta Oncol* 2006;45(3):280–284.
63. Jaeckle KA. Neurological manifestations of neoplastic and radiation-induced plexopathies. *Semin Neurol* 2004;24(4):385–393.
64. Schierle C, Winograd JM. Radiation-induced brachial plexopathy: review. Complication without a cure. *J Reconstr Microsurg* 2004;20(2):149–152.
65. Scully C, Epstein J, Sonis S. Oral mucositis: a challenging complication of radiotherapy, chemotherapy, and radiochemotherapy: part 1, pathogenesis and prophylaxis of mucositis. *Head Neck* 2003;25(12):1057–1070.
66. Scully C, Epstein J, Sonis S. Oral mucositis: a challenging complication of radiotherapy, chemotherapy, and radiochemotherapy. Part 2: diagnosis and management of mucositis. *Head Neck* 2004;26(1):77–84.
67. Marlow C, Johnson J. A guide to managing the pain of treatment-related oral mucositis. *Int J Palliat Nurs* 2005;11(7):338, 340–345.
68. Worthington HV, Clarkson JE, Eden OB. Interventions for preventing oral mucositis for patients with cancer receiving treatment. *Cochrane Database Syst Rev* 2006;(2):CD000978.
69. Denton AS, et al. Systematic review for non-surgical interventions for the management of late radiation proctitis. *Br J Cancer* 2002;87(2):134–143.
70. Colwell JC, Goldberg M. A review of radiation proctitis in the treatment of prostate cancer. *J Wound Ostomy Continence Nurs* 2000;27(3):179–187.
71. Jones K, et al. Treatment of radiation proctitis with hyperbaric oxygen. *Radiother Oncol* 2006;78(1):91–94.
72. Clarke RE, et al. Hyperbaric oxygen treatment of chronic refractory radiation proctitis: a randomized and controlled double-blind crossover trial with long-term follow-up. *Int J Radiat Oncol Biol Phys* 2008;72(1):134–143.
73. Malhotra V, Moryl N. *Palliative cancer care.* Sudbury, MA: Jones and Bartlett Publishers, 2006.
74. NCCN. *Practice guidelines in oncology: adult cancer pain (ver 1).* Available at: www.nccn.org (accessed December 15, 2011).
75. Society AP. *Principles of analgesic use in the treatment of acute pain and cancer pain.* Glenview, IL: International Association for the Study of Pain, 1999.

Palliative and Supportive Care

Chapter 97
Supportive Care and Quality of Life

Gary Deng and Barrie R. Cassileth

BASIC PRINCIPLES OF SUPPORTIVE CARE AND QUALITY OF LIFE

"Quality of life" entered the medical lexicon for the first time in 1976 with the groundbreaking publication by Priestman and Baum.[1] Attention was paid to quality of life increasingly throughout the 1980s, spurred in part by efforts to differentiate among numerous chemotherapeutic agents similar in their ability to treat malignancies. In 1989, the Institute of Medicine issued a Quality of Life and Technology Assessment document, supporting the importance of quality of life and its appropriate measurement with validated, patient-reported instruments.[2] Today, it is widely recognized that existing cancer treatments, in addition to affecting the disease itself, can negatively impact the patient's physical, psychosocial, cognitive, and other aspects of well-being, which, in the aggregate, we call quality of life.[3]

When assessing quality of life, the importance of patient-reported outcome is emphasized, as patients can best describe their symptoms and the consequent impact on their lives. The U.S. Food and Drug Administration published a useful document, "Guidance for Industry Patient-Reported Outcome Measures: Use in Medical Product Development to Support Labeling Claims" in December 2009.[4]

As the current voluminous literature suggests (there were 37,963 MEDLINE hits for "cancer quality of life" as of this writing), our understanding of what impairs cancer patients' well-being has expanded, and new ways to identify and manage these problems have emerged. As it became widely recognized that cancer patients have multiple concurrent symptoms from comorbidities as well as from cancer and its treatment, a new focus on symptom clusters, rather than on individual symptoms, has been stressed.[5,6] This important concept embodies a relation among concurrent symptoms based on a common etiology or mechanism or by producing outcomes different from those that would be produced by a single symptom alone. It also includes the idea of "symptom burden," the associated level of patient or survivor distress.

A joint report of the National Cancer Institutes of the United Kingdom, Canada, and the United States on supportive care emphasized the importance of assessing and treating multiple symptoms simultaneously. It indicates that some symptoms are more likely to cluster than others and thus may share a common cause (e.g., pain, fatigue, and depression).[7] Research on this topic began relatively recently and much more is required, but some data are beginning to emerge. Examples include an analysis of 25 symptoms from 922 patients with advanced cancer that revealed seven clusters: (a) fatigue or anorexia cachexia, (b) neuropsychological, (c) upper gastrointestinal (GI), (d) nausea and vomiting, (e) aerodigestive, (f) debility, and (g) pain. Many symptoms are associated with site of radiotherapy (RT). For example, emesis is most likely with radiation to the chest and upper abdomen, while diarrhea and other GI symptoms tend to occur with RT to the lower digestive tract.

It is widely agreed that recognition of symptom clusters should lead to better understanding of symptom pathophysiology, to targeted therapies, and improved quality of life. Using this approach may also reduce polypharmacy, lessen drug side effects, and produce pharmacoeconomic benefits.[8] A cancer anorexia-cachexia syndrome is described, consisting of a combination of anorexia, tissue wasting, malnutrition, weight loss, and loss of compensatory increase in feeding, the result of complex interaction between cancer growth and host response.[9] The statistical techniques used to identify symptom clusters remain an area of research. The potential clinical importance of symptom clusters are being actively investigated.[10,11]

CONSTITUTIONAL SYMPTOMS: FATIGUE AND RELATED MOOD DYSFUNCTION

Fatigue remains a major problem for cancer patients, even after treatment for underlying anemia and other contributing medical conditions.[12] RT-produced fatigue typically is short-lived and far less severe than chemotherapy-generated fatigue. This symptom is associated with depression and anxiety. It is also related to the areas of the body that are treated with RT. Although most surveys are careful to request information about cancer-related fatigue, it may not be possible for all patients to distinguish among various potential etiologies, including comorbidities or life problems.

It is necessary to bear in mind the complex, reciprocal relationship between physical dysfunction or distress, individual capacity to cope effectively, anxiety or depression, and sleep disturbance and fatigue. Moreover, the pathogenesis of fatigue, not yet well understood, is thought to play an important role. In most studies, fatigue returns to prediagnosis levels not long after completion of RT or chemotherapy. Prediagnosis levels are not necessarily minimal or no fatigue; rather, they reflect personality and coping characteristics as well as other life factors.

Prevalence and Severity of Fatigue Associated with Radiotherapy

In a prospective study of 28 men receiving radical external-beam RT for prostate cancer, the prevalence of moderate to severe fatigue increased from 7% at baseline to 32% at RT completion. Fatigue significantly interfered with walking ability, normal work, daily chores, and enjoyment of life, but only at the end of RT. Improvement occurred after completion of treatment, but at 6.5 weeks of follow-up remained higher than at baseline. Neither age, Gleason score, prostate-specific antigen, T-stage, hormone therapy duration, nor RT dose and fractions were significantly associated with fatigue scores.[13]

Similar results are seen in studies of breast cancer patients. In 38 women alive with no evidence of disease 2.5 years after adjuvant RT for localized breast cancer, there was no significant difference between chronic fatigue levels at 2.5 years after RT and pretreatment values. Neither age nor hormonal therapy was associated with fatigue levels, but cancer-related distress correlated closely with fatigue scores.

Personality patterns tend to be stable over time and typically predictive of how patients will react to cancer diagnosis and treatment. Patients with pretreatment elevated fatigue, anxiety, or depression are at risk for chronic fatigue. RT did not contribute to posttreatment fatigue in this patient sample. Field sizes (whole-breast vs. partial breast) and age in breast RT were positively associated with maximum radiation-induced fatigue.[14]

Compared with women who received adjuvant RT, women receiving adjuvant chemotherapy were more than twice as likely to develop fatigue during the course of therapy.[15] In a typical study, during and for 3 months after primary RT for breast cancer, fatigue increased from 33% to 93%, and gradual improvement occurred during the following 3 months.[16] Among 115 Taiwanese nasopharyngeal carcinoma patients, significantly higher symptom distress was seen for patients undergoing RT compared with those who completed RT 1 to 3 years previously.[17]

In patients with advanced cancer, fatigue levels initially worsened with RT, stabilized at week 8, and returned to baseline by week 27.[18] Patients with brain metastases who received whole-brain RT (69% of 104 patients) experienced severe fatigue and many problems with cognition, whereas only 34% of those receiving only radiosurgery reported side effects. Only 5% of radiosurgery patients reported fatigue.[19]

Treatment

Management of cancer-related fatigue (CRF) is challenging and will be maximally beneficial only when a multidisciplinary approach is applied. The National Comprehensive Cancer Network (NCCN) developed practice guidelines for the management of CRF. The most recent version, 1.2012, defines CRF as a distressing, persistent, subjective sense of physical, emotional, and/or cognitive tiredness or exhaustion related to cancer or cancer treatment that is not proportional to recent activity and that interferes with usual function.

When evaluating CRF, the nature of cancer, treatment history, comorbidities, concurrent medications, pain, emotional distress, anemia, sleep disturbance, nutritional imbalance, and decreased functional status should all be assessed as potential causes or contributing factors. The management approach progresses from education, to behavior changes, to nonpharmacologic, to pharmacologic interventions.

Education of patient and family members should form the foundation of CRF management. Patient should be counseled on self-monitoring of fatigue levels, energy conservation techniques, and the use of distraction. Simple behavioral changes in daily life, such as setting priorities, pacing daily activities, delegating as much as possible, scheduling activities at times of peak energy, and structuring a daily routine to promote quality of sleep can go a long way to reduce fatigue.

When specific interventions are warranted, nonpharmacologic interventions should be tried first. Initiation of an exercise program, referral to physical therapy, occupational therapy, or rehabilitation medicine may help enhance activity levels. Psychosocial interventions, such as cognitive behavioral therapy, educational therapy, and supportive expressive therapy, can be implemented to address depression, anxiety, and adjustment disorders. Nutrition deficits and imbalance often occur and may be overlooked in these patients. Weight, caloric intake, fluid intake, electrolyte abnormalities, and micronutrients deficiency from an imbalanced diet should be identified and nutritional counseling provided. One of the most common causes of fatigue is inadequate amount and poor quality of sleep. Control of stimulus, optimizing sleep environment, and promotion of sleep hygiene are all important. Massage therapy to reduce tension and stress is often helpful.

When nonpharmacologic interventions do not produce desired results, carefully selected pharmacologic interventions should be considered. Comorbidities and concurrent medications are taken into account. Psychostimulants, such as methylphenidate or modafinil, remain investigational and should be reserved for patients with severe symptoms and prescribed only after treatment and disease-specific morbidities have been characterized or excluded. Adequate treatment of pain, emotional distress, and anemia with pharmacologic agents should be achieved. Optimize treatment for sleep dysfunction, nutritional imbalance, and other comorbidities should also take place.

SALIVARY GLAND INJURY: XEROSTOMIA

Xerostomia, the subjective experience of dry mouth, is among the most common complaints experienced by cancer patients treated with RT to the head and neck area. It is caused by salivary gland dysfunction as a result of damage in the field of radiation. Histologically, irradiated salivary glands demonstrate acinar atrophy and chronic inflammation. Inflammatory changes and fibrosis are observed in periductal and intralobular areas, whereas the ductal system remains relatively intact.[20,21]

Salivary dysfunction develops immediately and predictably. A 50% to 60% decrease in salivary flow occurs during the first week. As RT continues and the total radiation dose increases, salivary function decreases accordingly in a dose-dependent fashion. After initial deterioration, a recovery phase may be seen, with patients reporting reduced xerostomia even though salivary flow remains depressed. This may result from adaptation to the sensation of xerostomia and compensatory response from surviving functional glandular tissues. However, salivary function usually continues to decline for 6 to 8 months after therapy, and many patients show no recovery even at 12 months.[22,23] In some patients, xerostomia may be permanent.

In addition to oral discomfort, radiation-induced salivary gland injury contributes to systemic problems, including loss of appetite, chronic esophagitis, gastroesophageal reflux, and sleep disruption due to the need for frequent mouth moistening and subsequent polyuria.[24] The lubricating, buffering, and antimicrobial effects of saliva maintain the integrity of oral tissue (dental and mucosal). Saliva also assists in speech, taste perception, mastication, bolus formation, and swallowing.[25] Decreased salivation can lead to dental caries, periodontal diseases, a shift of oral flora, poor tolerability to dental prosthesis and inflammation, and atrophy and ulceration of mucosa. As a result, radiation-induced xerostomia has a debilitating impact on health and overall quality of life in head and neck cancer patients and survivors.[26]

Prevention

The extent of radiation-induced salivary dysfunction is influenced by radiation field, radiation dose, and initial volume and function of the salivary gland. Several approaches have been developed to prevent or minimize injury to salivary glands. They include salivary gland transplantation, intensity-modulated RT, and amifostine therapy.[27]

In several earlier studies, surgical transfer of submandibular glands into the submental space prior to radiation therapy resulted in prevention of xerostomia.[28–30,31] A 2-year follow-up showed that 83% to 92% of patients reported no or minimal xerostomia.[31,32] Advances in three-dimensional conformal radiation therapy and intensity-modulated RT technology make it possible to conduct gland-sparing RT. Several studies showed that both subjective and objective measures of salivatory function are preserved. Limiting the mean dose of the parotid glands to ≤26 Gy decreases the risk of long-term xerostomia. Local treatment failure rates are not affected by intensity-modulated RT.[33–37,38]

Intravenous (IV) amifostine, a thiol-containing radio protectant, administered at 200 mg/m^2 daily 15 to 30 minutes before irradiation, reduced acute and chronic xerostomia in an open label phase III study. Antitumor treatment efficacy was preserved; however, mucositis was not reduced. Nausea, vomiting, hypotension, and allergic reactions were the most common side effects.[39] Subcutaneous administration of amifostine has been explored for reduced side effects.[40–42] A multicentered phase III randomized trial failed to show that subcutaneous amifostine is superior to IV amifostine in terms of patient compliance or efficacy.[43] Other agents are less promising. Pilocarpine during radiation therapy was compared to salivary gland transfer in prevention of xerostomia and found to be inferior.[44,45] Cevimeline, a muscarinic agonist, was evaluated in randomized controlled trial with conflicting results.[46,47]

Treatment

Current treatment of RT-induced xerostomia includes dietary and oral hygiene, saliva substitution, or stimulation of salivation by moistening agents or medications.[27,48,49] Cold, tepid, soft food, and beverages are preferred. Hard, spicy foods should be avoided. In patients without residual salivary function, saliva substitutes are used to relieve xerostomia. Water is commonly used and preferred by patients. Other types of mouthwash such as saline, bicarbonate, glycerol, or commercial formulations are available. Artificial saliva has been designed to mimic natural saliva. It may contain carboxymethylcellulose, porcine and bovine mucin, or xanthan gum. In patients with residual salivary function, increased flow of natural saliva can be achieved by stimulation with chewing gum, sucking ointment, sugarless candies, menthol, acid, vitamin C, or lozenges developed to provide antimicrobial enzymes.

Several sialogogues, defined as systemic salivary gland stimulants, have been tested with mixed results. They are typically muscarinic agonists such as pilocarpine, bethanechol, carbachol, or cevimeline. Other classes of agents include neostigmine, physostigmine, nicotinic acid, potassium iodide, bromhexine (a mucolytic), and anethole trithione.[21] Current data support the use of pilocarpine. Further studies are needed to determine the long-term efficacy and safety of cevimeline and bethanechol.[27]

The most extensively studied pharmacologic treatment for xerostomia is pilocarpine. Oral administration at 5 to 10 mg, 3 times daily, is the standard regimen. Several randomized, double-blind, placebo-controlled trials have shown clinical efficacy and safety of pilocarpine in treating radiation-induced xerostomia.[50–52] In a multicenter study, 54% of the 207 study subjects reported reduction in the overall severity of xerostomia. Only 25% of those receiving placebo reported improvement. Speaking ability improved in 33% of patients receiving pilocarpine versus 18% of those receiving placebo. Saliva production also improved, but this did not correlate with subjective symptom relief.[50] In another multicenter trial that involved 162 patients, both subjective symptom and objective measurement of saliva flow improved significantly in those receiving pilocarpine versus placebo. Best results were obtained with continuous treatment for 8 to 12 weeks.[51]

Some patients require pilocarpine treatment for 2 months or longer to achieve maximum effect. Sweating, the most common side effect, is experienced by 37% to 65% of patients. In one study, 6% and 29% of patients in the 5- and 10-mg groups, respectively, dropped out because of the adverse effects.[50] Because of the cholinergic activity of pilocarpine, it is not recommended for patients with cardiovascular disease, and it is contraindicated in patients with narrow-angle glaucoma and uncontrolled asthma.[53]

Acupuncture has been shown to stimulate saliva production.[54–56] It even shows some benefit in pilocarpine-resistant xerostomia.[57] Patients with more severe symptoms appear to benefit more from acupuncture treatment.[58] Acupuncture given concurrently with RT was shown to significantly reduce xerostomia and improve quality of life.[59] Yet an acupuncture-like transcutaneous electrical nerve stimulation given concomitantly with RT failed to do the same.[60] Acupuncture appears to modulate the function of the autonomic nervous system, which may stimulate salivary gland function and induce salivary flow.[61–64] Functional magnetic resonance imaging changes in the brain were associated with acupuncture treatment.[65] In summary, acupuncture appears to be a low-risk intervention that offers a potential future treatment for RT-induced xerostomia.[27,66]

MUCOSAL INJURY: ORAL MUCOSITIS, NAUSEA AND VOMITING, DIARRHEA, AND OTHER GASTROINTESTINAL TOXICITY

Radiation therapy causes mucosal injury. When such injury occurs in the oral cavity, as commonly seen in patients irradiated at the head and neck area, it is called *stomatitis* or *oral mucositis*. When the injury occurs in nonoral alimentary tract mucosa, it presents as esophagitis, gastritis, enteritis, colitis, or proctitis. These injuries manifest as pain, dysphagia, odynophagia, nausea, vomiting, and diarrhea, typically described as GI toxicity. Mucosal injuries by radiation appear to share the same underlying molecular pathogenesis, regardless of anatomic location.[67–69] Some favor the terminology of *alimentary mucositis* to describe the hierarchy and constellation of toxicity to the oral and GI mucosa.[70] Depending on the site of irradiation, dosage, and fractionation, patients' risks of mucositis vary. More than 50% of patients receiving radiation to the head and neck, abdomen, or the pelvis will experience moderate-to-severe mucositis. Accelerated fractionation increases the risk. Stem cell transplant recipients who received total-body irradiation have more severe and prolonged symptoms.[71] Graft-versus-host disease further exacerbates mucosal injury.

Recent research indicates that the pathogenesis of mucositis is not simply the result of nonspecific epithelial cell death. Rather it may involve a more complex pan–tissue process.[72–74] The complexity of the pathogenesis of mucositis reflects the dynamic interactions of all of the cell and tissue types that comprise the epithelium and submucosa. Genetic predisposition, circadian variables, epithelial type and characteristics, and local microbial environment all play a role in determining the risk of mucosal injury.[75,76,77] New therapies are being developed based on these new findings.[76,78]

A practice guideline developed in 2004 by the Multinational Association of Supportive Care in Cancer and International Society of Oral Oncology was updated in 2007.[73,79] Recommendations related to RT are summarized in Table 97.1.

Oral Mucositis Prevention

Midline mucosa-sparing blocks were shown to protect the aerodigestive tract and significantly reduce acute toxicity during RT for head and neck cancer without compromising tumor control.[80] Another technique is three-dimensional treatment planning with conformational dose delivery. It reduces the volume of mucosa exposed to irradiation.[81] Topical benzydamine, a drug with anti-inflammatory, analgesic, and antimicrobial effects, reduces the frequency and severity of oral ulcers and pain in several randomized controlled trial. It inhibits the production of proinflammatory cytokines, including tumor necrosis factor-α.[82,83] Chlorhexidine failed to prevent radiation-induced oral mucositis (Fig. 97.1).[84–86]

Basic oral care is the foundation of care for oral mucositis. There is a lack of evidence supporting one protocol over another. Therefore, feasibility, adherence, performance, and outcomes are more important than the use of specific agents. Three randomized and three nonrandomized trials showed that implementation of a systematic protocol improved outcome.[87–92] Protocols consisting of brushing, flossing, bland rinses, and moisturizers should be implemented for all patients. An interdisciplinary approach to oral care (nurse, physician, dentist, dental hygienist, dietician, pharmacist, and others as relevant) is preferred. Dental examinations and treatment are important prior to the start of cancer therapy, especially for those with head and neck cancer, and should continue throughout active treatment and follow-up.[79]

Studies testing amifostine for oral mucositis have been disappointing. Although it appeared useful in the prevention of

TABLE 97.1 RECOMMENDATIONS FOR PREVENTION AND TREATMENT OF ORAL AND GASTROINTESTINAL MUCOSITIS

	Oral Mucositis	*GI Mucositis*
Prevention	Use of midline radiation blocks and three-dimensional radiation treatment (recommendation).	Use 500 mg oral sulfasalazine twice daily to help reduce the incidence and severity of radiation-induced enteropathy in patients receiving external-beam radiotherapy to the pelvis (suggestion).
	Benzydamine for prevention of radiation-induced mucositis in patients with head and neck cancer receiving moderate-dose radiotherapy (recommendation).	Amifostine in a dose ≥ 340 mg/m² may prevent radiation proctitis in those receiving standard dose radiotherapy for rectal cancer (suggestion). Oral sucralfate should not be used. It does not prevent acute diarrhea in patients with pelvic malignancies undergoing external-beam radiotherapy; and, compared with placebo, it is associated with more GI side effects, including rectal bleeding (recommendation).
	Chlorhexidine should not be used to prevent oral mucositis in patients with solid tumors of the head and neck who are undergoing radiotherapy (recommendation). Antimicrobial lozenges should not be used for the prevention of radiation-induced oral mucositis (recommendation).	5-Aminosalicylic acid and its related compounds mesalazine and olsalazine should not be used to prevent GI mucositis (recommendation).
Treatment	Oral care protocols that include patient and staff education should be used in an attempt to reduce severity of oral mucositis from chemotherapy or radiation therapy (suggestion).	Use of sucralfate enemas to help manage chronic, radiation-induced proctitis in patients with rectal bleeding is suggested (suggestion).
	Protocol development should be multidisciplinary and the impact of the oral care and educational protocols should be evaluated (suggestion). The oral care protocol should include use of a soft toothbrush that is replaced on a regular basis (suggestion). Sucralfate should not be used for the treatment of radiation-induced oral mucositis (recommendation).	Use amifostine to reduce esophagitis induced by concomitant chemotherapy and radiotherapy in patients with non–small cell lung cancer (suggestion).

GI, gastrointestinal.

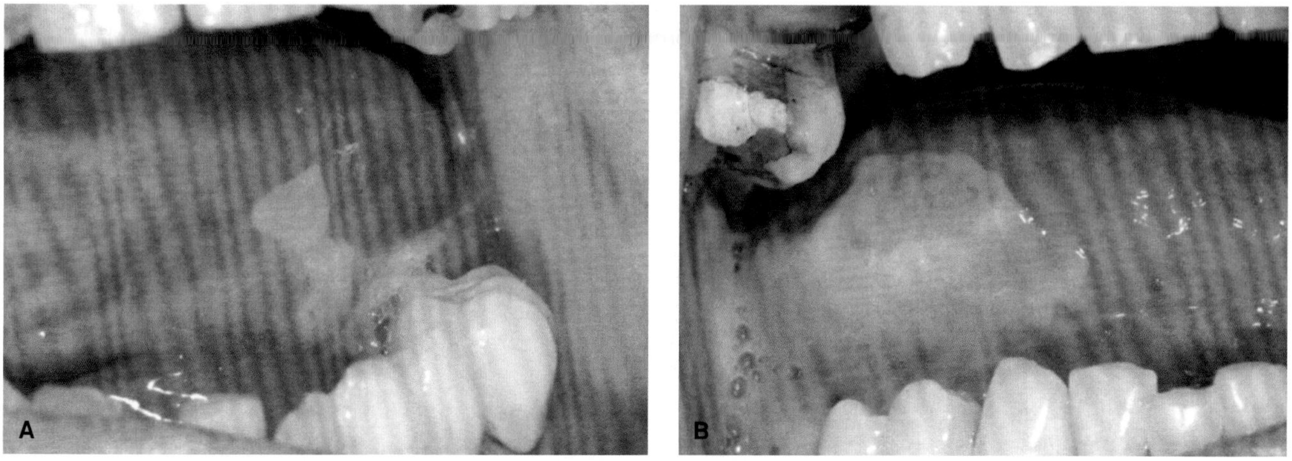

FIGURE 97.1. (A, B) Radiotherapy-induced oral mucositis.

xerostomia, inconsistent results have been reported for its use for oral symptoms.[93]

New classes of agents are being investigated. Recombinant human keratinocyte growth factor-1 (rhuKGF-1, palifermin) was shown to reduce mucositis in patients with hematologic malignancies receiving high-dose chemotherapy and total-body irradiation with autologous stem cell transplantation.[94] Palifermin reduces incidence of severe oral mucositis in head and neck cancer patients receiving definitive chemoradiotherapy and delays the onset of severe symptoms when compared to placebo. Yet the differences are not significant after multiplicity adjustment.[95] Its use in non–stem cell transplantation settings is not recommended based on current data.

On the other hand, a local granulocyte macrophage colony-stimulating factor mouthwash should *not* be used in efforts to prevent oral mucositis in the transplant setting. Other growth factors and cytokines are in early stage of development, including epidermal growth factor, transforming growth factor-β, glucagon-like peptide-2, lactoferrin, anti-inflammatory amino acid decapeptide, recombinant human interleukin-11, and insulin-like growth factor-1.[96] Natural product and dietary supplements such as glutamine, PV701 (milk-derived protein extract), several vitamins (A, B_{12}, E), folate, aloe vera (a plant extract), probiotics, and Curcumin, an extract from turmeric, were shown to hold promise in reducing radiation-induced mucositis. Most of the studies are not of sufficient quality to support a recommendation.

Oral Mucositis Treatment

Pain management is an important component of the management of oral mucositis. Most studies were done in the setting of chemotherapy-induced mucositis, instead of radiation-induced oral mucositis. Systemic and topical analgesics are used, as are coating agents. The use of opioids, nonopioids, and adjuvant medications is covered in more detail in Chapter 96. These agents can be given via oral, transmucosal, transdermal, or IV routes. Use of topical agents is widespread in practice, with practices and institutions using their own favorite formulation. Typically, these are compounded mixtures with nicknames such as "magic mouth wash." Common ingredients include viscous lidocaine, milk of magnesia, chlorhexidine, and diphenhydramine. Despite their popularity, there is no significant evidence supporting their effectiveness or tolerability.[86,97–102] A recent systematic review recommends against use of antibiotic lozenges or sucralfate for the prevention of radiation therapy–induced oral mucositis. Guidelines could not be generated because of conflicting data or insufficient evidence on topical anesthetics or analgesics (morphine, fentanyl).[103]

Gastrointestinal Mucositis Prevention

Several medications have been shown to significantly reduce the frequency and severity of radiation-induced GI mucositis, which usually presents as diarrhea and pain. Depending on the location, the GI mucositis may be termed *esophagitis, enteritis, colitis, proctosigmoiditis,* or *proctitis.* External-beam irradiation to the pelvis as part of treatment for prostate, rectal, or cervical cancer produces lower GI injury in the majority of patients.

In a randomized, controlled trial of pelvic irradiation, sulfasalazine, 1 g orally, twice daily, reduces GI toxicity from 93% to 80% and diarrhea from 86% to 55%, when compared with placebo. Grade 4 diarrhea was reduced from 16% of the patients to none.[104] Amifostine is an antioxidant that appears to protect normal cells from radiation injury preferentially to cancer cells.[105] Amifostine was shown in several studies to prevent proctitis in patients receiving standard-dose RT for rectal cancer.[93] The frequency, onset, and duration of acute rectal toxicity was reduced.[106–108] When used in patients receiving combined chemoradiation for non–small cell lung cancer, amifostine significantly reduced the need for morphine to control pain from severe esophagitis,[109] but its efficacy was mixed in other settings.[106,110,111] IV amifostine is not without side effects. Other routes of administration that might reduce side effects are under study.

Other agents that did not show significant benefit include glutamine,[110] oral sucralfate,[112,113] rectal administration of sucralfate,[114] and other anti-inflammatories commonly used in ulcerative colitis, such as 5-aminosalicylates,[115] mesalazine,[116] and olsalazine.[117] They should not be used to prevent radiation GI toxicity.

Gastrointestinal Mucositis Treatment

Nausea and Vomiting

In addition to measures discussed here that aim to treat the underlying pathology of radiation-induced mucosal injury, symptomatic treatment should also be provided. Radiation-induced nausea and emesis tend to be undertreated. Factors that influence radiation-induced emesis include single and total dose rate; fractionation; field-size and irradiated volume; site of irradiation and organs included in the radiation field; patient positioning; radiation technique, energy, and beam quality; previous or simultaneous influencing therapy; and general health status of the patient.[118] Evidence-based practice guidelines developed by national organizations differ in specific recommendations and in when recommendations apply, reflecting the limited amount of high-level evidence available to date. The updated guidelines from the

TABLE 97.2 GUIDELINES FOR PREVENTION AND TREATMENT OF RADIATION-INDUCED NAUSEA AND VOMITING

	Risk			
	High	*Moderate*	*Low*	*Minimal*
MASCC risk category	Total body	Upper abdomen, half body, upper body	Cranium (all), craniospinal, H&N, lower thorax region, pelvis	Breast, extremities
MASCC recommendation	Prophylaxis with 5-HT_3 receptor antagonists + dexamethasone	Prophylaxis with 5-HT_3 receptor antagonists + optional dexamethasone	Prophylaxis or rescue with 5-HT_3 receptor antagonists	Rescue with dopamine receptor antagonists or 5-HT_3 receptor antagonists
ASCO risk category	Total body, total nodal	Upper abdomen, upper body, half body	Cranium, craniospinal, H&N, lower thorax region, pelvis	Breast, extremities
ASCO recommendation	A 5-HT_3 receptor antagonist before each fraction and for at least 24 hours after; corticosteroid during faction 1–5	A 5-HT_3 receptor antagonist before each fraction; corticosteroid during faction 1–5	A 5-HT_3 receptor antagonist either as rescue or prophylaxis	Dopamine or 5-HT_3 receptor antagonists offered as rescue; if rescue is used, prophylactic therapy should be given until the end of RT
NCCN risk category	Total body	Upper abdomen/localized sites	–	–
NCCN recommendation	Prophylactic ondansetron, 8 mg oral twice or 3 times a day or granisetron, 2 mg oral daily ± dexamethasone, 4 mg oral every day	Same as in total body radiation	–	–
NCCN recommendation for breakthrough treatment	The same in chemo-induced nausea vomiting	The same in chemo-induced nausea vomiting	–	The same in chemo-induced nausea vomiting

MASCC, Multinational Association of Supportive Care in Cancer; H&N, head and neck; 5-HT_3, 5-hydroxytryptamine 3; ASCO, American Society of Clinical Oncology; RT, radiotherapy; NCCN, National Comprehensive Cancer Network.

Multinational Association of Supportive Care in Cancer,[119] American Society of Clinical Oncology,[120] and NCCN[121] are summarized in Table 97.2.

Diarrhea

Symptomatic management of radiation-induced diarrhea is similar to that of chemotherapy-induced diarrhea but may not require hospitalization.[122,123] Diarrhea usually occurs during the third week of fractionated abdomen or pelvic RT. Guidelines were developed by an expert panel and updated in 2004.[124]

For mild to moderate diarrhea, the initial management should include dietary modifications.[125] Patients should eat small, frequent, protein-rich meals. Adequate fluid intake (35 mL/kg/day) is necessary. Liquids should be taken primarily between meals. Soluble fibers such as oats, pectin, guar, and psyllium help retain stool consistency. Spices, alcohol, caffeine, high-osmolar beverages, and high-lactose food should be avoided.[125]

Loperamide remains the mainstay of pharmacologic treatment. It should be started at 4 mg followed by 2 mg every 4 hours or after every unformed stool (maximum, 16 mg per day). Unlike in chemotherapy, where loperamide may be discontinued after initial response, standard doses of loperamide should be continued for the duration of RT. This is because the long duration of fractionated radiation may cause repeated injury to the intestinal mucosa. The dose is increased to 2 mg every 2 hours if the diarrhea persists for more than 24 hours.

If diarrhea has not resolved after another 24 hours on the higher dose of loperamide, the drug should be continued and a second-line agent, such as tincture of opium (paregoric), an antimotility agent, can be added. Diphenoxylate and atropine can also be used, although they do not have as favorable a side effect profile as loperamide. The patient may require outpatient evaluation and IV fluid. Antibiotics and complete stool and blood workup are usually not necessary in the absence of signs of dehydration or infection. Octreotide and glutamine have been studied and found of no benefit.[126,127] Probiotic supplementation showed beneficial effect in the prevention and treatment of radiation-induced diarrhea in animal studies, but high-quality clinical studies are lacking. If diarrhea is severe, persistent, or complicated, hospitalization may be considered.[124]

SKIN INJURY: ACUTE DERMATITIS AND CHRONIC SKIN CHANGES

Radiation-induced skin injury can lead to acute dermatitis or chronic skin changes.[128,129] These changes can occur at both the entrance and exit site of the irradiation beam. Severity is determined by the dose, fractionation, beam, volume, and surface area. Patient-specific factors also play a role, such as poor nutrition status, pre-existing vascular condition or connective tissue disease, excessive skin folds, or genetics.[130] The pathophysiology is a combination of direct radiation injury and a subsequent inflammatory response. Free radicals from ionizing radiation cause alteration of DNA, proteins, lipids, and carbohydrates. Epithelial basal cells, vascular endothelial cells, and Langerhans cells are damaged. A cascade of proinflammatory cytokines, thrombotic factors, growth factors, and other molecules is activated.[131]

Acute skin changes may become visible after 10 to 14 hours. Grade 1 changes include mild generalized erythema and dry desquamation, pruritus, scaling, dyspigmentation, and hair loss. After 4 or 5 weeks of radiotherapy and radiation doses to the skin of 40 Gy or greater, grade 2 dermatitis may develop, with tender or edematous erythema, moist desquamation in skin folds, and considerable pain. They tend to peak 1 to 2 week after the last treatment and start healing 3 to 5 weeks after radiation. Complete healing may take 1 to 3 months. Occasionally, dermatitis may progress to grade 3, characterized by confluent moist desquamation, or even grade 4, with ulcers, hemorrhage, and necrosis.[128,132] Chronic changes may develop months or years after the initial exposure. Postinflammatory hypo- or hyperpigmentation, textural changes (xerosis and hyperkeratosis), loss of hair follicles and sebaceous glands, atrophy, telangiectasia, or subcutaneous fibrosis are among the manifestations. Fibrosis can result in tissue retraction, pain, and limitation of movement. Scalp appears more tolerant to radiation injury than the skin of the face, neck, trunk, and extremities. Affected skin can be predisposed to ulcers and skin breakdown.[133,134] In some patients, radiation recall dermatitis may occur. This happens when a patient who has completed RT encounters a drug and develops skin reaction similar to acute radiation dermatitis. The drugs are usually cytotoxic agents. It

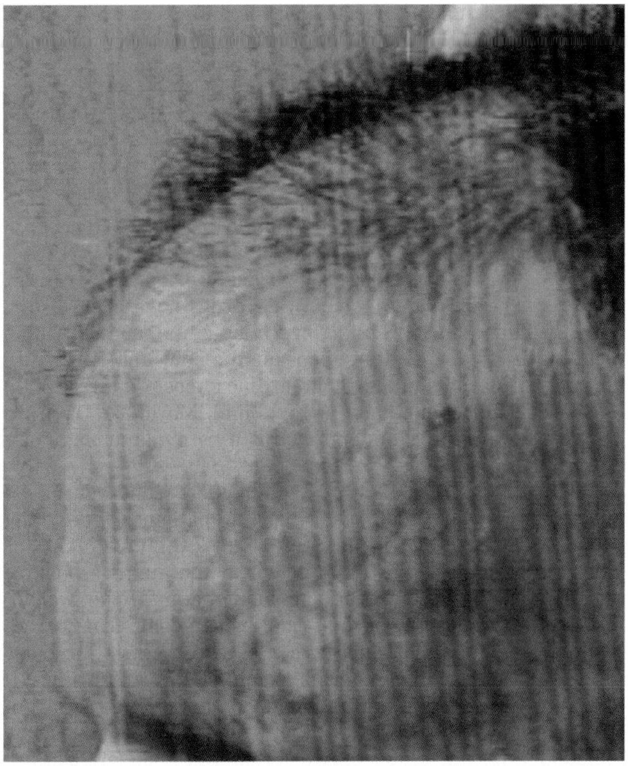

FIGURE 97.2. Acute dermatitis after whole-brain radiation.

is probably due to local cutaneous immunologic responses to the challenging agent (Fig. 97.2).[135]

Mild acute dermatitis is treated symptomatically. Washing with water, gentle cleansing with a mild agent, wearing loose, nonbinding clothing, and avoidance of irritants, antiperspirants, and ultraviolet exposure all help. When erythema and dry desquamation occurs, creams or ointments (petrolatum-based, castor oil, balsam of Peru, trypsin, trolamine) can be used. Topical sucralfate or hyaluronic acid was shown to be efficacious in some controlled studies.[136,137] In a phase III study in breast cancer patients receiving postoperative RT, an extract from the calendula plant significantly reduced the occurrence of moderate to severe acute dermatitis from 63% to 41% when compared with trolamine, a nonsteroidal agent.[138] Other topical agents containing aloe vera, D-panthenol, almond, or chamomile can also be tried. The use of these agents is supported only by uncontrolled studies or anecdotal evidence.[139,140]

The value of topical antioxidants has not been established, and topical steroids are controversial, with research producing conflicting results. There are concerns of infection and skin atrophy, known side effects of topical steroids. At best, steroids may ameliorate the symptoms, but they do not prevent the dermatitis.[141] Topical ascorbic acid lotion (vitamin C) did not show discernible benefit for the prevention of radiation dermatitis.[142]

When acute dermatitis becomes severe, usual wound care should be applied to the erosions and ulcerations. Key measures are keeping the site clean and moist, pain management, protection from contamination, debridement, and infection control.[134,143] During radiation treatment, hydrogel dressings, hydrocolloid dressing, burn pads, or foam dressings can be applied. If the wound is infected, ionic silver powder, topical antibiotics, cadexomer iodine, or maltodextrin powder can be added. Referral to wound care specialists should be made.[139] In recent years, more specific agents have been investigated, such as topical granulocyte-macrophage colony-stimulating factor, tacrolimus, pimecrolimus, and platelet-derived growth factor.[128]

Chronic skin changes from radiation injury are harder to treat. Chronic fibrosis is associated with high incidence of skin breakdown and infection. A team approach should be adopted that includes wound care, physical therapy, deep massage, and pain management to address cosmetic and quality of life issues. Pentoxifylline (Trental) appears to have an antifibrotic effect. Oral pentoxifylline (800 mg per day) and vitamin E (1,000 IU per day) for 6 months significantly reduce radiation-induced fibrosis.[144] Prophylactic use of pentoxifylline significantly reduces late skin changes, fibrosis, and soft tissue necrosis in a randomized controlled study, possibly through its protective effect against vascular pathology.[145] Intramuscular liposomal copper or zinc superoxide dismutase, subcutaneous interferon-γ, or hyperbaric oxygen therapy has also been used.

GENITOURINARY TRACT INJURY

Urinary Symptoms

Irradiation to the pelvic region as part of treatment for cancer of the prostate, uterus, ovary, cervix rectum, or urinary bladder can cause urinary problems due to injury to mucosa, vasculature, and smooth muscles.[146,147] Acute reactions occur within 3 to 6 months of treatment. Chronic changes occur later. Acute reactions present as dysuria, frequency, and urgency as a result of radiation cystitis. They are usually not as severe as some of the cystitis caused by chemotherapy. Strictures or fistula can develop during the years following RT.[148,149]

If infection is ruled out, symptomatic relief with phenazopyridine (Pyridium) is usually the first-line treatment for acute symptoms. It is given at 200 mg orally, 3 times a day. Phenazopyridine accumulates in the urine essentially unchanged and acts as a topical analgesic within the bladder. Patients should be warned that phenazopyridine turns the urine into a bright orange color and can stain clothing. If the symptoms are not adequately relieved, antispasmodics can be added. Oxybutynin (Ditropan) or flavoxate (Urispas) help relax the smooth muscles and reduce urinary urgency and frequency.[150] Tolterodine (Detrol) is a cholinergic antagonist that is also effective for overactive bladder. It causes less dry mouth but its response rate is lower.[151] Trospium (Sanctura) was documented to improve symptoms in radiation-induced cystitis and is significantly better tolerated than immediate-release oxybutynin.[152]

Intravesical infusion of hyaluronic acid or chondroitin sulfate, injection of botulinum toxin A into bladder wall, and hyperbaric oxygen therapy have shown benefit.[153–156] IV WF10 (tetrachlorodecaoxide), an immunomodulator, was reported to be beneficial.[157,158] In patients with severe pain, aggressive pain control with opioids may be needed.

Symptomatic management of chronic changes is similar to that of acute reactions. Dilatation or placement of a permanent catheter may be required for significant obstruction. Patients not responding to less-aggressive treatment may be candidates for reconstructive surgery to repair the stricture, sphincter failure, or fistula.

Female Sexuality

High-dose radiation to the pelvis causes varying degrees of sexual dysfunction related to injury to the ovaries and vagina.[159,160] Ovarian failure as a result of pelvis irradiation leads to postmenopausal changes. Acute injury occurs during the course of RT and the following few months. It usually presents as vaginal and vulval mucositis, pain, and ulceration. Chronic changes are less frequent than acute changes, which can develop more than 3 months after the completion of treatment. Chronic changes include fibrosis, loss of elasticity and sensation, susceptibility to trauma and infection, postcoital bleeding, and dyspareunia.[161–163]

Maintenance of local hygiene, aggressive treatment of infection, and regular dilatation of the vaginal canal help reduce the acute reaction. Hormone replacement therapy and application of lubricants for mucosal dryness can be used to treat acute injury. To prevent chronic changes, uses of vaginal dilators, lubricants, and supplemental estrogen were shown to be helpful. When fibrosis is established, treatment may require more drastic measures, such as hyperbaric oxygen therapy or surgical reconstruction. Although these are common options in clinical practice, the level of evidence supporting their use varies.[159]

Most studies of use of topical estrogen showed benefit.[164,165] Radiation causes damage to the epithelium, which may persist for another 3 to 6 months after therapy. Topical estrogen promotes epithelial regeneration. Benzydamine is an anti-inflammatory that also has analgesic, local anesthetic, and antimicrobial effects. It can be applied topically to achieve a higher local tissue concentration. It reduced both subjective symptoms and objective observation of vaginal mucositis.[166,167] There have been several uncontrolled studies of hyperbaric oxygen therapy in the treatment of established necrotic wound resulting from perineal and vaginal radiation; the strength of evidence is modest.[168,169] In women with severe radiation damage, such as perineal defect or obliteration of vagina, reconstructive surgery may be considered. All reported studies are retrospective.[159]

Male Sexuality

When planning RT for prostate cancer, its effect on male sexual function must be considered and discussed with the patient. Although the rate of erectile dysfunction (ED) is lower in patients receiving RT versus radical prostatectomy, sexual dysfunctions remain one of the most important posttreatment quality of life issues.[170] A survey showed that 68% of men aged 45 to 70 years were willing to trade off a 10% or greater advantage in 5-year survival to maintain sexual potency.[171] Onset of ED is gradual, usually beginning about 6 months posttreatment and continuing to deteriorate for 4 years.[172]

RT does not appear to reduce testosterone production or cause pelvic nerve injury.[173] In addition to psychological reasons, vascular changes after RT appear to be the predominant cause of postradiation male sexual dysfunction. As such, smoking and hypertension are risk factors.[174,175] With external-beam RT, the rates of ED vary from 7% to 72%, a wide range attributed to the study populations. Brachytherapy is associated with 2% to 89% of ED.[176] Diminished sexual desire, decreased orgasmic pleasure, and a reduced ejaculation volume are other problems reported by patients.[177]

Treatment of post-RT sexual dysfunction should take a multidisciplinary approach, including psychosocial evaluation and counseling, pharmacologic intervention, and exploration of the use of mechanical devices.[176,178] The mainstay of pharmacologic treatment is phosphodiesterase inhibitors in patients with arteriogenic ED. A randomized double-blinded, placebo-controlled crossover trail suggests a positive response to sildenafil (Viagra). Yet the overall response rate is low. Only 21% of patients improved during sildenafil treatment but not during placebo treatment.[179] Tadalafil (Cialis) is found beneficial in these patient populations too.[180,181]

Intracavernosal injection of prostaglandins or phentolamine papaverine is also effective. For patients who are refractory to pharmacologic intervention, implantation of a penile prosthesis can be considered. Minimal intraoperative and postoperative complications and an excellent patient satisfaction rate were reported.[182] Vacuum devices are another option.

NUTRITION

Nutritional support is very important for patients undergoing RT. Patients may be malnourished when they come for initial treatment. Cancer creates a catabolic state. Anorexia, early satiety, nausea and vomiting, and involvement of the alimentary tract by cancer all contribute to impaired nutrition intake, digestion, and absorption. Once RT is started, a patient's nutritional status can deteriorate, especially in those with GI toxicity. A weight loss of more than 20% of total body weight is associated with poorer outcome. Nutritional support measures include prescription of appetite enhancers, provision of a high-quality diet, ensuring adequate enteral intake via tube feeding, and hyperalimentation with parenteral nutrition.[183] A multidisciplinary approach should be taken with the involvement of GI physicians, nutritionists, and nursing staff.

A systematic review showed that only progestins (megestrol [Megace]) and corticosteroids (methylprednisolone, prednisolone, and dexamethasone) are supported by evidence for cancer-related anorexia. A number of other drugs have been tested. They include metoclopramide, cyproheptadine, pentoxifylline, melatonin, erythropoietin, eicosapentaenoic acid (fish oil), androgenic steroids (nandrolone or fluoxymesterone), ghrelin, interferon, and cannabinoid (dronabinol [Marinol]). Data are mixed. No strong recommendation can be made at this point regarding these agents.[184,185]

Cancer patients tend to have a higher protein turnover. Adequate protein intake is critical in patients undergoing cancer treatment. Daily intake of 1.5 to 2.0 g of protein per kilogram of ideal body weight generally maintains a positive nitrogen balance. Caloric intake help maintain the weight. Between 30% and 90% of total calories can come from carbohydrates. Fat provides energy, serves as a vehicle for other nutrients, and performs other important biological functions. It usually makes up around 30% of the content in enteral formulas. Vitamins, minerals, and other micronutrients should be included. Sufficient water intake is required to offset the 2.5-L daily fluid loss. Dietary counseling improves outcomes in selected populations.[186] Body weight and serum markers (albumin, transferrin, and prealbumin) can be monitored to assess whether the nutritional support is adequate.[187–189]

In patients with moderate to severe radiation-induced oral mucositis or esophagitis, oral nutritional support can be challenging. Tube feeding bypasses the injured tissues and provides direct access to the absorption surface. Nasogastric or nasojejunal tubes enable short-term access. For longer term access (>30 days), gastrostomy, gastrojejunostomy, and jejunostomy tubes can be placed endoscopically, radiologically, or surgically. Percutaneous endoscopic gastrostomy is increasingly the method of choice, often placed prophylactically when severe upper GI toxicity is anticipated.[190–193] Gastrostomy tube placement is not without risk. Some series suggest a 17% morbidity rate. In 3% of patients, serious complications such as peritonitis, sepsis, perforation, and dislodgement were reported.[194,195] Metastasis to percutaneous endoscopic gastrostomy site has also been reported, likely due to direct implantation of cancer cells. For patients with reflux esophagitis, gastroparesis, aspiration pneumonia, or limited stomach volume, a jejunostomy tube may be placed instead. The feeding tube should be cared for properly to prevent displacement or malfunctioning such as clogging.

When adequate nutrition intake can be achieved, enteral intake is preferred over parenteral support because it uses and helps maintain the existing alimentary functions. It is less expensive, safer, and associated with fewer side effects. However, in patients without a functioning GI tract because of obstruction, poor GI motility, intractable vomiting, severe diarrhea, short bowel syndrome, or severe pancreatitis, total parenteral nutrition may be appropriate. Implementation of total parenteral nutrition requires special expertise and is done in a concerted manner between the cancer-treating team and the nutrition support team.[196,197]

ACKNOWLEDGMENTS

The authors thank Dr. Joseph Huryn, Chief, Dental Service, and Dr. Liang Deng, Dermatology Service, at Memorial Sloan-Kettering Cancer Center for providing the photographs for this chapter, and Jyothirmai Gubili for expert editorial assistance.

SELECTED REFERENCES

A full list of references for this chapter is available online.

4. McLeod LD, et al. Interpreting patient-reported outcome results: US FDA guidance and emerging methods. *Expert Rev Pharmacoecon Outcomes Res* 2011;11(2):163–169.
7. Hagen NA, et al. The Birmingham International Workshop on Supportive, Palliative, and End-of-Life Care Research. *Cancer* 2006;107(4):874–881.
11. Kirkova J, et al. Cancer symptom clusters: clinical and research methodology. *J Palliat Med* 2011;14(10):1149–1166.
18. Brown P, et al. Will improvement in quality of life (QOL) impact fatigue in patients receiving radiation therapy for advanced cancer? *Am J Clin Oncol* 2006;29(1):52–58.
27. Jensen SB, et al. A systematic review of salivary gland hypofunction and xerostomia induced by cancer therapies: management strategies and economic impact. *Support Care Cancer* 2010;18(8):1061–1079.
31. Zhang Y, et al. Prevention of radiation-induced xerostomia by submandibular gland transfer. *Head Neck* 2012;34(7):937–942.
38. Little M, et al. Reducing xerostomia after chemo-IMRT for head-and-neck cancer: beyond sparing the parotid glands. *Int J Radiat Oncol Biol Phys* 2012;83(3):1007–1014.
43. Bardet E, et al. Subcutaneous compared with intravenous administration of amifostine in patients with head and neck cancer receiving radiotherapy: final results of the GORTEC 2000–02 phase III randomized trial. *J Clin Oncol* 2011;29(2):127–133.
44. Jha N, et al. Phase III randomized study: oral pilocarpine versus submandibular salivary gland transfer protocol for the management of radiation-induced xerostomia. *Head Neck* 2009;31(2):234–243.
45. Rieger JM, et al. Functional outcomes related to the prevention of radiation-induced xerostomia: oral pilocarpine versus submandibular salivary gland transfer. *Head Neck* 2012;34(2):168–174.
49. Kahn ST, Johnstone PA. Management of xerostomia related to radiotherapy for head and neck cancer. *Oncology (Williston Park)* 2005;19(14):1827–1832.
58. Pfister DG, et al. Acupuncture for pain and dysfunction after neck dissection: results of a randomized controlled trial. *J Clin Oncol* 2010;28(15):2565–2570.
59. Meng Z, et al. Randomized controlled trial of acupuncture for prevention of radiation-induced xerostomia among patients with nasopharyngeal carcinoma. *Cancer* 2012;118(13):3337–3344.
60. Wong RK, et al. Phase II randomized trial of acupuncture-like transcutaneous electrical nerve stimulation to prevent radiation-induced xerostomia in head and neck cancer patients. *J Soc Integr Oncol* 2010;8(2):35–42.
65. Deng G, et al. Functional magnetic resonance imaging (fMRI) changes and saliva production associated with acupuncture at LI-2 acupuncture point: a randomized controlled study. *BMC Complement Altern Med* 2008;8:37.
70. Peterson DE, et al. Alimentary tract mucositis in cancer patients: impact of terminology and assessment on research and clinical practice. *Support Care Cancer* 2006;14(6):499–504.
73. Sonis ST, et al. Perspectives on cancer therapy-induced mucosal injury: pathogenesis, measurement, epidemiology, and consequences for patients. *Cancer* 2004;100(9 Suppl):1995–2025.
74. Yeoh AS, et al. Nuclear factor kappaB (NFkappaB) and cyclooxygenase-2 (Cox-2) expression in the irradiated colorectum is associated with subsequent histopathological changes. *Int J Radiat Oncol Biol Phys* 2005;63(5):1295–1303.
75. Anthony L, et al. New thoughts on the pathobiology of regimen-related mucosal injury. *Support Care Cancer* 2006;14(6):516–518.
77. Peterson DE, Lalla RV. Oral mucositis: the new paradigms. *Curr Opin Oncol* 2010;22(4):318–322.
79. Keefe DM, et al. Updated clinical practice guidelines for the prevention and treatment of mucositis. *Cancer* 2007;109(5):820–831.
93. Bensadoun RJ, et al. Amifostine in the management of radiation-induced and chemo-induced mucositis. *Support Care Cancer* 2006;14(6):566–572.
94. Hensley ML, et al. American Society of Clinical Oncology 2008 clinical practice guideline update: use of chemotherapy and radiation therapy protectants. *J Clin Oncol* 2009;27(1):127–145.
95. Le QT, et al. Palifermin reduces severe mucositis in definitive chemoradiotherapy of locally advanced head and neck cancer: a randomized, placebo-controlled study. *J Clin Oncol* 2011;29(20):2808–2814.
96. von Bultzingslowen I, et al. Growth factors and cytokines in the prevention and treatment of oral and gastrointestinal mucositis. *Support Care Cancer* 2006;14(6):519–527.
115. Baughan CA, et al. A randomized trial to assess the efficacy of 5-aminosalicylic acid for the prevention of radiation enteritis. *Clin Oncol (R Coll Radiol)* 1993;5(1):19–24.
116. Resbeut M, et al. A randomized double blind placebo controlled multicenter study of mesalazine for the prevention of acute radiation enteritis. *Radiother Oncol* 1997;44(1):59–63.
117. Martenson JA Jr, et al. Olsalazine is contraindicated during pelvic radiation therapy: results of a double-blind, randomized clinical trial. *Int J Radiat Oncol Biol Phys* 1996;35(2):299–303.
118. Feyer PC, Stewart AL, Titlbach OJ. Aetiology and prevention of emesis induced by radiotherapy. *Support Care Cancer* 1998;6(3):253–260.
119. Feyer PC, et al. Radiotherapy-induced nausea and vomiting (RINV): MASCC/ESMO guideline for antiemetics in radiotherapy: update 2009. *Support Care Cancer* 2011;19(Suppl 1):S5–S14.
120. Basch E, et al. Antiemetics: American Society of Clinical Oncology clinical practice guideline update. *J Clin Oncol* 2011;29(31):4189–4198.
121. Urba S. Radiation-induced nausea and vomiting. *J Natl Compr Canc Netw* 2007;5(1):60–65.
122. Gwede CK. Overview of radiation- and chemoradiation-induced diarrhea. *Semin Oncol Nurs* 2003;19(4 Suppl 3):6–10.
123. O'Brien BE, Kaklamani VG, Benson AB 3rd. The assessment and management of cancer treatment-related diarrhea. *Clin Colorectal Cancer* 2005;4(6):375–383.
124. Benson AB 3rd, et al. Recommended guidelines for the treatment of cancer treatment-induced diarrhea. *J Clin Oncol* 2004;22(14):2918–2926.
125. Stern J, Ippoliti C. Management of acute cancer treatment-induced diarrhea. *Semin Oncol Nurs* 2003;19(4 Suppl 3):11–16.
126. Martenson JA, et al. Phase III, double-blind study of depot octreotide versus placebo in the prevention of acute diarrhea in patients receiving pelvic radiation therapy: results of North Central Cancer Treatment Group N00CA. *J Clin Oncol* 2008;26(32):5248–5253.
128. Hymes SR, Strom EA, Fife C. Radiation dermatitis: clinical presentation, pathophysiology, and treatment 2006. *J Am Acad Dermatol* 2006;54(1):28–46.
153. Shao Y, Lu GL, Shen ZJ. Comparison of intravesical hyaluronic acid instillation and hyperbaric oxygen in the treatment of radiation-induced hemorrhagic cystitis. *BJU Int* 2012;109(5):691–694.
154. Hazewinkel MH, et al. Prophylactic vesical instillations with 0.2% chondroitin sulfate may reduce symptoms of acute radiation cystitis in patients undergoing radiotherapy for gynecological malignancies. *Int Urogynecol J* 2011;22(6):725–730.
155. Smit SG, Heyns CF. Management of radiation cystitis. *Nat Rev Urol* 2010;7(4):206–214.
156. Chuang YC, et al. Bladder botulinum toxin A injection can benefit patients with radiation and chemical cystitis. *BJU Int* 2008;102(6):704–706.
159. Denton AS, Maher EJ. Interventions for the physical aspects of sexual dysfunction in women following pelvic radiotherapy. *Cochrane Database Syst Rev* 2003;1:CD003750.
176. Incrocci L, Slob AK, Levendag PC. Sexual (dys)function after radiotherapy for prostate cancer: a review. *Int J Radiat Oncol Biol Phys* 2002;52(3):681–693.
179. Watkins Bruner D, et al. Randomized, double-blinded, placebo-controlled crossover trial of treating erectile dysfunction with sildenafil after radiotherapy and short-term androgen deprivation therapy: results of RTOG 0215. *J Sex Med* 2011;8(4):1228–1238.
180. Ricardi U, et al. Efficacy and safety of tadalafil 20 mg on demand vs. tadalafil 5 mg once-a-day in the treatment of post-radiotherapy erectile dysfunction in prostate cancer men: a randomized phase II trial. *J Sex Med* 2010;7(8):2851–2859.
184. Davis MP, et al. Appetite and cancer-associated anorexia: a review. *J Clin Oncol* 2004;22(8):1510–1517.

SECTION V ECONOMICS, ETHICS, AND TECHNOLOGY ASSESSMENT

Chapter 98

Technology Assessment, Outcome Analysis Research, Comparative Effectiveness, and Evidence-Based Radiation Oncology

Carlos A. Perez, Edward C. Halperin, and Yolande Lievens

There is worldwide concern about rising medical costs. The problem is particularly acute in the United States, which has led to multiple efforts to institute health care reforms. Health care expenditures constitute about 17% of the U.S. gross domestic product, compared to 6% to 11% for Canada, Germany, Japan, and the United Kingdom.[1] The cost of administration of U.S. health care is approximately one-fourth of the total national expenditure on health care. Health care administrative costs in the United States exceed those in many other developed countries. In 2002 the administrative cost of the federal Medicare program was 3% of the program's total budget, whereas the administrative costs of the federal and state Medicaid programs was 6.7% compared to 12.8% of total revenues for private health insurance plans. One reason for the low administrative cost of Medicare is its lack of advertising and marketing expenses. Medicare pays for roughly 1 employee for 10,000 beneficiaries, whereas most large private insurers hire 15 or more employees per 10,000 enrollees. The Kaiser Foundation Health Plan, one of the largest and best-known group-health maintenance organizations (HMOs), has self-reported administrative costs of 4%.[2]

According to the 2011 report of the Organisation for Economic Co-operation and Development, the average annual growth rate in health care spending between 2000 and 2006 ranged from 1.4% in Germany to 10.7% in Korea. With health expenditure of $6,714 per person per year, the United States largely outspent the other countries surveyed.[3]

Borger et al.[4] projected that in 2015 the United States will spend >$4 trillion, about 20% of the gross domestic product, on health care. Over the last 30 years overall inflation in the United States was 106%, whereas health care costs grew by 251%.[5] It is estimated that >$100 billion are devoted yearly to research, development, and regulatory approval of new technologies, but <$1 billion is spent on assessment of these new technologies.[6] Concern over the magnitude and continued growth of expenditures for health care in the United States has led to economic pressure on health service providers to contain costs.

Powerful forces affect the assessment of new technologies in radiation therapy. Inventors and developers, medical equipment manufacturers, corporate stock holders, and equipment salespeople seek rapid entry of new technologies into the marketplace at a minimum cost for as rapid a financial return as possible. Radiation oncologists desire new technology either for a real or perceived improvement in health care, career development, competitiveness with other practitioners, and/or personal profit. Patients and family members hope to see an improvement in clinical outcomes. Third-party payers seek cost reductions or stabilization, stable budgetary expenditures, and a plausible explanation of the "medical necessity" of the new technology. Finally, policy makers seek to balance the competing pressures that they feel from medical equipment manufacturers, physicians, and patients and the overall need for cost containment.[7]

Historically, regulatory approval of new drugs and devices was reliant on well-funded developers with a significant revenue stream conducting and funding randomized, prospective clinical trials. Many new technologies in radiation therapy, however, are introduced by small startup companies that are smaller, less well capitalized, and often single-product vendors. They are not capable of funding randomized, prospective trials and they have a powerful financial impetus to bring their product to market as quickly and as profitably as possible.

In 1985 the Blue Cross Blue Shield Association adopted criteria that required "adequate scientific evidence" to determine that technology improved health outcomes. This approach quickly became the norm among public and private payers. In an interesting development, in 2005, the Centers for Medicare and Medicaid Services (CMS) posted on its website draft guidelines describing a new approach to the determination of coverage policies called "Coverage with Evidence Development."[7] This proposal argued that Medicare coverage of promising technologies or services could be linked directly to a requirement that the beneficiary be a participant in a trial or registry and that the CMS had statutory or regulatory authority for that requirement. In the United Kingdom there was a similar proposal for funding "only-in-research" programs. Such programs were used for the evaluation of laparoscopic surgery for colorectal cancer, photodynamic therapy for age-related macular degeneration, the National Emphysema Treatment Trial to determine whether lung reduction surgery was superior to pulmonary rehabilitation without surgery, a comparison of balloon angioplasty plus carotid artery stenting versus carotid endarterectomy in patients at high risk for stroke, and the role of positron emission tomography scanning in suspected dementia.[8]

ECONOMIC EVALUATION IN HEALTH CARE

Economic evaluation is routinely becoming an important criterion for evaluation of therapeutic strategies. Unfortunately, consistent criteria are not followed for evaluation of the economics of treatment, which reduces the usefulness and credibility of comparative cost and other financial data/statistics across studies or over time.[9]

Health technology assessment (HTA) plays an essential role in modern health care by supporting evidence-based decision making in policy and practice. HTA involves addressing five questions[10]:

1. Can a health care intervention achieve its expected goal when used in optimal circumstances? (Efficacy)
2. Does the intervention do more good than harm when used in routine practice? (Effectiveness)
3. What is the balance between the health outcome obtained and the resources required to deliver the intervention? (Efficiency or Cost-Effectiveness)
4. Is the supply of services matched to locations where they are accessible to persons that need them? (Availability)
5. Who gains and who loses by choosing to allocate resources to one health care program instead of another? (Distribution).

A full economic evaluation typically involves quantitative examination of both costs and outcomes, or consequences, of competing interventions possible, including no intervention. An appropriately performed economic evaluation is incremental, that is, it measures the extra cost incurred to obtain the incremental improvement in outcome. Drummond et al.[11] identified different types of full economic evaluation based on the denominator chosen (Table 98.1). The most widely used approach, *cost-effectiveness analysis* (CEA), compares the incremental costs of a new technology or intervention to the incremental gain or loss of clinical outcome of the new intervention,

TABLE 98.1 LEVELS OF EVIDENCE AND GRADING OF EVIDENCE FOR RECOMMENDATIONS

	Type of Evidence
Level	
I	Evidence obtained from meta-analysis of multiple, well-designed, controlled studies or from high-power randomized, controlled clinical trials
II	Evidence obtained from at least one well-designed experimental study or low-power randomized, controlled clinical trial
III	Evidence obtained from well-designed, quasi-experimental studies such as nonrandomized, controlled, single-group, pre/post, cohort, time, or matched case–control series
IV	Evidence from well-designed, nonexperimental studies, such as comparative and correlational descriptive and case studies
V	Evidence from case reports and clinical examples
Grade	
A	There is evidence of type I or consistent findings from multiple studies of type II, III, or IV
B	There is evidence of type II, III, or IV and findings are generally consistent
C	There is evidence of type II, III, or IV but findings are inconsistent
D	There is little or no systematic empirical evidence

Adapted from Drummond M, Sculpher MJ, Torrance GW, et al. *Methods for the economic evaluation of health care programmes.* Oxford: Oxford University Press, 2005.

ideally measured in life-years gained (LYG). Other potential denominators in a CEA are disease-free survival or number of cancers prevented or detected, but the use of such intermediary outcome measures hampers comparison among different CEAs and should therefore be discouraged. The evaluation will result in a ratio of the cost/outcome, for example, cost/life-year gained ($/LYG, €/LYG), called the incremental cost-effectiveness ratio.

When the outcome of the evaluated interventions is expected to be the same, the economic evaluation will be limited to a cost comparison called *cost-minimization analysis* (CMA). Assuming a well-defined comparison of two radiation therapy (RT) approaches and a sufficiently long follow-up, prolongation of life, life-years gained, can be measured, but it can be questioned whether this is the metric that has most relevance to patients. The third type of full economic evaluation, *cost–utility analysis* (CUA), acknowledges quality of life after anintervention by weighting the LYG with a "utility factor" typically ranging from 0 (death) to 1 (perfect health). For example, if a patient had a utility or preference for a health state of 0.5 and he survived in that state for 1 year, then he would have had a quality-adjusted survival of 6 months. A CUA employs quality-adjusted life years (QALYs) in the denominator, with the result expressed as cost/QALY. Utilities or patient preferences for a certain health outcome can be measured with instruments such as the Health Utilities Index III[12] and EuroQol[13] or tests such as Time-Trade Off or Standard Gamble.[14] CUAs are helpful in trying to compare nonsimilar health interventions, such as a prostate cancer–screening program with a child immunization program, for example.

The last type of full economic evaluation is *cost–benefit analysis,* in which both cost and outcome are valued in terms of currency. Where the benefit in monetary units is greater than the cost, the medical intervention is considered worthwhile. Putting a dollar value on the quantity and quality of a life is, however, a highly specialized and controversial area. Full economic evaluation in RT, requiring detailed input on short- and long-term costs and outcomes, can be difficult to perform. One such approach addresses costs and outcomes separately and leads to cost and outcome descriptions, respectively.[11] However, there are dangers with separating costs and outcomes, and one has to be cautious that the information generated will not be misused.

The most useful descriptions of outcome of a new treatment strategy, particularly from the patient's perspective, result from the conduct of clinical trials. Randomized and controlled phase III trials have been categorized as efficacy or effectiveness evaluations.[11] It can be argued, however, that such comparisons may indirectly lead to the increased cost of health care as funders come under pressure to broadly adopt new interventions with only marginal clinical benefit and no consideration of the opportunity cost. A pure cost comparison, in contrast, entails the opposite risk. If the tendency to reduce health care spending is strong, this might result in the simple choice of the cheapest approach, which may, in turn, lead to reduced quality, hence inferior outcome. Provided that there is sufficient evidence that the outcome of interest for the experimental treatment or intervention does not differ from the standard treatment, a CMA is undertaken (discussed earlier), that is, a mere cost comparison, with the intervention resulting in the lower cost being the favored one from a health economics' perspective.

In evaluating medical care, the term *efficacy* is not interchangeable with *effectiveness.* The maximum possible reduction in a disease due to the use of medical intervention is properly *termed efficacy,* which is generally measured with randomized, controlled trials, which will achieve the maximum possible benefit when patients are carefully selected and stratified, randomization arms are properly designed, compliance is high, and trial participants are often free of other diseases or conditions that might interfere with the intervention being evaluated. The benefits established in a randomized, controlled trial are only partially applicable to day-to-day practice in a general population. The value of a medical intervention in the general population is termed *effectiveness.* The difference between efficacy and effectiveness can be very large, and obtaining a realistic measurement of effectiveness is often difficult.[15]

There are three approaches to health economic evaluation for comparing two therapies: (a) cost minimization, in which one assumes or observes no difference in effectiveness, (b) incremental cost-effectiveness, and (c) incremental net benefit. The last can be expressed in units of either effectiveness or costs. When analyzing data from a clinical trial, expressing incremental net benefit in units of cost allows the investigator to examine all the approaches in a single graph, complete with the corresponding statistical inferences.[15a]

A computerized literature search of >14,000 articles published since 1994 having *cost* as a keyword was carried out. Criticisms of these costing studies focus on three areas:

1. Costs are not measured correctly[16–18] because most studies use charge or reimbursement dollars as a proxy for cost. This is an incorrect measure because neither value is representative of the resources consumed or foregone in the process of providing a good service; hence, it is not a cost; the former figure is a construct, and the latter is the result of a negotiation between a payer and a provider.
2. Costs are not compiled using a proper perspective and scope.[17,19] Most studies only tabulate the cost of the health care provider and not to the patient, the family, or society.
3. There is a lack of consistency in reporting results,[16,20,21] which prevents interstudy and interinstitutional comparison.[22]

As a result of these problems, the data and conclusions from many cost-based studies are suspect.[19]

Clearly, a better costing method is required. Russell[23] emphasized that to serve its purpose, a model must produce accurate predictions and low probability for substantial variation in the factors that influence costs and effects. He identified three aspects of modeling: validating effectiveness estimates, modeling costs, and the implications of common statistical forms. Validation procedures similar to those for effectiveness estimates are proposed for costs. Modelers need to pay more attention to ensuring that the events described by a model represent costs and effects. Modelers can also help improve the epidemiologic and clinical research on which cost-effectiveness analyses depend by showing the implications for resource allocation of the statistical forms conventionally used in these fields.

Comparative effectiveness research (CER) aims to improve the quality, effectiveness, and efficiency of health care and to help patients, health care professionals, and purchasers make informed decisions regarding various treatment options, particularly for chronic illnesses or cancer. CER is moving forward, with recently defined priorities and a newly funded Patient-Centered Outcomes Research Institute, which, it is hoped, will survive cost cutting in the U.S. Congress. Economic analyses are most valuable to health policy analysts and health care managers who must allocate resources and establish benefit packages. An economic health care analysis tries to directly relate the incremental cost of an intervention to its potential benefit. The intervention is always evaluated relative to an alternative form of treatment.[9]

Technology assessment, cost–benefit outcome analysis, clinical trials supported by evidence-based medicine, and comparative effectiveness together can enhance the rationale and quality of medical care provided to patients at a competitive cost.

TECHNOLOGY ASSESSMENT

Technological change is the key driver of health care expenditure growth because it is generally associated with increased rather than reduced cost. As the economist Henry Aaron is quoted as saying, "Rapid scientific advance always raises expenditures even as it lowers prices. Those who think otherwise need only to turn their historical eyes to automobiles, airplanes, television, and computers. In each case, massive technological advance drove down the price of services, the total outlay soared."[2] A good example in medicine of this phenomenon is laparoscopic cholecystectomy. Although the price of a laparoscopic procedure is less than the price of an open cholecystectomy, after the introduction of the new technology the rates of both types of surgery increased, and the growth in the quantity of services overwhelmed the impact of per-unit reduction in price. Similar examples can be found in the widespread use of magnetic resonance imaging, computer tomography, coronary artery bypass grafting, angioplasty, cardiac intensive care units, neonatal intensive care units, and positron emission tomography and the growth of radiation oncology facilities. Technology may also increase costs by either premature adoption of the technology without adequate evidence that it improves outcome or overuse of technology, regardless of value, to provide a competitive market advantage or to generate revenues.[24]

Technology assessment is undertaken to determine (a) the appropriateness of adopting a new procedure consistent with the health care organization's mission and strategic plan; (b) the safety, efficacy, and cost-effectiveness of the new technology; (c) distinctions between appropriate and inappropriate use for the new technology; and (d) quality improvement methods to optimize the use of the new technology.[25] Technology assessment is a complex process that involves financial considerations, therapeutic outcome (locoregional tumor control, amelioration of symptoms and survival), treatment-induced morbidity, quality of life, impact on caregivers, family, and coworkers, and lost-opportunity costs.

When new technology emerges and priorities for allocation of increasingly scarce resources are considered, it is imperative to carry out economic analyses and also to assess the positive effects to the population who will benefit from the new technology compared with standard treatment techniques. The U.S. Center for Medicare Management concluded that cost-effectiveness should be considered in approving reimbursement by Medicare for new technology procedures.

Halperin[26] pointed out the importance of technology assessment in determining the merits of new devices or modalities and the impact they may have on the cost of health care. In a provocative editorial, Lee[27] pointed out that although technology is ubiquitous in radiation oncology, it is our professional responsibility to critically evaluate the merits of new technological developments. Yet, technology assessment can be a thorny and complex subject. Many of the technological advances in radiation oncology have not undergone a strict test of worthiness in formal clinical trials. Simulation, positioning techniques, computed tomography scanning for treatment planning, online imaging, and even intensity-modulated radiation therapy have had multiple dosimetric validations, but no randomized trial has documented their impact on outcome of large numbers of patients. However, lack of this evidence would not lead us to discontinue any of these procedures, which have been shown to improve in some way (i.e., less toxicity) the quality of care provided to patients.

The profusion of new technologies in medicine is related to the number of specialists in an area. Specialists receive income from new technologies and prompt hospitals to invest in them. A hospital that is constructing innovative facilities may attract specialists to the community and improve its revenue. It is also likely that public attitudes are influenced by medical providers and suppliers that advertise new technologies through the mass media.

Many nations have agencies to conduct health technology assessment, and there is an international network of agencies for health technology assessment that can share such data. The United States, however, has no national coordinating body on health technology assessment. Assessments are conducted through organizations such as the Veterans Administration, the Blue Cross Blue Shield Association, and professional organizations like the American College of Radiology, the Medicare Coverage Advisory Committee, and HMOs.

Health care organizations use a variety of models to assess and acquire technology, some of which include outcome. Reliable data for such benchmarking is frequently scarce. Some compare new and emerging technology against existing technology, although reliable outcome data are rare. Most institutions or individuals buy what physicians, advocacy groups, philanthropists, or governing boards want and use manufacturers and physicians as the primary sources of technology information. Cowan and Berkowitz[24] pointed out several key mistakes that occur during the diffusion of technology:

1. Technologies are adopted simply because they are new, without assessing their impact on outcomes.
2. Equipment is replaced solely because of its age. To avoid overuse of technology, health care organizations must carefully match the capacity of existing technology with projected utilization in a world of limited resources.
3. Applications of technology expand without adequate justification based on outcome or cost considerations.
4. Numerous vendors are used, and numerous models of products with duplicative specifications are purchased. Reducing the number of brands and models of devices used may provide an opportunity to reduce purchasing and inventory costs, as well as maintenance and repair costs. On the other hand, competitive pressures in the marketplace may provide downward pressure on equipment prices and argue in favor of the existence of multiple vendors.
5. Economies of scale in regionalizing technology decisions are missed because of lack of consolidation of services. This is sometimes related to inadequate systems for patient transport to treatment centers.
6. Duplication of services sometimes adds cost without significant increase in work volume.

A number of studies on the costs of treating cancer patients with radiation therapy[28–31] used either relevant costs defined in a number of ways or different proxies for actual costs (billed charges, revenue received, Medicare allowable). Recent reviews illustrate the wide variety of cost information and cost methods used in the literature and call for a consistent method for estimating site- and intent-specific treatment costs.[9,18,19,22,32] In estimating costs of health care interventions, several decision tools, including cost analysis, cost-effectiveness, and cost–utility and cost–benefit analysis, seek to define a unit of health outcome per unit input of cost. Before employing any of these decision tools, proper definition and calculation of cost is essential. The literature on the cost-effectiveness of particle therapy for cancer is scarce, studies are often not comparable, and many studies are not performed according to standard health assessment criteria. Evidence on the cost-effectiveness of particle therapy is, therefore, limited. One would hope that adequate reimbursement can be found to support innovative yet costly treatment to learn whether it is truly more efficacious.

TYPES OF COST IN HEALTH CARE

Costs During Treatment

Direct medical costs include the value of all the goods and services consumed in the provision of an intervention or dealing with the side effects of treatment. These costs include the consumption of all capital and human resources such as professional time, diagnostics, treatment, and medications.

Direct non–health care costs include all costs as a consequence of undergoing a treatment but not related to the treatment itself. Examples are the cost of transportation while patients are receiving treatment. Other costs sometimes included are *changes in use of informal caregiver time* (including the cost of family or other providers to provide health care in the home or continuous nursing care for disabled individuals) and *patient time costs* (referring to the time patients spend receiving care, including the value of the time consumed in receiving the treatment as well as travel and waiting time).

Indirect medical costs include all costs in the time after the treatment has been terminated and include costs of late toxicity or related diseases. In RT, these costs can differ quite substantially between different approaches if the side effects are very different or if one of the interventions has a higher curative potential. Typically, however, these costs occur many years after termination of the treatment.

Indirect nonmedical costs refer to costs that are important for society, in that they measure loss of productivity due to long-term disability or premature death. Costs to the family or society can be substantial. These include the patient's travel costs, the patient's or care provider's time off from work, and the considerable strain on caregivers. There may also be "downstream" effects. If a caregiver is devoting time to an ill spouse, he or she is taking time away from work or child care responsibilities, for example.

Global cost estimates of the cost of RT are the aggregate costs of the human and capital resources consumed in the delivery of a RT service. They do not contain the fine detail required when comparing, say, one RT protocol with another. However, they can have value as a background to allocating national health care budgets between different classes of medical intervention.

The data show that even in countries with optimal infrastructure, the budget assigned to RT is roughly 5% of the total amount spent on cancer care.[33] In the early 1990s, the European Union estimated the average cost per course of RT at about 3,000€, compared to roughly 7,000€ and 17,000€ for surgical and chemotherapy treatments, respectively. However, in spite of the perception of high capital costs, it is the personnel cost that dominates the cost of the provision of the service (about 70%), with capital investment typically representing <30% of the total RT budget.[3,14,34]

Reimbursement-Based Costs

Whereas economic evaluation theoretically advocates the use of cost figures that reflect actual resource consumption, this is frequently not achievable, and charges for service are used as a proxy. It should, however, be realized that large discrepancies may exist between the reimbursement of treatments and the costs of resources consumed while delivering a treatment. Due to the fact that reimbursement often lags behind the introduction of novel technologies, in many countries there is a tendency for high-tech treatments to be underreimbursed. The inverse seems to hold for the United States, where the reimbursement is likely to be higher for new technologies, although it decreases with time.

Besides numerical differences between costs and charges, other, more practical and theoretical problems may arise when utilizing reimbursement figures for economic evaluation. This was observed by the Radiation Therapy Oncology Group when performing an economic evaluation based on combining clinical trial data with cost data obtained from Medicare for each patient.[35] The first problem was that Medicare-managed care products do not have individual claims because managed care companies receive capitated payments and therefore may not record and/or report individual claims to Medicare. A more accurate estimation of costs would result from using administrative claims data to calculate costs, provided that they contain all claims of care a patient received. Another potential problem is that an underestimation of costs could occur if codes with only a cancer diagnosis were used, thus neglecting costs related to treatment toxicity or indirect medical costs occurring in the further follow-up of the patient. It may also be difficult to generalize the results of an analysis based on Medicare patients older than 65 years to the general population. Finally, it is apparent that obtaining administrative claims data from Medicare can be a costly procedure in itself.[36]

ACTIVITY-BASED COST ANALYSIS

Activity-based costing (ABC) is a system widely used in manufacturing but rarely in health care. ABC dissects the process of providing patient care into a series of microlevel tasks and assigns costs to these tasks. As a result, ABC directly identifies resources consumed by cost objects (treatments, patients, or health care providers).[12] Tabulating these tasks and resources consumed allows for comparison of cost values across institutions and time in a consistent and credible way. From this, the economic impact of differences in operating policies can be quantified and the comparison of cost to health outcome will be improved.

The traditional cost models that hospitals have used are outdated and ill equipped to provide accurate information on costs of a specific medical procedure or global cost of medical care for a patient from initial diagnosis to death. Cost models break organizations into departments for financial oversight and budgetary control; the focus of these cost models is departmental budgets, and they are not specific for a patient or a procedure, when it is really patients and procedures, not the department, triggering costs. For example, the accounting system of a hospital may be able to provide a fair assessment of the total budget (cost) of its radiation oncology department. However, the same system is of little help in assessing the actual cost of treating a patient with, for instance, prostate cancer using radiation therapy. This lack of applicability of cost information at the patient or the procedure level often leads to faulty decision making because analysis of the whole department does not necessarily translate into data about an individual patient.

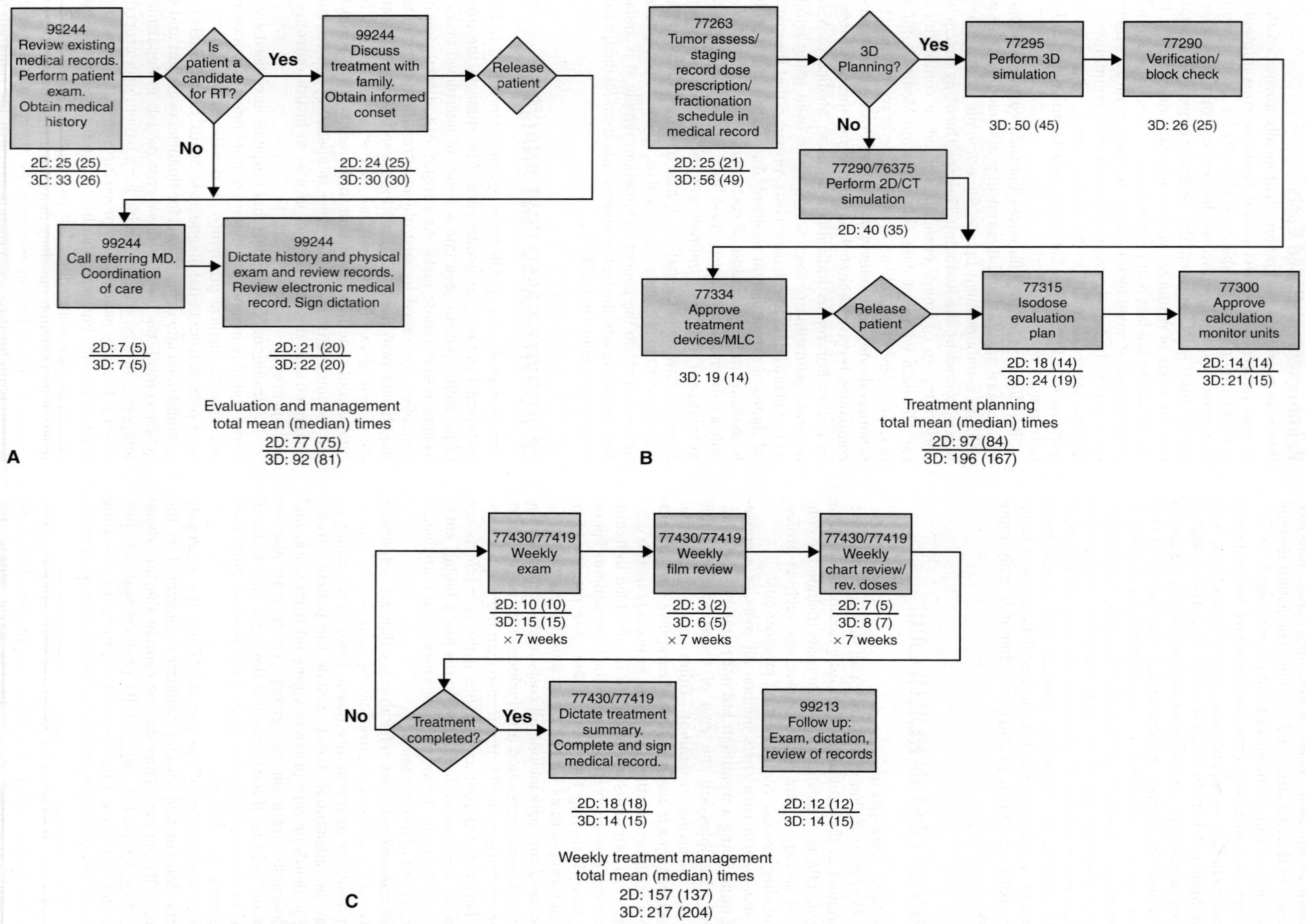

FIGURE 98.1. Process flow chart. Activity map and corresponding mean (median) times for definitive irradiation of cancer of prostate. **A:** Evaluation and management. **B:** Treatment planning. **C:** Weekly management.

ABC is concerned with measuring resource consumption by an individual patient. There are two general advantages of using ABC: increased accuracy of cost measurements and transparency of cost-incurring sections. The latter advantage—increased accounting transparency—means that there is a more lucid and readily apparent correlation between costs and actions. This allows managers to evaluate each step of the process, perceive inefficiencies in the system, and quantify economic benefits of process improvements.

The cost data of any technology should reflect the facilities and equipment costs (including depreciation and replacement), space (including housekeeping and utilities), and recorded time and effort of all professional staff on hospital payroll treating patients. Specific technical approaches should be identified, for example, in patients undergoing definitive radiation therapy, standard two-dimensional (2D) or three-dimensional (3D) conformal RT (CRT) or intensity-modulated RT (IMRT) or image-guided RT (IGRT). Time and effort observations for multiple tasks must be recorded by the respective staff members as they take place. The numbers of observations provide a representative sample of treatment procedures.

Technical cost is defined as the actual expenditures recorded in hospital accounting records. The total technical cost of a course of therapy includes staff time and effort, compensation including fringe benefits, space, utilities, maintenance, equipment depreciation, supplies, support services, liability cost, and administrative overhead. The ABC method[37–40] was used to derive technical (hospital) resource utilization costs for treatment procedures in treating localized prostate cancer.[9,30] The costing method consists of four major steps:

1. Creating a process flow map that identifies and defines all of the activities and steps associated with the treatment of patients with standard irradiation or with 3D CRT (Fig. 98.1).
2. Collecting and recording the staff time expended on each activity.
3. Identifying and accumulating all hospital costs from the general accounting ledger system related to the patients treated at a radiation oncology center in a given period.
4. Allocating actual cost to each activity to derive total specific costs of technical resource utilization for a course of 2D or 3D CRT, IMRT, or IGRT.

An example of an ABC cost-calculation model is the one developed in by Lievens et al.[34] Because it was felt that current RT protocols, with a shift toward more complex treatment planning and delivery techniques and more thorough quality assurance procedures, were no longer accurately captured within the original model, a novel version has recently been developed.[41] Because evolving technology over the last decade was more complex, it was found that the introduction of IMRT compared to 3D CRT translated into an almost doubling of procedure costs. ABC analysis allowed the authors to identify exactly where these extra costs were incurred. It was shown that the cost increase was the consequence not of the IMRT technique as such but of the combined effect of IMRT using more fields and delivering higher fraction numbers and, very important, the introduction of more, often daily, online imaging for position verification. If, however, techniques such as IMRT or gated radiotherapy delivery make it possible to reduce the number of fractions using simultaneous integrated boosts or accelerated hypofractionation, the resulting costs may decrease while yielding potentially improved treatment outcomes.[36]

Time and Effort Analysis

An integral phase of ABC is identifying process flow, listing each individual involved in the process and recording the actual amount of time spent to perform an activity by the staff using electronic or paper daily activity logs. Determining the participant's task time should follow the monopolizing rule: timing begins when a specific patient requires the participant's attention and stops when he or she is no longer doing so. Whether or not the patient is still present in the activity area is immaterial. For example, for an office visit, the nurse's time to prepare the patient's paperwork should be attributed to the patient, even before the patient arrives or after he or she has left the office. The actual activity time may be adjusted upward to recognize some normal unproductive time of activity participants, such as time spent in work breaks. Tables are generated to show the time and effort involved in each of the functions necessary to register and evaluate the patient, perform treatment planning, deliver external-beam irradiation, and supervise the management, as well as in preparation of the appropriate records to document all information, including quality assurance requirements.

Times are collected for each activity in the treatment process beginning with the initial consultation through the first follow-up visit after full treatment. These data points are analyzed and used to generate average times for patients treated with a specific technique along with the standard deviation of times.

RESOURCE UTILIZATION COSTS

Four types of resources should be catalogued and measured for each task:

1. Activity participants (e.g., radiation oncologists, physicists, therapists, dosimetrists, nurses, receptionists)
2. Physical resources (e.g., space, equipment, machines)
3. Supplies (e.g., x-ray films, office supplies)
4. Support services (e.g., administration, centralized information system)

Patient-related expenses include salaries and fringe benefits of the staff, Social Security contributions, retirement annuities, health, life disability and long-term care, dental insurance, tuition and childcare benefits, and disability insurance. Average hourly salary and related costs for each staff member are computed.

There are many supplies, such as office paper and latex gloves, for which the cost is trivial, and it is not economically worthwhile to track their specific use for individual patients. An average cost rate can be computed for such supplies by dividing their total cost by the total number of patients, which is applied to each patient. However, supplies used only by patients with specific diseases or procedures (e.g., contrast material, immobilization devices) need to be recorded for individual patients.

For hospital-based departments, indirect operating costs are classified into general hospital operating expenses and administrative overhead, which includes hospital liability insurance and administrative costs such as shared activities (administrative personnel for purchasing and payroll functions, human resources, public relations, and financial operations). The allocation of indirect operating costs among different departments of the hospital is complex. Models include allocating them as a proportion of personnel costs and many others. The allocation of cost among various units in a hospital can also be the source of pitched battles between different units. In many hospitals allocation of costs is a mechanism of cross-subsidization among different departments (e.g., the surgery department subsidizing primary care). Administrative cost can be determined by computing prorated allocation, dividing the total hospital indirect expenses by the proportion of the radiation oncology center technical budget to the total hospital annual budget.

Technical equipment expenses for treatment of patients are included using American Hospital Association standard depreciation schedules. The cost of depreciation of all equipment involved in the management of these patients, including treatment planning and delivery, should be accounted for on a prorated basis.

COST BENEFIT

If all that matters is minimizing expense, then the lowest-cost treatment (or no treatment) would be preferred. However, cost benefit, which incorporates the incremental impact of a new technology on outcome, and cost utility, which also relates additional costs to impact on survival as well as on the patient's quality of life and productivity, are important parameters in the assessment of new technology.[9] The projected cost of treating a patient who initially has control of the local tumor and no distant metastases is about one-third of that for a patient who develops a treatment failure.[42]

As a concomitant to an increasing proportion of the health insurance market being controlled by managed care, with its cost-cutting pressures, there may be a tendency to de-emphasize the importance of quality of care. However, it is critical, for instance, to document the alleged decreased morbidity of treatment with 3D CRT, IMRT, or protons in comparison with treatment of patients with carcinoma of the prostate[43] with conventional external-beam radiation therapy. This benefit, if it is real, is of great financial significance because treatment of major therapy complications may be costly.

Owen et al.[44] conducted economic studies for two phase III Radiation Therapy Oncology Group studies that compared different irradiation fractionation schedules (1-04 and 90-03, brain metastasis and head and neck cancer, respectively). Expected quantities of current procedural terminology codes and relative value units (RVUs) were modeled. Institutions retrospectively provided procedure codes, quantities, and components, which were converted to RVUs used for Medicare payments. The median and mean RVUs were within the range predicted by the model for all arms of one study and above the predicted range for the other study. The model predicted resource use well for patients who completed treatment per protocol. Actual economic data can be collected for critical cost items. Some institutions experienced difficulty collecting retrospective data, and prospective collection of data is necessary to validate these studies.

We must move from a fee-for-service mentality to a more critical and fiscally responsible health care system delivering high-quality care at a competitive cost. Based on current trends, 70% of hospital revenues will be capitated in a not-too-distant future. A challenge for future health care initiatives will be to strive for the lowest (optimally speaking, most competitive) cost with the highest value for the patient, including decreased morbidity of treatment and enhanced quality of life.[45]

The potential contribution of more complex and expensive procedures to the outcome of cancer therapy needs to be carefully evaluated.[46] Obviously, a significant portion of the increase in health care costs is linked to new technology; a great deal of this technology is welcome, but cost benefit should be demonstrated. Some technologic advances improve health care and can be justified economically if we document a positive impact on tumor control, patient survival, morbidity of treatment, and quality of life. The efficacy of diagnostic and therapeutic procedures can be related to outcome studies, and costs should be carefully evaluated based on both monetary and health-related considerations. Doubilet et al.[47] cautioned against the indiscriminate use of "cost-effectiveness" as the criterion on which medical decisions should be made, and thus we must carefully define the endpoints on which these studies are based.

Models can be constructed using a Markov model and available data on the natural history of a tumor, prognostic factors, efficacy and morbidity of a given therapeutic modality (based on outcome analysis), and reimbursement data for treating a specific patient population. When patterns-of-failure data are used, the cost differential can be calculated for a patient treated successfully in contrast to one who fails in a specific anatomic site (locoregional failure, distant metastasis, or combination), incorporating expenditures related to management of the treatment failure. The model can be made more complete (and complex) by adding costs of the morbidity of therapy. With the information and epidemiologic data currently available in the United States, annual costs of care can be computed and compared for various therapeutic modalities. Using Monte Carlo simulation, sensitivity analysis of cost-effectiveness may be performed.

Total cost-of-care projections should be carried out using a Markov-type analysis based on clinical experience, which will provide more accurate cost data for different management options. Providing cost–benefit information to patients (consumers) will be necessary when evaluating diagnostic and treatment options, particularly in carcinoma of the breast and prostate, in which great controversy exists regarding the merits of various modalities.

This information also will be very helpful in contract negotiations with health care organizations and third-party payers and in setting policies for establishing therapy guidelines and justification of health care expenditures.

Cost–utility analysis calculates the value of an intervention as the ratio of its incremental cost divided by its incremental survival benefit, with survival weighted by utilities to produce QALYs. Many studies are at variance with current standards; only 20% of studies took a societal perspective, more than one-third failed to discount both the costs and QALYs, and utilities were often simply estimates from the investigators or other physicians. There remains much room for improvement in the methodologic rigor with which utilities are measured. Considering quality-of-life effects by incorporating utilities into economic studies is particularly important in oncology, when many therapies obtain modest improvements in response or survival at the expense of nontrivial toxicity.

Stinnett and Mullahy[48] introduced the concept of net health benefit as an alternative to cost-effectiveness ratios for the statistical analysis of patient-level data on the costs and health effects of competing interventions. Net health benefit addresses a number of problems associated with cost-effectiveness ratios by assuming a value for the willingness-to-pay for a unit of effectiveness. Willan[49] extended the concept of net health benefit to demonstrate that standard statistical procedures can be used for the analysis power and sample size determines cost-effectiveness data. He showed that by varying the value of the willingness to pay, the point estimate and confidence interval for the increment cost-effectiveness ratio can be determined.

The benefit of 3D CRT, IMRT, or IGRT is hypothetically linked to improved local tumor control because of better coverage of the target volume with a specific dose of irradiation, less acute and late morbidity, and possibility of carrying out dose-escalation studies if morbidity is held to an acceptable level, resulting in improved survival.[42] Several institutions, the Radiation Therapy Oncology Group, and 10 institutions under cooperative agreement with the National Cancer Institute conducted phase I/II dose-escalation studies in carcinoma of the prostate and are carrying out a study on carcinoma of the lung. Depending on the results, the cost benefit of 3D CRT, IMRT, or IGRT must be further evaluated in dose-escalation and in larger multi-institutional phase III studies, comparing it with standard techniques to justify its somewhat higher initial cost. Cases that are most likely to benefit from 3D CRT, IMRT, or IGRT include patients with (a) tumors in sites with complex anatomy, (b) irregular-shaped tumors, (c) tumors adjacent to radiation-sensitive normal structures, (d) tumors that undergo significant changes in volume during treatment, and (e) small-volume or high-dose treatment.

The introduction of protons and heavy ions (hadrons) into the radiation therapy armamentarium has brought additional controversy in technology assessment because of the higher cost of facilities, equipment, and operation, with diverse opinions as to the cost-effectiveness of these innovative modalities. A 2008 review of the literature showed that only 17 publications (out of 777 on particle therapy) dealt with economic aspects, and only 5 of them were on cost-effectiveness.[50]

Many articles have been published on the physical advantages of protons or heavy ions in comparison to photons, resulting in better dose distribution in the target volume with less radiation administered to normal tissues, which may decrease morbidity and eventually the risk of second malignancies.[51,52] However there is a lack of randomized trials documenting superior clinical outcomes with these particles.

Opinions on the need for or ethical considerations to subjecting patients to prospective trials have been expressed.[53,54] Perrier et al.[55] used an ABC approach similar to the examples discussed previously to evaluate the cost of carbon-ion therapy. It allowed an in-depth definition of the cost of treatment preparation and the actual irradiation, depending on various parameters such as actual treatment time and patient setup time. The approach of Peeters et al.,[56] conversely, was more aggregate, using a spreadsheet model that assumes that treatment costs scale linearly with the number of fractions. This, obviously, is a somewhat simple approximation of reality, which results in less accurate estimates.[34]

Implementing new technologies in radiation oncology with advanced engineering, such as linear accelerators, cone beams, tomotherapy, treatment planning and delivery techniques, and accessories that enhance the efficiency and accuracy of operation, may decrease overall cost of treatment computed over the lifetime of the patient.

The American Society for Therapeutic Radiology and Oncology maintains the position that new technologies and modifications of existing technologies representing significant paradigmatic shifts in treatment approach should be implemented into clinical practice in such a manner as to ensure safety, efficacy, and, ideally, cost-effectiveness.[57]

EVIDENCE-BASED MEDICINE AND EVIDENCE-BASED ONCOLOGY

There have been significant scientific advances in biologic sciences and health care. At the same time, there has been increased accountability and in some instances attempts to ration services; as a mechanism to accomplish this, arbitrary clinical practice guidelines have been promulgated. A more rational effort to define optimal heath care should be based on identification of innovative approaches, outcome analysis in properly designed clinical trials, and careful assessment of current practice; more important, we have a dire need for solid and credible clinical research and evidence-based decision making in medicine.

The growth in basic and translational research data to guide medical practice has made it critical for clinicians to appraise and use published data for medical decisions. Evidence-based medicine (EBM) is the compelling idea that any recommendation of a specific medical procedure should be supported by empirical evidence for its superior efficacy/toxicity ratio compared with alternative treatment options in a patient with a given presentation.[43,58,59]

Evidence-based medicine helps correct an imbalance in contemporary medicine in which clinicians are being trained to maintain high standards of critical consciousness in methodologic domains but not in the broader historic and sociocultural domains that surround them.[60]

Evidence-based health care is the conscious use of current best evidence in making decisions about the care of individuals or the delivery of health services. Current best evidence is up-to-date information from relevant valid research about the effects of different forms of health care, the potential for harm from exposure to particular agents, the accuracy of diagnostic tests, and the predictive power of prognostic factors.

Evidence-based clinical practice is an approach to decision making in which the clinician uses the best evidence available, in the context of consultation with the patient, to decide on which option suits the patient best. Evidence-based medicine is a conscientious, explicit, and judicious use of current best evidence in making decisions about the care of individual patients.

Evidence-based medicine or evidence-based practice aims to apply the best available evidence gained from the scientific method to clinical decision making. It seeks to assess the strength of evidence of the risks and benefits of treatment or lack of treatment and diagnostic tests. Evidence quality can range from meta-analysis and systematic reviews of double-blind, placebo-clinical trials at the top end down to conventional wisdom at the bottom.

The systematic review of published research is the major method used for evaluating particular treatments. The Cochrane Collaborations are among the best known and respected examples of systematic reviews. Like other collections of systematic reviews, it requires authors to provide a detailed and repeatable plan of literature search and evaluation of the evidence. Once all the evidence is assessed, treatment is categorized as "likely to be beneficial," "likely to be harmful," or "evidence did not support either benefit or harm."

Evidence-based medicine categorizes different types of clinical evidence and rates or grades them according to the strengths of their freedom from the various biases that have beset medical research. The strongest evidence for therapeutic intervention is provided by systematic review of randomized, triple-blind, placebo-controlled trials with allocation concealment and complete follow-up involving a homogeneous patient population and medical condition. In contrast, patient testimonials, case reports, or even expert opinion have little value as proof because of the placebo effect, the biases inherent in observation in reporting cases, and difficulty in ascertaining who is an expert.

Randomized, controlled trials are highly desirable to answer questions about technology assessment, but there are alternatives. Carefully controlled observational studies are good predictors of the outcome of randomized trials as long as enough essential information is collected to ensure that the patients are standardized. It is equally important in an observational series to understand which patients have been excluded.[61]

The American College of Radiology (ACR) created a Task Force on Appropriateness Criteria. This task force incorporates attributes for developing exceptional medical practice guidelines that have been used by the Agency for Health Care Research and Quality as designated by the Institute of Medicine. The ACR adopted the AQA's[62] definition of appropriateness: "The concept of appropriateness, as applied to health care, balances risk and benefit of treatment, test, or procedure in the context of available resources for an individual patient with specific characteristics. Appropriateness criteria provides guidance to supplement the clinician's judgment as to whether a patient is a reasonable candidate for the given treatment, test, or procedure."

The ACR Task Force on Appropriateness Criteria established 20 expert panels. Ten are concerned with diagnostic radiology and 10 with radiation therapy. In this latter group there are panels for bone metastases, brain metastases, breast, gynecologic, head and neck malignancies, Hodgkin disease, and lung, prostate, and rectal/anal malignancies. Each expert panel is chaired by an individual who is deemed by the College to have leadership capabilities and a national recognition of expertise in the area of focus. Volunteer physicians are involved in the criteria development process. Expert panelists go through a process of literature searches, acquisition of scientific articles, drafting of evidence tables, dissemination of materials for the Delphi process, collation of results, conference calls, and documentation processing. For multiple radiation oncology treatments and procedures, there are published ACR appropriateness guidelines that one can consult to garner an opinion about the "consensus view."[62]

The Delphi methodology is a technique used to arrive at appropriateness ratings. A series of surveys is conducted to elicit members of the expert panel's interpretation of the evidence concerning the appropriateness of a therapeutic procedure for specific clinical scenario. The panelist receives a survey with an evidence table and narrative. Each panelist is asked to interpret the available evidence and rank each procedure. The survey is completed by each panelist without consulting fellow panel members. Ratings are done on a scale of 1 through 9, which is further divided into three categories, 1 to 3 is defined as usually not appropriate; 4 to 6 is defined as maybe appropriate; and 7 to 9 is defined as usually appropriate. Each panel member assigns one rating for each radiation therapy procedure or intervention per survey round. Surveys are collected and the results are tabulated, deidentified, and redistributed after each round. A maximum of three rounds is conducted. This modified Delphi technique enables each panelist to express individual interpretations of the evidence and his or her expert opinion without receiving bias from fellow panelists in a simple, standardized, and economical process. A consensus is defined as 80% agreement within a rating category.

Practicing evidence-based medicine requires recognition that, in most encounters with patients, questions arise that should be answered to provide the patient with the best available medical care. Appropriate and relevant clinical questions contain four elements: (a) a patient or problem, (b) an intervention, (c) a comparison intervention (if necessary), and (d) an outcome. Important practical steps in practicing evidence-based medicine include the following:

1. Formulation of the patient's clinical problem
2. Search of literature for relevant and reliable data
3. Evaluation of validity and usefulness of data
4. Integration of critical evaluation of evidence with clinical judgment
5. Implementation of useful information
6. Assessment of outcome to improve medical practice

Once the right questions have been formulated, the best source for finding most types of best evidence is by searching Medline (National Library of Medicine), PubMed (National Library of Medicine), OVID, the Cochrane Database, or a similar database by computer.

The quality (strength) of evidence is based on a hierarchy, proceeding from the most reliable results of systematic reviews of well-designed prospective clinical trials to results of one or more well-designed meta-analysis studies, results of large retrospective case series, expert opinion, and personal experience.[63] Once the best data have been found, the evidence-based medicine approach involves critically appraising the quality of the evidence, determining its magnitude and precision, and applying it to a specific patient.[64,65]

The Cochrane Collaboration was established in 1993 as an international network to help health care providers, policy makers, patients, their advocates, and their caregivers make well-informed decisions about health care by preparing, updating, and promoting the success of Cochrane reviews. More than 4,500 such reviews have been published so far online in the Cochrane Library.[66]

The Cochrane Collaboration traces its origins to a 1972 publication by the British epidemiologist A. Cochrane entitled *Effectiveness and Efficiency: Random Reflections on Health Services*.[67] This book called attention to the collective ignorance concerning the effects of health care. In 1979 Cochrane published an essay in which he suggested that "it is surely a great criticism of our profession that we have not organized a critical summary, by specialty or subspecialty, adapted periodically, of all relevant randomized controlled trials."[68] Responding to Cochrane's charge, the Cochrane Collaboration undertook such a crucial but enormous undertaking.

There are >28,000 people working within the Cochrane Collaboration in >100 countries. Its central functions are funded by royalties of its publisher, which comes from sales from subscription to the Cochrane Library. The individual entities of the Cochrane Collaboration are funded by a large variety of governmental, institutional, and private funding sources and are bound by organization policy limiting uses of funds from corporate sponsors.

Evidence-based medicine promotes rule-based behavior on the part of physicians in an effort, among other things, to eliminate variations in medical practice. However, professionals do not follow rules per se; they intuit what is right in a situation, including, sometimes, that it is right to defer to a rule.[69]

The practice of evidence-based medicine (careful clinical judgment in evaluating the "best available data") should be differentiated from the special collection of data regarded as "suitable evidence." The new collection of best available information has major constraints for the care of individual patients; derived almost exclusively from randomized trials and meta-analyses, the data do not include many types of treatments or patients seen in clinical practice, and the results show comparative efficacy of treatment for an "average" randomized patient, not for pertinent subgroups formed by such cogent clinical features as severity of symptoms, illness, comorbidity, and other clinical nuances. The intention-to-treat analyses in clinical trials reporting do not reflect important postrandomization events leading to altered treatment, and the results seldom provide suitable background data when therapy is given prophylactically rather than remedially. The authoritative aura given to the "collection of data" may lead to abuses that produce inappropriate guidelines or poorly supported doctrinaire dogmas for clinical practice.[70] There are a variety of mechanisms to apply evidence-based medicine to clinical practice, including formulation of treatment pathways, practice guidelines, appropriateness criteria, consensus conferences, patterns of care, and institutional peer review. A fundamental part of evidence-based medicine is the filtering of evidence through the clinical skill of the clinician. It is not easy to determine which level of evidence is required, and it is estimated that only 20% of medical procedures currently in practice can be justified by evidence-based medical standards. In addition, EBM has a dark companion: what Bentzen and Wasserman[58] called lack-of-evidence-based medicine (LEBM), a methodology used in the United Kingdom by the National Institute for Clinical Excellence to restrict access to a number of therapies on the National Health Service. Whereas evidence-based medicine is concerned with weighing level I evidence for or against a give intervention, LEBM is concerned with the systematic review of the lack-of-level I evidence on a given topic.

When does a new cancer therapy cease being experimental and become a component of the standard of care? This distinction is subject to powerful influences for for-profit pharmaceutical companies and medical equipment manufacturers wanting to increasing their sales and financial return to shareholders, advocacy groups, politicians, and a public anxiously awaiting the next "cancer breakthrough." A dispassionate set of systems for technology assessment of cancer therapies is essential to evidence-based oncology practice.

In 1993 in the United States the American Society of Clinical Oncology (ASCO) formed a Health Services Research Committee

(HSRC) to perform technology assessments and to develop guidelines for cancer treatment. The Committee is composed of clinical researchers and clinicians from academic centers and private practice and performs technology assessment after hearing from expert advisors. The committee does not develop guidelines; it assembles expert panels to develop guidelines.[71]

Among the most important initial tasks of the HSRC was to create an outcome working group to define the outcomes of cancer treatment that should be considered for technology assessment in forming cancer treatment guidelines. Not surprisingly, patients, physicians, researchers, payers, and policy makers all have different ideas about which outcomes of cancer treatment are important. The main purpose of ASCO's technology assessments and guidelines is to define what constitutes the best cancer treatment, not to inform policy development and payment decisions. The working group on outcomes, therefore, considered outcomes primarily from the perspective of the clinical investigators who produced evidence for the guidelines, individual doctors and patients who have to make decisions about treatment, and health services researchers who evaluate the quality and cost of care produced by the guidelines. Because it is clear that there are health policy implications of ASCO's technology assessments and guidelines, the working group also considered outcomes that would convince health policy makers that ASCO's technology assessment was sound and that its guidelines represented worthwhile treatment.[25,71] For technology assessment the ASCO working group is composed of members of the Health Service Research

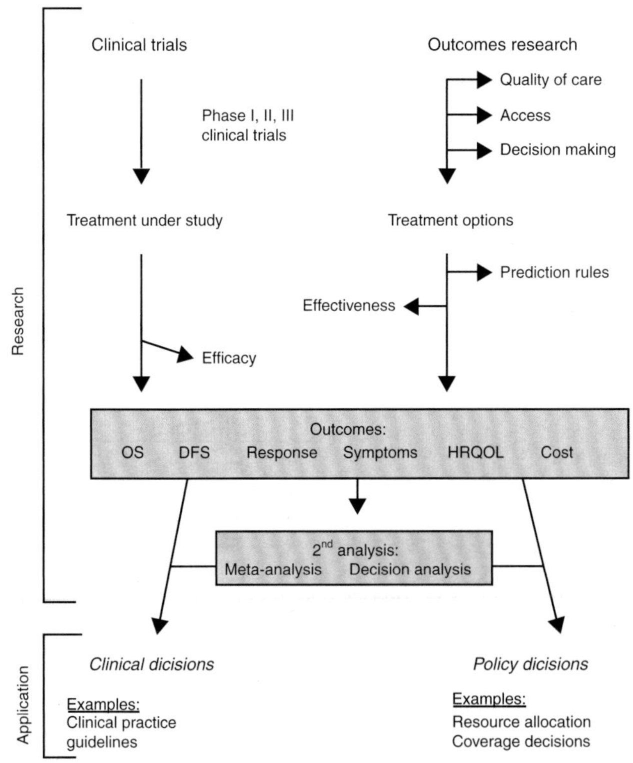

FIGURE 98.2. Conceptual framework of outcome research. Interaction is shown between research topics, endpoints, analytic techniques, and applications in defining outcomes research. Depicted in the upper left corner are the classic clinical trials and analytic techniques that are not outcomes research. In the upper right corner are shown the study topics, endpoints, and analytic techniques that are considered to be outcomes research. Outcomes depicted in the center box may or may not constitute outcomes research, depending on the context. For example, overall survival as measured in a phase III trial is not an outcomes study (efficacy), whereas it is if observed in a large community cohort (effectiveness). Symptoms have both efficacy and outcomes influences. Applications are indicated in italics and may emanate from either clinical trials or outcomes research. See text for further details. (From Lee SJ, Earle CC, Weeks JC. Outcomes research in oncology: history, conceptual framework, and trends in the literature. *J Natl Cancer Inst* 2000;92:195–204.)

Committee and selected members. They conduct a literature review and analyze the outcomes-based evidence. Testimony is collected from invited experts and interested parties. After evaluating the information, the working group defines specific questions and provides a report outlining conditions under which the proposed procedures are warranted to assist both physicians and patients in making informed decisions regarding the technologist or procedures.

The working group identifies specific questions to be addressed by the technology assessment, develops a strategy for completing the assessment, and reviews the available literature and evidence. The process may include face-to-face meetings of available working groups and members, circulation of draft forms of the technology assessment, and opportunities for comment. Working groups do not attempt to codify established practice. They review the available evidence and add their best clinical judgment to make final recommendations.

Making a treatment selection involves defining the patient's condition, identifying management options and outcome, collecting and summarizing evidence, and applying value judgments or preferences to arrive at an optimal course of action.[45] The randomized, controlled clinical trial has become the "gold standard" for evaluating the efficacy of health care intervention. In the 30-year period starting in 1966, >80,000 journal articles from randomized, controlled trials results were registered in the Medline database. The first 5 years of that period contributed <1% of the total number of articles, whereas the last half-decade contributed more than the previous 25 years combined. (For more detailed review of the principles of design in clinical trials, the reader is referred to Bentzen.[72]) A proposal for structured reporting of randomized clinical trials was described in the consolidation of standards for reporting trials guidelines[73] that have been accepted by many medical journals. For instance, the journal *Radiotherapy and Oncology* adopted a set of guidelines for reporting clinical research (Table 98.2).[72] Linking management options to known outcomes in clinical trials or obtained through systematic reviews is becoming a common procedure (Fig. 98.2).

Clinical decisions are complex and based on many sources of information (Fig. 98.3).[73] Patient management decisions are always a function of both scientific evidence and individual preferences (physicians, health care providers, patients). A development to improve the basis for clinical decision making is an international movement to improve the reporting of clinical research results, particularly in randomized, controlled trials and method analyses. New data on current molecular biology and genetics investigations have broadened the scope of evidence-based oncology.

Hunt et al.[74] reported on an analysis of 68 controlled medical trials, 40 of which were published since 1992, to assess the effects of computer-based clinical decision support systems on physician performance and patient outcome. They observed that, in 43 of 65 studies (66%) on physician performance, a benefit was found, including drug-dosing systems, use of diagnostic aids, preventive care assistance, and other medical care procedures. Only 6 of 14 studies assessing patient outcome found a benefit, indicating that the impact of clinical decision support systems on patient outcome has been insufficiently studied. Furthermore, very few reports dealt with cancer-related treatment issues; most reports centered on prevention, activities, and cancer screening.[75,76]

Although oncologists, patients, and national organizations recognize that communication is very important in cancer care, evidence-based data on the subject are scarce. Oncologists should use a patient-centered interview approach, ask patients what level of involvement they want in medical decision making, develop a caring attitude, and consider that patient–physician encounters should provide both cognitive data of patient understanding and feelings.[77]

TABLE 98.2 GUIDELINES FOR REPORTING CLINICAL OUTCOME STUDIES IN THE JOURNAL *RADIOTHERAPY AND ONCOLOGY*

Heading	*Subheading*	*Item*	*Was It Reported? Yes/No/NA[a]*	*If Yes, on What Page Number?*
Title		1. Identify the study as a randomized trial	____	____
Introduction		2. State the prospectively defined hypothesis, clinical objectives, and planned subgroup or covariate analyses	____	____
Methods	Study design	3. Define the patient population, inclusion and exclusion criteria	____	____
		4. Planned treatments and their timing	____	____
	Radiotherapy	5. Radiotherapy dose prescription method, dose-planning procedure	____	____
		6. Target volume definition, critical organs considered, simulation and verification procedures	____	____
		7. Dose fractionation details	____	____
		8. Planned radiotherapy quality assurance procedures	____	____
	Endpoints and analysis	9. Primary and secondary endpoints, specific follow-up procedures, the minimum clinically relevant difference, the target sample size and how it was decided	____	____
		10. Statistical analyses, their purpose and methods used, and whether the intention-to-treat principle was used.	____	____
		11. Trial monitoring, early-stopping rules	____	____
	Randomization	12. Method used for randomization	____	____
		13. Method of concealment and time of randomization	____	____
		14. Method to separate the generator of random treatment assignments from the treating physician	____	____
Results	Masking patient flow and follow-up analysis	15. Describe any blinding procedures (if relevant)	____	____
		16. Provide an overview of number of patients randomized, compliance with treatment, radiotherapy quality assurance results	____	____
		17. State the effect of treatment on primary and secondary tumor outcome measures, including effect estimates with confidence intervals	____	____
		18. Describe the incidence and grade of treatment-induced early and late toxicity by treatment group	____	____
		19. State frequencies as absolute numbers when feasible (e.g., 10/20 and not just 50%)	____	____
		20. Present summary data with appropriate statistics to permit alternative analyses or interpretations and comparisons with other trials on the same problem	____	____
		21. Describe prognostic variables by treatment group, check, if they were balanced, and if not describe attempts to adjust for them	____	____
		22. Describe protocol deviations from the study as planned, together with reasons	____	____
Discussion		23. State the interpretation of the study findings, including sources of bias and imprecision, and discuss how this trial compares with other similar studies	____	____
Conclusion		24. State the general interpretation of the trial in view of all available evidence in the literature	____	____

These guidelines meet the minimum criteria defined in the CONSORT statement for reporting of randomized clinical trials.

[a]NA, not applicable; certain items apply to randomized studies only.

From Bentzen SM. Towards evidence based radiation oncology: improving the design, analysis, and reporting of clinical outcome studies in radiotherapy. *Radiother Oncol* 1998; 46:5–18; with permission.

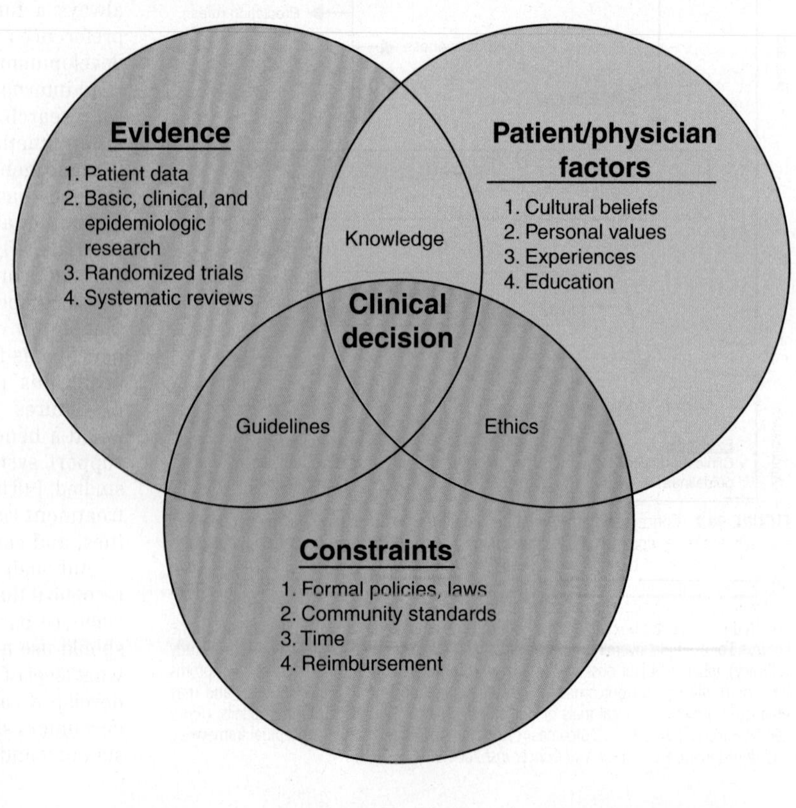

FIGURE 98.3. Factors that enter into clinical decisions. (From Mulrow CD, Cook DJ, Davidoff F. Systematic reviews; critical links in the great chain of evidence. In: *Systematic reviews: synthesis of best evidence for health care decisions.* Philadelphia: American College of Physicians, 1998:1–4.)

QUALITY OF MEDICAL CARE AND EVIDENCE-BASED MEDICINE

Continuous quality improvement emerged from the industrial sector as an effective means of reducing production errors. The quality of health care can be precisely defined and measured with a degree of scientific accuracy comparable to that of most measures in clinical medicine.[78] Health care quality problems can be classified into three categories:

1. *Underuse* is the failure to provide a health care service when it would have produced a favorable outcome for a patient, such as not administering irradiation in breast-conserving therapy.
2. *Overuse* occurs when a health care service is provided under circumstances in which its potential for harm exceeds the possible benefit—for example, prescribing postoperative pelvic irradiation to a patient with stage IA G1 endometrial carcinoma.
3. *Misuse* takes place when an appropriate service has been selected but a preventable complication occurs and the patient does not receive the full potential benefit of the service; avoidable complications of surgery, medications, or irradiation are important misuse problems.[79]

Other issues influencing the inadequate use of services include geographic variation in the rate of use, training of general practice or specialist physicians, the makeup of the nonphysician health care work force, and the effect of organization of medical services as a determinant of quality.

In health care, continuous quality improvement is most effective when used as an integral part of a scientific approach to improving clinical practice. A potential strength is the ability of motivate good performers to excel and to place emphasis on generating new methods for achieving improvement. Among its limitations are a too-narrow focus on administrative (as opposed to clinical) aspects of care and a lack of attention to problems of overuse or underuse. Several major strategies have been advocated to move the health care delivery system toward improving quality. The challenges are (a) to always provide effective care of those who could benefit from it, (b) to always refrain from providing inappropriate services, and (c) to eliminate all preventable complications.[80] Skeptics point out that no health care market currently competes on the basis of improving quality, and there is little theoretical basis in economics to predict that this success will occur.[79] Mendelson et al.[81] noted that there are many parties involved in outcome and effectiveness research (Fig. 98.4) and that payers and providers of health care may in the future use outcome research as a basis for coverage of services, including procedures, devices, or drugs.

OUTCOME RESEARCH

Outcome research focuses on identifying variations in medical procedures and associated health outcomes. Figure 98.2 illustrates the interplay of outcome research and clinical trials with clinical and policy decision making.

The term *outcome* is frequently used to describe a variety of endpoints or products of health care. Areas of specific focus of outcome analysis include the following:

1. Structure of care (such as features of health care facilities, staffing, equipment)
2. Process of care (such as type of studies performed, services provided)
3. Patient characteristics (gender, age, race, ethnic group)
4. Disease focus (such as location and type of tumor, histology, pathologic features)
5. Treatment-related factors (type of treatment, tumor response, disease-free survival, overall survival, morbidity of therapy)
6. Socioeconomics (such as cost benefit, quality of life, financial impact of the disease, recovery, and rehabilitation)

Meta-analysis is another mechanism to systematically research and collect published/unpublished randomized clinical trial data and quantitatively summarize results to obtain objective assessment of efficacy. The process should be (a) hypothesis driven, (b) protocol based, and (c) reproducible and comprehensive.

However, meta-analysis has some potential shortcomings, such as uncontrolled testing conditions, sample heterogeneity, unrecorded interventions, ambiguous endpoints, lack of independence of determinant factors, synergistic interactions, and sometimes contradictory experimental results.

Efforts have intensified during the last 20 years to promote outcome research in oncology, and there is a critical need to continue to support randomized, controlled studies. Patient and

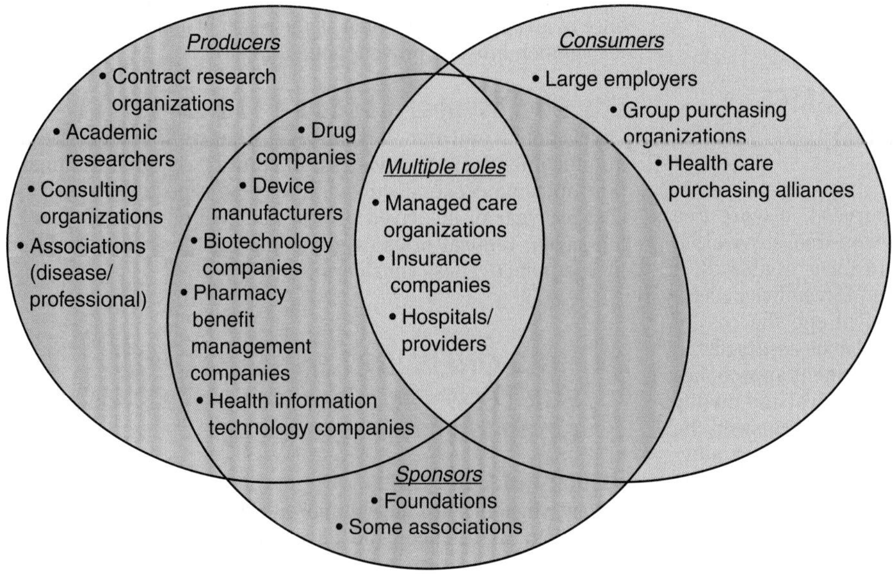

FIGURE 98.4. Stakeholders in outcomes and effectiveness research. (Adapted from Lewin Group. Outcomes and effectiveness research in the private sector: final report. Fairfax, VA: Lewin Group, 1997; and Mulrow CD, Cook DJ, Davidoff F. Systematic reviews; critical links in the great chain of evidence. In: *Systematic reviews: synthesis of best evidence for health care decisions.* Philadelphia: American College of Physicians, 1998:1–4.)

physician acceptance of participation in outcome research studies must be improved because only 10% to 20% of patients with newly diagnosed cancer participate in these important studies.[82] There is considerable variation in participation of patients in research studies as a function of patient age and disease site. In general, compliance with participation in studies is much higher among pediatric patients than adults.

Among the most commonly used data are those of the Surveillance, Epidemiology, and End Result (SEER) program. SEER is a continuing project of the biometry branch of the U.S. National Cancer Institute. The program draws data from several population-based cancer reporting systems covering approximately 14% of the total population of the United States. When linked to Medicare and other insurance administrative files, it has been extremely valuable in assessing the quality of care of the elderly and other insured populations. Although an excellent data source, SEER has been criticized as being inadequate to represent the diversity of systems of care throughout the country and in general does not have data that may more accurately define patient- or tumor-specific prognostic characteristics or treatment details.

The National Cancer Data Base, a joint project of the American College of Surgeons' Commission on Cancer and the American Cancer Society, holds information on more than half of all newly diagnosed cases of cancer in the United States and includes many of the demographic, clinical, and health systems data elements necessary to assess quality of care. A serious limitation of the National Cancer Data Base is the absence of complete information on outpatient care; its data have not been widely used to assess quality of care, but it has great potential for doing so.

An effective national system to collect this type of information should be established in the United States to collect data about the following:

1. Demographics of individuals with cancer (e.g., age, ethnic group, socioeconomic status, and insurance or health plan coverage)
2. Type of cancer (stage, histologic type, grade, comorbid conditions)
3. Treatment, including outcome of procedures, such as adjuvant chemotherapy and radiation therapy
4. Specialty training of care providers
5. Site of care delivery (such as community hospital or specialized cancer center)
6. Type of care delivery system (such as managed care, fee for service, government agency)
7. Outcomes (tumor control, survival, complications of treatment, quality of life, satisfaction with services provided)

THE WAYS TO MEASURE OUTCOMES INDICATIVE OF SURVIVAL AND TUMOR RESPONSE

Survival can be measured as overall survival, disease-free survival, progression-free survival, or event-free survival. It is clearly the most important outcome in cancer treatment. It is also clear, however, that survival alone is insufficient as a measure of outcome. The quality of survival and the cost of maintaining and improving survival must also be assessed.[83]

Making a choice between alternative treatment approaches often involves a tradeoff between length of survival and quality of life. A survival measurement alone might not answer the question of whether gains in survival justify toxicity. Quality-adjusted survival attempts to adjust the absolute length of life to reflect the patient's quality of life. Quality-adjusted survival provides a framework within which tradeoffs that influence treatment choices can be defined as in decision and cost-effective analysis to assess the effectiveness of alternative therapies.[71,73]

Quality-of-Life Outcome Measures

Quality of life considers the impact of cancer and its treatment on the physical, psychological, and social components of patient's lives. Cancer-related quality of life is a family of outcomes including the global quality of life as well as physical, psychological, and social dimensions, each one of which is a potentially separate outcome. Because of its subjective nature, the assessment of quality of life generally should include an evaluation by the patient. Quality-of-life measures should be characterized by reliability and validity.[73,81,84]

Toxicity Measures of Outcome

Toxicities are subjective, objective, or both. An example of a subjective toxicity would be a symptom such as nausea that is often not associated with overt signs or laboratory abnormalities. Evaluation of toxicities of this sort rest with the patient's report. Objective toxicities are measured by physical examination or laboratory tests. The common toxicity criteria use a system for categorizing toxicity from cancer treatment according to its severity. Such systems are widely used in cooperative group trials.

Measures of Cancer Response Outcomes

Measures of tumor response include complete response, response to radiation, and time to progression. Response may also be measured by biomarkers and changes in cancer-induced abnormalities and common blood tests. Some studies demonstrated the positive relationship between response rate and quality of life, but others did not. It is clear that freedom from progression may not be a convincing indication of the benefits of treatment if it does not predict significantly improved survival or cure. Freedom from progression is therefore not an adequate measure of quality of life.[82]

Comparative effectiveness research must be focused on patient outcomes. One cannot assume that a higher dose of radiation to a target field or a more conformal dose distribution will result in better survival or improved tolerance. Outcomes of significance to the patient such as survival, disease-free survival, quality of life, or specific side effects must be the focal points of research.[61] It is particularly important for radiation oncologists to remember that an improved dose distribution achieved through intensity-modulated radiotherapy, conformal techniques, or particle therapy is not the same as an improved outcome. The presence of an improved outcome as the result of a difference in dose distribution must be proven, not assumed.

Cost Effectiveness as a Cancer Outcome

Cost is not an outcome. It is, instead, what we spend to produce an outcome. Cost-effectiveness, in contrast, is often an important outcome. Cost-effectiveness may be reported in terms of cost per year of life saved or cost per quality adjusted year of life saved. Clinical practice guidelines are generally informed by cost-effectiveness considerations.[71,73]

HOW ONE MIGHT USE OUTCOMES FOR TECHNOLOGY ASSESSMENT AND GUIDELINE DEVELOPMENT

Priority of Outcomes

Patient outcomes are more important than cancer outcomes for technology assessment and development of cancer treatment guidelines. If a new technology or therapy is not ultimately shown to make patients live longer or feel better, then its use cannot be justified. Gathering the necessary data is not easy. Randomized, controlled trials are the gold standard for these comparisons but often fail to accrue enough patients. The reasons for failure to accrue include physicians who refuse to enroll patients because they believe one technology is superior, patients who refuse to be randomized because they have a treatment/technology preference, and the extra work necessary to enroll a patient in a trial.[61]

The Need to Use Multiple Outcomes

There is no single outcome that can represent the results of cancer treatment. Each of the various outcomes provides an unique perspective on treatment and has its own limitations. In general, multiple outcomes should be used for technology assessment.

Barriers to Progress in Cancer Outcome Research

Despite growing interest, there are numerous obstacles to overcome in health care outcome research, including the need to apply scientific disciplines that are different from the biomedical sciences (survey research, psychology, health services research, statistics, economics), the need for resources to collect additional data and information beyond that of standard clinical care, and limited coordination and collaboration among researchers working in the field. Other barriers are intrinsic to a specific cancer, including heterogeneity of patients, type of tumor, phases of the disease, and ethnic and socioeconomic characteristics. Furthermore, many institutions do not give a high priority to or adequately fund outcome research because this activity is considered a cost, not a revenue center, and there is a lack of conviction that this effort will reduce health care spending.[79,85]

Data sharing and increased collaboration in data collection and analysis should be promoted among health care providers and the various groups conducting outcome research. Creative approaches to educating providers and patients about outcome studies are needed, as well as mechanisms to ensure that patients and health professionals have ready access to the results of outcome research.

Making a treatment selection involves defining the patient's condition, identifying management options and outcome, collecting and summarizing evidence, and applying value judgments or preferences to arrive at an optimal course of action.[46] The randomized, controlled clinical trial, the first of which was published in 1952, has become the "gold standard" for evaluating the efficacy of health care intervention. Clinical decisions are complex and based on many sources of information (Fig. 98.3).[34] Patient management decisions are always a function of both scientific evidence and individual preferences (physicians, health care providers, patients).

Although oncologists, patients, and national organizations recognize that communication is very important in cancer care, evidence-based data on the subject are scarce. Oncologists should use a patient-centered interview approach, ask patients what level of involvement they want in medical decision-making, develop a caring attitude, and consider that patient–physician encounters should provide both cognitive data of patient understanding and feelings.[71]

The Complexity of Randomized, Prospective Clinical Trials

Randomized, prospective, controlled trials are held forth as the gold standard for determining the appropriateness of introducing technology into clinical practice. One must be cognizant, however, of adverse influences upon the generalizability of randomized, controlled trials. If the age, gender, severity of the disease, risk factors, comorbidity, ethnicity, or socioeconomic status of the patients in the randomized, prospective trial are not representative of the general population, it may be inappropriate to generalize the results of the clinical trial to that population. Similarly, if the dose, timing of administration, duration of therapy, quality of care, or comedications of the patients in the trial are not similar to those of the general population, the results may not be applicable.[23]

There is a long-standing joke that one does not need a randomized, prospective trial to ascertain the efficacy of a parachute. In medicine, there are long lists of new technologies that were introduced into general practice based on historical controls without randomized, prospective trials. These include, for example, the use of thyroxin for myxedema, insulin for diabetes, vitamin B12 for pernicious anemia, sulfonamides for puerperal sepsis, penicillin for lobar pneumonia, streptomycin for tuberculosis, defibrillation for ventricular fibrillation, and cisplatinum, vinblastine, and bleomycin for disseminated testicular cancer. The analysis of a randomized clinical trial has traditionally been based on a hypothesis that presumes that there is no difference between treatments. The hypothesis is tested by estimating the probability of obtaining a result as extreme as or more extreme than the one observed if the hypothesis is true. The hypothesis may be irrelevant if there had been previous studies demonstrating that the treatment had some benefits. Those who criticize randomized, prospective trials will quickly argue that "no one ever did a randomized trial to prove that a linear accelerator was better than a cobalt machine, that port films were necessary, or that simulation was preferable to a clinical setup." These arguments are, to some extent, true. One must remember, however, that there is a considerable financial difference between using and not using a port film compared to using a linear accelerator versus a $200 million proton machine.[76]

Nonetheless prospective, randomized clinical trials have come to occupy a prominent role in clinical research in radiation oncology. The most commonly used clinical endpoints are summarized in Table 98.3. Unfortunately, many published reports have unclear definitions or lack some of the fundamental endpoints.

Clinical trials are time consuming and costly. Randomization is the only method that may guarantee that comparisons of treatment outcome are, on average, unbiased. Not all clinical trials yield positive results, and not all new therapies are improvements compared with the standard therapy.[58,64] As an example, a recent analysis of outcome data from 57 randomized, controlled trials, including a total of 12,734 patients, conducted between 1968 and 2002 by the Radiation Therapy Oncology Group[63] showed that overall, experimental and standard radiotherapy were equally successful (odds ratio for survival, 1.01; $p = .5$); however, treatment-related mortality was significantly greater in the experimental arm of the trials (odds ratio, 1.76; $p = .008$) A drawback of randomized trials for the evaluation of a new technology in radiation oncology is that to detect small improvements in morbidity from, for example, an alleged improved dose distribution, an enormous number of patients will need to be accrued and followed for a considerable length of time. Radiation oncologists must, therefore, give serious consideration to the development of novel paradigms for health technology assessments without meeting, in some cases, the ideal requirement of randomization.[63]

Practice Guidelines

Guidelines for health services resulting from valid and appropriate outcome studies have the potential to promote consistency

TABLE 98.3 MOST COMMONLY USED CLINICAL ENDPOINTS IN RADIATION THERAPY TRIALS

Endpoint	Definition of Event	Comments
Local control	No evidence of disease at the primary site (T position)	Statistically this is the absence of an event (i.e., local recurrence); estimated at a given time as the local-recurrence-free rate
Local failure rate	Recurrence in T position	Estimated as 1 minus the local-recurrence-free rate
Locoregional control	No evidence of disease in T and N positions	See above, but for T or N recurrence, whichever comes first; sometimes defined as in-field control (i.e., control within the treated volume)
Survival or overall survival	Death irrespective of cause	–
Cancer-specific survival or cause-specific survival	Death of cancer	Often defined as death of cancer or with active disease
Disease-free survival	Any recurrence or death from any cause, whichever comes first	A composite endpoint combining survival and disease control
Local recurrence-free survival	Local recurrence or death from any cause, whichever comes first	As above, but with local recurrence as the relevant event
Disease-free rate	Any recurrence	Death without recurrence is a cause of censoring
Local relapse-free rate	Local recurrence	As above
Early reactions	Signs or symptoms of a specific early reaction; defined by measuring scale	Typically defined inside a time window; actuarial methods normally not used
Late reactions	Signs or symptoms of a specific late reaction; defined by measuring scale	Actuarial methods should be used
Palliation	Typically defined by measuring scale	May require special statistical considerations
Quality of life	Typically defined by measuring scale	May require special statistical considerations

All definitions involving local recurrence are defined for nodal recurrence (N position) or distant recurrence (M) by analogy.

From Bentzen SM. Towards evidence-based radiation oncology: improving the design, analysis, and reporting of clinical outcome studies in radiotherapy. *Radiother Oncol* 1998;46:5–18.

and quality of care. In the United States, clinical practice guidelines have been promulgated by the American Cancer Society, the American College of Radiology, the American Society of Clinical Oncology, the National Cancer Centers Network, and other professional organizations (Table 98.4).[61,84] Sisk[85] observed that for such guidelines to be successful, it is very important to involve local physicians in the process, to get their views and ultimately their support. The values of practice guidelines in medicine include minimizing inappropriate practice variations, providing reference points for education/practice, improving patient care and outcomes, providing criteria for self-evaluation, setting indicators for external quality review, assisting with service coverage and reimbursement, and decreasing overall cost of medical care. Perceived drawbacks to such guidelines include overregulation and loss of autonomy for both physicians and patients. The conflicting needs and motivations of physicians, patients, third-party carriers, and society bring into play a variety of ethical perspectives. Although contrasting ethical foundations likely will lead to significantly different solutions to the health care resource problem, it is only through educated and reasoned discussion that this problem can be tackled.[86]

Courts in the United States have ruled that guideline developers can be held liable for faulty guidelines and that doctors cannot pass off their liability by claiming that adherence to guidelines corrupted clinical judgment. Protocols and guidelines provide the courts with examples of clinical standards across a wide range of medical practice. However, adherence to guidelines has not automatically been equated with reasonable practice, and the courts seem unlikely to follow the standards enunciated in clinical guidelines without critically evaluating their authority, flexibility, and scope of application.[87]

TABLE 98.4 AMERICAN COLLEGE OF RADIOLOGY APPROPRIATENESS GUIDELINES LITERATURE EVIDENCE TABLE KEY

Strength of recommendation (quality of the study design)

- *Good* evidence to support recommendation that procedure be performed
- *Fair* evidence to support recommendation be performed
- *Poor* evidence to support recommendation, but may be made on other grounds
- *Fair* evidence to support recommendation not be performed
- *Good* evidence to support recommendation not be performed

From Leibel SA. ACR appropriateness criteria. Expert Panel on Radiation Oncology. American College of Radiology. *Int J Radiat Oncol Biol Phys* 1999;43:125–168.

The Patterns of Care Study in the United States

The basic concepts of the Patterns of Care Study are based on analysis of structure, process, and outcome.[88] Initially, all facilities in the United States that provided radiation therapy were identified, and a master list was developed; a statistically determined group of the facilities was selected to reflect the type of practice of radiation oncology throughout university hospitals, community hospitals, and free-standing facilities. Surveys were conducted to define the structure of the facilities, including equipment, staffing, and prevailing standards of practice. More than 1,000 institutions were surveyed in each period of study, and thousands of patients have been included in the database.

Ten diseases were chosen in which curative radiation therapy played a major role. Through extensive discussions with appropriate physicians, a consensus of the best current management was developed for each disease, and decision trees were designed that logically led to the appropriate application of radiation therapy. Process criteria were grouped into three categories, which included workup, treatment, and auxiliary services. Data were collected on individual patients (with appropriate safeguards of privacy), and later the institutions were resurveyed to record the results of treatment, including local/regional recurrence, disease outside the treated field, major complications of therapy, and so forth, leading to publication of several reports correlating process with treatment outcome. An example is a report on the practice of radiotherapy in carcinoma of the uterine cervix published by Eifel et al.[65]

Reports similar to those of the Patterns of Care studies in United States have been published in other countries, such as one by Ringborg et al.[31] in Sweden.

CONCLUSIONS

Technology assessment, outcome analysis, cost benefit, comparative effectiveness, and clinical trials supported by evidence-based medicine should be strengthened and fostered to enhance the rationale and quality of medical care provided to patients at a competitive cost. Basic and translational laboratory research and properly designed, relevant, and timely prospective clinical trials should be strongly promoted, and patient participation must be increased to acquire more accurate information to develop innovative therapeutic strategies in oncology. Methods for accurate cost accounting of medical care and comparative effectiveness studies need further development. Technology assessment will substantially contribute to better utilization of scarce health care resources and will be invaluable in determining the potential value of innovative therapeutic approaches.

REFERENCES

1. Doyle R. Health care costs. *Sci Am* 1999;280:36.
2. Bodenheimer T. High and rising health care costs. Part 2: Technologic innovation. *Ann Intern Med* 2005;142: 932–937.
3. Organisation for Economic Co-operation and Development. *OECD health data 2011.* Available at: http://www.oecd.org/document/16/o,3343,en_2649_34631_2085200_1_1_1_1, 00.html.
4. Borger C, Smith S, Truffer C, et al. Health spending projections through 2015: changes in the horizon. *Health Aff* (Millwood) 2006;25:w61–w73.
5. Forbes S. Dinosaur U. *Forbes* February 28, 2011, p. 13.
6. Emanuel EJ, Fuchs VR, Garber AM. Essential elements of a technology and outcome assessment initiative. *JAMA* 2007;298:1323–1325.
7. Centers for Medicare and Medicaid Services. Coverage with evidence development. Available at: http://www.cms.gov/Medicare/Coverage/Coverage-with-Evidence-Development/index.html.
8. Wallner PE, Konski A. A changing paradigm in the study and adoption of emerging health care technologies: coverage with evidence development. *J Am Coll Radiol* 2008;5:1125–1129.
9. Hayman J, Weeks J, Mauch P. Economic analyses in health care: an introduction to the methodology with an emphasis on radiation therapy. *Int J Radiat Oncol Biol Phys* 1996;35:827–841.
10. Detsky AS, Naglie IG. A clinician's guide to cost-effective analysis. *Ann Int Med* 1990;113:147–154.
11. Drummond M, Sculpher MJ, Torrance GW, et al. *Methods for the economic evaluation of health care programmes.* Oxford: Oxford University Press, 2005.
12. Harngren CT, Foster G, Datar SM. *Cost accounting. a managerial emphasis,* 9th ed. Upper Saddle River, NJ: Prentice-Hall, 1996.
13. EQ-5D. Available at: www.euroqol.org.
14. Perez CA. Methodology of research and practice for the third millennium: evidence-based medicine. *Rays* 2000;25:285–308.
15. Feeny D, Furlong W, Boyle M, et al. Multi-attribute health status classification systems. Health Utility Index. *Pharmacoeconomics* 1995;7:490–502.

15a. Meltzer MI. Introduction to health economics for physicians. *Lancet* 2001;358: 993–998.

16. Clancy CM, Kamerow DB. Evidence-based medicine meets cost-effectiveness analysis. *JAMA* 1996;276:329–330.
17. Neilson AR, Davies HT. Interpreting reported health-care costs. *Hosp Med* 1998; 59:803–806.
18. Siegel JE, Weinstein MC, Russell LB, et al. Recommendations for reporting cost-effectiveness analyses. Panel on Cost-Effectiveness in Health and Medicine. *JAMA* 1996;276:1339–1341.
19. Russell LB, Gold MR, Siegel JE, et al. The role of cost-effectiveness analysis in health and medicine. Panel on Cost-Effectiveness in Health and Medicine. *JAMA* 1996;276:1172–1177.
20. Rigby K, Silagy C, Crockett A. Health economic reviews. Are they compiled systematically?*Int J Technol Assess Health Care* 1996;12:450–459.
21. Smith JM. Effectively costing out options. *JAMA* 1996;276:1180.
22. Weinstein MC, Siegel JE, Gold MR, et al. Recommendations of the Panel on Cost-effectiveness in Health and Medicine. *JAMA* 1996;276:1253–1258.
23. Russell LB. Modelling for cost-effectiveness analysis. *Stat Med* 1999;18:3235–3244.
24. Cowan J, Berkowitz D. Technology assessment at work: part I—principles and a case study. *Physician Exec* 1996;22:5–6, 8–9.
25. Chlebowski RT, Collyar DE, Somerfield MR, et al. American Society of Clinical Oncology technology assessment on breast cancer risk reduction strategies: tamoxifen and raloxifene. *J Clin Oncol* 1999;17:1939–1955.
26. Halperin EC. Overpriced technology in radiation oncology. *Int J Radiat Oncol Biol Phys* 2000;48:917–918.
27. Lee WR. Technology assessment: vigilance required. *Int J Radiat Oncol Biol Phys* 2008;70:652–653.
28. Cotter GW. Surgery or radiation therapy: a comparative cost analysis for early carcinoma of the prostate and breast. *Appl Radiol* 1990;19:25–28.
29. Penn CR. Megavoltage irradiation in a district general hospital remote from a main oncology centre: the Torbay experience reviewed. *Clin Oncol (R Coll Radiol)* 1992;4:108–113.
30. Perez CA, Kobeissi B, Smith BD, et al. Cost accounting in radiation oncology: a computer-based model for reimbursement. *Int J Radiat Oncol Biol Phys* 1993; 25(5):895–906.
31. Ringborg U, Bergqvist D, Brorsson B, et al. The Swedish Council on Technology Assessment in Health Care (SBU) systematic overview of radiotherapy for cancer including a prospective survey of radiotherapy practice in Sweden 2001—summary and conclusions. *Acta Oncol* 2003;42:357–365.
32. Smith TJ, Hillner BE, Desch CE. Efficacy and cost-effectiveness of cancer treatment: rational allocation of resources based on decision analysis. *J Natl Cancer Inst* 993;85:1460–1474.
33. Norlund A. Cost of radiotherapy. *Acta Oncol* 2003;42:411–415.
34. Lievens Y, Van Den Bogaert W, Kesteloot K. Activity-based costing: a practical model for cost calculation in radiotherapy. *Int J Radiat Oncol Biol Phys* 2003; 57:522–535.
35. Konski A, Bhargavan M, Owen J, et al. Feasibility of economic analysis of Radiation Therapy Oncology Group (RTOG) 91-11 using Medicare data. *Int J Radiat Oncol Biol Phys* 2010;79:436–442.
36. Lievens Y, Dunscombe P, Konski A. Promises and pitfalls of health technology assessment. In: Levit SH, Purdy JA, Perez CA, et al., eds. *Technical basis of radiation therapy,* 5th ed. New York: Springer, 2012:549–564.
37. Antos J, Brimson JA. *Activity-based management for service industries, government entities and nonprofit organizations.* New York: Wiley, 1994.
38. Cooper R. *Elements of activity-based costing, emerging practices in cost management.* New York: Warren, Gorham & Lamont, 1990.
39. Cooper R, Kaplan RS. *The design of cost management systems.* Upper Saddle River, NJ: Prentice-Hall, 1991.
40. Foster G, Gupta M. Activity accounting: an electronics industry implementation. In: Kaplan RS, ed. *Measures for manufacturing excellence.* Boston: Harvard Business School Press, 1990:225–268.
41. Van der Werf E, Verstraete J, Lievens Y. The cost of radiotherapy in a decade of technology evolution. *Radiother Oncol* 2012;102(1):148–153.
42. Perez CA, Kobeissi BJ, Chao KSC, et al. *3-D conformal and intensity modulated radiation therapy: physics and clinical applications.* Madison, WI: Advanced Medical Publishing, 2001.
43. Sackett DL, Straus S, Richardson S, et al. *Evidence-based medicine: how to practice and teach EBM,* 2nd ed. London: Churchill Livingston, 2000.
44. Owen JB, Grigsby PW, Caldwell TM, et al. Can costs be measured and predicted by modeling within a cooperative clinical trials group? Economic methodologic pilot studies of the radiation therapy oncology group (RTOG) studies 90-03 and 91-04. *Int J Radiat Oncol Biol Phys* 2001;49:633–639.
45. Brook RH, Kamberg CJ, McGlynn EA. Health system reform and quality. *JAMA* 1996;276:476–480.
46. Fuchs VR, Garber AM. The new technology assessment. *N Engl J Med* 1990;323: 673–677.
47. Doubilet P, Weinstein MC, McNeil BJ. Use and misuse of the term "cost effective" in medicine. *N Engl J Med* 1986;314:253–256.
48. Stinnett AA, Mullahy J. Net health benefits: a new framework for the analysis of uncertainty in cost-effectiveness analysis. *Med Decis Making* 1998;18:S68–S80.
49. Willan AR. Analysis, sample size, and power for estimating incremental net health benefit from clinical trial data. *Control Clin Trials* 2001;22:228–237.
50. Pijls-Johannesma M, Pommier P, Lievens Y. Cost-effectiveness of particle therapy: current evidence and future needs. *Radiother Oncol* 2008;89:127–134.
51. Goitien M, Cox JD. Should randomized clinical trials be required for proton radiotherapy? *J Clin Oncol* 2008;26:175–176.
52. Lodge M, Pijls-Johannesma M, Stirk L, et al. A systematic literature review of the clinical and cost-effectiveness of hadron therapy in cancer. *Radiother Oncol* 2007;83:110–122.
53. Glatstein E, Glick J, Kaiser L, et al. Should randomized clinical trials be required for proton radiotherapy? An alternative view. *J Clin Oncol* 2008;26: 2438–2439.
54. Suit H, DeLaney T, Goldberg S, et al. Proton vs carbon ion beams in the definitive radiation treatment of patients with cancer. *Radiother Oncol* 2010;95:3–22.
55. Perrier L, Combs SE, Aurberger T, et al. A decision-making tool for a costly innovative technology. The case for carbon ion radiotherapy. *J Econ Med* 2007; 25:367–380.
56. Peeters A, Grutters JP, Pijls-Johannesma M, et al. How costly is particle therapy? Cost analysis of external beam radiotherapy with carbon-ions, protons and photons. *Radiother Oncol* 2010; 95:45–53.
57. Buyyounouski MK, Price RA, Harris EER, et al. Stereotactic body radiotherapy for primary management of early stage low to intermediate risk prostate cancer: report of ASTRO Emerging Technology Committee. *Int J Radiat Oncol Biol Phys* 2010;76:1297–1304.
58. Bentzen SM, Wasserman TH. Balancing on a knife's edge: evidence-based medicine and the marketing of new technology. *Int J Radiat Oncol Biol Phys* 2008;72: 12–13.
59. Bigby M. Evidence-based medicine in a nutshell. A guide to finding and using the best evidence in caring for patients. *Arch Dermatol* 1998;134:1609–1618.
60. Berkwits M. From practice to research: the case for criticism in an age of evidence. *Soc Sci Med* 1998;47:1539–1545.
61. Newcomer LN. Finding the answers we need: comparative effectiveness. *Pract Radiat Oncol* 2011;1:83–84.
62. Leibel SA. ACR appropriateness criteria. Expert Panel on Radiation Oncology. American College of Radiology. *Int J Radiat Oncol Biol Phys* 1999;43:125–168.
63. Guyatt GH, Sinclair J, Cook DJ, et al. Users' guides to the medical literature: XVI. How to use a treatment recommendation. Evidence-Based Medicine Working Group and the Cochrane Applicability Methods Working Group. *JAMA* 1999;281: 1836–1843.
64. Bentzen SM Randomized controlled trials in health technology assessment: overkill or overdue? *Radiother Oncol* 2008;86:142–147.
65. Eifel PJ, Moughan J, Erickson B, et al. Patterns of radiotherapy practice for patients with carcinoma of the uterine cervix: a pattern of care study. *Int J Radiat Oncol Biol Phys* 2004;60:1144–1153.
66. Cochrane collaboration. *Preparing, maintaining, and promoting the accessibility of systemic reviews of the effects of healthcare interventions.* Oxford: Cochrane Collaboration, 1999.
67. Cochrane A. *Effectiveness and efficiency: random reflection on health services.* London: Royal Society of Medicine Press Limited; 2004.
68. Cochrane AL. 1931–1971: A critical review, with particular reference to the medical profession. In: *Medicine for the year 2000.* London: Office of Health Economics; 1979:1–11.
69. Tanenbaum SJ. Evidence and expertise: the challenge of the outcomes movement to medical professionalism. *Acad Med* 1999;74:757–763.

70. Feinstein AR, Horwitz RI. Problems in the "evidence" of "evidence-based medicine". *Am J Med* 1997;103:529–535.
71. American Society of Clinical Oncology. Outcomes of cancer treatment for technology assessment and cancer treatment guidelines. *J Clin Oncol* 1996;14:671–670.
72. Bentzen SM. Towards evidence based radiation oncology: improving the design, analysis, and reporting of clinical outcome studies in radiotherapy. *Radiother Oncol* 1998;46:5–18.
73. Mulrow CD, Cook DJ, Davidoff F. Systematic reviews; critical links in the great chain of evidence. In: *Systematic reviews: synthesis of best evidence for health care decisions.* Philadelphia: American College of Physicians, 1998:1–4.
74. Hunt DL, Haynes RB, Hanna SE, et al. Effects of computer-based clinical decision support systems on physician performance and patient outcomes: a systematic review. *JAMA* 1998;280:1339–1346.
75. McAlister FA, Straus SE, Guyatt GH, et al. Users' guides to the medical literature: XX. Integrating research evidence with the care of the individual patient. Evidence-Based Medicine Working Group. *JAMA* 2000;283:2829–2836.
76. Rawlins M. De testimonio: on the evidence for decisions about the use of therapeutic interventions. *Clin Med* 8: 579–588, 2008.
77. Back A. Patient-physician communication in oncology: what does the evidence show? *Oncology* 2006;20:67–74.
78. Pommier P, Lievens Y, Feschet F et al. Simulating demand for innovative radiotherapies: an illustrative model based on carbon ion and proton radiotherapy. *Radiother Oncol* 2010;96:243–249.
79. Sisk JE. Increased competition and the quality of health care. *Milbank Q* 1998; 76:687–707, 512.
80. Chassin MR, Galvin RW. The urgent need to improve health care quality. Institute of Medicine National Roundtable on Health Care Quality. *JAMA* 1998;280:1000–1005.
81. Mendelson DN, Goodman CS, Ahn R, et al. Outcomes and effectiveness research in the private sector. *Health Aff* (Millwood) 1998;17:75–90.
82. Newman L, ed. *Medical outcomes and guidelines sourcebook.* New York: Faulkner & Gray, 1999.
83. Panek WC. Ethical considerations related to outcome studies-based clinical practice guidelines. *J Glaucoma* 1999;8:267–272.
84. American Society of Clinical Oncology. Recommended breast cancer surveillance guidelines. *J Clin Oncol* 1997;15:2149–2156.
85. Sisk JE. How are health care organizations using clinical guidelines? *Health Aff* (Millwood) 1998;17:91–109.
86. Bentzen S. Radiation oncology health technology assessment—the best is the enemy of the good. *Nat Clin Pract Oncol* 2008;5:563.
87. Hurwitz B. Clinical guidelines and the law: advice, guidance or regulation? *J Eval Clin Pract* 1995;1:49–60.
88. Kramer S. An overview of process and outcome data in the patterns of care study. *Int J Radiat Oncol Biol Phys* 1981;7:795–800.

Chapter 99
Ethics, Professional Values, and Legal Considerations in Radiation Oncology

Brian D. Kavanagh, Laurie J. Lyckholm, and Jeremy Sugarman

The medical profession experienced a rise in socioeconomic stature in the United States during the 20th century.[1] Physicians began to receive higher wages for their services and enjoy greater personal respect as providers of health. Although progress in medical science has improved the quality and duration of life for some patients with cancer and other serious illnesses, technical expertise alone does not fully account for the upsurge in the societal standing of medical doctors during the past 100 years.

High regard for physicians is contingent on the trust that doctors act unselfishly in a patient's best interests, a role sometimes called *moral fiduciary.*[2] Essential to this role are medical knowledge and a firm grasp of ethics. Derived from the Greek ἦθος (*ethos*), meaning *character,* ethics refers to the process of applying values and principles in professional interactions and particularly in medical decision making on behalf of patients. The curriculum of most medical schools now includes coursework in ethics, but many physicians practicing today completed their training without formal instruction in this topic. To foster an appreciation for the intellectual underpinnings of modern medical ethics, this chapter begins with an overview of scholarly approaches to ethics. Next is a discussion of selected proclamations and codes of ethics published by professional societies, federal commissions, and other authorities as guidelines for medical practice and research. Finally, common ethical issues in radiation oncology are addressed, including relevant medicolegal considerations.

CONCEPTUAL APPROACHES TO MEDICAL ETHICS

The term *bioethics,* coined in the early 1970s, refers to the academic inquiry and public policy movement addressing the application of science and medicine from a humanistic perspective.[3] Medical ethics may be most accurately viewed as a branch of bioethics, but the terms are commonly used interchangeably. Among the more influential theoretical approaches to ethics that are used in bioethics are *utilitarianism, deontology, casuistry, virtue theory,* and *principlism.*

Utilitarianism is based on the premise that, in any situation, the best course of action is the one that produces the maximum net positive value (or least negative value). Utilitarianism can be applied to an individual patient's case or to matters of health policy, in which decisions might be made to achieve the greatest overall benefit for the largest number of people.

Unlike utilitarianism, deontology is an ethical theory based on the morality of actions themselves rather than their net result. Deontology, sometimes called *Kantianism* in recognition of the influence of Immanuel Kant,[4] calls for consistent standards of behavior at all times, regardless of the consequences. One simple example of the difference between utilitarianism and deontology is the issue of educating patients about their diagnosis, especially if the prognosis is very poor. Whereas a deontologist would always feel obliged to tell the truth even at the risk of causing distress, a utilitarian considers whether telling a patient the complete truth about the disease does or does not really benefit the patient. In practice, there is obviously a need to find the right balance between purely utilitarian and purely deontologic perspectives in a situation like this one. Respect for the patient's autonomy, for example, is one of the *prima facie* ethical principles discussed further in the next section. Truth-telling is an integral component, and overriding this principle requires justification.

Casuistry is an approach to ethics that emphasizes inductive reasoning based on established precedents, and it is a common practice in both law and medicine. The proper course of action in any individual case is decided by recalling decisions made in prior similar cases. The major weakness of casuistry is the lack of a reference benchmark or settled opinion on novel technologies.

Virtue theory focuses on the character of moral agents, in this case physicians and other health care providers, focusing less on actions or outcomes. As such, virtue theory captures the way in which correct moral actions occur. For example, it is not only important to tell patients the truth about their diagnoses, but it is also critical to do so in a compassionate manner. In this case, the virtue is compassion. Accordingly, while virtue is a critical part of assessing moral action, virtues themselves have little guiding force.

Principlism is a system of applied ethics through which core principles ideally govern behavior in the absence of compelling reasons to override them. Principlism can be integrated with the other philosophical approaches already mentioned and serves as a unifying influence. Key features of principlism are addressed in the next section.

ETHICAL PRINCIPLES

A *prima facie* obligation may be defined as one that is "binding unless overridden or outweighed by competing moral obligations."[4] Four *prima facie* principles of bioethics are highlighted here: *respect for autonomy, beneficence, nonmaleficence,* and *justice.*

Respect for a patient's autonomy is based on respect for the right to individual liberty. A patient's voluntary decision to seek medical care or comply with referral to a specialist is the starting point of most patient–physician relationships, and competent patients should remain free to forgo therapy or change physicians at any time. The responsibility to respect patients' autonomy is established not only in ethics but also in law. An example is the requirement to obtain a patient's informed consent for proposed medical therapy. In a landmark case involving postmastectomy chest wall radiation therapy, a patient who sustained soft tissue necrosis won a lawsuit against her radiation oncologist for negligence and for lack of proper disclosure regarding possible treatment-related toxicity. The Kansas Supreme Court ruled that doctors should explain "in language as simple as necessary" the side effects associated with any recommended therapy.[5]

The principle of *beneficence* is intertwined with that of *nonmaleficence.* Some authors have offered nuanced distinctions between the two principles,[4] but the key point is that physicians should act for the benefit of patients and should not harm their patients. Beneficence and nonmaleficence are typically concordant objectives, but sometimes an intervention that is helpful also entails a high risk of adverse treatment-induced sequelae. For example, administering high-dose morphine to a patient severely dyspneic from an incurable lung malignancy can relieve symptoms but at the same time risks fatally suppressing respiratory drive. Here the quality of remaining life might be improved by a measure that also hastens death. Such an action can sometimes be justified by the principle of double effect, the earliest expression of which is generally attributed to St. Thomas Aquinas.[6] According to this concept, the benefit of an action might be valuable enough to outweigh a simultaneous significant risk of serious adverse event, as long as achieving benefit is the primary intent. High-dose chemotherapy, bone marrow transplant, and some high-complexity surgeries, such as Whipple procedures, are examples of cancer therapies in which potential burdens and risks might militate against potential benefits.

The principle of justice refers to fairness, typically the equitable distribution of health care resources. Justice-related questions often arise in regard to matters of public policy. Two examples are determining the means to allocate scarce organs for transplantation and selecting what types of research merit government funding. More globally relevant in the United States is the challenge of allocating federal dollars for health care. Distributive justice implies that persons ought to be afforded medical care according to their medical needs and the ability of the system to provide.

FORMAL OATHS AND CODES OF ETHICS

There are many published declarations of medical ethics authored by physicians. Not surprisingly, the tone and language of each reflect the social mores and sometimes historical events of the era in which it was composed.

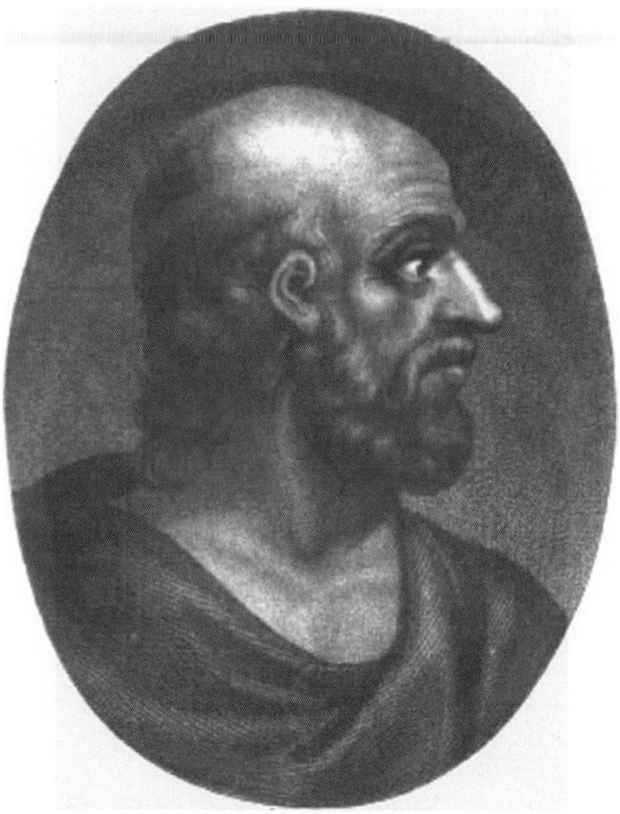

FIGURE 99.1. Early 19th-century engraving depicting a likeness of Hippocrates, closely resembling images of ancient coins found on the island of Cos bearing his likeness. (Courtesy of the National Library of Medicine.)

The Hippocratic Oath

> I will prescribe regimen for the good of my patients according to my ability and my judgment and never do harm to anyone

The *Corpus Hippocraticum* is a collection of medical treatises dating from around the fifth century BCE, believed to be the work of philosopher–physicians from the Greek island of Cos (Fig. 99.1). Contained within the *Corpus* is the well-known oath of Hippocrates, an ancient physician's pledge of professionalism. Curiously, the oath is inconsistent with some other sections of the *Corpus,* perhaps because it was added later. Comments about abortion and surgery, for example, are at variance with teachings elsewhere in the collected works.[7] Nevertheless, timeless themes are included, and the oath has survived in various modernized versions. The oath is often recited by medical students at the time of graduation—even if its contents are not always well remembered.[8,9]

Percival's Medical Ethics

> Hospital physicians and surgeons should minister to the sick, with due impressions of the importance of their office, reflecting that the ease, the health, and the lives of those committed to their charge depend on their skill, attention, and fidelity.

Thomas Percival (1740–1804) (Fig. 99.2) published *Medical Ethics* at a time when there were considerable tension among clinicians in his community.[10] In the 1760s, Manchester, England, was a prosperous urban society that comfortably supported public health initiatives, including an infirmary serving as a charity hospital and teaching institution. But as the city grew and became crowded by the 1790s, tensions arose between rival groups in the medical community. Percival was prompted to draft a code of ethics after a contentious dispute about enlarging the infirmary's staff, a threat to the controlling physician faction.[11]

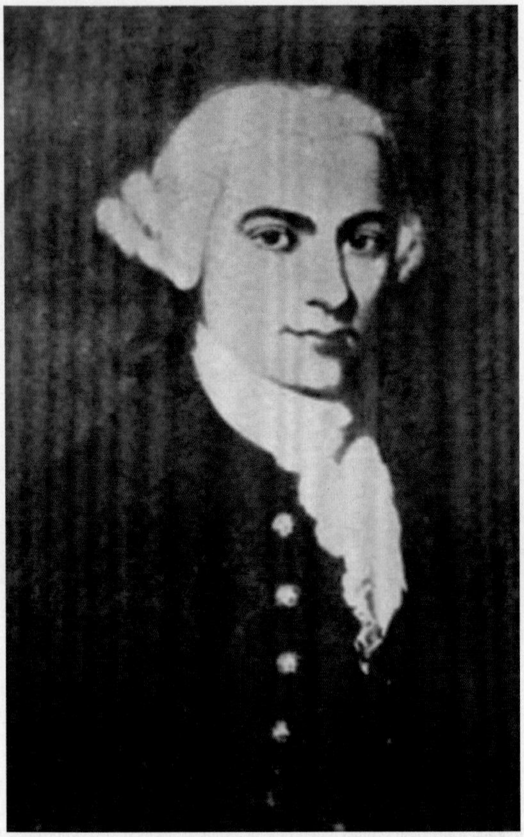

FIGURE 99.2. Thomas Percival (1740–1804). (From Brockbank EM. *Sketches of the lives and work of the honorary medical staff of the Manchester Infirmary, from its foundation in 1752 to 1830 when it became the Royal Infirmary*. Manchester, UK: Manchester University Press, 1904, with permission.)

When he began writing *Medical Ethics,* Percival was already a well-known writer and moralist whose *A Father's Instructions to His Children,* published in 1775, included essays promoting personal virtues and social awareness to young readers. While completing *Medical Ethics,* Percival suffered devastating personal tragedies, bereaving the untimely deaths of two of his own sons. The finished work was dedicated to a third son studying medicine at the time.

Ultimately, *Medical Ethics* provided a template for the codes of ethics adopted by the American Medical Association (AMA) and other societies in the 19th century. Early 20th-century pundits criticized Percival's work as merely a book of medical *etiquette* rather than medical *ethics*. However, revisionist historians have subsequently argued that although Percival focused on interprofessional relationships, he also taught that a physician's duty toward the patient outweighs obligations of civility toward other health care professionals. Furthermore, Percival advanced the enlightened view that indigent patients should receive the same quality of care as affluent patients.[12]

The American Medical Association Code of Ethics

The AMA first adopted a code of ethics at its inaugural meeting in 1847. The initial code was modeled on the work of Percival, but subsequent updates have reflected societal changes and technological progress. The 2004 version includes four components[13]:

a. *Principles of Medical Ethics;*
b. *Fundamental Elements of the Patient–Physician Relationship;*
c. *Current Opinions of the Council on Ethical and Judicial Affairs;* and
d. *Reports of the Council on Ethical and Judicial Affairs.*

The seven *Principles* are general instructions for a physician to maintain competence and integrity in the context of individual patient care and also in the larger view toward enhancing the standard of care in the community. The *Fundamental Elements* expand the concept of a collaborative interaction between physicians and patients, specifically mentioning the need for good communication and the need to protect patients' confidentiality. The AMA here advocates that all patients have a right to "necessary care," regardless of their ability to pay for that care, and that physicians should play a role in safeguarding this right. The *Current Opinions* and the *Reports of the Council on Ethical and Judicial Affairs* provide situational interpretations of the *Principles* and *Fundamental Elements,* and they are often referenced in legal proceedings.

The Nuremberg Code and the Declaration of Geneva

During World War II, odious crimes were committed by Nazi physicians who conducted horrific experiments on concentration camp prisoners who were coerced to submit. The Nuremberg Code was a formal response to these World War II–era human rights atrocities disguised as medical experiments.[14] Issued from the military tribunal that tried some of the Nazi doctors who conducted these experiments, the Nuremberg Code acknowledges that medical investigations are important. However, for a medical experiment to be morally permissible, it must meet 10 criteria, paraphrased as follows:

- Voluntary consent of the human subject
- Necessity to yield results helpful to society
- Appropriate design based on knowledge of the disease under study
- Avoidance of unnecessary physical and mental suffering and injury
- Absence of reason to believe that death or disabling injury will occur
- Overall degree of risk in proportion to the nature of the problem to be solved
- Adequate precautions against the possibility of the subject's injury, disability, or death
- Qualified persons conducting the study
- Unrestricted freedom of the subject to end the experiment if he or she reaches the physical or mental state where continuation of the experiment seems impossible
- Willingness of the investigator to discontinue the study at any time if there is reason to believe that continuing the experiment is likely to result in injury or death to the subject.

In the aftermath of the war, the international medical community was especially sensitized to the need for universal adherence to high standards of ethical behavior. The Declaration of Geneva was adopted in 1948 by the World Medical Association and has been updated since then. The text includes the physician's vow to ignore "considerations of age, disease or disability, creed, ethnic origin, gender, nationality, political affiliation, race, sexual orientation, or social standing" in the treatment of a patient and to uphold "even under threat . . . the utmost respect for human life."

Case Study

Despite publicity about the Nuremberg Code and the Geneva declaration, controversial large-scale, government-sponsored medical studies took place in the years following World War II. Experimentation on the effects of radiation exposure on humans was conducted in the United States during the Cold War, when fears of nuclear warfare prompted inquiry into the carcinogenic and other adverse health effects of environmental exposure to ionizing radiation. In response to public concern about thousands of federally funded studies conducted from the 1940s through 1970s without consent of the subjects, in

1994 President Bill Clinton established the Advisory Committee on Human Radiation Experiments (ACHRE). ACHRE was comprised of ethicists, radiation oncologists, and others with relevant expertise. It was charged with evaluating the experiments' ethical and scientific standards and recommending actions to ensure that any mistakes of the past would not be repeated. ACHRE reviewed all available documentation and also conducted an oral history project in which scientists described prevailing sentiments regarding human research ethics during the era of interest.

ACHRE found that government officials and investigators were in some cases culpable "for not having had policies and practices in place to protect the rights and interests of human subjects who ... could not possibly derive direct medical benefit."[15] One example was the observational study of uranium mine workers exposed to radon levels known to be hazardous, without warning and without efforts to reduce the radon levels by ventilating the mines. As a result, lung cancer developed in hundreds of workers, and appropriate compensation was recommended for the individuals affected.

The Belmont Report

In 1972 Jean Heller exposed the injustices of the U.S. Public Health Services (USPHS) Study of Untreated Syphilis in the Negro Male that was conducted in Tuskegee, Alabama.[16] During a 40-year period beginning in the 1930s, 399 indigent African American sharecroppers with syphilis and 200 without syphilis were subjects in a natural history study of the disease. The men mistakenly believed that diagnostic blood tests and lumbar punctures composed treatment for their "bad blood" when in reality these were done solely to monitor the course of the infection. Moreover, years later when penicillin was discovered and found to be effective in the treatment of syphilis, it was withheld intentionally from the men. Subsequently, public awareness of the USPHS study likely contributed to enduring reluctance among some members of minority groups to participate in clinical trials,[17,18] and the political backlash provoked action by the federal government.

The 1974 National Research Act established the National Commission for the Protection of Human Subjects of Biomedical and Behavioral Research. The commission met at the Belmont Conference Center in Maryland to develop ethical guidelines for the conduct of biomedical and behavioral research. In 1979 the commission published *Ethical Principles and Guidelines for the Protection of Human Subjects of Research,* commonly known as the Belmont Report.[19]

In the Belmont Report, a clear distinction is made between medical research and clinical practice. The term *practice* describes interventions intended "to enhance the well-being of an individual patient ... that have a reasonable expectation of success," whereas *research* is "designed to test an hypothesis, permit conclusions to be drawn, and ... contribute to generalizable knowledge." Sometimes a clinician uses good judgment and departs from standard methods for the benefit of an individual patient in special circumstances. However, if major innovations are proposed as replacement for standard techniques, then a formal investigation should be conducted to assess safety and efficacy. The National Commission embraced a principlist perspective in drafting the report, emphasizing in particular respect for persons, beneficence, and justice. The Belmont Report's definition of respect for persons incorporates respect for autonomy and special concern for individuals with diminished capacity to exercise their autonomy. Involving prisoners in research activity is cited as an example. Although it is inappropriate to deny prisoners the possible benefit of experimental interventions, any direct or indirect pressure on prisoners to participate in clinical studies must be avoided. For instance, a promise of clemency in return for study enrollment is unacceptable. The report also addresses the nature of justice in medical research, emphasizing that the process of selecting subjects for a research study must be carefully examined. Investigators should minimize the chance that socioeconomically disadvantaged groups are represented disproportionately as a result of a vulnerability to manipulation in the health care environment.

The American College of Radiation Oncology Code of Ethics

The American College of Radiation Oncology (ACRO) has published a code of ethics, contained within the organization's bylaws, which is available for review at the organization's website (www.acro.org). The principles expressed are concordant with accepted ethical standards and include respect of patient autonomy, the expectation that a radiation oncologist should always act in the best interests of the patient, and respect of patient confidentiality. The ACRO code also forbids deceptive billing arrangements, and members of ACRO who do not comply with the code of ethics are subject to disciplinary action by the organization.

National Electrical Manufacturers Association Code of Ethics

The makers of equipment and software used in the practice of radiation oncology are not required to demonstrate clinical efficacy of a new device or software through the same sort of clinical testing that is required by the U.S. Food and Drug Administration (FDA) for approval of a new drug or implantable medical device. Rather, most treatment devices are approved after demonstration of safety and substantial equivalence to an approved device that is already commercially available. A company that wishes to sell a new device submits a premarket notification to the FDA at least 90 days before commercial distribution is to begin, in accordance with Section 510(k) of the FDA Modernization Act of 1997. Because devices may be introduced into the market without proof of superiority in any given clinical situation, manufacturers may promote their products to physicians by emphasizing intuitively attractive features that might or might not provide meaningful clinical advantage to patients.

On January 1, 2005, members of the National Electrical Manufacturers Association (NEMA) adopted a code of ethics regarding interactions between makers of medical imaging and treatment equipment and physicians (www.nema.org). Individual sections of the NEMA code address member-sponsored product training and education, support for third-party educational conferences, sales and promotional meetings, arrangements with consultants, gifts, provision of reimbursement and other economic information, charitable donations, and research grants. The guidelines are essentially consistent with the AMA policy on gifts and applicable federal regulations. NEMA members are allowed to support educational conferences and advertise their wares in these venues, and also they may provide educational support for individual customers in the safe use of their products. However, hospitality provided by NEMA member at conferences and meeting should be "modest in value and ... subordinate in time and focus to the purpose of the meeting." When it is necessary to demonstrate nonportable equipment, members may pay for reasonable travel costs of attendees with a *bona fide* professional interest but not for their guests.[20]

COMMON ETHICAL ISSUES IN RADIATION ONCOLOGY

> Doctors wear a lot of hats these days; besides the usual physician role, we are expected to be a researcher, financial counselor, administrator, gatekeeper, patient advocate in the medicolegal system, ethicist, and Lord knows what else.
>
> —Thomas J. Smith[21]

Financial Relationships with Hospitals and Referring Physicians

Reimbursement for radiation oncology services or other procedure-intensive subspecialties can be a major revenue source for hospitals. At the same time, subspecialists depend on other physicians to refer patients for evaluation and management. These situations can tempt hospital administrators to reward subspecialists for practicing in their facility and might tempt the subspecialists to induce referrals with financial incentives. In either case, a conflict of interests emerges: Treatment recommendations can be influenced not only appropriately by patient-centered beneficence but also inappropriately by the physician's interest in personal gain. In the United States, the Anti-Kickback Statute and the Stark Law make it illegal to engage in such unscrupulous medical business practices.

The Anti-Kickback Statute (42 U.S.C. §1320a-7b) includes criminal penalties for acts involving Medicare or state health care programs. Section (b) makes it a felony punishable by a fine up to $25,000 and up to 5 years in prison to solicit or receive "any remuneration (including any kickback, bribe, or rebate) directly or indirectly ... in return for referring an individual to a person for ... any item or service" reimbursed in whole or in part through Medicare or a state health care program. The Anti-Kickback Statute also bans other fraudulent transactions supported through the same funding sources.

Named for its leading congressional author, Rep. Pete Stark of California, the Stark Law (42 U.S.C. §1395nn; "Limitation on certain physician referrals") bans other misconduct involving Medicare and Medicaid patients. The Stark Law prohibits a physician from referring a patient for a "designated health service" to a clinic or other facility with which the physician or an immediate family member of the physician has a financial relationship. Radiation therapy is considered a designated health service, but it is clarified that a request by a radiation oncologist for radiation therapy is considered integral to the consultation request from the (nonradiation oncologist) referring physician and does not constitute a self-referral *per se* in most situations. Sanctions for violations of the numerous Stark Law regulations may include civil prosecution.

Managed Care

By the early 1990s, more than 70% of Americans with health insurance were enrolled in some form of managed care plan[22] in which patients are restricted in their choices of physicians and medical services for the purpose of limiting the cost of the health care.[23] The idea has existed in the United States at least since the time of the Great Depression of 1929, when Dr. Michael Shadid of Oklahoma organized a prepay and copay system for surgical, medical, and dental services. To maintain profitability, managed care organizations influence the behavior of patients and physicians through strategies to minimize expenditures. Tactics directed toward patients are promotion of preventive medicine, limitation of access to medical specialists unless approved by a "gatekeeper" primary care physician, and restricted selection of physicians to those willing to accept lower reimbursements. Physicians are prompted to lower costs by capitation-based compensation packages and financial rewards to avoid excess resource utilization.

Managed care is ethically defensible insofar as it can provide equal access for participants and promote well-being through an emphasis on preventive medicine. However, managed care can also threaten the physician–patient relationship by undermining the patient's autonomy and creating a conflict of interest for the health care provider.[24] If the physician gatekeeper shares financial risk with the managed care organization, a patient with a difficult medical problem might be less likely to be referred to a specialist where higher costs would be expected to result.

Physicians' attitudes about managed care reflect concerns about ethics. A survey of primary care physicians revealed that most of them believed that managed care has a negative impact on the patient–physician relationships by interfering with patients' choices and compromising the physicians' ability to put the patients' interests first.[25] Medical students and residents frequently receive negative messages about managed care from their faculty mentors.[26]

Oncology services are often still provided by managed care organizations through fee-for-service contracts with independent practitioners. Nonetheless, there remain challenging patient management issues with regard to delivering radiation therapy in the setting of managed care that include the sometimes fragmented care and inconvenience for the patient, whose managed care organization might have contracted with several centers for various aspects of oncology care, and the administrative burdens associated with obtaining documentation of preapproval for patients' radiation treatments.[27]

Electronic Record-Keeping and Billing Practices

The principles of respect for autonomy and nonmaleficence oblige confidentiality in physician–patient communications. Publicizing private details of a patient's condition can create social and economic harms for the patient. With the advent of electronic medical records and Internet communication, there is a greater need for vigilance in this respect.

In the United States, the Health Insurance Portability and Accountability Act of 1996 (HIPAA) empowered the Department of Health and Human Services to codify standards for storage and transmission of an individual patient's health information. Penalties for violations vary in proportion to their severity. In the worst case of wrongful disclosure of information with intent to sell it, a fine of up to $250,000 and a prison term of up to 10 years can be imposed.

Submitting fraudulent claims to the government for reimbursement of health care services is illegal. The False Claims Act (31 U.S.C. §3729) provides that any person who knowingly presents fraudulent claims to the U.S. government may be fined $5,000 to $10,000 and may be liable for three times the amount of any damages sustained by the government.

Applications of New Technology

Innovative treatment-delivery technologies such as intensity-modulated radiation therapy and stereotactic body radiation therapy provide radiation oncologists freedom to exercise creativity in customizing treatment plans for each individual patient. Ideally, it is best that such innovations are tested in formal research protocols in which a clinical problem is identified and the new technology is proposed as a solution so that toxicity and efficacy can be monitored closely. A prospective clinical trial approved and monitored by an institutional review board affords the opportunity to advance knowledge in the field with ethical oversight.[28] It is inappropriate to apply a novel, more expensive technology to generate higher revenue in the absence of a sound clinical rationale. The AMA code of ethics proscribes superfluous therapy of no benefit to the patient.[29]

Clinical Trial Conduct

Instances of flagrantly improper clinical research taint the annals of medical history. The USPHS study of syphilis mentioned earlier and the human radiation experiments conducted during the Cold War without the consent of the participants are dark reminders of the need for ethical oversight of research.

Obtaining a participant's informed consent is of paramount importance in conducting most clinical research. Despite the recognized importance of informed consent, precisely how much information should be conveyed to a potential clinical trial participant is debatable. The Belmont Report offers this criterion: "the extent and nature of information should be such that persons, knowing that the procedure is neither necessary for their care nor perhaps fully understood, can decide whether they wish to participate" in the study. In certain situations the nature of a study requires that there is incomplete disclosure of information to the participant to sustain the integrity of the study. The Belmont Report condones such research only when "i) incomplete disclosure is truly necessary to accomplish the goals of the research, ii) there are no undisclosed risks to subjects that are more than minimal, and iii) there is an adequate plan for debriefing subjects, when appropriate, and for dissemination of research results to them." The federal rules governing research (45 CFR 46) reflect these arguments.

Advances in the biosciences, such as stem cell research, cloning, and manipulations of the human genome, have been associated with contentious public debate. Federal government and professional policies on such matters have sometimes been constructed as a compromise between scientific opportunity and political ideology.[30] Extra safeguards have been imposed in some settings; for example, the federal government requires an extra level of review for gene-transfer experiments.[31]

Genetics

The management of some cancer patients can involve assessment of genetic markers that might predict treatment response and also reveal a predisposition to the development of certain cancers among the patient's family members. The National Society of Genetic Counselors has published a guideline concerning genetic cancer risk assessment, counseling, and testing.[32] It is recommended that the process of obtaining informed consent for genetic testing should include, among other considerations, an explanation to the patient of possible implications on the ability to obtain health or disability insurance in the future.

Relationships with Industry Sponsors

Incentives from industry representatives to prescribe pharmaceuticals or purchase equipment threaten the fiduciary obligations physicians have to their patients. The AMA code of ethics allows that gifts of modest value with direct or indirect benefit to patients are acceptable.[33] Examples include textbooks or unrestricted educational grants for students or fellows. Subsidies for "modest meals or social events held as part of a conference" are permissible, as are honoraria for lectures or legitimate consulting services. However, cash or other valuable incentives intended to influence the decision to use a company's products are forbidden. Also unacceptable would be a blanket indemnification from liability for use of a product. Advertising items such as patient education pamphlets and anatomic models bearing a sponsor's name are commonly found in radiation oncology clinics.[34] Physicians should be aware of any real or perceived influence on the patient–physician relationships resulting from their tacit compliance with such marketing activities.

In recent years some pharmaceutical companies have been prosecuted for kickback schemes or other illegal enticements to physicians, and the civil and criminal penalties paid by the corporations held responsible have ranged up to hundreds of millions of dollars.[35] Brennan et al.[36] contend that voluntary self-regulation by physicians, industry, and government is an insufficient safeguard against the conflict of interests nurtured by close relationships between practicing doctors and sellers of pharmaceuticals and medical products. These authors argue that academic medical centers should set an example for the rest of the medical community by establishing policies that forbid gifts to physicians, funds for travel, unjustified consulting fees, participation in speakers' bureaus, and the practice of "ghostwriting" medical articles, among other things. Substantial attention has focused on implementing policies related to these issues.[37,38]

CASE-SPECIFIC DILEMMAS: THE ROLE OF AN ETHICS CONSULTANT OR COMMITTEE

The radiation oncology–related ethical issues discussed thus far relate primarily to general practice and research guidelines. However, individual cases can also pose uncertainties regarding the proper choice of action for a specific patient.

Case Study

A 37-year-old woman undergoes modified radical mastectomy for a pathologic T3N2M0 breast cancer; postoperative chemotherapy and locoregional radiation therapy are recommended. The patient wishes to receive the therapy only if she can periodically interrupt it to alternate with what she calls a "natural herbal" therapy.

In this case, respect for a patient's autonomy conflicts with what is believed to be in the patient's best interests, but a physician cannot ethically abrogate the fiduciary responsibility to a patient simply for reasons of unfamiliarity with alternative medicine or prejudice against its worth.[39] Similar situations may arise when patients are noncompliant with standard treatment recommendations because of a particular religious faith or cultural heritage. Although physicians must respect patients' choices, there is no strict obligation for a physician to accept a particular individual as a patient, especially if there are foreseeable personal conflicts that might adversely affect the patient–physician relationship.[40]

Pediatric oncology also requires special considerations. Parents are the chief decision makers, but sometimes their wishes can seem discordant with the best interests of the child. In a different context, what should be done if the adult children of a patient with a heritable trait for malignancy inquire of the patient's diagnosis, but the patient has instructed the physician not to reveal any information to them? The obligation to patient–physician confidentiality conflicts with a potentially overriding obligation toward the family members who might benefit from guidance toward screening.

In cases such as these in which it is difficult to choose between two defensible courses of action, individuals with experience in clinical medical ethics can provide the expertise needed to sort through the ethical, legal, and social issues involved.[41]

PALLIATIVE MEDICINE

Palliative medicine has become a well-established component of clinical practice, and numerous academic medical centers offer accredited fellowship programs in this field. Palliative medicine places emphasis on symptom management and on the goals of care, not only at the end of life but also in the treatment of serious illnesses. A palliative approach is ethically justified when fully aggressive therapy might be intolerable or futile.

Case Study

A 92-year-old woman presented with stage IVa maxillary sinus cancer. She complained of sinus fullness and a painful 4-cm neck node. Radical radiation therapy to the primary and neck was recommended, and the patient underwent placement of a percutaneous gastric feeding tube and full dental extraction. Midway through the course of treatment, the patient required a lengthy hospitalization for failure to thrive and severe mucositis.

In retrospect a less-aggressive course of radiation therapy intended to reduce the sinus and neck symptoms would have been a better choice for this patient, who was frail and unable to withstand intense treatment. Palliative medicine pays careful attention to a patient's individual needs, quality of life, and a discussion of goals of care. A recent randomized study demonstrated improved quality of life and overall survival when palliative care was given early alongside standard cancer treatment for metastatic lung cancer.[42] In many cases, aggressive symptom management and good communication among patient, family, and provider may result in better quality and, perhaps, quantity of life than would antineoplastic therapy that has little expectation of efficacy but significant risk of morbidity.[43]

ETHICS AND MEDICAL ERRORS

Soon after the discovery of x-rays by Wilhelm Röntgen more than 100 years ago, the first cases of malpractice involving the clinical use of radiation therapy were tried in the U.S. court system.[44] During the early 20th century, severe dermatitis was a frequent plaintiff's complaint—not surprising in view of the physical limitations of the low-energy machines available at the time.

In 1999, the Institute of Medicine published a report on medical errors, elevating the level of public awareness and stimulating inquiry into this topic.[45,46] Estimates of the number of Americans who die each year as a result of medical error have ranged from 44,000 to 98,000,[47,48] and the annual cost of preventable adverse events has been projected to be $17 billion to $29 billion.[49] In addition to encouraging efforts to improve patient safety, the Institute of Medicine recommended the development of confidential self-reporting programs and legislation to prevent voluntary reporting from legal discovery.[50]

Physicians are often reluctant to discuss errors. It has been suggested that doctors and patients "harbor deep within themselves the expectation that the physician will be perfect."[51] Other reasons for reticence include uncertainty about whether an event really is an error, concern for the patient's well-being, and fear of litigation.[52] Each of these items warrants comment.

First, if a patient has an undesirable treatment outcome, careful review of the case can help distinguish error from untoward but unsurprising occurrence. For example, severe pneumonitis after breast radiation therapy is uncommon but not necessarily proof of negligence. Second, concern that disclosing an error causes a patient undue anxiety is contradicted by studies revealing that patients prefer physicians to acknowledge errors[53] and they might even sue for lack of apology.[54] Finally, in cases of alleged or suspected error leading to injury, the institutional risk-management service should usually be contacted for advice. However, fear of litigation should be mitigated by the fact that a low overall percentage of patients who suffer negligent injuries actually file malpractice claims.[25,52]

Nondisclosure of error can weaken the trust at the core of the patient–physician relationship. The argument for disclosure is especially strong when there is a specific preventive intervention that might lessen the severity of possible future injury. Nevertheless, the question still remains: Are physicians ethically obliged to disclose an error, even if there is no immediate harm to the patient?

Case Study

A patient with T3N1M0 squamous cell carcinoma of the left retromolar trigone received concurrent cetuximab plus intensity-modulated radiation therapy to the gross disease, with elective coverage of adjacent nodal echelons. The intent was to give 54 Gy to adjacent uninvolved lymph nodes at a rate of 1.8 Gy per day and 66 Gy to the gross disease at a rate of 2.2 Gy per day using a synchronous integrated boost technique, with all treatment completed in 30 fractions. After the spinal cord was contoured as an organ at risk, the structure was inadvertently deleted on all planning computed tomography slices below the level of the gross disease. As a result, when the intensity-modulated radiation therapy inverse planning software optimized the dose distribution according to the constraint of limiting the maximum dose to the spinal cord to 50 Gy, the entire cross-section of a 6-cm length of cervical spinal cord received the full prescription dose, with some areas of the cord located in a "hot spot" region receiving more than 70 Gy. The error was not detected until 1 week after the patient completed treatment, during a routine quality assurance check.

In this example, no injury has yet occurred, but the patient is at increased risk for radiation myelitis. Although there is currently no available proven preventive measure, if the escalated risk of myelitis is unknown to the patient, he or she might later undergo misguided management by another physician if symptoms develop. For instance, if the patient develops arm and leg weakness, a magnetic resonance imaging scan showing nonspecific enhancement and edema in the cervical spinal cord might be interpreted as evidence of metastatic intramedullary or epidural tumor rather than radiation change. Unaware of the prior treatment error, the patient would be unable to inform the other physician involved about the high risk for radiation injury. As a result, the patient might be given only minimal supportive care on the assumption of incurable recurrent disease rather than appropriate efforts toward rehabilitation.

Evans and Decker[55] have offered practical suggestions on how to address the issue of a medical error in radiation oncology once the event has been recognized. They advise disclosure for any errors that result in a perceptible clinical effect, change in diagnosis or treatment course, or a chance of future harm. Their two-phase response recommendation involves initial attention to the patient's immediate needs and an apology that avoids giving an impression of defensiveness. Later, after a more thorough analysis of the situation has been completed with the involvement of the hospital's risk management team, a carefully prepared discussion with the patient and other interested parties can occur. Evans and Decker also encourage radiation oncologists to maintain a proactive process of practice self-review as one component of fostering a culture of safety and quality in patient care.

CONCLUSION

Society's view concerning medical ethics has shifted over time to adapt to the forces of advancing knowledge. Ethical guidelines have sometimes been constructed as formal documents or mandated as law, but no single system comprehensively predicts and resolves all situational dilemmas. The core principles of medical ethics remain essential foundations for the practice of medicine.

REFERENCES

1. Starr P. *The social transformation of American medicine.* New York: Basic Books, 1982.
2. Chervenak FA, McCullough LB. The moral foundation of medical leadership: the professional virtues of the physician as fiduciary of the patient. *Am J Obstet Gynecol* 2001;184:875–879.
3. Reich WT. The word "bioethics": its birth and the legacies of those who shaped it. *Kennedy Inst Ethics J* 1994;4:319–335.
4. Beauchamp TL, Childress JF. *Principles of biomedical ethics,* 4th ed. New York: Oxford University Press, 1994.
5. *Natanson v Kline,* 350 P. 2d 1093 (Kan 1960).
6. Aquinas T. *Summa Theologica* II-II, Q64, art. 7, "Of Killing." In: Baumgarth WP, Regan RJ, eds. *On law, morality, and politics.* Indianapolis: Hackett, 1988: 226–227.
7. Lyons AS. Hippocrates. In: Lyons AS, Petrucelli RJ, eds. *Medicine: an illustrated history.* Hong Kong: Abrams, 1987:207–217.
8. Halperin EC. Physician awareness of the contents of the Hippocratic Oath. *J Med Humanities* 1989;2:107–114.
9. Moffic HS, Coverdale J, Bayer T. The Hippocratic Oath and clinical ethics. *J Clin Ethics* 1992;1:287–289.
10. Leake CD, ed. *Percival's medical ethics.* Huntington, NY: Krieger, 1975.
11. Pickstone JV. Thomas Percival and the production of medical ethics. In: Baker R, Porter D, Porter R, eds. *The codification of medical morality: historical and philosophical studies of the formalization of Western medical morality in the eighteenth and nineteenth centuries, vol 1. Medical ethics and etiquette in the eighteenth century (Philosophy and Medicine, vol 45.)* Boston: Kluwer Academic, 1993:164–176.
12. Baker R. Deciphering Percival's code. In: Baker R, Porter D, Porter R, eds. *The codification of medical morality: historical and philosophical studies of the formalization of Western medical morality in the eighteenth and nineteenth centuries, vol 1. Medical ethics and etiquette in the eighteenth century (Philosophy and Medicine, vol 45).* Boston: Kluwer Academic, 1993:188–214.
13. American Medical Association Council on Ethical and Judicial Affairs. *Code of medical ethics: current opinions with annotations.* (Annotations prepared by the Southern Illinois University Schools of Medicine and Law). Chicago: AMA Press, 2004.

14. *Trials of War Criminals before the Nuremberg Military Tribunals under Control Council Law No. 10.* Nuremberg, October 1946–April 1949. Washington, DC: U.S. Government Printing Office, 1949–1953.
15. Advisory Committee on Human Radiation Experiments. *Final Report of the Advisory Committee on Human Radiation Experiments (stock number 061-000-00-848-9).* Washington, DC: Government Printing Office, 1995.
16. Heller J. Syphilis victims in the U.S. study went untreated for 40 years. *The New York Times.* July 26, 1972:1, 8. [The story was also reported in part in *The Evening Star and Washington Daily News.* July 25, 1972:A1.]
17. Corbie-Smith G, Thomas S, Williams M, et al. Attitudes and beliefs of African Americans toward participation in medical research. *J Gen Intern Med* 1999;14: 537–546.
18. Corbie-Smith G. The continuing legacy of the Tuskegee Syphilis Study: implications for clinical research. *Am J Med Sci* 1999;317:5–8.
19. National Commission for the Protection of Human Subjects of Biomedical and Behavioral Research. *Belmont Report: Ethical Principles and Guidelines for the Protection of Human Subjects of Research.* Available at: www.hhs.gov/ohrp/humansubjects/guidance/belmont.html. Accessed January 17, 2013.
20. National Electronic Manufacturers Association. *NEMA Code of Ethics on Interactions with Health Care Providers.* Adopted November 30, 2004. Available at:www.nema.org/news/Documents/nema+codeofethics-faq-adopted.pdf. Accessed January 17, 2013.
21. Smith TJ. A piece of my mind: which hat do I wear? *JAMA* 1993;270:1657–1659.
22. Glied S. Managed care. National Bureau of Economic Research Working Paper no. W7205, 1999.
23. Rodwin MA. Conflicts in managed care. *N Engl J Med* 1995;332:604–607.
24. Emanuel EJ, Dubler NN. Preserving the physician-patient relationship in the era of managed care. *JAMA* 1995;273:323–329.
25. Harvard Medical Practice Study Group. *Patients, doctors, and lawyers: medical injury, malpractice litigation, and patient compensation in New York.* Cambridge, MA: Harvard Medical Practice Study Group, 1990.
26. Simon SR, Pan RJD, Sullivan AM, et al. Views of managed care: a survey of students, residents, faculty, and deans at medical schools in the United States. *N Engl J Med* 1999;340:928–936.
27. Egan C, Jewler D. The impact of managed oncology care: integration or disintegration? *Oncol Issues* 1997;12:22–27.
28. Dunn CM, Chadwick G. *Protecting study volunteers in research: a manual for investigative sites.* Boston: CenterWatch, 1999.
29. Opinion 8.20 "Invalid medical treatment." *AMA Code of Medical Ethics.* Chicago: AMA Press, 2001:192.
30. Marwick C. President Bush sidesteps critics in stem cell debate. *BMJ* 2001;323:357.
31. *National Institutes of Health (NIH) Guidelines for Research Involving Recombinant DNA Molecules,* Appendix M. Washington, DC: Department of Health and Human Services, 2002.
32. Riley BD, Culver JO, Skrzynia C, et al. Essential elements of genetic cancer risk assessment, counseling, and testing: updated recommendations of the National Society of Genetic Counselors. *J Genetic Couns* 2012;21(2):151–161.
33. Opinion 8.061 "Gifts to physicians from industry." *AMA Code of Medical Ethics.* Chicago: AMA Press, 2001:160–163.
34. Hutchinson P, Halperin EC. The hidden persuaders: subtle advertising in radiation oncology. *Int J Rad Onc Biol Phys* 2002;54:989–991.
35. Studdert DM, Mello MM, Brennan TA. Financial conflict of interest in physician relationships with the pharmaceutical industry: self-regulation in the shadow of federal prosecution. *N Engl J Med* 2004;351:1891–1900.
36. Brennan TA, Rothman DJ, Blank L, et al. Health industry practices that create conflicts of interest: a policy proposal for academic medical centers. *JAMA* 2006; 295:429–433.
37. Wasserstein AG, Brennan PJ, Rubenstein AH. Institutional leadership and faculty response: fostering professionalism at the University of Pennsylvania School of Medicine. *Acad Med* 2007:82(11):1049–1056.
38. Coleman DL. Establishing policies for the relationship between industry and clinicians: lessons learned from two academic health centers. *Acad Med* 2008; 83(9):882–887.
39. Sugarman J, Burk L. Physicians' ethical obligations regarding alternative medicine. *JAMA* 1998;280:1623–1625.
40. Opinion 9.06 "Free choice." *AMA Code of Medical Ethics.* Chicago: AMA Press, 2001:207–209.
41. Lo B. *Resolving ethical dilemmas: a guide for clinicians,* 2nd ed. Philadelphia: Lippincott Williams & Wilkins, 2000.
42. Temel JS, Greer JA, Muzikansky A, et al. Early palliative care for patients with metastatic non-small-cell lung cancer. *N Engl J Med* 2010;363:733–742.
43. Ferris FD, Bruera E, Cherny N, et al. Palliative cancer care a decade later: accomplishments, the need, next steps—from the American Society of Clinical Oncology. *J Clin Oncol* 2009;27(18):3052–3058.
44. Halperin EC. X-rays at the bar, 1896–1910. *Invest Radiol* 1988;23:639–646.
45. Kohn LT, Corrigan JM, Donaldson MS, eds. *To err is human: building a safer health system* Washington, DC: Institute of Medicine, 1999.
46. Leape LL. Institute of medicine medical figures are not exaggerated. *JAMA* 2000; 284:95–97.
47. Brennan TA, Leape LL, Laird NM, et al. Incidence of adverse events and negligence in hospitalized patients: results of the Harvard Medical Practice Study I. *N Engl J Med* 1991;324:370–376.
48. Thomas EJ, Studdert DM, Burstin HR, et al. Incidence and types of adverse events and negligent care in Utah and Colorado. *Med Care* 2000;38:261–271.
49. Thomas EJ, Studdert DM, Newhouse JP, et al. Costs of medical injuries in Utah and Colorado. *Inquiry* 1999;36:255–264.
50. Kohn LT, Corrigan JM, Donaldson MS, eds. *To err is human: building a safer health system* Washington, DC: Institute of Medicine, 1999.
51. Hilfiker D. Facing our mistakes. *N Engl J Med* 1984;310:118–122.
52. Baylis F. Errors in medicine: nurturing truthfulness. *J Clin Ethics* 1997;8:336–340.
53. Whitman AB, Park DM, Hardin SB. How do patients want physicians to handle mistakes? A survey of internal medicine patients in an academic setting. *Arch Intern Med* 1996;156:2565–2569.
54. Vincent C, Young M, Phillips A. Why do people sue doctors? A study of patients and relatives taking legal action. *Lancet* 1994;343:1609–1613.
55. Evans SB, Decker R. Disclosing medical errors: a practical guide and discussion of radiation oncology-specific controversies. *Int J Radiat Oncol Biol Phys* 2011; 80(5):1285–1288.

Chapter 100
Economics of Radiation Oncology

Paul J. Schilling

ECONOMICS OF LOCOREGIONAL FAILURE

In 2012, 1,618,910 patients were diagnosed with cancer and 577,610 deaths were recorded.[1] Of those who succumbed to cancer, half had a component of local or regional failure. As systemic therapy improves, consequences of local failure become more pronounced.[2,3] Improving systemic therapy may lead to a longer lifetime free of systemic metastasis during which local failure can occur. This is one reason that postoperative radiation treatment improves survival in breast cancer, small cell lung cancer, prostate cancer, and rectal cancer.[1–3] The cost of regional failure in terms of human life and tragedy is staggering.

UNDERSTANDING MEDICARE

For patients who have Medicare as their primary insurance (these are the majority of radiation oncology patients), Medicare has a predetermined fee that is paid for each medical procedure, billed as a CPT (*Current Procedural Technology*) code. Medicare pays 80% of this allowable, and the patient's secondary insurance pays the remaining 20%. Charges are electronically billed, and turnaround time to receive payment can be as few as 14 days. Some secondary insurances will take between 6 and 9 months to pay the final 20%. Many secondary insurances must be billed using a paper claim sent through the mail instead of an electronic claim, thus delaying payment for up to 6 months.[4]

Hospital-owned, hospital-based radiation oncology practices bill under Medicare Part A. This provides for a technical component of radiation treatment delivery for the hospital; the professional component for physician services is billed separately by the radiation oncologist, also under Medicare Part A. The basis on which the technical component is paid to the hospital is called an ambulatory payment classification (APC). APC groups have different payments based on the complexity of radiation treatment delivery. The payments under the APC classification compared to those paid to outpatient free-standing facilities vary widely. For example, radiation treatment delivery for intensity-modulated radiation treatment, code 77418, is paid to the hospital under Medicare Part A at considerably less than the rate paid to free-standing centers under Medicare Part B. Alternatively, code 77370, special medical physics consultation, is paid to the hospital at approximately twice that paid to a free-standing facility.[4]

For a free-standing radiation oncology center, Medicare Part B is billed and a global fee is paid. This global fee combines both the professional fee to the physician and the technical fee to the equipment owner in one bundled payment. Some (CPT)

CPTCODE	Professional RVVIS	Technical RVVIS	Number	Professional RVUs Total	Technical RVUs Total
IMRT Prostate					
99205	5.86	0	1	5.86	0
77014	1.23	2.99	1	1.23	2.99
77263	4.65	0	1	4.65	0
77300	0.9	1.09	9	8.1	9.81
77301	11.57	46.74	2	23.14	93.48
77290	2.25	13.5	2	4.5	27
77470	3.02	2.08	1	3.02	2.08
77338	6.19	8.25	2	12.38	16.5
77418	12.84	0	45	0	577.8
77427	5.17	0	9	46.53	0
77336	1.37	0	9	12.33	0
77334	1.78	2.58	3	5.34	7.74
3 Dimensional Conformal Treatment Breast, Prostate			**Total**	127.08	737.4
99205	5.86	0	1	5.86	0
77263	4.65	0	1	4.65	0
77370	3.33	0	1	3.33	0
77014	1.23	2.99	2	2.46	5.98
77295	6.61	8.08	2	13.22	16.16
77315	2.25	1.79	1	2.25	1.79
77427	5.17	0	8	41.36	0
77414	7.95	0	40	0	318
77336	1.37	0	8	10.96	0
77470	3.02	2.08	1	3.02	2.08
Pauiative TX (Bone Metastasis)			**Total**	87.11	344.01
99205	5.86	0	1	5.86	0
77263	4.65	0	1	4.65	0
77300	0.9	1.09	5	4.5	5.45
77295	6.61	8.08	1	6.61	8.08
77427	5.17	0	2	10.34	0
77370	3.33	0	2	6.66	0
77414	7.95	0	10	0	79.5
77334	1.78	2.58	4	7.12	10.32
			Total	45.74	103.35
			Grand Total	259.93	1184.76

FIGURE 100.1. Medicare relative value units broken out by professional and technical classification per radiation treatment course.

codes have a professional component only, and some codes have a technical component only. Other codes have both professional and technical components, indicating that the physician and the equipment owner split this code based on their investment of physician time or equipment ownership. Calculating the professional/technical "split" in an outpatient facility can be difficult and depends on the payer mix, as well as the complexity of patients treated. The professional/technical split is calculated using the relative value units (RVUs) assigned to each CPT code. The RVUs are units of work assigned by Medicare, with each unit of work having a standard reimbursement. The RVUs in the professional/technical split are shown in Figure 100.1 and, as can be seen, vary depending on the complexity and objective of treatment. Calculating the professional/technical split is often difficult for physicians who are in free-standing centers and eligible to receive the professional component. In general, the professional component of global collections is approximately 11% to 35%, depending on the payer mix. If we consider equal rates of IMRT, 3D, and palliative treatment courses, the professional component of the global collections under Medicare Part B is 22%.

SUSTAINABLE GROWTH RATE VERSUS MEDICAL ECONOMIC INDEX

Medicare Part B (physician services) provides an annual update in allowable charges based on the gross domestic product called the sustainable growth rate (SGR). From the years 2000 through 2011, this has required a reduction in Medicare payment and thus Medicare-allowable fees. These cuts have been forestalled by Congress on multiple occasions.[5]

The Medicare Economic Index (MEI) is an annual update for Medicare Part A (hospital services) that is based on the rate of medical inflation. This has resulted in a yearly increase in payments to hospitals based on their self-reported rate of Medicare inflation.[6] If physician services were paid according to the MEI, we would be reimbursed at 40% more than we are now.

APPEALING DENIED MEDICARE CLAIMS FOR RADIATION ONCOLOGY

In January 2006 the Centers for Medicare and Medicaid Services (CMS) reduced the maximum time for adjudicating appeals for denied claims from a maximum of 1,000 days to 300 days. Nearly 20% of processed Medicare claims are denied. However, only 5% of denied Medicare claims are appealed.[7,8]

Physicians succeed in appealing payment denial in more than 60% of cases, indicating that the appeals process can be successful. If resubmitting the first rejection does not resolve the problem, the first level of appeal is called a *fair hearing,* and is usually conducted by telephone. You simply need to write a letter to the Medicare carrier requesting a fair hearing. The minimum denied amount needed to appeal a denied claim is $100. Multiple denied claims on different patients can be bundled together as long as the appeal amount is >$100. Include the appropriate documentation with the total amount appealed and CPT book definitions to describe what medical care was rendered and why you should be paid. Much to your surprise, most of the reviewers are not familiar with radiation oncology coding or the CPT coding books. Your job is to teach the reviewers to do their job and pay you.

For the carrier who habitually denies the same code, a previous favorable ruling may get the same code paid over and over again. In this situation, your goal is to use the last favorable ruling as evidence that the same denied code should be paid. This actually works, and sometimes the Medicare carrier will just pay the bill without the hearing as described earlier.[8]

For all fair hearings, the Medicare carrier is required to give you a written decision within 90 days. If the fair hearing process results in additional denial, the next step is a hearing before an administrative law judge. This is much more formal, and likely you should consider having legal representation. During the fair hearing process, the hearing officer will allow you to explain why a patient needed the (denied) care and provide documentation that you were able to help the patient based on available clinical evidence. During an administrative law hearing, the judge is only interested in whether the law allows you to be paid or not. Do not be afraid to try the appeals process if you feel the denial is inappropriate, and again, most often you will win.[7,8]

MEDICARE MEDICALLY UNLIKELY EDITS

A medically unlikely edit (MUE) is a limit on the number of units of a CPT code that would be reported for a patient in 1 day.[9] Medically unlikely edits were developed based on clinical judgment, and these were reviewed by insurance medical directors of Medicare and/or Medicare intermediary insurance companies. MUEs are used to screen out too many units of service done in a single day. For example, an appendectomy can only be done once on a patient in 1 day (or ever), and reporting two appendectomies in the same day of service would be impossible. Medicine as a profession can expect Medicare to pass more medically unlikely edits in the future.[9] These are often adopted by private insurance programs as well. MUEs apply to a number of procedures in radiation oncology, including dose calculations (code 77300), device charges (code 77334), and IMRT plans (code 77301), and for medical oncology limits in the total quantity of drugs that can be administered. If you find yourself the victim of not being paid due to medically unlikely edits, the first level of appeal as described earlier is a fair hearing, and the next level of appeal is an administrative law hearing. There is no prohibition for additional payments if clinically necessary.

BUNDLING EDITS

Medicare and some managed care organizations "bundle" procedures together so that only one charge is paid rather than two separate charges. For example, weekly physics management (code 77336) may not be able to be billed on the same day as special medical physics consultation (code 77370). The managed care organization may think that the special medical physics consultation is bundled into the weekly physics management.[10] It is essential to understand what these bundled codes are and where they conflict. Many times, this information is difficult to obtain during the contracting process. The best time to find out about bundling edits is before you sign an insurance contract. It is important to have a well-trained billing staff so that they can understand which codes are bundled, and decisions need to be made regarding a patient's care as to what specific service is required on a specific day. A sudden billing denial may herald new bundling edits.

Effective January 1, 2010, code 77338 replaced device charge 77334 used for each multileaf pattern for Medicare patients receiving IMRT. This code is used one time per IMRT plan (77301) and replaces multiple charges for multileaf patterns. Unfortunately, the reimbursement for this code is below what would be reimbursed under the prior system. Prior to 2010, if a head and neck cancer patient received a 10-beam, 10-gantry-angle IMRT treatment, code 77334 was billed for a quantity of 10 separate multileaf patterns used in treatment. Currently, code 77338 replaces *all* of these charges and can only be billed with a quantity of one, not 10. In Florida, in 2011, reimbursement for code 77338 is $459 and for code 77334 is $145. Thus, one charge of code 77338 represents 3.2 charges of code 77334, enough to pay for only 3.2 of the multileaf patterns for the aforementioned head and neck cancer patient.

INSURANCE REQUIREMENTS FOR PREAUTHORIZATION FOR RADIATION TREATMENT

A more recent feature of private insurers and Medicare HMOs is to require preauthorization for radiation treatment. This can be extraordinarily restrictive. Generally there are limitations on stereotactic radiosurgery as well as intensity-modulated radiation treatment. Often the patient will need to undergo simulation, and treatment can be delayed until a reviewer can decide if IMRT is warranted or three-dimensional (3D) conformal treatment will suffice. Needless to say, we do not get reimbursed for the treatment plans of both modalities, although they are requested by the insurer. There are various sets of guidelines developed by insurance companies to help their reviewers authorize or deny complex radiation oncology treatments. If denial occurs, again, it can be appealed, but the patient waits for treatment. Be sure to insist on a reviewer who is a board-certified radiation oncologist and not a retired general practitioner.

MEDICARE ADVANTAGE HEALTH MAINTENANCE ORGANIZATION INSURANCE PLANS

In 2007, Medicare Advantage Health Maintenance Insurance Programs were created. The insurance companies who administer Medicare HMOs are currently reimbursed up to 19%, more than traditional Medicare pays for each senior's care.[4,11] The seniors who sign up for Medicare Advantage plans often receive less care but pay higher copays and higher deductibles, and more than half of Medicare plans pay physicians below traditional Medicare rates. Many seniors do not realize that with a Medicare Advantage plan they need secondary insurance to pay for the additional costs that Medicare Advantage does not cover. More than 2,000 physicians responding to an American Medical Association survey on Medicare HMOs noted that Medicare HMOs routinely denied services typically covered by traditional Medicare plans including colonoscopies, prostate-specific antigen (PSA) blood tests, and other cancer screening procedures. A survey of patients enrolled in Medicare Advantage HMOs reported that 80% of them did not understand their plans and 60% did not realize they were actually giving up traditional Medicare.[11] Some seniors are being sold Medicare HMO plans through abusive marketing practices. CMS singled out insurers including United, Humana, Coventry, and Cigna for abusive marketing techniques, and these companies were advised to take steps to more closely scrutinize their sales personnel. Medicare Advantage plans have created an incentive for insurance companies who sponsor these plans to enroll healthy new patients. The bottom 50% of Medicare recipients spend only 3% of Medicare health dollars.[11] Insurance companies have found ingenious ways to enroll healthy seniors while making enrollment inconvenient to patients with many chronic diseases who might cost more. These incentives include offering free gym memberships to those enrolled (this appeals to the healthiest, most ambulatory seniors) and holding dinner seminars for prospective enrollees after dark in locations without access to public transportation or that require ascending several sets of stairs. An investigation by the Medicare Payment Advisory Commission in 2004 found that Medicare HMOs were designing their plans to avoid paying for kidney dialysis, chemotherapy drugs, home care, and radiation treatment. A *New England Journal of Medicine* article noted that currently enrolled Medicare HMO members spent only 66% of the average cost of non-Medicare HMO patients during the year prior to joining the HMO. This may indicate selection of the healthiest seniors. Seniors departing from Medicare HMOs went on to spend 180% of this average, indicating that sicker patients were leaving Medicare HMOs possibly due to higher out-of-pocket costs. Cancer treatment, unfortunately, continues to be extraordinarily expensive. We must keep informed as to where cost shifting is going in the future and educate our seniors.[11]

PATIENTS REQUIRING RADIATION TREATMENT WHO RESIDE IN SKILLED NURSING FACILITIES

Skilled nursing facilities are paid for by Medicare for seniors who need more care than a nursing home can provide but less care than an acute hospital provides. The skilled nursing facility is reimbursed by Medicare at a fixed rate per day for a patient's care. When patients residing in a skilled nursing facility require radiation treatment, if the radiation facility bills under Medicare Part B (physician and outpatient services), the skilled nursing facility is responsible for reimbursing the radiation oncology facility and physician out of the fixed amount of money that is received each day by the facility. Conversely, if a radiation facility is owned by a hospital and bills under Medicare Part A, a separate payment by Medicare Part A is made to the radiation oncology facility and thus does not cost the skilled nursing facility any portion of their daily fee. Because of this, there is a financial incentive to refer or divert patients who need radiation treatment to a hospital-based facility billing under Medicare Part A. Of course, skilled nursing facilities do not wish to generate a bill that would require payment by them for referring patients to a Medicare Part B facility. This places outpatient facilities at a distinct disadvantage and is certainly unfair. The radiation oncology community is lobbying to change this practice.

RADIATION TREATMENT OF PATIENTS ENROLLED IN HOSPICE

It is not unusual for patients in hospice care to require palliative radiation treatment for pain control, palliation of neurologic symptoms, and so forth. Under Medicare Part B, the outpatient facility can directly bill Medicare with a GV modifier. The GV modifier indicates that the radiation oncology facility is separate from hospice and that the physician who is consulting and overseeing radiation oncology care is not directly employed by the hospice facility. Hospice benefits do include radiation treatment if this is included in the hospice plan of care. Thus, if the hospice facility includes radiation treatment in its plan of care for a patient, it must pay for it out of its daily reimbursement, a fixed amount per day. Currently hospice services are paid for by Medicare with a daily fee. This is paid 7 days a week for a maximum of 6 months. However, hospices usually only provide care 1 to 3 days per week. Hospices are among the few patient care providers that receive reimbursement from Medicare, depend on volunteer services to provide some of the care, and receive charitable donations from the public. Consider this when donating your time or money to a for-profit or not-for-profit hospice.

MEDICAL PHYSICISTS: SHOULD THEY BILL MEDICARE DIRECTLY FOR THEIR SERVICES?

Many medical physicists maintain that they are board-certified professionals so should be able to bill Medicare directly; however, if they did so, their paychecks would shrink considerably. In 1960, lists of providers who could bill Medicare directly were formulated, and physicists were not among these professionals. Because of this, a congressional act is required to give billing status to medical physicists.[12] Currently there are only two codes recognized for the contribution of medical physicists: code 77336, continuing medical physicist services, and code 77370, special medical physics consultation. There are no other CPT codes in Medicare Part A or Part B that identify any medical physicist component of work.[12] At Florida Medicare rates, code 77336 is reimbursed at $50.43, and code 77370 is reimbursed at $105.55. In a busy department with 30 patients under continuous radiation treatment, there would be 30 continuing medical physicist services provided at a Medicare reimbursement level of $50.93 for 50 weeks per year, for a total reimbursement of $75,645. If 50% (this is high) of patients under treatment required a special medical consultation, this would mean a yearly reimbursement of $15,833. The total for these services, $91,478, is dramatically below what the average medical physicist makes in the United States.[12] In 2007, CPT code 77336 was submitted to CMS 475,000 times at a reimbursement of $50.93. This would yield total reimbursement for medical physicists of $24,191,750. During the same year, CPT code 77370 was submitted 25,000 times at a reimbursement of $105.55 for a total Medicare payment of $2,638,750. When we combine these two numbers we get a total reimbursement for physicist services of $26,593,000. There are currently 4,700 members of the American Association of Physicists in Medicine. It is uncertain as to how many medical physicists practice exclusively in radiation oncology; most estimate approximately 25% of the total. If we use the number of 1,000 medical physicists in the United States splitting the total reimbursement for physicist services delivered to Medicare patients in the United States, we get a per physicist rate of $26,593. Again, this is rather dramatically below what the average medical physicist makes in the United States. Professional self-determination appears to be important to medical physicists. If we examine published literature available to the public on the process of radiation treatment, very little mention is made to medical physicists being members of the patient care team. This is true of the National Cancer Institute's manual on radiation therapy and the American Cancer Society's publication on the process of care for radiation oncology. This is unfortunate. There is certainly room for improvement to include medical physicists in the process of care because they are an integral component. The patient should understand their role, and perhaps additional efforts can be directed toward recognizing the contributions of medical physicists in the care of our cancer patients.[12]

RADIATION ONCOLOGY NEGOTIATION WITH MANAGED CARE PLANS

In 1937, Dr. Sidney Garfield provided prepaid medical care for Henry J. Kiser's company in California, and this was the beginning of managed care in the United States. Managed care proliferated with the objective to reduce health care costs for workers covered by health care plans paid for by their employers.[4,10]

Many physicians have experience negotiating the rate of compensation for their contracts. However, a managed care company may be reluctant to disclose their fee schedule if other physicians in the area are contracted with them. Begin the negotiation by making an inquiry for 10 codes most commonly used for radiation oncology patients. Oftentimes, a managed care company will send the reimbursement for 10 codes total. From this it is possible to get an idea as to what the company's rate of payment is and whether you wish to continue the negotiation.[4,10]

Many private insurance contracts try to link reimbursement to a percentage of Medicare rates. Some managed care plans pay you based on 100% of the regional managed care company's usual and customary fees. Often, this is below Medicare rates, and it is imperative to know exactly how you are being paid.[4,10] Many managed care companies want you to take a fee reduction across the board for all radiation oncology CPT codes. Try to negotiate reduction in only a few codes (used less often), which may have a less deleterious effect on your practice. Always attach a comprehensive fee schedule to all contracts and make the insurance company sign off on this as an exhibit. This clearly prevents confusion later and locks in your rate of reimbursement instead of having it adjusted each year depending on Medicare rates.

Some managed care companies will try to get you to contract for a case-rate structure. In this scenario, for any patient who requires radiation treatment, a fixed dollar amount would be paid regardless of treatment complexity. Case-rate arrangements can sometimes be tiered, which allows two to three levels of complexity paid at a fixed rate. Case-rate reimbursements are difficult to manage and frequently do not increase year to year, while the complexity of treatment does increase. The physician is advised to use caution in accepting any case-rate structure.[10]

There are a few managed care companies that reimburse based on a capitation basis. Under this scenario, a certain amount of money is paid monthly to the radiation oncology group to provide services regardless of the covered population's average age or need for radiation treatment. These contracts are extraordinarily difficult to negotiate and manage. Ultimately, to remain solvent, you would need to know the age of the population insured, as well as their cancer incidence, cancer screening availability, and so forth. Unfortunately, this information usually resides with the insurer, and most likely they will not share this with the physician. Capitation rates can also be calculated from population-based data using Surveillance, Epidemiology, and End Results (SEER) data.[4] Nonetheless, these data underestimate the incidence of cancer and the volume of cancer treated with radiation.

For hospital-based practices, it may be necessary for the managed care company to have a contract with the hospital for the technical component of radiation treatment and a contract with the radiation oncologist for professional services. Pitfalls to watch out for include a provision that the codes with a professional/technical split must be billed on the same day by both the hospital and physician for either to obtain payment. This puts the physician in the position of auditing the hospital charge capture, a notoriously inefficient process.[4]

A contract with the managed care company should spell out emergency care provisions. Many times emergency treatment for spinal cord compression or brain metastasis, for example, will be provided and a managed care company will later indicate that this was a noncovered service, even on an emergency basis. Thus, an entire course of treatment may be denied in this way.[10]

The managed care organization may wish to retain the right to reduce current reimbursement to you for prior payments that were paid in error. Thus, they may "set off" current payments by past debts. Some states laws do not allow this. These clauses are often subject to abuse. For example, suddenly the managed care company decides that dose calculations (code 77300) are "bundled" or included in special medical physics consults (code 77370). They will be able to potentially audit the practices to disallow as many 77300 codes as you have and adjust the billing to create a debt for 3 years' worth of 77300 charges against which future payments are applied.

Audit provisions are similarly important to negotiate. Provisions on closing the claims process should apply equally to physician and managed care organizations. The time limit for auditing should be similar in time to which forfeiture of payment occurs. For example, if the managed care organization allows submission of bills up to 12 months after a service is rendered, you should negotiate an audit provision for only 12 months. Longer audit provisions may lead to abuse. Large-scale insurance companies routinely hire an auditing company on a contingency basis that is motivated to audit claims and recover payments. Occasionally audits are used to retaliate against physicians who request arbitration of unpaid claims.

It is important to assess your strengths and weaknesses during the negotiation process. Managed care companies realize that their contracts are subject to termination. Because of this, they usually do not depend on a single provider for medical care. Are you a second source of radioactive isotope therapy or radiopharmaceutical therapy? Are you one of only two providers of high–dose-rate brachytherapy in your area (which avoids a hospital stay)? Are you the only provider of intensity-modulated radiation treatment or the only practice that will treat children? All of these things count as strengths in negotiations and can be effective in setting the tone for negotiations with insurance companies.

SILENT PREFERRED PROVIDER ORGANIZATIONS

Because of the rise of managed care, a new process has been promulgated whereby a network in which a physician is contracted as a preferred provider is sold to another health plan without the physician's knowledge or consent.[13] This creates a *silent preferred provider organization (PPO)* in which a discount is extracted from the physician's usual and customary fees without the physician's consent. The net result is a secondary discount where an insurer (often with a low number of patients) pays the physician's discounted fee without the physician ever receiving the benefit of any additional patient volume. In most instances physicians become aware that they are victims of a silent PPO after providing services to a patient with indemnity insurance. When payment is made on behalf of an insurance company, the discount is applied even though the patient is not a member of the PPO and the physician is not a contracted member of that insurance organization. Unfortunately, there is no Health Insurance Portability and Accountability Act (HIPAA) statute governing selling lists of physicians and their associated contracted discounts. The American Medical Association estimates that $750 million to $3 billion is lost annually in the United States by physicians to silent PPOs.[13,14] The American Medical Association was successful in banning silent PPOs from all federal employee health insurance benefits contracts. However, currently state insurance boards generally provide insurance regulations. A few states including North Carolina, Louisiana, Oklahoma, California, and Texas have passed legislation banning this practice.[14] One simple step to combat this practice is to carefully read all contracts. Many health insurance contracts contain provisions that allow them to enter contracts with "other payers on the physician's behalf." If this language appears in your contract, insist on striking it. Additional language to protect yourself might include the prohibition of selling, renting, or leasing networks providing any information about a fee schedule to anyone without your express permission.[13] Currently the only recourse after an inappropriate discount has been applied and you have been paid inappropriately is to use the legal system. As always, "an ounce of prevention is worth a pound of cure," so be sure to look for the aforementioned clauses and lobby your state medical association to pass legislation that protects physician information.

ECONOMIC PROFILING: INSURANCE COMPANIES DETERMINE WHO PROVIDES THE LEAST EXPENSIVE CARE

Economic profiling tracks physician care expenditures including specialty referrals, laboratory testing, and utilization of other costly resources. Physicians are allowed to continue on the panel of certain insurance plans based on their level of utilization and cost to the insurance plan. Yet, expenditures to provide care to individual patients are variable.[15] Patients who have complex cancers have a higher average cost of care, which may institute multiple inquiries from the insurance company about specialist referral, prescribing habits, and overall resource utilization. Higher average costs of care may lead to deselection from insurance plans for "outlier" utilization. When comprehensive care is provided in a single geographic setting, insurance companies know that patient compliance in the stated plan of disease management is enhanced, leading to fewer episodes of missed testing or treatment. This "dropout rate" is calculated as care prescribed by a physician but not undertaken by a patient.[15] Physicians with high dropout rates reduce costs to the insurance company, but only temporarily.

ECONOMIC CREDENTIALING: HOSPITALS SEEK TO PREVENT PATIENT CHOICE

Economic credentialing is defined by the American Medical Association as the "use of economic criteria unrelated to the quality of care or professional competency to determine an individual physician's qualifications for granting or renewal of medical staff privileges."[16] The goal of economic credentialing in radiation oncology is to capture a revenue stream by denying hospital privileges to a group or terminating hospital privileges and thereby limiting competition. Hospital bylaws are considered by many states to be a contract between a hospital and medical staff, serving as a guideline for actions against physicians, as well as outlining due process provisions for physicians.[16] Read your hospital bylaws carefully and watch for hospital proposed changes. The medical staff should have its own legal representation, separate from the hospital, when hospital bylaws changes are proposed.

Hospitals may seek to institute differential credentialing to keep qualified physicians from becoming members of the medical staff, and thus limiting competition. One example is requiring radiation oncologists to complete 4 years of residency, whereas before 1994 radiation oncology residencies were only 3 years.[16]

Contracts between physician groups and hospitals establish a business relationship to provide radiation oncology services. Traditionally, exclusive contracts ensured patient access to care that would otherwise not be available. Because of increased access to cancer treatment in the United States, this is almost never the case today. Most hospitals enter into an exclusive contract strictly for financial reasons, which puts the physicians in the position of being controlled by the hospital master financial plan. Exclusive contracts may deprive patients of choices and limit the establishment of new physician practices. Some exclusive contracts contain "clean sweep" provisions, which stipulate that when a group loses an exclusive contract with a hospital, each physician simultaneously forfeits clinical privileges without the benefit of due process afforded by the hospital bylaws.[16]

The peer review process may be misused to further a hospital's economic goals. Because in most states peer review proceedings are protected from legal discovery, peer review affords an opportunity for physicians to evaluate their care and remediate their knowledge if necessary. Protection from legal discovery also invites hospitals to target and eliminate physicians who are economic threats to their service lines. This is particularly true for hospital-based specialists including radiation oncologists. Some radiation oncologists find themselves excluded from equipment or facilities when a health care institution changes radiation oncology from a hospital inpatient service to an outpatient service. This may occur with no change in location of building, equipment, or staffing. There is an entire consulting industry that teaches hospitals how to displace existing radiation oncologists and put their replacement physicians on salary. We are not the only target; physical medicine, diagnostic radiology, and cardiothoracic surgery are also vulnerable to these tactics.[16]

The American Medical Association has a long, continuous interest in fighting economic credentialing and has a litigation department with years of accumulated information and experience and will assist physicians who challenge health care institutions about these issues.[16]

RADIATION ONCOLOGY'S SOCIOECONOMIC TIES WITH DIAGNOSTIC RADIOLOGY

In previous years, delivery of radiation treatment was both crude and considerably simpler. "Therapeutic radiology" was a discipline of diagnostic radiology. As radiation treatment became more sophisticated and as megavoltage linear accelerators became available, it was clear that separate training was necessary for radiation oncologists to treat cancer patients. Eventually new CPT codes were created for radiation oncology and governmental payers began to recognize us as being separate from diagnostic radiology. Diagnostic radiologists seem to be embroiled in a campaign to close the "in-office ancillary exemption," which allows nonradiologist physicians to perform imaging within their offices. Currently, obstetricians perform pregnancy-related ultrasounds, cardiologists perform cardiac catheterizations and nuclear cardiac procedures, and family physicians perform bone densitometry and plain films within their offices. With the advent of image-guided radiation treatment, positron emission tomography (PET)/computed tomography (CT) simulators, and magnetic resonance imaging (MRI) simulators for treatment planning, radiation oncologists continue to fight for the ability to image our patients for diagnosis, staging, and treatment planning related to cancer. Our objective should be to show CMS that imaging is necessary for treating cancer patients appropriately.

In 2009, Medicare proposed a 95% "usage rate" for diagnostic imaging equipment and then proposed extending this to all medical equipment costing more than $1 million. This proposal was advanced by the Medicare Payment Advisory Commission and was based on a sample size of only six urban diagnostic radiology centers but, because of the cost of linear accelerators, was extended to radiation oncology.[17] Data collected by U.S. Oncology show that 50% of linear accelerators installed in the United States operate at a 50% utilization rate or less.[17] If this usage rate were enacted for radiation oncology, the technical reimbursement would be reduced with the assumption that more patients are being treated per day on each linear accelerator. A reduction in technical reimbursement would force the closure of many rural practices, making patients travel longer distances for cancer treatment. Fortunately, this proposal was defeated because radiation oncologists like you told Congress that we are different from diagnostic imaging. Radiation oncologists need to continue to show CMS that we treat cancer patients and are separate from diagnostic radiology.[17]

HEALTH CARE REFORM

In 2011, 48.6 million Americans did not have health insurance. According to census data taken in 2007, approximately one-third of those uninsured held jobs that offered health insurance coverage and had salaries 300% above the poverty level. This group chose not to pay for health insurance due to cost considerations. The Affordable Care Act will enroll currently uninsured patients into the Medicaid program. This will be a payment windfall for hospitals, which would be paid for emergency room visits for which they now do not receive reimbursement. Private practice physicians may not see more Medicaid patients due to low reimbursement, thus encouraging the use of emergency rooms for primary care.

The Congressional Budget Office estimated that tort reform with a $250,000 cap on noneconomic damages would save the United States $54 billion over 10 years and reduce national health care spending by 0.5% annually and save $41 billion in tests ordered due to physicians' needs to practice defensive medicine.[18] Medicaid expansion during a time when fewer doctors accept Medicare patients may not be an answer that is palatable to many physicians. The government has studied bundled "bulk" payments for hospital and physician care. One proposal would be to negotiate a bundled fee paid to hospitals for an episode of care (i.e., lung cancer). This led to the creation of accountable care organizations as part of the Affordable Care Act. The physicians would then negotiate with the hospital for their component of pay. As always, greater bargaining power is in the hands of the entity that receives the check.

ACCOUNTABLE CARE ORGANIZATIONS

Expenditures for health care in 2011 totaled $2.6 trillion. In the United States, we spend 17.6% of our gross domestic product on health care, which comes to $18,344 per person, while Japan spends 8.5% of its gross domestic product, accounting for $2,872 per person. Accountable care organizations (ACOs) promise to improve medical care coordination, with reductions in fragmented care, improvement in outcomes, and reductions in the cost of health care. Their successful operation is a priority in cost savings for the new Healthcare Reform Law. Under the Affordable Care Act, the minimum size of the population for Medicare beneficiaries for an ACO is 5,000 patients. ACO founders can be primary care physicians or independent practice associations. ACO participation includes hospital and physician specialists (like radiation oncologists). Patients are assigned to an ACO *retrospectively*. Thus, physicians providing care in an ACO do not know which patients do or do not belong to the ACO. Ostensibly, this is to encourage cost savings for all patients, not just those patients assigned to an ACO. Any savings achieved in the ACO population (actual medical care costs compared to expected medical care costs) are shared between Medicare and the ACO at a rate of 50%. If the cost of care for the population is more than 2% higher than Medicare expected, the ACO may need to repay this loss. Patients may self-refer to another Medicare provider physician outside their ACO, and care provided by that physician or that hospital counts against the ACO's cost goals.

Because ACOs are controlled by primary care physicians whose missions are cost savings, this may not bode well for the specialty of radiation oncology. Most primary care physicians have a difficult time understanding the benefits of radiation treatment, especially in palliative cases as well as in cases where the cure rate is <50%. Primary care physicians may leave the decision for radiation treatment to medical oncologists. This decision making by medical oncologists may diminish once primary care physicians realize that delivering chemotherapy is by far the most expensive portion of cancer treatment with the extremely high cost of cancer drugs. It is possible that patients for whom palliation is a goal will automatically be enrolled in hospice. We may see more hip fractures, intractable pain from metastatic disease, and brain metastases go untreated, all with the goal of cost savings, which individually benefits Medicare and the physician partners in the ACO. Primary care physicians need to be educated as to the benefits of radiation treatment. We should let them know that treating a hip metastasis may actually prevent a total hip arthroplasty, which is a more costly event. Preventing or palliating a spinal cord compression might prevent paralysis and a prolonged episode of bedridden care. Radiation treatment is dramatically more cost-effective than Mohs microsurgery and reconstruction, which costs more than $1,000 per stage. This will be our mission for the future, and given the change in the health care landscape, this will be challenging.[19]

There has been a tremendous push for independent practice of nurse practitioners (without physician supervision) and for nurse anesthetists.[20] The former may be provided to close the gap in primary care resulting from fewer primary care physicians choosing primary care as a profession due to low reimbursement.

The American Medical Association has requested insurance market reform with elimination of denials for pre-existing conditions, health insurance for all Americans, and health care decisions remaining in the hands of patients and their physicians, as well as repealing the Medicare sustainable growth formula that triggers deep cuts in Medicare and threatens seniors' access to care. The American Medical Association also desires proven medical liability reforms to reduce the cost of defensive medicine.[21,22]

RADIATION ONCOLOGISTS' LOBBYING AND POLITICAL ACTIVITY

Americans place a high value on the quality and availability of medical care. In this country, we have massive government programs that provide the funds to pay for the health care of the poor, disabled, and elderly. Unfortunately, payment rules are created by the legislature for a large portion of all physicians' practices in the United States.[4,20] The importance of interfacing with governmental payers, as well as in influencing the process that benefits our patients and brings them new technologies, cannot be underestimated. This can be accomplished through membership and in financial support of organized medicine at all levels. Select the organizations that you support carefully and specifically with an eye toward those which provide lobbying power for you and for your patients.[23–26] There are multiple organizations that interact with CMS. These include the American College of Radiation Oncology, the American Brachytherapy Society, the Association of Freestanding Radiation Oncology

Centers, and the American Society for Therapeutic Radiology and Oncology.[23–27]

STARTING A FREE-STANDING CANCER CENTER

Starting a free-standing cancer center requires substantial time, effort, and persistence. The population area served by the free-standing center must be clearly defined by the radiation oncologist. In an area where there is no cancer program, the population data for the area can be gathered, complete with the age range of the population and the number of each potential patient within defined age ranges. SEER data can then be applied using population-based cancer incidence. In 2010, the age-adjusted incidence of new cancers diagnosed was 5.4 cases per 1,000 men and 4.1 cases per 1,000 women.[4,28,29] The raw cancer incidence provided by the SEER data does not tell us how many patients may undergo radiation treatment during the course of their illness. Take the number of estimated patients and then apply a yield ratio of approximately 50%, which should estimate the total number of patients that the new cancer center would serve. An additional 25% of patients will need to be retreated for other metastases or other new primary cancers.[29] Model radiation oncology courses of treatment must be developed to estimate reimbursement per course of treatment (see Fig. 100.1).[4] A certain percentage of patients will receive a palliative treatment course, 3D conformal treatment, and intensity-modulated radiation treatment. If an average length of treatment (including palliative treatment and definitive treatment) is approximately 5 weeks, to have 20 patients under continuous treatment per day will require 200 new patients per year.

A second way to estimate the population served is to count the number of occupied beds of hospitals serving the area. Each permanently filled hospital bed yields approximately one cancer patient per year, of which half will require radiation treatment.

For a cancer center in a competitive market, one must establish exactly how many patients would be treated in the new cancer center and specifically how the physicians plan to obtain these referrals. If a hospital-based group of physicians builds its own free-standing cancer center, some of the patients may follow because referring physicians will continue to refer. There are always surprises and changes in referral patterns when hospital-based radiation oncologists open a competing free-standing center.[4]

Once the numbers of patients to be treated are established, along with their treatment length, the reimbursement for an "average course of treatment" can then be calculated. This average course of treatment should take into account intensity-modulated radiation treatment, palliative treatments, and 3D conformal therapy. When one uses a conservative estimate and sets the total reimbursement at Medicare rates, this seems to be a reasonable approach to many lending institutions. Once total collections for the population to be served are established, the total expenses need to be established, as well. This includes the costs of debt service, interest, principle, sales tax on equipment when installed, electric bills, costs of physics and dosimetry, costs of personnel including nursing and therapists, costs of water, building maintenance, professional liability, building insurance, employee benefits, physics equipment, accelerator maintenance, and so forth.

All of this can be packaged together as a pro forma to take to your financial institution. Generally, banks require a down payment between 5% and 20% of the total amount borrowed. In addition, working capital will be needed for approximately 6 months of operation.[4] The pro forma should be conservative. The goal should be to exceed the numbers that are projected, not just to meet them. This will give the bank a substantial amount of comfort as well. The carrying costs of maintaining a center, maintaining a competitive edge with equipment, and attracting and maintaining high-quality personnel are substantial. If you have never run a free-standing radiation center, you may substantially underestimate the costs of running one.[4] If medical oncology is to be added, the costs of the monthly drug bill need to be calculated.

MARKETING A RADIATION ONCOLOGY PRACTICE

Marketing for radiation oncology is directed toward the referring physician. Determine the physicians most likely to refer to you and make a list. *Any* physician can be a referring physician.[4,29] I have received two referrals from psychiatrists who had cancer patients that were unhappy with their care, underscoring this premise.

Presenting patient cases at cancer conferences at your local hospitals is a time-honored and useful form of individual marketing for your practice.[4,29] Nursing staff usually attend, and they can be a referral source. Radiation oncology images can be rewarding to present at tumor boards. Outlines of isodose plans and other imaging studies, MammoSite depictions, high-dose-rate brachytherapy plans, and so forth, form an image in referring physicians' minds that medical oncologists cannot accomplish.[29]

Giving talks to civic organizations and cancer support groups is also beneficial but requires patience for the long term.[4,29] Although I give multiple talks to groups, there has never been an instance where someone in the audience decided that he or she would change to me as a physician as the result of my presentation. Nonetheless, there have been multiple times when family members of new patients have said that they have heard me give a presentation. This underscored another physician's referral choice.

Advertising to the public generally does not yield new patients on its own. Advertising advanced technology may be helpful but usually only bolsters the understanding and familiarity with your physicians and facility when another primary physician makes a referral. In some larger urban markets, advertising advanced technology may make a difference or get some patients to call, ask questions, and possibly self-refer.

If your hospital has a teaching program, it is often rewarding to give a lecture or two within this program.[29] Physicians who attend will soon become your referring physicians, especially if they stay in the area to practice.

Develop a telephone answering on-hold message that showcases your technology, as well as the talents of your physicians. Thus, when the patients and physicians call, they are given an explanation of exactly what your practice does while they are waiting for the receptionist. Developing an immediate fax or e-mail form to briefly let referring physicians know what is being done for a new patient facilitates communication and gives them immediate information about the workup and progress of a patient you have seen.[4]

Internet website development can also be helpful. Again, this usually does not yield new patients, but rather reinforces the choice that other physicians have made to refer patients. Patients can find out about your practice on the Internet, as well as fill out their intake forms, and so forth. Some of these techniques may be helpful. But none of these techniques will be useful unless outstanding patient care is delivered, both socially and medically.

SELLING A FREE-STANDING CANCER CENTER

In recent years there has been much interest by private or publicly traded groups in purchasing radiation oncology centers. Publicly held or private corporations may seek to purchase radiation oncology centers to induce an economy of scale, dominate a certain region or state (and thereby exact additional reimbursement from the area insurers), or ultimately go public (issue stock certificates that can be purchased by the public). Generally a sale is based on earnings before depreciation, interest, taxes, and amortization (EBDITA). A multiple of this number is paid to the owner, generally in the 4 to 7.5 range. This range will decrease as cuts in reimbursement occur. Generally purchasers ask the owner to retain a minority percentage of the original cancer center he or she built. Sometimes this can be as small as a few percent, sometimes up to 49%. The purchasing entity may propose an automatic payout for the final percentage after 2 to 5 years of employment. It is important to negotiate how the buyout will be valued into the future. One potential problem is that an entity that owns more than 50% of your cancer center may dramatically reduce the profitability of this facility by allocating expenses incurred in the home office to your office, which actually is treating patients. This reduction in profitability likely will affect the buyout price in the end and will not adjust it upward. Sellers of radiation oncology practices should be aware of this potential and retain as small a percentage as possible or none at all. Some purchasers require a reduction in the ultimate purchase price based on the prospect of reduced reimbursement for some procedures. For example, an IMRT or stereotactic radiosurgery "earn-out" may be a reduction in payment price based on the future of reimbursement for these two modalities, with a portion of the purchase price paid at a later date. Predicting into the future of reimbursement is beyond the scope of most of our readers.

NONPROFIT HOSPITALS AND RADIATION ONCOLOGISTS

Earnings from many nonprofit hospitals have soared, with a combined income of the 50 largest nonprofit hospitals in the United States increasing eightfold to $4.27 billion between 2001 and 2006, according to a *Wall Street Journal* analysis updated from the American Hospital Directory. Nonprofit hospitals' "excess cash flow" (we call this profit in the for-profit sector) is spent on new facilities, generous executive pay, and often new and lavish cancer centers.[30] The largest nonprofit hospital chief executive officer pay ranged from $3.3 million to $16.4 million per year.[30] Historically, most nonprofit hospitals in America have been recognized as charitable organizations and exempt from taxes under Section 501(C)[3] of the U.S. tax code. In return for a generous tax exemption, the U.S. Internal Revenue Service (IRS) previously required nonprofit hospitals to provide a substantial amount of charity care for the poor. However, in 1965, when Medicare and Medicaid were created, the hospital industry felt there would not be enough demand for charity care to satisfy the IRS exemption standards. With substantial lobbying, the nonprofit hospital industry pushed for more flexible exemption that became known as the Community Benefits Standard adopted by the IRS in 1969. This allowed hospitals to provide local "community benefit" consistent with any other nonprofit hospital in their area.[30] Unlike for-profit hospitals, nonprofit hospitals do not pay dividends to shareholders. Instead, they use "excess cash flow" (profits), earned from operations, to pay for new facilities. Among these are proton treatment centers under construction in the Midwest, and located within minutes of each other, and various cancer centers being built by nonprofit hospitals without paying any taxes. These compete with those facilities that do pay taxes. While nonprofit hospitals have a charity obligation to the communities they serve, do they compete with physician practices by using an unfair tax advantage?

FEDERAL STARK REGULATIONS AFFECTING RADIATION ONCOLOGY

Current Stark laws prohibit self-referral to designated health services, which includes radiation oncology. Radiation oncologists who own their own facilities and equipment do not fall under violations of the Stark rule because it is not considered self-referral when the referring physician personally performs a designated health service in his or her own facility.[31]

There is also an in-office ancillary exemption, which applies to ownership and investment interest for ancillary services. The in-office ancillary service must be provided in a building in which the referring physician also furnishes substantial physician services.[31] This loophole has been exploited by some urologists to create a "group practice" with radiation oncologists and add a linear accelerator to their building. Curiously enough, the very radiation oncologists who join these ventures are often the displaced victims of hospital tactics of economic credentialing (see next section).

Congress made some of its conclusions and wrote portions of the Stark law based on studies that examined the effects of ownership of free-standing radiation oncology facilities by referring physicians who were not radiation oncologists and did not directly provide services. These "joint ventures" yielded a utilization rate 40% higher in these facilities than the rest of the United States, and a cost of radiation treatment that was 60% higher than the rest of the United States.[32] In addition, these studies showed that there was less access to poorly served populations without any reduction in mortality among cancer patients that indicated improved quality of care.[31,32] State laws may strengthen current existing federal laws, and it is important to understand the laws in your state concerning self-referral.[4,31,32]

"GROUP PRACTICES" INCLUDING RADIATION ONCOLOGY, UROLOGY, AND OTHER SPECIALTIES

Radiation oncologists have become increasingly concerned about the growing trend of self-referral for radiation treatment services by other specialty physicians seeking to create a group practice for apparent economic gain. Physician-driven financial arrangements may be consummated specifically to facilitate the delivery of intensity-modulated radiation treatment and have caused concern for the quality and cost of radiation treatment delivery. These arrangements have caused proliferation of "multispecialty groups" with the objective of delivering IMRT to prostate cancer patients that the group's urologist diagnoses. Prior to the initiation of the Stark laws, studies of radiation oncology facilities owned by referring physicians reported higher costs for cancer treatment without improved outcomes.[33] Radiation oncology is a designated health service under Section 1877 of the Social Security Act, which prohibits financial arrangements between the physicians and entities providing these services. Congress created an "in-office ancillary exemption" to protect medical services for which a service or test result is immediately needed for in-office patient care. As part of a program to address and study this growing trend, the American College of Radiation Oncology (ACRO) issued a physician statement on self-referrals specifically addressing the formation of urology and radiation oncology radiation groups for apparent financial reasons. ACRO then surveyed radiation oncologists who identified themselves as having a financial relationship with urologists. After telephone verification, there were 75 radiation oncologists who identified themselves as having a practice model that included urologists. The radiation oncologists were both employed in and a financial partner in the group. No radiation oncologists responded that their practice model included "block leasing" linear accelerator time to urologists. For all respondents, the radiation oncologists received the professional component of treatment. All 75 respondents either were economically displaced in a geographic region by an existing radiation oncology group or were economically displaced by a hospital in their region.[33]

All respondents were unable to achieve professional partnership status within a radiation oncology group, and 98.6% were unable to achieve any share of the technical component for radiation treatment within a radiation oncology group.

Sixty-six of 75 physicians provided a daily total of prostate cancer patients treated in their facility.[29] The range was one prostate cancer patient treated per day (newly started practice) to 48 patients per day (mature practice).[33] The mean was 17.1 prostate cancer patients treated per day. Eighty-six percent of radiation oncologists within this model were treating both prostate and nonprostate cancer patients. The average combined urology–radiation oncology practice treated 33 patients per day with nonprostate malignancies. Thus, the radiation oncologists responding to our survey who treated both prostate and nonprostate cancer patients treated 1.9 times more nonprostate cancer patients than prostate cancer patients.[33] This may possibly indicate that urologists seek radiation oncologists in an area where radiation oncologists already have an established referral base and bring nonprostate cancer referrals with them.[33] On August 19, 2008, the Office of the Inspector General (OIG) issued an opinion on the relationships between urologists and radiation oncologists that addressed leasing radiation equipment to provide IMRT to prostate cancer patients that urologists diagnose. The OIG expressed concern that urology groups are in a position to choose IMRT instead of other forms of radiation and ensure economic success of a joint venture while assuming minimal business risk. The radiation oncologist would then be able to reward the referring urologist with a profit. The opinion as written states, "We conclude the proposed arrangement could potentially generate prohibited remuneration under the anti-kickback statute."[33] Unfortunately, this opinion applies to equipment leasing arrangements only.

Some hospital medical oncologists, general surgeons, and neurosurgeons also choose a variation of this business model when they combine with radiation oncologists to provide radiation treatment including robotic radiosurgery.[33] Again, the radiation oncologist is in a position to reward the owners of equipment with a profit.

ECONOMIC ISSUES SPECIFIC TO NEW GRADUATES OF RESIDENCY PROGRAMS

Most new graduates are largely concerned about mastering the amount of medical knowledge necessary to become a specialist, as well as passing their radiation oncology boards. Few articles have been written on contracting specific to radiation oncology.[34] A contract is a promise between two parties that the law recognizes as a duty. Five elements are required to create a valid contract: two competent parties, mutual consent, consideration, a legal purpose and duty, and a mutual obligation. When evaluating a first contract, obtaining legal advice from a health care attorney is essential.

The terms and conditions of the contract should set forth working conditions, provision of nursing service, transcription, ancillary help, on-call arrangements, vacation time, and coverage. Arrangements should be spelled out for professional liability insurance coverage including term limits and a tail policy in the event that termination of employment occurs. Duties should be specific to the practice of radiation oncology and not be vaguely worded so the new physician is expected to "perform all duties as the board of directors may assign."[34] The employer should also spell out the terms of potential termination. Reasonable terms of automatic contract termination include loss of your medical license, loss of hospital privileges for patient care issues, loss of a drug enforcement agency license, loss of ability to prescribe controlled substances, conviction of a felony, and so forth. If there is a provision for termination of the contract prior to the end of the term, it should be clear and available to both parties. For example, "either party may terminate this agreement with 90 days written notice with or without cause."[34] Written performance reviews should be given at least quarterly. This assists the employer and the employee to identify potential areas of conflict and allow resolution.

Restrictive covenants protect employers by placing limitations on the rights of the employee to compete with the employer. They should include the period of time the restriction shall remain in effect, as well as the geographic restriction. Because some of these restrictive covenants are not enforceable in certain states, liquidated damages for terminating employment and remaining in an area to compete has also been used by some practices.[34] A liquidated damage clause provides a payment to the practice owner, negotiated in advance, that allows the employed physician to work in the area and compete after the contract is terminated.[34]

Associates are invited to become partners after some period of time, which varies from region to region. Traditionally, this has meant financial parody with the senior partners. Many physicians are being offered positions without a partnership track. Partnership has also traditionally meant voting and decision-making parody. Some groups offer graduated financial parody: the first 2 years may be salaried, and during the next 3 years they may gradually reach financial parody with senior partners in percentage increments. Formulas for buying into the practice are similarly variegated. In a hospital-based practice with an exclusive contract to provide professional services, the buy-in should be minimal, simply because the cost of maintaining the contract is minimal. There is no cost to maintain equipment. One should only purchase assets that have real value or cover the cost of maintaining the contract over time. The accounts receivable are usually generated by the physician during the years of nonpartnership. One questions a "buy-in" for these accounts receivable that the new physician helped to generate. Good will is augmented by the employed physician, who builds and contributes to practice expansion during the nonpartnership years. It is my opinion that accumulated practice goodwill is not worth a great deal financially.

Less than one-third of radiation oncologists are still in their first postresidency job 5 years later.[4,34] If negotiated into the contract, arbitration or mediation can be an effective and cost-efficient means to negotiate a dispute and avoid litigation between parties, should you decide to separate.[4,34]

ECONOMICS OF MEDICAL ONCOLOGY

As a way to achieve prescription drug coverage for our seniors, chemotherapy drug payments became the source of some revenue.[35] The target is huge: Medicare spends $70 billion each year for chemotherapy drugs. Compare that to the amount spent on radiation oncology professional and technical fees, which totals $7 billion per year, and our services appear very cost-effective.[35,36] Outpatient drug reimbursement has changed from paying a percentage of the average wholesale price (AWP) to paying a percentage of the average sales price (ASP). ASP is the sales price that is actually paid by outpatient practices with a tiny margin added, only 6%. Medical oncologists argue appropriately that the administration of chemotherapy does not cover the cost of nursing time, waste disposal, and supplies. Medicare responded to this reality by increasing the fee for administration of the first hour of chemotherapy infusion by over 270% between 2003 and 2004.[36] Because reimbursement for the first hour of chemotherapy has had the most dramatic increase in reimbursement for medical oncology, this makes any regimen that requires multiple days of therapy profitable for our medical oncology colleagues. These include daily or weekly chemoradiation protocols.[36] There is a new drug reimbursement update by Medicare every 12 weeks as the average sales price for chemotherapeutic drugs is recalculated by CMS. There continue to be proposals to reimburse chemotherapy drugs by Medicare at ASP plus 3%—a 50% cut in profit margin.

Consulting groups are letting medical oncologists know that they can profit from incorporating PET scanners, CT scanners, and radiation oncology equipment into their practices. Perhaps more realistically, medical oncologists will be looking for reduction in their overhead through combining with radiation oncologists and being able to enhance patient care by giving daily chemotherapy sensitization protocols within a combined cancer center. Do not build a new cancer center without at least considering adding space for medical oncologists.

MEDICAL ONCOLOGY SUPPLY AND DEMAND: HOW WILL THIS AFFECT RADIATION ONCOLOGY IN THE FUTURE?

The demand for medical oncologists will rise by 48% in the year 2020, but the supply will only rise 14%, creating a 34% shortfall in the number of medical oncologists needed in the workforce. These conclusions were drawn from a study performed by the American Association of Medical Colleges and reported in the *Journal of Oncology Practice.*[37,38] The number of patient visits for medical oncology was determined by the National Cancer Institute analysis of the SEER database. There was no adjustment for the ever-lengthening regimens of palliative or adjuvant chemotherapy, nor was there any adjustment for patients with metastatic cancer who may live longer as a result of palliative treatment and thus require increased patient visits in the future. In his article, Dr. Erickson Salsberg proposes increased use of nurse practitioners and physician assistants and delays in retirement for current medical oncologists. He also proposes increase use of primary care physicians to monitor patients during and after chemotherapy.[37,38] With the shortage of primary care doctors in the United States, this does not seem likely. One of our most respected mentors and long-time leader in radiation oncology, Dr. Luther Brady, teaches residents that we are first and foremost cancer physicians who use radiation as a tool to treat cancer patients. Radiation oncologists are trained in all aspects of solid tumor oncology and can easily direct medical care for cancer patients during their disease process. Given the need, there is every reason for radiation oncologists to see cancer patients for consultation and to design a program for biopsy, workup, and management of their malignancy, even if it does not include delivery of radiation treatment. We encourage radiation oncologists to step up to the plate and provide more consultative services, more direct patient care, more inpatient care, and more general oversight than ever before. This new role may be one of the most important challenges for our specialty. However, if realized, it will benefit countless cancer patients by the year 2020.[38]

PAY FOR PERFORMANCE

CMS continues to move toward pay for performance. Under this system, a physician practice meeting a certain benchmark of quality in patient care does not receive a reduction in Medicare payments. This movement, in its various combinations and permutations, including ACOs, started in 1999 when the Institute of Medicine released a report called *To Err Is Human.*[39] This report documented quality-of-care concerns in our health care system and pointed out that 98,000 people die each year due to preventable medical errors from health care professionals. Subsequently, a Rand study found that many hospital deaths were preventable.[40] In our legislators' minds, the findings of these studies sharpened their resolve to improve the quality of care delivered in our health care system. Pay for performance has the objective of improving the quality of care by linking physician reimbursement to quality measures and outcomes. Pay for performance was first instituted in hospitals. Under the Deficit Reduction Act of 2005, hospitals receive a 2% reduction if they do not report to CMS on 10 quality measures and have acceptable performance targets. This pilot project with hospitals has been viewed by Congress to be successful. The results of quality-of-care measures for these areas are available on the CMS website for any hospital that participates.

Certain specialties lend themselves better to pay-for-performance measures than others. For example, diabetic patients should have retina exams as a component part of their care, and not doing so would not be optimal care for them. The care of cancer patients is, however, quite variegated. As we all know, some patients with brain metastasis live only a few months, and others live for a year or more. Thus, outcome measures for patients who have cancer would probably not be appropriate. It is the physicians themselves within each specialty that should shape the compliance program linked to pay for performance. In this regard, likely the better measure of quality of care would be accreditation of radiation oncology practices. This has not been adopted by CMS to date but is currently required in several states in the United States.[41,42]

RADIATION ONCOLOGY DEPARTMENT: APPROPRIATE STAFFING AND PERSONNEL

Radiation treatment consists of a series of steps and involves a number of different professionals. Each radiation oncology department should establish a staffing program consistent with the level of patient care complexity and other factors within that department. Radiation oncologists can manage 30 to 40 patients per day under continuous radiation treatment. When considering new patient visits and simulation follow-up visits, this translates to 65 to 90 patient encounters per week and allows us sufficient time for treatment planning and clinical functions.[43] Medical physicists should be available when necessary for consultation with the radiation oncologists and to provide advice and direction of the technical staff when treatments are being planned or patient treatment initiated. Chart checks by the physicists should be performed at least once per week. Generally one medical physicist is needed for every 30 to 40 patients under continuous radiation treatment.[43] Medical dosimetrists act under the supervision of the radiation oncologist and medical physicist. There should be one full-time-equivalent dosimetrist per 40 patients under continuous treatment. More dosimetrists may be needed if a larger proportion of patients receive higher-complexity care. Radiation therapy technologists practice under the direction of the radiation oncologists. They should have achieved American Registered Radiologic Technologist (ARRT) certification in radiation oncology.[43,44] One radiation therapist is needed for 20 patients under continuous treatment.[43,44] It is ideal to have two therapists per treatment machine and to allow for vacations, meetings, absences, and so forth. Radiation oncology support staff may include radiation therapist treatment aides, who work under the direct supervision of the radiation therapist and radiation oncologist and are generally trained on site to assist and facilitate patient transport and patient flow.

RADIATION ONCOLOGY STAFF RECRUITING AND RETENTION

In the United States, currently there is a critical manpower shortage in radiation therapy personnel. Regional shortage of therapists, dosimetrists, and physicists creates a "musical chairs" job market: the bell rings and everyone changes position.[4] This situation is neither beneficial to patient care nor fiscally sound for our shrinking health care dollar. For those of us who have depended on temporary workers, we know that this is both an expensive proposition and seriously disruptive to employee morale.[44]

The U.S. Bureau of Labor statistics predicted that by the year 2010, there would be a shortage of 7,000 radiation therapists.[4,44,45] A shortage of this magnitude did not seem to materialize. One way to stabilize your workforce, create good will, and create excellence in our field is to start a scholarship program for radiation therapy professionals. Currently, most scholarship programs support radiographers to take 1 additional year of training to become radiation therapists. During the time of training, the student can receive a stipend, as well as have his or her tuition and books paid for. In exchange, the candidate agrees to work for the cancer center for a period of years after graduation. One source of candidates can be a local radiography training program. Contact the director of the program and let him or her know that you are offering a scholarship program to qualified candidates. For students who receive monthly stipend support, the best way to ensure that they are serious about accepting the obligation is to have them sign a promissory note. If they fail to honor their contract or pass the registry within a specified period of time, the amount that the practice advanced them becomes immediately due with interest.[4,44]

Although many dosimetrists today are trained "on the job," there are 1-year programs that enroll therapists in full-time dosimetry training. If you have a candidate willing to relocate to one of the cities that has these programs, it is worth the investment to train them outside of your facility and hopefully bring back some fresh ideas. For a radiation therapist who may have a baccalaureate degree in radiation therapy, and for the right individual who wishes to train in medical physics, this may be an opportunity to train a medical physicist for your program.

Opening your practice to scholarship programs and scholarship support creates a unique marketing opportunity for your facilities.[4,44] This also augments cancer center morale, where the seasoned employees can teach the new graduates the tricks of the trade.[4,44]

PRACTICE ACCREDITATION

Practice accreditation is a way to demonstrate the quality of radiation oncology practice to the public, as well as third-party payers. Practice accreditation may be one avenue whereby a practice demonstrates quality and distinguishes itself. Currently, ACRO and the American College of Radiology (ACR) are the two practice accreditation bodies for radiation oncology practices. Some states (Alabama, New Jersey, and New York) require practice accreditation for state certification.[4,41,45]

Most importantly, practice accreditation constitutes a mechanism to accomplish quality assurance and assess compliance with recognized standards for hospital or free-standing radiation oncology practices.[4,41,45] Practice accreditation can also be a value-added qualification for third-party payers; some will require it in the future.

Standards for accreditation should include external review of randomly selected radiation oncology treatment courses, peer review, and quality assurance activities performed regularly; physics and dosimetry standards consistent with drafted standards for external-beam radiation treatment and brachytherapy; and medical physics quality assurance.[41,42,45] An on-site verification visit by both physicists and physicians is essential to practice accreditation.[45]

ECONOMICS OF RADIATION ONCOLOGY: SELECTED INTERNATIONAL PERSPECTIVES

The rate of installation of megavoltage radiation therapy equipment was compared in Canada, Germany, and the United States.[4,46] Rublee[4,46] concluded that the higher proliferation of radiation equipment in the United States promoted rapid access to advanced medical services but was not necessarily associated with improved outcomes, more patient utilization, or efficient use of health care funds. He noted an average rate of growth of 10.3 radiation therapy units per million persons in the United States, 4.6 units per million persons in Germany, and 4.8 units per million persons in Canada.

Canada's socialized health care system creates some access problems for cancer patients. During the years 1982–1991, the waiting times for radiation treatment in Canada, specifically documented in Ontario, deteriorated. Prostate cancer patients waited longer than 3 months and larynx cancer patients waited longer than 1 month for treatment. During this time, patients often advanced a stage or required treatment that was more extensive than initially planned. This was well documented in a series of published articles indicating the waiting times for breast, cervix, larynx, and prostate cancers. The Canadian Association of Radiation Oncologists Commission on Standards recommended that intervals between treatment and consultation not exceed 2 weeks' time. This led to a scoring system that scores the severity of curative cancer patients and urgency in starting radiation treatment. Curable head and neck cancers received the highest score, whereas curable prostate cancers received the lowest. This system sorts access to radiation treatment.[47,48]

Radiation oncologists in China note that they have a single governmental payer system with socialized medicine and staggering cost increases. Patients in China who require chemotherapy are required to pay cash up-front for their medication prior to its delivery. With respect to radiation oncology, radiation oncologists note a dearth of intensity-modulated radiation treatment, image-guided radiation treatment, and access to 3D conformal radiation treatment.

Calvo and Santos[49] describe monetary limits on the investment in innovative radiation treatment techniques in Western Europe. These authors note that the need for cost containment in the public health care system in Western European countries has slowed investment in stereotactic radiosurgery, conformal radiation treatment, high–dose-rate brachytherapy, and intraoperative radiation treatment. They reported on cost–benefit analysis of each of these technologies. Their conclusion was that Western Europe was not adopting new technology rapidly enough.[49]

Radiation oncologists responding to our survey in England felt that access to curative radiation oncology was good. However, access to palliative radiation oncology was suboptimal.[4]

Radiation oncologists in the Netherlands felt that their cancer programs limited neither access nor the development of new technology. Dutch radiation oncologists reported limited waiting times for patients to start radiation treatment.[4]

Radiation oncologists in South America and Latin America cited too few radiation oncology installations particularly in Mexico, Bolivia, and Venezuela. They also noted a rapidly growing number of radiation oncology installations especially in Argentina.[50] The latter have tended to be for-profit centers. Deficiencies in radiation oncology services in Latin America are attributed to a shortfall of equipment. Approximately 100 more teletherapy machines are needed, increasing equipment need by 14%. There is currently less than one radiation oncologist per teletherapy machine and less than one radiation oncologist for 1,000 new radiation oncology patients.[50] A 69% increase in radiation oncologists would be needed to fill the void, and the number of radiation therapists would need to increase by 109% across Latin America. Currently, 69% of Latin American installations have no fluoroscopic or CT simulation.[50] However, Latin American radiation oncologists point with pride to the Latin American Association of Therapeutic Radiation and Oncology. This organization currently serves their needs and is trying to augment staffing and physicians and enroll more Latin American patients in cooperative randomized trials.

Radiation oncologists in the Scandinavian countries of Denmark and Sweden showcase their innovative, large, and integrated cancer centers. They do point out that they are geographically distant from each other, but there appears to be minimal to no limit in their access to new technology, nor long waiting times for patient treatment.[4]

Practice accreditation is uncommon internationally. However, ACRO currently has accredited a number of international facilities, and practice accreditation in other countries continues to be in greater demand and is growing.[4,45]

In general, countries with socialized medicine have certain defined limits on capital investment each year. As our technology grows ever more costly, these issues will need to be dealt with both at home and in the international community.[4]

REFERENCES

1. American Cancer Society. *Cancer prevention facts and figures 2012*. Atlanta, GA: American Cancer Society; 2012. Available at: www.cancer.org
2. Regaz J, Jackson SM, Le N. Adjuvant radiotherapy and chemotherapy in node-positive premenopausal woman with breast cancer. *N Engl J Med* 1997;337:956–962.
3. Gastrointestinal Study Group. Prolongation of the disease free interval in surgically treated rectal carcinoma. *N Engl J Med* 1985;312:1465–1472.
4. Schilling PJ. Economics of radiation oncology. In: Halperin EC, Perez CA, Brady LW, eds. *Perez and Brady's principles and practice of radiation oncology,* 5th ed. Philadelphia: Lippincott Williams & Wilkins, 2007:2043–2050.
5. Centers for Medicare and Medicaid Services. Sustainable growth rate. 2010. Available at: www.cms.gov
6. Centers for Medicare and Medicaid Services. Medical economic index. 2010. Available at: www.cms.gov
7. Schilling PJ. Managing the insurance denials and appeals process. In: *American College of Radiation Oncology practice management guide.* Bethesda, MD: American College of Radiation Oncology; 2004:67–69.
8. Schilling PJ. Tips on how to appeal denied medicare claims for radiation oncology. *ACROGRAM,* May 26, 2005.
9. Schilling PJ. Medically unlikely edits do not mean impossible reimbursement. *ACRO Alert*, 2009.
10. Schilling PJ. Radiation oncology negotiation for managed care. In: *American College of Radiation Oncology practice management guide.* Bethesda, MD: American College of Radiation Oncology; 2006:146–152.
11. Schilling PJ. Do Medicare HMOs cherry pick healthy seniors to enroll? *ACRO Alert,* 2010.
12. Schilling PJ. Should medical physicists bill governmental payers directly? *ACRO Alert.*
13. Schilling PJ. Beware of the silent preferred provider organization. *ACRO Alert,* 2006.
14. Tippet TN. Emergence of the silent preferred provider organization. *Fl Med Assoc Qtly J* 2006;6–7.
15. Schilling PJ. Code 77338 replaces 77434 multiple custom multileaf device charges for Medicare IMRT patients. *ACRO Alert,* 2010.
16. Schilling PJ. Economic profiling and economic credentialing: the increasing challenge for organized medicine. *Fl Med Assoc Qtly J* 2003;33–35.
17. Schilling PJ. More imaging limits: administration proposes a 95% usage rate for diagnostic imaging equipment; how will this affect radiation oncology? *ACRO Alert,* 2009.
18. Congressional Budget Office Department of Accounting.
19. Accountable care organizations: what does it mean for radiation oncologists and cancer patients? *ACRO Alert,* October 2011.
20. Schilling P. Nurse doctors. *ACRO Alert,* 2009.
21. AMA Meeting Policy, November 2009. AMA Meeting policy re-affirmed, June 2011.
22. Peady DN. American Medical Association Board of Trustees report 19-A-06 health plan and insurer transparency Chicago, IL: American Medical Association; 2006.
23. Rubenstein J. American College of Radiation Oncology: political activity. In: *American College of Radiation Oncology practice management guide.* Bethesda, MD: American College of Radiation Oncology; 2004:87–88.
24. Rubenstein J. ACRO responds to proposed CMS payment cuts. *ACRO Alert,* October 6, 2002.
25. Woods A. ACRO supports Quality Care Preservation Act. *ACRO Alert,* April 23, 2003.
26. Woods A. The American College of Radiation Oncology lobbies Washington: our specialty succeeds in reversing payment cuts. *ACROGRAM,* December 1, 2003.
27. Rubinstein J. Political activity. In: *American College of Radiation Oncology practice management guide.* Bethesda, MD: American College of Radiation Oncology; 2004:87–88.
28. National Cancer Institute Survey Epidemiology and End Results 2008 data. Available at: www.seer.cancer.gov.
29. Gillette R. Marketing a practice. In: *American College of Radiation Oncology practice management guide.* Bethesda, MD: American College of Radiation Oncology; 2005:39–46.
30. Schilling PJ. Nonprofit hospitals exploit tax breaks to outperform for-profit facilities. *ACRO Alert,* 2008.
31. Woods A. The impact of federal Stark laws on radiation therapy. In: *American College of Radiation Oncology practice management guide.* Bethesda, MD: American College of Radiation Oncology; 2004.
32. Mitchell JM. Consequences of physician ownership of healthcare facilities: joint ventures in radiation therapy. *N Engl J Med* 1992;327:1497–1501.
33. Schilling PJ. Formation of combined urology and radiation oncology practices: objective data from radiation oncologists for rationale. *Am J Clin Oncol* 2011; 34(3):289–291.
34. Schilling PJ, Woods A. Anatomy of a professional services' contract for radiation oncology. American College of Radiation Oncology website. Available at: www.acro.org
35. Schilling PJ. Radiation oncology and the prescription drug program: what does it mean to us? *ACROGRAM,* September 18, 2003.
36. Schilling PJ. AWP and ASP: what does the alphabet soup of medical oncology mean to the practicing radiation oncologist? *ACROGRAM,* June 2004.
37. Salsberg EC, Forte E, Bruinooge G,, et al. Future supply and demand for oncologists: challenges to assuring access to oncology service. *J Clin Oncol Pract* 2007;10–12.
38. Schilling PJ. Shortfall in the number of medical oncologists to reach 34% in the year 2020. *ACRO Alert.*
39. Kohn LT, Corrigan JM, Donalson MS, et al. *To err is human: building a safer healthcare system.* Washington, DC: National Academy Press, 1999.
40. Hayward RA, Hofer TP. Estimating hospital deaths due to medical errors. *JAMA* 2001;285:415–420.
41. American Society of Therapeutic Radiology and Oncology Government Relations update: pay for performance and quality of care. Alexandria VA: American Society of Clinical Oncology; 2006.
42. Dobelbower RR, Cotter GW, Schilling PJ, et al. Radiation oncology practice accreditation. *Rays* 2001;26(3):191–198.
43. Cotter GW, Dobelbower RR. *American College of Radiation Oncology red book: ACRO practice accreditation program, 2007–2008.* Bethesda, MD: American College of Radiation Oncology; 2008.
44. Schilling PJ. Your cancer center can benefit from starting a scholarship program for radiation therapy professionals. In: *American College of Radiation Oncology practice management guide.* Bethesda, MD: American College of Radiation Oncology; 2005.
45. Cotter GW, Dobelbower RR. The American College of Radiation Oncology practice accreditation program. *Crit Rev Oncol Hematol* 2005;55:93–102.
46. Rublee DA. Medical technology in Canada, Germany and the United States: an update. *Health Aff* 1994;113–117.
47. Mackillop WJ. Waiting for radiotherapy in Ontario. *Int J Radiat Oncol Biol Phys* 1994;30:221–228.
48. Brady LW. In response to waiting for radiotherapy in Ontario. *Int J Radiat Oncol Biol Phys* 1994;30:245–246.
49. Calvo FA, Santos M. Innovative techniques in modern radiation oncology: the economic and organizational impact. *Rays* 1999;24(3):379–389.
50. Zubizarreta EH, Poitevin A, Levin CV, et al. Overview of radiotherapy resources in Latin America: a survey by the International Atomical Energy Agency. *Radiother Oncol* 2004;73:97–100.

Index

Page numbers followed by "f" indicate figure, page numbers followed by "t" indicate table, and page numbers followed by "b" indicate box.

T